COMMON DRUG AND TOXIN-INDUCED VITAL SI

Hypothermia	Hyperthermia
Alpha-adrenergic agonists	Amphetamines
Beta-adrenergic antagonists	Anticholinergics
Carbon monoxide	Antihistamines
Ethanol and other alcohols	Antipsychotics (NMS)
General anesthetics	Cocaine and sympathomimetics
Hypoglycemic agents	Cyclic antidepressants
Opioids	Dinitrophenol
Phenothiazines	Lithium
Sedative-hypnotic agents	Monoamine oxidase inhibitors
	Phencyclidine
	Salicylates
	Sedative-hypnotic withdrawal
	Thyroxine

Hypoventilation/Bradypnea		
Botulinum toxin	Electrolyte abnormalities	Organic phosphorus compounds
Carbamates	Ethanol and other alcohols	Poison hemlock (coniine)
Clonidine	Gamma hydroxy-butyrate	Sedative-hypnotics
Colchicine	Neuromuscular blocking agents	Strychnine
Cyclic anti-depressants	Nicotine	Tetanus toxin
Elapid enveno-mation	Opioids	Tetrodotoxin

Hyperventilation/Tachypnea		
Amphetamines	Ethylene glycol	Pentachlorophenol
Anticholinergics	*Gyromitra* mush-rooms (mono-methyl hydrazine)	Phenformin
Caffeine	Hydrogen sulfide	Progesterone
Camphor	Iron	Salicylates
Carbon monoxide	Isoniazid	Sodium mono-fluoroacetate
Cocaine	Methanol	Theobromine
Cyanide	Metformin	Theophylline
Dinitrophenol	Methemoglobin inducers	
Ethanol (keto-acidosis)	Paraldehyde	

Hypotension	Hypertension
Alpha-adrenergic antagonists	Amphetamines
Angiotensin-converting enzyme inhibitors and antagonists	Cocaine
Antidysrhythmic agents	Ephedrine/pseudoephe-drine
Beta-adrenergic antagonists	Epinephrine
Carbamates	Lead
Calcium channel blockers	Monoamine oxidase in-hibitors (overdose and drug interaction)
Clonidine	Nicotine (early)
Cyanide	Phencyclidine
Cyclic antidepressants	Phenylpropanolamine
Disulfiram/ethanol	
Ethanol	
Iron	
Isopropanol	
Nitrates and nitrites	
Nitroprusside	
Opioids	
Organic phosphorus compounds	
Phenothiazines	
Sedative-hypnotic agents	
Theophylline	

Bradycardia	Tachycardia
Antidysrhythmic agents	Amphetamines
Alpha-adrenergic agonists	Carbamates
Baclofen	Anticholinergics
Beta-adrenergic antagonists	Antihistamines
Calcium channel blockers	Antipsychotic agents
Carbamates	Arsenic (acute)
Ciguatera	Caffeine
Clonidine	Carbamates
Digitalis glycosides	Carbon monoxide
Opioids	Cocaine
Organic phosphorus compounds	Cyclic antidepressants
Phenylpropanolamine	Disulfiram/ethanol
Sedative-hypnotic agents	Ephedrine/pseudephedrine
	Epinephrine
	Iron
	Organic phosphorus com-pounds
	Phencyclidine
	Sedative-hypnotic withdrawal
	Theophylline
	Thyroxine

GOLDFRANK'S
TOXICOLOGIC EMERGENCIES

7th EDITION

GOLDFRANK'S
TOXICOLOGIC EMERGENCIES

7th EDITION

Lewis R. Goldfrank, MD, FACEP, FAAEM, FAACT, FACMT, FACP

Director, Department of Emergency Medicine
Bellevue Hospital Center and New York University
    Medical Center
Professor of Clinical Medicine and Surgery
New York University School of Medicine
Medical Director, New York City Poison Center
New York, New York

Neal E. Flomenbaum, MD, FACP, FACEP

Emergency Physician-in-Chief
New York-Presbyterian Hospital,
    New York Weill Cornell Medical Center
Professor of Clinical Medicine
Weill Medical College of Cornell University
Consultant, New York City Poison Center
New York, New York

Neal A. Lewin, MD, FACP, FACEP, FACMT

Director, Didactic Education, Department of Emergency
    Medicine
Bellevue Hospital Center and New York University
    Medical Center
Associate Professor of Clinical Medicine
New York University School of Medicine
Consultant, New York City Poison Center
New York, New York

Mary Ann Howland, PharmD, DABAT, FAACT

Clinical Professor of Pharmacy, St. John's University
    College of Pharmacy
Consultant, Department of Emergency Medicine
Bellevue Hospital Center and New York University
    Medical Center
Consultant, New York City Poison Center
New York, New York

Robert S. Hoffman, MD, FACEP, FAACT, FACMT

Director, New York City Poison Center
Attending Physician, Department of Emergency Medicine
Bellevue Hospital Center and New York University
    Medical Center
Assistant Professor of Clinical Surgery/Emergency
    Medicine
New York University School of Medicine
New York, New York

Lewis S. Nelson, MD, FACEP, FACMT

Director, Medical Toxicology Fellowship Program
Associate Director, New York City Poison Center
Attending Physician, Department of Emergency Medicine
Bellevue Hospital Center and New York University
    Medical Center
Assistant Professor of Clinical Surgery/Emergency
    Medicine
New York University School of Medicine
New York, New York

With 116 contributors

McGraw-Hill
MEDICAL PUBLISHING DIVISION

New York / Chicago / San Francisco / Lisbon / London / Madrid / Mexico City /
Milan / New Delhi / San Juan / Seoul / Singapore / Sydney / Toronto

McGraw-Hill

A Division of The McGraw·Hill Companies

GOLDFRANK'S TOXICOLOGIC EMERGENCIES, 7/E

Copyright © 2002 by *The McGraw-Hill Companies,* Inc. All rights reserved. Printed in the United States of America. Except as permitted under the United States Copyright Act of 1976, no part of this publication may be reproduced or distributed in any form or by any means, or stored in a data base or retrieval system, without the prior written permission of the publisher.

The editors' and authors' royalties for this edition, as in the case of previous editions, are being donated to The New York City Poison Center to help care for poisoned patients.

Previous editions copyright © 1998, 1994, 1990, 1986, 1982, 1978 by Appleton & Lange.

23456789KGPKGP098765432

ISBN 0-07-136001-8

This book was set in Times Roman by Pine Tree Composition.
The editors were Andrea Seils, Susan R. Noujaim, and Karen G. Edmonson.
The production supervisor was Richard Ruzycka.
The design was done by Marsha Cohen/Parallelogram Graphics.
The index was done by Kathi Unger
Quebecor World Kingsport was the printer and binder.

The book is printed on recycled, acid-free paper.

Library of Congress Cataloging-in-Publication Data

Goldfrank's toxicologic emergencies/[edited by] Lewis R. Goldfrank . . . [et al.]; with 116 contributors.--7th ed.
    p.;cm.
  Includes bibliographical references and index.
  ISBN 0-07-136001-8
  1. Toxicological emergencies. 2. Toxicological emergencies--Case studies.
I. Title: Toxicologic emergencies. II. Goldfrank, Lewis R., 1941-
[DNLM: 1. Emergencies--Case Report. 2. Emergencies--Examination Questions.
3. Poisoning--Case Report. 4. Poisoning--Examination Questions. 5. Poisons--Case
Report. 6. Poisons--Examination Questions. QV 600 G618 2002]
RA1224.5.G65 2002
615.9--dc21
                                                     2001054422

DEDICATED TO

The staffs of our emergency departments,
who have worked with remarkable courage, concern, and understanding
in treating the patients discussed in this text
and many thousands more like them

The staff of the New York City Poison Center,
who have quietly and conscientiously integrated their skill with ours
to serve these patients and many others
who never needed a hospital visit because of their efforts

The ambulance staff,
who taught us a great deal about toxicology
and who had faith in our ability

To my children,
Rebecca, Jennifer, to Andrew and Joan,
to Michelle and James,
and my grandchildren, Benjamin, Adam, and Sarah
who have kept me acutely aware of the ready availability
of possible poisons, and
to my wife, partner, and best friend, Susan,
whose support was essential and
whose contributions will be found throughout the text (L.G.)

To my mother Mollie,
to the memory of my father, Lieutenant H. Stanley Flomenbaum
and to my wife, Meredith,
for all of the ways they have made my participation
in this book possible,
and to my children, Adam, David and Sari
who have competed with this text for my attention
but who have underscored the importance of these efforts (N.F.)

To my wife, Gail,
and to my children, Justin and Jesse,
for their support and patience and to my parents,
who made it possible (N.L.)

To my husband, Bob,
and children, Robert and Marcy,
and to my mother and to the loving memory of my father,
to family, friends, colleagues, and students for all their help
and continuing inspiration (M.A.H.)

To my friends, family, and colleagues
for their never-ending patience (R.H.)

To my wife, Laura,
for her support while I worked on this project;
to my children, Daniel, Adina and Benjamin,
for understanding when Daddy had to work and not play;
to my parents Dr. Irwin and Myrna,
for the foundation which they provided;
and to my family and friends
who keep me focused on what is important (L.N.)

CONTRIBUTORS

JUDITH C. AHRONHEIM, MD
Chief, Eileen E. Anderson Section of
Geriatric Medicine
Saint Vincent's Catholic Medical Centers -
St. Vincent's Manhattan
New York, New York
Chapter 107, "Geriatric Principles"

MICHAEL H. ALLEN, MD
Assistant Professor of Psychiatry
University of Colorado School of Medicine
Denver, Colorado
Chapter 114, "Psychiatric Principles"

DINA BEGAN, MD
Assistant Professor of Clinical Dermatology
New York University School of Medicine
New York, New York
Chapter 29, "Dermatologic Principles"

JEFFREY N. BERNSTEIN, MD, FACEP, FACMT
Medical Director, Florida Poison Information Center, Miami
Voluntary Associate Professor of Pediatrics
University of Miami School of Medicine
Attending Physician, Emergency Care Center
Jackson Memorial Hospital
Miami, Florida
Antidotes in Depth, "Antivenom (Scorpion and Spider)"

JOSEPH M. BETZ, PhD
Vice President for Scientific and Technical Affairs
American Herbal Products Association
Silver Spring, Maryland
Chapter 78, "Plants"

KENNETH E. BIZOVI, MD
Assistant Professor
Department of Emergency Medicine
Oregon Health Science University
Consultant, Oregon Poison Center
Portland, Oregon
Chapter 32, "Acetaminophen"

G. RANDALL BOND, MD, FACMT
Medical Director, Drug and Poison Information Center
Children's Hospital Medical Center
Professor of Pediatrics and Emergency Medicine
University of Cincinnati College of Medicine
Cincinnati, Ohio
Chapter 44, "Antimalarial Agents"

GEORGE M. BOSSE, MD
Associate Professor of Emergency Medicine
University of Louisville
Louisville, Kentucky
Chapter 40, "Antidiabetic and Hypoglycemic Agents"

EDWARD W. BOYER, MD, PhD
Director, Toxicology Fellowship Training Program
University of Massachusetts Medical Center
Worcester, Massachusetts
Assistant Professor, Children's Hospital
Clinical Instructor in Medicine
Children's Hospital, Boston
Clinical Instructor in Pediatrics
Harvard Medical School
Boston, Massachusetts
Chapter 43, "Antituberculous Agents"

KENNETH O. BRAMBILL, MSW, CSW
**Chapter 113, "Psychosocial Principles in
Assessment and Intervention"**

JEFFREY R. BRUBACHER, MD
Clinical Assistant Professor
Division of Emergency Medicine
Faculty of Surgery
University of British Columbia
Attending Physician
Vancouver General Hospital
Vancouver, British Columbia, Canada
Chapter 49, "β-Adrenergic Antagonists"

PAUL CALABRESI, MD, MACP
Professor of Medicine and Medical Science
   Chairman Emeritus
Brown University School of Medicine
Department of Medicine
Director, Division of Clinical Pharmacology
Rhode Island Hospital
Providence, Rhode Island
Chapter 47, "Antineoplastic Agents"

SUSAN CALLAGHAN-MONTELLA, RN, MA
Director of Education and Development
Emergency Care Institute
Department of Emergency Medicine
Bellevue Hospital Center
New York University Medical Center
New York, New York
Chapter 115, "Nursing Principles"

LOUIS R. CANTILENA, JR MD, PhD

Director, Division of Clinical Pharmacology and Medical Toxicology
Uniformed Services University of the Health Services
Bethesda, Maryland
Chapter 117, "Adverse Drug Events"

WILLIAM K. CHIANG, MD

Assistant Director, Department of Emergency Medicine
Bellevue Hospital Center
Assistant Professor of Clinical Surgery/Emergency Medicine
New York University School of Medicine
New York, New York
Chapter 28, "Otolaryngologic Principles"
Chapter 68, "Amphetamines"

JASON CHU, MD

Fellow in Medical Toxicology
Department of Clinical Surgery/Emergency Medicine
New York University School of Medicine
Bellevue Hospital Center
New York City Poison Center
New York, New York
Chapter 45, "Antimigraine Agents"
Chapter 30, "Genitourinary Principles"

JAMES E. CISEK, MD

Associate Professor of Emergency Medicine
Medical Director, Poison Control Center
Department of Emergency Medicine
Medical College of Virginia
Richmond, Virginia
Chapter 109, "Substance Users"

CATHLEEN CLANCY, MD

Associate Medical Director
National Capital Poison Center
Adjunct Assistant Professor
Department of Emergency Medicine
George Washington University Medical Center
Attending Physician
Department of Emergency Medicine
Georgetown University Medical Center
Washington, DC
Chapter 9, "Electrocardiographic Principles"

RICHARD F. CLARK, MD

Medical Director, San Diego Division California Poison Control System
Director, UCSD Division of Medical Toxicology
Associate Professor of Medicine
University of California, San Diego
San Diego, California
Chapter 88, "Insecticides: Organic Phosphorus Compounds and Carbamates"

STEVEN C. CURRY, MD

Director, Department of Medical Toxicology
Good Samaritan Regional Medical Center
Associate Professor of Clinical Medicine
University of Arizona College of Medicine
Phoenix, Arizona
Chapter 10 "Neurotransmitters"

KATHLEEN DELANEY, MD, FACP

Professor, Division of Emergency Medicine
University of Texas Southwestern Medical School
Medical Director, Parkland Memorial Hospital Emergency Department
Dallas, Texas
Chapter 13, "Biochemical Principles"
Chapter 14, "Hepatic Principles"
Chapter 16, "Carcinogens, Mutagens and Teratogens"
Chapter 18, "Thermoregulatory Principles"
Antidotes in Depth, "Dextrose"

FRANCIS DeROOS, MD

Residency Program Director
Department of Emergency Medicine
Hospital of the University of Pennsylvania
Assistant Professor
University of Pennsylvania School of Medicine
Philadelphia, Pennsylvania
Chapter 50, "Calcium Channel Blockers"
Chapter 51, "Miscellaneous Antihypertensives"

SUZANNE DOYON, MD

Medical Director
Maryland Poison Center
University of Maryland School of Pharmacy
Baltimore, Maryland
Chapter 41, "Anticonvulsants"

DONALD A. FEINFELD, MD, FACP

Director of Nephrology
Nassau University Medical Center, East Meadow, New York
Professor of Clinical Medicine
State University of New York at Stony Brook
Stony Brook, New York
Consultant New York City Poison Center
Chapter 23, "Renal Principles"

ROBERT P. FERM, MD, FAAP, FACEP, FACMT

Assistant Professor of Emergency Medicine
Division of Toxicology
Department of Emergency Medicine
University of Massachusetts Medical School
Director, Medical Toxicology Fellowship
Department of Emergency Medicine
University of Massachusetts Medical Center
Worcester, Massachusetts
Chapter 70, "Lysergic Acid Diethylamide and Other Hallucinogens"

JEFFREY S. FINE, MD

Assistant Professor of Clinical Pediatrics
New York University School of Medicine
Assistant Director
Pediatric Emergency Medicine
Bellevue Hospital Center
Consultant, New York City Poison Center
New York, New York
Chapter 105, "Reproductive and Perinatal Principles"
Chapter 106, "Pediatric Principles"

MARK FLOMENBAUM, MD, PhD

First Deputy Chief Medical Examiner
City of New York

Clinical Assistant Professor
Department of Forensic Medicine
New York University
New York, New York
Chapter 119, "Postmortem Toxicology"

MARSHA D. FORD, MD, FACEP, FACMT

Director, Division of Medical Toxicology
Carolinas Poison Center
Assistant Chairman, Department of Emergency Medicine
Carolinas Medical Center
Charlotte, North Carolina
Clinical Associate Professor of Emergency Medicine
School of Medicine
University of North Carolina—Chapel Hill
Chapel Hill, North Carolina
Chapter 79, "Arsenic"

PAUL D. FRANCIS, MD

Director, Pediatric Cardiology
Geisinger Medical Center
Danville, Pennsylvania
Chapter 57, "Cyclic Antidepressants"

FREDERICK W. FRAUNFELDER, MD

Cornea/Refractive Surgery
Casey Eye Institute
Portland, Oregon
Chapter 27, "Ophthalmic Principles"

E. JOHN GALLAGHER, MD

Professor and University Chair
Department of Emergency Medicine
Albert Einstein College of Medicine
Bronx, New York
Chapter 19, "Neurologic Principles"

FRANCIS A. GAUTIERI, MS, CSW, ACSW

Director, Social Work
Columbia Presbyterian Hospital
New York, New York
**Chapter 113, "Psychosocial Principles in Assessment and
    Intervention"**

BRETT GOLDBERG, MA

Associate Professor of Psychology
Department of Psychology
Hofstra University
Research Assistant Professor of Psychiatry
New York University School of Medicine
New York, New York
Chapter 114, "Psychiatric Principles"

DAVID S. GOLDFARB, MD

Assistant Chief, Nephrology Section
New York Harbor VA Medical Center
Associate Professor of Clinical Medicine and Urology
New York University School of Medicine
Consultant New York City Poison Center
New York, New York
**Chapter 6, "Principles and Techniques Applied to Enhance Elimina-
    tion of Toxic Compounds"**

KIMBERLIE A. GRAEME, MD

Fellowship Director
Department of Medical Toxicology
Good Samaritan Regional Medical Center
Phoenix, Arizona
Attending Physician
Department of Emergency Medicine
Mayo Clinic Hospital
Scottsdale, Arizona
Chapter 10, "Neurotransmitters"

MICHAEL I. GREENBERG, MD, MPH

Professor of Emergency Medicine and Public Health
Division of Occupational and Environmental Emergency Medicine
Allegheny University of the Health Sciences
MCP Hahnemann School of Medicine
Philadelphia, Pennsylvania
Chapter 110, "Healthcare Workers"

DAVID D. GUMMIN, MD

Associate Medical Director
Wisconsin Poison Center, Children's Hospital of Wisconsin
Assistant Clinical Professor of Emergency Medicine
Medical College of Wisconsin
Attending Emergency Physician
Infinity HealthCare Incorporated
Milwaukee, Wisconsin
Chapter 86, "Hydrocarbons"

JASON B. HACK, MD

Assistant Professor, Department of Emergency Medicine
Brody Medical School at East Carolina University
Associate Chief, Division of Toxicology
Department of Emergency Medicine
Pitt County Memorial Hospital
Greenville, North Carolina
Chapter 48, "Cardiac Glycosides"

IN-HEI HAHN, MD

Assistant Professor of Clinical Medicine
Columbia University
Associate Attending Emergency Physician
St. Luke's-Roosevelt Hospital Center
New York, New York
Chapter 102, "Arthropods"

RICHARD J. HAMILTON, MD

Associate Professor of Emergency Medicine
Program Director of Emergency Medicine
Service Chief of Emergency Medicine
MCP Hahnemann University
Philadelphia, Pennsylvania
Chapter 37, "Vitamins"
Chapter 72, "Substance Withdrawal"

FRED M. HENRETIG, MD

Professor of Pediatrics and Emergency Medicine
University of Pennsylvania School of Medicine
Medical Director, The Poison Control Center of Philadelphia,
    Pennsylvania
Director, Section of Clinical Toxicology
Division of Emergency Medicine
Children's Hospital of Philadelphia

Philadelphia, Pennsylvania
Chapter 80, "Lead"

GLENDON C. HENRY, MD
Medical Director, Harlem Hospital
Assistant Professor of Clinical Medicine
College of Physicians and Surgeons of Columbia University
New York, New York
Chapter 61, "Lithium"

ROBERT A. HESSLER, MD, PhD
Clinical Associate Professor Clinical Surgery/Emergency Medicine
New York University School of Medicine
Assistant Director
Department of Emergency Medicine
Bellevue Hospital Center
New York University Medical Center
New York, New York
Chapter 21, "Cardiovascular Principles"

ROBERT J. HOFFMAN, MD
Fellow in Medical Toxicology
Department of Clinical Surgery/Emergency Medicine
New York University School of Medicine
Bellevue Hospital Center
New York City Poison Center
New York, New York
Chapter 39, "Methylxanthines"

MICHAEL G. HOLLAND, MD, FACMT, FACOEM, FACEP
Assistant Professor of Emergency Medicine
Pennsylvania State University, College of Medicine
The Milton S. Hershey Medical Center
Hershey, Pennsylvania
Occupational and Environmental Toxicologist
Central Pennsylvania Poison Center
Hershey, Pennsylvania
Chapter 89, "Insecticides: Organochlorines, Pyrethrins, DEET"

JUDD E. HOLLANDER, MD
Clinical Research Director
Associate Professor
Department of Emergency Medicine
University of Pennsylvania
Philadelphia, Pennsylvania
Chapter 67, "Cocaine"

CHRISTOPHER P. HOLSTEGE, MD
Medical Director, Division of Medical Toxicology
Blue Ridge Poison Center
Assistant Professor, Department of Emergency Medicine
University of Virginia
Charlottesville, Virginia
Chapter 96, "Smoke Inhalation"

DANIEL HRYHORCZUK, MD, MPH, FACMT
Professor and Director
Great Lakes Centers for Occupational and Environmental Safety
   and Health
University of Illinois at Chicago
School of Public Health
Director of Toxikon Consortium
Chief of Clinical Toxicology
Cook County Hospital

Chicago, Illinois
Chapter 86, "Hydrocarbons"

OLIVER L. HUNG, MD
Attending Physician
Department of Emergency Medicine
Morristown Memorial Hospital
Morristown, New Jersey
Chapter 77, "Herbal Preparations"

GARY ISOM, PhD
Professor of Toxicology
Department of Medicinal Chemistry and Molecular Pharmacology
School of Pharmacy and Pharmaceutical Sciences, Purdue University
West Lafayette, Indiana
Chapter 98, "Cyanide and Hydrogen Sulfide"

PAUL A. JAMES, MD
IAFP Endowed Chair in Rural Medicine
Associate Professor
University of Iowa College of Medicine
Iowa City, Iowa
Chapter 111, "Farm Toxicology"

BRIAN KAUFMAN, MD
Associate Clinical Professor of Anesthesiology and Medicine
New York University School of Medicine
Director, Critical Care Section
Department of Anesthesiology
Medical Director, Respiratory Therapy
New York University Medical Center
New York, New York
Chapter 53, "Inhalational Anesthetics"
Chapter 54, "Neuromuscular Blocking Agents"
Chapter 55, "Local Anesthetics"

DEBRA KENNEDY MB, BS FRACP, HGSA
Director of Mothersafe
Staff Specialist in Clinical Genetics and Teratology
Royal Hospital for Women
Randwick, Australia
Conjoint Lecturer in Obstetrics and Gynecology
School of Women's and Children's Health
University of New South Wales
Sydney, Australia
Chapter 16, "Mutagens, carcinogens and Teratogens"

WILLIAM KERNS II, MD, FACEP, FACMT
Medical Toxicology Fellowship Director
Division of Medical Toxicology
Department of Emergency Medicine and Carolinas Poison Center
Carolinas Medical Center
Charlotte, North Carolina
Chapter 98, "Cyanide and Hydrogen Sulfide"
Antidotes in Depth, "Cyanide Antidotes"

CHRISTOPHER KEYES, MD, FACEP, FACMT
Chief, Section of Toxicology
Division of Emergency Medicine
University of Texas Southwestern Medical School
Dallas, Texas
Chapter 26, "Endocrine Principles"

MARK A. KIRK, MD

Medical Toxicology Fellowship Director
Methodist Hospital
Associate Director, Indiana Poison Center
Clinical Assistant Professor
Department of Emergency Medicine
Indiana University School of Medicine
Indianapolis, Indiana
Chapter 96, "Smoke Inhalation"
Chapter 98, "Cyanide and Hydrogen Sulfide"
**Chapter 104, "Use of the Intensive Care Unit for Poisoned
    Patients"**

LADA KOKAN, MD, FRCPC

Clinical Instructor
Department of Surgery
University of British Columbia
Vancouver, British Columbia, Canada
Chapter 60, "Monoamine Oxidase Inhibitors"

GIDEON KOREN, MD, FACMT, FRCPC

Professor, Division of Clinical Pharmacology and Toxicology
Departments of Pediatrics, Pharmacology, Pharmacy, and Medicine
University of Toronto
Director, Clinical Pharmacology, Toxicology and Motherisk Program
Department of Pediatrics
The Hospital for Sick Children
Toronto, Canada
Chapter 16, "Mutagens, Carcinogens and Teratogens"

EDWIN K. KUFFNER, MD

Attending Toxicologist
Rocky Mountain Poison and Drug Center
Denver, Colorado
Chapter 65, "Disulfiram and Disulfiramlike Reactions"
Chapter 85, "Camphor and Moth Repellents"

RICKY L. LANGLEY, MD, MPH

Medical Epidemiologist
North Carolina Department of Health and Human Services
Raleigh, North Carolina
Chapter 111, "Farm Toxicology"

DAVID C. LEE, MD, FAAEM

Director of Research
Department of Emergency Medicine
North Shore University Hospital
Manhasset, New York
Clinical Assistant Professor
Department of Clinical Surgery/Emergency Medicine
New York University
New York, New York
Chapter 63, "Sedative-Hypnotic Agents"

WALTER LeSTRANGE, RN, MPH, MS

Executive Director
United Medical Surgical PC
Staten Island, New York
Chapter 118 "Risk Management and Legal Principles"

ERICA L. LIEBELT, MD

Director, Pediatric Residency Program
Geisinger Medical Center
Danville, Pennsylvania
Chapter 57, "Cyclic Antidepressants"

FRANK LoVECCHIO, DO

Medical Director, Good Samaritan Regional Poison Center
Attending Physician, Maricopa Medical Center
Department of Emergency Medicine
Assistant Professor, Arizona College of Osteopathic Medicine
Phoenix, Arizona
Chapter 59, "Antipsychotics"

WILLIAM J. MEGGS, MD, PhD, FACEP

Professor and Vice Chair for Clinical Affairs
Chief, Division of Toxicology, Department of Emergency Medicine
Brody Medical School at East Carolina University
Greenville, North Carolina
Chapter 15, "Immunologic Principles"
Chapter 111, "Farm Toxicology"

MARIA MERCURIO-ZAPPALA, RPh, CSPI, MS

Managing Director
New York City Poison Center
New York, New York
Chapter 83, "Thallium"

KIRK C. MILLS, MD, FACEP, FACMT

Associate Residency Director
Emergency Medicine
Department of Emergency Medicine
Wayne State University
Detroit Receiving Hospital
Detroit, Michigan
Chapter 10, "Neurotransmitters"

SEAN P. NORDT, PharmD, DABAT

University College Dublin
School of Medicine
Dublin, Ireland
Chapter 56, "Pharmaceutical Additives"

RUEBEN OLMEDO, MD

Assistant Professor of Emergency Medicine
Mt. Sinai School of Medicine
Attending Physician
Mt. Sinai Hospital
New York, New York
Chapter 69 "Phencyclidine and Ketamine"

KEVIN C. OSTERHOUDT, MD

Assistant Professor of Pediatrics
University of Pennsylvania School of Medicine
Consultant Toxicologist,
    Children's Hospital of Philadelphia and
    Poison Control Center at Philadelphia
Research Fellow, Center for Clinical Epidemiology and Biostatistics
University of Pennsylvania
Philadelphia, Pennsylvania
Chapter 120, "Principles of Epidemiology and Research Design"

EDWARD J. OTTEN, MD, FACMT

Professor of Emergency Medicine and Pediatrics
Director, Division of Toxicology
University of Cincinnati College of Medicine
Cincinnati, Ohio
Chapter 71, "Marijuana"

Chapter 101, "Snakes and Other Reptiles"
Antidotes in Depth, "Antivenom: Crotaline and Elapid"

MARY PALMER, MD

Attending Physician
Department of Emergency Medicine
Landspitali University Hospital of Reykjavík
Reykjavík, Iceland
Chapter 78, "Plants"

JEANMARIE PERRONE, MD

Director, Division of Toxicology
Department of Emergency Medicine
University of Pennsylvania School of Medicine
Assistant Professor, Emergency Medicine, Pediatrics
    and Laboratory Medicine
University of Pennsylvania School of Medicine
Attending Physician, Emergency Department
Hospital of the University of Pennsylvania
Philadelphia, Pennsylvania
Chapter 36, "Iron"
Chapter 38, "Dieting Agents and Regimens"

SUSAN M. POND, MD, FRACP

Adjunct Professor
University of Queensland
Brisbane, Australia
Chapter 91, "Herbicides"

KEVIN PORTER, ESQ

Head of the Healthcare Practice Group
Thurm and Heller, LLP
Adjunct Professor of Health Care Regulation and Law
Milano Graduate School, Health Services Management and Policy
    Program
Chapter 118, "Risk Management and Legal Principles"

DENNIS PRICE, MD

Assistant Professor of Clinical Surgery/Emergency Medicine
New York University School of Medicine
Attending Physician
Department of Emergency Medicine
Bellevue Hospital Center
New York, New York
Chapter 94, "Methemoglobinemia"

PETRIE M. RAINEY, MD, PhD

Professor of Laboratory Medicine
University of Washington School of Medicine
Director, Clinical Chemistry and Toxicology Laboratories
University of Washington Medical Center
Seattle, Washington
**Chapter 7, "Laboratory Principles and Techniques for Evaluation
    of the Poisoned or Overdosed Patient"**

RAMA B. RAO, MD

Assistant Professor Clinical Surgery/Emergency Medicine and Forensic
    Medicine
New York University School of Medicine
Research Director
Department of Emergency Medicine
Attending Physician
Bellevue Hospital Center and New York University Medical Center
Consultant, New York City Poison Center

New York, New York
Chapter 82A, "Bismuth"
Chapter 87, "Caustics and Batteries"
Chapter 119, "Postmortem Toxicology"

JOSEPH RELLA, MD

Assistant Professor of Emergency Medicine
University of Medicine and Dentistry—New Jersey School
    of Medicine
Attending Physician
Department of Emergency Medicine
University of Medicine and Dentistry, New Jersey University Hospital
Newark, New Jersey
Chapter 99, "Radiation"

WENDY RIVES, MD [DECEASED]

Director, Comprehensive Emergency Psychiatric Program
Bellevue Hospital Center
Clinical Instructor, Department of Psychiatry
New York University School of Medicine
New York, New York
Chapter 114, "Psychiatric Principles"

JAMES R. ROBERTS, MD, FAAEM, FACMT

Professor and Vice Chair
Department of Emergency Medicine
Professor and Chief
Division of Toxicology
Director, Institute for the Treatment of Poisonous Bites and Stings
Allegheny University of the Health Sciences
MCP Hahnemann School of Medicine
Director, Division of Toxicology
Chairman, Department of Emergency Medicine
Mercy Health Systems
Philadelphia, Pennsylvania
Chapter 101, "Snakes and Other Reptiles"
Antidotes in Depth, "Antivenom (Crotaline and Elapid)"

MORTON E. SALOMON, MD, FACEP, FAAP

Professor of Clinical Emergency Medicine
Associate Professor of Pediatrics
Albert Einstein College of Medicine
Chairman, Department of Emergency Medicine
St. Vincent's Medical Center, Bridgeport, Connecticut
Chapter 73, "Nicotine and Tobacco Preparations"

DIANE SAUTER, MD, FACEP

Chairman, Department of Emergency Medicine
Greater Southeast Community Hospital
Washington, District of Columbia
Chapter 25, "Hematologic Principles"

DAVID T. SCHWARTZ, MD

Associate Professor of Clinical Surgery/Emergency Medicine
New York University School of Medicine
Attending Physician
Department of Emergency Medicine
New York University Medical Center/Bellevue Hospital Center
New York, New York
Chapter 8, "Diagnostic Imaging in Toxicology"

MARK SERPER, PhD

Associate Professor of Psychology
Hofstra University

Research Assistant Professor of Psychiatry
New York University School of Medicine
New York, New York
Chapter 114, "Psychiatric Principles"

ADHI N. SHARMA, MD
Fellow in Medical Toxicology
Department of Clinical Surgery/Emergency Medicine
New York University School of Medicine
Bellevue Hospital Center
New York City Poison Center
New York, New York
Chapter 66, "Toxic Alcohols"

MARTIN JAY SMILKSTEIN, MD
Associate Professor of Emergency Medicine
Department of Emergency Medicine
Associate Director, Toxicology Fellowship Program
Oregon Poison Center
Oregon Health Sciences University
Portland, Oregon
Chapter 22, "Gastrointestinal Principles"
Chapter 27, "Ophthalmic Principles"
Chapter 32, "Acetaminophen"

KEVIN SMOTHERS, MD, FACEP
Physician Director
Medicine Service Line
Franklin Square Hospital Center
Baltimore, Maryland
Chapter 108, "The HIV-Positive Patient—AIDS Pharmacology and Toxicology"

BARBARA E. SOPPET, RN, MA
Nurse Clinician
Division of Nursing
Emergency Department
Coney Island Hospital
Brooklyn, New York
Chapter 115, "Nursing Principles"

CHRISTINE M. STORK, PharmD, DABAT
Clinical Assistant Professor
Director, Central New York Poison Control Center
Department of Emergency Medicine
University Hospital, State University of New York Health Science Center
Syracuse, New York
Chapter 46, "Antibiotics"
Chapter 58, "Serotonin Reuptake Inhibitors and Atypical Antidepressants"

MARK SU, MD
Fellow in Medical Toxicology
Department of Clinical Surgery/Emergency Medicine
New York University School of Medicine
Bellevue Hospital Center
New York City Poison Center
New York, New York
Chapter 42, "Anticoagulants"

JEFFREY R. SUCHARD, MD
Assistant Clinical Professor, Division of Emergency Medicine
University of California Irvine Medical Center
Orange, California
Chapter 100, "Chemical and Biologic Weapons"

YOUNG-JIN SUE, MD
Assistant Clinical Professor
Division of Pediatric Emergency Medicine
Department of Pediatrics
Albert Einstein College of Medicine
Attending Physician
Division of Pediatric Emergency Services
Department of Pediatrics
Montefiore Medical Center
Bronx, New York
Chapter 81, "Mercury"

KENNETH M. SUTIN, MD
Assistant Professor of Clinical Anesthesiology and Surgery
New York University School of Medicine
Director of Critical Care
Bellevue Hospital Center
New York University Medical Center and Bellevue Hospital Center
Chapter 54, "Neuromuscular Blocking Agents"

STEPHEN R. THOM, MD, PhD
Associate Professor of Emergency Medicine
Department of Emergency Medicine
Chief of Hyperbaric Medicine
Institute for Environmental Medicine
University of Pennsylvania
Philadelphia, Pennsylvania
Antidotes in Depth, "Hyperbaric Oxygen"

CHRISTIAN TOMASZEWSKI, MD
Clinical Assistant Professor
Department of Emergency Medicine
University of North Carolina—Chapel Hill
Chapel Hill, North Carolina
Toxicology Fellowship Director
Medical Director, Hyperbaric Medicine
Department of Emergency Medicine
Carolinas Medical Center
Charlotte, North Carolina
Chapter 97, "Carbon Monoxide"

REBECCA L. TOMINACK, MD
Assistant Medical Director
Missouri Regional Poison Center
SSM Cardinal Glennon Children's Hospital
Associate Professor of Medicine and Pediatrics
Division of Toxicology
Saint Louis University Medical School
St. Louis, Missouri
Chapter 91, "Herbicides"

STEPHEN J. TRAUB, MD
Fellow in Medical Toxicology
Department of Clinical Surgery/Emergency Medicine
New York University School of Medicine
Bellevue Hospital Center
New York City Poison Center
New York, New York
Chapter 12, "Chemical Principles"
Chapter 82B, "Cadmium"

JEFFREY R. TUCKER, MD
Assistant Professor of Pediatrics and Emergency Medicine

University of Connecticut School of Medicine
Farmington, Connecticut
Attending Physician
Division of Emergency Medicine
Department of Pediatrics
Connecticut Children's Medical Center
Hartford, Connecticut
**Chapter 70, "Lysergic Acid Diethylamide
    and Other Hallucinogens"**

MICHAEL G. TUNIK, MD
Clinical Associate Professor of Pediatrics
New York University School of Medicine
Director of Research
Pediatric Emergency Medicine
Attending Physician
Department of Emergency Medicine
Bellevue Hospital Center
New York, New York
Chapter 74, "Food Poisoning"

SUSI U. VASSALLO, MD, FACEP, FACMT
Assistant Professor of Clinical Surgery/Emergency Medicine
New York University School of Medicine
Attending Physician
Department of Emergency Medicine
Bellevue Hospital Center and
New York University Medical Center
Consultant, New York City Poison Center
New York, New York
Chapter 18, "Thermoregulatory Principles"
Chapter 112, "Sports Toxicology"

LISA E. VIVERO, MD
Department of Pharmacology
Trinity College, School of Pharmacy
Dublin, Ireland
Chapter 56, "Pharmaceutical Additives"

STAFFAN WAHLANDER, MD
Assistant Professor of Anesthesiology
College of Physicians and Surgeons of Columbia University
Columbia Presbyterian Medical Center
New York, New York
Chapter 55, "Local Anesthetics"

PETER H. WALD, MD, MPH
Principal and Medical Director
WorkCare Incorporated
Orange, California
Chapter 92, "Industrial Poisoning: Information and Control"

FRANK G. WALTER, MD, FACEP, FACMT
Associate Professor of Emergency Medicine
Director, Medical Toxicology Fellowship
Department of Emergency Medicine
University of Arizona College of Medicine
Director of Clinical Toxicology
University Medical Center
Tucson, Arizona
**Chapter 93, "Hazmat Incident Response with Pre- and Interhospital
    Care of the Poisoned Patient"**

RICHARD Y. WANG, DO, FACEP
Director, Division of Medical Toxicology
Department of Emergency Medicine
Rhode Island Hospital
Brown University School of Medicine
Providence, Rhode Island
Chapter 47, "Antineoplastic Agents"

WILLIAM A. WATSON, PharmD, DABAT, FAACT, FAACP
Professor (Clinical), Department of Surgery
Managing Director, South Texas Poison Center
University of Texas Health Science Center At San Antonio
San Antonio, Texas
Chapter 34, "Nonsteroidal Antiinflammatory Agents"

PAUL M. WAX, MD, FACMT
Medical Toxicology Fellowship Director
Department of Medical Toxicology
Good Samaritan Regional Medical Center
Phoenix, Arizona
Chapter 1, "Historical Principles and Perspectives"
Chapter 2, "Toxicologic Plagues and Disasters in History"
Chapter 84, "Antiseptics, Disinfectants, and Sterilants"
Antidotes in Depth, "Antiquated Antidotes"
Antidotes in Depth, "Sodium Bicarbonate"

RICHARD S. WEISMAN, PharmD, DABAT, FAACT
Director, Florida Poison Information Center, Miami
Associate Research Professor of Pediatrics
University of Miami School of Medicine
Miami, Florida
**Chapter 4, "Principles and Techniques to Identify the Nontoxic
    Exposure"**
Chapter 35, "Antihistamines and Decongestants"
Chapter 103, "Marine Envenomations"

LESLIE R. WOLF, MD
Assistant Professor
Toxicology Coordinator
Department of Emergency Medicine
Wright State University School of Medicine
Dayton, Ohio
Chapter 30, "Genitourinary Principles"

LUKE YIP, MD
Attending Physician
Rocky Mountain Poison and Drug Center
Denver Medical Center
Department of Medicine, Section of Clinical Toxicology
Clinical Assistant Professor
University of Colorado Health Sciences Center
Department of Pharmaceutical Sciences
School of Pharmacy
Denver, Colorado
Chapter 64, "Ethanol"

TABLE OF ANTIDOTES IN DEPTH

Reader's of previous editions of Goldfrank's Toxicologic Emergencies are undoubtedly aware that the editors have always felt that an emphasis on general management of poisoning or overdoses coupled wth sound medical management is more important or as important as the selection and use of a specific antidote in the vast majority of cases. Nevertheless, there are some instances where nothing other than the timely use of a specific antidote or antagonist will save a patient. For this reason, and also because the use of such antidotes may be problematic, controversial, or unfamiliar to the practitioner (as new antidotes continue to emerge), we have included a section (or sections) at the end of each chapter where an in-depth discussion of such antidotes is relevant. The following "Antidotes in Depth" are included in this edition.

TABLE OF CONTENTS

Part D

THE CLINICAL BASIS OF MEDICAL TOXICOLOGY

SECTION I. CASE STUDIES IN TOXICOLOGIC EMERGENCIES

PREFACE

In this seventh edition of *Goldfrank's Toxicologic Emergencies,* we continue to proudly offer readers a case study approach to medical toxicology. Five new chapters in this edition are a reflection of some of the major advances, changes in our understanding and the ever expanding role of toxicologists.

We have tried to advance the usefulness of the basic sciences section by adding a chapter, Chemical Principles to serve as a foundation for many of the chapters that follow, particularly the Biochemical Principles chapter.

Critical medical events in the last decade have led to the development of four other new chapters: *Chemical and Biological Weapons, Sports Toxicology, Adverse Drug Events and Postmortem Toxicology.*

This new edition brings a major change in editorial leadership for our text. Richard Weisman, Pharm. D who played a role as editor for five editions, retains his role as author, but has chosen to devote a great deal of his creative efforts to other worthwhile toxicological activities. His substantial editorial contribution to our text will be missed.

Lewis S. Nelson, MD, the Director of our Fellowship Training Program in Medical Toxicology has joined our text as an editor as well as an author and his breadth of knowledge, immense energies and creative expression are already making a dramatic contribution to our efforts. The unifying style for the graphic expression of diverse toxicologic concepts that are evident throughout this edition are a clear example of his talents and his abilities to integrate his skills collaboratively with ours.

Goldfrank's Toxicologic Emergencies, originally a collection of clinical toxicology case discussions by two authors, is now a multi-authored text of more than 2,000 pages prepared under the direction of six author-editors who work at the New York City Poison Center. As the text has expanded in size and scope over the past two decades, we have sought to address issues in medical toxicology in unique and creative ways that would continue to make the book a valuable resource to the growing number of clinicians and researchers working in the field. In the second edition of our text (1982), we expanded the case study material to make the work a more comprehensive clinical resource. In the third edition (1986), we added an organ-system approach to medical toxicology and also began a series of *Antidotes-in-Depth* to provide specific detailed information about newer and, in some cases, experimental antidotes. In the fourth edition (1990), we expanded both of these newer sections and began to address such subjects as nursing care, medical-legal issues, and the toxicology of AIDS treatments. For the fifth edition (1994), we added a section addressing the needs of special populations including reproductive, perinatal, pediatric, and geriatric principles and intensive care unit patients; we also began to seriously consider basic science issues such as neurotransmitters and biochemical and metabolic pathways.

In the sixth and seventh editions we have continued our reflective approach by adding, fusing and splitting chapters based on the ever changing educational principles. For example the chapter on Anesthetics and Neuromuscular blocking agents that first appeared in the sixth edition has now been divided into three chapters: Inhalational Anesthetics, Neuromuscular Blocking Agents and Local Anesthetics. The single chapter on Heavy Metals has been divided into subchapters on Bismuth, Cadmium and Copper to focus on these agents in greater detail. The chapters on Hazardous Materials and their Decontamination and Prehospital and Interhospital Principles have been fused to emphasize the necessity of providing a continuum of care for these activities throughout the process of providing clinical care from the initial site through the hospitalization.

In this edition we reintegrated the Workbook sections of case studies and annotated multiple choice questions into the main text. Some cases are still relevant classical examples of toxicologic emergencies from previous editions and the remainder are new, extensively discussed cases from our regional monthly meetings. The wisdom of many of the current and former text authors has continued to be shared in these sessions for more than 20 years. Lewis Nelson and Robert Hoffman have analyzed these problems, distilled the discussions, and recreated the spirit of the meeting in these printed versions of the cases. Ten annotated multiple choice questions based on each chapter were developed by the respective chapter authors in an attempt to enhance self learning and meet the intellectual needs of our readers.

Work on the next edition of this text literally begins the day that the current edition is published. Although many of the chapters in this seventh edition may appear familiar to readers of previous editions, every single chapter without exception was discussed, analyzed, criticized, and dissected at our weekly editors' meetings and updated and rewritten accordingly by its old and/or new authors.

We have expanded the number of authors in this edition and have reassigned more than 20% of the chapters in an attempt to capture new and unique perspectives on toxicology.

After long and serious discussions, we have come to the conclusion that the format of utilizing cases to begin each chapter in Section I of *Part D: The Clinical Basis of Medical Toxicology* is an important and useful feature distinguishing our text from others and therefore should be retained. At the same time, it has become clear to us that the ease with which readers can find needed information in a traditionally organized comprehensive medical textbook is also valuable. We have therefore divided each chapter into standard sections to allow readers to find essential information when reviewing a topic or preparing for and treating a toxicologic emergency. Most chapters in this section are now initiated by a case followed by a brief Introduction, History and Epidemiology, Pharmacology, Pharmacokinetics and Toxicokinetics,

Pathophysiology, Clinical Manifestations, Diagnostic Testing, and Management concluding with a brief summary.

We hope that this chapter organization will further facilitate the usefulness of the index. The index has now been restructured in such a way that each chapter component will be listed according to the aforementioned subheads and will include almost all cross references from other chapters within these subheads. Of course, additional alphabetical listings of unique and important terms will also be retained.

Even more than previously, the rewriting and reorganization of this edition of the text has required an enormous personal effort by each author which we hope will facilitate your learning, reading and patient care.

Although "tearing down" and reconstructing the text between each edition may seem like an extreme exercise to some, only in this manner can we hope to prevent ourselves from accepting and promulgating unfounded treatments and outdated concepts. We hope that you agree that this exercise is worthwhile and that each

"new text" continues to serve you well. As always, we encourage your comments and thoughtful criticism, and we will do our best to incorporate your suggestions into future editions.

If this text helps to provide better patient care and stimulates interest in medical toxicology by students of medicine, nursing, and pharmacy; residents in emergency medicine, internal medicine, pediatrics, preventive health, critical care, family practice and others; and, of course, fellows in medical toxicology, our efforts will have indeed been worthwhile.

Lewis R. Goldfrank
Neal E. Flomenbaum
Neal A. Lewin
Mary Ann Howland
Robert S. Hoffman
Lewis S. Nelson

ACKNOWLEDGMENTS

We are grateful to Joan Demas, who not only helped manage this seventh edition's growth and development but also transformed scrawl into manuscript with precision and dedication.

The many letters and verbal communications we have received with the reviews of the previous editions of this book continue to improve our efforts. We are deeply indebted to our friends, associates, and students who stimulated us to begin this book with their questions and then faithfully criticized our answers.

We thank the many volunteers, students, librarians, and particularly the St. John's University College of Pharmacy students and drug information staff who provide us with vital technical assistance in our daily attempt to deal with toxicologic emergencies.

We appreciate the artistic skills of John Ruggeri and Pamela Ryder, FNP, who have added line drawings of important plants and mushrooms to assist the reader in the understanding of these botanical species.

No words can adequately express our indebtedness to the many authors who worked on earlier editions of many of the chapters in this book. As different authors write and rewrite topics with each new edition, we recognize that without the foundation work of their predecessors this book would not be what it is today.

We are forever indebted to the librarian of the New York City Health Department Shirley Chapin who has graciously, enthusiastically and methodically facilitated our efforts. We appreciate the conscientious and tireless work of James Semidey who has found so many essential articles and prepared so many copies for editorial review.

We appreciate the support of *Emergency Medicine* for publishing Lewis S. Nelson's reports of our monthly toxicology meeting at the NYC Poison Center as well as *Emergency Medicine's* willingness to permit us to use these same cases in the workbook section of this edition of the text.

We appreciate the calm, thoughtful and cooperative spirit of Karen Edmonson. Her intelligence and commitment to our efforts has been wonderful. We are pleased with the creative copyediting efforts of Richard Adin and Elissa Schiff. We greatly appreciate the compulsion and vigor that Kathi Unger has applied to our efforts to make this edition's index of unique value.

GOLDFRANK'S

TOXICOLOGIC EMERGENCIES

7th EDITION

CHAPTER 1

HISTORICAL PRINCIPLES AND PERSPECTIVES

Paul M. Wax

The term *poison* first appeared in the English literature around the year 1230 A.D. to describe a potion or draught that had been prepared with deadly ingredients.[109,136] The history of poisons and poisoning, however, dates back thousands of years. Throughout the millennia, poisons have played an important role in human history—from political assassination in Roman times to contemporary environmental concerns.

This chapter offers a perspective on the impact of poisons and poisoning on history. It also provides an historic overview of human understanding of poisons and the development of toxicology. The chapter follows the important events in the evolution of toxicology from antiquity to the present. The development of the modern poison control center, the genesis of the field of medical toxicology, and the recent increasing focus on medical errors are examined. An Antidote in Depth segment at the end of the chapter scrutinizes changes in poison management over the years, analyzing obsolete antidotes and other discarded therapeutic modalities. Chapter 2 describes poison plagues and disasters throughout history and examines the societal consequences of these unfortunate events. An appreciation of past successes and mistakes in dealing with poisons and poisoning promotes a keener insight and a more critical evaluation of present-day toxicologic issues, and helps in the assessment and management of future toxicologic problems.

POISONS, POISONERS, AND ANTIDOTES OF ANTIQUITY

The earliest poisons consisted of plant extracts, animal venoms, and minerals. They were used for hunting, waging war, and sanctioned and unsanctioned executions. The *Ebers Papyrus*, an ancient Egyptian text written about 1500 B.C., which is considered to be among the earliest medical records, describes many ancient poisons, including arsenic, antimony, lead, opium, mandrake, hemlock, aconite, wormwood, and cyanogenic glycosides.[91,136] These poisons were thought to have mystical properties, and their use was surrounded by superstition and intrigue. Some agents, such as the Calabar bean from the plant *Physostigma venenosum* containing physostigmine, were referred to as "ordeal poisons." Ingestion of these substances was believed to be lethal to the guilty and harmless to the innocent.[91] The "penalty of the peach" involved the administration of the ordeal poison of peach pits, which contain amygdalin that is metabolized to cyanide. Magicians, sorcerers, and priests were the poison experts of antiquity. The Sumerians, in about 4500 B.C., were said to worship the deity Gula, who was known as the "mistress of charms and spells" and the "controller of noxious poisons" (Table 1–1).[136]

Arrow and Dart Poisons

The prehistoric Masai hunters of Kenya, who lived 18,000 years ago, may have utilized arrow and dart poisons to increase the lethality of their weapons.[18] One of these poisons appears to have consisted of extracts of *Strophanthus* species, an indigenous plant that contains strophanthin, a digitalis-like substance.[91] Cave paintings of arrowheads and spearheads reveal that these weapons were crafted with small depressions at the end to hold the poison.[137] In fact, the term *toxicology* appears to be derived from the Greek terms *toxikos* ("bow") and *toxikon* ("poison into which arrowheads are dipped").[5,137]

References to arrow poisons are cited in a number of other important literary works. The ancient Indian text *Rg Veda*, written in the 12th century B.C., refers to the use of *Aconitum* species for arrow poisons.[18] In the *Odyssey*, Homer (ca. 850 B.C.) wrote that Ulysses anointed his arrows with a variety of poisons, including extracts of *Helleborus orientalis* (thought to act as a heart poison) and snake venoms.[106] Aristotle (384–322 B.C.) described how the Scythians prepared and used arrow poisons.[138] In the Book of Job 6:04, arrow poisons are also cited: "For the arrows of the Almighty pierce men, and my spirit drinks in their poison."[17] Finally, reference to weapons poisoned with the blood of serpents can be found in the writings of Ovid (43 B.C.–A.D. 18).[144]

The first attempts at poison identification and classification, and the introduction of the first antidotes, took place during Greek and Roman times. An early categorization of poisons divided them into fast poisons, such as strychnine, and slow poisons, such as arsenic. In his treatise, *Materia Medica*, the Greek physician Dioscorides (A.D. 40–80), categorized poisons by their origin: animal, vegetable, or mineral.[137] This categorization remained the standard classification for the next 1500 years.[137]

Animal Poisons

Animal poisons usually referred to the venom from poisonous animals. Although the venom from poisonous snakes has always been among the most commonly feared poisons, poisons from toads, salamanders, jellyfish, stingrays, and sea hares were also of concern. Nicander of Colophon (204–135 B.C.), a Greek poet and physician, and considered to be one of the earliest toxicologists, experimented with animal poisons on condemned criminals.[125] Nicander's poem *Theriaca*, which along with his other toxicologic verse *Alexipharmaca* is considered to be the earliest extant Greek toxicologic text, described the presentations and treatment of poisonings from animal toxins.[136] A notable fatality from the effects of an animal toxin was Cleopatra (69–30 B.C.), who reportedly committed suicide by deliberately falling on an African cobra.[72]

TABLE 1–1.   Important Early Figures in the History of Toxicology

Person	Date	Importance
Gula	ca. 4500 B.C.	First deity associated with poisons
Shen Nung	ca. 2000 B.C.	Chinese emperor who experimented with poisons and antidotes and wrote treatise on herbal medicine
Homer	ca. 850 B.C.	Wrote how Ulysses anointed arrows with the venom of serpents
Aristotle	384–322 B.C.	Described the preparation and use of arrow poisons
Theophrastus	ca. 370–286 B.C.	Referred to poisonous plants in *De Historia Plantarum*
Socrates	ca. 470–399 B.C.	Executed by poison hemlock
Nicander	204–135 B.C.	Wrote two poems that are among the earliest works on poisons: *Theriaca* and *Alexipharmaca*
King Mithridates VI	ca. 132–63 B.C.	Fanatical fear of poisons; developed mithradatum, one of first universal antidotes
Sulla	81 B.C.	Issued *Lex Cornelia,* first antipoisoning law
Cleopatra	69–30 B.C.	Committed suicide from deliberate cobra snake envenomation
Andromachus	A.D. 37–68	Refined the mithradatum, known as the Theriac of Andromachus
Dioscorides	A.D. 40–80	Wrote *Materia Medica,* which classified poison by animal, vegetable, and mineral
Galen	ca. A.D. 129–200	Prepared "Nut Theriac" for Roman Emperiors, a remedy against bites, stings, and poisons; wrote *De Antidotis I and II,* which provided recipes for different antidotes, including mithradatum and panacea
Ibn Wahshiya	9th century	Famed Arabic toxicologist. Wrote toxicology treatise *Book on Poisons,* combining contemporary science, magic, and astrology
Moses Maimonides	1135–1204	Wrote *Treatise on Poisons and Their Antidotes*
Petrus Abbonus	1250–1315	Wrote *De Venenis,* major work on poisoning

Vegetable Poisons

Theophrastus (ca. 370–286 B.C.) described vegetable poisons in his treatise *De Historia Plantarum.*[73] Notorious poisonous plants included *Aconitum* species (aconite), *Veratrum album* (hellebore), *Hyoscyamus niger* (henbane), *Mandragora officinarum* (mandrake), *Conium maculatum* (hemlock), and *Papaver somniferum* (opium). Aconite was among the most frequently encountered poisonous plants and has been described as the "queen mother of poisons."[136] Hemlock was the official poison used by the Greeks and was employed in the execution of Socrates (ca. 470–399 B.C.) and many others.[127] Poisonous plants used in India at this time included *Cannabis indica* (tetrahydrocannabinol), *Croton tiglium* (croton oil), and *Strychnos nux vomica* (strychnine).[73]

Mineral Poisons

The mineral poisons of antiquity consisted of the heavy metals: lead, mercury, arsenic, and antimony. Undoubtedly the most famous of these was lead. Lead was discovered as early as 3500 B.C. Although controversy continues to this day about whether an epidemic of lead poisoning among the Roman aristocracy contributed to the fall of the Roman Empire, lead was certainly used extensively during this period.[54,105] In addition to its considerable use in plumbing, lead was also utilized in the production of food and drink containers.[61] It was common practice to add lead directly to wine, or to intentionally prepare the wine in a leaden kettle to improve its taste. Not surprisingly, chronic lead poisoning became widespread. Nicander is credited with describing the first case of lead poisoning in the 2nd century B.C.[142] Dioscorides, writing in the 1st century A.D., noted that fortified wine was "most hurtful to the nerves."[142] Lead-induced gout ("saturnine gout") may have also been widespread among the Roman elite.[105]

Although not animal, vegetable, or mineral in origin, the toxic effects of gases were also appreciated during antiquity. In the 3rd century B.C., Aristotle commented that "coal fumes (carbon monoxide) lead to a heavy head and death"[70] and Cicero (106–43 B.C.) referred to the use of coal fumes in suicide and execution, a practice that continues 2000 years later.

Poisoners of Antiquity

Intentional poisoning was common during Roman times. In an attempt to curtail this practice, the Roman dictator Sulla issued the first law against poisoning, entitled the *Lex Cornelia,* in 81 B.C. According to its provisions, if convicted of poisoning, the perpetrator was sentenced to either loss of property and exile (if the perpetrator was of high rank) or exposure to wild beasts (if the perpetrator was of low rank). During this period, members of the aristocracy employed "tasters" to shield themselves from potential poisoners, a practice that was also in vogue during the reign of Louis XIV in 16th century France.[144]

One of the most infamous poisoners of Ancient Rome was Locusta, who was known to experiment on slaves with poisons that included arsenic, aconite, henbane, belladonna, and poisonous fungi. In A.D. 54, Nero's mother, Agrippina, hired Locusta to poison Claudius (Agrippina's husband and Nero's stepfather) and Britannicus (Nero's stepbrother) as part of a scheme to make Nero emperor. As a result of these activities, Claudius, who was a great lover of mushrooms, died from *Amanita phalloides* poisoning,[15] and in the next year, Britannicus also became one of Locusta's victims. In the case of Britannicus, Locusta managed to fool the taster by preparing unusually hot soup that required additional cooling after the soup had been officially tasted. At the time of cooling, the poison was unobtrusively slipped into the soup. Almost immediately after drinking the soup prepared in this manner, Britannicus collapsed and died. The exact identity of Locusta's choice of poison here remains debatable, but the rapidity of Britannicus's death suggests that it was a cyanogenic substance.[130]

Early Quests for the Universal Antidote

The recognition, classification, and use of poisons in Ancient Greece and Rome were accompanied by an intensive search for a universal antidote. In fact, many of the physicians of this period devoted significant parts of their careers to this endeavor.[136] Mystery and superstition surrounded the origin and source of these proposed antidotes. One of the earliest specific references to a protective agent can be found in Homer's *Odyssey,* when Ulysses is advised to protect himself by taking the antidote "moli." Recent speculation suggests that moli referred to *Galanthus nivalis*, a naturally occurring cholinesterase inhibitor. This agent could have been used as an antidote against poisonous plants such as *Datura stramonium*.[113]

Theriacs and the Mithradatum. The Greeks referred to the universal antidote as the *alexipharmaca* or *theriac*.[136] The term *alexipharmaca* was derived from the words *alexipharmakos* ("which keeps off poison") and *antipharmakon* ("antidote"). Over the years, *alexipharmaca* has been increasingly used to refer to a method of treatment, such as the induction of emesis by using a feather. *Theriac*, which originally had referred to poisonous reptiles or wild beasts, was later used to refer to the antidotes. Ingestion of the early theriacs (ca. 200 B.C.) was reputed to make people "poison-proof" against bites of all venomous animals except the asp. Their ingredients included wild thyme, apoponax, aniseed, fennel, parsley, meru, and anmi.[136]

The quest for the universal antidote was epitomized by the work of King Mithradates VI of Pontus (132–63 B.C.).[71] After repeatedly being subjected to poisoning attempts by his enemies during his youth, Mithradates channeled his fear of being poisoned into the development of universal antidotes. To find the best antidote, he performed acute toxicity experiments on criminals and slaves. The preparation he concocted, known as the "mithradatum," contained a minimum of 36 ingredients and was considered the best antidote in the Roman pharmacy at that time. This concoction was thought to be protective against spiders, scorpions, vipers, sea slugs, aconite, and all other poisonous substances.[71] Mithradates took his concoction every day. Ironically, as an old man, Mithradates attempted suicide by poison but supposedly was unsuccessful because he had become poison-proof. Having failed at self-poisoning, Mithradates was compelled to have a soldier kill him with a sword. Galen described Mithradates' experiences in a series of three books: *De Antidotis I, De Antidotis II,* and *De Theriaca ad Pisonem*.[71,140]

The Theriac of Andromachus, also known as the "Venice treacle" or "galene," is probably the most famous theriac. According to Galen, this preparation, formulated during the 1st century A.D., was considered an improvement over the mithradatum.[140] It was prepared by Andromachus (A.D. 37–68), physician to emperor Nero. Andromachus added to the mithradatum ingredients such as the flesh of vipers, squills, and generous amounts of opium.[146] Other ingredients were removed. Altogether, 73 ingredients were required. It was advocated to "counteract all poisons and bites of venomous animals," as well as a host of other medical problems, such as colic, jaundice, and dropsy, and it was used both therapeutically and prophylactically.[136,140] As evidence of its efficacy, Galen demonstrated that fowl receiving poison followed by theriac had a higher survival rate than fowl receiving poison alone.[136] It is likely, however, that the scientific rigor and methodology employed differed from current scientific practice.

By the Middle Ages, the Theriac of Andromachus contained more than 100 ingredients. Its synthesis was quite elaborate; the initial production period lasted months, followed by an aging process that lasted years, somewhat like vintage wine.[87] The final product was often more solid than liquid in consistency.

Other theriac preparations were named after famous physicians (Damocrates, Nicolaus, Amando, Arnauld, and Abano) who contributed additional ingredients to the original formulation. Over the centuries certain localities were celebrated for their own peculiar brand of theriac. Notable centers of theriac production included Cairo, Venice, Florence, Genoa, Bologna, and Istanbul. At times, theriac production was accompanied by great fanfare. For example, in Bologna, the mixing of the theriac could take place only under the direction of the medical professors at the university.[136]

Whether these preparations truly benefited anyone is debatable. Some have suggested that the theriac may have had an antiseptic effect on the gastrointestinal tract, while others have stated that theriac's sole benefit derived from its formulation with opium.[87] Theriacs remained in vogue throughout the Middle Ages and Renaissance, and it was not until 1745 that their efficacy was finally questioned by William Heberden in *Antitheriaka: An Essay on Mithradatum and Theriaca*.[71] Nonetheless, pharmacopeias in France, Spain, and Germany continued to list these agents until the last quarter of the 19th century and theriac was still available in Italy and Turkey into the early 20th century.[16,87]

Sacred Earth. Beginning in the 5th century B.C., an adsorbent agent called *terra sigillata* was promoted as a universal antidote. This agent, also known as the "sacred sealed earth," consisted of red clay that could be found on only one particular hill on the Greek island of Lemnos. Perhaps somewhat akin to the 20th-century "universal antidote," it was advocated as effective in counteracting all poisons.[136] With great ceremony, once per year, the terra sigillata was retrieved from this hill and prepared for subsequent use. According to Dioscorides, this clay was formulated with goat's blood to make it into a paste. At one time, it was included as part of the Theriac of Andromachus. Demand for terra sigillata continued into the 15th century. Similar antidotal clays were found in Italy, Malta, Silesia, and England. Later analysis revealed these clays to be a combination of iron, aluminum, magnesium, and silicates.[136]

Charms. Charms, such as toadstones, snakestones, unicorn horns, and bezoar stones, were also promoted as universal antidotes. Toadstones, found in the heads of old toads, were reputed to have the capability to extract poison from the site of a venomous bite or sting. In addition, the toadstone was supposedly able to detect the mere presence of poison by producing a sensation of heat upon contact with a poisonous substance.[136]

Likewise, snakestones extracted from the heads of cobras (known as *piedras della cobra de Capelos*) were also reported to have similar magical qualities.[13] The 17th-century Italian philosopher Athanasius Kircher (1602–1680) became an enthusiastic supporter of snakestone therapy for the treatment of snakebite after conducting experiments in the 1660s, demonstrating the antidotal attributes of these charms "in front of amazed spectators." Kircher attributed the snakestone's efficacy to the theory of "attraction of like substances," suggesting that the snakestone attracts magnetically and sympathetically toxic spirits from the snake bite that circulate in the victim's bloodstream. Francesco Redi (1626–1698), a court physician and contemporary of Kircher, debunked this quixotic approach. A harbinger of future experimental toxicologists, Redi was not willing to accept isolated case reports and field demonstrations as proof of the snakestone's utility. Using a considerably more rigorous approach, *provando et riprovando* (by testing and retesting), Redi performed multiple experiments assessing the antidotal efficacy of snakestone on different animal species and different toxins and failed to confirm any benefit from the use of snakestone.[13]

Much lore has surrounded the antidotal effects of the mythical unicorn horn. Ctesias, writing in 390 B.C., was the first to chronicle the wonders of the unicorn horn, claiming that drinking water or wine from the "horn of the unicorn" would protect against poison.[136] The horns were usually narwhal tusks or rhinoceros horns and were greatly valued. During the Middle Ages, the unicorn horn may have been worth as much as 10 times the price of gold. Similar to the toadstone, the unicorn horn was used both to detect poisons and to neutralize them. Supposedly a cup made of unicorn horn would sweat if a poisonous substance was placed in it.[85] To give further credence to its use, a 1593 study on arsenic-poisoned dogs reportedly showed that the horn was protective.[85]

Bezoar stones, also touted as universal antidotes, consisted of stomach or intestinal calculi formed by the deposition of calcium phosphate around a hair, fruit pit, or gallstone. They were removed from wild goats, cows, and apes and administered orally. The Persian name for the bezoar stone was *pad zahr* ("expeller of poisons"). The ancient Hebrews referred to them as *bel Zaard* ("every cure for poisons"). Over the years, regional variations of bezoar stones were popularized, including an Asian variety from wild goat of Persia, an Occidental variety from llamas of Peru, and a European variety from chamois of the Swiss mountains.[48,136]

Opium, Coca, and Hallucinogens in Antiquity

Although it was not until the mid-19th century that the peril of opiate addiction was first recognized, juice from the *Papaver somniferum* was known for its medicinal value in Egypt, at least as early as the writing of the *Ebers Papyrus* in 1500 B.C. Egyptian pharmacologists of that time reportedly recommended opium as a pacifier for children who exhibited incessant crying.[124] In Ancient Greece, Dioscorides and Galen were early advocates of opium as a therapeutic agent. During this time, it was also used as a means of suicide. Mithradates' lack of success in his own attempted suicide by poisoning may have been due to an opium tolerance that had developed from previous repetitive use.[124] One of the earliest descriptions of the abuse potential of opium is attributed to Epistratos (304–257 B.C.), who criticized the use of opium for earache because it "dulled the sight and is a narcotic."[124]

Cocaine use dates back to at least 300 B.C., when South American Indians reportedly chewed coca leaves during religious ceremonies.[99] Chewing coca to increase work efficacy and to elevate mood has remained commonplace in some South American societies for thousands of years. A recent study of an Egyptian mummy from about 950 B.C. revealed significant amounts of cocaine in the stomach and liver, suggesting oral use of cocaine during this time period.[103] High amounts of tetrahydrocannabinol (THC) were found in the lung and muscle of the same mummy. In another investigation of 11 Egyptian (1079 B.C.–A.D. 395) and 72 Peruvian (A.D. 200–1500) mummies, cocaine, thought to be indigenous only to South America, and hashish, thought to be indigenous only to Asia, were found in both groups.[112]

Other currently abused agents that were known to the ancients include peyote, hallucinogenic mushrooms, nutmeg, and cannabis. As early as 1300 B.C., Peruvian indian tribal ceremonies included the use of mescaline-containing San Pedro cacti.[99] The hallucinogenic mushroom, *Amanita muscaria,* known as "fly agaric," was used as a ritual drug and may have been known in India as "soma" around 2000 B.C. The use of cannabis dates back even further, to around 2700 B.C., when the Chinese used it. Known as the "liberator of sin," cannabis use during that period may have been both therapeutic and recreational.[99] In India and Iran, it was used as an intoxicant known as *bhang* as early as 1000 B.C.[102]

Early Attempts at Gastrointestinal Decontamination

Nicander's *Alexipharmaca* ("Antidotes for Poisons") recommended induction of emesis by one of several different methods: (a) ingesting warm linseed oil; (b) tickling the hypopharynx with a feather; or (c) "emptying the gullet with a small twisted and curved paper."[90] Nicander also advocated the use of suction to limit envenomation.[137] The Romans referred to the feather as the "vomiting feather" or "pinna." Most commonly, the feather was utilized after a hearty feast to avoid the gastrointestinal discomfort associated with overeating. At times, the pinna was dipped into a nauseating mixture to increase its efficacy.[90]

TOXICOLOGY DURING THE MEDIEVAL AND RENAISSANCE PERIODS

From the fall of Rome until the Renaissance, there is relatively little documented attention to the subject of poisons. Three of the most important medieval texts were written by Ibn Wahshiya (9th century), Moses Maimonides (12th century), and Petrus Abbonus (13th century) (Table 1–1). During the 9th century, a golden age of Arab toxicology, Arab scholars, including Jabir and Ibn Wahshiya, wrote several toxicology treatises entitled *Book of Poisons*.[82] Citing Greek, Persian, and Indian texts, Ibn Wahshiya's work combines contemporary science, magic, and astrology. In a lengthy treatise, Ibn Wahshiya discussed poison mechanisms (as they were understood at that time), symptomatology, antidotes, including his own recommendation for a universal antidote, and prophylaxis. He categorized poisons as lethal by sight, smell, touch, and sound, as well as by drinking and eating. For victims of an aconite-containing dart arrow, Ibn Wahshiya recommended excision, followed by cauterization and topical treatment with onion and salt.[82]

Another significant medieval contribution to toxicology can be found in Moses Maimonides' (1135–1204) *Treatise on Poisons and Their Antidotes.* In part one of this 1198 treatise, Maimonides discussed the bites of snakes and mad dogs, and the stings of bees, wasps, spiders, and scorpions.[122] He also discussed the use of cupping glasses for bites (a progenitor of the modern suctioning device), and was one of the first to differentiate the hematotoxic (hot) from the neurotoxic (cold) effects of poison. In part two, he discussed mineral and vegetable poisons and their antidotes. He described belladonna poisoning as causing a "redness and a sort of excitation."[122] He suggested that emesis should be induced by hot water, anethum, and oil, followed by fresh milk, butter, and honey. Although he rejected some of the popular treatments of the day, he advocated the use of the great theriac and the mithradatum as first- and second-line agents in the treatment of snakebite.[122]

Petrus Abbonus (1250–1315) wrote a very comprehensive textbook on toxicology that discussed in great detail animal, vegetable, and mineral poisonings and their treatment.[20] On the subject of oleander poisoning, Abbonus wrote that those who drink the juice, spines, or bark of oleander will develop anxiety, palpitations, and syncope. He described the clinical presentation of opium overdose as someone who "will be dull, lazy, and sleepy, without feeling, and he will neither understand nor feel anything, and if he does not receive succor, he will die." Although this "succor" is not defined, he recommended that treatment of opium intoxication include drinking the strongest wine, rubbing the extremities with alkali and soap, and olfactory stimulation with pepper. To treat snakebite, Abbonus suggested the immediate application of a tourniquet, as well as oral suctioning of the bite wound—preferably performed by a servant. Interestingly, from a 21st-century perspective, Abbonus also suggested that St. John's wort had the magical power to free anything from poisons and attributed this virtue to the influence of the stars.[20]

The Scientists

Paracelsus' (1493–1541) study on the dose-response relationship is usually considered the beginning of the scientific approach to toxicology (Table 1–2). He was the first to emphasize the chemical nature of toxic agents.[110] Paracelsus stressed the need for proper observation and experimentation regarding the true response to chemicals. He underscored the need to differentiate between the therapeutic and toxic properties of chemicals when he stated in his *Third Defense*, "What is there that is not poison? All things are poison and nothing [is] without poison. Solely, the dose determines that a thing is not a poison."[41]

Although Paracelsus is the best known Renaissance toxicologist, Ambroise Pare (1510–1590) and William Piso (1611–1678) also contributed to the field. Pare argued against the use of the unicorn horn and bezoar stone.[89] He also wrote an early treatise on carbon monoxide poisoning. Piso is credited as one of the first to recognize the emetic properties of ipecacuanha.[119]

Medieval and Renaissance Poisoners

Along with these advances in toxicologic knowledge, the Renaissance is mainly remembered as the age of the poisoner, a time when the art of poisoning reached new heights (Table 1–3). In fact, poisoning was so rampant during this time that King Henry VIII decreed in 1531 that convicted poisoners should be boiled alive.[50] From the 15th to 17th centuries, actual schools of poisoning existed in Venice and Rome. In Venice, poisoning services were provided by a group called the Council of Ten, whose members were hired to perform murder by poison.[144]

Members of the infamous Borgia family were credited with many poisonings during this period. They preferred to use a poison called "La Cantarella," a mixture of arsenic and phosphorus.[138] Rodrigo Borgia (1431–1503), who became Pope Alexander VI, and his son, Cesare Borgia, were reportedly responsible for the poisoning of cardinals and kings.

In the late 16th century, Catherine de Medici, wife of Henry II of France, introduced Italian poisoning techniques to France. She experimented on the poor, the sick, and the criminal. By analyzing the subsequent complaints of her victims, she is said to have learned the site of action and time of onset, the clinical signs and symptoms, and the efficacy of poisons.[55]

Murder by poison remained quite popular during the latter half of the 17th and the early part of the 18th centuries in Italy and France. A major center for poison practitioners was Naples, the home of the notorious Madame Giulia Toffana. She reportedly poisoned more than 600 people, preferring a particular solution of white arsenic (arsenic trioxide), better known as "aqua toffana,"

TABLE 1–2.   Important Figures in the Field of Toxicology from Paracelsus to the 1900s

Person	Date	Importance
Paracelsus	1493–1541	Introduced dose response concept to toxicology
Ambroise Pare	1510–1590	Spoke out against unicorn horns and bezoars as antidotes
William Piso	1611–1678	First to study emetic qualities of ipecacuanha
Bernardino Ramazzini	1633–1714	Father of occupational medicine; wrote *De Morbis Artificum Diatriba*
Richard Mead	1673–1754	Wrote English-language book dedicated to poisoning
Percivall Pott	1714–1788	First description of occupational cancer, relating the chimney sweep occupation to scrotal cancer
Felice Fontana	1730–1805	First scientific study of venomous snakes
Philip Physick	1767–1837	Early advocate of orogastric lavage to remove poisons
Baron Guillaume Dupuytren	1777–1835	Early advocate of orogastric lavage to remove poisons
Edward Jukes	1820	Self-experimented with orogastric lavage apparatus known as Jukes' syringe
M. Bertrand	1813	Demonstrated charcoal's efficacy in arsenic ingestion
P. Touery	1831	Demonstrated charcoal's efficacy in strychnine ingestion
A. Garrod	1846	First systematic study of charcoal in an animal model
B. Howard Rand	1848	First study of charcoal's efficacy in humans
Bonaventure Orfila	1787–1853	Father of modern toxicology; wrote *Traite Des Poisons;* first to isolate arsenic from humans organs
Robert Christison	1797–1882	Wrote *Treatise on Poisons,* one of the most influential texts in early 19th century
Francois Magendie	1783–1855	Discovered emetine and studied mechanism of cyanide and strychnine
Claude Bernard	1813–1878	Studied mechanism of toxicity of carbon monoxide and curare
O.H. Costill	1848	Wrote first book on symptoms and treatment of poisoning
Theodore Wormley	1826–1897	Wrote *Micro-Chemistry of Poisons;* first American book devoted exclusively to toxicology
James Marsh	1794–1846	Developed reduction test for arsenic
Hugo Reinsch	1842	Developed qualitative test for arsenic and mercury
Max Gutzeit	1847–1915	Developed method to quantitate small amounts of arsenic
Albert Nieman	1860	Isolated cocaine alkaloid
Rudolf Kobert	1854–1918	Studied digitalis and ergot alkaloids
Louis Lewin	1850–1929	Studied many toxins, including methanol, chloroform, snake venom, carbon monoxide, lead, opioids, and hallucinogenic plants
Alice Hamilton	1869–1970	Conducted landmark investigations associating worksite chemical hazards with disease; led reform movement to improve worker safety

TABLE 1–3. Notable Poisoners from Antiquity to the Present [130,136,138]

Poisoner	Date	Victim(s)	Poison(s)
Locusta	54–55 A.D.	Claudius and Britannicus	*Amanita phalloides,* cyanide
Cesare Borgia	1400s	Cardinals and kings	La Cantarella (arsenic and phosphorus)
Catherine de Medici	1519–1589	Poor, sick, criminals	Unknown agents
Hieronyma Spara	Died 1659	Taught women how to poison their husbands	Mana of St. Nicholas of Bari (arsenic trioxide)
Madame Giulia Toffana	Died 1719	>600 people	Aqua toffana (arsenic trioxide)
Marchioness de Brinvilliers	Died 1676	Hospitalized patients, husband, father	Arsenic, lead, mercury, antimony, copper
Catherine Deshayes	Died 1680	>2000 infants, many husbands	La poudre de succession (arsenic mixed with aconite, belladonna, and opium)
Mary Blandy	1752	Father	Arsenic
Anna Maria Zwanizer	1807	Random people	Arsenic, antimony
Marie Lefarge	1839	Husband	Arsenic (1st use of Marsh test)
John Tawell	1845	Mistress	Cyanide
William Palmer, MD	1855	Fellow gambler	Strychnine
Madeline Smith (acquitted)	1857	Lover	Arsenic
Edmond de la Pommerais, MD	1863	Patient and mistress	Digitalis
Edward William Pritchard, MD	1865	Wife and mother-in-law	Antimony
George Henry Lamson, MD	1881	Brother-in-law	Aconite
Adelaide Bartlett (acquitted)	1886	Husband	Chloroform
Florence Maybrick	1889	Husband	Arsenic
Thomas Neville Cream, MD	1891	Prostitutes	Strychnine
Johann Hoch	1892–1905	Serial wives	Arsenic
Cordelia Botkin	1898	Feminine rival	Arsenic (in chocolate candy)
Roland Molineux	1898	Acquaintance	Cyanide of mercury
Hawley Harvey Crippen, MD	1910	Wife	Hyoscine
Frederick Henry Seddon	1911	Boarder	Arsenic (fly paper)
Henri Girard	1912	Acquaintances	*Amanita phalloides*
Robert Armstrong	1921	Wife	Arsenic (weed killer)
Landru	1922	Many women	Cyanide
Suzanne Fazekas	1929	Supplied poison to 100 wives to kill husbands	Arsenic
Sadamichi Hirasawa	1948	Bank employees	Potassium cyanide
Christa Ambros Lehmann	1954	Friend, husband, father-in-law	E-605 (parathion)
Nannie Doss	1954	11 relatives including 5 husbands	Arsenic
Carl Coppolino, MD	1965	Wife	Succinylcholine
Graham Frederick Young	1971	Stepmother, coworkers	Thallium
Judias V. Buenoano	1971	Husband, son	Arsenic
Ronald Clark O'Bryan	1974	Son and neighborhood children	Cyanide (in Halloween candy)
Murderer of Georgi Markov	1978	Bulgarian diplomat	Ricin
Jim Jones	1978	911 people in mass suicide	Cyanide
Harold Shipman, MD	1974–1998	Patients (up to 297)	Heroin
Donald Harvey	1983–1987	Patients	Arsenic
"Tylenol" tamperer	1982	7 people	Extra Strength Tylenol laced with cyanide
George Trepal	1988	Family members	Thallium
Michael Swango, MD	1980s–1990s	Hospitalized patients	Succinylcholine, potassium chloride, arsenic

and dispensed under the guise of a cosmetic. Eventually convicted of poisoning, Madame Toffana was executed in 1719.[19]

In France, the Marchioness de Brinvilliers (1630–1676) and Catherine Deshayes (1640–1680) were two of the most notorious poisoners.[53] The Marchioness tested her poison concoctions on hospitalized patients and on her servants, and allegedly murdered her husband, father, and two siblings.[130] Among the favorite poisons of the Marchioness were corrosive sublimate (mercury bichloride), arsenic, lead, copper sulfate, and tartar emetic containing antimony.[138] Catherine Deshayes, a fortuneteller and sorcerer, was one of the last "poisoners for hire," and was implicated in countless poisonings, including the killing of more than 2000 infants.[55] Better known as "La Voisine," she reportedly sold poisons to women wishing to rid themselves of their husbands. Her particular brand of poison was a concoction of arsenic, aconite, belladonna, and opium known as "la poudre de succession."[138]

Ultimately, de Brinvilliers was beheaded and Deshayes was burned alive for their crimes. In an attempt to curtail these rampant poisonings, Louis XIV issued a decree in 1662 banning the sale of arsenic, mercury, and other poisons to customers not known to the apothecaries and requiring poison buyers to sign a register declaring the purpose for their purchase.[130]

EIGHTEENTH- AND NINETEENTH-CENTURY DEVELOPMENTS IN TOXICOLOGY

The development of toxicology as a distinct specialty began during the 18th and 19th centuries (see Table 1–2).[111] The poison mystique—mythologic and magical—was gradually replaced by an increasingly rational, scientific, and experimental approach to the study of these agents. Much of the poison lore that had survived for almost 2000 years was finally debunked and discarded. The 18th-century Italian Felice Fontana was one of the first to usher in the modern age. He was an early experimental toxicologist who studied the venom of the European viper and wrote the classic text *Traite sur le Venin de la Vipere* in 1781.[75] Through his exacting experimental study on the effects of venom, Fontana brought a scientific insight to toxicology that had previously been lacking, demonstrating that clinical symptoms are a result of the poison (venom) acting on specific target organs. During the 18th and 19th centuries, attention focused on the detection of poisons and the study of toxic effects of drugs and chemicals in animals.[104] Issues relating to adverse effects of industrialization and unintentional poisoning in the workplace and home environment were raised. Also during this time, early experience and experimentation with methods of gastrointestinal decontamination took place.

Development of Analytical Toxicology and the Study of Poisons

The French physician Bonaventure Orfila (1787–1853) has been called the father of modern toxicology.[104] He emphasized toxicology as a distinct, scientific discipline, separate from clinical medicine and pharmacology.[10] He also was an early medical-legal expert who championed the use of chemical analysis and autopsy material as evidence to prove that a poisoning had occurred. His treatise *Traite des Poisons* (1814)[108] had five editions and was regarded as the foundation of experimental and forensic toxicology.[143] This text classified poisons into six groups: astringents, corrosives, acrids, septics or putrefiants, stupefacients and narcotics, and narcoticoacrids.

A number of other landmark works on poisoning also first appeared during this period. In 1829, Robert Christison (1797–1882), a professor of medical jurisprudence and Orfila's student, wrote *A Treatise on Poisons*.[29] This work simplified Orfila's poison classification schema by categorizing poisons into three groups: irritants, narcotics, and narcoticoacrids. Less concerned with jurisprudence than with clinical toxicology, O.H. Costill's *A Practical Treatise on Poisons*, published in 1848, was the first modern clinically oriented text to emphasize the symptoms and treatment of poisoning.[34] In 1867, Theodore Wormley (1826–1897) published the first American book written exclusively on poisons. Entitled the *Micro-Chemistry of Poisons*,[145] this pioneering American contribution also expanded on methods of poison identification.[47]

During this time, important breakthroughs in the chemical analysis of poisons resulted from the search for a more reliable assay for arsenic. Arsenic was widely available and was the suspected etiology of a large number of deaths. In one study of 679 homicidal poisonings, arsenic was employed 31% of the time.[138] A reliable means of detecting arsenic was much needed by the courts.

Until the 19th century, poisoning was mainly diagnosed by symptoms rather than by analytic tests. The first use of a chemical test as evidence in a poisoning trial occurred in the 1752 trial of Mary Blandy, who was accused of poisoning her father with arsenic.[93] Although Blandy was convicted and hanged publicly, the test employed in this case was not very sensitive and depended in part on eliciting a garlic odor upon heating the gruel that the accused had fed to her father.

During the 19th century, James Marsh (1794–1846), Hugo Reinsch, and Max Gutzeit (1847–1915) all worked on this problem. Assays bearing their names are important contributions to the early history of analytic toxicology.[94,104] The "Marsh test" to detect arsenic was first used in a criminal case in 1839 during the trial of Marie Lefarge, who was accused of using arsenic to murder her husband.[130] Orfila's trial testimony that the victim's viscera contained minute amounts of arsenic helped to convict the defendant although subsequent debate suggested that contamination of the forensic specimen may have also played a role. In a further attempt to curtail criminal poisoning by arsenic, the British Parliament passed the Arsenic Act in 1851. This bill, which was one of the first modern laws to regulate the sale of poisons, required that the retail sale of arsenic be confined to chemists, druggists, and apothecaries, and that a poison book be maintained to record all arsenic sales.[14]

Homicidal poisonings remained common during the 19th and early 20th century. Infamous poisoners of the late 19th century and early 20th century included William Palmer, Edward Pritchard, Harvey Crippen, and Frederick Seddon.[138] Many of these poisoners were physicians who utilized their knowledge of medicine and pharmacology in an attempt to solve their domestic and financial difficulties by committing the "perfect" murder. Some of the poisons employed were strychnine (Palmer, Cream), antimony (Pritchard), hyoscine (Crippen), digitalis (Pommerais), aconite (Lamson, who was a classmate of Christison), cyanide (Molineux, Tawell), *Amanita phalloides* (Girard), as well as arsenic (Maybrick, Seddon, others) (Table 1–3).[22,136,138]

Systematic investigation into the underlying mechanisms of toxic substances also first took place during the 19th century. Much of this work was done in France and Germany. To cite just a few important accomplishments, Francois Magendie (1783–1855) studied the mechanisms of toxicity and sites of action of emetine, strychnine, and cyanide.[45] His student, Claude Bernard (1813–1878), the pioneering physiologist, made important contributions to the understanding of carbon monoxide and curare poisonings.[81] Rudolf Kobert (1854–1918) studied digitalis and ergot alkaloids, and also authored a textbook on toxicology.[106] His fellow German Louis Lewin (1850–1929) was the first person to intensively study the differences between the pharmacologic and toxicologic actions of drugs. Lewin studied chronic opium intoxication, as well as the toxicity of lead, carbon monoxide, snake venom, methanol, and chloroform. He also developed a classification system for psychoactive drugs, dividing them into euphorics, phantastics, inebriants, hypnotics, and excitants.[88]

Forensic investigation into suspicious deaths, including poisonings, was significantly advanced with the development of the medical examiner system that replaced the much-flawed coroner system that was subject to widespread corruption. In 1918, the first centrally controlled medical examiner system was established in New York City. Alexander Gettler, considered the father of forensic toxicology in the United States, established a toxicology laboratory within the newly created New York City Medical Examiner's Office. Gettler pioneered new techniques for the detection of a variety of substances in biologic fluids including carbon monoxide, chloroform, heavy metals, and cyanide.[46,104]

The Origin of Occupational Toxicology

The origins of occupational toxicology can be traced to the early 18th century and to the contributions of Bernardino Ramazzini

(1633–1714). Considered the father of occupational medicine, Ramazzini wrote *De Morbis Artificum Diatriba* (Diseases of Workers) in 1700, which was the first comprehensive text discussing the relationship between disease and workplace hazards.[52] Ramazzini's essential contribution to the care of the patient is epitomized by the addition of a question to the medical history, "What occupation does the patient follow?"[49] Altogether Ramazzini described diseases associated with 54 occupations, including mercury poisoning in mirror makers, pulmonary diseases in miners, and hydrocarbon poisoning in painters.

Sir Percivall Pott proposed the first association between workplace exposure and cancer in 1775 when he noticed a high incidence of scrotal cancer in English chimney sweeps. Pott's belief that the scrotal cancer was caused by prolonged exposure to tar and soot was confirmed by other investigation in the 1920s, indicating that the polycyclic aromatic hydrocarbons contained in coal tar (including benzo[*a*]pyrene) are carcinogenic.[68]

Another pioneer in occupational toxicology, whose rigorous scientific inquiry had a profound impact on linking chemical toxins with human disease was Dr. Alice Hamilton (1869–1970). A physician, scientist, humanitarian, and social reformer, Hamilton, who would become the first female professor at Harvard University, conducted groundbreaking studies of many different occupational exposures and problems, including wrist drop in lead workers, mercury poisoning in hatters, and carbon monoxide poisoning in steelworkers. Her overriding concerns about these "dangerous trades" and her commitment to improve the health of workers would lead to extensive voluntary and regulatory reforms in the workplace.[59,63]

Early Advances in Gastrointestinal Decontamination

Further experience with gastrointestinal decontamination also was gained during the late 18th and early 19th century. A stomach pump was first designed by Munro Secundus in 1769 to administer neutralizing substances to sheep and cattle for the treatment of bloat.[23] The American surgeon Philip Physick (1768–1837) and the French surgeon Baron Guillaume Dupuytren (1777–1835) were two of the first physicians to advocate gastric lavage for the removal of poisons.[23] As early as 1805, Physick demonstrated the use of a "stomach tube" for this purpose. Using brandy and water as the irrigation fluid, he performed stomach washings in twins to wash out excessive doses of tincture of opium.[23] Dupuytren performed gastric emptying by first introducing warm water into the stomach via a large syringe attached to a long flexible sound and then withdrawing the "same water charged with poison."[23] Edward Jukes, a British surgeon, was another early advocate of poison removal by gastric lavage. Jukes first experimented on animals, performing gastric lavage after the oral administration of tincture of opium. Attempting to gain human experience, he experimented on himself, by first ingesting 10 drams (600 g) of tincture of opium and then performing gastric lavage using a 25-inch-long, 0.5-inch-diameter tube, which became known as Jukes' syringe.[98] Other than some nausea and a 3-hour sleep, he suffered no ill effects, and the experiment was deemed a success.

The principle of using charcoal to adsorb poisons was first described by Scheele (1773) and Lowitz (1785), but the medicinal use of charcoal dates to ancient times.[33] The earliest reference to the medicinal uses of charcoal is found in the Egyptian Papyrus of ~1500 B.C.[33] The charcoal employed during Greek and Roman times, referred to as wood charcoal, was used to treat anthrax, chlorosis, vertigo, and epilepsy. By the late 18th century, topical application of charcoal was recommended for gangrenous skin ulcers, and internal use of a charcoal-water suspension was recommended for use as a mouthwash and in the treatment of bilious conditions.[33]

The first hint that charcoal might have a role in the treatment of poisoning came from a series of heroic self-experiments in France during the early 19th century. In 1813, the French chemist M. Bertrand publicly demonstrated the antidotal properties of charcoal by surviving a 5-g ingestion of arsenic trioxide that had been mixed with charcoal.[65] Eighteen years later, before the French Academy of Medicine, the pharmacist P.F. Touery survived an ingestion consisting of 10 times the lethal dose of strychnine mixed with 15 g of charcoal.[65] One of the first reports of charcoal used in a poisoned patient was by the American Hort, who successfully treated a mercury bichloride–poisoned patient with large amounts of powdered charcoal in 1834.[7]

In the 1840s, A. Garrod performed the first controlled study of charcoal when he examined its utility on a variety of poisons in animal models.[65] Garrod used dogs, cats, guinea pigs, and rabbits to demonstrate the potential benefits of charcoal in the management of strychnine poisoning. He also emphasized the importance of early utilization of charcoal and the proper ratio of charcoal to poison. Other toxic substances, such as aconite, morphine, mercury bichloride, and hemlock, were also studied during this period. The first charcoal efficacy studies in humans were performed by the American physician B. Rand in 1848.[65]

It was not until the early 20th century that an activation process was added to the manufacture of charcoal. In 1900, the Russian Ostrejko demonstrated that treating charcoal with superheated steam significantly enhanced its adsorbing power.[33] Despite this improvement and the favorable reports mentioned, charcoal was only occasionally used in gastrointestinal decontamination until the early 1960s, when Holt and Holz repopularized its use.[62]

The Increasing Recognition of the Perils of Drug Abuse

Opioids.   Although the medical use of opium was promoted by Paracelsus in the 16th century, the popularity of this agent was given a significant boost when the distinguished British physician Thomas Sydenham (1624–1689) formulated laudanum (tincture of opium). In addition to opium, this preparation contained sherry, saffron, cinnamon, and cloves. Sydenham also formulated a different opium concoction known as "syrup of poppies."[78] A third opium preparation used during this period was designed by Sydenham's protégé, Thomas Dover, and contained ipecac, as well as tartaric acid, saltpeter, licorice, and opium.

John Jones, the author of the 1700 text *The Mysteries of Opium Reveal'd,* was another enthusiastic advocate of the medicinal uses of opium.[78] A well-known opium user himself, Jones provided one of the earliest descriptions of opiate addiction. He insisted that opium offered many benefits if the dose was moderate, but that discontinuation or a decrease in dose, particularly after "leaving off after long and lavish use," would result in such symptoms as sweating, itching, diarrhea, and melancholy. His recommendation for the treatment of these withdrawal symptoms included decreasing the dose of opium by 1% each day until the drug was totally withdrawn. During this period, a number of English writers became well-known opium addicts, including Samuel Taylor Coleridge, Elizabeth Barrett Browning, and Thomas De Quincey. De Quincey, author of *Confessions of an English Opium Eater*, was an early advocate of the recreational use of opiates. The famed Coleridge poem, *Kubla Khan*, referred to opium as the "milk of paradise," while De Quincey's *Confessions* suggested that opium held the "key to paradise." In many of these cases, the initiation of opium use for medical reasons led to recreational use, tolerance, and dependence.[78]

Although opium was first introduced to Asian societies by Arab physicians some time after the fall of the Roman Empire, the use of opium in Asian countries grew considerably during the 18th and 19th centuries. In one of the more deplorable chapters in world history, China's growing dependence on opium was spurred on by the English desire to establish and profit from a flourishing drug trade.[124] Opium was grown in India and exported east. Despite Chinese protests and edicts against this practice, the importation of opium persisted throughout the 19th century, with the British going to war twice in order to maintain their right to sell opium. Not surprisingly, by the beginning of the 20th century, opium abuse in China was endemic.

In England, opium use continued to increase during the first half of the 19th century. During this period, opium was legal and freely available from the neighborhood grocer. To many, its use was considered no more problematic than alcohol.[57] The Chinese usually self-administered opium by smoking, a custom that was brought to the United States in the mid-19th century by Chinese immigrants, whereas the English use of opium was more often by ingestion, that is, "opium eating."

The liberal use of opiates as infant-soothing agents was one of the most unfortunate aspects of this period of unregulated opiate use.[79] Mrs. Winslow's Soothing Syrup, Godfrey's Cordial, Quietness, and Mother's Friend were among the most popular of children's opiates.[83] They were advertised as producing a natural sleep and recommended for teething and bowel regulation, as well as for crying. Because of the wide availability of opiates during this period, the number of acute opiate overdoses in children was consequential and would remain problematic until these unsavory remedies were condemned and removed from the market.

With the discovery of morphine in 1805 and Alexander Wood's invention of the hypodermic syringe in 1853, parenteral administration of morphine became the preferred route of opiate administration.[67] A legacy of the generous use of opium and morphine during the United States Civil War was "soldiers' disease," referring to a rather large veteran population that returned from the war with a lingering opiate habit.[117] One hundred years later, opiate abuse and addiction would become common among US military serving in the Vietnam War. Surveys indicated that as many as 20% of American soldiers in Vietnam were addicted to opiates during the war—in part because of its widespread availability in Vietnam.[121]

Growing concerns about opiate abuse in England led to the passing of the Pharmacy Act of 1868, which restricted the sale of opium to registered chemists. But in 1898, the Bayer Pharmaceutical Company of Germany would synthesize heroin from opium (Bayer also introduced aspirin that same year).[131] Although initially touted as a nonaddictive morphine substitute, problems with heroin use soon became evident and in the United States, the problems associated with uncontrolled use of all opiates became increasingly apparent.

Cocaine. Ironically, during the later part of the 19th century, Sigmund Freud and Robert Christison, among others, were enthu-

siastically recommending cocaine, the drug that would eventually compete with heroin for most notoriety, as a treatment for opiate addiction. After Albert Niemann's isolation of cocaine alkaloid from coca leaf in 1860, growing enthusiasm for cocaine as a panacea ensued.[74] Some of the most important medical figures of the time, including William Halsted, the famed Johns Hopkins surgeon, enthusiastically promoted the use of cocaine. In 1884, Freud wrote *Uber Cocaine*,[25] advocating cocaine as cure for opium and morphine addiction and as a treatment for fatigue and hysteria. Halsted championed the anesthetic properties of this drug, although his own use of cocaine and subsequent morphine use in an attempt to overcome his cocaine dependency would later take a considerable toll.[107]

During the last third of the 19th century, cocaine was added to many popular over-the-counter tonics of the day. In 1863, a Frenchman, Angelo Mariani, introduced a new wine, "Vin Mariani," that consisted of a mixture of cocaine and wine (6 mg of cocaine alkaloid per ounce) and was sold as a digestive aid and restorative.[99] In direct competition with the French tonic was the American-made Coca-Cola, developed by J.S. Pemberton. Coca-Cola was originally formulated with coca and caffeine and was marketed as a headache remedy and invigorator. With the public demand for cocaine increasing, patent medication manufacturers were adding cocaine to thousands of products including products for asthma. One such asthma remedy was "Dr. Tucker's Asthma Specific," which contained 420 mg of cocaine per ounce and was applied directly to the nasal mucosa.[74] By the end of the 19th century, the first great American cocaine epidemic was underway.[101]

Similar to what was occurring with opiates, the increasing use of cocaine led to a growing concern about its associated problems. In 1886, the first reports of cocaine-related cardiac arrest and stroke were published.[31] Reports of cocaine habituation occurring in patients using cocaine to treat their underlying opiate addiction also began to appear. In 1902, a popular book, *Eight Years in Cocaine Hell*, described some of these problems. *Century Magazine* called cocaine "the most harmful of all habit-forming drugs," and a report in the *New York Times* stated that cocaine was destroying "its victims more swiftly and surely than opium."[40] In 1910, President William Taft proclaimed cocaine Public Enemy Number 1.

In an attempt to curb the increasing problems associated with drug abuse and addiction, the 1914 Harrison Narcotics Act mandated stringent control over the sale and distribution of narcotics (defined as opium, opium derivatives, and cocaine).[40] It was the first federal law in the United States to criminalize the nonmedical use of drugs. The bill required doctors, pharmacists, and others who prescribed narcotics to register and to pay a tax. A similar law, the Dangerous Drugs Act, was passed in the United Kingdom in 1920.[57] To help enforce these drug laws in the United States, the Narcotics Division of the Prohibition Unit of the Internal Revenue Service (a progenitor of the Drug Enforcement Agency) was established in 1920. In 1924, the Harrison Act was further strengthened with the passage of new legislation that banned the importation of opium for the purpose of manufacturing heroin, essentially outlawing the medicinal uses of heroin. With the legal venues to purchase these drugs now eliminated, users were forced to buy from illegal street dealers, creating a burgeoning black market

Sedative-Hypnotics. The introduction to medical practice of the anesthetic agents nitrous oxide, ether, and chloroform during the 19th century was accompanied by the recreational use of these agents and the first reports of volatile substance abuse. Chloroform "jags," ether "frolics," and nitrous parties became a new type of entertainment.[51] Humphrey Davies was an early self-experimenter with the exhilarating effects associated with nitrous oxide inhalation.[51] In certain Irish towns, especially where the temperance movement was strong, ether drinking became quite popular.[96] Horace Wells, the American dentist who introduced chloroform as an anesthesic, became dependent on this volatile solvent and later committed suicide.

Until the last half of the 19th century, opium, aconite, hemlock, prussic acid (cyanide), and alcohol were the primary agents used for sedation.[30] During the 1860s, new, more specific sedative-hypnotics, such as chloral hydrate and potassium bromide, were introduced into medical practice. In particular, chloral hydrate was hailed as a wonder drug that was relatively safe, as compared to opium, and recommended for insomnia, anxiety, and delirium tremens, as well as for scarlet fever, asthma, and cancer. But within a few years, problems with acute toxicity of chloral hydrate, as well as its potential to produce tolerance and physical dependence, became apparent.[30] Mixing chloral hydrate with ethanol was noted to produce a rather powerful "knockout" combination that would be known as a "Mickey Finn." Abuse of chloral hydrate, as well as other new sedatives such as potassium bromide, would be a harbinger of 20th-century sedative-hypnotic abuse.

Hallucinogens. American Indians used peyote in religious ceremonies at least since the 17th century. Hallucinogenic mushrooms, particularly *Psilocybe* mushrooms, were also used in the religious life of Native Americans. These were called "teonanacatl," which means "God's sacred mushrooms" or "God's flesh."[114] Interest in the recreational use of cannabis also accelerated during the 19th century after Napoleon's troops brought the drug back from Egypt, where its use among the lower classes was widespread at the time. In 1843, several French Romantics, including Balzac, Hugo, Baudelaire, and Gautier, formed a hashish club called "Le Club des Hachichins" in the Parisian apartment of a young French painter. Fitz Hugh Ludlow's *The Hasheesh Eater*, published in 1857, was an early American text espousing the virtues of marijuana.[86]

Absinthe, an ethanol-containing beverage that was manufactured with an extract from wormwood (*Artemisia absinthium*), was very popular during the last half of the 19th century.[80] This emerald-colored, very bitter drink was memorialized in the paintings of Degas, Toulouse-Lautrec, and Van Gogh, and was a staple of French society during this period.[11] Thujone, a psychoactive component of wormwood, is thought to be responsible for the pleasant feelings, as well as for the hallucinogenic effects, hyperexcitability, and significant neurotoxicity associated with this drink. Given the increasing medical problems associated with its use, absinthe was banned throughout most of Europe by the early 20th century.

A more recent event that would have significant impact on modern-day hallucinogen use was the synthesis of lysergic acid diethylamide (LSD) by Albert Hofmann in 1938.[64] Working for Sandoz Pharmaceutical Company, Hofmann synthesized LSD while investigating the pharmacologic properties of ergot alkaloids. Subsequent self-experimentation by Hofmann led to the first description of its hallucinogenic effects and stimulated research into the use of LSD as a therapeutic agent. Hofmann is also credited with isolating psilocybin as the active ingredient in *Psilocybe mexicana* mushrooms in 1958.[99]

TWENTIETH-CENTURY EVENTS

Early Regulatory Initiatives

The development of the specialty of medical toxicology and the role of poison control centers began shortly after World War II. Prior to this time, serious attention to the problem of household poisonings in the United States had been limited to a few federal legislative antipoisoning initiatives (Table 1–4). The 1906 Pure Food and Drugs Act was the first federal legislation that sought to protect the public from problematic and potentially unsafe drugs and food. The driving force behind this reform was Dr. Harvey W. Wiley, the chief chemist at the Department of Agriculture. Beginning in the 1880s, Wiley investigated the problems of contaminated food. In 1902, he organized the "poison squad," which consisted of a group of volunteers who did self-experiments with food preservatives.[8] Revelations from the "poison squad," as well as the publication of Upton Sinclair's muckraking novel *The Jungle*[129] in 1906, exposing unhygienic practices of the meatpacking industry, led to growing support for legislative intervention. Samuel Hopkins Adams' reports about the patent (secret) medicine industry revealed that some drug manufacturers added opiates to soothing syrups for infants, and added to the call for reform.[118] Although the 1906 regulations were mostly concerned with protecting the public from adulterated food, regulations protecting against misbranded patent medications were also included.

The Federal Caustic Poison Act of 1927 was the first federal legislation to specifically address household poisoning. As early as 1859, bottles clearly demarcated "poison" were manufactured in response to a rash of unfortunate dispensing errors that occurred when oxalic acid was unintentionally substituted for a similarly appearing Epsom salts solution.[26] Prior to 1927, however, "poison" warning labels were not required on chemical containers, regardless of toxicity or availability. The 1927 Caustic Act was spearheaded by the efforts of Dr. Chevalier Jackson, an otolaryngologist, who showed that unintentional exposures to household caustic agents were an increasingly frequent cause of severe gastrointestinal burns. Under this statute, for the first time, lye and acid-containing products had to clearly display a "poison" warning label.[135]

The most pivotal regulatory initiative in the United States prior to World War II, and perhaps the most significant American toxicologic regulation of the 20th century, was the Federal Food, Drug, and Cosmetic Act of 1938. Although the Food and Drug Administration (FDA) had been established in 1930, and legislation to strengthen the 1906 regulations had been considered by Congress beginning with President Franklin Roosevelt's first inauguration in 1933, by 1938 proposed revisions still had not been passed. The Elixir of Sulfanilamide tragedy in 1938 (Chap. 2) claimed the lives of 105 people who ingested a prescribed liquid preparation of sulfanilamide dissolved in diethylene glycol. This event finally provided the catalyst for legislative intervention.[97,141] Prior to the elixir disaster, proposed legislation called only for the banning of false and misleading drug labeling and for the outlawing of dangerous drugs without mandatory drug safety testing. After the tragedy, the enacted 1938 proposal required assessment of drug safety prior to marketing.

The Development of Poison Control Centers

World War II led to the rapid proliferation of new drugs and chemicals in the marketplace and in the household.[37] At the same

TABLE 1–4. Protecting our Health: Important US Regulatory Initiatives Pertaining to Drugs and Toxins During the 20th Century

Date	Federal Legislation	Intent
1906	Pure Food and Drugs Act	Early regulatory initiative. Prohibits interstate commerce of misbranded and adulterated foods and drugs
1914	Harrison Narcotics Act	First federal law to criminalize the nonmedical use of drugs. Taxed and regulated distribution and sale of narcotics (opium, opium derivatives, and cocaine). It required doctors, pharmacists, and others who prescribed narcotics to register and pay a tax.
1927	Federal Caustic Poison Act	Mandated labeling of concentrated caustics.
1930	Food and Drug Administration (FDA) established	Successor to the Bureau of Chemistry; promulgation of food and drug regulations.
1937	Marijuana Tax Act	Applied controls over marijuana similar to narcotics.
1938	Federal Food, Drug, and Cosmetic Act	Required toxicity testing of pharmaceuticals prior to marketing.
1948	Federal Insecticide, Fungicide, and Rodenticide Act	Provided federal control for pesticide sale, distribution, and use.
1951	Durham-Humphrey Amendment	Restricted many therapeutic drugs to sale by prescription only.
1960	Federal Hazardous Substances Labeling Act	Mandated prominent labeling warnings on hazardous household chemical products.
1962	Kefauver-Harris Drug Amendments	Required drug manufacturer to demonstrate efficacy before marketing.
1963	Clean Air Act	Regulated air emissions by setting maximum pollutant standards.
1966	Child Protection Act	Banned hazardous toys where adequate label warnings could not be written.
1970	Comprehensive Drug Abuse and Control Act	Replaced and updated all previous laws concerning narcotics and other dangerous drugs. Emphasis on law enforcement.
1970	Poison Prevention Packaging Act	Mandated child-resistant safety caps on certain pharmaceutical preparations to decrease unintentional childhood poisoning.
1970	Environmental Protection Agency (EPA) established	Established and enforced environmental protection standards.
1970	Occupational Safety and Health Act (OSHA)	Enacted to improve worker and workplace safety. Created NIOSH as research institution for OSHA.
1972	Clean Water Act	Regulated discharge of pollutants into US waters.
1972	Consumer Product Safety Act	Established Consumer Product Safety Commission to reduce injuries and deaths from consumer products.
1972	Hazardous Material Transportation Act	Authorized the Department of Transportation to develop, promulgate, and enforce regulations for the safe transportation of hazardous materials.
1973	Drug Enforcement Administration (DEA) created	Succeeded predecessor Bureau of Narcotics and Dangerous Drugs; charged with enforcing federal drug laws.
1973	Lead-based Paint Poison Prevention Act	Regulated the utilization of lead in residential paint. Lead in some paints later banned by Congress in 1978.
1974	Safe Drinking Water Act	Set safe standards for water purity.
1976	Resource Conservation and Recovery Act	Authorized EPA to control hazardous waste from the "cradle-to-grave" including the generation, transportation, treatment, storage, and disposal of hazardous waste.
1976	Toxic Substance Control Act	Authorized EPA to track 75,000 industrial chemicals produced or imported into US. Required testing of chemicals that pose environmental or human health risk.
1980	Comprehensive Environmental Response, Compensation, and Liability Act (CERCLA)	Set controls for hazardous waste sites. Established trust fund (Superfund) to provide cleanup for these sites.
1983	Federal Anti-Tampering Act	Response to cyanide-Tylenol deaths. Outlawed tampering with packaged consumer products.
1986	Superfund Amendments and Reauthorization Act (SARA)	Amendment to CERCLA. Increased funding for the research and cleanup of hazardous waste sites.
1988	Labeling of Hazardous Art Materials Act	Required review of all art materials to determine hazard potential and mandated warning labels for hazardous materials.
1994	Dietary Supplement Health and Education Act	Permitted dietary supplements including many herbal preparations to bypass FDA scrutiny.
1997	FDA Modernization Act	Accelerated FDA reviews, regulated advertising of unapproved uses of approved drugs.

time, suicide as a leading cause of death from these agents was recognized.[134] Both of these factors led the medical community to develop a response to the serious problems of both unintentional and intentional poisonings. In Europe during the late 1940s, special toxicology wards were organized in Copenhagen and Budapest,[58] and a poison information service was begun in the Netherlands (Table 1–5).[139] An American Academy of Pediatrics study in 1952 revealed that more than 50% of childhood "accidents" in the United States were the result of unintentional poisonings.[60] This study led to the opening of the first US poison control center in Chicago in 1953, under the leadership of Dr. Edward Press.[115] Press believed that it had become extremely difficult for the individual physician to keep abreast of product information, toxicity, and treatment for the rapidly increasing number of poten-

tially poisonous household products. This initial center was organized as a cooperative effort among the departments of pediatrics at several Chicago medical schools, with the goal of collecting and disseminating product information to inquiring physicians—mainly pediatricians.[115]

By 1957, 17 poison control centers were operating in the United States.[36] With the Chicago center serving as a model, these early centers responded to physician callers by providing ingredient and toxicity information about drug and household products, and making treatment recommendations. Records were kept of the calls, and preventive strategies were introduced into the community. As more poison control centers opened, a second important function, providing information to callers from the general public, became increasingly commonplace. The physician pioneers in poi-

TABLE 1–5. 20th-Century Milestones in the Development of Medical Toxicology

Year	Milestone
1949	First toxicology wards open in Budapest and Copenhagen
1949	First poison information service begins in the Netherlands
1952	American Academy of Pediatrics study shows that 51% of children's "accidents" are the result of the ingestion of potential poisons
1953	First US poison control center opens in Chicago
1957	National Clearinghouse for Poison Control Centers established
1958	American Association of Poison Control Centers (AAPCC) founded
1961	First Poison Prevention Week
1963	Initial call for development of regional PCCs
1964	Creation of European Association for PCCs
1968	American Academy of Clinical Toxicology (AACT) established
1972	Introduction of microfiche technology to poison information
1974	American Board of Medical Toxicology (ABMT) established
1978	AAPCC introduces standards of regional designation
1983	First examination given for Specialist in Poison Information (SPI)
1985	American Board of Applied Toxicology (ABAT) established
1992	Medical Toxicology recognized by American Board of Medical Specialties (ABMS)
1994	First ABMS examination in Medical Toxicology
2000	ACGME approval of residency training programs in Medical Toxicology

son prevention and poison treatment were predominantly pediatricians who focused on unintentional childhood ingestions.[120]

During these early years in the development of poison control centers, each center had to collect its own product information, which was a laborious, and often redundant, task.[36] In an effort to coordinate poison control center operations and to avoid unnecessary duplication, Surgeon General Dr. James Goddard responded to the recommendation of the American Public Health Service and established the National Clearinghouse for Poison Control Centers in 1957.[95] This organization, placed under the Bureau of Product Safety of the Food and Drug Administration, disseminated 5-inch by 8-inch index cards containing poison information to each center to help standardize poison center information resources. The Clearinghouse also collected and tabulated poison data from each of the centers.

Between 1953 and 1972, a rapid, uncoordinated proliferation of poison control centers occurred in the United States.[92] In 1962, there were 462 poison control centers.[1] By 1970, this number had risen to 590,[84] and by 1978, there were 661 poison control centers in the United States, including 100 centers in the state of Illinois.[126] The nature of calls to centers changed as lay public–generated calls began to outnumber physician-generated calls. Recognizing the publicity value and strong popular support associated with poison centers, some hospitals started poison control centers for public relations reasons without adequately recognizing or providing for the associated responsibilities. Unfortunately, many of these centers offered no more than a part-time telephone service located in the back of the emergency department or pharmacy, staffed by poorly trained personnel.[126]

Despite the growing pains of the poison control services during this period, there were many significant achievements. A dedicated group of physicians and other healthcare professionals began devoting an increasing proportion of their time to matters pertaining to poisoning. In 1958, the American Association of Poison Control Centers (AAPCC) was founded to promote closer cooperation between poison centers, to establish uniform standards, and to develop educational programs for the general public and other healthcare professionals.[60] Annual research meetings were held, and important legislative initiatives were stimulated by the organization's efforts.[95] Examples of such legislation include the Federal Hazardous Substances Labeling Act of 1960, which improved product labeling; the Child Protection Act of 1966, which extended labeling statutes to pesticides and other hazardous substances; and the Poison Prevention Packaging Act of 1970, which mandated safety packaging. In 1961, in an attempt to heighten public awareness of the dangers of unintentional poisoning, the third week of March was designated as National Poison Prevention Week.

Another important organization, the American Academy of Clinical Toxicology (AACT), was founded in 1968 by a diverse group of toxicologists.[32] This group was "interested in applying principles of rational toxicology to patient treatment" and in improving the standards of care on a national basis.[123] The journal *Clinical Toxicology*, initially sponsored by AACT, also began publication in 1968. The first modern textbooks of clinical toxicology began to appear in the mid-1950s with the publication of Dreisbach's *Handbook of Poisoning* (1955),[43] Gleason, Gosselin, and Hodge's *Clinical Toxicology of Commercial Products* (1957),[56] and Arena's *Poisoning* (1963).[9]

Major advancements in the storage and retrieval of poison information were instituted during these years. Information regarding consumer products initially appeared on index cards distributed regularly to poison centers by the National Clearinghouse. By 1978, more than 16,000 individual product cards had been assembled.[126] The introduction of microfiche technology in 1972 enabled the storage of much larger amounts of data in much smaller spaces at the individual poison centers. Toxifile and POISINDEX, two large drug and poison databases employing microfiche technology, were introduced and gradually replaced the much more limited index card system.[126] During the 1980s, POISINDEX, which had become the standard database, was made more accessible by using CD-ROM technology. Sophisticated information about the most esoteric of toxins was now instantaneously available by computer at every poison center.

In 1978, the poison control center movement entered an important new stage in its development when AAPCC introduced standards for regional poison center designation.[92] By defining strict criteria, AAPCC sought to upgrade poison center operations significantly and to offer a national standard of service. These criteria included employing poison specialists dedicated exclusively to operating the poison control center 24 hours per day and serving a catchment area of between 1 and 10 million people. Not surprisingly, this professionalization of the poison center movement led to a rapid consolidation of services, and the number of centers decreased to 71 by 2000. Fifty-three of the 71 centers (75%) have obtained regional certification. An AAPCC credentialing examination for poison information specialists was inaugurated in 1983 to help ensure the quality and standards of poison center staff.[28]

In 2000, the Poison Control Center Enhancement and Awareness Act was passed by Congress and signed into law by President William Clinton. For the first time, federal funding became available to provide assistance for poison prevention and to stabilize the funding of regional poison control centers. As of October 2001 federal assistance has permitted the establishment of a single nationwide toll-free phone number (800-222-1222) to access poison centers.

A poison control center movement has also evolved in Europe over the last 35 years, but unlike the movement in the United States, from the beginning its growth focused on the development of strong centralized toxicology treatment centers. In the late 1950s, Dr. M. Gaultier in Paris developed an inpatient unit that was dedicated to the care of poisoned patients.[58] In Great Britain, the National Poison Information Service was developed at Guys Hospital in 1963 under Dr. Roy Goulding.[58] Dr. Henry Matthew initiated a regional poisoning treatment center in Edinburgh about the same time,[116] and in 1964, the European Association for Poison Control Centers was formed at Tours, France.[58]

The Rise of Environmental Toxicology and Further Regulatory Protection from Toxic Substances

The rise of the environmental movement during the 1960s can be traced, in part, to the publication of Rachel Carson's *Silent Spring* in 1962, which revealed the perils of an increasingly toxic environment,[27] and to the increasing awareness among those involved with the poison control movement of the growing menace of toxins in the home environment.[24] Battery casing fume poisoning, which resulted from the burning of discarded lead battery cases, and acrodynia, which resulted from exposure to a variety of mercury-containing products,[39] demonstrated that young children seemed particularly vulnerable to low-dose exposures from certain toxins. Worries about the persistence of pesticides in the ecosystem and the increasing number of chemicals introduced into the environment added to the concern that the environment was a potential source of illness, heralding a drive for additional regulatory protection.

Starting with the Clean Air Act in 1963, laws were passed to help reduce the toxic burden on our environment (see Table 1–4). The establishment of the Environmental Protection Agency in 1970 spearheaded this attempt at protecting our environment, and during the next 10 years, numerous protective regulations were introduced. Among the most important initiatives were the Occupational Safety and Health Act of 1970 that established the Occupational Safety and Health Administration (OSHA). This act mandated that employers provide safe work conditions for their employees. Specific exposure limits to toxic chemicals in the workplace were promulgated. The Consumer Product Safety Commission was created in 1972 to protect the public from consumer products that posed an unreasonable risk of illness or injury. Cancer-producing substances, such as benzene, vinyl chloride, and asbestos, have been banned from consumer products as a result of these new regulations. Toxic waste disasters at Love Canal, New York, and Times Beach, Missouri, led to the passing of the Comprehensive Environmental Response, Compensation, and Liability Act (known as the Superfund) in 1980. This fund would help to pay for cleanup of hazardous substance releases that posed a potential threat to public health.

Medical Toxicology Comes of Age

Over the last 25 years, the specialty of medical toxicologists has changed. The development of emergency medicine and preventive medicine as medical specialties led to the training of more physicians with a dedicated interest in toxicology. By the early 1990s, emergency physicians accounted for more than half of medical

toxicologists.[42] The increased diversity of medical toxicologists with primary training in emergency medicine, pediatrics, preventive medicine, or internal medicine has helped to broaden the goals of poison control centers and medical toxicologists beyond the treatment of acute unintentional childhood ingestions. The broad scope of medical toxicology now includes a much wider array of toxic exposures including acute and chronic, adult and pediatric, unintentional and intentional, occupational and environmental.

The development of medical toxicology as a medical subspecialty began in 1974, when AACT established the American Board of Medical Toxicology (ABMT) to recognize physician practitioners of medical toxicology.[4] From 1974 to 1992, 209 physicians obtained board certification from the ABMT. Formal subspecialty recognition of medical toxicology by the American Board of Medical Specialties (ABMS) was granted in 1992, and a conjoint board with representatives from the specialties of emergency medicine, pediatrics, and preventive medicine was created. The first ABMS-sponsored examination in medical toxicology was offered in 1994. By 2000, 254 physicians were board-certified in medical toxicology by the ABMT and/or ABMS. The American College of Medical Toxicology was founded in 1994 as an organization designed to advance clinical, educational, and research goals in medical toxicology. In 1999, the Accreditation Council of Graduate Medical Education (ACGME) in the United States formally recognized postgraduate education in Medical Toxicology, and resident program credentialing began in 2000.

During the 1990s in the United States, some medical toxicologists began to work on establishing regional toxicology treatment centers. Adapting the European model, toxicology treatment centers would serve as referral centers for patients requiring advanced toxicologic evaluation and treatment. Goals of such inpatient regional centers included enhancing care of the poisoned patient, strengthening toxicology training, and facilitating research. The evaluation of the clinical efficacy and fiscal viability of such programs is ongoing.

The professional maturation of nonphysicians with a primary interest in toxicology has also taken place over the past two decades. In 1985, AACT established the American Board of Applied Toxicology (ABAT), to administer a certifying examination for nonphysician practitioners of medical toxicology who meet certain rigorous standards.[3] By 2000, 69 toxicologists were certified by this board, most of whom held either a PharmD degree in pharmacy or a PhD in pharmacology.

Recent Poisonings and Poisoners

Although accounting for just a tiny fraction of all homicidal deaths (0.16% in the United States), notorious lethal poisonings continued throughout the 20th century (Table 1–3).[2] In 1982, deliberate tampering with nonprescription acetaminophen preparations with potassium cyanide caused seven deaths in Chicago.[44] Because of this tragedy, packaging of over-the-counter medications was changed to decrease the possibility of future product tampering.[100] The perpetrator(s) were never apprehended, and other deaths from over-the-counter product tampering were reported in 1991.[38]

In England, Graham Frederick Young developed a macabre fascination with poisons.[69] In 1971, at age 14 he killed his stepmother and other family members with arsenic and antimony. Sent away to a psychiatric hospital, he was released at age 24, when he was no longer considered to be a threat to society. Within months of his release he again engaged in lethal poisonings, killing several of his coworkers. Ultimately, he died in prison.

In 1978, a Bulgarian defector living in London developed multisystem failure and died 4 days after having been stabbed by an umbrella carried by an unknown assailant. The postmortem examination revealed a pin-sized metal sphere embedded in his thigh where he had been stabbed. Investigators speculated that this sphere had most likely carried a lethal dose of ricin into the victim.[35]

In 1998, Judias Buenoano, known as the "black widow," was executed for murdering her husband with arsenic in 1971 in order to collect insurance money. She was the first person executed in Florida in 150 years. The fatal poisoning remained undetected until 1983, when Buenoano was accused of trying to murder her fiancé with arsenic and by car bombing. Exhumation of the husband's body, 12 years after he died, revealed lethal amounts of arsenic in the remains.[6]

Healthcare providers have also been implicated in several poisoning homicides. An epidemic of mysterious cardiopulmonary arrests at the Ann Arbor Veterans Administration Hospital in Michigan, in July and August 1975, was attributed to the homicidal use of pancuronium by two nurses.[133] Intentional digoxin poisoning by hospital personnel may have explained some of the increased number of deaths on a cardiology ward of a Toronto pediatric hospital in 1981, but the exact cause of the high mortality rate was unclear.[21] In 2000, an English general practitioner was convicted of murdering 15 female patients with heroin and may have murdered as many as 297 patients during his 24-year career. These recent revelations prompted calls for strengthening the death certification process, for improving preservation of case records, and for better procedures for monitoring controlled drugs.[66] Also, in 2000, an American physician pleaded guilty to the charge of poisoning a number of patients under his care during his residency training. Succinylcholine, potassium chloride, and arsenic were some of the agents he used to kill his patients.[132] Attention to more careful physician credentialing and to maintenance of a national physician database arose from this case because the poisonings occurred at several different hospitals across the country.

By the end of the 20th century, 24 centuries after Socrates was executed by poison hemlock, the means of implementing capital punishment had come full circle. Government-sanctioned execution in the United States again favored the use of a "state" poison: this time, the combination of sodium thiopental, pancuronium, and potassium chloride.

Medical Errors

In late 1999, the problem of medical errors became a highly visible issue in the United States with the publication and subsequent reaction to an Institute of Medicine (IOM) report suggesting that 44,000 to 98,000 fatalities each year were the result of medical errors.[77] Many of these errors were attributed to preventable medication errors. The IOM report focused on the fact that errors usually resulted from system faults and not solely from the carelessness of individuals.

Several recent, highly publicized, medication errors received considerable public attention and provided a nidus for the initiation of change in policies and systems. Ironically, all of the cases occurred at nationally preeminent university teaching hospitals. In 1984, 18-year-old Libby Zion died from severe hyperthermia soon after hospital admission. While the cause of her death was likely multifactorial, drug-drug interactions, as well as the failure to rec-

ognize and appropriately treat her agitated delirium, also contributed to her death.[12] State and national guidelines for closer house staff supervision, improved working conditions, and a heightened awareness of consequential drug-drug interactions resulted from the medical, legislative, and legal issues of this case. In 1994, a prominent health journalist for the *Boston Globe*, Betsy Lehman, was the unfortunate victim of another preventable dosing error when she inadvertently received four times the dose of the chemotherapeutic agent cyclophosphamide as part of an experimental protocol.[76] Despite treatment at a world-renowned cancer center, multiple physicians, nurses, and pharmacists failed to notice this erroneous medication order. An overhaul of the medication-ordering system was implemented after this tragic event.

Another highly publicized death occurred in 1999, when 18-year-old Jesse Gelsinger died after enrolling in an experimental gene-therapy study. Mr. Gelsinger, who had ornithine transcarbamylase deficiency, died from multiorgan failure 4 days after receiving, by hepatic infusion, the first dose of an engineered adenovirus containing the normal gene. While this unexpected death was not the direct result of a dosing or drug-drug interaction error, the FDA review concluded that major research violations had occurred in this case, including failure to report adverse effects with this therapy in animals and earlier clinical trials, as well as failure to properly obtain informed consent.[128] Calls for additional safeguards to protect patients in research studies resulted from this case.

SUMMARY

Since the dawn of recorded history, toxicology has had a great impact on human events. And although over the millennia the important poisons of the day have changed to some degree, toxic substances continue to challenge our safety. The era of poisoners for hire may have long ago reached its pinnacle, but environmental poisons confront all of us, with no end in sight to this poisoning menace. Unfortunately, knowledge acquired by one generation is often forgotten or discarded inappropriately by the next generation, leading to a cyclical historic course. The ancients were undoubtedly much more knowledgeable than many current healthcare professionals about the benefits and drawbacks of medicinal and poisonous plants, lessons that would serve us well as additional herbal concoctions flood our marketplace, leading to some of our more challenging present-day poisonings. Gastrointestinal decontamination strategies and drug-abuse trends continue to evolve. This historic review is meant to describe the past and to better prepare toxicologists and society for the future.

REFERENCES

1. Adams WC: Poison control centers: Their purpose and operation. Clin Pharmacol Ther 1963;4:293–296.
2. Adelson L: Homicidal poisoning: A dying modality of lethal violence. Am J Forensic Med Pathol 1987;8:245–251.
3. American Board of Applied Toxicology: AACTion 1992;1:3.
4. American Board of Medical Toxicology: Vet Hum Toxicol 1987;29:510.
5. American Heritage Dictionary, 2nd college ed. Boston, Houghton Mifflin, 1991.
6. Anderson C, McGehee S: Bodies of Evidence: The True Story of Judias Buenoano: Florida's Serial Murderess. New York, St. Martins, 1993.

7. Anderson H: Experimental studies on the pharmacology of activated charcoal. Acta Pharmacol 1946;2:69–78.

8. Anderson OE: Pioneer statute: The pure food and drugs act of 1906. J Public Law 1964;13:189–196.

9. Arena JM: Poisoning: Chemistry, Symptoms, Treatments. Springfield, IL, Charles C. Thomas, 1963.

10. Arena JM: The pediatrician's role in the poison control movement and poison prevention. Am J Dis Child 1983;137:870–873.

11. Arnold WN: Vincent van Gogh and the thujone connection. JAMA 1988;260:3042–3044.

12. Asch DA., Parker RM. The Libby Zion case. One step forward or two steps backward? N Engl J Med 1988;318:771–775.

13. Baldwin M: The snakestone experiments: An early modem medical debate. Isis 1995;86:394–418.

14. Bartrip P: A "pennurth of arsenic for rat poison": The arsenic act, 1851 and the prevention of secret poisoning. Med Hist 1992;36:53–69.

15. Benjamin DR: Mushrooms: Poisons and Panaceas. New York, WH Freeman, 1995.

16. Berman A: The persistence of theriac in France. Pharm Hist 1970;12:5.

17. Bible. Job 6:04.

18. Bissett NG: Arrow and dart poisons. J Ethnopharmacol 1989;25:1–41.

19. Bond RT: Handbook for Poisoners: A Collection of Great Poison Stories. New York, Collier Books, 1951.

20. Brown HM: De Venenis of Petrus Abbonus: A translation of the Latin. Ann Med Hist 1924;6:25–53.

21. Buehler JW, Smith LF, Wallace EM, et al: Unexplained deaths in a children's hospital: An epidemiologic assessment. N Engl J Med 1985;313:211–216.

22. Burchell HB: Digitalis poisoning: Historical and forensic aspects. J Am Coll Cardiol 1983;1:506–516.

23. Burke M: Gastric lavage and emesis in the treatment of ingested poisons: A review and a clinical study of lavage in ten adults. Resuscitation 1972;1:91–105.

24. Burnham JC: How the discovery of accidental childhood poisoning contributed to the development of environmentalism in the United States. Environ Hist Rev 1995;19:57–81.

25. Byck R, ed: Cocaine Papers by Sigmund Freud (English translation). New York, Stonehill Publishing, 1975, pp. 48–73.

26. Campbell WA: Oxalic acid, Epsom salt, and the poison bottle. Hum Toxicol 1982;1:187–193.

27. Carson RL: Silent Spring. Boston, Houghton Mifflin, 1962.

28. Certification examination for poison information specialists. Vet Hum Toxicol 1983;25:54–55.

29. Christison R: A Treatise on Poisons. London, Adam Black, 1829.

30. Clarke MJ: Chloral hydrate: Medicine and poison? Pharm Historian 1988;18:2–4.

31. Cocaine deaths reported for century or more. JAMA 1992;267:1045–1046.

32. Comstock EG: Roots and circle in medical toxicology: A personal reminiscence. J Toxicol Clin Toxicol 1998;36:401–407.

33. Cooney DO: Activated Charcoal in Medical Applications. New York, Marcel Dekker, 1995.

34. Costill OH: A Practical Treatise on Poisons. Philadelphia, Grigg, Elliot, 1848.

35. Crompton R, Gall D: Georgi Markov: Death in a pellet. Med Leg J 1980;48:51–62.

36. Crotty J, Armstrong G: National clearinghouse for poison control centers. Clin Toxicol 1978;12:303–307.

37. Crotty JJ, Verhulst HL: Organization and delivery of poison information in the United States. Pediatr Clin North Am 1970;17:741–746.

38. Cyanide poisonings associated with over-the-counter medication, Washington State, 1991. MMWR Morb Mortal Wkly Rep 1991;40:161,167.

39. Dally A: The rise and fall of pink disease. Soc Hist Med 1997;10:291–304.

40. Das G: Cocaine abuse in North America: A milestone in history. J Clin Pharmacol 1993;33:296–310.

41. Deichmann WB, Henschler D, Holmstedt B, Keil G: What is there that is not poison? A study of the Third Defense by Paracelsus. Arch Toxicol 1986;58:207–213.

42. Donovan JW, Goldfrank LR: Medical toxicologist practice characteristics, specialty certifications and manpower needs [abstract]. Vet Hum Toxicol 1992;34:336.

43. Dreisbach RH: Handbook of Poisoning: Diagnosis and Treatment. Los Altos, CA, Lange, 1955.

44. Dunea G: Death over the counter. Br Med J 1983;286:211–212.

45. Earles MP: Early theories of mode of action of drugs and poisons. Ann Science 1961;17:97–110.

46. Eckert WG. Medicolegal investigation in New York City: History and activities 1918–1978. Am J Forensic Med Pathol 1983;4:33–54.

47. Eckert WG: Historical aspects of poisoning and toxicology. Am J Forensic Med Pathol 1981;2:261–264.

48. Elgood C: A treatise on the bezoar stone. Ann Med Hist 1935;7:73–80.

49. Felton JS: The heritage of Bernardino Ramazzini. Occup Med 1997;47:167–179.

50. Ferner RE: Forensic Pharmacology: Medicines, Mayhem, and Malpractice. Oxford, Oxford University Press, 1996.

51. Flanagan RJ, Ramsey JD: Humphry Davy (1778–1829) and Nitrous Phosoxyde (Nitrous Oxide): 200 Years of Volatile Substance Abuse. In press.

52. Franco G: Ramazzini and worker's health. Lancet 1999;354:858–861.

53. Funck-Brentano F: Princes and Poisoners: Studies of the Court of Louis XIV. London, Duckworth & Co, 1901.

54. Gaebel RE: Saturnine gout among Roman aristocrats. N Engl J Med 1983;309:431.

55. Gallo MA: History and scope of toxicology. In: Klaassen CD, ed: Casarett and Doull's Toxicology: The Basic Science of Poisons, 5th ed. New York, McGraw-Hill, 1996, pp. 3–11.

56. Gleason MN, Gosselin RE, Hodge HC: Clinical Toxicology of Commercial Products: Acute Poisoning (Home and Farm). Baltimore, Williams & Wilkins, 1957.

57. Golding AMB: Two hundred years of drug abuse. J R Soc Med 1993;86:282–286.

58. Govaerts M: Poison control in Europe. Pediatr Clin North Am 1970;17:729–739.

59. Grant, MP: Alice Hamilton: Pioneer Doctor in Industrial Medicine. London, Abelard-Schuman, 1967.

60. Grayson R: The poison control movement in the United States. Indust Med Surg 1962;31:296–297.

61. Green DW: The saturnine curse: A history of lead poisoning. South Med J 1985;78:48–51.

62. Greensher J, Mofenson HC, Caraccio TR: Ascendency of the black bottle (activated charcoal). Pediatrics 1987;80:949–950.

63. Hamilton A: Landmark article in occupational medicine: Forty years in the poisonous trades. Am J Indust Med 1985;7:3–18.

64. Hofmann A: How LSD originated. J Psychedelic Drugs 1979;11:53–60.

65. Holt LE, Holz PH: The black bottle: A consideration of the role of charcoal in the treatment of poisoning in children. J Pediatr 1963;63:306–314.

66. Horton R: The real lesson from Harold Frederick Shipman. Lancet 2001;357:82

67. Howard-Jones N. The origins of hypodermic medication. Sci Am 1971;224:96–102.

68. Hunter D: The Diseases of Occupations, 6th ed. London, Hodder & Stoughton, 1978.

69. Irvine A, Johnson H: R vs Young: Murder by thallium. Med Leg J 1974;42:76–90.

70. Jain KK: Carbon Monoxide Poisoning. St. Louis, Warren H. Green, 1990, pp. 3–5.

71. Jarcho S: Medical numismatic notes. VII: Mithradates IV. Bull N Y Acad Med 1972;48:1059–1064.

72. Jarcho S: The correspondence of Morgagni and Lancisi on the death of Cleopatra. Bull Hist Med 1969;43:299–325.

73. Jensen LB: Poisoning Misadventures. Springfield, IL, Charles C. Thomas, 1970.

74. Karch SB: The history of cocaine toxicity. Hum Pathol 1989;20:1037–1039.

75. Knoefel PK: Felice Fontana on poisons. Clio Medica 1980;15:35–66.

76. Knox RA: Doctor's orders killed cancer patient: Dana Farber admits drug overdose caused death of Globe columnist, damage to second woman. Boston Globe March 23, 1995, p. M1.

77. Kohn LT, Corrigan J, Donaldson MS, eds: To Err Is Human: Building a Safer Health System. Washington, DC, National Academy Press, 2000.

78. Kramer JC: Opium rampant: Medical use, misuse, and abuse in Britain and the West in the 17th and 18th centuries. Br J Addict 1979;74:377–389.

79. Kramer JC: The opiates: Two centuries of scientific study. J Psychedelic Drugs 1980;12:89–102.

80. Lanier D: Absinthe: The Cocaine of the Nineteenth Century. Jefferson, NC, McFarland, 1995.

81. Lee JA: Claude Bernard (1813–1878). Anaesthesia 1978;33:741–747.

82. Levey M: Medieval Arabic toxicology: The book on poison of Ibn Wahshiya and its relation to early Indian and Greek texts. Trans Amer Philosph Soc 1966:56:5–130.

83. Lomax E: The uses and abuses of opiates in nineteenth-century England. Bull Hist Med 1973;47:167–176.

84. Lovejoy FH, Alpert JJ: A future direction for poison centers: A critique. Pediatr Clin North Am 1970;17:747–753.

85. Lucanie R: Unicorn horn and its use as a poison antidote. Vet Hum Toxicol 1992;34:563.

86. Ludlow FH: The Hasheesh Eater Microform: Being Passages from the Life of a Pythagorean. New York, Harper, 1857.

87. Lyons AS: Medicine: An Illustrated History. New York, Abradale Press, 1978.

88. Macht DI: Louis Lewin: Pharmacologist, toxicologist, medical historian. Ann Med Hist 1931;3:179–194.

89. Magner LN: A History of Medicine. New York, Marcel Dekker, 1992.

90. Major RH: History of the stomach tube. Ann Med Hist 1934;6:500–509.

91. Mann J: Murder, Magic, and Medicine. New York, Oxford University Press, 1992.

92. Manoguerra AS, Temple AR: Observations on the current status of poison control centers in the United States. Emerg Med Clin North Am 1984;2:185–197.

93. Mant K: Forensic medicine in Great Britain: II. The origins of the British medicolegal system and some historic cases. Am J Forensic Med Pathol 1987;8:354–361.

94. Marsh J: Account of a method of separating small quantities of arsenic from substances with which it may be mixed. Edinb New Phil J 1836;21:229–236.

95. McIntire M: On the occasion of the twenty-fifth anniversary of the American Association of Poison Control Centers. Vet Hum Toxicol 1983;25:35–37.

96. Mead GO. Ether drinking in Ireland. JAMA 1891;16:391–392.

97. Modell W: Mass drug catastrophes and the roles of science and technology. Science 1967;156:346–351.

98. Moore SW: A case of poisoning by laudanum, successfully treated by means of Jukes's syringe. NY Med Phys J 1825;4:91–92.

99. Moriarty KM, Alagna SW, Lake CR: Psychopharmacology: An historical perspective. Psychiatr Clin North Am 1984;7:411–433.

100. Murphy DH: Cyanide-tainted Tylenol: What pharmacists can learn. Am Pharm 1986;26:19–23.

101. Musto DF: America's first cocaine epidemic. Wilson Q 1989;13:59–64.

102. Nahas GG: Hashish in Islam 9th to 18th century. Bull N Y Acad Med 1982;58:814–831.

103. Nerlich AG, Parsche F, Wiest I, et al: Extensive pulmonary haemorrhage in an Egyptian mummy. Virchows Arch 1995;427:423–429.

104. Niyogi SK: Historical development of forensic toxicology in America up to 1978. Am J Forensic Med Pathol 1980;1:249–264.

105. Nriagu JO: Saturnine gout among Roman aristocrats: Did lead poisoning contribute to the fall of the empire? N Engl J Med 1983;308:660–663.

106. Oehme FW: The development of toxicology as a veterinary discipline in the United States. Clin Toxicol 1970;3:211–220.

107. Olch PD: William S. Halsted and local anesthesia. Anesthesiology 1975;42:479–486.

108. Orfila MP: Traite des Poisons. Paris, Ches Crochard, 1814.

109. Oxford English Dictionary, 2nd ed, vol 18. Oxford, Clarendon Press, 1989, p. 328.

110. Pachter HM: Paracelsus: Magic into Science. New York, Collier, 1961.

111. Pappas AA, Massoll NA, Cannon DJ: Toxicology: Past, present, future. Ann Clin Lab Sci 1999;25:253–262.

112. Parsche F, Balabanova S, Pirsig W: Drugs in ancient populations. Lancet 1993;341:503.

113. Plaitakis A, Duvoisin RC: Homer's moly identified as *Galanthus nivalis:* Physiologic antidote to stramonium poisoning. Clin Neuropharmacol 1983;6:1–5.

114. Pollock SH: The psilocybin mushroom pandemic. J Psychedelic Drugs 1975;7:73–84.

115. Press E, Mellins RB: A poisoning control program. Am J Public Health 1954;44:1515–1525.

116. Proudfoot AT: Clinical toxicology: Past, present and future. Hum Toxicol 1988;7:481–487.

117. Quinones MA. Drug abuse during the Civil War (1861–1865). Int J Addictions 1975;10:1007–1020.

118. Regier CC: The struggle for federal food and drugs legislation. Law Contemp Prob 1933;1:3–15.

119. Reid DHS: Treatment of the poisoned child. Arch Dis Child 1970;45:428–433.

120. Robertson WO: National organizations and agencies in poison control programs: A commentary. Clin Toxicol 1978;12:297–302.

121. Robins LN, Helzer JE, Davis DH: Narcotic use in Southeast Asia and afterward: An interview study of 898 Vietnam returnees. Arch Gen Psychiatry 1975;32:955–961.

122. Rosner F: Moses Maimonides' treatise on poisons. JAMA 1968;205:98–100.

123. Rumack BH, Ford P, Sbarbaro J, et al: Regionalization of poison centers: A rational role mode. Clin Toxicol 1978;12:367–375.

124. Sapira JD: Speculations concerning opium abuse and world history. Perspect Biol Med 1975;18:379–398.

125. Scarborough J: Nicanders' Toxicology. Pharm Hist 1979;21:3–34.

126. Scherz RG, Robertson WO: The history of poison control centers in the United States. Clin Toxicol 1978;12:291–296.

127. Scutchfield FD, Genovese EN: Terrible death of Socrates: Some medical and classical reflections. Pharos 1997;60:30–33.

128. Silberner J: A gene therapy death. Hastings Cent Rep 2000;30:6.

129. Sinclair U: The Jungle. New York, Doubleday, 1906.

130. Smith S: Poisons and poisoners through the ages. Med Leg J 1952:20:153–167.

131. Sneader W: The discovery of heroin. Lancet 1998;352:1697–1699.

132. Stewart JB: Blind Eye: The Terrifying Story of a Doctor Who Got Away with Murder. New York, Touchstone, 1999.

133. Stross JK, Shasby M, Harlan WR: An epidemic of mysterious cardiopulmonary arrests. N Engl J Med 1976;295:1107–1110.

134. Suicide: A leading cause of death. JAMA 1952;150:696–697.

135. Taylor HM: A preliminary survey of the effect which lye legislation has had on the incidence of esophageal stricture. Ann Otol Rhinol Laryngol 1935;44:1157–1158.

136. Thompson CJ: Poisons and Poisoners. London, Harold Shaylor, 1931.

137. Timbrell JA: Introduction to Toxicology. London, Taylor & Francis, 1989.

138. Trestrail JH: Criminal Poisoning: Investigational Guide for Law Enforcement, Toxicologists, Forensic Scientists, and Attorneys. Totowa, NJ, Humana Press, 2000.

139. Vale JA, Meredith TJ: Poison information services. In: Vale JA, Meredith TJ, eds: Poisoning: Diagnosis and Treatment. London, Update Books, 1981: pp. 9–12

140. Watson G: Theriac and Mithradatum: A Study in Therapeutics. London, Wellcome Historical Medical Library, 1966.

141. Wax PM: Elixirs, diluents and the passage of the 1938 federal Food, Drug and Cosmetic Act. Ann Intern Med 1995;122:456–461.

142. Wells C: Lead poisoning in the ancient world. Med Hist 1973;17: 391–397.

143. Witthaus RA, Becker TC: Medical Jurisprudence: Forensic Medicine and Toxicology, vol. 1. New York, William Wood, 1894.

144. Witthaus RA: Manual of Toxicology, 2nd ed. New York, William Wood, 1911.

145. Wormley TG: Micro-Chemistry of Poisons. New York, William Wood, 1869.

146. Wright-St. Clair RE: Poison or medicine. N Z Med J 1970;71: 224–229.

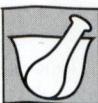

ANTIDOTES IN DEPTH

Antiquated Antidotes
Paul M. Wax

While the judicious use of certain antidotes (eg, *N*-acetylcysteine, naloxone, pyridoxine) is critically important in the management of select poisoned patients, other antidotes do not necessarily offer a distinct clinical advantage and may create additional problems (eg, flumazenil, physostigmine). A perpetual search for better and improved antidotes features prominently in the history of toxicology. Unfortunately, many of the "antidotal breakthroughs" over the years have not lived up to their promise (Table 1–6). A number of these antidotes, such as caffeine, are ineffective. Others, such as propylene glycol, were insufficiently tested or were replaced by "safer," more effective treatment such as paraldehyde.[11] Most troubling, the use of some of these agents, such as analeptics and copper sulfate, actually worsened the clinical situation. Unfortunately, just as the various classic theriac preparations remained popular into the 20th century, the use of many of these "modern antidotes" has persisted long after scientific investigation demonstrated their ineffectiveness. An emphasis on physiologic antagonism with antidotes, such as analeptics, has often taken precedence over good supportive care. Not surprisingly, the use of modern-day theriacs, such as the "universal antidote," persisted until quite recently, despite a lack of serious scientific support. This section highlights some of the critical changes in 20th-century poison management.

ANALEPTICS

One of the most interesting changes in poison management took place during the 1940s and 1950s with regard to the use of analeptics in the treatment of barbiturate overdose.[49] Analeptics are nonspecific arousal agents and include such stimulants as strychnine, camphor, caffeine, picrotoxin, pentylenetetrazol, nikethamide, amphetamine, and methylphenidate. Barbiturates, the first widely available sedative-hypnotics, were introduced in the early 20th century. Within a few years they became the most common cause of serious overdose.[5] In the 1920s, barbiturate overdose management recommendations still included blood-letting techniques.[34] By the next decade, as interest in principles of antagonism between stimulants and depressants became widespread, much attention was focused on the use of analeptic agents to combat the sedative effects of barbiturates. Proponents of analeptics argued that because the effects of cocaine intoxication appeared to be neutralized by barbiturates, a reciprocal approach—treating depressant overdoses with stimulants—should also be effective.[34] The principal goal of analeptic therapy was to awaken the patient as soon as possible.

Numerous analeptic agents have been recommended over the years. Prior to the development of the first synthetic analeptics in the late 1920s, naturally occurring stimulants, such as caffeine, lobeline, strychnine, cocaine, and camphor, were utilized for this purpose. According to Leschke's *Clinical Toxicology*, a standard textbook published in 1934, the most effective remedy for the treatment of a sedative-hypnotic overdose was the intrathecal injection of 10% camphorated oil.[31]

Picrotoxin, obtained from the berries of the *Cocculus indicus* plant, was first suggested as an antagonist to morphine in 1847.[29] After a series of animal studies in the early 1930s, picrotoxin was enthusiastically endorsed as the analeptic of choice.[35] Picrotoxin acts as a $GABA_A$ and $GABA_C$ receptor antagonist and as a glycine-receptor antagonist facilitating excitatory neurotransmission.[18] Although picrotoxin remains one of the most powerful central nervous system (CNS) and respiratory stimulants in our pharmacopeia, it also exhibits marked convulsive activity.

The subsequent introduction of synthetic analeptics, such as pentylenetetrazol (Metrazol, Cardiazol) and nikethamide (Coramine), increased the growing dependence on analeptics as the major treatment modality for barbiturate overdose.[25,28,36] During his search for an effective camphor substitute, Schmidt synthesized pentylenetetrazol, the first synthetic analeptic, in 1924, and it was initially introduced as a cardiac stimulant.[48] Mechanistically, it reduces GABA-ergic inhibition and interacts with picrotoxin-binding sites. It may also work by changing extraneuronal potassium permeability, thereby partially depolarizing neuronal membranes and increasing excitability. Pentylenetetrazol was employed as a CNS stimulant in the treatment of depressant overdoses from the 1930s through the 1960s,[16,25] but was considered less effective than picrotoxin or strychnine.

Nikethamide was also used as a cardiac and respiratory stimulant and was reputed to be helpful in overcoming the respiratory depression of morphine, sedative-hypnotics, and volatile anesthetics.[36] Further experience showed that it was a less efficacious analeptic than either picrotoxin or pentylenetetrazol.[20] Its exact mechanisms of enhancing excitation are unknown.

Analeptic treatment strategies were often referred to as "very energetic," because large doses of multiple analeptics were frequently utilized.[38] As recently as the 1950s, newer analeptics, such as bemegride, were being introduced as the "real antidote" to barbiturate overdoses.[45] During this time, methylphenidate was also used in the treatment of barbiturate overdoses. In 1967, one enthusiastic methylphenidate proponent emphasized, "Don't let comatose patients remain comatose [after barbiturate overdose]. Methylphenidate will waken them safely."[36] Toxicology textbooks published in the 1950s and 1960s continued to recommend caffeine, picrotoxin, and nikethamide as useful analeptic agents.[13,19,32] Subconvulsive electric shock therapy was also advocated as an alternative or adjunct to these chemical convulsants during this period.[42]

Unfortunately, many adverse effects occurred with the use of these analeptics, including hyperthermia, dysrhythmias, seizures, and psychoses.[27,36,41] It gradually became evident that analeptic therapy, despite its theoretic benefits, offered no real advantage, did not reduce mortality, and, placed the patient at risk for significant iatrogenic complications.[7] A different strategy was required.

Beginning in the mid-1940s, a distinctive approach to barbiturate overdose was pioneered by Eric Nilsson and Carl Clemmesen at the Bispebjergs Hospital in Copenhagen, Denmark.[7,39] This treat-

TABLE 1–6. Antiquated Antidotes

Type of Antidote	Therapeutic Agent	Uses	Adverse Effects
Analeptic	Amphetamine	Sedative overdose	Seizures, hyperthermia, aspiration
	Bemegride	Sedative overdose	Seizures, hyperthermia, aspiration
	Caffeine	Sedative overdose	Seizures, hyperthermia, aspiration
	Camphorated oil	Sedative overdose	Seizures, hyperthermia, aspiration
	Lobeline	Sedative overdose	Seizures, hyperthermia, aspiration
	Nikethamide (Coramine)	Sedative overdose	Seizures, hyperthermia, aspiration
	Pentylenetetrazol (Metrazol)	Sedative overdose	Seizures, hyperthermia, aspiration
	Picrotoxin	Sedative overdose	Seizures, hyperthermia, aspiration
	Strychnine	Sedative overdose	Seizures, hyperthermia, aspiration
Adsorbent	Universal antidote	Gastrointestinal decontamination	Ineffective; tannic acid hepatotoxicity
	Burnt toast	Gastrointestinal decontamination	Ineffective
Complexing agent	Sodium phosphate (Phospho-Soda)	Iron	Hyperphosphatemia
Emetic	Apomorphine	Gastric emptying	CNS depression, aspiration
	Copper sulfate	Gastric emptying	Caustic, increased copper load
	Mechanical stimulation	Gastric emptying	Oropharyngeal trauma; ineffective
	Mustard powder	Gastric emptying	Ineffective
	Saltwater	Gastric emptying	Hypernatremia
	Tartar emetic	Gastric emptying	GI toxicity
	Zinc sulfate	Gastric emptying	GI toxicity
Heavy metal antidote	Ascorbic acid	Lead, arsenic	Ineffective
	Calcium bromide	Lead	Ineffective
	Ferric hydroxide/magnesium hydroxide	Arsenic	Ineffective
	Potassium ferrocyanide	Copper	Ineffective
	Potassium iodide	Lead	Ineffective
	Sodium formaldehyde sulfoxylate	Mercury bichloride	Ineffective
Miscellaneous	Acetazolamide	Salicylate	Acidemia; increased CNS salicylate load
	Hypochlorites	Snakebites	Ineffective
	Potassium permanganate	Alkaloids (morphine, strychnine, aconite)	Caustic
	Propylene glycol	Phenolphthalein	
	Raw rabbit brain	*Amanita phalloides*	Ineffective
Neutralizing agent	Calcium carbonate	Acid	Exothermic reaction; gas formation; ineffective
	Hydrochloric acid	Alkali	Exothermic reaction; gas formation; ineffective
	Lemon juice	Alkali	Exothermic reaction; gas formation; ineffective
	Lime water	Acid	Exothermic reaction; gas formation; ineffective
	Magnesium hydroxide	Acid	Exothermic reaction; gas formation; ineffective
	Sodium bicarbonate	Acid	Exothermic reaction; gas formation; ineffective
	Vinegar	Alkali	Exothermic reaction; gas formation; ineffective
Sedative	Chloroform	Strychnine	Hepatotoxin, dysrhythmias
	Digitalis	Delirium tremens	Ineffective
	Ethanol	Delirium tremens	Difficult to titrate, metabolic abnormalities
	Ether	Agitation/seizures	Difficult to administer; irritating
	Paraldehyde	Delirium tremens	Acidosis; difficult to administer
	Sodium bromide	Delirium tremens	Difficult to use; bromism
	Tribromoethanol (Avertin)	Agitation/seizures	Sedation

ment regimen, known as *the Scandinavian method,* abandoned the use of analeptics in the treatment of barbiturate overdoses. Instead of primarily emphasizing the termination of coma, attention was directed at intensive supportive therapy with respiratory ventilation, oxygenation, and cardiovascular support. This strategy was analogous to the postanesthetic recovery room care provided to surgical patients. Using this "revolutionary" approach, barbiturate overdose mortality significantly dropped from about 20% with stimulation therapy to 1–2% with the Scandinavian method.[7]

EARLY TREATMENTS OF OPIOID OVERDOSES

Prior to the 1950s, opioid overdose was treated with many of the same analeptic agents. In the early 1950s, an important development in the history of poison management occurred when two specific opioid antidotes were introduced: nalorphine (Nalline) and levallorphan (Lorfan).[14] These drugs were capable of reversing the respiratory effects of an opioid overdose by blocking opioid receptors. Nalorphine was also routinely administered to determine the presence or absence of opioids in suspected opioid abusers. This test, known as the *Nalline test*, was used as a monitoring tool in drug abuse programs.[22] The test was considered positive if it precipitated signs of opioid withdrawal or pupillary dilatation.

Unfortunately, neither nalorphine nor levallorphan was a pure opioid antagonist. Instead, the mixed agonist/antagonist properties of these drugs significantly limited their usefulness. Respiratory depression could be potentiated, especially in opioid-free patients. This was most likely to occur when these drugs were administered to comatose patients with mild hypoventilation who had overdosed on sedative-hypnotics or ethanol.

Naloxone, which was introduced in the 1970s, is a much safer drug because of its pure opioid antagonistic properties. It has completely replaced nalorphine and levallorphan in the treatment of opioid overdoses.[15] Naloxone has no agonist properties, does not cause any additional respiratory depression, regardless of the ingestion, is short acting, and is safe to use for patients with coma following an undefined overdose. In addition, it is useful in treating patients with an overdose of other mixed agonist-antagonist opioids, such as pentazocine, who do not typically respond to nalorphine.

OUTDATED AND DANGEROUS EMETICS

The role of emetics in poison management, both in the home and at the hospital, has undergone significant transformation over the years. The antimony salt commonly known as tartar emetic had a long history of use as an emetic, as well as a sedative, expectorant, cathartic, and diaphoretic. During the 19th century, tartar emetic was one of the three most widely prescribed drugs, along with opium and calomel (mercurous chloride).[23] Tartar emetic is no longer recommended for any purpose because of its inherent toxicity and unreliability.[6]

Standard gastrointestinal decontamination recommendations during the 1960s included mechanical stimulation of the throat and the ingestion of saltwater emetics, or mustard water in the home, and copper sulfate, zinc sulfate, or apomorphine in the hospital.[1,26] Many authorities recommended mechanical stimulation of the pharynx (finger-down-the-throat technique) as a quick-and-easy home remedy when induction of emesis was desirable.[1,9] This method, however, is both ineffective and potentially traumatic, and is no longer encouraged.[9] Similarly, the use of saltwater emetics was abandoned after numerous cases of severe salt poisoning resulted from their administration.[3,12] Mustard powder has never been proved to be effective.[6] The use of copper sulfate as an emetic[26] also fell out of favor because of its caustic properties, its potential to cause acute copper poisoning, and its unreliability.[24,46] Zinc sulfate also is no longer used as an emetic.[6]

Until the 1980s, apomorphine was advocated as an emetic.[8,37] One reason for its use was the thought that it was safer and more effective than copper sulfate.[24] It was supposed to be particularly useful for the combative or uncooperative patient because of its rapid onset of action and parenteral administration, and in this setting, was frequently used instead of syrup of ipecac.[39] Apomorphine's propensity to cause CNS depression, however, increased the risk of subsequent aspiration and made its use potentially very dangerous. Moreover, a sterile injectable form of apomorphine has not been available in the United States for many years. For all of these reasons, enthusiasm for apomorphine gradually waned, leaving syrup of ipecac as the sole available emetic.[33]

THE UNIVERSAL ANTIDOTE

Two other "antidotes" that were once commonly used for decontamination but that have since fallen into disfavor are the "universal antidote" and burnt toast. For many years the universal antidote, sold under the trade names Unidote and Res-Q, was a medical tradition[40] and was advocated by many textbooks as part of the standard management of the poisoned patient.[13,19,32] Commercial preparations consisted of one part magnesium oxide, one part tannic acid, and two parts activated charcoal. An alternative home recipe consisted of milk of magnesia, strong tea, and burnt toast. Combination therapy of this sort was thought to offer a broader spectrum of action than activated charcoal alone. It was theorized that the magnesium oxide would neutralize acids and the tannic acid would precipitate alkaloids and metals.[32] The use of the universal antidote declined by the mid-1980s and is no longer available. Studies demonstrated that activated charcoal was superior to the universal antidote in decreasing absorption[10,40] and that the decreased efficacy of the universal antidote was caused by tannic acid interfering with activated charcoal's adsorbence of other toxins.[10] Furthermore, the potential hepatotoxicity of tannic acid was increasingly recognized.[40] Although burnt toast had been advocated as an activated charcoal substitute in the home,[2] its use was also abandoned because of its lack of significant adsorbent activity.[30]

OTHER ANTIQUATED ANTIDOTES

The use of drugs for the chemical restraint of agitated individuals has also undergone significant evolution during the past decades. Depressant agents, such as tribromoethanol (Avertin) and ether, are no longer used because of the availability of safer alternative agents. Likewise, paraldehyde and ethanol, which were commonly used for the treatment of alcohol withdrawal,[21] have been replaced by the much safer and less toxic benzodiazepines. The use of analeptics to treat the depressive effects of ethanol has also become obsolete.[47]

Another change in treatment involves the abandonment of neutralizing agents for caustic ingestions. Until the 1970s, typical recommendations for the treatment of alkali ingestions included the use of vinegar (acetic acid), lemon juice, or, in some cases, dilute hydrochloric acid.[32] Suggestions for neutralizing acid ingestions included the use of magnesium hydroxide, lime water, or calcium carbonate.[32] Because of the extremely rapid onset of action of caustic agents, concerns arose over whether it was already too late to reverse the caustic process. Furthermore, the addition of neutralizing agents could increase the exothermic reaction and/or gas production.[43] Such reactions in an already weakened hollow viscus may be poorly tolerated and lead to extension of the tissue injury or perforation. For all of these reasons, the use of neutralizing agents is no longer recommended.

Other abandoned antidotes include potassium iodide, which was used to enhance lead excretion, and ferric hydroxide (*antidotum arsenici*), which was used in the treatment of arsenic poisoning. Acetazolamide, which was advocated for alkalinizing the urine in salicylate poisoning,[44] causes a systemic acidemia that can worsen the salicylate toxicity, and is therefore no longer used. The use of sodium phosphate (Phospho-Soda) in the management of iron overdose in an attempt to create insoluble ferrous phosphate has also ceased because of problems with its marginal efficacy and resultant hyperphosphatemia.[17]

Finally, enthusiasm has waned for raw rabbit brain, which had been recommended as recently as the 1930s as a "chance of life" for patients with *Amanita phalloides* poisoning.[31] The raw brain approach was pioneered in the early 1800s after it was observed that rabbits could eat poisonous mushrooms without ill effects.[4] Postulating that rabbits had some sort of protective mechanism that neutralized the mushroom toxin, investigators formulated an antidotal concoction consisting of seven rabbit brains and three rabbit stomachs. The preparation was minced and ground into pellets and administered with a sweetener. When patients who received the rabbit brain antidote survived the mushroom poisoning, it was erroneously concluded that these uncontrolled observations provided proof of efficacy.[4]

Many of our current antidotes have not undergone rigorous scientific evaluation regarding efficacy and safety. In time, some of these antidotes will undoubtedly join this list of antiquated antidotes. Lessons learned from the past, such as the abandonment of analeptics, help to optimize present-day patient care and to better prepare us to investigate and evaluate the next generation of antidotes.

REFERENCES

1. Adams WC: Emetics in accidental poisoning. Pediatr Clin North Am 1961;8:351–352.
2. Arena J: Poisoning: Chemistry, Symptoms, Treatment. Springfield, IL, Charles C. Thomas, 1963.
3. Barer J, Hill L, Hill RM, Martinez WM: Fatal poisoning from salt used as an emetic. Am J Dis Child 1973;125:889–890.
4. Benjamin DR: Mushrooms: Poisons and Panaceas. New York, WH Freeman, 1995.
5. Berger FM: Drugs and suicide in the United States. Clin Pharmacol Therap 1967;8:219–223.
6. Cashman TM, Shirkey HC: Emergency management of poisoning. Pediatr Clin North Am 1970;17:525–534.
7. Clemmesen C, Nilsson E: Therapeutic trends in the treatment of barbiturate poisoning: The Scandinavian method. Clin Pharmacol Ther 1961;2:220–229.
8. Corby DG, Decker WJ, Moran MJ, Payne CE: Clinical comparison of pharmacologic emetics in children. Pediatrics 1968;42:361–364.
9. Dabbous IA, Bergman AB, Robertson WO: The ineffectiveness of mechanically induced vomiting. J Pediatr 1965; 66:952–954.
10. Daly JS, Cooney DO: Interference by tannic acid with the effectiveness of activated charcoal in "universal antidote." Clin Toxicol 1978; 12:515–522.
11. Decker WJ: Antidotes: Some ineffective, insufficiently tested, outmoded, and potentially dangerous therapeutic agents. Vet Hum Toxicol 1983;25:10–15.
12. DeGenaro F, Nyhan WL: Salt: A dangerous "antidote." J Pediatr 1971;78:1048–1049.
13. Deichmann WB, Gerarde HW: Signs, Symptoms and Treatment of Certain Acute Intoxications, 2nd ed. Springfield, IL, Charles C. Thomas, 1958.
14. Eckenhoff JE, Funderburg LW: Observations on the use of the opiate antagonists nalorphine and levallorphan. Am J Med Sci 1954; 228:546–553.
15. Evans LEJ, Roscoe P, Swainson CP, Prescott LF: Treatment of drug overdosage with naloxone, a specific narcotic antagonist. Lancet 1973;1:452–455.
16. Freund JD: Metrazol treatment of barbiturate poisoning. Psychosomatics 1968;9:172–174.
17. Geffner ME, Opas LA: Phosphate poisoning complicating treatment for iron ingestion. Am J Dis Child 1980;134:509–510.
18. Gilman AG, Goodman LS, Gilman A: Goodman and Gilman's The Pharmacological Basis of Therapeutics, 7th ed. New York, Macmillan, 1985.
19. Gleason MN, Gosselin RE, Hodge HC: Clinical Toxicology of Commercial Products: Acute Poisoning (Home & Farm), 2nd ed. Baltimore, Williams & Wilkins, 1963.
20. Goodman LS: The Pharmacological Basis of Therapeutics. New York, Macmillan, 1941.
21. Gower WE, Kersten H: Prevention of alcohol withdrawal symptoms in surgical patients. Surg Gynecol Obstet 1980;151:382–384.
22. Halbach H, Eddy NB: Tests for addiction of morphine type. Bull World Health Organ 1963;28:139–173.
23. Haller JS: The use and abuse of tartar emetic in the 19th century materia medica. Bull Hist Med 1975;49:235–259.
24. Holtzman NA, Haslam RH: Elevation of serum copper following copper sulfate as an emetic. Pediatrics 1968;42:189–193.
25. Jones AW, Dooley J, Murphy JR: Treatment of choice in barbiturate poisoning. JAMA 1950;143:884–888.
26. Karlsson B, Noren L: Ipecacuanha and copper sulfate as emetics in intoxications in children. Acta Pediatr Scand 1965;54:331–335.
27. Klaer-Larsen J: Delirious psychosis and convulsions due to Megimide. Lancet 1956;2:967–970.
28. Koppanyi T, Fazekas JF: Acute barbiturate poisoning: Analysis and evaluation of current therapy. Am J Med Sci 1950;220:559–576.
29. Koppanyi T, Linegar CR, Dille JM: Analysis of the barbiturate-picrotoxin antagonism. J Pharmacol Exper Therap 1936;58:199–228.
30. Lehman AJ: Substitution of burned toast for activated charcoal in the "universal antidote." Assoc Food Drug Official US Q Bull 1957;21:210–211.
31. Leschke E: Clinical Toxicology: Modern Methods in the Diagnosis and Treatment of Poisoning. Baltimore, William Wood, 1934.
32. Lucas GH: The Symptoms and Treatment of Acute Poisoning. Toronto, Canada, Clark Irwin, 1952.
33. MacLean WC: A comparison of ipecac syrup and apomorphine in the immediate treatment of ingestion of poisons. J Pediatr 1973;82:121–124.
34. Maloney AH, Fitch RH, Tatum AL: Picrotoxin as an antidote in acute poisoning by shorter-acting barbiturates. J Pharmacol Exp Ther 1931;41:465–482.
35. Maloney AH: A comparative study of the antidotal action of picrotoxin, strychnine and cocaine in acute intoxication by the barbiturates. J Pharmacol Exp Ther 1933;49:133–140.
36. Mark LC: Analeptics: Changing concepts, declining status. Am J Med Sci 1967;254:296–302.
37. Meester WD: Emesis and lavage. Vet Hum Toxicol 1980; 22:225–234.
38. Nilsson E, Eyrich B: On treatment of barbiturate poisoning. Acta Med Scand 1950;137:381–389.
39. Nilsson E: On treatment of barbiturate poisoning: Modified clinical aspects. Acta Med Scand 1951;139(Suppl 253):1–127.
40. Picchioni AL, Chin L, Verhulst HL, Dieterle B: Activated charcoal vs. "universal antidote" as an antidote for poisons. Toxicol Appl Pharmacol 1966; 8:447–454.
41. Reed CE, Driggs MF, Foote CC: Acute barbiturate intoxication: Study of 300 cases based on physiologic system of classification of severity of intoxication. Ann Intern Med 1952;37:290–303.
42. Robie TR: Treatment of acute barbiturate poisoning by nonconvulsive electrostimulation. Postgrad Med J 1951;253–256.
43. Rumack BH, Burrington JD: Caustic ingestions: A rational look at diluents. Clin Toxicol 1977;11:27–34.
44. Schwartz R, Fellers F, Knapp J, Yaffe S: The renal response to administration of acetazolamide (Diamox) during salicylate intoxication. Pediatrics 1959;23:1103–1114.

45. Shulman A, Shaw FH, Cass NM, Whyte HM: A new treatment of bar-
    biturate intoxication. Br Med J 1955;1:1238–1244.

46. Stein RS, Jenkins D, Korns ME: Death after use of cupric sulfate an
    emetic. JAMA 1976;235:801.

47. Taberner PV: Pharmacological treatment for alcohol dependence and
    withdrawal—An historical perspective. Alcohol 1993;S2:259–262.

48. Wang SC, Ward JW: Analeptics. Pharmacol Therapy 1977;3:
    123–165.

49. Wax PM: Analeptic use in clinical toxicology. A historical appraisal.
    J Toxicol Clin Toxicol 1997;35:203–209.

CHAPTER 2

TOXICOLOGIC PLAGUES AND DISASTERS IN HISTORY

Paul M. Wax

Throughout history mass poisonings have caused suffering and misfortune. From the ergot epidemics of the Middle Ages to contemporary industrial disasters, these plagues have had great political, economic, social, and environmental ramifications. Particularly within the last 100 years, as the number of toxins and potential toxins has risen dramatically, toxic disasters have become an increasingly common event. The sites of some of these events—Bhopal (India), Chernobyl (Ukraine), Jonestown (Guyana), Love Canal (New York), Minamata Bay (Japan), West Bengal (India)—have come to symbolize our increasingly toxic habitat. This chapter provides an overview of some of the most consequential and historically important toxin-mediated disasters.

GAS DISASTERS

Inhalation of toxic gases and oral ingestions resulting in food poisoning tend to subject the greatest number of people to adverse consequences of a toxic exposure. Toxic gas exposures may be the result of a natural disaster (volcanic eruption), unintentional mishap (industrial fire), chemical warfare, or intentional homicidal or genocidal endeavor (concentration camp gas chamber). Depending on the toxin, the clinical presentation may be acute, with a rapid onset of toxicity (cyanide gas), or subacute/chronic, with a gradual onset of toxicity (air pollution). Chemical toxins used in warfare include both gases (phosgene, chlorine) and liquids (mustard, organic phosphorus agents).

One of the earliest recorded toxic gas disasters resulted from the eruption of Mount Vesuvius near Pompeii, Italy, in A.D. 79 (Table 2–1). Poisonous gases generated from the volcanic activity reportedly killed thousands.[24] A much more recent natural disaster occurred in 1986 in Cameroon, when excessive amounts of carbon dioxide were mysteriously vented from Lake Nyos, the volcanic crater lake.[6] Seventeen hundred fatalities reportedly resulted from exposure to this asphyxiant.

A toxic gas leak at the Union Carbide pesticide plant in Bhopal, India, in 1984, resulted in one of the greatest civilian toxic disasters in modern history.[129] An unintended exothermic reaction at this carbaryl-producing plant caused the release of over 24,000 kg of methyl isocyanate. This gas was quickly dispersed through the air over the densely populated area surrounding the factory, resulting in at least 2500 deaths and 200,000 injuries.[78] The initial response to this disaster was greatly limited by a lack of pertinent information about the toxicity of this agent. A followup study 10 years later showed persistence of small-airway obstruction among survivors.[19] Calls for improvement in disaster preparedness and strengthened right-to-know laws regarding potential toxic exposures resulted from this tragedy.[24,129]

The release into the atmosphere of 26 tons of hydrofluoric acid at a petrochemical plant in Texas, in October 1987, resulted in 939 people seeking medical attention at nearby hospitals. Ninety-four people were hospitalized, but there were no deaths.[136]

More than any other single toxin, carbon monoxide has been involved with the largest number of toxic disasters. Catastrophic fires, such as the Cocoanut Grove Nightclub Fire in 1943, have caused hundreds of deaths at a time, many of them from carbon monoxide poisoning.[28] The 1990 fire at the Happy Land Social Club in the Bronx, New York, claimed 87 victims, including a large number of nonburn deaths.[71] Carbon monoxide poisoning was a major culprit in many of these deaths, although hydrogen cyanide gas and simple asphyxiation may also have contributed to the overall mortality. Another notable toxic gas disaster involving a fire occurred at the Cleveland Clinic in 1929, where a fire in the radiology department resulted in 125 deaths.[23] The burning of nitrocellulose radiographs produced nitrogen dioxide, cyanide, and carbon monoxide gases that were thought to be responsible for many of the fatalities.

Air pollution is another source of toxic gases causing significant disease and death. Known to Shakespeare, whose witches in Macbeth chant "fair is foul, and foul is fair: hover through the fog and filthy air," complaints about smoky air date back to at least 1272, when King Edward I banned the burning of sea-coal.[126] By the 19th century—the era of rapid industrialization in England—winter "fogs" became increasingly problematic. An 1873 London fog was responsible for 268 deaths from bronchitis. Excessive smog in the Meuse Valley of Belgium in 1930, and in Donora, Pennsylvania, in 1948, was also blamed for excess morbidity and mortality. Another dense sulfur dioxide–laden smog in London in 1952 was responsible for 4000 deaths.[69] Both the initiation of long overdue air-pollution reform in England and Parliament's passing of the 1956 Clean Air Act resulted from this later "fog."

CHEMICAL WARFARE

Exposure to toxic chemicals with the deliberate intent to inflict harm has claimed an extraordinary number of victims during the 20th century (Table 2–2). During World War I, chlorine and phosgene gases and the liquid vesicant mustard were used as battlefield weapons, with mustard causing about 80% of the chemical casualties.[113] Reportedly, 100,000 deaths and 1.2 million casualties were attributed to these chemical attacks during WWI.[24] These toxic exposures resulted in severe airway irritation, pulmonary edema, hemorrhagic pneumonitis, skin blistering, and ocular damage. Chemical weapons were used again in the 1980s during the Iran-Iraq war.

TABLE 2–1.   Gas Disasters

Toxin	Location	Date	Significance
Poisonous gas	Pompeii	A.D. 79	>2000 died from eruption of Mt. Vesuvius
Smog (SO_2)	London	1873	268 deaths from bronchitis
NO_2, CO, CN	Cleveland Clinic, Cleveland, OH	1929	Fire in radiology department, 125 deaths
Smog (SO_2)	Belgium, Meuse Valley	1930	64 deaths
CO, CN	Cocoanut Grove Night Club, Boston	1942	498 deaths from fire
CO	Salerno, Italy	1944	>500 deaths on train stalled in tunnel
Smog (SO_2)	Donora, PA	1948	20 deaths, thousands ill
Smog (SO_2)	London	1952	4000 deaths attributed to the fog/smog
Methyl isocyanate	Bhopal, India	1984	>2000 deaths; 200,000 injuries
Carbon dioxide	Cameroon	1986	>1700 deaths from release of gas from Lake Nyos
Hydrofluoric acid	Texas	1987	Atmospheric release, 94 hospitalized
CO, ? CN	Happy Land Social Club, Bronx, NY	1990	87 died in fire from toxic smoke

The Nazis utilized poisonous gases during World War II to commit mass murder and genocide. Initially, the Nazis employed carbon monoxide to kill. To expedite the killing process, Nazi scientists developed Zyklon B gas (hydrogen cyanide gas). As many as 10,000 people per day were killed by the rapidly acting cyanide, and millions of deaths were attributed to the use of these gases.

During recent wars, a variety of physical and neuropsychologic ailments were attributed to possible exposure to toxic agents.[47] Agent Orange was widely used as a defoliant during the Vietnam War. This herbicide consists of a mixture of 2,4,5-trichlorophenoxyacetic acid (2,4,5-T) and 2,4-dichlorophenoxyacetic acid (2,4-D), as well as small amounts of a contaminant, 2,3,7,8-tetrachlorodibenzo-*p*-dioxin (TCDD), better known as dioxin. Although a higher incidence of skin cancers has been found in veterans who handled Agent Orange, other possible dioxin-related adverse health effects, such as nonskin cancer, birth defects, and hepatic dysfunction, have not been observed.[22] An increase in non-Hodgkin lymphoma among Vietnam veterans has occurred, but this is not clearly attributable to herbicide exposure.[108]

Gulf War syndrome is a constellation of chronic symptoms, including fatigue, headache, muscle and joint pains, ataxia, paresthesias, diarrhea, skin rashes, sleep disturbances, impaired concentration, memory loss, and irritability, noted in thousands of Persian Gulf War veterans without a clearly identifiable cause. A number of etiologies have been advanced to explain these varied symptoms, including exposure to the smoke from burning oil wells; chemical and biologic warfare agents, including nerve agents; and

medical prophylaxis, such as the use of pyridostigmine bromide, anthrax, and botulinum toxin vaccines.[48] Other possible etiologies include pesticides such as DEET, infectious agents such as leishmaniasis, inhalation of sand contaminated with fungus, insect vectors, depleted uranium munitions, and posttraumatic stress disorder. Although organic phosphorous–induced delayed polyneuropathy may explain some of these clinical findings,[39] at present, the true etiology of this illness remains unknown.[30,47,49,62,125] "Emerging overlap syndromes," such as multiple chemical sensitivity, chronic fatigue syndrome, and fibromyalgia, may also play a role in Gulf War Syndrome, making this diagnosis particularly perplexing.[42,55]

Mass exposure to the very potent organic phosphorus compound sarin occurred in March 1995, when terrorists released this chemical warfare agent in three separate subway lines in Tokyo.[94] Eleven people were killed, and 5510 people sought emergency medical evaluation at more than 200 hospitals and clinics in the area.[114] Sarin exposure also resulted in several deaths and hundreds of casualties in Matsumoto, Japan, in June 1994.[83,91]

FOOD DISASTERS

Unintentional contamination of food and drink has led to numerous toxic disasters (Table 2–3). Ergot, produced by the fungus *Claviceps purpurea*, has caused a large number of deadly epidemics.[80] Epidemic ergotism occurred as the result of eating

TABLE 2–2.   Chemical Warfare Disasters

Toxin	Location	Date	Significance
Chlorine, phosgene, mustard gas	Ypres, Belgium	1915–1918	100,000 dead and 1.2 million casualties from chemicals during WWI
CN, CO	Europe	1939–1945	Millions murdered by Zyklon-B (HCN) gas
Agent Orange (2-4D, 2-4-5-T, TCDD)	Vietnam	1960s	Contains dioxin; excess skin cancer
Mustard gas	Iraq-Iran	1982	New cycle of war gas casualties
Toxic smoke?	Persian Gulf	1991	Gulf War syndrome—possible toxic etiology
Sarin	Matsumoto, Japan	1994	First of terrorist attacks in Japan using sarin
Sarin	Tokyo	1995	Subway exposure; 5510 people seek medical attention

TABLE 2–3. Food Disasters

Toxin	Location	Date	Significance
Ergot	Aquitania, France	A.D. 994	40,000 died in the epidemic
Ergot	Salem, Massachusetts	1692	Bizarre behavior may be attributable to ergot
Lead	Devonshire, England	1700s	Colic from production of cider
Arsenious acid	France	1828	40,000 cases of polyneuropathy from contaminated wine and bread
Lead	Canada	1846	134 men died during Franklin expedition, possibly due to contamination of food stored in lead cans
Cadmium	Japan	1939–1954	Itai-itai ("ouch-ouch") disease
Hexachlorobenzene	Turkey	1956	4000 cases of porphyria cutanea tarda
Methyl mercury	Minamata Bay, Japan	1950s	Organic mercury poisoning from fish
Triorthocresylphosphate	Meknes, Morocco	1959	Cooking oil adulterated with turbojet lubricant
Methylenedianiline	Epping, England	1965	Epping jaundice
Polychlorinated biphenyls	Japan	1968	Yusho ("rice oil disease")
Methyl mercury	Iraq	1971	>400 deaths from contaminated grain
Polybrominated biphenyls	Michigan	1973	97% of state contaminated through food chain
Polychlorinated biphenyls	Taiwan	1979	Yu-Cheng ("oil disease")
Rape seed oil (denatured)	Spain	1981	Toxic oil syndrome affected 19,000 people
Arsenic	Buenos Aires	1987	Malicious contamination of meat; 61 people underwent chelation
Polychlorinated biphenyls	Belgium	1999	Contamination of meat, dairy products; no reports of illness
Arsenic	Bangladesh and W. Bengal, India	1990s to present	Ground water contaminated with arsenic; millions exposed; 100,000s with symptoms; greatest mass poisoning in history

breads and cereals made from rye that had been contaminated by *C. purpurea*. In some epidemics, convulsive manifestations predominated, and in others, gangrenous manifestations predominated. Ergot-induced severe vasospasm was thought responsible for both types of presentations.[79] In A.D. 994, 40,000 people died in Aquitania, France, in such an epidemic.[67] Convulsive ergotism was initially described as a "fire which twisted the people," and the term "St. Anthony's fire" (*ignis sacer*) was used to refer to the excruciating burning pain experienced in the extremities that is an early manifestation of gangrenous ergotism. The events surrounding the Salem witchcraft trials have also been attributed to the ingestion of contaminated rye. The bizarre and psychotic behaviors exhibited by some of the individuals associated with this event may have been caused by the hallucinogenic properties of ergotamine, an LSD precursor.[12,76]

During the 20th century, unintentional mass poisoning from food and drink contaminated with toxic chemicals has become all too common. One of the more unusual poisonings occurred in 1956, in Turkey, when wheat seed treated with the fungicide hexachlorobenzene and intended for planting was inadvertently used for human consumption. Four thousand cases of porphyria cutanea tarda were attributed to the ingestion of this wheat seed.[106]

Another example of chemical food poisoning took place in Epping, England, in 1965. In this incident, a sack of flour became contaminated with methylenedianiline when the chemical unintentionally spilled onto the flour during transport to a bakery. Subsequent ingestion of bread baked with the contaminated flour produced hepatitis in 84 people. This outbreak of toxic hepatitis became known as Epping jaundice.[58]

The manufacture of polybromated biphenyls (PBBs) in a factory that also produced food supplements for livestock resulted in the unintentional contamination of a large amount of livestock feed in Michigan in 1973.[13] Significant morbidity and mortality among the livestock population resulted. Increased human tissue levels of PBBs were reported,[137] although human toxicity seemed limited to vague constitutional symptoms and abnormal liver function tests.[2]

The chemical contamination of a particular lot of rice oil in Japan in 1968 caused an illness called Yusho ("rice oil disease"). This occurred when heat-exchange fluid containing polychlorinated biphenyls (PCBs) and polychlorinated dibenzofurans (PCDFs) leaked from a heating pipe into the rice oil. More than 1600 people developed this new illness. Manifestations included chloracne, hyperpigmentation, increased incidence of liver cancer, and adverse reproductive effects. A similar illness after exposure to another batch of PCB-contaminated rice oil affected 2000 people in Taiwan in 1979. This latter epidemic was referred to as Yu-Cheng ("oil disease").[51] In 1999, toxic amounts of PCBs and dioxin were found in Belgian meat (particularly poultry), eggs, and other dairy products, as a result of the consumption of animal feed deliberately contaminated with motor oils.[9] The PCB/dioxin burden was considerably less than that found in the Yushu incident and no human illnesses linked to the contaminated feed were reported.

In another oil contamination epidemic, consumption of an illegally marketed cooking oil in Spain, in 1981, was responsible for a mysterious poisoning epidemic that affected more than 19,000 people and resulted in at least 340 deaths. Exposed patients developed a multisystem disorder referred to as toxic oil syndrome (or toxic epidemic syndrome), which was characterized by pneumonitis, eosinophilia, pulmonary hypertension, scleroderma-like features, and neuromuscular changes. Although this syndrome was associated with the consumption of rapeseed oil denatured with 2% aniline, the exact etiologic agent was never definitively identified.[54,123]

In 1999, an outbreak of Coca-Cola–related health complaints occurred in Belgium, when about 100 people, mostly children, complained of gastrointestinal symptoms, malaise, headaches, and palpitations, after consuming Coca-Cola. Many of those affected complained of an off taste or bad odor to the soft drink. Millions of cans and bottles were removed from the market at a cost of $900 million. Although a toxicologic cause was never identified in the drink, a hydrocarbon was found on the outside of the containers and it remains unclear whether the complaints should be solely attributable to mass sociogenic illness.[92,127]

Epidemics of heavy metal poisoning from contaminated food and drink have also occurred throughout history. Epidemic lead poisoning has been associated with many different vehicles of transmission, including leaden bowls, kettles, and pipes. A famous 18th-century epidemic was known as the Devonshire colic. Although the exact etiology of this disorder was unknown for many years, later evidence suggested that the ingestion of lead-contaminated cider was responsible.[130]

A more recent incident involving multiple cases of heavy-metal poisoning occurred in Buenos Aires in 1987, when vandals broke into a butcher's shop and poured an unknown amount of acaricide (45% sodium arsenite solution) over 200 kg of partly minced meat.[102] The contaminated meat was purchased by 718 people. Of 307 meat purchasers who submitted to urine sampling, 49 had urine arsenic levels of 76–500 μg/dL, and 12 had urine arsenic levels above 500 μg/dL.

At the end of the 20th century and into the 21st century, what some observers call the greatest mass poisoning in history is occurring in Bangladesh and the West Bengal State of India.[21,85,118] In Bangladesh alone, 60 million people are regularly drinking arsenic-contaminated ground water. At least 220,000 inhabitants of India's West Bengal have been diagnosed with symptoms of arsenic poisoning.[84] Reported symptoms include melanosis, depigmentation, hyperkeratosis, hepatomegaly, splenomegaly, squamous cell carcinoma, intraepidermal carcinoma, and gangrene.[21] In a country that was long plagued with dysentery, attempts to clean up the water supply led to the drilling of millions of wells into the superficial water table. Unbeknownst to the engineers, this water was naturally contaminated with arsenic leaving several thousand tube wells with extremely high concentrations of arsenic—up to 40 times the acceptable concentration. Although toxicity from arsenic-contaminated groundwater was previously reported from other areas of the world, including Argentina, China, Mexico, Taiwan (Black Foot's Disease), and Thailand, the number of people at risk in Bangladesh and West Bengal is by far the largest.

Methyl mercury, an organic mercurial, has been the etiologic agent for several recent poisoning epidemics. During the 1950s, a Japanese chemical factory that manufactured vinyl chloride and acetaldehyde routinely discharged mercury into Minamata Bay, resulting in contamination of the aquatic food chain. An epidemic of methyl mercury poisoning followed after the local people ate the poisoned fish.[100,124] Chronic brain damage, tunnel vision, deafness, and severe congenital defects were associated with this outbreak.[100] Another mass epidemic of methyl mercury poisoning occurred in Iraq in 1971, when the local population consumed homemade bread prepared from wheat seed treated with a methyl mercury fungicide.[4] Six thousand hospital admissions and more than 400 hospital deaths were associated with this disaster. As with the hexachlorobenzene exposure in Turkey 25 years previously, the treated grain, intended for use as seed, was instead used as food.

Contamination of the local water supply with the wastewater runoff from a zinc-lead-cadmium mine in Japan, from 1939 to 1954, was believed responsible for causing itai-itai ("ouch-ouch") disease, an unusual chronic syndrome manifested by extreme bone pain and osteomalacia. The local water was used for drinking and irrigation of the rice fields. Approximately 200 people who lived along the banks of the Jintsu River developed these peculiar symptoms, which were thought most likely to be due to the cadmium.[10]

THERAPEUTIC DRUG DISASTERS

Illness and death as a consequence of therapeutic drug use occur as sporadic events, usually affecting individual patients, or as mass disasters, affecting multiple (sometimes hundreds or thousands) patients. Sporadic single-patient medication-induced tragedies usually result from errors (Chap. 1) or unforeseen idiosyncratic reactions. Mass therapeutic drug disasters have generally occurred secondary to poor safety testing, a lack of understanding of diluents and excipients, drug contamination, or problems with unanticipated drug-drug interactions or drug toxicity (Table 2–4).

In September and October 1937, more than 100 deaths were associated with the use of one of the early sulfa preparations—elixir of sulfanilamide-Massengill—that contained 72% diethylene glycol as the vehicle for drug delivery. Little was known about diethylene glycol toxicity at the time, and many cases of renal failure and death occurred.[33] As a result of this catastrophe, animal drug testing was mandated by the Food, Drug, and Cosmetic Act of 1938 to avoid similar tragedies in the future.[131] Unfortunately, diethylene glycol continued to be sporadically used in other countries as a medicinal diluent, resulting in additional deaths in South Africa (1969), India (1986), Nigeria (1990), Bangladesh (1990–1992), and Haiti (1995–1996).[132] In the most recent disaster in Haiti at least 88 children died (case fatality rate 98% for those who remained in Haiti) after ingesting an acetaminophen elixir formulated with diethylene glycol–contaminated glycerin.[93,105]

A lesser-known drug manufacturing disaster, also involving an early sulfa antimicrobial, occurred in 1940–1941, when at least 82 people died from the therapeutic use of sulfathiazole that had been contaminated with phenobarbital (Luminal).[119] The responsible pharmaceutical company, Winthrop Chemical, produced both sulfathiazole and phenobarbital, and the contamination likely occurred during the tabletting process, because the tabletting machines for the two medications were adjacent to each other and were used interchangeably. Each contaminated sulfathiazole tablet contained about 350 mg of phenobarbital (and no sulfathiazole), and the typical sulfathiazole dosing regimen was several tablets within the first few hours of therapy. Twenty-nine percent of the production lot was contaminated. FDA intervention was required to assist with the recovery of the suspect sulfathiazole, although 22,000 contaminated tablets were never found.[119]

In the early 1960s, one of the greatest modern-day drug catastrophes occurred with the release of thalidomide as an antiemetic and sedative-hypnotic.[20] Its use as a sedative-hypnotic by pregnant women resulted in about 5000 babies born with severe congenital anomalies.[80] This tragedy was largely confined to Europe, Australia, and Canada, where the drug was initially marketed. Only the length of time required for review and the rigorous scrutiny of new drug applications by the FDA in the United States prevented a concurrent disaster here.[77]

Another major therapeutic drug misadventure that did occur in the United States involved the widespread use of diethylstilbestrol (DES) for the treatment of threatened and habitual abortions. Despite the lack of convincing efficacy data, as many as 10 million Americans received DES during pregnancy, or in utero, during a 30-year period, until use of the drug in pregnancy was prohibited in 1971. Adverse health effects associated with DES use include increased risk for breast cancer in "DES mothers" and increased risk of a rare form of vaginal cancer, reproductive tract anomalies, and premature births in "DES daughters."[35,41]

TABLE 2–4. Therapeutic Drug Disasters

Toxin	Location	Date	Significance
Thallium	US	1920s–1930s	Used for ringworm; 31 deaths
Tubercle bacilli	Germany	1930	Tubercle bacilli given to neonates instead of BCG; 72 deaths
Diethylene glycol	US	1937	Elixir of sulfanilamide; renal failure
Thorotrast	US	1930s–1950s	Hepatic angiosarcoma
Phenobarbital	US	1940–1941	Sulfathiazole contaminated with phenobarbital; 82 deaths
Hepatitis virus	US	1942	Yellow fever vaccine contamination; 28,000 military develop hepatitis
Diethylstilbestrol	US, Europe	1940s–1950s	Vaginal adenocarcinoma in daughters
Stalinon	France	1954	Severe neurotoxicity from triethyltin
Clioquinol	Japan	1955–1970	Subacute myelooptico neuropathy (SMON); 10,000 symptomatic
Thalidomide	Europe	1960	5000 cases of phocomelia (limb deformaties)
Pentachlorophenol	US	1967	Used in hospital laundry; 9 neonates ill, 2 deaths
HIV	US	1970s–1980s	Cryoprecipitate contaminated with HIV; 90% hemophilia A population seroconverted
Benzyl alcohol	US	1981	Gasping syndrome
Acetaminophen-cyanide	Chicago	1982	Tampering incident resulted in 7 homicides
Tryptophan	US	1989	Eosinophilia-myalgia syndrome
Diethylene glycol	Haiti	1996	Acetaminophen elixir contaminated; renal failure; >88 pediatric deaths
Fenfluramine/dexfenfluramine	US	1997	Fen-phen diet regimen associated with valvular heart disease
Phenylpropanolamine (PPA)	US	2000	OTC cold remedy removed from market due to association with hemorrhagic stroke

Drug disasters that have affected the greatest number of individuals have often occurred from infectious contamination of vaccines or other drug treatments. After the American entrance into World War II, 3 million troops received yellow fever immunization. It was the practice at the time to add human serum to the vaccine to preserve the attenuated yellow fever virus. In the spring of 1942, 28,000 cases of hepatitis and 62 deaths resulted from the yellow fever vaccination. Subsequent investigation traced this outbreak to viral hepatitis contamination of 9 of the 177 lots of vaccine administered.[104]

Another vaccine-related disaster occurred in 1930, when 207 of 251 newborn babies in Lubeck, Germany, who were given oral bacillus Calmette-Guérin (BCG) vaccination to prevent tuberculosis, ended up developing clinical tuberculosis; 72 newborns died. This tragedy occurred because a preparation containing nonattenuated human tubercle bacilli had been carelessly substituted for the nonvirulent BCG vaccine.[61]

A more recent infectious disaster attributed to medication has been the calamitous development of HIV infection in hemophiliacs who had received concentrated cryoprecipitate preparations. Approximately 90% of patients with hemophilia A seroconverted after receiving factor replacement treatments in the late 1970s and early 1980s. By the time HIV was first identified as the causative agent of AIDS, and routine screening for HIV on blood products was implemented, a profound impact on the hemophiliac community had already occurred.

Thorotrast (thorium dioxide 25%) is an intravenous radiologic contrast medium that was widely used between 1928 and 1955. Its use was associated with the delayed development of hepatic angiosarcomas, as well as skeletal sarcomas, leukemia, and "thorotrastomas"—malignancies at the site of extravasated thorotrast.[117,133]

The use of thallium to treat innocuous ringworm infections in the 1920s and 1930s also led to needless morbidity and mortality.[36] Understanding that thallium caused alopecia, dermatologists and other physicians prescribed thallium acetate, both as pills and as a topical ointment (Koremlu), to remove the infected hair. A 1934 study found 692 cases of thallium toxicity after oral and topical application and 31 deaths after oral use.[87] Medicinal thallium was subsequently taken off the market.

The "Stalinon affair" in France, in 1954, was another major toxicologic disaster that involved the unintentional contamination of a therapeutic agent. Stalinon was a proprietary oral medication that was marketed for the treatment of staphylococcal skin infections, osteomyelitis, and anthrax. Although it was supposed to contain diethyltin diiodide and linoleic acid, triethyltin, a potent neurotoxin and the most toxic of organotin compounds, and trimethyltin were present as impurities. Of the approximately 1000 people who received this medication, 217 patients developed symptoms, and 102 patients died.[5,116]

An unusual syndrome, featuring a constellation of abdominal symptoms (pain and diarrhea), followed by neurologic symptoms (peripheral neuropathy and visual disturbances including blindness), was experienced by approximately 10,000 Japanese between 1955 and 1970, resulting in several hundred deaths.[61] This presentation, subsequently labeled subacute myelo-opticoneuropathy (SMON), was associated with the use of the gastrointestinal disinfectant clioquinol, known in the West as Entero-Vioform and most often used for the prevention of travelers' diarrhea.[90] In Japan, this drug was referred to as "sei-cho-zai" ("active in normalizing intestinal function"). It was incorporated into more than 100 nonprescription proprietary medications and was used by millions of people, often for weeks or months. The exact mechanism of toxicity has not been determined, but recent investigators theorize that clioquinol may enhance the cellular uptake of certain heavy metals, particularly zinc, and that the clioquinol-zinc chelate may act as a mitochondrial toxin causing this syndrome.[3] New cases declined rapidly when clioquinol was banned in Japan.

In 1981, a number of premature neonates died with a "gasping syndrome," manifested by severe metabolic acidosis, respiratory depression with gasping, and encephalopathy.[34] Prior to the development of these findings, they had all received multiple injections of heparinized bacteriostatic sodium chloride solution (to flush their indwelling catheters) and bacteriostatic water (to mix medications), both of which contained 0.9% benzyl alcohol. Accumulation of large amounts of benzyl alcohol and its metabolite benzoic acid in the blood was thought responsible for this syndrome.[34]

A previous nursery mass poisoning occurred in 1967, when nine neonates developed extreme diaphoresis, fever, and tachypnea, without rash or cyanosis. Two fatalities resulted, although the others responded dramatically to exchange transfusion. The illness was traced to sodium pentachlorophenate that had been used as an antimildew agent in the hospital laundry.[97]

In 1989 and 1990, eosinophilia-myalgia syndrome, a debilitating syndrome somewhat similar to toxic oil syndrome, developed in more than 1500 people who had taken the dietary supplement L-tryptophan.[53,128] These patients presented with disabling myalgias and eosinophilia, often accompanied by extremity edema, dyspnea, and arthralgias. Skin changes, neuropathy, and weight loss sometimes developed. Intensive investigation revealed that all affected patients had ingested tryptophan produced by a single manufacturer, who had recently introduced a new process involving genetically altered bacteria to improve tryptophan production. A contaminant produced by this process probably is responsible for this syndrome.[7] The banning of L-tryptophan by the FDA set in motion the passage of the Dietary Supplement Health and Educa-

tion Act of 1994 that facilitated industry marketing of dietary supplements bypassing FDA scrutiny.

During the 1990s a growing number of therapeutic drugs, previously approved by the FDA, were withdrawn from the market because of concern about health risks. In a number of cases, the drugs that were withdrawn had been responsible for causing serious drug-drug interactions (astemizole, cisapride, mibefradil, terfenadine).[86] Other drugs were withdrawn because of a propensity to cause hepatotoxicity (troglitazone), anaphylaxis (bromfenac sodium), valvular heart disease (fenfluramine, dexfenfluramine), and hemorrhagic stroke (phenylpropanolamine). One of the most disconcerting drug problems to arise was the development of cardiac valvulopathy and pulmonary hypertension in patients taking the weight loss drug combination fenfluramine and phentermine (fen-phen) or dexfenfluramine.[17,112] The histopathologic features observed with this condition were similar to the valvular lesions associated with ergotamine and carcinoid. Interestingly, appetite suppressant medications, as well as ergotamine and carcinoid all increase available serotonin.

While many of these withdrawals involved drugs that had only recently been approved, the withdrawal of phenylpropanolamine in 2000 removed an omnipresent over-the-counter agent that for several decades had continually been consumed as a component of many cough and cold remedies. Despite the accumulation over the years of increasing numbers of case reports and case series of medical problems associated with phenylpropanolamine use, drug production was only halted after a well-designed case-control study demonstrated that phenylpropanolamine use was an independent risk factor for hemorrhagic stroke.[52]

ALCOHOL AND ILLICIT DRUG DISASTERS

Unintended toxic disasters have also resulted from the use of alcohol and other drugs of abuse (Table 2–5). Arsenical neuropathy developed in an estimated 40,000 people in France in 1828, when wine and bread were unintentionally contaminated by arsenious acid.[75] The use of arsenic-contaminated sugar in the production of beer in England in 1900 resulted in at least 6000 cases of peripheral neuropathy and 70 deaths (Staffordshire beer epidemic).[31]

TABLE 2–5. Alcohol and Illicit Drug Disasters

Toxin	Location	Date	Significance
Arsenic	Staffordshire, England	1900	Arsenic-contaminated sugar used in beer production
Triorthocresyl-phosphate	US	1930–1931	Jamaica ginger paralysis
Methanol	Atlanta, GA	1951	Epidemic from ingesting bootleg whiskey
Cobalt	Quebec City, Canada	1960s	Cobalt beer cardiomyopathy
Methanol	Jackson, MI	1979	Occurred in a prison
MPTP	San Jose, CA	1982	Drug-induced parkinsonism
3-Methyl fentanyl	Pittsburgh, PA	1988	"China-white" epidemic
Methanol	Baroda, India	1989	Moonshine contamination; 100 deaths
Fentanyl	New York, NY	1990	"Tango and Cash" epidemic
Methanol	New Delhi, India	1991	Antidiarrheal medication contaminated with methanol; >200 deaths
Methanol	Cuttack, India	1992	Methanol-tainted liquor; 162 deaths
Scopolamine	US East Coast	1995–1996	325 cases of anticholinergic poisoning in heroin users
Methanol	Cambodia	1998	>60 deaths

Another toxin-induced disorder, also associated with beer drinking, involved the addition of cobalt, as a foam stabilizer, to several brands of beer in the 1960s. Certain local breweries in Quebec City, Canada, Minneapolis, Minnesota, Omaha, Nebraska, and Louvain, Belgium, added 0.5–5.5 ppm cobalt to their beer. This resulted in epidemics of fulminant heart failure among heavy beer drinkers in these locales (cobalt-beer cardiomyopathy).[1,82]

During the early 20th century, and particularly during prohibition, the ethanolic extract of Jamaican ginger (sold as "the Jake") was a popular ethanol substitute in the southern and midwestern United States.[81] It was sold legally because it was considered a medical supplement to treat headaches and aid digestion and was not subject to prohibition. For years, the Jake was sold adulterated with castor oil, but in 1930, as the price of castor oil rose, the Jake was reformulated with an alternative adulterant, triorthocresyl-phosphate (TOCP). Little was previously known about the toxicity of this compound, but TOCP proved to be a potent neurotoxin. At least 50,000 people who drank the Jake developed TOCP poisoning from 1930 to 1931, which was manifested by upper and lower extremity weakness ("ginger Jake paralysis") and gait impairment ("Jake walk" or "Jake leg").[81] Thirty years later, in Morocco, the dilution of cooking oil with a turbojet lubricant containing TOCP caused an additional 10,000 cases of TOCP-induced paralysis.[115]

Epidemic methanol poisoning among those seeking ethanol and other inebriants has also been well described. In one such incident in Atlanta, in 1951, the ingestion of methanol-contaminated bootleg whiskey caused 323 cases of methanol poisoning, resulting in 41 deaths.[8] In another epidemic in 1979, 46 prisoners became ill after ingesting a methanol-containing diluent used in photocopy machines.[120]

In recent years, major mass methanol poisonings have continued to occur in third-world countries where store-bought alcohol is often prohibitively expensive. In the eastern Indian city of Baroda, in 1989, at least 100 people died and another 200 became ill after drinking a homemade liquor that was contaminated with methanol.[27] In New Delhi, India, in 1991, an inexpensive antidiarrheal medicine, advertised as containing large amounts of ethanol, was contaminated with methanol, and caused more than 200 deaths.[16] The following year, in Cuttack, India, 162 people died and an additional 448 were hospitalized after drinking methanol-tainted liquor.[121] More recently, a major epidemic of methanol poisoning occurred in Cambodia, in 1998, when rice wine was contaminated with methanol.[11] At least 60 deaths and 400 cases of illness were attributed to the methanol. Fomepizole was exported to Cambodia on an emergent basis to treat some of the victims.

So-called "designer drugs" are responsible for several toxicologic disasters. In 1982, several intravenous drug abusers living in San Jose, California, who had been using meperidine analog MPPP (1-methyl-4-phenyl-4-propionoxy-piperidine), developed a peculiar irreversible neurologic disease closely resembling parkinsonism.[64] Investigation revealed that these patients had unknowingly injected trace amounts of MPTP (1-methyl-4-phenyl-1,2,3,6-tetrahydropyridine), present as an inadvertent product of the clandestine MPPP synthesis. The subsequent metabolism of MPTP to MPP$^+$ resulted in a toxic moiety that selectively destroyed cells in the substantia nigra, causing severe irreversible parkinsonism. A result of the vigorous pursuit of the cause of this disaster was a better understanding of the pathophysiology of parkinsonism and the development of possible future treatment modalities.

Another example of a "designer-drug" mass poisoning occurred in the New York metropolitan area in 1991, when a sudden epidemic of opioid overdoses occurred among heroin abusers who bought envelopes labeled "Tango and Cash."[29] Expecting to receive a new brand of heroin, the drug abusers instead purchased the much more potent fentanyl. Increased toxicity from fentanyl resulted from the inability of the dealer to adjust ("cut") the dose properly. Some purchasers presumably received little or no fentanyl, while others received potentially lethal doses. A similar epidemic involving 3-methylfentanyl occurred in Pittsburgh in 1988.[73]

At least 325 cases of anticholinergic poisoning occurred among heroin users in New York City, Newark, Philadelphia, and Baltimore from 1995 to 1996.[107] The "street drug" used in these cases was contaminated with scopolamine. Whereas naloxone treatment was associated with increased agitation and hallucinations, physostigmine administration resulted in resolution of symptoms. Why the heroin was contaminated was unknown, although the use of an opiate-scopolamine mixture was reminiscent of the morphine/scopolamine combination therapy known as "twilight sleep" that was heavily used in obstetric anesthesia during the early 20th century.[98]

Another unexpected complication of heroin abuse was observed in the Netherlands in the 1980s, when 47 heroin abusers developed spongiform leukoencephalopathy, manifested by mutism and spastic quadriparesis.[138] In these cases, as well as in subsequent cases in Europe and the United States, the users inhaled heroin vapors after the heroin powder had been heated on aluminum foil, a drug administration technique known as "chasing the dragon."[59,138] The exact toxic mechanism has not been elucidated.

OCCUPATIONAL TOXIN EPIDEMICS

Unfortunately, occupation-related toxic epidemics have become increasingly common (Table 2–6). These poisoning syndromes tend to have an insidious onset and may not be recognized clinically until years after the exposure. A specific toxin may cause a myriad of problems; among the most worrisome being the carcinogenic and mutagenic potentials.

While the 18th-century observations of Ramazzini and Pott introduced the concept that certain diseases were a direct result of toxic exposures in the workplace, it was not until the height of the 19th-century industrial revolution that the problems associated with the increasingly hazardous workplace became apparent.[46] During the 1860s, a peculiar disorder, attributed to the effects of inhaling mercury vapor, was described among manufacturers of felt hats in New Jersey.[134] Mercury nitrate was used as an essential part of the felting process at the time. "Hatter's shakes" refers to the tremor that developed in an estimated 10–60% of hatters surveyed.[134] Extreme shyness, another manifestation of mercurialism, was also seen in many hatters in later studies. Five percent of hatters during this period died from renal failure.

Other notable 19th-century and early 20th-century occupational tragedies included an increased incidence of mandibular necrosis (phossy jaw) among workers in the match-making industry who were exposed to white phosphorus,[44] an increased incidence of bladder tumors among synthetic dye makers who used β-naphthylamine,[37] and an increased incidence of aplastic anemia

TABLE 2–6.　**Occupational Disasters**

Toxin	Location	Date	Significance
Polycyclic aromatic hydrocarbons	England	1700s	High incidence of scrotal cancer among chimney sweeps; first description of occupational cancer
Mercury	New Jersey	Mid- to late 1800s	Outbreak of mercurialism in hatters
White phosphorus	Europe	Mid- to late 1800s	Phossy jaw in matchmakers
β-Naphthylamine	Worldwide	Early 1900s	Increased bladder cancer in dye makers
Benzene	Newark, New Jersey	1916–1928	Aplastic anemia among artificial leather manufacturers
Asbestos	Worldwide	20th century	Millions at risk for asbestos-related disease
Vinyl chloride	Louisville, Kentucky	1960s–1970s	Increased cases of hepatic angiosarcoma among polyvinyl chloride polymerization workers
Chlordecone	James River, Virginia	1973–1975	Increased incidence of neurologic abnormalities among insecticide workers
1,2-Dibromo-chloropropane	California	1974	Infertility among pesticide makers

among artificial leather manufacturers who used benzene.[111] The epidemic of phossy jaw among match makers had an induction period of 5 years and a mortality rate of 20% and has been called the "greatest tragedy in the whole story of occupational disease."[14] The problem continued in the United States until Congress passed the White Phosphorus Match Act in 1912, which established a prohibitive tax on white phosphorus matches.[89]

Since antiquity, occupational lead poisoning has been a constant threat. Workplace exposure to lead was particularly problematic during the 19th century and early 20th century, because of the large number of industries that relied heavily on lead. One of the most notorious of the "lead trades" was the actual production of white lead and lead oxides. Palsies, encephalopathy, and death from severe poisoning were reported by Alice Hamilton from every worksite.[40] Other occupations that entailed dangerous lead exposures included pottery glazing, rubber industry, pigment manufacturing, painting, printing, and plumbing.[72] Given the increasing awareness of harm suffered in the workplace, the British Factory and Workshop Act was enacted in 1895, which required the notification of occupational diseases caused by lead, arsenic, and phosphorus poisoning, as well as of occupational diseases caused by anthrax.[66]

Exposure to asbestos during the 20th century has become one of the most consequential occupational and environmental disasters in recent memory.[18,88] Despite the fact that the first case of asbestosis was reported in 1907, asbestos was heavily utilized in the shipbuilding industries in the 1940s as an insulating and fireproofing material. Since the early 1940s, 8–11 million individuals were

occupationally exposed to asbestos,[68] including 4.5 million individuals who worked in the shipyards. Asbestos-related diseases include mesothelioma, lung cancer, and pulmonary fibrosis (asbestosis). A 3-fold excess of cancer deaths has been attributed to asbestos-exposed insulation workers, primarily as a consequence of excess lung cancer deaths.[109]

Other more recent occupational poisonings involve exposure to a variety of newly synthesized chemicals. In Louisville, Kentucky, in 1974, an increased incidence of angiosarcoma of the liver was first noticed among polyvinyl chloride polymerization workers who were exposed to vinyl chloride monomer.[26] In 1975, chemical factory workers exposed to the organochlorine insecticide chlordecone (Kepone) experienced a high incidence of neurologic abnormalities, including tremor and chaotic eye movements.[122] An increased incidence of infertility among male Californian pesticide workers exposed to dibromochloropropane (DBCP) was noted in 1977.[135]

ENVIRONMENTAL DISASTERS

Although the incidence of significant human toxicity from dioxin (2,3,7,8-tetrachlorodibenzodioxin) and other similar polychlorinated compounds remains controversial, the lethality of this agent in an animal model has caused considerable concern for acute and latent injury from human exposure to this and other environmental toxins (Table 2–7). The release of a dioxin-containing chemical

TABLE 2–7.　**Environmental and Radiation Disasters**

Toxin	Location	Date	Significance
Radium	Orange, New Jersey	1910s–1920s	Increase in bone cancer in dial-painting workers
Radium	United States	1920s	"Radithor" (radioactive water) sold as radium-containing patent medication
Radiation	Hiroshima and Nagasaki, Japan	1945	First atomic bombs dropped at end of WWII; clinical effects still evident today
Dioxin	Seveso, Italy	1976	Unintentional release of dioxin into environment; chloracne
Toxic waste	Times Beach, Missouri	1975	Public alarmed by dioxin-containing toxic waste
Toxic waste	Love Canal, New York	1978	Further concern and intense debate regarding toxic waste
Radiation	Chernobyl, Belarus and Ukraine	1986	Increase in childhood thyroid cancer; increase in other cancers anticipated
Cesium	Goiania, Brazil	1987	Acute radiation sickness and radiation burns
Radiation	Japan	1999	Nuclear event at a uranium processing plant; 2 deaths
Cyanide	Romania	2000	Cyanide contaminated Danube River, killing wildlife for hundreds of miles

cloud into the atmosphere from an explosion at a hexachlorophene production factory in Seveso, Italy, in 1976, resulted in one of the most serious exposures to dioxin.[43] Chloracne was the only significant clinical finding related to the dioxin exposure at 5-year followup.[110]

Large-scale toxic disasters have also increased because of mass exposure to toxic waste dumps. Previously inhabited, but now deserted sites, such as Times Beach, Missouri, and Love Canal, New York, conjure up the very worst consequences of our toxic environment. Although little scientific evidence has been offered to confirm adverse health effects from the Love Canal toxic dump, this event directed attention to the problems of how best to deal with environmental poisons and their disposal.[50,96]

A recent environmental disaster, called the greatest environmental catastrophe since Chernobyl, occurred in February 2000, when a gold mine in western Romania disgorged 100,000 gallons of cyanide-contaminated water into the Tisza River.[57] Within a few days the contaminated water flowed into the Danube River as well. The chemical spill eradicated all animal life for 250 miles along the rivers, resulting in 200 tons of dead fish. Adverse human health effects from this chemical spill were not reported.

RADIATION DISASTERS

A discussion of mass poisonings is incomplete without mention of a growing number of radiation disasters that have occurred during the 20th century (Table 2–7). The first significant mass exposure to radiation occurred among several thousand teenage girls and young women employed in the dial-painting industry.[15] These workers painted luminous numbers on watch and instrument dials with paint that contained radium. Exposure occurred by licking the paint brushes and inhaling radium-laden dust. Studies showed an increase in bone-related cancers, as well as aplastic anemia and leukemia, in exposed workers.[74,99]

At the time of the "watch" disaster, radium was also being sold as a nostrum touted to cure all sorts of ailments, including rheumatism, syphilis, multiple sclerosis, and sexual dysfunction. Referred to as "mild radium therapy," in order to differentiate it from the higher-dose radium that was used in the treatment of cancer at that time, such α-particle-emitting isotopes were hailed as a powerful natural elixir that acted as a metabolic catalyst by delivering direct energy transfusions.[70] During the 1920s, dozens of patent medications contained small doses of radium and were sold as radioactive tablets, liniments, or liquids. One of the most infamous preparations was Radithor. Each half-ounce bottle contained slightly more than 1 µCi of radium 228 and radium 226. This radioactive water was sold all over the world "as harmless in every respect" and was heavily promoted as a sexual stimulant and aphrodisiac, taking on the glamour of a recreational drug for the wealthy.[70] More than 400,000 bottles were sold. The 1932 death of a prominent socialite and Radithor connoisseur from chronic radiation poisoning drew increased public and governmental scrutiny to this unregulated radium industry and helped end the era of radioactive patent medications.[70]

Concerns about the health effects of radiation have continued to escalate since the dawn of the nuclear age in 1945. Long-term followup studies 50 years after the atomic bombings at Hiroshima and Nagasaki show an increased incidence of leukemia, other cancers, radiation cataracts, hyperparathyroidism, delayed growth and development, and chromosomal anomalies in exposed individuals.[56]

The unintentional nuclear disaster at Chernobyl, Ukraine, in April 1986, again forced us to confront the medical consequences of 20th-century scientific advances that brought us the atomic age.[32] The release of radioactive material resulted in the hospitalization of more than 200 people for acute radiation sickness and 31 deaths. In some areas with heavy contamination, the increase in childhood thyroid cancer has increased 100-fold.[103] In the long term, many more people will undoubtedly be affected, and the total number of Chernobyl-associated cancer cases is likely to be high.

Another serious radiation event occurred in Goiania, Brazil, in 1987. When an abandoned radiotherapy unit was opened in a junkyard, 244 people were exposed to cesium-137. Of those people exposed to cesium-137, 104 showed evidence of internal contamination, 28 had local radiation injuries, and 8 developed acute radiation syndrome. There were at least 4 deaths.[95,101]

In September 1999, a nuclear event at a uranium processing plant in Japan set off an uncontrolled chain reaction exposing 49 people to radiation.[25,60] Radiation measured outside the facility reached 4000 times the normal ambient level. Two workers died from the effects of the radiation.

MASS SUICIDE BY POISON

Toxic disasters have also manifested themselves as events of mass suicide. In 1978, in Jonestown, Guyana, 911 members of the Peoples Temple died when they ingested a beverage to which cyanide had been added.[38] Although the majority of these deaths may have been by suicide, some of them do not appear to have been voluntary.[65] More recently, in 1997, phenobarbital and ethanol (sometimes assisted by physical asphyxiation) was the suicidal method favored by 39 members of the Heavens Gate cult in Rancho Santa Fe, California. This means of suicide was recommended in the book *Final Exit*.[45] Apparently the cult members committed suicide in order to shed their bodies in hopes of hopping aboard an alien spaceship they believed was in the wake of Comet Hale-Bopp.[63]

SUMMARY

Unfortunately, toxicologic plagues and disasters have had an all too prominent role in our history. An understanding of the pathogenesis of these toxic plagues (eg, issues pertaining to drug, food, and occupational safety) is critically important if future disasters are to be prevented. Given the practical and ethical limitations in studying the effects of many specific toxins in humans, lessons from these unfortunate tragedies must be fully mastered and retained for future generations.

REFERENCES

1. Alexander CS: Cobalt-beer cardiomyopathy: A clinical and pathologic study of twenty-eight cases. Am J Med 1972;53:395–417.
2. Anderson HA, Wolff MS, Lilis R, et al: Symptoms and clinical abnormalities following ingestion of polybrominated-biphenyl-contaminated food products. Ann N Y Acad Sci 1979;320:684–702.
3. Arbiser JL. Kraeft SK. van Leeuwen R. et al: Clioquinol-zinc chelate: A candidate causative agent of subacute myelo-optic neuropathy. Mol Med 1998;4:665–670.

4. Baker F, Damluji S, Amin-Zaki L, et al: Methylmercury poisoning in Iraq. Science 1973;181:230–241.

5. Barnes JM, Stoner HB: The toxicology of tin compounds. Pharmacol Rev 1959;11:211–232.

6. Baxter PJ, Kapila M, Mfonfu D: Lake Nyos disaster, Cameroon, 1986: The medical effects of large-scale emission of carbon dioxide? BMJ 1989;298:1437–1441.

7. Belongia EA, Hedberg CW, Gleich GJ, et al: An investigation of the cause of the eosinophilia-myalgia syndrome associated with tryptophan use. N Engl J Med 1990;323:357–365.

8. Bennett IL, Cary FH, Mitchell GL, Cooper MN: Acute methyl alcohol poisoning: A review based on experiences in an outbreak of 323 cases. Medicine 1953;32:431–463.

9. Bernard A, Hermans C, Broeckaert F, et al: Food contamination by PCBs and dioxins. Nature 1999;401:231–232.

10. Cadmium pollution and itai-itai disease. Lancet 1971;2:382–383.

11. Cambodian mob kills two Vietnamese in poisoning hysteria. Deutsche Presse-Agentur September 4, 1998.

12. Caporael LR: Ergotism: The satan loosed in Salem. Science 1976; 192:21–26.

13. Carter LJ: Michigan PBB incident: Chemical mix-up leads to disaster. Science 1976;192:240–243.

14. Cherniack M: Diseases of unusual occupations: An historical perspective. Occup Med 1992;7:369–384.

15. Clark C: Radium Girls: Women and Industrial Health Reform. 1910–1935. Chapel Hill: University of North Carolina Press, 1997.

16. Coll S: Tainted foods, medicine make mass poisonings rife in India: Critics press for tougher inspection, more accurate labels. Washington Post, December 8, 1991, p. A36.

17. Connolly HM, Crary JL, McGoon MD, et al: Valvular heart disease associated with fenfluramine-phentermine. N Engl J Med 1997;337: 581–588.

18. Corn JK, Starr J: Historical perspective on asbestos: Policies and protective measures in World War II shipbuilding. Am J Indust Med 1987;11:359–373.

19. Cullinan P, Acquilla S, Dhara VR: Respiratory morbidity 10 years after the Union Carbide gas leak at Bhopal: A cross sectional survey. BMJ 1997;314:338–342.

20. Dally A: Thalidomide: Was the tragedy preventable? Lancet 1998: 351:1197–1199.

21. Das D, Chatterjee A, Mandal BK, et al: Arsenic in ground water in six districts of West Bengal, India: The biggest arsenic calamity in the world. Part 2. Arsenic concentration in drinking water, hair, nails, urine, skin-scale and liver tissue (biopsy) of the affected people. Analyst 1995;120:917–924.

22. DeStefano F: Effects of agent-orange exposure. JAMA 1995;273: 1494.

23. Easton WH: Smoke and fire gases. Ind Med 1942;11:466–468.

24. Eckert WG: Mass deaths by gas or chemical poisoning: A historical perspective. Am J Forensic Med Pathol 1991;12:119–125.

25. Efron S. Dozens hurt in Japan's worst nuclear accident. Los Angeles Times, October 1, 1999;A1.

26. Falk H, Creech JL, Health CW, et al: Hepatic disease among workers at a vinyl chloride polymerization plant. JAMA 1974;230:59–63.

27. Fatal moonshine in India. Newsday, March 6, 1989.

28. Faxon NW, Churchill ED: The Coconut Grove disaster in Boston. JAMA 1942;120:1385–1388.

29. Fernando D: Fentanyl-laced heroin. JAMA 1991;265:2962.

30. Ficarra BJ: Medical mystery: Gulf War syndrome. J Med 1995; 26: 87–94.

31. Final report of the Royal Commission on Arsenical Poisoning. Lancet 1903;2:1674–1676.

32. Geiger HJ: The accident at Chernobyl and the medical response. JAMA 1986;256:609–612.

33. Geiling EHK, Cannon PR: Pathological effects of elixir of sulfanilamide (diethylene glycol) poisoning: A clinical and experimental correlation—Final report. JAMA 1938;111:919–926.

34. Gershanik J, Boecler B, Ensley H, et al: The gasping syndrome and benzyl alcohol poisoning. N Engl J Med 1982;307:1384–1388.

35. Giusti RM, Iwamoto K, Hatch EE: Diethylstilbestrol revisited: A review of the long-term health effects. Ann Intern Med 1995;122: 778–788.

36. Gleich M: Thallium acetate poisoning in the treatment of ringworm of the scalp. JAMA 1931;97:851.

37. Goldblatt MW: Vesical tumours induced by chemical compounds. Br J Indust Med 1949;6:65–81.

38. Guyana tragedy: An international forensic problem. INFORM Rep 1979;11:2–8.

39. Haley RW, Kurt TL: Self-reported exposure to neurotoxic chemical combinations in the Gulf War. JAMA 1997;277:231–237.

40. Hamilton A: Landmark article in occupational medicine: Forty years in the poisonous trades. Am J Indust Med 1985;7:3–18.

41. Herbst AL, Ulfelder H, Poskanzer DC: Adenocarcinoma of the vagina. Association of maternal stilbestrol therapy with tumor appearance in young women. N Engl J Med 1971;284:878–881.

42. Hodgson MJ, Kipen HM: Gulf War illnesses: Causation and treatment. J Occup Environ Med 1999;41:443–452.

43. Holmstedt B: Prolegomena to Seveso. Arch Toxicol 1979;44: 211–230.

44. Hughes JP, Baron R, Buckland DH, et al: Phosphorus necrosis of the jaw: A present day study. Br J Indust Med 1962;19:83–99.

45. Humphry D: Final Exit. New York, Dell, 1991.

46. Hunter D: The Diseases of Occupations, 6th ed. London, Hodder & Stoughton, 1978.

47. Hyams KC, Wignall S, Roswell R: War syndromes and their evaluation: From the U.S. Civil War to the Persian Gulf War. Ann Intern Med 1996;125:398–405.

48. Iowa Persian Gulf Study Group: Self-reported illness and health status among Gulf War veterans. JAMA 1997;277:238–245.

49. Ismail K, Everitt B, Blatchley N, et al: Is there a Gulf War syndrome? Lancet 1999;353:179–182.

50. Janerich DT, Burnett WS, Feck G, et al: Cancer incidence in the Love Canal area. Science 1981;212:1404–1407.

51. Jones GRN: Polychlorinated biphenyls: Where do we stand now? Lancet 1989;2:791–794.

52. Kernan WN, Viscoli CM, Brass LM, et al: Phenylpropanolamine and the risk of hemorrhagic stroke. N Engl J Med 2000;343;1826–1832.

53. Kilbourne EM, de la Paz MP, Borda IA, et al: Toxic oil syndrome: A current clinical and epidemiologic summary, including comparisons with eosinophilia-myalgia syndrome. J Am Coll Cardiol 1991; 18: 711–717.

54. Kilbourne EM, Rigau-Perez JG, Heath C, et al: Clinical epidemiology of toxic-oil syndrome: Manifestations of a new illness. N Engl J Med 1983;309:1408–1414.

55. Kipen HM, Hallman W, Kang H, et al: Prevalence of chronic fatigue and chemical sensitivities in Gulf Registry veterans. Arch Environ Health 1999;54:313–318.

56. Kodama K, Mabuchi K, Shigematsu I: A long-term cohort study of the atomic-bomb survivors. J Epidemiol 1996;6:S95–S105.

57. Koenig R: Wildlife deaths are a grim wake-up call in Eastern Europe. Science 2000;287:1737–1738.

58. Koppelman H, Robertson MH, Saunders PG: The Epping jaundice. Br Med J 1966;1:514–516.

59. Kriegstein AR, Shungu DC, Millar WS, et al: Leukoencephalopathy and raised brain lactate from heroin vapor inhalation ("chasing the dragon"). Neurology 1999;53:1765–1773.

60. Lamar J: Japan's worst nuclear accident leaves two fighting for life. BMJ 1999;319:937.

61. Lambert ED: Modern Medical Mistakes. Bloomington, IN, Indiana University Press, 1978.

62. Landrigan PJ: Illness in Gulf War veterans: Causes and consequences. JAMA 1997;277:259–261.

63. Lang J: Heaven's gate suicide still a mystery 1 year later. The Arizona Republic, March 26, 1998, p. A11.

64. Langston JW, Ballard P, Tetrud JW, Irwin I: Chronic parkinsonism in humans due to a product of meperidine-analog synthesis. Science 1983;219:979–980.

65. Layton D: Seductive Poison: A Jonestown Survivor's Story of Live and Death in the Peoples Temple. New York, Anchor, 1998.

66. Lee WR: The history of the statutory control of mercury poisoning in Great Britain. Brit J Indust Med 1968;25:52–62.

67. Leschke E: Clinical Toxicology: Modern Methods in the Diagnosis and Treatment of Poisoning. Baltimore, William Wood, 1934.

68. Levin SM, Kann PE, Lax MB: Medical examination for asbestos-related disease. Am J Indust Med 2000;37:6–22.

69. Logan WPD: Mortality in the London fog incident, 1952. Lancet 1953;1:336–338.

70. Macklis RM: Radithor and the era of mild radium therapy. JAMA 1990;262:614–618.

71. Magnuson E: The devil made him do it. Time, April 9, 1990, p. 38.

72. Markowitz G, Rosner D: "Cater to the children": The role of the lead industry in a public health tragedy, 1900–1955. Am J Pub Health 2000:90:36–46.

73. Martin M, Hecker J, Clark R, et al: China white epidemic: An eastern United States emergency department experience. Ann Emerg Med 1991;20:158–164.

74. Martland HS: Occupational poisoning in manufacture of luminous watch dials. JAMA 1929;92:466-473, 552–559.

75. Massey EW, Wold D, Heyman A: Arsenic: Homicidal intoxication. South Med J 1984;77:848–851.

76. Matossian MK: Ergot and the Salem witchcraft affair. Am Sci 1982; 70:355–357.

77. McFadyen RE: Thalidomide in America: A brush with tragedy. Clin Med 1976;11:79–93.

78. Mehta PS, Mehta AS, Mehta SJ, Makjijani AB: Bhopal tragedy's health effects: A review of methyl isocyanate toxicity. JAMA 1990; 264:2781–2787.

79. Merhoff GC, Porter JM: Ergot intoxication: Historical review and description of unusual clinical manifestations. Ann Surg 1974;180: 773–779.

80. Modell W: Mass drug catastrophes and the roles of science and technology. Science 1967;156:346–351.

81. Morgan JP: The Jamaica ginger paralysis. JAMA 1982;248: 1864–1867.

82. Morin YL, Foley AR, Martineau G, Roussel J: Quebec beer-drinkers' cardiomyopathy: Forty-eight cases. Can Med Assoc J 1967;97:881–883.

83. Morita H, Yanagisawa N, Nakajima T, et al: Sarin poisoning in Matsumoto, Japan. Lancet 1995;346:290–293.

84. Mudur G: Arsenic poisons 220,000 in India. BMJ 1996;313:9.

85. Mudur G: Half of Bangladesh population at risk of arsenic poisoning [news]. BMJ 2000;320:822.

86. Mullins ME, Horowitz BZ, Linden DHJ, et al: Life-threatening interaction of mibefradil and beta blockers with dihydropyridine calcium channel blockers. JAMA 1998;280;157–158.

87. Munch JC: Human thallotoxicosis. JAMA 1934;102:1929–1934.

88. Murray R: Asbestos: A chronology of its origins and health effects. Br J Indust Med 1990;47:361–365.

89. Myers ML, McGlothin JD: Matchmakers "phossy jaw" eradicated. AIHAJ 1996;57:330–332.

90. Nakae K, Yamamoto A, Shigematsu I, et al: Relation between subacute myelo-optic neuropathy (S.M.O.N.) and clioquinol: Nationwide survey. Lancet 1973;1;171–173.

91. Nakajima T, Ohta S, Morita H, et al: Epidemiological study of sarin poisoning in Matsumoto City, Japan. J Epidemiol 1998;8:33–41.

92. Nemery B, Fischler B, Boogaerts M, Lison D: Dioxins, Coca-Cola, and mass sociogenic illness in Belgium [letter]. Lancet 1999;354:77.

93. O'Brien KL, Selanikio JD, Heedivert C, for the Acute Renal Failure Investigation Team: Epidemic of pediatric deaths from acute renal failure caused by diethylene glycol poisoning. JAMA 1998;279: 1175–1180.

94. Okumura T, Takasu N, Ishimatsu S, et al: Report on 640 victims of the Tokyo subway sarin attack. Ann Emerg Med 1996;28:129–135.

95. Oliveira AR, Hunt JG, Valverde NJL, et al: Medical and related aspects of the Goiania accident: An overview. Health Physics 1991; 60:17–24.

96. Paigen B: Controversy at Love Canal. Hastings Cent Rep 1982; 12:29–37.

97. Pentachlorophenol poisoning in newborn infants—St Louis Missouri, April-August 1967. MMWR Morb Mortal Wkly Rep 1996; 45:545–549.

98. Pitcock CD, Clark RB: From Fanny to Fernand: The development of consumerism in pain control during the birth process. Am J Obstet Gynecol 1992;167:581–587.

99. Polednak AP, Stehney AF, Rowland RE: Mortality among women first employed before 1930 in the U.S. radium dial-painting industry. Am J Epidemiol 1978;107:179–195.

100. Powell PP: Minimata disease: A story of mercury's malevolence. South Med J 1991;84:1352–1358.

101. Roberts L: Radiation accident grips Goiania. Science 1987;238: 1028–1031.

102. Roses OE, Fernandez JCG, Villaamil ED, et al: Mass poisoning by sodium arsenite. J Toxicol Clin Toxicol 1991;29:209–213.

103. Rytomaa T: Ten years after Chernobyl. Ann Med 1996;28:83–87.

104. Sawyer WA, Meyer KF, Eaton MD, et al: Jaundice in army personnel in the western region of the United Sates and its relation to vaccination against yellow fever. Am J Hygiene 1944;39:337–432.

105. Scalzo AJ: Diethylene glycol toxicity revisited: The 1996 Haitian epidemic. J Toxicol Clin Toxicol 1996;34:513–516.

106. Schmid R: Cutaneous porphyria in Turkey. N Engl J Med 1960;263: 397–398.

107. Scopolamine poisoning among heroin users—New York City, Newark, Philadelphia, and Baltimore, 1995 and 1996. MMWR Morb Mortal Wkly Rep 1996;45:457–460.

108. Selected Cancers Cooperative Study Group: The association of selected cancers with service in the U.S. military in Vietnam, I: non-Hodgkin's lymphoma. Arch Intern Med 1990;150:2473–2483.

109. Selikoff IJ, Hammond EC, Seidman H: Mortality experience of insulation workers in the United States and Canada, 1943–1976. Ann N Y Acad Sci 1979;330:91–116.

110. Seveso after five years. Lancet 1981;2:731–732.

111. Sharpe WD: Benzene, artifical leather and aplastic anemia: Newark, 1916–1928. Bull N Y Acad Med 1993;69:47–60.

112. Shively BK, Roldan CA, Gill EA, et al: Prevalence and determinants of valvulopathy in patients treated with dexfenfluramine. Circulation 1999;100:2161–2167.

113. Sidell FR, Takafuji ET, Franz DR, eds: Medical Aspects of Chemical and Biological Warfare. Washington, DC, Office of the Surgeon General, 1997.

114. Sidell FR: Chemical agent terrorism. Ann Emerg Med 1996;28: 223–224.

115. Smith HV, Spalding JM: Outbreak of paralysis in Morocco due to ortho-cresyl phosphate poisoning. Lancet 1959;2:1019–1021.

116. Stalinon: A therapeutic disaster. Br Med J 1958;1:515.

117. Stover BJ: Effects of thorotrast in humans. Health Physics 1983; 44(S1):253–257.

118. Subramanian KS, Kosnett MJ: Human exposures to arsenic from consumption of well water in West Bengal, India. Int J Occup Environ Health 1998;4:217–230.

119. Swann JP: The 1941 sulfathiazole disaster and the birth of good manufacturing practices. PDA J Pharm Sci Technol 1999;53: 148–153.

120. Swartz RD, Millman RP, Billi JE, et al: Epidemic methanol poisoning: Clinical and biochemical analysis of a recent episode. Medicine (Baltimore) 1981;60:373–382.

121. Tainted liquor kills 162, sickens 228. Los Angeles Times, May 10, 1992.

122. Taylor JR, Selhorst JB, Houff SA, Martinez AJ: Chlordecone intoxication in man. Neurology 1978;28:626–630.

123. Toxic Epidemic Syndrome Study Group: Toxic epidemic syndrome, Spain, 1981. Lancet 1982;2:697–702.

124. Tsuchiya K: The discovery of the causal agent of Minamata disease. Am J Indust Med 1992;21:275–280.

125. Unwin C, Blatchley N, Coker W, et al: Health of UK servicemen who served in Persian Gulf War. Lancet 1999;353:169–178.

126. Urbinato D: London's historic "pea-soupers." EPA J 1994, p. 59 (Summer).

127. Van Loock F, Gallay A, Demarest S, et al: Outbreak of Coca-Cola-related illness in Belgium: A true association [letter]. Lancet 1999; 354:680–681.

128. Vargas J, Uitto J, Jimenez SA: The cause and pathogenesis of the eosinophilia-myalgia syndrome. Ann Intern Med 1992;116:140–147.

129. Varma DR, Guest I: The Bhopal accident and methyl isocyanate toxicity. J Toxicol Environ Health 1993;40:513–529.

130. Waldron HA: The Devonshire colic. J Hist Med 1970;25:383-413.

131. Wax PM: Elixirs, diluents and the passage of the 1938 federal Food, Drug and Cosmetic Act. Ann Intern Med 1995;122:456–461.

132. Wax PM: It's happening again—another diethylene glycol mass poisoning. J Toxicol Clin Toxicol 1996;34:513–516.

133. Weber E, Laarbai F, Michel L, Donckier J: Abdominal pain: Do not forget Thorotrast! Postgrad Med J 1995;7:367–369.

134. Wedeen RP: Were the hatters of New Jersey "mad?" Am J Indust Med 1989;16:225–233.

135. Whorton MD, Krauss RM, Marshall S, Milby TH: Infertility in male pesticide workers. Lancet 1977;2:1259–1261.

136. Wing JS, Sanderson LM, Brender JD, et al: Acute health effects in a community after a release of hydrofluoric acid. Arch Environ Health 1991;46:155–160.

137. Wolff MS, Anderson HA, Selikoff IJ: Human tissue burdens of halogenated aromatic chemicals in Michigan. JAMA 1982;247: 2112–2116.

138. Wolters ED, van Wijngaarden GK, Stam FC: Leucoencephalopathy after inhaling "heroin" pyrolysate. Lancet 1982;2:1233–1237.

GENERAL APPROACH TO MEDICAL TOXICOLOGY

CHAPTER 3

PRINCIPLES OF MANAGING THE POISONED OR OVERDOSED PATIENT: AN OVERVIEW

Lewis R. Goldfrank / Neal E. Flomenbaum / Neal A. Lewin / Mary Ann Howland / Robert S. Hoffman / Lewis S. Nelson

For almost four decades, medical toxicologists and information specialists at poison centers have utilized a clinical approach to the poisoned or overdosed patient that emphasizes treating the patient rather than treating the poison. Too often in the past, patients were initially all but neglected while attention was focused on the list of ingredients on the container of the product(s). Although the astute clinician must always be prepared to administer a specific antidote immediately in those uncommon instances when nothing else will save a patient, all poisoned or overdosed patients will benefit from an organized, rapid clinical management plan (Fig. 3–1).

The initial management of all seriously ill patients begins with attention to the ABCs: *a*irway compromise, *b*reathing difficulties, and *c*irculatory problems. When a patient's mental status is abnormal, metabolic derangements, such as glucose and electrolyte abnormalities, and the possibilities of head and cervical spine trauma must be considered. In such cases, the cervical spine may need to be protected until injury can either be excluded or diagnosed and treated. The bedside assessment of the adequacy of respirations (frequency and depth) and a decision on the necessity of early intubation is followed by a determination of all of the vital signs and identification and treatment of life-threatening conditions such as hypotension, hypertension, bradycardia, tachycardia, dysrhythmias, hyperthermia, and hypothermia (Chap. 17). Accurate identification and treatment of conduction disturbances and dysrhythmias necessitate obtaining a 12-lead ECG and cardiac monitoring (Chap. 9). Similarly, an arterial blood gas analysis may be indicated to more accurately assess ventilation, oxygenation, some toxic-metabolic etiologies of altered mental status such as a wide anion gap metabolic acidosis, and, when appropriate, carbon monoxide poisoning (by cooximetry).

With the initiation of an IV infusion, blood samples can also be sent as indicated. If the patient has an altered mental status, there may be specific indications to test for CNS depressants and/or "drugs of abuse," but these tests rarely provide useful information. For the potentially suicidal patient, an acetaminophen level should routinely be requested along with tests affecting the management of any specific drug or toxin such as lithium, theophylline, iron, salicylates, and digoxin, as suggested by the history, physical examination, or bedside diagnostic tests.

Early treatment of a patient with a suspected toxicologic exposure and an altered mental status should typically include consideration or administration of (a) hypertonic dextrose, 0.5–1.0 g/kg as $D_{50}W$ for an adult or $D_{10-20}W$ for a child; (b) thiamine, 100 mg IV for an adult; (c) naloxone, 0.4–2 mg IV bolus for adults and children with respiratory compromise; and (d) oxygen, 100% at 8–10 L/min. Dextrose administration should be omitted when hypoglycemia can be definitely excluded, but hypoglycemia may be the sole or contributing cause of coma even when the patient manifests focal findings.

While focusing on probable or possible toxicologic etiologies, nontoxicologic conditions that may have similar presentations must be excluded. The physical examination, therefore, should include a careful search for any external signs of head, neck, or blunt abdominal trauma; abnormal or focal neurologic findings; abnormal pupillary responses; unusual breath or skin odors (Table 28–1); abnormal respiratory or cardiac sounds; as well as toxicologic syndromes or "toxidromes." Toxicologic etiologies of abnormal vital signs and physical findings are summarized in Tables 17–1 to 17–7. Toxidromes are summarized in Table 17–2 and other details of the physical assessment are provided in Chapter 31.

With stabilization of the patient's condition, attention can be addressed to the issues of gastrointestinal decontamination. A detailed discussion of these issues is found in Chapter 5. The indications, contraindications, precautions, and adverse effects associated with orogastric lavage, whole-bowel irrigation, administration of single- or multiple-dose activated charcoal, (MDAC), cathartics, and (in the conscious patient) emesis utilizing syrup of ipecac are summarized in Tables 31–1 to 31–5. Fully referenced descriptions of whole-bowel irrigation, activated charcoal, cathartics, and syrup of ipecac may be found in the respective Antidotes in Depth sections immediately following Chapter 31.

At the next stage in the management of a poisoned or overdosed patient, it is appropriate to consider various methods of eliminating absorbed toxins. Currently, available methods range from raising urinary pH (also known as "ion trapping") and MDAC to hemodialysis, hemoperfusion, hemofiltration, and exchange transfusion. All are described in Chapter 6.

Although the vast majority of toxicologic emergencies result from ingestion, injection, or inhalation, the eyes and skin are occasionally the route of systemic absorption or are the organs at risk. The management of toxic cutaneous and ophthalmic exposures are described along with a more detailed management approach to the unknown or suspected overdose in Chapters 27, 29, and 31.

Typically, in managing patients with toxicologic emergencies, there is both a necessity and an opportunity to obtain various diagnostic studies and ancillary tests interspersed with stabilizing the patient's condition (when establishing intravenous access, for example), obtaining the history, and performing the physical examination. Chapters 7 through 9 discuss the timing and indications for qualitative and quantitative diagnostic laboratory studies, the use and interpretation of the electrocardiogram, and radiologic and imaging procedures in diagnosing and managing the poisoned or overdosed patient.

A recommended stock list of antidotes and therapeutic agents for the treatment of poisonings and overdoses appears in Table 3–1.

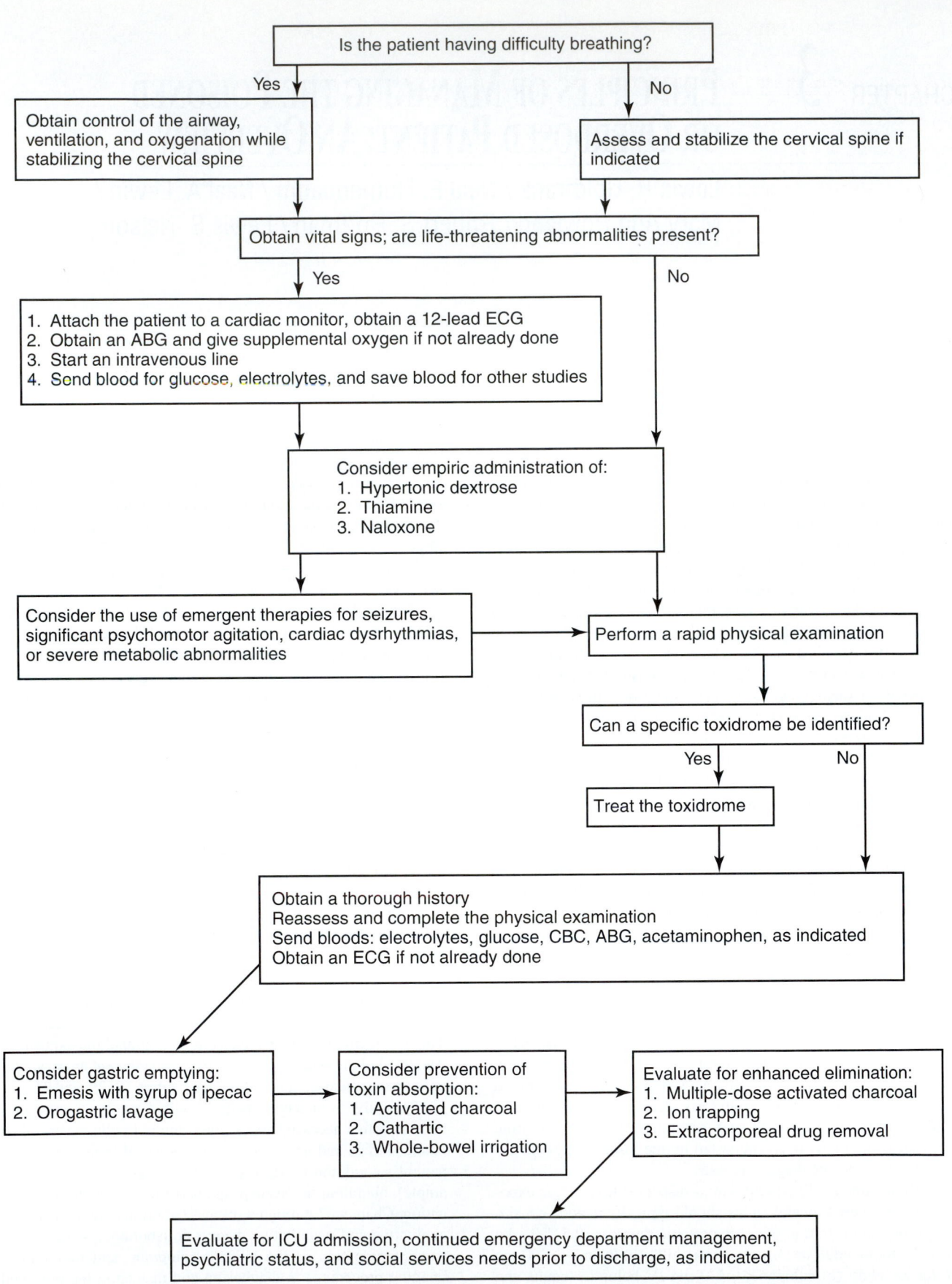

Figure 3–1. This algorithm is a basic guide to management of poisoned patients. A more detailed description of the steps in management may be found in the accompanying text and in Chapter 31. This algorithm is only a guide to actual management, which must, of course, consider the patient's clinical status.

TABLE 3–1.   Antidotes and Therapeutic Agents for the Treatment of Poisonings and Overdoses*

Therapeutic Agent**	Uses
Activated charcoal (p. 469)	Adsorbs toxin or drug in GI tract
Antivenom *(Crotalinae)* (p. 1568) Polyvalent	Crotaline snake envenomations
Antivenom *(Latrodectus mactans)* (p. 1589)	Black widow spider envenomations
Antivenom *(Elapidae)* (p. 1568)	Coral snake envenomations
Atropine (p. 1353)	Bradydysrhythmias, cholinesterase inhibitors (organic phosphorus agents, physostigmine) poisonings, muscarinic mushrooms *(Clitocybe, Inocybe)* ingestions
Botulinum antitoxin (ABE-Trivalent) (p. 1112)	Botulism (available from local health department or Centers for Disease Control)
Calcium chloride, calcium gluconate (p. 1341)	Oxalates, fluoride, hydrofluoric acid, ethylene glycol, calcium channel blockers, hypomagnesemia, β-adrenergic antagonists
Carnitine (p. 621)	Valproic acid
Cyanide kit (amyl nitrite, sodium nitrite, sodium thiosulfate) (p. 1511)	Cyanide poisoning
Deferoxamine mesylate (Desferal) (p. 558)	Iron ingestions
Dextrose in water (50% adults; 20% pediatrics; 10% neonates) (p. 606)	Hypoglycemia due to a variety of agents, to Dx or Rx patients with altered mental status
Diazepam (Valium) or lorazepam (Ativan) (p. 1011)	Seizures, severe agitation, stimulants, sedative-hyponotic withdrawal
Digoxin-specific antibody fragments (Digibind) (p. 735)	Digoxin, digitoxin, and digoxin-like cardiac glycosides of any origin (pharmaceuticals, plants, animals)
Dimercaprol (BAL, British Anti-Lewisite) (p. 1196)	Arsenic, mercury, gold, and lead poisoning
Diphenhydramine (p. 879)	Extrapyramidal drug reactions, allergic reactions
Edetate calcium disodium (Calcium disodium versenate, CaNa$_2$ EDTA) (p. 1235)	Lead, and other selected metal poisonings
Ethanol oral and parenteral dosage forms (p. 995)	Methanol and ethylene glycol poisoning
Flumazenil (Romazicon) (p. 946)	Pure benzodiazepine poisoning in a non-benzodiazepine-dependent patient
Folinic acid (p. 991)	Methotrexate toxicity, methanol poisoning
Fomepizole (Antizole) (p. 999)	Ethylene glycol, methanol poisoning
Glucagon (p. 758)	β-adrenergic antagonist and calcium channel blocker overdoses
Ipecac, syrup of (p. 465)	Induces emesis
Magnesium sulfate or magnesium citrate (p. 475)	Induces catharsis
Magnesium sulfate injection (p. 732)	Cardiac glycoside overdoses, hydrofluoric acid exposures, hypomagnesemia, ethanol withdrawal, torsades de pointes
Methylene blue (1% solution) (p. 1450)	Methemoglobinemia
N-Acetylcysteine (Mucomyst) (p. 502)	Acetaminophen overdoses, and other causes of liver failure
Naloxone hydrochloride (Narcan) (p. 924)	Opioid overdoses, clonidine overdoses
Norepinephrine (Levarterenol) (p. 858)	Hypotension (preferred for cyclic antidepressants), α-adrenergic antagonist overdoses
Octreotide (Sandostatin) (p. 611)	Oral hypoglycemic agent-induced hypoglycemia
Oxygen (oxygen, hyperbaric) (p. 1492)	Carbon monoxide, cyanide, hydrogen sulfide poisoning
D-Penicillamine (Cuprimine) (p. 1268)	Copper, lead poisoning
Phenobarbital (p. 1063)	Seizures, agitation, stimulants, sedative-hypnotic withdrawal
Phentolamine (p. 1011)	MAOI interactions; cocaine; epinephrine and ergot alkaloid overdoses
Physostigmine salicylate (Antilirium) (p. 544)	Anticholinergic toxicity
Polyethylene glycol electrolyte solution (p. 478)	Decontaminates GI tract
Pralidoxime chloride (2-PAM-chloride) (Protopam) (p. 1361)	Acetylcholinesterase inhibitor (organic phosphorus agents and carbamates) poisoning
Protamine sulfate (p. 651)	Heparin anticoagulation (agent reverses anticoagulation)
Pyridoxine hydrochloride (Vitamin B$_6$) (p. 667)	Ethylene glycol poisoning, isoniazid overdoses, gyromitrin-containing mushroom ingestions
Sodium bicarbonate (p. 519)	Ethylene glycol and methanol poisoning; salicylate, cyclic antidepressant, methotrexate, phenobarbital, quinidine, and chlorpropamide overdoses, drugs with type I antidysrhythmic toxicity; chlorphenoxy herbicide poisoning
Sorbitol (p. 475)	Induces catharsis
Starch (p. 1285)	Iodine poisoning
Succimer (Chemet) (p. 1228)	Lead, mercury, arsenic poisoning
Thiamine hydrochloride (p. 966)	Thiamine deficiency, ethylene glycol poisoning, chronic ethanol consumption ("alcoholism")
Vitamin K$_1$ (Aquamephyton) (p. 647)	Warfarin or rodenticide anticoagulant

*Each emergency department should have all the above agents readily available to its staff. Some of these antidotes may be stored in the pharmacy, and others may be available from the Centers for Disease Control and Prevention, but the precise mechanism for locating each one must be known by each staff member.
**A detailed analysis of each of these agents is found in the text, in the Antidotes in Depth section on the page cited to the right of each therapeutic agent listed.

CHAPTER 4

PRINCIPLES AND TECHNIQUES TO IDENTIFY THE NONTOXIC EXPOSURE

Richard Weisman

A large number of calls received by physicians and poison centers throughout the United States are for nontoxic exposures. During the past 5 years, greater than 40% of the exposures reported to the American Association of Poison Centers were judged by poison information specialists to be nontoxic exposures (Chap. 116 has further details). One of the most important skills that an emergency physician, poison information specialist, or medical toxicologist can develop is the ability to identify and appropriately triage exposures that are not likely to result in toxicity. This may prevent an unnecessary visit to the emergency department (or physician's office), or if the patient is in the emergency department, it may prevent unnecessary testing. Allowing patients with nontoxic exposures to be evaluated, observed, and followed up outside of the emergency department or physician's private office is cost effective, and a major justification for governmental funding for poison centers. Poison centers also render a substantial public health service in that they relieve the overcrowding common to many large inner-city emergency departments by keeping patients at home who do not require medical evaluation or interventions.

The patient with a potentially nontoxic exposure who telephones an emergency department, paramedic base station, or a poison center requires extensive evaluation by a healthcare provider with specialized training in toxicology. The analysis of nontoxic exposures can be divided into two major categories. The first and least problematic category is an exposure to products unlikely to result in toxicity at any dose by a particular route of administration. In such a situation, the physician or poison information specialist must only establish, by history, an absolute identity of the product and the route of administration. A product that is harmless at any dose by a particular route of exposure may nevertheless be toxic by another route. For example, pure talcum powder never causes a problem when applied dermally. If, however, during intentional ingestion or substantial inhalation the patient aspirates the powder, severe pulmonary complications or death may occur.[9]

The second type of nontoxic exposure is exposure to a nontoxic quantity of a product that is potentially toxic, for example, a patient with a 50-mg/kg exposure to acetaminophen.[11]

WHEN CAN AN EXPOSURE BE CONSIDERED NONTOXIC?

An exposure is considered nontoxic when a sufficient history regarding the exposure can be obtained, when the information is considered reliable, and when the exposure would still be considered nontoxic if the quantity was significantly underestimated. Before an exposure should be considered nontoxic, all of the criteria discussed below and listed in Table 4–1 should be met.[6–8]

PRODUCT IDENTIFICATION

For an exposure to be categorized as nontoxic, the product must be absolutely and completely identified. The product name, manufacturer, ingredients, quantities, concentrations, and production date are all essential in assessing the toxicity of the product. Manufacturers often change product ingredients (both active and inactive) without changing the product name. If there are any inconsistencies or missing information in the patient's exposure history, the ingestion cannot be classified as nontoxic. Patients often transfer medications into different containers. When unexplained symptoms occur, a manufacturing or labeling error or product tampering must be considered. In 1996, more than 70 Haitian children developed acute renal failure and neurologic toxicity when diethylene glycol was used instead of propylene glycol as the vehicle in acetaminophen syrup.[13]

SINGLE-PRODUCT EXPOSURE

Usually, for an exposure to be considered nontoxic, only a single product should be involved. Often, exposure to two nontoxic products will also be nontoxic. Synergistic or additional toxicity and/or toxic interactions may occur if multiple substances are involved and additional care must therefore be used in trying to assess this type of exposure. Nontoxic amounts of aspirin, ibuprofen, and iron ingested together would likely result in gastrointestinal toxicity. When evaluating patients who have ingested multiple substances, the most prudent plan is for the patient to be examined at either the

TABLE 4–1. General Guidelines for an Exposure to be Considered Nontoxic

1. Identification of the product and its ingredients is possible.
2. Usually only one product is involved with the exposure.
3. The exposure was unintentional. The patient is not suicidal or the victim of abuse or neglect.
4. The CPSC "signal words" CAUTION, WARNING, or DANGER do not appear on the product label.
5. The history permits a reliable approximation of the quantity involved with the exposure.
6. The history permits the routes of exposure to be determined.
7. The patient is asymptomatic.
8. Followup consultation with the patient or care provider is possible.

physician's office or at an emergency department. Unintentional exposures, particularly in children, typically involve small amounts of a single product. Concurrent exposure to multiple products should alert the physician to the possibility of an intentional ingestion, abuse, or neglect.[6,12] An ingestion that is not the patient's first "unintentional" poisoning may be a clue to a psychiatric disorder in the case of a child or a compromised adult, or to neglect or abuse.

UNINTENTIONAL EXPOSURE

An adult who has intentionally ingested a drug or toxin almost always requires evaluation in a healthcare facility. With the exception of therapeutic errors and mistakes from confusion, or mental, linguistic, or visual impairment, most ingestions in adults result from misuse, abuse, or suicidal intent. Identifying over the telephone adults who may require psychiatric or social interventions is not possible. Unintentional toxic exposures in adults may result from therapeutic errors and drug interactions, occupational or environmental exposures, and food poisonings.

Suicidal ingestions and ingestions by drug and alcohol users comprise the largest proportion (>90%) of intentional exposures. Both groups of patients may be difficult to adequately assess over the telephone; they give the least-accurate histories and are most likely to have a life-threatening exposure. Every effort should be made to expedite their transfer to a healthcare facility capable of providing medical, psychiatric, and social assistance. The emergency physician should be extremely reluctant to categorize an adult exposure as unintentional and nontoxic without a complete evaluation.

CONSUMER PRODUCT SAFETY COMMISSION SIGNAL WORDS

To be considered a nontoxic exposure, the product label must not contain a Consumer Product Safety Commission "signal word." These signal words include *Caution*, *Warning*, and *Danger*.[1] Patients who have been exposed to a product containing a signal word require assessment by a healthcare provider knowledgeable in toxicology and capable of providing both basic and advanced poison management.

AMOUNT OF EXPOSURE

A reliable approximation of the amount of product or toxin ingested must be possible in order to establish whether an exposure is nontoxic. The detail required in the history of the amount ingested is directly related to the potential toxicity of the product. A much more precise history will be required for the patient who unintentionally ingests digoxin tablets than for the patient who unintentionally ingests oral contraceptives. The margin of error acceptable in quantifying the amount ingested is inversely related to the toxicity of the product.

Several logical conclusions can be reached from the magnitude of the ingestion: The patient who ingests 4 ounces of automotive motor oil may require psychiatric evaluation and counseling, whereas the patient who unintentionally takes a sip of the same motor oil may not require any care.

Although the 4-ounce ingestion will probably not result in significantly greater toxicity than the sip, one is unintentional and the other may be representative of either a grave psychiatric impairment or of suicidal intent. The likelihood is also greater that other substances have been concurrently ingested with the larger ingestion. The larger ingestion requires referral to an emergency department or healthcare facility for immediate evaluation, including psychiatric assessment. Little, if any, poison management would be required for either ingestion unless aspiration occurred. If it can be established that an ingestion is unintentional, the amount ingested can often be used to calculate the nontoxic nature of the exposure.

For example, if a 3-year-old (15-kg) child drank liquid acetaminophen (160 mg/5 mL) from a bottle containing 60 mL, an accurate analysis can be made of the maximum possible exposure based upon knowledge of the quantity of acetaminophen remaining.[10] In this example, knowing that 30 mL remains of a 60 mL bottle containing 32 mg/mL of acetaminophen enables the healthcare provider to determine that a total of 960 mg of acetaminophen was ingested. A dose-per-body-weight-exposure calculation (mg/kg) enables the determination of an ingestion of 64 mg/kg of acetaminophen. Because the toxicity data for acetaminophen poisonings predict that an acute ingestion of less than 150 mg/kg is not associated with hepatotoxicity,[11] the clinician can confidently categorize this ingestion as nontoxic. To ensure that no toxicity ensues, it is also necessary to determine that the child has not received any other acetaminophen during the previous 12–24 hours. If these questions can be answered with confidence, the administration of activated charcoal would not be necessary, nor would a visit to a healthcare facility for an acetaminophen blood level be necessary. The child would have had to ingest approximately 2.5 times the amount reported by history to reach the predicted threshold for hepatotoxicity. The clinician's or poison information specialist's only intervention should be to counsel the child's parents about the basic skills necessary to poison-proof the child's environment.

The assessment of an exposure or ingestion cannot be quantitative when two children simultaneously share exposure to a toxin. It is also difficult to assess the actual amount ingested when a large amount of a liquid product has been partially ingested and partially spilled on or around the child. In both of these situations, the only safe approach is to develop a worst-case scenario. When it is possible to determine exactly how much of the product is unaccounted for, it is necessary to assume that each child ingested the entire amount that is missing. In the situation in which a product has been partially spilled and partially ingested, it is again necessary to assume that the entire missing amount was ingested. It is extremely difficult to estimate how much liquid the child's clothing absorbed or how much liquid is present in a puddle on the bathroom or kitchen floor. If the product is well absorbed through the skin, the contribution it may play in a combined ingestion and dermal exposure is impossible to predict. The problem can be further complicated if the product contains highly volatile substances such as acetone, ethyl acetate, or ethyl or isopropyl alcohol, which may lead to toxicity not only by gastric absorption, but also by dermal absorption and inhalation.[4]

In summary, if an accurate estimate of the amount of the ingestion cannot be established, the prudent approach is to assume the worst-case scenario and to provide a higher level of care and surveillance than might initially appear necessary.

ROUTE OF EXPOSURE

The route(s) of exposure can often be accurately assessed from the available history. Determination of the amount of toxicity that is likely to occur from an exposure is largely dependent on how the patient was exposed.[5] Household products such as bleach, laundry detergents, ammonia, or rubber cement are generally nontoxic following a dermal exposure, minimally toxic following an oral exposure, but can cause considerable morbidity following inhalation or upon ophthalmic exposure. As in the case of most other products, if such household products are aspirated, the consequences may be significant. A routine part of assessing a patient for a nontoxic exposure should include careful questioning to exclude the possibility of multiple routes of exposure.

AN ABSENCE OF CLINICAL EFFECTS

The presence of symptoms (related to the exposure) is a clue that some toxic effect is occurring and that further assessment may be warranted. If symptoms are present, the exposure cannot be considered nontoxic, but this does not necessarily mean that a patient must be evaluated in a healthcare facility. If the symptoms are minor in severity and unlikely to result in further illness or complications, further medical evaluation may not be needed. The ingestion of products such as household bleach (2–5% sodium hypochlorite) is usually not associated with significant toxicity such as burns of the skin, oropharynx, or esophagus.[3] Following an ingestion of household bleach, the patient should not have pain, dysphagia, drooling, or dyspnea (Chap. 87), but it is common for a patient to vomit once following the ingestion of household bleach. If the child continues to vomit or shows any involvement of the respiratory tract such as coughing, shortness of breath, or any other difficulty in breathing, immediate medical care is needed. If the caller cannot reliably perform this assessment, the patient should be evaluated in an emergency department or by a physician.

FOLLOWUP CONSULTATION

Most triage decisions are based on the premise that followup consultation is possible and that the parent or guardian is reliable. Care must be taken in establishing that an exposure is nontoxic or minimally toxic. There is always the possibility that an error in judgment can occur. The option of care in the home is only possible if the poison center, physician's office, or emergency department is capable of making a followup call to ascertain that the victim has remained asymptomatic or that minor symptoms are resolving. A parent, guardian, or other responsible adult (not the victim) must be capable of recontacting the healthcare provider when there is either a change in the history or a change in the patient's clinical condition. At the time of the initial contact, it is extremely important to assess the reliability and capacity to understand and comply with the directions needed to monitor the exposed individual. Whenever a failure in communications occurs, or when there is a high probability of a communications breakdown, the patient should be brought into the healthcare environment.

A list of household items that generally do not result in toxicity appears in Table 4–2.[2] The list specifically applies to oral exposures, not to ophthalmic, cutaneous, or inhalational exposures.

TABLE 4–2. Household Items Generally Regarded as Nontoxic Following Oral Exposure

Personal-Use Items
Antiperspirants
Baby soaps
Baby lotion (without alcohol)
Baby shampoo
Baby wipes (without alcohol)
Bar soap
Bath oils (beads)
Body conditioners
Bubble bath
Chewing gum
Cologne (low alcohol content)
Cosmetics
Deodorants
Eye makeup
Fingernail polish (dry)
Hair products (dyes, sprays, tonics)
Hand lotion
Hand soap
Lipstick
Lip balm
Mascara
Petroleum jelly
Rouge
Shampoo (small amounts)
Shaving cream
Shoe polish (white)
Suntan lotion
Sunscreen products
Thermometer (elemental mercury not toxic if ingested)
Toothpaste (without fluoride)
Vitamins (without fluoride, iron, and niacin)

Art Supplies
Acacia
Ballpoint pen ink (blue and black)
Chalk
Charcoal
Clay
Crayons (marked A.P., C.P.)
Cyanoacrylate
Erasers
Felt-tip pens (waterbase)
Glow stick/jewelry
Ink (without aniline dyes)
Pencils (graphite)
Photographs
Plaster
Starch
Styrofoam
Water colors
Wax
White glue, paste

Toys
Bathtub toys
Etch-a-Sketch
Mylar balloons
Play-Doh
Silly-Putty
Teething rings
Toy cosmetics

Medications
Antacids
Antibiotics (with exceptions such as Chloramphenicol, Isoniazid, Penicillin)
Antibiotic ointment
Calamine lotion
Carboxymethyl cellulose
Clotrimazole cream
Corticosteroids
Glycerol
Lactaid
Lanolin
Oral contraceptives
Titanium oxide
Zinc oxide

Miscellaneous
Abrasives
Air fresheners
Hand dish-washing liquid soaps (not electric dishwashing type)
Aluminum foil
Ashes, wood/fireplace
Book matches (one book)
Candles (paraffin wax)
Charcoal briquettes
Cigarette ashes
Dehumidifying packets (silica or charcoal)
Grease, motor oil
Gypsum
Incense
Latex paint
Lubricant
Lubricating oils
Newspaper
Putty
Rust
Sachets (essential oils, powder)
Sesame oil
Sheet rock
Silica gel
Soil
Spackle
Stick-em Glue Traps
Sweetening agents (saccharin, cyclamate)
Wallboard
Tallow

Any of those routes of exposure may lead to significant morbidity and even mortality. The products can be conveniently divided into five major categories: personal-use items, art supplies, toys, medications, and miscellaneous household items.

REFERENCES

1. Craft AW, Lawson CR, Williams H, Sibert JR: Accidental childhood poisoning with household products. Br Med J 1984;288:682.
2. Done AK: Poisoning from common household products. Pediatr Clin North Am 1970;17:569–581.
3. Edwards JN, Jenkins, HL, Volans GN: Hazards of household cleaning products. Hum Toxicol 1982;1:403–409.
4. Litovitz TL: The alcohols: Ethanol, methanol, isopropanol, ethylene glycol. Pediatr Clin North Am 1986;33:311–323.
5. Lovejoy FH JR, Flowers J, McGuigan MA: The epidemiology of poisoning from household products. Vet Hum Toxicol 1979; 21(Suppl):33–34.
6. McGuigan MA: Poisoning in childhood. Emerg Med Clin North Am 1983;1:187–200.
7. Mofenson HC, Greensher J, Caraccio TR: Ingestions considered nontoxic. Emerg Med Clin North Am 1984;2:159–174.
8. Mofenson HC, Greensher J: The nontoxic ingestion. Pediatr Clin North Am 1970;17:583–590.
9. Motomatsu K, Adachi H, Uno T: Two infant deaths after inhaling baby powder. Chest 1979;75:448–450.
10. Osborne SC, Garrettson LK: Perception of toxicity and dose by 3- and 4-year-old children. Am J Dis Child 1985;139:790–792.
11. Peterson RG, Rumack BH: Toxicity of acetaminophen overdose. JACEP 1978;7:202–205.
12. Rogers J: Recurrent childhood poisoning as a family problem. J Fam Pract 1981;13:337–340.
13. Scalzo AJ: Diethylene glycol toxicity revisited: The 1996 Haitian epidemic. J Toxicol Clin Toxicol 1996;34:513–516.

CHAPTER 5

TECHNIQUES USED TO PREVENT GASTROINTESTINAL ABSORPTION OF TOXIC COMPOUNDS

Martin J. Smilkstein

Limiting ongoing absorption of toxic compounds is a core principle of care for poisoned patients. Gastrointestinal decontamination is the most common issue considered and the topic of this chapter; however, an understanding of dermal, ophthalmic, and respiratory decontamination is also important. Dermal decontamination is discussed in Chapter 29, decontamination of the eye in Chapter 27, and considerations for inhalation exposures in Chapter 95.

Although gastrointestinal decontamination has been a critical and familiar part of therapy of the poisoned patient for some time, no other area of medical toxicology has generated as much recent and continuing controversy. [15,37,78,90,152,154] The controversy arises because the results of clinically relevant studies of gastric emptying, activated charcoal, and cathartics challenge many of the assumptions on which previous therapy was based. Studies of gastric emptying fail to show benefit, or find benefit only in limited circumstances. [4,91,108,128] Activated charcoal appears to be more effective than gastric emptying in many cases, [44,115] and often may enhance drug elimination in addition to decreasing absorption. [19,20,38] These findings are among many that have radically changed concepts about gastrointestinal decontamination. [70,78]

Despite these ongoing controversies, a great deal of information is available that can form the basis for a rational approach to gastrointestinal decontamination. For specific information on dosages and technical aspects of delivering gastrointestinal decontamination modalities, see Chapters 3 and 31 and these Antidotes in Depth: Syrup of Ipecac, Activated Charcoal, Cathartics, and Whole-Bowel Irrigation. This chapter discusses a conceptual approach to the use of those modalities that can be modified, as new data become available.

Because of variations in patient age, agent ingested, severity of symptoms, time since ingestion, presence of coingestants, and numerous other factors, it is inappropriate to create simplistic gastrointestinal decontamination guidelines. A single strategy may not always be logical, even in treating the same type of ingestion in two different patients. It is more useful to understand each intervention and its limitations, and then to consider each clinical situation individually using a logical approach. The first consideration is often whether or not to empty the stomach.

WHAT CONSIDERATIONS GUIDE APPROPRIATE GASTRIC EMPTYING DECISIONS?

The decision to utilize or forgo gastric emptying should be based on whether it is reasonable to expect that a beneficial amount of drug removal can be safely accomplished by gastric emptying.

Several factors must be considered: (a) the risk or potential danger to the patient caused by the ingestion; (b) the likelihood that gastric emptying will remove a clinically significant amount of the ingestion; (c) the benefits of removing that amount of agent; (d) the risks of gastric emptying; and (e) the availability and utility of alternative methods to limit absorption or effectively treat the poisoning.

What Factors Indicate That Ongoing Absorption May Be Dangerous?

An assessment of the risk to the patient includes a consideration of the amount and type of agent ingested and the clinical course since ingestion. If the clinician is confident that the ingestion was of a nontoxic agent or of a nontoxic amount of a potentially toxic agent, then obviously gastric emptying is not indicated.

If the history obtained suggests a toxic ingestion but the clinical course excludes toxicity, then gastric emptying is inappropriate. For example, consider an asymptomatic patient with a history of ingesting several diazepam tablets 6 hours earlier, with no access to other agents, and observed by family members to be asymptomatic throughout that 6-hour period. Regardless of the amount reportedly ingested, such a patient does not require gastric emptying. The absorption and onset of the clinical effects of diazepam occur rapidly, and the clinical course effectively excludes the ingestion. Such decisions require familiarity with the agent involved: 6 hours without symptoms is adequate to exclude significant iron poisoning, but it is inadequate to exclude poisoning by sustained-release verapamil or diltiazem, a sulfonylurea, or a monoamine oxidase inhibitor, each of which may cause delayed life-threatening symptoms.

Such an approach is appropriate only when other ingestants can be excluded. Because this is often not the case, many patients should be managed as though they have either a more recent, larger, or different (and potentially toxic) ingestion than that described to the healthcare practitioner. Another exception should be made for ingestions of extraordinarily high potential risk. Although the benefit of gastric emptying remains unproved for the majority of these high-potential-risk ingestions, patients with high-risk ingestions are either not specifically studied or are expressly excluded, and as is discussed later, some data suggest evidence of gastric emptying benefit in this group. Therefore, the safest course at this time is to perform gastric emptying on patients with undefined, potentially lethal ingestions or with recognized high-risk ingestions (eg, cyanide, colchicine, chloroquine, aspirin, cyclic antidepressants, verapamil), sometimes even if the patient is asymptomatic beyond the time that onset of toxicity would be expected by history.

Can Gastric Emptying Remove a Clinically Significant Amount of the Agent Ingested?

The likelihood that gastric emptying will effectively remove a clinically significant amount of the agent depends on whether any of the agent remains in the stomach and whether the gastric emptying technique chosen can in fact remove it. Absorption of many agents (eg, alcohols, most acetaminophen formulations) is so rapid that essentially no toxin remains in the stomach after a few hours,[22] and gastric emptying is therefore not indicated. Even for the many toxins that are more slowly absorbed, the yield of delayed gastric emptying is often unimpressive.[42] Uncontrolled clinical studies[41,42] suggest that other than anticholinergics, sedative-hypnotics, and opioids (drugs that slow gastrointestinal motility), drugs are unlikely to be recoverable by gastric emptying more than 2–4 hours after ingestion. These results, as in the case of other gastric emptying research, suggest little potential value of gastric emptying in most cases, but fail to resolve the question of benefit to the subset of individuals at very high risk.

Drugs with or without the ability to slow gut motility can also remain in the stomach if they tend to form adherent masses. Aspirin (especially enteric-coated),[21] iron,[58] meprobamate,[75] and phenobarbital[77] serve as examples of this phenomenon, although this may also occur following massive ingestion of many agents. Drugs such as aspirin that may cause pylorospasm also cause prolonged gastric retention. Clinical anecdotes including postmortem information clearly show that, in some cases, large amounts of drug can remain in the stomach for hours to days. Even rapidly absorbed drugs may remain in the stomach for unusually long periods under certain clinical conditions.[145] These observations continue to stimulate the use of delayed gastric emptying despite the lack of proven clinical efficacy.

The occurrence of antecedent spontaneous vomiting is often considered another determinant of whether or not an agent remains in the stomach. Although it is true that some drug may remain in the stomach after repeated episodes of spontaneous vomiting, it is unlikely that either lavage or emesis can subsequently remove a significant amount. To induce further emesis or to perform orogastric lavage is not only futile, it may increase the risk of complications, and in the case of the use of syrup of ipecac, makes subsequent administration of activated charcoal more difficult.[44] Any attempt to determine how much antecedent vomiting is sufficient to obviate gastric emptying is clearly speculative and a matter of clinical judgment. As is true for most issues related to gastrointestinal decontamination, the degree of risk to the patient from the ingestion must be considered along with the complications from the procedure. For example, it is logical to forego gastric emptying after a codeine ingestion if the patient has vomited two or three times, but orogastric lavage might be appropriate after the same amount of vomiting following a massive colchicine overdose.

What Clinical Benefits of Gastric Emptying Have Been Demonstrated?

Gastric emptying can result in removal of drug from the stomach of poisoned patients,[13,24,41] and volunteer studies demonstrate that drug absorption can be decreased,[144] but neither of these observations proves clinical benefit. Although a difficult issue to study, clinical benefit from gastric emptying is, to date, demonstrable only in patients with serious overdoses when gastric emptying is accomplished within 1 hour of the ingestion.[91] Other authors are unable to describe a benefit at all.[108,128] New guidelines emphasize these studies and conclude that gastric emptying should be entirely abandoned, or used only in extraordinary situations.[15,37,90,152,154] While these studies do demonstrate that the majority of patients can be treated effectively with activated charcoal alone, they clearly do not prove that either timely or delayed gastric emptying is ineffective in all cases.

It is worthwhile to examine how the limitations of these studies should affect their interpretation. The decision to perform gastric emptying should be largely based on speculation that the ingestion may lead to a clinically unstable, life-threatening condition for which even a small decrease in toxic exposure may be critical. The impact of gastric emptying on the clinical outcome of patients with the most dangerous exposures is therefore of greatest interest. Studies thus far include patients with a wide variety of overdoses and possible exposures, the vast majority of whom are expected to do well with supportive care alone. This is particularly true of those patients who had no actual exposure, but who were included in the study because of the technical difficulties in confirming most suspected poisonings. Clearly, it is difficult to show any therapeutic benefit in this situation, and study of this heterogeneous group of cases does not resolve the question in the most important subset. Understandably, no controlled study to date has included enough patients with confirmed life-threatening ingestions to adequately compare outcome with and without gastric emptying. It is also important to consider certain other drug subsets, such as sustained-release formulations, drugs likely to form aggregations or to cause pylorospasm, amounts of drug large enough to exceed the adsorptive capacity of activated charcoal, and agents not well adsorbed to activated charcoal. Although gastric emptying would seem most logical after these ingestions, either they were not studied separately or they were excluded from study altogether.[91,108]

In one study, in which the author concludes that gastric emptying is futile, the results actually appear to suggest benefit to gastric emptying in the highest-risk patients.[128] In 8 of 10 analyses of groups subdivided by severity or time to presentation and compared with regard to incidence of improvement and deterioration, results were better in the groups undergoing gastric emptying. Despite small subgroup size, these differences approached or achieved statistical significance in four of these analyses. The authors discount these observations as either a consequence of other factors or as not statistically significant. Power analysis indicated that the group size of the "severely" intoxicated group was only large enough to detect a 50% reduction in poor outcome from gastric emptying. Very few medical interventions provide such dramatic results, and lesser degrees of benefit may be important, particularly in patients very close to life-threatening thresholds of toxicity.

An earlier study demonstrated benefit to gastric emptying among the most ill, despite the fact that seven critically ill patients were excluded from the study.[91] Within any large sample of poisoned patients, the incidence of serious toxicity is low, and the ability to demonstrate benefit despite exclusion of a significant portion of the sickest patients is noteworthy. In combination with the above-mentioned recent data, such observations suggest that gastric emptying will continue to benefit a small, but critically important subset of patients.

An example of an analogous consideration is thrombolytic therapy for acute myocardial infarction. If thrombolytic therapy is assessed among all patients with chest pain, there is no evidence of benefit, and it is likely that harm will be evident because of treatment. If, instead, appropriate criteria are selected to define the patients at highest risk for consequential myocardial infarction and the conditions most likely to be associated with benefit, thrombolysis is an extraordinarily effective therapy. This effect, sometimes called the Pollyanna phenomenon, similarly explains why, as in the above studies, no benefit is identified from gastric emptying if all patients with actual or potential overdose are considered. What remains to be done is to define the characteristics of patients with overdoses most likely to benefit from gastric emptying, and to study those cases.

It is unlikely that gastric emptying decisions will ever be amenable to strict predetermined criteria. Instead, a case-by-case analysis considering the factors that make gastric emptying more or less logical is appropriate (Table 5–1). In most cases, gastric emptying is only suggested for patients with ingestions matching several of the listed features. In some cases, however, the potential lethality of the ingestion is so great that a single feature might appropriately prompt orogastric lavage.

Until these issues are better evaluated, the value of gastric emptying will remain controversial. Studies clearly support the use of a selective approach and result in decreased patient discomfort, complications, and cost from unnecessary gastric emptying. Nonetheless, it is inappropriate to generalize these findings to include patients at highest risk. Based on current studies, it is neither scientifically nor logically sound to withhold gastric emptying from patients with overdoses of cyanide, colchicine, cyclic antidepressants, and many other potentially lethal ingestions; or after large ingestions of aspirin, β-adrenergic antagonists, or calcium channel blockers and other agents with delayed and prolonged toxicity; or ingestions of lithium, iron, or other less adsorbable agents (see individual chapters for expanded discussion). To establish the appropriate indications for gastric emptying in the context of these observations, it is critical to consider the possible risks. As the benefits of other modes of gastrointestinal decontamination are identified, they may supplant or complement those of

gastric emptying. For example, whole-bowel irrigation has essentially displaced gastric emptying for patients with consequential sustained-release tablet ingestions.

What Are the Potential Complications of Gastric Emptying?

Gastric emptying is usually safe but can cause significant morbidity. Complications are very rare, and most are preventable by appropriate patient selection and the use of appropriate techniques (Chaps. 3 and 31). Orogastric lavage can cause esophageal tears or perforation.[91,161] In addition, following lavage, nasal, oral, and pharyngeal injury, pyriform sinus and gastric perforation, and tracheal aspiration can occur.[103] Other complications described following nasogastric tube placement in settings other than poisoning management, such as tracheal intubation, pulmonary hemorrhage, pneumothorax, and empyema, are all potential complications of orogastric lavage. Therapeutic use of syrup of ipecac may result in aspiration,[91,127] protracted vomiting,[35] Mallory-Weiss tears,[143] intracerebral hemorrhage,[87] pneumomediastinum and pneumoretroperitoneum,[159] and diaphragmatic rupture.[131] Attempts at gastric emptying may also propel ingested material beyond the pylorus, where many drugs are more readily absorbed.[134]

Perhaps the most common avoidable morbidity occurs in the somewhat combative patient who resists attempts at gastric emptying. If patient movement cannot be well controlled, alternatives to orogastric lavage must be considered. In the majority of such cases, there is little evidence for efficacy of gastric emptying, good evidence that activated charcoal will be effective (discussed later), and significant risk for injury to the patient or staff during the procedure. In the unusual case in which gastric emptying is deemed to be very important, persistent attempts at lavage may be indicated. Although the use of sedation or neuromuscular paralysis is common prior to orogastric lavage,[48] except to obtain airway control such measures are almost never indicated. Except in vanishingly rare circumstances, the risks of sedation and paralysis far outweigh the benefits of gastric emptying, and orogastric lavage can be avoided or delayed until clinical findings permit the procedure without additional risk.

Contraindications to gastric emptying include any situation when it is unnecessary or ineffective (see the earlier discussion) or potentially dangerous. For example, gastric emptying is illogical after ingestion of alkaline caustics (Chap. 87), which cause consequential local injury but carry little risk from systemic absorption. Gastric emptying cannot be safely undertaken in these cases, and would not be expected to be of any value. The advisability of gastric emptying is more controversial after ingestion of agents such as phenols and acids, which, although caustic, can also cause systemic toxicity by absorption (Chap. 87). With some caustic agents, such as mercuric chloride, the potential systemic toxicity is so great that gastric emptying seems clearly warranted despite the presence of probable gastric injury.

What Are the Appropriate Alternatives to Gastric Emptying?

Assessment of the risk/benefit ratio of gastric emptying should consider alternative treatments. Some authors suggest the use of no gastrointestinal decontamination at all;[108] however, the most important alternative to gastric emptying is the use of activated charcoal alone. In volunteer studies following small ingestions of agents well adsorbed to activated charcoal, activated charcoal is

---

TABLE 5–1. Factors that Cumulatively Increase the Appropriateness of Gastric Emptying*

- Substantial risk of consequential toxicity: eg, ingestion of aspirin, chloroquine, colchicine, cyclic antidepressants, calcium channel blockers
- Evidence of consequential toxicity: eg, repeated seizures, hypotension, cardiac dysrhythmias, apnea, acid-base or other metabolic disturbances
- Antidotal or adjunctive therapy ineffective or nonexistent: eg, colchicine, paraquat
- Recent ingestion (<1–2 h)
- Ingestion exceeds adsorptive capacity of initial activated charcoal dosing: eg, >100 mg/kg of pills such as aspirin, sustained-release verapamil, sustained-release theophylline
- Ingested agent not adsorbed by activated charcoal: eg, iron, lithium
- Ingested agent likely to form durable mass after overdose: eg, large amounts of aspirin, enteric-coated agents, iron, meprobamate
- Ingestions of extended or sustained-release formulations: eg, calcium channel blockers, theophylline
- No antecedent vomiting
- Gastric tube placement required for activated charcoal administration
- No contraindications to gastric emptying

*The explanations and examples that follow each factor are meant only to illustrate the concepts, and are not intended to be comprehensive. See text for further discussion.

more effective in preventing drug absorption than is gastric emptying.[44,106,116,149] Studies of actual drug overdoses find gastric emptying followed by activated charcoal to be no more effective than activated charcoal alone for the majority of poisoned patients.[91,108,128] Because the activated charcoal–to-drug ratio is one of the most important determinants of activated charcoal efficacy,[122] the amount of drug ingested may determine whether activated charcoal alone is likely to be adequate. For patients with small ingestions of agents well adsorbed to activated charcoal, there is good support for the use of activated charcoal alone.

An activated charcoal–to-drug ratio of 10:1 can serve to illustrate this important concept. This commonly mentioned ratio is a midrange value from in vitro studies[7] of uncertain clinical value, because ideal ratios vary by agent and GI conditions, but it serves as a useful conceptual guide. Using lorazepam as an example, to achieve a 10:1 activated charcoal–to-drug ratio in a patient who has ingested 100 tablets of 2 mg each requires only 2 g of activated charcoal. In an adult, a typical activated charcoal dose of 1 g/kg of body weight is likely to be effective in reducing further drug absorption. From another perspective, 2 g of activated charcoal theoretically treats an ingestion of one thousand 0.2-mg clonidine tablets (200 mg total), whereas even 100 g of activated charcoal is ineffective after an ingestion of only fifty 300-mg theophylline tablets (15 g total). Activated charcoal is still a critical part of management of patients with large ingestions, but gastric emptying may take on greater importance as an adjunct in these situations.

The availability of an antidote or adjunctive therapy may also affect the decision to forego gastric emptying. When there is no clear indication for gastric emptying, the risk of subsequent unexpected gastrointestinal absorption is more acceptable if there is a very effective treatment or antidote available. Antidotal therapy obviously should not replace gastric emptying if gastric emptying is clearly effective, but this is not usually the case. Consider a patient who reportedly ingested 25 tablets of acetaminophen with codeine 4.5 hours earlier. Absorption would probably be complete even if slowed by codeine. Because there is probably little or no benefit of gastric emptying at this point, and because there are effective antidotes for both acetaminophen (*N*-acetylcysteine) and codeine (naloxone), it is appropriate to forego gastric emptying.

Summary: Gastric Emptying

The use of gastric emptying should be a selective (Table 5–1), not a routine procedure. Gastric emptying is largely an unproved therapy that is, nevertheless, useful in some situations when it can be accomplished safely. The method chosen should consider the nature of the poison and the current and projected clinical status of the patient. Rarely, if ever, should the patient be placed at additional serious risk to empty the stomach.

WHEN GASTRIC EMPTYING IS INDICATED, WHICH TECHNIQUE SHOULD BE USED?

Until 1985, syrup of ipecac was routinely administered after ingestions unless the patient was comatose, or convulsing, or had lost the gag reflex; under these circumstances, orogastric lavage was recommended. Comparing the risks and benefits of these two methods, it became apparent that this approach was far too simplistic. While earlier debate focused primarily on which method removed more drug,[1,11,25] more recent work attempts to view these modalities in the context of the whole patient. Determining relative benefit includes consideration of the amount of drug removed, whether that removal is consequential, comparison of the potential complications of each gastric emptying technique, and the impact of each upon the use of other important treatment methods such as activated charcoal and oral antidotes. In most circumstances, comparison of induced emesis and orogastric lavage is only of historical interest; however, the analysis is instructive.

Is Either Emesis or Orogastric Lavage Superior in Prevention of Toxin Absorption?

Attempts to determine conclusively whether emesis or lavage removes more drug fail partly because of study design but more importantly because there may be no single correct answer. With respect to study design, studies of emesis or lavage recovery of liquid barium from puppies[1] or magnesium hydroxide solution from children[43] performed soon after ingestion may have little or no bearing on the potential to recover solid pill fragments 2–3 hours after overdose. Similarly, studies of lavage utilizing small-bore nasogastric tubes[25] do not provide useful information about the efficacy of lavage as practiced, using large-bore orogastric tubes. Other study design issues are evident in the literature and have led to a variety of conflicting and inaccurate conclusions.

Currently, no adequately controlled study shows either emesis or lavage as clearly superior in drug removal.[133] Both are probably equivalent overall, but in the clinical setting of an actual specific ingestion, the overall results are not relevant. The results of several gastric emptying studies emphasize this fact. Although children given a standard dose of a magnesium hydroxide marker immediately before syrup of ipecac–induced emesis vomited an average of 28% of the marker, the range was 0 to 78%.[43] In another study, syrup of ipecac and lavage each resulted in average removal of about half of the ingested material, but the range of retained material in the gastrointestinal tract was 0 to 100%.[134] Similar variability is noted in other controlled studies,[11] and the actual overdose setting certainly offers substantially more variables than these studies.

What Substances Will Pass Through an Orogastric Lavage Tube?

Another factor in considering whether emesis or lavage is preferable for a patient with a particular ingestion is the formulation of the substance (eg, liquid, tablet, capsule, enteric coating, size, shape) as it relates to the tube lumen size and the mechanics of orogastric lavage. Large drug packets, pills, or pill fragments (particularly enteric coated and sustained release), adherent masses of pills, and plant or mushroom fragments will not pass through even a 40-French lavage tube.[2] If gastric emptying is appropriate, ipecac-induced emesis may be more logical for this group of ingestions. This issue is even more important when the patient is a small child. Passing a very large-bore tube in an infant is impossible, and a 24-French tube is probably the largest that can safely be used. As a result, substances that might be effectively removed by lavage in an adult cannot be lavaged from a child. In many cases, however, although lavage may not return a substantial amount of solid material, syrup of ipecac–induced emesis may be contraindicated. In such cases, lavage should be considered for the removal of dissolved drug and small fragments as well as for the administration of activated charcoal.

When Is Emesis Contraindicated?

Deciding between syrup of ipecac–induced emesis and lavage is more often based on a consideration of potential risks than on efficacy. The most important of these risks is the aspiration of stomach contents into the tracheobronchial tree. Any patient who initially lacks the ability to protect his or her airway, or who is likely to lose airway-protective reflexes during the duration of action of syrup of ipecac, must not have emesis induced. Instead, if gastric emptying is indicated, such a patient should be lavaged after endotracheal intubation. An ingestion of any substance causing or capable of rapidly causing a decreased level of consciousness, seizure, cardiovascular collapse, or neuromuscular paralysis should be managed in this manner. Examples of substances that may preclude the use of syrup of ipecac are camphor, cyclic antidepressants, isoniazid, propoxyphene, and propranolol; but many, if not most, serious overdoses may fit this description. The limited potential benefit offered by emesis does not justify placing the patient at risk for aspiration.

Induction of emesis is also contraindicated following ingestions of foreign bodies likely to cause mechanical injury or upper airway obstruction and in patients with certain structural lesions or bleeding diatheses. Contraindications to emesis are summarized in Table 31–4 and should be considered in addition to contraindications to gastric emptying in general.

How Does the Anticipated Use of Activated Charcoal or Other Oral Antidotes Impact the Choice of Gastric Emptying Method?

The increasing appreciation of the efficacy of activated charcoal also has a profound effect on the approach to gastric emptying. In addition to replacing gastric emptying in many settings, activated charcoal is useful following gastric emptying in the vast majority of ingestions and is absolutely essential in some (see Antidotes in Depth: Activated Charcoal). Orogastric lavage can usually be accomplished rapidly and then followed quickly by administration of activated charcoal via the lavage tube. Syrup of ipecac results in significant delays in charcoal administration, as a consequence of the combination of delay to its onset of effect and a period of repeated emesis and subsequent nausea during recovery. Because delayed administration of activated charcoal decreases its efficacy, emesis has been largely abandoned or replaced by lavage in cases involving ingestions of toxic substances well adsorbed to activated charcoal.

The effective use of oral *N*-acetylcysteine and other oral agents can also be delayed by the use of syrup of ipecac. Patients poisoned with acetaminophen are often nauseated from the ingestion itself, making the effective use of oral *N*-acetylcysteine difficult. Using syrup of ipecac in this situation will increase their tendency to vomit, further preventing or delaying effective use of *N*-acetylcysteine. In summary, if *N*-acetylcysteine or other oral agents are needed within 2–3 hours and gastric emptying is indicated, orogastric lavage is the preferred method.

Are There Other Unique Considerations?

The at-home use of syrup of ipecac for children who are not subsequently treated at a healthcare facility, as often recommended by poison information specialists, represents an important clinical issue. Thus far, activated charcoal is not a widely available or a practical alternative in the home,[32,47,50,69,88,94,121] and studies of gastric emptying efficacy are largely irrelevant in the assessment of this form of intervention. Because of the nature of such exposures, the potential benefit of emesis in this setting would likely be avoidance of an emergency department visit, rather than avoidance of consequential clinical deterioration. Without the use of ipecac, would symptoms occur from the exposure that are not dangerous, but that are noticeable enough to prompt medical evaluation? Are other symptoms masked by, or misattributed to, ipecac-induced emesis? Does the induction of emesis provide reassurance to parents or poison center staff, facilitating home observation? Given the high incidence of minor, unintentional pediatric exposures (Chap. 106), these questions are extraordinarily important to resolve.

A much rarer gastric emptying challenge is the "body stuffer" (Chap. 67). Body stuffers are people who spontaneously, and without antecedent preparation, ingest packets containing illicit drugs, generally in an attempt to conceal evidence of drug possession. The amount ingested is often unclear, there is significant risk of drug container leakage, and there is no reliable early test to confirm and quantify the ingestion.[71] The drugs involved, typically cocaine or heroin, may cause abrupt clinical deterioration, but in the overwhelming majority of cases no identifiable toxicity occurs. Lavage is ineffective because of the size of the drug packages; syrup of ipecac-induced emesis is potentially dangerous because of the possibility of clinical deterioration before or during emesis; and observation alone means a lengthy hospitalization that is most often unnecessary and for which there is no clear endpoint. Some authors believe that ipecac-induced emesis deserves consideration if the ingestion involves a small amount of drug; if there is no evidence of drug leakage or drug effect by history or physical examination; if the drug containers are crack vials or sealed water-resistant bags that are less likely to result in early massive leakage; and if there is no contraindication to emesis. There is certainly no consensus on the management of these patients, but in our opinion, there is no role for syrup of ipecac–induced emesis in these cases. We feel that the risk of subsequent deterioration can never be predicted and thus favor the use of activated charcoal and whole-bowel irrigation (described later in this chapter).

Some sustained-release pharmaceutical preparations present a special problem because the bulk of the pill matrix remains largely intact even as the active drug is released. These dissolution characteristics result in a pill that persists for many hours, too large to pass through a lavage tube.[2] In this case, lavage is ineffective and emesis will significantly complicate effective activated-charcoal delivery, but such ingestions are often very serious and may be too massive to rely on activated charcoal alone. In many such cases, use of whole-bowel irrigation is logical, but questions related to gastric emptying may be pertinent. For example, consider a patient who presents within an hour of a massive ingestion of persistent-matrix theophylline or verapamil, without antecedent vomiting. Is induction of emesis a logical intervention?

Apomorphine is a morphine derivative with diminished analgesic action and potent emetic effects mediated by stimulation of the chemoreceptor trigger zone and possibly the vestibular apparatus.[100] It generally induces emesis within 3–5 minutes of a single subcutaneous dose. However, it produces concomitant central nervous system and respiratory depression, and holds the potential for severe or protracted vomiting. It is also currently unavailable in a premixed parenteral form. Although there are data to suggest that naloxone may reverse vomiting and at least some of the adverse effects associated with apomorphine,[23] it is unlikely that it will ever be used for this clinical indication. A related, more practical issue is the capability of newer potent antiemetics to reverse the emetic effects of syrup of ipecac.[109] Although these potential therapies are mentioned, they remain only areas of investigation and there are no data to support their use at this time.

Summary: Emesis versus Orogastric Lavage

In summary, when gastric emptying is indicated in a hospital, orogastric lavage is almost always preferable to syrup of ipecac–induced emesis. Emesis continues to be important following the ingestion of large pills that do not disintegrate, ingestions by infants and small children in whom large-bore tubes cannot be used safely, very recent ingestion of lithium or other agents that are not adsorbed by activated charcoal, and for home use. These guidelines are not absolute and always must be considered on an individual basis, recognizing potential contraindications and alternatives for a particular patient and a particular poison.

WHAT IS THE ROLE OF ACTIVATED CHARCOAL?

There is no question that activated charcoal is important in the management of toxicologic emergencies, but its role is still being defined. Like other treatment modalities, the appropriate use of activated charcoal should be determined by analysis of the relative risks and benefits of its use. Adverse effects are rare despite its widespread use, but in the absence of well-controlled studies in poisoned patients it is difficult to accurately assess its clinical benefit.

How Beneficial Is Activated Charcoal?

It is necessary to consider separately the two potential benefits of activated charcoal: preventing the absorption of toxic agents from the gastrointestinal tract and enhancing the elimination of agents already absorbed. For activated charcoal to prevent systemic absorption of toxic substances from the gastrointestinal tract effectively, the substance must be adsorbed by activated charcoal and still be present in the gastrointestinal tract at the time of activated charcoal administration. When both of these conditions are met, there is no doubt that activated charcoal results in diminished absorption, lower peak serum concentration, and decreased area under the concentration versus time curve. Activated charcoal has been studied with hundreds of substances in vitro, in animals, in human volunteers, and in patients with actual overdoses.[26,38,118,126] Although controlled studies showing clinical benefit are not available, these other data are convincing enough to warrant the use of activated charcoal soon after most ingestions.

Even substances not well adsorbed qualitatively to activated charcoal may nevertheless be adequately adsorbed from a quantitative perspective, and thus activated charcoal may be beneficial even following these exposures. For example, based on in vitro studies, cyanide is considered to be poorly adsorbed by activated charcoal, because 1 g of activated charcoal binds only 35 mg of potassium cyanide, far less than other toxic agents studied.[7] If the same ratio were to hold in an actual patient, then delivery of 60 g

of activated charcoal could adsorb 2.1 g of potassium cyanide, well above the expected lethal dose. In vivo efficacy of activated charcoal in the treatment of cyanide poisoning was demonstrated in an animal model,[93] suggesting that this logic is valid and that it may apply to other potentially lethal agents as well. As the amount ingested increases and the binding affinity decreases, the stoichiometric advantage is lost and this approach clearly becomes less effective. Typical ingestions of ethanol, lithium, or iron, for example, involve several grams of drug; thus, the very limited adsorption of each to activated charcoal makes this modality clinically insignificant. In fact, of all commonly ingested substances, ethanol, lithium, and iron are the only ones for which activated charcoal is documented to be completely ineffective.[119]

There are other substances described in qualitative terms as being poorly adsorbed to activated charcoal that are nevertheless adsorbed to an extent that may justify the administration of activated charcoal. Hydrocarbons are said to be poorly adsorbed, yet activated charcoal decreased gastrointestinal absorption of kerosene, benzene, and dichloroethane in rats.[92] Metals are similarly described as poorly adsorbed, but significant activated charcoal adsorption of mercuric chloride was first noted in the 1940s,[7] and its therapeutic use in mercury poisoning dates to the 19th century. For many agents, only in vitro data are available, which may or may not be applicable.

Regardless of the ingestion history, administration of activated charcoal may be appropriate due to the likelihood of inaccurate information or unrecognized coingestion of agents that are well adsorbed. For substances that are well adsorbed, activated charcoal decreases drug absorption from the gastrointestinal tract and enhances elimination of drug already absorbed; thus, its use is often appropriate regardless of the interval since ingestion. An initial dose of activated charcoal should be administered in nearly all cases of potentially toxic ingestions unless contraindicated.

Because of concerns that orogastric lavage might delay activated charcoal administration, or might increase drug absorption by dissolving a drug or pushing it out of the stomach into the small intestine, some have suggested that activated charcoal be administered prior to or during lavage.[30,134] Although theoretically appealing, this approach has obvious practical disadvantages and its true value remains to be determined. Although one volunteer study found that lavage forced marker past the pylorus,[134] another did not.[135] In addition, proper patient positioning[156] and proper lavage technique should limit drug passage beyond the pylorus. As a result, activated charcoal prior to or during lavage is rarely indicated, but it may be appropriate after particularly massive or dangerous ingestions.

Multiple-dose activated charcoal (MDAC) may also be indicated to prevent absorption in several circumstances when a significant amount of the agent is likely to remain in the gastrointestinal tract. Some ingestions are too massive to be effectively adsorbed by a single dose of activated charcoal. In other cases, the continuous release of drug from a sustained-release formulation or from concretion makes repeated doses of activated charcoal a logical choice. Only a few agents probably lead to formation of true concretions, but persistence of large quantities of undissolved drug in any form has similar clinical implications. Many substances slow gastrointestinal motility and are thus particularly likely to remain in the gastrointestinal tract, especially following large ingestions. Although cyclic antidepressants, calcium channel blockers, phenothiazines, anticholinergics, opioids, and sedative-hypnotics are usually associated with delayed gastrointestinal passage, many other substances are also capable of effectively delaying gastrointestinal passage directly or indirectly by altering electrolytes, changing blood pressure, causing mechanical obstruction or pylorospasm, or by other mechanisms. As a result, MDAC is often appropriate regardless of whether or not the ingested substance is known to slow motility or cause concretions.

MDAC is far more controversial as a method of enhancing elimination of toxic substances (see Antidotes in Depth: Activated Charcoal).[33,38,119,126,150] For it to be effective in enhancing elimination of a given substance, the substance must either undergo enterohepatic recirculation or, more often, be present to a significant extent in circulating blood (enteroenteric recirculation, or "gut dialysis") and be well adsorbed to activated charcoal. For some substances, such as theophylline, there is good evidence that MDAC substantially limits absorption and enhances elimination. For many other substances, MDAC alters drug kinetics favorably, but the change is small. In still other cases, despite in vitro adsorption, no effect is noted in volunteers.

Applying the results of these studies to the overdose setting remains difficult. There are profound differences between drug pharmacokinetics at doses used in therapeutic or volunteer studies and toxicokinetics in poisoned patients. Depending on whether the drug is likely to persist in the gastrointestinal tract and whether the elimination of the drug is zero-order, first-order, or Michaelis-Menten, the effect of activated charcoal in overdose may be less than, equal to, or more than that reported at a low drug dosage.[39] There is also uncertainty as to how much effect on drug kinetics is required to produce a clinical benefit.[150] For example, many authors argue that MDAC is not useful for treating salicylate overdose because it either has no effect[76] or only slightly augments salicylate elimination.[85,105] On the other hand, proponents of MDAC in this setting speculate that a small reduction in the area under the concentration versus time curve[80] might be enough to prevent some component of delayed clinical deterioration. On the basis of current information, utilization of MDAC is appropriate in many such potentially serious ingestions, when it can be accomplished safely.

Can Activated Charcoal Harm the Patient? Is It Ever Contraindicated?

Activated charcoal is generally safe and has few contraindications. Most patients with caustic ingestions who require endoscopy should not receive activated charcoal, because activated charcoal does not effectively adsorb most caustics. In addition, activated charcoal obscures the endoscopist's view. Although most patients tolerate activated charcoal well, at least some patients do vomit after receiving it. As a result, it is also contraindicated in patients with ingestions of pure petroleum distillates and other agents that are not well adsorbed to activated charcoal but that do carry a high risk of pulmonary aspiration. It should be noted that other toxic hydrocarbons (eg, benzene) and agents found in combination with hydrocarbons (eg, pesticides) are not well studied and may be at least partially adsorbed by activated charcoal, making its administration appropriate.

Minor adverse effects of activated charcoal, including nausea, vomiting, and constipation, are common.[1,5,119] Pulmonary aspiration is the most serious complication that may occur in the overdose setting. Activated charcoal is occasionally noted in the respiratory tract, and several cases of aspiration, including fatalities,[18,51,68,107] are described.[45,63,67,127] It is inappropriate to consider

these cases the result of activated charcoal use; instead, they illustrate failure to secure adequate airway protection or direct instillation of activated charcoal into the trachea after improper nasogastric or orogastric tube placement. In addition to massive consequential aspiration, trivial charcoal aspiration is very common. An endotracheal tube cuff does not provide a perfect seal, and small amounts of black-tinged secretions are occasionally suctioned from intubated patients with properly protected airways.[111] There is no evidence that the administration of oral activated charcoal increases the risk of aspiration in patients with intact airway protective reflexes. Although it increases lung microvascular permeability, causing acute lung injury in animal models,[12] there is no evidence that it causes more severe sequellae than equivalent aspiration of gastric contents without activated charcoal. In summary, if appropriate standards of airway protection and activated charcoal administration techniques are observed, there appears to be no increased risk of consequential pulmonary aspiration as a result of activated charcoal. This concern is therefore an inappropriate reason to forgo activated charcoal therapy.

Although there are few credible reports of other serious complications from a single dose of activated charcoal, cases of bowel obstruction or pseudo-obstruction are described following MDAC.[27,57,65,66,99,129,158] Although extraordinarily rare, these cases deserve consideration. Most cases involve the administration of repeated activated charcoal dosing at 3–6-hour intervals for 36–120 hours. As experience with MDAC continues, other cases may be reported. This rare but serious risk should be weighed against the potential benefits. In a patient with decreased gastrointestinal motility, MDAC might be continued despite the risk if there were good evidence of enhanced toxin elimination (eg, massive phenobarbital or theophylline overdose). On the other hand, if ileus is present, MDAC might not be warranted when there is little reason to expect much yield (eg, cyclic antidepressant overdose). Most reports of serious complications after MDAC are actually the result of multiple cathartic doses. Because so many commercial preparations combine both agents, it is of critical importance to specify activated charcoal without cathartic when ordering MDAC for a patient (cathartics are discussed later in this chapter).

Activated Charcoal: How Much, How Many Times, How Often?

There is no single correct dose of activated charcoal. As discussed earlier, in some cases, the expenditure of time, effort, and cost in administering large amounts or repeated doses of activated charcoal is not justifiable, but in other cases (eg, theophylline overdose), it should be considered a life-saving therapeutic maneuver of the highest priority. The maximum amount of activated charcoal that can be safely and successfully given is unknown and certainly varies with the patient. For example, to treat a severe theophylline overdose in an adult, as much as 100 g initially, followed by a continuous nasogastric tube infusion of 100 g/h, may be appropriate. It is unusual for both patient and staff to tolerate such a regimen. It is certainly unnecessary and unreasonable to give most patients the maximum possible dosage; although complications are rare, such dosing likely increases the risks. Although dosage is largely dictated by convention or packaging, a more rational approach is possible. It is certainly necessary to consider the age and size of the patient when determining activated charcoal dosage, but it is also critical to consider the type of agent involved and the amount ingested.

The optimum activated charcoal dose theoretically is the minimum dose that completely adsorbs the ingested toxic agent and, if relevant, that maximizes enhanced elimination. Because of variables such as the physical properties of the drug formulation ingested, the volume and pH of gastric and intestinal fluid, and the presence of other agents or foods adsorbed by activated charcoal,[8,9,101,117,121] the optimum dose cannot be known with certainty in any given patient. It is possible, however, to develop a logical approach to dosing based on available data. The results of in vitro studies show that ideal activated charcoal–to-drug ratios vary widely, but that 10:1 is a representative value for many typical drugs and is therefore useful in theoretical consideration of optimal activated charcoal dosing.[7,122]

As noted, achieving a large activated charcoal–to-drug ratio is often quite feasible for ingestions of drugs dispensed in small formulations, such as digoxin (0.25 mg), clonidine (0.2 mg), or levothyroxine (0.025–0.3 mg), but impossible for agents such as adult aspirin (325 mg), sustained-release theophylline (200–400 mg), or sustained-release verapamil (up to 240 mg). This should not be interpreted to mean that activated charcoal dosage should be decreased significantly for small ingestions; it seems logical to use the largest dose that can be easily and safely given (0.5–1 g/kg). Activated charcoal dosage should, however, be increased to treat certain ingestions. Maximal initial dosing (1.5–2 g/kg) is appropriate after massive ingestions of dangerous substances that are well adsorbed to activated charcoal (eg, theophylline, aspirin, sustained-release verapamil). Maximal activated charcoal dosing should also be used after ingestion of some lethal substances, even if they are poorly adsorbed, if a limited amount of adsorption to activated charcoal might be of significant clinical benefit (eg, cyanide). Thus, it is the total quantitative adsorption to activated charcoal relative to the amount of drug ingested and not the qualitative characteristics of the drug adsorption that determines the optimal dosing of activated charcoal.

The amount and frequency of MDAC dosing should vary based on considerations of risks and benefits as discussed. For cases less likely to benefit significantly from multiple doses, such as exposure to low-risk, rapidly absorbed, widely distributed substances, a low dose of MDAC, such as 0.5–1 g/kg every 4–6 hours, may be appropriate. More seriously poisoned patients should receive larger doses of activated charcoal, and patients for whom MDAC is critical, as in life-threatening overdoses of sustained-release theophylline, should be given as high a dose as they can tolerate, 1 g/kg or more per hour. Some patients tolerate "miniboluses" or continuous nasogastric infusions better than large intermittent doses. In many cases, antiemetics are necessary to accomplish aggressive activated charcoal dosing. Some drugs or agents, particularly the phenothiazines, possess the undesirable effects of decreasing gastrointestinal motility and, possibly, of lowering the seizure threshold. For this reason, metoclopramide or a serotonin agonist, such as ondansetron, may be most advantageous in poisoned patients. The appropriate endpoint for MDAC is also unstudied and may vary with the agent involved. The pharmacokinetics, toxicokinetics, and amount of the agent ingested all must be considered. In some cases, altered mental status or another toxic effect will persist long after the role of activated charcoal's has become minimal; in these cases multiple-dose therapy may be discontinued prior to clinical resolution. A number of studies suggest that activated charcoal may unbind a drug in the gastrointestinal tract, a process known as *desorption*. This drug then becomes available for systemic absorption.[14,56,117] If desorption from activated charcoal is likely, such as after massive salicylate ingestion, it may be appropriate to continue MDAC even after clinical improvement is evident. In most cases, significant clinical improvement and the passage of activated charcoal stools are adequate criteria for termination of MDAC.

Summary: Activated Charcoal

A single dose of activated charcoal is appropriate after nearly all suspected toxic ingestions. Exceptions include confirmed, single-substance ingestions of lithium, iron, ethanol, simple hydrocarbons, or acid or alkali caustics. With adequate airway protection, there is no serious risk associated with single-dose therapy. MDAC is warranted if there is evidence of a large amount of residual substance in the gastrointestinal tract, or to enhance the elimination of a drug or toxin already absorbed. Strong clinical evidence supporting the use of MDAC exists for only a few types of drug overdoses, but its use is often appropriate even in unproved circumstances.

In most instances, 0.5–1 g/kg is an appropriate initial dose of activated charcoal; doses of 1.5–2 g/kg should be used following particularly massive or dangerous ingestions. Dosing varies when using MDAC. To treat exposures to substances for which there are less data or rationale to support MDAC, 0.5 g/kg once or twice is probably adequate. When multiple-dose therapy is thought to be critical, activated charcoal doses as high as 1.5 g/kg/h may be justified. Other exposures warrant dosing between these extreme values, based on the factors discussed.

SHOULD A CATHARTIC BE USED?
Are Cathartics Beneficial?

Although cathartics are routinely used in the treatment of the poisoned patient, their efficacy remains unproved. Cathartics are used to increase gastrointestinal transit speed, and thus cathartics, theoretically, decrease the transit time during which drug absorption may occur. Cathartics may also counteract the constipating effect of activated charcoal. Another proposed reason to use cathartics is to promote rapid passage through the gastrointestinal tract to decrease time available for systemic absorption of a drug that has "desorbed" from activated charcoal.

Despite these theoretical advantages of cathartic use, it has been impossible to prove any consistent benefit. In fact, one study even suggests that use of cathartics alone may be deleterious, perhaps by increasing drug dissolution.[3] Most studies examine the possible effects of cathartics on the efficacy of activated charcoal. The addition of cathartic to activated charcoal is occasionally beneficial,[36,62,64,82,124] usually ineffective,[49,60,118,136] and infrequently alleged to reduce the efficacy of activated charcoal.[59,155]

Many cathartics are available, although only magnesium citrate, magnesium sulfate, and sorbitol are generally considered for use (Table 31–3). All are effective cathartics and, although sorbitol may produce a bowel movement more rapidly, none appears to be clinically superior or better tolerated.[89,141] Another clinically useful method of comparing cathartics is to investigate how different cathartics affect adsorption of a drug to activated charcoal. The results of such studies thus far offer conflicting results and no single cathartic significantly affects drug absorption. Although study design issues hinder direct comparison of the cathartics, some studies suggest that sorbitol is the most effective cathartic[74,89] (see Antidotes in Depth: Cathartics).

Do Cathartics Harm the Patient? Are Cathartics Ever Contraindicated?

In appropriate doses, and when contraindications to their use are excluded, there is no evidence that a single dose of cathartic is harmful. Following inadvertent overdosing or the use of repetitive, and therefore inappropriate, dosing, cathartics may have the potential for significant morbidity and mortality.

Use of sodium sulfate and sodium phosphate (Phospho-Soda) is associated with serious fluid and electrolyte disturbances.[46,104] The relative safety of magnesium cathartics may be a result of the limited absorption of magnesium ions compared to those of sodium.[1] Although no reports exist of magnesium toxicity following appropriate single-dose cathartic therapy in patients with normal renal function, cathartic-induced hypermagnesemia can occur, even in patients with normal renal function, after acute overdose or following multiple "appropriate" doses.[55,110,137,138]

All cathartics can cause dehydration from water loss in the stool or intraluminal "third-spacing." For example, although sorbitol is not significantly absorbed, severe fluid and electrolyte derangements, intravascular volume depletion, hypernatremia, shock, and acidosis are reported following excessive dosing. Although these abnormalities can occur in adults,[5] children, presumably because of their size, are at a particular risk.[54] Because sorbitol fermentation by gut flora results in gas production, it may also cause abdominal distension. Although this is usually without serious result, massive distension sufficient to result in respiratory embarrassment and death is reported.[10,53] Distension appears to be most common and problematic when there is decreased gut motility.

The incidence of all cathartic-induced fluid and electrolyte disturbances is probably increased by slow gastrointestinal transit; thus, obstruction and ileus should be considered at least relative contraindications to cathartic use. Conversely, the use of cathartics in patients with preexisting diarrhea is obviously also unnecessary and therefore contraindicated. Volume depletion should always be corrected before catharsis, and cathartic use should be minimized in infants because of the risk of causing significant fluid and electrolyte disorders. To avoid precipitating hypermagnesemia, magnesium-containing cathartics should not be used in patients with renal failure or decreased glomerular filtration rates from any cause, because of resultant impaired renal magnesium excretion.[142] Table 31–3 summarizes these contraindications.

What Is an Appropriate Cathartic Dose?

Cathartic dosing is largely empirical with the goal of safely speeding the passage of stool. An initial dose of sorbitol, 1 g/kg, is reasonable in adults receiving activated charcoal. Cathartic administration, however, should not be considered obligatory for all adult patients. Furthermore, given the lack of proven benefit and potential for increased risk in children, cathartics are relatively contraindicated for infants and young children with low-risk ingestions. For those with potentially serious ingestions in whom cathartic administration is desired, a single dose of 0.5 g/kg of sorbitol may be acceptable.

Repetitive cathartic administration is speculative and only rarely indicated. An adult patient who is receiving MDAC occa-sionally requires a second sorbitol dose of 0.5 g/kg if laxity does not occur and no ileus is present. More than one additional dose of cathartic is probably inappropriate and dangerous. Children should never receive additional cathartic doses, and if done inadvertently, they should have meticulous monitoring of their vital signs, their intravascular volume status, and their electrolytes. Inadvertent administration of multiple doses of cathartic during MDAC therapy is a frequent occurrence because premixed preparations combining activated charcoal and sorbitol are widely available.

Summary: Cathartics

Single doses of cathartics are generally safe and appropriate for adults, despite a lack of convincing evidence of efficacy. Although more than one dose of cathartic may sometimes seem logical, using multiple doses of any cathartic can cause significant toxicity, particularly in children. Repeat cathartic dosing should not be routine. If indicated in adults, repeat doses of cathartics should only be used if frequent fluid and electrolyte monitoring can be provided.

WHEN SHOULD WHOLE-BOWEL IRRIGATION BE USED?

Because cathartic administration is limited by the risk of serious fluid and electrolyte disturbances, other methods of gastrointestinal decontamination are gaining favor. One clinical advance is the use of whole-bowel irrigation by using isotonic polyethylene glycol electrolyte lavage solutions (PEG-ELS).[1,6,146] These solutions were originally introduced for preoperative bowel preparations, and were adapted for the management of poisoned or overdosed patients over the past 15 years. The components of these solutions are not absorbed, and because they are isotonic, there is no significant fluid shift into or out of the gastrointestinal tract. As a result, large volumes of PEG-ELS can be safely administered to patients with normal gastrointestinal function to "flush the gastrointestinal tract." Huge volumes over long durations are routinely used without any significant change in volume status, electrolytes, or other laboratory parameters.[72,79]

Rather than inducing diarrhea by drawing water into the stool or directly stimulating motility, the large volume of fluid administered during whole-bowel irrigation mechanically washes bowel contents through the gastrointestinal tract. The first successful use of whole-bowel irrigation for poisoning management occurred in patients with iron overdoses who had radiographic evidence of residual iron in their gastrointestinal tract.[151] Subsequently, studies of both human volunteers and animals show that whole-bowel irrigation reduces drug absorption after ingestion of ampicillin,[148] lithium,[139] and enteric-coated aspirin.[84] Other studies, however, have not found beneficial effects for whole-bowel irrigation.[29,127,132,142] Although case reports provide visually impressive radiographic or bedside evidence of gastrointestinal passage of arsenic,[96] iron,[52] lead,[112,130] or sustained-release calcium channel blockers,[28] they provide little useful data regarding either the clinical benefits achieved with the procedure or the outcome without it.

The apparent safety and efficacy of whole-bowel irrigation make it an intriguing tool, but its role is yet to be fully defined. Delivering and retrieving the large volumes of solution required can present significant problems and is certainly not warranted routinely. The greatest utility of whole-bowel irrigation probably is in the management of life-threatening ingestions of agents that are poorly adsorbed to activated charcoal (eg, iron, lithium), too massive for activated charcoal alone (eg, sustained-release calcium channel blockers, theophylline), or ostensibly foreign bodies (eg, in body packers and stuffers) that are impossible to remove safely and effectively by other means.

Other than practical issues related to the administration of whole-bowel irrigation, the most important concerns raised are about its effect on the adsorptive capacity of activated charcoal. Several in vitro studies demonstrate that PEG-ELS may interfere with activated charcoal efficacy.[73,86,102,132] Whether the magnitude of benefit from whole-bowel irrigation outweighs the risk from slightly decreased activated charcoal adsorption remains to be shown. In patients with massive ingestions of sustained-release drugs such as theophylline or verapamil, where whole-bowel irrigation may be of benefit and MDAC is essential, the potential for decreased efficiency of activated charcoal becomes an extremely important consideration. Perhaps simply increasing the amount, frequency, or duration of activated charcoal administration would effectively compensate for any decreased adsorption. Other important considerations for study include effects of whole-bowel irrigation–induced pH, intestinal fluid volume, and mechanical action on drug dissolution in massive overdose models.

An additional, related concern involves the institution of whole-bowel irrigation in patients who are already receiving oral activated charcoal. This is most consequential following overdose with sustained-release products, such as calcium channel blockers, under circumstances in which there is delayed recognition of the utility of whole-bowel irrigation. These patients may have large amounts of drug already adsorbed to the activated charcoal, which may be displaced by PEG-ELS. The liberated drug is available for subsequent absorption and may lead to acute decompensation of the patient.

Summary: Whole-Bowel Irrigation

Whole-bowel irrigation can reduce absorption and augment removal of toxic agents in the gastrointestinal tract, although, like many other modalities, its actual clinical benefit remains undefined and unproved. Until the clinical benefit and potential adverse effects are better understood, its use should be limited to patients who have ingested sustained-release pills or drug packets, or who have gastrointestinal drug bezoars.

ARE THERE OTHER GASTROINTESTINAL DECONTAMINATION MODALITIES TO CONSIDER?

What Other Binding Agents May Be Used?

In rare cases, oral or enteral administration of binding resins may be useful. Cholestyramine adsorbs organochlorine pesticides such as chlordecone (Kepone) and lindane, and may limit their absorption or enhance their fecal elimination,[40,61,81] but it is not known whether this is clinically beneficial. Elimination of digoxin and digitoxin is also enhanced by use of cholestyramine[31,125] or colestipol,[16,83] but the availability of the far more effective digoxin-specific antibodies and activated charcoal probably makes these other forms of therapy unnecessary. The possible efficacy of sodium polystyrene sulfonate (Kayexalate) to prevent gastroin-

testinal absorption and to increase elimination of lithium is demonstrated in human volunteer and animal studies,[17,97,153] but several study design issues limit the applicability of these results to poisoned patients. The resin-to-lithium ratios in these studies, which are very large, suggest that its value after actual poisoning will ultimately prove to be quite limited. In addition, the development of hypokalemia may prove problematic.[98]

Gastrointestinal administration of Prussian blue (potassium ferricyanoferrate) is advocated to exchange potassium for thallium, thus enhancing fecal thallium excretion (Chap. 83). Fuller's earth adsorbs paraquat and diquat, but there appears to be no reason to advocate its use over activated charcoal. Oral starch can be utilized both diagnostically and therapeutically after ingestion of concentrated iodine solutions.

When Should Endoscopic Removal Be Used?

Endoscopic removal of gastric contents is often considered but is rarely of practical value.[113] Endoscopic removal is logical when a substance remains in the stomach, is a significant threat to the patient, cannot be removed by another less invasive means, and can be safely removed in this manner. Unfortunately, on a practical basis, many of the agents likely to be considered for endoscopic removal do not meet these criteria. Drug masses due to iron, enteric aspirin, meprobamate, and others, despite their solid appearance on radiographs, cannot be effectively grasped through an endoscope. When life-threatening deterioration is likely or evident, it remains unresolved whether these masses are best left untreated, treated with whole-bowel irrigation, broken up, or surgically removed. There are no clinically relevant data regarding the use of these methods or others of theoretical value (eg, lithotripsy). In body packers and body stuffers (Chap. 67) only the most durable drug packets may be safely grasped in this manner;[72] others may rupture during removal, limiting the usefulness of endoscopy. In addition, removing multiple objects with an endoscope requires repeated passage of the endoscope and thus increases potential complications. Procedural complications, such as perforation, are expected to occur, but unexpected complications, such as gastrointestinal bleeding, are reported.[95] Nonetheless, in rare circumstances meeting the criteria given, endoscopic removal may be of value.

When Is Surgery Indicated?

Although exceptional, there are a few indications for surgical gastrointestinal decontamination. In rare instances, patients who ingest packets containing illicit drugs may require their surgical removal. Specifically, mechanical bowel obstruction, or bowel ischemia because of release of cocaine from drug packets, is an indication for surgery.[34] Rupture of the packets and resultant toxicity may be managed medically if the amount of drug is small, the agent is not potentially lethal (marijuana), or an effective antidote is available (opioids). However, if packets containing a large amount of cocaine rupture, immediate surgical removal of remaining drug is warranted following appropriate stabilization.[140]

Other agents that cause toxicity and that form large masses or that adhere to the gastrointestinal tract wall and are not removed by gastric emptying, activated charcoal, and cathartic or whole-bowel irrigation might require surgical removal. Although many agents are described as resulting in bezoar formation (eg, aspirin, bromide, meprobamate), in nearly all cases, gastric emptying and repetitive doses of activated charcoal are sufficient treatment. Patients with massive iron ingestions who have iron evident on radiograph after gastric emptying attempts and whole-bowel irrigation should be considered for gastrotomy if serious systemic toxicity or evidence of active gastrointestinal bleeding occurs.[58,151] Surgical intervention is frequently indicated for patients who ingest strong acids or bases, not for decontamination purposes, but to treat resultant gastrointestinal necrosis and perforation.

SUMMARY

Gastrointestinal decontamination is far from an exact science, and controversy and change are expected. The issues discussed in this chapter provide a framework on which to build and refine a clinical approach. As in all areas of medicine, it is expected that thoughtful analysis of further research, clinical experience, and the unique features of each case will suggest appropriate modifications of current thinking and lead to improved patient care.

REFERENCES

1. Abdallah AH, Tye A: A comparison of the efficacy of emetic drugs and stomach lavage. Am J Dis Child 1967;113:571–575.
2. Agocha A, Wang R, Longmore W, et al: Drug disintegration time and its value in orogastric lavage [abstract]. Vet Hum Toxicol 1986;28:493–494.
3. Al-Shareef AM, Buss DC, Allen EM, Routledge PA: The effects of charcoal and sorbitol (alone and in combination) on plasma theophylline concentration after a sustained-release formulation. Hum Exp Toxicol 1990;9:179–182.
4. Albertson TE, Derlet RW, Foulke GE, et al: Superiority of activated charcoal alone compared with ipecac and activated charcoal in the treatment of acute toxic ingestions. Ann Emerg Med 1989;18:56–59.
5. Allerton JP, Strom JA: Hypernatremia due to repeated doses of charcoal-sorbitol. Am J Kidney Dis 1991;17:581–584.
6. Ambrose N, Johnson M, Burdon D, et al: A physiologic approach of polyethylene glycol and a balanced electrolyte solution as bowel preparation. Br J Surg 1983;70:428–430.
7. Anderson AH: Experimental studies on the pharmacology of activated charcoal: I. Adsorption power of charcoal in aqueous solutions. Acta Pharmacol 1946;2:69–78.
8. Anderson AH: Experimental studies on the pharmacology of activated charcoal: II. The effect of pH on the adsorption by charcoal from aqueous solutions. Acta Pharmacol 1947;3:199–218.
9. Anderson AH: Experimental studies on the pharmacology of activated charcoal: III. Adsorption from gastric contents. Acta Pharmacol 1948;4:275–284.
10. Anker AL, Smilkstein MJ: Fatality from respiratory failure due to sorbitol-induced intestinal gas formation [abstract]. Vet Hum Toxicol 1993;35:334.
11. Arnold FJ, Hodges JB, Barta PA, et al: Evaluation of the efficacy of lavage and induced emesis in treatment of salicylate poisoning. Pediatrics 1959;23:286–301.
12. Arnold TC, Willis BH, Xiao F, et al: Aspiration of activated charcoal elicits an increase in lung microvascular permeability. J Toxicol Clin Toxicol 1999;37:9–16.
13. Auerbach P, Osterloh J, Braun O, et al: Efficacy of gastric emptying: Orogastric lavage versus emesis induced with ipecac. Ann Emerg Med 1986;15:692–698.
14. Augenstein WL, Kulig KW, Rumack BH: Delayed rise in serum drug levels in overdose patients despite multiple dose charcoal and after charcoal stools [abstract]. Vet Hum Toxicol 1987;29:491.
15. Barceloux D, McGuigan M, Hartigan-Go K. Position statement: Cathartics. American Academy of Clinical Toxicology; European

Association of Poisons Centres and Clinical Toxicologists. J Toxicol Clin Toxicol 1997;35:743–752.
16. Bazzano G, Bazzano GS: Digitalis intoxication: Treatment with a new steroid-binding resin. JAMA 1972;220:828–830.
17. Belanger DR, Tierney MG, Dickinson G: Effect of sodium polystyrene sulfonate on lithium bioavailability. Ann Emerg Med 1992;21:1312–1315.
18. Benson B, VanAntwerp M, Hergott T: A fatality resulting from multiple dose activated charcoal therapy. Vet Hum Toxicol 1989;31:335. Abstract.
19. Berg M, Berlinger W, Goldberg M, et al: Acceleration of the body clearance of phenobarbital by oral activated charcoal. Clin Pharmacol Ther 1983;33:351–354.
20. Berlinger WG, Spector R, Goldberg MJ, et al: Enhancement of theophylline clearance by oral activated charcoal. Clin Pharmacol Ther 1983;33:351–354.
21. Bogacz K, Caldron P: Enteric-coated aspirin bezoar: Elevation of serum salicylate level by barium study. Am J Med 1981;83:783–786.
22. Bond GR, Requa RK, Krenzelok EP, et al: Influence of time until emesis on the efficacy of decontamination using acetaminophen as a marker in a pediatric population. Ann Emerg Med 1993;22:1403–1407.
23. Bonuccelli U, Piccini P, Del Dotto P, et al: Naloxone partly counteracts apomorphine side effects. Clin Neuropharmacol 1991;14:442–449.
24. Bosse GM, Barefoot JA, Pfeifer MP, Rodgers GC: Comparison of three methods of gut decontamination in tricyclic antidepressant overdose. J Emerg Med 1995;13:203–209.
25. Boxer L, Anderson F, Rowe D: Comparison of ipecac-induced emesis with gastric lavage in the treatment of acute salicylate ingestion. J Pediatr 1969;74:800–803.
26. Bradberry SM, Vale JA: Multiple-dose activated charcoal: A review of relevant clinical studies. J Toxicol Clin Toxicol 1995;33:407–416.
27. Brubacher JR, Levine B, Hoffman RS: Intestinal pseudo-obstruction (Ogilvie's syndrome) in theophylline overdose. Vet Hum Toxicol 1996;38:368–370.
28. Buckley N, Dawson AH, Howarth D, Whyte IM: Slow-release verapamil poisoning. Use of polyethylene glycol whole-bowel lavage and high-dose calcium. Med J Aust 1993;158:202–204.
29. Burkhart KK, Wuerz RC, Donovan JW: Whole-bowel irrigation as adjunctive treatment for sustained-release theophylline overdose. Ann Emerg Med 1992;21:1316–1320.
30. Burton BT, Bayer MJ, Barron L, Aitchison JP: Comparison of activated charcoal and orogastric lavage in the prevention of aspirin absorption. J Emerg Med 1984;1:411–416.
31. Cady WJ, Rehder TL, Campbell J: Use of cholestyramine resin in the treatment of digitoxin toxicity. Am J Hosp Pharm 1979;36: 92–94.
32. Calvert W, Corby D, Herbertson L, Decker W: Orally administered activated charcoal: Acceptance by children. JAMA 1971;215:641.
33. Campbell J, Chyka P: Physiochemical characteristics of drugs and response to repeat dose activated charcoal. Am J Emerg Med 1992;10:208–210.
34. Caruana DS, Weinbach B, Goerg D, et al: Cocaine-packet ingestion: Diagnosis, management, and natural history. Ann Intern Med 1984;100:73–74.
35. Chafee-Bahamon C, Lacouture PG, Lovejoy FH Jr: Risk assessment of ipecac in the home. Pediatrics 1985;75:1105–1109.
36. Chin L, Picchioni A, Gillespie T: Saline cathartics and saline cathartics plus activated charcoal as antidotal treatments. Clin Toxicol 1981;18:865–871.
37. Chyka PA, Seger D. Position statement: Single-dose activated charcoal. American Academy of Clinical Toxicology; European Association of Poisons Centres and Clinical Toxicologists. J Toxicol Clin Toxicol 1997;35:721–741.
38. Chyka PA: Multiple-dose activated charcoal and enhancement of systemic drug clearance: Summary of studies in animals and human volunteers. J Toxicol Clin Toxicol 1995;33:399–405.

39. Chyka PA, Holley JE, Mandrell TD, Sugathan P: Correlation of drug pharmacokinetics and effectiveness of multiple-dose activated charcoal therapy. Ann Emerg Med 1995;25:356–362.

40. Cohn WJ, Boylan JJ, Blanke RV, et al: Treatment of chlordecone (Kepone) toxicity with cholestyramine. N Engl J Med 1978;298:243–248.

41. Comstock EG, Faulkner TP, Boisaubin E, et al: Studies on the efficacy of gastric emptying as practiced in a large metropolitan hospital. Clin Toxicol 1981;18:581–597.

42. Comstock EG, Boisaubin EV, Comstock BS, et al: Assessment of the efficacy of activated charcoal following orogastric lavage in acute drug emergencies. Clin Toxicol 1982;19:149–165.

43. Corby D, Decker W, Moran M, et al: Clinical comparison of pharmacologic emetics in children. Pediatrics 1968;42:361–364.

44. Curtis RA, Barone J, Giacona N: Efficacy of ipecac and activated charcoal and cathartic: Prevention of salicylate absorption in a simulated overdose. Arch Intern Med 1984;144:48–52.

45. Dammann KZ, Wiley SH, Tominack RL: Aspiration pneumonia following activated charcoal: A case report [abstract]. Vet Hum Toxicol 1988;30:353.

46. Davis R, Eichner J, Bleyer W, et al: Hypocalcemia, hyperphosphatemia, and dehydration following a single hypertonic phosphate enema. J Pediatr 1977;90:484–485.

47. Docksteder LL, Lawrence RA, Bresnick BL: Home administration of activated charcoal: Feasibility and acceptance [abstract]. Vet Hum Toxicol 1986;28:471.

48. Dronen SC, Merigian KS, Hedges JR, et al: A comparison of blind nasotracheal and succinylcholine-assisted intubation in the poisoned patient. Ann Emerg Med 1987;16:650–652.

49. Easom JM, Caraccio TR, Lovejoy FH Jr: Evaluation of activated charcoal and magnesium citrate in the prevention of aspirin absorption in humans. Clin Pharm 1982;1:154–156.

50. Eisen TF, Lacouture PG, Woolf A: The palatability of a new milk chocolate charcoal mixture in children [abstract]. Vet Hum Toxicol 1988;30:351–352.

51. Elliot CG, Colby TV, Kelly TM, et al: Charcoal lung: Bronchiolitis obliterans after aspiration of activated charcoal. Chest 1989;96:672–674.

52. Everson G, Bertaccini E, O'Leary J: Use of whole-bowel irrigation in an infant following iron overdose. Am J Emerg Med 1991;9:366–369.

53. Falkaw S, Mekalanos J: The enteric bacilli and Vibrio. In: Davis BD, Dulbecco R, Eisen HN, Ginsberg HS, eds: Microbiology, 4th ed. Philadelphia, Lippincott, 1990, pp. 561–587.

54. Farley TA: Severe hypernatremic dehydration after use of an activated charcoal-sorbitol suspension. J Pediatr 1986;109:719–722.

55. Fassler CA, Rodriguez DB, Badesch WJ, et al: Magnesium toxicity as a cause of hypotension and hypoventilation: Occurrence in patients with normal renal function. Arch Intern Med 1985;145:1604–1606.

56. Fillippone G, Fish S, Lacouture P, et al: Reversible adsorption (desorption) of aspirin from activated charcoal. Arch Intern Med 1987;147:1390–1392.

57. Flores F, Battle WS: Intestinal obstruction secondary to activated charcoal. Contemp Surg 1987;30:57–59.

58. Foxford R, Goldfrank LR: Gastrotomy: A surgical approach to iron overdose. Ann Emerg Med 1985;14:1223–1226.

59. Galey FD, Lambert RJ, Busse M, et al: Therapeutic efficacy of superactive charcoal in rats exposed to oral lethal doses of T-2 toxin. Toxicon 1987;25:493–499.

60. Galinsky RE, Levy G: Evaluation of activated charcoal-sodium sulfate combination for inhibition of acetaminophen absorption and repletion of inorganic sulfate. J Toxicol Clin Toxicol 1984;22:21–30.

61. Garrettson LK, Guzelian PS, Blanke RV: Subacute chlordane poisoning. J Toxicol Clin Toxicol 1984–85;22:565–571.

62. Gaudreault P, Friedman PA, Lovejoy FH Jr: Efficacy of activated charcoal and magnesium citrate in the treatment of oral paraquat intoxication. Ann Emerg Med 1985;14:123–125.

63. Givens T, Holloway M, Wason S: Pulmonary aspiration of activated charcoal: A complication of its misuse in overdose management. Pediatr Emerg Care 1992;8:137–140.

64. Goldberg M, Spector R, Park G, et al: The effect of sorbitol and activated charcoal on serum theophylline concentrations after slow release theophylline. Clin Pharmacol Ther 1987;41:108–111.

65. Gomez BIF, Brent JA, Munoz DC, et al: Charcoal stercolith with intestinal perforation in a patient treated for amitriptyline ingestion. J Emerg Med 1994;12:57–60.

66. Goulbourne KB, Cisek JE: Small-bowel obstruction secondary to activated charcoal and adhesions. Ann Emerg Med 1994;24:108–110.

67. Harris CR, Filandrinos D: Accidental administration of activated charcoal into the lung: Aspiration by proxy. Ann Emerg Med 1993;22:143–146.

68. Harsh HH: Aspiration of activated charcoal. N Engl J Med 1986;414:318.

69. Haulman J, Robertson WO: Syrup of ipecac in 1993 [editorial]. A personal perspective. Drug Safety 1993;9:79–84.

70. Hoffman RS: Does consensus equal correctness? J Toxicol Clin Toxicol 2000;38:689–690.

71. Hoffman RS, Chiang WK, Weisman RS, et al: Prospective evaluation of "crack vial" ingestion. Vet Hum Toxicol 1990;32:164–167.

72. Hoffman RS, Smilkstein MJ, Goldfrank LR: Whole-bowel irrigation and the cocaine body packer. Am J Emerg Med 1990;8:523–527.

73. Hoffman RS, Chiang WK, Howland MA, et al: Theophylline desorption from activated charcoal caused by whole-bowel irrigation solution. J Toxicol Clin Toxicol 1991;29:191.

74. James LP, Nichols MH, King WD: A comparison of cathartics in pediatric ingestions. Pediatrics 1995;96:235–238.

75. Jenis EH, Payne RJ, Goldbaum LR: Acute meprobamate poisoning: A fatal case following a lucid interval. JAMA 1969;207:361–365.

76. Johnson D, Eppler J, Giesbrecht E, et al: Effect of multiple-dose activated charcoal on the clearance of high-dose intravenous aspirin in a porcine model. Ann Emerg Med 1996;26:569–574.

77. Johnson WE: Massive phenobarbital ingestion with survival. JAMA 1967;202:1106–1109.

78. Juurlink DN, McGuigan MA. Gastrointestinal decontamination for enteric-coated aspirin overdose: What to do depends on who you ask. J Toxicol Clin Toxicol 2000;38:465–470.

79. Kaczorowski JM, Wax PM: Five days of whole-bowel irrigation in a case of pediatric iron ingestion. Ann Emerg Med 1996;27:258–263.

80. Karkkainen S, Neuvonen P: Pharmacokinetics of amitriptyline influenced by oral charcoal and urine pH. Int J Clin Pharmacol Ther Toxicol 1986;24:326–332.

81. Kassner JT, Maher TJ, Hull KM, Woolf AD: Cholestyramine as an adsorbent in acute lindane poisoning: A murine model. Ann Emerg Med 1993;22:1392–1397.

82. Keller RE, Schwab RA, Krenzelok EP: Contribution of sorbitol combined with activated charcoal in prevention of salicylate absorption. Ann Emerg Med 1990;19:654–656.

83. Kilgore TL, Lehmann CR: Treatment of digoxin intoxication with colestipol. South Med J 1982;75:1259–1260.

84. Kirshenbaum LA, Mathews SC, Sitar DS, Tenenbein M: Whole-bowel irrigation versus activated charcoal in sorbitol for the ingestion of modified release pharmaceuticals. Clin Pharmacol Ther 1989;46:264–271.

85. Kirshenbaum LA, Mathews SC, Sitar DS, et al: Does multiple dose charcoal therapy enhance salicylate excretion? Arch Intern Med 1990;150:1281–1283.

86. Kirshenbaum LA, Sitar DS, Tenenbein M: Interaction between whole-bowel irrigation solution and activated charcoal: Implications for the treatment of toxic ingestions. Ann Emerg Med 1990;19:1129–1132.

87. Klein-Schwartz W, Gorman RL, Oderda GM, et al: Ipecac use in the elderly: The unanswered question. Ann Emerg Med 1984;13:1152–1154.

88. Komberg AE, Dolgin J: Pediatric ingestions: Charcoal alone versus ipecac and charcoal. Ann Emerg Med 1991;20:648–651.

89. Krenzelok EP, Keller R, Stewart RD: Gastrointestinal transit times of cathartics combined with charcoal. Ann Emerg Med 1985;14: 1152–1155.

90. Krenzelok EP, McGuigan M, Lheur P: Position statement: Ipecac syrup. American Academy of Clinical Toxicology; European Association of Poisons Centres and Clinical Toxicologists. J Toxicol Clin Toxicol 1997;35:699–709.

91. Kulig KW, Bar-Or D, Cantrill SV, et al: Management of acutely poisoned patients without gastric emptying. Ann Emerg Med 1985;14: 562–567.

92. Laass W: Therapy of acute oral poisonings by organic solvents: Treatment by activated charcoal in combination with laxatives. Arch Toxicol 1980;4(Suppl):406–409.

93. Lambert RJ, Kindler BL, Schaeff DJ: The efficacy of superactivated charcoal in treating rats exposed to a lethal oral dose of potassium cyanide. Ann Emerg Med 1988;17:595–598.

94. Lamminpaa A, Vilska J, Hoppu K: Medical charcoal for a child's poisoning at home: Availability and success of administration in Finland. Hum Exp Toxicol 1993;12:29–32.

95. Lapostolle F, Finot MA, Adnet F, et al: Radiopacity of clomipramine conglomerations and unsuccessful endoscopy: Report of 4 cases. J Toxicol Clin Toxicol 2000;38:477–482.

96. Lee DC, Roberts JR, Kelly JJ, Fishman SM: Whole-bowel irrigation as an adjunct in the treatment of radiopaque arsenic [letter]. Am J Emerg Med 1995;13:244–245.

97. Linakis JG, Savitt DL, Wu TY, et al. Use of sodium polystyrene sulfonate for reduction of plasma lithium concentrations after chronic lithium dosing in mice. J Toxicol Clin Toxicol 1998;36:309–313.

98. Linakis JG, Hull KM, Lacouture PG, et al: Sodium polystyrene sulfonate treatment for lithium toxicity: Effects on serum potassium concentrations. Acad Emerg Med 1996;3:333–337.

99. Longdon P, Henderson A: Intestinal pseudo-obstruction following the use of enteral charcoal and sorbitol with mechanical ventilation with papaveretum sedation for theophylline poisoning. Drug Safety 1992;7:74–77.

100. MacLean W: A comparison of ipecac syrup and apomorphine in the immediate treatment of ingestion of poisons. J Pediatr 1973;82: 121–124.

101. Makosiev F, Hoffman RS, Howland MA: Cocaine adsorption to activated charcoal: The effects of pH [abstract]. Vet Hum Toxicol 1990; 32:350.

102. Makosiev FJ, Hoffman RS, Howland MA, Goldfrank LR: An in vitro evaluation of cocaine hydrochloride adsorption by activated charcoal and desorption upon addition of polyethylene glycol electrolyte lavage solution. J Toxicol Clin Toxicol 1993;31:381–395.

103. Mafiani PJ, Poole N: Gastrointestinal tract perforation with charcoal peritoneum complicating orogastric intubation and lavage. Ann Emerg Med 1993;22:606–609.

104. Martin R, Lisehora G, Braxton M, et al: Fatal poisoning from sodium phosphate enema: A case report and experimental study. JAMA 1987; 257:2190–2192.

105. Mayer AL, Sitar DS, Tenenbein M: Multiple dose charcoal and whole-bowel irrigation do not increase clearance of absorbed salicylate. Arch Intern Med 1992;152:393–396.

106. McNamara R, Aaron C, Gemborys M, Davidheiser S: Efficacy of charcoal versus ipecac in reducing serum acetaminophen in a simulated overdose. Ann Emerg Med 1988;17:243–246.

107. Menzies DG, Busuttel A, Prescott LF: Fatal pulmonary aspiration of oral activated charcoal. BMJ 1988;297:459–466.

108. Merigian KS, Woodard NM Jr, Hedges JR, et al: Prospective evaluation of gastric emptying in the self poisoned patient. Am J Emerg Med 1990;8:479–483.

109. Minton NA: Volunteer models for predicting antiemetic activity of 5-HT3-receptor antagonists. Br J Clin Pharmacol 1994;37: 525–530.

110. Mofenson H, Caraccio T: Magnesium intoxication in a neonate from oral magnesium hydroxide laxative. J Toxicol Clin Toxicol 1991;29: 215–222.

111. Moll J, Kerns W, Tomaszewski C, et al: Incidence of aspiration pneumonia in intubated patients receiving activated charcoal. J Emerg Med 1999;17:279–83.

112. Murphy DG, Gerace RV, Peterson RG: The use of whole-bowel irrigation in acute lead ingestion [abstract]. Vet Hum Toxicol 1991; 33:353.

113. Nelson L: As if there weren't enough controversies in gastrointestinal decontamination. J Toxicol Clin Toxicol 2000;38:483–484.

114. Neuvonen PJ: Clinical pharmacokinetics of oral activated charcoal in acute intoxications. Clin Pharmacokinet 1982;7:465–489.

115. Neuvonen PJ, Vartiainen M, Tokola O: Comparison of activated charcoal and ipecac syrup in prevention of drug absorption. Eur J Clin Pharmacol 1983;24:557–562.

116. Neuvonen PJ, Olkkola KT. Activated charcoal and syrup of ipecac in prevention of cimetidine and pindolol absorption in man after administration of metoclopramide as an antiemetic agent. J Toxicol Clin Toxicol 1984;22:103–114.

117. Neuvonen P, Olkkola K, Alanen T: Effect of ethanol and pH on the adsorption of drugs to activated charcoal: Studies in vitro and in man. Acta Pharmacol Toxicol 1984;54:1–7.

118. Neuvonen PJ, Olkkola KT: Effect of purgatives on antidotal efficacy of oral activated charcoal. Hum Toxicol 1986;5:255–263.

119. Neuvonen PJ, Olkkola KT: Oral activated charcoal in the treatment of intoxications: Role of single and repeated doses. Med Toxicol 1988;3:33–58.

120. Nordt SP, Manoguerra A, Williams SR, et al: The availability of activated charcoal and ipecac for home use. Vet Hum Toxicol 1999; 41:247–248.

121. Olkkola KT, Neuvonen PJ: Do gastric contents modify antidotal efficacy of oral activated charcoal? Br J Clin Pharmacol 1984;18: 663–669.

122. Olkkola KT: Effect of charcoal-drug ratio on antidotal efficacy of oral activated charcoal in man. Br J Clin Pharmacol 1985;19: 767–773.

123. Olsen KM, Ma FH, Ackerman BH, Stull RE: Low-volume whole bowel irrigation and salicylate absorption: A comparison with ipecac-charcoal. Pharmacotherapy 1993;13:229–232.

124. Picchioni A, Chin L, Gillespie T: Evaluation of activated charcoal-sorbitol suspension as an antidote. Clin Toxicol 1982;19:435–444.

125. Pieroni RE, Fisher JG: Use of cholestyramine resin in digitoxin toxicity. JAMA 1981;245:1939–1940.

126. Poisindex editorial staff: Activated charcoal/treatment. In: Rumack BH, ed: Poisindex Information System, Vol. 110. Denver, Micromedex, edition expired 12/31/01.

127. Pollack MM, Dunbar BS, Holbrook PR, et al: Aspiration of activated charcoal and gastric contents. Ann Emerg Med 1981;10:528–529.

128. Pond SM, Lewis-Driver DJ, Williams G, et al: Gastric emptying in acute overdose: A prospective randomised controlled trial. Med J Austral 1995;163:345–349.

129. Ray MJ, Padin DR, Condie JD, Halls JM: Charcoal bezoar: Small-bowel obstruction secondary to amitriptyline overdose therapy. Dig Dis Sci 1988;33:106–107.

130. Roberge RJ, Martin TG: Whole-bowel irrigation in an acute oral lead intoxication. Am J Emerg Med 1992;10:577–583.

131. Robertson WO: Syrup of ipecac associated fatality: A case report. Vet Hum Toxicol 1979;21:87–89.

132. Rosenberg PJ, Livingstone DJ, McLellan BA: Effect of whole-bowel irrigation on the antidotal efficacy of activated charcoal. Ann Emerg Med 1988;17:681–683.

133. Saetta JP, Quinton DN: Residual gastric content after orogastric lavage and ipecacuanha induced emesis in self-poisoned patients: An endoscopic study. J R Soc Med 1991;84:35–38.

134. Saetta JP, March S, Gaunt ME, Quinton DN: Gastric emptying procedures in the self-poisoned patient: Are we forcing gastric content beyond the pylorus? J R Soc Med 1991;84:274.

135. Shrestha M, George J, Chiu MJ, et al: A comparison of three gastric lavage methods using the radionuclide gastric emptying study. J Emerg Med 1996;14:413–418.

136. Sketris IS, Mowry JB, Czajka PA, et al: Saline catharsis: Effect on aspirin bioavailability in combination with activated charcoal. J Clin Pharmacol 1982;22:59–64.

137. Smilkstein MJ, Smolinske SC, Kulig KW, et al: Severe hypermagnesemia due to multiple dose cathartic therapy. West J Med 1987;148: 208–211.

138. Smilkstein MJ, Steedle D, Kulig KW, et al: Magnesium levels after magnesium-containing cathartics. J Toxicol Clin Toxicol 1988;26: 51–65.

139. Smith SW, Ling LJ, Halstenson CE: Whole-bowel irrigation as a treatment for acute lithium overdose. Ann Emerg Med 1991;20: 536–539.

140. Suarez CA, Arango A, Lester JL: Cocaine-condom ingestion: Surgical treatment. JAMA 1977;238:1391–1392.

141. Sue YJ, Woolf A, Shannon M: Efficacy of magnesium citrate cathartic in pediatric toxic ingestions. Ann Emerg Med 1994;24:709–712.

142. Swanson-Brearman B, Dean BS, Krenzelok EP: Failure of whole-bowel irrigation to decontaminate the GI tract following massive jequirity bean ingestion [abstract]. Vet Hum Toxicol 1992;34:352.

143. Tandberg D, Liechty EJ, Fishbein D: Mallory-Weiss syndrome: An unusual complication of ipecac-induced emesis. Ann Emerg Med 1981;10:521–523.

144. Tandberg D, Diven BG, McLeod JW: Ipecac-induced emesis versus orogastric lavage: A controlled study in normal adults. Am J Emerg Med 1986;4:205–209.

145. Tarling MM, Toner CC, Withington PS, et al: A model of gastric emptying using paracetamol absorption in intensive care patients. Intensive Care Med 1997;23:256–260.

146. Tenenbein M: Whole-bowel irrigation for toxic ingestions. J Toxicol Clin Toxicol 1985;23:177–184.

147. Tenenbein M: Whole-bowel irrigation in iron poisoning. J Pediatr 1987;111:142–145.

148. Tenenbein M, Cohen S, Sitar DS: Whole-bowel irrigation as a decontamination procedure after acute drug overdose. Arch Intern Med 1987;147:905–907.

149. Tenenbein M, Cohen S, Sitar DS: Efficacy of ipecac-induced emesis, orogastric lavage, and activated charcoal for acute drug overdose. Ann Emerg Med 1987;16:838–841.

150. Tenenbein M: Multiple doses of activated charcoal: Time for reappraisal? Ann Emerg Med 1991;20:529–531.

151. Tenenbein M, Wiseman N, Yatscoff RW: Gastrotomy and whole-bowel irrigation in iron poisoning. Pediatr Emerg Care 1991;7: 286–288.

152. Vale JA: Position statement: Orogastric lavage. American Academy of Clinical Toxicology; European Association of Poisons Centres and Clinical Toxicologists. J Toxicol Clin Toxicol. 1997;35: 711–719.

153. Tomaszewski C, Musso C, Pearson JR, et al: Lithium absorption prevented by sodium polystyrene sulfonate in volunteers. Ann Emerg Med 1992;21:1308–1311.

154. Vale JA: Position statement: Orogastric lavage. American Academy of Clinical Toxicology; European Association of Poisons Centres and Clinical Toxicologists. J Toxicol Clin Toxicol. 1997;35: 711–719.

155. Van de Graaf W, Thompson WL, Sunshine I, et al: Adsorbent and cathartic inhibition of enteral drug absorption. J Pharmacol Exp Ther 1982;221:656–663.

156. Vance MV, Selden BS, Clark RF: Optimal patient position for transport and initial management of toxic ingestions. Ann Emerg Med 1992;21:243–246.

157. Wald P, Stern J, Weiner B, et al: Esophageal tear following forceful removal of an impacted oral-orogastric lavage tube. Ann Emerg Med 1986;15:80–82.

158. Watson WA, Cremes KF, Chapman JA: Gastrointestinal obstruction associated with multiple-dose activated charcoal. J Emerg Med 1986;4:401–407.

159. Wolowodiuk OJ, McMicken DB, O'Brien P: Pneumomediastinum and retropneumoperitoneum: An unusual complication of syrup of ipecac-induced emesis. Ann Emerg Med 1984;13:1148–1150.

PRINCIPLES AND TECHNIQUES APPLIED TO ENHANCE THE ELIMINATION OF TOXIC COMPOUNDS

David S. Goldfarb

Enhancement of the elimination of a drug or toxin from a poisoned patient is a logical step after techniques to inhibit absorption such as orogastric gastric lavage, multiple-dose activated charcoal, or whole-bowel irrigation are initiated. Methods that may enhance elimination are listed in Table 6–1. Some of these techniques are described in more detail in other chapters that deal with specific drugs and poisons. In this chapter hemodialysis and hemoperfusion are considered *extracorporeal therapies* because drug and toxin removal occurs in a blood circuit outside the body. All of these methods are used infrequently because current methods of intensive supportive care keep the overall mortality rate low in poisoned patients who reach the hospital alive.[29] Because the elimination techniques are not without adverse effects and complications,[16,42,71] they are indicated in a relatively small number of patients.[29,72] Although undoubtedly underestimates, the number of instances in which enhancement of elimination was used in a cohort of 2.2 million patients in 1999 demonstrate the relative infrequency of their use: alkalinization of the urine was used 6247 times; hemodialysis was used 1049 times; hemoperfusion was used 33 times; and other extracorporeal procedures were used 25 times. Statistics regarding peritoneal dialysis, a slower modality that should have little or no role in such cases, are not reported (Chap. 116 and p. 1752).

There are very few prospective, randomized, controlled clinical trials to determine whether or not groups of patients actually benefit from enhanced elimination of various toxins. It is unlikely that these sorts of studies will ever be performed, given the relative scarcity of appropriate cases of sufficient severity and the many variables that would have to be controlled. Thus, anecdotal evidence predominates. We must still rely on our knowledge of the principles of the methods to identify the individual patients for whom enhanced elimination is indicated. Isolated case reports in which the kinetics are studied before, during, and after enhanced elimination are also very useful in establishing the efficacy of a method.

INDICATIONS FOR ENHANCED ELIMINATION

Enhanced elimination may be indicated in several types of patients:

- *Patients who fail to respond adequately to full supportive care.* Such patients may have intractable hypotension, heart failure, seizures, metabolic acidosis, or dysrhythmias. Hemodialysis or hemoperfusion are much better tolerated than in the past, and may be the only opportunities available to patients with life-threatening toxicity caused by theophylline, lithium, aspirin, or a toxic alcohol.

- *Patients in whom the normal route of elimination of the toxin is impaired.* Such patients may have renal or hepatic dysfunction, either preexisting or caused by the overdose. For example, a patient with chronic renal insufficiency associated with long-term lithium use is more likely to develop toxic drug levels and to require hemodialysis as therapy.

- *Patients in whom the amount of toxin absorbed or its high concentration in serum indicates that serious morbidity or mortality is likely.* Such patients may not appear acutely ill on presentation. Toxins in this group include arsenic trioxide, ethylene glycol, lithium, mercuric chloride, methanol, paraquat, salicylate, and theophylline.

- *Patients with concurrent disease or in an age group (very young or old) associated with increased risk of morbidity or mortality from the overdose.* Such patients are intolerant of prolonged coma, immobility, and hemodynamic instability. An example is a patient with severe underlying respiratory disease and chronic theophylline intoxication.

Ideally, these techniques will be applied to poisonings for which studies have suggested an improvement in outcome in treated patients as compared to patients not treated with extracorporeal removal. As previously mentioned, these data are rarely available.

The need for extracorporeal elimination is less clear for patients who are poisoned with drugs or toxins that are known to be removed by the various modalities of treatment, but which cause limited morbidity if supportive care is provided. Relatively high rates of endogenous clearance would also make extracorporeal elimination redundant. Examples of such toxins are ethanol and barbiturates. Both are subject to substantial rates of hepatic metabolism, and neither would be expected to lead to significant morbidity after an affected patient is intubated and ventilated. There may be instances of severe toxicity with these two substances in which enhanced elimination will reduce the length of ICU stays and the associated nosocomial risks; extracorporeal elimination may then be a reasonable option.[5,52]

CAN THE TOXIN BE REMOVED?

Effective removal by any of the procedures listed in Table 6–1 is limited by a large volume of distribution. The volume of distribution (Vd) relates the concentration of the toxin in the blood or

TABLE 6–1. Potential Methods of Enhancing Elimination of Toxic Compounds

Cerebrospinal fluid drainage and replacement
Chelation
Diuresis
Exchange transfusion
Hemodialysis
Hemofiltration
Manipulation of pH
Multiple doses of activated charcoal, cholestyramine, colestipol, Kayexalate, Prussian blue
Nasogastric suction
Peritoneal dialysis
Plasmapheresis
Sorbent hemoperfusion
Toxin-specific antibody fragments
Whole-bowel irrigation

serum to the total body burden. The Vd can be envisioned as the apparent volume in which a known total dose of drug is distributed after acute administration, and before metabolism and excretion occur:

$$Vd(L) = dose~(mg)/concentration~(mg/L)$$

The larger the Vd, the less the compound is available to the blood compartment for elimination. A drug with a relatively small Vd, considered amenable to extracorporeal elimination, would distribute in an apparent volume not much larger than total body water. Total body water is approximately 60% of total body weight, so that Vd equal to total body water is approximately 0.6 L/kg body weight.

Ethanol is an example of a toxin with a small Vd approximately equal to total body water. A substantial fraction of a dose of ethanol could be removed by hemodialysis. In contrast, an insignificant fraction of digoxin, with a large volume of distribution (Vd = 5–12 L/kg body weight), would be removed by this therapy. Lipid-soluble drugs and toxins, and those that are highly protein bound, have large volumes of distribution, which can exceed total body water, or even total body weight. These high apparent volumes of distribution imply that the drug is not available to extracorporeal removal because only a small portion of the substance would be in the extracorporeal circuit. In addition to the alcohols, other substances with relatively low Vd include acetaminophen, phenobarbital, lithium, salicylates, and theophylline. Conversely, those with a high Vd (up to 40 L/kg body weight), which would not be removed substantially by hemodialysis, include many β-adrenergic antagonists (with the possible exception of atenolol[64]), diazepam, organic phosphorus compounds, phenothiazines, quinidine, and the cyclic antidepressants.

Whether a toxin can be removed is also determined by the pharmacokinetics of the compound. Kinetic parameters after an overdose may differ from those after therapeutic or experimental doses.[62] For instance, carrier or enzyme-mediated elimination processes may be overwhelmed by higher levels of the drug or toxin in question, making extracorporeal removal potentially more useful. Alternatively, plasma protein- and tissue-binding sites may all be saturated at higher concentrations, making extracorporeal removal feasible in instances where it would have no role in less significant overdoses. An example is valproic acid, which may be poorly dialyzed at nontoxic levels associated with high rates of

protein binding. Higher, potentially toxic concentrations saturate protein-binding sites and lead to a higher proportion of the drug free in the serum and amenable to being removed at a clinically relevant rate by hemodialysis.[35] Estimates of the expected endogenous rates of elimination of a substance in the setting of an overdose should be made then, where possible, from knowledge of the pharmacokinetics obtained in relevant models of toxicity, not after therapeutic doses.

When assessing the efficacy of any technique of enhanced elimination, a generally accepted principle is that the intervention is worthwhile only if the total body clearance of the toxin is increased by at least 30%.[16] This substantial increase is easier to achieve when the compound has a low endogenous clearance. Examples of substances with low endogenous clearance (<4 mL/min/kg) include the toxic alcohols (when metabolism is blocked), atenolol, sotalol, lithium, paraquat, phenytoin, salicylate, and theophylline. Drugs with high endogenous clearances include many β-adrenergic antagonists, lidocaine, opioids, nicotine, and tricyclic antidepressants. Enhancement of elimination is expected to contribute more to the former group than the latter.

The efficacy of any technique of elimination can also be assessed by comparing the blood or plasma concentrations of the substance at the beginning and at the end of the procedure.[66] For example, a compound like theophylline, with one-compartment kinetics, is essentially limited to the extracellular space. The difference between the theophylline concentration before the procedure, minus the concentration at the end of the procedure, divided by the concentration at the beginning, is the fraction of the body burden of the compound that has been eliminated.

If the toxin is like lithium in that it distributes in part to the intracellular compartment and to the extracellular compartment, an equilibrium is established for the compound between the intracellular and extracellular compartments. The latter includes the blood from which elimination occurs. An increase in the elimination rate from the extracellular compartment, such as by hemodialysis, alters this equilibrium. If the rate of redistribution of the compound from the intracellular compartment into the now-dialyzed extracellular compartment is slower than the rate of clearance across the dialysis membrane, the dialysis clearance, or total-body clearance rate, can be limited. Thus, although plasma or blood concentrations may fall precipitously during the procedure, the total-body burden of the substance may not be affected significantly. This is demonstrated most clearly if the blood concentrations are monitored after discontinuation of the procedure and demonstrate rebounding serum levels, indicating postdialysis redistribution (Fig. 6–1). The magnitude of the rebound depends on total-body stores of the drug, as well as on whether there is ongoing absorption from the gastrointestinal tract.

Similarly, what appears to be efficient removal by hemodialysis or hemoperfusion may not indicate efficient removal of the total-body burden of a drug or toxin. Extraction ratios (discussed later) of 100% indicate that all of the substance passing through a hemoperfusion cartridge is removed. Yet, if the compound fails to redistribute from the intra- to extracellular compartment during the procedure, or is largely in the intracellular compartment to begin with, the total-body clearance may be quite low. An example is a 60-kg patient who ingests one hundred 25-mg amitriptyline tablets, a tricyclic antidepressant.[24] Assuming the drug is fully absorbed, the 2500 mg distributes in an apparent volume of 40 L/kg body weight, to achieve a plasma level of 1000 ng/mL, a potentially toxic level. If charcoal hemoperfusion is performed with a

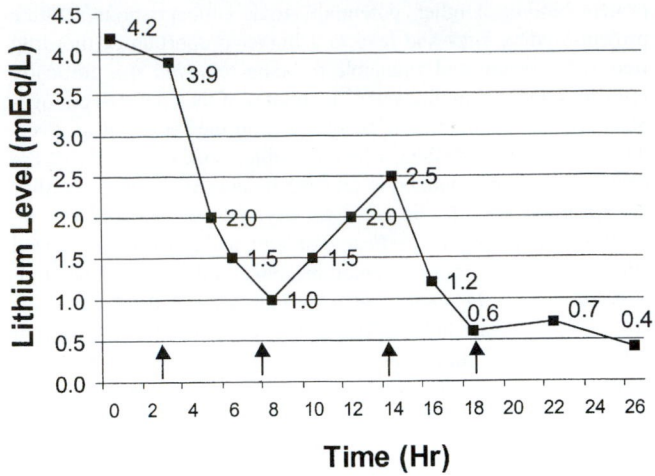

Figure 6–1. Repeated serum lithium concentrations after an acute ingestion. Arrows indicate beginning and end of hemodialysis. Following a 5-hour hemodialysis treatment, a significant rebound in serum concentration occurred, with recurrence of neurologic impairment. An additional 4-hour hemodialysis treatment was then begun.

blood flow rate of 350 mL/min (plasma flow rate of 200 mL/min), and the extraction ratio is 100%, the clearance of drug is 200 mL/min or 200 μg/min. In 4 hours (240 minutes) of treatment, 48 mg (48,000 μg), or less than 2% of the drug ingested, will be removed, which will have no effect on prognosis.

When assessing efficacy, the clinical response must be considered in addition to the evidence of enhanced elimination. In some instances, improvement has been observed that would not be predicted from data based on the kinetics of the parent compound. In severe cases of tricyclic antidepressant poisoning,[67] unexpected improvement during hemoperfusion could have been fortuitous because the toxicity is manifested early and ameliorates rapidly during the initial distribution phase. Beginning a procedure during the initial distribution phase may increase the fraction of body burden that can be removed. Later administration of extracorporeal treatment may have much lower clearance rates and benefits. Poisonings with paraquat and toxic mushrooms are other examples in which early, but not late, extracorporeal therapy *may* have benefit. An alternative explanation for unanticipated evidence of improvement is the removal of small amounts of the drug and active metabolites from a shallow "toxic effect" compartment. This theory has been advanced to explain the response of patients overdosed with the antipsychotic chlorprothixene,[38] or with a combination of diltiazem and metoprolol.[2] Such effects can lead to transient improvements that are not sustained as drug redistributes from one pool to another, leading to early benefit but eventual recurrence of symptoms. Much of the relevant literature fails to provide longterm followup to demonstrate prolongation of benefits after extracorporeal therapy is completed.

Other examples also demonstrate that removal of toxin is a poor surrogate for clinical benefit. Enhanced elimination of phenobarbital[56] or carbamazepine[70] by repeated oral activated charcoal did not affect clinical outcomes as compared to those of overdosed, untreated controls. In another study, no difference was observed between patients with lithium poisoning for whom hemodialysis was done and those for whom it was recommended by

a poison control center but not done.[6] The conclusion was that hemodialysis should be considered appropriate only for the more severe cases.

TECHNIQUES AVAILABLE TO ENHANCE REMOVAL OF TOXINS

Although controversies remain about the efficacy of, or need for, removal of many toxins, a consensus regarding the indications for a number of procedures has developed. This consensus has led to consistent application of several techniques for some toxic exposures that occur relatively frequently. The techniques to enhance toxin elimination most commonly applied over the last decade have been alkalinization of the urine for salicylates, hemodialysis for methanol, ethylene glycol, lithium, and salicylates; and hemoperfusion for theophylline.[29]

Forced Diuresis and Manipulation of Urinary pH

Forced diuresis by volume expansion with sodium-containing solutions, such as 0.9% NaCl or lactated Ringer solution, may increase renal clearance of some molecules. This would theoretically be most true for substances such as lithium for which the glomerular filtration rate (GFR) is an important determinant of excretion, and particularly in instances where extracellular fluid volume is contracted. In the latter circumstance, restoration of the extracellular fluid volume leads to an increase in GFR and augments drug excretion. An additional mechanism is to suppress tubular sodium reabsorption, which also leads to an increase in excretion of lithium, a drug whose absorption in the proximal tubule is augmented in states of sodium avidity. After the extracellular fluid volume is restored, continued infusion of saline increases urine volume proportionally more than GFR, which increases excretion of small molecules such as urea, but which has marginal efficacy in the case of poisonings. The significant risk of this therapy is extracellular fluid volume overload, manifested by pulmonary and cerebral edema. This complication may be particularly likely in patients with long-standing lithium use in whom chronic tubulointerstitial disease can lead to renal insufficiency that does not improve with fluid therapy. Knowing the result of recent serum creatinine concentrations may help distinguish acute from chronic renal insufficiency in such cases. Administration of diuretics such as furosemide along with saline may diminish the risk of extracellular fluid volume overload, but complicates the therapy and increases the risk of metabolic alkalosis and hypokalemia. The unproven efficacy of forced diuresis in the management of *any* overdose has led most experts to abandon its use. On the other hand, the repletion of extracellular fluid volume in the presence of depletion, as determined by the history and physical examination, is appropriate.

Many toxic compounds are weak acids or bases that are ionized in aqueous solution to an extent that depends on the pKa of the compound and the pH of the solution. Knowing these variables, the Henderson-Hasselbalch equation (Chap. 11) can be used to determine the relative proportions of the acids, bases, and buffer pairs. Cell membranes are relatively impermeable to ionized, or polar, molecules (such as an unprotonated salicylate anion), whereas nonionized, nonpolar forms (such as the protonated, noncharged salicylic acid) can cross more easily. As compounds pass through the kidney, they may be filtered, secreted, and reabsorbed. If the urinary pH is manipulated to favor the formation of the ionized form in the tubular lumen, the drug is trapped in the tubular fluid and not reabsorbed into the bloodstream. Hence the rate and extent of its elimination can be increased. To make manipulation of urinary pH worthwhile, the renal excretion of the compound must be a major route of elimination. Acidification of the urine by systemic administration of HCl or NH_4Cl to enhance elimination of weak bases, such as phencyclidine or amphetamines, is no longer considered useful. The technique has been abandoned because it does not significantly enhance removal of toxic compounds and is complicated by systemic metabolic acidosis. Alkalinization of the urine to enhance elimination of weak acids has a limited role for compounds such as salicylates,[50] phenobarbital,[40] chlorpropamide, formate, and the herbicide 2,4-dichlorophenoxyacetic acid [2,4-D].[58] These weak acids are ionized at alkaline urine pH and tubular reabsorption is thereby greatly reduced. Alkalinization is achieved by the intravenous administration of sodium bicarbonate, 1–2 mEq/kg every 3–4 hours. The goal is to increase urinary pH to 7–8.

This degree of alkalinization may be difficult, if not impossible, if metabolic acidosis and acidemia are present, as often is the case with salicylate poisoning. Administered sodium bicarbonate is consumed by titration of plasma protons before appearing in the urine. On the other hand, salicylate poisoning often causes respiratory alkalosis as well. In that case, where PCO_2 is low, raising serum bicarbonate may lead to profound, life-threatening alkalemia. Finally, the risk of volume overload with sodium bicarbonate administration is the same as with the administration of 0.9% NaCl. Hypernatremia after administration of hypertonic sodium bicarbonate may also ensue. Bicarbonaturia will also be associated with urinary potassium losses, so serum potassium concentration should be monitored frequently and KCl given liberally. If these complications can be identified and dealt with judiciously and safely, the renal clearance of salicylate can increase 4-fold as urine pH increases from 6.5 to 7.5 with alkalinization.[50] Alkali administration will also, by the same mechanism, favor movement of salicylate from the central nervous system (CNS) to the blood, thereby decreasing CNS toxicity (Chap. 33).

Increasing urine pH by administering carbonic anhydrase inhibitors such as acetazolamide is not recommended. Although elimination of the drug may be increased, metabolic acidosis will ensue unless ample sodium bicarbonate is also administered. In the case of salicylates, acidemia may cause increased distribution of drug into the central nervous system. As with $NaHCO_3$ administration, bicarbonaturia is accompanied by urinary potassium losses; hypokalemia can be profound. The role of urinary alkalinization in the management of salicylate poisoning is further discussed in Chapter 33.

Alkalinization with or without diuresis is also used to maintain renal elimination of methotrexate in patients given high-dose folinic acid rescue therapy.[14] Extracellular fluid volume expansion with 0.9% NaCl and $NaHCO_3$ administration also protects the kidneys from the toxic effects of myoglobinuria in patients with extensive rhabdomyolysis.

Peritoneal Dialysis

Peritoneal dialysis theoretically can be performed to enhance the elimination of a few water-soluble, low-molecular-weight, poorly protein-bound compounds with a low volume of distribution.[27]

Examples are the alcohols, lithium, salicylate, and theophylline. Clearance of compounds in the aqueous dialysate is related to dialysate flow rate, the surface area of the peritoneum, and the molecular weight (MW) of the compound. The highest clearances are achieved for molecules with MW <500 daltons. The efficacy of peritoneal dialysis is markedly decreased when the patient is hypotensive.

Although peritoneal dialysis is a relatively simple method to enhance drug elimination, it is too slow to be useful. Peritoneal dialysis is, therefore, never the method of choice unless hemodialysis and hemoperfusion are unavailable and transfer to a center that can offer these techniques is not feasible. It may be the only practical option in small children if experience with extracorporeal techniques in younger age groups is lacking, or until a child can be transported to an appropriate center.

Hemodialysis

Prompt consultation with a nephrologist is always indicated in the case of any poisoning with a substance that might benefit from extracorporeal removal. The nephrologist has to call in a nurse or technician, the dialysis machine requires preparation, and the vascular access catheter has to be inserted. A delay of several hours before hemodialysis can be instituted should be anticipated. If indicated, modalities of treatment such as ethanol or fomepizole should be administered and other modalities to enhance elimination such as urinary alkalinization or oral multiple-dose activated charcoal (MDAC) should be used where appropriate.

The technical details of the performance of hemodialysis for treatment of poisonings do not differ markedly from those used in the treatment of acute renal failure. Vascular access is best attained via the femoral vein. The subclavian and internal jugular veins are also acceptable, but probably have slightly higher complication rates such as pneumothorax and arterial puncture.[13] Hemostasis after catheter removal is also easily achieved at the femoral site. Hemodialysis and hemoperfusion (see below) are usually performed using a double-lumen catheter manufactured for dialysis, made of polyethylene, polyurethane, or Teflon. Blood is pumped from one lumen and returned to the venous circulation through the second lumen. Blood flow rates with these catheters can be as high as 450–500 mL/min, although 350 mL/min may sometimes be the maximum rate achieved .

The blood lines and artificial kidney should be primed with an appropriate volume of fluid to reduce or avoid hypotension when the procedure is started. Larger "high-efficiency" or "high-flux" artificial kidneys should be selected (discussed later). Full anticoagulation with heparin is usually required. A typical adult heparin dose would be 4000–5000 units as a bolus, followed by 400–500 units hourly. Alternatively, periodic flushes of the dialysis membrane with heparinized saline exposes the patient to very low doses of heparin and little risk of systemic anticoagulation. Regional anticoagulation of the dialysis circuit with citrate or protamine is possible if heparin is absolutely contraindicated, although these agents complicate the procedure. In poisoned patients, hemodialysis is usually performed for 4–8 hours. Assuming that serum potassium concentration is normal, a standard bicarbonate-based dialysate with a potassium concentration of 3 or 4 mEq/L and a calcium concentration of 3 mEq/L, flowing at 600–800 mL/min, is sufficient.

During conventional hemodialysis, blood traverses a semipermeable membrane, bathed by a dialysis solution, or dialysate.

Drugs and toxins diffuse across the membrane from blood into the dialysate along the concentration gradient (Fig. 6–2). The characteristics of compounds that make them amenable to hemodialysis are listed in Table 6–2. These requirements greatly reduce the number of substances that can be expected to be cleared by dialysis. During hemodialysis, clearance of a drug or toxin (Cl_H) can be calculated according to:

$$Cl_H = [Q_{in}(C_{in} - C_{out})] / C_{in}$$

where Q_{in} is the blood flow entering the dialyzer, C_{in} is the concentration of the drug or toxin in blood entering the system, and C_{out} is the concentration in blood leaving the system. The extraction ratio (ER) is a measure of the percentage of substance passing through the artificial kidney, or charcoal hemoperfusion cartridge. This can be calculated as:

$$ER = \frac{C_{in} - C_{out}}{C_{in}} \times 100$$

Hemodialysis is preferred to hemoperfusion to remove compounds such as bromides; chloral hydrate; trichloroethanol; ethanol, methanol, and ethylene glycol; lithium; and salicylate. In addition to removing these compounds, hemodialysis can correct abnormalities such as metabolic acidosis or alkalosis, hyperkalemia, and fluid overload. It is therefore preferred for poisonings characterized by these disorders, if clearance rates resulting from hemoperfusion and hemodialysis are relatively similar. An example is salicylates, poisoning with which is often associated with metabolic acidosis.[32]

Several recent technologic advances enable patients to tolerate dialysis with better clearances and much less hemodynamic instability than in the past. For instance, the source of base in dialysate routinely is now $NaHCO_3$ rather than sodium acetate; the latter caused hypotension and decreased cardiac output. Computerized machines allow fine control of ultrafiltration rates to limit volume losses; in the past, imprecise calculations and manipulations led to frequent episodes of hypotension. The sodium concentration of the dialysate can be programmed to promote hemodynamic stability as well, a technique called *sodium modeling*. Better hemodynamic stability and larger dual-lumen catheters allow use of higher blood flows, up to 400–500 mL/min. As a result of such innovations, treatment can be delivered in more instances than were previously possible. Clearance rates reported in the literature of the 1970s and 1980s may significantly underestimate currently achievable clearance rates.[52] Thus, there are few patients in whom hemodialysis should not at least be instituted, if indicated, and particularly when supportive measures have failed. Hypotension may still occur in critically ill patients. Saline, colloid, vasopressors, or inotropic agents may also be required in such patients, but if dialysis seems to offer the best chance for the patient's survival, it should usually be at least attempted.

Dialysis membrane composition has continued to evolve. The hollow-fiber dialyzer is by far the most commonly used design. It is composed of thousands of blood-filled capillary tubes held together in a bundle and bathed in the machine-generated dialysate. Conventional dialyzers are made of cellulose-derived polymers, typified by Cuprophane. High-efficiency dialyzers have larger surface areas and therefore larger clearances. Hemodialysis efficacy for poisonings with low-molecular-weight substances should improve with the use of larger membranes with larger clearances.

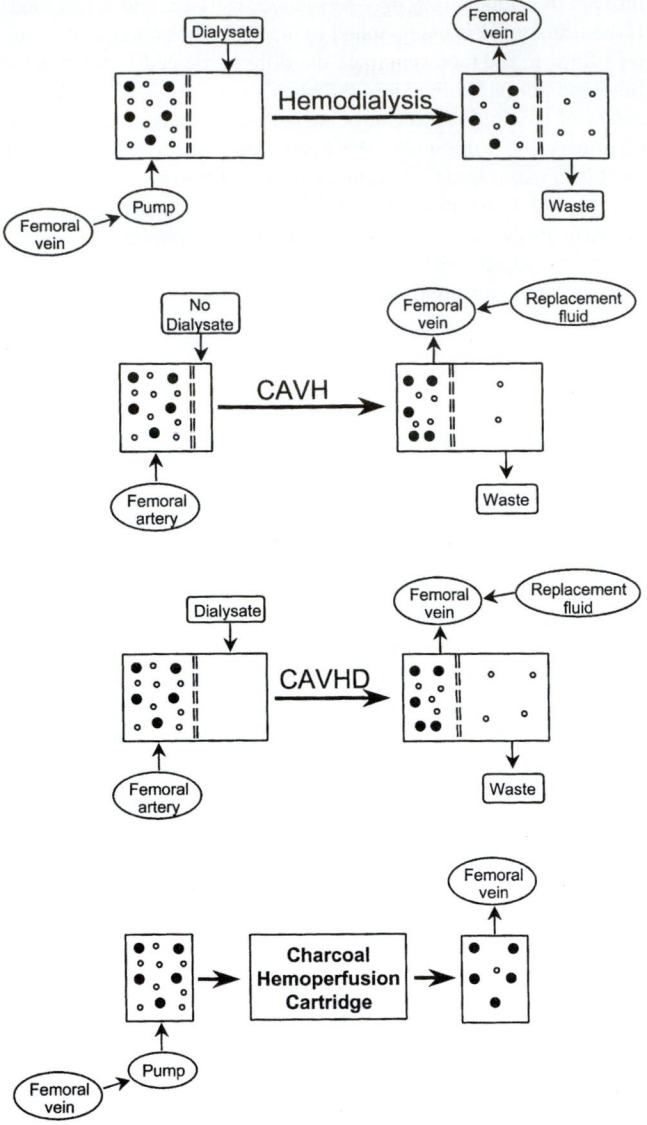

Figure 6–2. The comparative schematic layouts of HD (hemodialysis), CAVH (continuous arteriovenous hemofiltration), CAVHD (CAVH with dialysis), and HP (hemoperfusion). *Filled circles* are high-molecular-weight substances such as plasma protein; *open circles* are low-molecular-weight diffusible solutes such as urea or methanol. In dialysis, solute moves across a semipermeable membrane (*dashed lines*) from a solution in which it is present in a high concentration (blood) to one in which it is at a low concentration (dialysate). In CAVH and CAVHD, plasma moves across a similar membrane in response to hydrostatic pressures. CVVHD, continuous *venovenous* hemofiltration with dialysis, not pictured, is similar to CAVHD, except that it requires a blood pump because it does not have arterial pressure to drive hemofiltration. Availability of blood pumps has made arteriovenous modalities nearly obsolete. Charcoal hemoperfusion requires movement of blood through a sorbent-containing cartridge and does not include dialysis or hemofiltration.

TABLE 6–2. Characteristics of Compounds That Allow Clearance by Hemodialysis, Hemoperfusion, and Hemofiltration

For All Three Techniques
Low volume of distribution (<1 L/kg)
Single-compartment kinetics
Low endogenous clearance (<4 mL/min/kg)

For Hemodialysis
MW <500 daltons
Water soluble
Not bound to plasma proteins

For Hemoperfusion
Adsorption by activated charcoal
Plasma protein binding is not a contraindication

For Hemofiltration
MW <10,000 or 40,000 daltons, depending on filter used

"High-flux" dialyzers have larger pores that allow more clearance of larger molecules. The prototypical "middle molecule," the clearance of which is used to express a dialyzer's high-flux dialysance, is the β-2 microglobulin. Because these membranes also have higher water permeability, the capability to limit ultrafiltration rates, discussed earlier, allows their use. There are some instances in which high-flux dialyzers might be important in promoting clearance of larger molecules, such as vancomycin, which are not readily removed by conventional low-flux membranes.[25] Nonetheless, a sound pharmacologic basis for the efficacy of dialysis must still be present; no amount of increased clearance will eliminate a drug or toxin with a large volume of distribution or significant tissue binding. Definitive evidence is not available that hemodialysis for poisonings with larger-molecular-weight substances improves clinical outcomes.

High-flux, synthetic membranes composed of polysulfone (PS), polymethamethacrylate (PMMA), polyacrylonitrile (PAN), and other polymers also have better biocompatibility, as measured by the rate of activation of inflammatory mediators that include complement, white blood cells, and cytokines. Better biocompatibility means less activation of these potentially damaging mechanisms as compared with cellulose-derived, more bioincompatible membranes. The importance of biocompatibility for the treatment of chronic renal failure is currently being evaluated. Patients with chronic renal failure are exposed to these membrane materials at least 3 treatments a week for many years. It is unlikely that better biocompatibility will affect outcomes for dialysis of poisoned patients who will require only 1 or 2 treatments.

Complications of acute hemodialysis are relatively rare. Bleeding or thrombosis at the venous site used for vascular access is infrequent with normal hemostasis and adequate postprocedure tamponade of the catheter site. Bleeding in the gastrointestinal tract and elsewhere, caused by systemic anticoagulation with heparin, can be avoided if low doses of heparin are used. Nosocomial bacteremia can occur if central lines are left in place for prolonged periods; central lines should be removed after 5 days at most. In addition, hemodialysis increases the elimination of some drugs administered therapeutically, such as folic acid and other water-soluble vitamins and antibiotics. Doses of these drugs therefore need to be increased during dialysis or administered immediately afterwards. Ethanol infusions used in the treatment of toxic alcohol ingestions must be increased (see Antidotes in Depth: Ethanol). Ethanol removal can be limited in such cases by enriching the dialysate with ethanol to a concentration of 100 mg/dL.[17] Similarly, hypophosphatemia after more prolonged high-flux hemodialysis can be avoided by adding sodium phosphate salts, in the form of Fleet's Phospho-Soda, to the dialysate.[25] Use of angiotensin-converting enzyme inhibitors is associated with angioedema when PAN membranes are used for dialysis.[12]

The use of the REDY hemodialysis system in the management of poisonings should be discouraged. These units require no continuous water supply because they regenerate dialysate by adsorption of solute by activated charcoal and exchange resins, and generate HCO_3 from urea by urease. This machine is still sometimes used as a portable unit in some hospitals for the management of renal failure. However, dialysis clearance rates are too low for the management of poisoning. Although the activated charcoal may be specifically useful in adsorbing theophylline, the absence of sufficiently high urea concentrations in most poisoned patients will prevent bicarbonate regeneration from urea and lead to metabolic acidosis.[9]

Charcoal Hemoperfusion

In general, if a compound is adsorbed by activated charcoal, charcoal hemoperfusion clearance will exceed that of hemodialysis. During hemoperfusion, blood is pumped through a cartridge containing a very large surface area of sorbent, either activated charcoal or carbon (Fig. 6–2). The sorbent is coated with a very thin layer of cellulose acetate (Adsorba, made by Gambro), cellulose nitrate (Hemokart, made by Erika), or heparin-hydrogel (Biocompatible Hemoperfusion Systems, made by Clark), which prevents direct contact between blood and sorbent, improves biocompatibility, and helps to prevent charcoal embolization. There may be a further theoretical advantage to the heparin-hydrogel coating to diminish platelet aggregation. The adsorptive capacity of the cartridge is reduced with use because of deposition of cellular debris and blood proteins. Estimation of residual adsorptive capacity by serial serum levels is usually not practical because of time delays in obtaining results. The cartridge should therefore be changed after 2 hours. As with hemodialysis, patients must be anticoagulated with heparin, and regional heparinization of the cartridge is possible if full anticoagulation is undesirable. The technique can be used in adults[19,54,73] or children.[15,46,53] Hemoperfusion is usually performed for 4–6 hours at flow rates of 250–400 mL/min.

The characteristics of compounds that make them amenable to hemoperfusion (summarized in Table 6–2) differ from those for hemodialysis in the important respect that hemoperfusion is not limited by plasma protein binding. This is exemplified in a report in which hemoperfusion but not hemodialysis increased the elimination of the avidly protein-bound oral hypoglycemic agent chlorpropamide.[43] Some substances are poorly adsorbed by activated charcoal, including the alcohols, lithium, and many metals (see Antidotes in Depth: Activated Charcoal), making hemoperfusion inappropriate in their management. Hemoperfusion clearance is calculated in a manner similar to that for hemodialysis. Although hemoperfusion is the preferred method to enhance the elimination of carbamazepine, phenobarbital, phenytoin, and theophylline (Table 6–3), recent improvements in hemodialysis technology may make older comparisons of hemodialysis and hemoperfusion clearance rates obsolete.[52]

TABLE 6–3. Properties of Toxins Grouped by Efficacy of Extracorporeal Techniques for Elimination

Drug/Toxin	MW (daltons)	Water Soluble	Vd (L/kg)	Protein Binding (%)	Endogenous Clearance (mL/min/kg)	Preferred Method	Comments
Clinically Efficacious							
Bromide	35	Yes	0.7	0	0.1	HD	
Ethylene glycol	62	Yes	0.6	0	2.0	HD	Cl ↑ as dose ↓
Isopropanol	60	Yes	0.6	0	na	HD	
Lithium	7	Yes	0.6–1.0	0	0.4	HD	Cl ↓ in renal failure
Methanol	32	Yes	0.6	0	0.7	HD	
Salicylate	138	Yes	0.2	50	0.9	HD, HP	Cl and protein binding ↓ with ↑ dose; HD also corrects electrolytes, acid-base
Theophylline	180	Yes	0.5	56	0.7	HP>HD	HP & HD can also be combined
Valproic acid	144	Yes	0.13–0.22	90	0.1	HD, HP	↑ Levels associated with ↓ % protein binding
Possibly Clinically Efficacious							
Amanita toxin	373–990	Yes	0.3	0	2.7–6.2	HP	Possibly effective if performed in first 24 hours
Aminoglycosides	>500	Yes	0.3	1.5	<10	HD/HF	Cl ↓ with renal failure
Atenolol	255	Yes	1.0	2.5	<5	HD or HP	Useful if Cl ↓ due to renal failure
Carbamazepine	236	No	1.4	74	1.3	HP	Cl ↑ in patients on long-term therapy
Disopyramide	340	No	0.6	1.2	90	HP	Protein binding ↓ as concentration ↑
Meprobamate	218	Yes	0.5–0.8	0–30	Low	HP	Most drug eliminated in 24–36 hours
Methotrexate	454	Yes	0.4–0.8	50	1.5	HF	
Paraquat	186	Yes	1.0	6	24.0	HP	Tight tissue binding precludes efficacy, unless early in course
Phenobarbital	232	No	0.5	24	0.1	HP	Only for prolonged coma
Phenytoin	252	No	0.6	90	0.3	HP	Cl ↓ as dose ↑
Procainamide	272	Yes	1.9	16	8.0	HF	Cl ↓ in renal failure
Sotalol	272	Yes	2.0	2.0	<5	HD or HP	
Trichlorethanol	149	Yes	0.6	0.4	0.7	HD	Metabolite of chloral hydrate

Cl = clearance; na = not available.

Hemodialysis and hemoperfusion have been performed in series for procainamide, thallium, and carbamazepine overdoses, with greater apparent clinical efficacy than either procedure alone.[10,21,37] In this technique, blood circulates first through the hemodialysis membrane, and then through the charcoal cartridge. A hemoperfusion cartridge also has been inserted into an extracorporeal membrane oxygenation (ECMO) circuit through which the flow rate was >3 L/min in a patient who ingested 2 g of propranolol.[65] The plasma concentrations of propranolol decreased more rapidly during extracorporeal membrane oxygenation than after it was discontinued. The high flow rate through the cartridge may have led to substantial clearance of the drug.

A practical problem limiting the use of charcoal hemoperfusion is the availability of the cartridges. Many dialysis units do not routinely have them in stock. The cartridges are expensive ($350–$425 as compared to the maximal cost for a high-flux dialysis membrane at about $20–$23). Some have expiration dates, limiting shelf life. Others, such as the Clark system, have an indefinite shelf life but must be autoclaved before use, which may affect their availability in an emergency. Charcoal cartridges were more available in chronic hemodialysis units when they were needed for the treatment of chronic aluminum toxicity. This syndrome of aluminum-associated dementia and osteodystrophy was previously more prevalent in chronic hemodialysis units, but aluminum carbonate has been supplanted as a phosphate binder by calcium salts. The most frequent indication for acute charcoal hemoperfusion in the past was theophylline intoxication. Theophylline is no longer popular in the treatment of obstructive lung disease, so that charcoal hemoperfusion is less frequently utilized. In turn, the low incidence of theophylline poisoning contributes to poor stocking of the cartridges. All of these factors contribute to the poor availability of charcoal cartridges and the relative infrequency with which the procedure is performed.

Other adsorptive resins have been used for hemoperfusion, such as the synthetic Amberlite XAD-2 and XAD-4 and anion exchange resins such as Dow 1X-2. None of these columns is approved or available for use in the United States. The literature regarding their efficacy is scant and relatively anecdotal. Though there is in vitro evidence that these resins may have greater adsorptive capacities than activated charcoal, there are few, if any, meaningful comparisons in a clinical setting.

The complications of hemoperfusion are similar to those of hemodialysis. In addition, patients may develop thrombocytopenia, leukopenia, or hypocalcemia.[57] Better membrane encapsulation techniques have made embolization of charcoal particles extremely rare. As in the case of hemodialysis, doses of drugs used therapeutically may need to be increased if they are removed by hemoperfusion.

For theophylline toxicity, it may be advantageous to combine both hemoperfusion and hemodialysis by putting both the dialysis membrane and the activated charcoal cartridge "in series" in the blood circuit.[7,31] If blood traverses the dialysis membrane first, 50%

of the drug is dialyzed, and the activated charcoal cartridge has less drug to adsorb. The activated charcoal cartridge is exhausted more slowly, and higher extraction ratios are maintained. The dialysis membrane also enables correction of the acid-base and electrolyte disorders that frequently accompany theophylline toxicity.

Multiple-Dose Activated Charcoal: "Gastrointestinal Dialysis"

Oral administration of multiple doses of activated charcoal increases elimination of some drugs present in the blood. Avid adsorption of the drug by the activated charcoal maintains a concentration gradient across the intestinal epithelium. The drug then diffuses from blood, where it is present in higher concentration, to the intestinal lumen, where no drug is left unbound.

This technique was first clearly demonstrated to enhance elimination after parenteral administration of phenobarbital.[8] As in the case of hemoperfusion, the technique would be expected to be effective with compounds that are avidly bound by activated charcoal, have low volumes of distribution with little binding by plasma proteins, and properties that permit transmembrane diffusion across the intestinal epithelium. Theophylline is another drug for which this technique appears to be especially useful. Valproic acid is an example of a toxin cleared significantly by MDAC only when levels are high, as protein-binding sites become saturated and unbound drug in plasma becomes accessible to the enteric activated charcoal.[28] MDAC, often administered with a single dose of cathartic, such as sorbitol, may lead to bowel obstruction if not carefully observed. Diarrhea with sodium and water depletion may also complicate MDAC. MDAC is discussed in more detail in Chapter 5. In appropriate cases, MDAC should be continued if extracorporeal techniques are applied, as it represents another route of elimination.

Continuous Hemofiltration and Hemodiafiltration

Continuous modalities of dialytic therapy are still relatively experimental for the treatment of poisoning. These techniques have found relatively common and widespread usage in the treatment of acute renal failure in the intensive care unit, and in this context are referred to collectively as modalities of *continuous renal replacement therapies* (CRRT). The clearances of either urea or drugs that are achieved with these techniques are significantly lower than those achieved with hemodialysis. Despite many anecdotal reports demonstrating significant drug clearance, there are no data demonstrating that these techniques affect prognosis or mortality. There are several possible advantages of continuous modalities. One is the capability to continue therapy for 24 hours each day. Therefore, hemofiltration can be instituted after hemodialysis or hemoperfusion to further remove a drug or toxin after it redistributes from tissue to blood.[55] This is an attractive modality for slow, continuous removal of drugs, such as procainamide or lithium, that distribute slowly from tissue-binding sites or from the intracellular compartment (Fig. 6–1).[22,40] Other drugs with volumes of distribution that are large enough to preclude use of dialysis or hemoperfusion might also be eliminated with longer courses. The properties of toxins that make them amenable to hemofiltration are summarized in Table 6–2. However, the rate of removal with this form of therapy may be insufficient to benefit critically ill patients. Patients who can tolerate slower clearance rates, in other words, may not require therapy. Whether slow treatment to avoid

redistribution of intracellularly distributed lithium, for example, is preferable to repeating conventional hemodialysis is not at all clear.[47,68] The technique may be best suited for patients with severe hypotension who cannot tolerate conventional hemodialysis or hemoperfusion.[18] It may have the advantage over hemodialysis in being able to clear larger molecules such as methotrexate (MW 454.4).[22,26,49] There is growing evidence that a significant part of the clearance of many molecules occurs because of adsorption of the molecule to the synthetic membrane.[20] Another practical advantage is that the procedure is usually done now in intensive care units by ICU nurses, and, where available in such units, might not require dialysis personnel.

Hemofiltration, or ultrafiltration, refers to the movement of plasma across a semipermeable membrane in response to hydrostatic pressure gradients. In pure hemofiltration, sometimes called *slow continuous ultrafiltration* (SCUF), there is no dialysate solution on the other side of the dialysis membrane (see Fig. 6–2). Smaller solutes are transported across the membrane with plasma water, a mechanism known as *convective transport* or *bulk flow*. Larger solutes, depending on permeability characteristics of the membrane, are excluded. The extracellular fluid volume status of the patient determines whether replacement of all or some of the filtered plasma with physiologic electrolyte solution (lactated Ringer solution or other commercially available preparations) is indicated. Although this technique can be done intermittently using a hemodialysis machine, it has been adapted for use in intensive care units as a continuous form of treatment, particularly where removal of extracellular fluid is indicated. The clearance of low-molecular-weight solutes such as urea is relatively low. Solute clearance can be significantly enhanced by adding a diffusive mechanism (dialysis), thus permitting a dialysate solution to bathe the blood-filled capillaries running countercurrent to the blood flow. The combination of hemofiltration with dialysis is known as *hemodiafiltration*. Addition of dialysis also usually suffices to treat supervening acute renal failure or preexisting chronic renal failure.

Hemodiafiltration, like hemodialysis, requires that blood perfuse a hollow-fiber dialysis membrane, usually made of synthetic polysulfone, polyamide, or PMMA.[23,39] For all of these procedures, the patient must be fully anticoagulated, but some hemofilters are available that may not require anticoagulation. The hydrostatic pressure required for hemofiltration can be derived either from the patient or from a blood pump. In continuous arteriovenous hemofiltration (CAVH), blood is pumped through the filter by the patient's arterial pressure via a single-lumen femoral artery catheter returning to a femoral vein catheter. Arteriovenous modalities are less favored now because they require a large (eg, 16-French) catheter in the femoral artery while heparin is administered. In continuous venovenous hemofiltration (CVVH), a blood pump is required to maintain adequate flow rates, and arterial puncture with large-bore catheters is avoided. However, the need for a blood pump also necessitates an experienced ICU team to be continuously present for more than the 4–6 hours needed for acute hemodialysis or hemoperfusion. Both the expense and the complexity of a drug-removal procedure are thereby increased. The addition of a dialysate bathing solution to the hemofiltration apparatus changes CAVH and CVVH to the augmented CAVHD (CAVH with dialysis) and CVVHD (CVVH with dialysis), respectively (Fig. 6–2).

Ultrafiltrate flows of 100–6000 mL/h across the membrane can be achieved. Fluid and electrolyte losses must be replaced carefully. Depending on the filter, compounds with a molecular weight of <10,000 or <40,000 daltons, as well as water, urea, creatinine, and sodium, pass into the ultrafiltrate. Heparin, myoglobin, insulin, and vancomycin are examples of larger molecules cleared with relative efficiency.[23] Up to 50% of vancomycin doses may be removed by continuous hemofiltration.[45] The cellular components and molecules larger than the pore size of the membrane return to the circulation in the venous line. For instance, a hemofilter with a molecular weight cutoff of 40,000 daltons cannot remove digoxin-antibody complexes (MW 45,000–50,000).[59] Essential electrolytes lost in the ultrafiltrate are replaced by balanced IV fluids.

Attention must be paid to the undesirable removal of therapeutic drugs such as antibiotics via these continuous modalities. Drug clearances with different synthetic membranes have been measured and are available in the literature; the doses necessary to maintain therapeutic drug levels can also be determined.[11,20,61] Binding of some drugs to ultrafiltration membranes may be of substantial significance with regard to their clearance.

Plasmapheresis and Exchange Transfusion

Plasmapheresis and exchange transfusion are intended to eliminate molecules with large molecular weights that are not dialyzable. This would include substances with molecular weights greater than 15,000 daltons, typified by immunoglobulins. The substance should also have limited endogenous metabolism to make pheresis or exchange worthwhile. By removing plasma proteins, both techniques offer the consequent potential benefit of removal of protein-bound molecules such as *Amanita* toxins,[33] thyroxine, vincristine, or complexes of digoxin and antidigoxin antibodies. However, there is little evidence that either technique affects the clinical course and prognosis. Thyroxine or carbamazepine removal after poisoning, for example, is followed by significant rebound from tissue stores, so that reduction in serum levels is only transient.[30,36] While removal of digoxin-antibody complexes in patients with renal failure may lead to more rapid drug removal,[60] a simpler and more effective therapy may be to repeat administration of digoxin-specific antibody fragments.

Pheresis is particularly expensive, and both pheresis and exchange transfusion expose the patient to the risks of infection with plasma- or blood-borne diseases. Replacement of the removed plasma during plasmapheresis can be accomplished with fresh frozen plasma, albumin, or combinations of both. The former is associated with anaphylactic or allergic manifestations, such as fever, urticaria, wheezing, and hypotension, in as many as 21% of cases.[48]

A different setting in which exchange transfusion may be an appropriate technique is in the management of small infants or neonates in whom dialysis or hemoperfusion may be technically difficult or impossible. Anticoagulation and MDAC may be hazardous and therefore contraindicated in the neonatal nursery where the risk of intracerebral bleeding and necrotizing enterocolitis is high. In premature neonates, a single volume exchange appears to alleviate manifestations of theophylline toxicity.[4,51] The therapy has also been successfully used in this setting to treat salicylate poisoning.[44]

Toxicology of Hemodialysis

Unlike patients who receive acute hemodialysis once or twice in the management of poisoning, patients with chronic renal failure are repeatedly exposed to large volumes of water during the course of their hemodialysis treatments. If an "average" regimen consists of 3 treatments of 4 hours each week, with dialysate flows of 500 mL/min, patients will be exposed to 360 L of water separated only by a semipermeable membrane designed to allow solute passage in either direction. Misadventures in the generation of water for dialysate, therefore, have the potential to be lethal to this population by exposing this population to significant quantities of toxins. The quality of water used for dialysate generation is regulated in the United States by the Association for the Advancement of Medical Instrumentation (AAMI).[1] Water from the municipal supply is first treated with a water softener to remove calcium and magnesium; it is then run through an activated charcoal bed to adsorb chlorine and chloramine. Most commonly, water for dialysate is then generated by reverse osmosis, a process that requires that water cross a membrane that is relatively impermeable to solutes. The water movement occurs as a result of applied hydrostatic pressure, and leaves behind any solutes. Water can also be purified using deionization, a technique that runs water over an exchange resin, releasing hydroxyl ions in exchange for charged species in the water. Deionization is inferior to reverse osmosis for removal of aluminum, and may be associated with release of lethal levels of fluoride when exchange sites are exhausted.[3] General water chemistry testing is mandated annually, while testing for chlorine and chloramine is done daily.

Current requirements are that water be highly purified, but not sterile, because bacteria cannot cross from the dialysate into the blood. However, small quantities of endotoxin can cross, particularly in situations that include the use of high-flux membranes. Endotoxin is suspected of being responsible for activation of circulating cytokines, malnutrition, fever, and other syndromes such as carpal tunnel syndrome associated with chronic inflammation. Recommendations for the frequency of testing for and the allowable maximum amounts of endotoxin are currently under consideration. Water distribution systems are cleaned at least monthly with bleach, peracetic acid, and/or other sterilants. Unusual microbes have also been associated with serious toxicity. Untreated water at one center in Brazil demonstrated growth of Cyanobacteria (blue-green algae) and production of microcystins, cyclic peptides that cause serious hepatic toxicity; patients dialyzed with the contaminated water had a dramatic rate of death from liver failure.[34]

Water contamination should especially be suspected when multiple patients experience similar symptoms nearly simultaneously. Contamination of dialysate with potential toxins can occur at the source of the municipal water supply (either as a result of run-off of chemicals into reservoirs or after water treatment occurs) or because of contaminants derived from the dialysis unit. Chloramine is frequently added to municipal water supplies to control bacterial populations, and can cause nausea, vomiting, methemoglobinemia, and hemolytic anemia.[69] Recently, chloramine was blamed for decreased bone marrow sensitivity to erythropoietin. Aluminum is present in some municipal water supplies, and before it was recognized as a problem, aluminum led to encephalopathy characterized by seizures, myoclonus, and dementia; to osteomalacia; and to microcytic anemia. Dialysate distribution systems are always made of PVC or other inert plastics, rather than copper, which also can leach into the water and cause similar syndromes.

Besides water for dialysate, another source of poisoning in hemodialysis units is the process of reusing dialysis membranes. At least 70% of dialysis units in the United States reuse membranes because of cost considerations. Each dialysis membrane is sterilized with peracetic acid, formaldehyde, or glutaraldehyde. Careful quality assurance programs ensure that there is no significant exposure of the patients to these molecules during the dialysis procedure. Nonetheless, reuse programs have been associated with a variety of syndromes such as pyrogenic reactions attributed to patient exposure to germicides or endotoxin due to inadequate sterilization procedures.[63]

SUMMARY

Further discussion of some of techniques to enhance elimination, not discussed here, is found in Chapters 47 (cerebrospinal fluid drainage and replacement), 48 (toxin-specific antibodies), 80 (chelation), and 105 (exchange transfusion). All of these techniques have limited, very specific indications, and the effect of these interventions on the overall body burden of the intoxicant is usually small. Interruption of the enterohepatic circulation and/or gastrointestinal dialysis (Chap. 5) can be used concurrently with the techniques discussed.

MDAC, urinary alkalinization, and many of the other techniques listed in Table 6–1 can be instituted quickly in the emergency department. In contrast, the extracorporeal methods of toxin removal, including hemodialysis, sorbent hemoperfusion, and continuous hemofiltration, all require consultation with a nephrologist or intensivist. Timely utilization of these techniques requires mobilization of a competent team and preparation of the requisite equipment. Rapid identification of a toxic exposure for which these techniques are appropriate, and the presence of more ominous prognostic features, should lead to prompt notification of the appropriate consult services so that application of these techniques can proceed in an expeditious manner.

REFERENCES

1. AAMI WQD:1998—Water Quality for Dialysis. Arlington, VA, Association for the Advancement of Medical Instrumentation, 1998.
2. Anthony T, Jastremski M, Elliott W, et al: Charcoal hemoperfusion for the treatment of a combined diltiazem and metoprolol overdose. Ann Emerg Med 1986;15:1344–1348.
3. Arnow PM, Bland LA, Garcia-Houchins S, et al: An outbreak of fatal fluoride intoxication in a long-term hemodialysis unit. Ann Intern Med 1994;121:339–344.
4. Assael BM, Caccamo ML, Gerna M, et al: Effect of exchange transfusion in elimination of theophylline in premature neonates. J Pediatr 1977;91:331–332.
5. Atassi WA, Noghnogh AA, Hariman R, et al: Hemodialysis as a treatment of severe ethanol poisoning. Int J Artif Organs 1999;22:18–20.
6. Bailey B, McGuigan M. Comparison of patients hemodialyzed for lithium poisoning and those for whom dialysis was recommended by PCC but not done: What lesson can we learn? Clin Nephrol 2000; 54:388–392.
7. Benowitz NL, Toffelmire EB: The use of hemodialysis and hemoperfusion in the treatment of theophylline intoxication. Semin Dial 1993; 6:243–252.
8. Berg M, Berlinger W, Goldberg M, et al: Acceleration of the body clearance of phenobarbital by oral activated charcoal. N Engl J Med 1982;307:642–644.
9. Berns A, comment in Benowitz NL, Toffelmire EB: The use of hemodialysis and hemoperfusion in the treatment of theophylline intoxication. Semin Dial 1993;6:243–252.
10. Bock E, Keller E, Heitz J, Heinemeyer G: Treatment of carbamazepine poisoning by combined hemodialysis/hemoperfusion. Int J Clin Pharmacol Ther Toxicol 1989;27:490–492.
11. Bressolle F, Kinowski J, de la Coussaye JE, et al: Clinical pharmacokinetics during continuous haemofiltration. Clin Pharmacokinet 1994; 26:457–471.
12. Brunet P, Jaber K, Berland Y, Baz M: Analphylactoid reactions during hemodialysis and hemofiltration: Role of associating AN69 membrane and angiotensin 1-converting enzyme inhibitors. Am J Kidney Dis 1992;19:444–447.
13. Canaud B, Leray-Moragues H, Kamoun K, et al: Temporary vascular access for extracorporeal therapies. Ther Apher 2000;4:249–255.
14. Chan H, Evans WE, Pratt CB: Recovery from toxicity associated with high-dose methotrexate: Prognostic factors. Cancer Treat Rep 1977; 61:797–804.
15. Chavers BM, Kjellstrand CM, Weigand C, et al: Techniques for use of charcoal hemoperfusion in infants: Experience in two patients. Kidney Int 1980;18:386–389.
16. Cherskov M: Extracorporeal detoxification: Still debatable. JAMA 1992;247:3047.
17. Chow MT, DiSilvestro VA, Chun YY, et al: Treatment of acute methanol intoxication with hemodialysis using an ethanol-enriched, bicarbonate-based dialysate. Am J Kid Dis 1997;30:568–570.
18. Christiansson LK, Kaspersson KE, Kulling PE, Ovrebo S: Treatment of severe ethylene glycol intoxication with continuous arteriovenous hemofiltration dialysis. J Toxicol Clin Toxicol 1995;33:267–270.
19. Cutler RD, Forland SC, St. John PG, et al: Extracorporeal removal of drugs and poisons by hemodialysis and hemoperfusion. Ann Rev Pharmacol Toxicol 1987;27:169–191.
20. Davies JG, Kingswood JC, Sharpstone P, Street MK: Drug removal in continuous haemofiltration and haemodialysis. Brit J Hosp Med 1995; 54:524–528.
21. DeBacker W, Zachee P, Verpooten GA, et al: Thallium intoxication treated with combined hemoperfusion-hemodialysis. J Toxicol Clin Toxicol 1982;19:259–264.
22. Domoto DT, Brown WW, Bruggensmith P: Removal of toxic levels of N-acetylprocainamide with continuous arteriovenous hemofiltration or continuous arteriovenous hemodiafiltration. Ann Intern Med 1987;106:550–552.
23. Forni LG, Hilton PJ: Continuous hemofiltration in the treatment of acute renal failure. N Engl J Med 1997;336:1303–1309.
24. Garella S: Extracorporeal techniques in the treatment of exogenous intoxications. Kidney Int 1988;33:735–754.
25. Gatchalian RA, Popli A, Ejaz AA, et al: Management of hypophosphatemia induced by high-flux hemodiafiltration for the treatment of vancomycin toxicity: Intravenous phosphorus therapy versus use of a phosphorus-enriched dialysate. Am J Kid Dis 2000;36:1262–1266.
26. Golper TA, Bennett WM: Drug removal by continuous arteriovenous haemofiltration: A review of the evidence in poisoned patients. Med Toxicol 1988;3:341–349.
27. Golper TA: Drugs and peritoneal dialysis. Dial Transplant 1979;8: 41–43.
28. Graudins A, Aaron CK: Delayed peak serum valproic acid in massive divalproex overdose—Treatment with charcoal hemoperfusion. J Toxicol Clin Toxicol 1996;34:335–341.
29. Henderson A, Wright DM, Pond SM: Experience with 732 acute overdose patients admitted to an intensive care unit over six years. Med J Aust 1993;158:28–30.
30. Henderson A, Hickman P, Ward G, Pond SM: Lack of efficacy of plasmapheresis in a patient overdosed with thyroxine. Anaesth Intens Care 1994;22:463–464.
31. Hootkins R, Lerman MJ, Thompson JR: Sequential and simultaneous "in series" hemodialysis and hemoperfusion in the management of theophylline intoxication. J Am Soc Nephrol 1990;1:923–926.
32. Jacobsen D, Wiik-Larsen E, Bredesen J: Haemodialysis or haemoperfusion in severe salicylate poisoning? Hum Toxicol 1988;7: 161–163.

33. Jander S, Bischoff J, Woodcock BG. Plasmapheresis in the treatment of Amanita phalloides poisoning: II. A review and recommendations. Ther Apher 2000;4:308–312.

34. Jochimsen EM, Carmichael WW, Cardo DM, et al: Liver failure and death after exposure to microcystins at a hemodialysis center in Brazil. N Engl J Med 1998;338:873–878.

35. Johnson LZ, Martinez I, Fernandez MC, et al: Successful treatment of valproic acid overdose with hemodialysis. Am J Kidney Dis 1999; 33:786–789.

36. Kale PB, Thomson PA, Provenzano R, et al: Evaluation of plasmapheresis in the treatment of an acute overdose of carbamazepine. Ann Pharmacother 1993;27:866–870.

37. Kar PM, Kellner K, Ing RS, Leehey DJ: Combined high-efficiency hemodialysis and charcoal hemoperfusion in severe N-acetylprocainamide intoxication. Am J Kidney Dis 1992;10:403–406.

38. Koppel C, Schirop TH, Ibe K, et al: Hemoperfusion in severe chlorprothixene overdose. Intensive Care Med 1987;13:358–360.

39. Kramer P, ed: Arteriovenous Hemofiltration: A Kidney Replacement Therapy for the Intensive Care Unit. Berlin, Springer-Verlag, 1985, pp. 1–13.

40. Leblanc M, Raymond M, Bonnardeaux A, et al: Lithium poisoning treated by high-performance continuous arteriovenous and venovenous hemodiafiltration. Am J Kidney Dis 1996;3:365–372.

41. Linton AL, Luke RG, Briggs JD: Methods of forced diuresis and its application in barbiturate poisoning. Lancet 1967;2:377–379.

42. Lorch JA, Garella S: Hemoperfusion to treat intoxications. Ann Intern Med 1979;19:301–304.

43. Ludwig SM, McKenzie J, Faiman C: Chlorpropamide overdose in renal failure: Management with charcoal hemoperfusion. Am J Kidney Dis 1987;10:457–460.

44. Manikian A, Stone S, Hamilton R, et al: Exchange transfusion as an alternative to hemodialysis in severe infant salicylism [abstract]. J Toxicol Clin Toxicol 1996;34:585.

45. Matzke GR, O'Connell MB, Collins AJ, et al: Disposition of vancomycin during hemofiltration. Clin Pharmacol Ther 1986;40: 425–430.

46. Mauer SM, Chabers BM, Kjellstrand CM: Treatment of an infant with severe chloramphenicol intoxication using charcoal-column hemoperfusion. J Pediatr 1980;96:136–139.

47. Menghini VV, Albright RC. Treatment of lithium intoxication with continuous venovenous hemodiafiltration. Am J Kidney Dis 2000; 36:E21–34.

48. Mokrzycki MH, Kaplan AA: Therapeutic plasma exchange: Complications and management. Am J Kidney Dis 1994;23:817–827.

49. Molina R, Fabian C, Cowley B: Use of charcoal hemoperfusion with sequential hemodialysis to reduce serum methotrexate levels in a patient with acute renal insufficiency. Am J Med 1987;82:350–352.

50. Morgan AG, Polak A: The excretion of salicylate in salicylate poisoning. Clin Sci 1971;41:475–484.

51. Osborn HH, Henry G, Wax P, et al: Theophylline toxicity in a premature neonate: Elimination kinetics of exchange transfusion. J Toxicol Clin Toxicol 1993;31:639–644.

52. Palmer BF: Effectiveness of hemodialysis in the extracorporeal therapy of phenobarbital overdose. Am J Kidney Dis 2000;36:640–643.

53. Papadopoulou ZL, Novello AC: The use of hemoperfusion in children: Past, present, and future. Pediatr Clin North Am 1982;29: 1039–1052.

54. Park GD, Spector R, Roberts RJ, et al: Use of hemoperfusion for treatment of theophylline intoxication. Am J Med 1983;74:961–966.

55. Pond SM, Johnston SC, Schoof DD, et al: Repeated hemoperfusion and continuous arteriovenous hemofiltration in a paraquat poisoned patient. J Toxicol Clin Toxicol 1987;25:305–316.

56. Pond SM, Olson KR, Osterloh JD, Tong TC: Randomized study of the treatment of phenobarbital overdose with repeated doses of activated charcoal. JAMA 1984;251:3104–3108.

57. Pond SM, Rosenberg J, Benowitz NL, et al: Pharmacokinetics of haemoperfusion for drug overdose. Clin Pharmacokinet 1979;4: 329–354.

58. Prescott L, Park J, Darrien T: Treatment of severe 2,4-D and mecoprop intoxication with alkaline diuresis. J Clin Pharmacol 1979;7: 111–116.

59. Quaife EJ, Banner W, Vernon DD, Christensen DW: Failure of CAVH to remove digoxin-Fab complex in piglets. J Toxicol Clin Toxicol 1990;28:61–68.

60. Rabetoy GM, Price CA, Findlay JWA, Sailstad JM: Treatment of digoxin intoxication in a renal failure patient with digoxin-specific antibody fragments and plasmapheresis. Am J Nephrol 1990;10: 518–521.

61. Reetze-Bonorden P, Bohler J, Keller E: Drug dosage in patients during continuous renal replacement therapy. Clin Pharmacokinet 1993; 24:362–379.

62. Rosenberg J, Benowitz NL, Pond SM: Pharmacokinetics of drug overdose. Clin Pharmacokinet 1981;6:161–192.

63. Rudnick JR, Arduino MJ, Bland LA, et al: An outbreak of pyrogenic reactions in chronic hemodialysis patients associated with hemodialyzer reuse. Artif Organs 1995;19:289–294.

64. Saitz R, Williams BW, Farber HW: Atenolol-induced cardiovascular collapse treated with hemodialysis. Crit Care Med 1991;19:116–118.

65. Smith B, Sullivan MJ: Lifesaving use of extracorporeal membrane oxygenation. Aust J Cardiovasc Perf 1990;4:7–11.

66. Takki S, Gambertoglio JG, Honda DH, Tozer TN: Pharmacokinetic evaluation of hemodialysis in acute drug overdose. J Pharmacokinet Biopharm 1978;6:427–442.

67. Trafford JAP, Jones RK, Evans R, et al: Haemoperfusion with RB004 Amberlite resin for treating acute poisoning. BMJ 1997;2:1453–1455.

68. Van Bommel EF, Kalmeijer MD, Ponssen HH. Treatment of life-threatening lithium toxicity with high-volume continuous venovenous hemofiltration. Am J Nephrol 2000;20:408–411.

69. Ward DM. Chloramine removal from water used in hemodialysis. Adv Ren Replace Ther 1996;3:337–347.

70. Wason S, Baker RC, Carolan P, et al: Carbamazepine overdose: The effects of multiple dose activated charcoal. J Toxicol Clin Toxicol 1992;30:39–48.

71. Winchester JF: Evolution of artificial organs: Extracorporeal removal of drugs. Artif Organs 1986;10:316–323.

72. Winchester JF: Poisoning: Is the role of the nephrologist diminishing? Am J Kidney Dis 1989;13:171–183.

73. Woo OF, Pond SM, Benowitz NL, et al: Benefit of hemoperfusion of theophylline intoxication. J Toxicol Clin Toxicol 1984;22:411–424.

CHAPTER 7

LABORATORY PRINCIPLES AND TECHNIQUES FOR EVALUATION OF THE POISONED OR OVERDOSED PATIENT

Petrie M. Rainey

Toxicology may be thought of as the study of substances that harm living organisms by causing damage or disruption at the cellular and molecular levels. The field is broad, with many subdisciplines. It is often functionally subdivided into environmental toxicology, clinical or medical toxicology, occupational toxicology, forensic toxicology, experimental toxicology, and pharmaceutic toxicology. Similarly, toxicology laboratories generally have a primary focus, most commonly in environmental, medical, or forensic toxicology.

Environmental toxicology is focused on substances that cause harm through prolonged exposure at relatively low levels. These exposures often result from interaction with a contaminated environment. Typical poisons can be distributed rather widely, such as lead, or they can be limited to uniquely contaminated microenvironments, such as those occurring in various occupational settings. Environmental toxicology testing involves not only measurement of the concentration of implicated substances in individuals, but also concentrations in the environment. Because the duration of the exposure may be as important as the level of exposure, single measurements in individuals may be difficult to interpret. Moreover, some environmental poisons may accumulate slowly in the body and testing may be done intermittently. Consequently, toxicity may precede the finding of elevated blood or urine concentrations. Direct measurement of poisons in the environment offers greater opportunity to prevent, rather than merely detect, toxic exposures.

Medical toxicology addresses harm caused by acute and chronic exposures to excessive concentrations of a substance. The management of toxicologic emergencies is a major component of medical toxicology. Detecting the presence or measuring the concentration of various drugs and other acutely toxic substances is the primary activity of the medical toxicology laboratory. Such testing is closely intertwined with therapeutic drug monitoring, in which drug concentrations are measured as an aid to optimizing drug-dosing regimens. As Paracelsus noted long ago, the only difference between a medication and a poison is the size of the dose. In addition to drugs, measurements may be made of substances that lack a therapeutic purpose, for example, pesticides, herbicides, and naturally occurring plant and animal poisons. The unifying characteristic of the substances typically measured is their common association with a toxicologic emergency and the subsequent need for testing results within a relatively short time frame.

Forensic toxicology largely deals with the same substances that are encountered in medical toxicology. The primary difference is that this testing is done with a legal purpose rather than one of facilitating medical management. Thus, rapid results are not a priority, but the focus is on results that are accurate beyond a reasonable doubt. A practical difference is that medical toxicology limits itself to specimens that can be obtained with minimal risk to the subject, whereas forensic testing may involve measurement of drug concentrations in a variety of body tissues (Chap. 119). A characteristic of forensic testing is the maintenance of a chain of custody, which documents the location of the specimen and the person responsible for its integrity at all times between collection and generation of the final results (for further details see Chap. 118). While some medical toxicology laboratories also do some forensic testing (most commonly workplace drug testing), the majority do not. Laboratories that do both medical and forensic testing typically maintain chain of custody only for forensic specimens, due to the substantial additional costs. As a rule, forensic specimens should be submitted only to a laboratory that routinely performs forensic testing.

The remainder of this chapter focuses primarily on medical toxicology laboratories. Within this limited focus, there is still a remarkable variability in the range of testing available. Test menus may range from once-daily testing for routinely monitored drugs and common drugs of abuse to around-the-clock availability of a broad array of assays with the theoretic potential to identify several thousand substances. The first rule in effectively using the toxicology laboratory is to become familiar with the menu of tests that the laboratory offers.

ROUTINELY AVAILABLE TOXICOLOGY TESTS

There is no consensus on a recommended menu of toxicology tests but there is currently work in progress on guidelines. Many physicians will order a comprehensive toxicology screen on a poisoned patient, if one is readily available, but only about 4% of clinical laboratories provide comprehensive toxicology services (as estimated from proficiency testing data[15]). While comprehensive toxicology screens can identify most substances present in overdosed patients,[28] the results of comprehensive screens infrequently alter management or outcomes.[5,10,14,32,38,53,54] Consequently, many laboratories provide a more limited menu of toxicologically useful tests.

The choice of testing offered should be dictated by the types of cases seen and the resources available to the laboratory. Table 7–1 suggests three levels of toxicology testing. Level I includes tests for drugs that are commonly encountered in overdose situations and for which commercial reagents are available and usable with instrumentation already present in most clinical laboratories.

TABLE 7–1. Routinely Available Toxicology Assays

Level*	Serum (Quantitative) Tests	Urine (Qualitative) Tests
I	Acetaminophen; carbamazepine; digoxin; ethanol; iron; phenobarbital; phenytoin; salicylates; theophylline; tricyclic antidepressants (semiquantitative); valproic acid	Amphetamines; barbiturates; benzodiazepines; cocaine; opiates; phencyclidine; tricyclic antidepressants (if no serum assay)
II	Barbiturates, total; carboxyhemoglobin; lead; lidocaine; lithium; methemoglobin; osmolality; procainamide; quinidine	Thin-layer chromatography screen; methadone; propoxyphene
III	Cholinesterase; GC, HPLC, or GC/MS screens; thiocyanate; toxic alcohols (ethylene glycol, isopropanol, methanol); other specialized assays dictated by local use and abuse patterns (eg, γ-hydroxybutyrate)	Heavy metals (quantitative); LSD; GC/MS confirmation of abused drugs in urine

*Levels represent the complexity of the equipment available and the sophistication of the staff necessary for performance, with I being the lowest level.

Level II includes tests that are less frequently needed or that require specialized instrumentation that is relatively inexpensive and easy to use. Level III includes tests that are needed only in selected settings, require specialized instrumentation that is expensive, or require expert operators. Tests that are not offered should be available through a reference laboratory when clinically indicated.

Decisions on the menu of tests to be offered by any specific laboratory should be determined by the laboratory director in consultation with clinicians who will use the service, and should consider local patterns of use of prescription and illicit drugs, as well as resources available and competing priorities. However, a quantitative assay for acetaminophen should be considered mandatory. Acetaminophen is frequently taken in overdose, but it has no distinctive acute clinical presentation to signal its presence in toxic amounts. Serious overdoses require a specific antidote, *N*-acetylcysteine, which is often lifesaving. A timed serum concentration provides the best indicator of the need for antidotal therapy.

While there is no formal consensus on appropriate toxicology test menus, an operational consensus may be deduced from the numbers of laboratories participating in various types of proficiency testing. Result summaries from the 1999 series of proficiency surveys administered by the College of American Pathologists suggest that assays for digoxin, phenytoin, and theophylline, as well as screening tests for drugs of abuse in urine, are available in approximately two-thirds of laboratories that offer routine clinical testing. More than half of the participating laboratories also typically offer tests for ethanol, acetaminophen, salicylates, iron, phenobarbital, carbamazepine, and valproic acid. About one-third of laboratories offer lithium and osmolality measurements.[15]

In contrast to those tests that are routinely available and stratified as such in Table 7–1, there are certain stat toxicologic tests that should be readily available with a quick turnaround to aid the emergency department management of patients. The exact listing of these tests is under debate and recommendations under consideration can be found at http://www.nacb.org/emergency/Toxicol-

ogy. A preliminary list of quantitative serum concentrations that would be extremely helpful include acetaminophen, cooximetry (carboxyhemoglobin, methemoglobin), digoxin, ethanol, ethylene glycol, iron, lead, lithium, methanol, phenobarbital, theophylline, and valproic acid. Urine qualitative assays are less likely to be useful to the emergency department but may have utility in other situations (psychiatry, child abuse).

Only 4% of laboratories participated in proficiency testing for a relatively comprehensive menu of toxicologic testing. These laboratories typically offer quantitative assays for additional therapeutic drugs, particularly tricyclic antidepressants, as well as assays that are designated as toxicologic screens. About half of these full-service toxicology laboratories, or ~2% of all clinical laboratories, offer testing for volatile alcohols other than ethanol.[15]

While relatively few laboratories offer a wide range of in-house testing, most laboratories will send out specimens to reference laboratories that offer large toxicology menus. The turnaround time for such "send out" tests can range from a few hours to several days, depending on the proximity of the reference laboratory and the type of test requested.

Even in comprehensive toxicology laboratories, the test menu may vary substantially from institution to institution. Routinely available tests are usually listed in the laboratory manual. Laboratories with comprehensive services may be able to offer ad hoc chromatographic assays for additional substances that are not listed. Reference laboratory tests may also not be listed in the laboratory manual. The best way to know whether a test is available is to ask the laboratory.

Larger laboratories may offer one or more testing choices designated as "tox screens." There is as much variety in the range of compounds detected in toxicologic screens offered by various laboratories as there is in the total menu of toxicologic tests. Toxicology screens are discussed in greater depth later in this chapter.

USES OF THE TOXICOLOGY LABORATORY

The lack of comprehensive toxicology testing at many institutions argues that rapid comprehensive testing is rarely necessary for effective management of toxicologic emergencies. Supportive care is the mainstay of treatment for most patients with overdoses, and trainees are routinely admonished to "treat the patient, not the poison." Nonetheless, there are many indications for toxicologic testing, as well as additional benefits, as summarized in Table 7–2.

The most common function is to confirm or exclude toxic exposures suspected from the history and physical exam. A laboratory result provides a level of confidence not readily obtained otherwise and may avert other unproductive diagnostic investigations driven by the desire for completeness and medical certainty. Testing has been effective in increasing diagnostic certainty in 59–82% of cases.[5,12,32] In some instances, a diagnosis may be based primarily on the results of testing. This can be particularly important in poisonings with substances having delayed onset of clinical toxicity or in patients with ingestion of multiple substances. In these instances, characteristic clinical findings may have not yet developed at the time of presentation, or may be obscured or altered by the effects of coingestants.

Quantitative testing results have prognostic significance and can help to guide the management of certain poisoned patients.

TABLE 7–2. Indications and Benefits of Toxicologic Testing

Indications
  Make or confirm a diagnosis of poisoning
    Identify presence of substances with delayed manifestations of toxicity
    Identify multiple substance ingestions
    Exclude specific toxic exposures
  Guide the management of confirmed poisonings
    Determine the prognosis (from type and severity of exposure)
      Determine whether to observe or admit
      Anticipate level of supportive care
      Facilitate transfer and discharge planning
    Facilitate telephone consultation with poison center
    Determine need for specific antidotes and interventions
    Monitor effectiveness of treatments to increase elimination
    Determine when to stop antidotal therapy
    Anticipate possible withdrawal reaction (chronic substance users, neonates)
  Exclude pharmacologic basis or contribution to psychiatric disturbance
  Provide medicolegal documentation
    Confirm suspected substance use
    Monitor compliance for drug-abuse programs
    Confirm substance use for admission to detoxification programs
    Confirm brain death (exclude drugs as cause of flat EEG)
    Confirm pharmacologic child abuse/elder abuse

Additional Benefits
  Reassurance
    Reassure patient (or parent)
    Reassure caregivers
  Feedback
    Assess accuracy of clinical decisions
    Clarify unexpected findings and outcomes
    Quality assurance parameter
  Documentation
    Facilitate case studies and reviews
    Document concentration-response relationships at toxic levels
    Determine patterns of exposure
  Hypothesis testing

Serum drug concentrations can facilitate decisions to employ specific antidotes or specific interventions to hasten elimination. Laboratory results can also facilitate the management of poisoning for which only supportive care is available. Because supportive care is basically reactive, knowing what to expect can greatly increase the speed with which appropriate responses are instituted.

Testing can provide two key parameters that will have a major impact on the clinical course, namely, the poison involved and the intensity of the exposure. This information can assist in triage decisions, such as whether to admit a patient or to observe the individual for expectant discharge, and if admission seems indicated, whether admission should be to an intensive care unit. Well-defined exposure information can also facilitate provision of optimum advice by poison control centers, whose personnel do not have the ability to make decisions based on direct observation of the patient. Quantitative data have the greatest prognostic ability, but qualitative results can also facilitate anticipatory management. For example, a positive test for barbiturates can alert the physician to the possibility of a withdrawal reaction. Serum concentrations can be used to determine when to institute and terminate interventions such as hemodialysis or antidote administration, and can support the decision to transfer from intensive care or discharge from the hospital.

Toxicologic testing can also be important for patients presenting with psychiatric disturbances. It can be difficult to distinguish between an organic psychosis and a toxic psychosis on clinical findings alone. Yet the decision often determines whether an admission should be made to a psychiatric or a medical service.

Testing is also often indicated for medicolegal reasons. Diagnoses with legal implications should be established "beyond a reasonable doubt." While testing for illicit drugs is often done for medical purposes, it is almost impossible to dissociate such testing from legal considerations. Documentation is also important in malevolent poisonings, intentional or unintentional child abuse involving therapeutic or illicit drugs, and pharmacologic elder abuse. Where test results may be used to document clear criminal activity, consideration should be given to having testing done in a forensic laboratory maintaining full chain of custody.

An important benefit of toxicology testing is reassurance. This can be reassurance that an unintentional ingestion did not result in absorption of a toxic amount of drug, or that there are no common intoxications or no additional intoxications complicating a clinical presentation. There may be reassurance that the concentration of a drug is declining rather than increasing, or that there is no laboratory evidence for the presence of toxicity at a cellular level that has not yet become clinically apparent. Such reassurance enables a physician to avoid spending excessive time with patients who are relatively stable. It enables admissions to be made and interventions undertaken more confidently and efficiently than would be likely based solely on a clinical diagnosis. This is especially beneficial in a setting in which multiple cases are competing for the physician's attention.

The testing of patients thought to have suffered brain death provides a unique form of reassurance. Demonstration of the absence of central nervous system depressants provides reassurance that a flat electroencephalogram tracing and the interpretation of neurosensory evoked potentials actually reflect true brain death and not pharmacologic suppression of electrical activity.

The confirmation of a clinical diagnosis of poisoning provides an important feedback function, whereby the physician may evaluate the diagnosis against a "gold standard." Much of the art of clinical medicine is learned by making medical decisions and receiving feedback on the outcomes. Regular feedback on diagnostic accuracy provides a key piece of outcome data, one that is particularly valuable in the emergency department, because the patient's clinical course usually is observed elsewhere.

Another important function of toxicology testing is documentation. Results of testing in a central laboratory are almost invariably entered into the patient's medical record and can often provide definitive documentation of a problem. This documentation function has an importance that goes beyond the individual cases. Medical toxicology does not lend itself readily to experimental human investigation. Much of toxicologic knowledge has been derived from experiments of nature. Case reports and case series provide an empirical database for the derivation of medical knowledge. Relatively hard data, such as drug measurements, can serve as key quantitative variables in summarizing and correlating the data. That laboratory results can be reliably (and generally easily) found in the medical record makes them particularly valuable in retrospective reviews. Review of local patterns of exposure can also be used to determine an optimal toxicology testing menu.

Finally, the toxicology laboratory may carry out analyses in support of scientific investigations in medical toxicology. While all of these benefits of toxicologic testing appear to be logical and reasonable ones, there is little empiric evidence verifying this utility. However, lack of evidence of benefit is not evidence of lack of benefit, but only lack of investigation.

METHODS USED IN THE TOXICOLOGY LABORATORY

Most tests in the toxicology laboratory are directed toward the identification and/or quantitation of drugs and poisons. The primary techniques used include spot tests, spectrochemical tests, immunoassays, and chromatographic techniques. Mass spectrometry may also be used, usually in conjunction with gas chromatography. Table 7–3 compares the basic features of commonly used methodologies. Less common methodologies include ion-selective electrode measurements of lithium, atomic absorption spectroscopy or inductively coupled plasma mass spectroscopy for lithium and heavy metals, and anodic stripping methods for heavy metals. There are also many adjunctive tests that may be useful in the management of the poisoned patient. These measure a variety of nondrug substances, including glucose, electrolytes, metabolic products, and enzyme activities. The focus here is on the major methods used for measuring drugs and poisons.

Spot Tests

The simplest tests are spot tests. These rely on the rapid reaction of a drug with a chemical reagent to produce a colored product; for example, the formation of a colored complex between salicylates and ferric ions. Because the reagents may cause precipitation of serum proteins, spot tests are more commonly performed on urine specimens or gastric aspirates. Such tests were once a mainstay of toxicologic testing. Because of the limited selectivity of chemical reagents, as well as the significant variability in visual interpretation, these assays suffer from fairly frequent false-positive results and occasional false-negative results. As more sensitive and more specific methods have become available, spot tests have waned in popularity. Only a few are still in use, largely to fill gaps in a testing menu, or to rapidly exclude some common poisonings (Table 7–4). Although these tests are capable of producing rapid results, the reagents for most of them are dangerously corrosive (ferric chloride is an exception). Thus, they are not particularly suited for testing at the point of care. In the bedside setting, variation in operator technique and use of outdated reagents may also degrade performance. Moreover, the need to comply with federal regulations that govern all laboratory testing, regardless of site, has made bedside testing more demanding (see the later discussion on regulatory issues). The introduction of point-of-care testing devices that have better sensitivity and specificity and are designed to facilitate compliance with regulations is likely to further reduce the use of spot tests.

Spectrochemical Tests

Spectrochemical tests are sophisticated versions of spot tests. They also rely on a chemical reaction to form a light-absorbing substance. They differ in that the reaction conditions and reagent concentrations are carefully controlled and the amount of light absorbed is quantitatively measured at one or more specific wavelengths. The use of specific wavelengths enhances the sensitivity and particularly the specificity of the detection, and the measurement of the amount of light absorbed under controlled conditions allows quantitation of the substance.

When an analyte is intrinsically light absorbing, no reaction may be necessary. Cooximetry represents a sophisticated application of spectrophotometry to the measurement of various forms of hemoglobin in a hemolyzed blood sample. Measurement of light absorption at several wavelengths enables multiple hemoglobin species to be simultaneously quantitated. For mathematical reasons, the number of wavelengths used must be greater than the number of different types of hemoglobin present. This is why pulse oximetry, which uses only two wavelengths, yields spurious results in the presence of methemoglobin or carboxyhemoglobin (Chaps. 20 and 94).

Most analytes are neither as deeply colored nor as highly concentrated as hemoglobin species. Their detection requires the generation of an intensely light-absorbing product, as is done in spot tests. Most spot-test reactions have been used for spectrochemical assays, for example, salicylate assays using Trinder reagent[34] (a variation on ferric chloride). The difference between a spot test and a spectrochemical test lies in whether the colored product is visually observed or quantitatively measured in a spectrophotometer. Because spectrophotometers can also measure ultraviolet and infrared light, it is not necessary that the product have a visible color. Although early spectrochemical assays typically measured the absorption of light after completion of the reaction that produced the colored product, modern assays usually employ rate spectrophotometry, taking multiple measurements over a period of time to determine the rate of increase in light absorption as the reaction proceeds. During the initial phase of the reaction, this rate is constant and proportional to the initial concentration of the substance to be detected (Fig. 7–1). This approach reduces the time needed to obtain the result because the reaction does not have to proceed to completion. It also allows the averaging of multiple

TABLE 7–3.   Relative Comparison of Toxicology Methods

Method	Sensitivity	Specificity	Quantitation	Analyte Range	Speed	Cost
Spot test	+	±	No	Few	Fast	$
Spectrochemical	+	+	Yes	Few	Medium	$
Immunoassay	++	++	Yes	Moderate	Medium	$$
TLC	+	++	No	Broad	Slow	$$
HPLC	++	++	Yes	Broad	Medium	$$
GC	++	++	Yes	Broad	Medium	$$
GC/MS	+++	+++	Yes	Broad	Slow	$$$

TLC, thin-layer chromatography; HPLC, high-performance liquid chromatography; GC, gas chromatography; GC/MS, gas chromatography-mass spectroscopy.

TABLE 7–4.   Substances That Interfere with Spot Tests

Test	Drug or Drug Class	Interferences*
o-Cresol	Acetaminophen	*N*-acetylcysteine (–); ascorbic acid (–); phenols; phenacetin; ketonuria (–)
Diphenylamine	Ethchlorvynol	Phenothiazines; nitrate
Ferric chloride	Salicylates	Acetaminophen; phenothiazines
Forrest	Imipramine, desipramine	Phenothiazines
FPN	Phenothiazines	Desipramine; ketonuria; salicylates
Fujiwara	Chloral hydrate metabolite	Halogenated hydrocarbons
Meixner	Amatoxins	Terpenes
Trinder	Salicylate	Bilirubin; diflunisal; hippuric acid (toluene metabolite); ketonuria; phenothiazines; salicylamide; sulfonamides

*Interferences causing false-negative results are indicated by (–). Other interferences cause false-positive results.

measurements, improving precision. Furthermore, it is unaffected by nonreacting substances that also absorb light at the test wavelength. This is because light absorbance by nonreacting substances is constant and does not contribute to the change in absorbance over time.

Rate spectrophotometry remains subject to interference by substances that also react to produce a light-absorbing product, and falsely increased apparent concentrations may result. Falsely low results may occur when substances are present that inhibit the assay reaction. For example, ascorbic acid produces negative interference in many spectrophotometric assays that rely on oxidation reactions to generate colored products.

Cooximetry is generally relatively free of interferences because the concentrations of the hemoglobins are so much higher than other substances in the blood. However, the presence of intensely colored substances may lead to spurious answers. Methylene blue, which is used to treat methemoglobinemia, typically yields falsely increased measurements of methemoglobin when measured by cooximetry.[33] This interference is not seen when methemoglobin is measured by other methods, such as electrophoresis.

One way to improve the selectivity of a spectrochemical assay is to increase the selectivity of the reaction that generates the light-absorbing product. Enzymes, which can catalyze highly selective reactions, are often used for this purpose. For example, the most widely used assays for ethanol employ alcohol dehydrogenase to catalyze the oxidation of ethanol to acetaldehyde, with concomitant reduction of the cofactor NAD^+ to NADH. The initial rate of increase in light absorption produced by the conversion of NAD^+ to NADH is proportional to the concentration of ethanol. Although other alcohols, such as isopropanol and methanol, can also be oxidized by alcohol dehydrogenase, they are much poorer substrates with low rates of reaction and correspondingly low levels of interference (Fig. 7–1).

In addition to alcohol dehydrogenase–based assays, many other enzymatic assays rely on measuring the change in light absorption at 340 nm when NAD^+ is converted to NADH or vice versa. These include enzymatic assays for ethylene glycol, as well as some enzyme-linked immunoassays, such as EMIT (enzyme-multiplied immunoassay technique) assays (discussed later). All such assays are potentially subject to interference by specimens with high concentrations of lactate. Lactate dehydrogenase, which is naturally present in the serum, converts this lactate to pyruvate with the concomitant conversion of NAD^+ to NADH. However, after all of the NAD^+ in the serum is converted to NADH, this reaction can no longer continue. When the serum specimen is mixed

with assay reagents containing fresh NAD^+, the reaction resumes and contributes to the total rate of NADH production, thereby producing falsely increased results.[50,60]

Immunoassays

The need to measure very low concentrations of substances with a high degree of specificity led to the development of immunoassays. The combination of high affinity and high selectivity makes antibodies ideal assay reagents. There are two common types of immunoassays. In noncompetitive immunoassays, the analyte is

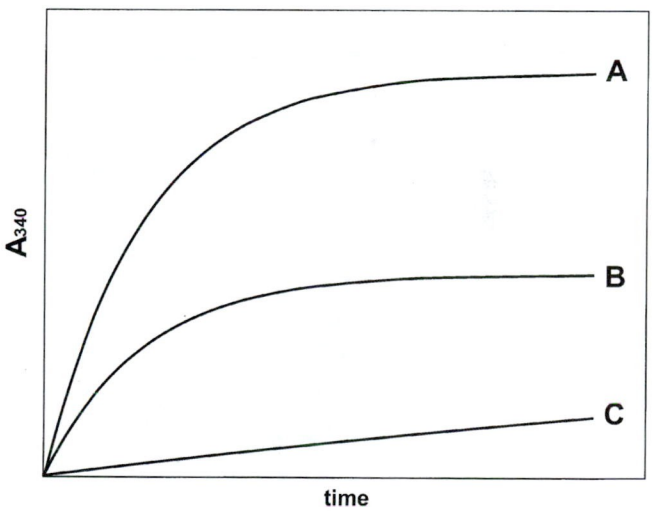

Figure 7–1. Spectrochemical determination of alcohol. Absorbance at 340 nm increases as NAD^+ is converted to NADH by the oxidation of ethanol by alcohol dehydrogenase ($CH_3CH_2OH + NAD^+ \rightarrow CH_3CHO + NADH + H^+$). The curves represent assays of specimens containing 100 mg/dL ethanol (**A**), 50 mg/dL ethanol (**B**), and 100 mg/dL isopropanol (**C**). The initial rate of increase (slope) for reaction A is twice that of B and 36 times that of C. In an assay based on the initial rate, isopropanol produces an interference of only 2.8%. The final absorbance for reaction A is also twice that of B but only 30% greater than reaction C. Complete oxidation of isopropanol (which takes much longer and is not shown on the graph) produces 77% as much NADH as produced by the same amount of ethanol, because of differences in the molecular weight. Thus, isopropanol could produce up to 77% interference in an end-point reaction. Usually, the interference would be less because oxidation is incomplete at the time the absorbance was read.

sandwiched between two antibodies, each of which recognizes a different epitope on the analyte. In competitive immunoassays, analyte from the patient competes for a limited number of antibody binding sites with a labeled version of the analyte provided in the reaction mixture. Because most drugs are too small to have two distinct antibody binding sites, drug immunoassays are usually competitive.

In competitive immunoassays, increasing the concentration of drug in the specimen results in increasing displacement of labeled drug from the antibodies. The amount of drug present in the specimen can be determined by measuring either the amount of label remaining bound to the assay antibody or the amount of label free in solution. In the earliest immunoassays, the label was a radioisotope, typically iodine-125, tritium, or carbon-14. The bound and free radioactivity were physically separated, for example, by using a second antibody to cross-link and precipitate the assay antibody, along with its bound radioactivity (Fig. 7–2), or by adsorbing the free label with activated charcoal. Today, radioimmunoassays are relatively uncommon because of problems with handling and disposing of radioactivity. They are primarily used for analytes with insufficient demand to justify the development costs of more sophisticated nonisotopic assays.

Nonisotopic immunoassays are currently the most widely used methodologies for the measurement of drugs. They offer high selectivity and good precision, and are readily adapted to automated analyzers, thereby decreasing both the cost and the turnaround

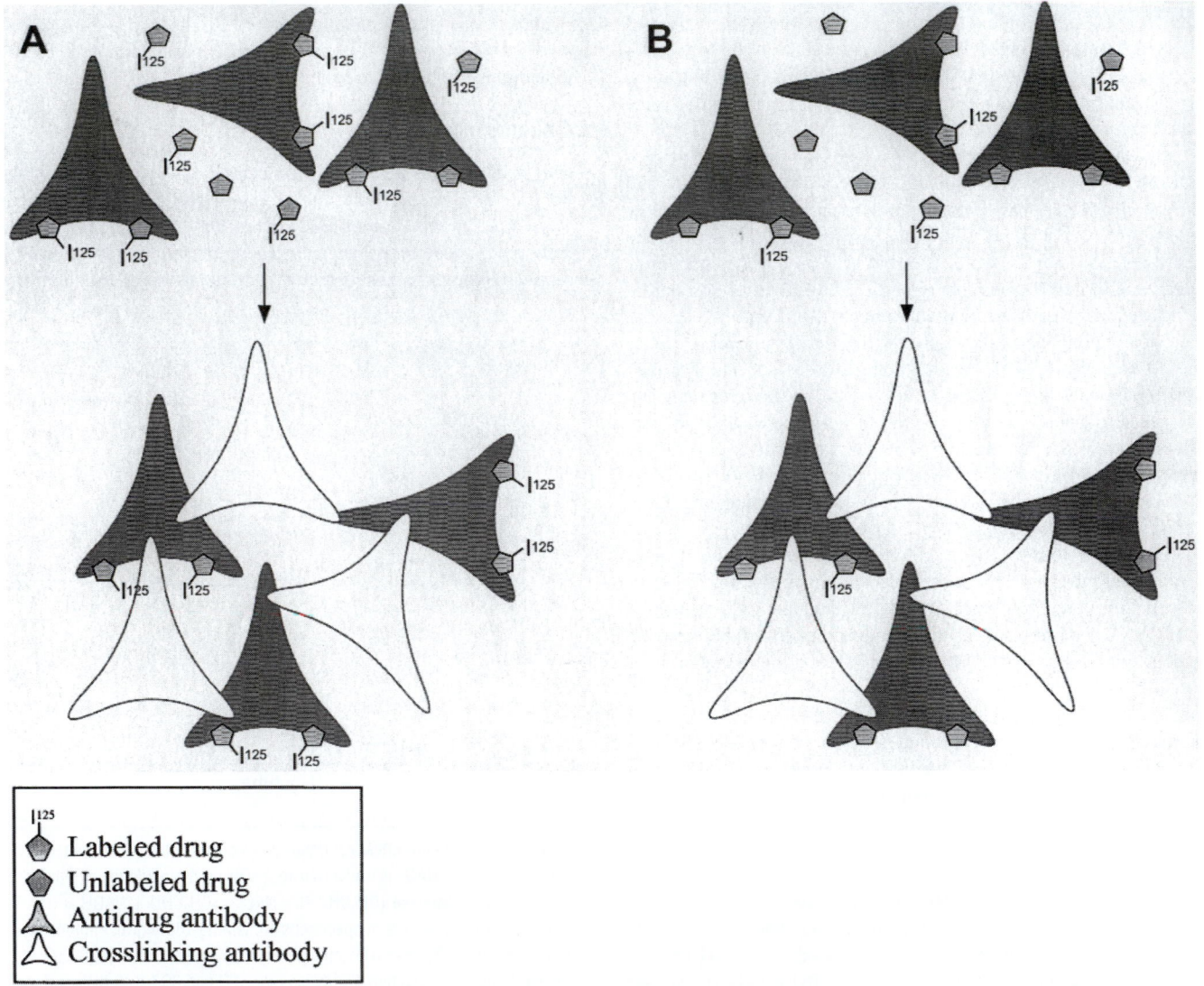

Figure 7–2.   Competitive radioimmunoassay. Radiolabeled drug competes with unlabeled drug from the specimen for binding to antidrug antibodies. Subsequently, the antibody-bound radiolabel is separated from the unbound radiolabel, in this instance, by cross-linking and precipitating the antidrug antibody with a second antibody. Either bound or free radioactivity may be measured, resulting in a calibration curve in which radioactivity decreases or increases, respectively, as the amount of drug from the specimen increases. In Panel **A,** no drug was present in the specimen to displace the labeled drug, and the precipitate contains a high level of radioactivity. In Panel **B,** there was unlabeled drug in the specimen, which displaced the labeled drug, resulting in lower radioactivity in the precipitate and more radioactivity in the supernatant.

time of the assays. The effort involved in developing these assays is substantial. Accordingly, the menu of drugs for which immunoassays are available is limited to those for which there is a high demand, such as widely monitored therapeutic drugs and drugs of abuse included in workplace drug screening. However, after assay development is complete, production costs are relatively low, enabling the tests to be widely distributed at reasonable prices.

The most widely used nonisotopic drug immunoassays are in the category of homogenous immunoassays. Homogenous immunoassays use functional rather than physical separation of bound and free label and therefore can be readily adapted to automated analysis. Homogenous techniques that are in wide use include EMIT (Fig. 7–3), fluorescence polarization immunoassay (FPIA; Fig. 7–4), kinetic inhibition of microparticles in solution (KIMS; Fig. 7–5), and cloned enzyme donor immunoassay (CEDIA; Fig. 7–6).[27]

Some of the newest immunoassays are again using physical separation techniques. In these assays, the detection antibody is physically attached to a solid support and separation occurs by a simple wash step. This wash step removes the patient's serum along with many potential interfering substances. Newer solid supports consist of fine glass fibers or latex microparticles. These

have very high total-surface areas that allow for rapid equilibration and short assay times. Older assays of this type used antibodies bound to large plastic beads or wells of microtiter plates, and required long incubation steps because of substantial times required for diffusion of the reactants to the antibodies. These new techniques are readily automated and allow the measurement of bound label with more sensitive methods than are available with homogenous immunoassays. This includes use of chemiluminescent, electroluminescent, and total fluorescence labels.

Another category of competitive immunoassays uses microparticle capture techniques. These types of assays are being widely incorporated into point-of-care devices for drugs of abuse, as well as other analytes. The specimen is introduced into a well that contains colored microparticles (latex or colloidal metal) attached to either the drug to be measured or to antidrug antibodies. The resulting mixture is drawn by capillary action along a nitrocellulose or similar membrane. On the membrane, there are bands where capture reagents have been immobilized. As the solution flows by these bands, the colored beads may or may not be captured, depending on the design of assay. This results in the formation of a colored band that may denote a positive test or a negative one. The use of multiple antibodies and multiple capture zones can allow several drugs to be detected with a single device.

Figure 7–7 illustrates a direct reading design in which a positive result is indicated by the formation of a colored band in the region of the strip containing immobilized antidrug antibodies. Another design uses an antidrug antibody bound to colored microparticles and a capture zone consisting of immobilized drug. When the amount of drug in the patient specimen exceeds the detection limit, all of the antibody sites will be occupied by patient drug and no labeled antibody will be retained in the capture zone. While simpler in design, this latter variation has the potential for causing confusion, since a positive result is indicated by the absence of a band.

Although immunoassays have a high degree of sensitivity and selectivity, they are also subject to interferences and problems with cross-reactivity. Cross-reactivity refers to the capability of the assay antibody to bind to molecules other than the target analyte. Molecules with similar chemical structures may be efficiently bound, which can lead to falsely elevated results. In some situations, cross-reactivity can be beneficially exploited. For example, some immunoassays effectively detect classes of drugs rather than one specific drug. Immunoassays for opiates employ antibodies that recognize various substances that are structurally related to morphine, including codeine, hydrocodone, and hydromorphone. However, they have little or no cross-reactivity with synthetic opioids such as meperidine or methadone. Immunoassays for the benzodiazepine class react with a wide variety of benzodiazepines, but are less sensitive to some benzodiazepines than to other benzodiazepines.[51] Lack of cross-reactivity for benzodiazepine glucuronides may cause false-negative results in some benzodiazepine immunoassays.[41]

Class specificity can be a two-edged sword. Assays for the tricyclic antidepressant family have similar reactivity with amitriptyline, nortriptyline, imipramine, and desipramine, and can be used to provide a semiquantitative estimate of the total concentration of any combination of these. However, a large number of other drugs with tricyclic structures also cross-react and give a positive detection, particularly at overdose concentrations. These include carbamazepine, many phenothiazines, and diphenhydramine. However,

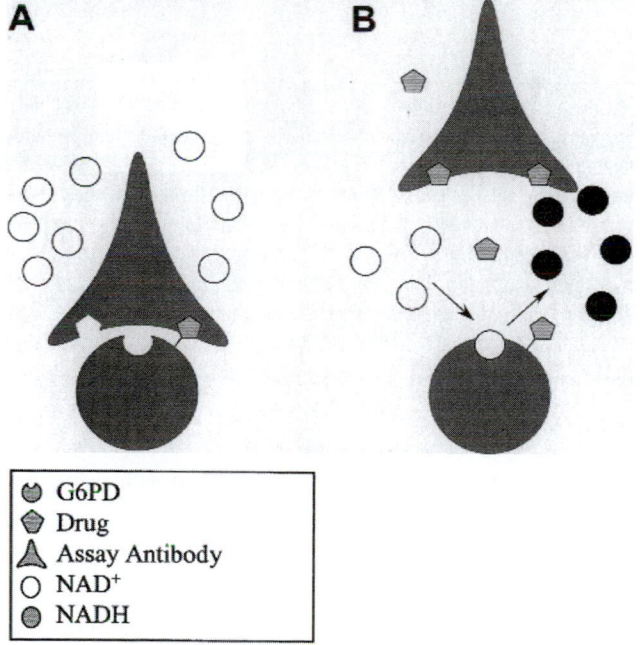

- ⬤ G6PD
- ⬠ Drug
- ▲ Assay Antibody
- ○ NAD⁺
- ◐ NADH

Figure 7–3.   EMIT immunoassay. The enzyme-multiplied immunoassay technique (EMIT) assays use the enzyme glucose-6-phosphate dehydrogenase (⬤) as the label. A molecule of the drug to be measured (⬠) is linked to the enzyme near this enzyme's active site. Addition of the substrates glucose-6-phosphate and NAD+ (○) results in production of NADH (◐), with an increase in light absorption at 340 nm. If the assay antibody (▲) is bound to the labeled drug, the bulky antibody reduces access to the enzyme active site and the rate of change in absorbance is low (Panel **A**). Increasing concentrations of unlabeled drug from the specimen displace the drug-enzyme conjugate from the antibody, thereby unblocking the active site and increasing the rate of reaction (Panel **B**).

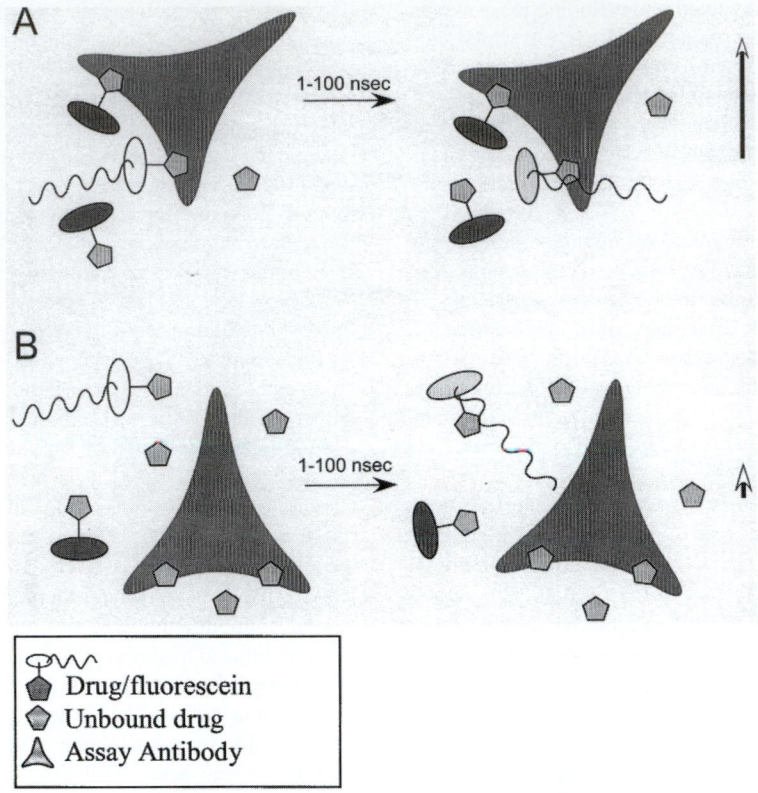

Figure 7–4. FPIA immunoassay. In the FPIA, drug labeled with fluorescein competes with unlabeled drug from the specimen for binding to the assay antibody. The fluorescein is then photoexcited with a brief flash of polarized light. Fluorescein moieties aligned with the plane of polarization can absorb the light, entering an excited state, as indicated by the white color. The excited fluorescein reemits the light a few nanoseconds later at a lower wavelength. Unaligned fluorescein, indicated by the darkened color, does not absorb any light and remains in an unexcited state. The polarization of the emitted light is determined by the orientation of fluorescein molecules at the time of the emission. Those fluorescein molecules that are tethered by the drug to the assay antibody move little during the reemission interval and emit light that is largely in the same plane of polarization as the excitation beam. On the other hand, unbound drug-fluorescein conjugates tumble freely and randomize their orientation prior to reemission, with resultant loss of polarization. Thus, when drug is absent from the specimen, the drug-fluorescein conjugate is primarily bound to antibodies and a high degree of polarization (shown by the *arrow* on the right) is detected in the emitted light (**A**). As specimen drug concentrations increase, the drug-fluorescein conjugate is displaced, with loss of ability to retain polarization. The amount of polarization in the emitted light decreases in inverse ratio to the drug concentration in the specimen (**B**).

the signal intensity generated by the cross-reacting drugs is generally well below the signal intensity generated by tricyclic antidepressant concentrations associated with toxicity.

Even when an antibody is selected to be specific to a single drug, it is not uncommon for metabolites of the target drug to show some cross-reactivity. This, too, may be beneficial. When the metabolite is an active one (for example, carbamazepine epoxide), the contribution of its cross-reactivity may yield results that correlate better with the drug effect than the true concentration.

Immunoassays are also subject to interference by substances that impair detection of the label. The mechanism by which elevated lactate concentrations may lead to spuriously increased drug concentrations in specimens tested by EMIT is described above. Immunoassays that rely on enzyme labels are particularly sensitive to nonspecific interference because enzyme activity is highly dependent on reaction conditions. A number of substances that can inhibit the enzyme reaction in EMIT assays are used to adulterate urine submitted for drug-abuse testing with the intent of producing false-negative results (see discussion of drug-abuse screening tests later in this chapter). Such adulteration may be detected when the rate of reaction is lower than the rate observed with a drug-free control.

Chromatography

Chromatography encompasses several related techniques in which analyte specificity is achieved by physical separation. The unifying mechanism for separation is the partition of substances between a stationary phase and a moving phase (mobile phase). In most instances, the stationary phase consists of very fine particles arranged in a thin layer or enclosed within a column. The mobile phase flows through the spaces between the particles. Analytes are in a rapid equilibrium between solution in the mobile phase and adsorption to the surfaces of the particles. They move when in the mobile phase and stop when adsorbed to the stationary phase. The average velocity of the analyte molecules depends on the relative time spent in the moving versus stationary phase. Molecules that partition primarily into the mobile phase have average velocities slightly less than the mobile phase velocity. Average velocity decreases as the proportion of time adsorbed to the stationary phase

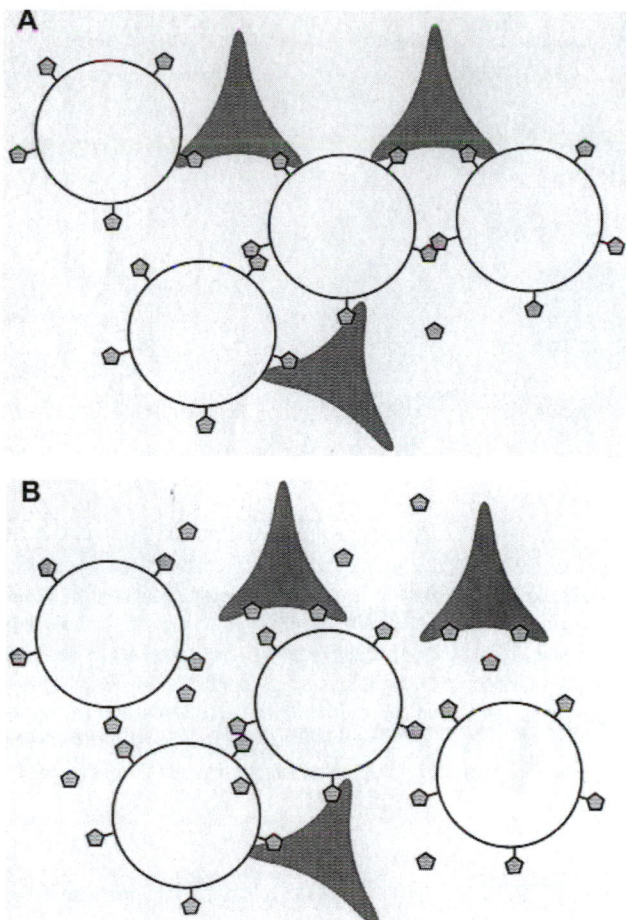

product using a postchromatographic chemical reaction. Chromatographic behavior is sufficiently reproducible that the failure to find a substance at a characteristic Rf value or retention time effectively excludes the presence of that substance in amounts greater than the detection limit. On the other hand, a number of different substances may have migration velocities that are identical or nearly so. A positive finding is, therefore, not completely specific. Definitive identification depends on having additional information, which may be obtained through selective detection techniques or by confirmatory testing using a second methodology.

A major advantage of chromatographic techniques is that multiple substances may be detected and measured in a single procedure. It is not always necessary to know in advance the specific material to be looked for. For this reason, chromatographic techniques have a major role in the performance of screening tests.

Most chromatographic procedures require separation and concentration of the substances to be analyzed prior to the chromatography. This is because the substances to be analyzed must be introduced in a narrow "band" so that the bands corresponding to substances with similar relative mobilities become completely resolved, or separated from one another, rather than overlapping. This also results in more intense signals as a band passes through the detector and increases sensitivity. Finally, this results in removal of proteins and other substances that may exhibit unfavorable interactions with either of the chromatographic phases. The separation and concentration of drugs is most commonly done by extraction with organic solvents, but "solid-phase" extraction is

Figure 7–5. KIMS immunoassay. In KIMS homogenous immunoassays, a suspension of latex microparticles having drug molecules bound to the surface is mixed with antidrug antibody and patient specimen. The antibodies cross-link and agglutinate the microparticles, resulting in decreasing turbidity of the suspension. If drug is present in the specimen, it competes for the antibody-binding sites and slows the agglutination process. The more drug there is in the specimen, the slower is the clearing of turbidity. In a qualitative variant of this approach, agglutination is read visually as an endpoint. Absence of agglutination implies the presence of the drug at a concentration exceeding the cutoff value.

increases. Under controlled conditions, these average velocities are highly reproducible. Substances may be provisionally identified based on their characteristic velocity, which is measured as the distance traveled relative to the solvent migration distance in thin layer chromatography, or the amount of time required to traverse the length of a chromatography column. These characteristic parameters are referred to as the *Rf value* and *retention time*, respectively.

Chromatography is a separation method and must be combined with a detection method to allow identification and measurement of the separated substances. The sensitivity of chromatographic methods depends on both the amount of specimen available and the sensitivity of the detection method. The detection limit may range from less than 10 ng with mass spectrometric detection to more than 10 μg when detection is achieved by forming a colored

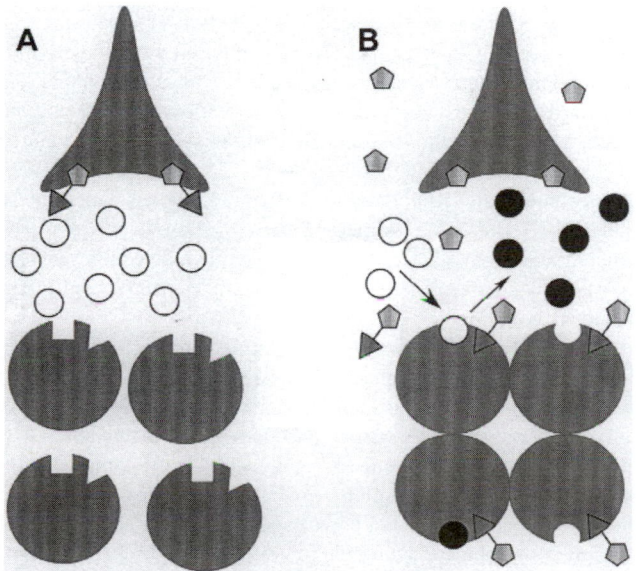

Figure 7–6. CEDIA immunoassay. CEDIA uses genetically engineered β-galactosidase that is missing a small peptide segment. The missing peptide is attached to the target drug. When drug from the specimen displaces the drug-peptide conjugate from the assay antibody, the peptide spontaneously combines with the large fragment to generate a reconstituted monomer. These monomers then reassemble to form an enzymatically active tetramer that can hydrolyze a colorless galactoside to yield a colored product. The rate of product formation is proportional to the concentration of drug in the specimen.

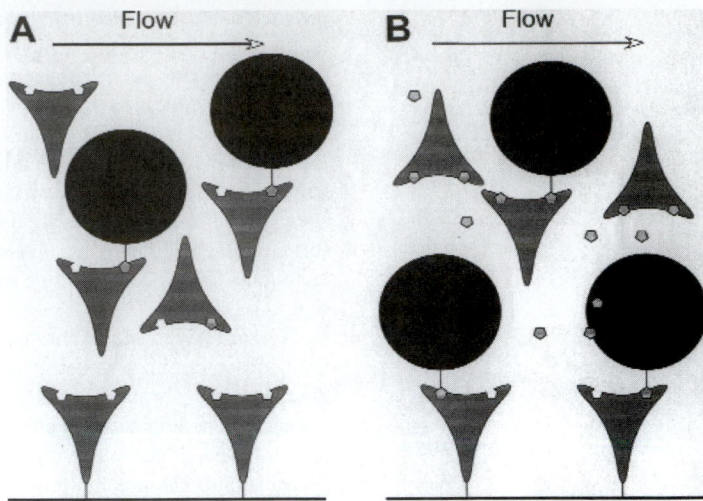

Figure 7–7.   Microparticle capture immunoassay. In a direct reading design, the specimen well contains drug-labeled colored microparticles and an excess of soluble antidrug antibody. The amount of excess defines a predetermined detection limit. The capture zone of the strip contains immobilized antidrug antibodies. There is also a control zone further down the strip with antibodies to the Fc portion of the soluble antidrug antibody. **A.** When drug from the patient specimen is less than the detection limit, all of the labeled drug remains bound to the soluble antibody and is unavailable for capture by the immobilized antibodies at the capture site. In this instance, no colored band forms. However, the complex is subsequently retained in the control zone by capture of the soluble antibody attached via the drug to the colored microparticles. A positive band in the control zone verifies the integrity of the reagents. **B.** If the patient specimen contains drug in excess of the detection limit, then some particle-labeled drug is displaced from the soluble antibody. This unbound, labeled drug is retained in the test capture zone and a colored band develops signifying a positive assay. Some drug-labeled microparticles remain bound to soluble antibodies, thereby crossing the assay zone to be captured and to create a second colored band in the control zone.

also popular.[25,36] Solid-phase extraction is a modified chromatographic procedure in which the mostly aqueous specimen is passed through a short chromatography column with a hydrophobic stationary phase. Most drugs are sufficiently hydrophobic that they partition almost completely into the stationary phase and are retained on the column. Subsequently, these substances are eluted with an organic solvent. The organic solvents from either extraction technique are evaporated to concentrate the substances to be analyzed. Because the extraction process allows analytes to be concentrated from a large volume of specimen, detection sensitivity can be increased if large-volume specimens can be readily obtained, as with urine.

Often there is a preextraction treatment to increase the hydrophobicity of the substances to be extracted. The most common manipulation is pH adjustment, either upward or downward, to convert charged forms of drugs into uncharged, extractable ones. In other instances, enzymatic or chemical hydrolysis may be employed to convert water-soluble glucuronide metabolites back to their more readily extracted parent compounds, for example, conversion of morphine glucuronide to morphine.

In thin-layer chromatography (TLC), the concentrated extracts are redissolved in a small amount of solvent and spotted onto a thin layer of silica gel that is supported on a glass or plastic plate, or embedded in a fiber matrix. A typical TLC plate has room for several different spots of extracts from samples and controls. The plates are placed vertically in closed tanks containing a shallow layer of an organic solvent mixture. As the solvent is drawn upward through the silica gel by capillary action, the substances are carried along at characteristic velocities determined by their partition between the moving organic solvent and the stationary silica gel (Fig. 7–8). Silica gel is polar, so hydrophobic substances migrate rapidly and hy-

drophilic ones more slowly. Adjusting the composition of the solvent allows optimization of the migration rates. After sufficient solvent migration, the plates are removed from the tanks, dried, and sprayed with a series of reagents that convert the drugs to be detected into various colored substances. The drugs are visualized as spots and identified by their migration distance (Rf value), as well as by the colors produced after each spray. Drugs that are metabolized can be further confirmed by the finding of additional spots corresponding to characteristic metabolites. Identifications can be most confidently made when an authentic sample of the drug has been included as a control on the plate.

TLC has the capability to identify the presence of a large number of drugs and is widely used in drug screens. Visualization as colored spots generally requires fairly large amounts of material. For this reason, TLC is usually applied to urine and gastric aspirate specimens, which typically have higher concentrations of many drugs than do corresponding serum specimens and are readily available in large volumes.

Drawbacks include the need for multiple steps: extraction, concentration, chromatography, and a series of detection reactions. This makes TLC a relatively slow and labor-intensive procedure. Interpretation of the spots requires a skilled technologist who knows the TLC behavior of commonly encountered drugs. Quantitation of the drugs detected is difficult and rarely attempted. Therefore, TLC is primarily used to demonstrate the presence of a substance. It is of limited value in identifying a substance not previously seen by the chromatographer, unless a possible candidate is suggested to the laboratory and an authentic sample can be obtained to verify the behavior of the substance in the TLC system. Drugs that have insignificant excretion in the urine are not readily detected.

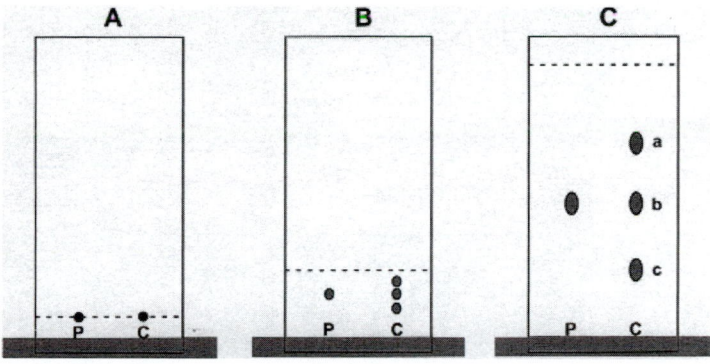

Figure 7–8.   Thin-layer chromatography . **A.** Concentrated extracts from patient and control specimens are dried in small spots on a plate coated with a thin layer of silica gel particles. The plate is then placed vertically into an organic solvent mixture. The solvent is drawn up the plate by capillary action, and the leading edge (or solvent front, shown by the *dotted line*) has just reached the extracts and begun to dissolve them. **B.** Various spots are moving at different rates depending on the relative time spent in the moving solvent (mobile phase) and adsorbed to the silica gel (stationary phase). **C.** The development of the chromatogram was stopped when the solvent front neared the top. Various spots are found at characteristic positions relative to the solvent front. The patient specimen contained a drug that can be tentatively identified as being compound *b* in the control mixture, based on its relative mobility. While shown as colored (black) spots here for clarity, most drugs are colorless and are visualized at the end of the chromatography by being dipped or sprayed with reagents that form colored products. The tentative identification of the unknown drug as compound *b* would require that it show the same behavior with the visualizing reagents.

In the past, full-service toxicology laboratories used classic TLC procedures to screen urine for a variety of drugs.[18] The introduction of a commercial kit for TLC of drugs in urine (Toxilab, Ansys, Inc., Lake Forest, CA) has reduced the time, labor, and expertise required, and has extended its practicability to a broader range of laboratories.[1,30] The use of a standardized procedure also enables tentative identification of a drug not previously encountered by comparison of its characteristics with those of a broad range of drugs provided by the manufacturer in a compendium. Identifications made solely based on such a comparison should be considered provisional until confirmed by additional testing.

In the related technique of high-performance liquid chromatography (HPLC), the stationary phase is packed into a column and the mobile phase is pumped through under high pressure (Fig. 7–9). This allows good flow rates to be achieved, even when solid phases with very small particle sizes are used. Smaller particle size increases surface area, decreases diffusion distances, and improves resolution, but the spaces between the particles are also smaller, increasing the resistance to flow. The use of high pressure and small particles allows better separations in a fraction of the time required for thin-layer chromatography.

Another way that HPLC often differs from TLC is that HPLC typically employs "reverse-phase" chromatography. Reverse-phase chromatography employs stationary phases in which the silica gel particles have had hydrocarbon molecules covalently linked to the outer surface. This reduces the surface charge on the silica, thereby reducing its hydrophilicity, and simultaneously coats the particles with a permanently bonded oil-like layer. At the same time solvent polarity is increased by using a primarily aqueous mobile phase with varying amounts of organic solvent. Because of these modifications, hydrophobic molecules are more strongly adsorbed by the stationary phase, whereas hydrophilic ones tend to remain in the mobile phase. This results in an order of elution from the column that is approximately the reverse of that seen with organic solvents and unmodified silica gel. Thus, the term *reverse-phase chromatography* is used. (Note that both TLC and HPLC can be done using either "normal phase" or "reverse phase" conditions. However, TLC

is more commonly done in normal phase and HPLC is more commonly done in reverse phase.) A variety of hydrocarbons can be used to derivatize the silica gel. By far the most common reverse-phase columns use an octadecyl hydrocarbon as the outer coating and are often referred to as C-18 columns.

In HPLC, the drugs are detected after they exit the chromatographic column. In this case, they are identified by their retention time (the characteristic time required to traverse the column). Because most drugs absorb ultraviolet light, detection is commonly done by ultraviolet spectroscopy that uses specially designed flow-through cuvettes. Measuring the amount of light absorbed allows the amount of the drug to be determined. Accuracy is often enhanced by comparing the amount of light absorbed by the target analyte with light absorption by an internal standard, that is, a compound with a unique retention time that is added in a fixed amount to all specimens. The ratio of the drug absorbance to the internal standard absorbance is proportional to the drug concentration in the specimen.

While most HPLC detectors allow a selection of the detection wavelength, only one wavelength can be used during a given run. Some detectors, however, allow absorbance at multiple wavelengths to be determined, either by rapidly and repeatedly scanning through a range of wavelengths, or by breaking the light into its component wavelengths only after it has passed through the detection cuvette and using an array of photodiode detectors to make measurements at a series of different wavelengths simultaneously.[36] These techniques enable the absorption spectrum of a compound to be determined as it elutes from the column. This information supplements the retention time and enables more specific identifications to be made. An automated HPLC system is available that employs multiple columns and solvents to effect both specimen extraction and chromatography (REMEDi HS, Bio-Rad Laboratories, Inc., Hercules, CA). The ultraviolet spectrum of each compound is determined on elution. Computerized comparison of the retention times and spectra with a library of known compounds enables potential identification of several hundred substances.[42]

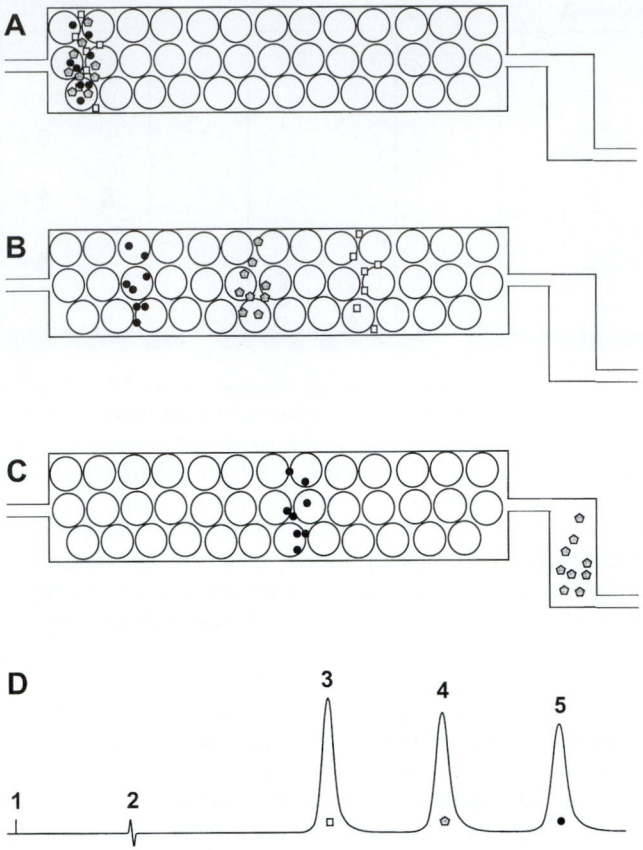

Figure 7–9. High-performance liquid chromatography. HPLC is schematically shown. **A.** A mixture of three compounds is injected into a column with a reversed-phase packing having a hydrophobic outer surface (large open circles). The black compound is the most hydrophobic and adsorbs strongly to the packing; the white compound is the least hydrophobic and remains largely in the mobile phase. **B.** The compounds are moving through the column at their characteristic speeds. None have yet reached the spectrophotometric detector at the end of the column. **C.** The most polar compound has passed through the detector already. The compound of intermediate polarity is in the detection cell; light passing through the detection cell is absorbed by the compound, generating a signal proportional to the concentration in the cell. The least polar compound is still moving through the column. **D.** An HPLC tracing that might result is illustrated. The mark at **1** indicates the time of injection. The artifact at **2** is the result of slight changes in solvent composition that occur when the injection solvent reaches the detector. This indicates the time required for an unretained substance to emerge from the column. The peaks at **3**, **4**, and **5** correspond to the separated substances. In a typical chromatogram, peak **4** might be the drug of interest, for example, amitriptyline. Peak **3** might be a more polar metabolite, for example, nortriptyline. Peak **5** could be a less polar internal standard, for example, *N*-ethylnortriptyline. Later emerging peaks are typically wider and shorter because of greater opportunity for diffusion and other dispersive forces to spread out the molecules in the peak.

TLC generally requires 1 or more hours to complete and provides qualitative identification of drugs present at concentrations of 1 mg/L or higher. HPLC can routinely provide quantitation of drugs at 10-fold lower concentrations in less than 1 hour (provided the calibration was done in advance). Thus, HPLC is often the method of choice for measuring serum concentrations of drugs for which no immunoassay is available. Relative disadvantages of HPLC in comparison with TLC are the much higher costs of the equipment, the inability to analyze multiple samples simultaneously, and a relative inability to analyze substances with a wide range of polarities with a single assay. The latter limitation limits the use of HPLC as a broad drug-screening technique.

Gas chromatography (GC) is similar in principle to HPLC, except that the moving phase is a gas, usually the inert gas helium, or occasionally nitrogen. The schematic illustration of HPLC in Fig. 7–9 is also applicable to GC. The low flow resistance of gas allows high flow rates that make possible substantially longer columns than are used in HPLC. This offers the dual advantages of high resolution and fast analysis. As was true in HPLC, most GC assays incorporate an internal standard to increase precision.

Because the inert carrier gas does not engage in intermolecular interactions, partition of the analytes into the moving gas phase depends primarily upon their intrinsic volatility. Elevated column temperatures are required to achieve sufficient volatility for analysis of most substances. The use of a temperature gradient (the column temperature is programmed to increase throughout the course of the analysis) enables compounds with a wide range of volatility to be analyzed in a single run. This feature makes GC suitable for screening assays encompassing a broad range of drugs.

Gas chromatography is limited to molecules that are reasonably volatile at temperatures below 300°C (572°F), above which the columns may begin to break down. Two principal attributes of a molecule limit its volatility: its size and its capability to form hydrogen bonds. Molecules that form hydrogen bonds via amino, hydroxyl, and carboxylate moieties can be made more volatile by replacing donor hydrogens on oxygen and nitrogen atoms with a nonbonding, preferably large, substituent. (Large substituents sterically hinder access to the acceptor electron pairs on the nitrogen and oxygen atoms.) A number of derivatizing agents can be used to add appropriate substituents. The most common derivatives involve the trimethylsilyl (TMS) group. Although derivatization with TMS substantially increases the molecular weight, the resulting derivative is much more volatile because of the loss of hydrogen bonding.

In traditional packed-column GC, the packing may consist of inert support particles with a fine coating of nonvolatile, high-molecular-weight oil that comprises the stationary phase. It is becoming more common for the stationary phase to be covalently bonded to the support particles. A highly useful variant of gas chromatography is capillary chromatography. A long, fine capillary tube of fused silica is coated on the inside with a covalently bonded stationary phase. The mobile gas phase flows through the tiny channel in the middle. These capillaries are flexible, allowing very long columns (10 m or more) to be coiled into a small space. The long column length, coupled with highly uniform conditions throughout the column, results in extremely high resolution. The fineness of the column allows rapid thermal equilibration and the use of steep temperature gradients that can speed analysis. The major drawback to capillary chromatography is a very limited column capacity. Special techniques are needed to restrict the amount of material introduced into the column and to avoid overloading it. High-sensitivity detectors are required to measure the small quantities that can be chromatographed.

A number of detectors are available for gas chromatography. The most common detector, particularly for packed columns, is the flame ionization detector. This involves directing the outflow of the column into a hydrogen flame. Organic substances emerging from the column are burned, creating charged combustion intermediates that can be measured as a current. The amount of current flow is largely determined by the mass of carbon that is being burned. Nitrogen-phosphorus detectors are also widely used in drug analysis. In this modification of a flame ionization detector, a heated bead coated with an alkali metal salt is used to selectively generate ions from compounds containing nitrogen or phosphorus. These devices detect broad ranges of substances, but do not identify them. The identity of the compounds detected must be inferred from the retention time.

The mass spectrometer can serve as a highly sensitive GC detector and possesses, in addition, the capability to generate highly characteristic mass spectra from the compounds it is detecting. A special requirement of the mass spectrometer is that it requires a high vacuum in order to prevent the ionic particles that it creates from interacting with other molecules or ions. This requires removal of the inert carrier gas and is easiest when there is a low total gas flow, such as occurs with capillary GC. The mass spectrometer, in turn, provides good sensitivity for the small amounts of analyte that can be accommodated in capillary GC.

This detection process also begins by generating ions from the analyte molecules. This is usually done using electron impact ionization. The gas phase analyte is separated from the bulk of the carrier gas and introduced into an ionization chamber, where it is bombarded by a stream of electrons. Electron impact can dislodge an electron from the analyte, creating a positively charged ion and frequently imparting sufficient energy to the ion to break it into pieces. If fragmentation occurs, conservation of charge requires

that one of the resulting fragments be a positively charged ion. The fragments into which a molecular ion breaks are characteristic of the molecule, as is the relative probability that a given fragment will carry the positive charge.

The mass spectrometer then uses electromagnetic filtering to direct only ions of a specified mass-to-charge (m/z) ratio to a detector. Because most of the ions produced have a single positive charge, the observed peaks generally correspond to the mass of the ions. The detector has sufficient electronic amplification so that a single ion could theoretically be detected, which accounts for the high sensitivity of mass spectrometric detection. By rapidly scanning through a range of masses that are sequentially allowed to reach the detector, a mass spectrum may be generated. The mass spectrum records the masses of the pieces produced by fragmentation of the parent ion, as well as the relative frequency with which these fragments are produced and detected. The highest mass observed in the spectrum usually corresponds to the mass of intact parent ions generated from collisions that were not energetic enough to cause fragmentation. Figure 7–10 shows the mass spectrum obtained from a gas chromatograph at a time when trimethylsilyl derivatives of the cocaine metabolite benzoylecgonine were emerging from the capillary column, as well as the mass spectrum of pure trimethylsilyl benzoylecgonine. The mass spectrum of any compound is highly distinctive and usually unique. The primary exception involves optical enantiomers, both of which have the same mass spectrum. Toxicologically significant examples of enantiomers include d-methamphetamine, a drug of abuse, and l-methamphetamine, found in Vicks decongestant inhalers, or dextrorphan, the major metabolite of the cough suppressant dextromethorphan, and levorphan (levorphanol), a controlled substance.

To avoid the need to scan the full range of masses in a typical mass spectrum, selected ion monitoring is often used. Here, the mass spectrometer is typically programmed to detect only three of the larger and more characteristic peaks in the spectrum. In the case of trimethylsilyl benzoylecgonine (TMS-BZE), the peaks at m/z 240, 256, and 361 are used. The amount of TMS-BZE is determined from the ratio of the peak height at m/z 240 to the peak height at m/z 243. The latter peak results from a corresponding fragment from a triply deuterium-labeled internal standard, d_3-TMS-BZE (Fig. 7–10). The specificity of the identification is verified by finding peaks at m/z 256 and m/z 361 as well, with intensities relative to the peak at m/z 240 comparable to those seen in authentic TMS-BZE. The detection at the correct retention time of a substance producing all three peaks in the correct ratios produces an extremely specific identification.

The high sensitivity and specificity afforded by gas chromatography/mass spectroscopy is further extended by the related hybrid technique of liquid chromatography/tandem mass spectroscopy, often abbreviated as LC/MS/MS. Initially restricted to research settings, the technique is now becoming available is some full-service toxicology laboratories.[24] In LC/MS/MS, a tandem mass spectrometer is used as the detector for an HPLC system. The initial ionization is done under conditions that do not promote fragmentation and that yield primarily the intact parent ions of the molecules emerging from the HPLC. The first mass spectrometer is used to selectively filter only those ions with the correct molecular mass. As the selected ions exit the first mass spectrometer, they are allowed to collide with molecules of an inert gas. These collisions cause the ions to break apart to create the mass spectrum that is detected by the second mass spectrometer. The additional

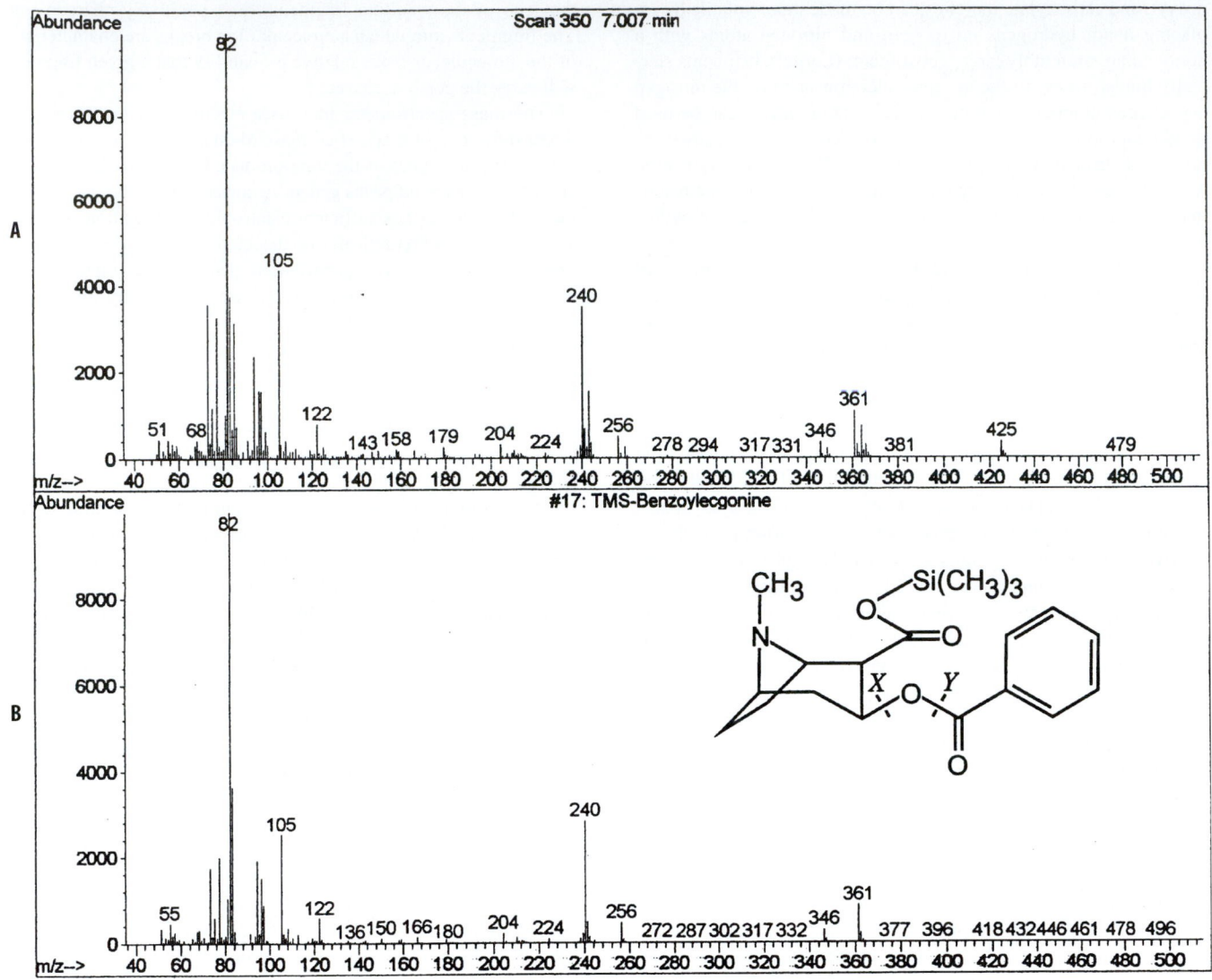

Figure 7–10.   Mass spectrum of the trimethylsilyl derivative of benzoylecgonine (TMS-BZE). **A.** Mass spectrum of effluent from a gas chromatography column at the retention time of TMS-BZE. The major peaks include the parent ion of TMS-BZE at *m/z* 361 and two fragment peaks at *m/z* 240 and 256. Additional peaks are derived from trideuterated TMS-BZE (*d₃*-TMS-BZE) added as an internal standard. The three deuterium atoms increase the mass by 3, yielding peaks at *m/z* 243, 259, and 364. Although TMS-BZE and *d₃*-TMS-BZE are emerging from the GC column simultaneously, the mass spectrometer can identify and measure each independently of the others by using the heights of the unique peaks for each compound. The peak at *m/z* 425 is a coeluting contaminant. **B.** Mass spectrum of pure TMS-BZE. The peak at *m/z* 361 is ionized, but otherwise intact TMS-BZE. The fragments at *m/z* 240 and 256 result from fracture of the bonds at X and Y, respectively, on the inset structure of TMS-BZE.

selection step provided by the first mass spectrometer greatly enhances specificity, and it also reduces background signal, enhancing sensitivity.

TOXICOLOGY SCREENING

A test unique to the toxicology laboratory is the toxicology screen, or "tox screen." Depending on the laboratory, this term may refer to a single testing methodology with the capability to detect multiple drugs, such as thin-layer or gas chromatography. It may refer to a panel of individual tests, such as a drug-abuse screen, or it may be a combination of broad-spectrum and individual tests. The

widespread use of the term *tox screen* is unfortunate, because this wrongly implies for many physicians the availability of a test that can exclude poisoning as a diagnosis. Unfortunately, no such test exists.

There are more toxic substances in the world than there are named diseases. However, a relatively limited number of substances account for most serious poisonings. As a result, in one study, a comprehensive toxicology screening protocol using multiple detection methods applied to both serum and urine specimens was capable of identifying more than 98% of implicated substances.[28] This suggests that a comprehensive tox screen can exclude poisoning with a substantial degree of reliability. However, this study was done some time ago when the rate of introduction of new drugs was much slower than is currently the case. Even the "comprehensive" screens currently in use might not identify many newer drugs.[61] Moreover, comprehensive toxicology screens typically do not detect ionic materials, including bromide, lithium, iron, lead, and other heavy metals. Nor do they necessarily detect substances that are toxic at extremely low concentrations, such as digoxin or fentanyl. Table 7–5 lists a number of substances encountered in emergency toxicology that may not be detected by routine toxicology screening.

It should be apparent that a negative toxicology screen cannot exclude poisoning. It is equally true that a positive finding does not necessarily make a diagnosis of poisoning. For assays that only detect the presence of a drug, it is not possible to distinguish benign or therapeutic levels from toxic ones. Quantitative tests rarely may falsely suggest toxicity when drug concentrations are measured during the drug's distribution phase, which may extend for several hours with drugs such as digoxin and lithium. Moreover, the phenomenon of tolerance may enable chronic drug users to be relatively unaffected by concentrations that would be quite toxic to a naïve individual. Because comprehensive drug screens may differ widely between institutions, and because patterns of exposure also show substantial regional variation, there is limited ability to draw meaningful conclusions from any study of the sensitivity and specificity of such screens for detecting or excluding poisoning.

The predictive power of the result of a toxicology screen depends on a number of factors, including the likelihood of poisoning prior to receiving the test results (the prior probability or the prevalence), the range of substances effectively detected, and the frequency of false-positive results. It should be noted that false-positive and false-negative results may be either analytical or clinical in origin. A clinical false-positive occurs when a drug is detected that is not contributing to the medical problem, for example, a therapeutic amount of acetaminophen. A clinical false-negative may occur when the wrong test is ordered, for example, a screen for drugs of abuse for a patient with acetaminophen poisoning.

Table 7–6 explores the positive and negative predictive values of a toxicology screen in several scenarios. The sensitivity and specificity of 98% each in one scenario reflects the sensitivity of a broadly comprehensive toxicology screen[28] and an achievable false-positive rate of 2%. The second scenario uses a sensitivity of only 80% and a specificity of 95%, and represents plausible, but

TABLE 7–5. Substances Often Undetected in Comprehensive Toxicology Screens

Antidysrhythmic drugs	Heavy metals
Anticholinergic drugs	Hypoglycemic drugs
Anticoagulant drugs	Iron
Antipsychotic agents	Isopropanol
β-Agonists and antagonists	Ketamine
Calcium channel blockers	Lithium
Carbon monoxide	LSD
Clonidine	MDA/MDMA
Cyanide	Methanol
Digoxin	Methemoglobin
Diphenhydramine	Serotonin reuptake inhibitors
Ethylene glycol	Solvents
Fentanyl	Strychnine
γ-Hydroxybutyrate	Toxins (plant or animal)

TABLE 7–6. Positive and Negative Predictive Values of Toxicology Screens

Sensitivity/Specificity (%/%)	Prior Probability		
	10%	50%	95%
Excellent (98/98)[a]	84%/99.8%	98%/98%	99.9%/72%
Mediocre (80/95)[b]	64%/98%	94%/83%	99.7%/20%

[a]The excellent laboratory has a comprehensive toxicology screen (98% sensitivity) and an overall false-positive rate of 2%.
[b]The mediocre laboratory has a screen that is positive in 80% of poisoning cases and that gives false-positive results in 5% of negative cases.

mediocre performance. Three sets of prior probabilities are used: 10%, 50%, and 95%. A prior probability of 10% might be seen if screening were indiscriminately applied to all patients in an emergency department, or in a scenario in which drugs were being excluded as secondary cause of lethargy in an older patient who fell and struck his or her head. Both laboratories do well at excluding drugs when their presence is already unlikely. However, a positive finding from either does not yield a fully convincing diagnosis of drug presence. A prior probability of 50% falls into the range of rates of positivity actually observed in patients for whom toxicology screens were ordered (see later). In this scenario of maximum uncertainty, both labs do a good job of diagnosing poisoning, but drug exclusion by the mediocre lab will be incorrect in 1 of 6 instances.

A prior probability of 95% represents testing where the clinical presentation strongly suggests poisoning, as in the investigation of lethargy in a known regular drug user. Although positive findings by either lab raise the probability to almost complete certainty, negative findings from the excellent lab are incorrect 1 time out of 4, whereas negative results from the mediocre lab are wrong 4 times out of 5. Overall, toxicology screens have better positive predictive value than negative predictive value. This observation should give pause to those who primarily order toxicology screens "to rule out poisoning."

Although only about 4% of laboratories offer comprehensive toxicology screening, most laboratories offer some sort of testing in response to a request for a tox screen. This may consist of a panel of immunoassays for drugs of abuse, or a urine TLC screen, or it may result in a comprehensive screening performed at a reference laboratory. Other laboratories may offer a focused, rather than comprehensive, screening panel.[2,6,58,59] Larger laboratories may have several types of tox screens available for use in different situations. Among laboratories that do not limit themselves exclusively to commercially available methods, it is likely that no two will have exactly the same menu of drugs that can be reliably detected. A recent survey of emergency physicians found that more than 75% were not fully aware of the range of drugs detected, and not detected, by their laboratory's toxicologic screens. The majority believed that the screen was more comprehensive that it actually was.[22]

Comprehensive toxicology screens typically require several hours of intense labor, particularly if confirmatory testing is also included. Given the trends toward increasing automation and decreasing personnel in clinical laboratories, it is relevant to ask what benefits may be derived from such testing. Studies show that comprehensive toxicologic screening has the potential to provide significant information, with utility varying with the indication for testing. The prevalence of positive results has ranged from 34–86% of specimens submitted for testing.[2,3,5,6,14,23,28,32,38,43–46,53] When drug exposure, as predicted from the history and physical, was compared with screening results, clinically unsuspected substances were found in 7–48% of the cases and clinically suspected substances were not found in 9–25% of cases.[5,6,14,28,32,43,46,56] However, limited utility is suggested by studies showing that the results of comprehensive screening affected management in less than 15% of the cases,[43] and in many instances, in less than 5% of cases.[5,6,32,38,46,53,54,56]

One reason for a limited effect on management is the substantial time delay before results of comprehensive screening are available. Generally, more than 3 hours are required for the report of a negative result, and even a longer time is required for a positive finding. By this time, many management decisions are already implemented. Another possible explanation for limited utility is that comprehensive screening is largely available only in major medical centers, where consultation from a medical toxicologist is more likely to be available. Such experts may be more able to make correct diagnoses and to initiate appropriate management relying on clinical findings alone.

Some laboratories address the issue of providing useful information in a timely fashion through the use of focused, rather than comprehensive, screening protocols.[2,3,58,59] These screens include drugs commonly implicated in local overdose cases and/or drugs for which there are specific interventions. The goal is typically to provide results within an hour, including quantitation of those substances where management decisions require concentration data. A combination of serum and urine tests is used. Table 7–7 suggests the possible composition of a focused screen. Such a screen should be supplemented with additional specific tests when indicated.

Unfortunately, limited screens have had limited investigations for their utility. One study compared a limited urine screen of immunoassays for drugs of abuse and spot tests for salicylates, phenothiazines, imipramine, and ethchlorvynol with a comprehensive screen and found that the comprehensive screen detected substances not found in the limited screen in 399 of 1734 cases (23%). Eighty-seven (22%) of the discrepancies were a result of omission of cocaine from the limited screen. Effect on management was not studied.[3] A study in children found that drugs detected in only 7 of 234 comprehensive screens (3%) were both

clinically significant and undetected by a limited urine screen that included drugs of abuse (including cocaine), as well as acetaminophen, salicylates, and ethanol. Management was not affected in any of these 7 cases.[6]

Several recently introduced point-of-care devices are capable of rapidly screening urine for the presence of drugs of abuse, as well as tricyclic antidepressants. Results are typically available in 20–30 minutes. In a small study of one such device, diagnosis was thought to have been aided in 82% of cases and clinical management was changed in 25%.[12] Additional studies are needed to ascertain the utility of point-of-care drug screening in emergency toxicology.

A useful alternative to the toxicology screen is the *toxicology hold*. This is a set of serum and urine specimens drawn at the time of presentation, when drug concentrations are likely to be near maximum levels, and initially held refrigerated or frozen without testing. A maxim for management of the poisoned patient is that an evaluation is not complete until it has been repeated over time. In many instances, observation will clarify the diagnosis, allowing toxicology screening to be dispensed with or to be replaced by a specific assay. On the other hand, the specimens remain available for subsequent testing if the diagnosis remains unclear, or if there are unexplained findings. Most laboratories will hold such specimens for several days, if necessary.

BEDSIDE TOXICOLOGY TESTS

Testing at the bedside is attractive for emergency toxicology. When a specific diagnosis is being considered, a bedside test can provide confirmation or exclusion quickly and cheaply, enabling appropriate management to be initiated. This benefit must be balanced against the generally poorer sensitivity and specificity of spot tests in comparison with testing in the clinical laboratory, the lack of quantitative information for most tests, the need to perform testing in accord with regulatory requirements (see later), and the erosion of the time advantage when multiple bedside tests are done on the same patient.

Table 7–8 lists some tests that can be conveniently performed at the bedside. The spot tests listed in Table 7–4 can also be done at the bedside, although most of these tests employ hazardous reagents that may not be suitable for use in many bedside settings. A major problem with bedside tests that are not done with commercial devices is that these are considered "highly complex" tests under federal regulations, although they may be very simple to perform. This classification results from the fact that they are not subject to the validation processes required for FDA-approved commercial devices. Meeting the regulations requires significant initial and ongoing investment of time. The Meixner test[8,37] and breath analysis are exempted from these regulations, because they do not involve human specimens. (See "Regulatory Issues Affecting Toxicology Testing" below.)

The Substance Abuse and Mental Health Services Administration (SAMHSA) evaluated the performance of 15 point-of-care drug-screening devices, as compared to a gold standard of GC/MS using SAMHSA-recommended cutoff values. The study was carried out with a disproportionately large number of specimens (approximately 50%) having concentrations within 25% of the cutoff value. In these samples, false-positives ranged from 25–50% of total positive results, whereas 15–30% of negative results were false-negatives.[13] In actual testing practice, specimens with con-

TABLE 7–7. Components of a Focused Toxicology Screen

Serum Tests	Urine Tests
Acetaminophen	Cocaine metabolite
Ethanol	Opiates
Salicylates	Tricyclic antidepressants[a]
Tricyclic antidepressants	
Consider inclusion:	
Barbiturates	Amphetamines
Carboxyhemoglobin[b]	Barbiturates[a]
Iron	Benzodiazepines
Lithium	Phencyclidine
Theophylline	Other locally prevalent agents
Volatile alcohols[c]	
Other locally prevalent substances	

[a]If not included in serum tests.
[b]Requires whole-blood specimen.
[c]Methanol, isopropanol (+ acetone).

TABLE 7–8. **Bedside Toxicology Tests**

Test	Substrate	Drug or Toxin	Comments
Alcohol dehydrogenase	Saliva	Ethanol	Other alcohols may interfere. Some tests are semiquantitative.
Anodic stripping	Blood	Lead	Requires fresh specimen. Confirmation of elevated results recommended.
Breath analysis	Breath	Carbon monoxide	Ethanol may interfere.
Breath analysis	Breath	Ethanol	Good cooperation required. Ethanol in oral cavity interferes. Calibrated to give whole-blood rather than serum concentration.
Ferric chloride	Urine	Salicylates	Acetaminophen and phenothiazines interfere.
Meixner	Mushroom	Amatoxins	Paper must contain lignin (use filter paper, which is lignin-free, as negative control). Requires strong acid. Some false-positives.
Microparticle agglutination	Urine	Drugs of abuse	KIMS variant with visual endpoint. Separate test for each drug.
Microparticle capture	Urine	Drugs of abuse	Single device detects one or more of the drugs listed in Table 7–9, in a variety of menus available from multiple manufacturers. Some multitest devices include tricyclic antidepressants. Higher false-positive and false-negative rates than for clinical laboratory testing.
Oxalate crystals	Urine	Ethylene glycol	Metabolic end-product. Not detected during early stages. Nonspecific.
Wood's lamp	Urine	Ethylene glycol	Detects fluorescein added to many (but not all) antifreeze products. Window of detection is brief. Alkalinize urine (only the fluorescein anion fluoresces).

centrations near the cutoff concentration should be less frequent, with many specimens having drug concentrations that are either quite high or zero. An extensive study using a more representative range of urine drug concentrations observed higher rates of correct results, but performance remained inferior to that of immunoassays performed with laboratory instrumentation.[23]

A clinical and methodologic issue with bedside drug-screening assays is whether positive results will subsequently be confirmed. The extra investment of labor needed to submit a specimen to the laboratory tends to discourage confirmatory testing. The argument for confirmation is that this has been the accepted standard of practice for screening assays that have lower false-positive rates than the point-of-care devices (see "Special Considerations for Drug-Abuse Screening Tests" later). The counterargument is that if testing is limited to populations with a high prior probability of drug exposure, the predictive value of a positive test will be high. This is an area in which policy might best be established by an institutional point-of-care testing committee (see "Regulatory Issues Affecting Toxicology Testing" below).

REGULATORY ISSUES AFFECTING TOXICOLOGY TESTING

Since 1992, medical laboratory testing has been governed by federal regulations (42 CFR part 405 et seq) issued under the authority of the Clinical Laboratory Improvement Amendments of 1988 (often referred to as CLIA-88 or simply CLIA). These regulations apply to all laboratory testing of human specimens for medical purposes, regardless of site. They include the universal requirement for possession of an appropriate certificate to perform even the simplest of tests. The remaining requirements depend on the complexity of the test. These regulations become important to the emergency toxicologist whenever testing is done at the bedside using spot tests or commercial point-of-care devices such as dipsticks, glucose meters, or urine drug-screening devices.

The regulations divide testing into three categories: waived, moderate complexity, and high complexity. Waived tests include a number of specifically designated simple tests, including urine dipsticks, urine pregnancy tests, and glucose measurements with a handheld monitor. The only legal requirements for performing waived testing are the possession of an appropriate CLIA certificate (certificate of waiver or higher) and performance of the test in accordance with the manufacturer's instructions.

There are substantial additional requirements for both moderate and highly complex testing, most of which simply represent good laboratory practice. The most significant of these requirements are listed in Table 7–9. Most assays performed with commercial kits or devices are classified as belonging to the moderately complex category. All tests not specifically classified as waived or moderately complex are considered highly complex. This includes essentially all noncommercial tests, including spot tests, because the testing materials have not been subject to review and approval by the Food and Drug Administration.

These regulations have had a substantial impact in all areas of laboratory testing. Some of the most significant effects have been on bedside testing, including spot tests and point-of-care devices. Although clinical laboratories had followed most of the required

TABLE 7–9.   Major CLIA-88 Requirements for Laboratory Testing

Waived Tests
Certificate of waiver
Follow manufacturer's instructions

Moderate-Complexity Tests
CLIA certificate
Record keeping
Documented method validation
Written procedure
Personnel educational requirements
Documented training of personnel
Annual competency testing
Two levels of controls daily
Participate in proficiency testing every 4 months
Biennial inspection and certification

High-Complexity Tests
All moderate-complexity requirements *plus*
Qualified on-site supervisor *or*
Daily review of all results by qualified supervisor

This table lists only the most significant requirements of the regulations implementing the Clinical Laboratory Improvement Amendments of 1988 (CLIA-88). These regulations continue to evolve. Regulatory agencies such as the Joint Commission on Accreditation of Healthcare Organizations (JCAHO) may have additional requirements. Consultation with the clinical laboratory or with an institutional point-of-care coordinator is recommended prior to implementing any testing. (See http://www.clianet.org/.)

practices prior to the implementation of the regulations, this was usually not the case for testing done at other sites. Most institutions have now established point of care testing programs to facilitate compliance with the regulations, as well as with additional requirements of accrediting agencies. Any toxicologic or other testing done at the point of care should be set up in consultation with the institutional program. Often, all point-of-care testing is done under a CLIA certificate held by the program. There is frequently a point-of-care testing coordinator who may make recommendations, or who may personally assist in efficiently addressing the assorted requirements.

A few tests that may be done at the bedside are not regulated by CLIA because no human specimen is involved. These include breath tests for ethanol and carbon monoxide (both considered to be patient monitoring) and the Meixner test,[8,37] which is done with a mushroom. However, such testing may be covered by state laws, or by institutional or accrediting agency policies.

Personnel unaccustomed to quality assurance practices may find the requirements initially burdensome. Compliance is nonetheless important. Following these practices may lead to a 3-fold reduction in incorrect results,[55] thereby improving the quality of care provided to the patient. Moreover, noncompliant testing is illegal under federal law, and usually under state laws as well.[4] Any untoward outcome associated with illegal testing creates a major risk management liability for both the institution and the individual. Additionally, billing for any testing which is not CLIA-compliant may be considered fraudulent.

Another area in which the CLIA regulations have impacted toxicology testing is in the provision of infrequently requested tests. Meeting regulatory requirements involves a substantial labor investment even when no patient specimens are being tested. Mounting pressures to reduce laboratory costs make it less likely that laboratories will continue to maintain such assays.

Another important regulation, although not part of the CLIA regulations, requires that the medical reason for ordering a test accompany the order. Federal regulations require that the ordering physician provide the diagnosis that establishes the medical necessity for the test, either by name or by diagnostic code (CPT code). Laboratories may not use a "best guess" to assign codes to undocumented test requests.

SPECIAL CONSIDERATIONS FOR DRUG-ABUSE SCREENING TESTS

Testing for drugs of abuse is a significant component of medical toxicology testing. Initial testing is usually done with a screening immunoassay. Positive results are often, but not always, confirmed by retesting using a nonimmunological test. The immunoassays were developed for use in workplace drug-screening programs and are not always optimal for medical purposes, but their wide availability in inexpensive, easy-to-use formats has led to their nearly universal adoption. Drug-abuse testing for nonmedical reasons is generally considered to be forensic testing.[21]

The most commonly tested-for drugs are amphetamines, cannabinoids, cocaine, opiates, and phencyclidine. These are often referred to as the NIDA 5, because they are the five drugs that were recommended by the National Institute on Drug Abuse in 1988 for drug screening of federal employees. (Responsibility for recommendations for federal drug testing has subsequently been passed to SAMHSA.) Drug-screening immunoassays are also frequently done for barbiturates and benzodiazepines, and less frequently for methadone and propoxyphene. Table 7–10 lists some of the general characteristics of these tests. There are also commercial urine immunoassays for LSD and methaqualone. Drug-screening immunoassays are available in a number of formats, which may differ in performance. All are designed to be used with urine specimens, because these can be obtained noninvasively and generally have higher drug concentrations than serum, thereby enhancing the sensitivity of the test.

Two drug-screening tests, for cannabinoids and cocaine, are directed toward inactive drug metabolites rather than toward the active parent compound. The active drugs, cocaine and tetrahydrocannabinol, are both short-lived and persist for no more than a few hours after use. The metabolites remain present substantially longer. Detection of the metabolites increases the ability to detect any recent drug use. However, this limits the utility of the assays for determining whether a patient is currently under the influence of the drug. Because the metabolites are rapidly formed, a negative test effectively excludes intoxication, but a positive test indicates only past use, not current intoxication.

To increase sensitivity for detection of less-recent drug use, substrates other than urine have been employed for drug screening, including hair and meconium. The latter is used to document intrauterine drug exposure (Chaps. 16 and 105). These tests have little utility for the management of toxicologic emergencies and are generally available only through reference laboratories.

The stigma attached to a positive test for an abused drug requires that special care be exercised in performing and reporting the tests. To protect citizen rights, many states have legislated specific requirements for workplace drug screening. In some states, the requirements apply only to screening in the workplace, whereas testing for medical purposes is exempt. Laws in other

TABLE 7–10.   Performance Characteristics of Common Drug-Abuse Tests[a]

Drug/Class	Detection Limits[b]	Confirmation Limits[b]	Detection Interval[c]	Comments
Amphetamines	1000 ng/mL	500 ng/mL	1–2 d (2–4 d)	Screening immunoassays may give false-positives with decongestants; MDA and MDMA are variably detected. Confirmation of methamphetamine requires detection of >500 ng/mL with >200 ng/mL of metabolite, amphetamine.
Barbiturates	200 ng/mL secobarbital		2–4 d	Phenobarbital may be detected up to 4 weeks.
Benzodiazepines	100–300 ng/mL		1–30 d	Benzodiazepines vary in reactivity and potency. Hydrolysis recommended to convert glucuronides to immunoreactive forms. False-positives with oxaprozin.
Cannabinoids	50 ng/mL; 20 ng/mL; 25 ng/mL; 100 ng/mL THCA	15 ng/mL THCA	1–3 d (>1 mo)	Screening assays detect inactive and active cannabinoids; confirmatory assay detects inactive metabolite tetrahydro-cannabinoic acid (THCA). Duration of positivity highly dependent on screening assay detection limits.
Cocaine	300 ng/mL BZE	150 ng/mL BZE	2 d (1 wk)	Screening and confirmatory assays detect inactive metabolite benzoylecgonine (BZE). False-positives unlikely.
Opiates	2000 ng/mL; 300 ng/mL	2000 ng/mL	1–2 d; 2–4 d (<1 wk)	>10 ng/mL of heroin metabolite 6-acetylmorphine is also confirmatory. Semisynthetic opiates derived from morphine show variable cross-reactivity. Fully synthetic opioids (eg, fentanyl, meperidine, methadone, propoxyphene, tramadol) have minimal cross-reactivity.
Methadone	300 ng/mL		1–4 d	Doxylamine may cross-react.
Phencyclidine	25 ng/mL	25 ng/mL	4–7 d (>1 mo)	Structural analogues (dextromethorphan) may cross-react.
Propoxyphene	300 ng/mL		3–10 d	Duration of positivity depends on cross-reactivity of metabolite norpropoxyphene.

[a]Based on data in references 19, 26, 39, 41, 51, 57, and 62. Performance characteristics vary with manufacturer and may change over time. For the most accurate information, consult the package insert of the current lot.
[b]SAMHSA recommendations shown as first value for amphetamine, cannabinoids, cocaine, opiate, and phencyclidine immunoassays, and as the only values for confirmatory assays. Other commercial immunoassay cutoffs are also listed; other GC/MS cutoffs are set by the laboratory.
[c]Values are after typical use; values in parentheses are after heavy or prolonged use.

states may apply to all drug screening. Although they are not always required, some workplace drug-screening practices are widely applied to all drug screening.

The use of specific cutoff concentrations is nearly universal. Test results are considered positive only when the concentration of drug in the specimen exceeds a predetermined threshold. This threshold should be set sufficiently high that false-positive results due to analytic variability or to cross-reactivity are extremely infrequent. They should also be low enough to consistently give a positive result in persons who are using drugs. Cutoff concentrations used will vary with the drug or drug class under investigation. In some drug-screening immunoassays, the laboratory has the option of selecting from several cutoff values.

The use of cutoff values sometimes creates confusion when a patient who is known to have recently used a drug has a negative result reported on a drug screen. In such instances, the drug is usually present, but at a concentration below the cutoff value. Another potential problem occurs when a patient's drug-screening test is positive after previously having become negative. This is usually interpreted as indicating renewed drug use, but it may be an artifact. Urine drug concentrations are directly proportional to the serum drug concentrations, but inversely proportional to the rate of urine production. The rate of the urine flow may vary up to 100-fold with a resulting possible 100-fold change in the urine drug concentration. This effect is often exploited by individuals who imbibe large quantities of water prior to taking a urine drug test. A decrease in the rate of urine production can result in a positive test following a negative test, despite no new drug exposure. A similar effect may be produced by changes in urine pH. Drugs containing a basic nitrogen may demonstrate ionic trapping, with increasing

concentrations as urine pH decreases. Similarly, excretion of the phenobarbital anion may increase with increasing pH. (This phenomenon is medically exploited by alkalinizing the urine to increase phenobarbital excretion.)

Another widely adopted practice is the confirmation of all positive screening results using an analytical methodology different from that used in the screen, such as an immunoassay screen followed by chromatographic confirmation. The possibility of simultaneous false-positive results by two distinct methods is quite low. The most common confirmatory method is GC/MS. The high specificity afforded by the combination of the retention time and the mass spectrum makes false-positive results extremely unlikely. GC/MS also has greater sensitivity than the screening immunoassays, minimizing failed confirmations because of drug concentrations below the sensitivity of the confirmatory assay. GC/MS confirmation is required by law for workplace drug screening in some states and may be legally required for all drug screening.

Immunoassay results can generally be obtained within 1 hour or less. Confirmatory testing usually requires at least several hours. This can create a problem when confirmation of initial immunoassay results is considered mandatory. Most laboratories will provide a verbal report of a presumptive positive result to facilitate medical management, but may not enter the result into a permanent record, such as the laboratory computer, until after confirmation has been completed.

The importance of confirmatory testing in workplace drug screening follows from the relatively low prevalence of positive results. A screening test with both sensitivity and specificity of 98% will produce two false-positive results per 100 subjects tested. A workforce with a 2% prevalence of illicit drug use will yield 2 true positive results per 100 subjects. The predictive value of a positive test will only be 50% (2 of 4). This is an unacceptable level of certainty for results that might be used to terminate employment.

The prevalence of positive results may be very different in drug screening applied to selected patients in medical settings. Rates of positivity of 34–86% have been reported in various emergency department populations such as trauma patients or persons suspected of illicit drug use.[2,3,5,6,14,23,28,32,38,43–46,53] Given a population with a 50% prevalence of recent drug use and a test with 98% sensitivity and specificity, the false-positive rate will be 0.02 of the 50% of subjects who have true negative findings, or 1%. The true positive rate will be 49% (0.98 × 50%). In this population, the predictive value of a positive test is 49/(49+1), or 98%.

A high prior probability of drug positivity for patients tested in medical settings results in a very high posterior probability after a positive test. Confirmatory testing is much less critical in such a setting, particularly because a positive finding infrequently has consequences that extend beyond the medical management of the patient. An exception may occur where results of testing performed on motor vehicle crash victims can be subsequently subpoenaed as evidence in legal proceedings. When confirmation is not legally required, some laboratories may report the results of screening immunoassays without a confirmation.

Many toxicology laboratories have a policy of confirmation by a distinct second method prior to a final positive report for drugs of abuse. If confirmation by GC/MS is not required, a common practice is to confirm screening immunoassays by TLC and vice versa. Positive findings by both methods provide a high degree of specificity. A disadvantage of the approach is the low sensitivity of TLC relative to immunoassays. True positive immunoassays may fail to be confirmed, leading to false-negative final results. Some laboratories accept this because false-negatives are unlikely in the presence of serious overdoses. Other laboratories may retest TLC-negative specimens with a more sensitive method, such as GC/MS. Often, confirmatory testing is done on positive results for illicit drugs, but not for legal drugs such as barbiturates, benzodiazepines, and ethanol.

One workplace drug-screening practice that is not widely followed in medical toxicology is maintenance of a chain of custody. Employers generally insist on chain of custody for workplace testing because actions taken in response to a positive result may be contested in court. A chain of custody provides results with maximum legal defensibility. Laboratories providing testing for medical purposes rarely keep a chain of custody, because it is quite expensive and does not benefit the patient. Additionally, the medical personnel responsible for obtaining the specimens are rarely trained in chain of custody requirements.

The lack of chain of custody can create problems when persons with no medical complaints present at an emergency department or other medical facility requesting the performance of a drug-screening test. Unless the facility is prepared to initiate the chain of custody at the time of specimen collection and the laboratory is prepared to maintain it, such persons should be redirected to a site maintained by a commercial laboratory that routinely performs workplace drug testing and that has appropriate procedures in place. Many laboratories have had the experience of unwittingly performing drug-abuse testing for nonmedical purposes because the reason for the testing is not always included on the test requisition. To avoid liability issues, the laboratory may choose to include a disclaimer with every drug-screening report indicating that the results are for purposes of medical management only.

Testing for various adulterants is another practice common in workplace testing, but rare in medical laboratories. Most workplace programs measure urinary creatinine to determine the possible dilution of the specimen (either physiologically achieved through water ingestion, or by direct addition of water to the specimen), as well as test for the presence of common additive adulterants (including acids, bases, bleach, glutaraldehyde, nitrite, detergents, and soap). Adulteration is rarely a problem in medical testing.

PERFORMANCE CHARACTERISTICS OF COMMON DRUG-SCREENING ASSAYS

Medical toxicologists, toxicology laboratory directors, and practicing physicians frequently are asked about the significance of drug-screening assays, particularly about the causes of false-positive results. Usually these questions are from an individual who has recently had a positive test. Drug-screening test performance characteristics are summarized in Table 7–10 and discussed in more detail below.

Immunoassays for opiates are directed toward morphine but have good cross-reactivity with a number of structurally similar natural and semisynthetic opiates. A positive immunoassay result may reflect multiple contributions from various opiates and opiate metabolites. Concentrations of morphine glucuronide in the urine may be up to 10-fold higher than the concentrations of unchanged morphine, and can contribute substantially to positive results. Because glucuronides are not readily extracted, enzymatic or chemical hydrolysis of glucuronides to parent substances is generally undertaken prior to confirmatory testing with a chromatographic method. Synthetic opioids show little or no cross-reactivity in opiate immunoassays. These include dextromethorphan, fentanyl, meperidine, methadone, naloxone, propoxyphene, and tramadol. Urine immunoassays specific for methadone and propoxyphene are available.

The duration of positivity of an opiate immunoassay after last use depends on the identity and amount of the opiate used, the specific immunoassay, the cutoff value, and the pharmacokinetics of the individual. Typically, the urine is positive for 2–4 days after last use with a cutoff of 300 ng/mL, or for 1–2 days with a cutoff of 2000 ng/mL. Currently, SAMHSA recommends a cutoff equivalent to 2000 ng/mL of morphine for workplace screening. This change was implemented after it was shown that ingestion of food products containing poppy seeds could, in rare instances, produce transient positive results with the lower cutoff value.[19] Most workplace screening programs now use the 2000 ng/mL cutoff, whereas most toxicology laboratories continue to use a 300 ng/mL cutoff.

Drug-screening assays for cocaine are actually assays for the inactive cocaine metabolite benzoylecgonine, which is eliminated more slowly than cocaine. As a result of testing for the metabolite, the duration of positivity after last use is extended from a few hours to 2 days. After prolonged heavy use, positive results may be observed for a week or more (rarely up to 3 weeks). The assay is extremely specific for benzoylecgonine. Even cocaine exhibits low cross-reactivity. Consequently, false-positive results are extremely uncommon. Because the assay is directed toward an inactive metabolite, positive results do not equate with intoxication but merely indicate recent exposure. In the past, true-positive results were recorded after ingestion of an herbal tea that actually contained small amounts of cocaine; however, these were clinically false-positives.[29] This tea is no longer available in the United States.[19]

Immunoassays for cannabinoids are also directed toward an inactive metabolite, in this case tetrahydrocannabinoic acid. These immunoassays exhibit cross-reactivity with other cannabinoids, but little else. Because cannabinoids are structurally unique and occur only in plants of the genus *Cannabis*, false-positives are uncommon. It is difficult, although possible, to become exposed to sufficient "second hand" or sidestream marijuana smoke to develop a positive urine test.[16] Legal hemp products include fiber, oil, and seedcake derived from *Cannabis* varieties with low levels of cannabinoids. Although hemp food products contain insufficient amounts of tetrahydrocannabinol to produce psychoactive effects, their ingestion may raise urinary cannabinoid concentrations above screening thresholds.[17]

Interpretation of a positive result for cannabinoids can be problematic. Urine may be positive for up to 3 days after occasional recreational use. However, with heavy or prolonged use, there may be significant accumulation of cannabinoids in adipose tissue. These stored cannabinoids are slowly released into the bloodstream and can produce positive findings for a month or more. Prolonged positivity is particularly likely when a cutoff value lower than the SAMHSA-recommended value of 50 ng/mL is used. Because of the possibility of prolonged detection of inactive metabolites, little can be concluded from a positive finding with regard to current intoxication by tetrahydrocannabinol. Medical false-positives (urine positive for the metabolite in the absence of current intoxication) are common. For this reason, and because tetrahydrocannabinol rarely is responsible for serious acute toxicity, some laboratories do not include cannabinoids in their menu of routinely performed urine drug tests.

Assays for amphetamines have the greatest problems with false-positive results. A number of structurally related compounds have significant cross-reactivity, including over-the-counter decongestants, such as phenylpropanolamine and pseudoephedrine, as well as *l*-ephedrine, which is found in a variety of herbal preparations. This cross-reactivity is beneficial from the point of view of the medical toxicologist, because all of these compounds may produce serious stimulant toxicity. But it is problematic in drug-abuse screening because of the widespread legitimate use of cold medications. Assays with greater selectivity for amphetamine and/or methamphetamine have been developed. Although these have fewer false-positive results caused by decongestant cross-reactivity, they are also less sensitive for the detection of other abused amphetamine-like compounds, including methylenedioxyamphetamine (MDA), methylenedioxymethamphetamine (MDMA, Ecstasy), and phentermine. Cross-reactivity patterns vary from assay to assay.[51] The manufacturer's literature should be consulted for specific details.

Testing for benzodiazepines is complicated by the wide array of benzodiazepines that differ substantially in their potency, cross-reactivity, and half-lives. This heterogeneity complicates the interpretation of benzodiazepine-screening assays. Results may be positive in persons using low therapeutic doses of diazepam, but negative after an overdose of a highly potent benzodiazepine such as clonazepam. False-negative results are also attributable to the fact that some benzodiazepines are excreted in the urine almost entirely as glucuronides. These glucuronides may have little cross-reactivity with antibodies directed toward an unmodified benzodiazepine. This is one reason for the poor detectability of lorazepam. This has led to the recommendation that specimens be treated with β-glucuronidase prior to analysis.[41] Because of the frequency of false-negative results, as well as the fact that benzodiazepines are relatively benign in overdose, not all toxicology laboratories include benzodiazepine immunoassays in their routine drug-screening protocols.

Barbiturates are comparable to benzodiazepines in heterogeneity of potency, cross-reactivity, and half-lives, although the differences are less substantial. Specific assays for serum phenobarbital can often help to clarify the significance of a positive barbiturate screen.

MEASUREMENT OF ETHANOL CONCENTRATIONS

Measuring ethanol may have ramifications beyond guiding medical management, particularly when performed on crash victims. Although testing for ethanol in urine is common in workplace drug screening, most testing in clinical laboratories is done using serum or plasma. Concentrations are most commonly measured enzymatically using alcohol dehydrogenase. Other alcohols exhibit much lower reaction rates with alcohol dehydrogenase than does ethanol, and rarely contribute substantially to the measured level. In larger toxicology laboratories, ethanol measurements are often done using a GC assay that also measures isopropanol and methanol, as well as the isopropanol metabolite, acetone. Alcohols with lower volatility, including ethylene and propylene glycol, are usually not detected. Because both enzymatic and chromatographic assays have substantial specificity for ethanol, confirmatory testing with a second method is uncommon.

Breath-alcohol analyzers may also be employed in assessing ethanol intoxication, as may point-of-care devices that measure salivary ethanol. These measurements are less precise than laboratory assays[31,52] and are more subject to interference by other alcohols because they are generally end-point methods (Fig. 7–1). They may also give false-positive results with other organic solvents.[9] Breath-alcohol analyzers require good cooperation from the patient to obtain an appropriate breath sample and are typically calibrated to give results approximating whole-blood alcohol concentrations, which underestimate serum alcohol concentrations (see below). For these reasons, confirmation of positive findings with a laboratory measurement may be desirable.

Alcohol concentrations are often informally interpreted by medical personnel in terms of legal criteria for driving under the influence, with levels in excess of 80 mg/dL interpreted as being legally "drunk" (Chap. 64). It should be noted that legal standards are written in terms of whole-blood alcohol concentrations, whereas clinical laboratories measure alcohol in serum or plasma. Serum and plasma alcohol concentrations are essentially identical, but both will be higher than the alcohol concentration measured in a whole-blood specimen obtained at the same time. This is a result of the lower concentration of alcohol in the red blood cells. The ratio of serum alcohol to whole-blood alcohol varies from individual to individual, with a median value of 1.15.[49] It is more likely than not that an individual with a serum alcohol concentration of 115 mg/dL has a whole-blood alcohol concentration of 100 mg/dL or greater (<0.10%, w/v).

QUANTITATIVE DRUG MEASUREMENTS

When properly used to guide dosing adjustments, drug concentration measurements improve medical outcomes.[20] However, many therapeutic drug measurements are made without an appropriate therapeutic question in mind, or are drawn at inappropriate times.[59] An essential requirement for interpretation of drug concentrations is that the relationship between drug concentrations and drug effects be known. Such knowledge is available for routinely monitored drugs and is often encapsulated in published ranges of effective concentrations and toxic concentrations.[7] Concentrations designated as "toxic" are usually higher than the upper end of the therapeutic range and typically represent concentrations at which toxicity is acute and potentially serious.

The relationships between toxic concentrations and effects cannot be systematically studied in humans, and consequently are often incompletely defined. They are largely derived from concentration and outcomes data obtained from overdose case reports and case series. The measurement of drug concentrations in overdose cases where concentration-effect relationships are not well defined may contribute more to the management of future overdosed patients than to the management of the current patient.

For the toxicologist, drug concentrations are especially useful in two ways. For drugs whose toxicity is either delayed or clinically inapparent during the early phases of an overdose, drug concentrations may have substantial prognostic value. These concentrations may be used to make decisions regarding the employment of antidotes or of interventions to hasten drug elimination, such as hemodialysis or hemoperfusion. Specific concentrations allow anticipation of the type or intensity of supportive care that may be needed. Properly timed drug measurements can also per-

mit estimation of the rate of elimination, facilitating anticipatory planning for stepdown of care intensity and for discharge.

Quantitative drug measurements are subject to various interferences, but these are less problematic than in qualitative assays. Signals generated by cross-reacting substances are weaker than signals from the target analyte, and are relatively unlikely to lead to a false diagnosis of toxicity, particularly if the target analyte is absent. Such cross-reactivity can be exploited in some instances to provide confirmatory evidence of a poison for which no specific assay is immediately available. For example, the immunoassay finding of apparent subtoxic levels of tricyclic antidepressants can help to confirm a diphenhydramine overdose, and the finding of a measurable digoxin concentration in an unexposed patient may suggest poisoning with other cardiac glycosides of plant or animal origin. Negative interferences are much less frequent. Table 7–11 summarizes some of the more common interferences in quantitative assays for drugs and poisons.

Interferences in chromatographic methods usually result from the presence of other compounds with migration rates similar to the target analyte. Because the migration rates are rarely exactly the same, the laboratory can usually recognize the presence of the interference as an overlapping peak when both substances are present. In such instances, the interference may impair accurate measurement of the drug concentration. When there is no target drug present, misidentification of the interfering peak as the target becomes much more likely, because a single peak is seen at approximately the expected position. Because interferences in chromatographic methods are generally unique to a specific method, information about these interferences should be obtained by asking the laboratory.

Drug measurements are unlike most other laboratory measurements in that the concentrations are highly dependent on the timing of the measurement. Knowledge of a drug's pharmacokinetics can substantially enhance the ability to draw meaningful conclusions. Some drugs alter their pharmacokinetic behavior at very high concentrations. Atypical pharmacokinetics observed at high concentrations are often referred to as *toxicokinetics*. They may be predictable from the mechanisms of drug clearance and the extent of plasma protein and the tissue binding (Chap. 11).

TABLE 7–11. Interferences in Quantitative Assays for Drugs and Poisons

Analyte	Technique	Interference
Acetaminophen	Spectrochemical	Bilirubin, phenacetin, renal failure, salicylates
	Immunoassay	Phenacetin
Carboxyhemoglobin	Spectrochemical	Fetal hemoglobin
Digoxin	Immunoassay	Other cardiac glycosides (oleander, red squill, Chan Su); endogenous digoxinlike substances (found in hepatic and renal failure, neonates, pregnancy); digoxin metabolites in renal failure; digoxin Fab may increase or decrease results
Ethylene glycol	Spectrochemical	High concentrations of lactate, glycerol
	GC	Propylene glycol, propionic acid
Iron	Spectrochemical	Deferoxamine and EDTA decrease iron, with variable effect on iron-binding capacity
Lithium	Electrochemical	Lithium heparin anticoagulant; abnormal serum sodium
Methemoglobin	Spectrochemical	Hyperlipidemia; methylene blue; sulfhemoglobin
Salicylate	Spectrochemical	Bilirubin, diflunisal, ketosis, salicylamide, salicylsalicylate
	Immunoassay	Diflunisal
Theophylline	Immunoassay	Caffeine

Knowledge of the relationship between drug concentrations and drug effects, or pharmacodynamics, is also important. Drug effects depend on local drug concentrations at the site of action, typically at cell membranes or intracellular locations. Serum or plasma drug concentrations can be correlated with drug effects only when these concentrations are in equilibrium with concentrations at the site of action. Table 7–12 lists several circumstances that may alter the normal ratio of measured drug concentrations to concentrations at the site of action, thereby altering the usual concentration-effect relationships. The concentration ratio has generally not reached its equilibrium value during the absorption and distribution phases, yet often, the only drug concentration measured after an acute overdose is the concentration obtained while absorption and distribution are still ongoing.

For drugs that bind significantly to plasma proteins, it is the concentration of drug that is not bound to proteins (the free drug concentration) that is in equilibrium with concentrations at the site of action. For most drugs at therapeutic levels, the free drug concentration is an approximately constant percentage of the total drug concentration, which is the concentration that is usually measured in the laboratory. Under these conditions, the ratio of total drug concentration to active site concentration is approximately constant, and a reasonable correlation between total drug concentrations and drug effects can be expected.

Increasing the percentage of drug in free form results in stronger effects than would be predicted from the total drug concentration. The free fraction of phenytoin may increase from its usual value of 10% when the number of albumin-binding sites are decreased, either by hypoalbuminemia, or by occupancy of the sites by other drugs, such as valproic acid, or by phenytoin metabolites that accumulate in renal failure. Saturation of protein-binding sites, as occurs with salicylate or valproic acid, also results in an increased percentage of drug in free form.

A major change in the free fraction occurs after treatment of digoxin toxicity with digoxin-immune Fab, when the free digoxin concentration falls from ~75% of the total concentration to less than 1%, as a result of digoxin binding by the antidigoxin antibody fragments. At the same time, there is extensive redistribution of digoxin from tissues to plasma, leading to substantial increases in total digoxin concentration. The complex of digoxin-immune Fab and digoxin results in interference with many digoxin immunoassays.[48]

Measurement of free drug concentrations can clarify such situations.[35] Assays for free phenytoin are available in many laboratories. Assays for other free drug concentrations may require special arrangements. Contact the laboratory to determine availability and expected turnaround time. For patients treated with digoxin-immune Fab, newer immunoassays that use antibodies attached to microparticles or glass fibers give results that can be used to set an upper bound on free digoxin concentrations and thereby verify adequacy of treatment.[47]

EFFECTIVE USE OF THE TOXICOLOGY LABORATORY

The toxicology laboratory is frequently an underappreciated resource. It may be viewed in much the same way as other clinical laboratories often are, that is, as a black box that converts orders into test results. Because toxicology testing volumes are relatively low and menus are extensive, it is not as highly automated as other laboratories. Many results may be "handmade the old-fashioned way." The downside of this may be longer turnaround times. But the upside is that toxicology personnel have the incentive and flexibility to develop substantial expertise, as well as the desire to share that expertise.

Communication is the key to getting the most from the toxicology laboratory. This begins with learning the laboratory's capabilities—which drugs can it reliably detect at all times, which drugs it can reliably detect if specifically requested, and which drugs it can't detect at all. The laboratory should also be able to provide approximate turnaround times for various tests. A key, often overlooked item of communication is noting any drugs that are particularly suspected on any request for a screening test. This knowledge enables the laboratory to set up the tests for those drugs first and possibly to adjust the protocols to increase sensitivity or specificity. This may save an hour or more in the time needed to receive the critical information.

Consultation with the laboratory regarding puzzling cases or unusual needs can allow consensus on an effective and feasible testing strategy. The full capabilities of a toxicology laboratory are not often apparent from published lists of tests available. Most laboratories devote substantial efforts to meeting reasonable requests. The laboratory also provides advice on special specimen collection requirements and may also advise on appropriate timing based on the relevant toxicokinetics. The toxicology laboratory, like the poison center, is one of the few medical services willing to offer extensive consultation at no charge.

The laboratory should also be contacted whenever results are inconsistent with clinical presentation. The most common causes for this are interferences and preanalytical errors. The laboratory is familiar with the common sources of these discrepancies. If the discrepancy is the result of a laboratory error, it is critical that the laboratory be informed so that steps can be taken to avoid a recurrence.

In the future, toxicology testing may be automated by using a chip-based array of miniaturized immunoassays and microelectrodes that detect or measure several dozen substances simultaneously. Given the relatively limited market that currently exists, the future may take some time to arrive. In the meanwhile, the toxicologist can rely on strong, collegial support from the toxicology laboratory.

TABLE 7–12. Factors That Might Alter Concentration/Effect Relationships

Factor	Effect	Examples
Measurement during absorption phase	Underestimation of eventual effects	Sustained-release preparations; large ingestions of poorly soluble drugs (eg, salicylates); drugs that slow gastric emptying (eg, tricyclic antidepressants)
Measurement during distribution phase	Overestimation of effects	Lithium, digoxin, tricyclic antidepressants
Decreased binding to proteins	Underestimation of effects	Phenytoin
Saturation of binding proteins	Underestimation of effects	Salicylate, valproic acid
Binding by antidote	Variable (see discussion)	Digoxin/digoxin-immune Fab

REFERENCES

1. Badcock NR, Zoanetti GD: Modifications to Toxi-Lab for the routine screening for drugs in paediatric toxicology. Ann Clin Biochem 1996; 33:75–77.
2. Bailey DN: Drug use in patients admitted to a university trauma center: Results of limited (rather than comprehensive) toxicology screening. J Anal Toxicol 1990;14:22–24.
3. Bailey DN: Results of limited versus comprehensive toxicology screening in a university medical center. Am J Clin Pathol 1996;105: 572–575.
4. Belanger AC: Alternate site testing. The regulatory perspective. Arch Pathol Lab Med 1995;119:902–906.
5. Belson MG, Simon HK, Sullivan K, Geller RJ: The utility of toxicologic analysis in children with suspected ingestions. Pediatr Emerg Care 1999;15:383–387.
6. Belson MG, Simon HK: Utility of comprehensive toxicologic screens in children. Am J Emerg Med 1999;17:221–224.
7. Benet LZ, Oie S, Schwartz JB: Design and optimization of dosage regimens: Pharmacokinetic data. In: Hardman JG, Limbird LE, Molinoff PB, et al, eds: The Pharmacological Basis of Therapeutics, 9th ed. New York, McGraw-Hill, 1996, pp. 1707–1792.
8. Beutler JA, Vergeer PP: Amatoxins in American mushrooms: Evaluation of the Meixner test. Mycologia 1980;72:1142–1149.
9. Biwasaka H, Tokuta T, Sasaki Y, et al: Application of Q.E.D. and Alco-Screen test kits to measurements of ethanol in forensic samples. Nippon Hoigaku Zasshi 2000;54:233–240.
10. Brett AS: Implications of discordance between clinical impression and toxicology analysis in drug overdose. Arch Intern Med 1988;148: 437–441.
11. Buchfuhrer LA, Radecki SE: Alcohol and drug abuse in an urban trauma center: Predictors of screening and detection. J Addict Dis 1996;15:65–74.
12. Buck C, Brunner D, Otten E, et al: Evaluation of rapid urine toxicological testing in patients with altered mental status in the emergency department [abstract]. J Toxicol Clin Toxicol 1999;37:597–598.
13. Center for Substance Abuse Prevention, Division of Workplace Programs: An evaluation of non-instrumented drug test devices. Washington, DC, Substance Abuse and Mental Health Services Administration, 1999, 22 pp.
14. Clark RF, Harchelroad F: Toxicology screening of the trauma patient: A changing profile. Ann Emerg Med 1991;20:151–153.
15. College of American Pathologists Participant Summaries: Toxicology Survey Set T-B; Therapeutic Drug Monitoring (General) Survey Set Z-B; Urine Toxicology Survey Set UT-B; Serum Alcohol/Volatiles Survey Set AL2-B; Chemistry Survey Set C4-B. Northfield, IL: College of American Pathologists, 1999.
16. Cone EJ, Johnson RE, Darwin WD, et al: Passive inhalation of marijuana smoke: Urinalysis and room air levels of delta-9-tetrahydrocannabinol. J Anal Toxicol 1987;11:89–96.
17. Costantino A, Schwartz RH, Kaplan P: Hemp oil ingestion causes positive urine tests for delta 9-tetrahydrocannabinol carboxylic acid. J Anal Toxicol 1997;21:482–485.
18. Davidow B, Petri NL, Quame B: A thin-layer chromatographic screening procedure for detecting drug abuse. Am J Clin Pathol 1968;50:714–719.
19. Department of Health and Human Services: Medical Review Officer Manual. http://www.health.org/workplace/mromanual.htm. (Last accessed 12/23/00.)
20. Destache CJ, Meyer SK, Rowley KM: Does accepting pharmacokinetic recommendations impact hospitalization? A cost-benefit analysis. Ther Drug Monit 1990;12:427–433.
21. Dubowski KM: The role of the scientist in litigation involving drug-use testing. Clin Chem 1988;34:788–792.
22. Durback LF, Scharman EJ, Brown BS: Emergency physicians perceptions of drug screens at their own hospitals. Vet Hum Toxicol 1998; 40:234–237.
23. Ferrara SD, Tedeschi L, Frison G, et al: Drugs-of-abuse testing in urine: Statistical approach and experimental comparison of immunochemical and chromatographic techniques. J Anal Toxicol 1994;18: 278–291.
24. Fitzgerald RL, Rivera JD, Herold DA: Broad spectrum drug identification directly from urine, using liquid chromatography-tandem mass spectrometry. Clin Chem 1999;45:1224–1234.
25. Franke JP, de Zeeuw RA: Solid-phase extraction procedures in systematic toxicological analysis. J Chromatogr B 1998;713:51–59.
26. Fraser AD, Howell P: Oxaprozin cross-reactivity in three commercial immunoassays for benzodiazepines in urine. J Anal Toxicol 1998;22: 50–54.
27. Henderson DR, Friedman SB, Harris JD, et al: CEDIA, a new homogeneous immunoassay system. Clin Chem 1986;32:1637–1641.
28. Hepler BR, Sutheimer CA, Sunshine I: The role of the toxicology laboratory in emergency medicine. II. Study of an integrated approach. J Toxicol Clin Toxicol 1984–85;22:503–528.
29. Jackson GF, Saady JJ, Poklis A: Urinary excretion of benzoylecgonine following ingestion of Health Inca Tea. Forensic Sci Int 1991; 49:57–64.
30. Jarvie DR, Simpson D: Drug screening: Evaluation of the Toxi-Lab TLC system. Ann Clin Biochem 1986;23:76–84.
31. Keim ME, Bartfield JM, Raccio-Robak N, et al: Accuracy of an enzymatic assay device for serum ethanol measurement. J Toxicol Clin Toxicol 1999;37:75–81.
32. Kellermann AL, Fihn SD, Logerfro JP, et al: Impact of drug screening in suspected overdose. Ann Emerg Med 1987;16:1206–1216.
33. Kelner MJ, Bailey DN: Mismeasurement of methemoglobin. Clin Chem 1985;31:168–169.
34. King JA, Storrow AB, Finkelstein JA: Urine Trinder spot test: A rapid salicylate screen for the emergency department. Ann Emerg Med. 1995;26:330–333.
35. Kwong TC: Free drug measurements: Methodology and clinical significance. Clin Chim Acta 1985;151:193–216.
36. Lai CK, Lee T, Au KM, Chan AY: Uniform solid-phase extraction procedure for toxicological drug screening in serum and urine by HPLC with photodiode-array detection. Clin Chem 1997;43:312–325.
37. Lampe KF, McCann MA: Differential diagnosis of poisoning by North American mushrooms, with particular emphasis on Amanita phalloides-like intoxication. Ann Emerg Med 1987;16:956–962.
38. Loiselle JM, Baker MD, Templeton JM Jr, et al: Substance abuse in adolescent trauma. Ann Emerg Med 1993;22:1530–1534.
39. Luebbert PP: Screening for drugs of abuse. Lab Med 1991;22: 881–883.
40. Manno JE, Manno BR: Experimental basis of alcohol-induced psychomotor performance impairment. In: Garriott JC, ed: Medicolegal Aspects of Alcohol. Tucson, AZ, Lawyers and Judges Publishing Co., 1996, pp. 303–340.
41. Meatherall R: Benzodiazepine screening using EMIT II and TDx: Urine hydrolysis pretreatment required. J Anal Toxicol 1994;18: 385–390.
42. Ohtsuji M, Lai JS, Binder SR, et al: Use of REMEDi HS in emergency toxicology for a rapid estimate of drug concentrations in urine, serum, and gastric samples. J Forensic Sci 1996;41:881–886.
43. Osterloh JD: Utility and reliability of emergency toxicologic testing. Emerg Med Clin North Am 1990;8:693–723.
44. Parker KM, White BN, Beattie DJ, Altmiller DH: Comprehensive drug screening for a pediatric population. Clin Chem 1988;34: 748–750.
45. Parran TV Jr, Weber E, Tasse J, et al: Mandatory toxicology testing and chemical dependence consultation follow-up in a level-one trauma center. J Trauma 1995;38:278–280.
46. Pohjola-Sintonen S, Kivisto KT, Vuori E, et al: Identification of drugs ingested in acute poisoning: Correlation of patient history with drug analyses. Ther Drug Monit 2000;22:749–752.
47. Rainey PM: Digibind and free digoxin. Clin Chem 1999;45:719.

48. Rainey PM: Effects of digoxin immune Fab (ovine) on digoxin immunoassays. Am J Clin Pathol 1989;92:779–786.

49. Rainey PM: Relationship between serum and whole-blood ethanol concentrations. Clin Chem 1993;39:2288–2292.

50. Roberts WL, Santos FS, Rainey PM, et al: Erroneous results with diluted EMIT reagents. Clin Chem 1994;40:1597–1598.

51. Shaw LM, Kwong TC, Orsulak PJ, et al, eds: Contemporary Practice in Clinical Toxicology, 2d ed. Washington, DC, AACC Press, 2000. pp. D.1 – D.10.

52. Simpson G: Accuracy and precision of breath-alcohol measurements for a random subject in the postabsorptive state. Clin Chem 1987;33: 261–268.

53. Sloan EP, Zalenski RJ, Smith RF, et al: Toxicology screening in urban trauma patients: Drug prevalence and its relationship to trauma severity and management. J Trauma 1989;29:1647–1653.

54. Sporer KA, Ernst AA: The effect of toxicologic screening on management of minimally symptomatic overdoses. Am J Emerg Med 1992; 10:173–175.

55. Stull TM, Hearn TL, Hancock JS, et al: Variation in proficiency testing performance by testing site. JAMA 1998;279:463–467.

56. Sugarman JM, Rodgers GC, Paul RI: Utility of toxicology screening in a pediatric emergency department. Pediatr Emerg Care 1997;13: 194–197.

57. Vega WA, Kolody B, Hwang J, Noble A: Prevalence and magnitude of perinatal substance exposures in California. N Engl J Med 1993; 329:850–854.

58. Warner AM: Cost-effective toxicology testing. Ther Drug Monit 1996;17:35–47.

59. Warner A: Setting standards of practice in therapeutic drug monitoring and clinical toxicology: A North American view. Ther Drug Monit 2000;22:93–97.

60. Wax P, Branton T, Cobaugh D, Kwong T: False-positive ethylene glycol determination by enzyme assay in patients with chronic acetaminophen hepatotoxicity [abstract]. J Toxicol Clin Toxicol 1999;37: 604.

61. Wiley JF II: Difficult diagnoses in toxicology. Poisons not detected by the comprehensive drug screen. Pediatr Clin North Am 1991;38: 725–737.

62. Young DS: Effects of Drugs on Clinical Laboratory Tests, 4th ed. Washington, DC, AACC Press, 2000, pp. 3.1–3.643.

CHAPTER 8

DIAGNOSTIC IMAGING IN TOXICOLOGY

David T. Schwartz

Diagnostic imaging plays an important role in many areas of clinical medicine, and in certain cases, it can help in the management of toxicologic emergencies. In some instances, radiographic studies visualize the toxin itself. In other cases, they reveal the toxin's effect on various organ systems (Table 8–1). Radiography can confirm a diagnosis, assist in therapeutic interventions such as monitoring gastrointestinal decontamination, and detect complications of the exposure.[148]

Conventional radiography is readily available in the Emergency Department (ED) and is the imaging modality most frequently used in acute patient management. However, many other imaging modalities are employed in toxicologic emergencies, including computed tomography (CT), enteric and intravascular contrast studies, ultrasound, magnetic resonance imaging (MRI), and nuclear scintigraphy.

VISUALIZING THE TOXIN

A number of toxins and medications are *radiopaque* and can potentially be detected radiographically. If ingested, the toxin may be seen on an abdominal radiograph. Injected toxins are also amenable to radiographic detection. If the toxic material itself is available for examination, it can be radiographed outside of the body to detect radiopaque contents (Fig. 85–1 and Case Studies Fig. 1–2).

The radiopacity of a toxin or drug is determined by several factors. First, the *intrinsic radiopacity* of a substance depends on its physical density (g/cm^3) and the atomic numbers of its constituent atoms. Biologic tissues are composed mostly of carbon, hydrogen, and oxygen, and have an average atomic number of approximately 6. Substances that are more radiopaque than soft tissues include bone, which contains calcium (atomic number 20); radiocontrast agents containing iodine (atomic number 53) and barium (atomic number 56); iron (atomic number 26); and lead (atomic number 82). Some medications and toxins have constituent atoms of high atomic number, such as chlorine (atomic number 17), potassium (atomic number 19), and sulfur (atomic number 16), that contribute to their radiopacity.

The thickness of an object affects its radiopacity. Small particles of a moderately radiopaque substance are often not visible on a radiograph. The radiographic appearance of the surrounding area also affects the detectability of an object. A moderately radiopaque tablet is easily seen against a uniform background, but in a patient, overlying bone or bowel gas often obscures the tablet.

Ingestion of an Unknown Toxin

Although an early clinical policy suggested that an abdominal radiograph be obtained in the unresponsive overdose patient in an attempt to identify the involved toxin,[1] the role of abdominal radiography in screening patients who have ingested an unknown substance is questionable. The number of potentially ingested substances that are radiopaque is limited. In addition, the radiographic appearance of an ingested substance is not sufficiently distinctive to determine its identity (Fig. 8–1).[168] However, when ingestion of a radiopaque substance such as iron tablets or heavy metals is suspected, abdominal radiographs are helpful.[2] In addition, knowledge of potentially radiopaque substances is useful in suggesting diagnostic possibilities when a radiopaque substance is discovered on an abdominal radiograph that was obtained for reasons other than suspected toxin ingestion, such as in a patient with abdominal pain (Fig. 8–2).[147,153]

Several investigators have studied the radiopacity of various medications.[36,43,59,66,76,120,144,156,163] The investigations used an in vitro water-bath model to simulate the radiopacity of abdominal soft tissues. These studies found that only a small number of medications exhibit some degree of radiopacity. A short list of the more consistently radiopaque substances is summarized in the mnemonic CHIPES—chloral hydrate, heavy metals, iron, psychotropics (phenothiazines), and enteric-coated and sustained-release preparations.

The CHIPES mnemonic has several limitations.[144] It does not include all of the pills that are radiopaque in vitro (eg, acetazolamide and busulfan). Most of these medications, however, are only moderately radiopaque and, when ingested, dissolve rapidly and become difficult or impossible to detect. Psychotropic medications include a wide variety of compounds of varying radiopacity.[120,144] For example, trifluoperazine (containing fluorine, atomic number 9) is radiopaque in vitro, whereas chlorpromazine (containing chlorine, atomic number 17) is not.[144] Finally, slow-release preparations and enteric coatings have variable composition and radiopacity. Pill formulations of fillers, binders, and coatings vary between manufacturers, and even a specific product can change depending on the date of manufacture. The insoluble matrix of some sustained-release preparations is radiopaque; however, when seen on a radiograph these pills may no longer contain active medication. Newer sustained-release cardiac medications such as verapamil and nifedipine have inconsistent radiopacity.[94,154,163]

In comparison to conventional radiography, *ultrasonography* theoretically is a useful tool for detecting ingested pills. Solid pills within the fluid-filled stomach have an appearance similar to gallstones within the gallbladder. In one in vitro study using a water-

TABLE 8–1.   Drugs and Toxins with Diagnostic Imaging Findings

Drug or Toxin	Imaging Study*	Finding	Page
Amiodarone	Chest	Phospholipidosis (interstitial and alveolar filling)	104, 108
Asbestos	Chest	Interstitial fibrosis (asbestosis), calcified pleural plaques, mesothelioma	104, 108
Beryllium	Chest	Acute: airspace filling; chronic: hilar adenopathy	106
Body packer	Abdominal Enteric contrast or abdominal CT	Ingested packets, ileus, bowel obstruction Retained packets	97, 101 110
Carbon monoxide	Head CT, MRI SPECT, PET	Bilateral basal ganglion lucencies, white matter demyelinization Cerebral dysfunction	113
Caustic ingestion	Enteric contrast	Esophageal perforation or stricture	110, 111
Chemotherapeutic agents (busulfan, bleomycin)	Chest	Interstitial pneumonitis	104
Cholinergic agents	Chest	Diffuse airspace filling (bronchorrhea)	106
Cocaine	Chest, abdominal Head CT, MRI SPECT, PET	Diffuse airspace filling, pneumomediastinum, aortic dissection ileus, bowel infarction, perforation SAH, intracerebral hemorrhage, infarction Cerebral dysfunction, dopamine receptor down-regulation	108, 109, 112
Corticosteroids	Skeletal	Avascular necrosis (femoral head)	105
Ethanol	Chest Head CT, MRI SPECT, PET	Dilated cardiomyopathy, aspiration pneumonitis Cortical atrophy, cerebellar atrophy, SDH (head trauma) Cerebellar and cortical dysfunction	106, 113
Fluorosis	Skeletal	Osteosclerosis, osteophytosis, ligament calcification	100
Heavy metals (Pb, Hg, Tl, As)	Abdominal	Ingested compound	96, 97
Hydrocarbons (low viscosity)	Chest	Aspiration pneumonitis	98, 107
Inhaled allergens	Chest	Hypersensitivity pneumonitis	104
Iron	Abdominal	Radiopaque tablets, gastric perforation (pneumoperitoneum)	96, 97
Irritant gases (low water solubility)	Chest	Diffuse airspace filling	106
IVDU (intravenous drug use)	Chest, skeletal, head CT	Septic emboli, pneumothorax, osteomyelitis (axial skeleton), AIDS-related infections	103, 104, 113
Lead	Skeletal Abdominal	Metaphyseal bands in children (proximal tibia, distal radius), bullets (dissolution near joints) Ingested leaded paint chips or other leaded compounds	97, 100
Mercury (elemental)	Abdominal, skeletal, or chest	Ingested, injected, or embolic deposits	96, 99
Nitrofurantoin	Chest	Hypersensitivity pneumonitis	106
Opioids	Chest Abdominal	Acute lung injury Ileus	107, 110
Phenytoin	Chest	Hilar lymphadenopathy	106
Procainamide, INH, hydrazine	Chest	Pleural and pericardial effusions (drug-induced lupus syndrome)	104, 106
Salicylates	Chest	Acute lung injury	103
Silica, coal dust	Chest	Interstitial fibrosis, hilar adenopathy (egg-shell calcification)	106
Thorium dioxide	Abdominal	Hepatic and splenic deposition	108, 111

*Plain radiography unless otherwise stated.

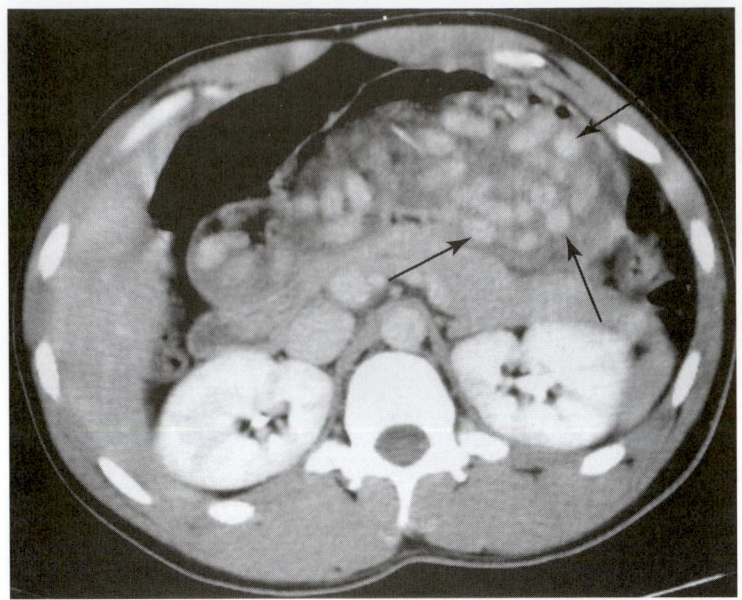

Figure 8–1. Ingestion of an unknown substance. A 46-year-old male presented to the ED with a depressed level of consciousness and the strong odor of an alcoholic beverage on his breath. Because he also complained of abdominal pain and mild diffuse abdominal tenderness, a CT scan of the abdomen was obtained. The CT revealed innumerable tablet-shaped densities within the stomach (*arrows*). The CT finding was suspicious for an overdose of an unknown medication. Orogastric lavage was attempted and the patient vomited a large amount of whole navy beans. CT is able to detect small, nearly isodense structures such as these, which cannot be seen using conventional radiography. However, the radiographic detection of tablets, or tablet-like densities, does not permit their pharmacologic identification. (*Courtesy of Earl J. Reisdorff, MD, Michigan State University, Lansing, Michigan.*)

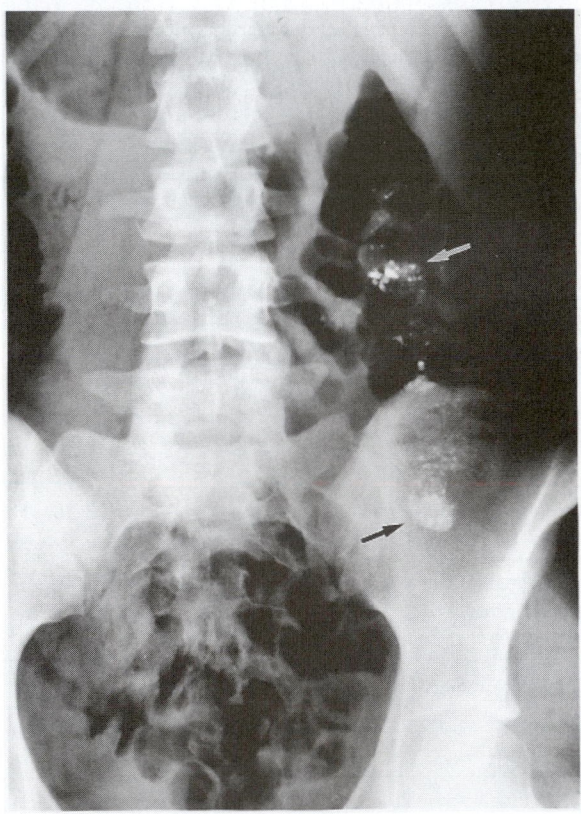

Figure 8–2. Detection of a radiopaque substance on an abdominal radiograph. An abdominal radiograph obtained on a patient with upper abdominal pain revealed radiopaque material throughout the intestinal tract (*arrows*). Is his abdominal pain because of an overdose of iron tablets or because of lead toxicity from eating paint chips? Is this retained barium from a previous upper GI series? Further questioning of the patient revealed that he had been consuming bismuth subsalicylate (Pepto-Bismol) tablets to treat his peptic ulcer (bismuth, atomic number 83). The identification of radiopaque material does not allow determination of the nature of the substance.

bath model, virtually all intact pills could be seen.[3] These authors were also successful at detecting pills within the stomachs of human volunteers who ingested pills. Nonetheless, reliably finding pills scattered throughout the gastrointestinal tract, which often contains air and feces that block the ultrasound beam, is a formidable task. Ultrasonography, therefore, has limited clinical practicality.

Exposure to a Known Toxin

When a substance that is known to be radiopaque is involved in a poisoning, radiography plays an important role in patient care.[2] Radiography can confirm the diagnosis of a radiopaque toxin exposure, quantify the approximate amount of toxin involved, and monitor its removal from the body.

Iron Tablet Ingestion. Ferrous sulfate tablets are readily detected radiographically because they are highly radiopaque and disintegrate slowly when ingested. Radiographs repeated after whole-bowel irrigation help to determine whether further gastrointestinal decontamination is needed (Figs. 8–3 and 22–3).[37,45,79,119,124,126,167] However, caution must be exercised in using radiography to exclude an iron ingestion. Some iron preparations are not radiographically detectable. Liquid, chewable, or encapsulated ("Spansule") iron preparations rapidly fragment and disperse after ingestion. Even when intact, these preparations are less radiopaque than ferrous sulfate tablets.[36]

Heavy Metals. Metals of high atomic number, such as lead, mercury, arsenic, and thallium, can be detected radiographically. Examples of heavy metal exposure include leaded ceramic glaze (Fig. 8–4);[138] paint chips containing leaded paint (Fig. 80–8);[88,106] mercuric oxide (Fig. 81–1); zinc sulfate (zinc, atomic number 30);[18] arsenic (atomic number 33; Fig. 8–5);[91,57] and thallium (atomic number 81; Case Studies Fig. 1–2).[31,107]

Mercury. Unintentional ingestion of elemental mercury can occur when a glass thermometer or a long intestinal tube breaks.

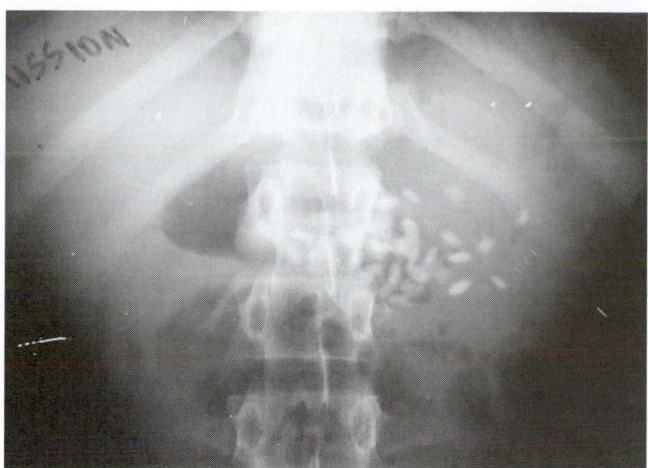

A

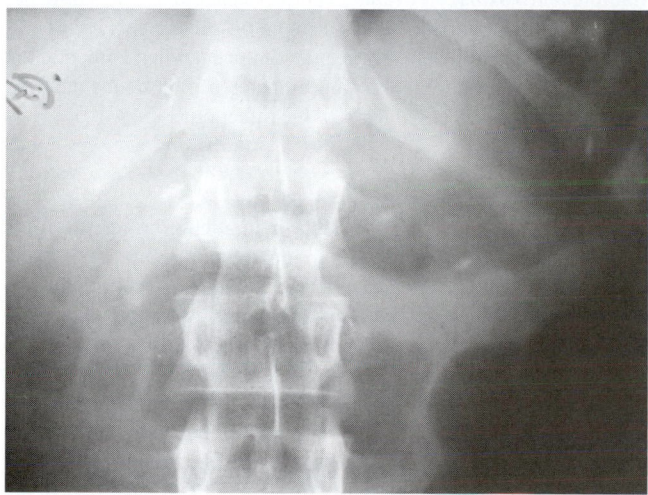

B

Figure 8–3. Iron tablet overdose. **A.** The identification of the large amount of radiopaque tablets confirms the diagnosis in a patient with a suspected iron overdose and permits rough quantification of the amount ingested. **B.** Following emesis and whole-bowel irrigation, a second radiograph revealed some remaining tablets and indicated the need for further intestinal decontamination. A third radiograph after additional bowel irrigation demonstrated clearing of the intestinal tract. (*Courtesy of the Toxicology Fellowship of the New York City Poison Control Center.*)

Liquid elemental mercury can be injected subcutaneously or intravenously. Radiographic studies assist débridement by detecting mercury that remains after the initial excision. Elemental mercury that is injected intravenously produces a dramatic radiographic picture of pulmonary embolization (Fig. 8–6).[20,99,116]

Lead. Unlike elemental mercury, metallic lead (eg, a bullet) embedded in soft tissues is not usually systemically absorbed. However, when the bullet is in contact with an acidic environment such as synovial fluid or CSF, there can be significant absorption. Over many years, mechanical and chemical action within the joint causes the bullet to fragment and to gradually dissolve (Fig. 8–7).[32,38,158,161]

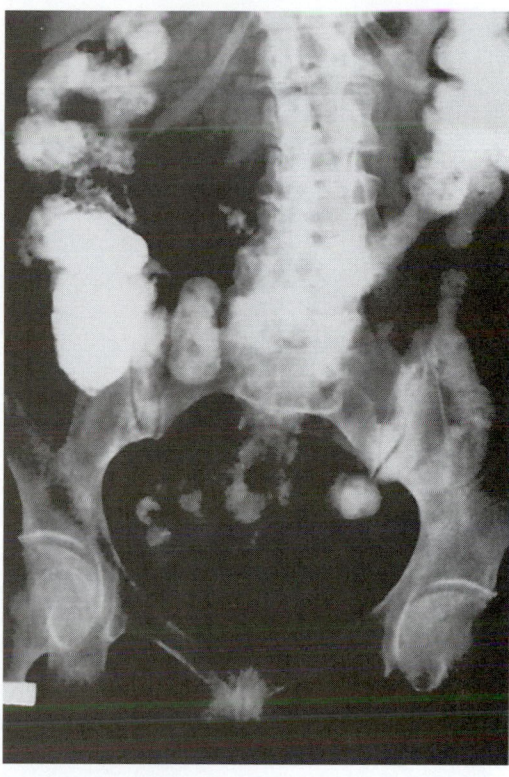

Figure 8–4. An abdominal radiograph of a patient who intentionally ingested ceramic glaze containing 40% lead. (*Courtesy of the Toxicology Fellowship of the New York City Poison Control Center.*)

Toxins in Containers. In some circumstances, ingested toxins can be seen even though they are of similar radiopacity to surrounding soft tissues. If a toxin is ingested in a container, the container itself may be visible (Fig. 22–2).

Body Packers. "Body packers" are individuals who smuggle large quantities of drugs across international borders in securely sealed packets.[12,13,19,41,75,85,98,105,150] The uniformly shaped oblong packets can be seen on plain abdominal radiographs either because there is a thin layer of air or metallic foil within the container wall or because the packets are outlined by bowel gas (Fig. 8–8 and Case Studies Fig. 1–9). In some cases, a "rosette" representing the knot at the end of the packet is seen.[150]

Because rupture of a single container can be fatal, care must be taken to ensure that all packets are removed. One or two retained packets can be difficult to detect on a plain radiograph, and an upper GI series with oral contrast can reveal any remaining packets (Fig. 22–3).[70] CT with enteric contrast is also capable of disclosing remaining packets.[121] However, in one reported case, a single retained packet was not seen on CT and was identified on a subsequent abdominal film with oral contrast.[58] The best study to detect retained packets is therefore uncertain. If one study does not reveal a suspected retained packet, the second study should be performed.

Body Stuffers. The "body stuffer" is an individual who, in an attempt to avoid imminent arrest, hurriedly ingests his contraband in less secure packaging.[140] The risk of leakage from such haphaz-

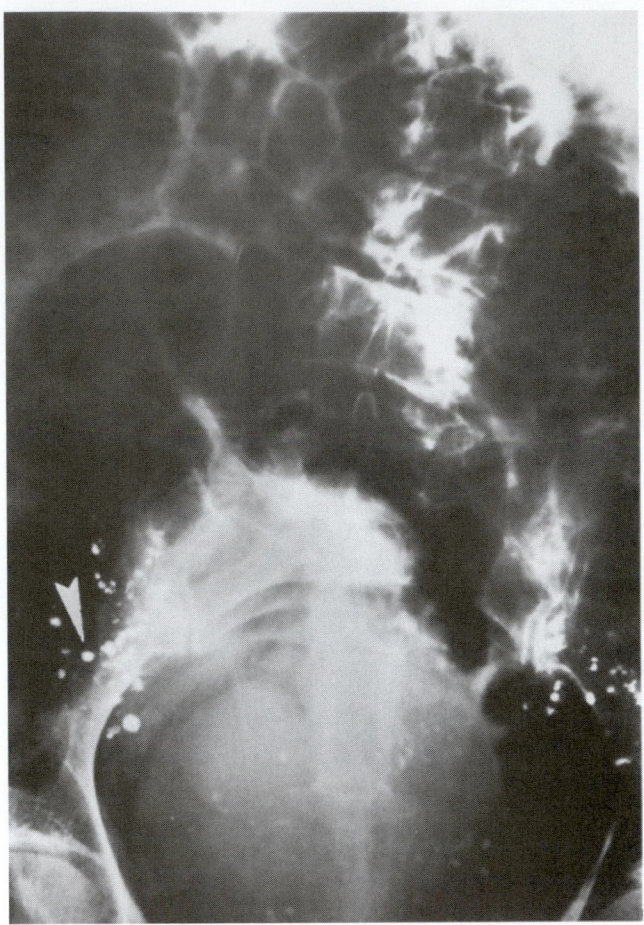

Figure 8–5. An abdominal radiograph in an elderly woman incidentally revealed radiopaque material in the pelvic region. This was residual from gluteal injection of antisyphilis therapy she had received 35–40 years earlier. The injections may have contained an arsenical. (*Courtesy of Dr. Emil J. Balthazar, Professor of Radiology, New York University.*)

ardly constructed containers is high. The patient usually denies having ingested any drugs, and, unfortunately, radiographic studies cannot reliably confirm or exclude an ingestion. In one series, none of 98 patients had a positive abdominal radiograph.[155]

Occasionally a radiograph will demonstrate the ingested material (Fig. 8–9). If the drug is in a glass or in a hard-plastic crack vial, the container may be seen on a plain film. However, only a small number of crack vials are detected radiographically, and the radiograph cannot determine whether the vial still contains any drug. In one series, crack vials were seen on abdominal radiographs in only 2 of 11 patients (18%).[69] If the body stuffer swallows soft plastic bags containing the drug, the containers are not usually visible. However, in three reported cases, "baggies" were visualized by abdominal CT.[61,80,129,148] Occasional reports have noted that some crack cocaine "rocks" can be detected by plain radiographs or by CT because they contain radiopaque contaminants.[27,61,64]

Halogenated Hydrocarbons. Some halogenated hydrocarbons can be visualized on plain radiographs.[28] Radiopacity is propor-

tionate to the number of chlorine atoms, and both carbon tetrachloride (CCl_4) and chloroform ($CHCl_3$) are radiopaque. Because these liquids are immiscible in water, a triple layer is seen within the stomach on an upright abdominal film: an uppermost air bubble, a middle radiopaque chlorinated hydrocarbon layer, and a lower gastric fluid layer. However, these ingestions are rare and the quantity ingested is usually too small to show this effect. Other halogenated hydrocarbons such as methylene iodide are highly radiopaque.[177]

Mothballs. Different types of mothballs can be distinguished by radiography. Relatively nontoxic paradichlorobenzene mothballs (containing chlorine, atomic number 17) are moderately radiopaque, whereas more toxic naphthalene mothballs are radiolucent.[159] Radiographs of mothballs outside of the patient can help distinguish these two types (Fig. 85–1).

Radiolucent Toxins. A radiolucent substance may be visible because it is less radiopaque than surrounding soft tissues. Hydrocarbons such as gasoline are relatively radiolucent when embedded in soft tissues. The radiographic appearance resembles subcutaneous gas as seen in a necrotizing soft tissue infection (Fig. 8–10).

Summary

Obtaining an abdominal radiograph in an attempt to identify pills or other toxins in a patient with an unknown ingestion is unlikely to be helpful and is, in general, not warranted. Radiography is most useful when the suspected substance is known to be radiopaque, as is the case with iron tablets and heavy metals. The toxin can be radiographed either within the patient's abdomen, elsewhere in the patient's body, or outside of the patient if the material is available. A "body packer" whose intestinal tract contains a large number of packets can also be reliably evaluated by plain radiography. Small numbers of retained radiolucent packets are better detected by using enteric contrast material.

Extravasation of Intravenous Contrast Material

Extravasation of radiographic contrast material is a common occurrence. In most cases, the volume extravasated is small and there are no clinical sequelae.[26,39] Rarely, there is an extravasation large enough to cause cutaneous necrosis and ulceration. In the past, the most common radiographic procedure associated with contrast extravasation was lower extremity venography. This is because in venography a small peripheral vein of an edematous leg or foot is injected and often a metal needle rather than a plastic intravenous cannula is used.

Recently, the incidence of sizable extravasations has increased because of the use of rapid-bolus automated power injectors for certain spiral CT studies. These CT studies are most often used to diagnose aortic dissection or pulmonary embolism. Fortunately, nonionic low-osmolality contrast solutions are usually used for these studies. These solutions are less toxic to soft tissues than older ionic high-osmolality contrast materials.

The treatment of contrast extravasation has not been studied in a large series of human subjects and is therefore controversial. Various strategies have been proposed. The affected extremity should be elevated to promote drainage. Although topical application of heat causes vasodilatation and could theoretically promote

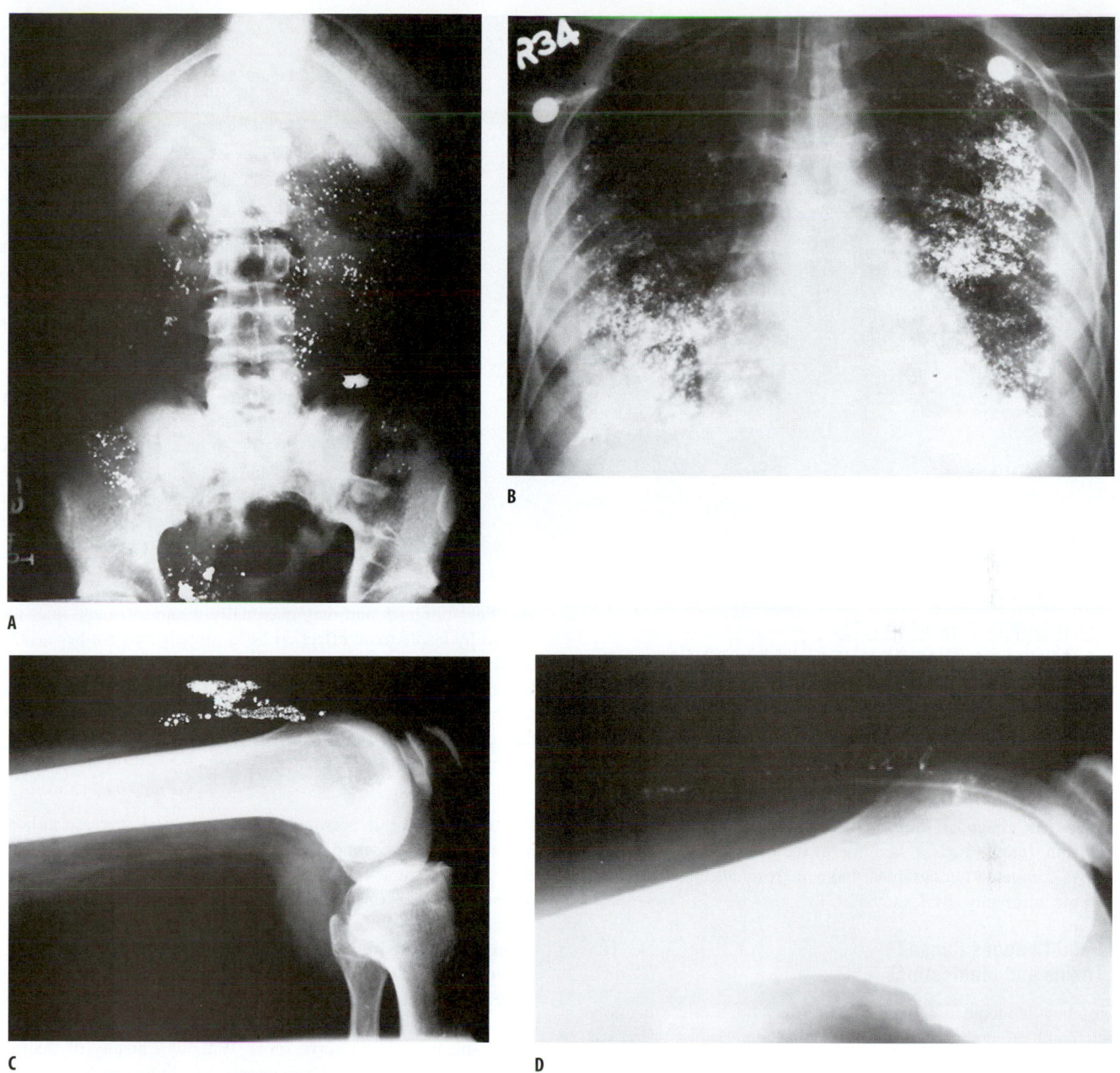

Figure 8–6.   Liquid elemental mercury exposures. **A.** Unintentional rupture of a Cantor intestinal tube distributed mercury throughout the bowel. Elemental mercury is not absorbed if the intestinal mucosa is intact. (*Courtesy of Dr. Richard Lefleur, Associate Professor of Radiology, New York University.*) **B.** The chest radiograph in a patient following intravenous injection of elemental mercury showing metallic pulmonary embolism. The patient developed respiratory failure, pleural effusions, and uremia, and expired despite aggressive therapeutic interventions. (*Courtesy of Dr. N. John Stewart.*) **C.** Subcutaneous injection of liquid elemental mercury is readily detected radiographically. Because mercury is systemically absorbed from subcutaneous tissues, it must be removed by surgical excision. (*Courtesy of the Toxicology Fellowship of the New York City Poison Control Center.*) **D.** A radiograph following surgical débridement reveals nearly complete removal of the mercury deposit. Surgical staples and a radiopaque drain are visible (*Courtesy of the Toxicology Fellowship of the New York City Poison Control Center.*)

resorption of extravasated contrast material, in some studies the intermittent application of ice packs has shown a lower incidence of ulceration.[26] Rarely, an extremely large volume of liquid is injected into the soft tissues, which requires surgical decompression. A radiograph of the extremity will demonstrate the extent of extravasation.[26]

Precautions should be taken to prevent extravasation. A recently placed, well-running intravenous catheter should be used. The distal portions of the extremities (hands, wrist, and feet) should be avoided. Patients at greater risk, such as infants, the elderly, debilitated patients, and those with an impaired ability to communicate, must be closely monitored if extravasation occurs.

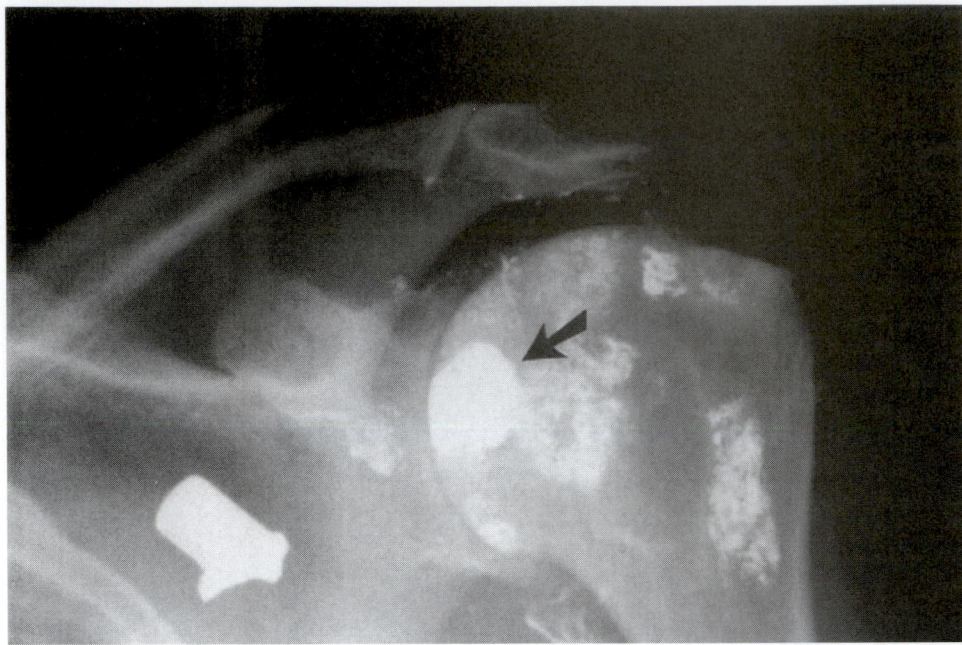

Figure 8–7. A "lead arthrogram" discovered many years after a bullet wound to the shoulder. At the time of the initial injury, the bullet was embedded in the articular surface of the humeral head (*arrow*). The portion of the bullet that protruded into the joint space was surgically removed, leaving a portion of the bullet exposed to the synovial space. A second bullet is embedded in the muscles of the scapula. Eight years after the injury, the patient presented with weakness and anemia. Extensive lead deposition throughout the synovium is seen. Lead level was 91 µg/dL. The patient was treated with dimercaptosuccinic acid (DMSA) chelation and surgical débridement of the synovium. (*Courtesy of the Toxicology Fellowship of the New York City Poison Control Center.*)

VISUALIZING THE EFFECTS OF A TOXIN ON THE BODY

The lungs, central nervous system, gastrointestinal tract, and skeleton are the organ systems most amenable to diagnostic imaging. Disorders of the lungs and skeletal system are seen by plain radiography. For abdominal pathology, contrast studies and computed tomography are usually more effective, although plain radiographs can diagnose intestinal obstruction, perforation, and radiopaque foreign bodies. Imaging of the central nervous system employs computed tomography, magnetic resonance imaging, and nuclear scintigraphy (PET and SPECT).

Skeletal Changes Caused by Toxins and Medications

A number of medications and toxins affect bone mineralization. Toxicologic effects on bone result in either increased or decreased density (Table 8–2). Some toxins produce a characteristic radiographic picture, although the exact diagnosis usually depends on correlation with the clinical scenario.[6,118] Furthermore, alterations in skeletal structure develop gradually and are usually not visible unless the exposure continues for at least 2 weeks.

Lead Poisoning. Skeletal radiography can support the diagnosis of lead poisoning before the blood lead level or erythrocyte protoporphyrin measurement is obtained. With lead poisoning, the metaphyseal regions of rapidly growing long bones develop transverse bands of increased density along the growth plate (Fig. 8–11).[16,132,135,143] Characteristic locations are the distal femur and proximal tibia. Flaring of the distal metaphysis also occurs. Lead lines are also seen in the vertebral bodies and iliac crest. Lead lines usually occur in children 2–9 years of age. Lead lines are detected in approximately 80% of children with a mean lead level of 49 ± 17 µg/dL.[16] It usually takes several weeks for lead lines to appear, although in very young infants (2–4 months old) lead lines can develop within days of exposure.[180] After exposure ceases, lead lines diminish and may eventually disappear. Lead lines are caused by lead's toxic effect on bone growth, and not because of the deposition of lead in bone. Lead impedes resorption of calcified cartilage in the zone of provisional calcification adjacent to the growth plate. This is termed *chondrosclerosis*.[16,34] Other toxins that cause metaphyseal bands are yellow phosphorus, bismuth, and hypervitaminosis D (Chap. 37).

Fluorosis. Fluoride poisoning causes a diffuse increase in bone mineralization. Endemic fluorosis occurs where drinking water contains very high levels of fluoride (at least 2 or more parts per million) or as an occupational exposure for aluminum workers handling cryolite (sodium-aluminum fluoride). The skeletal changes associated with fluorosis are osteosclerosis, osteophytosis, and ligament calcification. Fluorosis primarily affects the axial skeleton, especially the vertebral column and pelvis, as well as the teeth. Thickening of the vertebral column can cause compression of the spinal cord and nerve roots. Without a history of fluoride exposure, the clinical and radiographic findings can be mistaken for osteoblastic skeletal metastasis. The diagnosis of fluorosis is confirmed by histologic examination of the bone and measurement of fluoride levels in the bone and urine.[17,172]

Focal Loss of Bone Density. Skeletal disorders associated with focal diminished bone density (or mixed sclerosis and rarefaction) include osteonecrosis, osteomyelitis, and osteolysis. *Osteonecrosis*, also known as avascular necrosis, most often affects the femoral head, the humeral head, and proximal tibia.[100] There are many causes of osteonecrosis. Toxicologic causes include long-term corticosteroid use and alcoholism. Radiographically, there are focal skeletal lucencies and sclerosis, with loss of bone volume and collapse (Fig. 8–12A).

Acro-osteolysis refers to bone resorption of the distal phalanges and is associated with occupational exposure to vinyl chloride monomer. Protective measures have reduced its incidence since it was first described in the early 1960s.[136]

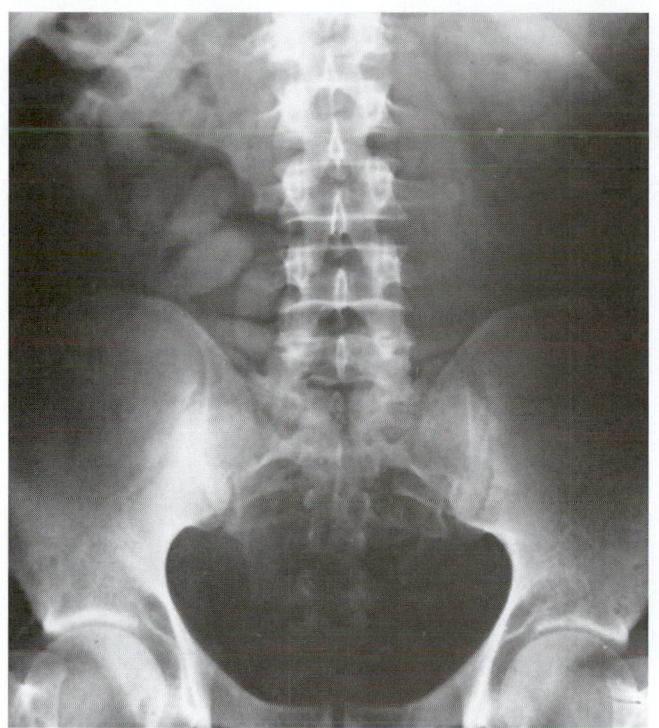

A

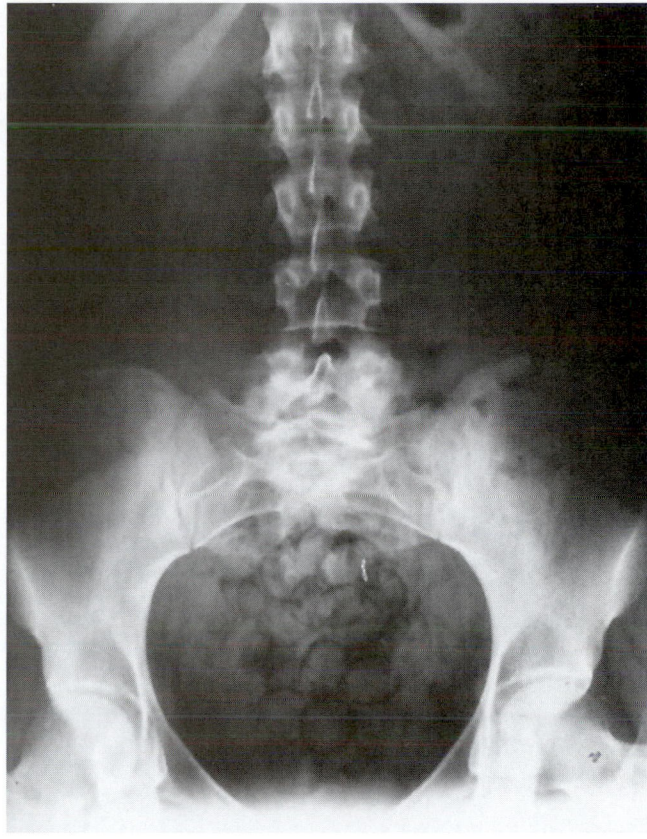

B

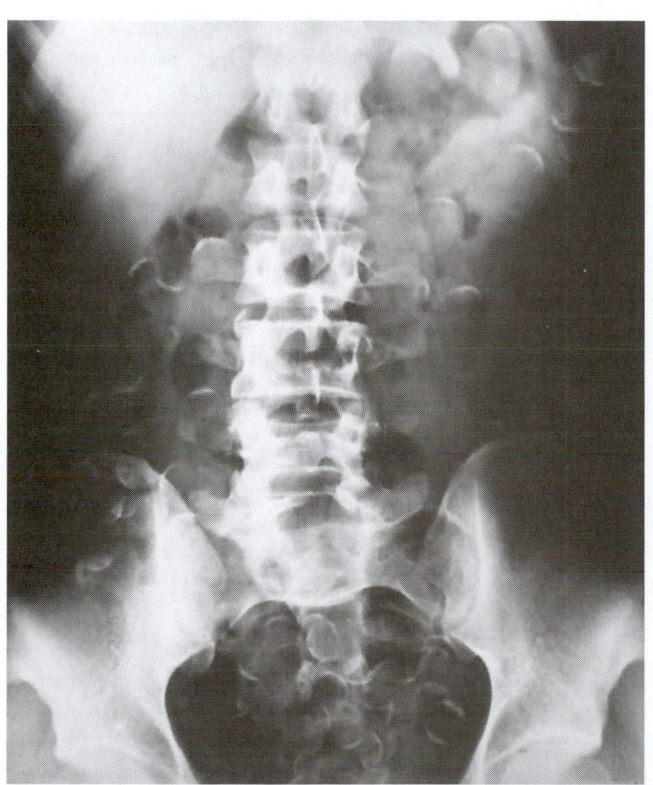

C

Figure 8–8. Radiographs of three "body packers" showing the various appearances of drug packets. Drug smuggling is accomplished by packing the gastrointestinal tract with large numbers of manufactured, well-sealed containers. **A.** Multiple oblong packages of uniform size and shape are seen throughout the bowel. **B.** The packets are visible in this patient because they are surrounded by a thin layer of air within the wall of the packet. **C.** Metallic foil is part of the packet's container wall in this patient. (*Courtesy of Dr. Emil J. Balthazar, Professor of Radiology, New York University.*)

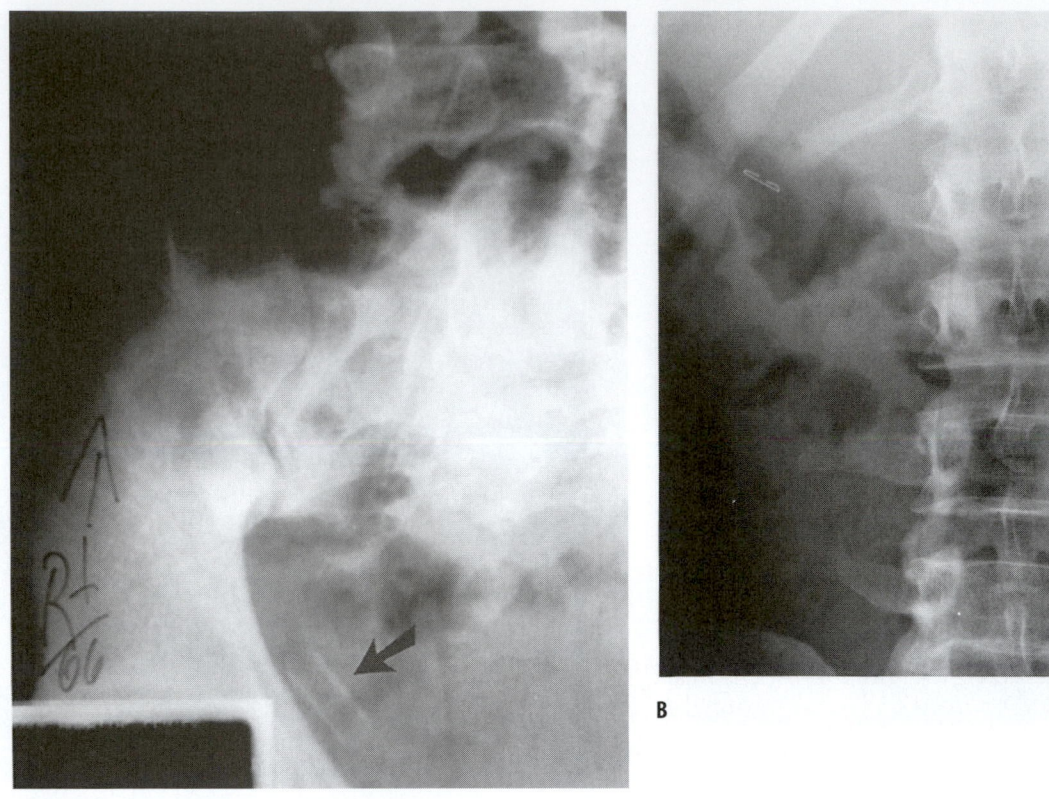

A

B

Figure 8–9. Two "body stuffers." Radiography infrequently helps with the diagnosis. **A.** An ingested glass crack vial is seen in the distal bowel (*arrow*). The patient had ingested his contraband several hours earlier at the time of a police raid. Only the tubular-shaped container, and not the drug, is visible radiographically. The patient did not develop signs of cocaine intoxication during 24 hours of observation. **B.** Another patient in police custody was brought to the ED for allegedly ingesting his drugs. The patient repeatedly denied this. The radiographs revealed "nonsurgical" staples in his abdomen. When questioned again, the patient admitted that he had swallowed several plastic bags that were stapled closed. (See also Fig. 22–1—esophageal obstruction due to a hashish-filled toy balloon.)

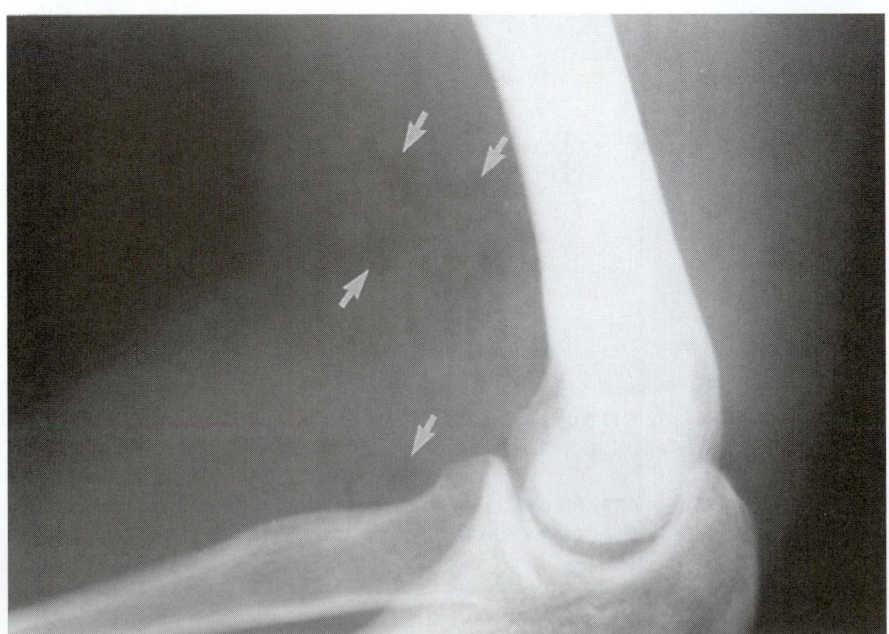

Figure 8–10. Subcutaneous injection of gasoline into the antecubital fossa. The radiolucent hydrocarbon mimics gas in the soft tissues that is seen with a necrotizing soft-tissue infection such as necrotizing fasciitis or gas gangrene (*arrows*). The patient presented with localized redness, warmth, swelling, and fever. Sterile fluid collections without gas or purulence were found during surgical débridement. (*Courtesy of the Toxicology Fellowship of the New York City Poison Control Center.*)

TABLE 8–2. Toxicologic Causes of Skeletal Abnormalities

Toxins Causing Increased Bone Density	Toxins Causing Diminished Bone Density (either diffuse osteoporosis or focal lesions)
Metaphyseal Bands (children) Lead, bismuth, phosphorus: Chondrosclerosis due to toxic effect on bone growth. **Diffuse Increased Bone Density** Fluorosis: Osteosclerosis, osteophytosis, ligament calcification. Usually involves the axial skeleton (vertebrae and pelvis) and can cause compression of the spinal cord and nerve roots. Hypervitaminosis A (pediatric): Cortical hyperostosis and sub-periosteal new bone formation. Diaphyses of long bones have an undulating appearance. Hypervitaminosis D (pediatric): Generalized osteosclerosis, cortical thickening, and meta-physeal bands.	Corticosteroids: Osteoporosis: diffuse. Osteonecrosis: focal lesions, eg, avascular necrosis of the femoral head; loss of volume with both increased and decreased bone density; osteonecrosis also occurs in alcoholism, bismuth arthropathy, Caisson disease (dysbarism), trauma. Hypervitaminosis D (adult): Focal or generalized osteoporosis. Intravenous drug use: Osteomyelitis (focal lytic lesions) due to septic emboli; usually affects vertebral bodies and sternomanubrial joint. Vinyl chloride monomer: Acro-osteolysis (distal phalanges).

Osteomyelitis is a serious complication of intravenous drug use. It usually affects the axial skeleton, especially the vertebral bodies, as well as the sternomanubrial and sternoclavicular joints (Fig. 8–12B). Back pain or neck pain in intravenous drug users warrants careful consideration. A spinal epidural abscess causing spinal cord compression can accompany vertebral osteomyelitis.[72,82,111] Plain films are negative early in the disease course, and the diagnosis is made by MRI (Fig. 8–12C).

Pulmonary and Other Thoracic Complications

Many toxicologic emergencies that affect intrathoracic organs can be detected on chest radiographs.[5,8,46,113] The lungs are most often involved, but the pleura, hilum, heart, and great vessels may also be affected. Chest radiographs should be obtained in patients with chest pain, respiratory distress, dyspnea, rales or rhonchi, and hypoxemia.[2] Patients with chest pain may have a pneumothorax, pneumomediastinum, or aortic dissection. Patients with fever with or without respiratory symptoms may have a focal infiltrate, pleural effusion, or hilar lymphadenopathy.

The chest radiographic findings will suggest certain diseases, although the diagnosis ultimately depends on a thorough clinical history. When a specific toxin exposure is known or suspected, the chest radiograph can confirm the diagnosis and assess its severity. If a history of toxin exposure is not obtained, a patient with an abnormal chest radiograph may initially be misdiagnosed as having pneumonia or another disorder that is more common than toxin-mediated lung disease.[136] Therefore, all patients with chest radiographic abnormalities must be carefully questioned regarding possible toxin exposures at work or at home, as well as about the use of medications or other drugs.

Many pulmonary disorders are radiographically detectable because they result in fluid accumulation within the normally air-filled lung. The fluid accumulates within the alveolar spaces or interstitial tissues of the lung, producing the two major radiographic patterns of pulmonary disease—airspace filling and interstitial lung disease (Table 8–3). Most toxins are widely distributed throughout the lungs and produce a diffuse rather than a focal radiographic abnormality.

Diffuse Airspace Filling. Overdose with various toxins, including salicylates, opioids, and paraquat, causes *acute lung injury,* which is characterized pathologically by leaky capillaries and radiographically by pulmonary edema (Figs. 8–13 and 91–2).[63,68,151,157,178] There are many other causes of acute lung injury, including sepsis, anaphylaxis, and major trauma.[174] Other toxin exposures resulting in diffuse airspace filling include inhalation of irritant gases that are of low water solubility such as phosgene ($COCl_2$), nitrogen dioxide (silo filler disease; Chap. 111), chlorine, and sulfur dioxide (Chaps. 95–98). Organic phosphorus insecticide poisoning causes cholinergic hyperstimulation, resulting in bronchorrhea (Chap. 88). Smoking "crack" cocaine is associated with diffuse intrapulmonary hemorrhage.[44]

Focal Airspace Filling. Most focal infiltrates are caused by bacterial pneumonia, although aspiration also causes localized airspace disease.[160] Aspiration of gastric contents can occur during a sedative drug or alcohol intoxication, or during a seizure. Low-viscosity hydrocarbons often enter the lungs when they are swallowed. This happens in children with unintentional ingestion of household products such as pine oil or kerosene, and in adults who have siphoned gasoline (Figs. 8–14 and 86–2). Because of the delay in development of radiographic abnormalities, the chest radiograph may not be abnormal until 6 hours after the ingestion.[4] During aspiration, the most dependent portions of the lung are affected. When the patient is upright at the time of aspiration, the lower lung segments are involved. When the patient is supine, the posterior segments of the upper and lower lobes are affected.

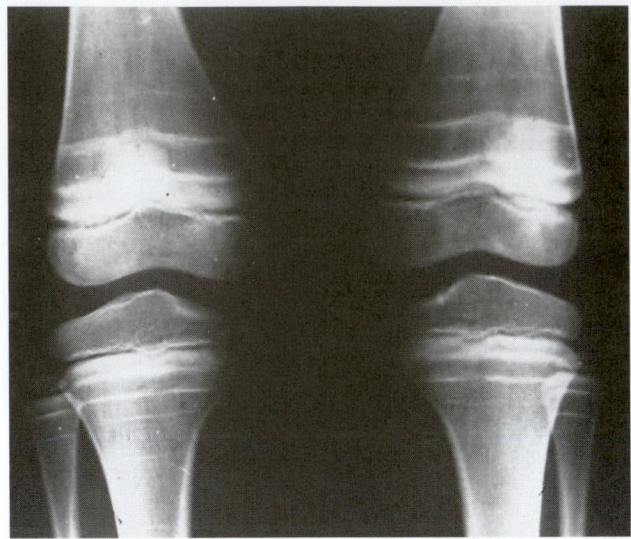

A

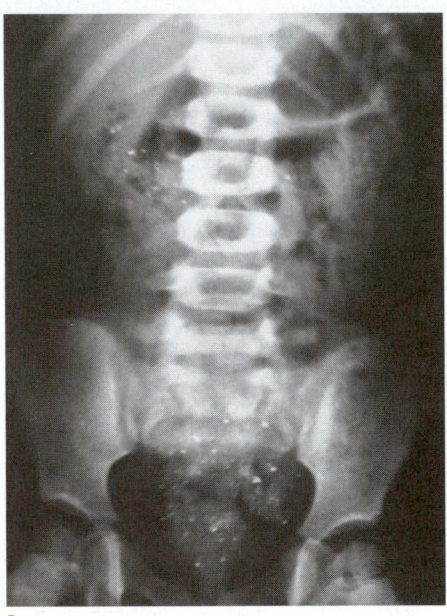

B

Figure 8–11. **A.** A radiograph of the knees of a child with lead poisoning. The metaphyseal regions of the distal femur and proximal tibia have developed transverse bands representing bone growth abnormalities caused by lead toxicity. The multiplicity of lines implies repeated exposures to lead. **B.** The abdominal radiograph of the child shows many radiopaque flakes of ingested leaded paint chips. Lead poisoning also caused abnormally increased cortical mineralization of the vertebral bodies, which gives them a boxlike appearance. (*Courtesy of Dr. Nancy Genieser, Professor of Radiology, New York University.*)

Multifocal Airspace Filling. Multifocal airspace filling occurs with septic pulmonary emboli, a complication of intravenous drug use and right-sided bacterial endocarditis. The foci of pulmonary infection often undergo necrosis and cavitation (Fig. 8–15).

Interstitial Lung Diseases. Toxicologic causes of interstitial lung disease include hypersensitivity pneumonitis, medications

with direct pulmonary toxicity, and inhalation or injection of inorganic particulates. Interstitial lung diseases can have an acute, subacute, or chronic course. On the chest radiograph, acute and subacute disorders cause a fine reticular or reticulonodular pattern (Fig. 8–16). Chronic interstitial disorders cause a coarse reticular "honeycomb" pattern.

Hypersensitivity Pneumonitis. Hypersensitivity pneumonitis is a delayed-type hypersensitivity reaction to an inhaled or ingested allergen.[29,137] Inhaled organic allergens such as those in moldy hay (farmer's lung) and bird droppings (pigeon breeder's lung) cause hypersensitivity pneumonitis in sensitized individuals. There are two clinical syndromes: an acute, recurrent illness and a chronic, progressive disease. The acute illness presents with fever and dyspnea. The chest radiograph is normal or may show fine interstitial or alveolar infiltrates. Chronic hypersensitivity pneumonitis causes progressive dyspnea. The radiograph shows interstitial fibrosis.

The most common medication causing hypersensitivity pneumonitis is nitrofurantoin. Respiratory symptoms occur after taking the medication for 1–2 weeks. Other medications that can cause hypersensitivity pneumonitis include sulfonamides and penicillins.

Chemotherapeutic Agents. Many chemotherapeutic agents, such as busulfan, bleomycin, cyclophosphamide, and methotrexate, cause pulmonary injury by their direct cytotoxic effect on alveolar cells.[30,48] The radiographic pattern is usually interstitial (reticular or nodular), but can include airspace filling or mixed patterns. The patient presents with dyspnea, fever, and pulmonary infiltrates that begins after several weeks of therapy. The clinical and radiographic findings must be distinguished from opportunistic infection, pulmonary carcinomatosis, pulmonary edema, and intraparenchymal hemorrhage. Symptoms usually resolve with discontinuation of the offending medication.

Amiodarone. Amiodarone toxicity causes phospholipid accumulation within alveolar cells. An interstitial radiographic pattern is seen, although airspace filling can also occur (Fig. 8–16).

Particulates. Inhaled inorganic particulates such as asbestos, silica, and coal dust cause *pneumoconiosis*. This is a chronic interstitial lung disease characterized by interstitial fibrosis and loss of lung volume.[110,176] The injection of illicit drugs that have particulate contaminants such as talc causes a chronic interstitial lung disease.[40]

Pleural Disorders. *Asbestos-related calcified pleural plaques* develop many years after asbestos exposure (Fig. 8–17). These lesions do not cause clinical symptoms and have only a minor association with malignancy and interstitial lung disease. Asbestos-related pleural plaques should not be called "asbestosis" because that term refers specifically to the interstitial lung disease caused by asbestos. Pleural plaques must be distinguished from a mesothelioma, which is not calcified, enlarges at a rapid rate, and erodes into nearby structures such as the ribs.

Pleural effusions occur in drug-induced systemic lupus erythematosus.[113] The medications most frequently implicated are procainamide, hydralazine, isoniazid, methyldopa, and chlorpropamide. The patient presents with fever and other symptoms of systemic lupus erythematosus.

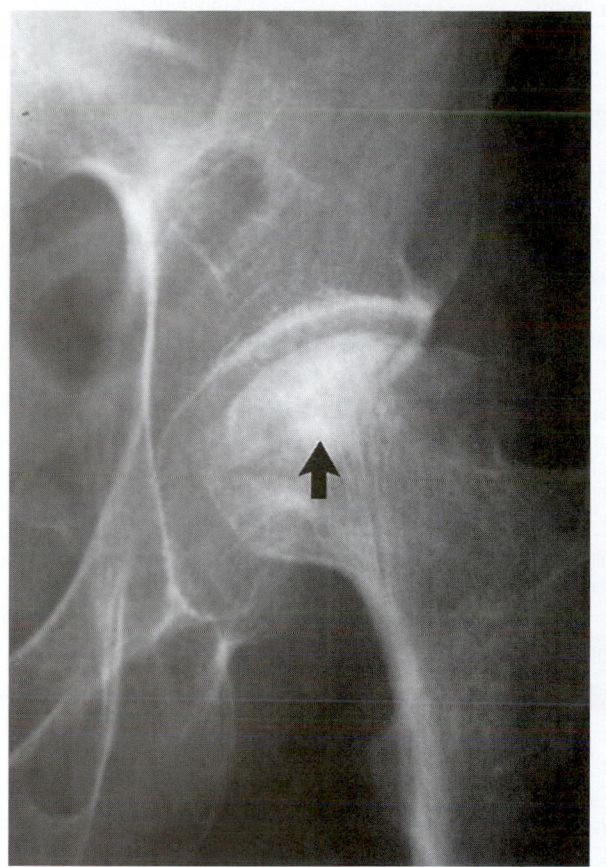

A

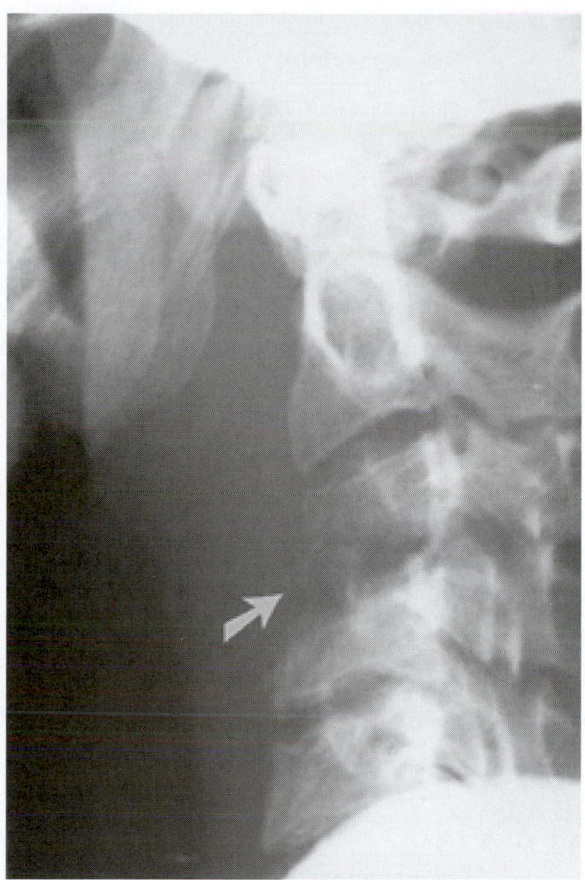

B

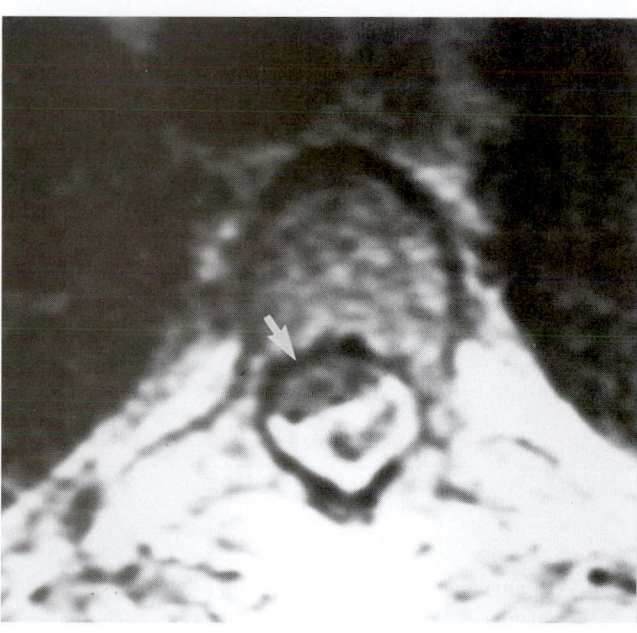

C

Figure 8–12. **A.** Avascular necrosis causing collapse of the femoral head in a patient with long-standing steroid-dependent asthma (*arrow*). **B.** A patient with vertebral body osteomyelitis complicating intravenous drug use. He presented with neck pain, fever, and signs of spinal cord compression that developed over 1–2 weeks. Destruction of the intervertebral disk and endplates of C_3 and C_4 are seen (*arrow*). He underwent surgical decompression, iliac crest bone graft, and stabilization by plates and screws. Operative culture of the bone grew *Staphylococcus aureus.* **C.** An intravenous drug user with thoracic back pain, leg weakness, and low-grade fever. Radiographs of the spine were negative. MRI showing an epidural abscess (*arrow*) compressing the spinal cord. The cerebral spinal fluid in the compressed thecal sac is bright white on this T2-weighted image. (*From Levitan R: Thoracolumbar spine. In: Schwartz DT, Reisdorff EJ, eds: Emergency Radiology. New York, McGraw-Hill, 2000, p. 343, with permission.*)

TABLE 8–3.   Chest Radiographic Findings in Toxicologic Emergencies

Radiographic Finding	Responsible Agents	Disease Processes
Diffuse Airspace Filling	Salicylates Opioids Paraquat Irritant gases (low and intermediate solubility): NO$_2$ (silo filler's disease), phosgene (COCl$_2$), Cl$_2$	Acute lung injury (leaky capillaries)
	Organic phosphorus agents, carbamates	Cholinergic stimulation (bronchorrhea)
	Alcoholic cardiomyopathy, cocaine, adriamycin, cobalt	Congestive heart failure
Focal Airspace Filling	Low-viscosity hydrocarbons Gastric contents aspiration: CNS depressants, alcohol, seizure	Aspiration pneumonitis
Multifocal Airspace Filling	IVDU	Septic emboli
Interstitial Patterns Fine or coarse reticular or reticulo-nodular pattern. Patchy airspace filling is seen in some cases.	Inhaled organic allergens: farmer's lung, pigeon-breeder's lung Nitrofurantoin	Hypersensitivity pneumonitis
	Chemotheraputic agents: busulfan, bleomycin	Cytotoxic lung damage
	Amiodarone	Phospholipidosis
	Talcosis (illicit drug contaminant)	Injected particulates
	Pneumoconiosis: asbestosis, silicosis, coal dust, berylliosis (chronic)	Inhaled inorganic particulates
Pleural Effusion	Procainamide, hydralazine, INH, methyldopa, chlorpropamide	Drug-induced systemic lupus erythematosus
Pneumomediastinum **Pneumothorax**	"Crack" cocaine and marijuana (forceful inhalation), ipecac and alcoholism (forceful vomiting), subclavian vein injection	Barotrauma
Pleural Plaques (calcified)	Asbestos exposure	
Lymphadenopathy	Phenytoin, methotrexate (rare)	Pseudolymphoma
	Silicosis (eggshell calcification), berylliosis	Pneumoconiosis
Cardiomegaly	Ethanol, adriamycin, cocaine (chronic), amphetamine (chronic)	Dilated cardiomyopathy
	Systemic lupus erythematosus (procainamide, hydrazine, INH)	Pericardial effusion
Aortic Enlargement	Cocaine	Aortic dissection

Pneumothorax and *pneumomediastinum* are associated with illicit drug use, and are related to the route of administration rather than to the particular drug. Barotrauma during the smoking of "crack" cocaine or marijuana results in pneumomediastinum (Fig. 8–18A).[35,123] Pneumomediastinum is one cause of cocaine-related chest pain that can be diagnosed by chest radiography. Forceful vomiting after ingestion of syrup of ipecac or alcohol can produce esophageal tears, pneumomediastinum, and mediastinitis.[179] Attempted injection into the subclavian and internal jugular veins is a cause of pneumothorax in intravenous drug users.[33]

Lymphadenopathy.   Phenytoin can cause drug-induced lymphoid hyperplasia with hilar lymphadenopathy.[113] The patient presents with a febrile illness, usually without respiratory symptoms. Chronic beryllium exposure results in hilar lymphadenopathy that mimics sarcoidosis, and granulomatous changes in the lung parenchyma. Silicosis is associated with "eggshell" calcification of hilar lymph nodes.

Cardiovascular Abnormalities.   *Dilated cardiomyopathy* occurs in chronic alcoholism and exposure to cardiotoxic medications

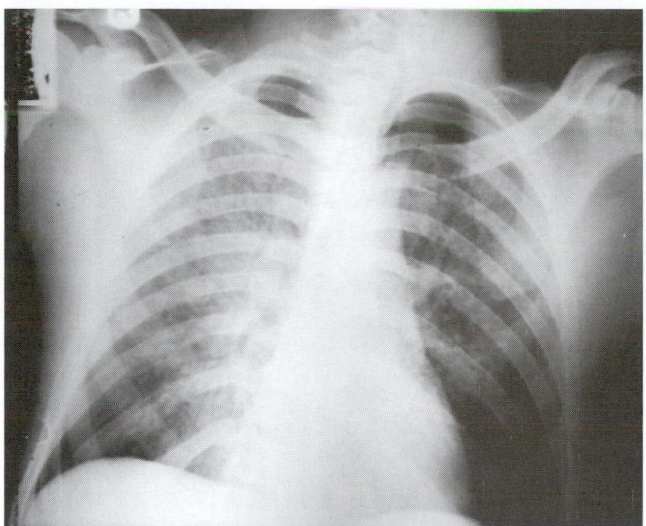

Figure 8–13. Diffuse airspace filling. The chest radiograph of a patient who had recently injected heroin intravenously presented with respiratory distress and pulmonary edema. The heart size is normal. Rapid resolution with clearing of the radiograph in 2 days is typical of heroin-induced acute lung injury. A salicylate overdose can produce a similar radiographic picture.

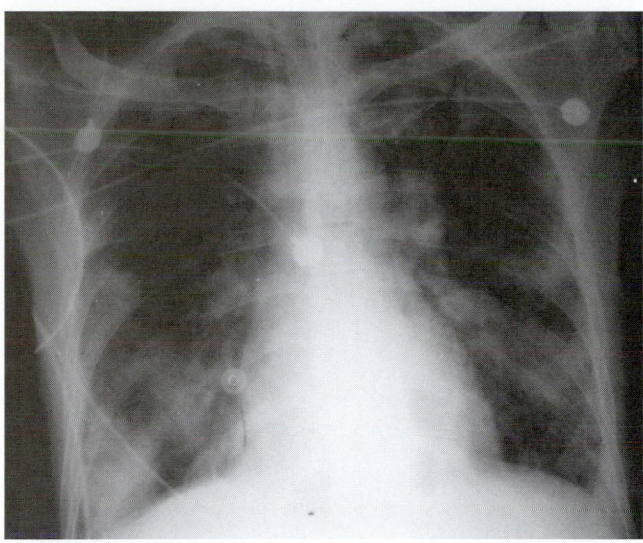

Figure 8–15. Multifocal airspace filling. The chest radiograph in an injection drug user who presented with high fever but without pulmonary symptoms. There are multiple ill-defined pulmonary opacities throughout both lungs, which are characteristic of septic pulmonary emboli. His blood cultures grew *Staphylococcus aureus*.

such as adriamycin. Enlargement of the cardiac silhouette can also be caused by a pericardial effusion, which can accompany a drug-induced systemic lupus erythematosus. *Aortic dissection* is associated with use of cocaine and is a serious cause of cocaine-related chest pain.[49,125,134] The chest radiograph may show an enlarged or indistinct aortic knob or ascending or descending aorta (Fig. 8–18B).

Abdominal Complications

Abdominal imaging modalities include conventional radiography, CT, GI contrast studies, and angiography.[51] Conventional radiography is limited in its capability to detect most intra-abdominal pathology because most pathologic processes involve soft-tissue structures that are not well seen by plain radiographs. However, plain radiography readily visualizes gas in the abdomen and is therefore able to diagnose pneumoperitoneum (free intraperitoneal air) and bowel distension caused by mechanical obstruction or diminished gut motility (adynamic ileus). Other abnormal gas collections, such as intramural gas associated with intestinal infarction, are seen infrequently. Abdominal radiography is also used to identify radiopaque foreign bodies such as ingested iron pills and heavy-metal compounds (Table 8–4).[56,95,101,109,153]

Pneumoperitoneum. Gastrointestinal perforation is diagnosed by seeing free intraperitoneal air under the diaphragm on an upright chest radiograph. Peptic ulcer perforation is associated with crack cocaine use.[23,83] Esophageal or gastric perforation can be a complication of large-bore orogastric tube placement and forceful emesis induced by syrup of ipecac or alcohol intoxication (Fig. 8–19).[179] Esophageal and gastric perforation can also occur following the ingestion of erosive and caustic substances such as iron, alkali, or acid (Figs. 87–1 and 87–2). Esophageal perforation causes pneumomediastinum and mediastinitis.

Obstruction and Ileus. Both mechanical bowel obstruction and adynamic ileus cause bowel distension. With mechanical obstruction, there is a greater amount of intestinal distension proximal to the point of obstruction and a relative paucity of gas and intestinal collapse distal to the point of obstruction. In adynamic ileus, the bowel distension is relatively uniform throughout the entire intestinal tract. On the upright abdominal radiograph, both mechani-

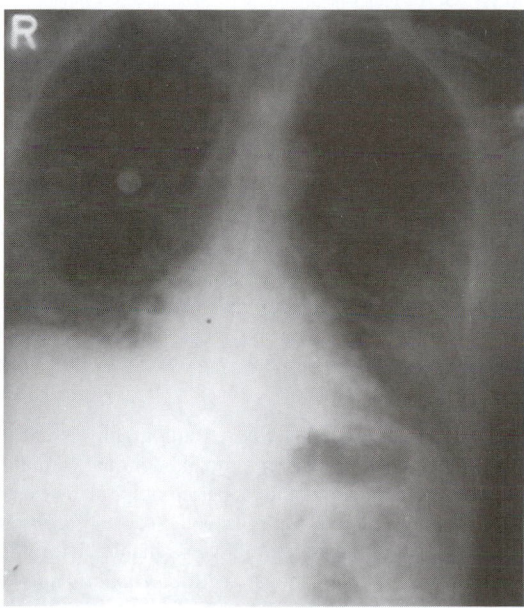

Figure 8–14. Focal airspace filling due to hydrocarbon aspiration. A 34-year-old male aspirated gasoline. The chest radiograph shows bilateral lower lobe infiltrates.

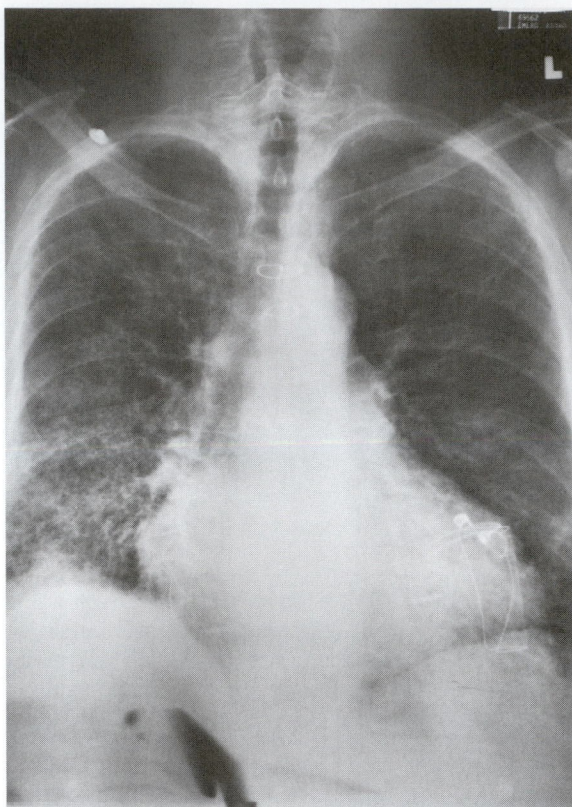

Figure 8–16. Reticular interstitial pattern. The chest radiograph of a patient with cardiac disease who presented to the ED with progressive dyspnea. The initial diagnostic impression was interstitial pulmonary edema. The patient was on amiodarone for malignant ventricular dysrhythmias (note the implanted automatic defibrillator). The lack of response to diuretics and the high-resolution CT pattern suggested that this was toxicity to amiodarone. The medication was stopped and there was partial clearing over several weeks. (*Courtesy of Dr. Georgeann McGuinness, Department of Radiology, New York University.*)

cal obstruction and adynamic ileus show air-fluid levels. In mechanical obstruction, air-fluid levels are seen at different heights and produce a "step-ladder" appearance.

Mechanical bowel obstruction can be caused by large intraluminal foreign bodies such as a body packer's packets or a medication bezoar.[47,162] Adynamic ileus can complicate ingestions of opioids, anticholinergics, and tricyclic antidepressants (Fig. 8–20).[12,51] Because adynamic ileus is seen in many diseases, the radiographic finding of an ileus is not helpful diagnostically. In some cases, adynamic ileus is difficult to distinguish radiographically from a mechanical obstruction. Abdominal CT can clarify the diagnosis.[108]

Mesenteric Ischemia. In most patients with intestinal ischemia, plain abdominal radiographs show only a nonspecific or adynamic ileus pattern. In a small proportion of patients with ischemic bowel (5%), intramural gas is seen.[12] Rarely, gas is also seen in the hepatic portal venous system. CT is better able to detect signs of mesenteric ischemia (Case Studies, Fig. 1–9).[11]

Intestinal ischemia and infarction are caused by cocaine or ergot alkaloids, which induce mesenteric vasoconstriction.[86,103]

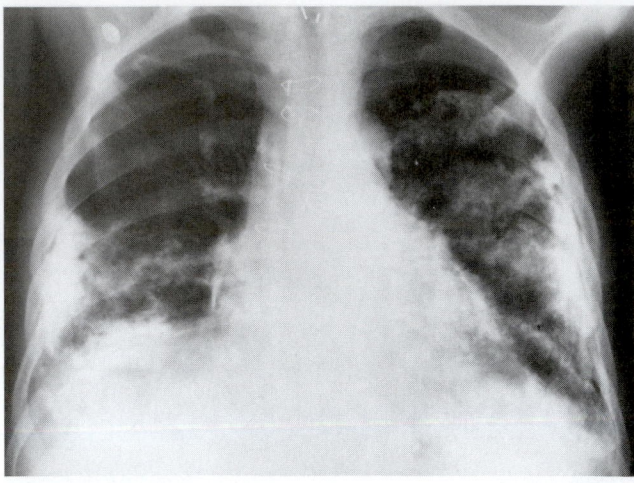

A

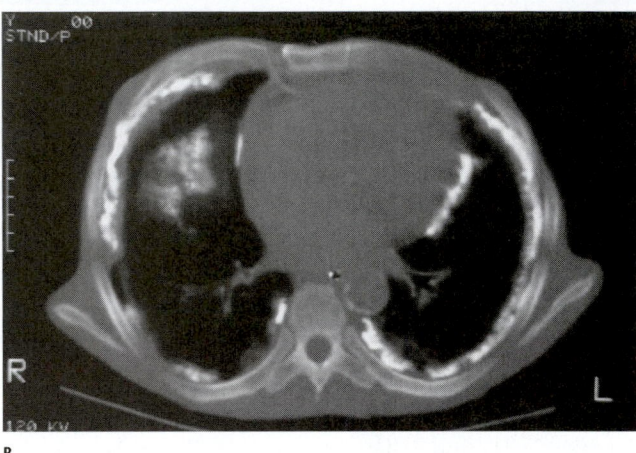

B

Figure 8–17. **A.** Calcified plaques typical of asbestos exposure are seen on the pleural surfaces of the lungs, diaphragm, and heart. The patient was asymptomatic; this was an incidental radiographic finding. **B.** The CT scan demonstrates that the opacities seen on the chest radiograph do not involve the lung itself. A lower thoracic image shows calcified pleural plaques (the diaphragmatic plaque is seen on the right). The CT confirms that there is no interstitial lung disease ("asbestosis").

Calcium channel blocker overdoses cause splanchnic vasodilatation and hypotension resulting in intestinal infarction.[175] Superior mesenteric vein thrombosis can be caused by hypercoagulability associated with oral contraceptives.

GI Hemorrhage and Hepatotoxicity. Radiography is not usually helpful in the diagnosis of such common abdominal complications as gastrointestinal bleeding and hepatotoxicity. However, radiographs can reveal ingested iron pills as the cause of gastrointestinal bleeding in a child too young to give a reliable history.

The now obsolete radiocontrast agent *thorium dioxide* (Thorotrast; thorium, atomic number 90) provides a unique example of pharmaceutic-induced hepatotoxicity. It was used as an angiographic contrast agent until 1947, when it was found to cause hepatic malignancies. The radioactive isotope of thorium has a half-life of 400 years. It accumulates within the reticuloendothelial

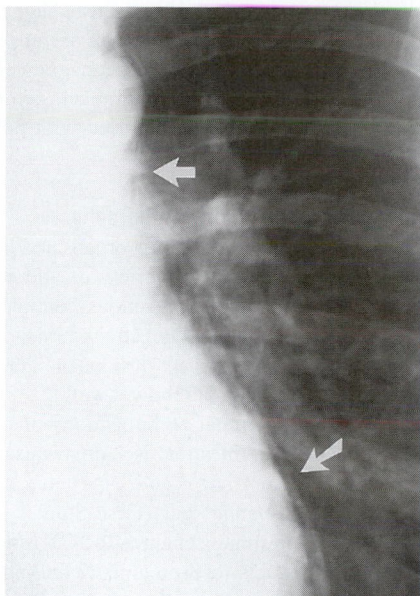

A

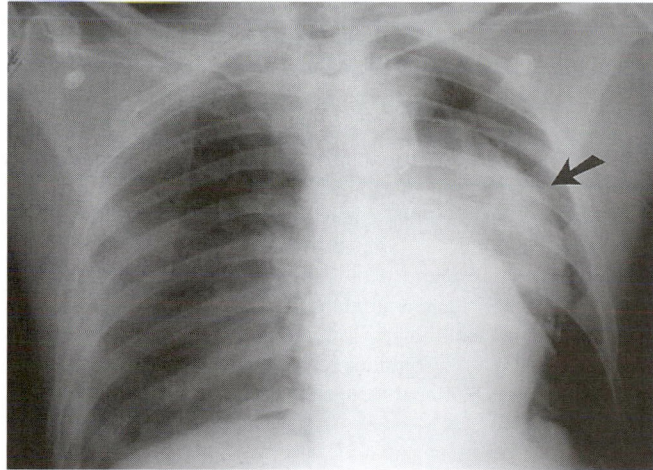

B

Figure 8–18. Two patients with chest pain following cocaine use. **A.** Pneumomediastinum after forceful inhalation while smoking "crack" cocaine. A fine white line representing the pleura elevated from the mediastinal structures is seen (*arrows*). The patient's chest pain resolved during a 24-hour period of observation. **B.** Thoracic aortic dissection and rupture following cocaine use. The patient presented with chest pain radiating to the back. Chest radiography reveals a wide and indistinct aortic contour (*arrow*). Hypotension and cardiac arrest occurred soon after arrival to the Emergency Department. (*Courtesy of the Toxicology Fellowship of the New York City Poison Control Center.*)

TABLE 8–4. **Plain Abdominal Radiography in Toxicologic Emergencies**

Radiographic Finding	Toxin or Drug
Pneumoperitoneum (hollow viscus perforation)	Caustics: iron, alkali, acids Cocaine GI decontamination (ipecac, lavage tube)
Mechanical obstruction (intraluminal foreign body) Intestinal Gastric outlet } Upper GI Esophageal } series	Foreign-body ingestion: body packer, enteric-coated pills (bezoar)
Ileus (diminished gut motility)	Opioids Anticholinergics Tricyclic antidepressants Mesenteric ischemia caused by cocaine, oral contraceptives Toxin-induced hypokalemia, hypomagnesemia
Intramural gas (intestinal infarction) Bowel wall thickening Hepatic portal venous gas (CT is more sensitive)	Cocaine Ergot alkaloids Oral contraceptives Calcium channel blockers Agents causing systemic hypotension
Foreign-body ingestion	Iron pills Heavy metals (Hg, Pb, Tl, As) Body packers and stuffers Bismuth subsalicylate Calcium carbonate Enteric-coated and sustained-release tablets Pica (calcareous clay)

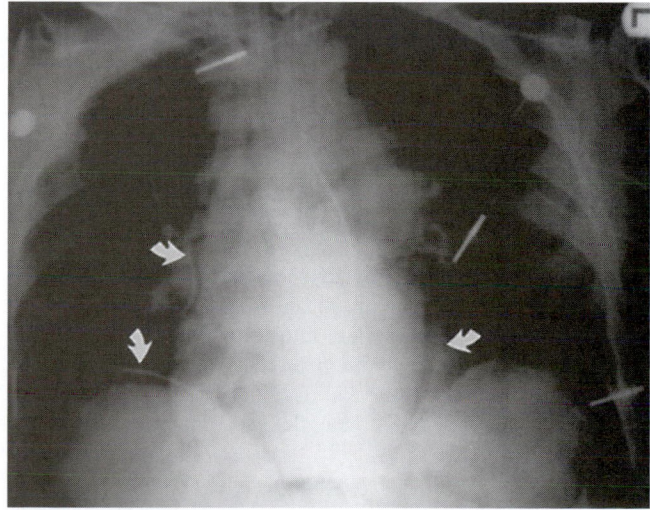

Figure 8–19. GI perforation following gastric lavage with a large-bore orogastric tube. The upright chest radiograph shows air under the right hemidiaphragm and pneumomediastinum (*arrows*). An esophagram with water-soluble contrast did not demonstrate the perforation. Laparotomy revealed perforation of the anterior wall of the stomach.

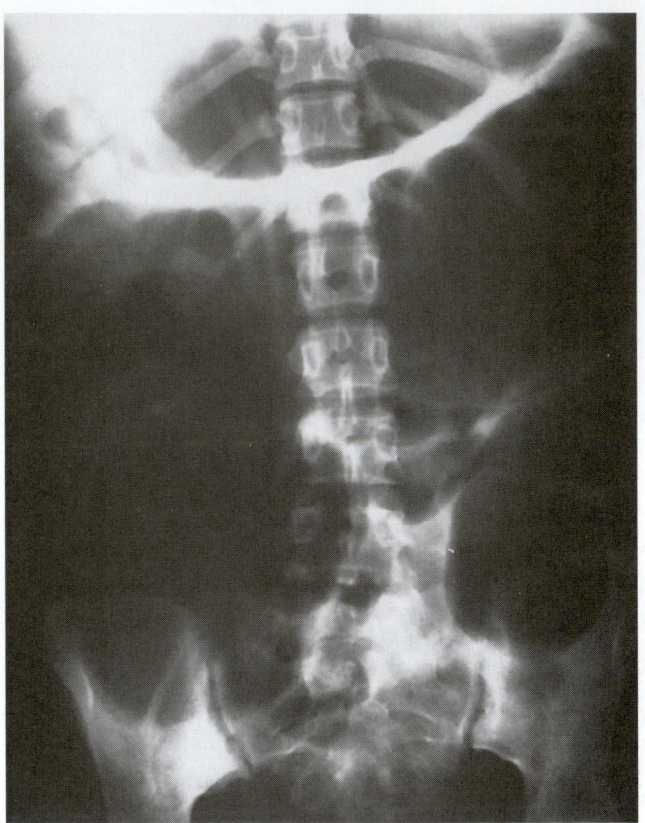

Figure 8–20. Methadone maintenance therapy causing marked abdominal distension. The radiograph reveals striking large bowel dilatation, termed colonic ileus, caused by chronic opioid use. A similar radiographic picture is seen with anticholinergic medications and distal large bowel obstruction due to a tumor, fecal impaction, or volvulus. A contrast enema can clarify the diagnosis. (*Courtesy of Dr. Emil J. Balthazar, Professor of Radiology, New York University.*)

system and remains there for the life of the patient. It has a characteristic radiographic appearance with multiple punctate densities in the liver, spleen, and lymph nodes (Fig. 8–21). These patients are at risk for hepatic malignancies and pneumococcal sepsis.[14,166]

Contrast Esophagram and Upper GI Series. Ingestion of a caustic substance can cause severe damage to the mucosal lining of the esophagus. This can be demonstrated by a contrast esophagram. However, in the acute setting, upper endoscopy should be performed because it provides more information about the extent of injury and prognosis.[87] In addition, administration of oral contrast will coat the mucosa, making endoscopy difficult. For later evaluation, a contrast esophagram identifies mucosal defects, scarring, and stricture formation (Figs. 8–22 and 87–3).[102]

The choice of radiographic contrast agent (barium or water-soluble material) depends on the clinical situation. If the esophagus is severely strictured and there is risk of aspiration, barium should be used because water-soluble contrast material is damaging to the pulmonary parenchyma. If, on the other hand, esophageal or gastric perforation is suspected, water-soluble contrast is safer because extravasated barium is highly irritating to mediastinal and peritoneal tissues.

Ingested objects can cause esophageal and gastric outlet obstruction. Esophageal obstruction because of a drug packet can be demonstrated by a contrast esophagram (Fig. 22–1). Concretions of ingested material in the stomach can cause gastric outlet obstruction. This has been reported with potassium chloride tablets and enteric-coated aspirin.[7,152]

Abdominal Computed Tomography. CT provides great anatomic definition of intra-abdominal organs and plays an important role in the diagnosis of a wide variety of abdominal disorders. In most cases, both oral and intravenous contrast are administered. Oral contrast delineates the intestinal lumen. Intravenous contrast is needed to reliably detect lesions in hepatic and splenic parenchyma, the kidneys, and bowel wall.

Certain abdominal complications of poisonings are amenable to CT diagnosis. Intestinal ischemia causes bowel wall thickening, intramural hemorrhage, and, at a later stage, intramural gas and hepatic portal venous gas (Case Studies Fig. 1–9).[11] In some patients with intestinal ischemia, the CT is nondiagnostic, and the diagnosis ultimately rests on clinical findings. Splenic infarction and splenic and psoas abscesses are complications of intravenous drug that can be diagnosed on CT.[12] Radiopaque foreign substances can be detected and accurately localized by CT such as intravenously injected elemental mercury.[99] Radiolucent foreign bodies, such as a body packer's packets, can be detected by using enteric contrast.[61,64] However, in one case, a retained packet was missed by CT and detected on an upper GI oral contrast study.[58]

Vascular Lesions. Angiography can detect such complications of injection drug use as venous thrombosis and arterial laceration causing pseudoaneurysm formation (Figs. 109–3 and 109–4). Intravenous injection of amphetamine, cocaine, or ergotamine causes necrotizing angiitis that is associated with microaneurysms, segmental stenosis, and arterial thrombosis. These lesions are seen in the kidneys, small bowel, liver, pancreas, and cerebral circulation (Fig. 8–23).[25,133] Complications include aneurysm rupture and visceral infarction. Renal lesions cause severe hypertension and renal failure.

Neurologic Complications

Imaging studies have revolutionized the diagnosis of central nervous system (CNS) disorders.[55] Both acute focal brain lesions and chronic degenerative changes can be detected (Table 8–5). A wide variety of toxins cause CNS dysfunction.[93] Some have a direct toxic effect on the CNS. In other instances, neurologic injury is an indirect sequela of toxin exposure due to hypoxia, hypotension, hypertension, cerebral vasoconstriction, head trauma, or infection.

Imaging Modalities. *Computed tomography* can directly visualize brain tissue and many intracranial lesions.[53] CT is the imaging study of choice in the emergency setting because it readily detects acute intracranial hemorrhage as well as parenchymal lesions that are causing mass effect. Infusion of intravenous contrast further delineates intracerebral mass lesions such as tumors and abscesses. CT is fast, widely available on an emergency basis, and can accommodate critical support and monitoring devices.

Magnetic resonance imaging has supplanted CT in nearly all areas of nonemergency neurodiagnosis. It offers greater anatomic discrimination of brain tissues and of areas of cerebral edema and demyelinization. However, in the emergency setting, the disad-

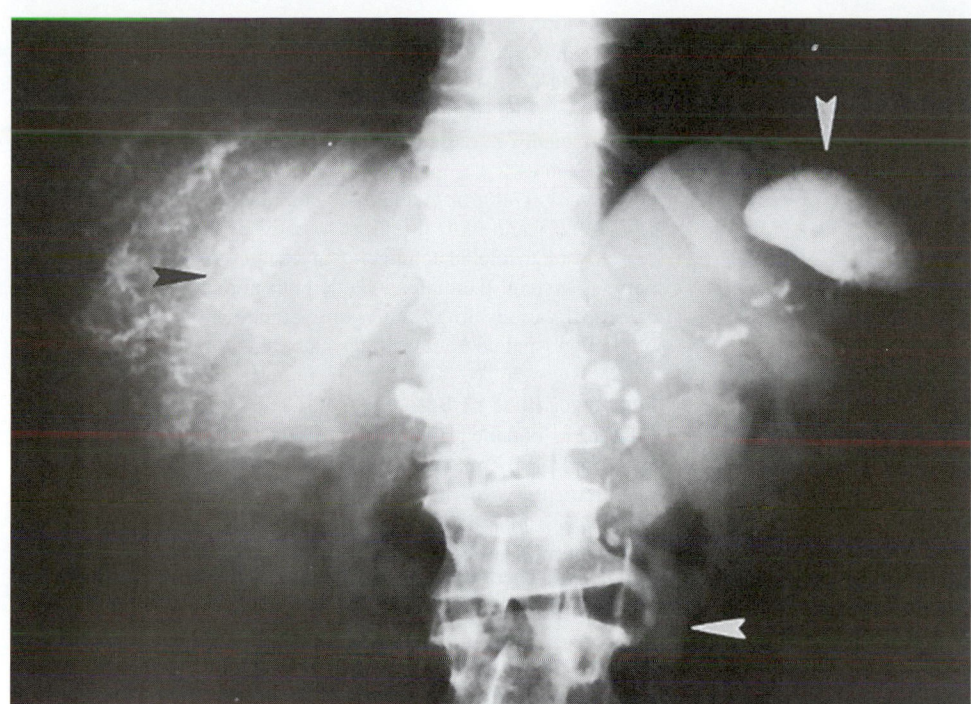

Figure 8–21. The abdominal radiograph of a patient who had received thorium dioxide (Thorotrast) for a radiocontrast study many years previously. The spleen (*vertical white arrow*), liver (*horizontal black arrow*), and lymph nodes (*horizontal white arrow*) are demarcated by thorium retained in the reticuloendothelial system. (*Courtesy of Dr. Emil J. Balthazar, Professor of Radiology, New York University.*)

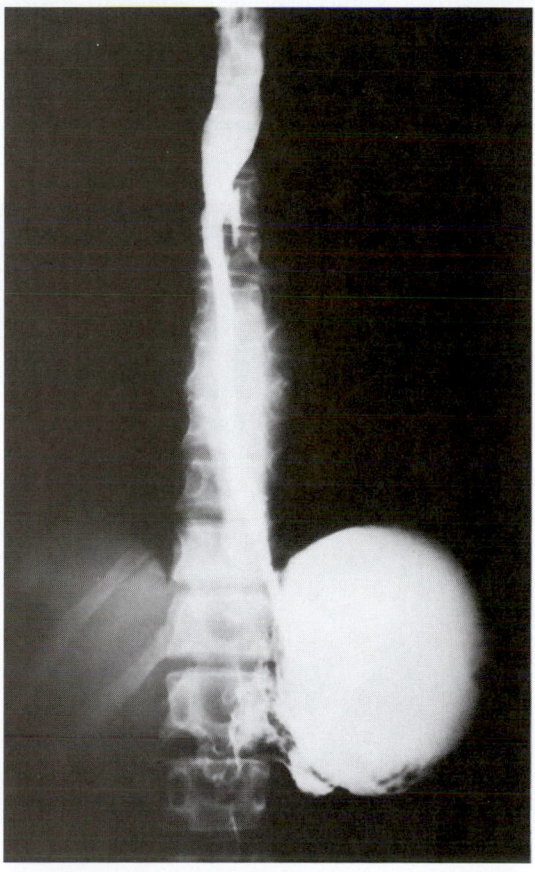

A

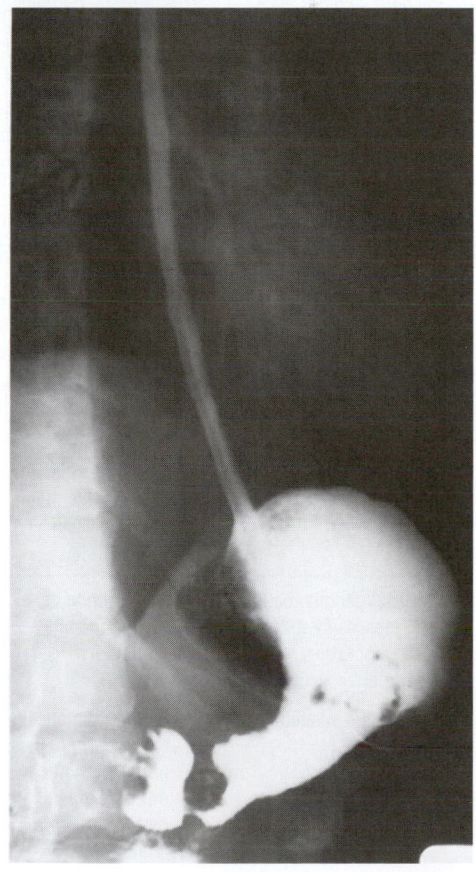

B

Figure 8–22.   A. A barium swallow performed several days after ingestion of liquid lye shows intramural dissection and extravasation of barium with early stricture formation. **B.** At 3 weeks postingestion, there is an absence of peristalsis, diffuse narrowing of the esophagus, and reduction in size of the fundus and antrum of the stomach as a result of scarring. (*Courtesy of Dr. Emil J. Balthazar, Professor of Radiology, New York University.*)

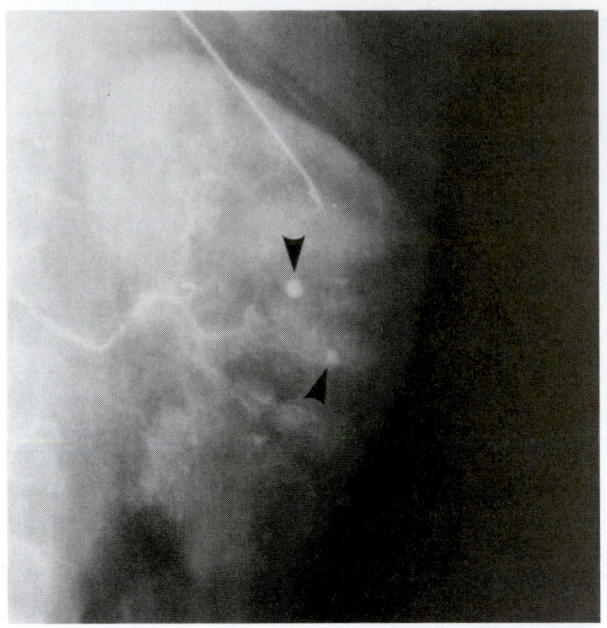

Figure 8–23. A selective renal angiogram in an intravenous methamphetamine user demonstrating multiple small and large aneurysms (*arrow*). (*Courtesy of Dr. Richard Lefleur, Associate Professor of Radiology, New York University.*)

vantages of MRI outweigh its strengths. MRI is no better than CT in detecting acute blood collections. Furthermore, MRI is usually not readily available on an emergency basis, image acquisition time is long, and supportive and monitoring devices that are essential for acutely ill patients are often incompatible with MR scanning machines.[96]

Nuclear scintigraphy that uses computed tomography technology (SPECT and PET, discussed later) is being employed as a research tool to elucidate functional characteristics of the central nervous system. Examples include both immediate and long-term effects of various drugs and toxins on regional brain metabolism, blood flow, and neurotransmitter function.[90,127]

Emergency Head CT Scanning. An emergency noncontrast head CT scan is obtained primarily to detect acute intracranial hemorrhage and focal brain lesions causing cerebral edema and mass effect. Patients with these lesions present with focal neurologic deficits, seizures, headache, or altered mental status. Toxicologic causes of intraparenchymal and subarachnoid hemorrhage include cocaine or other sympathomimetic drugs (Fig. 8–24).[89,92] Cocaine-induced vasospasm can cause acute ischemic infarction, although this is not seen by CT until 6–24 or more hours after onset of the neurologic deficit. Drug-induced CNS depression, most commonly ethanol intoxication, predisposes the patient to head trauma, which can result in a subdural hematoma or cerebral contusion (Fig. 8–25). Toxicologic causes of intracerebral mass lesions include septic emboli complicating intravenous drug use and HIV-associated CNS toxoplasmosis and lymphoma (Fig. 8–26).[15,122] On a contrast CT, such tumors and focal infections exhibit a pattern of "ring enhancement."

TABLE 8–5. **Head CT (Noncontrast) in Toxicologic Emergencies**

CT Finding	Brain Lesion	Toxicologic Etiology
Hemorrhage	Intraparenchymal hemorrhage Subarachnoid hemorrhage	Sympathomimetics: cocaine ("crack"), amphetamine, phenylpropanolamine, phencyclidine, ephedrine, pseudoephedrine Mycotic aneurysm rupture (IVDU)
	Subdural hematoma	Trauma secondary to alcohol, sedative-hypnotics, seizure. Anticoagulants
Brain lucencies	Basal ganglia focal necrosis (also subcortical white matter lucencies)	Carbon monoxide, cyanide, hydrogen sulfide, methanol
	Stroke—vasoconstriction	Sympathomimetics: cocaine ("crack"), amphetamine, phenylpropanolamine, phencyclidine, ephedrine, pseudoephedrine, ergotamine
	Mass lesion—tumor, abscess	Septic emboli, AIDS-related CNS toxoplasmosis or lymphoma
Loss of brain tissue	Atrophy—cerebral, cerebellar	Alcoholism, toluene

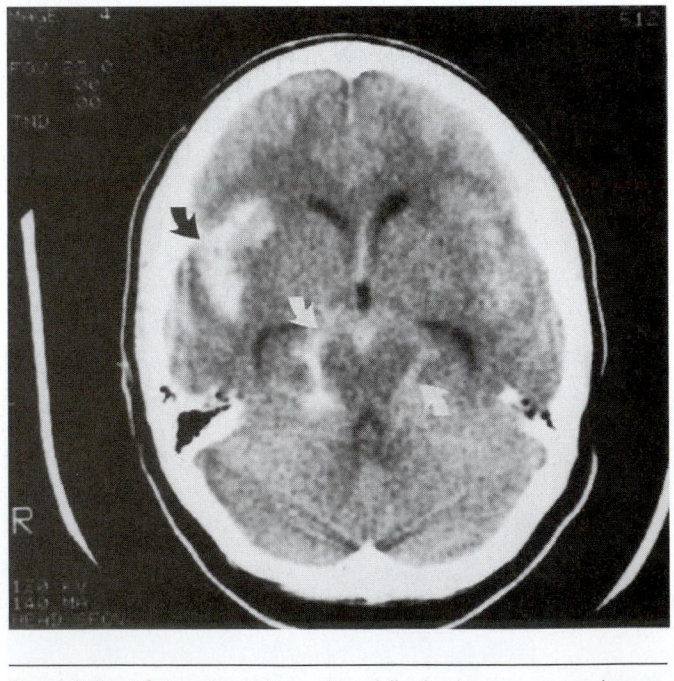

Figure 8–24. Subarachnoid hemorrhage following intravenous cocaine use. The patient had sudden severe headache followed by a generalized seizure. Extensive hemorrhage is seen surrounding the midbrain (*white arrows*) and in the right sylvian fissure (*black arrow*). Angiography revealed an aneurysm at the origin of the right middle cerebral artery. Rupture of the aneurysm was provoked by the acute elevation of blood pressure following cocaine use.

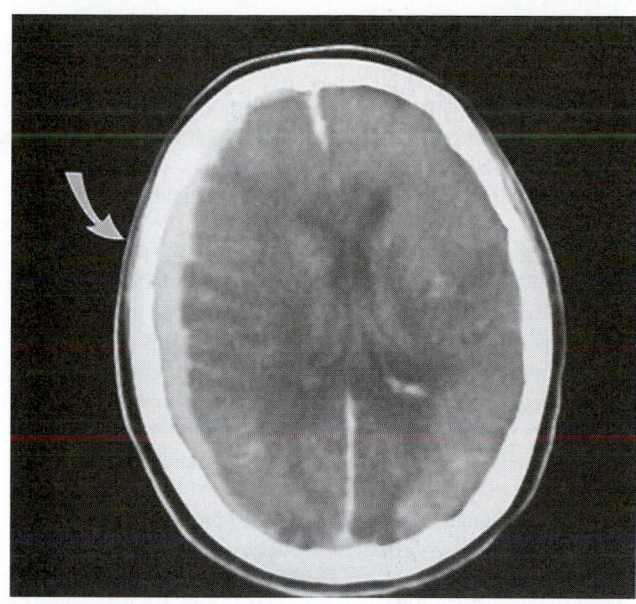

Figure 8–25. An acute subdural hematoma in an alcoholic patient following an alcohol binge. Although there were no external signs of head trauma, the patient's mental status did not improve during several hours of observation. A crescent-shaped blood collection is seen between the right cerebral convexity and the inner table of the skull (*arrow*).

Toxin-Mediated Neurodegenerative Disorders. A number of toxins directly damage brain tissue, which produces morphologic changes that are detectable with CT and MRI. Such changes include generalized atrophy, focal areas of neuronal loss, demyelinization, and cerebral edema. Imaging abnormalities can help establish a diagnosis or predict prognosis in a patient with neurologic dysfunction following a toxin exposure. In some cases, the imaging abnormality will suggest a toxicologic diagnosis in a patient with a neurologic disorder in whom a toxin exposure was not suspected clinically.[9,78,128]

Atrophy. Ethanol is the most widely used neurotoxin. With long-term ethanol use, there is a widespread loss of neurons with resultant atrophy. In some alcoholics, the loss of brain tissue is especially prominent in the cerebellum. However, the amount of cerebral or cerebellar atrophy does not always correlate with the extent of cognitive impairment or gait disturbance.[50,62,65,81,171,173] Chronic toluene exposure (occupational and illicit use) also causes diffuse cerebral atrophy.[73,141]

Focal Degenerative Lesions. Carbon monoxide poisoning produces focal degenerative lesions in the brain. In about half of patients with severe neurologic dysfunction following carbon monoxide poisoning, CT scans show bilateral symmetric lucencies in the basal ganglia, particularly the globus pallidus (Figs. 8–27 and 97–1).[22,74,78,114,130,131,145,146,149,164,169] Neuronal injury by carbon monoxide is a result of hypoxia, acidosis, hypoperfusion, and

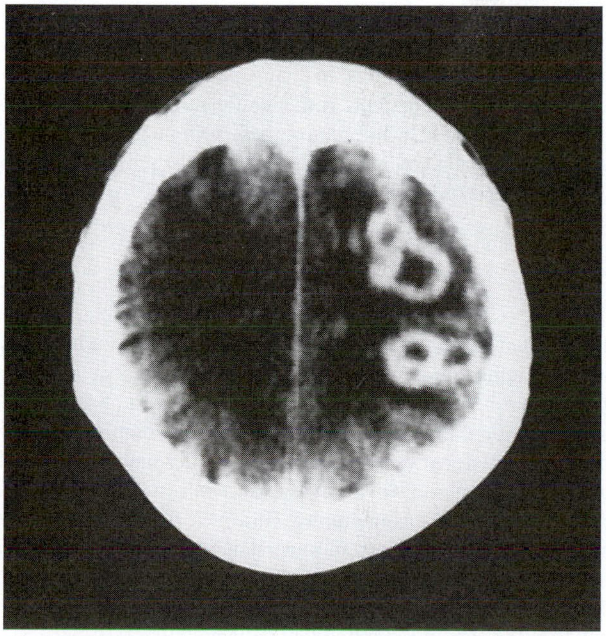

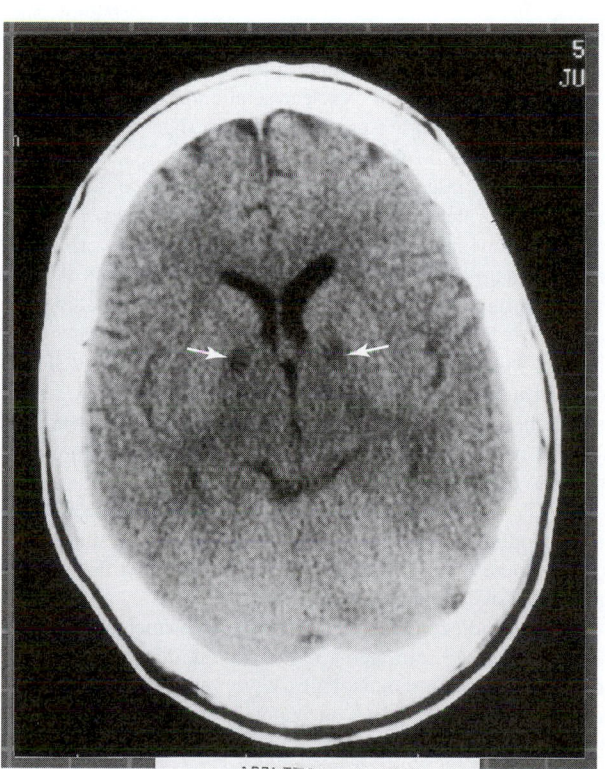

Figure 8–26. An intravenous drug user with ring-enhancing intracerebral lesions. The patient presented with fever and altered mental status. In this patient, the lesions represent multiple septic emboli complicating acute *Staphylococcus aureus* bacterial endocarditis. A similar ring-enhancing appearance is seen with lesions caused by toxoplasmosis or primary CNS lymphoma in patients with AIDS. This patient was HIV negative.

Figure 8–27. A head CT of a patient with mental status changes following carbon monoxide poisoning. The scan shows characteristic bilateral symmetrical lucencies of the globus pallidus (*arrows*). (*Courtesy Dr. Paul Blackburn, Maricopa Medical Center, Arizona.*)

binding of carbon monoxide to cytochrome oxidase. Ischemia and demyelinization produce lesions that may be reversible, whereas irreversible lesions are caused by necrosis. The basal ganglia are especially sensitive to hypoxic damage because of their limited blood supply and high metabolic requirements. Subcortical white matter lesions also occur following carbon monoxide poisoning. Although less frequent than lesions of the basal ganglia, white matter lesions are more clearly associated with poor neurologic outcome. Some patients with basal ganglion lesions and no white matter lesions experience significant clinical recovery. In general, patients with carbon monoxide poisoning who have normal CT scans have a better prognosis than patients with imaging abnormalities. MRI is more sensitive than CT at detecting these CNS lesions, especially at detecting white matter abnormalities.[22,131,164]

Occasionally, symmetric globus pallidus lesions are found on the CT scan of a patient with altered mental status in whom carbon monoxide poisoning was not suspected.[128] In one reported case, an elderly patient suspected of having had a stroke had actually been poisoned by his newly installed wood-burning stove. The CT scan showed bilateral basal ganglion lesions that led to the diagnosis of carbon monoxide poisoning.[78]

Basal ganglion lucencies, white matter lesions, and atrophy are caused by other toxins such as methanol (putamenal lesions),[8,52,60,115,139,142] ethylene glycol, cyanide,[42,112] hydrogen sulfide, inorganic and organic mercury,[104] manganese,[9] heroin,[84] barbiturates, solvents such as toluene,[73,141] and podophyllin.[21,117] Nontoxicologic disorders can also cause similar imaging abnormalities including hypoxia, hypoglycemia, and infectious encephalitis.[60,67]

Functional Brain Imaging. Both CT and MRI display cerebral anatomy, whereas nuclear medicine studies provide functional information about the brain. Nuclear scintigraphy uses radioactive isotopes that are bound to carrier molecules (ligands). The choice of ligand depends on the biologic function being studied. Brain cells take up the radiolabeled ligand in proportion to their physiologic activity or the regional blood flow. The radioactive emission from the isotope is detected by a scintigraphic camera, which produces an image showing the quantity and distribution of tracer. Better anatomic detail is provided by using computed tomography techniques to generate cross-sectional images. There are two technologies: *single photon emission computed tomography* (SPECT) and *positron emission tomography* (PET). These imaging modalities have been used in the research setting to study the neurologic effects of particular toxins and the mechanisms of toxin-induced neurologic dysfunction.

SPECT employs conventional isotopes such as technetium-99m and iodine-123.[90] These isotopes are bound to ligands that are taken up in the brain in proportion to regional blood flow, reflecting the local metabolic rate.

PET uses radioactive isotopes of biologic elements such as carbon-11, oxygen-15, nitrogen-13, and fluoride-18 (a substitute for hydrogen).[127] These radioisotopes have very short half-lives so that PET scanning requires an on-site cyclotron to produce the isotope. The isotopes are incorporated into molecules such as glucose, oxygen, water, various neurotransmitters, and drugs. Labeled glucose is taken up in proportion to the local metabolic rate for glucose. Uptake of labeled oxygen demonstrates the local metabolic rate for oxygen. Labeled neurotransmitters generate images reflecting their concentration and distribution within the brain.

Both PET and SPECT have been used to study the effects of various toxins on cerebral function. For example, although both CT and MRI can detect cerebellar atrophy in chronic alcoholics, there is a poor correlation between the magnitude of cerebellar atrophy and the clinical signs of cerebellar dysfunction. PET scans can demonstrate diminished cerebellar metabolic rate for glucose, which correlates more accurately with the patient's clinical status.[54,171]

In patients with severe neurologic dysfunction following carbon monoxide poisoning, SPECT regional blood flow measurements show diffuse hypometabolism in the frontal cortex.[24] In one patient, severe perfusion abnormalities improved slightly over several months in proportion with the patient's gradual clinical improvement.[77] In another patient treated with hyperbaric oxygen, a SPECT scan revealed increased blood flow in the frontal lobes, although the blood flow still remained significantly less than normal. These findings suggest a beneficial effect for hyperbaric oxygen therapy, although this patient did not improve clinically.[97]

In patients who chronically use cocaine, SPECT blood flow scintigraphy demonstrates focal cortical perfusion defects. The extent of these perfusion defects correlates with the frequency of drug use. Focal perfusion defects probably represent local vasculitis or small areas of infarction.[71,165] PET scanning has been used to demonstrate the effects of cocaine on cerebral blood flow and regional glucose metabolism. PET neurotransmitter studies show promise in elucidating potential mechanisms of action of cocaine. Using radiolabeled dopamine analogs, down-regulation of dopamine (D_2) receptors has been noted following a cocaine binge. This finding may be responsible for cocaine craving that occurs during cocaine withdrawal. Using ^{11}C-labeled cocaine, uptake of cocaine can be demonstrated in the basal ganglia, a region rich in dopamine receptors.[170]

Much remains to be learned about these imaging modalities before they can be applied to patient care. They are capable of demonstrating abnormalities in many patients with toxin exposures, although other patients with significant cerebral dysfunction have normal studies. In the future, these techniques may assist in the diagnosis, management, and assessment of prognosis following a toxic exposure.

SUMMARY

This chapter highlighted the variety of situations in which diagnostic imaging studies are useful in toxicologic emergencies. Imaging can be an important tool in establishing a diagnosis, assisting in patient management, or in detecting complications of a toxicologic emergency. The imaging modalities include plain radiography, CT, enteric or intravascular contrast studies, nuclear scintigraphy, and ultrasonography. However, the intelligent use of any diagnostic test requires an understanding of the clinical situations in which the test can be useful, thorough knowledge of the test's capabilities and limitations, and how the results should be applied to the care of the individual patient.

REFERENCES

1. American College of Emergency Physicians: Clinical policy for the initial approach to patients presenting with acute toxic ingestion or dermal or inhalation exposure. Ann Emerg Med 1995;25:570–585.

2. American College of Emergency Physicians: Clinical policy for the initial approach to patients presenting with acute toxic ingestion or dermal or inhalation exposure. Ann Emerg Med 1999;33:735–761.

3. Amitai Y, Silver B, Leikin JB, Frischer H: Visualization of ingested medications in the stomach by ultrasound. Am J Emerg Med 1992;10:18–23.

4. Anas N, Namasonthi V, Ginsberg CM: Criteria for hospitalizing children who have ingested products containing hydrocarbons. JAMA 1981;246:840–843.

5. Ansell G: The chest. In: Ansell G, ed: Radiology of Adverse Reactions to Drugs and Toxic Hazards. Rockville, MD, Aspen Publications, 1985, pp. 1–99.

6. Ansell G: Skeletal system and soft tissues. In: Ansell G, ed: Radiology of Adverse Reactions to Drugs and Toxic Hazards. Rockville, MD, Aspen Publications, 1985, pp. 254–326.

7. Antonescu CG: Potassium chloride and gastric outlet obstruction. Ann Intern Med 1989;111:855–857.

8. Aquilonius SM, Bergstrom K, Enolesson P, et al: Cerebral computed tomography in methanol intoxication. J Comput Assist Tomogr 1980;4:425–428.

9. Arjona A, Mata M, Bonet M: Diagnosis of chronic manganese intoxication by magnetic resonance imaging. N Engl J Med 1997;336:964–965.

10. Aronchick JM, Gefter WB: Drug-induced pulmonary disorders. Semin Roentgenol 1995:30;18.

11. Balthazar EJ, Hulnick D, Megibow AJ, Opulencia JF: Computed tomography of intramural intestinal hemorrhage and bowel ischemia. J Comput Assist Tomogr 1987;11:67–72.

12. Balthazar EJ, Lefleur R: Abdominal complications of drug addiction: Radiologic features. Semin Roentgenol 1983;18:213–214.

13. Beerman R, Nunez D, Wetli C: Radiographic evaluation of the cocaine smuggler. Gastrointest Radiol 1986;11:351–354.

14. Bensinger TA, Keller AR, Merrell LF, O'Leary DS: Thorotrast-induced reticuloendothelial blockade in man. Am J Med 1971;51:663–668.

15. Berger JR, Donovan-Post MJ, Levy RM: The acquired immunodeficiency syndrome. In: Greenberg JO, ed: Neuroimaging: A Companion to Adams and Victor's Principles of Neurology. New York, McGraw-Hill, 1995, chap. 18, pp. 413–434.

16. Blickman JG, Wilkinson RG, Graef JW: The radiologic "lead band" revisited. AJR Am J Roentgenol 1986;146:245–247.

17. Bruns BR, Tytle T: Skeletal fluorosis: A report of two cases. Orthopedics 1988;11:1083–1087.

18. Burkhart KK, Kulig KW, Rumack B: Whole-bowel irrigation as treatment for zinc sulfate overdose. Ann Emerg Med 1990;19:1167–1170.

19. Caruana DS, Weinbach B, Goerg D, Gardner LB: Cocaine-packet ingestion. Ann Intern Med 1984;100:73–74.

20. Celli B, Khan MA: Mercury embolism of the lung. N Engl J Med 1976;295:883–885.

21. Chan YW: Magnetic resonance imaging in toxic encephalopathy due to podophyllin poisoning. Neuroradiology 1991;33:372–373.

22. Chang KH, Han MH, Kim HS, et al: Delayed encephalopathy after acute carbon monoxide intoxication: MR imaging features and distribution of cerebral white matter lesions. Radiology 1992;184:117–122.

23. Cheng CLY, Svesko V: Acute pyloric perforation after prolonged crack smoking. Ann Emerg Med 1994;23:126–128.

24. Choi IS, Kim SK, Lee SS, Choi YC: Evaluation of outcome of delayed neurologic sequelae after carbon monoxide poisoning by technetium-99m hexamethylpropylene amine oxime brain single photon emission computed tomography. Eur Neurol 1995;35:137–142.

25. Citron BP, Halpern MM, McCarron M, et al: Necrotizing angiitis associated with drug abuse. N Engl J Med 1970;283:1003–1011.

26. Cohan RH, Ellis JH, Garner WL: Extravasation of radiographic contrast material: Recognition, prevention, and treatment. Radiology 1996;200:593–604.

27. Cranston PE, Pollack CV, Harrison RB: CT of crack cocaine ingestion. J Comput Assist Tomogr 1992:16;560–563.

28. Dally SL, Garnier R, Bismuth C: Diagnosis of chlorinated hydrocarbon poisoning by x-ray examination. Br J Indus Med 1987;44:424–425.

29. Dee P, Armstrong P: Inhalational lung diseases. In: Armstrong P, Wilson AG, Dee P, Hansell DM, eds: Imaging of Diseases of the Chest, 2nd ed. St. Louis, Mosby-Year Book, 1995, pp. 426–460.

30. Dee P: Drug- and radiation-induced lung disease. In: Armstrong P, Wilson AG, Dee P, Hansell DM, eds: Imaging of Diseases of the Chest, 2nd ed. St. Louis, Mosby-Year Book, 1995, pp. 461–483.

31. Desenclos JA, Wilder MH, Coppenger GW, et al: Thallium poisoning: An outbreak in Florida, 1988. South Med J 1992;85:1203–1206.

32. Dillman RO, Crumb CK, Lidsky MJ: Lead poisoning from a gunshot wound. Am J Med 1979;66:509–514.

33. Douglass RE, Levison MA: Pneumothorax in drug abusers: An urban epidemic? Am Surg 1986;52:377–380.

34. Edeiken J, Dalinka M, Karasick D: Edeiken's Roentgen Diagnosis of Diseases of Bone, 4th ed. Baltimore, Williams and Wilkins, 1990, pp. 1401–1406.

35. Eurman DW, Potash HI, Eyler WR, et al: Chest pain and dyspnea related to "crack" cocaine smoking: Value of chest radiography. Radiology 1989;172:459–462.

36. Everson GW, Oudjhane K, Young LW, Krenzelok EP: Effectiveness of abdominal radiographs in visualizing chewable iron supplements following overdose. Am J Emerg Med 1989;7:459–463.

37. Everson GW, Bertaccini EJ, O'Leary J: Use of whole-bowel irrigation in an infant following iron overdose. Am J Emerg Med 1991;9:366–369.

38. Farber JM, Rafii M, Schwartz D: Lead arthropathy and elevated serum lead levels after a gunshot wound of the shoulder. AJR Am J Roentgenol 1994;162:385–386.

39. Federle MP, Chang PJ, Confer S, Ozgun B: Frequency and effects of extravasation of ionic and nonionic CT contrast media during rapid bolus injection. Radiology 1998;206:637–640.

40. Feigen DS: Talc: Understanding its manifestations in the chest. AJR Am J Roentgenol 1986;146:295–301.

41. Felson B, Spitz HB: Unusual foreign bodies in bowel. JAMA 1977;237:2225–2226.

42. Finelli PF: Changes in the basal ganglia following cyanide poisoning. J Comput Assist Tomogr 1981;5:755–756.

43. Florez MV, Evans JM, Daly TR: The radiodensity of medications seen on x-ray films. Mayo Clin Proc 1998;73:516–519.

44. Forrester JM, Steele AW, Waldron JA, Parsens PE: Crack lung: An acute pulmonary syndrome with a spectrum of clinical and histopathological findings. Am Rev Respir Dis 1990;142:462–467.

45. Foxford R, Goldfrank L: Gastrotomy—A surgical approach to iron overdose. Ann Emerg Med 1985;14:1223–1226.

46. Fraser RO, Pare JAP, Pare PD, Fraser RS, Genereux GP: Drug- and poison-induced pulmonary disease. In: Fraser RO, Pare JAP, Pare PD, Fraser RS, Genereux GP, eds: Diagnosis of Diseases of the Chest, 3rd ed. Philadelphia, WB Saunders, 1991, pp. 2417–2479.

47. Freed TA, Sweet LN, Gauder PJ: Balloon obturation bowel obstruction: A hazard of drug smuggling. AJR Am J Roentgenol 1976;127:1033–1034.

48. Fulkerson WJ, Gockerman JP: Pulmonary disease induced by drugs. In: Fishman AP, ed: Pulmonary Diseases and Disorders, 2nd ed. New York, McGraw-Hill, 1988, pp. 793–811.

49. Gadaleta D, Hall MH, Nelson RL: Cocaine-induced acute aortic dissection. Chest 1989;96:1203–1205.

50. Gallucci M, Amicarelli I, Rossi A, et al: MR imaging of white matter lesions in uncomplicated chronic alcoholism. J Comput Assist Tomogr 1989;13:395–398.

51. Gatenby RA: The radiology of drug-induced disorders in the gastrointestinal tract. Semin Roentgenol 1995;30;62–76.

52. Gaul HP, Wallace CJ, Auer RN, Fong TC: MR findings in methanol intoxication. AJNR Am J Neuroradiol 1995;16:1783–1786.

53. Gibby WA, Zimmerman RA: X-ray computed tomography. In: Mazziotta JG, Gilman S, eds: Clinical Brain Imaging: Principles and Applications. Philadelphia, FA Davis, 1992, pp. 3–34.

54. Gilman S, Adams K, Koeppe RA, et al: Cerebellar and frontal hypometabolism in alcoholic cerebellar degeneration studied with positron emission tomography. Ann Neurol 1990;28:775–785.

55. Gilman S: Advances in neurology. N Engl J Med 1992;326: 1608–1616.

56. Ginaldi S: Geophagia: An uncommon cause of acute abdomen. Ann Emerg Med 1988;17:979–981.

57. Gray JR, Khalil A, Prior JC: Acute arsenic toxicity—an opaque poison. Can Assoc Radiol J 1989;40:226–227.

58. Hahn I, Hoffman RS, Nelson LS: Contrast CT fails to detect the last heroin packet [abstract]. J Toxicol Clin Toxicol 1999;37:644–645.

59. Handy CA: Radiopacity of oral non-liquid medications. Radiology 1971;98:525–533.

60. Hantson P, Duprez T, Mahieu P: Neurotoxicity to the basal ganglia shown by magnetic resonance imaging (MRI) following poisoning by methanol and other substances. J Toxicol Clin Toxicol 1997;35: 151–161.

61. Harchelroad F: Identification of orally ingested cocaine by CT scan. Vet Hum Toxicol 1992;34:350.

62. Haubek A, Lee K: Computed tomography in alcoholic cerebellar atrophy. Neuroradiology 1979;18:77–79.

63. Heffner JE, Harley RA, Schabel SI: Pulmonary reactions from illicit substance abuse. Clin Chest Med 1990;11:151–162.

64. Hibbard R, Wahl M, Kirshenbaum M, et al: Spiral CT imaging of ingested foreign bodies wrapped in plastic: A pilot study designed to mimic cocaine body stuffers [abstract]. J Toxicol Clin Toxicol 1999; 37:644.

65. Hillbom M, Mulronen A, Holm L, Hindmarsh T: The clinical versus radiological diagnosis of alcoholic cerebellar degeneration. J Neurol Sci 1986;73:45–53.

66. Hinkel CL: The significance of opaque medications in the gastrointestinal tract, with special reference to enteric coated pills. AJR Am J Roentgenol 1951;65:575–581.

67. Ho VB, Fitz CR, Chuang SH, Geyer CA: Bilateral basal ganglia lesions: Pediatric differential considerations. Radiographics 1993;13: 269–292.

68. Hoffman CK, Goodman PC: Pulmonary edema in cocaine smokers. Radiology 1989;172:463–465.

69. Hoffman RS, Chiang WK, Weisman RS, Goldfrank LR: Prospective evaluation of "crack-vial" ingestion. Vet Hum Toxicol 1990;32: 164–167.

70. Hoffman RS, Smilkstein MJ, Goldfrank LR: Whole-bowel irrigation and the cocaine body-packer. Am J Emerg Med 1990;8:523–527.

71. Holman BL, Mendelson J, Garada B, et al: Regional cerebral blood flow improves with treatment in chronic cocaine polydrug users. J Nucl Med 1993;34:723–727.

72. Holzman RS, Bishko F: Osteomyelitis in heroin addicts. Ann Intern Med 1971;75:693–696.

73. Hormes JT, Filley CM, Rosenberg NL: Neurologic sequelae of chronic solvent vapor abuse. Neurology 1986;36:698–702.

74. Horowitz AL, Kaplan R, Sarpel O: Carbon monoxide toxicity: MR imaging in the brain. Radiology 1987;162:787–788.

75. Horrocks AW: Abdominal radiography in suspected "body packers." Clin Radiol 1992;45:322–325; [comment]. 1993;47:219.

76. Jaeger RW, Decastro FJ, Barry RC, et al: Radiopacity of drugs and plants: In vivo limited usefulness. Vet Hum Toxicol 1981:23 (Suppl): 2–4 (suppl).

77. Jibiki I, Kurokawa K, Yamaguchi N: 123I-MP brain SPECT imaging in a patient with the interval form of CO poisoning. Eur Neurol 1991;31:149–151.

78. Jones JS, Lagasse J, Zimmerman G: Computed tomographic findings after acute carbon monoxide poisoning. Am J Emerg Med 1994;12: 448–451.

79. Kaczorowski JM, Wax PM: Five days of whole-bowel irrigation in a case of pediatric iron ingestion. Ann Emerg Med 1996;27:258–263.

80. Keys N, Wahl M, Aks S, et al: Cocaine body stuffers: A case series. J Toxicol Clin Toxicol 1995;33:517.

81. Koller WC, Glatt SL, Perlik S, et al: Cerebellar atrophy demonstrated by computed tomography. Neurology 1981;31:405–412.

82. Koppel BS, Tuchman AJ, Mangiardi JR, et al: Epidural spinal infection in intravenous drug abusers. Arch Neurol 1988;45:1331–1337.

83. Kram HB, Hardin E, Clark SR, Shoemaker WC: Perforated ulcers related to smoking "crack" cocaine. Am Surg 1992;58:293–294.

84. Kreigstein AR, Armitage BA, Kim PK: Heroin inhalation and progressive spongiform leukoencephalopathy. N Engl J Med 1997;336: 589–590.

85. Krishnan A, Brown R: Plain abdominal radiography in the diagnosis of the "body packer." J Accid Emerg Med 1999;16:381.

86. Krupski WC, Selzman CH, Whitehill TA: Unusual causes of mesenteric ischemia. Surg Clin North Am 1997;77:471–502.

87. Kuhn JR, Tunell WP: The role of cine-esophagography in caustic esophageal injury. Am J Surg 1983;146:804–806.

88. Kulshrestha MK: Lead poisoning diagnosed by abdominal x-rays. J Toxicol Clin Toxicol 1996;34:107–108.

89. Landi JL, Spickler EM: Imaging of intracranial hemorrhage associated with drug abuse. Neuroimaging Clin N Am 1992;2:187–194.

90. Lassen NA, Holm, S: Single photon emission computerized tomography. In: Mazzotta JG, Gilman S, eds: Clinical Brain Imaging: Principles and Applications. Philadelphia, FA Davis, 1992, pp. 108–134.

91. Lee DC, Roberts JR, Kelly JJ, Fishman SM: Whole-bowel irrigation as an adjunct in the treatment of radiopaque arsenic. Am J Emerg Med 1995;13:244–245.

92. Levine SR, Brust JCM, Futrell N, et al: Cerebrovascular complications of the use of the "crack" form of alkaloidal cocaine. N Engl J Med 1990;323:699–704.

93. Lexa FJ: Drug-induced disorders of the central nervous system. Semin Roentgenol 1995;30:7–17.

94. Linowiecki KA, Tillman DJ, Ruggles D, et al: Radiopacity of modified release cardiac medications: A case report and in vitro analysis [abstract]. Vet Hum Toxicol 1992;34:350.

95. Litovitz TL: Button battery ingestions: A review of 56 cases. JAMA 1983;249:2495–2500.

96. Lufkin RB: Magnetic resonance imaging. In: Mazziotti JG, Gilman S, eds: Clinical Brain Imaging: Principles and Applications. Philadelphia, FA Davis, 1992, pp. 36–69.

97. Maeda Y, Kawasaki Y, Jibiki I, et al: Effect of therapy with oxygen under high pressure of regional cerebral blood flow in the interval form of carbon monoxide poisoning: Observation from subtraction of technetium-99m HMPAO SPECT brain imaging. Eur Neurol 1991;31:380–383.

98. Mahoney MS, Kahn M: A medical mystery (images in clinical medicine). N Engl J Med 1998;339:745, 1333–1334.

99. Maniatis V, Zois G, Stringaris K: I.V. mercury self-injection: CT imaging. AJR Am J Roentgenol 1997;169:1197–1198.

100. Mankin HJ: Nontraumatic necrosis of bone (osteonecrosis). N Engl J Med 1992;326:1473–1479.

101. Maravilla AM, Berk RN: The radiographic diagnosis of pica. Am J Gastroenterol 1978;70:94–99.

102. Martel W: Radiographic features of esophagogastritis secondary to extremely caustic agents. Radiology 1972;103:31–36.

103. Martin TJ: Cocaine-induced mesenteric ischemia. N C Med J 1991; 52:429–430; [comment]. 591.

104. Matsumoto SC, Okajima T, Inayoshi S, Ueno H: Minamata disease demonstrated by computed tomography. Neuroradiology 1988;30: 42–46.

105. McCarron MM, Wood JD: The cocaine "body packer" syndrome. JAMA 1983;250:1417–1420.

106. McElvaine MD, DeUngria EG, Mattte TD, et al: Prevalence of radiographic evidence of paint chip ingestion among children with moderate to severe lead poisoning, St. Louis, Missouri, 1989 through 1990. Pediatrics 1992;89:740–742.

107. Meggs WJ, Hoffman RS, Shih RD, et al: Thallium poisoning from maliciously contaminated food. J Toxicol Clin Toxicol 1994;32: 723–730.

108. Megibow AJ, Balthazar EJ, Cho KC, et al: Bowel obstruction: Evaluation with CT. Radiology 1991;180:313–318.

109. Mengel CE, Carter WA: Geophagia diagnosed by roentgenograms. JAMA 1964;187:955–956.

110. Merchant JA, Schwartz DA: Chest radiography for assessment of the pneumoconioses. In: Rom WN, ed: Environmental and Occupational Medicine, 2nd ed. Boston, Little Brown, 1992, pp. 215–225.

111. Messer HD, Litvinoff J: Pyogenic cervical osteomyelitis. Arch Neurol 1976;33:571–576.

112. Messing B, Storch B: Computer tomography and magnetic resonance imaging in cyanide poisoning. Eur Arch Psychiatr Neurol Sci 1988;237:139–143.

113. Miller WT: Pleural and mediastinal disorders related to drug use. Semin Roentgenol 1995:30;35–48.

114. Miura T, Mitomo M, Kawi R, Harada K: CT of the brain in acute carbon monoxide intoxication: Characteristic features and prognosis. AJNR Am J Neuroradiol 1985;6:739–742.

115. Moral AR, Ayanoglu HO, Erhan E: Putamenal necrosis after methanol intoxication. Intensive Care Med 1997;23:234–235.

116. Naidich TP, Bartlett D, Wheeler PS, Stern WZ: Metallic mercury emboli. AJR Am J Roentgenol 1973;117:886–891.

117. Nelson DL, Batnitzky S, McMillan JH, et al: The CT and MRI features of acute toxic encephalopathies. AJNR Am J Neuroradiol 1987;8:951.

118. Neustadter LM, Weiss M: Medication-induced changes of bone. Semin Roentgenol 1995;30:88–95.

119. Ng RCW, Perry K, Martin DJ: Iron poisoning: Assessment of radiography in diagnosis and management. Clin Pediatr 1979;18: 614–616.

120. O'Brien RP, McGeehan PA, Helmeczi AW, Dula DJ: Detectability of drug tablets and capsules by plain radiography. Am J Emerg Med 1986;4:302–312.

121. Olmedo RE, Hoffman RS, Nelson LS: Limitations of whole bowel irrigation and laparotomy in a cocaine "body-packer" [abstract]. J Toxicol Clin Toxicol 1999;37:645.

122. Olsen WL, Cohen W: Neuroradiology of AIDS. In: Federle M, Megibow A, Nadich DP, eds: Radiology of Acquired Immune Deficiency Syndrome. New York, Raven Press, 1988, pp. 21–45.

123. Palat D, Denson M, Sherman M, Matz R: Pneumomediastinum induced by inhalation of alkaloidal cocaine. N Y State J Med 1988;438–439.

124. Palatnick W, Tenenbein M: Leukocytosis, hyperglycemia, vomiting, and positive x-rays are not indicators of severity of iron overdose in adults. Am J Emerg Med 1996;14:454–455.

125. Perron AD, Gibbs M: Thoracic aortic dissection secondary to crack cocaine ingestion. Am J Emerg Med 1997;15:507–509.

126. Peterson CD, Fifield GC: Emergency gastrotomy for acute iron poisoning. Ann Emerg Med 1980;9:262–264.

127. Phelps ME: Positron emission tomography. In: Mazziotti JS, Gilman S, eds: Clinical Brain Imaging: Principles and Applications. Philadelphia, FA Davis, 1992, pp. 71–106.

128. Piatt JP, Kaplan AM, Bond RO, Berg RA: Occult carbon monoxide poisoning in an infant. Pediatr Emerg Care 1990;6:21–23.

129. Pollack CV, Biggers DW, Carlton FB, et al: Two crack cocaine body stuffers. Ann Emerg Med 1992;21:1370–1380.

130. Pracyk JB, Stolp BW, Fife CE, et al: Brain computerized tomography after hyperbaric oxygen therapy for carbon monoxide poisoning. Undersea Hyperb Med 1995;22:1–7.

131. Prockop LD, Naidu KA: Brain CT and MRI findings after carbon monoxide toxicity. J Neuroimaging 1999;9:175–181.

132. Raber SA: The dense metaphyseal band sign. Radiology 1999;211: 773–774.

133. Ramchandani P, Pollack HM: Radiology of drug-related genitourinary disease. Semin Roentgenol 1995;30;77–87.

134. Rashid J, Eisenberg MJ, Topol EJ: Cocaine-induced aortic dissection. Am Heart J 1996;132:1301–1304.

135. Resnick D: Heavy metal poisoning and deficiency. In: Resnick D, ed: Diagnosis of Bone and Joint Disorders, 3rd ed. Philadelphia, WB Saunders, 1995, pp. 3353–3364.

136. Resnick D, Niwayama G: Osteolysis and chondrolysis. In: Resnick D, ed: Diagnosis of Bone and Joint Disorders, 3rd ed. Philadelphia, WB Saunders, 1995, pp. 4467–4469.

137. Richerson HB: Hypersensitivity pneumonitis (extrinsic allergic alveolitis). In: Fishman AP, ed: Pulmonary Diseases and Disorders, 2nd ed. New York, McGraw-Hill, 1988, pp. 667–674.

138. Roberge RJ, Martin TG: Whole-bowel irrigation in an acute oral lead intoxication. Am J Emerg Med 1992;10:577–583.

139. Roberge RJ, Srinivasa NS, Frank LR, et al: Putamenal infarct in methanol intoxication: Case report and role of brain imaging studies. Vet Hum Toxicol 1998;40:95–98.

140. Roberts JR, Price D, Goldfrank LR, Hartnett L: The body stuffer syndrome: A clandestine form of drug overdose. Am J Emerg Med 1986;4:24–27.

141. Rosenberg NL, Kleinschmidt-DeMasters BK, Davis KA, et al: Toluene abuse causes diffuse central nervous system white matter changes. Ann Neurol 1988;23:611–614.

142. Rubinstein D, Escott E, Kelly JP: Methanol intoxication with putamenal and white matter necrosis: MR and CT findings. AJNR Am J Neuroradiol 1995;16:1492–1494.

143. Sachs HK: The evolution of the radiologic lead line. Radiology 1981;139:81–85.

144. Savitt DL, Hawkins HH, Roberts JR: The radiopacity of ingested medications. Ann Emerg Med 1987;16:331–339.

145. Sawada Y, Ohashi N, Maemura K, et al: Computerized tomography as an indication of long term outcome after acute carbon monoxide poisoning. Lancet 1980;2:783–784.

146. Sawada Y, Sakamoto T, Nishide, et al: Correlation of pathological findings with computed tomographic findings after acute carbon monoxide poisoning. N Engl J Med 1983;308:1296.

147. Schabel SI, Rogers CI: Opaque artifacts in a health food faddist simulating ovarian neoplasm. AJR Am J Roentgenol 1978;130:789–790.

148. Schwartz DT: Toxicologic emergencies. In: Schwartz DT, Reisdorff EJ, eds: Emergency Radiology. New York, McGraw-Hill, 2000, pp. 627–648.

149. Silver DA, Cross M, Fox B, Paxton RM: Computed tomography of the brain in acute carbon monoxide poisoning. Clin Radiol 1996; 51:480–483.

150. Sinner WN: The gastrointestinal tract as a vehicle for drug smuggling. Gastrointest Radiol 1981;6:319–323.

151. Smith DA, Leake L, Loflin JR, Yealy DM: Is admission after intravenous heroin overdose necessary? Ann Emerg Med 1992;21: 1326–1330; [comment]. 1993;22:1638–1639.

152. Sogge MR, Griffith JL, Sinar DR, Mayes GR: Lavage to remove enteric-coated aspirin and gastric outlet obstruction. Ann Intern Med 1977;87:721–722.

153. Spitzer A, Caruthers S, Stables DP: Radiopaque suppositories. Diagn Radiol 1976;121:71–73.

154. Sporer KA, Manning JJ: Massive ingestion of sustained-release verapamil with a concretion and bowel infarction. Ann Emerg Med 1993;22:603–605.

155. Sporer KA, Firestone J: Clinical course of crack cocaine body stuffers. Ann Emerg Med 1997;29:596–601.

156. Staple TW, McAlister WH: Roentgenographic visualization of iron preparations in the gastrointestinal tract. Radiology 1964;83: 1051–1056.

157. Stern WZ, Spear PW, Jacobson HG: The roentgen findings in acute heroin intoxication. AJR Am J Roentgenol 1968;103:522–532.

158. Stromberg BV: Symptomatic lead toxicity secondary to retained shotgun pellets: Case report. J Trauma 1990;30:356–357.

159. Sue YJ, Saperstein A, Zawin J, et al: Radiopacity of para-dichlorobenzene-containing household products. Vet Hum Toxicol 1992;34:350.

160. Swartz MN: Approach to the patient with pulmonary infections. In: Fishman AP, ed: Pulmonary Diseases and Disorders, 2nd ed. New York, McGraw-Hill, 1988, pp. 1375–1759.

161. Switz DM, Elmorshidy ME, Deyerle WM: Bullets, joints and lead intoxication. Arch Intern Med 1976;136:939–941.

162. Tatekawa Y, Nakatani K, Ishil H, et al. Small bowel obstruction caused by a medication bezoar: Report of case. Surg Today 1996; 26:68–70.

163. Tillman DJ, Ruggles DL, Leiken JB: Radiopacity study of extended-release formulations using digitized radiography. Am J Emerg Med 1994;12:310–314.

164. Tom T, Abedon S, Clark RI, Wong W: Neuroimaging characteristics in carbon monoxide toxicity. J Neuroimaging 1996;6:161–166.

165. Tumeh SS, Nagel JS, English RJ, et al: Cerebral abnormalities in cocaine abusers: Demonstration by SPECT perfusion brain scintigraphy. Radiology 1990;176:821–824.

166. Velasquez G, Ward CF, Bohrer SP: Thorium dioxide: Still around. South Med J 1985;78:743–745.

167. Venturelli J, Kwee Y, Morris N, Cameron O: Gastrotomy in the management of acute iron poisoning. J Pediatr 1982;100:768–769.

168. Vernace MA, Bellucci AG, Wilkes BM: Chronic salicylate toxicity due to consumption of over-the-counter bismuth subsalicylate. Am J Med 1994;97:308–309.

169. Vieregge P, Klostermann W, Blumm RG, Borgis KJ: Carbon monoxide poisoning: Clinical, neurophysiological, and brain imaging observations in acute disease and follow-up. J Neurol 1989;236: 478–481.

170. Volkow ND, Fowler JS, Wolf AP: Use of positron emission tomography to investigate cocaine. In: Nahas GG, Latour C, eds: Physiopathology of Illicit Drugs: Cannabis, Cocaine, Opiates. Oxford, Pergamon Press, 1991, pp. 129–141.

171. Wang GJ, Volkow ND, Roque CT, et al: Functional importance of ventricular enlargement and cortical atrophy in healthy subjects and alcoholics as assessed with PET, MR imaging, and neuropsychologic testing. Radiology 1993;186:59–65.

172. Wang Y, Yin Y, Gilula LA, Wilson AJ: Endemic fluorosis of the skeleton: Radiographic features in 127 patients. AJR Am J Roentgenol 1994;162:93–98.

173. Warach SJ, Charness ME: Imaging the brain lesions of alcoholics. In: Greenberg JO, ed: Neuroimaging: A Companion to Adams and Victor's Principles of Neurology. New York, McGraw-Hill, 1995, chap. 18, pp. 503–515.

174. Ware LB, Matthay MA: The acute respiratory distress syndrome. N Engl J Med 2000;342:1334–1349.

175. Wax PM: Intestinal infarction due to nifedipine overdose. J Toxicol Clin Toxicol 1995;33:725–728.

176. Weill H, Jones RN: Occupational pulmonary diseases. In: Fishman AP, ed: Pulmonary Diseases and Disorders, 2nd ed. New York, McGraw-Hill, 1988, pp. 1465–1474.

177. Weimerskirch PJ, Burkhart KK, Bono MJ, et al: Methylene iodide poisoning. Ann Emerg Med 1990;19:1171–1176.

178. Williams MH: Pulmonary complications of drug abuse. In: Fishman AP, ed: Pulmonary Diseases and Disorders, 2nd ed. New York, McGraw-Hill, 1988, pp. 819–860.

179. Wolowodiuk OJ, McMicken DB, O'Brien P: Pneumomediastinum and pneumoperitoneum: An unusual complication of syrup of ipecac-induced emesis. Ann Emerg Med 1984;13:1148–1151.

180. Woolf DA, Riach CF, Derweesh A, Vyas H: Lead lines in young infants with acute lead encephalopathy: A reliable diagnostic test. J Trop Pediatr 1990;36:90.

CHAPTER 9

ELECTROCARDIOGRAPHIC PRINCIPLES

Cathleen Clancy

The electrocardiogram (ECG) is ubiquitous in emergency departments and intensive care units and its interpretation is widely understood by physicians of nearly all disciplines. It is certainly invaluable as a diagnostic tool for patients with acute cardiovascular complaints. However, it is also a ready source of information in poisoned patients and holds the potential to enhance or redirect their care. Although it seems obvious that an ECG would be required following exposure to a drug used for cardiovascular indications, many toxins with no overt cardiovascular effects with therapeutic dosing become cardiotoxic in overdose. In patients with undefined poisoning, the ECGs can suggest specific toxins or demonstrate electrolyte abnormalities, long before blood is even drawn on a patient. For example, oropharyngeal or dermal burns in a patient whose ECG has evidence of hyperkalemia or hypocalcemia suggests exposure to hydrofluoric acid.[43] Alternatively, a patient manifesting signs of the opioid toxidrome with runs of ventricular tachycardia might be exposed to propoxyphene.[23] Additionally, the ECG may have proven prognostic ability with regard to a complication such as a seizure following tricyclic antidepressant overdose. Therefore, an ECG should be critically examined early in the initial evaluation of any poisoned patient.

HISTORY

The knowledge of a relationship between electricity and muscular movement can be traced back to 1790, when Luigi Galvani electrically stimulated an in vitro preparation of the legs of a frog, and made them "dance." In 1887, Waller developed a "capillary electrometer" that transmitted electrical impulses from a man's skin to a capillary tube. Pulsations similar to the patient's heartbeat were visible in the tube.[38] In 1903, Willem Einthoven graphically displayed the electrical activity of the heart and even named the different waves—P, QRS, and T. He called this tracing an "elektrokardiogramme."[13] The acronym *EKG*, still employed by some authors, was derived from Einthoven's spelling. The acronym *ECG*, which is consistent with our current spelling of electrocardiogram, is used throughout this text.

Since this initial description, physicians have described the normal electrophysiology of the heart and catalogued the pharmacologic effects of various substances by their effect on the surface electrocardiogram. Despite the large number, diversity, and complexity of the various cardiac toxins, there are a far more limited number of possible electrocardiographic manifestations and many trends are apparent when the principles of electrophysiology and electrocardiography are understood and categorized.

BASIC ELECTROPHYSIOLOGY OF THE MYOCARDIAL CELL

The resting myocardial cell, or myocyte, is negatively charged, or polarized. When the myocytes in the sinus node depolarize, ion channels in the nearby myocardium open and admit a net influx of positive sodium and calcium ions. This influx raises the electrical potential of the cell toward and past neutral and initiates an impulse that propagates throughout the myocardium, producing electrical and mechanical systole. After a well-defined time period the myocardial membrane is repolarized by an outward current of potassium and an inward current of chloride and returns ultimately to the polarized state, or diastole (Table 9–1).

Figure 9–1 shows schematically the relationship of the major ion flux across the myocardial cell membrane, the phases of the action potential, and the surface ECG recording. A more detailed description of ion fluxes and channels may be found in Chapters 10 and 21.

BASIC ELECTROPHYSIOLOGY OF AN ELECTROCARDIOGRAM

Simplistically, a positive or upward deflection on the electrocardiogram represents an electrical force moving toward the implicated electrode and its length represents the magnitude (Fig. 9–2). In practical terms, however, the deflection on the tracing represents the sum of all forces in effect on the heart at the moment of the tracing. Only during depolarization or repolarization does the electrocardiogram tracing leave the isoelectric baseline, because it is only during these periods that current is actually flowing. During the other periods, mechanical effects are occurring in the myocardium, but current is not moving.

TABLE 9–1. Ions as Charge Carriers Across Cell Membranes

Ion	Charge	Direction of Passive Flux	Current Generated	Effect of Membrane Potential
Calcium	Positive	Inward	Inward	Depolarization
Sodium	Positive	Inward	Inward	Depolarization
Potassium	Positive	Outward	Outward	Repolarization
Chloride	Negative	Inward	Outward	Repolarization

Reproduced, with permission, from Katz AM: Cardiac ion channels. N Engl J Med 1993;328:1245.

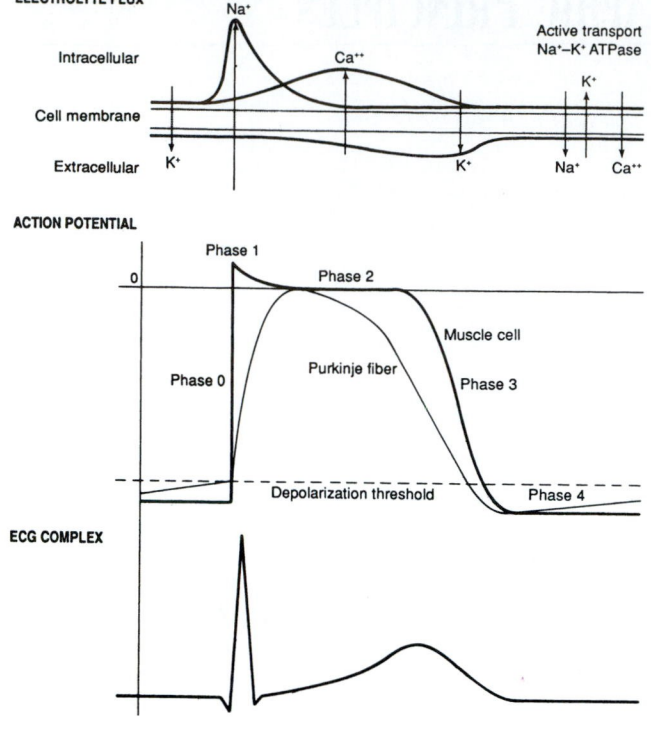

Figure 9–1. Relationship of electrolyte movement across the cell membrane to the action potential and the surface ECG recording.

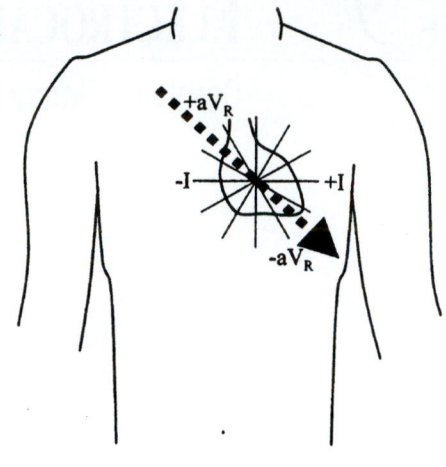

Figure 9–2. A simplistic correlation between cardiac anatomy and electrocardiographic representation.

Leads

Although the reading from a single electrocardiogram lead provides an immense amount of information, to visualize the heart in a nearly three-dimensional perspective, multiple leads must be assessed simultaneously. Given the cylindrical nature of both the heart and thorax, at any given moment some of these leads will record positive voltage and others negative. The lead placement that was described in 1913 forms the basis for the bipolar or limb leads, described as I, II, and III (Fig. 9–3).[13] Einthoven's triangle is an equilateral triangle formed by the sum of these leads. Unipolar limb leads and precordial leads were subsequently added to the standard electrocardiogram. Wilson and colleagues connected limb leads, called V_R, V_L, and V_F, to a common point where the sum of the potentials from leads I, II, and III was zero. A unipolar potential was measured.[39] The currently used, augmented (a) leads (aV_R, aV_L, and aV_F) are based on these unipolar leads (Fig. 9–4).[16] The precordial leads, called V_1 through V_6, are also unipolar measurements of the change in electric potential measured from a central point to the six anterior and left lateral chest positions (Fig. 9–5). If V_2 is placed over the right ventricle, part of the initial positive ventricular deflection (QRS complex) reflects right ventricular activation, with electrical forces moving toward the electrode. The majority of the subsequent terminal negative deflection reflects activation of other muscle tissue (septum, left ventricular wall) when the electrical forces are moving away from the electrode. Recordings from each of these 12 leads (I, II, III, aV_R, aV_L, aV_F, V_{1-6}) evaluate the heart from two different planes in 12 different positions, yielding a three-dimensional electrical "picture" of the heart, with respect to time and voltage.

A continuous cardiac monitor usually relies on recordings from one of two bipolar leads: a modified left chest (lead MCL_1) or a

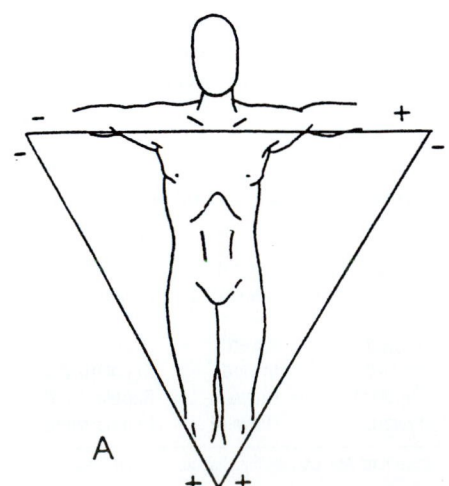

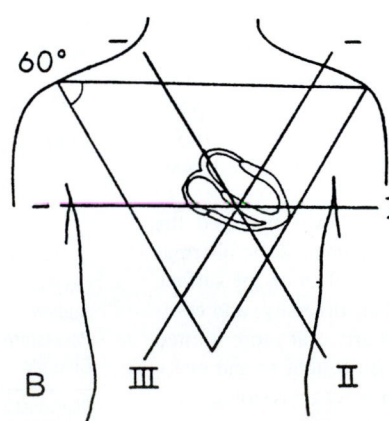

Figure 9–3. The relationships of the original three limb leads are illustrated. **A.** The equiangular (60°) Einthoven triangle formed by leads I, II, and III is shown with positive nd negative poles of each of the leads indicated. **B.** The Einthoven triangle is shown in relation to a schematic view of the heart. Leads I, II, and III are also presented as a triaxial reference system that intersects in the center of the ventricles. *(Reproduced, with permission, from Wagner GS: Cardiac electrical activity, recording the normal electrocardiogram. In: Wagner GS: Marriott's Practical Electrocardiography, 9th ed. Baltimore, Williams & Wilkins, 1994, p. 21.)*

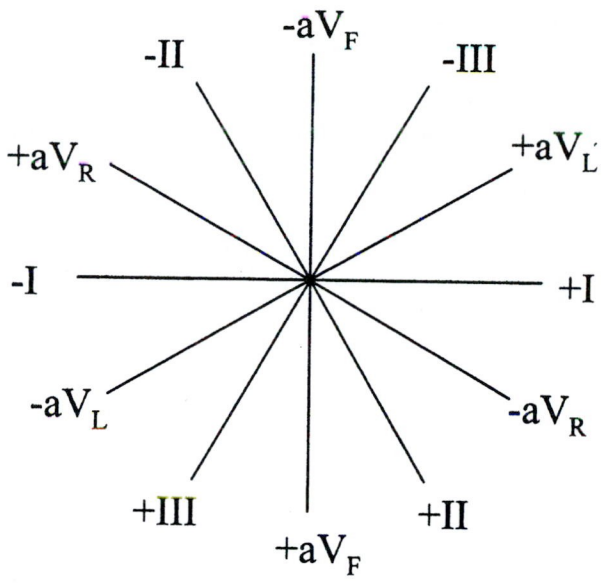

Figure 9–4. The hexaxial reference system derived from Einthoven's equilateral triangle defining the electrical potential vectors of electrocardiography.

lead II. The recording from an MCL₁ lead, in which the positive electrode is in the V₁ position, is similar in appearance to a V₁ recording on a 12-lead ECG. This lead visualizes ventricular activity well; however, lead II shows atrial activity (ie, the P wave) much more clearly.

The Various Intervals and Waves

The ECG tracing has specific nomenclature to define the characteristic patterns. Waves refer to positive or negative deflections from baseline (ie, P, T, or U wave). A segment is defined as the distance between two waves (ie, ST segment), and an interval measures the duration of a wave plus a segment (QT or PR interval). Complexes are a group of waves without intervals or segments between them (QRS). Electrophysiologically, the P wave and PR interval on the ECG tracing represent the depolarization of the atria. The QRS complex represents the depolarization of the ventricles. Repolarization is depicted by the ST segment, the T wave, the QT interval, and the U wave (Fig. 9–6).

The P Wave
Electrophysiology. The early, middle, and late portions of the P wave are represented sequentially by the electrical potential initiated by the sinus node. The impulse is propagated directly through the right atrial muscle, producing contraction, as well as by specialized conduction tissue across the interatrial septum to produce contraction of the left atrium. Additionally, internodal pathways rapidly conduct the impulse to the atrioventricular node (AV node). The electrical excitation of the sinus node differs from that of the ventricular myocardium in that current is mediated primarily by calcium ion influx via slow calcium channels, not by sodium entering through fast sodium channels. Furthermore, the vagus nerve exerts a profound suppressive influence on the nodal tissues.

The Abnormal P Wave. Clinically, abnormalities of the P wave occur with agents that depress automaticity of the sinus node, causing sinus arrest and nodal or ventricular escape rhythms (β-adrenergic antagonists, T-type calcium channel blockers). The P wave is absent in rhythms with sinus arrest, such as occurs with cardiac glycoside poisoning or drugs that enhance cholinergic tone. A notched P wave suggests delayed conduction across the atrial septum and is characteristic of quinidine poisoning. P waves decrease in amplitude as hyperkalemia becomes more severe until they become indistinguishable from the baseline.

The PR Interval
Electrophysiology. The PR interval is measured from the beginning of the P wave to the beginning of the QRS complex (normal is 120–200 msec). Despite rapid conduction by specialized conduction tissue from the SA to the AV node, the AV node delays transmission of the impulse into the ventricles ostensibly to allow for complete atrial emptying. Thus, the PR interval represents the interval between the onset of atrial depolarization and the onset of ventricular depolarization. Children usually have more rapid conduction and a shorter PR interval, and older adults generally have a longer PR interval. The segment between the end of the P wave and the beginning of the QRS complex reflects atrial contraction and is usually isoelectric. Atrial repolarization immediately follows, but its electrocardiographic findings, or atrial T waves, are obscured by the subsequent ventricular depolarization.

The Abnormal PR Interval. Agents that decrease interatrial or AV nodal conduction would initially cause marked lengthening of the PR segment until such conduction completely ceases. At this

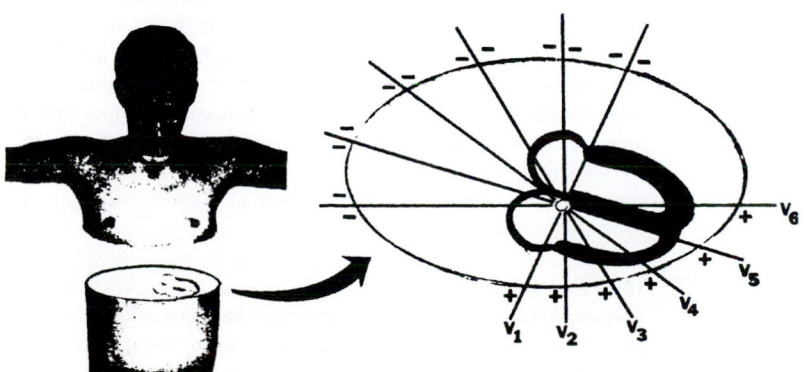

Figure 9–5. Each of the chest leads is oriented through the AV node and exits through the patient's back, which is negative. (*Reproduced, with permission, from Dubin D: Rapid Interpretation of EKG's, ed. V, Tampa, FL, Cover Publishing Co, 1996, p. 47.*)

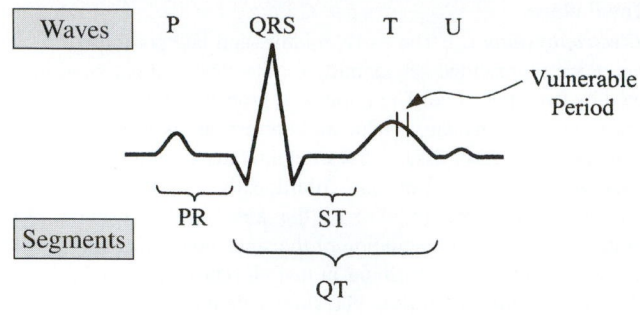

Figure 9–6.   The normal ECG: P wave, atrial depolarization; QRS, ventricular depolarization; ST segment and T wave, ventricular repolarization. The U wave is a small positive deflection.

point the P wave no longer relates to the QRS complex; this is AV dissociation or complete heart block. Some agents suppress AV nodal cells by blocking their calcium channels, such as magnesium, or antagonizing at the β-adrenergic receptors. Other drugs alter cellular repolarization through inhibition of their sodium-potassium pump (eg, digoxin). Although the therapeutic use of digoxin, as well as early cardiac glycoside poisoning, causes PR prolongation through vagotonic effects, direct electrophysiologic effects account for the bradycardia of poisoning. As the AV node becomes more refractory and the myocardium more "sensitized," ventricular ectopy occurs (see later in this chapter, as well as Chap. 48 and Antidotes in Depth: Digoxin-Specific Antibody Fragment).

The QRS Complex

Electrophysiology.   The QRS complex reflects the electrical forces generated by ventricular depolarization. Although under normal conditions both ventricles depolarize nearly simultaneously, the greater mass of the left ventricle causes it to contribute the majority of the electrical forces. Thus, the QRS complex is primarily positive in leads I and aV$_L$ on the surface ECG recording. This is because under normal conditions the depolarization vector is directed at 60° and is thus moving toward the positive electrodes in these leads. The normal range for the QRS axis in the frontal plane is between −30° and 105°, although most people will have values between 30° and 75°. This axis will vary with the weight and age of the patient. Alterations in myocardial function may also alter the electrical axis of the heart.

The simultaneous and rapid depolarization of the ventricles results in a very short period of electrical activity recorded on the electrocardiogram. Of course, mechanical systole lasts well past the end of the QRS complex and is maintained by continued depolarization during the plateau phase of the action potential. The return and maintenance of the baseline, or isoelectric potential, is simply a result of the fact that the entire heart is depolarized and there is no flow of current during this period. The normal QRS duration in adults varies between 60 and 120 msec.

The axis of the terminal 40 msec (0.04 seconds) of the QRS complex can be considered separately. This part of the QRS complex represents the late stages of ventricular myocardial depolarization and generally points in the direction of the overall axis. Thus, under normal conditions, most patients do not manifest any significant deflection at this point. This axis is simply determined

by examining the last box (0.04 seconds, or 40 msec) of the QRS complex on the electrocardiogram paper.

The Abnormal QRS Complex.   In the presence of a bundle branch block, the two ventricles depolarize sequentially rather than concurrently. Although conceptually conduction through either the left or right bundle may be affected, many drugs preferentially affect the right bundle. This drug effect typically results in the left ventricle depolarizing slightly more rapidly than the right. The consequence on the electrocardiogram is both a widening of the QRS complex and the appearance of the right ventricular electrical forces that were previously obscured by those of the left ventricle. When these changes are a result of the effects of a drug, agents that block fast sodium channels are predictably implicated. Examples include cyclic antidepressants, quinidine and other type IA and IC antidysrhythmic agents, phenothiazines,[2] amantadine, diphenhydramine,[9] carbamazepine, and cocaine. In the setting of tricyclic antidepressant poisoning, this finding has both prognostic and therapeutic value (Chap. 57).[14,18,19,31] Specifically, in a prospective analysis of ECGs the maximal limb lead QRS duration was prognostic of seizures (0% if <100 msec; 30% if greater) and ventricular dysrhythmias (0% if <160 msec; 50% if greater).[5]

This terminal 40-msec axis of the QRS complex contains critical information regarding the likelihood, not the extent, of poisoning by sodium channel blocking agents. Alteration of this axis from poisoning most commonly involves finding an R wave (positive deflection) in lead aV$_R$ and an S wave (negative deflection) in leads I and aV$_L$.[21] The interpretation of this finding is that the patient has a rightward deviation, greater than 120°, of this segment. The combination of a rightward axis shift in the terminal 40 msec of the QRS complex (Fig. 9–7) along with a prolonged QTc and a sinus tachycardia is highly specific and sensitive for cyclic antidepressant poisoning, and their absence, in one study at least, excluded tricyclic antidepressant poisoning.[28,40] Although not specifically studied, this finding may also hold value in patients with exposure to other toxins with sodium channel blocking effects. In addition, a prospective study suggests that an absolute height of the terminal portion of aV$_R$ that is greater than 3 mm predicted seizures or dysrhythmias in tricyclic antidepressant–poisoned patients.[20] In infants younger than 6 months old, however, a rightward deviation of the terminal 40-msec QRS axis is physiologic and not predictive of tricyclic antidepressant toxicity.[4] In older children, retrospective chart review of 37 children diagnosed with tricyclic antidepressant overdose and 35 controls (all younger than 11 years old) found such interpatient variability, unrelated to age, that a rightward deviation of the terminal 40-msec QRS axis could not distinguish between poisoned and healthy children.[4]

An apparent increase in QRS duration, which is actually an elevation or distortion of the J point called a J wave or an Osborn wave (Chap. 18, Fig. 18–2), is a common finding in patients with hypothermia.[29,35,37] Hypermagnesemia is also associated with an increase in the QRS duration and a slight narrowing of the QRS complex may occur with hypomagnesemia.[26] Abnormalities in the serum concentrations of potassium may also cause widening and distortion of the QRS complex.

The ST Segment

Electrophysiology.   The ST segment is the distance between the end of the QRS complex and the beginning of the T wave. This segment reflects the period of time between depolarization and the

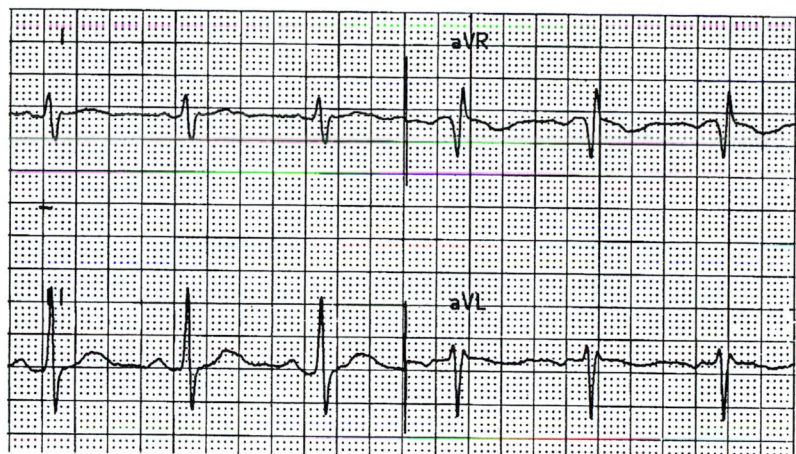

Figure 9–7. ECG showing leads I, II, aV$_R$, and aV$_L$ of a patient with a tricyclic antidepressant overdose. The prominent S wave in leads I and aV$_L$ and R wave in aV$_R$ demonstrate the terminal 40-msec rightward axis shift.

start of repolarization, or the plateau phase of the action potential. During this period, no currents flow within the myocardium, explaining why under normal circumstances the ST segment is isoelectric. Although both the degree of displacement from the baseline and the length of this segment are important, the ST segment duration is usually measured by its effects on the QT duration (see later). The J point is the site at which the T wave begins following the ST segment.

The Abnormal ST Segment. Displacement of the ST segment from its baseline characterizes myocardial ischemia or infarction (Fig. 9–8). The subsequent appearance of a Q wave is diagnostic of myocardial infarction. The electrocardiographic patterns of these entities reflect the different underlying electrophysiologic states of the heart. Ischemic regions are highly unstable and produce currents of injury because of inadequate repolarization, which is related to lack of energy substrate to power the Na$^+$-K$^+$ ATPase. Infarction represents the loss of electrical activity from the necrotic, inactive left ventricular tissue (typically), allowing right ventricular forces to be visualized. Patients who are poisoned by agents that commonly cause vasoconstriction, such as cocaine (Chap. 67), other α-adrenergic agonists, or the ergot alkaloids, are particularly prone to develop focal myocardial ischemia and infarction. The specific electrocardiographic manifestations help to identify the region injured and may, to some extent, be correlated with an arterial flow pattern: inferior (leads II, III, aV$_F$; right coronary artery); anterior (I, aV$_L$; left anterior descending artery); or lateral (aV$_L$, V$_{5-6}$; circumflex branch). However, any poisoning that results in profound hypotension or hypoxia may also result in ECG changes of ischemia, injury, and cellular death. In this situation, the injury may be more global, involving more than one arterial distribution. Diffuse myocardial damage may not be identifiable on the electrocardiogram because there are global, symmetric electrical abnormalities. In this situation, the diagnosis is made by other noninvasive testing, such as by echocardiogram.

Many young, healthy patients have ST segment abnormalities that may mimic those of myocardial infarction. The most common normal variant is termed "early repolarization" or "J-point elevation," and is identified as diffusely elevated, upwardly concave ST segments, located commonly in the patients' precordial leads and typically with corresponding T waves of large amplitude.[7] Because this electrocardiographic variant is common in patients with

cocaine-associated chest pain (Chap. 67),[17] its recognition is critical to avoid the administration of unneeded thrombolytic therapy.

Sagging ST segments, inverted T waves, and normal or shortened QT intervals are characteristic effects of cardiac glycosides on the electrocardiogram. These repolarization abnormalities are sometimes identified by their similar appearance to "Salvador Dali's mustache." As a group, these findings, along with PR prolongation, are commonly described as "digitalis effect." They are found in patients with therapeutic drug levels and in patients with cardiac glycoside poisoning. As the serum, or more precisely the

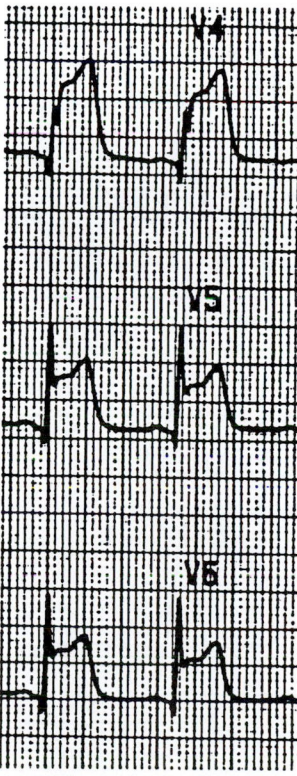

Figure 9–8. Leads V$_4$–V$_6$ are shown from the ECG of a 27-year-old with substernal chest pain after using crack cocaine.

tissue, digoxin concentration increases, clinical and electrocardiographic manifestations of toxicity will appear (Chap. 48).

Changes in the duration of the ST duration are frequently caused by abnormalities in the serum calcium concentration. Hypercalcemia causes shortening of the ST segment through enhanced calcium influx, although for practical purposes this effect is most commonly identified by reduction of the QTc interval (Fig. 9–9). In patients with hypercalcemia, the morphology and duration of the QRS complex and T and P waves remain essentially unchanged. Drug-induced hypercalcemia may result from exposure to antacids (milk alkali syndrome), diuretics (eg, hydrochlorothiazide), cholecalciferol (vitamin D), vitamin A, and other retinoids. Hypocalcemia causes prolongation of the QT interval (Fig. 9–9).

The T Wave

Electrophysiology.   The T wave represents ventricular repolarization. The polarity of repolarization generally proceeds in the same direction as depolarization and thus the deflection is usually in the same direction as the QRS complex.

The Abnormal T Wave.   Isolated peaked T waves are usually evidence of early hyperkalemia.[25] Hyperkalemia at levels less than 6.5 mEq/L causes tall, tented T waves with normal QRS, QTc, and P wave (Fig. 9–10). As the measured potassium rises to 6.5–8 mEq/L, the P wave diminishes in amplitude and the PR and QRS intervals prolong. Progressive widening of the QRS complex causes it to merge with the ST segment and T wave forming a sine wave. Electrocardiographic manifestations of hyperkalemia may occur following chronic exposure to numerous therapeutic agents including potassium sparing diuretics, angiotensin-converting enzyme inhibitors (Chap. 51), or potassium supplements. Either flu-

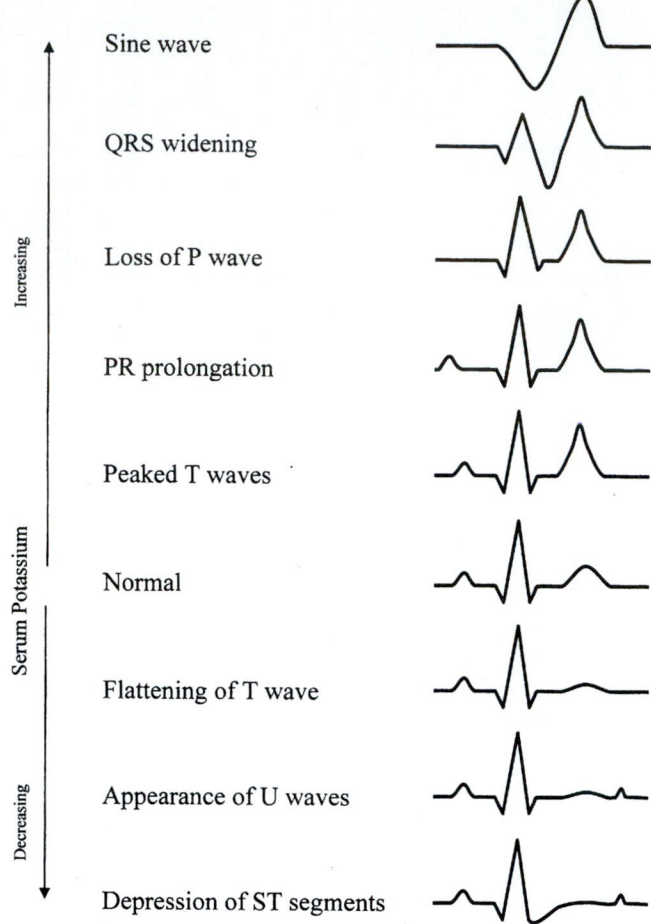

Figure 9–10. Electrocardiographic manifestations associated with changes in serum potassium.

oride or cardiac glycoside poisoning produces acute hyperkalemia, but the latter rarely produces hyperkalemic electrocardiogram changes (Chap. 24). Peaked T waves also occur following myocardial ischemia and may also be confused with early repolarization effects (see The ST Segment). Thus, the ability to properly identify electrolyte abnormalities by electrocardiography is often limited.[42]

Hypokalemia, on the other hand, typically reduces the amplitude of the T wave and, ultimately, the appearance of prominent U waves (Fig. 9–10). Its effects on the electrocardiogram are manifestations of altered myocardial repolarization. Lithium similarly affects myocardial ion fluxes and causes reversible changes on the electrocardiogram that may mimic mild hypokalemia, although documentation of low cellular potassium levels is lacking.[10,34] Patients chronically poisoned with lithium have more T-wave abnormalities than do those who are acutely poisoned.[22] T-wave flattening is the most commonly reported electrocardiographic abnormality.[6] Other findings include T-wave inversion, ST segment depression or elevation, and conduction abnormalities. The clinical significance of these reversible ECG findings is unclear. More serious cardiovascular manifestations, including ventricular dysrhythmias[12,41] and myocardial infarction,[30] are rare, but reportedly occur following serious lithium overdose.

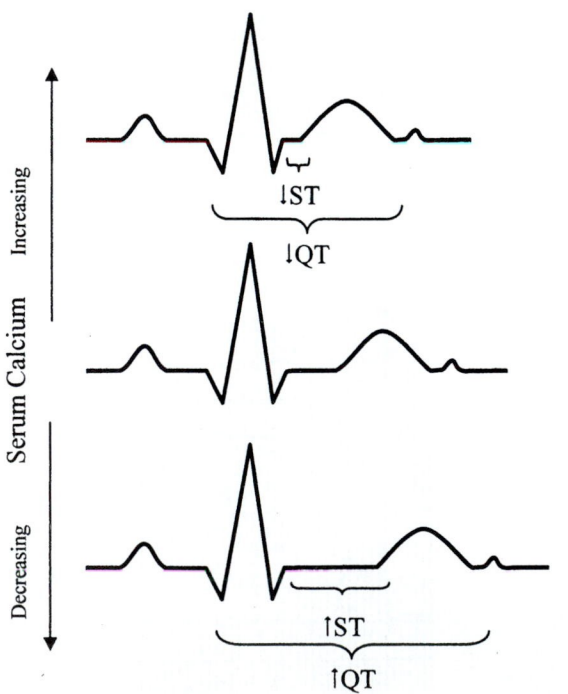

Figure 9–9. Electrocardiographic findings associated with changes in serum calcium.

The QT Interval

Electrophysiology. The QT interval represents the entire duration of ventricular systole and is measured from the beginning of the QRS complex to the end of the T wave. The bipolar limb lead with the largest T wave should be used for this measurement. As the normal QT interval varies with the heart rate, numerous formulas (such as $QT \div \sqrt{RR}$ interval) and tables are available to obtain the corrected QT interval (QTc).[15] Using the QTc allows the determination of the appropriateness of the QT interval independent of the heart rate. With slow heart rates, a prominent U wave can obscure the terminal portion of the T wave, and with fast heart rates, the subsequent P wave can obscure the terminal portion of the T wave. In these cases the QT interval should be estimated by following the downslope of the T wave.

The Abnormal QT Interval. A prolonged QT interval increases the time period that the heart is "vulnerable" to the initiation of ventricular dysrhythmias[32] (Fig. 9–6). This occurs because although some myocardial fibers are refractory during this time period, others are not. Early afterdepolarizations may be responsible for the lengthened repolarization time and ventricular tachydysrhythmias in long QT syndromes, and in patients with drug-induced torsades de pointes (Fig. 9–11 and Table 9–2).[27] An "early afterdepolarization" (EAD) occurs when an impulse reaches the myocardial cell before repolarization is complete (Fig. 9–12), and causes a depolarization leading to electrical chaos. This chaos may manifest as ventricular tachycardia, ventricular fibrillation, or torsades de pointes. There are two types of EADs that occur either when the membrane potential is decreased during phase 2 (type 1) and phase 3 (type 2) of the cardiac action potential. The ionic basis of EADs is unclear, but may be via the L-type calcium channel; EADs are suppressed by magnesium.[1,36]

Agents that cause sodium channel blockade, or Vaughan-Williams Class I antidysrhythmic agents (Chap. 52), prolong the QT duration by slowing cellular depolarization during phase 0. Thus, the QT duration increases due to a prolongation of the QRS complex duration, and the ST segment duration remains near normal. Agents that cause potassium channel blockade, or Class III antidysrhythmic agents, similarly prolong the QT interval, but through prolongation of the plateau and repolarization phases. This specifically prolongs the ST segment duration. Although at a cellular level these agents are antidysrhythmic, the multicellular effects may be prodysrhythmic.[32] Prolongation of the QT interval may be caused by numerous agents that affect ventricular repolarization.

Hypocalcemia is caused by a number of agents, including fluoride, calcitonin, ethylene glycol, phosphates, and mithramycin (Chap. 24, Table 24–9). Hypokalemia and hypomagnesemia alone do not usually prolong the QT interval. Arsenic poisoning may cause prolongation of the QT interval and torsades de pointes.[3] The mechanism is unknown, although either a direct dysrhythmogenic effect or an autoimmune myocarditis are postulated.

The U Wave

Electrophysiology. The U wave is a small deflection that occurs after the T wave and usually with a similar orientation. One theory is that the U wave represents afterpotentials, or incomplete repolarization, of the ventricular myocardium. Another proposed mechanism is that the U wave is caused by repolarization of the Purkinje fibers. Distinguishing a U wave from a notched T wave is difficult. The apices of a notched T wave are usually less than 150 msec apart, and the peaks of a TU complex are greater than 150 msec apart.

The Abnormal U Wave. Hypokalemia is the most common cause of prominent U waves (Chap. 24). As the serum potassium declines from the normal range, ECG findings include ST depression and a progressive decrease in the amplitude of the T wave. When the serum potassium decreases further, the amplitude of the U wave increases and eventually the U and T waves fuse. The amplitude and duration of both the QRS complex and the P wave increase as the PR interval lengthens. Ventricular tachycardia, torsades de pointes, ventricular fibrillation, and asystole may develop if proper therapy is not instituted. Hypokalemia is a common adverse effect of many medications and toxins including loop and thiazide diuretics, cathartics, toluene, soluble barium salts, and sympathomimetic agents (Chap. 24, Table 24–8). Transient U-wave inversion can be caused by myocardial ischemia or systemic hypertension.

The Abnormal QU Interval. The QU interval is the distance between the end of the Q wave and the end of the U wave. Differentiation between the QU and the QT intervals is difficult if the T and U waves are superimposed. When hypomagnesemia coexists with hypokalemia, as is usually the case, QU prolongation and torsades de pointes may occur.[36]

ELECTROCARDIOGRAM DISTURBANCES

The distinction between toxins that cause a rapid rate and those that cause a slow rate on the ECG is somewhat artificial, because many agents can do both. For example, patients poisoned by tricyclic antidepressants always develop sinus tachycardia, but most die with a wide complex bradycardic rhythm. Regardless, abnormalities in the pattern or rate on the electrocardiogram can provide

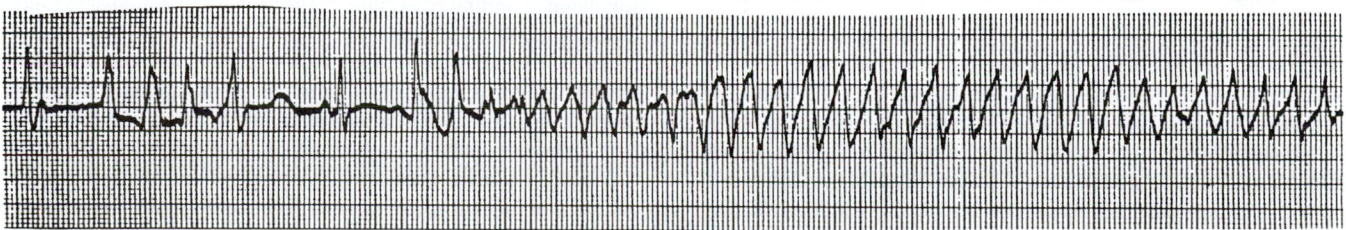

Figure 9–11. Torsades de pointes in a patient who ingested an unknown amount of thioridazine.

TABLE 9–2. Classification and Causes of an Acquired Long QT Interval

Antidysrhythmic drugs
  Class IA and IC drugs
  Class III drugs
Electrolyte disturbances
  Hypokalemia
  Hypomagnesemia
Nonantidysrhythmic drugs
  Psychotropic agents: phenothiazines, haloperidol, atypical antipsychotics tricyclic and tetracyclic antidepressants
  Antihypertensive agents: bepridil, ketanserin
  Antimicrobial agents: erythromycin, trimethoprim-sulfamethoxazole, pentamidine, amantidine, chloroquine
  Antifungal agents: ketoconazole, itraconazole
  Antihistaminic agents: terfenadine, astemizole
  Other drugs: cisapride, cocaine, organic phosphorus insecticides, arsenic, vasopressin
Other conditions
  Cardiac disorders: myocarditis, ventricular tumor
  Endocrine disorders: hypothyroidism, hypoparathyroidism, pheochromocytoma, hyperaldosteronism
  Intracranial disorders: subarachnoid hemorrhage, cerebrovascular accident, encephalitis, head injury
  Nutritional disorders: liquid protein diet, starvation
  Severe bradycardia

the clinician with immediate information about a patient's cardiovascular status. Any rhythm other than normal sinus rhythm is referred to as a dysrhythmia in this text. Electrocardiographic disturbances in many poisoned patients may be categorized in more than one manner (abnormal pattern, fast rate, slow rate). Regardless, when electrocardiographic abnormalities are detected, appropriate interpretation, evaluation, and therapy must be rapidly performed.

Tachydysrhythmias

The intrinsic pacemaker cells of the heart undergo spontaneous depolarization and reach threshold at a predictable rate. Under

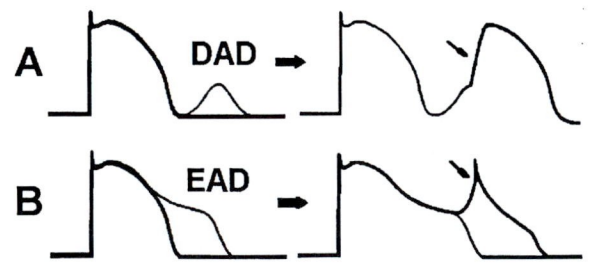

Figure 9–12. **A.** Delayed afterdepolarization (DAD) arising after full repolarization. A delayed afterdepolarization that reaches threshold results in a triggered upstroke (*arrow, right*). **B.** Early afterdepolarization (EAD) interrupting phase 3 repolarization. Under some conditions, a triggered beat can arise from an early afterdepolarization (*arrow, right*). (*Reproduced, with permission, from Roden DM: Antiarrhythmic drugs. In: Hardman JG, Limbird LE, Molinoff PB, Ruddon RW, Gilman AG, eds: Goodman and Gilman's The Pharmacological Basis of Therapeutics, 9th ed. New York, McGraw-Hill, 1996, p. 845.*)

normal circumstances the sinus node is the most rapidly firing pacemaker cell of the heart; because of this, it controls the heart rate. Spontaneous depolarization occurs during ion entry through potassium, sodium, and calcium channels during phase 4 of the action potential. Other potential pacemakers exist in the heart, but their rate of spontaneous depolarization is considerably slower than that of the sinus node. Thus, they are reset during depolarization of the myocardium and they never spontaneously reach threshold. Agents that speed the rate of rise of phase 4, or diastolic depolarization, speed the rate of firing of the pacemaker cells. As long as the sinus node is preferentially affected, it maintains the pacemaker activity of the heart. If the firing rate of another intrinsic pacemaker exceeds that of the sinus node, ectopic rhythms may develop. This effect may be either pathologic or lifesaving depending on the clinical circumstances.

Because the rate of impulse formation at the sinus node is regulated by the balance between parasympathetic and sympathetic tone, varying the influences of these parts of the autonomic nervous system is responsible for regulating the heart rate under normal conditions. Sympathomimetic agents, such as norepinephrine, cocaine, and amphetamines, increase sympathetic tone, producing sinus tachycardia and enhancing AV nodal conduction. Sinus tachycardia may be the first manifestation of exposure to a sympathomimetic agent. However, other supraventricular or ventricular dysrhythmias may develop if an abnormal rhythm is generated in another part of the heart. Similarly, agents that antagonize acetylcholine released from the vagus nerve onto the sinus node enhance the rate of firing, producing sinus tachycardia. Such agents include the belladonna alkaloids atropine and scopolamine, antihistamines, and the tricyclic antidepressants. Table 21–7 lists a wide variety of agents that often cause tachydysrhythmias.

Certain agents are more highly associated with ventricular tachydysrhythmias following poisoning. Those that alter myocardial repolarization and prolong the QT interval predispose to the development of R on T phenomena, which initiates ventricular tachycardia. If torsades de pointes is noted, this is undoubtedly the mechanism, and the QT interval should be carefully assessed and appropriate treatment initiated. Alternatively, agents that increase the adrenergic tone on the heart, either directly or indirectly, may cause ventricular dysrhythmias. Whether a result of excessive circulating catecholamines (eg, cocaine), myocardial sensitization (eg, halogenated hydrocarbons, thyroid hormone), or increased second messenger activity (eg, theophylline), the extreme inotropic and chronotropic effects cause dysrhythmias. Altered repolarization, increased intracellular calcium concentrations, or myocardial ischemia may cause the dysrhythmia. Additionally, drugs that produce focal myocardial ischemia, such as cocaine or ephedrine, may lead to malignant ventricular dysrhythmias. Finally, an uncommon cause of drug-induced ventricular dysrhythmias is persistent activation of sodium channels, as occurs following aconitine poisoning.[33] There are no distinguishing electrocardiographic findings.

Not all wide QRS complex tachydysrhythmias are ventricular in origin, but making this assumption is generally considered to be prudent. For example, in a patient known to be poisoned with tricyclic antidepressants, cocaine, or similar agents (see The QRS Complex), the differentiation of aberrantly conducted sinus tachycardia (common) from ventricular tachycardia (rare) is important, but difficult. Although guidelines for determining the origin of a wide complex tachydysrhythmia exist,[8] they are imperfect, difficult to apply, and unstudied in poisoned patients.

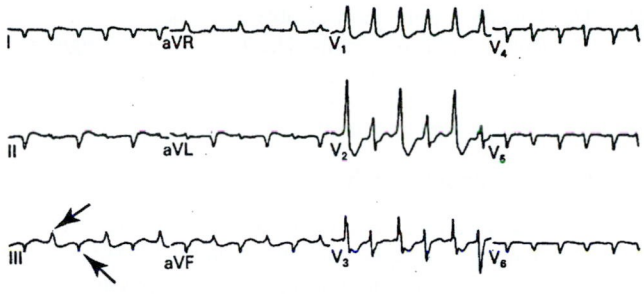

Figure 9–13. Digoxin-induced bidirectional ventricular tachycardia. A 71-year-old woman had recently undergone mitral-valve replacement after being treated with digoxin for 12 years for atrial fibrillation. After the operation, the same dose of digoxin was administered intravenously, despite rising creatinine levels. The 12-lead electrocardiogram shows an alternating QRS axis that is characteristic of bidirectional ventricular tachycardia (*arrows*), a dysrhythmia virtually diagnostic of digitalis toxicity. The serum digoxin level at the time of the electrocardiogram was 4.5 ng/mL (normal, 0.8–2.0 ng/mL). *(Reproduced, with permission, from Valent S, Kelly P: Images in clinical medicine: Digoxin-induced bidiretional ventricular tachycardia. N Engl J Med 1997;336:550.)*

Bidirectional ventricular tachycardia is particularly characteristic of severe cardiac glycoside toxicity and results from alterations of intraventricular conduction, junctional tachycardia with aberrant intraventricular conduction, or on rare occasions, alternating ventricular pacemakers (Fig. 9–13). The only other drug that is commonly associated with this dysrhythmia is aconitine, usually from traditional or alternative therapies (Chaps. 77 and 78).

Bradydysrhythmias

Bradycardia and asystole are the terminal events following fatal ingestions of many drugs, but some agents tend to cause sinus bradycardia (Table 21–9) and conduction abnormalities (Table 21–8) early in the course of toxicity. Sinus bradycardia with an otherwise normal electrocardiogram is characteristic of drugs that reduce central nervous system outflow. Examples include benzodiazepines, ethanol, and clonidine, and differentiating between these agents is not possible based on electrocardiographic criteria alone. Agents that directly affect ion flux across myocardial cell membranes cause abnormalities in AV nodal conduction. Calcium

channel blockers, β-adrenergic receptor antagonists, and cardiac glycosides (see Chaps. 48–51) are the leading causes of sinus bradycardia and conduction disturbances.

The electrocardiographic manifestations of calcium channel blocker and β-adrenergic antagonist overdoses are difficult to distinguish. In general, both drug classes cause decreased dromotropy (conduction), although the specific pharmacologic actions of the drugs differ even within the class (Chaps. 49 and 50). For example, most members of the dihydropyridine subclass of calcium channel blockers do not have any antidromotropic effect, whereas verapamil and diltiazem routinely produce PR prolongation. Similarly, while most β-adrenergic antagonists produce sinus bradycardia, certain members of this group, such as propranolol, may prolong the QRS complex through their sodium channel blocking abilities. Others, such as sotalol, which have properties of the class III agents, block myocardial potassium channels and prolong the QT interval duration. The bradycardia produced by cardiac glycosides is typically accompanied by signs of "digitalis effect" including PR prolongation and ST segment depression (Chap. 48).

Ectopy

Ectopy is the electrocardiographic manifestation of myocardial depolarization initiated from a site other than the sinus node. Ectopy may be lifesaving under circumstances in which the atrial rhythm cannot be conducted to the ventricles, as during high-degree AV blockade induced by cardiac glycosides. Alternatively, ectopy may lead to dramatic alterations in the physiologic function of the heart or deteriorate into lethal ventricular dysrhythmias (Fig. 9–14).

Several mechanisms by which ectopic rhythms may develop are noted. An impulse that occurs after completion of repolarization (phase 4) is called a "delayed afterdepolarization" (DAD) (Figs. 9–12 and 9–15 and Table 9–3). The mechanism of DADs is related to increases in intracellular calcium that activate a nonselective cation channel or an electrogenic Na^+-Ca^{2+} exchanger that causes a transient inward current carried primarily by sodium ions. This inward sodium current generates the DAD. The increased calcium concentrations may come from extensive sympathetic stimulation,[24] large doses of cardiac glycosides, or other abnormal physiologic conditions. Delayed afterdepolarizations are the likely cause of some dysrhythmias induced by cardiac glycoside poisoning (Chap. 48). Compared with EADs, DADs generally arise when the membrane potential is more negative.

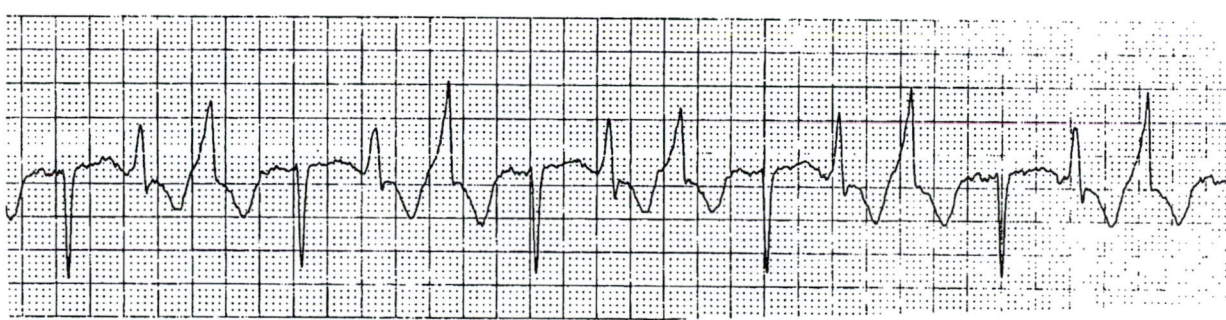

Figure 9–14. This rhythm strip shows ventricular ectopy in a patient following a chloral hydrate overdose. Following the administration of propranolol the ectopy resolved.

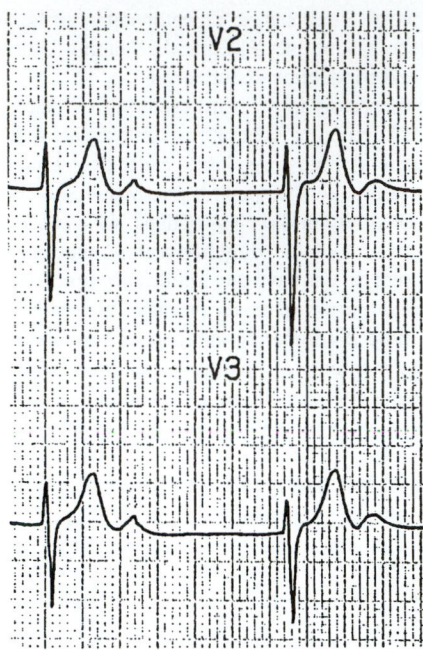

Figure 9–15. This ECG was recorded from a 20-year-old man who ingested an unknown quantity of digoxin. Delayed afterdepolarizations can be seen following the T waves.

THE PEDIATRIC ELECTROCARDIOGRAM

The Normal Pediatric ECG

The normal pediatric ECG differs in many ways from the normal adult ECG. The resting heart rate of infants and children is substantially higher than that of adults, and conduction, in general, is faster. In a term infant, the right ventricle is substantially larger than the left, and the ECG demonstrates prominent R waves in the right precordium and deep S waves in the left lateral precordium.[11] An adult ratio of left-right ventricular size is usually reached by the age of 6 months. In infants, Q waves commonly exist in the inferior and lateral precordial leads, but are abnormal in leads I and

aV$_L$. The T waves are the most notable difference between pediatric and adult electrocardiograms. The T waves in the right precordial leads in children are deeply inverted until age 7 and sometimes beyond (persistent juvenile T-wave pattern).

The Abnormal Pediatric ECG

Although congenital heart disease is the most common cause of electrocardiographic abnormalities in children, electrolyte disorders and drugs may also cause changes in electrophysiology that are reflected on the ECG. Abnormalities that are useful markers on the adult ECG may not always be as useful in the pediatric population.

SUMMARY

The electrocardiogram (ECG) is one of the few widely available diagnostic procedures that reveal immediate, useful clinical information. This has far-reaching implications in toxicology, where other diagnostic test results often return too late to effectively impact the care of an acutely poisoned patient.

REFERENCES

1. Baillie DS, Inoue H, Kaseda S, et al: Magnesium suppresses early depolarizations and ventricular tachyarrhythmias induced in dogs by cesium. Circulation 1989;77:1395–1402.
2. Banta TA, St Jean A: The effect of phenothiazines on the electrocardiogram. Can Med Assoc J 1964;91:537.
3. Beckman KJ, Bauman JS, Pimental PA, et al: Arsenic-induced torsades de pointes. Crit Care Med 1991;19:290–292.
4. Berkovitch M, Matsui D, Fogelman R, et al: Assessment of the terminal 40-millisecond QRS vector in children with a history of tricyclic antidepressant ingestion. Pediatr Emerg Care 1995;11:75–77.
5. Boehnert M, Lovejoy FH Jr: Value of the QRS duration versus the serum drug level in predicting seizures and ventricular arrhythmias after an acute overdose of tricyclic antidepressants. N Engl J Med 1985;313:474–479.
6. Brady HR, Horgan JH: Lithium and the heart: Unanswered questions. Chest 1988;93:166–169.
7. Brady WJ, Chan TC. Electrocardiographic manifestations: Benign early repolarization. J Emerg Med 1999;17:473–478.

TABLE 9–3.   The Electrophysiologic Basis for Delayed Afterdepolarization and Early Afterdepolarization

	Phase of Action Potential Affected by Depolarization	Clinical Effect	Mechanism
Delayed after-depolarization (DAD)	After repolarization is complete Phase 4	Cardiac glycoside–induced dysrhythmias	↑ intracellular Ca^{++} →→ Activation of a nonselective cation channel or Na$^+$ -Ca^{++} exchanger →→ Transient inward current carried mostly by Na$^+$ ions
Early after-depolarization (EAD)	During repolarization	↑ repolarization time Long QT syndrome (hereditary and acquired)	Possibly via L-type calcium channels
Type 1	Phase 2	Drug-induced torsades de pointes, ventricular tachycardia	Suppressed by magnesium
Type 2	Phase 3		

8. Brugada P, Brugada J, Mont L, et al: A new approach to the differential diagnosis of a regular tachycardia with a wide QRS complex. Circulation 1991;83:1649–1659.

9. Clark RF, Vance M: Massive diphenhydramine poisoning resulting in a wide-complex tachycardia: Successful treatment with sodium bicarbonate. Ann Emerg Med 1992;21:318–321.

10. Cooper R, LeGrady D, Nanas S, et al: Increased sodium-lithium countertransport in college students with elevated blood pressure. JAMA 1983;249:1030–1034.

11. Davignon A, Rautabarjo P, Boiselle E, et al: Normal ECG standards for infants and children. Pediatr Cardiol 1979;1:123.

12. Demers RG, Heninger G: Electrocardiographic changes during lithium therapy. Dis Nerv Syst 1970;31:674–677.

13. Einthoven W: Die galvanometrische Registrirung des menschlichen Elecktrokardiogramms, zugleich eine Beurteilung der Anwendung des Capillar-Elektrometers in der Physiologie. Arch f d g Physiol 1903;99:472.

14. Foulke GE: Identifying toxicity risk early after antidepressant overdose. Am J Emerg Med 1995;13:123–126.

15. Funck-Brentano C, Jaillon P: Rate-corrected QT interval: Techniques and limitations. Am J Cardiol 1993;72:17B–22B.

16. Goldberger E: A simple, indifferent, electrocardiographic electrode of aero potential and a technique of obtaining augmented, unipolar, extremity leads. Am Heart J 1942;23:483–492.

17. Hollander JE, Lozano M, Fairweather P, et al: "Abnormal" electrocardiograms in patients with cocaine-associated chest pain are due to "normal" variants. J Emerg Med 1994;12:199–205.

18. Hulten B-A, Adams R, Askenasi R, et al: Predicting severity of tricyclic antidepressant overdose. J Toxicol Clin Toxicol 1992;30:161–170.

19. Lavoie FW, Gansert GG, Weiss RE: Value of initial ECG findings and plasma drug levels in cyclic antidepressant overdose. Ann Emerg Med 1990;19:696–699.

20. Liebelt EL, Francis PD, Woolfe AD: ECG lead aVR versus QRS complex in predicting seizures and arrhythmias in acute tricyclic antidepressant toxicity. Ann Emerg Med 1995;26:195–201.

21. Liebelt EL: Serial electrocardiogram changes in acute tricyclic antidepressant overdoses. Crit Care Med 1997;25:1721–1726.

22. Linakis J, Woolf A: Clinical features of acute versus chronic lithium intoxication [abstract]. Vet Hum Toxicol 1989;31:370.

23. Madfsen PS, Strom J, Reiz S: Acute propoxyphene poisoning in 222 consecutive cases. Acta Anaesth Scand 1984;28:661–665.

24. Marchi S, Szabo B, Lazzara R: Adrenergic induction of delayed afterdepolarizations in ventricular myocardial cells: Beta induction and alpha modulation. J Cardiovasc Electrophysiol 1991;2:476.

25. Mattu A, Brady WJ, Robinson DA. Electrocardiographic manifestations of hyperkalemia. Am J Emerg Med 2000;18:721–729.

26. Miller JR, Van Dellen TR: Electrocardiographic changes following the intravenous administration of magnesium sulfate. J Lab Clin Med 1941;26:1116–1120.

27. Nguyen PT, Scheinman MM, Seger J: Polymorphous ventricular tachycardia: Clinical characterization, therapy, and the QT interval. Circulation 1986;74:340–349.

28. Niemann JT, Bessen HA, Rothstein RJ, et al: Electrocardiographic criteria for tricyclic antidepressant overdose. Ann Emerg Med 1986;57:1154–1159.

29. Osborn JJ: Experimental hypothermia: Respiratory and blood pH changes in relation to cardiac function. Am J Physiol 1953;175:389.

30. Perrier A, Martin P-Y, Fuvre H, et al: Very severe self-poisoning: Lithium carbonate intoxication causing a myocardial infarction. Chest 1991;100:863–865.

31. Shannon M: Duration of QRS disturbances after severe tricyclic antidepressant intoxication. J Toxicol Clin Toxicol 1992;30:377–386.

32. Starmer FC: The cardiac vulnerable period and reentrant arrhythmias: Targets of anti- and proarrhythmic processes. PACE 1997;20(pt II):445–454.

33. Tai YT, But PP-H, Young K, Cau C-P: Cardiotoxicity after accidental herb-induced aconite poisoning. Lancet 1992;340:1254–1256.

34. Tilkian AS, Schroeder JS, Kao JJ: Cardiovascular effects of lithium in man: A review of the literature. Am J Med 1976;61:665–670.

35. Trevino A, Razi B, Beller BM: The characteristic electrocardiogram of accidental hypothermia. Arch Intern Med 1971;127:470.

36. Tzivoni D, Keren A, Cohen AM, et al: Magnesium therapy for torsades de pointes. Am J Cardiol 1984;53:528–530.

37. Vassallo SU, Delaney KA, Hoffman RS, Slater W, Goldfrank LR: A prospective evaluation of the electrocardiographic manifestations of hypothermia. Acad Emerg Med 1999;6:1121–1126.

38. Waller AD: Demonstration on man of the electromotive changes accompanying the heart's beat. J Physiol 1887;8:229.

39. Wilson FN: Foreword. In: Barker JM: The Unipolar Electrogram: A Clinical Interpretation. New York, Appleton-Century-Crofts, 1952, p. xii.

40. Wolfe TR, Caravati EM, Rollins DE, et al: Terminal 40-ms frontal plane QRS axis as a marker for tricyclic antidepressant overdose. Ann Emerg Med 1989;18:348–351.

41. Worthley L: Lithium toxicity and refractory cardiac arrhythmias treated with intravenous magnesium. Anesth Intensive Care 1974;2:357–360.

42. Wrenn KD, Slovis BS, Slovis CM. The ability of physicians to predict electrolyte deficiency from the ECG. Ann Emerg Med 1990;19:580–583.

43. Yamaura K, Kao B, Iimori E, et al: Recurrent ventricular tachyarrhythmias associated with QT prolongation following hydrofluoric acid burns. J Toxicol Clin Toxicol 1997;35:311–313.

PART B

THE BIOCHEMICAL AND MOLECULAR BASIS OF MEDICAL TOXICOLOGY

CHAPTER 10 NEUROTRANSMITTERS

Steven C. Curry / Kirk C. Mills / Kimberlie A. Graeme

Many poisonous substances produce their primary toxic effects by affecting neurotransmission. This chapter reviews the normal physiology of neurotransmission, the molecular action and biochemistry of several major neurotransmitters and their receptors, and the toxicologic mechanisms by which numerous substances act at the molecular level. Neurotransmitters and neuromodulators of particular toxicologic interest that are discussed in this chapter are acetylcholine, norepinephrine, epinephrine, dopamine, serotonin, γ-aminobutyric acid, γ-hydroxybutyrate, glycine, glutamate, and adenosine.

When examining molecular actions of drugs and toxins on neurotransmitter systems, it is apparent that substances rarely possess single pharmacologic actions. For example, doxepin, in part, antagonizes voltage-gated sodium channels, histaminic H_1 and H_2 receptors, α-adrenoceptors, muscarinic acetylcholine receptors, dopamine D_2 receptors, and $GABA_A$ receptors; prevents potassium efflux; and inhibits norepinephrine, serotonin, and adenosine uptake. For obvious reasons, then, this chapter cannot include every action of every drug or toxin on the nervous system. Nor is it meant to be a complete discussion of toxic syndromes produced by various agents, as these are discussed in specific chapters. Rather, this chapter provides a general and basic understanding of the mechanisms of action of various toxic agents affecting neurotransmitter function and receptors, especially in the central nervous system. With this focus, the clinical effects produced by various toxins are more easily understood and predicted, and specific treatments aimed at reversing pharmacologic effects of the offending agents can be rationally undertaken.

Given the complexity of the nervous system and the numerous actions of a given drug, it is not always clear which neurotransmitter system is producing an observed effect during a particular toxicity. Therefore, pharmacologic agents discussed in this chapter may be found in several sections. In each section, an attempt is made to note what appears to be a drug or toxin's main mechanism of action, although other actions are noted when possible.

NEURON PHYSIOLOGY AND NEUROTRANSMISSION

Membrane Potentials, Ion Channels, and Nerve Conduction

Membrane-bound sodium-potassium ATPase moves three sodium ions (Na^+) from inside the cell to the interstitial space while pumping two potassium ions (K^+) into the cell. Because the cell membrane is not freely permeable to large, negatively charged molecules on the inside of the cell, such as proteins, an equilibrium results in which the inside of the neuron is negative with respect to the outside. This typical neuronal resting membrane potential is -65 mV.

Sodium, calcium (Ca^{2+}), K^+, and chloride (Cl^-) ions move into and out of neurons through ion channels. Ions always move passively down electrochemical gradients through ion channels, which are long polypeptides comprising several subunits that span the plasma membrane several times. Many different ion channels are structurally comparable, sharing similar amino acid sequences.[16] Channels for a specific ion can also vary in structure, depending on the specific subunits that have combined to form the channel. Because of structural similarity of different channels, it is not surprising that many drugs or toxins are able to bind to more than one type of ion channel.

More than 40 different ion channels have been described in various nerve terminals,[93] and it is estimated that a human being contains hundreds of different varieties of ion channels for Na^+, Cl^-, Ca^{2+}, and K^+. Most ion channels fall into two general classes: voltage-gated (voltage-dependent) ion channels and ligand-gated ion channels.[93] Voltage-gated channels open or close in response to changes in membrane potential. Ligand-gated channels open or close when a ligand (eg, neurotransmitter) binds to the channel to change its configuration.

A commonly accepted model describes voltage-gated Na^+ channels and other voltage-gated channels in three possible states. Using Na^+ channels as an example, the Na^+ channel is closed at rest and impermeable to sodium, preventing Na^+ from moving into the cell. When the channel undergoes activation, the channel opens, allowing Na^+ to move intracellularly, down its electrochemical gradient. The channel then undergoes a third conformational change by becoming inactivated, preventing further influx of Na^+. The term *recovery* describes the conversion of inactive channels back to the resting state, a process that requires repolarization of the cell membrane.

Depolarization of a neuron usually results from an initial inward flux of cations (Na^+ or Ca^{2+}), or prevention of K^+ efflux. The fall in membrane potential (movement toward 0 mV) results in further activation of these voltage-dependent Na^+ channels, allowing yet a greater influx of cations. When the membrane potential falls to threshold, Na^+ channels are activated en masse, and there is a large influx of Na^+.

Depolarization of a segment of the neurolemma causes the adjacent neuronal membrane to reach threshold, resulting in the propagation of an action potential down the neuron. Sodium channel activation is quickly followed by inactivation. Over the short term, repolarization of the neuron occurring after inactivation of

Na$^+$ channels mainly results from efflux of K$^+$ and some influx of Cl$^-$.

Neurotransmitter Release

Neurotransmitters are chemicals that are released from nerve endings into the synapse, where they produce effects by binding to receptors on postsynaptic and/or presynaptic cell membranes. The receptors may be on other neurons or effector organs such as smooth muscle. Concentrations of neurotransmitters in cytoplasm are usually low because of rapid degradation by various enzymes and because they diffuse out of the nerve ending. To provide a source of neurotransmitters that is protected from degradation and that can be rapidly released, neurotransmitters are concentrated and stored within vesicles in the axonal nerve terminal for release. As a wave of depolarization from Na$^+$ influx reaches the nerve ending, the membrane depolarization causes voltage-gated Ca^{2+} channels to open, allowing Ca^{2+} to move rapidly into the cell. This influx of Ca^{2+} triggers exocytosis of vesicle contents into the synapse. The voltage-gated Ca^{2+} channels responsible for inward Ca^{2+} currents that trigger neurotransmitter release are mainly of the N and P/Q subtypes.[97,114] Calcium channel blockers used in clinical practice (eg, verapamil, nifedipine) do not block this subtype of voltage-dependent Ca^{2+} channel, but rather block the L type. However, L-subtype Ca^{2+} channels reside elsewhere on neurons, which explains the ability of traditional Ca^{2+} channel blockers to affect some neurologic functions.

Vesicle Transport of Neurotransmitters

The pH inside neurotransmitter vesicles is about 5.5, much lower than that in the cytoplasm. An ATPase in the vesicular membrane is responsible for movement of H$^+$ into the vesicular lumen. Vesicular uptake pumps that move neurotransmitters or their precursors from the cytoplasm into the vesicle lumen, in turn, are powered by the electrochemical H$^+$ gradient—ie, the movement of an H$^+$ out of the vesicle into the cytoplasm is coupled to the movement of a neurotransmitter from the cytoplasm into the vesicle. The five main, structurally unique, vesicular uptake pumps identified thus far are relatively specific for glutamate, acetylcholine, catecholamines, glycine/γ-aminobutyric acid, and ATP.[2,16] All vesicle uptake pumps appear to consist of 12 transmembrane segments.

Neurotransmitters are confined within the vesicle, to a great extent, by ion trapping, as they are more ionized and less able to diffuse back out of the vesicle at the lower pH. Anything that causes a decrease in the pH gradient across the vesicle membrane results in the movement of neurotransmitters into the cytoplasm.[137] For example, amphetamines move into vesicles, where they buffer H$^+$ ions, causing the movement of biogenic amine neurotransmitters out of vesicles, and raising cytoplasmic concentrations of neurotransmitters.[137,138]

Neurotransmitter Uptake

Although acetylcholine is inactivated in the synapse by enzymatic degradation, most neurotransmitters have their synaptic effects terminated by active uptake into neurons and, frequently, into glial cells. These transporters are distinct from those transporters responsible for movement of neurotransmitters into vesicles within the cytoplasm. Cell membrane transporters (uptake pumps) for different neurotransmitters are Na$^+$-dependent transport proteins, in which the uptake of neurotransmitters is accompanied by the movement of Na$^+$ (sometimes with movement of other ions) across the synaptic membrane.[2]

Neurotransmitter uptake transporters have been subdivided into two main families.[2] One family includes structurally similar uptake pumps for γ-aminobutyric acid, glycine, norepinephrine, dopamine, and serotonin. They generally comprise 600–700 amino acids, and form loops spanning the plasma membrane 12 times. The second family comprises the glutamate uptake transporters, which appear to traverse the plasma membrane 10 times.

Several properties make transporter proteins of particular toxicologic significance. First, they are capable of moving neurotransmitters in either direction; when cytoplasmic neurotransmitter concentrations are significantly elevated, neurotransmitters can be transported back into the synapse. Second, these transporters are not always completely specific for a particular substance. For instance, the uptake transporter for norepinephrine can pump dopamine and other biogenic amines into the neuron. Third, a drug or toxin that acts at the level of the membrane transporter may affect functions of several different neurotransmitters, depending on its specificity for a particular transporter. As an example, fluoxetine is fairly specific at inhibiting uptake of serotonin, whereas cocaine inhibits the uptake of serotonin, norepinephrine, and dopamine.

Neurotransmitter Receptors

Channel Receptors. The first general class of neurotransmitter receptors comprise ligand-gated ion channels (channel receptors or ionotropic receptors) in which the receptor for the neurotransmitter is part of an ion channel. By binding to its receptor, the neurotransmitter allosterically changes the configuration of the ion channel so that ions can more easily traverse the channel and enter or leave the cell. As an example, the acetylcholine nicotinic receptor at the neuromuscular junction is a ligand-gated Na$^+$ channel. When acetylcholine binds to the nicotinic receptor, the channel's configuration changes, allowing Na$^+$ to move into the cell and trigger an action potential. (The action potential then propagates down muscle via voltage-gated Na$^+$ channels.) Other examples of channel receptors are found in Table 10–1.

G Protein Receptors. The second general class of neurotransmitter receptors are linked to G proteins, which are part of a superfamily of proteins with GTPase activity responsible for signal transduction across plasma membranes.[101] G proteins comprise three polypeptide subunits: α, β, and γ chains. These chains span

TABLE 10–1. Types of Neurotransmitter and Neuromodulator Receptors

Ion Channel	Linked to G Protein
ACh nicotinic	ACh muscarinic
GABA$_A$, GABA$_C$	GABA$_B$
Glycine (inhibitory)	Dopamine
Glutamate AMPA	Norepinephrine
Glutamate NMDA	5-HT$_{1,2,4-7}$
Glutamate kainate	Adenosine
5-HT$_3$	Glutamate metabotropic

ACh = acetylcholine; GABA = γ-aminobutyric acid; 5-HT = serotonin; AMPA = α=amino-3-hydroxy-5-methyl-4-isoxazole propionate; NMDA = N-methyl-D-aspartate.

the plasma membrane several times, and they associate with a separately transcribed neurotransmitter receptor that spans the cell membrane seven times, with an external binding site for neurotransmitters. Some receptors (eg, $GABA_B$ receptor) coupled to G proteins are dimers comprising two separate proteins, both of which must be present for activity.

Both the α subunit and the $\beta\gamma$ subunit of a G protein account for activity resulting from a neurotransmitter binding to its receptor. The α chain normally binds GDP in the cytoplasm and is inactive. When a neurotransmitter binds to its receptor on the outside of the cell membrane, GDP dissociates from the α chain and GTP binds in its place, activating the α subunit. The activated α chain then dissociates from receptor and from the β and γ chains. Historically, it was believed that the activated α subunit alone moved to an effector in the membrane to produce a physiologic effect; now, however, the consensus is that the $\beta\gamma$ subunits, in many instances, actually modulate effectors in the plasma membrane.[101] The effector influenced by α or $\beta\gamma$ subunits may be an enzyme that the subunits stimulate or inhibit (eg, adenylate cyclase) or an ion channel that is opened or closed directly or through other chemical reactions (eg, channel phosphorylation).[26] Intrinsic GTPase activity in the α chain eventually converts the GTP to GDP, inactivating the α subunit and allowing it to reassociate with the β and γ chains and the neurotransmitter receptor, terminating the action of the subunits.[65]

G proteins are mainly categorized by the type of α chain they contain. For examples, G_s (containing the α subunit α_s) is a positive allosteric effector of membrane-bound adenylate cyclase; activation of a neurotransmitter receptor coupled to G_s causes a rise in intracellular 3′,5′-cyclic adenosine monophosphate (cAMP) concentration.[82] Neurotransmitter receptors activating G_i (containing α_i) inhibit adenylate cyclase and can open K^+ channels to cause K^+ efflux. Receptors coupled to $G_{q/11}$ act through membrane-bound phospholipase C to increase intracellular calcium concentrations. These and other types of G proteins produce other effects as well.

Neurotransmitter receptors coupled to G proteins are noted in Table 10–1. A given neurotransmitter can activate different classes of receptors (eg, channel and G protein) or different types of receptors in the same class. For example, $GABA_A$ receptors are Cl^- channels, whereas $GABA_B$ receptors are coupled to G proteins. Dopamine D_1 receptors are linked to G_s, whereas D_2 receptors are linked to G_i or G_o.

Neuronal Excitation and Inhibition

Excitatory neurotransmitters usually act postsynaptically by causing Na^+ or Ca^{2+} influx, or by preventing K^+ efflux, triggering depolarization and an action potential (Fig. 10–1). These effects may be mediated by channel or G protein–coupled receptors.

Postsynaptic inhibition can be mediated by channel receptors or by receptors coupled to G proteins (Fig. 10–1). Inhibition is usually accomplished by movement of Cl^- into the neuron or by movement of K^+ out of the neuron. Both processes hyperpolarize the neuron and move membrane potential farther away from threshold, making it more difficult for a given stimulus to depolarize the membrane to threshold voltage.

Presynaptic inhibition, the prevention of neurotransmitter release, is usually mediated by receptors coupled to G proteins. When a neurotransmitter released from a neuron binds to a receptor on that same neuron to limit further neurotransmitter release, the receptor is termed an *autoreceptor*.[124] Autoreceptors reside on dendrites, cell bodies, axons, and presynaptic terminals. Autoreceptors on dendrites and cell bodies (somatodendritic autoreceptors) usually inhibit further neurotransmitter release by increasing K^+ efflux, hyperpolarizing the neuron away from threshold (Fig. 10–2). Conversely, activation of autoreceptors found on presynaptic terminals (terminal autoreceptors) usually limits increases in intracellular Ca^{2+} concentration by limiting Ca^{2+} influx or preventing release from intracellular Ca^{2+} stores, impairing exocytosis of neurotransmitter vesicles (Fig. 10–2). Types of neurotransmitter receptors that serve as autoreceptors also usually reside postsynaptically, where they may mediate different physiologic effects.

Presynaptic nerve terminal inhibition of neurotransmitter release is not limited to actions by autoreceptors. Presynaptic terminal inhibitory receptors for various neurotransmitters may be found on a single neuron (heteroreceptors). For example, not only does stimulation of an α_2 autoreceptor on a noradrenergic nerve limit norepinephrine release, but stimulation of presynaptic α_2 receptors found on postsynaptic parasympathetic nerve terminals prevents acetylcholine release.

Finally, stimulation of receptors on presynaptic nerve endings may enhance, rather than inhibit, neurotransmitter release. Such receptors also are usually coupled to G proteins. For example, stimulation of a β_2 receptor on an adrenergic nerve terminal enhances norepinephrine release.

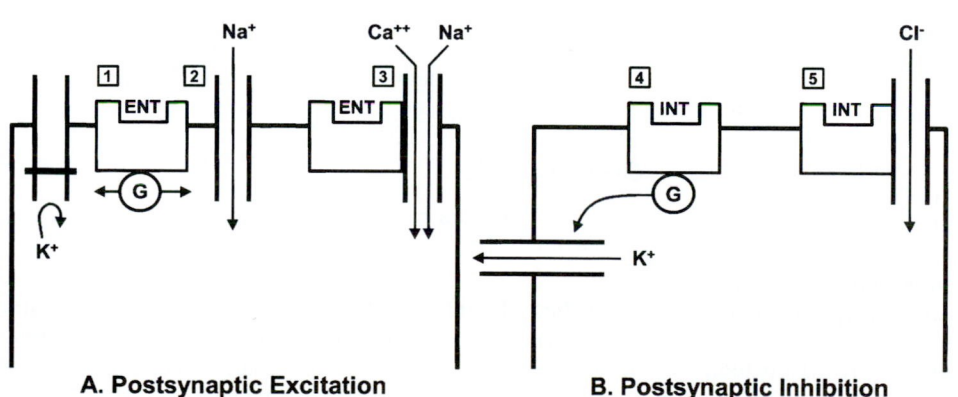

A. Postsynaptic Excitation   **B. Postsynaptic Inhibition**

Figure 10–1. Common mechanisms of postsynaptic excitation and inhibition. **A.** An excitatory neurotransmitter (ENT) binds to receptors linked to G proteins to prevent K^+ efflux [1] or to allow Na^+ influx [2], producing membrane depolarization. An ENT may bind to and activate a cation channel [3] to allow Na^+ and/or Ca^{2+} influx with resultant membrane depolarization. **B.** An inhibitory neurotransmitter (INT) hyperpolarizes the membrane (makes membrane potential more negative) by binding to receptors linked to G proteins to enhance K^+ efflux [4], or to Cl^- channels to allow Cl^- influx [5]. Some chloride channels are regulated by G proteins as well. G = G protein.

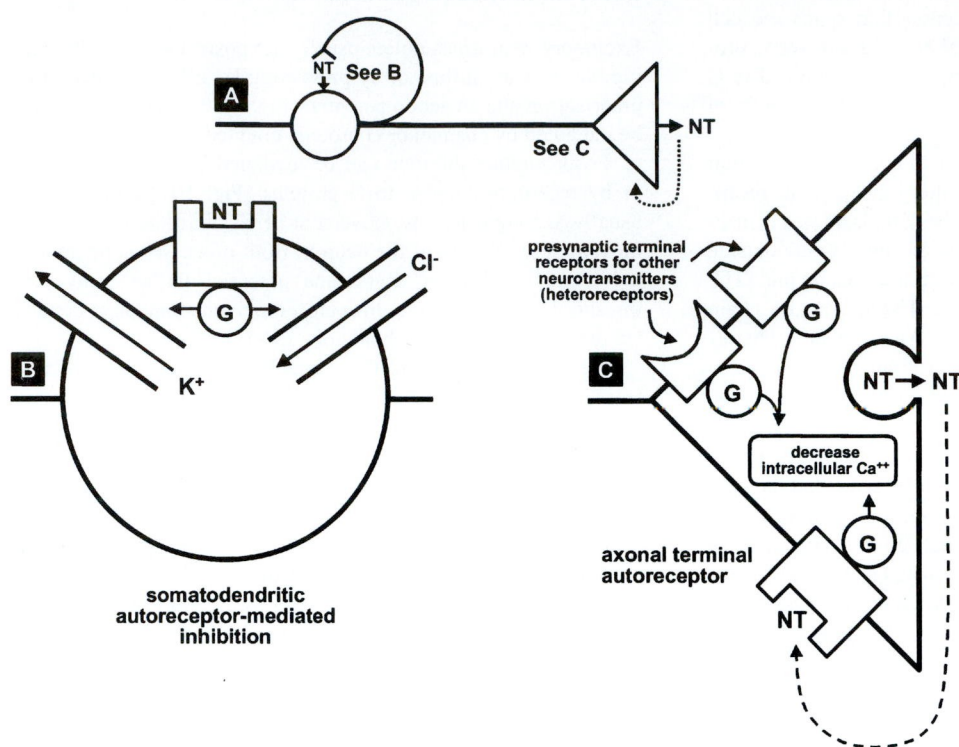

Figure 10–2. Common mechanisms of presynaptic inhibition (the inhibition of neurotransmitter [NT] release). **A.** Neuron A releases NT, which returns to activate receptors on the cell body or dendrites (somatodendritic autoreceptors), or on the axonal terminal (terminal autoreceptors). Such activation limits further release of NT by completing a negative feedback loop. **B.** At somatodendritic autoreceptors, NT binding produces activation of G proteins, which promote either K^+ efflux or Cl^- influx; both processes hyperpolarize the neuron away from threshold. **C.** At terminal autoreceptors, NT binding activates G proteins, which, through various mechanisms, lower intracellular Ca^{2+} concentrations to prevent exocytosis of NT vesicles, despite depolarization. Presynaptic inhibitory receptors for other types of NTs (heteroreceptors) are illustrated in C. Excitatory axonal terminal autoreceptors and heteroreceptors that serve to enhance (not inhibit) neurotransmitter release are not shown. G = G protein.

ACETYLCHOLINE

Acetylcholine (ACh) is a neurotransmitter of the central and peripheral nervous system. Centrally, it is found in both brain and spinal cord; cholinergic fibers project diffusely to the cerebral cortex. Peripherally, ACh serves as a neurotransmitter in autonomic and somatic motor fibers (Fig. 10–3).

Synthesis, Release, and Inactivation

Acetylcholine is synthesized from acetyl coenzyme A and choline. Acetylcholine moves into synaptic vesicles, where it is stored before release into the synapse by Ca^{2+}-dependent exocytosis. Acetylcholine undergoes degradation in the synapse to choline and acetic acid by acetylcholinesterase. An Na^+-dependent transporter in the neuronal membrane then pumps choline back into the cytoplasm to be used again as a substrate for ACh synthesis (Fig. 10–4). Pseudocholinesterase (plasma cholinesterase) is made in the liver and plays no role in the degradation of synaptic ACh metabolism. However, it does metabolize some drugs, including cocaine and succinylcholine.

Acetylcholine Receptors

Nicotinic Receptors. After release from cholinergic nerve endings, ACh activates two main types of receptors, nicotinic and muscarinic.[79] Nicotinic receptors (nAChRs) reside in the central nervous system (CNS; mainly in spinal cord), on postganglionic autonomic neurons (both sympathetic and parasympathetic), and at skeletal neuromuscular junctions, where they mediate muscle contraction (Fig. 10–3).

Nicotinic receptors at neuromuscular junctions (NMJ nAChRs) are part of an Na^+ channel made of five protein subunits and are

thus channel receptors. Stimulation of these receptors by ACh results mainly in Na^+ influx, depolarization of the endplate, and triggering of an action potential that is propagated down muscle by voltage-gated Na^+ channels.

Nicotinic receptors on central or peripheral neurons or in the adrenal gland are termed neuronal nAChRs. Neuronal nAChRs are also ion channels, although in some cases Ca^{2+} influx through the receptor may be more important than Na^+ influx. Neuronal nAChRs also comprise five protein subunits.

Muscarinic Receptors. Muscarinic receptors are found in the CNS (mainly in the brain) as receptors for postganglionic parasympathetic nerve endings and as postganglionic sympathetic receptors for most sweat glands (Fig. 10–4). At least five subtypes of muscarinic receptors, $M_{1–5}$, are recognized and linked to several G proteins. For example, in the heart, ACh released from the vagus nerve binds to M_2 receptors linked to G_i. G_i opens K^+ channels, allowing efflux of K^+ down its concentration gradient, which makes the inside of the cell more negative and more difficult to depolarize, slowing heart rate. Different subtypes of muscarinic receptors also act as autoreceptors in various locations, M_1 being the most common.

Chemical Agents

Table 10–2 provides examples of agents that affect cholinergic neurotransmission.

Modulators of Acetylcholine Release. Figure 10–4 illustrates sites of actions of numerous agents that influence the cholinergic nervous system. Botulinum toxins, some neurotoxins from pit vipers, and elapid β-neurotoxins prevent release of ACh from pe-

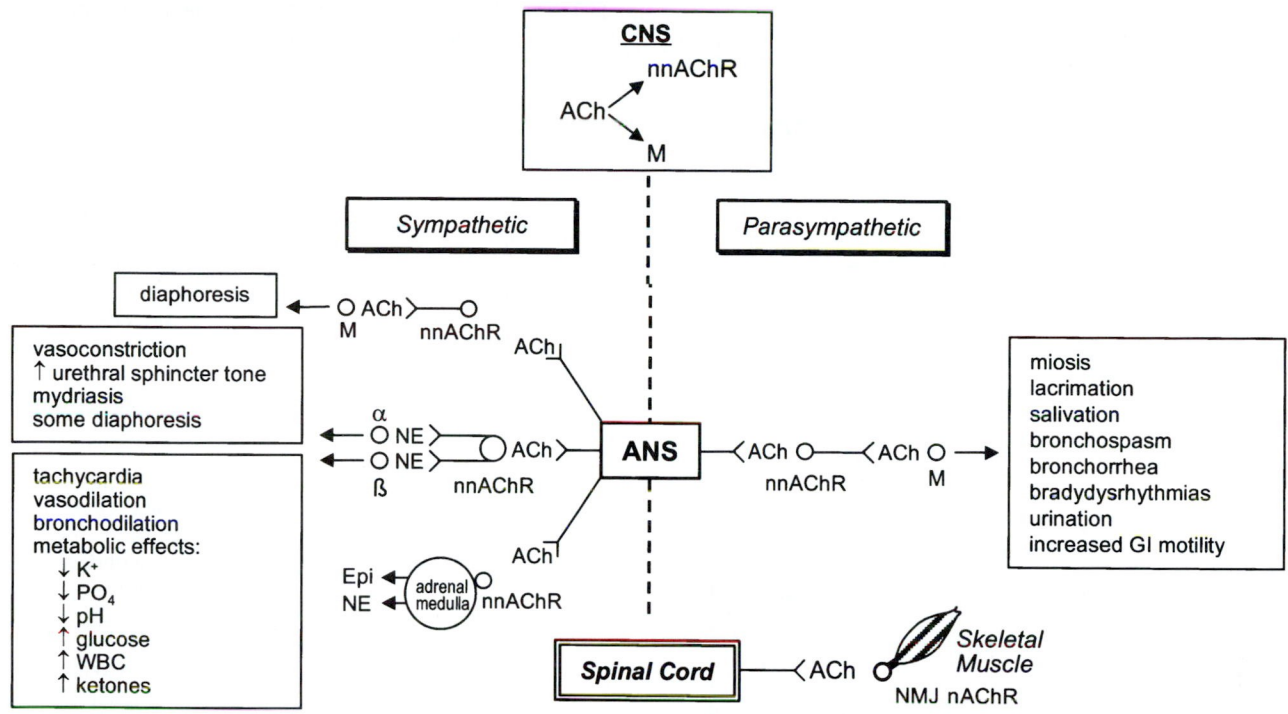

Figure 10–3. Diagram of the cholinergic nervous system, including adrenergic involvement in the autonomic nervous system. ACh binds to CNS, ganglionic, and adrenal neuronal nicotinic receptors (nnAChRs) and to neuromuscular junction nicotinic receptors (NMJ nAChRs). ACh also binds to various subtypes of muscarinic (M) receptors in the CNS and on effector organs innervated by postsynaptic parasympathetic neurons and to most sweat glands. NE and/or EPI released in response to ganglionic ACh stimulation of nnAChRs activates α- and β-adrenoceptors. ACh = acetylcholine; ANS = autonomic nervous system; CNS = central nervous system; EPI = epinephrine; NE = norepinephrine.

ripheral nerve endings.[58] This results in ptosis, other cranial nerve signs, weakness, and respiratory failure. Hypermagnesemia also inhibits acetylcholine release, probably by inhibiting Ca^{2+} influx into the nerve endings.[79]

Guanidine, aminopyridines, and black widow spider venom enhance the release of ACh from nerve endings. Guanidine has been unsuccessfully tried as a treatment for botulism. Aminopyridines block voltage-gated K^+ channels to prevent K^+ efflux; the resultant action potential widening (delayed repolarization) causes prolongation of Ca^{2+} channel activation, enhancing influx of Ca^{2+} and promoting neurotransmitter release. Aminopyridines have been used therapeutically in Lambert-Eaton syndrome, myasthenia gravis, multiple sclerosis, and experimentally in calcium channel blocker overdose.

Black widow spider venom causes acetylcholine release with resultant muscle cramping and diaphoresis.[6] Carbachol, a nicotinic and muscarinic agonist, also probably causes ACh release.

Nicotinic Receptor Agonists and Antagonists. Agents that bind to and activate nicotinic receptors may stimulate postganglionic sympathetic and parasympathetic neurons, skeletal muscle endplates, and neurons within the CNS (Fig. 10–3). Prolonged depolarization at the receptor eventually causes blockade of nicotinic receptors.[105] For example, poisoning by nicotine, both a neuronal and NMJ nAChR agonist, produces hypertension, tachycardia, vomiting, diarrhea, muscle fasciculations, and convulsions (excitation), followed by hypotension, bradydysrhythmias, paralysis, and coma (blockade). Nicotinic agonists include nicotine alkaloids (eg,

nicotine, coniine, arecoline, lobeline), carbachol (mainly muscarinic effects), and methacholine (slight effect). Succinylcholine is a neuromuscular blocking agent that initially stimulates and then blocks NMJ nAChRs.

Agents that block NMJ nAChRs without stimulation at skeletal neuromuscular junctions produce weakness and paralysis. Examples include curare and atracurium. α-Neurotoxins from elapids (eg, α-bungarotoxin) directly antagonize NMJ nAChRs, producing ptosis, weakness, and respiratory failure from paralysis.[148]

Chemicals blocking peripheral neuronal nAChRs produce autonomic ganglionic blockade. Trimethaphan is used as a pharmacologic ganglionic blocker; however, trimethaphan is not entirely specific for neuronal nAChRs. Occasional patients develop weakness and paralysis from NMJ nAChR blockade.

Recent studies demonstrate that the function of neuronal nAChRs can be modulated by a variety of compounds that do not bind to the ACh binding site, but bind instead to a number of distinct allosteric sites on the neuronal nAChR. For example, aside from their ability to inhibit acetylcholinesterase, physostigmine, tacrine, and galantamine bind to a noncompetitive allosteric activator site on neuronal nAChRs to enhance channel opening and ion conductance (there is evidence suggesting that serotonin may bind here as well). Conversely, a diverse range of compounds, including chlorpromazine, phencyclidine, ketamine, local anesthetics, and ethanol bind to a noncompetitive negative allosteric site(s) to inhibit inward ion fluxes without directly affecting ACh binding. Steroids can desensitize neuronal nAChRs by binding to yet an additional allosteric site. Finally, a dihydropyridine calcium

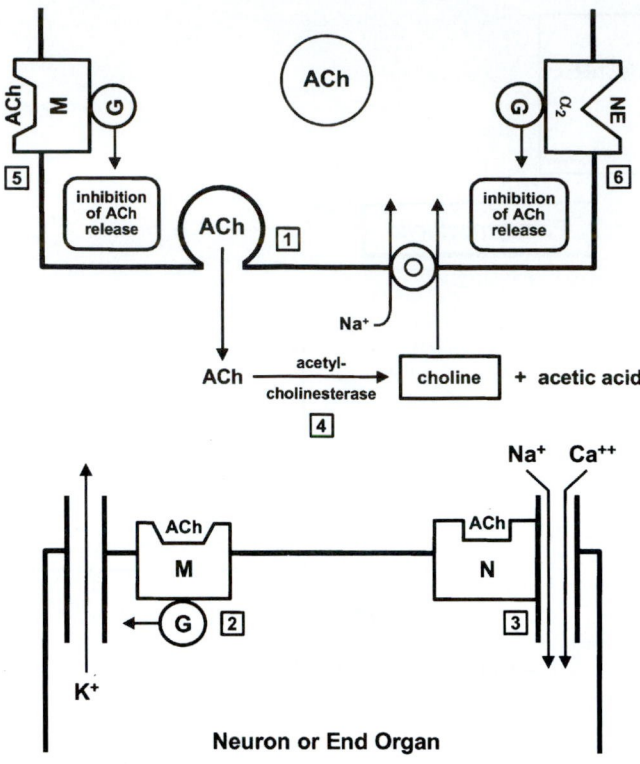

Neuron or End Organ

Figure 10–4. Cholinergic nerve ending. Activation of postsynaptic muscarinic receptors hyperpolarizes the postsynaptic membrane through G-protein-mediated enhancement of K^+ efflux. Several subtypes of muscarinic receptors coupled to various G proteins exist—a muscarinic receptor coupled to a G protein that opens K^+ channels is shown only as an example. Postsynaptic nicotinic receptor activation causes Na^+ influx and membrane depolarization. Importantly, Ca^{2+} influx appears to be the main cation involved with some neuronal nicotinic receptors. Presynaptic muscarinic and α_2-adrenoceptor activation prevents ACh release through lowering of intracellular Ca^{2+} concentrations. Agents in Table 10–2 may act to enhance or prevent release of ACh [1]; activate or antagonize postsynaptic muscarinic (M) receptors [2]; activate or antagonize nicotinic (N) receptors [3]; inhibit acetylcholinesterase [4]; prevent ACh release by stimulating presynaptic muscarinic autoreceptors [5] or α_2-adrenergic heteroreceptors [6]; or enhance ACh release by antagonizing presynaptic autoreceptors [5] or by antagonizing presynaptic α_2-adrenergic heteroreceptors [6] (on parasympathetic postganglionic terminals). ACh = acetylcholine; G = G protein; NE = norepinephrine.

channel blocker binding site has been described, but remains poorly understood.[107]

Muscarinic Receptor Agonists and Antagonists. Peripheral muscarinic agonists produce bradycardia, miosis, salivation, lacrimation, vomiting, diarrhea, bronchospasm, bronchorrhea, and micturition. Central muscarinic agonists produce sedation, extrapyramidal dystonias and rigidity, coma, and convulsions. Examples of direct muscarinic agonists include muscarine (from mushrooms), bethanechol, pilocarpine, carbachol, and methacholine.

Anticholinergic poisoning syndrome results from blockade of muscarinic receptors and is more appropriately referred to as an-

TABLE 10–2. Examples of Agents Affecting Cholinergic Neurotransmission

Cholinomimetic Agents	Coniine
Cause ACh release	Cytisine
α_2-Adrenergic antagonists[a]	Gallamine
Aminopyridines	Hexamethonium
Black widow spider venom	Lobeline
Carbachol	Mecamylamine
Guanidine	Nicotine
	Nondepolarizing neuromus-
Anticholinesterases	cular blocking agents
Echothiophate iodide	Succinylcholine[b]
Edrophonium	Trimethaphan
Galantamine	
N-methylcarbamate insecticides	Indirect neuronal nicotinic an-
Metrifonate	tagonists
Neostigmine	Chlorpromazine
Organic phosphorus insecticides	Corticosteroids
Physostigmine	Ethanol
Pyridostigmine	Ketamine
Rivastigmine	Local anesthetics
Tacrine	Phencyclidine
	Volatile anesthetics
Direct nicotinic agonists	
Arecoline	Direct muscarinic antagonists
Carbachol	Amantadine
Coniine	Antihistamines
Cytisine	Atropine
Lobeline	Benztropine
Nicotine	Carbamazepine
Succinylcholine (initial)[b]	Clozapine
	Cyclobenzaprine
Indirect neuronal nicotinic agonists	Disopyramide
Physostigmine	Glutethimide
Tacrine	Orphenadrine
Galantamine	Phenothiazines
	Procainamide
Direct muscarinic agonists	Quinidine
Bethanechol	Scopolamine
Carbachol	Tricyclic antidepressants
Methacholine	Trihexyphenidyl
Muscarine	
Pilocarpine	Inhibit ACh release
	α_2-Adrenergic agonists[d]
Cholinolytic Agents	Botulinum toxins
Direct nicotinic antagonists	Crotalinae venoms
α-Bungarotoxin[c]	Elapidae β-neurotoxins
Arecoline	Hypermagnesemia

ACh = acetylcholine.
[a]Antagonism of α_2-adrenoceptors enhances ACh release from parasympathetic nerve endings.
[b]Depolarizing neuromuscular blocking agent.
[c]α-Bungarotoxin exemplifies many elapid α-neurotoxins that produce paralysis and death from respiratory failure.
[d]Stimulation of presynaptic α_2-adrenoceptors on parasympathetic nerve endings prevents ACh release.

timuscarinic poisoning syndrome.[127] Central nervous system muscarinic blockade produces confusion, agitation, myoclonus, tremor, picking movements, abnormal speech, hallucinations, and coma. Peripheral antimuscarinic effects include mydriasis, anhidrosis, tachycardia, urinary retention, and ileus. Muscarinic antagonists number in the hundreds. Examples are listed in Table 10–2.

Acetylcholinesterase Inhibition. Agents inhibiting acetylcholinesterase raise ACh concentrations at both nicotinic and muscarinic receptors, producing a variety of CNS, sympathetic, parasympathetic, and skeletal muscle signs and symptoms.[28] Anticholinesterases include organic phosphorus compounds and *N*-methylcarbamates. Organic phosphorus compounds are usually encountered as insecticides, although topical medicinal organic phosphorus compounds are used for the treatment of glaucoma and lice. *N*-methylcarbamates are found as insecticides and pharmaceutics. Medicinal *N*-methylcarbamates include physostigmine, pyridostigmine, rivastigmine, and neostigmine. Edrophonium, galantamine, tacrine, and metrifonate are noncarbamate, reversible anticholinesterases.

α₂-Adrenoceptor Agonists and Antagonists. Agonists and antagonists of α₂-adrenoceptors are discussed in detail later. Briefly, stimulation of presynaptic α₂-adrenoceptors on postganglionic parasympathetic nerve endings decreases ACh release. Conversely, presynaptic α₂ antagonism increases ACh release (Fig. 10–4).

NOREPINEPHRINE AND EPINEPHRINE

Norepinephrine (NE), epinephrine (EPI), dopamine (DA), and serotonin (5-hydroxytryptamine; 5-HT) have historically been referred to as biogenic amines, and their neurotransmitter systems are similar in many respects. Neurotransmitter synthesis, vesicle transport and storage, uptake, and degradation share many enzymes and structurally similar transport proteins. Cocaine, reserpine, amphetamines, and monoamine oxidase inhibitors (MAOIs) affect all four types of neurons. In addition, these agents produce several different effects in the same system. For example, in the noradrenergic neuron, amphetamines work mainly by causing the release of cytoplasmic norepinephrine, but they also inhibit norepinephrine uptake and their metabolites inhibit monoamine oxidase. Actions of drugs that affect all biogenic amine neurotransmitters are described in the most detail for noradrenergic neurons. For the sake of brevity, similar mechanisms of action are simply noted in discussions of dopaminergic and serotonergic neurotransmission.

Norepinephrine is released from postganglionic sympathetic fibers (Fig. 10–3) and is also found in the CNS. The adrenal gland, acting as a modified sympathetic ganglion, releases epinephrine and lesser amounts of norepinephrine in response to stimulation of neuronal nAChRs. Epinephrine-containing neurons also reside in the brainstem.

The locus ceruleus is the main noradrenergic nucleus in the brain. Axons radiate from this nucleus out to all layers of the cerebral cortex, to the cerebellum, and to other structures. Norepinephrine demonstrates both excitatory and inhibitory actions in the CNS. Norepinephrine released from locus ceruleus projections in the hippocampus increases cortical neuron activity through β-adrenoceptor activation and G protein–mediated inhibition of K^+ efflux. Norepinephrine released in outer cortical areas produces inhibitory effects mediated by α-adrenoceptor agonism. At this level, norepinephrine produces slow cortical neuron hyperpolarization and decreased rates of spontaneous firing. Consistent with this, norepinephrine demonstrates anticonvulsant actions in animals; carbamazepine's anticonvulsant action may be partly due to inhibition of norepinephrine uptake.[41] Despite antagonistic actions on different cortical neurons, electrical stimulation of the locus

ceruleus produces widespread cortical activation and excitation. This overall effect probably explains a great deal of the hyperattentiveness and lack of fatigue that accompanies use of agents that mimic or increase noradrenergic activity in the brain.

Synthesis, Release, and Uptake

Figure 10–5 is a representation of a noradrenergic neuron. Tyrosine hydroxylase is the rate-limiting enzyme in norepinephrine synthesis and is sensitive to negative feedback by norepinephrine. Dopa undergoes decarboxylation by L-amino acid decarboxylase to dopamine. L-Amino acid decarboxylase (dopa decarboxylase) is not specific for dopa. For example, it also catalyzes the formation of serotonin from 5-hydroxytryptophan.

About one-half of cytoplasmic dopa is actively pumped into vesicles containing the enzyme dopamine-β-hydroxylase. The remaining dopamine is quickly deaminated. Two closely related vesicular membrane uptake pumps—VMAT1 and VMAT2—are selective for monoamines. Whereas VMAT1 is found in peripheral neuroendocrine cells, VMAT2 resides in neurons and in adrenal chromaffin cells.

In the vesicle, dopamine-β-hydroxylase converts dopamine to norepinephrine. Vesicles isolated from nerve endings contain dopamine, norepinephrine, dopamine-β-hydroxylase, and ATP. All of these substances are released into the synapse during Ca^{2+}-dependent exocytosis triggered by neuronal firing. In neurons containing epinephrine as a neurotransmitter, norepinephrine is released from vesicles into the cytoplasm, where it is converted to epinephrine. Epinephrine is then transported back into vesicles before synaptic release.[79]

Norepinephrine is removed from the synapse mainly by uptake into the presynaptic neuron by a norepinephrine transporter. While this transporter has great affinity for norepinephrine, it also transports other amines, including dopamine, tyramine, MAOIs, and amphetamines. Once pumped back into the cytoplasm, norepinephrine can either be transported back into vesicles for further storage and release, or can be quickly enzymatically degraded by monoamine oxidase (MAO), an enzyme expressed on the outer mitochondrial membrane.

MAO resides in sympathetic postganglionic neurons, intestinal mucosa, liver, kidney, lung, and brain. It comprises two isoenzymes, MAO-A and MAO-B,[92] each with relatively separate affinities for various substrates (Table 10–3). MAO possesses two main actions. First, neuronal MAO degrades cytoplasmic amines, including neurotransmitters, to prevent elevated cytoplasmic concentrations of biogenic amines. Second, hepatic and intestinal MAO prevent large quantities of dietary bioactive amines from entering the circulation and producing systemic effects. Catechol-*O*-methyltransferase (COMT) also metabolizes norepinephrine and epinephrine. However, little COMT resides in neurons. In other tissue, COMT metabolizes catecholamines, including those that have entered the systemic circulation.

Adrenergic Receptors

The two main types of adrenoceptors are α-adrenoceptors and β-adrenoceptors. All adrenoceptors are linked to G proteins.

β-Adrenoceptors. β-Adrenoceptors are divided into three major subtypes (β₁, β₂, and β₃) depending on their affinity for various agonists and antagonists.[23,64,65,82] β₁- and β₂-adrenoceptors are linked to G_s, and their stimulation raises cAMP concentration,

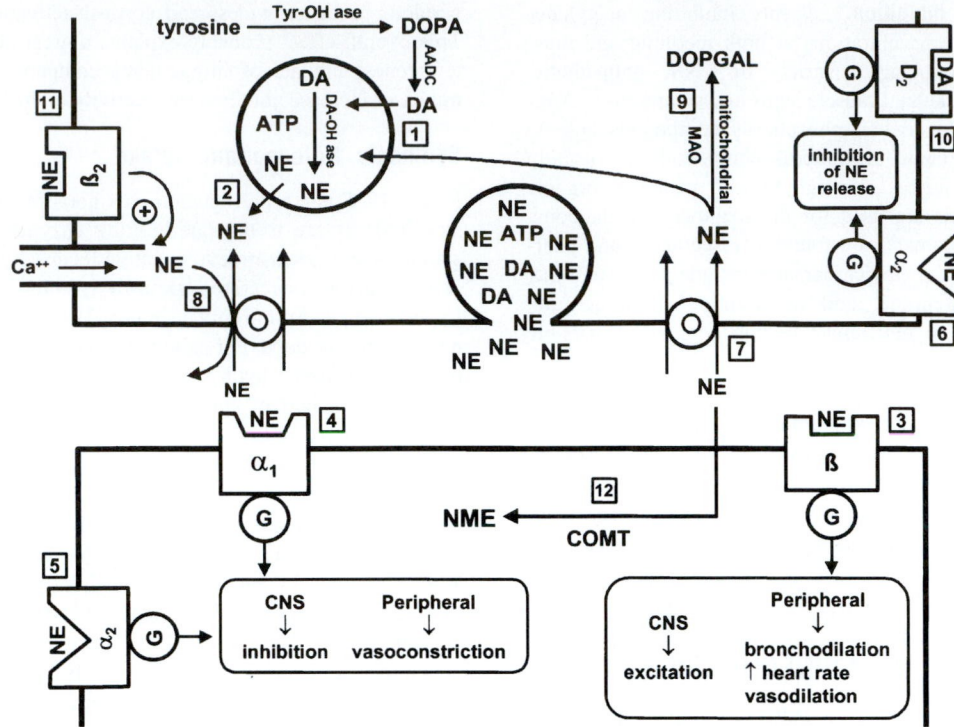

Figure 10–5. Noradrenergic nerve ending. The postsynaptic membrane may represent an end organ or another neuron in the CNS. Brief examples of effects resulting from postsynaptic receptor activation are shown. Agents in Tables 10–4 and 10–5 produce effects by inhibiting transport of dopamine (DA) or norepinephrine (NE) into vesicles [1]; causing movement of NE from vesicles into the cytoplasm [2]; activating or antagonizing postsynaptic α- and β-adrenoceptors [3–5]; modulating NE release by activating or antagonizing presynaptic α_2-autoreceptors [6], dopamine$_2$ (D$_2$) heteroreceptors [10], or β_2-autoreceptors [11]; blocking uptake of NE [7]; causing reverse transport of NE from the cytoplasm into the synapse by raising cytoplasmic NE concentrations [8]; inhibiting monoamine oxidase (MAO) to prevent NE degradation [9]; or inhibiting COMT to prevent NE degradation [12]. COMT is not found in neurons in large amounts. AADC = aromatic L-amino acid decarboxylase; ATP = adenosine triphosphate; DA-OHase = dopamine-β-hydroxylase; COMT = catechol-*O*-methyltransferase; CNS = central nervous system; DOPGAL = 3,4-dihydroxyphenylglycoaldehyde; G = G protein; NME = normetanephrine; Tyr-OHase = tyrosine hydroxylase.

TABLE 10–3.   Characteristics of Monoamine Oxidase (MAO) Isoenzymes

	MAO Isoenzymes	
	MAO-A	**MAO-B**
Location		
Brain	+	+++
Intestine	+++	+
Liver	++	++
Platelets	0	++++
Placenta	++++	0
Substrates		
Norepinephrine	++++	+
Epinephrine	++	++
Dopamine	++	++
Serotonin	++++	+
Tyramine	++	++

which in turn produces several effects, including regulation of ion channels. Preliminary data suggest that at least some β_3-adrenoceptors may be coupled to other G proteins.

The β-adrenoceptors are polymorphic, with genetic variation in the human population.[23] Polymorphism influences response to medications, regulation of receptors, and clinical course of disease.[23,65,82] In general, peripheral β_1-adrenoceptors are found mainly in the heart (along with β_2 receptors), whereas peripheral β_2-adrenoceptors also mediate additional adrenergic effects.[65] Presynaptic β_2-adrenoceptor activation causes release of norepinephrine from nerve endings (positive feedback). β_3-Adrenoceptors reside mainly in fat, but they also reside in skeletal muscle, gallbladder, and colon where they regulate metabolic processes. Activation of cardiac β_3-adrenoceptors might produce negative inotropic effects in some circumstances. β_3-Adrenoceptors' polymorphism may contribute to clinical expressions of non-insulin-dependent diabetes and obesity.[23,136,149]

α-Adrenoceptors.   α-Adrenoceptors are linked to G proteins that inhibit adenylate cyclase and lower cAMP levels, affect ion channels, increase intracellular calcium through inositol triphosphate and diacylglycerol production, or produce other actions. These receptors are divided into two main types, α_1 and α_2, and at least six subtypes, α_{1A}, α_{1B}, α_{1D}, α_{2A}, α_{2B}, and α_{2C}.[35,64]

In peripheral tissue, α_1-adrenoceptors reside on the postsynaptic membrane in continuity with the synaptic cleft. Stimulation of these receptors on vasculature results in vasoconstriction.

α_2-Adrenoceptors reside on both sides of the synapse. Presynaptic α_2-adrenoceptor activation mediates negative feedback, limiting further release of norepinephrine (Fig. 10–5). Postganglionic parasympathetic neurons (cholinergic) also contain presynaptic α_2-adrenoceptors that, when stimulated, prevent release of ACh (Fig. 10–4).

Postsynaptic α_2-adrenoceptors on vasculature also mediate vasoconstriction.[25] Initially, it was suggested that postsynaptic α_2-adrenoceptors resided mainly outside of the synapse and mediated vasoconstrictive responses to circulating α agonists such as norepinephrine, whereas postsynaptic α_1-adrenoceptors responded to norepinephrine released from nerve endings. However, it has been demonstrated that in at least some tissues (eg, saphenous vein), norepinephrine released following nerve stimulation produces vasoconstriction through action at α_2-adrenoceptors, making the previous differentiation not as distinct.[35,69] Because both α_1- and α_2-adrenoceptors on vasculature mediate vasoconstriction, a patient with hypertension from high circulating catecholamine concentrations (eg, pheochromocytoma or clonidine withdrawal) or from extravasation of norepinephrine from an intravenous line commonly needs both α_1- and α_2-adrenoceptor blockade to vasodilate adequately (eg, phentolamine). Stimulation of postsynaptic α_2-adrenoceptors in the brainstem inhibits sympathetic output and produces sedation (Fig. 10–6). In fact, dexmedetomidine, an imidazole and potent α_{2A}-adrenergic agonist, is utilized for sedation in intensive care patients, although hypotension and bradycardia occur as expected side effects.[11]

Chemical Agents

Chemicals producing pharmacologic effects that result in or mimic increased activity of the adrenergic nervous system are *sympathomimetics* (Table 10–4). Those with the opposite effect are *sympatholytics* (Table 10–5).

Sympathomimetics

Direct-Acting Agents. Drugs or chemicals whose sympathomimetic actions result from direct binding to α- or β-adrenocep-

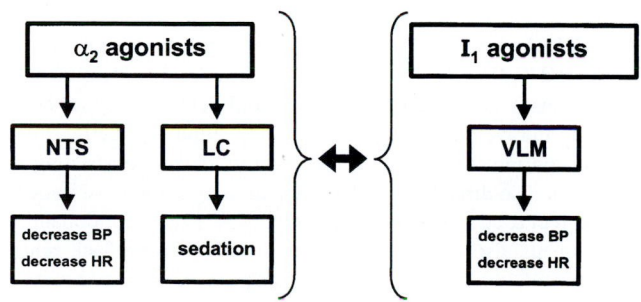

Figure 10–6. Central action of agents that activate α_2-adrenoceptors or that bind to type 1 imidazoline binding sites (I_1). There are poorly understood interactions between imidazoline binding sites and α_2-adrenoceptors that make delineation of specific effects difficult to attribute to specific receptor activation. BP = blood pressure; HR = heart rate; LC = locus ceruleus; NTS = nucleus tractus solitarius; VLM = ventrolateral medulla.

TABLE 10–4. Examples of Sympathomimetics

Direct-Acting	Mephentermine
β-Adrenoceptor agonists	Phenylpropanolamine
Albuterol	Pseudoephedrine
Dobutamine	
Epinephrine	**Selective α₂-Adrenoceptor Antagonists**
Isoproterenol	Idazoxan
Metaproterenol	Yohimbine
Norepinephrine	
Ritodrine	**Imidazoline Binding-Site Antagonists**
Terbutaline	Idazoxan
α-Adrenoceptor agonists	**MAOIs**
Dobutamine	Amphetamine metabolites
Epinephrine	Clorgyline[a]
Ergot alkaloids	Isocarboxazid
Methoxamine	Moclobemide[a]
Norepinephrine	Pargyline
Phenylephrine	Phenelzine
	Selegiline[b]
Indirect-Acting	Tranylcypromine
Amphetamines	
Cocaine	**Inhibit NE Uptake**
Fenfluramine	Amphetamines
MAOIs	Benztropine
Methylphenidate	Bupropion
Pemoline	Carbamazepine
Phencyclidine	Cocaine
Phenmetrazine	Diphenhydramine
Propylhexedrine	Orphenadrine
Tyramine	Pemoline
	Tramadol
Mixed-Acting	Tricyclic antidepressants
Dopamine	Trihexyphenidyl
Ephedrine	Venlafaxine

MAOIs = monoamine oxidase inhibitors; NE = norepinephrine.
[a]Mainly inhibit MAO-A at low doses.
[b]Mainly inhibit MAO-B at low doses.

tors are called direct-acting sympathomimetics. Most of these drugs do not cross the blood-brain barrier in significant quantities.

Indirect-Acting Agents. Agents that produce sympathomimetic effects by causing the release of cytoplasmic norepinephrine from the nerve ending in the absence of vesicle exocytosis are called indirect-acting sympathomimetics. Amphetamine is the prototype of indirect-acting agents and is used for the discussion of what is known about their mechanism of action. In general, mechanisms of indirect release of norepinephrine by amphetamines, cocaine, phencyclidine, MAOIs, and mixed-acting agents noted in Table 10–4 are similar in that their actions depend on their ability to produce elevated cytoplasmic norepinephrine concentrations.

Amphetamine and structurally similar indirect-acting agents move into the neuron by the membrane transporter that pumps norepinephrine into the neuron. (Lipophilic indirect-acting agents move into the neuron by diffusion.) From the cytoplasm, amphetamines are transported into neurotransmitter vesicles, where they buffer hydrogen ions to raise intravesicle pH. As noted earlier, much of the vesicle's ability to concentrate norepinephrine (and other neurotransmitters) is a result of ion trapping of norepinephrine at the lower pH. The rise in intravesicle pH produced by amphetamines causes norepinephrine to leave the vesicle and move

TABLE 10–5. Examples of Sympatholytics

α-Adrenoceptor Antagonists
  Clozapine
  Doxazosin
  Droperidol
  Ergot alkaloids
  Labetalol
  Olanzapine
  Phenothiazines
  Phenoxybenzamine
  Phentolamine
  Prazosin
  Quinidine
  Risperidone
  Terazosin
  Tolazoline
  Trazodone
  Tricyclic antidepressants
  Urapidil

Inhibit Dopamine-β-Hydroxylase
  Diethyldithiocarbamate
  Disulfiram
  MAOIs

β-Adrenoceptor Antagonists
  Acebutolol[a]
  Alprenolol[a]
  Atenolol
  Betaxolol
  Bisoprolol
  Carteolol
  Carvedilol
  Esmolol
  Labetalol
  Metipranolol[a]
  Metoprolol
  Nadolol
  Oxprenolol[a]

Penbutolol[a]
Pindolol[a]
Practolol[a]
Propranolol
Sotalol
Timolol

Prevent NE Release with Depolarization
  Bretylium[b]
  Reserpine[b]

α₂-Adrenoceptor Agonists[d]
  α-Methyldopa[c]
  Brimonidine
  Clonidine
  Dexmedetomidine
  Guanabenz
  Guanfacine
  Moxonidine
  Naphazoline
  Oxymetazoline
  Rilmenidine
  Tetrahydralazine
  Xylometazoline

Imidazoline Binding-Site Agonists[d]
  Clonidine
  Guanabenz
  Guanfacine
  Moxonidine
  Naphazoline
  Oxymetazoline
  Rilmenidine

Inhibitors of Vesicle Uptake
  Reserpine[b]
  Tetrabenazine

MAOIs = monoamine oxidase inhibitors; NE = norepinephrine.
[a]Partial β agonist.
[b]Causes transient NE release after initial dose.
[c]Metabolized to α-methylnorepinephrine, which activates α₂-receptors.
[d]Agents in these categories vary in their relative selectivity for α₂-adrenoceptors and imidazoline binding sites.

into the cytoplasm.[137,138] Such movement may be due to diffusion and/or reverse transport of norepinephrine by the vesicle membrane transporter. In the cytoplasm, amphetamines also compete with norepinephrine and dopamine for transport into vesicles, which further contributes to elevated cytoplasmic norepinephrine concentrations. In the case of amphetamines, the rise in cytoplasmic concentrations of norepinephrine is enhanced by the ability of amphetamine metabolites to inhibit MAO, which impairs norepinephrine degradation.

Every time the Na+-dependent transporter moves a bioactive amine (eg, tyramine) into the neuron where it is then released, a binding site for norepinephrine on the transporter transiently faces inward and becomes available for reverse transport of norepinephrine out of the neuron. The normally low concentration of cytoplasmic norepinephrine prevents significant reverse transport. In the face of elevated cytoplasmic norepinephrine concentrations produced by indirect-acting agents as described earlier, the Na+-

dependent neuronal membrane transporter moves norepinephrine out of the neuron and back into the synapse, where the neurotransmitter stimulates adrenoceptors (indirect action). This process is sometimes referred to as *facilitated exchange diffusion,* or *displacement,* of norepinephrine from the nerve ending. Evidence supporting reverse transport produced by amphetamines is that inhibitors of the transporter (eg, tricyclic antidepressants) prevent amphetamine-induced norepinephrine release.

While all indirect-acting agents cause reverse norepinephrine transport by increasing cytoplasmic norepinephrine concentrations, those that move into the neuron by the membrane transporter (eg, amphetamines, MAOIs, dopamine, tyramine) further enhance reverse transport because their uptake causes more norepinephrine binding sites on the transporter to face inward per unit time.

While cocaine's main adrenergic effect results from inhibition of the membrane uptake transporter, cocaine also causes some norepinephrine release. In fact, cocaine similarly lessens pH gradients across vesicle membranes[138] to raise cytoplasmic concentrations of norepinephrine. That cocaine produces less norepinephrine release than amphetamines is explained by cocaine-induced inhibition of the membrane transporter and by the fact that cocaine does not move into the neuron by active uptake (ie, does not increase the number of norepinephrine binding sites facing inward), but diffuses into the neuron.

Phencyclidine (PCP) is a hallucinogen that demonstrates multiple pharmacologic actions. Like toxicity from many hallucinogens, PCP toxicity is accompanied by increased adrenergic activity, which results from PCP-induced decreases in pH gradients across the vesicle membrane[138] and indirect release of norepinephrine. Like cocaine, PCP moves into the neuron by diffusion rather than uptake through the membrane transporter, at least partly explaining less PCP-induced norepinephrine release than is typically seen in amphetamine poisoning.

Reserpine, guanethidine, and bretylium cause neurotransmitter release with initial doses or early in overdose before their primary sympatholytic effects are observed. Presumably this is a result of transient rises in cytoplasmic norepinephrine concentrations.

In addition to causing acetylcholine release, black widow spider venom causes vesicle exocytosis of norepinephrine,[110] producing hypertension and diaphoresis over the palms, soles, upper lip, and nose. All of the aforementioned indirectly acting agents, except black widow spider venom, enter the CNS.

Mixed-Acting Agents. Mixed-acting sympathomimetics act directly and indirectly.[79] For example, phenylpropanolamine indirectly causes norepinephrine release and acts directly as an α-agonist. Intravenously administered dopamine indirectly causes norepinephrine release, explaining most of its vasoconstricting activity, but also directly stimulates dopaminergic and β-adrenoceptors. Direct α-agonism occurs at high doses. Except for dopamine, these agents also cross the blood-brain barrier to produce central effects.

Uptake Inhibitors. Inhibitors of norepinephrine uptake raise concentrations of norepinephrine in the synapse to produce excessive stimulation of adrenoceptors. Cocaine's main adrenergic effect results from this mechanism.

There are two main mechanisms of action for inhibitors of biogenic amine uptake: competitive and noncompetitive. Noncompetitive inhibitors, such as cyclic antidepressants, carbamazepine, methylphenidate, and cocaine, bind at or near the carrier site on the transporter to prevent the transporter from moving norepinephrine and other agents into or out of the neuron. These inhibitors are not transported into the neuron by this mechanism; lipophilic agents diffuse into the neuron. Various drugs used for their antimuscarinic effects also block norepinephrine uptake noncompetitively. These include benztropine, diphenhydramine, trihexyphenidyl, and orphenadrine.[99]

The second mechanism, competitive inhibition of uptake, characterizes most indirect-acting agents, including amphetamines and structurally similar compounds (eg, mixed-acting agents, MAOIs). These agents prevent norepinephrine uptake by competing with synaptic norepinephrine for binding to the carrier site on the membrane transporter, the mechanism by which these agents move into the neuron. In fact, an additional adrenergic action of amphetamines, mixed-acting agents, MAOIs, and tyramine is to raise synaptic norepinephrine concentrations by competing with norepinephrine for uptake, thereby compounding their indirect and/or direct actions.

MAOIs. MAOIs are transported by the norepinephrine transporter into the neuron, where they act through several mechanisms.[92] Inhibition of MAO, their main pharmacologic effect, results in increased cytoplasmic concentrations of norepinephrine and some indirect release of neurotransmitter into the synapse. As a minor effect they also may displace norepinephrine from vesicles by raising pH in a manner similar to amphetamines. These actions explain the initial hyperadrenergic findings following MAOI overdose and probably also account for occasional and unpredictable adrenergic crises in patients taking these agents, despite the patients' compliance with diet.

Nonspecific MAOIs inhibit both isozymes of MAO, preventing intestinal and hepatic degradation of bioactive amines as well. A person taking such an MAOI who then ingests food or receives drugs containing indirect-acting sympathomimetics (eg, tyramine, phenylpropanolamine, dopamine, amphetamines) has a much larger cytoplasmic concentration of norepinephrine to transport into the synapse and may therefore develop central and peripheral hyperadrenergic findings. Although MAO inhibitors specific for the MAO-B isozyme may be less likely to predispose to food or drug interactions by maintaining significant hepatic MAO activity, isozyme specificity is lost as the dose of the MAOI is increased. In fact, selegiline, currently marketed as a selective MAO-B inhibitor, partially inhibits MAO-A activity at therapeutic doses. Specificity may lack importance when indirect-acting agents are administered systemically (eg, intravenous dopamine or amphetamines). Several amphetamine metabolites are capable of inhibiting MAO, contributing to their sympathomimetic activity.

Occasionally, patients suffering from refractory depression respond to a combination of MAOIs and tricyclic antidepressants. This combination therapy is usually unaccompanied by excessive adrenergic activity because the inhibition of the membrane uptake transporter by the tricyclic antidepressant prevents excessive reverse transport of elevated cytoplasmic norepinephrine concentrations produced by MAOIs. In animals, tricyclic antidepressants that prevent norepinephrine uptake or cocaine, also an norepinephrine uptake inhibitor, protect against drug and food interactions with MAOIs by inhibiting the uptake transporter, thus inhibiting reverse transport. Nevertheless, some patients suffer severe toxicity and death when MAOIs and tricyclic antidepressants are combined.

COMT Inhibitors. Inhibitors of COMT are administered in the treatment of Parkinson disease to prevent the catabolism of concomitantly administered L-dopa. Entacapone only acts peripherally, whereas tolcapone also crosses the blood-brain barrier.

α-Adrenoceptor Antagonists. Yohimbine blocks α_2-adrenoceptors to produce a mixed clinical picture. Peripheral postsynaptic α_2 blockade produces vasodilatation. Blockade of presynaptic α_2-adrenoceptors on cholinergic nerve endings (Fig. 10–4) enhances ACh release, occasionally producing bronchospasm[77] and contributing to diaphoresis. Similar presynaptic actions on peripheral noradrenergic nerves enhance catecholamine release (Fig. 10–5). Blockade of central α_2-adrenoceptors in the locus ceruleus results in CNS stimulation, whereas blockade of postsynaptic α_2-adrenoceptors in the nucleus tractus solitarius may enhance sympathetic output (Fig. 10–6). The final result includes hypertension, tachycardia, agitation, mania, mydriasis, diaphoresis, and bronchospasm.[84] Yohimbine does not block imidazoline receptors (see discussion of imidazoline receptors later). One action of the antidepressant mirtazapine is α_2-adrenoceptor blockade.

Sympatholytics

Direct Antagonists. Direct α- and β-adrenoceptor antagonists are noted in Table 10–5. In overdose, and sometimes at therapeutic doses, any β-adrenoceptor selectivity becomes insignificant. Some β-adrenoceptor antagonists also are partial agonists.

Drugs That Prevent Norepinephrine Release. Drugs that prevent the release of norepinephrine, despite membrane depolarization, include guanethidine and bretylium. Both drugs initially cause release of norepinephrine and can produce transient sympathomimetic effects. Drugs that block the vesicle uptake transporter prevent the movement of norepinephrine into vesicles and deplete the nerve ending of this neurotransmitter, also preventing norepinephrine release after depolarization. Examples include rauwolfia alkaloids (reserpine), tetrabenazine, and guanethidine (in part). Reserpine and ketanserin inhibit both VMAT1 and VMAT2, whereas tetrabenazine only inhibits VMAT2. Like guanethidine, reserpine causes transient norepinephrine release with initial dosing or early in overdose. β-Adrenoceptor antagonists block presynaptic β_2-adrenoceptors to limit catecholamine release from nerve endings, although this does not appear to be their main mechanism of action.

Imidazoline and α_2-Adrenoceptor Agonists. Numerous imidazoline derivatives (eg, clonidine) and structurally similar compounds have been used as centrally acting antihypertensive agents or long-acting topical vasoconstrictors. These agents are currently divided into first-generation agents (eg, clonidine) that are thought to act at both α_{2A}-adrenoceptor and imidazoline binding sites, and into second-generation agents (eg, rilmenidine) that express much greater affinity for imidazoline binding sites than for α_{2A}-adrenergic receptors.

The ventromedial (depressor) and the rostral-ventrolateral (pressor) areas of the medulla (VLM) are responsible for the central regulation of cardiovascular tone and blood pressure. They receive afferent fibers from the carotid and aortic baroreceptors, which form the tractus solitarius via the nucleus tractus solitarius (NTS).[68]

The hypotensive actions of α_2-adrenoceptor agonists were previously attributed entirely to brainstem α_2-adrenoceptor activation, because stimulation of postsynaptic α_2-adrenoceptors in the NTS decreased sympathetic output (Fig. 10–6).[19] The discovery of imidazoline binding sites, however, led to a more complicated analysis. It was discovered that imidazolines and related substances produced hypotension when applied to the VLM, whereas catecholamines capable of activating α_2-adrenoceptors were claimed to be incapable of producing effects at this site. This led to the hypothesis that receptors specific for imidazoline-like compounds, different from α_{2A}-adrenoceptors, must exist. Decreased sympathetic output could result from activation of imidazoline binding sites in the VLM and from α_2-adrenoceptor activation in the NTS; sedation and respiratory depression were attributed to α_2-adrenoceptor activation in the locus ceruleus.[44]

Imidazoline binding sites have been characterized and subdivided into I_1, I_2 (with subtypes), and I_3.[38] I_1 binding sites reside on neuronal plasma membranes and are involved in controlling systemic blood pressure. I_2 sites are allosteric sites found on the external membrane of mitochondria and modulate MAO-A and MAO-B.[19,38] The putative I_3 sites are thought to modulate insulin secretion via ATP-sensitive potassium channels in β-islet cells.[38]

It has not been established whether imidazoline binding sites act through ion channels, through G proteins, or through some other mechanism. Naturally occurring ligand(s) for these receptors have yet to be elucidated. An endogenous ligand referred to as *clonidine-displacing substance* has been proposed. This ligand is capable of displacing clonidine from imidazoline sites; however, no biologic function has been ascribed to this ligand, and its identity remains elusive.[38]

Functional studies suggested that the hypotensive effects of clonidine-like drugs involved imidazoline binding sites, while most of the side effects involved α_{2A}-adrenoceptors.[44] Drugs such as rilmenidine, possessing much greater activity at imidazoline binding sites than at α_{2A}-adrenoceptors, were, therefore, developed. However, more recent functional evidence suggests that there is significant interaction between the imidazoline sites and α_{2A}-adrenoceptors, and that this interaction is necessary to trigger hypotensive effects.[18,44] As examples, there appears to be a close relationship between "presynaptic" imidazoline sites and "downstream" α_{2A}-adrenoceptors in the VLM mediating hypotension;[59] α_{2A}-adrenoceptors in the VLM appear to be activated as a consequence of imidazoline site activation. Although second-generation agents (rilmenidine and moxonidine) preferentially act via imidazoline binding sites, and although α_{2A}-adrenoceptors are important for the hypotension produced by first-generation agents (clonidine and α-methyldopa), hypotension produced by all of these agents is dependent on central noradrenergic pathways.[18,59] Some studies report that yohimbine, an α_2-adrenoceptor antagonist, reverses the hypotensive effect of both clonidine and rilmenidine-like drugs, when given at high doses.[18,38] Thus, it appears that there is significant interaction between imidazoline sites and α_{2A}-adrenoceptors, and that centrally acting antihypertensive agents with relatively high affinity for imidazoline binding sites may require both imidazoline-specific sites and functional α_{2A}-adrenoceptors to produce their hypotensive actions.[18,19,38,44,59]

Ingestions of agents that activate α_{2A}-adrenoceptors and imidazoline binding sites (Table 10–5) produce a mixed picture. Peripheral postsynaptic α_2-adrenoceptor stimulation produces vasoconstriction, pallor, and hypertension, often with reflex bradycardia (Fig. 10–5). Peripheral presynaptic α_2-adrenoceptor stimulation prevents norepinephrine release (Fig. 10–5), whereas central α_2-adrenoceptor stimulation in the locus ceruleus accounts for CNS and respiratory depression (Fig. 10–6). Stimulation of postsynaptic α_2-adrenoceptors in the NTS and, with some agents, stimulation of central I_1 receptors in the VLM are thought to inhibit sympathetic output and enhance parasympathetic tone, explaining hypotension with bradycardia (Fig. 10–6).[68] Both first- and second-generation agents produce dry mouth.[19,38]

Dopamine-β-Hydroxylase Inhibition. Inhibition of dopamine-β-hydroxylase (Fig. 10–5) prevents the conversion of dopamine to norepinephrine, resulting in less norepinephrine release and less α- and β-adrenoceptor stimulation with neuronal firing. Disulfiram produces such inhibition.[40] Because norepinephrine release mediates most of dopamine's ability to cause vasoconstriction, norepinephrine is the vasopressor of choice in a hypotensive patient taking disulfiram. Diethyldithiocarbamate, used in metal chelation and in some AIDS patients, is a disulfiram metabolite that produces similar actions. MAOIs and α-methyldopa also inhibit dopamine-β-hydroxylase, although this is not their main mechanism of action.[92]

Dopamine is relatively contraindicated in hypotensive patients who have overdosed on MAOIs. First, dopamine acts indirectly and its administration may produce an adrenergic storm. Second, even if an adrenergic storm does not occur, most of dopamine's α-mediated vasoconstriction is secondary to norepinephrine release. In the presence of MAOIs, norepinephrine synthesis may be impaired from concomitant dopamine-β-hydroxylase inhibition, and dopamine may not reliably raise blood pressure if cytoplasmic and vesicular stores have been depleted. In the presence of impaired norepinephrine release or α blockade by any cause, unopposed dopamine-induced vasodilatation from action on peripheral dopamine and β-adrenoceptors may paradoxically lower blood pressure further. Norepinephrine and epinephrine can be used to support blood pressure relatively safely in patients taking MAOIs, because these vasopressors have little or no indirect action and are metabolized by COMT when given intravenously.

DOPAMINE

Because dopamine is the direct precursor of norepinephrine, noradrenergic vesicles contain dopamine. The release of norepinephrine from peripheral sympathetic nerves, therefore, always results in release of some dopamine (Fig. 10–5), as does the release of norepinephrine and epinephrine from the adrenal gland, explaining the normal presence of dopamine in blood. In peripheral tissues, dopamine receptors cause vasodilatation of mesenteric, renal, and coronary vascular beds. Dopamine can also stimulate β-adrenoceptors and, at high doses, can directly stimulate α-adrenoceptors. When dopamine is administered intravenously, most vasoconstriction is caused by dopamine-induced norepinephrine release.

Dopamine accounts for about one-half of all catecholamines in the brain and is present in greater quantities than norepinephrine or 5-HT. In contrast to the diffuse projections of noradrenergic neurons, dopaminergic neurons and receptors are highly organized and concentrated in several areas, especially in the basal ganglia and limbic system.[76,126]

Excessive dopaminergic activity in the striatum and/or other areas from any cause (eg, increased release, impaired uptake, increased receptor sensitivity) may produce acute choreoathetosis[70] and acute Gilles de la Tourette syndrome, with tics, spitting, and cursing. Excessive dopaminergic activity in the limbic system and, perhaps, in other areas, produces paranoid psychosis that is indistinguishable from paranoid schizophrenia and is thought responsible for much of the drug craving and addictive behavior in patients abusing sympathomimetic drugs. Diminished dopaminergic tone (eg, impaired release, receptor blockade) in the basal ganglia produces various extrapyramidal disorders such as acute dystonias and parkinsonism.[116,134,143]

Synthesis, Release, and Uptake

The steps of dopamine synthesis and vesicle storage are the same as those for norepinephrine, except that dopamine is not converted to norepinephrine after transport into vesicles (Fig. 10–7). Dopamine is removed from the synapse via uptake by a neuronal membrane dopamine transporter. Like the norepinephrine transporter, this pump is not completely specific for dopamine, but transports drugs such as amphetamines and other structurally similar sympathomimetics.

Cytoplasmic dopamine has a fate similar to norepinephrine. It is pumped back into vesicles or degraded by MAO. COMT degrades dopamine that has entered the systemic circulation.

Dopamine Receptors

All dopamine receptors are linked to G proteins and are divided into two main groups, depending on whether they raise or lower cAMP concentrations. Dopamine D_1-like receptors (D_1 and D_5) are expressed as various subtypes and are linked to G_s to stimulate adenylate cyclase and to raise cAMP concentrations.[76] Dopamine is 5–10 times more potent at D_5 receptors as it is at D_1 receptors.[76] D_1 receptors are concentrated in the caudate putamen, nucleus accumbens, and olfactory tubercle, whereas D_5 receptors are concentrated in the olfactory tubercle, hippocampus, and mammillary nucleus.[76,126]

D_2-like receptors (D_2, D_3, D_4) are linked to G_i and G_o, and perhaps to other G proteins, to produce several actions, including inhibition of adenylate cyclase and the lowering of cAMP levels. Again, numerous subtypes of receptors exist (eg, D_{2S}, D_{2L}). D_2 receptors are concentrated in the basal ganglia and limbic system.

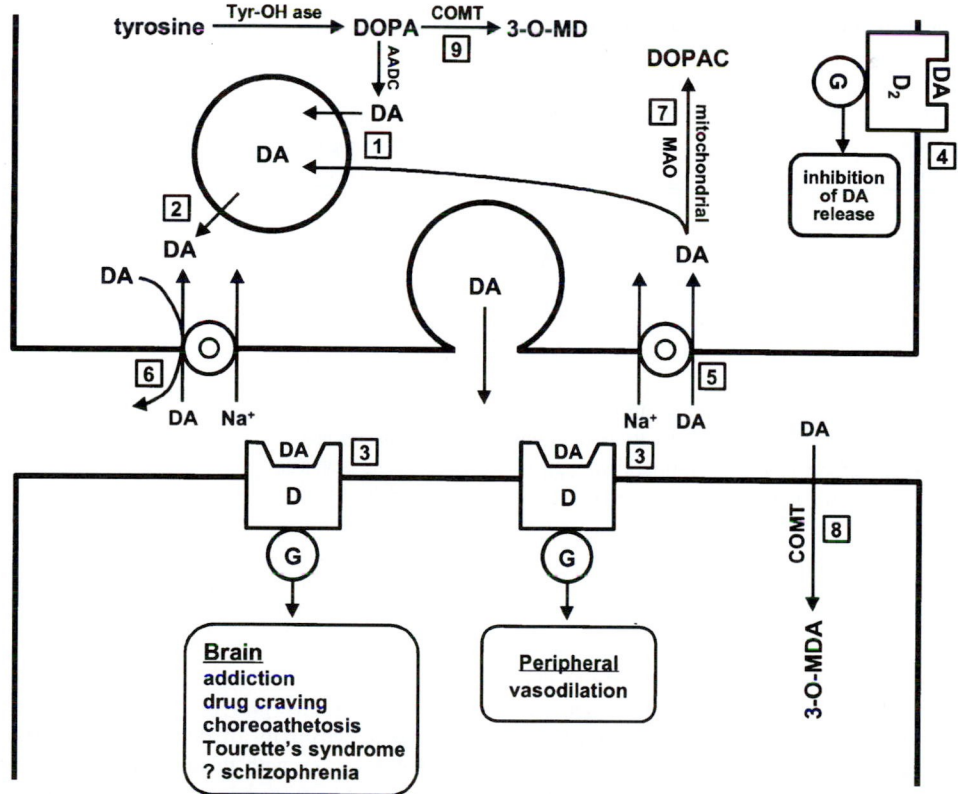

Figure 10–7. A dopaminergic nerve ending and postsynaptic membrane. Dopamine (DA) released from nerve endings binds to various postsynaptic DA receptors (D) on neurons or peripheral end organs. Stimulation of presynaptic D_2 receptors [4] lessens DA release. Agents in Table 10–6 may act to inhibit vesicle uptake [1]; cause DA to leave the vesicle and move into the cytoplasm [2]; activate or antagonize DA receptors [3,4]; inhibit DA uptake [5]; cause reverse transport of cytoplasmic DA into the synapse by raising cytoplasmic DA concentrations [6]; prevent DA degradation by inhibiting monoamine oxidase (MAO) [7]; prevent DA degradation by inhibiting catechol-*O*-methyltransferase (COMT) [8]; or prevent dopa metabolism by inhibiting COMT [9]. Importantly, physiologic actions of COMT inhibitors mainly result from COMT inhibition in nonneuronal tissue because only small amounts of COMT actually reside in neurons. Both DA and dopa are substrates for COMT. For purposes of illustration, dopa metabolism is shown presynaptically, and DA metabolism shown postsynaptically. 3-*O*-MD = 3-*O*-methyldopa; 3-*O*-MDA = 3-*O*-methyldopamine; AADC = L-aromatic amino acid decarboxylase; DOPAC = 3,4-dihydroxyphenylacetic acid; Tyr-OHase = tyrosine hydroxylase.

Some D_2 receptors also reside on presynaptic membranes, where their activation limits neurotransmitter release, including the peripheral release of norepinephrine (Figs. 10–5 and 10–7). D_3 receptors are concentrated in the hypothalamic and limbic nuclei. D_4 receptors are concentrated in the frontal cortex and limbic nuclei (rather than basal ganglia nuclei). Most agonists bind to the D_3 receptors with higher affinity than to D_2 receptors, whereas most antagonists bind preferentially to D_2 receptors.[76,126] Most agonists and antagonists express a lower affinity for D_4 receptors than they express for D_2 receptors; a notable exception is clozapine.

Chemical Agents

Table 10–6 provides examples of chemical agents that affect dopaminergic neurotransmission.

Dopamine Agonism

Indirect- and Mixed-Acting Agents. Most indirect- and mixed-acting sympathomimetics cause dopamine release. The mechanism of action is similar to that causing norepinephrine release. Benztropine, diphenhydramine, trihexyphenidyl, and orphenadrine cause dopamine release, perhaps contributing to their abuse potential, which is noted below.[99] Excessive dopaminergic activity following therapeutic doses or overdoses of decongestants (eg, pseudoephedrine), amphetamines, methylphenidate, and pemoline can produce acute choreoathetosis and Tourette syndrome.[21,85] Parkinsonian patients ingesting excessive doses of L-dopa (which is converted to dopamine) may present with similar symptoms.

Direct Agonists. Bromocriptine is an ergot derivative that directly activates dopamine receptors. Toxic effects include those described above for indirect-acting agents. Apomorphine directly activates D_2 receptors. Such action at the chemoreceptive triggering zone produces vomiting, whereas agonism in the basal ganglia explains apomorphine's use in the treatment of Parkinson disease. Fenoldopam is a D_1 agonist used as a vasodilator in the treatment of hypertensive emergencies.

D_1- and D_2-receptor activation is the predominant mediator of locomotor effects from dopamine agonists. Activation of either D_1- or D_2-like receptors, therefore, produces antiparkinsonian effects.[60,126] Cabergoline, ropinirole, and pramipexole are newer selective D_2-like agonists used to treat Parkinson disease.[8,42,60] Dihydrexidine is a D_1-like agonist under investigation for the same purpose.

Uptake Inhibition. Agents inhibiting dopamine uptake include cocaine, amphetamines, methylphenidate, and probably amantadine. Increased dopaminergic activity from cocaine toxicity may produce choreoathetosis ("crack dancing") and Tourette syndrome. In general, antidepressants are not strong dopamine uptake blockers. However, bupropion appears to be more active in this regard.[122]

As noted earlier, much of the drug craving and addiction produced by sympathomimetics probably results from excessive dopaminergic activity.[134] Interestingly, the anticholinergic drugs benztropine, diphenhydramine, trihexyphenidyl, and orphenadrine are also dopamine uptake inhibitors, possibly explaining their abuse.[99,131] In fact, benztropine is one of the most potent dopamine uptake inhibitors known. Amantadine, an antiparkinsonian agent that causes dopamine release and some inhibition of dopamine uptake (as well as being anticholinergic), is also abused.

TABLE 10–6. Examples of Chemical Agents That Affect Dopaminergic Neurotransmission

Dopamine Agonism	
Direct stimulation of dopamine receptors	Cocaine
Apomorphine	Diphenhydramine
Bromocriptine	Methylphenidate
Cabergoline	Orphenadrine
L-Dopa[a]	Pemoline
Fenoldopam	Trihexyphenidyl
Lisuride	
Pergolide	Increase dopamine-receptor sensitivity
Pramipexole	Amphetamines
Ropinirole	Antipsychotics
	Metoclopramide
Inhibit dopamine metabolism—MAOIs	Phenytoin
Clorgyline	
Isocarboxazid	
Moclobemide	**Dopamine Antagonism**
Pargyline	Block dopamine receptors
Phenelzine	Amoxapine
Selegiline	Buspirone
Tranylcypromine	Clozapine
	Droperidol
	Haloperidol
Inhibit dopamine metabolism—COMTIs	Loxapine
Entacapone	Metoclopramide
Tolcapone	Molindone
	Olanzapine
Indirect-acting	Phenothiazines
Amantadine	Pimozide
Amphetamines	Quetiapine
Benztropine	Risperidone
Decongestants	Thioxanthenes
Diphenhydramine	Trazodone
MAOIs	Tricyclic antidepressants[b]
Methylphenidate	
Orphenadrine	Ziprasidone
Pemoline	
Phencyclidine	Destroy dopaminergic neurons
Trihexyphenidyl	MPTP
Inhibit dopamine uptake	
Amantadine	Prevent vesicle dopamine uptake
Amphetamines	
Benztropine	Reserpine
Bupropion	Tetrabenazine

MAOIs = monoamine oxidase inhibitors; COMTIs = catechol-o-methyltransferase inhibitors; MPTP = 1-methyl-4-phenyl-1,2,3,6-tetrahydropyridine.
[a]Metabolized to dopamine, which acts as an agonist.
[b]Relatively weak D_2-receptor antagonists.

Increase of Receptor Sensitivity. Several drugs are thought to increase sensitivity of dopamine receptors, resulting in choreoathetosis, even with therapeutic doses (eg, phenytoin). Evidence exists that increased dopamine receptor sensitivity may be responsible for movement disorders resulting from amphetamines.[29] Tardive dyskinesia (discussed later) may also result from increased dopamine receptor sensitivity.

MAO Inhibition. MAOIs inhibit the breakdown of cytoplasmic dopamine. Part of the food and drug interactions with MAOIs results from excessive release of dopamine from nerve endings.

COMT Inhibition. Peripheral COMT inhibitors (eg, entacapone, tolcapone) are given with levodopa to patients with Parkinson disease to prevent peripheral degradation of levodopa to 3-*O*-methyl-dopa.[62,67] This allows more levodopa to traverse the blood-brain barrier and to be converted to dopamine by neuronal dopa decarboxylase. Tolcapone also inhibits COMT in the brain.[67] Other substrates of COMT include dopa, dopamine, norepinephrine, epinephrine, and their hydroxylated metabolites. COMT inhibitors might potentiate the effects of these drugs when administered intravenously.[67]

Dopamine Antagonism

Direct Receptor Blockade. Blockade of dopamine receptors is the specific aim when using many therapeutic agents. The neuroleptic actions of butyrophenones, phenothiazines, and other antipsychotics mainly correlate with their ability to block D_2 receptors, probably in the limbic system. Many phenothiazines block both D_1-like and D_2-like receptors, whereas haloperidol mainly blocks D_2-like receptors. Unfortunately, antipsychotics and metoclopramide also block dopamine receptors in the striatum, producing various extrapyramidal symptoms, including acute parkinsonism and dystonias.

In the last decade, several "atypical" antipsychotics were marketed that produce fewer extrapyramidal effects and are thought to carry less risk of producing tardive dyskinesia.[118] The relative affinity of an antipsychotic for $5-HT_{2A}$ receptors over D_2 receptors has predictive value for atypical agents with lower risk of extrapyramidal symptoms.[118] Such agents include clozapine, olanzapine, quetiapine, risperidone, and ziprasidone.

The ratio of muscarinic (M_1) blockade to D_2-receptor blockade is also important in limiting extrapyramidal symptoms. Antipsychotic agents exhibiting strong antimuscarinic effects (eg, olanzapine, clozapine, thioridazine) are also less likely to induce extrapyramidal symptoms.[118]

Buspirone, an antianxiety agent, antagonizes D_2 receptors, which explains the occasional extrapyramidal reactions. Various cyclic antidepressants, especially amoxapine, block D_2 receptors to some extent.

The chronic use of dopamine-blocking agents causes up-regulation of dopamine receptors. The continued use or, especially, withdrawal of dopamine antagonists (antipsychotics, metoclopramide, and occasionally antidepressants) may result in excessive dopaminergic activity and tardive dyskinesia, characterized by choreiform movements typical of excessive dopaminergic influence in the striatum.

The blockade of dopamine receptors by numerous agents, including butyrophenones, phenothiazines, and metoclopramide, can produce a poorly understood disorder called *neuroleptic malignant syndrome*. Neuroleptic malignant syndrome also follows acute withdrawal of dopamine agonists (eg, stopping L-dopa or bromocriptine in a patient prior to surgery). Neuroleptic malignant syndrome is characterized, in part, by mental status changes, autonomic instability, rigidity, and hyperthermia.

Indirect Antagonism. Reserpine and tetrabenazine prevent transport of dopamine into storage vesicles and deplete nerve endings of dopamine. 1-Methyl-4-phenyl-1,2,3,6-tetrahydropyridine (MPTP), a meperidine analog, undergoes activation by MAO to a metabolite that causes neuronal death. That MPTP causes isolated destruction of dopaminergic neurons is explained by its selective uptake by the membrane dopamine transporter. Both MAOIs and inhibitors of dopamine transporters prevent MPTP-induced destruction of dopaminergic neurons.

SEROTONIN

Serotonin (5-HT, 5-OH-tryptamine) is a ubiquitous indole alkylamine found in nature (animals, plants, venoms) that acts as a neurotransmitter centrally, but is also found peripherally. In fact, less than 2% of the body's 5-HT is found within the CNS.

In the CNS, serotonergic neurons lie in or in juxtaposition to numerous midline nuclei in the brainstem (9 raphe nuclei), from which they project to various parts of the brain, including the basal ganglia. Serotonin is involved with mood, personality, affect, appetite, motor function, temperature regulation, sexual activity, pain perception, sleep induction, and other basic functions. Serotonin is not essential for any of these processes but modulates their quality and extent. The serotonergic system is extremely diverse, with 14 types of receptors that act to stimulate or inhibit neurons, including those of other neurotransmitter systems. Serotonin is also the precursor for the pineal hormone melatonin.[46]

Peripherally, 5-HT is produced mainly in the enterochromaffin cells of the intestine. Local release may contribute to peristalsis, but the corelease of numerous other mediators makes serotonin's exact action difficult to discern. Platelets take up 5-HT while passing through the enteric circulation. Serotonin is released from activated platelets to interact with other platelet membranes (promote aggregation) and with vascular smooth muscle (vasoconstriction in most vascular beds).

Experimentally, 5-HT exhibits diverse effects on the cardiovascular and peripheral nervous systems, although the importance of these actions remains uncertain in the normal physiologic state. Serotonin vasoconstricts (stimulation of $5-HT_2$, $5-HT_{1D}$, and $5-HT_{1B}$ receptors) most vascular beds except for coronary arteries and skeletal muscle, where it produces vasodilatation in the presence of intact endothelium. $5-HT_{1B}$ and $5-HT_{1D}$ agonists (eg, sumatriptan) might produce coronary vasoconstriction as an adverse effect to their desired actions on cranial vasculature.[56]

Centrally, it is particularly difficult to ascribe a specific symptom or physical finding to serotonergic neurons because of the diversity of their physiologic actions. However, 5-HT definitely plays an important role in the action of many hallucinogenic or illusionogenic drugs, which act as partial agonists at cortical $5-HT_2$ receptors.[81] Proserotinergic agents are used to treat depression, whereas agents that antagonize 5-HT receptors ($5-HT_2$) have taken on greater importance in the management of schizophrenia.

Generally, 5-HT acts in opposition to dopamine. For example, 5-HT serves to increase prolactin, ACTH, and growth hormone secretion, whereas dopamine decreases prolactin secretion. As another example, activation of basal ganglial $5-HT_{2A}$ receptors inhibits dopamine release. However, well-known exceptions exist, such as cortical $5-HT_3$ receptors, whose activation promotes dopamine release.[81]

Synthesis, Release, and Uptake

Figure 10–8 illustrates 5-HT synthesis. Tryptophan-5-hydroxylase is the rate-limiting enzyme of 5-HT synthesis and is free from negative feedback influences by the end product, 5-HT. Thus increases in tryptophan are predictably accompanied by increased 5-HT production. L-Amino acid decarboxylase (dopa decarboxylase) converts 5-hydroxytryptophan to 5-HT. Cytoplasmic 5-HT is transported into vesicles, where it is concentrated by ion trapping before release by Ca^{2+}-dependent exocytosis. In contrast to vesicles containing dopamine or norepinephrine, 5-HT vesicles con-

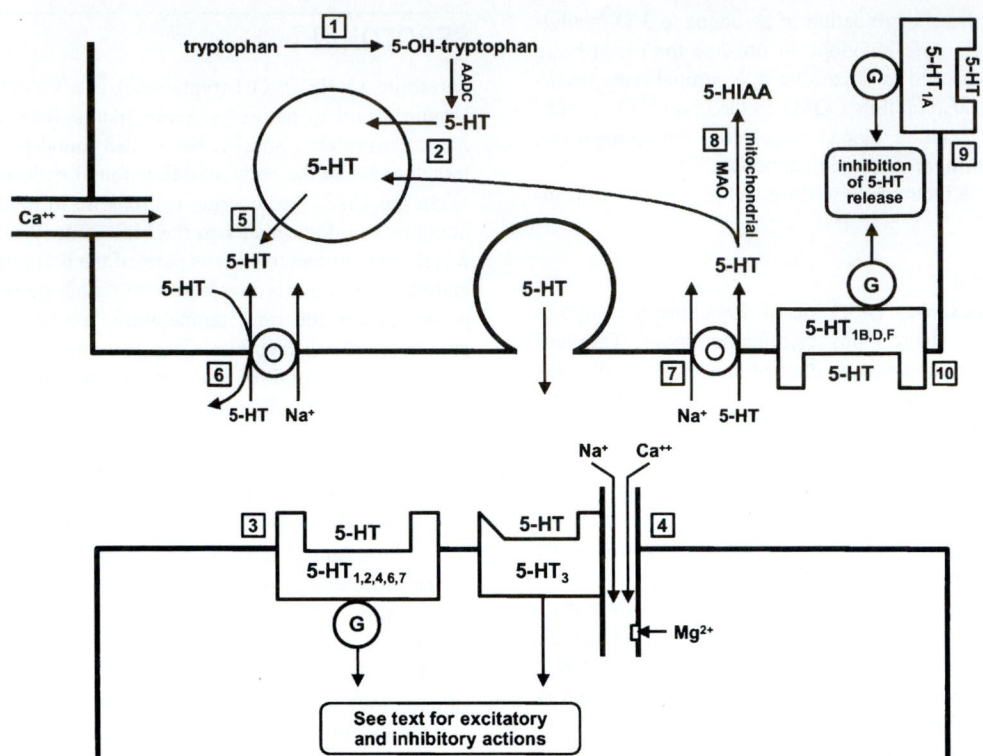

Figure 10–8. A serotonergic nerve ending and postsynaptic membrane. Tryptophan hydroxylase [1] converts tryptophan to 5-hydroxytryptophan (5-OH-tryptophan). Aromatic L-amino acid decarboxylase (AADC) then metabolizes 5-OH-tryptophan to serotonin (5-HT). Serotonin is concentrated within vesicles [2] before exocytosis. After uptake into the neuron [7], 5-HT is transported back into vesicles or undergoes degradation by monoamine oxidase (MAO) to an intermediate compound, which is converted to 5-hydroxy-indoleacetic acid (5-HIAA) [8]. $5\text{-HT}_{1,2,4,6,7}$ receptors [3,9,10] are coupled to G proteins, while 5-HT_3 receptors [4] are ligand-gated cation channels that may conduct Na^+ and/or Ca^{2+}. 5-HT_3 cation channels also appear to be blocked by Mg^{2+} until the cell is depolarized, allowing Mg^{2+} to dissociate—a mechanism similar to that found at NMDA glutamate receptors. In addition to residing on postsynaptic membranes, 5-HT_{1A}, 5-HT_{1B}, $5HT_{1D}$, and 5-HT_{1F} receptors serve as presynaptic autoreceptors that, when stimulated, decrease further release of 5-HT [9,10]. Presynaptic 5-HT_{1A} receptors mainly serve as somatodendritic autoreceptors, whereas presynaptic 5-HT_{1B}, 5-HT_{1D}, and 5-HT_{1F} receptors serve as terminal autoreceptors. Agents in Table 10–7 act to enhance 5-HT synthesis [1]; prevent vesicle uptake of 5-HT [2]; raise cytoplasmic concentrations of 5-HT, resulting in reverse transport of 5-HT into the synapse [6] by displacing 5-HT from vesicles [5] or inhibiting MAO [8]; activate or antagonize 5-HT receptors [3,4,9,10]; or by inhibiting 5-HT uptake [7]. G = G protein.

tain almost no ATP. After release into the synapse, a transporter in the neuronal membrane transfers 5-HT back into the neuron, where it reenters vesicles or is degraded by MAO.

Serotonin is preferentially metabolized by the MAO-A isozyme. Paradoxically, the serotonergic nerve terminal is almost devoid of MAO-A but contains abundant amounts of MAO-B. It has been hypothesized that the large amounts of MAO-B metabolize other agents that might inappropriately promote serotonin release (eg, dopa). However, the small amount of MAO-A found in serotonergic neurons provides adequate degradation of 5-HT.[46]

Serotonin Receptors

Serotonin receptor classification is complex and continuously evolving as new receptors are identified. Most authors identify seven major functioning receptors (5-HT_1 through 5-HT_7) and numerous subtypes.[7]

5-HT_1 Receptors. Receptors in the 5-HT_1 class are coupled to G proteins and commonly increase K^+ efflux and decrease cAMP concentrations. Members of the 5-HT_1 receptor class express

greatest affinity for 5-HT and are thus biologically active under normal physiologic conditions. 5-HT_{1A} receptors reside predominantly on raphe nuclei, where they act as somatodendritic autoreceptors. Hippocampal 5-HT_{1A} receptors reside postsynaptically, where they also inhibit through similar mechanisms.[78]

Central 5-HT_{1D} and 5-HT_{1B} receptors primarily act as inhibitory terminal autoreceptors and heteroreceptors. They are found less commonly on postsynaptic membranes. There has been a recent change in 5-HT_{1D} and 5-HT_{1B} receptor nomenclature. Originally, the 5-HT_{1B} receptor was not believed to exist in humans. However, most of the actions described in previous literature regarding 5-HT_{1D} receptors can now be attributed to 5-HT_{1B} receptors. Unfortunately, this distinction will continue to lead to confusion for some years to come. Ketanserin and ritanserin specifically antagonize 5-HT_{1D} receptors. Cranial blood vessels possess 5-HT_{1D} and 5-HT_{1B} receptors, whose activation produces vasoconstriction and decreased inflammation.[54,56]

5-HT_{1E} and 5-HT_{1F} receptors are the most recently discovered and characterized members of the 5-HT_1 receptor class. 5-HT_{1F} receptors reside on presynaptic membranes and may act in a similar fashion to 5-HT_{1D} and 5-HT_{1B} receptors.[7]

5-HT$_2$ Receptors. The three subtypes of 5-HT$_2$ receptors are coupled to G proteins, thus serving to decrease K$^+$ efflux and/or increase intracellular Ca^{2+} concentration by raising concentrations of inositol triphosphate and diacylglycerol.[121] The three subtypes of 5-HT$_2$ receptors are so similar in characterization that investigational agents have great difficulty in distinguishing the subtypes. 5-HT$_{2A}$ receptors are most concentrated in the cerebral cortex, where they serve as excitatory postsynaptic receptors. Their activation increases glutamate release from pyramidal cells.[1] 5-HT$_{2A}$ receptors also reside on platelets, where their activation produces platelet aggregation. 5-HT$_{2C}$ receptors (previously 5-HT$_{1C}$) reside on the choroid plexus, where they regulate cerebral spinal fluid production. Peripherally, 5-HT$_{2C}$ activation also promotes penile erection. Although 5-HT$_{2B}$ receptors have been identified and are abundant in the gastric fundus, their role remains ill defined.[7]

5-HT$_3$ Receptors. 5-HT$_3$ receptors are ligand-gated cation channels that are structurally similar to ACh nicotinic receptors and GABA$_A$ Cl$^-$ channels.[4] They have been localized to both presynaptic and postsynaptic membranes. Upon activation, they stimulate the neuron by opening the channel to cause depolarization through Na$^+$ and/or Ca^{2+} influx. In addition, these channels are normally blocked by Mg^{2+} in a voltage-dependent manner similar to glutaminergic NMDA receptors (see section on glutamate). Centrally, 5-HT$_3$ receptors are expressed diffusely, but are especially concentrated in the chemoreceptive triggering zone, where their activation induces emesis. In the cerebral cortex, their activation leads to increased release of dopamine and decreased release of ACh. Cortical 5-HT$_3$ receptors are frequently identified on GABA interneurons where they increase inhibitory, GABAergic tone. In contrast to cerebral actions, activation of peripheral 5-HT$_3$ receptors on cholinergic nerves in the gut enhances ACh release to increase gastrointestinal motility.[7,15]

5-HT$_4$ Receptors. 5-HT$_4$ receptors are coupled to G proteins (G$_s$). Their activation leads to increased cAMP concentrations. 5-HT$_4$ receptors are scattered diffusely throughout the brain, and their exact role remains undefined. Peripheral 5-HT$_4$ receptors reside in the heart and intestines, where their activation can be demonstrated to produce tachycardia and contraction of gut smooth muscle, respectively. Again, whether this action is important under normal physiologic conditions is not clear. Both central and peripheral 5-HT$_4$ receptors promote the release of acetylcholine.[37]

5-HT$_5$ Receptors. 5-HT$_5$ receptors exist in the form of at least two subtypes. Their mechanism of activation remains unknown. 5-HT$_5$ receptor agonists or antagonists are not readily available.[7]

5-HT$_6$ and 5-HT$_7$ Receptors. 5-HT$_6$ and 5-HT$_7$ receptors are positively coupled to cAMP formation through G proteins. Their distribution is poorly defined. However, many antidepressant and antipsychotic agents antagonize these receptors. They are currently a source of great interest because of the possibility of avoiding dopamine blockade to achieve antipsychotic activity. The 5-HT$_7$ receptor may be particularly important in regulating circadian rhythms.[73]

Chemical Agents

Table 10–7 provides examples of chemical agents that affect serotonergic meurotransmission.

TABLE 10–7. Examples of Agents That Affect Serotonergic Neurotransmission

Serotonin Agonism	Citalopram
Enhance 5-HT synthesis	Cocaine
L-Tryptophan	Dextromethorphan
5-Hydroxytryptophan	Fluoxetine
	Fluvoxamine
Direct 5-HT agonists	Lamotrigine
Buspirone	Meperidine
Cisapride	Nefazodone
Ergots and indoles (eg, LSD)[a]	Sertraline
Gepirone	Tramadol
Ipsapirone	Trazodone
mCPP	Tricyclic antidepressants[b]
Metoclopramide	Vanlafaxine
Naratriptan	
Phenylalkylamines (eg, mescaline)[a]	**Serotonin Antagonism**
Rizatriptan	Direct 5-HT antagonists
Sulpriride	Amisulpride
Sumatriptan	Clozapine
Urapidil	Cyproheptadine
Zolmitriptan	Ergots and indoles (eg, LSD)[a]
	Granisetron
Increase 5-HT release	Haloperidol
Amphetamines	Ketanserin
Cocaine	Mianserin
Codeine derivatives	Methysergide
Dexfenfluramine	Metoclopramide
Dextromethorphan	Mirtazapine
L-Dopa	Nefazodone
Fenfluramine	Olanzapine
MDMA	Ondansetron
Mirtazapine	Phenothiazines
Reserpine (initial)	Phentolamine
	Phenylalkylamines (eg, mescaline)[a]
Increase 5-HT tone by unknown mechanism	Pindolol
Lithium	Propranolol
	Quetiapine
Inhibit 5-HT breakdown (MAOIs)	Risperidone
Clorgyline	Ritanserin
Isocarboxazid	Sertindole
Moclobemide	Trazodone
Pargyline	Tricyclic antidepressants
Phenelzine	Tropisetron
Tranylcypromine	Ziprasidone
Selegiline	Zotepine
Inhibit 5-HT uptake	Inhibit vesicle uptake
Amoxapine	Reserpine
Amphetamines	Ketanserin
Carbamazepine	Tetrabenazine

5-HT = serotonin; LSD = lysergic acid diethylamide; MAOIs = monoamine oxidase inhibitors; mCPP = *m*-chlorphenylpiperazine (metabolite of trazodone and nefazodone); MDMA = methylenedioxymethamphetamine.
[a]Indoles and phenylalkylamines activate and antagonize various 5-HT receptors. Their hallucinogenic/illusionogenic effects mainly result from partial agonism at 5-HT$_2$ receptors.
[b]Clomipramine is the most potent 5-HT uptake inhibitor of the tricyclic antidepressants.

Serotonin Agonists.   The ingestion of tryptophan is thought to increase 5-HT production and was commonly used as an unproved sleep aid until it was associated with the eosinophilia myalgia syndrome. 5-Hydroxytryptophan (5-HTP) is the immediate precursor to 5-HT. 5-HTP is commonly available over-the-counter. The antianxiety agents buspirone, gepirone, and ipsapirone act as partial agonists at somatodendritic and postsynaptic 5-HT$_{1A}$ receptors.[7] Sumatriptan, an antimigraine agent, mainly activates 5-HT$_{1D}$ and 5-HT$_{1B}$ receptors. Sumatriptan's action may result from vasoconstriction of meningeal and other cranial, extracerebral vasculature; no impairment of cerebral blood flow follows the use of this agent. Other members of the triptan class of drugs include rizatriptan, zolmitriptan, and naratriptan.[56]

Metoclopramide and cisapride, prokinetic drugs, activate 5-HT$_4$ receptors to increase gut motility.[37,57] Activation of myocardial 5-HT$_4$ receptors explains tachycardia that sometimes occurs with therapeutic doses of these agents.

Numerous indoles and phenylalkylamines, including ergot alkaloids, LSD, psilocybin, and mescaline, exhibit both agonistic and antagonistic properties at multiple 5-HT receptors. Their hallucinogenic/illusionogenic action is best explained by partial agonism at 5-HT$_{2A}$ receptors. Some substituted amphetamines (eg, methylenedioxymethamphetamine) may directly stimulate serotonin receptors.[1,81]

Cocaine and indirect-acting sympathomimetics, especially amphetamines, cause serotonin release as previously described. Other releasing agents are dextromethorphan and codeine derivatives. Centrally, dopamine undergoes uptake into serotonergic neurons to displace 5-HT from the neuron. Ingestion of L-dopa or other agents that increase CNS dopamine concentrations can cause 5-HT release.[98]

Inhibitors of 5-HT uptake include amphetamines, cocaine, various antidepressants, meperidine, and dextromethorphan.[98] Several antidepressants specifically inhibit 5-HT uptake. Examples of selective serotonin reuptake inhibitors (SSRIs) include fluoxetine, sertraline, paroxetine, fluvoxamine, and citalopram.[49] The use of SSRIs sometimes produces extrapyramidal side effects[5] for reasons that remain unclear because of the numerous actions of 5-HT in the basal ganglia. Two anticonvulsants—carbamazepine and lamotrigine—appear to inhibit 5-HT uptake.[133] Again, reserpine and tetrabenazine prevent 5-HT uptake into vesicles.

MAO-A accounts for most 5-HT degradation, and nonspecific MAOIs and MAO-A inhibitors (clorgyline, moclobemide) both raise 5-HT levels and, through indirect action, probably cause 5-HT release.[49,98]

Serotonin Antagonists.   Trazodone and nefazodone act mainly as antagonists at 5-HT2 receptors, but are also weak uptake inhibitors. Both undergo metabolism to m-chlorophenylpiperazine (mCPP), which activates most 5-HT receptors, but is especially active at 5-HT2C receptors. Methysergide and cyproheptadine antagonize 5-HT1 and 5-HT2 receptors. 49,98

Mirtazapine exhibits complex actions, including antagonism of 5-HT$_2$ and 5-HT$_3$ receptors. Mirtazapine also indirectly increases 5-HT$_{1A}$ activity and enhances release of norepinephrine through antagonism of α_2-adrenoceptors. Mirtazapine also demonstrates potent antagonism of histaminic, muscarinic, and α-adrenoceptors.[49]

Most antipsychotics and tricyclic antidepressants antagonize 5-HT$_{2A}$ and, to a lesser extent, 5-HT$_{2C}$ receptors. In fact, investigators are interested in developing antipsychotic agents similar to

risperidone that possess potent antagonistic properties at 5-HT$_2$ receptors without accompanying dopamine receptor antagonism in order to limit extrapyramidal side effects. These investigations have resulted in the introduction of olanzapine, sertindole, ziprasidone, zotepine, quetiapine, and amisulpride.[14]

Ondansetron, granisetron, and tropisetron antagonize 5-HT$_3$ receptors.[42] Their antiemetic action is thought to be explained by several mechanisms. Central antagonism at the chemoreceptor triggering zone lessens vomiting. Peripheral 5-HT$_3$ receptor antagonism in the gut prevents ACh release, decreasing gut motility. Finally, antagonism of vagal 5-HT$_3$ receptors decreases afferent stimulatory signals to the vomiting center in the brainstem.[7] Ondansetron and other experimental 5-HT$_3$ antagonists are being studied in the treatment of schizophrenia because of their ability to prevent dopamine release. Metoclopramide antagonizes 5-HT$_3$ and D$_2$ receptors.

Serotonin Syndrome.   Excessive stimulation of 5-HT$_{1A}$ receptors and, to a lesser extent, 5-HT$_2$ receptors causes serotonin syndrome.[98] Briefly, this disorder is characterized by shivering, myoclonus, tremor, and rigidity (especially of legs), along with hyperthermia, tachycardia, diaphoresis, confusion, agitation, convulsions, and coma. This iatrogenic, idiosyncratic syndrome results most commonly from the combined use of two serotonergic drugs (eg, SSRI and lithium, SSRI and MAOI, MAOI and clomipramine). Recent reports indicate that serotonin syndrome may occur following the isolated use or overdose of a single serotonergic agent (eg, venlafaxine or fluvoxamine). Drugs that act to increase CNS dopamine concentrations, such as levodopa and bromocriptine, have potential to precipitate serotonin syndrome by indirect serotonin release.[98] Adverse effects (eg, rigidity, hyperthermia) resulting from interactions between MAOIs and meperidine, dextromethorphan, or codeine may result from excessive serotonergic activity, as well, because all of these agents enhance serotonergic tone (Table 10–7).[98]

γ-AMINOBUTYRIC ACID

γ-Aminobutyric acid (GABA) is one of two main inhibitory neurotransmitters of the central nervous system (glycine is discussed below). Drugs that enhance GABA activity are generally used as anticonvulsants, sedative-hypnotics, and general anesthetics. Agents that antagonize GABA activity typically produce CNS excitation and convulsions. GABA is synthesized from glutamate, the brain's main excitatory neurotransmitter.

In general, GABA inhibition predominates in the brain. In the spinal cord, through mono- and polysynaptic reflex pathways, GABA mediates a number of physiologically minor peripheral effects outside the CNS (eg, vasodilatation, bladder relaxation). Spinal cord GABA is important in attenuating skeletal muscle reflex arcs.[90]

Synthesis, Release, and Uptake

Figure 10–9 illustrates GABA synthesis. Glutamic acid decarboxylase (GAD) requires pyridoxal phosphate (PLP) as a cofactor. Pyridoxal phosphate is synthesized from pyridoxine (vitamin B$_6$) by the enzyme pyridoxine kinase (PK).[96] GABA is transported into vesicles and later released through Ca^{2+}-dependent exocytosis into the synapse.[90] Uptake of GABA from the synapse is mediated

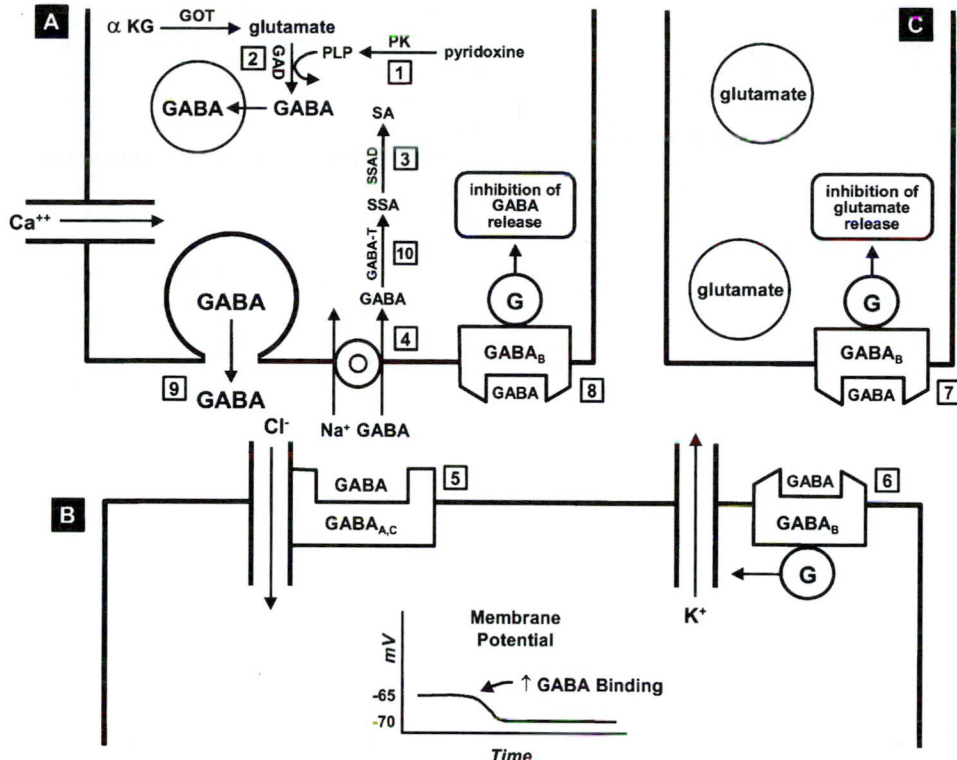

Figure 10–9.   GABAergic neurotransmission. GABA (γ-aminobutyric acid) released from neuron A binds to postsynaptic GABA$_A$, GABA$_B$, or GABA$_C$ receptors to hyperpolarize and inhibit neuron B [5,6] or to presynaptic GABA$_B$ heteroreceptors on neuron C [7] to inhibit neurotransmitter release by blocking Ca^{2+} influx (an excitatory glutamatergic neuron is shown as an example). Stimulation of GABA$_B$ autoreceptors on neuron A [8] also reduces further release of GABA. Acute falls in pyridoxal phosphate (PLP) lead to impaired glutamic acid decarboxylase (GAD) activity and low GABA concentrations. Although GABA-transaminase (GABA-T) also requires PLP, acute falls in PLP do not affect this enzyme as dramatically because of tight PLP binding to the GABA-T complex. Agents in Table 10–9 act to impair PLP formation by inhibiting pyridoxine kinase (PK) [1]; to increase GABA concentrations by either stimulating GAD [2] or inhibiting succinic semialdehyde dehydrogenase (SSAD) [3]; to inhibit GABA uptake [4]; to stimulate or block GABA receptors [5–8]; to cause GABA release [9]; or to inhibit GABA-T [10]. Glutamic-oxaloacetic transaminase (GOT), GABA-T, and SSAD are mitochondrial enzymes. G = G protein; α-KG = α-ketoglutarate; SA = succinic acid.

by a Na$^+$-dependent transporter.[90] Evidence also suggests that GABA is released into the synapse from cytoplasm by reverse transport under some conditions. Cytoplasmic GABA can be transported back into vesicles or degraded by GABA-transaminase (GABA-T) to succinic semialdehyde (SSA), part of which then undergoes oxidation to succinate. GABA-T also requires PLP as a cofactor.[103]

GABA Receptors

There are three main types of GABA receptors (Table 10–8).[17] GABA$_A$ receptors are Cl$^-$ channels that mediate postsynaptic inhi-

TABLE 10–8.   GABA Receptors and Their Characteristics

	GABA$_A$	GABA$_B$	GABA$_C$
Receptor	Cl$^-$ channel	G-protein-coupled	Cl$^-$ channel
Bicuculline antagonism	Yes	No	No
Baclofen agonism	No	Yes	No
Benzodiazepine agonism	Yes	No	No
Barbiturate agonism	Yes	No	No
Picrotoxin antagonism	Yes	No	Slight

bition by allowing Cl$^-$ to move into and hyperpolarize the postsynaptic neuron. Situated at various sites in relation to the GABA recognition site on the Cl$^-$ channel are sites for exogenous and endogenous modulatory agents (Fig. 10–10) where numerous excitatory and depressant drugs bind, and through which GABA$_A$ receptor responsiveness is regulated under normal physiologic conditions.[33,129,150] The common denominator for modulation at the GABA$_A$ complex is an increase or decrease in inward Cl$^-$ current.

Throughout the CNS there is regional variation in the expression of multiple subunit genes for the GABA$_A$ complex. GABA$_A$ receptors exist as pentamers, composed of at least an α, β, and γ subunit. At least 15 distinct subunits have been identified (six α, three β, three γ, one δ, one epsilon, and one π), and these combine to form various pentameric GABA$_A$ Cl$^-$ channels with different pharmacologic affinities for certain ligands, including anesthetics, benzodiazepines, and for GABA itself.[130]

In mammalian brain, the majority of receptor subtypes comprise α, β, and γ subunits. GABA binds to the β subunit. Both the α and γ subunits compose the benzodiazepine binding site.[130] The α subunit provides some selectivity for different pharmaceutic agents. Zaleplon and zolpidem are particularly effective at displacing benzodiazepines from GABA$_A$ receptors containing the α$_1$

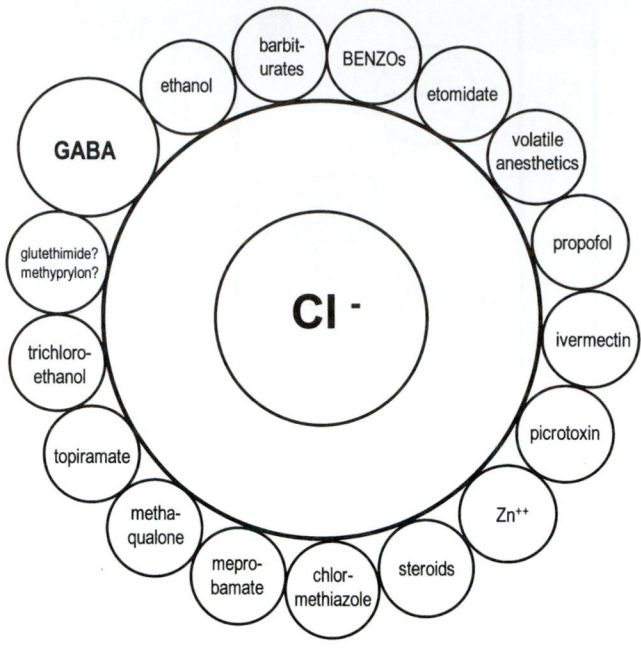

Figure 10–10. Representation of the GABA$_A$ Cl$^-$ channel receptor complex. Benzodiazepines (BENZOs), barbiturates, picrotoxin, steroids, and GABA (γ-aminobutyric acid) clearly bind to different sites on the channel. Although separate circles represent different agents capable of binding to and of modulating Cl$^-$ influx through the GABA$_A$ receptor complex, it is not always apparent where these agents bind on the channel. For example, general anesthetics and ethanol may produce their effects by interacting with the steroid binding site. Chloral hydrate undergoes metabolism to trichloroethanol, which interacts with the GABA$_A$ receptor complex. Zolpidem, zopiclone, and zaleplon are nonbenzodiazepines that bind to the benzodiazepine site. Given the structural similarity of glutethimide and methyprylon to barbiturates, it is speculated that their action may be mediated at GABA$_A$ receptors.

subunit, but are ineffective at GABA$_A$ receptors containing the α_5 subunit.[33,130] This selective binding is thought to account for relatively selective sedative properties of zaleplon and zolpidem at therapeutic doses, as compared to benzodiazepines.[33,53,61,142]

The second type of GABA receptor, GABA$_B$, was discovered when baclofen, a GABA analog now known to be a GABA$_B$-specific agonist, was surprisingly found to bind to presynaptic membranes. Baclofen does not bind to GABA$_A$ receptors. The GABA$_B$ receptors are heterodimers, with companion proteins linked to the receptors, and are coupled to G proteins (probably G_i or G_o) that mediate both presynaptic and postsynaptic inhibition.[20] Presynaptic inhibition results from preventing Ca^{2+} influx so as to impair exocytosis of neurotransmitter vesicles, including those containing excitatory amino acids (eg, glutamate). Postsynaptic inhibition is mediated by increasing K$^+$ efflux through K$^+$ channels, resulting in hyperpolarization of the membrane away from threshold.[20] Through presynaptic actions, GABA$_B$ receptors also serve as autoreceptors, where their activation in response to synaptic GABA provides feedback inhibition of further neurotransmitter release (Fig. 10–9).[17]

A third GABA receptor, GABA$_C$, has been localized in the mammalian retina, particularly in axon terminals of dendrites of

bipolar cells.[17] Like GABA$_A$, the GABA$_C$ receptor is a Cl$^-$ channel that, when activated, allows increased Cl$^-$ influx. GABA$_C$ receptors are composed of ρ-subunits (ρ1–ρ3). The GABA$_C$ receptors are thought to comprise five ligand-binding sites, whereas GABA$_A$ receptors have two ligand-binding sites.[17] GABA$_C$ receptors are insensitive to baclofen, bicuculline, benzodiazepines, barbiturates, and neuroactive steroids, and are less sensitive to picrotoxin (Table 10–8). GABA$_C$ receptors are activated at 40-fold lower GABA concentrations than GABA$_A$ receptors, are less liable to desensitization, and remain open longer than GABA$_A$ Cl$^-$ channels.

Chemical Agents

Table 10–9 provides examples of chemical agents that affect GABAergic neurotransmission.

TABLE 10–9. Examples of Agents That Affect GABAergic Neurotransmission

GABA Agonism	GABA Antagonism
Stimulate GAD	Direct GABA$_A$ antagonists
Valproate	Bicuculline
Gabapentin	Cephalosporins
	Ciprofloxacin
Direct GABA$_A$ agonists	Enoxacin
Muscimol	Imipenem
Progabide[a]	Nalidixic acid
	Norfloxacin
Indirect GABA$_A$ agonists	Ofloxacin
Avermectin	Penicillins
Barbiturates	
Benzodiazepines	Indirect GABA$_A$ antagonists
Chloral hydrate	Aztreonam
Chlormethiazole	Clozapine
Ethanol	Flumazenil
Etomidate	Lindane
Felbamate	MAOIs
Ivermectin	Maprotiline
Meprobamate	Organochlorine insecticides
Methaqualone	Penicillins
Propofol	Pentylenetetrazol
Steroids	Picrotoxin
Topiramate	Tricyclic antidepressants
Trichloroethanol	
Volatile anesthetics	Inhibit GAD
Zaleplon	Cyanide
Zolpidem	Domoic acid
Zopiclone	Hydrazines
	Isoniazid
Direct GABA$_B$ agonists	
Baclofen	Direct GABA$_B$ antagonists
Progabide[a]	Phaclofen[b]
	Saclofen[b]
Inhibit GABA-T	
Vigabatrin	Inhibit PK
	Hydrazines[c]
Inhibit GABA uptake	Isoniazid[c]
Guvacine	
Tiagabine	
Valproate	

GABA = γ-aminobutyric acid; GABA-T = GABA transaminase; GAD = glutamic acid decarboxylase; PK = pyridoxine kinase; MAOIs = monoamine oxidase inhibitors.
[a]Directly activate GABA$_A$ and GABA$_B$ receptors, as well as being metabolized to GABA.
[b]Thought not to cross blood-brain barrier in meaningful amounts.
[c]Major site of action is PK inhibition, although some direct GAD inhibition occurs.

Modulation of GABA Production and Degradation. Isoniazid (INH) and other hydrazines (eg, monomethylhydrazine from mushrooms) lower CNS GABA concentrations by several mechanisms. Most important, they compete with pyridoxine for binding to PK, impairing PLP production.[96] Pyridoxal phosphate binding to the GAD complex is easily reversible.[103] The acute decrease in PLP concentration, then, is rapidly accompanied by impaired GABA synthesis and a decrease in GABA concentration. Lack of normal GABA inhibition produces seizures typical of hydrazine intoxications. Although PLP is also required for GABA degradation by GABA-T, acute decreases in PLP do not affect this enzyme nearly as much, because PLP is more tightly bound to the GABA-T complex and remains associated with the enzyme.[103] To a lesser extent, isoniazid binds to the GAD-PLP complex to prevent GABA formation.

Cyanide inhibits numerous enzymes besides cytochrome oxidase. Inhibition of GAD with a resultant fall in GABA concentration may partly explain seizures that occur in cyanide-poisoned patients. Domoic acid (see section on glutamate) may inhibit GAD.[31]

The exact mechanism of valproate's anticonvulsant action is unknown. In vitro studies demonstrate its ability to increase brain GABA concentrations either by inhibition of succinic semialdehyde dehydrogenase or by activation of GAD.[66] Gabapentin's ability to increase the rate of GABA synthesis in the brain may result from stimulation of GAD, as well.[140] Vigabatrin, an anticonvulsant, acts by irreversibly inhibiting GABA-T.

GABA_A Agonism. Figure 10–10 illustrates the $GABA_A$ receptor complex. In general, substances that increase $GABA_A$ complex activity cause CNS depression, ranging from mild sedation and nystagmus to ataxia, stupor, coma, and even general anesthesia. Most indirect agonists that bind to the $GABA_A$ complex have no activity in the absence of GABA. With some exceptions, their pharmacologic actions require the binding of GABA to its receptor and do not result from a direct effect on Cl^- conductance exclusive of GABA binding. Many of these drugs demonstrate additional actions that are not mediated through the $GABA_A$ complex.

Direct GABA Agonists. The main direct GABA agonist of toxicologic interest is muscimol, found in some poisonous mushrooms. Muscimol binds to the GABA receptor on the $GABA_A$ complex to mimic the action of GABA.[104] Ibotenic acid, a direct glutamate agonist found in the same mushrooms, is decarboxylated to muscimol just as glutamate is decarboxylated to GABA.

Indirect GABA Agonists. Benzodiazepines bind to benzodiazepine receptors on $GABA_A$ complexes to increase the affinity of GABA for its receptor and to increase the frequency of Cl^- channel opening in response to GABA binding.[129] GABA also increases benzodiazepine receptor affinity for benzodiazepines (benzodiazepines also inhibit adenosine uptake apart from $GABA_A$ activity; see section on adenosine).

Various isoforms of $GABA_A$ Cl^- channels differ in their affinity for different benzodiazepines. The γ subunit must be present for benzodiazepine activity. Investigators have divided these benzodiazepine binding sites on the $GABA_A$ complex into at least two different types, depending on their affinity for various compounds. $GABA_A$ receptors containing the α_1 subunit in combination with the β_2 and γ_2 subunits are known as the BZ_1, or "type-1-selective" receptors and bind benzodiazepine ligands, as well as zolpidem and zaleplon.[33,130] BZ_1 receptor subtypes reside throughout the

brain, particularly on hippocampal and cortical interneurons. The BZ_2 receptor subtype is composed of the $\alpha_2\beta_3\gamma_2$ and $\alpha_3\beta\gamma_2/\gamma_3$ subtypes. BZ_2 receptors are rich in the hippocampus and other brain areas and respond to benzodiazepines and zopiclone, but are less responsive to zolpidem and zaleplon.

Numerous steroids, such as alphaxalone and naturally occurring analogues, bind to more than one site on the $GABA_A$ complex to inhibit or enhance the action of GABA.[51,129] Even large doses of intravenous cholesterol (containing a steroid nucleus) produce general anesthesia.

The synthesis of neuroactive steroids is regulated, in part, by benzodiazepine binding to mitochondrial benzodiazepine receptors (MBRs) apart from the $GABA_A$ complex.[75,129] These mitochondrial benzodiazepine binding sites are found both inside and outside the CNS and were originally called peripheral benzodiazepine receptors. Mitochondrial benzodiazepine binding sites comprise three subunits: a voltage-dependent anion channel; an adenine nucleotide carrier; and a binding site for PK 11195, an isoquinoline carboxamide derivative.[50] Benzodiazepines vary in their affinity for mitochondrial binding. Upon binding, benzodiazepines appear to enhance the movement of cholesterol into mitochondria to begin steroid synthesis. Some of carbamazepine's action may be a result of binding at mitochondrial benzodiazepine receptors.[41]

Barbiturates bind to the $GABA_A$ complex to produce several effects.[72,129] All barbiturates enhance the action of GABA. That is, they produce more Cl^- influx for a given amount of GABA binding by increasing the duration of Cl^- channel opening. Whereas phenobarbital does not change the affinity of GABA or benzodiazepines for their binding sites, depressant barbiturates, such as pentobarbital, do increase GABA and benzodiazepine receptor affinities for their ligands, further enhancing inward Cl^- currents. At high concentrations, at least some barbiturates directly open Cl^- channels to cause Cl^- influx.[72] In addition, barbiturates possess other actions that depress all excitable membranes, including cardiac and smooth muscle.

The intravenous anesthetics propofol and etomidate enhance inward $GABA_A$ Cl^- currents to produce their anesthetic actions.[3] Etomidate is selective for $GABA_A$ receptors comprising β_2 or β_3 subunits over those containing β_1 subunits. Volatile general anesthetics also directly activate $GABA_A$ channels.[83,129] Some of ethanol's action is mediated through binding to the $GABA_A$ complex.[129,150] At low concentrations, ethanol enhances the effect of GABA on Cl^- influx. In mouse neurons, ethanol concentrations as low as 230 mg/dL directly open the Cl^- channel. Methaqualone produces at least part of its pharmacologic effect through indirect $GABA_A$ activity. Little is known of glutethimide's and methyprylon's mechanism of action. Their structural similarity to barbiturates suggests that much or most of it resides at the $GABA_A$ receptor. Trichloroethanol, a metabolite of chloral hydrate, and chlormethiazole interact at the $GABA_A$ complex in a manner similar to barbiturates, although it is not clear whether they are binding to an identical site on the Cl^- channel.[150] Ivermectin, an anthelminthic, activates $GABA_A$ Cl^- channels by increasing GABA binding in rat brains. Meprobamate displays barbiturate-like action at the $GABA_A$ receptor, and, at high concentrations, is able to cause Cl^- influx in the absence of GABA.[117] High concentrations of felbamate also cause inward Cl^- currents in the presence of GABA, although this seems unimportant at therapeutic doses.[117] Part of topiramate's anticonvulsant action may result from enhanced Cl^- influx through binding to $GABA_A$ receptors.[128]

Inhibition of GABA Uptake. Valproate and the anticonvulsants guvacine and tiagabine work, in part, by inhibiting GABA uptake. Although valproate is structurally similar to GABA, its inhibition of the GABA transporter does not appear to be competitive, which suggests that valproate moves into the neuron by a different mechanism (eg, diffusion).[102]

GABA$_A$ Antagonism

Direct GABA$_A$ Antagonists. Substances that act by any mechanism to decrease GABA$_A$ activity can cause CNS excitation and convulsions by preventing inhibitory inward Cl$^-$ currents. Direct antagonists bind to the same site as GABA to prevent GABA binding, the prototype being the convulsant bicuculline. Various antibiotics interact with the GABA$_A$ receptor to antagonize the action of GABA. In a dose-dependent manner, both imipenem and cephalosporins appear to directly antagonize GABA binding and can produce seizures at high doses or at therapeutic doses in susceptible individuals.[147] Evidence suggests that penicillin may also directly antagonize GABA binding. Electrophysiologic and radioligand binding studies indicate that norfloxacin, ciprofloxacin, ofloxacin, and enoxacin all combine with the GABA binding site to prevent GABA binding.[147] Theophylline and at least some nonsteroidal antiinflammatory agents markedly enhance GABA antagonism by some fluoroquinolones in vitro.[147]

Indirect GABA$_A$ Antagonists. Penicillin is well known for producing convulsions at high doses (eg, >20 million units penicillin/day with renal insufficiency), and both penicillin and aztreonam, a monobactam, appear to block the Cl$^-$ channel to prevent GABA-mediated inward Cl$^-$ currents.[147]

Picrotoxin, from *Anamirta cocculus* (fish berries), and the experimental convulsant pentylenetetrazol bind to the picrotoxin site of the GABA$_A$ receptor complex to inhibit the action of GABA. Excessive doses produce CNS excitation and convulsions. Organochlorine insecticides (eg, lindane, chlordane, heptachlor) also inhibit the action of GABA by binding to what appears to be the picrotoxin site.[86] Convulsions characterize acute poisonings by these agents.

Flumazenil competitively antagonizes benzodiazepines, zolpidem, zaleplon, and zopiclone at their receptors to reverse their pharmacologic effects.[17,130] Paradoxically, large doses of flumazenil exhibit anticonvulsant activity in animals. This is explained by flumazenil's ability to inhibit adenosine uptake, not by its partial agonism at the benzodiazepine receptor (see later).[109]

Some investigators suggested that the efficacy of most antidepressants may be due to antagonism at the GABA$_A$ complex.[135] Cyclic antidepressants, including amoxapine and maprotiline, and at least two MAOIs (isocarboxazid and tranylcypromine) inhibit GABA-mediated Cl$^-$ influx at GABA$_A$ receptors.[89,135] Their potency at inhibiting Cl$^-$ influx correlates with the frequency of seizures that occur in patients taking therapeutic doses of these medications. Impaired GABA$_A$ activity may contribute to or be primarily responsible for seizures seen in patients who overdose on these agents. The exact binding site of these drugs on the GABA$_A$ receptor complex is not yet known, although some evidence suggests at least indirect activity at the picrotoxin binding site.

Some subtypes of GABA$_A$ receptors are susceptible to inhibition by zinc ions.[129] What role this plays in normal physiology or toxicology is not established.

GABA$_A$ Withdrawal. Chronic use of GABA$_A$ complex agonists leads to down-regulation of GABA$_A$ receptor activity. Acute withdrawal from all GABA$_A$ direct and indirect agonists appears almost identical except for time course; in all cases, the common mediator is impaired Cl$^-$ influx. Withdrawal of all GABA$_A$ agonists can cause tremor, hypertension, tachycardia, diaphoresis, agitation, hallucinations, and convulsions. Conversely, any GABA$_A$ complex agonist can stop withdrawal from another, because all increase Cl$^-$ influx. One exception might be that withdrawal from a triazolobenzodiazepine appears controllable only with a similar drug because of actions on certain subtypes of benzodiazepine receptors (ie, particular subtypes of GABA$_A$ chloride channels). Because of their GABA$_A$ action, benzodiazepines and barbiturates are effective in controlling GABA$_A$ withdrawal seizures. Phenytoin and carbamazepine do not stop GABA$_A$ withdrawal seizures because pharmacologic effects independent of GABA cause their anticonvulsant actions.

GABA$_B$ Agonists. The main GABA$_B$ receptor agonist of toxicologic significance is baclofen. Coma, hypothermia, hypotension, bradydysrhythmias, and seizures characterize its toxicity. The convulsions that occur in patients with baclofen overdose are thought to result from disinhibition (inhibition of inhibitory neurons). Carbamazepine's activation of GABA$_B$ receptors has been demonstrated, although this is not thought to explain most of its anticonvulsant action. As noted later, some of γ-hydroxybutyrate's actions following pharmacologic doses may be mediated through activation of GABA$_B$ receptors.

GABA$_B$ Withdrawal. Baclofen withdrawal is similar clinically to GABA$_A$ withdrawal. Hallucinations, agitation, tremor, increased sympathetic activity, and convulsions are the main characteristics of baclofen withdrawal. Reinstitution of baclofen therapy is the treatment for withdrawal.[90]

γ-HYDROXYBUTYRATE

γ-Hydroxybutyrate (GHB; γ-hydroxybutyric acid) was first synthesized in the 1960s as a water-soluble sedative agent able to cross the blood-brain barrier and was later found to occur naturally in mammalian brains.[43] Controversy exists as to whether GHB should be considered a neurotransmitter or simply a neuromodulator because it is unclear whether this substance is concentrated within vesicles for synaptic release. There is evidence demonstrating a sodium-dependent uptake transporter for GHB, and there are central GHB receptors.[43]

Specific interactions between GHB and dopamine are complex and not fully delineated.[9] GHB appears to influence dopaminergic activity, probably via GHB receptors.[43] GHB affects the firing rates of dopaminergic neurons, dopamine release, dopamine synthesis, and levels of dopamine and its major metabolites. GHB is thought to mediate sleep cycles, temperature regulation, cerebral glucose metabolism and blood flow, memory, and emotional control, and it may be neuroprotective.[80]

Several proposed pathways for endogenous GHB formation exist (Fig. 10–11).[9] Evidence exists for GHB's metabolism back to GABA, although this appears minimal at physiologic GHB concentrations.[43] However, pharmacologic effects resulting from GHB administration may result, in part, from secondary GABA formation.[9,43]

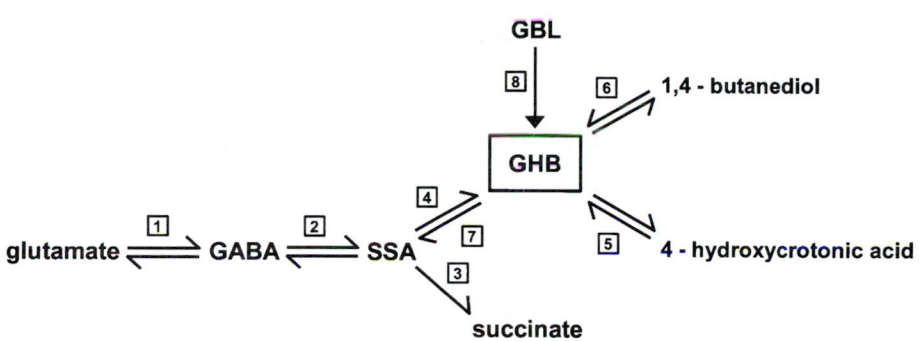

Figure 10–11. Potential pathways of GHB (γ-hydroxybutyrate) synthesis and degradation. GABA = γ-aminobutyric acid; GBL = γ-butyrolactone; SSA = succinic semialdehyde; [1] = glutamic acid decarboxylase; [2] = GABA-transaminase; [3] = succinic semialdehyde dehydrogenase; [4] = specific succinic semialdehyde reductase and/or NADPH-dependent aldehyde reductase 2; [5] = mitochondrial β oxidation; [6] = alcohol dehydrogenase and aldehyde dehydrogenase; [7] = GHB dehydrogenase; [8] = γ-lactonase.

Little is known of GHB receptors.[9] Receptors appear to be heterogeneously distributed throughout the brain, with highest concentrations in the cerebral cortex, limbic areas, and thalamus, as well as in regions innervated by dopaminergic terminals and dopaminergic nuclei. GHB receptors exist on neurons, mainly at the synaptic level, but are absent from glial or peripheral cells. GHB receptors may be metabotropic receptors linked to G_i or G_o proteins.

At least two general GHB receptors have been described thus far, based on binding affinity for GHB and other ligands.[9] High-affinity receptors for GHB do not respond to GABA, GABAergic agonists, γ-butyrolactone, or dopamine. Similarly, GHB does not activate $GABA_A$ Cl^- channels. Flumazenil and baclofen (a $GABA_B$ agonist) fail to antagonize GHB binding to its binding site.[9]

Although γ-butyrolactone (GBL) does not express affinity for GHB binding sites, GBL rapidly undergoes hydrolysis to form GHB by peripheral γ-lactonase.[9,88] 1,4-Butanediol undergoes conversion to GHB via alcohol dehydrogenase and aldehyde dehydrogenase.[88]

Although normal endogenous GHB concentrations are probably not high enough to activate $GABA_B$ receptors, such receptor activation may occur with exogenous administration of GHB. Furthermore, there appears to be functional interplay between GHB and $GABA_B$ receptors.[9]

Toxicologic interest in GHB stems both from its abuse and from its use for the treatment of narcolepsy.[9,43,80] GHB is rapidly absorbed and freely crosses the blood-brain barrier.[9,80] Toxicity resulting from ingestion of GHB is explained by GHB receptor and possibly $GABA_B$ receptor activation, and comprises agitation, tremor, rapid onset of coma, vomiting, bradycardia, hypotension, hypotonia, and apnea that usually resolve within several hours.[9,80] Although seizure activity has been noted in experimental animals, it is debated whether GHB causes true convulsive activity in human beings. Human experiments with "therapeutic" doses of GHB have not found EEG changes consistent with seizure activity.[80] Some authors have reported "generalized seizures" occurring in patients presenting after GHB overdose. Interestingly, patients with a rare inborn error of metabolism that disrupts the normal metabolism of GABA because of a deficiency in succinic semialdehyde dehydrogenase (SSAD) and that causes GHB to accumulate tend to experience seizures.[52] Valproate similarly elevates endogenous GHB concentrations by inhibiting SSAD.

Although GHB can suppress alcohol withdrawal, GHB is also addictive, and both tolerance and a withdrawal syndrome have been described with GHB use. Withdrawal is characterized by insomnia, cramps, tremor, and anxiety.[9]

GLYCINE AS AN INHIBITORY NEUROTRANSMITTER

Glycine acts as a postsynaptic inhibitory neurotransmitter in the spinal cord and lower brainstem. In the CNS, serine is converted to glycine by serine hydroxymethyltransferase (SHMT).

Release and Uptake

Glycine is transported into storage vesicles and undergoes Ca^{2+}-dependent exocytosis upon neuronal depolarization (Fig. 10–12). Glycine is removed from the synapse through uptake by a Na^+-dependent transporter.

Glycine Receptors

Like $GABA_A$, the glycine receptor is a Cl^- channel on the postsynaptic membrane. $GABA_A$ Cl^- channels and glycine Cl^- channels share significant amino acid homology. Glycine receptors are pentameric proteins made up of α and β subunits. Four isoforms of the α subunit and one isoform of the β subunit have been described.[95]

Glycine receptor activation causes an inward Cl^- current that hyperpolarizes the membrane. It appears that three glycine molecules must bind to sites on the Cl^- channel to produce inhibitory Cl^- influx.

Chemical Agents

Table 10–10 provides examples of chemical agents that affect inhibitory glycine chloride channels.

The amino acids D-alanine, taurine, L-alanine, L-serine, and proline can activate glycine chloride channels. Both ethanol and propofol potentiate glycine-mediated inward Cl^- currents through action at the α subunit of the glycine receptor, just as they do at $GABA_A$ Cl^- channels.[91,95]

Strychnine is the main toxicologic agent affecting glycinergic transmission. Strychnine binds to the α subunit of the glycine receptor to prevent glycine's action on Cl^- influx,[4] at least in part by decreasing glycine's binding to its receptors. Because glycine must bind to more than one site on the Cl^- channel for successful agonism, a plausible explanation is that strychnine may bind to one of glycine's binding sites. This physiologic antagonism of glycine's action produces increased muscle tone, rigidity, opisthotonus, trismus, and death from respiratory failure and rhabdomyolysis. Given the similarity in Cl^- channels, it is not surprising that strychnine binds to the $GABA_A$ complex in vitro. However, strychnine's affinity for this complex is less than that for glycine

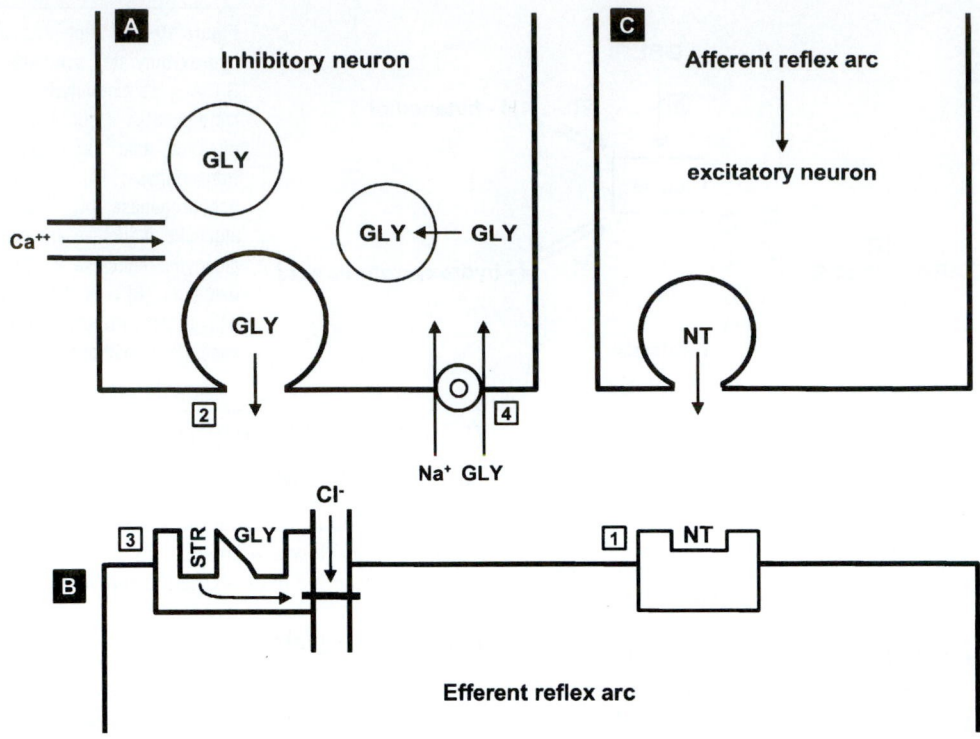

Figure 10–12.   Inhibitory glycinergic neurotransmission. Signals from the afferent limb of a reflex arc (neuron C) cause the release of an excitatory neurotransmitter (NT) that crosses the synapse to bind to neuron B in the efferent limb of the reflex arc [1]. To prevent excessive neuronal firing and motor activity, glycine [GLY] released from inhibitory neuron A [2] binds to glycine Cl⁻ channel receptors on neuron B [3] and causes inhibition by hyperpolarization. Synaptic glycine is transported back into the neuron [4]. Strychnine (STR) binds to the glycinergic Cl⁻ channel to decrease glycine's binding, which prevents Cl⁻ influx. Although strychnine is shown to bind to a separate site from glycine, there is evidence that these sites may overlap.

receptors, and most of its toxicologic action is a result of physiologic antagonism of glycine's inhibitory action.

Picrotoxin binds to the glycine receptor to impair Cl⁻ influx.[87] Tetanus toxin produces rigidity and trismus by preventing glycine release from nerve endings in the spinal cord and brainstem.

GLUTAMATE

Glutamate is the main excitatory neurotransmitter in the CNS. Aspartate displays similar actions although its exact role as a neurotransmitter is not as well defined because it is only active at certain types of glutamate receptors. Glutamate and aspartate are commonly referred to as excitatory amino acid (EAA) neurotransmitters. Glutamate is essential for memory, learning, perception, and locomotion.[34,71]

TABLE 10–10.   Examples of Agents That Affect Inhibitory Glycine Chloride Channels

Glycine Agonists	Glycine Antagonists
Ethanol	Strychnine
Propofol	Picrotoxin

Ethanol and propofol enhance Cl⁻ influx through glycine Cl⁻ channels, although they do not appear to act as direct agonists. Evidence exists for picrotoxin's direct antagonism at the glycine binding site(s) in contrast to GABAₐ Cl⁻ channels, where it acts at a site separate from where GABA (γ-aminobutyric acid) binds.

Glutamatergic neurotransmission has been a subject of intense research because of its role in mediating neuronal damage in degenerative neurologic diseases and during times of trauma, ischemia, hypoglycemia, and status epilepticus.[34] Although glutamate receptor stimulation is necessary for normal brain activity (eg, memory), excessive glutamate receptor activation endogenously or by glutamate agonists can produce convulsions, neuronal damage, and death. Conversely, glutamate antagonists demonstrate anticonvulsant activity and neuroprotective action in animal models of brain and spinal cord injury. Glutamate may also play an important role in the development of drug abuse and subsequent withdrawal symptoms. Glutamate antagonists decrease drug craving and withdrawal symptoms in patients addicted to ethanol, benzodiazepines, and opioids.[12]

Synthesis, Release, and Uptake

Glutamate is a nonessential amino acid that does not cross the blood-brain barrier. It must, therefore, be synthesized from products of glucose metabolism or other precursors that enter neurons. Glutamate is primarily synthesized from glutamine by the enzyme glutaminase located within the mitochondrial compartment. Other amino acids, such as aspartate, also serve as sources for glutamate production. Glutamate stored within vesicles is released into the synapse by Ca⁺²-dependent exocytosis.[34] Five different EAA uptake transporters have been identified, and glutamate undergoes uptake both by neuronal and glial cells.[125] Synaptic glutamate transported into glial cells undergoes conversion back to glutamine by the enzyme glutamine synthase. Glial cells then release glutamine back into the synapse for uptake by neurons and recycling back to glutamate and then into storage vesicles (Fig. 10–13). Reverse transport of glutamate from the cytoplasm into the synapse by the membrane transporter may occur under some circumstances.[34] Glutamate also serves as the precursor for GABA's synthesis.

Glutamate Receptors

The EAA receptor system is the most complex of all neurotransmitters. This complexity is necessary for protection against the devastating effects of uncontrolled excitatory neurotransmission. At present, 11 different glutamate receptors are recognized. Three

ionotropic glutamate receptors are cation channels, and 8 metabotropic receptors are linked to G proteins.[34]

A single neuron may express numerous types of glutamate receptors. Postsynaptic glutamate receptors are usually excitatory, although some inhibitory actions have been demonstrated. Presynaptic terminal glutamate receptors appear mainly to inhibit release of various neurotransmitters, including glutamate (Fig. 10–13).[111]

Ionotropic Glutamate Receptors. Three ionotropic glutamate receptors have been identified. All allow for excitation through cation influx. These receptors are further categorized and named by their abilities to be activated or antagonized by various substances: kainate, AMPA (α-amino-3-hydroxy-5-methyl-4-isoxazole propionate), and NMDA (*N*-methyl-D-aspartate).[34]

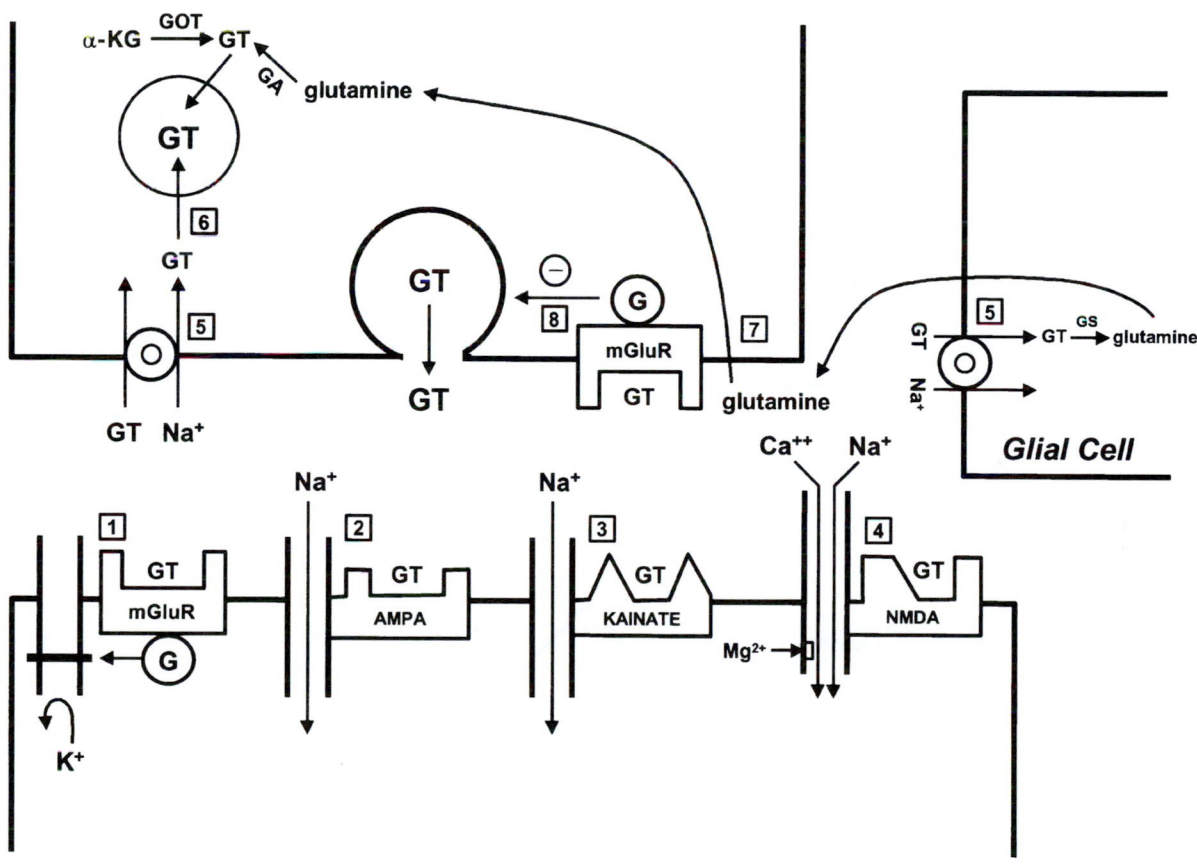

Figure 10–13. Glutamatergic neurotransmission. Glutamic-oxaloacetic transaminase (GOT) converts α-ketoglutarate (δ-KG) to glutamate (GT) in the mitochondria. Glutamate also forms from glutamine via glutaminase (GA). Glutamate is transported into vesicles for exocytotic release into the synapse [6]. Synaptic glutamate activates four main types of receptors. AMPA [2], kainate [3], and NMDA [4] receptors are cation channels. Membrane depolarization in response to their activation causes neuronal excitation through cation influx. Metabotropic receptors (mGluR) [1,8] are coupled to G proteins and are expressed on pre- and postsynaptic membranes. In addition, some mGluRs reside outside of the synapse. Postsynaptic mGluR excitation in this example [1] results from preventing K^+ efflux, but other mechanisms of excitation exist. Presynaptic mGluRs act to inhibit [8] glutamate (and other neurotransmitter) release through modulating intracellular Ca^{2+} concentrations. A more detailed illustration of the NMDA receptor is found in Figure 10–14. Excessive influx of Ca^{2+} through NMDA receptors (and through some AMPA and kainate receptors) causes neuronal damage and cell death. An Mg^{2+} ion normally blocks the NMDA receptor channel to prevent Ca^{2+} influx despite glutamate binding. However depolarization of the neuronal membrane by cation influx resulting from activation of any of the other receptors causes Mg^{2+} to dissociate from the NMDA receptor and to allow potentially damaging inward Ca^{2+} currents. Glutamate undergoes uptake by neurons and glial cells [5]. In glial cells, glutamate is converted to glutamine by glutamine synthase (GS), and then glutamine is released for uptake back into neurons [7] where glutamine undergoes conversion back to glutamate. Various agents in Table 10–11 affect glutaminergic neurotransmission, in part, by stimulating or blocking the various glutamate receptors [1–4,8] or by preventing glutamate uptake [5]. G = G protein.

Kainate receptors are named for their affinity for kainic acid found in seaweed. Activation allows Na$^+$ influx and a small amount of K$^+$ efflux, resulting in neuronal depolarization. Some kainate receptors in the hippocampus also appear to allow Ca^{2+} influx following activation. Kainate receptors are the only ionotropic glutamate receptors, to date, found presynaptically, although they are much more prevalent on postsynaptic neuronal membranes.[48]

The AMPA receptor is an ion channel structurally similar to the kainate receptor that also mediates Na$^+$ influx (and lesser amounts of K$^+$ efflux) on postsynaptic membranes, triggering neuronal depolarization.[10] The AMPA receptor is the most common ionotropic glutamate receptor found in the brain and appears to account for most glutamatergic excitation under normal conditions. A subtype of AMPA receptors in the hippocampus may also allow Ca^{2+} influx after activation.[119]

The NMDA receptor, the most studied of all glutamate receptors, is a Ca^{2+} channel whose activation allows for inward Ca^{2+} and Na$^+$ currents (and some K$^+$ efflux), resulting in neuronal depolarization and excitation (Fig. 10–14). Excessive stimulation of NMDA receptors by glutamate released during times of ischemia, trauma, hypoglycemia, or convulsions triggers damaging rises in intracellular Ca^{2+} concentrations, activation of numerous enzymes, and free radical formation, all of which incite cell death.[71] Antagonists of NMDA Ca^{2+} channels demonstrate anticonvulsant and neuroprotective activity during times of neuronal insult.

The NMDA Ca^{2+} channel is normally blocked by Mg^{2+} in a voltage-dependent manner, preventing Ca^{2+} influx despite glutamate binding (Fig. 10–14).[120] Only when the neuronal membrane is depolarized by at least 20–30 mV through some other mechanism (eg, activation of another type of glutamate receptor) will Mg^{2+} leave the channel and allow Ca^{2+} influx in response to glutamate binding. Thus, the NMDA glutamate receptor is both a ligand-gated and voltage-gated ion channel. Many neurons express both NMDA and non-NMDA receptors for glutamate. Excessive stimulation of kainate or AMPA receptors by glutamate causes cell damage through Na$^+$ (and in some instance, Ca^{2+}) influx, because the membrane depolarization they produce causes Mg^{2+} to leave the NMDA receptor and allows for potentially damaging inward Ca^{2+} currents.[34] Calcium ion influx through voltage-gated ion channels (including L subtype) on cell bodies that open in response to depolarization also contributes to accumulation of intracellular calcium and cell damage. Therefore, excessive activation of any excitatory glutamate receptor has the potential to produce neuronal cytotoxicity.[71]

Glutamate alone is incapable of activating NMDA receptors, even after Mg^{2+} has dissociated from the ion channel. Glycine also must bind to its specific receptor on the NMDA receptor complex for successful glutamate agonism (Fig. 10–14), making glycine an indirect agonist of excitatory neurotransmission.[34] Strychnine does not antagonize glycine's excitatory action at NMDA receptors, explaining why glycine NMDA receptors are also known as strychnine-insensitive glycine receptors.

Zinc ions normally bind to the NMDA receptor complex to antagonize the action of glutamate. Binding of spermine or spermidine to a polyamine binding site on the extracellular side of the NMDA receptor results in increased affinity of glycine and glutamate for their binding sites. However, polyamine agonism is not essential for glutamate activation of NMDA receptors.[63]

Metabotropic Glutamate Receptors. Metabotropic glutamate receptors (mGluRs) are linked to various G proteins on post- and presynaptic membranes (Fig. 10–13). Eight different receptors have been isolated to date.[94] In contrast to ionotropic glutamate receptors, mGluRs may excite or inhibit at postsynaptic membranes, and appear mainly to inhibit at presynaptic locations. Postsynaptic excitation most commonly results from prevention of K$^+$ efflux or activation of phospholipase C, which serves to raise intracellular

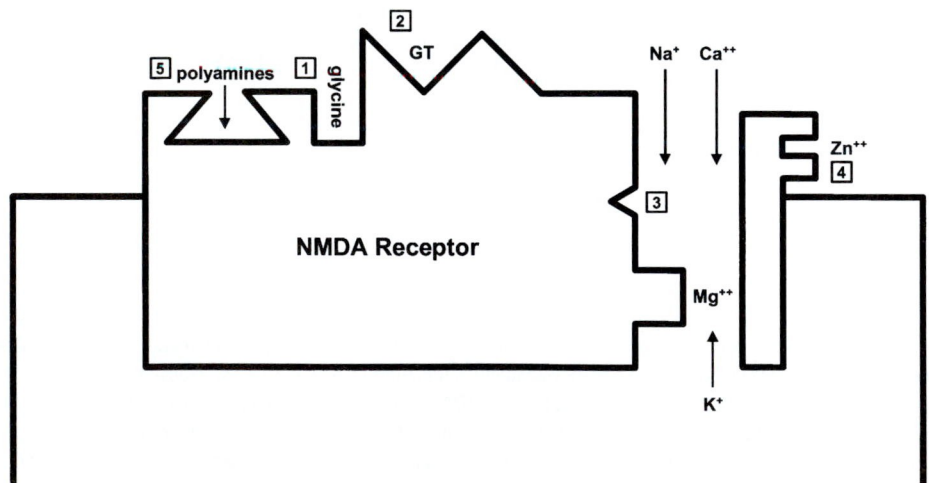

Figure 10–14.   Representation of the NMDA glutamate receptor. The NMDA receptor is a voltage-gated and ligand-gated Ca^{2+} channel. Glutamate (GT) binds to its receptor on the channel [2] to open the Ca^{2+} channel and to allow Ca^{2+} and Na$^+$ influx and lesser amounts of K$^+$ efflux. Mg^{2+} normally blocks the Ca^{2+} channel, preventing cation influx in response to glutamate binding. Mg^{2+} leaves the channel when the membrane is depolarized by 20–30 mV. Glycine must also bind to its site on the NMDA receptor complex for successful glutamate agonism. Polyamines bind on the extracellular surface of the receptor [5]. Zn^{2+} binds [4] to inhibit Ca^{2+} influx. The phencyclidine (PCP) binding site [3] lies within the channel. Agents in Table 10–11 may antagonize glycine binding [1]; block the Ca^{2+} channel by binding to the PCP binding site [3]; bind to the polyamine binding site [5]; or directly stimulate the glutamate binding site [2].

Ca^{2+} concentration. Postsynaptic inhibition usually results from enhanced K^+ efflux.[94]

Metabotropic glutamate receptors are commonly subdivided into three main groups based on their intracellular signaling mechanisms and response to specific experimental agonists. As a general rule, group I receptors reside postsynaptically; activation produces excitation through blockade of K^+ efflux or by activating phospholipase C, producing rises in intracellular Ca^{2+}.[139]

Group II and III receptors, conversely, most commonly serve as presynaptic autoreceptors and heteroreceptors and, when activated, inhibit adenylate cyclase activity. This, in turn, prevents Ca^{2+} influx and serves to inhibit release of neurotransmitters, including glutamate, GABA, dopamine, and adenosine. Group II presynaptic autoreceptors may play an especially important role in decreasing further glutamate release during pathologic conditions when the extracellular concentration of glutamate exceeds normal physiologic levels.[139]

Chemical Agents

Table 10–11 provides examples of chemical agents that affect glutamatergic neurotransmission.

Glutamate Agonism. Domoic acid produces amnestic shellfish poisoning, partly characterized by confusion, agitation, convulsions, memory disturbance, neuronal damage, and death.[55] The structural similarity between domoic acid and glutamate is thought to explain excessive activation of kainate receptors with secondary NMDA receptor activation and neuronal damage.[55]

Investigators hypothesize that other naturally occurring glutamate receptor agonists produce additional neurologic diseases. The neurogenic form of lathyrism results from using chickling peas (*Lathyrus sativus*) as a food staple. Chickling peas contain β-*N*-oxalylamino-L-alanine (BOAA), an agonist of AMPA receptors.[34,74] Neurogenic lathyrism was common in German concentra-

tion and prisoner of war camps in World War II and still occurs regularly in some parts of the world. Ibotenic acid, from poisonous mushrooms, activates NMDA and some metabotropic glutamate receptors.[34,74] It undergoes decarboxylation to muscimol, a direct agonist at $GABA_A$ receptors.

Because noncompetitive NMDA receptor antagonism reproduces many signs and symptoms of schizophrenia, investigators are directing efforts at increasing glutamate's activity at NMDA channels in an effort to treat the disease. After crossing the blood-brain barrier, milacemide undergoes conversion to glycine, which is required for NMDA receptor activation. D-Cycloserine also crosses the blood-brain barrier to stimulate glycine receptors on NMDA calcium channels.[34]

Glutamate Antagonism

Prevention of Glutamate Release. Riluzole, used for the treatment of amyotrophic lateral sclerosis, indirectly prevents release of glutamate. Lamotrigine diminishes glutamate release through blockade of voltage-gated Na^+ channels. Blockade of voltage-gated Ca^{2+} channels by nimodipine appears to impair glutamate release as well.[141]

NMDA Receptor Antagonists. Although some experimental agents and pharmaceutics antagonize the action of glutamate, most of our knowledge concerns antagonism at NMDA receptors. Phencyclidine and ketamine appear to bind within the ion channel (PCP binding site) to block Ca^{2+} influx following glutamate binding (Fig. 10–14).[71] Both agents possess other pharmacologic actions and can produce convulsions in overdose. However, in animal models of seizures and neuronal insult, both drugs are neuroprotective and anticonvulsant.

Dextromethorphan and its first-pass metabolite, dextrorphan, exhibit anticonvulsant activity in animals. Dextrorphan's anticonvulsant activity results, in part, from blockade of NMDA receptor Ca^{2+} channels by binding to the PCP binding site. Dextromethorphan does not bind to the NMDA complex but, like dextrorphan, can directly block N- and L-type voltage-dependent Ca^{2+} channels.[25]

Dizocilpine (MK-801) is an NMDA receptor antagonist that binds to the PCP binding site in the NMDA Ca^{2+} channel. Human trials of dizocilpine resulted in adverse effects similar to those produced by phencyclidine, preventing further use in humans as a neuroprotective agent. Amantadine, memantine, and orphenadrine act as low-affinity antagonists at the PCP site but are not associated with psychotomimetic adverse effects.[71] Part of amantadine's effectiveness in the treatment of Parkinson disease may be related to NMDA antagonism. Pentamidine also antagonizes glutamate binding at NMDA channels.[141]

Ethanol competitively inhibits NMDA receptor stimulation by an unknown mechanism, resulting in up-regulation of this glutamatergic system. It does not appear to act through currently recognized binding sites.[151] In some animal models of ethanol withdrawal seizures, NMDA receptor antagonists demonstrate better anticonvulsant action than $GABA_A$ agonists.

Glycine Antagonists. Felbamate's anticonvulsant activity may result, in part, from antagonism of glycine at NMDA receptors.[94] Kynurenic acid, a metabolite of L-tryptophan, prevents NMDA activation through glycine antagonism. Meprobamate also antagonizes NMDA glutamate receptors by a yet-to-be-determined

TABLE 10–11. Examples of Agents That Affect Glutamatergic Neurotransmission

Glutamate Agonism	Dextrorphan
Direct glutamate receptor agonists	Dizocilpine (MK-801)
BMAA	Ketamine
BOAA	Memantine
Domoic acid	Orphenadrine
Ibotenic acid	Pentamidine
Willardine	Phencyclidine
	Ethanol[a]
Glycine NMDA receptor agonists	
D-Cycloserine	NMDA glycine antagonists
Milacemide	Felbamate
	Kynurenic acid
Glutamate Antagonism	Meprobamate
Prevent glutamate release	
Lamotrigine	Polyamine antagonists
Nimodipine	Ifenprodil
Riluzole	Eliprodil
NMDA receptor antagonists	
Amantadine	

BMAA = α-amino-β-methylaminopropionic acid; BOAA = β-*N*-oxalylamino-L-alanine; NMDA = *N*-methyl-D-aspartate.
[a]Ethanol antagonizes glutamate's action at NMDA receptors through an unknown mechanism.

mechanism. However, given the structural similarity to felbamate, meprobamate may act by antagonizing the action of glycine.[117]

Polyamine Antagonism.   Ifenprodil and eliprodil antagonize glutamate's action at NMDA channels by preventing polyamine binding.[94]

ADENOSINE

The overall action of adenosine throughout the body is to lessen oxygen requirements and to increase oxygen and substrate delivery. In keeping with the paradigm, adenosine functions in the CNS as an extremely important inhibitory neuromodulator and vasodilator.

Synthesis, Release, and Uptake

Normal intracellular concentrations of adenosine range from 50 to 300 nM. A Na^+-dependent purine uptake transporter moves adenosine into the neuron (Fig. 10–15). During times of adequate oxygen delivery and oxidative phosphorylation, intracellular ATP concentrations are normally manyfold greater than those of adenosine. Adenosine begins conversion to ATP by adenosine kinase, but adenosine can also be metabolized to inosine by adenosine deaminase, a less important pathway.[22,113]

ATP is commonly coreleased with other neurotransmitters (eg, norepinephrine, ACh, glutamate) into the synapse where it can be degraded to AMP (Fig. 10–15). When oxygen delivery remains adequate to meet metabolic demands, most synaptic adenosine arises from the extracellular dephosphorylation of AMP by ectosolic 5-nucleotidase.[22]

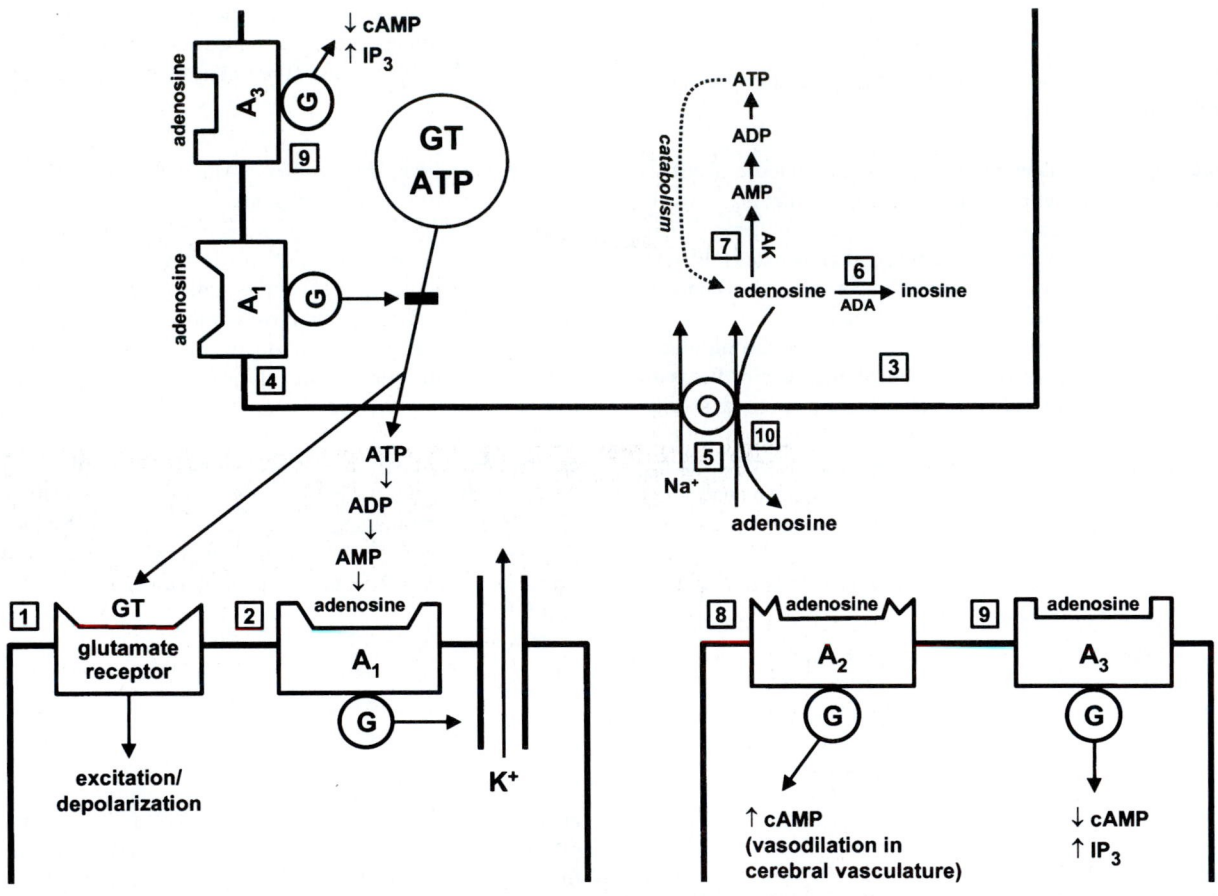

Figure 10–15.   Adenosine's role in regulating excitatory neurotransmission, using glutamate as an example. In this example, glutamate (GT) excites a postsynaptic neuron by activating glutamate receptors [1]. Adenosine triphosphate (ATP) enters the synapse when glutamate is released. Adenosine formed from metabolism of ATP within the synapse binds to postsynaptic A_1 receptors [2], which open K^+ channels to inhibit the neuron through hyperpolarization. Adenosine also activates presynaptic A_1 receptors [4] to lower intracellular Ca^{2+} concentrations, thereby impairing further glutamate release. After uptake [5], adenosine is acted upon either by adenosine kinase (AK) [7] to form adenosine monophosphate (AMP), or by adenosine deaminase (ADA) [6] to form inosine. Adenosine also binds to neuronal A_2 receptors (especially in the striatum) and to vascular A_2 receptors to cause vasodilatation [8]. A_3 receptors [9] are not activated by normal concentrations of adenosine. During times of excessive catabolism (eg, seizures, hypoglycemia, stroke) when intracellular adenosine concentrations rise markedly, adenosine moves into the synapse through reverse transport via the purine uptake transporter [10]. Resultant stimulation of A_1 and A_2 receptors results in inhibitory actions to decrease oxygen requirements and to increase substrate delivery through vasodilatation as described above. However, the resultant stimulation of A_3 receptors [9] may contribute to neuronal damage and death. Agents in Table 10–12 act to inhibit adenosine uptake [5]; to inhibit ADA [6]; to inhibit AK [7]; to increase adenosine release; and to antagonize A_1 [2,4] and A_2 [8] receptors. ADP = adenosine diphosphate; ATP = adenosine triphosphate; cAMP = cyclic-AMP; G = G protein; IP_3 = inositol triphosphate.

During increased cellular catabolism, especially during inadequate oxygen delivery, intracellular adenosine concentrations rapidly rise as phosphorylated adenosine species are degraded to adenosine. The rise in intracellular adenosine concentration results in reverse transport of adenosine into the synapse by the purine uptake transporter (Fig. 10–15). Synaptic adenosine, then, activates adenosine receptors on neuronal and nonneuronal tissue (eg, vasculature). Adenosine's actions are terminated by uptake into glial cells and neurons (Fig. 10–15).[22]

Exogenously administered adenosine used in the treatment of supraventricular tachycardia does not cross the blood-brain barrier and therefore is centrally inactive. The half-life of adenosine in the blood is less than 10 seconds.

Adenosine Receptors

The purine P_1 receptor family comprises four adenosine receptor subtypes linked to G proteins: A_1, A_{2A}, A_{2B}, and A_3.[115] In the central and autonomic nervous systems, A_1 receptors reside on presynaptic and postsynaptic membranes, where they serve as inhibitory modulators for numerous neurotransmitter systems; they are particularly prevalent in association with glutamatergic neurons in the CNS.[146] A_1 receptor stimulation produces sedation and is important in sleep regulation.[113] Other functions attributed to A_1 receptors include neuroprotection, anxiolysis, temperature reduction, anticonvulsant activity, and spinal analgesia.

Postsynaptic A_1 stimulation results in K^+ channel opening and K^+ efflux with subsequent hyperpolarization of the neuron (Fig. 10–15). Evidence suggests that G protein–mediated Cl^- influx may explain postsynaptic hyperpolarization by A_1 activation in some cases.

Presynaptic A_1 stimulation modifies voltage-dependent Ca^{2+} channels, lessening Ca^{2+} influx during depolarization, which limits exocytosis of neurotransmitter. Therefore, activation of A_1 receptors prevents release of neurotransmitters presynaptically and inhibits their response postsynaptically.[115,146]

In the CNS, A_{2A} receptors demonstrate limited distribution. They are concentrated on cerebral vasculature and produce vasodilatation when stimulated.[115,146] Additionally, A_{2A} receptors are especially prevalent on neurons in the striatum where they inhibit the activity of D_2 receptors.[45] Striatal A_{2A} receptors decrease GABA effects while enhancing cholinergic, glycinergic, and glutamatergic neurotransmission.[36]

A_{2B} receptors are expressed diffusely throughout the brain, and are most commonly identified on glial cells. A_{2B} receptors demonstrate low affinity for adenosine, and little is known of their physiologic role.[22] Both A_{2A} and A_{2B} receptors are coupled to G_s. The rise in cAMP concentration resulting from A_{2A} activation on cerebral vasculature and elsewhere explains vasodilatation.[115]

A_3 receptors reside diffusely throughout the CNS and express low affinity for adenosine. A_3 receptors act through G proteins to decrease adenylate cyclase activity and increase phospholipase C activity.[145] The low concentrations of adenosine found during normal metabolism minimally activate A_3 receptors to produce inhibitory effects. During times of excessive adenosine accumulation (eg, hypoxia, seizures), adenosine accumulates at and activates A_3 receptors to produce complex responses that appear to enhance ischemic cellular injury and death, at least in part through disinhibition of presynaptic metabotropic glutamate receptor responses. Thus, A_3 receptor antagonists are being examined for neuroprotective actions.[145]

Adenosine and Seizure Termination

In humans and in animal models of status epilepticus, including those from drugs and toxins, there are two alternating phases of electrical activity noted on electroencephalography. Periods of high-frequency spike activity accompanied by marked increases in cerebral oxygen consumption and metabolic requirements alternate with interictal periods of isolated spike waves during which metabolic demands are less. The high-frequency phase lasts only a few minutes before suddenly terminating, sometimes with a few seconds of electrocerebral silence. A gradual increase in electrical activity during the interictal phase eventually leads to a recurrence of high-frequency spike activity.

These periodic spontaneous self-terminations of high-frequency electrical activity initially occur before neurons exhaust oxygen and energy supplies. These punctuations result from adenosine release from depolarizing neurons (and probably glial cells).[39] Adenosine acts on presynaptic receptors to prevent further release of excitatory neurotransmitters and acts on postsynaptic receptors to inhibit their actions.

Any agent that directly or indirectly enhances adenosine's action at A_1 receptors in the brain will usually exhibit anticonvulsant activity. Conversely, A_1 receptor antagonists lower the seizure threshold and make seizure termination more difficult and less likely to respond to anticonvulsants.

Agents that antagonize A_{2A} receptors produce cerebral vasoconstriction and may limit oxygen delivery during times of increased demand. Antagonism of A_{2A} receptors in the striatum increases dopamine-mediated motor activity.

Chemical Agents

Table 10–12 provides examples of chemical agents that affect adenosine receptors.

Indirect Adenosine Agonists. Papaverine and dipyridamole inhibit adenosine uptake.[108] Like all agonists of adenosine's action, papaverine and dipyridamole demonstrate anticonvulsant activity

TABLE 10–12. Examples of Agents That Affect Adenosine Receptors

Adenosine Agonism	
Inhibit uptake	Inhibit AK
Acadesine	Acadesine
Acetate[a]	
Benzodiazepines	Increase adenosine release
Calcium channel blockers	Opioids
Carbamazepine	
Dipyridamole	**Adenosine Antagonism**
Ethanol[a]	A_1 blockade
Flumazenil	Caffeine
Indomethacin	Carbamazepine
Papaverine	Theophylline
Propentafylline	
Tricyclic antidepressants	A_2 blockade
	Caffeine
Inhibit ADA	Theophylline
Acadesine	
Dipyridamole	
Pentostatin	

ADA = adenosine deaminase; AK = adenosine kinase.
[a]Ethanol is metabolized to acetate, which inhibits adenosine uptake.

when injected into the CNS. Such actions are not achievable with safe systemic doses.

In addition to their actions at $GABA_A$ receptors, benzodiazepines inhibit adenosine uptake.[30,109] This may explain observations that methylxanthines, potent adenosine receptor antagonists, reverse benzodiazepine-induced sedation in humans. The potencies of benzodiazepines as inhibitors of adenosine uptake show good correlation with clinical anxiolytic and anticonflict potencies, suggesting that such inhibition contributes to their action. The anticonvulsant effect of large doses of flumazenil also results from inhibition of adenosine uptake. Carbamazepine inhibits adenosine uptake, although this is not thought to account for most anticonvulsive action.

Adenosine may mediate many of the acute and chronic motor effects of ethanol on the brain. Ethanol, probably through its metabolite, acetate, prevents adenosine uptake, raising synaptic adenosine concentrations.[24] Excessive stimulation of several adenosine receptors in the cerebellum may explain much of the motor impairment from low ethanol concentrations. In fact, animals made tolerant to ethanol develop cross-tolerance to adenosine agonists. In mice, adenosine receptor agonists increase ethanol-induced incoordination while adenosine antagonists decrease this intoxicating response.[32]

Numerous other agents are now recognized as inhibitors of adenosine uptake, including propentofylline, nimodipine, tricyclic antidepressants, and other calcium channel blockers.[106,108]

A_1 receptors located at the spinal cord level are important modulators of pain transmission by limiting release of substance P.[123] Tricyclic antidepressants have been reported to inhibit adenosine uptake, and this may explain some of their effectiveness in treating neuropathic pain.[123] The analgesic effectiveness of opioids can be partially attributed to their ability to increase the release of adenosine within the spinal cord.[132]

Dipyridamole inhibits adenosine deaminase, raising adenosine concentrations. During times of elevated adenosine levels that occur with cardiac or cerebral ischemia, acadesine further enhances adenosine's beneficial actions by three mechanisms: inhibition of AK, inhibition of ADA, and inhibition of adenosine uptake.[100]

Adenosine Antagonists. The main adenosine antagonists of toxicologic concern are methylxanthines. Theophylline and caffeine are selective P_1 antagonists, blocking both A_1 and A_2 receptors.[144] The response to methylxanthines by A_3 receptors varies widely depending on the species. Human A_3 receptors demonstrate very low affinity for methylxanthines.[145]

Peripherally, methylxanthines produce excessive release of catecholamines from peripheral nerve endings (and probably the adrenal gland) by blocking presynaptic A_1 receptors. In turn, catecholamine-mediated responses are exaggerated by blockade of inhibitory postsynaptic A_1 receptors on end organs.[47]

Centrally, enhanced release and actions of excitatory neurotransmitters (eg, glutamate) and resultant lack of periodicity probably explain convulsions that are frequently refractory to anticonvulsants in methylxanthine poisoning. The reasons why theophylline convulsions carry such a high mortality stem from a lack of self-termination (continual high-frequency spike activity and large metabolic demands) that has resulted from A_1 antagonism, compounded by A_2-blockade-mediated cerebral vasoconstriction.[112] $GABA_A$ receptor agonism, especially by barbiturates, most effectively prevents and terminates methylxanthine-induced

seizures. Phenytoin not only is ineffective in treating theophylline-induced seizures, but it actually increases likelihood of seizures and mortality.[13]

Like phenytoin, carbamazepine's major anticonvulsant effect results from Na^+ channel blockade. Unlike phenytoin, carbamazepine appears to antagonize A_1 receptors.[27,30] This may explain the higher frequency of seizures after carbamazepine overdose than after phenytoin overdose. The absence of A_2 blockade by carbamazepine theoretically allows for increases in cerebral blood flow to meet metabolic demands of the seizing brain.

SUMMARY

Neurotransmitter systems share common physiologic features, including neurotransmitter uptake, vesicle membrane pumps, ion trapping of neurotransmitters within vesicles, calcium-dependent exocytosis, and receptors coupled to either G proteins or to ion channels. It is not surprising, then, that a single pharmacologic agent frequently produces effects on several different neurotransmitter systems.

As the number of new drugs and toxins encountered by man continues to grow, an understanding of their molecular actions in the nervous system helps the physician to anticipate and better understand various pharmacologic and adverse effects resulting from therapeutic or toxic doses.

REFERENCES

1. Aghajanian GK, Marel GJ: Serotonin model of schizophrenia: Emerging role of glutamate mechanisms. Brain Res Brain Res Rev 2000;31:302–312.
2. Albers RW, Siegel GJ: Membrane transport. In: Siegel GJ, Agranoff BW, Albers RW, et al: Basic Neurochemistry, 6th ed. Lippincott Williams & Wilkins, Philadelphia, 1999, pp. 95–118.
3. Albertson TE, Walby WF, Joy RM: Modification of GABA-mediated inhibition by various injectable anesthetics. Anesthesiology 1992;77:488–499.
4. Aprison MH, Lipkowitz KB, Simon JR: Identification of a glycine-like fragment on the strychnine molecule. J Neurosci Res 1987; 17:209–213.
5. Arya DK: Extrapyramidal symptoms with selective serotonin reuptake inhibitors. Br J Psychiatry 1994;165: 728–733.
6. Baba A, Cooper JR: The action of black widow spider venom on cholinergic mechanisms in synaptosomes. J Neurochem 1980;34: 1369–1379.
7. Barnes NM, Sharp T: A review of central 5-HT receptors and their function. Neuropharmacology 1999;38:1083–1152.
8. Bennet JP, Piercey MF: Pramipexole—A new dopamine agonist for the treatment of Parkinson's disease. J Neurolog Sci 1999;163: 25–31.
9. Bernasconi R, Mathivet P, Bischon, et al: Gamma-hydroxybutyric acid: An endogenous neuromodulator with abuse potential? Trends Pharmacol Sci 1999;20:135–141.
10. Bettler B, Mulle C: AMPA and kainate receptors. Neuropharmacology 1995;34:123–139.
11. Bhana N, Goa KL, McClellan KJ: Dexmedetomidine. Drugs 2000; 59:263–268.
12. Bisaga A, Popik P: In search of a new pharmacological treatment for drug and alcohol addiction: N-methyl-D-aspartate (NMDA) antagonists. Drug Alcohol Depend 2000;59:1–15.
13. Blake KV, Massey KL, Hendeles L, et al: Relative efficacy of phenytoin and phenobarbital for the prevention of theophylline-induced seizures in mice. Ann Emerg Med 1988;17:1024–1028.

14. Blin O: A comparative review of new antipsychotics. Can J Psychiatry 1999;44:235–244.

15. Bloom FE, Morales M: The central 5-HT3 receptor in CNS disorders. Neurochem Res 1998;23:653–659.

16. Bloom FE: Neurotransmission and the central nervous system. In: Hardman JG, Limbird LE, Molinoff PB, Ruddon RW, Gilman AG, eds: The Pharmacological Basis of Therapeutics, 9th ed. McGraw-Hill, New York, 1995, pp. 267–293.

17. Bormann J: The "ABC" of GABA receptors. Trends Pharmacol Sci 2000;21:16–19.

18. Bousquet P, Bruban V, Schann S, et al: Participation of imidazoline receptors and alpha2-adrenoceptors in the central hypotensive effects of imidazoline-like drugs. Ann N Y Acad Sci 1999;881:272–278.

19. Bousquet P, Feldman J: Drugs acting on imidazoline receptors. Drugs 1999;58:799–812.

20. Bowery NG, Enna SJ: GABA-B receptors: First of the functional metabotropic heterodimers. J Pharmacol Exp Ther 2000;292:2–7.

21. Briscoe JG, Curry SC, Gerkin RD, Ruiz RR: Pemoline-induced choreoathetosis and rhabdomyolysis. Med Toxicol Adverse Drug Exp 1988;3:72–76.

22. Brundege JM, Dunwiddie TV: Role of adenosine as a modulator of synaptic activity in the central nervous system. Adv Pharmacol 1997;39:353–391.

23. Buscher R, Herrmann V, Insel PA: Human adrenoceptor polymorphisms: Evolving recognition of clinical importance. Trends Pharmacol Sci 1999;20:94–99.

24. Carmichael FJ, Orrego H, Israel Y: Acetate-induced adenosine mediated effects of ethanol. Alcohol Alcohol 1993;2(Suppl):411–418.

25. Carpenter CL, Marks SS, Watson DL, Greenberg DA: Dextromethorphan and dextrorphan as calcium channel antagonists. Brain Res 1988;439:372–375.

26. Clapham DE: Direct G protein activation of ion channels? Annu Rev Neurosci 1994;17:441–464.

27. Clark M, Post RM: Carbamazepine, but not caffeine, is highly selective for adenosine A_1 binding sites. Eur J Pharmacol 1989;164:399–401.

28. Clark RF, Curry SC: Organophosphates and carbamates. In: Reisdorff EJ, Roberts MR, Wiegenstein JG, eds: Pediatric Emergency Medicine. Philadelphia, WB Saunders, 1993, pp. 684–693.

29. Clements MR, Hamilton DV, Siklos P: Thyrotoxicosis presenting with choreoathetosis and severe myopathy. J R Soc Med 1981;74:459–460.

30. Czuczwar SJ, Szczepanik B, Wamil A, et al: Differential effects of agents enhancing purinergic transmission upon the antielectroshock efficacy of carbamazepine, diphenylhydantoin, diazepam, phenobarbital, and valproate in mice. J Neural Transm Gen Sect 1990;81:153–166.

31. Dakshinamurti K, Sharma SK, Sundaram M: Domoic acid induced seizure activity in rats. Neurosci Lett 1991;127:193–197.

32. Diamond I, Gordon AS: The role of adenosine in mediating cellular and molecular responses to ethanol. EXS 1994;71:175–183.

33. Doble A: New insights into the mechanism of action of hypnotics. J Psychopharmacol 1999;13(4 Suppl 1):S11–20.

34. Doble A: The role of excitotoxicity in neurodegenerative disease: Implications for therapy. Pharmacol Ther 1999;81:163–221.

35. Docherty JR: Subtypes of functional α_1- and α_2-adrenoceptors. Eur J Pharmacol 1998;361:1–15.

36. Edwards FA, Robertson SJ: The function of A2 adenosine receptors in the mammalian brain: Evidence for inhibition vs. enhancement of voltage dated calcium channels and neurotransmitter release. Prog Brain Res 1999;120:265–273.

37. Eglen RM: 5-hydroxytryptamine (5-HT4) receptors and central nervous system function: An update. Prog Drug Res 1997;49:9–24.

38. Eglen RM, Hudson AL, Kendall DA, et al: Seeing through a glass darkly: Casting light on imidazoline "I" sites. Trends Pharmacol Sci 1998;19:381–390.

39. Eldridge FL, Paydarfar D, Scott SC, Dowell RT: Role of endogenous adenosine in recurrent generalized seizures. Exp Neurol 1989;103:179–185.

40. Eneanya DI, Bianchine JR, Duran DO, Andresen BD: The actions and metabolic fate of disulfiram. Annu Rev Pharmacol Toxicol 1981;21:575–596.

41. Faingold CL, Browning RA: Mechanisms of anticonvulsant drug action. I. Drugs primarily used for generalized tonic-clonic and partial epilepsies. Eur J Pediatr 1987;146:8–14.

42. Fariello RG: Pharmacodynamic and pharmacokinetic features of cabergoline: Rationale for use in Parkinson's disease. Drugs 1998;55(Suppl 1):10–16.

43. Feigenbaum JJ, Howard SG: Gamma-hydroxybutyrate is not a GABA agonist. Prog Neurobiol 1996;50:1–7.

44. Feldman J, Greney H, Monassier L, et al: Does a second generation of centrally acting antihypertensive drugs really exist? J Auton Nerv Sys 1998;72:94–97.

45. Ferre S: Adenosine-dopamine interactions in the ventral striatum. Implications for the treatment of schizophrenia. Psycopharmacology (Berl) 1997;133:107–120.

46. Frazer A, Hensler JG: Serotonin. In: Siegel GJ, Agranoff BW, Albers RW, et al, eds: Basic Neurochemistry, 6th ed. Philadelphia, Lippincott Williams & Williams, 1999, pp. 263–292.

47. Fredholm BB, Duner-Engstrom M, Fastbom J, et al: Role of G proteins, cyclic AMP, and ion channels in the inhibition of transmitter release by adenosine. Ann N Y Acad Sci 1990;604:276–288.

48. Frerking M, Nicoll RA: Synaptic kainate receptors. Curr Opin Neurobiol 2000;10:342–351.

49. Gareri P, Falconi U, De Fazio P, et al: Conventional and new antidepressant drugs in the elderly. Prog Neurobiol 2000;61:353–396.

50. Gavish M: Hormonal regulation of peripheral-type benzodiazepine receptors. J Steroid Biochem Mol Biol 1995; 53:57–59.

51. Gee KW, McCauley LD, Lan NC: A putative receptor for neurosteroids on the $GABA_A$ receptor complex: The pharmacological properties and therapeutic potential of epalons. Crit Rev Neurobiol 1995;9:207–227.

52. Gibson KM, Hoffmann GF, Hodson AK, et al: 4-Hydroxybutyric acid and the clinical phenotype of succinic semialdehyde dehydrogenase deficiency, an inborn error of GABA metabolism. Neuropediatrics 1998;29:14–22.

53. Hajak G: A comparative assessment of the risks and benefits of zopiclone. Drugs 1999;21(6):457–469.

54. Hamel E: The biology of serotonin receptors: Focus on migraine pathophysiology and treatment. Can J Neurol Sci 1999;26:(Suppl 3):S2–S6.

55. Hampson DR, Manalo JL: The activation of glutamate receptors by kainic acid and domoic acid. Nat Toxins 1998;6:153–158.

56. Hargreaves RJ, Shepeard SL: Pathophysiology of migraine—New insights. Can J Neurol Sci 1999;26:(Suppl 3):S12–S19.

57. Hasler W: Serotonin receptor physiology. Dig Dis Sci 1999;44(Suppl 8):108S–113S.

58. Hawgood B, Bon C: Snake venom presynaptic toxins. In: Tu AT, ed: Reptile Venoms and Toxins: Handbook of Natural Toxins, Vol. 5. New York, Marcel Dekker, 1991, pp. 3–52.

59. Head GA, Chan CK, Burke SL: Relationship between imidazoline and alpha2-adrenoceptors involved in the sympatho-inhibitor actions of centrally acting antihypertensive agents. J Auton Nerv Sys 1998;72:163–169.

60. Hobson DE, Pourcher E, Martin WR: Ropinirole and pramipexole , the new agonists. Can J Neurol Sci 1999;26(Suppl 2):S27–S33.

61. Holm KJ, Goa KL: Zolpidem: An update of its pharmacology, therapeutic efficacy and tolerability in the treatment of insomnia. Drugs 2000;59:865–889.

62. Holm KJ, Spencer CM: Entacapone: A review of its use in Parkinson's disease. Drugs 1999;58:159–177.

63. Igarashi K, Kashiwagi K: Polyamines: Mysterious modulators of cellular functions. Biochem Biophys Res Commun 2000;271:559–564.

64. Insel PA: Adrenergic receptors—Evolving concepts and clinical implications. N Engl J Med 1996;334:580–585.

65. Johnson M: The β-adrenoceptor. Am J Resp Crit Care Med 1998; 158:S146–S153.

66. Joy RM, Albertson TE: In vivo assessment of the importance of GABA in convulsant and anticonvulsant drug action. Epilepsy Res 1992;8(Suppl):63–75.

67. Kaakkola S: Clinical pharmacology, therapeutic use and potential of COMT inhibitors in Parkinson's disease. Drugs 2000;59:1233–1250.

68. Khan ZP, Ferguson CN, Jones RM: Alpha-2 and imidazoline receptor agonists. Anaesthesia 1999;54:146–165.

69. Kiowski W, Hulthen UL, Ritz R, Buhler FR: α₂ Adrenoceptor-mediated vasoconstriction of arteries. Clin Pharmacol Ther 1983;34: 565–569.

70. Klawans HL, Weiner WJ: The pharmacology of choreatic movement disorders. Prog Neurobiol 1976;6:49–80.

71. Kornhuber J, Wiltfang J: The role of glutamate in dementia. J Neural Transm 1998;53(Suppl):277–287.

72. Korpi ER, Mattila MJ, Wisden W, Luddens H: GABA-A receptor subtypes: Clinical efficacy and selectivity of benzodiazepine site ligands. Ann Med 1997;29:275–282.

73. Kroeze WK, Roth BL: The molecular biology of serotonin receptors: Therapeutic implications for the interface of mood and psychosis. Biol Psychiatry 1998;44:1128–1142.

74. Krogsgaard-Larsen P, Hansen J: Naturally occurring excitatory amino acids as neurotoxins and leads in drug design. Toxicol Lett 1992;64/65:409–416.

75. Krueger KE, Papadopoulos V: Mitochondrial benzodiazepine receptors and the regulation of steroid biosynthesis. Annu Rev Pharmacol Toxicol 1992;32:211–237.

76. Lachowicz JE, Sibley DR: Molecular characteristics of mammalian dopamine receptors. Pharmacol Toxicol 1997;81:105–113.

77. Landis E, Shore E: Yohimbine-induced bronchospasm. Chest 1989; 96:1424.

78. Lanfumey L, Hamon M: Central 5-HT1A receptors: Regional distribution and functional characteristics. Nucl Med Biol 2000;27: 429–435.

79. Lefkowitz RJ, Hoffman BB, Taylor P: The autonomic and somatic motor nervous systems. In: Hardman JG, Limbird LE, Molinoff PB, Ruddon RW, Gilman AG, eds: The Pharmacological Basis of Therapeutics, 9th ed. New York, McGraw-Hill, 1995, pp. 105–139.

80. Li J, Arnaud-Stokes S, Woeckener A: A tale of novel intoxication: A review of the effects of gamma-hydroxybutyric acid with recommendations for management. Ann Emerg Med 1998;31:729–736.

81. Lieberman JA, Mailman RB, Duncan G, et al: Serotonergic basis of antipsychotic drug effects in schizophrenia. Biol Psychiatry 1998; 44:1099–1117.

82. Liggett SB: Molecular and genetic basis of β2-adrenergic receptor function. J Allergy Clin Immunol 1999;103:S42–S46.

83. Lin LH, Whiting P, Harris RA: Molecular determinants of general anesthetic action: Role of GABA_A receptor structure. J Neurochem 1993;60:1548–1553.

84. Linden CH, Vellman WP, Rumack B: Yohimbine: A new street drug. Ann Emerg Med 1985;14:1002–1004.

85. Lowe TL, Cohen DJ, Detlor J, et al: Stimulant medications precipitate Tourette's syndrome. JAMA 1982;247:1168–1169.

86. Lummis SC, Buckingham SD, Rauh JJ, Sattelle DB: Blocking actions of heptachlor at an insect central nervous system GABA receptor. Proc R Soc Lond [Biol] 1990;240:97–106.

87. Lynch JW, Rajendra S, Barry PH, Schofield PR: Mutations affecting the glycine receptor agonist transduction mechanism convert the competitive antagonist, picrotoxin, into an allosteric potentiator. J Biol Chem 1995;270:13799–13806.

88. Maitre M: The gamma-hydroxybutyrate signaling system in brain: Organization and functional implications. Prog Neurobiol 1997;51: 337–361.

89. Malatynska E, Knapp RJ, Ikeda M, Yamamura HI: Antidepressants and seizure-interactions at the GABA-receptor chloride-ionophore complex. Life Sci 1988;43:303–307.

90. Malcangio M, Bowery NG: GABA and its receptors in the spinal cord. Trends Pharmacol Sci 1996;17:429–465.

91. Mascia MP, Mihic SJ, Valenzuela CF: A single amino acid determines differences in ethanol actions on strychnine-sensitive glycine receptors. Mol Pharmacol 1996;50:402–406.

92. McDaniel KD: Clinical pharmacology of monoamine oxidase inhibitors. Clin Neuropharmacol 1986;9:207–234.

93. Meir A, Ginsburg S, Butkevich A, et al: Ion channels in presynaptic nerve terminals and control of transmitter release. Physiol Rev 1999; 79:1019–1088.

94. Meldrum BS, Chapman AG: Excitatory amino acid receptors and antiepileptic drug development. Adv Neurol 1999;79:947–963.

95. Mihic SJ: Acute effects of ethanol on GABA_A and glycine receptor function. Neurochem Int 1999;35:115–123.

96. Miller J, Robinson A, Percy AK: Acute isoniazid poisoning in childhood. Am J Dis Child 1980;134:290–292.

97. Miller RJ: Presynaptic receptors. Ann Rev Pharmacol Toxicol 1998; 38:201–227.

98. Mills KC: Serotonin syndrome: A clinical update. Crit Care Clin 1997;13:763–783.

99. Modell JG, Tandon R, Beresford TP: Dopaminergic activity of the antimuscarinic antiparkinsonian agents. J Clin Psychopharmacol 1989;9:347–351.

100. Muller CE, Scior T: Adenosine receptors and their modulators. Pharm Acta Helv 1993;68:77–111.

101. Nestler EJ, Duman RS: G proteins. In: Siegel GJ, Agranoff BW, Albers RW, et al: Basic Neurochemistry, 6th ed. Philadelphia, Lippincott Williams & Wilkins, 1999, p. 110, pp. 401–414.

102. Nilsson M, Hansson E, Rohnback L: Transport of valproate and its effects on GABA uptake in astroglial primary culture. Neurochem Res 1990;15:763–767.

103. Oja SS, Kontro P: Neurochemical aspects of amino acid transmitters and modulators. Med Biol 1987;65:143–152.

104. Olsen RW: The GABA postsynaptic membrane receptor-ionophore complex. Mol Cell Biochem 1981;39:261–279.

105. Palmer T: Agents acting at the neuromuscular junction and autonomic ganglia. In: Hardman JG, Limbird LE, Molinoff PB, Ruddon RW, Gilman AG, eds: The Pharmacological Basis of Therapeutics, 9th ed. New York, McGraw-Hill, 1995, pp. 177–197.

106. Parkinson FE, Rudophi KA, Fredholm BB: Propentofylline: A nucleoside transport inhibitor with neuroprotective effects in cerebral ischemia. Gen Pharmacol 1994;25:1053–1058.

107. Paterson D, Nordberg A: Neuronal nicotinic receptors in the human brain. Prog Neurobiol 2000;61:75–111.

108. Pelleg A, Porter RS: The pharmacology of adenosine. Pharmacotherapy 1990;10:157–174.

109. Phillis JW, O'Regan MH: The role of adenosine in the central actions of the benzodiazepines. Prog Neuropsychopharmacol Biol Psychiatry 1988;12:389–404.

110. Picotti GB, Bondiolotti GP, Meldolesi J: Peripheral catecholamine release by alpha-latrotoxin in the rat. Naunyn Schmiedebergs Arch Pharmacol 1982;320:224–229.

111. Pin JP, Bockaert J: Get receptive to metabotropic glutamate receptors. Curr Opin Neurobiol 1995;5:342–349.

112. Pinard E, Riche D, Puiroud S, Seylaz J: Theophylline reduces cerebral hyperaemia and enhances brain damage induced by seizures. Brain Res 1990;511:303–309.

113. Porkka-Heiskanen T: Adenosine in sleep and wakefulness. Ann Med 1999;31:125–129.

114. Pucilowski O: Psychopharmacological properties of calcium channel inhibitors. Psychopharmacology (Berl) 1992;109:12–29.

115. Ralevic V, Burnstock G: Receptors for purines and pyrimidines. Pharmacol Rev 1998;50:413–492.

116. Redgrave P, Prescott TJ, Gurney K: Is the short-latency dopamine response too short to signal reward error? Trends Neurosci 1999;22: 146–151.

117. Rho JM, Donevan SD, Rogawski MA: Barbiturate-like actions of the propanediol dicarbamates felbamate and meprobamate. J Pharmacol Exp Ther 1997;280:1383–1391.

118. Richelson E: Receptor pharmacology of neuroleptics: Relation to clinical effects. J Clin Psychiatry 1999;60(Suppl 10):5–14.

119. Rogawski MA, Donevan SD: AMPA receptors in epilepsy and as targets for antiepileptic drugs. Adv Neurol 1999;79:947–963.

120. Rogawski MA: The NMDA receptor, NMDA antagonists and epilepsy therapy. Drugs 1992;44:279–292.

121. Roth BL: Multiple serotonin receptors: Clinical and experimental aspects. Ann Clin Psychiatry 1994;6:67–78.

122. Rudorfer MV, Potter WZ: Antidepressants: A comparative review of the clinical pharmacology and therapeutic use of the "newer" versus the "older" drugs. Drugs 1989;37:713–738.

123. Sawynok J: Adenosine receptor activation and nociception. Eur J Pharmacol 1998;347(1):1–11.

124. Scholz KP: Introductory perspective. In: Dunwiddie TV, Lovinger DM, eds: Presynaptic Receptors in the Mammalian Brain. Boston, Birkhauser, 1993, pp. 1–11.

125. Seal RP, Amara SG: Excitatory amino acid transporters: A family in flux. Ann Rev Pharmacol Toxicol 1999;39:431–456.

126. Sealfon S: Dopamine receptors and locomotor responses: Molecular aspects. Ann Neurol 2000;47(Suppl 1):S12–S21.

127. Selden BS, Curry SC: Anticholinergics. In: Reisdorff EJ, Roberts MR, Wiegenstein JG, eds: Pediatric Emergency Medicine. Philadelphia, WB Saunders, 1993, pp. 693–700.

128. Shank RP, Gardocki JF, Streeter AJ, Maryanoff BE: An overview of the preclinical aspects of topiramate: Pharmacology, pharmacokinetics, and mechanism of action. Epilepsia 2000;41(Suppl 1):S3–S9.

129. Sieghart W: Structure and pharmacology of γ-aminobutyric acid$_A$ receptor subtypes. Pharmacol Rev 1995;47:181–234.

130. Sigel E, Buhr A: The benzodiazepine binding site of GABA-A receptors. Trends Pharmacol Sci 1997;18:425–429.

131. Smith MJ: Abuse of the antiparkinson drugs: A review of the literature. J Clin Psychiatry 1980;41:351–354.

132. Sollevi A: Adenosine for pain control. Acta Anaesthesiol Scand Suppl 1997;110:135–136.

133. Southam E, Kirkby D, Higgins GA, et al: Lamotrigine inhibits monoamine uptake in vitro and modulates 5-hydroxytryptamine uptake in rats. Eur J Pharmacol 1998;358:19–24.

134. Spanagel R, Weiss F: The dopamine hypothesis of reward: Past and current status. Trends Neurosci 1999;22:521–527.

135. Squires RF, Saederup E: Antidepressants and metabolites that block GABA$_A$ receptors coupled to 35S-t-butylbicyclophosphorothionate binding sites in rat brain. Brain Res 1988;441:15–22.

136. Strosberg AD: Association of β3-adrenoceptor polymorphism with obesity and diabetes: Current status. Trends Pharmacol Sci 1997;18: 449–454.

137. Sulzer D, Maidment NT, Rayport S: Amphetamine and other weak bases act to promote reverse transport of dopamine in ventral midbrain neurons. J Neurochem 1993;60:527–535.

138. Sulzer D, Rayport S: Amphetamine and other psychostimulants reduce pH gradients in midbrain dopaminergic neurons and chromaffin granules: A mechanism of action. Neuron 1990;5:797–808.

139. Takumi Y, Matsubara A, Rinvik E, Ottersen OP: The arrangement of glutamate receptors in excitatory synapses. Ann N Y Acad Sci 1999;868:474–481.

140. Taylor CP: Mechanisms of new antiepileptic drugs. In: Delgado-Escueta AV, Jasper HH, Herbert H, et al: Jasper's Basic Mechanisms of the Epilepsies, 3rd ed. Philadelphia, Lippincott William & Wilkins, 1999, p. 1018.

141. Thomas RJ: Excitatory amino acids in health and disease. J Am Geriatr Soc 1995;43:1279–1289.

142. Toner LC, Tsambiras BM, Catalano G, et al: Central nervous system side effects associated with zolpidem treatment. Clin Neuropharmacol 1999;23:54–58.

143. Vallone D, Picetti R, Borrelli E: Structure and function of dopamine receptors. Neurosci Biobehav Rev 2000;24:125–132.

144. von Lubitz DK, Carter MF, Beenhakker M, et al: Adenosine: A prototherapeutic concept in neurodegeneration. Ann N Y Acad Sci 1995;765:163–178.

145. von Lubitz DK, Ye W, McClellan J, et al: Stimulation of adenosine A3 receptors in cerebral ischemia. Neuronal death, recovery, or both? Ann N Y Acad Sci 1999;890:93–106.

146. von Lubitz KE: Adenosine and cerebral ischemia: Therapeutic future or death of a brave concept? Eur J Pharmacol 1999;371:85–102.

147. Wallace KL: Antibiotic-induced convulsions. Crit Care Clin 1997; 13:741–762.

148. Watt G, Theakston RDG, Hayes CG, et al: Positive response to edrophonium in patients with neurotoxic envenoming by cobras (*Naja naja philippinensis*). N Engl J Med 1986;315:1444–1448.

149. Weyer C, Gautier JF, Danforth E: Development of beta$_3$-adrenoceptor agonists for the treatment of obesity and diabetes—An update. Diabetes Metab 1999;25:11–21.

150. Whiting PJ, McKernan RM, Wafford KA: Structure and pharmacology of vertebrate GABA$_A$ receptor subtypes. Int Rev Neurobiol 1995;38:95–138.

151. Wirkner K, Poelchen LK, Muhlberg K, et al: Ethanol-induced inhibition of NMDA receptor channels. Neurochem Int 1999;35:153–162.

CHAPTER 11 PHARMACOKINETIC AND TOXICOKINETIC PRINCIPLES

Mary Ann Howland

The following basic definitions develop the principles used in this chapter. *Pharmacokinetics* is the study of the behavior of drugs including absorption, distribution, metabolism, and excretion. Mathematical models and equations are used to describe and to predict this behavior. *Pharmacodynamics* is the investigation of the relationship of drug concentration to clinical effect. *Toxicokinetics* is the study of the absorption, distribution, metabolism, and excretion of a xenobiotic under circumstances that produce toxicity or excessive exposure. *Xenobiotics* are foreign, natural, or synthetic chemicals, including drugs, pesticides, environmental agents, and industrial agents.[38] *Toxicodynamics* is the study of the relationship of toxic concentrations of xenobiotics to clinical effect.

Humans with overdoses provide many challenges to the mathematical precision of toxicokinetics and toxicodynamics because many variables (dose, time of ingestion, presence of vomiting, etc) are often unknown. In contrast to the therapeutic setting, atypical solubility characteristics are noted and saturation of enzymatic processes occurs. Alterations in enzymatic saturation and protein binding may lead to enhanced absorption (decreased first-pass effect), more free drug available in the serum because of saturation of plasma protein binding, or prolonged elimination because of saturation of hepatic enzymes or active tubular secretion. In addition, age, obesity, gender, genetics, chronopharmacokinetics (diurnal variations), and the effects of critical illness and compromised organ perfusion all further inhibit attempts to achieve precise analyses.[3,14,31,35,56,60] Poison management interventions may alter one or more kinetic parameters. There are numerous approaches to these obstacles that include obtaining historical information from the patient's family and friends, doing pill counts, procuring sequential serum concentrations during the toxic phases, and occasionally repeating a pharmacokinetic evaluation during therapeutic dosing of that same agent to obtain comparative data.

Toxicokinetic principles can, however, be applied to facilitate our understanding and to make certain predictions. These principles can help evaluate whether a certain antidote or extracorporeal method is appropriate for use, when the serum concentration might be expected to drop into the therapeutic range, what ingested dose might be considered potentially toxic, what the onset and duration of toxicity might be, and what the importance is of a specific serum concentration. With all of this in mind, the clinical status of the patient is paramount, and mathematical formulas and equations can never substitute for evaluating the patient! This chapter explains the principles, presents the mathematics in a "user-friendly" fashion,[66] and demonstrates the application of these principles and mathematics by way of examples and case illustrations.

ABSORPTION

Absorption is the process by which a xenobiotic enters the body. For an agent to cause a systemic effect, it must reach the bloodstream and then be distributed to the site or sites of action. Both the rate (k_a) and extent of absorption (F) are measurable and important determinants of toxicity. The rate of absorption often predicts the onset of action and relies on dosage form, while the extent of absorption (bioavailability) often predicts the intensity of the effect and depends in part on first-pass effects.[29,30] Figure 11–1 depicts how changes in the rate of absorption may affect toxicity when the bioavailability is held constant versus how toxicity may be affected by changes in bioavailability when the rate of absorption is held constant.

The route by which the xenobiotic enters the body significantly affects both the rate and extent of absorption. As an approximation, the rate of absorption proceeds in the following order from fastest to slowest: intravenous, inhalation > intramuscular, subcutaneous, intranasal, oral > cutaneous, rectal. Following the oral administration of 200 mg of cocaine hydrochloride, the onset of action is 20 minutes, with an average peak concentration of 200 ng/mL.[59] These results distinctly differ when smoking 200 mg of cocaine freebase, which has an onset of action of 8 seconds and a peak level of 640 ng/mL, or when administered intravenously as 200 mg cocaine hydrochloride, which then has an onset of action of 30 seconds and a peak level of 1000 ng/mL.[59]

A xenobiotic must diffuse through a number of membranes before it can reach its site of action. Figure 11–2 shows the number of membranes through which a xenobiotic typically diffuses. Membranes are predominantly composed of phospholipids and cholesterol in addition to other lipid compounds.[43] A phospholipid is composed of a polar head and a fatty acid tail, which are arranged in membranes so that the fatty acid tails are inside and the polar heads face outward in a mirror image.[47] Proteins (in a 1:5 ratio with lipids) are found on both sides of the membranes and may traverse the membrane.[43] These proteins may function as receptors and channels. Pores are found throughout the membrane. The principles relating to diffusion apply to absorption, distribution, certain aspects of elimination, and to each instance when a xenobiotic is transported through a membrane.

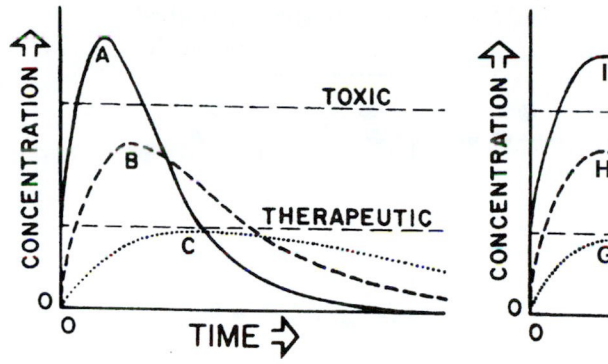 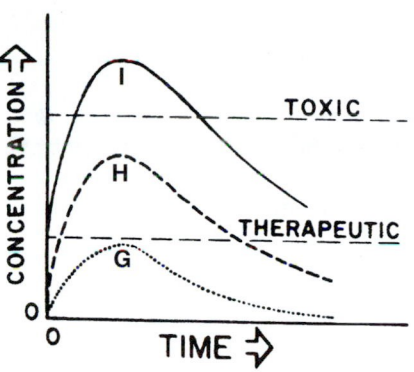

Figure 11–1. Effects of changes in k_a (rate of absorption) and F (bioavailability) on the blood concentration time graph and achieving a toxic threshold. In curves A, B, and C, F is constant as k_a is decreased. In curves G, H, and I, k_a is constant as F is increased. *(Reprinted, with permission, from Riviere JE: Absorption and distribution. In: Hodgson E, Levi P, eds: Introduction to Biochemical Toxicology. Norwalk, CT, Appleton & Lange, 1994, p. 22.)*

Transport through membranes occurs via passive diffusion, filtration (bulk flow is the major mechanism of transport which occurs with water directly through pores for small molecules with MW <100), active transport or facilitated transport, and rarely endocytosis (Fig. 11–3). Most xenobiotics traverse membranes via simple passive diffusion. The rate of diffusion is determined by Fick's Law of Diffusion (Eq. 11–1).

$$\text{Rate of diffusion} = \frac{dQ}{dt} = \frac{DAK(C_1 - C_2)}{h}$$

D = diffusion constant
A = surface area of the membrane
h = membrane thickness
K = partition coefficient
$C_1 - C_2$ = difference in concentrations of the xenobiotic at each side of the membrane

(Eq. 11–1)

The driving force for passive diffusion is the difference in concentration of the xenobiotic on both sides of the membrane. D is a constant for each xenobiotic and derived when the difference in concentrations between the two sides of the membrane is 1. The larger the surface area A, the higher the rate of diffusion. Most ingested xenobiotics are absorbed more rapidly in the small intestine than in the stomach because of the tremendous increase in surface area created by the presence of microvilli. The partition coefficient K represents the lipid-to-water partitioning of the xenobiotic. To a substantial degree, the more lipid soluble an agent is, the more easily the agent crosses membranes. Membrane thickness (h) is in-

versely proportional to the rate at which a xenobiotic diffuses through the membrane. Xenobiotics that are uncharged, nonpolar, of low molecular weight, and of sufficient lipid solubility have the highest rates of diffusion.

The extent of ionization of weak electrolytes (weak acids and weak bases) affects their rate of diffusion. Nonpolar and uncharged molecules penetrate faster. The Henderson-Hasselbalch relationship is used to determine the degree of ionization. An acid, by definition, gives up a hydrogen ion and a base accepts a hydrogen ion. RCOOH(HA) (ie, aspirin, phenobarbital) and $RNH_3^+(BH^+)$ are acids and $RCOO^-(A^-)$ and $RNH_2(B)$ (amphetamines, TCAs) are bases. The equilibrium dissociation constant K_a can then be described by Equations 11–2A and 11–2B.

$$\text{For weak acids: } HA = H^+ + A^- \quad K_a = \frac{[H^+][A^-]}{[HA]}$$

(Eq. 11–2A)

$$\text{For weak bases: } BH^+ = B + H^+ \quad K_a = \frac{[H^+][B]}{[BH^+]}$$

(Eq. 11–2B)

To work with the numbers in a more comfortable fashion, the negative log of both sides is determined and results in Equations 11–3A and 11–3B.

$$\text{For weak acids: } -\log K_a = -\log [H^+] - \log \frac{[A^-]}{[HA]}$$

(Eq. 11–3A)

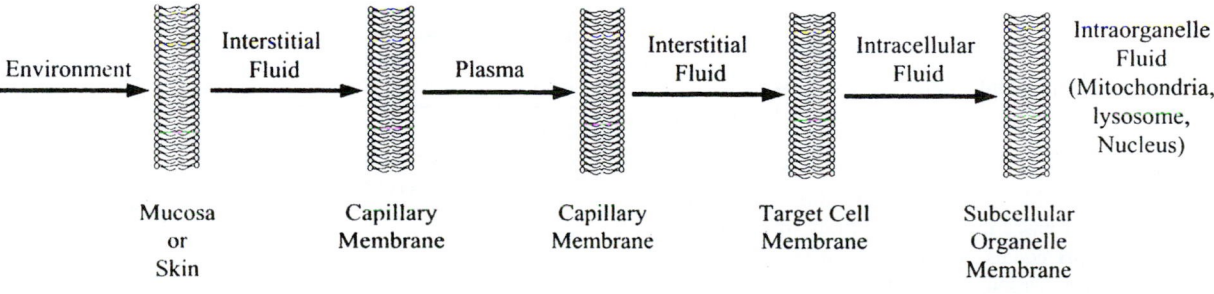

Figure 11–2. Illustration of the number of membranes encountered by a xenobiotic in the processes of absorption and distribution. *(Adapted from Riviere JE: Absorption and distribution. In: Hodgson E, Levi P, eds: Introduction to Biochemical Toxicology. Norwalk, CT, Appleton & Lange, 1994, p. 12.)*

Type of Transport	Example		Membrane	Absorbed molecule
Diffusion	Non-electrolytes (ethanol) and unionized forms of weak acids (salicylic acid) and bases (phenobarbital)			
Filtration and bulk flow	Molecules of varying sizes			
Endocytosis	Sabin polio virus vaccine			
Facilitated	5-Fluorouracil Lead Methyldopa Thallium			
Active	Thiamine Pyridoxine			

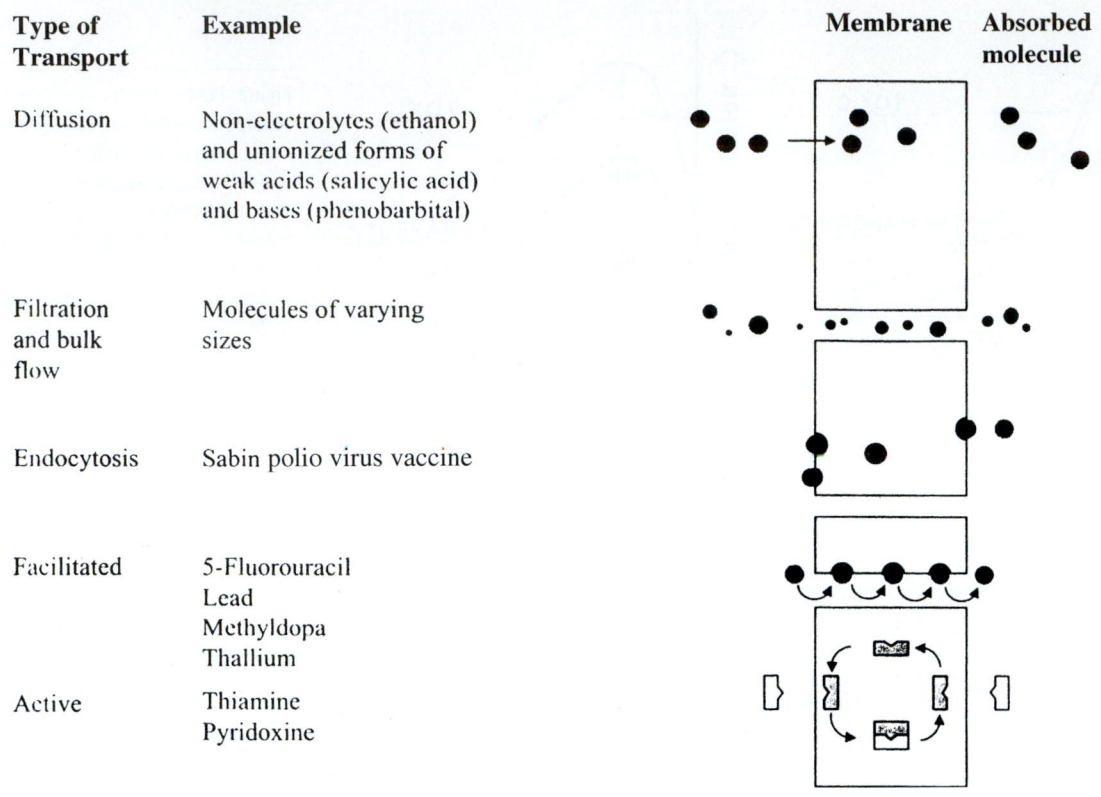

Figure 11–3. Illustration of transport mechanisms involved in the passage of xenobiotics across membranes. *(Adapted from Gram TE: Drug absorption and distribution. In: Craig CR, Stitzel RE, eds: Modern Pharmacology with Clinical Applications. Boston, Little, Brown, 1997, p. 17.)*

For weak bases:
$$-\log K_a = -\log [H^+] - \log \frac{[B]}{[BH^+]}$$
(Eq. 11–3B)

By definition, the negative log of $[H^+]$ is expressed as pH and the negative log of K_a is pK_a. Rearranging the equations gives the familiar forms of the Henderson-Hasselbalch equations as shown in Equations 11–4A, 11–4B, and 11–4C.

$$pH = pK_a + \log \frac{unprotonated\ species}{protonated\ species}$$
(Eq. 11–4A)

For weak acids:
$$pH = pK_a + \log \frac{[A^-]}{[HA]}$$
(Eq. 11–4B)

For weak bases:
$$pH = pK_a + \log \frac{[B]}{[BH^+]}$$
(Eq. 11–4C)

Because noncharged molecules traverse membranes faster, it is understood that weak acids cross membranes faster in an acidic environment and weak bases move more rapidly in a basic environment. When the pH equals the pK_a, half of the xenobiotic is charged and half is noncharged. An acid with a low pK_a is a strong acid while a base with a low pK_a is a weak base. For an acid, a pH less than the pK_a favors the protonated or noncharged species facilitating membrane diffusion, whereas for a base, a pH greater than the pK_a achieves the same result. The pH of selected body

fluids is given in Table 11–1 and the extent of charged versus non-charged xenobiotic is represented in Figure 11–4 at different pH and pK_a values.

Lipid solubility and ionization both have a distinct influence on absorption. These characteristics are demonstrated in Figure 11–5 for three different xenobiotics. Although the three agents have similar pK_a values, their different partition coefficients result in different degrees of absorption from the stomach.

Specialized transport mechanisms either require energy to transport xenobiotics against a concentration gradient (active transport) or they can be nonenergy requiring and lack the ability to transport against a concentration gradient (facilitated transport).

TABLE 11–1. pH of Selected Body Fluids

Fluids	pH
Gastric secretions	1.0–3.0
Small intestinal secretions: duodenum	5.0–6.0
Small intestinal secretions: ileum	8
Large intestinal secretions	8
Eye	7–8
Plasma	7.4
Cerebrospinal fluid	7.3
Urine	4.0–8.0

Reprinted, with permission, from Brody TM: Absorption, distribution, metabolism and elimination. In: Brody TM, Larner J, Minneman KP, Neu HC, eds: Human Pharmacology: Molecular to Clinical, 2nd ed. St. Louis, Mosby, 1994, p. 51.

pH	Aspirin (pK$_a$ = 3.5)	% nonionized	Methamphetamine (pK$_a$= 10)	% nonionized
1	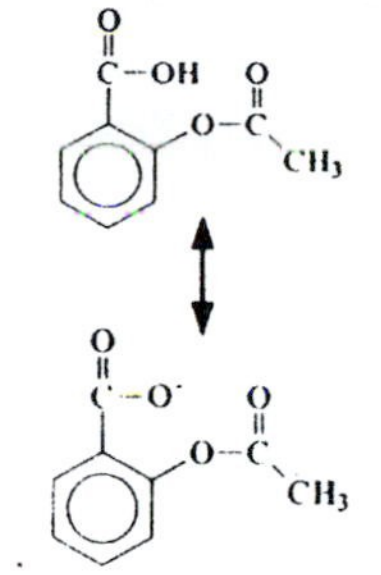	99.7		
2		97		
3		76		
3.5		50		
4		24	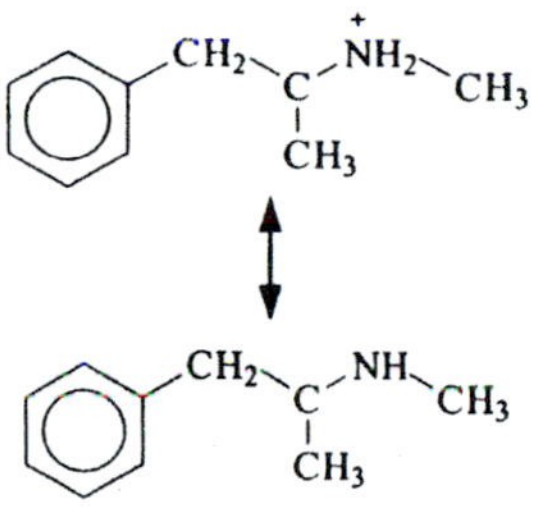	
5		3		0.001
6		0.315		0.01
7		0.032		0.1
10				50
11				90.9
12				99

Figure 11–4. Effect of pH on the ionization of aspirin (pK$_a$ = 3.5) and methamphetamine (pK$_a$ = 10).

These transport mechanisms are of importance in numerous areas including the intestines, liver, lung, renal, and biliary systems. These same principles apply to a small number of lipid-insoluble molecules that resemble essential endogenous agents.[22,52] For example, 5-fluorouracil resembles pyrimidine and is transported by the same system, whereas thallium and lead are actively absorbed by the endogenous transport mechanisms that absorb and transport iron and calcium, respectively.[22]

Currently *P-glycoprotein*, an ATP-dependent transporter, is being extensively investigated because of its role in controlling xenobiotic entry into the body and because of its contribution to drug interactions. The discovery of P-glycoprotein resulted from an investigation into why certain tumors exhibit multidrug resistance to many cancer chemotherapy agents. P-glycoprotein is located in the intestines, renal proximal tubule, hepatic bile canaliculi, and blood-brain barrier. First-generation inhibitors such

as amiodarone, ketoconazole, quinidine, and verapamil are responsible for increasing body levels of P-glycoprotein substrates such as digoxin, the protease inhibitors, Vinca alkaloids, and paclitaxel among others. St. John's wort is an inducer and lowers serum concentrations of these same agents. Second-generation reversal agents with a higher affinity are in development.[53]

Filtration is generally considered to be of limited importance for the absorption of most xenobiotics, but it is substantially more important with regard to elimination. Endocytosis, the act occurring when a cellular membrane encircles a xenobiotic, is responsible for the absorption of large macromolecules such as the oral Sabin polio vaccine.[52] Many of the same agents that affect CYP3A4 also affect P-glycoprotein.

Gastrointestinal absorption is affected by xenobiotic-related characteristics such as dosage form, degree of ionization, partition coefficient, and patient factors such as gastrointestinal blood flow, gastrointestinal motility, and the presence or absence of food, ethanol, or other interfering substances (Fig. 11–6).

The formulation of a xenobiotic is extremely important in predicting GI absorption. Disintegration and dissolution must precede passive absorption. Controlled-release, extended-release, and sustained-release formulations are designed to release the xenobiotic over a prolonged period of time in order to simulate the blood concentrations achieved with the use of a constant intravenous infusion. These formulations minimize blood level fluctuations, reduce peak related side effects, reduce dosing frequency, and improve patient compliance. A variety of products employ different pharmaceutic strategies, including dissolution control (encapsulation or matrix; Feosol), diffusion control (membrane or matrix; Slow K, Plendil ER), erosion (Sinemet CR), osmotic pump systems (Procardia XL, Glucotrol XL), and ion exchange resins (MS Contin suspension). Overdoses with controlled-release formulations result in a prolonged absorption phase, a delay to peak concentrations, and a prolonged duration.[7] Enteric-coated (ASA, divalproex sodium) formulations resist disintegration and delay the time to onset of effect.[6] Dissolution is affected by ionization, solubility, and the partition coefficient, as noted earlier. In the overdose setting, the formation of poorly soluble or adherent masses such as concretions (meprobamate) and bezoars (bromide) significantly delays the time to onset of toxicity[4,9,23,24] (Table 11–2).

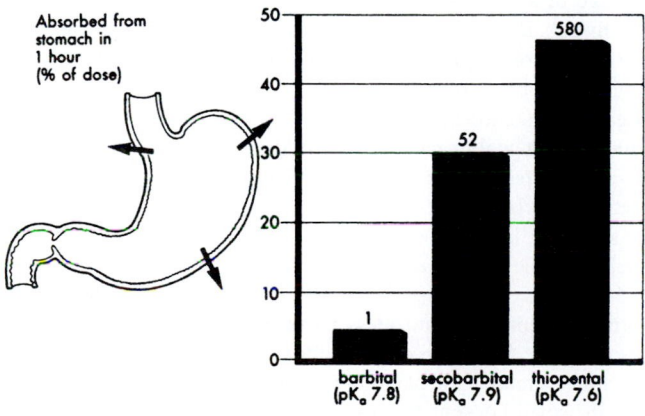

Figure 11–5. Influence of increasing lipid solubility on the amount of xenobiotic absorbed from the stomach for three xenobiotics with similar pK$_a$ values. The number above each column is the oil/water equilibrium partition coefficient. *(Reprinted, with permission, from Brody T: Absorption, distribution, metabolism and elimination. In: Brody TM, Larner J, Minneman KP, Neu HP, eds: Human Pharmacology: Molecular to Clinical, 2nd ed. St. Louis, Mosby, 1994, p. 50.)*

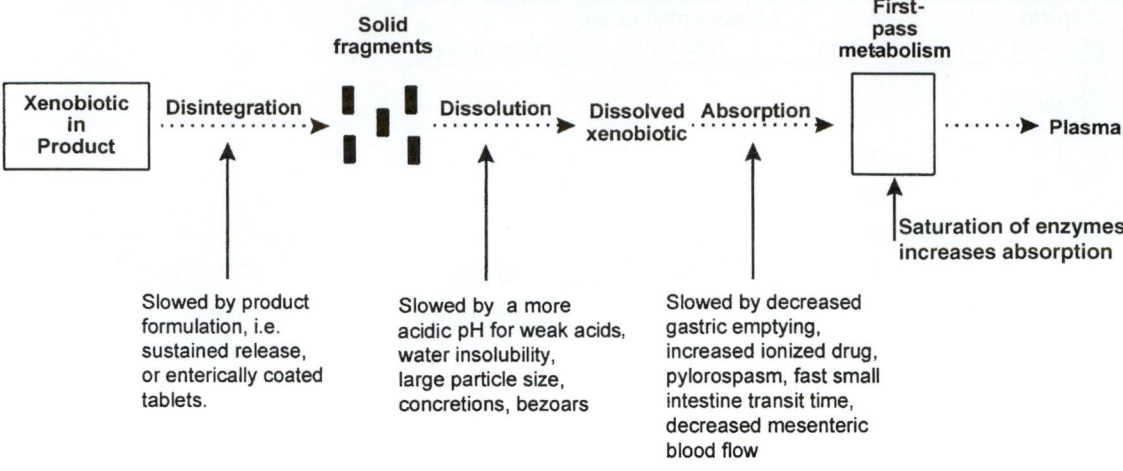

Figure 11–6. Determinants of absorption.

Most ingested xenobiotics are primarily absorbed in the small intestine as a result of the large surface area and extensive blood flow of the small intestines.[46] Critically ill patients who are hypotensive, who have a reduced cardiac output or who are receiving vasoconstrictors such as norepinephrine, have a decreased perfusion of vital organs, including the GI tract, kidneys, and liver.[3] Not only will absorption be delayed, but elimination will also be diminished.[46] Extremely short gastrointestinal transit times will reduce absorption. This change in transit time is the unproven rationale for the use of cathartics and whole-bowel irrigation. Any delays in emptying of the stomach delay absorption as a result of the delay in delivery to the small intestine. Delays in gastric emptying occur due to the presence of food, especially fatty meals, agents with anticholinergic, opioid, or antiserotonergic properties, ethanol, and any agent that results in pylorospasm (salicylates, iron).

Bioavailability is the extent of absorption (Eq. 11–5). The fractional absorption (F) of a xenobiotic is defined by the area under the curve (AUC) of the designated route of absorption as compared to the AUC of the intravenous route. The plasma concentration versus time curve (AUC) for each route represents the amount absorbed.

$$F = \frac{(AUC)_{\text{route under study}}}{(AUC)_{IV}} \qquad \text{(Eq. 11–5)}$$

Gastric emptying (orogastric lavage, syrup of ipecac) and activated charcoal are used to decrease the bioavailability of ingested xenobiotics. The oral administration of certain chelators (deferox-

amine, D-penicillamine) actually enhances the bioavailability of the complexed xenobiotic; although some chelators, such as succimer, may increase absorption, they increase urinary elimination even more.[25] A less soluble form of iron is not produced by the administration of sodium bicarbonate.[13]

Presystemic elimination may decrease or increase the bioavailability of a xenobiotic.[42] The GI tract contains microbial organisms that can metabolize or degrade xenobiotics such as digoxin and oral contraceptives by microbial metabolism, and insulin by peptidases.[43] However, in rare cases, gastrointestinal hydrolysis can convert a xenobiotic into a toxic metabolite such as amygdalin into cyanide, a metabolic step that does not occur following intravenous administration.[21] Venous drainage from the stomach and intestine delivers orally (and intraperitoneally) administered xenobiotics directly to the liver via the portal vein and avoids direct delivery to the systemic circulation. This venous drainage is referred to as the *first-pass effect*.[2,63] The hepatic extraction ratio is the percentage of xenobiotic metabolized in one pass of blood through the liver.[42] Drugs that undergo significant first-pass metabolism (eg, propranolol, verapamil) are used at much lower IV doses than oral doses. Some drugs are not administered by the oral route at all because of significant first-pass effect (eg, lidocaine, nitroglycerin).[4] Sublingual or rectal administration of agents such as nitroglycerin bypasses the portal circulation and avoids first-pass metabolism. In the overdose setting, presystemic elimination may be saturated, leading to an increased bioavailability of xenobiotics such as cyclic antidepressants, phenothiazines, opioids, and many β-adrenergic antagonists.[45] Hepatic metabolism usually transforms the xenobiotic into a less active metabolite, but occasionally results in the formation of a more toxic agent such as occurs with the transformation of parathion to paraoxon.[40] Biliary excretion into the small intestine usually occurs for these transformed xenobiotics of molecular weights >350 daltons and may result in a xenobiotic appearing in the feces, although it has not been administered orally.[27,43,55] Hepatic conjugated metabolites such as glucuronides may be hydrolyzed in the intestines to the parent form or to another active metabolite that can be reabsorbed by the enterohepatic circulation.[32,38,41,43] The enterohepatic circulation may result in what has been termed a double-peak phenomenon following the administration of certain xenobiotics.[52]

TABLE 11–2. **Drugs That Commonly Form Concretions or Bezoars, Delay Gastric Emptying, and/or Result in Pylorospasm**

Anticholinergic agents	Meprobamate
Barbiturates	Methaqualone
Bromides	Opioids
Enteric-coated tablets	Phenytoin
Glutethimide	Salicylates
Iron	

DISTRIBUTION

After the xenobiotic reaches the systemic circulation or central compartment, it is available for transport to peripheral tissue compartments. Both the rate and extent of distribution depend on many of the same principles discussed with regard to diffusion. Additional factors include affinity of the xenobiotic for plasma and tissue proteins, acid-base status of the patient (which affects ionization), and physiologic barriers to distribution (blood-brain barrier, placental transfer, blood-testis barrier).[18,28,47] Blood flow accounts for the initial phase of distribution, whereas xenobiotic affinities determine the final distribution pattern. Hypoperfusion in the critically ill affects absorption, distribution, and elimination.[61]

Plasma and serum concentrations are used essentially interchangeably. When a reference or calculation is made with regard to a concentration in the body, it is actually a plasma concentration. When concentrations are measured in the laboratory, a serum concentration (clotted and centrifuged blood) is often determined. In reality the laboratory measurements of most xenobiotics in serum or plasma are nearly equivalent. This is often not the case for whole-blood determination if the xenobiotic distributes into the erythrocyte, such as lead and most other heavy metals.

Volume of distribution (Vd) is the proportionality term used to relate the dose of the xenobiotic the individual receives and the resultant plasma concentration. Vd is an apparent or theoretic volume into which a drug distributes. It is a measure of how much drug is located inside and outside of the plasma compartment, because only the plasma compartment is assayed. In a 70-kg adult male, the total body fluid (TBF) is 60% of total body weight or 42 L with two-thirds (28 L) of that as intracellular fluid. Of the 14 L of extracellular fluid, 8 L are considered interstitial; 3 L, or 0.04 L/kg, is plasma; and 6 L, or 0.08 L/kg, is blood. If 42 g of a xenobiotic is administered and remained in the plasma compartment, the concentration is 14 g/L. If the distribution of the xenobiotic (of 42 g) approximated TBF (methanol), the concentration would be 100 mg/dL. These calculations can be performed by using Equation 11–6, where S equals the percent pure drug if a salt form is used.

$$V_d = \frac{S \times F \times \text{dose (mg)}}{C_0}$$

(Eq. 11–6)

Experimental determination of a Vd involves administering an IV dose of the xenobiotic and extrapolating the plasma concentration time curve back to time zero (C_0). If the determination takes place after steady state has been achieved, the volume of distribution is then referred to as the Vdss. For many xenobiotics the Vd is known and readily available in the literature (Table 11–3). When the Vd and the dose ingested are known, a maximum plasma concentration can be predicted, assuming all of the xenobiotic is absorbed and no elimination occured. This assumption usually overestimates the plasma concentration. Distribution is complex, and differential affinities for various storage sites (plasma proteins, liver, kidney, fat, and bone) in the body determine where a xenobiotic resides. A low Vd is often considered to be <1 L/kg. For some xenobiotics such as digoxin (Vd = 5 L/kg) or the cyclic antidepressants (Vd ≥10–15 L/kg), the Vd is much larger than the actual volume of the body. A large Vd indicates that the xenobiotic resides outside of the plasma compartment, but again it does not describe the site of distribution.

The site of accumulation of a xenobiotic may or may not be a site of action or toxicity. If the site of accumulation is not a site of toxicity, then the storage depot may be relatively inactive and the accumulation at that site may be theoretically protective to the biologic specimen.[47] Selective accumulation of xenobiotics occurs in certain areas of the body because of affinity for certain tissue-binding proteins. The kidney contains metallothionein, which has a high affinity for metals such as cadmium, lead, and mercury.[18] The retina contains the pigment melanin, which binds and accumulates chlorpromazine, thioridazine, and chloroquine.[18] Other examples of xenobiotics accumulating at primary sites of toxicity are carbon monoxide binding to hemoglobin and myoglobin and paraquat distributing to the lungs.[44] DDT, chlordane, and polychlorinated biphenyls are stored in fat, which can be mobilized following starvation.[64] Lead sequestered in bone[26] is not immediately toxic, but mobilization of bone through an increase in osteoclastic activity[47] (hyperparathyroidism, possibly pregnancy) may distribute lead to sites of toxicity (soft tissues, blood).

Several plasma proteins bind xenobiotics and act as carriers and storage depots. The percentage of protein binding varies among drugs as do their affinities and potential for reversibility. Once bound to plasma protein, a xenobiotic with high binding affinity will remain largely confined to the plasma until elimination occurs. However, dissociation and reassociation may occur if another carrier is available with a higher binding affinity. Most plasma measurements of xenobiotic concentration reflect total drug (bound plus unbound). Only the unbound drug is free to diffuse through membranes for distribution or for elimination. Albumin binds primarily to weakly acidic, poorly water-soluble xenobiotics, which include salicylates, phenytoin, and warfarin. α_1-Acid glycoprotein (a globulin of MW 44,000 daltons) usually binds basic xenobiotics including lidocaine, imipramine, and propranolol.[50] Transferrin, a β_1-globulin, transports iron, and ceruloplasmin carries copper.

Phenytoin is an example of a drug whose effects are significantly influenced by changes in concentration of plasma albumin. When albumin concentrations are in the normal range, approximately 90% of phenytoin is bound to albumin. As the albumin concentration decreases, however, more drug is free for distribution and a greater clinical response to the same phenytoin level is often observed. It is this free form of phenytoin that is active. The free plasma phenytoin concentration can be calculated based on the albumin concentration to achieve an appropriate interpretation of total phenytoin within the conventional therapeutic range of 10–20 mg/L of free plus bound phenytoin (Eq. 11–7).

$$\text{Adjusted phenytoin concentration} = \frac{\text{actual phenytoin concentration}}{(0.25 \times [\text{albumin}]) + 0.1}$$

(Eq. 11–7)

The clinical implications are that a malnourished patient with an albumin of 2 g/dL receiving phenytoin can manifest toxicity with a plasma phenytoin concentration of 14 mg/L. This measurement is total phenytoin (bound + unbound). Because the patient has a reduced albumin concentration, this actually represents a substantially higher proportion and absolute amount of active unbound phenytoin. Substitution into the above equation of 14 mg/L for actual plasma phenytoin concentration and 2 g/dL for albumin gives an adjusted plasma phenytoin concentration of 23.33 mg/L (therapeutic range 10–20 mg/L).

TABLE 11–3.   Pharmacokinetic Characteristics of Agents Associated with the Largest Number of Toxicologic Deaths

	Vd L/kg	Protein Binding %	Renal Elimination % Unchanged	Hepatic Metabolism (CYP)	Active Metabolite	Enterohepatic
Analgesics						
Acetaminophen	0.8–1	5–20	2	95% (CYP2E1-3–8%)	NAPQI	27–42% excreted in bile
Aspirin	0.15–0.2	50–80 (salicylic acid) saturable	10 (pH dependent)	Majority	Salicylic acid	None
Methadone	3.59	71–87	5–10	Majority (3A4, 2D6)	None?	Yes
Morphine	3–4	35	<10	n-Demethylation	15% Morphine-6-glucuronide 55% morphine-3-glucuronide	Yes
Propoxyphene	12–26	80	<10	>90% (3A4, 2D6)	Norpropoxyphene	Yes?
Antidepressants						
Amitriptyline	8.3±2	96	5	Yes (2C9)	Nortriptyline (2D6)	Yes
Desipramine	33–42	92	0.3–2.6	Yes (2D6)	None	Yes
Doxepin	20±8	—	0	Yes	Desmethyldoxepin	Yes
Imipramine	15±6	85	0–1.7	Yes (2D6)	Desipramine	Yes
Lithium	0.79	None	89–98	None	None	None
Cardiovascular Drugs						
Digoxin	5.1–7.4	20–25	57–80 in 6–12 h		Minor amount	Yes
Diltiazem	5.3	70–80	1–3	90% (3A)	Yes, many	No
Nifedipine	0.8–1.4	92–98	?	98% (3A4)	No	No
Propranolol	3.6	93	<0.5	>95% (2C19, 2D6)	No	No
Verapamil	4.7	83–92	3–4%	97% (3A4, 1A2, 2C9)	Norverapamil	No
Stimulants and Drugs of Abuse						
Amphetamine	6.11 in drug dependent 3.5–4.6	16	45 (pH dependent)	50%	Conjugated p-hydroxynor-ephedrine 0.3% Conjugated p-hydroxyam-phetamine 2–4%	No
Cocaine	1.96–2.7	8.7	9.5–20 (pH dependent)	5–10% (3A4)	Norcocaine; (?) others	No
Heroin	25	40	Minor		β-Acetylmorphine 1.3% Morphine 4.2%	No
Methamphetamine	3.2–3.7	pH dependent			Amphetamine 4–7% p-Hydroxymethamphet-amine 15%	No
Sedative/Hypnotics						
Chloral hydrate	0.75	70–80	Minor	Alcohol dehydrogenase	Trichloroethanol	No
Phenobarbital	0.88	40–50	20–50 pH dependent	Yes (2C9 × 2C19)	None	No
Alcohols						
Ethanol	0.5–0.6	None	Very little	95% Alcohol dehydrogenase	Acetaldehyde	No
Ethylene glycol	0.6–0.8	None	20		Many (oxalic acid)	No
Methanol	0.6–0.7	None	3–5	95% Alcohol dehydrogenase	Formic acid	No
Miscellaneous						
Cyanide	0.4	60	0		None	None
Theophylline	0.5	50–60	7	90% (1A2, 2E1 >3A4)	1,3-Dimethyluric acid Caffeine (in neonates)	No

(continued)

TABLE 11–3. **Pharmacokinetic Characteristics of Agents Associated with the Largest Number of Toxicologic Deaths (continued)**

	Vd L/kg	Protein Binding %	Renal Elimination % Unchanged	Hepatic Metabolism (CYP)	Active Metabolite	Enterohepatic
Organic Phosphorus Compounds						
Malathion	?	None		Metabolized by microsomal enzymes		No
Chlorpyrifos	?	None		Yes	3,5,6-Trichloro-2-pyridonol	No
Rodenticides						
Brodifacoum	0.985 (rats)	None		Yes		No
Strychnine	13	None	10–20 24 h	Yes		No

Although drug interactions are often attributed to the displacement of xenobiotics, the significance is overestimated. Displacement transiently increases the amount of unbound drug, making this drug available for elimination as well as distribution. Many instances in which protein displacement occurred were previously thought to result in toxicity; they are now attributed to simultaneous inhibition of metabolism.[48]

Saturation of plasma proteins may occur in the therapeutic range for agents such as valproic acid. Acute saturation of plasma protein binding following an overdose often leads to consequential effects. Salicylates and iron are examples of xenobiotics for which saturation of plasma protein binding in the overdose setting is an important factor in increasing toxicity caused by increased distribution to the CNS (salicylates) or to the liver, heart, and other tissues (iron).

Specific therapeutic maneuvers in the overdose setting are designed to alter xenobiotic distribution by inactivating and/or enhancing elimination to limit toxicity. These therapeutic maneuvers include (a) manipulation of serum or urine pH (salicylates); (b) use of chelators (lead); and (c) the use of antibodies or antibody fragments (digoxin).

The Vd permits predictions about plasma concentrations and also assists in defining whether an extracorporeal method of removal is beneficial for a particular toxin. If the Vd is large (>1 L/kg), it is unlikely that hemodialysis, hemoperfusion, or exchange transfusion would be effective because most of the xenobiotic resides outside of the plasma compartment. Plasma protein binding also influences this decision. If the xenobiotic is more tightly bound to plasma proteins than to activated charcoal, then hemoperfusion is unlikely to be beneficial even if the Vd is small. In addition, high plasma protein binding limits the effectiveness of hemodialysis, because only unbound xenobiotic will freely cross the dialysis membrane. Exchange transfusion and hemoperfusion can be effective for a xenobiotic with a small Vd and substantial plasma protein binding, because both bound and free xenobiotic are removed simultaneously.

ELIMINATION

Removal of a parent compound from the body (*elimination*) begins as soon as the xenobiotic is delivered to clearance organs such as the liver, kidneys, and lungs. Elimination begins immediately, but may not be the predominant kinetic process until absorp-

tion and distribution are substantially completed. As expected, the functional integrity of the major organ systems (cardiovascular, renal, hepatic) are major determinants of the efficiency of xenobiotic removal and of therapeutically administered antidotes. The xenobiotics themselves may cause renal or hepatic failure (acetaminophen), subsequently limiting their own elimination. Other factors influencing elimination include age (enzyme maturation), competition or inhibition of elimination processes by interacting xenobiotics, saturation of enzymatic processes, gender, genetics, and the physicochemical properties of the xenobiotic.[36]

Elimination can be accomplished by biotransformation to one or more metabolites, or by *excretion* from the body of unchanged xenobiotic. Excretion can occur via the kidneys, lungs, GI tract, and body secretions (sweat, tears, milk). Hydrophilic (polar) or charged xenobiotics and their metabolites, due to their water solubility, are generally excreted via the kidney. The majority of xenobiotic metabolism occurs in the liver but it also commonly occurs in the blood, skin, GI tract, placenta, or kidneys. Lipophilic (noncharged or nonpolar) xenobiotics are usually metabolized in the liver to hydrophilic metabolites, which are then excreted by the kidneys.[19,40] These metabolites are generally inactive, but if active may contribute to toxicity. Examples include the metabolism of amitriptyline to nortriptyline, procainamide to *N*-acetylprocainamide, and meperidine to normeperidine (Table 11–4).

Metabolic reactions catalyzed by enzymes categorized as either phase I or phase II generally result in pharmacologically active metabolites; frequently the latter have different toxicities than the parent compounds. *Phase I*, or preparative metabolism, which may or may not precede phase II, is responsible for introducing polar groups onto nonpolar xenobiotics by oxidation, reduction, and hydrolysis or dealkylation. The result of phase metabolism is commonly to add or expose polar groups.[17,38] *Phase II*, or synthetic reactions, conjugate the polar group with a glucuronide, sulfate or acetate (often a less polar metabolite, which is reabsorbed), methyl groups, glutathione (mercapturic acid synthesis), and amino acids (glycine, taurine, and glutamic acid).[12,17,38] Comparatively, phase II reactions produce a much larger increase in hydrophilicity than phase I reactions. The enzymes involved in these reactions have low substrate specificity, and those in the liver are usually localized to either the endoplasmic reticulum (microsomes) or the soluble fraction of the cytoplasm (cytosol).[38] The location of the enzymes becomes important if they form reactive metabolites that then concentrate at the site of metabolism and cause toxicity (Table 11–5). For example, acetaminophen causes centrilobular necrosis because the cytochrome P450 2E1 isoen-

TABLE 11–4.   Examples of Xenobiotics Activated by Human P450

CYP1A1	Benzene
Benzo[*a*]pyrene and other polycyclic aromatic hydrocarbons	Carbon tetrachloride
	Chloroform
CYP1A2	Dichloromethane
Acetaminophen	Ethylene dibromide
NNK[a]	Ethylene dichloride
CYP2A6	Ethyl carbamate
NNK[a]	*N*-Nitrosodimethylamine
CYP2B6	Trichloroethylene
CYP2C 8, 9, 18, 19	Vinyl chloride
None known	CYP3A4
CYP2D6	Acetaminophen
NNK[a]	Aflatoxin B and G
CYP2E1	Cyclophosphamide
Acetaminophen	Ifosphamide
Acrylonitrile	

[a]NNK: 4-(methylnitrosamino)-1-(3-pyridyl)-/-butanone, a tobacco-specific nitrosamine.
Adapted from Guengerich, FP: Reactions and significance of cytochrome P450 enzymes. J Biol Chem 1991;266:10019–10022.
Reprinted, with permission, from Parkinson A: Biotransformation of xenobiotics. In: Klaassen C, ed: Casarett & Doull's Toxicology: The Basic Science of Poisons, 5th ed. New York, McGraw-Hill, 1996, p. 154.

zymes, which form NAPQI, the toxic metabolite, are located in their highest concentration in that zone of the liver.

The enzymes that metabolize the largest variety of xenobiotics are heme-containing proteins referred to as *cytochrome P*(CYP) *450 monooxygenase enzymes.*[22,38] This group of enzymes, formerly called the mixed function oxidase system, is found in abundance in the liver's microsomal endoplasmic reticulum. These enzymes primarily catalyze the oxygenation of xenobiotics. However cytochrome P450 in a reduced state (Fe^{2+}) binds carbon monoxide, its discovery and initial name resulted from spectral identification of the CO-bound cytochrome P450, which absorbs light maximally at 450 nm. The cytochrome P450 system is composed of many enzymes grouped into gene families and subfamilies, of which approximately 39 of these functional human genes are sequenced. Members of a gene family have >40% similarity of their amino acid sequencing and subfamilies have >55% similarity. Toxicity may result from induction or inhibition of cytochrome P450 isoenzymes by another xenobiotic, resulting in a consequential drug interaction (Table 11–6). Many of these interactions are predictable based on the known xenobiotic affinities and their ability to induce or inhibit the P450 system.[10,33,38,39,54] However, *polymorphism* (individual genetic expression of isoenzymes),[1] stereoisomer variability[62] (enantiomers with different potencies and isozyme affinities), and the ability of a xenobiotic's metabolism to be performed by alternate pathways contribute to unexpected metabolic outcomes. The pharmaceutical industry is now exploiting the concept of chiral switching (marketing a single enantiomer instead of the racemic mixture) to alter efficacy or side effect profiles. Enantiomers are named either according to the direction in which they rotate polarized light (l or − for levorotatory, and d or + for dextrorotatory) or according to the absolute spatial orientation of the groups at the chiral center (S or R). Chiral means "hand" in Greek, and the latter designations refer to either sinister or left-handed or rectus or right-handed. There is no direct correlation between the direction light is polarized and the absolute configuration. Recent investigations precluded specific

drug marketing because of the unexpected toxicity of the enantiomer.[58]

Excretion is primarily accomplished by the kidneys, although, as mentioned earlier, biliary, pulmonary, and body fluid secretions contribute to lesser degrees. Urinary excretion occurs through glomerular filtration, tubular secretion, and passive tubular reabsorption. The glomerulus filters unbound xenobiotics of a particular size and shape in a manner that is not saturable subject to renal blood flow and perfusion. Passive tubular reabsorption accounts for the reabsorption of noncharged, lipid-soluble xenobiotics, and is therefore influenced by the pH of the urine and the pK_a of the xenobiotic. The principles of diffusion discussed earlier permit, for example, the ion trapping of salicylate ($pK_a = 3.5$) in the urine through urinary alkalinization. Tubular secretion is an active process subject to saturation and drug interactions (Table 11–7). Tubular secretion is often less developed in the neonate.

CLASSICAL VERSUS PHYSIOLOGIC COMPARTMENT TOXICOKINETICS

Models exist to study and describe the movement of xenobiotics in the body with mathematical equations. Traditional *compartmental* models (one or two compartments) are data based and assume that changes in plasma concentrations represent tissue concentrations[37](Fig. 11–7). Advances in computer technology facilitate the utilization of the classic concepts developed in the late

TABLE 11–5.   General Pathways of Xenobiotic Biotransformation and Their Major Subcellular Location

Reaction	Enzyme	Localization
	Phase I	
Hydrolysis	Carboxylesterase	Microsomes, cytosol
	Peptidase	Blood, lysosomes
	Epoxide hydrolase	Microsomes, cytosol
Reduction	Azo- and nitro-reduction	Microflora, microsomes, cytosol
	Carbonyl reduction	Cytosol
	Disulfide reduction	Cytosol
	Sulfoxide reduction	Cytosol
	Quinone reduction	Cytosol, microsomes
	Reductive dehalogenation	Microsomes
Oxidation	Alcohol dehydrogenase	Cytosol
	Aldehyde dehydrogenase	Mitochondria, cytosol
	Aldehyde oxidase	Cytosol
	Xanthine oxidase	Cytosol
	Monoamine oxidase	Mitochondria
	Diamine oxidase	Cytosol
	Prostaglandin H synthase	Microsomes
	Flavin-mono-oxygenases	Microsomes
	Cytochrome P450	Microsomes
	Phase II	
	Glucuronide conjugation	Microsomes
	Sulfate conjugation	Cytosol
	Glutathione conjugation	Cytosol, microsomes
	Amino acid conjugation	Mitochondria, microsomes
	Acylation	Mitochondria, cytosol
	Methylation	Cytosol

Reprinted, with permission, from Parkinson A: Biotransformation of xenobiotics. In: Klaassen CD, ed: Casarett & Doull's Toxicology: The Basic Science of Poisons, 5th ed. New York, McGraw-Hill, 1996, p. 114.

TABLE 11–6.   Xenobiotics as Substrates, Inhibitors, and Inducers of Various Hepatic Cytochrome Isoenzymes

Isoenzyme	Substrates	Inhibitors[b]	Inducers[c]	Isoenzyme	Substrates	Inhibitors[b]	Inducers[c]
CYP1A2	Acetaminophen (minor)	Cimetidine	Charcoal broiled foods	CYP2E1	Acetaminophen (major)	Disulfiram	Ethanol
	Aromatic amines	Diltiazem			Acrylonitrile	DMSO	Isoniazid
	Caffeine	Erythromycin	Cigarette smoke (not pure nicotine)		Alcohols	Fomepizole	
	Clozapine	Fluvoxamine			Aniline		
	Phenacetin	Mexiletine			Benzene		
	Polycyclic aromatic hydrocarbons	Quinolones	Omeprazole		Caffeine		
		Enoxacin	Piperonyl butoxide		Chloroform		
	Tacrine	Ciprofloxacin			Dapsone		
	TCAs (demelthylation)	Perfloxacin	TCDD (dioxin)		Ethylene dibromide		
	Amitriptyline	(NOT Ofloxacin or lomefloxacin)			Halothane		
	Clomipramine				Isoniazid		
	Imipramine				Theophylline		
	Theophylline				Vinyl chloride		
	Triorthocresylphos-phate			CYP3A4 (previously known as nifedipine oxidase)	Acetaminophen (minor)	Cimetidine	Carbamazepine
	R-warfarin				Aflatoxin B_1 & G_1	Clotrimazole	Dexamethasone
	Zileuton				Aldrin	Clarithromycin	Glucocorticoids
CYP2C9[a]	Amitriptyline (demethylation)	Amiodarone	Rifampin		Amiodarone	Diltiazem	Nevirapine (auto)
		Cimetidine			Astemizole	Erythromycin	Phenobarbital
	Diclofenac	Cotrimoxazole			Atorvastate		
	Ibuprofen	Fluconazole			Budesonide	Fluconazole	Phenytoin
	Imipramine	Metronidazole			Carbamazepine	(large dose)	Rifampin
	Phenytoin (4-OH)	Sulfinpyrazone			Cisapride	Fluoxetine	
	Piroxicam				Cyclosporine	(norfluoxetine)	
	Tolbutamide				Dapsone	Grapefruit juice	
	S-warfarin				Delavirdine	furanocoumal	
CYP2C19[a]	Diazepam	Felbamale	Rifampin		Diazepam	± (flavonoids)	
	Impiramine	Fluoxetine			Diltiazem	Itraconazole	
	Omeprazole	Fluvoxamine			Droperidol	Ketoconazole	
	Pentamidine	Omeprazole			Erythromycin	Miconazole	
	Phenytoin	Tranylcypromine			Felodipine	Nefazodone	
	Propranolol				Fentanyl	Omeprazole	
CYP2D6[a]	Amitriptyline	Amiodarone			Indinavir	Propoxyphene (?)	
	Captopril	Cimetidine			Imipramine	Protease inhibitors	
	Clomipramine	Fluoxetine			Lidocaine	Quinidine	
	Clozapine	Haloperidol			Losartin		
	Codeine (to morphine)	Paroxetine			Lovastatin		
	Debrisoquine	Propafenone			Methadone		
	Deprenyl	Quinidine			Mibefradil		
	Desipramine	(not quinine)			Midazolam		
	Dextromethorphan	Ritonavir			Neviripine		
	Doxepin	Sertraline			Nifedipine		
	Encainide	Thioridazine			Omeprazole		
	Flecainide	Yohimbine			Propoxyphene		
	Fluoxetine				Quinidine		
	Haloperidol (reduced)	Desipramine			Saquinavir		
	Imipramine (OH)				Sildenafil		
	Loratidine				Simvastatin		
	Meperidine				Sufentanyl		
	Methadone				Tacrolimus		
	Metoprolol				Tamoxifen		
	Mexiletine				Taxol		
	Nevirapine				Terfenadine		
	Nortriptyline (OH)				Theophylline		
	Ondansetron				Triazolam		
	Paroxetine				Verapamil		
	Perphenazine				R-Warfarin		
	Propafenone				Zonisamide		
	Propoxyphene						
	Propranolol (4-OH)						
	Quinidine						

(continued)

TABLE 11–6. Xenobiotics as Substrates, Inhibitors, and Inducers of Various Hepatic Cytochrome Isoenzymes (continued)

Isoenzyme	Substrates	Inhibitors[b]	Inducers[c]	Isoenzyme	Substrates	Inhibitors[b]	Inducers[c]
CYP2D6[a]	Risperidone Sparteine Tramadol Thioridazine Timolol Venlafaxine						

[a]2C subfamily subject to polymorphism. Genetic factors are responsible for producing poor metabolizers (5–10% of North American population), normal metabolizers (vast majority), and fast metabolizers (very minor). Antipyrine is used experimentally to define the genotype of poor metabolizers.

[b]Inhibitors reduce the metabolism of substrates and lead to elevated blood levels of substrates. The onset for inhibition occurs quickly in contrast to induction. Inhibitors may or may not be substrates for the enzyme they inhibit (competitive), or they may be noncompetitive (mechanism based or suicidal).

[c]Administration of inducers causes the creation of quantitatively more enzymes that can metabolize substrates leading to reduced blood levels of substrates. Induction is dose dependent and time dependent. Time is required for increased synthesis of the enzyme (delaying onset) and time is required for the inducers to be eliminated. Cigarette smoking is known to have an effect on theophylline metabolism for as long as 4 mo after cessation. Inducers do not necessarily cause autoinduction.

This is not meant to be an exhaustive listing and is adapted from references 5, 28, 29, and 43.

CYP	→	Cytochrome
Arabic numeral	→	Family
Capital letter	→	Subfamily
Arabic numeral eg, CYP1A2	→	Individual gene

1930s.[57] Physiologic models consider the movement of xenobiotics based on known or theorized biologic processes and are unique for each xenobiotic. This allows the prediction of tissue concentrations, while incorporating the effects of changing physiologic parameters, and affording better extrapolation from laboratory animals.[66] Unfortunately, physiologic modeling is still in its infancy and the mathematical modeling it entails is often very complex.[15] Regardless, the most commonly used mathematical equations are based on traditional compartmental modeling.

The *one-compartment model* is the simplest for analytic purposes and is applied to xenobiotics that rapidly enter and distribute throughout the body. This model assumes that changes in plasma concentrations will result in and reflect proportional changes in tissue concentrations. Many xenobiotics, such as digoxin, lithium, and lidocaine, do not instantaneously equilibrate with the tissues and are better described by a two-compartment model. In the *two-compartment model*, a xenobiotic is distributed instantaneously to highly perfused tissues (central compartment) and then is secondarily and more slowly distributed to a peripheral compartment. Elimination is assumed to take place from the central compartment.

If the rate of a reaction is directly proportional to the concentration of xenobiotic, it is termed *first order or linear*. Processes that are capacity limited or saturable are termed *nonlinear* (not proportional to the concentration of xenobiotic) and are described by the *Michaelis-Menten* equation, which is derived from enzyme kinetics. Calculus is used to derive the first-order equation, as done by Yang and Andersen.[66] Rate is directly proportional to concentration of xenobiotic as in Equation 11–8.

$$\text{Rate} \ \alpha \ \text{concentration (C)} \qquad \text{(Eq. 11–8)}$$

An infinitesimal change in concentration of a xenobiotic (dC) with respect to an infinitesimal change in time (dt) is directly proportional to the concentration (C) of the xenobiotic as in Equation 11–9.

$$\frac{dC}{dt} \ \alpha \ C \qquad \text{(Eq. 11–9)}$$

The proportionality constant k is added to the right side of the expression to mathematically allow the introduction of an equal sign. The constant k represents all of the bodily factors, such as metabolism and excretion, that contribute to the determination of concentration (Eq. 11–10).

$$\frac{dC}{dt} = kC \qquad \text{(Eq. 11–10)}$$

Introducing a negative sign to the left-hand side of the equation describes the "decay" or decreasing xenobiotic concentration (Eq. 11–11).

$$-\frac{dC}{dt} = kC \qquad \text{(Eq. 11–11)}$$

This equation is impractical because of the difficulty of measuring infinitesimal changes in C or t. Therefore, the use of calculus allows the integration or summing of all of the changes from one

TABLE 11–7. Xenobiotics Secreted by Renal Tubules

Organic Anion Transport	Organic Cation Transport
Acetazolamide	Acetylcholine
Bile salts	Amiodarone
Cephalosporins	Atropine
Indomethacin	Cimetidine
Hydrochlorothiazide	Digoxin
Furosemide	Diltiazem
Methotrexate	Dopamine
Penicillin G	Epinephrine
Probenecid	Morphine
Prostaglandins	Neostigmine
Salicylate	Procainamide
	Quinidine
	Quinine
	Triamterene
	Trimethoprim
	Verapamil

MODEL 1. One-compartment open model, IV injection.

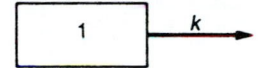

MODEL 2. One-compartment open model with first-order absorption.

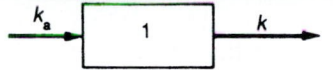

MODEL 3. Two-compartment open model, IV injection.

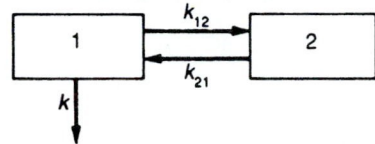

MODEL 4. Two-compartment open model with first-order absorption.

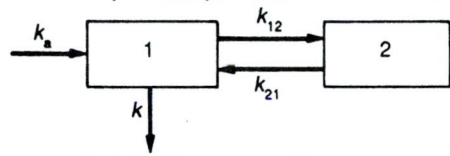

Figure 11–7. Various classical compartmental models. k = pharmacokinetic rate constants; 1 = plasma or central compartment; 2 = tissue compartment; k_{12} = rate constant into tissue from plasma; k_{21} = rate constant into plasma from tissue; k_a = absorption rate constant. *(Reprinted, with permission, from Shargel L, Yu A: Introduction to Pharmacokinetics: Applied Biopharmaceutics and Pharmacokinetics, 3rd ed. Norwalk, CT, Appleton & Lange, 1993, p. 40.)*

concentration to another beginning at time zero and terminating at time t. This relationship is mathematically represented by the integration sign ($\int$). $\int$ means to integrate the term from concentration at time zero (C_0) to concentration at a given time t (C_t). $\int$ means the same with respect to time, where t_0 = zero. Prior to this application, the previous equation is first rearranged (Eq. 11–12).

$$-\frac{dC}{C} = kdt$$

$$\int_{C_0}^{C_t} -\frac{dC}{C} = k \int_{t_0}^{t} dt \qquad \text{(Eq. 11-12)}$$

The integration of dC divided by C is the natural logarithm of C (ln C) and the integration of dt is t (Eq. 11–13).

$$-\ln C \Big|_{C_0}^{C_t} = kt \Big|_{t_0}^{t} \qquad \text{(Eq. 11-13)}$$

The vertical straight lines proscribe the evaluation of the terms between those two limits. The following series of manipulations are then performed (Eq. 11–14A–D).

$$-(\ln C_t - \ln C_0) = k(t-0) \qquad \text{(Eq. 11-14A)}$$

$$-\ln C_t + \ln C_0 = kt \qquad \text{(Eq. 11-14B)}$$

$$-\ln C_t = -\ln C_0 + kt \qquad \text{(Eq. 11-14C)}$$

$$\ln C_t = \ln C_0 - kt$$

Can be   Constant   Can be

measured   selected   (Eq. 11-14D)

Equation 11–14D can be recognized as taking the form of an equation of a straight line (Eq. 11–15), where the slope is equal to the rate constant k and the intercept is C_0.

$$y = b + mx \qquad \text{(Eq. 11-15)}$$

Instead of working with natural logarithms, an exponential form (the antilog) of Equation 11–14D may be used (Eq. 11–16).

$$C_t = C_0 e^{-kt} \qquad \text{(Eq. 11-16)}$$

Graphing the ln (natural logarithm) of the concentration of the xenobiotic at various times for a first-order reaction is a straight line. Equation 11–16 describes the events when only one first-order process occurs. This is appropriate for a one-compartment model (Fig. 11–8).

In this model, regardless of the concentration of the xenobiotic, the rate (percentage) of decline is constant. The absolute amount of xenobiotic eliminated changes continuously while the percent eliminated remains constant. k is reported in h^{-1}. A k of 0.10 h^{-1} means that the xenobiotic is being processed (eliminated) at a rate of 10% per hour. k is often designated as k_e and referred to as the elimination rate constant. The time necessary for the xenobiotic concentration to be reduced by 50% is called the *half-life*. The half-life is determined by a rearrangement of Equation 11–14D whereby C_2 becomes C at time t_2 and C_1 becomes C at t_1, and by rearrangement giving Equation 11–17.

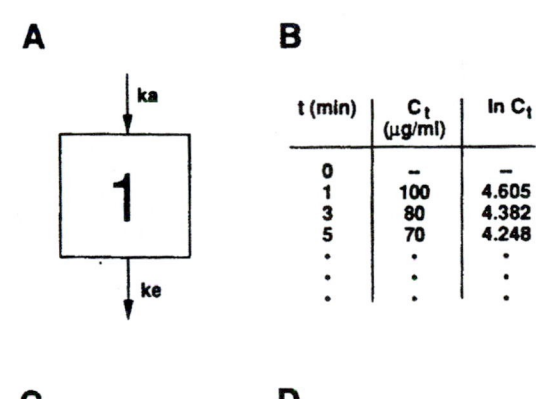

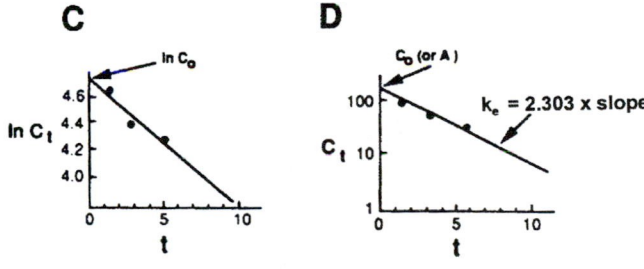

Figure 11–8. A one-compartment pharmacokinetic model demonstrating **(A)** Graphical illustration. **(B)** Hypothetical data set. **(C)** Linear plot. **(D)** Semilogarithmic plot. *(Modified and reprinted, with permission, from Yang R, Andersen M: Pharmacokinetics: In: Hodgson E, Levi P, eds: Introduction to Biochemical Toxicology. Norwalk, CT, Appleton & Lange, 1994, p. 54.)*

$$(t_1 - t_2) = \frac{(\ln C_1 - \ln C_2)}{k_e}$$

(Eq. 11–17)

Substitution of 2 for C_1 and 1 for C_2 or 100 for C_1 and 50 for C_2 gives Equation 11–18A and 11–18B.

$$t_{1/2} = \frac{(\ln 2 - \ln 1)}{k_e}$$

(Eq. 11–18A)

$$t_{1/2} = \frac{0.693}{k_e}$$

(Eq. 11–18B)

The use of semilog paper facilitates graphing the first-order equation. However, because semilog paper plots log (not ln) versus time, to retain appropriate mathematical relationships the rate constant or slope (k) must be divided by 2.303 (Fig. 11–8).

The mathematical modeling becomes more complex when more than one first-order process contributes to the overall elimination process. The equation that incorporates two first-order rates is used for a two-compartment model and is Equation 11–19.

$$C_t = Ae^{-\alpha t} + Be^{-\beta t}$$

(Eq. 11–19)

Figure 11–9 demonstrates a two-compartment model. α often represents the distribution phase, while β is the elimination phase.

The rate of reaction of a saturable process is not linear (not proportional to the concentration of xenobiotic) when saturation occurs (Fig. 11–10). This model is best described by the Michaelis-Menten equation used in enzyme kinetics (Eq. 11–20) in which v is the velocity or rate of the enzymatic reaction; C is the concentration of the xenobiotic; V_{max} is the maximum velocity of the reaction between the enzyme and the xenobiotic; and K_m is the affinity constant between the enzyme and the xenobiotic.[66]

$$v = \frac{V_{max} \times C}{K_m + C}$$

(Eq. 11–20)

Application of this equation to toxicokinetics requires v to become the infinitesimal change in concentration of a xenobiotic (dC) with respect to an infinitesimal change in time (dt) as previously discussed (Eq. 11–10). V_{max} and K_m both reflect the influences of diverse biologic processes. The Michaelis-Menten equation then becomes Equation 11–21, in which the negative sign again represents decay.

$$-\frac{dC}{dt} = \frac{V_{max} \times C}{K_m + C}$$

(Eq. 11–21)

When the concentration of the xenobiotic is very low ($C <<< K_m$), it can be dropped from the bottom right of the equation because its contribution becomes negligible and the resultant equation is described as a first-order process. (Eq. 11–22A and 11–22B). Conceptually, this is understandable, because at a very low xenobiotic concentration the process is not saturated.

$$-\frac{dC}{dt} = \frac{V_{max} \times C}{K_m}$$

(Eq. 11–22A)

Since V_{max} divided by K_m is a constant, K, then:

$$-\frac{dC}{dt} = kC$$

(Eq. 11–22B)

However, when the concentrations of the xenobiotic are extremely high and exceed the capacity of the system ($C >>> K_m$), the rate becomes fixed at a constant maximal rate regardless of the exact concentration of the xenobiotic, termed a zero-order reaction. Table 11–8A and 11–8B compares a first-order reaction to a zero-order reaction. In this particular example, zero order is faster, but if the fraction of xenobiotic eliminated in the first-order example were 0.4, then the amount of xenobiotic in the body would fall below 100 before the xenobiotic in the zero-order example. It is inappropriate to perform half-life calculations on a xenobiotic displaying zero-order behavior because the metabolic rates are continuously changing. Following overdoses enzyme saturation is a common occurrence as the capacity of enzyme systems are overwhelmed.

CLEARANCE

Clearance (Cl) is the relationship between the rate of transfer or elimination of a xenobiotic from a reference fluid (usually plasma) to the plasma concentration of the xenobiotic and is expressed in units of volume per unit time (ie, mL/min) (Eq. 11–23).[20,37,49]

$$Cl = \frac{\text{Rate of elimination}}{C}$$

(Eq. 11–23)

TWO-COMPARTMENT MODEL

$$C_t = Ae^{-\alpha t} + Be^{-\beta t}$$

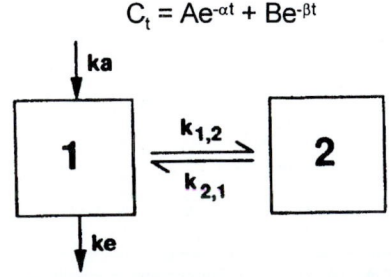

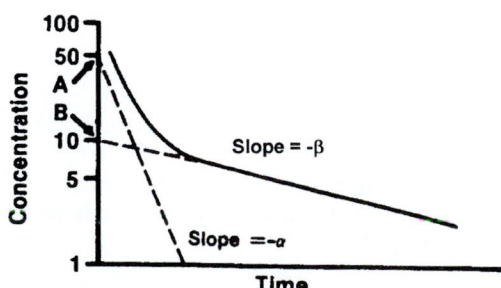

Figure 11–9. Mathematical and graphical forms of a two-compartment classical pharmacokinetic model. k_a represents the absorption rate constant, k_e represents the elimination rate constant, α represents the distribution phase, and β the elimination phase. *(Reprinted, with permission, from Yang R, Andersen M: Pharmacokinetics. In: Hodgson E, Levi P, eds: Introduction to Biochemical Toxicology. Norwalk, CT, Appleton & Lange, 1994, p. 55.)*

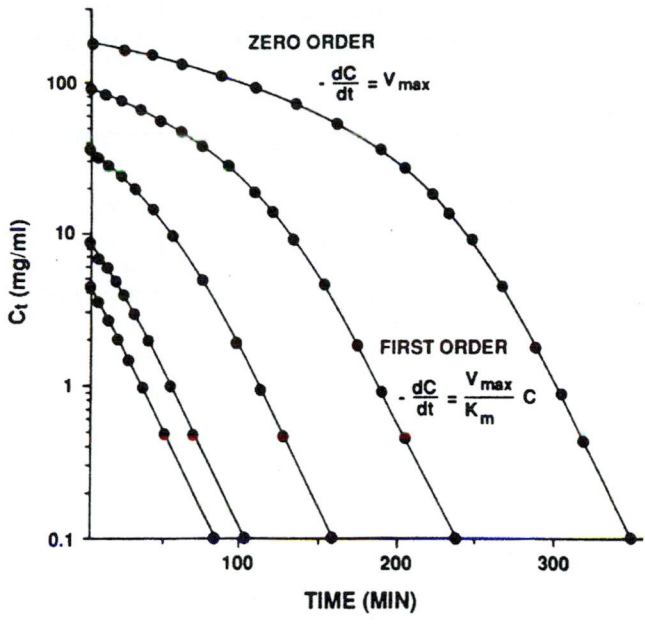

Figure 11–10. Concentration versus time curve for a xenobiotic showing nonlinear pharmacokinetics. *(Reprinted, with permission, from Yang R, Andersen M: Pharmacokinetics. In: Hodgson E, Levi P, eds: Introduction to Biochemical Toxicology. Norwalk, CT, Appleton & Lange, 1994, p. 57.)*

The determination of creatinine clearance is a well-known example of the concept of clearance. Creatinine clearance ($Cl_{creatinine}$) is determined by Equation 11–24,

$$Cl_{creatinine} = \frac{U \times V}{C}$$

(Eq. 11–24)

in which U is the concentration of creatinine in urine (mg/mL); V is the volume flow of urine (mL/min); C is the plasma concentration of creatinine (mg/mL); and the units for clearance are mL/min. A creatinine clearance of 100 mL/min means that 100 mL of plasma is completely cleared of creatinine each minute. Clearance for a particular eliminating organ or for extracorporeal elimination is calculated with Equation 11–25.

$$Cl = Q \times (ER) = Q \times \frac{(C_{in} - C_{out})}{C_{in}}$$

Cl = clearance for the eliminating organ or extracorporeal device

Q = blood flow to the organ or device

ER = extraction ratio

C_{in} = xenobiotic concentration in fluid (blood or serum) entering the organ or device

C_{out} = xenobiotic concentration in fluid (blood or serum) leaving the organ or device

(Eq. 11–25)

Clearance can be applied to any elimination process independent of the precise mechanisms (ie, first-order, Michaelis-Menten), and will represent the sum total of all of the rate constants for xenobiotic elimination. Total body clearance ($Cl_{total\ body}$) is the sum of the clearances of all of the individual eliminating processes, as seen in Equation 11–26.

$$Cl_{total\ body} = Cl_{renal} + Cl_{hepatic} + Cl_{intestinal} + Cl_{chelation} + \cdots$$

(Eq. 11–26)

For a first-order process (one-compartment model), clearance is given by Equation 11–27.

$$Cl = k_e Vd$$

(Eq. 11–27)

Experimentally, the clearance can be derived by examining the intravenous dose of xenobiotic in relation to the area under the plasma concentration (AUC) versus the time curve from time zero to time *t* (Eq. 11–28). The AUC is calculated using the trapezoidal rule or through integral calculus (units: eg, mg/mL) (Figs. 11–11 and 11–12.)

$$Cl = \frac{dose_{IV}}{AUC_{0-t}}$$

(Eq. 11–28)

STEADY STATE

When exposure to a xenobiotic occurs at a fixed rate, the plasma concentration of the xenobiotic gradually achieves a plateau level at a concentration at which the rate of absorption equals the rate of

TABLE 11–8A. Illustration of 1000 mg of Xenobiotic in Body Following First-Order Elimination

Time after Drug Administration (h)	Amount of Drug in Body (mg)	Amount of Drug Eliminated over Preceding Hour (mg)	Fraction of Drug Eliminated over Preceding Hour
0	1000	—	—
1	850	150	0.15
2	723	127	0.15
3	614	109	0.15
4	522	92	0.15
5	444	78	0.15
6	377	67	0.15

TABLE 11–8B. Illustration of 1000 mg of Xenobiotic in Body Following Zero-Order Elimination

Time after Drug Administration (h)	Amount of Drug in Body (mg)	Amount of Drug Eliminated over Preceding Hour (mg)	Fraction of Drug Eliminated over Preceding Hour
0	1000	—	—
1	850	150	0.15
2	700	150	0.18
3	550	150	0.21
4	400	150	0.27
5	250	150	0.38
6	100	150	0.60

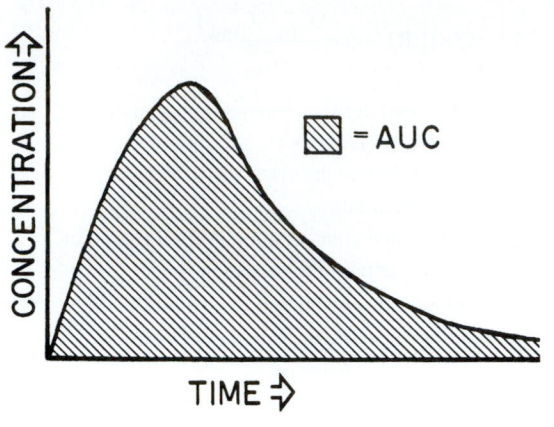

Figure 11–11. The area under the curve (AUC) of a concentration versus time profile obtained after extravascular administration of a xenobiotic. *(Reprinted, with permission, from Riviere JE: Absorption and distribution. In: Hodgson E, Levi P, eds: Introduction to Biochemical Toxicology. Norwalk, CT, Appleton & Lange, 1994, p. 21.)*

elimination and is termed *steady state*. The time to achieve 95% of steady-state concentration for a first-order process is dependent on the half-life and usually necessitates five half-lives. The concentration achieved at steady state depends on the Vd, the rate of exposure, and the half-life.

Iatrogenic toxicity can occur in the therapeutic setting when dosing decisions are based on plasma concentrations determined

Compartment model

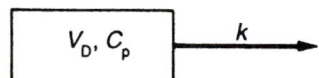

Static volume and first-order elimination is assumed. Plasma flow is not considered. $Cl_T = k\,V_D$.

Physiologic model

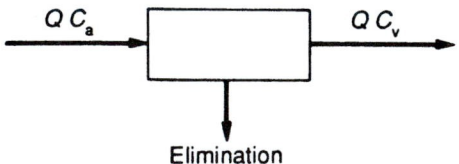

Clearance is the product of the plasma flow (*Q*) and the extraction ratio (ER). Thus, $Cl_T = Q\,ER$.

Model independent

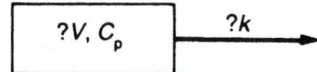

Volume and elimination rate constant not defined. $Cl_T = Dose/[AUC]_0^\infty$.

Figure 11–12. General approaches to clearance. *(Reprinted, with permission, from Shargel L, Yu A: Introduction to pharmacokinetics. In: Applied Biopharmaceutics and Pharmacokinetics, 3rd ed. Norwalk, CT, Appleton & Lange, 1993, p. 280.)*

prior to achieving a steady state. This adverse event is particularly common when using drugs with long half-lives such as digoxin[65] and phenytoin.

PEAK PLASMA CONCENTRATIONS

Peak plasma concentrations (C_{max}) of a xenobiotic occur at the time of peak absorption. At this point in time, the absorption rate is at least equal to the elimination rate. Thereafter, the elimination rate predominates and plasma concentrations begin to decline. Whereas the C_{max} depends on the dose, the *rate of absorption* (k_a), and *the rate of elimination* (k_e), whereas the *time to peak* (t_{max}) is independent of dose and only depends on the k_a and k_e. For the same dose of xenobiotic, if the k_e remains constant and the rate of absorption decreases, then the t_{max} will occur later and the C_{max} will be slightly lower. Controlled-release dosage forms or xenobiotics that form concretions and have a decreased rate of absorption may not achieve peak levels until many hours after an immediate-release preparation with rapid absorption. The AUC will remain the same. However if the k_a remains constant and the k_e is increased, then the t_{max} occurs sooner, the C_{max} decreases, and the AUC decreases[41] (Table 11–9).

In the overdose setting, gastric emptying, single-dose activated charcoal, and whole-bowel irrigation decrease k_a. Multiple-dose activated charcoal, manipulation of pH to promote ion trapping to facilitate elimination, and certain chelators (ie, DMSA, deferoxamine) increase k_e and are likely to decrease C_{max}, t_{max}, and AUC.

INTERPRETATION OF PLASMA CONCENTRATIONS

In order for plasma concentrations to have significance there must be an established relationship between effect and plasma concentration. For many medications such as phenytoin, digoxin, carbamazepine, and theophylline there is an established therapeutic

TABLE 11–9. **Pharmacokinetic Effects of the Absorption Rate Constant and Elimination Rate Constant[a]**

Absorption Rate Constant K_a (h^{-1})	Elimination Rate Constant K_e (h^{-1})	t_{max} (h)	C_{max} (μg/mL)	AUC (μg•h/mL)
0.1	0.2	6.93	2.50	50
0.2	0.1	6.93	5.00	100
0.3	0.1	5.49	5.77	100
0.4	0.1	4.62	6.26	100
0.5	0.1	4.02	6.69	100
0.6	0.1	3.58	6.99	100
0.3	0.1	5.49	5.77	100
0.3	0.2	4.05	4.44	50
0.3	0.3	3.33	3.68	33.3
0.3	0.4	2.88	3.16	25
0.3	0.5	2.55	2.79	20

[a]t_{max} = time to peak plasma concentration, C_{max} = peak xenobiotic concentration, AUC = area under the curve. Values are based on a single oral dose (100 mg) that is 100% bioavailable (F = 1) and has an apparent V_d of 10 L. The drug follows a one-compartment open model. The AUC is calculated by the trapezoidal rule from 0 to 24 h.
Reprinted, with permission, from Shargel L, Yu A: Pharmacokinetics of drug absorption. In: Applied Biopharmaceutics and Pharmacokinetics, 3rd ed. Norwalk, CT: Appleton & Lange, 1993, p. 183.

range. However, there are also many drugs for which there is no established therapeutic range (diazepam, propranolol, verapamil). Some agents exhibit *hysteresis* in which the effect increases as the plasma concentration is decreasing (eg, physostigmine). For many xenobiotics, there is very little information on toxicodynamics. Often, sequential plasma concentrations are collected for retrospective analysis in an attempt to correlate plasma concentrations and toxicity. Tolerance to drugs such as ethanol also influences the interpretation of plasma concentrations. *Tolerance* is an example of a pharmacodynamic or toxicodynamic effect as a result of cellular adaptation, and it occurs when larger doses of a xenobiotic are necessary to achieve the same clinical or pharmacologic result.

Other factors that influence the interpretation of plasma concentrations include chronicity of dosing (a single dose vs. multiple doses); whether absorption is still ongoing and therefore concentrations are still rising; whether distribution is still ongoing and therefore concentrations are uninterpretable (Figure 11–13); or whether the value is a peak, trough, or steady-state concentration. Clinical examples where interpretation varies dependent on the dosing pattern of a single dose versus multiple doses include theophylline, digoxin, lithium, and acetaminophen. Controlled-release preparations and those xenobiotics that delay gastric emptying or form concretions would be expected to have prolonged absorptive phases and require serial plasma concentrations to obtain a meaningful analysis of plasma concentrations (Chap. 7). Peak values and minimum inhibitory concentrations are consequential for monitoring antibiotics such as gentamicin.[8,34]

Pitfalls in interpretation arise when the units for a particular plasma concentration are not obtained or are unfamiliar (eg, mmol/L) to the clinician. In the overdose setting, the type of analysis used is not generally applied to such large concentrations, and the laboratory may make errors in dilution, or errors can be inherent in the assay (Chap. 7). In those cases, the director of the laboratory should be consulted for advice with regard to the need for a reference laboratory. The type of collection tube (eg, plasma or serum instead of whole-blood for certain metals) or receptacle or the conditions during delivery of the sample may give rise to inaccurate or inadequate information. When in doubt, the laboratory should be called prior to sample collection. The laboratory usually measures total xenobiotic (free plus bound), and for agents that are highly plasma protein bound, reductions in albumin increase free concentrations and alter the interpretation of the reported value (Eq. 11–7). Active metabolites may contribute to toxicity and may not be measured.[30] Collection of accurate data for analysis requires at least four data points during one elimination half-life. During extracorporeal methods of elimination, ideal criteria for determining the amount removed require assay of the dialysate or charcoal cartridge or multiple simultaneous serum concentrations going into and out of the device and not random serum concentrations. Clearance calculations for drugs such as lithium that partition significantly into the red cell are more accurate when measurements are taken on whole blood.[11,16] Patient weight and height and, when indicated, hemoglobin, creatinine, albumin, and other parameters to assess elimination pathways may be helpful.

CASE ILLUSTRATIONS

The following cases are designed to illustrate a number of pharmacokinetic and toxicokinetic principles. The cases demonstrate the applications of many of the mathematical models explained above.

Case 1. A 23-year-old, 90-kg female is seen in the emergency department 2 hours after the ingestion of 50 of her brother's Theo-Dur (300 mg) tablets. She is alert and oriented. Her vital signs are: a blood pressure of 130/75 mm Hg; a heart rate of 110 beats/min; a respiratory rate of 20 breaths/min; and a temperature of 99.7°F (37.6°C) rectally. Her initial theophylline serum concentration is 40 mg/L.

1. Estimate a peak serum concentration knowing that theophylline has a Vd of 0.5 L/kg, an $S = 1$ (not a salt form), and an $F = 1$ (100% bioavailable). Rearrange Equation 11–6.

$$C_0 = \frac{S \times F \times \text{dose (mg)}}{Vd}$$

$$C_0 = \frac{1 \times 1 \times 50 \times 300 \text{ mg}}{0.5 \text{L} / \text{kg} \times 90 \text{ kg}} = 333 \text{ mg} / \text{L}$$

2. If the history were correct what would prevent the patient from achieving this serum concentration?

Increasing the number of tablets of sustained-release dosage forms may alter release characteristics, delay absorption, and

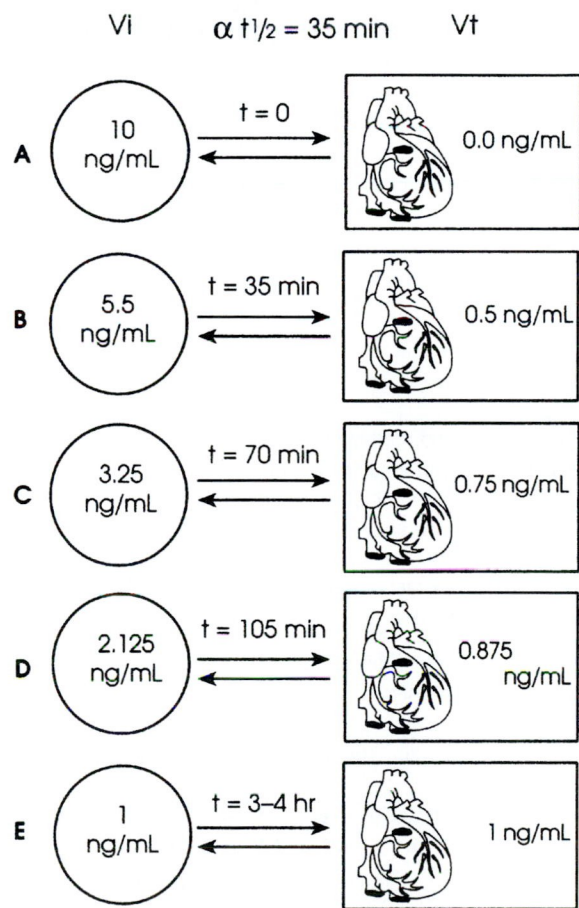

Figure 11–13. A theoretical two-compartment model for digoxin. *(Reprinted, with permission, from Winter ME: Digoxin. In: Koda-Kimble MA, Young LY, eds: Basic Clinical Pharmacokinetics, 3rd ed. Vancouver, WA, Applied Therapeutics, 1994; pp. 198–235.)*

reduce k_a (absorption rate constant). Elimination (k_e) occurs during the absorptive phase, so C_{max} and AUC are reduced. Vomiting typically occurs following theophylline ingestion and will decrease bioavailability.

3. How would treatment strategies affect the toxicokinetics of theophylline?

    Activated charcoal and whole-bowel irrigation decrease bioavailability. Multiple-dose activated charcoal, charcoal hemoperfusion, and hemodialysis enhance elimination.

4. Can the patient be considered medically clear at this time?

    No. Serum concentrations may continue to rise and may not achieve peak levels for 12–24 hours. Therefore, sequential serum concentrations should be analyzed frequently until concentrations start to fall, and then less frequent determinations are necessary as the concentration approaches the therapeutic range (Chap. 39).

Case 2. A 63-year-old, 60-kg female is brought to the emergency department by her family 30 minutes after ingesting 25 (0.25 mg) digoxin tablets. The patient complains of nausea, but is otherwise asymptomatic. Her physical examination is normal. Her vital signs are: a blood pressure of 130/85 mm Hg; a heart rate of 76 beats/min and irregular; a respiratory rate of 17 breaths/min; and a temperature of 98°F (36.6°C) rectally. The ECG shows controlled atrial fibrillation at a rate of 76.

1. Estimate this patient's plasma digoxin concentration. Assume a Vd = 5 L/kg, an S = 1, and an F = 0.8 (80%).

$$C_0 = \frac{S \times F \times dose}{Vd}$$

$$C_0 = \frac{1 \times 0.8 \times 25 \times 0.25 \text{ mg} \times 1000000 \text{ ng}/1 \text{ mg}}{5 \text{ L}/\text{kg} \times 1000 \text{ mL}/\text{L} \times 60 \text{ kg}} = 16.7 \text{ ng/mL}$$

2. Her serum digoxin concentration is reported to be 15 ng/mL (therapeutic = 0.8–2 ng/mL). Why doesn't this patient show more severe signs of digoxin toxicity?

    This patient does not show serious signs and symptoms of toxicity from digoxin because digoxin fits a two-compartment model with a long distribution half-life. Toxicity is related to the concentration in the peripheral (heart) compartment. However, in several hours she may demonstrate severe signs of toxicity (Fig. 11–13).

3. How does Digibind alter the toxicokinetics of digoxin?

    Digibind reduces the Vd of digoxin by binding digoxin in the plasma, thereby establishing a concentration gradient to remove digoxin from reversible myocardial binding sites. All digoxin bound to Digibind is inactive. The Digibind–digoxin complex is eliminated slightly faster than digoxin alone due to a reduced Vd.

4. How would you calculate the appropriate dose of Digibind?
    If the ingested dose is known:

$$\text{Total body load (TBL)} = S \times F \times dose$$
$$= 1 \times 0.8 \times 25 \times 0.25 \text{ mg} = 5 \text{ mg}$$
1 vial of Digibind binds 0.5 mg of digoxin

$$\text{No. vials Digibind} = \frac{\text{TBL (5 mg)}}{0.5 \text{ mg digoxin}/\text{vial Digibind}} = 10 \text{ vials}$$

If serum concentration is known:

$$\text{TBL (mg)} = C \text{ (ng/mL)} \times (1 \text{ mg}/1000000 \text{ ng})$$
$$\times V_d \text{(L/kg)}(1000 \text{mL/L}) \times \text{weight of patient (kg)}$$

$$= \frac{15 \text{ ng/mL} \times 5 \text{ L/kg} \times 60 \text{ kg}}{1000} = 45 \text{ mg}$$

$$\text{No. vials Digibind} = \frac{\text{TLB (45 mg) of digoxin}}{0.5 \text{ mg digoxin}/\text{vial Digibind}} = 9 \text{ vials Digibind}$$

OR a simplified version:

$$\text{No. vials Digibind} = \frac{C \text{(ng/mL)} \times \text{weight per patient (kg)}}{100}$$
$$= 9 \text{ vials Digibind}$$

The numbers of vials of Digibind calculated either by using the history of the amount ingested or based on the serum concentration are usually different because each formula has independent inherent errors.

Case 3. A patient receives a continuous infusion of pentobarbital for 3 days. The infusion is terminated, but the patient has not awakened after 6 hours. The reported duration of hypnotic action after a single IV dose is 1–4 hours. Is there a toxicokinetic explanation for the persistent somnolence?

    Yes. The short duration of action after a single dose of IV pentobarbital is attributed to redistribution. With chronic dosing, accumulation occurs and the elimination half-life becomes 15–48 hours. This patient may require several days to awaken.

Case 4. A 70-kg man with no history of alcoholism ingests methanol and is found to have a serum concentration of 100 mg/dL (1 g/L). The following information is available:

    Methanol: molecular weight 32 daltons; water soluble
    Specific gravity (sp gr) of absolute ethanol and methanol: 0.8 g/mL
    Vd of ethanol and methanol = 0.6 L/kg
    Protein binding of ethanol and methanol = negligible
    Bioavailability for ethanol and methanol = 100%
    Hemodialysis clearance of ethanol and methanol = 150 mL/min; assume hemodialysis is a first-order process
    Hemodialysis extraction ratio of ethanol and methanol = 100%
    V_{max} = 0.15 g/kg/h for ethanol for a naive person

1. How much methanol did the patient drink if he drank gas-line antifreeze which is 95% methanol?

$$C_0 = \frac{S \times F \times dose}{V_d} \quad \text{Rearranging: } S \times F \times dose = C_0 \times V_d$$
$$1 \times 1 \times dose = 1 \text{ g/L} \times 0.6 \text{ L/kg} \times 70 \text{ kg}$$
$$= 42 \text{ g of 100\% concentration}$$
$$(S = 1; \text{there is no salt form of an alcohol})$$
$$42 \text{ g} \times 1 \text{ mL}/0.95 \text{ g (95\% conc)} \times 1 \text{ mL}/0.8 \text{ g (sp gr)}$$
$$= 55 \text{ mL of 95\% methanol}$$

2. How much ethanol as vodka (80 proof = 40%) should be given to the patient as a loading dose to achieve a serum ethanol concentration of 100 mg% (100 mg/dL or 1 g/L)?

$$C_0 = \frac{S \times F \times dose}{Vd} \quad \text{Rearranging: } S \times F \times dose = C_0 \times Vd$$

$$1 \times 1 \times dose = 1\,g/L \times 0.6\,L/kg \times 70\,kg = 42\,g$$

$$42\,g \times 1\,mL/0.4\,g\,(40\%\,conc) \times 1\,mL/0.8\,g\,(sp\,gr)$$

$$= 131\,mL\ of\ 40\%\ ethanol$$

3. What maintenance dose of ethanol should be given to the patient to maintain an ethanol serum concentration of 100 mg/dL (1 g/L)?

The V_{max} of 0.15 g/kg/h is the maximum rate of elimination for a patient not tolerant to ethanol. The maintenance dose is designed to replace the amount of ethanol eliminated. Therefore:

$$0.15\,g/kg/h \times 70\,kg = 10.5\,g/h \times 1\,mL/0.1\,(10\%)$$

$$\times 1\,mL/0.8\,(sp\,gr) = 131.25\,mL/h\ of\ 10\%\ ethanol$$

$$(can\ be\ given\ PO\ or\ IV)$$

4. How many hours of hemodialysis are necessary to reduce the methanol serum concentration to 10 mg/dL (0.1 g/L)?

$$k_e = Cl/Vd; \quad Cl_{total\,body} = Cl_{HD} + Cl_{endogenous}$$

$$= Cl_{HD} + 0\ (\text{minimal endogenous clearance when}$$

$$\text{methanol metabolism is blocked with ethanol})$$

$$\frac{150\,mL/min \times 60\,min/h \times 1\,L/1000\,mL}{0.6\,L/kg \times 70\,kg}$$

$$= 0.214\,h^{-1} = 21.4\%\ per\ hour\ eliminated$$

$$t_{1/2} = 0.693/k_e = 0.693/0.214\,h^{-1} = 3.22\,h$$

$$t_1 - t_2 = \frac{\ln C_1 - \ln C_2}{k_e} = \frac{\ln 100 - \ln 10}{0.214\,h^{-1}}$$

$$= 10.74\ hours\ to\ go\ from\ 100\,mg/dL\ to\ 10\,mg/dL$$

Case 5. A 70-kg male is brought to the hospital with a serum concentration of phenytoin of 80 μg/mL (mg/L). Assume the ingestion occurred 2 days earlier and there is no ongoing absorption. Estimate how long it might take this patient to reach 20 μg/mL. The following information is available:

$$Vd = 0.7\,L/kg$$

$$V_m\ (\text{maximum metabolic capacity}) = 7\,mg/kg/d$$

K_m (serum concentration at which the metabolic rate is at one-half the maximum metabolic rate) = 4 mg/L

$$v = \frac{V_{max} \times C}{K_m + C} = \frac{7\,mg/kg/d \times 70\,kg \times 80\,mg/L}{4\,mg/L + 80\,mg/L}$$

$$= 466.6\,mg/day\ eliminated\ at\ zero\ order$$

Estimate the initial amount of phenytoin in body:

$$Dose = C \times Vd\ 80\,mg/L \times 0.7\,L/kg \times 70\,kg = 3920\,mg_0$$

Estimate the amount of phenytoin in body at 20 mg/L:

$$Dose = C \times Vd = 20\,mg/L \times 0.7\,L/kg \times 70\,kg = 980\,mg$$

$$3920\,mg - 980\,mg = 2940\,mg\ as\ the\ amount\ that\ needs$$

$$to\ be\ eliminated$$

At an elimination rate of 466.6 mg/d, it takes about 6.3 days for the serum phenytoin concentration of 80 mg/dL to fall to 20 mg/dL assuming neither ongoing absorption nor enhanced elimination from repeat dose activated charcoal occurs.

A similar result is found using the following formula

$$t = \frac{[(K_m)\,(\ln Cp_1/\ln Cp_2)] + (C_1 - C_2)}{V_m/Vd}$$

$$= \frac{(4\,mg/L) \times (4.38 - 3) + (80 - 20)}{7\,mg/kg/d \times 70\,kg \times 0.7\,L/kg \times 70\,kg}$$

$$= 6.55\,days$$

Case 6. Compare the utility of exchange transfusion, peritoneal dialysis, hemodialysis, and hemoperfusion for the ingestion of 2 g of either amitriptyline or theophylline in a 15-kg child.

The following information is available:

$$Vd\ of\ amitriptyline = 30\,L/kg;\ protein\ binding = high$$

$$Vd\ of\ theophylline = 0.5\,L/kg;\ protein\ binding = moderate$$

$$Blood\ volume = 85\,mL/kg;\ a\ double\ volume\ exchange$$

$$= 85\,mL/kg \times 2$$

Estimate that 300 mL of peritoneal fluid is administered over 10 min, that the equilibration time is 20 min, and that 300 mL is removed over 30 min for a total time of 60 min.

Assume HP clearance of 200 mL/min for theophylline.

1. Would exchange transfusion be reasonable for amitriptyline or theophylline removal?

$$Double\ volume\ exchange = 85\,mL/kg \times 2$$

$$In\ this\ child = 85\,mL/kg \times 15\,kg \times 2 = 2550\,mL = 2.55\,L$$

$$Vd\ for\ amitriptyline\ in\ this\ child = 30\,L/kg \times 15\,kg = 450\,L$$

$$450\,L/2.55\,L = 176\ double\text{-}exchange\ transfusions,$$

$$an\ unrealistic\ number!$$

$$Vd\ for\ theophylline\ in\ this\ child = 0.5\,L/kg \times 15\,kg = 7.5\,L$$

$$7.5\,L/2.55\,L = about\ 3\ double\ exchanges,\ a\ reasonable\ number!$$

2. Would peritoneal dialysis be reasonable for amitriptyline or theophylline removal? (For peritoneal dialysis, assume a 300-mL/h exchange which equals 7.2 L/d.)

No for both amitriptyline and theophylline.

For amitriptyline,

$$450\,L/7.2\,L/d = 62.5\,days$$

for theophylline,

$$7.5\,L/7.2\,L/d = 25\,hours$$

which is too long in a life-threatening situation.

3. Would hemodialysis be reasonable for amitriptyline or theophylline removal?

No, for amitriptyline; yes, for theophylline.

For hemodialysis, there is unlikely to be any benefit for amitriptyline removal because of the high protein binding and large Vd. Moderate protein binding of theophylline would be a limiting factor but a small Vd would be advantageous. The result would be acceptable for theophylline.

4. Would activated charcoal hemoperfusion be reasonable for amitriptyline or theophylline removal?

No, for amitriptyline; yes, for theophylline.

For hemoperfusion, protein binding may be of less importance if binding to activated charcoal is more substantial than protein binding.

$$k_e = Cl / Vd$$

Assume HP Cl = 200 mL/min × 60 min/h = 1.2 L/h and the endogenous clearance is minimal.

For amitriptyline:

$$1.2 \text{ L/h} / 30 \text{ L/kg} \times 15 \text{ kg} = 0.00266 \text{h}^{-1}$$

$t_{1/2} = 0.693/k_e = 0.693/.00266 = 260$ hours, which is clinically unreasonable

For theophylline:

$$1.2 \text{ L/h} / 0.5 \text{ L/kg} \times 15 \text{ kg} = 0.16 \text{h}^{-1}$$

$t_{1/2} = 0.693/k_e = 0.693/0.16 = 4.33$ hours, which is clinically reasonable

ACKNOWLEDGMENT

Some of these cases were used at workshops given at the NYCPCC and Christine Stork, PharmD, assisted with the development of some of these cases.

REFERENCES

1. Bertilsson L: Geographical/interracial differences in polymorphic drug oxidation. Clin Pharmacokinet 1995;29:192–209.
2. Blaschke TF, Rubin PC: Hepatic first-pass metabolism in liver disease. Clin Pharmacokinet 1979;4:423–432.
3. Bodenham A, Shelly MP, Park GR: The altered pharmacokinetics and pharmacodynamics of drugs commonly used in critically ill patients. Clin Pharmacokinet 1988;14:347–373.
4. Bosse GM, Matyunas NJ: Delayed toxidromes. J Emerg Med 1999; 17:679–690.
5. Boyes RN, Scott DB, Jebson PJ, et al: Pharmacokinetics of lidocaine in man. Clin Pharmacol Ther 1971;12:105–116.
6. Brubacher J, Dahghani P, McKnight D: Delayed toxicity following ingestion of enteric-coated divalproex sodium. J Emerg Med 1999;3: 463–467.
7. Buckley N, Dawson A, Reith D: Controlled-release drugs in overdose. Drug Safety 1995;12:73–84.
8. Burgess D: Pharmacodynamic principles of antimicrobial therapy in the prevention of resistance. Chest 1999;115:19S –23S.
9. Chaikin P, Adir J: Unusual absorption profile of phenytoin in a massive overdose case. J Clin Pharmacol 1987;27:70–73.
10. Ciummo PE, Katz NL: Interactions and drug metabolizing enzymes. Am Pharm 1995;9:41–51.
11. Clendenin N, Pond S, Kaysen G, et al: Potential pitfalls in the evaluation of the usefulness of hemodialysis for the removal of lithium. J Toxicol Clin Toxicol 1982;19:341–352.
12. Dauterman WC: Metabolism of toxicants: Phase II reactions. In: Hodgson E, Levi P, eds: Introduction to Biochemical Toxicology. Norwalk, CT, Appleton & Lange, 1994, pp. 113–132.
13. Dean B, Oehme FW, Krenzelok E: A study of iron complexation in a swine model. Vet Hum Toxicol 1988;30:313–315.
14. DeGeorge JJ: Food and drug administration viewpoints on toxicokinetics: The view from review. Toxicol Pathol 1995;23:220–225.
15. Engasser JM, Sarhan F, Falcoz C, et al: Distribution, metabolism and elimination of phenobarbital in rats: Physiologically based pharmacokinetic model. J Pharm Sci 1981;70:1233–1238.
16. Ferron G, Debray M, Buneaux F, et al: Pharmacokinetics of lithium in plasma and red blood cells in acute and chronic intoxicated patients. Int J Clin Pharmacol Therap 1995;33:351–355.
17. Gillette JR: Factors affecting drug metabolism. Ann N Y Acad Sci 1971;179:43–66.
18. Gram TE: Drug absorption and distribution. In: Craig CR, Stitzel RE, eds: Modern Pharmacology with Clinical Applications. Boston, Little, Brown, 1997, p. 13.
19. Guengerich FP, Liebler DC: Enzymatic activation of chemicals to toxic metabolites. Crit Rev Toxicol 1985;14:259–307.
20. Gwilt PR: Pharmacokinetics. In: Craig CR, Stitzel RE, eds: Modern Pharmacology with Clinical Applications. Boston, Little, Brown, 1997, pp. 49–58.
21. Hill HZ, Backer R, Hill GJ: Blood cyanide levels in mice after administration of amygdalin. Biopharm Drug Dispos 1980;1:211–220.
22. Hodgson E, Levi PE: Metabolism of toxicants phase I reactions. In: Hodgson E, Levi P, eds: Introduction to Biochemical Toxicology. Norwalk, CT, Appleton & Lange, 1994, pp.75–111.
23. Iberti T, Patterson B, Fisher C: Prolonged bromide intoxication resulting from a gastric bezoar. Arch Intern Med 1984;144:402–403.
24. Jenis EH, Payne RJ, Goldbaum LR: Acute meprobamate poisoning: A fatal case following a lucid interval. JAMA 1969;207:361–365.
25. Kapoor SC, Wielopolski L, Graziano JH, LoIacono NJ: Influence of 2,3-dimercaptosuccinic acid on gastrointestinal lead absorption and whole-body lead retention. Toxicol Appl Pharmacol 1989;97: 525–529.
26. Klaassen CD, Shoeman DW: Biliary excretion of lead in rats, rabbits and dogs. Toxicol Appl Pharmacol 1974;29:436–446.
27. Klaassen CD, Watkins JB: Mechanisms of bile formation, hepatic uptake, and biliary excretion. Pharmacol Rev 1984;36:1–67.
28. Klotz U: Pathophysiological and disease-induced changes in drug distribution volume: Pharmacokinetic implications. Clin Pharmacokinet 1976;1:204–218.
29. Koch-Weser J: Bioavailability of drugs. Part I. N Engl J Med 1974; 291:233–237.
30. Koch-Weser J: Bioavailability of drugs. Part II. N Engl J Med 1974; 291:503–506.
31. Lemmer B, Bruguerolle B: Chronopharmacokinetics, are they clinically relevant? Clin Pharmacokinet 1994;26:419–427.
32. Levine WG: Biliary excretion of drugs and other xenobiotics. Ann Rev Pharmacol Toxicol 1978;18:81–96.
33. Levy R, Thummel K, Trager W, et al, eds. Metabolic Drug Interactions. Philadelphia, Lippincott Williams & Wilkins, 2000.
34. Li R, Zhu M, Shentag J: Achieving optimal outcome in the treatment of infections. Clin Pharmacokinet 1999;37:1–16.
35. Marik P, Varon J: The obese patient in the ICU. Chest 1998;113: 492–498.
36. McCarthy J, Gram TE: Drug metabolism and disposition in pediatric and gerontological stages of life. In: Craig CR, Stitzel RE, eds: Modern Pharmacology with Clinical Applications. Boston, Little, Brown, 1997, pp. 43–48.
37. Medinsky MA, Klaassen CD: Toxicokinetics. In: Klaassen CD, ed: Casarett & Doull's Toxicology: The Basic Science of Poisons, 5th ed. New York, McGraw-Hill, 1996, pp. 187–198.
38. Parkinson A: Biotransformation of xenobiotics. In: Klaassen C, ed: Casarett & Doull's Toxicology: The Basic Science of Poisons, 5th ed. New York, McGraw-Hill, 1996, pp. 113–186.
39. Pharmacist's Letter: Stockton, CA, Pharmacy Information Services, University of the Pacific, June 1985.
40. Pirmohamed M, Kitteringham NR, Park BK: The role of active metabolites in drug toxicity. Drug Safety 1994;11:114–144.
41. Plaa OL: The enterohepatic circulation. In: Gillette JR, Mitchell JR, eds: Handbook of Experimental Pharmacology. New York, Springer, 1975, pp. 28, 130–140, 480.

42. Pond SM, Tozer TN: First-pass elimination: Basic concepts and clinical consequences. Pharmacokinetics 1984;9:1–25.

43. Riviere JE: Absorption and distribution. In: Hodgson E, Levi P, eds: Introduction to Biochemical Toxicology. Norwalk, CT, Appleton & Lange, 1994, pp.11–48.

44. Rose MS, Lock EA, Smith LL, Wyatt I: Paraquat accumulation: Tissue and species specificity. Biochem Pharmacol 1976;25:419–423.

45. Rosenberg J, Benowitz NL, Pond S: Pharmacokinetics of drug overdose. Clin Pharmacokinet 1981;6:161–192.

46. Rowland M, Tozer TN: Clinical Pharmacokinetics Concepts & Applications, 2nd ed. Philadelphia, Lea & Febiger, 1989.

47. Rozman KK, Klaassen CD: Absorption, distribution and excretion of toxicants. In: Klaassen CD, ed: Casarett & Doull's Toxicology: The Basic Science of Poisons. New York, McGraw-Hill, 1996, pp. 91–112.

48. Sansom LN, Evans AM: What is the true clinical significance of plasma protein binding displacement interactions? Drug Safety 1995;12:227–233.

49. Shargel L, Yu A: Drug clearance. In: Applied Biopharmaceutics and Pharmacokinetics, 3rd ed. Norwalk, CT, Appleton & Lange, 1993, pp. 265–292.

50. Shargel L, Yu A: Drug distribution and protein binding. In: Applied Biopharmaceutics and Pharmacokinetics, 3rd ed. Norwalk, CT, Appleton & Lange, 1993, pp. 77–110.

51. Shargel L, Yu A: Pharmacokinetics of drug absorption. In: Applied Biopharmaceutics and Pharmacokinetics, 3rd ed. Norwalk, CT, Appleton & Lange, 1993, pp. 169–192.

52. Shargel L, Yu A: Physiologic factors related to drug absorption. In: Applied Biopharmaceutics and Pharmacokinetics, 3rd ed. Norwalk, CT, Appleton & Lange, 1993, pp. 111–134.

53. Silverman J: P-Glycoprotein. In: Levy R, Thummel K, Trager W, et al, eds: Metabolic Drug Interactions. Philadelphia, Lippincott Williams & Wilkins, 2000, pp. 135–144.

54. Slaughter RL, Edwards DJ: Recent advances: The cytochrome P450 enzymes. Ann Pharmacother 1995;29:619–623.

55. Stowe CM, Plaa GL: Extrarenal excretion of drugs and chemicals. Annu Rev Pharmacol 1968;8:337–356.

56. Sue Y, Shannon M: Pharmacokinetics of drugs in overdose. Clin Pharmacokinet 1992;23:93–105.

57. Teorell T: Kinetics of distribution of substances administered to the body. Depart Med Chem Univ of Uppsala, Sweden 1937;205–225.

58. Tucker G: Chiral switches. Lancet 2000;355:1085–1087.

59. Verebey K, Gold MS: From coca leaves to crack: The effect of dose and routes of administration in abuse liability. Psychiatr Ann 1988;18:513–520.

60. Vesell ES: The model drug approach in clinical pharmacology. Clin Pharmacol Ther 1991;50:239–248.

61. Wagner B, O'Hara D: Pharmacokinetics and pharmacodynamics of sedatives and analgesics in the treatment of agitated critically ill patients. Clin Pharmacokinet 1997;33:426–453.

62. Welling PG: Differences between pharmacokinetics and toxicokinetics. Toxicol Pathol 1995;23:143–147.

63. Wilkinson GR: Influence of hepatic disease on pharmacokinetics. In: Evans WE, Schentag J, Justo W, eds: Applied Pharmacokinetics: Principles of Therapeutic Drug Monitoring. Spokane, WA, Applied Therapeutics, 1986, pp. 116–138.

64. Wilkinson GR: Plasma and tissue binding considerations in drug disposition. Drug Metab Rev 1983;14:427–465.

65. Winter ME: Digoxin. In: Koda-Kimble MA, Young LY, eds: Basic Clinical Pharmacokinetics, 3rd ed. Vancouver, WA, Applied Therapeutics, 1994; pp. 198–235.

66. Yang R, Andersen M: Pharmacokinetics. In: Hodgson E, Levi P, eds: Introduction to Biochemical Toxicology. Norwalk, CT, Appleton & Lange, 1994, pp. 49–73.

CHAPTER 12   CHEMICAL PRINCIPLES

Stephen J. Traub / Lewis S. Nelson

Chemistry is the science of matter; as such, it encompasses the structure, physical properties, and reactivities of atoms and their compounds. In many respects, toxicology is the science of the interactions of matter with physiologic entities; as such, chemistry and toxicology are intimately linked. The study of inorganic, organic, and biologic chemistry may lead to a deeper and more complete understanding of the effects of drugs and poisons on the human body. The principles or inorganic and organic chemistry offer important insight into the mechanisms and clinical manifestations of poisons and poisoning, respectively. This chapter reviews many of these tenets and provides relevance to the current practice of medical toxicology.

THE STRUCTURE OF MATTER

Basic Structure

Matter includes the substances of which everything is made. *Elements* are the foundation of matter, and all matter is made from one or more of the known elements. An *atom* is the smallest quantity of a given element that retains the properties of that element. Atoms consist of a nucleus, incorporating protons and neutrons, coupled with its orbiting electrons. The *atomic number* depicts the number of protons in the nucleus of an atom, and is a whole number that is unique for each element. Thus, elements with 6 protons are always carbon, and all forms of carbon have exactly 6 protons. However, although the vast majority of carbon nuclei have 6 neutrons in addition to the protons, accounting for a *mass number* (ie, protons plus neutrons) of 12 (^{12}C), a small proportion of naturally occurring carbon nuclei, called *isotopes*, have 8 neutrons and a mass number of 14 (^{14}C). Hence, the *atomic weight* of carbon displayed on the periodic table is 12.011 and actually represents the average mass numbers of all isotopes found in nature weighted by their frequency of occurrence. Moreover, ^{14}C is actually a *radioisotope*, which is an isotope with an unstable nucleus that emits radiation (particles and/or rays), presumably in an effort to attain a stable state (Chap. 99). The atomic weight, measured in grams/mole (g/mol), also indicates the molar mass of the element. That is, in 1 atomic weight (12.011 g for carbon) there exists 1 mole of atoms (6.023×10^{23} atoms).

Elements combine chemically to form *compounds*, which generally have physical and chemical properties different than those of the constituent elements. Furthermore, the elements in a compound can only be separated by chemical means that destroy the original compound. This occurs during the burning (ie, oxidation) of a hydrocarbon to release the carbon as carbon dioxide. This important property differentiates compounds from *mixtures*, which are combinations of elements or compounds that can be separated by physical means. This occurs, for example, during the distillation of petroleum into its hydrocarbon components or the evaporation of salt water to leave sodium chloride. With notable exceptions, such as the elemental forms of many metals or chlorine (eg, Cl_2), most toxins are compounds or mixtures.

Dimitri Mendeleev, a Russian chemist in the mid-19th century, recognized that when all of the known elements were arranged in order of atomic weight, certain patterns of reactivity became apparent. The result of his work was the Periodic Table of the Elements (Fig. 12–1), which, with some minor alterations, is still used today. All of the currently recognized elements are represented; those heavier than uranium are not known to occur in nature. Many of the symbols used to identify the elements refer to the Latin name of the element. For example, silver is Ag, for argentum, and mercury is Hg, for hydrargyrum, or silver water.

The reason for the periodicity of the table relates to the electrons that circle the nucleus in discrete orbitals. Although the details of quantum mechanics and electronic configuration are complex, it is important to review some aspects in order to predict chemical reactivity. Orbitals, or quantum shells, represent the energy levels in which electrons may exist around the nucleus. The orbitals are identified by various schemes, but the maximum number of electrons each shell may contain is calculated as $2x^2$, where x represents the numerical rank order of the shell. Thus, the first shell may contain 2 electrons, the second shell may contain 8, the third may contain 18, and so on. However, the outermost shell may only contain up to 8 electrons. This is irrelevant through element 20, calcium, because there is no pressure to fill the third-level orbitals. Even though the third shell may contain 18 electrons, once 8 are present, the fourth shell begins to fill. This occurs at element 21, scandium, and accounts for its chemical properties and those of the other transition elements. Note that hydrogen and helium are unique in needing only 2 electrons to complete their valence shell; all other elements require 8 to be complete. Also, because the inert gas elements, also known as noble gases, have complete outermost orbitals, they are completely unreactive under standard conditions.

In general, only electrons in unfilled shells, or *valence shells*, are involved in chemical reactions. This property relates to the fact that the most stable form of an element is when the configuration of its valence shell resembles that of the nearest noble gas, found in group 0 on the periodic table. This state can be obtained through either the gaining, losing, or sharing of electrons with other elements and is the basis for virtually all chemical reactions.

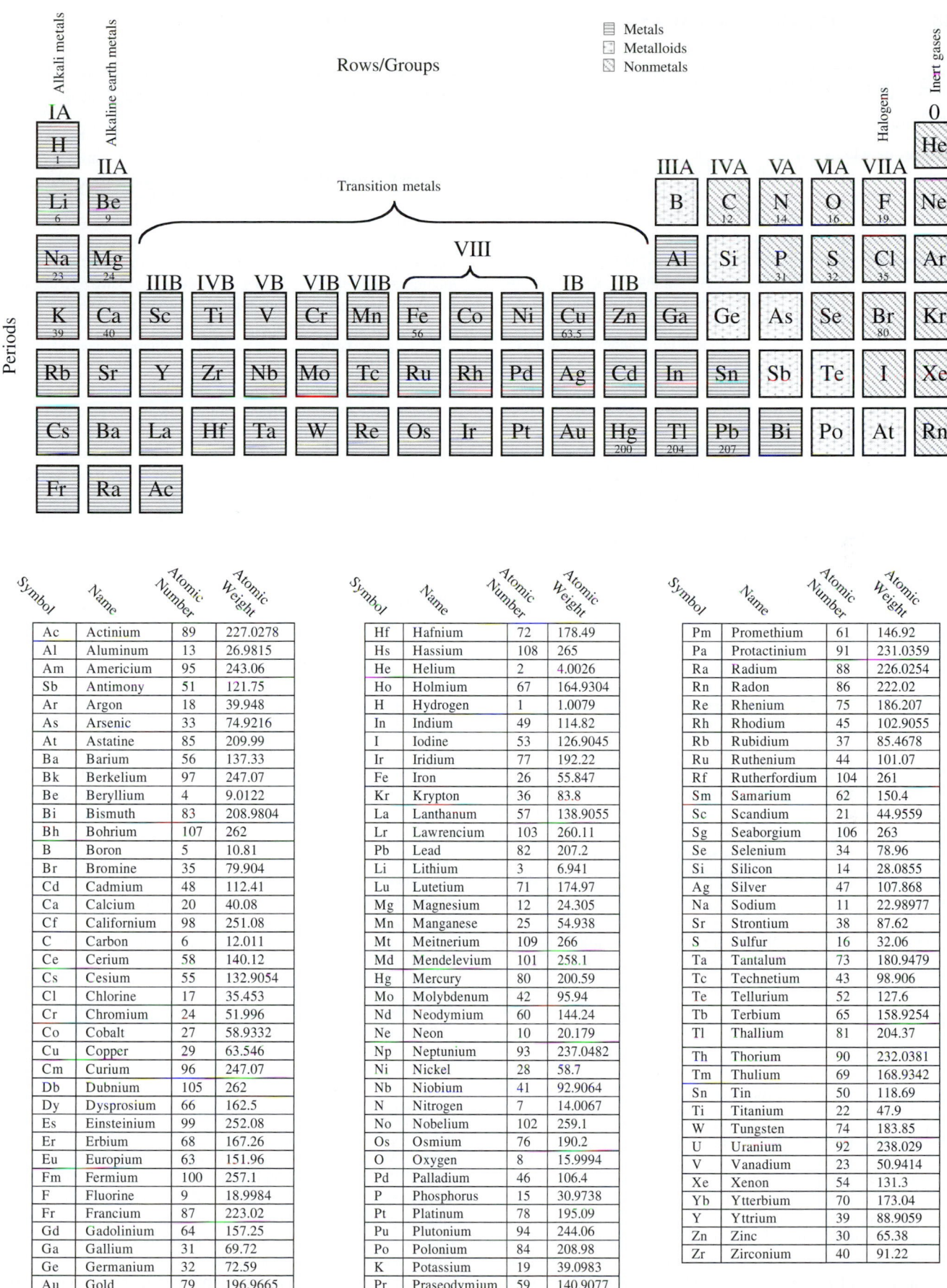

Figure 12–1. The periodic table of the elements.

INORGANIC CHEMISTRY

The Periodic Table

Chemical Reactivity. Broadly, the periodic table is divided into metals and nonmetals. Metals, in their pure form, are typically malleable solids that conduct electricity, whereas nonmetals are usually dull, fragile, nonconductive compounds (C, N, P, O, S, Se, halogens). The metals are found on the left side of the periodic table, and account for the majority of the elements, whereas the nonmetals are on the right side. Separating the two groups are the metalloids, which fall on a jagged line starting with boron (B, Si, Ge, As, Sb, Te, At). These agents have chemical properties that are intermediate between the metals and the nonmetals. Each column of elements is termed a family or group, and each row is a period. Although contrived and organized in periods, trends in the chemical reactivity, and therefore toxicity, typically exist within the groups.

The ability of any particular element to produce toxicologic effects relates directly to one or more of its many physicochemical properties. An understanding of the relationships of the elements may, to some extent, be predicted by their location on the periodic table. For example, the substitution of arsenate for phosphate in the mitochondrial production of adenosine triphosphate (ATP) creates adenosine diphosphate monoarsenate (Chap. 13). Because this compound is unstable, energy production by the cell fails; thus arsenic "uncouples" oxidative phosphorylation. Similarly, the existence of an interrelationship between Ca^{2+} and either Mg^{2+} or Ba^{2+} is predictable, although the actual effects are not. That is, under most circumstances, Mg^{2+} is a Ca^{2+} antagonist, and patients with hypermagnesemia present with neuromuscular weakness caused by blockade of myocyte calcium channels. Alternatively, Ba^{2+} mimics Ca^{2+} and closes Ca^{2+}-dependent K^+ channels in myocytes, producing life-threatening hypokalemia. Additionally, the chemical similarities between lithium (Li^+), potassium (K^+), and sodium (Na^+) are consistent with their physiologic relationship, whereas others, such as those between thallium (Tl^+) and K^+, are less consistent. Other than their monovalent nature (ie, +1 charge), it is impossible to predict the substitution of Tl^+ for K^+ in membrane ion channel functions.

The Alkali (Group IA: Li, Na, K, Rb, Cs, Fr) and Alkaline Earth (Group IIA: Be, Mg, Ca, Sr, Ba, Ra) Metals.
Alkali metals and hydrogen have a single outer valence electron and lose this electron easily to form compounds with a valence of 1+. The alkaline earth metals lose two electrons in forming their ionic bonds, and their cations have a 2+ charge. In their metallic form members of both of these groups react violently with water to liberate strongly basic solutions, accounting for their common names ($2Na^0 + 2H_2O \rightarrow 2NaOH + H_2$). The soluble ionic forms of sodium, potassium, or calcium, which are critical to survival, also produce life-threatening symptoms following excessive intake (Chap. 24). Toxins may interfere with the physiologic role of these key electrolytes. Li^+ may mimic potassium and enter neurons through K^+ channels, following which it appears to serve as a poor substrate for the repolarizing Na^+/K^+ ATPase. Thus, lithium interferes with cellular potassium homeostasis and alters neuronal repolarization. Similarly, the molecular effects of Mg^{2+} and Ba^{2+} may supplant that of calcium. More commonly though, the consequential toxicities ascribed to alkali or alkaline earth salts actually relate to the anionic component. In the case of NaOH or $Ca(OH)_2$, it is a hydroxide

anion (not the hydroxyl radical as discussed elsewhere), while it is a CN^- anion in patients poisoned with potassium cyanide.

The Transition Metals (Group IB to VIIIB). Unlike the alkali and alkaline earth metals, most other metallic elements are neither soluble nor reactive. This includes the transition metals, a large group that contains several ubiquitous metals such as iron (Fe) and copper (Cu). These elements, in their metallic form, are widely utilized both in industrial and household applications. Many also form brightly colored metal salts that find widespread applications including pigments for paints or fireworks. However, the ionic forms of these elements are typically highly reactive and toxicologically important. Because the transition metals have partially filled valence shells, they are capable of obtaining several, usually positive, oxidation states. This important mechanism explains the role of transition metals in redox reactions generally as electron acceptors (see Oxidation-Reduction below). This reactivity is utilized by living organisms in various metabolic and physiologic roles, such as at the active sites of enzymes or hemoglobin. Expectedly, the substantial reactivity of these transition metal elements is highly associated with cellular injury caused by the generation of reactive oxygen species. For example, manganese exposure is implicated in the free radical damage of the basal ganglia causing parkinsonism.

The Heavy Metals. *Heavy metal* is often loosely used to describe all metals of toxicologic significance, but in reality, the term should be reserved to describe only those metals in the lower period of the periodic table, particularly those with atomic masses greater than 200. The chemical properties and toxicologic predilection of this group vary among the agents, but electrophilic interference with nucleophilic sulfhydryl-containing enzymes appears to be their unifying toxicologic mechanism. Some of the heavy metals also participate in Fenton chemistry and liberate free radicals. The likely determinant of the specific toxicologic effects produced by each metal is the tropism for various physiologic systems, enzymes, or microenvironments; thus the lipophilicity, water solubility, ionic size, and other physicochemical parameters are undoubtedly critical. Also, because the chemistry of metals varies dramatically based on the chemical form (ie, organic, inorganic, or elemental), as well as the charge on the metal ion, prediction of an individual metal's clinical effects is often highly complex.

Mercury. Elemental mercury (Hg^0) is unique in that it is a metal in a liquid form at room temperature, and as such is capable of creating solid solutions, or amalgams, with other metals. As its high vapor pressure suggests, it is readily volatilized, converting it from a relatively innocuous physical state into one that is harmful because inhalation causes pulmonary mucosal irritation. In addition, the change in the route of exposure raises its systemic bioavailability. Absorbed, or incorporated, Hg^0 undergoes biotransformation in the erythrocyte and brain to the mercuric (Hg^{2+}) form, which has a high affinity for sulfhydryl-containing molecules including proteins. This causes a depletion of glutathione in organs such as the kidney, and also initiates lipid peroxidation. The mercurous form (Hg^+) is considerably less toxic than Hg^{2+}, perhaps because of its reduced water solubility. Organic mercurial compounds, such as monomethyl- and dimethylmercury, are environmentally formed by anaerobic bacteria containing the methylating agent methylcobalamin, a vitamin B_{12} analogue (Chap. 81).

Thallium. Another toxicologically important member of this group is thallium. Metallic thallium is used in the production of electronic equipment and is itself minimally toxic. Thallium ions, on the other hand, have physicochemical properties that most closely mimic potassium, causing it to alter various physiologic activities. This property is clinically utilized during a thallium-stress test, which is used to assess for myocardial ischemia or infarction. Because ischemic myocardial cells lack adequate energy for normal Na^+-K^+ ATPase function, they cannot uptake radioactive thallium, producing a "cold spot" in the ischemic areas on cardiac scintigraphy.

Lead. Although lead is not very abundant in the earth's crust (only 0.002%), exposure may occur during the smelting process or from one of its diverse commercial applications. Most of the useful lead compounds are inorganic lead (II) (Pb^{2+}) salts, but lead (IV) (Pb^{4+}) compounds are also available. The Pb^{2+} compounds are typically ionizable, releasing Pb^{2+} when dissolved in an appropriate solvent, such as water. Lead (II) ions are absorbed in place of Ca^{2+} ions by the gastrointestinal tract and replace calcium in certain physiologic processes. This mechanism is implicated in the neurotoxic effect of lead ions. Lead (IV) compounds tend to be covalent compounds that do not ionize in water. However, some of the Pb^{4+} compounds are oxidants. Although elemental lead is not itself toxic, it rapidly develops a coating of toxic lead oxide or lead carbonate upon exposure to air or water.

The Metalloids (B, Is, Ge, As, Sb, Te, At).

Although the metalloids share many physical properties with the metals, they are differentiated because of their propensity to form compounds with metals as well as carbon, nitrogen, or oxygen. Metalloids may be either oxidized or reduced in chemical reactions.

Arsenic. Toxicologically important inorganic arsenic compounds exist in either the pentavalent arsenite (As^{5+}) form or the trivalent arsenate (As^{3+}) form. The reduced water solubility of the arsenate compounds, such as arsenic pentoxide, accounts for the compounds' limited clinical toxicity when compared to trivalent arsenic trioxide. The trivalent form is primarily a nucleophilic toxin, binding sulfhydryl groups and interfering with enzymatic function (Chaps. 13 and 79).

The Nonmetals (C, N, P, O, S, Se, halogens).

The nonmetals are highly electronegative and, unlike the metals, may be toxic in either their compounded or their elemental form. The nonmetals with large electronegativity, such as O_2 or Cl_2, generally oxidize other elements in chemical reactions. Those with smaller electronegativity, such as C or H_2, behave as reducing agents.

The Halogens (F, Cl, Br, I, At).

In their highly reactive elemental form, which contains a covalent dimer of halogen atoms, the halogens carry the suffix -ine (eg, Cl_2, chlorine). Halogens require the addition of one electron to complete their valence shell; thus, halogens are strong oxidizing agents. Because they are highly electronegative, they form halides (eg, Cl^-, chloride) by abstracting electrons from less electronegative elements. Thus the halogen ions, in their stable ionic form, generally carry a charge of -1. The halides, although much less reactive than their respective elemental forms, are reducing agents. The hydrogen halides (eg, HCl, hydrogen chloride) are gases under standard conditions, but they ionize when dissolved in aqueous solution to form the hydro-

halidic acids (eg, HCl, hydrochloric acid). All hydrogen halides except HF ionize completely in water to release H^+ and are considered *strong acids*. Because of its small ionic radius, lack of charge dispersion, and intense electronegativity, hydrogen fluoride ionizes only slightly and is a *weak acid*. This specific property of HF has important toxicologic implications (Chap. 87).

Group 0 or VIII: The Inert Gases (He, Ne, Ar, Kr, Xe, Rn).

Inert gases maintain completed valence shells and are thus entirely unreactive. Under certain extreme circumstances that cannot exist concurrently with human life, these elements can be made to form compounds, but they have no known toxicologic implications. The inert gases themselves, despite their lack of chemical reactivity, are toxicologically important as simple asphyxiants. That is, because they displace ambient oxygen from a confined space, consequential hypoxia may occur, and the expected warning signs may be completely absent (Chap. 95). In addition, inert gases may produce anesthesia when breathed at high concentrations. Radon, although a chemically inert gas, is radioactive, and prolonged exposure is associated with the development of lung cancer.

Bonds

Electrons are not generally shared evenly between atoms when they form a compound. Instead, unless the bond is between the same elements, as in Cl_2, one of the elements exerts a larger attraction for the shared electrons. The degree to which an element draws the shared electron is determined by the element's *electronegativity* (Fig. 12–2). The electronegativity of each element was catalogued by Linus Pauling and relates to the ionic radius, or the distance between the orbiting electron and the nucleus, and the shielding effects of the inner electrons. The electronegativity rises toward the right of the periodic table, corresponding with the expected charge obtained on an element when it forms a bond. Flouride ion has the highest electronegativity of all elements, which explains many of its toxicologic properties.

Several types of bonds exist between elements when they form compounds. When one element gains valence electrons and another loses them, the resulting elements are charged and attract one another in an *ionic,* or *electrovalent,* bond. An example is NaCl, or table salt, in which the electronegativity difference between the elements is 1.9, or greater than the electronegativity of the sodium (Fig. 12–2). Thus the chloride wrests control of the electrons in this bond. In solid form, ionic compounds exist in a crystalline lattice, but when put into solution, as in the serum, the

IA								VIIA
H 2.20	IIA		IIIA	IVA	VA	VIA	VIIA	He
Li 0.98	Be 1.57		B 2.04	C 2.55	N 3.04	O 3.44	F 3.98	Ne
Na 0.93	Mg 1.31		Al 1.61	Si 1.90	P 2.19	S 2.58	Cl 3.16	Ar
K 0.82	Ca 1.00				As 3.18	Se 2.55	Br 2.96	Kr

Figure 12–2. Electronegativity of the common elements.

elements may separate and form charged particles, or *ions* (Na^+ and Cl^-). The ions are stable in solution, however, because their valence shells contain 8 electrons and are complete. Ions, however, have properties that differ from both the original atom from which the ion is derived and the noble gas with which it shares electronic structure.

It is important to recognize that when a mole of a salt, for example NaCl (molecular weight 58.45 g/mol), is put in solution, two moles of particles results. This is because NaCl ionizes fully; ie, it produces 1 mole of Na^+ (23 g/mol) and 1 mole of Cl^- (35.45 g/mol). For salts that do not ionize completely, less than the complete number of moles are released and this quantity can be predicted based on the defined solubility of the compound, or the solubility product constant (K_{sp}). For ions that carry more than a single charge, *equivalent* is often used to denote that the element will be complexed with more than an equimolar number of other particles. Thus, an equivalent weight of calcium ion in a calcium salt will typically be one-half of its molecular weight because calcium ions are divalent. Alternatively stated, a standard calcium chloride ($CaCl_2$) solution (10%) contains approximately 1.4 mEq/mL or 0.7 mmol/mL of Ca^{2+}.

Compounds formed by two elements of similar electronegativity have little ionic character because there is little impetus for separation of charge. Instead, these elements share pairs of valence electrons, a process known as *covalence*. The resultant molecule contains a *covalent bond*, which is typically very strong and generally requires a high-energy chemical reaction to disrupt it. There is wide variation in the extent to which the electrons are shared between the participants of a covalent bond, and the physicochemical and toxiciologic properties of any particular molecule are in part determined by its nature. Rarely is sharing truly symmetric, as in oxygen (O_2) or chlorine (Cl_2). If sharing is asymmetric and the electrons thus exist to a greater degree around one of the component atoms, the bond is *polar*. However, the presence of a polar bond does not mean that the compound is polar. For example, methane contains a carbon atom that shares its valence electrons with 4 hydrogen atoms, in which there is a small charge separation between the elements (electronegativity (EN) difference = 0.40). Furthermore, because the molecule is configured in a tetrahedral formation, there is no notable polarity to the compound; this compound is *nonpolar*. The lack of polarity suggests that methane molecules have little affinity for other methane molecules and they are held together only by weak intermolecular bonds. This explains why it is highly volatile under standard conditions.

Because the electronegativity differences between hydrogen (EN = 2.20) and oxygen (EN = 3.44) are greater (EN difference = 1.24), the electrons in the HO bonds in water are drawn toward the oxygen atom, giving it a partial negative charge and the hydrogens a partial positive charge. Futhermore, because H_2O is angular, not linear or symmetric, water is a polar molecule. Water molecules are held together by hydrogen bonds, which are stronger than intermolecular bonds. These hydrogen bonds have sufficient energy to open many ionic bonds and *solvate* the ions. In this process, the polar ends of the water molecule surround the charged particles of the dissolved salt. Thus, because there is little similarity between the nonpolar methane and the polar water molecules, methane is not water soluble. Similarly, salts cannot be solvated by nonpolar compounds, and thus a salt, such as sodium chloride, cannot dissolve in a nonpolar solvent, such as carbon tetrachloride.

Alternatively, the stability and irreversibility of the bond between an organic phosphorus insecticide and the cholinesterase enzyme are due to covalent phosphorylation of an amino acid at the active site of the enzyme. The resulting bond is essentially irreversible in the absence of another chemical reaction.

Compounds may share multiple pairs of electrons. For example, the two carbon atoms in acetylene (HC≡CH) share three pairs of double bonds between them, and each shares one pair with its own hydrogen. Carbon and nitrogen share three pairs of electrons in forming cyanide (C≡N).

Furthermore, complex ions are covalently bonded groups of elements that behave as a single element. For example, the hydroxide ion (OH^-) and sulfate (SO_4^{2-}) form sodium salts as if they were simply a chloride ion.

Noncovalent bonds, such as hydrogen or ionic bonds, are important in the interaction between ligands and receptors, ion channels and enzymes. These bonds are of low energy and therefore easily reversible.

Oxidation-Reduction

Redox (oxidation-reduction) reactions involve the movement of electrons from one atom or molecule to another, and actually comprise two dependent reactions: reduction and oxidation. *Reduction* is the gain of electrons by an agent that is thereby *reduced*. The electrons derive from a *reducing agent*, which in the process becomes *oxidized*. Oxidation is the loss of electrons from an agent, which is, accordingly, *oxidized*. An *oxidizing agent* accepts electrons, and in the process, is reduced. By definition, these chemical reactions involve a change in the valence of an atom. It is also important to note that acid/base and electrolyte chemical reactions involve electrical charge interactions but no change in valence of any of the involved components. The implications of redox chemistry for medical toxicology are profound. For example, the conversion of ferrous (Fe^{2+}) to ferric (Fe^{3+}) iron within the hemoglobin molecule changes the hemoglobin to a dysfunctional form called methemoglobin.

Also, metallic lead and elemental mercury are both intrinsically harmless metals but when oxidized to their cationic forms both produce devastating clinical effects. Additionally, the oxidation of methanol to formic acid involves a change in the oxidation state of the molecule. In this case, an enzyme, alcohol dehydrogenase, acting as a catalyst, oxidizes (ie, removes electrons from) the C-O bond and delivers the electrons to oxidized nicotinamide adenine dinucleotine (NAD^+), reducing it to the reduced form (NADH). As in this last example, *oxidation* is occasionally used to signify the gain of oxygen by a substance. That is, when elemental iron (Fe^0) undergoes rusting (to Fe_2O_3), it is said to oxidize. The use of this term is consistent because in the process of oxidation, oxygen abstracts electrons from the agent to which it is binding.

Reactive Oxygen Species. Free radicals are reactive molecules that contain one or more unpaired electrons, and may be anionic, cationic, or neutral. However, because certain toxicologically important reactive molecules do not contain unpaired electrons, such as hydrogen peroxide (H_2O_2), Δ singlet oxygen (O·), and ozone (O_3), the term *reactive species* is preferred (Fig. 12–3). The reactivity of these molecules directly relates to their desire to fill their outermost orbitals by receiving an electron. Reactive species are continually generated as a consequence of endogenous metabo-

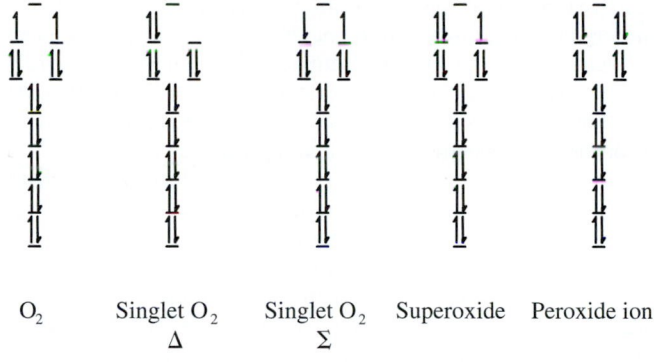

Figure 12–3. Electron structure of various reactive oxygen species.

TABLE 12–1. Structure of Important Reactive Oxygen and Nitrogen Species

Reactive Oxygen Species	Structure	Biologic $t_{1/2}$ (sec)
Free radicals		
Hydroxyl radical	OH·	10^{-9}
Alcoxyl radical	RO·	10^{-6}
Singlet oxygen (Σ)	[O] or $^1O_2$	10^{-5}
Peroxyl radical	ROO·	7
Superoxide radical	$O_2^{\cdot-}$ or O_2^-	Superoxide dismutase
Nonradicals		
Hydrogen peroxide	H_2O_2	Catalase
Hypochlorous acid	HOCl	
Singlet oxygen (Δ)	[O] or $^1O_2$	
Ozone	O_3	

Reactive Nitrogen Species

Free radicals		
Nitric oxide	NO·	1–10
Nitrogen dioxide	NO_2·	
Nonradicals		
Peroxynitrite anion	$ONOO^-$	0.051
Nitronium cation	NO_2^+	

Adapted from Bergendi L, Benes L, Durackova Z, et al: Chemistry, physiology and pathology of free radicals. Life Sci 1999;65:1865.

lism and, although they are a nuisance in some senses, they are also critical to survival. Under conditions of either excessive endogenous generation or exposure to exogenous reactive species, the physiologic defense against these toxic products is overwhelmed. Under these conditions, reactive species induce direct cellular damage as well as initiate a cascade of oxidative reactions that perpetuate the toxic damage.

Intracellular organelles, particularly the mitochondria, may also be disrupted by various reactive oxygen species. This causes further injury to the cell as energy failure occurs. This initial damage is compounded by the activation of the host inflammatory response by chemokines that are released from cells in response to reactive oxygen species–induced damage. This inflammatory response aggravates cellular damage. The resultant membrane dysfunction or damage causes cellular apoptosis or necrosis (Chap. 13).

The most important reactive oxygen species in medical toxicology are derived from oxygen, although those derived from nitrogen are also important. The important reactive oxygen species are listed with their biologic half-life in Table 12–1. In general, the more reactive molecules have shorter half-lives and greater biologic consequences.

Molecular oxygen itself fits the definition of a free radical in that it is a biradical, with two unpaired electrons in its outermost orbital (Fig. 12–3). This biradical nature explains both the physiologic and toxicologic importance of oxygen in biologic systems. Physiologically, the majority of oxygen is utilized by the body to serve as the ultimate electron acceptor in the mitochondrial electron transport chain (Chap. 13, Fig. 13–2). In this situation, four electrons are added to each molecule of oxygen to form two water molecules ($O_2 + 4 H^- + 4 e^- \rightarrow 2 H_2O$).

Superoxide is generated within neutrophil and macrophage lysosomes as part of the oxidative burst, a method of damaging and destroying infectious agents and damaged cells. Superoxide may subsequently be enzymatically converted, or dismutated, into hydrogen peroxide by superoxide dismutase. Hydrogen peroxide may be subsequently converted into hypochlorous acid by the enzymatic addition of chloride by myeloperoxidase. Both hydrogen peroxide and hypochlorite ion are more potent reactive oxygen species than superoxide. However, this lysosomal protective system may also be responsible for tissue damage following poisoning as the innate inflammatory response attacks toxin-damaged cells. Examples include acetaminophen-induced hepatotoxicity

(Chap. 32), carbon monoxide neurotoxicity (Chap. 97), and chlorine-induced pulmonary toxicity (Chap. 95), each of which may be altered, in experimental systems at least, by the addition of scavengers of reactive oxygen species.

Although superoxide and hydrogen peroxide are reactive oxygen species, it is their conversion into the hydroxyl radical (OH·) that accounts for their most consequential effects. The hydroxyl radical is generated by the Fenton reaction, in which superoxide and hydrogen peroxide combine in the presence of a transition metal. This catalysis typically involves Fe^{2+}, Cu^+, Cd^{2+}, Cr^{5+}, Ni^{2+}, or Mn^{2+} (Fig. 12–4). Superoxide dismutase (SOD), within the erythrocyte, contains an atom of Cu^{2+} that participates in the catalytic activity (SOD was originally called erythrocuprein).

Transition metal cations may bind to the cellular nucleus where they locally generate reactive oxygen species, most importantly hydroxyl radical. This results in DNA strand breaks and modification, accounting for the promutagenic effects of many transition metals.[2] In addition to the important role that transition metal chemistry plays following iron or copper salt poisoning, the long-term consequences of chronic transition metal poisoning are exemplified by asbestos. The iron contained in this mineral is the origin of the Fenton-generated hydroxyl radicals that are responsible for the pulmonary fibrosis and cancers associated with long-term exposure to this mineral.[2]

The most consequential toxicologic effects of reactive oxygen species occur on the cell membrane, and are caused by the initiation by hydroxyl radical of the lipid peroxidative cascade. The al-

$$Cu^+ + H_2O_2 \longrightarrow Cu^{2+} + OH^- + OH\cdot$$

Figure 12–4. The Fenton reaction.

teration of these lipid membranes ultimately causes membrane destruction. Identification of released oxidative products such as malondialdehyde is a common method of assessing lipid peroxidation.

Under normal conditions, there is a delicate balance between the formation and immediate endogenous detoxification of reactive oxygen species. For example, the conversion of superoxide radical to hydrogen peroxide via SOD is rapidly followed by the transformation of hydrogen peroxide to water by glutathione peroxidase or catalase. Furthermore, transition metals cannot be unattended in biologic systems and exist in "free" form in only minute quantities, presumably to minimize the formation of hydroxyl radicals through Fenton reactions. Thus, cells have developed extensive systems by which transition metal ions can be sequestered and rendered harmless. Ferritin (binds iron), ceruloplasmin (binds copper), and metallothionein (binds cadmium) are specialized proteins that safely shelter metal ions. Certain enzymes that contain transition metals at their active sites, such as hemoglobin or SOD, harness the activity of transition metal ions in a controlled fashion.

Detoxification of certain reactive species is difficult because of their extreme reactivity. Widespread antioxidant systems exist to trap these agents before they can damage tissues. Upon binding reactive oxygen species, antioxidants transform into stable radicals and prevent the initiation of successive redox reactions.

The key reactive nitrogen species is nitric oxide. At typical physiologic concentrations, this radical is responsible for vascular endothelial relaxation through stimulation of guanylate cyclase. However, during oxidative burst, high concentrations of nitric oxide are formed from L-arginine. At these concentrations, nitric oxide both has primarily damaging effects and reacts with superoxide radical to generate the peroxynitrite anion. This is particularly important because peroxynitrite may spontaneously degrade to form the hydroxyl radical. Peroxynitrite ion is implicated in the delayed neurologic effects of carbon monoxide poisoning.

Redox Cycling. Although transition metal chemistry is an important source of reactive species formation, certain xenobiotics are also capable of independently generating reactive species. Most do so through a process called *redox cycling*, in which the agent accepts an electron from a reductant and subsequently transfers that electron to oxygen, generating the superoxide radical. At the same time, this second reaction regenerates the parent compound, which itself can gain another electron and restart the process. In the case of paraquat, the toxicity of which is selectively localized to pulmonary endothelial cells, the result of redox cycling generation of reactive oxygen species is pulmonary toxicity (Chap. 91). A similar process, localized to the heart, occurs with anthracycline antineoplastic agents such as doxorubicin, which also undergo redox cycling.

ACID-BASE CHEMISTRY

Water is *amphoteric*, which implies that water can function as either an acid or a base, much the same way as the bicarbonate ion (HCO_3^-). In fact, because of the amphoteric nature of water, H^+, despite the nomenclature, does not ever actually exist in aqueous solution; rather, it is covalently bound to a molecule of water to form the hydronium ion (H_3O^+). However, the term H^+, or proton, is used for convenience.

Even in neutral solution, a tiny proportion of water is always undergoing ionization to form both H^+ and OH^- in exactly equal amounts. It is, however, the quantity of H^+ that concerns chemists, and this is the basis of using the pH to characterize a solution. At equilibrium, the concentration of H^+ ions in pure, neutral water is precisely 0.0000001, or 10^{-7}, moles per liter and that of OH^- is the same (Fig. 12–5). The number of H^+ ions increases when an acid is added to the solution and falls when an alkali is added. However, in an attempt to make this quantity more practical, the negative log of the H^+ concentration is calculated, which defines the *pH*. Thus, the negative log of 10^{-7} is 7, and the pH of a neutral aqueous solution is 7. In reality, however, the pH of standing water is actually around 6. This is because of dissolution of ambient carbon dioxide to form carbonic acid ($H_2O + CO_2 \rightarrow H_2CO_3$), which ionizes to form H^+ and bicarbonate (HCO_3^-).

There are many definitions of acid and base. The three commonly used definitions are those advanced by (a) Arrhenius, (b) Brønsted-Lowry, and (c) Lewis. Because the focus is on physiologic systems, which are aqueous, the original definition by the Swedish chemist Arrhenius is the most practical. In this view, an acid is any substance that releases hydrogen ions, or protons (H^+), in water. Similarly, a base is anything that produces hydroxyl ions (OH^-) in water. Thus, hydrogen chloride (HCl), a neutral gas under standard conditions, dissolves in water to liberate H^+, and is thus an acid.

For nonaqueous solutions the Brønsted-Lowry definition is preferable. An acid, in this schema, is a substance that donates a proton and a base is one that accepts a proton. Thus, any molecule that has a hydrogen in the 1+ oxidation state is technically an acid, and any molecule with an unbound pair of valence electrons is a base. Because most of the acids or bases of toxicologic interest have ionizable protons or available electrons, respectively, the Brønsted-Lowry definition is most often considered when discussing acid-base chemistry (ie, $HA + H_2O \rightarrow H_3O^+ + A^-$; $B^- + H_2O \rightarrow HA + OH^-$). However, this is not a defining property of all acids or bases. Thus, Lewis offered the least restrictive definition

[H$^+$] (mol/L)	[H$^+$] (mol/L)	pH
0.1	10^{-1}	1
0.01	10^{-2}	2
0.001	10^{-3}	3
0.0001	10^{-4}	4
0.00001	10^{-5}	5
0.000001	10^{-6}	6
0.0000001	10^{-7}	7
0.00000001	10^{-8}	8
0.000000001	10^{-9}	9
0.0000000001	10^{-10}	10
0.00000000001	10^{-11}	11
0.000000000001	10^{-12}	12
0.0000000000001	10^{-13}	13
0.00000000000001	10^{-14}	14

Figure 12–5. The relationship between hydrogen ion concentations [H$^+$] and pH of an aqueous solution.

of such substances. A Lewis acid is an electron acceptor and a Lewis base is an electron acceptor. These three systems are complementary, with the Arrhenius system being the most restrictive. In practice, acids are sour and turn litmus paper red, while bases are slippery and bitter and turn litmus paper blue.

Because acidity is determined by the number of available H^+ ions, or, conversely, the alkalinity of a solution, it is useful to classify chemicals by their effect on the H^+ concentration. Strong acids ionize completely in aqueous solution and very little of the parent compound remains. Thus, 0.001 (or 10^{-3}) mole of HCl, a strong acid, added to 1 L of water produces a solution with a pH of 3. Weak acids, on the other hand, obtain an equilibrium between parent and ionized forms, and thus do not alter the pH to the same degree as a similar quantity of a strong acid. Note that using this chemical notation, the strength or weakness of an acid does not necessarily relate to the pH of the solution it produces. Thus, a dilute strong acid may have a substantially less acid pH than a concentrated weak acid (Fig. 12–6).

The degree of ionization of a weak acid is determined by the pK_a, or the negative log of the *ionization constant*, which represents the pH at which an acid is half dissociated in solution. The same relationship applies to the pK_b of an alkali, although by convention the pK_b is expressed as the pK_a ($pK_a = 14 - pK_b$). The lower the pK_a, the stronger the acid; the converse is true for bases. Knowledge of the pK_a does not itself denote whether a substance is an acid or an alkali. This quality may to some extent be predicted by its chemical structure or reactivity, or obtained through direct measurement or from a reference source. The pK of a strong acid is clinically irrelevant because it is fully ionized under all but the most extreme acid conditions.

Because only uncharged compounds cross lipid membranes spontaneously, the pK_a has clinical relevance. Salicylic acid, a weak acid with a pK_a of 3, is nonionized in the stomach (pH 2) and passive absorption occurs (Chap. 11, Fig. 11–4). However, because it is predominantly in the ionized form (ie, salicylate) in blood, which has a pH of 7.4, little of the ionized bloodborne salicylate passively enters the tissues. However, because in overdose the serum salicylate rises considerably, under such conditions enough enters the tissue to have devastating clinical effects. Salicylate, a conjugate base of a weak acid and thus a strong base, equilibrates across the outer mitochondrial membrane. In the mitochondrial intermembrane space abundant protons exist, which are transported there via the electron transport chain of this organelle (Chap. 13). Because salicylate is a strong base, it protonates easily in this environment. In this nonionized form, some of the salicylic acid may pass through the inner mitochondrial membrane, into the mitochondrial matrix, and again establish equilibrium by losing a proton. The process just described uncouples oxidative phosphorylation, by dispersing the highly concentrated protons in the intermembrane space that are used to generate adenosine triphosphate. Uncoupling leads to anaerobic glycolysis and lactate production, resulting in a metabolic acidosis, and this shifts the blood equilibrium toward the nonionized, protonated form, enabling salicylic acid to cross the blood-brain barrier. Presumably, once in the brain, the salicylate uncouples the metabolic activity of neurons with the subsequent development of cerebral edema. Because the salicylate molecule cannot differentiate between metabolic acidosis and respiratory acidosis, intubation without explicit attention to maintaining appropriate hyperventilation causes a respiratory acidosis to develop and the pH to fall.

This is also the rationale for serum alkalinization in patients with aspirin overdose. Because increasing the pH increases ionization, it prevents salicylic acid from passively entering the central nervous system. Similarly, alkalinization of the patient's urine prevents reabsorption by maintaining ionization of all urinary salicylate. Because tricyclic antidepressants are organic bases, alkalinization of the urine reduces their ionization, which actually decreases the drug's urinary elimination. This phenomenon is of interest, but because the other beneficial effects of sodium bicarbonate in the management of cyclic antidepressant poisoning have more consequential clinical effects, alkalinization is strongly recommended.

ORGANIC CHEMISTRY

The study of carbon-based chemistry and the interaction of inorganic molecules with carbon-containing compounds is called *organic chemistry*, because the chemistry of living organisms is carbon based. *Biochemistry* (Chap. 13) is a subdivision of organic chemistry; it is the study of organic chemistry within biologic systems. This section reviews many of the salient points of organic chemistry, focusing on those with the most applicability to medicine and the study of toxicology. In particular, nomenclature, bonding, nucleophiles and electrophiles, stereochemistry, and functional groups are reviewed.

Chemical Properties of Carbon

Carbon, atomic number 6, has a molecular weight of 12.011 g/mol. With few exceptions (notably cyanide ion and carbon monoxide), carbon forms four bonds in stable organic molecules. In organic compounds, carbon is commonly bonded to other carbon atoms, as well as to hydrogen, oxygen, nitrogen, or halide (ie, fluorine, bromine, or iodine) atoms. Under certain circumstances,

Acid or Base	pH
HCl (hydrochloric acid)	1.1
H_2SO_4 (sulfuric acid)	1.2
H_2SO_3 (sulfurous acid)	1.5
H_3PO_4 (phosphoric acid)	1.5
HF (hydrofluoric acid)	2.1
CH_3CO_2H (acetic acid)	2.9
H_2CO_3 (carbonic acid) (saturated solution)	3.8
H_2S (hydrogen sulfide)	4.1
NH_4Cl (ammonium chloride)	4.6
HCN (hydrocyanic acid)	5.1
$NaHCO_3$ (sodium bicarbonate)	8.3
$NaCH_3CO_2$ (sodium acetate)	8.9
Na_2HPO_4 (sodium hydrogen phosphate)	9.3
Na_2SO_3 (sodium sulfite) ·	9.8
NaCN (sodium cyanide)	11.0
NH_3 (aqueous ammonia)	11.1
Na_2CO_3 (sodium carbonate)	11.6
Na_3PO_4 (sodium phosphate)	12.0
NaOH (sodium hydroxide, lye)	13.0

Figure 12–6.   pH of 0.10 M solutions of common acids and bases.

carbon can be bonded to metals, as is the case with methylmercury.

Nomenclature

The most rigorous method to name organic compounds is by standards adopted by the International Union of Pure and Applied Chemistry (IUPAC); these names are infrequently used, especially for larger molecules, and *alternative chemical names* are common. Alternative chemical names are those based on the structure of a molecule, but which do not adhere completely to IUPAC rules. The complete details of the IUPAC naming system are beyond the scope of this text and can be reviewed elsewhere, but a brief description of the fundamentals of this system is included here.

The carbon backbone serves as the basis of the chemical name. A list of prefixes used for carbon backbones containing 1–10 carbons is noted in Table 12–2. Once the carbon backbone has been identified and named, *substituents* (atoms or groups of atoms that substitute for hydrogen atoms) are identified, named, and numbered. The number refers to the carbon to which the substituent is attached. Some of the common substituents in organic chemistry are –OH (referred to as hydroxy), –NH2 (amino), –Br (bromo), –Cl (chloro), and –F (fluoro). Substituents are then alphabetized and placed as prefixes to the carbon chain.

As an example, consider the molecule 2-bromo-2-chloro-1,1,1-triflouroethane. The molecule has a 2-carbon backbone (ethane), 3 fluoride atoms on the first carbon, a bromine atom on the second carbon, and a chlorine atom on the second carbon (Fig. 12–7). Thus basic understanding of a few simple rules of nomenclature can help to quickly generate the molecular structure of a familiar compound, halothane, from what initially appeared to be an intimidating name.

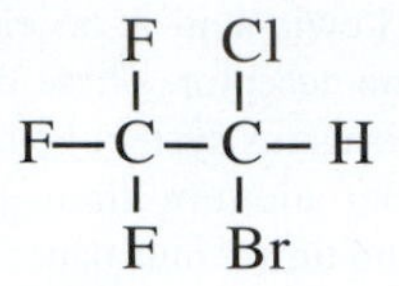

Although the above-mentioned rules suffice to name simple structures, they are inadequate to describe many others, such as molecules with complex branching or ring structures. The IUPAC rules for naming compounds such as [1R-(exo,exo)]-3-(Benzoyloxy)-8-methyl-8-azabicyclo[3.2.1]octane-2-carboxylic acid methyl ester (Fig. 12–8), for example, are too complex to include here. Fortunately, many compounds with complex chemical names have simpler names for day-to-day use; as an example, the molecule in Figure 12–8 is commonly referred to as cocaine.

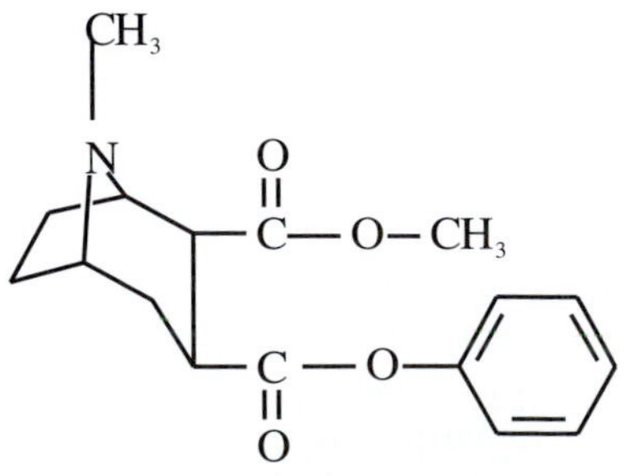

Cocaine is an example of a *common* or *trivial* name, that is, one without a rigorous scientific basis, but which is generally accepted as an alternative to (frequently unwieldy) proper chemical names. Common or trivial names may refer to the origin of the substance; for example, cocaine is derived from the coca leaf, and

Figure 12–7. 2-Bromo-2-chloro-1,1,1-trifluoroethane, or halothane.

wood alcohol (methanol) can be prepared from wood. Alternatively, a trivial name may refer to the way in which a compound is used; thus, "rubbing alcohol" is a common name for the liniment isopropanol.

Although a convenient shorthand, trivial names are often imprecise and may generate some confusion. For example, at the time of publication of this text the common name *ecstasy* refers to the stimulant 3,4-methylenedioxymethamphetamine (MDMA), which is most frequently consumed in pill form. It would stand to reason that *liquid ecstasy* might refer to a solution of MDMA; instead, this common name refers to the drug γ-hydroxy butyrate (GHB), a sedative-hypnotic agent with a completely different pharmacologic and toxicologic profile. Thus, although generally more convenient than chemical names, trivial names are often ambiguous and may have multiple meanings.

A final consideration must be given to *proprietary names*. Proprietary names are "trade names" under which a given compound might be marketed, and are frequently different from both their chemical name and trivial or common name. Thus, the inhalational anesthetic in Figure 12–7 has the chemical name *2-bromo-2-chloro-1,1,1-triflouroethane*, the common name *halothane*, and the trade name *Fluothane*. Table 12–3 lists some examples of the chemical, common, and proprietary names for some important toxicologic compounds.

Bonding in Organic Chemistry

Whereas much of the bonding in inorganic chemistry is ionic or electrovalent, the vast majority of bonding in organic molecules is *covalent*. Whereas electrons in ionic bonds are described as "belonging" to one atom or another, electrons in covalent bonds are shared between two atoms; this type of bonding occurs when the difference in electronegativity between two atoms is not great enough for one atom to wrest control of an electron from another.

There are two general types of bonds in organic molecules: *sigma* bonds, in which the electron density of the bond is maximal along the line which connects the two atoms, and *pi* bonds, in

TABLE 12–2. Prefixes for Carbon Backbones

One carbon	Meth-
Two carbons	Eth-
Three carbons	Prop-
Four carbons	But-
Five carbons	Pent-
Six carbons	Hex-
Seven carbons	Hept-
Eight carbons	Oct-
Nine carbons	Non-
Ten carbons	Dec-

Figure 12–8. [1R-(exo,exo)]-3-(benzoyloxy)-8-methyl-8-azabicyclo-[3,2,1]-octane-2-carboxylic acid methylester, or cocaine.

TABLE 12–3. Chemical, Common and Proprietary Names for Selected Compounds

IUPAC Name or Alternative Chemical Name	Common Name	Proprietary Name(s)
2-[o-chlorphenyl]-2 methylamino] cyclo-hexane hydrochloride	Ketamine	Ketalar
3-(10,11-dihydro-5H-dibenzo-[a,d] cyclohepten-5-ylidene)-N,N-dimethylpropylamine hydrochloride	Amitriptyline	Elavil, others
n-Dipropyl acetic acid	Valproic acid	Depakate, Depakene
4-Methylpyrazole	Fomepizole	Antizol
Acetyl salicyclic acid	Aspirin	Bayer, Anacin, others

which the electron density of the bond is maximal above and below the line that connects the two atoms. With very few exceptions, single bonds in organic chemistry are sigma bonds, double bonds consist of one sigma bond and one pi bond, and triple bonds consist of one sigma bond and two pi bonds. Figures 12–9A–C show examples of single, double, and triple bonds, and the sigma and pi components of these bonds.

Nucleophiles and Electrophiles

Many organic reactions of toxicologic importance can be described as the reaction of a *nucleophile* with an *electrophile*. *Nucleophiles* (literally, nucleus-loving) are species with increased electron density, frequently in the form of a lone pair of electrons (as is the case with cyanide ion and carbon monoxide). Nucleophiles, by virtue of this increased electron density, have an affinity for atoms or molecules which are electron deficient; such moieties are called *electrophiles* (literally, electron-loving). The electron deficiency of electrophiles can be described as absolute or relative. Absolute electron deficiency occurs when an electrophile is

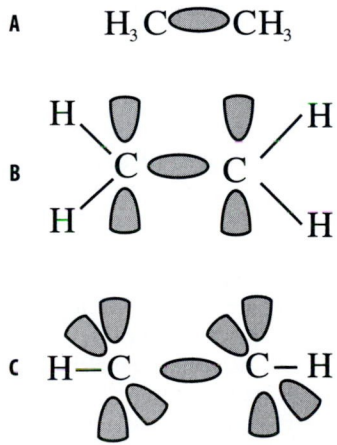

Figure 12–9. Orbital theory. **A.** A carbon-carbon sigma bond (electron density represented by shading). **B.** A carbon-carbon sigma bond and a carbon-carbon pi bond. **C.** A carbon-carbon sigma bond and two carbon-carbon pi bonds. The two sets of pi bonds are oriented at right angles to each other. All carbon-hydrogen bonds are represented by straight lines.

charged, as is the case with cations such as Pb^{2+} and Hg^{2+}. Relative electron deficiency occurs when one atom or group of atoms pulls electron density away from a second atom, making the second atom relatively electron deficient. This is the case for the neurotoxin 2,5-hexanedione (Fig. 12–10); the electronegative oxygen of the carbon-oxygen double bond pulls electron density away from the second and fifth carbon atoms of this molecule, making these carbon atoms electrophilic.

The reaction of a nucleophile with an electrophile involves the movement of electrons, forming and/or breaking bonds. This movement of electrons is frequently denoted by the use of curved arrows, which helps the reader to better understand how the nucleophile and electrophile interact. The interaction of acetylcholinesterase with acetylcholine, organic phosphorous pesticides, and pralidoxime hydrochloride provides an excellent example of the way in which nucleophiles and electrophiles interact, and of how the use of curved arrow notation can lead to better understanding of the reactions involved.

Under normal circumstances, the action of acetylcholine is terminated when the serine residue in the active site of acetylcholinesterase attacks this neurotransmitter, forming a transient serine-acetyl complex and liberating choline; this serine-acetyl complex is then rapidly hydrolyzed, producing an acetate ion and regenerating the serine residue for another round of the reaction (Fig. 12–11A). In the presence of organic phosphorus agents, however, this serine residue attacks the electrophilic phosphate atom, forming a stable serine-phosphate bond, which is not hydrolyzed (Fig. 12–11B). The enzyme, thus inactivated, can no longer break down acetylcholine, leading to an increase of this neurotransmitter in the synapse, and possibly to a cholinergic crisis.

The enzyme can be reactivated, however, by the use of another nucleophile. Pralidoxime hydrochloride (2-PAM) is referred to as a *site-directed nucleophile*. Because part of its chemical structure (the charged nitrogen atom) is similar to the choline portion of acetylcholine, this antidote is directed to the active site of acetylcholinesterase. Once in position, the nucleophilic oxime moiety (–NOH) of 2-PAM attacks the electrophilic phosphate atom; this displaces the serine residue, regenerating the enzyme (Fig. 12–11C). For a further discussion of organic phosphorus compound toxicity and the use of 2-PAM, see Chapter 88 and Antidotes in Depth: Pralidoxime.

A second toxicologically important electrophile is *N*-acetyl-*p*-benzoquinoneimine, or NAPQI (Fig. 12–12). NAPQI is formed when the endogenous detoxification pathways of acetaminophen metabolism are overwhelmed (Chap. 32). As a result of the electron configuration of this molecule, the carbon atoms adjacent to the *carbonyl carbon* (a carbonyl carbon is one that is double-bonded to an oxygen) are very electrophilic; the sulfur group of cysteine residues of hepatic proteins reacts with NAPQI to form a characteristic adduct, 3-(cystein-*S*-yl)acetaminophen, in a multi-

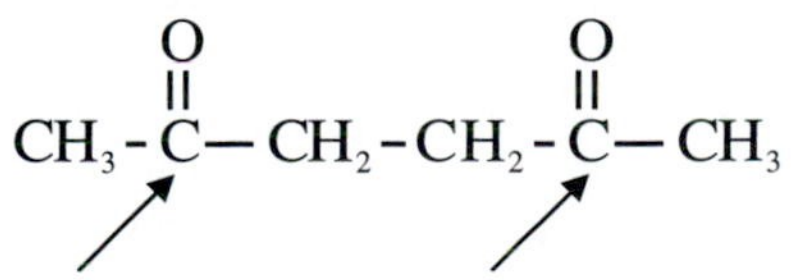

$$CH_3-\overset{\overset{\displaystyle O}{\|}}{C}-CH_2-CH_2-\overset{\overset{\displaystyle O}{\|}}{C}-CH_3$$

Figure 12–10. Chemical properties of 2,5-hexanedione. Arrows point to the electrophilic carbon atoms.

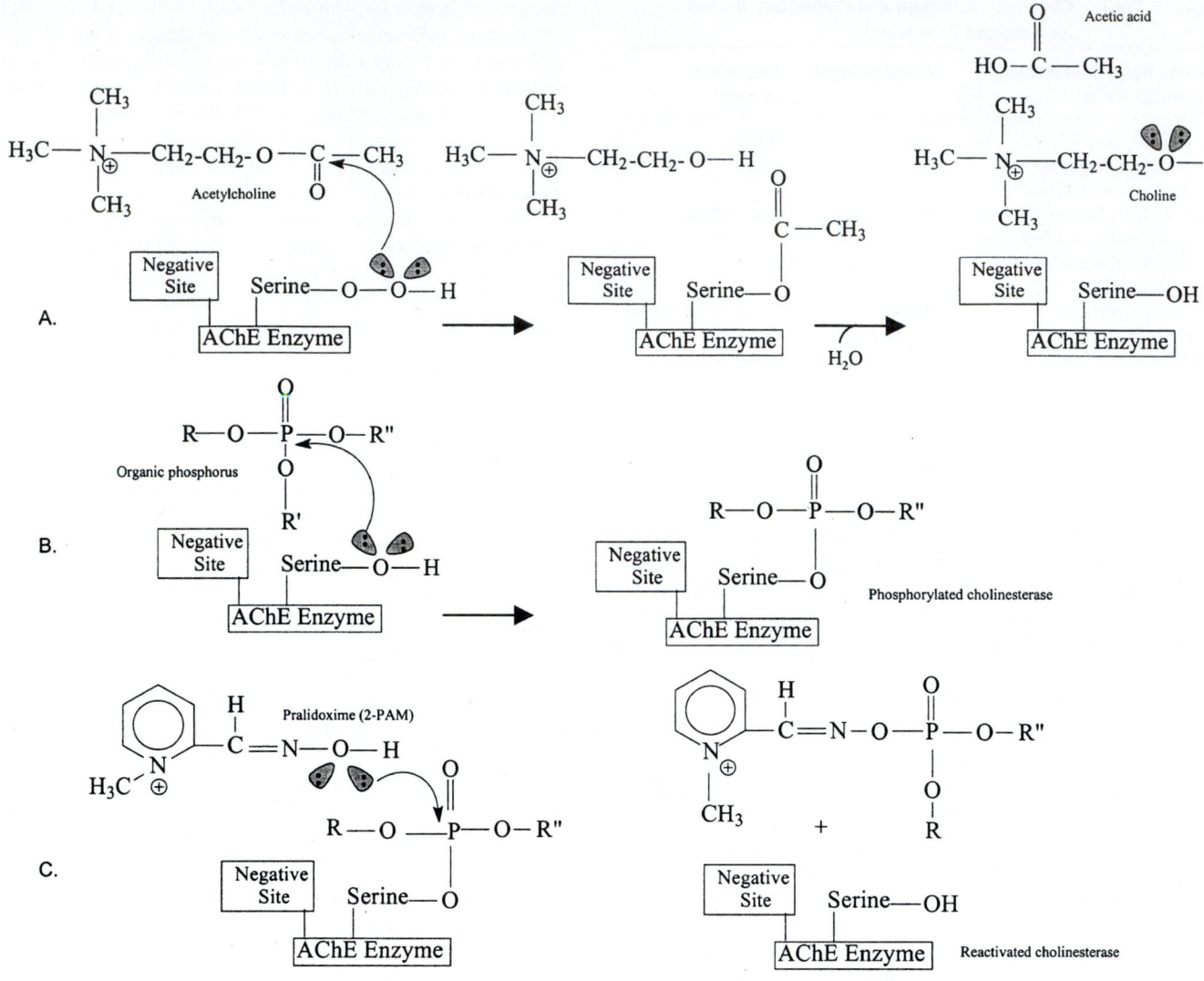

Figure 12–11. The reactions of acetylcholinesterase (AChE), organic phosphorus compounds, and pralidoxime (2-PAM). Curved arrows represent the movement of electrons as bonds are formed or broken. **A.** Normal hydrolysis of acetylcholine by acetylcholinesterase. **B.** Inactivation of acetylcholinesterase by organic phosphorus compounds. **C.** Regeneration of phosphorylated acetylcholinesterase by 2-PAM.

step process. These adducts are released as hepatocytes die, and can be found in the blood of patients with acetaminophen-related liver toxicity. Figure 12–12 diagrams the mechanism of the protein-NAPQI reaction.

Nucleophiles can be described by their strength; strength is related to the rate at which they react with a reference electrophile, CH_3I. Of more use in pharmacology and toxicology, however, are the descriptive terms "hard" and "soft." Although these are imprecise terms, the concept of "hard" versus "soft" helps to predict, on a qualitative level, how nucleophiles and electrophiles might interact with one another.

"Hard" species have a charge (or partial charge) that is highly localized. Hard nucleophiles are molecules in which the electron density or lone pair is tightly held; fluoride, a small atom that cannot spread its electron density over a large area, is an example. Similarly, hard electrophiles are species in which the positive charge cannot be spread over a large area; ionized calcium, a small ion, is a hard electrophile.

"Soft" species, on the other hand, are capable of diffusing their charge over a larger area, either because the atom is large or because the charge can be spread over a number of atoms within a given molecule. Soft nucleophiles can delocalize their electron density, either because the atom is large or not very electronegative; sulfur is the prototypical example of a soft nucleophile. Similarly, soft electrophiles are those in which the positive charge can be delocalized, either by dispersing the positive charge over a number of atoms, or by delocalizing the charge over a large atom, as is the case with the lead ion, Pb^{2+}.

The utility of this classification lies in the observation that hard nucleophiles tend to react with hard electrophiles, and soft nucleophiles with soft electrophiles. For example, one of the principal toxicities of fluoride ion intoxication is hypocalcemia; this is because the fluoride ions (hard nucleophiles) readily react with calcium ions (hard electrophiles), leading to hypocalcemia (Chap. 87). On the other hand, the soft nucleophile lead is effectively chelated by soft electrophiles such as the sulfur atoms in the

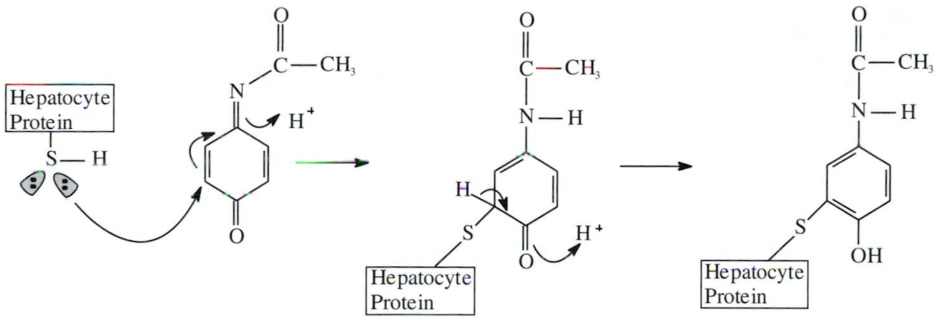

Figure 12–12. The reaction of cysteine residues with NAPQI.

chelating agents dimercaptopropanol and dimercaptosuccinic acid (Chap. 80 and Antidotes in Depth: Dimercaptosuccinic Acid, Succimer).

Isomerism

Isomerism describes the different ways in which molecules with the same chemical formula (that is, the same number and types of atoms) can be arranged to form different compounds. These different compounds are called *isomers*. Isomers always have the same chemical formula, but differ in the way that atoms are bonded to each other (*constitutional isomers*), or in the spatial arrangement of these atoms (*geometric isomers* or *stereoisomers*).

Constitutional isomers are conceptually the easiest to understand, because a quick glance shows them to be very different molecules. The chemical formula C_2H_6O, for example, can refer to either dimethyl ether or ethanol (Fig. 12–13). These molecules have very different physical and chemical characteristics, and have little in common other than the number and type of their atomic constituents (Table 12–4).

Stereoisomerism, also referred to as *geometric isomerism,* refers to the different ways in which atoms of a given molecule, with the same number and types of bonds, might be arranged. The most important type of stereoisomerism in pharmacology and toxicology is the stereochemistry around a *chiral carbon,* a carbon atom to which four different substituents are bonded.

Consider these two representations of halothane (Fig. 12–14): In Figure 12–14, the straight solid lines and the atoms to which they are bonded exist in the plane of the paper; the solid triangle and the atom to which it is bonded are coming out of the paper; and the dashed triangle and the atom to which it is bonded are receding into the paper. It is clear that, for the molecules in Figure 12–14A and B, no amount of rotation or manipulation will make these molecules superimposable. They are, therefore, different compounds.

The molecules in Figure 12–14A and B are *enantiomers* or *optical isomers*; they differ only in the way in which their atoms are bonded to the chiral carbon. It is important to define the stereochemical configuration of these two molecules, which can be done in one of two ways. In the first classification—the D(+)/L(−) sys-

tem—molecules are named empirically based on the direction in which they rotate plane-polarized light. Each enantiomer will rotate plane-polarized light in one direction; the enantiomer that rotates light clockwise (to the right) is referred to as D(+), or *dextrorotatory;* the L(−), or *levorotatory* enantiomer rotates plane-polarized light in a counterclockwise fashion (to the left).

Alternatively, enantiomers can be named using the *Cahn-Ingold-Prelog rules.* These rules establish priority for substituents, and then use these priorities to assign a configuration. Although the full description of these criteria is not presented here, the essence is that priority is based on the atomic weight of the first atom of the substituent; in the event that the first atom of two substituents is the same, the second (then third, fourth, etc) atoms are considered. After priorities are assigned, the molecule is rotated into a projection in which the chiral carbon is in the plane of the page, the lowest priority substituent is directly behind the chiral carbon (and therefore behind the plane of the page), and the other three substituents come out of the page toward the reader. Figure 12–15 assigns Cahn-Ingold-Prelog priority to the halothane enantiomers of Figure 12–8, and rearranges the molecules in the appropriate projections.

If the priority increases as one moves clockwise (to the right), the enantiomer is named R (Latin, *rectus* = right); if it increases as one moves counterclockwise, the enantiomer is named S (Latin, *sinister* = left). Thus, Figure 12–15A is the R halothane and Figure 12–15B is the S enantiomer.

Enantiomers have identical physical properties, such as boiling point, melting point, and solubility in different solvents; they differ from each other in only two significant ways. The first, as mentioned above, is that enantiomers rotate plane-polarized light in opposite directions; this point has no practical toxicologic importance. The second is that enantiomers may interact in very different ways with other three-dimensional structures (such as proteins and other cell receptors), which is of tremendous pharmacologic and toxicologic interest.

Perhaps the best analogy to explain the toxicologic and pharmacologic importance of stereochemistry is that of the way a hand (analogous to a molecule of drug or toxin) fits into a glove (analogous to the biologic site of activity). Consider the left hand as the

$$CH_3 — O — CH_3 \qquad CH_3 — CH_2 — OH$$

A   B

Figure 12–13. Two molecules with chemical formula C_2H_6O. **A.** Dimethylether. **B.** Ethyl alcohol.

TABLE 12–4.   Some Physical Properties of Dimethyl Ether and Ethanol

Property	Dimethyl Ether	Ethanol
Melting point °C (°F)	−141.50 (−222.7)	−114.1 (−173.38)
Boiling point, °C (°F)	−24.82 (−12.676)	78.5 (173.3)
Solubility in water	Negligible	Infinite

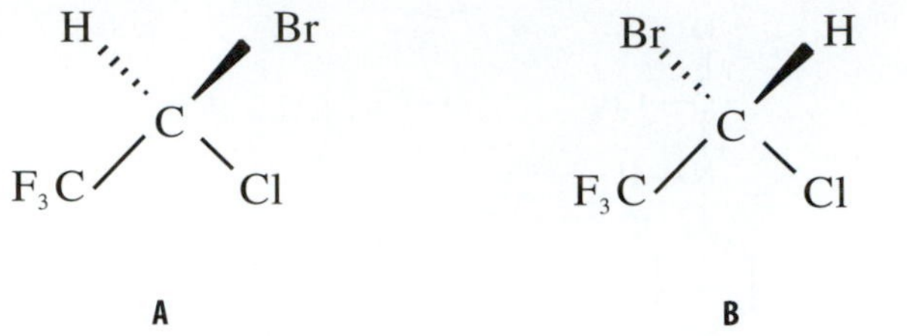

Figure 12–14. Two different ways to draw the molecule halothane.

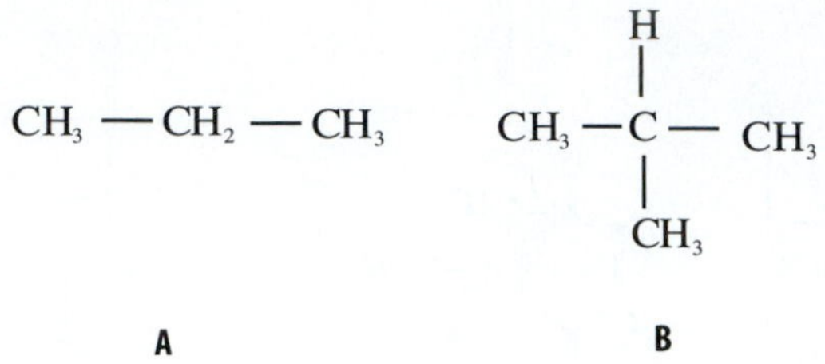

Figure 12–16. Two isomers of the 4-carbon alkane butane. **A.** *n*-Butane. **B.** Isobutane.

S enantiomer, and the right hand as the *R* enantiomer. There are, qualitatively, three different ways in which the hand can fit into (interact with) the glove.

First, if a glove is very pliable (such as a disposable latex glove), it can accept either the left hand or the right hand without difficulty; this is the case for halothane, whose **R** and *S* enantiomers possess equal activity. Second, if a glove is constructed with greater specificity, one hand will fit well and the other poorly; this is the case for many substances. Consider epinephrine and norepinephrine: the naturally occurring levorotatory enantiomers of these catecholamines are approximately 10-fold more potent than the synthetic dextrorotatory enantiomers. Finally, a glove can be made with exquisite precision, such that one hand fits perfectly, while the other hand does not fit at all. This is the case for physostigmine, in which the (−) enantiomer is biologically active, whereas the (+) enantiomer is not active at all.

Yet even the above analogy is overly simplified, as one enantiomer of a drug can be an agonist, while the other enantiomer is an antagonist. Dobutamine, for example, has one chiral carbon and thus two enantiomers. At the α_1 receptor, *l*-dobutamine is a potent agonist and *d*-dobutamine a potent antagonist; because dobutamine is marketed as a *racemic mixture* (a racemic mixture is a 1:1

mixture of enantiomers), however, these effects cancel each other out. Interestingly, at the β_1 receptor, both *d*- and *l*-dobutamine have agonist effects, but they are unequal, with *d*-dobutamine 10 times more potent than *l*-dobutamine.

Functional Groups

There is perhaps no concept in organic chemistry as powerful as that of the *functional group*. Functional groups are atoms or groups of atoms that confer similar reactivity on a molecule; of less importance is the molecule to which it is attached. Some representative functional groups in organic chemistry and toxicology are the *hydrocarbons* (*alkanes* and *alkenes*), *alcohols*, *carboxylic acids*, and *thiols*. These groups are discussed here because they illustrate important principles, not because this represents an exhaustive list of important functional groups in toxicology.

Hydrocarbons, as their name implies, consist of only carbon and hydrogen. *Alkanes* are hydrocarbons that contain no multiple bonds; they may be straight chain, usually designated by the prefix *n-* (Fig. 12–16A), or branched (isopropane, Fig. 12–16B). *Alkenes* contain carbon-carbon double bonds. *Alkynes*, which contain carbon-carbon triple bonds, are of limited toxicologic importance.

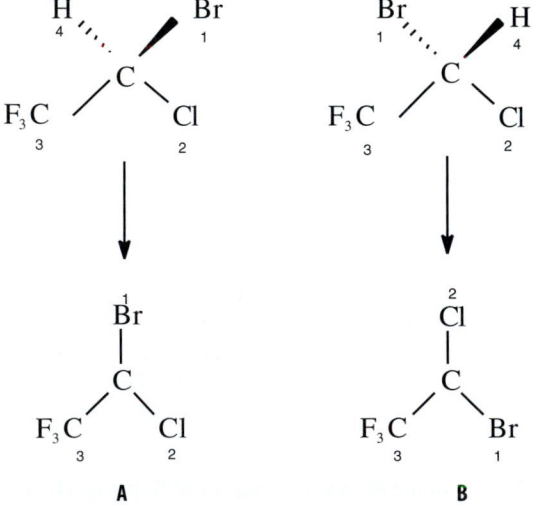

Figure 12–15. *R* and *S* enantiomers of halothane. **A.** The substituents increase in a clockwise fashion, so the configuration is *R.* **B.** The substituents increase in a counterclockwise fashion, so that the configuration is *S.* In this projection, hydrogen atoms are directly behind the carbon atoms. (See text for explanation).

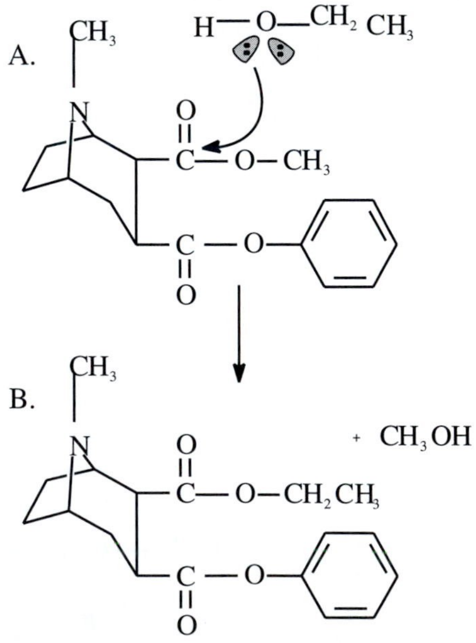

Figure 12–17. Reaction of cocaine with ethanol (Fig. 12–11A) to form cocaethylene (Fig. 12–11B).

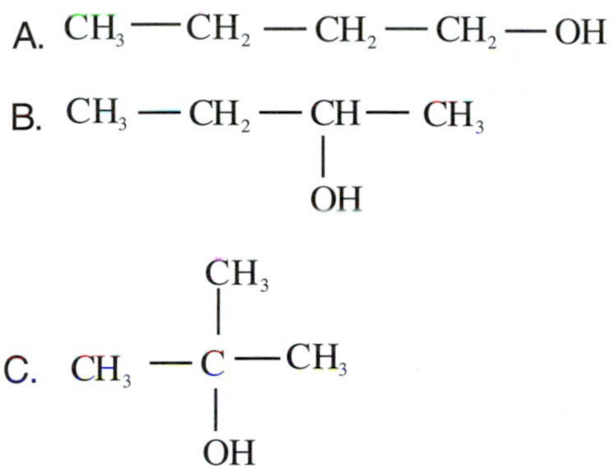

A. $CH_3—CH_2—CH_2—CH_2—OH$

B. $CH_3—CH_2—CH—CH_3$
            |
           OH

          CH_3
           |
C. $CH_3—C—CH_3$
           |
          OH

Figure 12–18. Primary (**A**), secondary (**B**), and tertiary (**C**) alcohols.

Butane (lighter fluid) is an alkane, and gasoline is a mixture of alkanes.

Hydrocarbons are of toxicologic importance for two reasons: they are widely abused as inhalational drugs of abuse (for their central nervous system depressant effects), and they can cause profound toxicity when aspirated. Although these effects are physiologically disparate, an understanding can be derived based on an understanding of the characteristics of the hydrocarbon functional group.

Hydrocarbons do not contain *polar groups*, or groups that introduce full or partial charges into the molecule; as such, they interact readily with other nonpolar substances, such as lipids or lipophilic substances. Hydrocarbons readily interact with the myelin of the central nervous system (CNS), disrupting normal ion channel function and causing CNS depression. When aspirated, hydrocarbons can dissolve the highly polar mixture of substances known as surfactant; the dissolution of surfactant can quickly lead to acute lung injury. Thus, a basic understanding of the alkane functional group and its potential reactivity leads to an understanding of the toxicity of this class of chemicals in vivo.

Alcohols are another functional group of toxicologic importance. Alcohols possess the hydroxyl (-OH) functional group, which adds polarity to the molecule and makes alcohols highly soluble in other polar substances, such as water. For example, ethane gas (CH_3CH_3) has negligible solubility in water, whereas ethanol (CH_3CH_2OH) is *miscible*, or infinitely soluble, in water. In

biologic systems, alcohols are generally CNS depressants; they can also act as nucleophiles, and the reaction of ethanol with cocaine to form cocaethylene is an important example (Fig. 12–17).

Alcohols can be primary, secondary, or tertiary, in which the reference carbon is bonded to 1, 2, or 3 carbons in addition to the hydroxyl group (Fig. 12–18). Methanol, in which the reference carbon is bonded to no other carbons, is also a primary alcohol. The difference between primary, secondary, and tertiary structures is important, because although the alcohol functional group imparts many qualities to the molecule, the degree of substitution can affect the chemical reactivity. Primary alcohols can undergo multistep oxidation to form carboxylic acids, whereas secondary alcohols generally undergo one-step metabolism to form ketones, and tertiary alcohols do not readily undergo oxidation. This is a point of significant toxicologic importance, and is discussed in more detail later.

Alcohols can be named in many ways; the most common is to add -ol or -yl alcohol to the appropriate prefix. If the alcohol group is bonded to an interior carbon, the number to which the carbon is bonded precedes the suffix.

Carboxylic acids contain the functional group -COOH. As their name implies, they are acidic, and the pKa of carboxylic acids is generally around 4 or 5, depending on the substitution of the molecule. Carboxylic acids are capable of producing a significant anion gap metabolic acidosis, which is true whether the acids are endogenous or exogenous. Examples of endogenous acids are β-hydroxybutyric acids and lactic acids; examples of exogenous acids are formic acid (produced by the metabolism of methanol) and glycolic, glyoxylic, and oxalic acids (produced by the metabolism of ethylene glycol). Carboxylic acids are named by adding -oic acid to the appropriate prefix.

Thiols contain a sulfur atom, which usually functions as a nucleophile. The sulfur atom of N-acetylcysteine can regenerate glutathione reductase, and can also react directly with NAPQI to detoxify this electrophile. The sulfur atom of many chelating agents, such as dimercaptopropanol and dimercaptosuccinic acid (as discussed earlier), are nucleophiles that are very effective at chelating electrophiles such as heavy metals. Thiols are generally named by adding the word *thiol* to the appropriate base. Thus, a 2-carbon thiol is ethane thiol.

Functional groups should be recognized as a crucial part of the molecule that confers both physical properties and chemical reactivity. Perhaps the most important point regarding functional

TABLE 12–5.   Physical Properties of Some Alkanes and Their Corresponding Alcohols

	MP, °C (°F)	BP, °C (°F)	State, STP	Water Solubility
Alkanes				
Methane	−182.6 (−296.68)	−161.4 (−258.52)	Gas	Negligible
Ethane	−172 (−277.6)	−88 (−126.4)	Gas	Negligible
Propane	−187.7 (−305.86)	−42 (−43.6)	Gas	Negligible
Alcohols				
Methanol	−97.8 (−144.04)	64.7 (148..46)	Liquid	Infinite
Ethanol	−114.1 (−173.38)	78.5 (173.3)	Liquid	Infinite
Ethylene glycol	−13 (8.6)	197.6 (387.68)	Liquid	Infinite
1-Propanol	−127 (−196.6)	97.2 (206.96)	Liquid	Infinite
Isopropanol	−88.5 (−127.3)	82.5 (180.5)	Liquid	Infinite

BP, boiling point; MP, melting point; STP, standard temperature and pressure. The disparity in MP and BP between ethylene glycol and the other alcohols is caused by the presence of the second hydroxyl (alcohol) group.

OH
|
CH_3
Methanol

OH
|
CH_3—CH_2
Ethanol

OH   OH
| |
CH_2—CH_2
Ethylene glycol

OH
|
CH_3-CH_2-CH_2
1-Propanol

OH
|
CH_3-CH—CH_3
Isopropanol

↓ *ADH*   ↓ *ADH*   ↓ *ADH*   ↓ *ADH*   ↓ *ADH*

O
||
CH_2
Formaldehyde

O
||
CH_3-CH
Acetaldehyde

OH   O
| ||
CH_2-CH
Glycoaldehyde

O
||
CH_3–CH_2–CH
Propylaldehyde

O
||
CH_3–C—CH_3
Acetone

Figure 12–19. Oxidation of selected alcohols by alcohol dehydrogenase (ADH).

groups is that *molecules with a given functional group often have more in common with molecules within the same functional group than they have in common with the molecules from which they were derived.*

As an example, consider the alkanes methane, ethane, and propane. All are straight chain hydrocarbons with similar properties. All are gases at room temperature, have almost no solubility in water, and have similar melting and boiling points. When these molecules are substituted with one or more hydroxide functional groups, they become alcohols: examples are methanol, ethanol, ethylene glycol (a *glycol* is a molecule that contains two alcohol functional groups), the primary alcohol 1-propanol, and the secondary alcohol 2-propanol (isopropanol). Each of these alcohols is a liquid at room temperature, and all are very water soluble. All have boiling points that are markedly different from the alkane from which they were derived, and quite close to each other. The physical properties of these alkanes and their corresponding alcohols are compared in Table 12–5.

In addition to conferring different physical properties on the molecule, the addition of the alcohol functional group also confers different chemical properties and reactivities. For example, methane, ethane, and propane are virtually incapable of undergoing oxidation in biologic systems. The alcohols formed by the addition of one or more hydroxide groups, however, are readily oxidized by alcohol dehydrogenase (Fig. 12–19). Acetaldehyde is

quickly metabolized to acetyl coenzyme A and enters into many normal biochemical processes. 1-Propanol is an infrequently encountered toxin. Neither is considered further in this section, leaving the toxic alcohols methanol, ethylene glycol, and isopropanol for discussion.

As Figure 12–19 indicates, the oxidation of the primary alcohols methanol and ethylene glycol results in the formation of *aldehydes* (an aldehyde is a functional group in which a carbon atom contains a double bond to oxygen and a single bond to hydrogen), whereas the oxidation of the secondary alcohol isopropanol resulted in the formation of a *ketone* (a ketone is a functional group in which a carbon is double-bonded to an oxygen atom and single-bonded to two separate carbon atoms). Although both aldehydes and ketones contain the *carbonyl group* (a carbon-oxygen double bond), aldehydes and ketones are distinctly different functional groups, and have different reactivity patterns. For instance, aldehydes can undergo enzymatic oxidation to carboxylic acids, whereas ketones cannot (Fig. 12–20).

It is here that recognition of functional groups helps us to understand the potential toxicity of an alcohol. Methanol, ethylene glycol, and isopropanol are all alcohols; as such, their toxicity before metabolism is expected to be (and in fact is) similar to that of ethanol, producing CNS sedation.

Because these toxins are primary and secondary alcohols, all three can be metabolized to a carbonyl compound, either an aldehyde or a ketone. Here, however, the functional groups on the molecules have changed; whereas aldehydes can be metabolized to carboxylic acids (which can, in turn, cause an anion gap acidosis), ketones cannot. It is for this reason that methanol and ethylene glycol can cause an anion gap acidosis, and isopropanol cannot.

The concept of functional groups, however useful, does have limitations. For example, although both formic acid and oxalic acid are organic acids, they have different patterns of organ system toxicity. Formic acid is a mitochondrial toxin, and exerts effects primarily in areas (such as the retina or basal ganglia) that poorly tolerate an interruption in the energy supplied by oxidative phosphorylation. Oxalic acid, on the other hand, readily precipitates calcium and is toxic to renal tubular cells, which accounts for the hypocalcemia and nephrotoxicity that are characteristic of severe ethylene glycol poisoning. Thus, although useful, the concept of the functional group is an aid to understanding chemical reactivity, not a substitute for a working knowledge of the effect of different toxins in living systems.

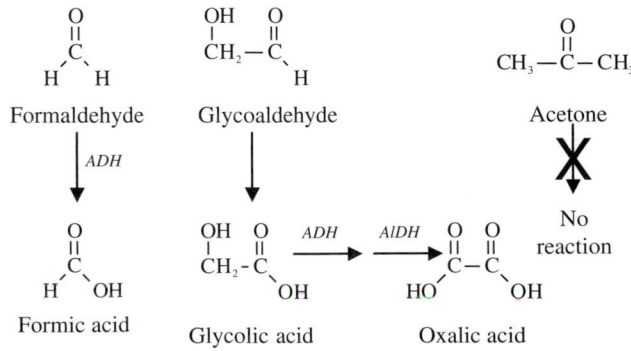

Figure 12–20. Oxidative fates of formaldehyde and glycoaldehyde. Note that acetone does not undergo further oxidation in vivo. ADH, alcohol dehydrogenase; AlDH, aldehyde dehydrogenase.

SUMMARY

Although not a substitute for a comprehensive knowledge of individual toxins, understanding key principles in inorganic and organic chemistry provides insight into the mechanisms by which poisons act.

REFERENCES

1. Bailey PS, Bailey CA: Organic Chemistry: A Brief Survey of Concepts and Applications, 5th ed. Englewood Cliffs, NJ, Prentice-Hall, 1995.

2. Kasprzak KS: Possible role of oxidative damage in metal-induced carcinogenesis. Cancer Invest 1995;13:411–430.

3. Loudon GM: Organic Chemistry, 3rd ed. Redwood City, CA, Benjamin/Cummings Publishing, 1995.

4. Manahan SE: Toxicologic Chemistry. Boca Raton, FL, Lewis Publishers, 1992.

5. McMurry J, Castellion ME: General, Organic, and Biological Chemistry, 2nd ed. Upper Saddle River, NJ, Prentice Hall, 1996.

6. Oulette RJ, Rawn JD: Organic Chemistry. Upper Saddle River, NJ, Prentice-Hall, 1996.

7. van der Vliet A, Cross CE: Oxidants, nitrosants, and the lung. Am J Med 2000;109:398–421.

CHAPTER 13   BIOCHEMICAL PRINCIPLES

Kathleen A. Delaney

Xenobiotics injure living organisms by interfering with critical metabolic processes, either causing structural injury to cells or by altering the cellular genetic material. The specific biochemical sites of actions that disrupt metabolic processes are well characterized for many xenobiotics although mechanisms of cellular injury are not. This chapter focuses on those general biochemical principles that are relevant to an understanding of the injurious effects of toxic xenobiotics, with references to a few well-characterized toxins whose mechanisms of action illustrate basic principles. It also reviews the clinical implications elucidated by recent studies of biotransformation enzymes. Mutagens and carcinogens are discussed in Chap. 16.

Knowing what a xenobiotic does at its site of action—for example, enzyme or receptor inhibition, DNA alteration, or lipid peroxidation—contributes only partly to understanding the injurious interaction between a xenobiotic and a living organism. How the xenobiotic is absorbed, distributed, and eliminated, and where it is activated or detoxified, all affect the form and concentration of the toxin in different tissues, and its capacity to produce injury. Damage may be confined to one organ by the mechanism of exposure, such as gastrointestinal or dermal injury by a caustic agent; hepatocellular injury following ingestion of a xenobiotic selectively delivered to the liver by the portal venous system; or pulmonary injury by an inhaled xenobiotic. In addition, the ability of a toxic substance to enter a particular organ is an important factor in toxicity. As an example, many potential central nervous system (CNS) toxins fail to produce injury because they cannot cross the blood-brain barrier. The negligible CNS effects of the mercuric salts when compared with organic mercury compounds are related to their inability to penetrate the CNS. Two potent biologic toxins—ricin (from *Ricinus communis*) and α-amanitin (from *Amanita phalloides*), both block protein synthesis through the inhibition of RNA polymerase. Their very different clinical effects are related to tissue accessibility. Ricin has a special binding protein that enables it to gain access to the endoplasmic reticulum in gastrointestinal (GI) mucosal cells where it inhibits cellular protein synthesis and causes severe diarrhea.[44] α-Amanitin is transported into hepatocytes by the bile salt transport systems, where inhibition of protein synthesis leads to cell death.[41,47]

The electrical charge on a toxin also affects its ability to enter a cell. Unlike ionized or charged toxins, uncharged, or lipophilic substances pass easily through lipid cell membranes to enter the systemic circulation. Depending on its pK_a, a molecule may be charged or uncharged in different pH environments. This affects the site of gastrointestinal absorption (see Chap. 11 for a more extensive discussion of basic principles of pharmacokinetics.)

TOXINS THAT INHIBIT CRITICAL BIOCHEMICAL PATHWAYS

When inhibition of a specific enzyme disrupts critically important biochemical pathways, rapid cellular death occurs. Such important metabolic pathways include glycolysis, the tricarboxylic acid or Krebs cycle, and oxidative phosphorylation.

Glycolysis results in the oxygen-independent, or anaerobic metabolism of glucose (Fig. 13–1). The tricarboxylic acid cycle and oxidative phosphorylation are the major pathways of oxidative metabolism (Fig. 13–2). These pathways are primarily responsible for the synthesis of adenosine triphosphate, or ATP, the metabolic fuel required for synthetic functions, active transport, and maintenance of electrolyte balance and membrane integrity. Oxidative phosphorylation also disposes of electrons or "reducing equivalents" generated by the oxidative metabolism of cellular fuels such as sugars and lipids. Oxidative metabolism is highly energy efficient, producing 36 moles of ATP for each mole of glucose metabolized, compared to the 2 moles of ATP produced by glycolysis. The following sections review the basics of cellular metabolism and those toxins that affect critical metabolic functions.[52]

Roles of NADH and NADPH in Metabolism

The pyridine nucleotides NADPH/NADP⁺ (nicotinamide adenine dinucleotide phosphate) and NADH/NAD⁺ (nicotinamide adenine dinucleotide) function in their reduced and oxidized forms to transport electrons in oxidation-reduction reactions. Oxidation involves the extraction of electrons from a substrate and their transfer to molecular oxygen or to another electron-seeking (electrophilic) substance. Reduction involves the transfer of electrons to a substrate. The reduction of NAD⁺ to NADH (or NADP⁺ to NADPH) requires two electrons plus a hydrogen ion (H⁺):

$$2e^- + H^+ + NAD^+ = NADH$$
$$2e^- + H^+ + NADP^+ = NADPH$$

NADH is primarily involved in the transfer of electrons extracted from catabolic processes by the 2-electron reduction of NAD⁺ to NADH and then to molecular oxygen through the mitochondrial cytochrome-mediated electron transport system. The ability to recycle NADH by "dumping" electrons picked up during the oxidation of various cellular fuels allows oxidative metabolism to proceed. This is the metabolic point where hypoxia exerts its deleterious effect (shown in Fig. 13–2).

202

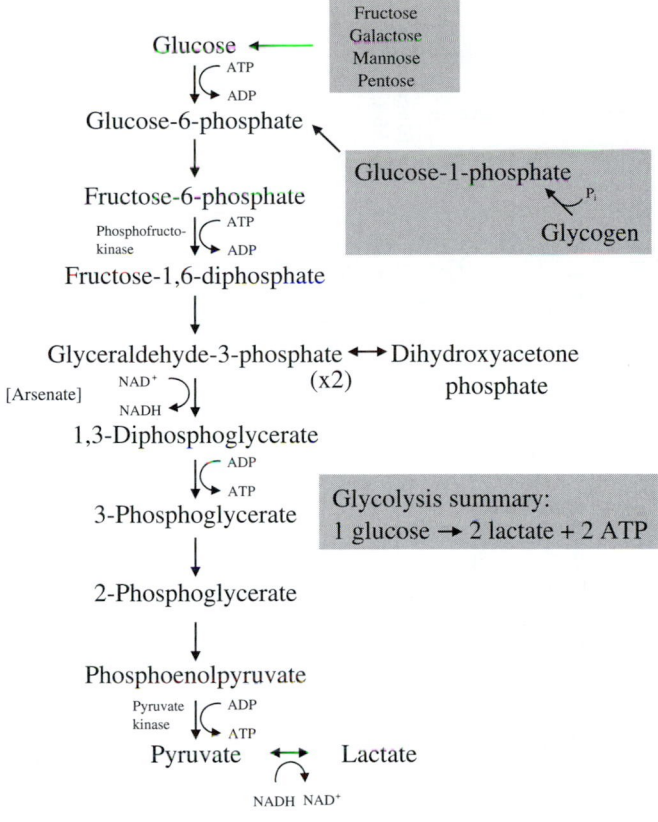

Figure 13–1. During glycolysis, the anaerobic metabolism of one mole of glucose to two moles of lactate results in the net production of 2 moles of ATP. Arsenic inhibits 3-phosphoglycerate dehydrogenase, which catalyzes the oxidation of glyceraldehyde-3-phosphate to 1,3-diphosphoglycerate.

NADPH serves primarily to carry electrons from the oxidative reactions of catabolism to the synthetic (anabolic) reactions of biosynthesis. It is also important in the cycling of oxidized glutathione to reduced glutathione, making an important contribution to the protection of cells from oxidative damage. It is present in significant amounts only in cells that are actively synthesizing new molecules, such as proteins, steroids, and fatty acids. The primary source of NADPH in the cell is the pentose phosphate pathway (also called the hexose-monophosphate shunt), an alternative pathway for the oxidation of glucose that produces NADPH and ribose-5-phosphate as a byproduct (Fig. 13–3).

Glycolysis

Glycolysis is the biochemical pathway responsible for the initial metabolism of glucose. Other sugars enter the glycolytic pathway after conversion to glycolytic intermediates (Fig. 13–1). The biochemical reactions depicted in Fig. 13–1 occur in the cytosol. Glycolysis results in the anaerobic production of two molecules of ATP for each molecule of glucose metabolized to pyruvate. Under anaerobic conditions, pyruvate is enzymatically reduced to lactate by lactate dehydrogenase in an NADH-requiring step that regenerates NAD^+. When NAD^+ and oxygen are available, pyruvate is converted by pyruvate decarboxylase to acetyl-CoA, which is

transported from the cytosol into the mitochondrion and condenses with oxaloacetate to form citrate and enter the Krebs cycle [37,52] (Fig. 13–2).

The toxicity of arsenic is caused in part by its effects on glycolysis, specifically on the enzyme 3-phosphoglyceraldehyde dehydrogenase (3-PGA), which catalyzes the oxidation of glyceraldehyde-3-phosphate to 1,3-diphosphoglycerate. This reaction normally results in the preservation of a high-energy phosphate bond that is used to synthesize ATP in the next step of glycolysis [15] (see Fig. 13–1). Arsenic effectively inhibits this step by forming an unstable intermediate that cannot be used in the synthesis of ATP. Arsenic substitutes for phosphate in the synthesis of 1,3-diphosphoglycerate, forming 3-phosphoglyceroyl arsenate. This unstable compound is rapidly hydrolyzed, resulting in interruption of glycolysis [56] (see Fig. 79–3).

The Krebs Cycle

Mitochondria contain all the enzymes essential to the function of the tricarboxylic acid or Krebs cycle (Fig. 13–2). These reactions are a major source of NADH and are critical to the aerobic production of ATP. The Krebs cycle oxidizes pyruvate, the end product of glycolysis, to ultimately form 1 molecule of CO_2, 1 molecule of GTP (guanosine triphosphate), and 5 molecules of NADH, which feed into the electron cytochrome transport chain and produce 15 molecules of ATP. In addition, the Krebs cycle provides intermediates for amino acid synthesis and for gluconeogenesis.[37]

Inhibitors of the Krebs cycle are significant toxins. Two powerful rodenticides—sodium fluoroacetate and fluoroacetamide—become incorporated into fluoroacetyl coenzyme-A and enter the Krebs cycle by condensation with oxaloacetate, forming fluorocitrate. This blocks the conversion of citrate to isocitrate by aconitase, resulting in the accumulation of large amounts of citrate in the mitochondria and inhibition of the cycle[83] (Fig. 13–2).

Thiamine is an important cofactor for Krebs cycle enzymes that carry out decarboxylation reactions. It is required for the conversion of pyruvate to acetyl-CoA by pyruvate decarboxylase and for the conversion of α-ketoglutarate to succinyl-CoA by α-ketoglutarate dehydrogenase.[85] The life-threatening effects of thiamine deficiency are likely related to impairment of these enzyme functions (see Antidotes in Depth: Thiamine).

The Electron Transport Chain and Oxidative Phosphorylation

The success of aerobic metabolism requires disposal of electrons generated by oxidative metabolism, so that new electrons can enter the pathway. The oxidative phosphorylation of adenosine diphosphate (ADP) to ATP captures energy generated by the oxidative reactions of the Krebs cycle in the high-energy phosphate bond of ATP (see Fig. 13–2). The electron transport chain consists of a series of cytochrome-enzyme complexes within the mitochondrial membrane. At various cytochrome steps, a hydrogen atom (H) is removed from NADH and split into a proton (H^+) and an electron (e^-). This occurs within the inner mitochondrial membrane. This process also regenerates oxidized NAD^+ from NADH, allowing oxidative metabolism to continue. The protons are pumped outside, setting up an energy gradient across the mitochondrial membrane. ATP synthase later captures the energy po-

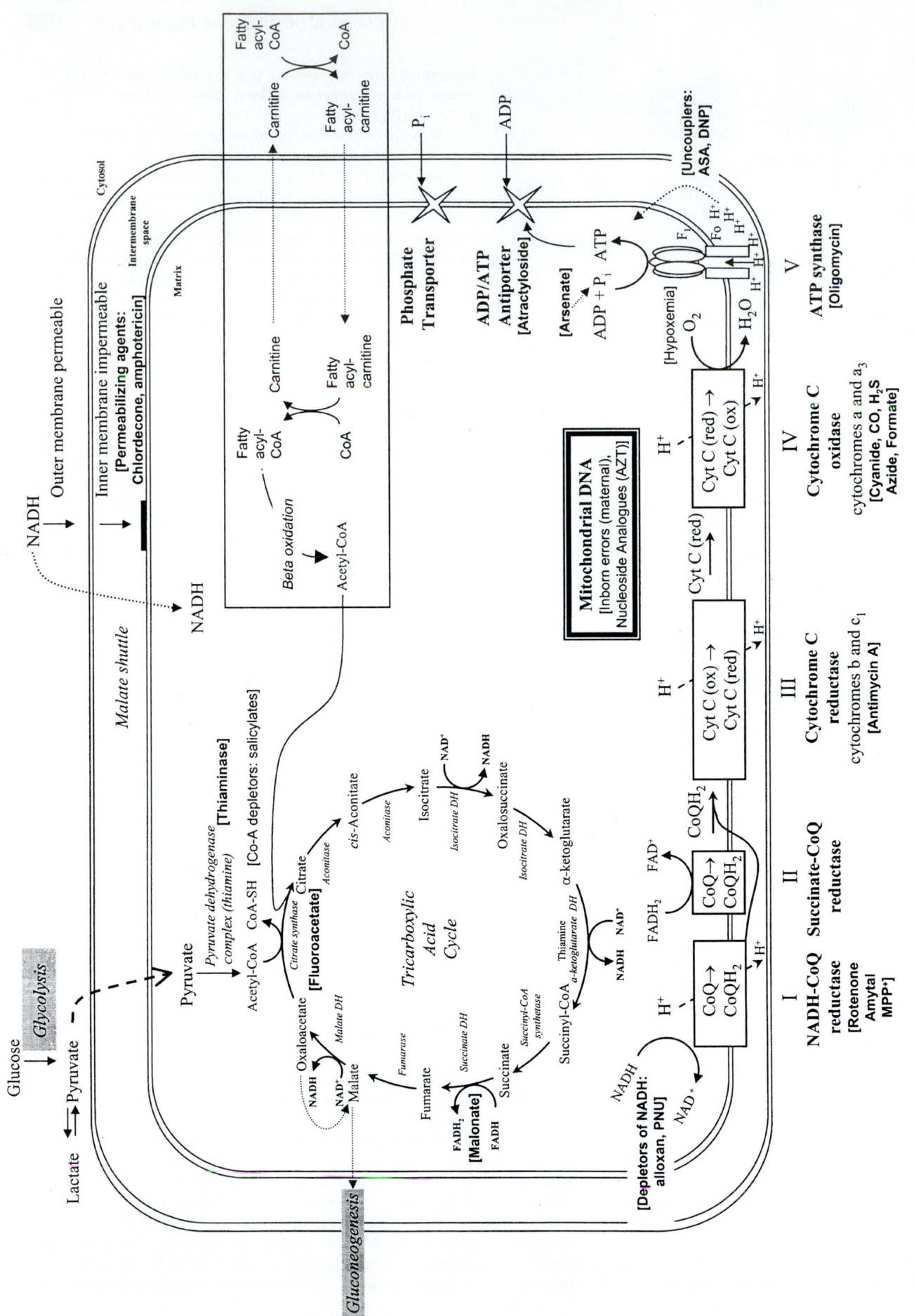

Figure 13–2. Pyruvate is converted to acetyl-CoA, which enters the Krebs cycle as shown. Reducing equivalents, in the form of NADH, and FADH donate electrons to a chain of cytochromes beginning with NADH dehydrogenase. These reactions "couple" the energy released during electron transport to the production of ATP. Ultimately, electrons combine with oxygen to form water. The sites of action of toxins that inhibit oxidative metabolism are shown. The sites where thiamine functions as a coenzyme are also illustrated. DH=Dehydrogenase.

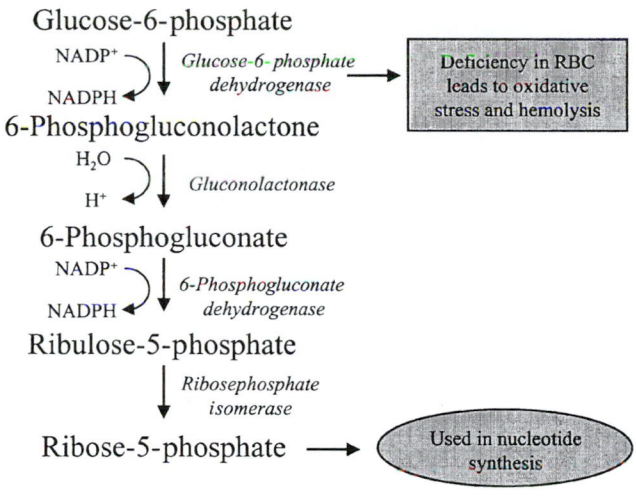

Glucose-6-phosphate

6-Phosphogluconolactone

6-Phosphogluconate

Ribulose-5-phosphate

Ribose-5-phosphate

Figure 13–3. The oxidation reactions of the pentose phosphate pathway are an important source of NADPH for reductive biosynthesis and for protection of cells against oxidative stress. Deficiency of the first enzyme in the pathway, G-6-PD, may result in RBC hemolysis during oxidative stress.

tential of this proton gradient in the high-energy bonds of ATP. The final step of oxidative phosphorylation, the reduction of molecular oxygen to water by cytochrome a-a3, enables perpetual regeneration of oxidized substrates. This last step also uses a proton, which increases the proton gradient across the mitochondrial membrane and helps to maintain the energy gradient.[52] (Fig. 13–2).

Toxins inhibit oxidative phosphorylation in two different ways. Inhibition of specific cytochromes shuts down the electron transport chain and causes a build up of reduced intermediates. Failure to regenerate oxidized substrates for the Krebs cycle shuts down oxidative metabolism. A second mechanism of interference occurs when toxins disrupt the coupling of the energy generated by electron transport to the synthesis of ATP. These are said to "uncouple" oxidative phosphorylation. Both of these mechanisms result in rapid depletion of cellular energy stores, followed by failure of ATP-dependent active transport pumps, loss of essential electrolyte gradients, and increases in cell volume.[52] Well-characterized toxins that block electron transport include cyanide, carbon monoxide, and hydrogen sulfide, which block the cytochrome a-a3–mediated reduction of O_2 to H_2O. The very dramatic clinical effects of significant cyanide exposure—rapid onset of seizures, profound lactic acidosis, myocardial depression, and rapid death—illustrate the importance of aerobic metabolism (Chap. 98). Other agents less commonly involved in poisoning also exert their toxic effects by inhibiting electron transport at various cytochrome steps: Sodium azide at cytochrome a-a3, antimycin A at the cytochrome b-c1 step, and rotenone (a toxic plant substance used by South American Indians to poison fish) at the NADH dehydrogenase-ubiquinone (CoQ) step.[6,7,75]

When the energy generated by electron transport cannot be coupled to ATP synthesis, it is released as heat. Various xenobiotics act as "uncouplers" of ATP synthesis. Fatal exposures of workers to dinitrophenol compounds used as weed killers and to pentachlorophenol, a wood preservative, are associated with severe hyperthermia that is attributed to heat generation by uncou-

pled electron transport.[49,51] Fatalities in rats following acute oral ingestion of dinitrophenol are also associated with significant hyperthermia.[79] In in vitro mitochondrial preparations, dinitrophenol stimulates increased glutamate oxidation associated with decreased ATP synthesis and no change in oxygen utilization, suggesting an uncoupling of oxidative phosphorylation from ATP synthesis.[61] More than 60 years ago, dinitrophenol was administered to patients for control of obesity. Although no reports of death can be found at the doses used, a significant incidence of cataracts was noted in patients who took as little as 2 mg/kg/d.[35] The hyperthermia and lactic acidosis resulting from severe salicylate poisoning are also attributed to its uncoupling of oxidative phosphorylation.[76]

OTHER METABOLIC PATHWAYS AFFECTED BY TOXINS
The Pentose Phosphate Pathway

The pentose phosphate pathway provides the only source of cellular NADPH. The reduction of $NADP^+$ to NADPH is accomplished by two enzymes in the pentose phosphate pathway, glucose-6-phosphate dehydrogenase (G6PD) and 6-phosphogluconate dehydrogenase[37,52] (Fig. 13–3). NADPH is used in cellular biosynthetic reactions and is also an important source of reducing power for the maintenance of sulfhydryl groups that protect the cell from free radical injury.[11] The cycling of oxidized glutathione to reduced glutathione, which is quantitatively the most important general antioxidant in cells, depends on the availability of NADPH. Red cells are especially vulnerable to deficiency of NADPH, which results in hemolysis during oxidative stress.

Another manifestation of oxidative stress in the red cell is the oxidation of the iron in hemoglobin from Fe^{2+} to Fe^{3+}, producing methemoglobin, which occurs both spontaneously and as a response to xenobiotics such as nitrites and aminophenols. Because the majority of reduction of methemoglobin is done by NADH-dependent methemoglobin reductase, which is not deficient in persons who lack G6PD, they do not develop methemoglobinemia under normal circumstances. However, when oxidative stress is severe and methemoglobinemia develops, persons who have G6PD deficiency have limited ability to utilize the alternative NADPH-dependent methemoglobin reductase that reduces methylene blue to leukomethylene blue to reduce methemoglobin.[86] In rare cases of severe G6PD deficiency, methylene blue, which has mild oxidative capabilities, may actually precipitate hemolysis (see Antidotes in depth: Methylene Blue).

Gluconeogenesis

Gluconeogenesis is the biochemical pathway localized predominantly in the liver that facilitates the conversion of amino acids and intermediates of the Krebs cycle to glucose. It is an important source of glucose during fasting, and enables maintenance of glycogen stores. The pathway is illustrated in Fig. 13–4. Most of the steps in the synthesis of glucose from pyruvate are simply the reverse of glycolysis, with three exceptions: (a) the conversion of glucose-6-phosphate to glucose, (b) the conversion of fructose-1,6-diphosphate to fructose-6-phosphate, and (c) the synthesis of phosphoenolpyruvate from pyruvate. The enzyme steps that catalyse these reactions in the direction of glycolysis are irreversible.

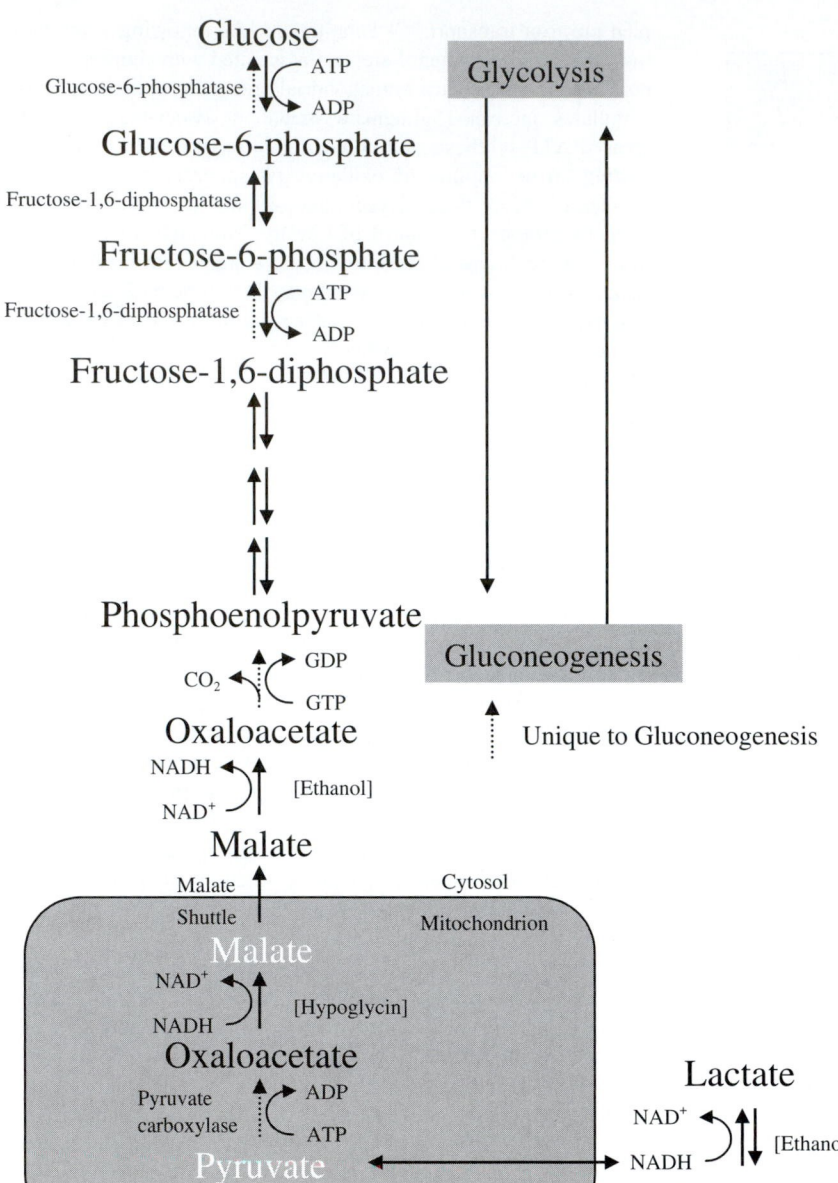

Figure 13–4. Gluconeogenesis reverses the steps of glycolysis, with the exception of the bypass of the three irreversible steps shown. The step from pyruvate to phosphoenolpyruvate involves both cytosolic and mitochondrial reactions that use ATP. Hypoglycin A inhibits the intramitochondrial conversion of oxaloacetate to malate by depleting NADH through interference with β-oxidation of fatty acids. Ethanol decreases cytosolic supplies of NAD+. Pyruvate kinase (PK) and phosphofructokinase (PFK), the enzymes whose activities are regulated by glucagon via cAMP-dependent phosphokinase, are shown.

While the first two gluconeogenic bypasses simply use different enzymes, the synthesis of phosphoenolpyruvate from pyruvate is more complex. Pyruvate is first converted to oxaloacetate within the mitochondria, then to malate, which is transported out of the mitochondria and converted in the cytosol back to oxaloacetate, then to phosphoenolpyruvate. Certain amino acids, notably alanine, glutamate and aspartate, are readily converted to Krebs cycle intermediates and can be used in the synthesis of glucose through this cycle.[37]

The regulation of gluconeogenesis is opposite to that of glycolysis. Both glucagon and catecholamines stimulate the synthesis of glucose by activating cAMP-dependent protein kinase A(PKA). PKA then phosphorylates two enzymes, phosphofructokinase (PFK) and pyruvate kinase. Phosphorylated PFK acts as a phosphatase, dephosphorylating fructose-1,6-diphosphate and pushing the reaction in the direction of gluconeogenesis. Phosphorylated

PFK activity is also affected by the ATP/ADP ratio. The rate of gluconeogenesis is highest when this ratio is high.[37] Phosphorylation of pyruvate kinase (PK) leads to inhibition of this important step of glycolysis, increasing activity in the gluconeogenesis pathway. PK is also inhibited by an increased ATP/ADP ratio.[37]

Gluconeogenesis depends on the presence of NAD+ in the cytosol, which is necessary to oxidize lactate to pyruvate. It also requires the presence of NADH within the mitochondria. Under conditions when the reducing potential (the NADH/NAD+ ratio) in the cytosol outside the mitochondria is high, gluconeogenesis is impaired.

A number of toxins impair gluconeogenesis, resulting in hypoglycemia when glycogen stores are depleted. Hypoglycin A, an unusual amino acid in unripe Akee fruit that is the cause of Jamaican vomiting sickness, causes profound hypoglycemia.[23,76,80] Its metabolite methylenecyclopropylacetic acid (MCPA) indirectly inhibits gluconeogenesis by blocking the oxidation of long-chain fatty acids, an important source of NADH in the mitochondrion. It also inhibits the metabolism of several glycogenic amino acids, including leucine, isoleucine, and tryptophan, and blocks their entrance into the Krebs cycle. MCPA may also prevent the transport of malate out of the mitochondria.[71,80–82]

Significant hypoglycemia occurs in fasting patients who are intoxicated with ethanol.[5,25] This is likely due to the impairment of gluconeogenesis by the increased cytosolic NADH/NAD$^+$ ratio associated with metabolism of ethanol by alcohol dehydrogenase. This inhibits the two steps that require NAD$^+$, the conversion of lactate to pyruvate and the conversion in the cytosol of malate to oxaloacetate.[5,45,68]

Fatty Acid Metabolism

Figure 13–5 illustrates the major reactions of fatty acid metabolism. Fatty acids mobilized in adipose tissue are taken into hepatocytes by passive diffusion. Under normal metabolic conditions their fate is determined by the metabolic needs of the cells. In energy-

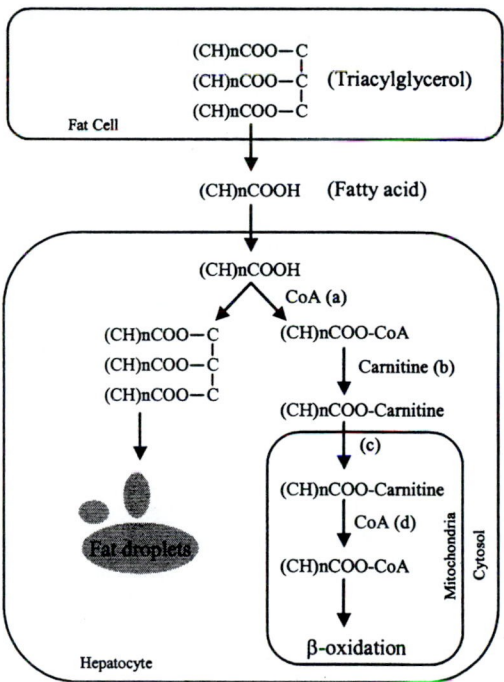

Figures 13–5. Steatosis, an accumulation of fat, results when toxins interfere with the oxidation of fatty acids. Other processes that may be associated with intracellular accumulation of fat include: (a) Impaired lipoprotein synthesis; (b) impaired lipoprotein release; (c) increased mobilization of free fatty acids; (d) increased uptake of circulating lipids; and (e) increased production of triglycerides. β-Oxidation takes place in the mitochondria after transport of fatty acids from the cellular cytosol across the mitochondrial membrane. The enzymes involved are (a) acyl-CoA synthetase; (b) carnitine palmitoyltransferase I; (c) carnitine acylcarnitine translocase; and (d) carnitine palmitoyltransferase II. Acyl-CoA is the intramitochondrial substrate for β-oxidation. Potential mechanisms of inhibition of β-oxidation include induction of carnitine deficiency, inhibition of the transferase or translocase, and increased NADH/NAD$^+$ ratio via increased utilization of NAD$^+$ or by inhibition of NADH utilization. The specific site of action is not defined for many toxins that cause steatosis.

repleted cells, fatty acids react with α-glycerol phosphate to form triacylglycerol, the first step in the synthesis of fat for storage. Triglycerides synthesized in the hepatocyte are then bound to lipoprotein to form very-low-density lipoprotein (VLDL), which is transported to and stored in adipocytes. In energy-depleted cells, fatty acids are transported into the mitochondrion where β-oxidation occurs. This is a complex process that requires the expenditure of cellular energy. The free fatty acid is converted to fatty acyl-CoA through an ATP-dependent reaction mediated by thiokinase, or acyl-CoA synthetase. The fatty acyl-CoA is then bound to carnitine by carnitine palmitoyltransferase forming fatty acylcarnitine, which is transported across the inner mitochondrial membrane. A reverse reaction catalyzed by a second carnitine palmitoyltransferase then reforms Acyl-CoA, which is a substrate for β-oxidation within the mitochondrion. This process is termed "β" oxidation because it involves the sequential removal of 2-carbon fragments of the fatty acid, each time acting at the β carbon position of the fatty acid. Each 2-carbon reaction produces 1 mole of NADH and 1 mole of flavin adenine dinucleotide (FADH$_2$), which enter oxidation phosphorylation, and 1 mole of acetyl-CoA, which enters the Krebs cycle and is oxidized to CO$_2$. This process produces 1.3 times more ATP per molecule of carbon metabolized than does the metabolism of glucose or other carbohydrates.[37]

Many xenobiotics interrupt fatty acid metabolism at various steps, resulting in accumulation of triglycerides in the liver. Table 13–1 lists toxins that are commonly associated with impaired fat metabolism. The mechanisms of the disruption of fatty acid metabolism are not well defined, although some agents have been shown to inhibit β-oxidation, at least indirectly, through effects on NADH levels. These include ethanol, hypoglycin, and nucleoside analogues (Chap. 14). Recently a syndrome of peripheral fat wasting, central adiposity, hyperlipidemia, and insulin resistance has been identified in patients taking protease inhibitors. A complex disturbance of regulation of fat metabolism by protease inhibitors is proposed, beginning with interference with the regulation of peripheral adipocyte differentiation, followed by impaired peripheral fat storage and the associated consequences of hyperlipidemia.[17]

The condition of alcoholic ketoacidosis is related in part to inhibition of gluconeogenesis in the alcoholic patient and in part to an exuberant response to nutritional needs by the fatty-acid machinery. Vomiting in the alcoholic patient leads to decreased intake of carbohydrate, which stimulates a starvation response with increases in serum glucagon, cortisol, growth hormone and epinephrine levels and depression of insulin. When the need for carbohydrate is not met by gluconeogenesis, lipolysis, which is normally inhibited by insulin, is intensified and fatty acid mobilization progresses. Glucagon stimulates mitochondrial carnitine acyltransferase, and β-oxidation of fatty acids is increased. The increased mitochondrial NADH/NAD+ ratio favors the production of β-hydroxybutyrate over acetoacetate, its oxidized form. The administration of glucose to the alcoholic patient leads to correction of this process.[70]

TABLE 13–1. Toxins that Interfere with Fatty Acid Metabolism

Aflatoxin	Nucleoside analogues (AZT, fialuridine)
Amiodarone	Protease inhibitors
Cereulide	Tetracycline
Cortisone	Valproic acid
Hypoglycin ("Ackee Fruit")	Vitamin A
Margosa oil	

MECHANISMS OF PHYSIOLOGIC INHIBITION BY TOXINS

Toxins That are Substrates for Synthetic Enzymes

Sometimes a toxin is mistaken for a natural substrate by synthetic enzymes, which act on it and facilitate its injurious effect. The incorporation of the rodenticide fluoroacetate into the Krebs cycle, described earlier, is an example of this mechanism of toxic injury (Fig. 13–2). Another example is illustrated by analogues of purine or pyrimidine bases that are phosphorylated and inserted into growing DNA or RNA chains, resulting in mutations and disruption of cell division. This mechanism is used therapeutically in the case of antitumor agents such as 5-fluorouracil (5-FU), a pyrimidine base analogue. When phosphorylated to 5-fluoro-dUTP and incorporated into growing DNA chains, the pyrimidine base analogue causes structural instability of the growing tumor cells[72] (Chap. 47).

TOXINS PRODUCED BY DETOXIFICATION REACTIONS

The ability to detoxify and eliminate both endogenous toxins and exogenous xenobiotics is crucial to the maintenance of physiologic homeostasis and normal metabolic functions for all organisms. A simple example is the necessity of detoxifying cyanide, a potent cellular poison that is ubiquitous in the environment and that is also a product of normal metabolism. Mammals have evolved the enzyme rhodanese, which combines cyanide with thiosulfate to create the less toxic, renally excreted compound thiocyanate.[84]

Enzymes that function to detoxify xenobiotics are ubiquitous in the body. Many of them facilitate the biotransformation of broad classes of substrates such as alcohols, aldehydes, esters, or amines, acting on many different substrates within these groups. The locations of these enzymes are often related to their function. Enzymes that act on more fat soluble, lipophilic xenobiotics are commonly found embedded in lipid membranes such as the endoplasmic reticulum. When cells are mechanically disrupted and centrifuged, these membrane-bound enzymes are found in the pellet or microsomal fraction, hence they are called microsomal enzymes. Enzymes located in the liquid matrix of cells are called cytosolic enzymes and are found in the supernatant when disrupted cells are centrifuged. Microsomal enzymes are found primarily in the liver, but also exist in the kidney, lung, gut, and urinary bladder. Cytosolic biotransformation enzymes are found in all tissues.[40] Many episodes of cellular injury occur during the metabolism and attempted detoxification of xenobiotics, representing the effects of cellular detoxification strategies gone awry. The following sections review the basic reactions involved in the detoxification of xenobiotics and discuss mechanisms of cellular injury related to these processes.

Mechanisms of Biotransformation of Xenobiotics

Phase I Reactions. The majority of xenobiotics have lipophilic properties that facilitate absorption through the skin, lungs, or mucosal surfaces. These require metabolic transformation to more water-soluble compounds before they can be excreted. These transformations are mediated by phase I and phase II biotransformation reactions. Phase I reactions result in the synthesis of a more chemically reactive metabolite of a lipophilic xenobiotic. In most cases, these are followed by phase II reactions that conjugate the product produced in the phase I reaction with another molecule that detoxifies it, renders it significantly more soluble, and facilitates its elimination.

Phase I reactions are primarily oxidation-reduction reactions. Oxidation involves the extraction of electrons from a substrate and their transfer to molecular oxygen or to another electron-seeking (electrophilic) substance such as NAD^+. Reduction involves the transfer of electrons to a substrate. Phase I reactions result in the addition of more polar, reactive groups such as hydroxyl (-OH), sulfhydryl (-SH), amino ($-NH_2$), aldehyde (-COH), or carboxyl (-COOH).[40] The most common biochemical oxidation-reduction reactions are mediated by three types of enzyme systems: (a) membrane bound iron-containing P450 cytochromes that are oxidized (Fe^{3+}) or reduced (Fe^{2+}) during their transfer of electrons from one substrate to another; (b) membrane-bound flavin-associated NADPH-dependent monooxygenases; and (c) cytosolic NADH or NADPH-linked dehydrogenases, which oxidize or reduce substrates by transfer of electrons between the oxidized (NAD^+, $NADP^+$) and reduced (NADH, NADPH) forms of these nucleotides.[28,42,46] Prostaglandin H synthase, found in abundance the renal tubules, participates in the biotransformation of xenobiotics. It metabolizes acetaminophen to a highly reactive semiquinoneimine.[22]

The cytochrome P450 enzymes, located primarily in the mitochondrial endoplasmic reticulum, are the most numerous and important of the enzymes involved in phase I oxidation reactions. They are heme proteins whose name derives from spectrophotometric characteristics of the heme molecule. When reduced cytochrome P450 (Fe^{2+}) binds to carbon monoxide, its maximal absorption spectrum occurs at 450 nm.[29] The cytochrome P450 system is actually a coupled system containing an NADPH-dependent reductase that facilitates the transfer of electrons from NADPH to the enzyme-substrate complex and a heme-containing cytochrome that then allows oxidation of the complex by molecular oxygen and transfer of electrons to oxygen to form a water molecule. These enzymes mediate many different types of oxidation reactions. A general example is illustrated by the oxidation of a foreign compound R-H to R-OH:

$$RH + NADH + O_2 \rightarrow NAD^+ + H_2O + ROH$$

This reaction occasionally proceeds through a reactive radical intermediate:

$$(FeO)^{3+} + RH \rightarrow [(FeOH)^{3+}R] \rightarrow Fe^{3+} + ROH$$

In other cases, electron transfer may result in the production of an activated metabolite:[29]

$$Fe^{3+} + ROOH \rightarrow RO^- + (FeOH)^{3+}$$

$$Fe^{3+} + ROOH \rightarrow RO + (FeOH)^{2+}$$

Reductive biotransformation is facilitated by the P450 system when the electrons donated by NADPH are transferred to the substrate, rather than to molecular oxygen. The reduction of a nitro group R-NO$_2$ to an amine R-NH$_2$ is an example of reductive bio-transformation. The clinical implications of the P450 system are discussed later.

Other important phase I reactions are mediated by the alcohol, aldehyde, and ketone oxidation system. These are predominantly cytosolic enzymes that depend on NAD$^+$ for oxidation reactions. A clinically familiar example is the metabolism of ethanol to ac-etaldehyde by alcohol dehydrogenase (ADH) followed by the rapid metabolism of acetaldehyde to acetic acid by aldehyde dehydrogenase (Fig. 13–6). Alcohol dehydrogenase (ADH) is a cyto-solic enzyme found in the liver, lungs, kidney, and gastric mucosa that oxidizes many different alcohols.[2,46] Gender-based differences in the activity of ADH in gastric mucosa may account for the greater observed effect of ethanol in women.[26] Atypical forms of ADH are responsible for the rapid oxidation of ethanol in Asian peoples, resulting in a characteristic flush as acetaldehyde, the product of ADH, accumulates. These persons may also be defi-cient in acetaldehyde dehydrogenase (ALDH), an enzyme that converts aldehydes to carboxylic acids, or, in this specific case, converts acetaldehyde to acetic acid.[2]

Pharmacokinetic properties of these enzymes determine the ex-tent of their involvement in the metabolism of a substrate. The ability of an enzyme to metabolize a substrate in a test tube does not predict its role in the cell. If two cellular enzymes are able to metabolize a substrate, but one requires a high concentration of the substrate in order to function, and needs only a low concentra-tion, the enzyme that works at the low concentration will be re-sponsible for most of the metabolism of that substrate. The K_m, which is defined as the concentration of enzyme that results in 50% of maximal enzyme activity, describes this property of en-zymes. For example, liver ADH has a very low K_m for ethanol, in-dicating that it is highly effective in metabolizing ethanol at very low concentrations, and is therefore the primary metabolic enzyme for ethanol.[46]

Ethanol may also be metabolized by an oxygen and NADPH-dependent cytochrome P450 enzyme named P4502E1. P4502E1 has a high K_m for ethanol, which means that it is functional only when ethanol levels are high. It accounts for only a small fraction of ethanol metabolism in those who drink modestly, but accounts for a significant fraction of ethanol metabolism in alcoholics. This enzyme is also inducible; that is, its concentration and activity in-crease in persons who chronically consume large amounts of ethanol.[46] The gene for this enzyme is named CYP2E1. P4502E1 also metabolizes other substrates such as acetaminophen and car-bon tetrachloride.[46]

Figure 13–6 illustrates the oxidation of ethanol to acetaldehyde by alcohol dehydrogenase and by P4502E1. In these reactions, NAD and NADP function in oxidation reactions in both their oxi-dized and reduced forms.

Conjugation (Phase II) Reactions. Conjugation with endoge-nous molecules such as glucuronic acid, glutathione, or sulfate, terminates pharmacologic activity and greatly increases the water solubility of the activated molecules resulting from phase I bio-transformation reactions. The resulting molecules are more readily excretable.[36,83] Phase II reactions are synthetic in nature and re-quire energy provided by the hydrolysis of high-energy phosphate compounds such as ATP.

Glucuronide formation is an important conjugation reaction. It occurs via glucuronyl transferase through conjugation of glu-curonic acid donated by uridine diphosphate glucuronic acid

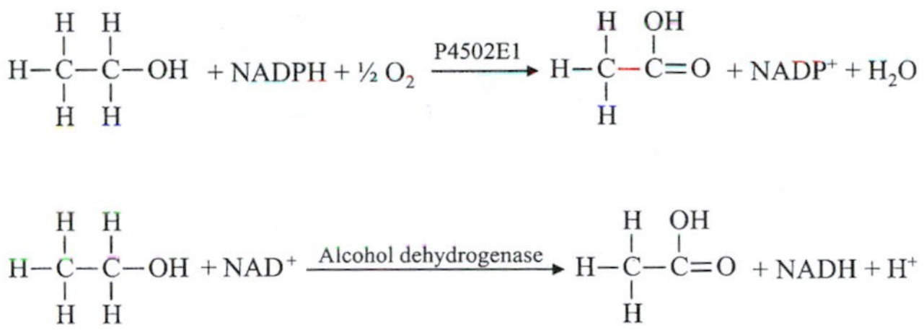

Figure 13–6. Conversion of ethanol to acetaldehyde by P4502E1 that uses reduced NADPH and oxygen and by alcohol dehydrogenase that uses oxi-dized NAD$^+$. This illustrates how NAD and NADP can function in oxidation reactions in both their oxidized and reduced forms. Alcohol dehydrogenase has a low K_m for ethanol and is the predominant metabolic enzyme in mod-erate drinkers.

(UDPG) with the nitrogen, sulfhydryl, hydroxyl, or carboxyl groups of foreign or endogenous compounds. The conjugated compounds are readily eliminated in the urine or bile, not only be-cause they are more polar, but because glucuronidation confers an ionized carboxyl group that is recognized by biliary and renal ac-tive transports systems for organic acids. The glucuronidation of aniline is illustrated in Fig. 13–7 and the glucuronidation of phe-nol and benzoic acid is illustrated in Fig. 13–8. Glucuronidation is an important mechanism for the detoxification of acetaminophen (Chap. 32).

Transfer of an inorganic sulfate group to the hydroxyl group of phenols or alcohols is another common mechanism for detoxifica-tion of compounds. The major donor for this reaction is oxidized cysteine. The sulfation of phenol illustrates an important concept in biotransformation (Fig. 13–7). The affinity of sulfate for phenol is very high, so that when low doses of phenol are administered, the predominant excretion product is the sulfate ester. However, the capacity of this reaction is readily saturated, so that when high doses of phenol are administered, glucuronidation becomes the main method of detoxification. Alternative biochemical pathways of metabolism are utilized when primary pathways are inaccessi-ble because of overwhelming concentrations of the toxin, deple-tion of important cofactors, or inhibition of the favored pathway

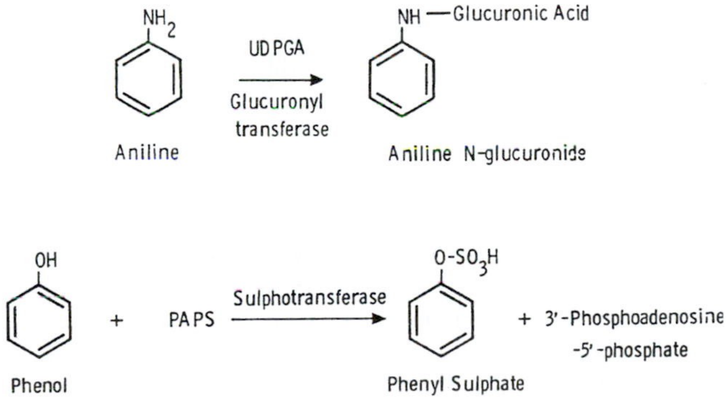

Figure 13–7. Examples of phase II conjugation reactions; aniline conjuga-tion with glucuronic acid, and phenol with sulfate. PAPS = 3′-phospho-adenosine-5′-phosphosulfate; UDPGA = uridine diphosphate glucuronic acid. (*Reprinted with permission from Timbrell JA: Principles of Biochemi-cal Toxicology. London, Taylor & Francis, 1987.*)

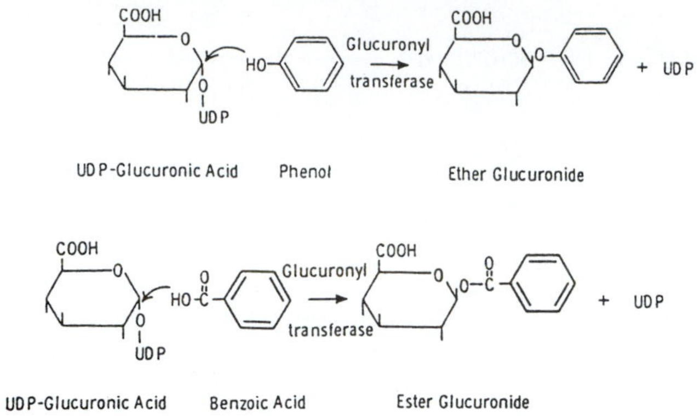

Figure 13–8. Formation of ether and ester glucuronides of phenol and benzoic acid, respectively. (*Reprinted with permission from Timbrell JA: Principles of Biochemical Toxicology. London, Taylor & Francis, 1987.*)

by another agent. This can result in the production of toxic metabolites that are not normally generated. A familiar example of this is the generation of the injurious electrophilic metabolite *N*-acetyl-*p*-benzoquinoneimine (NAPQI) during the metabolism of large amounts of acetaminophen (Chap. 32).

The glutathione-S transferases catalyze the conjugation of the tripeptide glutathione (glycine-glutamate-cysteine) with a diverse group of toxic compounds. The reactive compounds are electrophilic metabolites of P450 enzymes that initiate an electrophilic attack on the sulfur group of cysteine. The glycine and glutamate residues are then cleaved and the molecule acetylated, resulting in an *N*-acetylcysteine (mercapturic acid) conjugate that is readily excreted in the urine. This mechanism effectively detoxifies many reactive electrophiles produced by the P450 system. An important example of the clinical significance of this mechanism of detoxification in toxicology is the avid binding of NAPQI, the toxic metabolite of acetaminophen, by glutathione.[8,13] The importance of glutathione conjugation in the prevention of acetaminophen-induced liver injury is well appreciated.[53–55] The binding of glutathione to the epoxide metabolite of bromobenzene (Fig. 13–9) or naphthalene (Fig. 13–10) illustrates the broad importance of glutathione in the detoxification of a multitude of xenobiotics.

MECHANISMS OF CELLULAR INJURY

Ideally, reactive and potentially toxic metabolites produced by phase I reactions are detoxified during the phase II reaction. When detoxification goes awry, whether because of overproduction of a reactive intermediate or because of a deficiency of phase II substrates, toxic intermediates can cause cellular injury. Examples of agents that are transformed to more toxic agents by biotransformation are discussed in the following sections.

Injury by Metabolites at Distant Sites

Toxic metabolites may be synthesized at one site and transported to other target sites where they cause injury. Cyanide formed by the hepatic metabolism of acetonitrile nail removers acts at distant sites to produce toxicity.[16] This also appears to be the case for benzene, which is metabolized in the liver to benzoquinone and dihydroxybenzene intermediates that subsequently injure the

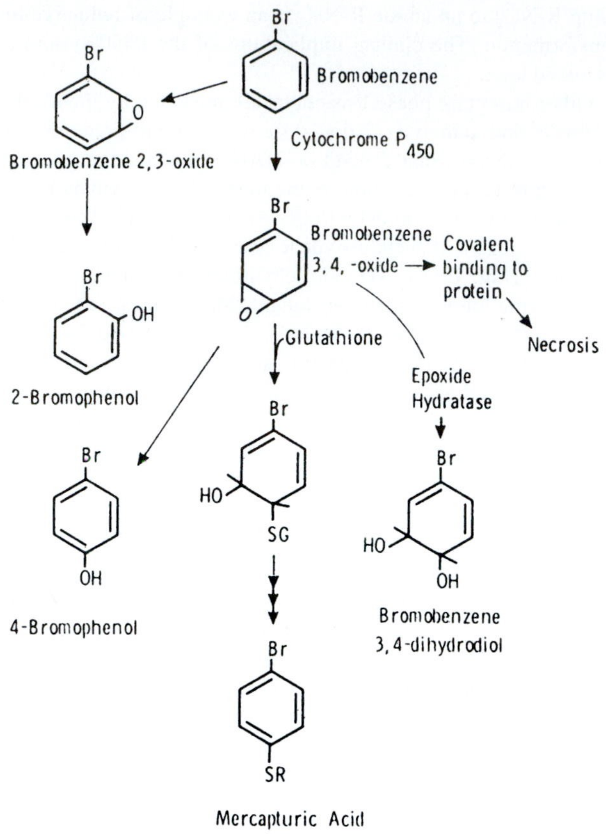

Figure 13–9. The metabolism of bromobenzene. Bromobenzene 2,3-oxide and 3,4-oxide may undergo chemical rearrangement to the 2- and 4-bromophenol, respectively. Bromobenzene 3,4-oxide may also be conjugated with glutathione and in its absence, react with tissue proteins. An alternative detoxification pathway is hydration to the 3,4-dihydrodiol via epoxide hydratase. (*Reprinted with permission from Timbrell JA: Principles of Biochemical Toxicology. London, Taylor & Francis, 1987.*)

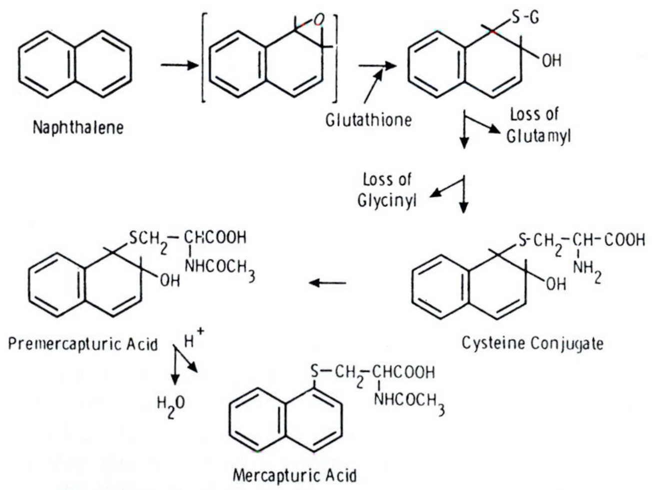

Figure 13–10. Conjugation of naphthalene-1,2 oxide with glutathione and formation of naphthalene mercapturic acid. (*Reprinted with permission from Timbrell JA: Principles of Biochemical Toxicology. London, Taylor & Francis, 1987.*)

bone marrow.[87] 2,5-Hexanedione, the neurotoxic metabolite of n-hexane and methyl-n-butyl ketone, is also produced in the liver, far from the site where injury occurs.[19]

The toxicity of ingested compounds may be altered by enzymatic activity or by bacterial flora in the GI tract. Laetrile (amygdalin) was used as an alternative treatment for cancer but caused deaths because of its metabolism to a cyanide. Amygdalin must be hydrolyzed in the gut to cyanide to exert its toxicity. When administered intravenously, amygdalin is not metabolized to cyanide and is not toxic.[33] Nitrates present in well water in farming communities are converted to nitrites by gut bacteria, leading to methemoglobinemia. A high gastric pH in very young infants allows the growth of enteric organisms in the stomach and makes them particularly susceptible to the toxic effects of ingested nitrates. Infants also have a reduced ability to detoxify nitrites.[69]

In Situ Injury by Metabolites of Biotransformation Reactions

The capacity of a tissue to metabolize certain toxins may be essential to the production of injury in that tissue. Highly reactive metabolites exert damage at the site where they are synthesized. Tissue injury by reactive metabolites occurs commonly in the liver, the major site of metabolism of foreign compounds, but occurs in other organs as well[28,77,89] (Chap. 14). The lungs, skin, kidneys, and gastrointestinal tract, even the nasal mucosa, have the capacity to convert xenobiotics to metabolites that result in local injury.[14,40] Cycasin, a naturally occurring carcinogen, is harmless when administered parenterally to animals. However, when administered orally, it is hydrolyzed by gut bacteria to methylazoxymethanol, a powerful carcinogen that causes colon cancers at the site of metabolism.[24,83] Similarly, following selective concentration in lung tissue, paraquat is transformed to an injurious free radical by enzymes in the nonciliated alveolar epithelial cells.[67]

Overdoses of acetaminophen lead to excessive hepatic production of the highly reactive electrophile NAPQI, which initiates a damaging covalent bond with hepatocytes (Chaps. 12 and 32). Acute renal tubular necrosis also occurs in patients with overdose of acetaminophen.[39] This is attributed to its metabolism by prostaglandin H synthase within renal tubular cells to a highly reactive semiquinoneimine.[22]

Monoamine oxidases (MAO) are mitochondrial enzymes present in many tissues. They oxidize a large number of different amines, including dopamine, epinephrine, and serotonin, and toxins such as primaquine and haloperidol. The metabolic activity of MAO was responsible for the outbreak of parkinsonism associated with the use of MPTP (methylphenyltetrahydropyridine), an unintended product of an attempt to synthesize a "designer" analog of meperidine, methylphenylpropionoxypiperidine (MPPP; Chap. 62). After crossing the blood-brain barrier, MPTP is transformed by MAO in glial cells to MPDP+ (methylphenyldiydropyridine), which is nonenzymatically converted to MPP$^+$. The MPP$^+$ is subsequently taken up by specific dopamine transport systems into dopaminergic neurons in the substantia nigra, resulting in neuronal death by inhibition of oxidative phosphorylation.[27]

Free Radical Formation

The mechanisms that lead to cellular injury by reactive metabolites are less well defined than those that result in metabolic impairment. Several mechanisms have been postulated. Free radicals are highly reactive molecules that have an unpaired electron in their outer orbits. They can be formed by homolytic cleavage of a covalent bond, illustrated by the reaction

$$AB \rightarrow A\cdot + B\cdot \text{ or } O_2 \rightarrow O\cdot + O\cdot$$

Free radicals are too reactive to be directly measured but their presence is implied by the products of their reactions. Oxygen free radicals are common products of metabolism, and "scavenging" enzymes such as superoxide dismutase and peroxidase are abundant in cells. In the presence of oxygen, certain toxins generate highly reactive free radicals that cause injury at the site of their formation. The ethanol-inducible P4502E1 likely has a significant role in the production of toxic injury by its substrates, including carbon tetrachloride, ethanol, and acetaminophen.[18] It produces significant amounts of superoxide and peroxide and, in the presence of iron, produces hydroxyl free radicals that readily initiate lipid peroxidation.[18] The most destructive oxygen free radical is the hydroxyl free radical, OH· which will react with any biologic molecule in the vicinity, causing damage to proteins, DNA, lipids, or carbohydrates. Free radicals are most destructive when they initiate chain reactions, such as occurs when a free radical attacks polyunsaturated fatty acids in cellular membranes, resulting in lipid peroxidation. (Chap. 12) Free radical attack on an unsaturated fatty acid in a lipid membrane removes a hydrogen atom from a methylene carbon and leaves an unpaired electron, causing the formation of a lipid radical that attacks other unsaturated fatty acid chains and results in a chain reaction, destroying the cellular membrane. Membrane destruction produces degradation products that initiate inflammatory reactions in the cell.[77] The formation of free radicals is implicated in the pulmonary injury caused by paraquat, the myocardial injury caused by doxorubicin, and the liver injury caused by carbon tetrachloride.[58,67,77] Paraquat reacts with NADPH to form a pyridinyl free radical, which, in turn, reacts with oxygen to generate the superoxide anion radical (Fig. 13–11). In the presence of iron, these superoxide radicals are converted to hydroxyl radicals that initiate lipid peroxidation in the lungs. Adriamycin is metabolized to a semiquinone free radical in the cardiac mitochondria, which in the presence of oxygen, forms a superoxide anion radical that initiates myocardial lipid peroxidation.[58] Carbon tetrachloride (CCl_4) is metabolized by the P4502E1 to the trichloromethyl radical ($\cdot CCl_3$), which binds covalently to cellular macromolecules. In the presence of oxygen, this is con-

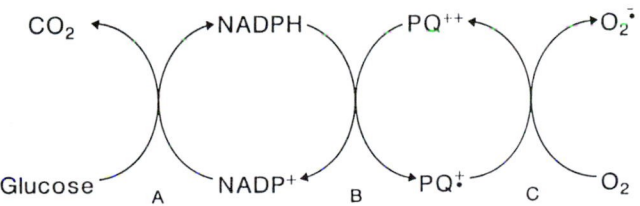

Figure 13–11. Formation of superoxide anion radical by oxidation-reduction of paraquat pyridynyl cation. The following reactions are involved in paraquat toxicity. **A.** Pentose phosphate pathway provides reducing equivalents in the form of NADPH. **B.** Paraquat pyridinyl cation (PQ^{++}) is reduced to cation radical ($\cdot$PQ$^+$). This reaction proceeds continuously being catalyzed by NADPH cytochrome P450 reductase. **C.** Oxidation-reduction cycling of pyridinyl cation radical reaction with molecular oxygen forms superoxide anion radical and pyridinyl cation. (*Reprinted with permission from Southern PA, Powis G: Free radicals in medicine: 1. Chemical nature of biologic reactions. Mayo Clin Proc 1988;63:381.*)

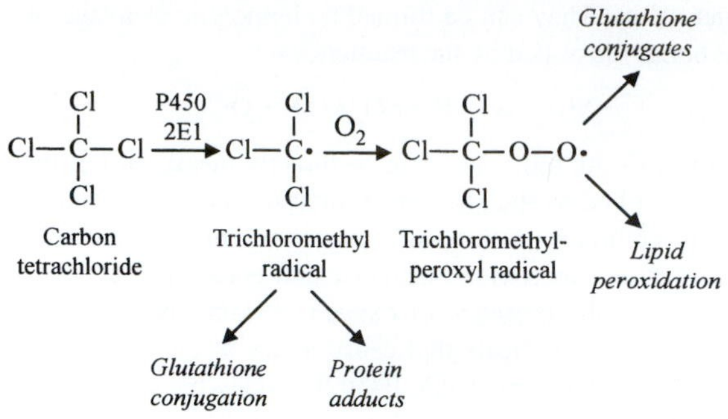

Figure 13–12. Carbon tetrachloride metabolism by the hepatocyte. Under hypoxic conditions, the CCl_3 radical is the predominant species formed. At higher oxygen tensions, CCl_3 radical is oxidized to the CCl_3OO radical, which is more readily detoxified by glutathione. Both free radicals bind to hepatocytes and cause cellular injury.

verted to the trichloromethylperoxyl radical ($\cdot CCl_3O_2$), which can initiate lipid peroxidation[68] (Fig. 13–12).

Adduct Formation

Activated xenobiotics formed by phase I biotransformation reactions may also injure cells by binding, or forming adducts, with cellular molecules. This occurs with hepatocellular injury by acetaminophen. How the binding of an activated toxin to a cellular macromolecule causes injury to the cell is not known. Interference with enzyme activity as a result of alteration of the conformational structure of adduct-bound proteins has been postulated.[8] Suicidal alkylation of P450 enzymes by activated substrates may stimulate lysosomal proteolysis.[29] In the case of acetaminophen-induced hepatotoxicity, cellular injury does not occur in the absence of demonstrable binding of NAPQI to cellular protein constituents; but again, the exact mechanism of injury is unknown.[9] Some cases demonstrate autoimmune mechanisms. The most likely mechanism by which a drug precipitates autoimmune injury is through the formation of an adduct with a cell, which then induces an immune response against the drug-macromolecule or against an immunologically altered cellular macromolecule. Cell destruction might then be mediated by complement or antibody directed lysis; by specific cell-mediated cytotoxicity; or by an inflammatory response induced by immune complexes and complement.[50,66] The idiosyncratic form of halothane hepatitis is associated with autoantibodies against a neoantigen formed by an adduct of halothane with an hepatoprotein (Chap. 14) Very recent studies have shown autoantibodies against the P450E1 enzyme in halothane hepatitis.[21] A trifluoroacetyl protein adduct similar to that associated with halothane hepatitis was detected in workers who developed hepatic necrosis following exposure to hydrochlorofluorocarbons.[34]

OTHER CLINICAL IMPLICATIONS OF BIOTRANSFORMATION REACTIONS: METABOLISM OF PHARMACEUTICS

The major enzyme participants in the phase I biotransformation of xenobiotics are the P450 enzymes. Information about these enzymes is accumulating rapidly. More than 200 genes coding for

P450 enzymes have been identified and classified into more than 30 families based on their amino acid sequences.[30] Enzymes that share less than 40% of their amino acid sequences are classified into different gene families (CYP1, CYP2, CYP3, etc), while enzymes that share 40–55% of their sequences are in different subfamilies (CYP1A, CYP1B, CYP1C, etc). Those that have greater than 55% homology of their amino acid sequences are in the same subfamilies (CYP1A1, CYP1A2, CYP1A3, etc). All of the P450 enzymes that have a role in metabolism of xenobiotics in humans belong to three gene families: CYP1, CYP2, and CYP3.[59] A great deal of information about the substrate selectivity and catalytic activity of the different P450 enzymes is known.[28] Most of these enzymes have low substrate specificity and can enzymatically alter a variety of substances.[28] The amount of the enzyme and the sensitivity of the enzyme for the substrate (its K_m) makes one P450 enzyme dominant over another.[28,30] Because many different P450 enzymes may catalyze the same reaction in vitro, it is sometimes difficult to determine which enzyme has the major role in vivo, that is, which has the lowest K_m and the fastest rate. In addition, the lack of specificity allows metabolism of a substance to occur in spite of deficiency of a specific enzyme. The effect of the K_m for ethanol on its metabolism by ADH and the P450 system was discussed earlier. As another example, diazepam is metabolized by both P4502C19 and P4503A4. However the affinity of P4503A4 for diazepam is so low (that is, the K_m is high) that the majority of diazepam is metabolized by P4502C19.[38] Omeprazole, which is also metabolized by P4502C19, competitively blocks the metabolism of diazepam and significantly prolongs its half-life.[63] Other P450 enzymes are highly selective. This is the case for P45021A2, a mitochondrial enzyme that specifically catalyzes the 21-hydroxylation of progesterone, an important step in steroid synthesis.[28]

The functional heterogeneity exhibited by these different enzymes has considerable impact on the potential toxicity of xenobiotics in an individual patient. Functional differences are related to the genetic polymorphism among human P450 systems and to alterations by concomitant exposure to other agents.

Genetic Effects on Drug Metabolism by P450 Enzymes

Nearly 90% of oxidative transformation of drugs is accomplished by 6 P450 enzymes, encoded by genes CYP1A2, CYP2C9, CYP2C19, CYP2D6, CYP2E1, and CYP34A.[74] Increasingly, isolated genetic mutations are associated with specific variations in the effects of drugs on individual patients. Important examples are illustrated by the impact of the genetically defined availability of P4502D6 and CYP2C9 on the toxicity of certain drugs (see the discussions of P4502D6 and CYP2C9 below).

Drug-Drug and Drug-Chemical Interactions with P450 Enzymes. Drugs metabolized by the same enzyme are shown to alter the metabolism of other drugs, resulting in adverse drug-drug interactions. Many of these are not apparent in initial drug studies, and are not predictable even when the P450 enzyme responsible for the metabolism of a drug is known, because of overlapping substrate specificities of many P450 enzymes. The life-threatening interactions between terfenadine and ketoconazole, both metabolized by P4503A4 (see below), were not defined or appreciated until 11 years after terfenadine was marketed.[74] Terbinafine, an oral antifungal agent that has been used in Canada for the past 8 years, was recently shown to strongly inhibit P4502D6, an enzyme responsible for the oxidation of 35 other drugs, including some β-adrenergic and calcium channel blocking drugs and tricyclic antidepressants. Drug interactions involving terbinafine have yet to be identified and defined despite this revelation, so that the clinical significance of this information is unknown.[3,74] Effects of environmental chemicals, such as the induction of P45 1A2 by smoking, or the inhibition of P4503A4 by grapefruit juice (discussed below) also result in alterations in drug metabolism that, although statistically significant, do not appear to be have great clinical consequences.[1] Serious clinical consequences result when impairment of metabolism results in large changes in drug level, or when the drug has a low toxic-therapeutic ratio.

The drug interactions of a single drug cannot be predicted by its class. The HMG-CoA inhibitors are an excellent example of this problem. Of the 5 statins currently on the market for treatment of dyslipidemia, 3 are metabolized by P4503A4, 1 is metabolized by P4502C9, and 1 is not metabolized at all. Detailed pharmacokinetic knowledge allows prediction of potentially serious drug interactions for some patients; for example, a renal transplant patient on cyclosporin or an AIDS patient on a protease inhibitor, both of which are powerful inhibitors of P4503A4, should avoid the use of a drug that is metabolized by P4503A4.[32]

Some well-defined examples of P450 enzymes and their effects are discussed below.

P4503A4. This is the most abundant P450 enzyme, comprising anywhere from 30–70% of the mass of hepatic P450 enzymes.[32] More than 150 drugs are known to be metabolized by P4503A4, many with significant potential for toxicity. These include dihydropine calcium channel blockers, cyclosporine, cisapride, many of the opioid analgesics, and many of the HMG-CoA reductase inhibitors.[32] An excellent example of an adverse drug interaction related to P450 enzyme characteristics is the discovery that patients taking terfenadine in combination with ketoconazole or erythromycin develop QT prolongation and spontaneous ventricular tachycardia. This is caused by inhibition of P4503A4 metabolism of terfenadine by these other enzyme substrates.[57,64,74] A substance in grapefruit juice also decreases the clearance of felodipine, nifedipine, terfenadine, and cyclosporin by P4503A, although the clinical implications of this remain unclear.[1,20] CYP3A4 does not exhibit genetic polymorphism.[64]

P4502D6. This enzyme was first detected as the enzyme responsible for the metabolism of the antihypertensive debrisoquine, hence it is sometimes referred to as debrisoquine hydrolase. About 8% of whites and 3% of blacks are deficient in this enzyme. Although it accounts for only 4% of hepatic P450 enzymes, it has a very important substrate profile that the metabolism of phenformin, several tricyclic antidepressants, the newer selective serotonin reuptake inhibitors (SSRIs), antiarrhythmics, and many others.[28,32,64] Perhexiline, an antianginal agent marketed in Europe in the 1980s, caused severe liver disease and peripheral neuropathy in persons with a demonstrated inability to metabolize debrisoquine.[73] Decreased activity of P4502D6 was implicated in the development of severe lactic acidosis in some patients taking phenformin.[60] This enzyme is inhibited by any substance that it metabolizes, an effect that resulted in a 10-fold decrease in the clearance of desipramine when coadministered with fluoxetine in one study. The toxic implications of this are clear.[10] Quinidine also inhibits P4502D6, although it is not a substrate for the enzyme.[10,64]

P4502E1. P4502E1 is a form of P450 that has significant toxicologic implications. It is inducible by a number of substances including ethanol, phenobarbital, isoniazid, phenytoin, and cigarette smoke.[43,88] It also actively produces free radicals such as hydroxyl (OH·), superoxide ($O_2\cdot^-$), peroxide (H_2O_2) and other reactive metabolites associated with adduct formation and lipid peroxidation. Free radical production has been extensively demonstrated in rat and rabbit livers, and in cultured human hepatocytes. It occurs during the metabolism of a number of substrates including carbon tetrachloride, ethanol, acetaminophen, paranitrophenol, aniline and *N*-nitrosomethylamine.[19] Induction of this enzyme is associated with increased liver injury by reactive metabolites of carbon tetrachloride (Chap. 14). It also increases liver injury by bromobenzene in rats.[31] Acute elevations of ethanol inhibit this enzyme. This effect is illustrated by the capacity of acute administration of ethanol to inhibit the metabolism of methadone by P4502E1, resulting in higher brain levels, while chronic ingestion hastens its metabolism. Cimetidine also inhibits P4502E1 and is protective against liver injury by acetaminophen in rats.[43,65,78] Acute ethanol ingestion inhibits the metabolism of acetaminophen by cytochrome P450 and may also be protective.[12]

Table 11–6 lists some of the defined human P450 enzymes and their substrates. For the reader who wishes more depth in this subject, Parkinson wrote a highly comprehensive review of the P450 enzymes and their roles.[62]

P4502C9. P4502C9 is the most abundant enzyme of the CYP2C family, which comprises approximately 20% of the P450 enzymes in the liver.[32] A recent study demonstrates a significant association between mutation of the CYP2C9 gene that codes for the enzyme responsible for the oxidative metabolism of the S-isomer of warfarin, and increased risk of bleeding. Patients with a very low daily dose requirement of 1.5 mg of warfarin per day or less had a 6.21% increase in the incidence of the mutated CYP2C9 allele and 5.97% increase in the risk of major bleeding complications, compared to a control group randomly selected from a coagulation clinic population.[4,48]

SUMMARY

Humans and animals are exposed to a wide variety of potential toxins. Some substances, including therapeutic drugs, are harmless at low doses and toxic only at high doses. The toxicity of those agents that interrupt important biologic functions or that result in cellular injury is dose-related and is manifested acutely. The diverse mechanisms of toxic injury have been discussed in general terms. The capacity of foreign chemicals to cause injury is clearly a function of many factors specific to the toxin, the tissue injured, and the individual animal or species.

REFERENCES

1. Abernethy DR: Grapefruits and drugs: When is statistically significant clinically significant? J Clin Invest 1997;99:2297–2298.
2. Agarwal DP, Goedde HW: Pharmacogenetics of alcohol dehydrogenase. In: Kalow W, ed: Pharmacogenetics of Drug Metabolism. New York, Pergamon, 1992, pp. 263–280.
3. Agdel-Rahman SM, Gotschall RR, Kauffman RE, et al: Investigations of terbinafine as a CYP2D6 inhibitor in vivo. Clin Pharmacol Ther 1999;65:465–472.

4. Aithal GP, Day CP, Kesteven PJ, Daly AK: Association of polymorphisms in the cytochrome P-450 CYP2C9 with warfarin dose requirement and risk of bleeding complications. Lancet 1999;353:717–719.

5. Arky RA, Freinkel N: Alcohol hypoglycemia. Arch Intern Med 1964;114:501–507.

6. Albert A: Fundamental aspects of selective toxicity. Ann N Y Acad Sci 1965;123:5–18.

7. Ariens EJ, Wius EW, Veringa EJ: Stereoselectivity of bioactive xenobiotics. Biochem Pharmacol 1988;37:9–18.

8. Badr MZ, Belinsky SA, Kauffman FC, Thurman RG: Mechanism of hepatotoxicity to periportal regions of the liver lobule due to allyl alcohol: Role of oxygen and lipid peroxidation. J Pharmacol Exp Ther 1986;238:1138–1142.

9. Bartolone JB, Beierschmitt WP, Birge RB, et al: Selective acetaminophen metabolite binding of hepatic and extrahepatic proteins: An in vivo and in vitro analysis. Toxicol Appl Pharmacol 1989;99:240–249.

10. Bergstrom RF, Peyton AL, Lemberger L: Quantification and mechanism of the fluoxetine and tricyclic antidepressant interaction. Clin Pharmacol Ther 1992;51:239–248.

11. Beutler E: Glucose-6-phosphate dehydrogenase deficiency. N Engl J Med 1991;324:169–174.

12. Black M, Raucy J: Acetaminophen, alcohol and cytochrome P450. Ann Intern Med 1986;104:427–429.

13. Boyland E, Chasseaud LF: The role of glutathione S-transferase in mercapturic acid biosynthesis. Adv Enzymol 1969;32:173–219.

14. Brittebo EB: Metabolism of xenobiotics in the nasal olfactory mucosa: Implications for local toxicity. Pharmacol Toxicol 1993;72:50–52.

15. Brown MM, Rhyne BC, Goyer RA, Fowler BA: Intracellular effects of chronic arsenic administration on renal proximal tubule cells. J Toxicol Environ Health 1976;1:505–514.

16. Caravati EM, Litovitz TL: Pediatric cyanide intoxication and death from an acetonitrile-containing cosmetic. JAMA 1988;260:3470–3473.

17. Carr A, Samaras K, Chisholm DJ, Cooper DA: Pathogenesis of HIV-1-protease inhibitor-associated peripheral lipodystrophy, hyperlipidaemia, and insulin resistance. Lancet 1998;351:1881–1883.

18. Dai Y, Rashba-Step J, Cederbaum AI: Stable expression of human cytochrome P4502E1 in HepG2 cells: Characterization of catalytic activities and production of reactive oxygen intermediates. Biochem J 1993;32:6928–6937.

19. DiVincenzo G, Kaplan CJ, DeDinas J: Characterization of the metabolites of methyl n-butyl ketone, methyl iso-butyl ketone, and methyl ethyl ketone in guinea-pig serum and their clearance. Toxicol Appl Pharmacol 1976;36:511–518.

20. Edgar B, Bailey D, Bergstrand R, et al: Acute effects of drinking grapefruit juice on the pharmacokinetics and dynamics of felodipine, and its potential clinical relevance. Eur J Clin Pharmacol 1992;42:313–317.

21. Eliasson E, Kenna JG: Cytochrome P4502E1 is a cell surface autoantigen in halothane hepatitis. Mol Pharmacol 1996;50:573–582.

22. Eling TE, Thompson DC, Foureman GL, et al: Prostaglandin H synthase and xenobiotic oxidation. Ann Rev Pharmacol Toxicol 1990;30:1-45.

23. Feng PC, Patrick SJ: Studies of the action of hypoglycin-A, an hypoglycaemic substance. Br J Pharmacol 1958;13:125–130.

24. Fiala ES, Caswell N, Sohn OS, et al: Nonalcohol dehydrogenase-mediated metabolism of methylazoxymethanol in the deer mouse, *Peromyscus maniculatus*. Cancer Res 1984;44:2885–2891.

25. Freinkel N, Singer DL, Arky RA, et al: Alcohol hypoglycemia. I. Carbohydrate metabolism of patients with clinical alcohol hypoglycemia and the experimental reproduction of the syndrome with pure ethanol. J Clin Invest 1963;42:1112–1133.

26. Frezza M, di Padova C, Pozzato G, et al: High blood alcohol levels in women: The role of decreased gastric alcohol dehydrogenase activity and first-pass metabolism. N Engl J Med 1990;322:95–99.

27. Gerlach M, Riederer P, Przuntek H, et al: MPTP mechanisms of neurotoxicity and their implications for Parkinson's disease. Euro J Pharmacol 1991;208:273–286.

28. Guegenrich FP: Catalytic selectivity of human cytochrome P450 enzymes: Relevance to drug metabolism and toxicity. Toxicol Lett 1994;70:133–138.

29. Guegenrich FP: Reactions and significance of cytochrome P-450 enzymes. J Biol Chem 1991;266:10019–10022.

30. Halpert JR, Guegenrich FP, Bend JR, et al: Selective inhibitors of cytochromes. Toxicol Appl Pharmacol 1994;125:163–175.

31. Hétu C, Dumont A, Joly J: Effect of chronic ethanol administration on bromobenzene liver toxicity in the rat. Toxicol Appl Pharmacol 1983;67:166–177.

32. Herman RJ: Drug interactions and the statins. Can Med Assoc J 1999;161:1281–1286.

33. Hill HZ, Backer R, Hill GJ: Blood cyanide levels in mice after administration of amygdalin. Biopharm Drug Dispos 1980;1:211–220.

34. Hoet P, Louise M, Graf M, et al: Epidemic of liver-disease caused by hydrochlorofluorocarbons used as ozone-sparing substitutes of chlorofluorocarbons. Lancet 1997;350:556–559.

35. Horner WD: Dinitrophenol and its relation to formation of cataracts. Arch Ophthalmol 1942;27:1097.

36. Jakoby WB, Bend JR, Caldwell J: Metabolic Basis of Detoxification: Metabolism of Functional Groups. New York, Academic Press, 1982.

37. King, MW: Medical biochemistry site at Indiana State University. Last updated 12/2000. http://web.indstate.edu/thcme/mwking/home.html.

38. Kato R, Yamazoe Y: The importance of substrate concentration in determining cytochromes P450 therapeutically relevant in vivo. Pharmacogenetics 1994;4:359–362.

39. Kleinman JG, Breittenfield RV, Roth DA: Acute renal failure associated with acetaminophen ingestion: Report of a case and review of the literature. Clin Nephrol 1980;14:201–205.

40. Krishna DR, Klotz U: Extrahepatic metabolism of drugs in humans. Clin Pharmacokinet 1994;26:144–160.

41. Kroncke KD, Fricker G, Meier PJ, et al: Alpha-amanitin uptake into hepatocytes. J Biol Chem 1986;261:12562–12567.

42. Lawton MP, Cashman JR, Cresteil T, et al: A nomenclature for the mammalian flavin-containing monooxygenase gene family based on amino acid sequence identities. Arch Biochem Biophys 1994;308:254–257.

43. Lee WM: Drug-induced hepatotoxicity. N Engl J Med 1995;333:1118–1127.

44. Lewis MS, Youle RJ: Ricin subunit association: Thermodynamics and the role of the disulfide bond in toxicity. J Biol Chem 1986;261:11571–11577.

45. Lieber CS: Alcohol and the liver: 1994 update. Gastroenterology 1994;106:1085–1105.

46. Lieber CS: Metabolic derangement induced by alcohol. Ann Rev Med 1967;18:35–54.

47. Lindell TJ, Weinberg F, Morris PW: Specific inhibition of nuclear RNA polymerase II by alpha-amanitin. Science 1970;170:447–449.

48. Mannucci PM: Genetic control of anticoagulation. Lancet 1999;353:688–689.

49. Mason MF, Wallace SM, Forster E, et al: Pentachlorophenol poisoning: Report of two cases. J Forensic Sci 1965;10:136–147.

50. Mehendale HM, Roth RA, Gandolfi AJ: Novel mechanisms in chemically induced hepatotoxicity. FASEB J 1994;8:1285–1295.

51. Menon JA: Tropical hazards associated with the use pentachlorophenol. BMJ 1958;1:1156.

52. Miller K: Metabolic pathways of biochemistry. 1998. http://www.gwu.edu/~mpb/index.html.

53. Mitchell JR, Jollow DJ: Metabolic activation of gas to toxic substances [review]. Gastroenterology 1975;68:392–394.

54. Mitchell JR, Thorleinsson SS, Potter WZ, et al: Acetaminophen-induced hepatic injury: Protective role of glutathione in man and rationale for therapy. Clin Pharmacol Ther 1974;16:676–683.

55. Mitchell JR, Jollow DJ, Potter WZ, et al: Acetaminophen induced hepatic necrosis. IV: Protection role of glutathione. J Pharmacol Exp Ther 1973;187:211–217.

56. Mitchell RA, Chang BF, Huang CH, DeMaster EG: Inhibition of mitochondrial energy-linked functions by arsenate: Evidence for a nonhydrolytic mode of inhibitor action. Biochem J 1971;10:2049–2053.

57. Monahan BG, Ferguson CL, Kelleavy ES, et al: Torsades de pointes occurring in association with terfenadine use. JAMA 1990;264:2788–2790.

58. Myers CD, McGuire WP, Liss RH: Adriamycin: The role of lipid peroxidation in cardiac toxicity and tumor response. Science 1977;197:165–167.

59. Nelson DR, Kamataki T, Waxman DJ, et al: The P450 superfamily: Update on new sequences, gene mapping, accession numbers, early trivial names, and nomenclature. DNA Cell Biol 1993;12:1–51.

60. Oates NS, Shah RR, Idle JR, Smith RL: Influence of oxidation polymorphism on phenformin kinetics and dynamics. Clin Pharmacol Ther 1983;34:827–834.

61. Parker VH: Effect of nitrophenols and halogenophenols on the enzymatic activity of rat liver mitochondria. Biochem J 1957;69:306–310.

62. Parkinson A: Biotransformation of xenobiotics. In: Klaassen CD, ed: Casarett & Doull's Toxicology, The Basic Science of Poisons. New York, McGraw-Hill, 1996, pp. 151–156.

63. Parkinson A, Hurwitz A: Omeprazole and the induction of human cytochrome P-450: A response to concerns about potential adverse effects. Gastroenterology 1991;100:1157–1164.

64. Peck CC, Temple R, Collins JM: Understanding consequences of concurrent therapies. JAMA 1993;269:1550–1552.

65. Pirotte JH: Apparent potentiation of hepatotoxicity from small doses of acetaminophen by phenobarbital. Ann Intern Med 1984;101:403.

66. Pohl LR: Drug-induced allergic hepatitis. Semin Liver Dis 1990;10:305–315.

67. Rose MS, Lock EA, Smith LL, Wyatt I: Paraquat accumulation: Tissue and species specificity. Biochem Pharmacol 1976;25:419–423.

68. Rosen GM, Rauckman EJ: Carbon tetrachloride induced lipid peroxidation: A spin trapping study. Toxicol Lett 1982;10:337–344.

69. Rosenfield AB, Huston R: Infant methemoglobinemia in Minnesota due to nitrates in well water. Minn Med 1950;33:787–796.

70. Rubinchik SM, Schade DS: Alcoholic ketoacidosis. 2001. http://www.emedicine.com/med/topic102.html.

71. Ruderman N, Shafrir E, Bressler R: Relation of fatty acid oxidation to gluconeogenesis: Effect of pentanoic acid. Life Sci 1968;7:1083–1089.

72. Santi DV, McHenry CS, Sommer A: Mechanism of interactions of thymidylate synthetase with 5-fluorodeoxyuridylate. Biochem J 1974;13:471–480.

73. Shah RR, Oates NS, Idle JR, et al: Impaired oxidation of brisoquine in patients with perhexiline neuropathy. B M J 1982;284:295–299.

74. Shapiro LE, Shear NH: Drug-drug interactions: How scared should we be? Can Med Assoc J 1999;161:1266–1267.

75. Shimkin MB, Anderson NN: Acute toxicities of rotenone and mixed pyrethrins in mammals. Proc Soc Exp Biol Med 1936;34:135–138.

76. Smith MHG, Jeffrey SW: The effects of salicylate on oxygen and carbohydrate metabolism in the isolated rat diaphragm. Biochem J 1956;63:524–529.

77. Southorn PA, Powis G: Free radicals in medicine: I. Chemical nature of biologic reactions. Mayo Clin Proc 1988;63:381–389.

78. Speeg KV, Mitchel MC, Maldonado AL: Additive protection of cimetidine and N-acetylcysteine treatment against acetaminophen induced hepatic necrosis in the rat. J Pharmacol Exp Ther 1985;234:550–554.

79. Spencer HC, Rowe VK, Adams EM, Irish DD: Toxicological studies on laboratory animals of certain alkyldinitrophenols used in agriculture. J Indian Hyg Toxicol 1948;30:10–25.

80. Tanaka K: On the mode of action of hypoglycin A. J Biol Chem 1972;247:7465–7478.

81. Tanaka K, Kean EA, Johnson B: Jamaican vomiting sickness. N Engl J Med 1976;295:461–467.

82. Tanaka K, Miller EM, Isselbacher KJ: Hypoglycin A: A specific inhibitor of isovaleryl CoA dehydrogenase. Proc Natl Acad Sci U S A 1971;68:20–24.

83. Timbrell JA: Principles of Biochemical Toxicology. London, Taylor & Francis, 1987.

84. Way JL: Cyanide intoxication and its mechanism of antagonism. Ann Rev Toxicol 1984;24:451.

85. Wilson JD: Vitamin Deficiencies. In: Harrison TR, Isselbacher KJ, eds. Harrison's Principles of Internal Medicine, 13th ed. New York, McGraw-Hill, 1994, pp. 472–479.

86. Wright RO, Lewander WJ, Woolf AD: Methemoglobienmia: Etiology, pharmacology, and clinical management. Ann Emerg Med 1999;34:646–656.

87. Yager JW, Eastmond DA, Robertson ML, et al: Characterization of micronuclei induced in human lymphocytes by benzene metabolites. Adv Cancer Res 1990;50:393–399.

88. Zand R, Nelson SD, Slattery JT, et al: Inhibition and induction of cytochrome P4502E1-catalyzed oxidation by isoniazid in humans. Clin Pharmacol Ther 1993;54:142–149.

89. Zedeck MS, Grab DJ, Sternberg S: Differences in the acute responses of the various segments of rat intestine to treatment with the intestinal carcinogen, methoxyazomethanol acetate. Cancer Res 1977;37:32–36.

CHAPTER 14 HEPATIC PRINCIPLES

Kathleen A. Delaney

The liver has an essential role in the maintenance of physiologic homeostasis. Its functions include the synthesis, storage, and breakdown of glycogen; the metabolism of lipids; the synthesis of albumin, clotting factors, and other important proteins; the synthesis of bile acids necessary for the absorption of lipids and fat-soluble vitamins; the metabolism of cholesterol; the excretion of metals, most importantly iron, copper, zinc, manganese, mercury, and aluminum; and the detoxification of products of metabolism such as bilirubin and ammonia.[23,44,85] Generalized disruption of these important functions results in familiar manifestations of liver failure: hyperbilirubinemia, coagulopathy, hypoalbuminemia, hyperammonemia, and hypoglycemia. Disturbances of more specific functions result in accumulation of fat, toxic metals, hypercholesterolemia, and fat-soluble vitamin deficiencies.[18]

The liver, which contains the highest concentration of enzymes involved in phase I oxidation-reduction reactions, is also the primary site of biotransformation and detoxification of exogenous toxins or xenobiotics.[23,34,54] Its interposition between the gut and systemic circulation makes it the first-pass recipient of toxins absorbed from the gastrointestinal tract into the portal vein. The liver also receives blood from the systemic circulation and participates in the detoxification and elimination of substances that reach the blood stream through other routes, such as inhalation or cutaneous absorption. The biliary tract provides an important route for the excretion of detoxified xenobiotics and products of metabolism.[45]

Many of these toxins are lipophilic, chemically inert substances that require chemical activation to make them sufficiently soluble to be eliminated. Although phase I activation followed by phase II conjugation usually results in detoxification of these compounds, it occasionally leads to the production of compounds with increased toxicity, which is often manifest at the site of their synthesis.[54] Owing to its location at the end of the portal system and its substantial complement of biotransformation enzymes, the liver is especially vulnerable to toxic injury. (Chapter 13 has a more in-depth discussion of the biotransformation reactions.)

MORPHOLOGY AND FUNCTION OF THE LIVER

Approximately 75% of the blood supply to the liver is derived from the portal vein, which drains the alimentary tract, spleen, and pancreas. This blood is enriched with nutrients and other absorbed agents and is poor in oxygen. The remainder of the hepatic blood flow comes from the hepatic artery, which delivers well-oxygenated blood from the systemic circulation.[18] Blood from the hepatic artery and portal vein mixes in the sinusoids where it comes in close contact with cords of hepatocytes before it exits through small holes in the wall of the vein.[18] Oxygen content diminishes several fold as blood flows from the portal area to the central vein.[5] The sinusoidal lining formed by endothelial cells is thin and fenestrated, allowing transfer of fluid, chylomicrons, and proteins across the space of Disse, an extrasinusoidal space filled with microvilli.[18] Macrophages (Kupffer cells) within the sinusoids scavenge particulate materials and cell debris. When immunologically activated by toxins, Kupffer cells contribute to the generation of oxygen free radicals and may also participate in the production of autoimmune injury to hepatocytes.[26] Ito cells, or "fat storage cells," found between the endothelial cells and hepatocytes are a primary site for the storage of vitamin A and fat.[33]

Bile acids, organic anions, bilirubin, phospholipids, xenobiotics and other constituents of bile are transported through the hepatocytes into the bile canaliculi by active transport systems that have specificity for acids, bases, and neutral compounds.[45] The hepatocyte plasma membranes have three active transport systems for bile acids: a sodium-dependent bile salt transporter in the sinusoidal membrane; an (adenosine triphosphate) ATP-dependent bile salt carrier across the canalicular membrane; and a canalicular membrane transport site driven by the membrane voltage potential.[12] Glucuronidated xenobiotics are substrates for the bile acid transport systems and are actively secreted into bile. Compounds with molecular weights greater than 350 daltons are also preferentially secreted into bile. Bile formation involves the production of a flow of fluid, in addition to the transport and concentration of constituents from the sinusoids and hepatocytes. Bile flow is an active process facilitated by ATP-dependent contractions of actin filaments that encircle the canaliculi.[60,126] Tight junctions separate the contents of the bile canaliculi from the sinusoids and hepatocytes, maintaining a rigid and functionally necessary compartmentalization. Bile flows from tiny canaliculi through increasingly larger conduits, finally into the gall bladder, common duct, and duodenum.[49] A physiologically necessary enterohepatic circulation facilitates the conservation of bile acids and some vitamins.[7] While most detoxified xenobiotics that are secreted into bile are eliminated in the feces, some are reabsorbed back into the systemic circulation, resulting in an enterohepatic circulation. Compounds most likely to be reabsorbed have a low molecular weight and are nonionized at intestinal pH. Nortriptyline and phencyclidine are examples of toxins that undergo enterohepatic recirculation. Methyl mercury also recirculates between the gall bladder and the systemic circulation, resulting in decreased clearance and prolonging toxicity.[23]

Two basic pathologic concepts, a structural one represented by the hepatic lobule, and a functional one represented by the acinus, are utilized to describe the appearance and function of the liver. The basic morphologic unit of the liver characterized by light microscopy is the hepatic lobule, a hexagon with the central vein at the center and the portal triads at the angles (Fig. 14–1). Cords of hepatocytes are oriented radially around the hepatic vein.[18] The acinus, or "metabolic lobule" is a functional unit of the liver.[18] Located between two central veins, it is bisected by terminal branches of the hepatic artery and portal vein that extend from the bases of the acini toward hepatic venules at the apices. The acinus is subdivided into three metabolically distinct zones. Zone 1 lies near the portal triad, zone 3 lies near the central vein, and zone 2 is intermediate. The different metabolic functions of these zones determine the cellular location of biotransformation reactions and affect the anatomic distribution of liver injury produced by toxins (Fig. 14–2; see later).

There is useful correlation between these anatomic and functional conceptualizations of the liver. Hepatocellular injury that occurs near the central vein is called centrilobular necrosis and describes injury that occurs in zone 3 of the liver acinus. The term "periportal necrosis" describes injury in zone 1.

FACTORS AFFECTING THE LOCALIZATION OF HEPATIC INJURY

Metabolic characteristics of the three zones of the acinus have important relevance to the anatomic distribution of toxic liver injury. Zone 1, which begins in the periportal area and is closest to the vascular supply, has a 2-fold higher oxygen content than does zone 3. Predictably, hepatic injury that results from the metabolic production of oxygen free radicals predominates in zone 1.[5] The tendency for centrilobular or zone 3 accumulation of fat in patients with alcoholic steatosis is attributed to the effect of relative hypoxia in the central vein area on the oxidation potential of the hepatocyte.[58] Other metabolic differences that may impact on the localization of injury by different toxins are described. Zone 1 has a higher concentration of glutathione, whereas zone 3 has a greater capacity for glucuronidation and sulfation.[121] The localization of enzymes involved in biotransformation also affects the site of injury. Zone 3 has higher levels of alcohol dehydrogenase and of the ethanol inducible P4502E1 cytochrome oxidase, so that injury caused by toxic metabolites of these enzymes results in centrilobu-

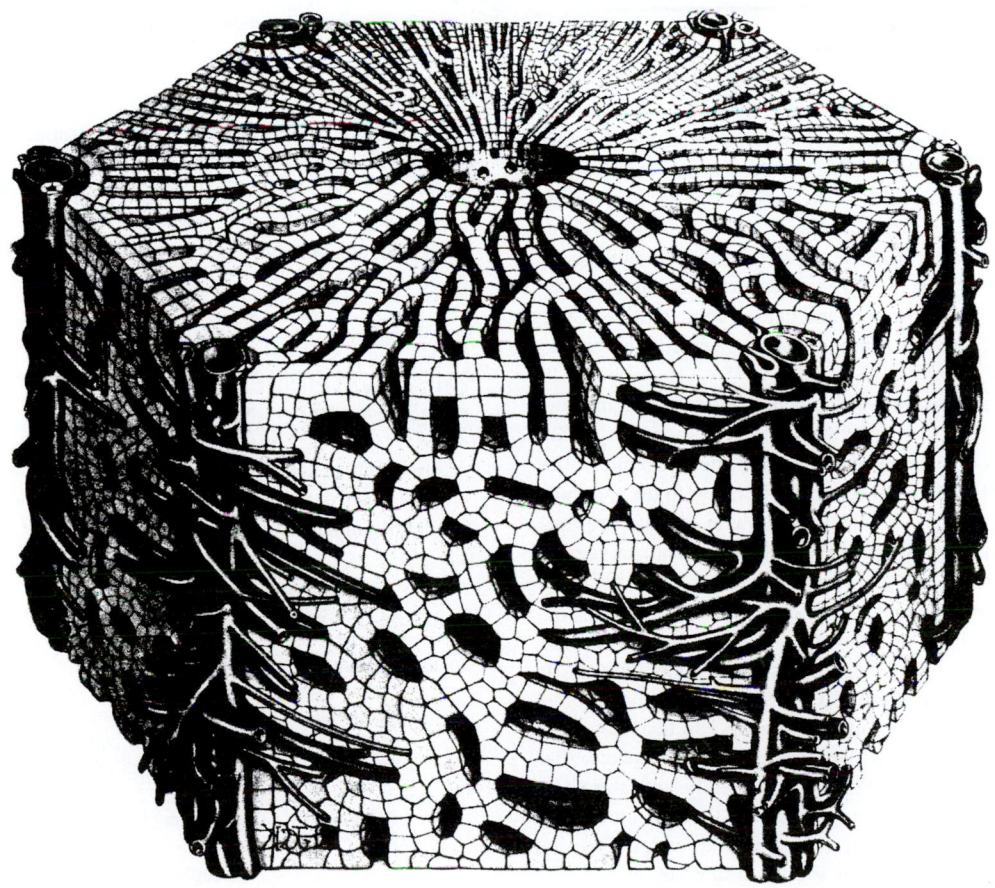

Figure 14–1. Liver lobule. The central vein lies in th center of the figure, surrounded by anastomosing cords of hepatocytes. Around the periphery are six evenly spaced "triads" that lie at an angle in the polyhedron lobule. Each triad consists of branches of the portal vein, hepatic artery, and bile duct. (*Used with permission from Weiss L: Cell and Tissue Biology. A Textbook of Histology, 6th ed., Fig 22–1. p 687.*)

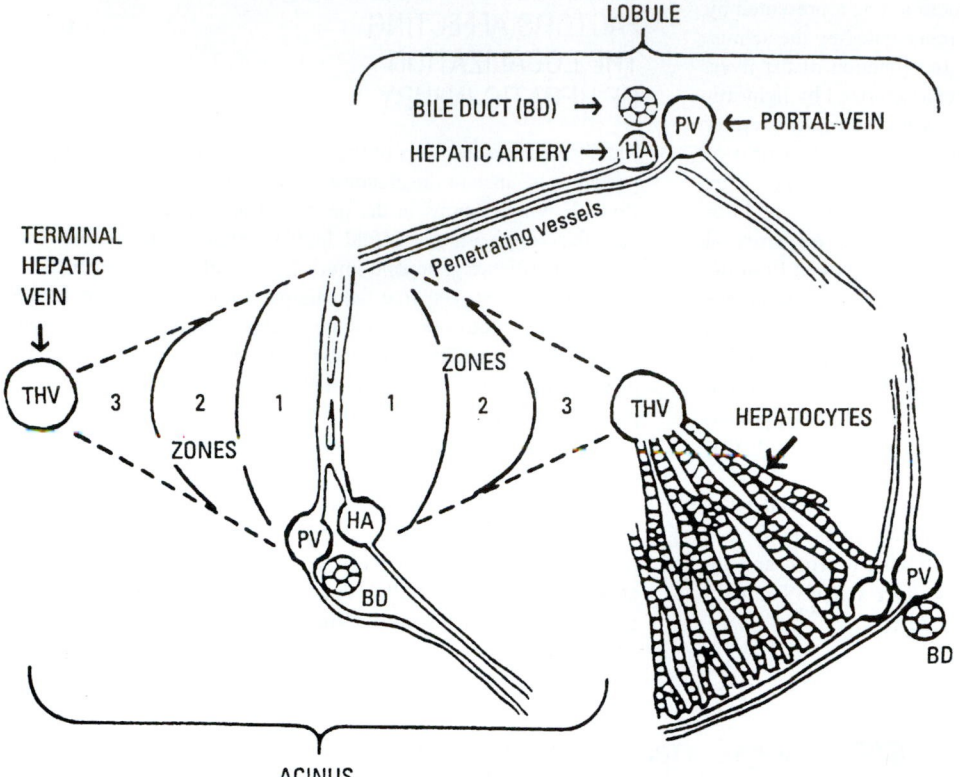

Figure 14–2. The liver lobule and the acinus. The hepatic lobule is a hexagonal structure with the hepatic vein at the center. The hepatic artery and portal vein are located at the base of the acinus. Blood flows from the base of the acinus through the sinusoids across zones 1, 2, and 3 of the acinus to exit in the hepatic vein. Zone 1 of the acinus corresponds with the periportal area of the lobule, while zone 3 of the acinus corresponds with the centrilobular area. (*Used with permission from Moslen MT: Toxic responses of the liver. In: Klaassen C, ed: Casarett & Doull's Toxicology, The Basic Science of Poisons. New York, McGraw-Hill, 1996:403.*)

lar necrosis.[37,58,59,79,121] In chronic alcoholics, demonstrable proliferation of the smooth endoplasmic reticulum in the centrilobular areas accompanies an increase in the activity of the ethanol inducible enzyme P4502E1 in the centrilobular areas. This may lead to increased production of toxic acetaldehyde at the centrilobular sites.[58,61] P4502E1 also has a significant capacity to convert acetaminophen, nitrosamines, benzene, and carbon tetrachloride (CCl$_4$) to reactive intermediates, resulting in selective centrilobular injury by these agents.

The formation of hepatic free radicals following the metabolism of CCl$_4$ has been extensively studied in the laboratory. CCl$_4$ is converted by P4502E1 in an (nicotinamide adenine dinucleotide phosphate) NADPH-dependent reduction reaction to the free radical ·CCl$_3$, which can form covalent bonds with cellular proteins, cause lipid peroxidation, or spontaneously react with oxygen to form the more reactive, and therefore more destructive, CCl$_3$OO· radical.[3] Because low oxygen tension and high P4502E1 activities are found in zone 3, there is a tendency to form the less reactive CCl$_3$· radical, whereas high oxygen tension in zone 1 results in formation of the more reactive CCl$_3$OO· radical. Although a more highly reactive metabolite is produced in zone 1, it does not result in greater injury because glutathione in zone 1 rapidly detoxifies the CCl$_3$OO· radical but does not react as readily with the CCl$_3$· radical.[14] Therefore zone 3 is subject to the greatest amount of liver injury. Hyperbaric oxygen increases the oxygen tension throughout the liver and has been shown in animals to decrease liver injury. This is thought to be due to formation of the CCl$_3$OO· radical in zone 3, and its subsequent detoxification by glutathione.[15]

The observed effects of isoniazid (an inhibitor of the enzyme P4502E1) and chronic ethanol intake (an inducer of the gene CYP2E1) on cellular injury in cultures of cells from the periportal

and centrilobular areas exposed to CCl$_4$ support the association of CCl$_4$ injury with the localization of P4502E1 activity. Acute exposure to isoniazid significantly decreases the injury associated with exposure of cultured zone 3 cells to CCl$_4$, whereas chronic treatment with ethanol significantly enhances it[59] (see Table 14–1).

FACTORS AFFECTING THE DEVELOPMENT OF HEPATOTOXICITY

Agents such as acetaminophen, CCl$_4$, or yellow phosphorous that produce liver damage in all humans in a predictable and dose-dependent manner are known as intrinsic hepatotoxins. Those that

TABLE 14–1. Metabolic Zones of the Acinus

Zone	Location	Biochemistry	Types of Injury
1	Periportal	High oxygen content High glutathione content	Oxygen free radical mediated necrosis
2	Intermediate	Shared functions zones 1/3	Shared functions zones 1/3
3	Central vein	Low oxygen content	Centrilobular necrosis caused by toxic metabolites of P4502E1 metabolites
		High capacity for glucuronidation and sulfation	
		High P4502E1, alcohol dehydrogenase	Increased CCl$_4$ and ethanol injury caused by reducing environment

cause liver damage in a small number of individuals, and whose effect is not apparently dose dependent or predictably reproducible, are known as idiosyncratic hepatotoxins (Table 14–2). The majority of hepatotoxins are idiosyncratic.[87] Some cause hepatotoxicity very rarely while others produce it commonly. The inhaled anesthetic agent halothane is both an intrinsic and an idiopathic hepatotoxin. A mild degree of hepatitis occurs in as many as 20% of patients exposed to halothane.[25,38] This form of halothane hepatitis, which can be reliably induced in animals pretreated with P450 inducers and then subjected to hypotension or hypoxia, is likely a result of direct toxicity.[25,104] A more severe idiosyncratic form is caused by an autoimmune response induced by halothane that targets liver proteins.[122]

An individual's susceptibility to a hepatotoxin depends on numerous factors, including the activity of biotransformation enzymes, the availability of substrates, and the immunocompetence of the individual. These, in turn, are affected by age, sex, diet, underlying diseases, concurrent exposure to other drugs or toxins, and genetic factors. Sporadic unpredicted hepatotoxicity is not really "idiosyncratic," but more likely a result of the combined effects of genetic and other factors that result in the overproduction or decreased clearance of toxic metabolites.[54]

TABLE 14–2.   Hepatotoxic Agents

Intrinsic
 Acetaminophen
 Carbon tetrachloride
 Cyclopeptide-containing mushrooms
 Ethanol
 Heavy metals
 Hydrocarbons (chlorinated)
 Methotrexate
 Phosphorus (yellow)

Idiosyncratic
 Allopurinol
 Amiodarone
 Bromfenac
 Chlorpromazine
 Chlorpropamide
 Disulfiram
 Diclofenac
 Erythromycin estolate
 Halothane
 Isoniazid
 Metformin
 Methyldopa
 Methylenedioxymethamphetamine (MDMA)
 Nitrofurantoin
 Oral contraceptives
 Pemoline
 Phenylbutazone
 Phenytoin
 Paroxetine
 Propylthiouracil
 Quinolines
 Rosiglitazone
 Tasmar
 Tetracycline
 Troglitazone
 Valproic acid
 Venlafaxine

Enzyme Polymorphism

Many enzymes involved in biotransformation show genetic polymorphism. For example, approximately 8% of whites are deficient in the enzyme P4502D6 (formally called debrisoquine hydroxylase), which is responsible for the metabolism of a number of drugs that include debrisoquine (an antihypertensive first identified as the substrate of this enzyme), several antidepressants and antidysrhythmics, some opioids, and phenformin.[54,83] Perhexiline, an antianginal agent marketed in Europe in the 1980s, caused severe liver disease and peripheral neuropathy in persons with a demonstrated inability to metabolize debrisoquine.[111] Patients with Gilbert syndrome, a congenital disorder that results in impairment of glucuronyl transferase, demonstrate decreased glucuronidation and increased bioactivation of acetaminophen during chronic therapeutic dosing.[21] This suggests an increased risk of hepatic injury following ingestions of acetaminophen.[21]

Effects of Other Drugs or Toxins on Enzyme Function

Changes in the activities of biotransformation enzymes that result in increased formation of hepatotoxic metabolites may increase susceptibility to hepatic injury in humans. As noted earlier, the chronic ingestion of ethanol induces the CYP2E1 gene, which results in a 5–10-fold increase in P4502E1 activity.[20,58] Chronic administration of isoniazid (INH) to slow acetylators also induces P4502E1 activity.[134] P4502E1 has a significant capacity to convert acetaminophen, nitrosamines, bromobenzene, and CCl_4 to reactive intermediates, increasing their potential toxicity. Anecdotal observations in humans suggest the possibility that hepatic toxicity because of solvents such as CCl_4, dimethylformamide, and bromobenzene, may be exacerbated by the chronic ingestion of ethanol.[4,93] Anecdotal reports also suggest that chronic ethanol use increases susceptibility to acetaminophen-induced hepatic injury in humans.[79,109]

The major studies that have described these interactions are done in experimental animals.[37,76] Studies of bromobenzene toxicity, an agent whose metabolism is similar to that of acetaminophen, show that chronic ethanol administration causes an earlier onset of bromobenzene hepatotoxicity in rats, with only a small increase in the extent of hepatic necrosis. The dose of bromobenzene required for hepatic injury to occur is not altered by pretreatment with ethanol.[37] Chronic administration of phenobarbital to rats results in a very significant increase in the hepatotoxic effects of bromobenzene.[95] The cultured hepatocytes of ethanol-treated rats show increased in vitro susceptibility to the hepatotoxic effects of CCl_4, which is also metabolized by P4502E1.[59] In rat studies, prior administration of phenobarbital or INH predisposes to acetaminophen toxicity at lower doses, whereas prior administration of cytochrome P450 inhibitors, such as cimetidine, may be protective.[84,115]

Some drug combinations increase the possibility of hepatotoxic reactions because one agent alters the metabolism of the other, leading to the production of toxic metabolites. This is the case with combinations of rifampin and INH; amoxicillin and clavulanic acid; and trimethoprim and sulfamethoxazole.[1,41,51,56,69,128]

Immune Responses

Several types of hypersensitivity reactions result in different forms of liver injury. An autoimmune etiology of hepatic toxicity is implied but not proven for many suspected agents. An immune mechanism is implied by the demonstration of autoantibodies, antibodies against the drugs, or activated T lymphocytes. The presence of eosinophilia, atypical lymphocytosis, fever, and rash suggest a hypersensitivity mechanism. A history of repeated exposure followed by illness that resolves with withdrawal of the agent and recurs with reexposure also suggests hypersensitivity. Phenytoin-induced hepatic necrosis and cholestasis occurs in association with a systemic response that includes rash, eosinophilia, atypical lymphocytosis and demonstrated serum immunoglobulin (IgG) antibodies against phenytoin.[46,114] Jaundice associated with fever, chills, rash, and eosinophilia occurs in 1% of patients treated with chlorpromazine 1–5 weeks after exposure. Readministration of the drug results in recurrence.[39] Erythromycin estolate causes fever, rash, and eosinophilia that begins 2–21 days after initiation of the drug and recurs with readministration.[22,128] An autoimmune mechanism was suspected in children treated with pemoline for attention deficit hyperactivity disorder (ADHD) who developed liver injury associated with positive antinuclear antibody (ANA) tests.[103] Similar reactions occur following exposure to diclofenac.[105]

A possible mechanism by which a drug initiates autoimmune injury to the liver is through the formation of an adduct with the hepatic cell. An adduct is formed when an activated metabolite becomes covalently bonded following an electrophilic attack on a cellular macromolecule. The adduct then acts as a hapten, inducing an immune response against the drug-macromolecule or against an immunologically altered cellular macromolecule. The formation of adducts requires activation of the drug because most are chemically inert in their ingested forms. Destruction of the hepatocyte might then be mediated by complement or antibody directed lysis; by specific cell-mediated cytotoxicity; or by an inflammatory response induced by immune complexes and complement.[68,87,88]

An immune mechanism was demonstrated in a rat model of experimental liver injury by α-napthylthiocyanate (ANIT), a toxin that causes acute cholangitis associated with polymorphonuclear cell (PMN) infiltration.[19] In in vitro studies, PMNs release cytotoxic lysosomal enzymes and oxygen free radicals in response to activation by ANIT.[19,68] Additionally, antibodies directed against circulating neutrophils decrease the extent of liver damage caused by ANIT, supporting the proposal that PMN activation is an important factor in this model.[19] Lymphocyte sensitization is also demonstrated in hepatitis caused by a number of drugs including INH, erythromycin, and floxacillin.[87,124] The idiosyncratic form of halothane hepatitis results in fulminant hepatic failure that is associated with autoantibodies, against a neoantigen formed by an adduct of halothane with an hepatoprotein, which may be a microsomal carboxylesterase[25,87,122] (Chap. 53). Studies show autoantibodies against the P450E1 enzyme in halothane hepatitis.[24,114] A trifluoroacetyl protein adduct similar to that associated with halothane hepatitis was detected in workers who developed hepatic necrosis following exposure to hydrochlorofluorocarbons.[38]

Availability of Substrates

The availability of substrates for detoxification may significantly affect the likelihood of hepatic injury. The metabolism of acetaminophen illustrates the delicate balance that the availability of glutathione exerts between detoxification and the production of injurious metabolites. In healthy adults taking therapeutic amounts of acetaminophen, 90% of hepatic metabolism results in formation of glucuronidated or sulfated metabolites.[21] The 10% that undergoes oxidative metabolism to the toxic electrophilic metabolite N-acetyl-p-benzoquinoneimine (NAPQI) is rapidly detoxified by conjugation with glutathione.[70,89] Excessive amounts of acetaminophen result in increased synthesis of NAPQI, which reacts avidly with hepatocellular macromolecules if glutathione is not available.[17,70] Glutathione may be depleted during the course of metabolism of acetaminophen by otherwise normal livers, or it may be decreased by starvation or liver disease.[52,113] An inverse correlation exists between the cellular concentration of glutathione and the demonstration of injurious covalent binding of NAPQI to liver cells.[17]

PATHOLOGIC AND BIOCHEMICAL MANIFESTATIONS OF HEPATIC INJURY

The liver responds to injury in a limited number of ways.[18] Cells may swell (ballooning degeneration) and accumulate fat (steatosis) or biliary material. They may necrose and lyse or undergo apoptosis, forming shrunken, nonfunctioning, eosinophilic bodies.[18] Necrosis may be focal or bridging, linking the periportal or centrilobular areas; zonal or panacinar, or it may be massive. An inflammatory cell response may precede or follow necrosis.[18,54] Injury to the bile ducts results in cholestasis. In addition, vascular injuries may cause obstruction to venous or arterial flow. Table 14–3 lists various morphologies of toxic hepatic injury and associated toxins. The difficulty in categorizing and characterizing all of the forms and causes of toxic hepatic injury is illustrated by the variety and spectrum of injury caused by azathioprine. This single agent is associated with most forms of injury, including mild asymptomatic liver test abnormalities, simple cholestasis, hepatitis, bile duct injury, and vascular injury.[29] All of these manifestations of toxic injury are discussed below (Fig. 14–3).

TABLE 14–3.   Morphology of Liver Injury

Hepatocellular Necrosis	Fatty Change (Steatosis)
Acetaminophen	Amiodarone
Arsenic	Corticosteroids
Carbon tetrachloride	Ethanol
Disulfiram	Tetracycline
Ethanol	Valproic Acid
Halothane	
Iron	**Neoplasms**
Isoniazid	Androgens
Methotrexate	Contraceptive steroids
Methyldopa	Vinly chloride
Phenytoin	
Phosphorus (yellow)	**Mitochondrial Failure**
Procainamide	Aflatoxin
Propylthiouracil	Cereulide
Tetracycline	Fialuridine
	Hypoglycin
Cholestasis	Margosa Oil
Chlorpromazine	Nucleoside analogues
Chlorpropamide	Tetracycline
Ethanol	Valproic Acid
Erythromycin estolate	
Nitrofurantoin	
Rifampin	

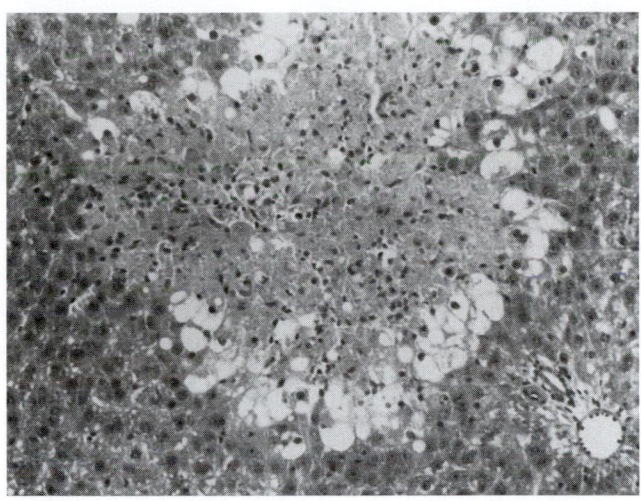

Figure 14–3. Centrilobular necrosis in a rat liver caused by bromobenzene administration. Note the polymorphonuclear infiltrate in the necrotic area surrounded by vacuolated hepatocytes. (*Reprinted with permission from Hétu C, Dumont A, Joly JG, et al: Effect of chronic ethanol administration on bromobenzene liver toxicity in the rat. Toxicol Appl Pharm 1983;67:166.*)

Acute Hepatocellular Necrosis

Acute necrosis of the hepatocyte disrupts all aspects of its function. Because there is a great deal of functional reserve in the liver, hepatic function may be preserved despite the development of focal necrosis. Extensive necrosis results in functional liver failure. Cell lysis is preceded by the formation of blebs in the lipid membrane and leakage of cytosolic enzymes, primarily aminotransferases and lactate dehydrogenase. Coalescence of blebs leads to rupture of the cellular membrane and acute irreversible cell death with disintegration of the nucleus and termination of all cellular function. Prior to membrane rupture, this injury is reversible by membrane repair processes.[18] The formation of activated metabolites that bind to cell macromolecules as well as the potential for immune-mediated cell injury are described. How these interactions, particularly the binding of electrophilic metabolites, lead to cell necrosis is not well known. One mechanism of rapid injury to the cell is that of initiation of a cascading lipid peroxidation reaction following attack by a free radical. The P4502E1 enzyme has a significant potential to produce oxygen free radicals, as do activated PMNs and Kupffer cells.[20,26,68,87] Intracellular rises in calcium ion precede the onset of cellular injury. This is proposed as a final common pathway of cell death, although this simple concept does not account for all observed processes.[29,61]

Many common drugs and toxins are shown to produce hepatic necrosis. Cl_4, halothane, and acetaminophen were previously described. Although the incidence is not clear, INH also results in severe hepatic necrosis, as indicated by a report of 10 patients who developed liver failure during INH treatment that resulted in death or transplantation.[71] A recent study of more than 11,000 patients exposed to isoniazid during preventive treatment showed that reversible hepatocellular injury occurred in 0.10% of those starting treatment, and in 0.15% of those completing treatment.[78] Risk factors for the development of hepatotoxicity from INH exposure are female sex, increasing age, coadministration with rifampin, and alcoholism.[48,56,78] This is discussed extensively in Chap. 43.

Recently, the new thiazolidinedione agents troglitazone and rosiglitazone, marketed for the treatment of type 2 diabetes, were associated with acute hepatocellular necrosis.[2,32] A significant number of cases attributed to troglitazone led to its withdrawal from the market in March 2000.[57] Table 14–2 summarizes the pharmacologic and toxic agents that have been reported to cause hepatic necrosis.

Herbal remedies are increasingly recognized as a cause of acute hepatocellular injury. Plants or plant products that are known or suspected to cause hepatic injury are listed in Table 14–4.

Steatosis

Steatosis is the abnormal accumulation of fat in hepatocytes. Two forms of steatosis are described: macrovesicular steatosis (Fig. 14–4), in which the nucleus is displaced by accumulation of intracellular fat, and microvesicular steatosis (Fig. 14–5), which is characterized by fat droplets that do not displace the nucleus. The intracellular fat accumulation reflects abnormal hepatocellular metabolism and may occur because of any one or more of these mechanisms: impaired synthesis of lipoproteins; increased mobilization of peripheral adipose stores; increased uptake of circulating lipids; increased triglyceride production; decreased binding of triglycerides to lipoprotein; decreased release of very-low-density lipoproteins from the hepatocytes; or decreased β-oxidation of fatty acids.[58] Steatosis is a sign of the underlying metabolic dysfunction that leads to cell injury and death, not a cause of it. It is reversible in nonfatal cases following withdrawal of the causative agent. Common toxins associated with macrovesicular steatosis include ethanol and amiodarone. The initial pathologic lesion seen in alcoholic liver disease is the development of reversible macrovesicular steatosis. Ethanol increases the uptake of fatty acids into hepatocytes and decreases lipoprotein secretion. Most

TABLE 14–4. Plants Associated With Liver Injury*

Pyrrolizidine Alkaloids Producing
Venoocclusive Disease
   Crotalaria sp
   Gordolobo yerba
   Heliotropium sp
   Ilex sp (Mate)
   Senecio sp
   Symphytum sp (Comfrey)

Hepatocellular Injury
   Amanita sp
   Aspergillus flavus → Aflatoxins
   Blighia sp (Ackee fruit)
   Bupleurum sp (Hare's Ear Root)
   Clove oil
   Cycas (Cycad nuts)
   Ephedra (Ma-huang)
   Gentianae sp (Gentian Root)
   Hedioma, Mentha sp (pennyroyal, squawmint)
   Larrea sp (Chaparral)
   Lycopodium sp (Jin Bu Huan)
   Paeonia sp (Red Peony Root)
   Sassafras
   Teucrium sp (Bermander)

*See references 13, 50, 51, 72, 74, 98, 107, 110, 118, 131, and 133.

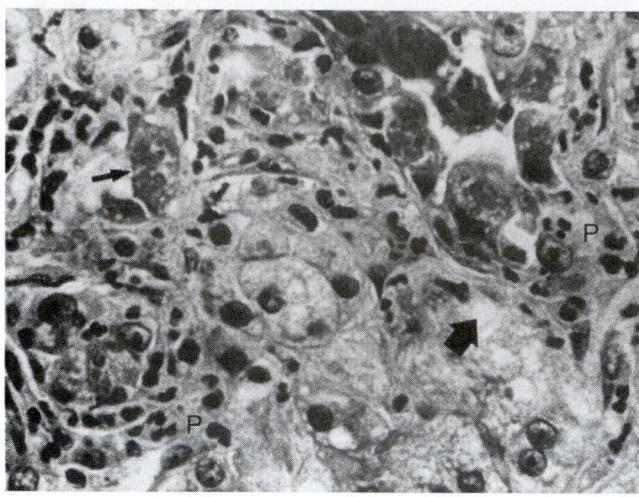

Figure 14–4.   Macrovesicular steatosis associated with the administration of amiodarone. The *small arrow* indicates the presence of Mallory bodies. The *large arrow* points to accumulated intracellular fat. The letter P indicates polymorphonuclear leukocytes. The nuclei are eccentric and are displaced by the accumulated intracellular fat. (*Reprinted with permission from Lee WM: Drug-induced hepatotoxicity. N Engl J Med 1995;333:1118.*)

importantly, the increased NADH/NAD⁺ ratio associated with hepatic metabolism of ethanol results in decreased oxidation of fatty acids and promotion of fatty acid synthesis.[58] Amiodarone is concentrated in the liver and may account for up to 1% of its wet weight during chronic therapy.[29] Amiodarone hepatic toxicity resembles that of alcoholic hepatitis, with steatosis, Mallory bodies, and potential of progression to cirrhosis. Lamellated intralysosomal phospholipid inclusion bodies were found in all cases in one study and seem to be specific for amiodarone toxicity.[99]

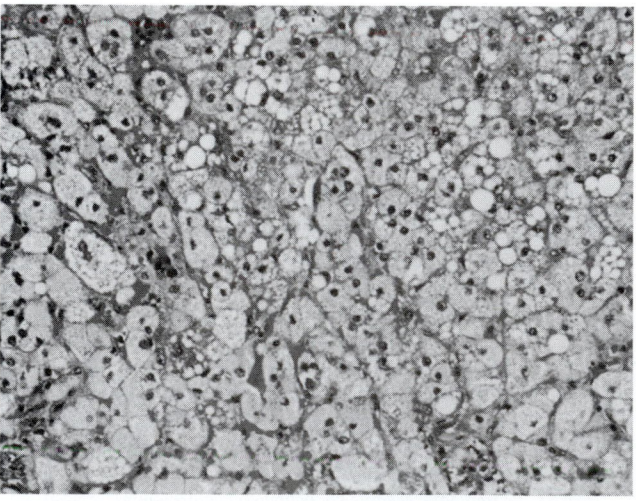

Figure 14–5.   This figure shows severe microvesicular steatosis in a patient treated with fialuridine. Note the central location of the nuclei. (*Reprinted with permission from McKenzie R, Fried MW, Sallie R, et al: Hepatic failure and lactic acidosis due to fialuridine (FIAU), an investigational nucleoside analogue for chronic hepatitis B. N Eng J Med 1995;333:1099.*)

Microvesicular steatosis is often associated with a more severe form of hepatocellular dysfunction and has, in some cases, been attributed to toxic impairment of β-oxidation of fatty acids and generalized failure of mitochondrial function.[106,108] High doses of tetracycline produce a microvesicular form of hepatic steatosis. This is associated with moderately elevated aminotransferase and alkaline phosphatase concentrations and markedly prolonged international normalized ratio (INR) with progression to fulminant hepatic failure.[108] Recently, microvesicular steatosis has been reported in patients taking antiviral nucleoside analogues (zidovudine, zalcitabine, and didanosine) for the treatment of HIV infection.[106,117] The nucleoside analogue fialuridine caused severe hepatotoxicity and several deaths during a study of its use in the treatment of chronic hepatitis B infection. Microscopic examinations of liver specimens showed marked accumulation of fat with minimal necrosis or structural injury. In these cases, severe acidosis with minimal elevation of hepatocellular enzymes and bilirubin, and failure of hepatic synthetic function suggested injury localized to the mitochondria. This was supported by a demonstrably abnormal appearance of the mitochondria on electron microscopic examination.[67] Microvesicular steatosis associated with defective β-oxidation of fatty acids, and also attributed to mitochondrial failure, was reported in a fatal case of *Bacillus cereus* food poisoning, in which high levels of the bacterial emetic toxin cereulide were found in the bile and liver. In this case, microvesicular steatosis was associated with extensive hepatocellular necrosis.[63] In all cases, lactic acidosis is a prominent biochemical manifestation of impaired energy production, whereas microvesicular steatosis reflects failure of fatty acid metabolism, which is likely also related to impairment of energy production.[31,106] In addition to cereulide, other toxins associated with mitochondrial failure are hypoglycin, the cause of Jamaican vomiting sickness, aflatoxin, and margosa oil.[106]

Sodium valproate causes mild elevations of aminotransferases in about 11% of patients, usually during the first few months of therapy. The earliest pathologic lesion is the production of microvesicular steatosis, which occurs in the absence of necrosis. A small percentage of patients progress to fulminant hepatic failure characterized by microvesicular steatosis and centrilobular necrosis.[135] The incidence of fatal hepatocellular injury is highest in children, approaching 1/800 under the age of 2 years.[91] Carnitine is an amino acid that has an essential role in the mitochondrial transport and β-oxidation of fatty acids. An association between deficiency of carnitine and the development of hyperammonemia is observed in children treated with valproic acid.[91,123] It is not yet known whether valproic acid causes carnitine deficiency that results in hepatic injury, or whether patients with preexisting metabolic errors that result in carnitine deficiency are at greater risk of liver injury.

Steatosis also occurs following exposure to the industrial solvent dimethylformamide. The mechanism of hepatotoxicity in humans is unknown. Liver biopsies in patients with acute illness show focal hepatocellular necrosis and microvesicular steatosis. More prolonged, less symptomatic exposures result in significant macrovesicular steatosis with mild aminotransferase elevations.[94]

Cholestasis

Cholestasis results from a number of toxic mechanisms. It may occur with or without associated hepatitis. The development of jaundice following hepatic necrosis is a manifestation of general failure of liver function. More specific mechanisms that are postulated to result in cholestasis include (a) impairment of the integrity of tight membrane junctions that functionally isolate the canaliculus from the hepatocyte and sinusoids; (b) failure of transport of bile components across the hepatocytes; (c) blockade of specific membrane active transport sites; (d) decreased membrane fluidity resulting in altered transport; and (e) decreased canalicular contractility resulting in decreased bile flow[49] (Fig. 14–6).

Estrogens cause intrahepatic cholestasis by altering the composition of the lipid membrane and inhibiting the rate of secretion of bile into the canaliculi.[49,57] Rifampin impedes the uptake of bilirubin into hepatocytes.[128] Methyltestosterone and C-17 alkylated anabolic steroids impair the secretion of bilirubin into canaliculi.[57] Cholestasis with periductal inflammation may follow exposure to chlorpromazine and may be caused by inhibition of Na^+-K^+ ATPase, which results in decreased canalicular contractility.[40,102] Cyclosporine inhibits sodium dependent uptake of bile salts across the sinusoidal membrane, and blocks ATP-dependent bile salt transport across the canalicular membrane.[12] Floxacillin, rifampin and erythromycin cause cholestasis with minimal inflammation or evidence of hepatocellular injury.[124,128] An experimental model that demonstrates a specific type of toxin-induced cholestasis is the exposure of rats to ANIT. A specific injury localized to the tight junctions that separate the hepatocyte from the canaliculi results in reflux of bile constituents into the sinusoidal space and increased access of sinusoidal molecules to the biliary tree.[49]

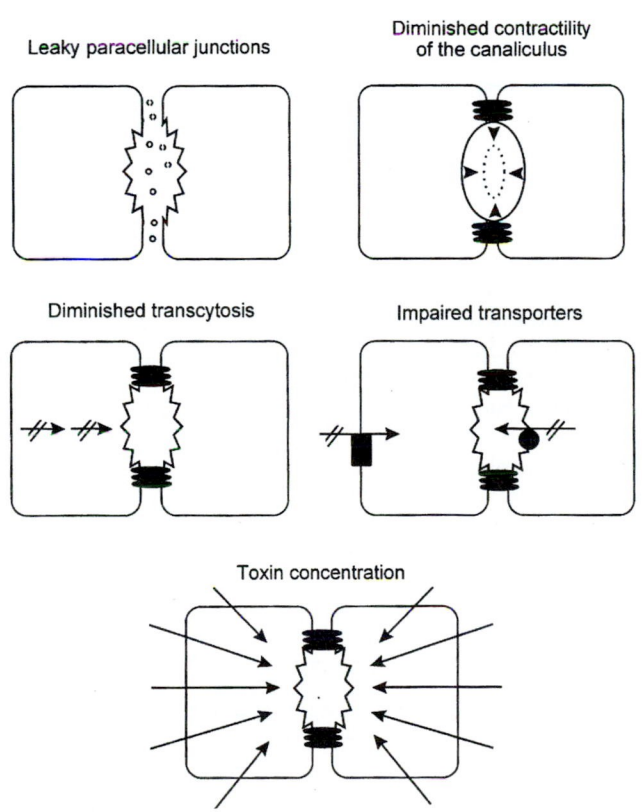

Figure 14–6. Potential mechanisms of toxin-induced cholestasis. (*Used with permission from Moslen MT: Toxic responses of the liver. In: Klaassen C, ed: Casarett & Doull's Toxicology, The Basic Science of Poisons. New York, McGraw-Hill, 1996:403.*)

Veno-Occlusive Disease

Hepatic veno-occlusive disease is caused by toxic injury to the endothelium of terminal hepatic venules that results in intimal thickening, edema, and nonthrombotic obstruction. Central and sublobular hepatic veins may also be narrowed by intimal edema and fibrosis. There is intense sinusoidal dilatation in the centrilobular areas associated with liver cell atrophy and necrosis. The gross appearance is that of a "nutmeg" liver.[50] Massive hepatic congestion and ascites ensues.[50,98] Hepatic veno-occlusive disease is rapidly fatal in 15–20% of cases.[107] It is associated with the use of cytotoxic drugs especially in patients undergoing bone marrow transplantation. A rapidly progressive form may follow high-dose treatment with cyclophosphamide.[66] Hepatic veno-occlusive disease has occurred in epidemic proportions after exposure to pyrrozolidine alkaloids found in herbal teas and in a variety of other plant preparations, primarily from Heliotrope, Senecio, and Crotalaria species.[50,98,130,131] The injury is caused by an activated pyrrole derivative produced by the cytochrome P450 system.[64,129] Outbreaks of hepatotoxicity have been reported in South Africa after the ingestion of flour contaminated with ragwort (Senecio); in Jamaica after the ingestion of "bush teas" (Crotalaria plants); and in India and Afghanistan when food was contaminated with *Heliotropium lasiocarpium* and *Crotalaria*.[13,72,110,118] Hepatic veno-occlusive disease has also been associated with the ingestion of comfrey tea (Symphytum species).[98,127] Herbal preparations associated with hepatic injury are listed in Table 14–4 (Chaps. 77 and 78).

Peliosis Hepatis

Peliosis hepatis is characterized by large blood-filled cavities associated with sinusoidal dilatation (Chap. 112). It is most frequently associated with the use of androgenic steroids.[6] Most patients are asymptomatic, but occasionally these dilated sinusoids rupture and cause hemoperitoneum.

Chronic Hepatitis

A form of chronic hepatitis clinically resembling that produced by indolent viral infections occurs with the chronic administration of some drugs such as methyldopa, nitrofurantoin, trazodone, nafcillin, diclofenac, and phenytoin.[55,62,65,96,101,105] In some cases, γ-globulins are elevated and there is a positive test for antinuclear antigens, suggesting an immune mechanism for chronic active hepatitis. Jaundice is prominent in these patients, with liver biopsy commonly revealing intrahepatic cholestasis as well as centrilobular inflammation. Hepatocellular enzymes are elevated 5–60-fold.

A long list of drugs is associated with the development of granulomatous hepatitis, an entity associated with chronic fatigue and histologic characteristics including caseating granulomata that resemble sarcoidosis[54] (Table 14–5).

Cirrhosis

Cirrhosis, which results in irreversible hepatic dysfunction and portal hypertension, is caused by progressive fibrosis and scarring of the liver. Fibrosis is related to increased production of collagen. In alcoholic cirrhosis, "activated" lipocytes in the centrilobular area appear to play a major role in the production of septal and perivenular collagen that correlates with collagen deposition in the space of Disse. Acetaldehyde also stimulates collagen production by lipocytes, as do other aldehydes that are products of lipid per-

TABLE 14–5.   Drugs Associated with Granulomatous Liver Disease

Allopurinol
Aspirin
Carbamazepine
Cephalexin
Diazepam
Diltiazem
Halothane
Hydralazine
Isoniazid
Methyldopa
Metolazone
Nitrofurantoin
Oxyphenbutazone
Penicillin
Phenytoin
Procainamide
Procarbazine
Quinidine
Sulfonamides
Sulfonylureas
Trichlormethiazide

Adaped from Lee WM: Drug-induced hepatotoxicity. N Engl J Med 1995;333:1118.

oxidation.[58] Alcoholic hepatitis generally precedes cirrhosis, although cirrhosis may develop in its absence.[61] Chronic ingestion of excessive amounts of vitamin A (25,000 U/d × 6 years or 100,000 U/d × 2.5 years) results in cirrhosis. The earliest lesions in vitamin A toxicity are a characteristic increase in the fat content of the sinusoidal fat storing cells, or Ito cells, with increasing degrees of collagen formation by the Ito cells (Chap. 37). The presence of portal hypertension may be early and striking.[33] Like vitamin A, methyldopa and methotrexate can cause a slow progressive development of cirrhosis with minimal clinical symptoms.[54,55] Methotrexate-induced hepatic fibrosis is dose dependent. Risk factors include associated alcohol intake and preexisting liver disease. Reduced dosing has largely overcome the risk of the development of cirrhosis in patients receiving methotrexate.[29]

Hepatic Tumors

There is persuasive evidence that the use of anabolic steroids increases the risk of hepatic adenomas.[29] Anabolic steroids are also associated with the development malignant tumors such as angiosarcomas and hepatocellular carcinomas. There is some weak evidence associating oral contraceptives with hepatocellular carcinoma. Most commonly, the contraceptive steroids are associated with the development of hepatic adenoma.[47] Angiosarcoma is strongly associated with exposure to vinyl chloride, in addition to arsenic, thorium dioxide, and steroid hormones.[16,28,29,42] Estrogens are weakly associated with much rarer hepatic malignancies such as cholangiocarcinoma.[29]

CLINICAL PRESENTATIONS

Two general types of clinical patterns occur with hepatic toxins: a chronic indolent progression of injury that may elude diagnosis, and a more acute, sometimes fulminant, progression of injury that is temporally related to exposure to the toxin.

Chronic injury is associated with an initially asymptomatic or minimally symptomatic clinical state, with mildly abnormal liver chemistries and slow progression to clinically evident liver dysfunction or cirrhosis.[54,124,128] Over a period of time ranging from months to years, jaundice, coagulopathy, encephalopathy, hepatomegaly, or signs of cirrhosis, such as spider angiomata, ascites, *caput medusa*, and gynecomastia, may be evident. An indolent progression to cirrhosis with minimal symptoms occurs in some patients with chronic exposures to vitamin A, methotrexate, ethanol, and methyldopa.[33,54,58,61] Cholestatic injury is manifested primarily by jaundice and pruritus.

Symptoms of acute liver injury include fever, anorexia, nausea, vomiting, and fatigue. Signs include coagulopathy, jaundice, percussion tenderness in the right upper quadrant, and encephalopathy. Rapid development of portal hypertension, ascites and death follows the onset of some cases of veno-occlusive disease.[50] Patients with acute, large exposures to CCl_4, yellow phosphorus, acetaminophen, and cyclopeptide-containing mushrooms present first with GI symptoms. This is followed by a period of well-being (1–3 days) and then by signs of acute hepatic and renal failure with fatigue, anorexia, and nausea followed by profound jaundice, hemorrhage, ascites, hepatic encephalopathy, and death.[53] Patients with significant acute occupational exposure to dimethylformamide present with abdominal pain, anorexia, and disulfiram-type reactions.[94,125]

Fulminant hepatic failure (FHF) is defined as liver injury that progresses to encephalopathy within 8 weeks of onset of illness in a patient without preexisting liver disease.[53,100] Table 14–6 defines the degrees of hepatic encephalopathy. Some patients may progress from health to death in as few as 2–10 days.[53,77] The prognosis of FHF is related to the time that passes between the onset of jaundice and the onset of encephalopathy. Perhaps sur-

TABLE 14–6.   Clinical Stages of Acute Hepatic Encephalopathy

Stage	Mental Status	Neurologic Signs	Electroencephalographic Changes
Subclinical	Work or driving may be impaired	Subtle psychometric changes	None
Stage I	Attention impaired, irritable, slowed mentation, personality change, depression	Tremor, incoordination	Usually lacking
Stage II	Drowsiness, poor memory, sleep disorder, inappropriate behavior	Asterixis, ataxia, slurred speech	Abnormal; generalized slowing
Stage III	Marked confusion, disorientation, somnolence	Hypoactive reflexes, clonus, rigidity	Abnormal
Stage IV	Stupor and coma	Decerebrate posturing, mydriasis	Abnormal

See Fitz G: Hepatic encephalopathy. In Feldman, M. Scharschmidt BF, Sleisenger M, eds: Sleisenger & Fordtran's Gastrointestinal and Liver Disease, 6th ed., Philadelphia, WB Saunders, 1998:1335; and Trey C, Burns DG, Saunders SJ: Treatment of hepatic coma by exchange blood transfusion. N Engl J Med 1966;274:473.

prisingly, a better prognosis is associated with shorter (2–4 weeks) jaundice to encephalopathy intervals.[100] Most cases of FHF are caused by toxins or viral hepatitis. FHF is usually associated with extensive necrosis, although it may occur in the absence of demonstrable necrosis, such as occurs in exposures to agents that injure mitochondria, including nucleoside analogues and *Bacillus cereus* toxin.[63,67,117] Toxins that have been associated with fulminant necrosis include *Amanita phalloides* mushrooms, acetaminophen, tetracycline, phosphorus, halogenated hydrocarbons, INH, methyldopa, and valproic acid.[53]

Complications from fulminant hepatic failure include encephalopathy, cerebral edema, coagulopathy, renal dysfunction, hypoglycemia, hypotension, pulmonary edema, sepsis, and death.[53,100]

THE EVALUATION OF THE PATIENT WITH LIVER DISEASE

The history is critical in establishing the diagnosis of the patient with liver disease. A medication history should include careful investigation of nonprescription agents, especially acetaminophen and the possible use of herbal therapies. Nearly all chronically used medications should be suspect. An occupational history may indicate exposure to vinyl chloride (plastics industry), dimethylformamide (leather industry) or other industrial solvents. Alcohol abuse is a common cause of acute hepatitis and the most common cause of cirrhosis in this country.[18,58] A history of male homosexual contacts, recent transfusion or intravenous drug use indicates the possibility of hepatitis B, whereas recent travel to an underdeveloped country suggests the possibility of hepatitis A. A history of significant pain and vomiting should suggest the possibility of cholelithiasis.

Clinical Laboratory

Aminotransferases. Laboratory tests are helpful and certain patterns may be suggestive of specific etiologies (Table 14–7). Elevation of hepatocellular enzymes, especially the aspartate aminotransferase (AST) and alanine aminotransferase (ALT), indicates hepatocellular injury, and within a given clinical context, has useful diagnostic significance. ALTs may be increased up to 500 times normal when hepatic necrosis is extensive, such as in severe acute viral or toxic hepatitis.[53] The degree of elevation does not always reflect the severity of injury because levels may decline as FHF progresses. Only moderately elevated, or occasionally normal aminotransferase levels occur in some patients with hepatic failure caused by mitochondrial failure, cirrhosis, or veno-occlusive disease.[33,50,135] Processes associated with intrahepatic cholestasis in the absence of hepatitis may not lead to significant aminotransferase elevation.[92] Patients with acute liver injury caused by work-related dimethylformamide exposure demonstrate aminotransferase concentrations elevated 2–30 times normal, and ALT greater than AST. Bilirubin and alkaline phosphatase concentrations were often normal.[94] In contrast to other forms of hepatitis, in alcoholic liver disease the AST level is 2–3 times greater than the ALT. This is attributed to impairment of ALT synthesis caused by pyridine-5-phosphate deficiency in the alcoholic patient. Elevation of either of these enzymes above 300 IU/L is inconsistent with injury caused by ethanol.[86] During acute extrahepatic obstruction of the biliary tract the AST or ALT may be as high as 1000 IU/L, indicating inflammation because of reflux of the obstructed flow of bile into the biliary tree.[86] The measurement of glutamyl transpeptidase (GGTP) is not very useful because it is present throughout the liver and its elevation is often nonspecific.[86] It is elevated in alcoholic liver disease.[61]

Alkaline Phosphatase. In patients with cholestasis, bile acids stimulate the synthesis of alkaline phosphatase by hepatocytes and biliary epithelium in response to a number of pathologic processes in the liver that affect both hepatocytes and the biliary tract. Elevations of the alkaline phosphatase as high as 10-fold may occur with infiltrative liver diseases, but are most commonly associated with extrahepatic obstruction.[86] Although the alkaline phosphatase may be normal or elevated only minimally in hepatocellular injury, it is unusual for obstruction to occur without some elevation of the alkaline phosphatase. Elevations of alkaline phosphatase and GGTP parallel each other in disease of the biliary tract.[86]

Bilirubin. Elevation of conjugated, or direct, bilirubin implies impairment of secretion into bile, whereas elevation of unconjugated, or indirect, bilirubin implies impairment of conjugation. Unconjugated hyperbilirubinemia occurs during hemolysis and in rare disorders of hepatic conjugation such as Gilbert or Crigler-Najjar syndrome. Except in cases of pure unconjugated hyperbilirubinemia, the fractionation of bilirubin in the case of

TABLE 14–7. Tests for the Evaluation of Liver Function

Disorder	Alkaline Phosphatase, Glutamyl Transferase, 5' Nucleotidase (AlkPhos/GGTP/5'NT)	Alanine Aminotransferase, Aspartate Aminotransferase (ALT, AST)	Albumin	INR	Bilirubin	Ammonia (NH$_3$)
Acute hepatocellular dysfunction (hepatitis)	↑	↑↑↑	N	N or ↑	↑↑	N
Chronic hepatic dysfunction (cirrhosis)	↑	N or ↑	N or ↓	N or ↑	N	N or ↑
Hepatic failure, acute	↑	↑↑↑	N or ↓	↑	↑↑↑	↑↑
Chronic infiltrative liver disease (tumor, fatty liver)	↑↑	↑	N	N	N	N

↑ = increase; ↓ = decrease

hepatobiliary disorders does not have any important diagnostic utility, and will not distinguish patients with parenchymal disorders of the liver from intrinsic or extrinsic cholestatsis.[86] The presence of bilirubin in the urine implies elevation of conjugated or direct bilirubin, and obviates the need for laboratory fractionation.

Urobilinogen is produced by the bacterial metabolism of bilirubin in the bowel lumen. It is absorbed and excreted in the urine. Its presence in the urine indicates the normal excretion of bilirubin in bile, whereas its absence is associated with complete biliary obstruction. Owing to more modern methods of detection of complete obstruction of the biliary tract, this test is mainly of historical interest.[86]

Serum Albumin. Quantitatively, albumin is the most important protein that is made in the liver. With a half-life of up to 20 days, the albumin is usually normal in the previously healthy patient with acute liver injury. In the absence of other disorders that affect albumin, such as nephrotic syndrome, protein-losing enteropathy, or starvation, a low serum albumin is a useful marker for the severity of chronic liver disease.[86]

Coagulation Factors. Impairment of coagulation is a marker of the severity of hepatic dysfunction in both acute and chronic liver disease. Unlike the serum albumin with its half-life of 20 days, the short half-lives of the vitamin K-dependent clotting factors II, VII, IX, and X make the INR (International Normalized Ratio) a useful early indicator of the severity of acute hepatic injury. Elevation of the INR in acute hepatitis is associated with a higher risk of FHF.[35,53,67] In addition to failure of hepatic synthesis, inadequate levels of factors II, VII, IX, and X may also result from ingestion of warfarin anticoagulants or malabsorption of vitamin K (Chap. 42).

Ammonia. Severe generalized impairment of hepatic function leads to a rise in the serum ammonia level, because of impairment of detoxification of ammonia produced during catabolism of proteins. The absolute level of elevation is not clearly associated with mental status alteration.[86] Elevations of serum ammonia levels occur in 60–80% of patients with hepatic encephalopathy, suggesting that ammonia may be a marker rather than a primary cause of CNS dysfunction.[30]

Some patients treated with valproic acid have developed alterations in mental status related to elevated ammonia levels, sometimes in the absence of other laboratory indicators of hepatic injury, and without demonstrable toxic levels of valproic acid. This is attributed to selective impairment of urea cycle enzymes ornithine transcarbamylase or carbamyl phosphate synthetase by pentanoic acid metabolites[27,90,119] (Chap. 41).

Other Laboratories

Serologic studies for the presence of markers of hepatitis A, B, and C should be done routinely in patients with hepatitis.

In the patient with severe liver injury, hypoglycemia is a major concern because of impairment of glycogen storage and gluconeogenesis. Hyperglycemia also occurs as a result of an inability of the liver to handle a large glucose load.[86] The arterial blood gas most commonly shows a respiratory alkalosis. Severe lactic acidosis is seen in patients with hepatic failure caused by mitochondrial injury. Measurements of serum lactate may be useful in identifying the cause of acidosis in a patient with suspected toxic liver injury.[63,67,106]

The CT or MRI scan are useful tests for evaluating parenchymal disease of the liver and will also demonstrate obstruction of the biliary tract. An ultrasound examination will also demonstrate extrahepatic etiologies of hyperbilirubinemia. The radionucleotide liver scan is used to diagnose cirrhosis and veno-occlusive disease, although MRI and CT scans are now used more commonly. Liver biopsy may be helpful but is not specifically diagnostic of drug-induced hepatic injury.

MANAGEMENT

Toxic liver injury often resolves with simple withdrawal of the offending toxin. In cases of severe injury, good supportive care in an intensive care environment is essential. Early referral to a transplant center for patients with evidence of severe or rapidly progressive toxic injury is indicated. See Chap. 32 for a discussion of the indications for the use of N-acetyl-cysteine.

Liver Transplantation

Prior to 1980, 1-year survival for orthotopic liver transplantation was 30% or less.[132] With the development of improved immunosuppressive agents and surgical modalities, liver transplantation is now a practical therapeutic option. Overall 1-year survival for liver transplantation in the 1980s was 80% and 5-year survival was 60–70%.[112] Current overall 1-year survival is greater than 85% at some centers.[132] Patients who require emergent transplantation for FHF generally have a poorer outcome than patients with more chronic disorders. This is likely related to the necessity of utilizing suboptimal grafts such as partial livers, or damaged or ABO-incompatible livers, and the frequent presence of encephalopathy, which has a poorer outcome in all cases.[9,10] The presence of encephalopathy was associated with only a 56% 1-year survival in one very experienced center.[9] Because complications that make transplantation difficult or contraindicated may develop quickly in toxin-induced hepatic failure, the decision to transplant needs to be made early and clinical criteria are needed to predict which patients will benefit. This prediction is extremely difficult. Patients who survive acute hepatic necrosis often recover completely so that one would hope to offer hepatic transplantation only to those patients who have little chance for survival without the procedure. A chance-of-survival rate of less than 20% is regarded as an acceptable cutoff point for this risk-benefit decision.[10,80,81] Currently, two sets of criteria are used to predict 20% survival in patients with FHF who do not receive a transplant. The Clichy criteria, derived from studies of patients with acute viral hepatitis, use a serum level of factor V that is less than 20% of normal in patients under 30, and a factor V level that is 30% of normal in patients over 30.[8,10] The King's College Criteria for patients with FHF caused by acetaminophen poisoning are listed in Table 14–8. For patients with FHF not caused by acetaminophen, the Kings College criterion is an INR >6.5 regardless of degree of encephalopathy.[132] These criteria for orthotopic liver transplant have been widely used and validated. They are highly reliable in predicting death, but their ability to predict survival is poorer.[82,100] Whether the improvement of extracorporeal devices designed to provide temporary support to the failing liver with potential for re-

TABLE 14–8. **Adapted King's College Criteria for Liver Transplantation of Patients with APAP-Induced FHF**

pH of <7.30 or
Grade III encephalopathy plus
creatinine >3.3 mg/dL or
prothrombin time >100 sec
or INR >6.5

Adapted from O'Grady JG, Warden J, Tan KC: Liver transplatation after paracetamol overdose. BMJ 1991; 303:221.

generation will alter decision-making in patients with FHF remains to be seen.[100]

The auxiliary partial orthotopic liver transplant is a new modality that may allow more patients with FHF caused by toxins to survive. This modality uses part of a donor liver as an auxiliary graft that keeps the patient alive until the native liver can regenerate. It provides a smaller mass of liver, making it less useful in treatment of patients with severe encephalopathy, and it is a more complex surgery. If successful, it allows withdrawal of immunosuppression. Although it is a theoretically attractive option, its role is still being defined.[11,73]

OTHER THERAPIES

Intravenous *N*-acetylcysteine benefits patients with fulminant hepatic failure caused by different etiologies and is also beneficial in the later phase of acetaminophen toxicity[36,43] (Chap. 32 and Antidotes in Depth: *N*-Acetylcysteine). The administration of glutathione also protects the rat liver against injury by CCl_4.[14]

Hyperbaric oxygen increases the oxygen tension throughout the liver and decreases liver injury by carbon tetrachloride in rats. Hyperbaric oxygen converts the $\cdot CCl_3$ radical produced by P4502E1 metabolism of CCl_4 to the $\cdot CCl_3OO$ radical, which, although highly reactive, is less toxic because it is rapidly detoxified by glutathione.[14,116] Hyperbaric oxygen was used in one human poisoning with a good outcome.[120]

SUMMARY

The primary role of the liver in the biotransformation of xenobiotics results in an increased risk of hepatotoxicity. The spectrum of liver injury includes combinations of cholestasis, steatosis, and hepatocellular necrosis. Injury may be a result of immunologic mechanisms, free radical initiation of lipid peroxidation, mitochondrial injury, or other less-well-defined mechanisms related to the formation of adducts. Disturbances in intracellular calcium levels likely play a role in the development of hepatocellular injury. Drug-induced liver injury can be dose-dependent and predictable, or idiosyncratic and unpredictable. Idiosyncratic injury is affected by host characteristics that include genetic makeup, concomitant or previous exposure to drugs and toxins, and the underlying condition of the liver.

REFERENCES

1. Alberti-Flor JJ, Hernandez ME, Ferrer JP, et al: Fulminant liver failure and pancreatitis associated with the use of sulfamethoxazole-trimethoprim. Am J Gastroenterol 1989;84:1577–1579.

2. Al-Salman J, Al-Salman J, Arjomand H, et al: Hepatocellular injury in a patient receiving rosiglitazone: A case report. Ann Intern Med 2000;132:121–124.

3. Ahr HJ, King LJ, Nastainczyk W, et al: The mechanism of chloroform and carbon monoxide formation from carbon tetrachloride by microsomal cytochrome P450. Biochem Pharm 1980;29: 2855–2861.

4. Babany G, Bernuau J, Cailleux A, et al: Severe monochlorobenzene-induced liver cell necrosis. Gastroenterology 1991;101:1734–1736.

5. Badr MZ, Belinsky SA, Kauffman FC, Thurman RG: Mechanism of hepatoxicity to periportal regions of the liver lobule due to allyl alcohol: Role of oxygen and lipid peroxidation. J Pharmacol Exp Ther 1986;238:1138–1142.

6. Bagheri SA, Boyer JL: Peliosis hepatis associated with androgenic-anabolic steroid therapy. Ann Intern Med 1974;81:610–618.

7. Bahar R J, Stolz A: Bile salts: Metabolic pathologic, and therapeutic considerations. Gastroenterol Clin 1999;28:27–58.

8. Bernuau J, Samuel D, Durand F, et al: Criteria for emergency liver transplantation in patients with acute viral hepatitis and factor V below 50% of normal: A prospective study. Hepatology 1991;14: 49A.

9. Bismuth H, Samuel D, Castaing D, et al: Orthotopic liver transplantation in fulminant and subfulminant hepatitis: The Paul Brousse experience. Ann Surg 1995;222:109–119.

10. Bismuth H: Liver transplantation in Europe for patients with acute liver failure. Semin Liver Dis 1996;16:415–425.

11. Bismuth H, Azoulay D, Samuel D, et al: Auxiliary partial orthotopic liver transplantation for fulminant hepatitis. The Paul Brousse experience. Ann Surg 1996;224:712–724.

12. Böhme M, Müller M, Leier I, et al: Cholestasis caused by inhibition of the adenosine triphosphate-dependent bile salt transporter in rat liver. Gastroenterology 1994;107:255–265.

13. Bras G, Jellife DB, Stuart KL: Veno-occlusive disease of liver with non-portal type of cirrhosis, occurring in Jamaica. Arch Pathol 1954; 57:285–300.

14. Burk RF, Lane JM, Patel K: Relationship of oxygen and glutathione in protection against carbon tetrachloride-induced hepatic microsomal lipid peroxidation and covalent binding in the rat: Rationale for the use of hyperbaric oxygen to treat carbon tetrachloride ingestion. J Clin Invest 1984;74:1996–2001.

15. Burk RF, Reiter R, Lane JM: Hyperbaric oxygen protection against carbon tetrachloride hepatotoxicity in the rat. Gastroenterology 1986;90: 812–818.

16. Carrasco D, Prieto M, Pallardo L: Multiple hepatic adenomas after long-term therapy with testosterone enenthate. J Hepatol 1985;1: 573–578.

17. Corcoran GB, Racz WJ, Smith CV, Mitchell JR: Effects of *N*-acetylcysteine on acetaminophen covalent binding and hepatic necrosis in mice. J Pharmacol Exp Ther 1985;232:864–872.

18. Crawford JM: The liver and the biliary tract. In: Cotran RS, Kuar V, Collins T, et al, eds: Robbins Pathologic Basis of Disease, 6th ed. Philadelphia, WB Saunders, 1999, pp. 845–891.

19. Dahm LJ, Schultze AE, Roth RA: An antibody to neutrophils attenuates napthylisothiocyanate-induced liver injury. J Pharmalcol Exp Ther 1991;256:412–420.

20. Dai Y, Rashba-Step J, Cederbaum AL: Stable expression of human cytochrome P4502E1 in HepG2 cells: Characterization of catalytic activities and production of reactive oxygen intermediates. Biochemistry 1993;32:6928–6937.

21. DeMorais SMF, Uetrecht JP, Wells PG: Decreased glucuronidation and increased bioactivation of acetaminophen in Gilbert's syndrome. Gastroenterology 1992;102:577–586.

22. Diehl AM, Latham P, Boitnott JK: Cholestatic hepatitis from erythromycin ethylsuccinate. Am J Med 1984;76:931–934.

23. Dutczak WJ, Clarkson TW, Ballatori N: Biliary-hepatic recycling of a xenobiotic: Gallbladder absorption of methyl mercury. Am J Physiology 1991;261:G873-G880.

24. Eliasson E, Kenna JG: Cytochrome P4502E1 is a cell surface autoantigen in halothane hepatitis. Mol Pharmacol 1996;50:573–582.

25. Elliott RH, Strunin L: Hepatotoxicity of volatile anaesthetics. Br J Anaesth 1993;70:339–348.

26. ElSisi AED, Earnest DL, Sipes IG: Vitamin A potentiation of carbon tetrachloride hepatotoxicity: Role of liver macrophages and active oxygen species. Toxicol Appl Pharmacol 1993;119:295–301.

27. Eze E, Workman M, Donley B: Hyperammonemia and coma developed by a woman treated with valproic acid for affective disorder. Psychiatr Serv 1998;49:1358–1359.

28. Falk H, Thomas LB, Popper H, et al: Hepatic angiosarcoma associated with androgenic-anabolic steroids. Lancet 1979;2:1120–1122.

29. Farrell GC: Liver disease caused by drugs, anesthetics and toxins. In: Feldman M, Scharschmidt BF, Sleisenger M, Zorab R, eds: Sleisenger & Fordtran's Gastrointestinal and Liver Disease, 6th ed. Philadelphia, WB Saunders, 1998, pp. 1221–1249.

30. Fitz G: Hepatic encephalopathy In: Feldman M, Scharschmidt BF, Sleisenger M, eds: Sleisenger & Fordtran's Gastrointestinal and Liver Disease, 6th ed. Philadelphia, WB Saunders, 1998, pp. 1335–1341.

31. Fromenty B, Pessayre D: Inhibition of mitochondrial beta-oxidation as a mechanism of hepatotoxicity. Pharmacol Ther 1995;67:101–154.

32. Gitlin N, Julie NL, Sputt CL, et al: Two cases of severe clinical and histologic hepatoxicity associated with troglitazone. Ann Intern Med 1998;129:36–38.

33. Guebel AP, DeGalocsy C, Alves N, et al: Liver damage caused by therapeutic vitamin A administration: Estimate of dose-related toxicity in 41 cases. Gastroenterology 1991;100:1701–1709.

34. Guegenrich FP: Catalytic selectivity of human cytochrome P450 enzymes: Relevance to drug metabolism and toxicity. Toxicol Lett 1994;70:133–138.

35. Harrison PM, O'Grady JG, Keays RT, et al: Serial prothrombin time as prognostic indicator in paracetamol induced fulminant hepatic failure. BMJ 1990;301:964–966.

36. Harrison PM, Wendon AE, Grimson AE: Improvement by *N*-acetylcysteine of hemodynamics and oxygen transport in fulminant hepatic failure. N Engl J Med 1991;324:1852–1857.

37. Hétu C, Dumont A, Joly JG: Effect of chronic ethanol administration on bromobenzene liver toxicity in the rat. Toxicol Appl Pharm 1983;67:166–167.

38. Hoet P, Louise M, Graf M, et al: Epidemic of liver-disease caused by hydrochlorofluorocarbons used as ozone-sparing substitutes of chlorofluorocarbons. Lancet 1997;350:556–559.

39. Hollister LE: Allergy to chlorpromazine manifested by jaundice. Am J Med 1957;23:870–879.

40. Ishak KG, Irey NS: Hepatic injury associated with phenothiazines: Clinicopathologic and follow-up study of 36 patients. Arch Pathol 1972;93:283–304.

41. Jenner PJ, Ellard GA: Isoniazid-related hepatotoxicity: A study of the effect of rifampicin administration on the metabolism of acetylisoniazid in man. Tubercle 1989;70:93–101.

42. Johnson FL, Lerner KG, Siegel M: Association of androgenic-anabolic steroids therapy with development of hepatocellular carcinoma. Lancet 1972;2:1273–1276.

43. Keays R, Harrison PM, Wendon JA: Intravenous acetylcysteine in paracetamol induced fulminant hepatic failure: A prospective controlled trial. BMJ 1991;303:1026.

44. Klaasen CD: Biliary excretion of metals. Drug Metab Rev 1976;5:165–193.

45. Klaasen CD, Watkins JB: Mechanisms of bile formation, hepatic uptake, and biliary excretion. Pharmacol Rev 1984;36:1–67.

46. Kleckner HB, Yakulis V, Heller P: Severe hypersensitivity of diphenylhydantoin with circulating antibodies to the drug. Ann Intern Med 1975;83:522–523.

47. Knowles DM, Casarella WJ, Johnson PM, et al: The clinical, radiologic, and pathologic characterization of benign hepatic neoplasms. Medicine 1978;57:223–239.

48. Kopanoff DE, Snider D, Caras GJ: Isoniazid-related hepatitis. Am Rev Respir Dis 1978;117:991–1001.

49. Krell H, Metz J, Jaeschke H, et al: Drug-induced intrahepatic cholestasis: Characterization of different pathomechanisms. Arch Toxicol 1987;60:124–130.

50. Kumana CR, Ng M, Lin HJ, et al: Herbal tea-induced veno-occlusive disease: Quantification of toxic alkaloid exposure in adults. Gut 1985;26:101–104.

51. Larrey D, Vial T, Micaleff A, et al: Hepatitis associated with amoxicillin-clavulanic acid combinations: Report of 15 cases. Gut 1992;33:368–371.

52. Lauterburg BH, Velez ME: Glutathione deficiency in alcoholics: Risk factor for paracetamol hepatotoxicity. Gut 1988;29:1153–1157.

53. Lee WM: Acute liver failure. N Engl J Med 1993;329:1862–1872.

54. Lee WM: Drug-induced hepatotoxicity. N Engl J Med 1995;333:1118–1127.

55. Lee WM, Denton WT: Chronic hepatitis and indolent cirrhosis due to methyldopa. The bottom of the iceberg? J S C Med Assoc 1989;85:75–79.

56. Lees AW, Allan GW, Smith J: Toxicity from rifampicin plus isoniazid and rifampin plus ethambutol therapy. Tubercle 1971;52:182–190.

57. Lewis JH: Drug-induced liver disease. Med Clin North Am 2000;84:1275–1311.

58. Lieber CS: Alcohol and the liver: 1994 update. Gastroenterology 1994; 106:1085–1105.

59. Lindros KO, Cai Y, Penttila KD: Role of ethanol-inducible cytochrome P-450 IIE1 in carbon tetrachloride-induced damage to centrilobular hepatocytes from ethanol-treated rabbits. Hepatology 1990;5:1092–1097.

60. Lira M, Schteingart CD, Steinbach JH, et al: Sugar absorption by the biliary ductular epithelium of the rat: Evidence for two transport systems. Gastroenterology 1992;102:563–571.

61. Maddrey WC: Alcohol-induced liver disease. Clin Liver Dis 2000; 4:116–130.

62. Maddrey WC, Boitnott JK: Severe hepatitis from methyldopa. Gastroenterol 1975;68:351–360.

63. Mahler H, Pasi A, Kramer JM, et al: Fulminant liver failure in association with the emetic toxin of *Bacillus cerreus*. N Eng J Med 1997;336:1142–1148.

64. Mattocks AR: Pyrrolic and N-oxide metabolites formed from pyrrolizidine alkaloids by hepatic microsomes in vitro: Relevance to in vivo hepatoxicity. Chem Biol Interact 1983;43:209–222.

65. Mazuryk H, Kastenberg D, Rubin R, Munoz SJ: Cholestatic hepatitis associated with the use of nafcillin. Am J Gastroenterol 1993;88:1960–1962.

66. McDonald GB, Hinds MS, Fisher LD, et al: Veno-occlusive disease of the liver and multiorgan failure after bone marrow transplantation: A cohort study of 355 patients. Ann Intern Med 1993;118:255–267.

67. McKenzie R, Fried MW, Sallie R, et al: Hepatic failure and lactic acidosis due to fialuridine (FIAU), an investigational nucleoside analogue for chronic hepatitis B. N Eng J Med 1995;333:1099–1105.

68. Mehendale HM, Roth RA, Gandolfi AJ: Novel mechanisms in chemically induced hepatotoxicity. FASEB J 1994;8:1285–1295.

69. Mitchell I, Wendon J, Fett S, et al: Anti-tuberculous therapy and acute liver failure. Lancet 1995;345:555–556.

70. Mitchell JR, Thorgeisson SS, Potter WZ: Acetaminophen-induced hepatic injury: Protective role of glutathione in man and rationale for therapy. Clin Pharmacol Ther 1974;16:676–684.

71. Centers for Disease Control: Severe isoniazid-associated hepatitis—New York, 1991–1993. Mort Morb Wkly Rep 1993;42:545–547.

72. Mohabbat O, Younos MS, Merzad AAA, et al: An outbreak of hepatic veno-occlusive disease in North Western Afghanistan. Lancet 1976;2:269–271.

73. Munro HM, Snider SJ, Magee JC: Halothane-associated hepatitis in a 6-year-old boy: Evidence for native liver regeneration following failed treatment with auxiliary liver transplantation. Anesthesiology 1998;89:524–527.

74. Nadir A, Agrawal S, King PD, Marshall JB: Acute hepatitis associated with the use of a Chinese herbal product, ma-huang. Am J Gastroenterol 1996;91:1436–1438.

75. Nair SS, Kaplan JM, Levine LH, Geraci K: Trimethoprim-sulfamethoxazole-induced intrahepatic cholestasis. Ann Intern Med 1980;92:511–512.

76. Nakajima T, Okino T, Sato A: Kinetic studies on benzene metabolism in the rat liver-possible presence of three forms of benzene metabolizing enzymes in the liver. Biochem Pharm 1987;36:2799–2804.

77. Nicolas F, Rodineau P, Rouzioux JM: Fulminant hepatic failure in poisoning due to ingestion of T 61, a veterinary euthanasia drug. Crit Care Med 1990;18:573–575.

78. Nolan CM, Goldberg SV, Buskin SE: Hepatotoxicity associated with isoniazid preventive therapy: A 7-year survey from a public health tuberculosis clinic. JAMA 1999;281:1014–1018.

79. O'Dell JR, Zetterman RK, Burnett DA: Centrilobular hepatic fibrosis following acetaminophen-induced hepatic necrosis in an alcoholic. JAMA 1986;255:2636–2637.

80. O'Grady JG, Alexander GJM, Hayllar KM, et al: Early indications of prognosis in fulminant hepatic failure. Gastroenterology 1989;97:439–445.

81. O'Grady JG, Wendon J, Tan KC: Liver transplantation after paracetamol overdose. BMJ 1991;303:221–223.

82. Pauwels A, Mostefa-Kara N, Florent C, et al: Emergency liver transplantation for acute liver failure: Evaluation of London and Clichy criteria. J Hepatol 1993;17:124–127.

83. Peck CC, Temple R, Collins JM: Understanding consequences of concurrent therapies. JAMA 1993;269:1550–1552.

84. Pirotte JH: Apparent potentiation of hepatotoxicity from small doses of acetaminophen by phenobarbital. Ann Intern Med 1984;101:403.

85. Podolsky KD, Isselbacher KJ: Derangements of hepatic metabolism. In: Fauci A, Braunwald E, Isselbacher KJ, Wilson J, eds: Harrison's Principles of Internal Medicine, 14th ed. New York, McGraw-Hill, 1999, pp. 1667–1672.

86. Podolsky KD, Isselbacher KJ: Evaluation of liver function. In: Fauci A, Braunwald E, Isselbacher KJ, Wilson, J, eds: Harrison's Principles of Internal Medicine, 14th ed. New York, McGraw-Hill, 1999, pp. 1663–1667.

87. Pohl LR: Drug-induced allergic hepatitis. Semin Liver Dis 1990;10:305–315.

88. Potter WZ, Davis DC, Mitchell JR, et al: Acetaminophen-induced hepatic necrosis: III. Cytochrome P-450 mediated covalent binding in vitro. J Pharm Exp Therap 1973;187:203–210.

89. Prescott LF: Paracetamol toxicity: Pharmacological consideration and clinical management. Drugs 1983;25:290–314.

90. Rawat S, Borkowski WJ, Swick HM:Valproic acid and secondary hyperammonemia. Neurology 1981;31:1173–1174.

91. Raskind JY, El-Chaar GM: The role of carnitine supplementation during valproic acid therapy. Ann Pharmacol 2000;34:630–638.

92. Reddy KR, Brillant P, Schiff ER: Amoxicillin-clavulanate potassium-associated cholestasis. Gastroenterology 1989;96:1135–41.

93. Redlich CA, Beckett WS, Sparer J, et al: Liver disease associated with occupational exposure to the solvent dimethylformamide. Ann Intern Med 1988;108:680–686.

94. Redlich CS, West AB, Fleming L: Clinical and pathological characteristics of hepatotoxicity associated with occupational exposure to demethylformamide. Gastroenterology 1990;99:748–757.

95. Reid WD, Christie B, Krishna G, et al: Bromobenzene metabolism and hepatic necrosis. Pharmacology 1971;6:41–55.

96. Reynolds TB, Peters RL, Yamada S: Chronic active and lupoid hepatitis caused by a laxative, oxyhenisatin. N Engl J Med 1971;285:813–820.

97. Rheinhart HH, Reinhart E, Korlipara P, Peleman R: Combined nitrofurantoin toxicity to liver and lung. Gastroenterology 1992;102:1396–1399.

98. Ridker PM, Phkuma S, McDermott W, et al: Hepatic veno-occlusive disease associated with the consumption of pyrrolizidine-containing dietary supplements. Gastroenterology 1985;88:1050–1054.

99. Rigas B, Rosenfeld LE, Barwick KW, et al: Amiodarone hepatotoxicity: A clinicopathologic study of five patients. Ann Intern Med 1986;104:348–351.

100. Riordan SM, Williams R: Fulminant hepatic failure. Clin Liver Dis 2000;4:25–45.

101. Rodman JS, Deutsch DJ, Grutman SI: Methyldopa hepatitis: A report of six cases and review of the literature. Am J Med 1976;60:941–948.

102. Ros E, Small DM, Carey MC: Effects of chlorpromazine hydrochloride on bile salt synthesis, bile formation and biliary lipid secretion in the rhesus monkey: A model for chlorpromazine-induced cholestasis. Eur J Clin Invest 1979;9:29–33.

103. Rosh JR, Dellert SF, Narkewicz M, et al: Four cases of severe hepatotoxicity associated with pemoline: Possible autoimmune pathogenesis. Pediatrics 1998;101:921–924.

104. Ross WT Jr, Daggy BP: Hepatic necrosis caused by halothane and hypoxia in phenobarbital-treated rats. Anethesiology 1979;51:321–326.

105. Sallie RW, McKenzie T, Reed WD, et al: Diclofenac hepatitis. Aust N Z J Med 1991;21:251–255.

106. Schafer F, Sorrell MF: Power failure, liver failure. N Engl J Med 1997;336:1173–1174.

107. Schiano TD: Liver injury from herbs and other botanicals. Clin Liver Dis 1998;2:607–626.

108. Schultz JC, Adamson JS, Workman WW, et al: Fatal liver disease after intravenous administration of tetracycline in high dosage. N Engl J Med 1963;269:999–1004.

109. Seef LB, Cuccherini BA, Zimmerman HJ, et al: Acetaminophen hepatotoxicity in alcoholics. Ann Intern Med 1986;104:399–404.

110. Selzer G, Parker RGF: Senecio poisoning exhibiting as Chiari's syndrome: A report on twelve cases. Am J Pathol 1951;27:885–907.

111. Shah RR, Oates NS, Idle JR, et al: Impaired oxidation of brisoquine in patients with perhexilene neuropathy. BMJ 1982;284: 295–299.

112. Sherlock S: Drugs and the liver. Diagnosis of the Liver and Biliary System, 8th ed. Oxford, Blackwell Scientific, 1989, pp. 372–409.

113. Slattery JG, Wilson JM, Kalhorn TF, Nelson SD: Dose-dependent pharmacokinetics of acetaminophen: Evidence of glutathione depletion in humans. Clin Pharmacol Ther 1987;41:413–418.

114. Smith GCM, Kenna JG, Harrison DW, et al: Autoantibodies to hepatic microsomal carboxylesterase in halothane hepatitis. Lancet 1993;342:963–964.

115. Speeg KV, Mitchel MC, Maldonado AL: Additive protection of cimetidine and N-acetylcysteine treatment against acetaminophen-induced hepatic necrosis in the rat. J Pharmacol Exp Ther 1985;234:550–554.

116. Stacey NH, Ottenwilder H, Kappus G: CCl_4-induced lipid peroxidation in isolated rat hepatocytes with different oxygen concentration. Toxicol Appl Pharmacol 1982;62:421–427.

117. Sundar K, Suarez M, Banogon PE, Shapiro JM: Zidovudine-induced fatal lactic acidosis and hepatic failure in patients with acquired immunodeficiency syndrome: Report of two patients and review of the literature. Crit Care Med 1997;25:1425.

118. Tandon BN, Tandon HD, Tandon RK, et al: An epidemic of veno-occlusive disease of liver in central India. Lancet 1976;2:271–272.

119. Thabet H, Brahmi N, Amamou M, et al: Hyperlactatemia and hyperammonemia as secondary effects of valproic acid poisoning. Am J Emerg Med 2000;18:508.

120. Truss CD, Killenberg PG: Treatment of carbon tetrachloride poisoning with hyperbaric oxygen. Gastroenterology 1982;82:767–769.

121. Tsutsumi M, Lasker JM, Shimizu M, et al: The intralobular distribution of ethanol-inducible P450IIE1 in rat and human liver. Hepatology 1989;10:437–446.

122. Vergani D, Mieli-Vergani G, Alberti A: Antibodies to the surface of halothane-altered rabbit hepatocytes in patients with severe halothane associated hepatitis. N Engl J Med 1980;303:66–71.

123. Verrotti A: Carnitine deficiency and hyperammonemia in children receiving valproic acid with and without other anticonvulsant drugs. Int J Clin Lab Res 1999;29:36–40.

124. Victorino RMM, Maria VA, Correia AP, et al: Floxacillin-induced cholestatic hepatitis with evidence of lymphocyte sensitization. Arch Intern Med 1987;147:987–989.

125. Wang JD, Lai MY, Chen JS: Dimethylformamide-induced liver damage among synthetic leather workers. Arch Environ Health 1991;46:161–166.

126. Watanabe M, Tsukada N, Smith CR, et al: Permeabilized hepatocyte couplets: Adensosine triphosphate-dependent bile canalicular contractions and a circumferential pericanalicular microfilament belt demonstrated. Lab Invest 1992;65:203–213.

127. Weston CF, Cooper BT, Davies JD, et al: Veno-occlusive disease of the liver secondary to ingestion of comfrey. BMJ 1987;295:183.

128. Westphal JF, Vetter D, Brogard JM: Hepatic side-effects of antibiotics. J Antimicrob Chemother 1994;33:387–401.

129. Williams DE, Reed RL, Kezierski B, et al: Bioactivation and detoxification of the pyrrolizidine alkaloid senecionine by cytochrome P-450 enzymes in rat liver. Drug Metab Dispos 1989;17:387–392.

130. Yeong ML, Clark SP, Waring JM, et al: The effects of comfrey derived pyrrolizidine alkaloids on rat liver. Pathology 1991;23:35–38.

131. Yeong ML, Swinburn B, Kennedy M, et al: Hepatic veno-occlusive disease associated with comfrey ingestion. J Gastroenterol Hepatol 1990;5:211–214.

132. Yoshida EM, Lake JR: Selection of patients for liver transplantation in 1997 and beyond. Clin Liver Dis 1997;1:247–261.

133. Yoshida EM, McLean CA, Cheng ES, et al: Chinese herbal medicine, fulminant hepatitis, and liver transplantation. Am J Gastroenterol 1996;91: 2647–2648

134. Zand R, Nelson SD, Slattery JT, et al: Inhibition and induction of cytochrome P4502E1-catalyzed oxidation by isoniazid in humans. Clin Pharmacol Ther 1993;54:142–149.

135. Zimmerman HJ, Ishak KG: Valproate-induced hepatic injury: Analysis of 23 fatal cases. Hepatology 1982;2:591–597.

CHAPTER 15 IMMUNOLOGIC PRINCIPLES

William J. Meggs

Immunology has impacted virtually every medical specialty with improved diagnostic tools, insights into pathophysiology of a host of diseases, and new treatments. Medical toxicology has been greatly advanced by modern immunology. Both diagnosis and treatment of poisonings can depend on immunologic techniques. Toxins can damage immune function resulting in immunodeficiencies and life-threatening infections. Autoimmune states can be activated by toxic exposures through several mechanisms. Toxins can induce allergic diseases such as asthma and rhinitis. A host of chemical irritants can induce inflammation and disease by neurogenic inflammation. Immunotoxicology is now an established interdisciplinary field of considerable importance.

Laboratory developments in immunology have brought new tools to the diagnosis and treatment of poisonings. Monoclonal and polyclonal antibodies are used to neutralize colchicine, digoxin, and venoms. Immune assays are used to provide qualitative and quantitative data on toxins in the body. This chapter gives a brief overview of the immune system and discusses the interaction between the immune and nervous systems and the role of neurogenic inflammation in disease; the role of toxins in immune deficiency, autoimmunity, and allergy; and the role of immunology in laboratory developments that are used to diagnose and treat poisonings.

THE IMMUNE SYSTEM: AN OVERVIEW

The immune system is a large and extended organ system with sentinels throughout the body. Bone marrow, lymphatic ducts, lymph nodes, thymus, and spleen are all intimately involved in immunity. Immune cells arise from the bone marrow and migrate throughout the body and are listed in Table 15–1. These cells communicate by the release of and response to a group of protein molecules called *interleukins* (Table 15–2). Immune cells have the ability to recognize specific protein markers on the surfaces of bacteria, fungi, and viruses. Host cells infected with viruses and cancer cells that have developed from host cells can also be recognized and destroyed. Antibody molecules are excreted that can locate and lead to the destruction of microorganisms (Table 15–3). The complement system consists of a groups of proteins produced by the liver, which can destroy bacteria by cell wall lysis (Table 15–4).

The immune system is controlled by T lymphocytes. T helper cells potentiate the response to a specific antigen, and T-suppressor cells suppress the response. T cells secrete protein messengers called cytokines that regulate the immune system and modulate inflammatory responses. Activation of one branch of the immune system shuts down the other branches through the production of inhibitory cytokines.

TH1 helper cells stimulate immunoglobulin E (IgE) production and suppress cellular immunity. TH2 helper cells stimulate cellular immunity and suppress IgE production. Human disease can arise from activation of the wrong type of immunity to a given pathogen, as evidenced in chronic *Candida* vulvovaginitis. Women with this disease make IgE against *Candida*, so that infections produce severe inflammation with swelling and pruritus, even with a small burden of pathogens. Cellular immunity, the only defense humans have against *Candida*, is inhibited, so the *Candida* infection cannot be cleared.[11] Immunotherapy with injections of *Candida* antigen cures chronic *Candida* vaginitis by the inhibition of IgE production and a concomitant activation of cellular immunity against *Candida*.[84]

Neurogenic Inflammation and the Immune System-Nervous System Interaction

The nervous system can induce inflammation in tissues throughout the body. This type of inflammation is known as *neurogenic inflammation*. Inflammatory mediators are released from sensory nerve C-fibers either by local stimulation or from retrograde propagation of a nerve impulse. Local stimulation arises when chemicals bind to chemoreceptors on the C-fibers and from mechanical stimulation of tissues. Sensory nerve C-fibers are found in subepithelial tissues of the respiratory tract, gastrointestinal tract, and skin. These fibers contain chemoreceptors that are triggered by chemical irritants. Examples of chemical irritants are cigarette smoke, gases such as sulfur dioxide and chlorine, solvents such as toluene diisocyanate and formaldehyde, and some fragrances, perfumes, and pesticides. When the irritants bind to the nerve fiber chemoreceptors, chemical mediators, including substance P, calcitonin gene-related peptide, and neurokinin A, are released. These substances produce vasodilatation and edema. In addition, the binding of irritants to the chemoreceptors triggers a nerve impulse that travels to the central nervous system.[70,72]

Neurogenic inflammation is of clinical importance. It is responsible for reactivity to chemical irritants in the skin and respiratory system and plays a role in systemic anaphylaxis. The importance of neurogenic inflammation in many inflammatory diseases is emerging through active research into this important and often neglected area of medicine.

Crossover Network

Immunogenic and the neurogenic inflammation are related. Human skin mast cells contain receptors for substance P,[11] and the

TABLE 15–1. Cells of the Immune System

Granulocytes	Bone marrow-derived cells with cytoplasmic granules and multilobed nucleii
Basophils	Granulocytes with surface IgE receptors, which release histamine and other mediators of anaphylaxis
Eosinophils	Granulocytes that destroy parasites by releasing major basic protein and can damage host tissues; activated in allergic reactions
Neutrophils	Granulocytes that phagocytize bacteria
Lymphocytes	Bone marrow-derived white blood cells that have a spherical nucleus and scant cytoplasm
T cells	
Helper cells	Regulate the immune system by producing lymphokines that control the actions of other cells
Cytolytic cells	Destroy host cells that are infected or cancerous; destroy transplants
B cells	Migrate into tissues and differentiate into plasma cells to produce antibody
Plasma cells	Antibody-producing cells
Natural killer cells	Bind to tumor cells and microbes; release chemicals that destroy the membranes of these cells
Monocytes	Migrate into tissues and differentiate into macrophages, which phagocytize bacteria, fungi, and mycobacterium
Mast cells	Fight parasites; found in connective tissues along nerves and blood vessels; have surface receptors for IgE; degranulate to release allergic mediators

binding of substance P to mast cells triggers mast cell degranulation and the release of mast cell mediators. Sensory nerve C-fibers have surface receptors for histamine. When histamine binds to the nerve fibers, substance P is released and an impulse is transmitted up the nerve fiber.[9] Figure 15–1 depicts the relationship between nerve fibers and mast cells. This crossover network leads to systemic anaphylaxis.

Neurogenic Switching

Most commonly, clinical symptoms appear at the site of inoculation with antigen or chemical irritant. In certain instances, the site of response can be switched to another site.[60] Examples include systemic anaphylaxis to ingestions of food and drugs, in which there is a rapid development of signs and symptoms in many organ systems. Food allergens most commonly cause gastrointestinal symptoms of diarrhea, nausea, vomiting, abdominal bloating, and cramping. Ingestion of a food to which one is allergic can result in urticaria, asthma, laryngeal edema, and systemic anaphylaxis. Patients with chemical irritant rhinosinusitis and asthma report headaches, musculoskeletal symptoms, and involvement of other organ systems when exposed to airborne chemicals. The site switching is thought to occur at the level of the central nervous system, with the response to the sensory nerve signal from the site of inoculation being rerouted to another peripheral location, leading to substance P release at the other location, as depicted in Figure 15–2. Evidence for neurogenic switching comes from animal studies in which systemic anaphylaxis can be blocked by ablating nerve pathways, even though histamine release still occurs at the inoculation site.[46,48] Evidence for neurogenic switching in chemically sensitive humans is provided by a recent blinded, placebo-controlled study that inoculated conjunctiva with perfume in patients breathing fresh air. Although there was no perfume exposure to the airway, respiratory symptoms were induced by perfume

TABLE 15–2. Interleukins and Interferons: Sources and Actions

	Sources(s)	Action(s)
Interleukin		
IL-1	Macrophages	T-cell stimulant; hematopoiesis; fever; inflammation
IL-2	Activated TH1 cells, NK cells	B cell and activated T cell proliferation; NK cells
IL-3	Activated T cells	Hematopoietic progenitor cell growth
IL-4	Mast cells, TH2 cells	Proliferation of B cells; growth and function of eosinophils and mast cells; B cell expression of IgE and class II MHC expression; monokine production inhibition
IL-5	Mast cells, TH2 cells	Growth and function of eosinophils
IL-6	Macrophages, activated TH2 cells	Proliferation of B cells; aids TNF and IL-1 action on T cells
IL-7	Thymic cells, marrow stromal cells	T-and B-cell lymphopoiesis
IL-8	Macrophages	Neutrophil and T-cell chemoattractant
IL-9	T cells	Affects hemato- and thymopoiesis
IL-10	T and B cells, CD8+ cells; macrophages; activated TH2 cells	B cell proliferation; antibody production inhibits cytokine production; cellular immunity, and mast cell growth
IL-11	Stromal cells	Affects hematopoiesis, thrombopoiesis
IL-12	Macrophages, B cells	NK cell proliferation; interferon production; cell-mediated immune function
IL-13	TH2 cells	Similar to IL-4
Interferons		
INF-α and -β	Macrophages, neutrophils	NK cell and macrophage activation; antiviral; class I MHC induction
INF-γ	NK and activated TH1 Cells	Class I MHC induction on somatic cells; class II MHC induction on antigen

TABLE 15–3. Human Antibody Molecule Isotypes

Isotype	Forms	Molecular Weight	Function
IgA	Monomer, dimer, trimer	150 kD, 300 kD, 400 kD	Secretory, mucosal immunity
IgD	Monomer	180 kD	Binds B-cell surface receptor Possible role in B-cell activation
IgE	Monomer	190 kD	Binds mast cell and basophil cell membranes; triggers degranulation
IgG	Monomer	150 kD	Binds to bacterial surfaces, leading to phagocytosis
IgM	Pentamer	950 kD	Earliest response to infection; binds complement; agglutination reactions

TABLE 15–4. Proteins of the Complement System

Classical Pathway
  C1
  C4
  C2
  C3
Alternate Pathway
  Factor B
  Factor D
  Properdin
  C3
Terminal Lytic Components
  C5
  C6
  C7
  C8
  C9

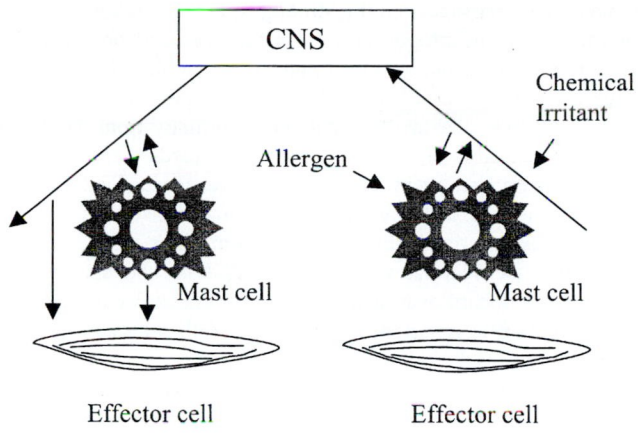

Figure 15–2. Sensory nerve fibers communicate an inflammatory response to the central nervous system.

but not placebo.[66] A study that isolated the upper and lower airways of intubated cats demonstrated that inoculating the upper airway with sulfur dioxide produced bronchospasm, even though there was no direct contact of the sulfur dioxide with the lower airway.

SYSTEMIC ANAPHYLAXIS

Systemic anaphylaxis, or anaphylactic shock, is a severe life-threatening allergic reaction that involves multiple organ systems. Onset occurs most often immediately after exposure to the triggering agent. Delayed reactions can occur several hours after exposure through late-phase mechanisms. Distinction is made between the clinically indistinguishable anaphylactic and anaphylactoid reactions by mechanism. Anaphylactic reactions are initiated by the degranulation of mast cells by antigen to which the victim has IgE antibody and requires prior sensitization. Anaphylactoid reactions occur when mast cell degranulation is initiated by a substance to which there is no IgE antibody and prior sensitization is not necessary. There is no different between treatment recommendations for anaphylactic and anaphylactoid reactions. Table 15–5 lists examples of substances that can trigger anaphylactic and anaphylactoid reactions.

Clinical manifestations of systemic anaphylaxis include urticaria, angioedema, and flushing of the skin. Swelling of the

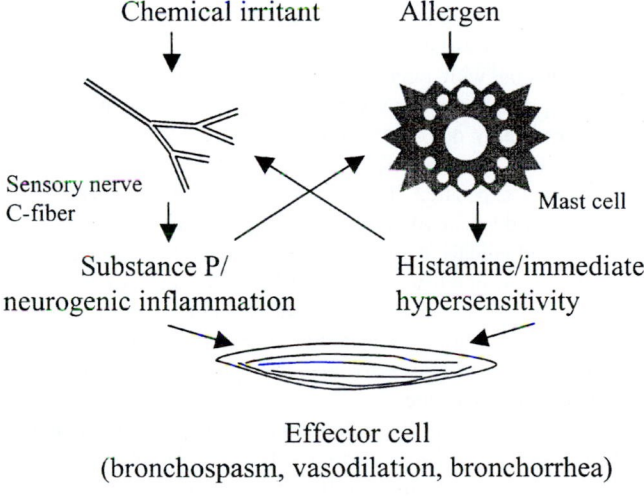

Figure 15–1. The mechanisms of neurogenic inflammation triggered by chemical irritants, immunogenic inflammation triggered by allergens, and their relationship is depicted. Chemical irritants bind sensory nerve C-fibers to release substance P and other inflammatory mediators, while antigen binds IgE molecules on mass cell surfaces to produce mast cell degranulation and the release of histamine and other mediators. Mast cells have receptors for substance P, whereas sensory nerve fibers have histamine receptors.

TABLE 15–5. Examples of Substances Known to Cause Anaphylactic and Anaphylactoid Reactions

Antibiotics	Rattlesnake
Ampicillin	Wasp
Cephalothin	Yellow jacket
Penicillin	
Streptomycin	**Foods**
Tetracycline	Beans
	Carrot
Autologous serum	Cotton seed meal
Horse serum	Egg
	Fish
Enzymes	Milk
Chymotrypsin	Nuts
Chymopapain	Peanuts
L-Asparginase	Shrimp
Penicillinase	
	Parenteral nutrients
Diagnostic agents	Vitamin E
Radiocontrast media	Iron dextran
Diagnostic/Therapeutic agents	**Nonsteroidal anti-inflammatory agents**
Allergy extracts	Aspirin
	Ibuprofen
Venoms	Indomethacin
Honey bee	Naprosyn
Hornet	

tongue, nasal passages, glottic structures, and vocal cords can be of life-threatening proportions. Bronchospasm and bronchorrhea compromise oxygenation. Gastrointestinal manifestations include nausea, vomiting, diarrhea, abdominal bloating, and abdominal pain. Cardiovascular involvement can be primary from the direct effect of mediators on the heart. Secondary cardiac effects result from hypoxia, treatment with cardioactive agents, and the vasodilatory effects of histamine released from mast cells and basophils. Cardiac dysrhythmias range from sinus tachycardia to ventricular tachycardia, ventricular fibrillation, and asystole. In extreme cases, cardiovascular collapse and shock occur. Myocardial infarction is reported in individuals with otherwise normal coronary arteries.[20,47]

The pathophysiology of systemic anaphylaxis is complex and involves multiple pathways and different initiating mechanisms. Protein antigens initiate anaphylaxis by cross-linking IgE antibodies on the surface of mast cells and basophils. A cascade of events leads to the release of preformed mediators. The degranulation process initiates the synthesis of other mediators. Table 15–6 lists mast cell mediators.

Activation of the complement system can initiate anaphylaxis because the C3a and C5a fragments of the degradation of complement proteins C3 and C5, respectively, bind to mast cells and trigger degranulation. Complement-initiated anaphylaxis occurs when the transfusion of mismatched blood products leads to the formation of immune complexes that activate complement. Individuals with IgA deficiency who are infused with immunoglobulin products can have anaphylactic reactions from the formation of IgG–IgA–anti-IgA immune complexes which then activate complement.

Some chemicals, including pharmaceutic products, directly degranulate mast cells through nonimmunologic mechanisms. Aspirin and other prostaglandin synthesis inhibitors can lead to anaphylaxis in susceptible individuals by blocking prostaglandin but not leukotriene synthesis. Because some prostaglandins antagonize the action of proanaphylactic leukotrienes, severe reactions can occur. Opioids, radiocontrast mediators, and vancomycin are examples of agents that are pharmacologically active against mast cells and that can lead to anaphylaxis without prior sensitization.

Table 15–7 outlines treatment of anaphylaxis. Epinephrine is the first-line agent and can be given by the intramuscular, subcutaneous, endotracheal, and intravenous routes, depending on the circumstances and severity of the attack. In an animal model, epinephrine is absorbed more rapidly by the intramuscular route

than the subcutaneous route, with plasma concentrations twice as high via the intramuscular route at 5 minutes[92] Airway control with endotracheal intubation is vital. In the instance of severe laryngeal edema, emergency tracheostomy may be necessary. H_1 and H_2 antihistamines are used. Although corticosteroids are not of immediate benefit, their use is essential to prevent recurrent or late-phase reactions and adverse consequences of the inflammatory medicators that are released in anaphylaxis.

THE TOXIC INDUCTION OF IMMUNE DEFICIENCIES

The hallmark of immune deficiency is a susceptibility to infections. A number of immune deficiency syndromes are defined, and the types of infections associated with each syndrome correlate with the branch of the immune system that is deficient. Many immune deficiency syndromes are genetic in origin and present in early childhood. Examples include severe combined immune deficiency syndrome (SCIDS) in which there is an absence of both B and T lymphocytes. Both cellular and antibody deficiencies occur, and death occurs in early childhood in the absence of a bone marrow transplant or extreme environmental isolation. Bruton disease is X-linked with B-lymphocyte lineage failure, no antibody production, and infections with encapsulated bacteria. Common variable immunodeficiency syndrome is an acquired loss of the ability to produce antibodies, with a susceptibility to sinusitis and pneumonia.

Table 15–8 gives examples of xenobiotics associated with immune suppression. The most devastating immune deficiency induced by toxins is aplastic anemia, in which all branches of the immune system are destroyed. A recent study in the United States, Europe, Israel, and Thailand found penicillamine, gold, and carbamazepine to be the pharmaceutical agents most strongly associated with the development of aplastic anemia[34] Recent case reports have linked aplastic anemia with both the antiplatelet agent ticlopidine[19,52,87,97,108] and the anticonvulsant felbamate.[2] A case of aplastic anemia associated with a herbal medicine was linked to contamination with phenylbutazone.[71] A French study found a vanishing role for toxins previously known to cause aplastic anemia, presumably due to preventive measures.[54] In 1897, benzene was reported to cause aplastic anemia with chronic occupational inhalational exposure. The estimated incidence is 1 per 100 exposed individuals at 100 parts per million (ppm) and 1 per 10,000 exposed individuals at 10–20 ppm.[94] Inhalation exposure to burning oil in Kuwait during the Persian Gulf War has also been associated with aplastic anemia,[88,89] and the organochlorine pesticide lindane has also been associated with aplastic anemia.[6] Agranulocytosis is most strongly associated with procainamide, antithyroid drugs, and sulfasalazine.[34]

Dioxins and furans may suppress cellular immunity in humans. The compound 2,3,7,8- tetrachlorodibenzo-p-dioxin (TCDD) suppresses T-helper cell function in exposed workers up to 20 years after exposure.[102] Workers exposed to a mixture of phenoxy herbicides contaminated with dioxins and furans have an increased total and respiratory cancer mortality relative to controls.[3] An increased total cancer mortality, and in particular cancer mortality from digestive and respiratory cancers, was found in workers exposed to TCDD.[74] This increase in cancer mortality may be a result of impaired cellular immunity against tumors.

The toxic suppression of antibody production leads to bacterial infections. IgG deficiency is associated with sinusitis, bronchitis,

---

TABLE 15–6.   Mast Cell Mediators

Preformed mediators
Histamine
Tryptase
Heparin
Proteoglycan
Chymase
Cathepsin G
Carboxypeptidase

Mediators synthesized after degranulation
Prostaglandin D2
Leukotriene C4
Platelet activating factor
Cytokines (IL-1, IL-4, IL-5, IL-6, TNG)
Colony stimulating factors (IL-3, GM-CSF)

TABLE 15–7.   Guidelines for Treatment of Anaphylaxis

Agent	Dose	Complications
Airway reactions: Goal: Maintain airway patency		
Initial Therapy		
Epinephrine	0.01 mL/kg (up to 0.5 mL) of 1:1000 dilution SQ every 10–20 min	Dysrhythmias, hypertension
Oxygen Inhaled	40–100%	None
β_2-adrenergic agonists	Through nebulizer 0.3–0.5 mL in 2.5 mL of 0.9% NaCl	Dysrhythmias, hypertension
Secondary Therapy		
Corticosteroids	125–250 mg of methylprednisolone or equivalent Q 6 hr for 2–4 doses	Hyperglycemia, fluid retention
H_1 antagonists	1 mg/kg of diphenhydramine or equivalent	Anticholinergic effects
H_2 antagonists	300 mg of cimetidine or equivalent	None
Cardiovascular reactions: Goal: Maintain hemodynamic stability		
Initial Therapy		
Intravenous fluids	10–30 mL/kg, titrated to effect	Congestive heart failure
Epinephrine	See Airway Reactions 1 mL of a 1:10,000 solution IV added to 9 mL of 0.9% NaCl to create a 1:100,000 solution infused slowly	Dysrhythmias, hypertension
Secondary Therapy		
Norepinephrine	2–12 µg/min IV in adults	Same as epinephrine
H_1 and H_2 antagonists	See Airway Reactions	See above
Glucagon	5–15 µg/min	Nausea, vomiting, hyperglycemia

and pneumonia. IgA deficiency is associated with upper respiratory infections and gastroenteritis. A number of xenobiotics suppress antibody production, and in many cases, the association was verified by rechallenge. One or more IgG subclass deficiencies are observed in 66.7% of asthmatics treated with chronic corticosteroids, but in only 6.7% of asthmatics not treated with chronic corticosteroids.[42] Carbamazepine produces hypogammaglobulinemia with absent B lymphocytes accompanied by agranulocytosis.[95] In workers occupationally exposed to lead, there is a decrease in immunoglobulin levels with increasing lead levels.[8] Sulfasalazine depresses IgG, IgM, and IgA in patients with inflammatory arthritis, with an incidence of 2%, 5%, and 3%, respectively.[21] Suppression of serum immunoglobulins by cigarette smoking and exposure to industrial solvents is synergistic.[68]

A number of studies link phenytoin to selective IgA deficiency, and the link has been verified in some reports by rechallenge.[31,90,99] Recurrent respiratory infections and decreases in serum levels of IgA, IgG_2, and IgG_4 are documented in patients on phenytoin, with clinical improvement and normalization of antibody levels with discontinuation of phenytoin.[5] Selective IgA deficiency is associated with captopril[27,107] and penicillamine.[29,79] Three patients with juvenile rheumatoid arthritis treated with aspirin developed an IgA deficiency that resolved with discontinuation of aspirin therapy.[43]

TABLE 15–8.   Examples of Xenobiotics Implicated in the Induction of Immunosupression

Agranulocytosis
Angiotension-converting enzyme inhibitors; antithyroid agents; phenothiazines

Aplastic anemia
Antineoplastic agents; arsenic; benzene; bismuth; carbamazepine; chlordane; chloramphenicol; DDT; felbamate; gold compounds; mercury; penicillamine; phenytoin; silver; sulfonamides; ticlopidine; trimethadione; zidovudine

Cellular immune impairment
Chlordane; DDT; lindane; malathion; HCDD; PBBs; TCDD; 2, 3, 7, 8-TCDF; phencyclidine

Hypogammaglobulinemia
Carbamazepine; cigarette smoke; corticosteroids; phenytoin; sulfasalazine; solvents

LABORATORY EVALUATION OF THE HUMAN IMMUNE SYSTEM

A tiered approach should be used in evaluating the human immune system for immune deficiency following a toxic exposure, with the tests ordered determined by the toxic exposure and the clinical consequences. A complete blood count with differential screens for "cytopenias" Should be obtained. Neutropenia can result from exposure to a number of drugs and toxins, and results in bacterial and fungal sepsis.[41] Lymphopenia is most notably associated with iatrogenic corticosteroid administration, and results in susceptibility to viral, fungal, and mycobacterial infections.[13] Recurrent

TABLE 15–9. Xenobiotic Induction of Autoimmunity

Autoimmune hemolytic anemia
Methyldopa; penicillin; pencillamine

Autoimmune thyroid disease
Polybrominated biphenyl; polychlorinated biphenyl; lithium; penicillamine; amiodarone

Autoimmune hepatitis
Methyldopa; oxyphenisatin; halothane

Immune complex glomerulonephritis
Cadmium; gold; mercury

Myasthenia gravis
Pencillamlne; tiopronine; trimethadione

Pemphigus
α-Mercaptopropionylglycine; captopril; penicllamine,

Polymyositis
Penicillamine

Scleroderma
Rapeseed oil contaminated with anilines; silica dust; vinyl chloride

Systemic lupus erythematosus
Hydralzaine; procainamide; phenytoin; hydrazine; tartrazine; alfalfa sprouts

---

respiratory infections including sinusitis is associated with hypogammaglobulinemias, which is assessed by ordering immunoglobulin levels. A total IgG level is insufficient to exclude IgG subclass deficiencies, which are associated with infections.

Integrity of cellular immunity can be assessed with delayed hypersensitivity skin tests to mumps, measles, and *Candida*. Intradermal injections of antigen should lead to erythema and induration at 24–48 hours. In vitro evaluation of cellular immunity may be determined by lymphocyte proliferation assays to specific antigens and mitogens. Deficiencies of cellular immunity are associated with viral, fungal, and mycobacterial infections, and are thought to impart an increased risk of cancer. Some toxins selectively decrease T-helper cell counts, and total T-helper and T-suppressor cell counts, as well as the ratio of helper to suppressor cells which can be determined by flow cytometry. Dioxin exposure lowers the helper-to-suppressor ratio[102] and is associated with an increased risk of cancer.[74]

THE TOXIC INDUCTION OF AUTOIMMUNITY

Autoimmune diseases are diseases in which an immune response is mounted against noninfected host tissues, leading to inflammation and tissue destruction. The toxic induction of autoimmunity is associated with some pharmaceutic and environmental chemicals. Table 15–9 provides examples of xenobiotics that are associated with the induction of autoimmune diseases.

There are several mechanisms by which a xenobiotic can induce autoimmune disease.

1. A chemical can bind to host tissue so that modified host tissue antigens are recognized as foreign and the tissue is destroyed. Autoimmune hemolytic anemia associated with penicillin results if an immune response is mounted against penicillin bound to red blood cell membranes.[24]

2. In a process termed *molecular mimicry*, an immune response can be mounted against an agent that is chemically similar to host tissue, and the host tissue can be secondarily destroyed. Examples in which infectious agents can induce autoimmunity by molecular mimicry include type I diabetes mellitus[26,33,101] and rheumatic heart disease.[15]

3. A chemical can alter the regulatory system that prevents the immune system from attacking self-antigens. Examples of this mechanism include autoimmune hemolytic anemia induced by the antihypertensive methyldopa,[40] which inhibits T-suppressor cell function. Procainamide stimulates T-helper cell function[65] and induces autoimmunity.

Epidemics of autoimmune disease have occurred when populations were exposed to an environmental chemical that induced autoimmunity. The Spanish Toxic Oil Syndrome began in May 1981, when street vendors in the region of Madrid, Spain, sold bottles of cooking oil which were later found to be rapeseed oil that was contaminated with anilines. Of approximately 100,000 exposed individuals, some 20,000 developed a disease with arthralgias and myalgias, gastrointestinal symptoms, fever, rash, pruritus, pneumonitis with dyspnea, often with laboratory abnormalities of eosinophilia, and thrombocytopenia.[73] The disease was self-limited in most individuals, but approximately 15% of those with illness developed a progressive collagen vascular disease with features of progressive systemic sclerosis, Sjörgen syndrome, Raynaud's phenomena, and pulmonary hypertension.[1,22] A revealing feature of this epidemic was that those who developed progressive autoimmune disease from the exposure were more likely to have HLA haplotypes associated with collagen vascular disease.[32,106] These data suggest that a combination of environmental exposure and genetic susceptibility can lead to the onset of some cases of autoimmune disease.

In 1960, an epidemic of erythema multiforme was associated with a margarine preparation, with approximately 20,000 of some 600,000 exposed individuals developing the disease.[50]

Systemic lupus erythematosus is commonly associated with xenobiotic exposure. Pharmaceutical agents that can induce lupus include hydralazine and procainamide, and, less commonly, phenytoin and isoniazid.[109] Inhalation of the laboratory reagent hydrazine has also lead to lupus.[81] Ingestion of alfalfa sprouts and the yellow coloring agent tartrazine[77] can also induce lupus. Many cases thought to represent idiopathic lupus may be related to environmental chemicals that induce the disease,[81] and careful environmental histories of exposures are essential for any patient presenting with lupus.

ALLERGIC DISEASES AND TOXINS

Disorders that may be triggered by exposure to allergens include asthma, rhinitis, sinusitis, gastroenteritis, migraine,[67,104] urticaria, and angioedema (see Table 15–10). Disease results from the combination of allergy and end-organ sensitivity. For example, an attack of allergic asthma occurs with a combination of exposure to an allergen in a host with asthmatic airways. Toxic exposures may

TABLE 15–10. Hypersensitivity Associated With Drugs and Chemicals

Cardiovascular
Myocarditis: amphetamine; cyclic antidepressants; hydrochlorthiazide; vaccines
Vasculitis: barbiturates; cephalosporins; dapsone; griseofulvin; insulin; penicillin; phenylbutazone; phenytoin; sulfonamides; vaccines; antivenoms

Hematologic
Hemolytic anemia: cephalosporins; methyldopa; procainamide; sulfonamides

Hepatic
Halothane; *p*-aminosalicylic acid; methyldopa; sulfonamides

Renal
Interstitial nephritis: methicillin; penicillins; phenytoin

Respiratory
Asthma: aspirin; cephalosporins; penicillin; sulfonamides; diisocyanates; phthalic anhydrides; trimellitic anhydrides; formaldehyde; cobalt salts; nickel salts; platinum salts

Skin
Contact dermatitis: benzocaine; beryllium salts; chlorpromazine; chromium salts; isoniazid; neomycin; nickel salts; phenols; pyrethrins; quinidine
Exanthems: numerous pharmaceutical agents
Erythema multiforme: penicillin; salicylates; phenytoin; phenylbutazone; sulfonamides
Fixed drug eruptions: barbiturates; phenolphthalein; quinine; sulfonamides; tetracycline
Cutaneous vasculitis: penicillins; phenytoin; pyrazalones; sulfonamides
Purpura: phenytoin; quinine; quinidine; sulfonamides
Erythema nodosum: oral contraceptives
Toxic epidermal necrolysis: allopurinol; mithramycin; phenytoin; sulfonamides

induce both antibody production against previously benign substances and induce end-organ sensitivity to allergic stimuli.

The reactive airways dysfunction syndrome (RADS) is described as an asthmalike illness occurring after a single high-dose irritant exposure that persists long after the initial exposure.[7] Substances reported to induce asthma include acetic acid;[80] ammonia;[23] chlorine;[25,28,37] ethylene oxide;[16] sulfur dioxide;[10] glacial acetic acid;[39] smoke; dust;[7] and toluene diisocyanate.[49] Patients with RADS have asthma attacks as well as constitutional symptoms associated with previously tolerated levels of chemical irritants.[61] Chronic inflammation with lymphocytic infiltrates is seen on pulmonary biopsy.[25]

Reactive upper-airways dysfunction syndrome (RUDS) refers to the induction of chronic rhinitis following an irritant exposure, and these individuals have a persistent intolerance to chemical irritants.[58] Nasal biopsy findings in patients with RADS and RUDS include proliferation of peripheral nerves, basement membrane thickening, chronic inflammation with lymphocytic infiltrates, and gaps in tight junctions.[61] These findings suggest a mechanism for the persistent reactivity to chemicals and inflammation seen in this patient population.[62]

Toxins can induce allergic diseases by acting as environmental adjuvants. An adjuvant is a substance that enhances the develop-

ment of immunity to a second substance. The branch of the immune system activated is specific for each adjuvant. Alum is an adjuvant that induces IgE antibody to a coinjected protein. Killed mycobacteria in oil (Freund's complete adjuvant) induces cellular immunity to a coinjected protein. Environmental adjuvants are chemicals found in the environment, which induce immune responses to other substances in the environment. Environmental adjuvants are thought to be responsible for the increasing prevalence of respiratory allergy in industrialized countries.[55–57] Diesel exhaust particles,[69] sulfur dioxide,[55–57,83] nitrogen dioxide,[55–57] and ozone[4,55–57] are verified inducers of IgE antibody to simultaneously inhaled proteins in experimental models.

Polyaromatic hydrocarbons in diesel exhaust particles enhance the production of IgE antibodies by B cells in vitro[98] and enhance the in vivo IgE production in the human upper airway.[18] After in vivo nasal challenge with diesel exhaust particles, cytokine production is increased in the human upper airway.[18] It is suggested that diesel exhaust particles may play a role in the worldwide increase in allergic respiratory disease.[78]

Both in vivo and in vitro tests are available for establishing hypersensitivity. Scratch tests are performed by placing an antigen-containing solution on the skin and puncturing the dermis with a needle. A wheel-and-flare reaction correlates with the presence of specific IgE against the antigen. Intradermal injection of antigen is used to establish both immediate and delayed hypersensitivity. Patch tests, in which a material is applied to the skin and covered with an occluding dressing, is used to test for contact dermatitis. Radioimmunoabsorbent tests (RAST) and related tests such as enzyme-linked immunosorbent assay (ELISA) are in vitro tests to detect specific IgE antibody. Intradermal skin testing is much more sensitive than in vitro tests for specific IgE.

Chemical Sensitivity

Many individuals have a heightened response to chemical irritants, the most common of which are listed in Table 15–11. Chemical sensitivity differs from allergy in the size of the molecules, the binding sites, and the mediators released. Chemical sensitivity when low-molecular-weight (<3000 daltons) chemical irritants interact with chemoreceptors on sensory nerves to release substance P and other mediators of neurogenic inflammation. Allergic reac-

TABLE 15–11. Exposures Associated with Chemical Sensitivity

Products of combustion
Gasoline- and diesel-powered vehicle exhaust
Emissions from natural gas appliances
Furnace fumes
Environmental tobacco smoke
Cleaning products
Ammonia
Bleach
Pine oil
Fragrances and perfumes
Indoor air contaminants
Volatile organic chemicals outgassing from building products, carpets, fabrics
Outgassing from office and electronic equipment
Pesticides
Organic solvents

tions occur when large molecular weight proteins (>10,000 daltons) react with IgE antibodies on mast cell surfaces to release histamine and other allergic mediators. Respiratory symptoms are very prominent in chemically sensitive individuals.[58] The majority of individuals with asthma or rhinosinusitis have some degree of chemical sensitivity.[59,89]

Chemical sensitivity is a general term that refers to individuals with sensitivity to chemical irritants and includes individuals with disorders that are exacerbated by exposures to chemical irritants, such as rhinosinusitis and asthma. The *multiple chemical sensitivity syndrome* is a term from the occupational medicine literature that refers to individuals with severe and disabling intolerance to multiple chemicals of diverse classes, with multiple organ system involvement.

Sick building syndrome is a disorder associated with poorly ventilated buildings, and symptoms are predominantly respiratory and neurologic. Workers in sick buildings complain of mucosal irritation, with cough, rhinosinusitis, and dry or burning eyes. Neurologic symptoms associated with sick building syndrome are headache, difficulty with concentration, and memory problems. *Environmental illness* and *20th century disease* are expressions used in the popular literature to refer to sensational cases of individuals who have retreated from the modern world because of an intolerance of indoor and outdoor air contaminants. *Idiopathic environmental intolerances* refers to a condition with no documentable abnormalities except a subjective intolerance of chemicals. It is important to note that individuals with asthma, rhinosinusitis, and dermatitis associated with exposures to a broad class of chemical irritants do not have idiopathic environmental intolerances.

There is considerable overlap between these disorders. Persons with chemical-irritant asthma and rhinosinusitis often have headaches and fatigue associated with chemical exposures, and hence meet case definitions for the multiple chemical sensitivity syndrome.[61] In sick building episodes, the most severely affected often become chronically ill with the multiple chemical sensitivity syndrome.[110] Persons with occupationally related asthma and rhinosinusitis are sometimes labeled as having noncompensable psychologic problems and idiopathic environmental intolerances by physicians testifying against workers seeking worker's compensation insurance benefits.

Chemical sensitivity is very common in general populations. A telephone survey by the California Department of Health found that 15.9% of the 4,046 adults residing in California reported being "allergic to or unusually sensitive to everyday chemicals," and 6.3% of those surveyed had been given a diagnosis of the multiple chemical sensitivity syndrome by a physician.[44] A general population telephone survey of 1446 households contacted in North Carolina found that chemical sensitivity was of comparable prevalence to allergy with 35% reporting allergies, 33% of adults reporting chemical sensitivity and 4% of this latter group affected daily.[63]

Early hypotheses considered chemical sensitivity to be a psychologic or psychiatric disorder, but these hypotheses have been thoroughly investigated and found to be incorrect. Controlled scientific studies have shown that although there is an increased incidence of anxiety and depression among those patients with chemical sensitivities relative to control groups, the majority of patients with chemical sensitivities do not have psychiatric illness.[91]

IMMUNOLOGIC THERAPY OF POISONINGS

There are two types of antibodies that can be administered to treat poisonings. Antibodies can bind directly to a toxin and neutralize its action. Alternatively catalytic antibodies enhance the metabolism of toxins to nontoxic chemicals. Table 15–12 lists the antibody therapies currently available in the United States. Scherrman and collaborators[85] have defined *immunotoxicotherapy* as the procedure to sequester, extract, or redistribute, and to eliminate a toxin from the body by the use of antibody molecule entities with *specific active binding sites* (SABS). A schematic of an antibody molecule is given in Fig. 15–3. The variable region V is the site on the antibody molecule that binds specific antigens. A fragment of an antibody molecule that contains a variable region should be as effective in neutralizing a toxin as the entire molecule. Nonmenclature for possible fragments of antibiotic molecules are given in Fig. 15–3.

Polyvalent sera contain antibodies to multiple binding sites. Polyvalent sera are produced by immunizing an animal and harvesting antibody without regard to specificity. The serum is collected and the globulin fraction is extracted for injection. This serum contains antibody against a host of substances, and also contains other serum proteins. Monovalent sera, which contains antibody to a specific substance, is purified from polyvalent serum by affinity chromatography. Monoclonal antibody is produced by a hybridoma, which is the fusion product of a plasma cell producing specific antibody and a tumor cell. Hybridomas produce large quantities of specific antibody in culture, and have provided a source of previously unimaginable quantities of specific antibody. Recombinant DNA technology can be used to insert the gene for a specific antibody into a bacterial cell, which then manufactures the antibody.

TABLE 15–12. **Immunotoxicotherapy for Poisoning Currently Available in the United States**

Toxin	Serum	Manufacturer/Supplier
Microcrura venom (coral snake)	Horse	Wyeth
Bark scorpion venom	Goat	University of Arizona
Lactrodectus mactans (Black widow spider) venom	Horse	Merck
Botulinum toxin	Horse	Centers for Disease Control
Crotalidae venom* (pit viper)	Horse	Wyeth
	Cro Tab (Fab fragment)	Protherics
Digoxin	Fab fragment of sheep antibody	GlaxoSmithKline
Loxoscles reclusa (brown recluse spider; experimental)	Rabbit immunoglobulin isolated with affinity chromatography	Vanderbilt University
Tetanus toxin	Human	Bayer Biological

*Antivenom for nonnative snakes can be obtained from zoologic parks. Consult poison centers for sources.

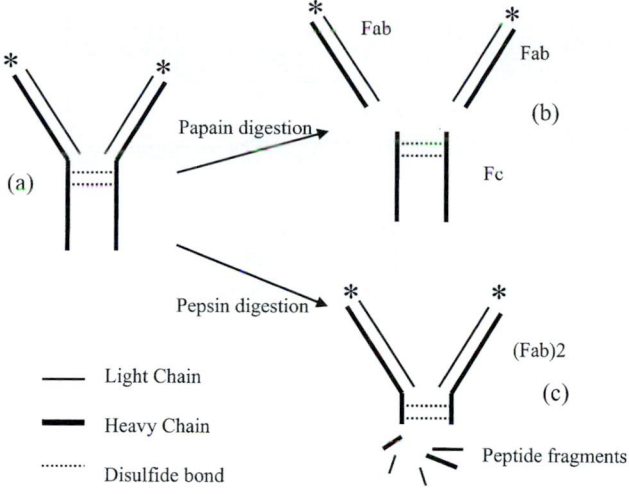

Figure 15–3. **A.** A monomeric antibody molecule consists of two light chains and two heavy chains joined by disulfide bonds. Antigen binding sites are marked with an asterisk. **B.** Papain digestion divides the antibody molecule into three fragments, with two Fab (fragment, antigen-binding) molecules and one Fc (fragment, crystalline) molecule. **C.** Pepsin digestion cleaves the molecule so that there is a (Fab)2 fragment with two antigen binding sites and small peptide fragments.

Fig. 15–4 depicts electrophoresis of four different antibody products. An affinity purified or monoclonal antibody against a single epitope would appear as a monoclonal spike in the gamma region of the electrophoretic spectrum. It can be seen from the figure that increasing levels of purification lead to a predominance of γ-globulins.

Cleaving the antibody molecules with enzymes produces antibody fragments. Fragments containing variable regions specific for a toxin are obtained. The advantage of treating poisoning with antibody fragments is that the reduced molecular weight of fragments results in a lower protein load. Fragments lack the Fc portions of antibody molecules that are associated with serum sickness, activation of complement, and allergic reactions. In a rat model, doses of Fab fragments up to several g/kg were well tolerated.[39] Humanized antibodies are prepared by combining antibody fragments containing variable regions from a nonhuman species with a human Fc fragment. Humanized antibodies have greater utility in the treatment of infectious diseases than in the treatment of poisonings because the human Fc portion aids in fighting infections by activating complement.

Adverse reactions to autologous sera include allergic reactions and serum sickness. Anaphylactic shock, urticaria, and bronchospasm can occur during the administration of sera. A positive skin test to the sera increases the probability of an allergic reaction. Treatment is with epinephrine, antihistamines, oxygen, fluid support, and corticosteroids, as given in Table 15–7. If a patient with known allergy to a serum has to be treated, the patient can be desensitized by beginning therapy with a dose too small to produce a reaction, and then progressively increasing the dose.

Serum sickness occurs 7–14 days after initial exposure to foreign protein such as those contained in sera. Urticaria, vasculitis, arthralgias, myalgias, fever, and, in some cases, glomerulonephri-

tis occur in serum sickness. With prior exposure, onset may be as early as 2 days. Serum sickness can be effectively treated with corticosteroids. Plasma apheresis is effective but seldom needed. Both anaphylaxis and serum sickness are avoided by using antibody fragments rather than whole-antibody molecules.

Factors that determine the clinical utility of an antibody or fragment specific for a toxin are the size of the product; the volumes of distribution of the toxin and antibody product; the kinetics of the binding of the toxin to the variable region; the kinetics of the binding of the toxin to active sites such as receptors; the stability of the product in vivo; and the elimination kinetics of the toxin-antibody complex.[85] The volume of distribution of IgM and IgG in humans is 5 L, whereas the volume of distribution of Fab fragments is 30 L. Volume of distribution of toxins varies greatly, and ideally the volume of distribution of the antibody product should equal that of the toxin. The rate at which the antibody product is distributed in tissue can also influence efficacy. IgG and (Fab)$_2$ equilibrates with interstitial fluid within 12–24 hours, whereas Fab equilibrates within 2–4 hours.[100]

To reverse toxicity, the specific antibody must have a high affinity for the toxin. Treatment of digoxin toxicity with monoclonal antibodies results in a marked redistribution of toxin, with total digoxin in plasma increasing by approximately 6-fold while free plasma digoxin falls dramatically.

The high molecular weight and small volume of distribution of antibody molecules limits their use to those substances that do not require large amounts of neutralizing antibody. Although factors in addition to stoichiometry play a role in determining the effective dose of an antibody or fragment, toxins with small lethal doses will generally require less neutralizing antibody. One antibody molecule has two binding sites for antigen, so from the standpoint of stoichiometry 1 antibody molecule and 1 (Fab)$_2$ fragment neutralizes 2 molecules of drug. A Fab fragment neutralizes 1 molecule of drug.

IMMUNOTOXICOTHERAPY OF DRUG OVERDOSES

A product currently available in the United States for treating drug overdoses is Digibind (GlaxoSmithKlein), which is a Fab fragment of specific antibody to digoxin from the sera of immunized sheep. The digoxin specific antibody is purified by affinity chromatography, and the Fab fragment is obtained by digestion of the antibody with papain. The molecular weight is 46,200. Digibind is a safe and effective treatment for digoxin poisoning (see Chap. 48 and Antidote in Depth: Digoxin Specific Antibody Fragments). DigiTab (Protherics) is another product that neutralizes digoxin. Colchicine poisoning has also been effectively treated with Fab antibody fragments.[86] Antibodies have been developed against and demonstrated to be effective in animal models for poisonings with desipramine. Ricin toxicity has been reversed by neutralizing monoclonal antibodies in a mouse model,[45] while phencyclidine has been studied in dogs.[75]

For substances in which ingestions of a large mass of drug occur, such as theophylline, antibody therapy is possible only if a small variable region fragment can be developed. Consider a 100-kg patient who ingests enough theophylline to develop a toxic blood level of 100 μg/mL. The amount of drug ingested would be

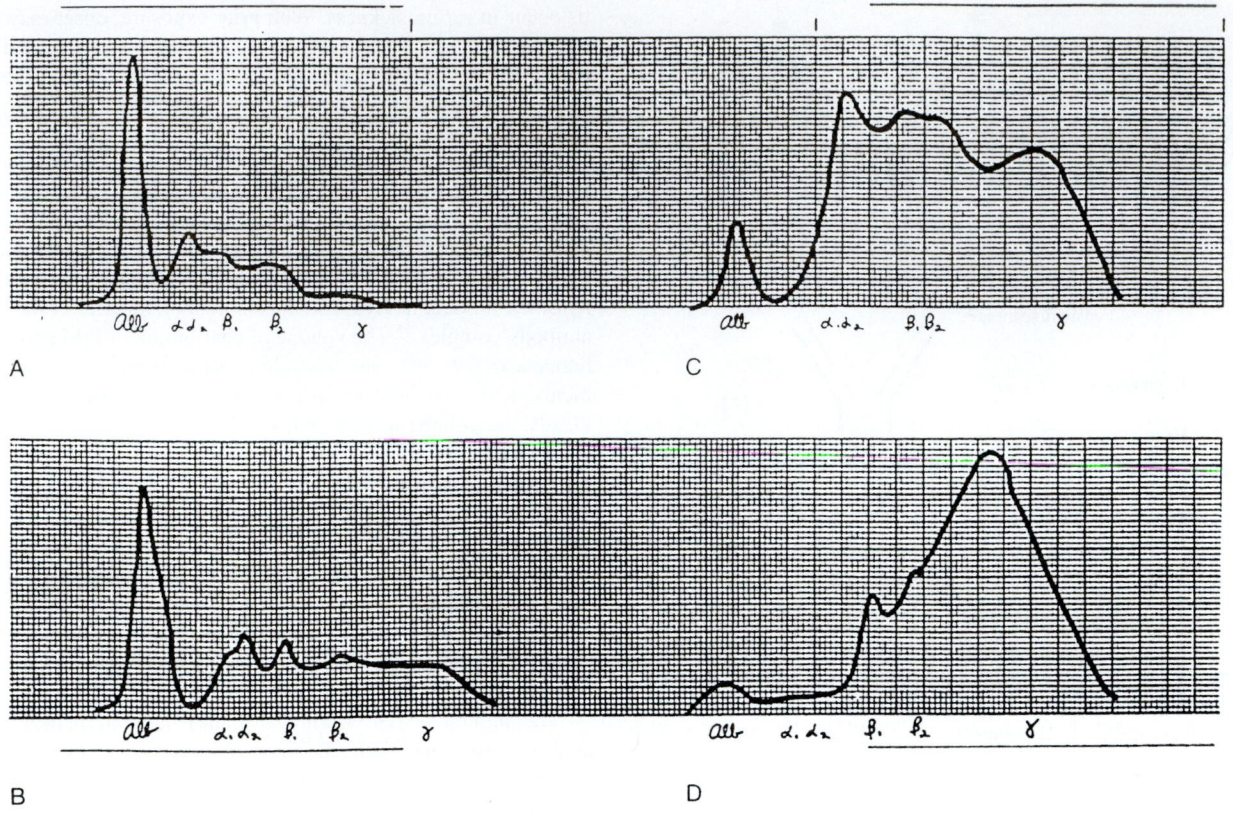

Figure 15–4. Protein electrophoresis of equine-derived (**A**) skin test material (normal serum; Merck Sharpe & Dohme); (**B**) *Latrodectus* antivenom (crude hyperimmune serum; Merck Sharpe & Dohme); (**C**) Crotalidae antivenom (ammonium sulfate precipitation, filtration; Wyeth); (**D**) *Latrodectus* antivenom (pepsin digestion, ammonium sulfate precipitation, filtration; Commonwealth Serum Laboratories). With increasing purification, a relative increase in immunoglobulins and decrease in other fractions can be seen.

Total drug (mg) =

serum drug concentration × Vd × weight in kg

$$= 100 \ \mu g \, / \, mL \times 0.5 \ L \, / \, kg \times 100 \ kg$$

$$= 5 \ g$$

The molecular weight of Fab needed to stoichiometrically bind 5 g of theophylline is

Ratio of Fab to drug needed = (molecular weight of Fab)/

(molecular weight of drug) = 261:1

The mass of Fab needed = 261 × 5g

$$= 2.81 \ kg.$$

Clearly it would be impossible to infuse this amount of Fab fragment into a person. Also, the cost would be prohibitive. This example illustrates that immunotoxicotherapy will probably be limited to those situations in which milligram amounts of the substance is toxic, unless small fragments containing variable regions can be developed.

Technical problems can impede the development of an antibody to specific drugs. The molecular weight of most drugs is too small for them to be immunogenic, so the drug must be conjugated to a protein. Antibodies have to be raised against the drug-protein conjugate. The affinity for antibody molecules raised against a drug-protein adduct to the drug alone varies with the specific epitope on the adduct that the antibody recognizes.

Monoclonal Fab fragments specific for phencyclidine reduces toxicity in rats.[103] Progress has been made in developing catalytic antibodies that hydrolyze the organic phosphorus compound VX.[35,105] This work gives hope that in the future, catalytic antibodies may be used to treat exposure to chemical warfare agents and other toxins. A catalytic antibody that metabolizes cocaine to nontoxic metabolites protected rats from cocaine-induced seizures and sudden death in a dose-dependent fashion, whereas a noncatalytic anticocaine antibody did not reduce toxicity.[64]

IMMUNOTOXICOTHERAPY OF ENVENOMATIONS

The venom of the various pit viper species in the United States is sufficiently similar that one product, Antivenin (Crotalidae) Polyvalent (equine origin; ACP, Wyeth Laboratories, Philadelphia, PA) is useful for all pit viper envenomations. This antivenin is derived from horse sera, contains whole-antibody molecules, and has a greater than 75% rate of hypersensitivity reactions.[12] Antivenom Polyvalent Crotalidae (Ovine) Fab (CroFab, Protherics, Inc.) is an affinity-purified sheep Fab fragment that was approved in October 2000 for use in the United States. In a murine model using lethality as an outcome, the Fab product was found to be 3.1–9.6 times more potent than the whole-antibody product when tested against the venom of 9 pit vipers indigenous to the United States.[12] Experience with other Fab products suggests that incidence of hypersensitivity reactions will be greatly reduced with the Fab product.

Internationally, a host of antivenoms are available for many local poisonous species. Envenomations by nonnative species occurs as a result of importation for research, display in zoos, and pets. Antivenom is stocked by zoos and other institutions and may be located by consulting a regional poison center.

IMMUNOTOXICOTHERAPY FOR BACTERIAL TOXINS

Antibody products are currently used to treat poisoning with Botulinum toxin (Chap. 75) and as a prophylaxis against tetanus toxin. Immunotoxicotherapy using monoclonal antibodies against the toxins and mediators of septic shock has not been successful. Immunotoxicotherapy directed against *Clostridium difficile* toxoids is successful against *C. difficile* enteritis for both in vitro and in vivo models. A case of severe pertussis treated with specific γ-globulin with high titers of antipertussis toxin antibody had a good clinical outcome.[30]

IMMUNE TECHNIQUES FOR DETECTING TOXINS

A number of techniques have been developed that use specific antibody against a substance to quantitate the amount of substance present in a specimen. Radioimmunoassay (RIA) heralded a new era in laboratory medicine. Techniques that followed include the ELISA, the enzyme-multiplied immunoassay technique (EMIT), and the fluorescence polarization immunoassay (FPIA). In the RIA method, a known amount of antibody against the substance to be measured (analyte) is incubated with the specimen, and then radiolabeled analyte of known quantity is added to the specimen. Determination of the amount of radioactivity bound to antibody allows a calculation of the amount of analyte in the original specimen. Disadvantages of RIA are expense, hazards of radioisotope use and disposal, and the long time required to complete assays. Its uses are limited to hormone assays, for which it was originally developed, and measurement of therapeutic drug levels.

In the ELISA assay, specific antibody against the analyte is conjugated to an enzyme, which changes the optical characteristics of a reagent. The specimen with unknown amount of analyte is mixed with the antibody-enzyme complex, the solution is cleansed by removal of excess complex, the reagent that undergoes an optical change in the presence of the enzyme is added, and quantitation of the color change allows a calculation of the amount of analyte in the original specimen. ELISA assays are used in Sweden to measure plasma levels of viper venom before and after administration of Fab antivenom[93] (Chap. 7).

Such technology is not as essential in the United States as it is in other countries, because the two groups of poisonous snakes found in the United States are easily distinguished. Immunodiagnosis following envenomation can be used to help determine the need for treatment after bites when there is delayed toxicity, such as envenomation by the coral snake and the Mohave rattlesnake. Because brown recluse spider bites have delayed toxicity and the spider is not always identified, the simultaneous availability of an antivenom and a diagnostic test would greatly impact treatment. EMIT and FPIA are similar to RIA, but fluorescein-labeled analyte is used instead of radiolabeled analyte. Advantages of the fluorescence assays over RIA are cost and avoidance of radioactive reagents. EMIT and FPIA are used in toxicologic screens to detect drugs of abuse and drugs associated with overdoses.

SUMMARY

An understanding of immunology is essential for new concepts in pathophysiology, diagnostic techniques, and treatment. Broad new advances in these areas will dramatically improve our comprehension of immunotoxicology.

REFERENCES

1. Alonso-Ruiz A, Zea-Mendoza AC, Salazar-Vallinas JM, et al: Toxic oil syndrome: A syndrome with features overlapping those of various forms of scleroderma. Semin Arthritis Rheum 1986;15:200–212.
2. Anonymous: Felbamate use linked to aplastic anemia. Warning issued on drug's use. Am J Hosp Pharm 1994;51:2324.
3. Becher H, Flesch-Janys D, Kauppinen T, et al: Cancer mortality in German male workers exposed to phenoxy herbicides and dioxins. Cancer Causes Control 1996;7:302–304.
4. Biagini RE, Moorman WJ, Lewis TR, et al: Ozone enhancement of platinum asthma in a primate model. Am Rev Respir Dis 1986;134:719–725.
5. Blanco A, Palencia R, Solis P, et al: Transient phenytoin induced IgA deficiency and permanent IgE icnreae. Allergologia Immunopathologia 1986;14:535–538.
6. Brahams D: Lindane exposure and aplastic anaemia: Lancet 1994;343:1092.
7. Brooks SM, Weiss MA, Bernstein IL: Reactive airways dysfunction syndrome (RADS): Persistent asthma syndrome after high-level irritant exposure. Chest 1985;88:376–384.
8. Castillo Mendez A, Rodriguez Diaz T, Leon Lobeck A, et al: Effect of occupational lead exposure on the immunoglobulin concentration and cellular immune function in man. Revista Alergia 1993;40:95–97.
9. Cavagnaro J, Lewis RM: Bidirectional regulatory circuit between the immune and neuroendocrine systems. Year Immunol 1989;4:241–252.
10. Charan NB, Myers CG, Lakshminarayan S, et al: Pulmonary injuries associated with acute sulfur dioxide inhalation. Am Rev Respir Dis 1979;119:555–560.
11. Church MK, el-Lati S, Caulfield JP: Neuropeptide-induced secretion from human skin mast cells. Int Arch All Appl Immunol 1991;94:310–310.
12. Consroe P, Egen NB, Russell FE, et al: Comparison of a new ovine antigen binding fragment (Fab) antivenin for United States Crotalidae with the commercial antivenin for protection against venom-induced lethality in mice. Am J Trop Med Hyg 1995;53:507–510.
13. Craddock CG: Corticosteroid induced lymphopenia, immunosuppression, and body defense. Ann Intern Med 1978;88:564–566.
14. Dart, RC, Sidki A, Sullivan JB Jr, et al: Ovine desipramine antibody fragments reverse desipramine cardiovascular toxicity in the rat. Ann Emerg Med 1996;27:309–315.
15. Dell A, Antoine SM, Gaunt CJ, et al: Autoimmune determinants of rheumatic carditis: Localization of epitopes in human cardiac myosin. Eur Heart J 1991;12(Suppl D):155–162.
16. Deschamps D, Rosenberg N, Soler P, et al: Persistent asthma after accidental exposure to ethylene oxide. Brit J Ind Med 1992;49:523–525.

17. Diaz-Sanchez D, Dotson AR, Takenaka H, Saxon A: Diesel exhaust particles induce local IgE production in vivo and alter the pattern of IgE messenger RNA isoforms. J Clin Invest 1994;94:1417–25, 1994.

18. Diaz-Sanchez D, Tsien A, Casillas A, et al: Enhanced nasal cytokine production in human beings after in vivo challenge with diesel exhaust particles. J Allergy Clin Immunol 1996;98:114–123.

19. Dunn P: Aplastic anemia with ticlopidine therapy in two Chinese patients [letter]. Ann Pharmacother 1996;30:547.

20. Engrav MB, Zimmerman M: Electrocardiographic changes associated with anaphylaxis in a patient with normal coronary arteries. West J Med 1994;161:602.

21. Farr M, Kitas GD, Tunn EJ, et al: Immunodeficiencies associated with sulphasalazine therapy in inflammatory arthritis. Brit J Rheum 1991;30:413–417.

22. Fernandez-Segoviano P, Esteban A, Martinez-Cabruja R: Pulmonary vascular lesions in the toxic oil syndrome in Spain. Thorax 1983; 38:724–729.

23. Flury KE, Ames DE, Rodarte JR, et al: Airway obstruction due to inhalation of ammonia. Mayo Clin Proc 1983;58:389–393.

24. Garratty G: Immune cytopenia associated with antibiotics. Transfus Med Rev 1993;7:255–267.

25. Gautrin D, Boulet L-P, Boutet M, et al: Is reactive airways dysfunction syndrome a variant of occupational asthma? J Allergy Clin Immunol 1994;93:12–22.

26. Gianani R, Sarvetnick N: Viruses, cytokines, antigens, and autoimmunity. Proc Natl Acad Sci U S A 1996;93:2257–2259.

27. Hammarstrom L, Smnith CI, Berg CI: Captopril-induced IgA deficiency [letter]. Lancet 1991;337:435.

28. Hasan FM, Geshman A, Fuleihan FJD: Resolution of pulmonary dysfunction following acute chlorine exposure. Arch Environ Health 1983;38:76–80.

29. Hjalmarson O, Hanson LA, Nilsson LA: IgA deficiency during D-penicillamine treatment. BMJ 1977;1:549.

30. Ichimaru T, Ohara Y, Hojo M, et al: Treatment of severe pertussis by administration of specific gamma globulin with high titers antitoxin antibody. Acta Paediatr 1993;82:1076–1078.

31. Ishizaka A, Nakinishi M, Kasahara E, et al: Phenytoin-induced IgG_2 and IgG_4 deficiencies in a patient with epilepsy. Acta Paediatr 1992; 81:646–648.

32. Kammuler ME, Bloksma N, Seinen W: Chemical-induced autoimmune reactions and Spanish toxic oil syndrome. Focus on hydantoins and related compounds. J Toxicol Clin Toxicol 1988;26:157–174.

33. Karges WJ, Ilonen J, Robinson BH, et al: Self and non-self antigens in diabetic autoimmunity: Molecules and mechanisms. Mol Aspects Med 1995;16:79–213.

34. Kaufman DW, Kelly JP, Jurgelon JM, et al: Drugs in the aetiology of agranulocytosis and aplastic anemia. Eur J Haematol Suppl 1996;60: 23–30.

35. Kawatsu K, Shibata T, Hamano Y: Application of immunoaffinity chromatography for detection of tetrodotoxin from urine samples of poisoned patients. Toxicon 1999;37:325–333.

36. Kelly CP, Pothoulakis C, Vavva F, et al: Anti-*Clostridium difficile* bovine immunoglobulin concentrate inhibits cytotoxicity and enterotoxicity of *C. difficile* toxins. Antimicrob Agents Chemother 1996; 40:373–379.

37. Kennedy SM, Enarson DA, Janssen RG, et al: Lung health consequences of reported accidental chlorine gas exposures among pulp mill workers. Am Rev Resp Dis 1991;143:74–79.

38. Kern DG: Outbreak of the reactive airways dysfunction syndrome after a spill of glacial acetic acid. Am Rev Respir Dis 1991;144: 1058–1064.

39. Keyler DE, Shelver WL, Landon J, et al: Toxicity of hig doses of polyclonal drug-specific antibody Fab fragments. Int J Immunopharm 1994;16:1027–1034.

40. Kirtland HH, Mohler DN, Horowitz DA: Methyldopa inhibition of suppressor-lymphocyte function: A proposed caused of autoimmune hemolytic anemia. N Engl J Med 1980;302:825–832.

41. Klastersky J: Febrile neutropenia. Support Care Cancer 1993;1: 233–239.

42. Klaustmeyer WB, Gianos ME, Kurchara ML, et al: IgG subclass deficiencies associated with corticosteroids in obstructive lung disease. Chest 1992;102:1137–1142.

43. Kondo N, Takao A, Ori T: Case report: immunoglobulin A deficiency in patients with juvenile rheumatoid arthritis treated with aspirin. Biotherapy 1993;7:59–62.

44. Kreutzer R, Neutra RR, Lashuay N: Prevalence of people reporting sensitivities to chemicals in a population-based survey. Am J Epidemiol 1999;150:1–12.

45. Lemley PV, Amanatides P, Wright DC: Identification and characterization of a monoclonal antibody that neutralizes ricin toxicity in vitro and in vivo. Hybridoma 1994;13:417–421.

46. Leslie CA, Mathe AA: Modification of guinea pig lung anaphylaxis by central nervous system (CNS) perturbations. J Allergy Clin Immunol 1989;83:94–101.

47. Levine HD: Acute myocardial infarction following a wasp sting: Report of two cases and survey of the literature. Am Heart J 1976; 91:365.

48. Levy RM, Rose JE, Johnson JS: Effect of vagotomy on anaphylaxis in rat. Clin Exp Immunol 1976;24:96–101.

49. Luo JC, Nelsen KG, Fischbein A: Persistent reactive airways dysfunction syndrome after exposure to toluene diisocyanate. Brit J Ind Med 1990;47:239–241.

50. Mali JW, Malten KE: The epidemic of polymorph toxic erythema in the Netherlands in 1960. The so-called margarine disease. Acta Derm Venereol 1966;46:123–135.

51. Malinow MR, Bardana EJ, Pirofsky B, et al: Systemic erythematosus in monkeys fed alfalfa sprouts: Role of a non-protein amino acid. Science 1982;216:415–417.

52. Mallet L, Mallet J: Ticlopidine and fatal aplastic anemia in an elderly woman. Ann Pharmacotherapy 1994;28:1169–1171.

53. Manzullo EF: Sepsis: The role of steroids and monoclonal antibodies in treatment. Oncology 1994;8:115–120.

54. Mary JY, Guiguet M, Baumelou E: Drug use and aplastic anaemis: The French experience. French Cooperative Groups for the epidemiological study of aplastic anemia. Eur J Haematol Suppl 1996;60: 35–41.

55. Matsumura Y: The effects of ozone, nitrogen dioxide, and sulfur dioxide on the experimentally induced allergic respiratory disorder in guinea pigs. I. The effects of sensitization with albumin through the airway. Am Rev Respir Dis 1970;102:430–437.

56. Matsumura Y: The effects of ozone, nitrogen dioxide, and sulfur dioxide on the experimentally induced allergic respiratory disorder in guinea pigs. II. The effects of ozone on the absorption and the retention of antigen in the lung. Am Rev Respir Dis 1970;102: 438–443.

57. Matsumura Y: The effects of ozone, nitrogen dioxide, and sulfur dioxide on the experimentally induced allergic respiratory disorder in guinea pigs. III. The effect on the recurrence of dyspnea attacks. Am Rev Respir Dis 1970;102:444–447.

58. Meggs WJ, Cleveland CH Jr: Rhinolaryngoscopic examination of patients with the multiple chemical sensitivity syndrome. Arch Environ Health 1993;48:14–18.

59. Meggs WJ: Health effects of indoor air pollution. N C Med J 1992; 53:354–358.

60. Meggs WJ: Neurogenic switching: A hypothesis for a mechanism for shifting the site of inflammation in allergy and chemical sensitivity. Environ Health Perspect 1995;103:54–56.

61. Meggs WJ, Elsheik T, Metzger WJ, et al: Nasal pathology and ultrastructure in patients with chronic airway inflammation (RADS and RUDS) following an irritant exposure. J Toxicol Clin Toxicol 1996; 34:383–396.

62. Meggs WJ: Hypothesis for the induction and propagation of chemical sensitivity based on biopsy studies. Environ Health Perspect 1997;105(Suppl 2):473–481.

63. Meggs WJ, Dunn KA, Bloch RM, et al: Prevalence and nature of allergy and chemical sensitivity in a general population. Arch Environ Health 1996;51:275–282.

64. Mets B, Winger G, Cabrera C, et al: A catalytic antibody against cocaine prevents cocaine's reinforcing and toxic effects in rats. Proc Natl Acad Sci U S A 1998;95:10176–10181.

65. Miller KB, Salem K: Immune regulatory disorders produced by procainamide. Transplant Proc 1982;73:487–492.

66. Millqvist E, Bengtsson U, Lowhagen O: Provocations with perfume in the eyes induce airway symptoms in patients with sensory hyperreactivity. Allergy 1954;54:495–499.

67. Monro J: Food-induced migraine. In: Brostoff J, Challacombe SJ, eds: Food Allergy and Intolerance. Bailliere Tindall, London. Chapter 37, 1987, p. 633.

68. Moszczynski P, Slowinski S, Moszczynski P: Synergistic effect of organic solvents and tobacco smoke on the indicators of humoral immunity in humans. Gigiena Truda i Professionalnye Zabolevaniia 1991;3:34–36.

69. Muranaka M, Suzuki S, Koizumi S, et al: Adjuvant activity of diesel-exhaust particulates for the production of IgE antibody in mice. J Allergy Clin Immun 1986;77:616–623.

70. Nadel JA: Neutral endopeptidase modulates neurogenic inflammation. Eur Respir J 1991;4:745.

71. Nelson L, Shih R, Hoffman R: Aplastic anemia induced by an adulterated herbal medication. J Toxicol Clin Toxicol 1995;33:467–470.

72. Nielsen GD: Mechanisms of activation of the sensory irritant receptor by airborne chemicals. Crit Rev Toxicol 1991;21:183–208.

73. Noriega AR, Gomez-Reino J, Lopez-Encouentra A, et al: Toxic epidemic syndrome, Spain, 1981. Lancet 1982;2:697–702.

74. Ott MG, Zober A: Cause specific mortality and cancer incidence among employees exposed to 2,3,7,8-TCDD after a 1953 reactor accident. Occup Environ Med 1996;53:606–612.

75. Owens SM, Mayersohn M: Phencyclidine-specific Fab fragments alter phencyclidine disposition in dogs. Drug Metab Dispos 1986;14:52–58.

76. Pentel PR, Ross CA, Landon J, et al: Reversal of desipramine toxicity in rats with polyclonal drug-specific antibody Fab fragments. J Lab Clin Med 1994;123:387–393.

77. Pereyo N: Hydrazine derivatives and induction of systemic lupus erythematosus. J Am Acad Dermatol 1986;14:514–515.

78. Peterson B, Saxon A: Global increases in allergic respiratory disease: The possible role of diesel exhaust particles. Ann Allergy Asthma Immunol 1996;77:26308.

79. Proesmans W, Jaeken J, Eeckels R: D-Penicillamine-induced IgA deficiency in Wilson's disease. Lancet 1976;2:804–805.

80. Rajan KG, Davies BH: Reversible airways obstruction and interstitial pneumonitis due to acetic acid. Br J Ind Med 1989;46:67–68.

81. Reidenberg MM, Durant PJ, Harris RA, et al: Lupus erythematosus-like disease due to hydrazine. Am J Med 1983;75:365–370.

82. Rees R, Campbell D, Reiger E, et al: The diagnosis and treatment of brown recluse spider bites. Ann Emerg Med 1987;16:945–949.

83. Riedel F, Kramer M, Scheibenbogen C, Rieger CH, Effects of SO_2 exposure on allergic sensitization in the guinea pig. J Allergy Clin Immunol 1988;82:527–534.

84. Riggs D, Miller MM, Metzger WJ: Recurrent allergic vulvovaginitis. Treatment with *Candida albicans* allergen immunotherapy. Am J Obstet Gynecol 1990;162:332–336.

85. Scherrman JM, Terrien N, Urtizberea M, et al: Immunotoxicotherapy: Present status and future trends. J Toxicol Clin Toxicol 1989; 27:1–35.

86. Scherrmann JM, Sabouraud A, Urtizberea M, et al: Clinical use of colchicine-specific Fab fragments in colchicine poisoning [abstract]. Vet Hum Tox 1992;34:334, 1992.

87. Shapiro CD, Walk D: Aplastic anemia associated with ticlopidine. Neurology 1996;47:300.

88. Shem SC, Kumar R, Roberts IA: Aplastic anaemia after exposure to burning oil. Lancet 1995;346:183.

89. Shim C, Williams MH Jr: Effect of odors in asthma. Am J Med 1986;80:18–22.

90. Shindo K, Kono T, Kitajima J, et al: Crusted scabies in acquired selective IgA deficiency. Acta Derm Venereol 1991;71:250–251.

91. Simon GE: Psychiatric symptoms in multiple chemical sensitivity. Toxicol Indus Health 1994;10:487–96.

92. Simons FER, Roberts JR, Gu X, Simons KJ: Epinephrine absorption after different routes of administration in an animal model. J Allergy Clin Immunol 1998;101:33–37.

93. Sjostrom L, Karlson-Stiber C, Persson H, et al: Development and clinical application of immunoassays for European adder (*Vipera berus berus*). Toxicon 1996;34:91–98.

94. Smith MT: Overview of benzene-induced aplastic anaemia. Eur J Haematol Suppl 1996;60:107–110.

95. Spickett GP, Gompeis MM, Saunders PW: Hypogammaglobulinaemia with absent B lymphocytes and agranulocytosis after carbamazepine treatment. J Neurol Neurosurg Psychiatry 1996;60:459.

96. Stern MA, Eckman J, Otterman MK: Aplastic anemia after exposure to burning oil [letter]. N Engl J Med 1994;331:358.

97. Su CC, Tseng CD, Hwang JJ, et al: Severe aplastic anemia induced by ticlopidine. Report of a case. J Formos Med Assoc 1995;94:689–691.

98. Takenaka H, Zhang K, Diaz-Sanchez D, et al: Enhanced IgE production results from exposure to the aromatic hydrocarbons from diesel exhaust: Direct effects on B-cell IgE production. J Allergy Clin Immunol 1995;95:103–115.

99. Talesnik E, Rivero SJ, Gonzalez B: Serum IgA deficiency induced by prolonged phenytoin treatment. Rev Invest Clin 1989;41:331–335.

100. Thanh-Barthet CV, Urtizberea M, Sabouraud AE, et al: Development of a sensitive radioimmunoassay for Fab fragments: Application to Fab pharmacokinetics in humans. Pharm Res 1993;10:692–696.

101. Tisch R, McDevitt H: Insulin dependent diabetes mellitus. Cell 1996;85:291–297.

102. Tonn T, Esser C, Schneider EM, et al: Persistence of decreased T-helper cell function in industrial workers 20 years after exposure to 2,3,7,8- tetrachlorodibenzo-p-dioxin. Environ Health Perspect 1996;104:422–426.

103. Valentine JL, Mayersohn M, Wessinger WD, et al: Antiphencyclidine monoclonal Fab fragments reverse phencyclidine-induced behavioral effects and ataxia in rats. J Pharmacol Exper Therap 1996; 278:709–716.

104. Vaughn R, Lyndon E: Neurologic reactions to foods and food additives. In: Metcalfe DD, Sampson HA, Simon RA, eds: Food Allergy. Oxford, Blackwell Scientific, 1991, pp. 355–369.

105. Vayron P, Renard PY, Taran F, et al: Toward antibody-catalyzed hydrolysis of organophosphorus poisons. Proc Natl Acad Sci U S A 2000;97:7058–7063.

106. Vicario JL, Serrano-Rios M, San Andres F, et al: HLA-DR3, DR4 increase in chronic stage of Spanish oil disease [letter]. Lancet 1982; 1:276.

107. Vil'chinskaia M, Nasonov EL, Zharova EA, et al: Immunological effects of captopril and ramipril in patients with hypertension. Klin Med (Mosk) 1990;68:61–64.

108. Weiner P, Zidan F, Paz R: Severe aplastic anemia due to ticlopidine. Isr J Med Sci 1995;31:444–445.

109. Weinstein A: Drug-induced lupus erythematosus. In: Schwartz RS, ed: Progress in Clinical Immunology, Vol 4. New York, Grune Stratton, 1980, pp.1–21.

110. Welch LS, Sokas R: Development of multiple chemical sensitivity after an outbreak of sick-building syndrome. Toxicol Indust Health 1992;8:47–50.

111. Witkens SS, Jeremias J, Ledger WJ: A localized allergic response to *Candida* in woman with recurrent vaginitis. J Allergy Clin Immunol 1988; 81:412–416.

CHAPTER 16 MUTAGENS, CARCINOGENS, AND TERATOGENS

Gideon Koren / Kathleen A. Delaney / Debra Kennedy

Toxins injure living organisms by interfering with critical metabolic processes, causing structural injury to cells, or altering the cellular genetic material. Many specific types of injury to the genome that may result in genetic mutations are described. Mechanisms of tumor formation or carcinogenesis are less clearly understood and documented. The general principles relevant to an understanding of the mechanisms of mutagenesis and carcinogenesis are outlined below.

The teratogenesis section of the chapter focuses on the different ways in which the extent of fetal xenobiotic exposure can be more accurately determined. The various biologic markers of fetal exposure that are currently available and the ways in which they may be used to counsel couples at risk, as well as to gain a more quantitative estimate of the true extent of fetal xenobiotic exposure, are also discussed.[32]

THE CHEMISTRY OF THE GENOME

DNA (deoxyribonucleic acid) is the primary genetic material of eukaryotic cells. It is composed of chains of nucleotide bases that pair with a second, complementary chain to form a double-stranded structure known as a double helix. The human genome is incorporated into 23 pairs of chromosomes (22 autosomes and 1 pair of sex chromosomes). All somatic cells contain a diploid number of chromosomes,[45] whereas germ cells contain a haploid number.[23]

DNA is transcribed into RNA (ribonucleic acid), which is then translated into amino acids, the building blocks of protein. In DNA, the purine bases adenine and guanine always pair with the pyrimidine bases thymine and cytosine, respectively. In RNA, the pyrimidine base uracil substitutes for thymine.

Figure 16–1 illustrates the structures of the nucleotide base precursors.

A typical hypothetical DNA sequence might be:

$$5' - AAATTGGGCCTACGGCTA - 3'$$
$$3' - TTTAACCCGGATGCCGAT - 5'$$

The 3'–5' section of this sequence would be transcribed into single-stranded messenger RNA (mRNA) with the following sequence:

$$5' AAAUUGGGCCUACGGCUA - 3'$$

When the mRNA strand is translated into protein, each set of three bases will code for a specific amino acid. The code is redundant, so that several different triplets may code for the same amino acid. This hypothetical segment of mRNA would code for a protein with the following amino acid sequence:

$$5' - AAA\ UUG\ GGC\ CUA\ CGG\ CUA - 3'$$
lysine - leucine - glycine - leucine - threonine - leucine

MUTAGENS

Mutagens are agents that produce alterations in DNA. They may interact with the DNA molecule in a number of ways to produce chemical injury. Not every alteration or mutation in DNA has an effect on gene expression.

For example, a DNA alteration such that the third base of mRNA in the above sequence is changed from A to G would have no effect on the protein synthesized, as both AAA and AAG code for the amino acid lysine. However, a change of the second base to guanine (A to G) would result in arginine being incorporated into the protein, as AGA codes for arginine. The significance of this change depends on the importance of that particular amino acid alteration to protein structure and function. Some amino acid changes have no clinical effect at all and are known as *polymorphisms*. Other changes have profound clinical effects and result in absent or abnormal protein (*gene product*). For example, the common genetic disorder sickle cell disease results from a single amino acid change in the hemoglobin molecule, which produces an abnormal hemoglobin called hemoglobin S.

In the above mRNA (AAAUUG), a mutation that would cause the fifth base (uracil) to change to adenine (U to A) would result in the codon UAG, which is a *stop codon* that signals the termination of protein synthesis, which could have a deleterious effect on the final protein product, depending on the part of the sequence where it occurred. Deletion or addition of a DNA base pair causes a *frameshift mutation*, which puts the triplet code out of sequence. Again, depending on where in the sequence it occurs, a frameshift may have a significant impact on the final protein product.

The following simple linguistic example illustrates the effect of a frameshift mutation:

CAN THE CAT EAT THE RAT

becomes:

CAN HEC ATE ATT HER AT

This makes no sense at all. A comparable effect would be seen in the protein product of mRNA transcribed from a frameshift mutation.

Other mutagens act on the chromosomes during cell division, causing large breaks and, consequently, deletions and rearrangements at the time of crossover during mitosis.[40] Mutations can occur both in somatic (body) cells and in germ (gonadal) cells. The implications of germ cell mutations are that these errors may be passed on to the individual's offspring and hence to subsequent generations.

A number of biochemical mechanisms may lead to the above-mentioned alterations in cellular DNA. Base-pair changes can result from a direct chemical action on a base. For example, nitrous acid (HNO_2) deaminates adenine to form hypoxanthine, which pairs with cytosine. This leads to an A:T to G:C mutation (Fig. 16–2). Alkylation of the N7 or O6 positions of guanine may cause a G:C to A:T change[40] (Fig. 16–2).

Incorporation of abnormal analogues into DNA occurs only when the cell is dividing and DNA is being replicated. These abnormal analogues may result in single base-pair mutations. For example, the keto form of 5-bromouracil closely resembles thymine and may be inserted as a nucleotide in place of thymidine triphosphate during DNA replication. It may then spontaneously convert to its enol form, which pairs more readily with guanine. Further replication would therefore result in an A:T to G:C base-pair mutation.[40] Frameshift mutations may be caused by interference in

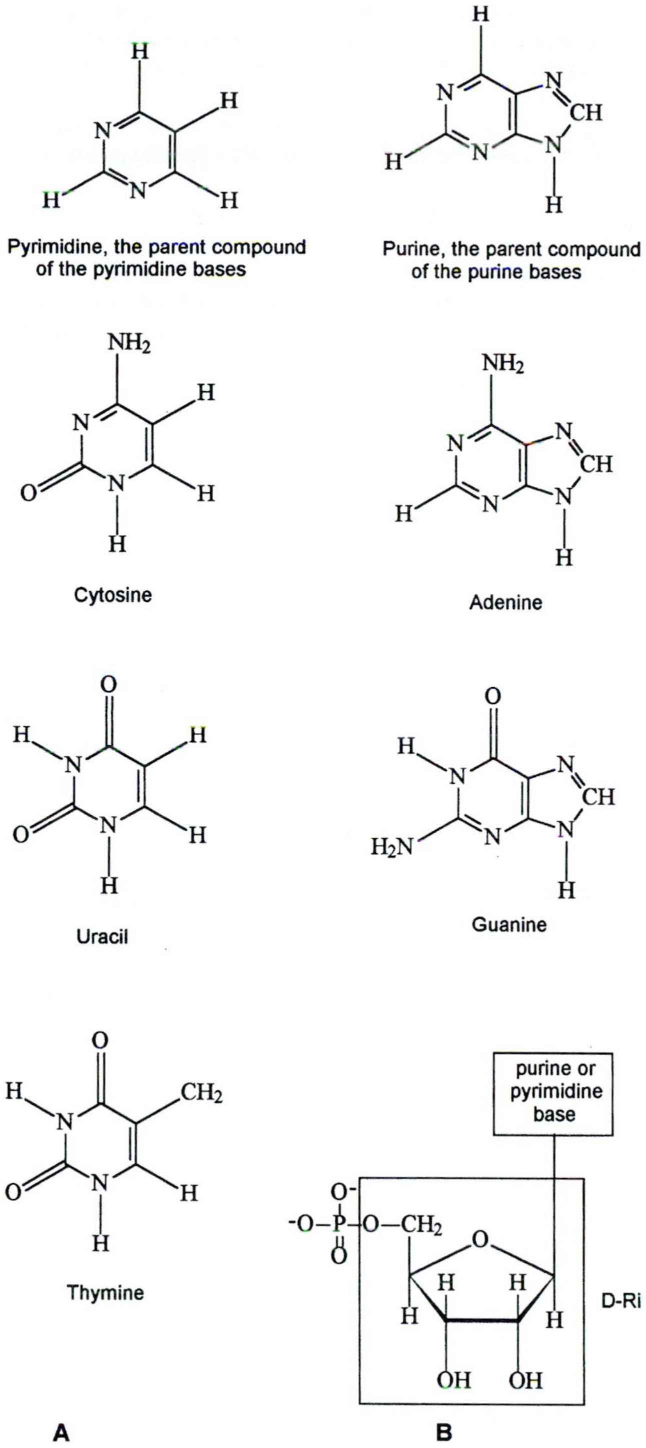

Figure 16–1. **(A)** The structures of the purine and pyrimidine bases. **(B)** The general structure of a nucleotide. *(Reprinted with permission from Lehninger AL: Principles of Biochemistry. New York, Worth 1982.)*

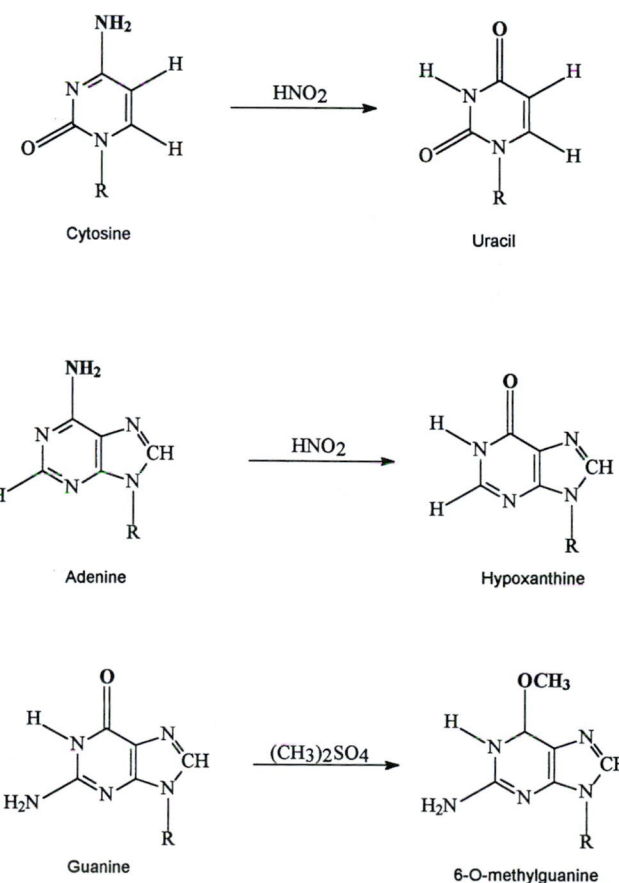

Figure 16–2. Deamination of cytosine and adenine by nitrous acid, a metabolite of nitrosamines. Methylation of guanine leads to faulty base-pairing. *(Reprinted with permission from Lehninger AL: Principles of Biochemistry. New York, Worth 1982.)*

the DNA chain by a foreign molecule prior to replication, such as noted with acridine. When the chain is replicated, an additional base is inserted opposite acridine. Alkylating agents may cause alteration of bases so that they cannot pair, leading to deletion of a base pair and a frameshift mutation. Alkylation and cross-linking of DNA strands during replication may also result in disruption of the chromosome during mitosis. These effects are more prominent in growing tissues, and this ability of alkylating agents is responsible for their therapeutic action of killing cancer cells as well as their carcinogenic property.

A simple in vitro measure of mutagenicity is the Ames test, which uses *Salmonella* bacteria that are unable to synthesize histidine. Mutagenic chemicals increase the likelihood of back mutations, which allow these bacteria to grow on histidine-free media. The number of colonies of altered bacteria growing on histidine-free media gives a quantitative measure of the capacity of the tested chemical to alter DNA.[1,2]

Mutagens that require metabolic activation are identified by the addition of liver homogenate to the Ames test. The Ames test is a good screening technique to determine whether a chemical has the potential to interact with DNA. However, it is clear that a simple in vitro test such as the Ames test cannot take into account all the complexities of the intact organism.

CARCINOGENS

Most classic carcinogens are also mutagens in that they alter DNA. When the Ames test is used as a predictor of carcinogenicity, approximately 90% of known carcinogens react positively. Although the biochemical mechanisms of alteration of DNA by foreign chemicals are fairly well characterized, the ultimate events leading to the unregulated growth of cells is not well understood.

Carcinogens such as estrogen and asbestos, which do not appear to affect DNA, are called *epigenetic* carcinogens. Their mechanisms of carcinogenicity are poorly understood and are not further addressed here. This section focuses on the toxicology of a number of well-studied mutagenic compounds known to be carcinogens.

The list of agents in Table 16–1 makes clear that carcinogens are found in a wide variety of chemical classes and that they may be naturally occurring or synthetic agents.[2] For example, aflatoxin B1 is a potent liver carcinogen that is formed by molds that contaminate improperly stored foodstuffs. Polycyclic aromatic amines, such as benzo(a)pyrene are generated by partial combustion processes such as the charcoal cooking of food and burning wood.[51]

TABLE 16–1. Examples of Agents Implicated in Human Carcinogenesis and the Specific Cancer Induced

Acetophenitidin (phenacetin), renal	Diethylstilbestrol (DES) — vaginal
Aromatic amines — bladder	Ionizing radiation — renal cell
Aflatoxins — liver	Phenytoin — neuroblastoma
Benzene — leukemia	Tars, soots, mineral oils — lung
Benzidine — bladder	Tobacco smoke — lung
Cadmium — lung	Ultraviolet radiation — skin
Carbon tetrachloride — liver	Vinyl chloride — liver
Chromium — lung	

There are no known simple structure-activity relationships that can be applied to determine whether a given compound can be designated as a carcinogen (or noncarcinogen) solely on the basis of its chemical structure.

Most mutagenic carcinogens interact with DNA in a way that may lead to persistent alteration of the cell's genome and its ability to normally regulate cell division. Whether or not the cellular DNA is permanently altered depends on a number of factors, including distribution, access to tissues, and biotransformation. Many mutations in DNA strands are recognized by the cell and are repaired before the damaged DNA is replicated and incorporated into new DNA or transcribed into RNA. The availability and efficiency of DNA repair systems in a particular tissue is an important factor influencing carcinogenicity. Replication of the cell with the unrepaired DNA still present is a requirement for permanent alteration of the genome.[47,69] Many DNA mutations are probably lethal to the cell carrying them. Individuals with conditions such as xeroderma pigmentosum in which there is a genetic deficiency of DNA-repair enzymes, exhibit an increased risk for the development of some, but not all, forms of cancer.

Carcinogenesis is a multistage biochemical and biologic process. In its simplest form, the process can be divided into two major events: initiation and promotion. Initiation or neoplastic transformation involves the covalent binding of the ultimate carcinogen to DNA, resulting in alteration of the genetic code. Initiation can occur after a single exposure to the putative agent. However, many chemicals known to cause cancer are not carcinogenic in the form in which they enter the body and require biotransformation to convert them from an inactive state into their ultimate carcinogenic form.[47] For example, polycyclic aromatic hydrocarbons such as benzo(a)pyrene are chemically inert in their parent form and are unable to form covalent bonds with DNA. Enzyme systems biotransform these nonreactive pro- or precarcinogens into chemically reactive (electron-deficient) products that can covalently bind with nucleophilic sites on cellular macromolecules. Metabolic activation generally requires more than one enzymatic step. Initial activation is often carried out by different enzymes of cytochrome P450, but activation by enzymes in the prostaglandin synthesis pathway, as well as by reductases and peroxidases, is also well established.[51]

Promotion refers to a poorly defined series of events that enable initiated cells to proliferate into tumors. Several chemicals that are not in themselves carcinogens are able to promote the development of tumors that have been initiated by other agents. Examples in experimental animals include phenol, DDT, cigarette smoke extracts, and polychlorinated biphenyls (PCBs). In contrast to initiating agents, promoting agents do not appear themselves to be mutagens.

In experimental settings, promoting agents must be given after treatment with the initiator and need to be given repeatedly over a prolonged period of time. The actions of promoters, unlike those of initiators, appear to be reversible, at least in the early stages of the process.

In recent years, there has been great interest in "cancer genes." As a general model, it is proposed that the conversion of proto-oncogenes into oncogenes is a key event in the initiation of tumors. Proto-oncogenes are normal cellular genes, most of which appear to code for cellular growth factors or growth factor receptors. When a proto-oncogene is damaged by a carcinogen (for example, undergoes mutation or chromosomal breakage and translocation) the resulting oncogene drives the abnormal cell division and differentiation that is typical of neoplasia.[68]

The site of tumor development is determined by the tissue- and species-specific DNA repair systems, tissue activation and deactivation, the structure of the carcinogen, as well as the dosage. For example, the symmetric dialkylnitrosamines (Fig. 16–3) cause tumors in rats according to the chemical structure of the R group. The dimethyl and diethyl compounds cause liver cancer, whereas the dibutyl compound causes bladder cancer, and lung cancer is associated with the diamyl compound.

Large single doses of dimethylnitrosamine in rats lead to renal rather than to hepatic carcinomas. Hamsters are deficient in a specific liver enzyme that repairs alkylated guanine bases in DNA, and are thus highly susceptible to the hepatic carcinogenic effects of dimethylnitrosamine. In contrast, diethylnitrosamine primarily causes lung tumors in hamsters. Asymmetric nitrosamines cause cancer of the esophagus in rats.[75] These effects are specific to the structure of the carcinogen, the tissue affected, and the species, and in a very general way, illustrate the enormous complexity of the interaction between living tissues and potential carcinogens.

TERATOGENS

Environmental insults that result in structural defects after fertilization are known as *teratogens.* The term is derived from the Greek words *teratos* (monster) and *gen* (producing). Those environmental influences that produce abnormalities of function rather than visible structural anomalies are termed *hadegens* (derived from Hades, the Greek god of the underworld, who wore a helmet to render himself invisible). A third term, *trophogen*, is used to describe environmental agents that alter growth. Constituents of tobacco smoke are an example. A given environmental agent may cause all three types of effects, or may cause different effects according to the gestational timing of the exposure.[25] For example, rubella infection is teratogenic, hadegenic, and trophogenic in the first trimester, whereas after 20 weeks' gestation it is only hadegenic.

For both medicolegal and scientific reasons, there has been increasing interest in the field of teratology, particularly with regard to the relatively new field of neurobehavioral teratology (hadegenic agents). There has also been increased emphasis on providing "proof" of human teratogenicity. Unfortunately, it may be difficult to prove that a particular insult or agent is teratogenic, hadegenic, or trophogenic. A number of approaches may be used to try and delineate potentially harmful fetal exposures.[6]

Qualitative Criteria for Proof of Teratogenicity

The first approach is to establish certain qualitative criteria for the proof of human teratogenicity.[67] Many recognized human teratogens do not fulfill all of the criteria shown in Table 16–2. For example, thalidomide, a major human teratogen, was not shown to be teratogenic in animal models. Therefore, these criteria can be used only as guidelines and need to be considered in conjunction with other relevant data.

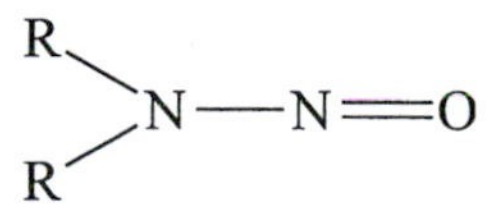

Another approach to attempt to qualify and/or quantify fetal exposure is to measure biologic markers of the putative teratogen in the fetus or neonate (or even in the mother), thereby gaining a semiquantitative estimate of the extent of teratogen exposure in utero. This approach may also yield a "fetal dose response" by estimating the dose and timing of a particular exposure.[25]

However, this approach is not universally applicable for several reasons:

1. Exposure may be too early in gestation to be measured at a later stage of pregnancy.
2. Appropriate biologic markers may not exist for the particular xenobiotic.
3. Suitable body fluid samples may not be readily obtainable.

There are also a number of ethical issues that go beyond the scope of this text involved in the measurement, particularly in neonates, of biologic markers of in utero exposure to xenobiotics, especially to illicit drugs such as cocaine and opioids.

It is clear that neither documentation of the extent of fetal exposure nor measurement of biologic markers alone can prove teratogenicity in a particular situation. A rational approach is to combine both the qualitative criteria and the biologic markers where available, in an attempt to provide the mother with the best possible information and risk estimate.

TABLE 16–2.   Criteria for the Establishment of Human Teratogenicity

1. There should be proof of exposure to the agent having occurred at a critical stage(s) in prenatal development (evidence from prescriptions, physicians' records, dates of ingestion).
2. There should be findings from appropriately controlled epidemiolgoic studies that show that exposure to the agent produces an increase in the occurrence of specific phenotypic effects, and a recognizable pattern of both major and minor malformations. A particular defect (eg, Ebstein's anomaly in association with lithium exposure) or constellation of defects (eg, fetal hydantoin syndrome) is particularly helpful.
3. There should be animal models of the exposure that mimic the effects in humans, ideally at clinically comparable doses.
4. There should be a dose-response relationship that has been demonstrated in either animal models or human exposures, such that the greater the exposure, the more severe the fetal phenotypic effects. It should be noted that dose-response has not been shown for any of the well-known human teratogens, including retinoic acid, thalidomide, and diethylstilbestrol.
5. There should be biologic plausibility for the mechanism of action of the putative teratogenic agent (eg, retinoic acid appears to interfere with normal neural crest cell function and migration).
6. There may be a subset of exposed individuals who are intrinsically predisposed to the teratogenic effects of a particular agent due either to an inborn error of metabolism or to some other genetic polymorphism. This would provide a biologic explanation for the clinically well-recognized variability of teratogenic effects.

Holmes L: Fetal environmental toxins. Pediatr Rev 1992;13:364 and Shephard TH: "Proof" of human teratogenicity. Teratology 1994;50:97.

Figure 16–3.   These symmetric dialkylnitrosamines cause tumors in rats, the type of which depends on the chemical structure of the R group.

PROBLEMS IN ASSESSING POSSIBLE FETAL EXPOSURE

Recall and Reporting Bias

A major limitation in risk assessment is the mother's recall of her xenobiotic exposure. There may be a number of reasons for this, including genuine inability to recall details, guilt, denial, or because the substances involved are illicit and admission of their use may result (in the mother's perception at least) in prosecution or the involvement of children's welfare agencies.

For example, women who have given birth to children with congenital defects tend to retrospectively minimize their history of alcohol ingestion as compared with their reported consumption when questioned antenatally.[15]

There is also a less-than-optimal recall not only of drug dosages and gestational timing of the exposure, but also of the actual agents, especially when there are multiple exposures. In addition, the manner in which the mother is questioned may alter her responses.[48] With regard to substance abuse, it has been shown that maternal history does not reliably predict fetal exposure, although actual drug abusers are more likely to admit use than infrequent drug users.[18,52]

Biologic Variability

Most human teratogens (including alcohol and thalidomide) affect only some of the fetuses exposed and there is considerable variability in phenotypic effects. Causes of this variability may include differences in placental transfer and metabolism as well as genetic polymorphisms in enzymatic function and expression. After a mother has had a child affected by in utero exposure to phenytoin, for example, she is more likely to have a second affected child than another mother whose first infant was not similarly affected. It has been proposed that the reason for this is that the child has inherited from at least one parent a gene that results in a diminished ability to deactivate a toxic metabolite, and therefore increases the likelihood of the drug's teratogenic effects.[69] In the future, it may be possible to predict which fetuses are at highest risk of teratogenicity, based on their drug-metabolizing genotype.[6] By performing analysis on neonatal samples such as hair, urine, blood, meconium, and amniotic fluid, a better understanding of the sources of mother-infant variability may be gained.[57] This can be useful in the study of environmental agents and drugs of abuse, as well as in the study of prescribed drugs and medicinal teratogens, such as warfarin and valproic acid, as well as fetotoxins such as captopril.[30]

BIOLOGIC MARKERS OF FETAL EXPOSURE

Blood

Cord blood is a readily available biologic fluid, collection of which does not entail invasive procedures. Frequently, however, cord-blood levels of a xenobiotic may have a very limited clinical applicability and the potential for analytic value may be restricted. For example, measurement of carboxyhemoglobin from cord-blood samples in the neonate reflects exposure to carbon monoxide only over the few hours immediately prior to delivery, a time when most women are in a hospital and therefore do not smoke.

Similarly, measurement of blood and urine levels of nicotine and cotinine reflect only very recent exposure. Tissue hypoxia causes increased production of erythropoietin, and elevated cord-blood erythropoietin levels occur in chronic fetal hypoxia in association with conditions such as maternal preeclampsia, diabetes, and Rh isoimmunization. Because maternal smoking affects fetal hemodynamics and increases the level of fetal carboxyhemoglobin, it is likely that a proportion of fetuses of smoking mothers are chronically hypoxic in utero. Erythropoietin and hemoglobin levels are indirect biologic markers of fetal exposure to maternal cigarette smoking.[72] About 20% of neonates whose mothers smoked during pregnancy had mean cord-blood erythropoietin concentrations higher than in infants whose mothers were nonsmokers, suggesting chronic hypoxia. There was also a positive correlation between cord-blood hemoglobin and erythropoietin concentrations.[72]

Lead is recognized as a neurodevelopmental toxin,[49] but it is only recently that concerns were raised about its teratogenic effects. An association between cord-blood lead levels greater than 10 μg/dL and lower cognitive achievements at 6, 12, 18, and 24 months of age has been demonstrated.[4] Of note, postnatal blood lead levels were not associated with low cognitive scores.[4]

Obstetric complications associated with elevated lead exposure include spontaneous abortion, premature rupture of the membranes, and preterm delivery.[50] Lead crosses the placenta freely, probably by both passive and active transport mechanisms. Transplacental transfer of lead occurs as early as 12–14 weeks of gestation with increasing amounts of lead being detected in fetal tissues with advancing gestation.[58] Lead also accumulates in fetal liver and bones. It is important to detect babies potentially exposed in utero to excess lead as early as possible. Several studies demonstrate good correlation between maternal and cord-blood lead levels.[3,22,48] However, lead exposure throughout pregnancy cannot be assumed from a single blood measurement, because of changes in maternal blood levels and placental permeability to lead. Thus, neonatal hair analysis (as discussed later) may be a more accurate way of assessing cumulative in utero lead exposure.[38]

Urine

Urine reflects only a very small window of time in terms of fetal exposure. For example, the cocaine metabolite, benzoylecgonine, is measurable in urine only 96–120 hours after the last exposure to cocaine; thus, urine analysis alone may underestimate the true extent of prenatal cocaine exposure. One group of researchers found that when sufficiently sensitive analytic methods were used, maternal urine, neonatal urine, and meconium analyses yielded similar results for detection of prenatal cocaine exposure.[8] Rapid mass screening techniques with high sensitivity and specificity (96% and 100%, respectively) have been developed to test urine and to identify neonates exposed in utero to cocaine.[74]

Meconium

Meconium is an ideal specimen for analysis of drugs and metabolites in the newborn period for these reasons:

1. The collection of meconium is simple and noninvasive.
2. Meconium is available for up to 3 days after delivery.
3. Initial testing can be performed with common laboratory techniques for mass screening, with confirmatory testing using gas chromatography-mass spectrometry (GC-MS).

4. Testing is sensitive and specific.
5. It is a window to the last 30 weeks of gestation.

Opioids and cannabinoids as well as cocaine and nicotine and their metabolites can all be measured in meconium, and several different analytic methods are validated.[9,46,53,54] Meconium is formed from a composite of desquamated intestinal and cutaneous epithelial cells, bile, pancreatic and intestinal secretions, and swallowed amniotic fluid. Fetal swallowing first occurs at around 12 weeks' gestation so that the accumulation of drugs in meconium via fetal urine production and swallowing of amniotic fluid should theoretically be demonstrable after this time.

Postmortem analysis of meconium from a fetus that was spontaneously aborted at 17 weeks gestation revealed the presence of cocaine, at a concentration that could be related to the amount and timing of maternal cocaine use during the pregnancy.[55]

A study of 59 infants showed that the analysis of newborn infants' hair by radioimmunoassay or of meconium by GC-MS was more sensitive than analysis by immunoassay of urine and can detect fetal exposure to cocaine during the last 2 trimesters of pregnancy.[7]

Another study of 1201 mother-infant pairs showed that meconium testing detected an additional 33% of exposed infants compared with urine testing.[65] Furthermore, cocaethylene, a metabolite of both cocaine and ethanol, accumulates in greater concentrations in meconium than in urine, and thus is a useful analyte for identifying both cocaine and ethanol exposure.[14,41,59]

A large-scale prospective drug screening study of over 3000 neonates using analysis of meconium for morphine (opioids), cocaine, and cannabinoids showed a 4-fold increase in the incidence of drug exposure in newborns as compared to the maternal self-report. This was particularly significant in the less-heavily-exposed group of neonates with no obvious manifestations at birth and whose mothers denied drug use during pregnancy, as compared with the more-heavily-exposed group who either had obvious clinical signs and/or mothers who were drug abusers (consistent and substantial users) and who were more likely to admit to drug use.[52]

The nicotine metabolites cotinine and trans-3′-hydroxycotinine can be measured in the meconium of infants of active smokers, and their concentrations are directly related to the degree of smoking by the mother. Similarly, metabolite levels are detected in the meconium of infants of passive smokers, with concentrations found to be comparable to those of infants whose mothers are light smokers.[54]

There are, however, a number of limitations to using meconium as opposed to hair samples to determine intrauterine drug exposure in a clinical setting. As yet no dose-response curves have been established with meconium (as opposed to hair). Meconium is present in only the first few days of life, so that if the exposure is not initially suspected or if the first specimen(s) of meconium are discarded, then analysis cannot be performed. It is also not clear how much of the drugs and their metabolites that are present in meconium result from the swallowing of amniotic fluid and how much results from the enterohepatic circulation.

Results of meconium analysis may be inaccurate if there is in utero passage of meconium and the infant is meconium-stained at birth (often a sign of fetal distress, which may or may not be related to the particular in utero exposure). In these situations, the first postnatal meconium specimen may contain less drug than the initial meconium, which was unaffected by exogenous feeding, but was passed in utero and therefore unable to be analyzed.[55]

After birth, the amount of drug measurable in meconium may be diluted as the baby feeds and new stool is formed. For example, although measurable in the first 3 meconium stools, the amount of cocaine metabolite diminishes significantly after the second stool.[62]

Another confounding issue is contamination of meconium specimens by neonatal urine. Thus, high concentrations of drug metabolites in meconium may actually represent urinary contamination.[42]

Hair

The hair that neonates are born with grows during the last 3–4 months of pregnancy. Thus, the presence of drugs or environmental toxins in neonatal hair reflects the xenobiotic milieu over the last trimester of gestation.[16,21]

Animal and human studies demonstrate that both maternal and fetal accumulation of cocaine and its major metabolite, benzoylecgonine, follow a linear pattern within clinically used doses, and thus hair measurements may be used to estimate maternal use.[17] Benzoylecgonine can also be measured in neonatal hair.[29] Pyrolysis of crack cocaine results in hair accumulation of cocaine, but not its benzoylecgonine metabolite as the accumulation is a result of environmental exposure. Additionally, external contamination with crack smoke is washable, whereas systemic exposure is not. Also, in the context of the neonate, "external contamination" is irrelevant, as fetal hair is in contact with amniotic fluid, which is swallowed and excreted via the urinary tract of the unborn baby.[34] Thus, measurement of fetal hair benzoylecgonine can distinguish between passive and active maternal crack cocaine exposure.

Maternal cigarette smoking is associated with negative obstetric outcome, including decreased birth weight, prematurity, spontaneous abortions, perinatal mortality, and the sudden infant death syndrome.[12] Infants of passive smokers are also at risk of measurable exposure to cigarette smoke.

Cigarette smoke emits numerous toxins, including nicotine, carbon monoxide, hydrogen cyanide, and benzo(a)pyrene. Because of its oxygen dissociation properties, fetal hemoglobin has a higher affinity for carbon monoxide than does normal adult hemoglobin; thus, levels of carboxyhemoglobin are higher in fetal than in maternal blood. This results in lower amounts of oxygen reaching developing fetal tissues, as well as reduced function of cytochrome enzymes and impaired cellular respiration.[43] There is also increasing evidence that intrauterine exposure to cigarette smoke and its toxic metabolites may result in neurobehavioral teratogenicity.[19,20,64] Accumulation of nicotine and cotinine in neonatal hair reflects chronic systemic exposure to these toxins and therefore may correlate with neonatal risks.

Because it is lipid soluble, nicotine has a large volume of distribution (2–3 L/kg) and readily permeates cell membranes. It is absorbed through the lungs and skin, as well as the mucous membranes of the gastrointestinal tract and nasal passages. Once absorbed, nicotine disappears rapidly from the bloodstream because of widespread tissue uptake and hepatic metabolism. Nicotine is filtered and actively secreted by the renal tubules. Nicotine's elimination half-life in adult humans is between 1 and 3 hours; thus, monitoring in the blood is unlikely to reflect the true extent of chronic smoking. Cotinine is the major metabolite of nicotine, formed by a double oxidation reaction catalyzed by cytochrome P450 and then by cytosolic aldehyde oxidase.[56] Cotinine has a considerably longer elimination half-life than nicotine (10–14 hours) and is predominantly excreted in the urine.[37] Accumulation of nicotine and its major metabolite, cotinine, may be measured in neonatal hair to estimate fetal exposure to maternal cigarette smoking.[13,27] A study measuring hair concentrations of both cotinine and nicotine in 94 mother-infant pairs, including mothers who were smokers, nonsmokers, and passive smokers, found significantly high concentrations of nicotine and cotinine in the hair of smokers and their infants when compared with nonsmoking mothers and their infants. Concentrations in passive smokers and their infants were also significantly higher than in nonsmokers and their infants. There was also a significant correlation between maternal and neonatal hair concentrations of both nicotine and cotinine.[13]

Unfortunately, maternal reporting of cigarette use in pregnancy is often inaccurate because of guilt, perception of fetal risk, and fear. It is probably for these reasons that reported use correlates poorly with hair accumulation of nicotine and cotinine in mother and infant. This highlights the importance of an independent biologic marker, such as hair nicotine and cotinine measurement, to more accurately evaluate fetal exposure to cigarette smoke.

Because there frequently is only a small amount of neonatal hair available for analysis, a method to detect both cocaine and nicotine in the same hair sample was developed.[28] This has clear benefits in quantifying specific exposures and in correlating potential neonatal effects, particularly as the majority of mothers who use cocaine also smoke cigarettes.

The tragic experience from Minamata Bay, Japan, (see Chapter 2 and 81) revealed the devastating neurotoxicity of methylmercury, with fetuses and infants showing particular susceptibility. Research supports that the developing nervous system is particularly vulnerable during the second and third trimesters of pregnancy and during early postnatal life. Methylmercury actually crosses the placental barrier and achieves higher concentrations in the fetus than in the mother.[60]

Methylmercury is distributed evenly throughout the body and is also incorporated into growing hair. Based on toxicokinetic and practical considerations, hair is the optimal biomarker of methylmercury exposure in both mothers and infants. Mercury levels in cord blood and in maternal scalp hair correlate well. However, dose-response relationships, particularly with regard to developmental neurotoxicity, are not completely known.[23–25] Methylmercury may also be transferred to neonates via breast milk, thus representing a further potential neurotoxic risk. Urinary mercury excretion is a good marker of inorganic mercury exposure but does not reflect methylmercury exposure.

Amniotic Fluid

It is well-documented in both animals and humans that drugs may be detected in amniotic fluid after maternal drug administration.[5,70] The appearance of drug in the amniotic fluid is usually delayed after a single dose of drug to the mother. However, with chronic drug use, the concentration in amniotic fluid gradually increases. Peak concentrations may greatly exceed simultaneously obtained concentrations in maternal and fetal plasma.[70] Many drug metabolites, as well as the parent compound, also appear in amniotic fluid; for example, cocaine and its metabolites benzoylecgonine, ecgonine methyl ester, and cocaethylene.[61] The fetus may be repeatedly exposed to the effects of these drugs via contact with amniotic fluid that contains these substances.[44]

In one study, amniotic fluid and urine samples were obtained from 23 subjects with documented cocaine abuse. Cocaine and benzoylecgonine were detected in 74% of amniotic fluid samples taken from the known cocaine abusers, while in the same subjects, conventional maternal and neonatal urine toxicology screens were positive in only 61% and 35%, respectively.[26] Other data suggest that measurement of cocaine and its metabolites in amniotic fluid offers no benefits over urinary drug evaluation.[10] Cotinine may be measured in amniotic fluid collected during routine second trimester amniocentesis. Although the mechanism is not understood, it appears that nicotine and its metabolites accumulate both in the fetus and in the amniotic fluid, as levels in neonatal cord blood and in amniotic fluid are found to be higher than in maternal blood.[63]

Ultrasonography

Another prenatal biologic marker of fetal exposure is ultrasound examination with particular emphasis on fetal biometry and specific structural defects, such as neural tube defects (for example in association with valproic acid or carbamazepine exposure). With improved ultrasound technology over the past decade, there has been an increased awareness and reporting of fetal anomalies associated with known or potential teratogen exposures detected on midtrimester ultrasound examination.[35,73]

There are reports of specific fetal anomalies being detected on midtrimester ultrasound, for example, radial ray defects, following valproic acid exposure,[39,66,76] as well as a major cardiac defect and hydrocephalus associated with first trimester retinoic acid exposure.[71]

COUNSELING ISSUES

The main aim of counseling women following potential teratogenic exposure is to present an accurate, up-to-date estimate of their specific risk in an easily understood, nondirective manner. Different women will perceive and interpret the same data very differently, partly because of their educational, ethnic, and social backgrounds, and partly because of their levels of fear, anxiety, and guilt. Hence, the counseling they receive should be specifically tailored to their needs, so that they are able to understand the particular issues concerning the teratogenic exposure during their pregnancy and in particular what should be done regarding the future of the pregnancy.

Perception of Risk and Decision Making

The major decision to be made by women exposed to a xenobiotic is whether or not to continue with their pregnancy. Clearly there may be several possible reasons why a woman (and her partner) would want to terminate a pregnancy, but incorrect perception of teratogenic risk is an important factor.[31]

Since the tragedy of thalidomide in the 1960s, there has been increased public and media awareness of the possibility of teratogenic effects of drugs and environmental agents, even though there are relatively few proven human teratogens. Both the mass media and reputable scientific publications tend to publish and emphasize the positive findings (ie, fetal abnormalities) and potentially harmful effects of xenobiotics rather than their safety and lack of documented teratogenicity.[11,33]

1. FEELING TOWARD TERMINATION OF PREGNANCY

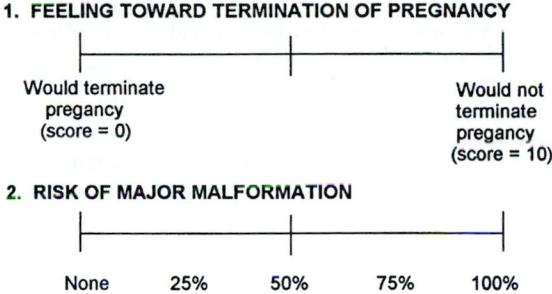

Would terminate
pregancy
(score = 0)

Would not
terminate
pregancy
(score = 10)

2. RISK OF MAJOR MALFORMATION

None   25%   50%   75%   100%

3. RISK OF MAJOR MALFORMATION IN THE GENERAL POPULATION

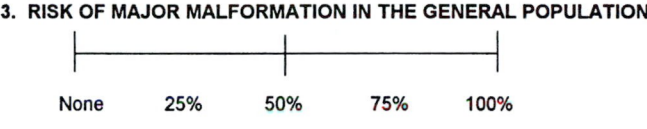

None   25%   50%   75%   100%

Figure 16–4. A visual analog scale depicting an individual's feeling about the need for termination of pregnancy and the individual's perception of the teratogenic risk for drug or chemical exposure.

One study, using the visual analogue scale depicted in Fig. 16–4, assessed the perception of teratogenic risk of 80 women attending an antenatal consultation clinic for drug and chemical exposure and found that women exposed to agents not known to be teratogenic assigned themselves a risk of 24% ± 2.8% (comparable to the risk of one of the major known teratogens—thalidomide). After they received appropriate counseling, their perception of risk was reduced to 14.5% ± 3%, and their tendency to terminate the pregnancy also decreased significantly after the consultation. In contrast, women exposed to known teratogens perceived their risk as being 36.2% ± 11.7% before the interview and did not change their perception afterwards. They also did not change their tendency toward terminating the pregnancy.[36]

Thus appropriate intervention (counseling) in early pregnancy can prevent unnecessary termination of pregnancy by correcting misinformation and misconceptions and thereby decreasing the unrealistically high perception of risk by women exposed to non-teratogens.

SUMMARY

Increasingly and predominantly because of medicolegal influences, it is necessary to determine as precisely as possible the nature of fetal xenobiotic exposure. The use of biologic markers is a way to semiquantitatively determine exposure to a number of these agents. In the future, it is likely that there will be more substances, both environmental and medicinal, that will be amenable to this form of analysis, and that new techniques will result in increased accuracy and improved quantification of the exposure.

Most human teratogens affect some fetuses while sparing others. It is possible that interpreting variability in the rate and extent of placental transfer of drugs is one source of variability in toxicologic response. Thus, neonatal hair and meconium analysis may enable a better understanding of the sources of variability that clearly exist between some mother-infant pairs. This approach may well have relevance not just for environmental agents and

drugs of abuse, but also for medicinal teratogens (eg, phenytoin) and fetotoxins (eg, captopril).

REFERENCES

1. Ames BN: Identifying environmental chemicals causing mutations and cancer. Science 1979;204:587–593.
2. Ames BN, Magaw R, Gold LS: Ranking possible carcinogenic hazards. Science 1987;236:271–280.
3. Angell NF, Lavery JP: The relationship of blood lead levels to obstetric outcome. Am J Obstet Gynecol 1982;142:40–46.
4. Bellinger D, Leviton A, Waternauz C, et al: Longitudinal analyses of prenatal and postnatal lead exposure and early cognitive development. N Engl J Med 1987;316:1037–1043.
5. Brien JF, Clarke DW, Smith GN, et al: Disposition of acute, multiple-dose ethanol in the near-term pregnant ewe. Am J Obstet Gynecol 1987;157:204.
6. Buehler BA, Delimont D, van Maes M, Finnell RH: Prenatal prediction of risk for the fetal hydantoin syndrome. N Engl J Med 1990;322:1567–1572.
7. Callahan CM, Grant TM, Phipps P, et al: Measurement of gestational cocaine exposure: Sensitivity of infants' hair, meconium, and urine. J Pediatr 1992;120:763–768.
8. Casanova OQ, Lombardero N, Behnke M, et al: Detection of cocaine exposure in the neonate. Analyses of urine, meconium, and amniotic fluid from mothers and infants exposed to cocaine. Arch Pathol Lab Med 1994;118:988–993.
9. Clark GD, Rosenweig IB, Raisys VA, et al: The analysis of cocaine and benzoylecgonine in meconium. J Anal Toxicol 1992;16:261–263.
10. DiGregorio GJ, Barbieri EJ, Ferko AP, Ruch EK: Prevalence of cocaethylene in the hair of pregnant women [letter]. J Anal Toxciol 1993;7:445–446.
11. Easterbrook PJ, Berlin JA, Copalan R, Matthews DR: Publication bias in clinical research. Lancet 1991;337:867–872.
12. Eh S: Cigarette smoking during pregnancy. Am J Obstet Gynecol 2000;183:1045–1046.
13. Eliopoulos C, Klein J, Phan MK, et al: Hair concentrations of nicotine and cotinine in women and their newborn infants. JAMA 1994;271:621–623.
14. Farre M, de la Torre R, Llorente M, et al: Alcohol and cocaine interactions in humans. J Pharmacol Exp Ther 1993;266:1364–1373.
15. Feldman Y, Koren G, Mattice D, et al: Determinants of recall and recall bias in studying drug and chemical exposure in pregnancy. Teratology 1989;40:37–45.
16. Forman R, Klein J, Meta D, et al: Prevalence of fetal exposure to cocaine in Toronto, 1990–1991. Clin Invest Med 1994;17:206–211.
17. Forman R, Schneiderman J, Klein J, et al: Accumulation of cocaine in maternal and fetal hair: The dose-response curve. Life Sci 1992;50:1333–1341.
18. Frank DA, Zuckerman BS, Amaro H, et al: Cocaine use during pregnancy: Prevalence and correlates. Pediatrics 1988;82:888–895.
19. Fried PA, O'Connel CM, Watkinson B: Sixty- and 72-month follow-up of children prenatally exposed to marijuana, cigarettes and alcohol: Cognitive and language assessment. Dev Behav Pediatr 1992;13:383–391.
20. Fried PA, Watkinson B, Gray BA: A differential effect-on-cognitive functioning in 9- to 12-year-olds prenatally exposed to cigarettes and marijuana. Neurotoxicol Teratol 1998;20:293–306.
21. Gerschanick J, Brooks G, Little J: Blood lead values in pregnant women and their offspring. Am J Obstet Gynecol 1974;119:508–511.
22. Graham K, Koren G, Klein J, et al: Determination of gestational cocaine exposure by hair analysis. JAMA 1989;262:3328–3330.
23. Grandjean P, Weihe P, Nielsen JB: Methylmercury: Significance of intrauterine and postnatal exposures. Clin Chem 1994;40:1395–1400.

24. Grant BF, Harford TC: Concurrent and simultaneous use of alcohol with cocaine: Results of a national survey. Drug Alcohol Depend 1990;25:97–104.

25. Holmes L: Fetal environmental toxins. Pediatr Rev 1992;13:364–370.

26. Jain L, Meyer W, Moore C, et al: Detection of fetal cocaine exposure by analysis of amniotic fluid. Obstet Gynecol 1993;81:787–790.

27. Klein J, Chitayat D, Koren G: Hair analysis as a marker for fetal exposure to maternal smoking. N Engl J Med 1993;328:66–67.

28. Klein J, Forman R, Eliopoulos C, Koren G: A method for simultaneous measurement of cocaine and nicotine in neonatal hair. Ther Drug Monit 1994;16:67–70.

29. Klein J, Karaskov T, Koren G: Clinical application of hair testing for drug abuse. Forensic Sci Int 2000;107:281–288.

30. Koren G: Measurement of drugs in neonatal hair: A window to fetal exposure. Forensic Sci Int 1995;70:77–82.

31. Koren G, Bologa M, Long D, et al: Perception of teratogenic risk by pregnant women exposed to drugs and chemicals during the first trimester. Am J Obstet Gynecol 1989;160:1190–1194.

32. Koren G, Pastuszak A, Ito S: Drugs in pregnancy. N Engl J Med 1998;338:1128–1137.

33. Koren G, Klein N: Bias against negative studies in newspaper reports of medical research. JAMA 1991;266:1824–1826.

34. Koren G, Klein J, Forman R, Graham K: Hair analysis of cocaine: Differentiation between systemic exposure and external contamination. J Clin Pharmacol 1992;32:671–675.

35. Koren G, Nulman I: Antenatal visualization of malformations associated with drugs and chemicals. Dev Brain Dysfunct 1993;6:305–316.

36. Koren G, Pastuszak A: Prevention of unnecessary pregnancy terminations by counselling women on drug, chemical, and radiation exposure during the first trimester. Teratology 1990;41:657–661.

37. Kyerematen GA, Vesel E: Metabolism of nicotine. Drug Metab Rev 1991;23:3.

38. Laker M: On determining trace element levels in man: The uses of blood and hair. Lancet 1982;2:260–262.

39. Langer B, Haddad J, Gasser B, et al: Isolated fetal bilateral radial ray reduction associated with valproic acid usage. Fetal Diagn Ther 1994;9:155–158.

40. Lehninger AL: Principles of Biochemistry. New York, Worth, 1982, pp. 879–886.

41. Lewis DE, Moore CM, Leikin JB: Cocaethylene in meconium specimens. J Toxicol Clin Toxicol 1994;32:697–703.

42. Lombardero N, Casanova O, Behnke M, et al: Comparison of specimens for GC/MS detection of prenatal cocaine exposure. Ann Clin Lab Sci 1993;23:385–394.

43. Longo L: The biological effects of carbon monoxide on the pregnant woman, fetus and newborn infant. Am J Obstet Gynecol 1977;129:69–103.

44. Mahone PR, Scott K, Sleggs G, et al: Cocaine and metabolites in amniotic fluid may prolong fetal drug exposure. Am J Obstet Gynecol 1994;171:465–469.

45. Marsh DO, Clarkson TW, Cox C, et al: Fetal methylmercury poisoning, relationship between concentrations in single strand of maternal hair and child effects. Arch Neurol 1987;44:1017–1022.

46. Maynard EC, Amuroso LP, Oh W: Meconium for drug testing. Am J Dis Child 1991;145:650–652.

47. Miller EC: Some current perspectives on chemical carcinogenesis: Presidential address. Cancer Res 1978;8:1479–1496.

48. Mitchell AE, Cottler LB, Shapira SP: Effect of questionnaire design on recall of drug exposure in pregnancy. Am J Epidemiol 1986;123:670–676.

49. Moore MR, McIntosh MJ, Bushnell JWR: The neurotoxicity of lead. Neurotoxicology 1986;7:541–546.

50. Nogaki K: On action of lead on body of lead refinery workers: Particularly conception, pregnancy and parturition in case of females and on vitality of their newborn. Excerpta Med 1958;4:2176.

51. Okey AB: Carcinogenesis and mutagenesis by xenobiotic chemicals. In: Kalant H, Roschlau WHE, eds: Principles of Medical Pharmacology, 5th ed. Toronto, Canada, Decker, 1989; pp. 632–643.

52. Ostrea EM: Testing for exposure to illicit drugs and other agents in the neonate: A review of laboratory methods and the role of meconium analysis. Curr Probl Pediatr 1999;29:37–56.

53. Ostrea EM, Matias O, Keane C, et al: Spectrum of gestational exposure to illicit drugs and other xenobiotic agents in newborn infants by meconium analysis. J Pediatr 1998;133:513–515.

54. Ostrea EM, Knapp DK, Romero A, et al: Meconium analysis to assess fetal exposure to nicotine by active and passive maternal smoking. J Pediatr 1994;124:471–476.

55. Ostrea EM, Romero A, Knapp DK, et al: Postmortem drug analysis of meconium in early gestation human fetuses exposed to cocaine: Clinical implications. J Pediatr 1994;125:477–479.

56. Pilotti A: Biosynthesis and mammalian metabolism of nicotine. Acta Physiol Scand 1980;479(Suppl):13–17.

57. Potter S, Klein J, Valilante G, et al: Maternal cocaine use without evidence of fetal exposure. J Pediatr 1994;125:652–654.

58. Rajegowda BK, Glass L, Evans HE: Lead concentration in newborn infants. J Pediatr 1972;80:116–117.

59. Randall T: Cocaine, alcohol mix in body to form even longer lasting, more lethal drug. JAMA 1992;267:1043–1044.

60. Reynolds WA, Pitkin RM: Transplacental passage of methylmercury and its uptake by primate fetal tissues. Proc Soc Exp Biol Med 1975;148:523–526.

61. Ripple MG, Goldberger BA, Caplan YH, et al: Detection of cocaine and its metabolites in human amniotic fluid. J Anal Toxicol 1992;16:328–331.

62. Rosengren S, Longobucco D, Bernstein B, et al: Meconium testing for cocaine metabolite: Prevalence, perceptions, and pitfalls. Am J Obstet Gynecol 1993;168:1449–1456.

63. Ruhle W, Graf von Ballestrem CL, Pult HM, Gnirs J: Correlation of cotinine levels in amniotic fluid, umbilical artery blood and maternal blood (in German). Geburtshilfe und Frauenheilkunde 1995;15: 156–159.

64. Rush D, Callahan KR: Exposure to passive cigarette smoking and child development. Ann N Y Acad Sci 1989;562:74–100.

65. Ryan RM, Wagner CL, Schultz JM, et al: Meconium analysis for improved identification of infants exposed to cocaine in utero. J Pediatr 1994;125:435–440.

66. Sharony R, Garber A, Viskochil D, et al: Preaxial ray reduction defects as part of valproic acid embryo fetopathy. Pregnant Diagn 1993;13:909–918.

67. Shephard TH: "Proof" of human teratogenicity. Teratology 1994;50:97–98.

68. Silva Lima B, Van der Laan JW: Mechanism of nongenotoxic carcinogenesis and assessment of the human hazard. Regul Toxicol Pharmacol 2000;32:135–143.

69. Strickler SM, Dansky LV, Miller MA, et al: Genetic predisposition to phenytoin-induced birth defects. Lancet 1989;2:746–749.

70. Szeto HH, Umans JG, McFarland JW: A comparison of morphine and methadone disposition in the maternal-fetal unit. Am J Obstet Gynecol 1982;143:700–706.

71. Van Maldergem L, Jauniaux E, Gillerot Y: Morphological features of a case of retinoic acid embryopathy. Prenat Diag 1992;12:699–701.

72. Varvarigou A, Beratis NG, Makri M, Vagenakis AG: Increased levels and positive correlation between erythropoietin and hemoglobin concentrations in newborn children of mothers who are smokers. J Pediatr 1994;124:480–482.

73. Viscarello RR, Ferguson DD, Nores J, Hobbins JC: Limb body wall complex associated with cocaine abuse: Further evidence of cocaine's teratogenicity. Obstet Gynecol 1992;80:523–526.

74. Welch E, Fleming LE, Peyser I, et al: Rapid cocaine screening of urine in a newborn nursery. J Pediatr 1993;123:468–470.

75. Williams GM, Weisburger JH: Chemical carcinogens. In: Amdur MO, Doull J, Klaassen CD, eds: Casarett and Doull's Toxicology: The Basic Science of Poisons. New York, Macmillan, 1991, pp. 127–200.

76. Ylagan LR, Budorick NE: Radial ray aplasia in utero: A prenatal finding associated with valproic acid exposure. J Ultrasound Med 1994;13:408–411.

THE PATHOPHYSIOLOGIC BASIS OF MEDICAL TOXICOLOGY: THE ORGAN SYSTEM APPROACH

CHAPTER 17 VITAL SIGNS AND TOXIC SYNDROMES

Lewis R. Goldfrank / Neal E. Flomenbaum / Neal A. Lewin /
Mary Ann Howland / Robert S. Hoffman / Lewis S. Nelson

Normal Vital Signs by Age

Age	Systolic BP mm Hg	Diastolic BP mm Hg	Pulse bpm	Respirations per min
Adult	90–140	<90	60–100	8–14
16 years	120	70	80	12–16
12 years	110	70	85	15–20
10 years	110	70	90	15–20
6 years	100	60	100	20–25
4 years	100	60	100	20–25
2 years	100	60	110	25–30
1 year	95	60	120	25–30
6 months	90	60	120	30
4 months	85	50	120	30–35
2 months	80	45	120	30–35
Newborn	60	40	125	35–40

The normal temperature is defined at 95–100.4°F or 35–38°C for all ages.

For more than 200 years the American medical community has attempted to standardize its approach to the assessment of patients.[2] At the New York Hospital in 1865, temperature, pulse, and respiratory rate were incorporated into the bedside chart and called "vital signs." Only in the early part of the 20th century, however, did the blood pressure determination also become routine.[8] In addition to their more widely appreciated role in assessing and monitoring the overall status of a patient, the vital signs can provide valuable physiologic clues pointing to the toxicologic etiology of an illness. Many toxic substances affect the autonomic nervous system, which, in turn, affects the vital signs via the sympathetic and parasympathetic pathways. Meticulous attention to initial as well as serial determinations of these clinical signs is of extreme importance in identifying a pattern of changes suggesting a particular drug or group of drugs. A description of the vital signs as "normal" or "stable" is too nonspecific to be meaningful, and therefore should never be accepted. Conversely, no patient should be considered too agitated for the physician to obtain a complete set of vital signs; indeed, the agitated patient most urgently needs a thorough evaluation including all of the vital signs.

The value of continually monitoring the vital signs is demonstrated by the patient who presents with an anticholinergic overdose and is then given physostigmine or, conversely, a patient poisoned by organic phosphorus compounds who is then given atropine. It is important to recognize when a sinus tachycardia becomes a sinus bradycardia (anticholinergic syndrome followed by physostigmine use or excess) or when a sinus bradycardia becomes a normal sinus rhythm or progresses to a sinus tachycardia (organic phosphorus compound overdose followed by atropine use). Meticulous attention to these changes assures that the therapeutic interventions can be modified or adjusted accordingly. A more commonly occurring situation, perhaps, is the patient who

overdoses on an opioid and is given the opioid antagonist naloxone (bradypnea to tachypnea and then to a more normal pattern). These analyses become exceedingly complicated when a patient is exposed to two or more substances, such as an opioid and cocaine. The effects of cocaine may be "unmasked" by the use of naloxone to counteract the opioid, and the clinician is then forced to differentiate opioid withdrawal from cocaine toxicity by analyzing a combination of information including history, vital signs determination, and physical examination. Careful observation helps to determine the success of a therapeutic intervention and guides the clinician in making the necessary adjustments to initial therapy.

The most typical toxic syndromes are described in Table 17–1. These autonomic syndromes are best described by a combination of the vital sign values (blood pressure, pulse, respiratory rate, temperature) and clinically obvious end-organ manifestations. The signs that prove most clinically useful are those of the central nervous system (mental status); ophthalmic system (pupil size); gastrointestinal system (peristalsis); dermatologic system: skin (dryness vs. diaphoresis) and mucous membranes (salivation vs. dryness); and genitourinary system (urinary retention). Among all of the vital signs, the most clinically sensitive indicators are typically the pulse and blood pressure. A detailed analysis of each toxic syndrome can be found in appropriate chapters throughout the text. In this chapter, the toxic syndromes are considered in their broadest sense to enable the reader to initiate an appropriate assessment and differential diagnosis.

Mofenson and Greensher[7] coined the term *toxidrome* from the words *toxic syndromes* to describe the groups of signs and symptoms that consistently result from particular toxins. The original toxidromes they listed, along with others, are listed in Table 17–2. This table includes many of the most commonly encountered toxins and their typical clinical manifestations. However, the reader

TABLE 17–1. Toxic Syndromes

Group	Vital Signs				Mental Status	Pupil Size	Peristalsis	Diaphoresis	Other
	BP	P	RR	T					
Adrenergic (α, β) agents	↑	↑	↑	↑	Altered	↑	↑	↑	Tremor
Anticholinergic agents	±	↑	±	↑	Altered	↑	↓	↓	Dry mucous membranes, flush, urinary retention
Cholinergic (muscarinic, nicotinic) agents	±	±	—	—	Altered	±	↑	↑	Salivation, lacrimation, urination, bronchorrhea, fasciculations, brady-cardia
Opioids	↓	↓	↓	↓	Altered	↓	↓	—	Hyporeflexia
Withdrawal of opioids	↑	↑	—	—	Normal	↑	↑	↑	Nausea, vomiting, hyper-activity, rhinorrhea, piloerection
Sedative-hypnotics or ethanol	↓	↓	↓	±	Altered	±	↓	—	Hyporeflexia
Withdrawal of sedative-hypnotics or ethanol	↑	↑	↑	↑	Altered	↑	↑	—/↑	Nausea, tremor, seizures

↑ = increases; ↓ = decreases; ± = variable; — = change unlikely

should always remember that the actual clinical manifestations of an ingestion or exposure are far more variable than the syndromes described in the table. Toxidromes are most useful when thinking about a clinical presentation and formulating the framework for assessment. Whereas some patients may present with "classic" cases, others will manifest combinations or *formes frustes* with fewer signs, nevertheless providing at least a partial clue to the correct diagnosis. Partial presentations do not necessarily imply less-severe disease and, therefore, are no less important to appreciate.

The broad range of values considered normal in adults should serve only as a guide. The complete assessment of each individual patient is essential in determining whether or not a particular value truly is clinically normal, rapid, or slow, or high or low. A table of normal vital sign values is particularly useful in assessing children. Knowing the variations in values that are considered normal at a particular age is essential. The very young as well as the very old may have thermoregulatory abnormalities that either inhibit responses or promote excessive responses. Blood pressure and pulse may vary significantly because of change in receptor responsiveness, degree of fitness, the presence of atherosclerosis, or general cardiovascular function.

In some instances, an unexpected combination of findings may be particularly helpful in identifying a toxin or a combination of toxins. For example, a dissociation between such typically paired changes as an increase in pulse with a decrease in blood pressure (cyclic antidepressants or phenothiazines), or a decrease in pulse with an increase in blood pressure (phenylpropanolamine), may be extremely helpful diagnostically, as the etiologies for an unexpected dissociation may include only a few possibilities. The use of these unexpected or atypical clinical findings is demonstrated in Chap. 21.

necessary, to treat these rapidly changing conditions. Proper cuff sizes for the obese adult (large) and for children (small) must be used, and determination of blood pressures in both arms and legs, if indicated, prevents serious diagnostic errors. Following this initial determination, a more dynamic evaluation of cardiovascular integrity can be made by obtaining orthostatic vital signs—both blood pressure and pulse in at least two different positions. This combined assessment is one of the most helpful bedside examinations that can be performed to assess a patient for either actual volume depletion or functional volume depletion secondary to peripheral vasodilatation (Chap. 21, Table 21–3). A rough estimation of volume deficits can be correlated with these changes. However, the response is also affected by other factors such as advanced age,[5] autonomic nervous system dysfunction (diabetes mellitus, tabes dorsalis, thiamine depletion, postsympathectomy states), and medications (Table 17–3 and Chap. 21).

Drugs and toxins cause hypotension by four major mechanisms: decreased peripheral resistance, decreased myocardial contractility, dysrhythmias, and intravascular volume depletion. Many drugs and toxins can initially cause severe orthostatic hypotension, without marked supine hypotension, and any drug or toxin that affects autonomic control of the myocardium or peripheral capacitance vessels may lead to orthostatic hypotension (Table 17–4 and Chap. 21). Hypertension and a concomitant decrease in heart rate is a common presentation noted with phenylpropanolamine ingestion. As a rule, hypertension resulting from drug overdoses is followed by hypotension.

Changing patterns of blood pressure often assist in the diagnostic evaluation: a patient with a monoamine oxidase inhibitor (MAOI) overdose characteristically results in an initially normal blood pressure, and then severe hypertension followed abruptly by severe hypotension.

BLOOD PRESSURE

Blood pressure and pulse should initially be assessed with the patient in the supine position. Accurate, consistently performed serial blood pressure determinations are essential to identify and, if

PULSE

Extremely useful clinical information can be obtained by evaluating the pulse for rate, regularity, and amplitude (Table 17–5 and Chap. 21). The carotid artery is usually easily palpated in children

TABLE 17–2. Specific Drugs or Toxins and Their Toxic Syndromes

Page	Toxin	Vital Signs	Mental Status	Signs and Symptoms	Clinical Findings
	Acetaminophen	Normal (early)	Normal	Anorexia, nausea, vomiting	RUQ tenderness, jaundice (late)
	Amphetamines	Hypertension, tachycardia, tachypnea, hyperthermia	Agitaion	Hyperalertness, panic, anxiety, diaphoresis	Mydriasis, hyperactive peristaltism, diaphoresis
	Antihistamines	Hypotension, hypertension, tachycardia, hyperthermia	Altered (agitation, lethargy to coma), hallucinations	Blurred vision, dry mouth, inability to urinate	Dry mucous membranes, mydriasis, flush, diminished peristaltism, urinary retention
	Arsenic (acute)	Hypotension, tachycardia	Alert to coma	Abdominal pain, vomiting, diarrhea, dysphagia	Dehydration
	Barbiturates	Hypotension, bradypnea, hypothermia	Altered (lethargy to coma)	Slurred speech, ataxia	Dysconjugate gaze, bullae, hyporeflexia
	β-Adrenergic antagonists	Hypotension, bradycardia	Altered (lethargy to coma)	Dizziness	Cyanosis, seizures
	Botulism	Bradypnea	Normal unless hypoxia	Blurred vision, diplopia, dysphagia, sore or dry throat, constipation	Ophthalmoplegia, mydriasis, ptosis, cranial nerve abnormalities, descending parlysis
	Calcium channel blockers	Hypotension, bradycardia	Altered (lethargy, confusion)	Nausea	
	Carbamazepine	Hypotension, tachycardia, bradypnea, hypothermia	Altered (lethargy to coma)	Hallucinations, extrapyramidal movements, seizures	Mydriasis, nystagmus
	Carbon monoxide	Often normal	Altered (lethargy to coma)	Headache, dizziness, nausea, vomiting	Seizures
	Clonidine	Hypotension, hypertension, bradycardia, bradypnea	Altered (lethargy to coma)	Dizziness, confusion	Miosis
	Cocaine	Hypertension, tachycardia, tachypnea, hyperthermia	Altered (anxiety, agitation, delirium)	Hallucinations, paranoia, panic, anxiety. restlessness	Mydriasis, nystagmus
	Cyclic antidepressants	Hypotension, tachycardia	Altered (lethargy to coma)	Confusion, dizziness, dry mouth, inability to urinate	Mydriasis, dry mucous membranes, distended bladder, flush, seizures
	Digitalis	Hypotension, bradycardia	Normal or altered	Nausea, vomiting, anorexia	None
	Disulfiram/ethanol	Hypotension, tachycardia	Normal	Nausea, vomiting, headache, vertigo	Flush, diaphoresis,
	Ethylene glycol	Tachypnea	Altered (lethargy to coma)	Abdominal pain	Slurred speech, ataxia
	Iron	Hypotension, tachycardia	Normal or lethargy	Nausea, vomiting, diarrhea, abdominal pain, hematemesis	
	Isoniazid	Often normal	Normal or altered (lethargy to coma)	Nausea, vomiting	Status epilepticus
	Isopropanol	Hypotension, tachycardia, bradypnea	Altered (lethargy to coma)	Nausea, vomiting	Hyporeflexia, ataxia, acetone odor on breath
	Lead	Hypertension	Altered (lethargy to coma)	Irritability, abdominal pain (colic), nausea, vomiting, constipation	Peripheral neuropathy, seizures, gingival pigmentation
	Lithium	Hypotension (late)	Altered (lethargy to coma)	Diarrhea, tremor, nausea	Weakness, tremor, ataxia, myoclonus, seizures
	Mercury	Hypotension (late)	Altered (psychiatric disturbances)	Salivation, diarrhea, abdominal pain	Stomatitis, ataxia, tremor
	Methanol	Hypotension, tachypnea	Altered (lethargy to coma)	Blurred vision, blindness, abdominal pain	Hyperemic disks, mydriasis
	Opioids	Hypotension, bradycardia bradypnea, hypothermia	Altered (lethargy to coma)	Slurred speech, ataxia	Miosis, decreased peristaltism
	Organic phosphorus compounds, carbamates	Hypotension/hypertension bradycardia/tachycardia, bradypnea/tachypnea	Altered (lethargy to coma)	Diarrhea, abdominal pain, blurred vision, vomiting	Salivation, diaphoresis, lacrimation, urination, bronchorrhea, defecation, miosis, fasciculations, seizures
	Phencyclidine	Hypertension, tachycardia, hyperthermia	Altered (agitation, lethargy to coma)	Hallucinations	Miosis, diaphoresis, myoclonus, blank stare, nystagmus, seizures
	Phenothiazines	Hypotension, tachycardia, hypothermia or hyperthermia	Altered (lethargy to coma)	Dizziness, dry mouth, inability to urinate	Miosis or mydriasis, decreased bowel sounds, dystonia

(*continued*)

TABLE 17–2. Specific Drugs or Toxins and Their Toxic Syndromes (continued)

Page	Toxin	Vital Signs	Mental Status	Signs and Symptoms	Clinical Findings
	Salicylates	Hypotension, tachycardia, tachypnea, hyperthermia	Altered (agitation, lethargy to coma)	Tinnitus, nausea, vomiting, hyperpnea	Diaphoresis, congestive heart failure
	Sedative-hypnotics	Hypotension, bradypnea, hypothermia	Altered (lethargy to coma)	Slurred speech, ataxia	Hyporeflexia, bullae
	Theophylline	Hypotension, tachycardia, tachypnea, hyperthermia	Altered (agitation)	Nausea, vomiting, diaphoresis, anxiety	Diaphoresis, tremor, seizures, dysrhythmias

and young adults; however, for reasons of safety and reliability, the brachial artery is preferred in infants and elderly adults. There is a direct correlation between heart rate and temperature in that heart rate increases approximately 8 beats/min for each 1°C (1.8°F) elevation in temperature.[4]

Because pulse rate is the net result of a balance between adrenergic and cholinergic (muscarinic and nicotinic) tone, any substance that exerts a therapeutic or toxic effect on these components can cause pulse abnormalities. The inability to differentiate easily between the adrenergics and anticholinergics by vital signs alone illustrates the principle that no single vital sign abnormality can definitively establish a toxicologic diagnosis or etiology. In trying to differentiate between adrenergic and anticholinergic exposure, remember that although a rapid pulse rate commonly results from both adrenergics and anticholinergics, diaphoresis and/or increased bowel sounds suggest adrenergic toxicity, whereas decreased sweating, absent bowel sounds, and urinary retention point to anticholinergic toxicity (Table 35–4).

Assessment of the amplitude of the pulse can be helpful in evaluating cardiac output. For example, the regularly occurring alternating force known as pulsus alternans results from myocardial dysfunction caused by digitalis poisoning.

RESPIRATIONS

As always, establishment of an airway and evaluation of respiratory status are the initial priorities in patient stabilization. Although respiration is typically assessed initially for rate alone, careful observation of the depth and pattern is essential (Table 17–6) for establishing the etiology of a systemic illness or toxic exposure.[3]

Hyperventilation may be characterized by tachypnea (an increased rate of breathing), or hyperpnea (an increase in tidal volume), or both. When hyperventilation results solely or predominantly from hyperpnea, the less-astute clinician may miss this important finding entirely and even incorrectly describe such a hyperventilating patient as *hypoventilating* if the rate is slow.

Tachypnea, an increase in breathing rate, may result from the direct effect of a CNS stimulant, salicylates, acting on the brainstem. Salicylate poisoning may result in only an increased tidal volume or hyperpnea without tachypnea. Aspiration of gastric contents is a common complication of toxic exposures to hydrocarbon products or CNS depressants. Pulmonary injury from any source may lead to hypoxemia with initial increase of the tachypnea, but may later lead to bradypnea and shallow breaths (hypop-

TABLE 17–3. Common Drug Groups and Important Toxins that Cause Orthostatic Hypotension

Antihypertensives
α-Adrenergic antagonists
Central α₂-adrenergic agonists
Angiotensin-converting enzyme inhibitors
  and antagonists
Vasodilators
  Hydralazine
  Nitrates

Antianginals
β-Adrenergic antagonists
Calcium channel blockers

Antidepressants
Cyclic antidepressants
MAO inhibitors

Antiparkinson agents
Bromocriptine
L-Dopa

Ciguatera toxin

Diuretics
Thiazides
Loop diuretics

CNS depressants
Ethanol
Opioids
Sedative-hypnotics

Antipsychotics
Phenothiazines
Butyrophenones

See Chap. 21 for additional agents that affect hemodynamic function.

TABLE 17–4. Common Drugs and Important Toxins that Affect Blood Pressure

Hypotension	Hypertension
α-Adrenergic antagonists	Amphetamines
Angiotensin-converting enzyme inhibitors and antagonists	Cocaine
	Ephedrine/pseudoephedrine
Antidysrhythmic drugs	Epinephrine
β-Adrenergic antagonists	Ergot alkaloids
Calcium channel blockers	Lead
Clonidine	Monoamine oxidase inhibitors
Cyanide	(overdose and drug interaction)
Cyclic antidepressants	Nicotine (early)
Disulfiram/ethanol	Phencyclidine
Ethanol	Phenylpropanolamine
Iron	
Isopropanol	
Nitrates and nitrites	
Nitroprusside	
Opioids	
Organic phosphorus compounds and carbamates	
Phenothiazines	
Sedative-hypnotic agents	
Theophylline	

See Chap. 21 for additional agents that affect hemodynamic function.

TABLE 17–5. Common Drugs and Important Toxins that Affect Pulse

Bradycardia	Tachycardia
Antidysrhythmic drugs	Amphetamines
α-Adrenergic agonists	Antihistamines
Baclofen	Atropine and other anticholinergics
β-Adrenergic antagonists	Arsenic (acute)
Calcium channel blockers	Caffeine
Ciguatera toxin	Carbon monoxide
Clonidine	Cocaine
Digitalis glycosides	Cyclic antidepressants
Opioids	Disulfiram/ethanol
Organic phosphorus compounds and carbamates	Ephedrine/pseudoephedrine
Phenylpropanolamine	Epinephrine
	Iron
	Organic phosphorus compounds and carbamates
	Phencyclidine
	Phenothiazines
	Sedative-hypnotic withdrawal
	Theophylline
	Thyroxine

See Chap. 21 for additional agents affecting heart rate.

nea). Bradypnea, or a decrease in breathing rate, may occur even sooner when a CNS depressant acts on the brainstem. A progression from fast to slow breathing may also occur with increasing levels of cyanide or carbon monoxide.

The alcohols methanol or ethylene glycol may transiently produce hypoventilation because of bradypnea (a decreased rate of breathing) or hypopnea (a decrease in tidal volume). In time, however, hyperventilation (tachypnea or hyperpnea) will predominate as (late-onset) metabolic acidosis develops. Typically, metabolic acidosis is accompanied by hyperventilation as a compensatory mechanism to maintain (or attempt to maintain) a normal pH. Drugs and toxins that routinely produce a metabolic acidosis include salicylates, methanol, and ethylene glycol, and sometimes ethanol when it results in alcoholic ketoacidosis.

It is important to note, however, that toxin- or drug-induced CNS dysfunction classically presents with a rostrocaudal *dissociation of neurologic signs* that do not correspond to a well-defined

TABLE 17–6. Common Drugs and Important Toxins that Affect Respiratory Rate

Bradypnea	Tachypnea
Barbiturates	Carbon monoxide
Botulinum toxin	Cyanide
Clonidine	Ethylene glycol
Ethanol	Hydrogen sulfide
Neuromuscular blockers	Isopropanol
Opioids	Methanol
Sedative-hypnotics	Methemoglobin producing agents
	Nicotine
	Organic phosphorus compounds and carbamates
	Salicylates
	Sympathomimetics
	Theophylline

See Chap. 20 for additional agents affecting respiratory rate.

lesion affecting a single locus or contiguous loci. The combination of ataxic breathing with intact pontine reflexes, such as reactive pupils, is a good example of the dissociative neurologic character of toxin-induced coma in contradistinction to a pontine hemorrhage in which a patient has pinpoint pupils and decreased respirations (Chap. 19).

TEMPERATURE

Temperature evaluation and control are critical. However, temperature assessment can be done only if safe and reliable equipment is used. The risks of inaccuracy are substantial when an oral temperature is taken in a tachypneic patient, an axillary temperature is taken in a patient found outdoors, or a tympanic temperature is taken in a patient with cerumen. Obtaining a rectal temperature utilizing a rubber protective probe is essential for an agitated individual. In this text reported temperatures are rectal determinations unless stated otherwise.

Both hypothermia (T <35°C; <95°F) and hyperthermia (T >38°C; >100.4°F) are common manifestations of a drug overdose. Hypothermia and hyperthermia, unless immediately recognized and managed appropriately, can result in grave complications and inappropriate or inadequate resuscitation efforts. Life-threatening hyperthermia (T >41.1°C; >106°F) from any cause can lead to extensive rhabdomyolysis and myoglobinuric renal failure as well as direct brain injury.

Hyperthermia can result from a distinct neurologic response to a signal demanding thermal up-regulation or from an externally imposed hyperthermia as seen in heat stroke, in cancer chemotherapy, or in an infant excessively swaddled in clothing.[10] Fevers higher than 41.1°C (106°F) are extremely rare unless normal feedback mechanisms are overwhelmed.[1] Hyperthermia of this extreme nature is usually attributed to heat stroke, malignant hyperthermia, or drug-related temperature disturbances.

Drug-induced fevers coincide with the administration of a drug and disappear within 48–96 hours of the drug's discontinuation.[6,9] A common drug-related hyperthermia pattern that occurs in the emergency department is defervescence after an acute temperature elevation resulting from agitation or seizure activity. In the case of a seizure, hyperthermia may persist for several hours, even in the

TABLE 17–7. Common Drugs and Important Toxins that Affect Body Temperature

Hyperthermia	Hypothermia
Amphetamines	Carbon monoxide
Anticholinergics	Ethanol and other alcohols
Antihistamines	Hypoglycemic agents
Cocaine	Opioids
Cyclic antidepressants	Phenothiazines
Monoamine oxidase inhibitors	Sedative-hypnotic agents
Phencyclidine	
Phenothiazines	
Salicylates	
Sedative-hypnotic withdrawal	
Thyroxine	

See Chap. 18 for a more complete listing.

absence of an infectious etiology for the elevation in body temperature. One-third of the patients may still be febrile at 48 hours.[11] Table 17–7 is a representative list of toxins that affect body temperature (see Chap. 18 for greater detail).

Hypothermia will impair the metabolism of many drugs at both toxic and therapeutic levels, leading to unpredictable delayed effects when the patient is warmed. Most importantly, a hypothermic patient should never be declared dead without both an extensive assessment and a full resuscitative effort, particularly if the body temperature remains less than 95°F (35°C). In addition, many drugs and toxins impair judgment and CNS function, thereby placing patients at great risk for becoming hypothermic from exposure to the cold of northern winter climates.

Continuous monitoring of the vital signs is as essential in medical toxicology as in any other type of emergency or critical care medicine. For this reason, the vital signs an essential part of the initial evaluation of every case, and repeated vital sign values are almost always necessary throughout the subsequent case management.

REFERENCES

1. Dubois EF: Why are fever temperatures over 106°F rare? Am J Med Sci 1949;217:361–368.
2. Fiore MC: The new vital signs: Assessing and documenting smoking status. JAMA 1991;266:3183–3189.
3. Gravelyn TR, Weg JG: Respiratory rate as an indicator of acute respiratory dysfunction. JAMA 1980;244:1123–1125.
4. Karajalainen J, Vitassalo M: Fever and cardiac rhythm. Arch Intern Med 1986;146:1169–1171.
5. Lipsitz LA: Orthostatic hypotension in the elderly. N Engl J Med 1989;321:952–957.
6. Lipsky BA, Hirschman JV: Drug fever. JAMA 1981;245:851–854.
7. Mofenson HC, Greensher J: The nontoxic ingestion. Pediatr Clin North Am 1970;17:583–590.
8. Musher DM, Dominguez EA, Bar-Sela A: Edouard Seguin and the social power of thermometry. N Engl J Med 1987;316:115–117.
9. Orringer CE, Eustace JC, Wunsch CD, Gardner LB: Natural history of lactic acidosis after grand mal seizures: A model for the study of an anion gap acidosis not associated with hyperkalemia. N Engl J Med 1977;297:796–799.
10. Styrt B, Sugarman B: Antipyresis and fever. Arch Intern Med 1990;150:1589–1597.
11. Wachtel TJ, Steele GH, Day JA: Natural history of fever following a seizure. Arch Intern Med 1987;147:1153–1155.

THERMOREGULATORY PRINCIPLES

Susi U. Vassallo / Kathleen A. Delaney

Despite exposure to wide fluctuations of environmental temperature, human body temperature is maintained within a narrow range.[14,109] Elevation or depression of body temperature occurs when (a) thermoregulatory mechanisms are overwhelmed by exposure to extremes of environmental heat or cold; (b) endogenous heat production is either inadequate, resulting in hypothermia, or exceeds the physiologic capacity for dissipation, resulting in hyperthermia; or (c) disease processes or drug effects interfere with normal thermoregulatory responses to heat or cold exposure.

METHODS OF HEAT TRANSFER

Heat is transferred to or away from the body through radiation, conduction, convection, and evaporation. *Radiation* involves the transfer of heat from a body to the environment, and from warm objects in the environment, for example, the sun, to a body. *Conduction* involves the transfer of heat to solid or liquid media in direct contact with the body. Water immersion or wet clothing in contact with the body conducts significant amounts of heat away from the body. This effect facilitates cooling in a swimming pool on a hot summer day, or may lead to hypothermia despite moderate ambient temperatures on a rainy day. The amount of heat lost through conduction and radiation depends on the temperature gradient between skin and surroundings, cutaneous blood flow, and insulation such as subcutaneous fat, hair, clothing, or fur in lower animals.[124] In the respiratory tract, heat is lost by conduction to water vapor or gas. In animals unable to sweat, this represents the primary method of heat loss. The amount of heat lost through the respiratory tract depends on the temperature gradient between inspired air and the environment, as well as the rate and depth of breathing.[124] *Convection* is the transfer of heat to the air surrounding the body. Wind velocity and ambient air temperature are the major determinants of convective heat loss. *Evaporation* is the process of vaporization of water, or sweat. Large amounts of heat are dissipated from the skin during this process, resulting in cooling. Ambient temperature, rate of sweating, air velocity, and relative humidity are important factors in determining how much heat is lost through evaporation. On a very humid day, sweat may pour off, rather than evaporate from a person exercising in a hot environment, thereby accomplishing little heat loss. In very warm environments, thermal gradients may be reversed, leading to transfer of heat to the body by radiation, conduction, or convection.[135,159]

PHYSIOLOGY OF THERMOREGULATION

In the normal human, stimulation of peripheral and hypothalamic temperature-sensitive neurons results in autonomic, somatic, and behavioral responses that lead to the dissipation or conservation of heat. Thermoregulation is the complex physiologic process that serves to maintain hypothalamic temperature within a narrow range of $37 \pm 0.4°C$ ($98.6 \pm 0.8°F$) known as the set point.[262] This hypothalamic set point is influenced by factors such as diurnal variation, the menstrual cycle and others. Maintaining, raising, or lowering the set point results in many outwardly visible physiologic manifestations of thermoregulation such as sweating, shivering, flushing, or panting. In the central nervous system, thermosensitive neurons are located predominantly in the preoptic area of the anterior hypothalamus, although some are found in the posterior hypothalamus. These neurons may be divided into those that are warm-sensitive, cold sensitive, or temperature-insensitive. About 30% of preoptic neurons are warm-sensitive. These increase their firing rate during warming and decrease their firing rate during cooling.[22] Warming of the hypothalamus in conscious animals results in vasodilatation, hyperventilation, salivation, and increases in evaporative water loss, as well as a reduction of cold-induced shivering and vasoconstriction.[106] Cooling of the hypothalamus in conscious animals causes shivering, vasoconstriction, and increased metabolic rate, even if the environment is hot.[98] How these temperature-sensitive neurons of the hypothalamus detect temperature changes and effect neuronal transmission is unclear. Altered action potential initiation and propagation due to temperature-dependent changes in membrane potential, changes in the ratios of Na^+ to Ca^{2+} ions which alter neuronal excitability and neurotransmitter release, or effects on the Na^+K^+-ATPase (adenosine triphosphatase) pump, may be involved.[124] Drugs that increase intracellular cyclic AMP increase the thermosensitivity of warm-sensitive neurons.[22] In the brainstem, warm- and cold-sensitive neurons are located in the medullary reticular formation, where information from cutaneous receptors, spinal cord, and preoptic area of the anterior hypothalamus is integrated.[109,113,116,185]

The spinal cord also manifests thermosensitivity. Heat- and cold-sensitive ascending spinal impulses are conducted in the spinothalamic tract. As in the hypothalamus, local heating or cooling of the spinal cord results in thermoregulatory responses.[106] In addition to the hypothalamus, brainstem, and spinal cord, there is evidence of thermosensitivity in the deep abdominal viscera.[94,106,208] Intra-abdominal heating or cooling results in thermoregulatory responses. Cold- and warm-sensitive afferent impulses can be recorded from the splanchnic nerves in animals.[94,210] Finally, the skin also contains heat and cold thermosensitive neurons. Cold receptors are free nerve endings that protrude into the basal epidermis, whereas warm-sensitive receptors protrude into the dermis.[107,108] Cutaneous thermoreceptor output is affected by the absolute temperature of the skin, rate of temperature change, and area of stimulation.[106] Cutaneous cold receptors are Aδ and C nociceptor afferent fibers. Aδ fibers are small-diameter thinly myelinated fibers that conduct at 5–30 m/sec, and C-fibers are small-diameter unmyelinated fibers that conduct at 0.5–2 m/sec.[122] Afferents from heat receptors are primarily C fibers. Cutaneous thermoreceptive neurons respond to external temperature change as well as rate of temperature change, sending early warning to the central nervous system (CNS) via afferent impulses, allowing rapid and transient thermoregulatory responses before brain temperature changes (Fig. 18–1).

VASOMOTOR AND SWEAT GLAND FUNCTION

Vasomotor responses to thermoregulatory input differ according to location. The normal thermoregulatory response to heat stress is mediated primarily by heat-sensitive neurons in the hypothalamus. Increased body-core temperature results in active vasodilatation in the extremities and is under noradrenergic control; increasing sympathetic stimulation results in vasoconstriction, and decreasing sympathetic control results in vasodilatation. Vasodilatation in the head, trunk, and proximal limbs is not a result of decreased sympathetic tone; instead, it is a result of an active process that is under the influence of cholinergic sudomotor nerves and local effects of temperature on venomotor tone. Sweat glands release local transmitters, such as vasoactive intestinal polypeptide (VIP) or bradykinins, and vasodilatation results. Areas of the body such as the forehead, where sweating is most prominent during heat stress, correspond to areas where active vasodilatation is greatest. The neurotransmitters involved in the regulation of relationships between vasodilatation and sweating as a response to heat stress are not fully elucidated, but animal evidence suggests the presence of specific vasodilator nerves.[106]

Sweat glands are controlled by sympathetic postganglionic nerve fibers, which are cholinergic, and large amounts of acetylcholinesterase as well as other peptides involved in neural transmission.[106,107]

NEUROTRANSMITTERS AND THERMOREGULATION

The neurotransmitters involved in thermoregulation include serotonin, norepinephrine, acetylcholine, dopamine, prostaglandins, β-endorphins, and intrinsic hypothalamic peptides such as argi-

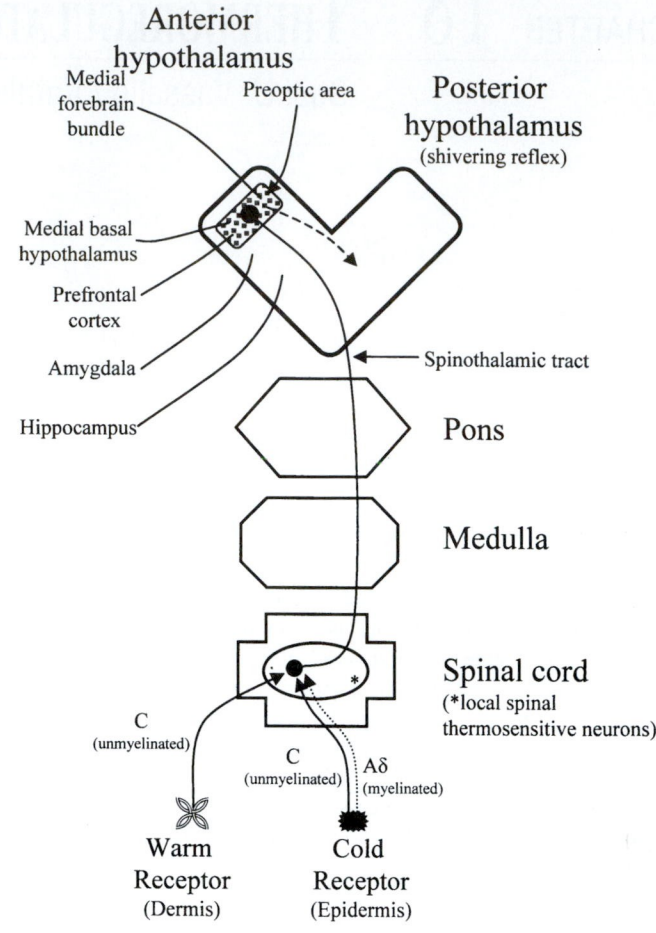

Figure 18–1. A schematic representation of the response of cutaneous thermoreceptive neurons to external termperature change as an early warning to the central nervous system.

nine vasopressin, adrenocorticotrophic hormone, thyrotropin releasing hormone, and α-melanocyte stimulating hormone.[40,195] Studies on the effects of individual neurotransmitters in thermoregulation yield contradictory results, depending on the animal species and the route of administration of the exogenous neurotransmitter. Refinements in techniques of microinjection of neurotransmitters into the hypothalamus of animals, rather than intraventricular instillation, have elucidated microanatomic sites where neurotransmitters are active. However, more research is necessary with regard to stimulation of thermoregulatory responses by individual neurotransmitters. Interspecies variation and theoretic differences in response to exogenous versus endogenous peptides makes this study difficult.

Apomorphine is a mixed dopamine agonist that has been shown to cause hypothermia in animals; studies using selective D_1- and D_2-receptor agonists and antagonists suggest that the hypothermic effect of apomorphine is a result of its effects on D_2 receptors, with some modulation by D_1 receptors in the hypothalamus.[173] Stimulation of D_2 receptors appears to mediate the hypothermia induced by the peptide sauvagine.[25] Dopamine D_3 receptors undoubtedly play a role, as well; stimulation of D_3 by specific agonists caused hypothermia in an animal model.[174,175] There appears to be a link between dopamine D_2 receptors and norepinephrine receptors in the hypothalamus, perhaps leading to vasodilatation and hypothermia. The effect of clozapine in producing hypothermia in the rat was demonstrated to be caused by D_1 and D_3 stimulation.[174,219] Lesser-known peptides appear to be involved in thermoregulation. For example, neuropeptide Y is an amino acid neurotransmitter that occurs in high concentrations in the preoptic area of the anterior hypothalamus. Administration of neuropeptide Y caused a reduction in core temperature when administered with adrenoceptor antagonists such as prazosin, an α_1 antagonist, propranolol, a β-adrenergic antagonist, and clonidine, a central α_2-adrenergic agonist.[70,218] The administration of synthetic cannabinoids induces hypothermia in animals, an effect that is antagonized by adrenergic agonists and enhanced by adrenergic antagonists.[203] Finally, studies on muscarinic receptors suggest the involvement of muscarinic M_2 and M_3 receptors in the production of hypothermia when agonists to these receptors are administered centrally.[220] Blockers of ATP-sensitive K^+ channels can reverse the effect of cholinomimetic drugs in producing hypothermia.[205]

DRUG EFFECTS ON THERMOREGULATION

Many drugs and toxins have pharmacologic effects that interfere with thermoregulatory responses[157,160,250] (Tables 18–1 and 18–2). α-Adrenergic agonist agents prevent vasodilatation in response to heat stress. Increased endogenous heat production in the setting of increased motor activity also occurs in patients poisoned with cocaine or amphetamines. Life-threatening hyperthermia has been associated with the use of these agents. β-Adrenergic antagonists and calcium channel blockers diminish the cardiac reserve available to compensate for heat-induced vasodilatation, whereas diuretics decrease cardiac reserve through their effects on intravascular volume.[54] β-Adrenergic antagonists also interfere with the capacity to maintain normothermia under conditions of cold stress, possibly related to their interference with the mobilization of substrates required for thermogenesis.[106,160] Opioids, and diverse sedative-hypnotics, depress hypothalamic function and predispose to hypothermia in the overdose setting.[72] Carbon monoxide poisoning must also be considered in the hypothermic patient. Organic phosphorous insecticides and other agents that cause cholinergic stimulation cause hypothermia by stimulation of inappropriate sweating and possibly through depression of the endogenous utilization of calorigenic substrates.[160] Drugs with anticholinergic effects decrease sweating and predispose to hyperthermia during environmental heat exposure or exercise. Phenothiazines appear to interfere with normal response to both heat and cold. Severe hyperthermia associated with the absence of sweating has been frequently described in patients on phenothiazines and may be a consequence of their anticholinergic effects.[221,264] Effects on cold tolerance are attributed to their α-adrenergic antagonist effects, which prevent vasoconstriction in response to cold stress.[158] In addition, hyperthermia associated with severe extrapyramidal rigidity may occur in patients on antipsychotic agents.[150] This rigidity is attributed to the dopamine-blocking effects of this class of drugs.

TABLE 18–1. Effects of Drugs and Toxins that Predispose to Hyperthermia

I. Impaired cutaneous heat loss
  A. Vasoconstriction through α-adrenergic stimulation
   Amphetamine and derivatives
   Cocaine
   Ephedrine
   Phenylpropanolamine
   Pseudoephedrine
  B. Sweat gland dysfunction by anticholinergic effects
   Antihistamines
   Belladonna alkaloids
   Cyclic antidepressants
   Phenothiazines

II. Myocardial depression
  A. Decreased cardiac output
   Antidysrhythmic agents
   β-Adrenergic antagonists
   Calcium channel blockers
  B. Reduced cardiac filling by dehydration
   Diuretics
   Ethanol

III. Hypothalamic depression
   Antipsychotic agents

IV. Impaired behavioral response
   Ethanol
   Opioids
   Phencyclidine
   Sedative-hypnotics
   Cocaine

V. Uncoupling of oxidative phosphorylation
   Pentachlorophenol
   Dinitrophenol
   Salicylates

VI. Increased muscle activity through agitation, seizures, or rigidity
   Amphetamine derivatives
   Caffeine
   Cocaine
   Isoniazid
   Lithium
   Monoamine oxidase inhibitors
   Phencyclidine
   Strychnine
   Sympathomimetic agents

VII. Dystonia
   Butyrophenones
   Phenothiazines

VIII. Withdrawal
   Dopamine agonist
   Ethanol
   Sedative-hypnotic

TABLE 18–2. Effects of Drugs and Toxins that Predispose to Hypothermia

Impaired nonshivering thermogenesis
β-Adrenergic antagonists
Cholinergic agents
Hypoglycemic agents

Impaired perception of cold
Carbon monoxide
Ethanol
Hypoglycemic agents
Opioids
Sedative-hypnotics

Impaired shivering by hypothalamic depression
Carbon monoxide
Ethanol
General anesthetic agents
Opioids
Phenothiazines
Sedative-hypnotics

Impaired vasoconstriction
α-Adrenergic antagonists
Ethanol
Phenothiazines

ETHANOL

The most common variable related to the occurrence of hypothermia in an urban setting is the use of ethanol.[51,257] The mechanism by which ethanol predisposes to hypothermia is said to be by virtue of its effects on CNS depression, vasodilatation, and blunting of behavorial responses to cold. However, thermoregulatory dysfunction associated with ethanol intoxication is undoubtedly more complex.

In animal models, ethanol leads to hypothermia, the extent of which is in part dependent on ambient temperature.[190,211,212] In mice, as the dose of ethanol increased, body temperature decreased and the rate of this decline in body temperature was faster at higher ethanol doses.[184] The decline in body temperature could be reversed by increasing ambient temperature; increasing ambient temperature to 36°C (96.8°F) caused an immediate rise in the body temperature.[184] The poikilothermic effect of ethanol was not due to hypoglycemia. Poikilothermia is the variation in body temperature >± 2°C (3.6°F) upon exposure to environmental temperature changes. Rats treated with equipotent amounts of sodium pentobarbital showed the same effects on body temperature as rats treated with ethanol, suggesting a similar central mechanism of central nervous system depression resulting in altered thermoregulation.[184]

Numerous mechanisms are involved in the "ethanol-induced depression of central nervous system function."[215] Genetic factors influence the role of ethanol in the production of hypothermia. Mouse strains bred for sleep times differed in sensitivity to ethanol's effect on temperature.[83,178,184] Mice can be selectively bred for genetic sensitivity or insensitivity to acute ethanol-induced hypothermia, and the differences appear to be mediated by the serotonergic systems.[73] Histidyl-proline dike-topiperazine (cyclo His-Pro or CHP), another neurotransmitter that is found in many animal species, acts at the preoptic-anterior hypothalamus to modulate body temperature.[32,117] Exogenous administration of this neuropeptide produced a dose-dependent decrease in ethanol-induced hypothermia. Attenuation of hypothermia resulted from passive immunization with CHP antibody.[32,117] Ethanol effects may be mediated through modulation of endogenous opioid peptides, as high-dose (10 mg/kg) naloxone reverses ethanol-induced hypothermia in animals.[200]

Pharmacokinetic characteristics of ethanol metabolism change in the presence of hypothermia. Hypothermic piglets infused with ethanol showed slower ethanol metabolism and a smaller volume of distribution and, as a result, higher ethanol levels than normothermic controls. Ethanol elimination and metabolism decreased as temperature fell.[141]

Tolerance develops to the effect of ethanol in producing hypothermia in all species.[74,190] The degree of tolerance is proportional to the dose and duration of treatment with ethanol and is not explained by the increased rate of metabolism with chronic exposure.[124] Age is a factor in the development of tolerance; older animals do not display the same degree of tolerance to the hypothermic effects of chronic ethanol administration as do younger animals.[182,199,261] The development of tolerance to ethanol-induced hypothermia is affected by genetic factors. Experimentally, tolerance to ethanol-induced hypothermia increases the incorporation of certain amino acids into proteins in the rat brain. The formation of new proteins in ethanol-tolerant rats suggests stimulation of gene expression related to the tolerant state.[124,253] Deficits in N-methyl-D-aspartate (NMDA) receptor systems may also be implicated in the development of ethanol tolerance. In addition, altered nicotinamide adenine dinucleotide (NADH) oxidation to NAD^+, diminished blood flow to the liver, or slowing of metabolism through the P450 microsomal enzyme system may be involved.[215]

Hypothermia alters the breath-ethanol partition in the alveolus, and the temperature of expired breath alters breath-alcohol analysis results. In patients with mild hypothermia, ethanol breath analysis results in lower values by 7.3% per degree centigrade (or 1.8°F) decrease in body temperature.[77] Whether breath-alcohol analysis is also affected by hyperthermia in the test subject remains to be studied.[77]

DISEASE PROCESSES AND THERMOREGULATION

Many disease processes interfere with normal thermoregulation, limiting an individual's capacity to prevent hypothermia or hyperthermia. Extensive dermatologic disease or cutaneous burns impair sweating and vasomotor responses to heat stress.[27] Patients with autonomic disturbances such as diabetes or peripheral vascular disease also have altered vasomotor responses that impair vasodilatation and sweating.[209] Extensive surgical dressings may preclude the evaporation of sweat in an otherwise normal patient. Heat-stressed persons with poor cardiac reserve may not be able to sustain a skin blood flow high enough to maintain normothermia.[64,239] Intense motor activity may lead to excessive endogenous heat production in patients with Parkinson disease or hyperthyroidism. Patients with agitated delirium or seizures also have significantly elevated rates of endogenous heat production. Hypothalamic injury caused by cerebrovascular accidents, trauma, or infection may disturb thermoregulation.[62,153] Hypothalamic dysfunction can lead to high, unremitting fevers and insufficient stimulation of heat loss mechanisms such as sweating. Hypothalamic damage may predispose to hypothermia by interference with centrally mediated heat conservation.[62,153,222,223] Fever, the normal response to stimulation of the hypothalamus by pyrogens, results in an elevated physiologic temperature set point and is a disadvantage in the heat-stressed individual.[106]

HYPOTHERMIA

Epidemiology

Hypothermia is defined as an unintentional lowering of the core body temperature to <95°F (<35°C). Between 1979 and 1995, at least 12,368 people died of hypothermia in the United States.[35] Hypothermia-related deaths decreased significantly in the United States between 1979 and 1996.[34] This downward trend was strongest for black males age >65 years, a group with one of the highest hypothermia-related death rates. Possible reasons for the decrease in hypothermia-related deaths in the United States include a change in reporting practices, milder winters, and better prevention measures, such as public education and outreach programs.[34]

Medical factors increase the risk in the elderly, including limited mobility, impaired shivering, chronic illness, confusion, decreased protective fat, and slower metabolic rates. Social isolation and deprivation, poor nutrition, and inadequate access to or use of indoor heating, often because of financial concerns, are additional factors associated with hypothermia.[37,111,131] Other risks associated with hypothermia in all groups are ethanol use, mental illness, use of antipsychotic medication, hypothyroidism, starvation, immobilization, dehydration, poverty, and homelessness[36] (Table 18–3).

Most hypothermic deaths occur in the winter months; however, mildly cool environments and windy wet conditions are also frequently associated with hypothermia. Of the 10 states with the greatest rate of hypothermia-related deaths, in only 2, Illinois and Alaska, are the deaths associated with severe winter weather. The other states that led the nation in hypothermia-related deaths between 1979 and 1982 are not commonly associated with severe winter conditions and include Alabama, Arizona, New Mexico, North Carolina, Oklahoma, South Carolina, Tennessee, and Virginia.[36]

Response to Cold

The normal physiologic response to cold is precipitated by stimulation of cold-sensitive neurons in the skin, so that the onset of the body's response to cold occurs prior to cooling of central blood. Cold-sensitive neurons in the skin send afferent impulses to the hypothalamus, resulting in shivering and piloerection. Shivering is the main thermoregulatory response to cold in humans, except in neonates, where nonshivering thermogenesis prevails. Shivering is initiated in the posterior hypothalamus when impulses from cold-sensitive thermoreceptors are integrated in the anterior hypothalamus and communicated to the posterior hypothalamus, or when cold-sensitive neurons in the posterior hypothalamus are activated directly. Efferent stimuli from the posterior hypothalamus travel through the midbrain tegmentum, pons, and lateral medullary reticular formation to the motor pathways of the tectospinal and rubrospinal tracts, resulting in shivering.[17] A mechanism of stimulation of shivering that usually occurs later when core temperature

TABLE 18–3. Factors Predisposing to Hypothermia

Advanced age
  Decreased metabolic rate
  Decreased temperature discrimination
  Decreased ability to shiver
  Reduced peripheral blood flow

Central nervous system depression
  Ethanol
  Hypothalamic dysfunction
  Infection
  Intracranial bleeding
  Stroke
  Toxins

Endocrine
  Diabetic ketoacidosis
  Hyperosmolar coma
  Hypopituitarism
  Hypothyroidism

Environmental
  Homelessness
  Unintentional

Hepatic failure

Immobilization
  Central nervous system dysfunction
  Illness
  Spinal cord injury
  Trauma

Nutritional
  Hypoglycemia
  Glycogen depletion
  Starvation
  Thiamine deficiency

Sepsis

Social
  Failure to use indoor heating
  Homelessness
  Inadequate indoor heating
  Poverty
  Social isolation

Uremia

drops is the local cooling of the spinal cord, which leads to shivering by increasing excitability of motor neurons.

Heat produced without muscle contraction is known as nonshivering thermogenesis.[26,106] Nonshivering thermogenesis is mediated by the sympathetic nervous system.[46] Catecholamines activate adenylate cyclase, increasing cyclic adenosine monophosphate (cAMP), resulting in mobilization of fat and glucose stores (β-adrenergic receptors).[160,217] Nonshivering thermogenesis is blocked by β-adrenergic receptor antagonism and increased by administration of norepinephrine. Brown adipose tissue is the most important site of nonshivering thermogenesis. In humans, brown fat is found primarily in neonates, although in cold-acclimatized people there may be small amounts found on autopsy.[26] Brown adipose tissue functions as a thermoregulatory effector organ, producing heat by the oxidation of fatty acids when the tissue is stimulated by norepinephrine.[31]

In addition to shivering and nonshivering thermogenesis, efferent sympathetic fibers from the hypothalamus stimulate peripheral vasoconstriction (α-adrenergic receptors). Piloerection and vasoconstriction result in decreased heat loss from the body. Intense vasoconstriction shunts blood away from the periphery to the core and antidiuretic hormone antagonism results in increased urine output and hemoconcentration.

Disease Processes and Hypothermia

Several disease processes commonly result in an inability to maintain a normal body temperature in a cool environment. Hypothermia may develop in association with sepsis,[151] hypothyroidism, hypoglycemia, uremia, hepatic failure, or poor nutrition.[206,209] Hypothalamic injury may result in chronic poikilothermia.[158] Thiamine deficiency adversely affects the hypothalamus, perhaps because of inefficient glucose metabolism, and leads to hypothermia.[139] Spinal cord transections above the first thoracic segment interrupt hypothalamic-sympathetic outflow pathways, resulting in hypothermia.[209] The elderly are at greater risk of hypothermia because of decreased vasomotor responses and decreased capacity to shiver.[46,49] Mentally and physically compromised patients may be unable to make appropriate behavioral responses to hot or cold environments.

Evaluations to determine the presence of underlying diseases are often difficult in the hypothermic patient.[75,151] The mental status may be markedly altered by hypothermia but is not usually abnormal until the temperature falls below 32°C (90°F). If normal mental status is not regained when the temperature reaches 32°C (90°F) during rewarming, underlying CNS structural, toxic, or metabolic problems must be considered.[75,206] Failure of the patient to rewarm quickly suggests the presence of underlying disease. In one study, hypothermic patients without underlying disease are reported to rewarm at a rate of 1.0–3.7°F/h (average, 2.1°F/h) (1.2°C/h), whereas patients with significant underlying disease (sepsis, GI hemorrhage, diabetic ketoacidosis, pulmonary embolus, myocardial infarction) warmed at a rate of 0.25–1.8°F/h (average, 1°F/h)(0.6°C/h).[256]

Alteration of Drug Metabolism in Hypothermia

Metabolism of drugs is altered in the setting of hypothermia. In hypothermic piglets, the volume of distribution and the clearance of fentanyl are decreased.[142] Similarly, in piglets given gentamicin, the volume of distribution and clearance rate decreased in direct proportion to the decrease in cardiac output and glomerular filtration rate.[140] Hypothermic puppies given intravenous lidocaine showed slower rates of disappearance of the drug than when normothermic.[179] Humans and animals given propranolol showed a reduced volume of distribution and decreased total body clearance, resulting in higher than expected propranolol levels.[168,187] Decreased hepatic metabolism of propranolol during hypothermia has been shown in vitro.[169] Hypothermia prolongs neuromuscular blockade with *d*-tubocurarine,[96] and increases neuromuscular blockade with suxamethonium.[259] Phenobarbital metabolism and volume of distribution decreased with hypothermia in children.[123] The lethal dose of digoxin was doubled in hypothermic dogs.[15] Digoxinlike substances are present during hypothermia.[80,110]

Reasons for altered metabolism in hypothermia include delayed distribution of the drug and altered enzyme function with temperature and pH changes. Volume of distribution changes, in part because of peripheral vasoconstriction. Cardiac output decreases,[196] leading to decreased liver perfusion and decreased delivery of drug to hepatic microsomal enzymes.[96,126,125,127] Plasma volume decreases as free water moves intracellularly, causing hemoconcentration and further decreasing organ perfusion.[260] Biliary excretion of atropine, procaine, and sulfanilamide decreases in vitro.[125–127] The glomerular filtration rate decreases in hypothermia.[23] In vitro, the activity of metabolic pathways including acetylation and hydrolysis decrease with cooling.[125,126]

Clinical Findings

The clinical effects of hypothermia are related to the membrane-depressant effects of cold, which result in ionic and electrical conduction disturbances in the brain, heart, peripheral nerves, and other major organs[112] (Table 18–4). Cold tissues are protected by decreases in tissue oxygen requirements. As body temperature decreases, metabolic activity will decline at about 7% per 1°C (1.8°F).[260] This effect provides significant protection to vital organs despite the potentially deleterious effects of membrane suppression.

Effects on the central nervous system are temperature-dependent and predictable. Mild hypothermia (32–35°C; 90–95°F) usually results in relatively benign clinical manifestations. Ataxia, slight clumsiness, slowed response to stimuli, and dysarthria are common.[75] As cooling continues, the mental status slowly deteriorates. In moderate hypothermia (27–32°C; 80–90°F), the patient is usually lethargic but still likely to respond verbally. In severe hypothermia (20–27°C; 68–80°F) the patient is unlikely to respond verbally, but will react purposefully to noxious stimuli.[75] In profound hypothermia (<20°C; 68°F), the patient is unresponsive to stimuli. Pupils may be fixed and dilated and the patient may appear dead.[103] However, standard criteria of brain death do not apply to hypothermic patients. The hypothermia itself protects against cerebral hypoxic damage.[112] Temperature drop inhibits the release of the excitatory neurotransmitter glutamate and attenuates the release of dopamine in brain ischemia animal models, suggesting a protective effect of hypothermia in brain injury.[30] Ventricular cerebrospinal fluid glutamate concentrations were lower in patients showing benefit from mild induced hypothermia after brain injury when compared to brain injured patients kept normothermic.[165] However, a subsequent report of 362 patients showed a lack of effect of induction of hypothermia after acute brain injury.[42,102,164]

Under controlled circumstances patients have survived with temperatures as low as 9°C (48.2°F).[78] Vigorous resuscitation is required for these patients. In particular, cardiac resuscitation should not be terminated in the field, where temperatures are seldom taken. The adage that a patient cannot be considered dead until the patient is warm and dead is critical to providing appropriate management. This approach may lead to hours of cardiopulmonary resuscitation in hypothermic patients with ventricular fibrillation, ventricular tachycardia, or asystole, but may be ultimately successful in patients initially presumed to be dead.[237]

The cardiac and hemodynamic effects of cold correlate closely with body temperature. As cooling begins there is a transient increase in cardiac output. Tachycardia develops secondary to shivering and sympathetic stimulation. At about 81°F (27°C) shivering

TABLE 18–4. Physiologic and Clinical Manifestations of Hypothermia

Cardiovascular
Normal, decreased, or increased cardiac output
Normal heart rate or tachycardia, then bradycardia
Vasoconstriction and central shunting of blood

ECG
Prolongation of intervals
Atrial fibrillation
Increased ventricular irritability
J-point elevation "Osborn waves"

Central nervous system
Mild: 32–35°C (90–95°F)
    Normal mentation or slightly slowed
Moderate: 27–32°C (80–90°F)
    Lethargic but verbally responsive
Severe: 20–27°C (68–80°F)
    Unlikely to respond verbally, purposefully to noxious stimuli
Profound: <20°C (<68°F)
    Unresponsive, may appear dead

Gastrointestinal tract
Decreased motility
Depressed hepatic metabolism

Hematologic
Hemoconcentration
Left shift of oxyhemoglobin dissociation curve

Kidneys
Cold-induced diuresis
Antidiuretic hormone antagonism

Lungs
Respiratory rate variable
Bronchorrhea

Metabolic
Metabolic acidosis
Increased glycogenolysis
Increased serum free fatty acids
Normal thyroid and adrenal function

ceases. Bradycardia develops with maintenance of a normal cardiac stroke volume.[28] This bradycardia is responsible for the decreased myocardial oxygen demand which may be protective in the setting of hypothermia.[28] In profound hypothermia, bradycardia may progress to asystole and death.

Unlike cerebral circulation, where autoregulation is preserved during cooling, coronary autoregulation is disturbed during hypothermia, and myocardial injury may ensue.[28] Attempts to maximize myocardial oxygenation through administration of oxygen and volume replacement to increase diastolic filling pressure are appropriate. Pharmacologic or electrical attempts to increase heart rate may dangerously increase myocardial oxygen demand.

The initial respiratory response to hypothermia is hyperventilation. As temperature continues to decrease, hypoventilation develops, which may progress to apnea and death. In animal models, this has been attributed to cold-induced failure of phrenic nerve conduction.[133]

The Electrocardiogram

The most common ECG abnormality in hypothermia is generalized, progressive depression of myocardial conduction. Because myocardial oxygen demand remains unchanged in spite of cooling, and stroke volume is preserved, the number of beats per minute decreases as a means of decreasing myocardial oxygen requirements. PR, QRS, and QTc intervals are all prolonged, and increasingly profound hypothermia may lead to gradual progression to asystole.[60,249] Ventricular fibrillation occurs in an irritable myocardium most commonly at temperatures less than 30°C (86°F) resulting in a high O_2 consumption dysrhythmia. Atrial fibrillation is the most common dysrhythmia occurring in hypothermia.[76,197,251] Shivering may not be clinically evident, but a fine muscular tremor frequently produces a mechanical artifact in the baseline of the electrocardiogram.[65] A deflection occurring at the junction of the QRS and ST segment is invariably present in patients with temperatures <30°C (86°F)[66] (Fig. 18–2). First described in a single patient in 1938,[245] the J-point deflection is commonly known as the *Osborn wave*.[201] The J-point deflection, thought to be a "current of injury" associated with CO_2 retention under hypothermic conditions, was believed to be a poor prognostic sign.[201] Subsequent study has refuted its prognostic significance, as the J-point deflection is invariably found in the hypothermic patient when multiple electrocardiographic leads are obtained.[65,66,247,251] The size of the J-point deflection increases as

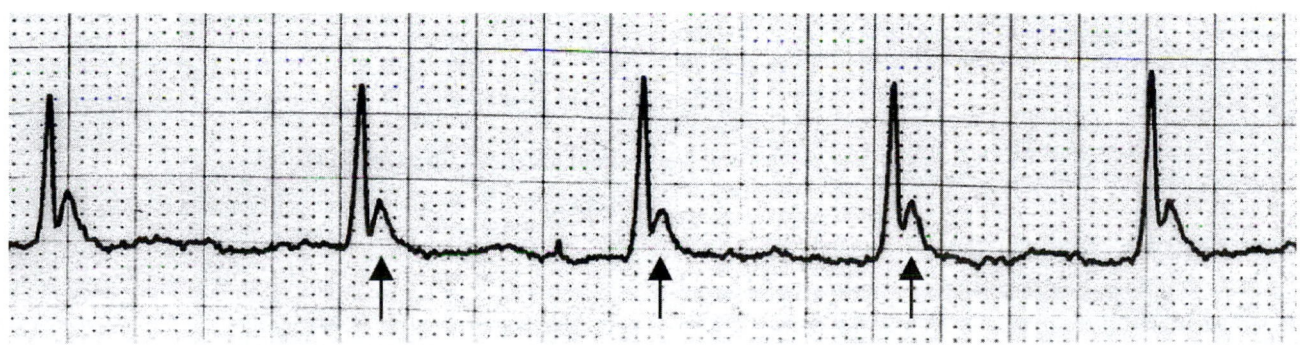

Figure 18–2. A characteristic electrocardiographic finding in the patient with profound hypothermia. The terminal phase of the QRS complex shows a typical elevation of the J-point Osborn wave (↑).

body temperature decreases.[197,251] Atrial dysrhythmias that occur in the absence of underlying heart disease invariably disappear solely with rewarming.

Management

After blood specimens have been drawn, the hypothermic patient should be given 0.5–1.0 g glucose/kg body weight as $D_{50}W$ and 100 mg of thiamine IV. If hypoglycemia is the cause of the hypothermia, the response to glucose may be dramatic, heralded by the onset of shivering and rapid return to normal body temperature. Wernicke's encephalopathy is uncommon, but may be associated with mild hypothermia; thermoregulation and normal ocular motion may return after the initiation of thiamine therapy.[139]

Hypothermia shifts the oxygen dissociation curve to the left (Chap. 20), resulting in decreased oxygen unloading to tissues; therefore, oxygen administration may be of benefit.[56] If clinically indicated for airway protection or inadequate ventilation or oxygenation, endotracheal intubation should be performed and can be done without complication.[51,147,176] However, there are case reports of ventricular fibrillation occurring during endotracheal intubation.[12,82,103,202,258] Every effort should be made to limit patient activity and stimulation during the acute rewarming period, as activity might increase myocardial oxygen demand or alter myocardial temperature gradients, increasing the risk of iatrogenic ventricular fibrillation. Although Swan-Ganz catheters and central venous lines have been placed without complications,[100,147] they should be avoided unless absolutely essential, so as not to precipitate ventricular dysrhythmias.[246] If a central venous catheter is considered necessary, it should not be allowed to touch the myocardium.[248] Patients who develop ventricular fibrillation are difficult to manage. In these instances, cardiopulmonary resuscitation (CPR) should be initiated, and the patient intubated and ventilated to maintain a pH of 7.40 uncorrected for temperature. Active internal rewarming should be instituted because standard therapy for ventricular fibrillation is often unsuccessful until rewarming is achieved. Patients should be supported, then defibrillated; if unsuccessful, defibrillation should not be attempted again until the patient has been warmed several degrees centigrade. Defibrillation may not be successful until the temperature exceeds 30°C (86°F); however, defibrillation can be successfully accomplished in animals and patients with temperatures of less than 30°C (86°F).[5,12,53,181] The oxygen-powered "thumper" and cardiopulmonary bypass devices are used successfully during prolonged hypothermic cardiopulmonary arrests.[12,45,149,238,246] Transesophageal echocardiographic examination of seven hypothermic patients demonstrated that the thoracic pump mechanism is important for forward blood flow during CPR. The thoracic pump theory states that forward blood flow is caused by blood forced out of the heart and thoracic aorta by a general increase in intrathoracic pressure. Doppler studies demonstrate forward blood flow across the open mitral valve during external chest compression.[162]

Arterial Blood Gas Physiochemistry

Assessment of the adequacy of ventilation and oxygenation in the hypothermic patient often poses a dilemma to clinicians, as chemical effects of cold on arterial pH and blood gases lead to confusion in the interpretation of arterial blood gas values. Cold inhibits the dissociation of water molecules, causing pH to increase as cooling occurs. In vitro, the pH change of blood as it is cooled increases

parallel to the pH change of neutral water. The partial pressures of CO_2 and O_2 decrease as cooling occurs, even as the blood content of those gases remains unchanged. Blood in a syringe taken from a patient whose body temperature is 98.6°F (37°C) yields a pH of 7.40 and a P_{CO_2} of 40 mm Hg in the blood gas machine at 98.6°F (37°C), but yields a pH of 7.72 and a P_{CO_2} of 14 mm Hg if the blood is cooled to 61°F (16°C) and the values were measured at that temperature. Specially calibrated laboratory equipment, not routinely available, is required to measure blood gas values directly at other than normal body temperature. A patient whose body temperature is 61°F (16°C) and whose actual in vivo blood gas values are pH 7.72 and P_{CO_2} 14 mm Hg will have values of pH 7.40 and P_{CO_2} 40 mm Hg when the blood is warmed to 98.6°F (37°C) and measured in the standard laboratory blood gas machine. Because the machine measures pH and blood gas pressures only in blood warmed to 98.6°F (37°C; the uncorrected values), the actual in vivo values in hypothermic patients can be approximated using mathematically derived corrected values. Because the pH of neutrality has also increased, it is unclear what clinical meanings these corrected values have. The uncorrected values indicate what the pH and P_{CO_2} would be if the patient were normothermic. At first glance, the clinician might be content to learn that a hypothermic patient at 61°F (16°C) has a corrected pH of 7.47 and P_{CO_2} of 40 mm Hg. However, the uncorrected values of pH 7.18 and P_{CO_2} 111 mm Hg indicate that the patient has a significant respiratory acidosis. Attempts to maintain a corrected pH of 7.40 may lead to hypoventilation and risk alveolar collapse and impairment of oxygenation. The preponderance of evidence in the anesthesia and cardiovascular surgery literature suggests that maintenance of ventilation is associated with a decreased incidence of myocardial injury and a decreased incidence of ventricular fibrillation.[56] Blood-gas values of pH and P_{CO_2} should be left uncorrected after the blood sample is warmed in the blood-gas machine and interpreted in the same way as in the normothermic patient.[56]

Hypotension

When hypotension occurs in hypothermia, it is usually due to the presence of bradycardia and the commonly associated volume depletion. Fluid depletion in hypothermia occurs as a result of a variety of mechanisms, including central shunting of blood by vasoconstriction and cold-induced diuresis. Cold diuresis occurs when increases in central blood volume result in inhibition of antidiuretic hormone. Impairment of renal enzyme activity and decreased renal tubular reabsorption contribute to the large quantities of dilute urine known as cold diuresis.[97,101,147,260] Normal saline should be given to expand intravascular volume. Urine output is an important indicator of organ perfusion and the adequacy of intravascular volume in the hypothermic patient, although the initial cold diuresis may lead to underestimation of fluid needs.[260]

Pharmacologic Interventions

Bretylium.   Bretylium tosylate is a benzyl quaternary ammonium compound with a biphasic action, initially causing release of norepinephrine and then blocking its release. This may cause transient hypertension, but hypotension is the most common result.[181,200] Hypothermic dogs given bretylium had significantly lower mean arterial pressures and systemic and pulmonary vascular resistance as compared to controls.[200] The mechanism of the antidysrhythmic effect of bretylium in normothermia may be related to its ability to increase the myocardial refractory period.[200]

Bretylium may be of benefit in the treatment of ventricular fibrillation in the hypothermic patient. The antidysrhythmic effect of bretylium is poorly understood. It prolongs the cardiac action potential and reduces heterogeneity of repolarization times.[214] The net effect seems to be stabilization of the cardiac rhythm. Bretylium is found to increase the fibrillation threshold in hypothermic cats given 50 mg/kg bretylium,[189] and in dogs given 15 mg/kg bretylium,[29] whereas 7.5 mg/kg was found to increase the threshold prior to cooling.[200] In a canine study,[181] cooling occurred and either a saline placebo or bretylium 40 mg/kg was administered prior to attempted induced ventricular fibrillation. Six of 11 dogs given placebo developed ventricular fibrillation, whereas only 1 of the 11 dogs pretreated with bretylium developed ventricular fibrillation following manipulation. In this study, 3 dogs receiving pretreatment with bretylium fibrillated during the infusion, prior to maneuvers. Of the 6 dogs given placebo that developed ventricular fibrillation, all were successfully resuscitated, although 4 required bretylium to do so. This study did not attain statistical significance, and bretylium infusion both resulted in ventricular fibrillation and was effective in chemical defibrillation of ventricular fibrillation.[181] A single case of successful chemical defibrillation with bretylium in an environmentally exposed patient with a core temperature of 29.5°C (85.1°F).[52] Given the difficulty of treating ventricular fibrillation once it occurs during hypothermia, the preponderance of evidence suggests a role for the use of bretylium.

Dopamine. Dopamine increases cardiac output, mean arterial pressure, heart rate, and stroke volume in dogs cooled to 25°C (77°F), and stabilizes pulmonary arterial wedge pressure.[186] In a canine hypothermia model, dopamine infusions provided some protection from ventricular fibrillation. Dopamine lowered the temperature at which ventricular fibrillation occurred and reduced the incidence of ventricular fibrillation, as did infusion of norepinephrine.[8] The added benefit of dopamine in hypothermia may be due to its renal and splanchnic vasodilating properties, increasing renal perfusion and supporting urine output.[85] Dopamine increases myocardial oxygen demand and decreases peripheral perfusion, potentially detrimental effects in the hypothermic patient.[8] Nevertheless, after the administration of intravenous fluids, dopamine infusion during hypothermia is indicated in the patient requiring blood pressure support.

Rewarming

Three types of rewarming modalities are used in the management of hypothermic patients.[48,152] *Passive external rewarming* involves covering the patient with blankets and protecting the patient from further heat loss. Passive external rewarming uses the patient's own endogenous heat production for rewarming and is most successful in healthy patients with mild to moderate hypothermia whose capacity for endogenous heat production is intact.[101] Passive external rewarming is reported to be successful in hypothermic patients with temperatures as low as 20.6°C (69°F).[244,251,257] Advocates of passive external rewarming argue that it allows vasoconstriction to persist and it decreases the afterdrop and shock from vasodilatation associated with active skin rewarming.[101,176,244]

Active external rewarming involves the external application of heat to the patient. There is disagreement about the possible detrimental effects of active external rewarming. For example, skin warming may lead to a physiologically detrimental suppression of shivering.[101] Acute vasodilatation of peripheral vessels could cause hypotension and an increased peripheral demand on the persistently cold myocardium. The return of cold blood from the extremities to the heart is suggested to exacerbate intramyocardial temperature gradients, which could cause ventricular irritability during hypothermia.[156] However, in pigs, blood returning to the heart was found to be warm before warming of central organs occurred.[87]

Afterdrop is the continuing decrease in temperature once rewarming begins. Some authors recommend (including the American Heart Association Advanced Cardiac Life Support (ACLS) guidelines)[1] that rewarming of the extremities should be delayed by application of heat to the trunk only, rather than to the trunk and extremities, in an attempt to avoid the complications of afterdrop and intramyocardial temperature gradients.[144] However, there is no scientific evidence to suggest that this drop in temperature is more dangerous than the very temperature that had existed originally.[155] In addition, there is no evidence of pooling of blood in the periphery, nor of increased flow during surface rewarming.[155,224] Flow studies in the hand, arm, calf, and foot demonstrate that afterdrop has already occurred and is completed before any increase in blood flow occurs in the limbs.[155,255] Initial experiments demonstrating afterdrop were done in inanimate objects and reflected continued cooling of central structures before heat from external sources reached the core.[87,155,255]

Treatment including complete submersion is available in some institutions. Eighteen patients with temperatures of 26–33°C (78.8–91.4°F) were successfully warmed in a Hubbard tank, although one fatality not associated with rewarming occurred.[263] Submersion must be used with caution, however, because of the inherent difficulties of controlling agitated patients and monitoring and resuscitating patients in water.

Mortality rates for active external rewarming are frequently reported to be higher than for passive external rewarming,[209] but case selection is not controlled in these series. It is possible that sicker patients who fail to rewarm passively are then actively rewarmed and have a higher mortality rate caused by their underlying disease, rather than by the method of therapy selected. The published series and case reports do not allow for an analysis of this hypothesis. Selection of either passive or active external rewarming in treatment of mild to moderate hypothermia does not appear to influence the prognosis as much as the presence or absence of underlying disease.[115,176,256] In our experience, active external rewarming has not resulted in mortality except in those patients with severe underlying disease.[251]

Active internal rewarming involves attempts to increase central core temperature directly, by warming the heart prior to the extremities or periphery. The administration of heated, humidified oxygen delivered by facemask is considered part of active internal rewarming. Additional minimally invasive modalities of active internal rewarming include endotracheal intubation with warmed, humidified oxygen,[104] and gastric lavage with warmed fluids. Transcutaneous pacing was successful in improving hemodynamic parameters and speeding rewarming in an animal model.[62] More invasive modalities, those procedures that are fundamental to the rewarming controversy, include peritoneal lavage with warmed dialysate,[121,192] and the rerouting of blood through external blood rewarming equipment via cardiopulmonary or femoral-femoral bypass and hemodialysis.[33,109,183] Heparin-coated bypass systems are available, which avoids systemic anticoagulation, thus decreasing the risk of bleeding complications. It is suggested that extracorporeal venovenous rewarming and continuous arteriovenous rewarming show improved rewarming rates when compared to standard techniques such as saline lavage of the bladder, stomach, or peritoneal cavity.[81] Extracorporeal methods of active internal rewarming should be reserved for severely hypothermic patients (<80°F or <27°F) or those with unstable cardiac rhythms (ventricular fibrillation or tachycardia, or asystole) attributed to hypothermia.[5,55,98] The evidence for the benefit of extracorporeal methods in those patients with stable rhythms is not yet available. In patients with stable rhythms, studies are essential to resolve the debate over the merits of passive or active external rewarming versus active internal rewarming.

Unfortunately, current ACLS guidelines for the management of hypothermia make several recommendations that are not supported by the literature. The most glaring area of controversy is the recommendation of extracorporeal rewarming for stable patients based on a temperature of 30°C (86°F) or less because passive rewarming is ineffective in the stable patient with severe hypothermia, which is defined as a temperature below 30°C (86°F). Many patients with temperatures below 30°C have been successfully treated with passive external rewarming with, at most, the addition of warm, humidified oxygen.[251,257] Patient temperature correlates poorly with outcome.[5,53,146,246,249] Stability of the vital signs and cardiac rhythm, and the underlying cause of hypothermia, are much more critical considerations in management. It is hard to imagine a patient with a stable cardiac rhythm and core temperature of 80–86°F (26.6–30°C) in whom extracorporeal rewarming with cardiopulmonary bypass is indicated.

Additionally, ACLS guidelines state that significant hyperkalemia may develop during rewarming, suggesting that this is a complication of rewarming. Hyperkalemia is not described as a consequence of rewarming.[51] In all of the evidence collected with regard to hyperkalemia, this abnormality was present as a consequence of the hypothermia and not the rewarming.[103,161,226]

These are ideal subjects for intensive evidence-based investigations to resolve the science versus myth in hypothermia resuscitation.

Prognosis in Hypothermia

Except in cases of profound hypothermia,[103] the prognosis is most closely correlated with the presence or absence of underlying disease.[115,176,198,256,257] In patients with hypothermia alone, in the absence of underlying disease, mortality is 0–10%. In the presence of an underlying disease, mortality rises to 75–90%. Morbidity results from associated frostbite and trauma.

Prolonged cardiopulmonary arrest and absolute temperature are not predictive of poor outcome.[5,53,146,246,249] In severely hypothermic patients, profound hyperkalemia (K$^+$ >10 mEq/L) is associated with unsuccessful resuscitation.[103,161,226]

Frostbite. Hypothermia may be accompanied by frostbite when patients are exposed to environmental temperatures that are less than −6.7°C (20°F).[177] Frostbite should be managed by rapid rewarming. The extremity involved may be placed in a large, soft basin of warm water (38–43°C; 100–108°F) for 30 minutes. The water temperature must be frequently adjusted, as the frozen extremity will have the effect of ice cubes, and with time cool the water in the basin. Parenteral analgesics may be necessary, as the rewarming process is often painful. Frostbitten areas should never be rubbed, as the tissue is particularly sensitive to trauma. Dex-

tran, alcohol, vasodilators, and anticoagulants have not proven useful. Sympathectomy in this situation is also of unproven benefit and remains highly controversial.[134,145,171]

Prevention. Because many patients may not wear (and may not possess) adequate clothing, it is essential that they be assessed for social services support after the acute episode is resolved. In addition, many of these patients live in substandard, inadequately heated (often unheated) housing. Patients should be advised to wear comfortable, warm clothing to prevent future episodes of hypothermia. Adequate clothing is particularly important for patients traveling by automobile during inclement weather conditions. The importance of adequate nutrition should also be stressed.

HYPERTHERMIA

Definition of Heatstroke

Heatstroke is defined by a rectal temperature greater than 106°F (41.1°C) in the setting of a neurologic disturbance manifested by psychosis, delirium, stupor, coma, and/or convulsions.[135] Temperature criteria cannot be absolute, as information regarding the patient's temperature is rarely available at the time of onset of heatstroke. In some instances the temperature may not be measured for several hours, during which time cooling may have been instituted or occurred spontaneously.[129,130] When appropriate environmental conditions prevail, the diagnosis of heatstroke should be made liberally. Although the absence of sweating was once thought to be an essential component of the definition of heatstroke,[43,193] many patients with heatstroke have been noted to maintain the ability to sweat on presentation.[50,163,232,252]

Epidemiology of Heatstroke

Hundreds of Americans die annually of heatstroke, and 80% of the victims are older than 50 years. Heatstroke is the second most common cause of death among high school athletes, exceeded only by spinal injuries. Several studies show mortality rates from heatstroke to be 30%–80%. Thousands of other victims survive with significant heat-related morbidity.[7,61,122,132] The high morbidity and mortality of heatstroke markedly contrast with those of profound hypothermia, in which the prognosis is related not to the temperature itself, but to the underlying etiology. The overall prognosis in heatstroke depends primarily on how long the temperature has been elevated prior to cooling, the maximum temperature reached, and the affected individual's health.

Heat-related deaths are preventable, and preparedness of cities and healthcare workers is essential. Mortality during heat waves is increased in urban areas where there has not been a heat wave for several years.[41,63,122,228] Socially isolated individuals or those with preexisting illness, as well as the frail and elderly, are at greatest risk of death during heat waves. Confinement to bed was the strongest predictor of death in the Chicago heat wave of 1995, and living alone doubled the risk of death. There were fewer deaths among people with working air conditioners or who had access to an air-conditioned environment.[229] In times of heat waves, preventive public health programs should encourage visiting nurses, housekeepers, and community service programs, such as Meals-on-Wheels, to increase the awareness of the danger of heat and identify those individuals most at risk.[227] A decreased risk of death was found among people with contacts from these agencies during the Chicago heat wave.[229]

High ambient temperature is associated with an increase in mortality from cocaine overdose.[166] The mean daily number of deaths from cocaine overdose was 33% higher when the ambient temperature exceeded 88°F (31°C). The media must alert the public and provide information on avoiding heat illness, as well as encourage individuals to help others to stay cool by assuring access to cooling measures.

The number of deaths from exposure-related illness has increased 3-fold in foreign transients attempting to enter the United States from Mexico. Because urban areas are more tightly patrolled, individuals attempting to cross into the United States illegally have turned to the harsh deserts and mountain ranges of the southwestern United States, increasing prolonged heat exposure and resulting in death.[69]

Thermoregulation and Heat Stress

The normal thermoregulatory response to heat stress is mediated primarily by heat-sensitive neurons in the hypothalamus. Increased body core temperature results in active dilatation of cutaneous vessels, and skin blood flow increases.[106,217] Increased skin blood flow is attained primarily by an increase in heart rate and stroke volume; therefore, the capacity to increase cardiac output is critical to cooling. Compensatory shifting of blood flow from the splanchnic and renal vessels to the skin further increases skin blood flow.[114,217] Sweat-gland function is activated by parasympathetic stimulation, and the combination of vasodilatation, increased skin blood flow, and increased sweating results in heat loss through convection and evaporation. Dehydration after profuse sweating increases plasma osmolarity. Heat-sensitive neurons in the preoptic anterior hypothalamus are inhibited by locally increased osmolarity and by input from distal hepatoportal osmoreceptors. The inhibition of heat-sensitive neurons results in decreased heat dissipation response.[40,195]

Types of Heatstroke

Heatstroke is commonly divided into two types: exertional and nonexertional. Nonexertional, or classic, heatstroke describes heatstroke occurring in the absence of extreme exertion. Nonexertional heatstroke is most commonly described during heat waves, and the victims are predominantly those persons least able to tolerate heat: infants,[11] the aged,[47] those with psychiatric disorders, and the chronically ill.

Exertional heatstroke occurs as a result of increased motor activity. It may occur in young, healthy individuals who are exercising, or in individuals whose increased motor activity results from other causes, such as seizures or agitation. Often a period of significant heat stress in exercising individuals precedes the development of heatstroke. Military recruits who develop heatstroke may sometimes present to the camp infirmary with vague complaints prior to collapse.[232] Published studies of heatstroke in miners, athletes, and military recruits describe several precipitating factors in heatstroke: fatigue associated with a recent deficit in sleep; poor physical conditioning; a recent febrile illness; recent heat-related symptoms such as thirst or weakness; relative volume depletion; failure to allow for acclimatization; and obesity. Symptoms of nausea, weakness, headache, diarrhea, or irritability often precede the development of heatstroke. Although rapid onset of symptoms and acute loss of consciousness are frequently reported in exer-

tional heatstroke, the preceding period of heat stress and insidious symptoms may go unrecognized. Although exertional heatstroke is more likely to occur during intense exertion in a hot, humid environment, it may also occur with moderately intense exercise early in the morning, when environmental conditions do not usually represent a thermoregulatory stress.[9]

Infants may suffer heatstroke under environmental conditions that would not be expected to place the child in danger. Well-meaning parents sometimes overinsulate children with clothing and blankets, inhibiting their cutaneous heat loss and placing them at risk.[11,118,119,188]

Differential Diagnosis of Hyperthermia

In addition to exposure and exertion, conditions that predispose to severe hyperthermia include primary hypothalamic lesions; intracranial hemorrhage; agitation; alcohol and sedative-hypnotic withdrawal; seizures; and the use of therapeutic and illicit drugs.[84,89–91,143,167,242] (Table 18–5). Included in the differential diagnosis of severe hyperthermia are the serotonin syndrome, malignant hyperthermia, and neuroleptic malignant syndrome, all of which may result in high temperature, altered mental status, and increased muscle tone.

Serotonin Syndrome. The serotonin syndrome results from excess stimulation of the serotonin receptor, primarily the $5-HT_{1A}$ subtype.[241] Drug interactions are most commonly the cause of the syndrome. Monoamine oxidase inhibitors used in conjunction with tricyclic antidepressants;[13] selective serotonin reuptake inhibitors;[71] L-tryptophan;[71,243] meperidine;[99] dextromethorphan;[213] amphetamines;[143,235] and sumatriptan have all been reported to lead to serotonergic hyperstimulation and severe symptoms.[86,241] The clinical condition resulting from excess serotonin includes alterations in consciousness, restlessness, increased muscle tone, tremor, gastrointestinal disturbance, and hyperthermia. Treatment of the syndrome focuses on control of hyperthermia by using aggressive cooling; muscle relaxation by using primarily benzodiazepines; or, in severe cases, endotracheal intubation and paralysis (Chap. 58).

Malignant Hyperthermia. Malignant hyperthermia is a very rare disorder that is associated with a congenital disturbance of calcium regulation in striated muscle. Malignant hyperthermia was first reported in 1960. Ten deaths occurred in a single family following general anesthesia.[59] Exposure to anesthetics, depolarizing muscle relaxants or, rarely, severe exertion precipitates uncontrolled calcium influx into the sarcoplasmic reticulum leading to severe muscle rigidity and hyperthermia.[92,120] The clinical setting of severe muscle rigidity and hyperthermia following general anesthesia usually is adequate to define the syndrome (Chap. 54).

Neuroleptic Malignant Syndrome. A severe extrapyramidal syndrome associated with muscle rigidity, autonomic dysfunction, and altered mental status was first described in 1968.[57] This disorder develops during the administration of antipsychotic drugs or the withdrawal of dopaminergic agents. Increased muscle tone because of dopaminergic blockade of the striatum, as well as central altered hypothalamic thermoregulation, leads to hyperthermia.[105] Temperature elevation and alteration of mental status occur after the onset of "lead pipe" muscle rigidity.[16,95] Laboratory findings are not specific and include marked elevation of CPK in some pa-

TABLE 18–5.   Differential Diagnosis of Hyperthermia

I. Increased heat production
- Increased muscle activity
  - Agitation
  - Catatonia
  - Ethanol withdrawal
  - Exercise
  - Infectious diseases
  - Malignant hyperthermia
  - Monoamine oxidase inhibitor drug interactions
  - Neuroleptic malignant syndrome
  - Parkinson disease
  - Sedative-hypnotic withdrawal
  - Seizures
  - Serotonin syndrome
  - Toxins
- Increased metabolic rate
  - Hyperthyroidism
  - Pheochromocytoma
  - Sympathomimetic agents

II. Impaired heat loss
- Environmental
  - Heat
  - Humidity
  - Lack of acclimatization
- Social disadvantage
  - Isolation
  - Poverty
  - Lack of air conditioning
  - Confinement to bed
- Medical illness
  - Cardiac insufficiency
  - Diabetes
  - Hypertension
  - Pulmonary
  - CNS dysfunction
- Dehydration
- Fatigue
- Limited behavioral response
  - Extremes of age
  - Psychiatric impairment
  - Mental retardation
  - Toxin-induced

tients and leukocytosis with a left shift. Neuroleptic malignant syndrome must be distinguished from the much more common cases of heatstroke in psychiatric patients that are caused by heat intolerance that is caused by the anticholinergic effects of antipsychotic drugs or antihistamines prescribed to control extrapyramidal symptoms[221,264] (Chap. 59).

Pathophysiologic Characteristics of Heatstroke

Hypotension and tachycardia in heatstroke are caused by a number of factors. The patient with heatstroke may have a reduced plasma volume secondary to dehydration. There is peripheral pooling of blood associated with an increase in cutaneous blood flow from 0.5 L/min to 7–8 L/min.[114,217] In addition, patients may manifest primary myocardial insufficiency.[138] Clinically, patients exhibit either a hypo- or hyperdynamic circulatory response. The observed circulatory response to heat stress is a function of the patient's cardiac reserve, volume status, and degree of myocardial

heat injury. The hyperdynamic condition is characterized by increased cardiac index and decreased systemic vascular resistance.[194] These hemodynamic characteristics occur in patients who are able to maintain a significantly increased cardiac output in response to the circulatory demand of heat stress.

Volume-depleted patients, or those patients with primary myocardial insufficiency, may exhibit a hypodynamic response. These patients have a decreased cardiac index and increased systemic vascular resistance.[194,240] Whether pulmonary vascular resistance is affected is unclear. High central venous pressures have been found in some patients, with evidence of right-heart failure and right-heart dilatation on autopsy.[163] This has led to the suggestion that pulmonary vascular resistance may be elevated.[194] In 22 of 34 patients (64%) with heatstroke, central venous pressures (CVPs) were greater than 3 cm H_2O. Twelve patients had a CVP ≤0, and 10 were >10 cm H_2O. These authors cautioned against injudicious infusion of large quantities of intravenous fluids and resulting complications of congestive heart failure and fluid overload. In the study, only 3 patients required more than 2 L of normal saline during cooling. Crystalloid infusion ranged from 500 to 2500 mL, and none of the patients developed associated fluid overload problems.[230]

A study of 13 cases of heatstroke in Mecca pilgrims monitored with pulmonary artery (Swan-Ganz) catheters demonstrated a good correlation of CVP with pulmonary capillary wedge pressures.[4] A study of elderly patients with heatstroke using pulmonary artery catheters showed that pulmonary vascular resistance was low or normal. Pulmonary capillary wedge pressures were not elevated.[239] Serial electrocardiograms in 51 religious pilgrims suffering from heatstroke showed normal sinus rhythm in 25%, sinus tachycardia in 52%, atrial fibrillation in 16%, and sinus bradycardia in 6%. ST segment depression and other ST-T wave changes were reported. The QT interval showed no abnormality. In some patients, echocardiography showed pericardial effusions and regional wall motion abnormalities, asymmetric septal hypertrophy, right ventricular dilatation, and left ventricular dilatation with impaired function.[3]

Autopsy studies of the heart demonstrate right-heart dilatation pericardial effusions, interstitial edema, degeneration and necrosis of myocardial fibers, and subendocardial hemorrhage.[130,163] Postmortem examination of the lungs revealed vascular congestion, pleural effusions, and parenchymal hemorrhages.[163,194]

Gastrointestinal hemorrhage, vomiting, and diarrhea occur frequently.[232] At autopsy, edema and hemorrhage of the bowel wall occur.[38] Liver injury occurs commonly and is not clinically manifest until the second or third day following the temperature increase.[129,232] Centrilobular changes, such as widening of central veins and adjacent sinusoids and pooling of blood, and varying degrees of hepatocellular degeneration, are demonstrated on liver biopsy. Repeat biopsies demonstrated that these changes resolve as the patient recovers.[129] In other cases, only congestion and fatty infiltration are reported.[38]

Neuropsychiatric impairment is, by definition, present in all cases of heatstroke. Length of coma correlates significantly with mortality.[10,232] Autopsy studies demonstrate a variety of structural and microscopic CNS injuries. Edema and venous congestion are evident. The number of cortical neurons is reduced, with concomitant glial proliferation. Striking cerebellar Purkinje cell deterioration occurs. The hypothalamus appears to be relatively spared, with limited edema of the neuronal nuclei. Hemorrhages occur throughout the brain.[38,163,232] Persistent cerebellar dysfunction occurs, as does lower motor neuron damage, manifested by areflexia and muscle wasting.[58,148] Higher cortical functions are spared in survivors.[172] Permanent neurologic sequelae are correlated with the degree and duration of hyperthermia.

Acute renal failure was the major cause of death in heatstroke victims before the advent of hemodialysis.[227,252] In addition to the direct effects of heat, volume depletion, and hypotension, myoglobinuria secondary to rhabdomyolysis results in further renal tubular injury. This is especially common in the agitated or exercising patient.[44,84,204] The mechanism by which myoglobin contributes to renal failure remains controversial. At autopsy the kidneys are enlarged, with numerous petechial hemorrhages.[163] Acute tubular necrosis is seen on biopsy.

Bleeding is associated with significant morbidity and mortality in many cases of heatstroke. Coagulation disturbances seen in patients with heatstroke appear to be multifactorial. Elevation of the prothrombin time may occur within 30 minutes of temperature elevation and is attributed to direct heat injury of clotting factors.[13] Liver damage may significantly contribute to the coagulation disturbances, although this is not manifested as acutely.[13,184,207] Evidence of diffuse capillary basement-membrane injury has been demonstrated by electron microscopy and is thought to precipitate consumptive coagulopathy in severe cases of heatstroke.[38,236] Thrombocytopenia is very common and occurs within 30 minutes of onset of heatstroke, frequently in the absence of other evidence of disseminated intravascular coagulation. Direct thermal injury leading to decreased platelet survival and megakaryocyte damage may play a role[163,184] (Table 18–6).

Clinical Findings in Heatstroke

Clinical evaluation of the hyperthermic patient begins with careful assessment of the vital signs. Vital sign abnormalities commonly include heart rates greater than 130 beats/min, hypotension, and an elevation of the respiratory rate, often above 30 breaths/min. Most importantly, temperature is elevated. After cooling, there is often a secondary rise in temperature that suggests persistent disturbances of thermoregulation.[163]

Neurologic examination reveals a confused, delirious, comatose, or seizing patient. Pupils may be normal, fixed and dilated, or pinpoint. Decerebrate or decorticate posturing may be evident. Muscle tone is increased, normal, or flaccid. The skin may be hot and dry or diaphoretic. Nasal and oropharyngeal bleeding may be present as a consequence of the acute coagulopathy. Examination of the lungs is often nonspecific, although heatstroke victims are at risk of pulmonary edema as a primary event associated with capillary endothelial damage or following overly aggressive fluid resuscitation. Cardiac auscultation may reveal a flow murmur secondary to high cardiac output or a right ventricular gallop. Neck vein distension indicates increased central venous pressure. Jaundice suggests hepatic injury and occurs on the second or third day following the onset of heatstroke.[39] Nasogastric aspiration or rectal examination may demonstrate gross bleeding. A petechial rash develops, probably secondary to capillary endothelial damage.

Laboratory Findings of Heatstroke

Lactic acid dehydrogenase (LDH) rises as a consequence of diffuse tissue injury. Early rises in aminotransferases (ALT, AST), which peak at 48 hours, are indicators of the liver damage that occurs during heatstroke.[129] Muscle enzymes were elevated in all pa-

TABLE 18–6. Physiologic and Clinical Manifestations of Heatstroke

Cardiovascular
Hypodynamic states in elderly
Hyperdynamic states in young healthy individuals
Electrocardiogram
  Nonspecific
  Widening of QRS due to underlying abnormality (eg, cocaine toxicity, hyperkalemia associated with rhabdomyolysis)

Central nervous system
Altered mental status
  Irritability, confusion, ataxia, seizures, coma
  Weakness, dizziness, headache
  Plantar extension, pupillary abnormalities, decorticate posturing
EEG
  Normal or diffuse slowing
CSF
  Normal or increased protein
  Lymphocytosis

Gastrointestinal
Vomiting, diarrhea, hematemesis

Hematologic
Bleeding diathesis
  Prolonged PT (INR) and PTT
  Disseminated intravascular coagulation
  Thrombocytopenia
  Petechiae
  Purpura
Leukocytosis

Hepatic
Hepatic insufficiency at 12–36 h
Elevated AST, ALT, LDH

Metabolic
Metabolic acidosis and respiratory alkalosis
Electrolyte disturbance
  Hypernatremia
  Hypokalemia
  Hypocalcemia
  Hypophosphatemia

Muscle
Rhabdomyolysis
Elevated CPK

Renal
Decreased renal perfusion
Myoglobinuria
Proteinuria
Oliguria
Acute tubular necrosis
Interstitial necrosis

tients in a study of exertional heatstroke[232] and in 86% of patients in one study of nonexertional heatstroke.[88] Nonspecific ST and T wave changes on ECG are common. Myocardial enzyme elevation occurs and correlates with ECG changes.[130] Results of lumbar puncture are nonspecific, are often normal, or may demonstrate elevated cerebrospinal fluid (CSF) protein and lymphocytosis.[232]

Other laboratory parameters are affected by heatstroke. Dehydration leads to hemoconcentration in patients exposed to elevated temperatures for a period of time. Hypokalemia is common, with potassium deficits as great as 500 mEq occurring during the early period of heat exposure.[137] Arterial blood-gas analysis may show a respiratory alkalosis secondary to direct stimulation of the respiratory center by heat or a metabolic acidosis secondary to lactic acid production.[50,240] Hypophosphatemia is common and is attributed to respiratory alkalosis, which causes intracellular shifts of phosphate. However, in 8 of 10 heatstroke patients with hypophosphatemia, none were alkalemic.[21] The hypophosphatemia in these cases was associated with increased phosphaturia and decreased tubular reabsorption of phosphorus, a finding which reversed after cooling.[136] Renal tubular damage may also lead to phosphate depletion.[93] Phosphate and potassium are elevated when significant muscle injury has occurred. Calcium is normal or low, the latter secondary to binding to damaged muscle tissue. Later, hypercalcemia occurs, possibly due to release of this bound calcium.[79,154]

Significant alterations occur in leukocyte subsets in heatstroke victims. One study reported an increased ratio of T-suppressor to T-cytotoxic cells, as well as increased natural killer cells. There was a significant decrease in the percentages of T, B, and T-helper cells. These changes correlated with the degree of hyperthermia.[19] Catecholamines are increased in heatstroke,[2] and may affect the distribution of the lymphocyte subsets.[19] It is possible that the increased susceptibility to infection described in heatstroke and the alterations in lymphocyte populations are related.[19]

Effects of Drugs in Heatstroke

Drugs predispose the individual to heatstroke by two primary mechanisms: increased production of heat as a result of drug action and interference with the body's ability to dissipate heat because of pharmacologic effects on thermoregulatory centers (see Table 18–5). Drug-drug interactions may cause life-threatening increases in temperature, such as the combination of monoamine oxidase inhibitors with meperidine or dextromethorphan resulting in the hyperserotonin syndrome. The uncoupling of oxidative phosphorylation by salicylate, pentachlorophenol, or dinitrophenol leads to the release of metabolic energy as heat, rather than trapping that energy in the form of high-energy phosphate bonds in ATP. Increased heat production occurs as a result of the stimulation of hepatic metabolism by sympathomimetic drugs and, of course, by the increased physical activity often associated with sympathomimetic drug use.

During heat stress, vasodilatation leads to increased cutaneous blood flow, resulting in an increased cardiac output. Parasympathetic stimulation results in increased sweating. Drugs that impair these physiologic mechanisms for heat dissipation predispose the individual to heatstroke. Drugs with anticholinergic effects, such as antihistamines, cyclic antidepressants, and antipsychotics interfere with sweating. Sympathomimetic drugs stimulate α-adrenergic receptors, impairing vasodilatation. Antihypertensives and antianginal drugs (most notably calcium channel blockers and β-adrenergic antagonists) with negative inotropic and chronotropic effects impair the heart's ability to meet the output requirements of increased skin blood flow. Diuretic induced volume depletion also limits cardiac output. Antipsychotics cause hypothalamic depression, altering the normal CNS response to heat stress. Finally, drugs such as ethanol, opioids, and sedative-hyp-

notics impair normal behavioral responses, and heat-related discomfort may go unnoticed.

Heatstroke and Subsequent Heat Intolerance

Whether heatstroke victims are subsequently unable to adapt to exercise in a hot environment remains unclear. Is the heatstroke victim genetically predisposed to heat intolerance, or does heatstroke occur as a result of environmental and host factors? Several studies have suggested that heatstroke leads to persistent heat intolerance. These studies have often used a single heat intolerance test.[68,231,233,234] A study of 10 previous heatstroke victims showed no difference in acclimatization responses, thermoregulation, whole-body sodium and potassium balance, sweat-gland function, and blood values when compared with controls.[9] The rate of recovery from exertional heatstroke probably differs among individuals. In this study, 1 of 10 patients was found to have recurrent heat intolerance 12 months after the study.[9] Resolution of heat intolerance was delayed for 5 months in an individual who had experienced heatstroke twice.[128]

Treatment of Heatstroke

Management must focus on the early recognition of hyperthermia. Body temperatures >106°F (41.1°C) place the patient at great risk for end-organ injury. Rapid cooling is the first priority. Successful treatment requires adequate preparation. Equipment needed for rapid cooling should be readily available in the ED and includes fans, ice and tubs for submersion. En route to the hospital, the patient's clothes should be removed and the patient should be covered with ice- and water-soaked sheets. Respiration and cardiovascular status should be stabilized and monitored. Oxygen should be administered. The cause of the heatstroke should be determined and appropriate measures initiated immediately. Pharmacologic agents, such as antihistamines, butyrophenones, and phenothiazines, and physical restraints that interfere with heat dissipation, such as camisoles and strait jackets, should not be used.[91] Light hand and foot restraints should be used to protect the patient from harming himself or herself. If light restraints are used, the patient should be monitored continuously. The patient who is hyperthermic in the setting of ethanol or sedative-hypnotic withdrawal should be treated with a benzodiazepine.[90] The patient should never be confined to a small, unventilated seclusion room. Adequate cooling, hydration, sedation, and electrolytes and substrate repletion should be ensured.[88]

In the Emergency Department, appropriate laboratory studies should be performed and an IV line placed. Administration of 0.5–1.0 g/kg glucose as $D_{50}W$ and 100 mg of thiamine should be considered. A rectal probe should be placed for continuous temperature monitoring. The patient should be immersed in an ice bath with a fan blowing over the patient if possible. In addition to the ice bath, iced gastric lavage may be effective.

Agitation, seizures, and cardiac dysrhythmias must be managed while cooling is accomplished. Benzodiazepines are the treatment of choice for agitation and seizures. Heatstroke patients may have significant volume needs, depending on the amount of fluid lost prior to the onset of heatstroke. Hypotension should be treated with fluids and cooling. Volume repletion should be monitored carefully by parameters such as blood pressure, pulse, central venous pressure, pulmonary wedge pressure, and urine output. As the temperature returns to normal, the hypotension may resolve if significant volume deficits are not present.[43,137,138] In patients with myoglobinuria, an attempt should be made to increase renal blood flow and urine output. The use of sodium bicarbonate and mannitol in the prevention of acute tubular necrosis in these cases is controversial.[67,79,216]

Phenothiazines should not be used in the treatment of heatstroke. Phenothiazines depress an already altered mental status, may produce hepatotoxicity in a compromised liver, lower the seizure threshold,[18] cause acute dystonic reactions, exacerbate hypotension, and interfere with thermoregulation and cooling by affecting the hypothalamus. However, although phenothiazines may theoretically reduce shivering and the possibility of rebound hyperthermia, their onset of action is slow.[193] When shivering occurs during cooling, we recommend the judicious use of a benzodiazepine. In addition, benzodiazepines treat ethanol and sedative-hypnotic withdrawal and cocaine intoxication, common causes of hyperthermia.

There is no role for antipyretic agents in the management of heatstroke. Aspirin and acetaminophen lower temperature by reducing the hypothalamic set point, which is only altered in a patient febrile from inflammation or endogenous pyrogens.[59] Heatstroke, however, occurs when cooling mechanisms are overwhelmed, and the hypothalamic thermoregulatory set point is not disturbed.[14,106]

Dantrolene sodium is the preferred drug in the treatment of malignant hyperthermia.[86,120,254] It acts directly on skeletal muscle and either inhibits the release of calcium or increases calcium uptake through the sarcoplasmic reticulum.[24] Its utility has not been demonstrated in other conditions associated with hyperthermia, and there is no evidence to support its administration for other conditions.[6] In a prospective, randomized double-blind, placebo-controlled study of 52 patients with heatstroke, IV dantrolene sodium at 2 mg/kg of body weight did not alter cooling time.[20] There was no significant difference in the mean number of hospital days necessitated by heatstroke victims who received dantrolene and cooling versus those who received cooling alone. It has been proposed that dantrolene may influence central dopaminergic metabolism in patients with neuroleptic malignant syndrome by affecting calcium-triggered neurotransmitter release in the central nervous system; however, further study is required.[191] Anecdotal reports of the efficacy of dopamine agonist agents such as bromocriptine and amantadine have appeared in descriptions of neuroleptic malignant syndrome.[170] No drug therapy should delay the institution of aggressive external cooling (Table 18–7).

Prevention of Heatstroke

In the young, active population, prophylaxis should be accomplished by gradual acclimatization. Active persons should select the coolest and least humid time of day to be outdoors. Exposure should be increased slowly, and work paced. Breaks should be frequent initially and later may be decreased in number and length. Overweight and underconditioned persons require even longer periods of acclimatization. Airy and cool clothing should be chosen. The practice of exercising in unventilated plastic clothing to increase weight loss leads to the loss of fluid, not fat, and defeats the body's cooling mechanisms, resulting in hyperthermia.

Athletes performing during hot, humid weather should increase drinking beyond their thirst.[180,225] All individuals who fatigue easily or manifest nausea, vomiting, cramps, weakness, dizziness, or collapse should limit their activity and must be watched carefully.

TABLE 18–7. Management of Heatstroke

Preparation
Ice and cooling fans available in Emergency Department
Monitor weather reports
Alert media

Upon Arrival
Rapid cooling
  Clear airway and administer oxygen
  Cover with ice- and water-soaked sheets
  Stabilize respiratory and cardiovascular status
  Cool as rapidly as possible

Intravenous access
  0.9% NaCl or Ringer lactate based on CVP or pulmonary artery catheter
  Administration of 0.5–1.0 g/kg dextrose, and 100 mg thiamine
  Benzodiazepines for agitation, shivering, seizures

Continous monitoring
  Remove from ice bath at 38.3°C (101°F)
  Watch for rebound hyperthermia

Cautions
  Antipsychotics may have serious adverse effects
  Antipyretic agents do not work
  Cooling blankets alone are inadequate

Anyone who takes illicit drugs, who takes medications, or who has a medical condition that may interfere with thermoregulation should be monitored closely for signs of heat intolerance or hyperthermia. Stopping or at least decreasing the dose of high-risk medications during heatstroke season should be strongly considered.

SUMMARY

The thermoregulatory processes responsible for the maintenance of normothermia are complex. Pharmacologic agents may disturb normal thermoregulation and result in the abnormal conditions of hyperthermia or hypothermia. These disturbances of homeostasis present significant clinical management challenges. In particular, recommendations for the treatment of hypothermia perpetuate themselves in the literature with little supportive scientific evidence. Although greater understanding is gained through research and thoughtful analysis, emphasis must be placed on prevention. Hypothermia and heatstroke are largely preventable conditions. During heat waves, many socioeconomically disadvantaged and elderly individuals are affected, and it is essential that cities be prepared and that the public be aware of the dangers of heat waves, to themselves and to others. Similarly, hypothermia is preventable by prudent preparation for harsh environmental conditions, and by policies that provide for shelter for those at greatest risk—the poor, the homeless and those with underlying medical and psychiatric illnesses.

REFERENCES

1. AHA: American Heart Association Advanced Cardiac Life Support Guidelines: Special challenges. Circulation 2000;102:229–232.
2. al-Hadramy MS, Ali F: Catecholamines in heat stroke. Mil Med 1989;154:263–264.

3. al-Harthi SS, Nouh MS, al-Arfaj H, et al: Non-invasive evaluation of cardiac abnormalities in heat stroke pilgrims. Int J Cardiol 1992; 37:151–154.

4. al-Harthi SS, Sharaf E-D, Aktar JN: Hemodynamic changes and intravascular hydration state in heat stroke. Ann Saudi Med 1989; 9:378–383.

5. Althaus U, Aeberhard P, Schupbach P, et al: Management of profound accidental hypothermia with cardiorespiratory arrest. Ann Surg 1982;195:492–495.

6. Amsterdam JT, Syverud SA, Barker WJ, et al: Dantrolene sodium for treatment of heatstroke victims: lack of efficacy in a canine model. Am J Emerg Med 1986;4:399–405.

7. Anderson RJ, Reed G, Knochel J: Heatstroke. Adv Intern Med 1983; 28:115–140.

8. Angelakos ET, Daniels JB: Effect of catecholamine infusions on lethal hypothermic temperatures in dogs. J Appl Physiol 1969;26: 194–196.

9. Armstrong LE, De Luca JP, Hubbard RW: Time course of recovery and heat acclimation ability of prior exertional heatstroke patients. Med Sci Sports Exerc 1990;22:36–48.

10. Austin MG, Berry JW: Observations on 100 cases of heatstroke. JAMA 1956;161:1525–1529.

11. Bacon C, Scott D, Jones P: Heatstroke in well-wrapped infants. Lancet 1979;1:422–425.

12. Baumgartner FJ, Janusz MT, Jamieson WR, et al: Cardiopulmonary bypass for resuscitation of patients with accidental hypothermia and cardiac arrest. Can J Surg 1992;35:184–187.

13. Beard ME, Hickton CM: Haemostasis in heat stroke. Br J Haematol 1982;52:269–274.

14. Bernheim HA, Block LH, Atkins E: Fever: pathogenesis, pathophysiology, and purpose. Ann Intern Med 1979;91:261–270.

15. Beyda EJ, Bellet S, Jung M: Effect of hypothermia on tolerance of dogs to digitalis. Circ Res 1961;9:129.

16. Birkhimer LJ, DeVane CL: The neuroleptic malignant syndrome: presentation and treatment. Drug Intell Clin Pharm 1984;18: 462–465.

17. Birzis L, Hemingway A: Descending brainstem connections controlling shivering in cat. J Neurophysiol 1956;19:37–43.

18. Blum K, Eubanks JD, Wallace JE, Hamilton H: Enhancement of alcohol withdrawal convulsions in mice by haloperidol. Clin Toxicol 1976;9:427–434.

19. Bouchama A, al Hussein K, Adra C, et al: Distribution of peripheral blood leukocytes in acute heatstroke. J Appl Physiol 1992;73: 405–409.

20. Bouchama A, Cafege A, Devol EB, et al: Ineffectiveness of dantrolene sodium in the treatment of heatstroke. Crit Care Med 1991;19: 176–180.

21. Bouchama A, Cafege A, Robertson W, et al: Mechanisms of hypophosphatemia in humans with heatstroke. J Appl Physiol 1991;71: 328–332.

22. Boulant A: Hypothalamic neurons. Mechanisms of sensitivity to temperature. Ann N Y Acad Sci 1998;856:108–115.

23. Boylan JW, Hong SK: Regulation of renal function in hypothermia. Am J Physiol 1966;211:1371–1378.

24. Britt BA: Dantrolene. Can Anaesth Soc J 1984;31:61–75.

25. Broccardo M, Improta G: Sauvagine-induced hypothermia: Evidence for an interaction with the dopaminergic system. Eur J Pharmacol 1994;258:179–184.

26. Bruck K: Non-shivering thermogenesis and brown adipose tissue in relation to age, and their integration in the thermoregulatory system. In: Lindberg O, ed: Brown Adipose Tissue. New York, Elsevier, 1970, pp. 117–154.

27. Buchwald I, Davis PJ: Scleroderma with fatal heat stroke. JAMA 1967;201:270–271.

28. Buckberg GD, Brazier JR, Nelson RL, et al: Studies of the effects of hypothermia on regional myocardial blood flow and metabolism during cardiopulmonary bypass. I. The adequately perfused beating, fibrillating, and arrested heart. J Thorac Cardiovasc Surg 1977;73: 87–94.

29. Buckley JJ, Bosch OK, Bacaner MB: Prevention of ventricular fibrillation during hypothermia with bretylium tosylate. Anesth Analg 1971;50:587–593.

30. Busto R, Globus MY, Dietrich WD, et al: Effect of mild hypothermia on ischemia-induced release of neurotransmitters and free fatty acids in rat brain. Stroke 1989;20:904–910.

31. Cannon B, Houstek J, Nedergaard J: Brown adipose tissue. More than an effector of thermogenesis? Ann N Y Acad Sci 1998;856: 171–187.

32. Carlton J, Khan SI, Haq W, et al: Attenuation of alcohol-induced hypothermia by cyclo (His-Pro) and its analogs. Neuropeptides 1995; 28:351–355.

33. Carr ME Jr, Wolfert AI: Rewarming by hemodialysis for hypothermia: Failure of heparin to prevent DIC. J Emerg Med 1988;6: 277–280.

34. Centers for Disease Control: Hypothermia-related deaths-Alaska, October 1998–April 1999, and trends in the United States, 1979–1996. MMWR Morb Mortal Wkly Rep 2000;49:11–14.

35. Centers for Disease Control: Hypothermia-related deaths, Georgia— January 1996–December 1997, and United States, 1979–1995. MMWR Morb Mortal Wkly Rep 1998;47:1037.

36. Centers for Disease Control: Hypothermia-related deaths—New Mexico, October 1993–March 1994. MMWR Morb Mortal Wkly Rep 1995;44:933–935.

37. Centers for Disease Control: Hypothermia-related deaths—Vermont, October 1994–February 1996. MMWR Morb Mortal Wkly Rep 1996;45:1093–1095.

38. Chao TC, Sinniah R, Pakiam JE: Acute heat stroke deaths. Pathology 1981;13:145–156.

39. Chobanian SJ: Jaundice occurring after resolution of heat stroke. Ann Emerg Med 1983;12:102–103.

40. Clark WG, Lipton JM: Brain and pituitary peptides in thermoregulation. Pharmacol Ther 1983;22:249–297.

41. Clarke JF: Some effects of the urban structure on heat mortality. Environ Res 1972;5:93–104.

42. Clifton GL, Miller ER, Choi SC, et al: Lack of effect of induction of hypothermia after acute brain injury. N Engl J Med 2001;344: 556–563.

43. Clowes GH Jr, O'Donnell TF Jr: Heat stroke. N Engl J Med 1974; 291:564–567.

44. Cogen FC, Rigg G, Simmons JL, Domino EF: Phencyclidine-associated acute rhabdomyolysis. Ann Intern Med 1978;88:210–212.

45. Cohen DJ, Cline JR, Lepinski SM, et al: Resuscitation of the hypothermic patient. Am J Emerg Med 1988;6:475–478.

46. Collins KJ. The autonomic nervous system and the regulation of body temperature. In: Bannister R, ed: Autonomic Failure: A Textbook of Clinical Disorders of the Autonomic Nervous System, 3rd ed. New York: Oxford University Press, 1992, pp. 212–230.

47. Collins KJ, Exton-Smith AN: 1983 Henderson Award Lecture. Thermal homeostasis in old age. J Am Geriatr Soc 1983;31:519–524.

48. Collis ML, Steinman AM, Chaney RD: Accidental hypothermia: An experimental study of practical rewarming methods. Aviat Space Environ Med 1977;48:625–632.

49. Cooper KE, Ferguson AV: Thermoregulation and hypothermia in the elderly. In: Pozos RS, Wittmers LE, eds: The Nature and Treatment of Hypothermia. Minneapolis, University of Minnesota Press, 1983, pp. 165–181.

50. Costrini AM, Pitt HA, Gustafson AB, Uddin DE: Cardiovascular and metabolic manifestations of heat stroke and severe heat exhaustion. Am J Med 1979;66:296–302.

51. Danzl DF, Pozos RS, Auerbach PS, et al: Multicenter hypothermia survey. Ann Emerg Med 1987;16:1042–1055.

52. Danzl DF, Sowers MB, Vicario SJ, et al: Chemical ventricular defibrillation in severe accidental hypothermia. Ann Emerg Med 1982; 11:698–699.

53. DaVee TS, Reineberg EJ: Extreme hypothermia and ventricular fibrillation. Ann Emerg Med 1980;9:100–102.

54. de Garavilla L, Durkot MJ, Ihley TM, et al: Adverse effects of dietary and furosemide-induced sodium depletion on thermoregulation. Aviat Space Environ Med 1990;61:1012–1017.

55. Delaney KA: Hypothermic sudden death. In: Paradis NA, Halaperin HR, Nowak RM, eds: Cardiac Arrest. The Science and Practice of Resuscitation. Baltimore, Williams and Wilkins, 1996, pp. 745–760.

56. Delaney KA, Howland MA, Vassallo S, Goldfrank LR: Assessment of acid-base disturbances in hypothermia and their physiologic consequences. Ann Emerg Med 1989;18:72–82.

57. Delay J, Deniker P. Drug-induced extrapyramidal syndromes. In: Vinkin PJ, Bruyn GW, eds: Handbook of Clinical Neurology: Diseases of the Basal Ganglia. Amsterdam, North Holland, 1969, pp. 248–266.

58. Delgado G, Tunon T, Gallego J, Villanueva JA: Spinal cord lesions in heat stroke. J Neurol Neurosurg Psychiatry 1985;48:1065–1067.

59. Dinarello CA, Wolff SM: Pathogenesis of fever in man. N Engl J Med 1978;298:607–612.

60. Durakovic Z, Misigoj-Durakovic M, Corovic N: The corrected Q-T interval in the elderly with urban hypothermia. Coll Antropol 1999; 23:683–689.

61. Eichler AC, McFee AS, Root HD: Heat stroke. Am J Surg 1969; 118:855–863.

62. el-Gamal N, Frank SM: Perioperative thermoregulatory dysfunction in a patient with a previous traumatic hypothalamic injury. Anesth Analg 1995;80:1245–1247.

63. Ellis FP: Mortality from heat illness and heat-aggravated illness in the United States. Environ Res 1972;5:1–58.

64. el-Sherif N, Shahwan L, Sorour AH: The effect of acute thermal stress on general and pulmonary hemodynamics in the cardiac patient. Am Heart J 1970;79:305–317.

65. Emslie-Smith D: Accidental hypothermia: A common condition with a pathognomonic electrocardiogram. Lancet 1958;2:492–495.

66. Emslie-Smith D, Sladden GE, Stirling GR: The significance of changes in the electrocardiogram in hypothermia. Br Heart J 1959; 21:343–351.

67. Eneas JF, Schoenfeld PY, Humphreys MH: The effect of infusion of mannitol-sodium bicarbonate on the clinical course of myoglobinuria. Arch Intern Med 1979;139:801–805.

68. Epstein Y, Shapiro Y, Brill S: Role of surface area-to-mass ratio and work efficiency in heat intolerance. J Appl Physiol 1983;54: 831–836.

69. Eschbach K, Hagan J, Rodriguez N. Causes and Trends in Migrant Deaths Along the U.S.-Mexico Border, 1985–1998. Houston, TX, University of Houston Center for Immigration Research, 2001.

70. Esteban J, Chover AJ, Sanchez PA, et al: Central administration of neuropeptide Y induces hypothermia in mice. Possible interaction with central noradrenergic systems. Life Sci 1989;45:2395–2400.

71. Feighner JP, Boyer WF, Tyler DL, Neborsky RJ: Adverse consequences of fluoxetine-MAOI combination therapy. J Clin Psychiatry 1990;51:222–225.

72. Fell RH, Gunning AJ, Bardhan KD, Triger DR: Severe hypothermia as a result of barbiturate overdose complicated by cardiac arrest. Lancet 1968;1:392–394.

73. Feller DJ, Young ER, Riggan JP, et al: Serotonin and genetic differences in sensitivity and tolerance to ethanol hypothermia. Psychopharmacology (Berl) 1993;112:331–338.

74. Finn DA, Boone DC, Alkana RL: Temperature dependence of ethanol depression in rats. Psychopharmacology (Berl) 1986;90: 185–189.

75. Fischbeck KH, Simon RP: Neurological manifestations of accidental hypothermia. Ann Neurol 1981;10:384–387.

76. Fleming PR, Muir FH: Electrocardiographic changes in induced hypothermia in man. Br Heart J 1957;19:59–66.

77. Fox GR, Hayward JS: Effect of hypothermia on breath-alcohol analysis. J Forensic Sci 1987;32:320–325.

78. Fruehan AE: Accidental hypothermia: Report of 8 cases of subnormal body temperature due to exposure. Arch Intern Med 1960;106: 218–229.

79. Gabow PA, Kaehny WD, Kelleher SP: The spectrum of rhabdomyolysis. Medicine (Baltimore) 1982;61:141–152.

80. Garvie AA, Howland MA, Brubacher JR, Hoffman RS: Endogenous digoxin-like substances in hypothermia patients. Acad Emerg Med 1999;6:376.

81. Gentilello LM, Cobean RA, Offner PJ, et al: Continuous arteriovenous rewarming: Rapid reversal of hypothermia in critically ill patients. J Trauma 1992;32:316; discussion 325–317.

82. Gillen JP, Vogel MF, Holterman RK, Skiendzielewski JJ: Ventricular fibrillation during orotracheal intubation of hypothermic dogs. Ann Emerg Med 1986;15:412–416.

83. Gilliam DM, Collins AC: Concentration-dependent effects of ethanol in long-sleep and short-sleep mice. Alcohol Clin Exp Res 1983;7:337–342.

84. Ginsberg MD, Hertzman M, Schmidt-Nowara WW: Amphetamine intoxication with coagulopathy, hyperthermia, and reversible renal failure. A syndrome resembling heatstroke. Ann Intern Med 1970; 73:81–85.

85. Goldberg LI: Cardiovascular and renal actions of dopamine: potential clinical applications. Pharmacol Rev 1972;24:1–29.

86. Goldberg LI: Monoamine oxidase inhibitors: Adverse reactions and possible mechanisms. JAMA 1964;190:456.

87. Golden FSC, Hervey GR: The "after-drop" and death after rescue from immersion in cold water. In: Adam JM, ed: Hypothermia Ashore and Afloat. Aberdeen, TX, Aberdeen University Press, 1981, pp. 37–56.

88. Graham BS, Lichtenstein MJ, Hinson JM, Theil GB: Nonexertional heatstroke. Physiologic management and cooling in 14 patients. Arch Intern Med 1986;146:87–90.

89. Granoff AL, Davis JM: Heat illness syndrome and lithium intoxication. J Clin Psychiatry 1978;39:103–107.

90. Greenblatt DJ, Gross PL, Harris J, et al: Fatal hyperthermia following haloperidol therapy of sedative-hypnotic withdrawal. J Clin Psychiatry 1978;39:673–675.

91. Greenland P, Southwick WH: Hyperthermia associated with chlorpromazine and full-sheet restraint. Am J Psychiatry 1978;135: 1234–1235.

92. Gronert GA: Controversies in malignant hyperthermia. Anesthesiology 1983;59:273–274.

93. Guntupalli KK, Sladen A, Selker RG, et al: Effects of induced total-body hyperthermia on phosphorus metabolism in humans. Am J Med 1984;77:250–254.

94. Gupta BN, Nier K, Hensel H: Cold-sensitive afferents from the abdomen. Pflugers Arch 1979;380:203–204.

95. Guze BH, Baxter LR Jr: Current concepts. Neuroleptic malignant syndrome. N Engl J Med 1985;313:163–166.

96. Ham J, Miller RD, Benet LZ, et al: Pharmacokinetics and pharmacodynamics of d-tubocurarine during hypothermia in the cat. Anesthesiology 1978;49:324–329.

97. Hamlet MP: Fluid shifts in hypothermia. In: Pozos RS, Wittmers LE, eds: The Nature and Treatment of Hypothermia. Minneapolis, University of Minnesota Press, 1983, pp. 94–99.

98. Hammel HT: Regulation of internal body temperature. Annu Rev Physiol 1968;30:641–710.

99. Hansen TE, Dieter K, Keepers GA: Interaction of fluoxetine and pentazocine. Am J Psychiatry 1990;147:949–950.

100. Harari A, Regnier B, Rapin M, et al: Haemodynamic study of prolonged deep accidental hypothermia. Eur J Intensive Care Med 1975; 1:65–70.

101. Harnett RM, Pruitt JR, Sias FR: A review of the literature concerning resuscitation from hypothermia: Part I—The problem and general approaches. Aviat Space Environ Med 1983;54:425–434.

102. Hartung J, Cottrell JE: Statistics and hypothermia. J Neurosurg Anesthesiol 1998;10:1–4.

103. Hauty MG, Esrig BC, Hill JG, Long WB: Prognostic factors in severe accidental hypothermia: Experience from the Mt. Hood tragedy. J Trauma 1987;27:1107–1112.

104. Hayward JS, Steinman AM: Accidental hypothermia: An experimental study of inhalation rewarming. Aviat Space Environ Med 1975; 46:1236–1240.

105. Heiman-Patterson TD: Neuroleptic malignant syndrome and malignant hyperthermia. Important issues for the medical consultant. Med Clin North Am 1993;77:477–492.

106. Hensel H: Neural processes in thermoregulation. Physiol Rev 1973; 53:948–1017.

107. Hensel H: Cutaneous thermoreceptors. In: Hensel H, ed: Handbook of Sensory Physiology. Berlin, Springer-Verlag, 1972:79–110.

108. Hensel H, Andres KH, von During M: Structure and function of cold receptors. Pflugers Arch 1974;352:1–10.

109. Hernandez E, Praga M, Alcazar JM, et al: Hemodialysis for treatment of accidental hypothermia. Nephron 1993;63:214–216.

110. Hexdall A, Greenblatt B, Garvie AA, Hoffman RS: Endogenous digoxin-like binding substance in cold cardioplegia. Acad Emerg Med 2000;7:467.

111. Hislop LJ, Wyatt JP, McNaughton GW, et al: Urban hypothermia in the west of Scotland. West of Scotland Accident and Emergency Trainees Research Group. BMJ 1995;311:725.

112. Hochachka PW: Defense strategies against hypoxia and hypothermia. Science 1986;231:234–241.

113. Hori T, Harada Y: Responses of Midbrain raphe neurons to local temperature. Pflugers Arch 1976;364:205–207.

114. Hubbard RW: The role of exercise in the etiology of exertional heatstroke. Med Sci Sports Exerc 1990;22:2–5.

115. Hudson LD, Conn RD: Accidental hypothermia. Associated diagnoses and prognosis in a common problem. JAMA 1974;227:37–40.

116. Inoue S, Murakami N: Unit responses in the medulla oblongata of rabbit to changes in local and cutaneous temperature. J Physiol 1976; 259:339–356.

117. Jacobs JJ, Prasad C, Wilber JF: Cyclo (His-Pro): Mapping hypothalamic sites for its hypothermic action. Brain Res 1982;250:205–209.

118. Jardine DS: A mathematical model of life-threatening hyperthermia during infancy. J Appl Physiol 1992;73:329–339.

119. Jardine DS, Haschke RH: An animal model of life-threatening hyperthermia during infancy. J Appl Physiol 1992;73:340–345.

120. Jardon OM: Physiologic stress, heat stroke, malignant hyperthermia—A perspective. Mil Med 1982;147:8–14.

121. Jessen K, Hagelsten JO: Peritoneal dialysis in the treatment of profound accidental hypothermia. Aviat Space Environ Med 1978;49: 426–429.

122. Jones TS, Liang AP, Kilbourne EM, et al: Morbidity and mortality associated with the July 1980 heat wave in St Louis and Kansas City, Mo. JAMA 1982;247:3327–3331.

123. Kadar D, Tang BK, Conn AW: The fate of phenobarbitone in children in hypothermia and at normal body temperature. Can Anaesth Soc J 1982;29:16–23.

124. Kalant H, Le AD: Effects of ethanol on thermoregulation. Pharmacol Ther 1983;23:313–364.

125. Kalser SC, Kelvington EJ, Randolph MM, Santomen DM: Drug metabolism in hypothermia II. C14-atropine uptake metabolism and excretion by isolated perfused rat liver. J Pharmacol Exp Ther 1965; 147:260.

126. Kalser SC, Kelvington EJ, Kunig R, Randolph MM: Drug metabolism in hypothermia. Uptake, metabolism and excretion of C14-procaine by the isolated, perfused rat liver. J Pharmacol Exp Ther 1968; 164:396–404.

127. Kalser SC, Kelvington EJ, Randolph MM: Drug metabolism in hypothermia. Uptake, metabolism and excretion of S35-sulfanilamide by the isolated, perfused rat liver. J Pharmacol Exp Ther 1968;159: 389–398.

128. Keren G, Epstein Y, Magazanik A: Temporary heat intolerance in a heatstroke patient. Aviat Space Environ Med 1981;52:116–117.

129. Kew M, Bersohn I, Seftel H, Kent G: Liver damage in heatstroke. Am J Med 1970;49:192–202.

130. Kew MC, Tucker RB, Bersohn I, Seftel HC: The heart in heatstroke. Am Heart J 1969;77:324–335.

131. Kilbourne EM: Illness due to thermal extremes. In: Last JM, ed: Maxcy-Rosenau Public Health and Preventive Medicine. Norwalk, CT, Appleton-Century-Crofts, 1986, pp. 711–714.

132. Kilbourne EM, Choi K, Jones TS, Thacker SB: Risk factors for heatstroke. A case-control study. JAMA 1982;247:3332–3336.

133. Kiley JP, Eldridge FL, Millhorn DE: The effect of hypothermia on central neural control of respiration. Respir Physiol 1984;58: 295–312.

134. Killian H. Cold and frost injuries. In: Frey R, Safer P, eds: Disaster Medicine. New York, Springer-Verlag, 1981, p. 9.

135. Knochel JP: Environmental heat illness. An eclectic review. Arch Intern Med 1974;133:841–864.

136. Knochel JP, Caskey JH: The mechanism of hypophosphatemia in acute heat stroke. JAMA 1977;238:425–426.

137. Knochel JP, Dotin LN, Hamburger RJ: Pathophysiology of intense physical conditioning in a hot climate. I. Mechanisms of potassium depletion. J Clin Invest 1972;51:242–255.

138. Knochel JP, Gerard ES, Beisel WR, et al: Renal, cardiovascular, hematologic and serum electrolyte abnormalities of heat stroke. Am Med J 1961;30:299.

139. Koeppen AH, Daniels JC, Barron KD: Subnormal body temperatures in Wernicke's encephalopathy. Arch Neurol 1969;21:493–498.

140. Koren G, Barker C, Bohn D, et al: Influence of hypothermia on the pharmacokinetics of gentamicin and theophylline in piglets. Crit Care Med 1985;13:844–847.

141. Koren G, Barker C, Bohn D, et al: Effect of hypothermia on the pharmacokinetics of ethanol in piglets. Ann Emerg Med 1989;18: 118–121.

142. Koren G, Barker C, Goresky G, et al: The influence of hypothermia on the disposition of fentanyl—human and animal studies. Eur J Clin Pharmacol 1987;32:373–376.

143. Krisko I, Lewis E, Johnson JE 3rd: Severe hyperpyrexia due to tranylcypromine-amphetamine toxicity. Ann Intern Med 1969;70: 559–564.

144. Kuehn LA: Introduction. In: Pozos RS, Wittmers LE, eds: The Nature and Treatment of Hypothermia. Minneapolis, University of Minnesota Press, 1983, xi–xxiii.

145. Lapp NL, Juergens JL: Frostbite. Mayo Clin Proc 1965;40:932.

146. Laufman H: Profound accidental hypothermia. JAMA 1951;147: 1201–1212.

147. Ledingham IM, Mone JG: Treatment of accidental hypothermia: a prospective clinical study. BMJ 1980;280:1102–1105.

148. Lefkowitz D, Ford CS, Rich C, et al: Cerebellar syndrome following neuroleptic induced heat stroke. J Neurol Neurosurg Psychiatry 1983;46:183–185.

149. Letsou GV, Kopf GS, Elefteriades JA, et al: Is cardiopulmonary bypass effective for treatment of hypothermic arrest due to drowning or exposure? Arch Surg 1992;127:525–528.

150. Levinson DF, Simpson GM: Neuroleptic-induced extrapyramidal symptoms with fever. Heterogeneity of the "neuroleptic malignant syndrome." Arch Gen Psychiatry 1986;43:839–848.

151. Lewin S, Brettman LR, Holzman RS: Infections in hypothermic patients. Arch Intern Med 1981;141:920–925.

152. Lilja P: Emergency treatment of hypothermia. In: Pozos RS, Wittmers LE, eds: The Nature and Treatment of Hypothermia. Minneapolis, University of Minnesota Press, 1983, pp. 143–151.

153. Lipton JM, Rosenstein J, Sklar FH: Thermoregulatory disorders after removal of a craniopharyngioma from the third cerebral ventricle. Brain Res Bull 1981;7:369–373.

154. Llach F, Felsenfeld AJ, Haussler MR: The pathophysiology of altered calcium metabolism in rhabdomyolysis-induced acute renal failure. Interactions of parathyroid hormone, 25-hydroxycholecalciferol, and 1,25-dihydroxycholecalciferol. N Engl J Med 1981;305:117–123.

155. Lloyd EL: The cause of death after rescue. Int J Sports Med 1992; 13:S196–199.

156. Lloyd EL, Mitchell B: Factors affecting the onset of ventricular fibrillation in hypothermia. Lancet 1974;2:1294–1296.

157. Lomax P. Neuropharmacological aspects of thermoregulation. In: Pozos RS, Wittmers LE, eds: The Nature and Treatment of Hypothermia. Minneapolis, University of Minnesota Press, 1983, pp. 81–94.

158. MacKenzie MA, Hermus AR, Wollersheim HC, et al: Poikilothermia in man: Pathophysiology and clinical implications. Medicine (Baltimore) 1991;70:257–268.

159. Maclean D, Emslie-Smith D: Accidental Hypothermia. London, Blackwell, 1977.

160. Maickel RP: Interaction of drugs with autonomic nervous function and thermoregulation. Fed Proc 1970;29:1973–1979.

161. Mair P, Kornberger E, Furtwaengler W, et al: Prognostic markers in patients with severe accidental hypothermia and cardiocirculatory arrest. Resuscitation 1994;27:47–54.

162. Mair P, Kornberger E, Schwarz B, Hoermann BM: Forward blood flow during cardiopulmonary resuscitation in patients with severe accidental hypothermia. An echocardiographic study. Acta Anaesth Scand 1998;42:1139–1144.

163. Malamud N, Haymaker W, Custer RP: Heatstroke: A clinicopathologic study of 125 fatal cases. Milit Surg 1946;99:397–444.

164. Marion DW: Response to "Statistics and hypothermia." J Neurosurg Anesthesiol 1998;10:120–123.

165. Marion DW, Penrod LE, Kelsey SF, et al: Treatment of traumatic brain injury with moderate hypothermia. N Engl J Med 1997;336: 540–546.

166. Marzuk PM, Tardiff K, Leon AC: Ambient temperature and mortality from unintentional cocaine overdose. JAMA 1998;279: 1795–1899.

167. McAllister RG Jr: Fever, tachycardia, and hypertension with acute catatonic schizophrenia. Arch Intern Med 1978;138:1154–1156.

168. McAllister RG, Jr., Bourne DW, Tan TG, et al: Effects of hypothermia on propranolol kinetics. Clin Pharmacol Ther 1979;25:1–7.

169. McAllister RG Jr, Tan TG: Effect of hypothermia on drug metabolism. In vitro studies with propranolol and verapamil. Pharmacology 1980;20:95–100.

170. McCarron MM, Boettger ML, Peck JJ: A case of neuroleptic malignant syndrome successfully treated with amantadine. J Clin Psychiatry 1982;43:381–382.

171. McCauley RL, Hing DN, Robson MC, Heggers JP: Frostbite injuries: A rational approach based on the pathophysiology. J Trauma 1983;23:143–147.

172. Mehta AC, Baker RN: Persistent neurological deficits in heat stroke. Neurology 1970;20:336–340.

173. Menon MK, Gordon LI, Kodama CK, Fitten J: Influence of D-1 receptor system on the D-2 receptor-mediated hypothermic response in mice. Life Sci 1988;43:871–881.

174. Millan MJ, Audinot V, Melon C, Newman-Tancredi A: Evidence that dopamine D3 receptors participate in clozapine-induced hypothermia. Eur J Pharmacol 1995;280:225–229.

175. Millan MJ, Audinot V, Rivet JM, et al: S 14297, a novel selective ligand at cloned human dopamine D3 receptors, blocks 7-OH-DPAT-induced hypothermia in rats. Eur J Pharmacol 1994;260: R3–5.

176. Miller JW, Danzl DF, Thomas DM: Urban accidental hypothermia: 135 cases. Ann Emerg Med 1980;9:456–461.

177. Mills W: Accidental hypothermia. In: Pozos RS, Wittmers LE, eds: The Nature and Treatment of Hypothermia. Minneapolis, University of Minnesota Press, 1983, pp. 182–193.

178. Moore JA, Kakihana R: Ethanol-induced hypothermia in mice: Influence of genotype on development of tolerance. Life Sci 1978;23: 2331–2337.

179. Morishima HO, Mueller-Heubach E, Shnider SM: Body temperature and disappearance of lidocaine in newborn puppies. Anesth Analg 1971;50:938–942.

180. Moroff SV, Bass DE: Effects of overhydration on man's physiological responses to work in the heat. J Appl Physiol 1965;20: 267–270.

181. Murphy K, Nowak RM, Tomlanovich MC: Use of bretylium tosylate as prophylaxis and treatment in hypothermic ventricular fibrillation in the canine model. Ann Emerg Med 1986;15:1160–1166.

182. Murphy MT, Lipton JM: Effects of alcohol on thermoregulation in aged monkeys. Exp Gerontol 1983;18:19–27.

183. Murray PT, Fellner SK: Efficacy of hemodialysis in rewarming accidental hypothermia victims. J Am Soc Nephrol 1994;5:422–422.

184. Myers RD: Alcohol's effect on body temperature: Hypothermia, hyperthermia or poikilothermia? Brain Res Bull 1981;7:209–220.

185. Nakayama T, Hardy JD: Unit responses in the rabbit's brainstem to changes in brain and cutaneous temperature. J Appl Physiol 1969;27: 848–857.

186. Nicodemus HF, Chaney RD, Herold R: Hemodynamic effects of inotropes during hypothermia and rapid rewarming. Crit Care Med 1981;9:325–328.

187. Nicodemus HF, Chaney RD, Herold R: Lidocaine/propranolol: hemodynamic effects during hypothermia and rewarming. J Surg Res 1981;30:6–13.

188. Nicoll KA, Davies L: How warm are babies kept at home? Health Visit 1986;59:113–114.

189. Nielsen KC, Owman C: Control of ventricular fibrillation during induced hypothermia in cats after blocking the adrenergic neurons with bretylium. Life Sci 1968;7:159–168.

190. Nikki P, Vapaatalo H, Karppanen H: Effect of ethanol on body temperature, postanaesthetic shivering and tissue monoamines in halothane-anaesthetized rats. Ann Med Exp Biol Fenn 1971;49: 157–161.

191. Nisijima K, Ishiguro T: Does dantrolene influence central dopamine and serotonin metabolism in the neuroleptic malignant syndrome? A retrospective study. Biol Psychiatry 1993;33:45–48.

192. O'Connor JP: Use of peritoneal dialysis in severely hypothermic patients. Ann Emerg Med 1986;15:104–105.

193. O'Donnell TF Jr: Acute heat stroke. Epidemiologic, biochemical, renal, and coagulation studies. JAMA 1975;234:824–828.

194. O'Donnell TF Jr, Clowes GH Jr: The circulatory abnormalities of heat stroke. N Engl J Med 1972;287:734–737.

195. Ogawa T, Low PA: Autonomic regulation of temperature and sweating. In: Low PA, ed: Autonomic Disorders. Evaluation and Management. Boston, Little, Brown, 1993, pp. 79–91.

196. Ohmura A, Wong KC, Westenskow DR, Shaw CL: Effects of hypocarbia and normocarbia on cardiovascular dynamics and regional circulation in the hypothermic dog. Anesthesiology 1979;50: 293–298.

197. Okada M: The cardiac rhythm in accidental hypothermia. J Electrocardiol 1984;17:123–128.

198. O'Keeffe KM: Accidental hypothermia: A review of 62 cases. J Am Coll Emerg Phy 1977;6:491–496.

199. Okuliczkorayn I, Mikolajczak P, Kaminska E: Tolerance to hypothermia and hypnotic action of ethanol in 3 and 14 months old rats. Pharmacol Res 1992;25:63–64.

200. Orts A, Alcaraz C, Goldfrank L, et al: Morphine-ethanol interaction on body temperature. Gen Pharmacol 1991;22:111–116.

201. Osborn JJ: Experimental hypothermia: Respiratory and blood Ph changes in relation to cardiac function. Am J Physiol 1953;175: 389–398.

202. Osborne L, Kamal El-Din AS, Smith JE: Survival after prolonged cardiac arrest and accidental hypothermia. BMJ 1984;289:881–882.

203. Ovadia H, Wohlman A, Mechoulam R, Weidenfeld J: Characterization of the hypothermic effect of the synthetic cannabinoid HU-210 in the rat. Relation to the adrenergic system and endogenous pyrogens. Neuropharmacology 1995;34:175–180.

204. Patel R, Das M, Palazzolo M, et al: Myoglobinuric acute renal failure in phencyclidine overdose: Report of observations in eight cases. Ann Emerg Med 1980;9:549–553.

205. Patel S, Hutson PH: Hypothermia induced by cholinomimetic drugs is blocked by galanin: Possible involvement of ATP-sensitive K+ channels. Eur J Pharmacol 1994;255:25–32.

206. Paton BC: Accidental hypothermia. Pharmacol Ther 1983;22: 331–377.

207. Perchick JS, Winkelstein A, Shadduck RK: Disseminated intravascular coagulation in heat stroke. Response to heparin therapy. JAMA 1975;231:480–483.

208. Rawson RO, Quick KP: Evidence of deep-body thermoreceptor response to intra-abdominal heating of the ewe. J Appl Physiol 1970; 28:813–820.

209. Reuler JB: Hypothermia: Pathophysiology, clinical settings, and management. Ann Intern Med 1978;89:519–527.

210. Riedel W: Warm receptors in the dorsal abdominal wall of the rabbit. Pflugers Arch 1976;361:205–206.

211. Ritzmann RF, Tabakoff B: Body temperature in mice: A quantitative measure of alcohol tolerance and physical dependence. J Pharmacol Exp Ther 1976;199:158–170.

212. Ritzmann RF, Tabakoff B: Dissociation of alcohol tolerance and dependence. Nature 1976;263:418–420.

213. Rivers N, Horner B: Possible lethal reaction between Nardil and dextromethorphan. Can Med Assoc J 1970;103:85.

214. Roden DM: Antiarrhythmic drugs. In: Hardman JG, Limbird LE, Molinoff PB, Ruddon RW, Gilman AG, eds: The Pharmacological Basis of Therapeutics. New York, McGraw-Hill, 1996, p. 862.

215. Romm E, Collins AC: Body temperature influences on ethanol elimination rate. Alcohol 1987;4:189–198.

216. Ron D, Taitelman U, Michaelson M, et al: Prevention of acute renal failure in traumatic rhabdomyolysis. Arch Intern Med 1984;144: 277–280.

217. Rowell LB: Cardiovascular aspects of human thermoregulation. Circ Res 1983;52:367–379.

218. Ruiz de Elvira MC, Coen CW: Centrally administered neuropeptide Y enhances the hypothermia induced by peripheral administration of adrenoceptor antagonists. Peptides 1990;11:963–967.

219. Salmi P, Karlsson T, Ahlenius S: Antagonism by SCH 23390 of clozapine-induced hypothermia in the rat. Eur J Pharmacol 1994; 253:67–73.

220. Sanchez C, Lembol HL: The involvement of muscarinic receptor subtypes in the mediation of hypothermia, tremor, and salivation in male mice. Pharmacol Toxicol 1994;74:35–39.

221. Sarnquist F, Larson CP Jr: Drug-induced heat stroke. Anesthesiology 1973;39:348–350.

222. Satinoff E: Disruption of hibernation caused by hypothalamic lesions. Science 1967;155:1031–1033.

223. Satinoff E: Impaired recovery from hypothermia after anterior hypothalamic lesions in hibernators. Science 1965;148:399.

224. Savard GK, Cooper KE, Veale WL, Malkinson TJ: Peripheral blood flow during rewarming from mild hypothermia in humans. J Appl Physiol 1985;58:4–13.

225. Sawka MN, Young AJ, Latzka WA, et al: Human tolerance to heat strain during exercise: Influence of hydration. J Appl Physiol 1992; 73:368–375.

226. Schaller MD, Fischer AP, Perret CH: Hyperkalemia. A prognostic factor during acute severe hypothermia. JAMA 1990;264: 1842–1845.

227. Schrier RW, Henderson HS, Tisher CC, Tannen RL: Nephropathy associated with heat stress and exercise. Ann Intern Med 1967;67: 356–376.

228. Schuman SH: Patterns of urban heat-wave deaths and implications for prevention: Data from New York and St. Louis during July 1966. Environ Res 1972;5:59–75.

229. Semenza JC, Rubin CH, Falter KH, et al: Heat-related deaths during the July 1995 heat wave in Chicago. N Engl J Med 1996;335:84–90.

230. Seraj MA, Channa AB, al Harthi SS, et al: Are heat stroke patients fluid depleted? Importance of monitoring central venous pressure as a simple guideline for fluid therapy. Resuscitation 1991;21:33–39.

231. Shapiro Y, Magazanik A, Udassin R, et al: Heat intolerance in former heatstroke patients. Ann Intern Med 1979;90:913–916.

232. Shibolet S, Coll R, Gilat T, Sohar E: Heatstroke: Its clinical picture and mechanism in 36 cases. Q J Med 1967;36:525–548.

233. Shvartz E, Shapiro Y, Magazanik A, et al: Heat acclimation, physical fitness, and responses to exercise in temperate and hot environments. J Appl Physiol 1977;43:678–683.

234. Shvartz E, Shibolet S, Meroz A, et al: Prediction of heat tolerance from heart rate and rectal temperature in a temperate environment. J Appl Physiol 1977;43:684–688.

235. Smilkstein MJ, Smolinske SC, Rumack BH: A case of MAO inhibitor/MDMA interaction: Agony after ecstasy. J Toxicol Clin Toxicol 1987;25:149–159.

236. Sohal RS, Sun SC, Colcolough HL, Burch GE: Heat stroke. An electron microscopic study of endothelial cell damage and disseminated intravascular coagulation. Arch Intern Med 1968;122:43–47.

237. Southwick FS, Dalglish PH Jr: Recovery after prolonged asystolic cardiac arrest in profound hypothermia. A case report and literature review. JAMA 1980;243:1250–1253.

238. Splittgerber FH, Talbert JG, Sweezer WP, Wilson RF: Partial cardiopulmonary bypass for core rewarming in profound accidental hypothermia. Am Surg 1986;52:407–412.

239. Sprung CL: Hemodynamic alterations of heat stroke in the elderly. Chest 1979;75:362–366.

240. Sprung CL, Portocarrero CJ, Fernaine AV, Weinberg PF: The metabolic and respiratory alterations of heat stroke. Arch Intern Med 1980;140:665–669.

241. Sternbach H: The serotonin syndrome. Am J Psychiatry 1991;148: 705–713.

242. Tavel ME, Davidson W, Batterto TD: A critical analysis of mortality associated with delirium tremens: Review of 39 fatalities in a 9-year period. Am J Med Sci 1961;242:18.

243. Thomas JM, Rubin EH: Case report of a toxic reaction from a combination of tryptophan and phenelzine. Am J Psychiatry 1984;141: 281–283.

244. Tolman KG, Cohen A: Accidental hypothermia. Can Med Assoc J 1970;103:1357–1361.

245. Tomaszewski W: Changements electrocardiographiques. Observes chez un homme mort de froid. Arch Mal Coeur 1938;31:525–528.

246. Towne WD, Geiss WP, Yanes HO, Rahimtoola SH: Intractable ventricular fibrillation associated with profound accidental hypothermia—successful treatment with partial cardiopulmonary bypass. N Engl J Med 1972;287:1135–1136.

247. Trevino A, Razi B, Beller BM: The characteristic electrocardiogram of accidental hypothermia. Arch Intern Med 1971;127:470–473.

248. Truscott DG, Firor WB, Clein LJ: Accidental profound hypothermia. Successful resuscitation by core rewarming and assisted circulation. Arch Surg 1973;106:216–218.

249. Tysinger DS, Grace JT, Gollan F: The electrocardiogram of dogs surviving 1.5 degrees centigrade. Am Heart J 1955;50:816–822.

250. Vassallo SU, Delaney KA: Pharmacologic effects on thermoregulation: Mechanisms of drug-related heatstroke. J Toxicol Clin Toxicol 1989;27:199–224.

251. Vassallo SU, Delaney KA, Hoffman RS, et al: A prospective evaluation of the electrocardiographic manifestations of hypothermia. Acad Emerg Med 1999;6:1121–1126.

252. Vertel RM, Knochel JP: Acute renal failure due to heat injury. An analysis of ten cases associated with a high incidence of myoglobinuria. Am J Med 1967;43:435–451.

253. Walczak DD: Biochemical correlates of alcohol tolerance: Role of cerebral protein synthesis. PhD Thesis. University of Toronto.

254. Ward A, Chaffman MO, Sorkin EM: Dantrolene. A review of its pharmacodynamic and pharmacokinetic properties and therapeutic use in malignant hyperthermia, the neuroleptic malignant syndrome and an update of its use in muscle spasticity. Drugs 1986;32:130–168.

255. Webb P: Afterdrop of body temperature during rewarming: An alternative explanation. J Appl Physiol 1986;60:385–390.

256. Weyman AE, Greenbaum DM, Grace WJ: Accidental hypothermia in an alcoholic population. Am J Med 1974;56:13–21.

257. White JD: Hypothermia: The Bellevue Experience. Ann Emerg Med 1982;11:417–424.

258. Wickstrom P, Ruiz E, Lija GP, et al: Accidental hypothermia: Core rewarming with partial bypass. Am J Surg 1976;131:622–625.

259. Wislicki L: Effects of hypothermia and hyperthermia on the action of neuromuscular blocking agents. I. Suxamethonium. Arch Int Pharmacodyn Ther 1960;126:68–78.

260. Wong KC: Physiology and pharmacology of hypothermia. West J Med 1983;138:227–232.

261. York JL, Chan AW: Age effects on chronic tolerance to ethanol hypnosis and hypothermia. Pharmacol Biochem Behav 1994;49: 371–376.

262. Young AA, Dawson NJ: Evidence for on-off control of heat dissipation from the tail of the rat. Can J Physiol Pharmacol 1982;60: 392–398.

263. Zachary L, Kucan JO, Robson MC, Frank DH: Accidental hypothermia treated with rapid rewarming by immersion. Ann Plast Surg 1982;9:238–241.

264. Zelman S, Guillan R: Heat stroke in phenothiazine-treated patients: A report of three fatalities. Am J Psychiatry 1970;126:1787–1790.

E. John Gallagher

GENERAL CONCEPTS

Neurotoxicology

The simplest conceptual approach to neurotoxicology is to think of the nervous system anatomically as a vertical neural axis. This cephalocaudad orientation divides the neuraxis into two highly interactive components: The central nervous system (CNS) and the peripheral nervous system (PNS), each of which is further subdivided into several different levels.

The CNS and PNS are differentially affected by toxins for several reasons. Although both are protected compartments, the characteristics of the blood-brain barrier and blood-nerve barrier differ. Thus, certain toxins that are able to gain access to one compartment may fail to gain access to the other, resulting in differential vulnerabilities. Furthermore the composition of the CNS is not uniform. Thus physical factors such as water, pigment and cell complement differ from to region. In addition, recovery from neurotoxic insult differs in the CNS and PNS. Although the entire nervous system is postmitotic and therefore not particularly well adapted to self-repair, axon regrowth following nerve injury is much more extensive in the PNS than in the CNS. Finally, CNS toxicity and PNS toxicity have different clinical presentations. Whereas CNS toxins commonly cause altered mental status, movement disorders, headache, or seizures, PNS toxicity characteristically presents as altered sensory and/or motor function together with normal cognition. Unfortunately, many toxins do not adhere to simple efforts at anatomic classification. A thorough understanding of neurotoxicology requires knowledge of the biochemical affinities of particular toxins for specific classes of neurons and glia, as well as a comprehension of the interactions of these toxins with neural tissue at the molecular level. These basic considerations are discussed in subsequent chapters targeted at specific toxins. This chapter focuses on general clinical neurologic principles that are specifically relevant to toxicology.

CENTRAL NERVOUS SYSTEM

Central nervous system toxicity presenting as acute changes in mentation may be characterized as abnormalities in either the level or content of consciousness. Alterations in level of consciousness, which represent quantitative abnormalities, may reflect a toxin-induced depression of consciousness, ranging from lethargy through stupor to coma. In contrast, alterations in the content of consciousness represent qualitative abnormalities, typically presenting as confusion or delirium, often with superimposed agitation. Because altered mental status is such a common component of a toxicologic emergency, the first part of this chapter focuses on a comprehensive approach to this clinical problem. This section is followed by a discussion of drug- and toxin-induced movement disorders. Finally, other manifestations of CNS toxicity, such as seizures and headache, are discussed.

Altered Mental Status

The practical problem confronting the physician in the evaluation of a patient with acute change in mental status is determining whether the cause is toxicologic, metabolic (including infectious), neurologic (structural), psychiatric, or a combination of one or more of these groups. For example, an agitated and apparently confused patient might be suffering from a sympathomimetic ingestion, hypoglycemia, subarachnoid hemorrhage, or acute schizophrenia. A patient presenting in coma might be suffering from a sedative-hypnotic ingestion, hepatic encephalopathy, or intracerebral hemorrhage. Only through the systematic application of basic neurologic principles can the differential diagnosis be narrowed to the point where rational management decisions can be made.

The first portion of this section discusses these basic principles with the intent of assigning patients with altered mental status to one of the four major categories listed above and displayed in Fig. 19–1. It is appropriate that this discussion should be undertaken in a toxicology text, because approximately 30% of all patients presenting with coma of unknown etiology will, on further investigation, be demonstrated to have been exposed to a toxin.[127] In addition to alteration of the level of consciousness, poisonings also commonly induce delirium. For both of these reasons, the physician must always consider a toxin in the differential diagnosis of a patient with an acutely altered mental status.

Initial Management. The first priority in the management of any patient with altered mental status is assessment and stabilization of the airway and vital signs (Chap. 3). Patients with a depressed level of consciousness and respiratory depression should receive 0.1–2.0 mg of naloxone IV (see Antidotes in Depth: Opioid Antagonists). Thiamine, 100 mg IV, can be given safely to any patient with an altered mental status, but is especially indicated for those who appear undernourished, particularly chronic alcoholics. Finally, 0.5–1.0 g/kg of dextrose should be administered to all patients with altered mental status with or without focal findings if the serum glucose is undetermined or if it is <150 mg/dL by rapid determination[10,26] (see Antidotes in Depth: Opioid Antagonists, Thiamine Hydrochloride, and Dextrose). All patients should have continuous vital sign monitoring and pulse oximetry.

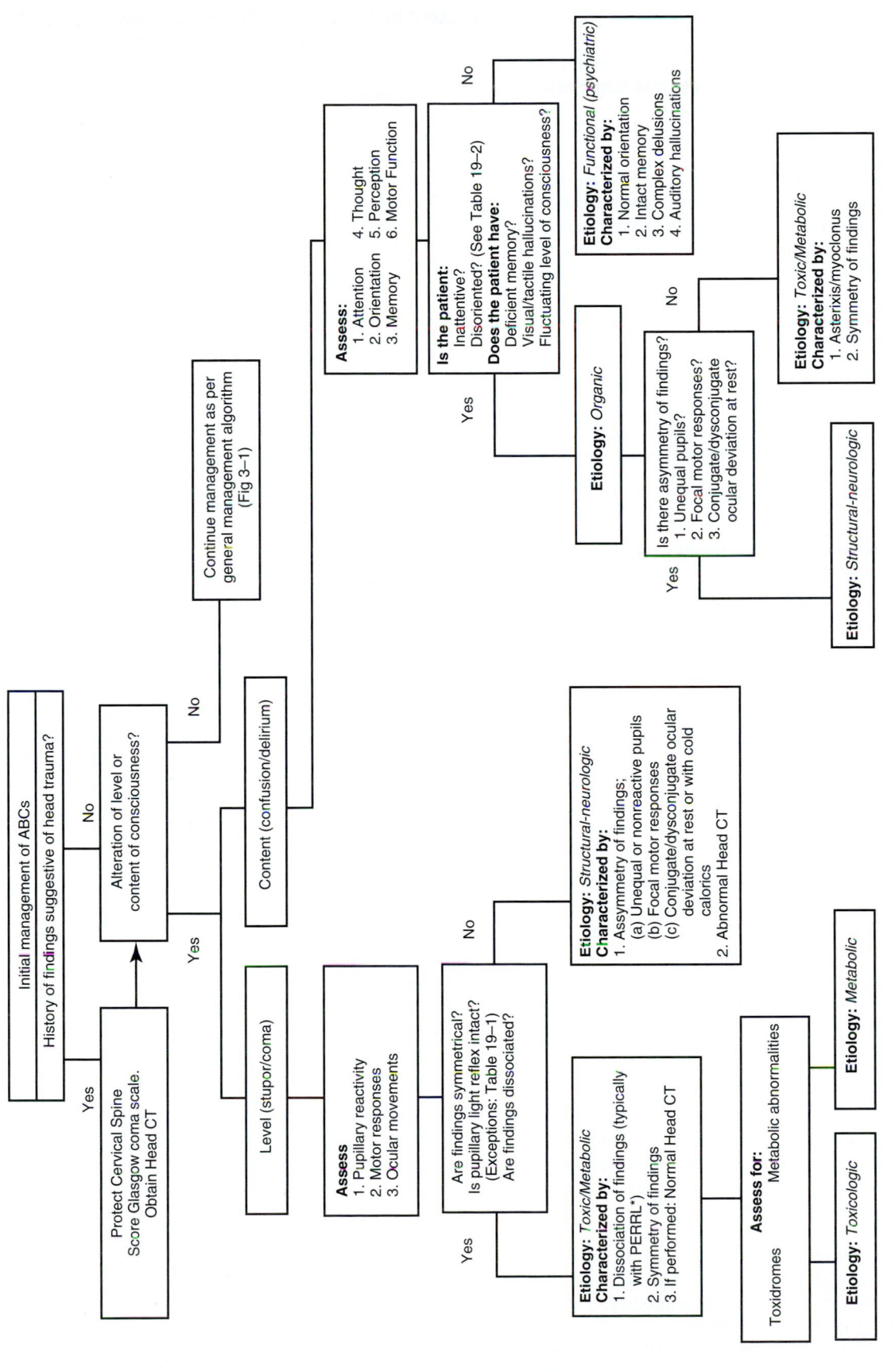

Figure 19–1. Essential aspects of the assessment of the patient with an altered level or content of consciousness. *PERRL = Pupils equal, round, reactive to light. Dissociated findings usually pair PERRL with another finding that cannot be explained anatomically, eg, with absent oculovestibular reflex or with absent motor response.

Additional tests that may be helpful in a patient with altered mental status include an electrocardiogram (ECG), electrolytes, blood, urea, nitrogen (BUN), blood ethanol, calcium, prothrombin timed, international normalized ratio (INR), and serum ketones, and a venous or arterial blood gas should be considered. Specific toxicologic tests are determined by the clinical findings (Chap. 7).

After these initial interventions and stabilization are accomplished, a "circumstantial" history is obtained (see detailed discussion in Chaps. 3 and 31). The patient is then examined as described below and categorized as probable toxicologic, metabolic, structural neurologic, or psychiatric. From this initial categorization, further management logically follows.

Alterations in the Level of Consciousness

The Comatose Patient. A significant alteration in the level of consciousness precludes meaningful evaluation of the content of consciousness. Coma, defined as unarousable unresponsiveness, is the prototypic alteration in level of consciousness. Stupor is defined as arousability only in response to a noxious stimulus. Although stupor and coma are often discussed as a single entity, the general principles mentioned below strictly pertain only to patients who are unarousable and therefore truly comatose. Much of the discussion that follows is a distillation of Plum and Posner's seminal work on the classification of disorders of consciousness.[127]

In a patient presenting to the Emergency Department (ED) in coma, it is of primary importance to distinguish between structural neurologic causes, such as cerebrovascular accidents and epidural/subdural hematomas, and toxic-metabolic derangements, such as sedative-hypnotic ingestions or hyperosmolarity. This can be accomplished with reasonable accuracy by the assessment of three clinical parameters: pupillary equality and reactivity to light, ocular position at rest and in response to provocative maneuvers, and motor response to noxious stimuli.

Pupillary Reflexes.
Assessment of pupillary reactivity requires a strong light source, and for small pupils may require examination under magnification. An otoscope or ophthalmoscope is usually available in an ED and is useful for detecting "microreactivity."

In coma caused by a toxic-metabolic process, the integrity of the pupillary light reflex remains intact. There are very few exceptions to this principle (Table 19–1). The vast majority of toxic and metabolic processes preserve the pupillary light reflex until the terminal (near apneic) stages of coma. The commonly used depolarizing agents, such as succinylcholine,[124] and nondepolarizing agents, such as pancuronium[41] and vecuronium,[21] do not represent exceptions to this general rule and do not impair the pupillary light reflex. These agents demonstrate nicotinic effects, whereas the pupil depends upon muscarinic control.

Asymmetric findings are the hallmark of structural neurologic disease. The pupils may react unequally to light. In striking contrast to the vast majority of patients with overdoses, coma caused by structural neurologic disease may be accompanied by pupillary abnormalities at some point in its evolution.

The hallmark of toxicologic coma, and indeed of all toxic-metabolic coma, is a dissociation of findings. With respect to the pupils, this means that pupillary reactivity is "dissociated from" other neuraxis dysfunction in a fashion that is not characteristic of

TABLE 19–1. Toxic-Metabolic Encephalopathies that May Cause Coma and Nonreactive Pupils

	Large/Fixed	Small/Fixed	Mid/Variable/Fixed
Anoxia	X		
Anticholinergics	X		
Barbiturates[a]			X
Cholinergics[b,c]		X	
Glutethimide			X
Hypothermia (<28°C; <82.4°F)			X
Opioids		X	

[a]Seen only with very large doses of barbiturates.
[b]Usually pupils are not truly fixed, but are "microreactive," requiring magnification to identify reactivity.
[c]Pilocarpine eye drops, although not causes of coma, are common causes of small, fixed pupils in older patients with wide-angle glaucoma who are comatose for reasons unrelated to cholinergic overdose.

structural brain disease. Thus, in addition to symmetric findings, patients whose coma originates from a toxicologic or metabolic cause typically have an intact and equal pupillary light reflex (see exceptions in Table 19–1) that may be paired with an absent oculovestibular response, an absent (flaccid) motor response to noxious stimuli, or hypoventilation requiring ventilatory support. This phenomenon of dissociation occurs with toxic-metabolic coma because other brainstem functions tend to be far more vulnerable to toxic and metabolic insult than are the pupillary light reflexes.

Provocative Maneuvers in the Assessment of Eye Movements.
Two provocative maneuvers are used to assess eye movements: The oculocephalic (*doll's eye[s]*) reflex and oculovestibular (*cold caloric[s]*) testing. The oculocephalic maneuver in patients not suspected of having a cervical spine injury is performed by gently rotating the patient's head first to the right, then pausing to observe whether "doll's eyes" are present. In this direction, conjugate movement of both eyes to the left, such that the limbus of the right eye is buried in its medial canthus and the limbus of the left eye is buried in its lateral canthus, indicates that the oculocephalic reflex is intact. The head is then rotated to the opposite side, in this example, to the left. If doll's eyes are present in this direction, the left eye will move into its medial canthus and the right eye into its lateral canthus. In order for doll's eyes to be declared fully present and equal, the conjugate deviation in response to head turning must occur bilaterally. The two other possible responses are asymmetry or absence (no movement) of doll's eyes. Both mandate performance of the cold caloric test for confirmation.

The cold caloric examination is performed by first confirming that the tympanic membranes are intact, and then gently irrigating the right ear with ice water. Cold calorics are defined as present in this direction if the eyes deviate fully in a conjugate fashion toward the irrigated ear. After waiting approximately 10 minutes for the irrigated right ear to warm up, cold water is injected into the left auditory canal. Cold calorics are present in this direction if the eyes move fully and conjugatively toward the irrigated ear. For cold calorics to be fully present, the ocular reflex must occur bilaterally. Asymmetry of movement strongly suggests a focal lesion rather than a toxicologic process. Absence of movement indicates that a component of the brainstem is not functioning. However, this observation must be paired with other findings to determine whether or not the combination is "dissociative," suggestive of a toxic-metabolic process or of a structural cause of coma.

With structural disease, the position of the eyes at rest may be asymmetric, demonstrating either conjugate or dysconjugate gaze deviation. In contrast, in toxic-metabolic processes the eyes are positioned within a few degrees of the midline, unless the patient is seizing or postictal or has an underlying strabismus. If these entities can be excluded with reasonable certainty, significant ocular divergence in a comatose patient is indicative of a structural brainstem lesion, although severe alcohol intoxication can cause divergence.[127]

In contrast, in coma caused by a toxic-metabolic process the eyes either respond or do not respond to provocative maneuvers, but in either case there is bilateral symmetry.

Motor Response to Noxious Stimuli.   Stimuli that are noxious but not harmful, in ascending order of discomfort, include nasal tickle with cotton wisp, pressure on the lunula of the nailbed with the side of a pen or tongue depressor, and pinching the loose skin on the inner aspect of the upper arm. The use of more painful stimuli is unnecessary and inappropriate.

The motor responses to a noxious stimulus in structural neurologic disease are often asymmetric or focal. When a comatose patient is given a noxious stimulus, one of three motor responses occurs: "appropriate," flaccid, or stereotypic. Stereotypic responses take one of two forms, abnormal flexor (decorticate posturing) or abnormal extensor (decerebrate posturing). Use of the abnormal flexor/extensor terminology is preferred, because this is less misleading anatomically and affords better interobserver concordance.[148] A comatose patient with a structural lesion might show abnormal flexion in one upper extremity and flaccidity or abnormal extension in the other. Alternatively, a patient with a toxicologic cause for coma may demonstrate any of the various motor responses, but in general should do so symmetrically and without evidence of focality.

Thus, by observing the pupillary reactivity, eye movements, and motor responses for evidence of asymmetry or dissociation, it is usually possible to decide whether a patient's coma is based on a structural neurologic or a toxic-metabolic etiology. From this decision, subsequent management logically follows.

There are exceptions to the above generalizations. Structural disease does not always produce focality. Mass lesions of the brain may cause compression of the brainstem bilaterally. In this dynamic process, neurologic signs that were originally asymmetric may become bilateral and symmetric by the time the physician sees the patient. Conversely, toxic-metabolic conditions such as hyperosmolar nonketotic hyperglycemia[127] or hypoglycemia[112] may produce focal deficits.

Alteration in the Content of Consciousness: the Patient with Delirium or Psychiatric Illness

Clinical assessment of the content of consciousness presupposes a certain arousability or level of consciousness. Acute alterations in the content of consciousness may be caused by either organic or "functional" etiologies. The term *organic* denotes toxic-metabolic or structural neurologic disease; the term *functional*, in contrast, refers to the major psychiatric disorders. The term *psychotic* describes patients with a nonorganic psychosis who are suffering from serious psychiatric illness.

This division between organic and functional disease is an artificial dichotomy that reflects our limited knowledge of the neurochemistry of psychiatric disorders. The psychoses are a diverse set of diseases of unknown etiology that are almost certainly organic in origin (perhaps reflecting defects in neurotransmission), but have not yet been clearly characterized as such.

Unlike the partitioning of coma into structural and toxic-metabolic categories, the organic versus functional construct has no firm anatomic or physiologic substrate. The basis for this division is that the current management of these two groups of illnesses is very different.[99]

In approaching a patient with an alteration in the content of consciousness, the physician must decide first whether the etiology is organic or functional, and if it is organic, whether it is toxic-metabolic or structural (see Fig. 19–1). This problem is analogous to that presented by the comatose patient. The major difference in the evaluation of the patient with an alteration in content (psychosis or delirium) rather than level of consciousness (coma) is that in the case of altered content, the clinical examination places great emphasis on meticulous assessment of the mental status. In the case of a severely altered level of consciousness, a mental status examination is not possible and attention is therefore directed toward the assessment of pupils, ocular movements, and motor response. The major difference is that psychiatric disease, which only rarely causes coma (1–2% of all cases of coma),[127] typically presents as an alteration in content of consciousness (Table 19–2).

In general, any middle-aged or elderly person presenting with acutely altered mentation, without an antecedent psychiatric history, should be presumed to have an organic etiology until proved otherwise. Table 19–2 lists the components of the mental status examination used for evaluating the patient with an alteration in content of consciousness.

Level of Alertness.   Initially, level of alertness is assessed by simple observation. Typically, a delirious patient demonstrates a clouded sensorium and fluctuating level of consciousness over time, whereas a patient with primary psychiatric illness generally has a more stable level of consciousness.

Attention.   Before evaluating higher cognitive function, the patient's attention span must be assessed. Just as a depressed level of consciousness precludes further testing of mental status, inattention makes it difficult to test orientation, memory, and other cognitive processes. Number repetition is the simplest means of testing attention, using a nonsequential, nonrepeating string of 7 digits such as 9207458. The numbers should be given to the patient at a rate of 1 per second. Inability to repeat at least 5 of the digits in the correct sequence is indicative of inattention,[147] an essential feature of delirium.[73] Attention may be impaired in patients with psychiatric disease who are actively hallucinating or severely depressed, but is more characteristically diminished in patients with organic confusion. A selective inattention toward one side of the body—usually the left—resulting from a nondominant parietal lobe lesion is virtually diagnostic of structural neurologic disease.

Orientation.   Disoriented patients must be assumed to have organic pathology until proved otherwise. Organically disturbed patients are typically disoriented as to time and place, but only rarely as to person. It is important to ask the patient to state as precisely as possible the day, month, and year, rather than to infer his or her

TABLE 19–2.   Typical Distinguishing Features of Alternations in the Content of Consciousness

| Clinical Feature | Organic | | Psychiatric | |
	Delirium	Dementia	Mood Disorder (Unipolar or Bipolar)	Schizophrenia
Onset	Acute	Insidious	Gradual/subacute	Gradual/subacute
Short-term temporal profile	Fluctuating	Stable	Stable	Stable
Age at onset	Any age	≥50 y	<40 y unless situational or involutional	<30 y
Level of alertness	Clouded (may be depressed or hyperalert)	Normal unless far advanced	Normal, slightly depressed or hyperalert	Normal or hyperalert
Attention	Impaired	Unimpaired unless far advanced	Unimpaired unless severe	Unimpaired unless distracted by hallucinations
Orientation	Disoriented	Disoriented unless early and mild	Oriented	Oriented
Memory	Globally impaired	Short-term more impaired than long-term	Intact	Intact
Thought processes	Disorganized, incoherent, rambling	Disorganized but less evident than in delirium	Delusions may be self-deprecatory or grandiose	Delusions typical, fixed, elaborate, paranoid, or grandiose
Perceptual distortions	Hallucinations commonly visual, tactile, or auditory	None	Hallucinations uncommon	Auditory hallucinations common
Asterixis	Suggestive of toxic metabolic encephalopathy	None	None	None
Outcome	Mortality or resolution	Deterioration if no treatable cause found	Resolution and recurrence; mortality associated with suicide	Resolution and recurrence, often with deterioration; mortality associated with command hallucinations

degree of orientation from conversation. Many patients, especially those with slowly progressive organic confusion such as dementia, can obscure their deficit quite skillfully in casual conversation. Unlike inattentiveness, disorientation is not an essential feature of delirium.[73]

Memory.   Memory requires sequential reception, retention, and retrieval of information. Short-term memory can be most readily assessed by asking the patient to recall 3 unrelated words after the passage of 3–5 minutes. Ability to recall 2 of 3 objects is the best cutpoint, but is only about 80% sensitive and 75% specific for the diagnosis of organic confusion.[49] Impairment of memory is characteristically seen only in organic conditions, although a severely psychotic patient may occasionally do poorly on memory testing because of preoccupation with intrusive hallucinations. Similarly, a severely depressed "pseudodemented" patient may appear to have poor recall simply because of a failure to make the required effort.[164]

Thought.   Assessment of the patient's thought process and content should be directed toward a search for delusions, often paranoid or grandiose in nature. Specific questions asked in a matter-of-fact manner—"Are you afraid someone is out to hurt you? Is anyone trying to control your mind? Do you have thoughts you cannot get out of your head? Do you possess any special powers?"—are often met with a surprisingly direct response. Patients with organic disease may be paranoid, but generally their delusions are not as intricate as those of schizophrenic patients.

It is also important to distinguish between a thought disorder and a language disorder. A true language disturbance (aphasia) represents a focal neurologic finding, usually localizing the pathology to the dominant hemisphere. When the aphasia is characterized by a paucity of speech (nonfluent aphasia), there is often an accompanying right-sided hemiparesis, and the diagnosis of a structural lesion is not difficult. Fluent aphasia, however, can easily be confused with delirium or psychosis. Typically, fluent aphasia can be distinguished from organic confusion by the presence of frequent agrammatical paraphasic errors that are not a prominent feature of most cases of delirium or dementia. Fluent aphasia can also be distinguished from psychosis by the frequency of neologisms, which tend to appear in agrammatically constructed sentences and, unlike the occasional neologisms of acute psychosis, are nonrepetitive (because they essentially represent random output of language). A psychotic neologism may have some symbolic meaning to the patient and is repeated over and over. Although an extensive discussion of the various forms of aphasia is beyond the scope of this chapter, it is important to remember that disjointed speech does not necessarily reflect disjointed thought.

Perception.   To determine whether the patient is actively hallucinating, the examiner must observe the patient carefully for repeated head turning, directed eye movements, staring, or incoherent mumbling. As in the assessment of thought content, the direct approach is often most rewarding. For example, one might ask: "Do you sometimes see things that you think may not be real? Do you ever feel things, like bugs, crawling on your skin? Do you sometimes hear voices calling you names or telling you to do something you do not want to do? Have you ever heard your name called and turned to find no one there?"

Well-formed auditory hallucinations are indicative of schizophrenia, although they sometimes also occur in major affective disorders. Poorly formed auditory hallucinations are not diagnostically distinctive. Visual hallucinations are suggestive, but not diagnostic, of delirium. Tactile, gustatory, and olfactory hallucinations, although relatively rare, usually indicate organic disease.

Motor. Just as in coma, focal motor findings here suggest structural neurologic disease until proved otherwise. Asterixis is an extremely helpful finding because it is highly suggestive of a toxic-metabolic cause of altered mentation. Movement disorders associated with drugs or toxins are discussed later in this chapter.

In practice, it is sometimes difficult to distinguish toxic-metabolic from structural neurologic disease. This occurs when a toxic-metabolic process produces focal findings (which is relatively uncommon),[99,112,147] or when an "extra-axial" structural lesion, such as a subdural hematoma or subarachnoid hemorrhage, produces minimal focality because the pathologic process is located outside brain parenchyma. In the former case, usually the patient undergoes an unnecessary CT or MRI scan but little harm is done. In the latter case, however, failure to perform a CT or MRI scan may have dire consequences.[42,60,79,102] It is for this reason that even the slightest suggestion of focality in an apparent overdose should prompt a neuroimaging procedure, as should any degree of diagnostic uncertainty generated either by the circumstances under which the patient was found such as at the foot of a flight of stairs or by evidence of head trauma on examination. If structural disease is suspected in a comatose or confused patient, a CT scan should be obtained immediately.

With the application of basic neurologic principles, it should be possible to determine, on the basis of history, clinical examination, and readily obtainable laboratory and radiographic data, whether a patient with an altered mental status is suffering from structural neurologic disease, a psychiatric disorder, or a toxic-metabolic derangement. On the basis of a categorical rather than specific diagnosis, a rational plan of management and further evaluation can then be formulated.[62,63]

Movement Disorders

Virtually all of the movement disorders caused by primary neurologic disease can be induced by a drug or toxin.[59,76] The drugs most frequently implicated in movement disorders are the antipsychotics,[54,117,132] the calcium channel blockers,[39,55,56,109,120] substituted benzamides such as metoclopramide and cisapride,[13,35,75] CNS stimulants,[6,58,106,158] antidepressants,[61,74,78,90] anticonvulsants,[8,50,123] and lithium.[52,111,149] These disorders can be classified as a decrease in movement (akinesia) and or as altered or abnormal movement (dyskinesia).[156] The akinesias that occur secondary to drugs and toxins primarily include the family of drug-induced parkinsonian syndromes. The dyskinesias that are most relevant to toxicology include tremor, chorea, ballismus, dystonia, akathisia, tardive dyskinesia, myoclonus, and asterixis.

Akinesia. Parkinson disease is characterized by tremor, rigidity, akinesia, and postural instability. Other common features include lack of spontaneous smiling and decreased frequency of blinking, giving the patient an expressionless appearance. Stooped posture, a shuffling gait, drooling, and micrographia are also common features.[113]

Drug-induced parkinsonism may be caused by agents that either destroy cells in the substantia nigra such as manganese, 1-methyl-4-phenyl-1,2,3,6-tetrahydropyridine [MPTP], or, much more commonly, agents that antagonize the effects of dopamine, either pre- or postsynaptically (see Table 19–3).

MPTP-induced parkinsonism was reported almost exclusively in individuals using a synthetic opioid.[40,93] The syndrome differs from that of idiopathic Parkinson disease in its rapidity of onset. In most patients, the effects appear to be permanent.[92] Because of the insights that MPTP toxicity has provided into the pathophysiology, treatment, and prevention of idiopathic Parkinson disease, it has received a great deal of attention. MPTP is discussed in greater detail in Chap. 62.

Antipsychotic drugs are the most common reversible cause of parkinsonism. The development of parkinsonism is dose dependent and seems to be related to the blockade of D_2 receptors and is correlated with the degree of D_2-receptor occupancy in the striatum. The halogenated and piperazine phenothiazines and butyrophenones are most likely to produce parkinsonism.[76]

Parkinsonism caused by antipsychotics and other drugs may be treated either by the addition of an anticholinergic medication, such as benztropine, or by discontinuation of the antipsychotic.[14,77] However, onset or aggravation of Parkinsonian signs has occurred with withdrawal of antipsychotics perhaps by causing degeneration of vulnerable nigrostriatal neurons through the generation of cytotoxic free radicals or accelerating neuronal firing rates.[76]

Toxins that damage the basal ganglia, such as carbon monoxide (Chap. 97), often result in cell death, with variable symptomatic response to dopaminergic medications such as levodopa and bromocriptine. Other treatment modalities, such as long-term chelation for patients whose parkinsonism is caused by manganese poisoning, have been used with some success but remain controversial.[38]

Dyskinesias.

Tremor. Tremor, an involuntary rhythmic oscillating movement resulting from contractions of reciprocally innervated antagonistic muscles,[86] is traditionally categorized into three groups: resting, sustension, and kinetic. These three categories of tremor, caused by primary neurologic disease, are distinguished, in part, because the management of each is different. For example, the treatment of Parkinson disease is not at all similar to management strategies for essential tremor (the most common form of tremor encountered in practice). However, when the cause of tremor is a drug or toxin, there is often a great deal of overlap among the three varieties of tremor. In particular, a drug-induced resting tremor often has a component of sustension tremor as well. Thus, virtually all of the antipsychotic medications listed in Table 19–3 are capable of producing sustension tremor. Likewise, many of the agents such as phenytoin that cause sustension tremor also cause kinetic tremor. Conversely, drugs such as alcohol, benzodiazepines and barbiturates that cause sustension tremor as a manifestation of withdrawal will typically cause a kinetic tremor and ataxia at toxicity.

Resting Tremor. The most characteristic feature of a resting tremor (static or parkinsonian tremor) is that it is most marked with the limb at rest and decreases with voluntary movement. It typically occurs in association with the akinetic movement disor-

TABLE 19–3. Drug and Toxin-Induced Tremor

Resting Tremor	Sustension Tremor	Kinetic Tremor
Calcium-channel blockers	Amiodarone	Amiodarone
Carbon disulfide	Amphetamine	Barbiturates
Carbon monoxide	Arsenic	Benzodiazepines
Captopril	β-Adrenergic agonists	Carbamazepine
Chlorpromazine	Caffeine	Chloral hydrate
Chlorprothixene	Carbon disulfide	Colistin
Clozapine	Carbon monoxide	Ethanol (chronic)
Cyanide	Chlorpromazine	Glutethimide
Droperidol	Chlorprothixene	Lithium
Ethanol (withdrawal)	Clozapine	Methaqualone
Fluphenazine	Cocaine	Methyl mercury
Haloperidol	Corticosteroids	Phenytoin
Lithium	Cyclic antidepressants	Piperazine
Loxapine	Droperidol	Valproic acid
Manganese	Ergotamine	
Methanol	Ethanol	
Methyldopa	Fluphenazine	
Metoclopramide	Haloperidol	
Mesoridazine	Lead	
Molindone	Levodopa	
MPTP[a]	Lithium	
Perphenazine	Loxapine	
Phenytoin	MAOIs (food interaction	
Pimozide	or drug)	
Prochlorperazine	Mesoridazine	
Reserpine	Methylbromide	
Tetrabenazine	Molindone	
Thioridazine	Monosodium glutamate	
Thiothixene	Perphenazine	
Trifluoperazine	Phencyclidine	
	Phenytoin	
	Pimozide	
	Sedative-hypnotics	
	Theophylline	
	Thioridazine	
	Thiothixene	
	Trifluoperazine	
	Valproic acid	

[a]1-Methyl-4-phenyl-1,2,3,6-tetrahydropyridine. Modified with permission from Weiner WJ, Lang AE: Movement Disorders: A Comprehensive Survey. Mt. Kisco, NY, Futura, 1989.

ders and is often produced by the drugs and toxins listed in Table 19–3.

Sustension Tremor. Sustension tremor (action or postural tremor) is present when the limbs are maintained in an outstretched position and during movement, and may increase slightly at the endpoint of a goal-directed motion. This type of tremor is much less apparent at rest and disappears entirely if the patient completely relaxes the limb. Table 19–3 lists the drugs and toxins most commonly responsible for the induction of a sustension tremor.

Kinetic Tremor. Kinetic tremor (intention, ataxic, or cerebellar tremor) is absent when the extremity is at rest and during the first part of voluntary movement, but it increases markedly in amplitude as the goal is approached.

Alcoholic cerebellar degeneration is among the most common toxic causes of kinetic tremor and ataxia.[154] This tremor is often

made worse by an accompanying sensory peripheral neuropathy that impairs proprioception. When seen initially, recent onset ataxia should be treated with thiamine, because the tremor may be a manifestation of Wernicke's encephalopathy.

Lithium is another common cause of tremor, whose mechanism may be adrenergically mediated. The best evidence supporting this is worsening of lithium tremor with β-adrenergic agonists and its response to treatment with β-adrenergic antagonists, such as propranolol. Although tremor is a frequent sign of toxicity, patients with therapeutic lithium levels may exhibit both sustension and kinetic tremors.[152] However, grossly irregular kinetic and resting tremors should be regarded as a sign of toxicity until proved otherwise.[128]

Although most patients with tremor secondary to valproic acid have a mild sustension tremor, the drug may also cause a resting or kinetic tremor, including a marked tremor of the head.[83] Similar to tardive dyskinesias seen with psychotropic agents, the tremor may not begin until months after the drug has been started, and it may worsen over time.[72] Tremor severity is not closely related to valproic acid blood levels, but it does respond to reduction or cessation of the drug.[82]

Exposure to methyl mercury causes destruction of the small internal granular cell neurons of the cerebellar cortex, producing atrophy, marked ataxia, and kinetic tremor[142] (Chap. 81). Amiodarone, an antidysrhythmic agent commonly causes resting, sustension, and kinetic tremors.[156] The associated ataxia is worsened by a concomitant distal polyneuropathy that affects proprioception.[125]

Finally, toxicity associated with ethanol, phenytoin, carbamazepine, barbiturates, chloral hydrate, glutethimide, methaqualone, or any benzodiazepine can produce a syndrome of dysarthria, horizontal and vertical nystagmus, ataxia, kinetic tremor, and asterixis. Peripheral neuropathies may also cause tremor, known as neuropathic tremor, attributable to either weakness[135] or loss of proprioception (see the section on peripheral neurotoxicity).[3] Table 19–3 summarizes the causes of kinetic tremor.

Chorea. Chorea is a series of abrupt, random, excessive, spontaneous movements and is associated with the drugs and toxins listed in Table 19–4. It is also associated with a variety of electrolyte and endocrine disorders, such as hyperglycemia; hypoglycemia; hypernatremia; hyponatremia; hypocalcemia; hypomagnesemia; hyperthyroidism; hypoparathyroidism; and Wernicke's encephalopathy. The prototypic neurologic diseases associated with chorea are Huntington's chorea and Wilson disease.

Dystonia.

Acute Dystonia. Acute dystonias are slower than choreiform movements and include a wide array of sustained spasms of muscle groups. Some of the more common of these sustained spasms are oculogyric crisis (eyes are forced into upward or upward/lateral gaze); blepharospasm; involuntary tongue movements; torticollis (head twisted to the side); retrocollis (neck hyperextended); dysphagia; dysarthria; opisthotonos (a particularly severe form, characterized by hyperextension of the spine and retrocollis); and, occasionally, stridor.[103] Acute dystonias appear early in the course of therapy. Half of them present within 2 days of starting the drug, and the vast majority present within the first week[16] (Chap. 59). Any of the neuroleptic or antiemetic drugs listed in Table 19–4 can produce acute dystonias. They can occur rarely as adverse effects of the 4-aminoquinoline antimalarials, such as chloroquine

TABLE 19–4.   Other Drug and Toxin-Induced Movement Disorders

Chorea	Dystonia	Dyskinesia	Akathisia
Anticholinergics	Anticonvulsants	Antipsychotics	Antidepressants
Anticonvulsants	Antiemetics	Calcium channel blockers	SSRIs[b]
Carbamazepine	Metoclopramide	Flunarizine	Cyclic antidepressants
Phenobarbital	Prochlorperazine	Cinnarizine	Phenelzine
Phenytoin	Antipsychotics	Fluvoxamine[a]	Antiemetics
Antiparkinsonians	Fluvoxamine[a]	Orthopramides and substituted	Metoclopramide
Amantadine	Levodopa	benzamides	Prochlorperazine
Bromocriptine		Clebopride	Antipsychotics
Levodopa		Metoclopramide	Calcium channel blockers
Pergolide		Sulpride	Flunarizine
Antipsychotics		Veralipride	Cinnarizine
Carbon monoxide			Dopamine storage and transport inhibitors
			α-Methyltyrosine
Corticosteroids			Reserpine
Ethanol			Tetrabenzine
Lithium			
Manganese			
Metoclopramide			
Oral contraceptives			
Sympathomimetics			
Thallium			
Toluene			

[a]Antidepressant.
[b]Selective serotonin reuptake inhibitors.

and hydroxychloroquine.[150] The pathophysiology of acute dystonias appears to be linked, in part, to an increase in cholinergic tone, but the role of dopaminergic transmission remains obscure.[119]

These movement disorders are often extremely uncomfortable and frightening to patients. Unfortunately, because they occur in psychiatric patients, many of whom are psychotic, and because the movements appear at times to be under voluntary control, acute dystonias may be misdiagnosed as "hysterical" or malingering. A reasonable approach to treatment is to give patients who have a dystonic reaction, and who do not appear to have anticholinergic toxicity, 1 mg/kg of diphenhydramine IV. If the dystonia resolves with the diphenhydramine, an additional dose of 1 mg/kg IM may be given, followed by 1 mg/kg orally every 6 hours for 48 hours to prevent recurrence.

In addition to the antipsychotics, several other drugs and toxins produce opisthotonos. These include tricyclic antidepressants; phenytoin; metaldehyde; brucine; water hemlock (cicutoxin); tremetol (a plant chemical); phencyclidine; cocaine; lithium; delphene (an insect repellent); and strychnine. Some of these dystonias may be short-lived, episodic "events" with a predominantly tonic phase.

Tardive Dystonia.   As its name implies, tardive dystonia typically occurs following continuous use of antipsychotic drugs for months to years. It occurs with use of metoclopramide, levodopa, and other antiparkinsonian medications, such as bromocriptine, and occasionally is a presenting feature of phenytoin or carbamazepine toxicity. Like acute dystonia, tardive dystonia primarily involves the craniocervical musculature causing acute torticollis, and may respond to anticholinergic drugs.[28] Like tardive dyskinesia, with which it is often grouped, it is a delayed complication of antipsychotic medication and is a chronic illness, with only about

10% of patients returning to baseline after discontinuation of the drug[80] (Chap. 59).

Tardive Dyskinesia.   One simple working definition of tardive dyskinesia is all involuntary movement disorders, other than tremor, that occur as a complication of chronic antipsychotic treatment. The movements of tardive dyskinesia are choreiform in frequency and amplitude, although they tend to be more stereotypic than other choreiform movements. The muscles of the mouth, face, and especially the tongue are involved early, producing the characteristic lingual-facial-buccal dyskinesia. Other components of tardive dyskinesia include chewing, sucking, or lip-smacking movements, which are frequently audible. Because tardive dyskinesia is so polymorphous, the following three criteria are suggested as prerequisites to the establishment of the diagnosis: (a) minimum of 3 months cumulative exposure to an antipsychotic; (b) moderate abnormal involuntary movements in at least one body part or mild abnormal involuntary movements in at least two body parts; and (c) absence of any other explanation for the movement disorder[139] (see Table 19–4).

Because treatment of established tardive dyskinesia is extremely difficult, early identification is particularly important.[53] If a tardive dyskinesia develops, the patient should be immediately referred to the patient's psychiatrist for withdrawal of any anticholinergic medication and for dose reduction of the patient's antipsychotic medication, if possible. Other medications used to control debilitating tardive dyskinesias include benzodiazepines and dopamine antagonists.

Akathisia.   Akathisia is a form of involuntary motor restlessness that results in an inability to remain still for any sustained period.[25] The common causes of akathisia are the antipsychotics and antiemetics listed in Table 19–4, as well as the antiparkinsonian and the sympathomimetic agents. Akathisia is a common extrapyramidal adverse effect caused by antipsychotics and typically occurs within 2–3 months of starting oral medication.[28] In contrast, depot injections may produce akathisia within a few days.[15]

Patients with akathisia do not manifest any particular movement and often appear merely restless, making it easy to confuse this entity with psychotic agitation. Indeed, it may be possible to distinguish newly developed akathisia from worsening psychosis only by increasing the dose of antipsychotic medication.[115] If the agitation worsens, this suggests that the problem is akathisic. Because this is a common and troubling symptom to many patients, it is important to consider akathisia in the differential diagnosis of agitation in any patient on antipsychotics.

Myoclonus and Asterixis.   Myoclonic movements are shocklike, jerking, involuntary movements of muscle groups. They are usually caused by sudden contractions of muscles ("positive" myoclonus), but in the case of asterixis, a related movement disorder, the cause is a transient relaxation of a muscle group resulting in a momentary loss of posture or position ("negative" myoclonus) Myoclonus represents muscle contraction and asterixis represents muscle relaxation (see Table 19–5).

Myoclonus.   Myoclonus can be classified in several different ways, based on clinical findings, presumed anatomic locus of the pathology in the nervous system, the neurotransmitters thought to mediate the movement disorder, or etiology. The most useful classification scheme in toxicology is an etiologic one that focuses on the toxic-metabolic cause.

Asterixis.   Asterixis is most easily elicited by asking the patient to extend the elbow and dorsiflex the wrist with the fingers extended and abducted, as if stopping traffic. After a brief latent period, the fingers begin to flex and extend involuntarily at the

TABLE 19–5   Toxic-Metabolic Causes of Asterixis and Multifocal Myoclonus

Metabolic
  Hepatic failure
  Hyperosmolarity
  Hypoosmolarity
  Postanoxic encephalopathy
  Renal failure
  Ventilatory failure

Toxic
  Anticholinergics
  Anticonvulsants
  Benzodiazepines
  Bismuth
  Crotaline venom
  Cyclic antidepressants
  DDT
  Ethanol
  Lead
  Levodopa
  Mercury
  Methylbromide
  Sedative-hypnotics

Modified, with permission, from Fahn S, Marsden CD, Van Woert MH: Definition and classification of myoclonus. Adv Neurol 1986;43:1–5.

metacarpal-phalangeal joints, as posture is alternately lost and regained. This is followed by sudden palmar flexion at the wrist, with a slower return to dorsiflexion.[94,140] Although asterixis was first described in patients with hepatic failure,[2] it has since been found in association with a large number of toxic-metabolic encephalopathies. It is also associated with structural disease, but far less commonly.[104]

Multifocal Myoclonus.   Multifocal myoclonus is a dysrhythmic contraction of various muscle groups throughout the body, especially affecting the facial and proximal muscles. When asterixis begins to spread and the patient appears to be twitching all over, it may be difficult to distinguish severe asterixis from multifocal myoclonus. Fortunately, it may not be necessary to do so, because either usually implies a toxic-metabolic encephalopathy, such as those listed in Table 19–5. These encephalopathies are typically accompanied by an alteration of mental status, although in mild cases the movement disorder, in particular asterixis, may be more prominent than the altered mental status.

Fasciculations.   Fasciculations are contractions of muscle fibers within an individual motor unit—a single motor nerve cell and the several hundred muscle fibers it innervates. Fasciculations, which appear as a visible twitch, frequently occur when a muscle is fatigued or the patient is cold. In this setting, fasciculations are not pathologic. When associated with a primary neurologic disorder, fasciculations may be attributable to disease of the motor neuron (amyotrophic lateral sclerosis), nerve root, peripheral nerve, neuromuscular junction, or the skeletal muscle itself.[133]

Fasciculations are not well understood. Although there is disagreement regarding their origin,[133,159] it appears that a low excitability threshold of the axonal membrane plays a role in their production.[133] Consequently, augmentation of cholinergic "tone" at the neuromuscular junction (as is seen with organic phosphorous compounds or nicotine toxicity) or increase in the irritability of skeletal muscle due to agents such as caffeine and theophylline both of which produce fasciculations. See Table 19–6 for a complete listing of toxicologic causes of fasciculations.

Neuroleptic Malignant Syndrome.   The signs of neuroleptic malignant syndrome can be divided into four major categories: autonomic instability (thermoregulation), altered mental status, movement disorder, and other neurologic dysfunction.[30,88] The movement disorders include tremor in about half of patients, severe akinetic rigidity in about one-third, and dystonia or chorea in about half.[114] Some patients have a combination of movement disorders. For further discussion, see Chaps. 18 and 59.

Headache

The International Headache Society Classification divides headache into 13 categories, with 129 subtypes.[122] Most headaches associated with toxic-metabolic disorders are poorly understood, particularly those once thought to be of "vascular" origin.[17,66] Because the pathogenesis of vascular headache is currently being challenged on both clinical and epidemiologic grounds, it can no longer be presumed that agents that produce the common toxic vascular headache necessarily act directly on the vasculature to produce pain. It is at least equally plausible that the headache is secondary to a toxin-induced alteration in the relationship between

TABLE 19–6. Toxicologic Causes of Fasciculations

Amphetamines
Arsenic
Barium salts
Black widow spider venom
Brucine
Caffeine
Camphor
Cholinergics (including succinylcholine, organic phosphorus compounds, carbamates)
Cocaine
Crotaline venom
Ergotamines
Fluorides
Hypoglycemic agents
Lead
Lithium
Manganese
Mercury
Nicotine
Phencyclidine
Quaternary ammonium compounds (including muscarinic mushrooms)
Saxitoxin (shellfish poisoning)
Scorpion venom
Strychnine
Tetrodotoxin poisoning (puffer fish)

neurotransmitters, particularly serotonin, and their many different receptors (Table 19–7).[136]

Seizures

Seizures represent episodic pathologic electrical activity in the brain that causes an array of short-lived neurologic signs and symptoms.[37] Seizures are classified into generalized and partial, according to an international taxonomy. Generalized seizures are further subdivided into tonic-clonic (grand mal, major motor, or convulsive), tonic, clonic, absence (minor motor, nonconvulsive, or petit mal), atonic, and myoclonic. Partial seizures are classified as simple or complex (psychomotor or temporal lobe), either of which may evolve into the other or secondarily generalize to a grand mal seizure.[37]

Unless there is underlying focal neurologic disease or epilepsy, most seizures caused by drugs and toxins are of the generalized tonic-clonic variety. Depending on the degree of toxicity, the seizures may be isolated, recurrent, or continuous, without an interictal period of regaining consciousness, which is one definition of status epilepticus.[44,134]

Status epilepticus represents a true emergency, because brain metabolism is markedly increased at the same time oxygen supply is reduced by recurrent apneic periods.[44] In addition, status epilepticus produces dysfunctional autoregulation, shunting blood away from ischemic-sensitive areas.[44] Excessive muscle activity can cause hyperthermia and myoglobinuric acute renal failure.

The most common form of drug-induced seizures is alcohol related. These seizures usually present as withdrawal seizures ("rum fits") and can occur in the withdrawal phase after as little as 6 hours of abstinence from drinking.[143] Cocaine (especially crack) commonly causes drug-induced seizures by producing an abrupt decrement in the seizure threshold[58] and by its effect on sodium channels. Some anticonvulsant drugs prolong the inactivation of

the sodium channels, thereby reducing the ability of neurons to fire at high frequencies. The activated channel remains open but it is blocked by an inactivation gate; carbamazepine, phenytoin, and valproic acid act by this mechanism. Some anticonvulsant drugs reduce the metabolism of γ-aminobutyric acid (GABA), others act at the $GABA_A$ receptor, enhancing chloride influx in a response to GABA, thus increasing membrane polarization and decreasing seizures. Gabapentin acts presynaptically to promote GABA release; benzodiazepines and barbiturates act at $GABA_A$ receptors, enhancing chloride influx by opening the chloride channels. Some anticonvulsant drugs, such as valproic acid and ethosuximide, reduce the flow of calcium through T-type calcium channels, reducing current that may trigger generalized absence seizures (Chaps. 41).

Table 19–8 lists the drugs and toxins that commonly cause seizures as a primary (direct reduction of seizure threshold) or secondary (eg, cellular hypoxia caused by carbon monoxide) event. Virtually any drug can cause seizures as a terminal event.

PERIPHERAL NERVOUS SYSTEM

It is imperative that a rigorous history of exposure to infectious agents as well as toxins be obtained in any patient presenting with a peripheral neuropathy. Diseases of peripheral nerves can be categorized in at least two ways. The first classification is based on distribution of the neuropathy: focal or diffuse. Focal neuropathies include both unifocal (mononeuropathy) and multifocal neuropathy, usually attributable to injury, ischemia, infiltration, or autoimmune disease. In diffuse neuropathies (polyneuropathy), signs and symptoms tend to be symmetric and generalized rather than focal. Toxins almost invariably cause polyneuropathy and are only rarely implicated in focal neuropathy.

The second classification scheme is based on anatomic locations of the pathologic process within the peripheral nerve and is therefore divided into four subtypes: (a) axonopathies, which are characterized by early involvement of the axon; (b) myelinopathies, which are characterized by initial involvement of the myelin sheath or Schwann cell, causing demyelination of the peripheral nerve; and (c) neuronopathies, which are characterized by the presence of early pathologic changes in the nerve cell body. The neuronopathies can be further subdivided into (i) motor (anterior horn cell), (ii) sensory (dorsal root ganglion), and (iii) autonomic neuropathies. (d) Transmission neuropathies, which are characterized by toxins interfering with the release of neurotransmitters from the nerve or propagation of electrical impulses.[137] This classification, which is depicted schematically in Fig. 19–2, serves as the basis for Table 19–9.

Axonopathies

Axonopathies are the most common form of drug- or toxin-induced peripheral neuropathy. They typically begin distally, where the axons are most vulnerable, and proceed proximally.[65] For unclear reasons, long and large-diameter fibers are preferentially affected. Clinically there is symmetric, diffuse, stocking-glove sensorimotor loss. Withdrawal of the toxic exposure is followed by a period of coasting, during which the clinical findings continue to worsen before improvement begins. Because axons regenerate at a rate of about 2 mm/d, recovery is prolonged and is often complicated by denervation atrophy.

TABLE 19–7. Chemicals, Drugs, and Toxins Associated with Headache

Analgesics and nonprescription (OTC) preparations
α-Adrenergic agonists (eg, pseudoephedrine)
Caffeine withdrawal
Indomethacin
Isobutyl nitrite
Vitamin A

Prescription medications
Anesthetics (halothane, ketamine, enflurane, d-tubocurare)
Antibiotics (nalidixic acid, tetracycline, minocycline, nitrofurantoin, metronidazole, sulfamethoxazole, griseofulvin)
Antihypertensives (hydralazine, nifedipine, prazosin, reserpine)
Corticosteroids and steroid withdrawal
Danocrine (Danazol)
Ergotamines
Hypogylcemic agents
Isosorbide dinitrate
Nitroglycerin (oral, transdermal)
Oral contraceptives
Quinine (cinchonism)

Psychopharmacologic agents
Monoamine oxidase inhibitors when ingested with:
    Tyramine-containing foods (red wine, aged cheese, bananas)
    Medication (phenylephrine, ephedrine)
Phenothiazines

Alcohol and drugs of abuse
Amphetamines
Cocaine
Disulfiram (when mixed with ethanol)
Ethanol ("hangover")
Ethylene glycol
Methanol
Phencyclidine

Food and drink
Aged cheese (cheddar, mozzarella, Gruyere, Stilton, brie, Camembert)
Caffeine

Chocolate
Ethanol
Fermented or pickled foods (herring, sour cream, yogurt, vinegar, marinated meats, smoked fish)
Fruits (bananas, plantain, avocado, figs, passion fruit, raisins, pineapple, oranges, citrus fruits)
Monosodium glutamate
Nitrite-containing meat (hot dogs, bologna, pepperoni, salami, pastrami, bacon, sausages, corned beef)
Sugar substitutes (diet drinks)
Sulfites (salad bars, shrimp, soft drinks, some wines)
Vegetables (onions, pods of broad beans [lima, navy], nuts)

Botanicals
Coprinus spp (disulfiramlike reaction if ingested with ethanol) (see Chap. 76)
Herbal preparation (Lobelia, Galega) (see Chap. 77)
Nicotine

Heavy metals
Lead, especially tetraethyl lead
Metal fume fever (caused by welding or smelting of brass, cadmium, chromium, cobalt, copper, iron, magnesium, manganese, nickel, tin, zinc)

Pesticides
Carbamates
Organic phosphorous compounds

Occupational and Environmental
Carbon monoxide
Cyanide
Hydrocarbons
Hydrogen sulfide
Methemoglobin inducers
Nitrites

Toxic envenomation and marine animal ingestion
Marine animals (Ciguatoxin [vertebrate fish], Scombroid [mahimahi flush], Gymnothorax poisoning [eels], Tetrodon [puffer fish]) (Chap. 74)

Acrylamide monomer is generally regarded as an experimental model for toxin-induced axonopathies.[144] Acrylamides are used in grouting and, through occupational exposure, produce weakness of the extremities distally, hyperhidrosis, and numbness of the hands and feet.[57] Features of this exposure that are not typical of distal axonopathy include diffuse loss of reflexes (rather than initial loss of ankle jerks alone) and ataxia that is disproportionate to proprioceptive loss, perhaps attributable to cerebellar toxicity. Because the exposure is often transdermal, there may be an associated contact dermatitis of the hands. Removal from exposure in the early stages results in complete recovery. If exposure is prolonged, residual weakness, sensory abnormalities, and ataxia may persist.

Chronic alcoholism causes a distal, symmetric, sensorimotor polyneuropathy with a predilection for the lower extremities, producing dysesthesias, weakness, and decreased reflexes. The ataxia often seen in chronic alcoholics should always be treated as thiamine deficiency, although it is usually due to a combination of diminished proprioception and midline cerebellar degeneration. The pathologic process of alcoholic peripheral neuropathy shows features of axonopathy accompanied by demyelination. It is prob-

ably related to a nutritional deficiency rather than to a direct effect of alcohol, although this has not been established with certainty.[153]

Allyl chloride, used in the manufacture of epoxy resin, produces a characteristic distal axonopathy with stocking-glove sensory deficit and loss of ankle jerks.[68]

Inorganic arsenic produces two different clinical findings, depending on the nature of the exposure. Massive but sublethal exposure, as in attempted suicide or homicide, causes vomiting, diarrhea, and shock. In individuals who survive, a distal, sensorimotor, symmetric axonopathy characterized by severe paresthesias develops within 1–3 weeks of ingestion.[97] Chronic exposure, as occurs in copper and lead smelters and in miners, is characterized by the development of gastrointestinal upset and constitutional symptoms, followed by mucocutaneous changes, and finally by a predominantly sensory distal neuropathy with dysesthesias of the hands and feet (Chap. 79).

Carbon disulfide (CS_2), used in the manufacture of rayon and cellophane, produces a distal axonopathy with numbness and loss of reflexes in the lower extremities, extending to the upper limbs with continued exposure.[155] Recovery is gradual and may be incomplete.

TABLE 19–8.   Drug- or Toxin-Induced Seizures

Analgesics and nonprescription (OTC) preparations
  Antihistamines
  Caffeine
  Mefenamic acid
  Phenylbutazone
  Salicylates
 	
Prescription medications
  Antihistamines
  Carbamazepine
  Chlorambucil
  Chloroquine
  Clonidine
  Digoxin
  Ergotamines
  Fenfluramine
  Isoniazid
  Lidocaine
  Methotrexate
  Phenytoin
  Procarbazine
  Quinine (cinchonism)
  Sulfonylureas
  Theophylline
 	
Psychopharmacologic medications
  Antiemetics
  Antipsychotics
  Cyclic antidepressants
  Lithium
  Methylphenidate
  Monoamine oxidase inhibitors (esp w/food or
    drug reaction)
  Opioids (propoxyphene, meperidine)
  Pemoline
  Sedative-hypnotic withdrawal
 	
Alcohols and drugs of abuse
  Amphetamines
  Cocaine
  Disulfiram reaction
  Ethanol withdrawal
  Ethylene glycol
  MDMA (methylenedioxymethamphetamine)
  Methanol
  Phencyclidine
	Botanicals
	  Ackee fruit
	  Coprinus spp (disulfiramlike reaction w/alcohol)
	  Daphne
	  Herbal preparations (lobelia, jimson weed, gaiega, mandrake, passion flower,
	    periwinkle, wormwood) (see Chaps. 77, 78)
	  Nicotine
	  Rhododendron
	
	Heavy metals
	  Arsenic
	  Copper
	  Lead
	  Manganese
	  Nickel
	
	Household toxins
	  Boric acid (chronic)
	  Camphor
	  Fluoride
	  Hexachlorophene
	  Phenol
	
	Pesticides
	  Organochlorines (lindane)
	  Organic phosphorous compounds
	  Pyrethrins
	  Rodenticides (thallium, sodium monofluoroacetate, strychnine, zinc phosphide, arsenic)
	
	Occupational and environmental toxins
	  Carbon disulfide
	  Carbon monoxide
	  Chlorphenoxy herbicides
	  Cyanide
	  Hydrocarbons
	    Simple asphyxiants (methane, ethane, propane, butane, natural gas)
	    High volatility (benzene, toluene, gasoline, naphtha, mineral spirits, light gas oil)
	    Halogenated (carbon tetrachloride, trichloroethane)
	  Hydrogen sulfide
	  Methyl bromide
	  Toxic inhalants (simple asphyxiants producing hypoxia — helium, nitrogen, nitrous oxide)
	  Triazine
	
	Toxic envenomation and marine animal ingestion
	  Marine animals (Gymnothorax, saxitoxin [shellfish])
	  Pit viper
	  Scorpion
	  Tick bite (*Rickettsia rickettsii*)

Ethylene oxide produces a distal sensorimotor axonopathy marked by numbness, weakness, and absent or diminished reflexes throughout.[47] Because ethylene oxide is used in gas sterilization and may be retained in dialysis tubing following the sterilization process, it is considered a potential contributor to neuropathy in long-term dialysis patients.[161]

Hexacarbons that produce axonopathy include *n*-hexane and methyl *n*-butyl ketone, both of which are metabolized to 2,5-hexanedione, which is thought to be the neuropathic agent, decreasing phosphorylation of neurofilaments and destroying the normal cytoskeletal matrix. The neurofilament proteins cause axonal swelling, which causes the axonopathy.[1,71] *n*-Hexane is a common solvent used in lacquers and glues. Analogous to arsenic neurotox-

icity, there is a relatively acute form seen with large, short-term exposures (glue sniffing) and a more chronic form associated with industrial exposure. In both varieties, distal sensory symptoms predominate initially, with less loss of reflexes than is seen in other polyneuropathies.[145] As the neuropathy progresses, motor symptoms develop and migrate proximally. Glue sniffers, in whom toluene may also play a role, may have findings of cranial nerve involvement and autonomic disturbances, such as excessive sweating of the hands and feet. In some patients who have massive exposures due to chronic glue sniffing, a quadriparesis may develop over a period of months, presenting a clinical picture similar to that of acute inflammatory demyelinating polyradiculoneuropathy (AIDP or Guillain-Barré syndrome).[7] The phenomenon of

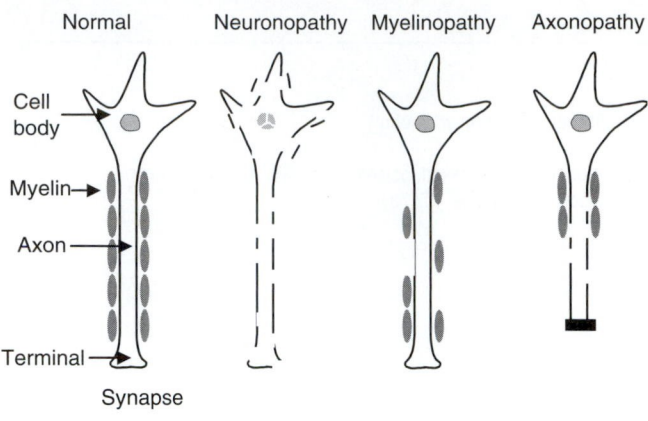

Figure 19–2. Schematic of a peripheral neuron and its three prototypic pathologic responses to toxic insults. Neuronopathies produce secondary axonopathic and myelinopathic changes, leading to degeneration of the entire peripheral nerve. Myelinopathies and axonopathies may occur separately or together. When the axon is involved, the prognosis is worse than with demyelination alone. Neuronopathies have the poorest prognosis of the three. *(Adapted from Chaudhry V: Multifocal motor neuropathy. Semin Neurol 1998;18:74; and Anthony DC, Montine TJ, Graham DG: Toxic responses of the nervous system. In: Klaassen CD, ed. Casarett and Doull's Toxicology, The Basic Science of Poisons, 5th ed. New York, McGraw Hill, 1996.*

coasting seen in other axonopathies is an extremely common feature of hexacarbon neurotoxicity. In mild industrial exposures, recovery is usually complete within a year. In glue sniffers with high-level exposure, residual neurologic deficits may persist indefinitely.

Most of the neurotoxicity of mercury involves the CNS rather than PNS. Mercury vapor and metallic mercury only rarely cause peripheral neuropathy.[4] Mercury vapor can cause an AIDP-like picture dominated by motor abnormalities.[162] Whether organic mercury causes peripheral neuropathy is unknown, although alkyl mercury can produce severe arm and leg dysesthesias (as in the Minamata Bay outbreak) through a CNS mechanism[96] (Chap. 81).

Methyl bromide is used as a refrigerant, insecticide, fumigant, and fire extinguisher. Exposure may produce both CNS and PNS disease. In the PNS, the findings are typical of an axonopathy with stocking-glove numbness, distal weakness, and loss of ankle jerks.[81] Ataxia of the upper and lower limbs may be caused by cerebellar toxicity, rather than by a sensory ataxia secondary to peripheral neuropathy.

Organophosphorus esters are used in plastics manufacturing, petroleum additives, flame retardants, and insecticides. Most of these agents interfere with the action of acetylcholinesterase. Those with potent anticholinesterase properties may produce fatal cholinergic poisoning. Others, of which triorthocresyl phosphate (TOCP) is the prototype, interfere only slightly with the action of acetylcholinesterase and produce a delayed polyneuropathy of the distal axonopathy type. In the mid-20th century there were outbreaks of polyneuropathies in the United States because of misuse of TOCP as an adulterant in Jamaican ginger extract (Jake leg paralysis).[12] With a single large exposure, a transient mild cholinergic syndrome occurs, followed in approximately 1 week by distal paresthesias and later by weakness and reflex loss, which may

migrate proximally. In contrast to the relatively gradual development of most other axonopathies, the neuropathy produced by TOCP becomes full-blown within 2 weeks of symptom onset. Although there is sensory involvement, the predominant symptom is marked weakness. As the peripheral neuropathy resolves, signs of previously masked CNS toxicity become apparent with the development of lower-extremity spasticity. Prognosis is related to severity of exposure, with some patients recovering fully and others remaining relatively disabled with a characteristic combination of upper and lower motor neuron findings.

Polychlorinated biphenyls (PCBs) have been reported to cause a neuropathy when ingested as contaminants of cooking oils.[36] The clinical findings are compatible with an axonopathy, presenting with distal numbness and dysesthesias with weakness and decreased or absent tendon reflexes.

Thallium produces acute, subacute, and chronic axonopathies, depending primarily on the quantity of the initial toxic exposure and the time elapsed since the exposure (Chap. 83). The acute variety begins within hours to a few days of poisoning. Distal dysesthesias and joint pain in the lower extremities, with minimal motor and reflex abnormalities follow this. Depression in level of consciousness reflects concomitant CNS toxicity, and death may occur within weeks due to cardiorespiratory failure[18] (Chap. 83). The subacute form develops a few weeks after exposure and, in contrast to acute toxicity, is characteristically accompanied by alopecia.[34] Severe, sometimes disabling dysesthesias dominate the clinical presentation, accompanied by mild weakness and preserved, though diminished, reflexes. Complete recovery can be expected. Chronic thallium toxicity is not well described, but it appears that tremor, chorea, and ataxia overshadow the signs and symptoms of the peripheral axonopathy. Most thallium toxicity that was seen in the United States was related to unintentional, suicidal, or homicidal ingestion, rather than to occupational exposure to a thallium-containing rodenticide or insecticide.

Ingestion of rodenticides containing Vacor (*N*-3-pyridylmethyl-*N'*-*p*-nitrophenyl urea; PNU) produces an acute axonopathy, marked by weakness and autonomic dysfunction, complicated by development of diabetes, often within hours of exposure[98] (Chap. 90).

Colchicine, when used as chronic prophylaxis against recurrent gouty arthritis, may cause a mild sensory distal axonopathy. However, an accompanying necrotizing myopathy with proximal muscle weakness and creatine kinase elevations usually dominates the clinical presentation, especially when the medication is given in patients with chronic renal failure.[1]

Dapsone has been used in the treatment of pneumocystis pneumonia (Chap. 108), brown recluse spider bites (Chap. 102), leprosy, and certain dermatologic conditions (Chap. 29). Prolonged treatment or massive ingestion produces a symmetric, distal, pure motor axonopathy followed by atrophy.[67]

Disulfiram, used in the treatment of alcoholism, may produce a sensorimotor distal axonopathy characterized by plantar dysesthesias, gait unsteadiness, weakness, and loss of ankle jerks. Return to baseline usually follows discontinuation of the drug.[23]

Isoniazid (Chap. 43), a widely used antituberculous medication, commonly produces a distal sensorimotor axonopathy through interference with pyridoxine and other vitamins of the B group.[19] For this reason, any patient taking isoniazid should also receive 50 mg of pyridoxine daily, as prophylaxis against isoniazid neuropathy (Chap. 43 and Antidotes in Depth: Pyridoxine).

TABLE 19–9. Classification of Selected Toxin- or Drug-Induced Peripheral Neuropathies

Neuronopathy	Axonopathy	Myelinopathy	Transmission Neuropathy
Acute toxic neuropathies			
Pyridoxine (S)	Hexacarbons (SMA)	Arsenic (SM)	Black widow spider
	Thallium (SM)	Diphtheria (SM)	Botulism
	Triorthocresyl		Ciguatoxin
	phosphate (SM)		Elapid and crotaline venoms
	Vacor (MA)		Gymnothoratoxin
			Saxitoxin
			Scorpion venom
			Tetradotoxin
			Tick paralysis
Subacute/chronic toxic neuropathies			
None convincingly	Acrylamide (SM)	Amiodarone (SM)	
demonstrated	Allyl chloride (SM)	Buckthorn	
	Arsenic (SM)	Diphtheria (SM)	
	Buckthorn (M)	Gold (SM)	
	Carbon disulfide (SM)	Trichlorethylene (SM)	
	Colchicine (S)		
	Disulfiram (SM)		
	Dapsone (M)		
	2'-3'-dideoxycytidine (ddC), ddI		
	Ethanol (M)		
	Ethambutol (S)		
	Ethionamide (S)		
	Ethylene oxide (SM)		
	Glutethimide (S)		
	Gold (SM)		
	Hexacarbons (SM)		
	Hydralzaine (SM)		
	Isoniazid (SM)		
	Methyl bromide (SM)		
	Mercury (M)		
	Metronidazole (SM)		
	Misonidazole (SM)		
	Nitrofurantoin (SM)		
	Nitrous oxide (S)		
	Nucleosides (S)		
	Organic phosphorous agents (SM)		
	Polychlorinated biphenyls (SM)		
	Phenytoin (SM)		
	Platinum (S)		
	Podophylin (SM)		
	Taxol (S)		
	Thallium (SM)		
	Vincristine (SM)		

S = sensory: M = motor: A = autonomic

Ethambutol, another antituberculous medication, appears to cause a mild sensory distal axonopathy characterized by numbness of the fingers and toes.[118] The optic neuropathy produced by ethambutol at doses exceeding 20 mg/kg/d is generally of greater concern because of the variable recovery of visual acuity following drug withdrawal.[126]

Ethionamide, which is much less widely used in treatment of tuberculosis than isoniazid or ethambutol, appears to produce a pe-

ripheral neuropathy similar to that caused by ethambutol, but has not been reported to produce optic neuropathy.[95]

Glutethimide is a sedative-hypnotic that causes a distal axonopathy in chronic, high-dose users. It is characterized by impairment of all sensory modalities, calf tenderness, mild ataxia, and loss of ankle jerks.[121]

Hydralazine, used occasionally in the management of hypertension in pregnancy and as a cardiac afterload-reducer, rarely produces a distal, predominantly sensory axonopathy. There is some evidence that this neuropathy is related to pyridoxine deficiency.[129]

Metronidazole, commonly used in the treatment of anaerobic and protozoal infections, causes a predominantly sensory axonopathy marked by distal dysesthesias and sensory ataxia caused by large-fiber proprioceptive involvement. Most cases follow prolonged exposure.[24]

Misonidazole, which is used to sensitize cancer cells in radiotherapy, causes a distal, predominantly sensory axonopathy, characterized by painful dysesthesias of the lower extremities.[108]

Nitrofurantoin is primarily used in the treatment of urinary tract infections. Peripheral neuropathy of the axonal type occurs within weeks to months of instituting the drug, beginning with distal numbness, followed by an unusually rapid development of severe motor and sensory symptoms.[43] Patients with diabetes or renal disease may be especially prone to develop nitrofurantoin neuropathy, although it has also been reported in patients without these underlying diseases.[163]

Nitrous oxide, widely used in emergency departments and dental offices as an analgesic, may produce a myeloneuropathy if abused. Moderate abuse produces a symmetric sensory axonopathy, sometimes accompanied by ataxia of the upper and lower extremities, presumably because of proprioceptive loss. Prolonged, high-level exposure causes, in addition to a severe peripheral neuropathy, lower-extremity spasticity, reflecting CNS involvement in the form of a myelopathy.[70] There is some evidence that this toxicity may be mediated through interference with vitamin B_{12} metabolism, thus accounting for the similarity between full-blown nitrous oxide toxicity and combined system disease.[9]

Nucleoside neuropathy is caused by a number of agents used to treat AIDS, particularly dideoxyinosine (ddI). The distal axonopathy is characterized by severe plantar dysesthesias that extend to the upper extremities if the drug is continued. There appears to be minimal motor involvement[110] (Chap. 108).

Phenytoin may rarely cause a mild peripheral neuropathy, characterized by stocking-glove dysesthesias and mild weakness that responds to drug withdrawal.[101]

Cisplatin (cis-diamine-dichlorplatinum II), a commonly used chemotherapeutic agent, produces a predominantly large-fiber sensory axonopathy, with marked diminution of proprioception and vibration sense, accompanied by minimal weakness with relative preservation of pain and temperature sense.[131]

Pyridoxine produces both acute and chronic forms of peripheral neuropathy by two different mechanisms. The acute form is a neuronopathy (discussed below). The chronic form is associated with high doses of pyridoxine and begins with acral numbness. This is followed by predominantly large-fiber proprioceptive involvement, producing an impairment of manual dexterity and a gait disturbance. Motor fibers appear to be spared. Distal tendon reflexes are diminished or absent because the afferent loop of the reflex arc is affected. In contrast to the acute pyridoxine-induced neuropathy, recovery is usually satisfactory following discontinuation of the drug[138] (Chap. 37 and Antidotes in Depth: Pyridoxine).

Organic gold, used in the treatment of rheumatoid arthritis, rarely causes a peripheral neuropathy with features of both axonopathy and myelinopathy. The clinical picture is one of distal numbness and, later, weakness in the lower extremities accompanied by loss of ankle jerks.[84]

Taxol is used in the treatment of solid tumors. Intravenous injection is followed by acral dysesthesias, loss of all sensory modalities, absent tendon reflexes, proximal spread, and preserved motor function. The neuropathy, which has pathologic features of both axonopathy and myelinopathy, worsens and then resolves in a few weeks.[100]

Vincristine is used as chemotherapy for a variety of malignancies. The axonopathy that this agent produces is unusual in that it begins with paresthesias in the hands prior to the feet, followed by weakness, which is initially more marked in the upper extremities. In general, motor abnormalities dominate the clinical picture and tend to resolve slowly following discontinuation of the drug.[32]

Podophyllin resin, used in the treatment of condylomata acuminata, appears to produce a severe distal axonopathy as well as CNS dysfunction. Neurotoxicity from a lipid-soluble mitotic spindle binder seems plausible, but it is rare and supported primarily by anecdotal case reports.[46]

A number of other drugs or toxins are associated with peripheral neurotoxicity, including lithium, amitriptyline, phenobarbital, penicillamine, cytosine arabinoside, and styrene.[137] However, these drugs have not convincingly been demonstrated to cause peripheral neuropathy.

Myelinopathies

Myelinopathies are characterized by diffuse demyelination that usually spares the axon. There is generalized weakness with mild sensory loss, presumably because the heavily myelinated, large motor axons are more severely affected than the small-diameter myelinated and unmyelinated sensory fibers. For this reason, the large sensory fibers that mediate proprioception, vibration, and touch are impaired, while pain, temperature, and autonomic function are relatively preserved. Because both the afferent and efferent limbs of the reflex arc are involved, the reflexes are symmetrically absent. Usually, areflexia in the lower extremities precedes reflex loss in the upper extremities. Because remyelination is a relatively rapid process compared to axonal regeneration, recovery may be dramatic once the toxin is removed.

Diphtheria neuropathy results from an exotoxin produced by *Corynebacterium diphtheriae*, usually following infection of the throat or skin. Diphtheria toxin inhibits the ability of Schwann cells to synthesize myelin, producing demyelination of the dorsal and ventral roots, with involvement of the dorsal root ganglion itself.[48] The disease produces two distinct forms of peripheral neurotoxicity. There is an early phase, characterized by weakness adjacent to the site of infection, due to local effects of the toxin. The pharyngeal variant of this syndrome follows throat infections. It is a cranial neuropathy characterized by palatal weakness, nasal speech, and palatal sensory loss, with a predominance of motor over sensory abnormalities. Blurred vision may develop as a consequence of paralysis of ocular accommodation, although the pupillary light reflexes are spared. In cutaneous diphtheria, weakness and numbness also occur contiguous to the site of infection. Both pharyngeal and cutaneous variants of the early phase have an excellent prognosis. The late manifestations include a generalized demyelinating neuropathy of rapid onset occurring about 5–8 weeks after infection, with distal sensorimotor findings and hyporeflexia. Recovery is usually complete in cases without myocardial involvement.[107]

Fruit from the buckthorn shrub, which is indigenous to the southwest United States, produces a subacute motor polyneuropathy that may cause death. One to 3 weeks following ingestion, survivors develop a diffuse segmental demyelination causing a rapidly ascending motor neuropathy, with minimal sensory findings.[29]

Lead polyneuropathy is now rare in the United States. Although it is difficult to classify, experimental models argue most strongly for a direct toxic effect on Schwann cells, leading to a myelinopathy.[146] Plumbism is a predominantly motor neuropathy with minimal sensory complaints. The previously reported focal motor variants of lead poisoning (wrist-drop, shoulder girdle weakness, hand intrinsic-muscle atrophy, peroneal muscle weakness, and laryngeal paralysis) are rare.[20] Current presentations are more often characterized by gastrointestinal complaints and constitutional symptoms associated with generalized distal weakness and atrophy, reflex loss, mild sensory abnormalities, and fasciculations[27] (Chap. 80).

Trichloroethylene is used in the rubber and dry cleaning industries and was once used as a general anesthetic. Industrial exposure produces a characteristic syndrome confined to the cranial nerves, especially the trigeminal nerve, producing loss of sensation on the face and difficulty chewing due to motor involvement. Cranial nerves III and VII are also sometimes involved. Trichloroethylene exposure is often associated with herpes simplex infection, suggesting that exposure reactivates the latent virus.[33] Although the neuropathology for this isolated neuropathy is unclear, the weight of evidence favors a myelinopathy.[45]

Amiodarone produces a distal polyneuropathy, with weakness of the lower extremities followed by dysesthesias.[125] Both sustension and kinetic tremor accompanied by ataxia have been reported. Although there are findings of both axonopathy and demyelination, nerve biopsies support histopathologic findings of a predominantly symmetric myelinopathy.

Neuronopathies

Toxic neuronopathies directly affect the neuron itself, especially the dorsal root ganglion.[87] The cell bodies for the trigeminal nerve, the sensory nerve for the face, have much in common with the dorsal root ganglion cells and often have similar vulnerabilities to neurotoxins. Because of this, the clinical findings are segmental; that is, they follow the course of a nerve root, either a dermatome or myotome. Abnormalities may be entirely sensory (if only the dorsal root ganglion is affected, as in herpes zoster), entirely motor (as in poliomyelitis, where only the anterior horn cell is affected), or mixed, with autonomic features. The neuronopathies are the least common and most poorly understood of the three types of peripheral neuropathy.

Acute pyridoxine neuronopathy is caused by massive doses of pyridoxine, which disrupts the cellular metabolism of the dorsal root ganglion. Presumably the fenestrated blood vessels at this site account for the selective vulnerability. The clinical findings demonstrate rapid to subacute development of widespread sensory loss with appendicular ataxia and autonomic instability. Because the pathologic process involves only the dorsal root ganglion, motor function is unimpaired. In contrast to the chronic form, the prognosis in the few patients studied is poor, with persistent, incapacitating sensory ataxia[5] (Chap. 37 and Antidotes in Depth: Pyridoxine).

Neuromuscular Junction Toxicity (Transmission Neuropathy)

The exotoxin of *Clostridium botulinum* binds to the presynaptic portion of the neuromuscular junction, preventing release of acetylcholine. The neurotoxic signs and symptoms are anticholinergic, with a predilection for involvement of the cranial neuromuscular junctions. Specific findings include abnormalities of extraocular movement, pupillary dilatation, ptosis, dysphagia, dysphonia, diplopia, descending motor paralysis, and respiratory failure, with preservation of mental status and sensation. Reflexes are also usually preserved until the end stage of the illness. Because the binding is irreversible, clinical recovery occurs slowly and only with the formation of new neuromuscular junctions. Chapter 75 discusses the presentation and management of botulism in greater detail.

Tetanus is a neurotoxin that involves the neuromuscular junction, sympathetic pathways, spinal cord, and brain. Tetanospasmin, the clinically important exotoxin of *Clostridium tetani*, travels from the point of entry, largely via the axon, to the central nervous system. There it blocks release of inhibitory neurotransmitters, producing disinhibited, widespread muscular spasm and autonomic instability. Tetanospasmin's effect on the neuromuscular junction, which is similar to that of botulism, is usually overshadowed by its central effects. Trismus is the most common presenting symptom, followed by generalized muscle spasm, which can be triggered by uninhibited afferent stimuli such as a noise, bright light, or touch. These spasms are produced by simultaneous and sustained contraction of agonist/antagonist muscles and may lead to laryngospasm, respiratory paralysis, and death. There are often accompanying fluctuations in vital signs and dysrhythmias, but the mental status is generally clear and unaltered.[157]

Among indigenous North American snakes, envenomation from the coral snake and from the Mojave rattlesnake can cause postsynaptic neuromuscular blockade. This produces ptosis (often the first sign of systemic toxicity), dysarthria, dysphagia, dysesthesias, and generalized weakness, which may culminate in death from respiratory failure.[85] Other Elapidae toxins may act presynaptically to prevent acetylcholine release or postsynaptically to produce competitive or noncompetitive acetylcholine receptor blockade. The majority of snakebites in the United States, however, are caused by pit vipers, and in these bites, the hematologic effects and local soft tissue reactions are most prominent (Chap. 101).

Black widow spider venom (Chap. 102) acts at the neuromuscular junction, causing release of acetylcholine from presynaptic vesicles.[64] This produces severe skeletal muscle cramping, frequently involving the chest or abdomen, depending on the site of envenomation. Fatalities are uncommon and tend to occur primarily in small children.

Tick paralysis is thought to be caused by presynaptic block of acetylcholine release at the neuromuscular junction.[116] The characteristic picture is one of an ascending paralysis, with reflex loss and intact sensation, closely resembling Guillain-Barré syndrome (AIDP). If the tick is not discovered and removed, death may occur secondary to paralysis of respiratory muscles. An unexplained ataxic variant of this syndrome has been reported that appears to implicate a separate central cerebellar effect of the toxin elaborated by the tick[89] (Chap. 102).

A number of marine neurotoxins interfere with neuromuscular transmission. These include ciguatoxin, gymnothoratoxin, tetrodotoxin, and saxitoxin. Initial symptoms of dysesthesias of the mouth, tongue, and perioral area are common to all four toxins, indicating that poisoning of the neuromuscular junction is neither the sole, nor, in many instances, the dominant effect of these toxins. Interference with neuromuscular transmission does, however, account for the mortality, which is attributable to respiratory paralysis. Ciguatoxin, the most commonly reported vertebrate fish-borne toxin, and gymnothoratoxin, found in certain eels, produce a similar clinical picture, dominated by sensory complaints. Ciguatoxin causes a unique, unexplained symptom of cutaneous temperature inversion (ie, warm feels cold and cold feels warm). Mortality is rare in both ciguatoxin and gymnothorax poisoning. In contrast, tetrodotoxin poisoning, which is secondary to ingestion of puffer-type fish, carries a high mortality. It is characterized by oral dysesthesias, followed by a rapidly ascending paralysis, which may culminate in respiratory failure. Saxitoxin is transmitted by shellfish, usually during the summer months when a red tide is present. Following onset of the characteristic dysesthesias described above, the patient may manifest several movement disorders, including both kinetic and sustension tremor, ataxia, lower cranial neuromuscular dysfunction, and cardiorespiratory symptoms, which may be fatal. Marine toxins are discussed in greater detail in Chaps. 74 and 103.

Organic phosphorus compounds and carbamates, which are frequently used as insecticides, produce cholinergic toxicity by binding to acetylcholinesterase, resulting in muscarinic (parasympathetic), nicotinic (striated muscle and autonomic ganglia), and CNS effects. Overstimulation of nicotinic receptors in the neuromuscular junction result in depolarizing neuromuscular blockade. (Chap. 88).

Table 19–10 lists drugs that act at the neuromuscular junction according to whether they are thought to act presynaptically, postsynaptically, or simultaneously at both sites.

TABLE 19–10. Drugs and Toxins that Act at the Neuromuscular Junction (Transmission Neuropathy)

Presynaptically acting drugs and toxins
ACTH, Corticosteroids
Azathioprine
Botulinum toxins
Crotaline venom
Elapidae β-neurotoxins
Lactrodectus mactans venom
Magnesium
Tick paralysis
Verapamil

Postsynaptically acting drugs and toxins
D-Penicillamine
Neuromuscular blocking agents
Nicotine alkaloids
Organic phosphorous compounds, carbamates
Phenothiazines
Trimethaphan

Pre- and postsynaptically acting drugs
Antibiotics
  Aminoglycosides
  Clindamycin
  Polymyxins
β-Adrenergic antagonists
Chloroquine
Lithium
Phenytoin
Procainamide
Quinidine

Myopathies

Diffuse Toxic Myopathies. Myopathies can be diffuse or focal. Diffuse myopathies present clinically with weakness, which must be distinguished from neuropathic weakness because further evaluation, management, and prognosis are quite different. Myopathic weakness typically is proximal, lacks sensory findings, and preserves deep tendon reflexes unless the myopathy is very far advanced.

Drugs and toxins may cause injury to skeletal muscle through a variety of mechanisms. Table 19–11 lists The drugs and mechanisms, which are discussed in detail elsewhere.[105]

TABLE 19–11. Myopathies Caused by Drugs and Toxins

Diffuse toxic myopathies
Necrotizing myopathy
  Aminocaproic acid
  Clofibrate
  Heroin
  Ipecac
  HMG-CoA reductase inhibitors ("statins")
  Phencyclidine
  Vincristine
  Zidovidine
Autophagic myopathy
  Amiodarone
  Chloroquine
Corticosteroids
Ethanol
Hypokalemia caused by
  Barium salts
  Cathartic abuse
  Emetic abuse
  Glycyrrhizic acid
Inflammatory myopathy (myositis)
  D-Penicillamine
  Eosinophilia-myalgia syndrome (L-tryptophan)
Other drugs
  β-Adrenergic antagonists
  Cimetidine
  Cyclosporine
  Doxylamine
  Ethchlorvynol
  Penicillin
  Propylthiouracil
  Rifampin
  Sulfonamides
Envenomation (species indigenous to North America)
Snakes
  Copperhead
  Rattlesnake
  Water moccasin
Spiders
  Brown recluse spider
Insects
  Hornets
  Wasps
Microbial myotoxins
  Clostridium perfringens
Focal toxic myopathies
Needle myopathy
Opioids

Necrotizing myopathy is caused by direct toxic action of a drug on muscle. The characteristic presentation is proximal weakness and myalgia, accompanied by creatine kinase elevations and, in severe cases, myoglobinuria. Toxins associated with a necrotizing myopathy include aminocaproic acid, clofibrate, HMG-CoA reductase inhibitors, heroin, phencyclidine, syrup of ipecac, vincristine, colchicine, and zidovudine.[11]

Chloroquine and amiodarone cause a relatively mild, painless, proximal "autophagic" myopathy with normal or slightly elevated creatine kinase. Both are associated with neuropathy, which usually dominates clinically, especially in the case of amiodarone-associated demyelination.[11]

Prolonged use of corticosteroids will produce a painless proximal myopathy. In asthmatics, systemic steroids produce skeletal muscle and diaphragmatic weakness,[22] whereas inhaled steroids may produce a localized myopathy of laryngeal muscles.[160]

Alcohol is among the most common causes of toxic myopathy. The acute form, which presents as widespread myalgia and proximal weakness with creatine kinase elevations, is less common than chronic alcoholic myopathy and is associated with binge drinking. In both animal models and in humans, there is a correlation between blood ethanol levels and creatine kinase elevations.[91] The chronic form of alcoholic myopathy is painless and proximal, with a predilection for the pelvic and shoulder girdles. It is accompanied by atrophy, normal creatine kinase levels, and, frequently, an alcoholic neuropathy. The pathology is not completely understood.

Hypokalemia may produce a myopathy ranging from mild to severe. When weakness is marked, there may be associated creatine kinase elevations and loss of reflexes. Causes include gastrointestinal losses as a result of chronic vomiting or diarrhea, often related to emetic or cathartic abuse. Patients with anorexia nervosa or bulimia may develop hypokalemic myopathy secondary to self-induced vomiting. Urinary losses occur with the use of diuretics and in individuals consuming large amounts of licorice, which contains glycyrrhizic acid, an aldosterone-like substance.[151] Glycyrrhizic acid is also found in traditional Chinese herbal medicines, snuff, and chewing tobacco.

A variety of agents may produce an inflammatory myopathy or myositis. These include D-penicillamine, which may produce a polymyositislike picture in some patients.[31]

Other drugs that are rarely associated with myopathy include β-adrenergic antagonists, rifampin, sulfonamides, penicillin, propylthiouracil, cimetidine, ethchlorvynol, and cyclosporin.

Eosinophilia-myalgia syndrome, first described in 1990, is associated with ingestion of a particular preparation of the amino acid L-tryptophan. The clinical picture is that of sudden onset of severe myalgia, cutaneous involvement, and peripheral eosinophilia. An ascending polyneuropathy has also been reported in some patients. Pathologically, this is an eosinophilic myositis and fasciitis.[69]

Envenomation with snakes, spiders, and wasps may produce serious myotoxicity. Among snakes indigenous to North America, pit viper venom (*Crotalidae sp.,* including the rattlesnake, copperhead, and water moccasin) produces more severe myonecrosis and rhabdomyolysis than the more neurotoxic coral snake venom (*Elapidae sp.*). Snake envenomation is discussed in further detail in Chap. 10. Among arthropods, brown recluse spider envenomation is associated with myonecrosis and rhabdomyolysis,[51] as have stings by wasps and hornets.[141]

Of the microbial myotoxins, those elaborated by *Clostridium perfringens* are among the best characterized. At least one of these toxins causes focal myonecrosis and gas gangrene, which is rapidly progressive and frequently fatal.

Focal Myopathies. Focal myopathies are caused by the combined effects of needle insertion and the local effects of the injected drug. Although many drugs are associated with focal myopathy, opioids are among the most important, especially in patients with sickle-cell disease. Because many of these patients lack venous access, they are given repeated intramuscular injections of opioids for painful crises, causing abscess formation, fibrosis, and muscle atrophy.

SUMMARY

This chapter introduces general neurologic principles pertinent to the assessment of a patient who may have suffered a neurotoxic exposure. Neurotoxins affect the CNS and PNS in very different ways.

CNS toxins commonly cause altered mental status, which may take the form of alterations in either the *level* of consciousness, such as coma, or its *content*, such as delirium. Movement disorders are also frequent manifestations of neurotoxicity, ranging from the akinesias, of which drug-induced Parkinsonism is the most common, to the large family of dyskinesias that include tremor, chorea, dystonia, akathisia, tardive dyskinesia, myoclonus, and asterixis. Other CNS neurotoxins may cause headaches or seizures.

PNS toxins, in contrast, cause alterations in sensorimotor function of the limbs, often accompanied by depressed or absent deep tendon reflexes. Whether the neurotoxin primarily attacks the myelin sheath surrounding the peripheral nerve (myelinopathy), the axon (axonopathy), or the neuronal cell body (neuronopathy) will determine the nature and extent of neurological signs and symptoms as well as the tempo of recovery.

In general, in both the CNS and PNS, symmetric, nonfocal neurologic abnormalities are more consistent with a neurotoxic etiology than are the focal findings that are the hallmark of structural damage to the nervous system.

REFERENCES

1. Abou-Donia MB: Solvents. In: Abou-Donia MB, ed: Neurotoxicology. Boca Raton, FL, CRC Press, 1992:395–421.
2. Adams RD, Foley JM: The neurological disorder associated with liver disease. Res Publ Assoc Res Nerv Ment Dis 1953;32:198–237.
3. Adams RD, Shahani BT, Young RR: A severe pansensory familial neuropathy. Trans Am Neurol Assoc 1972;98:67–69.
4. Albers JW, Cavender GD, Levine SP, et al: Asymptomatic sensorimotor polyneuropathy in workers exposed to elemental mercury. Neurology 1982;32:1168–1174.
5. Albin RL, Albers JW, Greenberg HS, et al: Acute sensory neuropathy-neuronopathy from pyridoxine overdose. Neurology 1987;37: 1729–1732.
6. Alburges ME, Hanson GR: Differential responses by neurotensin systems in extrapyramidal and limbic structures to ibogaine and cocaine. Brain Res 1999;818:96–104.

7. Altenkirch HJ, Mager J, Stoltenburg G, et al: Toxic polyneuropathies after sniffing a glue thinner. J Neurol 1977;214:137–152.

8. Alvarez-Gómez MJ, Vaamonde J, Narbona J, et al: Parkinsonian syndrome in childhood after sodium valproate administration. Clin Neuropharmacol 1993;16:451–455.

9. Amess JA, Burman JF, Rees GM, et al: Megaloblastic haematopoiesis in patients receiving nitrous oxide. Lancet 1978;1:339–342.

10. Anderson RE, Tan WK, Martin HS, Meyer FB: Effects of glucose and PaO_2 modulation on cortical intracellular acidosis, NADH redox state, and infarction in the ischemic penumbra. Stroke 1999;30:160–170.

11. Argov Z, Mastaglia FL: Drug-induced neuromuscular disorders in man. In: Walton JN, Karpati G, Hilton-Jones D, eds: Disorders of Voluntary Muscle, 6th ed. Edinburgh, Churchill Livingstone, 1994, pp. 989–1029.

12. Aring CD: The systemic nervous affinity of triorthocresyl phosphate (Jamaican ginger palsy). Brain 1942;65:34–47.

13. Avorn J, Bohn RL, Mogun H, et al: Neuroleptic drug exposure and treatment of parkinsonism in the elderly: A case-control study. Am J Med 1995;99:48–54.

14. Avorn J, Gurwitz JH, Bohn RL, et al: Increased incidence of levodopa therapy following metoclopramide use. JAMA 1995;274:1780–1782.

15. Ayd FJ: Side effects of depot fluphenazines. Compr Psychiatry 1974;15:277–284.

16. Ayd FJ: A survey of drug-induced extrapyramidal reactions. JAMA 1961;175:1054–1060.

17. Badran RH, Weir RJ, McGuiness JB: Hypertension and headache. Scot Med J 1970;15:48–51.

18. Bank WJ, Pleasure DE, Suzuki K, et al: Thallium poisoning. Arch Neurol 1972;26:456–464.

19. Blakemore WF: Isoniazid. In: Spencer PS, Schaumburg HH, eds: Experimental and Clinical Neurotoxicology. Baltimore, Williams & Wilkins, 1980,p. 476–489.

20. Boothby JA, DeJesus PV, Rowland LP: Reversible forms of motor neuron disease. Arch Neurol 1974;31:18–23.

21. Bowman WC: Non-relaxant properties of neuromuscular blocking drugs. Br J Anaesth 1982;54:147–160.

22. Bowyer SL, La Monthe MP, Hollister JR: Steroid myopathy: Incidence and detection in a population with asthma. J Allergy Clin Immunol 1985;76:234–242.

23. Bradley WG, Hewer RL: Peripheral neuropathy due to disulfiram. BMJ 1966;2:449–450.

24. Bradley WG, Karlsson IJ, Rasso ICG: Metronidazole neuropathy. BMJ 1977;2:610–611.

25. Braude WM, Barnes TR, Gore SM: Clinical characteristics of akathisia: A systematic investigation of acute psychiatric inpatient admissions. Br J Psychiatry 1983;143:139–150.

26. Browning RG, Olson DW, Steuven HA, Mateer JR: 50% dextrose: Antidote or toxin? Ann Emerg Med 1990;19:683–687.

27. Buchthal F, Behse F: Electrophysiological studies and nerve biopsy in men exposed to lead. Br J Ind Med 1979;36:135–147.

28. Burke RE, Fahn S, Jankovic J, et al: Tardive dystonia: Late-onset and persistent dystonia caused by antipsychotic drugs. Neurology 1982;32:1335–1346.

29. Calderon-Gonzalez R, Rizzi-Hernandez H: Buckthorn polyneuropathy. N Engl J Med 1967;277:69–71.

30. Caroff SN: The neuroleptic malignant syndrome. J Clin Psychiatry 1980;41:79–83.

31. Carroll GJ, Will RK, Peter JB, et al: Penicillamine-induced polymyositis and dermatomyositis. J Rheumatol 1987;14: 995–1001.

32. Casey EB, Jellife AM, LeQuesne PM, et al: Vincristine neuropathy: Clinical and electrophysiological observations. Brain 1973;96: 69–86.

33. Cavanagh JB, Buxton PH: Trichloroethylene cranial neuropathy: Is it really a toxic neuropathy or does it activate latent herpes virus? J Neurol Neurosurg Psychiatry 1989;52:297–303.

34. Cavanagh JB, Fuller NH, Johnson HR, et al: The effects of thallium salts, with particular reference to the nervous system changes. Q J Med 1974;43:293–319.

35. Chemnitius JM, Haselmeyer KH, Gonska BD, Kreuzer H, Zech R: Indirect parasympathomimetic activity of metoclopramide: reversible inhibition of cholinesterases from human central nervous system and blood. Pharmacol Res 1996;34:65–72.

36. Chia L, Chu F: Neurological studies on polychlorinated biphenyl (PCB)-poisoned patients. Am J Ind Med 1984;5:117–126.

37. Commission on Classification and Terminology of the International League Against Epilepsy: Proposal for the revised clinical and electroencephalographic classification of epileptic seizures. Epilepsia 1981;22:489–501.

38. Cook DG, Fahn S, Brait KA: Chronic manganese intoxication. Arch Neurol 1974;30:59–64.

39. Daniel JR, Mauro VF: Extrapyramidal symptoms associated with calcium-channel blockers. Ann Pharmacother 1995;29:73–75.

40. Davis GC, Williams AC, Markey SP, et al: Chronic parkinsonism secondary to intravenous injection of meperidine analogues. Psychiatry Res 1979;1:249–254.

41. Durant NN, Marshall IG, Savage DS, et al: The neuromuscular and autonomic blocking activities of pancuronium, Org NC 45 and other pancuronium analogues. J Pharm Pharmacol 1979;31:831–836.

42. Edelman RR, Warach S: Magnetic resonance imaging (first of two parts). N Engl J Med 1993;328:708–716.

43. Ellis FG: Acute polyneuritis after nitrofurantoin therapy. Lancet 1962;2:1136–1138.

44. Engel J Jr, Troupin AS, Crandall PH, et al: Recent developments in the diagnosis and therapy of epilepsy. Ann Intern Med 1982;97: 584–598.

45. Feldman RG, White RF, Currie JN, et al: Long-term follow-up after single toxic exposure to trichloroethylene. Am J Ind Med 1985;8: 119–126.

46. Filley CM, Graff-Richard NR, Lacy JR, et al: Neurologic manifestations of podophyllin toxicity. Neurology 1982;32:308–311.

47. Finelli PF, Morgan TF, Yaar I, et al: Ethylene oxide induced polyneuropathy. A clinical and electrophysiologic study. Arch Neurol 1983;40:419–421.

48. Fisher CM, Adams RD: Diphtheritic polyneuritis: A pathological study. J Neuropathol Exp Neurol 1956;15:243–268.

49. Folstein MF, Folstein SE, McHugh PR: The "mini-mental state": A practical method for grading the cognitive state of patients for the clinician. J Psychiatry Res 1975;12:189–198.

50. Froomes PR, Stewart MR: A reversible parkinsonian syndrome and hepatotoxicity following addition of carbamazepine to sodium valproate. Aust N Z J Med 1994;24:413–414.

51. Gabow PA, Kaehny WD, Kelleher SP: The spectrum of rhabdomyolysis. Medicine (Baltimore) 1982;61:141–152.

52. Gajkowski K, Werkowicz-Pelczyk D, Masiak I, et al. Neurologic symptoms in lithium poisoning. Neurol Neurochir Pol 1987;21: 412–414.

53. Ganzini L, Casey DE, Hoffman WF, et al: The prevalence of metoclopramide-induced tardive dyskinesia and acute extrapyramidal movement disorders. Arch Intern Med 1993;153:1469–1475.

54. Ganzini L, Heintz R, Hoffman WF, et al: Acute extrapyramidal syndromes in neuroleptic-treated elders: A pilot study. J Geriatr Psychiatry Neurol 1991;4:222–225.

55. García-Ruiz P, García de Yébenes, J, Jiménez-Jiménez FJ, et al: Parkinsonism associated to calcium channel blockers (CCB). A prospective follow-up study. Clin Neuropharmacol 1992;15:19–26.

56. García-Albea E, Jiménez-Jiménez FJ, Ayuso-Peralta L, et al: Parkinsonism unmasked by verapamil. Clin Neuropharmacol 1993;16: 263–265.

57. Garland TO, Patterson MW: Six cases of acrylamide poisoning. BMJ 1967;4:134–138.

58. Gawin FH, Ellinwood EH: Cocaine and other stimulants: Actions, abuse and treatment. N Engl J Med 1988;318:1173–1182.

59. Gershanik OS: Drug-induced movement disorders. Curr Opin Neurol Neurosurg 1993;6:369–376.
60. Gibby WA, Zimmerman RA: X-ray computed tomography. In: Mazziotta JC, Gilman S, eds: Clinical Brain Imaging: Principles and Applications. Philadelphia, FA Davis, 1992:3.
61. Gill HS, DeVane CL, Risch SC: Extrapyramidal symptoms associated with cyclic antidepressant treatment: A review of the literature and consolidating hypotheses. J Clin Psychopharmacol 1997;17:377–389.
62. Gilman S: Advances in neurology, Part I. N Engl J Med 1992;326:1608–1616.
63. Gilman S: Advances in neurology, Part II. N Engl J Med 1992;326:1671–1676.
64. Gorio A, Mauro A: Reversibility and mode of action of black widow spider venom on the vertebrate neuromuscular junction. J Gen Physiol 1979;73:245–263.
65. Griffin JW, Watson DF: Axonal transport in neurological disease. Ann Neurol 1988;23:3–13.
66. Gucer G, Vierstein: Long-term intracranial pressure recording in the management of pseudotumor cerebri. J. Neurosurg 1978;49:256–263.
67. Gutmann L, Martin JD, Welton W: Dapsone motor neuropathy: an axonal disease. Neurology (Minneap) 1976;26:514–516.
68. He F, Lu B, Zhang S, et al: Chronic allyl chloride poisoning: An epidemiological, clinical, toxicological, and neuropathological study. G Ital Med Lav Ergon 1985;7:5–15.
69. Hertzman PA, Blevins WL, Mayer J, et al: Association of the eosinophilia-myalgia syndrome with the ingestion of tryptophan. N Engl J Med 1990;322:869–873.
70. Heyer EJ, Simpson DM, Bodis-Wollner I, et al: Nitrous oxide: Clinical and electrophysiologic investigation of neurologic complications. Neurology 1986;36:1618–1622.
71. Holroyd S, Smith D: Disabling parkinsonism due to lithium: A case report [letter]. J Geriatr Psychiatry Neurol 1995;8:118–119.
72. Hyman NM, Dennis PD, Sinclair KG: Tremor due to sodium valproate. Neurology 1979;29:1177–1180.
73. Inouye SK, van Dyck CH, Alessi CA, et al: Clarifying confusion: The confusion assessment method. Ann Intern Med 1990;113:941–948.
74. Jansen Steur ENH: Increase of Parkinson disability after fluoxetine medication. Neurology 1993;43:211–213.
75. Jiménez-Jiménez FJ, Cabrera-Valdivia F, Ayuiso-Peralta L, et al: Persistent parkinsonism and tardive dyskinesia-induced by clebopride. Mov Disord 1993;8:246–247.
76. Jiménez-Jiménez FJ, Garcia-Ruis PJ, Molina JA: Drug-induced movement disorders. Drug Safety 1997;16:180–204.
77. Jiménez-Jiménez FJ, Ortí-Pareja M, Ayuso-Eralta L, et al: Drug-induced parkinsonism in a movement disorders unit. A four-year survey. Parkinsonism Rel Disord 1996;2:145–149.
78. Jiménez-Jiménez FJ, Tejeiro J, Martínez-Junquera G, et al: Parkinsonism exacerbated by paroxetine. Neurology 1994;45:2406.
79. Jones KM, Mulkern RV, Schwartz RB, et al: Fast spin-echo MR imaging of the brain and spine: Current concepts. AJR Am J Roentgenol 1992;158:1313–1320.
80. Kang UJ, Burke RE, Fahn S: Natural history and treatment of tardive dystonia. Mov Disord 1986;1:193–208.
81. Kantarjian AD, Shaheen AS: Methyl bromide poisoning with nervous system manifestations resembling polyneuropathy. Neurology (Minneap) 1963;13:1054–1058.
82. Karas BJ, Wilder BJ, Hammond EJ, et al: Treatment of valproate tremors. Neurology 1983;33:1380–1382.
83. Karas BJ, Wilder BJ, Hammond EJ, et al: Valproate tremors. Neurology 1982;32:428–432.
84. Katrak SM, Pollock M, O'Brien CP, et al: Clinical and morphological features of gold neuropathy. Brain 1980;103:671–693.
85. Kitchens CS, Van Mierop LH: Envenomation by the eastern coral snake (Micrurus fulvius fulvius). JAMA 1987;258:1615–1618.
86. Koller WC: Diagnosis and treatment of tremors. Neurol Clin 1984;2:499–514.
87. Krinke G, Schaumburg HH, Spencer P, et al: Pyridoxine megavitaminosis produces degeneration of peripheral sensory neurons (sensory neuronopathy) in the dog. Neurotoxicology 1980;2:13–21.
88. Kurlan R, Hamill R, Shoulson I: Neuroleptic malignant syndrome. Clin Neuropharmacol 1984;7:109–120.
89. Lagos JC, Thies RE: Tick paralysis without muscle weakness. Arch Neurol 1969;21:471–474.
90. Lambert MT, Trutia C, Petty F: Extrapyramidal adverse effects associated with sertraline. Prog Neuropsychopharmacol Biol Psychiatry 1998;22:741–748.
91. Lane RJM, Radoff FM: Alcohol and serum creatine kinase levels. Ann Neurol 1981;10:581–583.
92. Langston JW, Ballard P: Parkinsonism induced by MPTP: Implication for treatment and the pathogenesis of PD. Can J Neurol Sci 1984;11:160–165.
93. Langston JW, Ballard P, Tetrud JW, et al: Chronic parkinsonism in humans due to a product of meperidine-analog synthesis. Science 1983;219:979–980.
94. Leavitt S, Tyler HR: Studies in asterixis. Arch Neurol 1964;10:360–368.
95. Leggat PO: Ethionamide neuropathy. Tubercle 1962;43:95.
96. LeQuesne PM, Damluji SF, Rustam H: Electrophysiological studies of peripheral nerves in patients with organic mercury poisoning. J Neurol Neurosurg Psychiatry 1974;37:333–339.
97. LeQuesne PM, McLeod JG: Peripheral neuropathy following a single exposure to arsenic. J Neurol Sci 1977;32:437–451.
98. Lewitt P: The neurotoxicity of the rat poison Vacor. N. Engl J Med 1980;302:73–77.
99. Lipowski J: Update on delirium. Psychiatr Clin North Am 1992;15:335–346.
100. Lipton RB, Appel SC, Dutcher JP, et al: Taxol produces a predominantly sensory neuropathy. Neurology 1989;39:368–373.
101. Lovelace RE, Horwitz SJ: Peripheral neuropathy in long-term diphenylhydantoin therapy. Arch Neurol 1968;18:69–77.
102. Lufkin RB: Magnetic resonance imaging. In: Mazziotta JC, Gilman S, eds: Clinical Brain Imaging: Principles and Applications. Philadelphia, FA Davis, 1992, p. 39–68.
103. Marsden CD, Tarsy D, Baldessarini RJ: Spontaneous and drug-induced movement disorders in psychotic patients. In: Benson DF, Blemer D, eds: Psychiatric Aspects of Neurologic Disease. New York, Grune & Stratton, 1975, p. 219–226.
104. Masey EW, Goodman JC, Stewart C, et al: Unilateral asterixis: Motor integrative dysfunction in focal vascular disease. Neurology 1979;29:1180–1182.
105. Mastaglia RL, Walton LWD, eds: Skeletal Muscle Pathology, 2nd ed. Edinburgh, Churchill Livingstone, 1992, pp. 511, 599.
106. McCann UD, Wong DF, Yokoi F, et al: Reduced striatal dopamine transporter density in abstinent methamphetamine and methcathinone users: Evidence from positron emission tomography studies with [^{11}C]WIN-35,428. J Neurosci 1998;18:8417–8422.
107. McDonald WI, Kochen RS: Diphtheritic neuropathy. In: Dyck PJ, Thomas PK, Lambert EH, eds: Peripheral Neuropathy, Vol 2. Philadelphia, WB Saunders, 1984, p. 2010–2020.
108. Melgaard B, Hansen HS, Kamieniecka Z, et al: Misonidazole neuropathy: A clinical electrophysiological and histological study. Ann Neurol 1982;12:10–17.
109. Mena MA, Garcia de Yebenes MJ, et al: Effects of calcium antagonists on the dopamine system. Clin Neuropharmacol 1995;18:410–426.
110. Merigan T, Skowron G, Bozette SA, et al: Circulating p24 antigen levels and responses to dideoxycytidine in human immunodeficiency virus (HIV) infections. Ann Intern Med 1989;110:189–194.
111. Meyer-Lindenberg A, Krausnick B: Tardive dyskinesia in a neuroleptic-naive patient with bipolar-I disorder: Persistent exacerbation after lithium intoxication. Mov Disord 1997;12:1108–1109.

112. Montgomery BM, Pinner CA: Transient hypoglycemic hemiplegia. Arch Intern Med 1964;114:680–684.

113. Morgante L, Rocca WA, Di Rosa AE, et al: Prevalence of Parkinson's disease and other types of parkinsonism: A door-to-door survey in three Sicilian municipalities. The Sicilian Neuro-Epidemiologic Study (SNES) group. Neurology 1992;42:1901–1907.

114. Morris HH, McCormick WF, Reinarz JA: Neuroleptic malignant syndrome. Arch Neurol 1980;37:462–463.

115. Munetz MR, Cornes CL: Distinguishing akathisia and tardive dyskinesia: A review of the literature. J Clin Psychopharmacol 1983;3: 343–350.

116. Murnaghan MF: Site and mechanism of tick paralysis. Science 1960; 131:418–419.

117. Muscettola G, Barbato G, Pampallona S, Casiello M, Bollini P: Extrapyramidal syndromes in neuroleptic-treated patients: Prevalence, risk factors, and association with tardive dyskinesia. J Clin Psychopharmacol 1999;19:203–208.

118. Nair VS, LeBrun M, Kass I: Peripheral neuropathy associated with ethambutol. Chest 1980;77:98–100.

119. Neale R, Gerhardt S, Leibman JM: Effects of dopamine agonists, catecholamine depletors and cholinergic and GABAergic drugs on acute dyskinesias in squirrel monkeys. Psychopharmacology (Berl) 1984;82:20–26.

120. Negrotti A, Calzetti S: A long-term follow-up study of cinnarizine- and flunarizine-induced parkinsonism. Mov Disord 1997;12: 107–110.

121. Nover R: Persistent neuropathy following chronic use of glutethimide. Clin Pharmacol Ther 1967;8:283–285.

122. Oleson J: The classification and diagnosis of headache disorders. Neurol Clin 1990;8:793–799.

123. Onofrj M, Thomas A, Paci C: Reversible parkinsonism induced by prolonged treatment with valproate and lithium. J Neurol 1998;245: 794–796.

124. Paton WDM: The effects of muscle relaxants other than muscular relaxation. Anesthesiology 1959;20:453–463.

125. Pellissier JF, Pouget J, Cros D, et al: Peripheral neuropathy induced by amiodarone chlorohydrate. J Neurol Sci 1984;63:251–266.

126. Petrera JE, Fledelius HC, Trojaborg W: Serial pattern evoked potential recording in a case of toxic optic neuropathy due to ethambutol. Electroencephalogr Clin Neurophysiol 1988;71:146–149.

127. Plum F, Posner J: The Diagnosis of Stupor and Coma, 3rd ed. Philadelphia, FA Davis, 1982, pp. 2, 64, 255.

128. Prien RF: Lithium in the treatment of affective disorders. Clin Neuropharmacol 1978;3:113–131.

129. Raskin NH, Fishman RA: Pyridoxine-deficiency neuropathy due to hydralazine. N Engl J Med 1965;273:1182–1185.

130. Riggs JE, Schochet SS Jr, Gutman L, et al: Chronic human colchicine neuropathy and myopathy. Arch Neurol 1986;43: 521–523.

131. Roelofs RI, Hruskesky W, Rogin J, et al: Peripheral sensory neuropathy and cisplatin chemotherapy. Neurology 1984;34:934–938.

132. Rosebush PI, Mazurek MF: Neurologic side effects in neuroleptic-naive patients treated with haloperidol or risperidone. Neurology 1999;52:782–785.

133. Roth G: The origin of fasciculations. Ann Neurol 1982;12:542–547.

134. Rothner AD, Morris HH III: Generalized status epilepticus. In: Lueders H, Lesser R, eds: Epilepsy: Electroclinical Syndrome. New York, Springer-Verlag, 1987, p. 207–222.

135. Said G, Bathien N, Cesaro P: Peripheral neuropathies and tremor. Neurology 1982;32:480–485.

136. Saper JR, Silberstein SS, Gordon CD, Hamel RL: Handbook of Headache Management. Baltimore, Williams & Wilkins, 1993, pp. 6, 16.

137. Schaumburg HH, Berger AR, Thomas PK: Disorders of Peripheral Nerves, 2nd ed. Philadelphia, FA Davis, 1992, pp. 3, 257, 274, 314.

138. Schaumburg H, Kaplan J, Windelbank A, et al: Sensory neuropathy from pyridoxine abuse. N Engl J Med 1983;309:445–448.

139. Schooler NR, Kane JM: Research diagnoses for tardive dyskinesia. Arch Gen Psychiatry 1982;39:486–487.

140. Shahani BT, Young RR: Asterixis: A disorder of the neural mechanisms underlying sustained muscular contraction. In: Shahani M, ed: The Motor System: Neurophysiology and Muscle Mechanisms. New York, Elsevier, 1976:301.

141. Shilkin KB, Chen BT, Khoo OT: Rhabdomyolysis caused by hornet venom. BMJ 1972;1:156–157.

142. Shiraki H: Neuropathological aspects of organic mercury intoxication, including Minamata disease. In: Vinken PJ, Bruyn GW, eds: Handbook of Clinical Neurology, Vol. 36. Amsterdam, North-Holland, 1979, p. 83–145.

143. Simon RP: Alcohol and seizures [editorial]. N Engl J Med 1988; 319:715–716.

144. Spencer PS, Schaumburg HH: Central-peripheral distal axonopathy: The pathology of dying-back polyneuropathies. In: Zimmerman HM, ed: Progress in Neuropathology, Vol. 3. New York, Grune & Stratton, 1976, p. 253–295.

145. Spencer PS, Schaumburg HH, Sabri MI, et al: The enlarging view of hexacarbon neurotoxicity. Crit Rev Toxicol 1980;7:279–356.

146. Sobue G, Pleasure D: Experimental lead neuropathy: Inorganic lead inhibits proliferation but not differentiation of Schwann cells. Ann Neurol 1985;17:462–468.

147. Strub RL, Black FW: The Mental Status Examination in Neurology, 2nd ed. Philadelphia, FA Davis, 1985, p. 43.

148. Teasdale G, Jennett B: Assessment of coma and impaired consciousness. Lancet 1974;2:81–84.

149. Tyrer P, Alexander MS, Regan A, et al: An extrapyramidal syndrome after lithium therapy. Br J Psychiatry 1980;136:191–194.

150. Umez-Eronini EM, Eronini EA: Chloroquine-induced involuntary movements. BMJ 1977;1, pp. 945–946.

151. Valeriano J, Tucker P, Kattah J: An unusual cause of hypokalemic muscle weakness. Neurology (Cleveland) 1983;33:1242–1243.

152. Van Putten T: Lithium-induced disabling tremor. Psychosomatics 1978;19:27–31.

153. Victor M: Polyneuropathy due to nutritional deficiency and alcoholism. In: Dyck PJ, Thomas PK, Lambert EH, Bunfe RP, eds: Peripheral Neuropathy, 2nd edition. Philadelphia, WB Saunders, 1984, vol 1, pp. 1–43.

154. Victor M, Adams RD, Mancall E: A restricted form of cerebellar degeneration occurring in alcoholic patients. Arch Neurol 1959;1: 579–688.

155. Vigliani EC: Carbon disulfide poisoning in viscose rayon factories. Br J Ind Med 1954;11:235–244.

156. Weiner WJ, Lang AE: Movement Disorders: A Comprehensive Survey. Mt. Kisco, NY, Futura, 1989, p. 600.

157. Weinstein L: Tetanus. N Engl J Med 1973;289:1293–1296.

158. Westwood SC, Hanson GR: Effects of stimulants of abuse on extrapyramidal and limbic neuropeptide Y systems. J Pharmacol Exp Ther 1999;288:1160–1166.

159. Wettstein A: The origin of fasciculations in motor neuron disease. Ann Neurol 1979;5:295–300.

160. Williams AJ, Baghat MS, Stableforth DE, et al: Dysphonia caused by inhaled steroids: Recognition of a characteristic laryngeal abnormality. Thorax 1983;38:813–821.

161. Windebank AJ, Blexrud MD: Residual ethylene oxide in hollow fiber hemodialysis units is neurotoxic in vitro. Ann Neurol 1989;26: 63–68.

162. Windebank AJ, McCall JT, Dyck PJ: Metal neuropathy. In: Dyck PJ, Thomas PK, Lambert EH, Bunge RP, eds: Peripheral Neuropathy, Vol. 2, 2nd ed. Philadelphia, WB Saunders, 1984, p. 2150–2155.

163. Yiannikas C, Pollard JD, McLeod JG: Nitrofurantoin neuropathy. Aust N Z J Med 1981;11:400–405.

164. Yousef G, Ryan WJ, Lambert T, Pitt B, Kellett J: A preliminary report: A new scale to identify the pseudodementia syndrome. Int J Geriatr Psychiatry 1998;13:389–399.

CHAPTER 20

RESPIRATORY PRINCIPLES

Robert S. Hoffman

Essential Abbreviations

Po_2	Partial pressure of oxygen (in mm Hg; 1 mm Hg = 1 torr)
PAo_2	Alveolar Po_2
Pao_2	Arterial Po_2
Pco_2	Partial pressure of carbon dioxide (in mm Hg)
O_2 Sat	Hemoglobin oxygen saturation (in percent)
Fio_2	Percent oxygen in inspired air
CO	Carbon monoxide
COHb	Carboxyhemoglobin
MetHb	Methemoglobin

The primary function of the lung is to exchange gases. Specifically, this role can be divided into the transport of oxygen (O_2) into the blood, and the elimination of carbon dioxide (CO_2) from the blood. In addition, the lungs serve as minor organs of metabolism and elimination for a number of compounds, a source of insensible water loss, and a means of temperature regulation. Cellular oxygen utilization is dependent on many factors, including respiratory drive, percent oxygen in inspired air, airway patency, chest wall and pulmonary compliance, diffusing capacity, ventilation/perfusion mismatch, hemoglobin content, hemoglobin oxygen loading and unloading, cellular oxygen uptake, and cardiac output. Toxins have the unique ability to inhibit or impair each of these factors necessary for oxygen utilization and result in respiratory dysfunction. This chapter illustrates how toxins interact with the mechanisms of gas exchange and oxygen utilization, and concludes with a practical approach to assessing the poisoned patient.

PULMONARY MANIFESTATIONS OF TOXIN EXPOSURES

Respiratory Drive

Respiratory rate and depth are regulated by the need to maintain a normal Pco_2 and pH.[39] Most of the control for ventilation occurs at the level of the medulla, although this is modulated both by involuntary input from the pons and voluntary input from the higher cortices. Changes in Pco_2 are measured primarily by a central chemoreceptor, located near the exit for cranial nerves IX and X, which measures cerebral spinal fluid (CSF) pH, and secondarily by peripheral chemoreceptors in the carotid and aortic bodies, which actually measure Pco_2. Input with regard to Po_2 is obtained from carotid and aortic chemoreceptors. Stretch receptors relay information about pulmonary dynamics, such as the volume and pressure.

Toxins can affect respiratory drive in one of several ways: direct suppression of the respiratory center; alteration in the response of chemoreceptors to changes in Pco_2; direct stimulation of the respiratory center; increase in metabolic demands as a result of agitation or fever, which, in turn, increases total body oxygen consumption; or indirectly as a result of the creation of acid-base disorders. For example, opioids (Chap. 62) depress respiration by decreasing the responsiveness of chemoreceptors to CO_2 and by direct suppression of the pontine and medullary respiratory centers.[25,70,98] Any toxin that causes a decreased respiratory drive or a decreased level of consciousness can produce bradypnea (a decreased respiratory rate), hypopnea (a decreased tidal volume), or both, resulting in hypoventilation (Chap. 17).

Methylxanthines, cocaine, and other sympathomimetics may cause an increase in respiratory drive as well as an increase in oxygen consumption. Salicylates produce hyperventilation by both central and peripheral effects (ie, respiratory alkalosis and acidemia; Chaps. 24, 33, 39, and 67). The net consequence of increased respiratory drive, increased oxygen consumption, or metabolic acidosis is the generation of either tachypnea (an elevated respiratory rate), hyperpnea (an increased tidal volume), or both. Whether alone or in combination, tachypnea and hyperpnea produce hyperventilation. Toxins that commonly produce hypo- or hyperventilation are listed in Tables 20–1 and 20–2.

Decreased Inspired Fio_2

Barometric pressure at sea level ranges near 760 mm Hg. At this pressure, 21% of ambient air is comprised of oxygen (Fio_2 = 21%), and after subtracting for the water vapor normally present in the lungs, the PAo_2 is about 150 mm Hg. Any reduction in Fio_2 decreases the PAo_2, thereby producing signs and symptoms of hypoxemia (a low Pao_2). At an Fio_2 of 12–16%, patients experience tachypnea, tachycardia, and impaired coordination. A further decrease to an Fio_2 of 10–14% produces severe fatigue, and decreases to between 6 and 10% are associated with nausea, vomiting, and lethargy. An Fio_2 of less than 6% is incompatible with life.[64]

This effect on Fio_2 is typically observed as elevation increases above sea level, because barometric pressure falls. By 18,000 feet, barometric pressure is only 380 mm Hg, and the PAo_2 falls to below 70 mm Hg. At 63,000 feet, the barometric pressure falls to

TABLE 20–1. Drugs and Toxins that Produce Hypoventilation

Baclofen	Ethanol	Poison hemlock
Barbiturates	γ-Hydroxybutyrate	(coniine)
Botulinum toxin	Neuromuscular blocking	Sedative-hypnotics
Carbamates	agents	Strychnine
Clonidine	Nicotine	Tetanus toxin
Colchicine	Opioids	Tetrodotoxin
Cyclic antidepressants	Organic phosphorus	Toxic alcohols
Elapid envenomation	agents	
Electrolyte abnormalities		

TABLE 20–3. Simple Asphyxiants

Argon	Hydrogen
Carbon dioxide	Methane
Ethane	Nitrogen
Helium	Propane

47 mm Hg, a level where the PAO_2 equals 0 mm Hg. Although it is important to remember this relationship, altitude-induced decreases in FIO_2 are rarely important in clinical medicine, even in commercial airline flights, where the cabins are pressurized to a maximum of several thousand feet above sea level. However, in closed or low-lying spaces, oxygen may be replaced or displaced by other gases that intrinsically have no direct toxicity. Common examples of these gases, referred to as simple asphyxiants (Table 20–3), are found alone or in combination with more toxic gases. Because they have little or no toxicity other than their ability to replace oxygen, removal of the victim from exposure and administration of supplemental oxygen are curative if permanent injury due to hypoxia has not already developed (Chap. 95).

The potential magnitude of toxicity from simple asphyxiants was best exemplified by the disasters in Cameroon near the Lakes of Monoun and Nyos, in 1984 and 1986, respectively. For unclear reasons, Lake Nyos, a volcanic lake, released a cloud of carbon dioxide (CO_2) gas of approximately a quarter of a million tons. Because CO_2 is 1.5 times heavier than air, the gas cloud flowed into the surrounding low-lying valleys, killing by asphyxia more than 1700 people, and affecting countless more people because of hypoxia. Most survivors recovered without complications.[4,29,50]

Chest Wall

Hypoventilation can occur as a result of a decrease in either respiratory rate or tidal volume. Thus, even when the stimulus to breath is normal, adequate ventilation is dependent on the coordination and function of the muscles of the diaphragm and chest wall. Changes in this function can result in hypoventilation by two separate mechanisms; both muscle weakness and muscle rigidity may impair the patient's ability to expand the chest wall. Toxicologic causes of muscle weakness include botulinum toxin,[80] electrolyte abnormalities such as hypokalemia[51,99] or hypermagnesemia,[22] organic phosphorous compounds,[62,81] and neuromuscular blocking agents.[8,44] Patients with hypoventilation caused by muscle weak-

ness respond well to assisted ventilation and correction of the underlying problem (Chaps. 24, 54, 75, and 89). Chest-wall rigidity impairing ventilation can occur in strychnine poisoning,[9,55] tetanus,[14,48,86] and fentanyl use[13,16] (Chaps. 62 and 90). Often these patients are difficult to ventilate despite intubation and may require muscle relaxants, neuromuscular blocking agents, or naloxone (for fentanyl).

Airway Patency

The airway itself may be compromised in several ways. As a patient's mental status becomes impaired, the airway is often obstructed by the tongue.[33] Alternatively, drug- or toxin-induced vomitus, or aspiration of activated charcoal or a foreign body, can directly obstruct the trachea or major bronchi with resultant hypoxia.[33,58,73,79] Obstruction may also result from increased secretions produced during organic phosphorous compound poisoning. Laryngospasm may occur either as a manifestation of systemic reactions, such as anaphylaxis, as a result of edema from thermal or caustic injury[59] (Chaps. 87 and 96), or as a direct response to an irritant gas (Chap. 95). Similarly, the tongue can become swollen in response to thermal[59] or caustic injury or toxic exposure to plants such as *Dieffenbachia spp.*,[19] or as a result of angioedema from drugs such as angiotensin-converting enzyme inhibitors[24] (Chaps. 51, 78, 87, and 96). Regardless of the mechanism, upper airway obstruction results in hypoventilation, hypoxemia, and hypercapnia (hypercarbia) with the persistence of a normal A-a gradient (see discussion of A-a gradients later). Upper airway obstruction is often acute and severe and requires immediate therapy to prevent further clinical compromise. Bronchospasm may be a manifestation of anaphylaxis, as well as exposure to pyrolyzed cocaine,[35,78] smoke,[59] irritant gases[36,42,68] (Table 20–4), or dust (eg, cotton in byssinosis), or as a result of occupational asthma[54] and hypersensitivity pneumonitis[102] (Chaps. 95 and 96).

Airway collapse may result from pneumothorax caused by barotrauma, which more commonly results from the manner of administration of illicit drugs than from actual drug overdose (Chap. 109). One remarkable form of pneumothorax, or hydropneumothorax, results from an attempt to inject heroin or cocaine into the internal jugular vein, commonly referred to as a "pocket shot." A patient who attempts to direct a needle into the depression in the neck lateral to the sternocleidomastoid above the clavicle may instead lacerate the apical pleura. A predominance of left-sided pneumothoraces from pocket shots probably is related to the fact that most people are right-handed.[33] Barotrauma may also result from nasal insufflation or inhalation of drugs. This form of barotrauma occurs most often in cocaine (particularly in the form of "crack") and marijuana users, who either smoke or insufflate these drugs and then perform prolonged Valsalva maneuvers in an attempt to enhance the drug's effects[6,11,66,82,100] (Chaps. 67 and 71). The increased airway pressure leads to rupture of an alveolar bleb, and free air dissects along the peribronchial paths into the mediastinum and pleural cavities. The use of nitrous oxide is also noted

TABLE 20–2. Drugs and Toxins that Produce Hyperventilation

Amphetamines	Gyromitra mushrooms	Paraldehyde
Anticholinergics	(monomethyl	Pentachlorophenol
Caffeine	hydrazine)	Phenformin
Camphor	Hydrogen sulfide	Progesterone
Carbon monoxide	Iron	Salicylates
Cocaine	Isoniazid	Sodium monofluo-
Cyanide	Methanol	roacetate
Dinitrophenol	Metformin	Theobromine
Ethanol (ketoacidosis)	Methemoglobin inducers	Theophylline
Ethylene glycol		

TABLE 20–4. **Irritant Gases**

Ammonia	Isocyanates
Chloramine	Nitrogen dioxide
Chlorine	Ozone
Chloracetophenone (CN)	Phosgene
Chlorobenzylidene-malonitrile (CS)	Phosphine
Fluorine	Sulfur dioxide
Hydrogen chloride	

to cause barotrauma.[46] The medical profession has not been immune to this widespread abuse. Indeed, a study of medical and dental students from the 1970s found that between 8.5% and 20% of each enrolled class used nitrous oxide in social situations.[46] Although people who have access to nitrous oxide in the hospital or laboratory may siphon the agent from tanks meant for inhalation, at parties they inhale nitrous oxide that is used as a propellant in whipped cream cans. Tremendous pressure generated by the escaping gas is then transmitted to the airways, sometimes resulting in severe barotrauma (Chap. 53).

Under these circumstances a chest tube is inserted for a pneumothorax greater than 10–20% and/or when gas exchange is compromised.[30,37] Alternatively, insertion of a 14-gauge catheter into the pleural space with aspiration of the air may successfully treat the pneumothorax and avoid the occasional morbidity associated with chest tube insertion.[30] When hypoxia, hypotension, absent breath sounds, and tracheal deviation suggest tension pneumothorax, immediate intervention is required, prior to radiographic confirmation.

Ventilation-Perfusion Mismatch

Ventilation-perfusion (V/Q) mismatch is manifested at the extremes by aeration of the lung without arterial blood supply (as in pulmonary embolism from injected contaminants) and by a normal blood supply to the lung without any ventilation. Impaired blood supply to a normal lung and normal blood supply to an inadequately ventilated lung constitute an infinite number of gradations that exist between the extremes. The normal response to regional variations in ventilation is to shunt blood away from an area of lung that is poorly ventilated, thereby preferentially delivering blood to an area of the lung where gas exchange is more efficient. An hypoxia-induced reduction in local nitric oxide production appears to be responsible for the regional vasoconstriction that occurs.[1] This effect, commonly known as hypoxic pulmonary vasoconstriction, is best described in patients with chronic obstructive lung disease and facilitates compensation for the V/Q mismatch associated with that disorder. It is unclear whether toxin-induced alterations in pulmonary nitric oxide production are significant determinants in the V/Q mismatch that occurs in poisoning; research in this area is just beginning.

Toxin-induced V/Q mismatch more commonly results from perfusion of an abnormally ventilated lung, as may occur following aspiration of gastric contents, a frequent complication of many types of poisoning.[33] Although alterations in consciousness and loss of protective airway reflexes are predisposing factors, certain toxins, such as hydrocarbons, directly result in aspiration pneumonitis due to their specific characteristics of volatility, viscosity, and surface tension[32] (Chap. 86).

The diagnosis of aspiration pneumonitis often relies on the chest radiograph for confirmation. The location of the infiltrate de-

pends significantly on the patient's position when the aspiration occurred. Most commonly, aspiration occurs in the right mainstem bronchus, because the angle with the carina is not as acute as it is on the left side. When aspiration occurs in the supine position, the subsequent infiltrate is usually manifest in the posterior segments of the upper lobe and superior segments of the lower lobe. Aspiration not only involves vomitus; secretions, activated charcoal, teeth, dentures, food, and other foreign bodies are also frequently aspirated.

Diffusing Capacity Abnormalities

Severe impairment in diffusing capacity commonly results from local injury to the lungs in disorders such as interstitial pneumonia, aspiration, toxic inhalations, and near drowning, and from systemic effects of sepsis, trauma, and various other medical disorders.[5] When this process is acute and associated with clinical criteria including rales, hypoxemia (unspecified degree), and bilateral involvement on a chest radiograph demonstrating a normal heart size, it has been traditionally referred to as *noncardiogenic pulmonary edema*; throughout this chapter and text, however, the term *acute lung injury* (ALI) is used instead, which reflects current nomenclature.[5] ALI is the presence of increased intra-alveolar fluid in the lungs with a normal cardiac output.[74,103] More rigid criteria, such as a PaO_2/FIO_2 ratio <300 mm Hg (regardless of positive end-expiratory pressure (PEEP)), bilateral infiltrates on the chest radiograph, and either the pulmonary artery wedge pressure ≤18 mm Hg or no clinical evidence of left atrial hypertension, are used to define the ALI.[5] When these same criteria are met, but the patient's PaO_2/FIO_2 ratio is <200 mm Hg (regardless of PEEP), the term *acute respiratory distress syndrome* (ARDS) is used.[5,52] Approximately 150,000 Americans develop ARDS annually, many as a result of toxins; ARDS has a fatality rate of almost 50%.[12]

Commonly, patients are chronically exposed to toxins associated with reduced diffusing capacity by smoking tobacco and other substances, or working with asbestos, silica, and coal, which cause slow pulmonary fibrosis or promote emphysema. More recent work emphasizes the ability of chronically smoked cocaine to alter pulmonary function.[88] Acutely, ALI from opioids, salicylates, or phosgene and delayed severe fibrosis from paraquat can cause profound alterations in diffusion[63,74,103] (Chaps. 33, 62, 91, and 95). Associated parenchymal damage is almost always present and causes both reduction in lung volumes and V/Q mismatch. Intravenous injection of street drug contaminants such as talc[67] and septic emboli from right-sided endocarditis[45] may result in isolated vascular defects with reduction in diffusion capacity. Similarly, cocaine-induced pulmonary spasm can obstruct vascular channels and alter pulmonary function, creating V/Q mismatch.[18]

ALI with or without progression to ARDS is a common occurrence from poisoning. The edema fluid (and the resulting hypoxia, pulmonary rales, and radiographic abnormalities) may develop in part because of increased permeability of the alveolar and capillary basement membrane.[12,17,57,74,103] Proteinaceous fluid leaks from the capillaries into the alveoli and interstitium of the lung. Several mechanisms are proposed as the cause for ALI, although there is no single unifying mechanism for all of the drugs that have been implicated. Acute lung injury may result from exposure to toxins that produce hypoventilation by at least three different mechanisms: hypoxia may injure the vascular endothelial cells; autoregulatory vascular redistribution may cause localized capillary hypertension; or alveolar microtrauma may occur as alveolar units collapse, only to be reopened suddenly during reventilation.[74,103] These and other events may activate neutrophils and release inflammatory cytokines.[97] Other agents may be directly toxic to the capillary epithelial cells or may be partly responsible for the release of vasoactive substances.[74,103] The effects of salicylates and other nonsteroidal anti-inflammatory agents may be mediated via effects on prostaglandin synthesis. Finally, sympathomimetic stimulants may cause "neurogenic" pulmonary edema, which is thought to be mediated by massive catecholamine discharge. Elevated catecholamine levels are also noted in experimental opioid overdose, possibly supplying a link between hypoxia, hypercarbia, and the catecholamine hypothesis of acute lung injury.[61]

In the 1880s, William Osler described "pulmonary edema" in an opium user.[65] It is now recognized that there are many types of drugs and toxins that can cause ALI. The opioids, such as morphine, heroin, codeine, propoxyphene, and methadone, are still the most common causes (Chap. 62), but diverse drugs and toxins, such as the sedative-hypnotic agents, salicylates, cocaine, carbon monoxide, diuretics, and calcium channel blockers, are all associated with this entity.[20,21,23,27,28,34,40,43,49,69,71,77,83,85,104] Table 20–5 summarizes the causes of ALI. The route of administration is not usually the determining factor; ALI can result from oral, intravenous, and inhalational exposure. Because the source of the problem is increased pulmonary capillary permeability, patients with ALI have a normal pulmonary-capillary wedge pressure, unlike patients with cardiogenic pulmonary edema.

Cardiogenic pulmonary edema may also occur as the result of a drug overdose. Etiologies for this phenomenon include the ingestion of large amounts of a negative inotrope (β-adrenergic antagonists, type IA antidysrhythmics, etc), myocardial infarction (from cocaine), and, theoretically, the use of digoxin-specific antibodies to treat digoxin overdose in a patient with congestive heart failure. Because many overdoses are mixed overdoses, the distinction between cardiogenic pulmonary edema and ALI is often difficult to establish by physical examination and requires invasive monitoring techniques.

Although the treatments for cardiogenic pulmonary edema and ALI have many similarities, critical aspects of the therapy differ, and therefore an accurate diagnosis must be established. Most diagnostic tests are not helpful in differentiating between these two diseases. Physical examination reveals the presence of rales with both entities. An S_3 gallop, if present, suggests a cardiac cause of pulmonary edema, but its absence does not establish the diagnosis of ALI. In both entities, the arterial blood gas analysis demonstrates hypoxia and the chest radiograph shows perihilar, basilar, or diffuse alveolar infiltrates. The presence of "vascular redistribu-

tion" on the chest radiograph, however, is suggestive of a cardiogenic etiology; a normal-sized heart is more commonly associated with ALI, whereas an enlarged heart is more typical of cardiogenic pulmonary edema (see Fig. 8–13). Three diagnostic tests that may be useful in establishing the correct diagnosis are radionucleotide ventriculography ("gated-pool" scan), echocardiography, and pulmonary artery (Swan-Ganz) catheter pressure measurements. Although the radionucleotide scan accurately measures cardiac output, it is not routinely available in the emergency department (ED) or intensive care unit (ICU) and usually requires the transport of a critically ill patient to the nuclear medicine suite. Although echocardiography can be performed as a portable "bedside" technique, it is less sensitive and less specific for determinations of cardiac output. Therefore, the most definitive diagnostic procedure in the emergency setting is the insertion of a pulmonary artery catheter for hemodynamic monitoring. Cardiogenic pulmonary edema results from an elevated left-atrial filling pressure (elevated pulmonary-capillary wedge pressure) and a decreased cardiac output (measured by a thermodilution catheter). In patients with ALI, the pulmonary artery wedge pressure and the cardiac output are normal (Table 20–6).

The basic treatment for ALI and ARDS is supportive care while the toxin is eliminated and healing occurs in the pulmonary capillaries.[52] The most important specific therapeutic maneuver in patients with ALI/ARDS involves the use of low tidal-volume ventilation.[89,97] This results in reduced airway pressures which seem to "rest" the lung and allow healing to occur. Many critically ill patients require a pulmonary artery catheter to facilitate effective management. The pulmonary arterial wedge pressure should be kept below 10 mm Hg, and probably in the range of 2–4 mm Hg. However, an adequate cardiac output, blood pressure, and urine output must be maintained. Infusions of albumin or dextran to increase the plasma oncotic pressure and prevent fluid from exuding into the alveoli are not effective, unless the patient is hypoalbuminemic. The efficacy of jet ventilators or membrane oxygenators has not yet been well studied. Some studies suggested a potential role for extracorporeal membrane oxygenation in the treatment of ALI and ARDS.[47] PEEP may be particularly beneficial. The PEEP should be maintained as low as possible, in the range of 5–20 cm H_2O, to maintain a Po_2 of at least 55 mm Hg, or an oxygen saturation of 88%, with an inspired oxygen concentration of 40% or less. In patients who do not have a pulmonary artery catheter, the dynamic lung capacitance [tidal volume/(end-inspiratory pressure-end-expiratory pressure)] seems to correlate with the best PEEP for oxygenation. Higher PEEP settings are not always beneficial and may cause an increased incidence of pneumothorax or hypotension. An increase in PEEP may result in a modest increase in Po_2, but a larger decrease in venous return and decreased cardiac output. Therefore, with each change in PEEP, the resulting actual increase (or perhaps decrease) in oxygen delivery to the body should be determined. Chapter 21 discusses treatment of cardiogenic pulmonary edema.

Hemoglobin and the Chemical Asphyxiants

Disorders of hemoglobin oxygen content, as well as of hemoglobin loading and unloading, result in cellular hypoxia, which, in turn, results in hyperventilation. Anemia is a common complication of the infectious diseases associated with parenteral drug use. In addition, many toxins result in hemolysis or direct bone marrow suppression. Among the latter group are the heavy metals, lead,

TABLE 20–5. Toxicologic Causes of Acute Lung Injury

Amiodarone	Haloperidol
Amphetamines	Irritant gases
Amphotericin	Lidocaine
Bleomycin	Opioids
Calcium channel blockers	Protamine
Carbon monoxide	Salicylates
Chlordiazepoxide	Smoke inhalation
Cocaine	Streptokinase
Colchicine	Terbutaline
Cyclic antidepressants	Thiazide diuretics
Cytosine arabinoside	Vinca alkaloids
Ethchlorvynol	

TABLE 20–6.   Pulmonary Artery Catheter Values

	RA Mean (mm Hg)	RV S/D (mm Hg)	PA S/D (mm Hg)	PA Mean (mm Hg)	PAW (mm Hg)	CI (L/min/m²)
Normal	5	20/5	20/10	16	4–12	2.5–4.0
Cardiogenic pulmonary edema	N-H	N-H/H	H/H	H	H	L
ALI and ARDS	N	N/N	N/N	N	N	N

RA = right atrium; RV = right ventricle; PA = pulmonary artery; PAW = pulmonary capillary wedge; CI = cardiac index; S = systolic; D = diastolic; N = normal; H = high; L = low.

benzene, and ethanol. Hemolysis may occur in individuals exposed to lead, copper, or arsine gas, and in patients with G6PD deficiency exposed to oxidants (Chap. 25).

The oxygen-carrying capacity of blood declines in almost direct proportion to hemoglobin content, as seen in Figure 20–1. As shown in Figure 20–1A, under most normal conditions the dissolved oxygen content of the blood contributes little, and thus the

Oxygen content (O_2 content) = hemoglobin bound oxygen + dissolved oxygen

A. Normal conditions: hemoglobin (Hb) = 15 g/dL; P_{O_2} = 100 mm Hg, oxygen saturation (O_2 Sat) = 95%

O_2 content = [(Hb)(O_2 sat)(constant) + (another constant)(P_{O_2}]

$\quad$ = [(Hb)(O_2 sat)(1.39 mL O_2/g%)
$\qquad\qquad\qquad$ + (0.003 mL O_2/dL/mm Hg)(P_{O_2}]

$\quad$ =[(15 g/dL)(95%)(1.39 mL O_2/g%)
$\qquad\qquad\qquad$ + (0.003 mL O_2/dL/mm Hg)(100 mm Hg)]

$\quad$ = [$\qquad$ (19.8 mL O_2/dL) + $\qquad$ (0.3 mL O_2/dL)]

= 20.1 mL O_2/dL = 20.1 vol%

B. Anemia: Hb = 7.5 g/dL; P_{O_2} = 100 mm Hg, O_2 Sat = 95%

O_2 content = [(Hb)(O_2 sat)(1.39 mL O_2/g%)
$\qquad\qquad\qquad$ + (0.003 mL O_2/dL/mm Hg)(P_{O_2}]

$\quad$ = [(7.5 g/dL)(95%)(1.39 mL O_2/g%)
$\qquad\qquad\qquad$ + (0.003 mL O_2/dL/mm Hg)(100 mm Hg)]

$\quad$ = [$\qquad$ (9.9 mL O_2/dL) $\qquad$ + $\qquad$ (0.3 mL O_2/dL)]

= 10.2 mL/dL = 10.2 vol%

C. Hyperbaric oxygen: Hb = 15 g/dL; P_{O_2} = 1500 mm Hg, O_2 Sat = 100%

O_2 content = [(Hb)(O_2 sat)(1.39 mL O_2/g%)
$\qquad\qquad\qquad$ + (0.003 mL O_2/dL/mm Hg)(P_{O_2}]

$\quad$ = [(15 g/dL)(100%)(1.39 mL O_2/g%)
$\qquad\qquad\qquad$ + (0.003 mL O_2/dL/mm Hg)(1500 mm Hg)]

$\quad$ = [$\qquad$ (20.9 mL O_2/dL) $\qquad$ + $\qquad$ (4.5 mL O_2/dL)]

= 25.4 mL/dL = 25.4 vol%

Figure 20–1.   Oxygen content of the blood.

last portion of the equation can be eliminated. Anemia resulting in a decrease of the hemoglobin content to 7.5 g/dL (a hematocrit of approximately 22%) decreases the oxygen content of the blood to about 10.2 mL O_2/dL, as shown in Figure 20–1B. Because central cyanosis is only visible with a concentration of reduced deoxy-hemoglobin of at least 5 g/dL, unless an abnormal hemoglobin is present, anemia can significantly impair oxygen-carrying capacity without the development of this common physical manifestation (Chap. 94).

Similarly, as the P_{O_2} reaches higher values (as in hyperbaric oxygen chambers), the dissolved oxygen content becomes significant and may be of therapeutic value, particularly when the oxygen-carrying content of hemoglobin is compromised. The P_{O_2} corresponding to an FI_{O_2} of 100% is approximately 575 mm Hg. At 3 atm and 100% oxygen, P_{O_2} values in excess of 1500 mm Hg can be achieved.[56] Under these conditions, the dissolved oxygen content of the blood rises dramatically (to as much as 4.5 mL O_2/dL) and may be adequate to sustain life, even in the absence of any contribution from hemoglobin, as shown in Figure 20–1C.

The chemical asphyxiants that produce methemoglobin, carboxyhemoglobin, and sulfhemoglobin all interfere with oxygen loading and/or unloading to various degrees. Methemoglobin inhibits oxygen loading, producing cyanosis that is unresponsive to supplemental oxygen (Chap. 94). In addition, the oxyhemoglobin saturation curve is shifted to the left, interfering with unloading (see Fig. 20–2). Carboxyhemoglobin has similar effects on oxygen loading and unloading, but carboxyhemoglobin is not associated

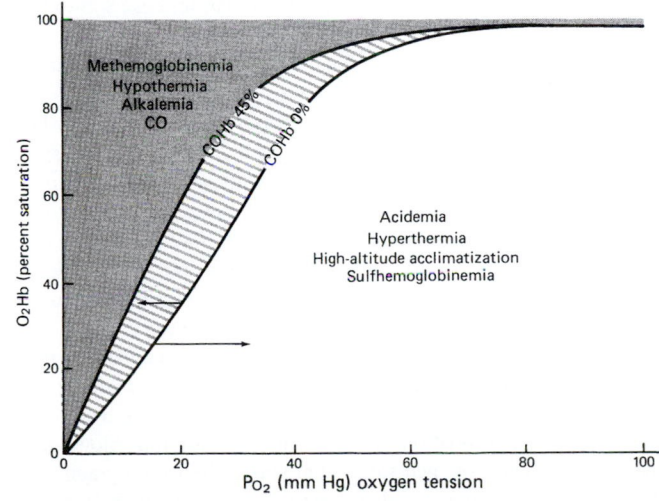

Figure 20–2.   Oxyhemoglobin dissociation curve at 37°C (98.6°F) and pH 7.40. (Hematocrit does not alter this relationship.)

with cyanosis (Chap. 97). Sulfhemoglobin has similar effects on oxygen loading, but actually shifts the oxyhemoglobin saturation curve to the right, favoring unloading. Cyanide, hydrogen sulfide, and sodium azide primarily affect oxygen utilization by interfering with the cytochrome oxidase system (Chap. 98).

Cardiac Output

Any toxin that causes a decreased cardiac output or hypotension may result in tissue hypoxia and tachypnea. This is seen most frequently with overdoses of β-adrenergic antagonists and calcium channel blockers, antidysrhythmics, cyclic antidepressants, and phenothiazines (Chap. 21).

APPROACH TO THE POISONED PATIENT

The initial assessment of every patient must involve the evaluation of upper airway patency. Adequacy of ventilation should then be determined. If concomitant injury is suspected, care must be taken to protect the cervical spine. When airway patency is in question, maneuvers to establish and protect the airway are of prime importance. Often this may simply involve repositioning the chin, jaw, or head, or suctioning secretions or vomitus from the airway. However, insertion of an oral or nasopharyngeal airway, or nasopharyngeal or endotracheal intubation, or surgical cricothyroidotomy may all be required as clinically indicated. After the airway is secured, high-flow supplemental oxygen should be provided and the depth, rate, and rhythm of respirations evaluated. An acceptable tidal breath is one that transports 12–15 mL of air/kg body weight.[92] Hypoventilation resulting from an inadequate respiratory rate or tidal volume is arbitrarily defined as P_{CO_2} greater than 44 mm Hg and leads to hypoxia and ventilatory failure.[31] The symptoms of hypoxia and or hypercarbia are nonspecific and resemble toxicity from many agents. Initially, patients appear restless and confused. Signs of sympathetic discharge, such as tachycardia and diaphoresis, may be noted. Later, patients may complain of headache, only to become sedated and subsequently comatose, as further deterioration occurs. Because these signs and symptoms are nonspecific, arterial blood-gas analysis must be used early in the assessment of patients who present with drug overdose and possible ventilatory failure.

A trial of naloxone, hypertonic dextrose, and thiamine may be indicated for the patient with an altered mental status and or respiratory compromise (Chap. 3). Because opioid overdose and hypoglycemia are rapidly reversible, potential causes of respiratory failure, these diagnoses should be addressed before most other interventions are considered. Failure to identify and reverse these conditions may result in unnecessary diagnostic and therapeutic interventions in addition to irreversible neurologic sequelae.

Having assured an acceptable airway, the remainder of the evaluation can proceed. A rapid assessment of the remainder of the vital signs (Chap. 17) should then occur. Obtaining a history and physical examination, pulse oximetry, arterial blood-gas analysis, measured oxygen saturation, and a chest radiograph are sufficient to determine the diagnosis of pulmonary pathology in most cases. However, adjuncts, such as invasive hemodynamic monitoring, evaluation of the arterial-venous oxygen difference, and xenon ventilation and technetium scanning, may be required.

History

A directed history must include questions on the nature, onset, and duration of symptoms; drug use and abuse; home and occupational exposures; and underlying pulmonary pathology. If the patient is suffering from a significant degree of respiratory compromise, most or all of the history may have to be obtained from friends, relatives, paramedics, coworkers, or others.

Physical Examination

The physical evaluation must include a detailed assessment of depth, rate, and rhythm of respirations, use of accessory muscles, direct evaluation of the oropharynx, position of the trachea, and presence and quality of breath sounds. Skin, nail bed, and conjunctival color must be observed for pallor or cyanosis. Funduscopic examination is a useful adjunct to the examination. Papilledema may be noted in the presence of acute hypercapnia. Additionally, because cyanide poisoning interferes with oxygen delivery to tissue, the venous oxygen saturation remains high. During the funduscopic examination this may appear as arteriolization of the retinal veins, where the veins take on a color more characteristic of arteries (Chap. 98).

Pulse Oximetry

Pulse oximeters have gained widespread acceptance as rapid, noninvasive indicators of hemoglobin oxygen saturation. As defined, hemoglobin oxygen saturation is the ratio of oxyhemoglobin to total hemoglobin. By using two light-emitting diodes, the pulse oximeter is able to measure absorbance at the peak wavelengths for oxy- and deoxyhemoglobin (typically at 940 and 660 nm, respectively). Thus the ratio of oxyhemoglobin to oxy- plus deoxyhemoglobin (total hemoglobin) can be calculated.[75] The clinician may then estimate the P_{O_2} from the oxygen saturation.

Some limitations of this approach require elaboration. Because the oxyhemoglobin saturation curve becomes quite flat above 90% saturation (Fig. 20–2), small changes in saturation over 90% may represent very large changes in P_{O_2}. Thus a decrease from 97% saturation to 95% saturation may represent a substantial change in P_{O_2}. Although a low saturation is an early indicator of hypoxic hypoxia, this is only one of many causes of tissue hypoxia. If total hemoglobin is low, oxygen-carrying capacity is inadequate even with good saturation, as shown in Fig. 20–1. Dyshemoglobinemias, such as carboxyhemoglobin, methemoglobin, and possibly sulfhemoglobin, interfere with the accuracy of pulse oximeter determinations and are of particular concern in the poisoned patient.[91,93] Specifically, using a standard pulse oximeter, the presence of elevated concentrations of methemoglobin will tend to make the saturation approach 84–86%.[3,76] Carboxyhemoglobin is falsely interpreted by the pulse oximeter as mostly oxyhemoglobin, thus readings tend to appear normal even with significant carbon monoxide poisoning, as Table 20–7 illustrates.

Accurate response by the pulse oximeter also requires adequate blood pressure, lack of strong venous pulsations (as might occur in a patient with tricuspid regurgitation), translucent nails (no nail polish), absence of circulating dyes (methylene blue), and a near normal temperature.[75] Finally, we are often more interested in P_{CO_2} than P_{O_2} because it is a better measure of ventilation. The pulse oximeter gives no information with regard to P_{CO_2}. Although the pulse oximeter may give early clues to the presence of hypoxic hypoxia, extrapolation of oxygen saturation to standard

TABLE 20–7. **Interpretation of Oxygen Saturations Reported from Various Sources**

Condition	Po$_2$ (mm Hg)	% Oxygen Saturation		
		ABG	Pulse oximeter	CO-oximeter
Normal	95	95	95	95
Anemia	95	95	95	95*
Methemoglobinemia (30%)	95	95	85	70
Carboxyhemoglobinemia (30%)	95	95	93	70
Hypoxemia	60	90	90	90

The table demonstrates limitations of the various methods for determining oxygen saturation (O$_2$ saturation). The arterial blood gas (ABG) calculates the O$_2$ saturation from the dissolved oxygen content (Po$_2$) and becomes abnormal only when the Po$_2$ falls. The pulse oximeter uses only two wavelengths of light and produces substantial errors in the presence of a dyshemoglobinemia. Because the CO-oximeter uses more wavelengths of light than the pulse oximeter, it can correctly identify the presence of carboxyhemoglobin and methemoglobin. The CO-oximeter has the additional advantage (*) of calculating the total hemoglobin and oxygen content, so that it is useful in the setting of anemia. All techniques are acceptable for the assessment of hypoxemia.

arterial blood-gas values may be difficult because of the many possible sources of error. Pulse oximetry is therefore best used as an initial screening tool for hypoxic hypoxia and later in combination with the initial arterial blood-gas measurement, as a determination of the patient's response to therapy.

Arterial Blood Gas

Arterial blood-gas analysis is an easy and rapid means of evaluating both acid-base status and the quality of gas exchange. Attention must be paid to the method for determining oxygen saturation, specifically whether it is measured or calculated from Po$_2$. If the measured O$_2$ saturation is lower than would be predicted from the Po$_2$ (the calculated O$_2$ saturation), the presence of carboxyhemoglobin or methemoglobin must be suspected. A normal calculated O$_2$ saturation does not exclude these disorders (see section on cooximetry).

Because it is easier to obtain, venous blood-gas analysis is occasionally used as a substitute for arterial blood-gas analysis. When compared to arterial values, venous pH and Po$_2$ are lower, while Pco$_2$ is higher. Errors can be introduced by increased muscle activity of the extremity being tested (eg, seizures) or placement of a tourniquet. Mixed venous blood, however, is required for accurate determination of the arterial-venous oxygen extraction (discussed later) and is an excellent indicator of acid-base status, cardiovascular function, and oxygen utilization. Unfortunately, a central venous catheter is required for sampling. When performing a peripheral venous blood-gas analysis, it is usually assumed that this is only an approximation of mixed venous blood.

The Po$_2$ is generally considered adequate only if it lies within the flat portion at the upper right of the sigmoidal-shaped oxyhemoglobin dissociation curve (Fig. 20–2). That portion of the curve includes the Po$_2$ range from 60 to 100 mm Hg, which corresponds to oxygen saturations greater than 90%. As mentioned earlier, within this flat portion there can be discernible changes in Po$_2$ with little change in oxygen saturation. For instance, an arterial Po$_2$ of 80 mm Hg corresponds roughly to an oxygen saturation of 95%. If the Po$_2$ falls to 60 mm Hg, the oxygen saturation falls to

90%, and this insignificant decrease in the oxygen-carrying capacity of the blood is of minimal clinical concern. If the Po$_2$ falls another 20 mm Hg, however, there is a more significant reduction in oxygen saturation, to about 70%. Thus, changes in Po$_2$ above 60 mm Hg are usually not of therapeutic significance, because the O$_2$ saturation is above 90%. These changes are, however, frequently of diagnostic significance.[31]

An exception to this concept applies to the patient who is under metabolic stress, as might result from low cardiac output, impaired vascular flow, anemia, or dyshemoglobinemia. Under these circumstances even the modest gain achieved by increasing both dissolved oxygen content and hemoglobin saturation above 90% may be desirable, as discussed in the section on hemoglobin and chemical asphyxiants. Also, even if a Po$_2$ greater than 60 mm Hg or an O$_2$ saturation greater than 90% is considered acceptable in most acute settings, it is still desirable to achieve greater values, when feasible, to create a safety zone in case of clinical deterioration.

Significance of a Decreased Po$_2$

In a patient with a diminished Po$_2$, five clinically relevant mechanisms for the hypoxemia should be considered: (a) alveolar hypoventilation; (b) V/Q mismatch; (c) shunting; (d) diffusion abnormality; and, rarely, (e) a decrease in inspired Fio$_2$. In most clinical circumstances, diffusion defects cannot be distinguished from V/Q mismatch. Usually the responsible mechanism can be identified by calculating the alveolar-arterial oxygen (A-a) gradient (discussed later in the chapter). In patients with alveolar hypoventilation, the A-a gradient is completely normal (15 mm Hg or less when breathing room air). Patients with V/Q mismatch have an A-a gradient that is increased but normalizes when 100% oxygen is administered for at least 20 minutes. A normal A-a gradient is less than 100 mm Hg on 100% oxygen. The arterial Po$_2$ on 100% oxygen reaches approximately 575 mm Hg. In contrast, a patient with a shunt will also have an increased A-a gradient while breathing room air, but when 100% oxygen is administered, the arterial Po$_2$ falls substantially below 575 mm Hg and the A-a gradient does not normalize.[90] Finally, in the case of a patient with hypoxia resulting from breathing in an environment in which the Fio$_2$ is less than 21%, the Po$_2$ should correct rapidly when the patient is removed from the environment or supplemental oxygen is delivered.

In general, as discussed previously, a low Po$_2$ can be improved by supplying supplemental oxygen. Although in this instance the patient's laboratory values correct, the underlying process still remains. It is important to remember that the laboratory correlate of hypoventilation is hypercapnia on the arterial blood-gas analysis. If hypercapnia is associated with a low arterial pH (less than 7.35), manual assistance or mechanical ventilation should be considered, regardless of whether the Po$_2$ corrects with supplemental oxygen.[31]

Use of the CO-oximeter

Routine analysis of an arterial blood-gas yields a measured pH, measured Po$_2$, and measured Pco$_2$. Ordinarily, the serum HCO$_3^-$, base excess, and percent oxygen saturation of hemoglobin are all calculated values. The oxygen saturation is of clinical significance because it usually correlates with the oxygen content of the blood, and thus the oxygen available to the tissues. However, implied in this relationship is a normal amount of functional hemoglobin. Because the oxygen saturation is calculated from the measured P_{O_2} using the oxyhemoglobin dissociation curve, it represents only the saturation of normal hemoglobin. Thus, in the presence of even a small percentage of abnormal hemoglobin, the calculated oxygen saturation overestimates the total oxygen content of the blood. For example, a patient with P_{O_2} of 95 mm Hg has a calculated oxygen saturation of 95%. If this patient also has a 30% methemoglobinemia, only 70% of the total hemoglobin is saturated to 95% and the actual saturation is only 67%. This is clinically important because, as stated earlier, hemoglobin saturations of less than 90% do not provide adequate oxygen delivery to the tissues. The CO-oximeter measures total hemoglobin, oxyhemoglobin, deoxyhemoglobin, carboxyhemoglobin, and methemoglobin spectrophotometrically, as shown in Figure 20–3. The resultant saturation is a measured oxygen saturation of the total hemoglobin by including four common hemoglobin variants, and thus correlates with the total oxygen content of the blood.

The difference between measured and calculated oxygen saturation represents the percentage of abnormal hemoglobin present. This gap is helpful in the diagnosis of methemoglobin and carboxyhemoglobin, and is useful in assessing the adequacy of therapy for these disorders. Common indications for cooximetry include cyanosis that is unresponsive to oxygen (methemoglobin and sulfhemoglobin), smoke inhalation (carboxyhemoglobin and possibly methemoglobin), and evaluation of therapy for cyanide toxicity (methemoglobin).

Like so many other tools, the CO-oximeter is not perfect. Its biggest limitation occurs when dealing with uncommon hemoglobins. Because only four wavelengths of light are used by most CO-oximeters, they have the ability to define only four hemoglobin variants. Rare dyshemoglobinemias, such as sulfhemoglobin, are therefore interpreted as one or a combination of the four common hemoglobin variants, giving erroneous results. This phenomenon is commonly noted in neonates, where fetal hemoglobin may

be interpreted as carboxyhemoglobin.[95,101] Although this error rarely adds more than 10% to the true carboxyhemoglobin value, this amount may become significant because of the difficulties in assessing the neuropsychiatric status of infants possibly exposed to carbon monoxide. Some newer CO-oximeters are not affected by fetal hemoglobin, and should be used in neonatal cases of suspected carbon monoxide poisoning.[96] Additionally, CO-oximeters tend to interpret low levels (<2.5%) of carboxyhemoglobin inconsistently.[60] Fortunately, this rarely has clinical implications.

Chest Radiograph

Radiographic detection of a pneumothorax or pneumomediastinum, cardiogenic pulmonary edema, ALI and ARDS, aspiration pneumonitis, or the presence of a foreign body is crucial, but can usually be delayed until the initial evaluation is completed. Confirmation of endotracheal tube placement is necessary but initially can be ascertained by auscultating bilateral breath sounds following compression of a bag valve mask. For patients with occupational disorders, the chest radiograph is essential to confirm and stage exposures to asbestos, silica, coal, and other causes of pneumoconiosis.

THERAPEUTIC OPTIONS

Supplemental Oxygen

Supplemental oxygen is indicated for all patients with suspected or confirmed respiratory insufficiency. While it is generally advisable to begin with high flow (12 L/min) via a nonrebreather mask, lower concentrations of oxygen may be used in more stable patients. It is important to remember that a normal saturation on pulse oximetry does not imply that there is no need for supplemental oxygen. This can be determined only after a more complete assessment. Initially, there should be little concern over worsening hypercapnia in patients with chronic obstructive pulmonary disease (COPD) and respiratory failure, as many of these patients will require intubation for their hypoventilation. If time and the patient's clinical condition permit, an arterial blood-gas analysis should be obtained prior to administering supplemental oxygen or mechanical ventilation so that the patient's intrinsic respiratory status can be adequately defined. In many situations, the patient's condition will not permit delay, and subsequent arterial blood-gas analyses will be needed to determine the ability to decrease the F_{IO_2} or the need for intubation. Hyperbaric oxygen is indicated for carbon monoxide poisoning and rarely other exposures (see Antidotes in Depth: Hyperbaric Oxygen).

Additional respiratory support can be offered from a newer technique. Bilevel positive airway pressure (BiPAP) is well known for its beneficial effects in patients with COPD. Some experimental evidence supports the use of BiPAP for patients with acute respiratory dysfunction in the Emergency Department.[72] Although this technique may be useful in overdose patients, it should be considered only a temporizing measure for patients who are expected to recover rapidly, or while preparing for intubation.

Intubation

After the decision for mechanical ventilation has been made, the route needs to be selected. We prefer oral intubation because it permits the use of a larger endotracheal tube—usually 8 mm or

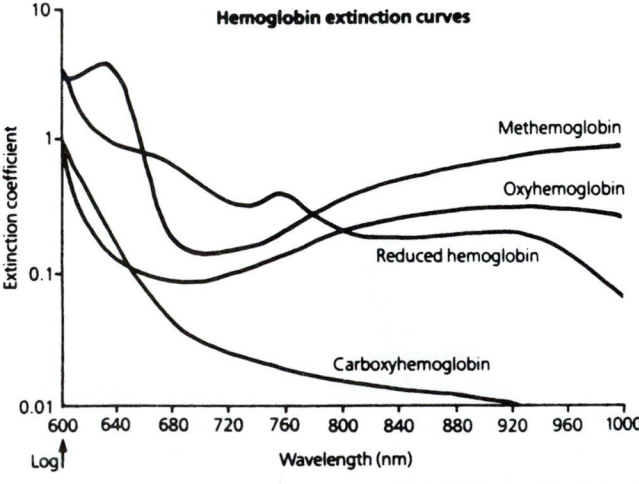

Figure 20–3. Normal and abnormal cooximetry curves. Transmitted light absorbance spectra are shown for four hemoglobin species: oxyhemoglobin, reduced (deoxy) hemoglobin, carboxyhemoglobin, and methemoglobin. (Adapted, with permission, from International Anesthesiology Clinics. Boston, Little Brown & Co., 1987; 25(3):138. Tremper KK, Barker SJ: Using pulse oximetry when dyshemoglobin levels are high. J Crit Illness 1998; 3:103–107.)

larger in adults—than does nasal intubation. If the patient later needs bronchoscopy, it can be done through the endotracheal tube. Some data suggest that bronchoscopy with bronchoalveolar lavage may be of both diagnostic[94] and therapeutic[53,59] benefit for selected poisoned patients. However, in an awake patient, nasotracheal intubation done blindly or with the aid of a flexible fiberoptic laryngoscope may be more easily performed. An advantage of nasotracheal intubation over oral intubation is that orogastric lavage can be performed more easily when the oral cavity is unimpeded. After the trachea is intubated, the tube should be checked to ensure that it is correctly positioned. If a patient breathing 100% oxygen has a P_{O_2} of 50 mm Hg, a 50% shunt exists. This may be caused by ARDS, but could also result from an endotracheal tube that is in the right mainstem bronchus and a left lung that is not being ventilated.[7,87] If the left lung is not being ventilated, the arterial blood-gas values can be restored to normal simply by pulling the endotracheal tube back above the level of the carina.

All patients who sustain drug overdoses and show signs or symptoms of respiratory insufficiency should have chest radiographs performed. Unfortunately, intubated patients usually have portable radiographs performed and the carina may be difficult to visualize because of the poor quality of the study. When seen, the carina is visualized between T-5 and T-7 in most patients. Thus, the tip of the endotracheal tube should be above T-5 for proper (safe) placement. When a portable chest radiograph is obtained, the patient's neck may be extended or flexed, altering the location of the endotracheal tube tip. The tip of the endotracheal tube may move up (with flexion) or down (with extension) by almost 2 cm. It is therefore essential to note the position of the neck during the radiograph.[7,84,88]

Mechanical Ventilation

After a patient is intubated for ventilatory support, the respirator mode—assist, control, or intermittent mandatory ventilation (IMV)—is selected. Patients with pure hypoventilation usually require a controlled fixed rate that can be easily adjusted based on serial arterial blood-gas analysis. Patients with pulmonary parenchymal processes, such as ALI, ARDS, or severe pneumonia, usually do well when placed on either assist or IMV mode. With the IMV mode, a given number of mandatory breaths is administered at the set tidal volume. The patient may take additional breaths without assistance, permitting lower mean airway pressure, which theoretically may reduce the risk of barotrauma and hemodynamic compromise.[39] Although the lower airway pressures associated with IMV are desirable, many authorities recommend the use of the assist mode because it eliminates the patient's work of breathing.[52]

The next step is to determine the appropriate FI_{O_2} to be delivered to the patient. A number of formulas have been devised. One simple approach is to intubate a patient, control breathing, administer 100% oxygen, and decrease to an FI_{O_2} of less than 50% as quickly as possible in an attempt to prevent oxygen toxicity.[52] Although the toxic effects of oxygen are well known for paraquat (Chap. 91), evidence suggests that oxygen may be an important mediator of other toxin-induced pulmonary injuries, such as with iron.[41] A P_{O_2} of 55 mm Hg or a measured oxygen saturation greater than 88% is generally acceptable; thus there is little reason to expose patients to much higher concentrations of oxygen once these conditions are met.[89,97] Many clinicians feel more comfort-

able establishing a "buffer" against deterioration by increasing the P_{O_2} somewhat above 55 mm Hg, but prolonged exposure to higher values is rarely indicated. In patients with pure alveolar hypoventilation, the tidal volume should be set at 12–15 mL/kg/breath. If oxygenation cannot be maintained with FI_{O_2} of 50% or less, PEEP may be used, with careful reassessment of serial arterial blood-gas analyses, changes in effective compliance, and hemodynamic data with each increment in PEEP. In patients with ALI or ARDS, however, lower tidal volumes (on the order of 6 mL/kg/breath) decrease both mortality and the total number of days on the ventilator.[89]

Pharmacologic Adjuncts

Only a few pharmacologic agents have a significant place in reversing toxin-induced respiratory dysfunction. Naloxone, as discussed earlier, may have the greatest role. Atropine and pralidoxime may be useful for respiratory dysfunction from cholinesterase inhibitors (Antidotes in Depth: Pralidoxime and Chap. 88). Elapid antivenom and botulism antitoxin are rarely used but may be lifesaving. Neostigmine can reverse muscle weakness from nondepolarizing neuromuscular blocking agents (Chap. 54). More commonly, clinicians are required to treat bronchospasm from exposure to pulmonary irritants. The use of β_2-selective adrenergic agonist bronchodilators is effective in these cases.[26] The role of corticosteroids remains controversial. An inhaled solution of 2% sodium bicarbonate may provide symptomatic relief for patients with exposure to hydrogen chloride or to chlorine.[15]

Exogenous nitric oxide has been considered for a variety of pulmonary conditions. Specifically, nitric oxide may be useful as a bronchodilator,[10] a means to reverse hypoxic pulmonary vasoconstriction,[2] and as a treatment for ARDS.[1] Unfortunately, controlled studies fail to demonstrate a benefit for nitric oxide in ALI/ARDS patients.[97] Similarly, the results are disappointing for glucocorticoids, surfactants, and a variety of anti-inflammatory agents.[97]

APPLICATIONS IN POISONED PATIENTS

Two 30-year-old patients who overdosed were brought to the ED. Each had ingested substantial amounts of barbiturates and diazepam. An arterial blood gas drawn from patient 1 while he was breathing room air revealed a pH of 7.18, P_{CO_2} of 70 mm Hg, P_{O_2} of 50 mm Hg, and a calculated bicarbonate of 24 mEq/L. An arterial blood gas drawn from patient 2, also breathing room air, revealed a pH of 7.31, P_{CO_2} of 50 mm Hg, P_{O_2} of 50 mm Hg, and a calculated bicarbonate of 25 mEq/L. Quick analysis showed that patient 1 was hypercapnic with a significant respiratory acidosis. Patient 2 did not appear as ill; his P_{CO_2} was not very elevated and his pH was not significantly reduced. The A-a gradients were calculated to be 12.5 mm Hg for patient 1 and 37.5 mm Hg for patient 2 (see Fig. 20–4A and B).

The A-a gradient should be no more than one-third of a patient's age.[38] Patient 1 has a normal A-a gradient (12.5 mm Hg). Therefore, the mechanism for his hypoxemia must be purely alveolar hypoventilation, because that is the only mechanism that does not disrupt gas exchange. The treatment is to reverse the hypoventilation by assisting the patient's ventilation. Mechanical ventilation will reduce the P_{CO_2}, increase the P_{O_2}, and stabilize the

A. Arterial P_{CO_2} approximates alveolar P_{CO_2} and is substituted as:

$$PA_{O_2} = PI_{O_2} - \frac{P_{CO_2}}{R}$$

$$PI_{O_2} = (FI_{O_2})\,(PB - PH_2O)$$

where PA_{O_2} is alveolar P_{O_2}, PI_{O_2} is partial pressure of inspired O_2, Pa_{CO_2} is arterial P_{CO_2}, and R is the respiratory exchange ratio. Therefore:

$$PA_{O_2} = [(FI_{O_2})(PB - PH_2O)] - \frac{P_{CO_2}}{R}$$

where FI_{O_2} is the inspired O_2 fraction, PH_2O is water vapor pressure, and PB is barometric pressure. On room air at sea level, $FI_{O_2} - 21\%$. At steady state, R = 0.8. At sea level, PB = 760 mm Hg and PH_2O = 47 mm Hg. Therefore:

$$PA_{O_2} = [(FI_{O_2})(PB - PH_2O)] - \frac{P_{CO_2}}{R}$$

$$= [(0.21)(760 - 47)] - \frac{P_{CO_2}}{R}$$

$$= 150 - [(1.25)(\Pi x O_2)]$$

Because the A-a gradient is equal to $PA_{O_2} - Pa_{O_2}$ it can be expressed as:

$$150 - [(1.25)(P_{CO_2})] - Pa_{O_2}\ \text{or}\ 150 - [(1.25)(P_{CO_2}) + Pa_{O_2}]$$

A normal A-a gradient is 10–15 mm Hg, but this increases with age. A rough estimate of the normal A-a gradient is one-third the patient's age.

B. Referring to the two overdosed patients above, the A-a gradient for patient 1 is:

$$150 - [(1.25)(70) + 50] = 12.5\ \text{mm Hg}$$

This calculation reveals a normal gradient, indicating that the etiology for hypoxemia and hypoventilation is extrinsic to the lung itself.

In patient 2 the A-a gradient is:

$$150 - [(1.25)(50) + 50] = 37.5\ \text{mm Hg}$$

This abnormally high A-a gradient is consistent with the pneumonia seen on the patient's chest radiograph.

Figure 20–4. **A.** Derivation of the definition of alveloar-arterial (A-a) oxygen gradients. **B.** Using the A-a gradients.

patient until he is no longer under the influence of the drugs he has ingested.

Alternatively, the A-a gradient of patient 2 (37.5 mm Hg) is significantly elevated. There are two possible mechanisms for this hypoxemia: V/Q mismatch or shunting. To discern which of these two mechanisms is responsible, the patient should be given 100% oxygen. In either case, however, the increased A-a gradient suggests that there is intrinsic pulmonary pathology causing the hypoxemia. On finding an increased A-a gradient, a chest radiograph should be examined for an intrinsic pulmonary cause of the gas

exchange abnormality. Patient 2 had a significant right lower-lobe infiltrate. He had aspirated and a pneumonia developed, which contributed to his hypoxemia. His treatment, therefore, included antibiotic therapy and respiratory support.

SUMMARY

Toxins adversely affect tissue oxygenation at every step required for oxygen delivery. This process begins with lowering the partial pressure of inspired oxygen (simple asphyxiants) and ends with inhibition or blockade of cytochrome oxidase (carbon monoxide, cyanide, hydrogen sulfide). Although the clinical manifestations of hypoxia are constant regardless of the etiology, the history, physical examination, and some simple laboratory testing will often allow the clinician to determine the specific mechanism of hypoxia. Once the specific mechanism for hypoxia is identified, potential etiologies can be appreciated, and specific treatments begun. While the diagnosis is being established, the first responses to tissue hypoxia always involve administration of supplemental oxygen, assisted ventilation if necessary, and assuring the adequacy of circulation.

ACKNOWLEDGMENT

Stuart Garay, MD, contributed to this chapter in a previous edition.

REFERENCES

1. Adnot S, Raffestin B, Eddahibi S: NO in the lung. Respir Physiol 1995;101:109–120.
2. Albertson TE, Walby WF, Allen RP, et al: The pharmacology and toxicology of three new biologic agents used in pulmonary medicine. J Toxicol Clin Toxicol 1995;33: 427–438.
3. Barker SJ, Tremper KK, Hyat J: Effects of methemoglobin on pulse oximetry and mixed venous oximetry. Anesthesiology 1989;70: 112–117.
4. Baxter PJ, Kapila, Mfonfu D: Lake Nyos disaster, Cameroon, 1986: The medical effects of large-scale emission of carbon dioxide. BMJ 1989;298:1437–1441.
5. Bernard GB, Artigas A, Brigham KL: The American-European consensus conference on ARDS: Definitions, mechanisms, relevant outcomes, and clinical trial coordination. Am J Respir Care Med 1994; 149:818–824.
6. Birrer RB, Calderon J: Pneumothorax, pneumomediastinum, and pneumopericardium following Valsalva's maneuver during marijuana smoking. N Y State J Med 1984;84:619–620.
7. Blanc VF, Tremblay NA: The complications of tracheal intubation. Anesth Analg 1974;53:202–212.
8. Book WJ, Abel M, Eisenkraft JB: Adverse effects of depolarizing neuromuscular blocking agents: Incidence, prevention and management. Drug Safety 1994;10:331–349.
9. Boyd RE, Brennan PT, Deng JF, et al: Strychnine poisoning: Recovery from profound lactic acidosis, hyperthermia, and rhabdomyolysis. Am J Med 1983;74:507–512.
10. Brett SJ, Evans TW: Nitric oxide: Physiologic roles and therapeutic implications in the lung. Br J Hosp Med 1996; 55:487–490.
11. Bush MN, Rubenstein R, Hoffman I, Bruno MS: Spontaneous pneumomediastinum as a consequence of cocaine use. N Y State J Med 1984;84:618–619.
12. Byrne K, Sugarman HJ: Experimental and clinical assessment of lung injury by measurement of extravascular lung water and trans-

capillary protein flux in ARDS: A review of current techniques. J Surg Res 1988;44:185–203.

13. Caspi J, Klausner JM, Safadi T, et al: Delayed respiratory depression following fentanyl anesthesia for cardiac surgery. Crit Care Med 1988;16:238–240.

14. Cherubin CE: Epidemiology of tetanus in narcotic addicts. N Y State J Med 1970;70:267–271.

15. Chisholm CD, Singletary EM, Okerberg CV, et al: Inhaled sodium bicarbonate therapy for chlorine inhalational injuries. Ann Emerg Med 1989;18;466.

16. Christian CM, Waller JL, Moldenhauer CC: Postoperative rigidity following fentanyl anesthesia. Anesthesiology 1983;58:275–277.

17. Cope DK, Grimbert F, Downey JM, Taylor AE: Pulmonary capillary pressure: A review. Crit Care Med 1992;20:1043–1056.

18. Delaney K, Hoffman RS: Pulmonary infarction associated with crack cocaine use in a previously healthy 23-year-old woman. Am J Med 1991;91:92–94.

19. Drach G, Maloney WH: Toxicity of the common houseplant *Dieffenbachia*. JAMA 1963;184:1047.

20. Duberstein JL, Kaufman DM: A clinical study of an epidemic of heroin intoxication and heroin-induced pulmonary edema. Am J Med 1971;51:704–714.

21. Ettinger NA, Albin RJ: A review of the respiratory effects of smoking cocaine. Am J Med 1989;87:664–668.

22. Fassler CA, Rodriguez N, Badesch DB, et al: Magnesium toxicity as a cause of hypotension and hypoventilation: Occurrence in patients with normal renal function. Arch Intern Med 1985;145:1604–1606.

23. Fein A, Grossman RF, Jones JG, et al: Carbon monoxide effect on alveolar epithelium permeability. Chest 1980;78:726–731.

24. Finley CJ, Silverman MA, Nunez AE: Angiotensin-converting enzyme inhibitor-induced angioedema is unrecognized. Am J Emerg Med 1992;10:550–552.

25. Florez J, McCarthy LE, Borison HL: A comparative study in the cat of the respiratory effects of morphine injected intravenously and into the cerebrospinal fluid. J Pharmacol Exp Ther 1968;163:448–455.

26. Flury KE, Dines DE, Rodarte JR, et al: Airway obstruction due to inhalation of ammonia. Mayo Clin Proc 1983;53:389–393.

27. Frand UI, Shim CS, Williams MH: Heroin-induced pulmonary edema. Ann Intern Med 1972;77:29–35.

28. Frand UI, Shim CS, Williams MH: Methadone-induced pulmonary edema. Ann Intern Med 1972;76:975–979.

29. Freeth KJ, Kay RLF: The Lake Nyos gas disaster. Nature 1987;325:104–105.

30. Frumpkin K, Wright SW: Tube thoracostomy. In: Roberts JR, Hedges JR, eds: Clinical Procedures in Emergency Medicine, 2nd ed. Philadelphia, WB Saunders, 1991, pp. 128–149.

31. Garay SM: Arterial blood gas analysis and pulmonary testing. In: Flomenbaum N, Goldfrank L, eds: Diagnostic Testing in the Emergency Department. Rockville, MD, Aspen, 1984, pp. 85–103.

32. Gerarde HW: Toxicological studies on hydrocarbons. IX: Aspiration hazard and toxicity of hydrocarbons and hydrocarbon mixtures. Arch Environ Health 1963;6:35–47.

33. Glassroth J, Adams GD, Schnoll S: The impact of substance abuse on the respiratory system. Chest 1987;91:596–602.

34. Glauser FL, Smith WR, Caldwell A, et al: Ethchlorvynol (Placidyl)-induced pulmonary edema. Ann Intern Med 1976;84:46–48.

35. Gordon K: Case report: Free-based cocaine smoking and reactive airway diseases. J Emerg Med 1989;7:145–147.

36. Griffith DE, Levin JL: Respiratory effects of outdoor air pollution. Postgrad Med J 1989;86:111–117.

37. Guenter CA: Chest trauma. In: Guenter CA, Welch MH, eds: Pulmonary Medicine, 2nd ed. Philadelphia, Lippincott, 1982, pp. 512–554.

38. Guenter CA: Respiratory function of the lungs and blood. In: Guenter CA, Welch MH, eds: Pulmonary Medicine, 2nd ed. Philadelphia, Lippincott, 1982, pp. 153–191.

39. Hedley-Whyte J, Burgess GE, Feeley TW, Miller MG: Applied Physiology of Respiratory Care. Boston, Little Brown, 1976.

40. Heffner JE, Sahn SA: Salicylate-induced pulmonary edema. Ann Intern Med 1981;95:405–409.

41. Howland MA: Risks of parenteral deferoxamine for acute iron poisoning. J Toxicol Clin Toxicol 1996;34:491–497.

42. Hu H, Fine J, Epstein P, et al: Tear gas: Harassing agent or toxic chemical weapon. JAMA 1989;262:660–663.

43. Humbert VH, Munn NJ, Hawkins RF: Noncardiogenic pulmonary edema complicating massive diltiazem overdose. Chest 1991;99:258–260.

44. Hunter JM: New neuromuscular blocking agents. N Engl J Med 1995;332:691–699.

45. Hussey HH, Katz S: Septic pulmonary infarction. Ann Intern Med 1945;22:526–542.

46. Joseph WL, Fletcher HS, Giordano JM: Pulmonary and cardiovascular implications of drug addiction. Ann Thorac Surg 1973;15:263–274.

47. Katz NM, Buchholz BJ, Howard E, et al: Venovenous extracorporeal membrane oxygenation for noncardiogenic pulmonary edema after coronary bypass surgery. Ann Thorac Surg 1988;46:462–464.

48. King WW, Cave DR: Use of esmolol to control autonomic instability of tetanus. Am J Med 1991;91:425–428.

49. Klein MD: Noncardiogenic pulmonary edema following hydrochlorothiazide ingestion. Ann Emerg Med 1987;116: 901–903.

50. Kling GW, Clark MA, Compton HR, et al: The 1986 Lake Nyos gas disaster in Cameroon, West Africa. Science 1987;236:169–175.

51. Knochel JP: Neuromuscular manifestations of electrolyte disorders. Am J Med 1982;72:521–535.

52. Kollef MH, Schuster DP: The acute respiratory distress syndrome. N Engl J Med 1995;332:27–37.

53. Kulling P: Hospital treatment of victims exposed to combustion products. Toxicol Lett 1992;64–65:283–289.

54. Lam S, Chan-Yeung M: Occupational asthma: Natural history, evaluation and management. In: Rosenstock L, ed: Occupational Medicine: State of the Art Reviews. Philadelphia, Hanley & Belfus, 1987, pp. 373–381.

55. Lambert JR, Byrick RJ, Hammeke MD: Management of acute strychnine poisoning. Can Med Assoc J 1981;124:1268–1270.

56. Leach RM, Rees PJ, Wilmshurst P: ABC of oxygen: Hyperbaric oxygen therapy. BMJ 1998;317:1140–1143.

57. Leeman D: The pulmonary circulation in acute lung injury: A review of some recent advances. Intensive Care Med 1991;17:354–360.

58. Little JW, Smith LH: Pulmonary aspiration. West J Med 1979;131: 122–129.

59. Liu D, Olson KR: Smoke inhalation. In: Hoffman RS, Goldfrank LR, eds: Contemporary Management in Critical Care: Critical Care Toxicology. New York, Churchill Livingstone, 1991, pp. 203–224.

60. Mahoney JJ, Vreman HJ, Stevenson DK, Van Kessel AL: Measurement of carboxyhemoglobin and total hemoglobin by five specialized spectrophotometers (CO-oximeters) in comparison with reference methods. Clin Chem 1993;39:1693–1700.

61. Mill CA, Flacke JW, Miller JD, et al: Cardiovascular effects of fentanyl reversed by naloxone at varying arterial carbon dioxide tensions in dogs. Anesth Analg 1988;67:730–736.

62. Minton NA, Murray SG: A review of organophosphate poisoning. Med Toxicol 1988;3:350–375.

63. Onyeama HP, Oehme FW: A literature review of paraquat toxicity. Vet Hum Toxicol 1984;26:494–502.

64. Osern LN: Simple asphyxiants. In: Rom WN, ed: Environmental and Occupational Medicine. Boston, Little, Brown, 1983, pp. 285–288.

65. Osler W: Edema of the left lung: Morphia poisoning. Mont Gen Hosp Rep 1880;1:291–292.

66. Palat D, Denson M, Sherman M, Matz R: Pneumomediastinum induced by inhalation of alkaloidal cocaine. N Y State J Med 1988;88:438–439.

67. Pare JAP, Fraser R, Hogg JC, et al: Pulmonary "mainline" granulomatosis: Talcosis of intravenous methadone abuse. Medicine (Baltimore) 1979;58:229–239.

68. Park S, Giammona ST: Toxic effects of tear gas on an infant following prolonged exposure. Am J Dis Child 1972; 123:245–246.

69. Parsons PE: Respiratory failure as a result of drugs, overdoses, and poisonings. Clin Chest Med 1994;15:93–102.

70. Pentiah P, Reilly F, Borison HL: Interactions of morphine sulfate and sodium salicylate on respiration in cats. J Pharmacol Exp Ther 1966;154:110–118.

71. Persky VW, Goldfrank LR: Methadone overdoses in a New York City hospital. J Am Coll Emerg Phys 1976;5:111–113.

72. Pollack C, Torres MT, Alexander L: Feasibility study of the use of bilevel positive airway for respiratory support in the emergency department. Ann Emerg Med 1996;27:189–192.

73. Pollack M, Dunbar B, Holbrook P, Fields A: Aspiration of activated charcoal and gastric contents. Ann Emerg Med 1981;10:528–529.

74. Reed CR, Glauser FL: Drug-induced noncardiogenic pulmonary edema. Chest 1991;100:1120–1124.

75. Reinhard M, Cuxem G: Pulse oximeters. Med Focus Int 1992;5:36–37.

76. Reynolds KJ, Palayiwa, E, Moyle JTB, et al: The effect of dyshemoglobins on pulse oximetry: Part I, theoretical approach and Part II, experimental results using an in vitro test system. J Clin Monitor 1993;9:81–90.

77. Richman SR, Harris RD: Acute pulmonary edema associated with Librium abuse. Radiology 1972;103:57–58.

78. Rubin RB, Neugarten J: Cocaine-associated asthma. Am J Med 1990;88:438–439.

79. Saba GP, James AE, Johnson BA, et al: Pulmonary complications of narcotic abuse. Am J Roentgenol 1974;122:733–739.

80. Schmidt-Nowara WW, Samet JM, Rasario PA: Early and late pulmonary complications of botulism. Arch Intern Med 1983;143:451–456.

81. Senanayake N, Karalliede L: Neurotoxic effects of organophosphorus insecticides: An intermediate syndrome. N Engl J Med 1987;316:761–763.

82. Shesser R, Davis D, Edelstein S: Pneumomediastinum and pneumothorax after inhaling alkaloidal cocaine. Ann Emerg Med 1981;10:213–215.

83. Sklar J, Timms RM: Codeine-induced pulmonary edema. Chest 1977;72:230–231.

84. Sladen A: Emergency endotracheal intubation [editorial]. Chest 1979;75:535–536.

85. Stern WZ: Roentgenographic aspects of narcotic addiction. JAMA 1976;236:963–965.

86. Sun KO, Chan YW, Cheung RTF, et al: Management of tetanus: A review of 18 cases. J R Soc Med 1994;87:11–13.

87. Taryle DA, Chandler JE, Good JT Jr, et al: Emergency room intubation: Complications and survival. Chest 1979;75:541–543.

88. Thadani PV: NIDA conference report on the cardiopulmonary complications of "crack" cocaine use: Clinical manifestations and pathophysiology. Chest 1996;110:1072–1076.

89. The Acute Respiratory Distress Syndrome Network: Ventilation with lower tidal volumes as compared with traditional tidal volumes for acute lung injury and the acute respiratory distress syndrome. N Engl J Med 2000;342:1301–1308.

90. Treacher DF, Leach RM: ABC of oxygen: Oxygen transport—1. Basic principles. BMJ 1998;317:1302–1306.

91. Tremper KK, Barker SJ: Using pulse oximetry when dyshemoglobin levels are high. J Crit Illness 1988;3:103–107.

92. Trunkey DD: Initial assessment and management. In: The American College of Surgeons Committee on Trauma, eds: Advanced Trauma Life Support Course. Chicago, American College of Surgeons, 1985, pp. 9–30.

93. Vegfors M, Lennmarken C: Carboxyhaemoglobinaemia and pulse oximetry. Br J Anaesth 1991;66:625–626.

94. Vijayan VK, Pandey VP, Sankaran K, et al: Bronchoalveolar lavage study in victims of toxic gas leak at Bhopal. Indian J Med Res 1989;90:407–414.

95. Vreman HJ, Ronquillo RB, Ariagno RL, et al: Interference of fetal hemoglobin with the spectrophotometric measurement of carboxyhemoglobin. Clin Chem 1988;34:975–977.

96. Vreman HJ, Stevenson DK: Carboxyhemoglobin determined in neonatal blood with a CO-oximeter unaffected by fetal oxyhemoglobin. Clin Chem 1994;40:1522–1527.

97. Ware LB, Matthay MA: The acute respiratory distress syndrome. N Engl J Med 2000;342;1334–1349.

98. Weil JV, McCullough RE, Kline JS, Sodal IE: Diminished ventilatory response to hypoxia and hypercapnia after morphine in normal man. N Engl J Med 1975;292:1103–1106.

99. Wetherill SF, Guarino MJ, Cox RW: Acute renal failure associated with barium chloride poisoning. Ann Intern Med 1981;95:187–188.

100. Wiener MD, Putman CE: Pain in the chest in a user of cocaine. JAMA 1987;258:2087–2088.

101. Wimberley PD, Siggaard-Anderson O, Fogh-Anderson N: Accurate measurements of hemoglobin oxygen saturation, and fractions of carboxyhemoglobin and methemoglobin in fetal blood using radiometer OSM3: Corrections for fetal hemoglobin fraction and pH. Scand J Clin Lab Invest 1990;50(Suppl 203):235–239.

102. Woodard ED, Friedlander B, Lesher RJ, et al: Outbreak of hypersensitivity pneumonitis in an industrial setting. JAMA 1988;259:1965–1969.

103. Zachariades N, Agouridakis P, Parker J: Adult respiratory distress syndrome: A review. J Oral Maxillofac Surg 1993;51:402–407.

104. Zimmerman GA, Clemmer TP: Acute respiratory failure during therapy for salicylate intoxication. Ann Emerg Med 1981;10:104–106.

CHAPTER 21 CARDIOVASCULAR PRINCIPLES

Robert A. Hessler

Toxins frequently produce deleterious effects on the cardiovascular system. The maintenance of adequate tissue perfusion depends on the volume status and vascular resistance, cardiac contractility, and cardiac rhythm. These components of the hemodynamic system are all vulnerable to the effects of drugs and toxins. Cardiovascular toxicity can be manifested by the development of (a) hypotension or hypertension; (b) congestive heart failure and pulmonary edema; (c) cardiac conduction abnormalities; or (d) dysrhythmias. The presence of these specific cardiovascular abnormalities can be helpful in determining the type of toxic exposure. Even when multiple cardiovascular abnormalities occur, the specific pattern of the anomalies can suggest a particular class or type of drug or toxin.

MECHANISMS OF CARDIOVASCULAR TOXICITY

An alteration in hemodynamic functioning may be caused by either indirect metabolic effects or by direct effects on the nervous system, heart, or blood vessels. Poisoning may lead to hemodynamic changes secondary to development of acidemia, alkalemia, hypoxia, or electrolyte abnormalities. In these patients, supportive care with ventilation, oxygenation, and fluid and electrolyte repletion will usually improve the cardiovascular status. These cardiovascular abnormalities are a result of metabolic changes and are generally not useful for identifying a specific toxic substance.

A xenobiotic may also cause specific hemodynamic abnormalities as a result of direct effects on the myocardial cells, the cardiac conduction system, or the arteriolar smooth muscle cells. These effects are frequently mediated by interactions with cellular ion channels or cell membrane receptors. To develop a rational approach to treatment of hemodynamic toxicity requires an understanding of the underlying pathophysiology of the neurohormonal receptors, membrane ion channels, intracellular calcium regulation, and the autonomic nervous system.

CARDIOVASCULAR REGULATION

Calcium is important for normal muscle function and contractility, for cell membrane conductance and electric impulse generation, for cardiac muscle contraction and rhythm generation, and for maintenance of vascular smooth muscle tone. The physiologic response to calcium channel blocking agents, and to agents that interact with the α- or β-adrenergic receptors, are both mediated through changes in the intracellular calcium. Thus, an understanding of the normal intracellular physiology of calcium is critical to the rational approach to therapy of overdose of these agents.

The inciting event in myocardial contraction is electrical depolarization of a single group of cells, known as the pacemaker. Following the opening of fast inward sodium channels on these cells, an inward flow of sodium ions carrying a positive current raises the intracellular potential toward the threshold potential. Reaching this threshold potential triggers myocyte contraction by opening voltage sensitive calcium channels that allow calcium ion movement down their concentration gradient into the cell. Maintaining the intracellular calcium ion concentration 5000–10,000 times lower than the extracellular concentration enhances the inward calcium flux. This immense resting gradient is maintained both by a calcium-sodium exchange mechanism and by ATP-dependent pumps in the membrane that together move calcium out of the cells.[92,93] These same mechanisms are also responsible for the extrusion of calcium during repolarization.

The voltage sensitive calcium channels are divided based upon their conductance (fast or slow) and their sensitivity to voltage changes.[101,116] The best characterized of these are the slow L-type channels and the fast N- and T-type channels. Most voltage-sensitive channels (including the calcium subtypes, potassium, and sodium channels) are composed of a large channel forming subunit termed α_1 along with associated subunits that control the entry of calcium through the channel.[101] Calcium channel blockers in clinical use block the L-type, voltage-dependent calcium channel, although their specificity for vascular versus myocardial calcium channels differs. Thus, patients poisoned by calcium channel blockers have less calcium ion entry during cardiac depolarization, which produces negative inotropy. Therefore, patients suffering from calcium channel blockade may benefit from intravenous administration of calcium chloride. This further increases the concentration gradient across the cell membrane and enhances flow through open calcium channels (see Antidotes in Depth: Calcium).

Only a small proportion of the calcium involved in myofibril contraction actually enters through the exterior cell membrane during depolarization. Instead, the contraction and relaxation cycle of the myocyte is controlled by the flux of calcium into and out of the sarcoplasmic reticulum (SR) into the cytoplasm.[4,69] When calcium enters the cell, channels open in the SR and release calcium from the intracellular stores into the cytoplasm. This phenomenon of calcium-induced calcium release results in rapid increase in the intracellular calcium concentration, and resulting rapid myosin and actin interaction and contraction. Increased activity of the SR associated calcium pump increases the rate of relaxation (ie, lusitropy) and enhances contractility (ie, inotropy). This SR-associated adenosine triphosphatase (ATPase) calcium pump is regulated by phospholamban, a cellular protein. The nonphosphorylated form of phospholamban binds to the calcium pump inhibiting its activity. As discussed later, β-adrenergic stimulation leads to phosphorylation of phospholamban, reducing its affinity for the calcium pump. When phosphorylated phospholamban dissociates from the pump, the activity of the pump, and thus the total SR calcium stores, increases.[34]

Cellular contraction occurs when myosin filaments interact with the actin-tropomyosin helix. Troponins act as regulators of the contraction. A complex of troponin T, troponin I, and troponin C binds to the actin helix near the myosin binding site. Troponin T binds the complex to the actin helix. Troponin I prevents the myosin from accessing the binding site on the actin and troponin C acts as the calcium trigger to initiate contraction. When the intracellular calcium concentration increases, 4 calcium ions bind to troponin C. A conformational shift occurs in the troponin complex and in the interaction between troponin T and the actin helix. Troponin I shifts and the myosin-binding site is exposed. Myosin binds to the site and myofibril contraction occurs.[6,33,52,98] This is shown in Fig. 21–1.

THE AUTONOMIC NERVOUS SYSTEM AND HEMODYNAMICS

In addition to the voltage-dependent channels, the cell membrane also contains channels that open in response to receptor binding of neurotransmitters or neurohormones.[92] A large number of drugs, hormones, and toxins exert their effects via interactions with membrane receptors. These receptor-binding agents include such diverse substances as pertussis and cholera toxins,[21] γ-aminobutyric acid (GABA),[70] nicotine,[24] calcium channel antagonists, and adrenergic agonist and antagonist agents. Understanding the func-

tion and structure of the membrane receptor system is crucial to understanding the normal and toxicologic response to these agents.

The hemodynamic effects of many xenobiotics are mediated by changes in the autonomic nervous system. The autonomic nervous system is functionally divided into the sympathetic (ie, adrenergic) and parasympathetic (ie, cholinergic) systems. These two systems, which share certain common features, function independently of one another. However, through complex feedback, the two systems provide the balance needed for existence under changing external conditions. This property of reflexive activation of one part of the autonomic nervous system to compensate for changes in the other is critical to understanding the effects that various xenobiotics have on the human body.

Anatomically both the sympathetic and parasympathetic systems originate in the central nervous system and synapse in ganglia outside of the brain or spinal cord. Drugs and toxins that interact with the adrenergic nervous system may (a) interfere with the synthesis of neurotransmitter; (b) affect the release of neurotransmitters into the synapse; (c) interfere with the normal reuptake or degradation of transmitters; (d) mimic neurotransmitters at the postsynaptic receptors; (e) block the postsynaptic receptors; or (f) alter the postsynaptic secondary messenger systems. (A detailed discussion of the normal physiology of neurotransmission, neurotransmitters, and receptors, and their interaction with toxins is found in Chap. 10.)

The parasympathetic system predominantly innervates the organs of digestion as well as the cardiovascular system. It utilizes acetylcholine as both its ganglionic and peripheral neurotransmitter. Parasympathetic stimulation produces profound increases in lacrimation, salivation, diaphoresis; parasympathetic antagonism has the opposite effects. Stimulation of cardiac parasympathetic innervation through the vagus nerve leads to a decrease in heart rate, contractility, conduction velocity, and to the development of various degrees of heart block. These effects at the autonomic effector organs are termed muscarinic effects, because they are mediated by acetylcholine receptors of the muscarinic (M) subtype. Stimulation of the muscarinic receptors on the vascular system causes minimal arteriolar dilatation. However, parasympathomimetic agents produce hypotension as a result of the vasodilatation, and accompanying bradycardia and decreased contractility. Acetylcholine receptors of the nicotinic subtype are located on the autonomic ganglia (N_N receptors), and at the neuromuscular junction of skeletal muscle (N_M receptors). Stimulation of the N_N receptors of the autonomic ganglia results in enhanced outflow from the parasympathetic, as well as the sympathetic, nervous system. For a discussion of cholinergic pharmacology see Chap. 10.

The sympathetic nervous system is primarily responsible for the maintenance of arteriolar tone and cardiac function. Although the ganglionic neurotransmitter of the sympathetic nervous system is acetylcholine, norepinephrine is its primary postganglionic neurotransmitter (Fig. 21–2). Norepinephrine is synthesized in the neuron and stored in vesicles in the nerve terminal. In response to neuronal depolarization, the vesicles fuse with the cell membrane and release norepinephrine into the synapse. Norepinephrine in the synapse binds to the postsynaptic adrenergic receptors to elicit an effect by the postsynaptic cell. The norepinephrine is subsequently reuptaken into the presynaptic terminal where it is either repackaged or metabolized by monoamine oxidase (MAO). Alternatively, the norepinephrine may diffuse out of the synapse and be

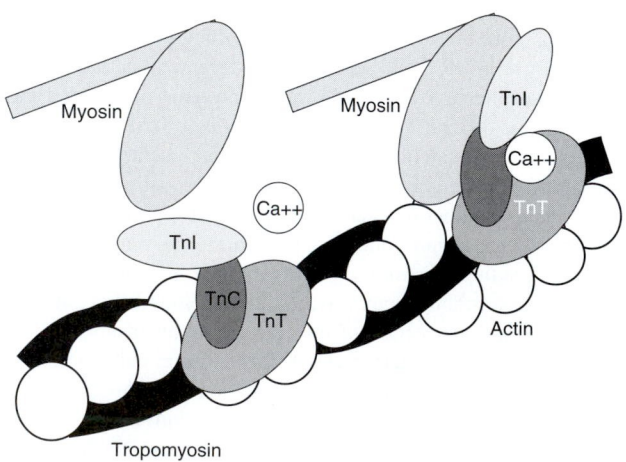

Figure 21–1. On the left, Troponin I (TnI) blocks the binding site for myosin on the tropomyosin–actin helix. On the right, calcium (Ca++) has bound to troponin C (TnC) and, due to conformational shifts in the troponin molecules, myosin is able to bind to the actin helix allowing myofibril contraction to occur.

naptic membrane. Activation of these postsynaptic α_2 receptors in the cardiovascular control centers in the medulla, and elsewhere in the central nervous system, decreases sympathetic outflow from the brain. Thus, α_2-adrenergic agonists cause decreased peripheral vascular resistance, decreased heart rate, and decreased blood pressure, even though some blood vessels have α_2-adrenergic receptors that mediate vasoconstriction. The α_1-adrenergic receptors are located on postsynaptic cells outside the central nervous system, primarily on blood vessels, and mediate arteriole constriction. The adrenergic receptors also interact with circulating catecholamines and other sympathomimetic agents. The effects that catecholamines produce vary based on the organ system. These diverse effects are due to variations in the adrenergic receptors and to differences in the cellular responses to the receptor interactions. In fact, at least 3 subtypes of each of the α-adrenergic receptors exist (α_{1A}, α_{1B}, α_{1D}, and α_{2A}, α_{2B}, α_{2C}), but distinctions in their clinical application, tissue location, and mechanisms of action is not well characterized.

The β-adrenergic receptors have been subclassified into 3 subtypes: β_1, β_2, and β_3 (Table 21–1). The physiology of the β_3 receptor has not yet been definitively characterized. The most prevalent β-adrenergic subtype in the heart is β_1, although β_2 and β_3 receptors are also present.[16,37,38,73,105] Stimulation of β_1-adrenergic receptors increases heart rate, contractility, conduction velocity, and automaticity. The β_2-adrenergic receptors is primarily responsible for relaxation of smooth muscle with resulting bronchodilation and arteriolar dilatation. The most recently identified β_3 receptor is located primarily on adipocytes where it plays a role in lipolysis and thermogenesis.[30,73] β_3-Adrenergic receptors in the heart may increase contractility,[124] but the bulk of evidence suggests that the β_3 receptors are mediators of negative inotropy.[38,81] Surprisingly, the β-adrenergic antagonists in current clinical use are ineffective at blocking β_3-adrenoreceptors and may even act as agonists at these receptor sites.[110]

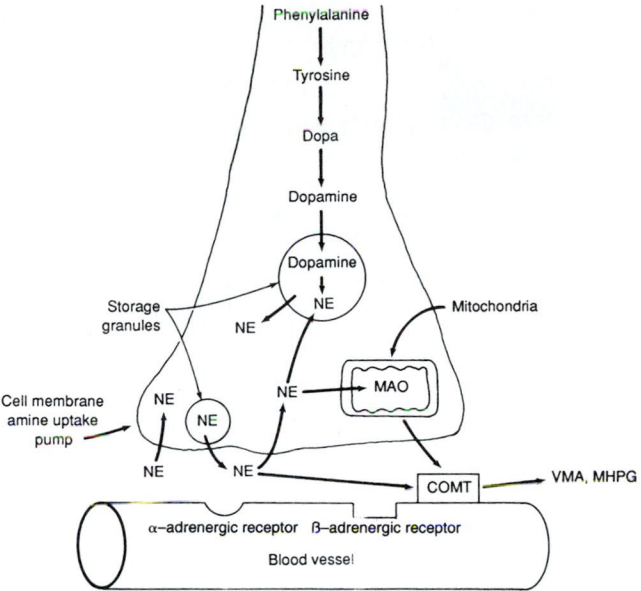

Figure 21–2. Postganglionic sympathetic neuron. Shown is the synthesis in storage granules, release, reuptake, and degradation of norepinephrine (NE). Norepinephrine is synthesized in storage vesicles in the nerve ending. These vesicles fuse with the nerve ending in response to stimulation and release the NE into the synaptic space. The NE then binds to postsynaptic receptors, undergoes active reuptake into the nerve ending, or is metabolized. MAO, monoamine oxidase; COMT, catechol-O-methyltransferase; VMA, 3-methoxy-4-hydroxymandelic acid; MHPG, methoxyhydroxyphenylglycol.

degraded by catechol-O-methyltransferase (COMT). Circulating catecholamines or drugs may also enter the synapse and bind to the receptors.

Xenobiotics may produce sympathomimetic effects through either direct or indirect interactions with postsynaptic adrenergic receptors. Direct-acting agents interact with the postsynaptic receptor, themselves. Alternatively, indirect-acting agents achieve their effects by increasing the release of presynaptic norepinephrine from the storage granules or by decreasing either the reuptake or degradation of neurotransmitter. However, as norepinephrine is eventually depleted from the nerve ending, the blood vessel may no longer constrict and the blood pressure would typically decrease.

ADRENERGIC RECEPTORS

In 1948, Ahlquist first proposed the existence of 2 types of adrenergic receptors—α and β—to explain the excitatory and inhibitory effects of catecholamines on different smooth-muscle tissue.[2] The α receptor was subsequently further subdivided into α_1 and α_2 when norepinephrine and other α-adrenergic agonists were found to inhibit the release of additional norepinephrine from neurons into the synapse. These "autoregulatory" receptors are the α_2 receptors and are primarily located on the presynaptic neuronal membrane. α_2-Adrenergic receptors are also found on the postsy-

TABLE 21–1. Types and Function of the β-Adrenergic Receptor

Type	Location	Function
β_1	Heart	Increase rate
		Increase inotropy
		Increase SA and AV node conduction
	Kidney	Increase renin
	Eye	Increase aqueous humor
	Adipose tissue	increase lipolysis
β_2	Heart	Increase rate (?)
		Increase inotropy
	Liver	Increase glycogenolysis
		Increase gluconeogenesis
	Skeletal muscle	Increase glycogenolysis
	Smooth muscle (bronchi, arterioles, GI tract, uterus)	Relaxation
β_3	Adipose tissue	Increase lipolysis
		Increase thermogenesis
	Heart	Decrease inotropy (?)
	Gall bladder	?
	Colon	?

Cellular Physiology of the Adrenergic Receptors

The effect of adrenergic agents on the cell is primarily mediated through a secondary messenger system of cyclic adenosine monophosphate (cAMP). The intracellular cAMP level is regulated by the membrane interaction of three components: the actual adrenergic receptor; a "G protein" complex; and adenyl cyclase, the enzyme that synthesizes cAMP in the cell.[39,55,95] These receptors are described in detail in Chap. 10.

The actual adrenergic receptor is a protein molecule with seven hydrophobic α-helical transmembrane domains. Catecholamines interact with the receptor at a pocket formed by these transmembrane helixes. Variations in these regions affect agonist and antagonist interactions.[35] The G protein serves as a "signal transducer" between the receptor molecule and the effector enzyme, adenyl cyclase. The G proteins consist of 3 subunits: α, β, and γ.[21,84,104] The α subunit of the G protein complex binds to the (carboxyl) COOH-terminal tail and to intracytoplasmic loops of the adrenergic receptor, and also binds to the adenyl cyclase enzyme. The α subunit of the G protein complex exists in several isomeric forms, depending upon their interactions with the adenyl cyclase enzyme. G_s proteins contain α_s subunits that stimulate adenyl cyclase when "activated" by adrenergic receptor interaction. The α_i subunits of G_i proteins inhibit the activity of adenyl cyclase. The β_1- and β_2-adrenergic receptors interact primarily with α_s subunits in stimulatory G_s protein complexes. β_2-Adrenergic receptors may also interact with G_i proteins. The α_2-adrenergic receptors interact with inhibitory G_i proteins. The α-adrenergic receptors interacts with a third form of a G protein, G_q. The G_q protein does not interact with adenyl cyclase, but interacts with phospholipase C to mediate cell response to α_1-adrenergic stimulation.

When not stimulated by the presence of a catecholamine, the receptor protein is bound to the α and βγ dimer of the G protein. Guanosine diphosphate (GDP) is bound to the α subunit. Catecholamine binding to the receptor causes a conformational change in the α subunit; GDP dissociates and guanosine triphosphate (GTP) binds to the α subunit. The α subunit then dissociates from the receptor and from the βγ dimer. This "activated" α subunit (with GTP bound) can now interact with adenyl cyclase or other effector enzymes. Interaction of the α_s subunit with adenyl cyclase increases the activity of the enzyme resulting in a rapid increase in the intracellular cAMP[21,72,83] (Fig. 21–3).

The cAMP acts as a secondary messenger in the cell. cAMP interacts with protein kinase A and other cAMP-dependent protein kinases to increase their protein phosphorylating activity.[71] In the absence of cAMP, protein kinase A is a tetramer of 2 regulatory and 2 catalytic subunits. cAMP binds to the regulatory subunits to release the active enzymatic units from the tetramer (Fig. 21–3). Protein kinase then transfers phosphate groups from adenosine triphosphate (ATP) to serine, as well as to threonine and tyrosine amino acids, of enzymes that are involved in intracellular regulation and activities. Phosphorylation may increase or decrease the activity of specific enzymes. And, specific protein kinases are highly selective in the proteins that they phosphorylate.[107]

Protein kinase A phosphorylates a variety of cellular proteins involved in calcium regulation, including the voltage-sensitive calcium channel, phospholamban, and troponin.[45,111] Phosphorylation of the L-type calcium channel increases the entry of calcium ions during membrane depolarization.[94,103] Phosphorylation of

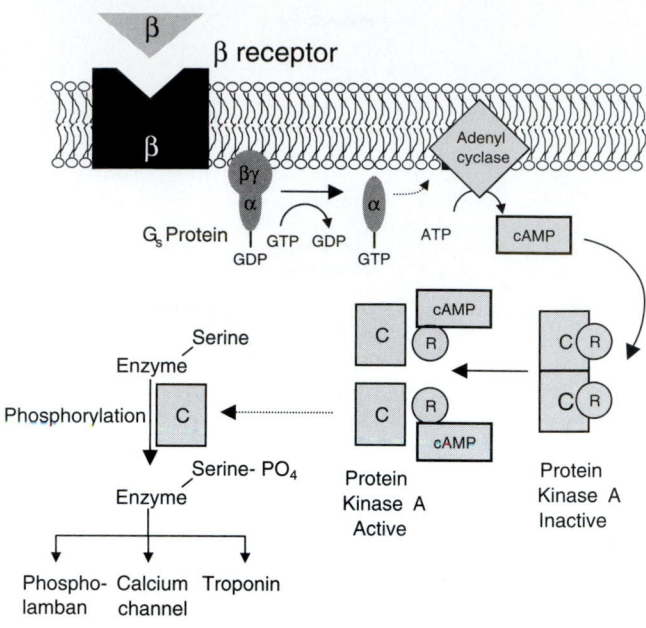

Figure 21–3. Cellular Physiology of β Adrenergic Receptor Interactions. Binding of ligand to the β receptor causes the Gs Protein to release bound ADP and bind ATP to activate the α subunit. This activates adenyl cyclase to produce cAMP. The cAMP interacts with protein kinase A to activate the enzyme, and phosphorylate thereby changing the activity of various cellular proteins (see text).

phospholamban decreases its inhibition of the calcium ATPase pump on the sarcoplasmic reticulum. This disinhibition increases the efficiency of the sarcoplasmic reticulum, which enhances both cellular contractility[4,34,94] and the relaxation of muscle fibers.[69]

Physiologic Effects of Adrenergic Receptors

The β_1-, β_2-, and α_2-adrenergic receptors all interact with G_s proteins and stimulate the adenyl cyclase enzyme. Differences in the resultant clinical effects are primarily related to the location and number of the different receptors in different tissues and to differences in the specificity of the protein kinases activated by cAMP. Table 21–1 shows the function and tissue distribution of the types of β receptors. Agonism at the β_1 receptor results in increased heart rate and increased contractility. However, the result of β_2 stimulation is relaxation, not contraction, of smooth muscle. Because both β-adrenergic receptor subtypes interact with stimulatory G_s proteins, their clinical effects appear to be paradoxical. However, there are two primary reasons for the effect. First, protein kinase A is not a single enzyme, but a group of related isoenzymes variably expressed in different tissues,[10,54,87] and the action and the substrates of the protein kinase isoenzymes may differ between β_1- and β_2-responsive tissues. Second, whereas β_1 stimulation results in cAMP-mediated effects throughout the cytoplasm, β_2 stimulation is compartmentalized within the cell. Thus, the effect of β_2 agonism of G_s type receptors is localized phosphorylation of the L-type calcium channels, increasing their activity.[25,64,130] β_2 Receptors are also coupled to G_i type receptors that inhibit adenyl cyclase and prevent the diffuse cytoplasmic increases in cAMP.[105,106,129] Additionally, β2-receptor stimulation does not result in phosphorylation of phospholamban[64] or troponins.[25]

The α2-adrenergic receptor interacts with a G_i protein that has an inhibitory interaction with adenyl cyclase. Binding of α2-adrenergic agents to the receptor results in inhibition (not stimulation) of adenyl cyclase and to a decrease in the intracellular cAMP.

The α1-adrenergic receptors also are associated with G proteins. However, unlike the β-adrenergic receptors that are associated with G_S proteins and adenyl cyclase, the α1-adrenergic receptors are associated with G_q proteins that are linked to phospholipase C. Binding to the receptor activates the hydrolysis of phosphatidyl inositol 4,5-bisphosphate (PIP_2) to 1,2-diacylglycerol (DAG) and inositol triphosphate (IP_3).[42] The IP_3, acting as an intracellular messenger, binds to receptors on the sarcoplasmic reticulum and initiates the release of calcium ion.[8] DAG activates protein kinase C, which phosphorylates slow calcium channels and other intracellular proteins, and increases the influx of calcium ion[45,94,103,111,113] (Fig. 21–4).

Many xenobiotics and antidotal agents interact with G protein membrane receptors and alter the intracellular cAMP or calcium concentration. β-Adrenergic antagonist overdose results decreased stimulation of adenyl cyclase by G_s proteins, decreased production of cAMP, decreased activation of the cAMP-dependent kinases, and decreased calcium release (Chap. 49). Similarly, by different mechanisms, calcium channel blocker overdose results in decreased cytoplasmic calcium concentration (Chap. 50). The therapy of these overdoses is targeted at reversal of the intracellular cAMP and calcium abnormalities. Table 21–2 lists the agents used to treat these toxic ingestions and their modes of action.

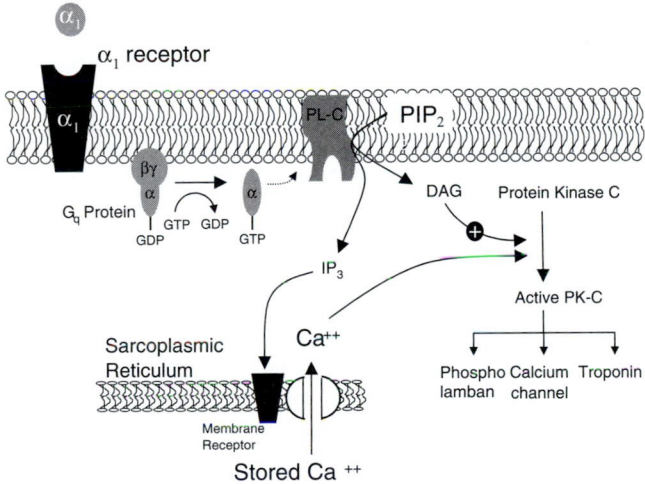

Figure 21–4. Cellular Physiology of α1 Adrenergic Receptor Interactions. Binding of ligand to the α1 receptor causes the Gq Protein to release bound ADP and bind ATP to activate the α subunit. This activates phospholipase C (PL-C) to catalyze the hydrolysis of phosphatidylinositol 4,5-bisphosphate (PIP_2) to produce 1,2-diacylglycerol (DAG) and inositol triphosphate (IP_3). IP_3 interacts with a membrane receptor on the sarcoplasmic reticulum to enhance release of calcium from the cellular stores. The calcium and DAG interact with protein kinase C (PK-C) to activate the enzyme. PK-C phosphorylates and changes the activity of various cellular proteins (see text).

TABLE 21–2. **Effects of Therapeutic Agents on Intracellular cAMP and Calcium**

Agent	Cellular Effect	Mode of Action
Glucagon	Increase cAMP	Glucagon receptor-mediated activation of adenyl cyclase Inhibition of phosphodiesterases
Phosphodiesterase inhibitors	Increase cAMP	Inhibit breakdown of cAMP
Calcium	Increase calcium	Increased membrane gradient increases cell Ca^{++}
Insulin + glucose	Increase cAMP? Increase calcium?	Mechanism not well characterized
Experimental: Forskolin	Increase cAMP	Direct activator of adenyl cyclase
Calcium channel activators	Increase calcium	Increase calcium entry through the cell membrane
Digoxin	Increase calcium	Not clinically useful because of potential side effects
β-Adrenergic agonists	Increase cAMP and calcium	Not clinically useful because of potential side effects

Glucagon receptors, which are similar to the β adrenergic receptors, are coupled to G_s proteins and stimulate adenyl cyclase activity.[40,51,53,62,89,96,121,131] Glucagon's activity to increase cAMP is further enhanced by its inhibitory activity on phosphodiesterase (preventing cAMP breakdown).[80] Phosphodiesterase inhibitors, such as amrinone, milrinone, and enoximone, exert at least some of their inotropic activity by preventing the degradation of cAMP and enhancing calcium cycling.[68,74,114] In a canine model, amrinone significantly increased inotropy, stroke volume, and cardiac output.[74] However, amrinone does not reverse the heart-rate depression caused by β-adrenergic antagonists. Therefore, it probably should be used together with either glucagon or a chronotropic agent.[48] Also, amrinone has significant β2-mediated vasodilatory properties and might result in worsening of hypotension. Therefore, phosphodiesterase inhibitors should be used with caution in poisoned patients and in combination with other antidotal therapies including chronotropic and vasopressor medications. These critically poisoned patients may require invasive hemodynamic monitoring.

Insulin therapy may be beneficial for those patients not responding to glucagon and calcium.[57,60,132] Insulin may simply enhance glucose movement into the cell and enhance general cell metabolism.[60] However, insulin may also have effects on cAMP and calcium.[3,32,79] The insulin receptor has tyrosine kinase activity, as opposed to the serine phosphorylation activity of protein kinase A.[31,117,125] However, this kinase activity may still lead to phosphorylation and activation or inhibition of proteins involved in calcium regulation. Additionally, a specific insulin-receptor-associated serine kinase may be present that is similar to the protein kinase A of the β-adrenergic receptor activity.[102] In addition to the protein kinase activity, insulin may cause activation of a specific phospholipase C that produces phosphatidylinositol-glycan and DAG.[75] These compounds are involved in modulation of several cellular activities, including the sarcoplasmic reticulum associated ATPase calcium pump and protein kinase A "deactivation" of the inhibitory effects of phospholamban (Fig. 21–4).

ANALYSIS OF THE HEMODYNAMIC EFFECTS OF TOXINS

A toxin that acts directly on the cardiovascular or nervous system may cause a characteristic alteration of blood pressure, heart rate (ie, chronotropy), and cardiac rhythm. Recognizing these patterns and understanding their etiology allows for specific rather than empiric therapy.

BLOOD PRESSURE

Blood pressure is dependent upon normal cardiac and vascular function. In fact, the blood pressure is directly related to the heart rate (HR), the stroke volume (SV), and the systemic vascular resistance (SVR): $BP = HR \times SV \times SVR$. The blood pressure measurement consists of both a systolic and a diastolic component. The systolic component is a reflection of the inotropic state of the myocardium, while the diastolic component reflects vascular tone. It is important to assess both portions of the blood pressure, because the many compensatory mechanisms within the cardiovascular system produce recognizable patterns of blood pressure alteration.

Many agents that affect blood pressure modulate the normal chemical interactions at the postganglionic sympathetic neurons. The interaction between these nerve endings and receptors on vascular and cardiac smooth muscle largely determines the patient's blood pressure. Toxins may initiate complex interactions resulting in hypotension or hypertension. In fact, a single drug can cause either hypotension or hypertension, depending on the dose and time.

Hypertension

Hypertension may be a result of an increase in inotropy (SV), or an increase in vasoconstriction (SVR), or both. For example, α_1-adrenergic receptor agonism causes hypertension through vasoconstriction and β_1-receptor agonism causes hypertension through enhanced myocardial contractility. Table 21–3 lists the xenobiotics that may cause hypertension along with their pharmacologic activities.

Because of the functional overlap of most sympathomimetic agents, physical examination alone seldom identifies the specific causative agent in any toxic exposure. However, a clinical constellation of signs and symptoms that is associated with this general class of agents can often be identified. For example, patients who ingest sympathomimetic amines (Chap. 17, Table 17–1), including amphetamines, typically have central nervous system stimulation. The presence of lethargy or coma in a patient suspected of cocaine or amphetamine overdose should suggest other possible diagnoses, including multiple-drug overdose, alternative drug ingestions, metabolic disorders, a postictal state, or either a central nervous system infection or hemorrhage.

The hemodynamic results of an overdose depend on the specific agent ingested and the relative action on the various types of β-adrenergic receptors (see Table 21–1). The pattern of blood pressure elevation might be helpful in determining the specific class of sympathomimetic agent ingested. For example, nonselective β-adrenergic agonists—that is, those that agonize at both β_1 and β_2—produce β_1-mediated systolic hypertension (ie, inotropy) with β_2-mediated diastolic hypotension (ie, vasodilatation). This

TABLE 21–3.   Drugs and Toxins that Commonly Cause Hypertension

Hypertensive effect mediated by α-adrenergic receptor interaction
Direct α-receptor binding agents
  Epinephrine
  Norepinephrine
  Phenylephrine
  Ergotamines
  Methoxamine
Indirect-acting agents[a]
  Amphetamines
  Bretylium
  Cocaine
  Monoamine oxidase inhibitors
  Phencyclidine
  Cyclic antidepressants
  Yohimbine
  Dexfenfluramine
Direct- and indirect-acting agents
  Dopamine
  Ephedrine
  Metaraminol
  Naphazoline
  Oxymetazoline
  Tetrahydrozoline
  Phenylpropanolamine[a]
  Pseudoephedrine

Hypertensive effects not mediated by α-adrenergic receptor interaction
Angiotensin
β-Adrenergic receptor agonist agents[b]
  Nonselective
    Isoproterenol
    Nylidrin
Cholinomimetics[a]
Corticosteroids
Nicotine[a]
Thromboxane A_2
Vasopressin

[a]These agents may cause transient hypertension followed by hypotension.
[b]These agents may also cause hypotension.

results in a widened pulse pressure, which is the numerical difference between the systolic and diastolic pressures.

β_1-Adrenergic receptors cause increased inotropy and chronotropy, whereas β_2-adrenergic receptors mediate bronchodilation and vasodilatation.[65] This would suggest that only agents with a predominant β_1-adrenergic effect would cause hypertension. However, recent work demonstrates that 10–50% of the heart's β-adrenergic receptors are actually of the β_2-adrenergic subtype.[14,15,17,133] And, in toxic ingestions, the relative specificity of the agents no longer is apparent. Thus, even selective β_2-adrenergic agents may cause increased inotropy and chronotropy. The resulting blood pressure would depend on the relative affinities of the drug for receptors in the heart that increase cardiac output and in the vasculature that decrease peripheral resistance.

Indirect-acting agents, such as cocaine and amphetamines, produce hypertension because of reuptake blockade or because of increased release of norepinephrine from presynaptic vesicles. Because norepinephrine is primarily an α_1- and β-adrenergic agonist, profound hypertension is the primary hemodynamic effect. However, with these indirect-acting agents, unlike with an intravenous norepinephrine infusion, the hypertensive effect may be transient because of depletion of the presynaptic supply of norepinephrine.

Empiric Approach to Patients with Xenobiotic-Induced Hypertension.

Treatment of xenobiotic-induced hypertension is required if the blood pressure is severely elevated or if the patient experiences cardiac, renal, or neurologic sequelae related to the hypertension. The recognition of "severe" elevations in blood pressure must be made from the perspective of the patient's baseline blood pressure. Patients with chronic hypertension may tolerate persistent elevations in blood pressure at levels that are intolerable in usually normotensive patients. This relates to the compensatory changes in cerebrovascular blood flow that occurs during autoregulation. All people autoregulate their cerebrovascular blood flow to a certain extent, but the range of tolerable blood pressure shifts upward in patients with chronic hypertension. To prevent excessive cerebrovascular blood flow, chronically hypertensive patients increase the arteriolar vascular tone to maintain a consistent flow of blood in the cranial space. When normotensive patients pharmacologically raise their intracranial blood pressure beyond their ability to autoregulate, the result may be cerebral edema or intracranial hemorrhage. Thus, previously normotensive patients may require antihypertensive therapy at blood pressures that are not of concern in patients with a history of chronic hypertension.

Knowledge of the mechanism and duration of a toxin's activity is important for deciding whether toxin-induced hypertension requires treatment and for choosing the appropriate antihypertensive agent. Because drug-induced hypertension may be transient, a relatively short-acting intravenous agent should be used in small initial doses to reduce the blood pressure to a safe level. Because the hypertension may recur or hypotension may result as the toxin is metabolized, careful blood-pressure monitoring must be continued until the toxic drug effect completely resolves.

Benzodiazepines are considered the agent of choice for treatment of hypertension caused by a centrally acting sympathetic stimulant such as cocaine. Sedative hypnotic agents are almost always successful in controlling the hypertension (and possible dysrhythmias) by reducing the central sympathetic stimulus[22,29,43] and the catecholamine excess state.[56] β-Adrenergic antagonists should be avoided in the treatment of hypertension caused by any sympathomimetic drug. Many sympathomimetic agents interact with the α-adrenergic receptors on the peripheral vasculature. Blocking any existing β$_2$-adrenergic receptor-mediated vasodilatation on these blood vessels may lead to "unopposed" α-adrenergic receptor stimulation, which produces increased arterial constriction and increased blood pressure (Chap. 67).

If benzodiazepines do not control the hypertension from a centrally acting agent, or if the hypertension is a result of a peripherally-acting agent (such as ephedrine), a direct dilating agent (eg, nitroprusside or nitroglycerin) or a pure α-adrenergic blocking agent (eg, phentolamine) should be used. Clinical experience with calcium channel blocking agents is limited and contradictory; results of their use in experimental animal models have shown the agents to be either protective[115] or harmful.[28]

Hypotension

An extremely large number of toxins are reported to cause hypotension. Frequently, the cause of hypotension is coexisting hypoxia, acidosis, anaphylaxis, volume depletion, or dysrhythmias.

In addition, the terminal event in any patient with massive poisoning may be cardiovascular collapse and hypotension.

Typically, hypotension in adults is arbitrarily defined as a systolic blood pressure of less than 90 mm Hg. However, this is not an adequate clinical parameter. Young children and adults with a small body habitus may have a normal systolic pressure that is less than 90 mm Hg (Chap. 17). Patients with hypothermia have decreased metabolic demands, and a lower blood pressure may be considered "normal" for these patients as well (Chap. 18). Most importantly, patients with long-standing hypertension may have inadequate tissue perfusion even with systolic pressures greater than 90 mm Hg. Chronically hypertensive patients lose their autoregulatory response because of atherosclerotic disease, arteriolar hypertrophy, or arteriolar smooth-muscle constriction. These narrowed arterioles may require a higher peripheral blood pressure to properly perfuse the brain. Because the tolerable blood pressure shifts upward in chronically hypertensive patients, they may manifest the clinical findings of hypotension at blood pressures in the "normal" range.

Hypotension is best clinically defined as inadequate tissue perfusion. The clinical assessment of tissue perfusion is based on the vital signs, skin color, capillary refill, mental status, urine output and concentration, and acid-base balance. However, a toxin often directly affects one or more of these clinical parameters. In these patients, the clinical assessment of volume and hemodynamic status may be difficult. Measurement of central venous pressure, cardiac filling pressure, cardiac output, systemic vascular resistance, and more precise arterial pressures may be necessary in critically ill patients.

Poor tissue perfusion may result from hypovolemia, decreased peripheral vascular resistance, myocardial depression, or dysrhythmias. A single toxin may exert several effects on the hemodynamic system. Appropriate treatment of the hypotension requires an understanding of the pathophysiologic consequences of the toxic ingestion and the resultant hemodynamic derangement.

A common mechanism responsible for hypotension in a poisoned patient is intravascular volume depletion. Intravascular volume may decrease as a result of gastrointestinal, urinary, or insensible losses. Additionally, fluid may redistribute from the intravascular space into the intracellular, interstitial, pleural, or peritoneal spaces ("third spacing" of fluid). Table 21–4 lists common toxins that can cause significant intravascular volume depletion.

Toxins that affect the venous tone may also cause hypotension. These agents result in an increase in venous capacitance, decrease in the venous pressure, and relative hypovolemia. The effects may be mediated via central effects on the sympathetic nervous system or direct effects on the peripheral vasculature. Sedative-hypnotic agents and central α$_2$-adrenergic agonists (eg, clonidine) decrease the central sympathetic outflow. Other toxins block peripheral α$_1$-adrenergic receptors or stimulate β$_2$-adrenergic receptors to produce vascular smooth-muscle relaxation and venodilatation. Tricyclic antidepressant agents, phenothiazines, theophylline, and cocaine may deplete catecholamines in the presynaptic nerve endings with resultant hypotension.

Assessment of Volume Status in the Poisoned Patient.

Assessment of volume status may be particularly difficult in the patient with a toxic exposure. The usual signs of dehydration include dry mucous membranes, dry skin, low blood pressure, tachycardia, narrowed pulse pressure, clouded sensorium, and decreased urine

TABLE 21–4.   Toxins that Cause Intravascular Volume Depletion

Gastrointestinal Losses	Insensible Losses	Urinary Losses	Interstitial Redistribution	Vascular Dilatation
Antibiotics	Amphetamines	Diabetes insipidus*	Caustics (acid or alkali)	Alcohols
Arsenic salts	Carbamate insecticides	Diuretics	Crotaline envenomation	Antihypertensives
Carbamate insecticides	Chlorphenoxy herbicides (2–4 D)	Ethanol	Iodine	Anticholinergic agents
Castor bean (ricin)	Cocaine	Lithium	Iron	Calcium channel blockers
Colchicine	Dinitrophenol	Mercury salts	Phenol	Cyclic antidepressants
Cyclopeptide mushroom toxin	Methylxanthines	Salicylates	Salicylates	Disulfiram reaction
Disulfiram reaction	Organic phosphorus insecticides	Tetracycline (outdated)		Diuretics
Iodine	Salicylates	Methylxanthines		Hydralazine
Iron		Vacor		Iron
Laxatives and cathartics				Methylxanthines
Lithium				Nitrates and nitrites
Mercury salts				Opioids
Methylxanthines				Phenothiazines
Nonsteroidal anti-inflammatory				Sedative-hypnotic agents
Opioid withdrawal				
Organic phosphorus insecticides				
Podophyllin				
Pokeweed (saponins)				
Rosary pea (abrin)				
Zinc phosphate				

*See Chap. 24 for toxins that cause diabetes insipidus.
Adapted and modified from Bania T, Hoffman R: Management of hemodynamic compromise in the poisoned patient. In: Hoffman RS, Goldfrank LR, eds: Contemporary Management in Critical Care. New York, Churchill Livingstone, 1991, pp. 181–183.

output. Unfortunately, various toxins can mimic any of these clinical findings in a euvolemic-poisoned patient (Chap. 17; Table 17–1). Moreover, hypovolemic patients may present with diaphoresis, flushed skin, hypertension, bradycardia, or increased urine output as a result of the effects of a toxic ingestion. This is particularly of concern in patients with sympathomimetic agent or cocaine ingestions, where inadequate initial fluid resuscitation may contribute to an eventual adverse outcome. A central venous or pulmonary artery pressure catheter may be required in some critically ill patients. But, in most cases, clinical assessment of central venous pressures and neck vein distension,[128] or empiric hydration of the patient, is adequate.

Additional information about the adequacy of the patient's volume status may be obtained by orthostatic vital sign testing (Chap. 17 and Table 17–3). Even with a 30% or greater volume loss, the supine blood pressure may remain normal in young, previously healthy patients. Normally, the cardiovascular system responds to sitting or standing with vasoconstriction and a slight increase in heart rate. Patients with hypovolemia will be unable to maintain adequate intravascular pressure when upright and will have either an exaggerated reflex increase in heart rate or a drop in blood pressure. Table 21–5 describes a generally accepted approach for testing orthostatic vital sign changes.[76,127]

A variety of toxins can produce orthostatic blood-pressure changes[76,127] (Table 21–6). Volume depletion is the most common cause of toxin-induced orthostatic vital sign changes. However, other toxins, such as α_1-adrenergic antagonists may prevent an adequate vasoconstrictor response or may block the normal slight heart rate increase, resulting in "positive" orthostatic vital sign testing. In these cases, cardiac output and blood pressure decrease when the patient is upright.

Agents that Cause Hypotension. Identification of a specific toxin that is causing hypotension in an overdosed or poisoned pa-

tient requires the integration of a detailed history, complete physical examination, and laboratory studies. The presence of volume depletion or orthostatic vital sign changes may be helpful. Other substances may produce a classic toxicologic syndrome (toxidrome) (Chap. 17). Certain medications exert their toxic hypotensive effects simply as their therapeutic effects are carried to an excessive degree. For example, the β_1-adrenergic antagonists cause decreased contractility and decreased heart rate with a resultant drop in cardiac output and blood pressure, and calcium channel blocking agents cause decreased contractility, decreased heart rate, and arterial dilatation. These effects are mediated through cAMP, intracellular calcium, and protein kinases (discussed earlier).

The cardiovascular changes that occur following overdose of either opioid (eg, morphine) or sedative-hypnotic agents (eg, ben-

TABLE 21–5.   Orthostatic Vital Signs ("Tilt" Testing)

1. After the patient is supine for 2 minutes, determine the blood pressure and pulse rate.
2. Stand the patient *for at least 1 minute* and determine the blood pressure and pulse rate again, and observe for any orthostatic symptoms, such as dizziness or light-headedness. If it is impossible for the patient to stand, have the patient sit up with feet dangling *for at least 2 minutes* before determining vital signs.

The test is positive if any *one* of the following is true:
   Systolic blood pressure decreases ≥20 mm Hg
   Diastolic blood pressure decreases ≥10 mm Hg
   Pulse increases ≥10 beats/min
   Develoment of clinical symptoms of hypovolemia (dizziness, syncope, light-headedness)

Significance of a positive test: 10–15 mL/Kg volume loss.
Adapted and modified from Williams T, Knopp R: The clinical use of orthostatic vital signs. In: Roberts JR, Hedges JR, eds: Clinical Procedures in Emergency Medicine. Philadelphia, WB Saunders, 1991, p. 445.

TABLE 21–6. Toxins that Cause Orthostatic Hypotension

Antihypertensives
Adrenergic antagonists
  Guanethidine
  Bretylium
Angiotensin-converting
  enzyme inhibitors
Central α_2-adrenergic
  agonists
  Clonidine
  Guanabenz
  Guanfacine
  Methyldopa
Ganglionic blockers
  Trimethaphan
Miscellaneous
  Reserpine
Peripheral α_1-adrenergic
  antagonists
  Prazosin
  Phenoxybenzamine
Vasodilators
  Hydralazine

Antianginals
β-Adrenergic antagonists
Calcium channel blockers
Nitrates

Antidepressants
Cyclic antidepressants
MAO inhibitors

Antiparkinson Agents
Bromocriptine
L-Dopa
Pergolide mesylate

Diuretics
Thiazides
Loop diuretics

CNS Depressants
Ethanol
Opioids
Sedative-hypnotics

Antipsychotics
Phenothiazines
Butyrophenones

Toxins that Cause Volume Depletion
See Table 21–4

zodiazepines, barbiturates, ethanol) are remarkably similar. Central nervous system depression is probably the common pathway by which these diverse drugs enact their hypotensive effects. Sedation results in a paralysis of neurocardiovascular regulation with a marked decrease in sympathetic impulses to the heart and peripheral vasculature. The heart rate decreases, cardiac contractility decreases, peripheral vasculature dilates, and hypotension results. In addition, some of these medications have mild direct effects on cardiac contractility, further contributing to the decreased blood pressure.

In addition to their sedative effects, opioids act directly on local vasculature to increase venous capacitance. This property is useful in the treatment of congestive heart failure, but potentiates the hypotensive effects of other drugs. Additionally, certain opioids induce vagal stimulation. This blocks the reflex sympathetic stimulation of the heart rate that would normally occur as a result of hypotension and a hemodynamically inappropriate bradycardia accompanies the low blood pressure. The bradycardia results from specific interaction of opioids with μ_2 opioid receptors in the brain,[46,86,90] resulting in vagal-afferent-mediated cardiovascular effects.

The identification of the toxin responsible for hypotension is often based on other physical findings associated with the drug. Some toxins that produce hypotension also exert specific cardiac effects that may help identify them as the causative agent (Table 21–7). The various medications may be separated into groups depending on their effects on the heart rate and the ECG. The presence of cardiac conduction abnormalities or dysrhythmias could implicate a particular class or group of medications. Likewise, the absence of specific pulse or ECG changes may help exclude, though not eliminate, a particular agent as the cause for the hypotension. While Table 21–7 lists common ECG manifestations

TABLE 21–7. Heart Rate and ECG Abnormalities of Drugs that Cause Hypotension

| Heart Rate | Characteristic ECG Abnormalities* | | |
	No Change	Heart Block or Prolonged Intervals	Dysrhythmia

Bradycardia	α_2-Adrenergic agonists
	Opioids
	Sedative-hypnotics
	Vancomycin
		β-Adrenergic antagonists
		Calcium channel blockers
		Cholinomimetic agents
		Digoxin
		Magnesium (severe)
		Propafenone
		Sotalol
			Digoxin
			Plant toxins
			  Aconitine
			  Andromedotoxin
			  Veratrine
			Propafenone
			Propoxyphene
			Sotalol

Tachycardia	Angiotonsin-converting enzyme inhibitors Arterial dilators Belladonna alkaloids Bupropion Cocaine Disulfiram Diuretics Iron Noncyclic antidepressants Yohimbine	Anticholinergic agents Antidysrhythmic agents Antihistamines Cocaine Cyclic antidepressants Phenothiazines Quinine/chloroquine	Anticholinergic agents Antidysrhythmic agents Antihistamines Arsenic Chloral hydrate Cocaine Cyclic antidepressants Methylxanthines Noncyclic antidepressants Phenothiazines Sympathomimetics

*The toxic ingestion of an agent does not always produce the characteristic ECG changes.

associated with particular toxins, individual toxins in specific cases may demonstrate different heart rate or ECG findings.

Empiric Treatment of Xenobiotic-Induced Hypotension. As with any significant abnormality in vital signs, hypotension must often be treated before the exact cause is known. The history, physical examination, laboratory evaluation, and treatment must proceed concomitantly. Treatment may include removal of the toxic agent from the gastrointestinal tract with orogastric lavage and activated charcoal and supportive care. Diagnostic studies should include an arterial blood-gas analysis, determinations of serum electrolytes and hematocrit, cardiac monitoring and a 12-lead ECG, chest radiography, and appropriate blood and urine toxicologic studies. If appropriate, orthostatic vital signs should be determined. A central venous pressure measurement may be useful in patients whose neck veins cannot be visualized. Patients who do not respond to clinical management may require echocardiography or the insertion of a pulmonary artery catheter for accurate determination of cardiac filling pressures and cardiac output.

As shown in Fig. 21–5, the empiric management of toxin-induced hypotension usually proceeds with the administration of intravenous fluids. However, in patients with evidence of fluid overload or congestive heart failure, a vasopressor or inotropic agent should be administered while further diagnostic studies are performed. A chest radiograph or measurement of pulmonary artery pressures may determine that the hypotension is not directly related to a toxin. For patients with distended neck veins, other diagnoses must be carefully considered, such as congestive heart failure (possibly related to the drug), myocardial infarction, cardiac tamponade, pulmonary embolism, tension pneumothorax, and valvular heart disease.

In general, if the precise toxin is unknown and if the hypotension is unresponsive to fluid infusion and other measures, a vasoconstrictor, or vasopressor, must be used. Choosing the most appropriate vasopressor requires an understanding of the pathophysiologic mechanisms causing the decrease in blood pressure. However, pressor agents should only be used until other more specific antidotal therapy is effective. In general, the first choice of vasopressor agent in most situations is either norepinephrine (Levophed) or phenylephrine (Neo-Synephrine). Because dopamine is an indirect-acting agent, it is dependent on the release of endogenous norepinephrine from the presynaptic nerve ending

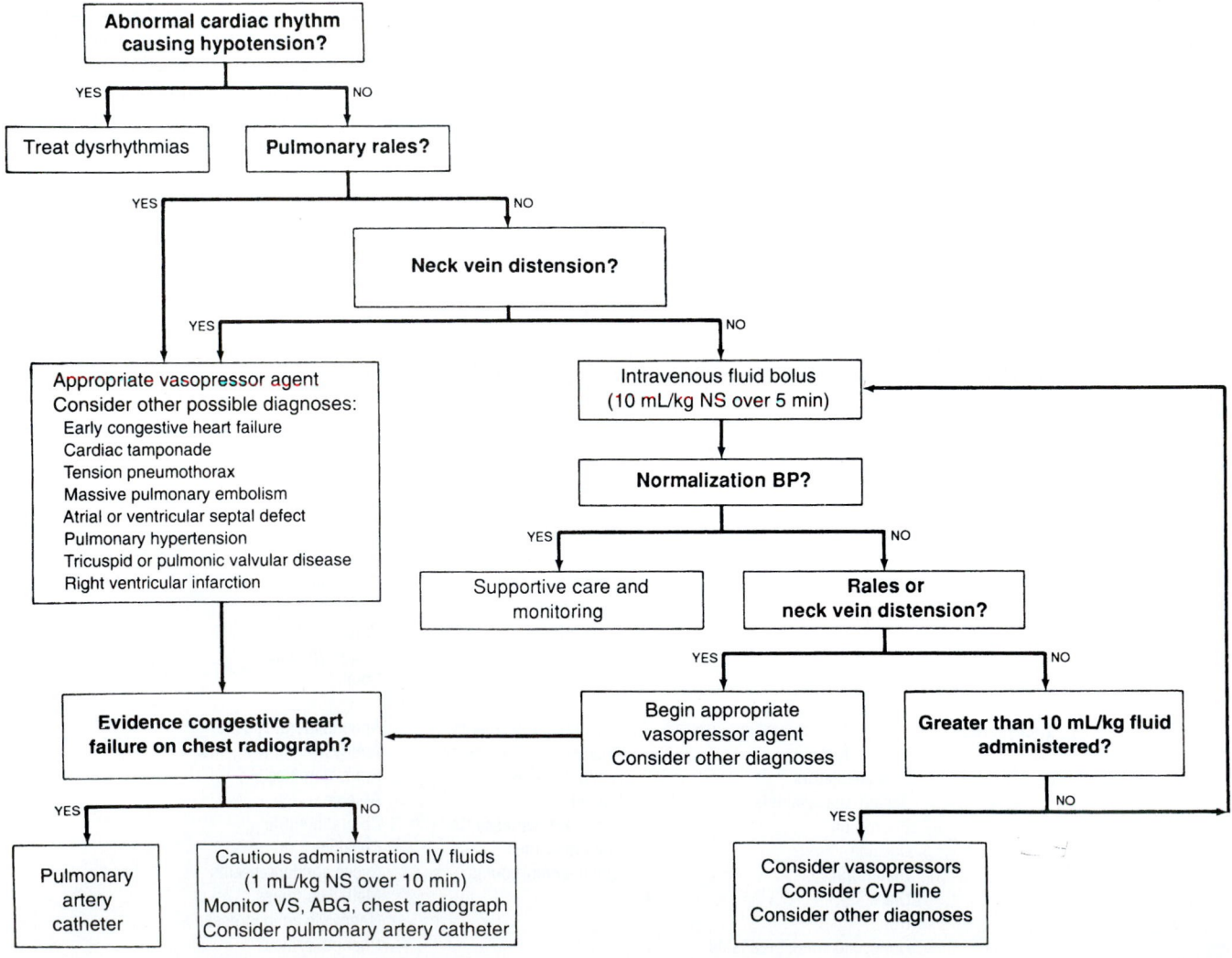

Figure 21–5. Management of drug-induced hypotension.

vesicles. If the toxin, such as a tricyclic antidepressant (Chap. 57), blocks the reuptake of norepinephrine into the presynaptic nerve ending, the presynaptic norepinephrine stores may be depleted and dopamine may be ineffective. Additionally, dopamine itself requires uptake into the presynaptic terminal to affect the release of norepinephrine. For both of these reasons, an indirect-acting agent, such as dopamine, may be relatively ineffective in the treatment of xenobiotic-induced hypotension. Furthermore, the β-adrenergic stimulatory effects of dopamine may predominate and lead to dysrhythmias and worsening of the hypotension (because of peripheral β-adrenergic-receptor-mediated vasodilatation).[1,7,19] However, in overdoses of agents that do not have α-adrenergic antagonist effects, dopamine may be the preferred vasopressor. At low doses, dopamine may preserve renal and gastrointestinal circulation via specific dopamine vasodilatory receptors in these organs.

The specific therapy of patients with β-adrenergic antagonist and calcium channel blocker poisoning are discussed in Chaps. 49 and 50, respectively (see Table 21–2).

CPR, TEMPORARY PACEMAKER, INTRA-AORTIC BALLOON PUMP, AND CARDIOPULMONARY BYPASS

Patients with hemodynamic compromise, bradycardia, or cardiogenic shock must receive aggressive hemodynamic support. Patients whose condition results from drug toxicity have a potentially completely reversible process. Every effort should be made to support the patient's hemodynamic status until the toxin can either be removed or metabolized. If the patient is bradycardic, a pacemaker may be indicated.[2,78,109,123] Patients have recovered completely even after prolonged cardiopulmonary resuscitation (CPR).[2,66] Extracorporeal membrane oxygenation[41,126] or an intra-aortic balloon pump can support life while specific therapy directed at the toxin is instituted.[19,27,36,47,66] In cases of severe cardiogenic shock or electromechanical dissociation, cardiopulmonary bypass[47,123] may sustain life until the toxin can be degraded by the normal metabolic pathways or removed by hemodialysis, hemofiltration, or the use of activated charcoal in the gastrointestinal tract.

CONGESTIVE HEART FAILURE

Toxins may produce cardiogenic pulmonary edema or acute lung injury ("noncardiogenic pulmonary edema"). In acute lung injury, there is increased intra-alveolar fluid in the lungs despite a normal cardiac output. The fluid, hypoxia, rales, and chest radiograph abnormalities result from increased permeability of the alveolar and capillary basement membrane. Proteinaceous fluid leaks from the capillaries into the alveoli and interstitium of the lung. Acute lung injury is a nonspecific response of the lung to insult and may result from many different exposures including solvents, salicylates, sedative-hypnotics, stimulants, nonsteroidal anti-inflammatory agents, and opioids (Chaps. 20 and 95).

Cardiogenic pulmonary edema generally occurs as a result of the toxin's direct effects on the contractility, or inotropy, of the heart. Acute cardiogenic pulmonary edema, resulting from a decreased cardiac output, occurs primarily in patients with calcium

channel blocking agent or β-adrenergic receptor antagonist overdoses. Other agents that can exert depressant effects on cardiac contractility include antihistamines, phenothiazines, antidysrhythmics, anticholinergics, and anesthetics. Pulmonary edema may also result from the fluid overload accompanying ingestion of large quantities of sodium-containing drugs (eg, sodium penicillin) or as a late consequence of drugs that cause renal failure. In addition, chronic exposure to some chemotherapeutic agents (eg, doxorubicin [Adriamycin]), cobalt, cocaine, and other drugs (eg, ethanol) may result in long-term cardiac toxicities.

In general, initial management of toxin-induced cardiogenic pulmonary edema is identical to that for other forms of cardiogenic pulmonary edema (eg, valvular or ischemic heart disease). The treatment modalities include agents to decrease preload and afterload, and agents to increase cardiac output.[13]

Three unique factors must be considered in the treatment of toxin-induced heart failure. First, interactions between the toxin and therapeutic agents, especially inotropic agents, may occur. Second, drugs that precipitate cardiogenic pulmonary edema (eg, calcium channel blocking agents and antihistamines) may also cause acute lung injury.[12,49,50] And, third, early invasive diagnostic and therapeutic interventions may be necessary. Patients with toxin-induced congestive heart failure or cardiogenic shock must receive aggressive hemodynamic support. Acutely toxic patients have a potentially completely reversible process and thus every effort must be made to support the patient's vital signs until the toxin can be removed or metabolized.

CARDIAC DYSRHYTHMIAS AND CONDUCTION ABNORMALITIES

Toxins may produce adverse effects on the electrical activity of the heart. These effects may be mediated by the sympathetic and parasympathetic nervous system or the toxin may act directly on the myocardial conduction system or other myocardial cells. Metabolic abnormalities, especially acidemia, hypotension, hypoxia, and electrolyte abnormalities, may further exacerbate the toxicity or may be the sole cause of the cardiovascular abnormalities. Therefore, correction of metabolic abnormalities must be a high priority in the treatment of patients with drug toxicity. The terminal phase of serious drug ingestions may include nonspecific hemodynamic abnormalities and cardiac dysrhythmias. However, many substances directly or primarily affect cardiac rhythm or conduction.

Mechanisms for Rhythm Generation and Conduction

Drugs that cause dysrhythmias or cardiac conduction abnormalities usually affect the myocardial cell membrane. They may act indirectly via the nervous system or directly on the myocardial cells, but the final result is an alteration in the functioning of the myocardial cellular membrane. The spontaneous generation of a normal or abnormal rhythm, and the conduction of the rhythm within the heart, depends on the maintenance of appropriate transmembrane potentials.

In most cases, the underlying mechanism responsible for a drug's cardiovascular toxicity is unknown. For some medications, such as calcium channel blocking agents and some antidysrhythmic agents, the toxicity appears to result from the same mechanism as their therapeutic effects. For other toxins, the mechanism seems to be an entirely unrelated effect on the cellular electrophysiology.

To understand the toxicity of drugs and to plan appropriate therapy, an understanding of the basic electrophysiology of the myocardial cell is essential. Figure 21–6 shows a typical action potential of myocardial cell depolarization, the electrolyte fluxes responsible for the action potential, and the resulting ECG complex. The action potentials of the contractile and the conductive cells are depicted. The action potential is divided into 5 phases: phase 0, depolarization; phase 1, overshoot; phase 2, plateau; phase 3, repolarization; and phase 4, resting. When the cell is excited either by a stimulus from an adjoining cell or by spontaneous depolarization of a pacemaker cell, selective channels in the membrane open, allowing sodium to enter the cell (phase 0). In the conductive cells of the heart, such as the Purkinje fibers, the sodium current during phase 0 contributes little to the overall action potential. During phase 1, these sodium channels begin to close, and the change in membrane potential opens L-type voltage-sensitive calcium channels. During phase 2, the inward depolarizing calcium current is balanced by an outward repolarizing potassium current, resulting in a plateau of the action potential. These outward repolarizing potassium currents are termed "delayed rectifier" currents. Over time, the current through the delayed rectifier channels increases and the inward calcium current decreases. Phase 3 occurs as the permeability of the membrane to sodium (Na^+) and potassium (K^+) and their intracellular concentrations return to resting levels. Phase 4 is a resting state, with active transport of sodium, potassium, and calcium to maintain the "predepolarization" concentrations and membrane potential. In pacemaker cells during phase 4, changes in potassium and sodium channels lead to a spontaneous, gradual increase in the resting potential and eventual spontaneous depolarization. Recent electrophysiologic studies of individual ion channels have identified multiple subtypes of the sodium, potassium, and calcium channels[97] (Chaps. 10 and 50).

During phases 0 to 2, the cell cannot be depolarized again with another stimulus; the cell is refractory. During phase 3, an electric stimulus of sufficient magnitude may cause another depolarization; the cell is relatively refractory. During phase 4, a stimulus that reaches the threshold level causes depolarization and phase 0 occurs.

Mechanisms of Dysrhythmias

Cardiac rhythms can be produced by three mechanisms: spontaneous depolarization (automaticity), afterdepolarization ("triggered automaticity"), and reentry pathways. In normal cardiac conduction system cells (eg, Purkinje fiber cells), the sodium channels play a much less significant role in generating the action potential (Fig. 21–4). During phase 4, the potassium current out of the cell and the inward sodium current gradually and spontaneously change until the threshold potential is reached (and the membrane undergoes depolarization). In normal myocardium, this spontaneous depolarization occurs most rapidly in the sinus node, the pacemaker for the heart. However, toxins can affect the membrane and cause other myocardial pacemaker cells or even cardiac muscle cells to depolarize more rapidly. This mechanism, increased automaticity, accounts for some of the dysrhythmias seen with cardiac glycoside and catecholamine toxicity.

Other dysrhythmias result from reentry phenomena. The dysrhythmias are usually generated when an early impulse (atrial premature contraction or ventricular premature contraction) reaches a branch point with a partial block to conduction in one of the branches (Fig. 21–7). The impulse is carried through only one of the branches and then spreads through the myocardial cells. After a short delay, the impulse reaches the distal end of the previously

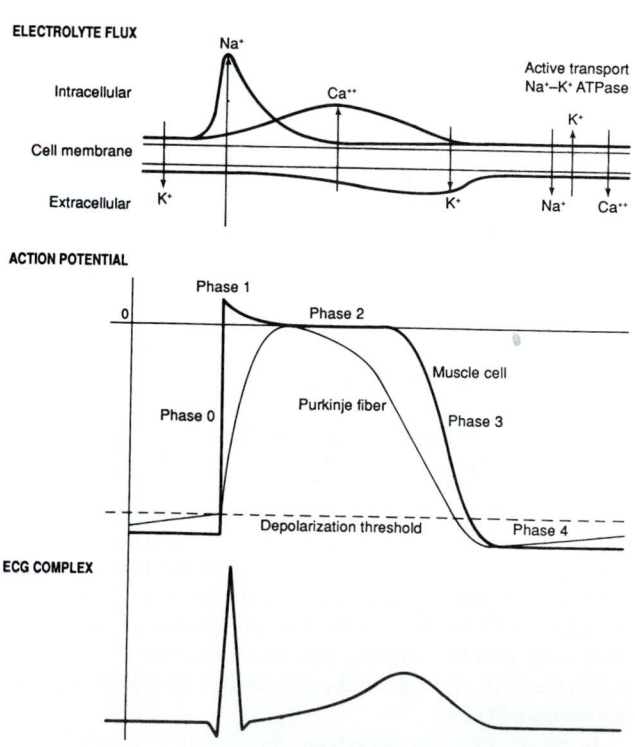

Figure 21–6.   Relationship of electrolyte movement across the cell membrane to the action potential and the ECG.

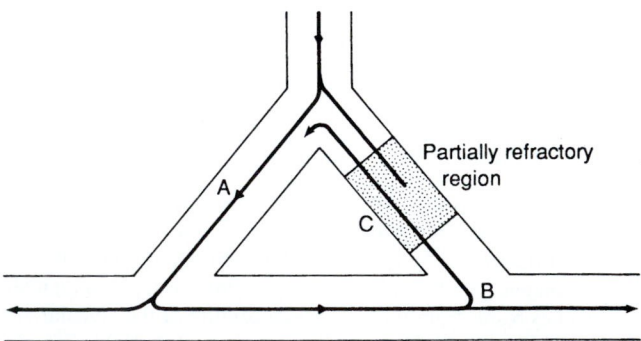

Figure 21–7.   Mechanism of reentry dysrhythmias. An impulse traveling down a conduction pathway reaches a branch point with one branch refractory (*C*). The impulse is conducted down the other branch (*A*) and spreads through the myocardium eventually to reach *B*, the distal end of the originally refractory branch. However, the branch (*C*) is no longer refractory, and the impulse is conducted retrograde up through branch *C*, again to be conducted down branch *A*. The myocardium is depolarized during each loop around the circuit as the impulse spreads from the distal end of branch *A*.

blocked pathway. By this time, the region is no longer refractory and conducts the impulse in a retrograde fashion. The impulse continues in a continuous circuit, depolarizing the heart with each passage. Reentry mechanisms appear to be responsible for most of the dysrhythmias attributable to overdose of antidysrhythmic agents.

Triggered dysrhythmias (or *afterdepolarizations*) result from oscillations and instability in the membrane potential during phase 4. The normal action potential is followed by an abnormal depolarization of lower amplitude. However, if the oscillation reaches the threshold potential, the membrane depolarizes and another action potential is generated. The initial normal action potential acts as a "trigger" for the abnormal oscillations. The mechanism is often termed *triggered automaticity*. Two major types of triggered automaticity occur. In *delayed afterdepolarization* (DAD), the normal action potential is followed by an oscillation during phase 4. DAD occurs primarily under conditions of increased intracellular calcium. These triggered rhythms are responsible for many of the dysrhythmias of cardiac glycoside toxicity. DAD amplitude increases with increased heart rate or cardiac pacing. This may explain why pacing may initiate dysrhythmias in digoxin toxic patients.[112] The second type of afterdepolarization is termed *early afterdepolarization* (EAD). The abnormal afterdepolarization occurs during the downslope of phase 3 of the action potential. EADs occur when the cardiac action potential is markedly prolonged. Specifically, antidysrhythmic and other drugs that prolong the action potential duration may result in EADs (Chap. 52). Torsades de pointes, discussed later, is typically caused by early afterdepolarizations (Chap. 9).

The cardiac toxicity of some drugs results from their effects on the propagation of the electric impulse through the conduction system of the heart. These drugs may cause conduction blocks, including first-, second-, and even third-degree (complete) heart block. The effects of these toxins on the AV node or His bundle cause the ECG abnormalities. Other drugs affect conduction by their action on the left-bundle or right-bundle branches by delaying depolarization of the myocardial cells. These effects are seen on the ECG directly as a widening of the QRS complex or indirectly as a prolongation of the QT interval. This is because toxins that cause conduction blocks usually affect phase 0 of the action potentials, which prolongs the action potential. These effects may result from overdoses of sodium channel blocking drugs such as the antidysrhythmic agents encainide or flecainide. Drugs and toxins that may cause conduction abnormalities are listed in Table 21–8. Frequently, drugs that cause conduction blocks may also set up the myocardium to participate in reentry dysrhythmias. Indeed, the presence of QRS or QT prolongation may portend the development of significant dysrhythmias from drugs such as antidysrhythmic or cyclic antidepressant agents.

Bradycardic Dysrhythmias

Bradycardia, heart block, and eventually asystole are frequently the terminal events in a massive overdose of any drug. In many cases, these effects are a result of the accompanying metabolic changes. For instance, severe hyperkalemia (or acidosis) results in a wide complex, sinusoidal bradycardic rhythm. Other drugs that usually produce tachycardia may, in massive overdoses or as a terminal event, produce bradycardia. These drugs include cyclic antidepressant, anticholinergic, and sympathomimetic agents. The bradycardia in these cases results either from profound depletion

TABLE 21–8. Medications and Toxins that Cause Conduction Abnormalities and/or Heart Block

α_1-Adrenergic antagonists
α_2-Adrenergic agonists
Amantidine
Antidysrhythmics
Astemizole
β-Adrenergic antagonists
Bupivacaine
Calcium channel blockers
Carbamazepine
Cardiac glycosides (digoxin)
Chloroquine and quinine
Cholinomimetics
Cocaine
Cyclic antidepressant agents
Cyclobenzaprine (Flexeril)
Electrolytes
    Potassium
    Magnesium
Heavy metal salts
    Arsenic
Pentamidine
Phenothiazines
Propoxyphene
Sympathomimetics
Terfenadine

of norepinephrine from peripheral sympathetic nerves or from severe conduction abnormalities.

Xenobiotics Causing Bradycardia. Several classes of drugs typically produce sinus bradycardia (Table 21–9). Several different mechanisms may account for drug-induced bradycardia. The toxin may affect the central or peripheral nervous system, or affect rhythm generation or conduction in the heart. Central nervous system (CNS)-mediated bradycardia is probably the most common drug-induced cause for mild sinus bradycardia. Most agents that cause CNS sedation usually decrease sympathetic outflow to the heart and produce a heart rate in the range of 40–60 beats/min. This includes the sedative-hypnotic agents, opioids, and α_2-adrenergic receptor agonist ("centrally acting") antihypertensive drugs. Blockade of the peripheral α_1-adrenergic receptors may also cause a relative bradycardia by decreasing sympathetic input to the heart. Drugs with these properties, such as methyldopa (Aldomet), are expected to cause only a mild bradycardia (in the range of 40–60 beats/min).

The most profound bradycardias result from overdoses of drugs that have direct effects on the myocardial pacemaker and conduction system cells. These drugs depress phase 4 spontaneous depolarization and result in reduced pacemaker activity. Examples of drugs with these effects include calcium channel blockers, β-adrenergic antagonists, and class Ia, Ib, and Ic antidysrhythmics (Table 21–10). The antidysrhythmics are divided into 4 classes based on their general properties: class I, sodium channel blockers; class II, β-adrenergic antagonists; class III, potassium channel blockers and membrane-active agents; and class IV, calcium channel blockers.[118,120] The class I antidysrhythmic agents are further divided into 3 classes based on their specific effects on both membrane ion channels and the action potential.[44,119] (See Table 21–10 and Chaps. 9 and 52).

TABLE 21–9. Medications and Toxins that Cause Bradycardia

α_1-Adrenergic antagonists (reflex bradycardia)
α_2-Adrenergic agonists
   Clonidine (Cataprses)
   Guanfacine (Tenex)
   Guanabenz (Wytensin)
   Methyldopa (Aldomet)
   Yohimbine (Locon)
Antidysrhythmics
β-Adrenergic antagonists
Cardiac glycosides (digoxin)
Cholinomimetics
   Carbamates or organophosphates
   Edrophonium (Tensilon)
   Neostigmine (Prostigmin)
   Physostigmine (Antilirium)
Ciguatera
Misoprostol
Opioids
Phenylpropanolamine
Plant Toxins
   Aconitine
   Andromedotoxin
   Cardiac glycosides
   Veratrine
   Jin bu huan[23]
Sedative hypnotic agents
Late presentations or massive exposures to
   Anticholinergics
   Cocaine
   Cyclic antidepressants
   Sympathomimetics

Asystole typically is the end result of progressive bradycardia and conduction system block. In massive overdoses, any toxin causing bradycardia could potentially cause asystole. β-Adrenergic antagonists, calcium channel blockers, cardiac glycosides, and the other antidysrhythmics are all reported to cause asystole and death.

Treatment of Toxin-Induced Bradycardia. The general treatment of toxin-induced bradycardia includes following the standard advanced cardiac life support (ACLS) guidelines. Symptomatic patients may initially be treated with atropine. Patients who do not respond to atropine should be treated with an intravenous infusion of epinephrine or dopamine. Isoproterenol should be avoided because of the potential for stimulation of vascular β_2-adrenergic receptors with resulting arteriolar dilatation and hypotension. Obviously, if the causative agent is known, specific therapy directed at removal or neutralization of the drug may be indicated. For example, digoxin-specific Fab antibodies (Digibind) should be administered early to patients with digoxin toxicity.

All patients with symptomatic bradycardia because of a toxic ingestion should have an external transcutaneous demand pacemaker placed. For severe symptomatic bradycardia, insertion of a transvenous pacemaker should be considered early. However, use of a temporary pacemaker must not delay or be substituted for more specific and effective therapy. For instance, in digitalis intoxication, cardiac pacing has a higher mortality than the use of Digibind (digoxin-specific antibodies), because of iatrogenic accidents associated with pacemaker placement, pacing-induced dys-

rhythmias, and limited effectiveness of the pacemaker in treating the underlying intoxication.[112] Patients who present with bradycardia or conduction delays must be considered to be at risk of progressing to asystole or to third-degree heart block if more drug is absorbed from the gastrointestinal tract or tissue concentrations increase.

Conduction Abnormalities and Heart Block

Table 21–8 lists the drugs and medications that cause cardiac conduction abnormalities. Most of these toxins are the same agents that cause bradycardia. The drugs and medications that decrease sympathetic tone usually only produce first-degree or second-degree Mobitz type I heart block via effects on innervation of the atrioventricular node. Rarely, these agents can produce second-degree Mobitz type II or even third-degree heart block. Anticholinergic and antihistaminic agents may also cause conduction delays. The more profound ECG interval abnormalities and the more serious degrees of heart block usually accompany overdoses with cardiac glycosides. (Chap. 9).

The cyclic antidepressants possess quinidinelike "membrane-stabilizing" activity identical to the class I antidysrhythmic agents. The result is slowed propagation of impulses through the ventricular myocardium. Figure 21–6 shows the action potential and the contribution of each phase to the ECG complex. Agents that depress phase 0 (sodium influx) produce widening of the QRS complex and slowing of conduction. Agents that prolong phase 2 or 3, produce prolongation of the QT interval and refractory period. Table 21–10 lists the classes of antidysrhythmic agents, their effects on action potential, and the ECG abnormalities they cause.

Tachycardic Dysrhythmias
Superventricular Tachycardia

Both supraventricular and ventricular tachydysrhythmias may occur in poisoning. Table 21–11 lists the common medications and toxins that can cause tachydysrhythmias. Indeed, the presence of either supraventricular or ventricular dysrhythmias often complicates the treatment of a patient with a toxic ingestion.

Sinus tachycardia is the most common tachycardic rhythm seen in the poisoned patient. Sinus tachycardia may result from such toxic effects as fever, stress, hypovolemia, catecholamine excess, or from direct effects of the toxin on the sinoatrial node. In general, the patient with sinus tachycardia is treated with supportive care and correction of any underlying metabolic or hemodynamic abnormalities. The tachycardia will resolve as the toxin is metabolized or removed from the body. In stimulant drug and sympathomimetic agent exposures, the sinus tachycardia may be extremely fast (greater than 150 beats/min) and may require treatment. In this case, sedation with benzodiazepines will usually control the tachycardia effectively.

Supraventricular tachycardias occur frequently in poisoned patients. The most common agents are medications or toxins with anticholinergic activity, the antidysrhythmics, and the sympathomimetic drugs. The drug's sympathomimetic effects often mediate the tachydysrhythmias. For instance, cocaine and amphetamines stimulate the β_1-adrenergic receptors on the myocardial cells. Much of the dysrhythmic potential of cyclic antidepressants, antihistamines, and theophylline appears to be mediated through indirect effects on the sympathetic system.

TABLE 21–10. Classes of Antidysrhythmic Agents

Class	Pharmacologic Effects			Examples	Effects on ECG Intervals		
	Sodium Channel	Potassium Channels	Calcium Channels		PR	QRS	QT
Sodium channel blockers							
Ia	++/+++	++	0	Diisopyramide Procainamide Quinidine	±	↑	↑
Ib	+/++	±	0	Lidocaine Phenytoin Mexiletine Tocainide	±	±	±
Ic	+++	++/+++	0	Encainide Flecainide Propafenone Moricizine	↑	↑	↑↑
β-Adrenergic antagonists							
II	0	0	+ (indirect)	Propranolol Atenolol Esmolol Metoprolol Timolol	↑	±	±
Potassium channel blockers							
III	+	++	0	Amiodarone Bretylium Sotalol Dofetilide Ibutilide*	↑	±	↑
Calcium channel blockers							
IV	0	0	+++	Verapamil Diltiazem Nifedipine Nicardipine	↑	±	±

+ = Mild blockade; ++ = moderate blockade; +++ = marked blockade; ↑ = increases; ± = no significanct effect

*Ibutilide actually activates a slow inward sodium channel rather than blocking outward potassium currents, but is classified as Class III (because of its increased action potential duration and atrial and ventricular refractoriness, which are typical of class III agents.

Treatment of Toxin-Induced Supraventricular Tachycardia (SVT). If the patient is unstable (hypotension, chest pain, or congestive failure), an attempt should usually be made to treat the dysrhythmia immediately with electric cardioversion. Unfortunately, because the toxic agent is still present, the dysrhythmia may recur. In these cases, repeated cardioversion is ineffective and pharmacologic therapy for the dysrhythmia should be considered.

Adenosine (Adenocard) would seem to be a potentially effective agent for toxin-induced supraventricular dysrhythmias. The drug has no hemodynamic effects when given as a 6–12-mg bolus, and the short half-life (less than 10 seconds) limits the duration of any adverse reactions. However, the short half-life could lead to rapid recurrence of the rhythm as the adenosine is quickly metabolized while the toxin is still present. If the dysrhythmia recurs, repeated boluses of adenosine would serve no useful purpose and should not be used; instead, an agent with a longer half-life should be considered. Additionally, a few potential drug interactions exist that must be considered when using adenosine for toxin-induced SVT. Most importantly, dipyridamole (Persantine) inhibits the uptake of adenosine into cells and prolongs and potentiates the effects of adenosine. Prolonged complete heart block or asystole may result. Adenosine may not be effective for dysrhythmias caused by methylxanthines, such as caffeine or theophylline. Methylxanthines competitively inhibit the effects of adenosine. Doses of adenosine higher than the usually recommended 6–12 mg may be effective in these cases. However, no clinical studies have been performed to assess the effectiveness or safety of higher doses of adenosine in methylxanthine toxicity.

Other antidysrhythmics may be employed, if necessary. Calcium channel blockers and β-adrenergic antagonists must not be administered to patients with wide complex dysrhythmias unless the rhythm is clearly demonstrated to not be ventricular tachycardia. Patients with ventricular tachycardia who are erroneously treated with verapamil for presumed supraventricular tachycardia with aberrancy develop profound hypotension in 44–100% of cases.[20,91,108] In suspected poisonings with a prolonged QRS or QT, the patient should be assumed to have ingested a cyclic antidepressant,[9,11,18,59,82,85,88,99,100] an antidysrhythmic,[58,61,122] or a phenothiazine.[63,77] Sodium bicarbonate (1–2 mEq/kg) should be administered and the ECG should be monitored. If the ECG inter-

TABLE 21–11.   Drugs and Toxins that Can Cause Ventricular and Supraventricular Dysrhythmias

Amantidine
Antidysrhythmics
 Class I, III
Anticholinergics
Antihistamines
Baclofen
Botanicals and plants (Chap. 78)
Carbamazepine (Tegretol)
Cardiac glycosides (Digoxin)
Catecholamines
Chloroquine and quinine
Cholinomimetics
 Physostigmine
Cyclic antidepressant agents
Cyclobenzaprine (Flexeril)
Flumazenil
Halogenated hydrocarbons
 Inhalational anesthetics
Hydrocarbons and solvents
Jellyfish venom
Metal salts
 Arsenic
 Lithium
 Magnesium
 Potassium
Pentamidine
Phenothiazines
Phosphodiesterase inhibitors
 Amrinone
 Methylxanthines
Propoxyphene
Sedative hypnotic agents
 Chloral hydrate
 Ethanol
Sympathomimetics
 α Adrenergic agonists
 Amphetamines
 β-Adrenergic agonists
 Cocaine
 Phencyclidine
Thyroid hormone preparations

vals improve, additional sodium bicarbonate should be infused to maintain the serum pH at approximately 7.50–7.55 (see Antidotes in Depth: Sodium Bicarbonate and Chap. 9).

If the patient is hemodynamically stable, frequently the best action is careful monitoring until the toxin is removed or metabolized or an antidote is administered.

Xenobiotics that Cause Ventricular Tachycardia. "Ventricular Tachycardia" Ventricular dysrhythmias frequently accompany hypotension, hypoxia, acidemia, electrolyte abnormalities, and other metabolic derangements that occur in critically ill patients. It is often impossible to determine whether the dysrhythmia is a result of the toxin or other underlying metabolic abnormalities. Some common drugs clearly can cause ventricular dysrhythmias; Table 21–11 lists them. The rarity of published reports detailing a particular drug's toxicity may reflect either the rarity of toxicity or infrequency of patient's exposure to the drug. Halogenated hydrocarbons including chloral hydrate "sensitize" the my-

ocardium to the effects of catecholamines. In the presence of halogenated hydrocarbons, ventricular tachycardia or ventricular fibrillation may occur with much lower levels of endogenous epinephrine or exogenous β-adrenergic stimulants.

Management of Drug-Induced Ventricular Dysrhythmias. Ventricular dysrhythmias should be managed much like those occurring in association with a myocardial infarction. In addition to the usual supportive measures (including oxygen, ECG monitoring, and blood tests such as hematocrit, electrolytes, and blood, urea, nitrogen (BUN)), antidysrhythmic drugs are frequently indicated. The choice of agent depends somewhat on the toxin. Class Ia and Ic, and possibly class III, antidysrhythmics should be avoided if the patient is poisoned with any drug with quinidinelike activities, or if the ECG shows any conduction delays. Using these drugs would only potentiate the conduction system toxicity of the drug originally ingested. If the QRS or QT interval is prolonged, the dysrhythmia should be presumed to be secondary to the quinidine-like activity of a cyclic antidepressant,[9,11,18,59,82,85,88,99,100] and sodium bicarbonate administered. If the QT itself is prolonged, in the absence of QRS prolongation, sodium bicarbonate should not be used because it induces hypokalemia, which may further prolong the QT interval. If sodium bicarbonate is ineffective for these dysrhythmias, a class Ib agent, such as lidocaine, would be an appropriate therapeutic agent and may be effective for treating cyclic antidepressant-induced ventricular dysrhythmias.[5,67]

Torsades de pointes is a unique type of polymorphic ventricular tachycardia in which the ECG resembles a sinusoidal wave of increasing and decreasing magnitude, undulating above and below the baseline (See Figure 9–11). The dysrhythmia may propagate from numerous simultaneous ventricular tachycardia reentry foci scattered throughout the ventricles. The QRS complexes change as these various foci compete to depolarize the ventricle. The pathophysiology of torsades de pointes is usually related to development of EAD in the setting of a myocardium primed for reentry. Myocardial cells with long refractory periods (phases 2 and 3 of the action potential curve, Fig. 21–4) are predisposed to both EADs and reentry.

Patients with either hereditary prolonged QT syndrome or acquired prolongation caused by drugs or metabolic effects are at increased risk of developing torsades de pointes. The QT interval corresponds to phases 2 and 3 of the action potential curve. Therefore, agents that affect the potassium or calcium channels and currents would be expected to cause torsades de pointes. However, drugs and antidysrhythmic agents that effect primarily sodium channels also may prolong the QT intervals and cause torsades de pointes. Some sodium channels may remain open during phase 2 and contribute to the plateau phase duration of the action potential. (See Figure 9–11.)

Metabolic and electrolyte abnormalities, particularly hypocalcemia, hypomagnesemia, and hypokalemia, may interfere with the ion channel currents and may cause of torsades de pointes. However, the most common cause is drug toxicity. Any drug that causes QT prolongation may cause torsades de pointes. The most frequent cause of drug-involved torsades de pointes are class Ia, Ic & III antidysrhythmics, and the antipsychotics. However, many diverse types of drugs and chemicals may cause QT prolongation and torsades de pointes. Class Ib agents, such as lidocaine, have no significant effect on QT interval and would not be expected to cause torsades de pointes. Treatments for torsades de pointes involve cardioversion, Magnesium^{2+} or overdrive pacing.

SUMMARY

Drugs and toxins may interact with the heart or blood vessels to produce hypotension or hypertension, congestive heart failure, dysrhythmias, or cardiac conduction delays. The occurrence of these abnormalities, individually or in combination, may suggest a particular toxin or class of drugs as the etiologic agent and may dictate initial treatment. Significant abnormalities in vital signs often must be corrected even before the toxin is identified. Only by understanding both the pharmacology of the toxic drug and the physiology of the heart and vasculature can appropriate treatment be delivered.

Definitive care of the poisoned patient with hemodynamic compromise or a dysrhythmia begins with recognition that a toxic agent may be present. Although structural and metabolic etiologies must always be considered, the toxic effects of drugs must also be included in the differential diagnosis. A variety of clinical clues, when present, should heighten the physician's suspicion that a toxic drug effect may be responsible for the hemodynamic or dysrhythmic problem. Table 21–12 lists some of these clues.

TABLE 21–12. Clues that an Unanticipated Toxin May Be the Cause of Hemodynamic Compromise or Dysrhythmias

History
New-onset, concomitant seizure
Gastrointestinal disturbances (colicky pain, nausea, vomiting, diarrhea)
Prior ingestion of medications
Depression
Suspected myocardial ischemia in patient <35 years old or without risk factors

Past Medical History
Treatment with *any* cardiac medications
History of psychiatric illness, asthma, or hypertension
History of drug use or abuse

Physical Examination Vital Signs
Heart rate
   Sinus tachycardia without apparent identified cause
Respiratory rate
   Any unexplained depression or elevation in rate
Temperature
   Elevation but especially if >106°F (>41.1°C)
   Hypothermia
Dissociation between typically paired changes, for example:
   Hypotension and bradycardia (tachycardia expected)
   Fever and dry skin (diaphoresis expected)
   Depressed mental status and tachypnea (decreased respirations common)
Relatively rapid changes in vital signs
   Initial hypertension becomes hypotension

General
Alteration in consciousness, such as depressed mental status, confusion, or agitation
Findings usually not associated with cardiovascular diseases
   Ataxia, bullae, dry mucous membranes, lacrimation, miosis or mydriasis, nystagmus, unusual odor, flushed skin, salivation, tinnitus, tremor, visual disturbances
Findings consistent with a toxidrome (Table 17–2)
   Anticholinergic, or sympathomimetic agents

Laboratory Tests
Any unexpected or unexplained laboratory result, especially:
   Metabolic acidosis
   Respiratory alkalosis
   Hypokalemia or hyperkalemia
   Hyperglycemia
ECG
   Prolonged QRS complex or QT interval
   Any heart block
   Supraventricular tachycardia rate >240 beat/min
   Occurrence of any uncommon dysrhythmia
   Occurrence of more than one type or class of dysrhythmia

REFERENCES

1. Addy JA: Dopamine not effective for treatment of hypotension in chlorpromazine overdose: First case report. J Emerg Nurs 1995;21:99–101.
2. Ahlquist RP: A study of the adrenotropic receptors. Am J Physiol 1948;153:586–600.
3. Amano T, Matsubara T, Watanabe J, et al: Insulin modulation of intracellular free magnesium in heart: Involvement of protein kinase C. Br J Pharmacol 2000;130:731–8.
4. Arai M: Function and regulation of sarcoplasmic reticulum Ca+2-ATPase, advances during the past decade and prospects for the coming decade. Jpn Heart J 2000;41(1):1–13.
5. Bain DJG, Turner T: Imipramine poisoning. Arch Dis Child 1971;46:887.
6. Barry WH, Bridge JHB: Intracellular calcium homeostasis in cardiac myocytes. Circulation 1993;87:1806–1815.
7. Benowitz NL, Rosenberg J, Becker CE: Cardiopulmonary catastrophes in drug-overdosed patients. Med Clin North Am 1979;63:127–140.
8. Berridge, MJ: Inositol trisphosphate and calcium signaling. Nature 1993;361:315–325.
9. Bessen HA, Niemann JT, Haskell RJ, et al: Effect of respiratory alkalosis in tricyclic antidepressant overdose. West J Med 1983;139:373–376.
10. Blackshear PJ, Nairn AC, Kuo JF: Protein kinases 988: A current perspective. FASEB J 1988;2:2957–2969.
11. Boehnert M, Lovejoy FH: Value of the QRS duration versus the serum drug level in predicting seizures and ventricular arrhythmias after an acute overdose of tricyclic antidepressants. N Engl J Med 1985;313:474–479.
12. Brass BJ, Winchester-Penny S, Lipper BL: Massive verapamil overdose complicated by noncardiogenic pulmonary edema. Am J Emerg Med 1996;14:459–461.
13. Braunwald E: Approach to the patient with heart disease. In Braunwald E, Isselbacher KJ, Fauci AS, et al., eds: Harrison's Principles of Internal Medicine. New York: McGraw-Hill, 1998, pp. 1229–1231.
14. Bristow MR, Ginsberg R: β_2 Receptors on myocardial cells in human ventricular myocardium. Am J Cardiol 1986;57:3F–6F.
15. Bristow MR: The β-adrenergic receptor: Configuration, regulation, mechanism of action. Postgrad Med 1988;29:19–26.
16. Brodde OE: The functional importance of β_1 and β_2 adrenoceptors in the human heart. Am J Cardiol 1988;62:24C–29C.
17. Brown JE, McLeod AA, Shand DG: In support of cardiac chronotropic β_2 adrenoceptors. Am J Cardiol 1986;57:11F–16F.
18. Brown TCK, Barker GA, Dunlop ME, et al: The use of sodium bicarbonate in the treatment of tricyclic antidepressant induced arrhythmias. Anesth Int Care 1973;1:203–210.
19. Buchman AL, Dauer J, Geiderman J: The use of vasoactive agents in the treatment of refractory hypotension seen in tricyclic antidepressant overdose. J Clin Psychopharmacol 1990;10:409–413.

20. Buxton AE, Marchlinski FE, Doherty JU, Flores B: Hazards of intravenous verapamil for sustained ventricular tachycardia. Am J Cardiol 1987;59:1107–1110.

21. Casey PJ, Gilman AG: G protein involvement in receptor-effector coupling. J Biol Chem 1988;263:2577–2580.

22. Catravas JD, Waters IW: Acute cocaine intoxication in the conscious dog: Studies on the mechanism of lethality. J Pharmacol Exp Ther 1981;217:350–356.

23. Centers for Disease Control and Prevention (CDC). Jin bu huan toxicity in adults—Los Angeles, 1993. MMWR Morb Mortal Wkly Rep 1993;42:920–922.

24. Changeux JP: The acetylcholine receptor: its molecular biology and biotechnological prospects. Bioessays 1989;10:48–54.

25. Chen-Izu Y, Xiao RP, Izu LT, et al: G(i)-dependent localization of β(2)-adrenergic receptor signaling to L-type Ca(2+) channels. Biophys J 2000;79:2547–2556.

26. Clemessy JL, Taboulet P, Hoffman JR, et al: Treatment of acute chloroquine poisoning: A 5-year experience. Crit Care Med 1996;24:1189–1195.

27. Crome P: Poisoning due to tricyclic antidepressant overdosage: Clinical presentation and treatment. Med Toxicol 1986;1:261–285.

28. Derlet RW, Albertson TE: Potentiation of cocaine toxicity with calcium channel blockers. Am J Emerg Med 1989;7:464–468.

29. Derlet RW, Albertson TE: Diazepam in the prevention of seizures and death in cocaine-intoxicated rats. Ann Emerg Med 1989;18:542–546.

30. Enocksson S, Shimizu M, Lonnqvist F, et. al: Demonstration of an in vivo functional β₃-adrenoceptor in man. J Clin Invest 1995;95:2239–2245.

31. Fantl WJ, Johnson DE, Williams LT. Signalling by receptor tyrosine kinases. Annu Rev Biochem 1993;62:453–481.

32. Farah AE, Alousi AA. The actions of insulin on cardiac contractility. Life Sci 1981;29:975–1000.

33. Farah CS, Reinach FC: The troponin complex and regulation of muscle contraction. FASEB J 1995;9(9):755–67.

34. Frank K, Kranias EG: Phospholamban and cardiac contractility. Ann Med 2000;32(8):572–578.

35. Frielle T, Daniel KW, Caron MG: Structural basis of β-adrenergic receptor subtype specificity studied with chimeric β1/β2-adrenergic receptors. Proc Natl Acad Sci U S A 1988;85:9494–9498.

36. Frierson J, Bailly D, Shultz T, et al: Refractory cardiogenic shock and complete heart block after unsuspected verapamil SR and atenolol overdose. Clin Cardiol 1991;14:933–935.

37. Gautier C, Lablais B, Kobzic L, et. al: The negative inotropic effect of β₃-adrenoreceptor stimulation is mediated by activation of a nitric oxide synthase pathway in human ventricle. J Clin Invest 1998;102:1377–1384.

38. Gautier C, Tavernier G, Charpentier F, Langin D, LeMarec, H: Functional β₃-adrenoreceptor in the human heart. J Clin Invest 1996;98:556–562.

39. Gilman AG: The Albert Lasker Medical Awards: G proteins and regulation of adenylyl cyclase. JAMA 1989;262:1819–1825.

40. Glick G, Parmley W, Wechsler A, Sonnenblick E: Glucagon: Its enhancement of cardiac performance in the cat and dog and persistence of its inotropic action despite β receptor blockade with propranolol. Circ Res 1968;22:789–799.

41. Goodwin DA, Lally KP, Null DM Jr: Extracorporeal membrane oxygenation support for cardiac dysfunction from antidepressant overdose. Crit Care Med 1993;21:625–627.

42. Graham RM, Perez DM, Hwa J, Piasik MT: α₁ Adrenergic receptor subtypes: Molecular structure, function, and signaling. Circ Res 1996;78:737–749.

43. Guinn MM, Bedford JA, Wilson MC: Antagonism of intravenous cocaine lethality in nonhuman primates. Clin Toxicol 1980;16:499–508.

44. Harrison DC: Current classification of antiarrhythmic drugs as a guide to their rational clinical use. Drugs 1986;31:93–95.

45. Hartzell HC, Hirayama Y, Petit-Jacques J: Effects of protein phosphatase and kinase inhibitors on the cardiac L-type calcium current suggests two sites are phosphorylated by protein kinase A and another protein kinase. J Gen Physiol 1995;106:393–414.

46. Hassen AH, Broudy EP: Selective autonomic modulation by mu- and kappa-opioid receptors in the hindbrain. Peptides 1988;9:63–67.

47. Hendren WG, Schieber RS, Garrettson LK: Extracorporeal bypass for the treatment of verapamil poisoning. Ann Emerg Med 1989;18:984–987.

48. Hoeper MM, Boeker KH: Overdose of metoprolol treated with enoximone. N Engl J Med 1996;335:1538.

49. Howarth DM, Dawson AH, Smith AJ, et al: Calcium channel-blocking drug overdose: An Australian series. Hum Exp Toxicol 1994;13:161–166.

50. Humbert VH, Munn NJ, Hawkins RF: Noncardiogenic pulmonary edema complicating massive diltiazem overdose. Chest 1991;99:258–260.

51. Ilingworth R: Glucagon for β blocker poisoning. Lancet 1980;1:86.

52. Katz AM, Lorell BH: Regulation of cardiac contraction and relaxation. Circulation 2000:102(20 Suppl 4):IV69–IV74.

53. Jacobsen D, Helgeland A, Koss A: Treatment of β blocker poisoning. Lancet 1980;2:1031–1032.

54. Jaken S: Protein kinase C isozymes and substrates. Curr Opin Cell Biol 1996;8:168–173.

55. Johnson GL, Dhanasekaran N: The G-protein family and their interaction with receptors. Endocr Rev 1989;10:317–331.

56. Karch SB: Serum catecholamines in cocaine intoxicated patients with cardiac symptoms. Ann Emerg Med 1987;16:481–483.

57. Kerns W, Schroeder D, Williams C, et al: Insulin improves survival in a canine model of acute β-blocker toxicity. Ann Emerg Med 1997;29:748–757.

58. Kim SY, Benowitz NL: Poisoning due to class Ia antiarrhythmic drugs quinidine, procainamide, and disopyramide. Drug Saf 1990;5:393–420.

59. Kingston ME: Hyperventilation in tricyclic antidepressant poisoning. Crit Care Med 1979;7:550–551.

60. Kline JA, Raymond RM, Leonova ED, et al: Insulin improves heart function and metabolism during non-ischemic cardiogenic shock in awake canines. Cardiovasc Res 1997;34:289–298.

61. Koppel C, Oberdisse U, Heinemeyer G: Clinical course and outcome in class Ic antiarrhythmic overdose. J Toxicol Clin Toxicol 1990;28:433–444.

62. Kosinski E, Malindzak G: Glucagon and isoproterenol in reversing propranolol toxicity. Arch Intern Med 1973;132:840–843.

63. Krikler DM, Curry PVL: Torsades de pointes, an atypical ventricular tachycardia. Br Heart J 1968;38:117–120.

64. Kuschel M, Zhou YY, Cheng H, et al: G(i) protein-mediated functional compartmentalization of cardiac β(2)-adrenergic signaling. J Biol Chem 1999;274(31):22048–22052.

65. Lands AM, Arnold A, McAuliff SP: Differentiation of receptor systems activated by sympathomimetic amines. Nature 1967;214:597–598.

66. Lane AS, Woodward AC, Goldman MR: Massive propranolol overdose poorly responsive to pharmacologic therapy: Use of the intra-aortic balloon pump. Ann Emerg Med 1987;16:1381–1383.

67. Langou RA, Van Dyke C, Tahan SR, et al: Cardiovascular manifestations of tricyclic antidepressant overdose. Am Heart J 1980;100:458–464.

68. Lee KC, Canniff PC, Hamel DW, et al: Cardiovascular and renal effects of milrinone in β-adrenoreceptor blocked and non-blocked anaesthetized dogs. Drugs Exp Clin Res 1991;18:145–158.

68. Lennon NJ and Ohlendieck K: Impaired Ca²⁺-sequestration in dilated cardiomyopathy [review]. Int J Mol Med 2001;7(2):131–41.

70. Levitan ES, Schofield PR, Burt DR, et al: Structural and functional basis for GABAA receptor heterogeneity. Nature 1988;335:76–79.

71. Levitzki A, Marbach I, Bar-Sinai A: The signal transduction between β receptors and adenyl cyclase. Life Sci 1993;52:2093–2100.

72. Limbird LE: Receptors linked to inhibition of adenylate cyclase: Additional signaling mechanisms. FASEB J 1988;2:2686–2695.

73. Lonnqvist F, Krief S, Strosberg AD, et al: Evidence for a functional β3 adrenoceptor in man. Br J Pharmacol 1993;110:929–936.

74. Love JN, Leasure JA, Mundt DJ, Janz TG: A comparison of amrinone and glucagon therapy for cardiovascular depression associated with propranolol. J Toxicol Clin Toxicol 1992;30:399–412.

75. Low MG, Saltiel AR: Structural and functional roles of glycosyl-phosphatidylinositol in membranes. Science 1988;239:268–275.

76. Mader SL: Orthostatic hypotension. Med Clin North Am 1989;73:1337–1349.

77. Marrs-Simon P, Zell-Kanter M, Kendzierski DL, et al: Cardiotoxic manifestations of mesoridazine overdose. Ann Emerg Med 1988;17:1074–1078.

78. Marshall JB, Forker AD: Cardiovascular effects of tricyclic antidepressant drugs: Therapeutic usage, overdose, and management of complications. Am Heart J 1982;103:401–414.

79. Mathe L, Vallerand D, Haddad PS: Insulin induces cation fluxes and increases intracellular calcium in the HTC rat hepatoma cell line. Can J Gastroenterol 2000;14:389–396.

80. Mery PF, Brechler V, Pavoine C, et al: Glucagon stimulates the cardiac Ca(+2) current by activation of adenyl cyclase and inhibition of phosphodiesterase. Nature 1990;345:158–161.

81. Moniotte S, Kobzik L, Feron O, Trochu JN, et al: Upregulation of β(3)-adrenoceptors and altered contractile response to inotropic amines in human failing myocardium. Circulation 2001;103(12):1649–1655

82. Nattel S, Mittleman M: Treatment of ventricular tachyarrhythmias resulting from amitriptyline toxicity in dogs. J Pharmacol Exp Ther 1984;231:430–435.

83. Neer EJ: Heterotrimeric G proteins: Organizers of transmembrane signals. Cell 1995;80:249–257.

84. Neer EJ, Clapham DE: Roles of G protein subunits in transmembrane signaling. Nature 1988;333:129–134.

85. Niemann JT, Bessen HA, Rothstein RH, et al: Electrocardiographic criteria for tricyclic antidepressant cardiotoxicity. Am J Cardiol 1986;57:1154–1159.

86. Paakkari P, Paakkari I, Peuerstein G, Siren AL: Evidence for differential opioid mu 1- and mu 2-receptor-mediated regulation of heart rate in the conscious rat. Neuropharmacology 1992;31:777–782.

87. Panayotou G, Waterfield MD: Cell surface receptors for polypeptide hormones, growth factors and neuropeptides. Curr Opin Cell Biol 1989;1:167–176.

88. Pentel PR, Benowitz NL: Tricyclic antidepressant poisoning: Management of arrhythmias. Med Toxicol 1986;1:101–121.

89. Peterson C, Leeder S, Sterner S: Glucagon therapy for β blocker overdose. Drug Intell Clin Pharm 1984;18:394–398.

90. Randich A, Robertson JD, Willinghan T: The use of specific opioid agonists and antagonists to delineate the vagally mediated antinociceptive and cardiovascular effects of intravenous morphine. Brain Res 1993;603:186–200.

91. Rankin AC, Rae AP, Cobbe SM: Misuse of intravenous verapamil in patients with ventricular tachycardia. Lancet 1987;2:472–474.

92. Rasmussen H: The calcium messenger system. N Engl J Med 1986;314:1094–1102.

93. Reiter M: Calcium mobilization and cardiac inotropic mechanisms. Pharmacol Rev 1988;40:189–217.

94. Reuter H, Porzig H: β-Adrenergic actions on cardiac cell membranes. Adv Myocardiol 1982;3:87–93.

95. Robishaw JD, Foster KA: Role of G proteins in the regulation of the cardiovascular system. Annu Rev Physiol 1989;51:229–244.

96. Robson R: Glucagon for β blocker poisoning. Lancet 1980;2:1356–1357.

97. Roden DM: Antiarrhythmic drugs. In: Hardman JG, Limbird LE, Molinoff PB, Ruddon RW, Gilman AG, eds: Goodman & Gilman's The Pharmacological Basis of Therapeutics, 9th ed. New York, McGraw-Hill, 1996, pp. 839–843.

98. Ruegg JC: Cardiac contractility: How calcium activates the myofilaments. Naturwissenschaften 1998;85:575–582.

99. Sasyniuk BI, Jhamandas V: Mechanism of reversal of toxic effects of amitriptyline on cardiac Purkinje fibers by sodium bicarbonate. J Pharmacol Exp Ther 1984;231:387–394.

100. Sasyniuk BI, Jhamandas V, Valois M: Experimental amitriptyline intoxication: Treatment of cardiac toxicity with sodium bicarbonate. Ann Emerg Med 1986;15:1052–1059.

101. Schwartz A: Molecular and cellular aspects of calcium channel antagonism. Am J Cardiol 1992;70:6F–8F.

102. Smith DM, King MJ, Sale GJ: Two systems in vitro that show insulin-stimulated serine kinase activity towards the insulin receptor. Biochem J 1988;250:509–519.

103. Sperelakis N, Xiong Z, Haddad G, et al: Regulation of slow calcium channels of myocardial cells and vascular smooth muscle by cyclic nucleotides and phosphorylation. Mol Cell Biochem 1994;140:103–117.

104. Spiegel AM: Signal transduction by guanine nucleotide binding proteins. Kidney Int Suppl 1987;23:S14–S42.

105. Steinberg SF: The molecular basis for distinct β-adrenergic receptor subtype actions in cardiomyocytes. Circ Res 1999;85:1101–1111.

106. Steinberg SF: The cellular actions of β-adrenergic receptor agonists: Looking beyond cAMP. Circ Res 2000;87:1072–1079.

107. Sunahara R, Dessauer C, Gilma A: Complexity and diversity of mammalian adenylyl cyclases. Annu Rev Pharmacol Toxicol 1996;36:461–480.

108. Stewart RB, Bardy GH, Greene HL: Wide complex tachycardia: Misdiagnosis and outcome after emergent therapy. Ann Intern Med 1986;104:766–771.

109. Stinson J, Walsh M, Feely J: Ventricular asystole and overdose with atenolol. BMJ 1992;305:693.

110. Strosberg AD: Structure, function, and regulation of the three β-adrenergic receptors. Obes Res 1995;3(Suppl 4):501S–505S.

111. Sulakhe PV, Vo XT: Regulation of phospholamban and troponin-I phosphorylation in the intact rat cardiomyocytes by adrenergic and cholinergic stimuli: Roles of cyclic nucleotides, calcium, protein kinases, and phosphatases and depolarization. Mol Cell Biochem 1995;149/150:103–126.

112. Taboulet P, Baud FJ, Bismuth C, Vicaut E: Acute digitalis intoxication: Is pacing still appropriate? J Toxicol Clin Toxicol 1993;31:261–273.

113. Talosi L, Kranias EG: Effect of α-adrenergic stimulation on activation of protein kinase C and phosphorylation of proteins in intact rabbit hearts. Circ Res 1992;70:670–678.

114. Travill CM, Pugh S, Noble MIM: The inotropic and hemodynamic effects of intravenous milrinone when reflex adrenergic stimulation is suppressed by β-adrenergic blockade. Clin Ther 1994;16:783–792.

115. Trouve R, Nahas GG, Maillet M: Nitrendipine as an antagonist to the cardiac toxicity of cocaine. J Cardiovasc Pharmacol 1987;9:S49–S53.

116. Tsien RW, Lipscombe D, Madison DV, et al: Multiple types of neuronal calcium channels and their selective modulation. 1988;11:431–438.

117. Ullrich A, Schlessinger J: Signal transduction by receptors with tyrosine kinase activity. Cell 1990;61:203–212.

118. Vaughan-Williams EM: In: Sandoe E, Ellen FJ, Olesen KH, eds: Symposium on Cardiac Arrhythmias. Helsingor, Denmark, Sodertalje Press, 1970.

119. Vaughn-Williams EM: Subgroups of class I antiarrhythmic drugs. Eur Heart J 1984;5:96–98.

120. Vaughn-Williams EM: A classification of antiarrhythmic actions reassessed after a decade of new drugs. J Clin Pharmacol 1984;24:129–147.

121. Ward DE, Jones B: Glucagon and β blocker toxicity. BMJ 1976;1:151.

122. Wasserman F, Brodsky L, Dick MM, et al: Successful treatment of quinidine and procainamide intoxication. N Engl J Med 1958;259:797–802.

123. Watling SM, Crain JL, Edwards TD, Stiller RA: Verapamil overdose: Case report and review of the literature. Ann Pharmacother 1992;26:1373–1378.

124. Wheeldon NM, McDevitt DG, Lipworth BJ: Investigation of putative β₃ adrenoceptors in man. Q J Med 1993;86:255–261.

125. White MF, Kahn CR: The insulin signaling system. J Biol Chem 1994;269:1–4.

126. Williams JM, Hollingshed MJ, Vasilakis A, et al: Extracorporeal circulation in the management of severe tricyclic antidepressant overdose. Am J Emerg Med 1994;12:456–458.

127. Williams T, Knopp R: The clinical use of orthostatic vital signs. In: Roberts JR, Hedges JR, eds: Clinical Procedures in Emergency Medicine. Philadelphia, WB Saunders, 1991, pp. 445–449.

128. Winson T, Burch GE: Clinical assessment of central venous pressure. Am Heart J 1946;31:387–391.

129. Xiao RP: Cell logic for dual coupling of a single class of receptors to G(s) and G(i) proteins. Circ Res 2000;87:635–637.

130. Xiao RP, Cheng, H, Zhou YY, et al: Recent advances in cardiac β(2)-adrenergic signal transduction. Circ Res 1999;85(11):1092–1100.

131. Yagami T: Differential coupling of glucagon and β-adrenergic receptors with the small and large forms of the stimulatory G protein. Mol Pharmacol 1995;48:849–854.

132. Yuan TH, Kerns WP, Tomaszewski CA, et al: Insulin-glucose as adjunctive therapy for severe calcium channel antagonist poisoning. J Toxicol Clin Toxicol 1999;37:463–474.

133. Zerkowski HR, Ikezono K, Rohm N, et al: Human myocardial β adrenoceptors: Demonstration of both β₁ and β₂ adrenoceptors mediating contractile responses to β agonists on the isolated right atrium. Arch Pharmacol 1986;332:142–147.

GASTROINTESTINAL PRINCIPLES

Neal E. Flomenbaum / Martin J. Smilkstein

The role of the gastrointestinal (GI) tract in toxicologic emergencies is usually defined by its relationship to the absorption of toxic agents; as a result, GI decontamination is a major focus of clinical practice, research, and controversy (Chap. 5). However, the GI tract should also be recognized as an important *site* of toxic effects, both as a result of decontamination procedures (Table 22–1) and, more importantly, the action of drugs and poisons. GI manifestations of toxic exposures range from incidental to life-threatening, and result from both direct and indirect mechanisms.[5] Direct effects alter GI tract function and/or structure. Direct effects that disrupt function without causing immediate structural changes may do so by extrinsic mechanisms (eg, cholinergic excess) or by intracellular mechanisms (eg, colchicine); direct effects that do cause immediate structural changes inevitably result in functional impairment (eg, caustics). An example of an *indirect* effect is vomiting caused by an agent that only stimulates the chemoreceptor trigger zone, and has no direct effect on the gastric mucosa (as with digoxin or apomorphine).[42]

In some cases of altered GI function, such as the increased gut motility resulting from opioid withdrawal, function is not seriously impaired and the change is often useful in establishing a diagnosis. Conversely, the decreased gut motility caused by cyclic antidepressants or other anticholinergics, the severe constipation or obstipation sometimes caused by opioids,[42] and the pseudo-obstruction caused by the antipsychotics, butyrophenones, and phenothiazines can harm the patient or complicate management. Because there are no structural changes associated with either of these types of altered GI function, there is no significant local injury. Such agents as salicylates, iron, and other metals, however, are capable of causing both serious systemic effects and life-threatening GI hemorrhage, perforation, or delayed stricture. Finally, alkalis typify substances that result in little or no systemic absorption or toxicity while causing morbidity or mortality from direct GI injury.

TOXINS WITH WIDESPREAD EFFECTS ON THE GASTROINTESTINAL TRACT

Caustics, ionizing radiation, and ethanol (and other alcohols) constitute a group of toxins that adversely affect the GI tract in many locations by a variety of mechanisms. Before considering specific sections of the GI tract, the gastrointestinal toxicity of these three classes of agents is reviewed.

Caustics

Without question, caustics are the most serious source of direct toxicity to the upper GI tract from lips to small intestines. Caustics are discussed extensively in Chap. 87, but a brief review of the patterns of destruction associated with alkalis and acids illustrates the type of structural damage the GI tract is subject to. Alkaline caustics such as sodium hydroxide (NaOH), also known as lye, drain cleaner, and oven cleaner, produce a liquefactive destruction of the mucosa that may destroy and perforate all layers, depending on the strength, form (liquid, crystal), amount, and duration of contact. After the ingestion of an alkaline caustic, the primary sites of destruction are the lips, mouth, oropharynx, and esophagus. When perforation does not occur, healing is characterized by scarring and strictures that can be so severe as to require colon interposition to replace the affected esophagus.[34,103]

In contrast to the alkalis, strong acids are said to be most damaging to the stomach and duodenum, and to skip or spare the esophagus. However, in India, where strong acids are commonly available as toilet cleansers, one study of a large number of acid ingestions demonstrated that the esophagus was as frequently involved as the stomach and duodenum. The author noted that in Western studies of caustic ingestions, acids only account for about 5% of reported cases and that this may explain, in part, the misconception that acids do not affect the esophagus.[110]

When acids injure the esophagus, the damage may not be as great as the esophageal damage caused by strong alkalis, perhaps as a result of the coagulation necrosis produced by acids in that location. However, the damage to the stomach and the systemic effects of acid ingestion may be devastating: Strong acids produce acidemia—normal (non) anion gap type initially, in the case of hydrochloric acid, and wide anion gap type in all other cases. Because of its tendency to perforate the stomach, acid ingestion results in widespread damage to other abdominal organs including the spleen, pancreas, and biliary tract (Chap. 87 and Fig. 8–22). In addition to causing the same type of late effects seen after alkaline ingestions, acid ingestions may cause esophageal pseudodiverticuli, gastric atony, decreased acid secretion, and gastric outlet obstruction.[15,48,75] Both acid and alkali ingestions are linked to squamous cell carcinoma of the esophagus and stomach, particularly at the gastroesophageal junction, years after the ingestion.[2,21,39,47]

The pattern of damage caused by hydrofluoric acid differs significantly from other acids: Although its pK_a would suggest that it is a weak acid, hydrofluoric acid is able to penetrate tissues much

TABLE 22–1. Gastrointestinal Complications of Gastric Decontamination Measures

Procedure	Adverse Effect
Orogastric lavage	Emesis Esophageal tears or perforation (Mallory-Weiss or Boerhaave syndromes) Gastric perforation Hemorrhage
Activated charcoal	Constipation Diarrhea Intestinal obstruction or pseudo-obstruction (especially after repetitive doses in the setting of dehydration or prior bowel adhesions) Vomiting and aspiration
Cathartics	Abdominal cramping (sorbitol) Diarrhea and frequent watery stools (sorbitol) Electrolyte imbalance: increased Mg^{2+}, decreased K^+ and Na^+, (also increased PO_4^{3-} and decreased Ca^{2+} and K^+ from phosphate enemas) Nausea and vomiting Rectal prolapse Volume depletion and consequent metabolic alkalosis
Emesis with syrup of ipecac	Delayed emesis after loss of gag reflex Diarrhea Electrolyte imbalance with chronic use Esophageal (Mallory-Weiss) tears Gastric rupture or herniation Intractable vomiting and aspiration
Whole-bowel irrigation	Bloating Colonic perforation (in the presence of severe diverticulitis) Rectal itching (from excessive wiping) Vomiting, especially with rapid administration

more effectively than other acids. This trait and its other unique properties make hydrofluoric acid the deadliest of all acids. Ingested, hydrofluoric acid primarily affects the stomach initially, but systemic absorption and consequent toxicity rapidly follow and ingestions of large amounts of highly concentrated solutions are almost always fatal (Chap. 87).[10,57,100]

Other commonly available substances that are corrosive to the GI tract include ammonium hydroxide (ammonia), automatic dishwasher detergents, sodium hypochlorite (bleach),[3] alcohols, and phenol.

Ionizing Radiation

Acute radiation syndrome is a symptom complex that develops after whole-body radiation exposure and is divided into 4 phases, 2 of which involve the gastrointestinal tract.[17,81] An initial phase of nausea, vomiting, intestinal cramps, diarrhea, salivation, and dehydration follows exposures to over 1 Gy. Onset of vomiting within 2 hours indicates exposure to doses over 6 Gy. Vomiting that begins within minutes usually indicates a lethal exposure;

within 1 hour, a near-lethal dose; and within 1–5 hours, a significant dose. Following the initial period of toxic effects, there is a latent period of days to weeks, unless the exposure is massive. The third phase is characterized by the additional gastrointestinal effects of electrolyte disturbances and dehydration and by such hematopoietic effects as pancytopenia (Chaps. 25 and 99). Death can occur within 2 weeks of an exposure to more than 10 Gy and within 2 days of an exposure to more than 20 Gy. Long-term effects such as neoplasms, sterility, and cataract formation characterize the fourth phase.[81]

The acute pathologic changes of the GI tract associated with acute radiation syndrome have been most extensively studied in the large bowel, and consist of crypts with bizarre-appearing nuclei, mucin depletion, eosinophils in the lamina propria, and eosinophilic crypt abscesses.[8,73,85,108] In the small bowel, exposure to more than 30 Gy results in loss of villi and inflammatory cells in the lamina propria.[85,101]

Late pathologic changes include mucin depletion, telangiectatic vessels in the mucosa and submucosa, mucosal atrophy, decreased number and distorted architecture of crypts, edema, fibrinous exudates, and fibrosis.[85]

Ethanol and Other Alcohols

Ethanol is often painful to the oropharynx and esophagus upon ingestion, but its major gastrointestinal toxicity occurs in the stomach (Table 22–2). Alcohol-induced lesions tend to occur after acute ingestions of 8% or higher concentrations,[85] and alcohol-in-

TABLE 22–2. Gastrointestinal Effects of Alcohol

Mouth
Nutritional stomatitis
Cheilosis

Esophagus
Esophagitis
Diffuse esophageal spasm
Mallory-Weiss tear
Rupture with mediastinitis

Stomach
Acute gastritis
Chronic hypertrophic gastritis
Peptic ulcer
Hematemesis

Small and Large Intestines
Malabsorption
Diarrhea

Liver
Steatosis
Alcoholic hepatitis
Cirrhosis

Pancreas
Acute pancreatitis
Chronic pancreatitis
Pancreatic pseudocyst

Adapted from West LF, Maxwell DS, Noble EP, Solomon DH: Alcoholism. Ann Intern Med 1984;100:412–420.

duced erosive gastritis (sometimes with the concomitant use of as-pirin and/or NSAIDS) may be responsible for more than half the cases of upper GI hemorrhages in some series.[18,46,85] As commonly used, the term "alcoholic gastritis" describes the gastric erosions and subepithelial hemorrhages with or without inflammatory cell infiltrates seen (endoscopically) in alcoholics.[51,107] When *H. pylori* is identified in alcoholics with chronic antral gastritis, eradication of the organism, and not abstinence or antacid treatment alone, is necessary to eliminate the lesions.[106]

Alcohol increases the secretion of gastric juice;[69,85] reduces the transmucosal potential difference, allowing back diffusion of hy-drogen ions;[29,85] and increases gastric mucosal permeability.[97] Mi-croscopically, alcohol-induced lesions initially alter cell cytoplasm and nuclei,[20] which is followed by widening of the intracellular space, focal separation of the tight junctions, and disruption of the apical membrane.[19,85]

Although most studies of small intestinal mucosa show only minimal light microscopic changes induced by alcohol,[65,85,90] pa-tients who drink large amounts of alcohol acutely or chronically, typically experience diarrhea for several reasons: rapid transit from enhanced propulsive movements,[58] decreased intestinal di-saccharidase activity,[77] decreased bile secretion from alcoholic liver disease,[55,88] and decreased pancreatic exocrine function or steatorrhea.[26,65] Markedly decreased absorption of fluid and elec-trolytes[49] together with ileal and colonic fluid malabsorption are also partly responsible for the diarrhea.[26]

Other gastrointestinal effects of ethanol include reflux esophagitis resulting from reduced lower esophageal sphincter pressure,[44] esophageal and gastric tears from vomiting (Mallory-Weiss and Boerhaave syndromes) after acute alcohol ingestion, and pancreatitis, hepatitis, and cirrhosis. In a Scandinavian study of 591 first episodes of acute alcoholic pancreatitis, 260 (46%) of the 562 patients who survived the episode developed recurrent dis-ease. The overwhelming majority of patients were men (503) and 80% of the first relapses occurred within 4 years.[76]

LIPS, MOUTH, AND OROPHARYNX

Edema and Obstruction

The loose connective tissue and rich vascularity of the lips, mouth, and oropharynx predispose this region to edema formation from both local and systemic exposures (Table 22–3). Angioedema caused by many agents may present in this manner.[31] Because swelling about the mouth may be the first recognized symptom of a systemic immediate hypersensitivity reaction, it is important to consider and prepare for the possibility of impending systemic anaphylaxis in addition to assessing the local findings.[4] Angio-edema of the face, tongue, soft palate, and uvula is a fairly com-mon adverse reaction to angiotensin-converting enzyme (ACE) inhibitors. Most cases of ACE inhibitor-induced angioedema may be successfully managed without airway intervention, but airway compromise has been described.[96] In addition to reactions following systemic exposures, substances that directly injure the mucosa or submucosa may also cause localized edema. Edema of the lips, mouth, and tongue is common after ingestion of caustic chemicals[103] or irritants such as oxalate-containing plants.[62] The latter category should not be regarded lightly, as deaths have oc-curred as a result of such ingestions, particularly by infants.[62] It is obviously imperative to establish and maintain an airway when

TABLE 22–3.   **Toxic Effects on the Lips, Mouth, and Oropharynx**

Type of Effect	Mechanism	Example
Gingivitis, stomatitis (loose teeth)	Inflammation and irritation	Caustics Chemotherapeutic agents Ciguatera (tooth pain) Ionizing radiation Metals (arsenic trioxide, mercuric chloride, lead, thallium, zinc chloride) Oxalates Phenol Phenytoin Phosphorous
Edema	Allergic Angioedema	Penicillin Angiotensin-converting en-zyme inhibitors
	Mechanical irritation and injury	Caustics Oxalate-containing plants
Pain and ulceration	Early	Caustics Paraquat
	Delayed	Daunorubicin Fluorouracil Methotrexate
Drooling	Increased saliva	Aminopyridine Cholinesterase inhibitors Nicotine Phencyclidine
	Dysphagia	Foreign bodies (drug pack-ets, batteries)
Dry mouth	Decreased saliva Direct	Anticholinergics Botulism
	From hypovolemia Diuresis	Diuretics Lithium
	Insensible loss	Salicylates CNS stimulants
	Decreased fluid intake	CNS depressants
	Increased GI fluid losses	Cathartics Colchicine
Tongue discoloration	Direct toxic effects	Blue — methylene blue Brown — bromide, bis-muth Green — vanadium

there is evidence of obstruction, but endotracheal intubation is also often indicated for patients without current airway compromise who may be expected to experience rapid swelling and consequent airway compromise.

Ulceration and Pain

Probably the most common sign of toxic exposure to the mouth and oropharynx is ulceration from the ingestion of caustic sub-stances, which the patient experiences as pain. In addition to the caustics already mentioned, paraquat ingestions result in lip, tongue, and pharyngeal pain and ulceration. A unique feature of paraquat ingestions is the formation of a pseudomembrane in the pharynx said to resemble that of diphtheria.[99] Lip, mouth, and pharyngeal ulcerations may also occur several days after exposure to agents that prevent regeneration of normal mucosa by interfering with the epithelial cell cycle. Examples of this second group include methotrexate[40] and ionizing radiation.

Drooling and Dry Mouth

Toxicologic causes of drooling include agents such as organic phosphorus compounds and carbamates that lead to increased production of saliva,[70] those that cause irritation of mucous membranes[82] as well as those that prevent normal swallowing because of pain (caustics),[24,32] obstruction (body stuffers),[71,87] or neurologic dysfunction (tetrodotoxin poisoning).[104]

Dry mouth may result from decreased production of saliva as a result of anticholinergic drugs (Chap. 35), exposure to other agents, such as botulism,[91] and, of course, intravascular volume depletion resulting from other sequelae of toxic exposures, such as decreased liquid intake during periods of altered consciousness, increased insensible water loss during fever or hyperpnea, increased GI or urinary losses, or a combination of exposures.

Tongue Discoloration

Discoloration of the mouth and tongue is associated with many conditions and exposures,[79] but few of these associations are specific or consistent enough to be of diagnostic value. Disturbances of normal taste are very common either from local oral exposure (eg, cocaine) or systemic effects (eg, crotalid envenomation). Extensive lists of taste alterations attributed to toxic exposures are available.[80,89] Again, a lack of specificity limits the applicability of these observations in the setting of toxicologic emergency care (Chap. 28).

ESOPHAGUS

The normal esophagus acts primarily as a conduit between the mouth and stomach. To accomplish this function, the esophagus consists of a layer of inner stratified squamous cell epithelium with mucous glands to provide lubrication, surrounded by layers of smooth muscle that contract in a coordinated manner to propel food distally into the stomach by peristalsis.[33] Afferent nerve pain fibers sense injury to the protective mucosa and submucosa, while fibers within and around the muscular layer sense excessive stretch or tension. As a result of this relatively simple structure and function, pain and difficulty swallowing are essentially the only esophageal signs and symptoms resulting from toxic exposures (Table 22–4).

Pain

Retrosternal pain from endothelial or submucosal injury is most often burning in quality and fairly well localized. Regardless of cause, direct stimulation of afferent esophageal pain fibers results in this "heartburn" perception.[33] Intermittent periods of sharp, severe chest pain often indicate alterations in esophageal muscle tension from spasm, contraction against resistance, or mechanical stretch from foreign bodies. Esophageal injury causes local spasm. Serious injury to the mucosa and submucosa can stimulate sustained, diffuse spasm,[33] without any obvious intermittent or waxing and waning character. Acids, alkalis, other caustics, corro-

TABLE 22–4.   **Drugs and Toxins that Effect the Esophagus**

Type of Effect	Mechanism	Examples
Pain — retrosternal	Pain fiber stimulation	Alcohol Caustics

	Increased muscle tension caused by
	    Obstruction
	
	    Spasm
		
		Foreign body/drug packets
		Caustics

	Mediastinitis/esophageal perforation	Caustics Emetics Foreign body
Dysphagia/odynophagia	Neuromuscular	Botulism Diphtheria Strychnine Thallium Tetrodotoxin Paralytic shellfish
	Mechanical — obstruction	Diphtheria Foreign body (drug packets) Large pill size or large number of pills
	Mechanical — irritation and injury	Caustics Iodine Mercuric chloride Paraquat, diquat

sives, and solvents cause the most significant esophageal injuries (Chap. 87), and may cause any combination of these pain patterns.

Dysphagia and Obstruction

Hastily swallowed drug packets (Fig. 22–1) and batteries (Fig. 22–2) may be considered toxicologic causes of difficulty swallowing caused by foreign body obstruction of the esophagus.[71,87] Drug packets may subsequently leak with disastrous consequences, and button batteries that obstruct may also leak or fragment causing electrochemical burns and caustic contact with the esophagus resulting in perforation, fistulae or stenosis.[52,56,59] Dysphagia may also be caused by esophageal spasm from local injury,[24,32,103] primarily from caustics.

The normal swallowing function of the striated muscle of the hypopharynx can be similarly affected and can cause dysphagia by interference with normal transfer of swallowed material into the esophagus. In addition, striated muscle function can be altered by agents that disrupt normal neuromuscular transmission, such as botulism.[91] Esophageal stricture is a late complication of caustic exposure, which may also result in pain and difficulty swallowing. Because of its delayed occurrence, it is not an important immediate treatment consideration, but it is important to anticipate this possibility and evaluate the patient for stricture development during follow-up (Chap. 87).

Esophageal stricture may occur after unrecognized esophageal injury from a variety of medications.[9] A common cause of both erosive esophagitis and esophageal strictures is the use of non-

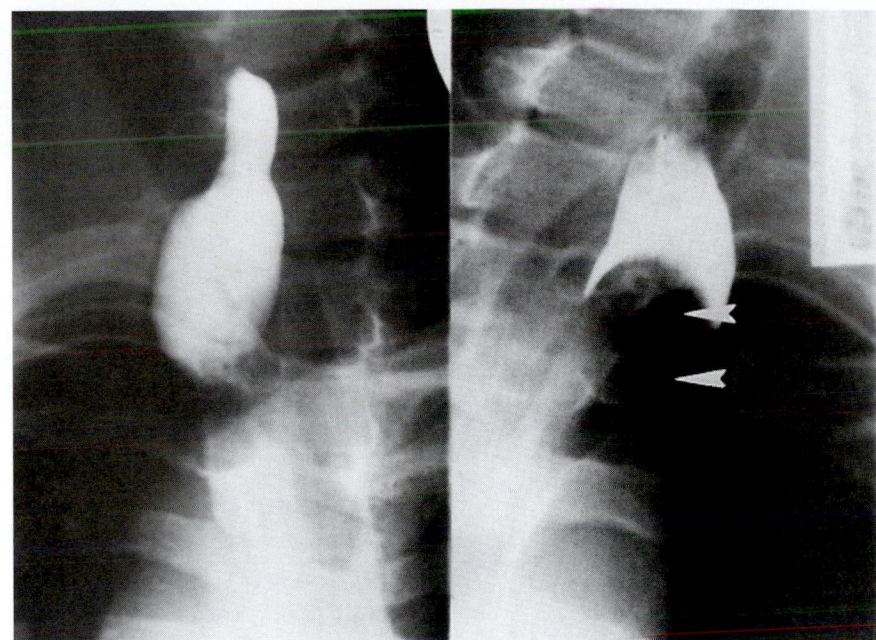

Figure 22–1. This barium swallow demonstrates an esophageal obstruction. It is part of a study done on a prisoner who had a contact visit with his wife. Shortly thereafter he became short of breath with severe neck pain and was unable to swallow water. After the barium study, a large toy balloon (*arrows*) filled with hashish was removed by endoscopy.

steroidal anti-inflammatory drugs (NSAIDs).[22] In a study of 101,366 patients with a variety of connective tissue and musculoskeletal diseases, 92,860 presented with esophagitis and 14,201 with esophageal stricture. The authors concluded that a large variety of diseases treated by NSAIDs are associated with significantly increased risk of esophageal erosion or strictures. Both direct and indirect mechanisms probably account for the contribution of NSAIDs to esophageal pathology: (a) Direct cellular toxicity is caused by lipid-soluble forms of NSAIDs formed in the acidic pH at the lower end of the esophagus in patients with gastroesophageal reflux disease (GERD); and (b) age, recumbent position (particularly from taking medications at bedtime), decreased

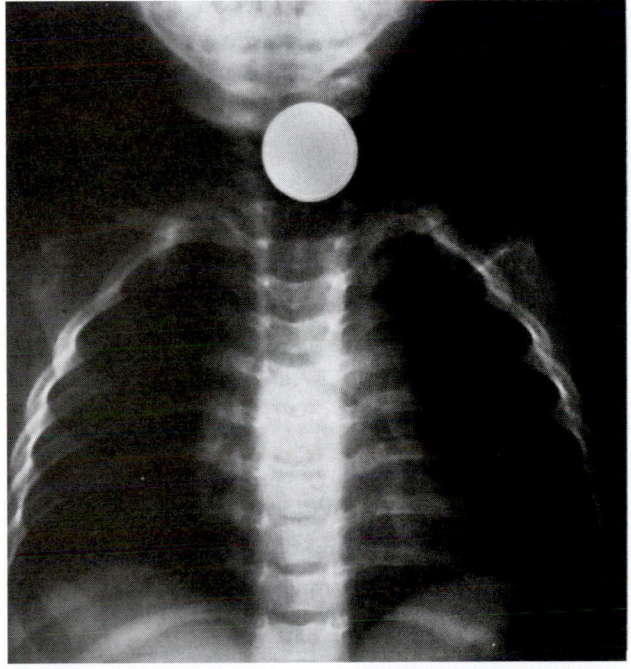

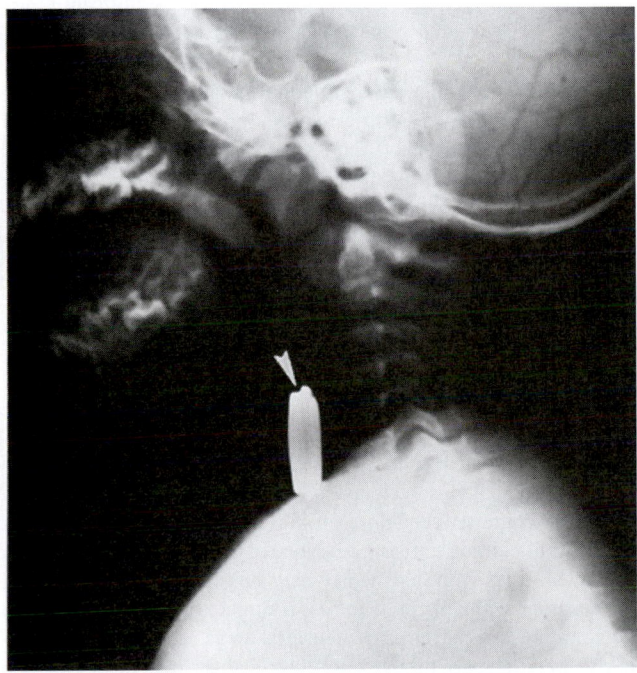

A

B

Figure 22–2. **A.** Posterior-anterior view. **B.** Lateral neck view. The large button battery demonstrated here (notice crimp [*arrow*]) provoked significant pain and was lodged in the esophagus at the level of the cricopharyngeus. Endoscopic removal of the battery was possible. (*Courtesy of Nancy Genieser, MD, Professor of Radiology, New York University.*)

saliva, and GERD-related motility disturbances all may result in prolonged contact of NSAIDs with the esophageal mucosa.[22] Such contact injuries may be caused by the caustic coatings of some pills, as well as from the active ingredients.[43]

NSAIDs are not the only medications associated with drug-induced esophageal disorders (DIED). More than 70 different drugs have been reported to cause esophageal pathology, with antibacterials such as tetracycline, doxycycline, and clindamycin responsible for more than half of the cases. Other drugs implicated in DIED include aspirin, KCl, FeSO₄, quinidine, alprenolol, steroids, and the NSAIDs.[43]

Although endoscopy is not indicated acutely for every patient, it tends to be abnormal in almost every patient in whom it is performed. The usual endoscopic findings are discrete focal erosions or ulcerations without stenosis or, in some cases, only focal erythema.[12] Typically, symptoms disappear within 10 days of stopping the drug.[12]

STOMACH

Pain and Ulceration

In general, the results of direct chemical injury to the stomach are similar to those of esophageal injury,[64] although several features make the clinical presentation somewhat different (Table 22–5). The location of pain is epigastric rather than retrosternal. Unremitting pain radiating to the back should suggest posterior penetration; severe diffuse abdominal pain and tenderness suggest possible gastric wall perforation and peritonitis,[54,74] but serious injury may be present without early tenderness.[72,83] Because of its horizontal position and restricted outlet at the pylorus, substances that pass quickly through the esophagus without significant injury may pool in the stomach and cause damage after prolonged contact.

The unique chemical and structural environment of the stomach also may make the gastric mucosa more susceptible to injury by acids and other agents (Chap. 87). Probably all gastric mucosal injury is compounded by the back-diffusion of gastric acid after disruption of the normal mucosal barrier.[33,95] Ingested foreign bodies may become obstructed throughout the GI tract as demonstrated both by plain radiography and/or contrast studies[61] (Fig. 22–3). Ingested drug packets and medication bezoars may cause significant complications from obstruction, as well as from the effects of the medications within the bezoar.[102]

Vomiting

The forceful, coordinated contraction of circumferential gastric smooth muscle against a closed pylorus results in regurgitation, an extremely common sequela of toxic exposure. Vomiting results from stimulation of the vomiting center in the floor of the fourth ventricle.[33] The vomiting center may be stimulated by either of two separate mechanisms. The first is direct afferent nerve input to the vomiting center from any of several areas. The GI tract, particularly the first part of the duodenum, gives rise to many such fibers. Many drugs and chemicals cause vomiting by direct action on these GI tract fibers.[33] The second mechanism is stimulation of the chemoreceptor trigger zone also in the area postrema of the fourth ventricle. This area lacks afferent fibers, and its electric stimulation does not cause vomiting. Rather, the chemoreceptors respond to certain agents in blood or cerebrospinal fluid, resulting

TABLE 22–5.   Drugs and Toxins that Effect the Stomach

Type of Effect	Mechanism	Examples
Pain	Epigastric pain fiber stimulation	Alcohols Antimetabolites Arsenic Caustics Colchicine Iron Mercuric chloride NSAIDs Podophyllin Salicylates
	Perforation (peritonitis)	Caustics Salicylates Pill concretions
	Obstruction	Bezoars Foreign body NSAIDs Salicylates
Vomiting	Local stimulation	Caustics Colchicine Detergents/soap (strong) Fluoride Metals (iron, mercury, thallium, arsenic) Mushrooms Salicylates Solvents Staphylococcal exotoxin Zinc chloride
	Central chemoreceptor trigger zone	Cardiac glycosides CO (?) Opioids Nicotine
	Local and central	Methylxanthines (theophylline, caffeine) Syrup of ipecac
	Increased intracranial pressure Toxin-induced hemorrhage Edema Hemorrhage or infarct Hypertension Hypotension Coagulopathy	 Amphetamine Cocaine Phenylpropanolamine Vitamin A Postanoxic brain injury Anticoagulants
Hematemesis	Direct mucosal injury	Alcohols (ethanol, isopropyl) Caustics Metals Plants Radiation Salicylates and NSAIDs Zinc chloride
	Coagulopathy	Anticoagulants Hepatic failure

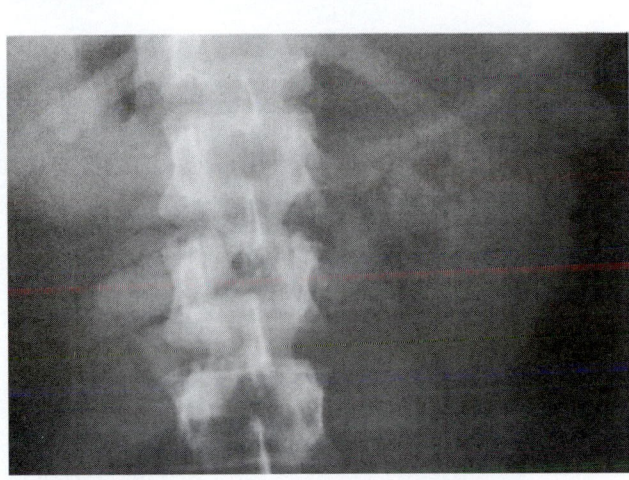

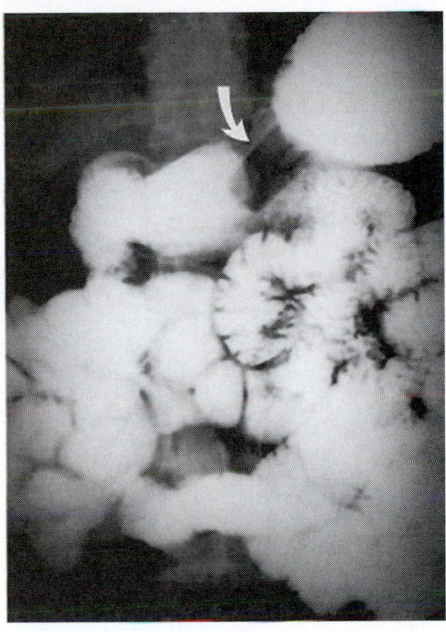

A   B

Figure 22–3. Use of GI radiocontrast agents to aid in the diagnosis of radiolucent foreign bodies. A "body packer" attempting to smuggle cocaine was arrested at the airport by customs agents alerted to his mission. **A.** Initial radiographs demonstrated multiple packets in the bowel, visible because of the thin layer of air trapped between layers of latex in the packet wall. Whole-bowel irrigation eliminated multiple packets in the fecal effluent and repeat plain radiographs were "negative." **B.** However, a subsequent upper GI contrast study with small-bowel follow-through revealed one remaining packet in the stomach (*arrow*), which was then removed using flexible endoscopy.

in efferent stimulation of the vomiting center. Some substances are capable of stimulating vomiting by stimulating both GI tract fibers and the chemoreceptor trigger zone. Also, secondary effects of toxic exposure may include increased intracranial pressure or brainstem ischemia or hemorrhage, all of which are very potent causes of vomiting.

The color of the emesis often has diagnostic value. In most cases, the color of the ingested agent determines the color of the emesis; occasionally, however, the emesis may have a characteristic color not reflective of the ingestant itself. Examples include blue-green emesis after ingestion of copper sulfate, blue-brown emesis if starch is present in the stomach after ingestion of iodine, and the smoking, luminescent stools with a "garlic-like" odor after a yellow-phosphorus ingestion.

Hematemesis

Hematemesis, sometimes massive, may occur after ingestion of any agent that disrupts the gastric mucosa such as caustics, mercuric chloride, or iron,[63,74] or as a result of toxic coagulopathy.[16,35,38]

SMALL AND LARGE INTESTINES

Normal intestinal function includes secretion of digestive enzymes, gentle mechanical mixing and propulsion of intestinal contents, and absorption of nutrients and water.[33] Each of these functions can be impaired by toxic exposures and result in signs and symptoms (Table 22–6).

Pain

Abdominal pain most commonly results from abnormally forceful or frequent intestinal smooth muscle contractions, which, in turn, results from local irritation, cholinergic stimulation, or contraction against a foreign body.[105] This type of pain is colicky and variable in intensity, frequency, and location. The frequency of intestinal contraction and the site of pain referral varies depending on the region of intestine affected.[94] Persistent pain associated with reproducible abdominal tenderness should suggest serosal or peritoneal involvement from intestinal perforation. Another form of pain, ischemic pain, results from cocaine use.[13,37,66,68] Gastrointestinal perforation may follow, particularly with the use of crack cocaine,[23,53] although bowel obstruction may be easier to demonstrate than perforation on plain radiography (Fig. 22–4).

Diarrhea

Diarrhea is a common GI manifestation of poisoning and accounts for about 7% of all adverse drug effects; more than 700 drugs have been implicated in causing diarrhea.[14] Drugs and toxins cause diarrhea by several distinct mechanisms: Direct injury to intestinal mucosa stimulates increased motility and results in impaired secretion of digestive enzymes as well as impaired absorption across the mucosa, all of which result in diarrhea.[1,25,26] Toxin-related diarrhea in the absence of structural injury may result from cholinergics, from inhibition of membrane proteins responsible for critical digestive or transport functions,[25] or from osmotically active agents such as cathartics.[50] Other toxic causes of diarrhea include colchicine, mercuric chloride, endogenous and exogenous bacter-

TABLE 22–6.   Drugs and Toxins that Effect the Small and Large Intestines

Type of Effect	Mechanism	Examples
Pain	Increased contraction Local irritation	Caustics Colchicine Metals Mushrooms Solanine-containing plants Stimulant cathartics
	Cholinergic stimulation	Cholinesterase inhibitors Opioid withdrawal
	Obstruction	Foreign body/drug-containing packets
Diarrhea	Mechanical irritation and injury	Bacterial endo- and exotoxins (food poisoning) Cathartic stimulants Caustics Colchicine Metals Mushrooms Solanine-containing plants
	Failure of mucosal regeneration	Colchicine Daunorubicin Etoposide Fluorouracil Ionizing radiation Podophyllin
	Cholinergic stimulation	Cholinesterase inhibitors Nicotine Opioid withdrawal
	Other mechanisms	Theophylline
Constipation	Local effects	Fluid and electrolyte depletion
	Central effects	Anticholinergics Infant botulism Opioids and other CNS depressants

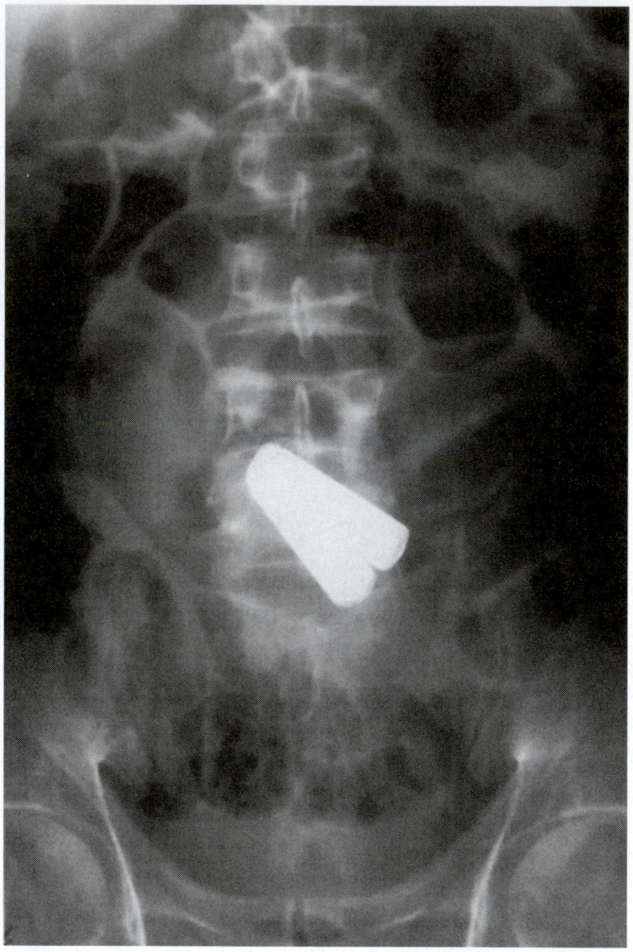

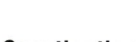

Figure 22–4.   Bowel obstruction, perforation, and peritonitis occured after ingestion of 2 AA batteries by a patient who had prior abdominal surgery. Plain films demonstrate the batteries and distended loops of bowel, but there is no evidence of free intraperitioneal air.

ial toxins (food poisoning), and plants such as pokeweed. Antimicrobials cause 25% of drug-induced diarrhea, which ranges in severity from "benign diarrhea" to pseudomembranous colitis.[14] Malabsorption can result from changes in intraluminal pH or binding of nutrients in a nonabsorbable form.

Melena

Melena and hematochezia result from the same substances that cause hematemesis but may also follow cocaine-related bowel ischemia[23,53,66,68,109] or antimetabolite poisoning. Many forms of stool discoloration have been described.[7,78] As in emesis, the color of the feces results from the color of the ingested material or from upper or lower GI bleeding. Black stools do not always indicate bleeding because they may also result from iron ingestion, senna, or bismuth subsalicylate (Pepto-Bismol) use. Rarely, a unique color change in the stools occurs, such as pink stools from phenolphthalein in alkaline medium, or smoking, phosphorescent stools with a garlic odor after phosphorus ingestion.

Constipation

Constipation results from several types of poisoning such as opioids, cyclic antidepressants, and infant botulism, which cause decreased GI motility;[28,92] phenothiazines causing pseudo-obstruction; and such indirect causes as drug-induced electrolyte disorders.[60]

PANCREAS

The remaining components of the digestive system include the liver, gallbladder, and pancreas. Hepatobiliary principles are considered in Chap. 14; pancreatic toxicity is considered briefly here (Table 22–7). Although the definitive diagnosis of acute pancreatitis is pathologic and therefore only possible after surgical intervention or postmortem examination, the combination of severe upper abdominal pain, elevated pancreatic enzymes (serum amylase, serum lipase), and perhaps diagnostic and ultrasound or CT

TABLE 22–7.   Drug and Toxins Associated with Pancreatitis

Exocrine Pancreas	Endocrine (Islets of Langerhans) Pancreas
Alcohols	**Alpha Cells**
Ethanol	Cobalt salts
Methanol	Decamethylene diquaindine
	Phenylethyldiquanide
Analgesics and NSAIDs	
Acetaminophen	**Beta Cells**
Opioids	Alloxan
Salicylates*	Androgens
Sulindac	Cyclizine
	Cyproheptadine
Antibiotics	Diazoxide
Pentamidine	Dihydromorphanthridine
Rifampin	Epinephrine
Sulfonamides	Glucagon
Tetracycline	Glucocorticoids
	Growth hormone
Anticonvulsants	Pentamidine
Valproic acid	Streptozocin
	Sulfonamides
Antihypertensives	Vacor
ACE inhibitors	Zinc chelators
α-Methyldopa*	
Diazoxide*	
	Delta Cells
Antimitotics	None known
Azathioprine	
L-Asparaginase	
Mercaptopurine	
Diuretics	
Chlorthalidone*	
Ethacrynic acid*	
Furosemide	
Thiazides	
Hormones	
Corticosteroids	
Estrogens	
Others	
Organic phosphorous compounds	
Phenformin	

*Based on single or rare case reports.
From Riddell RH, Strauss FH: The pancreas. In: Riddell RH, ed: Pathology of Drug-Induced and Toxic Diseases. New York, Churchill Livingstone, 1982, pp. 611–629.

findings, is usually sufficient to establish a clinical diagnosis.[6,41,98] Acute pancreatitis may occur either as isolated or recurrent attacks; it is distinguished from chronic pancreatitis by the absence of continuing inflammation, irreversible structural changes, or permanent impairment of exocrine and endocrine function.[98] In the United States, alcohol is responsible for at least 30% of cases of acute pancreatitis and is the most common cause of chronic pancreatitis.[6] When acute pancreatitis is induced by alcohol, small amounts of activated trypsin associated with disproportionately high concentrations of protein, zymogens, and trypsin inhibitor may be found within the ducts[84,86] along with hypertriglyceridemia.[86] An elevated blood-ethanol level is also associated with an acutely decreased hemoglobin oxygen saturation in the pancreas, but not the stomach or kidney, suggesting that alcohol may injure the pancreas by causing a functional impairment of pancreatic microperfusion.[27] Alcoholic pancreatitis is considered a form of chronic pancreatitis, but clinically an acute exacerbation more typically resembles and is treated as an acute pancreatitis.[98]

Unless further defined, *pancreatitis* tends to be used to describe dysfunction of the *exocrine* pancreas. The drugs and substances that are toxic to the exocrine pancreas differ from those that damage the *endocrine* pancreas. Sulfonamides, thiazides, furosemide, estrogens, and tetracycline are among drugs most strongly associated with dysfunction of the exocrine pancreas. More than 100 cases of pancreatitis induced by ACE inhibitor have been reported to the FDA, including 1 case caused by lisinopril, which appears to represent an unintentional rechallenge followed by a more significant adverse reaction than previously.[30] Agents that reduce or destroy β cells include the poisons alloxan, streptozocin, and Vacor,[45] and the antimicrobial pentamidine.[11,36,67,93] All of these substances may cause permanent diabetes mellitus. Other medications toxic to the endocrine pancreas include sulfonamides and diazoxide. Table 22–7 lists the drugs and substances toxic to both the exocrine and the endocrine pancreas.

SUMMARY

Except when injured or perforated by agents such as caustics, ionizing radiation, and alcohol, or obstructed by drug-containing packets or batteries, the gastrointestinal tract is typically not regarded as a significant site of drug toxicity. Nevertheless, because of both its potential as a site of severe local or systemic effects and the role that gastrointestinal signs and symptoms play in various diagnostic toxidromes, the gastrointestinal tract is an important consideration in almost any toxicologic emergency.

ACKNOWLEDGMENTS

Howard Mofenson, MD and Thomas Carraccio, PharmD contributed material to Table 22–3, and Mark Pochapin, MD was kind enough to review the manuscript.

REFERENCES

1. Anderson WM, Mason RE, Brinson RR, Schwartz GR: Diarrhea. In: Schwartz GR, Cayten CG, Mangelsen MA, et al, eds: Principles and Practice of Emergency Medicine, 3rd ed. Philadelphia, Lea & Febiger, 1992, pp. 463–471.
2. Appleqvist P, Salmo S: Lye corrosion carcinoma of the esophagus: A review of 63 cases. Cancer 1980;45:2655–2685.
3. Ashcraft KW, Padula RT: The effect of dilute corrosives on the esophagus. Pediatrics 1974;53:226–232.
4. Austen KF: The anaphylactic syndrome. In: Samte M, Talmage DW, Frank MM, et al, eds: Immunological Disease, 4th ed. Boston, Little, Brown, 1988, pp. 1119–1133.
5. Balthazar EJ, Lefleur R: Abdominal complications of drug addiction: Radiologic features. Semin Roentgenol 1983;18:213–220.
6. Banks PA: Acute and chronic pancreatitis. In: Feldman M, Scharschmidt BF, Sleisenger MH, eds: Sleisenger and Fordtran's Gastrointestinal and Liver Disease, 6th ed. Philadelphia, WB Saunders, 1998, pp. 809–886.
7. Baran RB, Rowles B: Factors affecting coloration of urine and feces. J Am Pharm Assoc 1973;13:139–142.
8. Berthrang M, Fajardo LF: Radiation injury in surgical pathology. Part II: Alimentary tract. Am J Surg Pathol 1981;5:153–178.

9. Bonavina L, DeMeester TR, McChesney L, et al: Drug-induced esophageal stricture. Ann Surg 1987;206:173–183.

10. Bost RO, Springfield A: Fatal Hydrofluoric acid ingestion: A suicide case report. J Anal Toxicol 1995;19:535–536.

11. Bouchard P, Sai P, Reach G, et al: Diabetes mellitus following pentamidine-induced hypoglycemia in humans. Diabetes 1982;31: 40–45.

12. Boyce HW Jr: Drug-induced esophageal damage: Diseases of medical progress. Gastrointest Endosc 1998;47:547–550.

13. Caruana DS, Weinbach B, Goerg D, Gardner LB: Cocaine packet ingestions: Diagnosis, management and natural history. Ann Intern Med 1984;100:73–74.

14. Chassany O, Michaux A, Bergmann JF: Drug-induced diarrhoea. Drug Saf 2000;22:53–72.

15. Chaudhary A, Puri AS, Dhar P, et al: Elective surgery for corrosive-induced gastric injury. World J Surg 1996;20:703–706.

16. Clark R, Rake MO, Flute PT, Williams R: Coagulation abnormalities in acute liver failure; pathogenetic and therapeutic implications. Scand J Gastroenterol 1973;8(Suppl 19):63–70.

17. Conklin JJ, Walker RL, Hirsch EF: Current concepts in the management of radiation injuries and associated trauma. Surg Gynecol Obstet 1985;156:809–826.

18. Dagradi AE, Lee ER, Brosco DL, Stampien SJ: The clinical spectrum of hemorrhagic erosive gastritis. Am J Gastroenterol 1973;60: 30–46.

19. Dinoso VP, Chuarg J, Marthy SNS: Changes in mucosal and venous histamine concentrations during installation of ethanol in the canine stomach. Am J Digest Dis 1976;21: 93–97.

20. Eastwood ME, Erdmann KR: Effects of ethanol on canine gastric epithelial ultrastructure and transmucosal potential difference. Am J Digest Dis 1978;23:429–435.

21. Eaton H, Tennekoon GE: Squamous carcinoma of the stomach following corrosive acid burns. Br J Surg 1972;59:382–387.

22. El-Serag HB, Sonnenberg A: Association of esophagitis and esophageal strictures with diseases treated with nonsteroidal anti-inflammatory drugs. Am J Gastroenterol 1997;92:52–56.

23. Endress C, Kling GA: Cocaine-induced small bowel perforation. Am J Radiol 1990;154:1346–1347.

24. Estrera A, Taylor W, Mills LJ, Platt MR: Corrosive burns of the esophagus and stomach: A recommendation for an aggressive surgical approach. Ann Thorac Surg 1986;41:276–283.

25. Field M, Rao MC, Chang EB: Intestinal electrolyte transport and diarrheal disease. N Engl J Med 1989;321:800–806, 879–883.

26. Fine KD: Diarrhea. In: Feldman M, Scharschmidt BF, Sleisinger MH, eds: Sleisenger and Fordtran's Gastrointestinal and Liver Disease, 6th ed. Philadelphia, WB Saunders, 1998, p. 128–137.

27. Foitzik T, Fernández-del Castillo MD, Rattner DW, et al: Alcohol selectively impairs oxygenation of the pancreas. Arch Surg 1995; 130:357–361.

28. Frommer DA, Kulig KW, Marx JA, Rumack BH: Tricyclic antidepressant overdose. JAMA 1987;257:521–526.

29. Geall MG, Phillips SF, Summerskill WHJ: Profile of gastric potential difference in man. Effects of aspirin, alcohol, bile, and endogenous acid. Gastroenterology 1970;58:437–443.

30. Gershon T, Olshaker JS: Acute pancreatitis following lisinopril rechallenge. Am J Emerg Med 1998;16:523–524.

31. Gigli I, Sheffer AL, Austen KF: Angioedema. In: Samte M, Talmage DW, Frank MM, et al, eds: Immunological Disease, 4th ed. Boston, Little, Brown, 1988, pp. 1205–1220.

32. Gorman RL, Khin-Maung-Gyi MT, Klein-Schwartz W, et al: Initial symptoms as predictors of esophageal injury in alkaline corrosive ingestions. Am J Emerg Med 1992;10:189–194.

33. Greenberger NJ: Gastrointestinal Disorders: A Pathophysiologic Approach, 4th ed. Chicago, Year Book, 1990.

34. Haller JA, Andrews HG, White JJ, et al: Pathophysiology and management of acute corrosive burns of the esophagus: Results of treatment in 285 children. J Pediatr Surg 1971;6:578–584.

35. Hardy DL: Fatal rattlesnake envenomation in Arizona: 1969–1984. J Toxicol Clin Toxicol 1986;24:1–10.

36. Hauser L, Sheehan P, Simpkins H: Pancreatic pathology in pentamidine-induced diabetes in acquired immunodeficiency syndrome patients. Hum Pathol 1991;22:926–929.

37. Hoffman RS, Smilkstein MJ, Goldfrank LR: Whole-bowel irrigation and the cocaine "body packer": A new approach to a common problem. Am J Emerg Med 1990;8:523–527.

38. Hoffman RS, Smilkstein MJ, Goldfrank LR: Evaluation of coagulation factor abnormalities after long-acting anticoagulant overdose. J Toxicol Clin Toxicol 1988;26:233–248.

39. Hopkins RA, Postlethwait RW: Caustic burns and carcinoma of the esophagus. Ann Surg 1981;194:146–148.

40. Hung DZ, Deng JF, Tsai WJ, et al: Methotrexate intoxication in a uremic patient [abstract]. European Association of Poison Centers and Clinical Toxicologists XV Congress, Istanbul, May 24–27, 1992, p. 95.

41. Jacobson S: Gastrointestinal testing. In: Flomenbaum N, Goldfrank L, Jacobson S, eds: Emergency Diagnostic Testing, 2nd ed. St. Louis, Mosby-Yearbook, 1995, pp. 258–264.

42. Jaffe JH, Martin WR: Opioid analgesics and antagonists. In: Gilman AG, Rall TW, Nies AS, Taylor P, eds: The Pharmacological Basis of Therapeutics, 8th ed. New York, Pergamon, 1990, pp. 485–521.

43. Jaspersen D: Drug-induced oesophageal disorders: Pathogenesis, incidence, prevention and management. Drug Saf 2000;22:237–249.

44. Kaufman SE, Kaye MD: Induction of gastro-oesophageal reflux by alcohol. Gut 1979;19:336–338.

45. Kenney RM, Michaels IAL, Flomenbaum NE, Yu GSM: Poisoning with N-3-pyridylmethyl-N^1-p-nitrophenyl urea (vacor). Arch Pathol Lab Med 1981;105:367–370.

46. Khodadoost J, Glass GBJ: Erosive gastritis and acute gastroduodenal ulceration as source of upper gastrointestinal bleeding in liver cirrhosis. Digestion 1972;7:129–138.

47. Kivrianta VK: Corrosion carcinoma of the esophagus. Acta Otolaryngol 1952;42:89–95.

48. Kocchar R, Mehta SK, Nagi B, Goenka MK: Corrosive acid-induced esophageal intramural pseudodiverticulosis—A study of 14 patients. J Clin Gastroenterol 1991;13:371–375.

49. Krasner N, Cochran KM, Russell RI, et al: Alcohol and absorption from the small intestine. I: Impairment of absorption from the small intestine in alcoholics. Gut 1976;17:245–248.

50. Krenzelok EP, Keller R, Stewart RD: Gastrointestinal transit times of cathartics combined with charcoal. Ann Emerg Med 1985;14: 1152–1155.

51. Laine L, Weinstein WM: Histology of alcoholic hemorrhagic "gastritis." A prospective evaluation. Gastroenterology 1988;94:1254–1262.

52. Laugel V, Beladdale J, Esconde B, Simeoni U: Accidental ingestion of button battery. Arch Pediatr 1999;6:1231–1235.

53. Lee HS, LaMaute HR, Prizzi WF, et al: Acute gastrointestinal perforations associated with use of crack. Ann Surg 1990;211:15–17.

54. Lewin KJ, Riddell RH, Weinstein WM: Stomach and proximal duodenum: Inflammatory and miscellaneous disorders. In: Lewin KJ, Riddell RH, Weinstein WM, eds: Gastrointestinal Pathology and Its Clinical Implications. New York, Igaku-Shoin, 1992, p. 506.

55. Linscheer WG: Malabsorption in cirrhosis. Am J Clin Nutr 1970; 23:488–492.

56. Litovitz T, Schmitz BF: Ingestion of cylindrical and button batteries: An analysis of 2382 cases. Pediatrics 1992;89:747–757.

57. Manoguerra AS, Neuman TS: Fatal poisoning from acute hydrofluoric acid ingestion. Am J Emerg Med 1986;4:362–363.

58. Martin JL, Justus PG, Mathias JA: Altered mutility of the small intestine in response to ethanol (ETOH): An explanation for the diarrhea associated with the consumption of alcohol [abstract]. Gastroenterology 1980;78:1218.

59. Maves MD, Carithers JS, Birck HG: Esophageal burns secondary to disc battery ingestion. Ann Otol Rhinol Laryngol 1984;93:364–369.

60. McAlister NH, Abrams HB, Schlosser R, Sturtridge W: Unintentional self-intoxication with inorganic calcium. J Intern Med 1990;228:193–195.

61. McCarron MM, Wood JD: The cocaine body packer syndrome. JAMA 1983;250:1417–1420.

62. McIntire MS, Guest JR, Porterfield JF: Philodendron: An infant death. J Toxicol Clin Toxicol 1990;28:177–183.

63. McLauchlan GA: Acute mercury poisoning. Anaesthesia 1991;46:110–112.

64. Meredith JW, Kon ND, Thompson JN: Management of injuries from liquid lye ingestion. J Trauma 1988;28:1173–1180.

65. Mezey E, Jow E, Slavin RE, Tobon F: Pancreatic function and intestinal absorption in chronic alcoholism. Gastroenterology 1970;59:657–664.

66. Mizrahi S, Laor D, Stamler B: Intestinal ischemia induced by cocaine abuse [letter]. Arch Surg 1988;123:394.

67. Murphey SA, Josephs AS: Acute pancreatitis associated with pentamidine therapy. Arch Intern Med 1981;141:56–58.

68. Nalbandian H, Sheth N, Dietrich R, et al: Intestinal ischemia caused by cocaine ingestion: Report of two cases. Surgery 1985;97:374–376.

69. Nalin DR, Levine MM, Rhead J, et al: Cannabis, hydrochlorohydria and cholera. Lancet 1978;2:859–861.

70. Namba T, Nolte C, Jackrel J, Grob D: Poisoning due to organophosphate insecticides. Am J Med 1971;50:475–492.

71. Nandi P, Ong GB: Foreign body in the esophagus: Review of 2,394 cases. Br J Surg 1978;65:5–9.

72. Nicosia JF, Thronton JP, Folk FA, Saletta JD: Surgical management of corrosive gastric injuries. Ann Surg 1974;180:139–143.

73. Novak JM, Collins JT, Donowitz M, et al: Effects of radiation on the human gastrointestinal tract. J Clin Gastroenterol 1979;1:9–39.

74. Oakes DD, Sherck JP, Mark JBD: Lye ingestion: Clinical patterns and therapeutic implications. J Thorac Cardiovasc Surg 1982;83:194–204.

75. Ochi K, Ohashi T, Sato S, et al: Surgical treatment for caustic ingestion injury of the pharynx, larynx and esophagus. Acta Otolaryngol 1996;522(Suppl):116–119.

76. Pelli H, Sand J, Laippala P, Nordback I: Long-term follow-up after the first episode of acute alcoholic pancreatitis: Time course and risk factors for recurrence. Scand J Gastroenterol 2000;35:552–555.

77. Perlow W, Baraona E, Lieber CS: Symptomatic intestinal disaccharidase deficiency in alcoholics. Gastroenterology 1977;72:680–684.

78. Poisindex editorial staff: Fecal discoloration by agent. In: Toll L, Hurlbut KM, eds: Poisindex System Micromedex. Greenville Village, CO, edition expires 7/01;108.

79. Poisindex editorial staff: Oral changes. In: Rumack BH, Spoerke DG, eds: Poisindex Information System. Denver, CO, Micromedex, edition expires 8/93;77.

80. Poisindex editorial staff: Disorders of Taste. In: Toll L, Hurlbut KM, eds: Poisindex System. Greenville Village, CO, Micromedex, edition expires 7/01;108.

81. Pons P, Sullivan JB: Radiation and radioactive emergencies. In: Sullivan JB, Krieger GR, eds: Hazardous Materials Toxicology. Baltimore, Williams & Wilkins, 1992, pp. 441–450.

82. Raikhlin-Eisenkraft B, Bentur Y: *Ecbalium elaterium* (squirting cucumber)—Remedy or poison? J Toxicol Clin Toxicol 2000;38:305–308.

83. Ray JF III, Myers WO, Lawton BR, et al: The natural history of liquid lye ingestion. Arch Surg 1974;109:436–439.

84. Renner IG, Rinderknecht H, Douglas AP: Profiles of pure pancreatic secretions in patients with acute pancreatitis: The possible role of proteolytic enzymes in pathogenesis. Gastroenterology 1978;75:1090–1098.

85. Riddell RH: The gastrointestinal tract. In: Riddell RH, ed: Pathology of Drug-Induced and Toxic Diseases. New York, Churchill-Livingstone, 1982, pp. 515–606.

86. Riddell RH, Strauss FH: The pancreas. In: Riddell RH, ed: Pathology of Drug-Induced and Toxic Diseases. New York, Churchill-Livingstone, 1982, pp. 607–629.

87. Roberts J, Price D, Goldfrank L, Hartnett L: The body stuffer syndrome: A clandestine form of drug overdose. Am J Emerg Med 1986;4:21–27.

88. Roggin GM, Iber FL, Linscheer WG: Intraluminal fat digestion in the chronic alcoholic. Gut 1972;13:107–111.

89. Rollin H: Drug-related gustatory disorders. Ann Otol Rhinol Laryngol 1978;87:37–42.

90. Rubin G, Rybak BJ, Linden J, et al: Ultrastructural changes in the small intestine induced by ethanol. Gastroenterology 1972;63:801–814.

91. Schmidt-Nowara WW, Samet JM, Rosario PA: Early and late pulmonary complications of botulism. Arch Intern Med 1983;143:451–456.

92. Schmidt RD, Schmidt TW: Infant botulism: A case series and review of the literature. J Emerg Med 1992;10:713–718.

93. Schwartz MS, Cappell MS: Pentamidine-associated pancreatitis. Dig Dis Sci 1989;34:1617–1620.

94. Silen W: Cope's Early Diagnosis of the Acute Abdomen, 18th ed. New York, Oxford University Press, 1991, pp. 146–153.

95. Silen W, Skillman JJ: Stress ulcer, acute erosive gastritis and the gastric mucosal barrier. Adv Intern Med 1974;19:195–212.

96. Slater EE, Merrill DD, Guess HA, et al: Clinical profile of angioedema associated with angiotensin converting-enzyme inhibition. JAMA 1988;260:967–970.

97. Smith BM, Skillman JJ, Edwards BG, Silen W: Permeability of the human gastric mucosa. Alteration by acetylsalicylic acid and ethanol. N Engl J Med 1971;285:716–721.

98. Soergel KH: Acute pancreatitis. In: Sleisinger MH, Fordtran JS, eds: Gastrointestinal Disease, 5th ed. Philadelphia, WB Saunders, 1993, pp. 1628–1655.

99. Stephens DS, Walker DH, Schaffer W, et al: Pseudodiphtheria. Ann Intern Med 1981;94:202–204.

100. Stremski ES, Grande GA, Ling LJ: Survival following hydrofluoric acid ingestion. Ann Emerg Med 1992;21:1396–1399.

101. Tarpila S: Morphological and functional response of human small intestine to ionizing radiation. Scand J Gastroenterol 1971;6(Suppl):9–48.

102. Taylor JR, Streetman DS, Castle SS: Medication bezoars: A literature review and report of a case. Ann Pharmacother 1998;32:940–946.

103. Thompson JN: Corrosive esophageal injuries. I. A study of nine cases of concurrent accidental caustic ingestion. Laryngoscope 1987;97:1060–1068.

104. Torda TA, Sinclair E, Ulyatt DB: Puffer fish (tetrodotoxin) poisoning: Clinical record and suggested management. Med J Aust 1973;1:599–602.

105. Trent MS, Kim U: Cocaine packet ingestions: Surgical or medical management. Arch Surg 1987;122:1179–1181.

106. Uppal R, Lateef SK, Korsten MA, et al: Chronic alcoholic gastritis. Roles of alcohol and *Helicobacter pylori*. Arch Intern Med 1991;151:760–764.

107. Weinstein WM: Other types of gastritis and gastropathies, including Ménetriér's disease. In: Feldman M, Scharschmidt BF, Sleisenger MH, eds: Sleisinger and Fordtran's Gastrointestinal and Liver Disease, 6th ed. Philadelphia, WB Saunders, 1998, pp. 713–714.

108. Weisbrot IM, Liber AF, Gordon BS: The effects of therapeutic radiation on colonic mucosa. Cancer 1975;36:931–940.

109. Yang RD, Han MW, McCarthy JH: Ischemic colitis in a crack abuser. Dig Dis Sci 1991;36:238–240.

110. Zargar SA, Kochar R, Nagi B, et al: Ingestion of corrosive acids: Spectrum of injury to upper gastrointestinal tract and natural history. Gastroenterology 1989;97:702–707.

CHAPTER 23 RENAL PRINCIPLES

Donald A. Feinfeld

OVERVIEW OF RENAL FUNCTION

The kidneys maintain the constancy of the extracellular fluid by creating an ultrafiltrate of the plasma that is virtually free of cells and larger macromolecules, and then processing that filtrate, reclaiming what the body needs and letting the rest escape as urine. Every 24 hours, an adult's kidneys filter about 180 L of water (total body water is ~25–60 L) and 25,000 mEq of sodium (total body Na$^+$ is ~1200–2800 mEq). Under normal circumstances the kidneys regulate these two substances independently of each other, depending on the body's needs. Only about 1% of the filtered water and 0.5–1% of the filtered Na$^+$ are excreted.

Renal function begins with filtration at the glomerulus, a highly permeable capillary network stretched between two arterioles in series. The relative constriction or dilatation of these vessels normally controls the glomerular filtration rate (GFR). Under normal circumstances, about 20% of the plasma water in the blood entering the glomeruli actually goes through the filter, carrying with it electrolytes, small metabolites such as glucose, amino acids, lactate, and urea; leaving behind the blood cells and nearly all the larger proteins, including albumin and globulins. The filtrate then enters a series of tubules that reabsorb most of it and secrete certain substances, such as organic acids and bases, into the urinary space. The proximal tubule performs bulk reabsorption, reclaiming isotonically 65–70% of the filtrate; distal to that are the loop of Henle, which controls concentration and dilution of the urine, and the distal nephron, which does the fine-tuning in the balance between excretion and reclamation. Reabsorption of sodium is controlled proximally by hydrostatic and oncotic pressures in the peritubular capillaries, and distally by hormones such as aldosterone. Water reclamation depends on function of the loop of Henle, which makes the medullary interstitium hypertonic, and the level of antidiuretic hormone (ADH), which inserts water-reabsorbing channels (aquaporins) into the membranes of the final nephron segments (collecting ducts). The kidneys also regulate balance for potassium and hydrogen ion (both of which are influenced by the effect of aldosterone on the distal nephron) and calcium and phosphate (both of which are influenced by the blood level of parathormone).

Injury to either the glomeruli or the tubules may lead to renal dysfunction; that is, to a decrease in glomerular filtration. As the kidneys fail, serum levels of the marker substances urea and creatinine increase. However, the relationship between these levels and the level of GFR is hyperbolic, not linear, so a small elevation in serum levels of these substances denotes a large decrease in renal function. By the time blood urea nitrogen (BUN) or serum creatinine exceeds the upper limit of normal, GFR is already reduced by more than 50%.

Many substances cause or aggravate renal dysfunction. The kidneys are particularly susceptible to toxic injury for four reasons;[141] (a) They receive 20–25% of cardiac output yet make up less than 1% of total body mass; (b) they are metabolically active, and thus vulnerable to agents that disrupt metabolism; (c) they remove water from the filtrate and may build up a high concentration of toxic substances; and (d) the glomeruli and interstitium are susceptible to attack by the immune system. Many factors, such as renal perfusion, may affect an individual's reaction to a particular nephrotoxin.[12] The clinician should be aware of these factors and, when possible, alter them to minimize the adverse effect after a toxic exposure.

Functional Toxic Renal Disorders

Although most toxic renal injury results in decreased renal function, there are 3 functional disorders that upset body balance despite normal GFR in anatomically normal kidneys: renal tubular acidosis; syndrome of inappropriate secretion of antidiuretic hormone; and nephrogenic diabetes insipidus.

Renal tubular acidosis (RTA) is a loss of ability to reclaim the filtered bicarbonate (proximal RTA) or a decreased ability to generate new bicarbonate to replace that lost in buffering the daily acid load (distal RTA). In either case, there is a nonanion gap metabolic acidosis, usually accompanied by hypokalemia. Proximal RTA often occurs as part of the *Fanconi syndrome* (proximal RTA plus aminoaciduria, renal glycosuria, and hyperphosphaturia).

Syndrome of inappropriate antidiuretic hormone (SIADH) occurs when the body produces ADH despite a fall in plasma osmolality, which normally inhibits ADH secretion. Although this most often occurs as a complication of intracranial lesions or from ectopic ADH production by a tumor or in a diseased lung, certain medications (eg, chlorpropamide, antidepressants, vincristine, opioids, and methylenedioxymethamphetamine (MDMA, or Ecstasy) can also cause inappropriate ADH release.

Nephrogenic diabetes insipidus is the reverse of SIADH. It denotes inability of the kidneys to respond to ADH stimulation despite severe losses of body water. Lithium, demeclocycline, foscarnet, clozapine, and methoxyflurane may cause this syndrome (Chap. 24).

MAJOR TOXIC SYNDROMES OF THE KIDNEY

Most nephrotoxicity involves histologic renal injury. Although toxins may affect any part of the nephron (Fig. 23–1), there are three major syndromes of toxic renal injury: (a) chronic renal fail-ure; (b) nephrotic syndrome; and especially, (c) acute renal failure (Table 23–1). For purposes of continuity, acute renal failure is dis-cussed last. Nephrotoxins usually affect the most metabolically active segment of the nephron—the tubules; therefore, most nephrotoxicity involves either acute or chronic tubular injury, al-though glomerular injury may sometimes result from drugs or chemicals. These processes are not mutually exclusive, and toxic

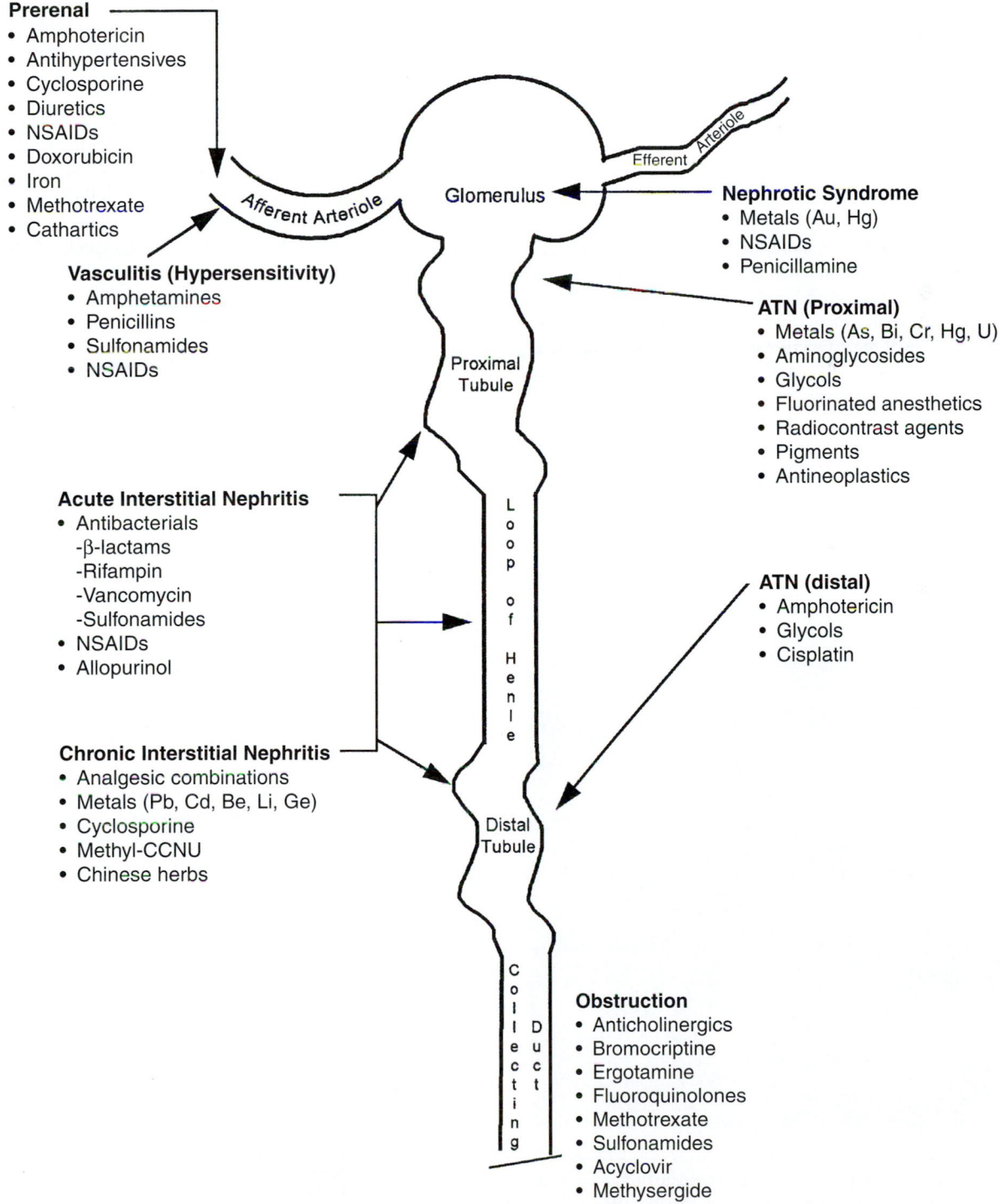

Prerenal
- Amphotericin
- Antihypertensives
- Cyclosporine
- Diuretics
- NSAIDs
- Doxorubicin
- Iron
- Methotrexate
- Cathartics

Vasculitis (Hypersensitivity)
- Amphetamines
- Penicillins
- Sulfonamides
- NSAIDs

Acute Interstitial Nephritis
- Antibacterials
  -β-lactams
  -Rifampin
  -Vancomycin
  -Sulfonamides
- NSAIDs
- Allopurinol

Chronic Interstitial Nephritis
- Analgesic combinations
- Metals (Pb, Cd, Be, Li, Ge)
- Cyclosporine
- Methyl-CCNU
- Chinese herbs

Nephrotic Syndrome
- Metals (Au, Hg)
- NSAIDs
- Penicillamine

ATN (Proximal)
- Metals (As, Bi, Cr, Hg, U)
- Aminoglycosides
- Glycols
- Fluorinated anesthetics
- Radiocontrast agents
- Pigments
- Antineoplastics

ATN (distal)
- Amphotericin
- Glycols
- Cisplatin

Obstruction
- Anticholinergics
- Bromocriptine
- Ergotamine
- Fluoroquinolones
- Methotrexate
- Sulfonamides
- Acyclovir
- Methysergide

Afferent Arteriole · Efferent Arteriole · Glomerulus · Proximal Tubule · Loop of Henle · Distal Tubule · Collecting Duct

Figure 23–1. Schematic diagram showing the major nephrotoxic processes and the sites on the nephron that they chiefly affect.

TABLE 23–1.   Major Nephrotoxic Syndromes

> **Chronic Renal Failure** (slowly increasing azotemia)
> Chronic interstitial nephritis
> Papillary necrosis
> Chronic glomerulosclerosis
>
> **Nephrotic Syndrome** (proteinuria, low albumin, edema)
> Minimal glomerular change
> Membranous nephropathy
> Focal segmental glomerulosclerosis
>
> **Acute Renal Failure** (rapidly increasing azotemia)
> Acute prerenal failure
> Acute urinary obstruction
> Acute tubular necrosis
> Acute interstitial nephritis
> Acute vasculitis

nephropathy may impinge on more than one part of the nephron (eg, nonsteroidal anti-inflammatory drug (NSAID)-induced acute renal failure and nephrotic syndrome).

Chronic renal failure refers to any disease process that causes progressive decline of renal function over a period of years. There is usually a gradual rise in BUN and serum creatinine as glomerular filtration falls; often there are no symptoms other than nocturia (indicating loss of urinary concentrating ability).

The most common lesion of nephrotoxic chronic renal failure is chronic interstitial nephritis (Fig. 23–1). This involves destruction of tubules over a prolonged period,[74] with tubular atrophy, fibrosis, and a variable cellular infiltrate (Fig. 23–2), sometimes

accompanied by papillary necrosis. Acute interstitial nephritis (see later) may progress to chronic interstitial nephritis if exposure to the allergen or toxin is prolonged.[201] The onset is usually insidious and relatively asymptomatic, often presenting as secondary hypertension or unexplained chronic azotemia. The major symptom is nonspecific nocturia. Papillary necrosis may lead to ureteral colic. There is mild to moderate proteinuria that remains well under the nephrotic range (see later). Unlike other chronic renal disorders, interstitial nephritis is characterized by failure of the diseased tubules to adapt to the renal impairment, resulting in metabolic imbalances such as hyperchloremic metabolic acidosis, sodium wasting, and hyperkalemia early in the disease course.[70] Injury to erythropoietin-secreting cells may produce a disproportionate anemia.

Nephrotic syndrome is characterized by massive proteinuria (>3 g/d in the adult), hypoalbuminemia, hyperlipidemia, and the edema that usually prompts the patient to seek medical attention. Although the relationships among these findings are not completely understood, the underlying event is injury to the glomerular barrier that normally prevents macromolecules from passing from the capillary lumen into the urinary space. Albumin loss usually exceeds urinary excretion as a result of renal tubular catabolism of filtered protein. The tubules also retain sodium, causing expansion of the extracellular space and edema. The glomerular lesion may progress to renal failure if the pathologic process continues. Toxins induce nephrotic syndrome (Table 23–2) either (a) by releasing hidden antigens into the blood, leading to immune deposits in the glomerular basement membrane and to changes in the basement membrane (eg, gold; Fig. 23–3); or (b) by upsetting immunoregulatory balance (eg, NSAIDs). A less-common glomerular lesion is hypersensitivity vasculitis.

Acute renal failure is defined as any abrupt decline in renal function that impairs the kidney's capacity to maintain metabolic balance. The 3 main categories of acute renal failure are prerenal, postrenal, and intrinsic renal failure.

Prerenal failure involves impaired renal perfusion, such as in volume depletion, shock, or congestive heart failure. Hence, toxic events that cause bleeding (overdose of anticoagulants), volume depletion (diuretics, cathartics, or emetics), cardiac dysfunction (β-adrenergic antagonists), or hypotension may lead to acute prerenal failure (see later).[66]

Postrenal failure, such as urinary tract obstruction, may result from crystalluria (eg, oxalosis in ethylene glycol poisoning) or blocked urinary flow (eg, bladder dysfunction from anticholinergic drugs). However, the most common nephrotoxic lesions are *intrinsic renal injuries*, particularly acute tubular necrosis and acute interstitial nephritis (see Table 23–1).[5]

Acute tubular necrosis (Table 23–3), the most common nephrotoxic event, is characterized pathologically by patchy necrosis of tubules, usually the proximal segments (Fig. 23–4). This lesion

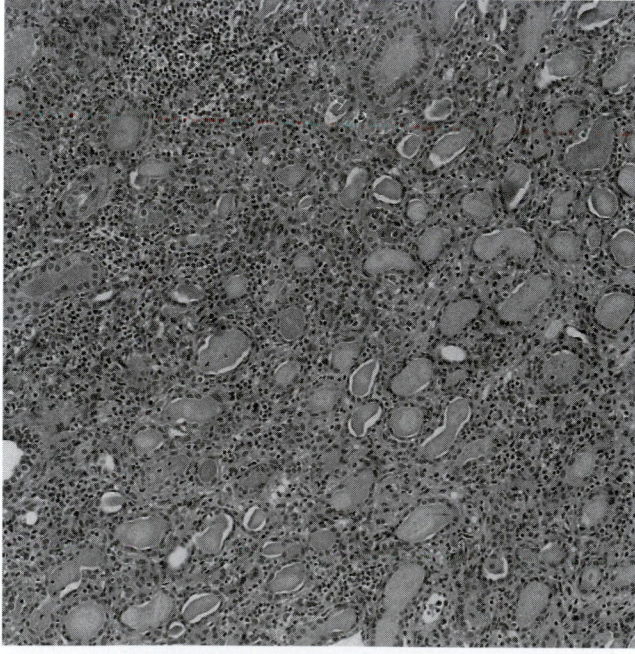

Figure 23–2. Chronic interstitial nephritis (secondary to NSAIDs). Interstitial fibrosis, lymphocytic infiltration, and tubular atrophy. (H&E × 225.) *(Courtesy of Dr. Rabia Mir.)*

TABLE 23–2.   Substances Commonly Causing Nephrotic Syndrome

> Captopril
> Drugs of abuse (heroin, cocaine)
> Metals (gold, mercury)
> NSAIDs
> Penicillamine

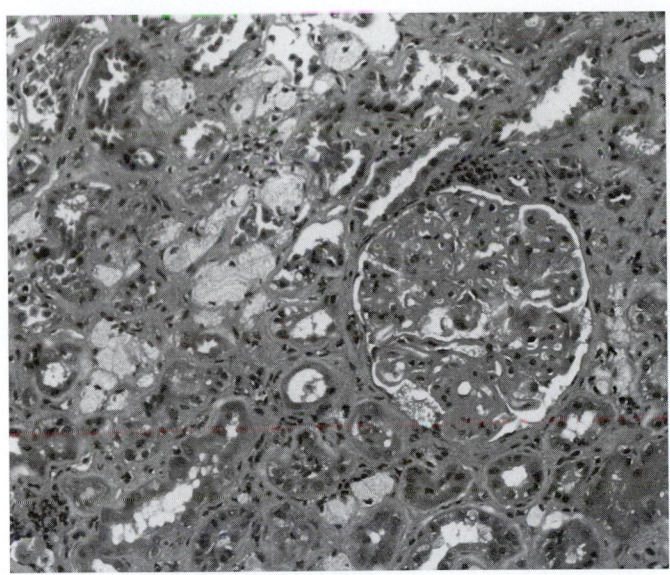

Figure 23–3. Membranous glomerulonephropathy (secondary to gold), a cause of nephrotic syndrome. Globally thickened glomerular capillaries and interstitial foam cells are seen. (H&E × 450.) *(Courtesy of Dr. Rabia Mir.)*

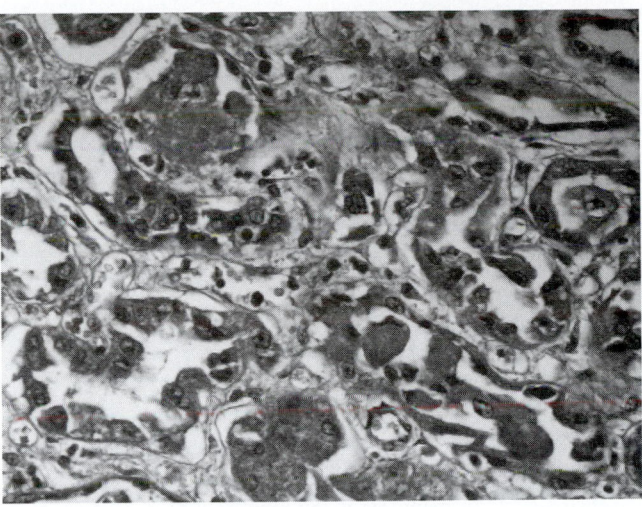

Figure 23–4. Acute tubular necrosis (secondary to mercury). Proximal tubular epithelial necrosis and sloughing are associated with interstitial edema. (H&E × 450.) *(Courtesy of Dr. Rabia Mir.)*

TABLE 23–3. Substances That Commonly Cause Acute Tubular Necrosis

Acetaminophen
Antibacterials
    Aminoglycosides
    Amphotericin
    Pentamidine
    Polymyxins
Antineoplastic Drugs
    Cisplatin
    Iphosphamide
    Methotrexate
    Mithramycin
    Streptozotocin
Fluorinated anesthetics
Glycols
    Ethylene glycol
    Diethylene glycol
Halogenated hydrocarbons
Metals
    Arsenic
    Bismuth
    Chromium
    Mercury
Mushrooms
    Cortinarius spp.
    Amanita smithiana
Pigments
    Myoglobin
    Hemoglobin
Radiocontrast agents
Toxins that cause hypotension or hypovolemia

is associated with three different processes: direct toxic injury, ischemic injury from renal hypoperfusion, and pigmenturia.[166]

Direct toxins affect different segments of the renal tubules; for example, uranium attacks the proximal tubule and amphotericin the distal tubule (see Fig. 23–1). However, the clinical pattern of rapidly declining renal function, often accompanied by oliguria, is identical in all forms of tubular necrosis. Direct toxicity accounts for about 35% of all cases of acute tubular necrosis.[124,218]

Poisoning may also lead to ischemic tubular necrosis if hypotension or cardiac failure causes ischemia of nephron segments (proximal straight tubule and inner medullary collecting duct) that are particularly vulnerable to hypoxia.

Pigmenturia refers to either myoglobinuria from rhabdomyolysis (skeletal muscle necrosis) or hemoglobinuria from massive hemolysis.[59] Either pigment may cause tubular injury and necrosis by precipitating in the tubular lumen.[72,166]

Although there is controversy as to how a tubular lesion leads to glomerular shutdown, it is generally felt that tubular obstruction, back-leak of filtrate across injured epithelium, renal hypoperfusion, and decreased glomerular filtering surface combine to impair glomerular filtration.[215] Recent evidence suggests that prolonged medullary ischemia, perhaps caused by an imbalance in the production of vasoconstrictors such as endothelin and vasodilators such as nitric oxide, plays a role in prolonging the renal dysfunction after the tubular injury develops.[133]

Clinically, acute tubular necrosis presents as a rapid deterioration of renal function, usually first noted as azotemia. Muddy brown casts or renal tubular cells may be seen in the urinary sediment, but hematuria and leukocyturia are unusual. Disorders of metabolic balance, such as hyperkalemia and metabolic acidosis, are also common. Although tubular sodium reabsorption is decreased, the fall in glomerular filtration usually leads to positive sodium and water balance, as renal output of these substances is fixed.[147]

Acute interstitial nephritis (Table 23–4) is clinically similar to acute tubular necrosis and often must be diagnosed by renal

TABLE 23–4. Substances That Cause Acute Interstitial Nephritis

More Common	Less Common
Allopurinol	Anticonvulsant drugs
Antibacterials	Carbamazepine
β-Lactams, especially ampicillin,	Phenobarbital
methicillin, penicillin	Phenytoin
Rifampin	Captopril
Sulfonamides	Diuretics
Vancomycin	Furosemide
Azathioprine	Thiazides
NSAIDs	

biopsy, which shows a cellular infiltrate separating tubular structures (Fig. 23–5). Nearly all acute interstitial nephritis is due to hypersensitivity.[219] In many cases the renal failure is accompanied by manifestations of systemic allergy such as fever, rash, or eosinophilia, and finding eosinophils in the urine is consistent with this disorder.[164] However, about 25% of patients with drug-induced interstitial nephritis have no signs of hypersensitivity. Unlike those with tubular necrosis, most patients with acute interstitial nephritis have hematuria and leukocyturia,[11] particularly eosinophiluria.[12] Secondary fever at the onset of azotemia is common, and flank pain or arthralgia may be present. The lesion usually improves once the drug is discontinued. Corticosteroids may hasten recovery;[9,89,136] many physicians use this treatment only if the renal failure does not improve promptly when the drug is stopped.

DIFFERENTIAL DIAGNOSIS OF ACUTE RENAL FAILURE

Patients who present with acutely deteriorating renal function often represent a difficult diagnostic challenge. Not only are there three major etiologic categories, but each category has several subdivisions; and more than one factor may be present. For example, a patient with an opioid overdose may have neurogenic hypotension (prerenal) together with muscle necrosis causing myoglobinuric renal failure (intrinsic renal) and opioid-induced urinary retention (postrenal). Because renal, prerenal, and postrenal processes are not mutually exclusive and require different interventions, all three should always be considered, even when one appears to be the most obvious cause of the renal failure.

Prerenal failure (renal hypoperfusion) initiates a sequence of events leading to renal salt and water retention.[14] Renin is released, causing production of angiotensin, which both enhances proximal tubular sodium reabsorption and stimulates adrenal aldosterone release, thus increasing distal sodium reabsorption. Prerenal failure is therefore accompanied by low urinary sodium excretion (Table 23–5). Release of antidiuretic hormone increases water and urea retention. Unresolving renal hypoperfusion may cause tubular necrosis.

Drugs may decrease renal blood flow without necessarily causing intrinsic renal injury (Fig. 23–1). Diuretics or cathartics can decrease blood volume and antihypertensive agents can excessively reduce blood pressure. Some drugs (eg, cyclosporine, amphotericin, methotrexate) cause prerenal vasoconstriction. NSAIDs lower filtration rate by inhibiting production of vasodilatory

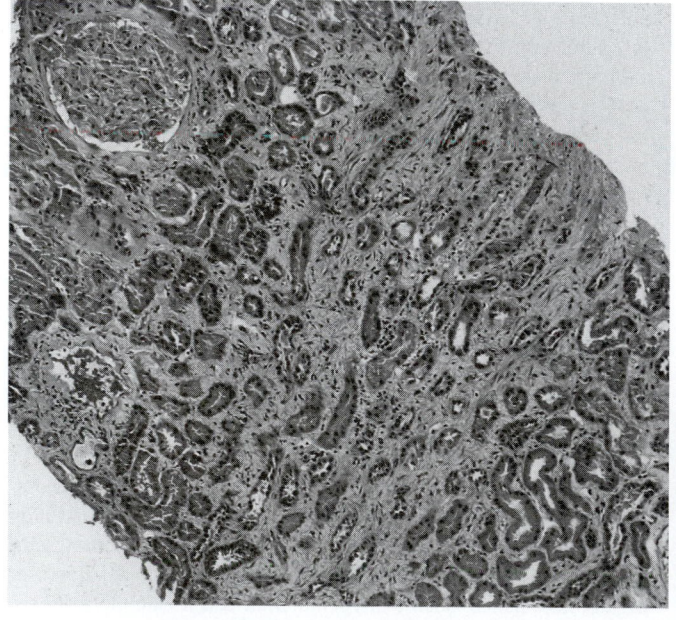

A

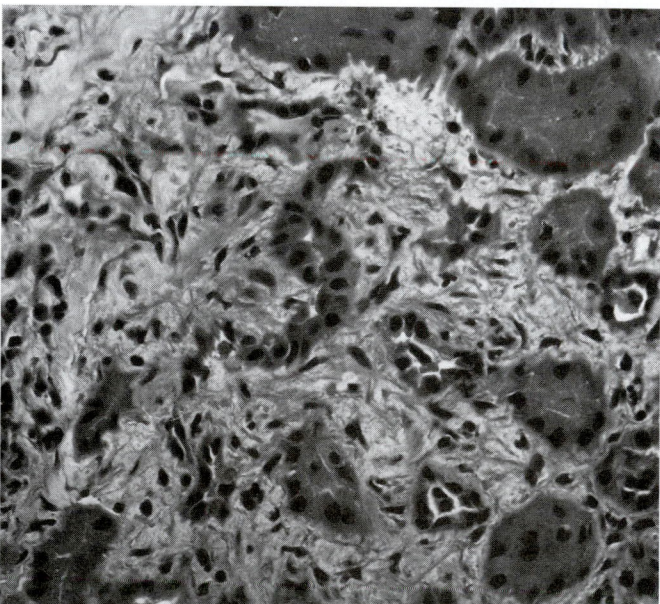

B

Figure 23–5. Acute interstitial nephritis (secondary to rifampin). Interstitial edema and patchy lymphocyte, plasma cell, and eosinophil infiltration occurs without fibrosis. Tubular epithelium shows degenerative and regenerative changes and mononuclear cell infiltration (tubulitis). (**A,** H&E × 112; **B,** H&E × 450.) *(Courtesy of Dr. Rabia Mir.)*

TABLE 23–5.   Tests of Renal Function

Acute

To differentiate prerenal failure from acute tubular necrosis:

1. BUN:Creatinine ratio: usually >20:1 in prerenal failure.
2. Urine sodium: usually <20 mEq/L in prerenal failure; usually >40 mEq/L in acute tubular necrosis.
3. Fractional sodium excretion (FE_{Na}) is the most reliable test:[12,13]

$$\frac{Urine\ [Na]/Plasma\ [Na]}{Urine\ [creatinine]/Plasma\ [creatinine]} \times 100$$

FE_{Na} is <1% (ie, normal) in prerenal failure if the patient has not received diuretics or large infusions of sodium, which increase fractional excretion of sodium despite normal tubular function. In tubular necrosis or interstitial nephritis, renal sodium absorption is decreased, and FE_{Na} is >1%. This is correct except in the case of pigmenturic or iodinated radiocontrast-associated renal failure, when the test is of no benefit.

Chronic

Creatinine clearance is U × V/P (normal range 90–130 ml/min, where *U* is urine creatinine concentration, *V* is urine flow in mL/min, and *P* is plasma creatinine. Urine collection must be complete and U and P must be in the same units.

---

prostaglandins in the afferent arteriole. Finally, cardiotoxins, such as doxorubicin, may cause severe heart failure. Some drugs cause a hypersensitivity vasculitis (Fig. 23–1).

Urinary tract obstruction should always be considered when the kidneys fail rapidly. Although complete obstruction leads to anuria, partial obstruction, which is more common, is usually associated with alternating oliguria and polyuria. Continued production of urine in the presence of obstruction leads to distension of the urinary tract above the blockage. Calyceal dilatation is common. Obstruction of the bladder outlet or urethra may distend the bladder.

Obstruction may be caused by medications (Table 23–6).[74] Most do so by impairing contraction of the bladder through anticholinergic action (atropine, tricyclic antidepressants). Rarely, certain drugs, particularly methysergide,[213] cause retroperitoneal fibrosis and ureteral constriction. Finally, a few drugs lead to crystalluria and intratubular obstruction. Sometimes the drug itself forms precipitates (sulfonamides[47], crixivan, or methotrexate) or causes excretion of a precipitating chemical such as oxalate (fluorinated anesthetics).

TABLE 23–6.   Substances That Cause Urinary Obstruction

Bladder Dysfunction	Crystal Deposition
Anticholinergics	Crixivan
Antihistamines	Ethylene glycol
Antidepressants (tricyclic)	Fluorinated anesthetics
Atropine	Fluoroquinolone antibacterials
Scopolamine	Heme pigments
Antipsychotics	Methotrexate
Butyrophenones	Phenylbutazone
Phenothiazine	Sulfonamides
Bromocriptine	
CNS depressants	**Retroperitoneal Fibrosis**
	Ergotamines (Methysergide)
	Chinese herbs (*Stephania*)

PATIENT EVALUATION

Evaluation of a patient with suspected toxic renal injury should include extrarenal as well as renal factors. The kidney's response to toxins is affected by previous renal function, renal blood flow, and the presence of urinary tract obstruction that can exert back pressure on the nephrons, all of which must be taken into consideration.

History

A past history of renal disease or conditions that can affect the kidney (eg, diabetes, hypertension, cardiovascular disease) should be noted. Flank pain, hematuria, or any abnormal pattern of urine output are important symptoms. The patient's intravascular volume status affects renal perfusion. Thus, a history of heart disease or a disorder that lowers plasma volume such as vomiting or diarrhea is important. Prior cancer chemotherapy with drugs such as cisplatin or methyl-CCNU should be noted. All current medications should be evaluated for potential renal effects, both directly toxic drugs and drugs such as diuretics that may enhance the toxicity of other substances.[92] The patient's intake of alcohol and drugs of abuse should be explored. Careful occupational history and assessment of hobbies and lifestyle are crucial, with emphasis on exposure to nephrotoxic chemicals, metals, and solvents.

Physical Examination

The patient's hemodynamics should be carefully assessed. Postural changes in pulse and blood pressure and either engorgement or decreased filling of the neck veins give important information about the intravascular volume. The skin should be examined for lesions. Pupillary abnormalities may suggest a toxic exposure. Funduscopy may reveal evidence of chronic hypertension or diabetes. All aspects of cardiac function should be noted, including presence or absence of edema. Injuries or scars in the suprapubic area or evidence of past urologic or retroperitoneal surgery may suggest obstruction, as may a palpable or percussible bladder.

Laboratory Evaluation

Nephrotoxic injury is not always apparent clinically, so the laboratory is exceedingly important. Acute loss of renal function may be suspected if urine output decreases, but oliguria is not universal. The most important parameter of renal function is glomerular filtration. Because urea and creatinine are largely excreted by this route, serum levels of these substances are used as markers of renal function. However, the blood level of any substance depends on both production and excretion. Azotemia—elevation of BUN or creatinine—is a standard indication of renal insufficiency. However, BUN or creatinine in the normal range does not exclude a substantial degree of renal impairment because of the previously discussed hyperbolic relationship between these parameters and GFR. In addition, decreased production of urea (starvation or liver failure) or creatinine (amputation, muscle wasting) may result in a normal-appearing BUN or creatinine in the presence of significant renal impairment. On the other hand, decreased renal perfusion (prerenal failure) is often associated with a disproportionate rise in BUN as compared to the rise in creatinine, because urea is partially reabsorbed along with salt and water, whose reabsorption is increased when the kidneys are underperfused. Thus, a BUN:creatinine ratio >20 should make one suspect prerenal failure (Table

23–5). Because many nephrotoxic drugs are associated with non-oliguric acute renal failure (urine volume >400 mL/d), progressive azotemia without oliguria should always raise suspicion of a drug-related cause. Tubular injury, especially in lead poisoning and myoglobinuria, may cause hyperuricemia from decreased tubular secretion of uric acid.

Certain drugs alter measured levels of urea and creatinine in the absence of any change in renal function.[159] The most obvious is exogenous creatinine taken to build muscle mass. Cefoxitin, nitromethane, and ketones absorb light at the same frequency as the creatinine reaction product, thus artifactually increasing the measured level. Nitromethane, a component of rocket model fuel, produces extreme elevation of creatinine through similer means. Drugs that block renal creatinine secretion, such as cimetidine and trimethoprim, may also increase serum creatinine. BUN may be raised independently of renal function by tetracycline or corticosteroids, which increase protein catabolism.

In patients with chronic renal insufficiency or failure, it is necessary to assess the remaining renal function in order to manage the patient properly. Clearance measurements are generally used to determine glomerular filtration rate. The most common is endogenous creatinine clearance (see Table 23–5).

In acute renal failure it is not helpful to determine creatinine clearance, as the accuracy of a clearance implies a steady state. Changing GFR during a clearance time period distorts the resulting estimation. There is also a lag period between changes in kidney function and changes in BUN or creatinine levels. In general, a patient with acute renal failure should be treated as if glomerular filtration were <10 mL/min. In patients with acute renal failure, a random sample of urine may be sent promptly to the laboratory for sodium and creatinine measurements to determine fractional sodium excretion, which may help differentiate prerenal azotemia from tubular necrosis (see Table 23–5).

Examination of the urine is of paramount importance in cases of poisoning. Even if urine is sent to the laboratory, it can also be examined carefully by the physician. Standard dipsticks will detect albumin and glucose. The dipstick test for blood is useful for confirming the presence of small amounts of blood or myoglobin, but it is not a substitute for careful microscopic examination of the sediment. Evaluation should look not only for red or white cells but also for crystals, tubular elements, casts, and bacteria. If acute interstitial nephritis is a consideration, a fresh urine sample should be stained for eosinophils.[164]

Further evaluation of the patient with acute renal failure should include tests for obstruction, which can be caused by a number of substances (see Table 23–6). Renal ultrasonography should be performed to look for hydronephrosis. Postvoiding residual urine volume may be measured as appropriate by catheterization; a volume in excess of 75–100 mL may make one suspect bladder dysfunction or obstruction.

NEPHROTOXICITY OF SPECIFIC SUBSTANCES

Metals

Table 23–7 summarizes the nephrotoxic effects of metals. In general, metals are toxic in their salt form, not their elemental form unless otherwise noted. *Antimony* caused transient acute renal failure in a child treated with high doses of the metal.[36] *Arsenic* commonly causes acute renal failure by binding to sulfhydryl-containing proteins. Renal failure may be caused in part by circulatory collapse or volume depletion from diarrhea, but arsenate is a direct distal tubule toxin.[225] Arsine gas induces hemolysis and also attacks both proximal and distal tubules, causing interstitial inflammation;[155] the resultant hemoglobinuria contributes to the renal failure.[129] Very severe arsenic-induced acute renal failure leads to chronic interstitial fibrosis.[224]

TABLE 23–7.　Nephrotoxic Effects of Metals

	Toxic ATN	Shock ATN	Hemolysis	AIN	CIN	Tub Dys	NS	GN
Antimony	+							
Arsenic	+++	+++	++	+	+			
Barium	+							
Beryllium					++			
Bismuth	++			+		+	+	
Cadmium					+++	+++		
Chromium	+++							
Copper		+	+					
Gadolinium	+							
Germanium					+			
Gold	+						+++	
Iron		++			+			
Lead	+		+		+++	+++		
Lithium	+				++	++		
Mercury	+++	+				+	+	
Platinum (cisplatin)	++				++	++		
Silicon								+
Silver	+							
Thallium	+			+				
Uranium	+							

ATN = acute tubular necrosis; AIN = acute interstitial nephritis; CIN = chronic interstitial nephritis; Tub Dys = tubular dysfunction; NS = nephrotic syndrome; GN = glomerulonephritis. +++ = common; + = uncommon.

Barium may cause acute renal failure.[234] Because this metal inhibits potassium exit from cells,[190] barium nephropathy may be accompanied by severe hypokalemia, which is otherwise unusual in acute renal failure (Chap. 90).

Beryllium, a known pulmonary toxin, may also cause chronic interstitial nephritis, with granulomas and glomerulosclerosis.[18]

Bismuth causes dose-related injury to the proximal tubule. Low doses lead to tubular dysfunction; higher doses cause oliguric acute renal failure from tubular necrosis with interstitial inflammation.[23,217] Nephrotic syndrome is reported after medicinal administration of bismuth (Chap. 82).[22]

Cadmium damages proximal tubular segments.[232] Initial changes are functional; pathologic changes occur after chronic exposure. As many as 80% of individuals exposed chronically to cadmium develop low-molecular-weight proteinuria[80] or Fanconi syndrome (amino aciduria, phosphaturia, renal glycosuria, proximal renal tubular acidosis, and hyperuricosuria).[1,118] The latter may be associated with urolithiasis.[118] Eventually, chronic interstitial nephritis with progressive renal failure supervenes (Chap. 82).

Chromium is nephrotoxic as chromate or dichromate ion; it injures the proximal segments of the proximal tubule.[166] Very low doses may lead to hyposthenuria or glycosuria.[229]

Copper was linked to two fatal cases of acute tubular necrosis secondary to volume depletion from vomiting, diarrhea, and sulfhemoglobinemic hemolysis (Chap. 82).[195]

Gadolinium is discussed later in this chapter under Radiocontrast Agents.

Germanium may cause chronic interstitial nephritis.[165]

Gold, generally administered in an organified form, may cause nephrotic syndrome, often with hematuria, which usually reverses over several months after gold is discontinued and chelation instituted. Pathologic examination shows membranous glomerulopathy (see Fig. 23–3) with subepithelial immune deposits.[222] Gold deposits in proximal tubular cells and occasionally in glomerular epithelium.[8] This lesion may be a human counterpart to experimental Heymann nephritis, in which reaction to a tubular antigen leads to epimembranous immune complex nephropathy;[222] this has been reproduced by injecting gold salts into rats.[161] Gold-induced tubular necrosis is also reported.[56]

Iron poisoning, particularly in children, may cause acute renal failure from renal ischemia as a result of GI bleeding, vomiting, diarrhea, and shock.[42,221] Large doses of iron are not nephrotoxic in animals, but chronic interstitial nephritis occurs in patients with hemochromatosis,[143] so long-term tubular iron deposition may have a toxic effect.

Lead inhibits sulfhydryl-dependent enzymes and replaces calcium in biochemical systems; its effect is cumulative. Lead slowly injures proximal tubular cells,[7,111] causing chronic interstitial nephritis with fibrosis, exacerbated by hypertension. Because progression of the disease is insidious, it is important to evaluate for prior or current lead exposure in patients with unexplained renal failure.

Like cadmium, lead causes functional impairment of proximal tubules, with Fanconi syndrome and tubular proteinuria.[39] Subclinical tubular impairment is reported in lead workers, some of whom had tubular fibrosis on biopsy.[233] Impaired uric acid secretion is characteristic of lead nephropathy, with hyperuricemia and clinical gout.[16] The combination of gout, hypertension, and chronic renal failure should raise the suspicion of lead exposure.[21,65] Confirmatory studies include whole blood lead levels, evaluation of heme synthesis (eg, δ-aminolevulinic acid levels),

and lead mobilization studies (24-hour urine lead excretion before and after 0.5–1 g of IV calcium disodium ethylenediaminetetraacetic acid (EDTA)).[35,45,65] Acute lead poisoning, characterized by jaundice, colic, and hemolytic anemia, is also reported to cause acute renal failure.[49]

Lithium commonly causes polyuria without pathologic changes,[205] from increased thirst or nephrogenic diabetes insipidus (Chap. 24). Some patients develop distal renal tubular acidosis (inability to lower urine pH <5.4 after an acid load). These derangements usually disappear when lithium is discontinued. A few patients treated chronically with lithium may develop decreased renal function[103] with chronic interstitial nephritis on biopsy.[102] The role of lithium in this disease was challenged by a study that showed a high incidence of interstitial nephritis in psychiatric patients not receiving the drug, for unclear reasons.[53] However, rats given lithium develop distal tubular lesions,[78] suggesting that there may be a risk of this complication in humans. There are occasional reports of both acute renal failure[130] and nephrotic syndrome[4] associated with lithium therapy.

Mercury has a strong affinity for renal tissue, especially as mercuric ion, although organic mercury and elemental mercury vapor are also nephrotoxic. Mercury necroses proximal tubular cells[166] (see Fig. 23–4) by attacking sulfhydryl groups of mitochondrial proteins.[185] Swelling of poisoned tubular cells may be a factor in renal failure.[83] Oliguric acute renal failure with tubular cell casts is typical. Tubular functional abnormalities (glycosuria, aminoaciduria) occurs rarely.

Animals given very low doses of mercury develop nephrotic syndrome[3] caused by low-grade tubular injury, which releases sequestered tubular antigens into the circulation and triggers an immune nephritis. A human equivalent is the membranous nephropathy reported in a few patients using topical mercury-containing preparations,[25] or chronic low-grade industrial exposure to mercury.[223] This disorder is probably analogous to the membranous nephropathy seen with gold toxicity.

Platinum metal is relatively innocuous, but some of its compounds, such as the antitumor drug cisplatin, are nephrotoxic, predominantly to distal tubules.[90,192] Functional renal defects related to cisplatin include loss of urinary concentrating ability and renal magnesium wasting, which precede acute renal failure from tubular necrosis. Pretreatment hydration with saline or mannitol ameliorates this,[95] but there is still a risk of renal failure; the dose must be carefully adjusted and the patient closely followed after treatment. The newer congener carboplatin is less nephrotoxic, but may injure the kidneys,[207] as can the industrial chemical carboplatinite.[236]

Chronic renal failure from tubulointerstitial disease has been reported in patients previously treated with cisplatin.[90] Even with hydration, enough cisplatin may be taken up by tubular cells to produce subsequent tubular atrophy.[192]

Exposure to *silicon* is felt to be a risk factor for development of rapidly progressive glomerulonephritis.[116]

Silver salts cause tubular lesions in animals[143] and (rarely) acute tubular necrosis in humans.[140]

Thallium poisoning is associated with loss of urinary concentrating ability and albuminuria and sometimes acute renal failure with tubular necrosis and interstitial inflammation.[199]

Uranium selectively injures the middle segment of the proximal tubule in experimental models of acute tubular necrosis,[166] but human cases of uranium-induced acute renal failure are rare.[172]

Solvents

Carbon tetrachloride (CCl₄), known for its hepatotoxicity, is also a nephrotoxin. Acute liver failure associated with CCl$_4$ poisoning may cause renal shutdown via the hepatorenal syndrome, but direct renal tubular injury is also common, with necrosis of the proximal tubule and loop of Henle.[166] Swelling of the glomerular basement membrane and parietal epithelial cells is also frequently seen.[209] CCl$_4$ is converted to trichloromethyl and trichloromethylperoxyl (see Fig. 13–12) free radicals by cytochrome P450 enzymes in proximal tubules. These free radicals are the probable causes of cell necrosis.[206] Clinical findings include oliguric acute renal failure, hematuria with red cell casts, moderate proteinuria, and crystalluria.[143] The lesion is usually reversible if the patient recovers from the hepatic injury.

Tetrachloroethylene poisoning resembles that of CCl$_4$, with hepatotoxicity predominating but occasionally acute renal failure from tubular necrosis.[199]

Trichloroethylene can cause acute tubular necrosis when sniffed.[15]

Toluene causes hippuric acidosis, a high anion gap acidosis. It can also produce a distal renal tubular acidosis, which may cause severe hypokalemia.[184]

Glycols

Ethylene glycol is itself nonnephrotoxic and is cleared fairly well by the kidneys.[37] However, it is hepatically metabolized to glycolic acid and then oxalic acid. Subsequent deposition of calcium oxalate crystals in the tubules causes obstruction and acute renal failure.[171] The crystals also provoke severe interstitial inflammation, which adds to the renal impairment and causes hematuria and proteinuria, followed by oliguria or anuria. The renal shutdown worsens the metabolic acidosis produced by the metabolites.

Diethylene glycol directly causes necrosis of proximal and distal tubular cells.[166] Hyperoxaluria may also complicate poisoning with this chemical.[96] Renal failure is often severe, especially if bilateral cortical necrosis supervenes.

Propylene glycol is relatively nontoxic but may cause acute hemolysis when injected and has caused hemoglobinuric acute renal failure in animals.[121]

Antimicrobial Agents

Aminoglycosides are still a leading cause of drug-induced renal failure. With the exception of streptomycin, all antibiotics in this group cause tubular necrosis and renal failure. Aminoglycosides are taken up by proximal tubular cells, and incorporated into lysosomes, inactivating them.[28] Dose-related tubular necrosis is attributed to lysosomal failure and subsequent damage to mitochondria.[204]

The incidence of nephrotoxicity in patients treated with aminoglycosides such as gentamicin varies from 1 to 30%. Risk factors for this complication include preexisting renal impairment, renal hypoperfusion, rising trough levels of the drug, and frequent dosage.[169] Infants are particularly at risk: a misplaced decimal point in a child's gentamicin order may lead to administration of a toxic dose. Tubular cell uptake of gentamicin, which determines the amount of cellular injury, appears to be saturable; hence, administration of infrequent large doses gives less net renal accumulation than more frequent, smaller doses.[54] A recent study confirms that once-daily aminoglycoside dosing is as effective as divided doses in treating infection but is much less likely to cause renal injury.[191]

Gentamicin is probably more nephrotoxic than tobramycin[210] or amikacin;[131] however, all of these drugs can cause renal failure. Aminoglycoside nephropathy presents clinically as nonoliguric acute renal failure,[109] which usually resolves 1–3 weeks after the drug is discontinued. Renal magnesium and potassium wasting may occur. In addition to tubular necrosis, aminoglycosides may rarely cause allergic acute interstitial nephritis.[152,193]

The *penicillins* are not nephrotoxic but can cause acute interstitial nephritis. This is most frequent with methicillin, followed by ampicillin and penicillin, but may occur with any drug in this group.[11] The hypersensitivity reaction is not dose related, although the majority of patients have received the drug for 10 days or more.[11] Many patients with penicillin-associated interstitial nephritis have no prior history of penicillin allergy.

The penicillins may rarely cause hypersensitivity vasculitis, leading to acute glomerular inflammation and renal failure.[157]

Cephalosporins, like penicillins, can cause allergic interstitial nephritis, either directly[12] or from cross-sensitivity to penicillins.[123]

Some cephalosporins have intrinsic nephrotoxicity. Cephaloridine, the most toxic, is transported into tubular cells, becomes trapped, and causes necrosis;[77] it is no longer used in the United States. Cephalothin, the first available cephalosporin, rarely caused acute tubular necrosis, in the absence of additional risk factors such as excessive dosage or concomitant use of other nephrotoxic agents.[77] The newer cephalosporins are much less nephrotoxic; acute renal failure with their use is nearly always a result of hypersensitivity.

Sulfonamides were the first drugs associated with acute interstitial nephritis.[150] There is a cellular infiltrate, sometimes with granulomas. Trimethoprim/sulfamethoxazole also causes acute interstitial nephritis.[136]

In the early reports of sulfonamide-associated renal failure, the failure was caused by tubular obstruction from precipitation of the drug in the urine,[58] which is still sometimes seen with sulfadiazine.[47] Newer sulfonamides, such as sulfisoxazole and sulfamethoxazole, are much more soluble than their predecessors, and crystalluria is now exceedingly rare. The sulfonamides, like the penicillins, are occasionally associated with hypersensitivity vasculitis.[157]

Tetracyclines may elevate BUN because of their catabolic activity, which leads to breakdown of endogenous proteins and excess production of urea.[178] There are scattered reports of acute tubular necrosis associated with tetracycline in patients with prior renal dysfunction, which decreases excretion of the drug, causing excessively high blood and tissue levels.[202] The most notorious functional renal defect associated with tetracycline is Fanconi syndrome, reported during the 1960s[81] after exposure to outdated medication containing citric acid stabilizer, which is no longer used; hence, this complication is historical. Tetracycline may also, albeit rarely, cause allergic acute interstitial nephritis.[230]

Vancomycin was once a common cause of acute tubular necrosis. It is now felt that much of the early toxicity from vancomycin was caused by incomplete purification of the drug.[10] Vancomycin-associated renal failure is relatively uncommon and is a result of allergic interstitial nephritis.[62]

Rifampin is also associated with acute interstitial nephritis (see Fig. 23–5) but nearly always occurs either with intermittent dosage (eg, twice weekly)[180] or after the drug is stopped and resumed,[162] such as when a patient with tuberculosis is lost to follow-up after discharge and restarted on rifampin when recrudescence occurs. The nephritis is often accompanied by systemic symptoms such as fever, flank pain, and nausea, and patients frequently develop hematuria and oliguria.[162] The pathologic lesion usually resolves after the drug is stopped and may not respond to steroid treatment.[183]

Polymyxins (polymyxin B and colistin), which are now rarely used, are potent renal tubular toxins that often caused nonoliguric acute tubular necrosis.[125] Acute interstitial nephritis is also reported with polymyxin.[26]

Amphotericin has many adverse effects on the kidney.[38] It creates channels in the luminal membrane of the distal nephron,[6] which allows back-leakage of secreted H^+ and leakage of cellular K^+ into the lumen. Nearly all patients given the drug develop distal renal tubular acidosis and hypokalemia.[144] Renal magnesium wasting, seen in patients receiving more than 200 mg of amphotericin, exacerbates potassium loss.[20] Equally concerning is loss of urinary concentrating ability, which can cause dehydration.

Decreased renal function is also frequent with amphotericin. Following intravenous infusion of the drug there is an acute reduction in glomerular filtration rate, caused by prerenal vasoconstriction, with transient oliguria followed by a short polyuric phase.[38] Renal dysfunction may persist for days. Acute tubular necrosis because of both toxic and hemodynamic effects on the kidney is common after administration of amphotericin, and is both dose-related and cumulative. Permanent renal damage occurs in many patients receiving more than 4 g of amphotericin. Limiting the dosage and correcting volume deficits promptly may prevent amphotericin nephrotoxicity. Prophylactic volume expansion with saline may ameliorate amphotericin toxicity,[98] but vasodilators and mannitol are felt to be ineffective. A new lipid-emulsion form of amphotericin has been reported to be less nephrotoxic than the unemulsified drug.[19]

Fluoroquinolones (levofloxacin, ciprofloxacin, ofloxacin, and cinoxacin) may cause acute tubular necrosis or interstitial nephritis.[88,211] In addition, there is a risk of crystalluria from these drugs.

Nitrofurantoin may rarely cause acute interstitial nephritis.[156]

Pentamidine, which is used to treat *Pneumocystis carinii* infections, can cause acute renal failure, often associated with hypoglycemia.[212]

Phenazopyridine is not antibacterial but is used to relieve dysuria in urinary tract infections. Overdose of the drug can cause acute tubular necrosis, accompanied by a yellow tinge to the skin and methemoglobinemia.[76]

Acyclovir may cause acute renal failure due to precipitation of the drug in the renal tubules,[32] or, rarely, acute tubular necrosis.[24]

Foscarnet can cause nephrotoxic acute renal failure.[33]

Ritonavir, a protease inhibitor used to treat HIV infection, has been reported to cause acute renal failure.[55]

Indinavir, another protease inhibitor, may precipitate in the renal tubules or collecting system; the resulting crystalluria may causes stones or acute interstitial nephritis.[115]

Nonsteroidal Anti-Inflammatory Agents

NSAIDs, which are widely used, range from over-the-counter agents such as aspirin, acetaminophen, naproxen, and ibuprofen to prescription drugs.[44] Because their nephrotoxicity is related to their common mechanism of action, they are discussed as a group.

NSAIDs inhibit cyclooxygenase (COX), the enzyme family that produces precursors to the prostaglandins, a family of 20-carbon fatty acids that act as local regulators of tissue function. As prostaglandin production decreases, production of leukotrienes, derived from the same fatty acid source but with different actions, is enhanced.[197]

A number of functional renal abnormalities accompany the use of NSAIDs. Prostaglandins dilate afferent renal arterioles in the presence of renal vasoconstrictor substances such as angiotensin. Patients with high angiotensin levels (eg, in chronic renal failure, volume depletion, or congestive heart failure) may have hemodynamically mediated decreases in renal perfusion when given NSAIDs,[84] causing both prerenal azotemia and retention of sodium, with edema or aggravated heart failure. Prostaglandins mitigate the effect of antidiuretic hormone on the collecting duct, so water retention and hyponatremia may result from NSAID use.[44] Prostacyclin, a renal prostaglandin, stimulates renin, and the NSAIDs compete with aldosterone for binding sites. These events make hyperkalemia a common complication of NSAID use;[197] this is usually well tolerated, but may become life-threatening, particularly in the elderly or in those with chronic renal disease or hypoaldosteronism.[84]

NSAIDs also cause parenchymal renal disease, possibly because of a loss of the anti-inflammatory effects of prostaglandins, which attenuate lymphokine activity.[44] The most common renal disease from NSAIDs is acute interstitial nephritis. The pathology closely resembles that of allergic interstitial nephritis, but without eosinophilia.[31] The resulting renal failure is usually exacerbated by the hemodynamic effects of prostaglandin deficiency. Nephritis usually occurs after the drug has been used for several months or more but may happen after shorter exposure. It generally resolves after the drug is discontinued, although prolonged exposure may lead to chronic interstitial nephritis (see Fig. 23–2).

Nephrotic syndrome often accompanies the interstitial nephritis caused by NSAIDs if the proteinuria is massive,[31] and may also occur as an isolated complication of NSAID use.[75,231] The glomerular lesion resembles "minimal-change" nephropathy—no abnormalities are seen on light or immunofluorescence microscopy. In addition to the renal toxicity described, *naproxen* and *fenoprofen* may also cause hypersensitivity vasculitis, which usually improves within a few weeks after the drug is stopped.

Acetaminophen can be directly nephrotoxic. Acetaminophen overdose is usually associated with hepatocellular necrosis. However, because the cytochrome P450 enzymes that convert the drug to a toxic metabolite are also present in kidney (CYP, 1A2, 2E1), tubular cell injury leading to renal failure may result from acetaminophen overdose (Chap. 32).[34] It has been suggested that acetaminophen's nephrotoxicity, unlike its hepatotoxicity, may not respond to N-acetylcysteine.[52]

Sulindac may be less nephrotoxic than other NSAIDs because of a weaker effect on renal prostaglandins.[41] It has not been associated with interstitial nephritis but can cause nephrotic syndrome.[231]

COX-2 (cyclooxygenase-2) inhibitors are a newly introduced class of NSAIDs. Two COX-2 inhibitor drugs, *celecoxib* and *rofecoxib*, are currently in use. These drugs spare COX-1, which protects gastric mucosa, and are less likely to cause gastric bleeding. However, because the kidneys contain inducible COX-2,[60] it is to be expected that the kidneys will be vulnerable to COX-2 inhibitors despite the sparing of the gastrointestinal tract. Cases of acute renal failure associated with use of these agents are reported.[174] At least one observer has noted reversible nephrotic syndrome in patients taking these medications (L. Mailloux, personal communication).

Chronic interstitial nephritis with papillary necrosis is a major complication of chronic NSAID use known as analgesic nephropathy.[194] The toxicity of these drugs is cumulative—a minimum of 2 kg is needed to cause renal injury. The lesion begins as inflammation around the renal papillae and culminates in nephron loss and interstitial fibrosis.[143] The papillae may slough and cause ureteral colic; more often there is insidious progressive renal failure with mild low-molecular-weight proteinuria and leukocyturia. Because patients are often reluctant to admit taking large quantities of nonprescription drugs, not only is a careful history important, but other clues, such as gastric irritation from aspirin or methemoglobinemia from phenacetin, must be sought. In addition to aspirin, other NSAIDs may rarely cause papillary necrosis.[197] Combinations of these drugs are far more nephrotoxic than individual agents,[64] although caution should be observed whenever any NSAID is prescribed. It was reported that daily consumption of acetaminophen, the first metabolite of phenacetin, may be a risk factor for chronic renal failure.[194] However, a position paper on analgesic use concludes that the main risk for analgesic nephropathy is the use of combinations, and that usual doses of acetaminophen are probably safe.[99]

Other Antiarthritis Agents

Allopurinol, which lowers uric acid, is a potent allergen that can cause interstitial nephritis.[85]

Sulfinpyrazone, a uricosuric agent, also causes allergic interstitial nephritis with nonoliguric acute renal failure and eosinophilia.[107,136]

Probenecid, another uricosuric drug, may cause nephrotic syndrome; pathology shows membranous nephropathy.[101]

Penicillamine, used to treat rheumatoid arthritis and to chelate toxic metals, is a well-documented cause of membranous nephropathy and nephrotic syndrome.[188]

Colchicine may cause acute renal failure, possibly due to muscle necrosis and myoglobinuria.[214]

5-Aminosalicylate, used to treat ulcerative colitis, is rarely associated with chronic interstitial nephritis.[2]

Diuretics

The commonly used diuretics are usually categorized as *loop diuretics*, which act at the loop of Henle (ethacrynic acid, furosemide, bumetanide, and torsemide); *distal tubule diuretics* (thiazides and quinazolines); and *potassium-sparing diuretics* (spironolactone, triamterene, and amiloride). Although these drugs are not generally nephrotoxic, they may cause functional or parenchymal renal injury.

Loop diuretics and distal tubule diuretics cause prerenal failure by contracting extracellular fluid volume. Both groups of diuretics may also be associated with allergic acute interstitial nephritis, often accompanied by drug fever and eosinophilia.[136,141] A renal granuloma was found in one such case.[142]

Potassium-sparing diuretics are minimally nephrotoxic but may cause life-threatening hyperkalemia and acidosis by inhibiting renal K^+ and H^+ secretion.[71]

Mannitol is the most commonly administered osmotic diuretic. Because it holds water and solute in the tubular lumen, it may be used acutely to prevent myoglobinuric acute tubular necrosis in cases of severe rhabdomyolysis. However, the drug may cause

acute renal failure when given in prolonged high doses, probably because of prerenal vasoconstriction.[93] In addition to its paradoxical vasoconstrictor activity, mannitol appears to enhance radiocontrast nephropathy in diabetic patients.[29]

Antihypertensive Agents

Antihypertensive drugs rarely cause nephrotoxicity and are generally given to protect the kidneys from hypertensive nephropathy. Excessive dosage, of course, causes prerenal failure because of decreased renal perfusion from the low blood pressure.

Captopril may rarely cause nephrotic syndrome,[182] with membranous nephropathy. This complication has not been reported to date with the newer angiotensin-converting enzyme inhibitors, which lack captopril's sulfhydryl group. Captopril may also cause allergic interstitial nephritis.[216]

Methyldopa rarely causes acute interstitial nephritis and acute renal failure.[235] There is one reported case of urinary obstruction from retroperitoneal fibrosis associated with methyldopa.[112]

Anticonvulsant Agents

Phenytoin is a well-documented cause of acute interstitial nephritis.[11] One such case was associated with antibodies to tubular basement membrane.[110]

Carbamazepine can cause interstitial nephritis; it activates the patient's cultured lymphocytes.[106]

Phenobarbital has rarely been associated with interstitial nephritis and acute renal failure.[167]

Trimethadione and *paramethadione*, which are used to treat petit mal epilepsy, may cause membranous nephropathy with nephrotic syndrome,[17] which usually regresses when the drug is discontinued.

Anesthetic Agents

General anesthesia may cause acute renal failure by producing hypotension. However, the fluorinated hydrocarbons are directly nephrotoxic because of the release of fluoride from the parent molecule.

Methoxyflurane is the most nephrotoxic anesthetic. Two functional renal disturbances are seen following prolonged methoxyflurane anesthesia. Nephrogenic diabetes insipidus is characterized by postanesthesia polyuria and hyperoxaluria, which may worsen the renal injury. Acute tubular necrosis with renal failure and oliguria may follow the polyuria after 2–3 days.[168] Although this process is usually reversible, repeated exposure to methoxyflurane can lead to chronic renal failure with interstitial fibrosis and calcification, accompanied by distal renal tubular acidosis.[94]

Halothane is much less nephrotoxic than methoxyflurane, as it releases less fluoride, but is associated with acute renal failure.[86]

Enflurane is less lipid-soluble than methoxyflurane, but may also rarely cause acute renal failure.[61]

Antineoplastic Agents

Of all the antineoplastic medications, cisplatin (see the Metals section earlier in the chapter) is the most nephrotoxic. However, a number of other drugs in this category can also cause renal damage.

Methotrexate, a folic acid analog, can cause dose-related acute renal failure. During administration of methotrexate, there is a transient fall in glomerular filtration rate, particularly in pediatric patients.[135] Although vasospasm is usually the cause, methotrexate may also precipitate in renal tubules, causing obstruction.[179] At low doses of methotrexate, this problem can usually be prevented by adequate hydration and alkalinization of the urine. However, direct tubular toxicity from methotrexate is also reported, with proximal tubular necrosis and interstitial infiltration.[46]

Streptozocin can damage kidney cells as well as pancreatic islets. The first indication of the drug's nephrotoxicity is proteinuria.[198] If the drug is continued, tubular injury ensues, starting as Fanconi syndrome and loss of urinary concentrating ability, followed by azotemia and oliguric acute renal failure, which usually resolves if the drug is stopped.

The *nitrosoureas (BCNU, CCNU,* and *methyl-CCNU)* are associated with long-term cumulative nephrotoxicity, most frequently in patients receiving more than 1.5–2 g/m^2 of the drug.[63,201] Methyl-CCNU is the most toxic of the three. The pathologic lesion is chronic interstitial nephritis, with irreversible fibrosis and glomerulosclerosis.

Mithramycin toxicity often includes acute tubular necrosis and renal failure.[120]

Mitomycin C primarily injures the glomerulus, and high doses are associated with glomerulosclerosis.[137] The drug may also cause hemolytic-uremic syndrome with microangiopathic hemolytic anemia.[173]

Azacytidine is a tubular toxin and can give rise to Fanconi syndrome, as well as to acute proximal and distal tubular necrosis.[177]

Iphosphamide may cause acute renal failure, particularly in young children.[203]

Immunosuppressive Agents

Azathioprine is not directly nephrotoxic but is associated with acute allergic interstitial nephritis.[208]

Cyclosporine is nephrotoxic. The earliest renal effect is prerenal vasoconstriction, with decreased glomerular filtration from renal hypoperfusion,[108,175] which usually responds to reduction of the dose. Some patients treated with cyclosporine develop acute renal failure, unrelated to rejection, that does not resolve with decreased dosage. Renal biopsy shows tubular injury with inclusion bodies,[146] confirmed by urinary appearance of a tubular cytosolic enzyme.[73] The renal ischemia may exacerbate this lesion. In kidney transplant patients, an interstitial infiltrate is reported.[146]

Chronic renal failure in patients receiving long-term cyclosporine treatment is from selective damage to medullary segments, fibrosis, and atrophy of the outer stripe that may then progress to end-stage disease.[160] This lesion is reported both in patients with renal homografts and with nonrenal transplants where the kidneys were initially normal.

Tacrolimus (FK-506) causes acute and chronic nephrotoxicity similar to that of cyclosporine, which is also related to prerenal vasoconstriction.[161] Animal studies suggest that both drugs, although chemically different, have a common toxic pathway because of their binding of the intracellular enzyme calcineurin phosphatase.[218] Tacrolimus may also cause distal renal tubular acidosis.[97]

Radiocontrast Agents

Acute renal failure caused by iodinated radiocontrast media usually begins within 24 hours of administration, and is often followed by an oliguric phase. Renal function usually begins to improve within a week, but dialysis is sometimes necessary.

Contrast agents deliver an osmotic load, and their injection leads to a period of volume expansion and diuresis,[154] accompanied by profound vasodilatation. This is followed by intense vasoconstriction, which suggests that ischemia plays a role in the pathogenesis of contrast nephropathy.[153] During the oliguric phase, fractional excretion of sodium is often low,[67] despite the fact that the pathologic lesion is acute tubular necrosis with vacuolization and cell swelling.[228] This lesion has been called *osmotic nephropathy*, because it occurs after injection of other hyperosmotic substances. Lower-osmolality contrast agents may be less nephrotoxic than the older high-osmolality dyes.[181] However, lower-osmolality contrast media can cause similar pathologic lesions[151] and severe renal failure.[13] The osmolality may be less important than a direct toxic or ischemic effect on tubular cells. One study suggests that oxygen free radicals may play a role in the renal dysfunction in contrast nephropathy.[117] Conditions that increase the risk of acute renal failure after radiocontrast agents include preexisting renal insufficiency, particularly from diabetes, Bence Jones proteinuria, renal hypoperfusion, and injection of a large amount of dye. Prevention of hypovolemia and saline or mannitol loading appear to reduce the risk of radiocontrast nephropathy,[165] except in diabetics.[29]

Gadolinium is used as a contrast agent for magnetic resonance imaging. Although it is renally excreted, it is felt to be safe to use even in the presence of renal failure.[200] However, there are two recent reports of worsening of chronic renal failure by gadolinium contrast media,[87,104] so it would be prudent to monitor renal function after MRI in patients with renal failure if gadolinium is used.

Miscellaneous Drugs And Substances

A number of other drugs may cause allergic interstitial nephritis, including *cimetidine*,[136,145] *ranitidine*,[79] *phenylpropanolamine*,[27] *clofibrate*,[50] and *ticlopidine*.[187]

Paraquat and *diquat*, two toxic herbicides, may cause acute renal failure in addition to damaging other organs (Chap. 91).[227]

Bromate poisoning may cause acute renal failure and deafness in children.[91]

Bromocriptine may cause urinary tract obstruction as a result of retroperitoneal fibrosis.[30]

Aluminum phosphide, used as a pesticide in granaries, is associated with acute renal failure.[122]

Deferoxamine overdose is reported to cause acute renal failure.[42]

Inhaled *mycotoxins*, such as *ochratoxin*, may cause acute renal failure.[57]

Overdose of *epinephrine* may lead to acute renal failure in the neonate.[132]

The bisphosphonate *etidronate* is associated with acute renal failure when given intravenously.[168]

Extremely high consumption of *Worcestershire sauce* was reported to cause renal stones and aminoaciduria.[158]

Drug-Abuse Nephropathy

Chronic self-injection of *heroin* or *cocaine* is recognized as a cause of chronic renal failure (CRF) and nephrotic syndrome; this has been confirmed epidemiologically.[51] There is generally a history of years of daily drug injections, most often with heroin. Renal biopsy shows focal segmental glomerulosclerosis,[51,138] but unlike patients with idiopathic focal sclerosis, drug abusers usually present with renal insufficiency or failure and progress rapidly to end-stage renal disease. Rarely do patients with drug abuse nephropathy improve or stabilize after discontinuing the drug.[138]

There is much speculation as to the etiology of drug-abuse nephropathy. It has been suggested that the contaminants, rather than the drug, cause the damage. In one study, animals injected with pure heroin had no renal lesions, whereas those injected with street heroin developed glomerulosclerosis.[149] Drug-abuse nephropathy is associated with marked interstitial fibrosis in addition to the glomerular lesion, which may explain the rapid progression to renal failure.[127]

Individuals who chronically inject drugs subcutaneously may develop renal amyloidosis secondary to chronic skin abscesses and granulomas with lymphedema and suppuration, similar to amyloid in patients with other chronic inflammatory conditions.[113] Like those drug users with focal segmental glomerulosclerosis, they often present with advanced renal dysfunction. One patient with renal amyloidosis because of drug abuse improved when the drug use was terminated.[48]

Lysergic acid diethylamide (LSD) is not nephrotoxic but has been linked to retroperitoneal fibrosis, like the related ergotamines methysergide and bromocriptine.[213]

Amphetamines may cause a polyvasculitis that leads to proteinuria, hematuria, and chronic renal failure.[43] Intravenous injection of amphetamines[100,119] or cocaine[189] may also cause myoglobinuric acute renal failure.

Pigment Nephropathy

Both myoglobinuria and hemoglobinuria can cause acute renal failure, and either of these conditions may complicate poisoning or overdose. Tubular injury results from precipitation of the pigment in the renal tubules.[166] However, the conditions that produce them may be different.

Myoglobinuria sufficient to cause renal damage usually occurs following necrosis of striated muscle. Alcohol can be directly myotoxic in some individuals,[176] as can HMG Co-A reductase inhibitors (the statins) used to lower blood cholesterol levels.[105] Drugs that produce profound hypokalemia (eg, diuretics and laxatives) or predispose to hyperthermia (antipsychotics) can cause muscle necrosis on this basis. Most commonly, poisoning leads to muscle breakdown from pressure necrosis following prolonged unconsciousness (opioids and sedative-hypnotics), excessive muscle contraction (cocaine), or grand mal seizures (alcohol withdrawal, theophylline).[82] Myoglobinuric acute renal failure has also accompanied poisoning with carbon monoxide, copper sulfate, and zinc phosphate.[35,124,139]

Myoglobin passes the glomerular filter and is normally excreted without causing toxicity. A study of patients with rhabdomyolysis suggested that the actual concentration of myoglobin in the urine may be a factor in the development of acute renal failure.[72] If myoglobin becomes inspissated in the lumen due to renal hypoperfusion and high tubular water absorption, the myoglobin molecule dissociates in an acidic environment, releasing hematin, which is tubulotoxic,[59] possibly as a result of production of oxygen free radicals. Because many intoxications are associated with intravascular volume depletion and acidosis, the poisoned patient with rhabdomyolysis is at risk to develop this complication.

Myoglobinuric renal failure is diagnosed by the development of acute renal failure in the presence of a condition causing muscle breakdown and a simultaneous elevation of muscle enzymes in the serum, especially creatinine kinase and aldolase. A positive ortho-tolidine test of the urine is seen in the absence of erythrocytes in the sediment, and urine myoglobin may be detected. However, because primary renal failure may itself result in detectable myoglobinuria that does not worsen renal function,[70] finding myoglobin in the urine does not necessarily establish the diagnosis.

The renal failure associated with myoglobinuria can be prevented by early intervention. Volume expansion is quite effective if renal injury has not yet occurred.[186] Alkalinizing the urine may prevent dissociation of the myoglobin molecule and minimize tubular necrosis. However, massive rhabdomyolysis may be associated with severe hypocalcemia caused by the release of large amounts of phosphorus from necrosing muscle into the blood. Alkalemia in this setting may cause tetany or seizures, which would worsen the muscle injury.[124] Hence, the risk of alkalinization must be weighed against the benefit. Early alkalinization, before the renal failure becomes irreversible and before electrolyte abnormalities occur, is more likely to be of benefit.

Hemoglobinuria follows hemolysis, which can be caused by a number of poisons, including snake and spider venoms and many chemicals, such as cresol, phenol, aniline, arsine, naphthalene, and methylene chloride. Sensitivity reactions to drugs (hydralazine, quinine) may also cause hemolysis.[59]

The pathophysiology of hemoglobinuric renal failure is similar to that seen with myoglobinuria. The pigment deposits in the tubules and dissociates, and necrosis occurs.[166] Volume depletion and acidosis are also precipitating factors in this disorder. Conversely, volume expansion may help prevent renal failure in hemolysis, as in myoglobinuria. Because phosphate release does not occur significantly with hemoglobinuria, the urine should be alkalinized as well.

Mushroom Poisoning

Two kinds of mushrooms have been reported to cause acute tubular necrosis. *Cortinarius spp* mushrooms may cause oliguric acute renal failure.[128] *Amanita* poisoning has also been associated with renal failure, in addition to its hepatic and GI toxicity.[148] In the United States, *Amanita smithiana* poisoning is now a recognized cause of renal failure, probably because of the toxin allelic nor-leucine, which is also present in *A. abrupta* (Chap. 76).

Alternative Medical Treatments

In recent years, there has been an interest in "alternative" or "complementary" medical treatments; the National Institutes of Health has established a Branch of Alternative Medicine. However, some of these remedies may have toxic effects on the kidneys.

Chinese herbal medicine sometimes employs the herbs *Stephania tetrandra* and *Magnolia officinalis* in weight-loss programs. Both have caused irreversible interstitial nephritis and fibrosis.[68,226] These herbs may also cause urinary obstruction from retroperitoneal fibrosis.[121]

Gallbladder of the grass carp, eaten by Chinese hoping to promote well being, causes acute tubular necrosis and toxic hepatitis.[134]

Disodium edetate (EDTA) is injected intravenously to chelate calcium in the hope of leaching the calcium out of atheromatous plaques. Although the major adverse effect of disodium edetate is profound hypocalcemia, there are two reports of acute renal failure associated with "chelation therapy."[45,68] In the second case, renal biopsy showed acute tubular necrosis, a complication more commonly seen with calcium disodium edetate.[35]

Hypericum and *Ledum*, administered to promote healing, have been associated with acute interstitial nephritis.[68]

SUMMARY

The kidneys' position as a primary defense against harmful substances that may enter the blood stream often results in their being exposed to exogenous or endogenous toxins. The environment, the workplace, and, especially, the administration of medications, all represent potential sources of nephrotoxicity. It is thus important to determine, by history and observation, to what drugs and chemicals a patient may have been exposed and to be aware of their potential to harm the kidneys. It is equally crucial to work the other way when a patient presents with renal dysfunction: review all medications, both conventional and "alternative," all substance exposures, and any conditions that can adversely affect renal function.

REFERENCES

1. Adams RG, Harrison JF, Scott P: The development of cadmium-induced proteinuria, impaired renal function and osteomalacia in alkaline battery workers. Q J Med 1969;38:425–443.
2. Agharazii M, Marcotte J, Boucher D, et al: Chronic interstitial nephritis due to 5-aminosalicylic acid. Am J Nephrol 1999;19: 373–376.
3. Albini B, Glurich I, Andres GA: Mercuric chloride-induced immunologically mediated diseases in experimental animals. In: Porter GA, ed: Nephrotoxic Mechanisms of Drugs and Environmental Toxins. New York, Plenum, 1982, pp. 413–423.
4. Alexander F, Martin J: Nephrotic syndrome associated with lithium therapy. Clin Nephrol 1981;15:267–271.
5. Anderson HL Jr, Feinfeld DA: Mechanisms of drug-induced renal failure. Hosp Physician 1987;23:27–40.
6. Andreoli T: On the anatomy of amphotericin B-cholesterol pores in lipid bilayer membranes. Kidney Int 1973;4:337–345.
7. Angevine JM, Kappas A, DeGowin RL, et al: Renal tubular nuclear inclusions of lead poisoning: A clinical and experimental study. Arch Pathol 1962;73:486–494.
8. Antonovych TT: Gold nephropathy. Ann Clin Lab Sci 1981;11: 386–391.
9. Appel GB: A decade of penicillin-related interstitial nephritis: More questions than answers. Clin Nephrol 1980;13:151–154.
10. Appel GB, Given DB, Levine LR, et al: Vancomycin and the kidney. Am J Kidney Dis 1986;8:75–80.
11. Appel GB, Kunis CL: Acute tubulointerstitial nephritis. Contemp Issues Nephrol 1983;10:151–185.
12. Appel GB, Neu HC: Acute interstitial nephritis induced by beta-lactam antibiotics. In: Fillastre JH, Whelton A, Tulkens P, eds: Antibiotic Nephrotoxicity. Paris, INSERM, 1982, pp. 195–212.
13. Aron NB, Feinfeld DA, Peters AT, et al: Acute renal failure associated with ioxaglate, a low-osmolality radiocontrast agent. Am J Kidney Dis 1989;13:189–193.
14. Badr KF, Ichikawa I: Prerenal failure: A deleterious shift from renal compensation to decompensation. N Engl J Med 1988;319:623–629.
15. Baerg RD, Kimberg DV: Centrilobular hepatic necrosis and acute renal failure in "solvent sniffers." Ann Intern Med 1970;73:713–720.
16. Ball BU, Sorensen LB: Pathogenesis of hyperuricemia in saturnine gout. N Engl J Med 1969;280:1199–1202.
17. Bar-Khayim Y, Teplitz C, Garella S, et al: Trimethadione (Tridione)-induced nephrotic syndrome. Am J Med 1973;54:272–280.
18. Barnett RN, Brown DS, Cadorna CB, et al: Beryllium disease with death from renal failure. Conn Med 1961;25:142–147.
19. Barquist E, Fein E, Shadick D, et al: A randomized prospective trial of amphotericin B lipid emulsion versus dextrose colloidal solution in critically ill patients. J Trauma 1999;47:336–340.
20. Barton CH, Pahl M, Vaziri N, et al: Renal magnesium wasting associated with amphotericin B therapy. Am J Med 1984;77:471–474.
21. Batuman V, Maesaka JK, Haddad B, et al: The role of lead in gouty nephropathy. N Engl J Med 1981;304:520–523.
22. Beattie JW: Nephrotic syndrome following sodium bismuth tartrate therapy in rheumatoid arthritis. Ann Rheum Dis 1953;12:144–146.
23. Beaver DL, Burr RE: Bismuth inclusions in the human kidney: A long-term autopsy study. Arch Pathol 1963;76:89–94.
24. Becker BN, Fall P, Hall C, et al: Rapidly progressive acute renal failure due to acyclovir: Case report and review of the literature. Am J Kidney Dis 1993;22:611–615.
25. Becker CG, Becker EF, Maher JF, et al: Nephrotic syndrome after contact with mercury: A report of five cases, three after the use of ammoniated mercury ointment. Arch Intern Med 1962;110:178–186.
26. Beirne GJ, Hansing CE, Octaviano GW, et al: Acute renal failure caused by hypersensitivity to polymyxin B sulfate. JAMA 1967;202: 156–158.
27. Bennett WM: Hazards of the appetite suppressant phenylpropanolamine [letter]. Lancet 1979;2:42–43.
28. Bennett WM, Gilbert DN, Houghton D, et al: Gentamicin nephrotoxicity: Morphologic and pharmacologic features. West J Med 1977; 126:65–68.
29. Better OS, Winaver JM, Knochel JP: Mannitol therapy revisited (1940–1997). Kidney Int 1997;51:886–894.
30. Bowler JV, Ormerod IE, Legg NJ: Retroperitoneal fibrosis and bromocriptine [letter]. Lancet 1986;2:466.
31. Brezin JH, Katz SM, Schwartz AB, et al: Reversible renal failure and nephrotic syndrome associated with non-steroidal anti-inflammatory drugs. N Engl J Med 1979;301:1271–1273.
32. Brigden D, Rosling AE, Woods NC: Renal function after acyclovir intravenous injection. Am J Med 1982;73:182–185.
33. Cacoub P, Deray G, Baumelou A, et al: Acute renal failure induced by foscarnet. Clin Nephrol 1988;29:315–318.
34. Campbell NR, Baylis B: Renal impairment associated with an acute paracetamol overdose in the absence of hepatotoxicity. Postgrad Med J 1992;68:116–118.
35. Catsch A, Harmuth-Hoene AE: The chelation of heavy metals. In: Levine WG, ed: International Encyclopedia of Pharmacology and Therapeutics. New York, Pergamon, 1979, pp. 107–224.
36. Charlas R, Benabadji A: Néphrite azotémique au cours du traitement par l'antimoine d'un cas de leishmaniase viscérale infantile. Maroc Méd 1962;41:1180–1182.
37. Cheng JT, Beysolow TD, Kaul B, et al: Clearance of ethylene glycol by kidneys and hemodialysis. J Toxicol Clin Toxicol 1987;25: 95–108.
38. Cheng JT, Feinfeld DA: Amphotericin B and the kidney. Hosp Physician 1988;24:68–72.
39. Chisolm JJ Jr, Harrison HC, Eberlein WR, et al: Aminoaciduria, hypophosphatemia, and rickets in lead poisoning. Am J Dis Child 1955;89:159–168.
40. Chugh KS, Nath IV, Ubroi HS, et al: Acute renal failure due to nontraumatic rhabdomyolysis. Postgrad Med J 1979;55:386–392.
41. Ciabbatoni G, Cinotti GA, Pierucci A, et al: Effects of sulindac and ibuprofen in patients with chronic glomerular disease. N Engl J Med 1984;310:279–283.
42. Cianciulli P, Sorrentino F, Forte L, et al: Acute renal failure occurring during intravenous desferrioxamine therapy: Recovery after hemodialysis. Haematologica 1992;77:514–515.
43. Citron BP, Halpern M, McCarron M, et al: Necrotizing angiitis associated with drug abuse. N Engl J Med 1970;283:1003–1011.
44. Clive DM, Stoff J: Renal syndromes associated with non-steroidal anti-inflammatory drugs. N Engl J Med 1984;310: 563–572.

45. Collet JT: EDTA-chelation therapy. Ned Tijdschr Geneeskd 1992; 136:191–192.

46. Condit PT, Chanes PE, Joel W: Renal toxicity of methotrexate. Cancer 1969;23:126–131.

47. Crespo M, Quereda C, Pascual J, et al: Patterns of sulfadiazine acute nephropathy. Clin Nephrol 2000;54:68–72.

48. Crowley S, Feinfeld DA, Janis R: Resolution of nephrotic syndrome and lack of progression of heroin-associated renal amyloidosis. Am J Kidney Dis 1989;13:333–335.

49. Crutcher JC: Clinical manifestations and therapy of acute lead intoxication due to the ingestion of illicitly distilled alcohol. Ann Intern Med 1963;59:707–715.

50. Cumming A: Acute renal failure and interstitial nephritis after clofibrate treatment. Br Med J 1980;281:1529–1530.

51. Cunningham EE, Brentjens JR, Zielezny MA, et al: Heroin nephropathy: A clinicopathologic and epidemiologic study. Am J Med 1980;68:47–53.

52. Davenport A, Finn R: Paracetamol (acetaminophen) poisoning resulting in acute renal failure. Nephron 1988;50:55–56.

53. Davies B, Kincaid-Smith P: Renal biopsy studies of lithium and pre-lithium patients and comparison with cadaver transplant kidneys. Neuropharmacology 1979;18:1001–1002.

54. DeBroe ME, Giuliano R, Verpooten G: Choice of drug and dosage regimen: Two important risk factors for aminoglycoside nephrotoxicity. Am J Med 1986;80:115–118.

55. Deray G, Bochet M, Katlama C, et al: Nephrotoxicity of ritonavir. Presse Med 1998;27:1801–1803.

56. Derot M, Kahn J, Mazalton A, et al: Néphrite anurique aigue mortelle après traitement aurique, chrysocyanose associée. Bull Mém Soc Méd Hôp Paris 1954;70:234–239.

57. Di Paolo N, Guarnieri A, Loi F, et al: Acute renal failure from inhalation of mycotoxins. Nephron 1993;64:621–625.

58. Dorfman LE, Smith JP: Sulfonamide crystalluria: A forgotten disease. J Urol 1970;104:482–483.

59. Dubrow A, Flamenbaum W: Acute renal failure associated with myoglobinuria and hemoglobinuria. In: Brenner BM, Lazarus JM, eds: Acute Renal Failure, 2nd ed. New York, Churchill Livingstone, 1988, pp. 279–293.

60. Dunn MJ: Are Cox-2 selective inhibitors nephrotoxic? Am J Kidney Dis 2000;35:976–977.

61. Eichhorn JH, Hedley-White J, Steinman TI, et al: Renal failure following enflurane anesthesia. Anesthesiology 1976;45:557–560.

62. Eisenberg ES, Robbins N, Lenci M: Vancomycin and interstitial nephritis [letter]. Ann Intern Med 1981;95:658.

63. Ellis ME, Weiss RB, Kuperminc M: Nephrotoxicity of lomustine. Cancer Chemother Pharmacol 1985;15:174–175.

64. Elseviers MM, De Broe ME: Analgesic nephropathy: Is it caused by multianalgesic abuse of single substance use? Drug Saf 1999;20: 15–24.

65. Emmerson BT: Chronic lead nephropathy: The diagnostic use of calcium EDTA and the association with gout. Australas Ann Med 1963;12:310–324.

66. Espinel CH, Gregory AW: Differential diagnosis of acute renal failure. Clin Nephrol 1980;13:73–77.

67. Fang LS, Sirota RA, Ebert TH, et al: Low fractional excretion of sodium with contrast media-induced acute renal failure. Arch Intern Med 1980;140:531–533.

68. Farrell J, Campbell E, Walshe JJ: Renal failure associated with alternative medical therapies. Ren Fail 1995;17:659–664.

69. Feinfeld DA, Ansari N, Nuovo M, et al: Tubulointerstitial nephritis associated with minimal self reexposure to rifampin. Am J Kidney Dis 1999;33:E3.

70. Feinfeld DA, Briscoe AM, Nurse HM, et al: Myoglobinuria in chronic renal failure. Am J Kidney Dis 1986;8:111–114.

71. Feinfeld DA, Carvounis CP: Fatal hyperkalemia and hyperchloremic acidosis: Association with spironolactone in the absence of renal impairment. JAMA 1978;240:1516.

72. Feinfeld DA, Cheng JT, Beysolow TD, et al: A prospective study of urine and serum myoglobin levels in patients with acute rhabdomyolysis. Clin Nephrol 1992;38:193–195.

73. Feinfeld DA, D'Agati V, Benvenisty A, et al: Cyclosporin A and urine glutathione-S-transferase. Proc EDTA-ERA 1985;22: 561–565.

74. Feinfeld DA, Nurse HM, Hotchkiss JL, et al: The clinical spectrum of chronic interstitial nephritis. Hosp Physician 1985;21:102–104.

75. Feinfeld DA, Olesnicky L, Pirani CL, et al: Nephrotic syndrome associated with the use of non-steroidal anti-inflammatory drugs. Nephron 1984;37:174–179.

76. Feinfeld DA, Ranieri R, Lipner HI, Avram MM: Renal failure in phenazopyridine overdose. JAMA 1978;240:2661.

77. Foord RD: Cephaloridine, cephalothin and the kidney. J Antimicrob Chemother 1975;1(Suppl 3):119–133.

78. Forrest JN Jr, Marcy TW, Biemesderfer D, et al: Cytoskeletal defect in cortical collecting duct cells in lithium-induced polyuria [abstract]. Kidney Int 1981;19:200.

79. Freeman HJ: Ranitidine-associated interstitial nephritis in a patient with celiac sprue. Can J Gastroenterol 1988;2:35.

80. Friberg L: Chronic cadmium poisoning. Arch Ind Health 1959;20: 401–407.

81. Frimpter GW, Timpanelli AE, Eisenmenger WJ, et al: Reversible "Fanconi syndrome" caused by degraded tetracycline. JAMA 1963; 184:111–113.

82. Gabow PA, Kaehny WD, Kelleher SP: The spectrum of rhabdomyolysis. Medicine (Baltimore) 1982;61:141–152.

83. Gade R, Feinfeld DA, Gade MF: A microradiographic study of nephrons in mercuric chloride-induced acute renal failure in the rabbit. Invest Radiol 1983;18:183–188.

84. Galler M, Folkert VW, Schlondorff D: Reversible acute renal insufficiency and hyperkalemia following indomethacin therapy. JAMA 1981;246:154–155.

85. Gelbart DR, Weinstein AB, Fajardo LF: Allopurinol-induced interstitial nephritis. Ann Intern Med 1977;86:196–198. Letter.

86. Gelman ML, Lichtenstein N: Halothane-induced nephrotoxicity. Urology 1981;17:323–327.

87. Gemery J, Idelson B, Reid S, et al: Acute renal failure after arteriography with gadolinium-based contrast agent. Am J Roentgenol 1998; 171:1277–1278.

88. Gerritsen WR, Peters A, Henny FC, et al: Ciprofloxacin-induced nephrotoxicity [letter]. Nephrol Dial Transplant 1987;2:382–383.

89. Gilbert DN, Gourley R, d'Agostino A, et al: Interstitial nephritis due to methicillin, penicillin, and ampicillin. Ann Allergy 1970;28: 378–385.

90. Goldstein RS, Mayor GH: The nephrotoxicity of cisplatin. Life Sci 1983;32:685–690.

91. Gradus D, Rhoads M, Bergstrom LB, et al: Acute bromate poisoning associated with renal failure and deafness presenting as hemolytic-uremic syndrome. Am J Nephrol 1984;4:188–191.

92. Greven J, Klein H: Renal effects of furosemide in glycerol-induced acute renal failure of the rat. Pflügers Arch 1976;365:81–87.

93. Gudallah MF, Lynn M, Work J: Case report: Mannitol nephrotoxicity syndrome. Am J Med Sci 1995;309:219–222.

94. Halpren BA, Kempson RC, Coplon NS: Interstitial fibrosis and chronic renal failure following methoxyflurane anesthesia. JAMA 1973;233:1239–1242.

95. Hayes DM, Cvitkovic E, Golbey RB, et al: High dose cisplatinum diamine dichloride: Amelioration of renal toxicity by mannitol diuresis. Cancer 1977;39:1372–1381.

96. Hébert JL, Auzépy P, Durand A: Acute human and experimental poisoning with diethylene glycol. Sém Hôp Paris 1983;59: 344–349.

97. Heering P, Ivens K, Aker S, et al: Distal renal tubular acidosis induced by FK-506. Clin Transplant 1998;12:465–471.

98. Heidemann HT, Gerkens JF, Spickard WA, et al: Amphotericin B nephrotoxicity in humans decreased by salt repletion. Am J Med 1983;75:476–481.

99. Henrich WL, Agodoa LE, Barrett B, et al: Analgesics and the kidney: Summary and recommendations to the scientific advisory board of the National Kidney Foundation from an ad hoc committee of the National Kidney Foundation. Am J Kidney Dis 1996;27: 162–165.

100. Henry JA, Jeffreys KJ, Dawling S: Toxicity and deaths from 3,4-methylenedioxyamphetamine ("ecstasy"). Lancet 1992;340: 384–387.

101. Hertz P, Yager H, Richardson JB: Probenecid-induced nephrotic syndrome. Arch Pathol 1972;94:241–243.

102. Hestbech J, Aurell M: Lithium-induced uremia [letter]. Lancet 1979; 1:212–213.

103. Hestbech J, Hansen HE, Amdisen A, et al: Chronic renal lesions following long-term treatment with lithium. Kidney Int 1977;12: 205–213.

104. Heuck A, Reiser M: Nephrotoxicity of contrast medium in magnetic resonance tomography. Internist (Berl) 1997;38:1234–1235.

105. Hill MD, Bilbao JM: Case of the month: February 1999—54-year-old man with severe muscle weakness. Brain Pathol 1999;9: 607–608.

106. Hogg RJ, Sawyer M, Hecox K, et al: Carbamazepine-induced acute tubulointerstitial nephritis. J Pediatr 1981;98:830–832.

107. Howard T, Hoy RH, Warren S, et al: Acute renal dysfunction due to sulfinpyrazone therapy in post-myocardial infarction: Cardiomegaly, reversible hypersensitivity, interstitial nephritis. Am Heart J 1981;102:294–295.

108. Humes HD, Jackson NM, O'Connor RP, et al: Pathogenetic mechanisms of nephrotoxicity: Insights into cyclosporine nephrotoxicity. Transplant Proc 1985;17(Suppl 1):51–62.

109. Humes HD, Weinberg JM, Knauss TC: Clinical and pathophysiologic aspects of aminoglycoside toxicity. Am J Kidney Dis 1982; 2:5–29.

110. Hyman LR, Ballow M, Knieser MR: Diphenylhydantoin interstitial nephritis: Roles of cellular and humoral immunologic injury. J Pediatr 1978;92:915–920.

111. Inglis JA, Henderson DA, Emmerson BT: The pathology and pathogenesis of chronic lead nephropathy occurring in Queensland. J Pathol 1978;124:65–76.

112. Iversen BM, Nordahl E, Thunold S, et al: Retroperitoneal fibrosis during treatment with methyldopa. Lancet 1975;2:302–304.

113. Jacob H, Charytan C, Rascoff JH, et al: Amyloidosis secondary to drug abuse and chronic skin suppuration. Arch Intern Med 1978;138: 1150–1151.

114. Jadoul M, de Plaen J-F, Cosyns J-P, et al: Adverse effects from traditional Chinese medicines. Lancet 1993;341:892–893.

115. Jaradat M, Phillips C, Yum MN, et al: Acute tubulointerstitial nephritis attributable to indinavir therapy. Am J Kidney Dis 2000; 35:E16.

116. Kallenberg CGM: Renal disease—Another effect of silica exposure. Nephrol Dial Transplant 1995;10:1117–1119.

117. Katholi RE, Woods WT Jr, Taylor GJ, et al: Oxygen free radicals and contrast nephropathy. Am J Kidney Dis 1998;32:64–71.

118. Kazantzis G: Renal tubular dysfunction and abnormalities of calcium metabolism in cadmium workers. Environ Health Perspect 1979;28: 155–159.

119. Kendrick WC, Hull, AR, Knochel JP: Rhabdomyolysis and shock after intravenous amphetamine administration. Ann Intern Med 1977;86:381–387.

120. Kennedy BJ: Metabolic and toxic effects of mithramycin during tumor therapy. Am J Med 1970;49:494–503.

121. Kesten HD, Mulinos MG, Pomerantz L: Pathologic effects of certain glycols and related compounds. Arch Pathol 1939;27:447.

122. Khosla SN, Nand N, Khosla P: Aluminium phosphide poisoning. J Tropic Med Hyg 1988;91:196–198.

123. Kleinknecht D, Vanhille P, Morel-Maroger L: Acute interstitial nephritis due to drug hypersensitivity: An up-to-date review with a report of 19 cases. Adv Nephrol 1983;12:277–308.

124. Knochel JP: Rhabdomyolysis and myoglobinuria. In: Suki WN, Eknoyan G, eds: The Kidney in Systemic Disease, 2nd ed. New York, Wiley, 1981, pp. 263–284.

125. Koch-Weser J, Sidel V, Federman ER, et al: Adverse effects of sodium colistimethate: Manifestations and specific reaction rates during courses of therapy. Ann Intern Med 1970;72:857–868.

126. Koren G: The nephrotoxic potential of drugs and chemicals: Pharmacologic basis and clinical relevance. Med Toxicol 1989;4:59–72.

127. Kunis C, Olesnicky L, Nurse H, et al: Heroin nephropathy: Clinical-pathological correlations [abstract 102A]. Ninth International Congress on Nephrology, Los Angeles CA, June 11–16, 1984.

128. Lampe KF: Toxic effects of plant toxins. In: Klaassen CD, Amdur MO, Doull J, eds: Casarett and Doull's Toxicology, 3rd ed. New York, Macmillan, 1986, pp. 757–770.

129. Landrigan PJ: Arsenic. In: Rom WN, ed: Environmental and Occupational Medicine. Boston, Little, Brown, 1983, pp. 473–480.

130. Lavender S, Brown JN, Berrill WT: Acute renal failure and lithium intoxication. Postgrad Med J 1973;49:277–279.

131. Lerner SA, Schmitt B, Seligsohn R, et al: Comparative study of ototoxicity and nephrotoxicity in patients randomly assigned to treatment with amikacin or gentamicin. Am J Med 1986;80:90–104.

132. Levine DH, Levkoff AH, Pappu LD, et al: Renal failure and other serious sequelae of epinephrine toxicity in neonates. South Med J 1985;78:874–877.

133. Lieberthal W: Biology of acute renal failure: therapeutic implications. Kidney Int 1997;52:1102–1115.

134. Lim PS, Lin JL, Hu SA, et al: Acute renal failure due to ingestion of the gallbladder of grass carp: Report of 3 cases with review of literature. Ren Fail 1993;15: 639–644.

135. Link DA, Fosburg MT, Ingelfinger JR, et al: Renal toxicity of high dose methotrexate [abstract]. Pediatr Res 1976;10:455.

136. Linton AL, Clark WF, Drieger AA, et al: Acute interstitial nephritis due to drugs: Review of the literature with a report of nine cases. Ann Intern Med 1980;93:735–741.

137. Liu K, Mittelman A, Sproul EE, et al: Renal toxicity in men treated with mitomycin C. Cancer 1971;28:1314–1320.

138. Llach F, Descoeudres C, Massry SG: Heroin-associated nephropathy: Clinical and histological studies in 19 patients. Clin Nephrol 1979;11:7–12.

139. Loughridge LW, Leader LP, Brown DAL: Acute renal failure due to muscle necrosis in carbon monoxide poisoning. Lancet 1958;2: 349–351.

140. Lucké B: Lower nephron nephrosis: The renal lesions of crush syndrome of burns, transfusions and other conditions affecting the lower segment of the nephrons. Mil Surg 1946;99:371–396.

141. Lyons H, Pinn VW, Cortell S, et al: Allergic interstitial nephritis causing reversible renal failure in four patients with idiopathic nephrotic syndrome. N Engl J Med 1973;288:124–128.

142. Magil AB, Ballon HS, Cameron ECC, et al: Acute interstitial nephritis associated with thiazide diuretics: Clinical and pathological observations in three cases. Am J Med 1980;69:939–943.

143. Maher JF: Toxic nephropathy. In: Brenner BM, Rector FC Jr, eds: The Kidney. Philadelphia, WB Saunders, 1976, 1355–1395.

144. McCurdy DK, Frederic M, Elkinton JR: Renal tubular acidosis due to amphotericin B. N Engl J Med 1968;278:124–130.

145. McGowan WR, Vermillion SE: Acute interstitial nephritis related to cimetidine therapy. Gastroenterology 1980;79:746–749.

146. Mihatsch MJ, Thiel G, Spichtin HD, et al: Morphological findings in kidney transplants after treatment with cyclosporine. Transplant Proc 1983;15:2821–2835.

147. Miller TJ, Anderson RJ, Linas SL, et al: Urinary diagnostic indices in acute renal failure: A prospective study. Ann Intern Med 1978; 89:47–50.

148. Mitchel DH: Amanita mushroom poisoning. Annu Rev Med 1980; 31:51–57.

149. Moody C, Kaufman R, McGuire D, et al: The role of adulterants in heroin nephropathy. Abstr Natl Kidney Found 1985;15:A12.

150. More RH, McMillan GC, Duff GL: The pathology of sulfonamide allergy in man. Am J Pathol 1946;22:703–705.

151. Moreau JF, Droz D, Noel LH: Tubular nephrotoxicity of water soluble iodinated contrast media. Invest Radiol 1980;15 (suppl 6): S54–S60.

152. Morin JP, Viotte G, Vandewalle A, et al: Gentamicin-induced nephrotoxicity: A cell biology approach. Kidney Int 1980;18: 583–590.

153. Mudge GH, Meier FA, Ward KK: Pathogenesis of renal impairment induced by radiocontrast drugs. In: Solez K, Whelton A, eds: Acute Renal Failure. New York, Marcel Dekker, 1984, pp. 361–388.

154. Mudge GH: Nephrotoxicity of urographic radiocontrast drugs. Kidney Int 1980;18:540–552.

155. Muehrcke RC, Pirani CL: Arsine induced anuria: A correlative clinicopathologic study with electron microscopic observations. Ann Intern Med 1968;68:853–866.

156. Muehrcke RC, Pirani CL, Kark RM: Interstitial nephritis: A clinicopathological renal biopsy study. Ann Intern Med 1967;66:1052.

157. Mullick FG, McAllister HA Jr, Wagner BM, et al: Drug-related vasculitis: Clinicopathologic correlations in 30 patients. Hum Pathol 1979;10:313–325.

158. Murphy KJ: Bilateral renal calculi and aminoaciduria after excessive intake of Worcestershire sauce. Lancet 1967;2:401–403.

159. Muther RS: Drug interference with renal function tests. Am J Kidney Dis 1983;3:118–120.

160. Myers BD, Ross J, Newton L, et al: Cyclosporine-associated chronic nephropathy. N Engl J Med 1984;311:699–705.

161. Nagi AH, Alexander F, Barbas AZ: Gold nephropathy in rats: Light and electron microscopic studies. Exp Mol Pathol 1971;15:354–362.

162. Nessi R, Bonoldi GL, Redaelli B, et al: Acute renal failure after rifampicin: A case report and survey of the literature. Nephron 1976; 16:148–159.

163. Neylan J, Whelchel J, Laskow D, et al: Adverse events in the comparative dose finding trial of FK-506 in primary renal transplantation. Am Soc Transplant Phys 1993;12:154.

164. Nolan CR, Anger MS, Kelleher SP: Eosinophiluria: A new method of detection and definition of the clinical spectrum. N Engl J Med 1986;315:1516–1519.

165. Obara K, Saito T, Sato H, et al: Germanium poisoning: Clinical symptoms and renal damage caused by long-term intake of germanium. Jpn J Med 1991;30:67–72.

166. Oliver J, MacDowell M, Tracy A: The pathogenesis of acute renal failure associated with traumatic and toxic injury: Renal ischemia, nephrotoxic damage and the ischemic episode. J Clin Invest 1951; 30:1307–1351.

167. Ooi BS, First MR, Pesce AJ, et al: IgE levels in interstitial nephritis. Lancet 1974;1:1254–1256.

168. O'Sullivan TL, Akbari A, Cadnapaphornchai P: Acute renal failure associated with the administration of parenteral etidronate. Ren Fail 1994;16:767–773.

169. Paller MS: Drug-induced nephropathies. Med Clin North Am 1990; 74:909–916.

170. Panner BJ, Freeman, RB, Roth-Mayo VA, et al: Toxicity following methoxyflurane anesthesia. JAMA 1970;214:86–90.

171. Parry MF, Wallach R: Ethylene glycol poisoning. Am J Med 1974; 57:143–150.

172. Pavlakis N, Pollack CA, McLean G, et al: Deliberate overdose of uranium: Toxicity and treatment. Nephron 1996;72:313–317.

173. Pavy MD, Wiley EL, Abeloff MD: Hemolytic-uremic syndrome associated with mitomycin therapy. Cancer Treat Rep 1982;66: 457–461.

174. Perazella MA, Eras J: Are selective COX-2 inhibitors nephrotoxic? Am J Kidney Dis 2000;35:937–940.

175. Perico N, Ruggenenti P, Gaspari P, et al: Daily renal hypoperfusion induced by cyclosporine in patients with renal transplantation. Transplantation 1992;54:56–60.

176. Perkoff GT, Dioso MM, Bleisch V, et al: A spectrum of myopathy associated with alcoholism. I. Clinical and laboratory features. Ann Intern Med 1967;67:493–510.

177. Peterson BA, Collins AJ, Vogelzang NJ, et al: 5-Azacytidine and renal tubular dysfunction. Blood 1981;57:182–185.

178. Phillips ME, Eastwood JB, Curtis JR, et al: Tetracycline poisoning in renal failure. Br Med J 1974;2:149–151.

179. Pitman SW, Parker LM, Tattersall MHN, et al: Clinical trials of high-dose methotrexate with citrovorum factor: Toxicologic and therapeutic observations. Cancer Chemother Rep 1975;6:43–49.

180. Poole G, Stradling P, Worlledge S: Potentially serious side effects of high-dose twice-weekly rifampicin. Br Med J 1971;3:343–347.

181. Porter GA: Radiocontrast-induced nephropathy. Nephrol Dial Transplant 1994;9(Suppl 4):146–156.

182. Prins EJL, Hoorntje SJ, Weening JJ, et al: Nephrotic syndrome in patients on captopril [letter]. Lancet 1979;2:306–307.

183. Qunibi WY, Godwin J, Eknoyan G: Toxic nephropathy during continuous rifampin therapy. South Med J 1980; 73:791–792.

184. Reisin E, Teicher A, Jaffe R, et al: Myoglobinuria and renal failure in toluene poisoning. Br J Ind Med 1975;32:163–164.

185. Rodin AE, Crowson CN: Mercury nephrotoxicity in the rat. II. Investigation of the intracellular site of mercury nephrotoxicity by correlated serial time histologic and histoenzymatic studies. Am J Pathol 1962;41:485–499.

186. Ron D, Taitelman MD, Michaelson MD, et al: Prevention of acute renal failure in traumatic rhabdomyolysis. Arch Intern Med 1984; 144:277–280.

187. Rosen H, El-Hennawy AS, Greenberg S, et al: Acute interstitial nephritis associated with ticlopidine. Am J Kidney Dis 1995;25: 934–936.

188. Ross JH, McGinty F, Brewer DG: Penicillamine nephropathy. Nephron 1980;26:184–186.

189. Roth D, Alarcon FJ, Fernandez JA, et al: Acute rhabdomyolysis associated with cocaine intoxication. N Engl J Med 1988;319: 673–677.

190. Roza O, Berman LB: The pathophysiology of barium: Hypokalemic and cardiovascular effects. J Pharmacol Exp Ther 1971;177: 433–439.

191. Rybak MJ, Abate BJ, Kang SL, et al: Prospective evaluation of the effect of an aminoglycoside-dosing regimen on rates of observed nephrotoxicity and ototoxicity. Antimicrob Agents Chemother 1999; 43:1549–1555.

192. Safirstein R, Winston J, Goldstein M, et al: Cisplatin nephrotoxicity. Am J Kidney Dis 1986;8:356–367.

193. Saltissi D, Pulsey CD, Rainford DJ: Recurrent acute renal failure due to antibiotic-induced interstitial nephritis. Br Med J 1979;1: 1182–1183.

194. Sandler DP, Smith JC, Weinberg CR, et al: Analgesic use and chronic renal disease. N Engl J Med 1989;320:1238–1243.

195. Sanghvi LM, Sharma R, Mirsa SN, et al: Sulfhemoglobinemia and acute renal failure after copper sulfate poisoning: Report of two fatal cases. Arch Pathol 1957;63:172–175.

196. Schacht RG, Feiner HD, Gallo GR, et al: Nephrotoxicity of nitrosoureas. Cancer 1981;38:1328–1334.

197. Scharschmidt LA, Feinfeld DA: Renal effects of nonsteroidal antiinflammatory drugs. Hosp Physician 1989;25:29–33.

198. Schein PS, O'Connell MJ, Blom J, et al: Clinical antitumor activity and toxicity of streptozotocin. Cancer 1974;34:993–1000.

199. Schreiner GE, Maher JF: Toxic nephropathy. Am J Med 1965;38: 409–449.

200. Schuhmann-Giamperi G, Krestin G: Pharmacokinetics of Gd-DTPA in patients with chronic renal insufficiency. Invest Radiol 1991; 26:975–979.

201. Schwarz A, Krause PH, Kunzendorf U, et al: The outcome of acute interstitial nephritis: risk factors for the transition from acute to chronic interstitial nephritis. Clin Nephrol 2000;54:179–190.

202. Shils ME: Renal disease and the metabolic effects of tetracycline. Ann Intern Med 1963;58:389–408.

203. Shore R, Greenberg M, Geary D, et al: Iphosphamide-induced nephrotoxicity in children. Pediatr Nephrol 1992;6:162–165.
204. Simmons CF, Bogusky RT, Humes HD: Inhibitory effects of gentamicin on renal mitochondrial oxidative phosphorylation. J Pharmacol Exp Ther 1980;214:709–715.
205. Singer I: Lithium and the kidney. Kidney Int 1981;19:374–387.
206. Sipes IG, Krishna G, Gillette JR: Bioactivation of carbon tetrachloride, chloroform, and bromotrichloromethane: Role of cytochrome. Life Sci 1977;20:1541–1548.
207. Sleijfer DTH, Smit EF, Meijer S, et al: Acute and cumulative effects of carboplatin on renal function. Br J Cancer 1989;60:116–120.
208. Sloth K, Thomsen AC: Acute renal insufficiency during treatment with azathioprine. Acta Med Scand 1971;189:145–148.
209. Smetana H: Nephrosis due to carbon tetrachloride. Arch Intern Med 1939;63:760–777.
210. Smith CR, Lipsky JJ, Laskin OL, et al: Double-blind comparison of the nephrotoxicity and auditory toxicity of gentamicin and tobramycin. N Engl J Med 1980;302:1106–1109.
211. Solomon NM, Mokrzycki MH: Levofloxacin-induced allergic interstitial nephritis [letter]. Clin Nephrol 2000;54:356.
212. Stahl-Bayliss CM, Kalman CM, Laskin OL: Pentamidine-induced hypoglycemia in patients with the acquired immune deficiency syndrome. Clin Pharmacol Ther 1986;39:271–275.
213. Stecker JF Jr, Rawls HP, Devine CJ, et al: Retroperitoneal fibrosis and ergot derivatives. J Urol 1974;112:30–32.
214. Stefanidis I, Bohm R, Hagel J, et al: Toxic myopathy with kidney failure as a colchicine side effect in familial Mediterranean fever. Dtsch Med Wochenschr 1992;117:1237–1240.
215. Stein JH, Lifschitz MD, Barnes LD: Current concepts of the pathophysiology of acute renal failure. Am J Physiol 1978;234:F171–F181.
216. Steinman TI, Silva P: Acute renal failure, skin rash, and eosinophilia associated with captopril therapy. Am J Med 1983;75:154–156.
217. Sterne TL, Whitaker C, Webb CH: Fatal cases of bismuth intoxication. J La State Med Soc 1955;107:332–335.
218. Su Q, Weber L, Lettir M, et al: Nephrotoxicity of cyclosporin A and FK-506: Inhibition of calcineurin phosphatase. Ren Physiol Biochem 1995;18:128–139.
219. Ten RM, Torres VE, Milliner DS, et al: Acute interstitial nephritis: Immunologic and clinical aspects. Mayo Clin Proc 1988;63:921–930.
220. Thadhani R, Pascual M, Bonventre J: Medical progress: Acute renal failure. N Engl J Med 1996;334:1448–1460.
221. Thompson J: Ferrous sulfate poisoning: Its incidence, symptomatology, treatment, and prevention. Br Med J 1950;1:645–646.
222. Tornroth T, Skrifvars B: Gold nephropathy prototype of membranous glomerulonephritis. Am J Pathol 1974;75:573–590.
223. Tubbs RR, Gephardt GN, McMahon JT, et al: Membranous glomerulonephritis associated with industrial mercury exposure. Am J Clin Pathol 1982;77:409–413.
224. Uldall PR, Khan HA, Ennis JE, et al: Renal damage from industrial arsine poisoning. Br J Ind Med 1970;27:372–377.
225. Vallee BL, Ulmer DD, Wacker WEC: Arsenic toxicology and biochemistry. Arch Ind Health 1960;21:132–151.
226. Vanherweghem JL, Depierreux M, Tielemans C, et al: Rapidly progressive interstitial renal fibrosis in young women: association with slimming regimen including Chinese herbs. Lancet 1993;341:387–391.
227. Vanholder R, Colardyn F, De Reuck J, et al: Diquat intoxication: Report of two cases and review of the literature. Am J Med 1981;70:1267–1271.
228. VanZee BE, Hoy WE, Talley TE, et al: Renal injury associated with intravenous pyelography in nondiabetic and diabetic patients. Ann Intern Med 1978;89:51–54.
229. Varma A, Jha V, Ghosh AK, et al: Acute renal failure in a case of fatal chromic acid poisoning. Ren Fail 1994;16:653–657.
230. Walker RG, Thomson NM, Dowling JP, Ogg CS: Minocycline-induced acute interstitial nephritis. Br Med J 1979;1:524.
231. Warren GV, Korbet SM, Schwartz MM, et al: Minimal change glomerulopathy associated with nonsteroidal anti-inflammatory drugs. Am J Kidney Dis 1989;13:127–130.
232. Wedeen RP, Batuman V: Tubulo-interstitial nephritis induced by heavy metals and metabolic disturbances. Contemp Issues Nephrol 1983;10:211–241.
233. Wedeen RP, Maesaka JK, Weiner B, et al: Occupational lead nephropathy. Am J Med 1975;59:630–641.
234. Wetherill SF, Guarine MJ, Cox RW: Acute renal failure associated with barium chloride poisoning. Ann Intern Med 1981;95:187–188.
235. Wilson M, Brown DJ, Brown RW, et al: Renal failure from alphamethyldopa therapy. Aust N Z J Med 1974;4: 415–416.
236. Woolf AD, Ebert TH: Toxicity after self-poisoning by ingestion of potassium chloroplatinite. J Toxicol Clin Toxicol 1991;29:467–472.

CHAPTER 24 FLUID, ELECTROLYTE, AND ACID-BASE PRINCIPLES

Robert S. Hoffman

Normal Laboratory Values

Electrolyte	Conventional Units	S.I. Units
Sodium	135–145 mEq/L	135–145 mmol/L
Potassium	3.5–5.0 mEq/L	3.5–5.0 mmol/L
Calcium	8.4–10.2 mg/dL (4.2–5.1 mEq/L)	2.10–2.55 mmol/L
Magnesium	1.3–2.1 mEq/L	0.65–1.05 mmol/L

Although many discussions of fluid, electrolyte, and acid-base abnormalities present guidelines for evaluating blood chemistries strictly on a numerical basis, a meaningful analysis must be based on the clinical characteristics of each patient. Specifically, although a rigorous appraisal of these laboratory parameters often yields the correct differential diagnosis, essential information can be gained from the history and physical examination, and this information often provides the data necessary to refine the differential diagnosis appropriately. Thus, the evaluation always begins with an overall assessment of the patient's status. (Many of the issues discussed here overlap with Chaps. 17, 20, and 21.)

INITIAL PATIENT ASSESSMENT

History

The history should include clinical complaints associated with fluid and electrolyte abnormalities. Common manifestations of toxin exposure result in fluid losses through the respiratory system (hyperpnea and tachypnea), the gastrointestinal system (vomiting and diarrhea), the skin (diaphoresis and fever), and the kidneys (polyuria). Patients with volume depletion may complain of thirst or even polydipsia.

A history of exposure to over-the-counter and prescription medications, toxins, and premorbid conditions is important to assess volume status. Also, the time of year, ambient temperature, and humidity should always be considered.

Physical Examination

The vital signs offer the first markers of gross alterations in volume status. Whereas hypotension and tachycardia may herald life-threatening volume depletion, an initial increase of the heart rate and a narrowing of the pulse pressure may be earlier findings. Patient abnormalities may be recognized through a dynamic evaluation, realizing that the measurement of a single set of supine vital signs offers useful information only when grossly abnormal. The addition of orthostatic pulse and blood pressure measurements provides a more meaningful determination of functional volume status (Chaps. 17 and 21).

The respiratory rate and pattern can give clues to the patient's metabolic status. When metabolic acidosis is present, hyperventilation (manifested as tachypnea, hyperpnea, or both) usually is noted. Although hypoventilation (bradypnea or hypopnea) is present in patients with metabolic alkalosis, it is rarely clinically significant, and it is usually only detected by arterial blood-gas analysis.

The skin should be evaluated for turgor, moisture content, and presence of edema. The moisture content of the mucous membranes can also provide valuable information. These are general parameters and may not necessarily directly correlate with the status of hydration. This dissociation is especially true with toxin exposure, as many drugs and toxins alter skin and mucous membrane findings without necessarily altering volume status. Antihistamines and anticholinergics commonly dry mucous membranes and skin without producing volume depletion. Conversely, patients exposed to sympathomimetic agents (cocaine) or cholinergic agents (organic phosphorus insecticides) may have quite moist skin and mucous membranes even in the setting of significant fluid losses. These dissociative characteristics further reinforce the need to assess the patient in his/her entirety to identify a unifying perspective for the clinical presentation.

The physical findings associated with electrolyte abnormalities are often nonspecific. Hypo- and hypernatremia, hypercalcemia, and hypermagnesemia all can produce a depressed mental status. Neuromuscular excitability (tremor, hyperreflexia, etc) is noted with hypocalcemia, hypomagnesemia, hyponatremia, and hyperkalemia. Multiple electrolyte disorders can produce confusing clinical presentations, or patients may appear normal. Rarer diagnostic findings, such as Chvostek and Trousseau signs (found in hypocalcemia), may be useful in assessing patients with potential toxin exposures.

Rapid Diagnostic Tools

The electrocardiogram (ECG) is a useful tool for Emergency Department (ED) screening of some common electrolyte abnormalities (Chap. 9). It is easy to perform, rapid, inexpensive, and routinely available. In this context, the ECG is used most often for evaluation of changes in potassium and calcium (discussed later). Unfortunately, because both poor sensitivity (0.43) and specificity (0.86) were demonstrated when ECGs were used to diagnose hyperkalemia, in actuality, the test is of limited value.[166]

In most patients, bedside assessment of urine specific gravity by dipstick analysis can provide valuable information about volume status.[88] A high urine specific gravity (greater than 1.020) signifies concentrated urine and usually correlates with volume depletion. However, when direct renal impairment is the source of the volume loss, the specific gravity is usually normal (1.010). Thus, many toxins interfere with this test's utility. Examples of this phenomenon include the patient with lithium-induced diabetes insipidus whose urine remains dilute (low specific gravity) despite consequential volume depletion and the patient with methylenedioxymethamphetamine (MDMA)-induced syndrome of inappropriate antidiuretic hormone secretion whose urine remains concentrated (high specific gravity) in the presence of a normal to high volume status.

The urine dipstick is also useful for rapidly determining the presence of ketones, which are often associated with specific toxicologic problems (eg, salicylates, alcoholic ketoacidosis) and common causes of metabolic acidosis (eg, diabetic ketoacidosis, salicylates, alcoholic ketoacidosis). The urine ferric chloride test rapidly detects exposure to salicylates with a high sensitivity and specificity (Chap. 33).

Laboratory Studies

A simultaneous determination of the serum electrolytes, blood urea nitrogen (BUN), glucose, and arterial blood gas is adequate to determine the nature of most common acid-base, fluid, and electrolyte abnormalities. More complex clinical problems may require determinations of urine and serum osmolalities, urine electrolytes, serum ketones, lactic acid concentrations, or other tests to assist in diagnosis. A systematic approach to common problems is discussed below.

ACID-BASE ABNORMALITIES

Definitions

The terminology of acid-base disorders often leads to confusion and error. The following definitions provide the appropriate frame of reference for the remainder of the chapter.

The terms *acidosis* and *alkalosis* refer to processes that tend to change pH in a given direction. By definition a patient is said to have:

- A *metabolic acidosis* if his or her serum bicarbonate (HCO_3^-) is less than 24 mEq/L. Because compensation is inherent, metabolic acidosis is normally accompanied by a PCO_2 less than 40 mm Hg and a pH less than 7.40 unless another primary process is present.

- A *metabolic alkalosis* if his or her serum HCO_3^- is more than 24 mEq/L. Because of inherent compensation, metabolic alkalosis is normally accompanied by a PCO_2 greater than 40 mm Hg and a pH greater than 7.40 unless another primary process is present.

- A *respiratory acidosis* if his or her partial pressure of carbon dioxide (PCO_2) is greater than 40 mm Hg. Because of inherent compensation, respiratory acidosis is normally accompanied by a serum HCO_3^- greater than 24 mEq/L and a pH less than 7.40 unless another primary process is present.

- A *respiratory alkalosis* if his or her PCO_2 is less than 40 mm Hg. Again, because of inherent compensation, respiratory alkalosis is normally accompanied by a serum HCO_3^- less than 24 mEq/L and a pH greater than 7.40 unless another process is present.

Any combination of acidoses and alkaloses can be present in any one patient at any given time.

The terms *acidemia* and *alkalemia* refer only to the resultant pH of blood (acidemia being less than 7.40 and alkalemia being greater than 7.40). These terms do not describe the process or processes that led to the alteration in pH. Thus a patient with acidemia may have both an acidosis and an alkalosis present at the same time. Although in reality a range exists for normal pH values, serum bicarbonate concentration, and partial pressure of carbon dioxide, accepting a single value as normal greatly simplifies the analysis without distorting the results.

The following case discussions illustrate the approach to acid-base disorders.

Patient 1 A 27-year-old man was found unconscious at home with a suicide note and some empty pill containers. A history of injection drug use was assumed by the paramedics because of the presence of track marks on his skin. The initial assessment was notable for a blood pressure of 140/90 mm Hg, a pulse of 120 beats/min, and a respiratory rate of 18 breaths/min. The patient was placed on high-flow oxygen and transported to the ED. En route to the ED, an IV line was inserted and blood samples were obtained for later analysis.

On arrival at the ED the patient was intermittently agitated and deeply lethargic with a blood pressure of 120/90 mm Hg, a pulse rate of 110 beats/min, labored respirations of 18 breaths/min, and a rectal temperature of 38.1°C (100.6°F). His skin was slightly diaphoretic and was notable for multiple track marks of various ages. His head was without signs of trauma. Pupils were 4 mm in size, equal, and round, but sluggishly reactive to light. His neck was supple, without signs of meningeal irritation. His chest was clear to auscultation and percussion, and heart sounds were normal. His abdomen was soft, without organomegaly, and with good bowel sounds. Rectal tone was normal, and stool was negative for occult blood. Neurologic assessment revealed good motor strength, intact corneal and oculocephalic reflexes, and brisk but symmetric deep tendon reflexes. Plantar flexion was present.

The blood specimens obtained by the paramedics were sent to the laboratory for electrolytes, glucose, BUN, CBC, and acetaminophen level. Two serum tubes were placed aside for future studies as indicated. An arterial blood-gas analysis was obtained on room air, and an ECG showed sinus tachycardia with no evidence of PR, QRS, QT abnormalities, or ectopy. After a gag reflex was confirmed, the patient was placed in the left lateral decubitus position and was lavaged with a 40-French orogastric tube. When the lavage fluid was clear, a slurry of 60 g of activated charcoal in water and 70 g of sorbitol was instilled and the tube was removed.

The arterial blood gas analysis showed a pH of 7.30, P_{CO_2} of 15 mm Hg, and P_{O_2} of 120 mm Hg.

Determining the Acid-Base Abnormality

By definition, the low P_{CO_2} is indicative of a respiratory alkalosis, which can be either primary or in response to a metabolic acidosis. In an acute respiratory alkalosis, the relationship between the fall in P_{CO_2} and the rise in pH is demonstrated[114] in Equation 24–1:

For every fall of 10 mm Hg in the P_{CO_2}, there should be a rise of 0.08 in the pH:

$$\Delta pH = [-0.008]\Delta P_{CO_2} \qquad \text{(Eq. 24–1)}$$

Thus for this patient, the fall in the P_{CO_2} of 25 mm Hg (from 40 mm Hg to 15 mm Hg) would be expected to produce a rise of 0.20 in the pH. Because the pH is lower than the predicted value of 7.60, a metabolic acidosis is present. If only one primary process affecting acid-base balance is present (meaning the other is compensatory), the primary process can be identified by the pH. Specifically, it is generally assumed that overcompensation from either a renal or a pulmonary perspective cannot occur.[109,114] That is, if the primary process is a metabolic acidosis, a respiratory alkalosis tends to raise the pH toward normal, but never to greater than 7.40. If the primary process is a respiratory alkalosis, a compensatory metabolic acidosis tends to lower the pH toward normal, but never to less than 7.40. The same is true for primary metabolic alkalosis and primary respiratory acidosis. Further assessment requires an evaluation of the serum electrolytes.

The laboratory studies of patient 1 returned as follows: sodium (Na^+), 133 mEq/L; potassium (K^+), 3.6 mEq/L; chloride (Cl^-), 99 mEq/L; bicarbonate (HCO_3^-), 12 mEq/L; BUN, 12 mg/dL; creatinine (Cr), 0.9 mg/dL; and glucose (Glu), 120 mg/dL.

The next step in the analysis involves a calculation of the anion gap.

Calculating the Anion Gap

The law of electroneutrality states that the net positive and negative charges of the serum must be equal. Although the concept of the anion gap is said to have arisen from the "Gamblegram" originally described in 1939,[51] its use was not popularized until the determination of serum electrolytes became routinely available. Simply put, because all of the negative charges present in the serum must equal all of the positive charges present in the serum, then the sum of the positive charges minus the sum of the negative charges must equal zero.

The problem that immediately arises is that all charged species are not routinely measured. Normally present but unmeasured cations consist of calcium and magnesium, whereas normally present but unmeasured anions consist of phosphate, sulfate, albumin, and organic acids.[41,49,116] Sodium and potassium normally account for 95% of extracellular cations, whereas chloride and bicarbonate account for 85% of extracellular anions.[41] Thus, because more cations than anions are measured, subtracting the anions from the cations normally yields a positive number, known as the anion gap. The anion gap is therefore derived as shown in Equation 24–2:

$$Na^+ + K^+ + \text{unmeasured cations } (U_c) = Cl^- + HCO_3^-$$
$$+\text{unmeasured anions } (U_a)$$
$$\text{Anion gap} = U_a - U_c$$

or

$$\text{Anion gap} = (Na^+ + K^+) - (Cl^- + HCO_3^-)$$
$$\text{(Eq. 24–2)}$$

Because K^+ is largely an intracellular cation and rarely alters the anion gap, it is often deleted from the equation for simplicity. Most authors[41,49,116] prefer this approach, yielding Equation 24–3:

$$\text{Anion gap} = (Na^+) - (Cl^- + HCO_3^-) \qquad \text{(Eq. 24–3)}$$

Using Equation 24–3, the normal anion gap was initially determined to be 12 ± 4 mEq/L.[41,164] More recent data demonstrated that as a result of a change in laboratory instrumentation and higher chloride values than previously reported, the range for a normal anion gap fell to 7 ± 4 mEq/L.[163]

A variety of pathologic conditions may result in a rise or fall of the anion gap. High anion gaps result from increased presence of unmeasured anions or decreased presence of unmeasured cations (Table 24–1).[41,49,138] Similarly, a low anion gap results from an increase in unmeasured cations or a decrease in unmeasured anions (Table 24–2).[41,49,63,148] Because hypoalbuminemia is a common cause of a decreased anion gap, it should be noted that for every fall of 1 g/dL in the albumin, the anion gap falls by 2.5 mEq/L.[47]

The popularity of the anion gap revolves around its ability to help diagnose disorders responsible for the generation of a metabolic acidosis. When a metabolic acidosis is present, as in the case described earlier, it should be further categorized as being a high- or normal-anion-gap type. A high anion gap metabolic acidosis results from the absorption or generation of an acid paired with an unmeasured anion (eg, lactic acid). Normal anion gap acidoses result from processes that produce bicarbonate loss and chloride retention (eg, diarrhea). Causes of high and normal anion gap metabolic acidoses are shown in Tables 24–3 and 24–4. The patient described above has an anion gap of 22 mEq/L [133 − (99 − 12)], and thus is said to have a high-anion-gap metabolic acidosis.

TABLE 24–1. Causes of a High Anion Gap

Increased unmeasured anions
  Metabolic acidosis (see Table 24–3)
  Dehydration
  Therapy with sodium salts of unmeasured anions
    Sodium citrate
    Sodium lactate
    Sodium acetate
  Therapy with certain antibiotics
    Carbenicillin
    Sodium penicillin
  Alkalosis

Decrease in unmeasured cations
  Simultaneous hypomagnesemia, hypocalcemia, and hypokalemia

TABLE 24–2.   Causes of a Low Anion Gap

Increase in unmeasured cations
Hypercalcemia
Hypemagnesemia
Hyperkalemia
Lithium intoxication
Multiple myeloma

Decrease in unmeasured anions
Hypoalbuminemia
Dilution

Overestimation of the chloride
Bromism
Iodism
Nitrate excess

Anion Gap Reliability

Several authors considered the utility of the anion gap determination.[20,50,75] When 57 hospitalized patients were studied to determine the cause of elevated anion gaps, in those patients whose anion gap was greater than 30 mEq/L the cause was always lactic acidosis or ketoacidosis.[50] In patients with smaller elevations of the anion gap, the ability to define the cause of the elevation diminished; in only 14% of patients with anion gaps of 17–19 mEq/L could the etiology be defined. Another study determined that although the anion gap is often used as a screening test for hyperlactacidemia (as a sign of poor perfusion), only those patients with the highest serum lactate concentrations had elevated anion gaps.[75] Finally, in a sample of 571 patients, those with higher anion gaps tended to have an increased severity of illness, resulting in a higher admission rate, a greater percentage of whom both required admission to intensive care units, and had a higher mortality.[20] Thus, although the absence of an anion gap does not exclude significant illness, when the anion gap is very elevated it usually can be attributed to a specific etiology and associated with consequential illness.

TABLE 24–3.   Causes of a High Anion Gap Metabolic Acidosis

Carbon monoxide
Cyanide
Ethylene glycol
Hydrogen sulfide
Isoniazid
Iron
Ketoacidoses (diabetic, alcoholic, and starvation)
Lactate
Metformin
Methanol
Paraldehyde
Phenformin
Salicylates
Sulfur (inorganic)
Theophylline
Toluene
Uremia

Note: Many clinicians rely on the mnemonic **MUDPILES** to help remember this differential diagnosis where M represents Methanol, U (Uremia), D (Diabetic Ketoacidosis), P (Paraldehyde), I (Iron), L (Lactic Acidosis), E (Ethylene Glycol), and S (Salicylates).

TABLE 24–4.   Causes of a Normal Anion Gap Metabolic Acidosis

Drugs
Acetazolamide
Acidifying agents
Ammonium chloride
Arginine hydrochloride
Hydrochloric acid
Lysine hydrochloride
Cholestyramine
Sulfamylon

Gastrointestinal bicarbonate loss
Diarrhea
Pancreatic fistula

Miscellaneous
Hyperalimentation
Posthypocapnia
Rapid IV hydration with 0.9% NaCl
Renal tubular acidosis
Ureteroenterostomy

Narrowing the Differential Diagnosis of a High Anion Gap Metabolic Acidosis

The ability to diagnose the etiology of a high anion gap metabolic acidosis is an essential skill in clinical medicine. The following discussion provides a rapid and cost-effective approach to the problem. As always, the clinical history and physical examination may provide essential clues to the diagnosis. For example, iron poisoning is virtually always associated with significant GI symptoms. The absence of which essentially excludes the diagnosis of this poisoning (Chap. 36). Furthermore, when iron overdose is suspected, an abdominal radiograph may show the presence of tablets. The acidosis associated with isoniazid (INH) toxicity results from seizures, the absence of which excludes INH as the cause of a metabolic acidosis (Chap. 43). Methanol toxicity may be associated with visual complaints or an abnormal funduscopic examination (Chap. 66). Paraldehyde has a characteristic odor (Chap. 28). When these findings are absent, the laboratory analysis must be relied on.

1. Begin with the electrolytes: An elevated BUN and creatinine are essential to diagnose uremia. Similarly, hyperglycemia should raise the possibility of diabetic ketoacidosis. The absence of an elevated glucose does not, however, exclude the possibility of euglycemic diabetic ketoacidosis,[77] or alcoholic or starvation ketoacidosis, which are often associated with normal or even low serum glucose concentrations. If complete electrolytes are not immediately available, a rapid glucose reagent test should be performed to help confirm or exclude the possibility of hyperglycemia.

2. Proceed to the urinalysis: Do not wait for the laboratory results, as all of these studies are easily accomplished. In addition, if there is a suspicion of high-anion-gap metabolic acidosis, and only the arterial blood gas analysis is completed, the evaluation may begin here, while the electrolyte determination is pending. A urine dipstick for glucose and ketones helps with the diagnosis of diabetic ketoacidosis and other ketoaci-

doses. The absence of urinary ketones does not exclude a diagnosis of alcoholic ketoacidosis (Chap. 64) and ketones are often present in severe salicylism (Chap. 33) or biguanide-associated metabolic acidosis (Chap 40). The urine of a patient who has ingested fluorescein-containing antifreeze (ethylene glycol) may fluoresce when exposed to a Wood's lamp. Also, because ethylene glycol is metabolized to oxalate, calcium oxalate crystals may be present in the urine of a poisoned patient. Both fluorescent and calcium oxalate-containing urine are useful findings if present, but their absence does not exclude ethylene glycol poisoning (Chap. 66). Finally, a urine ferric chloride test should be performed. This test is unfortunately neither 100% sensitive nor specific for the diagnosis of salicylism (Chap. 33). When the ferric chloride test is positive, a serum salicylate level must be obtained. Unfortunately a negative ferric chloride test may not definitively exclude salicylism in the correct clinical setting.

3. An arterial or central venous blood lactate level can be helpful. In theory, if the lactate (measured in mmol/L or mEq/L) can entirely account for the fall in serum bicarbonate, then the cause of the anion gap can be attributed to lactic acidosis.

When the above analysis is not productive, the diagnosis is usually toxic alcohol ingestion, starvation, alcoholic ketoacidosis (with minimal urine ketones), or a multifactorial process involving small amounts of lactate and other anions. One approach is to provide the patient with 1–2 hours of intravenous hydration, dextrose, and thiamine. If the acidosis resolves, the etiology is either keto- or lactic acidosis. Alternatively, a more detailed search for the toxic alcohols, involving either the osmol gap or specific levels, should be initiated (discussed later).

In patient 1, urinalysis revealed trace amounts of protein, small ketones, and large glucose (after dextrose administration). There were no crystals or fluorescence, but a ferric chloride test was positive. A lactate level was not obtained.

Further Refinement of the Differential Diagnosis

The most striking laboratory abnormality in this patient is the HCO_3^- of 12 mEq/L. This value not only confirms the presence of a significant metabolic acidosis, but also allows for a better definition of the nature of the disturbance.

Winters' equation[5] enables a prediction of the degree of the respiratory compensation (fall of the P_{CO_2}) in acute metabolic acidosis if the serum bicarbonate is known, as Equation 24–4 illustrates:

$$P_{CO_2} = [1.5 \times HCO_3^-] + 8 \pm 2 \qquad \text{(Eq. 24–4)}$$

Thus, because this patient has a HCO_3^- of 12 mEq/L, it can be predicted that the P_{CO_2} should be determined as shown in Equation 24–5:

$$(1.5 \times 12) + 8 \pm 2$$

or

$$26 \pm 2 \text{ mm Hg} \qquad \text{(Eq. 24–5)}$$

Because the P_{CO_2} of patient 1 was substantially lower than would have been predicted by Winters' equation, it can be concluded that both a primary metabolic acidosis and a primary respiratory alkalosis were present. As shown by Narins and Emmett, it

is empirically true that in a pure compensated metabolic acidosis, the P_{CO_2} is usually the same as the last two digits of the pH.[114] For example, a pH of 7.26 would correlate with a P_{CO_2} of 26 mm Hg. In this case the P_{CO_2} of 15 mm Hg is much lower than would be predicted from the last two digits of the pH (7.30 or 30), suggesting a second primary process.

The single disorder in the differential diagnosis of a high-anion-gap metabolic acidosis that is commonly associated with the presence of primary metabolic acidosis and primary respiratory alkalosis is salicylism (Chap. 33). Thus with the positive ferric chloride test, the presence of urinary ketones, and the acid-base abnormalities noted, salicylate toxicity is essentially confirmed.

The patient's serum salicylate level was later reported as 97 mg/dL, and he underwent hemodialysis with complete recovery.

The Osmol Gap

The osmol gap is defined as the difference between the measured osmolality and the calculated osmolarity.[148] Osmolarity is a measure of the total number of particles in 1 L of solution. Osmolality differs from osmolarity only in that the number of particles is expressed per kilogram of solution. Thus osmolarity and osmolality represent molar and molal concentrations of solutes, respectively.[56] Also, in clinical medicine, osmolarity is usually calculated, whereas osmolality is usually measured.

Calculating osmolarity requires a summing of the known particles in solution. Because molarity and milliequivalents are particle-based measurements, unlike weight or concentration, the known constituents of serum have to be converted to molar values. Assumptions are required based on the extent of dissociation of polar compounds (such as sodium chloride), the water content of serum, and present but rarely included species (calcium, magnesium). The nature and limitations of these assumptions is beyond the scope of this chapter. The reader is referred to several reviews for more details.[59,69,118] Many equations have been used and evaluated for calculating osmolarity. One investigation that used 13 different methods to evaluate sera from 715 hospital patients[36] concluded that the most accurate calculation could be determined by using Equation 24–6:

$$1.86(Na^+ \text{ in mEq} / L) + (\text{glucose in mg/dL}) / 18$$
$$+ (\text{BUN in mg/dL}) / 2.8 \qquad \text{(Eq. 24–6)}$$

Obvious sources of potential error in this calculation include laboratory error in determining any of the measured parameters and the failure to account for a number of osmotically active particles.

The measurement of serum osmolality has the potential for error as well, which stems from the use of different laboratory techniques. A 1989 survey of clinical laboratory methodology demonstrated that while more than 80% of facilities studied offered osmometry, 11% used the vapor pressure method exclusively (as opposed to the freezing point method).[40] Furthermore, half of the laboratory supervisors questioned failed to recognize that the vapor pressure technique was likely to produce an erroneously low serum osmolality for serum containing methanol, ethanol, or isopropanol.[40] This error results from the fact that these alcohols will boil out of solution before the boiling point of water is reached.

The mathematic and theoretical errors in determining osmolarity and osmolality are potentially additive when the two values are mathematically combined to determine the osmol gap. In addition, a conceptual error is also present. In methanol poisoning the uncharged particle has osmotic activity that is not calculated, but does not produce an anion gap until it is metabolized to formate. Although the metabolite also has osmotic activity, its activity is accounted for by sodium in the osmolarity calculation, because it is largely dissociated, existing as sodium formate. Thus, at least in theory, an early ingestion is marked by an elevated osmol gap and a normal anion gap, whereas later, the anion gap increases and the osmol gap decreases. This effect is highlighted by several case reports.[7,30,151] Despite these limitations, a determination of the osmol gap is commonly proposed as a diagnostic adjunct when considering ingestions of toxic alcohols. To qualify as a good screening test, the osmol gap should predict toxic alcohol ingestion with a low frequency of false-negative results (have a high sensitivity). To exclude a diagnosis of toxic alcohol ingestion, the determination of an osmol gap should have a low frequency of false-positive results (high specificity). As a first step, the range of normal values (and its variability) must be known. Using the formula for osmolarity shown above, the previously mentioned study determined that the "normal" osmol gap was 10 ± 6 mOsm.[36] However, when more than 300 adult samples were studied, the more commonly used equation (Equation 24–7):

$$2(Na^+ \text{ in mEq}/L) + (\text{glucose in mg}/dL)/18$$
$$+ (\text{BUN in mg}/dL)/2.8 \qquad \text{(Eq. 24–7)}$$

yielded normal values of -2 ± 6 mOsm and ranged from -5 to $+15$ mOsm with other commonly used equations.[69] Almost identical results are reported in children.[104] While the concept of a negative osmol gap might be disconcerting, the numerous approximations used to calculate osmolarity may not be valid. Also, although ethanol is the most common cause of elevated osmolality in varied groups of patients,[21,25,119,129] a serum ethanol measurement was not included for any of the patients used in the reference that serves as the standard to define osmol gaps.[36] The relatively recent inclusion of ethanol in the osmolarity formula in a systematic evaluation of normal values predictably increased the calculated osmolarity in patients in whom ethanol was present, making the osmol gap smaller than previously suggested, or even negative.[69] Furthermore, recent work has shown a slight rise in measured sodium.[163] If this is related to changes in laboratory determination, it will also lead to a lowering of the osmol gap. In fact, other investigations have concluded that the mean osmol gap in control (presumably ethanol-free) populations was a negative value.[59,76,137] Thus, the commonly used "normal" value of less than 10 mOsm, often attributed to two earlier works,[56,148] is clearly "arbitrary" and erroneous in the authors' own words and should be abandoned.

The largest limitation of the osmol gap calculation comes from the documented large standard deviation around a small "normal" number.[36,69,76,137] This variability may result from true population variability, in which case, the standard deviation is never reduced. Alternatively, an error of 1 mEq/L in the determination of the serum sodium may result in an error of 2 mOsm in the calculation of the osmol gap. As a result of this variability, the molecular weight of the toxins in question (ethylene glycol level of 50 mg/dL contributes only 7.8 mOsm/L), and the predicted fall in osmol gap as metabolism occurs, small or even negative osmol gaps never exclude toxic alcohol ingestion.[58,69] This overall concept is illustrated by the case of a patient with an osmol gap of 7.2 mOsm who

ultimately required hemodialysis for severe ethylene glycol poisoning.[151] Furthermore, although large osmol gaps may be suggestive of toxic alcohol ingestions, common conditions such as alcoholic ketoacidosis, lactic acidosis, renal failure, and shock are all associated with elevated osmol gaps.[76,137,145] Because lactate, acetoacetate, and β-hydroxybutyrate should not account for any increase in the osmol gap because they are charged, these conditions are probably associated with the accumulation of small uncharged molecules in the serum. Thus, because both the negative and positive predictive values of this test are inadequate, its utility as a screening tool must be questioned. However, in the presence of very high osmolar gaps (>50–70 mOsm), the diagnosis of toxic alcohol ingestion is usually confirmed (Chap. 66).

Differentiating a Normal Anion Gap Metabolic Acidosis

Although the differential diagnosis for a normal anion gap metabolic acidosis is extensive (Table 24–4), most cases result from either urinary or GI bicarbonate losses: renal tubular acidosis (RTA) or diarrhea, respectively. When the history and physical examination are unable to narrow the differential diagnosis, the use of a urinary anion gap has been suggested.[13]

The urinary anion gap (as shown in Equation 24–8):

$$(Na^+ + K^+) - (Cl^-) \qquad \text{(Eq. 24–8)}$$

correlates with ammonium (NH_4^+) excretion.[62] As ammonium elimination increases, the urinary anion gap narrows, because ammonium serves as an unmeasured cation and is accompanied by chloride. The normal anion gap metabolic acidosis that is associated with diarrhea results from GI bicarbonate loss. During this process the kidney's ability to eliminate ammonium is undisturbed and in fact increases as a normal response to the acidosis. Thus with GI bicarbonate losses the urinary anion gap should be low. Alternatively, the patient with RTA has lost the ability either to resorb bicarbonate or to increase ammonium excretion in response to an acidosis, and the urinary anion gap should be elevated. When the urinary anion gap was calculated in patients with diarrhea or RTA, it was found that those patients with diarrhea had a mean negative gap (-20 ± 5.7 mEq/L), as compared to a positive gap (23 ± 4.1 mEq/L) in those with RTA.[62] Therefore, when evaluating the patient with a normal-gap metabolic acidosis, the determination of a urinary anion gap should help to determine the source of the disorder.

METABOLIC ALKALOSIS

Patient 2 A 2-week-old boy was brought to the ED by his parents because of a 36-hour history of fever, diarrhea, and lethargy. The child was born at 39 weeks gestation via normal spontaneous vaginal delivery and had Apgar scores of 9 and 10. The baby and the mother were discharged from the hospital at the usual time, and the baby remained well until 36 hours prior to presentation in the ED. Physical examination was remarkable for an irritable child who was inconsolable, even by his parents. Vital signs were blood pressure, 60/40 mm Hg; irregular pulse, 160 beats/min; respiratory rate, 28 breaths/min; rectal temperature, 38.3°C (100.9°F). His skin was dry and without a rash. His anterior fontanel was depressed, and his capillary refill was delayed. The remainder of the physical assessment was unremarkable.

The child was placed on a cardiac monitor that showed frequent premature ventricular contractions (confirmed by 12-lead ECG). An intravenous catheter was inserted, and blood was drawn for culture, electrolytes, glucose, and CBC. An arterial blood gas sample was obtained on room air and supplemental oxygen was administered. The child was given dextrose (1 g/kg) and a 20-mL/kg bolus of 0.9% saline IV. A lumbar puncture was performed and the child was started on broad-spectrum antibiotics.

The laboratory studies returned. Arterial blood-gas values were pH, 7.76; P_{CO_2}, 40 mm Hg; P_{O_2}, 96 mm Hg. Electrolytes were Na^+, 154 mEq/L; K^+, 3.1 mEq/L; Cl^-, 86 mEq/L; HCO_3^-, 43 mEq/L; BUN, Cr, and glucose, were normal. The lumbar puncture revealed a normal cell count and chemistry, with a negative Gram's stain.

Adverse Effects of Metabolic Alkalosis

Life-threatening metabolic alkalosis is rare but can result in tetany (from decreased ionized calcium),[94] weakness (from decreased potassium),[105] altered mental status leading to coma,[89] seizures,[60] and cardiac dysrhythmias.[83] In addition, metabolic alkalosis shifts the oxyhemoglobin dissociation curve to the left, impairing tissue oxygenation (Chap. 20). The expected compensation for a metabolic alkalosis is a respiratory acidosis, which is produced by hypoventilation and increased P_{CO_2}. Standard discussions of metabolic alkalosis suggest that the respiratory compensation is irregular and inadequate at best, invoking a teleologic argument to suggest that hypoventilation and hypoxia are more undesirable than metabolic alkalosis.[114] However, several authors have demonstrated that cases of severe hypoventilation and respiratory failure can occur in response to metabolic alkalosis, suggesting a real, although uncommon risk.[105,121]

Approach to the Patient with Metabolic Alkalosis

Metabolic alkalosis results from GI or urinary loss of acids, administration of exogenous bases, or renal bicarbonate retention (impaired bicarbonate loss). Causes of metabolic alkalosis are listed in Table 24–5. By comparison, metabolic alkalosis is less common and less toxicologically consequential than high anion gap metabolic acidosis.

The etiologies of metabolic alkalosis can be characterized therapeutically as chloride-responsive or chloride-resistant. Chloride-responsive etiologies (diuretics, vomiting and nasogastric suction, chloride diarrhea, etc) are usually associated with a low urinary chloride excretion (<10 mEq/L).[66,83] These disorders respond rapidly to infusion of sodium chloride when concomitant therapy addresses the underlying problem. Chloride-resistant disorders (hyperaldosteronism, severe potassium depletion, etc) are characterized by urinary chlorides greater than 10 mEq/L and tend to be resistant to sodium chloride therapy.[53,66] These disorders often require potassium repletion or agents that reduce mineralocorticoid effects (spironolactone) before correction can occur.[53] When volume loading (sodium chloride repletion) is ineffective, or emergent correction of the alkalosis is required, some authors have suggested infusions of lysine or arginine hydrochloride, or dilute hydrochloric acid.[105]

Further history revealed that patient 2 was being fed oral baking soda several times per day as part of a folk remedy. Urinary chloride was 6 mEq/L. He was treated with intravenous normal

TABLE 24–5. Causes of Metabolic Alkalosis

Gastrointestinal acid loss
Chloride diarrhea (congenital)
Nasogastric suction (protracted)
Vomiting (protracted)

Urinary acid loss
Common
  Diuretics
Rare
  Adrenogenital syndrome
  Bartter syndrome
  Cushing syndrome
  Hyperaldosteronism (primary)
  Hypercalcemia
  Licorice (glycyrrhizic acid)
  Little syndrome
  Magnesium deficiency

Base administration
Acetate (dialysis or hyperalimentation)
Bicarbonate
Carbonate (antacids)
Citrate (posttransfusion)
Milk alkali syndrome

Renal bicarbonate retention
Hypercapnia (chronic)
Hypochloremia
Hypokalemia
Volume contraction

saline with a subsequent resolution of clinical and laboratory abnormalities. The parents were educated about the risks of prescription and nonprescription medications and alternative therapies.

THE DELTA (Δ) GAP

Many patients have mixed acid-base disorders such as a simultaneous metabolic acidosis and metabolic alkalosis. Depending on their relative effects, the patient may have significant acidemia or alkalemia, minor alterations in pH, or even a "normal" pH.

A typical example might be the patient with diabetic ketoacidosis (DKA) and vomiting. Although DKA would be expected to produce a classic high anion gap metabolic acidosis, the vomiting could raise the serum bicarbonate producing a normal value. The toxicologic clinical correlate of the patient with a mixed acid-base disorder might be the iron-poisoned patient with refractory vomiting and a multifactorial high-anion-gap metabolic acidosis (Chap. 36). Another example might be the patient with alcoholic ketoacidosis and vomiting. In both cases, it is conceivable that the patient with two clinically obvious disorders could have a pH of 7.40, a P_{CO_2} of 40 mm Hg, and a serum bicarbonate level of 24 mEq/L. In most circumstances, one process predominates, and its significance is minimized if the second process goes undiagnosed.

In the patient with a simple anion gap metabolic acidosis, each decrease of 1 mEq/L in the serum bicarbonate should be associated with a rise of 1 mEq/L in the anion gap.[114] This occurs because the unmeasured anion is paired with the acid that is titrating the bicarbonate. Any deviation from this direct relationship may be an indication of a mixed acid-base disorder.[64,114,120] Thus, the ratio of the change in the anion gap (ΔAG) to the change in the serum bicarbonate (Equation 24–9) evolved:

$$\text{Anion gap ratio} = \Delta AG / \Delta HCO_3^- \qquad \text{(Eq. 24–9)}$$

A ratio close to 1 would suggest a pure high anion gap metabolic acidosis. When the ratio is greater than 1, there is a relative increase in bicarbonate (suggesting a mixed disorder) that can result only from a concomitant metabolic alkalosis or a respiratory acidosis. Alternatively, when the ratio is less than 1, the added presence of either hyperchloremic (normal anion gap) metabolic acidosis or compensated (chronic) respiratory alkalosis is suggested. One author[165] suggested the use of the gap in the anion gap, as shown in Equation 24–10:

$$\text{Gap of the gap} = \Delta AG - \Delta HCO_3^- \qquad \text{(Eq. 24–10)}$$

where a gap in the gap greater than 6 mEq/L would suggest metabolic alkalosis and a gap in the gap less than 6 mEq/L would suggest hyperchloremic acidosis.

Several authors have evaluated the utility of the relationship between the change in the anion gap and the change in the serum bicarbonate.[34,117,120,133] Although supported strongly by some authors,[117,120] others suggest that it is often flawed and frequently misleading.[34,133] The next section summarizes the discussion.

For the fall in bicarbonate to be either proportionally or linearly related to the rise in the anion gap the following criteria should be met:

1. All of the acid formed should be titrated by bicarbonate. In fact, there are many nonbicarbonate buffer systems, and the duration of acidosis alters the relative contributions of these systems.[139]
2. The volumes of distribution of the proton, its associated anion, and bicarbonate should be the same. This is not always true. For example, in the case of lactic acidosis, lactate ions remain extracellular while some of the lactic acid is buffered intracellularly, such that the increase in the anion gap (from lactate) is less than the decrease in bicarbonate.[132]
3. Elimination of the anion and regeneration of bicarbonate should be equal. For example, in the patient with a ketoacidosis, acetoacetate, β-hydroxybutyrate and acetone are often cleared quickly when renal function is normal and poorly when renal function is impaired.[2]
4. Acidosis and alkalosis should not alter the anion gap themselves. As pH changes, the charges on serum proteins change, such that acidemia tends to decrease the anion gap and alkalemia tends to increase the gap.[1] This change is related to the generation of lactate and a change in the charges on albumin (an unmeasured anion).
5. There must be no concurrent process other than the metabolic acidosis in question that is affecting the anion gap.

For these reasons, we support the statements of one author,[34] who appears to be correct in concluding that "the exact relationship between the $-\Delta AG$ and $-\Delta HCO_3$ in a high anion gap acidosis is not readily predictable and deviation of the $\Delta AG/\Delta HCO_3^-$ ratio from unity does not necessarily imply the diagnosis of a second acid-base disorder." However, very large deviations from a value of 1 probably suggest the presence of a second disorder.

DRUGS AND TOXIN-INDUCED ALTERATIONS OF FLUID BALANCE

Significant fluid abnormalities occur commonly in the setting of toxin exposure. Gastrointestinal losses in the form of vomiting, diarrhea, GI hemorrhage, and third spacing (from GI burns) result from a variety of toxic exposures and their management (emetics and cathartics). Renal losses result from the ability of many toxins to increase glomerular filtration rate (inotropes), impair resorption (diuretics), or enhance urine volume in response to an obligate solute load (salicylates). Finally, insensible losses occur through increased sweating (sympathomimetics, cholinergics, and uncouplers of oxidative phosphorylation) and pulmonary losses as a result of increased minute ventilation (salicylates and sympathomimetics) or bronchorrhea (cholinergics). This section focuses on two specific entities: the syndrome of inappropriate secretion of antidiuretic hormone (SIADH) and diabetes insipidus (DI). Other specific fluid issues are discussed in Chaps. 22 and 23 and in chapters relating to individual toxins.

Diabetes Insipidus

Plasma osmolality is maintained through a complex interaction between the hypothalamus, pituitary gland, and kidney. Extensive discussions of these mechanisms[12,111,112,159] are summarized below. Osmolality is sensed by a group of neurons (known as osmoreceptors) located in the anterior hypothalamus. Changes in osmolality are mediated through changes in thirst and urinary concentration of solutes; the latter is controlled by the hormone arginine vasopressin (antidiuretic hormone; ADH). ADH is synthesized in the hypothalamus and released by the posterior pituitary gland in response to stimulation from the osmoreceptors. As plasma osmolality rises, ADH is released, reaching its maximum at a serum osmolality of about 295 mOsm/kg. Antidiuretic hormone is transported to the kidney via the bloodstream, where it increases the synthesis of cyclic adenosine monophosphate (cAMP). This increase in cAMP increases the permeability of the distal convoluted tubule and collecting duct (by opening aquaporin channels) such that water is reabsorbed and urine becomes more concentrated (urine osmolality may be as high as 800 mOsm/kg). Alternatively, as plasma osmolality falls, ADH release is diminished. This results in a decrease in renal cAMP generation, with the distal convoluted tubule and collecting duct becoming less permeable to water, and a net production of dilute urine.

Diabetes insipidus (hypotonic polyuria) may be termed neurogenic (resulting from failure to sense a rising osmolality, or from a failure to release ADH) or nephrogenic (resulting from failure of the kidney to respond appropriately to ADH). Although there are many nontoxicologic causes for DI (eg, trauma, tumor, sarcoid, idiopathic, vascular, and congenital), toxins have the ability to interfere with ADH effects through both central and peripheral mechanisms. Ethanol, opioid antagonists, and α-adrenergic agonists all suppress ADH release.[7,111] Lithium,[24,96,144] demeclocycline,[143] methoxyflurane,[99] propoxyphene,[15] foscarnet,[115] mesalazine,[97] streptozotocin,[28] amphotericin,[71] glufosinate,[154] lobenzarit,[132] rifampin,[125] and colchicine[159] are all associated with nephrogenic DI (see Table 24–6).

Of these agents, lithium has been the most extensively evaluated. Although polyuria is a common finding with lithium therapy (occurring in 20–70% of patients on maintenance therapy),[12] the exact incidence of DI is unclear. Estimates range from 10–20%[96] to as high as 80%.[24]

Signs, Symptoms, and Diagnosis Patients with DI complain of polyuria and polydipsia. Urine volumes typically exceed 30 mL/kg/d[159] and may be as high as 9 L/d with nephrogenic DI[96] and 12–14 L/d with neurogenic (central) DI.[113] Nocturia, fatigue, and decreased work performance are noted.[159] Neurogenic DI resulting from hypothalamic or pituitary damage is typically associated with other signs of neuroendocrine dysfunction.[113]

Urine specific gravity is low (<1.010) and serum sodium is usually elevated. Nephrogenic DI may be associated with hypokalemia and hypercalcemia.[159] Further diagnostic evaluation should begin with simultaneous determination of the urine and serum osmolality. The diagnosis of diabetes insipidus is established by the occurrence of dilute urine (urine osmolality ≤300 mOsm/kg) in the presence of concentrated electrolytes (plasma osmolality ≥295 mOsm/kg).[159] Following this determination, a trial of desmopressin (DDAVP), an arginine vasopressin analog, helps to differentiate between neurogenic and nephrogenic DI. If the etiology of the DI is neurogenic, the patient promptly responds to DDAVP and urine osmolality increases.[159]

Treatment The initial approach to the patient with DI involves the repletion of intravascular volume and the restoration of electrolyte balance. If a reversible cause for the DI can be established, it should be corrected. Patients with neurogenic DI should be maintained on either vasopressin or DDAVP. The latter is usually preferred because of the lack of vasopressor effects. In the past, patients were occasionally treated with oral agents known to produce SIADH (see below). Patients with nephrogenic DI can be treated with thiazide diuretics,[37] prostaglandin inhibitors,[33,71,91] or amiloride.[14]

SIADH

In a sense, the SIADH may be thought of as the opposite of DI. In SIADH hyponatremia and plasma hypotonicity result from continued production or release of ADH in the setting of low plasma osmolality.[12] Early reviews claimed that SIADH was a disorder of volume overload, based largely on evidence of weight gain.[111] The consistent absence of edema, however, and the fact that the decrease in sodium cannot be accounted for by the fluid gain (weight gain) suggest that fluid retention is only a minor part of the mechanism.[86]

The clinical presentation of SIADH is that of hyponatremia.[12,113] Symptoms are related to both the absolute fall in serum sodium concentration and its rate of decline. Irritability, lethargy, weakness, and muscle cramps may be noted.[113] In more severe cases, coma and seizures develop.[12,113]

There are many nontoxicologic etiologies of SIADH, most of which involve pulmonary or intracranial processes. Common causes include infections, malignancies, and surgery.[12,86,111,113] Table 24–6 summarizes drugs and toxins known to produce SIADH. The oral hypoglycemics, including agents from both the sulfonylurea (eg, chlorpropamide) and biguanide (eg, metformin) classes produce hyponatremia more commonly than the other agents.[112] Their actions are multifactorial and can include both the potentiation of endogenous ADH and the stimulation of ADH release.[112] Many psychiatric medications including the selective serotonin reuptake inhibitors, cyclic antidepressants, antipsychotics, and others are implicated in causing SIADH.[24,26,84,93,150,157] Evidence suggests that complex interactions between the dopaminergic and noradrenergic systems control ADH release.[150] Additional evidence supports a role of serotonin in drug induced SIADH. Serotonin (specifically 5-HT$_2$ and/or 5-HT$_{1C}$) stimulates ADH release[8,79] and stimulates water intake.[74] An important role of serotonin is supported by the occurrence of SIADH with hallucinogenic amphetamine (MDMA) use.[73,162]

Diagnosis and Treatment The diagnosis of SIADH is based on establishing the presence of hyponatremia, low plasma osmolality, and impaired urinary dilution. More simply stated, SIADH is present when urine osmolality is high in the setting of low plasma osmolality. In addition, evidence of edema, hypotension, hypovolemia, and adrenal or thyroid deficiency must be lacking.[86] Other atypical causes of hyponatremia such as psychogenic polydipsia need to be excluded.[128,134] Uric acid also falls and is a good marker of SIADH in cases in which the diagnosis is unclear.[31,149]

Treatment begins with fluid restriction.[12] Because the goal of this therapy is to establish a negative fluid balance, careful attention to intake and output is required. If an offending agent can be identified, it should be eliminated. Although most cases resolve in 1–2 weeks,[12,86,113] the syndrome occasionally persists. If this occurs, therapy with demeclocycline or lithium may be helpful, because severe fluid restriction is often intolerable. One author[48] suggested that demeclocycline was more efficacious than lithium when the two agents were compared in a small series of patients with SIADH. When hyponatremia is associated with life-threatening clinical presentations, most authorities recommend the careful infusion of hypertonic (3%) saline.[4,12,86] Formulas are available to

TABLE 24–6. Causes of SIADH and Diabetes Insipidus (DI)

SIADH	DI
Amiloride	Amphotericin
Amitriptyline	Colchicine
Biguanides	Demeclocycline
Carbamazepine (oxcarbamazepine)	Ethanol
Cisplatin	Foscarnet
Clofibrate	Glufosinate
Cyclophosphamide	Lithium
Desmopressin	Lobenzarit disodium
Diazoxide	Methoxyflurane
Imipramine	Mesalazine
Indapamide	Minocycline
Indomethacin	Propoxyphene
MDMA	Rifampin
Nicotine	Streptozotocin
Oxytocin	
Selective serotonin reuptake inhibitors	
Sulfonylureas	
Thioridazine	
Tranylcypromine	
Vasopressin	
Vincristine (vinblastine)	

help calculate the tonicity and rate of desired replacement fluids (Equation 24–11).[3,4]

When one liter of fluid is infused:

$$\text{The change in the serum Na}^+ = \frac{\text{infusate Na}^+ - \text{serum Na}^+}{\text{total body water} + 1 \text{ liter}}$$

Where infusate Na$^+$ concentrations in mEq/L equal:

3% sodium chloride	513
0.9% sodium chloride	154
Lactated Ringer solution	130
0.45% sodium chloride	77
0.33% sodium chloride	51

(Eq. 24–11)

DRUG- AND TOXIN-INDUCED ELECTROLYTE ABNORMALITIES

Sodium

Sodium concentration in the extracellular space is intrinsically related to extracellular fluid balance. Because serum sodium concentration is greater than that of any other electrolyte, it serves as the major osmotic agent. Thus, the osmoreceptors used to maintain fluid balance are, in a practical sense, sodium receptors. As the free-water deficit increases, the serum sodium rises. This results in an increase in serum osmolality, which releases antidiuretic hormone in an attempt to restore fluid balance by minimizing urinary water losses. Sodium balance is maintained by complex interactions between dietary intake, obligate losses in urine and stool, natriuretic factors, overall fluid balance, and effects of hormones such as antidiuretic hormone and adrenal mineralocorticoids.[19] Any perturbation in these normal regulatory pathways can potentially result in the development of hypo- or hypernatremia (depressed or elevated serum sodium concentration).

Hyponatremia results from sodium loss, fluid retention in excess of sodium retention, or both mechanisms. Because ADH controls the relative relationship between the amount of fluid and sodium in the urine, all drugs and toxins associated with SIADH produce hyponatremia. In addition to these agents, drugs such as the thiazide diuretics reduce the serum sodium through ADH effects. Although patients with diuretic-induced hyponatremia have elevated levels of ADH, the presence of a metabolic alkalosis and hypokalemia distinguishes them from patients with SIADH.[46] A complex mechanism for this effect is proposed, including interference with maximal urinary dilution and free water retention in response to decreased extracellular fluid volume.[46] Lithium also produces a renal sodium-wasting syndrome that seems to be unrelated to ADH effects.[106]

Other, non-ADH systems can contribute to hyponatremia. Ingestion of licorice, which contains glycyrrhizic acid, produces a syndrome of hyponatremia, hypokalemia, and hypertension resembling mineralocorticoid excess. Although the exact mechanism is debated, one report suggested that a glycyrrhizic acid-induced reduction in 11-β-hydroxysteroid dehydrogenase activity could account for the findings.[39,42]

Although psychogenic polydipsia is well described,[61,128] drug- and toxin-induced free-water excess is quite uncommon. An example occurs during urologic procedures, such as transurethral prostatic resection (TURP), where large volumes of irrigation solution are required. Because of the need to cauterize wounds electrically, these fluids cannot contain conductive electrolytes, such as sodium. Although sorbitol, dextrose, and mannitol have been used to maintain the osmolality of irrigating solutions, their optical characteristics are undesirable. Thus, it is currently common to irrigate with a glycine-containing solution. When this solution is absorbed through the prostatic venous plexus, a rapid reduction in sodium results due to a physiologic attempt to maintain a normal osmolality (the glycine solution has significant osmotic activity, but no sodium).[68,107] A similar complication is described during hysteroscopy.[122,141]

Finally, sodium loss via nonrenal or GI mechanisms is also uncommon. Hyponatremia in burn patients treated with the topical applications of silver nitrate cream results from the diffusion of sodium through permeable skin into the hypotonic dressing.[27] Table 24–7 summarizes these and other causes of hyponatremia.

The clinical manifestations of hyponatremia are dependent on both the absolute sodium concentration and its rate of decline.[10] Chronic, slow depression of sodium is usually well tolerated, while rapid decline may be associated with catastrophic events. Symptoms include lethargy, depression, apathy, and mental status changes that result from swelling of cells in the CNS. Although treatment is usually as described above, concern exists over the rapidity of the rate of correction of hyponatremia and the associated risk of irreversible CNS damage (central pontine myelinolysis).[4,11,152,]

Drug- and toxin-induced hypernatremia results from relative free water losses (DI and agents that produce significant GI and dermal fluid loss), the parenteral administration of sodium-containing drugs, and excessive oral sodium intake. Toxins that cause hypernatremia are summarized in Table 24–7.

Oral sodium chloride and oral sodium citrate have been used as emetics and antiemetics, respectively. As might be expected, both have produced severe hypernatremia.[19] One case of fatal hypernatremia resulted from gargling with a supersaturated salt solution.[108] Similarly, massive ingestion of sodium hypochlorite bleach is associated with hypernatremia.[67,131]

Agents that produce significant diarrhea, such as lactulose or cholestyramine, can cause hypernatremia through free-water loss. This is of grave concern with the use of cathartics in the management of poisonings. Multiple doses of sorbitol have been reported

TABLE 24–7. Causes of Altered Serum Sodium

Hyponatremia	Hypernatremia
Agents that cause SIADH: see Table 24–6	Agents that cause DI: see Table 24–6
Arginine	Antacids (baking soda)
Captopril and other ACE inhibitors	Cholestyramine
Diuretics	Glycerol
Glycine (transurethral prostatectomy syndrome)	Lactulose
Lithium	Mannitol
Nonsteroidal antiinflammatory drugs	Povidone-iodine
Silver nitrate	Sodium salts (bicarbonate, chloride, citrate, hypochlorite)
Water	Sorbitol
	Urea

to produce severe hypernatremic dehydration and death in both children and adults.[22,43,55] Given the limited evidence in support of routine administration of cathartics, the risk of diarrhea should contraindicate the use of multiple doses of cathartics in all but the rarest of situations. One survey demonstrated that a large percentage of EDs stocked only premixed activated charcoal preparations containing sorbitol.[160] The presence of sorbitol in this preparation creates the potential for iatrogenic cathartic poisoning from multiple-dose activated charcoal.

Water loss can also occur through the skin. Although diffuse diaphoresis resulting from cocaine or organophosphorus toxicity has the potential to produce hypernatremia, this rarely, if ever, occurs. However, application of a burn remedy containing hyperosmolar povidone-iodine to the skin of burn patients has been reported to produce significant water losses and hypernatremia.[140]

The symptoms of significant hypernatremia consist largely of altered mental status ranging from confusion to coma and neuromuscular weakness resulting in respiratory paralysis and eventually death. If hypernatremia is associated with volume depletion, cardiovascular findings consisting of tachycardia and orthostatic and eventually supine hypotension can occur. Treatment consists of replacing the relative water deficit. As in the case of hyponatremia, rapid correction of hypernatremia is potentially dangerous, resulting in cerebral edema. Although most sources suggest that 0.9% saline infusion is adequate regardless of the magnitude of the free-water deficit, recent emphasis has been placed on the use of hypotonic fluids in most cases of hypernatremia.[3]

Potassium

Drug- and toxin-induced alterations in serum potassium probably occur more commonly than do alterations in the other electrolytes, because of potassium's critical role in a variety of homeostatic processes and its large intracellular store. Potassium balance is complicated.[123,135] The total body potassium content of an average adult is about 53–55 mEq/kg, of which only 2% is located in the intravascular space. The large intracellular store of potassium is maintained by a variety of systems, the most important of which is the Na^+-K^+-ATPase pump. The relationship between total body stores and serum potassium is not linear, such that small changes in the total body potassium may result in dramatic alterations in serum concentrations.

Americans ingest 50–150 mEq/d of potassium, about 90% of which is subsequently eliminated in the urine. Although potassium undergoes free glomerular filtration, the majority is reabsorbed by the time the urine reaches the proximal tubule. The body has two major defenses against a potassium load: the ability to increase urinary elimination by decreased resorption and increased distal tubular secretion (to a maximum of 600–700 mEq/d), and the ability to transfer potassium intracellularly. In addition, GI absorption of potassium is decreased as serum potassium increases.

Hypokalemia (a decrease in serum potassium) results from decreased oral intake, GI losses secondary to repeated vomiting or diarrhea, urinary losses through increased secretion or decreased resorption, and processes that shift potassium into the intracellular compartment.[18,19,142] Table 24–8 summarizes drugs and toxins commonly associated with hypokalemia.

The neuromuscular manifestations of hypokalemia are extensively reviewed elsewhere.[85] Patients with hypokalemia are often asymptomatic when the decrease in serum potassium is mild (serum levels of 3.0–3.5 mEq/L). Occasionally, polyuria is noted,

TABLE 24–8.   Causes of Altered Serum Potassium

Hypokalemia	Hyperkalemia
Amphotericin	Amiloride
Barium (soluble salts)	Angiotensin-converting enzyme inhibitors
β-Adrenergic agonists	β-Adrenergic antagonists
Bicarbonate	Cardiac glycosides
Caffeine	Fluoride
Carbonic anhydrase inhibitors	Heparin
Cathartics	Nonsteroidal antiinflammatory drugs
Chloroquine	Penicillin (potassium)
Dextrose	Spironolactone
Hydroxychloroquine	Succinylcholine
Insulin	Triamterene
Licorice (glycyrrhizic acid)	Trimethoprim
Loop diuretics	
Oral hypoglycemics	
Osmotic diuretics	
Quinine	
Salicylates	
Sodium polystyrene sulfate	
Sympathomimetics	
Theophylline	
Thiazide diuretics	
Toluene	

as hypokalemia interferes with renal concentrating mechanisms. With more significant potassium deficits (serum levels of 2.0–3.0 mEq/L), generalized malaise and weakness become evident. As potassium levels fall (to less than 2 mEq/L), weakness becomes prominent and areflexic paralysis and respiratory failure may occur, necessitating intubation and mechanical ventilation.[85,161] Rhabdomyolysis is also likely. These neuromuscular manifestations are so prominent that prior to obtaining the serum electrolytes, these manifestations of hypokalemia may be erroneously attributed to a primary neuromuscular syndrome such as Guillain-Barré. Other findings may include GI symptoms (hypoperistalsis) or symptoms related to associated electrolyte abnormalities (depending on the etiology).

Electrocardiographic changes are common, even with mild potassium depletion, although the absence of ECG changes should never be used to exclude significant hypokalemia. Common ECG findings of hypokalemia include sagging of the ST segment, decreased T-wave amplitude, and increased U-wave amplitude (Chap. 9). These findings may herald life-threatening rhythm disturbances.[72,92]

Treatment of hypokalemia involves removing the offending agent and correcting the potassium deficit. Potassium supplementation may be given orally or intravenously or both. The debate over the maximum safe infusion rate for intravenous potassium is summarized elsewhere.[87] Based on experience with more than 1300 infusions, one group concluded that under intensive care monitoring, intravenous administrations of 20 mEq/h (by central or peripheral vein) were well tolerated. They also found that each 20 mEq of potassium administered correlated with an average increase in serum potassium of 0.25 mEq/L. Other authors have used significantly larger doses (up to 100 mEq/h) in life-threatening circumstances.[32,100]

Hyperkalemia (an increase in serum potassium) results from decreased elimination (renal insufficiency, potassium sparing diuretics, hypoaldosteronism), increased intake (either oral or IV), or redistribution from tissue stores.[19] The last mechanism is of major toxicologic importance: in overdose both the cardiac glycosides (Chap. 48) and the β-adrenergic antagonists (Chap. 49) cause hyperkalemia by allowing potassium to be released from its intracellular reservoir. Blockade of the Na^+-K^+-ATPase pump with digitalis toxicity produces hyperkalemia that may be not only diagnostic but also of prognostic importance[15] (Chap. 48). Intracellular potassium concentration is maintained in part through catecholamine-mediated uptake of potassium in liver and muscle cells.[95,130] Thus, with overdose of a β-adrenergic antagonist, some of the stores are released, producing a moderate rise of serum potassium (usually to the level of 5.0–5.5 mEq/L) (Chap. 49). Other drugs and toxins that cause hyperkalemia are listed in Table 24–8.

After oral ingestions of potassium salts, patients routinely present complaining of nausea and vomiting. Ileus, local irritation with bleeding, and GI perforation may complicate the clinical course.[135] In the absence of ingestion, GI symptoms of hyperkalemia are usually very mild. Neuromuscular manifestations include weakness with an ascending flaccid paralysis and respiratory compromise, with intact sensation and cognition.[85,123,102] The cardiac manifestations of hyperkalemia are the most prominent and life-threatening. Electrocardiographic patterns progress through characteristic changes.[135,136] Although the progression of ECG changes is very reproducible, there is tremendous individual variation with respect to the absolute potassium concentration at which these ECG findings occur. Initially, the only ECG finding may be the presence of tall, peaked T waves. As the potassium increases, the QRS complex tends to blend into the T waves, the P-wave amplitude decreases, and the PR-interval prolongs. Next, the P wave is lost and ST-segment depression occurs. Finally, the distinction between the S and T waves becomes blurred and the ECG takes on a sine wave configuration (Chap. 9). Hemodynamic instability and cardiac arrest result. As the patient's potassium falls, these ECG changes resolve in a reverse fashion.

The treatment of severe hyperkalemia includes standard airway management, methods to reverse the ECG effects, methods to move potassium intracellularly, and methods to enhance potassium elimination. Pharmacologic interventions, extensively discussed elsewhere,[135] are summarized here. Calcium works almost immediately to protect the myocardium against the effects of hyperkalemia but does not change the serum potassium concentration. A potentially life-threatening interaction occurs, however, when the patient with cardiac glycoside toxicity is given calcium (Chap. 48); thus, this modality should be used with some caution. The administration of insulin and hypertonic dextrose or of sodium bicarbonate moves potassium intracellularly. Cationic exchange resins, such as sodium polystyrene sulfonate, work slowly to enhance GI potassium loss. Hemodialysis or peritoneal dialysis may be useful, especially when significant renal impairment is present. β-Adrenergic agonist inhalation therapy is also suggested to increase the intracellular potassium concentration.[6]

Calcium

Calcium is the most abundant mineral in the human body and 98–99% of it is located in bone. Approximately half of the remaining 1–2% of the body's calcium is bound to plasma proteins (mostly albumin) and most of the rest is complexed to various anions, with free calcium representing a very small fraction of extraosseous stores. Calcium concentration is maintained through interactions between dietary intake and renal elimination, modulated by vitamin D activity, parathyroid hormone, and calcitonin. More extensive discussions of calcium physiology are found elsewhere.[124]

Drug- and toxin-induced hypercalcemia is uncommon and usually relates to agents that increase calcium in the diet (antacids) or decrease its elimination (thiazides).[19] Cholecalciferol, available as a rodenticide, can increase serum calcium by increasing its release from bone, increasing GI absorption, and decreasing renal elimination (Chap. 90). Vitamin D toxicity from excessive supplementation of milk can also cause hypercalcemia.[80] Table 24–9 lists other causes of hypercalcemia.

Symptoms of hypercalcemia consist of lethargy, muscle weakness, nausea, vomiting, and constipation. Life-threatening manifestations include complications from altered mental status (aspiration), ECG changes (Chap. 9), and cardiac dysrhythmias. Treatment of clinically significant hypercalcemia focuses on removing the offending agent when possible, decreasing GI absorption, increasing distribution into bone, and enhancing elimination through forced diuresis.[124,153]

Drug- and toxin-induced hypocalcemia is more common than hypercalcemia. Minor, often clinically insignificant, decreases in serum calcium occur in association with anticonvulsant[90] and aminoglycoside therapy.[19] Severe, life-threatening hypocalcemia can occur, however, from ethylene glycol poisoning (Chap. 66) or as a manifestation of fluoride toxicity from either fluoride salts or hydrofluoric acid (Chap. 87).[38,155] Direct complex formation with fluoride or oxalate ions are responsible for the rapid production of hypocalcemia in these settings. Similar effects occur with excess phosphate[158] or citrate.[101,156] This mechanism is distinct when compared to other drugs and toxins (Table 24–9) that produce hypocalcemia by decreased absorption, enhanced renal loss, or redistribution.

Symptoms of hypocalcemia consist largely of neuromuscular findings, including paresthesias, cramps, carpopedal spasm, tetany, and seizures. Although ECG abnormalities are common (Chap. 9), life-threatening dysrhythmias are rare. Treatment strategies focus on calcium replacement. When hypomagnesemia or hyperphosphatemia is present, these abnormalities must be corrected or calcium replacement will fail.[124]

TABLE 24–9. Causes of Altered Serum Calcium

Hypocalcemia	Hypercalcemia
Aminoglycosides	Aluminum
Bicarbonate	Androgens
Biphosphonates	Antacids (magnesium containing)
Calcitonin	Antacids (calcium containing)
Citrate	Cholecalciferol and other Vitamin D analogues
Ethanol	
Ethylene glycol	Glucocorticoids
Fluoride	Tamoxifen
Furosemide	Thiazide diuretics
Mithramycin	Lithium
Neomycin	Vitamin A
Phenobarbital	
Phenytoin	
Phosphate	
Theophylline	
Valproate	

Magnesium

Magnesium is the fourth most abundant cation in the body (after calcium, sodium, and potassium), with a normal total body store of about 2020 mEq in a 70-kg human.[126] Approximately 50% of magnesium is stored in bone, with most of the remainder distributed in the soft tissues. Only about 1–2% of magnesium is located in the extracellular fluid; therefore, serum levels correlate poorly with total body stores.[127] Magnesium homeostasis is maintained through dietary intake and renal and GI losses, modulated by hormonal effects.

Clinically significant hypermagnesemia is uncommon in the absence of renal failure, except when massive parenteral infusions of magnesium salts overwhelm renal compensatory mechanisms. This has been reported with inadvertent intravenous infusion,[16,23,70,110] urologic procedures involving irrigation with magnesium salts,[44,81] and ingestion of large quantities of magnesium-containing antacids[103] and cathartics.[45,52,57] The greatest concern is iatrogenic overdose from the use of magnesium-containing cathartics as part of routine poison management.[54,82,146] In a series of poisoned patients, single-dose magnesium cathartic failed to produce any demonstrable rise in serum magnesium concentrations.[147] However, patients who received three doses of magnesium sulfate over 8 hours had a statistically significant increase in their magnesium concentration.[147] Thus, as with sorbitol use, the potential for iatrogenic toxicity exists, mandating cautious use of magnesium-containing cathartics, especially in patients with renal insufficiency. Table 24–10 lists other causes of hypermagnesemia.

The symptoms of hypermagnesemia correlate roughly with serum concentrations but depend somewhat on the rate of increase and host factors. At magnesium concentrations of about 3–10 mEq/L, patients feel weak, nauseated, flushed, and thirsty. Bradycardia, hypotension, and decreased deep tendon reflexes are noted. As levels increase, hypoventilation, muscle paralysis, and ventricular dysrhythmias occur. Magnesium levels greater than 10 mEq/L, especially those greater than 15 mEq/L, are often associated with fatal events.

Hypermagnesemia should be considered a life-threatening disorder. When significant neuromuscular or ECG manifestations are noted, parenteral administration of calcium will reverse some of the toxicity.[65] Further therapy should focus on enhancing elimination with fluid resuscitation and loop diuretics.[65] Hemodialysis rapidly corrects hypermagnesemia when renal function is inadequate.

Drug- and toxin-induced hypomagnesemia is common, but rarely life threatening. Renal losses (from diuretics and renal tubular acidosis), GI losses (from ethanol), intracellular shifts from insulin[98] or β-adrenergic agonists, and complexation (from fluoride or hyperphosphatemia) are common. Table 24–10 lists other causes of hypomagnesemia. These are the same mechanisms that produce other electrolyte abnormalities, so when hypomagnesemia is suspected or discovered, other electrolyte abnormalities are usually present.

The symptoms of hypomagnesemia are lethargy, weakness, fatigue, neuromuscular excitation (tremor and hyperreflexia), nausea, and vomiting.[29,35] Dysrhythmias can occur, especially during therapy with cardiac glycosides. Signs and symptoms consistent with hypocalcemia and hypokalemia may also be present.

Treatment involves removing the offending agent (if it can be identified) and restoring magnesium balance. Although either oral or parenteral supplementation is usually acceptable for mild hypo-

TABLE 24–10. Causes of Altered Serum Magnesium

Hypomagnesemia	Hypermagnesemia
Aminoglycosides	Antacids (magnesium containing)
Amphotericin	Cathartics (magnesium containing)
Cisplatin	Lithium
Cyclosporine	
DDT	
Ethanol	
Fluoride	
Insulin	
Laxatives	
Loop diuretics	
Methylxanthines	
Osmotic diuretics	
Phosphates	
Strychnine	
Theophylline	
Thiazide diuretics	

magnesemia, parenteral therapy is required when significant clinical effects are present. Most authors suggest that in the absence of renal insufficiency a safe dose of magnesium sulfate in the adult is 16 mEq (2 g) infused over several minutes,[29,78] to a maximum of 1 mEq/kg of magnesium in a 24-hour period (1 g of magnesium sulfate contains about 8 mEq of magnesium). During any substantial magnesium infusion, frequent serum magnesium determinations should be obtained and the presence of reflexes documented. If hyporeflexia occurs, the magnesium infusion should be discontinued.

SUMMARY

The evaluation of fluid, electrolyte, and acid-base status is a fundamental component of the management of the poisoned or overdosed patient. A clear appreciation of the pathophysiologic causes of these abnormalities and a rational approach to their correction is essential for reducing the mortality and morbidity from poisoning. In addition, many fluid and electrolyte abnormalities result from adverse drug reactions and therefore become part of the routine patient evaluation.

REFERENCES

1. Adrogue HJ, Brensilver J, Madias NE: Changes in the plasma anion gap during chronic metabolic acid-base disturbances. Am J Physiol 1978;235:291–297.
2. Adrogue HJ, Madias NE: Hypernatremia. N Engl J Med 2000; 342:1493–1499.
3. Adrogue HJ, Madias NE: Hyponatremia. N Engl J Med 2000;342:1581–1589.
4. Adrogue HJ, Wilson H, Boyd AE, et al: Plasma acid-base patterns in diabetic ketoacidosis. N Engl J Med 1982;307:1603–1610.
5. Albert MD, Dell RB, Winters RW: Quantitative displacement of acid-base equilibrium in metabolic acidosis. Ann Intern Med 1967;66:312–322.
6. Allon M, Dunlay R, Copkney C: Nebulized albuterol for acute hyperkalemia in patients on hemodialysis. Ann Intern Med 1989;110:426–429.

7. Ammar KA, Heckerling PS: Ethylene glycol poisoning with a normal anion gap caused by concurrent ethanol ingestion: Importance of the osmolal gap. Am J Kidney Dis 1996;27:130–133.

8. Anderson IK, Martin GR, Ramage AG: Central administration of 5-HT activates 5-HT$_{1A}$ receptors cause sympathoexcitation and 5-HT$_2$/5-HT$_{1C}$ receptors to release vasopressin in anaesthetized rats. Br J Pharmacol 1992;107:1020–1028.

9. Andreoli TE: The posterior pituitary. In: Wyngaarden JB, Smith LH, eds: Cecil's Textbook of Medicine, 18th ed. Philadelphia, WB Saunders, 1988, pp. 1305–1313.

10. Ayus JC, Arieff AI: Symptomatic hyponatremia: Making the diagnosis rapidly. J Crit Ill 1990;5:846–856.

11. Ayus JC, Krothapalli RK, Arieff AI: Treatment of symptomatic hyponatremia and its relation to brain damage: A prospective study. N Engl J Med 1987;317:1190–1195.

12. Barter FC: The syndrome of inappropriate secretion of antidiuretic hormone (SIADH). Dis Mon 1973;Nov:1–47.

13. Battle DC, Hizon M, Cohen E, et al: The use of the urinary anion gap in the diagnosis of hyperchloremic metabolic acidosis. N Engl J Med 1988;318:594–599.

14. Battle DC, von Riotte AB, Aviria M, Grup M: Amelioration of polyuria by amiloride in patients receiving long-term lithium therapy. N Engl J Med 1985;312:408–414.

15. Bismuth C, Gaultier M, Conso F, et al: Hyperkalemia in acute digitalis poisoning: Prognostic significance and therapeutic implications. Clin Toxicol 1973;6:153–162.

16. Bourgeois FJ, Thiagarajah S, Harbert GM, et al: Profound hypotension complicating magnesium therapy. Am J Obstet Gynecol 1986;154: 919–920.

17. Bower BR, Wegienka LC, Forsham PH: In vitro studies of mechanism of polyuria induced by dextropropoxyphene (Darvon). Proc Soc Exp Biol Med 1965;120:155–157.

18. Brambilla G, Cenci T, Franconi F, et al: Clinical and pharmacological profile in a clenbuterol epidemic poisoning of contaminated beef meat in Italy. Toxicol Lett 2000;114:47–53.

19. Brass EP, Thompson WL: Drug-induced electrolyte abnormalities. Med Toxicol 1982;24:207–228.

20. Brenner BE: Clinical significance of the elevated anion gap. Am J Med 1985;79:289–296.

21. Britten JS, Myers RA, Benner C, et al: Blood ethanol and serum osmolality in the trauma patient. Am Surg 1982;48:451–455.

22. Caldwell JW, Nava AJ, DeHaas DD: Hypernatremia associated with cathartics in overdose management. West J Med 1987;147:593–596.

23. Cao Z, Bideau R, Valdes R, Elin RJ: Acute hypermagnesemia and respiratory arrest following infusion of MgSO$_4$ for tocolysis. Clin Chim Acta 1999;285:191–193.

24. Catalano G, Kanfer SN, Catalano MC, Alberts VA: The role of sertraline in a patient with recurrent hyponatremia. Gen Hosp Psychiatry 1996;18:278–283.

25. Champion HR, Baker SP, Benner C, et al: Alcohol intoxication and serum osmolality. Lancet 1975;1:1402–1404.

26. Chan TY: Indapamide-induced severe hyponatremia and hypokalemia. Ann Pharmacother 1995;29:1124–1128.

27. Connelly DM: Silver nitrate, ideal burn wound therapy? N Y State J Med 1970;70:1642–1644.

28. Cox M, Singer I: Lithium and water metabolism. Am J Med 1975;59:153–157.

29. Cronin RE, Knochel JP: Magnesium deficiency. Adv Intern Med 1983;28:509–533.

30. Darchy B, Abruzzese L, Pitiot O, et al: Delayed admission for ethylene glycol poisoning: Lack of elevated serum osmol gap. Intensive Care Med 1999;25:859–861.

31. Decaux G, Schlesser M, Coffernils M, et al: Uric acid, anion gap and urea concentration in the diagnostic approach to hyponatremia. Clin Nephrol 1994;42:102–108.

32. DeFronzo RA, Bia M: Intravenous potassium chloride therapy [letter]. JAMA 1981;245:2446.

33. Delaney V, de Pertuz Y, Nixon D: Indomethacin in streptozocin-induced nephrogenic diabetes insipidus. Am J Kidney Dis 1987;9:79–83.

34. DiNubile MJ: The increment in the anion gap: Overextension of a concept. Lancet 1988;2:951–952.

35. Dirks JH: The kidney and magnesium regulation. Kidney Int 1983;23:771–777.

36. Dorwart WV, Chalmers L: Comparison of methods for calculating serum osmolality from chemical concentrations, and the prognostic value of such calculations. Clin Chem 1975;21:190–194.

37. Earley LE, Orloff J: The mechanism of antidiuresis associated with administration of hydrochlorothiazide to patients with vasopressin resistant diabetes insipidus. J Clin Invest 1962;41:1988–1997.

38. Edelman P: Hydrofluoric acid burns: State of the art review. Occup Med 1986;1:89–103.

39. Edwards CRW: Lessons from licorice. N Engl J Med 1991;325:1242–1243.

40. Eisen TF, Lacouture PG, Woolf A: Serum osmolality in alcohol ingestions: Differences in availability among laboratories of teaching hospital, nonteaching hospital, and commercial facilities. Am J Emerg Med 1989;7:256–259.

41. Emmet M, Narins RG: Clinical use of the anion gap. Medicine 1977;56:38–54.

42. Farese RV, Biglieri EG, Shackleton CHL: Licorice induced hypermineralocorticoidism. N Engl J Med 1991;325:1223–1227.

43. Farley TA: Severe hypernatremic dehydration after use of an activated charcoal-sorbitol suspension. J Pediatr 1986;109:719–722.

44. Fassler CA, Rodriguez M, Badesch DB, et al: Magnesium toxicity as a cause of hypotension and hypoventilation: Occurrence in patients with normal renal function. Arch Intern Med 1985;145:1604–1606.

45. Ferdinandus J, Pederson JA, Whang R: Hypermagnesemia as a cause of refractory hypotension, respiratory depression, and coma. Arch Intern Med 1981;141:669–670.

46. Fichman MP, Vorherr H, Kleeman CR, et al: Diuretic-induced hyponatremia. Ann Intern Med 1971;75:853–863.

47. Figge J, Jabor A, Kazda A, Fencl V: Anion gap and hypoalbuminemia. Crit Care Med 1998;26:1807–1810.

48. Forrest JN, Cox M, Hong C, et al: Superiority of demeclocycline over lithium in the treatment of chronic syndrome of inappropriate secretion of antidiuretic hormone. N Engl J Med 1978;298:173–177.

49. Gabow PA: Disorders associated with an altered anion gap. Kidney Int 1985;27:472–483.

50. Gabow PA, Kaehny WD, Fennessey PV, et al: Diagnostic importance of an increased serum anion gap. N Engl J Med 1980;303:854–858.

51. Gamble JL: Chemical Anatomy, Physiology, and Pathology of Extracellular Fluids: A Lecture Syllabus, 6th ed. Cambridge, MA, Harvard University Press, 1960, p. 131.

52. Garcia-Webb P, Bhagat C, Oh T, et al: Hypermagnesaemia and hypophosphataemia after ingestion of magnesium sulfate. Br Med J 1984;288:759.

53. Garella S, Chazan JA, Cohen JJ: Saline-resistant metabolic alkalosis or "chloride wasting nephropathy." Ann Intern Med 1970;73:31–38.

54. Garrelts JC, Watson WA, Holloway KD, et al: Magnesium toxicity secondary to catharsis during management of theophylline poisoning. Am J Emerg Med 1989;7:34–37.

55. Gazda-Smith E, Synhawsky A: Hypernatremia following treatment of theophylline toxicity with activated charcoal and sorbitol. Arch Intern Med 1990;150:689–690.

56. Gennari FJ: Serum osmolality: Uses and limitations. N Engl J Med 1984;310:102–105.

57. Gerard SK, Hernandez C, Khayam-Bashi H: Extreme hypermagnesemia caused by an overdose of magnesium-containing cathartics. Ann Emerg Med 1988;17:728–731.

58. Glasser DS: The utility of the serum osmol gap in the diagnosis of methanol or ethylene glycol ingestion. Ann Emerg Med 1996;27:343–346.

59. Glasser L, Sternglanz PD, Combie J, Robinson A: Serum osmolality and its applicability to drug overdose. Am J Clin Pathol 1973;60:695–699.

60. Goldman MA, Lisak R, Matz R, et al: Hypochloremic alkalosis with symptoms of seizure disorder. N Y State J Med 1970;70:306–308.

61. Goldman MB, Luching DJ, Robertson GL: Mechanisms of altered water metabolism in psychotic patients with polydipsia and hyponatremia. N Engl J Med 1988;318:397–403.

62. Goldstein MD, Bear R, Richardson RMA, et al: The urine anion gap: A clinically useful index of ammonium excretion. Am J Med Sci 1986;292:198–202.

63. Goldstein RJ, Lichtenstein NS, Souder D: The myth of the low anion gap. JAMA 1980;243:1737–1738.

64. Goodkin OH, Krishna GG, Narins RG: The role of the anion gap in detecting and managing mixed acid-base disorders. Clin Endocrinol Metab 1984;13:333–349.

65. Graber TW, Yee AS, Baker FJ: Magnesium: Physiology, clinical disorders and therapy. Ann Emerg Med 1981;10:49–57.

66. Harrington JT: Metabolic alkalosis. Kidney Int 1984;26:88–97.

67. Hilbert G, Bedry R, Cardinaud JP, Benissan GG: Euro bleach: Fatal hypernatremia due to 13.3% sodium hypochlorite [letter]. J Toxicol Clin Toxicol 1997;35:635–636.

68. Hoekstra PT, Kahnoski R, McCamish MA, et al: Transurethral prostatic resection syndrome—A new perspective: encephalopathy with associated hyperammonemia. J Urol 1983:130:704–707.

69. Hoffman RS, Smilkstein MJ, Howland MA, Goldfrank LR: Osmol gaps revisited: Normal values and limitations. J Toxicol Clin Toxicol 1993;31:81–93.

70. Hoffman RS, Smilkstein MJ, Rubenstein F: An "amp" by any other name: The hazards of intravenous magnesium dosing [letter]. JAMA 1989;261:557.

71. Hohler T, Teuber G, Wanitschke R: Indomethacin treatment in amphotericin B induced nephrogenic diabetes insipidus. Clin Invest 1994;72:769–771.

72. Hohnloser SH, Verrier RL, Lown B, et al: Effect of hypokalemia on susceptibility to ventricular fibrillation in the normal and ischemic canine heart. Am Heart J 1986;112:32–35.

73. Holden R, Jackson MA: Near-fatal hyponatraemic coma due to vasopressin over-secretion after "ecstasy" (3,4-MDMA) [letter]. Lancet 1996;347:1052.

74. Hubbard JI, Lin N, Sibbald JR: Subfornical organ lesions in rats abolish hyperdipsic effects of isoproterenol and serotonin. Brain Res Bull 1989;23:41–45.

75. Iberti TJ, Leibowitz AB, Papadakos PJ, Fischer EP: Low sensitivity of the anion gap as a screen to detect hyperlactatemia in critically ill patients. Crit Care Med 1990;18:275–277.

76. Inaba H, Hirasawa H, Mizuguchi T: Serum osmolality gap in postoperative patients in intensive care. Lancet 1987;1:1331–1335.

77. Ireland JT, Thomson WS: Euglycemic diabetic ketoacidosis. Br Med J 1973;3:107.

78. Iseri LT, Freed J, Bures AR: Magnesium deficiency and cardiac disorders. Am J Med 1975;58:837–845.

79. Ivoino M, Steardo L: Effect of substances influencing brain serotonergic transmission on plasma vasopressin levels in the rat. Eur J Pharmacol 1985;113:99–103.

80. Jacobus CH, Holick MF, Shao Q, et al: Hypervitaminosis D associated with drinking milk. N Engl J Med 1992;326:1173–1177.

81. Jenny DB, Goris GB, Urwiller RD, et al: Hypermagnesemia following irrigation of renal pelvis: cause of respiratory depression. JAMA 1978;240:1378–1379.

82. Jones J, Heiselman D, Dougherty J, et al: Cathartic-induced magnesium toxicity during overdose management. Ann Emerg Med 1986;15:1214–1218.

83. Kassirer JP, Berkman PM, Lawrenz DR, Schwartz WB: The critical role of chloride in the correction of hypokalemic alkalosis in man. Am J Med 1965;38:172–189.

84. Kessler J, Samuels SC: Sertraline and hyponatremia [letter]. N Engl J Med 1996;335:524.

85. Knochel JP: Neuromuscular manifestations of electrolyte disorders. Am J Med 1982;72:521–535.

86. Kovacs L, Robertson GL: Syndrome of inappropriate antidiuresis. Endocrinol Metab Clin North Am 1992;21:859–875.

87. Kruse JA, Carlson RW: Rapid correction of hypokalemia using concentrated intravenous potassium chloride infusions. Arch Intern Med 1990;150:613–617.

88. Kulberg A: Urinalysis and urine culture. In: Flomenbaum N, Goldfrank LR, eds: Diagnostic Testing in the Emergency Department. Rockville, MD, Aspen, 1984, pp. 19–29.

89. Lavie CH, Crocker EF, Key KJ, et al: Marked hypochloremic metabolic alkalosis with severe compensatory hypoventilation. South Med J 1986;79:1296–1299.

90. Lee WL, Yang CC, Deng JF, et al: A case of severe hyperammonemia and unconsciousness following sodium valproate intoxication. Vet Hum Toxicol 1998;40:346–348.

91. Libber S, Harison H, Spector D: Treatment of nephrogenic diabetes insipidus with prostaglandin synthesis inhibitors. J Pediatr 1986;108:305–311.

92. Lichstein E, Chadda K, Fenig S: Atrial pacing in the treatment of refractory ventricular tachycardia associated with hypokalemia. Am J Cardiol 1972;30:550–553.

93. Liu BA, Mittmann N, Knowles SR, Shear NH: Hyponatremia and the syndrome of inappropriate secretion of antidiuretic hormone associated with the use of selective serotonin reuptake inhibitors: A review of spontaneous reports. Can Med Assoc J 1996;155:519–527.

94. Lubash GD, Cohen BD, Young CW, et al: Severe metabolic alkalosis with neurologic abnormalities. N Engl J Med 1958;258: 1050–1052.

95. Lundberg P: The effect of adrenergic blockade on potassium concentrations in different conditions. Acta Med Scand 1983;672 (Suppl): 121–152.

96. Lydiard RB, Gelenberg AJ: Hazards and adverse effects of lithium. Annu Rev Med 1982;33:327–344.

97. Masson EA: Mesalazine associated nephrogenic diabetes insipidus presenting as weight loss. Gut 1992;33:563–564.

98. Matsumura M, Nakashima A, Tofuku Y: Electrolyte disorders following massive insulin overdose in a patient with type 2 diabetes. Intern Med 2000;39:55–57.

99. Mazze RI, Trudell JR, Cousins MJ: Methoxyflurane metabolism and renal dysfunction: Clinical correlation in man. Anesthesiology 1971; 35:247–252.

100. McCarron D: Correcting potassium depletion. Drug Ther 1979;4:65–72.

101. McCarthy LJ, Danielson CF, Skipworth EM, Thompson CF: Hypocalcemia secondary to citrate toxicity [letter]. Ther Apher 1998;2:249.

102. McCarty M, Jagoda A, Fairweather P: Hyperkalemic ascending paralysis. Ann Emerg Med 1998;32:104–107.

103. McGuire JK, Kulkarni MS, Baden HP: Fatal hypermagnesemia in a child treated with megavitamin/megamineral therapy. Pediatrics 2000;105:E18.

104. McQuillen JJ, Anderson AC: Osmol gaps in the pediatric population. Acad Emerg Med 1999;6:27–30.

105. Mennen M, Slovis CM: Severe metabolic alkalosis in the emergency department. Ann Emerg Med 1988;17:354–357.

106. Mercado R, Michelis MF: Severe sodium depletion syndrome during lithium carbonate therapy. Arch Intern Med 1977;137:1731–1733.

107. Mizutani AR, Parker J, Katz J, et al: Visual disturbances, serum glycine levels and transurethral resection of the prostate. J Urol 1990;144:697–699.

108. Moder KG, Hurley DL: Fatal hypernatremia from exogenous salt intake: Report of a case and review of the literature. Mayo Clin Proc 1990;65:1587–1594.

109. Morganroth ML: Six steps to acid-base analysis: Clinical applications. J Crit Ill 1990;5:460–469.

110. Morisaki H, Yamamoto S, Morita Y, et al: Hypermagnesemia-induced cardiopulmonary arrest before induction of anesthesia for emergency cesarean section. J Clin Anesth 2000;12:224–226.

111. Moses AM, Miller M, Streeten DHP: Pathophysiologic and pharmacologic alterations in the release and action of ADH. Metabolism 1976;25:697–721.

112. Moses AM, Miller M: Drug-induced dilutional hyponatremia. N Engl J Med 1974;291:1234–1239.

113. Moses AM, Notman DD: Diabetes insipidus and syndrome of inappropriate antidiuretic hormone secretion (SIADH). Adv Intern Med 1982;27:73–100.

114. Narins RG, Emmett M: Simple and mixed acid-base disorders: A practical approach. Medicine 1980;59:161–187.

115. Navarro JF, Quereda C, Quereda C, et al: Nephrogenic diabetes insipidus and renal tubular acidosis secondary to foscarnet therapy. Am J Kidney Dis 1996;27:431–434.

116. Oh MS, Carroll HJ: Current concepts: The anion gap. N Engl J Med 1977;297:814–817.

117. Oster JR, Perez GO, Masterson BJ: Use of the anion gap in clinical medicine. South Med J 1988;81:229–237.

118. Osterloh JD, Kelly TJ, Khayam-Bashi H, Romeo R: Discrepancies in osmolal gaps and calculated alcohol concentrations. Arch Pathol Lab Med 1996;120:634–641.

119. Pappas AA, Gadsden RH, Taylor EH: Serum osmolality in acute intoxication: A prospective study. Am J Clin Pathol 1985;84:74–79.

120. Perez GO, Oster JR: Acid–base disorders: II. Use of $\Delta AG/\Delta HCO_3$ in evaluating mixed acid-base disorders—A patient management problem. South Med J 1986;79:882–886.

121. Perrone J, Hoffman RS: Compensatory hypoventilation in metabolic alkalosis. Acad Emerg Med 1996;3:981–982.

122. Phillips DR, Milim SJ, Nathanson HG, et al: Preventing hyponatremic encephalopathy: Comparison of serum sodium and osmolality during operative hysteroscopy with 5.0% mannitol and 1.5% glycine distention media. J Am Assoc Gynecol Laparosc 1997;4:567–576.

123. Ponce SP, Jennings AE, Madias NE, et al: Drug-induced hyperkalemia. Medicine (Baltimore) 1985;64:357–370.

124. Potts JT: Diseases of the parathyroid gland and other hyper- and hypocalcemic disorders. In: Wilson JD, Braunwald E, Isselbacher KJ, et al, eds: Harrison's Principles of Internal Medicine, 12th ed. New York, McGraw-Hill, 1991, pp. 1902–1921.

125. Quinn BP: Nephrogenic diabetes insipidus and tubulointerstitial nephritis during continuous therapy with rifampin. Am J Kidney Dis 1989;14:217–220.

126. Randall RE, Cohen MD, Spray CC, et al: Hypermagnesemia in renal failure: Etiology and toxic manifestations. Ann Intern Med 1964;61:73–88.

127. Reinhart RA: Magnesium metabolism: A review with special reference to the relationship between intracellular content and serum levels. Arch Intern Med 1988;148:2415–2420.

128. Riggs AT, Dysken MW, Kim SW, Opsahl JA: A review of disorders of water homeostasis in psychiatric patients. Psychosomatics 1991;32:133–148.

129. Robinson AG, Loeb JN: Ethanol ingestion: Commonest cause of elevated plasma osmolality? N Engl J Med 1971;284:1253–1255.

130. Rosa RM, Silva P, Young JB, et al: Adrenergic modulation of extrarenal potassium disposal. N Engl J Med 1980;302:431–434.

131. Ross MP, Spiller HA: Fatal ingestion of sodium hypochlorite bleach with associated hypernatremia and hyperchloremic metabolic acidosis. Vet Hum Toxicol 1999;41:82–86.

132. Sakane N, Yoshida T, Umekawa T, Miyazaki R: Nephrogenic diabetes insipidus induced by lobenzarit disodium treatment in patients with rheumatoid arthritis. Intern Med 1996;35:119–122.

133. Salem MM, Mujais SK: Gaps in the anion gap. Arch Intern Med 1992;152:1625–1629.

134. Santonastaso P, Sala A, Favaro A: Water intoxication in anorexia nervosa: A case report. Int J Eat Disord 1998;24:439–442.

135. Saxena K: Clinical features and management of poisoning due to potassium chloride. Med Toxicol Adverse Drug Exp 1989;4: 429–433.

136. Saxena K: Death from potassium chloride overdose. Postgrad Med 1988;84:97–102.

137. Schelling JR, Howard RL, Winter SD, Linas SL: Increased osmolal gap in alcoholic ketoacidosis and lactic acidosis. Ann Intern Med 1990;113:580–582.

138. Schwartz SM, Carroll HM, Scharschmidt LA: Sublimed (inorganic) sulfur ingestion. A cause of life-threatening metabolic acidosis with a high anion gap. Arch Intern Med 1986;146:1437–1438.

139. Schwartz WB, Orning KJ, Porter R: The internal distribution of hydrogen ions with varying degrees of metabolic acidosis. J Clin Invest 1957;36:373–382.

140. Scoggin C, McClellan JR, Cary JM: Hypernatraemia and acidosis in association with topical treatment of burns [letter]. Lancet 1977;1: 959.

141. Scott SM: Pulmonary edema and hyponatremia during hysteroscopic resection of uterine fibroids: Case report. CRNA 1998;9:113–117.

142. Sigue G, Gamble L, Pelitere M, et al: From profound hypokalemia to life-threatening hyperkalemia: A case of barium sulfide poisoning. Arch Intern Med 2000;160:548–551.

143. Singer I, Rotenberg D: Demeclocycline-induced nephrogenic diabetes insipidus. Ann Intern Med 1973;79:679–683.

144. Singer I, Rotenberg D: Mechanisms of lithium action. N Engl J Med 1973;289:254–260.

145. Sklar AH, Linas SL: The osmolal gap in renal failure. Ann Intern Med 1983;98:481–482.

146. Smilkstein MJ, Smolinske SC, Kulig KW, et al: Severe hypermagnesemia due to multiple-dose cathartic therapy. West J Med 1988; 148:208–211.

147. Smilkstein MJ, Steedle D, Kulig KW, et al: Magnesium levels after magnesium-containing cathartics. J Toxicol Clin Toxicol 1988;26: 51–65.

148. Smithline N, Gardner KD: Gaps: Anionic and osmolal. JAMA 1976; 236:1594–1597.

149. Sonnenblick M, Rosin A: Increased uric acid clearance in the syndrome of inappropriate secretion of antidiuretic hormone. Isr J Med Sci 1988;24:20–23.

150. Spigset O, Hedenmalm K: Hyponatremia and the syndrome of inappropriate antidiuretic hormone (SIADH) secretion induced by psychotropic drugs. Drug Saf 1995;12:209–225.

151. Steinhart B: Case report: Severe ethylene glycol intoxication with normal osmolal gap—"A chilling thought." J Emerg Med 1990;8: 583–585.

152. Sterns RH, Riggs JE, Schochet SS: Osmotic demyelination syndrome following correction of hyponatremia. N Engl J Med 1986; 314:1535–1542.

153. Suki WN, Yium JJ, Von Minden M, et al: Acute treatment of hypercalcemia with furosemide. N Engl J Med 1970; 283:836–840.

154. Takahashi H, Toya T, Matsumiya N, Koyama K: A case of transient diabetes insipidus associated with poisoning by a herbicide containing glufosinate. J Toxicol Clin Toxicol 2000;38:153–156.

155. Tepperman PB: Fatality due to acute systemic fluoride poisoning following a hydrofluoric acid skin burn. J Occup Med 1980;22: 691–692.

156. Uhl L, Maillet S, King S, Kruskall MS: Unexpected citrate toxicity and severe hypocalcemia during apheresis. Transfusion 1997;37: 1063–1065.

157. Van Amelsvoort T, Bakshi R, Devaux CB, Schwabe S: Hyponatremia associated with carbamazepine and oxcarbazepine therapy: A review. Epilepsia 1994;35:181–188.

158. Vincent JC, Sheikh A: Phosphate poisoning by ingestion of clothes washing liquid and fabric conditioner. Anaesthesia 1998;53: 1004–1006.

159. Vokes TJ, Robertson GL: Disorders of antidiuretic hormone. Endocrinol Metab Clin North Am 1988;17:281–299.

160. Wax PM, Wang R, Mercurio M, et al: The prevalence of sorbitol in repetitive dose activated charcoal regimens in emergency departments. Ann Emerg Med 1993;22:1807–1812.

161. Wetherill SF, Guarino MJ, Cox RW: Acute renal failure associated with barium chloride poisoning. Ann Intern Med 1981;95:187–188.

162. Wilkins B: Cerebral oedema after MDMA ("ecstasy") and unrestricted water intake. Hyponatraemia must be treated with low water input [letter]. BMJ 1996;313:689–690.

163. Winter SD, Pearson R, Gabow PA, et al: The fall of the serum anion gap. Arch Intern Med 1990;150:311–313.

164. Witte DL, Rodgers JL, Barrett DA: The anion gap: Its use in quality control. Clin Chem 1976;22:643–646.

165. Wrenn K: The delta gap: An approach to mixed acid-base disorders. Ann Emerg Med 1990;19:1310–1313.

166. Wrenn KD, Slovis CM, Slovis BS: The ability of physicians to predict hyperkalemia from the ECG. Ann Emerg Med 1991;20:1229–1232.

Diane Sauter

Exposure to toxins may interfere with any morphologic or functional aspect of the blood and blood-forming organs. Depressed cell formation, increased destruction, alteration of hemoglobin, and impairment of coagulation can all result from exposure to a large variety of toxic agents. The response to an exogenous toxin depends upon the nature and quantity of the agent, and the capacity of the system to respond to the insult. Because of individual variation, often no clear and predictable dose-response relationship can be determined. For example, healthy individuals may tolerate exposure to naphthalene in low levels, whereas individuals with glucose-6-phosphate dehydrogenase deficiency may develop massive hemolysis when similarly exposed. Even the ability of healthy individuals to detoxify naphthalene may be overwhelmed, resulting in hemolysis following substantial exposure.

HEMATOPOIESIS

Stem Cells

The majority of the cells of the blood system may be classified as either lymphoid (B, T, and natural-killer lymphocytes) or myeloid (erythrocytes, megakaryocytes, granulocytes, and macrophages).[88] All of these cells are descended from a small common pool of totipotent cells called *hematopoietic stem cells*.[139] A stem cell is capable of self-renewal as well as of reconstituting long-term hematopoiesis after marrow ablation.[88] The stem cell pool occupies a very small compartment (0.01% of the bone marrow), and the majority is usually quiescent. The surface phenotype includes the presence of the CD34 antigen (discussed later).[35] Stem cells are found in umbilical cord, bone marrow, and peripheral blood.[43] These cells are capable of self-renewal and of differentiation into other multipotential or committed progenitor cells with progressively limited differentiation potential.[88] With subsequent division and maturation these cells progressively display the antigenic, biochemical and morphologic features characteristic of mature cells of the appropriate lineages, and lose their capacity for self-renewal. It appears that multiple steps are involved in the commitment of less differentiated cells to more mature cell lines (see Fig. 25–1). The first step separates lymphoid from myeloid cell lines. The second step separates granulocyte/macrophage potential from erythroid/megakaryocyte potential until each descendent cell has only one lineage capability. The final steps in the maturation of blood cells involve extensive remodeling, the restructuring of cellular membranes, the accumulation of specialized proteins (such as hemoglobin), and the loss of nuclei and organelles. In the case of granulocytes, granules containing proteolytic enzymes are formed in cell cytoplasm, and the nucleus condenses to form the multilobulated nucleus of the mature cell. Megakaryocyte cytoplasm demarcates into units that are eventually split off as platelets.[12]

Growth Factors

Growth factors are glycoproteins necessary for the differentiation and maturation of individual or multiple cell lines.[57,63,64,80,84] More than 30 have been identified and characterized.[12] They fall into two families of ligands and receptors based on structural and functional features. The ligands of the cytokine receptor family include growth hormone, interleukin-2 (IL-2), macrophage colony-stimulating factor (CSF-1), granulocyte-macrophage colony stimulating factor (GM-CSF), interferon-γ, and granulocyte colony-stimulating factor (GCSF), to name a few. The second group, the tyrosine kinase family, includes Kit ligand and IGF1R, a member of the insulin family. The complete development of all of the mature blood cells from stem cells or multilineage progenitors requires the action of growth factors, either alone or in combination, for successful differentiation and final maturation.[12]

The effect of growth factors on hematopoiesis is modulated, in part through interactions with another family of molecules known as chemokines. Originally named for their ability to act as chemotactic cytokines for mature blood cells, more than 50 chemokines have been identified. Among their many functions are the modulation of hematopoiesis and directing the movement of stem cells.[16]

CD34 Antigen

The CD34 antigen (cluster designation 34) is a 115-kilodalton (kDa) glycoprotein. It is believed to be a differentiation antigen that is selectively expressed by primitive myeloid, lymphoid, and erythroid progenitors and stem cells.[122] The CD34 antigen identifies essentially all unipotent myeloid- and erythroid-forming cells, as well as multipotential cells. It is absent from mature T and B lymphocytes, although evidence suggests that both lymphoid lineages arise from CD34+ precursors.[122] The precursors of the stromal system share the expression of CD34 antigen, although they are otherwise phenotypically and functionally distinct cell types.

CD34 may function as an adhesion molecule.[39] It is in the class of molecules known as addressins. Addressins are molecules present on endothelial venules that bind circulating lymphocytes and mediate their homing to specific sites. CD34 antigen belongs to the rhodopsin superfamily (ie molecules sharing 50% or less sequence similarity) of cell membrane proteins.[98]

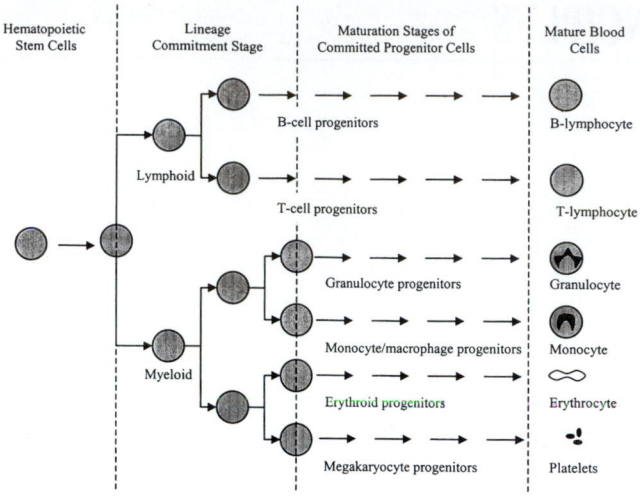

Figure 25–1. Principles of hematopoiesis.

BONE MARROW

In the normal adult, the bone marrow is the principle organ for mature blood cell formation. Its main function is to adjust the supply of cells to match the demand for cells. The functional requirements of the bone marrow are exceedingly complex. Mature marrow is capable of producing 2.5 billion red cells, 2.5 billion platelets, and 1 billion granulocytes per kilogram of body weight per day. It must also maintain a pool of undifferentiated cells that may be rapidly recruited in response to acute stresses such as hemolysis or infection.[88,90]

Embryology and Development of Erythropoiesis

The sites of hematopoiesis are established early in embryogenesis, and change several times until birth.[12] By day 8 of embryonic life, the yolk sac and fetal liver begin carrying out erythropoiesis. Lymphoid precursors also develop by day 8 in the yolk sac.[31,97] Anatomic sites other than the yolk sac and fetal liver give rise to other cellular elements of blood. The para-aortic splanchnopleura gives rise to B cell progenitors.[41] The aorto-gonad-mesonephros region contains pluripotential stem cells during embryogenesis.[83]

Marrow spaces within bone begin to form in humans at about the 5th fetal month and become the sole site of granulocyte and megakaryocyte proliferation.[1] Erythropoiesis moves from the liver to the marrow by the end of the last trimester. Cellular morphology, and the specific make-up of the hemoglobin produced in embryonic hematopoietic sites, changes as the location of hematopoiesis changes. This observation led to speculation that the stem cells of these various periods may be of separate origins.[12]

Embryologically, hemoglobin is produced with information from two different genetic loci. The α globin gene cluster codes for ζ globulin, an embryonic globulin, and α globulin, the adult form.[59] The β globulin gene family codes for the embryonic globulins ε and λ, in addition to the two adult globulins Δ and β. The expression of genes in each family changes during embryonic, fetal, neonatal, and adult development.[55] Until 8 weeks of intrauterine life, λ, α, ε, and ζ chains are produced and assembled in

various combinations. These hemoglobins are produced in red cells that originate in yolk sac-derived erythrocytes. With the shift in erythropoiesis from yolk sac to fetal liver and spleen, embryonic hemoglobin is no longer detectable.[55] The α and λ globin chains pair up to produce fetal hemoglobin (HgbF). Red cells containing HgbF have a higher O_2 affinity than does adult hemoglobin, conferring a survival advantage on the fetus in the relatively hypoxic intrauterine environment.[5]

Bone Marrow Anatomy

The arterial blood supply of the bone marrow comes from nutrient arteries, which penetrate the outer cortex and form periosteal capillaries (see Fig. 25–2). Blood from these two systems mixes and enters the marrow sinus system, from which blood drains into the systemic circulation via emissary veins.[74]

In mammals, blood formation takes place in marrow spaces between the venous sinuses. The developing blood cells are closely and systematically related to the sinuses and must traverse the wall of the sinus before entering the general circulation.[88] The sinus wall is composed of a layer of endothelial cells, a thin basement membrane and a layer of adventitial reticular cells that form the outer layer and the cell layer in closest approximation to the hematopoietic spaces.[73] A central arteriole runs along the hematopoietic spaces. Granulopoietic cells are distributed along the walls of the central arteriole. Erythropoietic cells are distributed in a continuous network of cords around the sinus wall.[88] In this setting, erythrocytes are found closely associated with

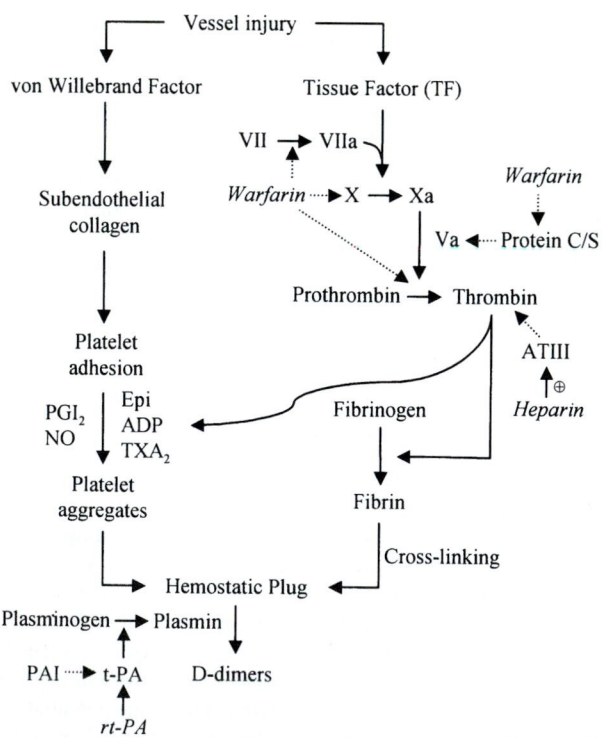

Figure 25–2. The relationships between thrombosis, coagulation and fibrinolysis. Although these pathways are shown independently, they are intricately linked as outlined in the text. Dotted lines indicate inhibition; drug effects are shown in italics. ATIII, antithrombin III; PAI, plasminogen activator inhibitor; t-PA, tissue plasminogen activator; rt-PA, recombinant t-PA.

macrophages whose function may be to phagocytose extruded nuclear material resulting from red cell and megakaryocyte development.[74] Megakaryocytes exist in close proximity to the surface of the sinus wall.[73] Mature cells apparently enter the systemic circulation by passing through the cytoplasm of the endothelial cells.[146] Progenitor cells must interact with a supportive microenvironment to sustain hematopoiesis. The hematopoietic stroma consists of macrophages, fibroblasts, adipocytes, and endothelial cells.[74] The extracellular matrix is composed of various fibrous proteins, glycoproteins, and proteoglycans, which are produced by the stromal cells and include collagen, fibronectin, laminin, hemonectin, thrombospondin, and proteoglycans.[12,70,73] Hematopoietic progenitor cells have receptors that bind to particular matrix molecules. The extracellular matrix provides a structural network to which the progenitors are anchored. As the cells approach maturity, they lose their surface receptors, presumptively allowing them to leave the hematopoietic space and enter the venous sinuses. Blood cell release depends upon the development of a pressure gradient that drives mature cells through channels in endothelial cell cytoplasm.[22,146] Pressure within the marrow is increased by erythropoietin and by GCSF.[57,58]

Aplastic Anemia

Aplastic anemia is a disease of the blood characterized by pancytopenia on peripheral smear and a hypocellular marrow. It is generally defined by numbers of circulating cells, particularly a granulocyte count of less than 500 cells/mm³, platelets of less than 20,000/mm³, and reticulocytes of less than 1%. Approximately 1000 new cases are diagnosed yearly in the United States. The incidence is much higher in Asia, presumably because of the greater prevalence of the hepatitis B virus. The fatality rate, while much improved over the previous century, remains at about 50%.[132] Aplastic anemia may be inborn (as in Fanconi's anemia) or acquired. Specific etiologies of acquired aplastic anemia include certain medications (see Table 25–1), radiation, benzene, pregnancy, viruses, and some rheumatic syndromes, such as rheumatoid arthritis and eosinophilic fasciitis.[14,151] While much of the pathophysiology of aplastic anemia has been defined over the past 30 years, there remain some gaps in our understanding. Generally speaking, the mechanism is believed to include the acquisition of intrinsic defects of the hematopoietic stem cells, and abnormal humoral and cellular immune control of hematopoiesis. Stem cells may be reduced to less than 1% of normal in patients with aplastic anemia.[152] The bone marrow stroma is not defective and produces normal or increased amounts of growth factors.[152] Since the 1970s it has been recognized that the immunosuppressive regimen used in preparation for bone marrow transplantation has resulted in improvements in the pancytopenia in patients with acquired aplastic anemia.[19,77,152]

Drug-Induced Immune-Mediated Causes of Aplastic Anemia. It is now believed that the majority of cases of aplastic anemia previously determined to be idiosyncratic are caused by immunologically mediated tissue specific destruction of CD34+ hematopoietic progenitor cells.[150,152] Following an exposure to an inciting antigen, T cells and cytokines act destructively on stem cells, reducing their numbers so that normal levels of circulating mature leukocytes, erythrocytes and platelets fall to dangerously low levels.[150] Toxicity may be mediated through intermediate metabolites that bind covalently to protein and DNA.[150] These reactive metabolites

TABLE 25–1. Chemical and Physical Agents Associated with the Development of Aplastic Anemia

Analgesics	Acetaminophen
	Acetylsalicylic acid
	Diclofenac
	Dipyrone
	Indomethacin
	Phenylbutazone
Antibiotics	Azothymidine
	Chloramphenicol
	Mephloquine
	Penicillin
Anticonvulsants	Carbamazepine
	Felbamate
Antidysrhythmics	Tocainide
Antihistamines	Cimetidine
Antiplatelet agents	Ticlopidine
Antipsychotics, sedatives	Chlorpromazine
	Clozapine
	Methyprylon
Antirheumatics	D-Penicillamine
	Gold salts
	Methotrexate, low dose
Antithyroid agents	Propylthiouracil
Diuretics	Acetazolamide
	Metazolone
Occupational Agents	Arsenic
	Benzene
	Cadmium
	Copper
	Pesticides
Agents that will predictably produce marrow hypoplasia or aplasia with a large enough exposure	Antibiotics (daunorubicin, adriamycin)
	Antimetabolites (purine and pyrimidine analogues)
	Antimitotics (colchicine, vincristine, vinblastine)
	Arsenic, inorganic
	Benzene
	Radiation, ionizing
	Sulfur or nitrogen mustard

are formed and degraded by complex metabolic pathways; genetic variation in the enzyme systems involved may contribute to the rarity of idiosyncratic drug reactions.[151] HLA DR2 is overrepresented among European and American patients with aplastic anemia. Clozapine-induced agranulocytosis is associated with the HLA B38, DR4, and the DQ3 haplotypes, underlining a genetic predisposition to acquired aplastic anemia.[91]

The peripheral blood and bone marrow of patients with aplastic anemia produces a soluble factor identified as interferon-γ (INF-γ) that inhibits hematopoiesis; normal lymphocytes can be stimulated to produce the same factor.[8,153] Both the blood and bone marrow of patients with aplastic anemia contain increased numbers of activated cytotoxic lymphocytes. The numbers and activity of activated cells decreases with immunosuppressive therapy.[67,103] The T cells of patients with aplastic anemia overproduce INF-γ and tumor necrosis factor (TNF).[140] Both cytokines are capable of suppressing proliferating early and late hematopoietic progenitor and stem cells.[119] In addition to the inhibition of the mitotic cycle, it is likely that the pathology includes the induction of programmed cell death through the induced expression (by TNF and INF-γ) of the Fas receptor on CD34+ progenitor cells. Fas (cluster designation 95 or CD95) is a receptor molecule that mediates signal transduction for apoptosis, or programmed cell death. Apoptosis is a morphologic pattern of genetically programmed cell death marked by cell shrinkage, condensation of chromatin, the formation of cytoplasmic blebs, and the fragmentation of the cell into membrane bound bodies that are eliminated by phagocytosis. It is a physiologic mechanism for cell deletion in the regulation of cell populations. Fas is a member of the TNF receptor family. Engagement of the Fas receptor by another cell surface molecule triggers apoptosis in the Fas-expressing cell. The initial focus of immune attack may be limited, however, as tissues are damaged, the exposure of previously hidden cellular antigens increases the range of immune targets in a process known as antigenic spread.[35] In normal individuals, Fas is rarely expressed on CD34+ cells. In patients with aplastic anemia, CD34+ bone marrow cells express Fas receptors to a much greater extent, resulting in anti-Fas antibody-mediated inhibition of hematopoiesis.[75,89] The genes for INF-γ and TNF are overexpressed in the marrow and blood cells of patients with aplastic anemia. The expression of Fas is also associated with infection by viruses implicated in marrow suppression such as the human immunodeficiency virus (HIV) and hepatitis C.[92] INF-γ expression is eliminated in patients successfully treated with immunosuppressive therapy, usually with antithymocyte globulin, cyclosporine, or cyclophosphamide. INF-γ again becomes detectable in those patients who have relapsed following therapy. It is not detectable in patients with Fanconi's anemia.[92]

Benzene

The toxicity of benzene very likely involves a combination of direct toxic as well as immune-mediated mechanisms. A ubiquitous solvent, it is a component of gasoline and a constituent of engine emissions and tobacco smoke.[149] The first cases of benzene toxicity to the hematopoietic system were reported in 1897.[126] Benzene is absorbed into the blood, and translocated to the liver where it is metabolized by the cytochrome P4502E1 enzyme system to its major metabolite, phenol. Susceptibility to benzene induced injury may be increased by high liver cytochrome P4502E1 activity and a low intake of folic acid.[126] Phenol is further oxidized by the same enzyme system to hydroquinone and catechol.[129] Phenol and hydroquinone can partition into blood and distribute to other tissues, including bone marrow. Benzene has relatively little hepatic toxicity but is highly toxic to the bone marrow. It appears that benzene metabolites are kept in their reduced, relatively nontoxic state in the liver, whereas the bone marrow contains high levels of enzymes capable of oxidizing benzene metabolites to reactive intermediates. In bone marrow, secondary activation to toxic quinones and free radicals by peroxidase enzymes results in the induction of apoptosis, damage to the DNA of bone marrow cells, altered differentiation in early progenitor pools and the depletion of the stem cell pool.[126] In addition, benzene may directly damage the hematopoietic microenvironment.

Ionizing Radiation

Immature and rapidly dividing cells are sensitive to injury from ionizing radiation. Stem cells and progenitor cells are injured and fail to proliferate with doses of greater than 1.5–2 Gy (Chap. 99). Following a significant exposure, nondividing cells, such as mature erythrocytes, neutrophils, and platelets, disappear from circulation at a rate that is determined by their natural life span. Neutrophils begin to disappear within 4 days, platelets within

7 days, and red cells within 120 days. For unknown reasons, lymphocytes, which are an exception to this general rule, are rapidly lysed and undergo interphase death. Whole-body radiation rapidly produces profound lymphopenia and immunosuppression. Death from this bone marrow syndrome generally occurs 14–28 days after exposure from infection related to lymphopenia, granulocytopenia, or hemorrhage from thrombocytopenia.[23]

THE RED CELL

The mature erythrocyte is a highly specialized cell composed of a phospholipid bilayer membrane surrounding a solution of electrolytes and protein. Hemoglobin constitutes 95% of the dry weight of the erythrocyte; the remaining 5% is composed of enzymes for energy production and for the maintenance of hemoglobin in its reduced, oxygen-carrying state. The red cell lacks cytoplasmic organelles and is incapable of reproduction or the synthesis of new protein. It contains no mitochondria so it cannot carry out the oxidative energy producing reactions that take place in most highly oxygenated cells. Rather, it has to rely on the anaerobic conversion of glucose to lactate, and glucose oxidation through the pentose phosphate pathway for energy production[137] (Chap. 13).

The red cell is shaped like a biconcave disc. This architecture maximizes the ratio of surface area to volume, and ensures the efficient transfer of gases.[69] It gives the red cell the property of deformability, thereby optimizing movement within the microvasculature.[17,117] Elastic and electrostatic forces within the membrane, surface tension, and osmotic and hydrostatic pressures maintain the shape of the erythrocyte. The limiting membrane is a double layer of phospholipids with globular proteins floating within it.[123,131] The majority of the lipids are phospholipids and cholesterol. Cholesterol markedly decreases membrane fluidity and increases viscosity.[30] The major blood group antigens are carried on membrane ceramide glycolipids and proteins, particularly glycophorin A and the Rh proteins.[21] Some membrane proteins serve as ion-exchange pumps or channels. Others, such as actin and spectrin, are essential for the maintenance of normal red cell structure.[116] Ankyrin serves as an anchor for the attachment of the cytoskeletal proteins.[66] Other essential structural proteins include tropomyosin, tropomodulin, and adducin. Absence or abnormalities of any of these proteins results in abnormal red cell shapes such as spherocytes and elliptocytes.[137]

Transport Proteins

Many specialized transport proteins are embedded in the red cell membrane. These include anion and cation transporters, glucose and urea transporters, and water channels.[4,86,95,136] Band 3 anion-exchange protein plays an important role in the chloride-bicarbonate exchanges that occur as the red cell moves between the lung and tissues.[137] Glucose, the sole source of energy of the red cell, crosses the membrane by facilitated diffusion mediated by a transmembrane protein designated as the glucose transporter.[86] The erythrocyte membrane is relatively impermeable to ion flux. The major intracellular cation is potassium, with sodium present in a much lower concentration. As the plasma is much higher in sodium and lower in potassium, an active transport mechanism must exist to maintain this transmembrane gradient. Passive diffusion tends to drive sodium inward and potassium outward.

Sodium-potassium ATPase Na$^+$-K$^+$ ATPase works against diffusion, pumping sodium out of the erythrocyte and potassium into the cytoplasm.[52,109] For every 3 sodium ions pumped out, 2 potassium ions are pumped in and 1 molecule of ATP is consumed. This results in a net loss of 1 positive charge, which is compensated for by the extrusion of a chloride ion. The cardiac glycosides bind to and inhibit the activity of (Na$^+$-K$^+$ ATPase). One result of this is the extracellular accumulation of K$^+$, and the potential for hyperkalemia when cardiac glycosides are present at toxic concentrations. Acute fluoride intoxication increases intracellular calcium and stimulates potassium efflux through effects on the calcium-dependent potassium channels.[82] This may contribute to the potentially lethal hyperkalemia that may result from fluoride toxicity.[32]

Membrane-Associated Enzymes

At least 50 membrane-bound or -associated enzymes are known to exist in the human erythrocyte. Acetylcholinesterase is an externally oriented red cell bound enzyme whose role in the function of the erythrocyte remains obscure.[26] Its absence, with other glycosyl phosphatidyl inositol-linked proteins, is associated with paroxysmal nocturnal hemoglobinuria, apparently resulting from an abnormal susceptibility of erythrocytes to complement mediated lysis.[26,27,113] Its function is inhibited by certain poisons, most notably the organic phosphorus insecticides, and can be used as a marker for exposure to these chemicals. Membrane-bound enzymes required for the production and consumption of energy include aldolase, glyceraldehyde-3-phosphate dehydrogenase and phosphoglycerate kinase. Adenyl cyclase, protein kinases, and adenosine triphosphatases catalyze the conversion of ATP to cyclic AMP. In turn, cyclic AMP activates a number of membrane-bound protein kinases, and serves as a second messenger in the regulation of certain metabolic processes, including the action of many peptide hormones.

Hemolysis

Glucose-6-Phosphate Dehydrogenase Deficiencies.

Glucose-6-phosphate dehydrogenase (G6PD) catalyzes the first step of the pentose phosphate shunt: the conversion of G6PD to phosphogluconolactone. In the process, NADP$^+$ is reduced to NADPH, a chemical that is necessary to maintain the supply of reduced glutathione. Glultathione provides the red cells' main defense against oxidation. In the presence of powerful oxidant drugs or chemicals, the supply of glutathione becomes exhausted and an attack on free sulfhydryl groups occurs. Intermediates implicated in this process include H$_2$O$_2$ and superoxide anion radicals.[28] Hemoglobin and other cellular elements may become denatured. Heme is released from globin, and the protein chain unfolds and precipitates within the erythrocyte as insoluble aggregates or Heinz bodies. The Heinz bodies attach to red cell membranes, compromising deformability and resulting in removal by liver or spleen reticuloendothelial cells.[10]

A large number of variants of G6PD exist, which results in differences in enzyme activities among individuals. Deficient activity of G6PD may result from decreased enzyme synthesis, altered catalytic activity, or reduced stability of the enzyme. The gene that encodes for G6PD is X-linked, thus males are affected more severely than females. In females, because of the random nature of X-chromosome inactivation, the blood of heterozygotes may have

a range of G6PD activity between 0 and 100%, and the severity of hemolysis varies.[62]

Clinically, hemolysis may ensue in susceptible individuals beginning 2–4 days following the ingestion of an offending agent (see Table 25–2). Jaundice, pallor, and dark urine may occur with abdominal and back pain. A decrease in the concentration of hemoglobin occurs. The peripheral smear demonstrates cell fragments and cells that have had Heinz bodies "bitten" from them. Bone marrow stimulation results in a reticulocytosis and an increased red cell mass. Newly formed cells have the highest activity of G6PD, and therefore are more resistant to hemolysis. In general, a normal bone marrow can compensate for ongoing hemolysis, and can return the hemoglobin concentration to normal. During an episode of hemolysis, the cells with the least G6PD activity (those with a genetically determined deficiency and those that are senescent) are hemolyzed first. The cells with adequate G6PD activity survive; thus, the measurement of the activity of G6PD following a hemolytic episode may be misleading.[50] Drugs and toxins that represent oxidative stressors for red cells are listed in Table 25–2.

Immune-Mediated Hemolytic Anemia

The immune-mediated hemolytic anemias occur when ingested drugs or environmental toxins trigger an antigen antibody reaction (see Table 25–3). In general, drug molecules are too small to be sensitizing agents. Antigenicity is acquired following the binding of drug molecules to carrier proteins in blood. The particulars of the drug carrier immune activation sequence form the basis for the classification of this group of hemolytic anemias.[121]

The first class of reaction occurs when the drug acts as a hapten and binds to membrane proteins on the surface of the red cell. This results in the fixation of complement by IgG, and subsequent splenic sequestration and hemolysis.[121] The hemolytic anemia triggered in certain patients by penicillin represents the prototype of this reaction.[40]

The second class of reaction is mediated by immune complexes and occurs with drugs that have a low affinity for cellular membranes. Small doses of drugs result in hemolysis, and red cell injury is primarily mediated by complement. Complexes of drug and IgM are implicated as the complement trigger in this second process.[121]

The third class of reaction occurs when the presence of drug induces the formation of antibody to cellular components (as with α-methyldopa).[68] This is a true autoantibody reaction directed

TABLE 25–2. Drugs and Chemicals That Cause Hemolytic Anemia in Patients with G6PD Deficiency

Acetanilid
Diphenylsulfone (Dapsone)
Methylene blue
Nalidixic acid
Naphthalene
Niridazole
Nitrofurantoin
Pamaquine
Pentaquine
Primaquine

Adapted from Beutler E, Lichtman MA, Coller BS, et al, eds: William's Hematology, 5th ed. New York, McGraw-Hill, 1995.

TABLE 25–3.   Etiologies of Hemolysis

Immune Mediated
  Type I: Drug–red cell complex; IgG triggers complement
  Type II: Immune complex mediated; IgM triggers complement
  Type III: True autoimmune to red cell membrane

Nonimmune Mediated
  Arsine gas
  Copper sulfate
  G6PD deficiency
  Hypo-osmolality
  Hypophosphatemia
  Lead
  Snake venoms
  Spider venoms

against red cell surface antigen.[9] The severity of hemolysis is variable. In certain cases, transfusion is required to replace red cells. In general, resolution of the hemolytic process is complete with withdrawal of the responsible agent.

Nonimmune-Mediated Nonoxidant Causes of Hemolysis

Arsine.   Arsine is a colorless, odorless, nonirritating gas that is 2.5 times denser than air (Chap. 79). It is produced by the action of water on a metallic arsenide. Poisonings are associated with the admixture of acids and crude metals that contain arsenic as an impurity. Workers involved in galvanizing, soldering, etching, lead plating, and computer microchip processing are at risk for poisoning. Acute toxicity is associated with a 25% mortality rate.[18] Clinical signs and symptoms appear 2–24 hours after exposure and may include headache, malaise, dyspnea, abdominal pain with nausea and vomiting, hepatomegaly, hemolysis with hemoglobinuric renal failure, and death.[18,102] The peripheral smear of arsine-poisoned patients shows all of the typical abnormalities associated with hemolytic anemia. The mechanism of hemolysis is believed to involve the fixation of arsine by hemoglobin.[44] The oxidation of arsine apparently yields arsenic dihydride as an intermediate, and finally elementary arsenic. Either of these products could be the hemolytic agent.

All heavy metals, including arsenic, have an affinity for sulfhydryl groups. One author proposed that the complexing of arsenic derivatives with red cell sulfhydryl groups results in an impairment of the Na^+-K^+-ATPase that is necessary for cell membrane stability.[72] It appears that chronic exposure to low levels of arsine can produce clinically significant disease. Chronic low-grade hemolysis is reported in workers exposed to arsine during the cyanide extraction of gold.[18] Arsine poisoning should, therefore, be included in the differential diagnosis of hemolytic anemia (Chap. 79).

The treatment of choice is cessation of exposure and possibly exchange transfusion in severe cases. Adequate hydration and, possibly, alkalinization of the urine may be useful to protect against hemoglobin cast formation.

Copper Sulfate.   Copper sulfate is widely used in India in the whitewashing and leather industries. Although no data are available on the incidence of this poisoning in the United States, in India its availability results in its frequent ingestion both accidentally and in suicide attempts.

Symptoms following ingestion include a metallic taste, nausea, vomiting, epigastric burning, and gastrointestinal hemorrhage. Methemoglobinemia, hemolysis, renal failure, and death are frequently reported[134] (Chap. 82).

An in vitro study in which human erythrocytes were incubated with copper sulfate showed a 10-fold enhancement in oxidation of NADPH, inhibition of glycolysis in the pentose phosphate shunt, and inhibition of G6PD.[37] Similar results were found after incubating red cells with cupric acetate.[33] Each of these phenomena probably contributes to the hemolytic effect of copper sulfate. Treatment is supportive with transfusions, volume replacement, and hemodialysis performed as indicated. Table 25–3 summarizes the causes of immune and nonimmune-mediated hemolysis.

Hemoglobin

Hemoglobin is the major constituent of the cytoplasm of the red cell. Hemoglobin is a conjugated protein with a molecular weight of 64,500 daltons. Each molecule is composed of 4 protein or globin chains, each attached to a porphyrin ring called *heme*. An iron molecule is complexed at the center of the porphyrin ring. The assembly and integrity of the molecule depends upon electrostatic forces.[120] Hemoglobin is so efficient at binding and carrying oxygen that it enables blood to transport 100 times as much oxygen as could be carried by plasma alone. In addition, the capacity of hemoglobin to bind oxygen under different conditions of oxygen availability and demand allows adaptation to a wide variety of environments and energy use patterns. Three complex metabolic pathways are required for the formation of hemoglobin. These include globin synthesis, heme synthesis, and iron absorption, transport, and incorporation into the porphyrin ring.

Globin Synthesis.   The active genetic regions that encode the structure of globin constitute the euchromatin of nuclear material of the erythroblast. Globin is transcribed from genetic loci, translated by ribosomal messenger RNA (mRNA), and the polypeptide chains assembled as other proteins. The rate of globin synthesis is increased in the presence of heme, and inhibited in its absence.[79] Distinct structural genetic loci exist for all of the known normal hemoglobins. These include α, β, γ, Δ, and ϵ loci. As the globin chains are released from the ribosomes, they spontaneously assemble into α/β dimers and α_2/β_2 tetramers. Vitamins B_{12} and folate are essential for DNA synthesis. They serve as cofactors in the methylation of deoxyuridine monophosphate to deoxythymidine monophosphate. A deficiency of B_{12} or folate may result from nutritional factors, or the use of the folate antagonists methotrexate and trimethoprim. Typically, the result is a macrocytic anemia.[108] The thalassemias, a group of inherited disorders, result from defective synthesis of one or more of the globin chains. Clinically this results in a hypochromic, microcytic anemia.[45,79]

Heme Synthesis.   Heme is the iron complex of protoporphyrin IX. Protoporphyrin IX is a tetramer composed of 4 porphyrin rings joined in a closed ring structure. All animal cells can synthesize heme, with the exception of mature erythrocytes.[106] Hemoproteins are involved in a multitude of biologic functions, including oxygen binding (hemoglobin, myoglobin), oxygen metabolism (oxidases, peroxidases, catalases, and hydroxylases), and electron transport (cytochromes).[13,107] Large amounts of heme are synthesized in liver and erythroid cells, where it is utilized for hemoglobin, as well as mitochondrial cytochromes, and as prosthetic groups for cytochrome P450. Erythroid cells synthesize 85% of total body heme. Hemoglobin is the most abundant hemoprotein, containing 70% of total body iron.[106]

The first step in the synthesis of heme takes place in the mitochondrion and is the condensation of glycine and succinyl CoA to form Δ-aminolevulinic acid (ΔALA) (see Fig. 80–5).[13,79] Succinyl CoA is produced by the oxidative decarboxylation of α-ketoglutarate via the Krebs cycle. The formation of ΔALA is catalyzed by ALA synthase (ALAS). Two isoforms of ALAS are known to exist, ALAS 1 and ALAS 2. Erythroid cells contain the ALAS 2 isoform. Nonerythroid cells contain the ALAS 1 isoform. This enzyme appears to control the rate of heme biosynthesis in the liver through heme-mediated negative feedback inhibition.[106] Pyridoxal phosphate (vitamin B_6) serves as a cofactor in this reaction. The clinical consequences of pyridoxine deficiency may include a hypochromic, microcytic anemia, iron overload, and neurologic impairment. Medications that increase the rate of synthesis of ΔALA (Table 25–4) may precipitate an inducible porphyric crisis.[34,107] This may occur in hepatocytes through drug-mediated induction in the rate of transcription of the ALAS 1 gene.[79] The result is an accumulation of porphyrins, which may result in a clinical syndrome of abdominal pain and neuropsychiatric symptoms.

Following synthesis, ΔALA is transported from the mitochondria to the cytosol in preparation for the next step in heme biosynthesis. It is likely that specific heme binding proteins are involved in the intracellular transport of heme. Some proteins that may mediate this transport include liver fatty-acid-binding protein and glutathione-S-transferase.[107] The next step in the synthesis of hemoglobin is the formation of the monopyrrole porphobilinogen via the condensation of 2 molecules of ALA. This reaction is catalyzed by ALA dehydratase. This enzyme requires zinc and free sulfhydryl groups for its normal activity and is inhibited by lead.

TABLE 25–4. Medications Known to be Unsafe in Patients with Inducible Porphyria

Aminoglutethimide
Barbiturates
Carbamazepine
Carisprodol
Chloroquine
Chlorpropamide
Danazol
Diclofenac
Ergot alkaloids
Ethanol
Ethchlorvynol
Glutethimide
Griseofulvin
Mephenytoin
Meprobamate
Methyprylon
Phenytoin
Primidone
Progestins
Pyrazolones
Sulfonamides
Tolbutamide
Trimethadione
Valproic acid

Porphobilinogen is excreted in large quantities by patients with acute intermittent porphyria. The breakdown product, porphobilinogen, colors the urine a deep red wine color.[13]

In the next two steps in heme synthesis, 4 molecules of porphobilinogen condense to form the ring open macrocycle, hydroxymethylbilane. This reaction is catalyzed by hydroxymethylbilane synthase. The loss of an amino group closes the ring to form uroporphyrinogen III, a reaction catalyzed by uroporphyrinogen III synthase.

Enzymatic decarboxylation of the four acetic side chains of uroporphyrinogen III results in coproporphyrinogen III. This reaction is catalyzed by uroporphyrinogen decarboxylase. Coproporphyrinogen III is transported back into the mitochondrion by an unknown mechanism. Oxidative decarboxylation of coproporphyrinogen III by coproporphyrinogen oxidase results in the formation of protoporphyrinogen III. Protoporphyrinogen III is oxidized to protoporphyrin IX by a mitochondrial oxidizing enzyme, protoporphyrinogen IX oxidase. The final step is the insertion of iron into protoporphyrin IX, a reaction that is catalyzed by ferrochelatase to form heme. In red blood cells this last reaction is the likely site of feedback inhibition of heme, thus controlling the rate of heme synthesis.[13,106]

Most steps in the heme biosynthetic pathway are inhibited by lead (Chap. 80). ALA dehydratase is the most sensitive, followed by ferrochelatase, coproporphyrinogen oxidase, and PBG deaminase. As a consequence, urinary ALA is greatly increased.

Erythropoietin. Erythropoietin (EPO) is a glycoprotein hormone of molecular weight (MW) 34,000 daltons that is produced in the epithelial cells lining the peritubular capillaries in the normal kidney. Anemia and hypoxemia stimulate its synthesis.[2,3] EPO receptors have been identified in human erythroid cells, megakaryocytes, and fetal liver. EPO promotes erythroid differentiation, the mobilization of marrow progenitor cells, and the premature release of marrow reticulocytes.[2] The cell most sensitive to EPO is a cell between the erythroid colony-forming unit (CFU-E) and the proerythroblast.[3] In the absence of EPO, rapid DNA cleavage, in a pattern characteristic of apoptosis, results in erythroid cell death.

Iron Metabolism. Total body iron content is about 55 mg/kg in adult men and about 45 mg/kg in adult women.[105] Very little iron is lost from the body; only in epithelial cells sloughed from the gastrointestinal tract, and in women during times of menstrual bleeding and pregnancy. Iron is not excreted; unbound plasma iron is rapidly distributed to hepatic parenchymal cells and to other tissues regardless of their need for iron. The average daily iron loss is estimated at no more than 4 mg. The control of total body iron content takes place at the level of absorption.[29] Unless appropriately chelated, excess iron (not bound by transport or storage proteins) can play a key role in the formation of harmful oxygen radicals that can damage cellular structures (Chap. 12).[105] As such, iron must be bound at all times to the transfer protein, transferrin, or stored in the form of ferritin. Exposure of ferritin to ionizing radiation, redox recycling xenobiotics such as paraquat, doxorubicin, and alloxan, or to high levels of nitric oxide can liberate iron. Iron and superoxide may initiate lipid peroxidation as well as DNA damage.[81]

Iron is absorbed from the gut passively during times of dietary excess.[142] When iron intake is less, active mechanisms are used. Two absorptive mechanisms are employed: one for the absorption of heme iron (dietary iron derived from meat products), and another for inorganic iron. Ingested hemoglobin is degraded to heme and globin. The globin degradation products apparently play a role in solubilizing heme so that it remains available for absorption. In this state, it enters the intestinal mucosal cell as an intact metalloporphyrin.[141] Unlike other nucleated cells, the luminal surfaces of absorptive cells contain no transferrin receptors. Ferric iron is chelated to surface mucin, crosses the luminal membrane in association with a duodenal surface integrin and becomes bound by the cytoplasmic proteins mobilferritin and paraferritin.[29,141] It may, over the next few hours be mobilized into plasma or incorporated into mucosal ferritin where, if not mobilized, it is lost in 3–4 days when the cell is sloughed. The amount of iron transported through plasma depends on total body iron stores and the rate of erythropoiesis. It is likely that transferrin bound iron is a regulator of heme synthesis.[3,106] The formation of ALAS in human erythroid cells is limited by the availability of iron. Normally, transferrin is about 30% bound with iron.[105,106]

The only physiologically active chelate that can provide iron for hemoglobin synthesis is transferrin.[106] Iron bound to transferrin is delivered to the hemoglobin-producing erythroid cells. The iron-transferrin complex binds to transferrin receptors on the surface of developing erythroid cells in bone marrow. Internalization of the iron-transferrin complex by receptor-mediated endocytosis is followed by cleavage of iron from the transferrin complex. The receptor returns the transferrin molecule to the cell surface, where it is released into the extracellular compartment.[2] Iron in the erythroid cell is used for hemoglobin synthesis or is stored in the form of ferritin. Lead limits the delivery of iron to ferrochelatase. The surrogate metal, zinc, is inserted into protoporphyrin, resulting in the accumulation of zinc protoporphyrin, and contributing to the anemia of lead poisoning.

After the red cell life span is complete at 120 days, it is engulfed by splenic macrophages. Heme is degraded by heme oxygenase to carbon monoxide and biliverdin, and the iron is extracted from hemoglobin.[105] Some iron may remain in macrophages in the form of ferritin or hemosiderin. Most is delivered back to the plasma where it is again bound to transferrin. Lead increases the rate of red cell destruction by inhibiting membrane Na^+-K^+-ATPase, resulting in the loss of intracellular K^+ and increased mechanical fragility.

Oxygen-Carbon Dioxide Exchange.   The binding of oxygen to one of the iron molecules in heme results in conformational changes that facilitate binding of oxygen at the other three sites. This phenomenon is known as cooperativity, which also facilitates the unbinding of oxygen at tissue sites. The phenomenon of cooperativity results in the sigmoidal shape of the oxyhemoglobin dissociation curve (Chap. 20). It assures the ease of oxygen unbinding in conditions of pH and oxygen tension found in tissues. The affinity of oxygen for hemoglobin is affected by pH. The oxyhemoglobin dissociation curve shifts to the left in lungs, where the level of carbon dioxide, and thus carbonic acid, are kept relatively low as a result of ventilation, an effect that promotes oxygen binding. The curve shifts to the right in tissues where cellular respiration keeps the level of CO_2 relatively high. This phenomenon, known as the *Bohr effect*, promotes the release of oxygen at tissue sites.[7,111] A by-product of the Rapoport-Luebering shunt is 2,3 diphosphoglycerate (2,3-DPG). 2,3-DPG binds to hemoglobin and decreases its O_2 affinity resulting in greater oxygen unbinding at tissue sites.[24] This is one mechanism of adaptation to

high-altitude environments in which the ambient O_2 tension is lower than at sea level.

Carbon dioxide transport does not involve direct binding to hemoglobin. Carbon dioxide diffuses into red cells where, to overcome its low water solubility, it is hydrated through the action of carbonic anhydrase, which spontaneously dissociates to H^+ and HCO_3^-. The hydrogen ion liberated in this reaction is accepted by deoxyhemoglobin. The band 3 anion exchange transporter located in the red cell membrane, mediates the rapid exchange of bicarbonate with plasma chloride, a process known as the *chloride shift*.[136] The bicarbonate is carried in plasma to the lungs where the relatively low CO_2 tension facilitates the reverse reaction, the formation of CO_2 from bicarbonate, and its subsequent elimination.[137]

Abnormal Hemoglobins

Methemoglobin.   Methemoglobin is an abnormal hemoglobin in which the iron is in the oxidized or ferric (Fe^{+3}) valence state. Normally, in deoxygenated hemoglobin, the heme iron is in the "high spin" or ferrous (Fe^{+2}) valence state. In this state, there are 6 electrons in the outer shell, 4 of which are unpaired. When oxygen is bound, one of these electrons is partially transferred to it and the iron is reversibly oxidized. When O_2 is released, the electron is transferred back to heme iron, yielding the normal reduced state. Sometimes, the electron remains with the O_2 yielding a superoxide anion ($O_2\cdot$) rather than molecular oxygen. In this case heme iron is left in the Fe^{+3} or oxidized state and is unable to release another electron to bind oxygen.[137] It is normally reduced by a set of enzymes in the red cell, including cytochrome b5 methemoglobin reductase, also known as NADH methemoglobin reductase, an enzyme that requires the presence of the electron carrier NADH.[56] Minor pathways are also involved in methemoglobin reduction, including NADPH methemoglobin reductase, which normally reduces only about 5% of the methemoglobin, and vitamin C, a direct reducing agent. The activity of NADPH methemoglobin reductase may be significantly accelerated by the presence of the electron donor methylene blue (see Antidotes in Depth: Methylene Blue and Chap. 94) or riboflavin.[60] Many chemicals and pharmaceutic agents are capable of increasing the rate of hemoglobin oxidation as much as 1000-fold. Nitrites, nitrates, chlorates, and quinones are capable of directly oxidizing hemoglobin. The mechanism of toxicity is not well understood but is related to the production of an oxidative stress that overwhelms normal cellular mechanism for reduction. Some compounds are metabolized in vivo to active intermediates that oxidize hemoglobin, including acetanilide, phenacetin, and aniline dyes.

Fetal hemoglobin is more susceptible to oxidation as compared with adult hemoglobin. Hgb-F also has a limited capacity to reduce methemoglobin caused by a significant decrease in soluble NADH-cytochrome b5 reductase. Levels of this enzyme reach adult levels by about 6 months of age.[25]

Carboxyhemoglobin.   Carbon monoxide (CO) is a ligand that binds reversibly to heme iron in the ferrous state. The affinity of CO for hemoglobin is 200–300 times that of oxygen. It thereby occupies oxygen-binding sites, acting as a cellular asphyxiant. In addition, CO binding with hemoglobin results in the loss of the cooperative unbinding of oxygen. The oxyhemoglobin dissociation curve is shifted to the left, reflecting the fact that oxygen is more tightly bound by hemoglobin, depriving tissues of oxygen. In addition, CO binds to myoglobin and to cytochromes, interfering with cellular respiration, exacerbating the clinical symptoms of hypoxia.[46] For further details see Chapter 97.

Sulfhemoglobin. Sulfhemoglobin, which is derived from the oxidative denaturation of hemoglobin, is a green-pigmented molecule that contains an extra sulfur atom in one or more of the porphyrin rings. It is believed that the sulfur atom is attached to a β carbon in the porphyrin ring, not at the normal oxygen-binding site. It has a spectrophotometric absorption band at approximately 618 nm. It is ineffective in oxygen transport and clinically produces cyanosis. Sulfhemoglobin results from the irreversible oxidation of hemoglobin by certain drugs and chemicals, most notable acetanilide, phenacetin, the sulfonamides, and certain chemical exposures, such as hydrogen sulfide. Sulfhemoglobin may be produced from methemoglobin in the presence of sulfur. The oxygen affinity of sulfhemoglobin is approximately 100 times less than that of oxyhemoglobin, shifting the oxyhemoglobin dissociation curve to the right, in favor of O_2 unbinding. Thus, the symptoms of hypoxia are not as severe with sulfhemoglobinemia as with carboxy- or methemoglobinemia[99] (Chap. 94).

NEUTROPHILIC LEUKOCYTES

Neutrophils (polymorphonuclear leukocytes or PMNs) provide the primary defense against the invasion of bacterial and fungal pathogens. Neutrophilic response does not depend upon prior exposure to pathogens. These cells emerge from bone marrow with the biochemical and metabolic machinery needed for the efficient killing of microorganisms. Neutrophils are activated when circulating cells detect low levels of chemokines released from sites of inflammation.[76] Upon activation by invading organisms, they undergo conformational and biochemical changes that transform them from resting cells into powerful host defenders.[78] These changes may be divided into several stages: rolling along the endothelial lining of postcapillary venules, chemotaxis, or migration toward the site of inflammation, adherence to the endothelium, migration through the endothelium to tissue sites, ingestion, killing, and digestion of the inciting agent.[78]

The Myeloid Colony-Stimulating Factors

The myeloid colony-stimulating factors (CSFs) are potent stimulators of mature neutrophils, monocytes, and eosinophils. They are glycoprotein hormones that regulate the differentiation and proliferation of myeloid progenitor cells, and the function of mature red blood cells (RBCs). They also augment platelet and red cell elaboration.[42] The major sources of CSFs are activated lymphocytes, monocytes, macrophages, endothelial cells, and fibroblasts. Upon activation, these cells produce endotoxin, IL-1, and TNF. Granulocyte-macrophage colony stimulating factor (GM-CSF) stimulates the production of monocytes, eosinophils, neutrophils, and megakaryocytes. Granulocyte colony-stimulating factor (GCSF) stimulates the production of neutrophils, whereas macrophage CSF stimulates mononuclear phagocyte development. IL-3 is active earlier in stem cell development. It also stimulates the production of platelets and basophils. The biologic effects of the CSFs are mediated through binding to specific receptors on the surface of target cells, including the myeloid precursor cells.[42] In addition to promoting cellular differentiation, stimulation with CSFs results

in prolonged survival, increased ruffling of the neutrophil membrane, increased expression of adhesion molecules and increased synthesis of proteins active in intracellular killing. These are all important functions involved in neutrophil defense against pathogens. Several of the CSFs have been produced through recombinant DNA technology and are in use as therapeutic agents for patients with AIDS and chemotherapy induced neutropenia.[100]

Activation and Chemotaxis

Neutrophils migrate to sites of infection along gradients of chemoattractant mediator (see Fig. 25–6). Some of these mediators include N-formylated peptides (NFP), the fifth component of complement (C5a), leukotriene B4, and IL-8.[11] IL-8 also effects the migration and activation of monocytes, T cells, eosinophils, basophils, and endothelial cells.[87] An acute inflammatory stimulus leads to the accumulation of PMNs along the endothelium of postcapillary venules.[15] The major molecules involved in this process fall into a few basic superfamilies: the selectins and their mucin ligands, the integrins and their extracellular matrix, or immunoglobulin (IG) superfamily ligands. The expression of P-selectin increases rapidly on the plasma membrane of endothelial cells after stimulation with mediators of inflammation, such as thrombin or histamine and by cytokines.[15] P-selectin on endothelium interacts with P-selectin glycoprotein ligand-1 (PSGL-1), a transmembrane mucin, on neutrophils resulting in the phenomenon known as *leukocyte rolling*.[76] Loose adhesions between PMNs and endothelium are made and broken, resulting in the slow movement of leukocytes along endothelium and a more intense exposure of neutrophils to activating factors.

Chemotactic stimuli cause dramatic changes in the shape and cytoskeletal organization of PMNs. Chemotaxis requires responses involving actin polymerization-depolymerization adhesion events mediated by integrins and resulting in changes in cell shape.[11] The cells develop a broad anterior lamellipodium, which takes the form of a delicate sheetlike extension of cytoplasm. This cellular projection forms transient adhesions with substrate, and waves, resulting in movement. The lamellipodium enclose a dense meshwork of microfilaments. Microfilaments are also prominent in the posterior uropods (cytoplasmic footlike processes that trail behind locomoting leukocytes), which serve as a point of attachment in cell-to-cell interactions. Microfilament membrane interactions likely control surface geometry, which may determine the distribution of membrane proteins.[94] The drug colchicine, used for acute attacks of gouty arthritis works by depolymerizing microfilaments, causing the dissolution of the fibrillar microtubules in granulocytes and other motile cells, impairing cellular function.

The next phase of the inflammatory response involves the migration of PMNs through the vascular endothelium. Chemotactic gradients across endothelial cell monolayers promote the transmigration of neutrophils.[125] Cytokine-stimulated endothelial cells produce the factors necessary to induce transendothelial migration of neutrophils, eosinophils, monocytes, and T cells. Leukocytes pass through endothelial cell junctions and into the subendothelial matrix. The molecular mechanisms of transendothelial migration are not completely understood, but it appears that CD11b/CD18-dependent adhesion plays a major role.[125]

Opsonized particles, immune complexes, and chemotactic factors activate neutrophils in tissues by binding to cell surface receptors.[128] The neutrophil makes tight contact with its target, and the plasma membrane surrounds the organism completely enclosing it. Phagocytosing neutrophils undergo a burst of oxygen consumption caused by an NADPH oxidase complex that assembles at the phagosomal membrane. Electrons are transferred from cytoplasmic NADPH to oxygen on the phagosomal side of the membrane, generating superoxide, hydrogen peroxide (formed by the dismutation of the superoxide radical), hydroxyl radical, singlet oxygen, hypochlorous acid, chloramines, nitric oxide and peroxynitrite.[48] Cytoplasmic granules within the PMN fuse with the phagosome and empty their contents into it. There are at least 4 different classes of granules.[48] The components of these granules include myeloperoxidase (MPO), elastase, lipases, metalloproteinases, and a pool of CD11b/CD18 proteins, which must be rapidly mobilized upon neutrophil activation for adhesion and migration.[110] Finally, the phagocytized organism is digested and eliminated by the PMN.

Central nervous system injury following CO exposure is believed to be a type of postischemic reperfusion injury mediated by leukocytes.[138] CO enhances the random migration and activation of neutrophils resulting in lipid peroxidation.[143] Myeloperoxidase activity is markedly enhanced in rats following CO exposure, indicating sequestration of leukocytes in the microvasculature.[148] This process produces oxidative stress manifested by peroxynitrite deposition in vascular endothelium. CO also binds to cytochrome aa_3, disrupting intracellular oxygen utilization, resulting in neurotoxicity and contributes to hippocampal cellular death through apoptosis.[147]

Neutropenia

Neutropenia is commonly defined for adults and children older than 1 year of age as a reduction in circulating PMN and band form neutrophils with an absolute neutrophil count of less than 1.5×10^9/L. Neutropenia can result from decreased production, increased destruction or retention of neutrophils in the various storage pools.[47] The chemotherapeutic agents will predictably cause neutropenia. Table 25–5 lists the pharmaceutics that are implicated in idiosyncratic drug-induced neutropenias.[110]

Agranulocytosis

Agranulocytosis develops as a result of a hypersensitivity reaction in patients previously exposed to the inciting antigen.[135,148] Multiple mechanisms for developing agranulocytosis have been postulated, including direct cell lysis, agglutination, and splenic sequestration and destruction.[49]

The onset of the disorder may be abrupt or may develop insidiously. It is twice as common in females as in males.[49] Typically, the patient develops a severe pharyngitis followed in rapid succession by prostration, agranulocytosis, sepsis, and death. Most reported cases of agranulocytosis are associated with the use of aminopyrine and dipyrone.[104] Table 25–6 lists other agents that may be associated with this syndrome.

Neonatal Considerations

Newborn infants have peripheral blood neutrophil counts similar to older children and adults. However, their response to bacterial sepsis differs from that of adults: whereas adults develop a neutrophil leukocytosis, neonates frequently become neutropenic. Immaturity of granulopoiesis results in a low neutrophil cell mass and a limited capacity for increasing progenitor proliferation. This results in neutropenia during episodes of sepsis.[20]

TABLE 25–5.   Idiosyncratic Drug-Induced Neutropenia

Analgesic/antiinflammatory agents
  Aminopyrine
  Indomethacin
  Phenylbutazone
Antimicrobials
  Cephalosporins
  Chloramphenicol
  Penicillin
  Sulfonamides
Anticonvulsants
  Carbamazepine
  Phenytoin
Antirheumatics
  Gold
  Levamisole
  Penicillamine
Antipsychotics
  Phenothiazines
Antithyroid agents
  Propylthiouracil
Cardiovascular agents
  Hydralazine
  Procainamide
  Quinidine
Diuretics
  Acetazolamide
  Hydrochlorthiazide
Hypoglycemic agents
  Chlorpropamide
Sedative-hypnotics
  Barbiturates
  Benzodiazepines

Adapted from Haddy TB, Rana SR, Castro O: Benign ethnic neutropenia: What is a normal absolute neutrophil count? J Lab Clin Med 1999;133:15–22.

Functional abnormalities of neonatal neutrophils include reduced chemotaxis. Neutrophils from newborns migrate at about half the speed traveled by adult cells. Neonatal neutrophils appear to interact to a lesser degree with endothelial cells than adult cells. Rolling adhesion is diminished, fewer cells attach to activated endothelium and fewer cells migrate to the subendothelial tissue.[20] These differences in function appear to result from the abnormal expression and dynamics of the β_2 integrins and the selectins, and immaturity of the cytoskeleton of neonatal PMNs. Transendothelial migration in neonates is reduced due to the reduced expression of P-selectin on endothelium.[20]

THROMBOSIS AND COAGULATION

In the absence of pathology, blood remains in a liquid, flowing form with cells in suspension. In response to injury, the processes of coagulation and thrombosis are triggered. The result, including clot formation, retraction, and dissolution involves an interaction between the vessel endothelium, soluble constituents of the coagulation system and receptors and intracellular proteins contained on the surface of and within platelets. Platelet function is influenced by the physical properties of flowing blood, as well as by the chemical constituents within it. Platelets respond to signals within their immediate environment and from injured components of the distant microcirculation.

TABLE 25–6. Drugs Associated with the Development of Agranulocytosis

Analgesic/antiinflammatory agents
  Acetaminophen
  Aminopyrine
  Diclofenac
  Dipyrone
  Ibuprofen
  Indomethacin
  Pentazocine
  Piroxicam
Antimicrobials
  β-Lactams
  Cephalosporins
  Chloroquine
  Cotrimoxazole
  Mebendazole
  Penicillins
  Pyrimethamine + dapsone
  Rifampicin
  Salazosulfapyridine
  Sulfonamides
  Trimethoprim
  Vancomycin
Anticonvulsants
  Carbamazepine
Antirheumatics
  Levamisole
  Penicillamine
Antithyroid agents
  Thiouracils
Cardiovascular agents
  Captopril
  Enalapril
  Nifedipine
Diuretics
  Acetazolamide
  Furosemide
  Hydrochlorthiazide
  Spironolactone
Hypoglycemic agents
  Chlorpropamide
Psychiatric agents
  Antipsychotics
  Clozapine
  Cyclic antidepressants
  MAO inhibitors
  Mianserin
Sedative-hypnotics
  Barbiturates
  Benzodiazepines

Platelets

In the resting state, platelets maintain a discoid shape. The platelet membrane is a typical trilaminal membrane with glycoproteins, glycolipids, and cholesterol embedded in a phospholipid bilayer.[130] The plasma membrane is in direct continuity with a series of channels, the surface-connected canalicular system (SCCS), which is sometimes referred to as the open canalicular system. The SCCS provides a route of entry and exit for various molecules, a storage pool for platelet glycoproteins, and an internal reservoir of membrane that may be recruited to increase platelet surface area.[93] This facilitates platelet spreading and pseudopod formation during the process of cell adhesion.

The glycocalyx, or outer coat, is heavily invested with glycoproteins that serve as receptors for a wide variety of stimuli. The β_1 integrin family includes receptors that mediate interactions between cells and mediators in the extracellular matrix, including collagen, laminin, and fibronectin.[124] The β_2 integrin receptors are present in inflammatory cells and platelets and are important in immune activation. The β_3 integrin receptors (also known as cytoadhesins) include the glycoprotein IIb-IIIa (GP IIb-IIIa) fibrinogen receptor, as well as vitronectin.[51] Vitronectin has binding sites for other integrins, collagen, heparin, and components of complement. All of the integrins are active in the process of platelet adhesion to surfaces. Platelet aggregation is mediated by the GP IIb-IIIa receptors.[51]

The submembrane region contains actin filaments that stabilize the platelets discoid shape and are involved in the formation and stabilization of pseudopods. They also generate the force needed for the movement of receptor-ligand complexes from the outer plasma membrane to the SCCS. These mobile receptors are important in the spreading of platelets on surfaces, and for binding fibrin strands and other platelets.[130] Platelet cytoplasm contains three types of membrane bound secretory granules.[51] The α granules contain β-thromboglobulin, which mediates inflammation, binds and inactivates heparin, and blocks the endothelial release of prostacyclin. In addition, platelet factor-4, which inactivates heparin, and fibrinogen are contained within the α granules. Dense granules store adenine nucleotides, serotonin, and calcium, which are secreted during the release reaction.[51] Platelet lysosomes contain hydrolytic enzymes. Stimulation by platelet agonists causes the granules to fuse with the channels of the SCCS, driving the contents out of the platelets and into the surrounding media.

Platelet Adhesion. In the vessel wall, collagen, von Willebrand factor (vWF), and fibronectin are the adhesive proteins that play the most prominent role in the adhesion of platelets to vascular subendothelium.[124] Upon the exposure of collagen (as following a laceration or the rupture of an atherosclerotic plaque), platelet adhesion is triggered. Under conditions of high shear (flowing blood), platelet adhesion is mediated by the binding of GP Ib-IX receptors on platelet membranes to vWF in the vascular subendothelium.[51,124] Following adherence of platelets to subendothelial vWF, a conformational change in GP IIb-IIIa on platelet membrane occurs, activating this receptor complex to ligate vWF and fibrinogen. The result is the amplification of platelet adhesion and aggregation.[51] An important interaction occurs between thrombosis and inflammation. Platelet-activating factor (PAF), is synthesized and coexpressed with P-selectin on the surface of the endothelium in response to mediators such as histamine or thrombin. PAF interacts with a receptor on the surface of neutrophils that activates the CD11/CD18 adhesion complex, and results in adhesion of PMNs to endothelium and to platelets. This results in the synthesis of leukotrienes and other mediators of inflammation.

Platelet Activation. Thrombin, collagen, and epinephrine may activate platelets. In response to thrombin, α granules fuse with each other and with elements of the SCCS to form secretory vesicles.[93] These vesicles are believed to fuse with the surface membrane, releasing their contents into the surrounding medium. The membranes of the secretory granules become incorporated into the platelet surface membrane.

Platelet Aggregation. Following activation, GP IIb-IIIa is expressed in active form on platelet surface. This receptor binds exogenous calcium and fibrinogen. GP IIb-IIIa, ligates fibrinogen along with fibronectin, vitronectin, and vWF, resulting in the binding of platelets to other platelets, and ultimately the formation of the platelet plug. Collagen induced platelet aggregation is mediated by ADP and thromboxane A2 (TXA2). Thromboxane A2 is formed from arachidonic acid by the action of cyclooxygenase (COX). It is a potent vasoconstrictor and inducer of platelet aggregation and release reactions.[51] Platelets participate in triggering the coagulation cascade by binding coagulation factors II, VII, IX, and X to membrane phospholipid, a calcium-dependent process.

Thrombocytopenia

Thrombocytopenia is the most common manifestation of an acquired bleeding disorder. The mechanism generally is immune mediated. Drug-induced platelet antibodies are reported to occur in 1 in 100,000 drug exposures.[71]

The development of antiplatelet antibodies occurs in association with the use of multiple medications (see Table 25–7). Most commonly, IgG is the antibody implicated, although some reports have identified IgA (associated with acetaminophen use) and IgM.[36,115]

As in the case of immune-mediated red cell destruction, multiple mechanisms may operate.[61,71] Drugs may act as haptens. Subsequent interactions between drug, antibody, and platelets result in platelet damage and removal by the reticuloendothelial system.[133] Alternatively, drugs may complex with plasma proteins or another carrier. Antibody forms to the complex, complement becomes fixed, and "innocent bystander" destruction of platelets ensues.

Thrombocytopenia develops within 12 hours of a repeated exposure to a sensitizing agent. In patients ingesting the drug for the first time, 7 days are required for the development of the immune response. Clinically, fever, chills, pruritus, and lethargy may occur.[61] The onset of bleeding may be abrupt. Hemorrhagic vesicles may be seen in the oral mucosa.[36,61] Life-threatening hemorrhage may develop. Laboratory investigations will demonstrate an absence of platelets on peripheral smear, prolongation of the bleeding time, deficient clot retraction, and an abnormal prothrombin consumption test. Bone marrow aspiration will demonstrate normal or increased numbers of megakaryocytes and immature forms will be seen.[61] Various laboratory methodologies are avail-

TABLE 25–7. Drugs Associated with the Development of Antiplatelet Antibodies

Acetaminophen
Ampicillin
Cephalosporin
Clonazepam
Heparin
Quinidine
Quinine
Rifampin
Stibophen
Valproic acid

able for confirmation of the presence of antiplatelet antibodies. Other than general supportive measures, treatment includes the transfusion of blood products as indicated, the use of steroids, as well as withdrawal of the involved agent.[61]

Platelet destruction that is not immunologically mediated was seen in association with the use of ristocetin, an antituberculous drug no longer in clinical use. It promotes the attachment of vWF to a platelet receptor and initiates direct platelet to platelet interactions and agglutination. Table 25–7 lists the drugs that are associated with the development of antiplatelet antibodies.

Heparin-Induced Thrombocytopenia. An immune response to heparin, manifested clinically by the development of thrombocytopenia, and, in some cases, by the development of venous thrombosis, is now recognized to result from antibodies to a complex of heparin and platelet factor 4 (PF4). The antibodies may be of the IgG, IgM and IgA isotypes.[6] The binding of antibodies to this complex on the platelet surface could directly induce platelet activation and thrombosis. IgM complexes may activate complement, resulting in platelet destruction and thrombocytopenia.[6]

Clinically, heparin-induced thrombocytopenia (HIT) is defined by a decrease in the platelet count to less than 150,000/μL in patients with previously normal counts or numbers of platelets, with the return to normal within days of the discontinuation of heparin. In previously unexposed patients, thrombocytopenia usually develops within 10 days of the initiation of anticoagulant therapy. In those previously exposed, the delay in the development of thrombocytopenia may be as little as 2 days. Thrombosis may occur in as many as 20% of patients with HIT, resulting in a mortality rate as high as 30%.[6]

The incidence of antibody formation is less in patients treated with low-molecular-weight heparin (LMWH). Cross-reactivity between antibodies to unfractionated heparin (UFH) with LMWH is high, eliminating LMWH as an alternative anticoagulant in patients who develop HIT.[6] Once the development of HIT is apparent, immediate discontinuation of heparin is essential.

When continued anticoagulation is necessary, a rapidly acting alternative to heparin must be used. Warfarin has significant disadvantages in this setting. The slow onset of anticoagulant effect, which takes a minimum of 5 days, is one drawback. In addition, and potentially more serious, is the potential for the development of venous limb gangrene. Pathologically, persistent thrombin generation and a decrease in protein C activity characterize this syndrome. This may result in limb necrosis and loss.[144,145]

Ancrod is a defibrinating agent derived from the venom of the Malayan pit viper; it is currently under investigation for use as an anticoagulant. It triggers the release of tissue plasmin activator (t-PA) or urokinase from vascular endothelium. The onset of action is slow, and use may be associated with the development of venous limb gangrene in patients with HIT.[145]

Hirudin is a direct thrombin inhibitor that is extracted from the salivary glands of leeches. Hirudin binds with and irreversibly inactivates thrombin. It has benefit in patients with HIT, but is itself immunogenic and cannot be used in patients with renal dysfunction.[144] Argatroban, a synthetic thrombin inhibitor is currently FDA approved and may have some value in the treatment of HIT.

Danaparoid sodium, a combination of heparan sulfate and dermatan sulfate has antithrombotic activity mediated primarily by AT3 inhibition of factor Xa. This agent successfully inhibits platelet aggregation in patients with HIT and appears to be the best available anticoagulant in this setting.[96]

Antithrombotic Agents.

Aspirin. Aspirin inhibits cyclooxygenase COX by acetylation of an active group on an amino acid serine within the COX molecule. Aspirin inhibition of the COX-1 isoform of this enzyme is 100–150 times more potent than its inhibition of the COX-2 isoform. The inhibition of COX-1 results in the irreversible inhibition of thromboxane A_2 formation. Platelet activation by other mechanisms, such as thrombin, remain intact, therefore thrombosis may develop despite aspirin therapy[118] (Chap. 33).

GP IIb-IIIa Antagonists. The GP IIb-IIIa antagonist abciximab is a human monoclonal antibody that binds the GP IIb-IIIa receptor of platelets and megakaryocytes. Two synthetic GP IIb-IIIa receptor antagonists have been developed: eptifibatide and tirofiban. These agents are used primarily in patients undergoing elective percutaneous coronary interventions for unstable angina.[51]

Coagulation

Two basic pathways are involved in the initiation of coagulation. Activation of the intrinsic system occurs when blood is exposed to tissue factor (TF) in damaged blood vessels or on the surface of activated leukocytes. TF binds factor VIIa forming the intrinsic tenase complex. The resulting TF-VIIa complex activates factors IX and X. Factor IXa binds to the surface of activated platelets together with VIIIa and calcium, forming the extrinsic tenase complex. Factor X, which is activated by extrinsic and intrinsic tenase binds to factor Va on the surface of activated platelets forming the prothrombinase complex. The prothrombinase complex activates prothrombin, which results in the generation of thrombin activity. Thrombin activates platelets, promotes its own generation by activation factors V, VIII, and XI, and converts fibrinogen to fibrin[51] (Chap. 42).

Drug-Induced Defects in Coagulation.

Warfarin. The recognition of a hemorrhagic disease in cattle in the 1920s and the isolation of the causative agent dicoumarol from spoiled sweet clover in the 1940s resulted in the development of the warfarin-type anticoagulants (Chap. 42). This group of anticoagulants indirectly inhibits hepatic synthesis of coagulation factors II, VII, IX, X, and proteins C and S.[101] Hepatic γ-carboxylation of glutamic acid residues by vitamin K-dependent carboxylase results in the formation of the vitamin K-dependent clotting factors. Vitamin K must be available in its reduced form, vitamin KH_2, to effectively catalyze this reaction. The carboxylation reaction oxidizes vitamin KH_2 to vitamin $K_{2,3}$ epoxide, which must be reduced to vitamin K by reductase enzymes. The warfarin anticoagulants inhibit the reductase that is responsible for the regeneration of vitamin K from vitamin K epoxide. As vitamin K is no longer available in its active form, vitamin KH_2, the synthesis of the vitamin K-dependent proteins is impaired.[65,127]

Heparin

Heparin is a highly sulfated glycosaminoglycan normally present is tissues. Commercial unfractionated heparin (UFH) is either bovine or porcine in origin, and consists of a mixture of polysaccharides with molecular weights ranging from 4000–30,000 Da. It is used extensively for the prophylaxis and treatment of venous thrombosis and thromboembolism. It is ineffective orally because it cannot cross membranes. This same property makes it safe for use during pregnancy because heparin cannot cross the placenta.[114] The anticoagulant activity of heparin is through its catalytic activation of antithrombin III (ATIII). ATIII is a serine protease that complexes with and inactivates thrombin and factor X.[85]

The LMWHs are considered more efficacious, safer, and more convenient to use than the UFHs. Commercial preparations have a mean molecular weight of 4000–6000 Da.[51] The pharmacokinetics and bioavailability of the LMWHs are more predictable, eliminating the need for close monitoring. They exhibit lower protein binding and a longer half-life, making them more convenient to use.[85]

Fibrinolysis

The coagulation system is opposed by three major inhibitory systems. As with the coagulation cascade, components of the fibrinolytic system circulate as zymogens, activators, inhibitors, and cofactors.[38] Plasminogen can be activated to plasmin by an intrinsic pathway involving factor XII, prekallikrein, and high-molecular-weight kininogen. This produces the degradation products and fibrin monomers that are found in disseminated intravascular coagulation. The extrinsic pathway involves the release of t-PA from tissues, and urokinase plasminogen activator (u-PA) from secretions.[38] Once activated, plasmin can degrade fibrinogen, fibrin, and coagulation factors V and VIII. The degradation of cross-linked fibrin strands results in the formation of D dimers.

Several inhibitors, including α_2-antiplasmin, α_2-macroglobulin, both of which oppose plasmin activity, and plasminogen activator-inhibitors (PAI) 1 and 2, which oppose t-PA, oppose the fibrinolytic system. PAI-1 and -2 are opposed by activated protein C (APC) and protein S. APC is activated by thrombin. Congenital deficiencies of protein C and S may result in pathologic venous thrombosis. Decreased fibrinolytic activity may result from decreased synthesis or release of t-PA or from an elevation of the PAI-1 level. Both conditions have been observed postoperatively, with the use of oral contraceptives, in the third trimester of pregnancy, and in obesity. An increase in the activity of α_2-antiplasmin and α_2-macroglobulin are increased in pulmonary fibrosis, malignancy, infection, and myocardial infarction, and in thromboembolic disease.[38]

Drug-Induced Defects in Fibrinolysis.
Table 25–8 lists agents associated with an acquired defect of fibrinolysis. The antitumor

---

TABLE 25–8. Agents Associated with an Acquired Fibrinolytic Disorder Resulting in Thrombosis

Anticancer agents
  Anthracyclines
   L-Asparaginase
  Mithramycin
Aprotinin and other antifibrinolytics
Coagulation factors
Cytokines
  Erythropoietin
  Thrombopoietin
Hormones

Adapted from Fareed J, Hoppensteadt DZ, Jeske WP, et al: Acquired defects of fibrinolysis associated with thrombosis. Semin Thromb Hemost 1999;25: 367–374.

agents may result in a reduction in serine protease inhibitors such as antithrombin. L-asparaginase has been associated with a reduction in circulating t-PA levels. Methotrexate can damage vascular endothelium, which may trigger thrombosis[38] (see chapter 47).

SUMMARY

The mechanisms of toxic injury to the blood are extremely varied and complex. The response to injury may be idiosyncratic, as in many drug-related causes of agranulocytosis and aplastic anemia, or predictable, as in the case of significant exposures to ionizing radiation or to benzene. Injury may depend on the presence of certain host factors, such as G6PD deficiency. Toxins may directly injure cellular elements, as occurs with red cell destruction following exposure to arsine gas, or damage supporting systems, such as the hematopoietic microenvironment. Injury may occur to mature cells or to the stem cell pool, thus prohibiting the development of mature cells. Toxicity, or injury may result from the amplification of a potentially therapeutic intervention, such as occurs with many chemotherapeutic agents and anticoagulants. It may result from an intentional attempt at injury, a therapeutic intervention, or an industrial or household exposure. It is therefore important for healthcare providers to be aware of and vigilant in the investigation of toxic etiologies of injury to the blood.

REFERENCES

1. Abboud CN, Lichtman MA: Structure of the marrow. In: Buetler E, Lichtman MA, Coller BS, Kipps TJ, eds: Williams Hematology, 5th ed. New York, McGraw-Hill, 1995, pp. 25–38.
2. Adamson J: Erythropoietin, iron metabolism, and red blood cell production. Semin Hematol 1996;33:5–9.
3. Adamson JW: Regulation of red blood cell production. Am J Med 1996;101(Suppl 2A):4S–6S.
4. Agre P, Preston GM, Smith BL, et al: Aquaporin CHIP: The archetypal molecular water channel. Am J Physiol 1993;265:F463–F476.
5. Allen DW, Wyman J, Smith CA: The oxygen equilibrium of foetal and adult hemoglobin. J Biol Chem 1953;203:81–87.
6. Alving BM, Krishnamurti C: Recognition and management of heparin-induced thrombocytopenia (HIT) and thrombosis. Semin Thromb Hemost 1997;23:569–574.
7. Astrup P: Red-cell pH and oxygen affinity of hemoglobin. N Engl J Med 1970;283:202–204.
8. Bacigalupo A, Podesta M, Frassone F, et al: Generation of CFU-C suppressor T cells in vitro. V. A multistep process. Br J Haematol 1982;52:421–427.
9. Bakemeier RF, Leddy JD: Erythrocyte autoantibody associated with alpha-methyldopa: Heterogeneity of structure and specificity. Blood 1968;32:1–14.
10. Beutler E: The mechanism of glutathione destruction and protection in drug-sensitive and non-sensitive erythrocytes. J Clin Invest 1957; 36:617–628.
11. Bokoch GM: Chemoattractant signaling and leukocyte activation. Blood 1995;86:1649–1660.
12. Bondurant MC, Koury MJ: Origin and development of blood cells. In: Lee GR, Foerster J, Lukens J, et al, eds: Wintrobe's Clinical Hematology, 10th ed. New York, Lippincott-Williams and Wilkins, 1999, pp. 145–168.
13. Bottomley SS, Muller-Everhard UM: Pathophysiology of heme synthesis. Semin Hematol 1988;25:282–302.
14. Brodsky RA: Biology and management of acquired severe aplastic anemia. Curr Opin Oncol 1998;10:95–99.
15. Brown E: Neutrophil adhesion and the therapy of inflammation. Semin Hematol 1997;34:319–326.
16. Broxmeyer HE, Kim CH: Regulation of hematopoiesis in a sea of chemokine family members with a plethora of redundant activities. Exp Hematol 1999;27:1113–1123.
17. Bull BS, Brailsford JD: The biconcavity of the red cell: An analysis of several hypotheses. Blood 1973; 41:833–844.
18. Bulmer FMR, Rothwell HE, Polack SS, et al: Chronic arsine poisoning among workers employed in the cyanide extraction of gold: A report of fourteen cases. J Ind Hygiene Tox 1940;22:111–124.
19. Camitta BM, Storb F, Thomas D: Aplastic anemia: Pathogenesis, diagnosis, treatment, and prognosis part 1. N Engl J Med 1982;306: 645–651.
20. Carr R: Neutrophil production and function in newborn infants. Br J Haematol 2000;110:18–28.
21. Cartron JP: Defining the Rh blood group antigens. Biochemistry and molecular genetics. Blood Rev 1994;8.199–212.
22. Chamberlain JK, Weiss L, Weed RI: Bone marrow sinus cell packing: A determinant of cell release. Blood 1075;46:91–102.
23. Champlain RE: Radiation accidents and nuclear energy: Medical consequences and therapy. Ann Intern Med 1988;109:730–44.
24. Chanutin A, Curnish RR: Effect of organic and inorganic phosphates on the oxygen equilibrium of human erythrocytes. Arch Biochem Biophys 1967;121:96–102.
25. Choury D, Reghis A, Pichard AL, Kaplan JC: Endogenous proteolysis of membrane-bound red cell cytochrome-b5 reductase in adults and newborns: Its possible relevance to the generation of the soluble "methemoglobin reductase." Blood 1983;61:894–898.
26. Chow FL, Telen MJ, Rosse WF: The acetylcholinesterase defect in paroxysmal nocturnal hemoglobinuria: Evidence that the enzyme is absent from the cell membrane. Blood 1985;66:940–945.
27. Cohen CM, Gascard P: Regulation and post-translational modification of erythrocyte membrane and membrane-skeletal proteins. Semin Hematol 1992;29:24–29.
28. Cohen G, Hochstein P: Generation of hydrogen peroxide in erythrocytes by hemolytic agents. Biochemistry 1964;3:895–900.
29. Conrad ME, Umbreit JN, Moore EG: Iron absorption and transport. Am J Med Sci 1999;318:213–229.
30. Cooper RA: Influence of increased membrane cholesterol on membrane fluidity and cell function in human red blood cells. J Supramol Struct 1978;8:413–430.
31. Cumano A, Furlonger C, Paige CJ: Differentiation and characterization of B-cell precursors detected in the yolk sac and embryo body of embryos beginning at the 10- to 12-somite stage. Proc Natl Acad Sci U S A 1993;90:6429–6433.
32. Cummings CC, McIvor ME: Fluoride-induced hyperkalemia: The role of Ca2+ dependent K+ channels. Am J Emerg Med 1988; 6:1–3.
33. Deiss A, Lee GR, Cartwright GE: Hemolytic anemia in Wilson's disease. Ann Intern Med 1970;73:413–418.
34. De Matteis F: Toxicological aspects of liver heme biosynthesis. Semin Hematol 1988;25:321–329.
35. Dexter M, Allen T: Multi-talented stem cells? Nature 1992;360: 709–710.
36. Eisner EV, Shahidi NT: Immune thrombocytopenia due to a drug metabolite. N Engl J Med 1972;287:376–381.
37. Fairbanks VF: Copper sulfate-induced hemolytic anemia. Arch Intern Med 1967;120:428–432.
38. Fareed J, Hoppensteadt DA, Jeske WP, et al: Acquired defects of fibrinolysis associated with thrombosis. Semin Thromb Hemost 1999;25:367–374.
39. Fina L, Molgaard HV, Robertson D, et al: Expression of the CD34 gene in vascular endothelial cells. Blood 1990;75:2417–2426.
40. Funicella T, Weinger RS, Moake JL, et al: Penicillin-induced immunohemolytic anemia associated with circulating immune complexes. Am J Hematol 1977;3:219–223.

41. Godin IE, Garcia-Porrero JA, Coutinho A, et al: Para-aortic splanchnopleure from early mouse embryos contains B1a cell progenitors. Nature 1993;364:67–70.

42. Golde DW: Overview of myeloid growth factors. Semin Hematol 1990;27:1–7.

43. Gordon MY: Physiology and function of the haematopoietic microenvironment. Brit J Haematol 1994;86:241–243.

44. Graham AF, Crawford TBB, Marian GF: The action of arsine on blood: Observations on the nature of the fixed arsenic. Biochem J 1946;40:256–260.

45. Grosveld F, DeBoer E, Dillon N, et al: The dynamics of globin gene expression and gene therapy vectors. Ann N Y Acad Sci 1998; 850:18–27.

46. Haab P: The effect of carbon monoxide on respiration. Experientia 1990;46:1202–1203.

47. Haddy TB, Rana SR, Castro O: Benign ethnic neutropenia: What is a normal absolute neutrophil count? J Lab Clin Med 1999;133:15–22.

48. Hampton MB, Kettle AJ, Winterbourne CC: Inside the neutrophil phagosome: Oxidants, myeloperoxidase, and bacterial killing. Blood 1998;92:3007–3017.

49. Hartl W: Drug allergic agranulocytosis (Schultz's disease). Semin Hematol 1965;2:313–337.

50. Herz F, Kaplan E, Scheye ES: Diagnosis of erythrocyte glucose-6-phosphate dehydrogenase deficiency in the Negro male despite hemolytic crisis. Blood 1970;35:90–93.

51. Hirsh J, Weitz I: Thrombosis and anticoagulation. Semin Hematol 1999;36:118–132.

52. Hoffman JF, Kaplan JH, Callahan TJ: The Na:K pump in red cells is electrogenic. Fed Proc 1979;38:2440–2441.

53. Hord JD, Lukens JN: Anemias unique to infants and young children. In: Lee GR, Foerster J, Lukens J, et al, eds: Wintrobe's Clinical Hematology, 10th ed. New York, Lippincott-Williams and Wilkins, 1999, pp. 1518–1537.

54. Hudson G: Bone-marrow volume in the human foetus and newborn. Brit J Haematol 1965;2:446–452.

55. Huehns ER, Dance N, Beaven GH, et al: Human embryonic haemoglobins. Nature 1964;201:1095–1097.

56. Hultquist DE, Passon PG: Catalysis of methaemoglobinemia reduction by erythrocyte cytochrome B5 and cytochrome B5 reductase. Nat New Biol 1971;229:252–254.

57. Iversen PO, Nicolaysen G, Benestad HB: Blood flow to bone marrow during development of anemia or polycythemia in the rat. Blood 1992;79:594–601.

58. Iversen PO, Nicolaysen G, Benestad HB: The leukopoietic cytokine granulocyte colony-stimulating factor increases blood flow to rat bone marrow. Exper Hematol 1993;21:231–235.

59. Kamuzora H, Lehmann H: Human embryonic hemoglobins including a comparison by homology of the human β and α chains. Nature 1975;256:511–513.

60. Kaplan JC, Chirouze M: Therapy of recessive congenital methaemoglobinaemia by oral riboflavin. Lancet 1978;2:1043–1044.

61. Karpatkin S: Drug-induced thrombocytopenia. Am J Med Sci 1971; 262:68–78.

62. Kattamis CA: Glucose-6-phosphate dehydrogenase deficiency in female heterozygotes and the X-inactivation hypothesis. Acta Pediatr Scand 1967;172(Suppl):103–109.

63. Kaushansky K: Thrombopoietin and hematopoietic stem cell development. Ann N Y Acad Sci 1999;872:314–319.

64. Kaushansky K: Thrombopoietin. N Engl J Med 1998;339:746–754.

65. Keller C, Matzdorff AC, Kemkes-Matthes B: Pharmacology of warfarin and clinical implications. Semin Thromb Hemost 1999;25: 13–16.

66. Lambert S, Bennett V: From anemia to cerebellar dysfunction. A review of the Ankyrin gene family. Eur J Biochem 1993;211:1–6.

67. Laver J, Castro-Malaspina H, Kernan NA, et al: In vitro interferon-gamma production by cultured T-cells in severe aplastic anaemia:

Correlation with granulomonopoietic inhibition in patients who respond to anti-thymocyte globulin. Brit J Haematol 1988;69:545–550.

68. Leddy JD: Erythrocyte autoantibody associated with alpha-methyldopa: Heterogeneity of structure and specificity. Blood 1968;32: 1–14.

69. Lenard JG: A note on the shape of the red cell. Bull Math Biol 1974;36:55–58.

70. Lerat H, Lissitzky JC, Singer JW, et al: Role of stromal cells and macrophages in fibronectin biosynthesis and matrix assembly in human long-term marrow cultures. Blood 1993;82:1480–1492.

71. Levine SP: Thrombocytopenia caused by immunologic platelet destruction. In: In Lee GR, Foerster J, Lukens J, et al, eds: Wintrobe's Clinical Hematology, 10th ed. New York, Lippincott-Williams and Wilkins, 1999, 1583–1611.

72. Levinsky WJ, Smalley RV, Hillger PN: Arsine hemolysis. Arch Environ Health 1970;20:436–440.

73. Lichtman MA, Chamberlain JK, Simon W, Santillo PA: Parasinoidal location of megakaryocytes in marrow: A determinant of platelet release. Am J Hematol 1978;4:303–312.

74. Lichtman MA: The ultrastructure of the hemopoietic environment of the marrow: A review. Exp Hematol 1981;9:391–410.

75. Maciejewski JP, Selleri C, Sato T, et al: Increased expression of Fas antigen on bone marrow CD34+ cells of patients with aplastic anaemia. Brit J Haematol 1995;91:245–252.

76. Malech HL, Nauseef WM: Primary inherited defects in neutrophil function: Etiology and treatment. Semin Hematol 1997;34:279–290.

77. Mathe G, Amiel FL, Schwarzenberg L, et al: Bone marrow graft in man after conditioning by antilymphocyte serum. Br Med J 1970; 18:131–136.

78. Matzner Y: Acquired neutrophil dysfunction and diseases with an inflammatory component. Semin Hematol 1997;34:291–302.

79. May BK, Bawden MJ: Control of heme biosynthesis in animals. Semin Hematol 1989;26:150–156.

80. Mayer P, Fred-Jochen W, Lam C, Besemer J: In vitro and in vivo activity of human recombinant granulocyte colony-stimulating factor in dogs. Exp Hematol 1990;18:1026–1033.

81. McCord JM: Iron, free radicals, and oxidative injury. Semin Hematol 1998;35:5–12.

82. McIvor, ME: Sodium fluoride produces a K+ efflux by increasing intracellular Ca2+ through Na+-Ca2+ exchange. Toxicol Lett 1987;38: 169–176.

83. Medvinsky AL, Samoylina NL, Muller AM, Dzierzak EA: An early pre-liver intraembryonic source of CFU-S in the developing mouse. Nature 1993;364:64–67.

84. Miyazaki H, Kato T: Thrombopoietin: biology and clinical potentials. Int J Hematol 1999;70:216–225.

85. Mousa SA: Comparative efficacy of different low-molecular-weight heparins (LMWHs) and drug interactions with LMWH: Interactions for management of vascular disorders. Semin Thromb Hemost 2000; 26(Suppl 1):39–46.

86. Mueckler M, Caruso C, Baldwin SA, et al: Sequence and structure of a human glucose transporter. Science 1985;229:941–945.

87. Murphy PM: Neutrophil receptors for interleukin-8 and related CXC chemokines. Semin Hematol 1997;34:311–318.

88. Naito K, Tamahashi N, Tamihiko C, et al: The microvasculature of the human bone marrow correlated with the distribution of hematopoietic cells. A computer-assisted three-dimensional reconstruction study. Tohoku J Exp Med 1992;166:439–450.

89. Nakao S, Yamaguchi M, Shiobara S, et al: Interferon gamma gene expression in unstimulated bone marrow mononuclear cells predicts a good response to cyclosporine therapy in aplastic anemia. Blood 1992;79:2532–2535.

90. Nardi NB, Alfonso ZZC: The hematopoietic stroma. Braz J Med Biol Res 1999;32:601–609.

91. Nimer SD, Ireland P, Meshkinpour A, Frane M: An increased HLA DTR2 frequency is seen in aplastic anemia patients. Blood 1994; 84:923–927.

92. Nistico A, Young NS: Gamma-interferon gene expression in the bone marrow of patients with aplastic anemia. Ann Intern Med 1994; 120,463–469.

93. Nurden P, Heilman E, Paponneau A, Nurden A: Two-way trafficking of membrane glycoproteins on thrombin-activated human platelets. Semin Hematol 1994;31:240–250.

94. Oliver JM, Berlin RD: Surface and cytoskeletal events regulating leukocyte membrane topography. Semin Hematol 1983;20:282–304.

95. Olives B, Neau P, Bailly P, et al: Cloning and functional expression of a urea transporter from human bone marrow cells. J Biol Chem 1994;269:31649–31652.

96. Ortel TL, Chong BH: New treatment options for heparin-induced thrombocytopenia. Semin Hematol 1998;35(Suppl 5):26–34.

97. Palacios R, Samaridis J: Bone marrow clones representing an intermediate stage of development between hematopoietic stem cells and pre-T-lymphocyte or pro-B-lymphocyte progenitors. Blood 1993;81: 1222–1238.

98. Paraskevas F: Clusters of differentiation. In: Lee GR, Foerster J, Lukens J, et al, eds: Wintrobe's Clinical Hematology, 10th ed. New York, Lippincott-Williams and Wilkins, 1999, pp. 72–97.

99. Park CM, Nagel RL: Sulfhemoglobinemia: Clinical and molecular aspects. N Engl J Med 1984;310:1579–1584.

100. Peters WP: The myeloid colony-stimulating factors: Introduction and overview. Semin Hematol 1991;28:1–5.

101. Pindur G, Morsdorf S, Schenk JF, et al: The overdosed patient and bleedings with oral anticoagulation. Semin Thromb Hemost 1999; 25:85–88.

102. Pinto SS: Arsine poisoning: Evaluation of the acute phase. J Occup Med 1976;18:633–635.

103. Platanias L, Gascon P, Bielory L, et al: Lymphocyte phenotype and lymphokines following anti-thymocyte globulin therapy in patients with aplastic anaemia. Brit J Haematol 1987;66:437–443.

104. Plum P: Etiology of Agranulocytosis in Clinical and Experimental Investigations in Agranulocytosis. London, 1937, p. 95–165.

105. Ponka P, Beaumont C, Richardson DR: Function and regulation of transferrin and ferritin. Semin Hematology 1998;35:35–54.

106. Ponka P: Tissue-specific regulation of iron metabolism and heme synthesis: Distinct control mechanisms in erythroid cells. Blood 1997;89:1–25.

107. Ponka P: Cell biology of heme. Am J Med Sci 1999;318:241–256.

108. Provan D, Weatherall D: Red cell II: Acquired anaemias and polycythaemia. Lancet 2000;355:1260–1268.

109. Proverbio F, Hoffman JF: Membrane compartmentalized ATP and its preferential use by the Na, K-ATPase of human red cell ghosts. J Gen Physiol 1977;69:605–632.

110. Rainger GE, Rowley AF, Nash GB: Adhesion-dependent release from human neutrophils in a novel flow-based model: Specificity of different chemotactic agents. Blood 1998;92:4819–4827.

111. Riggs A: Functional properties of hemoglobins. Physiol Rev 1965; 45:619–673.

112. Rosse C, Kraemer MJ, Dillon TL, al: Bone marrow cell populations of normal infants: The predominance of lymphocytes. J Lab Clin Med 1977;89:1225–1240.

113. Rosse WF: Phosphatidylinositol-linked proteins and paroxysmal nocturnal hemoglobinuria. Blood 1990;75:1595–1601.

114. Samama MM, Gerotziafas GT: Comparative pharmacokinetics of LMWHs. Semin Thromb Hemost 2000;26(Suppl 1):31–38.

115. Sandler RM, Emberson C, Roberts GE, et al: IgM platelet autoantibody due to sodium valproate. Br Med J 1978;2:1683–1684.

116. Schafer DA, Cooper JA: Control of actin assembly at filament ends. Annual Rev Cell Dev Biol 1995;11:497–518.

117. Schmid-Schonbein H, Wells Jr: Rheological properties of human erythrocytes and their influence upon the "anomalous" viscosity of blood. Ergeb Physiol 1971;63:146–219.

118. Schror K: Aspirin and platelets: The antiplatelet action of aspirin and its role in thrombosis and treatment prophylaxis. Semin Thromb Hemost 1997;23:349–356.

119. Selleri C, Sato T, Anderson S, et al: Interferon-γ and tumor necrosis factor-α suppress both early and late stages of hematopoiesis, and induce programmed cell death. J Cell Physiol 1995;165:538–546.

120. Shaeffer JR, Kingston RE, McDonald MJ, Bunn HF: Electrostatic interactions in the assembly of human hemoglobin. Nature 1983; 306–498.

121. Shulman NR: A mechanism of cell destruction in individuals sensitized to foreign antigens and its implications in autoimmunity. Ann Intern Med 1964;60:506–521.

122. Simmons PJ, Torok-Storb B: CD34 expression by stromal precursors in normal human adult bone marrow. Blood 1991;78:2848–2853.

123. Singer SJ, Nicholson GL: The fluid mosaic model of the structure of cell membranes. Science 1972;175:720–731.

124. Sixma J, van Zanten H, Banga JD, et al: Platelet adhesion. Semin Hematol 1995;32:89–98.

125. Smith CW: Leukocyte-endothelial cell interactions. Semin Hematol 1992;30:45–55.

126. Smith MT: Overview of benzene-induced aplastic anaemia. Eur J Haematol 1996;57(Suppl):107–110.

127. Smith RE: The INR: A perspective. Semin Thromb Hemost 1997;23: 547–549.

128. Smolen JE: Neutrophil signal transduction: Calcium kinases, and fusion. J Lab Clin Med 1992;120:527–532.

129. Snyder R, Witz G, Goldstein BD: The toxicology of benzene. Environ Health Perspect 1993;100:293–306.

130. Stenberg PE, Hill RJ: Platelets and megakaryocytes. In: Lee GR, Foerster J, Lukens J, et al, eds: Wintrobe's Clinical Hematology, 10th ed. New York, Lippincott-Williams and Wilkins, 1999, pp. 615–660.

131. Stoeckenius W, Engelman DM: Current models for the structure of biological membranes. J Cell Biol 1969;42:613–646.

132. Storb R: Aplastic anemia. J Intravenous Nurs 1997;20:317–322.

133. Stricker RB, Shuman MA: Quinidine purpura: Evidence that glycoprotein V is a target platelet antigen. Blood 1986;67:1377–1381.

134. Susarala S, Nagaraj MV, Rao PV: Copper sulphate poisoning, hemolysis and methemoglobinemia. J Assoc Physicians India 1985;33: 308–309.

135. Taetle R, Lane TA, Mendelsohn J: Drug-induced agranulocytosis: In vitro evidence for immune suppression of granulopoiesis and a cross-reacting lymphocyte antibody. Blood 1979;54:501–512.

136. Tanner MLA: Molecular and cellular biology of the erythrocyte anion exchanger (AE1). Semin Hematol 1993;30:34–57.

137. Telen MJ, Russel KE: The mature erythrocyte. In: Lee GR, Foerster J, Lukens J, et al, eds: Wintrobe's Clinical Hematology, 10th ed. New York, Lippincott-Williams and Wilkins, 1999, pp. 193–227.

138. Thom SR: Leukocytes in carbon monoxide-mediated brain oxidative injury. Toxicol Applied Pharmacol 1993;123:234–247.

139. Till JE, McCulloch EA: A direct measurement of the radiation sensitivity of normal mouse bone marrow cells. Radiat Res 1961;14: 213–222.

140. Tong J, Bacigalupo A, Piaggio G: In vitro response of T cells from aplastic anemia patients to antilymphocyte globulin and phytohemagglutinin: Colony stimulating activity and lymphokine production. Exp Hematol 1991;19:312–316.

141. Umbreit JN, Conrad ME, Moore EG, Latour LE: Iron absorption and cellular transport: The mobilferrin/paraferritin paradigm. Semin Hematol 1998;35:13–26.

142. Uzel C, Conrad ME: Absorption of heme iron. Semin Hematol 1998; 35:27–34.

143. VanUffelen BE, de Koster BM, VanSteveninck J, et al: Carbon monoxide enhances human neutrophil migration in a cyclic GMP-dependent way. Biochem Biophys Res Commun 1996;226:21–26.

144. Warkentin TE: Clinical presentation of heparin-induced thrombocytopenia. Semin Hematol 1998;35(Suppl 5):9–16.

145. Warkentin TE: Limitations of conventional treatment options for heparin-induced thrombocytopenia. Semin Hematol 1998;35:17–25.

146. Waugh RE, Sassi M: An in vitro model of erythroid egress in bone marrow. Blood 1986;68:250–257.

147. Weaver LK: Carbon Monoxide poisoning. Crit Care Med 1999; 15: 297–317.

148. Weitzman SA, Stossel TP: Drug-induced immunological neutropenia. Lancet 1978;2:1068–1072.

149. Yardley-Jones A, Anderson D, Parke DV: The toxicity of benzene and its metabolism and molecular pathology in human risk assessment. Brit J Indust Med 1991;48:437–444.

150. Young NS, Maciejewski J: Mechanisms of disease: The pathophysiology of acquired aplastic anemia. N Engl J Med 1997;336: 1356–1372.

151. Young NS: Drugs and chemicals. In: Young NS, Alter BP, eds: Aplastic Anemia, Acquired and Inherited. Philadelphia, WB Saunders, 1994, p. 100–131.

152. Young NS: Hematopoietic cell destruction by immune mechanisms in acquired aplastic anemia. Semin Hematol 2000;37:3–14.

153. Zoumbos NC, Djeu, Young NS: Interferon is the suppressor of hematopoiesis generated by stimulated lymphocytes in vitro. J Immunol 1984;133:769–774.

CHAPTER 26 ENDOCRINE PRINCIPLES

Christopher Keyes

Endocrine glands produce substances secreted into the systemic circulation to regulate activities in various parts of the body. These hormones include steroids, prostaglandins, catecholamines, and proteins or polypeptides. Hormones act primarily by modulating protein synthesis or activating cyclic adenosine monophosphate (cAMP) at receptor sites located on the cell walls of the target organs. The focus in this chapter is on the hypoglycemic agents, thyroid toxicology, and steroid and androgenic agents, all of which are important toxicologic concerns.

Endocrine physiology is a delicate homeostasis of hormone antagonists and corresponding feedback mechanisms. Toxins usually impact the endocrine system by changing the effect of a hormone on a target organ, by changing the response of that organ or substituting for it, or by altering the feedback mechanism necessary for homeostasis. Understanding basic organ function is necessary to predict the response evoked by a toxin.

APPROACH TO THE PATIENT WITH ENDOCRINE TOXICITY

Managing a patient's potential endocrine toxicity begins with obtaining a thorough medical history, including the pharmaceutical agents to which the person was exposed. Particular attention should be given to previous or ongoing endocrine therapy. This history may reveal important information about hormonal supplementation or other medications that the patient is receiving. Drug interactions may result as one health practitioner is unaware of the agents prescribed by another. A patient may not know the importance of these interactions. Diagnostic measures may include laboratory testing, an electrocardiogram, and other methods with regard to the specific agents. Pregnancy testing is always prudent in patients who are of childbearing potential, both for consideration of the health of the fetus and the hormonal effects specific to pregnancy.

HYPOGLYCEMIA AND HYPOGLYCEMIC AGENTS

Diabetes mellitus is the fourth leading cause of mortality in the United States.[50] Agents used in the treatment of this disease are therefore commonly prescribed, usually with the objective of long-term lowering of blood glucose.

Treatment of chronically increased blood glucose is an important objective to prevent the complications of diabetes mellitus. The Diabetes Control and Complications Trial (DCCT) was a multicenter trial that provided direct evidence of the benefits of maintaining close control of blood sugar for patients with insulin-dependent diabetes mellitus.[22] Patients who maintained an intensive treatment regimen had a reduced incidence of both microvascular and neuropathic complications. Unfortunately, this cohort had approximately a 3-fold increase in hypoglycemic episodes. The American Diabetes Association recommends the same targets for glycemic control for both type 1 and type 2 diabetics.[60] As a result of this study, many clinicians and their patients now emphasize closer control of blood glucose. Hypoglycemic reactions are common in most emergency departments. Some elderly patients, or those who are not intellectually competent or responsible, are at particular risk of hypoglycemia because of errors in the control of their own treatment. A hypoglycemic episode is commonly referred to as an "insulin reaction" by patients taking this hormonal replacement. Oral agents designed to control hyperglycemia are common today, and often require a different management from an overdose of insulin. The sulfonylureas usually have a much longer duration of action as compared to regular insulin, and hence require prolonged observation and admission to the hospital. The specific characteristics of these agents are discussed in Chapter 40.

Hypoglycemia effects all tissues, but clinically the most evident site of toxicity is the brain. This organ utilizes almost two-thirds of the circulating glucose. The brain is not able to make use of free fatty acids as an energy substrate and is therefore especially susceptible. Synthesis of glucose is essential during the early phases of hypoglycemia in order to preserve the integrity of the central nervous system. The hepatic process of *gluconeogenesis* involves the use of amino acids as primary precursors. Acetoacetic acid and β-hydroxybutyric acid can be used as energy substrates by the brain, but these substances require time to synthesize and are not available in the early phases of hypoglycemia.[93] Symptoms of neuroglycopenia may be mistaken for neuropsychiatric disease.[18]

GLUCOSE METABOLISM AND ENDOCRINE REGULATION

Carbohydrates constitute more than half of the usual dietary caloric intake. Starches are hexose polymers, and these are broken down to oligosaccharides and disaccharides by pancreatic amylase. Disaccharides are broken down to single hexose units by the *disaccharidases*. The α-*glucosidases* are disaccharidases that break down maltose and sucrose to their component monomers fructose and glucose. These glucosidases are located in the brush border of the small intestine. Glucose is readily absorbed across the intestinal lining. Facilitated by insulin, glucose is taken up into the bloodstream, and utilized by tissues throughout the body. It is then either oxidized by the glycolytic pathway (see Fig. 13–1) and the Krebs cycle (see Fig. 13–2) to provide energy for cellular metabolism, or saved by conversion to adipose tissue or glycogen.

GLUCONEOGENESIS

When blood sugar is decreased below normal levels, glucose production is stimulated. This occurs through the conversion of glycogen into glucose, or by the process of gluconeogenesis. Stimulated by glucagon, gluconeogenesis is the process of creating glucose by conversion from various substrates. In the gluconeogenic pathway, the reactions of glycolysis are reversed, with the exception of 3 steps that are irreversible. These irreversible metabolic reactions of glycolysis include those catalyzed by specific enzymes: the *hexokinases, phosphofructokinase* and *pyruvate kinase* (see Fig. 13–1). The first bypass step is from pyruvate to phosphoenolpyruvate (PEP). To accomplish this, pyruvate enters the Krebs cycle through conversion to oxaloacetate (OAA), a reaction catalyzed by *pyruvate carboxylase.* OAA is then converted to PEP by the enzyme *phosphoenolpyruvate carboxykinase.* The second bypass step occurs when fructose-1,6-diphosphate is converted to fructose-6-phosphate. This hydrolysis is catalyzed by *fructose-1,6-diphosphatase.* Finally, glucose-6-phosphate is converted to glucose, catalyzed by *glucose-6-phosphatase* (see Fig. 13–4).

A variety of substrates are used for glucose synthesis via gluconeogenesis. A prominent source is lactate, generated by anaerobic metabolism in the muscle tissues. Here pyruvate is reduced to lactate by *lactate dehydrogenase.* The lactate diffuses into the bloodstream traveling to the liver, where it is extracted and converted via gluconeogenesis to glucose. The glucose then enters the bloodstream and is available for use by brain, muscle, and other tissues. Conversion of tissue lactate to glucose by the liver occurs in what is called the Cori cycle. The gluconeogenic portion of the cycle requires net utilization of ATP. Any amino acid that can be converted to pyruvate, oxaloacetate, or α-ketoglutarate may serve as a glucose substrate in this pathway.

Triglycerides are made up of fatty acids and glycerol. Fatty acids enter the citric acid cycle via acetyl coenzyme A, but cannot be used to synthesize glucose. Glycerol, however, can be used after it is metabolized to dihydroxyacetone phosphate (DHAP).

GLYCOGEN UTILIZATION

The liver is able to store approximately 70 g of glucose in the form of glycogen. A much greater amount is stored in skeletal muscle. Glycogenolysis occurs between meals, and particularly during relatively long fasting periods such as sleep. Glucose residues are removed from α-1–4 linkages by *phosphorylase.* Activation of *glycogen phosphorylase* is subject to important hormonal regulation and is discussed later. Branches in glycogen require a *debranching enzyme* to remove further glucose residues. The resulting glucose-1-phosphate is catalyzed to glucose-6-phosphate by the enzyme *phosphoglucomutase,* then by the action of glucose-6-phosphatase to glucose. Although muscle contains the bulk of glycogen in the body, it lacks this last enzyme, hence glucose is not released into the bloodstream by this tissue.[77] Liver and intes-tine, however, have glucose-6-phosphatase, permitting them to release glucose to the circulation.

When there is a decrease in blood glucose, the liver is able to initiate glycogenolysis and gluconeogenesis to provide this essential substrate to the circulation. This process of glucose generation is inhibited by the presence of large amounts of insulin, but stimulated by the action of epinephrine, norepinephrine, and glucagon.

INSULIN: A MODULATOR OF ANABOLIC METABOLISM

Glucose permeability normally occurs in the brain even in the absence of insulin. Insulin, secreted by the β cells of the pancreatic islets, promotes glucose use by muscle, adipose tissue, and liver. Insulin causes these tissues to utilize more glucose by increasing their cellular permeability to this substrate while promoting glycogen formation and fatty acid synthesis (Fig. 26–1A). The enzyme *insulinase,* present in liver, kidney, and muscle, rapidly degrades insulin,[92] causing it to have a normal half-life of only 5–6 minutes. This time may be prolonged in diabetic individuals who have developed anti-insulin antibodies.[47]

Insulin acts somewhat differently in each of the major tissues. Glycogen formation and fatty acid synthesis are enhanced by insulin in adipose tissue. The conversion of glucose to glycerol, a precursor to triglyceride formation, is also promoted. Breakdown of triglycerides is blocked by insulin's inhibition of *hormone-sensitive lipase,* the enzyme responsible for hydrolysis of these molecules.[62]

Glucose transport into muscle tissue is enhanced by insulin (Fig. 26–1B). Insulin also increases *hexokinase* activity, which phosphorylates glucose to glucose-6-phosphate, transiently trapping the glucose inside the cell. Glycogen formation is then enhanced. The remainder of glucose is oxidized with the formation of energy for cellular metabolism. Protein synthesis is stimulated.

In the setting of insulin hypersecretion and hypoglycemia, glucose utilization by muscle, adipose, and other tissues is enhanced even at the expense of the brain. Glycogenolysis is suppressed, as is intrahepatic gluconeogenesis.

GLUCAGON AND MAINTENANCE OF NORMOGLYCEMIA

Glucagon is a polypeptide that contains 29 amino acids. It is secreted by the α cells of the pancreatic islets and serves to *sustain* adequate blood glucose in the setting of hypoglycemia, an effect opposite to that of insulin. Its metabolic action is almost entirely limited to the liver. Glucagon initiates a chain of events, through cAMP, to activate *phosphorylase,* the rate-limiting enzyme in the degradation of glycogen to glucose-1-phosphate. After dephosphorylation, glucose is released from the liver into the bloodstream. In addition, glucagon promotes glucose synthesis via gluconeogenesis.

Glucagon secretion is greatly stimulated by hypoglycemia, epinephrine, and norepinephrine. Conversely, insulin, glucose, and free fatty acids inhibit α cell release of glucagon. In addition to stimulating glucagon release, epinephrine also directly stimulates liver gluconeogenesis, although to a lesser extent than glucagon. Unlike glucose, amino acids stimulate *both* insulin and glucagon. When protein is ingested, glucagon may protect against the hypo-

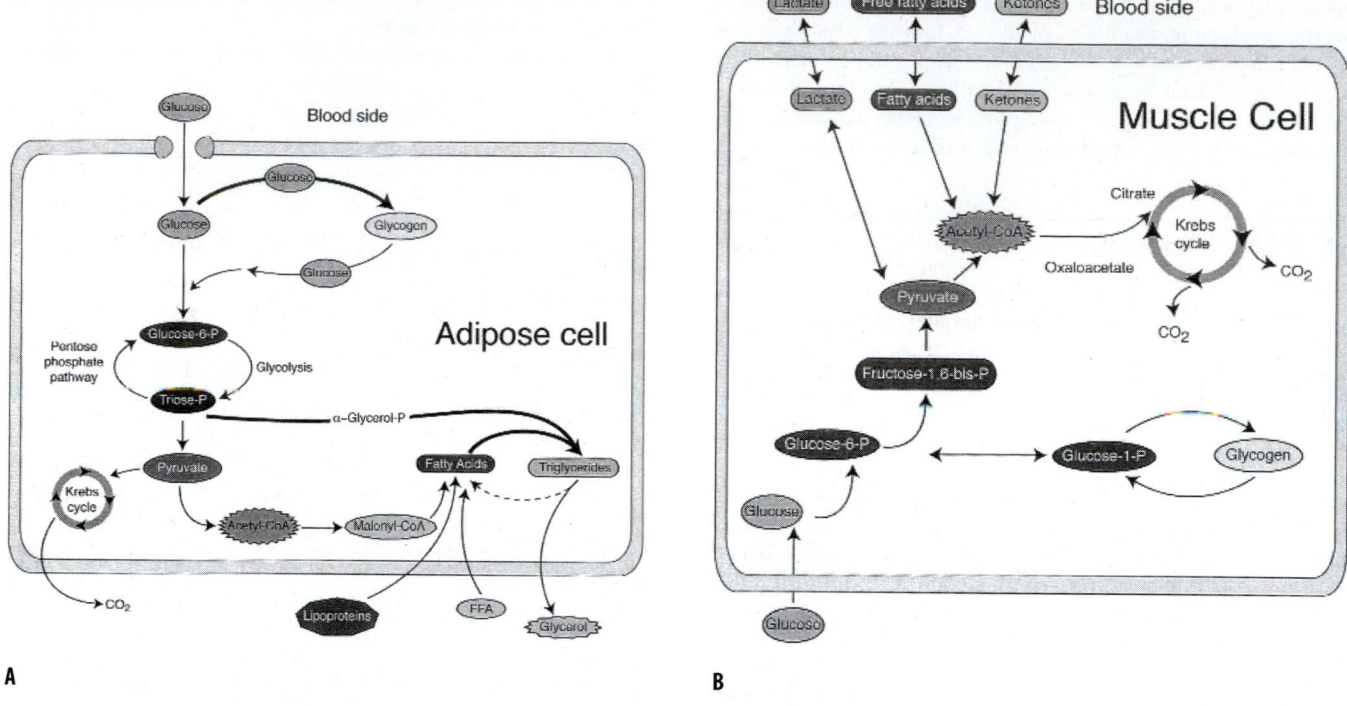

A

B

Figure 26–1. A. Adipose metabolism of carbohydrate and lipids. (*Reprinted with permission of Southwestern Medical School Medical Illustration Department.*) **B.** Muscle metabolism of carbohydrate and lipids. (*Reprinted with permission of Southwestern Medical School Medical Illustration Department.*)

glycemia caused by simultaneous insulin secretion. This is especially important for a low-carbohydrate meal. The balance of insulin and glucagon in the serum determines which processes will prevail intrahepatically: glucose utilization and storage (insulin effect predominates) or glucose production (glucagon effect predominates).[87,116]

Another hormone, somatostatin, inhibits the release from both α cells (glucagon) and β cells (insulin) of the pancreas, growth hormone, TSH, and gastrointestinal peptide hormones.[94] Somatostatin's suppression of glucagon is much more potent than with insulin, but it is also much more transient. Somatostatin is secreted by the δ cells of the pancreas, which appear to be downstream with respect to blood circulation from the α and β cells in this tissue. It is thought, therefore, that somatostatin must exert its effects through the systemic circulation.[99] The precise role of somatostatin remains to be elucidated. Its effects in different tissues are mediated by a variety of receptors. Researchers are seeking somatostatin analogues with more specific end-organ effects. This polypeptide is also found in other tissues of the body.[27]

In the diabetic patient, duration of illness is an important factor when considering the response to hypoglycemia. Early in the course of the disease, both glucagon and epinephrine action remain intact, and the response to hypoglycemia is effective.[96,97] Later in the illness, even secretion of epinephrine is diminished in response to hypoglycemia. There is evidence that with very strict control of type I diabetes, as evidenced by maintenance of glycosylated hemoglobin close to normal levels, brain uptake of glucose may be normal even in the setting of hypoglycemia, thus preserving cerebral metabolism.[12] Also the type of diabetes is important. Patients with noninsulin-dependent diabetes mellitus retain the

glucagon response as compared with insulin-dependent diabetics.[9,10] Hence, glucagon may be relatively less effective in treatment of sulfonamide-induced hypoglycemia, because these patients may have near-maximal stimulation of glucagon prior to the initiation of therapy.

AUTONOMIC NERVOUS SYSTEM AND CARBOHYDRATE METABOLISM

The autonomic nervous system (ANS) has important interactions with carbohydrate metabolism. Substances activate the ANS by interacting with proteins on the cell membrane. These occur in a specific sequence: the receptor is stimulated, a G protein is activated, and cell messenger enzymes or ion channels are "switched on."[98] G-proteins are membrane bound structures that allow very versatile and varied responses through complex interactions on the cell membrane.[38–40,110] Activated by the receptors, these proteins then regulate various cellular effectors such as adenyl cyclase and ion channels on the cell membrane.

β-Adrenergic agonist action stimulates insulin secretion, as does parasympathetic stimulation. α-Adrenergic receptor stimulation inhibits secretion. Epinephrine stimulates glucagon secretion and can also directly increase gluconeogenesis, although not as strongly as glucagon. The catecholamines also increase substrate availability for gluconeogenesis, and inhibit insulin secretion.[90] The catecholamines are dependent on a basal level of cortisol in order to exert their gluconeogenic action.[102] This is also true of glucagon. Cortisol therefore has a permissive effect on the action of these hormones.

Therapy with β-adrenergic antagonists can worsen hypoglycemia in diabetic patients. Epinephrine's effect on increasing hepatic glucose release is mediated by β_2-adrenergic stimulation.[23,89] When diabetics are given β-adrenergic antagonists, catecholamine induced gluconeogenesis and glycogenolysis are impaired. These agents are to be avoided whenever possible in diabetic patients on insulin or sulfonylurea therapy. A newly recognized β_3-adrenergic receptor exists, which may enhance breakdown of adipose tissue; the exact function of this receptor remains to be elucidated.[69,76]

HYPOGLYCEMIA

Insulin and sulfonylureas use are commonly associated with episodes of hypoglycemia (see Chap. 40 for an extensive discussion of this topic). Many diabetics are accustomed to recognizing these reactions, and are able to initiate replacement of glucose rapidly. Some individuals are not able to do so, and are therefore at greater risk of prolonged hypoglycemia if, for example, insulin control is too aggressive. The sulfonylureas have afforded an alternative to injection therapy, and are used primarily by patients who have decreased responsiveness to insulin. The latter condition is commonly associated with obesity. The biguanides work by decreasing production of glucose by the liver[108] and increasing peripheral utilization.[3] Currently the only biguanide available in the U.S. is metformin.

Troglitazone and rosiglitazone are two examples of a new thiazolidinedione class of agents that work primarily by increasing end-organ response to insulin.[35,63,68] These "insulin sensitizers" act by activating the peroxisome proliferator-activated receptor (PPAR-γ) which is responsible for regulating the transcription of genes involved in insulin-mediated glucose uptake in peripheral tissues.[4,73,8] Troglitazone (Rezulin) was removed from the US market by the FDA in March 2000 because of numerous reports of severe hepatotoxicity.[56]

XENOBIOTICS CAUSING HYPOGLYCEMIA

Many drugs may cause hypoglycemia (see Table 40–1). The mechanisms vary considerably, but attention to the basic principles discussed earlier helps in understanding how a decrease in circulating glucose occurs.

Ethanol may cause a decrease in serum glucose, particularly in the setting of previously depleted glycogen stores. Clinically significant hypoglycemia is uncommon, however.[29,105,109] Ethanol inhibits hepatic gluconeogenesis by decreasing the NAD+/NADH ratio, thus promoting oxaloacetate transformation to malate. This blocks the gluconeogenic step leading to phosphoenolpyruvate, stopping glucose synthesis. It is therefore understandable that hypoglycemia only occurs when glycogen stores are depleted. This may be the principal mechanism involved in the development of alcohol-induced hypoglycemia of children under the age of 5 years.[7,20,124]

Pentamidine causes hypoglycemia, and later hyperglycemia, by destroying pancreatic islet β cells.[101] Patients with renal failure are at particular risk of pentamidine-induced hypoglycemia.[2] Acetaminophen is not a direct inducer of hypoglycemia; however, in the event of extensive liver necrosis of any cause, glucose storage and metabolism are impaired, making glucose monitoring essen-

tial. Salicylates cause increased glucose utilization and may cause hypoglycemia, especially in children (Chap. 33). This may occur within the CNS even without peripheral hypoglycemia. For this reason it is recommended that serum glucose be determined with initial laboratory assessment and also whenever alteration in mental status is noted. β Adrenergic antagonists have an effect opposite to that of epinephrine, causing hypoglycemia and hyperkalemia in overdose (Chap. 49).

TREATMENT OF HYPOGLYCEMIA

Treatment of hypoglycemia is discussed in Chapter 40. Administration of dextrose is the mainstay of such treatment. Glucagon is sometimes used as a temporizing measure to treat hypoglycemia in patients who have no intravenous access because it can be administered intramuscularly.[113] It acts rapidly, and can maintain serum glucose at life-sustaining levels while glycogen stores continue to be available. When administered intravenously, glucagon action is transient, with a plasma half-life of only 3–6 minutes.[61,88] When used for the treatment of hypoglycemia usually 1–2 mg are administered parenterally. Glucagon's action to raise serum glucose is largely dependent on adequate glycogen stores in the liver. These stores may be depleted in chronic alcoholism, prolonged fasting, or with certain hormonal deficiencies (eg, cortisol, growth hormone) and hence glucagon may be ineffective in these circumstances.[13,15] Glucose supplementation should always follow its use. In the presence of high insulin levels, the ability of glucagon to raise blood glucose is decreased. Glucagon should not be used when intravenous dextrose is available in these situations.

Diazoxide is not recommended for treatment of hypoglycemia because it is minimally effective and is associated with hypotension. Somatostatin, which inhibits glucose-stimulated β-cell insulin release, has been used to control hypoglycemia, but it is not practical for clinical use due to its short half-life (4–5 minutes). Octreotide, a long-acting somatostatin analogue (half-life of 72 minutes) is effective in preventing recurrence of hypoglycemia in patients with sulfonylurea overdoses.[11] Octreotide also prevents hypoglycemia in patients with quinine overdoses[88] and in those patients with insulinomas.[53] Patients with recurrent hypoglycemia should be admitted and monitored with serial blood sugar measurements for a minimum of 1–2 days as clinically warranted (see Antidotes in Depth: Octreotide).[11,83]

THE BIGUANIDES AND LACTIC ACIDOSIS PRODUCTION

Even though phenformin and metformin were introduced in the late 1950s, their mechanism of action is poorly understood.[100] They are currently thought to act primarily by decreasing hepatic output of glucose, but they also improve peripheral insulin sensitivity. Insulin sensitivity is a result of metformin's augmentation of insulin-dependent glucose transport by the translocation of the glucose transporters GLUT-1 and GLUT-4. Numerous studies show efficacy for the use of metformin in type 2 diabetes mellitus, allowing control of serum glucose similar to the sulfonylureas, but without causing hypoglycemia.[24,117] Phenformin was removed from the market in the 1970s because of multiple reports of lactic acid production. Lactic acidosis is the most serious complication of biguanide use.[121] Lactic acidosis is classified as either type A (anaerobic) or type B (aerobic). The lactic acidosis from biguanides is type B. Phenformin is much more likely to cause lactic acidosis, with an estimated incidence of 0.64 cases per 1000 patient-years, as compared to 0.03 cases per 1000 patient-years for metformin.[108] The most important factor in the occurrence of lactic acidosis involves the improper prescribing of these agents to patients with contraindications. These contraindications include hepatic insufficiency, renal failure, cardiac or pulmonary disease, and chronic alcohol abuse. Chronic renal insufficiency is an important contraindication, because it results in the accumulation of metformin, and therefore presents a greatly increased risk of lactic acidosis. It is unclear whether the cause of lactic acidosis is entirely a result of metformin accumulation or a result of associated disease states.[108]

THE THYROID

Physiology

To properly understand the impact of thyroid supplements and inhibitory agents on the function of the human body, the interaction of these hormones with the following sites must be examined: (a) the hypothalamus; (b) the pituitary gland; (c) the thyroid gland;

and (d) the target organs for the thyroid hormones (Fig. 26–2). As in the case of many other endocrine relationships, feedback loops are very important in determining the function of these organs.

The hypothalamus is an intermediate between cerebral centers and the pituitary gland. When the hypothalamus receives specific neurotransmitter stimulation, thyroid-releasing hormone (TRH) is produced. TRH is transported through the venous sinusoids to the pituitary, where thyroid-stimulating hormone (TSH) is released. When TSH enters the circulation, it stimulates thyroid hormone production and its release.

Thyroid physiology is an excellent example of the concept of feedback control of hormonal function. Most endocrine organs tend to produce an excess of hormone. When the desired effect is achieved, inhibition of the secretory gland occurs. When thyroid hormones are released, they exert an inhibitory influence on the pituitary gland, which diminishes the production of TSH. This suppression of TSH is a frequently used laboratory marker in the evaluation of hyperthyroidism.

Thyroid hormones consist of tyrosine molecules with iodine substitutions. Two forms of the hormone are physiologically active: triiodothyronine and tetraiodothyronine (Fig. 26–2). The synthesis of thyroid hormones is a multiple-step process. Tyrosine is concentrated in the follicles of the thyroid gland, which consist of

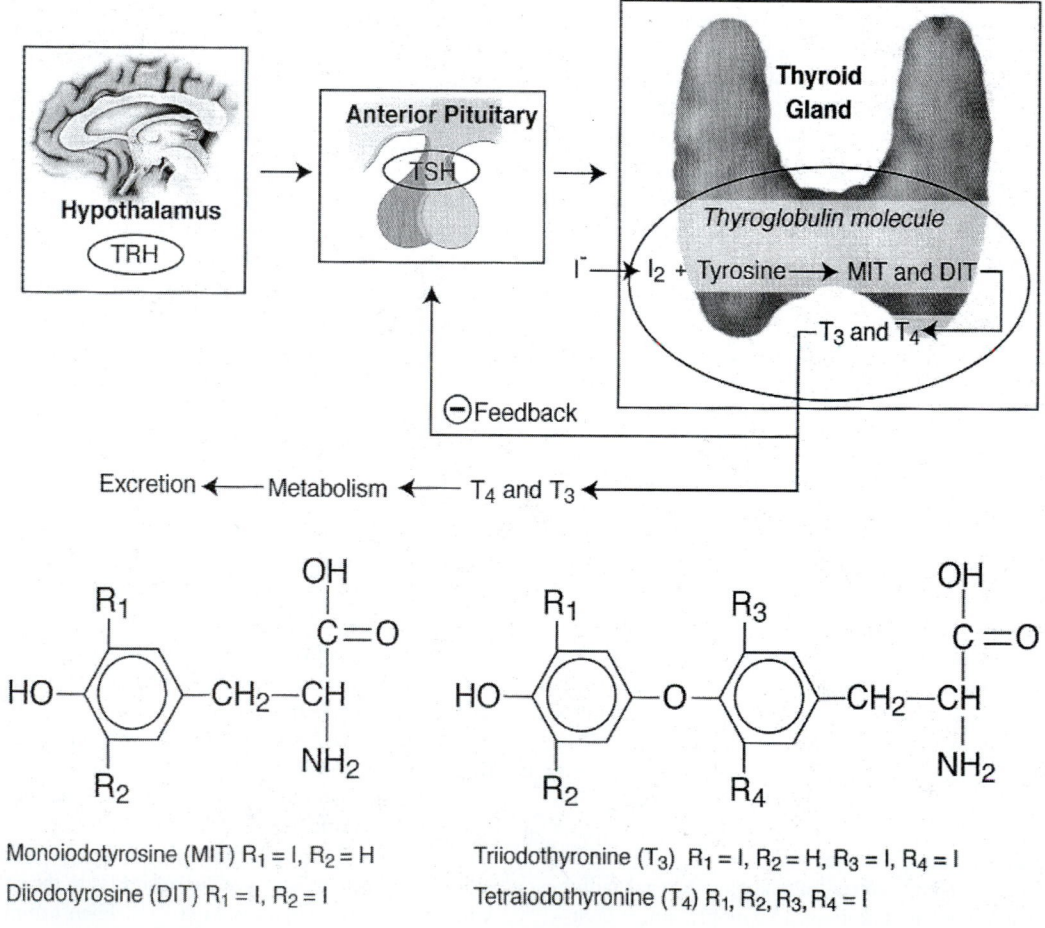

Figure 26–2. Thyroid hormone synthesis: its control, metabolism and molecular structures. (*Reprinted with permission of Southwestern Medical School Medical Illustration Department.*)

an epithelial layer surrounding a proteinaceous colloidal substance called thyroglobulin. Thyroglobulin contains a large amount of tyrosine. After iodide is absorbed from the circulation, it is concentrated in the thyroid cells that surround the follicles, by a process of active transport. It is thought that the enzyme *iodide peroxidase* catalyzes the formation of tyrosine and iodide free radicals, which then combine to form monoiodotyrosine (MIT) and diiodotyrosine (DIT). The substituted tyrosine molecules thus formed combine to form triiodothyronine (T_3) and tetraiodothyronine (T_4). T_3 and T_4 are taken up by the endothelial cells by endocytosis and broken down in the lysosomes. T_3 and T_4 (thyroxine), the thyroid hormones, are subsequently released into the circulation. Of the two thyroid hormones, T_3 is the more active, having approximately 3 times as great a thyroid hormonal effect as thyroxine (T_4). Only 15% of T_3 is secreted directly by the thyroid. The remaining T_3 is formed by the peripheral deiodination of T_4, which occurs mainly in the liver and kidney by the enzyme, 5'-deiodinase. The action of T_4 may be explained completely by its conversion to T_3 outside of the thyroid gland.

Thyroid Hormone Function and Hyperfunction

Thyroxine and T_3 exert their action intracellularly, where they are ultimately metabolized. Sequential deiodination accounts for approximately two-thirds of hormonal inactivation. Most of the remaining hormone is eliminated intrahepatically by glucuronidation or sulfation.

Cytochrome P450 inducers such as phenobarbital and phenytoin increase the rate of clearance of thyroid hormones, but there is no perceptible decrease in circulating hormone, presumably because of feedback stimulation of thyroid secretion.

Thyroid hormones act through nuclear receptors, regulating gene transcription and synthesis of specific proteins. These proteins act by stimulating Na^+/K^+-ATPase, thereby increasing oxygen consumption. Thyroid function is the most important determinant of basal metabolic rate (BMR). Most aspects of carbohydrate metabolism are increased in the presence of thyroid hormone excess, as is protein metabolism. Lipid metabolism is increased, and there is an increase in cholesterol synthesis. Cholesterol levels are actually lowered, however, because of thyroxine stimulation of bile acid secretion. Thyroid action exercises a permissive effect on many hormones to exert their action, including the catecholamines and insulin.

Thyroxine and T_3 are highly bound to proteins in the serum, approximately 99.97% in the nonpregnant adult. Thyroxine-binding globulin (TBG) binds approximately two-thirds of the circulating thyroid hormones, while albumin and other proteins bind the remainder. The amount of hormone bound to proteins can vary greatly, increasing in pregnancy and decreasing in chronic disease, for example. Such changes in protein binding must be considered when measuring total thyroxine in the blood.

When an excess of active thyroid hormone exists, the condition is known as hyperthyroidism. The clinical picture consists of the manifestations of increased metabolism, along with tachycardia, tremor, anxiety and other behavioral changes, and sometimes cardiovascular effects such as atrial fibrillation.[37] This constellation of symptoms is called *thyrotoxicosis,* and may result from overproduction of the hormone, activation of circulating hormone from T_4 to T_3 or from exogenous administration of thyroid supplements. The most common condition causing the thyroid to secrete excess hormone is Graves disease, a diffuse increase in thyroid gland volume that accounts for approximately two-thirds of cases. Graves disease is often accompanied by exophthalmos and is autoimmune in nature. Hyperfunction of the thyroid can be manifested by thyrotoxicosis, which was described earlier. If it is especially severe and accompanied by decompensation of the patient, it is called *thyroid storm* or *thyrotoxic crisis.* The most common causes of this condition involve primary pathology of the thyroid gland itself.

Chronic excess thyroid hormone ingestion is a relatively common occurrence. Thyroid supplementation for treatment of hypothyroidism is widespread. It is estimated that Synthroid, the commercial name of the most common form of levothyroxine (T_4), is the fifth most commonly prescribed drug in the United States. Acute overdoses with this agent are also common, particularly among children, but they are almost universally benign[75] and no deaths have been reported. Significant ingestions of levothyroxine usually do not manifest clinically until a week after the exposure. This is caused by the delay in peripheral conversion of thyroxine to the metabolically active T_3. Overdoses of preparations containing T_3 often manifest in the first several days after exposure.

Chronic exposures to thyroid supplementation can lead to more severe disease, and patients may present with thyrotoxicosis or thyroid storm. *Thyrotoxicosis factitia* is a chronic ingestion of thyroid hormone, often by healthcare workers.[48] The objective of such ingestion may be to achieve weight loss. This syndrome of thyrotoxicosis generally occurs in patients who have access to thyroid medications being taken by relatives or friends, or who can obtain the medications at their place of employment.[78,111] Ground meat from the neck of animals has resulted in symptoms of thyroid excess, dubbed *hamburger thyrotoxicosis*.[54] Administration of excessive thyroid supplement chronically may also result in accelerated osteoporosis.[85]

Persons who ingest these hormones chronically may develop severe manifestations such as cardiac dysrhythmias, including atrial flutter or atrial fibrillation, tachycardia, and even cardiac failure. Thyroid storm may occur as a result of intercurrent illness in the setting of thyrotoxicosis. Tachycardia is often disproportionate to fever. The patient may become unresponsive and death can occur in up to 20% of patients with thyroid storm.

Thyroid Laboratory Testing

Until recently, thyroid testing was undertaken using combinations of measurements of total T_3 and/or T_4 and some measurement of hormone binding. Recently, direct measurement of free hormone concentrations using radioimmunoassay was developed for commercial use. A newer, rapid TSH test, with very increased sensitivity, that uses monoclonal antibodies is now widely available. This supersensitive TSH test may be used in the emergent diagnosis and management of thyroid disorders. The most common application is in thyroid hormone excess, where TSH is usually nondetectable (<0.1 mU/L) in most assays.

Management of Thyroid Excess

In most cases of patients who overdose acutely with thyroid supplement medications, the management consists of home observation. Decontamination is recommended in those patients who ingest greater than 5 mg of levothyroxine, but the evidence is only exposure based.[115] In cases in which children have ingested larger doses, syrup of ipecac is usually recommended within the first hour after the ingestion. In cases in which the levothyroxine dose is greater than 4 mg, it has been suggested that the patient be followed by regular telephone contact for 10 days.[68] Thyroxine levels may be elevated but provide no clinically useful information. Treatment should be based on the development of symptoms.[43]

Treatment for thyroid storm includes hydration, antipyretics, antithyroid drugs, and addressing the underlying causes. β-Adrenergic antagonists are the usual treatment for suppression of the symptoms of thyrotoxicosis, and are successful in reducing heart rate, palpitations, anxiety, and tremor. Propranolol is the most commonly employed agent, but this is based on tradition and other β-adrenergic antagonists are also used. In those instances in which β-adrenergic antagonists are relatively contraindicated, such as in asthma, verapamil may be considered.[54]

Antithyroid Drugs

Antithyroid drugs are used to decrease the amount of thyroid hormone in hyperthyroidism, most commonly for Graves disease. Methimazole is a thioamide derivative that decreases production of thyroid hormone, most likely by inhibiting the activity of *thyroid peroxidase*.[112] Propylthiouracil, also a thioamide, is a more commonly used agent which in addition to this diminution of thyroid hormone synthesis also inhibits conversion of T_4 to the metabolically more active T_3. This results from PTU inactivation of 5'-deiodinase, an effect that methimazole does not have.[31,74] Methimazole can cause agranulocytosis, an effect not reported with propylthiouracil.[82] Agranulocytosis is apparently dose related. This potentially life-threatening adverse effect can now be treated by administration of granulocyte colony-stimulating factor.[5] No other serious sequelae have been associated with thioamides in acute overdose. These antithyroid drugs are not usually administered to victims of thyroid overdose.

Other Drugs that Alter Thyroid Function

A variety of drugs have secondary effects on thyroid physiology. It is uncommon for these agents to cause clinically significant disease related to thyroid function. Lithium therapy is an exception to this, causing goiter in as many as 37% of patients, and hypothyroidism in 5–15% of patients.[41] Thyroid function tests should be performed upon initiation of lithium treatment, and at regular intervals thereafter. Iodine can have a substantial impact on thyroid function, but this is usually transient. Small doses may stimulate thyroid hormone secretion. With larger iodine exposure (over 10 mg/d), thyroid hormone release is decreased, usually within the first day. This effect is maximal after about 2 weeks, but with time this effect does not continue.[52] Iodinated contrast media has also been reported to have this effect.

Hyperthyroidism resulting from amiodarone has been divided into two types. Type 1 is caused by iodine excess resulting in stimulation of thyroid production.[14,46] This typically occurs in patients who have preexisting goiters resulting from low iodine intake.[64,65] These patients can be treated with antithyroid drugs or radioiodine. Type 2 amiodarone hypothyroidism is associated with thyroid inflammation, has low radioiodine uptake, and usually occurs in patients who do not have goiter.[64] These patients may be treated with prednisone which is tapered after several weeks when thyroid function normalizes.

Amiodarone also may cause hypothyroidism as a result of inhibition of peripheral conversion of thyroxin to T_3. Hypothyroidism results in as many as 25% of patients treated with amiodarone.[49,64,120] Treatment is the same as for other causes of hypothyroidism. There is generally no need for discontinuation of the antiarrhythmic agent.

STEROIDS AND ANABOLIC SUPPLEMENTS

When corticotropin-releasing factor (CRF) is produced by the hypothalamus, it results in the release of adrenocorticotropin (ACTH), a polypeptide from the anterior pituitary gland. ACTH is produced from a larger precursor molecule, pro-opiomelanocortin (POMC), from which other important peptides are produced. Other peptides derived from POMC include the endorphins and melanocyte-stimulating hormones.[70] ACTH stimulates adrenal steroid synthesis, a process initiated by uptake of cholesterol to form an undifferentiated steroid nucleus. Three divergent metabolic pathways may then follow to produce C-19 steroids with androgenic function and 17-ketosteroids, or C-21 steroids with mineralocorticoid or glucocorticoid properties (Fig. 26–3). The more central zone is the *fasciculata-reticularis,* where cortisol and androgen synthesis occurs, whereas peripherally aldosterone and adrenal androgens are formed in the *glomerulosa*. As in the case of the thyroid hormones, steroid hormones circulate largely bound to serum proteins. Metabolism of the steroids occurs in the liver, largely by glucuronidation.

The major adrenally secreted androgen is dehydroepiandrosterone (DHEA). Other androgenic steroids secreted include 11-β-hydroxyandrostenedione and testosterone. In the male, the testes produce a smaller, yet significant proportion of androgenic steroids, whereas in the female, almost all are derived from the adrenals.

Steroids exert their action through a cAMP-mediated cascade, after diffusing passively across cell membranes. The action that results depends on the initiating molecule. Glucocorticoids are so named because they tend to increase blood glucose levels by promoting gluconeogenesis. The glucocorticoid receptor has been delineated, and amino acid sequences in the binding domain are now identified. DNA enhancement of transcription is normally inhibited by the receptor. When the glucocorticoid binds, the receptor is disinhibited.[36,58] Levels of hydrocortisone respond rapidly to stressors such as trauma or hypoglycemia. When hydrocortisone levels are diminished, stresses such as these may cause hypotension and death, hence the importance of substitution of this steroid agent in the setting of adrenal insufficiency. Levels of both the carrier proteins and free cortisol also increase in pregnancy.

Glucocorticoid effects are well known to most practitioners because of their widespread use. These effects are dependent upon the relative potency of a given agent being administered, and to the duration of therapy. They modulate carbohydrate, lipid, and nucleic acid metabolism. The most important role of glucocorticoids is in carbohydrate metabolism, where they act to preserve glucose availability to the brain. Gluconeogenesis is enhanced, while peripheral utilization is inhibited. This is particularly noticeable in the setting of starvation, where the absence of glucocorticoids results in hypoglycemia. With long-term exposure to supraphysiologic doses of glucocorticoids, a condition resembling diabetes ensues. This is manifested by fasting hyperglycemia and insulin resistance.[80] Cushing syndrome is the manifestation of glucocorticoid excess, which also effects lipid metabolism. Fat is deposited in a specific pattern in the back of the neck, a pattern

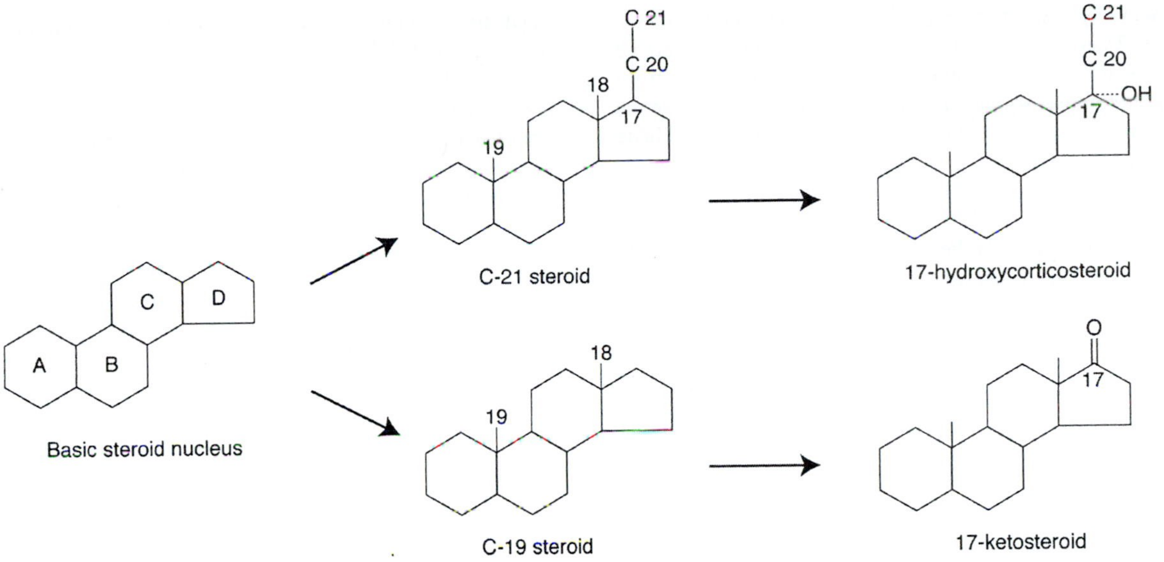

Figure 26–3. Structures of the major steroids. (*Reprinted with permission of Southwestern Medical School Medical Illustration Department.*)

which is referred to as "buffalo hump," and a pattern which in the face, is referred to as "moon facies." With acute administration of glucocorticoids, an increase in circulating polymorphonuclear leukocytes is seen, resulting from demargination from vessel walls. Over time, there is a decrease in the number of circulating eosinophils, lymphocytes, monocytes, and basophils. Leukocyte function is also impaired, which is the major reason that glucocorticoids possess immunosuppressive and anti-inflammatory effects.[16] In contrast, the red blood cell mass increases in Cushing syndrome, while a normochromic, normocytic anemia is characteristic of Addison disease (hypoadrenal state) (see Table 26–1).

Patients with glucocorticoid excess may develop mood elevation and CNS excitability. Some may become overtly psychotic. The mechanism of this "steroid psychosis" is unknown, but these agents may play a role in the control of local neuronal excitability.[81]

Mineralocorticoids increase extracellular fluid volume by causing renal distal tubular reabsorption of sodium. Aldosterone is the most important mineralocorticoid, which also acts to increase the secretion of potassium. Its major stimulus is the renin-angiotensin system. If angiotensin-converting enzyme (ACE) inhibitors are taken, activation of angiotensin is blocked, and synthesis of aldosterone is decreased. This has the effect of lowering blood pressure and retaining potassium. Treatment of ACE inhibitor overdose is undertaken primarily by intravenous volume repletion.

Other agents can also inhibit steroid genesis. One such agent that is used frequently in the emergency department is etomidate. Etomidate has occasionally been associated with suppression of the adrenal axis and decreased serum cortisol, especially when sedation with this agent has been prolonged. Hydrocortisone should be administered in these cases.[118]

Androgenic and Anabolic Steroid Use

Androgens stimulate male secondary sexual characteristics by binding to receptors in target tissue cytoplasm. As early as 1938, it was observed that removing the testes in guinea pigs abolished the larger skeletal muscle size in males.[86] Plasma concentrations of testosterone are increased in males during the neonatal period and remain elevated after puberty.[45] Feedback inhibition of the pituitary becomes minimal at puberty.[123]

Anabolic steroids are used for medical purposes for such indications as osteoporosis, anemia, breast cancer treatment, or hypogonadism.[19] There is a continual pursuit of newer agents that minimize the androgenic (masculinizing) effects while maintaining the anabolic (growth) effects. Use of anabolic steroids by athletes is an epidemic in the United States. Estimates based on the National Household Survey on Drug Abuse suggest that there are more than 1 million current or former users of anabolic steroids in the United States.[125] The users typically wish to increase athletic performance or muscle mass by using these agents. Muscle mass may be increased by use of these agents in some cases, but aerobic capacity is probably not increased.[1,51]

TABLE 26–1. **Adverse Effects Associated with Chronic Administration of Glucocorticoids**

Cardiovascular	Increased risk of coronary heart disease
	Acute myocardial infarction
	Increased blood pressure
Muscle	Increased muscle mass
Adipose	Truncal obesity
	Prominent supraclavicular and dorsal cervical fat pads
	Increased cholesterol
Liver	Cholestatic jaundice
	Abnormal liver function
	Hepatic tumors
	Gynecomastia
Skin	Increased acne
	Hair loss
Genitourinary	Testicular shrinkage
Behavior	Severe mood disorders
	Psychotic reactions
	Increased episodes of violence and rage
Development	Decreased height

The method of use of these agents varies considerably among individuals. Testosterone has had a resurgence in recent years because of the difficulty in distinguishing this molecule from endogenous hormone. It has a very short duration of action, however, and is not practical for those seeking the presumed benefits of anabolic steroids. Other agents fall into two general classes, based on the substitutions at the 17α position with alkyl or carboxylic acid side groups. The alkyl substitution results in agents that are well absorbed orally, because of their resistance to hepatic first-pass metabolism. These agents are associated with hepatotoxicity.[30,34,84] The 17α-carboxylic acid substitution results in agents that are poorly absorbed orally and that are used parenterally. The carboxylic side group must be hydrolyzed prior to becoming active biologically. Agents are often taken in large doses for short periods of time, and several different agents may be taken simultaneously. The latter phenomenon is referred to as *stacking.*[111] Other patterns of use include *plateauing,* where different steroids are taken in overlapping patterns to prevent tolerance. *Pyramiding* is the practice whereby anabolic steroids are taken for finite periods of time alternating with periods of abstinence.[44] These drugs have been taken in cycles of 12–18 weeks to minimize adverse effects such as testicular atrophy (Chap. 112).

Numerous side effects have been attributed to the anabolic steroids, and these are reviewed elsewhere.[57] In males, these hormones result in a negative feedback, causing a decrease in testosterone, luteinizing hormone (LH), and follicle-stimulating hormone (FSH).[17,95,103] This occurs even with long-term low-dose use of an agent such as the very commonly used methandrostenolone (Dianabol).[95] Testicular atrophy,[107] decreased spermatogenesis,[59] and gynecomastia often ensue, and may be the result of inadequate breakdown of estrogen by a less-efficient liver.[122]

Premature epiphyseal closure is an important musculoskeletal system effect in children. An increased susceptibility to cartilaginous and ligamentous injury has also been described with the use of these agents.[104] Levels of low-density lipoprotein (LDL) cholesterol are increased, with simultaneous decreases in high-density lipoprotein (HDL) cholesterol. These findings may explain a relationship between anabolic steroid use and an increased risk of stroke and myocardial infarction in athletes using these agents.[32,33]

In women, a variety of androgenic effects—including amenorrhea, acne, hirsutism, and reduction in breast size—become evident even at therapeutic doses.[57] Baldness, clitoral hypertrophy, deepening of the voice, and facial hairs are usually irreversible.

The most serious toxicity of the anabolic steroids is associated with the 17α-alkylated (oral) agents, which may cause severe hepatotoxicity. Elevated aminotransferase levels are often transient, but may persist and culminate in severe liver disease.[32] Hepatic cholestasis is occasionally fatal.[95] *Peliosis hepatis* is a common finding following anabolic steroid use, consisting of blood-filled sacks in the peripheral zone of the hepatic lobule.[72] Hepatic neoplasms have been reported extensively in association with anabolic steroid use. In one review, the majority of these were hepatocellular carcinomas or angiosarcomas, with the remaining being hepatomas or other benign tumors.[57] Although most patients with hepatocellular carcinoma rapidly succumb, some of these neoplasms may remit with cessation of the drug.[119]

Testing for anabolic steroid use has been an ongoing concern by those responsible for competitive athletic events. The International Olympic Committee has issued standards for such testing, indicating that gas chromatography/mass spectrometry (GC/MS) analysis is the only method that consistently does not report false-positive results.[57,61,104]

Other hormonal agents have also been used by athletes in an effort to enhance performance. Growth hormone is one such agent that has been used because of the inability of urine tests to detect this protein. No problems with short-term use have been noted, but no benefits are derived from such misuse of this hormone (Chap. 112).

ESTROGENIC AGENTS AND ORAL CONTRACEPTIVES

The estrogens are the hormones responsible for female secondary sexual characteristics. They exert their actions mostly on specific tissues that respond to their presence. These include the mammary glands, vagina, uterus, and fallopian tube. Of greatest importance, estrogens cause endometrial hyperplasia. Along with progesterone, estrogen regulates the reproductive cycle in females. Estrogen supplementation is very common. It is frequently prescribed in postmenopausal women to manage symptoms of menopause and later to prevent osteoporosis. Approximately one of five women in their childbearing years uses combinations of estrogens with progesterone to prevent conception.

Estrogens contain the cyclopentanophenanthrene ring characteristic of steroids, with an essential phenol present in the A ring. Nonsteroidal estrogens exist that also possess the phenol structure. The most widely known of these nonsteroidal agents is diethylstilbestrol (DES). Estradiol is produced in the liver and adipose tissue by oxidation of estradiol-17β, secreted by the ovary. Estradiol is subsequently hydrated to form estriol. Androstenedione is converted to estradiol-17βα through conversion to testosterone, and aromatization of the A ring. This accounts for up to one-third of estrogen production after menopause. In addition to conversion to estriol, estrogens can undergo glucuronidation and sulfation. These mechanisms increase their water solubility and renal excretion.

Estrogens taken in large quantities frequently cause nausea. Gynecomastia and feminization may be seen in males, especially after prolonged administration. If estrogens are administered for a long period and then withdrawn, uterine bleeding may be severe as a result of endometrial hyperplasia. Endometrial hyperplasia is also considered a risk factor for adenocarcinoma.

The nonsteroidal stilbene derivatives such as DES are metabolized via quinone and semiquinone intermediates, which may be related to the teratogenic and carcinogenic effects of these drugs. These agents are orally active and have a relatively long duration of action. DES has been associated with vaginal clear-cell adenocarcinoma in the offspring of women who received DES during their first trimester of pregnancy. Other vaginal and cervical structural abnormalities have also been identified in these daughters of DES users.

In addition to the physiologic role of the estrogens, they are often used in combination with progestins to inhibit ovulation. Progestins are substances related to progesterone, the endogenous hormone produced by the corpus luteum during pregnancy (by the placenta) and during the normal menstrual cycle (by the corpus luteum). Numerous synthetic derivatives of progesterone have been developed.

The tissue targets of progesterone action include the mammary gland and uterus. Receptors for progesterone in these tissues are dependent on a permissive effect of estrogen. This hormone is responsible for maintaining pregnancy and decreasing the contractility of the endometrium. Progesterone is necessary for breast development and postpartum lactation, mediated by prolactin. The progestins are used principally in conjunction with estrogen as oral contraceptive agents. These agents can cause androgenic sequelae when used in large doses, including hirsutism and acne. Progestins are thought to decrease the risk of endometrial cancer and perhaps breast cancer when used with estrogen in postmenopausal women.

Oral contraceptive pill use results in an increased risk of thromboembolic phenomena.[53] Carbohydrate and lipid metabolism are also influenced in many patients. Glucose intolerance may occur, especially in those patients who develop diabetes during their gestation. Serum triglyceride levels increase markedly, and depend on the progestin content of the preparation. Perhaps through this increase in triglycerides, HDL cholesterol levels are reduced. Estrogens tend to increase HDL levels.

Overdose with oral contraceptive pills is rarely reported, perhaps because of the benign nature of the increased dosage. Vaginal spotting may occur, and edema of the thighs has been reported with estradiol implant overdose.[28,106]

ENDOCRINE DISRUPTERS

In the 1970s, a marked increase in the number of vaginal adenocarcinomas was noted. It was subsequently found that these cases resulted from the exposure of women in the 1950s to DES, which was incorrectly thought to be effective at preventing spontaneous abortion.[55] Currently, the possibility that many environmental chemicals may result in endocrine modulation, such as fertility problems, cancer involving the testes, prostate, or breast, thyroid effects, and even behavioral changes,[42] is being investigated. These substances, or xenoestrogens as they are sometimes called, are the object of much scientific and regulatory interest. The United States Environmental Protection Agency has established the Endocrine Disrupter Screening and Testing Advisory Committee to investigate the impact of both estrogenic and antiestrogenic impact on human health.[79,91] At this time, more data is necessary to establish the clear environmental impact of these agents.[67,21]

SUMMARY

Diabetic agents are relatively frequent causes for toxicity, and the practitioner is often quite familiar with the management of these patients. Glucose is an essential substrate for energy production and measurement with bedside techniques has become an essential part of managing the patient who presents confused or in coma. Other endocrinopathies are uncommon causes of concern for the medical toxicologist or emergency practitioner. To make the correct diagnosis and properly manage these patients, it is necessary to give proper attention to the relevant history and physical findings, and to maintain a high index of suspicion. The basic physiology is directly applicable to the management of the patient with toxin-induced hypo- or hyperthyroidism, or with the steroid-based agents.

ACKNOWLEDGMENTS

Special thanks to Richard Sahadi, medical illustrator at the University of Texas Southwestern Medical Center for his important contribution to this chapter.

REFERENCES

1. American College of Sports Medicine: Position on the use of anabolic-androgenic steroids in sports. Am J Sports Med 1984;12:13–18.
2. Assan R, Perronne C, Assan D, et al: Pentamidine-induced derangements of glucose homeostasis. Determinant roles of renal failure and drug accumulation. A study of 128 patients. Diabetes Care 1995;18:47–55.
3. Bailey CJ: Biguanides and NIDDM. Diabetes Care 1992; 15: 755–772.
4. Balfour JA, Plosker GL: Rosiglitazone. Drugs 1999;57:921–930; discussion 931–932.
5. Bartalena L, Bogazzi F, Martino E: Adverse effects of thyroid hormone preparations and antithyroid drugs. Drug Saf 1996;15:53–63.
6. Bartalena L, Brogioni S, Grasso L, et al: Treatment of amiodarone-induced thyrotoxicosis, a difficult challenge: Results of a prospective study. J Clin Endocrinol Metab 1996;81:2930–2933.
7. Beattie JO, Hull D, Cockburn F: Children intoxicated by alcohol in Nottingham and Glasgow, 1973–84. Br Med J 1986;292:519–521.
8. Berger JP, Bailey CJ: Thiazolidinediones produce a conformational change in peroxisomal proliferator-activated receptor-gamma: Binding and activation correlate with antidiabetic actions in db/db mice. Endocrinology 1996;137:4189–4195.
9. Boden G, Soriano M, Hoeldke R, et al: Counterregulatory hormone release and glucose recovery after hypoglycemia in noninsulin-dependent diabetic patients. Diabetes 1983;32:1055–1059.
10. Bolli G, Tsahkian E, Haymond M, et al: Defective glucose counterregulation after subcutaneous insulin in noninsulin-dependent diabetes mellitus. J Clin Invest 1984;73:1532–1541.
11. Boyle PJ, Justice K, Krenz AJ, et al: Octreotide reverses hyperinsulinemia and prevents hypoglycemia induced by sulfonylurea overdoses. J Clin Endocrinol Metab 1993;76:752–756.
12. Boyle PJ, Kempers SF, O'Connor AM, et al: Brain glucose uptake and unawareness of hypoglycemia in patients with insulin-dependent diabetes mellitus. N Engl J Med 1995;333:1726–1731.
13. Cahill GF: Action of adrenal cortical steroids on carbohydrate metabolism. In: Christy NP, ed: The Human Adrenal Cortex. New York, Harper & Row, 1971, pp. 205–240.
14. Cappiello E, Boldorini R, Tosoni A, et al: Ultrastructural evidence of thyroid damage in amiodarone-induced thyrotoxicosis. J Endocrinol Invest 1995;18:862–868.
15. Cherrington AD: Gluconeogenesis: Its regulation by insulin and glucagon. In: Brownlee M, ed: Handbook of Diabetes Mellitus. Vol. 3. Intermediary Metabolism and Its Regulation. New York, Garland STPM Press, 1981, pp. 49–117.
16. Chrousos GP: The hypothalamic-pituitary-adrenal axis and immune-mediated inflammation. N Engl J Med 1995;332:1351–1362.
17. Clerico A, Ferdeghini M, Palombo C, et al: Effect of anabolic treatment on the serum levels of gonadotropins, testosterone, prolactin, thyroid hormones and myoglobin of male athletes under physical training. J Nucl Med Allied Sci 1981;23:79–84.
18. Cortesao L, Saraiva AM, Guerreiro L: The endocrine pancreas. Acta Med Port 1995;8(Suppl 1):S47–S53.
19. Council on Scientific Affairs, American Medical Association: Drug abuse in athletes. Anabolic steroids and human growth hormone. JAMA 1988;259:1703–1705.
20. Cummins LH: Hypoglycemia and convulsions in children following alcohol ingestion. J Pediatr 1961;58:23–26.

21. Daston GP, Gooch JW, Breslin NJ, et al: Environmental estrogens and reproductive health: A discussion of the human and environmental data. Reprod Toxicol 1997;11:465–481.

22. DCCT Research Group: The effect of intensive treatment of diabetes on the development and progression of long-term complications in insulin-dependent diabetes mellitus. N Engl J Med 1993;333:541–549.

23. DeFeo P, Bolli G, Periello G, et al: The adrenergic contribution to glucose counterregulation: Dependency on alpha-cell function and mediation through beta-adrenergic receptors. Diabetes 1983;32:887–893.

24. DeFronzo RA, Goodman AM: Efficacy of metformin in patients with non-insulin-dependent diabetes mellitus. The Multicenter Metformin Study Group. N Engl J Med 1995;333:541–549.

25. Dong BJ, Hauck WW, Gambertoglio JG, et al: Bioequivalence of generic and brand-name levothyroxine products in the treatment of hypothyroidism. JAMA 1997;277:1205–1213.

26. Drummond R: Thyroid storm [editorial]. JAMA 1997;277:1238–1243.

27. Dubois MP: Immunoreactive somatostatin is present in discrete cells of the endocrine pancreas. Proc Natl Acad Sci USA 1975;72:1340–1343.

28. Eden J: Too much of a good thing? Two cases of oestrogen overdosage associated with oestradiol implants [letter]. Med J Aust 1990;152:558.

29. Ernst AA, Jones K, Nick TG, et al: Ethanol ingestion and related hypoglycemia in a pediatric and adolescent emergency department population. Acad Emerg Med 1996;1:46–49.

30. Farrell GC, Joshua DE, Uren RF, et al: Androgen-induced hepatoma. Lancet 1975;1:430–432.

31. Farwell AP, Braverman LE: Thyroid and antithyroid drugs. In: Hardman JG, Limbird LE, Molinoff PB, Ruddon RW, eds: Goodman & Gilman's The Pharmacological Basis of Therapeutics, 9th ed. New York, McGraw-Hill, 1996, pp. 1383–1409.

32. Ferenchick GS: Drug abuse and stroke. Ann Internal Med 1991;114:431–432.

33. Ferenchick GS: Are androgenic steroids thrombogenic? N Engl J Med 1990;322:476–477.

34. Foss GL, Simpson SL: Oral methyltestosterone and jaundice. Br Med J 1959;1:259.

35. Fujita T, Sugiyama Y, Taketomi S, et al: Reduction of insulin resistance in obese and/or diabetic animals by 5-[4-(1-methylcyclonhexylmethoxy)benzyl]-thiazolidine-2,4-dione IADD-3878, U-63, 287, ciglitazone), a new antidiabetic agent. Diabetes 1983;32:804–810.

36. Funder JW: Adrenal steroids: New answers, new questions. Science 1987;237:236–237.

37. Gavin LA: Thyroid crisis. Med Clin North Am 1991;75:179–193.

38. Gilman AG: Nobel lecture. G proteins and regulation of adenyl cyclase. Biosci Rep 1995;15:65–97.

39. Gilman AG: G proteins: Transducers of receptor-generated signals. Annu Rev Biochem 1987;56:615–649.

40. Gilman AG: G proteins and dual control of adenylate cyclase. Cell 1984;36:577–579.

41. Gittoes NJ, Franklyn JA: Drug-induced thyroid disorders. Drug Saf 1995;13:46–55.

42. Golden RJ, Noller KL, Titus-Ernstoff L, et al. Environmental endocrine modulators and human health: An assessment of the biological evidence. Crit Rev Toxicol 1998;28:109–227.

43. Golightly LK, Smolinske SC, Kulig KW, et al: Clinical effects of accidental levothyroxine ingestion in children. Am J Dis Child 1985;141:1025–2110.

44. Graham W, Kennedy M: Recent developments in the toxicology of anabolic steroids. Drug Saf 1990;5:548–476.

45. Griffin JE, Wilson JP: The testes. In: Bondy PK, Rosenberg LE, eds: Metabolic Control and Disease, 7th ed. Philadelphia, WB Saunders, 1980, pp. 1535–1578.

46. Guyetant S, Wion-Barbot N, Rousselet MC: C-cell hyperplasia associated with chronic lymphocytic thyroiditis: A retrospective quantitative study of 112 cases. Hum Pathol 1994;25:514–521.

47. Hachiya HL, Treves ST, Kahn CR, et al: Altered insulin distribution and metabolism in type I diabetics assessed by I-insulin scanning. J Clin Endocrinol Metab 1987;64:801–808.

48. Hamolsky MW: Truth is stranger than factitious. N Engl J Med 1982;307:436–437.

49. Harjai KJ, Licata AA: Effects of amiodarone on thyroid function. Ann Intern Med 1997;126:63–73.

50. Harris MI, Flegal KM, Cowie CC, et al: Prevalence of diabetes, impaired fasting glucose, and impaired glucose tolerance in U.S. adults. The Third National Health and Nutrition Examination Survey, 1988–1994. Diabetes Care 1998;21:518–524.

51. Haupt HA: Anabolic steroids: A review of the literature. Am J Sports Med 1984;12:469–484.

52. Haynes RC: Thyroid and antithyroid drugs. In: Gilman, AG, Rall TW, Nies AS, Taylor P, eds: Goodman & Gilman's The Pharmacological Basis of Therapeutics, 8th ed. New York, McGraw-Hill, 1990, pp. 1361–1383.

53. Hearn PR, Ahmed M, Woodhouse NJY: The use of SMS 201–995, (somatostatin analogue) in insulinomas. Horm Res 1988;29: 211–213.

54. Hedbert CW: An outbreak of thyrotoxicosis caused by the consumption of bovine thyroid gland in ground beef. N Engl J Med 1987;316:993–998.

55. Herbst AL, Ulfelder H, Poskanzer DC: Adenocarcinoma of the vagina. Association of maternal stilbestrol therapy with tumor appearance in young women. N Engl J Med 1971;284:878–881.

56. HHS News, US Department of Health and Human Services: "Rezulin to be Withdrawn from the Market," March 21, 2000 (http://www.fds.gov/bbs/topics/NEWS/NEW00721.html).

57. Hickson RC, Ball KL, Falduto MT: Adverse effects of anabolic steroids. Med Toxicol Adverse Drug Exp 1989;4:254–271.

58. Hollenberg SM, Giguere V, Segui P, et al: Co-localization of DNA binding and transcriptional activation functions in the human glucocorticoid receptor. Cell 1987;49:39–46.

59. Holma P: Effect of an anabolic steroid (methandienone) on central and peripheral blood flow in well-trained male athletes. Ann Clin Res 1977;9:215–221.

60. American Diabetes Association: Implications of the Diabetes Control and Complications Trial. Diabetes 1993;42:1555–1558.

61. Johnson FL: The association of oral androgenic-anabolic steroids and life-threatening disease. Med Sci Sports 1975;7:284–286.

62. Kahn RC, Shecter Y: Insulin, oral hypoglycemic agents and the pharmacology of the endocrine pancreas. In: Gilman AG, Rall TW, Nies AS, Taylor P, eds: Goodman & Gilman's The Pharmacological Basis of Therapeutics, 8th ed. New York, McGraw-Hill, 1990, p. 1463–1495.

63. Kellerer M, Kroder G, Tippmer S, et al: Troglitazone prevents glucose-induced insulin resistance insulin receptor in Rat-1 fibroblasts. Diabetes 1994;43:447–453.

64. Klein I, Becker DV, Levey GS: Treatment of hyperthyroid disease. Ann Intern Med 1994;121:281–288.

65. Klein I, Ojamaa K: Thyroid hormone and the cardiovascular system. N Engl J Med 2001;344:501–509.

66. Kleiner SM: Performance-enhancing aids in sports: Health consequences and nutritional alternatives. J Am Coll Nutr 1991;10:163–176.

67. Korach, KS: Surprising places of estrogenic activity. Endocrinology 1993;132:2277–2278.

68. Kosaka K, Kuzuya K, Akanuma Y, et al. Clinical evaluation of a new oral hypoglycemic drug CS-045 in patients with noninsulin-dependent diabetes mellitus poorly controlled by sulfonylureas: A double-blind, placebo-controlled study. J Clin Ther Med 1993;3:61–93.

69. Krief S, Lonqvist F, Raimbault S, et al: Tissue distribution of β3-adrenergic receptor mRNA in man. J Clin Invest 1993;1:344–349.

70. Krieger DT, Martin JB: Brain peptides. N Engl J Med 1981;304: 944–951.

71. Lalau JD, Lacroix C, Compagnon P, et al: Role of metformin accumulation in metformin-associated lactic acidosis. Diabetes Care 1995;18:779–784.

72. Lamb DR: Anabolic steroids in athletics: How well do they work and how dangerous are they? Am J Sports Med 1984;12:31–38.

73. Lehmann JM, Moore LB, Smith-Oliver TA, et al: An antidiabetic thiazolidinedione is a high affinity ligand for peroxisome proliferator-activated receptor gamma (PPAR-gamma). J Biol Chem 1995;270(22):12953–12956.

74. Leonard JL, Visser TJ: Biochemistry of iodination. In: Hennemann G, ed: Thyroid Hormone Metabolism. New York, Marcel Dekker, 1986, pp. 189–230.

75. Litovitz TL, White J: Levothyroxine ingestions in children: An analysis of 78 cases. Am J Emerg Med 1985;3:297–300.

76. Lonqvist F, Krief S, Strosberg AD, et al: Evidence for a functional β3-adrenergic receptor in man. Br J Pharmacol 1993;110:929–936.

77. Luckner R, Challis A, West D, et al: A problem in the radiochemical assay of glucose-6-phosphate in muscle. Biochem J 1984;218: 649–651.

78. Mariotti S, Marino E, Cupin C, et al: Low serum thyroglobulin as a clue to the diagnosis of thyrotoxicosis factitia. N Engl J Med 1982; 307:410–412.

79. Marty MS, Crissman JW, Carney EW. Evaluation of the EDSTAC female pubertal assay in CD rats using 17β-estradiol, steroid biosynthesis inhibitors, and a thyroid inhibitor. Toxicol Sci 1999;52:269–277.

80. McMahon M, Gerich J, Rizza R: Effects of glucocorticoids on carbohydrate metabolism. Diabetes Metab Rev 1988;4:17–30.

81. Mellon SH: Neurosteroids: Biochemistry, modes of action, and clinical relevance. J Clin Endocrinol Metab 1994;78:1003–1008.

82. Meyer-Gessner M, Bender G, Lederbogen S, et al: Antithyroid drug-induced agranulocytosis: Clinical experience with ten patients treated at one institution and review of the literature. J Endocrinol Invest 1994;17:29–36.

83. Moore DF, Wood DF, Volans GN: Features, prevention and management of acute overdose due to antidiabetic drugs. Drug Saf 1993; 9:218–229.

84. Mosbach EH, Shefer S, Abell LL: Identification of the fecal metabolites of 17β-methyltestosterone in the dog. J Lipid Res 1968,9: 93–97.

85. Nuovo J, Ellsworth A, Christensen DB, et al: Excessive thyroid hormone replacement therapy. J Am Board Fam Pract 1995;8:435–439.

86. Papanicolau GN, Falk EA: General muscular hypertrophy induced by androgenic hormones. Science 1938;87:238–239.

87. Peterson DR, Carone FA, Oparil S, et al: Differences between renal tubular processing of glucagon and insulin. Am J Physiol 1989;38: 1217–1229.

88. Philips RE, Looareesuwan S, Bloom SR, et al: Effectiveness of SMS 210–995, a synthetic long-acting somatostatin analogue, in treatment of quinine-induced hyperinsulinemia. Lancet 1986;1:713–714.

89. Popp D, Shah S, Cryer P: Role of epinephrine mediated adrenergic mechanisms in hypoglycemic glucose counter-regulation and post-hypoglycemic hyperglycemia in insulin-dependent diabetes mellitus. J Clin Invest 1982;69:315–326.

90. Porte D: A receptor mechanism for the inhibition of insulin release by epinephrine in man. J Clin Invest 1967;45:86–94.

91. Purchase IF: Ethical review of regulatory toxicology guidelines involving experiments on animals: The example of endocrine disrupters. Toxicol Sci 1999;52:141–147.

92. Rabkin R, Hamik A, Yagil C, et al: Processing of ^{125}I-insulin by polarized cultured kidney cells. Exp Cell Res 1996;224:136–142.

93. Randle P, Hales C, Garland P, et al: The glucose fatty acid cycle. Its role in insulin sensitivity and the metabolic disturbances of diabetes mellitus. Lancet 1963;1:785–789.

94. Reichlin S: Somatostatin (parts I and II). N Engl J Med 1983;309: 1495–1503; 1556–1563.

95. Remes K, Vuopio P, Jarinenen M, et al: Effect of short-term treatment with an anabolic steroid (methandienone) and dehydro-epiandrosterone sulphate on plasma hormones, red cell volume and 2,3-diphosphoglycerate in athletes. Scand J Clin Lab Invest 1977; 37:577–586.

96. Rizza RA, Cryer PE, Gerich JE: Role of glucagon, catecholamines and growth hormone in human glucose counterregulation. Effect of somatostatin and combined alpha- and beta-adrenergic blockade on plasma glucose recovery and glucose flux rates after insulin-induced hypoglycemia. J Clin Invest 1979;64:62–71.

97. Rizza R, Cryer P, Haymond M, et al: Adrenergic mechanism for the effect of epinephrine on glucose production and clearance in man. J Clin Invest 1980;65:682–689.

98. Ross EM: G proteins and receptors in neuronal signaling. In: Hall ZW, ed: An Introduction to Molecular Neurobiology. Sunderland, MA, Sinaver, 1992, pp. 181–206.

99. Samols E, Bonner-Weir S, Weir GC: Intra-islet insulin-glucagon somatostatin relationships. J Clin Endocrinol Metab 1986;15:53–58.

100. Samos LF, Roos BA: Diabetes mellitus in older persons. Med Clin North Am 1998;82:791–803.

101. Sands M, Kron MA, Brown RB: Pentamidine: A review. Rev Infect Dis 1985;7:625–634.

102. Scully R: Case records of the Massachusetts General Hospital. N Engl J Med 1984;310:580–587.

103. Shephard RJ, Killinger D, Fried T: Responses to sustained use of anabolic steroids. Br J Sports Med 1977;11:170–173.

104. Smith DA, Perry PJ: The efficacy of ergogenic agents in athletic competition. I: Androgenic-anabolic steroids. Ann Pharmacother 1992;26:520–528.

105. Sporer KA, Ernst AA, Conte R, et al: The incidence of ethanol-induced hypoglycemia. Am J Emerg Med 1992;10:403–405.

106. Stadel BV: Oral contraceptives and cardiovascular disease. N Engl J Med 1981;305:672–677.

107. Strauss RH: Anabolic steroids. Clin Sports Med 1984;3:743–748.

108. Stumvoll M, Nurjan N, Perillo G, et al: Metabolic effects of metformin in non-insulin-dependent diabetes mellitus. N Engl J Med 1995;33:550–554.

109. Sucov A, Woolard RH: Ethanol-associated hypoglycemia is uncommon. Acad Emerg Med 1995;2:185–189.

110. Tang WJ, Gilman AG: Type-specific regulation of adenyl cyclase by G protein beta gamma subunits. Science 1991;254:1500–1503.

111. Tatro DS: Use of steroids by athletes. Drug Newsletter 1985;4: 33–34.

112. Taurog A, Dorris ML: Peroxidase-catalyzed bromination of tyrosine, thyroglobulin, and bovine serum albumin: Comparison of thyroid peroxidase and lactoperoxidase. Arch Biochem Biophys 1991;287: 288–296.

113. Taylor JR, Sherratt HJA, Davies DM: Intramuscular or intravenous glucagon for sulphonylurea hypoglycemia. Eur J Clin Pharmacol 1978;14:125–127.

114. Taylor WN: Anabolic Steroids and the Athlete. Jefferson, NC, Mc-farland, 1982.

115. Tunget CL, Clark RF, Turchen SG, et al: Raising the decontamination level for thyroid hormone ingestions. Am J Emerg Med 1995; 13:9–13.

116. Unger RH: Glucagon physiology and pathophysiology in the light of new advances. Diabetologia 1985;28:574–578.

117. United Kingdom Prospective Diabetes Study (UKPDS) Group. 13: Relative efficacy of randomly allocated diet, sulphonylurea, insulin, or metformin in patients with newly diagnosed non-insulin-dependent diabetes followed for three years. BMJ 1995;310:83–88.

118. Wagner RL, White PF, Kan PB, et al: Inhibition of adrenal steroidogenesis by the anesthetic etomidate. N Engl J Med 1984;310: 1415–1421.

119. Wakabayashi T, Onda H, Tada T, et al: High incidence of peliosis hepatis in autopsy cases of aplastic anemia with special reference to anabolic steroid therapy. Acta Pathol Jpn 1984;34:1079–1086.

120. Wiersinga WM: Amiodarone and the thyroid: In: Weetmen AP, Grossman A, eds. Handbook of Pharmacology. Vol. 128: Pharmacotherapeutics of the Thyroid Gland. Berlin, Springer-Verlag, 1997, pp. 225–287.

121. Wildasin EM, Skaar, DJ, Kirchain WR, Hulse M. Metformin, a promising oral antihyperglycemic for the treatment of noninsulin-dependent diabetes mellitus. Pharmacotherapy 1997;17:62–73.

122. Wilson JD, Griffin JE: The use and misuse of androgens. Metabolism 1980;29:1278–1295.

123. Wilson JD: Androgens. In: Hardman JG, Limbird LE, Molinoff PB, Ruddon RW, eds: Goodman & Gilman's The Pharmacological Basis of Therapeutics, 9th ed. New York, McGraw-Hill, 1996, p. 1441–1457.

124. Wright J: Alcohol-induced hypoglycemia. Br J Alcohol Alcoholism 1979;14:174–176.

125. Yesalis CE, Kennedy NJ, Kopstein AN, et al: Anabolic-androgenic steroid use in the United States. JAMA 1933;270:1217–1222.

Martin J. Smilkstein / Frederick W. Fraunfelder

The visual system is an essential consideration in toxicologic emergencies, and the clinician must perform a thorough ophthalmic examination if management is to be effective. Examination of the eye not only provides clues to the diagnosis of certain toxic exposures, but may also lead to timely detection of life-threatening nontoxicologic problems, such as intracranial hemorrhage. In addition to providing diagnostic clues, the visual system is the target of many toxins that threaten normal vision. The eye may be injured by direct contact with a number of agents, may provide a portal of entry for agents with systemic toxicity, and may itself be adversely affected by many systemic exposures. Understanding these principles can be lifesaving or sightsaving, and is essential to efficient, systematic patient care.

OPHTHALMIC EXAMINATION FINDINGS

Before considering specific toxic exposures in detail, it is important to briefly consider normal visual function and how dysfunction leads to clinical signs and symptoms.

Visual Acuity and Color Perception

Decreased acuity can result from abnormalities anywhere in the visual system that affect either light transmission or neural elements.[4,16,30] Corneal injury or edema from any cause may result in blurring of vision, characteristically described as "halos" around lights. Toxicologic causes of corneal abnormalities include direct exposure to chemicals, failure of corneal protective reflexes because of local anesthetic effects or a profoundly decreased level of consciousness, and incomplete eyelid closure during coma. Mydriasis, also a common feature of acute xenobiotic exposure (Table 27–1) may interfere with the pupillary constriction component of the near reflex, resulting in decreased acuity for near objects. Lens clouding or cataract formation causes blurred vision and decreased light perception, as does blood or other deposits in the aqueous or vitreous humors. Drug-induced lens abnormalities due to chronic exposures are well described[23,30,39] (Table 27–2), but are not important in the evaluation of toxicologic emergencies. Even if light reaches the retina without distortion, abnormal reception or transmission can result from ischemia or injury to any neural element from the retina to the optic cortex. Direct, acute visual neurotoxic injury is rare and is caused almost exclusively by methanol or quinine. Indirect injury following drug-induced central nervous system (CNS) ischemia or hypoxia is far more common. Alterations in color perception generally result from abnormalities in retinal or optic nerve function. Color vision abnormalities are attributed to hundreds of agents, but unlike those caused by chronic drug ex-

posure such abnormalities are rare and inconsistent features of acute toxicity.[23,30]

Pupil Size and Reactivity

Normally, the pupils are equal to each other in size, 3–4 mm under typical light conditions, round, and react directly and consensually to increased light intensity by constricting. Pupillary constriction also occurs as part of the near reflex when a person attempts to focus on near objects. All of these characteristics result from the balance between cholinergic innervation of the iris sphincter (constrictor) by cranial nerve III and sympathetic innervation of the radial muscle of the iris (dilator).[16] Pupillary dilation (mydriasis) can result from increased sympathetic stimulation by endogenous catecholamines or from systemic (eg, cocaine, amphetamines) or ocular (eg, phenylephrine) exposures to sympathomimetic drugs. Mydriasis can also result from inhibition of muscarinic cholinergic-mediated pupillary constriction and is the mechanism for mydriasis caused by systemic or ocular exposures to anticholinergic agents (Chap. 35). Neurologic injury resulting in either midbrain or cranial nerve III dysfunction (eg, increased intracranial pressure) is a more ominous etiology of the mydriasis, caused by loss of constrictor function. Because pupillary constriction in response to light is a major determinant of normal pupil size, blindness from ocular, retinal, or optic nerve disorders also leads to mydriasis (eg, methanol, quinine). Reactivity of mydriatic pupils to light varies with the etiology of the mydriasis.[30] Although often difficult to appreciate, constriction to light can usually be elicited after sympathomimetic exposures because constrictor function is preserved, whereas this is often not the case when mydriasis results from anticholinergic excess. Light reactivity is absent in cases of complete blindness caused by retinal or optic neurologic injury, but may be preserved if there is some remaining light perception (Chap. 19).

Pupillary constriction (miosis) can result from increased cholinergic stimulation (eg, opioids, pilocarpine, anticholinesterases such as organic phosphorus agents) or inhibition of sympathetic dilation (eg, clonidine, pontine hemorrhage). There are conflicting reports regarding the pupillary effects of many drugs. Depending on the stage and severity of toxicity, the presence of coingestants or coexistent hypoxemia, and numerous other factors, many individual substances (eg, phencyclidine, barbiturates) are reported to cause both mydriasis and miosis.[30,40] For some substances, the pupillary examination provides consistent information (Table 27–1), but many factors are involved and the significance of the pupil size and reactivity must always be considered in the context of the remainder of the patient evaluation.

TABLE 27–1. Ophthalmic Findings Due to Acute Toxic Exposures

Miosis
  Increased cholinergic tone
    Anticholinesterases (carbamates, organic phosphorus compounds, physostigmine)
    Carbachol
    Muscarine
    Nicotine
    Pilocarpine
  Decreased sympathetic tone
    Clonidine
    Guanabenz
    Methyldopa
  Opioids
  Coma from sedative-hypnotic agents (barbiturates, benzodiazepines, ethanol)
  Pontine hemorrhage

Mydriasis
  Decreased cholinergic tone
    Antihistamines
    Belladonna alkaloids
    Cyclic antidepressants (inconsistent finding)
    Postanoxic encephalopathy (many causes)
  Increased sympathetic tone
    Amphetamines
    Cocaine
    Phenylephrine and other sympathomimetics
    Ethanol and sedative-hypnotic withdrawal

Nystagmus
  Carbamazepine
  Ethanol
  Monoamine oxidase inhibitors
  Phencyclidine
  Phenytoin
  Sedative-hypnotic agents
  Thiamine deficiency

Disconjugate Gaze
  Botulism
  Elapid envenomation
  Neuromuscular blocking agents
  Paralytic shellfish poisoning
  Tetrodotoxin
  Thiamine deficiency
  Secondary to decreased level of consciousness (many causes)

Funduscopic Abnormalities
  Carbon monoxide (red)
  Cocaine (vasoconstriction)
  Cyanide (retinal vein arteriolization)
  Ergot alkaloids (vasoconstriction)
  IV drug use (embolic)
  Methanol (disc and retinal pallor or hyperemia)
  Methemoglobin (cyanotic)

Papilledema
  See causes of pseudotumor cerebri (Table 37–2)

TABLE 27–2. Examples of Ocular Abnormalities Caused by Chronic Systemic Exposures[a]

Corneal/Conjunctival Inflammation
  Cytosine arabinoside (Ara-C)
  Isotretinoin[b]
  Mercury (acrodynia)
  Practolol[c]

Uveitis
  Cidofovir
  Pamidronate
  Rifabutin
  Sulfonamides

Corneal Deposits
  Amiodarone[b]
  Chloroquine
  Chlorpromazine
  Copper[d]
  Gold
  Mercury[d]
  Silver (argyria)[d]
  Vitamin D

Cataracts
  Busulfan[c]
  Corticosteroids[b]
  Dinitrophenol (internal use)[d]
  Trinitrotoluene[d]

Lens Deposits
  Amiodarone[b]
  Chlorpromazine
  Copper[d]
  Iron
  Mercury[d]
  Silver[d]

Myopia[c]
  Acetazolamide
  Diuretics (chlorthalidone, thiazides, spironolactone)
  Sulfonamides

Retinal Injury
  Carbon disulfide[d]
  Carmustine[c]
  Chloramphenicol[c]
  Chloroquine
  Cinchona alkaloids (quinine)[b]
  Deferoxamine[c]
  Digitalis[c]
  Ethambutol
  Thallium
  Vincristine[c]

Retrobulbar and Optic Neuropathy
  Carbon disulfide[d]
  Chloramphenicol[d]
  Dinitrobenzene[d]
  Dinitrochlorobenzene[d]
  Dinitrotoluene[d]
  Disulfiram
  Ethambutol[b]
  Isoniazid[c]
  Lead[c]
  Thallium
  Vincristine[c]

Cortical Blindness
  Cisplatin
  Cyclosporine
  Interleukin[c]
  Tacrolimus (FK506)
  Methylmercury compounds[d]

[a]This list includes only selected examples and is not intended to be comprehensive.
[b]Particularly important example.
[c]Reported, but extremely rare from this exposure.
[d]Mostly historical interest — associated with patterns of use no longer common.

Extraocular Movement, Diplopia, and Nystagmus

Maintenance of normal eye position and movement requires coordinated function of a complex circuit involving bilateral frontal and occipital cortices, multiple brainstem nuclei, cranial nerves, extraocular muscles, and connecting fibers between each.[2,16] Because of the many elements necessary for normal function, abnormalities of eye movement can result from several causes and are extremely common.[30] Probably the most common abnormality is reversible nystagmus or rhythmic oscillations of the globes (Table 27–1). Drug-induced nystagmus may take many forms, but is most commonly jerk nystagmus, as opposed to pendular, or horizontal and symmetric. The nystagmus may be evident at rest but is accentuated by visual pursuit and extreme lateral gaze. These features are unique to drug-induced causes. Drug-induced vertical nystagmus rarely occurs, except as a result of phencyclidine, ketamine, or dextromethorphan toxicity, and when present should initially suggest a structural lesion of the CNS. Loss of conjugate gaze commonly results from CNS depression of any cause, including many sedative-hypnotic overdoses. Except after extremely rare neurotoxin exposures (Table 27–1), diplopia without decreased level of consciousness should not be attributed to acute toxicologic causes. In addition to the transient effects of some overdoses, other agents (eg, thallium, carbon disulfide, carbon monoxide) may cause sustained gaze disorders due to residual cranial nerve and CNS injury.[30] Nystagmus and ophthalmoplegia caused by thiamine deficiency usually improve after therapy, but nystagmus may not resolve completely.[61]

OCULAR CAUSTIC EXPOSURES: FIRST AID AND INITIAL APPROACH

The initial approach to all patients with ocular chemical exposures should be immediate decontamination by irrigation, using copious amounts of the most immediately available safe aqueous solution.[12,62] Irrigation is intended to accomplish at least four objectives: immediate dilution of the offending agent, removal of the agent, removal of any foreign body, and in some cases, normalization of anterior chamber pH. Water, normal saline, lactated Ringer solution, and balanced salt solution (BSS) are all appropriate choices. In theory, BSS is ideal, because it is both isotonic and buffered to physiologic pH. Lactated Ringer solution (pH 6–7.5) and normal saline (pH 4.5–7) are also isotonic and therefore theoretically preferable to water. There is no convincing evidence that the choice significantly affects outcome, and although lactated Ringer solution, normal saline, and water cause more discomfort than BSS,[34] an ocular topical anesthetic is usually required for effective irrigation, thus negating this concern. As delays of even seconds can dramatically affect outcome,[30] there is no justification for waiting for another solution if water is the first available agent. Irrigation must include the conjunctival recesses, internal and external palpebral surfaces, and cornea and bulbar conjunctiva. Effective irrigation includes lid retraction and eversion or use of a scleral shell or other irrigating device. After irrigation, visual acuity testing, inspection of the eye, and slit-lamp examination should be completed. Fluorescein examination demonstrates the area of corneal epithelial defects but not depth of the burn,[62] corneal edema, or anterior chamber involvement, and by itself is an unacceptable alternative to slit-lamp examination.

Exposure-Specific Irrigating Solutions

Much has been written about ideal irrigating agents and specific antidotes, but it is clear that simple dilution and mechanical removal by immediate, copious irrigation with water or other safe aqueous solutions is always appropriate.[12,54,62] Despite theoretical concern, there is probably no toxic exposure for which standard aqueous solutions are contraindicated. Of greatest theoretical concern are agents such as white or yellow phosphorus, metallic sodium, and metallic potassium that may react violently in the presence of water, leading to heat, mechanical injury, and, in the latter two cases, generation of sodium hydroxide and potassium hydroxide, respectively.[30] Although not well-studied, irrigation with large amounts of water probably dissipates the heat of the ini-

tial hydration reaction with conjunctival moisture more than it initiates a thermochemical reaction. In addition to removing the offending material, irrigation serves to dilute and remove the alkaline byproducts formed by reaction with conjunctival water.

The use of special irrigating solutions for more common exposures, including hydrofluoric acid and phenols, is also debated.

Hydrofluoric Acid. For hydrofluoric acid exposures (Chap. 87), experimental irrigation with calcium salt solutions was too irritating to the eye, but isotonic magnesium chloride solutions were effective and not irritating.[41,42] From a practical standpoint, however, normal saline is equally effective, and thus there is no reason to use less readily available solutions.

Phenol. For phenol exposure, topical low-molecular-weight polyethylene glycol (PEG) solutions are effective for treatment of experimental skin exposure; for eyes, copious water irrigation appears to be as effective as PEG.[10] There is, however, a report of superior efficacy of PEG-400 over water in treatment of human phenol eye burns.[36] Although PEG-400 may be readily available at work sites where phenols are used, it is not a realistic option in the emergency department, and there should be no hesitation to use water, normal saline, lactated Ringer solution, or BSS as lavage solutions.

Cyanoacrylate Adhesives. Ocular exposures to cyanoacrylate adhesives such as Super Glue and Krazy Glue commonly result in rapid adherence between upper and lower eyelids that may persist for days. Such occurrences may be associated with corneal abrasions,[17,22] but are otherwise relatively harmless. Management is problematic, as acetone or ethanol, which are often effective in dermal-to-dermal adhesions caused by cyanoacrylates, cannot be used safely on the eye. Application of gauze pads soaked with mineral oil is successful but requires 36 hours of treatment.[59]

Other agent-specific treatments have been tried experimentally or clinically,[31] but none should be considered prior to or instead of copious irrigation, most are not advocated, and consideration of such agents should be vanishingly rare.

Duration of Irrigation. In order to accomplish the goals of irrigation, as described, the appropriate duration varies with the exposure. Most solvents, for example, do not penetrate deeper than the superficial cornea, and brief (10–20 minutes) irrigation is generally sufficient.[30] After exposure to acids or alkalis, normalization of the conjunctival pH is often suggested as a useful endpoint. Testing of pH should be done in every case of acid or alkali exposure, but the limitations of testing must be understood. When measured by sensitive experimental methods, normal pH of the conjunctival surface is 6.5–7.6.[1] This is highly method-dependent, however, and normal values in the literature range from 5.2 to 8.6.[14] When measured by touching pH-sensitive paper to the moist surface of the conjunctival cul-de-sac, normal pH is most often near 8.[3] Therefore, after irrigation following alkali burns, pH should not be expected to reach 7 and is more likely to stabilize near 8.[30] In this setting, lower pH values may indicate the pH of the irrigant, rather than the ocular surface. Waiting for an interval of several minutes between irrigation and pH testing will allow washout of any residual irrigant.[15] Choice of testing paper is important, as some are intended for use at extremes of pH and lack sensitivity in the clinically useful range.

Despite these limitations, a logical role for pH assessment can be described: probably a minimum of 2 L of irrigant per affected eye should be used before any assessment of pH; and then, after 7–10 minutes, the pH of the lower fornix conjunctiva should be checked. Thereafter, cycles of 10–15 minutes of irrigation followed by rechecks should be continued until the pH is 7.5–8. This is certainly adequate for exposures to weak acids, which do not penetrate well, and for minor alkaline exposures.

For major alkaline, concentrated acid, or for hydrofluoric acid exposures with apparent eye abnormalities, normal surface pH is a minimum but not an adequate endpoint (see the section on Alkali later in the chapter). After these burns, irrigation should be continued for at least 2–3 hours, regardless of surface pH, in an attempt to correct anterior chamber pH,[30,54,62] and immediate ophthalmologic consultation is mandatory. Following this lengthy irrigation, it is important to verify that conjunctival pH has normalized. If not, irrigation must be continued, sometimes for 24–48 hours.

Other General Measures

There is a wide array of options for adjunctive therapy of chemical burns of the eye. In all cases in which serious injury is evident, the treatment plan must include consultation with an ophthalmologist. Generally, patients with corneal injury should be treated with an ocular topical antibiotic providing antistaphylococcal and antipseudomonal coverage. Cycloplegics not only reduce pain from ciliary spasm, but also decrease the likelihood of posterior synechiae formation. Eye patches, to a limited extent, and systemic analgesics also improve patient comfort. It is never appropriate to dispense topical ophthalmic anesthetic agents, because repeated use of these agents leads to further corneal disruption both by direct chemical effects and by eliminating corneal protective reflex sensation.

OCULAR CAUSTIC EXPOSURES: SPECIFIC AGENTS

The effect of any chemical on the eye depends on the inherent properties of the agent (eg, solvents, detergents); the amount, concentration, and pH of the agent; and the duration of exposure. The end result of ocular exposure to these agents depends on the extent of damage to the cornea, particularly the integrity and function of the stroma; chemical penetration into the anterior chamber and the resulting injury to its structures; and resultant inflammatory reaction.[30,62] Because similar chemicals tend to produce similar reactions, they can be conveniently grouped for discussion into acids, alkalis, and others.

Acids

Fortunately, weak acids do not penetrate the cornea well.[30,62] The hydrogen ion causes damage by lowering pH, while the anion precipitates ocular proteins on contact, causing coagulation and thereby somewhat limiting the extent of penetration. The dehydrating effect of some acids, the heat of hydration, and the affinity of each anion for corneal tissues all affect the extent of injury. Intense pain usually results from stimulation of exposed nerve endings in the corneal epithelium. Corneal defects are common, but in many cases the damaged epithelium is swept away, revealing

healthy Bowman's layer, over which epithelium resurfaces the cornea. Strong acids can penetrate the stroma, damage deeper tissue and structures of the anterior chamber, and lead to the more serious sequelae, such as those that often occur after alkali burns.[30,62] Prolonged exposure to weaker acids may result in significant extension of the injury and thus immediate irrigation is mandatory.

Hydrofluoric acid may cause unexpectedly severe injury because of its ability to penetrate deep into the eye.[7,41,42,53] Damage is generally concentration dependent with severe injury expected after exposure to 20% or higher, but even dilute formulations have led to persistent abnormalities. On the basis of anecdotal reports, repeated instillation of calcium gluconate eye drops is advocated by some[60] to bind free fluoride, but there is no evidence that this is beneficial.[5] Furthermore, topical instillation of calcium reverses the benefit of ascorbate and increases ulceration after alkali burns (see below).[33] For these reasons, we do not advocate the use of calcium or magnesium solutions for irrigation or instillation after hydrofluoric acid eye exposure.

Alkalis

Alkali burns of the eye represent an ophthalmic emergency. A rational approach to care is based on an understanding of the complex pathophysiology of these injuries.[62] The hydroxyl ion saponifies lipid membranes, directly disrupting cells, while the penetration of the alkali is determined by the cation. Cations react with and hydrate stromal components, causing loss of clarity. For this reason, once the damaged epithelium is swept away, any haziness of the underlying stroma is evidence of alkali penetration and potential serious sequelae. If injury is limited only to destruction and lysis of corneal epithelium, with clear stroma, rapid and complete resolution is expected. Large amounts of high-concentration strong bases (eg, sodium hydroxide), agents that penetrate rapidly (eg, ammonium hydroxide), and prolonged exposure all promote deeper injury.[30,52,62] Penetration into corneal stroma may destroy keratocytes, alter collagen structure, and damage the endothelium.[62] Paradoxically, more extensive burns may be less painful, because of destruction of corneal nerve endings and resultant anesthesia. In addition to indicating an increased depth of the burn, stromal and endothelial injuries often impair the ability of the cornea to regenerate later and to maintain an adequate epithelium. Further penetration can cause the pH of the anterior chamber to rise significantly within 2–3 minutes.[48,62] Ammonium hydroxide is especially destructive by this mechanism, as it penetrates far more rapidly than other alkalis. Experimentally, 8.5% ammonium hydroxide increases anterior chamber pH within 15 seconds.[30] As a result, the sequelae of these exposures are severe and may be out of proportion to both pH and the degree of surface injury.

The increase in intraocular pH is injurious to the trabecular meshwork, iris, lens, and ciliary body and also triggers a sudden contraction of corneal and scleral collagen, leading to increased intraocular pressure and exacerbation of pain. A less dramatic but more sustained increase in intraocular pressure then ensues, resulting from intraocular prostaglandin release.[62]

In addition to these direct effects, further injury results from the inflammatory response to the initial injury. Dysfunction of the normal blood-aqueous humor barrier results in exudation of protein and inflammatory cells into the anterior chamber, leading to a severe fibrinous reaction. Fibrosis in turn can lead to permanent angle closure and glaucoma. At the opposite extreme, permanent dysfunction of the ciliary body, which produces the aqueous humor, can result in visual loss due to collapse of the eye (phthisis bulbi).[30,62]

The full extent of injury may not be evident for 48–72 hours. In the ensuing days to weeks, outcome is determined by the balance between degradation and repair of the stromal matrix, the quantity and quality of corneal reepithelialization, and the extent of inflammatory cell infiltration. After severe burns, normal repair is distinctly rare and extensive scarring is the rule. The goal of therapy is to prevent corneal ulceration, ocular perforation, and glaucoma while preserving the eye for possible secondary surgical revision or repair.

The mainstay of treatment is immediate and copious irrigation following the guidelines discussed. After exposures to calcium hydroxide (lime) from mortar or cement splashes, any adherent material must be found and removed. A sterile cotton-tipped applicator soaked in 0.05 mol/L edetate disodium (Na_2 EDTA) may aid this process.[30,52,62] Follow-up is essential in all cases of alkali eye burns. Emergent consultation with an ophthalmologist should be obtained for all suspected severe burns. For isolated, very superficial corneal defects this is not necessary; however, if there is pain unrelieved by topical anesthetics, evident corneal opacification, increased intraocular pressure, or any slit-lamp examination evidence of deep corneal burn, corneal edema, or anterior chamber cell or flare, immediate consultation is essential.

Not only is comprehensive early evaluation important, but the advisability of several adjunctive treatments should be determined in conjunction with the ophthalmologist. Emergent needle paracentesis and lavage of the anterior chamber, when done early, removes alkali and returns pH to normal and also decreases intraocular pressure.[30,48,62] Animal studies suggest that this technique is useful if performed within minutes, but its benefit is not proved in human exposures, possibly because of delay in patient presentation and limited availability of expertise in the technique. In addition to topical antibiotics and cycloplegics, topical steroids, topical citrate, topical and systemic ascorbate, topical and systemic tetracyclines, and antiglaucoma medications may all be indicated. Early steroid treatment may decrease the inflammatory response, but continued use inhibits fibroblast function and healing.[18,62] Ophthalmologists therefore suggest steroids only for the first 7 days.

Well-controlled research supports the use of ascorbate and citrate.[49–51] The aqueous humor has ascorbate concentrations 15–20 times higher than blood. After alkali exposure, intraocular ascorbate concentrations decrease precipitously, suggesting that the local deficiency might result in impaired collagen synthesis and poor healing. In animals, both topical and systemic administration of ascorbate decreases the incidence of corneal ulceration after alkali burns. Apparently by chelation of calcium and magnesium,[33] citrate appears to inhibit chemotaxis, phagocytosis, and enzyme release by polymorphonuclear neutrophils. Experimentally, the instillation of calcium or magnesium reverses this benefit of citrate. In rabbits, the combination of topical citrate and ascorbate was more effective against corneal ulceration than citrate alone.[50] Clinical trials of combinations of oral and topical ascorbate, citrate, and placebo have been initiated, but no results have yet been reported.

Tetracyclines, particularly doxycycline, inhibit collagenase activity by chelating zinc and reduce corneal ulceration.[13,56] In addition, they also inhibit leukocyte activity. These treatments have supplanted less-effective earlier collagenase inhibitors (cysteine, acetylcysteine, penicillamine, EDTA), and many other previously used approaches. Investigational agents include fibronectin, epidermal growth factor, hyaluronate, and retinoic acid to promote regrowth of epithelium; and medroxyprogesterone and nonsteroidal anti-inflammatory drugs (NSAIDs) to limit inflammation without inhibiting stromal repair and collagen formation. Many surgical interventions are investigational and may be indicated, including limbal stem cell and conjunctival transplantation, among others.[62]

Other Chemical Exposures

Most solvents cause immediate pain and superficial injury because of dissolution of corneal epithelial lipid membranes, but do not penetrate or react significantly with deeper tissue.[30] The epithelial defect may be large or complete, but the limited depth of injury usually allows rapid regeneration of normal epithelium. Detergents and surfactants cause variable injury, ranging from minor irritation from soaps to extensive injury from cationic agents such as concentrated benzalkonium chloride.[31] Ocular exposure to A-200 pyrinate pediculicide shampoo causes typical detergent-surfactant injury, leading to extensive loss of corneal epithelium but with normal underlying stroma, and therefore complete healing within days. Lacrimators (tear gas), such as chloroacetophenone, stimulate corneal nerve endings and cause pain, burning, and tearing but produce no structural injury at low concentrations. At high concentrations, these agents can produce significant corneal injury. Specific information on thousands of agents is readily available if needed.[30,59]

SYSTEMIC ABSORPTION AND TOXICITY FROM OCULAR EXPOSURES

Systemic absorption from ocular exposures has caused serious toxicity, morbidity, or death.[20,35] Although the patterns of toxicity are characteristic of the agents involved, recognition may be delayed as a result of a failure to appreciate the eye as a significant route of absorption. There is limited transcorneal diffusion, substantial nasal mucosal absorption after nasolacrimal drainage, and absorption via conjunctival capillaries and lymphatics, which is markedly increased during conjunctival inflammation. Unlike the gastrointestinal route of absorption, there is no significant first-pass hepatic removal after ocular absorption and, therefore, bioavailability is much greater.[20,35,57] If nasolacrimal outflow is normal, up to 80% of instilled drug may be absorbed systemically.[20] By the time toxicity is apparent, there is no role for ocular decontamination to prevent further absorption. After instillation of eye drops, absorption is generally complete within 7 minutes.

Children appear to be at greatest risk, possibly because of the higher relative drug dose they experience when systemic absorption does occur.[8,20,47,57] Diligent attempts to comply with prescribed dosing in a struggling, crying infant may also result in excessive dosing. Because eyedrop size (40–50 μL) exceeds ocular cul-de-sac capacity (30 μL), overflow often occurs and is assumed to represent a failed instillation, which leads to unnecessary reinstillation. Also, as doses of ocular medications are typically not adjusted based on patient weight, the consequences of equivalent degrees of systemic absorption are much greater for an infant than for an adult. Toxicity from eye drops is also a problem among the elderly, probably due to the combination of greater use of potentially toxic ophthalmic medications and the presence of comorbid conditions.

Prevention of systemic toxicity from topical ophthalmic medications requires recognition of the risk, careful history taking before prescribing, use of the lowest effective concentration and dose, patient education, and proper administration. To minimize inadvertent absorption, instill no more than two drops of any eyedrop solution at one time in the superolateral corner of the eye and use gentle finger compression of the medial canthus to limit nasolacrimal drainage.[20,35]

Mydriatics

Mydriatics are used almost exclusively to dilate the pupils prior to diagnostic evaluation of the eyes. This extraordinarily common practice is not generally considered to be potentially dangerous; however, the risk may be substantial if the precautions outlined are not considered. Anticholinergic poisoning (Chap. 35), including substantial morbidity and mortality, is well described after ocular use of atropine (eg, Isopto Atropine), cyclopentolate (eg, Cyclogyl), or scopolamine (eg, Isopto Hyoscine) eyedrops, especially in infants.

The use of the α-adrenergic agonist phenylephrine (eg, Neo-Synephrine) eyedrops, in a 10% solution, may cause severe hypertension, subarachnoid hemorrhage, ventricular dysrhythmias, and myocardial infarction. Fortunately, these effects are rare if the 2.5% ocular phenylephrine is used. Mydriatics can also precipitate acute angle-closure glaucoma in susceptible individuals.

Miotics and Other Antiglaucoma Drugs

Maintaining miosis to prevent angle closure is an important part of glaucoma therapy. Cholinesterase inhibitors used for this purpose, such as echothiophate (eg, Phospholine), exacerbate asthma, parkinsonism, peptic ulcer, and cardiac disease. If neuromuscular blockade is required for patients using ocular cholinesterase inhibitors, an agent not metabolized by plasma cholinesterase (eg, atracurium, pancuronium, vecuronium, or tubocurarine) must be used. Succinylcholine and mivacurium are cleared by plasma cholinesterase and have profoundly prolonged effects when a cholinesterase inhibitor is present.[35] Because of their long duration of action and resultant risk of accumulation after repeated dosing, anticholinesterase agents are associated with the highest incidence of adverse reactions among susceptible patients.

Miosis can also be produced by use of direct cholinergic agonists, such as pilocarpine (eg, Isopto Carpine), which have a much shorter duration of action. Although absorption is limited, nausea and abdominal cramps can occur at recommended doses. After excessive dosing, salivation, diaphoresis, bradycardia, and hypotension may occur.

β-Adrenergic antagonists, such as timolol (eg, Timoptic), levobunolol, metipranolol, carteolol, and betaxolol, are used to lower intraocular pressure but cause a variety of adverse effects, including bradycardia, hypotension, myocardial infarction, syncope, transient ischemic attacks, congestive heart failure, exacerbation of asthma, status asthmaticus, and respiratory arrest. Timolol has exacerbated symptoms in patients with myasthenia gravis and is

implicated in both causing and masking symptoms of hypoglycemia in diabetics. Nonspecific complaints of anorexia, anxiety, depression, fatigue, hallucinations, headache, and nausea are also described after use of timolol eyedrops. Despite the cardioselectivity of betaxolol, respiratory toxicity has been reported.[20]

Dipivefrin, an esterified epinephrine derivative sometimes used to treat glaucoma, can cause adrenergic systemic effects, although much less than those of epinephrine. Ophthalmic formulations of highly selective α₂-adrenergic agonists, brimonidine (eg, Alphagan) and apraclonidine, have now been introduced to treat glaucoma.[20,63] Apraclonidine is expected to have less potential toxicity because of limited CNS absorption. Systemic absorption of brimonidine eye drops in a child has led to bradycardia, hypotension, and decreased level of consciousness, similar to the central effects of other α₂-adrenoceptor agonists (eg, clonidine),[8] apparently mediated through both α₂-adrenoceptors and imidazoline receptors.[11]

Antimicrobials

Life-threatening reactions to ophthalmic antimicrobials are unusual but do occur. Episodes of aplastic anemia have occurred after prolonged use of chloramphenicol (eg, Chloromycetin) eye preparations,[21] and Stevens-Johnson syndrome was reported after short-term use of ophthalmic sulfacetamide (eg, Sulamyd) in a patient with a history of allergy to sulfa drugs.[29]

TOXICITY TO OCULAR STRUCTURES FROM NONOCULAR EXPOSURES

Ocular toxicity from systemic agents is almost always the result of chronic exposure, and the manifestations develop over a prolonged period of time. Thousands of substances are implicated, affecting every element of the visual system from the cornea to the optic cortex. Thorough discussion of this topic is beyond the scope of this text, but examples of causative agents are listed in Table 27–2.[23,30] Many topical and systemic medications are associated with causing inflammation of the eye, including uveitis.[24] Unlike many other ocular abnormalities caused by drugs, uveitis should prompt immediate ophthalmologic consultation. Because many of these are commonly prescribed medications, adverse drug reactions should always be considered when patients present with visual abnormalities or unusual ocular findings on examination.

In the setting of emergency care, toxin-induced disturbances of normal vision from systemic exposures take many forms. Impaired near-vision from mydriasis, and diplopia or nystagmus from interference with normal control of extraocular movements, are examples of common, usually harmless, visual effects. Serious effects generally result from injury or dysfunction of the neural elements from the retina to the cortex. Such toxicity can be direct (neurotoxic) or indirect (hypoxia, ischemia). Many agents historically reported to cause acute visual loss directly are no longer available (Table 27–3).[30] Methanol and quinine are currently the most important agents that cause direct visual toxicity after acute oral poisoning. Many agents capable of causing vasospasm, hypotension, or embolization also cause acute visual loss (Table 27–3).[58] Hypoxia or ischemia can cause visual impairment, and many instances are reported after serious toxic exposures. Blindness and other visual defects are described following recovery from severe toxicity with barbiturates and other sedative-hyp-

TABLE 27–3. Agents Reported to Cause Visual Loss After Acute Exposures

Direct Causes
Caustics
Methanol
Quinine
Lead[a]
Mercuric chloride[a]

Indirect Causes[b]
Amphetamines
Cocaine
Embolization of foreign material (parenteral injection)
Cisplatinum
Combined endocrine agents (TRH with GnRH and glucagon)
Ergot alkaloids
Hypotension (eg, calcium channel blockers)

Agents No Longer in Use[c]
Arsanilates
Arsenicals (organic)
Aspidium (*Dryopteris filix-mas*)
Cinchona derivatives (cinchonine, cinchonidine, ethyl hydrocupriene, isoamyl hydrocupriene)
Cortex granati (pomegranate bark)
Hexamethonium
Iodates
Phenazone (antipyrine)
Phodomyrtus (finger cherries)

[a]Distinctly rare with these poisonings.
[b]Distinctly rare with use of these agents; visual loss often instantaneous, secondary to sudden hypotension, vascular spasm, or embolization.
[c]Well-documented causes of visual loss, but no cases in recent decades.
Adapted, with permission, from Smilkstein MJ, Kulig KW, Rumack BH: Acute toxic blindness: Unrecognized quinine poisoning. Ann Emerg Med 1987;16:98–101.

notics, opioids, carbon monoxide, and many other drugs and toxins.[30]

Methanol

Formate, the byproduct of methanol metabolism (Chap. 66), is the cause of visual toxicity from methanol poisoning. Although interspecies differences complicate the analysis, it appears that the primary event in ocular toxicity is the metabolism of methanol by retinal glial cells, which results in local elevation of formate concentration.[19,27,28,38,46] The exact effects of formate remain to be defined, but formate is postulated to interfere with mitochondrial cytochrome oxidase and succinate-cytochrome-c reductase, and possibly with the Na^+-K^+-ATPase system in the fibers of the optic nerve head.[37] Although the retina is the likely primary site of toxicity,[19,27,28,38,45,46] injury to the retinal ganglion cells and the retrobulbar optic nerve are also described, possibly as secondary effects. The visual signs and symptoms of methanol-induced visual disturbance include blurred or misty vision, "snowfield" vision, spots, central and peripheral scotomata, decreased light perception, and complete blindness.[6] The physical examination is consistent with the mechanism described: although in many patients with only mild visual impairment the examination may be normal, the most consistent finding in severe cases is initial hyperemia of the optic head, which later becomes edematous. The extension of the edema

to the surrounding retina correlates with central scotomata, which are common. In severe cases, the edema may extend to large areas of the retina. In the most severe cases, when light perception is lost, the pupils may be widely dilated and unreactive.

In severe cases, histopathologic examination reveals injury to the retinal ganglion cell layer and extension of the optic nerve injury to the retrobulbar nerve fibers.[28] Optic atrophy often follows, and although central scotomata and peripheral visual field constriction are common, more complete visual loss may then occur. It is not currently possible to predict which patients will develop residual visual impairment, but the constellation of severe initial impairment, dilated and unreactive pupils, and widespread retinal edema implies a particularly poor visual prognosis.

The concentration and duration of formate exposure also appears to be critical to the development of retinal toxicity, but there are not yet reliable estimates or practical methods of determining these variables after human poisoning. Therefore, any patient with acidemia after methanol poisoning is assumed to be at risk for retinal damage. As discussed in Chapter 66, the risk can be reduced by the administration of folate or folinic acid to enhance the elimination of formate and to prevent retinal folate depletion[27,28] (see Antidote in Depth: Folic Acid and Leucovorin [Folinic Acid] and Sodium Bicarbonate).

Quinine

The mechanism of quinine-induced visual impairment is less well understood, but it is known to involve neurotoxic injury to the optic nerve and perhaps retinal ganglion cells.[32] Visual symptoms may include blurred vision, central and peripheral scotomata, and complete blindness.[9] The onset of visual impairment varies, but sudden visual loss can occur as late as 14 hours or more after overdose.[58] Physical examination reveals pupils that are dilated and unreactive in proportion to the degree of visual impairment. Funduscopic examination is often completely normal but may show edema of the optic nerve, retina, or both, and retinal arteriolar constriction.[30] Retinal vasoconstriction was previously thought to be the cause of visual injury, and therapies such as vasodilators and stellate ganglion block were used in an attempt to reverse the vasospasm. Further study clearly shows both complete blindness with normal vessels, and recovery in patients with vasospasm.[26,58] Thus, retinal vasoconstriction is no longer thought to be of primary importance, although there is still speculation that vasospasm may have a modifying effect on outcome. Currently, there is no role for vasodilator therapy in these cases.

Recovery is often very rapid, but residual impairment is common in severe cases. In a study of 225 cases of quinine poisoning, 70 patients developed visual impairment. Of 31 patients whose worst ocular manifestation was blurred vision, all had complete visual recovery. However, of 39 patients who developed complete blindness, only 17 had full recovery.[9] The most common residual effects are peripheral field defects and central scotomata. Impaired color vision and complete blindness may also persist, but this is less common. Varying degrees of visual impairment (quinine amblyopia) have resulted from quinine exposure in many forms, but complete blindness is reported only after oral ingestion of large amounts of quinine. As in methanol poisoning, it is difficult to predict which patients will develop quinine amblyopia, but it does appear to be dose related. Although it certainly occurs at lower levels, complete blindness should be expected if quinine serum levels exceed 20 mg/mL in the first 10 hours after ingestion (Chap. 44).[9]

OCULAR COMPLICATIONS OF DRUG ABUSE

In addition to the well-known ocular pupillary signs of opioid, cocaine, amphetamine, and phencyclidine toxicity, a number of complications may result from short- or long-term use of these and other agents.[43] Quinine amblyopia (see the preceding section) caused by intravenous use of quinine-containing heroin is one of many ocular complications caused by injection of contaminants. Talc retinopathy was first described after prolonged intravenous use of methylphenidate,[25] but has subsequently been noted after intravenous use of heroin, methadone,[44] codeine, meperidine, and pentazocine. Talc retinopathy develops only after extensive intravenous drug use. In one study of intravenous methadone abusers, only patients who had injected more than 9000 tablets developed this complication.[44] Infectious complications, such as fungal (*Candida, Aspergillus*) or bacterial (*Staphylococcus spp., Bacillus cereus*) endophthalmitis, are well known as both direct effects of intravenous drug use and secondary complications of acquired immunodeficiency syndrome (AIDS). In addition to AIDS-related ophthalmic infections such as cytomegalovirus, cryptococcus, toxoplasmosis retinitis, and choroidal *Mycobacterium avium intracellulare*, other disorders include retinal cotton-wool spots, conjunctival Kaposi's sarcoma, and ocular motility disorders caused by infectious or neoplastic meningitis. Corneal defects have been noted after smoking cocaine alkaloid ("crack eye").[55] Cocaine that is either volatilized or inadvertently introduced by direct contact, probably results in corneal anesthesia and loss of corneal protective reflex sensation. Minor trauma, such as eye rubbing, then leads to corneal epithelial defects. In addition, there appears to be an increased incidence of infectious keratitis and corneal ulceration in these patients. The ability of local anesthetics to interfere with corneal epithelial adhesion may also play a role.

SUMMARY

Both systemic and local toxicologic emergencies occur in the ophthalmic system. The discussion focuses on the research in the treatment of damage to the eye caused by chemical agents. While these obvious physical injuries are most apparent to the clinician, the more subtle clues to the toxicologic mechanisms that involve the ophthalmic and neurologic systems are made by a meticulous examination of the eye. A careful ophthalmic examination often leads to early recognition of a toxicologic emergency.

REFERENCES

1. Abelson MB, Udell IJ, Weston JH: Normal human tear pH by direct measurement. Arch Ophthalmol 1981;99:301.
2. Adams RD, Victor M: Disorders of ocular movement and pupillary function. In: Adams RD, Victor M, eds: Principles of Neurology, 5th ed. New York, McGraw-Hill, 1993, pp. 225–246.
3. Adler IN, Wlodyga RJ, Rope SJ: The effects of pH on contact lens wearing. J Am Optom Assoc 1968;39:1000–1001.
4. Albert DM, Jakobiec FA, eds: Principles and Practice of Ophthalmology, 2nd ed. Philadelphia, WB Saunders, 2000.
5. Beiran I, Miller B, Bentur Y: The efficacy of calcium gluconate in ocular hydrofluoric acid burns. Hum Exp Toxicol 1997;16:223–228.
6. Benton CD, Calhoun FP: The ocular effects of methyl alcohol poisoning: Report of a catastrophe involving 320 persons. Am J Ophthalmol 1953;36:1677–1685.
7. Bentur Y, Tannenbaum S, Yaffe Y, Halpert M: The role of calcium gluconate in the treatment of hydrofluoric acid eye burn. Ann Emerg Med 1993;22:1488–1490.
8. Berlin R, Sing K, Lee U, Steiner R: Toxicity from the use of brimonidine ophthalmic solution in an infant and reversal with naloxone [abstract]. J Toxicol Clin Toxicol 1997;35:506.
9. Boland ME, Brennand Roper SM, Henry JA: Complications of quinine poisoning. Lancet 1985;1:384–385.
10. Brown VKH, Box VL, Simpson BJ: Decontamination procedures for skin exposed to phenolic substances. Arch Environ Health 1975;30: 1–6.
11. Burke J, Kharlamb A, Shan T, et al: Adrenergic and imidazoline receptor-mediated responses to UK-14,304–18 (brimonidine) in rabbits and monkeys. A species difference. Ann N Y Acad Sci 1995;763: 78–95.
12. Burns FR, Paterson CA: Prompt irrigation of chemical eye injuries may avert severe damage. Occup Health Saf 1989;58:33–36.
13. Burns FR, Stack MS, Gray RD, Paterson CA: Inhibition of purified collagenase from alkali burned rabbit cornea. Invest Ophthalmol Vis Sci 1989;30:1569–1575.
14. Carney LG, Hill RM: Human tear pH: Diurnal variations. Arch Ophthalmol 1976;94:821–824.
15. Chen FS, Maurice DM: The pH in the precorneal tear film and under a contact lens measured with a fluorescent probe. Exp Eye Res 1990;50: 251–259.
16. Davson H: Physiology of the Eye, 5th ed. New York, Pergamon Press, 1990.
17. Dean BS, Krenzelok EP: Cyanoacrylates and corneal abrasions. J Toxicol Clin Toxicol 1989;27:169–172.
18. Donshik PC, Berman MB, Dohlman CH, et al: Effect of topical corticosteroids on ulceration in alkali-burned corneas. Arch Ophthalmol 1978;96:2117–2120.
19. Eells JT, Salzman MM, Lewandowski MF, Murray TG: Formate-induced alterations in retinal function in methanol-intoxicated rats. Toxicol Appl Pharmacol 1996;140:58–69.
20. Flach AJ: Systemic toxicity associated with topical ophthalmic medications. J Fla Med Assoc 1994;81:256–260.
21. Fraunfelder FT, Bagby GC, Kelly DJ: Fatal aplastic anemia following topical administration of ophthalmic chloramphenicol. Am J Ophthalmol 1982;93:356–360.
22. Fraunfelder FT, Fraunfelder FW: Management of inadvertent cyanoacrylate tissue adhesives to the eyelid and eye. Arch Ophthalmol 2001, in press.
23. Fraunfelder FT, Fraunfelder FW, Grove JA, eds: Drug-Induced Ocular Side Effects and Drug Interactions, 4th ed. Philadelphia, PA, Lippincott Williams & Wilkins, 2001.
24. Fraunfelder FW, Rosenbaum JT: Drug induced uveitis incidence, prevention and treatment. Drug Saf 1997;17:197–207.
25. Friberg TR, Gragoudas ES, Regan CDJ: Talc emboli and macular ischemia in intravenous drug abuse. Arch Ophthalmol 1979;97: 1089–1091.
26. Friedman L, Rothkoff L, Zaks U: Clinical observations on quinine toxicity. Ann Ophthalmol 1980;12:640–642.
27. Garner CD, Lee EW, Terzo TS, Louis-Ferdinand RT: Role of retinal metabolism in methanol-induced retinal toxicity. J Toxicol Environ Health 1995;44:43–56.
28. Garner CD, Lee EW, Louis-Ferdinand RT: Muller cell involvement in methanol-induced retinal toxicity. Toxicol Appl Pharmacol 1995;130: 101–107.
29. Gottschalk HR, Stone Orville J: Stevens-Johnson syndrome from ophthalmic sulfonamides. Arch Dermatol 1976;112:513–514.

30. Grant WM, Schuman JS: Toxicology of the Eye, 4th ed. Springfield, IL, Charles C. Thomas, 1993.

31. Grant WM, Schuman JS: Toxicology of the Eye, 4th ed. Charles C. Thomas, Springfield, IL, 1993, p. 1531.

32. Grant WM: The peripheral visual system as a target. In: Spencer PS, Schaumberg HH, eds: Experimental and Clinical Neurotoxicology. Baltimore, Williams & Wilkins, 1980, pp. 77–91.

33. Haddox JL, Pfister RR, Slaughter SE: An excess of topical calcium and magnesium reverses the therapeutic effect of citrate on the development of corneal ulcers after alkali injury. Cornea 1996;15: 191–195.

34. Herr RD, White GL, Bernhisel K, et al: Clinical comparison of ocular irrigation fluids following chemical injury. Am J Emerg Med 1991; 9:228–231.

35. Hugues FC, Le Jeunne C: Systemic and local tolerability of ophthalmic drug formulations. An update. Drug Saf 1993;8:365–380.

36. Lang K: Treatment of phenol burns of the eye with polyethyleneglycol-400. Z Aerztl Fortbild (Jena) 1969;63:705–708.

37. Martin-Amat G, Tephly TR, McMartin KE, et al: Methyl alcohol poisoning: II. Development of a model for ocular toxicity in methyl alcohol poisoning using the Rhesus monkey. Arch Ophthalmol 1977;95: 1847–1850.

38. Martinasevic MK, Green MD, Baron J, Tephly TR: Folate and 10-formyltetrahydrofolate dehydrogenase in human and rat retina: Relation to methanol toxicity. Toxicol Appl Pharmacol 1996;141: 373–381.

39. Mattox C: Table of toxicology. In: Albert DM, Jakobiec FA, eds: Principles and Practice of Ophthalmology, 2nd ed, Philadelphia, WB Saunders, 2000, 496–507.

40. McCarron MM, Schulze BW, Thompson GA, et al: Acute phencyclidine toxicity: Incidence of clinical findings in 1,000 cases. Ann Emerg Med 1981;10:237–242.

41. McCulley JP: Ocular hydrofluoric acid burns: Animal model, mechanism of injury and therapy. Trans Am Ophthalmol Soc 1990;88: 649–684.

42. McCulley JP, Whiting DW, Petitt MG, Lauber SE: Hydrofluoric acid burns of the eye. J Occup Med 1983;25:447–450.

43. McLane NJ, Carroll DM: Ocular manifestations of drug abuse. Surv Ophthalmol 1986;30:298–311.

44. Murphy SB, Jackson WB, Dare JA: Talc retinopathy. Can J Ophthalmol 1977;95:861–868.

45. Murray TG, Burton TC, Rajani C, et al: Methanol poisoning: A rodent model with structural and functional evidence of retinal involvement. Arch Ophthalmol 1991;109:1012–1016.

46. Neymeyer VR, Tephly TR: Detection and quantification of 10-formyltetrahydrofolate deydrogenase (10-FTHFDH) in rat retina, optic nerve, and brain. Life Sci 1994;54:PL395–399.

47. Palmer EA: How safe are ocular drugs in pediatrics? Ophthalmology 1986;93:1038–1040.

48. Paterson CA, Pfister RR, Levinson RA: Aqueous humor pH changes after experimental alkali burns. Am J Ophthalmol 1975;79:414–419.

49. Petroutsos G, Pouliquen Y: Effect of ascorbic acid on ulceration in alkali-burned corneas. Ophthalmic Res 1984;16:185–189.

50. Pfister RR, Haddox JL, Yuille-Barr D: The combined effect of citrate/ascorbate therapy in alkali-injured rabbit eyes. Cornea 1991;10: 100–104.

51. Pfister RR, Paterson CA, Spiers JW, Hayes SA: The efficacy of ascorbate treatment after severe experimental alkali burns depends on the route of administration. Invest Ophthalmol Vis Sci 1980;19: 1526–1529.

52. Rozenbaum D, Baruchin AM, Dafna Z: Chemical burns of the eye with special reference to alkali burns. Burns 1991;17:136–140.

53. Rubenfeld RS, Silbert DI, Arentsen JJ, Laibson PR: Ocular hydrofluoric acid burns. Am J Ophthalmol 1992;114:420–423.

54. Saari KM, Leinonen J, Aine E: Management of chemical eye injuries with prolonged irrigation. Acta Ophthalmol 1984;161(Suppl 16): 52–59.

55. Sachs R, Zagelbaum BM, Hersh PS: Corneal complications associated with the use of crack cocaine. Ophthalmology 1993;100:181–191.

56. Seedor JA, Perry HD, McNamara TF, et al: Systemic tetracycline treatment of alkali-induced corneal ulceration in rabbits. Arch Ophthalmol 1987;105:268–271.

57. Shell JW: Pharmacokinetics of topically applied ophthalmic drugs. Surv Opthalmol 1982;26:207–217.

58. Smilkstein MJ, Kulig KW, Rumack BH: Acute toxic blindness: Unrecognized quinine poisoning. Ann Emerg Med 1987;16:98–101.

59. Toll LL, Hurlbut KM, eds: POISINDEX System. Englewood, CO, MICROMEDEX, 2000.

60. Trevino MA, Herrmann GH, Sprout WL: Treatment of severe hydrofluoric acid exposures. J Occup Med 1983;25:861–863.

61. Victor M, Adams RD: The effect of alcohol on the nervous system. Res Publ Assoc Res Nerv Ment Dis 1953;32:526–573.

62. Wagoner MD: Chemical injuries of the eye: Current concepts in pathophysiology and therapy. Surv Ophthalmol 1997;41:275–312.

63. Walters TR: Development and use of brimonidine in treating acute and chronic elevations of intraocular pressure: A review of safety, efficacy, dose response, and dosing studies. Surv Ophthalmol 1996; 41(Suppl 1):S19–S26.

CHAPTER 28

OTOLARYNGOLOGIC PRINCIPLES

William K. Chiang

Many toxins adversely affect the special senses of olfaction, gustation, and cochlear-vestibular functions. These toxic effects are not life-threatening and frequently not considered of substantial importance. Because of the lack of standardized diagnostic techniques and normal parameters, particularly for olfactory and gustatory functions, it is likely that such adverse effects will be overlooked and dismissed by healthcare providers, despite significant patient distress and dysfunction. This chapter delineates the effects of xenobiotics on these senses and examines the significant diagnostic information these senses contribute to the detection of xenobiotics. Understanding the effects of these agents on the senses may allow for early detection, which can occasionally be lifesaving.

OLFACTION

Physiology

Olfactory receptors are bipolar neurons located in the superior nasal turbinates and the adjacent septum. There are 10–20 million cells per nasal chamber, and the receptor portion of the cell undergoes continuous renewal from the olfactory epithelium.[105,108] Renewed olfactory receptors regenerate neural connections to the olfactory bulb. Olfactory receptor neurons are distinctive in their ability to regenerate.[25] The axons of these cells form small bundles that traverse the fenestrations of the cribriform plate of the ethmoid bone to the dura. Within the dura, these bundles form connections with the olfactory bulb. Neural projections then connect to the olfactory cortex. There are extensive central interconnections to other parts of the brain, such as the hippocampus, thalamus, hypothalamus, and frontal lobe, suggesting effects on other biologic functions.[105] Although primary odor detection is a function of the olfactory cranial nerve (CN I), some irritant odors, such as ammonia and acetone, are transmitted through the trigeminal cranial nerve (CN V) and its receptors.[43,140]

The actual olfactory receptor sites are structurally similar to taste receptors of the mouth and photoreceptors of the retina. The receptor is a single polypeptide chain consisting of approximately 350 amino acids, which folds back and forth on itself to transverse the cellular membrane seven times. The outer end of the polypeptide contains an amine group (*N*-terminal) and the cytosol end contains a carboxyl group (C-terminal). The transmembranous portions determine the receptor shape and characteristics of the binding site. When a molecule binds to a specific receptor site, the resultant conformational change leads to the activation of the G-protein system, and calcium and/or sodium channel activation and neurotransmission.[73]

Smelling is an extremely sensitive detector of certain substances. Olfactory receptors can detect as little as a few molecules of certain agents with a sensitivity that is superior to some of the most sophisticated laboratory detection instruments.[67]

Limitations of the Olfactory Senses

A number of problems result from the impact of smell as a toxicologic warning system. Human olfaction is a variable trait.[5,115,165] For example, 40–45% of people have specific anosmia for cyanide (a bitter almond smell).[44,87,115] There are limited data on the inheritance characteristics or genetic basis of these specific forms of anosmia. While some studies suggest that the ability to detect the odor of cyanide is a sex-linked recessive trait,[57] other studies yield conflicting results.[5,20,89] Females have a greater ability to detect androsterone, which is also prominent in human underarm secretion.[67] Human olfaction usually can distinguish a mixture of no more than four substances,[93] and therefore specific odors may be masked by other stimuli.

Olfactory fatigue is the process of olfactory adaptation following exposure to a stimulus for a variable period of time. This leads to a temporal diminution of the smell. Unfortunately, this adaptation may lead to a false sense of security with continued exposure to a toxin. For example, hydrogen sulfide, a toxin that inhibits cytochrome oxidase, is readily detectable as a distinct and offensive substance at the very low concentration of 0.025 ppm. At the higher and potentially toxic concentration of 50 ppm, the odor is less offensive, and recognition may disappear after 2–15 minutes of exposure.[8,144] At an even higher concentration, when toxicity is likely, the onset of olfactory fatigue is even more rapid. The combination of the rapid onset of olfactory fatigue and toxicity at high concentrations of hydrogen sulfide exposure has contributed to numerous fatalities[1,27] (Chap. 98).

In industrial settings, it is important to be aware of impaired olfactory function in any worker who may be exposed to chemical vapors or gases.[71,148] Such workers are at increased risk for toxic injury. The National Institute for Occupational Safety and Health (NIOSH) requires that an individual using an air-purifying respirator be capable of detecting a compound's odor at levels below those producing toxicity.[6,148] Sensory perception at this level ensures that the individual can detect filter cartridge "breakthrough" (ie, failure) at a safe level.[148] The odor safety factor refers to the ratio of the time-weighted average (TWA) threshold limit value (TLV) to the odor threshold for a given compound. A chemical with a high odor safety factor can be detected despite prolonged exposure.[6] Nontoxic agents, such as ethyl mercaptan, with a very high odor safety factor, can be added to agents that are odorless with lower safety factors, so that olfactory detection is predictable. This enhanced sensory awareness is the basis for the addition of mercaptans to the odorless natural gases used in the home so as to limit the potential for unrecognized hazardous exposure.

Clinical Use of Odor Recognition

The recognition of odors has traditionally been considered an important diagnostic skill in clinical medicine. Diseases can occasionally be diagnosed solely by a recognizable associated odor. Characteristic odors are described: diabetic ketoacidosis—fruity; diphtheria—sweet; scurvy—putrid; typhoid fever—fresh-baked brown bread; and scrofula—stale beer.[38] More recently, odors have been described for disorders of amino acid and fatty acid metabolism, such as phenylketonuria, maple syrup urine disease, hypermethioninemia, and isovaleric acidemia.[38]

The recognition of odors continues to be an important diagnostic skill for the rapid detection of toxins (Table 28–1). To increase the awareness of odors of toxic products, a simple and inexpensive "sniffing bar" may be prepared (Table 28–2).[62] Substances that simulate the odors of toxic products are placed in test tubes, numbered, and inserted in a test tube rack for circulation among staff. The sniffing bar, along with short descriptions of clinical presentations, and a table of diagnostic odors (Table 28–1), may be used to teach the recognition of odors in medical toxicology.[62]

Etiology of Olfactory Impairment

There are different types of olfactory dysfunction. Anosmia, the inability to detect certain odors, and hyposmia, a decrease in the perception of certain odors, are the most common forms of olfactory impairment. The etiology of olfactory impairment may be classified as conductive, from anatomic obstruction of inspired air, or perceptive, from dysfunction of the olfactory receptors or signal transmission. Most conductive olfactory dysfunction results in hyposmia, because the obstruction is usually incomplete.[105,137]

The most common causes of anosmia and hyposmia are viral infections, trauma, xenobiotics, tumors, and congenital and psychiatric disorders (Table 28–3).[43,125,130,137,140] Viral infections may result in olfactory impairment either by obstructing nasal airflow or by causing damage to the olfactory epithelium.[74] Trauma to the head or nose can shear fragile olfactory nerves crossing the cribriform plate. In fact as many as 5% of patients with head trauma have some olfactory dysfunction.[140,158]

Chronic exposures to numerous xenobiotics are associated with olfactory dysfunction (Table 28–3). The most common toxic mechanism related is perceptive olfactory dysfunction. This may be a result of a direct injury or of a structural alteration of the receptor, or its components such as G-proteins, adenylate cyclase, or receptor kinase.[72,73] Anosmia or hyposmia from hydrocarbons, formaldehyde, heavy metals such as cadmium, and antineoplastic agents such as cytarabine result from direct effects on the receptor sites.[47,73,78] Local effects on the epithelium and the receptors from antibiotic nose drops may lead to temporary anosmia and hyposmia.[84,164] Inhaled corticosteroids may have local effects on the epithelium, as well as direct effects on both G proteins and adenylate cyclase.[73] Cocaine insufflation causes direct local effects as well as effects on receptor functions.[65,73] Because of local effects of most xenobiotics and the regenerative ability of the olfactory receptor neurons, most xenobiotic-induced olfactory dysfunction is reversible.

Most people with anosmia have congenital anosmia to selected individual molecules, such as hydrogen cyanide, N-butyl mercaptan, trimethylamine, and isovaleric acid.[7,43] Some extreme forms of congenital anosmia are associated with other abnormalities, such as Kallmann syndrome, a hereditary form of anosmia associated with hypogonadotropic hypogonadism. Agenesis of the olfactory bulbs and incomplete development of the hypothalamus causes this form of anosmia.[43,140]

Dysosmia (or parosmia) is the distorted perception of smell (Table 28–3). Subclassifications of dysosmia include the perception of foul smell (cacosmia), the sensation of smell without a stimulus (phantosmia), and the sensation of the smell of a burnt or metallic material (torqosmia).[137] The etiologies are classified as peripheral or central. Peripheral etiologies include abnormalities of the nose, sinuses, and upper respiratory tract. Central etiologies may be related to disorders such as Addison disease, hypothyroidism, temporal lobe epilepsy, and psychosis, or to conditions such as pregnancy.[43,105,138] How these conditions actually alter the perception of smell is unclear. A number of xenobiotics with similar effects are listed in Table 28–3. Bromocriptine exerts its effect by affecting dopaminergic transmission and inhibiting adenylate cyclase. Levodopa also affects the dopaminergic transmission and chelates zinc, which is important in the maintenance of normal receptor functions.[73]

Evaluation of Patients with Olfactory Impairment

General evaluation of olfactory function should include a detailed history, focusing on types, duration, and progression of symptoms, recent illnesses, head and nose trauma, sinus problems, family history, occupational history, hobbies, medications, and drug history.[39,66] A complete physical examination and detailed examina-

TABLE 28–1. Diagnostic Odors

Characteristic Odor (Resembles)	Responsible Toxin
Acetone (sweet, fruity)	Lacquer, ethanol, isopropanol, chloroform, trichloroethane, paraldehyde, chloral hydrate, methylbromide
Bitter almond	Cyanide
Carrots	Cicutoxin (water hemlock)
Disinfectants	Phenol, creosote
Eggs (rotten)	Hydrogen sulfide, carbon disulfide, mercaptans, disulfiram, N-acetylcysteine
Fish or raw liver (musty)	Zinc phosphide, aluminum phosphide
Fruit	Nitrites (amyl, butyl, etc)
Garlic	Phosphorus, tellurium, arsenic, organic phosphorus compounds, selenium, thallium, dimethyl sulfoxide (DMSO)
Hay	Phosgene
Mothballs	Naphthalene, p-dichlorobenzene, camphor
Pepper	O-chlorobenzylidene malonitrile
Rope (burned)	Marijuana, opium
Shoe polish	Nitrobenzene
Tobacco	Nicotine
Vinegar	Acetic acid
Vinyl	Ethchlorvynol (Placidyl)
Violets	Turpentine (metabolites excreted in urine)
Wintergreen	Methyl salicylate

TABLE 28–2.   Case Studies for "Sniffing Bar"

Tube 1

Case history:	A lethargic 28-year-old woman was brought to emergency department with an altered mental status.
Odor:	Vinyl smell
Toxin:	Ethchlorvynol
Contents of tube:	Liquid contents of Placidyl capsule

Tube 2

Case history:	A 34-year-old man in cardiopulmonary arrest found in a chemical plant near several gas cylinders.
Odor:	Bitter almond
Toxin:	Cyanide
Contents of tube:	Macerated seeds from inside of peach pit

Tube 3:

Case history:	A 5-year-old child ingested unknown rodenticide, presented to emergency department with orthostatic hypotension, hyperglycemia, ketoacidosis. A small sample of rodenticide had this odor.
Odor:	Peanuts
Toxin:	Vacor. (Odor is from a flavoring agent used in commercially available products.)
Contents of tube:	Macerated peanuts

Tube 4

Case history:	A 27-year-old man was brought to emergency department with necrotic burns on his oral mucosa after gargling with an unknown liquid germicide. The patient thought that it would help his sore throat. The pH of the germicide was 5.
Odor	White paste (glue)
Toxin:	Phenol
Contents of tube:	Phenol (liquefied) (<1% concentration)

Tube 5

Case history:	A comatose 35-year-old man employed as sanitary engineer was pulled out of sewer by fellow worker. CPR was initiated. When he was brought to emergency department, the patient smelled like rotten eggs.
Odor:	Rotten eggs
Toxin:	Hydrogen sulfide
Contents of tube:	Sulfurated potash

Tube 6

Case history:	A photographer was brought to the emergency department after unintentionally ingesting a chemical used in developing film. On presentation, patient was drooling and grasping his throat in considerable distress. On examination the patient's mouth and throat were erythematous and he smelled "like a salad."
Odor:	Vinegar
Toxin:	Glacial acetic acid
Contents of tube:	Vinegar

Tube 7

Case history:	A crop duster was brought to the emergency department in acute respiratory distress. The patient had hypersalivation, miotic pupils (2 mm), a very unpleasant breath odor, and coarse rhonchi in both lung fields.
Odor:	Garlic
Toxin:	Organic phosphorus insecticide
Contents of tube:	Garlic

Tube 8

Case history:	A 4-year-old child was brought to the emergency department with a temperature of 39.7°C (103.5°F), a respiratory rate of 32 breaths/min, and markedly altered mental status. Laboratory tests on admission showed a high anion gap metabolic-acidosis. The patient smelled like a "wintergreen candy."
Odor:	Wintergreen
Toxin:	Methyl salicylate
Contents of tube:	Oil of wintergreen

Tube 9

Case history:	A 3-year-old was brought to the emergency department in considerable pain. On examination, the child exhibited dysphagia and dysphonia, the oral mucosa appeared blistered and erythematous. The child's mother stated that he must have gotten into cleaning supplies.
Odor:	Ammonia
Toxin:	Ammonia
Contents of tube:	Ammonia (diluted household)

Tube 10

Case history:	A 2-year-old was brought to the emergency department after vomiting and having what was described as a grand mal seizure. The child had been playing several minutes earlier in a storage closet.
Odor:	Moth balls
Toxin:	Camphor
Contents of tube:	Camphor

Reprinted with permission, from Goldfrank LR, Weisman R, Flomenbaum N: Teaching the recognition of odors. Ann Emerg Med 1982;11:685.

tion of the nasopharynx and sinuses should be performed to assess the potential for inflammation or structural abnormality. A simple set of olfactory stimulants, such as ground coffee, almond extract, peppermint extract, and musk, should be used to test each nostril individually with the patient's eyes closed.[66,140] Trigeminal stimulants such as ammonia, acetone, and menthol may be used to identify malingerers denying all odors. Because these agents depend not on olfactory (CN I) nerve function but on the trigeminal (CN V) nerve, a patient who has olfactory nerve damage should be able to detect these substances. Conversely, a malingerer may deny detection of these substances also.[66,140,164] If a drug-mediated mechanism is suspected, the offending agent should be discontinued. Radiographs of the sinuses and nose or CT scan of the nose, sinuses, and brain may be required if structural abnormalities are suspected.[140,164] Gas chromatographic analysis of the urine may be useful in patients with fish odor syndrome associated with

TABLE 28–3. Differential Diagnosis of Toxicologic Disorders of Smell

Hyposmia/Anosmia	Dysosmia/Cacosmia/Phantosmia
Acrylic Acid	Amebicides/antihelminthics: Metronidazole
Antihyperlipidemics: Cholestyramine, clofibrate, gemfibrozil, HMG-CoA reductase inhibitors	Anesthetics, local: Varied
Cadmium	Anticonvulsants: Carbamazepine, phenytoin
Chlorhexidine	Antihistamines
Cocaine (local effect)	Antihypertensives: ACE inhibitors, diazoxide
Formaldehyde	Antimicrobials
Gentamicin nose drops (local effect)	Antiinflammatory/antirheumatics: Allopurinol, colchicine, gold, D-penicillamine
Hereditary	
Hydrocyanic acid	Antiparkinson agents: Levodopa, bromocriptine
Hydrogen sulfide	
Hydrocarbons (volatile)	Antithyroid agents: Methimazole, methylthiouracil, propylthiouracil
Methylbromide	
Nutritional	β-Adrenergic antagonists
Vitamin B$_{12}$ deficiency	Calcium channel blockers
Zinc deficiency	Dental: Tooth pastes
Pentamidine	Diuretics: Ethacrynic acid
Sulfur dioxide	DSMO (dimethylsulfoxide)
	Insecticides
	Lithium
	Nicotine
	Opioids: Varied
	Sympathomimetics: Varied
	Vitamin D

Definitions: Anosmia, The loss of smell; Cacosmia, Sensation of a foul smell; Dysosmia, A distorted perception of smell; Hyposmia, A decreased perception of smell; Phantosmia, Sensation of smell without stimulus.

trimethylaminuria.[94,146] Complicated cases and patients with significant impairment should be referred to an otolaryngologist or neurologist.

GUSTATION

Physiology

Taste, the sensory interpretation of orally ingested materials, is determined by taste buds on the tongue, palate, throat, and upper third of the esophagus. The cells in the taste buds are constantly renewed, and have a life span of 10 days.[11,137] The taste buds on the anterior two-thirds of the tongue and the palate are innervated by the facial (CN VII) nerve, those on the posterior one-third of the tongue by the glossopharyngeal (CN IX) nerve, and those on the laryngeal and epiglottal regions by the vagus (CN X) nerve. There are at least 13 known chemical taste receptors responsible for the four primary taste sensations, sweet, sour, bitter, and salty: 2 sodium receptor types; 2 potassium receptor types; 1 chloride receptor; 1 adenosine receptor; 1 inosine receptor; 2 sweet receptor types; 2 bitter receptor types; 1 glutamate receptor; and 1 hydrogen ion receptor.[68] One substrate will typically activate multiple taste receptors, the combined effects of these stimulated receptors determine the taste of the substance.[55]

The structure of the taste receptors is similar to that of the olfactory receptors mentioned earlier, as they are coupled to G pro-

teins and sodium and calcium channels permitting neural stimulation. The pH of the substance determines sour or acid taste, whereas sodium or potassium concentrations determine salty taste. Many substances , such as sugars, glycols, aldehydes, ketones, amides, amino acids, inorganic salts of lead, and bretylium, activate the sweet receptors. Bitter taste may be the result of long-chain organic substances containing nitrogen, or alkaloids, including quinine, strychnine, caffeine, and nicotine.[68] Salivary proteins, such as zinc-containing gustin and ebnerin, are important in the regulation of taste sensation.[73,75,77,95,145] These molecules may serve as binding proteins and growth factors for the regeneration of taste receptors. Taste is also affected significantly by the appreciation of aromas or odors and, to a lesser extent, by visual perception.[138]

Etiology of Gustatory Impairment

Types of gustatory dysfunction include: ageusia—inability to perceive taste; hypogeusia—diminished sensitivity of taste; and dysgeusia—distortion of normal taste. There are several variations of dysgeusia, such as cacogeusia, which is a perceived foul, perverted, or metallic taste.[68,108] Taste impairment is commonly related to direct damage to the taste receptors, adverse effects on their regeneration, or effects on receptor mechanisms.[73] These effects can result from various pharmacologic and toxicologic agents, diseases, aging, and nutritional disorders (Table 28–4).[61,68,129,137,154] Any abnormality that interferes with either the direct contact of a substance with the gustatory cells of the tongue or cranial nerves VII, IX, or X dramatically affects taste.[137] Most common forms of xenobiotic-induced dysgeusia are related to direct effects on the taste receptor site or effects related to receptor mechanisms such as G proteins, adenylate cyclase, and calcium channels.[92] Other forms of dysgeusia may result from direct stimulation of chemical receptors by xenobiotics.[68,73]

Angiotensin-converting enzyme (ACE) inhibitors commonly cause gustatory impairment, usually hypogeusia and dysgeusia.[19,63,104,166] ACE inhibitors work by inhibiting zinc-dependent ACE, and chelating zinc from taste receptors and salivary proteins resulting in taste dysfunction. Calcium channel blockers act by inhibiting calcium channels of the taste receptor mechanisms.[68] Many diuretics cause zinc depletion by enhancing zinc elimination in the urine.[73] In addition, furosemide and spironolactone may also chelate zinc. Numerous other substances also cause gustatory dysfunction through variable degrees of zinc chelation, such as amrinone, ethambutol, hydralazine, methyldopa, the nonsteroidal anti-inflammatory drugs (NSAIDs), the antithyroid agents, penicillamine, and phenytoin.[68,73,167] Heavy metals such as arsenic, mercury, chromium, and lead may either chelate zinc or replace zinc in salivary proteins because of a higher level of affinity. Antineoplastic agents and antimicrotubular agents, such as colchicine, inhibit cellular division and taste receptor regeneration.[70] The oral antiseptic agent chlorhexidine directly alters taste-receptor function.[54] Acetazolamide causes cacogeusia when carbonated beverages are consumed. The exact mechanism is unclear, but is postulated to be a result of the inhibition of carbonic anhydrase causing carbon dioxide accumulation and an increased tissue bicarbonate.[73,85,106]

Taste-Aversive Agents and Poison Prevention

Nontoxic taste-aversive agents are frequently added to products such as shampoo, cosmetics, cleaning products, automotive prod-

TABLE 28–4. Xenobiotic Alterations of Taste

Hypogeusia/Ageusia
Local:
  Chemical burn
  Radiation therapy
Systemic:

ACE inhibitors	DMSO (dimethyl-sulfoxide)	Phenylbutazone
Amiloride		Propranolol
Amrinone	Gasoline	Pyrethrins
Captopril	Hydrochlorothiazide	Smoking
Carbon monoxide	Methylthiouracil	Spironolactone
Cocaine	Nitroglycerin	Triazolam
	Penicillamine	

Dysgeusia
Local:
  Chemical burn
  Radiation therapy
Systemic:

ACE inhibitors	DMSO (dimethyl-sulfoxide)	Naproxen
Adriamycin	5-Fluorouracil	Nicotine
Amphotericin B	Griseofulvin	Nifedipine
Botulism (in recovery)	Ibuprofen	Phenylthiourea (hereditary)
Bretylium	Isotretinoin	Quinine
Carbamazepine	Levodopa	Zinc deficiency

Metallic Taste

ACE inhibitors	Ethambutol	Metronidazole
Acetaldehyde	Ferrous salts	Pentamidine
Allopurinol	Flurazepam	Procaine penicillin
Arsenicals	Iodine	Propafenone
Cadmium	Lead	Snake envenomation
Ciguatoxin	Levamisole	Tetracycline
Copper	Lithium	
Coprinus spp.	Mercury	
Dipyridamole	Methotrexate	
Disulfiram	Metoclopramide	

ucts, and rubbing alcohol to discourage ingestion.[70] Except in the case of rubbing alcohol, this is done primarily to prevent poisoning in children. The most common taste-aversive agents are the denatonium salts, particularly denatonium benzoate (Bitrex, benzyldiethyl[(2,6-xylylcarbamoyl)methyl] ammonium benzoate), one of the most bitter tasting substances known.[26,42] The bitter taste of denatonium benzoate can be detected at 50 parts per billion (ppb). This agent is used in concentrations of 6–50 parts per million (ppm), typically 6 ppm in cosmetic products and ethanol and 30–50 ppm in methanol and ethylene glycol.[16,116] Only limited data are available on the utility of taste-aversive agents for prevention of poisoning. Denatonium benzoate added to liquid detergent and orange juice can decrease the amount ingested by children.[13,149] However, the degree of taste aversion is not universal; in one study, some children were noted to take more than one sip of denatonium benzoate-laced orange juice.[149] Taste aversion is partially a learned response; frequently young children do not find bitter taste as offensive as do adults.[14] It seems unlikely that taste-aversive agents will eliminate unintentional ingestions in children, because oral ingestion is required for aversive effects to occur. Taste-aversive agents may be most beneficial in the prevention of poisoning by moderately toxic and nonaversive products, such as ethylene glycol, methanol, paraquat, certain pesticides, acetoni-

trile, and bromate-containing cosmetics where more than one or two sips of the product must be ingested to cause toxicity. Taste-aversive agents are not and cannot be substitutes for other poison prevention modalities (Chap. 116).

HEARING

Physiology

Normal hearing begins when sound waves are captured by the external auricle and traverse the external auditory canal. They are then conducted to the tympanic membrane, the auditory ossicles of the middle ear, and through the oval window to the perilymph in the scala vestibuli of the cochlea (Figs. 28–1 and 28–2). The wave is then transferred through Reissner's membrane at the roof of the cochlear duct, to the endolymph and the organ of Corti.[51,150] The specialized hair cells of the organ of Corti convert mechanical waves into neurologic signals. The hair cells contain cross-linked stereocilia projections that detect transmitted shear forces, this leads to the influx of potassium from the endolymph through opened potassium channels.[41,96] Depolarization of the hair cells result in calcium influx and neurotransmitter release to the cochlear nerve. Neurologic signals from the cochlear nerve are conducted to the cochlear nucleus of the pons; bilateral projections are sent to the superior olivary nucleus of the midbrain, nuclei of lateral lemnisci, inferior colliculus, medial geniculate body of the thalamus, and then to the auditory cortex of the temporal lobe.[150] Interruption or damage to any part of the hearing mechanism may lead to auditory impairment.

The anatomy and physiology of the cochlea and its importance in the biomechanics of hearing are reviewed to understand the potential for toxicologic injury. The word "cochlea" is derived from the Greek word *kochlias*, meaning snail, and describes its general structure of a 2.5-turn spirally wound tube. The cochlea is further divided into 3 inner tubular structures, the upper tube or scala vestibuli, the middle tube or cochlear duct, and the lower tube or scala tympani. The scala vestibuli and the scala tympani contain the perilymph fluid. The cochlear duct contains endolymph fluid, Reissner's membrane at the roof, and the organ of Corti.[150] The cochlear fluids serve multiple functions: to conduct sound waves to the hair cells, to provide nutrients and remove waste for the cells lining the cochlear duct, to control pressure distribution in the cochlea, and to maintain an electrochemical gradient for the function of the hair cells. The sodium concentration of the perilymph is similar to that of the extracellular fluid, and the potassium concentration of the endolymph is similar to that of the intracellular fluid.[53] Any significant alterations of the sodium or potassium concentrations will depress the cochlear potential and function. The stria vascularis controls the production of the cochlear fluids and the repolarization of the hair cells, and maintains the electrochemical gradient between the endolymph and the perilymph. The stria vascularis contains a high concentration of the oxidative enzymes, Na^+-K^+-ATPase, adenylate cyclase, and carbonic anhydrase, which are highly susceptible to toxins.[21,79,135]

Although human speech is composed of sounds in the frequency of 250–3000 Hz, humans can normally detect sounds in the frequency range of 20–20,000 Hz.[114] The cochlea is a "tuned" structure with varying width and stiffness, such that different regions can receive different sound waves. The stiffer and wider base of the cochlea serves as a receptacle for higher-frequency

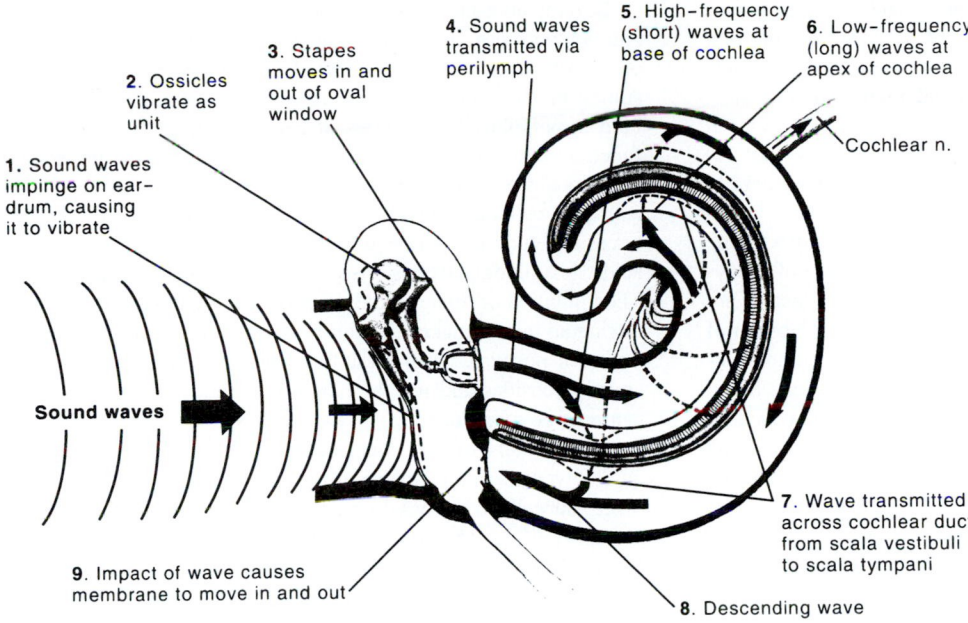

1. Sound waves impinge on eardrum, causing it to vibrate

2. Ossicles vibrate as unit

3. Stapes moves in and out of oval window

4. Sound waves transmitted via perilymph

5. High–frequency (short) waves at base of cochlea

6. Low–frequency (long) waves at apex of cochlea

Cochlear n.

Sound waves

7. Wave transmitted across cochlear duct from scala vestibuli to scala tympani

8. Descending wave

9. Impact of wave causes membrane to move in and out

Figure 28–1. Pathways of sound conduction in the ear. *(Reproduced, with permission, from Silverstein H, Wolfson RJ, Rosenberg S: Diagnosis and management of hearing loss. Clin Symposia 1994;44:3.)*

sounds, whereas the apex is responsible for receiving the lower-frequency sounds.[51] Because various regions of the cochlea are susceptible to different forms of injury, appropriate audiologic testing should be tailored specifically to each patient.[29]

Xenobiotic-Induced Ototoxicity

Quinine and salicylates were widely recognized in the 1800s and streptomycin in the 1940s as etiologies of ototoxicity.[79,131] Several hundred xenobiotics have been implicated as ototoxins, some of which cause reversible ototoxicity and others, irreversible toxicity (Table 28–5).[24,83,90,111] Ototoxic agents primarily affect two different sites in the cochlea: the organ of Corti (particularly the hair cells) and the stria vascularis. Because of the limited regenerative capacity of the sensory hair cells and other supporting cells, when significant cellular damage occurs, the loss is often permanent.[45,51,79,147] Evidence supports the concept that xenobiotic-related injury can be potentiated by loud noises and other ototoxic agents.[21,24,79,83] While the actual cellular mechanisms for many forms of ototoxicity remain unclear,[163] some of the mechanisms are known.[58] Loop diuretics, such as furosemide, bumetanide, and ethacrynic acid, cause physiologic dysfunction and edema at the stria vascularis, resulting in reversible hearing loss.[79,100] The underlying mechanisms appear to be the inhibition of potassium pumps and G proteins associated with adenyl cyclase.[9] Physiologic studies of loop diuretics demonstrate decreased potassium

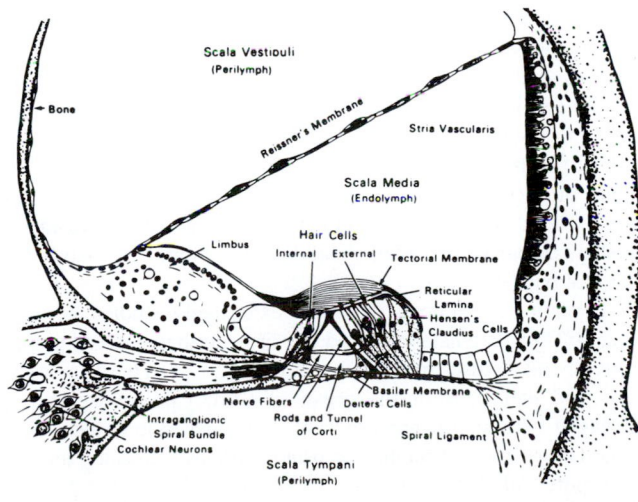

Figure 28–2. Cross-section of the organ of Corti. *(Reproduced, with permission, from Davis H: Advances in the neurophysiology and neuroanatomy of the cochlea. J Acoust Soc Am 1962; 34:1379.)*

TABLE 28–5. Xenobiotics Etiologies of Hearing Loss

Primarily Reversible
Antimicrobials: Chloroquine, erythromycin, quinine
Carbon monoxide
Diuretics: Acetazolamide, bumetanide, ethacrynic acid, furosemide, mannitol
NSAIDs
Salicylates

Primarily Irreversible
Aminoglycosides
Antineoplastics: Bleomycin, cisplatin, nitrogen mustard, vincristine, vinblastine
Bromates
Heavy metals: Arsenic, lead, mercury
Hydrocarbons: Styrene, toluene, xylene

activity in the endolymph and a decreased endocochlear potential.[132] Permanent hearing loss associated with furosemide and ethacrynic acid is also reported, and may be related to direct interference with oxidative metabolism in the outer hair cells.[91,100,132]

Salicylates are a well-known cause of ototoxicity. Aspirin (acetylsalicylic acid)-induced hearing impairment was first reported in 1877.[86] Salicylate-induced hearing loss is generally mild to moderate (20–40 dB loss) and is generally reversible.[18,81] Animal studies demonstrate immediate hearing impairment with the use of high doses of salicylates.[17,102,120] The mechanism of salicylate-induced ototoxicity is unclear, although multiple factors are postulated. The effect on prostaglandin synthesis (ie, inhibition of cyclooxygenase) may interfere with Na^+-K^+-ATPase pump function at the stria vascularis, and also decrease cochlear blood flow.[31,48,86] Reversible decrease in outer hair cell turgor secondary to membrane permeability changes may impair otoacoustic emissions.[121,124] In support of these theories, pretreatment of animals with leukotriene antagonists and α-adrenergic receptor antagonists attenuates or prevents salicylate-induced ototoxicity.[86]

Nonsteroidal antiinflammatory drugs (NSAIDs) and the cinchona alkaloid quinine also cause reversible hearing loss, particularly at the higher frequencies.[33,79] Occasionally, quinine-induced hearing loss may be permanent.[79,136] The primary mechanism is related to prostaglandin inhibition.[86] The NSAIDs inhibit cyclooxygenase, which converts arachidonic acid to prostaglandin G_2 and prostaglandin H_2. Quinine inhibits phospholipase A_2 enzyme, which converts phospholipids to arachidonic acid. Quinine also inhibits calcium channels that interact with prostaglandins.[86]

Antineoplastic agents, such as cisplatin, vinblastine, and vincristine, can cause permanent ototoxicity.[79] Cisplatin is the most toxic of the group, with clinically apparent hearing loss noted in 30–70% of the patients receiving doses of 50–100 mg/m². Children may be even more susceptible to ototoxicity. These agents typically damage the outer hair cells but may also affect the stria vascularis.[79] The underlying mechanisms may be related to the inhibition of adenyl cyclase in the stria vascularis, the inhibition of protein synthesis, and the formation of oxygen free radicals.[9,79,141] The generation of oxygen free radicals and the depletion of antioxidants is a significant mechanism in the irreversible damage to the hair cells.[50] Furthermore, cranial radiation will cause synergistic toxicity if radiation precedes cisplatin therapy. Various antioxidants and free radical scavengers prevent cisplatin-induced ototoxicity in animals.[109,126,133,152,162] Neurotrophic agents also prevent cisplatin-induced toxicity in animals, perhaps preventing oxidative injury induced apoptosis to hair cells. Amifostine (WR-2721), a precursor to a thiol free radical scavenger, is available to prevent cisplatin-induced nephrotoxicity. However, amifostine does not appear to prevent cisplatin-induced ototoxicity.[134a]

The aminoglycosides are the best known group of drugs associated with irreversible ototoxicity.[119] Neomycin and kanamycin are the most ototoxic of these agents, although all aminoglycosides are potentially toxic.[91] With the development of newer aminoglycosides and drug monitoring, the incidence of aminoglycoside-related ototoxicity appears to be decreasing. The reported rates of ototoxicity for the more commonly used aminoglycosides gentamicin and tobramycin are between 5 and 8%.[99] In China, where aminoglycosides are readily available over the counter, as much as 66% of deaf-mutism may be secondary to aminoglycoside toxicity.[56,97] Aminoglycosides are not concentrated in the cochlear or the renal cells. The endolymph concentration of gentamicin is approximately 10% of that in the serum.

Several mechanisms of ototoxicity have been postulated. Aminoglycosides antagonize calcium channels of the outer hair cells of the cochlea, blocking transduction of the hair cells and resulting in acute reversible hearing deficits. Aminoglycosides also bind to polyphosphoinositides of cell membranes and alter their functions. Polyphosphoinositides are essential for the generation of second messengers diacylglycerol and inositol trisphosphate and their cellular functions, for the maintenance of lipid membrane structure and permeability, and as a source for arachidonic acid.[159] Aminoglycosides also inhibit ornithine decarboxylase. The inhibition of this enzyme, important for cellular recovery following an injury, makes the cell more susceptible to toxicity.[135] It has been postulated that toxicity is related to the metabolites of aminoglycosides and not the parent compounds because toxicity can only be reproduced in in vivo models and not in vitro.[135] The outer hair cells of the cochlea are increasingly susceptible to aminoglycosides and damage progresses from the inner row of the outer hair cells to the basal turn of the cochlea, and, ultimately, to the apex.[4,7,91,128] The risks of ototoxicity are increased with prolonged duration of therapy (greater than 10 days), concomitant use of other ototoxic agents, and elevated serum levels.[7,52,134] Loop diuretics increase aminoglycoside toxicity by increasing aminoglycoside penetration into the endolymph. In animal models, certain free radical scavengers, such as glutathione, WR-2721, and deferoxamine, decrease aminoglycoside-induced ototoxicity.[59,136,153] Fosfomycin, a phosphonic antibiotic, has limited efficacy in reducing aminoglycoside-induced ototoxicity and salicylates are also suggested to reduce ototoxicity.[113,144] Further studies are required to elucidate their applicability to humans.

Other antibiotics are also implicated as causing ototoxicity, particularly erythromycin, vancomycin, and their respective analogues. There are a number of human reports of hearing loss following erythromycin therapy and an animal study supporting the ototoxic potential. Most human deficits are transient, although several cases of permanent hearing loss are reported.[22,23] The mechanisms of toxicity remain unclear although the proposed effects are on the central auditory pathways. Erythromycin-induced hearing loss occurs at both lower and higher frequencies for speech, allowing for recognition in the early stages of ototoxicity.[22] Ototoxicity from the newer macrolide antibiotics has not been reported.

The evidence for vancomycin-induced ototoxicity is less convincing. Although numerous cases of presumed vancomycin-related ototoxicity are reported, concomitant use of other ototoxic antibiotics was common or audiometric studies were not performed. In limited animal studies, vancomycin alone did not induce ototoxicity, but the agent increased ototoxicity when administered concomitantly with an aminoglycoside. Vancomycin analogues such as teicoplanin and daptomycin probably have similar ototoxic potentials.

Bromates are among the most extensively studied ototoxic agents.[36,98,122] Bromates are used in hair neutralizers, bread preservatives, and as fuses in explosive devices.[80,122,155] The stria vascularis and hair cells of the organ of Corti can be irreversibly damaged with significant exposure.[122] Bromates may also cause renal failure with substantial exposure, perhaps increasing the ototoxic potential.[80,122]

It is intriguing that agents such as the bromates and aminoglycosides primarily affect both the cochlea and the kidneys. One possible explanation is that the stria vascularis and the renal tubules have similar functions in maintaining electrochemical gradients.[122,123] However, renal tubules may regenerate while damage to the hair cells and the stria vascularis of the cochlea is more likely to be permanent.

Other agents also implicated as ototoxins are carbon monoxide, lead, arsenic, mercury, toluene, xylene, and styrene.[76,148] However, both human and animal data are quite limited. A number of chemicals, such as carbon disulfide, carbon tetrachloride, and trichloroethylene, are suspected of being ototoxic, but toxicity has not been demonstrated in humans.[76,148] Because exposures to chemicals and toxins are frequently occupational, they are of great concern as they may potentiate or be additive to other types of occupational hearing impairments.[88,127]

High-frequency hearing is most vulnerable, and early or limited impairment may not be noticeable unless audiometry (especially at 8 kHz and above) is performed.[159] These hearing tests can be performed in infants using the measurement of auditory brainstem response.[12]

Noise-Induced Hearing Impairment

Noise-induced hearing impairment had been recognized for hundreds of years, but became of great concern and prevalent with the discovery of gunpowder and the industrial revolution.[51] Some of the anatomic changes in the organ of Corti and the audiometric features of noise-induced hearing impairment were well described by 1900.[2,3,103] Unfortunately, few longitudinal studies on noise-induced hearing impairment have been performed.

Although noises of sufficient magnitude may cause hearing impairment with limited exposure, most noise-induced hearing losses result from preventable prolonged cumulative occupational exposure. The NIOSH has estimated that up to 1.7 million workers in the United States between 50 and 59 years of age have significant occupational hearing loss.[114] Noise can be defined as any unwanted sound, which can be further characterized by duration, time pattern (continuous, intermittent, or impulsive), frequency, and intensity. The intensity is measured in sound pressure levels (SPL) and expressed in a logarithmic scale in decibels (dB). The intensity of a normal conversation is approximately 65 dB (Table 28–6).[114] The risk of noise-induced hearing loss is related to cumulative duration of exposure, intensity, and individual susceptibility.[112,117,161] Much of the risk assessment of noise-induced hearing loss is inexact. Most authorities agree that sounds with

maximal intensity below 75–80 dB will not cause hearing impairment, regardless of the duration of exposure.[112] At higher intensity, the risk of hearing impairment increases with increased duration of exposure. Continued occupational exposure at 90–94 dB typically causes some high-frequency hearing loss in approximately 10 years.[2,117] Further exposure results in hearing loss in the lower-frequency range. The Occupational Safety and Health Administration (OSHA) established guidelines for permissible occupational noise exposure based on an analysis of the average intensity and duration of exposure (Table 28–7).[2,161]

The pathophysiology of noise-induced hearing impairment is related to an excessive energy impact on the cochlea, but the exact biochemical changes are unclear. Exposure to short duration of excessive noises results in a temporary hearing impairment (temporary threshold shift) with a duration of hours to weeks. However, prolonged exposure results in a permanent threshold shift or hearing impairment.[3,51,161] Initially, outer hair cells are lost, but with more significant exposures damage to both inner and outer hair cells and all supporting structures in the organ of Corti results. Cochlear nerve fibers degenerate after hair cell damage.[51,161] The section of the cochlea most at risk from loud noises is at the 9–13 mm region (the total length is 32 mm).[103] This region is responsible for hearing at the 3–6 kHz range, corresponding to the typical noise-induced hearing loss pattern.

Much of the clinical assessment and monitoring of noise-induced hearing loss is based on pure tone hearing loss, demonstrating an audiometric deficit at 3–6 kHz.[114,161] This typical pattern occurs in other conditions and becomes less typical with aging.[117] Although human speech is composed mainly of low-frequency sounds, the ability to perceive the higher frequency sounds is extremely important in speech recognition. For this reason, the major impairment in patients with noise-induced hearing loss is an inability to discriminate speech, particularly from background noise.[2,40] Currently, the science of the investigation of speech discrimination is limited with extensive areas for research.

Blast injury to the ear is an exposure of extremely short duration, but very high-intensity sound waves (usually greater than 140 dB). Military personnel are particularly at risk.[32,118,157] Hearing loss from blast injury may be related to rupture of the tympanic membrane, disruption of the ossicles, temporary cochlear dysfunction, and permanent cochlear dysfunction from labyrinthine fistulae and basilar membrane rupture.[30] When a large tympanic membrane rupture or disruption of the ossicles occurs, surgical intervention may be required to treat hearing impairment.[30]

TABLE 28–6. Typical Sound Levels on the Decibel Scale

Sound	Decibels
Weakest sound that humans can detect	10
Quiet bedroom, soft whisper	20
Broadcast studio	25–30
Insulated lounge	50
Normal conversation	65
Television-audio	70
Vacuum cleaner	80
Machine press, subway car (35 mph)	95
Spray painting, snowmobile	105
Power saw	110
Car horn	115
Armored personnel carrier; ear pain begins	120
Jet plane engine, gunshot	145
Highest sound level that can occur	194

TABLE 28–7. OSHA Standard for Permissible Noise Exposure

dBA[a]	Duration of Exposure (hr)
85	16
90	8
92	6
95	4
97	3
100	2
102	1.5
105	1
110	0.5
115	0.25 or less

[a]Decibels using the A-scale filter.

Prevention of any type of noise-induced hearing loss remains the best solution. Various hearing-protection devices are available if the noise exposure cannot be reduced. Better monitoring and more longitudinal studies are required on noise-induced hearing loss. Exposure to xenobiotics that can impair hearing may have synergistic effects with noise-induced hearing loss.[88,90] These factors should be considered when noise exposure is evaluated. Furthermore, noise exposure is not limited to the workplace. Significant noise exposure may occur at home or from leisure activities, such as power tools, stereo, and ambient exposure.[15,37,69,117] The impact of noise exposure outside of the workplace has only recently attracted the attention of investigators.

Etiology of Tinnitus

Tinnitus is the sensation of sound not resulting from mechano-acoustic or electric signals. Virtually all humans experience tinnitus in their lifetime. The exact mechanism or mechanisms resulting in tinnitus are largely unknown.[139] Several theories are proposed, but none is completely satisfactory. Tinnitus may result from spontaneous neurologic discharges when the hair cells or cochlear nerve are injured. Altered sound perception may result from local or central effects when feedback mechanisms are interrupted.[46,49,82,101] Severing the cochlear nerve terminates tinnitus in less than half of affected patients, suggesting important central mechanisms.[10] Furthermore, certain etiologies of tinnitus, such as migraine headache and temporal lobe seizures, do not affect hearing directly. Xenobiotics including salicylate may cause hair cell dysfunction and may modify neurotransmission centrally in both the cochlear nucleus and the inferior colliculis.[60,160] Although the probable sites involved in tinnitus may be classified as peripheral [external ear, middle ear, or cochlear (CN VIII)], central, or extra-auditory (vascular, nasopharyngeal), some etiologies may affect peripheral and central sites, and many etiologies remain unknown.[35,49,101]

Tinnitus may result from trauma or disease or as a manifestation of xenobiotic toxicity. Tinnitus is most commonly related to any mechanism that affects hearing. Excessive cerumen, fluid, or a foreign body in the external canal, perforated tympanic membrane, acoustic trauma resulting from exposure to excessive noise, otosclerosis, acoustic neuroma, and otitis media may produce tinnitus. However, the only otologic problem that always results in tinnitus is Meniere's disease. Other etiologies for tinnitus include diabetes, hypertension, autoimmune disease, hypothyroidism, and arteriovenous aneurysms.[34,101]

Numerous xenobiotics are associated with tinnitus (Table 28–8), but the incidence is probably low and the implied relationships have usually been supported only by case reports.[34,142,143] Tinnitus may or may not be associated with transient or permanent hearing loss. It is probable that these agents also associated with hearing loss affect cochlear function, while those that produce tinnitus without hearing loss probably act on the central nervous system. Xenobiotics that frequently produce tinnitus are streptomycin, neomycin, indomethacin, doxycycline, ethacrynic acid, furosemide, heavy metals, and high doses of caffeine.[64,142,143] Only a few drugs, such as quinine and salicylates, consistently cause tinnitus at toxic doses.[17,49] These two drugs also serve as examples of how the presence of tinnitus may be an indicator of drug toxicity.

Tinnitus associated with salicylates usually begins at the high therapeutic or low toxic level (approximately 20–40 mg/dL).[107]

TABLE 28–8.   Xenobiotics that Cause Tinnitus

Antifungal agents: Amphotericin B
Anticonvulsants: Carbamazepine
Antidepressants: Cyclic antidepressants, amoxapine, lithium, trancylcypromine
Antihistamines
Antimicrobials: Aminoglycosides, vancomycin, dapsone, doxycycline, tetracycline, sulphonamide, sulfasoxazole, sulphamethoxazole, metronidazole, thiabendazole, clindamycin
Antineoplastics: Cisplatin, nitrogen mustard, 6-aminonicotinamide, methotrexate
Antiparasitics: Chloroquine, hydroxychloroquine
Antipsychotics: Haloperidol, molindone
β-Adrenergic antagonists
Bromates
Cinchona alkaloids: Quinine, quinidine, salicylates
Diuretics: Furosemide, ethacrynic acid, bumetanide
Hydrocarbons: Benzene
Local anesthetics: Mepivacaine, bupivacaine, lidocaine
Nonsteriodal antiinflammatory drugs
Oral contraceptives
Sympathomimetics: Caffeine, theophylline, metaproterenol, albuterol, methylphenidate

Before the wide availability of salicylate serum measurements, physicians treating gout or rheumatoid arthritis often titrated the salicylate dosage until tinnitus developed.[37] Tinnitus and other signs and symptoms of salicylism (Chap. 33) should be sufficient for physicians to diagnose salicylate toxicity before serum salicylate levels are available. However, tinnitus may not be evident in elderly patients with hearing impairment despite significantly elevated salicylate concentrations.[107] The classic constellation of symptoms of quinine and salicylate toxicity, called cinchonism, includes nausea, vomiting, tinnitus, and visual disturbances.[4,28,110] Because serum quinine levels are not readily available, symptoms of quinine toxicity remain a clinical diagnosis (Chap. 44).[151]

SUMMARY

Numerous drugs and toxins commonly affect the sense of smell, taste, and hearing. They may cause significant patient morbidity. Some of the events may be foreseeable, whereas others will require monitoring and appropriate testing. Significant patient risk and discomfort may be avoided by an understanding of the basic pathophysiology of the otolaryngologic organs and by a heightened suspicion on the part of healthcare providers. Current knowledge and sophistication on the pathophysiology of toxins and these special organs at the molecular level is expanding rapidly. It is particularly encouraging and exciting to be able to witness the development of potential therapeutic agents.

REFERENCES

1. Adelson L, Sunshine I: Fatal hydrogen sulfide poisoning. Report of three cases occurring in a sewer. Arch Pathol 1966;81:375–380.
2. Alberti PW: Noise induced hearing loss. Br Med J 1992;304:522.
3. Alberti PW: Occupational hearing loss. In: Ballenger JJ, ed: Diseases of the Nose, Throat, Ear, Head, and Neck, 14th ed. Philadelphia, Lea & Febiger, 1991, pp. 1053–1068.

4. Alvan G, Karlsson KK, Villen T: Reversible hearing impairment related to quinine blood concentration in guinea pigs. Life Sci 1989; 45:751–755.

5. Amoore JE: Olfactory genetics and anosmia. In: Beidler LM, ed: Handbook of Sensory Physiology, vol 4. Chemical Senses, part I. Berlin, Springer-Verlag, 1971, pp. 145–156.

6. Amoore JE, Hautala E: Odor as an aid to chemical safety: Odor thresholds compared with threshold limit values and volatilities for 214 industrial chemicals in air and water diluted. J Appl Toxicol 1983;3:272–290.

7. Assael BM, Parini R, Rusconi F: Ototoxicity of aminoglycoside antibiotics in infants and children. Pediatr Infect Dis 1982;1:357–365.

8. Audeau FM, Gnanaharan C, Davey K: Hydrogen sulfide poisoning: Associated with pelt processing. NZ Med J 1985;98:145–147.

9. Bagger-Sjoback D, Filipek CS, Schacht J: Characteristics and drug responses of cochlear and vestibular adenylate cyclase. Arch Otorhinolaryngol 1980;228:217–222.

10. Barrs DM, Brackmann DE: Translabyrinthine nerve section: Effect on tinnitus. J Laryngol Otol 1984;98(S9):287–293.

11. Beidler LM: Renewal of cells within taste buds. J Cell Biol 1965;27: 263–272.

12. Bergstorm L, Thompson PL: Ototoxicity. In: Brown RD, Daigneault EA, eds: Pharmacology of Hearing: Experimental and Clinical Basis. New York, Wiley, 1981, pp. 119–134.

13. Berning CK, Griffith JF, Wild JE: Research on the effectiveness of denatonium benzoate as a deterrent to liquid detergent ingestion by children. Fundam Appl Toxicol 1982;2:44–48.

14. Bernstein IL, Webster MM: Learned taste aversions in humans. Physiol Behav 1980;25:363–366.

15. Bess FH, Poynor RE: Noise-induced hearing loss and snowmobiles. Arch Otol 1974;99:45–51.

16. Bitrex Product Information. Edinburgh, Macfarlan Smith, 1989.

17. Boettcher FA, Bancroft BR, Slvi RJ, et al: Effects of sodium salicylate on evoked-response measures of hearing. Hearing Res 1989;42: 129–142.

18. Boettcher FA, Salvi RJ: Salicylate ototoxicity: Review and synthesis. Am J Otol 1991;12:33–47.

19. Boyd O: Captopril induced taste disturbance. Lancet 1993;342:304.

20. Brown KS, Robinette RR: No simple pattern of inheritance in ability to smell solutions of cyanide. Nature 1967;215:406–408.

21. Brown RD, Penny JE, Henley CM, et al: Ototoxicity drugs and noise. In: Evered D and Lawrenson G, eds, Tinnitus. Ciba Foundation Symposium 85. London, Pitman, 1981, pp. 151–171.

22. Brummett RE: Ototoxicity of erythromycin and analogues. Otolaryngol Clin North Am 1993;26:811–819.

23. Brummett RE: Ototoxicity of vancomycin and analogues. Otolaryngol Clin North Am 1993;26:821–827.

24. Brummett RE, Traynor J, Brown R, et al: Cochlear damage resulting from kanamycin and furosemide. Acta Otolaryngol 1975;80:86–92.

25. Buckland ME, Cunninghamb AM: Alterations in the neurotrophic factors BDNE, GDNF and CNTF in the regenerating olfactory system. Ann N Y Acad Sci 1998;855:260–265.

26. Budavari S, O'Neil MJ, Smith A, et al, eds: The Merck Index: An Encyclopedia of Chemicals, Drugs, and Biologicals, 11th ed. Rahway, NJ, Merck, 1989, pp. 454–455.

27. Burnett WW, King EG, Grace M, et al: Hydrogen sulfide poisoning: Review of 5 years' experience. Can Med Assoc J 1977;117: 1277–1280.

28. Burst JCM, Richter RW: Quinine amblyopia related to heroin addiction. Ann Intern Med 1971;74:84–86.

29. Campbell KCM, Durrant J: Audiologic monitoring for ototoxicity. Otol Clin North Am 1993;26:903–914.

30. Casler JD, Chait RH, Zajtchuk JT: Treatment of blast injury to the ear. Ann Otol Rhinol Laryngol 1989;98:13–22.

31. Cazals Y, Li XQ, Aurousseau C, et al: Acute effects of noradrenaline related vasoactive agents on the ototoxicity of aspirin: An experimental study in guinea pigs. Hear Res 1988;36:89–96.

32. Chait R, Casler J, Zajtchuk JT: Blast injury of the ear: Historical perspective. Ann Otol Rhinol Laryngol 1989;98:9–12.

33. Chapman P: Naproxen and sudden hearing loss. J Laryngol Otol 1982;96:163–166.

34. Ciba Foundation Symposium 85: A central or peripheral source of tinnitus. In: Evered D, Lawrenson G, eds: Tinnitus. London, Putnam, 1981, pp. 279–294.

35. Ciba Foundation Symposium 85: Appendix I: Definition and classification of tinnitus. London, Pitman, 1981, pp. 300–302.

36. Chiu JJ, Hsu CJ, Lin-Shiau SY: The detrimental effects of potassium bromate and thioglycolate on auditory brainstem response of guinea pig. Chin J Physiol 2000;30:91–96.

37. Clark WW: Noise exposure from leisure activities. J Acoust Soc Am 1991;90:175–181.

38. Cone TE Jr: Diagnosis and treatment: Some diseases, syndromes, and conditions associated with an unusual odor. Pediatrics 1968;41: 993–995.

39. Davidson TM: The loss of smell. Emerg Med 1988;20:104–116.

40. Davignon DD, Leshowitz BH: The speech-in-noise test: A new approach to the assessment of communication capability of elderly persons. Int J Aging Hum Dev 1986;23:149–160.

41. Davis H: Advances in the neurophysiology and neuroanatomy of the cochlea. J Acoust Soc Am 1962;34:1377–1385.

42. DeCourcy Hinds M: Mother fights to ruin the taste of poison. New York Times, May 20, 1989.

43. Doty RL: A review of olfactory dysfunctions in man. Am J Otol 1979;1:57–79.

44. Drewnowski A: Genetics of taste and smell. World Rev Nutr Diet 1990;63:194–208.

45. Duckert LG, Rubel EW: Current concepts in hair regeneration. Otolaryngol Clin North Am 1993;26:873–901.

46. Eggermont JJ: On the pathophysiology of tinnitus: A review and a peripheral model. Hear Res 1990;48:111–123.

47. Emmett EA: Parosmia and hyposmia induced by solvent exposure. Br J Ind Med 1976;3:196–198.

48. Escoubet B, Amsallem P, Ferrary E, et al: Prostaglandin synthesis by the cochlea or the guinea pig. Influence of aspirin, gentamicin, and acoustic stimulation. Prostaglandins 1985;29:589–599.

49. Evans EF: Chairman's closing remarks. In: Evered D, Lawrenson G: eds, Tinnitus. Ciba Foundation Symposium 85. London, Putman, 1981, pp. 295–302.

50. Evans P, Halliwel B: Free radicals and hearing. Cause, consequence, and criteria. Ann N Y Acad Sci 1999;884:19–40.

51. Falk SA: Pathophysiological responses of the auditory organ to excessive noise. In: Lee DHK, Falk HL, Geiger SR, eds: Handbook of Physiology: Reactions to Environmental Agents. Bethesda, MD, American Physiological Society, 1977, pp. 17–30.

52. Fee WE Jr: Aminoglycoside ototoxity in the human. Laryngoscope 1980;90(Suppl 24):1–19.

53. Feldman AM: Cochlear fluids: Physiology, biochemistry, and pharmacology. In: Brown RD, Daigneault EA, eds: Pharmacology of Hearing. Experimental and Clinical Basis. New York, Wiley, 1981, pp. 81–97.

54. Flotra L, Gjermo P, Rolla G, et al: Side effects of chlorhexidine mouth washes. J Dent Res 1971;79:119–125.

55. Froloff N, Faurion A, MacLeod P: Multiple human taste receptor sites: A molecular modeling approach. Chem Senses 1996;21: 425–445.

56. Fu DM: Survey of 1583 deaf mutes. Qinghai Med J 1985;1:105–112.

57. Fukumoto Y, Nakajima H, Uetake M, et al: Smell ability to solution of potassium cyanide and its inheritance. Jpn J Hum Genet 1957; 2:7–16.

58. Gao W: Role of neurotrophins and lectins in prevention of ototoxicity. Ann N Y Acad Sci 1999;884:312–327.

59. Garetz SL, Altschuler RA, Schacht J: Attenuation of gentamicin ototoxicity by glutathione in the guinea pig in vivo. Hear Res 1994; 77:81–87.

60. Gerken GM: Central tinnitus and lateral inhibition: An auditory brainstem model. Hear Res 1996;97:75–83.

61. Glover J, Dibble S, Miaskoski C, et al: Changes in taste associated with intravenous administration pentamidine. J Assoc Nurses AIDS Care 1995;6:43–48.

62. Goldfrank LR, Weisman R, Flomenbaum N: Teaching the recognition of odors. Ann Emerg Med 1982;11:684–686.

63. Gomez HJ, Cirillo VJ, Irvin JD: Enalapril: A review of human pharmacology. Drugs 1985;30S:13–24.

64. Goodey RJ: Drugs in the treatment of tinnitus. In: Evered D, Lawrenson G, eds.: Tinnitus. Ciba Foundation Symposium 85. London, Putnam, 1981, pp. 263–278.

65. Gordon AS, Moran DT, Jafek BW, et al: The effect of chronic cocaine abuse on human olfaction. Arch Otolaryngol Head Neck Surg 1990;116:1415–1418.

66. Gordon CB: Practical approach to the loss of smell. Am Fam Physician 1982;26:191–193.

67. Gorman W: The sense of smell. Eye Ear Nose Throat 1964;43: 54–58.

68. Griffin JP: Drug-induced disorder of taste. Adv Drug React Rev 1992;11:229–239.

69. Grumet GW: Pandemonium in the modern hospital. N Engl J Med 1993;322:433–437.

70. Hansen SR, Janssen C, Beasley VR: Denatonium benzoate as a deterrent to ingestion of toxic substances: Toxicity and efficacy. Vet Hum Toxicol 1993;35:234–236.

71. Hastings L: Sensory neurotoxicology: Use of the olfactory system in the assessment of toxicity. Neurotoxicol Teratol 1990;12:455–459.

72. Henkin RI: Concepts of therapy in taste and smell dysfunction: Repair of sensory receptor functions as primary treatment. In: Kurihara K, Suzuki N, Ogawa H, eds: Olfaction and Taste. Tokyo, Springer-Verlag, 1994, pp. 568–570.

73. Henkin RI: Drug-induced taste and smell disorders. Incidence, mechanisms and management related primarily to treatment of sensory receptor dysfunction. Drug Saf 1994;11:318–377.

74. Henkin RI, Larson AL, Powell RD: Hypogeusia, dysgeusia, hyposmia, and dysosmia following influenza-like infection. Ann Otol Rhinol Laryngol 1975;84:672–682.

75. Henkin RI, Lippoldt RE, Bilstad J, et al: A zinc protein isolated from human parotid saliva. Proc Natl Acad Sci USA 1975;72:488–492.

76. Hetu R, Phaneuf R, Marien C: Non-acoustic environmental factor influences on occupational hearing impairment: A preliminary discussion. Paper presented at the second international conference on the combined effects of environmental factors, Kanazama, Japan, 1986, pp. 17–31.

77. Heyneman CA: Zinc deficiency and taste disorders. Ann Pharmacother 1996;30:186–187.

78. Hotz P, Tschopp A, Soderstrom D, et al: Smell or taste disturbances, neurological symptoms, and hydrocarbon exposure. Int Arch Occup Environ Health 1992;63:525–530.

79. Huang MY, Shacht J: Drug-induced ototoxicity: Pathogenesis and prevention. Med Toxicol 1989;4:452–467.

80. Hymes LC, Bruner BS, Rauber AP: Bromate poisoning from hair permanent preparations. Pediatrics 1985;76:975–978.

81. Jardini L, Findlay R, Burgi E, et al: Auditory changes associated with moderate blood salicylate levels. Rheumatol Rehab 1978;14: 233–236.

82. Jastreboff PJ: Phantom auditory perception (tinnitus): Mechanisms of generation and perception. Neurosci Res 1990;8:221–254.

83. Jobe PC, Brown RD: Auditory pharmacology. Trends Pharmacol Sci 1980;1:202–206.

84. Jojart G: Sense of smell after gentamicin nose-drops. Lancet 1992; 339:313.

85. Joyce PW: Taste disturbance with acetazolamide [letter]. Lancet 1990;336:1446.

86. Jung TTK, Rhee CK, Lee CS, et al: Ototoxicity of salicylate, nonsteroidal anti-inflammatory drugs, and quinine. Otolaryngol Clin North Am 1993;26:791–810.

87. Kare MR, Mattes RD: A selective overview of the chemical senses. Nutr Rev 1990;48:39–48.

88. Keeve JP: Ototoxic drugs and the workplace. Am Fam Physician 1988;38:177–181.

89. Kirk RL, Stenhouse NS: Ability to smell solutions of potassium cyanide. Nature 1953;171:698–699.

90. Kisiel DL, Bobbin RP: Miscellaneous ototoxic agents. In: Brown RD, Daigneault EA, eds: Pharmacology of Hearing: Experimental and Clinical Basis. New York, Wiley, 1981, pp. 231–269.

91. Koegel L: Ototoxicity: A contemporary review of aminoglycosides, loop diuretics, acetylsalicylic acid, quinine, erythromycin, and cisplatinum. Am J Otol 1985;6:190–199.

92. Kusakabe Y, Abe K, Tanemura K, et al: GUST27 and closely related G-protein-coupled receptors are localized in taste buds together with Gi-protein alpha-subunit. Chem Senses 1996;21:335–340.

93. Laing DG, Francis GW: The capacity of humans to identify odors in mixtures. Physiol Behav 1989;46:809–814.

94. Leopold DA, Preti G, Mozell MM, et al: Fish-odor syndrome presenting as dysosmia. Arch Otolaryngol Head Neck Surg 1990;116: 354–355.

95. Li XJ, Snyder SH: Molecular cloning of ebnerin, a von Ebner's gland protein associated with taste buds. J Biol Chem 1995; 270: 17674–17679.

96. Lim DJ: Functional structure of the organ of Corti: A review. Hear Res 1986;22:117–146.

97. Lu YF: Cause of 611 deaf mutes in schools for deaf children in Shanghai. Shanghai Med J 1987;10:159.

98. Matsumoto I, Morizona T, Paparella MM: Hearing loss following potassium bromate: Two case reports. Otolaryngol Head Neck Surg 1980;88:625–629.

99. Matz GJ: Aminoglycoside cochlear ototoxicity. Otolaryngol Clin North Am 1993;26:705–736.

100. Matz GJ: The ototoxic effects of ethacrynic acid in man and animals. Laryngoscope 1976;86:1065–1086.

101. McFadden D: Tinnitus: Facts, Theories, and Treatment. Washington, DC, National Academy Press, 1982, pp. 10–24.

102. McFadden D, Plattsmier HS: Aspirin abolishes spontaneous otoacoustic emissions. J Acoust Soc Am 1984;76:443–448.

103. McGill TJ, Schuknecht HF: Human cochlear changes in noise induced hearing loss. Laryngoscope 1976;86:1293–1302.

104. McNeil JJ, Anderson A, Christophidis N, et al: Taste loss associated with oral Captopril treatment. Br Med J 1979;15:1555–1556.

105. Meyerhoff WL: Physiology of the nose and paranasal sinuses. In: Paparella MM, Schumrick DA, eds: Otolaryngology: Basic Sciences and Related Disciplines, Vol. 1. Philadelphia, WB Saunders, 1980, pp. 308–311.

106. Miller LG, Miller SM: Altered taste secondary to acetazolamide. J Fam Pract 1990;31:199–200.

107. Mongan E, Kelly P, Nies K, et al: Tinnitus as an indication of therapeutic serum salicylate levels. JAMA 1973;226:142–145.

108. Mott AE, Leopold DA: Disorders of taste and smell. Med Clin North Am 1991;75:1321–1353.

109. Muldoon LL, Pagel MA, Kroll RA, et al: Delayed administration of sodium thiosulfate in animal models reduces platinum ototoxicity without reduction of antitumor activity. Clin Cancer Res 2000; 6:309–315.

110. Myers EN, Bernstein JM: Salicylate ototoxicity. Arch Otolaryngol 1965;82:483–493.

111. Nadol JB Jr: Hearing loss. N Engl J Med 1993;329;1092–1102.

112. National Institute of Health: Noise and hearing loss. Consensus Development Conference Statement. JAMA 1990;263:3185–3190.

113. Ohtani I, Ohtsuki K, Aikawa T, et al: Mechanism of protective effect of fosfomycin against aminoglycoside ototoxicity. Auris Nasus Larynx 1984;11:119–124.

114. Olishifski JB: Occupational hearing loss, noise, and hearing conservation. In: Zenz C, ed: Occupational Medicine: Principles and Practical Applications. Chicago, Year Book, 1988, pp. 274–323.

115. Patterson PM, Lauder BA: The incidence and probable inheritance of "smell blindness." J Hered 1948;39:295–297.

116. Payne HAS, Smalley HM, Tracy MJ: Denatonium benzoate as a bitter aversive additive in ethylene glycol and methanol-based automotive products. SAE Technical Paper Series, Presented 23rd International Conference on Environmental Systems, Colorado Springs, CO. July 1993, pp. 125–131.

117. Phaneur R, Hetu R: An epidemiological perspective of the causes of hearing loss among industrial workers. J Otolaryngol 1990;19:31–40.

118. Phillips YY, Zajtchuk JT: Blast injuries of the ear in military operations. Ann Otol Rhinol Laryngol 1989;98:3–4.

119. Prazma J: Ototoxicity of aminoglycoside antibiotics. In: Brown RD, Daigneault EA, eds: Pharmacology of Hearing: Experimental and Clinical Basis. New York, Wiley, 1981, pp. 155–193.

120. Puel JL, Bobbin RP, Fallon M: Salicylate, meclofenamate, and quinine on cochlear potentials. Otolaryngol Head Neck Surg 1990;102:66–73.

121. Puel JL, Bobbin RP, Fallon M: Salicylate abolishes cochlea potentials through a mechanism that does not involve prostaglandin synthesis and is different than quinine. Otolaryngol Head Neck Surg 1988;99:154.

122. Quick CA, Chole RA, Mauer SM: Deafness and renal failure due to potassium bromate poisoning. Arch Otolaryngol 1975;101:494–495.

123. Quick CA, Fish A, Brown C: The relationship between cochlea and kidney. Laryngoscope 1973;83:1469–1482.

124. Ramsden RT, Latif A, O'Malley S: Electrocochleographic changes in acute salicylate overdosage. J Laryngol Otol 1985;99:1269–1273.

125. Razani J, Murphy C, Davidson TM, et al: Odor sensitivity is impaired in HIV-positive cognitively impaired patients. Physiol Behav 1996;59:877–881.

126. Reser D, Rho M, Dewan D, et al: L- and D-methionine provide equivalent long-term protection against CDDP-induced ototoxicity in vivo, with partial in vitro and in vivo retention of antineoplastic activity. Neurotoxicology 1999;20:731–748.

127. Riggs LC, Brummett RE, Guitjens SK, et al: Ototoxicity resulting from combined administration of cisplatin and gentamicin. Laryngoscope 1996;106:401–406.

128. Roche RJ, Silamut K, Pukrittayakamee S, et al: Quinine induces reversible high-tone hearing loss. Br J Clin Pharmacol 1990;29:780–782.

129. Rollin H: Drug-related gustatory disorders. Ann Otol 1978;87:37–42.

130. Rose CS, Heywood PG, Costanzo RM: Olfactory impairment after chronic occupational cadmium exposure. J Occup Med 1992;34:600–605.

131. Rutka J, Alberti PW: Toxic and drug-induced disorders in otolaryngology. Otolaryngol Clin North Am 1984;17:761–774.

132. Rybak LP: Ototoxicity of loop diuretics. Otolaryngol North Am 1993;26:829–844.

133. Rybak LP, Husain K, Whitworth C, et al: Dose dependent protection by lipoic acid against cisplatin-induced ototoxicity in rats: Antioxidant defense system. Toxicol Sci 1999;47:195–202.

134. Rybak MJ, Abate BJ, Kang SL, et al: Prospective evaluation of the effect of an aminoglycoside dosing regimen on rates of observed nephrotoxicity and ototoxicity. Antimicrob Agents Chemother 1999;43:1549–1555.

134a. Santini V, Giles FJ: The potential of amifostine: From cytoprotective to therapeutic agent. Hematologia 1999;84:1035–1042.

135. Schacht J: Biochemical basis of aminoglycoside ototoxicity. Otolaryngol Clin North Am 1993;26:845–856.

136. Schacht J: Molecular mechanisms of drug-induced hearing loss. Hear Res 1986;22:297–304.

137. Schiffman SS: Taste and smell in disease (part 1). N Engl J Med 1983;308:1275–1279.

138. Schiffman SS: Taste and smell in disease (part 2). N Engl J Med 1983;308:1337–1343.

139. Schleuning AJ: Management of the patient with tinnitus. Med Clin North Am 1991;75:1225–1237.

140. Schneider BA: Anosmia: Verification and etiologies. Ann Otol 1972;81:272–277.

141. Schweitzer VG: Ototoxicity of chemotherapeutic agents. Otolaryngol Clin North Am 1993;26:759–789.

142. Seidman MD, Jacobson GP: Update on tinnitus. Otolaryngol Clin North Am 1996;29:455–465.

143. Seligmann H, Podoshin L, Ben-David J, et al: Drug-induced tinnitus and other hearing disorders. Drug Saf 1996;14:198–212.

144. Sha SH, Schacht J: Salicylate attenuates gentamicin-induced ototoxicity. Lab Invest 1999;79:807–813.

145. Shatzman AR, Henkin RI: Metal-binding characteristics of the parotid salivary protein gustin. Biochim Biophys Acta 1980;623:107–118.

146. Shelley WB: A diagnosis you can smell. Emerg Med 1992;24:232–235.

147. Shulman A: The cochleovestibular system/ototoxicity/clinical issues. Ann N Y Acad Sci 1999;884:433–436.

148. Shusterman DJ, Sheedy JE: Occupational and environmental disorders of the special senses. Occup Med 1992;7:515–542.

149. Sibert JR, Frude N: Bittering agents in the prevention of accidental poisoning: Children's reactions to denatonium benzoate (Bitrex). Arch Emerg Med 1991;8:1–7.

150. Silverstein H, Wolfson RJ, Rosenberg S: Diagnosis and management of hearing loss. Clin Symposia 1994;44:1–32.

151. Smilkstein MJ, Kulig KW, Rumack BH: Acute toxic blindness: Unrecognized quinine poisoning. Ann Emerg Med 1987;16:98–101.

152. Smoorenburg GF, De Groot JC, Hamers FP, et al: Protection and spontaneous recovery from cisplatin-induced hearing loss. Ann N Y Acad Sci 1999;884:192–210.

153. Song BB, Schacht J: Variable efficacy of radical scavengers and iron chelators to attenuate gentamicin ototoxicity in guinea pig in vivo. Hear Res 1996;94:87–93.

154. Stevens JC, Cruz LA, Hoffman JM, et al: Taste sensitivity and aging: High incidence of decline revealed by repeated threshold. Chem Senses 1995;20:451–459.

155. Stewart TH, Sherman Y, Politzer WM: An outbreak of food-poisoning due to a flour improver, potassium bromate. South Afr Med J 1969;200–202.

156. Stine R, Slosberg B, Beacham BE: Hydrogen sulfide intoxication. Ann Intern Med 1976;85:756–758.

157. Sullivan P: MD launches study to determine amount of job-related hearing loss in military. Can Med Assoc J 1992;146:2061–2062.

158. Sumner D: Post-traumatic anosmia. Brain 1964;87:107–120.

159. Tange RA, Dreschler WA, van der Hulst RJ: The importance of high-tone audiometry in monitoring for ototoxicity. Arch Otorhinolaryngol 1985;242:77–81.

160. Wallhauser-Frank E, Braun S, Langner G: Salicylate alters 2–DG uptake in the auditory system: A model for tinnitus? Neuroreport 1996;7:1585–1588.

161. Ward WD: Noise-induced hearing loss. In: Northern JL, ed: Hearing Disorder, 2nd ed. Boston, Little, Brown, 1984, pp. 143–152.

162. Watanabe KI, Hess A, Bloch W, et al: Nitric oxide synthase inhibitor suppresses the ototoxic side effects of cisplatin in guinea pig. Anticancer Drugs 2000;11:401–406.

163. Willems PJ: Genetic causes of hearing loss. N Engl J Med 2000;342:1101–1109.

164. Wright HN: Characterization of olfactory dysfunction. Arch Otolaryngol Head Neck Surg 1987;113:163–168.

165. Wysocki CJ, Gilbert AN: The National Geographic Smell Survey: The effects of age are heterogenous. Ann N Y Acad Sci 1989;561:12–28.

166. Zazgornick J, Kaiser W, Biesenbach G: Captopril induced dysgeusia [letter]. Lancet 1993;341:1542.

167. Zeller JA, Machetanz J, Kessler C: Ageusia as an adverse effect of phenytoin. Lancet 1998;351:1101.

Dina Began

The skin serves as a protective barrier to shield internal organs from harmful agents in the environment as well as to maintain internal organ integrity. When toxic exposure occurs, whether it is ingested, injected, or inhaled from an external source, the skin can express its effects. Dermal exposures account for 8% of the cases and for 1.3% of the fatalities reported to the American Association of Poison Control Centers (AAPCC) (see Chap. 116 and p. 1752). Dermatitis is among the most common occupational diagnoses. Cutaneous toxin effects are of great concern because the adult skin covers an average surface area of 2 m^2.[10] Despite its outwardly simple structure and function, the skin is actually extraordinarily complex. The microanatomic composition of the skin provides the foundation on which to understand the cutaneous effects of the toxins. It should be noted, however, that different agents may produce clinically similar skin changes and many agents may produce a repertoire of dermal lesions.

SKIN ANATOMY AND PHYSIOLOGY

The skin has three main anatomic components: the epidermis, the dermis, and the subcutis or hypodermis. The primary physiologic role of the epidermis, the most external layer of the skin, is to maintain water homeostasis and to establish immunologic surveillance. It is composed of five layers: the horny, transitional, granular, spinous, and basal layers (see Fig. 29–1). The thin stratum corneum, or horny layer, is predominantly responsible for the protective function of the skin. Disruption or inadequate formation of the stratum corneum leads to a breakdown of this barrier function and many disease processes. The cells of the stratum corneum serve as a buffer to acidic and alkaline substances. Barrier function is also maintained in part by the granular layer. In this layer, there are Odland bodies, also known as membrane-coating granules, lamellar granules, and keratinosomes. The contents of these organelles provide a barrier to water loss while mediating stratum corneum cell cohesion.[12]

The stratum corneum is covered by a surface film composed of sebum emulsified with sweat and breakdown products from the horny layer.[1] The role of the surface film, however, is only negligible in regard to percutaneous absorption.[21]. The major barrier molecules in the skin are lipids called *ceramides*. Diseases characterized by dry skin, such as atopic dermatitis and psoriasis, are caused by decreased levels of ceramide in the stratum corneum allowing increased toxin penetration because of barrier degradation.[11] Similarly, hydrocarbon solvents, such as gasoline or methanol, or detergents, commonly produce a "defatting dermatitis" by dissolving the surface lipids or keratolysis.

The degree of barrier function of the epidermis varies with its thickness as well. Differences in thickness are observed on different regions of the body. The epidermis varies from 1.5 mm on the palms and soles to 0.1 mm on the eyelids. The cells of the basal layer control the renewal of the epidermis. The basal layer contains stem cells and transient amplifying cells which are the proliferative cells resulting in new epidermal formation, which occurs every 59–75 days. As the basal cells migrate toward the skin surface they flatten, lose their nuclei, and develop keratohyalin granules, and eventually develop into the horny layer. Patients with cutaneous diseases, such as psoriasis, have a significantly shortened epidermal renewal or turnover time resulting in a thicker epidermis and less direct penetration of toxin.[2] The basal layer is adjacent to the basement membrane zone and is also populated by melanocytes and Langerhans cells. Melanocytes contain melanin, which is the major chromophore in the skin that is responsible for absorbing ultraviolet and other light energies. They are primarily responsible for the coloration of the skin. The Langerhans cells are bone marrow-derived cells with a primary role in immunosurveillance including primary contact sensitization. Langerhans cells function in the recognition, uptake, processing, and presentation of antigens to sensitized T lymphocytes. Langerhans cells may also carry antigens via dermal lymphatics to regional lymph nodes.

The basement membrane zone, which consists of three layers—the lamina lucida, the lamina densa, and the sublamina densa—separates the epidermis from the dermis. It provides a site of attachment for keratinocytes and permits epidermal-dermal interaction.

The dermis is deep to the epidermis and contains the adnexal structures, blood vessels, and nerves. The dermis provides a structural scaffold as well as houses many important appendageal structures. The support is provided by collagen and elastin fibers embedded in glycosaminoglycans, such as chondroitin A and hyaluronic acid. Mature dermis is predominantly type I collagen. The collagen accounts for 70% of the dry weight of the skin, while elastic fibers are equivalent to 1–2%. Several important cells, including fibroblasts and mast cells, are present in the dermis. Traversing the dermis are venules, capillaries, arterioles, nerves, and glandular structures.

The arteriovenous framework of the skin consists of a deep plexus in the region of the subcutaneous dermal junction. From this deep plexus, smaller arteries transverse upward to the junction of the reticular and papillary dermis, where they form the superficial plexus. Capillary-venules form superficial vascular loops that ascend into and descend from the dermal papillae. These communicating blood vessels provide channels in which toxins applied to the skin can be carried internally. In addition they transport inter-

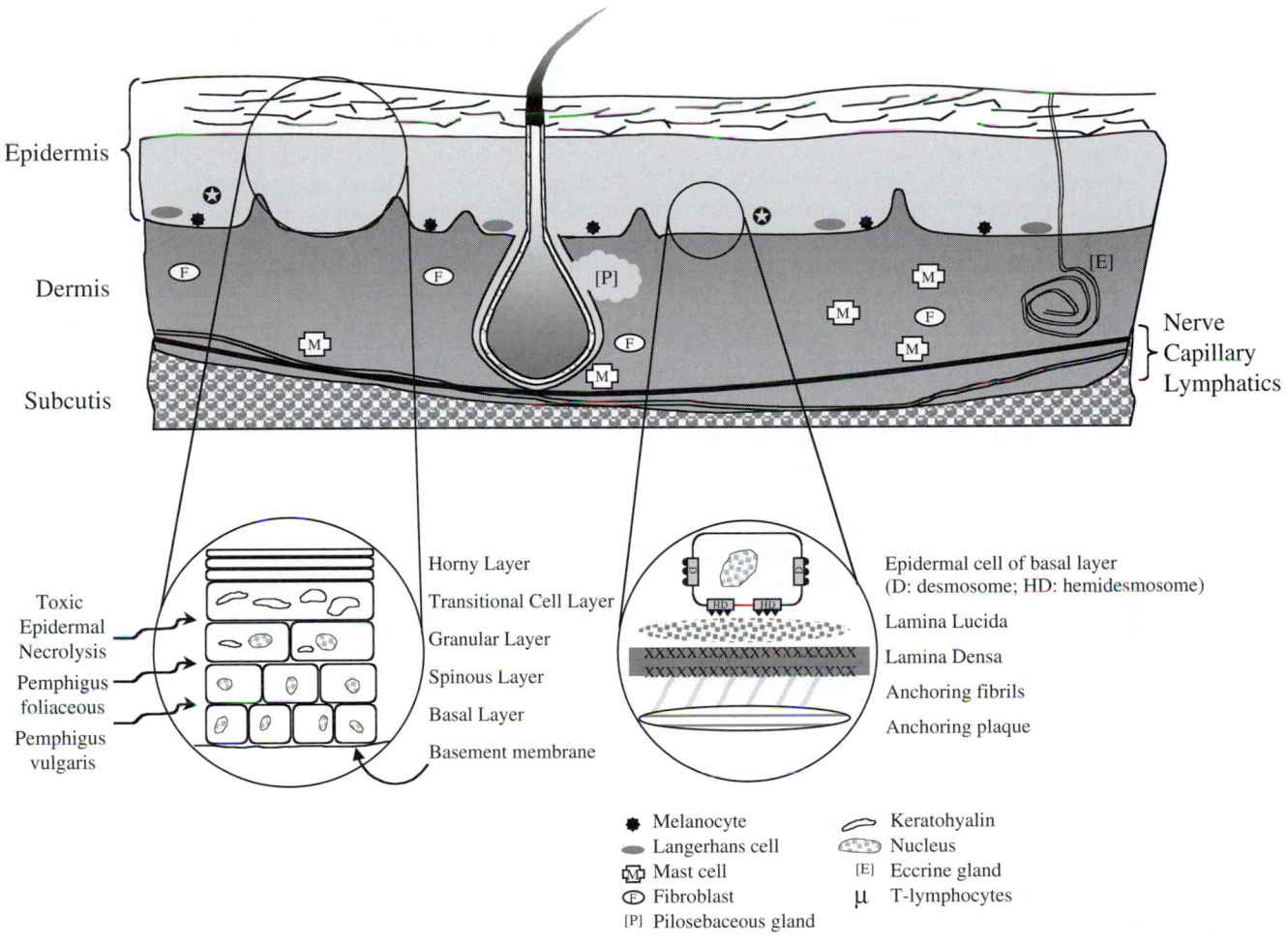

Epidermis

Dermis

Subcutis

Nerve
Capillary
Lymphatics

Toxic
Epidermal
Necrolysis

Pemphigus
foliaceous

Pemphigus
vulgaris

Horny Layer
Transitional Cell Layer
Granular Layer
Spinous Layer
Basal Layer
Basement membrane

Epidermal cell of basal layer
(D: desmosome; HD: hemidesmosome)
Lamina Lucida
Lamina Densa
Anchoring fibrils
Anchoring plaque

Melanocyte   Keratohyalin
Langerhans cell   Nucleus
Mast cell   [E] Eccrine gland
Fibroblast μ T-lymphocytes
[P] Pilosebaceous gland

Figure 29–1. Skin histology and pathology. Intraepidermal cleavage sites in various drug-induced blistering diseases. In pemphigus foliaceous, the cleavage is below or within granular layer, whereas in pemphigus vulgaris, it is suprabasilar. This accounts for the differing types of blisters found in the two diseases.

nally absorbed toxins to the skin. The vessels also allow the cells of the immune system to travel to the skin.

Parallel to the vasculature are cutaneous nerves, which serve the dual function of receiving sensory input as well as carrying sympathetically-mediated autonomic stimuli. Toxins and withdrawal in patients dependent on certain toxins which effect the sympathetic nervous system, have overt cutaneous effects, including piloerection, gooseflesh, and sweating.[15]

The apocrine glands consist of secretory coils and intradermal ducts ending in the follicular canal. The secretory coil is located in the subcutis and consists of a large lumen surrounded by columnar to cuboidal cells with eosinophilic cytoplasm.[15] Apocrine glands, which are located in select areas of the body such as the axilla, produce secretions that are rendered odoriferous by bacteria.

The eccrine glands, in contrast, produce an isotonic to hypertonic secretion that is modified by the ducts and emerges on the skin surface as sweat. The eccrine unit consists of the secretory gland, intradermal duct and intraepidermal duct. The coiled secretory gland is located in the area of the deep dermis and subcutis. Toxins can be concentrated in the sweat with increased skin reactions at the sites of sweat secretion. Certain antineoplastic agents,

such as cytarabine or bleomycin, directly damage the eccrine sweat glands, resulting in anhidrosis.

Sebaceous glands also lie in the dermis. They produce oily, lipid-rich secretions that function as emollients for the hair and skin. The glands can be reservoirs of noxious environmental toxins. Pilosebaceous follicles, which are present all over the body, consist of a hair shaft, hair follicle, sebaceous gland, sensory end organ, and erector pili. Certain halogenated aromatic chemicals, such as polychlorinated biphenyls (PCBs) and 2,4-dichlorophenoxyacetic acid, are excreted in the sebum and cause hyperkeratosis of the follicular canal. This produces a syndrome that looks like acne vulgaris known as chloracne because of plugging of the duct. Similar syndromes result from brominated and iodinated compounds, known as bromoderma and ioderma, respectively.[33]

The hair follicle is divided into three portions. The lower portion of the hair follicle contains the bulb with matrix cells. These matrix cells are mitotically active with a rapid metabolic rate and often the target of cytotoxic toxins. The rate of growth and the type of hair are unique for different body sites. Hair growth proceeds through three distinct phases: the active prolonged growth phase or anagen phase during which time matrix cell mitotic activity is high; a short involutional or catagen phase; and a resting phase or telogen phase.[15]

The nail, which is often considered analogous to the hair, is also a continuously growing structure. Fingernails grow at average of 0.1 mm/d and toenails grow at about one-third that rate. The mitotically active cells of the nail matrix can be subject to toxic injury. This affects the appearance of the growth of the nail plate. Because nail growth is consistent, location of an abnormality in the plate can predict the timing of exposure (eg Mees lines).

Where a toxin acts on the skin determines the morphology and the severity of the reaction pattern it induces. Examples include vesicular, bullous, papulosquamous, or purpuric lesions (see Table 29–1). Also, the body site will influence the overall clinical outcome. To properly characterize a reaction pattern, the proper terminology regarding the description of the cutaneous process is paramount. When the physician characterizes a cutaneous lesion, particular attention should be given to the color, surface change, morphology, and location. These findings often permit classification of a reaction pattern into a disease category, avoiding the need for a skin biopsy. When the diagnosis is not entirely clear from the clinical examination, a skin biopsy should be performed.

PRINCIPLES OF DERMAL DECONTAMINATION

Upon contact with a toxin the skin should be thoroughly cleansed to prevent direct effects and systemic absorption. In general, a copious amount of water is the decontamination agent of choice for skin irrigation. Soap should be used when adherent materials are involved. Following exposures to airborne toxins, the mouth, nasal cavities, eyes, and ear canals should also be irrigated. For nonam-

TABLE 29–1. **Dermatologic Diagnostic Descriptions of Lesions of the Skin**

Primary Cutaneous Lesions

Bulla: a circumscribed collection of free fluid more than 0.5 cm in diameter

Comedone: open and closed dilated pores (black heads and white heads)

Macule: a circumscribed flat variation of color that may be brown, blue, yellow, red, or hypopigmented (no thickness)

Nodule: a circumscribed elevation of 0.5 cm in diameter

Papule: an elevation of up to 0.5 cm in diameter

Plaque: a circumscribed elevation of more than 0.5 cm in diameter

Pustule: a circumscribed collection of leukocytes and free fluid that vary in size

Tumor: an elevation of greater than 0.5 cm in diameter

Vesicle: a circumscribed collection of free fluid up to 0.5 cm in diameter

Wheal: a firm edematous plaque resulting from infiltration of the dermis with fluid

Secondary Cutaneous Lesions

Erosion: a loss of the epidermis up to the full thickness of the epidermis but not through the basement membrane

Hypertrophy: a thickening of the skin

Lichenification: a secondary process with noted accentuation of skin surface markings

Scale: flaking which is separate from the original surface of a lesion

Scar: a thickened, often discolored, surface

Ulcer: a loss of full-thickness epidermis and papillary dermis, reticular dermis, or subcutis

bulatory patients, the decontamination process may need to be conducted using special collection litters if available.[7]

There are only a few situations in which water should not be used for skin decontamination. This includes contamination involving the reactive metallic forms of the alkali metals, sodium, potassium, lithium, cesium, and rubidium, which react with water to form strong bases. The dusts of pure magnesium, sulfur, strontium, titanium, uranium, yttrium, zinc, and zirconium will ignite or explode when contacted by water. Thus, following exposure to these metals, any residual metal should be removed with forceps, gauze, or towels and stored in mineral oil. Phenol has a tendency to thicken and become difficult to remove following exposure to water. Suggestions for phenol decontamination include high-flow water or polyethylene glycol solution. Lime, or CaO, also thickens and forms $Ca(OH)_2$ following wetting.[7,9]

TOPICAL TOXICITY

Exposure to myriad industrial or environmental chemicals may result in skin "burns." Although the majority of these chemical agents injure the skin through chemical reactivity rather than thermal damage, the clinical appearances of the two are often identical. Chemicals may act as oxidizing or reducing agents, corrosives, protoplasmic poisons, desiccants, or vesicants. Often an injury may initially appear to be mild or superficial with only faint erythema, blanching, or discoloration of the skin. Over the next 24–36 hours there may be progression to extensive necrosis of the skin and its underlying tissues.

Acids are water-soluble and readily penetrate into the subcutaneous tissue. The damaged tissue coagulates and forms a thick leathery eschar that limits the spread of the agent. The histopathologic finding following acid injury is termed *coagulative necrosis*. Alkali, on the other hand, characteristically produce liquefactive necrosis, which allows continued penetration of the corrosive material. For this reason, injury following alkali exposure is typically more severe than after equivalent magnitude acid exposure.[8]

Thermal damage may also be the result of a toxicologic exposure. For example, the exothermic reaction generated by the wetting of elemental phosphorus or sodium, may result in a burn. In these circumstances, the products of reactivity—phosphoric acid and sodium hydroxide—may produce secondary chemical injury. Alternatively, skin exposure to a rapidly expanding gas, such as nitrous oxide (eg, from whipped cream cartridges) or compressed liquefied nitrogen, or to frozen substances, such as dry ice (ie, carbon dioxide), may produce freezing injury, or frostbite.

Hydrocarbon-based solvents are typically liquids that are capable of dissolving nonwater-soluble solutes. Thus, when a hydrocarbon such as gasoline has prolonged contact with the skin, it can dissolve the lipids of the stratum corneum, resulting in a "defatting dermatitis," which presents as erythema or irritation.[8]

ABSORPTION

In addition to producing topical injuries, many toxins undergo percutaneous absorption by passive diffusion. Lipid solubility is the most important factor determining dermal absorption, although concentration, duration of exposure, molecular weight and specific skin characteristics are also important determinants. Thus, although metal ions such as Hg^+ have virtually no skin penetration, the addition of a methyl group, to form methylmercury, increases the systemic absorption. Dimethylmercury, formed by the addition of another methyl group, may produce life-threatening systemic effects with only a single drop (Chap. 87). Similarly, the nonionized component of the weakly acidic hydrofluoric (HF) acid is able to penetrate deeply. The proton (H^+) and fluoride ion (F^-) are unable to penetrate the skin lipids because of their charged nature. Once in the dermis, the HF acid may ionize and cause both acid-induced tissue necrosis and fluoride-induced hypocalcemia[5] (Chap. 87).

The vehicle also influences absorption and transdermal drug delivery systems are based on their ability to alter the skin partition coefficient through the use of an optimized vehicle. Similarly, through localized dermal occlusion, transdermal systems hydrate the skin and raise its temperature to increase the permeability. Despite these techniques to enhance drug delivery, transdermal systems still require that large amounts of drug be present externally to maximize the transcutaneous gradient.[30] Typically, much of the drug intentionally remains in the patch when it is discarded. Some of these drugs, such as nicotine or fentanyl, may present a hazard for children, while others, such as estradiol or nitroglycerin are less concerning.

If a percutaneously absorbed substance is capable of interfering with a physiologic process, it may produce systemic, even life-threatening, toxicity. Morbidity and mortality are reported with the topical application of podophyllin, camphor, phenol, organic phosphorus insecticides, ethanol, organochlorines (eg, lindane), nitrates, or salicylic acid. Children are particularly at risk for toxicities from percutaneous absorption because their skin is more penetrable than that of an adult and specific anatomic sites, such as the face, often represent larger percentage of body surface areas than in the adult.[29] Furthermore, there is enhanced absorption on anatomic parts of the body with thinner skin, such as the mucous membranes and the eyelids, and in areas where skin touches skin, such as the body folds. Under certain circumstances, the stratum corneum may serve a depot function leading to continued systemic exposure despite apparent removal of the toxin.[16]

DERMATOLOGIC SIGNS OF NONDERMATOLOGIC DISEASE

Cyanosis

Normal skin coloration is caused by several factors, one of which is the visualization of the capillary beds through the translucent dermis and epidermis. Cyanosis manifests as darkening or characteristic "bluing" of the skin. It occurs when the light-absorbing characteristics of hemoglobin are altered either through hypoxia or by oxidation of its iron moiety to the ferric state to form methemoglobin (Chap. 94). Thus, skin discoloration is caused by the presence of the more deeply colored blood within the dermal plexus and is most pronounced on the skin surfaces with the least overlying tissue, such as the mucous membranes or fingernails.

Jaundice

Jaundice, or a yellow discoloration of the skin, is typically a sign of hepatocellular failure or hemolysis. Bilirubin released from the damaged hepatocytes circulates in the blood-stream and dissolves in the subcutaneous fat resulting in the yellowish color of the skin. Yellow discoloration of the skin also occurs in patients with

carotenemia, which is caused by excessive consumption of either carrots or the vitamin A precursor carotene. True jaundice is differentiated from carotenemia by the presence of scleral icterus in patients with hyperbilirubinemia and the removal of the discoloration of carotenemia by wiping the skin with alcohol. Lycopenemia, a similar entity to carotenemia, is caused by the excessive consumption of tomatoes. Also, topical exposure to dinitrophenol or picric acid produces localized yellow discoloration of the skin.

Urticarial Drug Reactions

Urticarial drug reactions are characterized by transient, pruritic, edematous, pink papules, or wheals frequently associated with central clearing. This reaction pattern is representative of a type I, or IgE-dependent, immune reaction and commonly occurs as part of clinical anaphylaxis. Widespread urticaria may occur following systemic absorption of an allergen or following a minimal localized exposure in patients highly sensitized to the allergen (Chap. 15). Following limited exposure, a localized form of urticaria also may occur. Regardless of the specific clinical presentation, this reaction occurs when immunologic recognition occurs between IgE molecules and a foreign substance, triggering immediate degranulation of mast cells, which are distributed along the dermal blood vessels, nerves and appendages. The release of histamine, complements C3a and C5a, and other vasoactive mediators, result in leakage of fluid from dermal capillaries as their endothelial cells contract. This produces the characteristic urticarial lesions described above. Activation of the nearby sensory neurons produces pruritis. Nonimmunologically mediated mast cell degranulation producing an identical urticarial syndrome may also occur following exposure to various toxins, including jellyfish or benzoic acid.

Pruritis, or itching, is a common manifestation of urticarial reactions but it may also be of nonimmunologic origin. Patients with hepatocellular disease frequently suffer from pruritis, which is often considered as related to the release of bile acids. In addition, pruritis in patients with chronic liver disease and obstructive jaundice may be caused by central mechanisms, as suggested by elevated central nervous system (CNS) opioid peptide levels. Pruritis may also be caused by topical exposure to the urticating hairs of Tarantula spiders, spines of the Stinging Nettle plant (*Urtica sp.*), or certain chemicals such as capsaicin.[14]

Drugs also may evoke a type III immune reaction that causes mast cells to degranulate. The cellular inflammatory response to released chemotactic factors leads to increased vascular permeability.

Flushing

Vasodilation of the dermal arterioles leads to the reddening of the skin, which is called flushing. Flushing may occur following autonomically mediated vasodilatation, as occurs with stress or anger, or it may be chemically induced by vasoactive compounds. Agents that cause histamine release through a type I hypersensitivity reaction are the most frequent cause of toxin-induced flush. Histamine poisoning itself, most frequently caused by the consumption of scombrotoxic fish, may cause epidemic flushing. Flushing after the consumption of ethanol is common in patients of Asian descent and is similar to that following ethanol consumption in patients exposed to disulfiram or similar agents (Chap. 65). The inability to efficiently metabolize acetaldehyde, the initial metabolite of ethanol, as well as its increased production results in the characteristic syndrome of vomiting, headache, and flushing.

Niacin causes flushing through an arachidonic acid mediated pathway that may be inhibited by aspirin.[31]

Skin Moisture

Drug-induced diaphoresis, or sweating, may be part of a physiologic response to heat generation or may be pharmacologically mediated as it is following sympathomimetic drug use. The eccrine sweat glands are responsible for sweat production and they are uniquely innervated by acetylcholine-containing neurons within the sympathetic nervous system. Because the postsynaptic receptor on the eccrine glands is muscarinic, most muscarinic agonists are capable of stimulating sweat production. The latter most commonly occurs following exposure to cholinesterase-inhibiting insecticides, such as organic phosphorus compounds, but it may also occur with direct-acting muscarinic agonists such as pilocarpine. Alternatively, antimuscarinic agents, such as atropine or diphenhydramine, reduce sweating and produce dry skin.

Metallic Pigmentations

Discolorations in the skin can result from the deposit of fine metallic particles. These particles can be ingested and carried to the skin by the blood, or may permeate into the skin from topical applications. Argyria, a slate-colored pigmentation of the skin resulting from the systemic deposition of silver particles in the skin, can be localized or widespread. The discoloration tends to be most prominent in areas exposed to sunlight, probably secondary to the fact that silver stimulates melanocyte proliferation. Histologically, fine black granules are found in the basement membrane zone of the sweat glands, blood vessel walls, the dermoepidermal junction, and along the erector pili muscles. Gold, which is used parenterally in the treatment of rheumatoid arthritis, may cause a blue or slate-gray pigmentation known as chrysiasis. The pigmentation is also accentuated in light exposed areas but, unlike in argyria, sun-protected areas do not histologically demonstrate gold. Also, melanin is not increased in the areas of hyperpigmentation. The hyperpigmentation is probably secondary to the gold itself, but the cause of its distribution pattern remains unknown. Histologically, the gold is distributed in a perivascular pattern in the dermis with granules accentuated at the basement membrane zone of sweat glands.

Bismuth, historically important but still used, produces a characteristic oral finding of the metallic deposition in the gums known as bismuth lines. Arsenic, which is found in certain pesticides and in contaminated well water, causes cutaneous hyperpigmentation with areas of scattered hypopigmentation. Chronic lead poisoning can produce a characteristic "lead hue" with pallor. Lead also deposits in the gums causing the characteristic "lead line." Iron can cause staining of the skin resulting in pigmentation similar to that seen in tattoos.[13]

SPECIFIC SYNDROMES

Although the ability to describe lesions accurately is an important skill, the ability to recognize specific patterns allows a more focused approach to the clinical practice of dermatology. Several cutaneous reaction patterns account for the majority of those occurring in patients with drug-induced dermatotoxicity (Table 29–2).

Toxic Epidermal Necrolysis and Related Syndromes

Toxic epidermal necrolysis (TEN) is a rare, life-threatening dermatologic emergency. Its incidence is estimated at 0.4–1.2 cases per million population, and medications are causally implicated in 80–95% of the cases. The cutaneous reaction pattern is characterized by tenderness and erythema of the skin and mucosa, followed by extensive cutaneous and mucosal exfoliation.[27]

Classically, the eruption occurs within days of the exposure to the implicated substance and is preceded by malaise, headache, fever, myalgias, arthralgias, nausea, vomiting, diarrhea, chest pain, or cough. Initially, a macular erythema develops that subsequently becomes raised and morbilliform. The face, neck, and central trunk are usually the initial areas affected. The disease generally progresses to involve the extremities and the remainder of the body. Individual lesions are reminiscent of target lesions due to their dusky centers. The entire thickness of the epidermis, including the nails, becomes necrotic and may slough off. The mucosal surfaces of the lips, oropharynx, conjunctiva, vagina, urethra, and anus may show erythema and sloughing. Typically, a Nikolsky sign, consisting of sloughing of the epidermis when shearing pressure is exerted on the skin, occurs.[3] While suggestive, this sign is not pathognomonic of TEN and occurs in a variety of other dermatoses. If the diagnosis is suspected, a biopsy should be performed and treatment initiated immediately. The histopathology typically shows eosinophilic dermatitis and cleavage in the junction zone. Removal of the inciting agent and transfer to a burn center for sterile wound care are widely accepted initial management strategies. Although glucocorticoids are not generally recommended, there is emerging support for the use of immunosuppressive or immunomodulatory agents such as intravenous immunoglobulins, cyclophosphamide, and cyclosporine. Reported mortality is as high as 30%, particularly in those patients with gastrointestinal and tracheobronchial involvement.[27]

Toxic epidermal necrolysis is often considered to be the most severe manifestation of the spectrum of syndromes represented by erythema multiforme. Erythema multiforme is characterized by target-shaped, erythematous macules and patches on the palms and soles, as well as the trunk and extremities. The Nikolsky sign is negative. The etiology of erythema multiforme minor appears to be predominantly associated with recurrent herpes simplex virus infections. Progesterone may play a role in triggering recurrent erythema multiforme. Contact sensitization to sulfonamides, antihistamines, dinitrochlorobenzene (DNCB), diphencyclopropenone (DPCP), isopropyl-p-phenylenediamine (IPPD), Rosewood, and Rhus may elicit erythema multiforme. The Stevens-Johnson syndrome is similarly considered to be an overlap reaction with erythema multiforme when greater than 30% body surface area is involved. It is differentiated from TEN by characteristic clinical and histologic findings.

Blistering Reactions

Drug-related cutaneous blistering reactions may be clinically indistinguishable from autoimmune blistering reactions, such as pemphigus. Certain topically applied agents cause blistering by disrupting the anchoring filaments of basal cell desmosomes at the dermal-epidermal junction. In high concentrations, this can lead to both necrosis of skin and mucous membranes. Other agents cause

TABLE 29–2.   Agents Commonly Associated with Various Cutaneous Reaction Patterns

Acneiform
ACTH
Amoxapine
Androgens
Azathioprine
Bromides
Corticosteroids
Danazol
Dantrolene
Iodides
Isoniazid
Lithium
Oral contraceptives
Phenytoin

Alopecia
Anticoagulants
Chemotherapeutic agents
Hormones
NSAIDs
Phenytoin
Retinoids

Contact dermatitis
Bacitracin
Balsam of Peru
Benzocaine
Carba mix
Catechol (allergen found in plant sap;
    responsible for poison ivy and poison
    oak)
Cobalt
Diazolidinyl urea
Ethylenediamine dihydrochloride
Formaldehyde
Fragrance mix
Imidazolidinyl urea
Lanolin
Methylchloroisothiazolinone/
    methylisothiazolinone
Neomycin sulfate
Nickel sulfate
p-Tert-butylphenol formaldehyde resin
p-Phenylenediamine
Quaternium-15
Rosin (colophony)
Sesquiterpene lactones
Thimerosal

Erythema multiforme
Antibiotics
Allopurinol
Barbiturates
Carbamazepine
Cimetidine
Codeine
Gold
Glutethimide

Estinyl estradiol
Furosemide
Ketoconazole
Methazualone
NSAIDs
Nitrogen mustard
Phenolphthalein
Phenothiazines
Phenytoin
Sulfonamides
Thiazides

Fixed drug eruptions
Acetaminophen
Allopurinol
Barbiturates
Captopril
Carbamazepine
Chloral hydrate
Chlordiazepoxide
Chlorpromazine
Erythromycin
D-Penicillamine
Fiorinal
Gold
Griseofulvin
Lithium
Phenacetin
Phenolphthalein
Methaqualone
Metronidazole
Minocycline
Naproxen
NSAIDs
Oral contraceptives
Salicylates
Sulindac

Maculopapular reactions
Antibiotics
Anticonvulsants
Antihypertensive agents
Antiinflammatory agents

Photosensitivity reactions
Amiodarone
Benoxaprofen
Chlorpromazine
Ciprofloxacin
Darcabazine
5-Fluorouracil
Furosemide
Griseofulvin
Hydrochlorothiazide
Hematoporphyrin
Levofloxacin
Nalidixic acid
Naproxen

Piroxicam
Psoralen
Sulfanilamide
Tetracyclines
Tolbutamide
Vinblastine

Photoirritant contact dermatitis
Celery
Dispense blue 35
Eosin
Fig
Fragrance materials
Lime
Parsnip
Pitch

Toxic epidermal necrolysis
Allopurinol
L-Asparaginase
Amoxapine
Bactrim
Mithramycin
Nitrofurantoin
NSAIDs
Penicillin
Phenytoin
Prazocin
Pyrimethamine–sulfadoxine
Streptomycin
Sulfonamides
Sulfasalazine

Vasculitis
Allopurinol
Cimetidine
Gold
Hydralazine
Levamisole
NSAIDs
Penicillin
Phenytoin
Propylthiouracil
Quinidine

Vesiculobullous
Amoxapine
Barbiturates
Captopril
Chemotherapeutic agents
Dipyridamole
Furosemide
Griseofulvin
Penicillamine
Penicillin
Rifampin
Sulfonamides

a similar reaction pattern mediated by the production of antibody directed against the cells at the dermal-epidermal junction.

A number of medications can induce pemphigus foliaceous, a superficial blistering disorder in which the blister is at the level of the stratum corneum, or pemphigus vulgaris, in which blistering occurs at the suprabasalar level (Fig. 29–1). Other agents produce the tense bullae that resemble bullous pemphigoid. Immunofluorescence studies may show epidermal intracellular immunoglobulin deposits at the dermal-epidermal junction. Treatment options include immunosuppressive agents. The reaction may persist for up to 6 months after the offending agent has been withdrawn.

"Coma bullae" are flaccid bullae that occur in patients with sedative-hypnotic overdoses, particularly phenobarbital, or significant carbon monoxide poisoning. Although these blisters are thought to result from pressure-induced epidermal necrosis, they occasionally occur in nonpressure-dependent areas, suggesting a systemic mechanism. An intraepidermal or subepidermal blister may occur. There is accompanying eccrine duct and gland necrosis.

Bullous Drug Eruptions

Multiple, large, ill-defined, dull, purplish-livid patches sometimes accompanied by large flaccid blisters characterize these eruptions. Typical locations include acral extremities, genitals and intertriginous sites, and the process may be confused with toxic epidermal necrolysis if widely confluent. However, bullous drug eruptions spare the patient's mucous membranes. This reaction pattern is generally not life-threatening. Bullous fixed-drug reactions result from the ingestion of a variety of medications. Prior to its removal from the market, phenolphthalein, an ingredient in over-the-counter laxatives, was commonly sited as the cause of this reaction.

Hypersensitivity Syndrome

The skin may be involved with systemic drug-induced immunologic diseases. The hypersensitivity syndromes are characterized by erythroderma, and facial and periorbital edema, and are typically accompanied by high fevers, elevated liver function tests, lymphadenopathy and peripheral eosinophilia. The syndrome typically occurs 2–7 weeks after starting therapy with an anticonvulsant (Chap. 41) or sulfa-based drugs. Management of this syndrome is supportive following elimination of the offending substance.[19,32]

Exfoliative Erythrodermas

Exfoliative erythrodermic eruptions result from medications as well as toxins characterized by widespread erythema and scale. The process may persist for months. Such patients with exfoliative erythrodermas require aggressive fluid, electrolyte, and nutrition management. They are at risk for multisystem organ failure. Boric acid toxicity is well known to cause a bright red eruption followed usually within 1–3 days by a generalized exfoliation. The mechanism of toxicity is unknown.

Vasculitis

Hypersensitivity vasculitis is characterized by purpuric, nonblanching macules that may become raised and palpable. The purpura tends to occur predominantly on gravity-dependent areas, including the lower extremities, feet, and buttocks. Sometimes the reaction pattern can have edematous purpuric wheals (urticarial vasculitis), hemorrhagic bullae, or ulcerations. The underlying pathology consistently shows a leukocytoclastic vasculitis with fibrin deposition in the vessel walls and a perivascular infiltrate with intact and fragmented neutrophils (nuclear dust). This reaction pattern may be limited to the skin, or may be more serious and involve other organ systems particularly the kidneys, joints, liver, lungs, and brain. The purpura results from circulating immune complexes, which form as a result of a hypersensitivity to a xenobiotic.

Purpura

Purpura is the multifocal extravasation of blood into the skin or mucous membranes. Ecchymoses are therefore considered to be purpuric lesions. Cytotoxic agents that either diffusely suppress the bone marrow or specifically depress platelet counts below $30,000/mm^3$ predispose to intradermal hemorrhage resulting in petechiae or purpuric macules. Drugs that interfere with platelet aggregation, including valproic acid, aspirin, clopidogrel, and ticlopidine, may cause purpura. Also, anticoagulants, such as heparin or coumarin, may also result in purpura (Chaps. 25 and 42).

Coumarin Necrosis

Skin necrosis from coumarin may occur from day 3 to day 10 after the initiation of treatment. The necrosis is secondary to thrombus formation in vessels of the dermis and subcutaneous fat. There may be blisters, ecchymosis, ulcers, and massive subcutaneous necrosis usually in areas of abundant subcutaneous fat such as the breasts, buttocks, abdomen, thighs, and calves. It may be associated with protein C deficiency.[20]

Contact Dermatitis

When a chemical contacts the skin, it can result in either allergic contact dermatitis or irritant dermatitis. Contact dermatitis is characterized by inflammation of the skin with spongiosis, or intercellular edema, of the epidermis that results from the interaction of a chemical with the skin. Clinically, erythema, induration, pruritis, or blistering is noted on areas in direct contact with the drug and remaining areas are spared.

Allergic contact dermatitis fits into the classic delayed hypersensitivity, or type IV immunologic reaction. The development of this reaction requires prior sensitization to an allergen, which, in most cases, acts as a hapten by binding with an endogenous molecule that is then presented to an appropriate immunologic T cell. Upon reexposure, the hapten diffuses to the Langerhans cell, is chemically altered, bound to a HLA-DR and the complex is expressed on the Langerhans cell surface. This complex interacts with primed T cells either in the skin or lymph node, causing the Langerhans cells to make interleukin-1 and the activated T-cells to make interleukin-2 and interferon-γ. This subsequently activates the keratinocytes to produce cytokines and eicosanoids that activate mast cells and macrophages, leading to an inflammatory response[17,18] (Fig. 29–2).

Many allergens are associated with contact dermatitis, and a complete list is beyond the scope of this chapter. Among the most common sensitizers are the urushiols (eg, poison ivy), the sesquiterpene lactones (eg, ragweed), and tuliposide A (eg, tulip bulbs). Metals, in particular nickel, are commonly implicated. Several industrial chemicals, such as thiurams (eg, rubber) and

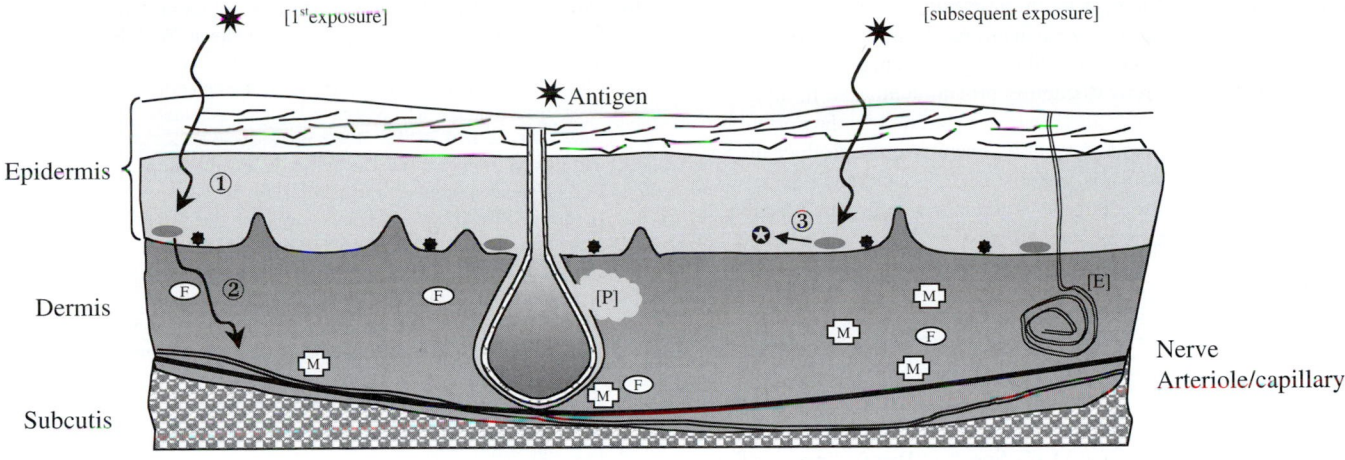

Figure 29–2. Contact dermatitis. (1) Causative chemical, typically a hapten of <500 daltons, diffuses through stratum corneum and binds to receptor on Langerhans cell. (2) The antigen is processed with HLA-DR receptor site, presented to T-helper lympocytes, and carried through the lymphatics to regional lymph nodes. There it undergoes the sensitization phase by producing memory, effector, and suppressor T lymphocytes. (3) Upon reexposure to the same, or to a cross-reactive antigen, the Langerhans cell represents the antigen to T lymphocytes, which are now sensitized. This initiates an inflammatory process that appears as indurated, scaly patches.

urea formaldehyde resins (eg, plastics) account for the majority of occupational contact dermatitis. Medications, particularly topical medications such as neomycin, commonly cause contact dermatitis.

Irritant dermatitis, while clinically indistinguishable, results from direct damage to the skin and does not require prior antigen sensitization. Still, the inflammatory response to the initial mild insult is the cause of the majority of the damage. Irritant chemicals include acids, bases, solvents, and detergents, many of which, in their concentrated form or following prolonged exposure, may produce direct cellular injury. The specific site of the toxin's damage varies with the chemical nature of the agent. Many toxins can affect the lipid membrane of the keratinocyte, whereas others can actually diffuse through the membrane injuring the lysosomes, mitochondria, or nuclear components. When the cell membrane is injured, phospholipases are activated and affect the release of arachidonic acid and the synthesis of eicosanoids. The second-messenger system is then activated leading to the expression of genes and the synthesis of various cell surface molecules and cytokines. Interleukin-1 is secreted, which can activate T cells directly and indirectly by stimulation of granulocyte-macrophage colony stimulating factor (GM-CSF) production.

Photosensitivity Reactions

Photosensitivity drug reactions are adverse reactions to nonionizing radiation, particularly ultraviolet A (320–400 nm) and less often to ultraviolet B (280–320 nm). There are generally two types of reaction patterns: phototoxic and photoallergic. Phototoxic reactions occur within 24 hours of the first dose and are dose-related. The clinical findings include erythema and edema in a light-exposed distribution, and resemble an exaggerated sunburn. Photoallergic reactions occur less frequently and may occur following even small exposures. The eruption, which may involve areas that are not exposed to light, ranges from lichenoid papules to eczematous changes. A contact dermatitis referred to as pho-

toallergic contact dermatitis may occur.[4] If this is suspected, then the patient should be referred for photopatch testing. Both phototoxic and photoallergic reactions are managed with symptomatic therapy, including topical or, if needed, systemic corticosteroids. The patient should be advised to avoid sun exposure or wear a sunscreen that blocks both ultraviolet A and ultraviolet B with a sun protection factor (SPF) of 15 or greater.

Sclerodermalike Reactions

A number of environmental chemicals are associated with a localized or diffuse sclerodermalike reaction. Sclerodermatous changes refer to tightened indurated surface change of the skin. These typically occur on the face, hands, forearms, and trunk. This may be accompanied by facial telangiectasias and Raynaud syndrome. Raynaud syndrome consists of skin color changes of white, red, and blue accompanied by intense pain with exposure to cold. The fibrotic process usually does not remit with removal of the external stimulus. The association of sclerodermalike reactions with polyvinyl chloride manufacture is likely related to exposure to vinyl chloride monomer. Similar reports of this syndrome have been noted in those exposed to trichloroethylene and perchlorethylene which are structurally similar to vinyl chloride.

Widespread cutaneous sclerosis in patients exposed to imported rapeseed oil mixed with an aniline denaturant occurred in Spain and became known as the "toxic oil syndrome." A similar syndrome following ingestion of impure L-tryptophan as a dietary supplement resulted in the eosinophilia-myalgia syndrome.[6,23]

Hair

Agents that produce anagen effluvium produce rapid hair loss, while those causing telogen effluvium may not produce hair loss for weeks. Anagen toxicity is the most common mechanism, as for instance with chemotherapeutic agents or thallium.[25] Many antineoplastic drugs reduce the mitotic activity of the rapidly dividing hair matrix cells, leading to the formation of a thin shaft that breaks easily. Thallium, a toxin classically associated with hair loss, causes alopecia by two mechanisms. Thallium distributes intracellularly like potassium inhibiting mitochondrial oxidative phosphorylation thereby disrupting protein synthesis. In addition, by binding sulfhydryl groups, thallium also inhibits the normal incorporation of cysteine into keratin. Selenium may produce alopecia by similar mechanisms. Soluble barium salts, such as barium sulfide, are applied topically as a depilatory to produce localized hair loss. The mechanism is undefined.

Nail

Nail findings may serve as important clues to toxic exposures that have occurred recently or in the remote past. Matrix keratinization leads to the formation of the nail plate. This keratinization is programmed and occurs uniformly in a scheduled pattern. The observed changes in nails like Mee's lines and Beau's lines can thus be used to predict the timing of a toxic exposure because of the reliability of rate of growth of the nails. Arsenic poisonings can accurately be dated by the position of growth of the Mee's line as nails grow approximately at an average rate of 0.1 mm/d. Thallium also causes Mee's lines.[22]

SUMMARY

Skin is constantly exposed to toxins. Whether the exposure occurs via ingestion, airborne, or topical routes, its effects are manifest in the skin. Prompt attention and diagnosis is imperative in treating such toxic exposures. The skin will provide clues as to the route and nature of the toxic agent. With careful history, clinical examination, and referencing of the agent, the etiology and nature of the reaction can be revealed and treated in an effective manner.

REFERENCES

1. Alberts B, Bray D, Lewis J, et al, eds: The cytoskeleton. In: Molecular Biology of the Cell, 2nd ed. New York, Garland Publishing, 1989, pp. 661–666, 797–798, 816–817.
2. Baden HP: Biology of the epidermis and pathophysiology of psoriasis and certain ichthyosiform dermatoses. In Soter NA, Baden HP, eds: Pathophysiology of Dermatologic Diseases, 2nd ed. New York, McGraw-Hill, 1991, pp. 131–158.
3. Bastuji-Garin S, Rzany B, Stern RS, et al: Clinical classification of cases of toxic epidermal necrolysis, Stevens-Johnson syndrome, and erythema multiforme. Arch Dermatol 1993;129:92–96.
4. Beijersbergen van Henegouwen GM: (Systemic) phototoxicity of drugs and other xenobiotics. J Photochem Photobiol 1991;10:183–210.
5. Bertolini JC: Hydrofluoric acid: A review of toxicity. J Emerg Med 1992;10:163–168.
6. Breathnack SM, Hintner H: Scleroderma-like reactions. In: Breathnack SM, Hintner H, eds: Adverse Drug Reactions and the Skin. London, Blackwell Scientific, 1992, pp. 118–122.
7. Burgess JL, Kirk M, Borron SW, Cisek J: Emergency department of hazardous materials protocol for contaminated patients. Ann Emerg Med 1999; 34:205–212.
8. Cartotto RC, Peters WJ, Neligan PC, et al: Chemical burns. Can J Surg 1996;39:205–211.
9. Christoph RA: General protocol for dermatologic poisoning. In: Noji EK, Kelen GD, eds: Manual of Toxicologic Emergencies. Chicago, Year Book, 1989, pp. 119–121.
10. Dover JS, Jackson BA, Junkins-Hopkins JM, et al: Pocket Guide to Cutaneous Medicine and Surgery. Philadelphia: W.B. Saunders Co., pp. 1.
11. Elias JJ: The microscopic structures of the epidermis and its derivatives. In: Bronaugh RL, Maibach HI, eds: Percutaneous Absorption. New York, Marcel Dekker, 1989, pp. 1–26.
12. Fartasch M, Diepgen TL: The barrier function in atopic dry skin. Acta Derm Venereol Suppl (Stockh) 1992;176:26–31.
13. Granstein RD, Sober AJ: Drug- and heavy-metal induced hyperpigmentation. J Am Acad Dermatol 1981;5:1–18.
14. Harvell J, Bason M, Maibach HI: Contact urticaria (immediate reaction syndrome). Clin Rev Allergy 1992;10:303–323.
15. Hood AF, Mihm MC, Horn TD, Kwan TH: Normal histology of the skin. In: Primer of Dermatopathology, 2nd ed. Boston, Little, Brown and Company, 1993, pp. 3–39.
16. Kao J, Carver MP: Skin Metabolism. In: Marzuli FN, Maibach HI, eds: Dermatotoxicology, 4th ed. New York Hemisphere, 1991, pp. 143–200.
17. Keyman AM: The spectrum of contact urticaria: Wheals, erythema and pruritus. Dermatol Clin 1990;8:57–60.
18. Marks JG, DeLeo VA, eds: Allergic and irritant contact dermatitis In: Contact and Occupational Dermatology. St. Louis, Mosby Year Book, 1997, pp. 3–13.
19. Morkunas AR, Miller MD: Anticonvulsant hypersensitivity syndrome. Crit Care Clin 1997;13:727–739.
20. Peterson CE, Kwaan HC: Current concepts of warfarin therapy. Arch Intern Med 1986;146:581–584.
21. Rook AJ, Champion RH, eds: Progress in Biological Sciences in Relation to Dermatology, 2nd ed. Cambridge, Cambridge University Press, 1964, pp. 245–261.
22. Scher RK, Daniel CR: Nails: Therapy, Diagnosis, Surgery. Philadelphia, WB Saunders, 1997, pp. 26–27, 221–222, 255–256.
23. Silver R, Heyes P, Jaize J, et al: Scleroderma, fasciitis and eosinophilia associated with the ingestion of tryptophan. N Engl J Med 1990;322:874–878.
24. Stoner JG, Rasmussen JE: Plant dermatitis. J Am Acad Dermatol 1983;9:1–15.
25. Susser W, Whitaker-Worth DL, Grant-Kels JM: Mucocutaneous Reactions to Chemotherapy. J Am Acad Dermatol 1999;40:367–398.
26. US Department of Health and Human Services, National Institute for Occupational Safety and Health: Registry of the Toxic Effects of Chemical Substances, 1981–82, DHHS (NIOSH), publ. no. 83–107. Washington, DC: US Government Printing Office, 1983.
27. Virad I, Wehrli P, Bullani R: Inhibition of toxic epidermal necrolysis by blockade of CD95 with human intravenous immunoglobulin. Science 1998;282:490–493.
28. VonBlomberg BME, Bruynzeel DP, Scheper RJ: Advances in mechanisms of allergic contact dermatitis: In vitro and in vivo research. In: Moschella SL, Hurley HJ, eds: Dermatotoxicology. Philadelphia, WB Saunders, 1992, pp. 255–362.
29. Webster RC, Maibach HI: Percutaneous absorption of drugs. Clin Pharmacokinet 1992;23:253–266.
30. Webster RC, Maibach HI: In vivo percutaneous absorption: Critical factors in transdermal transport. In: Marzulli FN, Maibach HI, eds: Dermatotoxicology, 4th ed. New York, Hemisphere, 1991, pp. 1–36.
31. Wilkin JK: The red face: Flushing disorders. Clin Dermatol 1993; 11:211–223.
32. Wolverton SE: Update on cutaneous drug reactions. Adv Dermatol 1997;13:65–84.
33. Zugerman C: Chloracne: Clinical manifestations and etiology. Dermatol Clin 1990;8:209–213.

Jason Chu / Leslie R. Wolf

The genitourinary system encompasses two major organ systems: the reproductive and the urinary systems. Successful reproduction requires interaction between two sexually mature individuals. Fecundity is an individual's or a couple's capacity to produce children, and fertility is the successful production of children. Fertility is a complex biologic phenomenon. Toxicant exposures of either individual can have adverse impacts on a couple's fertility. Laboratory tests used to evaluate fertility are relatively unreliable, clinical endpoints are unclear, exposure is difficult to monitor, and indicators of biologic effects are indefinite. Because of these factors, well-designed, conclusive epidemiologic studies are uncommon. Therefore, the role of occupational and environmental exposures in the development of infertility is difficult to define.[7,37,95,100] The negative impact on fertility as an adverse effect of drugs or chemicals is often ignored, but the evaluation of infertility is incomplete without a thorough drug and occupational history. Differences in toxicity of agents in individuals may be sex- and/or age-related. Drug-related, primary infertility may be the result of effects on the hypothalamic-pituitary-gonadal axis or of a direct toxic effect on the gonads.[82] Fertility is also affected by exposures that cause abnormal sexual performance. See Table 30–1 for a list of agents associated with infertility.

Aphrodisiacs are used to heighten sexual desire and to counteract sexual dysfunction. Historically, humans have continued to search for the perfect aphrodisiac, from oysters to toads. Efficacy is variable, and toxic consequences occur commonly. Various treatments have been evaluated for male sexual dysfunction, but the perfect remedy remains a mystery.

While many people search for a cure for impotence or infertility, many others explore drugs and plants that can be used as abortifacients. Routes of administration vary from oral to parenteral to intravaginal, with an end result of pregnancy termination. Toxicity results not only in the termination of pregnancy but also from the systemic effects of the various agents.

This chapter examines all of these issues, as well as the impact of toxicants on the urinary system, specifically, urinary retention and incontinence and abnormalities detected in urine specimens. Renal (Chap. 23), teratogenic, and carcinogenic (Chap. 16) principles are discussed in further detail elsewhere in this text.

MALE FERTILITY

The male reproductive system is comprised of the male gonads and the endocrine organs that provide the hormonal controls. Disruption of normal function at any part of the system affects fertility. There are a multitude of toxicants that adversely affect spermatogenesis and sexual function.

Spermatogenesis

Central to the male reproductive system is the process of spermatogenesis in the testes. The bulk of the testes consist of seminiferous tubules with germinal spermatogonia and Sertoli cells. The remainder of the gonadal tissue is interstitium with blood vessels, lymphatics, supporting cells, and Leydig cells. Spermatogenesis begins with the maturation and differentiation of the germinal spermatogonia. The process is controlled by the secretion of gonadotropin-releasing hormone (GnRH) from the hypothalamus, which stimulates the pituitary to release follicle-stimulating hormone (FSH) and luteinizing hormone (LH). FSH stimulates the development of Sertoli cells in the testes, which are responsible for the maturation of spermatids to spermatozoa. LH promotes production of testosterone by Leydig cells. Testosterone levels must be maintained to ensure the formation of spermatids.[18] Both FSH and testosterone are required for initiation of spermatogenesis, but testosterone alone is sufficient to maintain the process.

Testicular Toxicants. Toxicants can affect any part of the male reproductive tract, but, invariably, the end result is decreased sperm production defined as oligospermia or azoospermia. Spermatogenesis is an ongoing process throughout life, as compared to oogenesis in women, and can be inhibited by decreases in FSH and/or LH or Sertoli cell toxicity. Spermatogenic capacity is evaluated by semen analysis, including sperm count, motility, sperm morphology, and penetrating ability.[18,110] The normal sperm count is above 40 million sperm/mL semen, and a count below 20 million/mL is indicative of infertility.[18,114] Decreased motility (asthenospermia) below 40% of normal or abnormal morphology (teratospermia) of more than 40% of the total number of sperm also indicates infertility.[18,114]

Antineoplastic Agents

Oligospermia and azoospermia are reported with cyclophosphamide, chlorambucil, and methotrexate when used as single agents.[18,112] Combination therapies with procarbazine, vinca alkaloids, or any of the above agents also decrease sperm production and fertility with variable recovery rates.[18]

Hormonal Agents. Diethylstilbestrol exposure in utero can lead to testicular hypoplasia in men, but may not lead to infertility or sexual dysfunction.[18,129] Work-related exposure to estrogens and progestins in the oral contraceptive industry may result in decreased libido, impotence, and gynecomastia caused by hyperestrogenism.[114] Anabolic steroid use can result in decreased libido, azoospermia, and decreased testicular size.

TABLE 30–1. Drugs and Toxins Associated with Infertility

Men		Women	
Agent	**Effects**	**Agent**	**Effects**
Anabolic steroids	↓ LH, oligospermia	Antineoplastic agents	Gonadal toxicity
Androgens	Suppress testosterone production	Cyclophosphamide	Ovarian failure
Antineoplastic agents	Gonadal toxicity	Busulphan	Amenorrhea
Cyclophosphamide	Oligospermia	Combination therapy	Amenorrhea
Chlorambucil	Oligospermia	(MOPP, MVPP)	
Methotrexate	Oligospermia	Diethylstilbestrol	Spontaneous abortions
Combination therapy	Oligospermia	Ethylene oxide	Spontaneous abortions
(COP, CVP, MOPP, MVPP)		Lead	Spontaneous abortions, still births
Carbon disulfide	↓ FSH, ↓ LH, ↓ spermatogenesis	Oral contraceptives	Affect hypothalamic-pituitary axis, end-
Cimetidine	Oligospermia		organ resistance to hormones, amenorrhea
Chlordecone	Asthenospermia, oligospermia	Thyroid hormone	↓ Ovulation
DBCP	Azoospermia, oligospermia,		
Diethylstilbestrol	Testicular hypoplasia		
Ethanol	↓ Testosterone production, Leydig cell damage, asthenospermia, oligospermia, teratospermia		
Ethylene oxide	Asthenospermia (monkeys), oligospermia		
Ionizing radiation	↓ Spermatogenesis		
Opioids	↓ LH, ↓ testosterone		
Lead	↓ Spermatogenesis, asthenospermia, teratospermia		
Nitrofurantoin	↓ Spermatogenesis		
Sulfasalazine	↓ Spermatogenesis		
Tobacco	↓ Testosterone		

Radiation therapy. Treatment of neoplasms with ionizing radiation leads to dose-dependent oligospermia and azoospermia. Time to recovery is dependent on dose and duration of exposure.[4]

Occupational Exposures

1,2-Dibromo-3-chloropropane. A soil fumigant used in agriculture to control nematodes, 1,2-dibromo-3-chloropropane (DBCP) provides the clearest example of occupational exposure resulting in testicular toxicity and human reproductive dysfunction. In one series, 7 of 10 patients who were exposed to DBCP had decreased or absent spermatogenic activity on testicular biopsy. This correlated with duration of exposure and was most consistently observed after inhalation exposure. A selective decrease or loss of spermatogenic activity was observed without any other consistent testicular defect, and all stages of differentiation were affected. In the most severe cases, the seminiferous tubules were devoid of germ cells.[10]

The mechanism of toxicity of DBCP is unknown but may be the result of transformation of the parent compound to an alkylating agent. Testosterone levels remain normal, although testicular size is decreased. After removal from exposure, improvement in sperm counts occurred in most oligospermic men, but those who had developed azoospermia showed no recovery of spermatogenic function.[128]

Lead. Painters and artisans are commonly exposed to inorganic lead, which is also a hazard in the smelting and battery industries.[69] Lead is a proven spermicide, and lead exposure is associated with decreased libido, asthenospermia, oligospermia,

teratospermia, and testicular atrophy. An increase in the frequency of stillbirths and spontaneous abortions results when the male partner is a lead worker.[131] Lead levels of 35–50 µg/dL are associated with direct spermatogenic toxicity. Indirect effects result from the inhibition of general metabolic processes by lead (Chaps. 12 and 80).[131]

Ethylene Glycol Ethers. Ethylene glycol ethers are used as fuel deicers and as components in paints, varnishes, thinners, and printing inks. Animal studies with methoxymethanol and ethoxyethanol showed oligospermia, azoospermia, and testicular atrophy. One study documented decreased sperm counts in human workers exposed to ethylene glycol ether.[99]

Male Sexual Dysfunction

Sexual dysfunction can be a result of decreased libido (sexual desire), impotence, diminished ejaculation, and erectile dysfunction. Categories of drugs known to affect male sexual function include drugs of abuse, CNS depressants, antihypertensive agents, anticholinergics, psychotropic drugs, exogenous hormones, antibiotics,[113] and chemotherapeutic agents.[130] Libido can be decreased by drugs that block dopamine or testosterone production, or by those producing dysphoria. Agents that affect spinal reflexes can cause diminished ejaculation and erectile dysfunction.[130]

Approximately 30 million men in the United States suffer from erectile dysfunction, with an increased prevalence in older men.[56] Erectile dysfunction can be divided into the following classifications: psychogenic; vasculogenic; neurologic; endocrinologic; and drug-induced. Drug-induced erectile dysfunction is associated with the use of ganglion blockers or any drug that diverts blood flow from the penis. Treatment of the disorder is varied and includes vacuum-constriction devices, penile prostheses, vascular surgery, intracavernosal vasoactive agents, and oral agents.

The next section contains a discussion of the physiology of erection followed by a discussion of agents that cause sexual dysfunction in men, agents that are used to treat erectile dysfunction, and priapism.

Physiology of Erection. In the flaccid state, sympathetic efferents maintain helicine resistance arteriole constriction primarily through norepinephrine induced α-adrenergic agonism. Other vasoconstrictors, such as endothelin, prostaglandin $F_{2\alpha}$, and thromboxane A_2 play a role in maintaining corpus cavernosal smooth muscle tone in relaxation, which results in a flaccid state.[88]

Normal penile erection is a result of both neural and vascular effects leading to smooth muscle relaxation and increased blood flow into the erectile tissue of the penis. Psychogenic neural stimulation arising from the cerebral cortex is mediated through the thoracolumbar sympathetic and sacral parasympathetic tracts. In animals, CNS dopamine and CNS nitric oxide play a role in erection.[88] Reflex stimulation can also occur from the sacral spinal cord. The afferent limb of the reflex arc is supplied by the pudendal nerves and the efferent limb by the nervi erigentes (pelvic splanchnic nerves).

The internal pudendal arteries supply blood to the penis via four branches. Multiple emissary veins drain into the dorsal vein of the penis and plexus of Santorini. Within the penis, the corpora cavernosa share vascular supply and drainage due to extensive arteriolar, arteriovenous, and sinusoidal anastomoses.[135] When penile blood flow is above 20–50 mL/min, erection occurs. Maintenance of tumescence occurs with flow rates of 12 mL/min. The tunica albuginea limits the absolute size of erection.

Penile erection depends on corpus cavernosal smooth muscle relaxation and involves parasympathetic dominance, either by stimulation of parasympathetic receptors or inhibition of the sympathetic axis. Smooth-muscle relaxation is mediated by both cyclic guanosine monophosphate (cGMP) and cyclic adenosine monophosphate (cAMP) pathways. Cholinergic nerves release acetylcholine, which stimulates endothelial cells via M_3 receptors to produce nitric oxide and prostaglandin E_2 (PGE). PGE and nerves containing vasoactive intestinal peptide (VIP) and calcitonin gene-related peptide (CGRP) increase cellular cAMP to potentiate smooth-muscle relaxation. Nonadrenergic-noncholinergic nerves and endothelial cells produce nitric oxide, which activates guanylate cyclase conversion of guanosine triphosphate (GTP) to cGMP. Increasing levels of cGMP acts as a second messenger, mediating arteriolar and trabecular smooth-muscle relaxation to enable increased cavernosal blood flow and penile erection.[88] α-Adrenergic receptor agonism in the erectile tissues decreases cAMP and results in detumescence, while α-adrenergic antagonism can result in pathologic erection (priapism) as a consequence of parasympathetic dominance.[135]

Antihypertensive Drugs. Erectile dysfunction is reported as an adverse effect with all antihypertensive agents and may be caused, in part, by a decrease in hypogastric artery pressure, which impairs blood flow to the pelvis.[128] Methyldopa and clonidine both are centrally acting α_2-adrenergic agonists that inhibit sympathetic outflow from the brain. Sexual dysfunction is reported in 26% of patients taking methyldopa and in 24% of those patients receiving clonidine.[9,91] Erectile dysfunction associated with thiazide diuretics may be related to decreased vascular resistance, diverting blood from the penis.[20] Spironolactone acts as an antiandrogen by inhibiting the binding of dihydrotestosterone to its receptors. Impotence related to use of the β-adrenergic antagonist, propranolol, is well documented[21,60,83,125] and may be caused by unopposed α-mediated vasoconstriction resulting in reduced penile blood flow.

Ethanol. Ethanol is toxic to Leydig cells. Chronic alcohol abuse causes decreased libido, erectile dysfunction, and is associated with testicular atrophy. Liver disease in alcoholics contributes to sexual dysfunction because of decreased testosterone and increased estrogen production. Alcoholics also can have autonomic neuropathies affecting penile nerves and subsequent erection. Heavy drinkers suffer more from erectile dysfunction as compared to episodic drinkers.[127]

Psychotropic Agents. Individuals who take psychotropic agents therapeutically have varying levels of sexual dysfunction related to both their underlying disease and psychotropic medications. All psychotropic agents are associated with sexual dysfunction to some degree. Monoamine oxidase inhibitors (MAOIs), cyclic antidepressants (CAs), antipsychotics, and selective serotonin reuptake inhibitors (SSRIs) are associated with decreased libido and erectile dysfunction in men.[26] Thioridazine is associated with significantly lower LH and testosterone levels in men compared to other antipsychotics.[18] Table 30–2 lists other agents associated with sexual dysfunction.

Agents Used in the Treatment of Erectile Dysfunction.
Intracavernosal Agents. The three most commonly use intracavernosal agents used for erectile dysfunction are papaverine, prostaglandin E_1, and phentolamine. Papaverine is a benzylisoquinoline alkaloid derived from the poppy plant *Papaver somniferum*. It exerts its effects through nonselective inhibition of phosphodiesterase, leading to increased cAMP and cGMP levels and subsequent cavernosal vasodilation. Papaverine was used for the treatment of cardiac and cerebral ischemia but had limited results. Presently, it is used as intracavernosal therapy, either alone or in conjunction with phentolamine for erectile dysfunction. Systemic side effects include dizziness, nausea, vomiting, hepatotoxicity, lactic acidosis with oral administration, and cardiac dysrhythmias with intravenous use. Intracavernosal administration is associated with penile fibrosis as a dose-related phenomenon

TABLE 30–2. Drugs and Toxins Associated with Sexual Dysfunction (Particularly Diminished Libido and Impotence)

Agent	
Anabolic steroids	Lithium
Anticholinergics*	Monamine oxidase inhibitors*
Antihypertensives	Opioids (high dose)
Cimetidine	Oral contraceptives
Cyclic antidepressants	Phenothiazines
Ethanol	Selective serotonin reuptake
Lead	inhibitors

*Associated with erectile dysfunction.

but fibrosis can also occur with limited use.[29] More concerning is the development of priapism with papaverine use.

Prostaglandin E$_1$ (Alprostadil) is a nonspecific agonist of prostaglandin receptors resulting in increased levels of intracavernosal cAMP. It is effective via intracavernosal administration as a single agent, and an intraurethral form is available as well but has lower efficacy. Penile fibrosis can occur but the incidence is lower compared to papaverine. Other adverse effects include penile pain, secondary to its effects as a nonspecific prostaglandin receptor agonist, and priapism.

Phentolamine is a competitive α-adrenergic antagonist at α$_1$ and α$_2$ receptors. It effects erection by inhibiting the normal resting adrenergic tone in cavernosal smooth muscle, thus allowing increased arterial blood flow and erection. Intracavernosal use can cause systemic hypotension, reflex tachycardia, nasal congestion, and gastrointestinal upset. Penile fibrosis and priapism are also reported.

Sildenafil. Sildenafil is an orally available selective inhibitor of cGMP phosphodiesterase type 5 (PDE5) for male erectile dysfunction.[11] It increases nitric oxide induced cGMP levels by preventing cGMP breakdown, thus promoting penile vascular relaxation and erection. After oral administration, sildenafil is rapidly absorbed with a bioavailability of 40% and a median peak plasma concentration of 60 minutes. Its mean volume of distribution is 105 L, and its elimination half-life is approximately 4 hours. Metabolism is primarily by the P450 CYP3A4 pathway with some minor metabolic activity via the CYP2C9 pathway. Plasma levels of sildenafil are increased in patients older than 65 years, hepatic dysfunction, severe renal dysfunction (creatinine clearance <30 mL/min), and P450 CYP3A4 inhibitors (macrolide antibiotics, cimetidine, antifungal agents, protease inhibitors).[24]

An initial pilot study of 12 male patients with erectile dysfunction showed significantly improved erectile response to visual stimulation.[11] Since then, multiple studies with larger groups of patients showed significant improvement in erectile and sexual function over placebo.

The most common adverse effects are headache, flushing, dyspepsia, and rhinitis, which are related to sildenafil's PDE5 inhibitory effects on extracavernosal tissue.[56] Blurred vision, increased light perception and transient blue-green tinged vision are also reported and are related to sildenafil's weak PDE6 inhibition in the retina.[56]

More serious reported adverse effects are myocardial infarction, priapism, and optic ischemia.[42,64,115]

When taken alone, sildenafil's vasodilatory effects cause a modest decrease in systemic blood pressure. However, because of its mechanism of action via cGMP inhibition and vascular vasodilation, sildenafil can have synergistic interactions with the vasodilatory effects of nitrates or nitrites resulting in profound hypotension.[11] A study of healthy male volunteers taking sildenafil demonstrated significantly less tolerance to a glyceryl trinitrate infusion as compared to placebo.[126] Because of this interaction, the avoidance of nitrate therapy in patients taking sildenafil with acute myocardial ischemic syndromes is recommended.[24]

Yohimbine. Yohimbine, an indole alkylamine alkaloid from the West African yohimbe tree (*Corynanthe yohimbe*), is an α$_2$-adrenergic antagonist with cholinergic activity used to treat erectile dys-

function and postural hypotension associated with anticholinergic drugs.[73] It is structurally similar to reserpine. Other names for yohimbine include Aphrodyne, corynine, hydroaergotocin, quebrachine, and the street name "yo-yo."[74] Its use in the treatment of impotence is based on the theory that erection is linked to cholinergic stimulation and α$_2$ antagonism, resulting in an increase inflow and decrease outflow of blood to the penis. Although the agent Aphrodex, which contained 5 mg yohimbine, 5 mg methyltestosterone, and 5 mg strychnine, was shown to improve performance in males with erectile failure,[78] its distribution was halted in 1973 because of safety concerns.[109]

Yohimbine can be obtained by prescription, but extracts are also available in "health food" products marketed as "vitalizing agents for men."[35] Yohimbine can also be extracted from the Rauwolfia root.[46] The "therapeutic" dose is 2–6 mg 3 times daily. The drug is rapidly absorbed, with peak serum levels occurring in 45–60 minutes. The half-life is 36 minutes, and clearance is by hepatic metabolism without renal excretion.[96] Maximum pharmacologic effects occur 1–2 hours after ingestion and effects persist for 3–4 hours.[74]

Because the erectile process involves various neurotransmitters, a single agent would be expected to only have a partial effect. In a double-blind study of 100 males with erectile failure treated with 18 mg/d of yohimbine, 42.6% of the treatment group and 27.6% of the placebo group reported some improvement in erectile function, which was not statistically significant.[87] Another study that compared a higher dose of yohimbine and placebo in 82 elderly males showed a statistically significant improvement with treatment.[119]

Adverse effects can occur with relatively low doses of yohimbine. Tachycardia, hypertension, mydriasis, diaphoresis, lacrimation, salivation, nausea, vomiting, and flushing can occur following intravenous administration.[48,61] Ten milligrams of yohimbine can elicit manic symptoms in patients with bipolar disorder,[105] and 15 mg/d is associated with bronchospasm[68] and a lupuslike syndrome.[111] A 16-year-old female who ingested 250 mg of yohimbine powder, purchased for its purported aphrodisiac activity, developed an acute dissociative reaction with weakness, paresthesias, headache, nausea, palpitations, and chest pain. She also developed tachycardia, tachypnea, diaphoresis, tremors, and a rash. Her symptoms resolved without treatment after 36 hours.[74] Another case report describes a 62-year-old male who ingested 200 mg of yohimbine and developed tachycardia, hypertension, and a brief period of anxiety that resolved without treatment.[46] Symptomatic patients who ingest yohimbine should receive activated charcoal and should be observed until asymptomatic. Clonidine has been recommended for treatment of yohimbine's central and peripheral effects.[74] β-Adrenergic antagonists may attenuate some of the peripheral toxicity, but may also result in unopposed α$_1$-adrenergic activity and worsening of hypertension, and should be avoided. Benzodiazepine administration may be sufficient for the treatment of agitation and sympathomimetic effects related to yohimbine.

Priapism

Priapism is prolonged involuntary erection, which is painful, unassociated with sexual stimulation, and can result in impotence if prolonged. It most commonly occurs during the third and fourth decades of life and is caused by inflow of blood to the penis in excess of outflow. The corpora cavernosa become firm and the corpus spongiosum flaccid. Intracavernosal pressures can exceed arterial systolic pressure, resulting in cell death. Priapism can occur from an imbalance in neural stimuli, interference with venous outflow, or as a result of drug-induced inhibition of penile detumescence. α-Adrenergic antagonist agents prevent constriction of blood vessels supplying erectile tissue, resulting in priapism.[135] One per 10,000 patients taking trazodone develop priapism, which is thought to be related to its α-adrenergic antagonist effects.[109] A common cause of priapism is iatrogenic, resulting from the injection of papaverine for the treatment of impotence.[120] Other agents associated with drug-induced priapism include prazosin, labetalol, guanethidine, hydralazine, phenothiazines, androgens, anticoagulants, ethanol, marijuana, and cantharidin[63,120,135] (see Table 30–3).

The goal in treatment of priapism is detumescence with retention of potency. Initial therapy includes sedation and analgesia with benzodiazepines and opioids. Urology consultation should also be obtained. Aspiration and normal saline irrigation of the corpora cavernosa may be effective. If priapism occurs secondary to α-adrenergic antagonism, an α-adrenergic agonist (2–4 mg metaraminol, 0.02 mg norepinephrine, or 0.2 mg phenylephrine) diluted with normal saline to 10 mL volume can be instilled by placing a 19-gauge butterfly needle into the corpora cavernosa. If the above measures fail, operative venous shunt placement may be required.[120,135]

FEMALE FERTILITY

The female reproductive system consists of the female gonadal organs and the respective hormonal system. Female fertility encompasses the reproductive system, the process of oocyte fertilization and gestation. Female infertility may result from changes in hormone levels, direct toxicity to the ovum, interference with the transport of the ovum, or inhibition of implantation of the ovum in the uterus. Females usually notice reproductive abnormalities more quickly than males, because menses may be affected, although infertility may occur while normal menses persists. Evaluation of female fertility is more difficult owing to the complexity of the systems involved and the inaccessibility of the female germ cell, but it is feasible and involves investigations of the anatomy and hormonal levels. The following is a discussion of oogenesis, agents that disrupt oogenesis, and agents that affect early embryo gestation.

TABLE 30–3.   Drugs Associated with Priapism

Agent	
Androgens	Antipsychotics
Anticoagulants	Cantharidin
Antihypertensives	Cocaine
Guanethidine	Diazepam
Hydralazine	Ethanol
Labetalol	Marijuana
Phentolamine	Papaverine
Prazosin	Risperidone
Reserpine	Sildenafil
	Trazodone

Oogenesis

In contrast to men, women have a limited number of reproductive cells (ovarian follicles). Follicles are most numerous while the fetus is in utero, with the number decreasing to approximately 2 million at birth. By the time a woman reaches puberty, the majority of follicles have degenerated, leaving 300,000–400,000 ova, of which only about 400 will eventually produce mature ova during a woman's reproductive years. In contrast, men produce millions of spermatozoa a day. The process of oogenesis requires secretion of GnRH from the hypothalamus, resulting in production of LH and FSH from the pituitary, which are required for ovarian follicle maturation.[18] FSH induces early maturation by stimulating granulosa and thecal cell proliferation and estrogen production. LH is required for ovulation and for the formation of the corpus luteum. The corpus luteum continues estrogen production and produces progesterone, which stimulates the uterus to develop an endometrium receptive to any fertilized ovum. Successful ovulation requires not only hormone secretion but appropriate cyclic secretion as well.

Agents That Decrease Female Fertility

Antineoplastic Agents.   Alkylating agents are well described as causing oocyte destruction and disruption of the hypothalamic-pituitary-ovarian axis in women. Ovarian failure with menstrual cycle disruptions and amenorrhea are reported with cyclophosphamide and busulphan as single agents.[18,124] Combination therapies with alkylating agents and vinca alkaloids are also reported to cause menstrual irregularities.

Hormonal Agents.   Diethylstilbestrol in utero exposure can lead to cervical and vaginal abnormalities in women.[18] Oral contraceptive agents can produce persistent infertility in women, particularly in those women who are nulliparous, following their discontinuation. Prolonged infertility is more common with the use of the combined preparations as opposed to the use of sequential estrogen/progesterone contraceptives.[18] Medroxyprogesterone acetate depot administration is associated with transient ovulatory dysfunction of variable duration after cessation of therapy. These agents may affect the hypothalamic-pituitary axis, gonadotropin release, or end-organ sensitivity to hormonal stimulation.

Psychotropic Agents.   As in men, all psychotropic agents can cause sexual dysfunction. MAOIs and TCAs are associated with the highest rates of sexual dysfunction, followed by antipsychotics and SSRIs.[26] These drug classes decrease libido and cause orgasmic dysfunction. Bupropion and nefazodone have the lowest rates of sexual dysfunction and are used to reverse SSRI-induced sexual dysfunction.[134] One study reported amenorrhea in 50% of women on thioridazine with return of menstruation after 6 months.

Environmental Agents.   Chlorinated hydrocarbons are a large group of chemicals that include polychlorinated biphenyls (PCB), dichlorodiphenyltrichloroethane (DDT), pentachlorophenol, and hexachlorocyclohexane. PCBs were widely used prior to the 1970s and often released into the environment where they continue to exist and contaminate the food chain. Studies of the effect of PCBs on fertility are mixed. Some show no association with PCB exposure whereas others show increased levels of PCBs in women with endometriosis. The same study showed increased levels of hexachlorocyclohexane and pentachlorophenol in women with miscarriages and decreased conception rates with increasing DDT levels.[99]

Abortifacients.   An abortifacient is defined as an agent that affects early embryo gestation and induces abortion. These substances may act by flushing the zygote from the fallopian tube, blocking the uterine horn, inhibiting implantation, inducing fetal resorption, or by producing oxytocin like activity that results in uterine irritation and contraction. Abortifacients may also indirectly affect pregnancy by altering hormonal levels. Inhibition of HCG or progesterone production by the placenta or interference with progesterone receptors can also induce abortion. In a US poison center study, 5 of 43 pregnant patients intentionally overdosed on known abortifacients, including quinine, misoprostol, methylergonovine, and oral contraceptives. Four of these patients developed vaginal bleeding and cramping, but no short-term (1–3 days) fetal demise was reported.[102] The use of these agents is more common in underdeveloped countries and in populations without access to safer methods for termination or prevention of pregnancy.

Misoprostol is a synthetic prostaglandin E_1 methyl analog indicated for the prevention of gastric ulcers caused by nonsteroidal anti-inflammatory drugs. It was approved for marketing in Brazil in 1985 and in the United States in 1988. The abortifacient properties of prostaglandins are well established,[77] and misoprostol can produce uterine contractions, uterine bleeding, and expulsion of the products of conception.[106] Common adverse effects are nausea, vomiting, diarrhea, abdominal pain, chills, shivering, and fever. In one case, overdose with 6000 μg of misoprostol resulted in abortion, hyperthermia, rhabdomyolysis, hypoxemia, and an acid-base disorder.[53] Cases of congenital abnormalities (scalp and skull defects, cranial nerve palsies, limb defects such as talipes equinovarus) are reported when misoprostol did not terminate pregnancy.[32] This drug has been extensively misused in Brazil to induce abortion.[27,30,101] In 1991, an estimated 10% of mothers giving birth at public hospitals in Rio de Janeiro were exposed to misoprostol.[30,101] Although the rate of successful pregnancy termination with this agent is 11–50%, abortion can occur after amounts just above the recommended therapeutic dose.[66,106]

Mifepristone, or RU-486, an antiprogesterone agent legally used in Europe and recently FDA approved for use in the United States, is an effective abortifacient, especially when used in conjunction with a prostaglandin.[97,108] RU-486 is a steroid compound with a 5-fold greater affinity for progesterone receptors than progesterone. Upon complexing with the receptors, it causes downregulation of progesterone-dependent genes, decidual necrosis, cervical dilation, and consequent expulsion of the products of conception.[32] The sensitivity of the uterus to prostaglandins is also increased.[8] Adverse effects include excessive blood loss and fatigue, gynecomastia, alopecia, nausea, vomiting, and abdominal pain.[47,57] Data on toxicity in overdose is not known.

Methotrexate is a folic acid analogue that is used in conjunction with a prostaglandin in medical terminations of pregnancy. It competitively inhibits dihydrofolate reductase and decreases nucleic acid synthesis, which is necessary in rapidly dividing cells such as trophoblasts. Common adverse effects are nausea, vomiting, diarrhea, fever, and chills.[32] Large doses or decreased clearance of methotrexate can lead to clinical toxicity, which includes stomatitis and esophagitis, renal failure, and myelosuppression, and can be ameliorated with folinic acid administration. (See Chapter 47 for a more in-depth discussion of methotrexate toxicity and Antidotes is Depth: Folinic Acid.)

Many abortifacients are derived from plants and their extracts (Table 30–4). Not only are these agents toxic to the mother, but because many are ineffective in producing abortion, possible teratogenicity is a concern. Trichosanthin is an abortifacient protein extracted from the root of *Trichosanthes kirilowii*, a Chinese medicinal plant. The root is powdered and is used as a folk remedy to induce menstrual bleeding and to expel the fetus.[122] The active ingredient, trichosanthin, has abortifacient activity in animals and in

TABLE 30–4.   Drugs and Toxins Used as Abortifaciens

Substance	Source	Country of origin or use	Miscellaneous/Toxicity
Acanthospermum hispidum	*Acanthospermum hispidum* (whole plant)	Brazil	Preimplantation effects
Adhatoda vascia	*Adhatoda vascia*	India	100% abortifacient in rats
α-Momorcharin	*Momordica charantia*	China	Similar to trichosanthin
Cajanus cajan	*Cajanus cajan* (fresh leaves)	Brazil	Preimplantation effects
Devil's claw	*Ranunculus sp.* (root)	South Africa	Similar to pennyroyal oil
Dong quai	*Angelica polymorpha*	—	Anticoagulant effects, photodermatitis
Ergotamines	*Claviceps purpurea*	—	Oxytocic
Legenaria breviflora Robert	*Legenaria breviflora* Robert (fruit juice)	Nigeria	Anti-implantation, oxytocic
Lysol disinfectant	—	—	Death after intrauterine administration
Methotrexate	—	—	Medical use
Methylcytisine	*Caulophyllum thalictroides* (blue cohosh)	—	Toxicity similar to nicotine
Misoprostol	—	—	Medical use
Moringa oleifera	*Moringa oleifera*	India	100% abortifacient in rats
Prostaglandin E analogue	Misoprostol	Brazil, US	Marketed as Cytotec for gastric ulcers
Pulegone	*Hedeoma pulegeoides*, pennyroyal oil or tea	—	Hepatotoxicity; NAC may be effective
Quinine	Cinchona bark	—	Antimalarial
Rue	*Ruta graveolens*	Mexico	Preimplantation effects and oxytocic in animals
RU-486	Mifepristone	France, US	Marketed as an abortion pill; administered with prostaglandins
Tricosanthin (compound Q)	*Trichosanthes kirilowii*	China	Inhibits protein synthesis, ↓ HCG, ↓ progesterone

humans when injected or applied intravaginally.[122] The mechanism is unknown, but may be related to inhibition of protein synthesis by preventing the incorporation of leucine.[122] Trichosanthin's injurious effect on trophoblasts has been demonstrated, and it may also inhibit human chorionic gonadotropin (HCG) and progesterone production by the placenta.[122] Hypersensitivity occurs in some patients, limiting its clinical usefulness.

Pennyroyal oil is a volatile oil extracted from the leaves of *Mentha pulegium* and *Hedeoma pulegeoides* and contains the ketone pulegone (Chap. 77). Preparations also include a tablet, tea, essence of pennyroyal, and leaves. There are several reports of its use as an emmenagogue and illicit abortifacient. Pulegone depletes glutathione stores in the liver and is a direct hepatotoxin. The epoxide metabolite menthofuran may also contribute to hepatotoxicity. Fulminant hepatic failure can occur after ingestion of 2 ounces of pennyroyal oil.[2,6] Renal failure is also described.[118] *N*-Acetylcysteine has been successfully used to prevent pulegone-induced hepatotoxicity.[19]

Because of its oxytocic action, the cinchona alkaloid quinine has been used intravenously to induce labor in cases of fetal death.[90] It has also been used as an illicit abortifacient.[132,133] Because it is ineffective when ingested orally for this purpose, it may be taken in repeated doses leading to toxicity (Chap. 44).

Black cohosh root (*Cimicifuga racemosa*) extract is an herbal preparation used to induce abortion and primarily results in gastrointestinal toxicity after ingestion. Blue cohosh (*Caulophyllum thalictroides*) is also used and has methylcytosine, which causes toxicities similar to nicotine—nausea, vomiting, muscle paralysis, seizures, tachycardia, and hypotension.

TOXICITY OF APHRODISIACS

Aphrodisiacs are defined as substances that heighten sexual desire, pleasure, and/or performance and include agents from the plant, animal, and mineral kingdoms.[33] The search for an effective aphrodisiac has continued for thousands of years by a variety of societies. Ancient fertility cults used *Datura,* belladonna, and henbane as aphrodisiacs. Yohimbine has been used by African cultures to enhance sexual prowess, and mandrake was used in medieval Europe. Other substances recommended include oysters, vitamin E, and ginseng. Because there are no measurable objective parameters, research in this area is lacking. Most published studies evaluating aphrodisiacs have been conducted in male rodents, and little information is available in humans.

Dopamine, nitric oxide, oxytocin, and adrenocorticotrophic hormone (ACTH) all facilitate sexual behavior. Dopamine stimulates the forebrain and midbrain and leads to an increase in sexual response and arousal. In animals, dopamine agonists, such as apomorphine and quinpirole, have proerectile effects through stimulation of dopamine pathways, increasing nitric oxide in the paraventricular nucleus in the hypothalamus, and releasing oxytocin.[88] Other preparations tested for the treatment of impotence include bromocriptine,[1,12] glyceryl trinitrate,[89] zinc,[3] oxytocin,[72] and LH.[71] Endogenous opioids, GABA, and norepinephrine are associated with decreased sexual behavior. Serotonin is generally inhibitory to sexual function but the effects are dependent on the receptor subclass. 5-HT$_{1A}$ receptor stimulation inhibits erection but facilitates ejaculation in rats, whereas 5-HT$_{2C}$ receptors facilitate male sexual behavior.[88] Various serotonergic drugs, including tra-

zodone, nefazodone, bupropion, and clomipramine, are reported to improve sexual dysfunction.[109,134]

Lead

Some "aphrodisiacs" in Asian countries contain lead and are associated with toxicity. In a British report, a 50-year-old male from Pakistan presented with anorexia, abdominal pain, and anemia with basophilic stippling. A whole-blood lead level was 96 µg/dL. He reported ingestion of a yellow-white powder provided to him by a traditional Asian practitioner for the treatment of impotence, which contained 84% elemental lead by weight.[38] A 24-year-old male from Bangladesh presented to a London hospital with similar complaints and a whole-blood lead level of 102 µg/dL after chronic ingestion of an aphrodisiac containing 46% lead.[14] Traditionally, aphrodisiacs from the Indian subcontinent contain silver and/or gold, but occasionally lead is substituted. The indications for chelation therapy are the same as in other cases of lead poisoning (Chap. 80).

Topical Agents

Spanish Fly. Spanish fly is a cantharidin derived from crushed blister beetles (*Cantharis vesicatoria*) and is used to enhance sexual potency.[63] A 1% topical solution available for use in wart removal has also been marketed in adult sex shops and by mail order as an aphrodisiac. Adverse effects are a consequence of the vesicant properties of the agent, and gastrointestinal, dermatologic, genitourinary, renal, cardiac, pulmonary, neurologic, and hematologic effects are all described (Chap. 102).

Following absorption, ingested cantharidin is bound to albumin and excreted by the kidney.[104] Symptoms generally occur 2–6 hours after ingestion. Gastrointestinal and genitourinary signs include dysuria, oral pain, dysphagia, nausea, hematemesis, and hematuria. Blistering of mucous membranes also occurs, and patients commonly develop hemorrhagic mucositis of the mouth, esophagus, and stomach. Fatal gastrointestinal hemorrhage has been reported, and the lethal dose varies from 10 to 80 mg in adults.[31,92,104] Blister formation in the urinary tract, tubular necrosis, and glomerular damage all result in gross hematuria, which can continue for 2 weeks after ingestion. Proteinuria is common, and death from acute tubular necrosis and renal failure can occur.[121] Dermal exposure can result in blistering, ulceration, and systemic toxicity. Hemorrhage occurs in the ureters, bladder, and urethra, and hemorrhagic bullae may be noted in the bladder. Priapism, ovarian engorgement, and vaginal bleeding can also occur.[94] Sinus tachycardia is the most common cardiac manifestation of toxicity, but pericardial and subendocardial hemorrhage are also described. Patients may also develop dysrhythmias, ST segment elevation, and T-wave changes.[94] Pulmonary effects are rare and include pulmonary edema and bronchial hemorrhage. Disseminated intravascular coagulation has been reported and may be caused by vesicant-related vascular injury. Neurologic symptoms are rare. No specific antidote is available and treatment is supportive. Cantharidin exposure should be considered in the differential diagnosis of unexplained hematuria or gastrointestinal hemorrhage.

Bufotoxin. "Stone," "love stone," "black stone," and "rock hard" all refer to topical aphrodisiac preparations made from dried toad venom that contains bufalin, cinobufalin, cinobufagin, and other cardioactive steroids in the bufadienolide class. A 90-year-old male presented with bradycardia and a history of syncope after ingesting Yixin Wan, a nonprescription Chinese medication containing toad venom, ginseng, pearl, and musk.[67] Chan Su is a traditional Chinese medication produced from the venom of *Bufo bufo gargarizans,* which contains several cardiac glycosides, a topical anesthetic, and bufotenine.[16] Kyushin is another popular Asian traditional medication that contains dried toad venom. The cardiac glycosides have a similar structure and action to digoxin. Digoxin immunoassay may be positive after exposure to these agents, although the level may not correlate with toxicity. Four deaths were reported between 1993 and 1995 following ingestion of these topical aphrodisiacs. The patients presented with bradycardia and measurable digoxin levels. Hyperkalemia also occurred. One patient was successfully treated with digoxin-specific Fab fragments.[15,17] An animal study evaluating the usefulness of digoxin specific fragments in mice intoxicated with Chan Su demonstrated survival in 8 of 15 mice treated with digoxin-specific Fab, as compared with no survivors in the control group.[15] Digoxin Fab (10 vials) should be administered to any patient with a suspected cardioactive steroid overdose with hyperkalemia and/or dysrhythmia (Chap. 48 and Antidotes in Depth: Digoxin Specific Antibody Fragments).

Inhaled Agents

Nitrites. Alkyl (amyl, butyl, and isobutyl) nitrites are aliphatic esters of nitrous acid and are yellow, highly volatile, sweet-smelling liquids administered by inhalation. Glass capsules typically contain 0.3 mL and are enclosed in a gauze jacket of woven absorbent covering that can be crushed and held to the nostrils. The capsules are called "poppers" because of the sound produced when they are broken.[59,76] The vasodilatory effects produced by inhalation of amyl nitrite were first described in 1859, and amyl nitrite was first used for the treatment of angina in 1867. Amyl nitrite was originally marketed as a prescription drug in 1937, but the FDA removed the requirement for a prescription in 1960. After 1960, nitrates replaced nitrites in the treatment of angina. Because abuse of inhaled nitrites became widespread in the 1960s, particularly by healthy young males, the FDA reinstated the prescription requirement for amyl nitrite in 1968.[59] Since that time, isobutyl and butyl nitrite have been legally marketed as "room deodorizers" in bottles containing 10–30 mL.[52]

Amyl nitrite and other alkyl nitrites are especially popular aphrodisiacs among men who have sex with other men. They are inhaled during foreplay to obtain a "high" and to produce anal sphincter relaxation, or just before orgasm to heighten and prolong the climax.[43] Butyl nitrite is also popular among teens who seek a "high." In a 1986 survey by NIDA, 8.6% of 3000 US high school seniors and 9% of teens between 12 and 17 years old reportedly used nitrites, with 0.5% using them daily.[59]

Nitrites are absorbed via the skin, lungs, mucus membranes, and the gastrointestinal tract. They are metabolized in the liver and excreted, partially unchanged, in the urine.[76] In mice, butyl nitrite undergoes rapid hydrolysis to nitrite ion and butyl alcohol. The half-life is 2–3 seconds, and metabolism is by first-order kinetics.[59] The relaxation of vascular smooth muscle results in potent vasodilation and hypotension. Blood pressure can decrease significantly within 30 seconds of inhalation. Inhalation of as little as 5 drops can result in hypotension and reflex tachycardia.[76] Cardiovascular collapse can occur, especially if nitrites are injected intravenously. Vasodilation of cerebral blood vessels results in increased intracranial pressure, and cerebral aneurysm rupture has been reported after amyl nitrite inhalation.[93]

A feeling of warmth and palpitations are frequently described after nitrite inhalation.[59] Headache, nausea, and syncope are also common. Nitrite use can be dangerous in patients with glaucoma due to a transient increase in intraocular pressure.[43] Nitrites can cause methemoglobinemia[40] (Chap. 94), which can be fatal. Successful treatment of nitrite-induced methemoglobinemia with methylene blue is well reported. Hemolytic anemia is also reported[13,76] and is probably a result of the oxidizing effects of nitrites. "Popper dermatitis" is a characteristic rash that can be noted around the nose, lips, face, penis, and scrotum, and presents as erythematous, edematous, and crusted lesions.[43,75,76] It may have a similar appearance to impetigo and seborrheic dermatitis. The rash usually clears within 10 days, but reappears with repeat nitrite inhalation.[43] A generalized allergic dermatitis can also occur.[34]

The carcinogenic and immunosuppressive effects of amyl nitrite are not adequately tested in animals, although it is mutagenic with the Ames test.[41] There are some data to suggest that nitrites may be immunosuppressive in the setting of repeated viral antigenic stimulation.[52] It is postulated that this may contribute to the high frequency of Kaposi's sarcoma in men who have sex with other men. In one study, amyl nitrite was the only drug that 100% of patients with Kaposi's sarcoma reported using.[80] Concern for carcinogenicity associated with amyl nitrite has resulted in a recent decline in its use among men who have sex with other men.

URINARY SYSTEM

The urinary system is composed of the kidneys, ureters, bladder, and urethra. Many toxicants are concentrated by the kidneys and eliminated in the urine. The following discusses the effect of toxicants on the bladder and urine. See Chapter 23 for further discussion on toxicants affecting the kidneys.

Bladder Anatomy And Physiology

The bladder is a hollow, muscular reservoir composed of two parts, the body and the neck, and stores 350–450 mL of urine in adults. A smooth muscle, the detrusor muscle, makes up the bulk of the body and contracts in urination. Urine from the ureters enters the bladder at the uppermost part of the trigone, an area in the posterior wall of the bladder, and leaves via the neck and the posterior urethra. Surrounding the neck and posterior urethra is smooth muscle interlaced with elastic tissue to form the internal sphincter. Sympathetic innervation from S2 to S4 of the sacral spinal cord to the internal sphincter maintains smooth muscle contraction. Distal to the internal sphincter is an area with voluntary skeletal muscle that forms the external sphincter.

Nerve supply and neurophysiology involve interplay by the sympathetic and parasympathetic nervous systems arising from the sacral portion of the spinal cord (S2 to S4). Figure 30–1 illustrates the physiology of micturition. Norepinephrine is released by sympathetic postganglionic fibers, whereas parasympathetic pre- and postganglionic fibers release acetylcholine. β-Adrenergic receptors supply the bladder wall, and agonism facilitates filling. α-Adrenergic receptors predominate in the internal sphincter and the bladder neck. Consequently, stimulation of α or β-adrenergic receptors results in sphincter contraction and bladder outlet resistance, resulting in retention of urine.[28] Stimulation of acetylcholine receptors results in parasympathetic-mediated detrusor

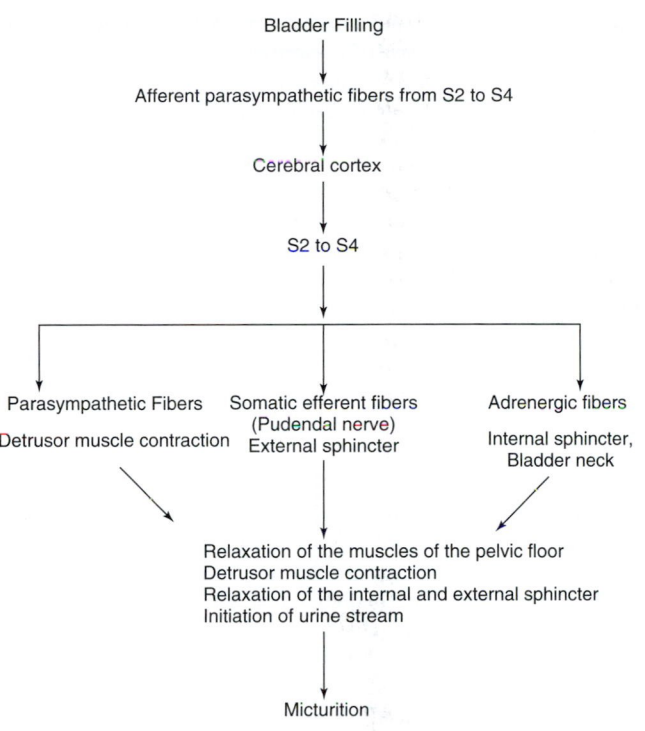

Bladder Filling

Afferent parasympathetic fibers from S2 to S4

Cerebral cortex

S2 to S4

Parasympathetic Fibers — Detrusor muscle contraction

Somatic efferent fibers (Pudendal nerve) External sphincter

Adrenergic fibers — Internal sphincter, Bladder neck

Relaxation of the muscles of the pelvic floor
Detrusor muscle contraction
Relaxation of the internal and external sphincter
Initiation of urine stream

Micturition

Figure 30–1. A schematic description of the physiology of micturition.

muscle contraction and bladder emptying. Conversely, anticholinergic drugs prevent bladder emptying and result in urinary retention.[22,23,25,45,51,86]

Urinary Abnormalities

Urinary incontinence is common in the elderly population. As age increases, bladder size decreases, resulting in more frequent emptying. Early detrusor contraction, even with low bladder volumes, occurs more commonly in the elderly causing a sense of urgency. There are many etiologies for urinary incontinence, including various drug exposures (Table 30–5). General or regional anesthesia, bladder instrumentation, and medications may produce bladder atony leading to incontinence.[25] Functional incontinence can also result from use of any medication that causes impaired cognition or decreased mobility (sedative/hypnotics, opioids, etc).[25] Urinary retention can occur as a side effect or with toxicity of various agents, including sympathomimetics, anticholinergics, antidysrhythmics (quinidine, procainamide, disopyramide), and hormonal agents (progesterone, estrogen, testosterone).[25,45]

Abnormalities in Urinalysis

Abnormalities of the urinalysis are often useful in identifying drug or chemical exposures. Color change or the presence of crystals may aid in diagnosis. The urinalysis in patients who ingest ethylene glycol often (but not always) reveals calcium oxalate or hippurate crystals. Calcium oxalate crystals are monohydrates (prism- or needlelike) or dihydrates (envelope shaped). Hippurate crystals are needle shaped.[98] Crystalluria is present in 50% of cases of ethylene glycol poisoning (Chap. 66, Fig. 66–4). Hexagonal crystals are noted after massive primidone poisoning and result from pre-

TABLE 30–5. **Drugs that Cause Incontinence**

Drug	Action
α-Adrenergic agonists	Increase internal sphincter tone
α-Adrenergic antagonists	Decrease internal sphincter tone
Anticholinergic agents	Impair detrusor contraction
Calcium channel blockers	Decrease detrusor contraction
Diuretics	Overflow of bladder
Opioids	Impair detrusor contraction
Sedatives-hypnotics	Decrease sensorium

Reprinted with permission from Chutka DS, Fleming KC, Evans MP, et al: Urinary incontinence in the elderly population. Mayo Clin Proc 1996;71:93–101.

cipitation of primidone in the urine.[123] Crystalluria is also described after therapeutic doses of salicylate, phenacetin, sulfonamide, and quinolones. After large ingestions, crystals can be seen with methotrexate, amoxicillin, cephalexin, ampicillin, and indinavir. Urine color is dependent on several factors, including pH, concentration, natural pigments, and length of time exposed to air.[55] Dilute urine secondary to diuretic use, diabetes mellitus, diabetes insipidus, or overhydration can appear colorless, whereas concentrated urine is usually orange. The presence of fluorescein, detected by illumination of the urine with a Wood's lamp, suggests ethylene glycol (commercial antifreeze) ingestion. Table 30–6 notes other causes of colored urine.

There are multiple causes of hematuria.[79] It can occur with drug-induced interstitial nephritis, a condition distinguished by fever, rash, eosinophilia, azotemia, and oliguria.[36] Hemorrhagic cystitis is a more frequent cause of hematuria, and is associated with a number of drugs. The clinical presentation of hemorrhagic cystitis includes hematuria, dysuria, and urinary frequency. Criteria for diagnosis include a history of gross hematuria, laboratory findings of gross hematuria (>5 RBC/HPF), platelet count above 50,000/mm^3, and a negative urine culture.[107] When in doubt, the diagnosis may be confirmed by cystoscopy, which reveals an inflamed, hyperemic, and sometimes ulcerated bladder mucosa.

Cyclophosphamide-related hemorrhagic cystitis was first described in 1959,[85] and is the best-documented type of drug-induced hemorrhagic cystitis.[49] As many as 46% of patients receiving cyclophosphamide will develop hemorrhagic cystitis.[39,62,65,70] Acrolein, the causative agent, is a metabolite of cyclophosphamide that damages the urothelium when excreted. There is no sex or age predilection, and symptoms can occur months after exposure. Hemorrhagic cystitis is described after oral doses exceeding 100 g and after a single intravenous dose of cyclophosphamide.[117] Sloughing of the bladder mucosa occurs, and 5% of patients die from intractable hemorrhage.[58,103] Patients at highest risk are those who are dehydrated, receive cyclophosphamide intravenously, or who have previous or concomitant exposure to busulfan or radiotherapy.[85] Treatment with cyclophosphamide is also associated with a dose-related increase (9–45-fold) in the risk of subsequent bladder cancer (Chap. 47).[102,117]

Prophylaxis against cyclophosphamide-induced hemorrhagic cystitis includes bladder catheterization and drainage, bladder irrigation, hydration, forced diuresis, and administration of oral sodium 2-mercaptoethanesulfonate (MESNA).[85] MESNA binds to acrolein in the urine to form an inert, nontoxic thioester, reducing the incidence of hemorrhagic cystitis by 85%.[117] Bladder irrigation with alum, silver nitrate, prostaglandins, and formalin[5] has also

TABLE 30–6. Drugs, Toxins, and Other Materials that Cause Colored Urine

Milky
Chyle
Lipids
Neutrophils

Reddish-Brown
Anthraquinone
Bilirubin
Chloroquine
Ibuprofen
Levadopa
Methyldopa
Phenacetin
Phenazopyridine
Phenothiazines
Phenytoin
Porphyrins
Trinitrophenol

Reddish-Orange
Aminopyrine
Aniline dyes
Antipyrine
Chlorzoxazone
Doxorubicin
Ibuprofen
Mannose
Phenacetin
Phenazopyridine
Phenothiazines
Phenytoin
Rifampin
Salicylazosulfapyridine

Red
Anthraquinones
Beets
Blackberries
Eosin
Erythrocytes
Hemoglobin
Myoglobin
Porphyrins
Rhubarb

Yellow-Brown
Aloe
Anthraquinones

Chloroquine
Fava beans
Nitrofurantoin
Primaquine
Rhubarb
Sulfamethoxazole

Yellow
Fluorescein
Phenacetin
Quinacrine
Riboflavin
Santonin

Yellow-Orange
Aminopyrine
Anisindione
Carrots
Sulfasalazine
Vitamin A
Warfarin

Black
Alcaptonuria
Homogentisic acid
Melanin
p-Hydroxyphenylpyruvic acid

Brown-Black
Cascara
Iron
Methyldopa
Phenylhydrazine
Senna

Greenish-Blue
Amitriptyline
Anthraquinones
Biliverdin
Chlorophyll breath mints
Flavin derivatives
Indicans

Indigo blue
Magnesium salicylate
Methylene blue
Phenol
Thymol

been used to treat cyclophosphamide-induced hemorrhagic cystitis.[85] In an animal model, pretreatment with hyperbaric oxygen reduces the incidence of hemorrhagic cystitis.[58] In severe cases, hypogastric artery ligation and/or cystectomy may be required to control bleeding.[58]

An outbreak of hemorrhagic cystitis occurred in workers in a packaging plant after exposure to chlordimeform, a formamidine insecticide used to control mites and insects on cotton. Nine workers developed abdominal pain, dysuria, urgency, and hematuria, with biopsy-proven hemorrhagic cystitis.[44] Eight young adults developed painful hematuria after consuming "bootleg" methaqualone. The cause was orthotoluidine, a compound utilized in the

synthesis of methaqualone, and the symptoms occurred within 6 hours of ingestion.[54] Cases of hemorrhagic cystitis have also been described with ticarcillin,[81] nafcillin, penicillin G, carbenicillin, piperacillin, isoniazid, indomethacin, tiaprofenic acid, and busulphan.[50,84,116]

SUMMARY

Toxicologic evaluation of the reproductive and urinary system is difficult. Reproduction is an intermittent phenomenon. Adverse effects from toxicant exposures to both the male and female reproductive systems may not be noticed until fertility is desired. Toxicants can affect the hormonal controls or the gametogenesis organs. Sexual dysfunction, whether psychogenic or toxin-induced, negatively impacts fertility. Agents used to treat sexual dysfunction, aphrodisiacs, can have adverse systemic effects. Adverse effects on the genitourinary tract are often overlooked when evaluating the toxicologic potential of various agents. Few physical findings, laboratory tests, or ancillary studies will aid in diagnosis. A thorough history including past and present medications, illicit drug use, occupational and environmental exposures, or the use of herbal or alternative therapies is mandatory in the evaluation of patients with genitourinary complaints.

REFERENCES

1. Ambrosi B, Bara R, Travaglini P, et al: Study of the effects of bromocriptine on sexual impotence. Clin Endocrin 1977;7:417–421.
2. Anderson IB, Mullen WH, Meeker JE, et al: Pennyroyal toxicity: Measurement of toxic metabolite levels in two cases and review of the literature. Ann Intern Med 1996;124:726–734.
3. Antomiou LD, Shalhoub RJ, Sudbaker T, Smith JC: Reversal of uraemic impotence by zinc. Lancet 1977;2:895–898.
4. Ash P: The influence of radiation on fertility in man. Br J Radiology 1980;53:271–278.
5. Axelsen RA, Leditschke JF, Burke JR: Renal and urinary tract complications following the intravesical instillation of formalin. Pathology 1986;18:453–458.
6. Bakerink JA, Gospe SM, Dimand RJ, et al: Multiple organ failure after ingestion of pennyroyal oil from herbal tea in two infants. Pediatrics 1996;98:944–947.
7. Baranski B: Effects of the workplace on fertility and related reproductive outcomes. Env Health Perspect 1993;101(Suppl 2):81–90.
8. Baulieu EE: RU–486 as an antiprogesterone steroid: From receptor to contragestion and beyond. JAMA 1989;262:1808–1814.
9. Beeley L: Drug-induced sexual dysfunction and infertility. Adv Drug React Pois Rev 1984;3:23–42.
10. Biava CG, Smuckler EA, Whorton D: The testicular morphology of individuals exposed to dibromochloropropane. Exp Mol Pathol 1978;29:448–458.
11. Boolell M, Allen MJ, Ballard SA, et al: Sildenafil: An orally active type 5 cyclic GMP-specific phosphodiesterase inhibitor for the treatment of penile erectile dysfunction. Int J Impot Res 1996;8:47–52.
12. Bommer J, Ritz E, del Pozo E, Bommer G: Improved sexual function in male hemodialysis patients on bromocriptine. Lancet 1979; 2:496–497.
13. Brandes JC, Bufill JA: Amyl nitrite-induced hemolytic anemia. Am J Med 1989;86:252–254.
14. Brearly RL, Forsythe AM: Lead poisoning from aphrodisiacs: Potential hazard in immigrants. Br Med J 1978;2:1748–1749.
15. Brubacher JR, Lachmanen D, Ravikumar PR, et al: Treatment of toad venom poisoning with digoxin-specific Fab fragments. Chest 1996;110:1282–1288.

16. Brubacher JR, Lachmanen D, Ravikumar PR, Hoffman RS. Efficacy of digoxin specific Fab fragments (Digibind) in the treatment of toad venom poisoning. Toxicon 1999;37:931–942.

17. Brubacher JR, Ravikumar PR, Hoffman RS: Deaths associated with a purported aphrodisiac—New York City, February 1993–May 1995. MMWR Morb Mortal Wkly Rep 1995;44:853–854.

18. Buchanan JF, Davis LJ: Drug-induced infertility. Drug Intell Clin Pharm 1984;18:122–132.

19. Buechel DW: Pennyroyal oil ingestion: Report of a case. J Am Osteopath Assoc 1983;2:793–794.

20. Buffum J: Pharmacosexology updates: Prescription drugs and sexual function. J Psychoactive Drugs 1986;18:97–102.

21. Burnett WC, Chahine RA: Sexual dysfunction as a complication of propranolol therapy in men. Cardiovasc Med 1979;5:811–815.

22. Castleden CM, Duffin HM, Gulati RS: Double-blind study of imipramine and placebo for incontinence due to bladder instability. Age Ageing 1986;15:299–303.

23. Chapple CR, Parkhouse H, Gardener C, et al: Double-blind, placebo-controlled, crossover study of flavoxate in the treatment of idiopathic detrusor instability. Br J Urol 1990;66:491–494.

24. Cheitlin MD, Hutter AM, Brindis RG, et al: Use of sildenafil (Viagra) in patients with cardiovascular disease. ACC/AHA Expert Consensus Document. Circulation 1999;99:168–177.

25. Chutka DS, Fleming KC, Evans MP, et al: Urinary incontinence in the elderly population. Mayo Clin Proc 1996;71:93–101.

26. Clayton DO, Shen WW: Psychotropic drug-induced sexual function disorders: Diagnosis, incidence, and management. Drug Saf 1998; 19:299–312.

27. Coelho HLL, Teixeira AC, Santos AP, et al: Misoprostol and illegal abortion in Fortaleza, Brazil. Lancet 1993;341:1261–1263.

28. Collste L, Lindskog M: Phenylpropanolamine in treatment of female stress urinary incontinence: Double-blind placebo controlled study in 24 patients. Urology 1987;30:398–403.

29. Corriere JN, Fishman IJ, Benson GS, et al: Development of fibrotic penile lesions secondary to the intracorporeal injection of vasoactive agents. J Urol 1988;140:615–617.

30. Costa SH, Vessey MP: Misoprostol and illegal abortion in Rio de Janerio, Brazil. Lancet 1993;341:1258–1261.

31. Craven JD, Polak A: Cantharidin poisoning. Br Med J 1954;2: 1386–1389.

32. Christin-Maitre S, Bouchard P, Spitz IM: Medical termination of pregnancy. N Engl J Med 2000;342:946–956.

33. Czajka P, Field J, Novak P, Kunnecke J: Accidental aphrodisiac ingestion. Tenn Med 1978;71:747–750.

34. Dax EM, Lange WR, Jaffe JH: Allergic reactions to amyl nitrite inhalation. Am J Med 1989;86:732.

35. DeSmet PA, Smeets OS: Potential risks of health food products containing yohimbe extracts. Br Med J 1994;309:958.

36. Ditlove J, Weidmann P, Bernstein M, et al: Methicillin nephritis. Medicine 1977;56:483–491.

37. Dlugosz L, Bracken MB: Reproductive effects of caffeine: A review and theoretical analysis. Epidemiol Rev 1992;14:83–100.

38. Dolan G, Blumsohn A, Brown MJ, et al: Lead poisoning due to Asian ethnic treatment for impotence. R Soc Med 1991;84:630–631.

39. Droller MJ, Saral R, Santos G: Prevention of cyclophosphamide-induced hemorrhagic cystitis. Urology 1982;20:256–258.

40. Ducker TE, Fleet WF, Morgan HJ: A case of cyanosis without hypoxemia. Tenn Med 1990;83:22.

41. Dunkel VC, Rogers-Back AM, Lawlar TE, et al: Mutagenicity of some alkyl nitrites used as recreational drugs. Environ Mol Mutagen 1989;14:115–122.

42. Egan R, Pomeranz H: Sildenafil (Viagra) associated anterior ischemic optic neuropathy. Arch Ophthalmol 2000;118:291–292.

43. Fisher AA: "Poppers" or "Snappers" dermatitis in homosexual men. Cutis 1984;34:120–122.

44. Folland DS, Kimbrough RD, Cline R, et al: Acute hemorrhagic cystitis. JAMA 1978;239:1052–1055.

45. Fontanarosa PB, Roush WR: Acute urinary retention. Emerg Med Clin North Am 1988;6:419–437.

46. Friesen K, Palatnick W, Tenenbein M: Benign course after massive ingestion of yohimbine. J Emerg Med 1993;11:287–288.

47. Gaillard RC, Herrmann W: Clinical use of RU-486: Control of the menstrual cycle and effect on the hypophyseal-adrenal axis. Ann Endocrinol 1983;44:345–346.

48. Garfield SL, Gershon S, Sletten F, et al: Chemically induced anxiety. Int J Neuropsychiatry 1967;3:426–433.

49. Gellman E, Kissane J, Frech R, et al: Cyclophosphamide cystitis. J Can Assoc Radiol 1969;20:99–101.

50. Ghose K: Cystitis and nonsteroidal antiinflammatory drugs: An incidental association or an adverse effect? N Z Med J 1993;106: 501–503.

51. Gilja I, Radej M, Kovacic M, Parazajder J: Conservative treatment of female stress incontinence with imipramine. J Urol 1984;132: 909–911.

52. Goedert JJ, Neuland CY, Wallen WC, et al: Amyl nitrite may alter T lymphocytes in homosexual men. Lancet 1982;1:412–415.

53. Goldberg AB, Greenberg BS, Darney PD: Misoprostol and pregnancy. N Engl J Med 2001;344:38–47.

54. Goldfarb M, Finelli: R Necrotizing cystitis secondary to "Bootleg" methaqualone. Urology 1974;3:54–55.

55. Goldfrank L, Osborn H: Rainbow urine. Hosp Phys 1978;3:22–26.

56. Goldstein I, Lue TF, Padma-Nathan H, et al: Oral sildenafil in the treatment of erectile dysfunction. N Engl J Med 1998;338: 1397–1404.

57. Grunberg SM, Weiss MH, Spitz JM, et al: Treatment of unresectable meningiomas with the antiprogesterone agent mifepristone. J Neurosurg 1991;74:861–866.

58. Hader JE, Marzella L, Myers RA, et al: Hyperbaric oxygen treatment for experimental cyclophosphamide-induced hemorrhagic cystitis. J Urol 1993;149:1617–1621.

59. Haverkos HW, Dougherty J: Health hazards of nitrite inhalants. Am J Med 1988;84:479–482.

60. Hogan MJ, Wallin JD, Baer RM: Antihypertensive therapy and male sexual dysfunction. Psychosomatics 1980;21:234–237.

61. Holmberg G, Gershon S: Autonomic and psychic effects of yohimbine hydrochloride. Psychopharmacologia 1961;2:93–106.

62. Jayalakshmamma B, Pinkel D: Urinary-bladder toxicity following pelvic irradiation and simultaneous cyclophosphamide therapy. Cancer 1976;38:701–707.

63. Karras DJ, Farrell SE, Harrigan RA, et al: Poisoning from "Spanish fly" (cantharidin). Am J Emerg Med 1996;14:478–483.

64. Kassim AA, Fabry ME, Nagel RL: Acute priapism associated with the use of sildenafil in a patient with sickle cell trait. Blood 2000; 95:1878–1879.

65. Klein FA, Smith MJV: Urinary complications of cyclophosphamide therapy. South Med J 1983;76:1413–1416.

66. Kotsonis FN, Dood DC, Regnier B, et al: Preclinical toxicology profile of misoprostol. Dig Dis Sci 1985;30:142S–146S.

67. Kwan T, Palusco AD, Kohl L: Digitalis toxicity caused by toad venom. Chest 1992;102:949–950.

68. Landis E, Shore E: Yohimbine-induced bronchospasm. Chest 1989; 96:1424.

69. Landrigan PJ: Current issues in the epidemiology and toxicology of occupational exposure to lead. Environ Health Perspect 1990;89: 61–66.

70. Lawrence HJ, Simone J, Aur RJA: Cyclophosphamide-induced hemorrhagic cystitis in children with leukemia. Cancer 1975;36: 1572–1576.

71. Levitt NS, Vinik AL, Sive AA, et al: Synthetic leutenizing hormone in impotent male diabetics: A double-blind cross-over trial. S Afr Med J 1980;57:701–704.

72. Lidberg L, Sternthal V: A new approach to the hormonal treatment of impotentia erectonis. Pharmacopsychiatry Neuropsychopharmacol 1977;10:21–25.

73. Lin SC, Hsu T, Fredrickson PA, Richelson E: Yohimbine- and tranylcypromine-induced postural hypotension. Am J Psychiatry 1987;144:119.

74. Linden CH, Vellman WP, Rumack B: Yohimbine: A new street drug. Ann Emerg Med 1985;14:1002–1004.

75. Lycka B: Amyl and butyl nitrites and telangiectasias in homosexual men. Ann Intern Med 1987;106:476.

76. Machabert R, Testud F, Descotes J: Methaemoglobinaemia due to amyl nitrite inhalation: A case report. Hum Exp Toxicol 1994;13: 313–314.

77. MacKenzie IZ, Davies AJ, Embrey MP, Guillebaud J: Very early abortion by prostaglandins. Lancet 1978;1:1223–1226.

78. Margolis R, Prieto P, Stein L, Chinn S: Statistical summary of 10,000 male cases using aphrodex in treatment of impotence. Curr Ther Res 1971;13:616–621.

79. Marks LB, Carroll PR, Dugan TC, Anscher MS: The response of the urinary bladder, urethra, and ureter to radiation and chemotherapy. Int J Radiat Oncol Biol Phys 1995;31:1257–1280.

80. Marmor M, Friedman-Kein AE, Laubenstein LL, et al: Risk factors for Kaposi's sarcoma in homosexual men. Lancet 1982;1: 1083–1087.

81. Marx CM, Alpert SE: Ticarcillin-induced cystitis. AJDC 1984;138: 670–672.

82. Mattison DR, Plowchalk DR, Meadows MJ, et al: Reproductive toxicity: Male and female reproductive systems as targets for chemical injury. Med Clin North Am 1990;74:391–411.

83. Medical Research Council Working Party: Adverse reactions to bendrofluazide and propranolol for the treatment of mild hypertension. Lancet 1981;2:539–543.

84. Millard RJ: Busulphan haemorrhagic cystitis. Br J Urol 1978;50:210.

85. Miller LJ, Chandler SW, Ippoliti CM: Treatment of cyclophosphamide-induced hemorrhagic cystitis with prostaglandins. Ann Pharmacother 1994;28:590–594.

86. Moore KH, Hay DM, Imrie AE, et al: Oxybutynin hydrochloride (3 mg) in the treatment of women with idiopathic detrusor instability. Br J Urol 1990;66:479–485.

87. Morales A, Condra M, Owen JA, et al: Is yohimbine effective in the treatment of organic impotence? Results of a controlled trial. J Urol 1987;137:1168–1172.

88. Moreland RB, Hseih G, Nakane M, et al: The biochemical and neurologic basis for the treatment of male erectile dysfunction. J Pharmcol Exp Ther 2000;296:225–234.

89. Mudd JW: Impotence responsive to glyceryl trinitrate. Am J Psychiatry 1977;134:922–925.

90. Mukherjee B, Bhose IN: Induction of labour and abortion with quinine infusion in intrauterine foetal death. Am J Obstet Gynecol 1968; 101:853–854.

91. Newman RJ, Salerno HR: Sexual dysfunction due to methyldopa. Br Med J 1974;4:106.

92. Nickolis LC, Teare D: Poisoning by cantharidin. Br Med J 1954;2: 1384–1388.

93. Nudelman RW, Saleman M: The birth of the blues II: Blue movie. JAMA 1987;257:3230.

94. Oaks WW, DiTunno DJ, Magnani T, et al: Cantharidin poisoning. Arch Intern Med 1960;105:574–582.

95. Olsen J: Is human fecundity declining—And does occupational exposure play a role in such a decline if it exists? Scand J Work Environ Health 1994;20:72–77.

96. Owen JA, Nakatsu SL, Fenemore J, et al: The pharmacokinetics of yohimbine in man. Eur J Clin Pharmacol 1987;32:577–582.

97. Paeyron R, Aubeny E, Targosz V, et al: Early termination of pregnancy with mifepristone (RU-486) and the orally active prostaglandin misoprostol. N Engl J Med 1993;328:1503–1513.

98. Parry MF, Wallach R: Ethylene glycol poisoning. Am J Med 1974; 57:143–150.

99. Paul M, Himmelstein J. Reproductive hazards in the workplace: What the practitioner needs to know about chemical exposures. Obstet Gynecol 1988;71:921–938.

100. Paumgartten FJ, Castilla EE, Monteleone-Neto R, et al: Risk assessment in reproductive toxicology as practiced in South America. In: Neubert D, Kavlock RJ, Merker HJ, Klein J, eds: Risk Assessment of Prenatally Induced Adverse Health Effects. Berlin, Springer-Verlag, 1992, pp. 163–179.

101. Paumgartten FJR, Magalhaes-de-Souza CA, de-Carvalho RR, Chahoud I: Embryotoxic effects of misoprostol in the mouse. Braz J Med Biol Res 1995;28:355–361.

102. Perrone J, Hoffman RS: Toxic ingestions in pregnancy: Abortifacient use in a case series of pregnant overdose patients. Acad Emerg Med 1997;4:206–209.

103. Plotz PH, Klippel JH, Decker JL, et al: Bladder complications in patients receiving cyclophosphamide for systemic lupus erythematosus or rheumatoid arthritis. Ann Intern Med 1979;91:221–223.

104. Polettini A, Crippa O, Ravagli A, Saragoni A: A fatal case of poisoning with cantharidin. Forensic Sci Int 1992;56:37–43.

105. Price LH, Charney DS, Heninger GR: Three cases of manic symptoms following yohimbine administration. Am J Psychiatry 1984;141:1267–1268.

106. Rabe T, Basse H, Thuro H, et al: Wirkung des PGE-1-Methylanalogons Misoprostol auf den schwangeren Uterus im ersten Trimester. Geburtshilfe Frauenheilkol 1987;47:324–331.

107. Relling MV, Schunk JE: Drug-induced hemorrhagic cystitis. Clin Pharm 1986;5:590–597.

108. Reproductive health and mifepristone [editorial]. Lancet 1990;336: 1480–1481.

109. Rosen RC, Ashton AK: Prosexual drugs: Empirical status of the "new aphrodisiacs." Arch Sex Behav 1993;22:521–543.

110. Rosoff MH, Cohen MV: Profound bradycardia after amyl nitrite in patients with a tendency to vasovagal episodes. Br Heart J 1986;55: 97–100.

111. Sandler B, Aronson P: Yohimbine-induced cutaneous drug eruption, progressive renal failure, and lupus-like syndrome. Urology 1993; 41:343–345.

112. Schilsky RL, Lewis BJ, Sherins RJ, et al: Gonadal dysfunction in patients receiving chemotherapy for cancer. Ann Intern Med 1980;93: 109–114.

113. Schlegel PN, Chang TK, Marshall FF: Antibiotics: Potential hazards to male fertility. Fertil Steril 1991;55:235–242.

114. Schrag SD, Dixon RL: Occupational exposures associated with male reproductive dysfunction. Annu Rev Pharmacol Toxicol 1985;25: 567–592.

115. Shah PK: Sildenafil in the treatment of erectile dysfunction. N Engl J Med 1998;339:699.

116. Shieh C, Chen B, Lin K: Late onset hemorrhagic cystitis after allogeneic bone marrow transplantation. Taiwan I Hsuen Hui Tsa Chih 1989;88:508–511.

117. Stillwell TJ, Benson RC: Cyclophosphamide-induced hemorrhagic cystitis. Cancer 1988;61:451–457.

118. Sullivan JB, Rumack BH, Thomas H, et al: Pennyroyal oil poisoning and hepatotoxicity. JAMA 1979;242:2873–2874.

119. Susset JG, Tessier CD, Wincze J, et al: Effect of yohimbine hydrochloride on erectile impotence: A double-blind study. J Urol 1989;141:1360–1363.

120. Tackett RE: Priapism. In: Stine RJ, Chudnofsky CR, eds: A Practical Approach to Emergency Medicine, 2nd ed. Boston, Little, Brown, 1994, pp. 710–711.

121. Till JS, Majmudar BN: Cantharidin poisoning. South Med J 1981; 74:444–447.

122. Tsao SW, Ng TB, Yeung HW: Toxicities of trichosanthin and alphamomorcharin, abortifacient proteins from Chinese medicinal plants, on cultured tumor cell lines. Toxicon 1990;28:1183–1192.

123. Van Jeijst ANP, de Jong W, Seldenrijk R, et al: Coma and crystalluria: A massive primidone intoxication treated with hemoperfusion. J Toxicol Clin Toxicol 1983;20:307–318.

124. Warne GL, Fairley KF, Hobbs JB, et al: Cyclophosphamide-induced ovarian failure. N Engl J Med 1973;289:1159–1162.

125. Warren SC, Warren SG: Propranolol and sexual impotence [letter]. Ann Intern Med 1977;86:112.

126. Webb DJ, Freestone S, Allen MJ, et al: Sildenafil citrate and blood-pressure-lowering drugs: Results of drug interaction studies with an organic nitrate and a calcium antagonist. Am J Cardiol 1999;83: 21C–28C.

127. Wetterling T, Veltrup C, Driessen M, et al: Drinking pattern and alcohol-related medical disorders. Alcohol 1999;34:330–336.

128. Whorton MD, Foliart DE: Mutagenicity, carcinogenicity, and reproductive effects of dibromochloropropane (DBCP). Mutat Res 1983; 123:13–30.

129. Wilcox AJ, Baird DD, Weinberg CR, Hornsby PP, et al: Fertility in men exposed prenatally to diethylstilbestrol. N Engl J Med 1995; 332:1411–1416.

130. Wilson B: The effect of drugs on male sexual function and fertility. Nurse Pract 1991;16:12–24.

131. Winder C: Reproductive and chromosomal effects of occupational exposure to lead in the male. Reprod Toxicol 1989;3:221–233.

132. Winek CL, Davis ER, Collom WD, Shanon SP: Quinine fatality—Case report. Clin Toxicol 1974;7:129–132.

133. Wolf LR, Otten EJ, Spadafora MP: Cinchonism: Two case reports and review of acute quinine toxicity and treatment. J Emerg Med 1992;10:295–301.

134. Woodrum ST, Brown CS. Management of SSRI-induced sexual dysfunction. Ann Pharmacother 1998;32:1209–1215.

135. Yealy DM, Hogya PT: Priapism. Emerg Med Clin North Am 1988; 6:509–520.

THE CLINICAL BASIS
OF MEDICAL TOXICOLOGY

I. CASE STUDIES IN TOXICOLOGIC EMERGENCIES

CHAPTER 31 MANAGING THE SYMPTOMATIC PATIENT WITH A POSSIBLE TOXIC EXPOSURE

Neal E. Flomenbaum, Lewis R. Goldfrank, Neal A. Lewin,
Mary Ann Howland, Robert S. Hoffman, and Lewis S. Nelson

Emergency Medical Services (EMS) was dispatched to the house of an 18-year-old male described by his mother as "barely arousable." When the paramedics arrived, the patient was lethargic, seemingly disoriented, hyperventilating, and "intermittently shaking" or shivering. In the patient's bedroom, the paramedics found empty medication containers labeled "erythromycin 500 mg", "Tylenol with Codeine #3", and "Robitussin DM". Upon questioning, the patient told the paramedics that he was trying to kill himself. His mother informed the paramedics that her son had been diagnosed as "asthmatic" as a child, but she did not believe that he had been using any asthma medications recently. After obtaining a blood pressure (BP) of 130/70 mm Hg, a pulse rate of 120 beats/min, and a respiratory rate of 24–36 breaths/min, the paramedics started an IV of D_5W to keep the vein open (KVO), and then transported the patient and the empty medication containers to the Emergency Department (ED).

In the ED, the patient was arousable to voice and was able to follow simple commands. Vital signs upon arrival were BP—120/80 mm Hg; pulse rate—96–108 beats/min; respiratory rate—20 breaths/min; and rectal temperature—98.4°F (36.9°C). The initial physical evaluation revealed a young adult male with no evidence of head or body trauma; pupils that were equal, round, and reactive to light; a poor gag reflex; a supple neck; clear breath sounds bilaterally; regular rapid heart sounds without murmurs, rubs, or gallops; a soft abdomen without scars or organomegaly; and normal extremities without clubbing, cyanosis, or edema. A bedside determination revealed a blood glucose of 100 mg/dL.

Based on their initial evaluation, the ED staff considered a differential diagnosis that included toxic exposures, sepsis, metabolic disorders, and structural and nonstructural cerebrovascular compromise. Information obtained from the patient and his mother regarding the possibilities of asthma, suicidal ideation, and exposure to particular medications such as antibiotics, antipyretics, and asthma medications, led the staff to request tests in addition to the few toxicologic and nontoxicologic tests routinely ordered for patients with suspected toxicologic exposures: routine tests are blood glucose and acetaminophen levels. In this case, the staff elected to draw blood samples for complete blood count (CBC), blood urea nitrogen (BUN), glucose, electrolytes, acetaminophen, salicylates, theophylline, and ethanol levels.

A portable chest radiograph was requested and an electrocardiogram (ECG) was obtained, which revealed a supraventricular tachycardia with narrow complexes (QRS = 0.08 sec) at a rate of 120–140 beats/min and a right-axis deviation. Because the patient was no longer arousable to voice, a decision was made to intubate him to protect his airway and to allow for safe orogastric lavage and instillation of activated charcoal (AC). While being intubated, the patient began having generalized tonic-clonic seizures, requiring a total of 20 mg of diazepam IV to achieve control. After the seizure activity ended, the patient was intubated, lavaged, and given activated charcoal. The pink lavage fluid contained white pill fragments. Urine obtained by catheterization was odorless and appeared normal in color. A portable chest radiograph revealed clear lungs and endotracheal and orogastric tubes that appeared to be correctly placed. The patient remained comatose throughout the time he spent in the ED prior to transfer to the Intensive Care Unit (ICU).

The CBC revealed a white blood [cell] count (WBC) of 18,000/mm³ with a normal differential and a normal hemoglobin. Urinalysis was within normal limits as were the prothrombin time (PT) and partial thromboplastin time (PTT). Blood glucose was 134 mg/dL and K^+ was 3.1 mEq/L. BUN and all other electrolytes tested, including Ca^{2+} and Mg^{2+}, were normal. The blood ethanol level was 75 mg/dL. Salicylate and theophylline levels were negative. The initial acetaminophen level was 40 µg/mL. The (arterial blood gases ABG) specimen, planned prior to the seizure to assess oxygenation and ventilation was instead drawn immediately after cessation of seizure activity and revealed a pH of 7.29, Pco_2 of 45.5 mm Hg, and Po_2 of 370 mm Hg on 100% Fio_2. One hour later, repeat ABG values were pH 7.49, Pco_2 31.7 mm Hg, and Po_2 307 mm Hg.

After the patient was extubated the next morning, he told the psychiatric consultant that he was depressed and had tried to commit suicide. He spoke of ingesting unknown quantities of erythromycin, Tylenol with Codeine, Robitussin DM, and several other pills from his medicine cabinet at home that he could not identify. He also confirmed that he had not been using any asthma medications for the past several years and had no symptoms of lung or airway problems. He denied the use of any other medications or illicit drugs.

On the second hospital day, the patient was transferred from the ICU to a "med-psych" floor and on day 5 he was transferred to the psychiatric service.

This case illustrates many of the problems clinicians face in managing ill patients with possible toxic exposures. Rarely, if ever, are all of the circumstances of a toxic exposure known: the history may be incomplete, unreliable, or unobtainable; multiple drugs, medications, or toxins may be involved; and even when a drug etiology is identified, it may not be easy to determine whether we are dealing with an overdose, an allergic or idiosyncratic reaction, or a drug-drug interaction. Similarly, it is sometimes difficult or impossible to differentiate between adverse effects of a correct dose of medication or the consequences of a deliberate or unintentional overdose. The patient's presenting signs and symptoms may force us to intervene at a time when we have almost no information about the etiology of the patient's condition and therefore therapeutic agents often must be thoughtfully chosen empirically to treat or diagnose a condition without exacerbating the situation. What is the initial management of a patient with an unknown overdose? What constitutes a "primary survey" and primary treatment for a comatose patient suspected of a drug overdose? What is an adequate "secondary survey," and what further interventions are required early on? When should attempts be made to eliminate absorbed toxins from the body, and what methods to do so are available? What are the management pitfalls to be avoided?

Conscious patients, asymptomatic patients, and pregnant patients with possible toxic exposures raise additional management issues, as do the victims of toxic cutaneous or ophthalmic exposures. This chapter represents our efforts to formulate a logical approach to managing the ill patient with a probable or actual toxic exposure.

Probably the most frequent toxicologic emergency that clinicians deal with is the patient with a suspected toxic exposure, sometimes referred to as *an unknown overdose*. Considering not only the patient with an altered mental status but those patients who are suicidal, those who use illicit drugs, and those who are exposed to medications or substances that they are unaware of, the majority of toxicologic emergencies at least partially fall under this category.

To effectively manage the patient with a suspected toxicologic exposure, clinicians must be able to utilize the principles developed in Part A of this text, "General Approach to Medical Toxicology." In that section, a basic principle of modern toxicologic management was described, which is that **for the vast majority of patients with toxic exposures, the clinical condition of the patient, rather than the specific ingredients of the exposure, dictates the management.** In other words, **treat the patient, not the poison, and do no harm**. Such an approach does not preclude identifying and treating specifically for certain toxins and/or toxic syndromes. But even in these situations, basic clinical management techniques must never be neglected.

When the principle of treating the patient, not the poison, is applied to managing the patient with a suspected toxicologic exposure, the answers to several early management questions become apparent. For example, when an unconscious patient presents, how do we know that we are dealing with an overdose? If the patient has obvious trauma, how do we know the patient has not also been exposed to a toxic substance? Clearly what is required is an approach that will identify and treat or exclude toxicologic etiologies of the patient's condition and, in any case, cause no harm to the patient.

INITIAL MANAGEMENT OF A PATIENT WITH A SUSPECTED TOXIC EXPOSURE

Similar to the management of any seriously compromised patient, the clinical approach to the patient who was exposed to a toxin begins with the recognition and treatment of life-threatening conditions: *a*irway compromise, *b*reathing difficulties, and *c*irculatory problems such as hypotension and serious dysrhythmias. Once the ABCs are addressed, the patient's level of consciousness should be assessed, as this helps to determine the techniques to be used for further management of the exposure.

"PRIMARY SURVEY" FOR THE PATIENT WITH AN ALTERED MENTAL STATUS AND SUSPECTED TOXIC EXPOSURE

After the airway is clear, and either cervical spine trauma is excluded or the cervical spine is protected, an initial bedside assessment should be made regarding the adequacy of respiration. If a qualitative bedside assessment of depth and rate is not possible, then at least the presence or absence of regular breathing should be determined. In this setting, any irregular breathing pattern should be considered a possible sign of the incipient cessation of breathing requiring hyperventilation with 100% oxygen by bag-valve-mask followed as soon as possible by tracheal intubation. Tracheal intubation is probably indicated for most cases of coma resulting from a toxic exposure, not only to insure and maintain control of the airway but also to enable safe performance of procedures to prevent gastrointestinal absorption or eliminate previously absorbed toxins. As soon as practicable, an ABG determination should be made because it will more accurately define the adequacy of oxygenation (PO_2, O_2 saturation) and ventilation (PCO_2), and because it might also alert the physician to possible toxic-metabolic etiologies of coma (pH, PCO_2). In addition, when clinically indicated, a carboxyhemoglobin determination is necessary to diagnose or exclude carbon monoxide poisoning.

After the patient's respiratory status is assessed and treated, the strength, rate, and regularity of the pulse should be evaluated, the blood pressure determined, and a rectal temperature obtained. Both a 12-lead ECG and continuous ECG monitoring are essential. Monitoring will alert the clinician to dysrhythmias that are directly or indirectly (via hypoxemia, electrolyte imbalance) related to toxic exposures. A 12-lead ECG demonstrating QRS widening and axis deviation might indicate a life-threatening cyclic antidepressant (or type IA or IC antidysrhythmic agent) exposure, enabling the physician to anticipate such serious sequelae as ventricular tachydysrhythmias, seizures, and cardiac arrest, and suggesting both the early use of specific treatment and antidotes such as intravenous sodium bicarbonate and the avoidance of some medications such as procainamide, quinidine, and other IA and IC antidysrhythmics that could exacerbate the situation. Other ECG changes such as PR and QTc lengthening or shortening, baseline changes, and T and U-wave abnormalities may point to cardioactive drug toxicity and serious electrolyte abnormalities.

Extremes of core body temperature must be addressed early in the evaluation and treatment of a comatose patient. Life-threatening hyperthermia (temperature ≥105°F or ≥40.5°C) is usually appreciated when the patient is touched. Regardless of the etiology, such temperatures must be immediately reduced to about 101.5°F (38.7°C) by ice water immersion or by fan-mist treatment to prevent catastrophic complications or death (Chap. 18). Hypothermia is probably easier to miss than hyperthermia, especially in northern states during winter months, when most arriving patients feel cold to the touch. Early recognition of hypothermia, however, helps to avoid administering a variety of medications that may be ineffective until the patient becomes relatively euthermic, at which time iatrogenic drug toxicity may result.

For the hypotensive patient with clear lungs and an unknown overdose, a fluid challenge with 0.9% NaCl or lactated Ringer solution may be started. At the time the IV line is secured, blood samples for glucose, electrolytes, BUN, a CBC, and toxicologic analysis should be drawn. **In the vast majority of cases, the blood tests that are most useful in diagnosing toxicologic emergencies are not the toxicologic assays but the nontoxicologic tests such as BUN, glucose, electrolytes, and ABG.** If the patient remains hypotensive or cannot tolerate fluids, a vasopressor or an inotrope may be indicated.

Drug or toxin-related seizures may broadly be divided into three categories: (a) those that respond to standard anticonvulsant treatment, typically a benzodiazepine (eg, ethanol withdrawal); (b) those that either require specific antidotes to control seizure activity or that do not respond consistently to standard anticonvulsant treatment (eg, isoniazid-induced seizures requiring pyridoxine administration); and (c) those that may *appear* to respond to initial treatment with cessation of tonic-clonic activity, but which leave the patient exposed to the underlying, unidentified toxin or to continued electrical seizure activity in the brain (eg, carbon monoxide or hypoglycemia of any etiology).

"PRIMARY TREATMENT" FOR THE PATIENT WITH AN ALTERED MENTAL STATUS RESULTING FROM A SUSPECTED TOXIC EXPOSURE

Within the first 5 minutes of managing a patient with altered mental status, four therapeutic agents should either be administered or considered: (a) dextrose 0.5–1.0 g/kg of $D_{50}W$ for an adult, or a more dilute dextrose solution ($D_{10}W$ or $D_{25}W$) for a child, to diagnose and to treat, or to exclude, hypoglycemia; (b) thiamine 100 mg IV for an adult (usually unnecessary for a child) to prevent or treat Wernicke's encephalopathy; (c) naloxone 0.4–2 mg IV for adults and children with respiratory compromise; and (d) high-flow oxygen (8–10 L/min).

"SECONDARY SURVEY" FOR A PATIENT WITH AN ALTERED MENTAL STATUS RESULTING FROM A SUSPECTED TOXIC EXPOSURE

While examining a patient with an altered mental status (AMS) for clues to the etiology of a presumably toxic-metabolic form of AMS, it is especially important to search for any indication that trauma may have caused, contributed to, or resulted from the patient's condition.

The remainder of the physical examination should be performed rapidly, but reasonably thoroughly. In addition to evaluating the level of consciousness, the physician should note abnormal posturing (decorticate or decerebrate), abnormal or unilateral withdrawal responses, and pupil size and reactivity. Pinpoint pupils suggest exposure to opioids or organic phosphorus insecticides, and widely dilated pupils suggest anticholinergic or sympathomimetic poisoning. The presence or absence of nystagmus, abnormal reflexes, and any other focal neurologic findings may provide important clues to a structural cause of AMS. Assigning the patient a Glasgow Coma Score (GCS); if not already done during the first survey provides a useful measure for assessing any changes in neurologic status, but the GCS should never be used for prognostic purposes, because complete recovery from properly managed toxic-metabolic coma despite a low GCS is the rule rather than the exception.

Characteristic breath or skin odors frequently identify the etiology of coma. The fruity odor of ketones on the breath suggests diabetic or alcoholic ketoacidosis, but also the possible ingestion of acetone, or isopropyl alcohol, which is metabolized to acetone. The pungent, minty odor of oil of wintergreen on the breath or skin suggests methyl salicylate poisoning. The odors of other substances such as cyanide ("bitter almonds"), hydrogen sulfide ("rotten eggs"), and organic phosphorus compounds ("garlic") are described in detail in Chapter 28.

"SECONDARY SURVEY" FOR *ALL* PATIENTS WITH A SUSPECTED TOXIC EXPOSURE

Reauscultation of breath sounds, particularly after a fluid challenge has been initiated, helps to diagnose pulmonary edema, or acute lung injury, or an aspiration pneumonia, if present. Coupled with an abnormal breath odor of hydrocarbons or organic phosphorus compounds, for example, crackles and rhonchi may point to a pulmonary *etiology* (which is important, because the administration of cardiac medications may be inappropriate or dangerous in these circumstances).

Heart murmurs in an intravenous drug user, especially when accompanied by fever, may indicate bacterial endocarditis. Bradydysrhythmias and tachydysrhythmias may suggest overdoses or inappropriate use of cardioactive medications (digoxin, β-adrenergic antagonists, calcium channel blockers, cyclic antidepressants).

Abdominal examination may reveal signs of trauma or alcohol-related hepatic disease. The presence or absence of bowel sounds helps to exclude or to diagnose anticholinergic toxicity, and is important in considering whether to manipulate the gastrointestinal tract in an attempt to remove toxin.

Examination of the extremities might reveal clues to current or former drug use (track marks, skin-popping scars), poisoning (Mees lines, arsenical dermatitis), and the presence of cyanosis or edema suggesting preexisting cardiac, pulmonary, or renal disease.

Reevaluation of the patient suspected of an overdose is essential in identifying new or developing findings or toxidromes, and in early identification and treatment of a deteriorating condition. Until the patient is completely recovered or considered no longer at risk for the consequences of a toxic exposure, frequent reassessment must be provided, even as the procedures described below are carried out.

SECONDARY TREATMENT FOR THE PATIENT WITH A SUSPECTED TOXIC EXPOSURE: THE ROLE FOR GASTROINTESTINAL EVACUATION TECHNIQUES

A series of individualized treatment decisions must now be made. Although many patients may benefit from gastrointestinal (GI) evacuation, those patients who show evidence of possible structural neurologic problems should probably have a head CT scan as well as hyperventilation and intubation, *prior* to any stressful procedure such as gastric intubation or lavage that might raise intracranial pressure.

As the discussion in Chapter 5 demonstrates, even the decision to evacuate the GI tract and/or administer activated charcoal can no longer be considered an automatic or generalized form of care. Instead, the decision should be based on the type of ingestion; estimated quantity and size; time since ingestion; concurrent ingestions; ancillary medical conditions; age and size of the patient; and so forth.

The indications, contraindications, and procedures for performing orogastric lavage and for administering whole-bowel irrigation, single or multiple-dose activated charcoal (AC; MDAC), cathartics, and, in the conscious patient, syrup of ipecac to induce emesis, are listed in Tables 31–1 through 31–5 and discussed in detail in Chapter 5 and in the specific antidotes in depth.

ELIMINATING ABSORBED TOXINS FROM THE BODY

After the decision regarding intervention to prevent absorption of toxic compounds is made, the clinician must next consider the applicability of techniques available to eliminate toxic compounds already absorbed. Detailed discussions of the indications and techniques of manipulating urinary pH (ion trapping), forced diuresis, hemodialysis, hemoperfusion, hemofiltration, and exchange transfusion are found in Chapter 6. Briefly, patients who may benefit are those who have ingested substances amenable to one of these techniques and whose clinical condition is both serious (or potentially serious) and unresponsive to supportive care, or whose physiologic route of elimination (liver-stools, kidney-urine) is impaired.

TABLE 31–1. Orogastric Lavage

Indications

Life-threatening exposures when the toxin is still expected to be accessible in the stomach and evacuation is expected to contribute to an improved outcome.

Tube Type and Size

Adults/adolescents: 36–40 French
Children: 22–28 French

Procedure

1. If there is potential airway compromise, endotracheal or nasotracheal intubation should precede orogastric lavage. Vomiting commonly follows lavage.
2. The patient should be kept in the left lateral decubitus position.
3. Prior to insertion, the proper length of tubing to be passed should be measured and marked on the tube. After the tube is introduced, confirmation that the distal end of the tube is in the stomach is essential.
4. Withdraw any material present and consider instillation of AC (see Table 31–2).
5. Via a funnel (or lavage syringe) 250-mL aliquots of a saline lavage solution should be instilled in an adult, and 10–15 mL/kg aliquots—not to exceed 250 mL — instilled in a child.
6. Lavage should continue for at least several liters in an adult and for 500 mL to 1 L in a child *or* until no particulate matter returns and the effluent lavage solution is clear.
7. Following lavage the same tube should be used to instill AC and a cathartic, if indicated (see Tables 31–2 and 31–3).

Contraindications

Caustic ingestions
Sharp materials
Drug-packet ingestions
Significant hemorrhagic diathesis, esophageal and gastric varices, thrombocytopenia (relative contraindication)
Prior significant emesis
Nontoxic ingestions

Adverse Effects

Inadvertent tracheal intubation and/or airway trauma
Aspiration pneumonitis
Emesis
Gastrointestial hemorrhage and/or perforation

Alkalinization of the urinary pH for acidic substances has limited applicability. Commonly, sodium bicarbonate can be used to alkalinize the urine (as well as the blood) and enhance salicylate, phenobarbital, chlorpropamide, formate, or methotrexate elimination. (see sodium bicarbonate: Antidotes in Depth). Acidification for alkaline substances is difficult to accomplish, probably useless, and possibly dangerous, and therefore has no role in poison management. *Forced diuresis* has no indication and may endanger the patient by causing pulmonary or cerebral edema. If a form of extracorporeal elimination is contemplated, consider *hemodialysis* for salicylates, methanol, ethylene glycol, lithium, and drugs that are both dialyzable and cause fluid and electrolyte problems; consider *hemoperfusion* for theophylline, phenobarbital, phenytoin and carbamazepine (though rarely, if ever, for the last three). *Peritoneal dialysis* is too ineffective to be of practical utility, and *hemofiltration* is not as efficacious. At times, both *hemodialysis* and *hemoperfusion in series* may be considered for life-threatening

TABLE 31–2.   Activated Charcoal (See Antidotes in Depth, page 469)

Indications

Single dose (AC):

Ingestions of drugs or toxins that bind to AC when no contraindication exists and an improved outcome is expected.

Multiple dose (MDAC)

Ingestions of drugs or toxins that bind to AC (a) when a prolonged absorption phase is expected; (b) when potential toxicity is great; and (c) when gastrointestinal dialysis is expected to be beneficial.

Drugs with a small volume of distribution (<1.0 L/kg), low endogenous clearance, low plasma-protein binding, biliary or gastric secretion of drug, or active metabolites that recirculate are most amenable to gastrointestinal dialysis.

Initial Dose (AC, MDAC), orally or via orogastric or nasogastric tube

Adults and children: 1 g/kg body weight or 10:1 ratio of activated charcoal: drug, whichever is greater. Following massive ingestions, 2 g/kg may be indicated, if such a large dose can be easily administered and tolerated.

Repeat Doses (MDAC), orally or via orogastric or nasogastric tube

Adults and children: 0.25–0.5 g/kg body weight q1–6h, in accordance with the dose and dosage form of drug ingested (larger doses or shorter dosing intervals may occasionally be indicated).

Procedure

1. Add 8 parts of water to the selected amount of powdered form. All formulations, including prepacked slurries, should be shaken well for at least 1 minute to form a transiently stable suspension prior to drinking or instillation via orogastric or nasogastric tube.
2. AC can be administered with a cathartic, *for the first dose only.*
3. If the patient vomits the dose of AC, it should be repeated. Smaller, more frequent doses, or continuous nasogastric administration may be better tolerated. An antiemetic may be needed.
4. If a nasogastric or orogastric tube is utilized for MDAC administration, time should be allowed for the last dose to pass through the stomach before suctioning all remaining AC prior to removing the tube. The suctioning may prevent subsequent charcoal aspiration.

Contraindications

Patients at risk for aspiration who have an unprotected airway. Caustic ingestions (activated charcoal is not only ineffective as an adsorbent, but may accumulate in burned areas, interfering with endoscopy).

Ileus: (a contraindication for MDAC).

Adverse Effects

Aspiration pneumonitis

Emesis

Obscuring of gastrointestinal mucosa (for endoscopist)

Constipation

TABLE 31–3.   Cathartics (See Antidotes in Depth, page 475)

Indications

Drugs or toxins that remain in the gastrointestinal tract and that may continue to be absorbed (or desorbed from AC) if not rapidly eliminated. Cathartics should be used only with the first dose of AC (or MDAC) and not repeated. Cathartics should not be used routinely and may pose a particular risk of serious fluid and electrolyte disturbances to children.

Types and Doses (adults and children)

Magnesium citrate (Mg citrate)	4 mL/kg, to a maximum of 300 mL
Magnesium sulfate (MgSO$_4$)	250 mg/kg, to a maximum of 30 g
Sorbitol	Adult 1–2 mL/kg of 70% solution
	Children 4 mL/kg of 35% solution

Precautions

Cathartics are not warranted for routine management of patients with trivial ingestions.

Cathartics should not be used more than once for any ingestion—beware of packaging and labelling of AC and cathartic (sorbitol) combinations that appear similar to AC alone.

Sorbitol should not be administered to children routinely; if used at all, strict attention to fluid and electrolyte status is mandatory.

Phosphosoda preparations should not be used either in children or adults.

Oil-based cathartics should not be used because of the risks of aspiration and enhanced toxin absorption.

Contraindications

Abdominal trauma

Intestinal obstruction

Adynamic ileus

Renal failure (a contraindication for MgSO$_4$ or Mg citrate cathartics).

Diarrhea

Adverse Effects

Volume depletion

Emesis

Electrolyle imbalance (hypermagnesemia, hypokalemia, hypernatremia)

Diarrhea

AVOIDING PITFALLS IN MANAGING A PATIENT WITH A SUSPECTED TOXIC EXPOSURE

The history alone is not a reliable indication of which patients require naloxone, hypertonic dextrose (D$_{50}$W), thiamine, and oxygen. Instead, these therapies should be considered for all patients with altered mental status unless specifically contraindicated. The physical examination should be used to guide the use of naloxone. If dextrose or naloxone is indicated, sufficient amounts should be administered to exclude and/or treat hypoglycemia or opioid toxicity.

The use of vasopressors in the initial management of hypotension should be avoided in a patient with a suspected or unknown overdose prior to using fluids or inserting a pulmonary artery (Swan-Ganz) catheter and an arterial line.

The possibility of concomitant trauma in cases of suspected drug overdose or poisoning should always be considered. Conversely, the possibility of a drug ingestion or toxic-metabolic dis-

overdoses (salicylates). When hemoperfusion is the method of choice (as for a theophylline overdose) but not available, hemodialysis is a logical, effective, alternative and certainly preferable to delaying treatment until hemoperfusion becomes available.

The indications for qualitative and quantitative diagnostic laboratory studies, and the use and interpretation of the ECG and radiologic and imaging procedures in diagnosing and managing the poisoned or overdosed patient are discussed fully in Chapters 7, 8, and 9.

TABLE 31–4. Emesis with Syrup of Ipecac (See Antidotes in Depth, page 465)

Indications

Early treatment for a potentially toxic ingestion—particularly for children at home, when there are no contraindications (see below).

Dose

Adult   30 mL (2 tbsp)

Children

6–12 months	5–10 mL (1–2 tsp)
1–12 years	15 mL (1 tbsp)
Older than 12 years	30 mL (2 tbsp)

One additional dose may be given if the patient has not vomited within 30 min.

Contraindications

Caustic ingestions
Sharp materials
An easily aspirated substance; ie, a pure petroleum distillate with little systemic toxicity in the amount ingested
Comatose patients
Seizing patients
Patients expected to deteriorate rapidly
Patients with a compromised gag reflex
Patients with a hemorrhagic diathesis, esophageal and gastric varices, thrombocytopenia
Children younger than 6 months of age
Significant prior vomiting or when vomiting will delay the timeliness of oral antidote or AC administration
Nontoxic ingestions

Adverse Effects

Intractable vomiting
Mallory-Weiss tears
Gastric rupture
Pneumothorax and/or pneumomediastinum
Aspiration
Delayed emesis after patient loses consciousness
Diarrhea (with chronic use)
Electrolyte abnormalities (with chronic use or abuse)
Cardiac and neurologic manifestations (with chronic use or abuse)

TABLE 31–5. Whole-Bowel Irrigation (See Antidotes in Depth, page 478)

Description

Whole-bowel irrigation with polyethylene glycol electrolyte lavage solution may be helpful in managing poisonings and overdoses when it is desirable or necessary to (a) rapidly clear the entire GI tract without emesis or causing fluid or electrolyte disturbances or (b) to prepare the GI tract for visualization. It is not to be substituted for activated charcoal (AC) when the latter is indicated.

Indications

Sustained-release medications
Slowly dissolving substances (eg, iron tablets, paint chips, bezoars, concretions)
Drug packets (eg, heroin, crack vials, cocaine) swallowed by "body packers" or "body stuffers"
Drugs or toxins not adsorbed by AC (eg, lithium, iron)

Dose orally or via nasogastric tube

Adults: 2 L/h for 4–6 hr, or until the rectal effluent is clear
Children: 0.5 L/h for 4–6 hr, or until the rectal effluent is clear
Note: AC should be administered before and during whole-bowel irrigation if a charcoal adsorbable drug or toxin is involved. (An antiemetic such as metoclopramide or a serotonin antagonist may be indicated to achieve compliance.)

Contraindications

Gastrointestional pathology: ileus, perforation, obstruction
Caustic ingestions
Patients at risk for pulmonary aspiration

Adverse effects

Rectal itching
Vomiting (especially with rapid administration)
Bloating
Decreased efficacy of AC
Desorption of toxin from AC

---

order in the patient with obvious head trauma should not be neglected. In any case, the GCS should not be used as a determinant for therapy.

Attributing altered mental status to an alcohol odor on a patient's breath is potentially dangerous and misleading. Small amounts of alcohol and its congeners generally produce the same breath odor as do intoxicating amounts. Conversely, even when an extremely high blood-ethanol level is *confirmed* by the laboratory, it is dangerous to ignore other possible etiologies of altered mental status; chronic alcoholics may be awake and seemingly alert with ethanol levels in excess of 500 mg/dL, a level that would result in coma and possibly apnea and death in a nonalcoholic.

As a general rule, a supposedly "inebriated" comatose patient still "sleeping it off" 3–4 hours after arrival should be considered to have structural CNS (central nervous system) damage (head trauma) and/or another toxic-metabolic etiology for the alteration in consciousness, until proven otherwise. Careful neurologic reevaluation supplemented by a head CT scan is frequently indicated in such a case. The metabolism of ethanol is fairly consistent

at 15–30 mg/dL/h, and regardless of the initial level, the patient who is comatose from ethanol alone should be more awake 3–4 hours after arrival. This is especially important in dealing with a patient who appears to have a minor bruise and who appears to be "intoxicated," as the early treatment of a subdural or epidural hematoma is critical to a successful outcome.

MANAGEMENT OF A PATIENT WITH A *NORMAL MENTAL STATUS* AND A SUSPECTED TOXIC EXPOSURE

As in the case of the patient with AMS, vital signs must be obtained and recorded. Initially, an assumption may have been made that the patient was breathing adequately, and if the patient is alert, talking, and in no respiratory distress, all that remains to document is the respiratory rate and rhythm. Because the patient is alert, additional history should be obtained, keeping in mind that information regarding the number and types of substances ingested, time elapsed, whether or not the patient vomited previously, and other critical information may be unreliable, depending in part on whether the ingestion was deliberate or unintentional.

If possible, another history should be privately and independently obtained from a friend or relative after the patient is initially stabilized. Speaking to the friend or relative may provide an opportunity to learn useful and reliable information regarding the ingestion, the patient's frame of mind, a history of previous ingestions, and the type of support that is available should the patient be discharged from the ED. At times, it may be essential to separate the patient from any relatives or friends initially, as the patient may not cooperate in their presence. Also, although friends or relatives may be clinical assets, their anxiety may interfere with therapy. As unreliable as the history taken from a patient with an overdose may be, it may nevertheless provide a clue to an overlooked possibility or a second ingestant, or may reveal the patient's mental and emotional condition. As is often true of the history, physical examination, or laboratory assessment in other clinical situations, the information obtained may confirm but never exclude possible etiologies.

At this point in the management of the conscious patient, a focused physical examination should be performed, concentrating on breath and heart sounds, and on an abdominal examination. A neurologic survey should emphasize reflexes and/or any focal findings.

APPROACHING THE PATIENT WITH AN INTENTIONAL TOXIC EXPOSURE

Initial efforts at establishing rapport with the patient, such as advising the patient that you are concerned about the problems that led up to the ingestion and that help is available after the drug or toxin is removed, will ultimately make management easier. At the same time, the appropriate options for gastrointestinal decontamination must be firmly explained. The patient should be reassured that after the chosen procedure is accomplished there will be time to discuss related problems and obtain additional appropriate care. These considerations are especially important in managing the patient with a deliberate overdose.

SPECIAL CONSIDERATIONS FOR MANAGING THE PREGNANT PATIENT WITH A TOXIC EXPOSURE

In general, a successful outcome for both mother and fetus is dependent on optimum management of the mother. Proven effective treatment for a potentially serious toxic exposure to the mother should never be withheld based on theoretical concerns regarding the fetus.

Physiologic Factors

A pregnant woman's total blood volume and cardiac output are elevated through the second trimester and into the later stages of the third trimester. This means that signs of hypoperfusion and hypotension will manifest later than they would in a woman who is not pregnant, and when they do, uterine blood flow might already be compromised. For these reasons, hypotension must be more aggressively identified and treated in the pregnant woman. Maintaining the patient in the left-lateral decubitus position will prevent supine hypotension resulting from impairment of systemic venous

return; this position is also the preferred position for orogastric lavage.

Because the tidal volume is increased in pregnancy, the baseline P_{CO_2} will normally be lower by approximately 10 mm Hg. Appropriate adjustment should be made for this effect when interpreting arterial blood gas results.

Use of Antidotes

Few data are available on the use of antidotes in pregnancy. In general, antidotes should not be used if the indications for use are equivocal. On the other hand, antidotes should not be withheld if their use might reduce potential morbidity and mortality. Risks and benefits should be considered. For example, reversal of opioid-induced respiratory depression calls for the use of naloxone, but if the woman is opioid dependent, the naloxone may precipitate acute withdrawal, including uterine contractions and possible induction of labor. Very slow, careful titration, starting with 0.05–0.1 mg naloxone, might be indicated, unless apnea is present, cessation of breathing appears imminent, or the P_{O_2} or O_2 saturation is already grossly inadequate. In these instances, naloxone may have to be administered in the usual manner, or assisted ventilation used, or a combination of assisted ventilation and small doses of naloxone.

Carbon monoxide (CO) poisoning is particularly threatening to fetal survival. The normal P_{O_2} of the fetal blood is about 15–20 mm Hg. Oxygen delivery to fetal tissues is impaired by the presence of carboxyhemoglobin, which shifts the O_2 hemoglobin dissociation curve to the left, potentially compromising an already tenuous balance. For this reason, we recommend hyperbaric oxygen for much lower carboxyhemoglobin levels in pregnancy (Chap. 97 and Antidotes-in-Depth: Hyperbaric Oxygen). Early notification of the obstetrician and close cooperation between physicians are essential for the best results.

MANAGEMENT OF TOXIC CUTANEOUS EXPOSURES

The chemicals that people are commonly exposed to externally include household cleaning materials; organic phosphorus compounds or carbamate insecticides from crop dusting, gardening, or roach extermination; acids from exploding batteries; alkalis, such as lye; and lacrimating agents which are used in crowd control. In all cases, the principles of management are:

1. The staff should avoid secondary exposures by wearing protective (rubber or plastic) gowns, gloves, and shoe covers. Many severe cases of secondary poisoning have occurred because emergency personnel were exposed to toxins such as organic phosphorus compounds merely by touching the victim or the victim's clothing.
2. The patient's clothing should be removed and placed in a plastic bag.
3. The patient should be washed with soap and copious amounts of water *twice*, no matter how much time has elapsed since the exposure.
4. No attempt should be made to neutralize an acid with a base, or vice versa.

5. The use of all greases or creams should be avoided. These will only keep the toxin in close contact with the skin and ultimately make removal more difficult.

MANAGEMENT OF TOXIC OPHTHALMIC EXPOSURES

The eyes should be irrigated with lids fully retracted for no less than 20 minutes. A drop of anesthetic such as proparacaine in each eye facilitates irrigation. Lids may be held open with a lid retractor. An adequate irrigation stream may be obtained by running 1 L of normal saline through regular IV tubing held a few inches from the eye or by using an irrigating lens. Checking the lid fornices with pH paper strips is important to ensure adequate irrigation; the pH should normally be 6.5–7.6 if accurately tested, although when using paper test strips, the measurement is often near 8 (Chap. 27).

ASSURING OPTIMAL OUTCOME FOR THE PATIENT WITH A SUSPECTED TOXIC EXPOSURE

As demonstrated by the case at the beginning of this chapter, one way to assure an optimal outcome for the patient with a suspected toxic exposure is to apply the *principles* of basic and advanced life support in conjunction with a "primary" and "secondary" survey, always bearing in mind that a toxicologic etiology or coetiology for any abnormal conditions necessitates modifying whatever standard approach one brings to the bedside. For example, it is extremely important to recognize that toxin-induced dysrhythmias and cardiac instability require alterations in standard protocols that assume a primary cardiac or non-toxicologic etiology (Chap. 21).

Typically, only some of the substances a patient was exposed to will ever be confirmed by the laboratory. In the case at the beginning of this chapter, the acetaminophen was confirmed whereas the erythromycin and other possible ingestants were either not tested for or remained undetermined throughout the hospitalization. Nevertheless, a successful outcome was in no way compromised. In addition to the general management techniques applicable to all patients with toxic exposures, the careful use of specific treatments or antidotes clinically indicated by the presentation may be reasonable even if not ultimately beneficial.

The thoughtful combination of stabilization, general management, and specific treatment when indicated, will result in successful outcomes in the vast majority of patients with actual or suspected toxic exposures.

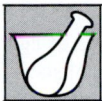 ## ANTIDOTES IN DEPTH

Syrup of Ipecac
Mary Ann Howland

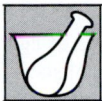

Emetine

Syrup of ipecac is an emetic that has been in use for the management of poisonings since the 1950s and has been available over the counter since the late 1960s. Ipecac is derived from the dried rhizome and roots of plants found in Brazil belonging to the family *Rubiaceae*, such as *Cephaelis acuminata* or *Cephaelis ipecacuanha*.[45] Cephaeline and emetine are the two alkaloids largely responsible for the production of nausea and vomiting, with cephaeline being the more potent.[23] Each 15-mL dose of the syrup of ipecac contains 16–21 mg of cephaeline and 6.4–21 mg of emetine, giving a cephaeline-to-emetine ratio of between 1:1 and 2.5:1.[45] Syrup of ipecac also contains a small amount of psychotrine, which is of minor importance. Syrup of ipecac induces vomiting in two ways: local activation of peripheral sensory receptors in the gastrointestinal tract, and central stimulation of the chemoreceptor trigger zone that serves as a sensory area with subsequent activation of the central vomiting center.[41] Recent evidence suggests that $5HT_3$ receptors mediate the nausea and vomiting produced by syrup of ipecac. This mechanism was demonstrated in 40 volunteers by administering a specific $5HT_3$ antagonist 30 minutes prior to administration of the syrup of ipecac which prevented or attenuated the nausea and vomiting in a dose-dependent fashion.[14]

The role of syrup of ipecac has changed dramatically in the last decade. Once the mainstay of poison management for children and adults, a critical evaluation of animal, volunteer, and a limited number of clinical studies suggests that ipecac administration should be reserved for a few selected circumstances rather than being administered on a routine basis.[3] The rationale for this change is based on the fact that (a) most poisonings in children are benign; (b) most adults overdose with toxins that rapidly cause an altered mental status thus constituting a contraindication to the administration of ipecac; (c) ipecac-induced vomiting may be delayed and/or persistent causing a delay in the administration of activated charcoal. Therefore only a few patients are considered appropriate candidates for the use of the syrup of ipecac. The remaining candidates include: (a) patients who overdose on toxins that do not cause a rapid change in mental status, such as acetaminophen or salicylates; (b) patients who consume massive amounts of a toxin that may exceed the binding capacity of activated charcoal, such as salicylates; or (c) those who ingest a toxin not bound to activated charcoal, such as lithium. Under these circumstances, if the overdose has occurred within a time frame during which, the presence of unabsorbed drug in the stomach remains a potential then ipecac use is appropriate. This time frame is usually within the first hour or two following ingestion.

In one of the earliest studies evaluating the delay in onset between administration of syrup of ipecac and vomiting, 214 children were given 20 mL of syrup of ipecac and copious amounts of water.[36] Eighty-eight percent of the children vomited within 30 minutes or less (mean of 18.7 minutes).[36] Toxicity secondary to syrup of ipecac was not noted. Subsequent studies demonstrate similar findings.[4,9,10,12,16,22,24,42,44]

The onset of emesis does not appear to be affected by fluid administration before or after the administration of syrup of ipecac, by the temperature of the fluids, or by gentle patient motion or walking.[12,13,16,40] Therefore, it is inadvisable to force fluids. Similarly, milk should not be given with the syrup of ipecac, as the onset of emesis may be delayed, although the actual incidence of vomiting does not appear to be affected.[13] Because the peripheral emetic sensory receptors are located in the proximal small intestine, this delay is consistent with the ability of milk to delay gastric emptying.[46] Syrup of ipecac is absorbed so quickly that vomiting still occurred in the majority of overdose patients given activated charcoal 10 minutes after syrup of ipecac administration.[15]

The average number of episodes of vomiting is 3, with a range of 1 to 8.[22] The duration of syrup of ipecac-induced vomiting reportedly averages 23–60 minutes in the United States,[22,34] although investigators in Finland report longer times (3–4 hours).[30] In spite of this variable data, it is probably reasonable to assume that persistent vomiting for more than 2 hours is unrelated to syrup of ipecac and another cause should be sought. This warning is of particular importance when syrup of ipecac is used in the home.

Many studies assessed the effectiveness of syrup of ipecac-induced emesis in decreasing absorption of an ingestion, and compared the results to other methods of gastric decontamination, such as gastric lavage or activated charcoal.[30,31,37] There appears to be a wide range of results, largely caused by differences in study design, including time to administration of the various techniques and the particular substance or marker used to assess efficacy. Older volunteer studies using small lavage tubes were further limited because of the quantity of drug that was administered and recovered.

Numerous studies support the concept that the sooner syrup of ipecac is administered after an ingestion, the greater the amount of the ingested substance that will be recovered. In a small, well-quantified study, when 6 adult volunteers were given 20 mL of syrup of ipecac at 5 or 30 minutes after acetaminophen ingestion, absorption was inhibited by 65% and 0%, respectively.[32] In this same volunteer model, absorption was inhibited by 80% and 40% when 50 g of activated charcoal was given at 5 and 30 minutes postingestion.[32]

A subsequent investigation demonstrated that the reduction in the area under the concentration-time curve was equivalent for patients treated with syrup of ipecac-induced emesis and patients treated with activated charcoal plus a cathartic following the ingestion of 40 mg/kg of acetaminophen 60 minutes prior to treatment.[27] Comparison of orogastric lavage, syrup of ipecac-induced emesis, and activated charcoal, all given at 60 minutes after ingestion of ampicillin by adult volunteers, showed reductions of 32%, 38%, and 57%, respectively.[44] Adult volunteers given syrup of ipecac 5 minutes after 30 capsules containing a radionucleotide marker demonstrated a mean 54% removal (range, 21–89%) as compared to a mean removal of 35.5% (range, 1–71%) with orogastric lavage.[49] Other researchers demonstrated recoveries from 0% to 85%.[4,10,11,42] Children given a magnesium hydroxide marker before administration of syrup of ipecac demonstrated a mean recovery of 28%, although the range was 0–78%.[10]

In a study of self-poisoned adults randomized to receive either syrup of ipecac or orogastric lavage with a 33-French lavage tube, all patients had subsequent endoscopy.[37] Thirteen patients were given syrup of ipecac and vomited within 23 minutes (range, 11–25 min). Two of these patients had tablets in the vomitus. Upon endoscopy, only those 2 patients had residual tablets in the stomach. Ten of 17 patients who were lavaged had tablets in the lavage fluid. All of these patients had tablets in the stomach at the time of endoscopy. Two additional patients also had residual tablets in the stomach. This study suggests that the presence of tablets in the vomitus or lavage fluid supports the presence of additional tablets in the stomach.[37]

This same group of investigators subsequently used barium-marked 3-mm³ pellets to evaluate the effectiveness of gastric emptying.[38] Forty self-poisoned patients were given 20 pellets on admission and randomized immediately to therapy with either orogastric lavage or syrup of ipecac-induced emesis. About 50% of the pellets were removed in both the orogastric lavage and the syrup of ipecac groups. Two patients in the lavage group and 1 in the syrup of ipecac group had 100% removal of pellets, and 2 patients in the lavage group had no removal.[38]

A large Emergency Department (ED) study addressed whether gastric emptying with either syrup of ipecac or orogastric lavage followed by activated charcoal was more effective than activated charcoal alone in overdosed patients.[21] Syrup of ipecac did not affect the outcome of patients who arrived awake and alert.

Three subsequent studies (2 adult and 1 pediatric) failed to show a benefit of gastric emptying before activated charcoal administration[2,29] compared with the administration of activated charcoal alone.[19] Furthermore, aspiration was more common in patients who had the combined regimen.[2,29]

Logically, the sooner that syrup of ipecac is administered after an ingestion, the more effective it may be in reducing absorption of the agent. For this reason syrup of ipecac should retain its role in toxicologic management in the home setting.[5] Activated charcoal has a role in the home setting as well, and the increased availability of more appealing products will increase its utility. Syrup of ipecac has lost favor in the ED for the care of adults because the sickest patients are lavaged and given activated charcoal, while others receive activated charcoal alone. Administration of syrup of ipecac to children in the ED setting delays time to activated charcoal administration by 100 minutes (2.6 vs. 0.9 hours),[19] and therefore is rarely recommended. Although syrup of ipecac may still be useful for toxins not adsorbed to activated charcoal, whole-bowel irrigation is generally preferred.

Syrup of ipecac should *not* be administered to patients who have ingested acids or alkalis, are younger than 6 months of age, are expected to deteriorate rapidly, have a depressed mental status, have a compromised gag reflex, have ingested objects such as batteries or sharps, or have a need for rapid gastrointestinal evacuation to prevent absorption. It should *not* be administered to those in whom the hazards of vomiting and aspiration of the ingested substance outweigh the risks associated with systemic absorption (eg, hydrocarbons), those who have significant prior vomiting, or when vomiting will delay administration of an oral antidote, or to those with a hemorrhagic diathesis, or to patients with nontoxic ingestions.

Considering the number of times syrup of ipecac has been administered without incident in this country, it must be considered a relatively safe drug when given in therapeutic doses and when no contraindications exist. Uncommon problems that have occurred after therapeutic doses include a Mallory-Weiss esophageal tear in an adult given 30 mL of syrup of ipecac for a multidrug overdose;[43] herniation of the stomach into the left chest in a child who had a previously unrecognized underlying congenital defect of the diaphragm;[35] intracerebral hemorrhage;[18] and pneumomediastinum.[47] Additional problems include aspiration of stomach contents, aspiration of a volatile hydrocarbon or foreign body, and the time delay before it is possible to perform a necessary therapeutic intervention (activated charcoal) or administer an antidote (*N*-acetylcysteine). Another reported problem is the emesis-induced vagal response of bradycardia.[28]

Administration of very large doses of ipecac, such as by giving the fluid extract of ipecac (no longer available), which is 14 times more potent than syrup of ipecac; or repeated and frequent doses of syrup of ipecac (as in patients with anorexia and bulimia), has resulted in substantial morbidity including congestive cardiomyopathy and mortality.[1,6,23,25,33,39,48] When emetine was used for the treatment of amebiasis in the early 1900s, cardiovascular and neuromuscular toxicity ensued. Similarly, inadvertent administration of the fluid extract of ipecac produces violent and protracted vomiting; diarrhea; seizures; cardiac toxicity (PR prolongation, T-wave abnormalities, QRS abnormalities, atrial dysrhythmias, premature ventricular beats, and ventricular fibrillation); neuromuscular toxicity (weakness and neuropathy); shock; and death.[23]

Surreptitious chronic intentional ipecac poisoning of children (Münchausen syndrome by proxy) is reported.[7,26] The findings in these children included vomiting, diarrhea, lethargy, irritability, hypothermia, and hypotonia. These children were referred by their parents for atypical patterns of vomiting and had multiple unsuccessful clinical evaluations. When surreptitious use of ipecac is suspected as the cause of chronic vomiting, screening the urine and vomitus for emetine (thin-layer chromatography screen—Toxi-Lab) may be useful.[26]

The dose of syrup of ipecac is 15 mL in children 1–12 years old and 30 mL in older children and adults. If vomiting does not ensue after the first dose, the same dose may be repeated once in 20–30 minutes. For children 6–12 months of age, ipecac use should be limited to a maximum single dose of 10 mL.[8,20] Water can be offered, but is not essential for success. Vomiting will occur in most patients. Home users should be warned that persistent vomiting for more than 2 hours may indicate toxicity from the primary substances ingested and not the antidote, and will necessitate medical evaluation.

Parents should still be encouraged to keep syrup of ipecac at home as a potential first aid measure, but they should be cautioned to use it only on the advice of their regional poison center or physician. In fact, there are very few cases in which syrup of ipecac is indicated and recommended in the home setting because either the ingestion is nontoxic or conversely of such consequence that an imminent deterioration in mental status would be expected to contraindicate its administration. Activated charcoal appears to be gaining acceptance as the first and sometimes only gastric decontamination procedure in the ED, whereas the role of syrup of ipecac is becoming extremely limited. The data seem adequate to consider administering syrup of ipecac to a child who arrives in the ED shortly after the ingestion of a large number of poorly soluble tablets of a size unlikely to be removed by lavage, as well as for the patient who has taken such a large amount of a highly toxic substance that a favorable activated-charcoal-to-drug ratio cannot be attained with certainty. Whole-bowel irrigation is probably a suitable alternative in either case.

REFERENCES

1. Adler AG, Walinsky P, Krall RA, Cho SY: Death resulting from ipecac syrup poisoning. JAMA 1980;243:1927–1928.
2. Albertson TE, Derlet RW, Foulke GE, et al: Superiority of activated charcoal alone compared with ipecac and activated charcoal in the treatment of acute toxic ingestions. Ann Emerg Med 1989;18:56–59.
3. American Academy of Clinical Toxicology, European Association of Poison Center and Clinical Toxicologists: Position statement; Ipecac syrup. J Toxicol Clin Toxicol 1997;35:699–709.
4. Auerbach P, Osterloh J, Braun O, et al: Efficacy of gastric emptying: Gastric lavage versus emesis induced with ipecac. Ann Emerg Med 1986;15:692–698.
5. Banner W, Veltri J: The case of ipecac syrup [editorial]. Am J Dis Child 1988;142:596.
6. Bennett H, Spiro A, Pollack M, et al: Ipecac-induced myopathy simulating dermatomyositis. Neurology 1982;32:91–94.
7. Berkner P, Kaster T, Skolnick L: Chronic ipecac poisoning in infancy: A case report. Pediatrics 1988;82:384–386.
8. Boehnert M, Lewander W, Gaudreault P, et al: Advances in clinical toxicology. Pediatr Clin North Am 1985;32:193–211.
9. Boxer L, Anderson F, Rowe D: Comparison of ipecac-induced emesis with gastric lavage in the treatment of acute salicylate ingestion. J Pediatr 1969;74:800–803.
10. Corby D, Decker W, Moran M, et al: Clinical comparison of pharmacologic emetics in children. Pediatrics 1968;42:361–364.
11. Curtis R, Barone J, Giacona N: Efficacy of ipecac and activated charcoal and cathartic: Prevention of salicylate absorption in a simulated overdose. Arch Intern Med 1984;144:48–52.
12. Dean B, Krenzelok E: Syrup of ipecac: 15 mL versus 30 mL in pediatric poisonings. J Toxicol Clin Toxicol 1985;23:165–170.
13. Eisenga B, Meester W: Evaluation of the effect of motility on syrup of ipecac-induced emesis [abstract]. Vet Hum Toxicol 1978;20:462.
14. Forster ER, Palmer JL, Bedding AW, Smith JTL: Syrup of ipecacuanha-induced nausea and emesis is medicated by $5HT_3$ receptors in man. J Physiol (London) 1994;477:72.
15. Freedman G, Pasternak S, Krenzelok E: A clinical trial using syrup of ipecac and activated charcoal concurrently. Ann Emer Med 1987;16:164–166.
16. Grande G, Ling L: The effect of fluid volume on syrup of ipecac emesis time. J Toxicol Clin Toxicol 1987;25:473–481.
17. Isner JM: Effects of ipecac on the heart. N Engl J Med 1986;314:1253.
18. Klein-Schwartz W, Gorman R, Oderda G, et al: Ipecac use in the elderly: The unanswered question. Ann Emerg Med 1984;13:1152–1154.
19. Kornberg AE, Dolgen J: Pediatric ingestions: Charcoal alone versus ipecac and charcoal. Ann Emerg Med 1991;20:648–651.
20. Krenzelok K, Dean B: Syrup of ipecac in children less than one year of age. J Toxicol Clin Toxicol 1985;23:171–176.
21. Kulig K, Bar-Or D, Cantrill SV, et al: Management of acutely poisoned patients without gastric emptying. Ann Emerg Med 1985;14:562–567.
22. MacLean W: A comparison of ipecac syrup and apomorphine in the immediate treatment of ingestion of poisons. J Pediatr 1973;82:121–124.
23. Manno B, Manno J: Toxicology of ipecac. Clin Toxicol 1977;10:221–242.
24. Manoguerra A, Krenzelok E: Rapid emesis from high dose ipecac syrup in adults and children intoxicated with antiemetics and other drugs. Am J Hosp Pharm 1978;35:1360–1362.
25. Mateer J, Farrell B, Chou SM, Gutman L: Reversible ipecac myopathy. Arch Neurol 1985;42:188–190.
26. McClung H, Murray R, Braden N, et al: Intentional ipecac poisoning in children. Am J Dis Child 1988;142:637–639.
27. McNamara R, Aaron C, Gemborys M, Davidheiser S: Efficacy of charcoal versus ipecac in reducing serum acetaminophen in a simulated overdose. Ann Emerg Med 1988;17:243–246.
28. Meester W: Emesis and lavage. Vet Hum Toxicol 1981;22:225–234.
29. Merigian KS, Woodard M, Hedges JR, et al: Prospective evaluation of gastric emptying in the self-poisoned patient. Am J Emerg Med 1990;8:479–483.
30. Neuvonen P: Clinical pharmacokinetics of oral activated charcoal in acute intoxications. Clin Pharmacokinet 1982;7:465–489.
31. Neuvonen P, Olkkola K: Activated charcoal and syrup of ipecac in the prevention of cimetidine and pindolol absorption in man after administration of metoclopramide as an antiemetic. J Toxicol Clin Toxicol 1984;22:103–114.
32. Neuvonen P, Vartiainen M, Tokola O: Comparison of activated charcoal and ipecac syrup in prevention of drug absorption. Eur J Clin Pharmacol 1983;24:557–562.
33. Palmer E, Guay A: Reversible myopathy secondary to abuse of ipecac in patients with major eating disorders. N Engl J Med 1985;313:1457–1459.
34. Rauber A, Maroncelli R: The duration of emetic effect of ipecac; Duration and frequency of vomiting [abstract]. Vet Hum Toxicol 1982;24:281.
35. Robertson WO: Syrup of ipecac associated fatality: A case report. Vet Hum Toxicol 1979;21:87–89.
36. Robertson WO: Syrup of ipecac: A slow or fast emetic? Am J Dis Child 1962;103:136–139.
37. Saetta JP, March S, Gaunt ME, Quinton DN: Gastric emptying procedures in the self-poisoned patient: Are we forcing gastric content beyond the pylorus? J R Soc Med 1991;84:274–277.
38. Saetta JP, Quinton DN: Residual gastric content after gastric lavage and ipecacuanha induced emesis in self-poisoned patients: An endoscopic study. J R Soc Med 1991;84:35–38.
39. Schiff R, Wurzel C, Brunson S, et al: Death due to chronic syrup of ipecac use in a patient with bulimia. Pediatrics 1986;78:412–416.
40. Spiegel R, Addouch I, Munn D: The effect of temperature on concurrently administered fluid on the onset of ipecac-induced emesis. Clin Toxicol 1979;14:281–284.
41. Stewart J: Effects of emetic and cathartic agents on the gastrointestinal tract and the treatment of toxic ingestion. J Toxicol Clin Toxicol 1983;20:199–253.
42. Tandberg D, Diven B, McLeod J: Ipecac-induced emesis versus gastric lavage: A controlled study in normal adults. Am J Emerg Med 1986;4:205–209.
43. Tandberg D, Liechty E, Fishbein D: Mallory-Weiss syndrome: An unusual complication of ipecac-induced emesis. Ann Emerg Med 1981;10:521–523.
44. Tenenbein M, Cohen, Sitar D: Efficacy of ipecac-induced emesis, orogastric lavage, and activated charcoal for acute drug overdose. Ann Emerg Med 1987;16:838–841.

45. United States Pharmacopeia 21 and National Formulary 16: Suppl 2. Rockville, MD, US Pharmacopeial Convention, 1985.

46. Varipapa RJ, Oderda GM: Effect of milk on ipecac-induced emesis. J Am Pharm Assoc 1977;17:510.

47. Wolowodiuk O, McMicken D, O'Brien P: Pneumomediastinum and pneumoretroperitoneum: An unusual complication of syrup of ipecac induced emesis. Ann Emerg Med 1984;13:1148–1151.

48. Woolf AD, Grew JM: Acute poisonings among adolescents and young adults with anorexia nervosa. Am J Dis Child1990;144: 785–788.

49. Young WF, Bruin SMG: Evaluation of gastric emptying using radionucleotides: Gastric lavage versus ipecac-induced emesis. Ann Emerg Med 1993;22:1423–1427.

ANTIDOTES IN DEPTH

Activated Charcoal

Mary Ann Howland

Activated charcoal, a fine, black, odorless powder, has been recognized for almost two centuries as an effective adsorbent of many substances. In 1930, the French pharmacist Touery dramatically demonstrated his belief in the powerful adsorbent qualities of activated charcoal by ingesting several times the lethal dose of strychnine mixed with 15 g of activated charcoal in front of colleagues; he suffered no ill effects.[8] An American physician, Holt, first used activated charcoal to save a patient from mercury bichloride poisoning in 1934.[8] However, it was not until the 1940s that Anderson began to systematically investigate the adsorbency of activated charcoal[3–5] and unquestionably demonstrated that activated charcoal is an excellent broad-spectrum gastrointestinal adsorbent. However its current role in the management of overdosed patients is being redefined by examining the rationale for its use with evidence based medicine.[4] Clearly, activated charcoal should not be administered to every overdosed patient without weighing the benefits versus the risks. Although the benefits include inactivating a potentially toxic ingestion, the risks include vomiting and aspiration. The merits of activated charcoal as a decontamination strategy are discussed in detail in Chapters 5 and 31.

Activated charcoal is produced in a two-step process beginning with the pyrolysis of various carbonaceous materials such as wood, coconut, or peat followed by treatment at high temperatures with a variety of activating (oxidizing) agents such as steam or carbon dioxide to increase the adsorptive capacity of the agent through the formation of an internal maze of pores with a huge surface area.[48,95,118] The rate of adsorption depends on external surface area, while the adsorptive capacity is dependent on the far larger internal surface area.[23,86,93] The actual adsorption is believed to rely on hydrogen bonding, ion-ion, dipole, and van der Waals' forces suggesting that most drugs are best adsorbed in their dissolved, nonionized form: Strongly ionized and dissociated salts like sodium chloride are not adsorbed, whereas iodine and mercuric chloride are adsorbed; nonpolar, poorly water soluble organic substances are more likely to be adsorbed, and adsorption is enhanced with an increase in size in comparison to small, polar, water-soluble organic substances. Among the organic molecules, aromatics are better adsorbed than aliphatics, branched chains better than straight chains, and molecules containing nitro groups are better adsorbed than those containing hydroxyl, amino, or sulfonic groups.[23] In vitro studies demonstrate that adsorption begins within about 1 minute of administration of activated charcoal but may not reach equilibrium for 10–25 minutes.[24,83]

Activated charcoal decreases the systemic absorption of a number of drugs, including aspirin, acetaminophen, barbiturates, glutethimide, phenytoin, theophylline, cyclic antidepressants, and most inorganic and organic materials.[37,83,97] Notable exceptions to the beneficial effects of activated charcoal are the alcohols, strong

acids and alkalies, iron, and lithium. Efficacy of activated charcoal is inversely related to the time elapsed following ingestion of the substance to be adsorbed and directly related to the amount of activated charcoal administered. The effect of the activated charcoal-to-drug ratio on adsorption was demonstrated both in vitro and in vivo with para-aminosalicylate (PAS): In vitro the fraction of unadsorbed PAS decreased from 55% to 3% as the activated charcoal-to-PAS ratio increased from 1:1 to 10:1 at pH 1.2.[92] In human volunteers, as the activated charcoal-to-PAS ratio increased from 2.5:1 to 50:1, the total 48-hour urinary excretion decreased from 37% to 4%.[93] Presumably because more of the drug was adsorbed by activated charcoal in the lumen of the gastrointestinal tract rather than being absorbed systemically. These studies demonstrate activated charcoal saturation at low ratios of activated charcoal to drug.

The role of timing in determining the overall effectiveness of activated charcoal depends largely on the rate of absorption of the drug. For example, early administration is much more important with rapidly absorbed drugs. The rate of absorption of a drug depends on many factors. In general, lipid solubility and rapid passage of a drug into the intestine speeds absorption, whereas sustained-release dosage forms, drugs that have anticholinergic properties and drugs that are co-ingested with food are more slowly absorbed.[94] However, the presence of food also decreases the adsorptive capacity of activated charcoal.[6,64]

As noted above, drugs are best adsorbed to activated charcoal in their undissociated form. According to the Henderson-Hasselbalch equation, weak bases are best adsorbed at basic pHs and weak acids are best adsorbed at acid pHs. For example, cocaine, a weak base, binds to activated charcoal with a maximum adsorptive capacity of 273 mg of cocaine per gram of activated charcoal at pH 7.0; this capacity is reduced to 212 mg of cocaine per gram of activated charcoal at pH 1.2.[68]

The adsorption of weakly dissociated metallic salts to activated charcoal decreases with decreasing pH because the number of complex ions increases.[7] Accordingly, desorption may occur, especially for weak acids, as the charcoal-drug complex passes from the stomach through the intestine and the pH changes from acidic to basic.[11,38,89,93,117] Desorption may lead to systemic absorption of larger total amounts of drug over several days; in this case, the elimination half-life of the drug appears to increase, but peak levels remain unaffected.[89] Desorption can be minimized by giving a large enough dose of activated charcoal to overcome the decreased affinity of the drug secondary to pH change and by utilizing multiple-dose activated charcoal. A cathartic should reduce gastrointestinal transit time and can possibly increase drug elimination. However, in spite of numerous human volunteer studies[55,76,87,98,111] this effect has been demonstrated only in a single study.[55] Despite the number of such studies, the importance of these negative results remains in question, as the overdose setting may not be clinically comparable to these study settings.

Although ethanol and other solvents are minimally adsorbed by activated charcoal, they nonetheless may decrease the adsorptive capacity of activated charcoal for a coingested drug by competing for activated charcoal binding with that drug.[89,93]

Activated charcoal is best administered as a water slurry. At present, activated charcoal is often the sole gastrointestinal intervention in patients for whom removal of gastric contents is deemed unnecessary or contraindicated. Activated charcoal may also be used following emesis induced by syrup of ipecac, shortly after ipecac administration but prior to vomiting (which will still occurs in 50–100% of activated charcoal-treated individuals),[40] or following orogastric lavage. The use of activated charcoal is relatively safe, although vomiting (especially after rapid administration), constipation, and diarrhea are all noted following administration:[86] constipation and diarrhea when they occur most probably result from the ingestion rather than the activated charcoal. Serious adverse effects of activated charcoal include the lethal complications that may result from the simultaneous aspiration of activated charcoal alone or with gastric contents,[9,35,42,45,46,52,77,83,99,110] peritonitis from spillage of activated charcoal into the peritoneum from gastrointestinal perforation caused by orogastric lavage,[70] and intestinal obstruction and pseudo-obstruction, especially following repeated doses of activated charcoal in the presence of dehydration[16,65,79,104,121] and prior bowel adhesions.[43] The incidence of aspiration of activated charcoal following endotracheal intubation varies from 4% to 25%, depending on the nature of the study. A significant number of patients aspirate prior to endotracheal intubation and administration of activated charcoal. This phenomenon was reflected in the retrospective study that found a 4% incidence of aspiration. The prospective study that found a 25% incidence of aspiration identified activated charcoal in bronchial secretions, although the outcomes of patients with or without charcoal secretions were similar. Rarely, activated charcoal may become entrapped in the distal esophagus and stomach, and present incidentally as a granulomatous lesion upon endoscopy. Presumably, a traumatic gastric lavage followed by the instillation of activated charcoal years earlier gave rise to the reaction.

The black and gritty nature of activated charcoal has led to many formulations to increase palatability and patient acceptance. Bentonite, carboxymethyl cellulose, and starch[44,82,109] have been used as thickening agents; and cherry syrup, chocolate syrup, sorbitol, sucrose, saccharin, ice cream, and sherbet[26,63,69,123] have been used as flavoring agents. The thickening agents do not appear to decrease the antidotal efficacy of activated charcoal if the mixtures are fluidlike rather than gelatinous in consistency.[25,71] In fact, a 20% activated charcoal slurry prepared with 70% sorbitol was more effective than activated charcoal alone.[98] Ice cream and sherbet decreased the adsorptive capacity of activated charcoal in one study,[63] but contradictory results were reported for chocolate syrup.[44,82] The other flavoring agents used produced no adverse effects on the adsorptive properties of activated charcoal. However, improvement in palatability and acceptance was minimal or nonexistent with all of these formulations. A milk chocolate formulation evaluated by a group of children was rated superior in palatability as compared to standard activated charcoal preparations,[34] but it was never marketed.

The acceptance of a dose of activated charcoal given as a water slurry in a paper cup was studied in 50 young children.[18] The children were told to drink the contents, that the substance did not taste bad, and that it would make them feel better and not sick. Eighty-six percent of the children readily drank the activated charcoal slurry, and 76% of them consumed 95–100% of the total dose.

Other attempts at getting children to ingest activated charcoal were not as successful. Difficulty was noted in 70% of attempts to administer a standard dose of activated charcoal to children in the home setting.[32] Similarly, only 30% of children drank the activated charcoal in the emergency department setting, with the remainder requiring placement of a nasogastric tube to instill the activated charcoal.[57]

A marketed activated charcoal product with cherry flavoring was rated by adult human volunteers as preferable over plain activated charcoal and a statistically significant larger quantity of the flavored activated charcoal was ingested.[22] This novel formulation utilized the instillation of a very small quantity of cherry flavoring to the straw as the activated charcoal slurry was being ingested, and resulted in improved acceptance of the activated charcoal without loss of its adsorptive capacity.[22] However in adult overdosed patients, this was not the case, as most patients consumed the entire bottle of activated charcoal with or without cherry flavoring. The subjects did not like the taste and surprisingly preferred the plain activated charcoal.[51] Two recent studies in adult overdose patients compared different brands of activated charcoal to determine the quantity of charcoal ingested.[15,39] In the British study, approximately half of the 50 g of charcoal offered was ingested and 7% of the patients vomited.[15] In the US study, 60 g of activated charcoal in 340 mL was offered and approximately 95% was consumed in 20 minutes. There was no difference in the amount consumed even though the palatability of the granular form of activated charcoal was rated higher.[39]

In the United States at present, activated charcoal is supplied either as a powder in a container to which sufficient water must be added to make it watery in consistency (8:1 water-to-charcoal ratio), or premixed with water or sorbitol. Currently, many activated charcoal products are available commercially, differing in the source of activated charcoal, amount per container, activated charcoal surface area, presence or absence of sorbitol, and cost.[73] Activated charcoal products used outside the United States may contain other additives, such as sodium bicarbonate.[105]

The relationship between activated charcoal surface area and adsorption capacity was studied in vitro and in vivo in animals and in humans. In vitro studies demonstrated significant differences in maximum binding capacities (MBC) and binding affinities. The enhanced MBC of petroleum-based activated charcoal preparations results from the physical structure, which is described as a nearly random array of graphite sheets with micropores. When surface area is large, capacity is increased, but affinity is decreased because van der Waals' forces and hydrophobic forces are diminished.[120] The net result in most studies is that the activated charcoal preparation with the largest surface area can decrease the absorption of drugs about 2.5–3 times more than that of standard activated charcoals.[27–29,58,120] Superactivated charcoals, which are petroleum-based and have the largest surface areas (approximating 3150 m^2/g), have the greatest MBC; binding affinities show an inverse relationship with MBC.[120] All of the superactivated charcoal preparations available in the United States prior to 1986 were subsequently removed from the market because of impurities thought to be carcinogenic. However, in 1996, a new superactivated charcoal free of such impurities and with a surface area approximately double the current activated charcoal formulations was marketed. Both in vitro and in vivo studies of this preparation indicate a greater MBC.[26,106,107]

ACTIVATED CHARCOAL PLUS CATHARTICS OR WHOLE BOWEL IRRIGATION

The question of the role of cathartics on activated charcoal is not completely resolved. However, most of the evidence suggests that activated charcoal alone is about as effective as activated charcoal plus a single dose of cathartic (sorbitol or magnesium citrate).[3,55,71,72,76,82,86,96] There may be some theoretical benefit, however, in combining multiple-dose activated charcoal (MDAC) with whole-bowel irrigation (WBI) in overdoses of delayed or sustained-release drugs. If a cathartic is used, it should be used only once as repeated doses of magnesium-containing cathartics are associated with reports of hypermagnesemia[80,113] and repeated doses of all types of cathartics are associated with severe fluid and electrolyte problems. Deaths have been reported following repeated doses of sorbitol containing activated charcoal mixtures.[36] Because WBI with a nonabsorbable polyethylene glycol electrolyte lavage solution (PEG-ELS) alone or in combination with activated charcoal is not known to be associated with morbidity, further study may indicate that WBI in sequence with activated charcoal is the preferred technique in certain circumstances.

WBI with PEG-ELS significantly decreases the in vitro adsorptive capacity of activated charcoal; this effect is most pronounced when the WBI and activated charcoal are premixed (in vitro) together.[47] In particular, the decreased adsorptive capacity for cocaine is pH dependent and more pronounced at pH 1.2 than at pH 7.0.[68] The osmolar characteristics of PEG-ELS do not appear to be affected by the admixture.[56]

ACTIVATED CHARCOAL AND N–ACETYLCYSTEINE

The standard treatment of an acute recent acetaminophen ingestion in overdose includes gastric decontamination and *N*-acetylcysteine (NAC). The role of activated charcoal for this ingestion has been questioned because of the concern that it may adsorb substantial quantities of the administered NAC, but this intervention remains a standard. The debate is developed extensively in Chapter 32.

MULTIPLE-DOSE ACTIVATED CHARCOAL (MDAC)

In 1982, a report concluded that orally administered MDAC enhanced the total body clearance (nonrenal clearance) of 6 healthy volunteers given 2.85 mg/kg of intravenous phenobarbital.[12] The serum half-life of phenobarbital decreased from 110 ± 8 to 45 ± 6 hours. An accompanying editorial suggested that MDAC enhanced the diffusion of phenobarbital from the blood into the gastrointestinal tract and trapped it there, to be excreted later in the stool. In this manner, activated charcoal was said to perform as an "infinite sink" allowing for "gastrointestinal dialysis" to take place.[62] These findings were subsequently confirmed by studies in

dogs and rats using IV aminophylline.[31,74] An isolated vascularly perfused rat small intestine elegantly demonstrated this concept of gastrointestinal dialysis.[74] Activated charcoal dramatically affected the pharmacokinetics of theophylline, producing a constant intestinal clearance that was approximately equivalent to intestinal blood flow. MDAC increases the elimination of digitoxin;[100] phenobarbital;[102] carbamazepine;[14] phenylbutazone;[84] dapsone;[85] nadolol;[33] theophylline;[13,67,116] salicylate;[103] cyclosporine;[49] propoxyphene;[54] nortriptyline; and amitriptyline, but clinical utility must be defined.[53,114] Extensive lists of adsorptive capacities for these and other agents are available.[5,19,20,23,75]

An analysis of 28 volunteer studies involving 17 drugs was unable to correlate the physiochemical properties of a particular drug with the ability of MDAC to decrease the plasma half-life of that drug.[19] Although the half-life was not thought to be the best marker of enhanced elimination, it was the only variable consistently mentioned in all of the studies that substantially differed with one another in design. The drugs with the longest intrinsic plasma half-lives seemed to demonstrate the largest percent reduction in plasma half-life when MDAC was utilized. A subsequent pig study of therapeutic doses of four simultaneously administered intravenous drugs (acetaminophen, digoxin, theophylline, and valproic acid) clarified the role of pharmacokinetics on the effectiveness of activated charcoal.[19] Theophylline, acetaminophen, and valproic acid all have small volumes of distribution. Only valproic acid is highly protein-bound at the doses employed, which probably accounted for the inability of activated charcoal to increase its clearance. The three other drugs all responded to MDAC with an increased clearance. The quickest and most dramatic effect was demonstrated with theophylline. Although digoxin has a large volume of distribution, it requires several hours to distribute from the blood to the tissues. MDAC is beneficial before distribution is complete, while the digoxin is still accessible in the blood compartment.

The benefits of MDAC undoubtedly depend on a number of patient variables and drug factors. Most important to remember, however, is that volunteer studies do not accurately reflect the overdose situation[75] in which saturation of plasma protein binding, saturation of liver enzymes, and acid-base disturbances may make more free drug available for an enteroenteric effect.

MDAC may also be beneficial to decrease drug absorption when large amounts of drugs are ingested and dissolution is delayed (masses, bezoars), when drugs exhibit a delayed or prolonged release phase (enteric coated, sustained release), or when reabsorption can be prevented (enterohepatic circulation of active drug, active metabolites, or conjugated drug hydrolyzed by gut bacteria to active drug). Once drug absorption is complete, MDAC may be most useful when free drug in the plasma is substantial enough to permit an enteroenteric effect. For this effect to be of clinical importance the drug or metabolite must possess a lengthy elimination phase, as MDAC is given every 2–6 hours. Drugs with a small volume of distribution or which fit a two compartment model with a prolonged initial distribution phase, and low or saturable plasma protein binding are theoretically most accessible.

MDAC appears to enhance gastrointestinal elimination of many drugs by interfering with enteroenteric circulation, interrupting enterohepatic circulation, and/or minimizing desorption. Shortening the half-life of a drug in overdose logically benefits the patient clinically by limiting the time of associated central nervous system (CNS) depression, risk of aspiration, intensive care, nursing hours, and hospitalization, although the actual proof of this is currently lacking. In a randomized clinical study of this potential benefit, some patients who overdosed with phenobarbital were given a single dose of activated charcoal, while others were given multiple doses.[102] Although the half-life of phenobarbital was significantly decreased in the multiple-dose group (36 vs. 93 hours), the length of intubation time required by each group did not differ from one another. This study has been criticized as being too small, having unevenly matched groups, and focusing on a single endpoint (extubation) that may be dependent on factors other than patient condition (such as the time of day) to determine potential clinical benefit. The adverse effects of MDAC include diarrhea (only when sorbitol-containing charcoal preparations are used), constipation, vomiting with a subsequent risk of aspiration, intestinal obstruction, and reduction of serum concentrations of therapeutically employed drugs.[79,83,99]

To prevent aspiration pneumonitis, it is imperative that the patient's airway be protected. Prior to administration of activated charcoal, gastrointestinal motility should be determined by the auscultation of bowel sounds and by an absence of abdominal distension. When bowel function is lost, the stomach should be decompressed to decrease the risk of subsequent vomiting and aspiration. An initial loading dose of activated charcoal should be administered to adults and children in an activated charcoal-to-drug ratio of 10:1 or 1–2 g/kg of body weight (if drug dose is unknown). The correct dose of activated charcoal for multiple dosing, when it is indicated, is best tailored to the dose and dosage form of the drug ingested, seriousness of the overdose, potential lethality of the ingestant, and the patient's ability to tolerate activated charcoal. Benefit should always be weighed against risk. Doses of activated charcoal for multiple dosing have varied considerably in the past, ranging from 0.25 to 0.5 g/kg every 1–6 hours, to 20–60 g for adults every 1, 2, 4, or 6 hours. The total dose administered may be more important than frequency of administration.[50,119] In some cases, continuous nasogastric administration of activated charcoal can be employed, especially when vomiting is a problem.[38,91,119]

In conclusion, when administration is timely activated charcoal is a very effective nonspecific adsorbent. It should be of benefit to a patient with a potentially life threatening ingestion involving a toxin adsorbable by activated charcoal and in whom no contraindications exist. Oral MDAC can decrease the elimination half-lives of a variety of drugs through diverse mechanisms, including gastrointestinal dialysis, making treatment applicable even to some nonoral drug overdoses. Care must be taken to avoid pulmonary aspiration and intestinal obstruction. Prehospital administration of activated charcoal by emergency medical services may offer a significant advantage in facilitating the administration of charcoal to occur closer to the time of overdose.[2,122] Home availability of activated charcoal should be encouraged, and as more palatable forms of activated charcoal are developed children may accept this agent more readily.[60,61]

REFERENCES

1. Albertson TE, Derlet RW, Foulke GE, et al: Superiority of activated charcoal alone compared with ipecac and activated charcoal in the treatment of acute toxic ingestions. Ann Emerg Med 1989;18:56–59.
2. Allison T, Gough J, Brown L, Thoms S: Potential time savings by prehospital administration of activated charcoal. Prehosp Emerg Care 1997;1:73–75.
3. Al-Shareef AM, Buss DC, Allen EM, Routledge PA: The effects of charcoal and sorbitol (alone and in combination) on plasma theophylline concentration after a sustained release formulation. Hum Exp Toxicol 1990;9:179–182.
4. American Academy of Clinical Toxicology & European Association of Poison Centers and Clinical Toxicologists: Position statement: Single-dose activated charcoal. Clin Toxicol 1997;35: 721–741.
5. American Academy of Clinical Toxicology & European Association of Poison Centers and Clinical Toxicologists: Position statement and practice guidelines on the use of multi-dose activated charcoal in the treatment of acute poisoning. J Toxicol Clin Toxicol 1999;37: 731–751.
6. Anderson H: Experimental studies on the pharmacology of activated charcoal. Acta Pharmacol 1948;4:275–284.
7. Anderson H: Experimental studies on the pharmacology of activated charcoal. II. The effect of pH on the adsorption by charcoal from aqueous solutions. Acta Pharmacol 1947;3:199–218.
8. Anderson H: Experimental studies on the pharmacology of activated charcoal. I. Adsorption power of charcoal in aqueous solutions. Acta Pharmacol 1946;2:69–78.
9. Anderson I, Ware C: Syrup of ipecacuanha [letter]. Br Med J 1987; 294:578.
10. Auerbach PS, Osterloh J, Braun O, et al: Efficacy of gastric emptying: Gastric lavage versus emesis induced with ipecac. Ann Emerg Med 1986;15:692–698.
11. Augenstein WL, Kulig KW, Rumack BH: Delayed rise in serum drug levels in overdose patients despite multiple dose charcoal and after charcoal stools [abstract]. Vet Hum Toxicol 1987;29:491.
12. Berg M, Berlinger W, Goldberg M, et al: Acceleration of the body clearance of phenobarbital by oral activated charcoal. N Engl J Med 1982;307:642–644.
13. Berlinger WG, Spector R, Goldberg MJ, et al: Enhancement of theophylline clearance by oral activated charcoal. Clin Pharmacol Ther 1983;33:351–354.
14. Boldy DAR, Heath A, Ruddock C, et al: Activated charcoal for carbamazepine poisoning [letter]. Lancet 1987;1:1027.
15. Boyd R, Hanson J: Prospective single-blinded randomized controlled trial of two orally administered activated charcoal preparations. Acad Emerg Med 1999;16:24–25.
16. Brubacher JR, Levine B, Hoffman RS: Intestinal pseudo-obstruction (Ogilvie's syndrome) in the theophylline overdose. Vet Hum Toxicol 1996;38:368–370.
17. Burton BT, Bayer MJ, Barron L, Aitchison JP: Comparison of activated charcoal and gastric lavage in the prevention of aspirin absorption. J Emerg Med 1984;1:411–416.
18. Calvert W, Corby D, Herbertson L, Decker W: Orally administered activated charcoal: Acceptance by children. JAMA 1971;215:641.
19. Campbell J, Chyka P: Physiochemical characteristics of drugs and response to repeat dose activated charcoal. Am J Emerg Med 1992;10:208–210.
20. Chyka PA: Multiple dose activated charcoal and enhancement of systemic drug clearance: Summary of studies in animals and human volunteers. J Toxicol Clin Toxicol 1995;33:399–405.
21. Chyka PA, Holley JE, Mandrell TD, Sugathan P: Correlation of drug pharmacokinetics and effectiveness of multiple-dose activated charcoal therapy. Ann Emerg Med 1995;25:356–362.
22. Cohen V, Howland MA, Hoffman RS: Palatability of Insta-Char with cherry flavoring: A human volunteer study [abstract]. J Toxicol Clin Toxicol 1996;34:635.
23. Cooney D, ed: Activated Charcoal in Medical Applications. New York, Marcel Dekker, 1995.
24. Cooney D: In vitro adsorption of phenobarbital, chlorpheniramine maleate, and theophylline by four commercially available activated charcoal suspensions. J Toxicol Clin Toxicol 1995;33:213–217.
25. Cooney D: Effect of type and amount of carboxymethyl-cellulose on in vitro salicylate adsorption by activated charcoal. Clin toxicol 1982;19:367–376.

26. Cooney D: Palatability of sucrose-sorbitol and saccharin sweetened activated charcoal formulations. Am J Hosp Pharm 1980;37: 237–239.

27. Cooney D: "Superactive" charcoal adsorbs drugs as fast as standard antidotal charcoal. Clin Toxicol 1980;16:123–125.

28. Cooney D: A "superactive" charcoal for antidotal use in poisonings. Clin Toxicol 1977;11:387–390.

29. Curd-Sneed C, Parks K, Bordelon J, et al: In vitro adsorption of sodium phenobarbital by Superchar, USP, and Darco G-60 activated charcoals. J Toxicol Clin Toxicol 1987;25:1–11.

30. Curtis RA, Barone J, Giacona N: Efficacy of ipecac and activated charcoal/cathartic: Prevention of salicylate absorption in a simulated overdose. Arch Intern Med 1984;144:48–52.

31. DeVries MH, Rademaker C, Geerlings C, et al: Pharmacokinetic modelling of the effect of activated charcoal on the intestinal secretion of theophylline, using the isolated vascularly perfused rat small intestine. J Pharm Pharmacol 1989;41:528–533.

32. Docksteder LL, Lawrence RA, Bresnick HL: Home administration of activated charcoal: Feasibility and acceptance [abstract]. Vet Hum Toxicol 1986;28:471.

33. DuSoeuch P, Caille G, Larochelle P: Reduction of nadolol plasma half-life by activated charcoal and antibiotics in man [letter]. Clin Pharmacol Ther 1982;31:222.

34. Eisen TF, Grbcich PA, Lacouture PG, Woolf A: The adsorption of salicylates by a milk chocolate-charcoal mixture. Ann Emerg Med 1991;20:143–146.

35. Elliot CG, Colby TV, Kelly TM, et al: Charcoal lung: Bronchiolitis obliterans after aspiration of activated charcoal. Chest 1989;96: 672–674.

36. Farley T: Severe hypernatremic dehydration after use of an activated charcoal-sorbitol suspension. J Pediatr 1986;109:719–722.

37. Farrar HC, Herold DA, Reed M: Acute valproic acid intoxication enhanced drug clearance with oral activated charcoal. Crit Care Med 1993;21:299–301.

38. Fillippone G, Fish S, Lacouture P, et al: Reversible adsorption (desorption) of aspirin from activated charcoal. Arch Intern Med 1987;147:1390–1392.

39. Fisher T, Singer A: Comparison of the palatabilities of standard and superactivated charcoal in toxic ingestions: A randomized trail. Acad Emerg Med 1999;6:895–899.

40. Freedman G, Pasternak S, Krenzelok E: A clinical trial using syrup of ipecac and activated charcoal concurrently. Ann Emerg Med 1987;16: 164–166.

41. Gadgil SD, Damle SR, Advani SH, Vaidya AB: Effect of activated charcoal on the pharmacokinetics of high dose methotrexate. Cancer Treat Rep 1982;66:1169–1171.

42. Givens T, Holloway M, Watson S: Pulmonary aspiration of activated charcoal: A complication of its misuse in overdose management. Pediatr Emerg Care 1992;8:137–140.

43. Goulbourne KB, Cisek JE: Small bowel obstruction secondary to activated charcoal and adhesions. Ann Emerg Med 1994;24:108–110.

44. Gwelt P, Perrier D: Influence of thickening agents on the antidotal efficacy of activated charcoal. Clin Toxicol 1976;9:89–92.

45. Harris CR, Filandrinos D: Accidental administration of activated charcoal into the lung: Aspiration by proxy. Ann Emerg Med 1993;22:143–146.

46. Harsch H: Aspiration of activated charcoal [letter]. N Engl J Med 1986;314:318.

47. Hoffman RS, Chiang WK, Howland MA, et al: Theophylline desorption from activated charcoal caused by whole-bowel irrigation. J Toxicol Clin Toxicol 1991;29:191–202.

48. Holt E, Holz P: The black bottle. J Pediatr 1963;63:306–314.

49. Honcharik N, Anthone S: Activated charcoal in acute cyclosporin overdose. Lancet 1985;1:1051.

50. Ilkhanipour K, Yealy D, Krenzelok E: The comparative efficacy of various multiple dose activated charcoal regimens. Am J Emerg Med 1992;10:298–300.

51. Jaggi M, Cohen V, Howland M, Hoffman R: Activated charcoal versus Insta-Char with cherry flavoring in adult overdose patients [abstract]. J Toxicol Clin Toxicol 1997;35:544.

52. Justiniani F, Hippalgaonkar R, Martinez L: Charcoal-containing empyema complicating treatment for overdose. Chest 1985;87: 404–405.

53. Karkkainen S, Neuvonen P: Pharmacokinetics of amitriptyline influenced by oral charcoal and urine pH. Int J Clin Pharmacol Ther 1986;24:326–332.

54. Karkkainen S, Neuvonen PJ: Effect of oral charcoal and urine pH on dextropropoxyphene pharmacokinetics. Int J Clin Pharmacol Ther Toxicol 1985;23:219–225.

55. Keller R, Schwab R, Krenzelok E: Contribution of sorbitol combined with activated charcoal in prevention of salicylate absorption. Ann Emerg Med 1990;19:654–656.

56. Kirshenbaum LA, Sitar DS, Tenenbein M: Interaction between whole-bowel irrigation solution and activated charcoal: Implications for the treatment of toxic ingestions. Ann Emerg Med 1990;19: 1129–1132.

57. Kornberg AE, Dolgin J: Pediatric ingestions: Charcoal alone versus ipecac and charcoal. Ann Emerg Med 1991;20:648–651.

58. Krenzelok E, Heller M: Effectiveness of commercially available aqueous activated charcoal products. Ann Emerg Med 1987;16; 1340–1343.

59. Kulig KW, Bar-Or D, Cantrill SV, et al: Management of acutely poisoned patients without gastric emptying. Ann Emerg Med 1985;14: 562–567.

60. Lamminpaa A, Vilska J, Hoppu K: Medical activated charcoal for a child's poisoning at home: Availability and success of administration in Finland. Hum Exp Toxicol 1993;12:29–32.

61. Lee RJ: Ancient antidote ignored. Activated charcoal is an underused antidote to a variety of drugs and chemicals, says this author. Am Pharm 1992;32:34–35.

62. Levy G: Gastrointestinal clearance of drugs with activated charcoal [editorial]. N Engl J Med 1982;307:676–678.

63. Levy G, Soda GM, Lampman TA: Inhibition by ice cream of the antidotal efficacy of activated charcoal. Am J Hosp Pharm 1975;32: 289–291.

64. Levy G, Tsuchiya T: Effect of activated charcoal on aspirin absorption in man. Clin Pharmacol Ther 1972;13:317–322.

65. Longdson P, Henderson A: Intestinal pseudo-obstruction following the use of enteral charcoal and sorbitol with mechanical ventilation with papaverum sedation for theophylline poisoning. Drug Saf 1992; 7:74–77.

66. Lopes de Freitas J, Ferreira MG, Brito MJ: Charcoal deposits in the esophageal and gastric mucosa. Am J Gastroenterol 1997;92: 1359–1360.

67. Mahutte CK, True RJ, Michiels TN, et al: Increased serum theophylline clearance with orally administered activated charcoal. Am Rev Resp Dis 1983;128:820–822.

68. Makosiej F, Hoffman RS, Howland MA, et al: An in vitro evaluation of cocaine hydrochloride adsorption by activated charcoal and desorption upon addition of polyethylene glycol electrolyte solution. J Toxicol Clin Toxicol 1993;31:381–386.

69. Manes M, Mann JF: Easily swallowed formulations of antidote charcoals. Clin Toxicol 1974;7:355–364.

70. Mariani PJ, Poole N: Gastrointestinal tract perforation with charcoal peritoneum complicating orogastric intubation and lavage. Ann Emerg Med 1993;22:606–609.

71. Mathur LK, Jaffe JM, Colaizzi JL, Moriarity RW: Activated charcoal-carboxymethylcellulose gel formulation as an antidotal agent for orally ingested aspirin. Am J Hosp Pharm 1976;33:717–729.

72. Mayersohn M, Perrier D, Picchioni A: Evaluation of a charcoal-sorbitol mixture as an antidote for oral aspirin overdose. Clin Toxicol 1977;11:561–567.

73. McFarland A, Chyka P: Selection of activated charcoal products for the treatment of poisonings. Ann Pharmacother 1993;27:358–361.

74. McKinnon RS, Desmond PV, Harmon PJ, et al: Studies on the mechanisms of action of activated charcoal on theophylline pharmacokinetics. J Pharm Pharmacol 1987;39:522–525.

75. McLuckie A, Forbes AM, Ilett KF: Role of repeated doses of oral activated charcoal in the treatment of acute intoxications. Anesth Intens Care 1990;18:375–384.

76. McNamara R, Aaron C, Gemborys M: Sorbitol catharsis does not enhance efficacy of charcoal in simulated acetaminophen overdose. Ann Emerg Med 1988;17:243–246.

77. Menzies DG, Busuttel A, Prescott LF: Fatal pulmonary aspiration of oral activated charcoal. BMJ 1988;297:459–466.

78. Merigian KS, Woodard M, Hedges JR, et al: Prospective evaluation of gastric emptying in the self poisoned patient. Am J Emerg Med 1990;8:479–483.

79. Mezutani T, Waits H, Oohashi W: Rectal ulcer with massive hemorrhage due to activated charcoal treatment in oral organophosphate poisoning. Hum Exp Toxicol 1991;10:385–386.

80. Mofenson H, Caraccio T: Magnesium intoxication in a neonate from oral magnesium hydroxide laxative. J Toxicol Clin Toxicol 1991;29:215–222.

81. Moll J, Kerns W, Tomaszewski C: Incidence of aspiration pneumonia in intubated patients receiving activated charcoal. J Emerg Med 1999;17:279–283.

82. Navarro R, Navarro K, Krenzelok E: Relative efficacy and palatability of three activated charcoal mixtures. Vet Hum Toxicol 1980;22:6–9.

83. Neuvonen PJ: Clinical pharmacokinetics of oral activated charcoal in acute intoxications. Clin Pharmacokinet 1982;7:465–489.

84. Neuvonen PJ, Elonen E: Effect of activated charcoal on absorption and elimination of phenobarbitone, carbamazepine, and phenylbutazone in man. Eur J Clin Pharmacol 1980;17:51–57.

85. Neuvonen PJ, Elonen E, Mattila MJ: Oral activated charcoal and dapsone elimination. Clin Pharmacol Ther 1980;6:823–827.

86. Neuvonen PJ, Olkkola K: Oral activated charcoal in the treatment of intoxications. Med Toxicol 1988;3:33–58.

87. Neuvonen PJ, Olkkola K: Effect of purgatives on antidotal efficacy of oral activated charcoal. Hum Toxicol 1986;5:255–263.

88. Neuvonen PJ, Olkkola K: Activated charcoal and syrup of ipecac in prevention of cimetidine and pindolol absorption in man after administration of metoclopramide as an antiemetic agent. J Toxicol Clin Toxicol 1984;22:103–114.

89. Neuvonen PJ, Olkkola K, Alanen T: Effect of ethanol and pH on the adsorption of drugs to activated charcoal: Studies in vitro and in man. Acta Pharmacol Toxicol 1984;54:1–7.

90. Neuvonen PJ, Vartiainen M, Tokola O: Comparison of activated charcoal and ipecac syrup in the prevention of drug absorption. Eur J Clin Pharmacol 1983;24:557–562.

91. Ohning B, Reed M, Blumer J: Continuous nasogastric administration of activated charcoal for the treatment of theophylline intoxication. Pediatr Pharmacol 1986;5:241–245.

92. Olkkola K: Effect of charcoal-drug ratio on antidotal efficacy of oral activated charcoal in man. Br J Clin Pharmacol 1985;19:767–773.

93. Olkkola K: Factors affecting the antidotal efficacy of oral activated charcoal. Dissertation. University of Helsinki, 1985.

94. Olkkola K, Neuvonen P: Do gastric contents modify antidotal efficacy of oral activated charcoal? Br J Clin Pharmacol 1984;18:663–669.

95. Osol A, ed: Remington's Practice of Pharmacy, 16th ed. Easton, PA, Mack Publishing, 1980.

96. Park G, Spector R, Goldberg M, et al: Effect of the surface area of activated charcoal on theophylline clearance. J Clin Pharmacol 1984;24:289–292.

97. Picchioni A: Activated charcoal: A neglected antidote. Pediatr Clin North Am 1970;17:535–543.

98. Picchioni A, Chin L, Gillespie T: Evaluation of activated charcoal-sorbitol suspension as an antidote. Clin Toxicol 1982;19:435–444.

99. Pollack M, Dunbar B, Holbrook P, Fields A: Aspiration of activated charcoal and gastric contents. Ann Emerg Med 1981;10;528–529.

100. Pond SM, Jacobs M, Marks J, et al: Treatment of digitoxin overdose with oral activated charcoal. Lancet 1982;2:1177–1178.

101. Pond SM, Lewis-Driver DJ, Williams G, et al: Gastric emptying in acute overdose: A prospective randomised controlled trial. Med J Aust 1995;163:345–349.

102. Pond SM, Olson KR, Osterloh JD, Tong TG: Randomized study of the treatment of phenobarbital overdose with repeated doses of activated charcoal. JAMA 1984;251:3104–3108.

103. Prescott L, Hillman R: Treatment of salicylate poisoning with repeated oral charcoal. Br Med J 1985;291:1472.

104. Ray MJ, Padin DR, Condie JD, Halls JM: Charcoal bezoar: Small bowel obstruction secondary to amitriptyline overdose therapy. Dig Dis Sci 1988;33:106–107.

105. Reynolds JEF, ed: Martindale: The Extra Pharmacopoeia, 29th ed. London, Pharmaceutical Press, 1989, p. 835.

106. Roberts JR, Gracely EJ: High surface area oral activated charcoal has superior clinical properties. Acad Emerg Med 1996;3:419–420.

107. Roberts J, Gracely E, Schoffetall J: Advantage of high surface area activated charcoal for GI decontamination in a human acetaminophen ingestion model. Acad Emerg Med 1997;4:167–174.

108. Roy TM, Ossorio MA, Cipolla LM, et al: Pulmonary complications after tricyclic antidepressant overdose. Chest 1989;96:852–856.

109. Scholtz E, Jaffe J, Colaizzi J: Evaluation of five activated charcoal formulations for inhibition of aspirin adsorption and palatability in man. Am J Hosp Pharm 1978;35:1355–1359.

110. Siberman H, Davis SM, Lee A: Activated charcoal aspiration. NC Med J 1990;51:79–80.

111. Sketris I, Mowry J, Czajka P, et al: Saline catharsis: Effect on aspirin bioavailability in combination with activated charcoal. J Clin Pharmacol 1982;22:59–64.

112. Smilkstein MJ, Knapp GL, Kulig KW, Rumack BH: Efficacy of oral N-acetylcysteine in the treatment of acetaminophen overdose: Analysis of the National Multicenter Study (1976–1985). N Engl J Med 1988;319:1557–1562.

113. Smilkstein MJ, Smolinske S, Kulig KW, et al: Severe hypermagnesemia due to multiple-dose cathartic therapy. West J Med 1988;148:208–211.

114. Swartz C, Sherman A: The treatment of tricyclic antidepressant overdose with activated charcoal. J Clin Psychopharmacol 1984;4:336–340.

115. Tenenbein M, Cohen S, Sitar DS: Efficacy of ipecac induced emesis, orogastric lavage and activated charcoal for acute drug overdose. Ann Emerg Med 1987;16:838–841.

116. True RJ, Berman JN, Mahutte CK: Treatment of theophylline toxicity with oral activated charcoal. Crit Care Med 1984;12:113–114.

117. Tsuchiya T, Levy G: Relationship between effect of activated charcoal on drug adsorption characteristics in vitro. J Pharm Sci 1972;61:586–589.

118. United States Pharmacopeial Convention: The United States Pharmacopoeia, 20th rev. The National Formulary, 15th ed. Easton, PA, Mack Publishing, 1980.

119. Vale JA, Proudfoot AT: How useful is activated charcoal? BMJ 1993;306:78–79.

120. Van de Graaf W, Thompson WL, Sunshine I, et al: Adsorbent and cathartic inhibition of enteral drug adsorption. J Pharmacol Exp Ther 1982;221:656–663.

121. Watson WA, Cremes KF, Chapman JA: Gastrointestinal obstruction associated with multiple dose activated charcoal. J Emerg Med 1986;4;401–407.

122. Wax P, Cobaugh D: Prehospital gastrointestinal decontamination of toxic ingestions: A missed opportunity Am J Emerg Med 1998;16:114–116.

123. Yancy RE, O'Barr TP, Corby DG: In vitro and in vivo evaluation of the effect of cherry flavoring on the adsorptive capacity of activated charcoal for salicylic acid. Vet Hum Toxicol 1980;22:163–165.

ANTIDOTES IN DEPTH

Cathartics

Mary Ann Howland

Drugs that promote intestinal evacuation are referred to as *laxatives, cathartics*, or *purgatives*. Laxatives promote a soft-formed or semifluid stool within 6 hours to 3 days, depending on the agent and the dose employed. Cathartics promote a rapid watery evacuation within 1–3 hours.[4] Purgatives imply an even stronger evacuation. The same drug may accomplish any or all of these tasks, depending on the dose.

The traditional classification of laxatives into the five categories of bulk-forming, stimulant or irritant, softeners, saline or osmotic, and lubricant is largely empirical.[3] Additional investigation is needed to determine how laxatives affect gastrointestinal motility and fluid and electrolyte movement.[3]

Traditionally, the effects of saline cathartics, such as magnesium citrate and sulfate salts, were attributed to the fact that they were relatively nonabsorbable anions and cations that established an osmotic gradient and drew water into the gut. The increased water retention led to increased intestinal pressure and a subsequent increase in intestinal motility.[6] This hypothesis, however, is probably overly simplistic.[3] Recent evidence shows that magnesium releases cholecystokinin, a gastrointestinal hormone, from the duodenal mucosa, which stimulates intestinal motor activity and alters fluid movement.[3,36] Magnesium decreases transit time while paradoxically decreasing smooth muscle contractility in the ileum.[3,36] In animals, saline cathartics may delay gastric emptying, which may affect the rate of absorption but not necessarily the extent of absorption of some drugs.[36] Bisacodyl and phenolphthalein are stimulant cathartics whose action is at least partially linked to the induction of nitric oxide synthase and an increased production of nitric oxide.[10]

Sorbitol (D-Glucitol) is naturally found in many ripe fruits and prepared industrially from glucose. Sorbitol is about 60% as sweet as glucose, and upon metabolism yields the same 4 calories per gram as glucose. It is slowly absorbed from the GI tract with some conversion to glucose, but the majority is converted to carbon dioxide. Sorbitol presumably works by an osmotic action, but little is known about the mechanisms of action of this drug. Sorbitol is not even mentioned as a laxative or cathartic in numerous reviews.[3,4,6,36,38,39]

Cathartics have been recommended for basic poison management for many years. Intuitively, the advantages of cathartics appear to be decreasing the potential for constipation or obstruction from activated charcoal, hastening the delivery of activated charcoal to the small intestine, and hastening the elimination of poorly absorbed or sustained-released drugs or toxins before they can be absorbed. A 1981 review of cathartic use in toxic ingestions confirmed frequent utilization, but found little evidence for their efficacy.[32] This analysis remains true today.[43]

Given alone, cathartics such as sorbitol or sodium sulfate may decrease peak and/or total absorption of some drugs, but in no study has this effect achieved the results reported with activated charcoal alone.[2,5,22,30,40] When comparing the efficacy of a single dose of activated charcoal alone with that of activated charcoal plus a single dose of cathartic, studies suggest the combination to be as good as,[2,24,29,30,33] a little better than,[5,14] or even a little worse than activated charcoal alone.[22,40] A study of a sustained-release theophylline preparation found that a combination of activated charcoal and sorbitol decreased total absorption a little more than activated charcoal alone when given at 6 and 8 hours after ingestion.[11]

In contrast to studying effects on total amount of drug absorbed, some studies have compared cathartic use with respect to time to first stool and number of stools. These studies used a variety of products and doses.[12,17,25,26,37] In general, sorbitol produced stools in the shortest amount of time but with the highest incidence of nausea and vomiting. When comparing gram doses of sorbitol, the specific gravity of 1.285 g/mL, the concentration, and the mL amount must be used in the calculation. For example, 70 mL of sorbitol 70% is equivalent to 62.965 g (70 mL × 70% × 1.285 g/mL).[42] The lack of precise calculations has led to inaccurate estimates of g/kg doses of sorbitol in some studies.

In nonpoisoned adult volunteers, four regimens were used, each including 50 g of activated charcoal administered as a water slurry with 300 mL ginger ale. Given alone it was the first regimen. Other groups had 70% sorbitol (240 mL), 300 mL magnesium citrate (17.45 g), or 30 mL 50% magnesium sulfate (15 g) added. The times to first charcoal stool were 23.5, 0.9, 4.2, and 9.3 hours, respectively.[17] Sorbitol produced 10–15 watery stools, the most abdominal cramping before catharsis, and its taste was rated second to that of magnesium citrate because of its nauseating sweetness. In a study of 6 adult volunteers, the ingestion of 30 g activated charcoal in 150 mL of 70% sorbitol resulted in severe diarrhea with mild to moderate abdominal cramping and gurgling.[26] The first charcoal stool was noted in 89 minutes, 12 hours ± 10 hours of diarrhea occurred, and 62 hours of black stools were reported.[26] There were no effects on routinely measured laboratory values.

A study of catharsis in poisoned children 1–5 years of age compared 4 mL/kg of sorbitol (50%; actually 2.48 g/kg, although reported as 2.57 g/kg), magnesium citrate (233 mg/kg), magnesium sulfate (250 mg/kg) and water, each added as a slurry with activated charcoal (1 g/kg) and delivered via a nasogastric tube.[12] Sorbitol produced the shortest time to first stool at 8.48 hours compared to magnesium citrate at 12.84 hours, water at 14 hours, and magnesium sulfate at 22.65 hours. Forty-two percent of patients using sorbitol vomited, whereas only 17% of patients vomited with the other regimens. The mean number of stools in 24 hours produced with sorbitol was 2.97; with magnesium citrate it was 1.79; with water it was 1.75; and with magnesium sulfate it was 1.65 stools.

The risks associated with cathartics are dehydration, absorption of magnesium or other salts and hypokalemia and metabolic alkalosis from dehydration and activation of the renin-angiotensin-aldosterone system. In two elderly patients, rectal prolapse occurred.[16] Nausea, vomiting, abdominal cramping, and frequent watery stools are common complaints after sorbitol administration.[14,15,28]

Hypocalcemia, hyperphosphatemia, and hypokalemia were reported following the use of hypertonic phosphate enemas.[7,9,19,20,31,35] In some of these cases, the recommended dose was used.[7] Consequential morbidity and mortality were reported in previously healthy children as well as in those with bowel abnormalities who received phosphosoda. In none of the case reports were the enemas used as part of basic poison management; nonetheless, hypertonic phosphate enemas or oral solutions of phosphosoda should never be used in children as part of poison management.

Because of the demonstrable efficacy of repetitive doses of activated charcoal in certain overdoses, some clinicians mistakenly assume that repetitive doses of cathartics should be given concomitantly.[21] Significant toxicity results from the repetitive administration of either magnesium or sorbitol-containing cathartics. A patient who received 300-mL doses of magnesium citrate every 4 hours for approximately 72 hours developed neuromuscular toxicity and coma and had a magnesium level of 11.4 mEq/L.[13] The patient was treated with intravenous calcium chloride and hemodialysis. A 25-day-old girl was given 8 teaspoons of milk of magnesia each day for 3 days (not in the management of an overdose). She became limp and difficult to arouse and had a serum magnesium level of 7.6 mEq/L.[27] A study investigating the effect of single versus two or three doses of 30 g of magnesium sulfate in suspected overdose patients revealed increasingly elevated serum magnesium levels after the second and third doses, with a resultant mean peak of 2.6 mEq/L.[34] These increases occurred in patients with normal renal function. Clinical signs and symptoms of hypermagnesemia were not reported. Multiple-dose activated charcoal regimens used to facilitate "gastrointestinal dialysis" have resulted in severe cathartic-related adverse effects in four case reports.[1,8,18,23] In each instance the activated charcoal preparations used also contained 70% sorbitol and repeat-dose sorbitol presumably led to severe dehydration and hypernatremia, with neurologic sequelae in one instance.[1,8,23] The retention of sorbitol after repetitive doses in an aperistaltic gut may lead to significant morbidity due to the gas formation and abdominal distention as a result of the digestive action of gut bacteria.[18] Highlighting the potential for toxicity from repetitive activated charcoal dosing was a survey revealing that 16% of those hospitals surveyed only stocked activated charcoal premixed with sorbitol.[41]

Contraindications to the use of cathartics include an adynamic ileus, preexisting or anticipated diarrhea or volume depletion or intestinal perforation, abdominal trauma, and intestinal obstruction. Renal failure is a contraindication to the use of magnesium-containing cathartics. Oil-based cathartics such as mineral oil should not be used because of the risks associated with aspiration and the possibility for enhancing the absorption of certain lipid-soluble toxins.

Cathartics should no longer be considered part of the routine management of overdose in either children or adults. There is no evidence to indicate that single doses of cathartics alone without activated charcoal are more effective than activated charcoal alone at decreasing absorption or enhancing elimination of substances capable of binding to activated charcoal. Cathartics should never be used as a substitute for activated charcoal when drugs that are adsorbed to activated charcoal are involved. When total drug absorption is evaluated, a single dose of a cathartic given with activated charcoal appears to be only as efficacious as activated charcoal given alone.

Giving a cathartic for the sake of producing a faster onset of charcoal stools has never been shown to produce a better clinical outcome. In adults, when large amounts of drugs have been ingested or when desorption from charcoal may be an important consideration (such as ASA), a single dose of a cathartic, preferably magnesium citrate or sorbitol, may be given with the activated charcoal. When multiple-dose activated charcoal is used, if cathartics are used they should only be employed with the first dose. Patients should be administered sufficient fluids orally to avoid inspissation and dehydration. Whole-bowel irrigation, unless contraindicated, is preferable to repetitive dose cathartics for the evacuation of sustained-release or poorly soluble drugs or toxins not adsorbed to activated charcoal.

The dose of sorbitol is 1–2 mL/kg of the 70% solution in adults and 4 mL/kg of a 35% solution in children. The dose of magnesium citrate as a 10% solution is 250 mL in adults or 4 mL/kg in children.

REFERENCES

1. Allerton J, Strom J: Hypernatremia due to repeated doses of charcoal-sorbitol. Am J Kidney Dis 1991;7:581–584.
2. Al-Shareef AH, Buss DC, Allen EM, Routledge PA: The effects of charcoal and sorbitol (alone and in combination) on plasma theophylline concentration after a sustained release formulation. Hum Exp Toxicol 1990;9:179–182.
3. Binder H: Pharmacology of laxatives. Annu Rev Pharmacol Toxicol 1977;17:355–367.
4. Brunton LL: Laxatives. In: Goodman LS, Gilman AG, Rall TW, Murad F, eds: The Pharmacological Basis of Therapeutics, 7th ed. New York, Macmillan, 1985, pp. 994–1003.
5. Chin L, Picchioni A, Gillespie T: Saline cathartics and saline cathartics plus activated charcoal as antidotal treatments. Clin Toxicol 1981;18:865–871.
6. Darlington RC: Laxatives. In: Griffenhagen GB, Hawkins LL, eds: Handbook of Nonprescription Drugs. Washington, DC, American Pharmaceutical Association, 1973, pp. 62–76.
7. Davis R, Eichner J, Bleyer W, et al: Hypocalcemia, hyperphosphatemia, and dehydration following a single hypertonic phosphate enema. J Pediatr 1977;90:484–485.
8. Farley T: Severe hypernatremic dehydration after use of an activated charcoal-sorbitol suspension. J Pediatr 1986;109:719–722.
9. Forman J, Baluarte J, Gruskin A: Hypokalemia after hypertonic phosphate enemas. J Pediatr 1979;94:149–151.
10. Gaginella TS, Mascolo N, Izzo AA, et al: Nitric oxide as a mediator of bisacodyl and phenolphthalein laxative action: Induction of nitric oxide synthase. J Pharm Exp Ther 1994;270:1239–1245.
11. Goldberg M, Spector R, Park G, et al: The effect of sorbitol and activated charcoal on serum theophylline concentrations after slow release theophylline. Clin Pharmacol Ther 1987;41:108–111.
12. James LP, Nichols MH, King WD: A comparison of cathartics in pediatric ingestions. Pediatrics 1995;96:235–238.
13. Jones J, Heiselman D, Dougherty J, et al: Cathartic-induced magnesium toxicity during overdose management. Ann Emerg Med 1986;15:1214–1218.
14. Keller R, Schwab R, Krenzelok E: Contribution of sorbitol combined with activated charcoal in prevention of salicylate absorption. Ann Emerg Med 1990;19:654–656.
15. Kirshenbaum CA, Mathews SC, Sitar DS, Tenenbein M: Whole-bowel irrigation versus activated charcoal in sorbitol for the ingestion of modified-release pharmaceuticals. Clin Pharmacol Ther 1989;46:264–271.

16. Korkis A, Miskowitz P, Kurt R, Klein H: Rectal prolapse after oral cathartics. J Clin Gastroenterol 1992;14:339–341.

17. Krenzelok EP, Keller R, Stewart RD: Gastrointestinal transit times of cathartics combined with charcoal. Ann Emerg Med 1985;14:1152–1155.

18. Longdon P, Henderson A: Intestinal pseudo-obstruction following the use of enteral charcoal and sorbitol and mechanical ventilation with papaveretum sedation for theophylline poisoning. Drug Saf 1992;7:74–77.

19. Loughnan P, Mullins G: Brain damage following a hypertonic phosphate enema. Am J Dis Child 1977;131:1032.

20. Martin R, Lisehora G, Braxton M, et al: Fatal poisoning from sodium phosphate enema: A case report and experimental study. JAMA 1987;257:2190–2192.

21. Massanari MJ, Hendeles L, Hill E, et al: The efficacy of sorbitol and activated charcoal in reducing theophylline absorption from a slow release formulation. Drug Int Clin Pharm 1986;20:471.

22. Mayersohn M, Perrier D, Picchioni A: Evaluation of a charcoal-sorbitol mixture as an antidote for oral aspirin overdose. Clin Toxicol 1977;11:561–567.

23. McCord M: Toxicity of sorbitol-charcoal suspension. J Pediatr 1987;110:307–308.

24. McNamara R, Aaron C, Gemborys M: Sorbitol catharsis does not enhance efficacy of charcoal in simulated acetaminophen overdose. Ann Emerg Med 1988;17:243–246.

25. Minocha A, Krenzelok EP, Spyker D: Dosage recommendations for activated charcoal—sorbitol treatment. J Toxicol Clin Toxicol 1985;23:579–587.

26. Minocha A, Merold DA, Bruns DE, et al: Effect of activated charcoal in 70% sorbitol in healthy individuals. J Toxicol Clin Toxicol 1984–85;22:529–536.

27. Mofenson HC, Caraccio TR: Magnesium intoxication in a neonate from oral magnesium hydroxide laxative. J Toxicol Clin Toxicol 1991;29:215–222.

28. Muller-Lissner SA: Adverse effects of laxatives: Fact and fiction. Pharmacol 1993;47(Suppl 1):138–145.

29. Neuvonen P, Olkkola K: Effect of purgatives on antidotal efficacy of oral activated charcoal. Vet Hum Toxicol 1986;5:255–263.

30. Picchioni A, Chin L, Gillespie T: Evaluation of activated charcoal-sorbitol suspension as an antidote. Clin Toxicol 1982;19:435–444.

31. Reedy J, Zwiren G: Enema-induced hypocalcemia and hyperphosphatemia leading to cardiac arrest during induction of anesthesia in an outpatient surgery center. Anesthesiology 1983;59:578–579.

32. Riegel J, Becker C: Use of cathartics in toxic ingestions. Ann Emerg Med 1981;10:254–258.

33. Sketris I, Mowry J, Czajka P, et al: Saline catharsis: Effect on aspirin bioavailability in combination with activated charcoal. J Clin Pharmacol 1982;22:59–64.

34. Smilkstein MJ, Steedle D, Kulig KW, et al: Magnesium levels after magnesium containing cathartics. J Toxicol Clin Toxicol 1988;26:51–65.

35. Sotos J, Cutler E, Finkel M, et al: Hypocalcemic coma following two pediatric phosphate enemas. Pediatrics 1977;60:305–307.

36. Stewart J: Effects of emetic and cathartic agents on the gastrointestinal tract and the treatment of toxic ingestions. Clin Toxicol 1983;20:199–253.

37. Sue YJ, Woolf A, Shannon M: Efficacy of magnesium citrate cathartic pediatric toxic ingestions. Ann Emerg Med 1994;24:709–712.

38. Tedesco F: Laxative use in constipation. Am J Gastroenterol 1985;80:303–309.

39. Thompson WG: Laxatives: Clinical pharmacology and rational use. Drugs 1980;19:49–58.

40. Van de Graff W, Thompson L, Sunshine I, et al: Absorbent and cathartic inhibition of enteral drug absorption. J Pharmacol Exp Ther 1982;221:656–663.

41. Wax PM, Wang RY, Hoffman RS, et al: Prevalence of sorbitol in multiple-dose activated charcoal regimens in emergency departments. Ann Emerg Med 1993;22:1807–1812.

42. Weaver WR: Calculating sorbitol dosage. Ann Emerg Med 1988;17:661–662.

43. American Academy of Clinical Toxicology and European Association of Poison Centers and Clinical Toxicologists: Position statement: Cathartics. Clin Toxicol 1997;35:743–752.

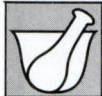 **ANTIDOTES IN DEPTH**

Whole-Bowel Irrigation

Mary Ann Howland

Rapid ingestion of a large volume of fluid can achieve the quality of bowel evacuation necessary for surgery. Absorbable solutions previously employed for this purpose consisted of normal saline or balanced electrolytes but they led to significant sodium and water retention.[8] A nonabsorbable solution is readily available, composed of polyethylene glycol and electrolytes lavage solution (PEG-ELS), which causes only minimal net water and electrolyte shifts.[8] Many studies demonstrate patient acceptance, effectiveness, and safety when used for bowel preparation.[1,4,9,10,26,36,37]

As mentioned, whole-bowel irrigation with PEG-ELS flushes out the gastrointestinal tract without causing fluid and electrolyte shifts, and the hope is to reduce drug or toxin bioavailability by decreasing the time available for drug absorption. However, there is some concern that moving drug from the stomach to the small intestine, or increasing the dissolution of a previously saturated solution, may increase absorption. Once absorption has occurred, it is unlikely that whole-bowel irrigation can play a prominent role. Although animal models suggest whole-bowel irrigation may enhance systemic clearance via gastrointestinal dialysis, much like multiple-dose activated charcoal,[20] low flow rates, the typical delay in administering whole-bowel irrigation (WBI) in actual clinical situations, and the inconvenience of this procedure make it highly unlikely that the effect can be achieved in humans.

Early forms of whole-bowel irrigation with saline and potassium chloride were used for two cases of drug overdoses.[26] As expected, fluid and electrolyte abnormalities did occur; nevertheless, the author concluded that the technique was safe in pediatric patients.[26] Whole-bowel irrigation was later applied to a series of 8 patients with toxic ingestions, including 4 patients who swallowed disk batteries.[33] Efficacy was difficult to prove in this series, and one patient who was given lactated Ringer solution developed peripheral edema. A volunteer study evaluated the ingestion of 5 g of ampicillin followed by whole-bowel irrigation with PEG-ELS.[34] After 234 minutes and 7.71 L of fluid, there was a 67% decrease in ampicillin absorption without any significant changes in fluid or electrolytes.

In a dog model involving sustained-release theophylline, and in a volunteer study involving enteric-coated aspirin, whole-bowel irrigation was shown to be as effective as, or slightly more effective than, a single dose or repeated doses of activated charcoal (with a single dose of sorbitol).[7,16] In another volunteer study involving sustained-release lithium preparations, whole-bowel irrigation significantly decreased peak lithium serum concentration and lithium bioavailability.[30] However, whole-bowel irrigation was inferior to activated charcoal when administered following 650 mg of immediate-release aspirin.[28] Once aspirin was absorbed, whole-bowel irrigation was unable to enhance systemic clearance.[23]

There are reports of the use of whole-bowel irrigation in the management of overdoses of iron,[11,22,32,35] sustained-release theophylline,[15] sustained-release verapamil,[5] zinc sulfate,[6] lead,[25,27] ar-senic-containing herbicide,[19] delayed-release fenfluramine,[24] and for body packers.[14,39]

Two case reports and 1 volunteer study question the efficacy of whole-bowel irrigation.[6,29,31] Whole-bowel irrigation for 5 hours following ingestion of 10 fluorescent coffee beans by 7 volunteers led to the removal of an average of only 4 beans (range, 1–8), for a 40% efficiency rate.[29] The coffee bean, because of its physical characteristics (density, solubility, size), might not be representative of substances amenable to whole-bowel irrigation. However, we are aware of anecdotal instances when whole-bowel irrigation has not evacuated all of the drug packets in a body packer either because of inadequate dosing, partial obstruction, or the nature of the procedure.

Several in vitro studies have demonstrated that the addition of PEG-ELS to activated charcoal significantly decreases the adsorptive capacity of activated charcoal.[13,21] The interaction was affected by pH and magnified by high ratios of PEG-ELS to activated charcoal.[3,17,21] However, the osmolality of the PEG-ELS did not seem to be affected at simulated clinical ratios.[17] Whole-bowel irrigation in an animal model appeared to have an adverse effect by washing the activated charcoal away from the sustained-release theophylline.[7]

Adverse effects include vomiting (especially with rapid administration) which is of concern in patients with potential airway compromise. Other adverse affects include abdominal bloating and anal itching (from excessive wiping); the patient will need to remain on a commode for 4–6 hours. Two unusual adverse effects are also reported following PEG-ELS use for bowel preparation. One is the exacerbation of congestive heart failure in an unstable patient with cardiac and renal dysfunction.[12] The other complication is colonic perforation, which occurred in a patient with severe diverticulitis.[18]

The recommended dose of PEG-ELS is 0.5 L/h for small children and 1.5–2 L/h for adolescents and adults. PEG-ELS solution may be administered orally to a patient or administered through a nasogastric tube for 4–6 hours or until the rectal effluent becomes clear. Vomiting may occur and appears to be related to the rate of delivery. An antiemetic such as metoclopramide or a serotonin antagonist may be required, particularly if an emetic agent has been ingested or syrup of ipecac was previously given.

Contraindications to whole-bowel irrigation include significant gastrointestinal pathology or dysfunction, such as ileus, perforation, hemorrhage and obstruction, an unprotected compromised airway, and hemodynamic instability.[2,32] Whole-bowel irrigation was used successfully in 2 pregnant women at 38 and 26 weeks of gestation.[38,40]

The role of PEG-ELS in the overdosed patient remains to be defined. There are no controlled clinical studies assessing outcome. Theoretically, ingestions of sustained-release drugs (theophylline, verapamil), drugs not adsorbed by charcoal (iron, sustained-release lithium, lead), and drug packets (in body packers) may be amenable to the use of PEG-ELS for whole-bowel irrigation. An added advantage may be that if these patients subsequently require endoscopy, diagnostic radiography, or surgery, after whole-bowel irrigation, the gastrointestinal tract mucosa may be easily visualized and, each intervention will be facilitated. Activated charcoal should be given to those patients for whom it is indicated, and a comparable dose of activated charcoal should be given following PEG-ELS administration to prevent or overcome the potential drug/toxin/activated charcoal desorption with its potential for further systemic absorption. The interaction between activated charcoal and PEG-ELS requires further study.

REFERENCES

1. Ambrose N, Johnson M, Burdon D, et al: A physiologic approach of polyethylene glycol and a balanced electrolyte solution as bowel preparation. Br J Surg 1983;70:428–430.

2. American Academy of Clinical Toxicology and European Association of Poison Centers and Clinical Toxicologists: Position statement: Whole-Bowel Irrigation. J Toxicol Clin Toxicol 1997;35:753–762.

3. Atta-Politou J, Macheras P, Koupparis M: The effect of polyethylene glycol on the charcoal adsorption of chlorpromazine studied by ion-selective electrode potentiometry. J Toxicol Clin Toxicol 1996;34: 307–316.

4. Beck D, Harford F, diPalma J, et al: Bowel cleansing with polyethylene glycol electrolyte lavage solution. South Med J 1985;78: 1414–1416.

5. Buckley N, Dawson A, Howarth D, Whyte I: Slow release verapamil poisoning. Med J Aust 1993;158:202–204.

6. Burkhart KK, Kulig KW, Rumack BH: Whole-bowel irrigation as adjunctive treatment for zinc sulfate overdose. Ann Emerg Med 1990;19:1167–1170.

7. Burkhart KK, Wuerz R, Donovan JW: Whole-bowel irrigation as adjunctive treatment for sustained release theophylline overdose. Ann Emerg Med 1992;21:1316–1320.

8. Davis G, Santa Ana C, Morawsk S, et al: Development of a lavage solution associated with minimal water and electrolyte absorption or secretion. Gastroenterology 1980;78:991–995.

9. DiPalma J, Brady C, Stewart D, et al: Comparison of colon cleansing methods in preparation for colonoscopy. Gastroenterology 1984;86: 856–860.

10. Erstoff J, Howard D, Marshall J, et al: A randomized blinded clinical trial of a rapid colonic lavage solution (GoLYTELY) compared with standard preparation for colonoscopy and barium enema. Gastroenterology 1983;84:1512–1516.

11. Everson G, Bertaccini E, O'Leary J: Use of whole-bowel irrigation in an infant following iron overdose. Am J Emerg Med 1991;9:366–369.

12. Granberry MC, White LM, Gardner SF, et al: Exacerbation of congestive heart failure after administration of polyethylene glycol-electrolyte lavage solution. Ann Pharmacother 1995;29:1232–1235.

13. Hoffman RS, Chiang WK, Howland MA, et al: Theophylline desorption from activated charcoal caused by whole-bowel irrigation. J Toxicol Clin Toxicol 1991;29:191–202.

14. Hoffman RS, Smilkstein MJ, Goldfrank LR: Whole-bowel irrigation and the cocaine body packer. Am J Emerg Med 1990;8:523–527.

15. Janss GJ: Acute theophylline overdose treated with whole bowel irrigation. S D J Med 1990;43:7–8.

16. Kirshenbaum L, Mathews SC, Sitar DS, Tenenbein M: Whole-bowel irrigation versus activated charcoal in sorbitol for the ingestion of modified release pharmaceuticals. Clin Pharmacol Ther 1989;46: 264–271.

17. Kirshenbaum LA, Sitar DS, Tenenbein M: Interaction between whole-bowel irrigation solution and activated charcoal: Implications for the treatment of toxic ingestions. Ann Emerg Med 1990;19;1129–1132.

18. Langdon DE: Colonic perforation with volume laxatives. Am J Gastroenterol 1996;91:622–623.

19. Lee DC, Roberts JR, Kelly JJ, Fishman SM: Whole-bowel irrigation as an adjunct in the treatment of radiopaque arsenic. Am J Emerg Med 1995;13:244–245.

20. Lenz K, Oroz R, Kleinberger G, et al: Effect of gut lavage on phenobarbital elimination in rats. J Toxicol Clin Toxicol 1983;20:147–157.

21. Makoseij F, Hoffman RS, Howland MA, Goldfrank LR: An in vivo evaluation of cocaine hydrochloride adsorption by activated charcoal and desorption upon addition of polyethylene glycol electrolyte lavage solution. J Toxicol Clin Toxicol 1993;31:381–395.

22. Mann K, Picciotti M, Spevack T, Durban D: Management of acute iron overdose. Clin Pharm 1989;8:428–440.

23. Mayer L, Sitar DS, Tenenbein M: Multiple-dose charcoal and whole-bowel irrigation do not increase clearance of absorbed salicylate. Arch Intern Med 1992;152:393–396.

24. Melandri R, Re G, Morigi A, et al: Whole-bowel irrigation after delayed release fenfluramine overdose. J Toxicol Clin Toxicol 1995;33:161–163.

25. Murphy DG, Gerace RV, Peterson RG: The use of whole-bowel irrigation in acute lead ingestion [abstract]. Vet Hum Toxicol 1991; 33:353.

26. Postuma R: Whole-bowel irrigation in pediatric patients. J Pediatr Surg 1982;17:350–352.

27. Roberge RJ, Martin T, Michelson EA, et al: Whole bowel irrigation in acute lead ingestion [abstract]. Vet Hum Toxicol 1991;33:353.

28. Rosenberg PJ, Livingston DJ, McLellan B: Effect of whole bowel irrigation on the antidotal efficacy of oral activated charcoal. Ann Emerg Med 1988;17:681–683.

29. Scharman EJ, Lembersky R, Krenzelok EP: Efficiency of whole-bowel irrigation with and without metoclopramide pretreatment. Am J Emerg Med 1994;12:302–305.

30. Smith S, Ling L, Halstenson C: Whole-bowel irrigation as a treatment for acute lithium overdose. Ann Emerg Med 1991;20:536–539.

31. Swanson-Brearman B, Dean BS, Krenzelok EP: Failure of whole-bowel irrigation to decontaminate the GI tract following massive jequirity bean ingestion [abstract]. Vet Hum Toxicol 1992;34:352.

32. Tenenbein M: Whole-bowel irrigation as gastrointestinal decontamination procedure after acute poisoning. Med Toxicol 1988;3:77–84.

33. Tenenbein M: Whole-bowel irrigation for toxic ingestions. J Toxicol Clin Toxicol 1985;23:177–184.

34. Tenenbein M, Cohen S, Sitar DS: Whole-bowel irrigation as a decontamination procedure after acute drug overdose. Arch Intern Med 1987;147:906–907.

35. Tenenbein M, Wiseman N, Yatscoff RW: Gastrotomy and whole-bowel irrigation in iron poisoning. Pediatr Emerg Care 1991;7: 286–288.

36. Thomas G, Brozinsky S, Isenberg J: Patient acceptance and effectiveness of a balanced lavage solution (GoLYTELY) versus the standard preparation for colonoscopy. Gastroenterology 1982;82:435–437.

37. Tuggle D, Hoelzer D, Tunell W, et al: Safety and cost-effectiveness of polyethylene glycol electrolyte solution bowel preparation in infants and children. J Pediatr Surg 1987; 22:513–515.

38. Turk J, Aks S, Ampuero F, et al: Successful therapy of iron intoxication in pregnancy with intravenous deferoxamine and whole-bowel irrigation. Vet Hum Toxicol 1993;35:441–444.

39. Utecht M, Stone A, McCarron M: Heroin body packers. J Emerg Med 1990;11:33–40.

40. Van Ameyde K, Tenenbein M: Whole-bowel irrigation during pregnancy. Am J Obstet Gynecol 1989;160:646–647.

A. ANALGESICS AND NONPRESCRIPTION MEDICATIONS

CHAPTER *32* ACETAMINOPHEN

Kenneth E. Bizovi / Martin J. Smilkstein

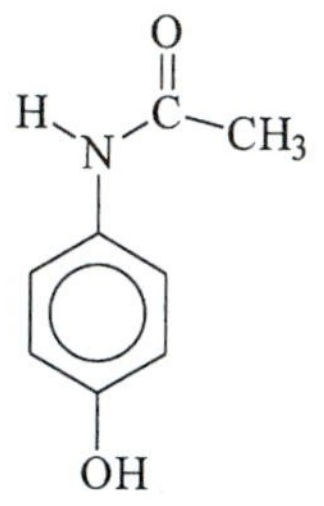

Acetaminophen

MW	= 151 daltons
Therapeutic serum level	= 10–30 µg/mL
	= 66–199 µmol/L
4-hour action level	= ≥150 µg/mL
	= ≥993 µmol/L

Values greater than or equal to the action level necessitate clinical intervention. Values less than this level may necessitate intervention based on the clinical characteristics of the patient.

A 21-year-old woman was brought to the Emergency Department (ED) by her boyfriend when he learned that she had ingested approximately thirty 325-mg acetaminophen tablets in an attempted suicide. He was unaware of any previous significant medical or psychiatric illness, but reported that she was seen in another ED several days earlier for persistent headaches. He said that she did not abuse alcohol or any other drugs.

The patient was able to provide a history. She admitted to taking about 30 tablets approximately 3 hours before coming to the hospital. She stated that she wanted to kill herself. She said shortly after taking the tablets she developed a bad "stomachache" and felt extremely nauseated, vomiting once. She denied taking any other medications or alcohol in the suicide attempt.

On physical examination the woman was diaphoretic, pale, and appeared uncomfortable. Her vitals signs were: blood pressure, 95/70 mm Hg; pulse, 100 beats/min; respiratory rate, 20 breaths/min; and oral temperature, 98.6°F (37°C). Examination of the head, eyes, ears, nose, and throat was unremarkable. The neck was supple and the lungs clear, and the cardiac examination was within normal limits. Examination of the abdomen revealed only moderate midepigastric tenderness without peritoneal signs. Bowel sounds were normoactive. Cranial nerves were grossly intact and reflexes were 2+ bilaterally. She was oriented to time, place, and person. She was given 50 g of oral activated charcoal along with 40 mL of 70% sorbitol. A 4-hour serum acetaminophen concentration was 215 µg/mL.

Acetaminophen (*N*-acetyl-*p*-aminophenol) is used far more than any other analgesic-antipyretic; consequently, overdose and toxic-ity are common considerations. The Toxic Exposure Surveillance System of the American Association of Poison Control Centers reports well over 100,000 calls to United States poison centers each year resulting from acetaminophen exposures, and there are more hospitalizations reported after acetaminophen overdose than after overdose of any other common pharmaceutic agent (Chap. 116).

Despite enormous experience with acetaminophen toxicity and long-standing dogma about its management, many controversies and challenges remain unresolved. In order to best understand the continuing evolution in approach to acetaminophen toxicity, it is critical to start with an analysis of certain fundamental principles and then to apply these principles to both typical and atypical presentations in which acetaminophen toxicity must be considered.

HISTORY AND EPIDEMIOLOGY

Although first synthesized[125] and used clinically[80] late in the 19th century, it was only 50 years ago that acetaminophen (a metabolite of phenacetin) was rediscovered.[26] Acetaminophen was first used clinically in the United States in 1950. The well-known toxicity of phenacetin led to unfounded concerns about acetaminophen safety that delayed widespread acceptance of acetaminophen until the 1970s. Acetaminophen has since proven to be a remarkably safe drug at appropriate dosage, a fact that, in combination with concerns about salicylate toxicity and association with Reye's syndrome, has resulted in the selection of acetaminophen as the analgesic-antipyretic of choice in most circumstances. Acetaminophen is available alone in myriad single-agent dose formulations and delivery systems, or in combination with opioids, other analgesics, sedatives, decongestants, and antihistamines. The diversity and wide availability of acetaminophen products dictate that acetaminophen toxicity be considered not only after identified acetaminophen exposures, but also after exposure to unknown or multiple drugs in settings of drug overdose, drug abuse, and therapeutic misadventures.

PHARMACOLOGY

Acetaminophen's action is attributed to central inhibition of prostaglandin synthetase.[40] It is an analgesic and antipyretic with weak anti-inflammatory properties.[84] Analgesic activity is reported with a serum acetaminophen concentration ([APAP]) of 10 μg/mL.

PHARMACOKINETICS

Following oral ingestion, regular release acetaminophen is rapidly absorbed with time to peak [APAP] of approximately 45 minutes.[54] Liquid acetaminophen has a time to peak of 30 minutes.[54] Extended-release acetaminophen has a time to peak of 1–2 hours, but by 5 hours, 95% of the drug is absorbed. Time to peak is delayed by food. Acetaminophen bioavailability is 60–98%. Peak [APAP] after recommended dose ranges from 8–32 μg/mL. After administration of rectal suppositories in children, the time to peak ranged from 107 to 288 minutes with bioavailability of 30–40%. Peak [APAP] after single 20-mg/kg doses given rectally varied from 8.8 to 11 mg/L. Acetaminophen has total protein binding of 10–30% with therapeutic dosing. It crosses both the placenta and the blood-brain barrier.[102]

First-pass metabolism removes 25% of the therapeutic dose. Once absorbed, approximately 90% of acetaminophen normally undergoes hepatic glucuronide (40–67%) and sulfate (20–46%) conjugation to form inactive, harmless metabolites, which are eliminated in urine. A small fraction of unchanged acetaminophen (<5%) and other minor metabolites reach the urine, but are not thought to be clinically relevant.[143] The remaining fraction, usually ranging from 5 to 15%, is oxidized by the CYP2E1, CYP1A2, and CYP3A4 subfamilies of the P450 mixed-function oxidase system, resulting in the formation N-acetyl-p-benzoquinoneimine (NAPQI).[42] Glutathione quickly combines with NAPQI; the resulting complex is then converted to nontoxic cysteine or mercaptate conjugates, which are then eliminated in urine (see Fig. 32–1).[117,122] The elimination half-life of acetaminophen is 2–4 hours. Biliary excretion is minimal. Breast milk contains less than 2% of the maternal dose.

TOXICOKINETICS

Even after overdose the majority of acetaminophen absorption occurs within 2 hours. Peak plasma concentrations generally occur within 4 hours, although later peaks have been documented in overdoses.[141,188] After clinically significant overdose, saturation of the normal nontoxic routes of metabolism becomes important in the development of toxicity.[139] The amount of NAPQI formed is increased out of proportion to the acetaminophen dose because the fraction of acetaminophen metabolized to NAPQI is increased as maximal rates of glucuronidation and sulfation are exceeded (see

Fig. 32–1).[48] In addition to an increase in the formation of toxic metabolite, elimination may become prolonged as these enzyme systems become saturated.

A more exact understanding of P450 metabolism, which is fundamental to assessing the relationship between ethanol or medication use and acetaminophen toxicity, is still being developed. The proportion of acetaminophen metabolized by CYP2E1, CYP1A2, and CYP3A4 varies with individual host factors and may vary with dosage.[152,185]

PATHOPHYSIOLOGY

After the earliest reports,[46,184] a flurry of subsequent case reports, and the first reported series of acetaminophen toxicity,[108,149,150] an intensive research effort clarified the metabolic basis for both the pharmacologic safety and the toxicologic danger of acetaminophen[89,120,121,138] (see Fig. 32–1).

The safety of appropriate acetaminophen dosing results from the availability of electron donors such as reduced glutathione (GSH) and other thiol-containing compounds. After appropriate acetaminophen dosing, GSH supply far exceeds that which is required to detoxify NAPQI, and no toxicity occurs. After overdose, the rate and quantity of NAPQI formation may outstrip GSH supply and regeneration, resulting in free NAPQI rapidly binding to hepatocyte constituents. In animal experiments of acetaminophen overdose, hepatic toxicity becomes evident only when hepatic GSH falls to 30% or less of baseline.[120] This affords acetaminophen a remarkably safe therapeutic index. Although a therapeutic acetaminophen dose is only 10–15 mg/kg, significant toxicity after single acute overdose generally involve doses of 150 mg/kg or higher.[140]

Once NAPQI formation overwhelms the supply of thiol-containing compounds, it covalently binds and arylates critical cell proteins, inducing a series of events that may result in cell death.[89] Once thought to be an irreversible process resulting directly from covalent binding of NAPQI, it is now clear that the events leading to cell death are far more complex, and, importantly, that the process can be prevented, interrupted, and even reversed after binding has occurred.[27,52,70,136] The potential for intervention after NAPQI binding represents one of the most important advances in understanding of acetaminophen toxicity.

Which, if any, single event is critical and commits the cell to death is still unknown. NAPQI-induced oxidation of enzymes alters normal cell functions and impairs cell defenses against endogenous reactive oxygen species, resulting in further oxidation of vital proteins.[190] Selective arylation of critical cell proteins is likely to be more important than total covalent binding as a determinant of toxicity. Subsequent intracellular calcium dyshomeostasis[124,189] and lipid peroxidation[202] have each been demonstrated, but neither of these processes is consistently required or sufficient to result in cell death.[24,73,75] Critical, possibly irreversible, events in cell death include DNA fragmentation[167] and mitochondrial injury,[55] but further work is required to reliably define the trigger or triggers of acetaminophen-induced cell death. The final pathway of cell death may also vary, with evidence for apoptosis and direct necrosis both demonstrated experimentally.[153]

Macrophages and inflammatory cells infiltrate after necrosis, and destruction caused by secondary inflammation[211] and impairment of microcirculation[119] are demonstrated, although, again, neither appears to be necessary for hepatic injury.[85,201]

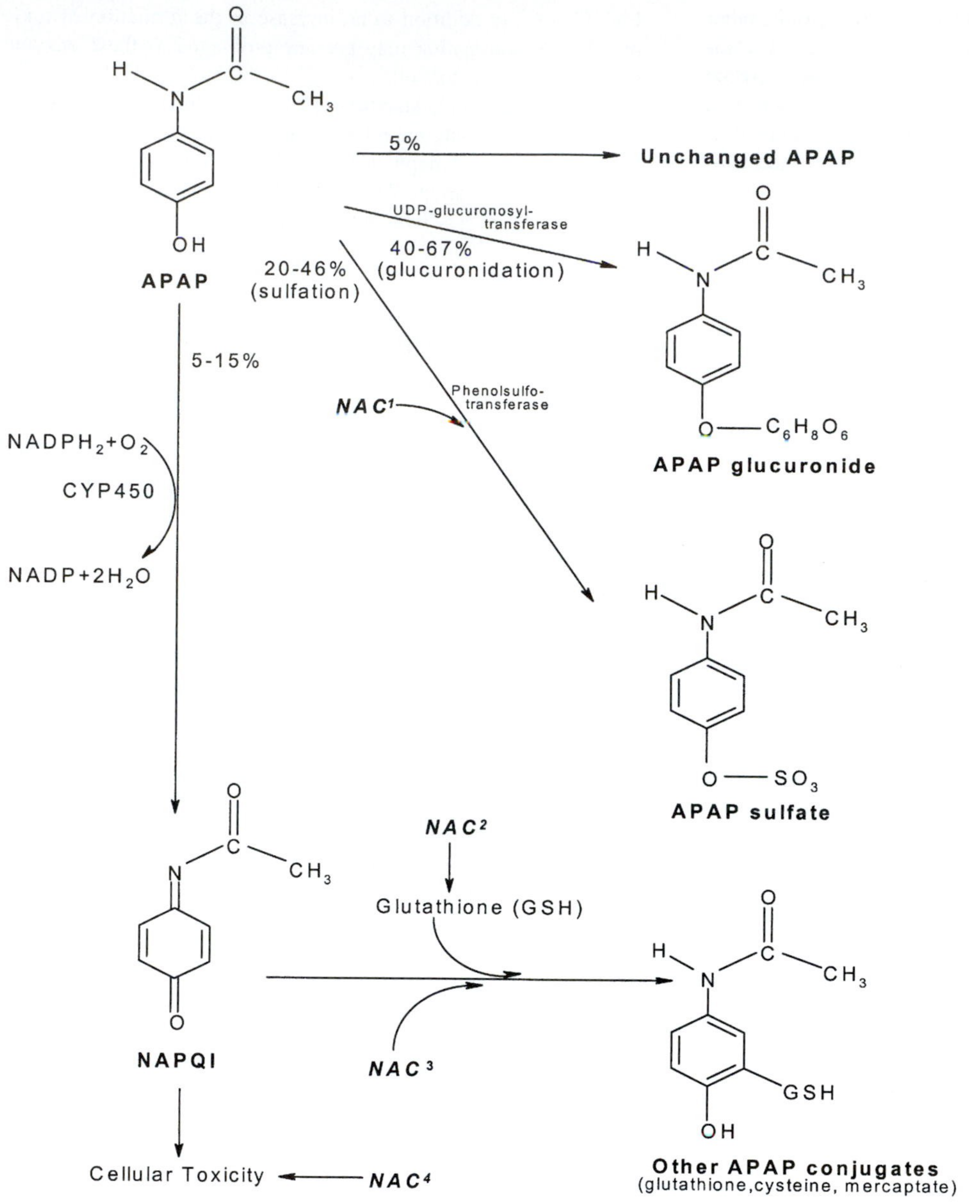

Figure 32–1. Important routes of acetaminophen metabolism in man and mechanisms of N-acetylcysteine (NAC) hepatoprotection. NAC[1] is glutathione (GSH) precursor; NAC[2] is GSH substitute; NAC[3] augments nontoxic sulfation; and, NAC[4] improves multiorgan function during hepatic failure and possibly limits extent of hepatocyte injury.

Factors that may predispose patients to hepatotoxicity include increased frequency of acetaminophen dosing, prolonged duration of excessive dosing, increased capacity for P450 activation to NAPQI, decreased GSH availability, or decreased capacity for glucuronidation and sulfation. Despite experimental evidence for each, clinical consideration of these factors is complex and controversial, and is discussed later.

The pathophysiology of most organ dysfunction resulting directly from acetaminophen is a result of the local formation of destructive acetaminophen metabolites. Normally, most oxidative drug metabolism is concentrated in hepatic zone III (centrilobular), and this zone is first and most profoundly affected by acetaminophen toxicity (Chap. 14). In more severe cases, however, necrosis may extend into zones I and II to destroy the entire liver parenchyma. In perhaps 25% of cases with significant hepatic enzyme elevation, clinically evident renal injury may also occur.[140] Renal P450 formation of NAPQI is the likely cause of acute proximal renal tubular necrosis after acute overdose;[22,63,81] however,

several other nephrotoxic mechanisms are proposed.[78] Conversion of acetaminophen to nephrotoxic p-aminophenol[32] and renal conversion of hepatically derived acetaminophen-GSH,[123] both demonstrated in selected animal models, appear unlikely to be significant.[62,64,115] NAPQI formation via renal prostaglandin synthetase[196] or prostaglandin-mediated renal medullary ischemia[146] is suspected of contributing to chronic analgesic nephropathy from acetaminophen in combination with other analgesics.[162] In addition, volume depletion and hepatorenal syndrome are often cofactors.

Injury to other organs is rarely reported. It remains controversial whether the etiology of these injuries is caused by local or circulating toxic metabolites. The mechanism causing myocardial damage, reported in some patients with acetaminophen-induced fulminant hepatic failure, is thought to be part of multisystem organ failure rather than being acetaminophen-specific.[23,106] Pancreatic injury from acetaminophen, experimentally produced in mice, appears not to be the result of NAPQI formation,[68] and the paucity of human cases prevent analysis of the specific toxic mechanism. Glutathione depletion in rat brain[33] is suggested as a possible cause of central nervous system effects of acetaminophen, but this finding is inconsistent[12] and the mechanism of early coma associated with massive acetaminophen doses remains undefined. Similarly, acetaminophen-induced alterations in intermediary metabolism[181] are presumed to cause metabolic acidosis with elevated lactate concentrations that accompany altered mental status in extraordinary cases,[69] but this too is speculative.

The remaining sequelae of severe toxicity are secondary effects of fulminant liver failure, rather than direct acetaminophen effects, and the pathophysiology of these complex multisystem problems is well-described elsewhere.[99] The ability of *N*-acetylcysteine (NAC) to ameliorate secondary multiorgan failure via extrahepatic mechanisms (see below) suggests that oxidation of vital thiols and loss of normal microvascular function is an important component of secondary organ failure.[77]

CLINICAL MANIFESTATIONS

Early recognition and treatment of patients with acetaminophen poisoning are essential in order to minimize morbidity and mortality. This task is made difficult by the lack of predictive clinical findings early in the course of acetaminophen poisoning, and clinicians should not feel reassured by a patient's lack of symptoms soon after ingestion. The first symptoms after acetaminophen overdose may be those of hepatic injury, which develop many hours after the ingestion, when antidotal therapy is already less effective.

Table 32–1 summarizes the clinical course of acute acetaminophen toxicity. During stage I of toxicity, hepatic injury has not yet occurred and even patients who ultimately develop hepatotoxicity may be asymptomatic at this stage. Clinical findings, when present are nonspecific, such as nausea, vomiting, malaise,

pallor, and diaphoresis. Laboratory indices of liver function are normal. In extremely rare cases of massive overdose, decreased level of consciousness and metabolic acidosis may occur during this stage in the absence of hepatotoxicity, and may be caused directly by the effects of acetaminophen.[69,95,210] These findings are so uncommon that they should never be attributed to acetaminophen alone without thorough evaluation of other possible causes.

Stage II represents the onset of liver injury, which occurs in only a fraction of those who overdose. Onset is most common within 24 hours after ingestion, but is nearly universal by 36 hours.[168] Symptoms and physical signs during stage II vary with the severity of liver injury but mimic other causes of hepatocellular injury such as infectious hepatitis. Aspartate aminotransferase (AST) is the most sensitive, widely available measure to detect the onset of hepatotoxicity, and AST abnormalities always precede evidence of actual liver dysfunction (elevated international normalized ratio [INR], elevated bilirubin, hypoglycemia, and metabolic acidosis). Although uncommon, AST elevations may occur as early as 8–12 hours after ingestion in the most severely poisoned patients.

Stage III, defined as the time of maximal hepatotoxicity, is most common between 72 and 96 hours after ingestion. The clinical manifestations vary from absent to fulminant hepatic failure with encephalopathy, coma, or exsanguinating hemorrhage. Laboratory studies are also variable: AST and alanine aminotransferase (ALT) values above 10,000 IU/L are common, even in patients without evidence of liver failure. The highest reported ALT caused by acetaminophen toxicity is over 100,000 IU/L.[131] Much more important than the degree of aminotransferase elevation, abnormalities of INR, bilirubin, glucose, and pH indicate the degree of liver failure and are essential determinants of prognosis and treatment.

Fatalities from fulminant hepatic failure generally occur between 3 and 5 days after overdose. Death results from either single or combined complications of multiorgan failure, including hemorrhage, acute respiratory distress syndrome (ARDS), sepsis, and, most importantly, cerebral edema.[110] Patients who survive this period reach stage IV, defined as the recovery phase. Hepatic regeneration becomes complete in survivors; there are no reported cases of chronic hepatic dysfunction solely because of acetaminophen poisoning. The rate of recovery varies; in most cases, laboratory evaluation is normal by 5–7 days after overdose; but recovery may take much longer in severely poisoned patients, and microscopic histologic abnormalities may persist for months.[101,112,137]

Renal function abnormalities are rare overall,[74,140] but occur in as many as 25% of cases with significant hepatotoxicity,[45,148] and in more than 50% of those with hepatic failure.[110,205] Renal abnormalities may be more common after sustained repeated excessive dosing.[142] Overt renal failure necessitating hemodialysis occurs, nearly always among patients with marked hepatic injury.[31] In cases of acetaminophen-induced fulminant hepatic failure, the incidence of acute renal failure is nearly the same as among patients with hepatic failure of other causes.[205]

Serious clinical manifestations other than hepatic and renal injury are unusual. Electrocardiographic and histologic evidence of myocardial injury, first noted in early case reports,[39,134] is most often noted in patients with fulminant hepatic and multisystem failure, but never as an isolated problem.[106] Hyperamylasemia and pancreatitis, both presumed[57] and proven,[71] are attributed to acetaminophen overdose alone or in combination with ethanol abuse.[66]

TABLE 32–1. Phases of Acetaminophen Poisoning

Phase I (0.5–24 h)
Patients experience anorexia, nausea, malaise, pallor, vomiting, and diaphoresis. The patient may appear normal.

Phase II (24–72 h)
The symptomatology of phase I becomes less pronounced. Right-upper-quadrant pain may be present secondary to hepatic damage. Blood chemistries become abnormal, with elevation of liver enzymes, International Normalized Ratio (INR), and bilirubin. Renal function may begin to deteriorate, but BUN usually remains low as a result of decreased hepatic urea formation.

Phase III (72–96 h)
Characterized by the sequelae of hepatic necrosis such as hepatic encephalopathy. Coagulation defects, jaundice, renal failure, and myocardial pathology may be present. Liver biopsy at this time reveals centrilobular necrosis. Nausea and vomiting may reappear. Death is related to hepatic failure and is frequently preceded by anuria and coma.

Phase IV (4 d–2 wk)
If the damage done during phase III is reversible, complete resolution of hepatic dysfunction will occur.

Adapted from Linden CH, Rumack BH: Acetaminophen overdose. Emerg Clin North Am 1984;2:103–119.

Clinical findings in these rare cases are typical of acute pancreatitis.

DIAGNOSTIC TESTING

Assessing Risk of Toxicity: Principles that Guide the Diagnostic Approach

Fatalities from acetaminophen overdose are common, but preventable by timely diagnosis and treatment with N-acetylcysteine, (NAC). At the same time, the overwhelming majority of acetaminophen exposures result in no toxicity. Therefore, an appropriate approach must avoid the enormous costs of unnecessary overtreatment while minimizing patient risk. To balance these seemingly divergent goals, the clinician must understand the basis for and sensitivity of current toxicity screening methods.

When considering risk determination, it is useful to separate different categories of acetaminophen exposure. For acute overdose in typical circumstances, there is an extensive body of experience and literature, permitting a more systematic approach with demonstrated efficacy. For issues related to repeated excessive acetaminophen dosing, uncertain circumstances, patients with possible predisposition to toxicity, new acetaminophen formulations, and many other permutations, there is an important conceptual framework for decision making, but little in the way of validated strategies. For these challenges, the central concepts and one approach are presented, with the understanding that these are dynamic and that more than one approach may have validity. Tables 32–2 and 32–3 present an overview summary of risk determination.

The amount and rate of NAPQI formation, the availability of hepatic GSH, and the capacity for nontoxic metabolism are major

---

TABLE 32–2.   A Risk Determination Strategy After Acute Acetaminophen Ingestion

A. Assess for risk of [APAP] toxicity:
1. If there is a history of acetaminophen overdose and the amount is >7.5 g in adults, >150 mg/kg in children, unknown, or the history is unreliable
2. If there is no history of acetaminophen ingestion, but another overdose is suspected, and there is an alteration in mental status, evidence of oral opioid exposure, or unreliable history
3. If there are signs or symptoms of hepatic injury

B. Initial laboratory assessment should consist of:
1. [APAP] 4 h after ingestion, or as soon as possible thereafter
2. AST[a] if [APAP] is above the treatment line, or signs or symptoms suggest hepatic injury
3. INR, electrolytes, glucose, BUN, and creatinine if very ill-appearing or marked elevation of AST.

C. On the basis of the initial laboratory assessment, consider the patient at risk:
1. If [APAP] is on or above the treatment line, or
2. If the AST is elevated, or
3. If the [APAP] is >10 µg/mL and the time of ingestion is completely unknown

[a]Early in the clinical course of toxicity, and particularly in certain subgroups, the AST may exceed ALT; therefore, AST is listed as the preferred measure. In most circumstances, however, ALT can be substituted for AST in patient assessment, particularly if nonhepatic sources of AST (eg, rhabdomyolysis) are suspected.

TABLE 32–3.   A Risk Determination Strategy After Repeated Excessive Acetaminophen Dosing

A. Assess for risk of acetaminophen toxicity:
1. If there are signs or symptoms of hepatic injury, or
2. If the patient is a child with antecedent/concurrent febrile illness, and has received >75 mg/kg acetaminophen in any 24-h period, or
3. If there is evidence of chronic use of alcohol, anticonvulsants, or isoniazid; or malnourishment in a patient who has received >4 g acetaminophen in any 24-h period, or
4. If the patient is not in one of the above groups and has received >7.5–10 g acetaminophen (adults) or >150 mg/kg acetaminophen (children) in any 24-h period

B. Initial laboratory assessment should consist of:
1. [APAP] immediately if symptomatic or if time of last dose unknown; otherwise, 4 h after last acetaminophen dose or as soon as possible thereafter
2. AST[a]
3. INR, electrolytes, glucose, BUN, and creatinine if very ill-appearing or marked elevation of AST

C. On the basis of the initial laboratory assessment, consider the patient at risk (also see below for risk subgroups):
1. If the AST is elevated, or
2. If the [APAP] is >10 µg/mL

D. Determination of risk subgroups:
1. Consider the patient at *higher-risk* if any of the following occur:
   a. If [APAP] is above the treatment line when plotted on the acetaminophen nomogram
   b. If the patient is symptomatic and AST > normal
   c. If the AST > twice normal
   d. If the AST > normal and [APAP] >10 µg/mL
   e. If [APAP] > expected for the appropriate dose
2. Consider the patient at risk, but at *low-risk* if either of the following occur:
   a. If there are no symptoms, [APAP] <10 µg/mL, and AST < twice normal
   b. If AST is normal and [APAP] consistent with appropriate dose
3. Consider the patient at *minimal-risk* if the patient has [APAP] <10 µg/mL and AST is normal

[a]Early in the clinical course of toxicity, and particularly in certain subgroups, the AST may exceed ALT; therefore, AST is listed as the preferred measure. In most circumstances, however, ALT can be substituted for AST in patient assessssment, particularly if nonhepatic sources of AST (eg, rhabdomyolysis) are suspected.

---

determinants of toxicity,[118] thus the ideal model for determining risk after acetaminophen overdose assesses each of these. At present, none of these measures is available to clinicians. The profile of urinary acetaminophen metabolites may reflect increased NAPQI formation,[48] but there is no indication that measurement is of any predictive value in any given case. Plasma GSH can be measured, but has an uncertain relationship to hepatic GSH availability.[176] Protein adducts, indicating binding of NAPQI to hepatocyte proteins, can be determined experimentally and are a marker of covalent binding[151,200] but are unlikely to prove useful as a screening measure. Because some degree of hepatocyte necrosis must precede the appearance of measurable serum adducts, the early warning value of the test is limited. Prior to actual hepatotoxicity, there are no reliable indirect measures of acetaminophen excess. Therefore, the clinician must rely solely upon the ingestion history and measurement of [APAP] in the patient to assess the risk for subsequent toxicity and thus the need for treatment.

Risk Determination after Acute Overdose

Acute overdose is usually considered to be a single ingestion, although, in fact, many patients consume the overdose in increments over some period. For purposes of this discussion, a single acute overdose is arbitrarily defined as one in which the entire ingestion occurs within a single 4-hour period. Figures of 7.5 gm in an adult or 150 mg/kg in a child are widely disseminated as the lowest acute dose capable of causing toxicity.[3,105] Although these standards have stood the test of time as sensitive markers, they are not based on human data and are quite conservative. Historical data suggest that toxicity generally occurs only above 150 mg/kg.[140] Although there is wide interspecies variation in susceptibility to acetaminophen,[142] animal data suggests that a single dose of at least 15 g would be required to cause consequential GSH depletion in an adult.[122]

Higher dose cutoffs for consideration of risk would improve specificity; however, the value of improving specificity has not been weighed against the current, sensitive lower cutoff. In the face of an enormous variety of potential outliers, the near-absence of screening failures is almost certainly due to the use of these standards as well as a very sensitive screening nomogram (see below). The adult standard is less controversial than that for children (see below) because massive ingestions, unreliable histories, and factors that might predispose to toxicity occur primarily in adults, justifying continued use of 7.5 g as a screening amount as a "safety net" to avoid missing serious toxicity.

The dose history should be used in the assessment of risk only if there is reliable corroboration or direct evidence of validity. Therefore, dose estimates may be useful in determining risk in many cases of unintentional or therapeutic acetaminophen exposures, but this information is not adequately reliable in most patients with ingestion due to self-harm attempts or drug abuse. When history does suggest possible risk, however, this is not sufficient evidence on which to base treatment decisions, and risk should then be assessed using determination of [APAP].

Interpretation of [APAP] after acute exposures is based on adaptation of the Rumack-Matthew nomogram (see Fig. 32–2),[159] which itself is an adaptation of previous data.[145] The original nomogram was based on the observation that patients who subsequently developed AST or ALT values greater than 1000 IU/L could be separated from those who did not on the basis of initial [APAP]. It was known that acetaminophen elimination followed first-order kinetics, that absorption is generally complete within 4 hours, and that the elimination half-life in those without toxicity is generally less than 4 hours. On the basis of these facts and observations, these authors constructed the original nomogram line on a plot of ln [APAP] versus time since ingestion. The line chosen started at an [APAP] of 200 µg/mL, 4 hours postingestion; declined with a 4-hour half-life through 50 µg/mL, 12 hours postingestion; and ended at 6.25 µg/mL, 24 hours after the overdose.

It is important to realize that the line was based on aminotransferase elevation rather than on hepatic failure or death, and was positioned to be very sensitive, with little regard to specificity. Without antidotal therapy, 60% of those with initial [APAP] above this original line will develop hepatotoxicity as defined by aminotransferase values above 1000 IU/L,[144] but the risk is not the same for all such patients. Aminotransferase elevation develops in virtually all patients with [APAP] far above the line, and serious hepatic dysfunction occurs frequently, whereas the incidence of

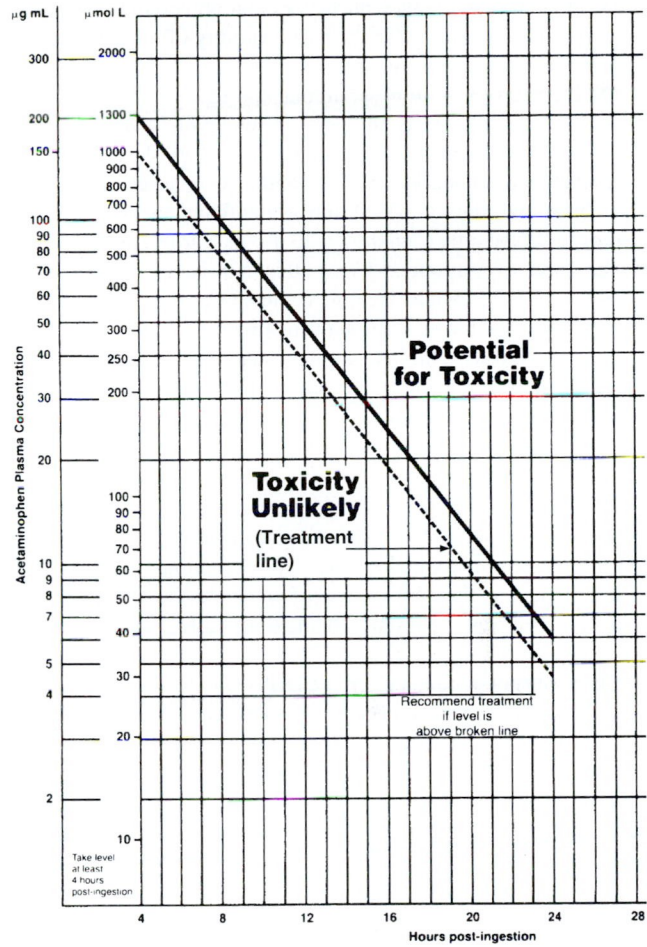

Figure 32–2. Acetaminophen nomogram: serum acetaminophen concentration versus time after ingestion. *(Reprinted from* Management of Acetaminophen Overdose. *McNeil Consumer Products Co., 1986.)*

hepatotoxicity among cases with [APAP] values immediately above the line is very low, and the risk of hepatic failure or death far less still.[140,144]

The original line is still used in the United Kingdom and other locations; however, the line used in the United States runs parallel to the original, but has been arbitrarily lowered by 25% in order to add even greater sensitivity.[160] The lower line, subsequently referred to as the *Treatment Line*, starts at an [APAP] of 150 µg/mL, 4 hours postingestion; declined with a 4-hour half-life; and ended at 4.7 µg/mL, 24 hours after the overdose. The Treatment Line is one of the most sensitive screening tools used in medicine. The incidence of nomogram failures in the United States, using the lower line, approaches zero.[171] A vanishingly small number of anecdotal cases of nomogram failure involve either special circumstances of increased risk,[36,114,127] questionable facts, or both.[171]

Cases of nomogram failure using the higher original line in the United Kingdom are published. Some of these patients are without any potentially predisposing factors such as malnutrition, alcoholism, or enzyme-inducing drugs.[25] Some authors suggest that the incidence of nomogram failures may be higher in the United Kingdom, and recommend that the nomogram in use there is not sensitive enough for cases with factors that potentially predispose patients to hepatotoxicity.[21,25,47,192] The validity of this observation has not been adequately studied.

On the basis of these observations and more than 20 years of use, the Treatment Line is an adequate screening device in nearly all cases and is reliable when rigorously followed. When using the acetaminophen nomogram, it is essential to precisely define the time "window" during which the acetaminophen exposure occurred, and if the time is unknown, to use the earliest possible time as the time of ingestion. Using this approach, patients with [APAP] values below the Treatment Line, even if only slightly so, do not require further evaluation or treatment for their acute acetaminophen overdose. This also applies to most patients with factors that may predispose them to acetaminophen induced hepatotoxicity, as well. There appears to be adequate experience with acute acetaminophen overdose in the settings of potentially predisposing factors such as chronic alcohol abuse, chronic medication with CYP450-inducing drugs, or inadequate nutrition to recommend that no special approach is required in such cases. Further study is needed to determine whether there are exceptions. Isolated case reports[127] suggest that chronic use of isoniazid, for example, may uniquely predispose patients for toxicity after acetaminophen overdose.[65,209]

The goal should be to determine [APAP] at the earliest point at which it will be meaningful in decision making. Measurement of [APAP] 4 hours after ingestion or as soon as possible thereafter is used to *confirm* risk of toxicity, and thus the need to initiate NAC. There are no established guidelines for the use of determinations made less than 4 hours after ingestion, and because of variability in absorption such values will have less predictive value. Furthermore, there is no advantage to earlier initiation of therapy because there is no improvement in NAC efficacy when started earlier than 4 hours after the overdose.[173] In light of these facts, there is no advantage to assessing [APAP] earlier in any case in which there is strong suspicion of a significant acetaminophen overdose. Factors that complicate the diagnostic decision making after acute overdose include situations that prevent the measurement of [APAP] prior to 8 hours post-ingestion, inability to establish the time of ingestion, presentation greater than 24 hours postingestion, and new formulations of acetaminophen.

Only if the results of [APAP] determination cannot be obtained within 8 hours of the overdose should history alone be considered adequate to consider the patient at risk and as an indication to start NAC. In such cases, [APAP] should still be determined as soon as possible. When the result becomes available it should be interpreted according to the treatment line on the acetaminophen nomogram, and NAC either continued or discontinued on the basis of this result. In the unusual circumstance that no determination of [APAP] can be obtained, evidence of possible risk by history alone is sufficient to initiate and complete a course of NAC therapy.

Early Measurement of [APAP]. To *exclude* toxicity and the need for antidotal therapy, [APAP] determination less than 4 hours after ingestion may sometimes be useful. This is irrelevant in most cases because the delay to presentation and time required to complete medical clearance usually exceeds 4 hours. If there is little evidence to suggest a substantial acetaminophen exposure, and it is feasible and desirable to facilitate more evaluation, determination of [APAP] less than 4 hours after exposure may then be considered. Assays obtained within 1 hour of ingestion are of no

value, but between 1 and 4 hours after ingestion, a negligible [APAP] may be sufficient to exclude risk of toxicity without further assessment in many cases. In cases with subsequent [APAP] above the Treatment Line, values obtained between 1 and 4 hours after ingestion already exceed 100 µg/mL in nearly all cases.[59] These data, studied retrospectively, include several outliers for which early levels were not predictive, however, and thus preclude establishment of firm guidelines. Until further prospective study, it is reasonable to include a safety margin when utilizing early [APAP] determinations. Therefore, when suspicion of consequential acetaminophen overdose is low and there is a compelling reason to obtain early [APAP], an [APAP] of 50 µg/mL or less obtained between 1 and 4 hours after exposure is adequate to exclude risk of toxicity if there are no extenuating circumstances such as sustained-relief formulation, coingestion of agents that delay gastric emptying and gut motility, or other factors. Early determination of [APAP] in pediatric patients is considered elsewhere in the chapter.

Determination of Risk when the Acetaminophen Nomogram is not Applicable

Risk Determined when Time of Ingestion Is Unknown. Another challenging variation on risk determination is the case in which the time of ingestion simply cannot be determined. Although this is a common initial concern, it is unusual after thoughtful questioning of the patient, family, and others. It is almost always possible to at least establish a time window during which the exposure must have occurred and then use the earliest possible time as the time of ingestion for risk-determination purposes. If this time window cannot be established or is so broad that it encompasses a span of more than 24 hours, the following approach is suggested. Determine both the [APAP] and the AST. If the AST is elevated, regardless of [APAP], treat with NAC as discussed below. If the [APAP] is below the lower level of detection and the AST is normal, there is no evidence that subsequent consequential hepatic injury is possible and NAC is unnecessary. Although some authors speculate that subsequent liver injury could follow an interval during which [APAP] was negligible and AST was normal, this does not appear to occur. There are no documented cases of serious hepatotoxicity from acetaminophen with normal AST and undetectable [APAP]. In all cases there has been either elevation of AST and or prolonged acetaminophen elimination resulting in a measurable [APAP] beyond 24 hours.

In the remaining cases, in which the time of ingestion is completely unknown, and [APAP] is detectable, it is prudent to assume that the patient is at risk. Treatment with NAC should be initiated, but consideration of a shorter course of therapy is appropriate, according to the protocols discussed below.

Risk Assessment After Extended Release Acetaminophen. Previously, acetaminophen formulations were all immediate-release acetaminophen (IR acetaminophen) preparations and exposures to these agents formed the basis for the nomogram and a successful diagnostic and therapeutic approach. A new product, Extended Relief Tylenol, Tylenol Arthritis Pain (ER acetaminophen), consists of an outer 325 mg IR acetaminophen dose of acetaminophen and an inner 325 mg dose designed for delayed dissolution. These dissolution characteristics give rise to concern about whether the nomogram is an appropriate method to evaluate patients with suspected overdosage of this new agent.

The manufacturer has initially recommended measurement of [APAP] with three possible results.[184] If nondetectable, risk of toxicity is excluded. If above the nomogram line, the patient is considered at risk, and NAC initiated. If a detectable value below the nomogram is obtained, the recommendation is to repeat the [APAP] determination in 4–6 hours, treating with NAC if the second value is above the nomogram, and excluding toxicity if the value is below the line.

This approach, and most analyses that have followed, are based on concern that an initial [APAP] below the line could be followed by a subsequent value above the line, and place the patient at risk for hepatotoxicity. Critical evaluation of the available information confirms that such nomogram "crossing" is indeed likely; however, despite intuitive concerns, there is no evidence of risk to the patient.

Whether or not [APAP] is above the Treatment Line is far less relevant than assessment of the temporal pattern and magnitude of the elevation of [APAP]. The critical threshold for acetaminophen toxicity is dependent on the rate, amount, and duration of NAPQI formation balanced against the supply and regeneration of GSH. The nomogram serves as a marker for risk of reaching that threshold after IR acetaminophen overdoses. To compare the risk after ER acetaminophen overdose, it is conceptually useful to separate the first few hours from the subsequent hours in the analysis.

IR acetaminophen results in early, rapid, massive peaks in [APAP], usually within the first 2 hours, which decline steadily thereafter. Volunteer studies clearly show that peak [APAP] and area-under-the [time-versus-concentration] curve (AUC) after ER acetaminophen are far less in the first 4 hours.[58,181] On the basis of time versus concentration curves after actual overdoses of ER acetaminophen, the same appears to be true.[34,193] Therefore, considering for the moment only the NAPQI formation and GSH depletion that occurs in the first few hours, the risk associated with any given 4-hour [APAP] after ER acetaminophen is likely to be far less than for the same [APAP] after IR acetaminophen.

Next, it is important to consider whether subsequent ER acetaminophen metabolism is likely to generate late risk after an initial [APAP] below the Treatment Line. This would require either delayed massive elevation of [APAP] or delayed sustained moderate elevations of [APAP] sufficient to result in GSH depletion. Neither seems likely to occur. Between 4 and 8 hours, [APAP] declines more slowly after ER acetaminophen than after IR acetaminophen, and nomogram "crossings" clearly occur, but subsequent elimination is identical to IR acetaminophen. The duration and magnitude of this *delayed* increased [APAP] after *ER* acetaminophen appears to be quantitatively far less than the duration and magnitude of *early* increased [APAP] after *IR* acetaminophen. Cases of sustained, delayed elimination attributed to ER acetaminophen are reported,[72] but are no different from what occurs after serious IR acetaminophen overdoses, with delayed elimination resulting from a combination of a very large dose and early acetaminophen-induced liver dysfunction. Thus far, only one reported case fails to fit these reassuring observations.[13] In this case, a dramatic late rise in [APAP] was noted after an overdose of ER acetaminophen, IR acetaminophen, nonsteroidal anti-inflammatory drugs (NSAIDs), and an anticholinergic agent, suggesting that coingestants may have played a role in the unique [APAP] profile. The actual risk to the patient is difficult to assess because

the impressive late rise in [APAP] was brief with rapid decline, and the patient was receiving NAC at the time.

Given the paucity of data regarding ER acetaminophen, it is instructive to look at the IR acetaminophen experience for perspective. First of all, the course of [APAP] after IR acetaminophen does not always follow a typical pattern. When serial levels are obtained, as many as 5% of cases with initial [APAP] below the Treatment Line may have subsequent determinations above the line (author's unpublished data). Because most patients with an initial [APAP] below the line are medically cleared without a repeat assay, it seems certain that among the thousands of cases screened by this method, many potential nomogram "crossers" have been medically cleared without treatment and without reported subsequent serious toxicity. In almost all cases of patients who "cross" the nomogram after IR acetaminophen or ER acetaminophen overdose, [APAP] is only slightly above the lower line, in a range associated with little or no serious toxicity after untreated IR acetaminophen overdose.[140] Additionally, when the formulation of ER acetaminophen is considered, it is evident that its pharmacokinetics closely mimic repeated doses of IR acetaminophen separated by a short interval. Considering the similarity between these exposures, it is reassuring that the nomogram proves effective in cases of repeat overdoses of IR acetaminophen, without reported cases of failure to detect serious risk.

In summary, when considering use of the nomogram as a screening tool for ER acetaminophen overdose, it is unimportant whether reliance upon an initial [APAP] below the line would fail to detect a patient whose subsequent [APAP] would be above the line. What is important is whether reliance upon an initial [APAP] below the line would fail to detect a patient who might develop consequential liver injury. It is evident that a single [APAP] will miss nomogram "crossing," which occurs in a small fraction of ER acetaminophen cases, but because of limited early absorption of acetaminophen and lack of late sustained elevations in [APAP], it is very unlikely that such cases are at risk for toxicity. Therefore, the approach suggested by the manufacturer and described above would certainly be expected to be safe, and it is likely that, unless unusual circumstances are evident, a single [APAP] determination, plotted on the nomogram, is adequate to exclude the need for antidotal therapy after ER acetaminophen overdose. This conclusion will require ongoing evaluation, and any new delayed-release acetaminophen formulations needs to be evaluated separately.

[APAP] Elimination Half-Life: Utility in Risk Assessment. There is a clear relationship between the elimination half-life of acetaminophen and hepatotoxicity; therefore, some authors advocate determination of half-life as a method of determining risk. A more detailed analysis shows that this is an invalid approach. This concept originated from work showing that among 30 patients with acetaminophen overdose, acetaminophen half-life was greater than 4 hours in all individuals who developed hepatotoxicity, and less than 4 hours in all those who did not.[149]

There are several features that limit the applicability of these data as justification for use of half-life for screening. Measurement of only a few [APAP] may not accurately reflect metabolic events that take hours to occur. Certainly, observation and serial [APAP] determinations cannot be justified over many hours without initiation of NAC in the interim. Once NAC is initiated, it alters acetaminophen elimination, making comparison with the previous data impossible.

Finally, this method offers no improved predictive value over a single value plotted against the nomogram when the time of ingestion is unknown. To equal the sensitivity of the nomogram, a half-life of 2.5 hours, not 4 hours, must be used.[175] A study using high-dose acetaminophen chemotherapy illustrates the variability of half-life after overdose.[94] Despite acetaminophen doses from 200–670 mg/kg and 4-hour [APAP] as high as 473 mg/mL, the mean elimination half-life was just under 4 hours with some patients exhibiting very short half-lives. When time, expense, patient discomfort, and predictive value are considered, there is no reason to consider using half-life determination when the nomogram can be used instead.

Patients with Signs or Symptoms of Hepatic Injury After Acute Ingestion.

Patients who present with signs or symptoms of hepatic injury after acute acetaminophen ingestion should have AST and [APAP] measured. Those patients with [APAP] above the Treatment Line should receive NAC, but those with an elevated AST and an [APAP] that is below the Treatment Line represent a potential pitfall. These patients require that the history be reviewed with specific questions regarding the timing of the ingestion and repeat excessive acetaminophen dosing. They should have evaluation for hepatic failure as well as other causes of elevated AST, and they should be treated with NAC.

Risk Determination After Chronic Acetaminophen Exposure

There are no proven guidelines for risk determination after repeated acetaminophen exposures; nonetheless, there is information that can make these difficult decisions less arbitrary (see Table 32–3). First, hepatotoxicity from repeated dosing is remarkably rare given the extent of acetaminophen use. Second, despite such patients being only a small fraction of those using acetaminophen, nearly all cases of reported "chronic" acetaminophen toxicity occur among patients with factors that potentially predispose them to the acetaminophen induced hepatic injury: infants with febrile illness who receive excessive dosing;[30,35,38,50,60,79,129,177,183] chronic alcohol users;[7,10,165,212] and patients taking P450-inducing medications chronically.[18,21] Short-term fasting is also suggested as a factor;[204] however, it is impossible to determine whether fasting is causal, or merely a marker of the severity of other associated conditions. It is striking that outside of these groups, the incidence of serious acetaminophen toxicity after repeated doses is negligible and appears to only follow massive dosing[100,107,113,199] or prolonged excessive dosing.[11,20] Less-serious hepatic abnormalities with atypical clinical or histologic features indicating other pathophysiologic mechanisms are reported at lower doses taken for months to years.[5,15,88]

Thus far, it has been impossible to establish an upper limit for safe repeated dosing. Unlike acute dosing, not only is the total dose important, but the interval between dosing and the duration of dosing also appear to be important. When interindividual variations such as P450 activity, GSH supply, and regeneration capacity are considered, predicting the dose that will reach the critical threshold for the development of toxicity becomes impossible. Analysis is further complicated by the likelihood of unreliable information. A substantial proportion of these cases involve parental dosing errors, iatrogenic errors, alcoholics, litigants in product liability cases, and other situations in which those providing the history may be unable or unwilling to accurately describe the dosing. Furthermore, because acetaminophen use is common after liver injury from alcoholism, acute infectious illnesses, and even other medication use, it is unclear in which cases acetaminophen is causative, contributory, or completely unrelated to the hepatotoxicity. Analysis of these cases if further complicated, because liver injury from any cause may lead to slowed metabolism and persistent elevation of [APAP]. Ultimately, resolution of this problem will require development of "gold standard" laboratory markers of impending or actual acetaminophen induced toxicity, but no such methods are yet available.

When there is concern about toxicity risk after repeated excessive acetaminophen dosing, many approaches are suggested, but none adequately studied. Conceptually, the goal should be to select patients at risk on the basis of dosing history and other risk factors, and then to use limited laboratory testing to determine need for NAC. A logical screening laboratory evaluation consists of determination of [APAP] and AST, with additional testing as indicated by these results and other clinical features. As discussed below (see treatment), the objective is to identify the two conditions that would warrant NAC therapy: remaining acetaminophen yet to be metabolized, or potential serious liver injury. The predictive value of this approach depends almost entirely on proper selection of patients at risk.

Role of History and Physical Examination.

The first consideration when evaluating a patient with a history of repeated excessive acetaminophen dosing is the presence or absence of signs or symptoms of hepatotoxicity. Regardless of risk factors or dosing history, such findings should prompt laboratory evaluation. This is particularly important since most reported cases of serious toxicity after repeated dosing are symptomatic for more than 24 hours prior to diagnosis, and earlier diagnosis should improve outcome. In the asymptomatic patient, the next consideration should be the presence or absence of factors that potentially predispose the patient to toxicity. In fact, it is likely that the adult dosing threshold for laboratory evaluation of asymptomatic patients without potentially predisposing factors should be at least 7.5 g, and perhaps as high as 10–12 g, in any 24-hour period.[109]

Despite the lack of verifiable data, logic and respect for anecdotal reports justify use of a lower threshold in patients with potentially predisposing factors. Although some retrospective series and some reports from litigation suggest that toxicity can occur after recommended dosing,[164] this is not supported by other major studies or personal experience. Therefore, it is reasonable to use the recommended upper limit of daily acetaminophen dosing (4 g in adults; 75 mg/kg in children) as a cutoff for considering laboratory evaluation of asymptomatic, high-risk patients. The duration of dosing, any occurrence of large bolus dosing, the presence of multiple potentially predisposing factors, and other features almost certainly affect risk, but until they can be factored in, the lowest logical risk cutoff seems appropriate. These amounts are almost certainly substantially less than that required to cause toxicity,[109] but it is prudent to start from this sensitive cutoff while better screening strategies are developed. We currently use this approach in alcoholics, patients taking anticonvulsants or isoniazid, and infants and young children with febrile illnesses. Others deserving similar consideration include those with chronic malnutrition, HIV infection, or other conditions that lead to GSH depletion.

Role of Laboratory Evaluation. Using the strategy described here, patients with elevated AST values are considered at risk, regardless of [APAP]. Therefore, the [APAP] in this setting is useful in patients with normal AST values as a tool to determine only whether there is sufficient remaining acetaminophen to lead to subsequent NAPQI formation and delayed hepatotoxicity. In most cases, this is essentially a qualitative assessment of the presence or absence of acetaminophen, because the numerical value of [APAP] is usually difficult to interpret. In rare cases of repeated dosing, [APAP] will be above the Treatment Line when plotted as if the case were an acute overdose. If so, obviously NAC is indicated. In other cases, [APAP] will be nondetectable, obviating the need for NAC if the AST is normal.

In most cases of repeated excessive dosing, however, [APAP] is usually intermediate between these two conditions. When this is the case, [APAP] is used only to dichotomize between patients with significant remaining acetaminophen and those who have completed acetaminophen metabolism. Because there is no evidence in the literature or experience that a patient with [APAP] <10 μg/mL and a normal AST has the potential to develop subsequent consequential liver injury, this value is appropriate as a sensitive cutoff to define presence or absence of remaining acetaminophen.

Although the above approach is not studied, the decision to treat patients who have any remaining acetaminophen or any elevation of AST is likely to prove very conservative (ie, sensitive but not specific), particularly because of recent acetaminophen dosing and comorbidity likely to elevate AST (eg, ethanol use, infectious illness). An alternative strategy in reliable patients after repeated ingestions may be to treat only patients with substantially elevated AST or [APAP] that may lead to consequential production of NAPQI. These and other possible approaches require thoughtful study.

An interim definition of [APAP] with potential consequence is above 10 μg/mL, and greater than would be expected for an appropriate acetaminophen dose. After ingestion of a normal dose of acetaminophen the peak [APAP] should be <30 μg/mL, 30–90 minutes after ingestion, and <10 μg/mL by 4–6 hours after ingestion.

Determination of Risk Subgroups. Using a strategy that describes risk in a relative manner, we consider patients to be at *higher risk* in these situations: symptomatic with any AST elevation; the AST is greater than twice normal even if asymptomatic; AST above normal with [APAP] >10 μg/mL; or [APAP] is greater than expected after an appropriate dose. For these cases, treatment with NAC is recommended. Patients who are asymptomatic with [APAP] <10 μg/mL and AST less than twice normal, or with normal AST and detectable [APAP] that is consistent with an appropriate dose are considered *low risk*. Follow-up by phone or repeat visit in 24 hours is recommended for *low-risk* patients. They should be given discharge instructions to return immediately for any symptoms of hepatic injury such as nausea, vomiting, abdominal pain, or constitutional symptoms. Treatment is only recommended for low-risk cases without adequate follow up. Those patients with normal AST and [APAP] <10 μg/mL, represent *minimal risk* and NAC is not recommended. *Minimal risk* patients should be instructed to return immediately if symptoms of hepatic injury arise.

Unlike the acute overdose setting, patients at risk for toxicity after repeated excessive dosing are more likely to already be symptomatic upon presentation because of time elapsed during the days of their ingestion period. Such cases will not be missed by a thoughtful evaluation. Careful history, physical examination, and the laboratory approach described above should include nearly all patients at risk. The theoretical patient with impending toxicity but without signs or symptoms of toxicity, who might be missed by the above approach, can still be detected in a timely manner by appropriate patient discharge instruction and follow-up.

Pediatric Acetaminophen Exposure

Serious hepatotoxicity after acute overdose is clearly less common in children than in adults, but it is unclear whether this reflects relative hepatoprotection or merely results from differences in the characteristics of poisoning in children. Although some data suggest that children are relatively protected from toxicity after acute overdose, closer evaluation shows this to be unresolved. Serious hepatotoxicity or death after acute acetaminophen overdose is reported in children, but is extremely rare.[4,104,157] When all cases with initial [APAP] above the Treatment Line are considered, the incidence of hepatotoxicity is lower in children under 5 years of age than in adults.[157] This comparison is valid only if the two groups are comparably stratified by [APAP] and delay to NAC, but despite the enormous number of reported pediatric acetaminophen exposures, there are insufficient documented cases with very high [APAP] and comparable delays to NAC to allow this comparison.

Although limited by methodology, recent studies advocate increasing the threshold acetaminophen dose for screening after pediatric acute overdose.[2,14] Similarly, because of the paucity of reported toxicity, some recommend that children be screened using the original, higher, nomogram. Although both of these suggestions are statistically likely to be safe, we advocate continued use of 150 mg/kg as the risk-defining dose and use of the Treatment Line for [APAP] screening until valid data demonstrate children to be selectively protected, or accumulated experience with 200 mg/kg as a dose threshold for screening proves safe.

If, in fact, children are protected after acute overdose, several theories have been advanced to account for it. In adults, acetaminophen glucuronidation exceeds sulfation (60% to 30%); in young children, sulfation is much greater and the ratio may even be reversed. The relatively greater proportion of sulfate conjugation in young children[117] has been suggested as protective; however, the sulfation/glucuronide ratio itself should not make a difference unless it results in less oxidative metabolism to NAPQI; this has not been shown.[195] A more likely explanation would be the increased glutathione supply and regenerative capacity of children.[97]

Following excessive repeated acetaminophen dosing, there is no evidence that children are relatively protected; in fact, infants and children with acute febrile illnesses comprise one of the few groups in which toxicity after repeated excessive dosing has been described.[30,35,38,50,60,79,129,177,183] Common sources of dosing errors include substitution of adult for pediatric preparations; substitution of drops (100 mg/mL) for elixir (32 mg/mL); overzealous dosing by amount or frequency in attempts to maximize effect; and failure to read the label and dose carefully. As in all examples of repeated dosing toxicity, the precise dosing pattern required to produce risk is unclear. In nearly all cases, the reported doses associated with toxicity are more than 150 mg/kg/d and generally much higher. Particularly in reports of lesser dosing, confounding factors make dose determination and acetaminophen attribution extremely difficult.

Toxicity after repeated excessive dosing in febrile children may simply reflect that this is the most common setting for pediatric acetaminophen use and that children are at greater relative risk for excessive dosing because of their size. In the absence of pediatric cases outside this group, and in light of the paucity of toxicity in normal adults after repeated excessive dosing, it is appropriate to consider whether acute febrile illness predisposes to toxicity. It is logical that oxidative drug metabolism and glutathione supply would be affected by inflammatory oxidant stress and short-term fasting during febrile infectious illnesses, but this relationship is complex and not well-defined. Chronic infectious diseases, particularly HIV-related, are associated with glutathione depletion, but this is not evident during acute illness.[142] Among reported cases, it is likely that hepatic injury is the result of the infectious illness in some, the result of acetaminophen in others, and the result of both in still others. The relative contributions of the underlying illness and acetaminophen in these cases is currently difficult to determine and an area of important research.

Although extremely rare, reports of serious hepatotoxicity in children necessitate vigilance and the need to develop a reasonable strategy for screening. Because acute febrile illness is an important feature, and because there is no credible evidence that recommended therapeutic dosing of acetaminophen poses a risk, a preliminary strategy can be proposed. Our practice is to consider measurement of [APAP] and AST in any child with acute febrile illness and reported dosing that exceeds 75 mg/kg in any 24-hour period, or if symptoms or signs of hepatotoxicity are evident, regardless of dosing. This suggested cutoff for screening is well below an amount actually expected to produce toxicity in order to provide a sensitive screening strategy. Results of this screening are used as in the case of multiple dosing described earlier.

Ethanol and Risk Determination

The effect of ethanol on acetaminophen toxicity is complex and best described by clearly separating experimental animal data from actual human overdose, acute from chronic ethanol abuse, and acute from repeated excessive acetaminophen dosing. Although not entirely consistent, most animal data indicate that acute ethanol coadministration with acetaminophen may be somewhat hepatoprotective,[186,191] presumably by competitive inhibition of P450 acetaminophen metabolism to NAPQI. Chronic ethanol dosing in animal models, however, increases risk from acute acetaminophen dosing,[103,165,191] on the basis of induced P450 acetaminophen metabolism or decreased GSH supply or regeneration.[98]

After acute acetaminophen overdose, these factors appear to be of little importance.[156,174,187] There is no evidence that chronic ethanol use should alter the approach after acute overdose. Because of failure of the higher original nomogram to adequately screen alcoholics and those chronically taking anticonvulsants, some authors suggest that a much lower standard should be used.[36,47,192] There is only one reported case of nomogram "failure" in an alcoholic using the Treatment Line, and the actual events of the case are unclear.[36,171] Furthermore, unpublished data from a large series revealed no difference in incidence of hepatotoxicity among groups identified as chronic, acute, or acute and chronic ethanol users, and ethanol nonusers.[174] These observations indicate that the Treatment Line is adequately sensitive for screening after acute overdose, regardless of ethanol use.

Chronic ethanol abuse does appear to impact toxicity after repeated excessive acetaminophen dosing.[7,10,165,212] Characterization of this relationship is complicated by the challenges of obtaining accurate histories in alcoholics, failure to exclude non-APAP causes of hepatotoxicity, and other factors in many cases. These limitations prevent valid definition of the acetaminophen dosing likely to cause toxicity, but the literature and personal experience confirm increased risk in alcoholics after excessive acetaminophen dosing. An approach to screening is discussed above (see Risk Determination After Chronic Acetaminophen Exposure).

Given the prevalence of both ethanol and acetaminophen use, this remains perhaps the most important unresolved issue in risk determination after acetaminophen. Resolution will require innovative methods of risk determination, but also clear case definition and meticulous recording of relevant clinical data. A public health issue of this importance deserves a careful and deliberate approach to study.

A Final Comment Regarding Difficult Risk Determination

Although early NAC is optimum, there is now clear evidence that delayed treatment is beneficial.[91] Therefore, even when a decision not to treat with NAC is made, careful discharge instructions and appropriate short-term follow-up to detect early signs of hepatotoxicity serve as an additional safety net for patients. This is particularly important in the case of those possibly at higher risk after repeated excessive dosing (eg, alcoholics, those taking P450-inducing medications, fasted or malnourished patients, febrile young children) and when the ingestion involves new delayed-release acetaminophen formulations. While further data are gathered and the approach to atypical presentations is refined and validated, the current lack of proven guidelines dictates the wisdom of assuring close follow-up when admission and treatment are not indicated.

Assessing Actual Toxicity: Critical Components of the Diagnostic Approach

Earlier protocols and guidelines recommended extensive and ongoing laboratory assessment after acetaminophen overdose.[105,160] On the basis of the pathophysiology and time course of toxicity, a simplified and far more cost-effective approach is logical.

Initial Testing. As outlined above, patients with acute acetaminophen overdose and no indication of evident hepatotoxicity should have [APAP] measured, but require no other initial laboratory assessment. Patients found to be at risk by use of the nomogram or by history (in the case of repeated excessive dosing), or those suspected to already have mild hepatotoxicity by history and physical examination should then have AST measured. The first AST determination serves as a screen to detect already established serious liver injury, which may require closer monitoring, and, as mentioned, is also a key component of decision making after repeated excessive dosing and other unusual circumstances.

Unless there is evident serious hepatotoxicity, AST is sufficient, and no additional testing is initially needed. Death of hepatocytes, resulting in release of measurable hepatic enzymes, precedes all cases of serious liver dysfunction. Abnormalities of other markers are suggested to precede AST elevation, but there is no evidence that their detection benefits the patient.[9] Renal toxicity may occur without significant hepatotoxicity; however, at least minimal AST elevation nearly always precedes evidence of nephrotoxicity.[1,41] Exceptions[33,92,148] are so rare that routine screening of renal function in the absence of AST elevation is unnecessary.

Many cases occur in which minor hepatic abnormalities such as elevated bilirubin or INR are noted in patients with normal AST after acetaminophen overdose. Preexisting conditions, laboratory error, and possible interference with the INR assay by NAC[86] make it unclear in these sporadic cases whether these abnormalities are related to acetaminophen effects. Even in these cases, if consequential liver injury does develop, AST elevation precedes serious liver dysfunction.

Ongoing Monitoring and Testing. If no AST elevation is noted, repeated AST determination every 24 hours until completion of treatment is sufficient, without other biochemical testing. If AST elevation is noted, then INR should be measured and repeated every 24 hours, or more frequently if clinically indicated. Other liver tests such as γ-glutamyltransferase (GGT), alkaline phosphatase, lactic acid dehydrogenase (LDH), and bilirubin, which are useful when determining the etiology of liver abnormalities, will be abnormal in cases of serious acetaminophen-induced hepatotoxicity but provide little additional useful information if the etiology is certain.

If AST exceeds 1000 IU/L, or if INR elevation is noted, then monitoring blood urea nitrogen (BUN) and creatinine is warranted. If evidence of actual liver failure is noted, then careful monitoring of blood glucose and acid-base status is important, in addition to meticulous bedside evaluation to detect and document vital signs, neurologic status, and evidence of bleeding. Many additional tests may be useful in the setting of liver failure, on the basis of clinical condition and local protocols. Testing for other rare acetaminophen-associated conditions by electrocardiograph, amylase determination, or other studies should be on a case-by-case basis only.

Assessing Prognosis. The availability and success of liver transplantation after acetaminophen-induced liver failure creates an important unmet need for early prognostic assessment. Survival without transplantation is certain if AST is normal at the time of NAC initiation,[173] but while this identifies patients at the lowest risk, the converse is of no value in identifying those who will not survive without transplant. Earlier reports described poor prognostic features that are sensitive but inadequately specific, and based on findings too late in the course to be useful.[39] Efforts to determine earlier or more specific markers of poor prognosis have improved our understanding; however, accurate early prediction of need for transplant remains one of the greatest challenges related to acetaminophen toxicity.

A method for prediction of hepatic encephalopathy has been developed.[163] The probability of hepatic encephalopathy is determined using the time until treatment with NAC, INR, and platelet count. These data are used to determine the prognostic index and subsequently the probability of hepatic encephalopathy. Though not predictive of need for transplant alone this prognostic tool may be clinically useful. Hepatic encephalopathy requires increased supportive care, merits monitoring for progression of liver failure, and assessment for liver transplantation.

One strategy for prognostication utilizes a combination of clinical features of fulminant hepatic failure. The single criteria of pH <7.30 after fluid and hemodynamic resuscitation or the combina-

tion of a PT $\geq 1.8 \times$ control, creatinine >3.3 mg/dL, and grade III or IV encephalopathy is extremely predictive of a patient who will die without transplant.[109,130] Any patient meeting or approaching these criteria should be considered for transplant. Other prognostic strategies use only the coagulation profile, in an attempt to simplify the approach, and, more importantly to allow earlier intervention. Using this approach, a markedly abnormal INR that continues to rise on the fourth day after overdose indicates a very poor prognosis.[76] In most cases, other poor prognostic criteria is evident by that time, but occasionally time is saved. For earlier screening, other authors suggest that any patient whose PT in seconds exceeds the number of hours since ingestion should be considered at extreme risk.[128] Attempts to correlate individual clotting factor levels or ratios show promise; however, these correlates appear to offer no benefit over use of INR alone.[19,133]

Interpretation of INR must include awareness of therapy with vitamin K, or fresh-frozen plasma (FFP). Use of vitamin K does not confuse interpretation. If it is effective, it implies that transplant is unnecessary because viable liver remains. If vitamin K is ineffective, INR can be used as above. Transfusion of exogenous clotting factors, such as FFP, obviously alters interpretation because improvement in INR may not indicate any improvement in liver function. Depending on the volume of factors transfused, the subsequent decline in factors must be considered when interpreting INR values. The prognostic importance of monitoring INR in this setting suggests that FFP should be given only for evidence of bleeding, risk of bleeding from known concomitant trauma, or prior to invasive procedures, but not merely on the basis of the INR value. As mentioned earlier, survivors regenerate normal liver; as a result, no long-term laboratory monitoring is indicated after return to adequate function is demonstrated.

MANAGEMENT

Limiting Gastrointestinal Absorption

Decisions regarding gastrointestinal (GI) decontamination are discussed elsewhere (Chap. 5) and these principles apply to acetaminophen overdose. In cases of very early presentation (<1 hour), ingestion of delayed-release formulations, or coingestion of agents that delay GI absorption, there may be rare patients for whom gastric emptying is appropriate. In general, however, gastric emptying is rarely a consideration for patients with isolated acetaminophen overdose because of the very rapid gastrointestinal absorption of acetaminophen and the availability of an effective antidote (see Table 32–4).

The administration of activated charcoal appears to decrease the number of patients who have [APAP] above the Treatment Line.[28] The role of activated charcoal after acetaminophen overdose was controversial because of concern that activated charcoal, administered to adsorb acetaminophen, might also adsorb orally administered NAC enough to limit its antidotal effect (see Antidotes in Depth: Activated Charcoal). This led many to recommend that activated charcoal not be used following acetaminophen overdose. Closer examination of the issue suggests that this concern is unfounded for several reasons.

In a large fraction of cases, there should be no potential conflict because the time period after ingestion during which activated charcoal would be used does not overlap with administration of NAC. There is no known value to the use of activated charcoal as

TABLE 32–4. **Suggested NAC Treatment Approach After Risk Determination as Described in Tables 32–2 and 32–3**

This approach applies to patients with either acute or repeated [APAP] dosing.

I. **For patients not at risk by criteria in Table 32–2 or** *minimal risk* **in Table 32–3:**
 A. They may be medically cleared relative to [APAP] toxicity
 B. Advise the patient to return immediately if he/she develops signs or symptoms consistent with hepatic injury

II. **For patients in** *low-risk* **subgroup after repeated ingestions as described in Table 32–3:**
 A. Advise the patient to return immediately if he/she develops signs or symptoms consistent with hepatic injury.
 B. Arrange phone or clinic follow-up, as appropriate, in 24 h
 C. If signs or symptoms do subsequently develop, initiate laboratory assessment and reassess for risk as described in Table 32–3.

III. **For all other patients at risk as described in Table 32–2 or** *higher risk* **in Table 32–3:**
 A. Initiate oral/enteral NAC
 B. Consider IV NAC[a]
  1. If the patient exhibits hepatic failure
  2. If the patient is pregnant[a,b]
  3. If 8 or more hours have elapsed since the [APAP] ingestion and the patient is unable to retain oral/enteral NAC
 C. At time of admission and every 24 h: Determine AST. Assess PT/INR and other chemistries as indicated by the clinical condition
 D. If all preceding AST values are normal: Determine AST and [APAP] 36 h after the time of the most recent [APAP] ingestion[a]

IV. **Selection of NAC treatment protocol:**
 A. Standard United States protocol: 17 doses (68 h) oral/enteral NAC following the loading dose (see Antidotes in Depth: *N*-Acetylcysteine)
 B. Appropriate circumstances for consideration of alternative protocols.[a]
  1. Short-course NAC: On the basis of assessment done 36 h after most recent APAP ingestion, if the [APAP] <10 μg/mL, AST is normal, the patient is not pregnant; discontinue NAC; otherwise continue NAC[c]
  2. Modified traditional course NAC: On the basis of daily assessment, if, at any time, the AST is elevated but no hepatic failure develops, and the patient is not pregnant, treat with NAC until the AST returns to normal or for 17 doses (68 h) — whichever is first[c]
  3. Long-course NAC: If the patient develops hepatic failure, treat with IV NAC until the INR is <2 and encephalopathy, if present, is resolving

[a]Denotes controversial elements that differ from the traditional approach in the United States. See text for discussion.
[b]*Editors' Note:* Currently there is inadequate scientific evidence to justify routine deviation from the use of oral NAC in pregnancy.
[c]*Editors' Note:* Currently there is inadequate scientific evidence to justify routine deviation from the 72-hour oral NAC regimen.

a method of speeding acetaminophen elimination, so in this setting, its only role is to limit GI absorption, and use of activated charcoal is logical only if ongoing acetaminophen absorption is likely. In nearly all isolated IR acetaminophen overdoses, GI absorption can be considered complete by 4 hours after ingestion; thus, there is no value to activated charcoal beyond that point. Because there is no loss of NAC efficacy unless started more than

8 hours after ingestion,[173] there is no difficulty in separating an activated charcoal dose from the initial NAC dose.

If delayed or repeated activated charcoal dosing is indicated because of suspected delayed absorption or because of coingestants, then the strategy of separating any NAC and activated charcoal doses by 1–2 hours is logical, as long as it can be accomplished safely. NAC is quickly well absorbed high in the GI tract and unlikely to interact with activated charcoal if the doses are not simultaneous.

In unusual cases, as a result of coingestants and timing of presentation, it may be important to administer NAC and activated charcoal simultaneously; it is these cases that pose theoretical concerns. There is clear in vitro evidence of activated charcoal to NAC binding,[37,93,161] and volunteer data suggest that activated charcoal causes statistically significant decreases in NAC absorption;[61] however, there is no evidence that this interaction is clinically significant.[180] There is no study of patients with serious acetaminophen overdose designed to investigate this issue; however, indirect information is available which suggests that even simultaneous activated charcoal and NAC is unlikely to cause consequential decrease in NAC availability.

Animal data demonstrate that the amount of NAC needed is dependent on the amount of acetaminophen ingested.[135] If the NAC dose given were very close to the threshold of efficacy, then adsorption of a fraction of the NAC to activated charcoal is likely to be significant. It appears, however, that the dosing protocol routinely used in the United States far exceeds the NAC dose actually needed, suggesting that partial adsorption of NAC by activated charcoal would still result in an effective dose. This is suggested by the observation that all patients treated with NAC within 8 hours of overdose have similar excellent outcome, with no decrease in efficacy even after massive overdose. In fact the incidence of hepatotoxicity is the same whether the initial [APAP] is below the Treatment Line or is above 500 μg/mL.[173]

Supportive Care

General supportive care consists primarily of control of nausea and vomiting. There are no well-controlled studies to determine choice of optimal antiemetic agent and dose. Because of the time-critical nature of NAC dosing, the choice of agent and dose may differ from other circumstances in which a stepwise trial of increasing antiemetic potency and dose might be appropriate. After acetaminophen overdose, patients with very high [APAP] who are approaching or beyond 8 hours from ingestion but still vomiting are placed at greater risk by subsequent delays in NAC administration. These patients should be treated with a potent antiemetic at moderate or high dose if oral NAC is to be tried. If oral NAC is then vomited, a loading dose of IV NAC should be considered, despite the lack of a formulation intended for IV use in the United States (see below). Unless significant liver injury is already evident, vomiting generally resolves within 12–16 hours after ingestion, so that subsequent oral dosing can be accomplished.

The remaining general treatment issues relate to the management of hepatic injury, renal dysfunction, and the other rare manifestations listed above. Treatment of these problems is based on general principles and is not acetaminophen-dependent. Discussion of the management of liver failure is clearly beyond the scope of this chapter; however, certain aspects deserve mention. Monitoring for and treatment of hypoglycemia due to liver failure is critical and represents one of the most readily treatable of the life-threatening effects of liver failure. If there are adequate viable hepatocytes, vitamin K may produce some improvement in coagulopathy; thus, trial dosing is logical as liver injury develops and as it resolves. As mentioned earlier, administration of FFP should be based on specific indications rather than upon the INR alone.

Bioartificial liver has been used in patients that meet indications for orthotopic liver transplant.[51] This treatment has a role as supportive care for those patients who are awaiting transplant and primary therapy in patients who have contraindications that preclude transplantation. This case series demonstrates improved outcome when compared to historical controls and improved metabolic parameters.

One of the most important advances in care is the use of NAC to treat fulminant hepatic failure, which is discussed in detail below. Parenteral NAC, other advances in supportive care, and successful liver transplantation programs appear to have substantially improved survival.[109]

Antidotal Therapy with NAC

Mechanism of Action of NAC. Conceptually, it is helpful to think of NAC as serving two separate roles. During the metabolism of acetaminophen to NAPQI, NAC *prevents* toxicity by limiting the formation of NAPQI. More important, however, is that it does so by increasing the capacity to detoxify NAPQI that is formed (see Fig. 32–1). In fulminant hepatic failure NAC *treats* toxicity through nonspecific mechanisms that preserve multiorgan function.

NAC prevents toxicity by serving as a glutathione precursor, leading to increased GSH availability.[96] NAC can also serve as a GSH substitute, combining with NAPQI and being converted to cysteine and mercaptate conjugates, just as GSH is converted.[29] NAC may also lead to increased substrate for nontoxic sulfation, allowing increased metabolism by this route and less metabolism by oxidation to NAPQI.[169] In a mouse model, NAC may actually reverse NAPQI oxidation,[42] but there is no evidence of this process in humans.

Each of these preventive mechanisms must be in place early, and none is of benefit after NAPQI has initiated cell injury. Time is required to saturate nontoxic metabolism, form excessive NAPQI, and deplete GSH; thus there is a window of opportunity after overdose during which NAC can be initiated prior to the onset of liver injury, without any loss of efficacy. Based on large clinical trials, it appears that NAC efficacy is nearly complete as long as it is initiated within 8 hours of the overdose.[173] In fact, there is no evident difference in efficacy between NAC started 0–2 hours, as compared to 2–4, 4–6, or 6–8 hours after ingestion.[172] Therefore, delays in NAC initiation that might result from gastrointestinal decontamination or awaiting results of [APAP] determination pose no harm to the patient, as long as NAC can be started within 8 hours of the overdose.

Although no side-by-side comparative studies have been done, historical comparisons indicate that all suggested NAC treatment protocols, as well as earlier methionine or cysteamine protocols appear to be equally effective if started within 8 hours of overdose.[144,147,170,173] Efficacy then decreases in a stepwise fashion with further delays. Compared with historical controls, late methionine and cysteamine is ineffective and possibly harmful, and there is no benefit to the 20-hour IV NAC protocol if started more than 15 hours after the overdose.[144] These findings presumably reflect the time course of events that are preventable by early NAC and led to the conclusion that later treatment was of no value.

Several subsequent observations illustrated that NAC has other mechanisms of action that are effective even after NAPQI formation and binding. In a large clinical trial of the 18-dose oral NAC protocol,[174] it was noted that the severity of hepatotoxicity among high-risk patients first treated with NAC between 16 and 24 hours after overdose was far less than had been observed in untreated historical controls or patients treated with the 20-hour IV NAC protocol.[144] Other experimental work showed that even after cell injury is initiated, late interventions could diminish hepatocyte injury.[27] Most significantly, in a prospective, randomized trial, British investigators found that even after fulminant hepatic failure was evident, starting IV NAC diminished the need for vasopressors, as well as the incidences of cerebral edema and death.[91]

These dramatic findings were accompanied by a fascinating observation. Despite improved organ function and survival in the NAC-treated group, there was no apparent difference in the degree of hepatic injury. Enzyme elevations and INR were equivalent in the two groups, suggesting that much of the NAC benefit may not be derived from lessening of hepatic injury. Initial investigations supported this hypothesis, showing that oxygen delivery and utilization were enhanced by NAC.[53,77,179] This proposed mechanism of action has been challenged,[90,197,198] but there are no subsequent studies that reevaluate or negate the impact of NAC on outcome.

Whether on the basis of its nonspecific antioxidant effects, enhanced GSH supply, or, more likely, its role in mediating microvascular tone, NAC may result in improved organ function in several organs affected by multisystem failure,[44,53,194] and has been suggested to be the agent of choice for cerebral edema after liver failure.[203] With aggressive hemodynamic treatment, hemodialysis and availability of blood products, cerebral edema remains the most feared and most lethal manifestation of liver failure. In this setting, NAC may preserve cerebral blood flow and perfusion better than traditional therapies such as mannitol and hyperventilation, which may actually be detrimental.

Duration of NAC Treatment. Known mechanisms of action and the observation that all studied durations of NAC are effective, when started early, suggest that shorter courses of treatment are effective when NAC is used for its early, preventive actions (see Table 32–4). In contrast, both the oral NAC data and the liver failure study seem to confirm the importance of longer duration of NAC when treating already established liver injury. In fact, except for duration of treatment, the IV NAC dosing protocol that demonstrated late benefit in liver failure[91] is the same as that previously found to be of no value after 15 hours.[144] In the earlier study, NAC was stopped after 20 hours; in the liver-failure study, it was continued until resolution of hepatic failure or death. These observations suggest that, rather than a single duration of therapy for all patients, it is appropriate to utilize varying treatment protocols, selected on the basis of the clinical course of the patient.

All available information indicates that the conceptual basis for discontinuing NAC should be the completion of acetaminophen metabolism and the absence or resolution of consequential liver injury. The challenge lies in translating these concepts into reliable practical guidelines and in the lack of formal study of such guidelines. In the United States, only the 18-dose oral NAC regimen has been studied or used on a large scale. Results from the traditional use of the 20-hour IV NAC protocol in the United Kingdom,[144] a 48-hour IV NAC protocol studied in the United States,[170] and other "short-course" dosing protocols[206,207] indicate that NAC therapy of shorter duration than the current United States standard is safe and effective in many patients.

Currently, the only formally studied standard treatment protocols are those listed above, all of which are based on a standard predetermined duration of NAC. In the United States, only the 18-dose (72-hour) oral NAC protocol is traditionally used (see Table 32–5). The alternative approach described below uses the clinical course of the patient to define the length of NAC therapy. It has been used for several years by the author, but it is a departure from routine guidelines. Preliminary studies suggest it is safe and effective.[132] It is presented here as an alternative in current use and to introduce important conceptual features that should form the basis for future protocol refinement.

The first criterion for discontinuation of NAC should be the completion of acetaminophen metabolism, and measurement of [APAP] is the only widely available method to make this assessment. Although it is theoretically possible that intrahepatic acetaminophen might remain after circulating [APAP] is negligible, there is no evidence that this is consequential. Therefore, [APAP] less than 10 μg/mL is adequate to practically define the completion of acetaminophen metabolism and exclude risk of subsequent substantial conversion of acetaminophen to NAPQI.

The second criterion for discontinuation of NAC should be the determination that there is no consequential hepatotoxicity and that none will develop, or, if it has developed, that it has resolved. As described above, the most practical measure for confirmation or exclusion of liver injury is AST, whereas the measures of liver function such as INR are more appropriate to confirm resolution of serious hepatotoxicity.

Risk of serious hepatic injury can be excluded in patients who show no elevation of AST, if adequate time has passed to exclude the possibility of subsequent significant AST rise. Defining this time point is controversial. There are anecdotal descriptions of the time course of AST rise[140,158] and some case series data;[168] however, there are *no comprehensive studies to define the latest point at which liver injury may become evident*. On the basis of these reports and extensive experience, we use the conservative figure of 36 hours after ingestion as the time at which all cases of AST elevation should be evident. While it is likely that serious liver injury is always evident sooner than this, a conservative approach seems warranted until further study because of the need to provide a safety net for outliers, errors in history or laboratory timing, and other factors.

Regardless of the acuity or chronicity of the ingestion, the risk characteristics of the patient, the delay to presentation, or other factors that may have impact on outcome, the above criteria should apply. Therefore, in any patient determined to be at risk and treated with NAC, clearance of measurable acetaminophen and continued normal AST values 36 hours after the most recent ingestion seem adequate to exclude risk of serious hepatotoxicity and adequate to justify discontinuation of NAC. Depending on circumstances and the delay to presentation, this may represent a duration of NAC treatment ranging from 0 to 36 hours. Many authors who use predetermined 20-hour or 24-hour dosing protocols instead recommend reevaluation at the completion of therapy, resulting in a similar net result in most cases. Refinement and validation of these guidelines will be an important area of research.

The aminotransferases of approximately half of all NAC-treated patients with [APAP] above the Treatment Line will remain below 100 IU/L.[172] Therefore, the use of a "short-course" of NAC may be appropriate in a large proportion of cases, substantially shortening hospital stays without subjecting the patient to any increased risk.

In contrast, for patients with liver failure, IV NAC is recommended (see below) to be continued until the INR is less than 2 and encephalopathy, if present, is nearly resolved.[109] This approach usually results in NAC dosing that continues well beyond other traditional endpoints.

Current information indicates that short-course NAC may be appropriate for those with no hepatotoxicity and that very long-course NAC is appropriate for those who develop liver failure. The most difficult approach to define is that for those in between, with increased AST but no liver failure. For these cases, short-course therapy seems inappropriate given the superiority of the 18-dose oral protocol over the 20-hour IV protocol for high-risk cases. Among patients without liver failure, there are no reports of deterioration after completion of the 18-dose protocol; thus, there is no indication that such cases benefit from NAC beyond the 18-dose duration. Because of the proven safety and efficacy of the 18-dose duration of NAC, use of this protocol seems the most logical for these patients. In the author's practice, on the basis of daily laboratory testing, NAC is discontinued sooner if all liver abnormalities completely resolve and treatment is extended until resolution if liver failure develops.

Given the current understanding of these issues and the extensive experience outside the United States, using a shorter course of NAC for appropriate patients is easily justified. Nonetheless, it must be recognized that definitive comparative studies have not been done. As a result, a thoughtful, circumspect analysis is always warranted. Use of a longer course of therapy is safe, and it is appropriate in any case in which there is suspicion of unusual circumstances. For example, there are theoretical reasons why pregnancy should be considered a contraindication to short-course therapy. Maternal course may not reflect the condition of the fetus,[74,154] and there is suspicion that NAC may provide limited sulfhydryls to the fetus.[87,166] It seems prudent, therefore, to continue therapy for the full 17-dose duration.

Intravenous Versus Oral Administration. As with many issues related to acetaminophen toxicity, the choice of oral versus intravenous NAC is not a simple one. Available information suggests that there are advantages and disadvantages to each, and settings

---

TABLE 32–5. Administration of Oral *N*-Acetylcysteine (Mucomyst) in Acetaminophen Overdose

How supplied
As 10% (10 g/100 mL) solution

Dosing

Loading	140 mg/kg
Maintenance	70 mg/kg every 4 h for an additional 17 doses

Administration
Dilute each dose 1:4 (for 20% concentration with water, carbonated beverage, or fruit juice to make a 5% concentration (chilled is more palatable)).
Repeat dose if patient vomits within 1 h of administration.
Try antiemetic (eg, metoclopramide) if vomiting persists.
Use nasogastric tube if vomiting persists.

in which each may be preferable. Understanding the risks and benefits of each route is necessary to a rational approach.

Safety is the best understood of these issues; oral NAC is clearly safer. Nausea or vomiting, common prior to NAC, is present in about half of patients treated with oral NAC and diarrhea is also prevalent, but there is no credible evidence of more serious complications.[116] Reports of skin rash and extraordinary complications occur but are so rare as to be insignificant.[126] In contrast, intravenous NAC is clearly associated with anaphylactoid reactions including rash, bronchospasm, hypotension, and death.[8,49,56,67,111,170,208] Fortunately, these serious complications are now known to be dose and concentration dependent and eliminated by slow administration of dilute NAC.[56,170,208] With the rapid 15-minute initial infusion originally recommended in the 20-hour IV protocol, such reactions were common. The same dose, or similar dose, diluted and given slowly appears to be entirely safe. Given in this manner, approximately 15% of patients develop a transient rash during the loading dose, without more serious sequelae unless a dosing or administration error occurs. The rash does not generally require treatment, rarely recurs, and does not preclude subsequent doses.[6,170,208] Reactions to NAC with urticaria, angioedema, and respiratory symptoms have been treated and NAC restarted with a very low incidence of recurrence.[6] Although proper dosing of IV NAC is very safe, it must still be considered more dangerous because of the risk of dosing errors. For any medication there is an expected incidence of dosing errors; with intravenous NAC this may be life-threatening. One additional safety concern is administration of large volumes of free water to pediatric patients.[182]

Because there have been no controlled side-by-side studies comparing IV and oral NAC, conclusions about relative benefit of each is more speculative; nonetheless, several observations are relevant. The theoretical, albeit unproven, advantage of oral NAC is that direct delivery via the portal circulation might yield higher concentration of NAC ([NAC]) in the liver. Because of this first-pass clearance, oral NAC results in circulating [NAC] 20–30-fold lower than after IV dosing;[16,82] higher blood [NAC] and consistent delivery regardless of vomiting represent the theoretical advantages of IV NAC.

Despite theoretical considerations and strong viewpoints of proponents of each, for patients without liver failure there is no evidence of superiority of one route over the other. The advantage of oral delivery is not evident, because each appears equivalent if treatment is started within 8 hours of ingestion. The apparent superiority of oral NAC over IV NAC when started 16–24 hours after overdose is almost certainly related to the duration of NAC therapy, rather than the route. Similarly, the concern about delays in oral NAC administration because of vomiting is not borne out by the apparently equivalent outcome. In fact, there is no evidence of any worsening of outcome among patients who required additional NAC doses because of vomiting of NAC doses within an hour of administration (author's unpublished data). This counterintuitive observation may be accounted for by partial NAC absorption prior to vomiting, but this remains speculative.

Lower costs of care are emphasized as an advantage of oral NAC. Avoidance of IV administration costs can reduce inpatient costs, and oral dosing allows the option of outpatient dosing. Whether this is appropriate requires further analysis, but it must be considered in any cost-effectiveness evaluation of this issue.

Until a formulation intended for IV use is available in the United States, these considerations indicate to us that oral NAC

should be the treatment of choice for most patients. In other countries where IV NAC is readily available, patient comfort and ease of administration suggest that IV NAC may be preferable, as long as it is carefully administered.

There is no proven advantage to either of the best-known IV-dosing protocols. One protocol involves dosing identical to oral NAC: 140 mg/kg loading dose followed by 70 mg/kg every 4 hours for 17 doses.[160,173] The other protocol provides a loading dose of 150 mg/kg, followed by 50 mg/kg over 4 hours, followed by a continuous infusion of 6.25 mg/kg/h for 16 hours.[109,144] We use the intermittent-dosing protocol rather than the continuous infusion protocol because of familiarity, lower published incidence of adverse effects, and the substantially higher total dose of NAC given.

In the United States, currently available formulations do not undergo the routine testing and documentation that is required for drugs listed for parenteral use. Thus, the manufacturers do not guarantee that the drug is sterile and pyrogen-free. This does not indicate that the product is not sterile, only that it is not documented to be so. In fact, sterility is expected in light of NAC use for inhalation by patients with a variety of lung diseases. Extensive IV use of these products indicates that there is no evidence of infectious or febrile consequences of its use.[17] Because these products are not intended for parenteral use, they should never be used intravenously unless there is good reason to believe that the patient may be harmed by failure to administer IV NAC. In such cases, however, we believe that the potential benefits of IV NAC outweigh the risk of parenteral use of nonparenteral formulations. It is customary to use an in-line 0.22-μm filter, although there is no evidence that this is necessary.

Using IV NAC. Despite the lack of an available parenteral form, there are three situations in which the available information suggests that IV NAC is preferable; fulminant hepatic failure, inability to tolerate oral NAC, and acetaminophen poisoning in pregnancy. Each requires further study to validate, but all three seem well supported by current information.

Fulminant hepatic failure is an important indication for IV NAC. The choice of IV over oral or enteral NAC is based on several observations. Most importantly, IV is the only route that has been studied in liver failure. Oral NAC may prove effective, but this has not yet been shown. Second, the evidence that the benefit of NAC in liver failure is extrahepatic suggests that IV is preferable. Intravenous NAC results in manyfold higher blood [NAC], which presumably leads to more NAC delivery to critical organs. Finally, concomitant GI bleeding, use of lactulose, and other factors make IV NAC more practical.

A more common indication for IV NAC is the patient with a very high [APAP] approaching or beyond 8 hours since ingestion who is unable to tolerate oral NAC after a brief, aggressive trial of antiemetic therapy. To avoid further delays and resultant loss of NAC efficacy, IV NAC is logical, even without proof that continued vomiting significantly limits NAC absorption.

The most controversial indication for IV NAC is pregnancy. Fetal toxicity is rare, but clearly can occur, with adverse outcomes documented at all stages of pregnancy. Because maternal condition and thiol depletion certainly affect the fetus, the relative contribution to toxicity of fetal NAPQI production at various stages of pregnancy remains hard to define. Fetal oxidation of acetaminophen has been demonstrated and is thought to increase with advancing fetal age, but little else is known.[155] There is every indication that NAC is both safe and effective to treat the mother,[154] but there are inadequate data to evaluate efficacy in the fetus. Fetal outcome has generally been excellent after maternal treatment with oral NAC,[154] but concern exists about those at greatest risk.

One case series examined [NAC] in cord or neonatal blood after oral maternal NAC administration.[83] The [NAC] in this study approached or equalled those seen in patients treated with oral NAC. This, however, does not prove adequacy of therapy. Unlike the neonates studied, patients treated with oral NAC have extensive first pass hepatic uptake prior to NAC entry into the serum where [NAC] was measured.[16,82] It remains uncertain if the serum [NAC] in the neonates studied reflects any significant hepatic NAC delivery. Other studies demonstrate that placental transfer of NAC to the fetus is limited.[87,166] To maximize the maternal-to-fetal gradient for NAC or, perhaps more importantly, other thiol-containing NAC metabolites, IV NAC is logical. In the United States, lacking availability or study of IV NAC in this setting, oral NAC is routinely used; however, it is the author's view that IV NAC is warranted, particularly in the later stages of pregnancy. In addition, because lack of maternal toxicity may or may not exclude fetal toxicity it is logical to continue NAC for 72 hours (the duration of the 17-dose protocol), and to not use short-course protocols.

Other Antidotes. Glutathione and cysteine were used experimentally, but subsequently abandoned. Oral glutathione bioavailability is minimal, intracellular penetration is limited even after parenteral administration, and its efficacy to prevent serious hepatotoxicity is poor. IV cysteine is equivalent to that of cysteamine or methionine, but without apparent advantage. In short, no other available glutathione precursor or substitute matches NAC in safety or efficacy.

Methods to decrease NAPQI formation have focused primarily on inhibition of P450 metabolism, and thus have not demonstrated a logical role in treatment. Such antidotes would be effective only prior to NAPQI covalent binding and arylation of hepatocyte proteins, at a stage when NAC has already proven to be safe and essentially completely effective. Inhibitors of P450 metabolism such as cimetidine are effective after massive dosing prior to experimental acetaminophen overdose,[178] but there is no evidence or rationale to suggest significant efficacy against serious human acetaminophen overdose,[43] particularly when compared to NAC.

CRITICAL DECISIONS

There are several key concepts that will help the clinician manage acetaminophen effectively. When managing intentional overdose the measurement of [APAP] should be considered as part of the patient's initial evaluation. In those cases in which risk assessment for acetaminophen toxicity is merited, treatment with NAC should be initiated within 8 hours from the time of ingestion, or as soon as possible if more than 8 hours has elapsed since ingestion. IV NAC should be used for fulminant hepatic failure, and when the patient is unable to tolerate oral NAC. It should also be considered for management of acetaminophen exposure in the pregnant patient. Patients who present with repeated excessive dosing should be assessed for evidence of hepatic injury, and potential for ongoing production of NAPQI. Factors that potentially predispose patients to hepatotoxicity after repeated dosing should be taken into account when deciding which patients to assess for hepatic injury.

Patients showing evidence of severe hepatotoxicity, hepatic encephalopathy, as well as those at risk for fulminant hepatic failure may need to be admitted to an ICU bed. These patients require frequent neurologic checks, monitoring of vital signs, and laboratory studies. Contact with a regional poison center, gastroenterology consultant, and regional transplant center is important to guide treatment strategies and to coordinate transplantation when needed. Early psychiatric consultation can be helpful in assessing transplant eligibility. Absolute indications for transplantation vary and should be discussed early with local transplant centers, poison control center, and hepatologists.

SUMMARY

Although our understanding of acetaminophen toxicity has advanced, there are many remaining important challenges. To accurately determine risk of toxicity in atypical patients, high-risk patients, after repeated dosing, after sustained-release formulations, and in other settings, an entirely new method of toxicity screening needs to be developed. Ongoing study of antidotal therapy dosing protocols is needed to assess the validity of many assumptions. Improved methods to determine need for liver transplantation in a timely manner are very important. These and other issues indicate that further changes are likely. The principles and current strategies presented in this chapter should serve as a strong foundation for these important future advances.

REFERENCES

1. Akca S, Suleymanlar I, Tuncer M, et al: Isolated acute renal failure due to paracetamol intoxication in an alcoholic patient. Nephron 1999;83:270–271.
2. Anderson BJ, Holford NHG, Armishaw JC, et al: Predicting concentrations in children presenting with acetaminophen overdose. J Pediatr 1999;135:290–295.
3. Anker AL, Smilkstein MJ: Acetaminophen: Concepts and controversies. Med Clin North Am 1994;12:335–349.
4. Arena JM, Rourk MHJ, Sibrack CD: Acetaminophen: Report of an unusual poisoning. Pediatrics 1978;61:68–72.
5. Arthurs Y, Fielding JR: Paracetamol and chronic liver disease. J Irish Med Assoc 1980;73:273–27.
6. Bailey B, McGuigan MA: Management of anaphylactoid reactions to intravenous N-acetylcysteine. Ann Emerg Med 1998;31:710–715.
7. Barker JD, deCarle DJ, Anuras S: Chronic excessive acetaminophen use of liver damage. Ann Intern Med 1977;87:299–301.
8. Bateman DN, Woodhouse KW, Rawlins KW: Adverse reactions to N-acetylcysteine. Hum Toxicol 1984;3:393–398.
9. Beckett GJ, Donovan JW, Hussey AJ, et al: Intravenous N-acetylcysteine, hepatotoxicity and plasma glutathione S-transferase in patients with paracetamol overdosage. Hum Exp Toxicol 1990;9:183–186.
10. Benson GD: Acetaminophen in chronic liver disease. Clin Pharmacol Ther 1983;33:95–101.
11. Bidault I, Lagier G, Garnier R, et al: Les hepatites par toxicite subaigue du paracetamol existent-elles? Therapie 1987;42:387–388.
12. Bien E, Vick K, Skorka G: Effects of exogenous factors on the cerebral glutathione in rodents. Arch Toxicol 1992;66:279–285.
13. Bizovi JE, Aks SE, Paloucek F, et al: Late increase in acetaminophen concentration after overdose of Tylenol Extended Relief. Ann Emerg Med 1996;28:549–551.
14. Bond GR, Krenzelok EP, Normann SA, et al: Acetaminophen ingestion in childhood—Cost and relative risk of alternative referral strategies. J Toxicol Clin Toxicol 1994;32:513–525.

15. Bonkowsky HL, Mudge GH, McMurtry RJ: Chronic hepatic inflammation role of intracellular calcium in paracetamol toxicity. Lancet 1978;1:1016–1018.

16. Borgstrom L, Kagedal B, Paulsen O: Pharmacokinetics of N-acetylcysteine in man. Eur J Clin Pharmacol 1986;31:217–222.

17. Borys DJ, Jackson TW, Jacobs MR, et al: Intravenous N-acetylcysteine. Use of an unapproved drug product. A two-year retrospective review [abstract]. Vet Hum Toxicol 1992;34:350.

18. Brackett CC, Bloch JD: Phenytoin as a possible cause of acetaminophen hepatotoxicity: Case report and review of the literature. Pharmacotherapy 2000;20:229–233.

19. Bradberry SM, Hart M, Bareford D, et al: Factor V and Factor VII:V ratio as prognostic indicators in paracetamol poison. Lancet 1995;1:646–647.

20. Bravo-Fernandez EF, Reddy KR, Jeffers L, et al: Hepatotoxicity after prolonged use of acetaminophen: A case report. Bol Assoc Med P R 1988;80:417–419.

21. Bray GP, Harrison PM, O'Grady JG, et al: Long-term anticonvulsant therapy worsens outcome in paracetamol-induced fulminant hepatic failure. Hum Exp Toxicol 1992;11:265–270.

22. Breen K, Wandscheer JC, Peignoux M, Pessayre D: In situ formation of the acetaminophen metabolite covalently bound in kidneys and lung: Supportive evidence provided by total hepatectomy. Biochem Pharmacol 1982;31:115–116.

23. Brent JA: New ways of looking at an old molecule. J Toxicol Clin Toxicol 1996;34:149–153.

24. Brent JA, Rumack BH: Role of free radicals in toxic hepatic injury. II. Are free radicals the cause of toxin-induced liver injury? J Toxicol Clin Toxicol 1993;311:173–196.

25. Bridger S, Henserson K, Glucksman E, et al: Lesson of the week, Deaths from low-dose paracetamol poisoning. BMJ 1998;316:1724–1725.

26. Brodie BB, Axelrod J: The fate of acetanilide in man. J Pharmacol Exp Ther 1948;94:29–38.

27. Bruno MK, Cohen S, Khairallah EA: Antidotal effectiveness of N-acetylcysteine in reversing acetaminophen-induced hepatotoxicity: Enhancement of the proteolysis of arylated proteins. Biochem Pharmacol 1988;37:4319–4325.

28. Buckley NA, Whyte IM, O'Connell DL: Activated charcoal reduces the need for N-acetylcysteine treatment after acetaminophen (paracetamol) overdose. J Toxicol Clin Toxicol 1999;37:753–757.

29. Buckpitt AR, Rollins DE, Mitchell JR: Varying effects of sulfhydryl nucleophiles on acetaminophen oxidation and sulfhydryl adduct formation. Biochem Pharmacol 1979;28:2941–2946.

30. Calvert LJ, Linder CW: Acetaminophen poisoning. J Fam Pract 1978;7:953–956.

31. Campbell NR, Baylis B: Renal impairment associated with an acute paracetamol overdose in the absence of hepatotoxicity. Postgrad Med J 1992;68:116–118.

32. Carpenter HM, Mudge GH: Acetaminophen nephrotoxicity: Studies on renal acetylation and deacetylation. J Pharmacol Exp Ther 1981;218:161–167.

33. Cerretani D, Micheli L, Fiaschi AI, et al: MK-801 potentiates the glutathione depletion induced by acetaminophen in rat brain. Curr Ther Res 1994;55:707–717.

34. Cetaruk EW, Dart RC, Horowitz RS, et al: Extended-release acetaminophen overdose [letter]. JAMA 1996;275:686.

35. Chao TC: Adverse drug reactions: Tales of a forensic pathologist. Ann Acad Med Singapore 1993;22:86–89.

36. Cheung L, Potts R, Meyer K: Acetaminophen treatment nomogram. N Engl J Med 1994;330:1907–1908.

37. Chinouth RW, Czajka PA, Peterson RG: N-Acetylcysteine absorption by activated charcoal. Vet Hum Toxicol 1980;22:392–394.

38. Clark JH, Russell GJ, Fitzgerald JF: Fatal acetaminophen toxicity in a 2-year-old. J Indiana State Med Assoc 1983;76:832–835.

39. Clark R, Thompson RPH, Borirakchanyavat V, et al: Hepatic damage and death from overdose of paracetamol. Lancet 1973;1:66–70.

40. Clissold SP: Paracetamol and phenacetin. Drugs 1986;32S:46–59.

41. Cobden I, Record CO, Ward MK, et al: Paracetamol-induced acute renal failure in the absence of fulminant liver damage. Br Med J 1982;284:21–22.

42. Corcoran GB, Mitchell JR, Vaishnav YN, et al: Evidence that acetaminophen and N-hydroxyacetaminophen form a common arylating intermediate, N-acetyl-p-benzoquinoneimine. Mol Pharmacol 1980;18:536–542.

43. Critchley JAJH, Dyson EH, Scott AW, et al: Is there a place for cimetidine or ethanol in the treatment of paracetamol poisoning? Lancet 1983;1:1375–1376.

44. Cuzzocrea S, Constantino G, Mazzon E, et al: Protective effect of N-acetylcysteine on multiple organ failure induced by zymosan in the rat. Crit Care Med 1999;27:1524–1532.

45. Davenport A, Finn R: Paracetamol (acetaminophen) poisoning resulting in acute renal failure without hepatic coma. Nephron 1988;50:55–56.

46. Davidson DGD, Eastham WN: Acute liver necrosis following overdose of paracetamol. BMJ 1966;2:497–499.

47. Davie A: Acetaminophen poisoning and liver function [letter]. N Engl J Med 1994;331:1311.

48. Davis M, Simmons CJ, Harrison NG, et al: Paracetamol overdose in man: Relationship between pattern of urinary metabolites and severity of liver damage. Q J Med 1976;45:181–191.

49. Dawson AH, Henry DA, McEwan J: Adverse reactions to N-acetylcysteine during treatment for paracetamol poisoning. Med J Aust 1989;150:329–331.

50. Day A, Abbott GD: Chronic paracetamol poisoning in children: A warning to health professionals. N Z Med J 1994;107:201.

51. Detry O, Arkavopoulos N, Ting P, et al: Clinical use of bioartificial liver in the treatment of acetaminophen-induced fulminant hepatic failure. Am Surg 1999;65:934–938.

52. Devalia JL, Ogilvie RC, McLean AE: Dissociation of cell death from covalent binding of paracetamol by flavones in a hepatocyte system. Biochem Pharmacol 1982;31:3745–3749.

53. Devlin J, Ellis AE, McPeake J, et al: N-Acetylcysteine improves indocyanine green extraction and oxygen transport during hepatic dysfunction. Crit Care Med 1997;25:236–242.

54. Divoll M, Greenblatt DJ, Ameer B, et al: Effect of food on acetaminophen absorption in young and elderly subjects. J Clin Pharmacol 1982;22:571–576.

55. Donnelly PG, Walker RN, Racz WJ: Inhibition of mitochondrial respiration in vivo is an early event in acetaminophen-induced hepatotoxicity. Arch Toxicol 1994;68:110–118.

56. Donovan JW, Jarvie DR, Prescott LF, et al: Adverse reactions of N-acetylcysteine and their relation to plasma levels. Vet Hum Toxicol 1987;29:470.

57. Douglas AP, Hamlyn AN: Controlled trial of cysteamine in treatment of acute paracetamol (acetaminophen) poisoning. Lancet 1976;1:111–115.

58. Douglas DR, Sholar JB, Smilkstein MJ: A pharmacokinetic comparison of acetaminophen products (Tylenol Extended Relief vs. regular Tylenol). Acad Emerg Med 1996;3:740–744.

59. Douglas DR, Smilkstein MJ, Rumack BH: APAP levels within 4 hours: Are they useful? [abstract]. Vet Hum Toxicol 1994;36:350.

60. Douidar SM, Al-Khalil I, Habersang RW: Severe hepatotoxicity, acute renal failure, and pancytopenia in a young child after repeated acetaminophen overdosing. Clin Pediatr 1994;33:42–45.

61. Ekins B, Ford DC, Thompson MIB, et al: The effect of activated charcoal on N-acetylcysteine absorption in normal subjects. Am J Emerg Med 1987;5:483–487.

62. Emeigh Hart SG, Beierschmitt WP, Bartolone JB, et al: Evidence against deacetylation and for cytochrome P450-medicated activation in acetaminophen-induced nephrotoxicity in the CD-1 mouse. Toxicol Appl Pharmacol 1991;107:1–15.

63. Emeigh Hart SG, Beierschmitt WP, Wyand DS, et al: Acetaminophen nephrotoxicity in CD-1 mice. I. Evidence of a role for in

situ activation in selective covalent binding and toxicity. Toxicol Appl Pharmacol 1994;126:267–275.

64. Emeigh Hart SG, Birge RB, Cartun RW, et al: In vivo and in vitro evidence for situ activation and selective covalent binding of acetaminophen (APAP) in mouse kidney. Adv Exp Med Biol 1991; 283:711–716.

65. Epstein MM, Nelson SD, Slatterly JT, et al: Inhibition of the metabolism of paracetamol by isoniazid. Br J Clin Pharmacol 1991;31: 139–142.

66. Erickson RA, Runyon BA: Acetaminophen hepatotoxicity associated with alcoholic pancreatitis. Arch Intern Med 1984;144:1509–1510.

67. Falk JL: Oral N-acetylcysteine given intravenously for acetaminophen overdose: We shouldn't have to, but we must. Crit Care Med 1998;26:7.

68. Ferguson DV, Roberts DW, Han-Shu H, et al: Acetaminophen-induced alterations in pancreatic B cells and serum insulin concentrations in B6C3F1 mice. Toxicol Appl Pharmacol 1990;104: 225–234.

69. Flanagan RJ, Mant TGK: Coma and metabolic acidosis early in severe acute paracetamol poisoning. Hum Toxicol 1986;5:256–259.

70. Gerber JG, MacDonald JS, Harbison RD, et al: Effect of N-acetylcysteine on hepatic covalent binding of paracetamol (acetaminophen). Lancet 1977;1:657–658.

71. Gilmore JT, Tourvas E: Paracetamol-induced acute pancreatitis. Br Med J 1977;1:753–754.

72. Graudins A, Aaron CK, Linden CH: Overdose of extended-release acetaminophen [letter]. N Engl J Med 1995;333:196.

73. Grewal KK, Racz WJ: Intracellular calcium disruption as a secondary event in acetaminophen-induced hepatotoxicity. Can J Physiol Pharmacol 1993;71:26–32.

74. Hamlyn AN, Douglas AP, James O: The spectrum of paracetamol (acetaminophen) overdose: Clinical and epidemiological studies. Postgrad Med J 1978;54:400–404.

75. Harman AW, Mahar SO, Burcham PC, et al: Level of cytosolic free calcium during acetaminophen toxicity in mouse hepatocytes. Mol Pharmacol 1992;41:665–670.

76. Harrison PM, O'Grady JG, Keays RT, et al: Serial prothrombin time as prognostic indicator in paracetamol induced fulminant hepatic failure. BMJ 1990;310:964–966.

77. Harrison PM, Wendon JA, Gimson AES, et al: Improvement by acetylcysteine of hemodynamics and oxygen transport in fulminant hepatic failure. N Engl J Med 1991;324:1852–1857.

78. Hart SG, Beierschmitt WP, Wyand DS, et al: Acetaminophen nephrotoxicity in CD-1 mice. Evidence of a role for in situ activation in selective covalent binding and toxicity. Toxicol Appl Pharmacol 1994;126:216–275.

79. Henretig FM, Selbst SM, Forrect C, et al: Repeated acetaminophen overdosing: Causing hepatotoxicity in children. Clin Pediatr 1989; 28:267–275.

80. Hinsberg O, Treupel G: Ueber die physiologische wirkung des p-amidophenols und einiger derivate desselben. Archiv fur experimentell Pathologie und Pharmakologie 1894;22:216–250.

81. Hoivik DJ, Manautou JE, Tviet A, et al: Gender-related differences in susceptibility to acetaminophen-induced protein arylation and nephrotoxicity on the CD-1 mouse. Toxicol Appl Pharmacol 1995; 130:257–271.

82. Holdiness MR: Clinical pharmacokinetics of N-acetylcysteine. Clin Pharmacokinet 1991;20:123–134.

83. Horowitz RS, Dart RC, Jarvie DR, et al: Placental transfer of N-acetylcysteine following human maternal acetaminophen toxicity. J Toxicol Clin Toxicol 1997;35:447–451.

84. Insel PA: Analgesic-antipyretic and anti-inflammatory agents and drugs employed in the treatment of gout. In: Hardman JG, Limbird LE, eds: Goodman and Gilman's The Pharmacological Basis of Therapeutics, 9th ed. New York, McGraw-Hill, 1995, pp. 631–633.

85. Jaeschke H, Smith SW: Role of neutrophils in acetaminophen-induced liver injury. Toxicologist 1991;11:32.

86. Jepsen S, Hansen AB: The influence of N-acetylcysteine on the measurement of prothrombin time and activated partial thromboplastin time in health subjects. Scand J Clin Lab Invest 1994;54:11–32.

87. Johnson D, Simone C, Koren G: Transfer of N-acetylcysteine by the human placenta [abstract]. Vet Hum Toxicol 1993;35:365.

88. Johnson GK, Tolman KG: Chronic liver disease and acetaminophen. Ann Intern Med 1977;87:302–304.

89. Jollow DJ, Mitchell JR, Potter WZ, et al: Acetaminophen-induced hepatic necrosis. II. Role of covalent binding in vivo. J Pharmacol Exp Ther 1973;187:195–202.

90. Jones AL: Mechanism of action and value of N-acetylcysteine in the treatment of early and late acetaminophen poisoning: A critical review. J Toxicol Clin Toxicol 1998;36:277–285.

91. Keays R, Harrison PM, Wendon JA, et al: Intravenous acetylcysteine in paracetamol induced fulminant hepatic failure: A prospective controlled trial. BMJ 1991;303:1026–1029.

92. Kher K, Makker S: Acute renal failure due to acetaminophen ingestion without concurrent hepatotoxicity. Am J Med 1987;82: 1280–1281.

93. Klein-Schwartz W, Oderda GM: Adsorption of oral antidotes for acetaminophen poisoning (methionine and N-acetylcysteine) by activated charcoal. J Toxicol Clin Toxicol 1981;18:283–290.

94. Kobrinsky NO, Hartfield D, Horner H, et al: Treatment of advanced malignancies with high-dose acetaminophen. Cancer Invest 1996;14: 202–210.

95. Koulouris Z, Tierney MG, Jones G: Metabolic acidosis and coma following a severe acetaminophen overdose. Ann Pharmacother 1999;33:1191–1194.

96. Lauterburg BH, Corcoran GB, Mitchell JR: Mechanism of action of N-acetylcysteine in the protection against hepatotoxicity of acetaminophen in rats in vivo. J Clin Invest 1983;71:980–991.

97. Lauterburg BH, Vaishnav Y, Stillwell WG, et al: The effect of age and glutathione depletion on hepatic glutathione turnover in vivo determined by acetaminophen probe analysis. J Pharmacol Exp Ther 1980;213:54–58.

98. Lauterburg BH, Velez ME: Glutathione deficiency in alcoholics: Risk factor for paracetamol hepatotoxicity. Gut 1988;29:1153–1157.

99. Lee WM: Acute liver failure. N Engl J Med 1993;329:135–138.

100. Leibowitz J, Huhn JA: Acetaminophen overdosage: A case presentation and review of current therapy. Del Med J 1980;52:135–138.

101. Lesna M, Watson AJ, Douglas AP, et al: Evaluation of paracetamol-induced damage in liver biopsies. Virchows Arch 1976;370: 333–344.

102. Levy G, Garrettson L, Soda D: Evidence of placental transfer of acetaminophen [letter]. Pediatrics 1974;55:895.

103. Lieber CS, Lasker JM, Alderman J, et al: The microsomal ethanol oxidizing system and its interaction with other drugs, carcinogens, and vitamins. Ann N Y Acad Sci 1987;492:11–24.

104. Lieh-Lai MW, Sarnaik AP, Newton JF, et al: Metabolism and pharmacokinetics of acetaminophen in a severely poisoned young child. J Pediatr 1984;105:125–128.

105. Linden CH, Rumack BH: Acetaminophen overdose. Emerg Med Clin North Am 1984;2:102–119.

106. Lip GYH, Vale JA: Does acetaminophen damage the heart? J Toxicol Clin Toxicol 1996;34:145–147.

107. Litovitz TL, Smilkstein MJ, Felberg L, et al: 1996 Annual report of the American Association of Poison Control Centers Toxic Exposure Surveillance System. Am J Emerg Med 1997;15:447–500.

108. MacLean D, Peters TJ, Brown RAG, et al: Treatment of acute paracetamol poisoning. Lancet 1968;2:849–852.

109. Makin AJ, Wendon J, Williams R: A 7-year experience of severe acetaminophen-induced hepatotoxicity (1987–1993). Gastroenterology 1995;109:1907–1916.

110. Makin AJ, Williams R: The current management of paracetamol overdosage. Br J Clin Prac 1994;48:144–148.

111. Mant TGK, Tempowski JH, Volans GN, et al: Adverse reactions to acetylcysteine and effects of overdose. Br Med J 1984;289:217–219.

112. Mathew J, Hines JE, James OFW, et al: Non-parenchymal cell responses in paracetamol (acetaminophen)-induced liver injury. J Hepatol 1994;20:537–541.

113. Mathis RD, Walker JS, Kuhns DW: Subacute acetaminophen overdose after incremental dosing. J Emerg Med 1988;6:37–40.

114. McClements BM, Hyland M, Callender ME, et al: Management of paracetamol poisoning complicated by enzyme induction due to alcohol or drugs. Lancet 1990;335:1526.

115. McCrae TA, Furuhama K, Roberts DW, et al: Evaluation of 3-(cystein-S-yl) acetaminophen in the nephrotoxicity of acetaminophen in rats. Toxicologist 1989;9:47.

116. Miller LF, Rumack BH: Clinical safety of high oral doses of N-acetylcysteine. Semin Oncol 1983;10(Suppl 1):76–85.

117. Miller RP, Roberts RJ, Fischer LJ: Acetaminophen elimination kinetics in neonates, children, and adults. Clin Pharmacol Ther 1976;19:676–684.

118. Mitchell JR: Host susceptibility and acetaminophen liver injury. Ann Intern Med 1977;87:377–378.

119. Mitchell JR: Acetaminophen toxicity. N Engl J Med 1988;319:1601–1602.

120. Mitchell JR, Jollow DJ, Potter WZ, et al: Acetaminophen-induced hepatic necrosis. I. Role of drug metabolism. J Pharmacol Exp Ther 1973;187:185–194.

121. Mitchell JR, Jollow DJ, Potter WZ, et al: Acetaminophen-induced hepatic necrosis. IV. Protective role of glutathione. J Pharmacol Exp Ther 1973;187:211–217.

122. Mitchell JR, Thorgeirsson SS, Potter WZ, et al: Acetaminophen-induced hepatic injury: Protective role of glutathione in man and rationale for therapy. Clin Pharmacol Ther 1974;16:676–684.

123. Moller-Hartmann W, Siegers CP: Nephrotoxicity of paracetamol in the rate-mechanistic and therapeutic aspects. J Appl Toxicol 1991;11:141–146.

124. Moore M, Thor H, Moore G, et al: The toxicity of acetaminophen and N-acetyl-p-benzoquinoneimine in isolated hepatocytes is associated with thiol depletion and increased cytosolic CA^{2+}. J Biol Chem 1985;260:13035–13040.

125. Morse HN: Ueber eine neue Darstellungsmethode der Acetylamidophenole. Berichte der Deutschen Chemischen Gesellschaft 1878;11:232–233.

126. Mroz LS, Krenzelok EP: Angioedema with oral N-acetylcysteine. Ann Emerg Med 1997;30:240–241.

127. Murphy R, Swartz R, Watkins PB: Severe acetaminophen toxicity in a patient receiving isoniazid. Ann Intern Med 1990;113:799–800.

128. Mutimer DJ, Ayres RC, Neuberger JM, et al: Serious paracetamol poisoning and the results of liver transplantation. Gut 1994;35: 809–814.

129. Nogen AG, Bremner JE: Fatal acetaminophen overdosage in a young child. J Pediatr 1978;92:832–833.

130. O'Grady JG, Alexander GJM, Hayllar KM, et al: Early indicators of prognosis in fulminant hepatic failure. Gastroenterology 1989;97:439–445.

131. Ohtani N, Matsuzaki M, Anno Y, et al: A case of myocardial damage following acute paracetamol poisoning. Jpn Circ J 1989;53:278–282.

132. Parker SJ, Bizovi KE, Smilkstein MJ: A variable duration NAC treatment protocol for acetaminophen overdose [abstract]. J Toxicol Clin Toxicol 1999;37:643.

133. Pereira LMMB, Langley PG, Hayllar KM, et al: Coagulation factor V and VII/V ratio as predictors of outcome in paracetamol induced fulminant hepatic failure: Relation to other prognostic indicators. Gut 1992;33:98–102.

134. Pimstone BL, Uys CJ: Liver necrosis and myocardiopathy following paracetamol overdosage. S Afr Med J 1968;42:259–262.

135. Piperno E, Berssenbruegge DA: Reversal of experimental paracetamol toxicosis with N-acetylcysteine. Lancet 1976;2:738–739.

136. Piperno E, Mosher AH, Berssenbruegge DA, et al: Pathophysiology of acetaminophen overdosage toxicity: Implications for management. Pediatrics 1978;62(Suppl):880–889.

137. Portmann B, Talbot IC, Day DW, et al: Histopathological changes in the liver following a paracetamol overdose: Correlation with clinical and biochemical parameters. J Pathol 1975;117:169–181.

138. Potter WZ, Davis DC, Mitchell JR, et al: Acetaminophen-induced hepatic necrosis. III. Cytochrome P450-mediated covalent binding in vitro. J Pharmacol Exp Ther 1973;187:203–210.

139. Prescott LF: Kinetics and metabolism of paracetamol and phenacetin. Br J Clin Pharmacol 1980;10(Suppl 2):291S–298S.

140. Prescott LF: Paracetamol overdosage: Pharmacological considerations and clinical management. Drugs 1983;25:290–314.

141. Prescott LF: Absorption of paracetamol. In: Prescott LF, ed: Paracetamol (acetaminophen), A Critical Bibliographic Review. London, Taylor & Francis, 1996, pp. 708.

142. Prescott LF: Factors influencing paracetamol metabolism. In: Prescott LF, ed: Paracetamol (acetaminophen). A Critical Bibliographic Review. London, Taylor & Francis, 1996, pp. 103–106.

143. Prescott LF: The metabolism of paracetamol. In: Prescott LF, ed: Paracetamol (acetaminophen). A Critical Bibliographic Review. London, Taylor & Francis, 1996, pp. 67–102.

144. Prescott LF, Illingworth RN, Critchley JAH: Intravenous N-acetylcysteine: The treatment of choice for paracetamol poisoning. Br Med J 1979;2:1097–1100.

145. Prescott LF, Matthew H: Cysteamine for paracetamol overdosage. Lancet 1974;1:998.

146. Prescott LF, Mattison P, Menzies DG, et al: The comparative effects of paracetamol and indomethacin on renal function in healthy female volunteers. Br J Clin Pharmacol 1990;29:403–412.

147. Prescott LF, Park J, Sutherland GR, et al: Cysteamine, methionine and penicillamine in the treatment of paracetamol poisoning. Lancet 1976;2:109–114.

148. Prescott LF, Proudfoot AT, Cregeen RJ: Paracetamol-induced acute renal failure in the absence of fulminant liver damage. Br Med J 1982;284:421–422.

149. Prescott LF, Wright N, Roscoe P, et al: Plasma-paracetamol half-life and hepatic necrosis in patients with paracetamol overdosage. Lancet 1971;1:519–522.

150. Proudfoot AT, Wright N: Acute paracetamol poisoning. Br Med J 1970;3:557–558.

151. Pumford NR, Hinson JA, Potter DW, et al: Immunochemical quantitation of 3-(cystein-S-yl) acetaminophen adducts in serum and liver proteins of acetaminophen-treated mice. J Pharmacol Exp Ther 1989; 248:190–196.

152. Raucy JL, Sker JML, Lieber CS, et al: Acetaminophen activation by human liver cytochromes P-450 IIE1 and P-450 IA2. Arch Biochem Biophys 1989;271:270–283.

153. Ray SD, Mumaw VR, Raje RR, et al: Protection of acetaminophen-induced hepatocellular apoptosis and necrosis by cholesteryl hemisuccinate pretreatment. J Pharmacol Exp Ther 1996;279:1470–1483.

154. Riggs BS, Bronstein AC, Kulig K, et al: Acute acetaminophen overdose during pregnancy. Obstet Gynecol 1989;74:247–253.

155. Rollins DE, Von Bahr C, Glaumann H, et al: Acetaminophen: Potentially toxic metabolite formed by human fetal and adult liver microsomes and isolated fetal liver cells. Science 1979;205:1414–1416.

156. Rumack BH: Acetaminophen overdose. Am J Med 1983;75(Suppl 5A):104–112.

157. Rumack BH: Acetaminophen overdose in young children: Treatment and effects of alcohol and other additional ingestants in 417 cases. Am J Dis Child 1984;138:428–433.

158. Rumack BH, Matthew H: Acetaminophen overdose: Incidence, diagnosis and management in 416 patients. Pediatrics 1978;62(Suppl):898–903.

159. Rumack BH, Peterson RG: Acetaminophen poisoning and toxicity. Pediatrics 1975;55:871–876.

160. Rumack BH, Peterson RG, Koch GG, et al: Acetaminophen overdose. 662 cases with evaluation of oral acetylcysteine treatment. Arch Intern Med 1981;141:380–385.

161. Rybolt TR, Burrell DE, Shults JM, et al: In vitro coadsorption of acetaminophen and N-acetylcysteine onto activated carbon powder. J Pharm Sci 1986;75:904–906.

162. Sandler DP: Analgesic use and chronic renal disease. N Engl J Med 1989;320:399–404.

163. Schiodt FV, Bondesen S, Tygstrup N, et al: Prediction of hepatic encephalopathy in paracetamol overdose: A prospective and validated study. Scand J Gastroenterol 1999;7:723–728.

164. Schiodt FV, Rochling FA, Casey DL, et al: Acetaminophen toxicity in an urban county hospital. N Engl J Med 1997;337:1112–1117.

165. Seeff LB, Cuccherini BA, Zimmerman HJ, et al: Acetaminophen hepatotoxicity in alcoholics. A therapeutic misadventure. Ann Intern Med 1986;104:309–404.

166. Selden BS, Curry SC, Clark RF, et al: Transplacental transport of N-acetylcysteine in an ovine model. Ann Emerg Med 1991;20:1069–1072.

167. Shen W, Kamendulis LM, Ray SD, et al: Acetaminophen-induced cytotoxicity in cultured mouse hepatocytes: Effects of CA^{2+}-endonuclease, DNA repair, and glutathione depletion inhibitors on DNA fragmentation and cell death. Toxicol Appl Pharmacol 1992;112:34–40.

168. Singer AJ, Carracio TR, Mofenson HC: The temporal profile of increased transaminase levels in patients with acetaminophen-induced liver dysfunction. Ann Emerg Med 1995;26:49–53.

169. Slattery JT, Wilson JM, Kalhorn TF, et al: Dose-dependent pharmacokinetics of acetaminophen: Evidence for glutathione depletion in humans. Clin Pharmacol Ther 1987;41:413–418.

170. Smilkstein MJ, Bronstein AC, Linden C, et al: Acetaminophen overdose: A 48-hour intravenous N-acetylcysteine treatment protocol. Ann Emerg Med 1991;20:1058–1063.

171. Smilkstein MJ, Douglas DR, Daya MR: Acetaminophen poisoning and liver function. N Engl J Med 1994;330:1310–1311.

172. Smilkstein MJ, Knapp GL, Kulig KW, et al: Acetaminophen overdose: How critical is the delay to N-acetylcysteine [abstract]? Vet Hum Toxicol 1987;29:486.

173. Smilkstein MJ, Knapp GL, Kulig KW, et al: Efficacy of oral N-acetylcysteine in the treatment of acetaminophen overdose: Analysis of the national multicenter study (1976–1985). N Engl J Med 1988;3190:1557–1562.

174. Smilkstein MJ, Knapp GL, Kulig KW, et al: N-Acetylcysteine in the treatment of acetaminophen overdose. N Engl J Med 1989;320:1418.

175. Smilkstein MJ, Rumack BH: Elimination half-life as a predictor of acetaminophen-induced hepatotoxicity [abstract]. Vet Hum Toxicol 1994;36:337.

176. Smith CV, Jones DP, Guenther TM, et al: Compartment of glutathione: Implications for the study of toxicity and disease. Toxicol Appl Pharmacol 1996;140:1–12.

177. Smith DW, Isakson G, Frankel LR, et al: Hepatic failure following ingestion of multiple doses of acetaminophen in a young child. J Pediatr Gastroenterol Nutr 1986;5:822–825.

178. Speeg KV, Mitchel MC, Maldonado L: Additive protection of cimetidine and N-acetylcysteine treatment against acetaminophen-induced hepatonecrosis in the rat. J Pharmacol Exp Ther 1985;234:550–554.

179. Spies CD, Reinhart K, Witt I, et al: Influence of N-acetylcysteine on indirect indicators of tissue oxygenation in septic shock patients. Crit Care Med 1994;22:1738–1746.

180. Spiller HA, Krenzelok EP, Grande GA, et al: A prospective evaluation of the effect of activated charcoal before oral N-acetylcysteine in acetaminophen overdose. Ann Emerg Med 1994;23:519–523.

181. Strubelt O, Younes M: The toxicological relevance of paracetamol-induced inhibition of hepatic respiration and ATP depletion. Biochem Pharmacol 1992;44:163–170.

182. Sung L, Simons JA, Dayneka NL: Dilution of N-acetylcysteine as a cause of hyponatremia. Pediatrics 1997;100:389–391.

183. Swetnam SM, Florman AL: Probable acetaminophen toxicity in an 18-month-old infant due to repeated overdosing. Clin Pediatr 1984;23:104–105.

184. Temple AR: "Dear Doctor" Tylenol ER letter. Fort Washington, PA, McNeil Consumer Products Company, 1995.

185. Thummel KE, Lee CA, Kunze KL, et al: Oxidation of acetaminophen to N-acetyl-p-benzoquinone imine by human CYP3A4. Biochem Pharmacol 1993;45:1563–1569.

186. Thummel KE, Slattery JT, Nelson SD: Mechanism by which ethanol diminishes the hepatotoxicity of acetaminophen. J Pharmacol Exp Ther 1988;245:129–136.

187. Thummel KE, Slattery JT, Nelson SD, et al: Effect of ethanol on hepatotoxicity of acetaminophen in mice and on reactive metabolite formation by mouse and human liver microsomes. Toxicol Appl Pharmacol 1989;100:391–397.

188. Tighe TV, Walter FG: Delayed toxic acetaminophen level after initial 4-hour nontoxic level. J Toxicol Clin Toxicol 1994;32:431–434.

189. Tirmenstein MA, Nelson SD: Subcellular binding and effects on calcium homeostasis produced by acetaminophen and a non-hepatotoxic regioisomer, 3-hydroxyacetoanilide in mouse liver. J Biol Chem 1989;264:9814–9819.

190. Tirmenstein MA, Nelson SD: Acetaminophen-induced oxidation of protein thiols: Contributions of impaired thiol-metabolizing enzymes and the breakdown of adenosine nucleotides. J Biol Chem 1990;265:3059–3065.

191. Tredger JM, Smith HM, Read RB, Williams R: Effects of ethanol ingestion on the metabolism of a hepatotoxic dose or paracetamol in mice. Xenobiotica 1986;16:661–670.

192. Vale JA, Proudfoot AT: Paracetamol (acetaminophen) poisoning. Lancet 1996;346:547–552.

193. Vassallo S, Khan AN, Howland MA: Use of the Rumack-Matthew nomogram in cases of extended-release acetaminophen toxicity [letter]. Ann Intern Med 1996;125:940.

194. Vaughan D, Yanay O, Zimmerman JJ: Deciphering the oxyradical inflammation rosetta stone: O_2-NO, OONO-, polymorphonuclear neutrophils, poly(ADP-ribose) synthetase, systemic inflammatory response syndrome, and multiple organ dysfunction syndrome. Crit Care Med 1999;27:1666–1669.

195. Volans GN: Antipyretic analgesic overdosage in children. Comparative risks. Br J Clin Prac 1991;70(Suppl):26–29.

196. Walker RJ, Fawcett JP: Drug nephrotoxicity—The significance of cellular mechanisms. Prog Drug Res 1993;41:51–94.

197. Walsh TS, Hopton P, Philips BJ, et al: The effect of N-acetylcysteine on oxygen transport and uptake in patients with fulminant hepatic failure. Hepatology 1998;27:1332–1340.

198. Walsh TS, Lee A: N-acetylcysteine administration in the critically ill. Intensive Care Med 1999;25:432–434.

199. Ware AJ, Upchurch KS, Eigenbrodt EH, et al: Acetaminophen and the liver. Ann Intern Med 1978;88:267–268.

200. Webster PA, Roberts DW, Benson RW, et al: Acetaminophen toxicity in children: Diagnostic confirmation using a specific antigenic biomarker. J Clin Pharmacol 1996;36:397–402.

201. Welty SE, Smith CV, Benzick AE, et al: Investigation of possible mechanisms of hepatic swelling and necrosis caused by acetaminophen in mice. Biochem Pharmacol 1993;45:449–458.

202. Wendel A, Feuerstein S, Konz KH: Acute paracetamol intoxication of starved mice leads to lipid peroxidation in vivo. Biochem Pharmacol 1979;28:2051–2055.

203. Wendon JA, Harrison PM, Keays R, et al: Cerebral blood flow and metabolism in fulminant liver failure. Hepatology 1994;19:1407–1413.

204. Whitcomb DC, Block GD: Association of acetaminophen hepatotoxicity with fasting and ethanol use. JAMA 1994;272:1845–1850.

205. Wilkinson SP, Moodie H, Arroyo VA, et al: Frequency of renal impairment in paracetamol overdose compared with other causes of acute liver damage. J Clin Pharmacol 1977;30:220–224.

206. Woo OF, Anderson IB, Kim SY, et al: Shorter duration of *N*-acetylcysteine for acute acetaminophen poisoning [abstract]. J Toxicol Clin Toxicol 1995;33:508.

207. Woo OF, Mueller PD, Olson KR, et al: Shorter duration of oral *N*-acetylcysteine therapy for acute acetaminophen overdose. Ann Emerg Med 2000;35:363–368.

208. Yip L, Dart R, Hurlbut KM: Intravenous administration of oral *N*-acetylcysteine. Crit Care Med 1998;26:40–43.

209. Zand R, Nelson SD, Slattery JT, et al: Inhibition and induction of cytochrome P4502E1—Catalyzed oxidation by isoniazid in humans. Clin Pharmacol Ther 1993;54:142–149.

210. Zezulka A, Wright N: Severe metabolic acidosis early in paracetamol poisoning. Br Med J 1982;285:851–852.

211. Zieve L, Anderson WR, Dozeman R, et al: Acetaminophen liver injury: Sequential changes in two biochemical indices of regeneration and their relationship to histologic alterations. J Lab Clin Med 1985;105:619–624.

212. Zimmerman HJ, Maddrey WC: Acetaminophen (paracetamol) hepatotoxicity with regular intake of alcohol: Analysis of instances of therapeutic misadventure. Hepatology 1995;22:767–773.

ANTIDOTES IN DEPTH

N-Acetylcysteine
Mary Ann Howland

N-acetylcysteine

Glutathione

Methionine

Cysteamine

N-acetylcysteine (NAC) is the cornerstone of therapy for the potentially lethal acetaminophen overdose. Early in the course of exposure, NAC can prevent nearly totally acetaminophen-induced toxicity. Later in the course, it can ameliorate toxicity. NAC has a role in the care of patients with poisonings where glutathione depletion and free radical formation are thought responsible for the toxicity such as carbon tetrachloride, chloroform, and pennyroyal oil.[11] NAC has a role in the management of fulminant hepatic failure caused by acetaminophen and most likely other toxicologic and nontoxicologic etiologies. Its beneficial effects are under investigation in critically ill patients with a variety of stress-induced disorders,[70] in the prevention of further renal impairment in patients with chronic renal insufficiency administered a radiographic-contrast agent, and in those with hepatorenal syndrome.[26,58,67]

HISTORY

Shortly after the first case of acetaminophen toxicity was reported, Mitchell and coworkers described the protective effect that glutathione exerts as acetaminophen is metabolized in the liver.[39] Prescott first suggested the possible use of NAC for acetaminophen poisoning in 1974.[44] Early experiments demonstrated that NAC could prevent acetaminophen-induced toxicity in mice when treatment was initiated within 4.5 hours of ingestion and that the oral and intravenous (IV) routes were equally efficacious when treatment was initiated within 1 hour of ingestion.[43] Rumack and

Peterson advanced research with oral NAC in 1978, and Prescott used IV NAC in 1979.[56] The United States Food and Drug Administration approved oral NAC in 1985.

BACKGROUND

Ninety percent of a therapeutic dose of acetaminophen is metabolized to the nontoxic glucuronide (approximately 60%) and sulfate (approximately 30%) conjugates.[45] Only 4% is metabolized by the cytochrome P450 mixed-function oxidase system (3A4 at low doses; 2E1 predominantly at high doses)[38] to a potentially toxic reactive intermediate, *N*-acetyl-*p*-benzoquinoneimine (NAPQI). This intermediate is then conjugated with glutathione to form nontoxic cysteine and mercapturic acid conjugates. After acetaminophen overdose, both the fraction and the total amount of drug undergoing P450 metabolism increases, leading to glutathione depletion, persistence of the highly reactive intermediate, and resultant hepatic centrilobular necrosis.[12] Cysteamine, methionine, and NAC all have been used successfully to prevent hepatotoxicity, but cysteamine and methionine both produce more adverse effects, and methionine is a less effective treatment modality. Therefore, NAC has emerged as the preferred treatment.[48,60,68]

CHEMISTRY

NAC is a thiol-containing compound that is deacetylated in the body to cysteine. Cysteine is a thiol-containing amino acid that is used intracellularly along with the plentiful amino acids glycine and glutamate to synthesize glutathione.[55] The availability of cysteine becomes the rate-limiting step in the synthesis of glutathione and NAC is effective in replenishing diminished supplies of cysteine.

MECHANISM OF ACTION

When administered shortly following acetaminophen exposure, NAC acts to prevent toxicity. Later in the clinical course NAC modifies the subsequent toxin induced inflammatory response. NAC effectively prevents acetaminophen-induced hepatotoxicity if administered before glutathione stores are depleted to 30% of normal. This level of depletion occurs approximately 8 hours after a toxic acetaminophen ingestion.[47,53,63] NAC prevents the binding of NAPQI to hepatocytes by acting as a precursor for the synthesis of glutathione (major)[32] and sulfate,[62] by acting intracellularly as a glutathione substitute and directly binding to NAPQI,[9] and by enhancing the reduction of NAPQI to APAP.[32]

After NAPQI covalently binds to hepatocytes, presumably through the formation of a 3-(cystein-5-yl) APAP (acetaminophen) protein adduct,[53] NAC appears to modulate the subsequent cascade of inflammatory events in a variety of ways.[23] This inflammatory response is presumed secondary to the generation of "oxidants" or "electrophiles" (electron acceptors containing an unpaired electron in an orbital) or, more specifically, "reactive oxygen species." These reactive oxygen species deplete thiols, including glutathione, endothelium-derived relaxant factor, NAD, and ATP, and cause lipid peroxidation, ultimately increasing intracellular calcium and activating proteases and phospholipases and causing additional cellular damage.[3,21,61] This inflammatory damage can occur in many tissues including the liver, lung, and heart. Antioxidants function as electron donors and are oxidized preferentially to relatively less reactive and destructive species.[3] Examples of endogenous antioxidants include vitamins C and E, and reduced glutathione. Glutathione serves as the body's protection against many stressors, including electrophilic compounds, by forming thioether bonds through conjugation, and as a reducing agent and antioxidant.[55] Glutathione reduction to 30% of normal levels sets in motion a cascade of inflammatory events that allows cytotoxic damage and possibly cell death to occur. Glutathione replenishment may protect against further cell damage but is incapable of completely restoring damaged tissues. In this second stage, NAC may act directly as an antioxidant, act as a reservoir for thiol groups, increase nitric oxide synthase to improve blood flow, may combine with nitric oxide to form s-nitrosothiol, which is a potent vasodilator, increase formation of essential endogenous antioxidants (ie, glutathione), and increase substances depleted by the oxidant stress (ie, endothelium-derived relaxant factor).[19,23,58] In this manner NAC can modulate the inflammatory cascade while improving oxygen delivery and extraction in extrahepatic organs such as the brain and heart and kidney.

CLINICAL USE

NAC is most effective if administered within 8 hours of the ingestion. Therefore, if the patient history suggests an acute acetaminophen ingestion ≥150 mg/kg and the results of blood tests will not be available within 8 hours of ingestion, or if plasma [APAP] concentration falls on or above the Rumack-Matthews nomogram, NAC should be instituted expeditiously. Chronic overdoses occur in adults who ingest more than the recommended maximum daily dose of 4 g or children who ingest more than 75 mg/kg/d. NAC should be administered when hepatotoxicity is manifest by symptoms or liver enzyme elevations, or probably when the acetaminophen serum concentration is above 10 μg/mL 4 hours after the last ingestion (Chap. 32). Interpretation of acetaminophen levels in these chronic overdoses is difficult, and the acetaminophen nomogram cannot be applied.

Some patients who are at increased risk of acute or chronic acetaminophen poisoning may require the administration of NAC at a lower threshold. Unfortunately, this threshold has not yet been defined. Glutathione-deficient patients such as the malnourished, the chronic alcoholic, those with anorexia, or those with AIDS, and those on cytochrome P450-inducing agents such as phenobarbital, phenytoin, or carbamazepine or those on isoniazid should theoretically be at increased risk for acetaminophen toxicity.[6,24,33,63] A recent analysis of a small number of patients who received anticonvulsants or chronically ingested alcohol did not demonstrate these to be a risk independent of acetaminophen dose.[36] It appears that the nomogram is sufficiently sensitive to assess risk to patients following an acute overdose, whereas in the presence of chronic acetaminophen poisoning, these risk factors may be more important and might necessitate lowering the threshold for the evaluation of hepatic enzymes.

PHARMACOKINETICS

Oral NAC is rapidly absorbed, but the bioavailability is low (10–30%) because of significant first-pass metabolism.[19,46] Intact NAC has a relatively small volume of distribution (0.5 L/kg).[71] Serum concentrations after intravenous administration of an initial loading dose of 150 mg/kg over 15 minutes are about 500 mg/L.[46] A steady-state plasma concentration of 35 mg/L (10–90 mg/L) is reached in about 12 hours following the loading dose with a continuous infusion of 50 mg/kg over 4 hours and 100 mg/kg over the next 16 hours.[46] Its elimination half-life is 5.7 hours. Severe liver damage does not appear to affect NAC elimination.[46] Pharmacokinetics and pharmacodynamics of oral NAC were determined in a phase 1 trial in 26 adult volunteers at risk for new onset or recurrent cancer.[41] Oral NAC is being studied as a potential chemopreventive agent. Absorption of NAC is rapid, with a mean time to maximum peak concentration of 1.4 ± 0.7 hours and a mean elimination half-life of 2.5 ± 0.6 hours that is linear with increasing dose up to 3200 mg/m^2/d given as a single daily dose. Intersubject plasma NAC levels vary 10-fold from a maximum concentration of 1.7–20.8 mg/L at a dose of 800 mg/m^2/d. Chronic administration leads to a decrease in plasma concentrations from a C_{max} of 8.9 mg/L at the end of 1 month to 5.1 mg/L at the end of 6 months.[41]

NAC is present in plasma in the reduced or oxidized state and is either free or bound with other thiols (ie, N-acetylcysteine-cysteine). NAC is metabolized to many sulfur-containing compounds (eg, cysteine, glutathione, methionine, cystine).[19,41,46] Thus the pharmacokinetic study of NAC is very complex.

ORAL N-ACETYLCYSTEINE VERSUS INTRAVENOUS N-ACETYLCYSTEINE

The 20-hour intravenous NAC protocol (150 mg/kg loading dose over 15 minutes, followed by an additional dose of 50 mg/kg over 4 hours and then 100 mg/kg over 16 hours—total dose 300 mg/kg) used in the United Kingdom and Canada is effective in preventing hepatic damage when given within 8 hours of acetaminophen ingestion.[47] A 48-hour intravenous regimen (140 mg/kg, then 70 mg/kg every 4 hours—total dose 980 mg/kg) studied in the United States appears to be superior to the 20-hour regimen if the first dose is administered 16–24 hours after ingestion, but this approach remains experimental.[63] The 72-hour oral NAC regimen (140 mg/kg loading dose followed by 70 mg/kg for 17 additional doses—total dose 1330 mg/kg) also appears superior to the 20-hour intravenous NAC protocol when begun at 16–24 hours postingestion. The question of which is better, the short (20 hours) or long (48 hours) intravenous course, or the oral course (72 hours) of NAC,[64] will not be settled until additional studies are completed. Although there has never been a direct comparison between these approaches when either is administered within 8 hours they seem to confer equal protection. Perhaps most patients who receive their first dose of NAC within 8 hours will require only the short course because the inflammatory cascade will not be initiated, whereas those whose treatment is delayed will benefit from a longer course of therapy and the associated benefits of the antiinflammatory/antioxidant effects of NAC. Some authors recommend a 36-hour course in low-risk patients with careful evaluation and follow-up, but this recommendation has not been adequately studied. The IV route assures delivery, but rate-related anaphylactoid reactions are possible. Most authors now recommend infusing the loading dose over 1 hour rather than over 15 minutes.

Only the IV route has been studied in hepatic failure. The IV route achieves higher serum concentrations than the oral route. It is unclear whether oral or intravenous dosing results in superior drug delivery to the liver and whether the higher hepatic concentrations enhance the efficacy.[42] Theoretically higher serum levels may be helpful for extrahepatic effects while the oral route might provide higher intrahepatic concentrations. The oral route often produces vomiting and requires antiemetics to complete therapy, but is not usually associated with other serious adverse effects.

DRUG INTERACTIONS

Conflicting in vitro[10,30,57] and in vivo[40,49] data regarding the concomitant use of activated charcoal suggest that the resultant bioavailability of NAC is either decreased or unchanged. A study involving 19 healthy volunteers compared peak and total absorption of NAC given alone as a loading dose and when it was followed by 100 g of activated charcoal. The authors demonstrated a statistically significant decrease in peak NAC and a 40% reduction in total absorption of NAC.[18] The issue not addressed by any study, however, is the critical amount of NAC necessary to prevent acetaminophen-induced liver damage. The current dose of NAC used is effective for even the largest acetaminophen overdoses, suggesting that current dosage has a built-in safety margin, and thus a small decrease in available NAC secondary to activated charcoal may not be of clinical importance.[64] In reality, activated charcoal is most effective when administered within an hour of acetaminophen ingestion and may continue to be beneficial up to 4 hours following an acetaminophen ingestion, whereas NAC is effective if absorbed within 8 hours.[8] In most circumstances, the administration of the two agents can be easily separated in time. If activated charcoal is being given as MDAC for its gastrointestinal dialysis effects it seems prudent to separate NAC and activated charcoal doses by 1–2 hours, if possible.

USE IN PREGNANCY AND NEONATES

Although teratogenicity data are unavailable for NAC, it appears that untreated acetaminophen toxicity is a far greater threat to the fetus than NAC treatment.[51] The risk of not treating pregnant women almost certainly far exceeds any potential risk to the developing fetus if a toxic ingestion has occurred. Although an earlier sheep model suggested otherwise, human data demonstrate that NAC traverses the placenta and produces cord blood levels comparable to maternal blood levels.[27]

There are very limited data on managing neonatal acetaminophen toxicity.[1,34,54,59] Both IV and oral NAC have been used safely.[1] IV administration has the advantage of assuring adequate antidotal delivery. Oral administration is associated with necrotizing enterocolitis.

OTHER INDICATIONS

NAC is being investigated as a treatment for a number of agents associated with free radical or reactive metabolite toxicity. Some of these toxins and chemotherapeutic agents include chloroform,

carbon tetrachloride, 1,2-dichloropropane, acrylonitrile, doxorubicin, and cyclophosphamide.[11,19] A theoretical role for the use of NAC in carbon monoxide poisoning has been suggested.[19]

NAC is under study as a chemopreventive agent against cancer, lung injury, and cardiac injury, as well as in other glutathione depletion clinical situations.[15,16,55,65] NAC has extracellular antimutagenic effects, enhances repair of nuclear DNA damaged by carcinogens, and inhibits malignant cell invasion and metastases.[16] NAC rescue is also being studied with high-dose acetaminophen (≤ 20 g/m^2) in patients with advanced malignancies.[31] The use of NAC in these settings may further enhance our understanding of its beneficial effects both in the early and late phases of acetaminophen poisoning.

ADVERSE EFFECTS AND SAFETY ISSUES

Anaphylactoid reactions described after intravenous dosing[4,5,13,14,17,20,25,37,46,50,69,71] of NAC are not noted after oral therapy and may be either rate related or related to high serum NAC levels.[17,46]

Administration of oral NAC via the IV route using the 48-hour IV protocol and infusing over 1 hour resulted in 4 patients with cutaneous reactions and 1 patient with an "anaphylactoid reaction" in a 76-patient study. None of these patients developed adverse hemodynamic effects.[72] A retrospective and prospective poison center study attempted to develop and then validate guidelines for management of NAC-induced anaphylactoid reactions, but deviations from the protocol limited recommendations.[2] Iatrogenic overdoses with intravenous NAC have resulted in significant morbidity and mortality.[14,17,37]

Intravenous NAC decreases clotting factors and increases the prothrombin time in healthy volunteers.[28] This effect occurred within the first hour, stabilized after 16 hours of continuous IV NAC, and rapidly returned to normal when the infusion was stopped.[28] Because the prothrombin time international normalized ratio (INR) is used as a marker of the severity of toxicity and is one of the criteria for transplantation, this adverse effect of NAC should always be considered when evaluating the patient's condition.

DOSING

When NAC is administered, the patient should receive a 140-mg/kg loading dose either orally or by enteral tube. Starting 4 hours after the loading dose, 70 mg/kg should be given every 4 hours for an additional 17 doses. The solution should be diluted to 5% with a soft drink to enhance palatability. If any dose is vomited within 1 hour of administration, it should be repeated.[35] Antiemetics (such as metoclopramide or a serotonin antagonist) should be used to ensure absorption. If the acetaminophen level is above the nomogram line, the patient should receive a full course of therapy, regardless of subsequent levels (Chap. 32 details deviation from this procedure). This regimen may need to be continued if hepatic failure intervenes. When fulminant hepatic failure occurs, NAC should be administered until the patient has a normal mental status (recovers from encephalopathy),[23] the patient's INR becomes <2,[52] or the patient receives a liver transplant.[7,22,29] However, the route of administration is problematic. Only oral NAC is

FDA approved, and only intravenous NAC has been used in these transplantation studies. Currently, oral NAC is preservative free and pyrogen free (communication with manufacturer), suggesting that it is safe to administer parenterally.

Intravenous administration is not FDA approved but is utilized when either the oral route is not feasible or hepatic failure has developed. The most commonly studied 20 hour British IV protocol is cited above. Most authors, however, now recommend infusing the loading dose over 60 minutes to reduce the potential for a life-threatening anaphylactoid reaction. Thereafter the dose for patients with fulminant hepatic failure is 150 mg/kg in D_5W infused over 24 hours until the aforementioned endpoints are attained. Some authors recommend using a 0.22-micron filter as a precaution.[72] When a 4.58% NAC concentration is prepared, it is isosmotic and isotonic. In children, a final concentration of NAC of about 4% in D_5W will avoid the administration of excess free water and the potential for hyponatremia.[66]

AVAILABILITY

NAC is available in 10-mL vials of 10% and 20% for oral administration.

ACKNOWLEDGMENT

Martin Jay Smilkstein, MD contributed to this Antidotes in Depth in a previous edition.

REFERENCES

1. Aw MM, Dhawan A, Baker AJ, Mieli-Vergani G: Neonatal paracetamol poisoning. Arch Dis Child Fetal Neonatal Ed 1999;81:F78.
2. Bailey B, McGuigan M: Management of anaphylactoid reactions to intravenous N-acetylcysteine. Ann Emerg Med 1998;31:710–715.
3. Bast A, Haenen G, Doleman C: Oxidants and antioxidants: State of the art. Am J Med 1991;91:2–13.
4. Bateman DN, Woodhouse KW, Rawlins MD: Adverse reactions to N-acetylcysteine. Hum Toxicol 1984;3:393–398.
5. Bonfiglio M, Traeger S, Hulisz D, et al: Anaphylactoid reaction to IV acetylcysteine associated with electrocardiographic abnormalities. Pharmacotherapy 1992;26:22–25.
6. Bray G, Harrison P, O'Grady J, et al: Long-term anticonvulsant therapy worsens outcome in paracetamol induced fulminant hepatic failure. Hum Exp Toxicol 1992;11:265–272.
7. Bromley PN, Cottam SJ, Hilmi I, et al: Effects of intraoperative N-acetylcysteine in orthotopic liver transplantation. Br J Anaesth 1995;75:352–354.
8. Buckley N, Whyte I, O'Connell DL, Dawson A: Activated charcoal reduces the need for N-acetylcysteine treatment after acetaminophen (paracetamol) overdose. J Toxicol Clin Toxicol 1999;37:753–757.
9. Buckpitt AR, Rollins DE, Mitchell JR: Varying effects of sulfhydryl nucleophiles on acetaminophen oxidation and sulfhydryl adduct formation. Biochem Pharmacol 1979;28:2841–2946.
10. Chinough R, Czajka P: N-Acetylcysteine adsorption by activated charcoal. Vet Hum Toxicol 1980;22:392–394.
11. Chyka P, Butler A, Holliman B, Herman M: Utility of acetylcysteine in treatment poisonings and adverse drug reactions. Drug Saf 2000;2:123–148.
12. Corcoran GB, Mitchell JR, Vaishnav YN, Horning EC: Evidence that acetaminophen and N-hydroxyacetaminophen form a common arylating intermediate, N-acetyl-p-benzoquinoneimine. Mol Pharmacol 1980;18:536–542.
13. Dawson A, Henry D, McEwen J: Adverse reactions to N-acetylcysteine during treatment for paracetamol poisoning. Med J Aust 1989;150:329–331.
14. Death after N-acetylcysteine [editorial]. Lancet 1984;1:1421.
15. De Backer WA, Amsel B, Jorens PG, et al: N-Acetylcysteine pretreatment of cardiac surgery patients influences plasma neutrophil elastase and neutrophil influx in bronchoalveolar lavage fluid. Intensive Care Med 1996;22:900–908.
16. De Flora S, Cesarone CE, Balansky RM, et al: Chemopreventive properties and mechanisms of N-acetylcysteine. The experimental background. J Cell Biochem 1995;22(Suppl):33–41.
17. Donovan JW, Jarvie DR, Prescott LF, et al: Hypersensitivity reactions to N-acetylcysteine: A concentration dependent phenomenon. Presented to European Association of Poison Control Congress, Edinburgh, September 1988.
18. Ekins B, Ford D, Thompson M, et al: The effect of activated charcoal on N-acetylcysteine absorption in normal subjects. Am J Emerg Med 1987;5:483–487.
19. Flanagan R, Meredith TJ: Use of N-acetylcysteine in clinical toxicology. Am J Med 1991;91:131–139.
20. Gervais S, Lussier-Labelle F, Beaudet G: Anaphylactoid reaction to acetylcysteine. Clin Pharm 1984;3:586–587.
21. Halliwell B: Reactive oxygen species in living systems: Source, biochemistry and role in human disease. Am J Med 1991;91:14–22.
22. Harrison P, Keays R, Bray G, et al: Improved outcome of paracetamol-induced fulminant hepatic failure by late administration of acetylcysteine. Lancet 1990;335:1572–1573.
23. Harrison P, Wendon J, Gimson A, et al: Improvement by acetylcysteine of hemodynamics and oxygen transport in fulminant hepatic failure. N Engl J Med 1991;324:1852–1857.
24. Henry JA: Glutathione and HIV. Lancet 1990;335:235–236.
25. Ho SW, Beilin JJ: Asthma associated with N-acetylcysteine infusion and paracetamol poisoning: Report of two cases. Br Med J 1983;287:876–877.
26. Holt S, Goodier D, Marley R, et al: Improvement in renal function in hepatorenal syndrome with N-acetylcysteine. Lancet 1999;353: 294–295.
27. Horowitz R, Dart R, Jarvie D, et al: Placental transfer of N-acetylcysteine following human maternal acetaminophen toxicity. J Toxicol Clin Toxicol 1997;35:447–451.
28. Jepsen S, Hansen AB: The influence of N-acetylcysteine on the measurement of prothrombin time and activated partial thromboplastin time in healthy subjects. Scand J Clin Lab Invest 1994;54:543–547.
29. Keays R, Harrison P, Wendon J, et al: Intravenous acetylcysteine in paracetamol-induced fulminant hepatic failure: A prospective controlled trial. BMJ 1991;303:1026–1029.
30. Klein Schwartz W, Oderda G: Adsorption of oral antidotes for acetaminophen poisoning (methionine and N-acetylcysteine) by activated charcoal. Clin Toxicol 1981;18:283–290.
31. Kobrinsky NL, Hartfield D, Horner H, et al: Treatment of advanced malignancies with high-dose acetaminophen and N-acetylcysteine rescue. Cancer Invest 1996;14:202–210.
32. Lauterburg BH, Corcoran GB, Mitchell JR: Mechanism of action of N-acetylcysteine in the protection against the hepatotoxicity of acetaminophen in rats. J Clin Invest 1983;71:980–991.
33. Lauterburg BH, Velez M: Glutathione deficiency in alcoholics: Risk factor for paracetamol hepatotoxicity. Gut 1988;29:1153–1157.
34. Lederman S, Fysh WJ, Tredger M, Gamsu HR: Neonatal paracetamol poisoning: treatment by exchange transfusion. Arch Dis Child 1983;58:631–633.
35. Linden CH, Rumack BH: Acetaminophen overdose. Emerg Med Clin North Am 1984;2:103–119.
36. Makin AJ, Wendon J, Williams R: A 7-year experience of severe acetaminophen-induced hepatotoxicity (1987–1993). Gastroenterology 1995;109:1907–1916.
37. Mant TGK, Tompowski JH, Volans GN, Talbot JC: Adverse reactions to acetylcysteine and effects of overdose. Br Med J 1984;289: 217–219.

38. Manyike P, Kharasch E, Kalhorn T, Slattery J: Contribution of CYP2E1 and CYP3A to acetaminophen reactive metabolite formation. Clin Pharmacol Ther 2000;67:275–282.

39. Mitchell JR, Thorgeirsson SS, Potter WZ, et al: Acetaminophen-induced hepatic injury: Protective role of glutathione in man and rationale for therapy. Clin Pharmacol Ther 1974;16:676–684.

40. North D, Peterson RG, Krenzelok E: Effect of activated charcoal administration on acetylcysteine serum levels in humans. Am J Hosp Pharm 1981;38:1022–1024.

41. Pendyala L, Creaven PJ: Pharmacokinetic and pharmacodynamic studies of N-acetylcysteine, a potential chemopreventive agent during a phase 1 trial. Cancer Epidemiol Biomarkers Prev 1995;4:245–251.

42. Peterson RG, Rumack BH: Treating acute acetaminophen poisoning with N-acetylcysteine. JAMA 1977;237:2406–2407.

43. Piperno E, Berssenbruegge DA: Reversal of experimental paracetamol toxicosis with N-acetylcysteine. Lancet 1976;2:738–739.

44. Prescott LF, Newton RW, Swainson CP, et al: Successful treatment of severe paracetamol overdosage with cysteamine. Lancet 1974;1:588–592.

45. Prescott LF: Paracetamol toxicity: Pharmacological considerations and clinical management. Drugs 1983;25:290–314.

46. Prescott LF, Donovan JW, Jarvie DR, et al: The disposition and kinetics of intravenous N-acetylcysteine in patients with paracetamol overdosage. Eur J Clin Pharmacol 1989;37:501–506.

47. Prescott LF, Illingworth RN, Critchley JAJH, et al: Intravenous N-acetylcysteine: The treatment of choice for paracetamol poisoning. Br Med J 1979;2:1097–1100.

48. Prescott LF, Sutherland GR, Park J, et al: Cysteamine, methionine, and penicillamine in the treatment of paracetamol poisoning. Lancet 1976;2:109–113.

49. Renzi F, Donovan J, Morgan L, et al: Concomitant use of activated charcoal and N-acetylcysteine. Ann Emerg Med 1985;14:568–572.

50. Reynard K, Riley A, Walker BE: Respiratory arrest after N-acetylcysteine for a paracetamol overdose [letter]. Lancet 1992;340:675.

51. Riggs BS, Bronstein AC, Kulig KW, et al: Acute acetaminophen overdose during pregnancy. Obstet Gynecol 1989;74:247–253.

52. Riordan SM, Williams R: Fulminant hepatic failure. Clin Liver Dis 2000;4:25–45.

53. Roberts DW, Bucci TJ, Benson RW, et al: Immunohistochemical localization and quantification of the 3 (cystein-5-yl) acetaminophen protein adduct in acetaminophen hepatotoxicity. Am J Pathol 1991;138:359–371.

54. Roberts I, Robinson M, Mughal MZ, et al: Paracetamol metabolites in the neonate following maternal overdose. Br J Clin Pharmacol 1984;18:201–201.

55. Ruffmann R, Wendel A: GSH rescue by N-acetylcysteine. Klin Wochenschr 1991;69:857–862.

56. Rumack BH, Peterson RG: Acetaminophen overdose: Incidence, diagnosis and management in 416 patients. Pediatrics 1978;62(Suppl)898–903.

57. Rybolt T, Burrell D, Shults J, Kelley A: In vitro coadsorption of acetaminophen and N-acetylcysteine onto activated carbon powder. J Pharm Sci 1986;75:904–905.

58. Safirstein R, Andrade L, Vieira J: Acetylcysteine and nephrotoxic effects of radiographic contrast agents—A new use for an old drug. N Engl J Med 2000;343:210–212.

59. Sharma A, Howland MA, Hoffman RS, et al: The dilemma of NAC therapy in a premature infant. J Toxicol Clin Toxicol 2000;38:57.

60. Shriner K, Goetz M: Severe hepatotoxicity in a patient receiving both acetaminophen and zidovudine. Am J Med 1992;93:94–96.

61. Sies H: Oxidative stress: From basic research to clinical application. Am J Med 1991;91:31–38.

62. Slattery JT, Wilson JM, Kalhorn TF, Nelson SD: Dose-dependent pharmacokinetics of acetaminophen: Evidence of glutathione depletion in humans. Clin Pharmacol Ther 1987;41:413–418.

63. Smilkstein MJ, Bronstein AC, Linden CH, et al: Acetaminophen overdose: A 48-hour intravenous N-acetylcysteine protocol. Ann Emerg Med 1991;20:1058–1063.

64. Smilkstein MJ, Knapp GL, Kulig KW, et al: Efficacy of oral N-acetylcysteine in the treatment of acetaminophen overdose. Analysis of the national multicenter study (1976–1985). N Engl J Med 1988;319:1557–1562.

65. Sochman J, Vrbska J, Musilova B, et al: Infarct size limitation: Acute N-acetylcysteine defense (ISLAND) trial. Start of the study [letter]. Int J Cardiol 1995;49:181–182.

66. Sung L, Simons J, Dayneka N: Dilution of intravenous N-acetylcysteine as a cause of hyponatremia. Pediatrics 1997;100:389–391.

67. Tepel M, VanDer Giet M, Schwarzfeld C, et al: Prevention of radiographic-contrast-agent-induced reductions in renal function by acetylcysteine. N Engl J Med 2000;343:180–184.

68. Vale JA, Meredith TJ, Goulding R: Treatment of acetaminophen poisoning. The use of oral methionine. Arch Intern Med 1981;141:394–396.

69. Vale JA, Wheeler DC: Anaphylactoid reactions to N-acetylcysteine [letter]. Lancet 1982;2:988.

70. Walsh TS, Lee A: N-Acetylcysteine administration in the critically ill. Intensive Care Med 1999;25:432–434.

71. Walton NG, Mann TN, Shaw KM: Anaphylactoid reaction to N-acetylcysteine [letter]. Lancet 1979;2:1298.

72. Yip L, Dart R, Hurlbut K: Intravenous administration of oral N-acetylcysteine. Crit Care Med 1998;26:40–43.

Neal E. Flomenbaum

Acetyl salicylic acid   **Methyl salicylic acid**

Salicylic Acid

MW	=	138 daltons
Therapeutic serum level	=	15–30 mg/dL
	=	1.1–2.2 mmol/L
Action level for hemodialysis	=	100 mg/dL
	=	7.2 mmol/L

Values greater than or equal to the action level necessitate clinical intervention. Values less than this level may necessitate intervention based on the clinical characteristics of the patient.

Case

A 22-year-old woman came to the Emergency Department (ED) complaining of abdominal pain, nausea, and vomiting. She had a history of depression, but stated that she was not currently being treated by a psychiatrist or taking any psychiatric medications. Upon further questioning, the patient said that 6 hours prior to admission she became severely depressed and ingested at least one-half bottle of aspirin tablets in a suicide attempt. She said that she had vomited once shortly afterwards. The patient denied tinnitus but said that she was short of breath. She also denied any other significant past medical or surgical problems.

On physical examination, the patient appeared to be well developed, well nourished, and diaphoretic. Vital signs were: blood pressure, 120/60 mm Hg; pulse, 110 beats/min; respiratory rate, 30 breaths/min; and rectal temperature, 37.9°C (100.2°F). Examination of the head, eyes, ears, nose, and throat was unremarkable. The neck was supple and there was no jugular venous distension. The chest was clear to auscultation and percussion. Cardiac examination revealed normal heart sounds and no murmurs, rubs, or gallops. Bowel sounds were normal but the abdomen was diffusely tender, without guarding; stools were negative for occult blood. There was no clubbing, cyanosis, or edema. The patient was alert and fully oriented. No cranial nerve abnormalities were noted; deep tendon reflexes were intact and symmetric with plantar flexion of the toes; and motor and sensory testing was normal. An intravenous catheter was inserted and blood was drawn and sent for blood urea nitrogen (BUN), glucose, electrolytes, a complete blood count, coagulation studies, and salicylate and acetaminophen levels. Cardiac monitoring was instituted and an arterial blood gas (ABG) specimen was obtained from the patient prior to administering supplemental oxygen. A Foley catheter was inserted and a bedside ferric chloride test of the urine was positive. With the patient in the left lateral decubitus position, orogastric lavage was performed using a 40-French lavage tube. After food and particulate matter were recovered and a total of 2 L of fluid instilled and removed, the lavage fluid was clear. Sixty grams of activated charcoal in a slurry of water and 60 g sorbitol were administered next, after which the lavage tube was removed.

The initial laboratory data revealed a urine pH of 5.5; specific gravity of 1.025; 1+ protein; 2+ ketones; no red blood cells (RBCs)

or white blood cells (WBCs). ABG values on room air were: pH, 7.51; Pco_2, 11 mm Hg; and Po_2, 134 mm Hg. Serum electrolytes were Na^+ 144 mEq/L; K^+ 3.8 mEq/L; HCO_3^- 8 mEq/L; Cl^- 98 mEq/L; BUN was 23 mg/dL, creatinine 0.9 mg/dL, and glucose 88 mg/dL; calcium was 9.6 mg/dL; and a urine pregnancy test was negative.

A bolus of 88 mEq of sodium bicarbonate was administered and a bicarbonate drip consisting of 132 mEq of $NaHCO_3$ in 1 L of D_5W was started at a rate of 250 mL/h. Potassium replacement was also initiated.

Two and one-half hours later, the patient's pulse had increased to 140 beats/min and her blood pressure dropped to 106/64 mm Hg. Although the salicylate level was not yet available, a nephrology consultation was requested. Fluid rates were increased and a second dose of activated charcoal was administered. A repeat ABG determination revealed a pH of 7.48, a Pco_2 of 13.9 mm Hg, and a Po_2 of 116 mm Hg.

About 1 hour later (4 hours after presentation), a third ABG analysis on room air revealed: pH, 7.44; Pco_2, 14 mm Hg; and Po_2, 93 mm Hg. At this time the initial salicylate level was reported to be 107 mg/dL and the acetaminophen level was 0 μg/mL. Arrangements for hemodialysis were made. Another ABG determination on room air 30 minutes later revealed: pH, 7.37; Pco_2, 24 mm Hg; and Po_2, 64 mm Hg; at this time, rales could be auscultated at both bases. The bicarbonate infusion was reduced to 125 mL/h, and a third dose of activated charcoal was administered.

The patient became agitated shortly thereafter. A fifth ABG determination on 4 L of nasal O_2 revealed: pH, 7.20; Pco_2, 46 mm Hg; and Po_2, 92 mm Hg. The ABG determination was immediately repeated and the results were: pH, 7.10; Pco_2, 63 mm Hg; and Po_2, 80 mm Hg.

Because of her rapidly deteriorating condition, the patient was intubated and hyperventilated, but her systolic blood pressure fell to 80 mm Hg by palpation and did not respond to a fluid bolus of 1 L of normal saline. A postintubation ABG determination revealed: pH, 6.90; Pco_2, 41 mm Hg; and Po_2, 182 mm Hg. Ventilation was increased, a second bolus of 88 mEq of bicarbonate was administered, and an intravenous dopamine infusion was started. Systolic blood pressure was maintained at approximately 100 mm Hg while hemodialysis was started in the medical intensive care unit.

After 4 hours, the patient's salicylate level was 22 mg/dL and her ABG was: pH, 7.42; Pco_2, 36 mm Hg; and Po_2, 190 mm Hg. Eight hours later with hemodialysis completed, the patient appeared to be significantly improved clinically. A psychiatric consultation was obtained the next day; 3 days later the patient was transferred to the psychiatric service from which she was later discharged home. One week after discharge the patient returned to her job.

EPIDEMIOLOGY

Each year the American Association of Poison Control Centers (AAPCC)/ Toxic Exposure Surveillance System (TESS) reports over 200,000 analgesic exposures and about 240 analgesic related deaths in the US (see Chap. 116 and p. 1752). Among the substances most frequently involved in human exposures, "analgesics" consistently rank second only to cleaning substances, and among the categories responsible for the largest number of deaths, "analgesics" ranks first. Of the average 240 analgesic-related deaths per year reported, acetaminophen, alone or in combination, accounts for about 50% and aspirin, alone or in combination, accounts for about 18%. If "aspirin, alone or in combination with other analgesics" were listed as a separate category, it would be the seventh or eighth most common cause of death from toxic exposures recorded by AAPCC/TESS.

Safety packaging, the increasing use of nonsteroidal antiinflammatory drugs (NSAIDs), acetaminophen, or other alternatives to aspirin for adults, and the use of acetaminophen instead of aspirin for children to avoid Reye syndrome,[9,46] have contributed to decreasing the incidence of unintentional salicylate poisoning. On the other hand, the historic widespread availability of salicylate preparations without prescription,[57] the increasing confusion regarding specific ingredients suggested by product names and brand names, and the toxicity caused by small increments in salicylate dosage when used chronically, make salicylate poisoning a very common and sometimes fatal occurrence.[51]

In recent years, popular brand and product names previously associated exclusively with salicylates or acetaminophen have been applied to other analgesic-containing products. For example, the names Alka-Seltzer, Anacin, and Excedrin, which had once been used exclusively for salicylate-containing products, now are used as brand names for products containing either aspirin or acetaminophen, or both. Bayer, a company once associated exclusively with aspirin, now markets, in addition to its aspirin products, a line of products called Bayer Select, which contains ibuprofen or acetaminophen. Clinicians should be aware that parents and healthcare providers seeking to use acetaminophen for children with viral illnesses to avoid Reye syndrome may inadvertently select a product containing aspirin either alone or in combination with acetaminophen, and an overdose in this setting might involve aspirin. Another source of confusion associated with salicylate toxicity concerns correct dosage: Terminology such as grains and milligrams, and "baby", "children's", "junior", and "adult" aspirin are confusing and often misinterpreted. Maximum doses of aspirin should never be based on age range; instead, doses should always be based on body weight.

Unintentional salicylate toxicity may occur in patients who are unaware that fixed-dose cold preparations often contain aspirin and then ingest additional aspirin tablets.[57] Another popular medication, Pepto Bismol, or bismuth subsalicylate, contains 8.7 mg of salicylic acid/mL[27] and travelers using large quantities (200–300 mL) of this antidiarrheal may expose themselves to high doses of salicylates.

Salicylate poisoning, particularly in children, but also in adults, may result from the extensive application of salicylate-containing ointments, keratolytic agents, or other agents containing methyl salicylate (oil of wintergreen).[14] Liniments and products used in hot vaporizers contain high concentrations of methyl salicylate (up to 30% in liniments and 100% in pure oil of wintergreen). The intentional or unintentional *ingestion* of such topicals is usually disastrous: approximately 1–2 teaspoons (5–10 mL) of methyl salicylate can be lethal for a young child.[15] In Hong Kong, medicated oils containing methyl salicylate accounted for 48% of acute salicylate poisoning cases treated in one hospital.[15]

Also, it should be noted that salicylates continue to be frequently used as antipyretics for children in developing countries. In one study in Kenya, 94% of 250 mothers who purchased drugs for a febrile child purchased nonprescription drugs containing salicylates and 21% administered a dose exceeding the recommended maximum daily dose. More than one salicylate preparation was given to 27% of children of whom 35% received a dose higher than the recommended maximum.[25]

Serious adolescent and adult salicylate overdoses frequently result from suicide attempts. Even in this setting, rapid diagnosis and appropriate therapy initiated quickly may reduce mortality. Salicylism must be considered in all patients who have focal and nonfocal neurologic abnormalities, tachypnea, acid-base disorders, and pulmonary edema, particularly in older patients and children and adults who are candidates for chronic iatrogenic salicylate poisoning.

PHARMACOKINETICS

Ingested salicylates (in the form of aspirin tablets) are rapidly absorbed from the stomach, as the pK_a of 3.5 leaves approximately 50% of salicylate nonionized in the acid stomach.[20,42,82] Absorption is less efficient in the small bowel, but because of its large surface area, absorption is rapidly effected there as well.[82] The dosage form (effervescent, enteric-coated) often influences the absorption rate.[79,97] Delayed absorption may result from salicylate-induced pylorospasm, pyloric stenosis,[37,79] gastric outlet obstruction,[83] or bezoar formation.[11] Protein-binding abnormalities, urine and plasma pH variations, and delayed absorption all influence the maximum salicylate levels and the rates of decline.[68]

After therapeutic doses of immediate release salicylates are ingested, significant levels are achieved in 30 minutes, and maximum levels are often attained in less than 1 hour.[20] Salicylates historically were typically prescribed in doses of 15 mg/kg as two regular strength (325 mg × 2 = 650 mg) aspirin tablets every 4 hours to achieve an antiinflammatory effect for chronic conditions such as rheumatoid arthritis. The goal of such dosing is to achieve blood salicylate levels of 15–30 mg/dL, which are considered to be in the therapeutic range,[60] as levels beyond 30 mg/dL are associated with signs and symptoms of toxicity. The Food and Drug Administration Advisory Panel on Internal Analgesic and Antirheumatic Products recommends that the maximum adult maintenance dose of aspirin not exceed 3900 mg in 24 hours for more than 10 days in a 70-kg person. No more than 650 mg should be given every 4 hours, except for the initial dose, which should not exceed 1000 mg.

In overdosage, peak serum levels may not be reached for 4–6 hours or longer. Salicylates also have substantially longer apparent half-lives at toxic levels than at therapeutic levels.[20,61] As the concentration increases, 2 of the 5 pathways of elimination—those for salicyluric acid and the salicylic phenolic glucuronide—become saturated and exhibit zero-order kinetics (Fig. 33–1 and Chap. 11). The result of this saturation changes overall salicylate elimination from the initial first-order kinetics to zero-order kinetics.[59] The half-life of salicylate is 2–4 hours at therapeutic levels, but the apparent half-life is as long as 20 hours at toxic levels.[22,61] There is also a decrease in protein binding from 90% at therapeutic levels to less than 75% at toxic levels,[1,12,26] and the apparent volume of distribution simultaneously increases (from 0.2 L/kg at low levels to more than 0.3 L/kg at higher levels).[62,86] Elimination varies with concentration and is complex, as first-order metabolism is initially substantial until some of the pathways become saturated with higher doses, as noted above (see "Alkaline Diuresis and Achieving Alkalinization: 'Ion Trapping'" later in this chapter).

Topical salicylates used as keratolytics or liniments are only rarely responsible for salicylate poisoning when used in the intended manner, ie, topically, as absorption through normal skin is very slow.[14] After 30 minutes of contact time only 1.5–2.0% of a dose is absorbed; even after 10 hours of contact with methyl salicylate, only 12–20% of the salicylates are systemically absorbed.[14,78] Although heat, occlusive dressings, young age, in-

flammation, and psoriasis all increase absorption, the real danger of salicylate toxicity associated with salicylate-containing topicals results from intentional or unintentional *ingestion*.[16] Methyl salicylate is rapidly absorbed from the gastrointestinal tract and much but not all of the ester is rapidly hydrolysed to free salicylates. Onset of symptoms usually occurs within 2 hours of ingestion.[16] When ingested, 1 mL of 98% methyl salicylate is as potent as 1.4 g of acetyl salicylic acid. In a 10-kg child, the minimum toxic salicylate dose of approximately 150 mg/kg body weight can almost be achieved with 1 mL of oil of wintergreen, which results in 140 mg/kg of salicylates (Chap. 106).

PATHOPHYSIOLOGY

Acid-Base Patterns of Salicylate Poisoning: Differences Between Adult and Pediatric Patients

Salicylates stimulate the respiratory center in the brainstem, leading to hyperventilation and respiratory alkalosis.[90] In addition, salicylates are weak acids and in toxic concentrations replace 2–

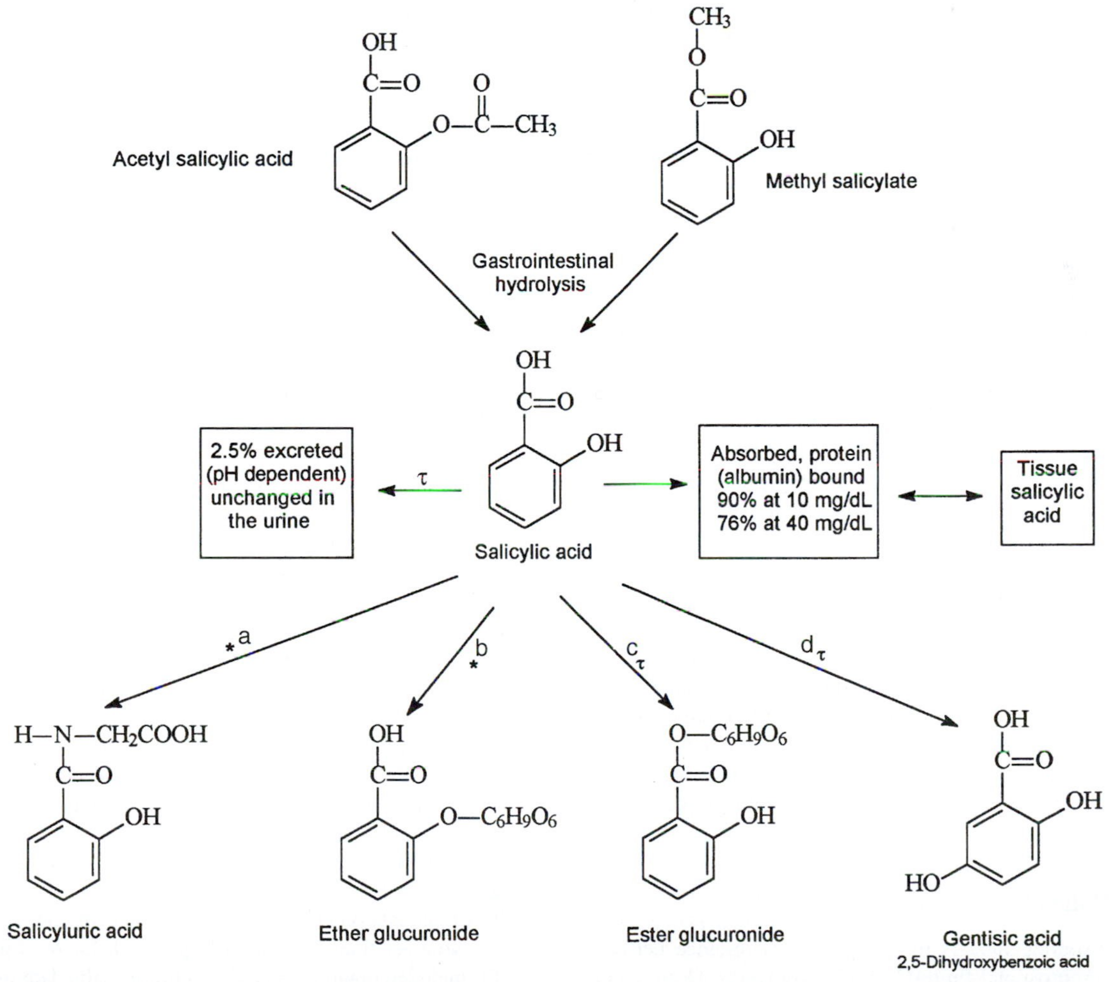

Figure 33–1. Salicylate metabolism. At excessive doses, the a, b, c, and d mechanisms are overloaded, leading to increased tissue binding, decreased protein binding, and increased excretion of unconjugated salicylic acid. * = Michaelis-Menten kinetics; τ = first-order kinetics.

3 mEq per liter of plasma bicarbonate. Impaired renal function resulting from salicylate toxicity leads to accumulation of sulfuric and phosphoric acids, both strong metabolic acids.[47] Salicylates also interfere with the Krebs cycle, limiting production of ATP,[49] and uncouple oxidative phosphorylation causing accumulation of pyruvic and lactic acids and generating large amounts of heat.[55] Salicylate-induced increased fatty acid metabolism generates ketone bodies—β-hydroxybutyric acid, acetoacetic acid, and acetone. The net result of these metabolic processes is a wide anion gap metabolic acidosis (Chaps. 24 and 66).

Although the metabolic acidosis begins with the earliest stages of toxicity, the respiratory alkalosis predominates initially and at the time that an adult patient typically presents to the hospital after an acute salicylate overdose, this mixed respiratory alkalosis and metabolic acidosis is discernible chiefly by astute ABG and serum electrolyte analysis.[34] It is important to understand that the respiratory alkalosis of salicylate poisoning is not merely compensatory for the metabolic acidosis (or vice versa), but that adults acutely poisoned by salicylates characteristically present with a mixed acid-base disturbance initially.[34]

In children, the initial predominant respiratory alkalosis may be missed, and at the time of presentation, the metabolic acidosis may already be quite significant,[35,87] either because the exposure to salicylates per body weight is so large or because children do not respond to salicylate poisoning with the same degree of sustained hyperventilation as do adults, or because children tend to present later after an exposure. (This presentation led some to incorrectly suggest that pediatric salicylate poisoning produces only a metabolic acidosis.) Although some children may present with a mixed acid–base disturbance and a normal pH, most present with acidemia.[35]

Mixed respiratory alkalosis and metabolic acidosis is found in the majority of adults with serum salicylate levels greater than 40 mg/dL[34] and, as noted above, respiratory alkalosis initially predominates. This pattern is so characteristic of adult salicylate poisoning that any adult who presents early on with a respiratory acidosis almost certainly has either salicylate-induced acute lung injury (salicylate induced pulmonary edema), central nervous system (CNS) depression from a mixed overdose, or severe fatigue from the strenuous exercise of hyperventilating for a prolonged period. Mixed drug overdoses in the adult population are fairly common, as demonstrated by one study that found that one-third of patients with a presumed primary salicylate overdose had taken other drugs;[34] benzodiazepines, barbiturates, alcohol, and cyclic antidepressants all appear to blunt the centrally induced hyperventilatory response to salicylates, resulting in either an actual respiratory acidosis (P_{CO_2} >40 mm Hg) or a metabolic acidosis without the appropriate respiratory compensation (P_{CO_2} <40 mm Hg, but inappropriately high for the concomitant pH). The combination of metabolic *and* respiratory acidosis from salicylate poisoning in an adult resulting in severe and worsening acidemia indicates an exceedingly grave prognosis and is almost invariably a preterminal event.[74]

Glucose Metabolism

Salicylate poisoning appears to produce a discordance between plasma and cerebrospinal fluid (CSF) glucose levels. Despite normal plasma glucose, CSF glucose fell 33% in salicylate-poisoned mice as compared to controls.[91] In other words, the rate of CSF glucose used exceeded the rate of supply, even in the presence of normal serum glucose. There was also a marked increase in oxygen consumption in mice, even with low salicylate levels.[40] A case report of refractory hypoglycemia secondary to poisoning from topical salicylate absorption underscores the problems of glucose metabolism caused by salicylates.[75]

Hepatic Effects

The effects of salicylates on the liver have been studied in mice.[40] Salicylate-poisoned mice had a marked decrease in glycogen and a dramatic increase in lactate compared to controls. Increased glycolysis apparently compensates for the uncoupling of oxidative phosphorylation.[66] In humans, the increased metabolic demands resulting from salicylate poisoning stimulate peripheral use of glucose and fat with resultant hypoglycemia and ketosis.

Salicylate-induced hepatitis occurred in children being treated with high (average level, 30.9 mg/dL) or chronic doses of salicylates for rheumatic fever and rheumatoid arthritis.[36,63,81] Another form of liver disease associated with salicylates, also primarily seen in children, is Reye syndrome, which is characterized by nausea, vomiting, hypoglycemia, elevated liver enzymes [aspartate aminotransferase (AST), alanine aminotransferase (ALT)], fatty infiltration of the liver, and coma following a viral illness, usually influenza or varicella.[6,9] Although the nature of the link between Reyes syndrome and salicylates has never been fully elucidated, the incidence of Reye syndrome in the United States has fallen steadily concomitantly with the decreased use of salicylates in children.[9,76,94] From December 1980 through November 1991, 1207 cases of Reye syndrome were reported in the United States in patients under age 18 with a peak incidence of 555 cases in 1980. Since 1994 (through 1997), no more than 2 cases have been reported each year.[9]

Pulmonary Effects

When a patient with salicylate poisoning presents with the clinical and radiographic manifestations of pulmonary edema, major etiologies that must be considered include aspiration pneumonitis, viral and bacterial infections, postictal and neurogenic acute lung injury (neurogenic pulmonary edema), and salicylate-induced acute lung injury (salicylate-induced pulmonary edema or noncardiogenic pulmonary edema)[44,50] (Chap. 20).

Many different causes of acute lung injury (ALI) result in increased pulmonary capillary permeability and subsequent exudation of high-protein edema fluid into the interstitial or alveolar spaces. Severe traumatic CNS injuries and elevation of intracranial pressure may be responsible for a form of "central" ALI.[45] Hypothalamic lesions from trauma, or increased intracranial pressure, or salicylate poisoning may be the critical factor, with resultant adrenergic overactivity producing a shift of blood from the systemic to the pulmonary circulation, loss of left ventricular compliance with left atrial and pulmonary capillary hypertension, and subsequent pulmonary edema (Chap. 20).

In 111 consecutive patients with peak salicylate levels >30 mg/dL, salicylate-induced pulmonary edema (SIPE) occurred in 35% of patients older than 30 years of age and none of the 55 patients younger than 16 years of age. Risk factors for developing SIPE included cigarette smoking, chronic salicylate ingestion, and the presence of neurologic symptoms on admission. The average arterial blood pH was 7.37 ± 0.022 in the 6 adult patients with SIPE and 7.46 ± 0.010 in the 30 adults without it. There was no significant difference in salicylate levels, which were approximately 57 mg/dL in both groups.[95]

Although the exact mechanism for salicylate-induced SIPE is obscure, hypoxia may be an important factor.[43,44] Hypoxia can result in pulmonary arterial hypertension and also a local release of vasoactive substances. Severe salicylate poisoning has also been identified as a distinct cause of ALI in children as well as adults.[30]

Hematologic Effects

Hematologic effects of salicylate poisoning include hypoprothrombinemia and platelet dysfunction.[33] Anemia in patients who chronically abuse salicylates may be a result of the effects of both platelet dysfunction and gastric mucosal barrier breakdown,[33] particularly in the elderly.[5,19] Hemolysis is unusual and alterations in leukocyte function are of no apparent clinical significance.[80]

Gastrointestinal Effects

Gastrointestinal manifestations include nausea, vomiting, hemorrhagic gastritis, decreased gastric motility, and pylorospasm.[79] Again, the effects appear more pronounced or consequential in the elderly.[51]

Musculoskeletal Effects

Rhabdomyolysis after pure salicylate overdoses is probably another result of the dissipation of heat and energy from uncoupling oxidative phosphorylation.[58,66,67]

Otolaryngologic Effects

Hearing loss preceded by tinnitus typically occurs with serum salicylate concentrations of 20–45 mg/dL or higher.[13,70] The mechanism of ototoxicity may include the biochemical effects of salicylates on glucose and protein metabolism affecting the endolymph and perilymph, which, in turn, result in electrophysiologic changes in the inner ear and eighth cranial nerve impulse transmission. Drug accumulation and vasoconstriction in the stria vascularis may also contribute to ototoxicity.[13]

CLINICAL MANIFESTATIONS OF ACUTE AND CHRONIC SALICYLATE POISONING

Acute Toxicity

The earliest signs and symptoms of salicylate toxicity include nausea, vomiting, diaphoresis, and tinnitus, which is a subjective sensation of ringing or hissing, with or without hearing loss.[13,33,87] As CNS salicylate levels increase, tinnitus is rapidly followed by diminished auditory acuity that sometimes leads to deafness.[13] Other early CNS effects may include vertigo and hyperventilation as well as hyperactivity, agitation, delirium, hallucinations, convulsions, lethargy, and stupor. Coma is rare and generally occurs only after massive ingestions (serum salicylate levels greater than 100 mg/dL) or mixed overdoses (Table 33–1).[33] A marked elevation in temperature resulting from the uncoupling of oxidative phosphorylation caused by salicylate poisoning[66] is an indication of severe toxicity and typically a preterminal condition. Unfortunately, many of the signs and symptoms of salicylate toxicity may be mis-

TABLE 33–1. Clinical and Laboratory Manifestations of Salicylate Toxicity

Acid-base and electrolyte disturbances	**Hepatic**
Anion gap increased	Abnormal liver enzymes
Metabolic acidosis	Altered glucose
Metabolic alkalosis (vomiting)	metabolism
Respiratory alkalosis (predominates early)	
Respiratory acidosis (late grave prognosis)	**Metabolic**
Hyponatremia or hypernatremia	Hyperthermia
Hypokalemia	Hypoglycemia
	Hyperglycemia
CNS	Hypoglycorrhachia
Tinnitus	Ketonemia
Diminished auditory acuity	Ketonuria
Vertigo	
Hallucinations	**Pulmonary**
Agitation	Hyperpnea
Hyperactivity	Tachypnea
Delirium	Respiratory alkalosis
Stupor	Acute lung injury (non-
Coma	cardiogenic pulmonary
Lethargy	edema; salicylate-
Convulsions	induced pulmonary
Cerebral edema	edema)
Syndrome of inappropriate secretion of antidiuretic hormone	**Renal**
	Tubular damage
Coagulation abnormalities	Proteinuria
Hypoprothrombinemia	NaCl and water retention
Inhibition of factors V, VII, X	Hypouricemia (hyper-
Platelet dysfunction	uricemia)
Gastrointestinal	**Volume status**
Nausea	Nausea
Vomiting	Vomiting
Hemorrhagic gastritis	Perspiration
Decreased motility	
Pylorospasm	

takenly attributed to the illness for which the salicylates were administered, with disastrous consequences.[18,87]

Chronic Toxicity

Chronic salicylate poisoning most typically occurs in the elderly as a result of unintentional overdosing on salicylates used to treat chronic conditions such as rheumatoid arthritis or osteoarthritis.[4,24,51] Although neither age nor gender appears to affect the absorption rate or plasma clearance of acute therapeutic doses of aspirin (900 mg) administered to healthy adults,[68] when used chronically, a small increase in dosage (eg, in response to increasing pain) or a small decrease in metabolism or renal function can result in substantial increases in serum salicylate levels.[51]

Presenting signs and symptoms of *chronic* salicylate poisoning include hearing loss and tinnitus, nausea, vomiting, dyspnea and hyperventilation, tachycardia, hyperthermia, and neurologic manifestations such as confusion, agitation, hyperactivity, slurred speech, hallucinations, seizures, and coma.[3,33] Although there is considerable overlap with some of the presenting signs and symptoms of *acute* salicylate poisoning, the slow onset and less-severe appearance of some of these signs of chronic poisoning in the elderly frequently cause delayed recognition of the true etiology of the patient's presentation.[18]

Typically, ill patients who suffer from chronic salicylate poisoning may be misdiagnosed as having delirium, dementia, encephalopathy of undetermined origin, diseases such as sepsis (fever of unknown origin), alcoholic ketoacidosis, respiratory failure, or cardiopulmonary disease—especially congestive heart failure, acute pulmonary edema, or even unstable angina.[3,7,18,25,33]

In a study of 73 consecutive adults hospitalized with salicylate intoxication, 27% were not correctly diagnosed for as long as 72 hours after admission.[3] These patients manifested toxicity with standard or excessive therapeutic regimens and had significant associated diseases without a history of previous overdoses. In this group, 60% had had a neurologic consultation before the diagnosis of salicylism was established. When diagnosis is delayed in the elderly, the morbidity and mortality associated with salicylate poisoning is high. Mortality was reported to be as high as 25% in the 1970s,[3] and there is no reason to believe from clinical experience that survival after delayed diagnosis is substantially better today (Table 33–2).

In one study of all children admitted to a district hospital in Kenya over a 3-month period with the primary diagnosis of severe malaria, 90% had detectable blood salicylate levels and 6 of 143 had plasma levels of 20 mg/dL or higher. All 6 had neurologic impairment and metabolic acidosis, and 4 had developed hypoglycemia, suggesting that salicylates may cause or contribute to those complications of malaria associated with high mortality.[25]

DIAGNOSTIC TESTING

Rapid Confirmation of Salicylate Use

Although serum salicylate levels are relatively easy to obtain in most hospital laboratories, salicylate *use* may be rapidly confirmed qualitatively with a simple point-of-care ferric chloride ($FeCl_3$) test. To perform the test, several drops of 10% $FeCl_3$ are added to 1 mL of urine. A purple color indicates the presence of salicylic acid, acetoacetic acid, or phenylpyruvic acid[96] (Fig. 33–2). This test is extremely sensitive to very small quantities of

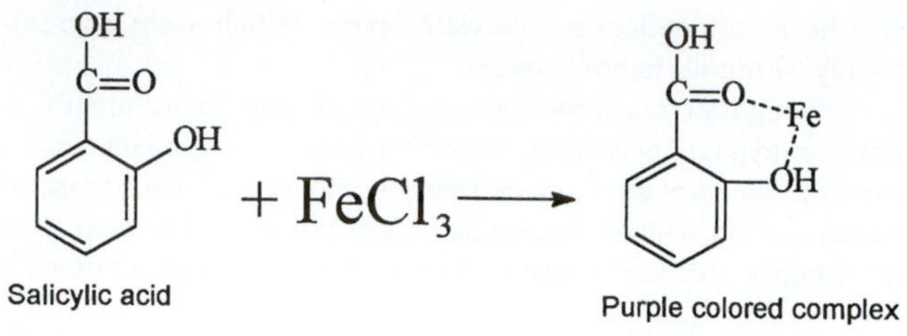

Figure 33–2. The formation of the purple-colored salicylic acid–iron complex is the result of the bedside ferric chloride test.

salicylates, and for this reason a positive test result indicates only salicylate usage and not necessarily poisoning or overdosage. Because the test is only a qualitative test, a positive $FeCl_3$ test must be confirmed with an actual serum salicylate determination. False-negative results of $FeCl_3$ testing do not occur, or are exceedingly rare—a single published abstract noted three false-negative results in tested specimens from 187 patients.[31] False-positive tests may occur when a small quantity of urine that has been used for dipstick analysis with the N-Multistix or Bili Labstix is then used for $FeCl_3$ testing. Presumably, in these cases, some impregnated chemical from the dipstick dissolves in the urine and then causes a false-positive reaction.

Another rapid point-of-care urine test for salicylate usage is known as the urine Trinder spot test.[53] This test utilizes a premixed reagent consisting of mercuric chloride, ferric nitrate, deionized water, and concentrated hydrochloric acid. When 1 mL of urine containing salicylates is mixed with 1 mL of Trinder reagent, it will turn violet or purple instantly. The sensitivity of the test was 100% when applied to urine collected 2–4 hours after oral ingestion of 975 mg of salicylate by volunteers.[53]

Other "point-of-care" determinations that may help rapidly establish the presence of salicylate poisoning are: (a) a positive urine ketone determination reflecting ketogenesis from increased fatty acid metabolism[41] (and perhaps the ketone forms of salicylates present); (b) a whole-blood glucose and electrolyte determination performed on a handheld analyzer (I-stat and others) demonstrating a decreased HCO_3^- (indicating a possible wide anion gap metabolic acidosis) and other characteristic glucose and electrolyte abnormalities; and (c) a whole-blood ABG determination performed on a handheld analyzer indicating acid-base disturbance(s) characteristic of salicylate poisoning.

Serum Salicylate Levels and Correlation with Toxicity

Serum salicylate levels should be requested when clinically significant salicylate exposures are suspected and not as part of a general toxicologic screen. The confusion in correctly identifying aspirin and acetaminophen products and the consequent possibility that either or both may be used in a suicide attempt, coupled with the initial absence (acetaminophen) or unreliability (salicylates) of clinical findings associated with these poisonings, make toxicologic analysis for both salicylates and acetaminophen reasonable when either one is implicated in an intentional poisoning.

This recommendation however, is not shared by the authors of two studies who concluded that universal salicylate screening is not indicated for patients with acute self-poisonings (Hong

TABLE 33–2. Differential Characteristics of Acute and Chronic Salicylate Poisoning

	Acute	Chronic
Age	Younger	Older
Etiology	Overdose rarely unintentional	Therapeutic misadventures; iatrogenic
Diagnosis	"Classic"	Frequently unrecognized
Other disease states	None	Underlying disorders (especially chronic pain conditions, etc)
Suicidal ideation	Typical	No
Clinical differences	Rapid progression of signs	Acute lung injury (ALI)* CNS abnormalities*
Serum concentrations	Marked elevation	Intermediate elevation
Mortality	Uncommon when recognized, unless ingestion massive	Approximately 25%

*More common

Kong)[17] or patients with suicidal ingestions or altered mental status (United States).[84] The latter study found that 0.16% of patients with suicidal ingestions had a toxic salicylate exposure *not* suggested by history, as compared to 0.3% of patients with potentially toxic acetaminophen exposures not suggested by history. Although these authors recommended universal acetaminophen screening in evaluating patients with suspected ingestions, they concluded that such screening was unnecessary for salicylates because severe salicylate exposures are less frequent and are usually accompanied by an elevated anion gap and an altered mental status.[84]

Except in certain narrowly defined situations, the toxicity of salicylates correlates poorly with serum levels. The Done Nomogram,[22] first published in 1960, continues to be used despite severely limited applicability: It was based on data from a predominantly pediatric population and intended to be applied only 6 hours or more after a single acute ingestion of nonenteric-coated, orally ingested aspirin. Moreover, the patient's blood pH must be approximately 7.4 or higher. Such conditions rarely apply to serious acute and chronic salicylate overdoses and poisonings. As an example of the shortcomings of the nomogram, a patient who presents with lethargy and/or a coagulation abnormality associated with salicylism can be classified on the nomogram as "mild" or "moderate," although such a patient must be considered severely poisoned. The poor predictive value of the nomogram when applied retrospectively to a group of 55 predominantly adult salicylate intoxications is evident from a 1989 study.[24]

Patients with acute ingestions whose initial serum salicylate determinations are either considered "acceptable," low, or moderate, sometimes deteriorate rapidly thereafter. For this reason, careful observation of the patient, correlation of the serum salicylate values with blood pH values, and repeat testing of serum salicylate levels every 2–4 hours are essential until the patient is clinically improving and has a low salicylate level in the presence of a normal or high blood pH. Methyl salicylate exposures have resulted in deaths in less than 6 hours, emphasizing the need for early salicylate determinations in addition to frequent testing after such exposures. In all cases, once a peak salicylate level has been reached, at least one additional level should be obtained in several hours and even more frequent levels obtained in managing the seriously ill patient, to assess efficacy of treatment and possible need for hemodialysis.

The reason that a concurrent arterial blood pH should be determined when a blood salicylate level is obtained is that in the presence of acidemia, more salicylic acid leaves the blood and enters the CSF and other tissues (Fig. 33–3), increasing the toxicity. Therefore, meaningful interpretation of *serum* salicylate levels must take into account the effect of the blood pH on salicylate distribution, unless the serum salicylate level is so high that hemodialysis is indicated regardless of the pH. A decreasing serum salicylate concentration may also be difficult to interpret as it can reflect either an increased tissue distribution with increased toxicity or an increased clearance with decreased toxicity: A decreasing serum salicylate level accompanied by a decreasing or low blood pH should be presumed to reflect a serious or worsening situation, not a benign or improving one.

When the patient's clinical signs and symptoms are given the highest priority and the serum salicylate level is interpreted in conjunction with a simultaneously obtained arterial blood pH, the severity of toxicity can usually be predicted and the need for hemodialysis accurately determined.

PRIOR TO ALKALINIZATION

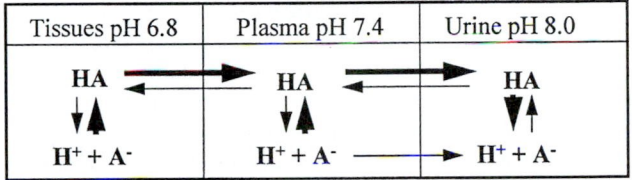

AFTER ALKALINIZATION

Figure 33–3. Rationale for alkalinization. Alkalinization of the plasma with respect to the tissues and alkalinization of the urine with respect to plasma shifts the equilibrium to the plasma and urine and away from the tissues (including the brain). This equilibrium shift has been called "ion trapping." *(Adapted, with permission, from Temple AR: Acute and chronic effects of aspirin toxicity and their treatment. Arch Intern Med 1981;141:367.)*

Errors in Reporting Serum Salicylate Levels

Laboratory errors are probably more common and problematic in reporting serum salicylate levels as compared to other drug level determinations. Analyzing and reporting results as mg/L when the clinician is accustomed to receiving results as mg/dL or inadvertently reporting mg/L results as mg/dL will multiply the true concentration by 10 and suggest a toxic level in a patient whose serum salicylate levels are within the therapeutic range (for example 165 instead of 16.5). Most errors can be eliminated prior to the initiation of such aggressive therapy as hemodialysis by determining whether the reported salicylate level is consistent with the clinical presentation and ABG results, and, when time permits, repeating the salicylate analysis with appropriate consideration for methodology and conversion calculations.

Correlation Between CSF and Serum Salicylate Levels

Although peak serum salicylate levels may provide useful clinical correlations at a normal or high blood pH, serum salicylate determinations not reflecting the peak level may be of limited value. Experimentally, there appeared to be a critical CSF salicylate level that correlated closely with mortality.[40] In addition, the CSF salicylate level correlated best with the peak serum salicylate level and reequilibrated more slowly than the serum salicylate level. As noted above, a serum salicylate level in the presence of acidemia may have little or no correlation with the CSF salicylate level. However, even if CSF salicylate levels in humans are more accurate predictors of toxicity, their use in clinical management is currently impractical.

MANAGEMENT

Gastric Decontamination and the Use of Activated Charcoal

The use of gastric decontamination and activated charcoal (AC) are discussed throughout this text, but their effects on absorption and elimination of salicylates have probably been studied more extensively than with any other drug or medication. In vitro studies suggest that each gram of AC can adsorb approximately 550 mg of salicylic acid.[62,71] In vitro, aspirin is adsorbed to AC with moderate efficacy. In humans, AC reduces the absorption of therapeutic aspirin doses by 50–80%, effectively binding enteric-coated and sustained-release preparations in addition to immediate-release tablets.[62] The sooner AC is given after the salicylate ingestion, the more effective it is in reducing absorption. A 10:1 ratio of AC to salicylate ingested appears to result in maximal efficiency. Although peak serum levels are markedly decreased from predicted concentrations, aspirin desorption from the aspirin-AC complex may diminish the impact on total absorption.[29,64,71] The addition of a cathartic to the initial dose of AC has been questioned and largely abandoned for most drugs, but the benefits of adding sorbitol to AC in achieving salicylate adsorption have been demonstrated in one study.[52]

Repetitive or multiple dosing of activated charcoal (MDAC) appears to increase the elimination of unabsorbed salicylates over that achieved by single-dose AC,[8,41] although the charcoal used in one of these studies contained "substantial amounts of sodium bicarbonate."[2,41] MDAC probably prevents desorption, which may reduce the level of initially absorbed salicylate to only 15–20%.[29] It is not clear however, that MDAC enhances the excretion of salicylates already systemically absorbed.[2,48]

In one volunteer study involving 2800 mg of aspirin followed by 25 g of activated charcoal at 4, 6, 8, and 10 hours after the ingestion, salicylate excretion from the body increased 9–18% but was not considered statistically significant.[54] The authors hypothesized that MDAC might be more effective in enhancing salicylate excretion in the *overdose* situation, when more salicylate is available because of decreased protein binding. However, in another study of the effects of MDAC on the clearance of high-dose intravenous aspirin in a porcine model, MDAC did not enhance the clearance of salicylates under alkaline conditions; that is, when the venous bicarbonate was kept at ≥15 mEq/L and urine pH kept at ≥7.5.[48] In contrast to the findings of both of these studies, two pediatric patients with salicylate overdoses were successfully treated with MDAC given every 4 hours for 36 hours, and the authors concluded that MDAC is effective in an overdose situation, even after alkalinization.[92]

Theoretical support may be found for using whole-bowel irrigation (WBI) consisting of polyethlyene glycol-electrolyte solution (PEG-ELS) in addition to AC to diminish potential desorption, particularly for enteric-coated aspirin preparations.[89] Moreover, the effectiveness of WBI alone in preventing absorption of other drugs has been suggested. However, the addition of WBI to MDAC did not increase the clearance of *absorbed* salicylate.[64]

In summary, although the value of MDAC in enhancing salicylate elimination is controversial, and the AACT/EAPCCT position statement concludes that data are presently insufficient to recommend MDAC for salicylate poisoning,[2] MDAC is probably warranted to decrease gastrointestinal absorption of salicylate overdoses (see Antidotes in Depth: Activated Charcoal).

Fluid Replacement

There is a need to differentiate between restoration of fluid and electrolyte balance in salicylate-poisoned patients as opposed to increasing the fluid load presented to the kidneys in an attempt to achieve "forced diuresis": Fluid losses from salicylate poisoning are prominent, especially in children, and can be attributed to tachypnea, vomiting, fever, a hypermetabolic state, hyperpnea, and insensible perspiration.[88] The kidneys also respond to salicylate poisoning by excreting an increased solute load, including large quantities of bicarbonate, sodium, potassium, and organic acids, but renal tubular damage leading to renal failure is rare. Ketoacidosis, hypoglycemia, or hyperglycemia may occur.[4] For all of these reasons the patient's volume status must be adequately assessed and corrected if necessary along with any glucose and electrolyte abnormalities. As in other cases, accurate management of volume status in the poisoned patient may require invasive monitoring with a central venous pressure monitor or, preferably, a pulmonary artery catheter, especially in patients with cardiac disease, acute lung injury, or renal compromise.

Increasing fluids *beyond* restoration of fluid balance in order to achieve a forced diuresis is a practice that has been inappropriately emphasized in the past. Although forced diuresis, theoretically, will increase renal tubular flow and reduce the urine tubular cell diffusion gradient for reabsorption, the renal excretion of salicylate depends much more on urine pH than on flow rate, and the use of forced diuresis alone is not effective regardless of whether diuretics, osmotic agents, or fluid volumes were used to achieve the diuresis.[73] Although renal salicylate clearance varies in direct proportion to flow rate, its relation to pH is logarithmic.[56] In summary, although fluid imbalance must be corrected, forced saline diuresis does little more than oral fluids to enhance elimination over a 24-hour period[73] and subjects the patient to the hazards of fluid overload.

Alkaline Diuresis and Achieving Alkalinization: "Ion Trapping"

Because salicylic acid is a weak acid (pK_a 3.5) it will be ionized in an alkaline milieu and, as a result, "trapped." For this reason, concomitant alkalinization of the blood and the urine will both keep salicylates away from the brain and in the blood and, in addition, enhance urinary excretion. Alkalinization for salicylate poisoning is the best clinical example of the concept of ion trapping, which in this instance results in enhanced excretion of the ionized acid form of salicylate in the alkaline urine, although at least one investigator maintains that ion trapping alone does not account for the increased excretion caused by $NaHCO_3$.[65] In any case, the renal excretion of salicylic acid is very dependent on the urinary pH[73,93] (Fig. 33–3; see Antidotes in Depth: Sodium Bicarbonate).

Alkalinization increases free salicylate secretion from the proximal tubule, but does not affect the renal elimination of free salicylate conjugates. In an alkaline urine with therapeutic serum salicylate levels, free salicylate represents more than 30% of total salicylate elimination as compared to an acidic urine, in which free salicylate represents as little as 2% of total elimination.[47] The percentage of a single dose of 1.5 g of sodium salicylate administered to volunteers, excreted unchanged, increased from 2.3 ±

1.5% under acidic conditions to 30.5 ± 9.1% under alkaline conditions. When urine acidity was maintained using ammonium chloride, salicylic acid had a terminal plasma $t_{1/2}$ value of 3.29 ± 0.52 hours, which was significantly reduced to 2.50 ± 0.41 hours when an alkaline urine was maintained with sodium bicarbonate treatment. The total body clearance of salicylic acid was significantly less under acidic urine conditions (1.38 ± 0.43 L/h) than under alkaline urine conditions (2.27 ± 0.83 L/h).[93]

Alkalinizing the urine from a pH of 5–8 logarithmically increased *renal* salicylate clearance from 1.3 mL/min to 100 mL/min.[69] Assuming an overdose V_d of 0.5 L/kg, this increased clearance would decrease renal salicylate half-life from 310 hours to 4 hours. However, alkalinizing the urine from a pH of 5 to a pH of 8 has a more modest effect on *serum* salicylate clearance:[73] The apparent serum half-life decreased from 48 hours to 6 hours at a fixed rate of 2 hours per unit pH change. This difference between serum and renal half-lives reflects the fact that renal clearance only applies to free salicylate, whereas serum clearance applies to both free and protein-bound salicylate.

Because acidemia enhances salicylate transfer into tissue, and particularly into the brain, it must be treated aggressively by raising the blood pH as compared to the brain pH, thereby shifting the equilibrium from the tissues to the plasma[38] (Fig. 33–3). To accomplish this, hyperventilation alone should not be relied upon and $NaHCO_3^-$ but not acetazolamide should be used for alkalinization. Although the administration of acetazolamide, a noncompetitive carbonic anhydrase inhibitor, results in the formation of a bicarbonate-rich alkaline urine, it, unfortunately, also causes a systemic metabolic acidosis and acidemia.[28,38] The effect of acetazolamide is usually self-limited and mild but nevertheless increases the concentration of freely diffusible nonionized molecules of salicylic acid, thereby increasing the volume of distribution and most probably enhancing the penetrance of salicylate into the CNS.[61] Because salicylate also appears to inhibit acetazolamide plasma protein binding and acetazolamide renal tubular secretion, older patients with diminished protein binding and renal function may be at even greater risk for significant metabolic acidosis from acetazolamide use.[38,85]

Hyperventilation versus NaHCO₃: Risks Associated with Assisting Ventilation

Endotracheal intubation of a salicylate poisoned patient poses a particular risk and may contribute to mortality in some instances. Although early endotracheal intubation to *maintain* hyperventilation may aid in the management of patients whose respiratory efforts are faltering after hours of hyperventilation, few healthcare providers are trained or skilled at maintaining the appropriate level of hypocarbia and hyperventilation that is necessary for managing a salicylate-poisoned patient receiving assisted ventilation (ie, on a respirator). Even when successful, a respiratory alkalosis sustained by hyperventilation (assisted or unassisted) should *never* be considered a substitute for the use of $NaHCO_3$—to achieve both alkalemia and alkalinuria—and, if indicated, hemodialysis. $NaHCO_3$ does not easily cross the blood-brain barrier whereas CO_2 does and, therefore, $NaHCO_3$ will create an environment conducive to keeping salicylates in the blood and away from the brain and liver.

For all of these reasons, alkalinization with intravenous $NaHCO_3$, should be considered for patients whose serum salicylate level exceeds 35 mg/dL, and for clinically suspected cases of serious salicylism, until a salicylate level and simultaneously obtained blood pH are available to guide treatment. Patients on therapeutic regimens of salicylates who feel well with salicylate levels of 30–40 mg/dL and who do not manifest toxicity do not require intervention. Oral bicarbonate administration should never be substituted for intravenous bicarbonate to achieve alkalinization, because the oral route may increase salicylate absorption from the gastrointestinal tract by enhancing dissolution.

Hemodynamically stable adults and children with significant salicylate levels may be alkalinized with a bolus of 1–2 mEq/kg, followed by an intravenous infusion of 3 ampules of $NaHCO_3$ (132 mEq) in 1 L of D_5W, to run at 1.5–2 times maintenance fluid range. Urine pH must be maintained at 7.5–8.0 to achieve maximum ion trapping and maximum excretion. Volume load should remain modest while repleting previous losses. Early hemodialysis must be considered when a patient cannot tolerate the increased solute load that results from alkalinization because of congestive heart failure, renal failure, or cerebral edema, but even when the decision has been made to hemodialyze a patient, alkalinization, when possible, helps to achieve a more rapid initial reduction in blood levels.[39]

Hypokalemia

Hypokalemia is a common complication of salicylate poisoning and prevents urinary alkalinization unless corrected. Hypokalemia results from the movement of potassium into cells in exchange for hydrogen ions in the presence of alkalemia, from potassium loss in the urine, and from vomiting, with subsequent metabolic alkalosis and bicarbonaturia.[33] If urinary alkalinization cannot be achieved easily, hypokalemia, excretion of organic acids, and volume depletion should be considered as possible reasons. Calcium should also be monitored, as decreases in both ionized[23] and total serum calcium[32] are also complications of bicarbonate therapy.

Frequent blood-gas monitoring is required for all patients exposed to significant amounts of salicylates. Although maintaining alkalemia is clearly essential for treatment, arterial pH should probably not be allowed to rise above 7.55, as alkalemia shifts the oxyhemoglobin dissociation curve to the left and may be otherwise detrimental and difficult to treat. It should be noted, however, that even when the blood pH is 7.45–7.50, large amounts of bicarbonate may be given to patients with severe salicylism without necessarily resulting in a further increase in pH. Frequent reassessment of blood pH (and fluid status) almost always allows administration of more $NaHCO_3$ than was initially thought possible.

Extracorporeal Measures for Severe Salicylate Poisoning

Extracorporeal measures are indicated if the patient is very ill, has a very high serum salicylate level, has severe fluid or electrolyte disturbances, or is unable to eliminate the salicylates (Table 33–3). In most instances of severe salicylate poisoning, hemodialysis is the extracorporeal technique of choice, allowing not only for clearance of the drug but also for rapid correction of fluid, electrolyte and acid–base disorders that are not correctable by hemoperfusion alone. Hemoperfusion provides a better clearance (57–116 mL/min) than hemodialysis (35–80 mL/min) and is acceptable if (1) hemodialysis is unavailable, (2) a mixed overdose might be better treated with hemoperfusion, or (3) severe hypernatremia is present. The combination of hemodialysis and hemoper-

TABLE 33–3. Indications for Hemodialysis in the Salicylate-Poisoned Patient

Renal failure
Congestive heart failure (relative)
Acute lung injury
Persistent CNS disturbances
Progressive deterioration in vital signs
Severe acid-base or electrolyte imbalance, despite appropriate treatment
Hepatic compromise with coagulopathy
Salicylate level (acute) >100 mg/dL

fusion in series is feasible and may be useful for treating severe or mixed overdoses,[21] but is rarely used.

A combination of therapies that is both useful and practical is to insure effective alkalinization (with $NaHCO_3$) while a patient is awaiting and then undergoing hemodialysis. In one unique case report, a patient who overdosed twice on salicylates within a 2-month period was treated in the first instance with 4 hours of hemodialysis, but no effective alkalinization; and in the second instance, with $NaHCO_3$ alkalinization but no hemodialysis. In both instances, blood levels of salicylates were over 5 mmol/L ($\approx$ over 65 mg/dL). Although similar salicylate levels were achieved with either technique, the rate of decline during the first 4 hours was faster with alkalinization.[39] Combining the two therapies makes sense even if part of the reason for the increased early effectiveness of $NaHCO_3$ treatment may be related to the rapidity with which it can be achieved compared to the 2–4 hours required to institute hemodialysis after a patient presents even under the most favorable circumstances.[39]

Although peritoneal dialysis had often been suggested in the past as a simpler extracorporeal procedure for eliminating salicylates in the setting of hemodynamic compromise, a coagulopathy, or the inability to perform hemoperfusion or hemodialysis, peritoneal dialysis is only 10–25% as efficient as hemoperfusion or hemodialysis and not even as efficient as renal excretion itself. The 24-hour clearance of salicylates with peritoneal dialysis is less than the 4-hour clearance of salicylates by hemoperfusion or hemodialysis; therefore, peritoneal dialysis is not recommended. (See Chap. 6 for further discussion.)

Pregnancy

Although considered to be a rare event, salicylate poisoning during pregnancy poses a particular hazard to the fetus because of the acid-base and hematologic characteristics of the fetus and placental circulation—salicylates cross the placenta and are present in higher concentrations in the fetus than in the mother. The respiratory stimulation that occurs in the mother after toxic exposures, does not occur in the fetus which has a decreased capacity to buffer acid. The ability of the fetus to metabolize and excrete salicylates are also less than in the mother. In addition to its toxic effects on the mother, including coagulation abnormalities, acid-base disturbances, tachypnea, and hypoglycemia, repeated exposure to salicylates late in gestation displaces bilirubin from protein binding sites.

A case report describing fetal demise in a woman who claimed to ingest 50 aspirin tablets per day for several weeks during the third trimester of pregnancy, supports the conclusion that the fetus is at greater risk from salicylate exposures than is the mother and

that emergent delivery of near-term fetuses of salicylate poisoned mothers should be considered very seriously[72] (Chap. 105).

SUMMARY

Initial assessment of a patient who has ingested excessive amounts of salicylates includes a determination of the vital signs, particularly the depth and frequency of respiration, along with the temperature. The clinical presentation of a salicylate overdose is characterized by the early onset of nausea, vomiting, abdominal pain, blood-tinged vomitus or gross hematemesis, tinnitus, and lethargy. The presence of hyperventilation, hyperthermia, confusion, coma, seizures, and any other nonspecific neurologic presentation should further heighten suspicion of salicylate poisoning (Tables 33–1 and 33–2). If either salicylism or salicylate poisoning is suspected, a bedside ferric chloride ($FeCl_3$) test will confirm salicylate *exposure* (see Fig. 33–2). Using a combination of symptoms, signs, bedside laboratory studies, and characteristic ABG findings, the clinician can rapidly confirm a significant salicylate ingestion, institute immediate alkalinization with $NaHCO_3$, achieve gastric decontamination by orogastric lavage (if indicated), AC, and MDAC (if indicated), and consider the need for hemodialysis early in the course of management.

For the patient who presents severely ill, maintenance of the airway requires an extremely careful approach because during initial airway management, death has occurred following sedation.[10] Moreover, in patients with pulmonary and CNS manifestations of salicylate toxicity, the protective nature of the hyperpnea or hyperventilation in maintaining alkalemia must be recognized, as maintaining a high pH ($\geq$7.5) at all times is of paramount importance. Urinary alkalinization with $NaHCO_3$ to eliminate salicylates by ion trapping is important, even though the use of $NaHCO_3$ may further complicate electrolyte abnormalities. Fluid and electrolyte replacement (especially potassium) is essential.

ACKNOWLEDGMENTS

Eddy A. Bresnitz, MD and Lorraine Hartnett, MD contributed to this chapter in a previous edition and the author gratefully acknowledges the contributions of Oliver Hung, MD, to the Alkaline Diuresis Section of the current edition.

REFERENCES

1. Alvan G, Bergman V, Gustafsson L: High unbound fraction of salicylate in plasma during intoxication. Br J Clin Pharmacol 1981;11: 625–626.
2. American Academy of Clinical Toxicology and European Association of Poisons Centers and Clinical Toxicologists: Position statement and practice guidelines on the use of multi-dose activated charcoal in the treatment of acute poisoning. J Toxicol Clin Toxicol 1999;37: 731–751.
3. Anderson RJ, Potts DE, Gabow PA, et al: Unrecognized adult salicylate intoxication. Ann Intern Med 1976;85:745–748.
4. Arena FP, Dugowson C, Saudek CD: Salicylate-induced hypoglycemia and ketoacidosis in a nondiabetic adult. Arch Intern Med 1978;138:1153–1154.
5. Armstrong CP, Blower AL: Non-steroidal anti-inflammatory drugs and life-threatening complications of peptic ulceration. Gut 1987;28: 527–532.
6. Arrowsmith JB, Kennedy DL, Kuritsky JN, et al: National patterns of aspirin use and Reye syndrome reporting. United States 1980 to 1985. Pediatrics 1987;79:858–863.

7. Bailey RB, Jones SR: Chronic salicylate intoxication: A common cause of morbidity in the elderly. J Am Geriatr Soc 1989;37:556–561.

8. Barone J, Raia J, Huang YC: Evaluation of the effects of multiple-dose activated charcoal on the absorption of orally administered salicylate in a simulated toxic ingestion model. Ann Emerg Med 1988;17:34–37.

9. Belay ED, Bresee JJ, Holman RC et al: Reye's syndrome in the United States from 1981 through 1997. N Engl J Med 1999;340:1377–1382.

10. Berk WA, Anderson JC: Salicylate associated asystole: Report of two cases. Am J Med 1989;86:505–506.

11. Bogazc K, Caldron P: Enteric-coated aspirin bezoar: Elevation of serum salicylate level by barium study. Am J Med 1981;83:783–786.

12. Borga O, Odar-Cederlof I, Ringberger V-A, et al: Protein binding of salicylate in uremic and normal plasma. Clin Pharmacol Ther 1976;20:464–475.

13. Brien J: Ototoxicity associated with salicylates. Drug Saf 1993;9:143–148.

14. Brubacher JR, Hoffman RS: Salicylism from topical salicylates: Review of the literature. J Toxicol Clin Toxicol 1996;34:431–436.

15. Chan TYK: Medicated oils and severe salicylate poisoning: Quantifying the risk based on methyl salicylate content and bottle size. Vet Human Toxicol 1996;38:133–134.

16. Chan TYK: Potential dangers from topical preparations containing methyl salicylate. Hum Exp Toxicol 1996;15:747–750.

17. Chan TYK, Chan AYW, Ho CS: The clinical value of screening for salicylates in acute poisoning. Vet Human Toxicol 1995;37:37–38.

18. Chui PT: Anesthesia in a patient with undiagnosed salicylate poisoning presenting as intraabdominal sepsis. J Clin Anesth 1999;11:251–253.

19. Coggon D, Langman MJS, Spiegelhalter D: Aspirin, paracetamol, hematemesis and melena. Gut 1982;23:340–344.

20. Davison C: Salicylate metabolism in man. Ann N Y Acad Sci 1971;179:249–268.

21. DeBroe ME, Verpooten GA, Christiaens ME, et al: Clinical experience with prolonged combined hemoperfusion-hemodialysis treatment of severe poisoning. Artif Organs 1981;5:59–66.

22. Done AK: Salicylate intoxication: Significance of measurements of salicylate in blood in cases of acute ingestion. Pediatrics 1960;26:800–807.

23. Done AK, Temple AR: Treatment of salicylate poisoning. Mod Treat 1971;8:528–551.

24. Dugandzic RM, Tierney MG, Dickinson GE, et al: Evaluation of the validity of the Done nomogram in the management of acute salicylate intoxication. Ann Emerg Med 1989;18:1186–1190.

25. English M, Marsh V, Amukoye E et al: Chronic salicylate poisoning and severe malaria. Lancet 1996; 347:1736–1737.

26. Ekstrand R, Alvan A, Borga O: Concentration dependent plasma protein binding of salicylate in rheumatoid patients. Clin Pharmacokinet 1979;4:137–143.

27. Feldman S, Chen SL, Pickering LK: Salicylate absorption from bismuth subsalicylate preparation. Clin Pharmacol Ther 1981;29:788–792.

28. Feuerstein RC, Finberg L, Fleishman BS: The use of acetazolamide in the therapy of salicylate poisoning. Pediatrics 1960;25:215–227.

29. Fillippone G, Fish S, Lacouture P, et al: Reversible adsorption (desorption) of aspirin from activated charcoal. Arch Intern Med 1987;147:1390–1392.

30. Fisher CJ, Albertson TE, Foulke GE: Salicylate induced pulmonary edema. Clinical characteristics in children. Am J Emerg Med 1985;3:33–37.

31. Ford M, Tomaszewski C, Kerns W, et al: Bedside ferric chloride urine test to rule out salicylate intoxication [abstract]. Vet Hum Toxicol 1994;36:364.

32. Fox GN: Hypocalcemia complicating bicarbonate therapy for salicylate poisoning. West J Med 1984;141:108–109.

33. Gabow PA: How to avoid overlooking salicylate intoxication. J Crit Illness 1986;1:77–85.

34. Gabow PA, Anderson RJ, Potts DE, Schrier RW: Acid-base disturbances in the salicylate poisoning in adults. Arch Intern Med 1978;138:1481–1484.

35. Gaudreault P, Temple AR, Lovejoy FH Jr: The relative severity of acute versus chronic salicylate poisoning in children: A clinical comparison. Pediatrics 1982;70:566–569.

36. Hamdan JA, Manasra K, Ahmed M: Salicylate-induced hepatitis in rheumatic fever. Am J Dis Child 1985;139:453–455.

37. Harris FC: Pyloric stenosis: Holdup of enteric-coated aspirin tablets. Br J Surg 1973;60:979–981.

38. Heller I, Halevy J, Cohen S, et al: Significant metabolic acidosis induced by acetazolamide: Not a rare complication. Arch Intern Med 1985;145:1815–1817.

39. Higgins RM, Connolly JO, Hendry BM: Alkalinization and hemodialysis in severe salicylate poisoning: Comparison of elimination techniques in the same patient. Clin Nephrol 1998;50:178–183.

40. Hill JB: Salicylate intoxication. N Engl J Med 1973;288:1110–1113.

41. Hillman RJ, Prescott LF: Treatment of salicylate poisoning with repeated oral charcoal. Br Med J 1986;291:1472.

42. Hogben CAM, Schanker LS, Jocco DJ, Brodie BB: Absorption of drugs from the stomach. II: The human. J Pharmacol Exp Ther 1957;120:540–545.

43. Hormaechea E, Carlson RW, Rogove H, et al: Hypovolemia, pulmonary edema and protein changes in severe salicylate poisoning. Am J Med 1979;66:1046–1050.

44. Hrnicek G, Skelton J, Miller W: Pulmonary edema and salicylate intoxication. JAMA 1974;230:866–867.

45. Huff RW, Fred HL: Postictal pulmonary edema. Arch Intern Med 1966;117:824–828.

46. Hurwitz ES, Barrett MJ, Bregman D, et al: Public Health Service study on Reye's syndrome and medications: Report of the pilot phase. N Engl J Med 1985;313:849–857.

47. Insel PA: Analgesic-antipyretic and anti-inflammatory agents and drugs employed in the treatment of gout. In: Harmon JG, Limbird LE, eds: Goodman & Gilman's The Pharmacological Basis of Therapeutics, 9th ed. New York, McGraw-Hill, 1996, pp. 617–657.

48. Johnson D, Eppler J, Giesbrecht E, et al: Effect of multiple-dose activated charcoal on the clearance of high-dose intravenous aspirin in a porcine model. Ann Emerg Med 1995;26:569–574.

49. Kaplan E, Kennedy J, David J: Effects of salicylate and other benzoates on oxidative enzymes of the tricarboxylic acid cycle in rat tissue homogenates. Arch Biochem Biophys 1954;51:47–61.

50. Karliner J: Noncardiogenic forms of pulmonary edema. Circulation 1972;46:212–215.

51. Karsh J: Adverse reactions and interactions with aspirin—Considerations in the treatment of the elderly patient. Drug Saf 1990;5:317–327.

52. Keller RE, Schwab RA, Krenzelok EP: Contribution of sorbitol combined with activated charcoal in prevention of salicylate absorption. Ann Emerg Med 1990;19:654–656.

53. King JA, Storrow AB, Finkelstein JA: Urine Trinder spot test: A rapid salicylate screen for the emergency department. Ann Emerg Med 1995;26:330–333.

54. Kirshenbaum LA, Mathews SC, Sitar DS, Tenenbein M: Does multiple-dose charcoal therapy enhance salicylate excretion? Arch Intern Med 1990;150:1281–1283.

55. Krebs HG, Woods HG, Alberti KG: Hyperlactatemia and lactic acidosis. Essays Med Biochem 1975;1:81–103.

56. Lawson AAH, Proudfoot AT, Brown SS, et al: Forced diuresis in the treatment of acute salicylate poisoning in adults. Q J Med 1968;149:31–48.

57. Leist ER, Banwell JC: Products containing aspirin. N Engl J Med 1974;291:710–712.

58. Leventhal LJ, Kuritsky L, Ginsburg R, et al: Salicylate-induced rhabdomyolysis. Am J Emerg Med 1989;7:409–410.

59. Levy G: Clinical pharmacokinetics of salicylates: A reassessment. Br J Clin Pharmacol 1980;10:285S–290S.

60. Levy G: Clinical pharmacokinetics of aspirin. Pediatrics 1978;62 (Suppl):867–872.

61. Levy G: Pharmacokinetics of salicylate elimination in man. J Pharm Sci 1965;54:959–967.

62. Levy G, Tsuchiya T: Effect of activated charcoal on aspirin absorption in man. Clin Pharmacol Ther 1972;13:317–322.

63. Manso C, Taranta A, Nydick I: Effect of aspirin administration on serum glutamic oxaloacetic and glutamic pyruvic transaminases in children. Proc Soc Exp Biol Med 1956;93:84–88.

64. Mayer AL, Sitar DS, Tenenbein M: Multiple-dose charcoal and whole-bowel irrigation do not increase clearance of absorbed salicylate. Arch Intern Med 1992;152:393–396.

65. Macpherson CR, Milne MD, Evans BM: The excretion of salicylate. Br J Pharmacol 1955;10:484–489.

66. Miyahara JT, Karler R: Effect of salicylate on oxidative phosphorylation and respiration of mitochondrial fragments. Biochem J 1965;97:194–198.

67. Montgomery H, Porter JC, Bradley RD: Salicylate intoxication causing a severe systemic inflammatory response and rhabdomyolysis. Am J Emerg Med 1994;12:531–532.

68. Montgomery PR, Berger LG, Mitenko PA, Sitar DS: Salicylate metabolism: Effects of age and sex in adults. Clin Pharmacol Ther 1986;39:571–576.

69. Morgan AG, Polak A: The excretion of salicylate in salicylate poisoning. Clin Sci 1971;41:475–484.

70. Myers EN, Bernstein JM, Fostiropolous G: Salicylate ototoxicity. N Engl J Med 1965;273:587–590.

71. Neuvonen PJ, Elfving SM, Elonen E: Reduction of absorption of digoxin, phenytoin, and aspirin by activated charcoal in man. Eur J Clin Pharmacol 1978;13:213–218.

72. Palatnick W, Tenenbien M: Aspirin poisoning during pregnancy: Increased fetal sensitivity. Am J Perinatol 1998;15:39–41.

73. Prescott LF, Balali-Mood M, Critchley JA, et al: Diuresis or urinary alkalinization for salicylate poisoning. Br Med J 1982;285:1383–1386.

74. Proudfoot AT, Brown SS: Acidaemia and salicylate poisoning in adults. Br Med J 1969;2:547–550.

75. Raschke R, Arnold-Capell P, Richeson R, Curry SC: Refractory hypoglycemia secondary to topical salicylate intoxication. Arch Intern Med 1991;151:591–593.

76. Reye's syndrome surveillance—United States 1989. Morb Mortal Wkly Rep 1991;40:88–89.

77. Roberts MS, Cossum PA, Kilpatrick D: Implications of hepatic and extrahepatic metabolism of aspirin in selective inhibition of platelet cyclooxygenase. N Engl J Med 1985;312:1388–1389.

78. Roberts MS, Favretto WA, Meyer A, et al: Topical bioavailability of methyl salicylate. Aust N Z J Med 1982;12:303–305.

79. Romankiewicz JA, Reidenberg MM: Factors that modify drug absorption. Ration Drug Ther 1978;12:1–6.

80. Rothschild BM: Hematologic perturbations associated with salicylate. Clin Pharmacol Ther 1979;26:145–150.

81. Schaller JG: Chronic salicylate administration in juvenile rheumatoid arthritis: Aspirin "hepatitis" and its clinical significance. Pediatrics 1978;62(Suppl):916–925.

82. Schanker LS, Tocco DJ, Brodie BB, Hogben CAM: Absorption of drugs from the rat's small intestine. J Pharmacol Exp Ther 1958;123:81–88.

83. Sogge MR, Griffith JL, Sinar DR, Mayes GR: Lavage to remove enteric-coated aspirin and gastric outlet obstruction. Ann Intern Med 1977;87:721–722.

84. Sporer KA, Khayam-Bashi H: Acetaminophen and salicylate serum levels in patients with suicidal ingestion or altered mental status. Am J Emerg Med 1996;14:443–447.

85. Sweeney KR, Chapron DJ, Brandt JL, et al: Toxic interaction between acetazolamide and salicylate: Case reports and a pharmacokinetic explanation. Clin Pharmacol Ther 1986;40:518–524.

86. Swintosky JV: Illustrations and pharmaceutical interpretations of first-order drug elimination rate from the bloodstream. J Am Pharm Assoc 1956;45:395–400.

87. Temple AR: Acute and chronic effects of aspirin toxicity and their treatment. Arch Intern Med 1981;141:364–369.

88. Temple AR, George DJ, Done AK, Thompson JA: Salicylate poisoning complicated by fluid retention. Clin Toxicol 1976;9:61–68.

89. Tenenbein M: Whole-bowel irrigation as a gastrointestinal decontamination procedure after acute poisoning. Med Toxicol 1988;3:77–84.

90. Tenney SM, Miller RM: The respiratory and circulatory action of salicylate. Am J Med 1955;19:498–508.

91. Thurston JH, Pollock PG, Warren SK, Jones EM: Reduced brain glucose with normal plasma glucose in salicylate poisoning. Clin Invest 1970;49:2139–2145.

92. Vertrees JE, McWilliams BC, Kelly HW: Repeated oral administration of activated charcoal for treating aspirin overdose in young children. Pediatrics 1990;85:594–597.

93. Vree TB, Van Ewuk-Beneken Kolmer EWJ, Verwey-Van Wissen CPWGM, Hekster YA. Effect of urinary pH on the pharmacokinetics of salicylate acid, with its glycine and glucuronide conjugates in human. Int J Clin Pharm Ther 1994;32:550–558.

94. Waldman RJ, Hall WN, McGee H, Van Amburg G: Aspirin as a risk factor in Reye's syndrome. JAMA 1982;247:3089–3094.

95. Walters JS, Woodring JH, Stelling CB, et al: Salicylate-induced pulmonary edema. Radiology 1983;146:289–293.

96. Weisberg HF: Water and electrolytes. In: Davidsohn I, Wells BB, eds: Clinical Diagnosis by Laboratory Methods. Philadelphia, WB Saunders, 1962, p. 500.

97. Wortzman DJ, Grunfeld A: Delayed absorption following enteric-coated aspirin overdose. Ann Emerg Med 1987;16:434–436.

ANTIDOTES IN DEPTH

Sodium Bicarbonate
Paul M. Wax

Sodium bicarbonate ($NaHCO_3$) is one of the most useful agents available for the treatment of the poisoned patient. Unlike more specific antidotes in which utility is usually limited to antagonizing a single drug or toxin, sodium bicarbonate is a nonspecific antidote effective in the treatment of a variety of poisonings by means of a number of distinct mechanisms (see Table 33–4). It is most commonly employed in the treatment of tricyclic antidepressant (TCA) and salicylate poisonings. Sodium bicarbonate may also have a role in the treatment of phenobarbital, chlorpropamide, and chlorophenoxy herbicide poisonings, and wide complex tachydysrhythmias induced by Type IA and Type IC antidysrhythmics and cocaine. Correcting the life-threatening acidosis generated by methanol and ethylene glycol poisoning and enhancing formate elimination are other important indications for sodium bicarbonate. Alkalinization of the urine for patients with drug- or toxin-associated myoglobinuria may also be useful. The use of sodium bicarbonate in the treatment of common nontoxicologic problems, such as lactic acidosis, cardiac resuscitation, and diabetic ketoacidosis is more questionable.[1] Studies suggest much less utility for sodium bicarbonate in the treatment of these nontoxicologic disorders than previously thought,[62, 90,96] but its use in these situations remains controversial.[24,92]

ALTERED DRUG IONIZATION RESULTING IN ALTERED DRUG DISTRIBUTION

Tricyclic Antidepressants

Sodium bicarbonate's most important role in toxicology appears to be its ability to reverse potentially fatal cardiotoxic effects of the tricyclic antidepressant drugs and other Type IA and IC antiarrhythmics. The use of sodium bicarbonate for TCA overdose developed as an extension of sodium bicarbonate use in the treatment of other cardiotoxic exposures. Noting similarities in electrocardiographic findings between hyperkalemia and quinidine toxicity (ie, QRS widening), investigators in the 1950s began to use sodium lactate, which is metabolized to sodium bicarbonate by cellular oxidative activity, for the treatment of quinidine toxicity.[2,6,95] In a dog model, quinidine-induced electrocardiographic changes and hypotension were consistently reversed by the infusion of sodium lactate.[5] Clinical experience confirmed this benefit.[6] Similar efficacy in the treatment of procainamide cardiotoxicity was also reported.[95]

With the introduction of the tricyclic antidepressants during the late 1950s and early 1960s, significant conduction disturbances, dysrhythmias, and hypotension were reported. Extending the use of sodium lactate from the Type I antidysrhythmics to the TCAs, uncontrolled observations in the early 1970s showed a decrease in mortality from 15% to less than 3% when sodium lactate was administered to patients with TCA poisoning.[27] In 1976, the first report of clinical success with the use of sodium bicarbonate in the treatment of a series of TCA-induced dysrhythmias in children was reported.[13] In this series, 9 of 12 children who had developed multifocal premature ventricular contractions (PVCs), ventricular tachycardia, or heart block reverted to normal sinus rhythm with sodium bicarbonate therapy alone. An early animal experiment at this time in amitriptyline-poisoned dogs demonstrated resolution of dysrhythmias upon alkalinization of the blood to a pH above 7.40.[13] Other methods of alkalinization, including hyperventilation and administration of a nonsodium buffer, tris(hydroxymethyl) aminomethane (THAM), also appeared effective in reversing the dysrhythmias.[14,42]

A better understanding of the mechanism and utility of sodium bicarbonate has come about through a series of additional animal experiments during the 1980s. In amitriptyline-poisoned dogs, it was shown that sodium bicarbonate reversed conduction slowing and ventricular dysrhythmias and suppressed ventricular ectopy.[64] When comparing sodium bicarbonate, hyperventilation, hypertonic sodium chloride, and lidocaine, sodium bicarbonate and hyperventilation proved most efficacious in reversing ventricular dysrhythmias and narrowing QRS interval prolongation. Although lidocaine transiently antagonized dysrhythmias, this antagonism was demonstrated only at nearly toxic lidocaine levels and was associated with hypotension. In these studies, hypertonic sodium chloride failed to reverse dysrhythmias. Furthermore, prophylactic alkalinization protected against the development of dysrhythmias in a pH-dependent manner.

In desipramine-poisoned rats, the isolated use of sodium chloride was also effective in decreasing QRS duration, as well as the use of sodium bicarbonate.[69] Both sodium bicarbonate and sodium chloride also increased mean arterial pressure, but hyperventilation or direct intravascular volume repletion with mannitol did not. In further experimental studies, in vivo and on isolated cardiac tissue, both alkalinization and sodium concentration modulated TCA effects on cardiac conduction.[80,81] Although hypocapnia and sodium chloride each independently improved conduction velocity, this effect was greater when sodium bicarbonate was administered.

Another study on amitriptyline-poisoned rats demonstrated that treatment with sodium bicarbonate was associated with shorter QRS interval, longer duration of sinus rhythm, and increased survival rates.[44] This study also investigated the effects of inotropic drug treatment, and treatment with epinephrine plus sodium bicarbonate was associated with a significantly higher survival rate than sodium bicarbonate by itself.

Because TCAs are weak bases (high pK_a), alkalinization increases the proportion of nonionized drug. This may decrease drug-receptor binding possibly due to a redistribution of drug from the central compartment to the periphery because of less ion trapping in the blood, thus diminishing the TCA effect on cardiac conduction. Decreased ionization should not significantly decrease the rate of TCA elimination because of the small contribution of renal pathways to overall TCA elimination (less than 5%).

TABLE 33–4. Sodium Bicarbonate in Toxicology: Mechanisms, Site of Action, and Uses

Mechanism	Site of Action	Uses
Altered interaction between drug and sodium channel (also altered sodium gradient)	Heart	Amantadine Carbamazepine Cocaine Encainide Flecainide Mesoridazine Procainamide Quinidine Quinine Thioridazine Tricyclic antidepressants
Altered drug ionization leads to altered tissue distribution	Brain	Formic acid Phenobarbital Salicylates
Altered drug ionization leads to enhanced drug elimination	Kidneys	Chlorophenoxy herbicides Chlorpropamide Formic acid Methotrexate Phenobarbital Salicylates
Correct acidosis	Metabolic	Cyanide Ethylene glycol Isoniazid Methanol
Increase drug solubility	Kidneys	Methotrexate
Prevent myoglobin dissociation	Kidneys	Rhabdomyolysis
Neutralization	Lungs	Chlorine gas Hydrogen chloride Phosgene

Sodium bicarbonate seems to work independently of initial blood pH. Animal studies showed that cardiac conduction improved after treatment with sodium bicarbonate or sodium chloride in both normal pH and acidemic animals.[69] Clinically, TCA-poisoned patients who are already alkalemic have also responded to repeat doses of sodium bicarbonate.[59]

Although several authors have suggested that sodium bicarbonate's efficacy is modulated via a pH-dependent change in protein binding that decreases the proportion of free drug,[14,49] further study failed to support this hypothesis.[71] The administration of large doses of a binding protein α_1-acid glycoprotein (AAG) (to which TCAs show great affinity) to desipramine-poisoned rats only minimally decreased cardiotoxicity. Although the addition of AAG increased the concentration of total desipramine and protein-bound desipramine in the serum, the concentration of active free desipramine did not decline significantly. A redistribution of TCA from peripheral sites may have prevented lowering of free desipramine. The persistence of other TCA-associated toxicity, such as the anticholinergic effects and seizures, also argues against changes in protein-binding modulating toxicity. In vitro studies performed in a protein-free bath further support that sodium bicarbonate's efficacy is independent of protein binding.[80]

Hence, sodium bicarbonate appears to have a crucial antidotal role in TCA poisoning by partially reversing the fast sodium channel blockade caused by these drugs, thereby decreasing QRS prolongation, reducing the frequency of ventricular dysrhythmias, and reducing hypotension.[64,69,80] The animal evidence supports two distinct and additive mechanisms for this effect: (a) a pH-dependent effect manifested by the production of an increased fraction of the more freely diffusible nonionized drug that can be liberated from the sodium channel; and (b) a sodium-dependent effect manifested by increasing the sodium gradient across the partially closed sodium channels. The actual contribution of each mechanism requires further clarification. Sodium bicarbonate reverses the quinidine-like effects that produce the major, life-threatening cardiovascular manifestations of TCA overdose. Other effects caused by the anticholinergic, α-adrenergic antagonism, reuptake inhibition, and direct central nervous system (CNS) properties of the TCAs are not affected by the administration of sodium bicarbonate.

Although there are many anecdotal accounts supporting the efficacy of sodium bicarbonate in treating TCA cardiotoxicity in humans,[35] these reports are all uncontrolled observations; controlled studies are not available. In one of the largest retrospective observational studies involving 91 patients who received sodium bicarbonate after TCA overdose, QRS prolongation corrected in 39 of 49 patients who had QRS duration greater than 0.12 seconds, and hypotension corrected within 1 hour in 20 of 21 patients who had systolic blood pressure <90 mm Hg.[36] The use of sodium bicarbonate was not associated with any complications in this study.

Prospective validation of treatment criteria for the use of sodium bicarbonate after TCA overdose has not been performed. The most common indications are conduction delays manifested by QRS >0.10 sec, $R_{avr} \geq 3$ mm, or right bundle branch block, wide-complex tachydysrhythmias, and hypotension.[50] Because studies show that there is a critical QRS duration at which ventricular dysrhythmias may occur (≥ 0.16 sec),[10] it seems reasonable that narrowing the QRS interval through the use of sodium bicarbonate or hyperventilation may prophylactically prevent the development of dysrhythmias. Controversy exists, however, over the use of sodium bicarbonate in situations in which the QRS interval is less than 0.16 sec. Although sodium bicarbonate has no proven efficacy in either the treatment or prophylaxis of TCA-induced seizures, seizures often cause acidemia, which rapidly increases the risks of conduction disturbances and ventricular dysrhythmias. Administering sodium bicarbonate in situations in which the QRS duration is 0.10 sec or greater may establish a theoretical margin of safety, in the event that the patient suddenly deteriorates, by lessening the likelihood of subsequent dysrhythmias, without adding significant demonstrable risk. In situations in which the QRS duration is less than 0.10 sec (given the negligible risk of seizures or dysrhythmias), prophylactic use of sodium bicarbonate is not indicated.

Because cardiotoxicity may worsen during the first few hours after ingestion, sodium bicarbonate should be started immediately if QRS interval widens to greater than 0.10 sec. Because TCA-induced hypotension also responds to sodium bicarbonate in experimental models, hypotension is another indication for sodium bicarbonate. However, there is no evidence to support a role for sodium bicarbonate in a TCA-poisoned patient who presents with an altered mental status or seizures without QRS widening or hypotension.

Because the potential benefits of alkalinization in TCA overdose usually outweigh the risks, sodium bicarbonate should be administered regardless of whether the patient has an acidemic or normal pH. Sodium bicarbonate is usually administered as a hypertonic solution. The most commonly used preparations are an

8.4% solution (1 M), containing 1 mEq each of sodium and bicarbonate ions per milliliter (calculated osmolarity of 2000 mOsm/L) and a 7.5% solution, containing 0.892 mEq each of sodium and bicarbonate ions per milliliter (calculated osmolarity of 1786 mOsm/L). Fifty-milliliter ampules of the 8.4% and 7.5% solutions contain 50 mEq and 44.6 mEq of $NaHCO_3$, respectively. One to 2 mEq of sodium bicarbonate per kg body weight should be administered intravenously as a bolus over a period of 1–2 minutes.[68] Greater amounts may be required to treat unstable ventricular dysrhythmias. Sodium bicarbonate can then be repeated as needed to achieve a blood pH of 7.50–7.55.[70,84] The endpoint of treatment is a narrowing of the QRS interval. Excessive alkalemia (pH >7.55) and hypernatremia should be avoided. Because sodium bicarbonate has a brief duration of effect, a continuous infusion is usually required after the intravenous bolus. One to three 50-mL ampules may be placed in 1 L of fluid and run at maintenance, or more than maintenance, depending on the fluid requirements and blood pressure of the patient. If a multiple-ampule infusion is contemplated, the sodium bicarbonate should be placed in a hypotonic solution, such as 5% dextrose in water, in order to limit the sodium load. Frequent evaluation of fluid status should also be performed to avoid precipitating pulmonary edema. Optimal duration of therapy has not been established. A recent study found that the time to resolution of conduction abnormalities during continuous bicarbonate infusion significantly varied, ranging from several hours to several days.[51] Sodium bicarbonate infusion is usually discontinued once there is improvement in hemodynamics, cardiac conduction, and resolution in altered mental status, although controlled data supporting such an approach is lacking.

The administration of 7.5% hypertonic saline may also prove beneficial in reversing QRS prolongation and hypotension after TCA overdose.[56] A study of nortriptyline-poisoned swine suggested that hypertonic saline may actually be more effective than sodium bicarbonate in reducing QRS duration and increasing blood pressure.[55] Significant clinical experience with this approach, however, is lacking, and safety issues concerning the potential for hyperosmolarity have not been adequately addressed. Despite suggestions that hyperventilation may be a useful alternative to sodium bicarbonate in reversing TCA cardiotoxicity, the swine study cited above reported no effect with such an approach.

Other Cardiotoxic Drugs

Sodium bicarbonate may also be useful in treating cardiotoxicity from other drugs with "quinidine-like effects" that impair sodium channel functioning, manifested by widened QRS complexes, dysrhythmias, and hypotension. Isolated case reports provide the bulk of the evidence in these situations. Demonstrable utility of sodium bicarbonate in treating Type IA antidysrhythmics, such as quinidine and procainamide, has already been shown.[5,95] The use of sodium bicarbonate in the successful treatment of conduction disturbances from an overdose of quinine (an optical isomer of quinidine) has also been reported.[9] Studies on dogs poisoned with the Type IC antidysrhythmics flecainide and encainide show reversal of the conductance slowing with sodium bicarbonate.[3,78] Clinical cases of severe cardiotoxicity from flecainide overdose and encainide overdose have also shown great improvement after sodium bicarbonate administration.[28,52,70] Sodium bicarbonate has also proven effective in narrowing the QRS complex in the setting of a diphenhydramine-[18] and propoxyphene-[87] induced wide complex dysrhythmias. The use of sodium bicarbonate in the treatment of

an amantadine overdose manifested by prolongation of the QRS and QTc intervals was associated with a narrowing of the QTc, but not the QRS interval.[22] Although sodium bicarbonate has also been reported to be useful in reversing QRS widening associated with fluoxetine-induced cardiac conduction delay,[29] sodium channel disturbances are not typical of specific serotonin reuptake inhibitor (SSRI) overdose, and routine use of alkalinization therapy in SSRI overdose is unwarranted. Sodium bicarbonate may also help in the management of other ingestions associated with Type IA-like cardiac conduction abnormalities and dysrhythmias, such as the phenothiazines, thioridazine and mesoridazine, and carbamazepine, but documentation of such benefit is lacking.

Cocaine (a local anesthetic with membrane-stabilizing properties resembling other Type I antidysrhythmics) may also cause similar conduction disturbances. In a dog model, sodium bicarbonate successfully reversed cocaine-induced QRS prolongation.[4,67] Similar findings were demonstrated in cocaine-treated guinea pig hearts.[98] Also, patients with pH-dependent cocaine-induced cardiotoxicity responded to treatment with sodium bicarbonate.[41,94] The simultaneous treatment with sedation, active cooling, and hyperventilation, in many of these cases, confounds the contribution of the sodium bicarbonate to overall recovery.

ALTERED DRUG IONIZATION RESULTING IN ENHANCED ELIMINATION

Salicylates

Although there is no known specific antidote for salicylate toxicity, judicious use of sodium bicarbonate is an essential treatment modality of salicylism. Sodium bicarbonate, through its ability to change the concentration gradient of the ionized and nonionized fractions of salicylates, is useful in decreasing tissue (eg, brain) levels of salicylates and in enhancing urinary elimination of salicylates. This therapy may also limit the need for more invasive treatment modalities, such as hemodialysis.

Salicylate is a weak acid with a pK_a of 3.0. According to the Henderson-Hasselbalch equation, at a pH of 3.0, equal concentrations of nonionized and ionized salicylate exist. As pH increases, more of the drug is in the ionized form. This change in ionization occurs in a logarithmic fashion such that 90% of the molecules are ionized at a pH of 4.0, and 99% are ionized at a pH of 5.0. Ionized molecules penetrate lipid-soluble membranes less rapidly than nonionized molecules because of the presence of polar groups on the ionized form. Consequently, weak acids, such as salicylates, may accumulate in an alkaline milieu, such as an alkaline urine, when the ionized forms predominate.[57,85]

Although alkalinizing the urine to increase salicylate elimination is certainly an important intervention in the treatment of salicylate poisoning, increasing the serum pH in patients with severe salicylism may prove even more consequential by protecting the brain from a lethal CNS salicylate burden. Using sodium bicarbonate to "trap" salicylate in the blood (keeping it out of the brain) may prevent clinical deterioration of the salicylate-intoxicated patient. Salicylate lethality is directly related to primary central nervous system dysfunction, which, in turn, corresponds to a "critical brain salicylate level."[33] At physiologic pH, where a very small proportion of the salicylate is in the nonionized form, a small change in pH will be associated with a significant change in amount of nonionized molecules (eg, at a pH of 7.4, 0.004% of the salicylate molecules are in the nonionized form; at a pH of 7.2, 0.008% of the salicylate is in the nonionized form). In experimental models, lowering the blood pH by inhaling a mixture of 20% carbon dioxide and 80% oxygen, or by infusing ammonium chloride, produces a shift of salicylate into the tissues.[15] Hence, the metabolic acidemia that is observed in significant salicylate poisonings can be devastating.

Fortunately, in salicylate poisonings, the earliest and most common acid-base disturbance is a respiratory alkalosis. Alkalemia slows the entrance of salicylate into the brain by widening the arterial-cerebral spinal fluid pH difference. In salicylate-poisoned rats, increasing the blood pH with sodium bicarbonate produced a shift in salicylate out of the tissues and into the blood.[34] This change in salicylate distribution did not result from enhanced urinary excretion because occlusion of the renal pedicles failed to alter these results. Acidemia, with resultant aciduria, however, tends to further inhibit elimination of salicylates, thus prolonging toxicity and possibly leading to worsening acidemia.

Trapping the ionized salicylate moiety in the urine may also provide great benefit. Salicylate elimination at low therapeutic concentrations consists predominantly of first-order hepatic metabolism. At these low concentrations, without alkalinization, only about 10–20% of salicylate is eliminated unchanged in the urine. With increasing concentrations, enzyme saturation occurs (Michaelis-Menten kinetics); thus, a larger percentage of elimination occurs as unchanged free salicylate. Under these conditions, in an alkaline urine, urinary excretion of free salicylate becomes even more significant, accounting for 60–85% of total elimination.[30,75]

The exact mechanism of pH-dependent salicylate elimination has generated controversy. The pH-dependent increase in urinary elimination was initially ascribed to "ion trapping": the filtering of both ionized and nonionized salicylate, while reabsorbing only the nonionized salicylate.[83] Other authorities, however, argue that limiting reabsorption of the ionizable fraction of filtered salicylate cannot be the primary mechanism responsible for enhanced elimination produced by sodium bicarbonate.[53] Because the quantitative difference between the percentage of molecules trapped in the ionized form at a pH of 5.0 (99% ionized) and a pH of 8.0 (99.999% ionized) is small, decreases in tubular reabsorption cannot fully explain the rapid increase in urinary elimination seen above a pH of 7.0.

"Diffusion theory" offers a reasonable alternative explanation. Fick's Law of Diffusion states that the rate of flow of a diffusing substance is proportional to its concentration gradient. A large concentration gradient between the nonionized salicylate in the peritubular fluid (and blood) and the tubular luminal fluid is found in alkaline urine. Because at a higher urinary pH a greater proportion of secreted nonionized molecules quickly becomes ionized upon entering the alkaline environment, more salicylate (ie, nonionized salicylate) must pass from the peritubular fluid into the urine in an attempt to reach equilibrium with the nonionized fraction. In fact, as long as nonionized molecules are rapidly converted to ionized molecules in the urine, equilibrium in the alkaline milieu will never be achieved. The concentration gradient of peritubular nonionized salicylates to urinary nonionized salicylates continues to increase with rising urinary pH. Hence, increased tubular secretion, not decreased reabsorption, probably accounts for most of the increase in salicylate elimination observed in the alkaline urine.[53]

Controversies regarding the indications for alkalinization in the treatment of salicylism have persisted. Although urinary alkalinization undoubtedly works to lower serum salicylate levels and enhance urinary elimination, the risks associated with alkalinization in the management of salicylism have generated concern. Questions regarding excessive alkalemia, hypernatremia, fluid overload, hypokalemia, and hypocalcemia, as well as the potential delay in achieving alkalinization with sodium bicarbonate (as opposed to more rapid response achieved with hyperventilation), have all been raised.[25,48,68,75,83] It has been suggested that the administration of sodium bicarbonate to adolescents and adults with prolonged hyperventilation and hypocapnia, who have a pure respiratory alkalosis, may result in tetany, encephalopathy, and death.[83] Patients with pure respiratory alkalosis often have alkaluria, as well as alkalemia, and do not require urinary alkalinization. In the more common scenario in which patients present with a mixed respiratory alkalosis and metabolic acidosis, sodium bicarbonate must be administered cautiously. The young child, who rapidly develops a metabolic acidosis, often requires alkalinization, but should be at less risk for complications of this therapy.[66]

Sodium bicarbonate is indicated in the treatment of salicylate poisoning for most patients with evidence of significant systemic toxicity. Although some authors have suggested alkali therapy for asymptomatic patients with levels above 30 mg/dL,[97] there are limited data to support this approach. For patients suffering from chronic poisoning, levels are not as helpful and may be misleading; clinical criteria remain the best indicators for therapy. A chest radiograph and arterial blood gas analysis to determine the alveolar-arterial oxygen gradient may be helpful in evaluating more subtle cases of acute or chronic poisonings. Patients with contraindications to sodium bicarbonate use, such as renal failure or pulmonary edema, may benefit from hyperventilation; extracorporeal removal may be required in some instances.

Dosing recommendations depend on the acid-base status of the patient. For the patient with acidemia, rapid correction is indicated with intravenous administration of 1–2 mEq/kg body weight of sodium bicarbonate.[88] Once the blood is alkalinized, or if the patient has already presented with an alkalemia, continued titration with sodium bicarbonate over 4–8 hours is recommended until the urine pH reaches 7.5–8.0.[86,88] Alkalinization can be maintained with a continuous sodium bicarbonate infusion of 100–150 mEq in 1 L of 5% dextrose in water at 150–200 mL/h (or about twice the maintenance requirements in a child). Obtaining a urinary pH of 8.0 is difficult but is considered to be the goal. Fastidious attention to the changing acid-base status is required. Systemic pH should be kept below 7.55 to prevent complications of alkalemia. Acetazolamide (Diamox) should not be used in the treatment of salicylate poisoning.[88] Although recommended in the past because of its ability to alkalinize the urine,[61,75] acetazolamide produces a systemic and possibly cerebrospinal fluid (CSF) acidosis that may potentiate salicylate poisoning.[19,31]

Hypokalemia can make urinary alkalinization particularly problematic.[48,82] In the hypokalemic patient, regardless of total body potassium stores, the kidney will preferentially reabsorb potassium in exchange for hydrogen ions. Alkalinization will be unsuccessful as long as hydrogen ions are excreted into the urine. Thus, appropriate potassium supplementation to achieve normokalemia may be required in order to alkalinize the urine.[99]

In the past, proper urinary alkalinization was thought to require forced diuresis in order to maximize salicylate elimination.[20,48] Suggestions included administering enough fluid (2 L/h) to produce a urine output of 500 mL/h. This method of alkalinization, however, often leads to fluid retention. Excess fluid may be of particular concern in salicylate-poisoned patients who present with, or who are at high risk of acute lung injury (ALI)-acute respiratory distress syndrome (ARDS), cerebral edema, and renal failure.[38,86,89,100] A significantly higher urinary pH was obtained with sodium bicarbonate alone (pH 8.10), as compared to forced alkaline diuresis.[73] Because forced alkaline diuresis appears unnecessary and is potentially harmful as a result of its unnecessarily large fluid load, alkalinization at a rate of approximately twice maintenance requirements to achieve a urine output of 3–5 mL/kg/h is the goal.

Phenobarbital

Although cardiopulmonary support is the most critical intervention in the treatment of severe phenobarbital overdose, sodium bicarbonate may be a useful adjunct to the general supportive care. The utility of sodium bicarbonate may be particularly important considering the long plasma half-life (about 100 hours) of phenobarbital. Phenobarbital is a weak acid (pK_a of 7.24) that undergoes significant renal elimination. As in the case of salicylates, alkalinization of the blood and urine may reduce the severity and duration of toxicity. In a mouse study, the median anesthetic dose for mice receiving phenobarbital increased by 20%, with the addition of 1 g/kg of sodium bicarbonate (raising the blood pH from 7.23 to 7.41), suggesting decreased tissue levels associated with increased pH.[93] Extrapolating the animal evidence to humans, it has been suggested that phenobarbital-poisoned patients in deep coma might develop a respiratory acidosis, secondary to hypoventilation, with the acidemia enhancing the entrance of phenobarbital into the brain, thus worsening central nervous system and respiratory depression. Alternatively, increasing the pH with bicarbonate and/or ventilatory support would enhance the passage of phenobarbital out of the brain, thus lessening toxicity. Given the relatively high pK_a of phenobarbital, significant phenobarbital accumulation in the urine is evident only when urinary pH is raised above 7.5.[8] As the pH approaches 8.0, a 3-fold increase in urinary elimination occurs. The urine-to-serum ratio of phenobarbital, while much higher in alkaline urine than in acidic urine, remains less than unity, thereby suggesting less of a role for tubular secretion than in salicylate poisoning.

Unfortunately, clinical studies examining the role of alkalinization in phenobarbital poisoning have been inadequately designed. Many are poorly controlled and fail to examine the effects of alkalinization, independent of coadministered diuretic therapy. In one uncontrolled study, a 59–67% decrease in duration of unconsciousness in patients with phenobarbital overdoses occurred in patients administered alkali, when compared to nonrandomized controls.[58] In other older studies, treatment with sodium lactate and urea reduced mortality and frequency of tracheotomy to 50% of controls, enhanced elimination, and shortened coma.[47,63] In a more recent human volunteer study, urinary alkalinization with sodium bicarbonate was associated with a decrease in phenobarbital elimination half-life from 148 hours to 47 hours. However, this beneficial effect was less than the effect achieved by multiple-dose activated charcoal, which reduced the half-life to 19 hours.[26] Sodium bicarbonate therapy does not appear warranted in the treatment of ingestions of other barbiturates, such as pentobarbital and secobarbital, each of which has a pK_a above 8.0 and is predominantly eliminated by the liver.

Chlorpropamide

Alkalinization enhances the renal elimination of chlorpropamide.[65] Chlorpropamide is a weak acid (pK_a of 4.80) and has a long half-life (30–50 hours). Because patients who ingest this agent in overdose are at risk for prolonged hypoglycemia, enhancing the elimination should shorten the duration of poisoning and lessen the risk of complications. In a human study using therapeutic doses of chlorpropamide, urinary alkalinization with sodium bicarbonate significantly increased renal clearance of the drug.[65] This study showed that nonrenal clearance was the more significant route of elimination at a urinary pH of 5.0–6.0 (only slightly above pK_a), while at a pH of 8.0, renal clearance was 10 times that of nonrenal clearance. Alkalinization reduced the area under the curve almost 4-fold and shortened elimination half-life from 50 hours to 13 hours; acidification increased the area under the curve by 41% and increased the half-life to 69 hours. While not a study in overdose patients, this report suggests that sodium bicarbonate may be useful in the management of patients with chlorpropamide overdose. The effect of alkalinization on elimination of other sulfonylureas is unknown.

Chlorophenoxy Herbicides

Alkalinization is also indicated in the treatment of poisonings from the weed killers that contain chlorophenoxy compounds, such as 2,4-dichlorophenoxyacetic acid (2,4-D), or 2–4-chloro-2-methylphenoxy propionic acid (MCPP).[74] Poisoning results in muscle weakness, peripheral neuropathy, coma, hyperthermia, and acidemia. These compounds are weak acids (pK_a of 2.6 and 3.8 for 2,4-D and MCPP, respectively) that are excreted largely unchanged in the urine. In an uncontrolled case series of 41 patients poisoned with a variety of chlorophenoxy herbicides, 19 of whom received sodium bicarbonate, alkaline diuresis significantly reduced the half-life of each compound by enhancing renal elimination.[23] In one patient, resolution of hyperthermia and metabolic acidosis and improvement in mental status were associated with a transient elevation of serum levels of these compounds, perhaps reflecting chlorophenoxy compound redistribution from the tissues into the more alkalemic blood. The limited data suggest that the increased ionized fractions of the weak-acid chlorophenoxy compounds produced by alkalinization appear to be trapped in both the blood and the urine (as demonstrated with salicylates and phenobarbital), thus ameliorating toxicity and shortening duration of effect.

CORRECTING METABOLIC ACIDOSIS
Toxic Alcohols

Sodium bicarbonate has two important roles in treating toxic alcohol ingestions. As an immediate temporizing measure, administration of sodium bicarbonate may reverse the life-threatening acidemia associated with methanol and ethylene glycol ingestions. In rats poisoned with ethylene glycol, the administration of sodium bicarbonate alone resulted in a 4-fold increase in median lethal dose, perhaps because of decreased calcium excretion.[11] Clinically, titrating the exogenous acid with bicarbonate may be of great assistance in reversing the consequences of the severe acidemia, such as hemodynamic instability and multiorgan dysfunction.

The second role for bicarbonate in the treatment of toxic alcohol poisoning involves its ability to favorably alter the distribution and elimination of certain toxic metabolites.[76] In cases of methanol poisoning, the proportion of ionized formic acid can be increased by administering bicarbonate, thereby trapping formate in the blood compartment.[40,54] Consequently, decreased visual toxicity may result from the removal of the toxic metabolite from the optic nerve. In cases of formic acid (pK_a 3.7) ingestion, sodium bicarbonate may also decrease tissue penetration of the formic acid and enhance urinary elimination.[60] Further investigation is required to delineate the beneficial effects of sodium bicarbonate in the treatment of toxic alcohol ingestions.

Early treatment of acidemia with sodium bicarbonate is strongly recommended in cases of methanol and ethylene glycol poisoning.[32] Sodium bicarbonate should be administered to toxic alcohol-poisoned patients with an arterial pH below 7.30.[46] More than 400–600 mEq of sodium bicarbonate may be required in the first few hours.[39] In cases of ethylene glycol toxicity, sodium bicarbonate administration may worsen hypocalcemia; therefore, serum calcium should be monitored. Combating the acidemia, however, is not the mainstay of therapy, and concurrent administration of intravenous ethanol or fomepizole and preparation for possible hemodialysis are almost always indicated.

INCREASING DRUG SOLUBILITY

Methotrexate

Urinary alkalinization with sodium bicarbonate is also routinely employed during high-dose methotrexate cancer chemotherapy therapy. Methotrexate is predominantly eliminated unchanged in the urine. Unfortunately, it is poorly water soluble in acidic urine. Under these conditions, tubular precipitation of the methotrexate may occur, leading to nephrotoxicity and decreased elimination, increasing the likelihood of methotrexate toxicity. The administration of sodium bicarbonate (as well as intensive hydration) during high-dose methotrexate infusions increases methotrexate solubility as well as increasing the elimination of methotrexate.[17,79]

PREVENTING MYOGLOBIN DISSOCIATION

Rhabdomyolysis

Skeletal muscle injury (rhabdomyolysis) is a frequent complication of significant poisoning. This occurs as a direct toxic effect (eg, doxylamine, heroin) or indirect manifestation of muscle ischemia (eg, barbiturates, cocaine, carbon monoxide, ethanol withdrawal). Subsequent myoglobinuria may lead to renal injury and accounts for approximately 10% of cases of acute renal failure.[45] Animal evidence suggests that renal injury from myoglobinuria is dependent on the pH of the urine.[72] At or below urine pH of 5.60, myoglobin dissociates into ferrihemate and globin; ferrihemate is apparently toxic to the renal tubule.

Routine urinary alkalinization in patients with rhabdomyolysis, as a means of preventing renal impairment and hyperkalemia, has been suggested.[7] In an uncontrolled retrospective study, forced alkaline diuresis (with an intravenous infusion of 25 g of mannitol and 100 mEq of sodium bicarbonate in 1 L of 5% dextrose in water at a rate of 250 mL/h for 4 hours, as soon as possible after admission, and after obvious volume deficits have been replaced) might prevent development of renal injury in some patients with rhabdomyolysis.[21] Urinary pH, however, was not measured. In a case series of traumatic rhabdomyolysis, a similar protocol appeared to prevent renal damage in patients who achieved a urine pH above 6.5.[77]

Given the lack of strong clinical data, some authors question the necessity for sodium bicarbonate, as long as the urine pH is kept above 6.0.[37,43] Fluid repletion and mannitol may increase the urine flow to 200–300 mL/h, thus creating alkaline urine simply from a dilution effect. The use of sodium bicarbonate may also precipitate tetany in patients already at risk for hypocalcemia.[43] If it is not possible to keep the urine pH above 6.0 with fluid resuscitation and mannitol alone, however, alkalinization with sodium bicarbonate is indicated. Large amounts (eg, 300 mEq/d) may be required.

NEUTRALIZATION

Chlorine Gas

Nebulized sodium bicarbonate may serve as a useful adjunct in the treatment of pulmonary injuries resulting from chlorine gas inhalation.[16,91] Inhaled sodium bicarbonate is purported to neutralize the hydrochloric acid that is formed when the chlorine gas reacts with the water in the respiratory tree. Although oral sodium bicarbonate is not recommended to neutralize acid ingestions because of the problems associated with the exothermic reaction and production of carbon dioxide in the relatively closed gastrointestinal tract, in the lungs the rapid exchange of air with the environment should facilitate heat dissipation. In a chlorine-inhalation sheep model, animals treated with 4% nebulized sodium bicarbonate solution demonstrated higher P_{O_2} and lower P_{CO_2} than did the normal, saline-treated animals.[16] There was no difference, however, in 24-hour mortality or pulmonary histopathology. Anecdotal experience suggests that nebulized bicarbonate therapy may lead to improvement of symptoms.[91] In a retrospective review, 86 cases of chlorine gas inhalation were treated with nebulized sodium bicarbonate.[12] Sixty-nine patients were sent home from the Emergency Department, 53 of whom had clearly improved. Such uncontrolled observations do not provide convincing evidence for the efficacy of such an approach, but the nebulized sodium bicarbonate was well tolerated. Further clinical studies are required to further assess the efficacy and safety of this treatment.

SUMMARY

Despite the increasing tendency to avoid sodium bicarbonate administration in the critically ill acidemic patient, sodium bicarbonate remains an important agent in the treatment of a wide variety of drug and toxin exposures. In fact, its utility in the poisoned patient continues to expand. Not only is sodium bicarbonate effective in the treatment of poisonings by tricyclic antidepressants, salicylates, and phenobarbital, but it also shows promise in the treatment of toxicity from newer antidysrhythmics, cocaine, chlorophenoxy herbicides, and chlorine gas. In the severely poisoned patient, such as those manifesting quinidine-like effects, sodium bicarbonate is specific therapy. In the more common causes of metabolic acidosis (eg, lactic acidosis), specific therapy such as antibiotics, volume resuscitation, and inotropic support usually takes precedence over bicarbonate administration.

REFERENCES

1. Ardrogue HJ, Madias NE: Medical progress: Management of life-threatening acid-base disorders: First of two parts. N Engl J Med 1998;338:26–34.
2. Bailey DJ: Cardiotoxic effects of quinidine and their treatment. Arch Intern Med 1960;105:37–46.
3. Bajaj AK, Woosley RL, Roden DM: Acute electrophysiologic effects of sodium administration in dogs treated with O-desmethyl encainide. Circulation 1989;80:994–1002.
4. Beckman KJ, Parker RB, Harmtan RJ, et al: Hemodynamic and electrophysiological actions of cocaine. Effects of sodium bicarbonate as an antidote in dogs. Circulation 1991;83:1799–1807.
5. Bellet S, Hamdan G, Somiyo A, Lara R: The reversal of cardiotoxic effects of quinidine by molar sodium lactate: An experimental study. Am J Med Sci 1959;237:165–176.
6. Bellet S, Wasserman F: The effects of molar sodium lactate in reversing the cardiotoxic effect of hyperpotassemia. Arch Intern Med 1957;100:565–581.
7. Better OS, Stein JH: Early management of shock and prophylaxis of acute renal failure in traumatic rhabdomyolysis. N Engl J Med 1990;322:825–829.
8. Bloomer HA: A critical evaluation of diuresis in the treatment of barbiturate intoxication. J Lab Clin Med 1966;67:898–905.
9. Bodenhamer JE, Smilkstein MJ: Delayed cardiotoxicity following quinine overdose: A case report. J Emerg Med 1993;11:279–285.
10. Boehnert MT, Lovejoy FH: Value of the QRS duration versus the serum drug level in predicting seizures and ventricular arrhythmias after an acute overdose of tricyclic antidepressants. N Engl J Med 1985;313:474–479.
11. Borden TA, Bidwell CD: Treatment of acute ethylene glycol poisoning in rats. Invest Urol 1968;6:205–210.
12. Bosse GM: Nebulized sodium bicarbonate in the treatment of chlorine gas inhalation. J Toxicol Clin Toxicol 1994;32:233–241.
13. Brown TCK: Sodium bicarbonate treatment for tricyclic antidepressant arrhythmias in children. Med J Aust 1976;2:380–382.
14. Brown TCK, Barker CA, Dunlop ME, Loughnan PM: The use of sodium bicarbonate in the treatment of tricyclic antidepressant-induced arrhythmias. Anaesth Intensive Care 1973;1:203–210.
15. Buchanan N, Kundig H, Eyberg C: Experimental salicylate intoxication in young baboons. J Pediatr 1975;86:225–232.
16. Chisholm CD, Singletary EM, Okerberg CV, Langlinais PC: Inhaled sodium bicarbonate therapy for chlorine inhalation injuries [abstract]. Ann Emerg Med 1989;18:466.
17. Christensen ML, Rivera GK, Crom WR, et al: Effect of hydration on methotrexate plasma concentrations in children with acute lymphocytic leukemia. J Clin Oncol 1988;6:797–801.
18. Clark RF, Vance MV: Massive diphenhydramine poisoning resulting in a wide-complex tachycardia: Successful treatment with sodium bicarbonate. Ann Emerg Med 1992;21:318–321.
19. Cowan RA, Hartnell GG, Lowdell CP, et al: Metabolic acidosis induced by carbonic anhydrase inhibitors and salicylates in patients with normal renal function. Br Med J 1984;289:347–348.
20. Dukes DC, Blainey JD, Cumming G, Widdowson G: The treatment of severe aspirin poisoning. Lancet 1963;2:329–331.
21. Eneas JF, Schoenfeld PY, Humphreys MH: The effect of infusion of mannitol-sodium bicarbonate on the clinical course of myoglobinuria. Arch Intern Med 1979;139:801–805.
22. Farrell S, Lee DC. McNamara RM: Amantadine overdose: Considerations for the treatment of cardiac toxicity [abstract]. J Toxicol Clin Toxicol 1995;33:516–517.
23. Flanagan RJ, Meridith TJ, Ruprah M, et al: Alkaline diuresis for acute poisoning with chlorophenoxy herbicides and ioxynil. Lancet 1990;335:454–458.
24. Forsythe SM, Schmidt GA: Sodium bicarbonate for the treatment of lactic acidosis. Chest 2000;117:260–267.
25. Fox GN: Hypocalcemia complicating bicarbonate therapy for salicylate poisoning. West J Med 1984;141:108–109.
26. Frenia ML, Schauben JL, Wears RL, et al: Multiple-dose activated charcoal compared to urinary alkalinization for the enhancement of phenobarbital elimination. J Toxicol Clin Toxicol 1996;34:169–175.
27. Gaultier M: Sodium bicarbonate and tricyclic antidepressant poisoning [letter]. Lancet 1976;2:1258.
28. Goldman MJ, Mowry JB, Kirk MA: Sodium bicarbonate to correct widened QRS in a case of flecainide overdose. J Emerg Med 1997;15:183–186.
29. Graudins A, Vossler C, Wang R: Fluoxetine-induced cardiotoxicity with response to bicarbonate therapy. Am J Emerg Med 1997;15:502–503.
30. Gutman AB, Sirota JH: A study by simultaneous clearance techniques of salicylate excretion in man: Effect of alkalinization of the urine by bicarbonate administration; effect of probenecid. J Clin Invest 1955;34:711–722.
31. Heller I, Halevy J, Cohen S, et al: Significant metabolic acidosis induced by acetazolamide, not a rare complication. Arch Intern Med 1985;145:1815–1817.
32. Herken W, Rietbrock N: The influence of blood pH on ionization, distribution, and toxicity of formic acid. Naunyn Schmiedebergs Arch Pharmacol 1968;260:142–143.
33. Hill JB: Salicylate intoxication. N Engl J Med 1973;228:1110–1113.
34. Hill JB: Experimental salicylate poisoning: Observations on the effects of altering blood pH on tissue and plasma salicylate concentrations. Pediatrics 1971;47:658–665.
35. Hoffman JR, McElroy CR: Bicarbonate therapy for dysrhythmia and hypotension in tricyclic antidepressant overdose. West J Med 1981;134:60–64.
36. Hoffman JR, Votey SR, Bayer M, Silver L: Effect of hypertonic sodium bicarbonate in the treatment of moderate-to-severe cyclic antidepressant overdose. Am J Emerg Med 1993;11:336–341.
37. Honda N: Acute renal failure and rhabdomyolysis. Kidney Int 1983;23:888–898.
38. Hormaechea E, Carlson RW, Rogove H, et al: Hypovolemia, pulmonary edema and protein changes in severe salicylate poisoning. Am J Med 1979;66:1046–1050.
39. Jacobsen D, McMartin KE: Methanol and ethylene glycol poisonings: Mechanism of toxicity, clinical course, diagnosis, and treatment. Med Toxicol Adverse Drug Exp 1986;1:309–334.
40. Jacobsen D, Webb R, Collins TD, McMartin KE: Methanol and formate kinetics in late-diagnosed methanol intoxication. Med Toxicol Adverse Drug Exp 1988;3:418–423.
41. Kerns W, Garvey L, Owens J: Cocaine-induced wide complex dysrhythmia. J Emerg Med 1997;15:321–329.
42. Kingston ME: Hyperventilation in tricyclic antidepressant poisoning. Crit Care Med 1979;7:550–551.
43. Knochel ,JP: Rhabdomyolysis and myoglobinuria. Annu Rev Med 1982;33;435–443.
44. Knudsen K, Abrahamsson J: Epinephrine and sodium bicarbonate independently and additively increase survival in experiential amitriptyline poisoning. Crit Care Med 1997;24:669–674.
45. Koppel C: Clinical features, pathogenesis, and management of drug-induced rhabdomyolysis. Med Toxicol Adverse Drug Exp 1989;4:108–126.
46. Kulig KW, Duffy JP, Linden CH, Rumack BH: Toxic effects of methanol, ethylene glycol, and isopropyl alcohol. Top Emerg Med 1984;6:14–28.

47. Lassen NA: Treatment of severe acute barbiturate poisoning by forced diuresis and alkalinization of the urine. Lancet 1960; 2:338–342.

48. Lawson AAH, Proudfoot AT, Brown SS, et al: Forced diuresis in the treatment of acute salicylate poisoning in adults. Q J Med 1969;149:31–48.

49. Levitt MA, Sullivan JB, Owens SM, et al: Amitriptyline plasma protein binding: Effect of plasma pH and relevance to clinical overdose. Am J Emerg Med 1986;4:121–125.

50. Liebelt EL: Toxicology reviews: Targeted management strategies for cardiovascular toxicity from tricyclic antidepressant overdose: The pivotal role for alkalinization and sodium loading. Pediatr Emerg Care 1998;14:293–298.

51. Liebelt EL, Ulrich A, Francis PD, et al: Serial electrocardiogram changes in acute tricyclic antidepressant overdoses. Crit Care Med 1997;25:1721–1726.

52. Lovecchio F, Berlin R, Brubacher JR, Sholar JB: Hypertonic sodium bicarbonate in an acute flecainide overdose. Am J Emerg Med 1998;16:534–537.

53. MacPherson CR, Milne MD, Evans BM: The excretion of salicylate. Br J Pharmacol 1955;10:484–489.

54. Martin-Amat C, McMartin KE, Hayreh MS, Tephly TR: Methanol poisoning: Ocular toxicity produced by formate. Toxicol Appl Pharmacol 1978;45:201–208.

55. McCabe JL, Cobaugh DJ, Menegazzi JJ, Fata J: Experimental tricyclic antidepressant toxicity: A randomized, controlled comparison of hypertonic saline solution, sodium bicarbonate, and hyperventilation. Ann Emerg Med 1998;32:329–333.

56. McCabe JL, Menegazzi JJ, Cobaugh DJ, Auble TE: Recovery from severe cyclic antidepressant overdose with hypertonic saline/dextran in a swine model. Acad Emerg Med 1994;1:111–115.

57. Milne MD, Scribner BR, Crawford MA: Non-ionic diffusion and the excretion of weak acids and bases. Am J Med 1958;24:709–729.

58. Mollaret P, Rapin M, Pocidalo JJ, Monsallier JF: Treatment of acute barbiturate intoxication through plasmatic and urinary alkalinization. Presse Med 1959;67:1435–1437.

59. Molloy DW, Penner SB, Rabson J, Hall KW: Use of sodium bicarbonate to treat tricyclic antidepressant-induced arrhythmias in a patient with alkalosis. Can Med Assoc J 1984;130:1457–1459.

60. Moore DF, Bentley AM, Dawling S, Henry JA: Folinic acid and enhanced renal elimination in formic acid intoxication. J Toxicol Clin Toxicol 1994:32:199–204.

61. Morgan AG, Polak A: Acetazolamide and sodium bicarbonate in treatment of salicylate poisoning in adults. Br Med J 1969;1: 16–19.

62. Morris LR, Murphy MB, Kitabchi AE: Bicarbonate therapy in severe diabetic ketoacidosis. Ann Intern Med 1986;105:836–840.

63. Myschetzky A, Lassen NA: Urea-induced, osmotic diuresis and alkalization of urine in acute barbiturate intoxication. JAMA 1963;185:936–942.

64. Nattel S, Mittleman M: Treatment of ventricular tachyarrhythmias resulting from amitriptyline toxicity in dogs. J Pharmacol Exp Ther 1984;231:430–435.

65. Neuvonen PJ, Karkkainen S: Effects of charcoal, sodium bicarbonate, and ammonium chloride on chlorpropamide kinetics. Clin Pharmacol Ther 1983;33:386–393.

66. Oliver TK, Dyer ME: The prompt treatment of salicylism with sodium bicarbonate. Am J Dis Child 1960;99:553–564.

67. Parker RB, Beckman KJ, Hariman RJI, et al: The electrophysiologic and arrhythmogenic effects of cocaine [abstract]. Pharmacotherapy 1989;9:176.

68. Pentel PR, Benowitz NL: Tricyclic antidepressant poisoning: Management of arrhythmias. Med Toxicol Adverse Drug Exp 1986: 1:101–121.

69. Pentel PR, Benowitz NL: Efficacy and mechanism of action of sodium bicarbonate in the treatment of desipramine toxicity in rats. J Pharmacol Exp Ther 1984;230:12–19.

70. Pentel PR, Goldsmith SR, Salerno DM, et al: Effect of hypertonic sodium bicarbonate on encainide overdose. Am J Cardiol 1986;57:878–880.

71. Pentel PR, Keyler DE: Effects of high dose alpha-1-acid glycoprotein on desipramine toxicity in rats. J Pharmacol Exp Ther 1988;246:1061–1066.

72. Perri GC, Gorini P: Uraemia in the rabbit after injection of crystalline myoglobin. Br J Exp Pathol 1952;33:440–444.

73. Prescott LF, Balali-Mood M, Critchley A, et al: Diuresis or urinary alkalinization for salicylate poisoning. Br Med J 1982;285: 1383–1386.

74. Prescott LF, Park J, Darrien 1: Treatment of severe 2,4-D and mecoprop intoxication with alkaline diuresis. Br J Clin Pharmacol 1979:7:111–116.

75. Reimold EW, Worthen HG, Reilly TP: Salicylate poisoning: Comparison of acetazolamide administration and alkaline diuresis in the treatment of experimental salicylate intoxication in puppies. Am J Dis Child 1973;125:668–674.

76. Roe O: Methanol poisoning: Its clinical course, pathogenesis, and treatment. Acta Med Scand 1946;126(Suppl 182):1–253.

77. Ron D, Taitelman U, Michaelson M, et al: Prevention of acute renal failure in traumatic rhabdomyolysis. Arch Intern Med 1984; 144:277–280.

78. Salerno DM, Murakami MM, Johnston RB, et al: Reversal of flecainide-induced ventricular arrhythmias by hypertonic sodium bicarbonate in dogs. Am J Emerg Med 1995:13:285–293.

79. Sand TE, Jacobsen S: Effect of urine pH and flow on renal clearance of methotrexate. Eur J Clin Pharmacol 1981;19:453–456.

80. Sasyniuk BI, Jhamandas V: Mechanism of reversal of toxic effects of amitriptyline on cardiac Purkinje fibers by sodium bicarbonate. J Pharmacol Exp Ther 1984;231:387–393.

81. Sasyniuk BI, Jhamandas V, Valois M: Experimental amitriptyline intoxication: Treatment of cardiac toxicity with sodium bicarbonate. Ann Emerg Med 1986;15:1052–1059.

82. Savege TM, Ward JD, Simpson BR, Cohen RD: Treatment of severe salicylate poisoning by forced alkaline diuresis. Br Med J 1969;1:35–36.

83. Segar WE: The critically ill child: Salicylate intoxication. Pediatrics 1969;44:440–444.

84. Smilkstein MJ: Reviewing cyclic antidepressant cardiotoxicity: Wheat and chaff. J Emerg Med 1990;8:645–648.

85. Smith PK, Gleason HL, Stoll CC, et al: Studies on the pharmacology of salicylates. J Pharmacol Exp Ther 1946;87:237–255.

86. Snodgrass W, Rumack BH, Peterson RG, Holbrook ML: Salicylate toxicity following therapeutic doses in children. J Toxicol Clin Toxicol 1981;18:247–259.

87. Stork CM, Redd JT, Fine K, Hoffman RS: Propoxyphene-induced wide QRS complex dysrhythmia responsive to sodium bicarbonate—A case report. J Toxicol Clin Toxicol 1995;33:179–183.

88. Temple AR: Acute and chronic effects of aspirin toxicity and their treatment. Arch Intern Med 1981;141:364–369.

89. Temple AR, George DJ, Done AK, Thompson JA: Salicylate poisoning complicated by fluid retention. J Toxicol Clin Toxicol 1976;9:61–68.

90. Viallon A, Zeni F, Lafond P, et al: Does bicarbonate therapy improve the management of severe diabetic ketoacidosis: Crit Care Med 1999;27:2690–2693.

91. Vinsel PJ: Treatment of acute chlorine gas inhalation with nebulized sodium bicarbonate. J Emerg Med 1990;8:327–329.

92. Vukmir RB, Bircher N, Safar P: Sodium bicarbonate in cardiac arrest: A reappraisal. Am J Emerg Med 1996;14:192–206.

93. Waddell WI, Butler TC: The distribution and excretion of phenobarbital. J Clin Invest 1957:36:1217–1226.

94. Wang RY: pH-dependent cocaine-induced cardiotoxicity. Am J Emerg Med 1999;17:364–369.

95. Wasserman F, Brodsky L, Dick MM, et al: Successful treatment of quinidine and procainamide intoxication. N Engl J Med 1958; 259:797–802.

96. Weil MH, Ruiz CE, Michaels S, Rackow EC: Acid-base determinants of survival after cardiopulmonary resuscitation. Crit Care Med 1985;13:888–892.

97. Whitten CE, Kesaree NM, Goodwin JF: Managing salicylate poisoning in children. Am J Dis Child 1961;101:178–194.

98. Winecoff AP, Hariman RJ, Grawe JJ: Reversal of the electrocardiographic effects of cocaine by lidocaine. Part 1: Comparison with sodium bicarbonate and quinidine. Pharmacotherapy 1994;14:698–703.

99. Yip L, Dart RC, Gabow PA: Concepts and controversies in salicylate toxicity. Emerg Med Clin North Am 1994;12:351–364.

100. Zimmerman GA, Clemmer TP: Acute respiratory failure during therapy for salicylate intoxication. Ann Emerg Med 1981;10:104–106.

CHAPTER 34 NONSTEROIDAL ANTIINFLAMMATORY AGENTS

William A. Watson

Ibuprofen

Following an argument with his girlfriend, a 26-year-old male ingested an unknown number of ibuprofen 800-mg tablets and subsequently became unresponsive. His girlfriend stated that he used heroin and cocaine whenever he could get them, but otherwise had no significant past medical history. The patient was responsive only to painful stimuli. Noting the patient's pinpoint pupils the paramedics administered 0.8 mg naloxone IV without subsequent improvement of his mental status. On arrival at the Emergency Department (ED) his vital signs were: blood pressure, 115/70 mm Hg; heart rate, 140 beats/min; respiratory rate, 16 breaths/min; and temperature, 97.5°F (36.4°C). On physical examination in the ED, the patient's pupils were approximately 5 mm, equal round, with normal response to light. His neck was supple and his skin was normal.

Following the brief examination the patient was lavaged with an orogastric tube and given activated charcoal (50 g). Stool and vomitus were negative for the presence of occult blood. Specimens for plasma acetaminophen and salicylate levels were collected and sent to the laboratory. Urine was negative for ketones and myoglobin.

The patient vomited 30 minutes after receiving a dose of activated charcoal and was subsequently intubated for further airway protection. Preintubation arterial blood gases with the patient breathing 100% oxygen by nonrebreather mask revealed a pH of 7.25, a P_{CO_2} of 44.3 mm Hg, and a P_{O_2} of 162 mm Hg, which were interpreted as respiratory and metabolic acidosis and an increased alveolar-arterial gradient. His sodium was 138 mEq/dL; potassium, 3.5 mEq/dL; chloride, 102 mEq/L; and bicarbonate, 19.9 mEq/L, with an anion gap of 16. Two hours later, the repeat electrolytes were sodium, 132 mEq/L; potassium, 3.3 mEq/L; chloride, 104 mEq/L; and bicarbonate, 11.2 mEq/L, with an anion gap of 17. His blood urea nitrogen (BUN) was 12 mg/dL; creatinine, 1.4 mg/dL; glucose, 153 mg/dL; and lactic acid level returned at 7.5 mmol/L. The ethanol level was 135 mg/dL. Complete blood count and calcium were normal. Salicylate and acetaminophen levels were undetectable.

During his hospital course renal function decreased by the morning of the second hospital day as the BUN rose to 60 mg/dL, the creatinine to 2.8 mg/dL, and the potassium to 5.1 mEq/L. Hepatic aminotransferases and the international normalized ratio (INR) remained normal. Stool specimens remained negative for occult blood. The patient's BUN and creatinine levels returned to baseline over a 2-day period without any treatment.

An ibuprofen level was reported as 1220 mg/dL by a specialty laboratory whose typical therapeutic reference range for steady-state trough plasma concentrations was reported to be 20–30 µg/mL.

HISTORY AND EPIDEMIOLOGY

Exposures and overdoses involving nonsteroidal antiinflammatory drugs (NSAIDs) are common, most likely because of their widespread availability and use. More than 73 million NSAID prescriptions are written annually.[1] Since the inception of the Toxic Exposure Surveillance System (TESS) in 1983, nonsteroidal exposures have become increasingly common, currently accounting for more than 3% of all reported cases (see p. 1752 and Chap. 116), and are second only to acetaminophen among the pharmaceutical products reported. In May 1984, ibuprofen became the first prescription NSAID approved for nonprescription status,[40] but this change in status did not increase the proportion of NSAID cases that are ibuprofen exposures; ibuprofen consistently accounts for 70–80% of all NSAID cases reported to TESS. Three NSAIDs (ibuprofen, naproxen, and ketoprofen) are currently available as both prescription and nonprescription products, both individually and in combination products such as symptomatic relief cough and cold products. Additionally, NSAIDs are available as veterinary products, and are occasionally identified in patent herbals.[44]

PHARMACOLOGY

The NSAID class includes at least 20 drugs that share the common mechanism of cyclooxygenase (COX) inhibition (Table 34–1). Competitive inhibition of COX produces both the therapeutic and certain of the systemic toxic effects of this group of drugs. Salicylates differ from the other NSAIDs in that they irreversibly bind to COX and produce an effect that lasts for the life of the cell unless it can produce more enzyme. Some of the NSAIDs, including diclofenac and indomethacin, also inhibit various lipoxygenase enzymes and decrease the production of leukotrienes in animals.[18,23] Acetaminophen inhibits COX in the central nervous system, but does not have clinical anti-inflammatory effects. Salicylates and acetaminophen are covered separately in this text (Chaps. 32 and 33).

COX inhibition prevents the formation of prostaglandins, prostacyclins, and thromboxane, but not leukotrienes and other eicosanoids[23,65] (Fig. 34–1). There are two isoforms of COX, which are labeled COX-1 and COX-2.[59] Inhibition of COX-2 is associated with both the analgesic and antiinflammatory actions of the NSAIDs and this discovery led to the introduction of COX-2 specific inhibitors. The action of COX-1 is described as cellular and organ homeostasis, and the adverse effects and probably the

TABLE 34–1. Classes of Nonsteroidal Antiinflammatory Agents

COX-1 and COX-2 inhibitors
    Salicylates
        Acetyl salicylic acid (aspirin)
        Nonacetylated derivatives (metabolized to salicylic acid)
            Salicylsalicylic acid (salsalate)
            Sodium salicylate
            Choline salicylate
            Magnesium salicylate
            Magnesium choline salicylate
        Diffunisal (Dolobid; not metabolized to salicylic acid)

    Pyrazolones
        Phenylbutazone

    Fenamates (anthranilic acids)
        Meclofenamate (Meclomen)
        Mefenamic acid (Ponstel)

    Acetic acids
        Diclofenac (Voltaren)
        Etodolac (Lodine)
        Indomethacin (Indocin)
        Ketorolac (Toradol)
        Nabumetone (Relafen)
        Sulindac (Clinoril)
        Tolmetin (Tolectin)

    Propionic acids
        Carprofen (Rimadyl)
        Fenoprofen (Nalfon)
        Flurbiprofen (Ansaid)
        Ibuprofen (Motrin, Advil, Medipren)[b]
        Ketoprofen (Orudis)[b]
        Naproxen (Naprosyn, Anaprox)[b]
        Oxaprozin (Daypro)

    Oxicams
        Piroxicam (Feldene)

COX-2 selective inhibitors
    Celecoxib (Celebrex)
    Meloxicam[a]
    Rofecoxib (Vioxx)

[a]COX-2 preferential
[b]Nonprescription

acute toxicity of the NSAIDs are primarily associated with the inhibition of COX-1.

Currently available COX-2 inhibitors demonstrate this property only at therapeutic doses; at very high concentrations the COX-2 specificity is lost.

PHARMACOKINETICS AND TOXICOKINETICS

Nonsteroidal antiinflammatory agents are rapidly absorbed from the gastrointestinal tract, with peak levels occurring within 2 hours after oral dosing for most agents. Sustained-release indomethacin, the enteric-coated diclofenac, mefenamic acid, piroxicam, and the prodrugs sulindac and nabumetone require 2–5 hours to reach peak levels.[5,61] All of these drugs are weakly acidic and highly protein-bound (>90%), with volumes of distribution of approximately 0.1–0.2 L/kg. The NSAIDs cross the blood-brain barrier and are found in cerebrospinal fluid (CSF) and brain tissue. Peak CSF concentrations lag behind serum concentrations by at least 2 hours, and the relative ability of different NSAIDs to cross the blood-brain barrier is determined by lipophilicity.[3,38] Hepatic metabolism is important for the elimination of NSAIDs,[23] with renal elimination of unchanged drug accounting for less than 10% of clearance (except indomethacin at 10–20%). The elimination half-life is less than 8 hours for the majority of NSAIDs. Phenylbutazone and piroxicam have very long half-lives (30 hours) and diflunisal, nabumetone, naproxen, and sulindac have half-lives of between 8 and 30 hours.

In patients with renal failure the conjugated metabolites of some drugs may be in equilibrium with the parent compound (ketoprofen, fenoprofen, naproxen, diflunisal). Although some NSAIDs undergo extensive biliary-fecal elimination (carprofen, indomethacin, piroxicam, sulindac), and therefore theoretically should be susceptible to enhanced excretion with multiple-dose activated charcoal, toxicity is rarely severe enough to warrant this therapy.

The ingestion of a large dose of an NSAID alters the kinetics of some NSAIDs. The absorption rate of naproxen is slower with larger doses, with peak concentrations from 3–4 hours after the ingestion of 12 of the 250-mg naproxen tablets.[55] Similar findings are suggested with ibuprofen, where determination of serum concentrations in poisoning and overdose patients demonstrated continued absorption over at least the first 2 hours after ED presentation in some patients.[19,40]

Because NSAIDs are primarily bound to plasma proteins, it is likely that with increasingly larger doses the percentage of unbound drug will increase, in turn resulting in a larger volume of distribution.[46] Theoretically, this, in turn, could result in a greater proportion of the dose available to distribute into tissue and the central nervous system, resulting in a nonlinear dose-toxicity curve.

The metabolism and excretion of naproxen is not saturated at doses up to 4 g and the half-life of elimination remains constant.[55] Renal elimination may be increased in overdose: in 16 healthy volunteers, excretion tended to increase in rate as naproxen levels rose.[55] In overdose, ibuprofen elimination remains similar to that of therapeutic doses, or is only slightly prolonged.[19,25]

PATHOPHYSIOLOGY

The adverse effects of chronic NSAID therapy provides a guide to the potential toxicity associated with acute NSAID overdoses. There are numerous reviews of adverse effects associated with NSAIDs[12,54,64,67] (Table 34–2). NSAIDs both directly irritate the gastrointestinal mucosa as well as inhibit formation of the cytoprotective prostaglandins PGI_2 and PGE_2 mediated by the COX-1 enzyme. The importance of the systemic effect is demonstrated by the perforation and bleeding that occurs with topical[15,70] or parenteral NSAID administration. The nonselective NSAIDs increase the relative risk of a serious gastrointestinal hemorrhage by approximately threefold compared to control populations.[7,17,69]

The NSAIDs are infrequently associated with hepatic damage. While transient asymptomatic increases of hepatic aminotrans-

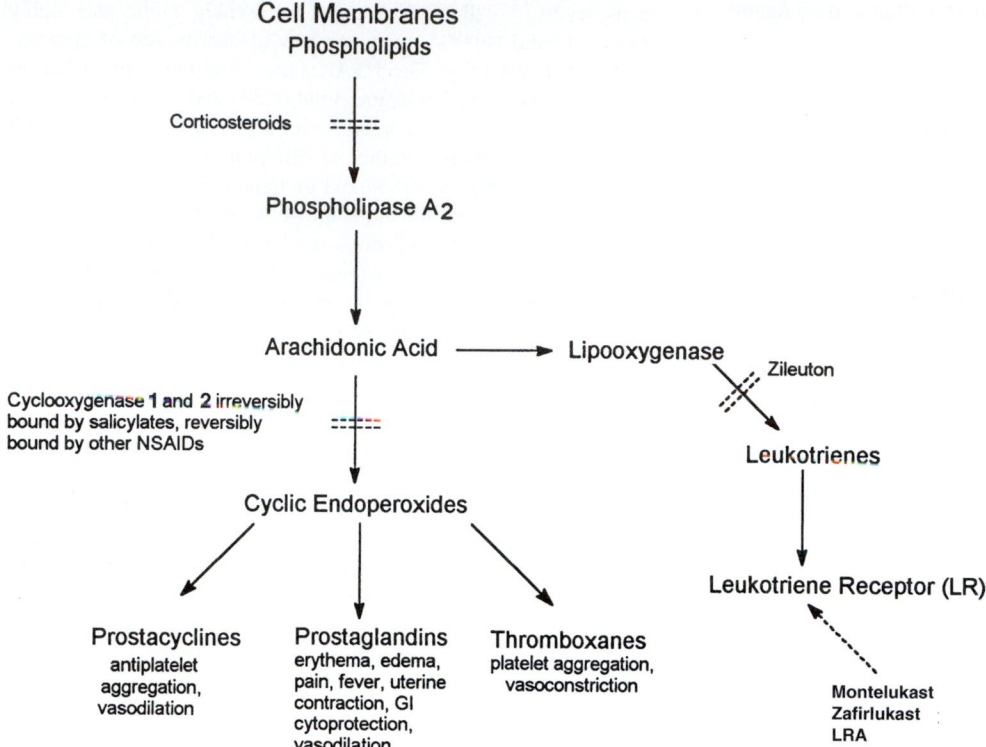

Figure 34–1. Mechanism of action of NSAIDs. Cyclooxygenase-1 (COX-1) is present in the kidney and GI tract. Cyclooxygenase-2 (COX-2) is induced by inflammatory mediators such as cytokines and endotoxin, and produces prostaglandins at the site of inflammation. Most NSAIDs block these enzymes nonselectively, with the exception of the newer COX-2 inhibitors. Leukotrienes and other products of lipooxygenase are blocked by corticosteroids but not salicylates or the newer COX-2 inhibitors. Leukotrienes may be involved in the sensitivity or asthmatic reactions produced by NSAIDs. Leukotriene receptor antagonists (LRAs) are designed to alleviate the effects of leukotrienes.

ferases occur in about 25% of NSAID users, hepatocellular necrosis and cholestatic jaundice occurs infrequently with the available NSAIDs.[30] A single case of fulminate hepatic failure has been described after the ingestion of 9.6 g of ibuprofen.[32] This suggests that the mechanism is more likely an idiosyncratic reaction associated with either the NSAID or its metabolites, and not associated with COX inhibition. Some NSAIDs, such as benoxaprofen, ibufenac, and sudoxicam, were withdrawn from use because of serious hepatotoxicity. There are some differences in hepatotoxicity among the different NSAIDs when both frequency and severity of toxicity are considered. The most hepatotoxic agents, such as benoxaprofen, fenclofenac, and ibufenac, are no longer available. Lower risk is associated with ibuprofen, indomethacin, and naproxen, and an intermediate risk is associated with diclofenac, phenylbutazone, and sulindac.[53]

The acidosis associated with NSAID overdoses occurs infrequently, and is usually a metabolic acidosis with increased serum lactic acid, an increased anion gap, and decreased serum bicarbonate. It appears to result from mechanisms including the formation of NSAID metabolites that are weak acids, hypotension, and relative hypoxia. There is no information to indicate that inhibition of COX is associated with the production of the metabolic acidosis.

Prostaglandins produce local dilation of renal arterioles in the presence of renal vasoconstrictor substances such as angiotensin.[18,43] In patients with the normal mechanisms of maintaining renal blood flow, NSAIDs have little effect on renal blood flow and renal function because there are low concentrations of angiotensin. However, in the setting of high angiotensin and low intravascular volume such as can occur in patients with congestive heart failure, cirrhosis, intrinsic renal disease, or hypovolemia, an NSAID-induced decrease in prostaglandins results in a decrease in renal blood flow and the rate of glomerular filtration. These, in turn, are also associated with retention of sodium, water, and hyperkalemia. All of these effects are usually reversible upon discontinuing NSAID therapy. At present the impact of the COX-2 selective inhibitors on renal function is not clear.[34]

Acute and chronic forms of interstitial nephritis and nephrotic syndrome occur in NSAID users.[8,29,42] In patients with significant analgesic use, the risk for papillary necrosis (69 out of 259 patients) may be higher than previously presumed.[58] Sulindac was initially believed to be renal sparing. Sulindac's active sulfide metabolite is not renally excreted and was not expected to be present in the kidneys at high enough concentrations to inhibit renal prostaglandin formation. However, sulindac is able to transiently decrease renal function in a manner similar to other NSAIDs, although this may occur less commonly than is recognized for other NSAIDs.

The NSAIDs have numerous hematologic effects. Inhibition of COX-1 results in decreased formation of thromboxane A_2. Thromboxane A_2 stimulates platelet aggregation and causes vasoconstriction. The effect of NSAIDs results in decreased platelet aggregation. The COX-2 selective inhibitor celecoxib does not suppress platelet aggregation.[33] NSAIDs are associated with other hematologic abnormalities including aplastic anemia (phenylbutazone, indomethacin, and etodolac), agranulocytosis (naproxen, phenylbutazone), hemolytic anemia (mefenamic acid), neutropenia (indomethacin), and thrombocytopenia (eg, indomethacin, ibuprofen, and naproxen).[11,48,49,56] These effects are idiosyncratic reactions.

The most common central nervous system (CNS) signs and symptoms associated with the use of NSAIDs are delirium, confusion, and headache.[28] Although seizures are very rarely reported as an adverse effect of therapeutic dosing, they are somewhat more common following overdose. Triphasic waves have been de-

TABLE 34–2. Selected Adverse Effects of Nonsteriodal Antiinflammatory Drugs

Gastrointestinal
Indigestion
Ulceration
Perforation
Hemorrhage
Elevated hepatic aminotransferases (transient)
Hepatocellular injury (rare)

Renal
Acute renal failure
Fluid and electrolyte retention
Interstitial nephritis
Nephrotic syndrome
Papillary necrosis

Hypersensitivity/pulmonary
Asthma exacerbation
Anaphylactoid reaction
Pneumonitis

Hematologic
Increased bleeding time
Agranulocytosis
Aplastic anemia
Thrombocytopenia
Neutropenia
Hemolytic anemia

Central nervous system
Headache
Aseptic meningitis
Delirium
Cognitive dysfunction, especially in the elderly
Hallucinations

Drug interactions
Anticoagulants: NSAIDs increase risk of GI bleeding
Antihypertensives (especially diuretics, β-adrenergic antagonists, and ACE inhibitors): NSAIDs reduce antihypertensive effects
Sulfonylureas: NSAIDs increase hypoglycemic effect
Lithium: NSAIDs increase risk of lithium toxicity
Digoxin: NSAIDs increase risk of digoxin toxicity
Aminoglycosides: NSAIDs increase risk of aminoglycoside toxicity

Life-threatening anaphylactoid reactions can occur after NSAID administration and should be treated like anaphylaxis from any other cause. Up to 25% of adult asthmatics with nasal polyps or chronic urticaria develop acute bronchospasm minutes to hours after NSAID exposure.[63] The asthma is often accompanied by flush of the head and neck, rhinorrhea, conjunctivitis, and/or angioedema. The probable mechanism is inhibition of COX, resulting in an increased production of leukotrienes LTC_4, LTD_4, and LTE_4.[57] There is no clear distinction among the NSAIDs, although anaphylactoid reactions are more frequently reported with tolmetin. There is cross-sensitivity among all NSAIDs despite their chemical diversity. Blockade of 5-lipoxygenase with zileuton or the use of leukotriene receptor antagonists (LTRAs) such as zafirlukast or montelukast may prevent symptoms and signs of aspirin intolerance[1,24] (Fig. 34–1). This suggests that the mechanism is not immunologically based, but involves some portion of the cyclooxygenase pathways. Zafirlukast and zileuton are now marketed for the treatment of chronic asthma.[1] About 2.5% of patients allergic to tartrazine dyes are also allergic to NSAIDs.

CLINICAL MANIFESTATIONS

The toxicity produced by the different NSAIDs is generally similar in poisoning and overdose. While there may be differences in severity and frequency of some manifestations, all the NSAIDs appear to cause similar effects. The clinical manifestations of NSAID poisoning and overdose tend to be minimal. The most common toxic effects are gastrointestinal distress (nausea, vomiting, epigastric pain, gastrointestinal hemorrhage) and mild central nervous system depression. Uncommon toxic effects include acidemia, respiratory depression, hypotension, hypothermia, acute renal failure, mild liver toxicity, elevated INR, confusion, hallucinations and seizures.

Complicating attempts to accurately assess the relative toxicity of NSAIDs is the significant reporting bias associated with different NSAIDs (Chap. 116). Reporting bias may result in the false impression that certain NSAIDs more commonly cause severe toxicity. Reports that focus on one NSAID must be carefully evaluated before being used to determine whether the toxicity caused is unique to that NSAID. More likely the toxicity is an unusual effect that can occur with all of the NSAIDs.

Propionic Acids

Ibuprofen toxicity is well described in the literature.[19,20] In a comparative survey of adults who ingested ibuprofen, salicylates, or acetaminophen, fewer adults required hospitalization after ibuprofen ingestions than after either of the other nonprescription agents.[66] In a retrospective case series of 126 ibuprofen overdoses, 19% of patients developed symptoms, predominantly CNS depression and gastrointestinal distress such as abdominal pain, nausea, and vomiting, usually within 4 hours of the ingestion.[19] This retrospective report was confirmed by a prospective study of 45 adults and 39 pediatric patients. Serious manifestations of coma, apnea, and/or metabolic acidosis developed in 9% of adults and 5% of children.[20] Patients who ingested more than 400 mg/kg of ibuprofen by history (especially children) were more likely to have seizures, apnea, hypotension, bradycardia, metabolic acidosis, and renal and hepatic dysfunction. Clinical effects occur within

scribed on an electroencephalogram in one case of naproxen toxicity, similar to changes seen with CNS depressant overdoses.[6] Aseptic meningitis in patients with and without autoimmune disorders are reported with ibuprofen, sulindac, and tolmetin use.[9,49] Some agents can cause tinnitus (ibuprofen, naproxen, fenoprofen, sulindac, tolmetin) or transient loss of hearing (ibuprofen, indomethacin, phenylbutazone).[23,49]

Various visual disturbances are associated with NSAID use, including toxic amblyopia, blurred vision, and colored spots. The causality and mechanism by which these effects are produced is unclear, although it has also been reported with COX-2 selective agents.[36]

Because uterine production of prostaglandins E and F increases dramatically in the hours before parturition, NSAIDs are used as tocolytics.[41] However, NSAID use may be associated with untoward intrauterine closure of the fetal ductus arteriosus, renal failure, and oligohydramnios in neonates.[26]

4 hours of ingestion.[22,35,61] Atrial fibrillation, possibly related to NSAID-induced acidemia, is also reported.[39]

Only a few cases of fenoprofen overdose are reported. One case series noted that 12 of 16 patients developed symptoms with 1 patient death after the ingestion of unknown amounts of fenoprofen.[10] The remaining 11 patients developed drowsiness, ataxia, tinnitus, nausea, hypotension, tachycardia, and/or Kussmaul respirations. Five children exhibited only drowsiness.

Most reported patient overdoses of naproxen develop only mild symptoms such as nausea, abdominal pain, or drowsiness.[16] Renal failure is also reported following overdose.[31,37] A 15-year-old who ingested approximately 50 naproxen sodium tablets developed metabolic acidosis and seizures.[37]

Similarly, ketoprofen poisoning is associated with mild gastrointestinal symptoms and drowsiness, and, rarely, seizures.[4,10] Little information is available about overdoses of carprofen except that rare but serious photosensitivity reactions may occur, as well as transient asymptomatic elevations in liver aminotransferases.[48] Coma and respiratory depression were reported in a single patient who overdosed on flurbiprofen.[10]

Pyrazolones

Historically, phenylbutazone is associated with the majority of the severe toxicity attributed to NSAIDs. In a review of 99 cases, phenylbutazone overdoses were characterized by early GI symptoms, acid-base and electrolyte disturbances, pulmonary edema, dizziness, seizures, coma, hypotension, and respiratory and cardiac arrest.[10,51] Acute signs may be followed by renal, hepatic, and hematologic dysfunction 2–7 days later. An overdose involving the veterinary formulation (1000-mg tablets) resulted in seizure, coma, hemodynamic instability, acute lung injury, and acute renal failure with hepatic dysfunction. Recovery took 5 weeks.[45] At least 50 phenylbutazone related fatalities have occurred in children.[50] The fatal dose in a 1-year-old was reported to be 2 g, with serious symptoms occurring in adults after ingestions of more than 4 g.[10,52,62]

Therapeutic doses of phenylbutazone are associated with aplastic anemia and agranulocytosis. Although the pyrazolones were withdrawn from the US market in the 1970s, phenylbutazone is still available from veterinary sources and from other countries.[44]

Anthranilic Acids

Mefenamic acid (Ponstel) and meclofenamate (Meclomen) are the two drugs in this category currently available in the United States. There are no reported cases of meclofenamate overdose, but because its structure is similar to that of mefenamic acid, the toxicity is probably similar. Muscle twitching and seizures are characteristic of symptomatic overdose.[2,10] Muscle twitching may be focal or generalized and in one series lasted 3–10 minutes with 20% of 54 patients progressing to grand mal seizures 2–7 hours postingestion.[2] Gastrointestinal distress including vomiting or diarrhea was noted in 15% of these patients. Seizures were responsive to benzodiazepines and all patients recovered. Reported doses as low as 2 g in a child and 6 g over 24 hours in an adult were implicated in the production of seizures.

Acetic Acids

Indomethacin or diclofenac toxicity appears to be relatively benign, resulting in nausea, abdominal pain, drowsiness, headache, and tinnitus.[10] Renal compromise was also reported in 1 case of diclofenac and in 9 cases of sulindac overdose.[31] Little is known about toxicity from etodolac, ketorolac, nabumetone, and tolmetin, the other agents in the acetic acid category. There are very few reported cases and almost all of these patients were asymptomatic.

Oxicams

The single drug currently available in this category is piroxicam (Feldene). Thirteen of 16 patients who ingested piroxicam alone remained asymptomatic and 2 patients developed dizziness and blurred vision.[10] One patient, who by history ingested 600 mg, developed coma with recovery within 24 hours.

There are no reports of exposures and overdoses with either of the available selective COX-2 inhibitor NSAIDs. As noted previously the COX-2 receptor selectivity is lost at high concentrations and therefore overdoses are expected to cause toxicity similar to the nonselective NSAIDs.

DIAGNOSTIC TESTING

Measurement of serum NSAID concentrations is unnecessary for the clinical assessment and management of NSAID exposures. Although a nomogram is available describing ibuprofen serum concentrations and their relationship to toxicity,[21,25] it is not clinically useful. Serum ibuprofen assays are generally unavailable, and most toxicity is mild and transient in nature.

In symptomatic patients, serum electrolytes, serum creatinine, and BUN should be considered as baseline parameters. Hyperkalemia and increased serum creatinine or BUN identify patients who are at increased risk for renal toxicity. These patients should have their renal function monitored more closely. A serum pregnancy test should be obtained for women of child-bearing age who have ingested NSAIDs. If significant respiratory or CNS toxicity is present, arterial blood gases should be obtained to evaluate both pulmonary and acid-base status. A serum acetaminophen concentration should be obtained to determine whether there is concurrent acetaminophen ingestion, especially in patients with a history of recent painful or febrile conditions.

At least two NSAIDs will produce a color change on ferric chloride testing of the urine (phenylbutazone and diflunisal) and these should be considered in the differential diagnosis if this qualitative bedside test is positive[47] (Chap. 33). The NSAIDs are generally identifiable using thin-layer chromatography methods. NSAID metabolites in the urine may produce false-positive drug screens using specific immunoassays. The question of false-positive test results is addressed by using information that is available for the specific assay in question.

MANAGEMENT

Otherwise healthy patients with a history of NSAID poisoning generally require only gastrointestinal decontamination with activated charcoal, fluid and electrolyte replacement, and supportive management of airway, breathing, and circulation as necessary. Those patients who may have ingested a large dose of a NSAID, and who present with CNS or cardiovascular toxicity, or who have known risk factors for organ system toxicity associated with NSAIDs, should be considered at higher risk for complications.

Orogastric lavage is most appropriate for patients with phenylbutazone or mefenamic acid overdoses in view of their greater potential toxicity. All patients require basic poison management including consideration of coingestants, evaluation for toxidromes, screening for acid-base disturbances, as well as fluid and electrolyte disorders, and psychosocial support. Most NSAID toxicity resolves with supportive care.

The high degree of protein binding characteristics of all NSAIDs makes hemodialysis ineffective in overdose and experience with hemoperfusion is insufficient to determine its utility.

Several therapeutic interventions have been tried to prevent the adverse gastrointestinal effects resulting from loss of cytoprotection from prostaglandins; use of proton pump inhibitors has shown some success,[13,68] whereas H_2-receptor blockade was unsuccessful in 1920 patients.[60] Concurrent administration of misoprostol, a PGE analogue, may also be effective in preventing GI side effects of NSAIDs. Other experimental efforts have involved the coadministration of nitric oxide[14] or substance P inhibitors.[27] These approaches to minimizing adverse effects have not been utilized as treatment of NSAID overdoses.

The specific NSAID involved in an ingestion should be identified and the presence or absence of concurrent acetaminophen serum levels documented. The possible ingestion of additional agents should be excluded, especially in the patient with evidence of clinically significant toxicity. Patients should always be evaluated to determine whether any concurrent disease states may increase the risk of toxicity (eg, renal, hepatic, gastrointestinal disease), or whether current medical therapy may interact with the NSAID (such as lithium or methotrexate).

SUMMARY

The NSAIDs are a large class of drugs that share similar clinical toxicity based on their ability to inhibit COX. The toxicity that results from overdose is usually minimal and consists of epigastric pain, nausea or vomiting, and mild CNS depression. Uncommonly, severe overdoses can result in acidosis, CNS toxicity including tinnitus, ataxia, seizures, confusion, delirium, and coma, transient decreases in renal function, apnea, hypotension, bradycardia, or tachycardia. Some notable differences are present among NSAIDs, with phenylbutazone associated with more severe toxicity and mefenamic acid associated with muscle fasciculations.

The specific NSAID involved should be identified and the presence or absence of acetaminophen documented by measurement of serum acetaminophen. The potential presence of additional agents should be evaluated. Patients should be evaluated to determine whether they have concurrent disease states that may increase the risk of toxicity (eg, renal, hepatic, gastrointestinal disease), or are receiving medical therapy that may interact with the NSAID (eg, lithium, methotrexate).

Necessary clinical management is usually limited to general supportive care, assessment for the presence of additional substances (especially acetaminophen), and risk factors for organ system toxicity. Activated charcoal is indicated as gastrointestinal decontamination if it can be administered within the first few hours after the ingestion of large doses of NSAIDs. The presence of significant CNS effects or risk factors mandates a more comprehensive evaluation of acid-base, fluid, renal, and electrolyte status.

ACKNOWLEDGMENT

Mary Ann Howland and Mary E. Palmer contributed to this chapter in a previous edition.

REFERENCES

1. Anonymous. Zafirlukast for asthma. Med Lett 1996;38:111–112.
2. Balali-Mood M, Proudfoot AT, Critchley J, et al: Mefenamic acid overdosage. Lancet 1981;2:1324–1356.
3. Bannwarth B, Netter P, Pourel J, et al: Clinical pharmacokinetics of nonsteroidal anti-inflammatory drugs in the cerebrospinal fluid. Biomed Pharmacother 1989;43:121–126.
4. Bond G, Curry S, Arnold-Cappel P, et al: Generalized seizures and acidosis after ketoprofen overdose [abstract]. Vet Hum Toxicol 1989;31:369.
5. Bond WS: Nonsteroidal antiinflammatory drugs: Are there significant differences? Facts Comp Drug Newsletter 1992;11:81–83.
6. Bortone E, Bettoni L, Buzio S, et al: Triphasic waves associated with acute naproxen overdose: A case report. Clin Electroencephalogr 1998;29:142–145.
7. Carson JL, Willett LR: Toxicity of nonsteroidal antiinflammatory drugs. An overview of the epidemiology evidence. Drugs 1993;46 (Suppl 1):243–248.
8. Clive DM, Stoff J: Renal syndromes associated with nonsteroidal anti-inflammatory drugs. N Engl J Med 1984;310:563–572.
9. Chez M, Sila CA, Ransohoff RM, et al: Ibuprofen-induced meningitis: Detection of intrathecal IgG synthesis and immune complexes. Neurology 1989;39:1578–1580.
10. Court H, Volans G: Poisoning after overdose with nonsteroidal antiinflammatory drugs. Adv Drug React Ac Pois Rev 1984;3:1–21.
11. Cramer RL, Aboko-Cole VC, Gualtieri RJ: Agranulocytosis associated with etodolac. Ann Pharmacother 1994;28:428–460.
12. Cryer B, Kimmey MB: Gastrointestinal side effects of nonsteroidal anti-inflammatory drugs. Am J Med 1998;105(1B):20S–30S.
13. Dajani EZ, Agrawal NM: Prevention of ulcers induced by nonsteroidal antiinflammatory drugs: An update. J Physiol Pharmacol 1995;46:3–16.
14. Elliott SN, McKnight W, Cirino G, Wallace JL: A nitric oxide-releasing nonsteroidal anti-inflammatory drug accelerates gastric ulcer healing in rats. Gastroenterology 1995;109:524–530.
15. Evans JM, McMahon AD, McGilchrist MM, et al: Topical nonsteroidal antiinflammatory drugs and admission to hospital for upper gastrointestinal bleeding and perforation: A record linkage case-control study. BMJ 1995;311:22–26.
16. Fredell E, Strand L: Naproxen overdose [letter]. JAMA 1977;238:938.
17. Gabriel SE, Jaakimainen L, Bombardier C: Risk for serious gastrointestinal complications related to use of nonsteroidal antiinflammatory drugs: A meta-analysis. Ann Intern Med 1991;115:787–796.
18. Garella S, Matarese R: Renal effects of prostaglandins and clinical adverse effects on nonsteroidal antiinflammatory agents. Medicine 1984;63:165–181.
19. Hall AH, Smolinske SC, Conrad FL, et al: Ibuprofen overdose: 126 cases. Ann Emerg Med 1986;15:1308–1312.
20. Hall AH, Smolinske SC, Kulig KW, at al: Ibuprofen overdose: A prospective study. West J Med 1988;48:653–656.
21. Hall AH, Smolinske SC, Stover B, et al: Ibuprofen overdose in adults. J Toxicol Clin Toxicol 1992;30:23–37.
22. Halpern SM, Fitzpatrick R, Volans GN: Ibuprofen toxicity. A review of adverse reactions and overdose. Adverse Drug React Toxicol Rev 1993;12:107–128.
23. Insel PA: Analgesic-antipyretic and antiinflammatory agents and drugs employed in the treatment of gout. In: Hardman JG, Limbird LE, Molinoff PB, et al, eds: Goodman and Gilman's The Pharmaco-

logical Basis of Therapeutics. New York, McGraw-Hill, 1996, pp. 617–657.

24. Israel E, Fischer AR, Rosenberg MA, et al: The pivotal role of 5-lipoxygenase products in the reaction of aspirin-sensitive asthmatics to aspirin. Am Rev Respir Dis 1993;148:1447–1451.

25. Jenkinson ML, Fitzpatrick R, Streete PJ, et al: The relationship between plasma ibuprofen concentrations and toxicity in acute ibuprofen overdose. Hum Toxicol 1988;7:319–324.

26. Kaplan BS, Restaino I, Raval DS, et al: Renal failure in the neonate associated with in utero exposure to nonsteroidal antiinflammatory agents. Pediatr Nephrol 1994;8:700–704.

27. Kataeva G, Argo A, Stanisz AM: Substance P-mediated intestinal inflammation: Inhibitory effects of CP 96,345 and SMS 201–995. Neuroimmunomodulation 1994;1:350–356.

28. Kertesz A: Neurological complications of nonsteroidal antiinflammatory agents. In: Borda I, Koff R, eds: Nonsteroidal Antiinflammatory Drugs: A Profile of Adverse Effects. Philadelphia, Hanley & Belfus, 1992:147–155.

29. Kincaid-Smith P: Effects of non-narcotic analgesics on the kidney. Drugs 1986;32(Suppl 4):109–128.

30. Koff RS: Liver disease induced by nonsteroidal antiinflammatory drugs. In: Borda I, Koff R, eds: Nonsteroidal Antiinflammatory Drugs: A Profile of Adverse Effects. Philadelphia, Hanley & Belfus, 1992:133–146.

31. Kulling PE, Backman EA, Skagius AS: Renal impairment after acute diclofenac, naproxen, and sulindac overdoses. Clin Toxicol J Toxicol 1995;33:173–177.

32. Laurent S, Rahier J, Geubel AP, et al. Subfulminant hepatitis requiring liver transplantation following ibuprofen overdose. Liver 2000;20:93–94.

33. Lefkowith JB: Cyclooxygenase-2 specificity and its clinical implications. Am J Med 1999;106(5B):43S–50S.

34. Lipsky PE: The clinical potential of cyclooxygenase-2-specific inhibitors. Am J Med 1999;106(5B):51S–57S.

35. Linden CH, Towsend PL: Metabolic acidosis after acute ibuprofen overdosage. J Pediatr 1987;111:922–925.

36. Lund BC, Neiman RF. Visual disturbance associated with celecoxib. Pharmacotherapy 2001;21:114–155.

37. Martinez R, Smith D, Frankel L: Severe metabolic acidosis after acute naproxen sodium ingestion. Ann Emerg Med 1989;18:1102–1104.

38. Mataga M, Pehourcq F, Lagrange F, et al: Influence of molecular lipophilicity on the diffusion of arylpropionate non-steroidal anti-inflammatory drugs into the cerebrospinal fluid. Arzneimittelforschung 1999;49(1):477–482.

39. McCune KH, O'Brien CJ: Atrial fibrillation induced by ibuprofen overdose. Postgrad Med J 1993;69:325–356.

40. McElwee NE, Veltri JC, Bradford DC, Rollins DE. A prospective, population-based study of acute ibuprofen overdose: Complications are rare and routine serum levels not warranted. Ann Emerg Med 1990;19:657–662.

41. Moise KJ, Huhta JC, Sharif DS, et al: Indomethacin in the treatment of premature labor: Effects on the fetal ductus arteriosus. N Engl J Med 1988;319:327–331.

42. Murray MD, Brater DC: Renal toxicity of the nonsteroidal antiinflammatory drugs. Annu Rev Pharmacol Toxicol 1993;33:435–465.

43. Murray MD, Brater DC: Adverse effects of nonsteroidal antiinflammatory drugs on renal function. Ann Intern Med 1990;112:559–560.

44. Nelson L, Shih R, Hoffman R: Aplastic anemia induced by an adulterated herbal medication. J Toxicol Clin Toxicol 1995;33:467–470.

45. Newton T, Rose R: Poisoning with equine phenylbutazone in a racetrack worker. Ann Emerg Med 1991;20:204–207.

46. Niazi SK, Alam SM, Ahmad SI: Dose-dependent pharmacokinetics of naproxen in man. Biopharm Drug Dispos 1996;17:355–361.

47. Nordt SP: Diflunisal cross-reactivity with the Trinder method from salicylate determination. Ann Pharmacother 1996;30:1041–1042.

48. O'Brien WM, Bagby GF: Carpofen: A new nonsteroidal anti-inflammatory drug. Pharmacology clinical efficacy and adverse effects. Pharmacotherapy 1987;7:16–24.

49. O'Brien WM, Bagby GF: Rare adverse reaction to nonsteroidal anti-inflammatory drugs. J Rheumatol 1985;12:785–790.

50. Okada H, Suzuki H, Awaya N, et al: Serious adverse effects induced by simultaneous administration of two nonsteroidal antiinflammatory drugs. South Med J 1993;86:1266–1268.

51. Okoneke S: Intoxication with pyrazolones. Br J Clin Pharmacokinet 1982;7:465–489.

52. Prescott L, Critchley J, Balali-Mood M: Phenylbutazone overdosage: Abnormal metabolism associated with hepatic and renal damage. Br Med J 1980;281:1106–1107.

53. Prescott LF: Liver damage with non-narcotic analgesics. Med Toxicol 1986;1(Suppl 1):44–56.

54. Raskin JB: Gastrointestinal effects of nonsteroidal anti-inflammatory therapy. Am J Med 1999;106(5B):3S–12S.

55. Runkel R, Chaplin M, Savelium H, et al: Pharmacokinetics of naproxen overdoses. Clin Pharmacol Toxicol 1976;20:269–277.

56. Ryback M: Hematologic effects of nonsteroidal antiinflammatory drugs. In: Borda I, Koff R, eds: Nonsteroidal Anti-Inflammatory Drugs: A Profile of Adverse Effects. Philadelphia, Hanley & Belfus, 1992:113–132.

57. Schapowal AG, Simm HU, Schmitz-Schumann M: Phenomenology, pathogenesis, diagnosis and treatment of aspirin-sensitive rhinosinusitis. Acta Otorhinolaryngol Belg 1995;49:235–250.

58. Segasothy M, Samad SA, Zulfigar A, Bennett WM: Chronic renal disease and papillary necrosis associated with the long-term use of nonsteroidal anti-inflammatory drugs as the sole or predominant analgesic. Am J Kidney Dis 1994;24:17–24.

59. Seibert K, Masferrer JL, Jiyi F, et al: The biochemical and pharmacological manipulation of cellular cyclooxygenase (COX) activity. Adv Prost Thromb Leuk Res 1990;21:45–51.

60. Singh G, Ramey DR, Morfeld D, et al: Gastrointestinal tract complications of nonsteroidal antiinflammatory drug treatment in rheumatoid arthritis. A prospective observational cohort study. Arch Intern Med 1996;156:1530–1536.

61. Smolinske S, Hall A, Vandenberg S, et al: Toxic effects of nonsteroidal antiinflammatory drugs in overdose. Drug Saf 1990;5:252–274.

62. Strong J, Wilson J, Douglas J, et al: Phenylbutazone self-poisoning treated by charcoal hemoperfusion. Anesthesiology 1979;34:1038–1040.

63. Szczeklik A, Gryglewshi R, Czerniawska-Myski G: Clinical patterns of hypersensitivity to nonsteroidal antiinflammatory drugs and their pathogenesis. J Allergy Clin Immunol 1997;60:276–284.

64. Tolman KG. Hepatotoxicity of non-narcotic analgesics. Am J Med 1998;105(1B):13S–19S.

65. Vane JR, Botting RM: New insights into the mode of action of antiinflammatory drugs. Inflamm Res 1995;44:1–10.

66. Veltri JC, Rollins DE: A comparison of the frequency and severity of poisoning cases for ingestion of acetaminophen, aspirin, and ibuprofen. Am J Emerg Med 1988;6:104–107.

67. Whelton A: Nephrotoxicity of nonsteroidal anti-inflammatory drugs: Physiologic foundations and clinical implications. Am J Med 1999;106(5B):13S–24S.

68. Wilde MI, McTavish D: Omeprazole. An update of its pharmacology and therapeutic use in acid-related disorders. Drugs 1994;48:91–132.

69. Willet LR, Carson JL, Strom BL: Epidemiology of gastrointestinal damage associated with nonsteroidal antiinflammatory drugs. Drug Saf 1994;10:170–181.

70. Zimmerman J, Siguencia J, Tsvang E: Upper gastrointestinal hemorrhage associated with cutaneous application of diclofenac gel. Am J Gastroenterol 1995;90:2032–2034.

Richard S. Weisman

$$CH_2CH_2NH_2$$

Histamine

An 18-year-old male was brought to the emergency department after informing his family that he ingested 100 (50 mg) diphenhydramine capsules in a suicide attempt 3 hours previously. An empty bottle was found on the floor. Upon initial evaluation, the patient was lethargic, had garbled speech, and became agitated when aroused. His initial vital signs were blood pressure, 200/90 mm Hg; pulse, 140 beats/min; respirations, 18 breaths/min; and rectal temperature of 101.2° F (38.4°C). His skin was dry and flushed. Examination of the head, eyes, ears, nose, and throat was remarkable only for pupils that were 6–7 mm and sluggishly reactive to light. His neck was supple. The chest and heart examination was normal and the abdominal examination was normal except for absent bowel sounds. The patient's neurologic status was notable for periods of lethargy alternating with agitation, disorientation to time and place, and myoclonic jerks. There was no evidence of tremor, asterixis, or meningeal irritation. Deep tendon reflexes were symmetric, and plantar flexion was elicited.

Oxygen was administered via nasal cannula at 8 L/min and a cardiac monitor was connected to the patient. Intravenous 0.9% sodium chloride was administered at a rate of 200 mL/h. Blood was sent to the laboratory for a complete blood count, electrolytes, glucose, and an acetaminophen level. A nasogastric tube was inserted for administration of 60 g of activated charcoal and 60 g of sorbitol. A Foley catheter was inserted and 700 mL of clear urine was immediately drained. An ECG revealed a sinus tachycardia at 140 beats/min with a QRS complex duration of 0.08 sec and a normal QTc interval of 0.3 sec.

One milligram of physostigmine was given intravenously over 5 minutes without a subsequent change in the patient's mental status or vital signs. However, his facial flush faded. There were no signs of salivation, lacrimation, or bronchorrhea from the physostigmine administration. Five minutes later the patient's vital signs were blood pressure, 180/110 mm Hg; pulse, 130 beats/min; and respirations 16 breaths/min. Bowel sounds remained absent. A repeat 1-mg dose of physostigmine was given intravenously over 5 minutes. The patient became alert and oriented over the next 3–5 minutes. His blood pressure and pulse fell to 140/90 mm Hg and 120 beats/min, respectively. Abdominal auscultation now revealed active bowel sounds. Laboratory analysis demonstrated a normal complete blood cell count (CBC), electrolytes, and glucose, and a zero acetaminophen level. The patient was admitted for observation, monitoring, and psychiatric assessment.

Twelve hours after initial presentation the patient remained alert and oriented, with no facial flushing. Vital signs were blood pressure, 146/88 mm Hg; pulse, 110 beats/min; respirations, 16 breaths/min;

rectal temperature, 100.0°F (37.8°C). At this time the Foley catheter was removed after which the patient was able to void spontaneously.

HISTORY AND EPIDEMIOLOGY

The H_1-receptor antagonists are the first group of antihistamines that were used to alleviate histamine-mediated symptoms of allergic reactions.[4] In contrast, the primary physiologic activity of the H_2 receptor antagonists is to reduce gastric acidity and treat urticaria. The receptors for a third group of antihistamines and antagonists, the H_3 receptors are located in the central nervous system. The agonists and antagonists which act at the H_3 receptors do not currently have therapeutic indications and are not further discussed.[3]

Antihistamines are available worldwide and many do not require a prescription.[5] Antihistamines are often used for the symptomatic relief of cold and allergy symptoms, as well as being found in nonprescription sleeping aids. Frequently ingested in suicide attempts, probably due to their ready availability,[13] unintentional exposures to antihistamine preparations are also very common with greater than 14,000 cases reported annually involving children younger than 6 years of age.[51] Although ingestion is usually the route of exposure, it is important to remember that toxicity can result from exposure to topical preparations that contain antihistamines. Those H_1 receptor antagonists that penetrate the blood-brain barrier more readily than others have been termed "first-generation antihistamines." Second-generation H_1-receptor antagonists are further classified by the US Food and Drug Administration as sedating or nonsedating.[70]

In February 1997, the US Food and Drug Administration suggested withdrawing the approval of all medications containing the second-generation H_1-blocker terfenadine because these agents predisposed to torsades de pointes and safer alternatives were available. In February 1998, the manufacturers voluntarily withdrew these agents. In June 1999, Janssen Pharmaceutica voluntarily withdrew Hismanal from the United States as a result of numerous similar adverse drug interactions that produced cardiac dysrhythmias. A review of the literature and databases of the FDA reveals that a much higher percentage of women than men develop torsades de pointes, and it has been hypothesized that gender differences in specific cardiac ion current densities are at least partly responsible.[23] Hismanal is still available in Canada, Mexico, and the Middle East.

The H_2 receptor antagonists became available shortly after the characterization of the H_2 receptor in 1972.[7] They are presently in widespread use for the treatment of peptic and duodenal ulcer disease, and acid hypersecretory states including Zollinger-Ellison syndrome. Less common indications include systemic mastocytosis and multiple endocrine adenomatosis. H_2 receptor antagonists also play a secondary role in the management of urticaria and anaphylaxis.

Decongestants are sympathomimetic agents that act on α-adrenergic receptors to produce vasoconstriction, to shrink swollen mucous membranes, and to improve ventilation. Ephedrine, the first agent of this class to be used pharmaceutically, can be extracted from various plants and was used in China for at least 2000 years before it was introduced in Western medicine in 1924.[14] Phenylephrine was first studied in 1910, but was not introduced into clinical medicine until the 1930s. The 20th century saw ephedrine used as a stimulant anorexiant usually in conjunction with caffeine and aspirin. The Food and Drug Administration does not approve its use for the treatment of obesity because of concerns over its safety profile and potential for abuse.

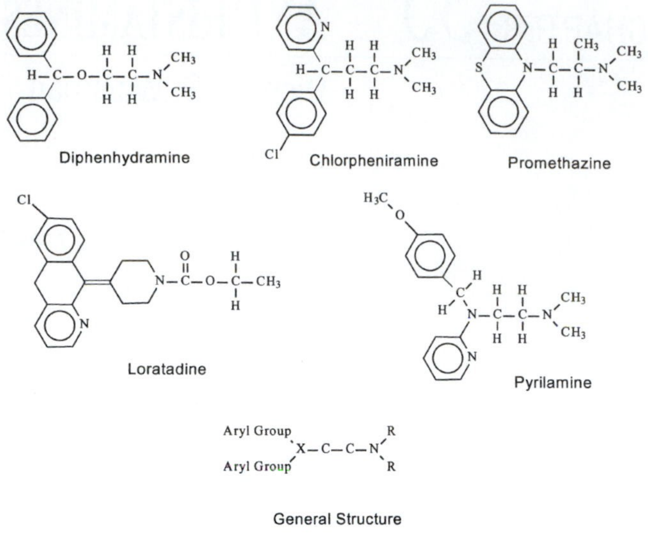

Figure 35–1. Structures of diverse H_1 receptor antagonists.

PHARMACOLOGY

H₁ Receptor Antagonists

There are histamine antagonists or antihistamines for each of the three different histamine-modulated receptor sites (H_1, H_2, H_3), allowing histamine to interact with G proteins in the plasma membranes.[30] The stimulation of H_1 receptors results in an increased synthesis of inositol-1,4,5-triphosphate and several diacylglycerols (DAGs) from phospholipids located in cell membranes. Inositol-1,4,5-triphosphate causes a release of calcium, which then activates calcium-calmodulin-dependent myosin light-chain kinase, resulting in enhanced cross-bridging and contraction.[52] The reaction at the H_1 receptors is mediated by phospholipase C.[3] H_2 receptor stimulation is mediated by adenyl cyclase activation of cyclic AMP-dependent protein kinase in smooth muscle and in parietal cells of the stomach and results in increased gastric acidity through stimulation of a H^+-K^+ ATPase pump.

There are six major classes of antihistamines. These include the first-generation derivatives of ethylenediamine, ethanolamine, the alkylamines, phenothiazines, and piperazines, and the peripherally selective or second-generation H_1 antagonists. Many of the older antihistamines are substituted ethylamine structures with a tertiary amino group linked by a 2- or 3-carbon chain with two aromatic groups.[30] This structure differs from histamine by the absence of a primary amino group and the presence of a single aromatic moiety. The structures of the pharmacologic classes of the antihistamines appear in Figure 35–1. Table 35–1 describes the peripheral selectivity of the antihistamines which is principally defined by the presence of diminished anticholinergic and sedative properties of the H_1 antagonists.

Some second-generation H_1 receptor antagonists, such as azelastine, a phthalazinone derivative, do not easily fit the standard classification scheme.[17,79,80,91] Cetirizine, fexofenadine, loratadine, azelastine (nasal spray), and ebastine share a distinct pharmacologic principle in that they all bind more selectively to peripheral rather than central H_1 receptors and have lower binding affinities for the cholinergic, α- and β-adrenergic receptor sites than do the first-generation antihistamines. This specificity for the peripheral histamine receptor sites eliminates many of the anticholinergic side effects, including central nervous system depression, blurred vision, dry mouth, tachycardia, and gastrointestinal effects. The relative incidence of anticholinergic and central nervous system adverse effects caused by these agents is similar to that produced by placebo.[2,17] However, sedation has been reported by some patients, especially if higher-than-recommended dosages are taken.[17]

H₂ Receptor Antagonists

These histamine congeners are very selective and competitively inhibit the H_2 receptor site. The original compound in this class, which retains the imidazole ring of histamine, is cimetidine (see Fig. 35–2). Although the newer compounds, such as ranitidine and famotidine, have replaced this ring with a furan or thiazole group, respectively, they retain significant similarity to the structure of histamine.[9]

Endogenous histamine is one of the triggers for gastric acid secretion by interaction with the H_2 receptor located on the gastric parietal cells. This results in an increase in adenylyl cyclase and cAMP, with activation of the H^+-K^+ ATPase pump and ultimately in the release of H^+ into the gastric lumen. In the treatment of peptic ulcer disease and gastroesophageal reflux disease (GERD), these H_2 receptor antagonists block the effects of histamine on the H_2 receptor. Their effectiveness is improved further by their concomitant alteration in the response of the parietal cell to acetylcholine and gastrin, two other stimulants for gastric acid secretion (Fig. 35–3). Important to note is that H_2 receptor antagonists have little effect elsewhere in the body, and that these drugs have weak central nervous system (CNS) penetration secondary to their hydrophilic properties.[9]

Decongestants

Decongestants are pharmacologically active following topical or oral administration. Absorption is rapid from the gastrointestinal

TABLE 35–1.   Antihistamines

Antihistamine	Anticholinergic Class	Sedation	Duration of Action	Typical Adult Dose
Acrivastine	Alkylamine	+	6–8 h	8 mg tid
Azatadine	Piperidine	+	12 h	1–2 mg bid
Brompheniramine	Alkylamine	++	4–6 h	4 mg qid
Buclizine	Piperazine	++	4–6 h	50 mg bid
Carbinoxamine	Ethanolamine	++++	3–6 h	4–8 mg qid
Cetirizine	Piperazine	+	12 h	5–10 mg qid
Chlorpheniramine	Alkylamine	++	4–6 h	4 mg qid
Clemastine	Ethanolamine	++++	12–24 h	2 mg bid
Dexbrompheniramine	Alkylamine	++	12 h	3–12 mg bid
Dexchlorpheniramine	Alkylamine	++	3–6 h	4–6 mg tid
Dimenhydrinate	Ethanolamine	++++	4–6 h	50–100 mg qid
Dimethindene	Alkylamine	++	8 h	1–2 mg tid
Diphenhydramine	Ethanolamine	++++	4–6 h	25–50 mg qid
Doxylamine	Ethanolamine	++++	6 h	7.5–12.5 mg qid
Fexofenadine	Piperidine	+	12 h	60 mg bid
Hydroxyzine	Piperazine	++	6–8 h	25 mg qid
Loratadine	Piperidine	+	8–12 h	10 mg qd
Meclizine	Piperazine	++	6–8 h	25 mg tid
Pheniramine	Alkylamine	++	4–6 h	5–15 mg q4h
Phenyltoloxamine	Ethanolamine	++++	4–8 h	7.5–25 mg tid
Promethazine	Phenothiazine	++++	4–6 h	12.5–25 mg qid
Trimeprazine	Phenothiazine	++++	4–6 h	2.5 mg qid
Tripelennamine	Ethylenediamine	+++	4–6 h	25–50 mg qid
Triprolidine	Alkylamine	++	4–6 h	2.5 mg qid

tract with peak blood levels occurring within 2–4 hours of ingestion. Oral decongestants can affect the cardiovascular, urinary, central nervous, and endocrine systems.[8,11,20] The decongestants phenylephrine, pseudoephedrine, ephedrine, and phenylpropanolamine (see Fig. 35–4) reduce nasal congestion by stimulating the α-adrenergic receptor sites on vascular smooth muscles.[47] This results in the constriction of dilated arterioles and reduces blood flow to engorged nasal vascular beds. The α_1-mediated decrease in volume ultimately lowers resistance to airflow. Prolonged topical administration may produce rebound congestion upon discontinuation, possible mechanisms of which include the desensitization of receptors and mucosal damage. This damage is thought to be caused by the α_1-mediated arteriolar constriction resulting in a decrease in the nutritional supply to the mucosa. Therefore, selective α_1 agonists may cause less mucosal damage.[42]

Phenylephrine is a powerful α-adrenergic receptor agonist with very little β-adrenergic agonist activity.[6] Pseudoephedrine and ephedrine are direct acting nonspecific $\alpha_{1,2}$- and $\beta_{1,2}$-adrenergic receptor stimulants. Pseudoephedrine is the *d*-isomer of ephedrine and has only 25% of the adrenergic receptor activity of ephedrine.[21] Phenylpropanolamine is an $\alpha_{1,2}$-adrenergic receptor stimulant devoid of any β-adrenergic receptor activity. Phenylpropanolamine can directly stimulate $\alpha_{1,2}$ receptors and can indirectly stimulate these receptors by causing a release of norepinephrine (see Table 35–2).

The imidazoline category of sympathomimetics are generally reserved for topical application and their local effects in the nasal passages and the eye. The more common medications include oxymetazoline hydrochloride, tetrahydrozoline hydrochloride, and naphazoline hydrochloride (see Fig. 35–5).[42] Their vasoconstrictor effects are mediated by their actions as α-adrenergic agonists, with binding to $\alpha_{1,2}$ receptors on blood vessels. The α_1-mediated vasoconstriction is complemented by an additive effect of a preferential binding to α_2 receptors located on resistance vessels regulating blood flow. In addition, these compounds show high affinity for imidazoline receptors, which are located in the ventrolateral medulla and some peripheral tissues. Stimulation of imidazoline receptors produces a sympatholytic effect with resultant bradycardia and hypotension (Chap. 10).

All imidazoline preparations have a relatively rapid onset of action, with 60% of maximum effectiveness after only 20 minutes. Oxymetazoline is the only compound with a duration of action greater than 8 hours; the other preparations average a duration of action of approximately 4 hours.[41]

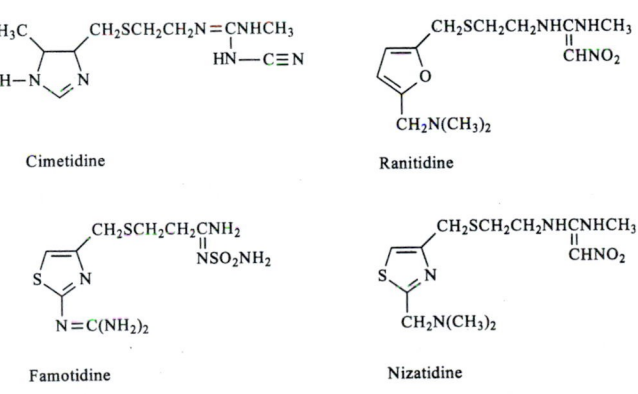

Figure 35–2.   Structures of H_2 receptor antagonists.

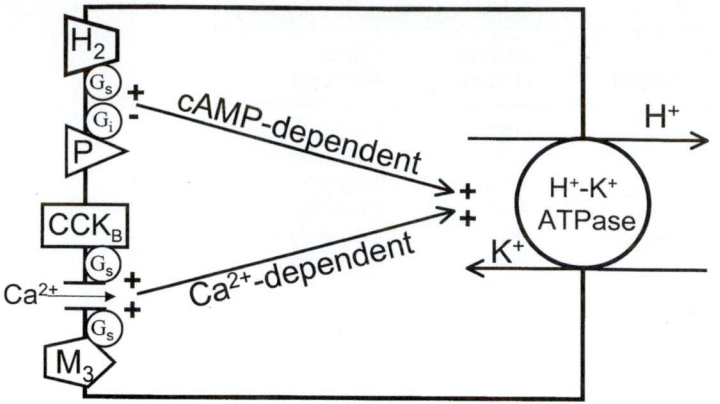

Figure 35–3. Schematic representation of a gastric parietal cell demonstrating the mechanism of hydrogen ion secretion into the lumen. Gastric acid is modulated by both calcium dependent and cyclic adenosine monophosphate (cAMP) dependent pathways. Histamine binding to the H_2 receptor increases gastric acidity by increasing cAMP through a stimulatory G protein (G_s). Prostaglandins decrease gastric acidity by decreasing cAMP through an inhibitory G protein (G_i). Both acetylcholine and gastrin increase gastric acidity by increasing the influx of calcium through G_s interactions. Acetylcholine binds at the muscarinic$_3$ (M_3) receptor, while gastrin binds at the cholecystokinin$_B$ (CCK_B) receptor.

PHARMACOKINETICS AND TOXICOKINETICS

H$_1$ Receptor Antagonists

The antihistamines are generally well-absorbed following oral administration and most achieve peak plasma concentrations within 2–3 hours. Although less-well studied, dermal absorption appears to be consequential, especially with extensive or prolonged application to abnormal skin. The maximum antihistaminic effect, however, occurs several hours after peak serum concentrations. The duration of action ranges from 3 hours to more than 24 hours; much longer than would be predicted from the extremely variable serum elimination half-life values of the antihistamines.[79] Hepatic metabolism is the primary route of metabolism for the antihistamines.[71] Many Asian patients can acetylate therapeutic concentrations of diphenhydramine to a nontoxic metabolite twice as rapidly as patients of caucasian descent, making Asians much less sensitive to both the psychomotor and sedative effects.[82]

Terfenadine and astemizole are extensively metabolized by the cytochrome P450 isoenzyme CYP3A4 to the active metabolites terfenadine carboxylate and desmethylastemizole, respectively. Terfenadine carboxylate, which possesses peripheral antihistaminic activity, is further metabolized via carboxylate oxidation to produce an inactive metabolite with a terminal half-life of 17 hours.[26] The active metabolite desmethylastemizole has a much longer half-life of 19 days.[35,54] Drugs, such as those listed in Table 11–6 which inhibit the cytochrome P450 isoenzyme CYP3A4,

delay metabolism, causing accumulation of both terfenadine and astemizole.[43] These parent compounds block potassium efflux, and can result in life-threatening cardiac dysrhythmias, particularly torsades de pointes.[16,19, 22,33,62,74,83,84,86] Although no longer available in the United States, these compounds are still sold in Europe and South America.

H$_2$ Receptor Antagonists

Cimetidine is the prototypical H_2 receptor antagonist. Table 35–3 lists the other available H_2 receptor antagonists. Cimetidine is rapidly and completely absorbed following oral administration. Cimetidine has a volume of distribution of approximately 2 L/kg with 13–25% protein binding.[1] Up to 75% of cimetidine is eliminated unchanged in the urine, 15% is metabolized by the liver, and 10% is found unchanged in the stool.[69] The elimination half-life in patients with normal renal function is approximately 2 hours but this is substantially prolonged with impaired renal function.[1] Cimetidine is responsible for numerous drug-drug interactions because it can inhibit cytochrome P450 activity, thereby impairing hepatic drug metabolism, and it can reduce hepatic blood flow, resulting in decreased clearance of drugs highly extracted by the liver (Chap. 11).[81] None of the other currently available H_2 receptor antagonists inhibit the cytochrome P450 oxidase system.[33] Additionally, by altering gastric pH, cimetidine and all the other H_2 antagonists may alter the absorption of acid-labile drugs. Finally, cimetidine is associated with myelosuppression if administered with drugs capable of causing bone marrow suppression.[75]

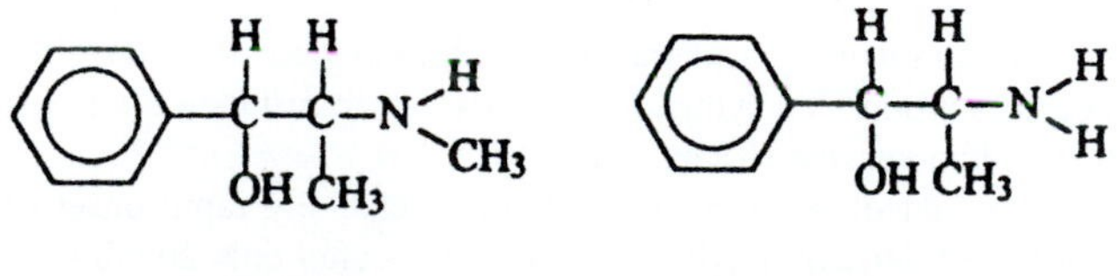

Figure 35–4. Structures of ephedrine and phenylpropanolamine.

Ephedrine

Phenylpropanolamine

TABLE 35–2. Decongestants

Decongestant	Class	Duration of Action	Alpha/Beta Activity
Ephedrine	Sympathomimetic	3–5 h	$\alpha_{1,2}$ and $\beta_{1,2}$
Naphazoline	Imidazoline	8 h	α_2
Oxymetazoline	Imidazoline	6–7 h	α_2
Phenylephrine	Sympathomimetic	1 h	$\alpha_{1,2}$
Phenylpropanolamine	Sympathomimetic	12 h (sustained release)	$\alpha_{1,2}$
Pseudoephedrine	Sympathomimetic	3–4 h	$\alpha_{1,2}$ and $\beta_{1,2}$
Tetrahydrozoline	Imidazoline	4–8 h	α_2
Xylometazoline	Imidazoline	5–6 h	α_2

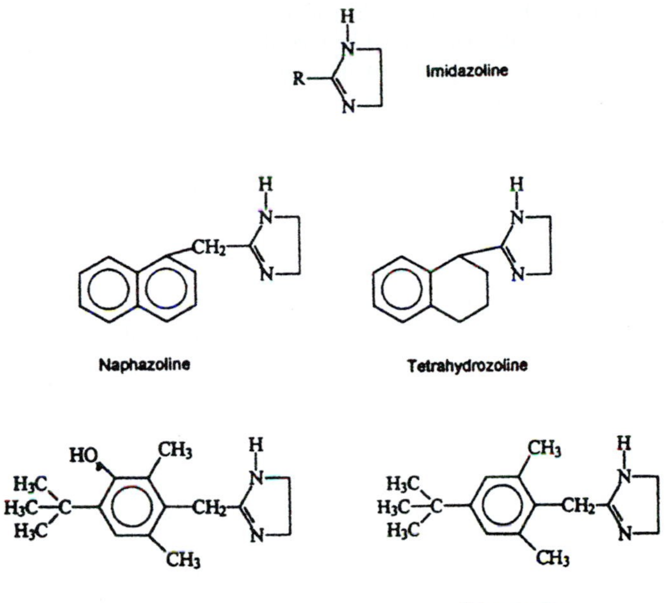

Figure 35–5. Structures of imidazoline decongestants naphazoline, tetrahydrozoline, oxymetazoline, and xylometazoline.

Decongestants

The imidazoline decongestants such as oxymetazoline and naphazoline are pure central and peripheral α_2-adrenergic receptor agonists; tetrahydrozoline stimulates α_2-receptors and H_2 receptors. These medications are primarily used as nasal decongestants. Tetrahydrozoline is available without prescription as an ophthalmic preparation to decrease eye irritation and redness. The imidazolines are rapidly absorbed from both the gastrointestinal tract and mucous membranes. The elimination half-lives of these agents range from 2–4 hours.

CLINICAL MANIFESTATIONS

H₁ Receptor Antagonists

The clinical manifestations of H_1 receptor antagonist overdose are largely extensions of adverse effects noted with therapeutic use of these agents. Although dry mouth and mydriasis are common, se-

dation is the most serious adverse effect at therapeutic dosing, with recent data demonstrating that therapeutic antihistamine use is as incapacitating as ethanol intoxication in a model of motor vehicle operation.[36] Following exposure to an excessive amount of a first-generation H_1 antihistamine, most patients present with CNS depression and excessive anticholinergic symptoms. These typically include mydriasis, tachycardia, fever, dry mucous membranes, urinary retention, diminished bowel sounds, and disorientation (Table 35–4). The patient's skin may appear flushed and warm and even if the patient is agitated there will be a notable absence of sweat. Agitation concomitant with the inability to sweat potentially results in hyperthermia that can be correlated with the extent of agitation, the ambient temperature and humidity, and the length of time during which the patient has been unable to dissipate heat. Patients who have ingested the second-generation antihistamines cetirizine, fexofenadine, or loratadine usually do not have significant CNS depression or anticholinergic symptoms.

In a review of 136 patients with diphenhydramine overdose, somnolence, lethargy, or coma occurred in approximately 55% of patients, whereas 15% experienced a catatonic stupor.[53] Several reports suggest that young children experience more respiratory complications,[76] CNS stimulation, anticholinergic symptoms, and seizures than do adult patients.[93] In a placebo-controlled study comparing the CNS effects of first- and second-generation H_1-receptor antagonists, the second-generation agents caused less cognitive dysfunction and somnolence.[17,44] This finding was corroborated in the simulated driving model, in which loratadine produced significantly less impairment than diphenhydramine.[36] Elderly patients are more susceptible to adverse events, because renal and hepatic dysfunction, which is more common in the elderly, delays metabolism of the antihistamines.[44]

Mydriasis develops at both therapeutic and toxic doses with most patients describing blurred vision and/or diplopia. Both vertical and horizontal nystagmus occur in diphenhydramine overdose.[18] Other symptoms of overdose may include adverse drug reactions associated with diphenhydramine. These include central nervous system effects such as seizures, hallucinations, acute extrapyramidal movement disorders, and psychoses.[50,57,58,93]

Sinus tachycardia is a consistent finding following an overdose of an antihistamine with anticholinergic effects. Both hypotension and hypertension may occur with sinus tachycardia.[61] These findings probably relate more to the patient's age, volume status, and vascular tone than to a specific class of antihistamines. As a result of the sodium channel blockade following a large diphenhydramine overdose, prolongation of both the QRS complexes and QT intervals may occur.[38,65,73]

TABLE 35–3. Pharmacology of Histamine H₂ Receptor Antagonists

Drug	Typical Adult Dose (mg)	Volume of Distribution (L/kg)	Protein Binding (%)	Half-Life (hours)	Urinary Elimination (%)
Cimetidine	800	1.0	19	2.0	62
Ranitidine	300	1.3	15	2.1	69
Nizatidine	300	1.2	28	1.3	61
Famotidine	40	1.3	17	2.6	67

TABLE 35–4. Anticholinergic Symptoms

Central	Peripheral
Agitation	Hypertension
Hallucinations	Tachycardia
Confusion	Hyperthermia
Sedation	Mydriasis
Coma	Dry, flushed skin
Seizures	Urinary retention

Rhabdomyolysis can occur in patients with extreme agitation or seizures following an H_1 antihistamine overdose. Rhabdomyolysis was reported in 7 patients with doxylamine overdoses in the absence of trauma or any of the other common etiologies such as seizures, shock, or crush injuries. Rhabdomyolysis is also reported as a rare adverse event following diphenhydramine overdose.[27,28,63]

H_2 Receptor Antagonists

Acute toxic effects appear to be extremely rare even following large (20 g) oral ingestions of cimetidine.[46] One patient developed tachycardia, dilated and sluggishly reactive pupils, and slurred speech following a 12-g ingestion of cimetidine.[69] Bradycardia, hypotension, and cardiac arrest have followed rapid intravenous administration of cimetidine in seriously ill patients.[78] Famotidine and ranitidine produce even fewer dose-related toxicities in overdose, and they are less likely to induce or inhibit the cytochrome P450 enzyme system, thereby producing fewer drug-drug interactions.[45,66]

Decongestants

Following a decongestant overdose, most patients will present with central nervous system stimulation, hypertension, tachycardia, or reflex bradycardia (in response to pure α-adrenergic agonist-induced hypertension only). Approximately 4–5 times the recommended dose of pseudoephedrine[21] or phenylpropanolamine is required to cause hypertension.[25] An increase in sinus dysrhythmias is reported in adults with the ingestion of 120 mg of pseudoephedrine and moderate exercise.[8,11,15] Headache was the most common initial symptom (39%) reported by patients who later developed severe toxicity.[55] Approximately 36% of patients with phenylpropanolamine overdoses present with central nervous system depression.[56] In more severe exposures, seizures,[20] myocardial infarction,[59] bradycardia, atrial and ventricular dysrhythmias, ischemic bowel infarction,[48] and cerebral hemorrhages are reported.[24,64] In 45 patients who developed hypertensive encephalopathy from the ingestion of phenylpropanolamine, 24 patients developed intracranial hemorrhages, 15 developed seizures, and 6 died.[55] In a review of 500 reports of adverse reactions from patients who had ingested ephedrine and such associated stimulants as dietary supplements, 8 fatalities from myocardial infarction and cerebral hemorrhage were reported.[72] Symptoms of toxicity from decongestants usually resolve within 8–16 hours. However, symptoms may persist for greater than 24 hours if a sustained-release product has been ingested.

Decongestants rarely cause systemic toxicity because of poor absorption. When ingested the imidazoline decongestants naphazoline, oxymetazoline, tetrahydrozoline, and xylometazoline are potent central and peripheral α_2-adrenergic and imidazoline receptor stimulants, and in overdose, can cause central nervous system depression, hypotension, bradycardia, and respiratory depression.[40] Children are particularly sensitive to the effects of the imidazoline decongestants.[49]

MANAGEMENT
General

On initial presentation the patient who is likely to develop a severe complication may not be easily distinguished from the patient who will have a benign course. The patient's vital signs must be monitored. The individual should be placed on a cardiac monitor, observed for the development of seizures and dysrhythmias, and treated when appropriate. Once intravenous access is established, blood should be obtained for an acetaminophen level because many cough and cold products combine an antihistamine or decongestant with acetaminophen. Early recognition of those at high risk for toxicity can be determined only by performing serial assessments of vital signs and mental status. Particular attention should be given to the patient's temperature and heart rate, as these findings are usually indicative of increasing toxicity. The patient who will require more than supportive care will have unstable vital signs or a mental status that either fails to improve or that deteriorates after several hours. The potential for clinical deterioration necessitates that the patient be managed in a critical care environment where gastrointestinal decontamination can be performed and where life support is immediately available if stabilization of the airway, cardiovascular, or thermoregulatory systems becomes necessary.

A patient with an abnormal neuropsychiatric examination following the ingestion of a decongestant should be evaluated for cerebral hemorrhage by a noncontrast head CT scan and subsequently a lumbar puncture if indicated.[55]

Specific Therapy

H_1 Receptor Antagonists. Most patients with antihistamine overdose will present with central nervous system depression and tachycardia, which can be managed initially with supportive care. The induction of emesis with syrup of ipecac is not recommended for patients with antihistamine overdoses. The administration of syrup of ipecac delays the administration of activated charcoal, which may be the most beneficial therapeutic intervention. A slurry of 1 g/kg of body weight of activated charcoal mixed in water and administered by mouth, is appropriate in the management of patients with antihistamine overdose when the drug is still expected to be accessible in the stomach. If the patient has significant CNS depression, lacks a gag reflex, or is unable to protect the airway, endotracheal intubation should be considered and the activated charcoal should be administered through a nasogastric tube. Orogastric lavage is rarely indicated to decontaminate the GI tract except for a massive antihistamine overdose. Multiple doses of activated charcoal are recommended for adjunctive treatment of significant antihistamine overdose because anticholinergic-induced alterations in gastrointestinal motility may greatly prolong time to peak drug serum concentrations.[32]

If the patient is hypotensive, 0.9% sodium chloride or lactated Ringer's solution should be administered and the patient should receive supplemental high-flow oxygen to maintain an adequate oxygen saturation level. If the desired increase in blood pressure is not attained, dopamine or norepinephrine may be titrated to achieve an acceptable blood pressure. In one instance, cardiogenic shock and myocardial depression resulting from a 10 g ingestion of pyrilamine maleate could only be reversed with an intra-aortic balloon counterpulsation device.[29] This approach represents a rarely needed but potentially useful intervention.

The sodium channel blocking (type IA antidysrhythmic) properties of diphenhydramine may lead to wide complex dysrhythmias that resemble cyclic antidepressant overdose (see Chaps. 52 and 57).[38,73] While not well characterized, this manifestation of toxicity is usually only associated with consequential toxicity. As would be expected based on theoretical grounds, recent work demonstrates that hypertonic sodium bicarbonate can reverse diphenhydramine-associated conduction abnormalities.[77]

Agitation, hallucinations, and psychosis can often be treated with the administration of either physostigmine or a benzodiazepine such as diazepam (see Antidotes in Depth: Physostigmine). If the ECG manifests a wide QRS complex, or if there is uncertainty about the safety of using physostigmine, it should not be used; instead, agitation should be managed with an intravenous benzodiazepine such as diazepam 5–10 mg (0.1 mg/kg). In a retrospective comparison of physostigmine and benzodiazepines, physostigmine was found to be safer and more effective for treating anticholinergic agitation and delirium when used in patients who did not have intraventricular conduction delays.[10]

Physostigmine can be an extremely effective antidote for anticholinergic toxicity. Physostigmine can be used safely when the patient has both peripheral and central anticholinergic effects (see Table 35–4), a narrow QRS complex on an ECG, and no history of exposure to other agents (IA and IC antidysrhythmics) that may cause intraventricular conduction delays. Physostigmine use is contraindicated with the class IA or IC sodium-channel-blocking antidysrhythmic agents include carbamazepine, cocaine, cyclic antidepressants, mesoridazine, propoxyphene, or thioridazine.

The anticipated benefits of physostigmine must outweigh the potential risks prior to use. Benefits of physostigmine include, restoring gastrointestinal motility and eliminating agitation, thereby obviating the need for a CT scan or lumbar puncture when normal mental status returns.

To safely administer physostigmine the patient should be connected to a cardiac monitor and secure intravenous access should be established. Physostigmine (1–2 mg adults; 0.5 mg children) should then be administered by *slow* intravenous push with continuous monitoring of vital signs, breath sounds, and oxygen saturation by pulse oximetry. The initial dose of physostigmine may be repeated at 5–10-minute intervals if anticholinergic symptoms are not reversed and cholinergic symptoms such as salivation, diaphoresis, bradycardia, lacrimation, urination, or defecation do not develop. When improvement occurs as a result of physostigmine, it may be necessary to readminister the physostigmine at 30–60-minute intervals. With each readministration, the minimum dose to reverse anticholinergic toxicity must be determined. A dose of intravenous atropine that is one-half of the dose of physostigmine should be available at the patient's bedside to treat cholinergic toxicity if it occurs (see Antidotes in Depth: Physostigmine).

The presence of agitation should heighten the awareness that hyperthermia may be present or may develop. When the patient's temperature is 40.5°C (104.9°F) or higher, or if the temperature is rising rapidly, immediate cooling with ice bath or cold water mist and fan is indicated.

Grand mal seizures should be treated with an intravenous benzodiazepine such as diazepam 10 mg (0.1–0.2 mg/kg in children) or lorazepam with repeated dosing as necessary. Seizures refractory to the benzodiazepine, should be treated with phenobarbital or general anesthesia and paralysis with a neuromuscular blocking agent if necessary. Additionally, proper fluid management is necessary to prevent the precipitation of myoglobin as a result of rhabdomyolysis.

H$_2$ Receptor Antagonists. Patients who have overdosed on an H$_2$ antihistamine need only be given 1 g/kg of body weight of activated charcoal mixed for gastrointestinal decontamination. H$_2$-antihistamine antagonists rarely result in significant toxicity and therefore do not warrant exposure to the risks of complications from orogastric lavage or emesis.

Decongestants. Patients who have overdosed on a decongestant generally should only receive 1 g/kg of body weight of activated charcoal; syrup of ipecac should rarely be used in the home, and orogastric lavage should be reserved only for life-threatening ingestions within the previous hour.

Extreme agitation, seizures, tachycardia, hypertension, and psychosis should initially be treated with the administration of oxygen and a benzodiazepine such as diazepam 5–10 mg (0.1 mg/kg in children). Intravenous benzodiazepines may be repeated as necessary until agitation is controlled and the patient is resting comfortably. A patient who remains hypertensive may be treated with phentolamine, an α-adrenergic antagonist, or nitroprusside, a venous and arterial vasodilator.

General anesthesia and or paralysis with a neuromuscular blocking agent may be necessary to treat seizures that are refractory to IV benzodiazepines and phenobarbital.

Ventricular dysrhythmias from decongestant ingestions should be treated with standard doses of lidocaine.[85] If the dysrhythmia fails to respond to lidocaine, propranolol can be administered.[60]

Phenylpropanolamine ingestions may cause hypertension with a reflex bradycardia with an atrioventricular block that is responsive to standard doses of atropine.[87] Atropine must be used with caution because it can cause a dangerous increase in blood pressure as the reflex bradycardia is reversed. Therefore, a direct acting vasodilator such as phentolamine or nitroprusside is preferred, because by reversing the hypertension, the stimulus for the bradycardia is also corrected.

SUMMARY

The popularity and availability of antihistamines and decongestants make them readily accessible for deliberate or unintentional ingestions in both adults and children. Fortunately, almost all patients exposed to excessive doses of both of these types of medications and treated with activated charcoal, continuous assessment and management of abnormal vital signs, electrocardiogram, and mental status will have an excellent outcome and no adverse sequelae. Familiarity with the more severe complications of antihistamine and decongestant overdoses will result in early and appropriate interventions to reduce both morbidity and mortality from these exposures.

REFERENCES

1. Abate MA, Hyneck ML, Cohen IA, et al: Cimetidine pharmacokinetics. Clin Pharm 1982;1:225–233.
2. Ament PW, Paterson A: Drug interactions with the nonsedating antihistamines [review]. Am Fam Physician 1997;56:223–231.
3. Arrang JM, Garbarg M, Lacelot JC, et al: Highly potent and selective ligands for histamine H$_3$ receptors. Nature 1987;327:117–123.
4. Ash ASF, Schild HO: Receptors mediating some actions of histamine. Br J Pharmacol 1966;27:427–439.
5. Ashworth L: Is my antihistamine safe? Home Care Provider 1997;2:117–120.
6. Barger G, Dale HH: Chemical structure and sympathomimetic action of amines. J Physiol (London) 1910;41:19–59.

7. Black JW, Duncan WAM, Durant CJ, et al: Definition and antagonism of histamine H_2 receptors. Nature 1972;236:385–390.

8. Bright TP, Sandage BW Jr, Fletcher HP: Selected cardiac and metabolic responses to pseudoephedrine with exercise. J Clin Pharmacol 1981;21:488–492.

9. Brunton LB: Agents for control of gastric acidity and treatment of peptic ulcers. In: Hardman JG, Limbird CE, Molinoff PB, Ruddon RW, eds: Goodman and Gilman's The Pharmacologic Basis of Therapeutics, 9th ed.. New York, McGraw-Hill, 1996, pp. 901–907.

10. Burns MJ, Linden CH, Graudins A, et al: A comparison of physostigmine and benzodiazepines for the treatment of anticholinergic poisoning. Ann Emerg Med 2000;35:374–381.

11. Burton BT, Rice M, Schmertzler LE: Atrioventricular block following overdose of decongestant cold medication. J Emerg Med 1985;2:415–419.

12. Cavero I, Mestre M, Guillon JM, et al: Preclinical in vitro cardiac electrophysiology—A method of predicting arrhythmogenic potential of antihistamines in humans? Drug Saf 1999;21:19–31.

13. Cetaruk EW, Aaron CK: Hazards of nonprescription medications. Curr Controv Toxicol 1994;12:483–510.

14. Chen KK, Schmidt CF: Ephedrine and related substances. Medicine (Baltimore), 1930;9:1–117.

15. Conway EE, Walsh CA, Palomba AL: Supraventricular tachycardia following the administration of phenylpropanolamine in an infant. Pediatr Emerg Care 1989;5:173–174.

16. Davies AJ, Harinda V, McEwan A, Ghose RR: Cardiotoxic effect with convulsions in terfenadine overdose. BMJ 1989;298:325.

17. Day J: Pros and cons of the use of antihistamines in managing allergic rhinitis [review]. J Allergy Clin Immunol 1999;103:S395–S399.

18. Daya L, Spyker DA, Hendin P, et al: Massive diphenhydramine overdose: A case report and comparison of pharmacokinetic models [abstract]. Vet Hum Toxicol 1991;33:357.

19. Delpon E, Valenzuela C, Tamargo J: Blockade of cardiac potassium and other channels by antihistamines [review]. Drug Saf 1999;21:11–18.

20. Dilsaver SC, Votolato NA, Alessi NE: Complications of phenylpropanolamine. Am Fam Physician 1989;39:201–206.

21. Drew CDM, Knight GT, Hughes DTD: Comparison of the effects of D-ephedrine and L-pseudoephedrine on the cardiovascular and respiratory systems in man. Br J Clin Pharmacol 1978;6:221–225.

22. Dubuske LM: Second-generation antihistamines—The risk of ventricular arrhythmias [review]. Clin Ther 1999;21:281–295.

23. Ebert SN, Liu XK, Woosley RL: Female gender as a risk factor for drug-induced cardiac arrhythmias—Evaluation of clinical and experimental evidence [review]. J Womens Health 1998;7:547–557.

24. Edwards M, Russo L, Harwood-Nuss A: Cerebral infarction with a single oral dose of phenylpropanolamine. Am J Emerg Med 1987;5:163–164.

25. Ekins BR, Spoerke DG: An estimation of the toxicity of non-prescription diet aids from seventy exposure cases. Vet Hum Toxicol 1983;25:81–85.

26. Eller MG, Okerholm RA: Effect of cimetidine on terfenadine and terfenadine metabolite pharmacokinetics. Pharm Res 1991;7:206–210.

27. Emadian SM, Caravati EM, Herr RD: Rhabdomyolysis—A rare adverse effect of diphenhydramine overdose. Am J Emerg Med 1996;14:574–576.

28. Frankel D, Dolgin J, Murray BM: Non-traumatic rhabdomyolysis complicating antihistamine overdose. J Toxicol Clin Toxicol 1993;31:493–496.

29. Freedberg RS, Friedman GR, Palu RN, Feit F: Cardiogenic shock due to antihistamine overdose: Reversal with intra-aortic balloon counterpulsation. JAMA 1987;257:660–661.

30. Ganellin CR, Parsons ME, eds: Pharmacology of Histamine Receptors. Bristol, MA, Wright/PSG, 1982, pp. 1–43.

31. Gras J, Llenas J: Effects of H_1 antihistamines on animal models of QTc prolongation. Drug Saf 1999;21:39–44.

32. Guay DR, Meatherall RC, Macaulay PA, et al: Activated charcoal adsorption of diphenhydramine. Int J Clin Pharmacol Ther Toxicol 1984;22:395–400.

33. Hansten PD. Drug interactions of gastrointestinal drugs. In: Lewis JH, ed: A Pharmacologic Approach to Gastrointestinal Disorders. Baltimore, Williams & Wilkins, 1994, pp. 47–74.

34. Hardin AS, Padilla F: Agranulocytosis during therapy with a brompheniramine medication. J Ark Med Soc 1978;75:206–208.

35. Heidemann SM, Sarnaik AP: Arrhythmias after astemizole overdose. Pediatr Emerg Care 1996;12:102–104.

36. Hennessy S, Strom BL: Non-sedating antihistamines should be preferred over sedating antihistamines in patients who drive. Ann Intern Med 2000;132:405–407.

37. Henry DA, Lowe JM, Donelly T: Jaundice during cyproheptadine treatment. Br Med J 1978;1:753.

38. Hestand HE, Teske DW: Diphenhydramine hydrochloride intoxication. J Pediatr 1977;90:1017–1018.

39. Heyman SN, Mevorach D, Ghanem J: Hypertensive crisis from chronic intoxication with nasal decongestant and cough medications. Ann Pharmacother 1991;25:1068–1070.

40. Higgins GL, Campbell B, Wallace K, et al: Pediatric poisoning from over-the-counter imidazoline-containing products. Ann Emerg Med 1991;20:655–658.

41. Hochban W, Althoff H, Ziegler A: Nasal decongestion with imidazoline derivatives: Acoustic rhinometry measurements. Eur J Clin Pharmacol 1999;55:7–12.

42. Hoffman BB, Lefkowitz RJ: Catecholamines, sympathomimetic drugs, and adrenergic receptor antagonists. In: Hardman JG, Limbird CE, Molinoff PB, Ruddon RW, eds: Goodman and Gilman's The Pharmacologic Basis of Therapeutics, 9th ed. New York, McGraw-Hill, 1996, pp. 221–224.

43. Honig PK, Woosley RL, Zamini K, et al: Changes in the pharmacokinetics and electrocardiographic pharmacodynamics of terfenadine with concomitant administration of erythromycin. Clin Pharmacol Ther 1992;52:231–238.

44. Horak F, Stubner UP: Comparative tolerability of second generation antihistamines. Drug Saf 1999;20:385–401.

45. Humphries TJ, Merritt GJ: Review article: Drug interactions with agents used to treat acid-related diseases. Aliment Pharmacol Ther 1999;13(Suppl 3):18–26.

46. Illingworth RN, Jarvie DR: Absence of toxicity in cimetidine overdosage. Br Med J 1979;1:453–454.

47. Johnson DA, Hricik JG: The pharmacology of alpha-adrenergic decongestants. Pharmacotherapy 1993;13:110S–115S.

48. Johnson DA, Stafford PW, Volpe RJ: Ischemic bowel infarction and phenylpropanolamine use. West J Med 1985;142:399–400.

49. Jones DG, Osterhoudt K, Stone M, et al: Sinoatrial node dysfunction following tetrahydrozoline (Visine) ingestion. J Toxicol Clin Toxicol 1996;34:564.

50. Jones IH, Stevenson J, Jordan A, et al: Pheniramine as an hallucinogen. Med J Aust 1973;1:382–386.

51. Jumbelic MI, Hanzlick R, Cohle S: Alkylamine antihistamine toxicity and review of pediatric toxicology registry of the National Association of Medical Examiners. Report 4: Alkylamines. Am J Forensic Med Pathol 1997;18:65–69.

52. Kamm KE, Stull JT: The function of myosin and myosin light-chain kinase phosphorylation in smooth muscle. Annu Rev Pharmacol Toxicol 1985;25:593–620.

53. Koppel C, Ibe K, Tenczer J: Clinical symptomatology of diphenhydramine overdose: An evaluation of 136 cases, 1982 to 1985. J Toxicol Clin Toxicol 1987;25:53–70.

54. Krestansky PM, Cluxton RJ Jr: Astemizole: A long-acting nonsedating antihistamine. Drug Intell Clin Pharm 1987;21:947–953.

55. Lake CR, Gallant S, Masson E, et al: Adverse drug effects attributed to phenylpropanolamine: A review of 142 case reports. Am J Med 1990;89:195–208.

56. Larson WL, Rogers A: Overdosage from phenylpropanolamine: Experience of the Hennepin Regional Poison Center. Vet Hum Toxicol 1986;28:546–548.

57. Lavenstein BL, Cantor FK: Acute dystonia: An unusual reaction to diphenhydramine. JAMA 1976;236:291.

58. Leighton KM: Paranoid psychosis after abuse of Actifed. Br Med J 1982;284:789–790.

59. Leo PJ, Hollander JE, Shih RD, Marcus SM: Phenylpropanolamine and associated myocardial infarction. Ann Emerg Med 1996;28: 359–362.

60. Liddle GG: Phenylpropanolamine induced dysrhythmias. JAMA 1973;223:324–326.

61. Llenas J, Cardelus I, Heredia A, et al: Cardiotoxicity of histamine and the possible role of histamine in the arrhythmogenesis produced by certain antihistamines. Drug Saf 1999;21:33–38.

62. MacConnell TJ, Stanner AJ: Torsades de pointes complicating treatment with terfenadine [letter]. BMJ 1991;302:1469.

63. Mendoza FS, Atiba JO, Krensky AL, et al: Rhabdomyolysis complicating doxylamine overdose. Clin Pediatr 1987;26:595–597.

64. Mesnard B, Ginn DR: Excessive phenylpropanolamine ingestion followed by subarachnoid hemorrhage. South Med J 1984;77:939.

65. Milgrom H, Bender B: Adverse effects of medications for rhinitis. Ann Allergy Asthma Immunol 1997;78:439–444.

66. Mills JG, Koch KM, Webster C, et al: The safety of ranitidine in over a decade of use. Aliment Pharmacol Ther 1997;11:129–137.

67. Monahan BP, Ferguson CL, Killeavy ES, et al: Torsade de pointes occurring in association with terfenadine use. JAMA 1989;264: 2788–2790.

68. Moss AJ: The QT interval and torsades de pointes [review]. Drug Saf 1999;21:5–10.

69. Nelson PG: Cimetidine and mental confusion [letter]. Lancet 1977; 2:928.

70. Nolen TM: Sedative effects of antihistamines—Safety, performance, learning, and quality of life [review]. Clin Ther 1997;19:39–55.

71. Patan DM, Webster DR: Pharmacokinetics of the H₁ receptor antagonists (the antihistamines). Clin Pharmacokinet 1985;10:477–497.

72. Perrotta DM, Coody G, Culmo C: Adverse events associated with ephedrine-containing products—Texas, December 1993–September 1995. Morb Mortal Wkly Rep 1996;45:689–693.

73. Rinder CS, D'Amato SL, Rinder HM: Survival in complicated diphenhydramine overdose. Crit Care Med 1988;16:1161–1162.

74. Sakeuir H, Vannata B: Torsades de pointes induced by astemizole in a patient with prolongation of the QT interval. Am Heart J 1993;125: 1436–1438.

75. Sawyer D, Conner CS, Scalby R: Cimetidine adverse reactions and acute toxicity. Am J Hosp Pharm 1981;38:188–197.

76. Schuller DE: The spectrum of antihistamines adversely affecting pulmonary function in asthmatic children. J Allergy Clin Immunol 1983; 71:147.

77. Sharma AN, Hexdall AH, Nelson L, Hoffman RS: Diphenhydramine-induced wide-complex tachycardia responds to bicarbonate [abstract]. J Toxicol Clin Toxicol 2000;38:572.

78. Shaw RG, Mashford MI, Desmond PV: Cardiac arrest after intravenous injection of cimetidine. Med J Aust, 1980;2:629–630.

79. Simons FE: New H1–receptor antagonists—Clinical pharmacology. Clin Exp Allergy 1990;20:19–24.

80. Simons FE, Simons KJ: Second-generation H₁-receptor antagonists [abstract]. Ann Allergy 1991;66:5–16,19.

81. Sorkin EM, Darvey DL: Review of cimetidine drug interactions. Drug Intell Clin Pharmacol 1983;17:110–120.

82. Spector R, Choudhury AK, Chiang CK, et al: Diphenhydramine in Orientals and Caucasians. Clin Pharmacol Ther 1980;28:229–234.

83. Tobin JR, Doyle TP, Ackerman AD, Brenner JI: Astemizole-induced cardiac conduction disturbances in a child. JAMA 1991;266: 2737–2740.

84. Tzivoni D, Banai S, Schuger C, et al: Treatment of torsade de pointes with magnesium sulfate. Circulation 1988;77:392–397.

85. Weesner KM, Denison M, Roberts RJ: Cardiac dysrhythmias in an adolescent following ingestion of an over-the-counter stimulant. Clin Pediatr 1982;21:700–701.

86. Wiley JF, Gelber ML, Henretig FM, et al: Cardiotoxic effects of astemizole overdose in children. J Pediatr 1992;120:799–802.

87. Woo OF, Benowitz NL, Baily FW: Atrioventricular conduction block caused by phenylpropanolamine. JAMA 1985;253:2646–2647.

88. Woodward JK: Pharmacology and toxicology of nonclassical antihistamines. Cutis 1988;42:5–9.

89. Woosley RL: Cardiac actions of antihistamines. Annu Rev Pharmacol Toxicol 1996;36:233–252.

90. Woosley R, Darrow WR: Analysis of potential adverse drug reactions—A case of mistaken identity. Am J Cardiol 1994;74:208–209.

91. Wyngaarden JB, Seevers MH: Toxic effects of antihistamines. JAMA 1951;145:277–288.

92. Yang T, Prakash C, Roden DM, Snyders DJ: Mechanism of block of a human cardiac potassium channel by terfenadine racemate and enantiomers. J Pharmacol 1995;115:267–274.

93. Zavitz M, Lindsay C, McGuigan MA: Acute diphenhydramine ingestion in children. Vet Hum Toxicol 1989;31:349.

ANTIDOTES IN DEPTH

Physostigmine
Mary Ann Howland

Physostigmine is a carbamate that reversibly inhibits cholinesterases both in the periphery and in the central nervous system (CNS).[39] This action inhibits the metabolism of acetylcholine, thereby allowing acetylcholine to accumulate. This indirect action of acetylcholine accumulation is used to antagonize the anticholinergic effects of drugs such as atropine, scopolamine,[44] and diphenhydramine. Although physostigmine was previously employed as an antagonist to the anticholinergic effects of the tricyclic antidepressants and the phenothiazines, this is no longer recommended due to a poor risk-benefit ratio given the potential for exacerbation of life-threatening quinidine-like effects. Similarly, it's likely that physostigmine will also have a poor risk-benefit ratio in the management of presumed γ-hydroxybutyrate (GHB) toxicity. Physostigmine's tertiary amine structure permits CNS penetration and differentiates it from neostigmine and pyridostigmine, which are quaternary amines.

HISTORY

The history of physostigmine dates to antiquity and the Efik people of Old Calabar in Nigeria.[15,18,20,39] There, the chiefs used a poisonous concoction made from the beans of an aquatic leguminous perennial plant found in the area to deliver the *esere ordeal*. Esere was the word used to represent both the bean and the ritual used to test the innocence or guilt of an accused person. It was also believed that the esere had the power to detect and kill those practicing witchcraft. Supposedly the innocent swallowed the poison quickly, causing immediate emesis.[20] Vomiting allowed them to survive on their own or to be given an antidote of excrement in water. The guilty, however, hesitated swallowing, leading to speculation that sublingual absorption led to severe systemic symptoms without the benefit of vomiting. They were noted to develop mouth fasciculations and died foaming at the mouth. Daniell, a British medical officer stationed in Calabar, brought samples of the bean and the plant back to England in 1840.[20] John Balfour, a professor of medicine and botany at the Edinburgh Medical School, is credited with characterizing the plant, which became known as *Physostigma venenosum Balfour* (family *Leguminoseae*) in 1857. The active alkaloid that was isolated from the Old Calabar, or ordeal bean, by Jobst and Hesse in 1864 was named physostigmine. Independently, a year later Vee and Leven also isolated the active alkaloid and named it eserine.

Christison performed the first toxicologic studies including self-experimentation with increasing doses of the seed. Fraser, Christison's student and later successor, originated the concept of antagonism from his experiments with physostigmine and atropine. Fraser plotted the dose relationships between the effects of atropine versus physostigmine on various organs such as the eye and the heart demonstrating that up to a certain dose, atropine

acted as an antidote to the lethal effects of physostigmine.[15] Experiments with physostigmine paved the way for Anderson, in 1906, to propose the existence of a transmitter to explain the mechanism of action of physostigmine. In the 1920s, Loewi proposed and then proved the theory of neurohumoral transmission. Stedman and Burger established the chemical structure of physostigmine in 1925. Julian and Pikl synthesized physostigmine in 1935. At this time physostigmine was employed as a miotic agent for patients with glaucoma, as a treatment for patients with myasthenia gravis, as a reversal agent to the paralytic effects of curare, as an antidote to atropine, and as a prototypical insecticide. In summary, physostigmine, a prototypical carbamate insecticide, was instrumental in the development of a bioassay for acetylcholine, concepts of neurohumoral transmission, mapping of cholinergic nerves, the concept of antagonism, the kinetics of enzyme inhibition, and an improved understanding of the blood brain-barrier.[18]

CHEMISTRY AND AFFINITY FOR CHOLINESTERASE

The general formula for carbamate inhibitors is shown in Figure 35–6A. Figures 35–6B and C show the chemical structures of physostigmine ($C_{15}H_{21}O_2N_3$), a tertiary amine, and neostigmine, a quaternary amine agent. Like acetylcholine, physostigmine is a substrate for the cholinesterases: erythrocyte acetylcholinesterase and plasma or pseudocholinesterase. Both acetylcholine and physostigmine bind to the cholinesterase enzymes to form a complex. Then a part of the substrate known as the leaving group (ie, choline for acetylcholine) is removed, and the remaining acetylated (for acetylcholine) or carbamoylated (for physostigmine) enzyme is hydrolyzed, regenerating the enzyme and freeing the acetate or carbamate groups, respectively (see Fig. 88–2). For acetylcholine, the process is extremely quick, with a turnover time of 150 ms, whereas the half-life for hydrolysis of the carbamoylated enzyme is 15–30 minutes.[39] The I_{50} (molar concentration that inhibits 50% of the enzyme) of physostigmine is 2.3×10^{-7} M for acetylcholinesterase, which is much weaker than other carbamates at 1×10^{-10} M or many organic phosphorus compounds at 1×10^{-11} M.[21] Only the (s) isomer inhibits cholinesterases, with plasma cholinesterase just a little more sensitive than acetylcholinesterase.[4] Newer agents with more selectivity for the CNS and for acetylcholinesterase (donepezil, rivastigmine, galantamine) are in use or under study for Alzheimer disease, but have not been studied for reversal of anticholinergic poisoning.[23,34]

PHARMACOKINETICS

Physostigmine is poorly absorbed orally, with a bioavailability of <5–12%.[1,2] Cholinesterases (choline ester hydrolases) cleave the ester linkage and very little drug is eliminated unchanged in the urine. Pharmacokinetic parameters following IV administration of 1.5 mg over 60 minutes in 9 patients with Alzheimer disease

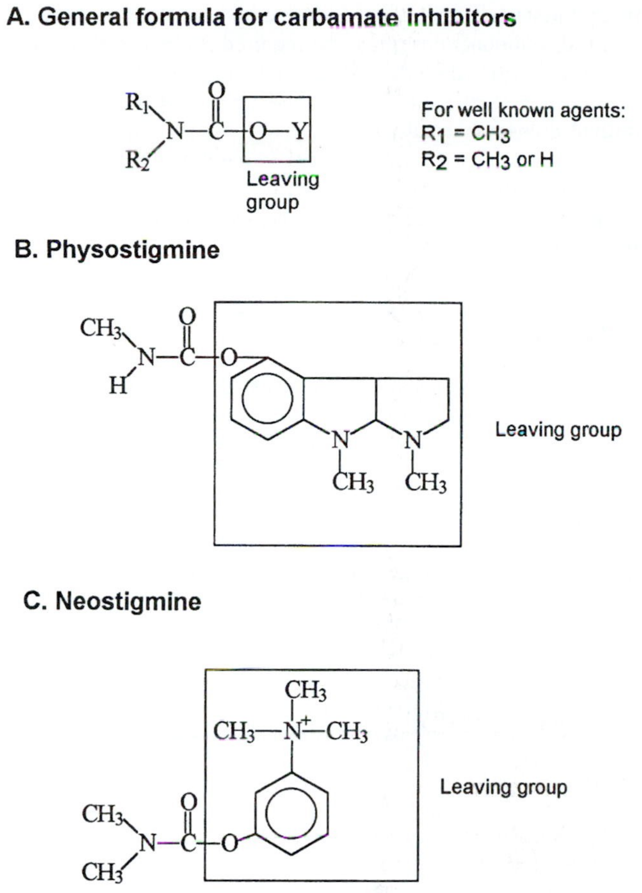

A. General formula for carbamate inhibitors

For well known agents:
$R_1 = CH_3$
$R_2 = CH_3$ or H

Leaving group

B. Physostigmine

Leaving group

C. Neostigmine

Leaving group

Figure 35–6. **A.** General formula for carbamate inhibitors. **B.** Structure of physostigmine. **C.** Structure of neostigmine.

demonstrated the following: V_d 2.4 ± 0.6 L/kg; $t_{1/2}$ 16.4 ± 3.2 minutes; peak plasma concentration 3 ± 0.5 ng/mL; clearance 0.1 L/min/kg (7.7 L/min). There was a 3-fold interindividual variability in plasma physostigmine concentrations. Plasma cholinesterase concentrations demonstrated inhibition within 2 minutes of initiating the physostigmine infusion; the half-time of plasma cholinesterase inhibition was 83.7 ± 5.2 minutes, with full recovery within 3 hours of the termination of the physostigmine infusion. A graph of physostigmine concentration versus either percent plasma or acetylcholinesterase inhibition demonstrated hysteresis.[3,22] The effects on plasma cholinesterase inhibition last about 5 times longer than the half-life of physostigmine. In this study, memory enhancement by physostigmine was directly related to plasma cholinesterase inhibition. All patients experienced varying degrees of diaphoresis, nausea, vomiting, headache, and generalized fatigue despite pretreatment with 2.5 mg methscopolamine.[3] The mouse LD_{50} (median lethal dose) for physostigmine is 0.47 mg/kg IV and 2.5 mg/kg po.[21]

CLINICAL USE

Physostigmine was first used as an antidote in 1864 to counteract severe atropine poisoning.[29] Today its role remains primarily in the treatment of antimuscarinic agents. More than 600 anticholinergic agents respond to physostigmine.[10] Anticholinergic agents fall into the categories of antimuscarinic (atropine, scopolamine, propantheline, benztropine, trihexyphenidyl), neuromuscular blockers (eg, curare), and ganglionic blockers (eg, trimethaphan). Other agents have anticholinergic properties that are not their primary therapeutic actions and are often considered as side effects (such as antihistamines: diphenhydramine; antipsychotics: chlorpromazine; and antidepressants: amitriptyline).

There has been a rise and fall of physostigmine use.[36] Enamored with its ability to cause CNS arousal, physostigmine was used in the 1970s to reverse the CNS effects of a large number of anticholinergic and nonanticholinergic agents.[16,27,28,30,32] The success with regard to anticholinergic agents is directly antidotal by virtue of its inhibition of cholinesterase. Effects for agents such as the benzodiazepines, opioids,[24,33,42] and GHB,[6] are attributable either to acetylcholine's direct action on the reticular activating system or as a result of interdependence of central neurotransmitters.[30] Remarkably few serious adverse effects are reported.[41] However, asystole followed the administration of physostigmine in 2 patients with tricyclic antidepressant overdose.[31] This led to the realization that toxicity from tricyclic antidepressants is complex and consists of more than just anticholinergic effects.[31] Sodium channel blockade causes myocardial depression, QRS and QT interval prolongation, and ventricular dysrhythmias. Physostigmine probably augments vagal effects, thus contributing to a decreased cardiac output and cardiac conduction defects. A reevaluation must conclude that the risks of physostigmine use for agents that are not primarily antimuscarinic often outweighs the benefits.

This analysis will probably hold true for GHB as well. GHB is rarely used alone and its effects are very variable with recovery occurring spontaneously in about 2 hours (16 minutes to 6 hours).[6,7,12,25,40] Three patients in whom a presumptive diagnosis of GHB toxicity was made were treated with physostigmine.[6] The 3 patients had an improved mental status within 5–15 minutes, with 1 patient relapsing and then fully awakening 40 minutes later. This patient was incontinent of feces, an adverse effect likely caused by the physostigmine.[6] A closer look at the descriptions of the patients reveals that all 3 improved with stimulation prior to physostigmine. Justification for use based upon a study done in the 1970s in the operating room when GHB was first being evaluated as an anesthetic appears illogical when caring for those who illicitly use GHB.[17]

INDICATIONS

Indications for the use of physostigmine include the presence of peripheral and central anticholinergic manifestations without evidence of QRS prolongation. Peripheral manifestations include dry mucosa, dry skin, flushed face, mydriasis, hyperthermia, decreased bowel sounds, urinary retention, and tachycardia. Central manifestations include agitation, delirium, hallucinations, seizures, and coma.[14,26] The peripheral and central findings usually occur together. It is uncommon to solely recognize central manifestations, although they are often more remarkable.[2,5,8,11,13,19,35,38] The central findings may persist longer than the peripheral findings, particularly when a patient is recovering from an overdose of an antimuscarinic agent.

ADVERSE EFFECTS AND SAFETY ISSUES

An excess of physostigmine results in the accumulation of acetylcholine at muscarinic, nicotinic (skeletal muscle, autonomic ganglia, adrenal glands), and the CNS sites.[21] Muscarinic effects produce the stimulation of smooth muscle and glandular secretions (respiratory, gastrointestinal, genitourinary) and the inhibition of contraction of most vascular smooth muscle. Nicotinic effects are stimulatory at low doses and depressant at high doses. For example, weakness and paralysis follow muscle fasciculations. The effect on the CNS results in anxiety, dizziness, tremors, confusion, ataxia, coma, and seizures.[21] The electroencephalogram (EEG) demonstrates desynchronous discharges followed by higher voltage discharges and a pattern similar to tonic-clonic seizures.[21] The cardiac effects are dose dependent and directly related to the presence of the diverse muscarinic and nicotinic effects. Small doses produce a rise in blood pressure, whereas moderate doses decrease heart rate and produce varying degrees of arteriovenous (AV) block.[21] At large doses, AV block appears de novo, the P wave is often absent, and the T waves are large and of variable shapes.[21] In addition to its inhibition of cholinesterase, physostigmine has direct actions on the nicotinic acetylcholine-receptor ionic channel on the neuromuscular junction, and it results in a decrease in GABA in the striatum.[37]

Physostigmine toxicity results when physostigmine is given in overdose, when it is used in the absence of an antimuscarinic agent, or when an excess is administered in relation to the antimuscarinic agent. Patients overdosed with physostigmine should be managed with intensive supportive care including mechanical ventilation if needed, intravenous atropine[43] titrated to reverse bronchial secretions, and rarely, pralidoxime to reverse the skeletal muscle findings.[9]

The relative contraindications to physostigmine use include bronchospastic disease, peripheral vascular disease, intestinal or bladder obstruction, intraventricular conduction defects, and AV block. Little information is available regarding the effects of physostigmine in pregnancy. Transient muscular weakness occurred in 10–20% of neonates whose mothers received anticholinesterases for the treatment of their myasthenia gravis.[1]

Drug interactions with cholinergic agonists (eg, pilocarpine), depolarizing neuromuscular blocking agents, or other anticholinesterase agents (carbamates, organic phosphorous compounds, pyridostigmine) are expected to be at least additive when taken concomitantly with physostigmine. The actions of drugs metabolized by plasma cholinesterases (eg, cocaine, succinylcholine, mivacurium) are expected to be prolonged.

DOSING

The dose of physostigmine is 1–2 mg in adults and 0.02 mg/kg (max, 0.5 mg) in children intravenously infused over at least 5 minutes. The onset of action is usually within minutes.[19] This dose can be repeated in 10–15 minutes if an adequate response is not achieved and muscarinic effects are not noted. Rapid administration may cause bradycardia, hypersalivation leading to respiratory difficulty, and possibly seizures. Although the half-life of physostigmine is about 16 minutes, its duration of action is usually much longer (about 5 times) and directly related to the duration of cholinesterase inhibition.[3] After anticholinergic reversal is achieved, additional doses may be required if clinical relapse occurs. The effective dose depends upon the ingested dose and duration of action of the antimuscarinic agent, although a total of 4 mg in divided doses is usually sufficient in most clinical situations.[14] However, significant interindividual variability exists. Atropine should be at the bedside and should be administered at one-half the physostigmine dose should excessive cholinergic toxicity (bronchorrhea) develop.

AVAILABILITY

Physostigmine is available as Antilirium in 2-mL ampules with each milliliter containing 1 mg of physostigmine salicylate. The vehicle contains sodium bisulfite and benzyl alcohol.

REFERENCES

1. McEvoy CK, ed: American Hospital Formulary Service (AHFS) 1997. Bethesda, Maryland: American Society of Health-System Pharmacists, 1997, pp. 902–904.
2. Aquilonius S, Hartvig P: Clinical pharmacokinetics of cholinesterase inhibitors. Clin Pharmacokinet 1986;11:236–249.
3. Asthana S, Greig NH, Hegedus L, et al: Clinical pharmacokinetics of physostigmine in patients with Alzheimer's disease. Clin Pharmacol Ther 1995;58:299–309.
4. Atack JR, Yu Q-S, Soncrant TT, et al: Comparative inhibitory effects of various physostigmine analogs against acetyl and butyrocholinesterases. J Pharmacol Exp Ther 1989;249:194–202.
5. Beaver KM, Gavin TJ: Treatment of acute anticholinergic poisoning with physostigmine. Am J Emerg Med 1998;16:505–507.
6. Caldicott DGE, Kuhn M: Gamma-hydroxybutyrate overdose and physostigmine: Teaching new tricks to an old drug? Ann Emerg Med 2001;37:99–102.
7. Chin RL, Sporer KA, Cullison B, et al: Clinical course of γ-hydroxybutyrate overdose. Ann Emerg Med 1998;31:716–722.
8. Crowell EB, Ketchum JS: The treatment of scopolamine-induced delirium with physostigmine. Clin Pharmacol Ther 1967;8:409–414.
9. Cumming G, Harding LK, Prowse K: Treatment and recovery after massive overdose of physostigmine. Lancet 1968;20:147–149.
10. Daunderer M: Physostigmine salicylate as an antidote. Int J Clin Pharmacol Ther Toxicol 1980;18:523–535.
11. Duvoisin R, Katz R: Reversal of central anticholinergic syndrome in man by physostigmine. JAMA 1968;206:1963–1965.
12. Eckstein M, Henderson SO, DelaCruz P, Newton E: Gamma-hydroxybutyrate (GHB): Report of a mass intoxication and review of the literature. Prehosp Emerg Care 1999;3:357–361.
13. El-Yousef MK, Janowsky D, Davis JM, Sekerke HJ: Reversal of antiparkinsonian drug toxicity by physostigmine: A controlled study. Am J Psychiatry 1973;130:141–145.
14. Forrer GR, Miller JJ: Atropine coma—A somatic therapy in psychiatry. Am J Psychiatry 1958;115:455–458.
15. Fraser TR: On the characters, action and therapeutic uses of the bean of Calabar. Edinburgh Med J 1863;9:36–56; 235–245.
16. Giannini AJ, Castellani S: A case of phenylcyclohexylpyrrolidine (PHP) intoxication treated with physostigmine. J Toxicol Clin Toxicol 1982;19:505–508.
17. Henderson RS, Holmes CM: Reversal of the anaesthetic action of sodium gamma-hydroxybutyrate. Anaesth Intensive Care 1976;4:351–354.
18. Holmstedt BO: The ordeal bean of old Calabar: The pageant of *Physostigmine venenosum* in medicine. In: Swain T, ed: Plants in the Development of Modern Medicine. Cambridge, MA, Harvard University Press, 1975, pp. 303–360.

19. Holzgrate RE, Vondrell JJ, Mintz SM: Reversal of postoperative reactions to scopolamine with physostigmine. Anesth Analg 1973;52: 921–925.

20. Karczmar AG: History of the research with anticholinesterase agents. In: Karczmar AG, ed: International Encyclopedia of Pharmacology and Therapeutics, Vol. I. Oxford, Pergamon Press, 1970, pp. 1–44.

21. Karczmar AG: Pharmacology of anticholinesterase agents. In: Karczmar AG, ed: International Encyclopedia of Pharmacology and Therapeutics, Vol. I. Oxford, Pergamon Press, 1970, pp. 45, 363.

22. Knapp S, Wardlow ML, Albert K, et al: Correlation between plasma physostigmine concentrations and percentage of acetylcholinesterase inhibition over time after controlled release of physostigmine in volunteer subjects. Drug Metab Dispos 1991;19:400–404.

23. Krall WJ, Sramck JJ, Cutler NR: Cholinesterase inhibitors: A therapeutic strategy for Alzheimer disease. Ann Pharmacother 1999;33: 441–450.

24. Larson GF, Hurbert BJ, Wingard DW: Physostigmine reversal of diazepam-induced depression. Anesth Analg 1977;56:348–351.

25. Li J, Stokes SA, Woeckener A: A tale of novel intoxication: Seven cases of γ-hydroxybutyric acid overdose. Ann Emerg Med 1998;31: 723–728.

26. Longo VG: Behavioral and electroencephalographic effects of atropine and related compounds. Pharmacol Rev 1966;18:965–996.

27. Manoguerra AS: Poisoning with tricyclic antidepressant drugs. Clin Toxicol 1977;10:149–158.

28. Nattel S, Bayne L, Ruedy J: Physostigmine in coma due to drug overdose. Clin Pharmacol Ther 1979;25:96–102.

29. Nickalls RWD, Nickalls EA: The first use of physostigmine in the treatment of atropine poisoning. Anesthesiology 1988;43:776–779.

30. Nilsson E: Physostigmine treatment in various drug-induced intoxications. Ann Clin Res 1982;14:165–172.

31. Pentel P, Peterson CD: Asystole complicating physostigmine treatment of tricyclic antidepressant overdose. Ann Emerg Med 1980;9: 588–590.

32. Rumack BH: 707 cases of anticholinergic poisoning treated with physostigmine [abstract]. Presented at annual meeting of American Academy of Clinical Toxicology, Montreal, Quebec, Canada, 1975.

33. Rupreht J, Dworacek B, Oosthoek H, et al: Physostigmine versus naloxone in heroin overdose. J Toxicol Clin Toxicol 1983–84;21: 387–397.

34. Shepherd G, Klein-Schwartz W, Edwards R: Donepezil overdose: A tenfold dosing error. Ann Pharmacother 1999;33:812–815.

35. Smiler BG, Bartholomew EG, Sivak BJ, et al: Physostigmine reversal of scopolamine delirium in obstetric patients. Am J Obstet 1973; 116:326–329.

36. Smilkstein MJ: Physostigmine [editorial]. J Emerg Med 1991;9: 275–277.

37. Somani SM, Dube SN: Physostigmine—An overview as pretreatment drug for organophosphate intoxication. Int J Clin Pharmacol Ther Toxicol 1989;27:367–387.

38. Sopchak CA, Stork CM, Cantor RM, O'Hara PE: Central anticholinergic syndrome due to Jimson Weed physostigmine: Therapy revisited? J Toxicol Clin Toxicol 1998;36:42–45.

39. Taylor P: Anticholinesterase agents. In: Hardman JG, Limbird CE, Molinoff PB, Ruddon RW, eds: Goodman and Gilman's The Pharmacologic Basis of Therapeutics, 9th ed. New York, McGraw-Hill, 1996, pp. 161–176.

40. Viera AJ, Yates SW: Toxic ingestion of gamma-hydroxybutyric acid. South Med J 1999;92:404–405.

41. Walker WE, Levy RC, Hanenson IB: Physostigmine—Its use and abuse. JACEP 1976;5:436–439.

42. Weinstock M, Davidson JT, Rosin AJ, et al: Effect of physostigmine on morphine-induced postoperative pain and somnolence. Br J Anesth 1982;54:429–443.

43. Weiss S: Persistence of action of physostigmine and the atropine-physostigmine antagonism in animals and in man. J Pharmacol Exp Ther 1925;27:181–188.

44. Young SE, Ruiz RS, Falletta J: Reversal of systemic toxic effects of scopolamine with physostigmine salicylate. Am J Ophthalmol 1971; 72:1136–1138.

CHAPTER 36 IRON

Jeanmarie Perrone

Iron

MW	=	55.85 daltons
Serum normal	=	80–180 µg/dL
	=	14–32 µmol/L
Action level	=	> 500 µg/dL
	=	> 90 µmol/L

Values greater than or equal to the action level necessitate clinical intervention. Values less than this level may necessitate intervention based on the clinical appearance of the patient.

A 17-month-old toddler was found by his mother playing with a bottle of iron supplements. The mother noted greenish discoloration around the child's lips and pill fragments in his mouth and brought him to the Emergency Department (ED). En route to the hospital, spontaneous vomiting of pill fragments and hematemesis occurred. In the ED, he was noted to be lethargic with these vital signs: blood pressure, 95/55 mm Hg; heart rate, 130 beats/min; respiratory rate, 35 breaths/min; temperature, 96.9°F (36°C). Supplemental oxygen was given, IV access obtained, and fluid resuscitation (20 mL/kg) initiated. An abdominal radiograph revealed a large number of radiopaque fragments in the stomach. Orotracheal intubation, orogastric lavage (with removal of more green pill fragments), and whole-bowel irrigation were initiated. An arterial blood gas following intubation revealed a severe mixed metabolic and respiratory acidosis: pH 7.15; P_{CO_2}, 34 mm Hg; P_{O_2}, 441 mm Hg.

Chelation with deferoxamine (15 mg/kg/h) was begun at 135 mg/h intravenously. Transfer of the patient to a tertiary care pediatric intensive care unit (ICU) was arranged. Other significant laboratory values were: WBC (white blood [cell] count), 22,000/mm³ hemoglobin, 11.6 g/dL; serum bicarbonate, 10 mEq/L; glucose, 384 mg/dL; international normalized ratio (INR), 4.5; iron, 18,570 µg/dL; ALT, 700 IU/mL. Upon arrival in the tertiary care pediatric ICU (3.5 hours after initial presentation), the patient had a pulse of 188 beats/min and he was hypotensive with a systolic blood pressure of 70 mm Hg. Additional fluid boluses and transfusions of fresh-frozen plasma and 2 units of packed red blood cells were administered. A repeat abdominal radiograph revealed persistent radiopaque pill fragments in the gut lumen (Fig. 36–1). Lavage was performed again with upper gastrointestinal (GI) endoscopy, but pill fragments were adherent to the gastric mucosa. The patient was taken to the operating room and a gastrotomy was performed for removal of all remaining pill fragments (Fig. 36–2). Ten hours postingestion, his oxygenation and hemodynamic status deteriorated, despite maximal support. Acute lung injury was demonstrated by increasing arterial-alveolar oxygen gradient and subsequent chest radiograph; oxygenation difficulties worsened, and increasing hypotension developed in spite of vasopressors and further transfusions of red blood cells and fresh-frozen plasma. A fatal cardiac arrest ensued, approximately 20 hours postingestion. His terminal serum iron level was 4000 µg/dL.

HISTORY AND EPIDEMIOLOGY

Iron has been used therapeutically for thousands of years, and continues to be available both with and without prescription for the prevention and treatment of iron-deficiency anemia in all ages. Despite this long history of use, the first reports of iron toxicity only occurred in the mid-20th century. Since then, numerous cases of iron poisoning and fatalities have been reported, many of them in children. In 1997, the Food and Drug Administration (FDA) mandated warning labels about the danger of pediatric iron poisoning on all iron-containing preparations.[22] In addition to the warning labels, the FDA also launched an educational campaign to alert caregivers of the potential toxicity of iron-containing medications.[2] Prevention of iron poisoning is pivotal in decreasing its morbidity and mortality.

The clinical consequences of untreated iron toxicity are described in the early case reports of pediatric iron poisoning. Despite the absence of laboratory or radiologic corroboration, the clinical manifestations are similar to those seen today. A British paper from the 1950s describes children found playing with a bottle of improperly stored iron pills who upon arrival in the ED the were pale, lethargic, and vomiting, often with hematemesis. A myriad of gastric-emptying procedures are described in this paper, including emesis with salt and water or "syrup of figs," and orogastric lavage with bismuth bicarbonate, sodium bicarbonate, magnesium hydroxide, or deferoxamine. Although lethargy ensues and "breathing [is] heavy," gastrointestinal symptoms diminish. Most children recover, but a few "become cyanosed, with moist accompaniments at both bases" and "choke on inspiration." Previous authors described a warning on the package by the "fersolate" manufacturer in 1950: "Excessive doses of iron can be dangerous. Do not leave these tablets within reach of young children, who may eat them as sweets with harmful results."[85]

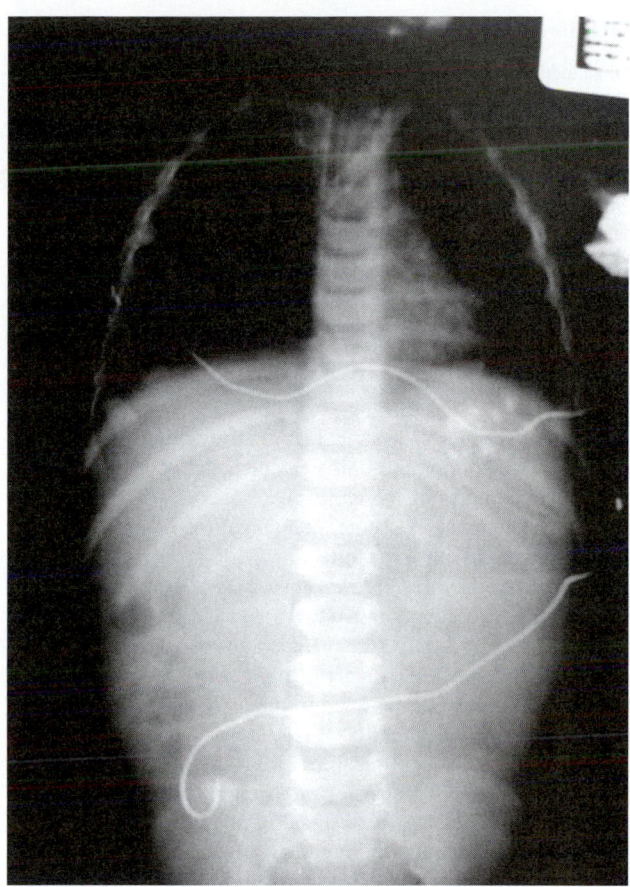

Figure 36–1. A 17-month-old toddler presented with lethargy and hematemesis following a large ingestion of iron supplement pills. Despite orogastric lavage and whole-bowel irrigation, iron pills and fragments can be visualized in the stomach 4 hours postingestion.

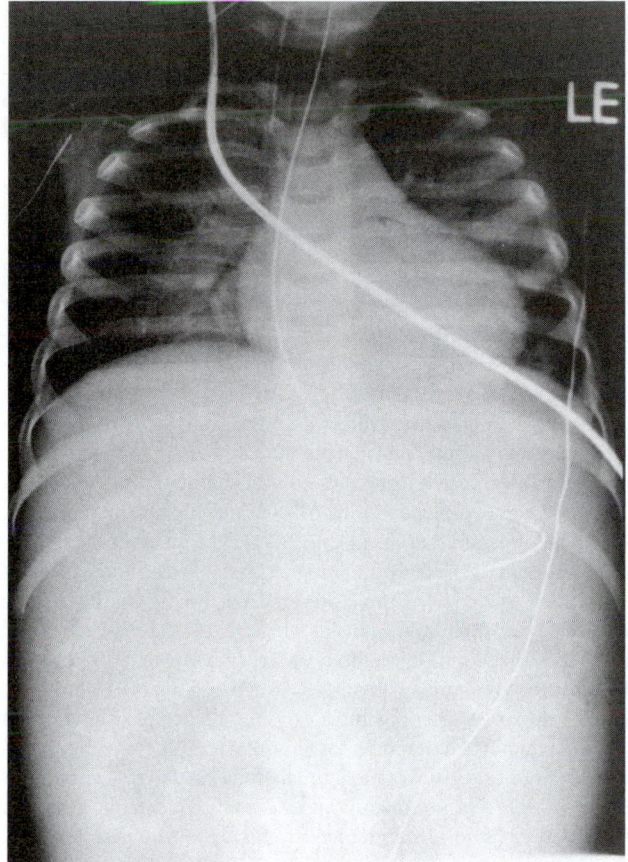

Figure 36–2. Ten hours postingestion; persistent iron pills were removed from the stomach by gastrotomy. No further radiopaque fragments can be visualized; however, acute lung injury is now visible.

Although the incidence of iron exposures continued to increase in the 1980s, it became the leading cause of poisoning deaths in children younger than 6 years of age only in the last decade. This tragic finding was publicized by a case series of fatalities involving 5 toddlers in Los Angeles in a 6-month period in 1992; all cases involved prenatal vitamins with iron.[92] This association highlights the paradoxical availability of these potentially lethal medications in the homes of families with young children, resulting from prescribing iron to treat anemia during pregnancy and in the postpartum period. Although FDA-mandated warning labels have been in place since 1997, their impact on poisoning epidemiology is unclear. Further improvements in packaging, including unit dosing (blister packs) of these prescriptions containing more than 30 mg of elemental iron, as well as limiting numbers of pills dispensed (ie, maximum 30-day supply) are predicted to enhance preventive efforts.[55] Education of patients by pharmacists and obstetricians prescribing prenatal vitamins with iron or iron supplements may also prevent poisoning. Isolated fatalities continue to occur,[56] although the trend in American Association of Poison Control Centers (AAPCC) Toxic Exposure Surveillance System (TESS) data suggests they are becoming less common (see p. 1752 and Chap. 116). Iron poisoning may occur following the ingestion of other iron salts such as ferric chloride used in industry or other commercial enterprises.[99]

PHARMACOLOGY AND TOXICOKINETICS

Iron supplementation is indicated when iron stores in the body are inadequate, or when iron requirements are increased. Iron is a versatile and critical element to organ function because of its capacity to accept and donate electrons easily, shifting from ferric (Fe^{3+}) to ferrous (Fe^{2+}) states (Chap. 12). This redox interchange allows iron to fulfill a critical role in multiple protein and enzyme complexes, including cytochromes and myoglobin, although it is principally found incorporated into hemoglobin in erythrocytes. Insufficient iron availability results in anemia, while excess total body iron results in hemochromatosis, a pathologic condition of iron overload. The body can neither synthesize nor excrete iron and thus must finely regulate iron absorption from the gastrointestinal tract. Iron absorption, which occurs predominantly in the duodenum, is determined by iron requirements of the body. In iron deficiency, iron uptake into intestinal mucosal cells may increase from a normal of 10–35% to as much as 80–95%. Following uptake into these cells, iron is either stored as ferritin and lost when the cell is shed, or released to transferrin, a serum iron-binding protein. In overdose, some of these processes become saturated and absorption may be limited. However, oxidative and corrosive effects of iron on gastrointestinal mucosa lead to dysfunction of this regulatory balance and, perhaps, in overdose, passive absorption of iron down its concentration gradient also may occur.[79] Once transferrin is saturated with iron, "free" iron, or iron not bound safely to transport protein, may become available in the patient's blood. Under these conditions iron may participate in various oxidative processes (Chap. 12).

Iron supplements are available as the iron salts, ferrous gluconate, ferrous sulfate, and ferrous fumarate, and as the nonionic preparations carbonyl iron and polysaccharide-iron. Additional sources of significant quantities of iron are vitamin preparations, especially prenatal vitamins (Table 36–1). The quantity of elemental iron in each of these formulations is variable and is the primary determinant of toxicity (Table 36–2). Their relative safety relates to the fact that their iron is in the elemental unreactive form and must be oxidized within the body to become effective. Children's chewable multivitamins contain less iron per tablet (10–18 mg elemental iron/tablet as compared to 65 mg elemental iron/tablet in prenatal vitamins) but severe toxicity may result from the ingestions of large quantities. One animal study actually demonstrates higher iron levels following ingestion of equivalent doses of chewable versus solid iron tablets.[58] This was attributed in part to the limited gastric irritation associated with the chewable iron preparations and consequently less vomiting. The polysaccharide-iron complex and carbonyl iron may be safer formulations despite comparable elemental iron content.[43]

Toxic effects of iron poisoning occur at doses of 10–20 mg/kg elemental iron. Significant gastrointestinal symptoms have been demonstrated in human adult volunteers who have ingested 10–20 mg iron/kg.[11,48] In one volunteer study, 6 subjects who ingested 20 mg/kg elemental iron developed nausea and voluminous diarrhea within 2 hours, and 5 of the 6 subjects had serum iron levels above 300 μg/dL.[11] Recommendations for the hospital referral of toddlers who had ingested iron ranged from those with potential exposures to >20 mg/kg[6] up to 60 mg/kg.[44] These wide ranges probably result from the interpretation of retrospective studies in possibly "exposed" toddlers because the doses were estimated. Many authors suggest that those who subsequently did not develop toxicity presumably had an overestimation of exposure (Chap. 116).

TABLE 36–1. Common Iron Formulations and Their Elemental Iron Equivalents

Contents	Product Name	Elemental Iron (%)
Ferrous chloride	Ferro-66	28
Ferrous fumarate	Chromagen, Nephro-Fer, Fetrin	33
Ferrous gluconate	Mission prenatal, Iromin-G	12
Ferrous lactate	Ferro-drops	19
Ferrous sulfate	Feosol, Slow-Fe, Irospan, Fero-Folic-500	20

TABLE 36–2. Determining Toxicity

A 10-kg toddler ingests 10 ferrous sulfate tablets. Is this ingestion consequential?

325-mg tablets ferrous sulfate × 20% elemental iron/tablet = 65 mg elemental iron/tab

65 mg elemental iron/tab × 10 tablets = 650 mg iron ingested

650 mg iron/10 kg toddler = 65 mg/kg

Following a 65-mg/kg ingestion, significant toxicity is expected.

PATHOPHYSIOLOGY

Iron toxicity manifests through local and systemic effects. The pathophysiology of iron poisoning can be better understood by analyzing the etiologies of the concomitant metabolic acidosis. Initial toxicity, including vomiting, abdominal pain, and diarrhea, is the result of direct corrosive effects on the gastric and intestinal mucosa, which may result in hematemesis, melena, or hematochezia.[83] Such profound gastrointestinal toxicity is analogous to other metal salt ingestions, such as mercury or arsenic exposures, where gastrointestinal effects are also severe (Chaps. 79 and 81). Intestinal ulceration, edema, transmural inflammation, and, in some extreme cases, small-bowel infarction and necrosis may occur.[23,70,83] Hypotension resulting from gastrointestinal losses contributes to tissue hypoperfusion, lactate formation, and metabolic acidosis. Other gastrointestinal effects include hepatotoxicity. Postmortem examination of patients with fatal iron ingestions reveals hemorrhagic periportal necrosis of the liver.[50] This pattern of hepatic injury was experimentally reproduced in rabbits given lethal doses of iron[50] and is thought to result from high tissue levels of iron absorbed from the gastrointestinal tract and carried to the liver via the portal vein. Formation of reactive oxygen species in the hepatocytes is likely responsible for the hepatocellular damage.

Absorption of iron also contributes to metabolic acidosis. Following absorption, ferrous iron is converted to ferric iron and an unbuffered hydrogen ion is liberated.[69] Also, high concentrations of intramitochondrial iron disrupt oxidative phosphorylation. A subsequent buildup of unused hydrogen ions normally incorporated into the synthesis of ATP leads to a liberation of H+ and further systemic acidosis (Chap. 13). Iron is a potent catalyst of reactive oxygen species formation which leads to oxidation of membrane-bound lipids and loss of cellular integrity (Chap. 12).[69,72] These factors exacerbate metabolic acidosis and contribute to cell death and tissue injury at the organ level.

In animals, multiple cardiovascular effects can be demonstrated, including decreased cardiac output contributing to shock.[89,97] Although this finding was initially solely attributed to decreased venous filling pressures, decreased preload, and a relative bradycardia,[89] a direct negative inotropic effect of iron on the myocardium can be demonstrated in animal models.[3] Reports of early coagulopathy unrelated to hepatotoxicity prompted investigations into the effect of iron on clotting.[81] Free iron was shown to inhibit the formation of thrombin and thrombin's effect on fibrinogen in vitro.[73]

Finally, autopsy studies support the significance of both local and systemic toxicity of iron. Postmortem studies reveal congestion, edema, necrosis, and iron deposition in the gastric and intestinal mucosa, as well as hemorrhage and congestion in the lungs.[29,31,50] A postmortem series of 11 fatal iron ingestions substantiated these findings with measurements of elevated iron levels in most major organs examined: stomach, liver, brain, heart, lung, small bowel, and kidney.[64]

CLINICAL MANIFESTATIONS

It is suggested that there are five clinical stages of iron toxicity, which have their basis in the pathophysiology of iron poisoning.[6,39,67] Although these stages are useful teaching tools, they are of little benefit to the clinician managing a poisoned patient, and should not be used to assign a clinical stage based on the number of hours postingestion, as patients do not necessarily follow the same temporal course through these stages. The first stage of iron toxicity is characterized by nausea, vomiting, abdominal pain, and diarrhea. The "local" toxic effects of iron predominate, and subsequent dehydration secondary to volume loss contributes to the ill appearance of the iron-poisoned patient. Occasionally, hematemesis, melena, or hematochezia may cause hemodynamic instability. Patients with large ingestions may progress directly from gastrointestinal symptoms (stage 1) without a latent period (stage 2) to signs of systemic toxicity (stage 3). Gastrointestinal symptoms always follow significant overdose; conversely, the absence of symptoms, specifically vomiting, in the first 6 hours following ingestion essentially excludes serious toxicity.

The "latent" or "second stage" of iron poisoning refers to the period of 6–24 hours following the resolution of gastrointestinal symptoms and before overt systemic toxicity develops. The delineation of this stage may have evolved from early case reports of patients whose gastrointestinal symptoms had seemingly resolved and then suddenly deteriorated.[85] There is controversy over whether this second stage is a true quiescent phase, or whether it represents the failure to recognize ongoing toxicity.[6] Although patients who remain asymptomatic from the time of ingestion are clearly not in this quiescent stage, clinicians should be cautious not to misinterpret the absence of gastrointestinal symptoms in significantly exposed patients with delayed presentations as being benign. During stage 2, hypovolemia and poor tissue perfusion resulting from the gastrointestinal effects of iron may produce a worsening metabolic acidosis if volume resuscitation is not adequate. Conversely, for many patients with lesser iron ingestions, gastrointestinal toxicity will resolve and they will recover. In summary, patients who are well since ingestion and who have stable vital signs, a normal mental status, and a normal acid-base balance, and who tolerate oral fluids, are not significantly poisoned.

Patients who progress to the third or shock stage of iron poisoning by definition have profound toxicity. This stage may occur in the first few hours after a massive ingestion or 12–24 hours after a more moderate ingestion. The etiology of shock may be multifactorial, resulting from hypovolemia, vasodilation, and poor cardiac output,[89,97] with decreased tissue perfusion and an ongoing metabolic acidosis. An iron-induced coagulopathy may worsen bleeding and hypovolemia.[81] Systemic toxicity exacerbates worsening CNS effects with lethargy, hyperventilation, seizures, or coma.

The fourth stage of iron poisoning is characterized by hepatic failure, which may occur 2–3 days following the ingestion.[29] The hepatotoxicity is directly attributed to uptake of iron by the reticuloendothelial system in the liver, where it causes oxidative damage.[25,98]

The fifth stage of iron toxicity rarely occurs. Gastric outlet obstruction secondary to strictures and scarring from the initial corrosive injury can develop 2–8 weeks following ingestion.[28,33,83]

Patients with chronic iron overload are at increased risk of *Yersinia enterocolitica* infection. Iron is a required growth factor for *Y. enterocolitica;* however, it lacks the siderophore to solubilize iron and to transport it intracellularly. Deferoxamine is a siderophore that fosters the growth of *Y. enterocolitica*. Patients with chronic iron overload or acute poisoning have developed *Yersinia* infection or sepsis as a complication of iron poisoning or deferoxamine therapy.[12,52,54,77] *Yersinia* infection should be suspected in patients who experience abdominal pain, fever, and diarrhea following resolution of iron toxicity. In this setting, cultures should be obtained and appropriate antibiotic therapy initiated.

DIAGNOSTIC TESTING

Radiography

Iron is available in many forms and different preparations vary with respect to radiopacity on abdominal radiography.[76] Factors such as time since ingestion and amount of elemental iron also play a role.[57,76] Liquid iron formulations and chewable iron tablets are typically not radiopaque, but may be responsible for significant poisonings because of their pleasant taste.[20] A retrospective review of pediatric iron ingestions revealed that abdominal radiographs were positive in only 1 of 30 patients ingesting chewable vitamins.[20] Because adult preparations have a higher elemental iron content, they tend to be more consistently radiopaque.[57] Finding radiopaque pills on an abdominal radiograph is helpful in guiding and following gastrointestinal decontamination.[34] However, their absence is not a reliable indicator to exclude potential toxicity[57,63] (Chap. 8).

Laboratory

Many different laboratory studies are used to assess iron poisoning. An anion gap metabolic acidosis accounted for primarily by lactate is a common finding in patients with serious iron ingestions. Serial electrolyte measurements can assess progression and response to volume replacement. Anemia may result from gastrointestinal blood loss, but may not be evident initially because of hemoconcentration secondary to plasma volume loss.

Other tests, such as the WBC and blood glucose, have been extensively examined for their ability to predict serious iron toxicity. Although one small retrospective study of iron-poisoned children found that a WBC >15,000/mm³ or a blood glucose >150 mg/dL was 100% predictive of an iron level >300 μg/dL,[47] three subsequent studies that examined this issue in a similar manner were unable to validate this association.[13,45,63] In practice, an elevated WBC or glucose should raise concern about an elevated iron level; however, iron poisoning is a clinical diagnosis, and an assessment of the signs and symptoms of the patient is more reliable than specific laboratory parameters.

Notwithstanding the statement that iron poisoning is a clinical diagnosis, serum iron levels can be used effectively to gauge toxicity and the success of treatment.[6] In the previously mentioned human volunteer study of 6 adults who ingested 20 mg/kg elemental iron, all 6 adults demonstrated significant gastrointestinal toxicity, and the 4 who required intravenous fluid resuscitation had peak serum iron levels in the range of 300 μg/dL between 2 and 4 hours after ingestion.[11] Serum iron levels between 300 and 500 μg/dL usually correlate with significant gastrointestinal toxicity and modest systemic toxicity. Levels between 500 and 1000 μg/dL are associated with pronounced systemic toxicity and shock,[93] and levels above 1000 μg/dL are associated with significant morbidity and mortality.[93] Although elevated levels may be an additional indicator of potentially serious toxicity, lower levels cannot be used to exclude the possibility of serious toxicity. A single serum iron level may not represent a peak level, or may be falsely lowered by the presence of deferoxamine, unless an atomic absorption technique is used for measurement.[27,32] Peak levels of iron are thought to occur 2–6 hours after ingestion, depending on the iron preparation.[11,48] In a study of human volunteers ingesting 5–10 mg/kg elemental iron in the form of chewable vitamins, peak serum iron levels occurred between 4.2 and 4.5 hours in all subjects.[48]

Total iron-binding capacity (TIBC) is a measurement of the total amount of iron that can be bound by transferrin in a given volume of serum.[21] Twenty years ago, it was taught that iron toxicity would not occur if the serum iron level was less than the TIBC because there would not be enough circulating "free" iron to cause tissue damage. While this is conceptually true, further research has clarified the limitations of the TIBC values. Most importantly, the in vitro value of TIBC factitiously increases as a result of iron poisoning and thus has a tendency to apparently rise above a concurrently measured serum iron level.[11,84] False elevations in TIBC can be corrected by adding excess magnesium carbonate reagent during the laboratory process, but this technique is rarely employed in clinical practice. Yet another confounding variable occurs when a patient is treated with deferoxamine, which also may falsely elevate the TIBC.[8] A recent laboratory investigation concluded that none of 3 different TIBC methods examined were accurate for measuring iron or TIBC in a simulated acute iron overdose.[71] In patients with hemochromatosis and chronic iron overload, iron-induced myocardial and hepatic injury occurs even when the TIBC remains higher than the serum iron level. In summary, TIBC has little or no value in the assessment of the iron-poisoned patient as it is analyzed today.

MANAGEMENT

Initial Approach

As with any serious ingestion, initial stabilization must include supplemental oxygen, an assessment of airway, and establishment of intravenous access. Evidence of hematemesis or lethargy following an iron exposure may be a manifestation of significant toxicity. Intravenous fluid rehydration should begin while considering orogastric lavage and whole-bowel irrigation. In any lethargic patient who is likely to deteriorate progressively, early orotracheal intubation may facilitate gastrointestinal decontamination measures. An abdominal radiograph may be used to estimate the iron burden in the gastrointestinal tract. Laboratory values including chemistries, hemoglobin, iron level, coagulation, and hepatic profiles are necessary in the sickest patients. An arterial blood gas will rapidly detect a metabolic acidosis. Patients who are well appearing, or who have had 1–2 brief episodes of vomit-

ing, should have a chemistry panel and perhaps a serum iron level measured.

Limiting Absorption

Following stabilization of the patient's condition, gastrointestinal decontamination procedures should be initiated. Gastric emptying may have added value following ingestion of substances such as iron which are not bound to activated charcoal. Although little benefit is expected from administration of syrup of ipecac in a child or adult who has already vomited spontaneously several times, syrup of ipecac may prove beneficial in the first hour prior to emesis. Similarly, orogastric lavage may not be effective for large-sized iron tablets or after several hours have elapsed since ingestion.[40] The location of radiopaque pills on the abdominal radiograph may guide the use of lavage. When many pills remain in the stomach, lavage may be used to remove some; occasionally orogastric lavage is ineffective in removing iron adherent to gastric mucosa.[23,88] Similarly, when iron pills have moved further along in the gastrointestinal tract, lavage or emesis is unlikely to be successful and whole-bowel irrigation may be more effective (Figs. 36–1 and 36–2).

Perhaps because of the lack of efficacy of activated charcoal, many different substances have been investigated for use as lavage solutions. A review of these different irrigants is helpful in understanding our current approach. Studies in the 1960s investigated the utility of adding the iron chelator deferoxamine in the lavage solution, thereby chelating iron as ferrioxamine before it was absorbed. In a canine model of iron poisoning, ferrioxamine toxicity was attributed to increased absorption of this iron-deferoxamine complex.[95,96] A small human volunteer trial was unable to demonstrate the efficacy of oral deferoxamine in decreasing iron absorption following 5 mg/kg of iron.[38] However, in another volunteer trial, oral deferoxamine in a premixed slurry of activated charcoal was effective in decreasing absorption of simultaneously administered ferrous sulfate.[30] At least one in vitro study also demonstrated that activated charcoal may be effective in binding ferrioxamine.[101] This concept requires further study because the possibility of systemic toxicity from simultaneous ferrioxamine absorption must be investigated to define this potential risk.

Another former practice of performing orogastric lavage with sodium bicarbonate or phosphosoda was based on the premise that these solutions produced insoluble iron salts and prevented its absorption. An in vitro model revealed a minimal reduction in iron solubility with the use of sodium bicarbonate.[16] In a rat model of iron poisoning, neither lavage with sodium bicarbonate nor sodium dihydrogen phosphate had any effect on subsequent serum iron levels as compared to control animals lavaged with water.[17] Additionally, reports of hyperphosphatemia and other electrolyte imbalances were reported following the use of phosphate lavage.[4,26] Magnesium hydroxide was effective in decreasing serum iron levels in a dog model, but elevated magnesium levels were also noted.[14] Magnesium hydroxide administered 1 hour following a simulated mild iron overdose in a human volunteer study resulted in a 50% reduction in iron absorption, although serum magnesium levels were not measured. This study used a 5:1 ratio of magnesium hydroxide to elemental iron. It is unclear whether this benefit would safely be realized in the setting of an actual iron overdose where this ratio may not be attained.[91] A subsequent investigation of magnesium hydroxide failed to show a significant decrease in iron absorption for 7 hours after subjects received magnesium hydroxide and 10 mg/kg ferrous sulfate, although there was a trend toward lower iron levels in the treatment group.[75] Sodium polystyrene sulfonate appeared to bind iron from ferrous sulfate solutions when investigated in a preliminary in vitro binding study.[59] In summary, although many solutions have been used for gastric lavage and although some actually demonstrate limited efficacy, the possible associated risks with their use mandate at this time that only normal saline or tap water be used for orogastric lavage.

The use of whole-bowel irrigation (WBI) in patients with iron poisoning is supported primarily by case reports and one uncontrolled case series.[19,40,80,87] However, the rationale for its use is logical, especially considering the limitations of other gastric decontamination modalities in iron poisoning. The usual dose of WBI with polyethylene glycol electrolyte lavage solution is 500 mL/h in children and 2 L/h in adults. This rate is best achieved by starting slowly and increasing as tolerated, often utilizing a nasogastric tube to administer the large volumes. Antiemetics such as metoclopramide or serotonin antagonists can be used to treat nausea and vomiting. A large volume (44 L) of WBI was administered safely over 5 days to a child who had persistent iron tablets on serial abdominal radiographs[40] (Antidotes in Depth: Whole-Bowel Irrigation).

For patients who demonstrate persistent iron in the gastrointestinal tract despite orogastric lavage and WBI, upper endoscopy or gastrotomy and surgical removal of iron tablets adherent to the gastric mucosa may be lifesaving.[23,65,88]

Deferoxamine

Deferoxamine, also known as desferrioxamine, has been available since the 1960s as a specific chelator for acute iron overdose, as well as for chronic iron toxicity resulting from multiple transfusions in patients with diseases such as thalassemia major. Deferoxamine is derived from culture of *Streptomyces pilosus* and has high affinity and specificity for iron. In the presence of ferric iron (Fe^{3+}), deferoxamine forms the complex ferrioxamine, which is then excreted by the kidneys,[41] imparting a reddish-brown discoloration to the urine. Deferoxamine chelates both free iron and iron transported between transferrin and ferritin,[49,66] but not the iron present in hemoglobin, hemosiderin, or ferritin.[41] In addition, it appears that deferoxamine cannot remove iron once it is bound to transferrin.[5] There is sufficient evidence to suggest that deferoxamine can reach intracytoplasmic and mitochondrial free iron, thereby limiting intracellular toxicity from excess iron.[49] Deferoxamine may work by other mechanisms in addition to binding excess iron. Because 100 mg of deferoxamine mesylate chelates approximately 8.5 mg of ferric iron, therapeutic dosing of deferoxamine does not account for a significant amount of chelated iron excretion in the urine, yet it produces dramatic clinical results (Antidotes in Depth: Deferoxamine).

Administration of deferoxamine should be considered in iron-poisoned patients with any of the following findings: metabolic acidosis, repetitive vomiting, toxic appearance, lethargy, hypotension, gastrointestinal bleeding, or signs of shock. Intravenous deferoxamine administration should also be considered in any patient with iron levels greater than 500 µg/dL. In patients manifesting serious signs and symptoms of iron poisoning, deferoxamine should be initiated as an intravenous infusion, starting slowly and gradually increasing to a dose of 15 mg/kg/h. Hypotension is the rate-limiting factor with more rapid infusions.[94,95] Intra-

muscular administration of deferoxamine, although once a popular method of administration and part of the "deferoxamine challenge" test, is rarely indicated.

The deferoxamine challenge test consisted of a 1–2 g (90 mg/kg) IM dose of deferoxamine followed by subsequent collection of urine samples searching for a "vin rose" urine-color change. When this urine-color change occurs, it represents toxic free iron being excreted as the colored compound ferrioxamine. Following a "positive" deferoxamine challenge test, a patient would then be treated with either additional IM deferoxamine every 4 hours or an intravenous regimen as described previously. Patients whose urine did not change color following the challenge were considered not to be significantly poisoned, and no further deferoxamine was administered. There are several problems with this approach. A single dose of deferoxamine is an unreliable indicator of toxicity because patients with high serum iron levels may rarely show no detectable urine-color change.[24] In addition, intramuscular administration of deferoxamine leads the clinician to manage patients without adequate intravenous access or the ability to administer adequate volume therapy. Overlooking this critical resuscitation measure in a seriously poisoned toddler or adult may result in hemodynamic instability and potentially devastating outcomes. Patients who appear toxic and/or have levels above 500 µg/dL serum iron should be treated with deferoxamine intravenously. Patients who have levels lower than 500 µg/dL or who do not appear toxic should be treated supportively without the administration of parenteral deferoxamine (Fig. 36–3).

Because of concern for possible deferoxamine toxicity, clinicians have attempted to define the earliest clear endpoints for deferoxamine therapy. In one report, a urine iron to creatinine ratio (U_I/Cr) was used to determine if free iron continued to be excreted in the urine during deferoxamine therapy.[100] This is a more objective measure of the presence of ferrioxamine in the urine than the less reliable and more subjective use of urine-color change.[18,44,90] This method, however, must be further studied clinically before it can be advocated for use. Most authors agree that deferoxamine therapy should be discontinued when the patient appears clinically well, the anion gap acidosis has resolved, and there is no further urine-color change.[53] In patients with signs and symptoms of serious toxicity after 24 hours of intravenous deferoxamine, continuing therapy should be undertaken cautiously and perhaps at a lower dose (Antidotes in Depth: Deferoxamine).

Patient Disposition

Fortunately, many patients who are exposed to iron do not develop significant toxic effects. If a toddler remains asymptomatic and develops minimal or no gastrointestinal manifestations after an observation period of 6 hours in the ED, discharge to an appropriate home situation can be considered. Patients who develop gastrointestinal symptoms and signs of mild poisoning (vomiting, diarrhea) should be observed as inpatients on regular hospital services. Patients who manifest signs and symptoms of significant iron poisoning such as metabolic acidosis, potential hemodynamic instability, and/or lethargy should be monitored and treated in an intensive care unit.

Pregnant Patients

The frequent diagnosis of iron deficiency anemia during pregnancy has lead to several reports of serious, and even fatal, iron ingestions in pregnant women.[10,42,60,68,86] Although in all cases of

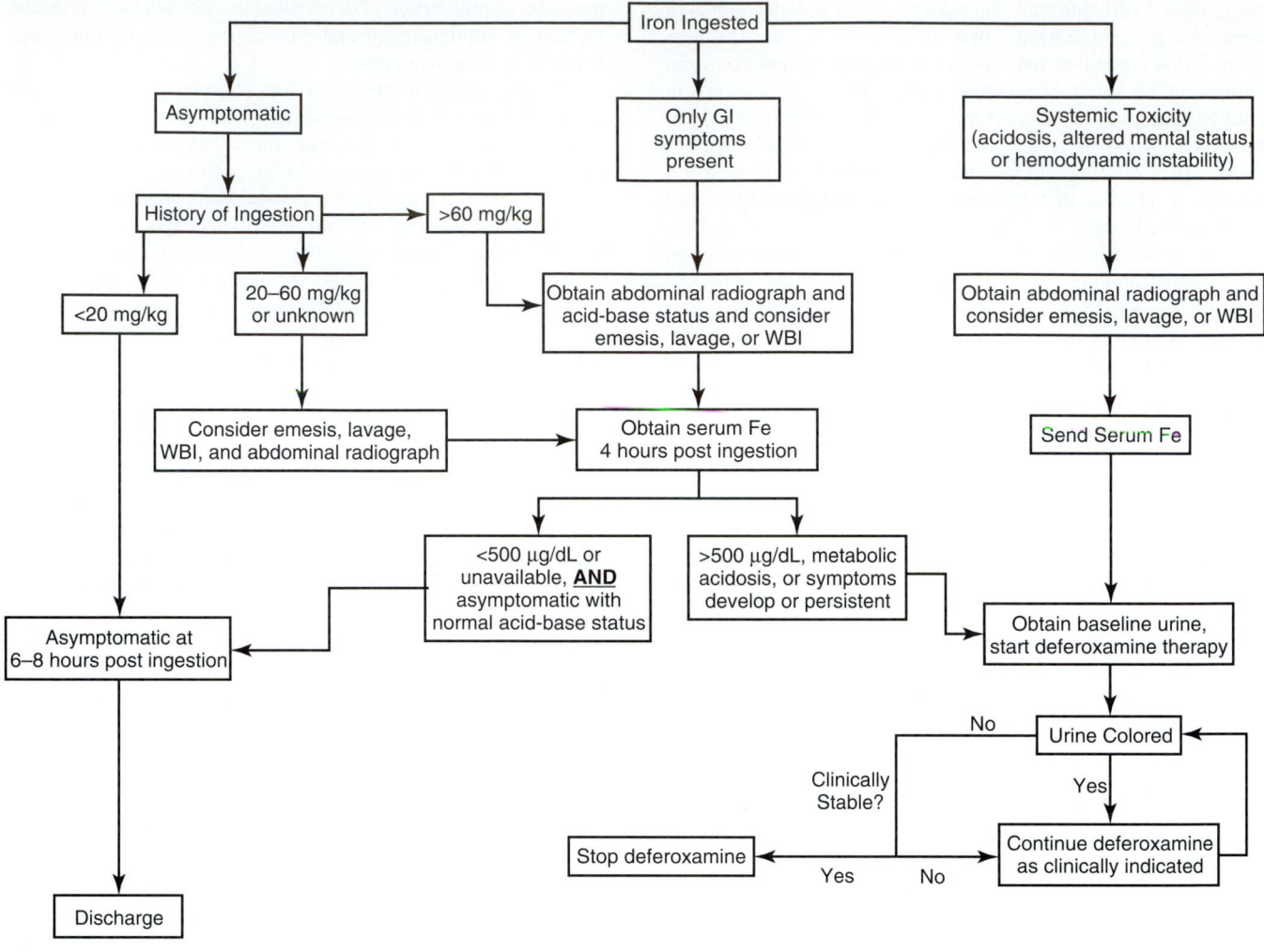

Figure 36–3. Algorithm for decision analysis following iron ingestion.

toxic exposures during pregnancy maternal resuscitation should always be the primary objective, unfounded concerns regarding deferoxamine toxicity in the fetus have inappropriately and at times disastrously delayed therapy.[60,78] This theoretical consideration of fetal deferoxamine toxicity is not supported in either human or animal studies.[15,51] A well-designed animal study demonstrated that in pregnant ewes near term poisoned with iron and treated with deferoxamine, fetal serum iron levels were not elevated and fetal deferoxamine levels could not be detected. In other words, neither iron nor deferoxamine is transferred to the fetus in appreciable quantities. Because fetal demise under these circumstances presumably results from maternal iron toxicity and not from a direct iron toxicity to the fetus, deferoxamine should be used to treat serious maternal iron poisoning and not withheld because of unfounded concern for fetal exposure to deferoxamine.

Adverse Effects of Deferoxamine

Most adverse effects of deferoxamine are reported in the setting of chronic administration for the treatment of hemochromatosis.[61,74] These same effects, such as pulmonary toxicity and acute respira-

tory distress syndrome (ARDS), however, are also described after treatment for acute iron overdose.[82] Four patients with serum iron levels ranging from 430 to 620 µg/dL developed ARDS following intravenous administration of deferoxamine for 32–72 hours. An animal study revealed significantly increased pulmonary toxicity when high-dose deferoxamine therapy was administered in the presence of high concentrations of oxygen (75–80% FIo_2).[1] The authors suggested that this effect was mediated via an oxygen free radical mechanism.

Administration of higher dose of deferoxamine has been suggested for the first 24 hours following serious iron poisoning, which occurs prior to tissue distribution of iron, and then subsequently decreasing the dose or limiting the duration of deferoxamine therapy to 24 hours.[35,37] The rationale is that high doses should be administered initially before free iron has been distributed to tissues and while it is available to bind to the deferoxamine. Pulmonary toxicity occurs 40 hours after a severe iron ingestion during very-low-dose deferoxamine (5 mg/kg) administration.[37] As suggested by the early iron-ingestion case reports cited above, pulmonary toxicity is a late manifestation of severe iron poisoning. The contribution of deferoxamine therapy to the acute lung injury that occurs in iron-poisoned patients is unclear. Pulmonary toxicity may be the result of iron-induced cardiovascular compromise or of a direct effect of deferoxamine in inactivating the iron-containing enzyme catalase. Catalase is responsible for the metabolism of certain reactive oxygen species. In either case, excessive dose and duration of deferoxamine therapy appear to contribute to toxicity. Further studies are needed to determine the optimal dosing regimen of deferoxamine therapy in the setting of iron poisoning. We would reserve the administration of higher doses of deferoxamine (up to 45 mg/kg) to those patients manifesting severe toxicity including signs of shock, metabolic acidosis, and hemodynamic instability.

Alternative Therapies

Many patients with conditions causing chronic iron overload are dependent on long-term chelation therapy. The use of the new orally active iron chelator 1,2-dimethyl-3-hydroxypyridin-4-one (deferiprone) may prove beneficial. In a small group of patients with thalassemia major, oral deferiprone was effective in decreasing and sustaining lower hepatic iron concentrations.[61] Deferiprone appears to be rapidly absorbed from the stomach, metabolized, and excreted as a glucuronide and iron complex in the urine.[46] Oral deferiprone was recently shown to be effective in reducing mortality in a rodent model of acute iron poisoning,[9] although an earlier study with deferiprone in iron-poisoned mice was unsuccessful.[36] Further study is needed to determine the safety and efficacy of deferiprone in human iron overdose.

One other treatment modality used experimentally for iron intoxication is continuous arteriovenous hemofiltration (CAVH). In a study of five iron-poisoned dogs, increased elimination of ferrioxamine in the ultrafiltrate was demonstrated when increasing doses of deferoxamine were infused into the arterial side of the system.[7] This technique is not described in iron-poisoned humans.

In toddlers with severe poisoning, it is theorized that exchange transfusion may help to physically remove free iron from the blood while replacing it with normal blood. Exchange transfusion in children is effective for poisonings such as theophylline, where the volume of distribution of the drug is small and removal from the blood compartment can be expected. However, iron-poisoned patients tend to have hemodynamic instability, so that removing blood volume may not be well tolerated.

SUMMARY

Despite FDA-mandated warnings on iron preparations, morbidity and mortality secondary to iron exposures continue to occur. A toddler presenting to the ED after presumed exposure with evidence of gastrointestinal toxicity and lethargy is at high risk for significant iron toxicity and possibly death. Although iron is available in multiple formulations (prenatal vitamins, ferrous gluconate supplements), toxicity is determined by the amount of elemental iron present; signs and symptoms occur following ingestions of 20 mg/kg elemental iron. Following stabilization of the patient, gastrointestinal decontamination, including orogastric lavage and whole-bowel irrigation (polyethylene glycol electrolyte lavage solution), should be initiated when indicated because activated charcoal is ineffective in binding iron. An abdominal radiograph may be helpful in determining the iron burden in the GI tract. After iron is absorbed, gastrointestinal symptoms of nausea, vomiting, diarrhea, hematemesis, and abdominal pain are prominent. Systemic iron toxicity leads to metabolic acidosis, hypotension, coagulopathy, and multiorgan system failure. Diagnosis and treatment of shock and acidosis, as well as chelation with deferoxamine, may be lifesaving. Education of parents, caregivers, and prescribers may decrease the incidence of serious iron exposures in the future.

REFERENCES

1. Adamson IY, Sienko A, Tenenbein M: Pulmonary toxicity of deferoxamine in iron poisoned mice. Toxicol Appl Pharmacol 1993;120: 13–19.
2. Anonymous. Preventing iron poisoning in children. FDA backgrounder—Current and useful information from the Food and Drug Administration, BG 97–1, amended 1/12/99. Available at http://www.fda.gov/opacom/backgrounders/ironbg.html. (Accessed April 16, 2000.)
3. Artman M, Olson RD, Boerth RC: Depression of myocardial contractility in acute iron toxicity in rabbits. Toxicol Appl Pharmacol 1982; 66:329–337.
4. Bachrach L, Correa A, Levin R, Grossman M: Iron poisoning: Complications of hypertonic phosphate lavage therapy. J Pediatr 1979;94: 147–149.
5. Balcerzak SP, Jensen WN, Pollack S: Mechanism of action of desferrioxamine on iron absorption. Scand J Haematol 1966;3:205–212.
6. Banner W, Tong TG: Iron poisoning. Pediatr Clin North Am 1986; 33:393–409.
7. Banner W, Vernon DD, Ward RM, et al: Continuous arteriovenous hemofiltration in experimental iron intoxication. Crit Care Med 1989;17:1187–1190.
8. Bentur Y, Klein J, Koren G: Misinterpretation of the iron-binding capacity in the presence of deferoxamine. J Pediatr 1991;118: 139–142.
9. Berkovitch M, Livne A, Lushkov G, et al: The efficacy of oral deferiprone in acute iron poisoning. Am J Emerg Med 2000;18:36–40.
10. Blanc P, Hryhorczuk D, Danel I: Deferoxamine treatment of acute iron intoxication in pregnancy. Obstet Gynecol 1984;64:125–145.
11. Burkhart KK, Kulig KW, Hammond KB, et al: The rise in the total iron-binding capacity after iron overdose. Ann Emerg Med 1991;20: 532–535.
12. Chiesa C, Pacifico L, Renzulli F, et al: *Yersinia* hepatic abscesses and iron overload [letter]. JAMA 1987;257:3230–3231.
13. Chyka PA, Butler AY: Assessment of acute iron poisoning by laboratory and clinical observations. Am J Emerg Med 1993;11:99–102.
14. Corby DG, McCullen AH: Effect of orally administered magnesium hydroxide in experimental iron intoxication. J Toxicol Clin Toxicol 1985;23:489–499.
15. Curry SC, Bond GR, Raschke R, et al: An ovine model of maternal iron poisoning in pregnancy. Ann Emerg Med 1990;19:632–638.
16. Czajka PA, Konrad JD, Duffy JP: Iron poisoning: An in vitro comparison of bicarbonate and phosphate lavage solutions. J Pediatr 1981;98:491–494.
17. Dean BS, Krenzelok EP: In vivo effectiveness of oral complexation agents in the management of iron poisoning. J Toxicol Clin Toxicol 1987:25:221–230.
18. Eisen TF, Lacouture PG, Woolf A: Visual detection of ferrioxamine color changes in urine. Vet Hum Toxicol 1988;30:369–370.
19. Everson GW, Bertaccini EJ, O'Leary JO: Use of whole-bowel irrigation in an infant following iron overdose. Am J Emerg Med 1991;9: 366–369.
20. Everson GW, Oudjhane K, Young LW, Krenzelok EP: Effectiveness of abdominal radiographs in visualizing chewable iron supplements following overdose. Am J Emerg Med 1989;7:459–463.
21. Finch CA, Huebers H: Perspectives in iron metabolism. N Engl J Med 1982;306:1520–1528.

22. Food and Drug Administration: Iron-containing supplements and drugs: Label warning statements and unit-dose packaging requirements. Fed Reg 1997;62:2217.

23. Foxford R, Goldfrank L: Gastrotomy: A surgical approach to iron overdose. Ann Emerg Med 1985; 14:1223–1226.

24. Freeman DA, Manoguerra AS: Absence of urinary color change in a severely iron-poisoned child treated with deferoxamine [abstract]. Vet Hum Toxicol 1981;23:351.

25. Ganote CE, Nahara G: Acute ferrous sulfate hepatotoxicity in rats. Lab Invest 1973;28:426–436.

26. Geffner ME, Opas LM: Phosphate poisoning complicating treatment for iron ingestion. Am J Dis Child 1980;134:509–510.

27. Gervitz NR, Wasserman LR: The measurement of iron and iron-binding capacity in plasma containing deferoxamine. J Pediatr 1966; 68:802–804.

28. Ghandi R, Robarts F: Hourglass stricture of the stomach and pyloric stenosis due to ferrous sulfate poisoning. Br J Surg 1962:49: 613–617.

29. Gleason WA, de Mello DE, de Castro FJ, et al: Acute hepatic failure in severe iron poisoning. J Pediatr 1979;95:138–140.

30. Gomez HF, McCLafferty HH, Flory D, et al: Prevention of gastrointestinal iron absorption by chelation from an orally administered premixed deferoxamine charcoal slurry. Ann Emerg Med 1997;30: 587–592.

31. Gold H, Cattell M, Hoppe JO, et al: Progress of medical science: A review of the toxicity of iron compounds. Am J Med Sci 1955; 558–571.

32. Helfer RE, Rodgerson DO: The effect of deferoxamine on the determination of serum iron and iron-binding capacity. J Pediatr 1966;68: 804–806.

33. Henretig FM, Karl SR, Weintraub WH: Severe iron poisoning treated with enteral and intravenous deferoxamine. Ann Emerg Med 1983;12:306–309.

34. Hosking CS: Radiology in the management of acute iron poisoning. Med J Aust 1969;1:576–579.

35. Howland MA: Risks of parenteral deferoxamine for acute iron poisoning. J Toxicol Clin Toxicol 1996;34:491–497.

36. Hung O, Manoach S, Howland MA, et al: Deferiprone for acute iron poisoning. J Toxicol Clin Toxicol 1997;35:565.

37. Ioannides AS, Panisello JM: Acute respiratory distress syndrome in children with acute iron poisoning: The role of intravenous desferrioxamine. Eur J Pediatr 2000;159:158–159.

38. Jackson TW, Ling LJ, Washington V: The effect of oral deferoxamine on iron absorption in humans. J Toxicol Clin Toxicol 1995;33: 325–329.

39. Jacobs J, Greene H, Gendel BR: Acute iron intoxication. N Engl J Med 1965;273:1124–1127.

40. Kaczorowski JM, Wax PM: Five days of whole-bowel irrigation in a case of pediatric iron ingestion. Ann Emerg Med 1996:27:258–263.

41. Keberle M: The biochemistry of desferrioxamine and its relation to iron metabolism. Ann N Y Acad Sci 1964;119:758–768.

42. Khoury S, Odeh M, Oettinger M: Deferoxamine treatment for acute iron intoxication in pregnancy. Acta Obstet Gynecol Scand 1995:74: 756–757.

43. Klein-Schwartz W: Toxicity of polysaccharide-iron complex exposures reported to poison control centers. Ann Pharmacother 2000;34: 165–169.

44. Klein-Schwartz W, Oderda GM, Gorman RL, et al: Assessment of management guidelines: Acute iron ingestion. Clin Pediatr 1990;29: 316–321.

45. Knasel AL, Collins-Barrow MD: Applicability of early indicators of iron toxicity. J Natl Med Assoc 1986;78:1037–1040.

46. Kontoghiorghes GJ, Goddard JG, Bartlett AN, Sheppard L: Pharmacokinetic studies in humans with the oral iron chelator 1,2-dimethyl-3-hydroxypyridine-4-one. Clin Pharmacol Ther 1990;48:255–261.

47. Lacouture PG, Wason S, Temple AR, et al: Emergency assessment of severity in iron overdose by clinical and laboratory methods. J Pediatr 1981;99:89–91.

48. Ling LJ, Hornfeldt CS, Winter JP: Absorption of iron after experimental overdose of chewable vitamins. Am J Emerg Med 1991;9: 24–26.

49. Lipschitz D, Dugard J, Simon M, et al: The site of action of desferrioxamine. Br J Haematol 1971;20:395–404.

50. Luongo MA, Bjornson SS: The liver in ferrous sulfate poisoning: A report of three fatal cases in children and an experimental study. N Engl J Med 1954;251:996–999.

51. McElhatton PR, Roberts JC, Sullivan FM: The consequences of iron overdose and its treatment with desferrioxamine in pregnancy. Hum Exp Toxicol 1991;10:251–259.

52. Melby K, Slordahl S, Gutterberg T, et al: Septicemia due to *Yersinia enterocolitica* after oral overdoses of iron. Br Med J 1982;285: 467–468.

53. Mills KC, Curry SC: Acute iron poisoning. Emerg Med Clin North Am 1994;12:397–413.

54. Mofenson HC, Caraccio TR, Sharieff N: Iron sepsis: *Yersinia enterocolitica* septicemia possibly caused by an overdose of iron. N Engl J Med 1987;316:1092–1093.

55. Morris CC: Pediatric iron poisonings in the United States. South Med J 2000;93;352–358.

56. Morse SB, Hardwick WE, King WD: Fatal iron intoxication in an infant. South Med J 1997;90:1043–1047.

57. Ng RCW, Perry K, Martin DJ: Iron poisoning: Assessment of radiography in diagnosis and management. Clin Pediatr 1979;18: 614–616.

58. Nordt SP, Williams SR, Behling C, et al: Comparison of the toxicities of two iron formulations in a swine model. Acad Emerg Med 1999;6:1104–1108.

59. O'Connor TA, Gruner BA, Gehrke JC, et al: In vitro binding of iron with the cation exchange resin sodium polystyrene sulfonate. Ann Emerg Med 1996;28:504–507.

60. Olenmark M, Biber B, Dottori O, Rybo G: Fatal iron intoxication in late pregnancy. J Toxicol Clin Toxicol 1987;25:347–359.

61. Olivieri NF, Brittenham GM, Matsui D, et al: Iron-chelation therapy with oral deferiprone in patients with thalassemia major. N Engl J Med 1995;332:918–922.

62. Olivieri NF, Buncic JR, Chew E, et al: Visual and auditory neurotoxicity in patients receiving subcutaneous deferoxamine infusions. N Engl J Med 1986;314:869–873.

63. Palatnick W, Tenenbein M: Leukocytosis, hyperglycemia, vomiting, and positive x-rays are not indicators of severity of iron overdose in adults. Am J Emerg Med 1996;14:454–455.

64. Pestaner JP, Ishak KG, Mullick FG, Centeno JA: Ferrous sulfate toxicity: A review of autopsy findings. Biol Trace Elem Res 1999;69: 191–198.

65. Peterson CD, Fifield GC: Emergency gastrotomy for acute iron poisoning. Ann Emerg Med 1980:9:262–264.

66. Propper R, Nathan D: Clinical removal of iron. Ann Rev Med 1982; 33:509–519.

67. Proudfoot AT, Simpson D, Dyson EH: Management of acute iron poisoning. Med Toxicol 1986;1:83–100.

68. Rayburn WF, Donn SM, Wolf ME: Iron overdose during pregnancy: Successful therapy with deferoxamine. Am J Obstet Gynecol 1983; 147:717–718.

69. Reissman KR, Coleman TJ: Acute intestinal iron intoxication. II: Metabolic, respiratory and circulatory effects of absorbed iron salts. Blood 1955;10:46–51.

70. Roberts RJ, Nayfield S, Soper R, et al: Acute iron intoxication with intestinal infarction managed in part by small bowel resection. Clin Toxicol 1975;8:3–12.

71. Roberts WL, Smith PT, Martin WJ, Rainey PM: Performance characteristics of three serum iron and total iron binding capacity methods in acute iron overdose. Am J Clin Pathol 1999:112:657–664.

72. Robotham JL, Troxler RF, Lietman PS: Iron poisoning: Another energy crisis. Lancet 1974;2:664–665.

73. Rosenmund A, Haeberli A, Struab PW: Blood coagulation and acute iron toxicity. J Lab Clin Med 1984:103:524–533.

74. Scanderbeg AC, Izzi GC, Butturini A, Benaglia G: Pulmonary syndrome and intravenous high-dose desferrioxamine [letter]. Lancet 1990;336:1511.

75. Snyder BK, Clark RF: Effect of magnesium hydroxide administration on iron absorption after a supratherapeutic dose of ferrous sulfate in human volunteers: A randomized controlled trial. Ann Emerg Med 1999;33:400–405.

76. Staple TW, McAlister WH: Roentgenographic visualization of iron preparations in the gastrointestinal tract. Radiology 1964;83: 1051–1056.

77. Stein ZL, Barkin RL: *Yersiniae* and iron intoxication [letter]. Drug Intell Clin Pharm 1987;21:661.

78. Strom RL, Schiller P, Seeds AE, ten Bensel R: Fatal iron poisoning in a pregnant female. Minn Med 1976;483–489.

79. Tenenbein M: Toxicokinetics and toxicodynamics of iron poisoning. Toxicol Lett 1998;102–103:653–656.

80. Tenenbein M: Whole-bowel irrigation in iron poisoning. J Pediatr 1987;111:142–145.

81. Tenenbein M, Israels SJ: Early coagulopathy in severe iron poisoning. J Pediatr 1988;113:695–697.

82. Tenenbein M, Kowalski S, Bowden DH, Adamson IYR: Pulmonary toxic effects of continuous desferrioxamine administration in acute iron poisoning. Lancet 1992;339:699–701.

83. Tenenbein M, Littman C, Stimpson RE: Gastrointestinal pathology in adult iron overdose. J Toxicol Clin Toxicol 1990;28:311–320.

84. Tenenbein M, Yatscoff RW: The total iron-binding capacity in iron poisoning. Is it useful? Am J Dis Child 1991;45:437–439.

85. Thomson J: Ferrous sulphate poisoning: Its incidence, symptomatology, treatment and prevention. Br Med J 1950;1:645–646.

86. Tran T, Wax JR, Steinfeld JD, Ingardia CJ: Acute intentional iron overdose in pregnancy. Obstet Gynecol 1998;92:678–680.

87. Turk J, Aks S, Ampuero F, Hryhorczuk DO: Successful therapy of iron intoxication in pregnancy with intravenous deferoxamine and whole-bowel irrigation. Vet Hum Toxicol 1993;35:441–444.

88. Venturelli J, Kwee Y, Morris N, et al: Gastrotomy in the management of acute iron poisoning. J Pediatr 1982;100:768–769.

89. Vernon DD, Banner W Jr, Dean JM: Hemodynamic effects of experimental iron poisoning. Ann Emerg Med 1989;18:863–866.

90. Villalobos D: Reliability of urine-color changes after deferoxamine challenge [abstract]. Vet Hum Toxicol 1992;34:330.

91. Wallace K, Curry SC, LoVecchio F, Raschke RA: Effect of magnesium hydroxide on iron absorption following simulated mild iron overdose in human subjects. Acad Emerg Med 1998;5:961–965.

92. Weiss B, Alkon E, Weindlar F, et al: Toddler deaths resulting from ingestion of iron supplements—Los Angeles, 1992–1993. MMWR Morb Mortal Wkly Rep 1993;42:111–113.

93. Westlin WF: Deferoxamine as a chelating agent. Clin Toxicol 1971; 4:597–602.

94. Westlin W: Deferoxamine in the treatment of acute iron poisoning: Clinical experiences with 172 children. Clin Pediatr 1966;5: 531–535.

95. Whitten CF, Gibson GW, Good MH, et al: Studies in acute iron poisoning. I. Desferrioxamine in the treatment of acute iron poisoning: Clinical observations, experimental studies, and theoretical considerations. Pediatrics 1965;36:322–335.

96. Whitten CF, Chen YC, Gibson GW: Studies in acute iron poisoning: II. Further observations on desferrioxamine in the treatment of acute experimental iron poisoning. Pediatrics 1966; 38:102–110.

97. Whitten CF, Chen YC, Gibson GW: Studies in acute iron poisoning III. The hemodynamic alterations in acute experimental iron poisoning. Pediatr Res 1968:2:479–485.

98. Witzleben CL, Chaffey NJ: Acute ferrous sulphate poisoning: A histochemical study of its effect on the liver. Arch Pathol Lab Med 1966;82:454–460.

99. Wu ML, Yang CC, Ger J, Deng JF: A fatal case of acute ferric chloride poisoning. Vet Human Toxicol 1998;40:31–34.

100. Yatscoff RW, Wayne EA, Tenenbein M: An objective criterion for the cessation of deferoxamine therapy in the acutely iron poisoned patient. J Toxicol Clin Toxicol 1991;29:1–10.

101. Yonker J, Banner W, Picchioni A: Absorption characteristics of iron and deferoxamine onto charcoal. Vet Hum Toxicol 1980;22 (Suppl):75.

ANTIDOTES IN DEPTH

Deferoxamine

Mary Ann Howland

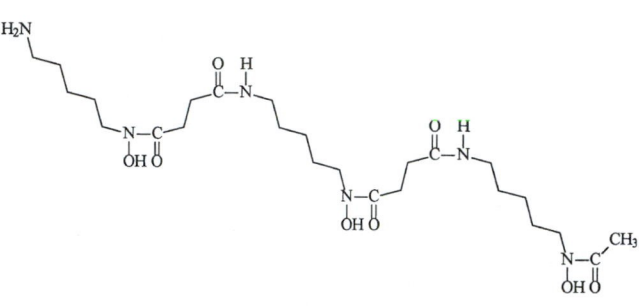

Deferoxamine is the parenteral chelator of choice for iron poisoning.

Although deferoxamine has been used to treat acute iron overdose for many years, there are no controlled studies that evaluate efficacy or dosing. Much of our knowledge comes from animal studies and case series in the 1960s and early 1970s, and from limited case reports throughout the ensuing years. Deferoxamine is also used in the chelation of aluminum in patients with chronic renal failure.

DISCOVERY OF DEFEROXAMINE

Iron toxicity was recognized as early as the 1800s, forgotten, and subsequently rediscovered.[28] The development of deferoxamine was initiated by the analysis of the metabolites of actinomycetes. Keberle isolated ferrioxamine B from the organism *Streptomyces pilosus*.[33] Ferrioxamine is a brownish-red compound containing trivalent iron (ie, ferric, Fe^{3+}) and 3 molecules of trihydroxamic acid. Deferoxamine (desferrioxamine B) is the colorless compound that results when the trivalent iron is chemically removed from ferrioxamine B (Fig. 36–4).[33]

CHEMISTRY

Deferoxamine (DFO) is a water-soluble hexadentate chelator with a molecular weight of 561 daltons. The commercial formulation is the mesylate salt with a molecular weight of 657 daltons. One mole of DFO binds 1 mole of Fe^{3+}; therefore, theoretically, 100 mg of DFO can bind 10 mg of Fe^{3+} or 8.5 mg as the mesylate salt.

DFO has a far greater affinity constant for iron (10^{31}) than for zinc, copper, nickel, magnesium, or calcium (10^2–10^{14}).[33] Therefore, at physiologic pH values, deferoxamine complexes almost exclusively with ferric iron.[24,67]

MECHANISM OF ACTION

DFO binds Fe^{3+} at the three N–OH sites, forming an octahedral iron complex (Fig. 36–4). Once bound, the resultant ferrioxamine is very stable. Deferoxamine appears to be of benefit to patients with iron poisoning by chelating free iron (nontransferrin-plasma-iron) and iron in transit between transferrin and ferritin (chelatable labile iron pool),[27,39,53] while not directly affecting the iron of hemoglobin, hemosiderin, or ferritin.[33] In vitro studies suggest that DFO removes iron from ferritin and transferrin and only very little from hemosiderin.[44] However, in vivo experiments demonstrate that DFO cannot remove iron once it is bound to transferrin.[4] Deferoxamine does bind "free iron" found in the plasma as nontransferrin-plasma-iron after transferrin is saturated. This situation occurs in the overdose setting or chronic iron overload syndromes.[27] In vitro studies demonstrate that deferoxamine chelates and inactivates cytoplasmic and mitochondrial iron, preventing disruption of mitochondrial function and injury.[39] In chronic iron overload, deferoxamine chelates iron deposited in the reticuloendothelial cells found in the spleen, liver, and bone marrow and excretes it in the urine as ferrioxamine.[27] It is unclear whether DFO actually chelates the iron within the reticuloendothelial cells or after liberation into the plasma. In vitro studies demonstrate that the liver can donate iron to deferoxamine and chelation may lead subsequently to biliary excretion and fecal elimination.[27,43]

PHARMACOKINETICS

DFO has a volume of distribution that ranges from 0.6 to 1.33 L/kg.[33,36,50] The initial distribution half-life of DFO is approximately 1 hour in the dog,[50] and about 5–10 minutes in humans.[35,57] DFO is probably metabolized in the plasma to metabolites (A-F), of which metabolite B may be toxic.[33,36,50] Unchanged DFO undergoes glomerular filtration and tubular secretion.[43] The terminal elimination half-life of DFO is approximately 6 hours in healthy patients,[2] but about 3 hours in patients with thalassemia.

Ferrioxamine has a smaller volume of distribution than DFO. In nephrectomized dogs, the volume of distribution of ferrioxamine was calculated to be 19% of body weight whereas it was about 50% of body weight for DFO,[33] implying that DFO has a wider tissue distribution. This different pharmacokinetic pattern may be related to the potential for penetrance of the straight-chain molecule deferoxamine when compared to that of the octahedral ferrioxamine. Experiments in dogs demonstrate that intravenous (IV) ferrioxamine is entirely eliminated by the kidney within 5 hours,[33] through glomerular filtration and partial reabsorption.[43]

The pharmacokinetics of DFO and ferrioxamine differ between healthy and iron-overloaded patients. Plasma concentrations of DFO in healthy patients are about twice the level noted in patients with thalassemia, while in these patients ferrioxamine concentrations are 5 times greater than those found in healthy patients.[33,58]

Some investigators suggest that DFO can be continued and hemodialysis performed to remove ferrioxamine in the presence of

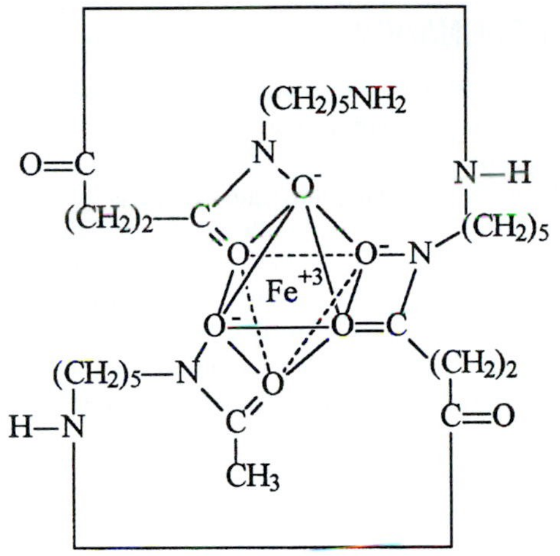

Figure 36–4. Ferrioxamine.

renal failure.[68] Although both hemodialysis[14,57] and hemoperfusion[14] are effective in ferrioxamine removal, it is unclear whether these interventions are indicated.

ANIMAL STUDIES

Studies in guinea pigs given LD_{50} (median lethal dose) and LD_{100} (lethal dose in all exposed subjects) oral doses of ferrous sulfate show dramatic improvement in survival rates after oral DFO was given in a dose calculated to bind most of the iron, which is substantially less DFO than is given clinically.[44] Mortality rates in this study, and in a similar study in swine,[18] directly correlate with the delay in DFO administration.[44]

Subsequent studies were carried out in dogs. In two different studies by the same authors, dogs receiving the iron-DFO complex orally had a 40–100% mortality.[67,68] When both oral and intravenous DFO were administered to 9 dogs poisoned with iron, 3 survived.[66] A similar follow-up study demonstrated a 50% survival rate in dogs given a lethal dose (225 mg/kg) of iron followed by oral DFO (2.6 g) and intravenous DFO (0.75–1.5 mg/kg/min for 8–12 hours).[68] These studies have limited any substantial interest in the use of oral DFO despite the more favorable results in noncanine species.[5,29,44,62]

EARLY HUMAN USE AND HISTORY OF DOSING RECOMMENDATIONS

In one of the earliest case series, 172 children who were not severely poisoned and who were hemodynamically stable were treated with 5–10 g of oral DFO and either 1 or 2 g of DFO IM every 3–12 hours.[66] One gram administered intravenously at no more than 15 mg/kg/h every 4–12 hours was continued for 2–3 days as necessary for those patients in shock or severely ill. Of the 28 patients who developed coma, shock, or both, only 3 died, 1 of whom received late treatment with DFO.

This case series was expanded to 472 patients and, based on this clinical experience, guidelines for DFO dosing were formulated.[65] The IM dose of DFO was suggested as 1 g initially, followed by 0.5 g 4 and 8 hours later and then every 4–12 hours as necessary, without exceeding 6 g in 24 hours. Intravenous DFO was recommended for patients in shock at a rate not to exceed 15 mg/kg/h, with an initial dose not to exceed 1 g, followed by two 0.5-g doses separated by 4 hours and a total dosage not to exceed 6 g in 24 hours. These recommendations for total dosages were not scientifically developed and appear to be based on arbitrary assumptions. However, the manufacturer continues to recommend these doses.[19]

URINARY COLOR CHANGE

In an attempt to further define the role of DFO, investigators turned to urinary examinations. A vin rosé color of the urine following DFO was indicative of 10–30 mg of urinary iron excretion per 24 hours.[44] In a review of 107 patients with acute iron poisoning who had received 5 g of DFO orally and 90 mg/kg IV at a rate not greater than 15 mg/kg/h,[41] the appearance of a vin rosé color in urine or a serum iron level greater than 500 μg/dL prompted chelation for at least 24 hours. Further studies have investigated the correlation between urinary iron concentrations and systemic toxicity.[70] Most data suggest that following DFO administration the absence of a urine color change indicates that very little ferrioxamine is being excreted renally.[23] When a baseline urine is not obtained prior to DFO administration, post-DFO administration comparisons of urine color are inadequate. No relationship between urinary iron excretion, clinical iron toxicity, and the effectiveness of DFO has been established.

IM VERSUS IV ADMINISTRATION

Prior to 1976, patients were given IM DFO and only received IV DFO if they were in shock. However, when transfusion-induced iron overload was studied, and IM and IV DFO administration were compared, IV DFO significantly enhanced urinary iron elimination.[54] This study provided compelling arguments against IM dosing, as did data showing higher peak concentrations and more stable levels with IV infusions. A single patient was given 425 mg/kg IV over 24 hours without incident, although the increase in urinary iron excretion seen when the DFO dose increased from 4 to 16 g/d appeared to be of limited consequence.

DURATION OF DOSING

How long DFO should be administered is unknown. In dogs, serum iron levels peak within 3–5 hours and then fall quickly as iron is transported out of the blood into the tissues.[63,69] In one human study, patients with initial iron levels of about 500 μg/dL fell to approximately 100 μg/dL within 12 hours.[37] Other case reports also suggest that by 24 hours most of the easily accessible iron is distributed out of the blood compartment.[20] Although severely poisoned patients have received DFO for more than 24 hours without difficulty, pulmonary toxicity has been associated with prolonged DFO infusions.[26,48,60] Intuitively, in patients with acute iron overdose DFO should be administered early and for a shorter duration while the iron is easily accessible in the blood. In patients with chronic iron overdoses prolonged infusions of smaller doses of DFO are necessary to act as a sink to slowly remove iron from the labile pool and tissue stores.[30]

ADVERSE EFFECTS

When administered to patients with acute iron overdose, DFO is associated with rate-related hypotension, pulmonary toxicity, and infection. When administered to patients with chronic iron overload, DFO is associated with auditory, ocular, and pulmonary toxicity and infection.[30]

Significant hypotension was first noted in 1965, in 2 children, when approximately 80–150 mg/kg of DFO was administered intravenously over 15 minutes.[67] Three dogs receiving 54–85 mg/kg/h of DFO also developed hypotension.[66] The mechanism for the rate-related hypotension is not fully understood, although histamine release is implicated. Elevated histamine levels were documented in a canine experiment, but pretreatment with diphenhydramine was not protective.[68] Intravascular volume depletion due to iron toxicity also contributes to the hypotension. No experiment has ever determined a maximum safe rate of administration of DFO. Adverse effects of DFO were noted when DFO was infused rapidly. These adverse effects included tachycardia, hypotension, shock, erythema, and urticaria.[66] These adverse effects led to the current recommendations for intravenous administration of not more than 15 mg/kg/h as mentioned earlier.[66–68] Currently suggested intravenous infusion rates are empiric, have never been scientifically determined, and higher rates are administered successfully, particularly in the critically ill.[11,15,20]

Acute lung injury (ALI) has been described in the setting of acute iron overdoses following IV administration of DFO (15 mg/kg/h) therapy for greater than 24 hours.[3,32,60] Usually there was a return to therapeutic iron levels in these patients after 24 hours, and the rationale for continued administration of DFO was not reported. Examination of the nontoxicologic literature reveals other instances of ALI occurring in patients receiving continuous IV DFO for hemosiderosis and malignancies.[13,22,64] Common to all these patients was the administration of continuous IV doses of DFO for prolonged (>24 hours) periods of time. The mechanism for the development of pulmonary toxicity after DFO is unknown. The pulmonary toxicity may result from excessive DFO chelation of intracellular iron and the depletion of catalase, resulting in subsequent oxidant damage[25] or the generation of free radicals.[1]

Deferoxamine therapy may lead to infection with a number of unusual organisms, including *Yersinia enterocolitica*, *Zygomycetes*, and *Aeromonas hydrophilia*. The virulence of these organisms is facilitated when the DFO-iron complex acts as a siderophore for their growth.[38,42,45] Most cases have occurred when DFO was employed for aluminum toxicity in patients receiving chronic hemodialysis.[43] Several cases of *Yersinia* sepsis are reported following acute iron overdose.[42,45]

Ocular toxicity characterized by decreased visual acuity, night blindness, color blindness, and retinal pigmentary abnormalities has occurred in patients who received continuous IV DFO for thalassemia and other nonacute iron- and aluminum-excess conditions.[8,12,17,47,49] Ototoxicity documented by abnormal audiograms indicating partial or total deafness has also been reported.[52] However, neither ocular nor ototoxicity has been reported in the toxicology literature.

USE IN PREGNANCY

A recent review of the literature identified 61 cases of intentional iron overdose in pregnant women.[61] Serious iron toxicity with organ involvement is associated with spontaneous abortion, preterm delivery, and maternal death. There is no evidence that deferoxamine is teratogenic.[61] Neither iron nor deferoxamine appears to cross the ovine placenta.[16] A case report of a pregnant woman with thalassemia and review of 40 other pregnant patients with thalassemia treated extensively with DFO found no evidence of teratogenicity.[56] Deferoxamine should be administered to pregnant women with acute iron overdose for the same indications as for nonpregnant women.

ADDITIONAL IRON CHELATORS

New iron chelators are being investigated. Pyridoxal isonicotinyl-hydrase and pyridoxal benzoylhydrazone are potent lipophilic chelators. Lipophilicity increases iron mobilization but may also increase toxicity. Deferiprone is a bidentate oral iron chelator. Three moles of deferiprone are required to bind 1 mole of ferric ion to form a stable complex.[27] Inappropriate ratios of drug to iron may be ineffective or even harmful due to the formation of potentially toxic intermediates.[27] Preliminary animal studies in acute toxicity are contradictory.[10,21,31,34] The effectiveness and long-term safety of deferiprone for chronic iron overload associated with thalassemia has been questioned.[7,35,46] Other hexadentate drugs and prodrugs are under investigation.[27]

INDICATIONS AND DOSING

The indications and dosage schedule for DFO are largely empiric because a controlled study has never been performed.[6,55] Systemic toxicity associated with acute iron poisoning manifested by coma, shock, or metabolic acidosis warrants intravenous infusion of DFO. The duration of therapy should probably be limited to 24 hours to maximize effectiveness while minimizing the risk of pulmonary toxicity. Some have suggested that more than the recommended dose of 15 mg/kg/h be employed in the first 24 hours for life-threatening iron toxicity, but this recommendation must be validated.[30] Although patients with mild toxicity may be treated with IM injections of DFO at 90 mg/kg (maximum, 1 g in children or 2 g in adults), this volume of antidote cannot be given intramuscularly with ease or painlessly in children. Therefore, few clinicians administer DFO IM and most prefer the IV route (Chap. 36). The total daily parenteral dose is limited by the infusion rate in children (if the manufacturer's recommendations are adhered to). In adults conservative recommendations limit the dose to 6–8 g/d, although doses as high as 16 g/d with diverse dosing regimens have been administered without incident.[15,20,40,48,54,59]

AVAILABILITY

Deferoxamine mesylate (Desferal) is available in vials containing 500 mg or 2 g of sterile, lyophilized powder. Addition of 5 mL or 20 mL of sterile water for injection to either the 500-mg or the 2-g vials, respectively, results in a solution of 100 mg/mL. This solution is isotonic, clear, and colorless to slightly yellowish.[19] The resulting solution can be further diluted with 0.9% NaCl, glucose in water, or Ringer lactate solution for intravenous administration. For IM administration, a smaller volume of solution is preferred and 2 mL or 8 mL of sterile water for injection can be added to the 500-mg or 2-g vials, respectively. This results in a stronger yellow-colored solution containing 250 mg/mL.

REFERENCES

1. Adamson I, Sienko A, Tenenbein M: Pulmonary toxicity of deferoxamine in iron-poisoned mice. Toxicol Appl Pharmacol 1993;120: 13–19.
2. Allain P, Mauras Y, Chaleil D, et al: Pharmacokinetics and renal elimination of desferrioxamine and ferrioxamine in healthy subjects and patients with hemochromatosis. Br J Clin Pharmacol 1987;24: 207–212.
3. Anderson KJ, Rivers PRA: Desferrioxamine in acute iron poisoning [letter]. Lancet 1992;339:1602.
4. Balcerzak SP, Jensen WN, Pollack S: Mechanism of action of desferrioxamine on iron absorption. Scand J Haematol 1966;3:205–212.
5. Banner W: Of iron and ancient mariners. Ann Emerg Med 1997;30: 687–688.
6. Banner W, Tong T: Iron poisoning. Pediatr Clin North Am 1986;33: 393–409.
7. Barman Balfour JA, Foster RH: Deferiprone: A review of its clinical potential in iron overload in beta-thalassaemia major and other transfusion-dependent diseases. Drugs 1999;58:553–578.
8. Bene C, Manzler A, Bene D, et al: Irreversible ocular toxicity from a single "challenge" dose of deferoxamine. Clin Nephron 1989;31: 45–48.
9. Bentur Y, McGuigan M, Koren G: Deferoxamine (desferrioxamine), new toxicities for an old drug. Drug Saf 1991;6:37–46.
10. Berkovitch M, Livne A, Lushkov G, et al: The efficacy of oral deferiprone in acute iron poisoning. Am J Emerg Med 2000;18:36–40.
11. Berland Y, Charhon SA, Olmer M, et al: Predictive value of desferrioxamine infusion test for bone aluminum deposit in hemodialyzed patients. Nephron 1985;40:433–435.
12. Blake D, Winyard P, Lunec J, et al: Cerebral and ocular toxicity induced by desferrioxamine. Q J Med 1985;219:345–355.
13. Castriota Scanderberg A, Izzi G, Butturini A, Benaglia G: Pulmonary syndrome and intravenous high-dose desferrioxamine [letter]. Lancet 1990;336:1511.
14. Chang TMS, Barne P: Effect of desferrioxamine on removal of aluminum and iron by coated charcoal hemoperfusion and hemodialysis. Lancet 1983;2:1051–1053.
15. Cheney K, Gumbiner C, Benson B, et al: Survival after a severe iron poisoning treated with intermittent infusions of deferoxamine. J Toxicol Clin Toxicol 1995;33:61–66.
16. Curry SC, Bond GR, Raschke R, et al: An ovine model of maternal iron poisoning in pregnancy. Ann Emerg Med 1990;19:632–638.
17. Davies S, Hungerford J, Arden G, et al: Ocular toxicity of high-dose intravenous desferrioxamine. Lancet 1983;2:181–184.
18. Dean B, Oehme FW, Krenzelok E, Hines R: A study of iron complexation in a swine model. Vet Hum Toxicol 1988;30:313–315.
19. Desferal. Package Insert. Novartis 2000.
20. Douglas D, Smilkstein M: Deferoxamine-iron induced pulmonary injury and N-acetylcysteine. J Toxicol Clin Toxicol 1995;33:495.
21. Fassos FF, Berkovitch M, Daneman N, et al: Efficacy of deferiprone in the treatment of acute iron intoxication in rats. J Toxicol Clin Toxicol 1996;34:279–287.
22. Freedman M, Grisaru D, Oliveri NF, et al: Pulmonary syndrome in patients with thalassemia major receiving intravenous deferoxamine infusions. Am J Dis Child 1990;144:565–569.
23. Freeman DA, Manoguerra AS: Absence of urinary color change in severely iron poisoned child treated with deferoxamine [abstract]. Vet Hum Toxicol 1981;23(Suppl 1):49.
24. Goodwin JF, Whitten CF: Chelation of ferrous sulfate solution by deferoxamine B. Nature 1965;205:281–283.
25. Helson L, Helson C, Braverman S, et al: Desferrioxamine in acute iron poisoning [letter]. Lancet 1992;339:1602–1603.
26. Henretig F, Karl S, Weintraub W: Severe iron poisoning treated with enteral and intravenous deferoxamine. Ann Emerg Med 1983;12: 306–309.
27. Hershko C, Link G, Cabantchik I: Pathophysiology of iron overload. Ann N Y Acad Sci 1998;850:191–201.
28. Hoppe JO, Marcell GMA, Tainter ML: A review of the toxicity of iron compounds. Am J Med Sci 1955;230:558–571.
29. Hoskin CS: A pharmacologic investigation of acute iron poisoning and its treatment. Aust Paediatr J 1970;6:92–96.
30. Howland MA: Risks of parenteral deferoxamine. J Toxicol Clin Toxicol 1996;34:491–497.
31. Hung O, Manoach S, Howland MA, et al: Deferiprone for acute iron poisoning. J Toxicol Clin Toxicol 1997;35:565.
32. Ioannides AS, Panisello JM: Acute respiratory distress syndrome in children with acute iron poisoning: The role of intravenous desferrioxamine. Eur J Pediatr 2000;159:158–159.
33. Keberle M: The biochemistry of desferrioxamine and its relation to iron metabolism. Ann N Y Acad Sci 1964;119:758–768.
34. Kontoghiorgher GJ: New concepts of iron and aluminum chelation therapy with oral L1 (deferiprone) and other chelators. Analyst 1995; 120:845–851.
35. Kowdley K, Kaplan M: Iron chelation therapy with oral deferiprone—Toxicity or lack of efficacy. N Engl J Med 1998;339:468–469.
36. Lee P, Mohammed N, Marshal L, et al: Intravenous infusion pharmacokinetics of desferrioxamine in thalassemic patients. Drug Metab Dispos 1993;21:640–644.
37. Leikin S, Vossough P, Mochiv-Fatemi F: Chelation therapy in acute iron poisoning. J Pediatr 1969;71:425–430.
38. Lin S, Shieh S, Lin Y, et al: Fatal *Aeromonas hydrophilia* bacteremia in a hemodialysis patient treated with deferoxamine. Am J Kidney Dis 1996;27:733–735.
39. Lipschitz D, Dugard J, Simon M, et al: The site of action of desferrioxamine. Br J Haematol 1971;20:395–404.
40. Lovejoy F: Chelation therapy in iron poisoning. J Toxicol Clin Toxicol 1982;19:871–874.
41. McEnery J: Hospital management of acute iron ingestion. Clin Toxicol 1971;4:603–613.
42. Melby K, Slordahl S, Gutteberg TJ, Nordbo SA: Septicemia due to *Yersinia enterocolitica* after oral doses of iron. Br Med J 1982; 285:487–488.
43. Mersko C, Hersko C, Weatherall D: Iron chelating therapy. Crit Rev Clin Lab Sci 1988;26:303–340.
44. Moeschlin S, Schnider U: Treatment of primary and secondary hemochromatosis and acute iron poisoning with a new potent iron eliminating agent (desferrioxamine-B). N Engl J Med 1963;269:57–66.
45. Mofenson HC, Caraccio TR, Sharieff N: Iron sepsis: *Yersinia enterocolitica* septicemia possibly caused by an overdose of iron. N Engl J Med 1987;316:1092–1093.
46. Olivieri NF, Brittenham GM, McLaren CE, et al: Long-term safety and effectiveness of iron-chelation therapy with deferiprone for thalassemia major. N Engl J Med 1998;339:417–423.
47. Olivieri N, Buncic J, Chew E, et al: Visual and auditory neuro-toxicity in patients receiving subcutaneous deferoxamine infusions. N Engl J Med 1986;314:869–873.
48. Peck M, Rogers J, Riverbach J: Use of high doses of deferoxamine (Desferal) in an adult patient with acute iron overdosage. J Toxicol Clin Toxicol 1982;19:865–869.
49. Pengloan J, Dantal J, Rossazza M, et al: Ocular toxicity after a single dose of desferrioxamine in two hemodialysis patients. Nephron 1987; 46:211–212.
50. Peter G, Keberle M, Schmid K: Distribution and renal excretion of desferrioxamine and ferrioxamine in the dog and in the rat. Biochem Pharmacol 1966;15:93–109.

51. Porter JB, Faherty A, Stallibrass L, et al: A trial to investigate the relationship between DFO pharmacokinetics and metabolism and DFO-related toxicity. Ann N Y Acad Sci 1998;30:483–487.

52. Porter J, Jaswon M, Huehns E, et al: Desferrioxamine ototoxicity: Evaluation of risk factors in thalassemic patients and guidelines for safe dosage. Br J Haematol 1989;73:403–409.

53. Propper R, Nathan D: Clinical removal of iron. Annu Rev Med 1982; 33:509–519.

54. Propper R, Shurn S, Nathan D: Reassessment of the use of desferrioxamine B in iron overload. N Engl J Med 1976;294:1421–1423.

55. Robotham J, Lietman P: Acute iron poisoning. Am J Dis Child 1980; 134:875–879.

56. Singer ST, Vichinsky EP: Deferoxamine treatment during pregnancy: Is it harmful? Am J Hematol 1999;60:24–26.

57. Stivelman J, Schulman G, Fosburg M, et al: Kinetics and efficacy of deferoxamine in iron overloaded hemodialysis patients. Kidney Int 1989;36:1125–1132.

58. Summers MR, Jacobs A, Tudway D, et al: Studies in desferrioxamine and ferrioxamine metabolism in normal and iron loaded subjects. Br J Haematol 1979;42: 547–555.

59. Tenenbein M: Benefits of parenteral deferoxamine for acute iron poisoning. J Toxicol Clin Toxicol 1996;34:485–489.

60. Tenenbein M, Kowalski S, Sienko A, et al: Pulmonary toxic effects of continuous administration in acute iron poisoning. Lancet 1992;339: 699–701.

61. Tran T, Wax JR, Philput C, et al: Intentional iron overdose in pregnancy—Management and outcome. J Emerg Med 2000;18:225–228.

62. Tripod JA: Pharmacologic comparison of the binding of iron and other metals. In: Gross F, ed: Iron Metabolism. International Symposium on Iron Metabolism. Berlin, Springer-Verlag, 1964, pp. 503–524.

63. Vernon DD, Banner W Jr, Dean JM: Hemodynamic effects of experimental iron poisoning. Ann Emerg Med 1989;18:863–866.

64. Weitman S, Buchanan G, Kamen B: Pulmonary toxicity of deferoxamine in children with advanced cancer. J Natl Cancer Inst 1991;83: 1834–1835.

65. Westlin W: Deferoxamine as a chelating agent. Clin Toxicol 1971;4: 597–602.

66. Westlin W: Deferoxamine in the treatment of acute iron poisoning: Clinical experiences with 172 children. Clin Pediatr 1966;5:531–535.

67. Whitten C, Gibson G, Good M, et al: Studies in acute iron poisoning: Desferrioxamine in the treatment of acute iron poisoning—Clinical observations, experimental studies and theoretical considerations. Pediatrics 1965;36:322–335.

68. Whitten C, You-chen C, Gibson G: Studies in acute iron poisoning: II. Further observations on deferoxamine in the treatment of acute experimental iron poisoning. Pediatrics 1966;38:102–110.

69. Whitten CF, Chen YC, Gibson GW: Studies in acute iron poisoning III: The hemodynamic alterations in acute experimental iron poisoning. Pediatr Res 1968;2:479–485.

70. Yatscoff RW, Wayne EA, Tenenbein M: An objective criterion for the cessation of deferoxamine therapy in the acutely poisoned patient. J Toxicol Clin Toxicol 1991;29:1–10.

Richard J. Hamilton

A 19-year-old woman came to the Emergency Department (ED) complaining of severe headaches and double vision. She had been in relatively good health, with no significant past medical or psychiatric history. For several weeks, however, she had been experiencing generalized headaches that were increasing in severity and duration. In addition, she noted the recent onset of diplopia, which was more marked on lateral gaze. Other complaints included anorexia, arthralgias, dryness and cracking of the lips, muscular stiffness and soreness after prolonged exercise, and a tendency to tire easily. She had acne vulgaris for several years, for which she was taking vitamins and topical agents prescribed by a local healthcare clinic. There were no menstrual irregularities, no symptoms of thyroid dysfunction, no history of recent viral syndrome, and no history of head trauma. She was a full-time college student with no exposure to toxins, and had no known drug or alcohol abuse. The family history was unremarkable.

Physical examination revealed a slender, well-nourished young woman in no acute distress. Blood pressure, pulse, respirations, and temperature were within normal limits. Her scalp hair was coarse, with diffuse alopecia. Pubic and axillary hair were scant. Her skin was dry, and there was superficial facial acne vulgaris. Her lips were scaled and cracked, and there were small fissures at the corners of her mouth. Her heart and lungs were unremarkable. Her liver was enlarged to 13 cm, extended 3 cm below the right costal margin, and was smooth and nontender. There was no splenomegaly. Mild to moderate pressure on the long bones elicited moderately severe pain. No other musculoskeletal abnormalities were noted. Neurologic examination revealed bilateral sixth nerve palsies, normal pupillary responses, and blurred and slightly elevated disk margins, with no spontaneous venous pulsations. There were no gross visual field defects. There was no motor weakness, sensory disturbance, abnormal reflexes, or signs of meningeal irritation. Cognitive testing was normal. The multisystem disease process coupled with her use of vitamins to treat acne vulgaris suggested vitamin A toxicity.[25,59,65] A normal CT scan eliminated intracranial mass or bleeding as a cause for her headaches.

Laboratory data revealed the complete blood cell count, glucose, blood urea nitrogen (BUN), electrolytes, and liver function to be within normal limits. Radiographs of the chest, hands, and legs did not disclose any abnormalities. A lumbar puncture revealed the opening pressure to be 320 mm H_2O (normal, 50–180 mm H_2O). The spinal fluid was clear and colorless, with no cells and with normal glucose and protein. These findings were consistent with the diagnosis of hypervitaminosis A with idiopathic intracranial hypertension.

VITAMIN A

MW = 272.43 daltons
Therapeutic serum level = 65–275 IU/dL
16.6–83.3 µg/dL

Action level = unknown

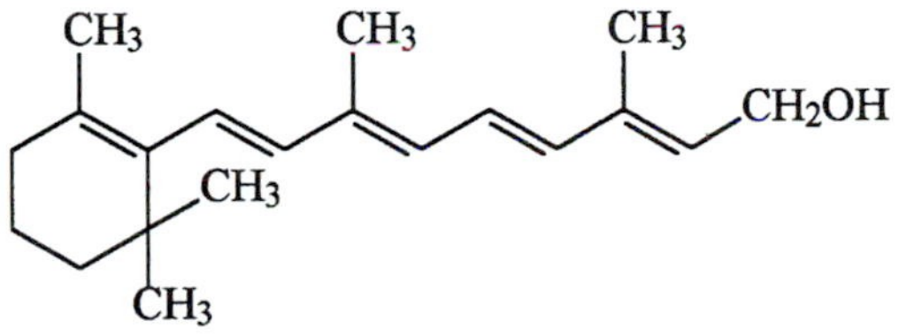

Vitamin A (retinol) is a fat-soluble vitamin. Little is known about its fundamental metabolic action, except in the retina, where it is required for the regeneration of the photosensitive chromoprotein rhodopsin. Vitamin A appears to be necessary for glycoprotein synthesis by mucus-secreting cells and for mucopolysaccharide homeostasis.[54,67] The vast majority of vitamin A is ingested as retinyl esters, the storage form of retinol. Vitamin A is a significant growth-promoting factor. It is obtained from the diet in two forms: preformed vitamin A from animal sources, particularly liver, and vitamin A precursors, carotenoids, found in vegetables, particularly carrots.[54,67] The average American diet provides about half of its vitamin A activity as carotene and the other half as preformed vitamin A.[18] Several fish-liver oils, such as swordfish and Black Sea bass, may contain more than 180,000 IU of vitamin A per gram of oil. In contrast, vitamin A precursors are converted rather inefficiently to vitamin A in the intestinal wall, where they are absorbed. Massive doses of carotene are not converted rapidly enough to induce vitamin A toxicity. Excess carotene does accumulate in the body, producing a yellow-orange skin discoloration, which can be differentiated from jaundice by the absence of scleral icterus. Absorption depends on the presence of bile and absorbable fat in the intestinal tract. Following absorption, retinol-binding protein produced by the liver transports vitamin A to the liver.

Epidemiology

Vitamin A toxicity is uncommon but should be considered in the differential diagnosis of all patients with hepatic and cutaneous diseases. Patients with chronic renal failure requiring hemodialysis who take even the small amount of vitamin A in multivitamin preparations are at increased risk for hypercalcemia.[23] Hypervitaminosis A usually occurs in adults who have initially been treated with large doses of this vitamin for a variety of dermatologic conditions, such as acne vulgaris, and who subsequently continue using the vitamin without medical supervision.[60,77] Hypervitaminosis A has also been reported in (a) food faddists who ingest large doses of fat-soluble vitamin preparations in their daily dietary regimens; (b)in an adult who had chronically ingested beef liver in large doses; and (c) among Inuits, whose diet may include polar bear liver.[41]

Vitamin A toxicity may be an occult illness. In fact, several reports demonstrate the unmasking of chronic hypervitaminosis A by intercurrent disease such as hepatitis and protein malnutrition.[36,79] Rat studies demonstrate that modest amounts of vitamin A may become hepatotoxic when combined with ethanol intake.[63] Although prolonged and continuous consumption of doses "theoretically in the therapeutic range" is reported to cause life-threatening hepatotoxicity and cirrhosis, the doses employed were actually 4–80 times the recommended daily allowance (RDA).[17,41]

Women should avoid daily doses of 25,000 IU or more unless they have severe documented deficiency of vitamin A. Doses of this magnitude taken for an extended time pose a risk, particularly to pregnant women and fetuses.[49] Much lower doses may also be a risk to women of childbearing age. Often critical periods of organogenesis occur before a woman knows that she is pregnant. Studies in pregnant animals have shown that large doses of vitamin A produce central nervous system (CNS) anomalies with hydrocephalus, encephalocele, and other teratogenic effects in the offspring.[68]

Isotretinoin (Accutane), a retinoic acid-vitamin A analogue, is effective in the management of severe nodulocystic acne. However, since the release of isotretinoin, extremely severe teratogenicity and complications such as spontaneous abortions, mucocutaneous abnormalities, idiopathic intracranial hypertension, corneal opacities, hypercalcemia, hyperuricemia, musculoskeletal symptoms, liver function abnormalities, and elevated triglycerides have occurred with alarming frequency.[1,27,28 34,35] A major problem arises in that 38% of the users of isotretinoin cited in the National Disease and Therapeutic Index reports are women aged 13–19 years. The risk of pregnancy in this group and the high risk of teratogenicity of this compound further underscore the need to inform all users of the contraindications to the drug's use during pregnancy as well as the need to demonstrate the absence of pregnancy before initiating therapy and the need to have the patient consider the consequences of unintentionally becoming pregnant while taking isotretinoin. The teratogenicity as well as all of the other adverse effects typical of hypervitaminosis A should lead to restraint in the prescription of this drug (Chaps. 16 and 29).

Toxicokinetics

Approximately 90% of the total vitamin A content of the mammalian body is stored in the liver, primarily as retinyl ester. The adrenal cortex also concentrates the vitamin. Because vitamin A is insoluble in water but soluble in fats, increased intake does not initially lead to elevated blood levels; rather, it leads to hepatic accumulation. When insufficient amounts of vitamin A are consumed, fairly constant blood levels are maintained at the expense of hepatic reserves, which may be sufficient to prevent symptoms of vitamin A deficiency for several months. The normal plasma level of retinol is about 30–70 μg/dL.[74] (Table 37–1 contains the RDAs of vitamin A.)

Transretinoic acid is a metabolite found in tissues or bound to albumin or in blood. Clinical toxicity correlates well with total body vitamin A content and is thus a function of dosage and duration of administration. As little as 25,000–50,000 IU/d for as few as 30 days can induce signs of increased intracranial pressure.[14,65] There is, however, considerable individual variability with respect to the cumulative intake necessary to produce toxicity. As a general guide, acute toxicity requires a single massive ingestion of a medicinal preparation containing in excess of 25,000 IU/kg body weight, and chronic toxicity requires 4000 IU/kg body weight daily for 6–15 months.

Pathophysiology

The skin, hair, bones, liver, and brain are all affected by hypervitaminosis A. The exact mechanism of action is unclear, although vitamin A may have hormonelike properties. Some authors suggest that the retinoids influence gene expression at the level of nuclear DNA, resulting in cell turnover, differentiation, and protein synthesis. Others suggest varied DNA- or RNA-related influences on gene expression.[14,17,60]

In the skin, vitamin A normally assists in epithelial maturation and membrane stability. However, excessive concentrations lead to increased permeability and decreased stability of lipoprotein membranes. These effects may result from unbound retinol and its esters. In excessive dosage, decreased keratinization and sebum production result in extreme thinning of epithelial tissue, manifested as brittle nails, thin rough skin, excessive desquamation, and alopecia.

Asynchronous growth patterns of long bones occur in children treated with vitamin A for keratinizing disorders. Bone resorption, hypercalcemia, and cartilaginous matrix degradation result in cortical hyperostosis, bony exostoses, metaphyseal flare, and epiphyseal premature closure. Radiographic findings may consist of pericapsular, ligamentous, and subperiosteal calcifications. Areas of new bone formation may be particularly prominent in the shafts of the long bones. Bone demineralization has also been reported.

Adult bony abnormalities are associated with oversupplementation, as well as with excessive dietary intake. In northern Europe, the region with the highest incidence of osteoporotic fractures, dietary intake of vitamin A is also high. Recent evidence suggests that in

TABLE 37–1. Recommended Daily Allowances (RDA) for Vitamin A (Regardless of Form) in International Units (IU)

Adult men		3300
Adult women		2700
Pregnant women	Second and third timesters	3300
Lactating women		4000
Children	Infants to 12 months	1350
	1–3 y	1350
	4–6 y	1650
	7–10 y	2300
	11–14 y	2700–3300

1 retinol equivalent (μg) = 3.3 IU = 1 μg all transretinols = 6 μg of β-carotene.

this population, the risk of first hip fracture increased by 68% for every 1 mg increase in retinol equivalent intake (3300 IU or the equivalent of the RDA). Compared to intake of less than 0.5 mg/d, intake greater than 1.5 mg/d reduced bone mineral density by 10% at the femoral neck, 14% at the lumbar spine, and 6% for the total body, and doubled the risk for hip fracture.[56] These results are supported by animal, human, and in vitro data from other studies.[10]

Idiopathic intracranial hypertension (formerly known as benign intracranial hypertension or pseudotumor cerebri) is a syndrome of uncertain etiology that is found in conjunction with a number of unrelated disorders. The syndrome is defined by the presence of intracranial hypertension without evidence of localizing neurologic findings. In more than 50% of cases, no cause can be identified; however, obese women, usually in their third or fourth decade, represent 75% of these cases.[1,71,80] Idiopathic intracranial hypertension (IIH) occur in patients with altered endocrine function, systemic diseases, impaired cerebral venous drainage, or ingestion of various drugs or toxins.[3] Of these ingestions, vitamin A is the most common. Recent evidence suggests that the link between IIH and vitamin A may be more substantial than originally thought, and appears not to necessarily require an increased intake of the vitamin. Serum retinol concentrations in patients with IIH are significantly elevated when compared to controls even after adjusting for age and body mass index despite similar dietary intakes of vitamin A.[43] Further study is necessary to determine if this is an effect of elevated retinol binding capacity or an epiphenomenon of another variable. Table 37–2 lists the drugs and toxins that are associated with intracranial hypertension.

Acute promyelocytic leukemia (APL) is now treated with a combination therapy that includes high-dose tretinoin (all-*trans* retinoic acid). Retinoic acid syndrome is the major adverse effect of tretinoin and occurs in 25% of treated APL patients in the absence of appropriate prophylactic measures. Cytokine release by maturing blast cells appears to be an important component in the development of this condition. The clinical manifestations of the retinoic acid syndrome are body weight gain, respiratory distress, serous effusions, and cardiac and renal failure. Adding dexamethasone to this regimen decreases the incidence of this syndrome to about 15% and its mortality to 1%.[26]

Manifestations of liver disease and outcome are associated with the amount of vitamin A ingested.[32] Cirrhosis, mild chronic hepatitis, noncirrhotic portal hypertension, and "increased storage" are all possible results of hypervitaminosis A. Death from causes related to liver diseases can be expected in the patients with cirrhosis during the 5 years after diagnosis.

Hepatotoxicity results from excessive deposition of vitamin A in the Ito cells of the liver.[52] Ito cells normally function as fat-storage cells and are found in the perisinusoidal space of Disse. They appear responsible, among other things, for maintaining the normal hepatic architecture (Chap. 14). Hypertrophy of Ito cells with vitamin A, retinol, and lipids leads to enhanced collagen production and scarring (Fig. 37–1). Extracellular cholestasis occurs without bile duct proliferation. Liver injury from vitamin A is histologically defined as cirrhosis. There appears to be a correlation between the dose of vitamin A and the characteristics of the liver disease that develop. With exposure to large doses cirrhosis develops and invariably progresses to portal hypertension, esophageal varices, jaundice, and ascites.[21,32,46] Liver function studies are frequently normal, even in the presence of hepatomegaly, although hepatotoxicity and cirrhosis may be manifested by elevations in bilirubin, aminotransferases, and alkaline phosphatase.

Clinical Manifestations

The initial symptoms are usually minor gastrointestinal manifestations and headache. The main manifestations of an acute ingestion include drowsiness or irritability, vomiting, and increased intracranial pressure. These findings are usually followed in 24–72 hours by extensive desquamation. Headache, nausea, and vomiting ensue.[6,29]

Headaches, blurred vision, and diplopia are the most characteristic initial symptoms of idiopathic intracranial hypertension. The most common ocular complaint is visual blurring, a manifestation of papillitis. Visual loss may be minimal, despite severe chronic papilledema; however, blindness may result from optic atrophy.[53] Visual field assessment may demonstrate blind spot enlargement, scotomata, and peripheral field constriction. A complaint of

TABLE 37–2. Drugs and Toxins Associated with Intracranial Hypertension

Drugs
Antibiotics: nalidixic acid, tetracycline, ampicillin, minocycline, nitrofurantoin, sulfamethoxazole, metronidazole
Corticosteroid therapy (oral and intranasal) and cessation
Griseofulvin
Lithium
Oral contraceptives and progestational drugs
Phenothiazines
Phenytoin
Vitamin A

Toxins
Lead

Anesthetics
Enflurane
Halothane
Ketamine
d-Tubocurare

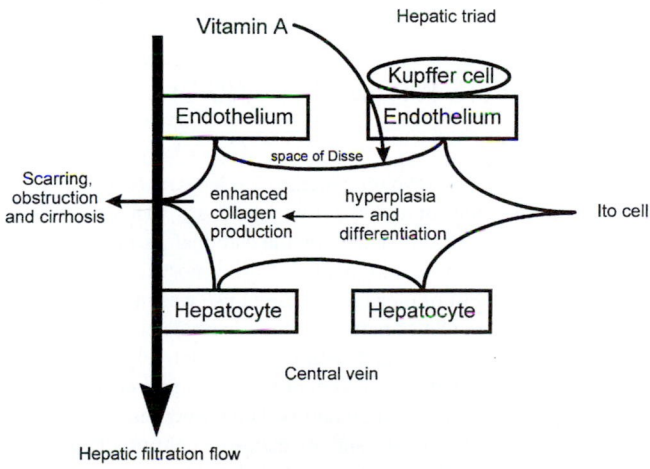

Figure 37–1. A schematic demonstration of hepatotoxicity resulting from excessive deposition of vitamin A in the Ito cells of the liver.

diplopia may result from sixth nerve palsy secondary to increased intracranial pressure.[70]

Diagnostic Testing

The only consistent laboratory abnormality is the elevation of the serum vitamin A level to a value ranging from 80 to 200 μg/dL. It is important to remember that in chronic toxicity a proportional relationship does not exist between the amount of vitamin A stored in the liver and the serum level. During initial stages of toxicity, much of the vitamin is stored in the liver, and the serum level may remain normal or disproportionately low. After the capacity for storage is exhausted, the serum level increases rapidly in an apparent nonlinear fashion. Hepatotoxicity may occur prior to the elevation of serum vitamin A levels. For this reason, serum levels may be high if a relatively minor excessive amount is given for a sufficiently long time. The serum level may remain low if large amounts are given for a short period of time. Histologic evidence of fat-storing cell hyperplasia with fluorescent vacuoles on liver biopsy supports the diagnosis.[32]

Treatment

The immediate management after an acute overdosage rarely requires more than gastrointestinal decontamination. Treatment of idiopathic intracranial hypertension consists of withdrawal of vitamin A and appropriate supportive care. Most signs and symptoms begin to resolve within 1 week, although papilledema and skeletal abnormalities may persist for several months after clinical recovery. Under certain circumstances more aggressive therapy to relieve pressure must be initiated by daily lumbar puncture, an initial dose of 40 mg of IV furosemide, 1 g of mannitol/kg body weight, 250 mg of acetazolamide 4 times a day, and a short course of prednisone, depending on the severity and resistance of the syndrome. The acetazolamide decreases cerebrospinal fluid (CSF) formation after a variable but transient increase in CSF pressure. These approaches must be individualized with regard to risk-to-benefit ratio, as remission is usually spontaneous. Visual impairment secondary to optic atrophy is the only major long-term central nervous system sequela of vitamin A toxicity.

Vitamin A-induced hypercalcemia associated with nausea and vomiting may respond to loop diuretics with intravenous fluids, and prednisone (20 mg daily).[8]

ANTIOXIDANTS (VITAMINS E AND C)

Epidemiology

The megadose theory of vitamin therapy has led Americans to spend phenomenal amounts of money for vitamin doses 10 to hundreds of times the amounts recommended by the National Academy of Science as daily dietary requirements.[62,64] The most frequently promoted health benefit of megadose vitamin use was muscle growth. However, recent evidence has identified ascorbic acid (vitamin C), α-tocopherol (vitamin E), and β-carotene (a relatively safe precursor of vitamin A) as having potential benefit in prevention of carcinogenic mechanisms via their antioxidant properties.[12]

Nutritional supplements and megadose vitamins often come packaged in tablet form and are labeled to advertise their purported benefits, for example, "Energy Pak." Many unusual and unidentifiable ingredients are included; 22.2% of the products ad-

vertised had no ingredients listed and no toxicologic data were available on 59% of the ingredients.[62] More than 90% of these vitamins and supplements are purchased without a prescription and used without supervision of a physician.[38,68] A 1983 demographic analysis of vitamin use determined that persons older than 65 years of age consumed more supplements than those in younger groups, and people with the highest educational levels had the highest consumption rates.[11,31] The incidence of vitamin overdoses in children appears directly related to the number of vitamin preparations used by their families.[42]

Antioxidant vitamins are used to disrupt the peroxidation and epoxidation of DNA that are often essential steps in mutagenesis and to prevent the oxidation of low-density lipoprotein, which is considered an important determinant in atherosclerosis. However, cancer prevention studies report mixed benefits of antioxidant vitamins. The Iowa Women's Health Study found no association between dietary antioxidants and breast cancer risk, although a statistically insignificant reduction was noted in those patients who took vitamin supplements.[47] Studies have noted lower antioxidant vitamin levels in cohorts of patients with coronary artery disease when compared to controls matched for age, gender, blood pressure, smoking, alcohol use, serum lipids, and body mass index.[45] The benefits of antioxidants may also include a reduction in markers of severity of myocardial infarction such as creatine kinase fractions and left ventricular dysfunction.[75] A prospective study of a cohort of postmenopausal women demonstrated a protective effect of consumption of vitamin E in the diet but no additional effect was obtained by using vitamin E supplements. Vitamins A and C appeared to have no protective effect.[48] A conclusive discussion of the efficacy of these vitamins in disease prevention is beyond the scope of this chapter. However, patients find sufficient evidence to take high-dose vitamins and, hence, the potential for toxicity exists. Fortunately, these antioxidant vitamins are relatively safe at the range of recommended doses (vitamin C, 1000 mg/d; vitamin E, 400 mg/d; β-carotene, 25 mg/d).[22,28]

Almost every scientific group that has issued a statement on vitamin usage concluded that healthy adult men and nonpregnant, nonlactating women who eat a normal varied diet do not require supplemental vitamins.[4] Most available preparations contain less than twice the RDA. These RDAs have long been established at approximately 2 standard deviations above the mean requirement, and therefore encompass the needs of 97% of the population.[4,24] While vitamins may have important roles in disease prevention, the question of the efficacy and safety of high-dose supplementation remains to be answered.

Vitamin E (α-Tocopherol)

MW = 430.69 daltons
Therapeutic serum level = 0.5–2.0 mg/dL
Action level = unknown

Vitamin E has a wide margin of safety even when taken in doses as high as 400 mg/d (which is 10 times the RDA).[5] Reports of adverse symptoms from large doses are anecdotal, with nausea, diarrhea, and flatulence as typical gastrointestinal (GI) manifestations. Numerous other symptoms and toxic effects are reported. In animals, absorption of vitamins A and K is impaired by large doses of vitamin E.[9,66] In addition, vitamin E appears to enhance the epoxidation of vitamin K to its inactive form (Fig. 42–3).[5] This can enhance the anticoagulant effect of warfarins, and clinicians should consider vitamin E supplementation as a cause for unexpected elevation of the INR in patients who are taking Coumadin.

A severe epidemic of low-birth-weight infants who manifested thrombocytopenia, renal dysfunction, cholestasis, ascites, and death occurred following the intravenous use of E-Ferol (a vitamin E supplement).[13] This product was removed from the market, and the emulsification of lipids and fat-soluble vitamins using polyoxyethylene sorbitan monolaurate and monooleate (polysorbate 20 and polysorbate 80, respectively) were implicated as the cause for this syndrome—not the vitamin E.

Vitamin C (Ascorbic Acid)

MW = 176.12 daltons
Therapeutic serum level = 0.4–2.0 mg/dL
Action level = unknown

On the basis of its action as a hydrogen donor for the detoxification of peroxy radicals, vitamin C has long been used as a panacea for cancer prevention, to treat or prevent the common cold, to increase mental attentiveness, and to treat minor wounds, cancer, and stress. This belief is so widely held that one study found that 67% of the residents in a California retirement community were using vitamin C, and 6% were taking greater than 2 g/d.[31] An extensive review of 14 studies of the role of ascorbic acid in the treatment of the common cold, however, suggested that only 8 were truly valid investigations and none demonstrated any therapeutic benefit.[16] Controlled valuations of the role of vitamin C in cancer therapy also demonstrate no advantage in survival over placebo.[19,58] Chronic doses in excess of 2 g/d of ascorbic acid may result in diarrhea and urinary cystine or oxalate nephrolithiasis. This results from the metabolism of ascorbic acid to oxalic acid. In addition, ascorbic acid can be oxidized in vitro to oxalate. Subsequently, oxalate crystals precipitate in the renal tubules.[78] Nephropathy and renal failure appear to be associated with single 40–50 g intravenous doses.[50,55]

Vitamin B₆ (Pyridoxine)

MW = 169 daltons
Therapeutic serum level = 3.6–18 ng/mL
Action level = unknown

For many years, pyridoxine was thought to be harmless because of its rapid excretion, until a single collection of case reports demonstrated that excessive doses of water-soluble vitamins could be toxic.[72] Seven patients taking pyridoxine at a daily dose of 2–6 g (minimum daily requirement is 2–4 mg) for 2–40 months developed sensory neuropathies. The 7 adults studied had normal CNS function but had progressive sensory ataxia and profound distal limb impairment of position and vibration sense. Touch, pain, and temperature sensation were minimally impaired. All tendon reflexes were diminished or absent. Nerve conduction and somatosensory studies showed dysfunction of distal portions of sensory peripheral nerves, and nerve biopsy showed widespread, nonspecific axonal degeneration, defined as a toxic sensory neuropathy of the distal axon and neuron. Fortunately, these patients improved over several months with abstinence from pyridoxine.

Since that initial report, other cases have been described with lower, but excessive, pyridoxine doses. Pyridoxine is widely available in tablet forms containing 50–500 mg of the drug and is promoted for body building and premenstrual syndrome (PMS). Additionally, use of pyridoxine is advocated in the treatment of schizophrenia, childhood autism, and attention deficit hyperactivity disorder. Later reports suggest that daily doses as low as 200–500 mg of pyridoxine may prove neurotoxic. In these studies early recognition of symptoms and withdrawal of supplementation have prevented permanent disability in most.[61] Pyridoxine supplementation is important in isoniazid therapy to prevent pyridoxine deficiency, a condition which can also lead to neuropathy.

Single, large, intravenous doses of pyridoxine may also cause acute neurotoxicity. A husband and wife who ingested *Gyromitra esculenta* mushrooms were inadvertently treated with 183 g and 132 g, respectively, of pyridoxine as a result of prescribing error and developed permanent dorsal root and sensory ganglia deficits as a consequence.[2]

A prospective study of pyridoxine neurotoxicity in volunteers characterized the pathophysiology of this syndrome.[7] The investigators administered 1 or 3 g/kg of pyridoxine to 5 healthy volunteers and closely followed clinical signs and symptoms, serum pyridoxal phosphate levels, quantitative sensory thresholds (QSTs), and sural nerve electrophysiologic determinations. The quantitative sensory threshold is a sensitive measure of toxicity that can be determined prior to changes in nerve conduction studies. Pyridoxine was discontinued at the first sign of either a clinical or laboratory abnormality. In all subjects, sensory symptoms and QST abnormalities occurred simultaneously. Those who received higher doses developed symptoms before those receiving lower doses. Elevation of thermal QSTs preceded or exceeded that for vibration in the low-dose subjects, whereas vibration and thermal QST became abnormal simultaneously in the high-dose subjects. Symptoms continued to progress ("coast") for 2–3 weeks after discontinuation of pyridoxine and the return of serum pyridoxal phosphate to normal levels (Antidote in Depth: Pyridoxine).

Vitamin D (Cholecalciferol)

MW	=	384.62 daltons
Therapeutic serum level	=	10–50 ng/mL
Action level	=	unknown

Vitamin D may be more appropriately thought of as a hormone than as a dietary nutrient, because it is manufactured in the skin from cholesterol with the aid of sunlight. It appears that even casual exposure of cutaneous tissues to ultraviolet light during the summer months produces adequate vitamin D for storage for winter months.[33] A series of British studies[15] of hypercalcemic patients in the 1950s demonstrated that chronic exposure to relatively small amounts of vitamin D in excess of the RDA can be toxic in children and adults. The manifestations that ensue are directly related to the increased physiologic response to vitamin D, resulting in increased calcium absorption and increased 25-hydroxy vitamin D leading to increased metabolism of calcium (Fig. 37–2). Children and especially infants appear to be susceptible to oversupplementation by vitamin D and will develop cardiovascular, CNS, and renal damage. Symptoms include anorexia, nausea, vomiting, hypertension, and renal compromise associated with hypercalcemia.[73] Hypervitaminosis D should be considered in children with nephrocalcinosis and hypercalciuria even if the serum calcium and phosphorus are normal.[57] Adults have similar systemic manifestations of anorexia, weakness, malaise, nausea, vomiting, hypertension, renal compromise, and even death. Calcium homeostasis is markedly altered, with hypercalcemia and hyperphosphatemia, resulting in polyuria, polydipsia, nephrolithiasis, renal failure, vascular calcifications, and ectopic calcification.[40]

Hypervitaminosis D as a consequence of fortified milk forced a reassessment of the appropriate amount of vitamin D necessary to achieve normal skeletal development and mineralization without causing toxicity.[44] This is particularly important in view of the unreliability of fortification of milk and infant formulas. Fortified milk may contain vitamin D_3 (cholecalciferol) and not vitamin D_2 (ergocalciferol). In addition, the quantities of vitamin D can vary from amounts that would be too small to prevent deficiencies to amounts excessive enough to cause toxicity.[30,39]

The elderly and the chronically ill who consume less vitamin D–fortified foods and milk and who have little exposure to sunshine may still benefit from food fortification monitored by regulatory agencies for safety. Vitamin D_3 is also currently widely available as a rodenticide (Chap. 90).

The decision to treat patients with hypervitaminosis D depends largely on the serum calcium and the severity of associated symptoms. Patients with severe hypercalcemia benefit from loop diuretics and hydration, but hormonal therapy with calcitonin or pamidronate may be indicated. In a single case report, an elderly lethargic patient who was oversupplemented with vitamin D was found to have a serum calcium of 21 mg/dL. Following unsuccessful diuretic therapy and the development of congestive heart failure, pamidronate was successful in the resolution of hypercalcemic symptoms without the need for hemodialysis.[51]

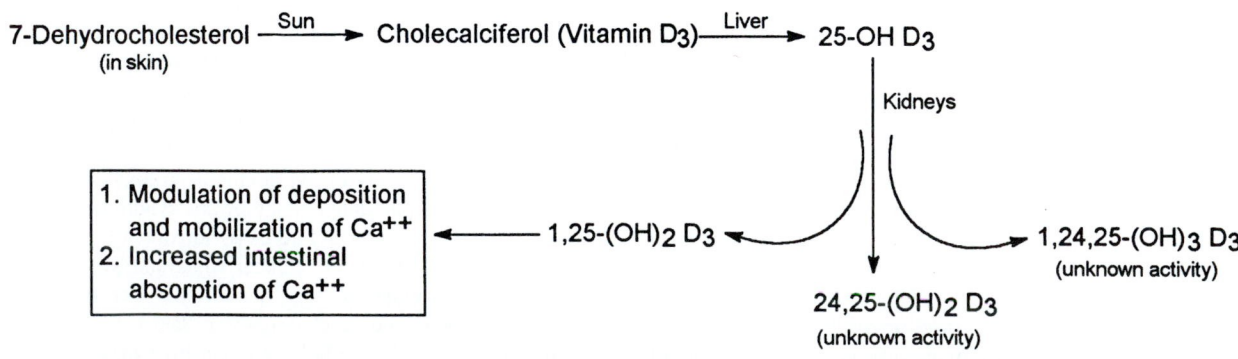

Figure 37–2. A schematic representation of the increased physiologic response to vitamin D resulting in increased calcium absorption and increased 25-hydroxy vitamin D_3.

Nicotinic Acid (Niacin)

MW	= 123 daltons
Therapeutic levels	= ?
Action level	= unknown
RDA	= 16 mg

Nicotinic acid is still used today as therapy for hyperlipidemias in doses 10–100 times the RDA. Regular-release formulations can cause extensive flushing, vasodilation, headache, and pruritus—an effect that is prostaglandin-mediated. The symptoms are usually transient and rarely require therapy. A single aspirin taken 30 minutes before ingestion of nicotinic acid diminishes the flush response.[81] Niacin can also cause amblyopia, hyperglycemia, hyperuricemia, coagulopathy, myopathy, and hyperpigmentation.[37] Excessive doses may result in nausea, diarrhea, and epigastric distress.

Niacin-induced hepatitis appears to be more frequent and more severe among those with hyperlipidemias treated with sustained-release preparations than those receiving crystalline or immediate-release niacin. Hepatotoxicity is consistent with centrilobular cholestasis and parenchymal necrosis. These manifestations appear to be dose related and not hypersensitivity responses.[20,63]

Patients typically develop tolerance to nicotinic acid flushing as plasma levels of 9α–11β prostaglandin F_2, a stable metabolite of prostaglandin D_2, become undetectable in most subjects. Tolerance is not associated with decreased nicotinic acid level nor tolerance to the prostaglandin mediator, but rather to decreased mediator levels. Flushing appears to occur because of the predilection for the skin as a source of prostaglandin D_2 production after niacin ingestion.[76]

SUMMARY

Patients perceive vitamins to be a source of wellness, not illness, and may ingest excessive amounts of supplements. Although the therapeutic/toxic threshold is wide, toxicity generally occurs when large doses are taken for sustained periods. Clinicians should consider hypervitaminosis in the differential diagnosis of varied presentations of illnesses. A thorough history, with special emphasis on dietary self-supplementation or physician-prescribed therapy, is important.

REFERENCES

1. Adverse effects with isotretinoin. FDA Drug Bull 1983;13:1–3.
2. Albin RL, Alpers JW, Greenberg HS, et al: Acute sensory neuropathy-neuronopathy from pyridoxine overdose. Neurology 1987;37:1729–1732.
3. Allain HJ, Weintraub M: Drug-induced headache. Ration Drug Ther 1980;14:1–6.
4. AMA Council on Scientific Affairs: Vitamin preparations as dietary supplements and as therapeutic agents. JAMA 1987;257:1929–1936.
5. Bendich A, Machlin LJ: Safety of oral intake of vitamin E. Am J Clin Nutr 1988;48:612–619.
6. Bergen S, Roels O: Hypervitaminosis A. Am J Clin Nutr 1965;16:265–269.
7. Berger AR, Schaumburg HH, Schroeder C, et al: Dose response, coasting and differential fiber vulnerability in human toxic neuropathy: A prospective study of pyridoxine neurotoxicity. Neurology 1992;42:1367–1370.
8. Bergman SM, O'Mailia J, Krane NK, Wallin JD: Vitamin A-induced hypercalcemia: Response to corticosteroids. Nephron 1988;50:362–364.
9. Bieri JG, Corash L, Hubbard VS: Medical uses of vitamin E. N Engl J Med 1983;308:1063–1071.
10. Binkley N, Krueger D: Hypervitaminosis A and bone. Nutr Rev 2000;58:138–144.
11. Block G, Cox C, Madans J, et al: Vitamin supplement use by demographic characteristics. Am J Epidemiol 1988;27:297–309.
12. Block G, Patterson B, Sklar A: Fruit, vegetables, and cancer prevention: A review of the epidemiological evidence. Nutr Cancer 1992;18:1–29.
13. Bove KE, Kosmetatos N, Wedig KE, et al: Vasculopathic hepatotoxicity associated with E-Ferol syndrome in low-birth-weight infants. JAMA 1985;254:2422–2430.
14. Boyd AS: An overview of the retinoids. Am J Med 1989;86:568–574.
15. British Pediatric Association: Hypercalcemia in infants and vitamin D. Br Med J 1956;2:149.
16. Chalmers TC: Effect of ascorbic acid in the common cold: An evaluation of the evidence. Am J Med 1975;58:532–536.
17. Chytil F, Sherman DR: How do retinoids work? Dermatologica 1987;175:8–12.
18. Committee on Recommended Dietary Allowances: Report of Food and Nutritional Board, 10th ed. Washington, DC, National Academy of Sciences, National Research Council, 1989, pp. 62–63.
19. Creagan ET, Moertel CG, O'Fallon JR, et al: Failure of high-dose vitamin C (ascorbic acid) therapy to benefit patients with advanced cancer: A controlled clinical trial. N Engl J Med 1979;301:687–690.
20. Dalton TA, Berry RS: Hepatotoxicity associated with sustained release niacin. Am J Med 1992;93:102–104.
21. Davis BH, Vucic A: The effect of retinol on Ito cell proliferation in vitro. Hepatology 1988;8:788–793.
22. Diplock A: Safety of antioxidant vitamins and beta-carotene. Am J Clin Nutr 1995;62:1510S–1516S.
23. Farrington K, Miller P, Varghese Z, et al: Vitamin A toxicity and hypercalcemia in chronic renal failure. Br Med J 1981;282:1999–2002.
24. FDA Consumer Memo: Nutrition Labels and US RDA Publication (FDA) 81–2146, US Department of Health and Human Services, 1981.
25. Feldman M, Schlezinger N: Benign intracranial hypertension associated with hypervitaminosis A. Arch Neurol 1970;22:1–7.
26. Fenaux P, De Botton S: Retinoic acid syndrome: Recognition, prevention and management. Drug Saf 1998;18:273–279.
27. Flynn WJ, Freeman PG, Wickboldt LG: Pancreatitis associated with isotretinoin-induced hypertriglyceridemia. Ann Intern Med 1987;106:63.
28. Garewal HS, Diplock AT: How "safe" are antioxidant vitamins? Drug Saf 1995;13:8–14.
29. Gerber A, Raab A, Sobel A: Vitamin A poisoning in adults. Am J Med 1954;16:729–745.
30. Giunta JL: Dental changes in hypervitaminosis D. Oral Surg Oral Med Oral Pathol Oral Radiol Endod 1998;85:410–413.

31. Gray GE, Paganini-Hill A, Ross RK: Dietary intake and nutrition supplement use in a southern California retirement community. Am J Clin Nutr 1983;38:122–128.

32. Guebel AP, de Galocsy C, Alves N, et al: Liver damage caused by therapeutic vitamin A administration: Estimate of dose related toxicity in 41 cases. Gastroenterology 1991;100:1701–1709.

33. Haddad JG: Vitamin D: Solar rays, the milky way or both? N Engl J Med 1992;326:1213–1215.

34. Hall JG: Vitamin A teratogenicity [letter]. N Engl J Med 1984;311:797–798.

35. Hall JG: Vitamin A: A newly recognized human teratogen-harbinger of things to come? J Pediatr 1984;105:583–584.

36. Hatoff DE, Gertler SL, Miyai K, et al: Hypervitaminosis A unmasked by acute viral hepatitis. Gastroenterology 1982;82:124–128.

37. Henkin Y, Oberman A, Hurst DC, Segrest JP: Niacin revisited: Clinical observations on an important but underutilized drug. Am J Med 1991;91:239–246.

38. Herbert V: The vitamin craze. Arch Intern Med 1980;140:173–176.

39. Holick MF, Shao Q, Liu WW, Chen TC: The vitamin D content of fortified milk and infant formula. N Engl J Med 1992;326:1178–1181.

40. Howard JE, Meyer RJ: Intoxication by vitamin D. J Clin Endocrinol Metab 1948;8:895–910.

41. Inkeles SB, Connor WE, Illingworth DR: Hepatic and dermatologic manifestations of chronic hypervitaminosis A in adults: Report of two cases. Am J Med 1986;80:491–496.

42. Issenman RM, Slack R, MacDonald L, Taylor W: Children's multiple vitamins: Overuse leads to overdose. Can Med Assoc J 1985;132:781–784.

43. Jacobson DM, Berg R, Wall M, Digre KB, Corbett JJ, Ellefson RD. Serum vitamin A concentration is elevated in idiopathic intracranial hypertension. Neurology 1999;53:1114–1118.

44. Jacobus CH, Holick MF, Shao Q, et al: Hypervitaminosis D associated with drinking milk. N Engl J Med 1992;326:1173–1177.

45. Kim SY, Lee-Kim YC, Kim MK, et al: Serum levels of antioxidant vitamins in relation to coronary disease: A case control study of Koreans. Biomed Environ Sci 1996;9:229–235.

46. Kowalski TE, Falestiny M, Furth E, Malet PF: Vitamin A hepatotoxicity: A cautionary note regarding 25,000 IU supplements. Am J Med 1994;97:523–528.

47. Kushi LH, Fee RM, Sellers TA, et al: Intakes of vitamins A, C, and E and postmenopausal breast cancer. The Iowa Women's Health Study. Am J Epidemiol 1996;144:165–174.

48. Kushi LH, Folsom AR, Prineas RJ, et al: Dietary antioxidant vitamins and death from coronary heart disease in postmenopausal women. N Engl J Med 1996;334:1156–1162.

49. Lammer EJ, Chen DT, Hoar RM, et al: Retinoic acid embryopathy. N Engl J Med 1985;313:837–841.

50. Lawton JM, Conway LT, Crosson JT, et al: Acute oxalate nephropathy after massive ascorbic acid administration. Arch Intern Med 1985;145:950–951.

51. Lee DC, Lee GY: The use of pamidronate for hypercalcemia secondary to acute vitamin intoxication. J Toxicol Clin Toxicol 1998;36:719–721.

52. Leo MA, Arai M, Sato M, Lieber CS: Hepatotoxicity of moderate vitamin A supplementation in the rat. Gastroenterology 1982;82:194–205.

53. Lysak WR, Svien HJ: Long term follow-up on patients with diagnosis of pseudotumor cerebri. J Neurol Surg 1966;25:284–287.

54. Marcus R, Coulston AM: Fat-soluble vitamins. In: Gilman AG, Rall TW, Nies AS, Taylor P, eds: The Pharmacological Basis of Therapeutics, 8th ed. New York, Pergamon Press, 1990, pp. 1553–1563.

55. McAllister OJ, Scowden EB, Dewberry FL, et al: Renal failure secondary to massive infusion of vitamin C [letter]. JAMA 1984;252:1684.

56. Melhus H, Michaelsson K, Kindmark A, et al: Excessive dietary intake of vitamin A is associated with reduced bone mineral density and increased risk for hip fracture. Ann Intern Med 1998; 129:770–778.

57. Misselwitz J, Hesse V, Markestad T: Nephrocalcinosis, hypercalciuria and elevated serum levels of 1,25-dihydrovitamin D in children. Acta Paediatr Scand 1990;79:637–643.

58. Moertel CG, Fleming TR, Creagan ET, et al: High-dose vitamin C versus placebo in the treatment of patients who have no prior chemotherapy: A randomized double blind comparison. N Engl J Med 1985;312:137–141.

59. Morrice G, Havener W, Kapetansky F: Vitamin A intoxication as a cause of pseudotumor cerebri. JAMA 1960;173:1802–1805.

60. Muenter M, Perry H, Ludwig J: Chronic vitamin A intoxication in adults. Am J Med 1971;50:129–136.

61. Parry GJ, Bredesen DE: Sensory neuropathy with low dose pyridoxine. Neurology 1985;35:1466–1468.

62. Philen RM, Ortiz DI, Auerbach SB, Falk H: Survey of advertising for nutritional supplements in health and body-building magazines. JAMA 1992;268:1008–1011.

63. Rader JI, Calvert RJ, Hathcock JN: Hepatic toxicity of unmodified and time-release preparations of niacin. Am J Med 1992;92:77–81.

64. Read MH, Graney AS: Food supplement usage by the elderly. J Am Diet Assoc 1982;80:250–253.

65. Restak R: Pseudotumor cerebri, psychosis, and hypervitaminosis A. J Nerv Ment Dis 1972;15:572–575.

66. Roberts HJ: Perspective of vitamin E as therapy. JAMA 1981;246:129–131.

67. Roels O: Vitamin A physiology. JAMA 1970;214:1097–1102.

68. Rosa FW, Wilk AL, Kelsey FO: Teratogen update: Vitamin A congeners. Teratology 1986;33:355–364.

69. Rudman D, William PJ: Megadose vitamins: Use and misuse. N Engl J Med 1983;309:488–489.

70. Rush JA: Pseudotumor cerebri: Clinical profile and visual outcome in 63 patients. Mayo Clin Proc 1980;55:541–546.

71. Saul RF, Hamburger HA, Selhorst JB: Pseudotumor cerebri secondary to lithium carbonate. JAMA 1985;253:2869–2870.

72. Schaumburg H, Kaplan J, Windebank A, et al: Sensory neuropathy from pyridoxine abuse: A new megavitamin syndrome. N Engl J Med 1983;309:445–448.

73. Seelig, MS: Vitamin D and cardiovascular, renal and brain damage in infancy and childhood. Ann N Y Acad Sci 1969;147:537–582.

74. Silverman AK, Ellis CN, Vorrhees JJ: Hypervitaminosis A syndrome: A paradigm of retinoid side effects. J Am Acad Dermatol 1987;16:1027–1039.

75. Singh RB, Niaz MA, Rastogi SS, et al: Usefulness of antioxidant vitamins in suspected acute myocardial infarction (the Indian experiment of infarct survival-3). Am J Cardiol 1996;77:232–236.

76. Stern RH, Spence JD, Freeman DJ, Parbtani A: Tolerance to nicotinic acid flushing. Clin Pharmacol Ther 1991;50:66–70.

77. Stimson W: Vitamin A intoxication in adults. N Engl J Med 1961;265:369–373.

78. Swartz RD, Wesley JR, Sommermeyer MG, et al: Hyperoxaluria and renal insufficiency due to ascorbic acid administration during total parenteral nutrition. Ann Intern Med 1984;100:530–531.

79. Weber FL, Mitchell GE Jr, Powell DE, et al: Reversible hepatotoxicity associated with hepatic vitamin A accumulation in a protein-deficient patient. Gastroenterology 1982;82:118–123.

80. Weisberg L: The syndrome of increased intracranial pressure without localizing signs: A reappraisal. Neurology 1975;25:85–88.

81. Whelan AM, Price SO, Fowler SF, Hainer BL: The effect of aspirin on niacin-induced cutaneous reactions. J Fam Pract

CHAPTER 38 DIETING AGENTS AND REGIMENS

Jeanmarie Perrone

A 34-year-old male presented to the emergency department complaining of intermittent palpitations for one day. He denied a prior cardiac history and previous palpitations and was not on any medications. He drank several cups of coffee daily without prior symptoms and had no recent increase in caffeine intake. Physical examination was significant for a slightly overweight male who looked generally comfortable. Vital signs were: pulse, 130 beats/min, which was noted to be irregular; blood pressure, 120/74 mm Hg; temperature, 97°F (36.1°C); respiratory rate, 16 breaths/min; pulse oximetry, 96% saturation on room air. There was no jugular venous distension or thyromegaly; heart and lungs were normal; there was no peripheral edema; and distal pulses were intact. An electrocardiogram (Fig. 38–1) revealed atrial fibrillation with a ventricular rate of 115 beats/min. No acute ischemia or ST segment abnormalities were noted. Upon further questioning, the patient admitted to using a dietary supplement called Xenadrine twice a day for the past 3 days for weight loss and energy supplementation. Contact with the regional poison control center identified the supplement as containing 20 mg ephedrine and 200 mg caffeine/tablet.

Dieting aids are conceptually very simple, yet include an expansive list of modalities to assist in the quest of taking in less energy than needed or expending more than taken (ie, increase metabolic rate) to produce a net calorie deficit and thus weight loss. Some dieting aids are anorexiants, designed to decrease appetite and calorie intake. Anorexiants may be sympathomimetics (amphetamines and derivatives) or serotonergic agents. Some anorexiants, such as ephedrine, are available in "herbal" form, which is minimally regulated and monitored by the Food and Drug Administration. Like ephedrine, γ-hydroxybutyrate (GHB) was also initially sold as a dietary supplement (Chap. 63) and promoted for weight loss and energy under the guise that it helps "burn fat into muscle." Although GHB and some congeners are now Schedule I drugs and illegal, other GHB prodrugs continue to be used. Clenbuterol is a long-acting β₂-agonist with stimulant properties that has been abused by body builders for energy and as an anorectic.[37,64] Other agents that inhibit absorption or prevent energy mobilization from ingested food, such as "starch blockers" and "fat blockers" (orlistat; Xenical), as well as dinitrophenol, are taken with regular calorie intake and block the potential for caloric yield from an ingested meal. Other treatments, including gelatin or fiber diet pills, act by absorbing large amounts of water and expanding in the stomach and intestinal tract, thus producing the satiety sensation of a large meal. Very-low-calorie diets or those containing high-protein liquid supplements advocate the intake of 300–800 calories per day and are associated with sudden cardiac death. The extremes of dieting toxicity continue to be manifest in the many people who suffer from anorexia nervosa and bulimia.

Leptin and the leptin gene have been explored as a basis for obesity and as a therapeutic strategy. Although genetically created leptin-deficient mice are obese and leptin supplementation allows them to lose weight, screening for leptin deficiency in obese humans fails to correlate with human obesity.[19] Subcutaneous leptin supplementation induces weight loss in lean and obese adults.[36] Since β₃-adrenergic receptors mediate lipolysis in brown and white adipose tissue, β₃ agonists are also under investigation as weight loss agents.[68] Neuropeptide Y, a peptide found in the arcuate and paraventricular nucleus of the hypothalamus, is a potent central appetite stimulant. Future drug therapy may target these genes, receptors, and proteins to modify metabolism. As obesity research proceeds and the biologic basis for obesity is defined, new approaches and mechanisms for drug therapy may be revealed.

HISTORY AND EPIDEMIOLOGY

Americans are the most overweight people in the world. One in 3 adults is obese, as are 20% of all children—that is, the amount of their body weight that is fat exceeds 25 percent (for males) or 30 percent (for females). The proportion of Americans who are obese has grown almost 10% since 1980,[47] representing 58 million Americans and accounting for 325,000 deaths annually.[3] Americans spend $33 billion per year toward weight loss annually. In addition, dieting fads and obsessions influence far more people than those who are truly obese.

Although obesity and attempts at weight loss may have existed since antiquity, one of the earliest accounts of weight loss therapy is described in 10th century Spain. King Sancho I, who was obese, underwent successful treatment with a "Theriaca," thought to contain plants, and possibly opiates, and administered with wine and oil. In addition, he was closely supervised and treated by a physician, who was able to direct his therapy.[38]

The Dietary Supplement and Health Education Act of 1994 created a new category, separate from food and drugs, that includes vitamins, minerals, herbs, and amino acids, and that is virtually free from FDA regulations. The result of this law has been an increased incidence of diet-related toxicity, especially with ephedrine-containing products.[33,35]

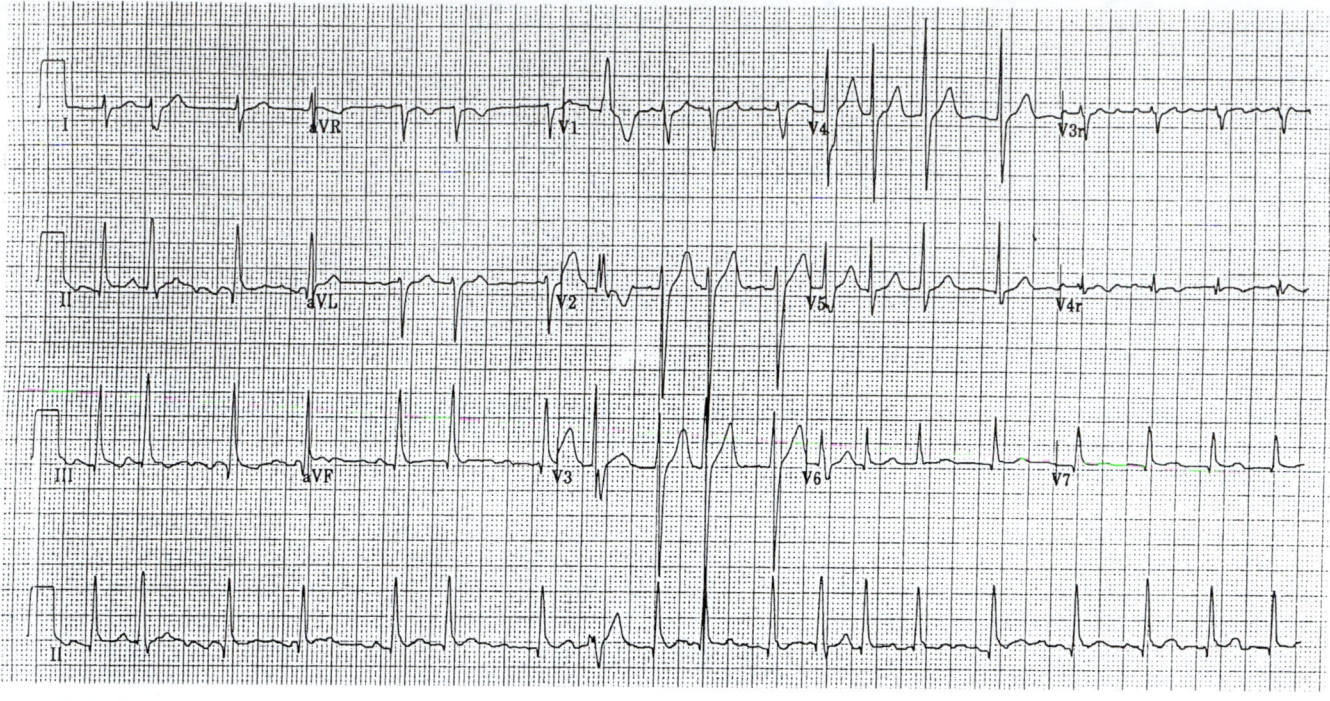

Figure 38–1. Electrocardiograph of a patient consuming ephedrine and caffeine, demonstrating atrial fibrillation.

PHARMACOLOGY

Sympathomimetics

Phentermine

Phenylpropanolamine

Ephedrine

Amphetamines were noted to cause weight loss soon after their introduction in the 1930s. Interestingly, these early observations prompted investigations to characterize whether the weight loss resulted from increased activity (stimulant effects), increased basal metabolic rate, or decreased intake. The net anorexiant effect of amphetamines was well demonstrated in early studies in animals, although tolerance to the anorectic effects was also noted.[75] Anorectic effects of the amphetamine class are mediated via β-adrenergic and dopaminergic effects on the hypothalamus (Chap. 68).

Although controversial, certain sympathomimetic amines are still "indicated" for short-term weight reduction according to physician prescribing information (Table 38–1).[5] Adverse side effects, dependence, and tolerance to their anorectic effects limit their net efficacy and use. A diet-drug therapy known colloquially as "phen-fen" refers to a two-drug prescription regimen of phentermine (an amphetamine derivative) and fenfluramine (a serotoninergic agent; see below). This regimen was once popular because of the improved side-effect profile achieved with lower doses of each, and better long-term weight control.[81]

TABLE 38–1.   Anorexiants

Serotonergic Agents	Noradrenergic Agents
Fluoxetine (Prozac) (not other SSRIs)	Dextroamphetamine (Dexedrine)
Mindazol (Sanorex)	Diethylpropion (Tenuate)
Sibutramine (Meridia)	Phendimetrazine (Bontril)
	Phenmetrazine (Prelu-2)
	Phentermine (Fastin, Ionamin)

Phenylpropanolamine, another sympathomimetic amine, was available until recently as a nonprescription diet aid. It is both a direct-acting agent, via stimulation of α-adrenergic receptors, and an indirect-acting agent, through release of norepinephrine. Both actions tend to cause a net increase in blood pressure when given in high doses. Phenylpropanolamine was available in various dosage forms, from 25 to 75 mg, including a sustained-release preparation. Phenylpropanolamine-induced anorexia may be mediated via α-adrenergic receptors within the hypothalamus.[83]

Ephedrine, or *ma huang* in Chinese herbal nomenclature, is a very popular health food supplement. Experts estimate that 12 million people used ephedrine-containing supplements in 1999.[35] Ephedrine is an indirect-acting sympathomimetic amine that has pharmacologic indications in the treatment of asthma, hypotension, and nasal decongestion. It is not indicated or available for treatment of obesity in proprietary form; however, it has been abused for its stimulant and anorectic properties.

Serotonergic Agents

Dexfenfluramine

Dexfenfluramine, the *d*-isomer of fenfluramine, was approved in 1995 for treatment of obesity and maintenance of weight loss.[6] Dexfenfluramine stimulates serotonin release and inhibits reuptake from presynaptic neurons. It is metabolized to *d*-norfenfluramine, which binds to a serotonin receptor on the postsynaptic neuron, increasing activity.[74]

Sibutramine, a newer anorexiant, and its two active amine metabolites are potent inhibitors of serotonin and norepinephrine reuptake, and weak inhibitors of dopamine reuptake. Although it does not directly release norepinephrine, blood pressure elevation can occur.

PATHOPHYSIOLOGY

"Fen-phen" gained notoriety in the 1990s when cardiac valvular abnormalities were observed in some users. The initial case series described valvular heart disease in 24 women treated with fenfluramine-phentermine who had no history of cardiac disease.[18] These women either presented with cardiovascular symptoms or solely with a heart murmur. They all had either right- or left-sided valvular abnormalities of morphology or regurgitation. Eight of these women also had newly documented pulmonary hypertension. Several of the patients had had cardiovascular surgery, which demonstrated plaquelike encasement of the leaflets and chordal structures, while preserving intact valve structure. These pathologic findings were identical to those that occur in patients with the carcinoid syndrome or those associated with ergotamine-induced valvular disease. In 1997, the FDA withdrew its approval of fenfluramine and reiterated that the use of the combination of fenfluramine-phentermine had never been approved. Although subse-

quent studies have corroborated this association the magnitude of the risk posed by these drugs was variable.[41,42,82] There is anecdotal evidence that regression of these valvular lesions occurred with removal of the drug[16] and that valvular effects were more mild than initially described.[29]

Following the recall of these agents, liability lawsuits resulted in a large settlement designated for the ongoing free medical evaluations of patients who received these drugs.

Another toxicity associated with therapeutic use of these amphetamine and serotonergic anorexiants is an increased incidence of primary pulmonary hypertension. In a multicenter case-control study of patients with primary pulmonary hypertension in Europe, an increased risk of this condition was associated with the use of anorectic drugs such as dexfenfluramine and fenfluramine, as well as phendimetrazine.[1] The risk of primary pulmonary hypertension was 30 times higher in patients using the drug for more than 3 months as compared to obese nonusers.[1] Primary pulmonary hypertension has been reported in association with fenfluramine since 1981.[7,12,15,23,59,65] A similar outbreak of primary pulmonary hypertension in Europe was described with the anorexiant aminorex fumarate in the 1960s.[34]

Several theories exist with regard to the mechanism of pulmonary toxicity of these agents.[15] Serotonin constricts isolated pulmonary arteries in dogs and humans.[11,56] In addition, serotonin-mediated platelet aggregation and vasoconstriction in the lungs may lead to microembolization, elevated pulmonary vascular resistance, and pulmonary hypertension.[56]

The amphetamine derivative phenylpropanolamine (PPA) was available as an over-the-counter diet preparation until October 2000, when the FDA recalled all products containing PPA in response to growing reports of cerebrovascular and cardiovascular complications associated with phenylpropanolamine use. A case-control study examined the use of PPA in the setting of hemorrhagic stroke and found that PPA was an independent risk factor for stroke in women.[44] Although the recall initiated by the FDA banned further sales of products containing PPA, this drug may still be available to patients from previously purchased products. A large number of cases of toxicity have been reported in patients receiving therapeutic dosing; cases of severe hypertension following "therapeutic" and toxic doses of PPA are published, some resulting in intracranial hemorrhage and death.[21,26,32,39,43,58] Additionally, hypertensive adverse drug interactions between PPA and drugs such as monoamine oxidase inhibitors and nonsteroidals are reported.[52,72] A comprehensive review of more than 100 case reports of adverse drug effects involving PPA summarized 24 intracranial hemorrhages, 8 seizures, and 8 fatalities between 1965 and 1990.[49] Many other patients suffered severe hypertension, headaches, and/or encephalopathy. Some of these adverse events occurred following ingestion of diet preparations that contained both PPA and caffeine.[45] Cardiac toxicity, although less common, was reported in 2 young patients who suffered myocardial injury following both therapeutic daily dosing and an acute overdose.[53]

CLINICAL MANIFESTATIONS

Toxic effects from all of the sympathomimetic amines are similar. Cardiovascular and cerebrovascular toxicity can be anticipated as a therapeutic misadventure or secondary to overdose (Chap. 68). Specific cases associated with the use of amphetamine derivatives for weight loss have been described.[46,66] Acute toxicity data with the serotonergic drugs are limited. A young female who ingested 60 times the therapeutic dose of dexfenfluramine in overdose developed coma and muscle rigidity refractory to benzodiazepine therapy, as well as metabolic acidosis and creatine phosphokinase (CPK) elevation. [55] This case most likely represents a serotonin syndrome variant. Drug interactions with other serotonergic drugs, and especially with monoamine oxidase inhibitors, must be avoided. In another case report, a 19-year-old woman, without prior psychiatric history, developed acute psychosis following a 3-month regimen of sibutramine for weight loss.[78] Psychosis resolved and did not recur after cessation of therapy.

Patients with PPA toxicity may experience anxiety, agitation, psychosis, seizures, palpitations, chest pain, or headache.[62] Although hypertension is common following overdose, some patients may also present with confusion and altered mental status as a result of hypertensive encephalopathy. Reflex bradycardia may accompany the hypertension and may be a clue to the diagnosis. Adolescents comprise a large group who may be using these agents; unintentional or intentional overdose in this population may result in seemingly mild elevations in blood pressure. However, even this mildly elevated blood pressure may be poorly tolerated in patients with a normal baseline blood pressure. Hypertension should be treated aggressively, either with phentolamine, a rapidly acting α-adrenergic antagonist, or nitroprusside. Analogous to cocaine toxicity, β-adrenergic antagonists should be avoided because the resultant unopposed α-adrenergic agonism may lead to increased vasoconstriction and increased hypertension.[2] Toddlers with unintentional ingestions may be at especially high risk for hypertensive episodes due to the relatively significant dose on a mg/kg basis.

Adverse events associated with the use of ephedrine dietary supplements include myocardial and cerebral infarctions and deaths.[63,79,84] Other manifestations include chest pain, palpitations, tachycardia, syncope, hypertension, mania,[17,24] psychoses, convulsions and coronary vasospasm.[13,63] Although many of these cases have been attributed to ephedrine use, an FDA-sponsored review of 140 adverse events reported to MedWatch following use of ephedrine were independently examined to assess causation.[35] In this study, thirty-one percent of the cases were considered to be definitely or probably related to the use of ephedrine supplements and 31% were deemed possibly related, including 10 strokes, 7 seizures, and 10 fatalities. Abuse in two adolescents of a concentrated ephedrine supplement led to hepatitis,[59] severe hypertension,[60] and life-threatening drug interactions with monoamine oxidase inhibitors.[21]

Herbal Weight-Loss Regimens

"Herbal phen-fen," a currently available combination of ephedrine and St. John's wort (*Hypericum perforatum),* has been linked to the initial popularity of the pharmaceutical "fen-phen" product. Other herbal weight-loss regimens may contain ephedrine in combination with caffeine and plant-derived diuretics such as juniper (*Juniperus communis*), goldenrod (*Solidago*), and parsley *(Petroselinum crispum).* Germander (*Teucrium chamaedrys*) supplements for weight loss resulted in 7 cases of hepatotoxicity following use in France.[51] A "slimming regimen" in Belgium produced an epidemic of renal failure and urothelial cancer when botanical misidentification led to substitution of a nephrotoxic plant.[80] A case of profound digitalis toxicity occurred from a laxative regimen contaminated with *Digitalis lanata.*[71]

OTHER APPROACHES
Starch Blockers

Amylase inhibitors, or so-called "starch blockers," were proposed as diet aids for the prevention of the absorption of carbohydrates by blocking their breakdown into sugars. These starch blockers were widely sold over-the-counter and in health food stores in the early 1980s. However, scientific evidence supporting their efficacy was lacking. In an elegant study in human volunteers, fecal calorie excretion following a high-starch meal of spaghetti and white bread was measured with and without the use of a starch-blocker tablet. The study showed no difference in net calorie excretion, and proposed that the lack of efficacy was because of the ability of the pancreas to secrete amylase in excess of that which is needed to digest any one meal.[9]

Dinitrophenol

One of the earliest attempts at a pharmaceutical treatment for obesity occurred in the 1930s, when dinitrophenol (DNP) was popularized as a weight-loss adjuvant.[77] DNP alters metabolism by uncoupling oxidative phosphorylation and thus leads to decreased functional caloric yield from ingested meals.[20] Since this net calorie loss is manifest as heat, elevated temperature and occasionally life-threatening hyperthermia are reported.[76] In addition, yellow-skin discoloration, cataracts, hepatotoxicity, and fatalities related to overdose were seen and eventually DNP use was abandoned.[10,31,48,76] Interestingly, epidemic use of DNP occurred in Texas in the 1980s where a chemist processed industrial DNP into tablets and began to distribute them in his weight loss center. Unfortunately, it was not until the hyperthermic death of a wrestler using this product that authorities became involved and were able to prevent further distribution and sales.[48]

Guar Gum

Guar gum is derived from the bean of the *Cyamopsis psorabides* plant. It was marketed in pill or tablet form as Cal-Ban 3000 until it was banned in 1992. These pills contained the hygroscopic guar gum polysaccharide that expanded 10–20-fold in the stomach, forming a gelatinous mass. The ingestion of guar led to gastric distension and the sensation of satiety in the dieter and, thus, decreased appetite and intake. Guar gum also resulted in multiple reports of adverse effects, including esophageal and small-bowel obstruction.[54,67] Initially, these cases of esophageal obstruction were reported in patients with predisposing anatomic lesions such as strictures.[30,69] Subsequent reports to the FDA of 26 patients with obstruction secondary to guar gum ingestion revealed that only half had normal gastrointestinal anatomy.[54]

Hypocaloric Diets

A variety of extreme calorie-restricted diets resulting in profound weight loss were very popular in the late 1970s. Reports followed shortly thereafter of a possible association with sudden death in patients on these diets.[70] Hypokalemia, torsades de pointes, and ventricular dysrhythmias[70,73] were described in some of the patients. Autopsies were available in 16 cases. Myocardial atrophy was the most common and consistent finding noted. Several authors have proposed that the cause of death was secondary to the effects of protein-calorie malnutrition on the heart,[25,73] while other authors postulated that a diet-induced ECG repolarization abnormality predisposed to these dysrhythmias.[70]

Following many of these negative reports and FDA warnings, most of the enthusiasm for the liquid-protein diets waned. A current regimen advocates intake of high protein, high fat, and low carbohydrates, limiting carbohydrates to 20 g daily, while allowing unlimited amounts of meat, fish, eggs, and cheeses. This lack of carbohydrates induces ketosis, which results in diuresis and dehydration, yielding the appearance of rapid weight loss. With rehydration and resumption of a normal diet, weight gain recurs. In addition, dehydration and water loss have been associated with orthostatic hypotension and ureterolithiasis.[4] Atherosclerosis and hypercholesterolemia may occur as a result of substitution of high-calorie, high-fat foods for carbohydrates.

MEDICATIONS ABUSED BY PATIENTS WITH EATING DISORDERS

Although many forms of eating disorders are described, the extent of medication abuse is remarkable.[14] Starvation, as well as abuse of laxatives, syrup of ipecac, diuretics, and anorexiants, has led to many fatalities, often in young patients.[28,40] Additionally, these agents have been used by abusing parents or caretakers to produce factitious chronic illnesses in patients termed Munchausen syndrome by proxy (Chap. 106). Eating disorders should be considered particularly in the high-risk group of young women with unexplained dehydration, syncope, or electrolyte disturbances.

Chronic use of syrup of ipecac to induce emesis in patients with anorexia has lead to the development of cardiomyopathy, subsequent dysrhythmias, and death.[28,61] Emetine, which is toxic to skeletal and cardiac muscle cells, is considered the alkaloid responsible for the severe myopathy in these patients. In addition, chronic administration of syrup of ipecac leads to tolerance of the emetic effects and increased systemic absorption of emetine.[61] Emetine can be detected in serum by high-pressure liquid chromatography or thin-layer chromatography, and persists for weeks to months after ingestion.

Laxatives are also commonly abused by patients with eating disorders. Although not as toxic as syrup of ipecac, chronic laxative abuse results in a vicious cycle of drug tolerance and the subsequent need for increasing doses to achieve catharsis. There is no net effect of cathartics on decreasing food absorption, and thus, these agents actually have limited effects on weight control.[9] However, chronic laxative abuse results in diarrhea, hypokalemia, metabolic alkalosis, dehydration, and an atonic colon.[8] Various screening methods can be used to detect laxative abuse.[22] Phenolphthalein can be detected as a pink or red coloration to stool or urine following alkalinization. Colonoscopy will reveal the benign, pathognomonic "melanosis coli," dark staining of the colonic mucosa secondary to anthraquinone laxative abuse.

Diuretics are also used to decrease body water and weight. Many diets, especially "herbal" plans, emphasize the use of some naturally occurring diuretics to encourage the dieter and suggest successful weight loss in the first few days of dieting. Like laxatives, diuretics cannot produce a net weight loss when used chronically. The toxicity of these herbal diuretics is dependent on their active ingredients (Chap. 77).

SUMMARY

Although obesity is a major health consideration and a tremendous cause of preventable morbidity and mortality, unproven cures are fraught with failure and toxicity. There is no current substitute for increasing the deficit between calories taken in and those utilized through activity and exercise. The safest approach to weight loss is one that incorporates nutritional counseling, behavioral therapy, and an appropriate exercise regimen to permanently alter lifestyle factors that are contributing to obesity. Clinicians should be aware of the lack of regulation of many available diet remedies and should report adverse events involving these products to poison centers and to the FDA MedWatch so that appropriate regulations may be sought.

REFERENCES

1. Abenhaim L, Moride Y, Brenot F, et al: Appetite suppressant drugs and the risk of primary pulmonary hypertension. N Engl J Med 1996; 335:609–616.
2. Albertson TE, Dawson A, De Latorre F, et al: Tox-ACLS: Toxicologic-oriented advanced cardiac life support. Ann Emerg Med 2001; 37;S78–S90.
3. Allison DB, Fontaine KR, Manson JE, et al: Annual deaths attributable to obesity in the United States. JAMA 1999;282:1530–1538.
4. Anonymous. The Atkins Diet. Med Lett Drugs Ther 2000;42:52.
5. Anonymous. Physician's Desk Reference. Montvale, NJ, Medical Economics, 2000, p. 54.
6. Anonymous: Dexfenfluramine for obesity. Med Lett Drugs Ther 1996;38:64–65.
7. Atanassoff PG, Weiss BK, Schmid ER, Tornic M: Pulmonary hypertension and dexfenfluramine. Lancet 1992;339:436–437.
8. Baker EH, Sandle GI: Complications of laxative abuse. Annu Rev Med 1996;47:127–134.
9. Bo-Linn GW, Santa Ana CA, Morawski SG, Fordtran JS: Starch blockers—Their effect on calorie absorption from a high-starch meal. N Engl J Med 1982;307:1413–1416.
10. Boardman WW: Rapidly developing cataract after dinitrophenol. JAMA 1935;105:108–110.
11. Boe J, Simonsson BG, Stahl E: Effect of histamine, 5-hydroxytryptamine, and prostaglandins on isolated pulmonary arteries. Eur J Respir Dis 1980;61:12–19.
12. Brenot F, Herve P, Petitprez P, et al: Primary pulmonary hypertension and fenfluramine use. Br Heart J 1993;70:537–541.
13. Bruno A, Nolte KB, Chapin J: Stroke associated with ephedrine use. Neurology 1993;43:1313–1316.
14. Bulik C: Abuse of drugs associated with eating disorders. J Subst Abuse 1992;4:69–90.
15. Cacoub P, Dorent R, Nataf P, et al: Pulmonary hypertension and dexfenfluramine. Eur J Clin Pharmacol 1995;48:81–83.
16. Cannistra LB, Cannistra AJ: Regression of multivalvular regurgitation after the cessation of fenfluramine and phentermine treatment. N Engl J Med 1998;339;771.

17. Capwell RR: Ephedrine induced mania from an herbal diet supplement [letter]. Am J Psychiatry 1995;152:647.

18. Connolly HM, Crary JL, McGoon MD, et al: Valvular heart disease associated with fenfluramine-phentermine. N Engl J Med 1997;337: 581–588.

19. Considine RV, Sinha MK, Heiman ML, et al: Serum immunoreactive leptin concentrations in normal-weight and obese humans. N Engl J Med 1996;334:292–295.

20. Cutting WC, Mehrtens HG, Tainter ML: Actions and uses of dinitrophenol. JAMA 1933;101:193–195.

21. Dawson JK, Earnshaw SM, Graham CS: Dangerous monoamine oxidase inhibitor interactions are still occurring in the 1990s. J Accid Emerg Med 1995;12:49–51.

22. De Wolff FA, Edelbroek PM, De Haas EJM, Vermeij P: Experience with a screening method for laxative abuse. Hum Toxicol 1983;2: 385–389.

23. Douglas JG, Munro JF, Kitchin AH, et al: Pulmonary hypertension and fenfluramine. Br Med J 1981;283:881–882.

24. Doyle H, Kargin M: Herbal stimulant containing ephedrine has also caused psychosis. BMJ 1996;313:756.

25. Drott C, Lunholm K: Cardiac effects of caloric restriction-mechanisms and potential hazards. Int J Obes Relat Metab Disord 1992:16: 481–486.

26. Edwards M, Russo L, Harwood-Nuss A: Cerebral infarction with a single oral dose of phenylpropanolamine. Am J Emerg Med 1987;5: 163–164.

27. Fallis RJ, Fisher M: Cerebral vasculitis and hemorrhage associated with phenylpropanolamine. Neurology 1985;35:405–407.

28. Friedman EJ: Death from ipecac intoxication in a patient with anorexia nervosa. Am J Psychiatry 1984;141:702–703.

29. Gardin J, Schumacher D, Ginger C, Davis K, Leung C, Reid C: Valvular abnormalities and cardiovascular status following exposure to dexfenfluramine or phentermine/fenfluramine. JAMA 2000;283; 1703–1709.

30. Gebhard RL, Albrecht J: The diet pill that worked. N Engl J Med 1990;322:702.

31. Geiger JC: A death from dinitrophenol poisoning. JAMA 1933;101: 1333–1334.

32. Glick R, Hoying J, Cerullo L, Perlman S: Phenylpropanolamine: An over-the-counter drug causing central nervous system vasculitis and intracerebral hemorrhage. Neurosurgery 1987;20:969–974.

33. Gurley BJ, Wang P, Gardner SF: Ephedrine-type alkaloid content of nutritional supplements containing *Ephedra sinica* (Ma-huang) as determined by high performance liquid chromatography. J Pharm Sci 1998;87:1547–1553.

34. Gurtner HP: Aminorex and pulmonary hypertension. Cor et Vasa 1985;27:160–171.

35. Haller CA, Benowitz NL: Adverse cardiovascular and central nervous system events associated with dietary supplements containing ephedra alkaloids. N Engl J Med 2000;343:1833–1838.

36. Heymsfield SB, Greenberg A, Fujioka K, et al: Recombinant leptin for weight loss in obese and lean adults: A randomized controlled, dose-escalation trial. JAMA 1999;1568–1575.

37. Hoffman RJ, Hoffman RS, Freyberg C, et al: Clenbuterol ingestion causing prolonged tachycardia, hypokalemia, and hypophosphatemia with confirmation by quantitative levels. J Toxicol Clin Toxicol 2001;39:339–344.

38. Hopkins KD, Lehmann ED: Successful medical treatment of obesity in 10th century Spain. Lancet 1995;346:452.

39. Horowitz JD, Lang WG, Kowes LG, et al: Hypertensive responses induced by PPA in anorectic and decongestant preparation. Lancet 1980;1:60–61.

40. Isner JM, Roberts WC, Heymsfield SB, Yager J: Anorexia nervosa and sudden death. Ann Intern Med 1985;102:49–52.

41. Jick H, Vasilakis C, Weinrauch LA, et al: A population based study of appetite-suppressant drugs and the risk of cardiac valve regurgitation. N Engl J Med 1998;339:719–724.

42. Khan MA, Herzog CA, St. Peter JV, et al: The prevalence of cardiac valvular insufficiency assessed by transthoracic echocardiography in obese patients treated with appetite suppressant drugs. N Engl J Med 1998;339:713–718.

43. Kase CS, Foster TE, Reed JE, et al: Intracerebral hemorrhage and phenylpropanolamine use. Neurology 1987;37:399–404.

44. Kernan WN, Viscoli C, Brass LM, et al: Phenylpropanolamine and the risk of hemorrhagic stroke. N Engl J Med 2000;343:1826–1832.

45. Kikta DG, Devereaux MW, Chandar K: Intracranial hemorrhages due to phenylpropanolamine. Stroke 1985;16:510–512.

46. Kokkinos J, Levine SR: Possible association of ischemic stroke with phentermine. Stroke 1993;24:310–313.

47. Kuczmarski RJ, Flegal KM, Campbell SM, Johnson CL: Increasing prevalence of overweight among US adults. JAMA 1994;272: 205–211.

48. Kurt TL, Anderson R, Petty C, et al: Dinitrophenol in weight loss: The poison center and public safety. Vet Hum Toxicol 1986;28: 574–575.

49. Lake CR, Gallant S, Masson E, Miller P: Adverse drug effects attributed to phenylpropanolamine: A review of 142 case reports. Am J Med 1990;89:195–208.

50. Lake CR, Rosenberg DB, Gallant S, et al: Phenylpropanolamine increases plasma caffeine levels. Clin Pharmacol Ther 1990;47: 675–685.

51. Larrey D, Vial T, Pauwels A, et al: Hepatitis after Germander (*Teucrium chamaedrys*) administration: Another instance of herbal medicine hepatotoxicity. Ann Intern Med 1992;117:129–132.

52. Lee KY, Vandongen R, Beilin LJ: Severe hypertension after ingestion of an appetite suppressant (phenylpropanolamine with indomethacin). Lancet 1979;2:1110–1111.

53. Leo PJ, Hollander JE, Shih RD, Marcus SM: Phenylpropanolamine and associated myocardial injury. Ann Emerg Med 1996;28:359–362.

54. Lewis JH: Esophageal and small bowel obstruction from guar gum-containing "diet pills": Analysis of 26 cases reported to the Food and Drug Administration. Am J Gastroenterol 1992;87:1424–1428.

55. LoVecchio F, Curry SC: Dexfenfluramine overdose. Ann Emerg Med 1998;32:102–103.

56. McGoon MD, Vanhoutte PM: Aggregating platelets contract isolated canine pulmonary arteries by releasing 5-hydroxytryptamine. J Clin Invest 1984;74:828–833.

57. McMurray J, Bloomfield P, Miller HC: Irreversible pulmonary hypertension after treatment with fenfluramine. Br Med J 1986;292: 239–240.

58. Mesnard B, Ginn DR: Excessive phenylpropanolamine ingestion followed by subarachnoid hemorrhage. South Med J 1984;77:939.

59. Nadir A, Agrawal S, King P, Marshall JB: Acute hepatitis associated with the use of a Chinese herbal product, Ma-huang. Am J Gastroenterol 1996;91:1436–1438.

60. Pace S: Ma Huang food supplement toxicity in two adolescents [abstract]. J Toxicol Clin Toxicol 1996;34:598.

61. Palmer EP, Guary AT: Reversible myopathy secondary to abuse of ipecac in patients with major eating disorders. N Engl J Med 1985; 313:1457–1459.

62. Pentel P: Toxicity of over-the-counter stimulants. JAMA 1984;252: 1898–1903.

63. Perrotta DM, Coody G, Culmo C: Adverse events associated with ephedrine-containing products—Texas, December 1993–September 1995. MMWR Morb Mortal Wkly Rep 1996;45:689–693.

64. Ramon MF, Ballesteros S, Martinez-Arrieta R, et al: Anabolic substances: Anabolic steroids, clenbuterol and GHB reported to Spanish Control Poison Centre. J Toxicol Clin Toxicol 2000;38:174–175.

65. Rosche N, Labrune S, Braun JM, Huchon GJ: Pulmonary hypertension and dexfenfluramine. Lancet 1992;339:436–437.

66. Rostagno C, Caciolli S, Felici M, et al: Dilated cardiomyopathy associated with chronic consumption of phendimetrazine. Am Heart J 1996;131:407–409.

67. Roach J, Martyak T, Benjamin G: Anhydrous pill ingestion: A new cause of esophageal obstruction. Ann Emerg Med 1987;16:913–914.

68. Rosenbaum M, Leibel RL, Hirsche J: Obesity. N Engl J Med 1997;337:396–407.

69. Seidner DL, Roberts IM, Smith MS: Esophageal obstruction after ingestion of a fiber-containing diet pill. Gastroenterology 1990;99: 1820–1822.

70. Singh BN, Gaarder TD, Kanegae T, et al: Liquid protein diets and torsade de pointes. JAMA 1978;240:115–119.

71. Slifman NR, Obermeyer WR, Aloi BK, et al: Contamination of botanical dietary supplements by *Digitalis lanata*. N Engl J Med 1998;339: 806–811.

72. Smookler S, Bermudez AJ: Hypertensive crisis resulting from an MAO-inhibitor and an over-the-counter appetite suppressant. Ann Emerg Med 1982;11:482–484.

73. Sours HE, Frattali VP, Brand CD, et al: Sudden death associated with very-low-calorie weight-reduction regimens. Am J Clin Nutr 1981;34: 453–461.

74. Spedding M, Ouvry C, Millan M, et al: Neural control of dieting. Nature 1996;380:488.

75. Tainter ML: Actions of benzedrine and propadrine in control of obesity. J Nutr 1944;27:89–105.

76. Tainter ML, Cutting WC: Febrile, respiratory and some other actions of dinitrophenol. J Pharmac Exp Ther 1933;48;410–429.

77. Tainter ML, Stockton AB, Cutting WC: Dinitrophenol in the treatment of obesity. JAMA 1935;105:332–337.

78. Taflinski T, Chojnacka J: Sibutramine associated psychotic episode. Am J Psychiatry 2000;157:2057–2058.

79. Traub SJ, Hoyek W, Hoffman RS: Dietary supplements containing ephedra alkaloids. N Engl J Med 2001;344:1096.

80. Vanherweghem JL, Depierreux M, Tielemans C, et al. Rapidly progressive interstitial renal fibrosis in young women: Association with slimming regimen including Chinese herbs. Lancet 1993;341(8842): 387–391.

81. Weintraub M, Sundaresen PR, Madan M, et al: Long-term weight control study I (weeks 0–34). Clin Pharmacol Ther 1992;51:586–594.

82. Weissman NJ, Tighe JF, Gottdiener JS, et al: An assessment of heart-valve abnormalities in obese patients taking dexfenfluramine, sustained-release dexfenfluramine, or placebo. N Engl J Med 1998;339: 725–732.

83. Wellman PJ: Overview of adrenergic anorectic agents. Am J Clin Nutr 1992;55:193S–198S.

84. Zahn KA, Li RL, Purssell RA: Cardiovascular toxicity after ingestion of "herbal ecstacy." J Emerg Med 1999;17:289–291.

B. PRESCRIPTION MEDICATIONS

CHAPTER **39** **METHYLXANTHINES**

Robert J. Hoffman

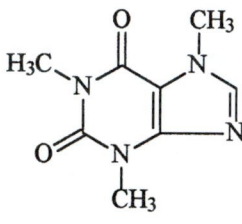

**Caffeine
(1,3,7-trimethylxanthine)**

**Theophylline
(1,3-dimethylxanthine)**

Caffeine

MW	=	194.22 daltons
Therapeutic serum level	=	1–10 µg/mL
Toxic serum level	=	> 25 µg/mL
	=	> 129 µmol/L

Theophylline

MW	=	180.17 daltons
Therapeutic serum level	=	5–15 µg/mL
S.I. units	=	10 µg/mL
	=	55.5 µmol/L
Toxic level	=	> 20 µg/mL
Action levels		
Multiple dose activated charcoal:	=	> 20 µg/mL
Extracorporeal removal (acute):	=	> 90 µg/mL
Extracorporeal removal (chronic):	=	> 40 µg/mL

Values greater than or equal to the action level necessitate clinical intervention. Values less than this level may necessitate intervention based on the clinical characteristics of the patient.

A 17-year-old girl presented to the Emergency Department reporting that she ingested 35 (200 mg) tablets of caffeine approximately 2 hours earlier. She complained of nausea, vomiting, and palpitations. Her vital signs were blood pressure, 115/66 mm Hg; heart rate, 142 beats/min; respiratory rate, 20 breaths/min; and temperature, 100.2°F (37.9°C). The patient was attached to a cardiac monitor. She was anxious and confused, but cooperative. Significant physical findings included mydriasis, tachycardia, tremor, and diaphoresis. A 12-lead ECG demonstrated a sinus tachycardia with frequent premature ventricular contractions (PVCs). Fifty grams of activated charcoal with sorbitol was given orally, but she immediately vomited. Metoclopramide (10 mg IV) was administered, and activated charcoal with sorbitol was again orally administered, but she again vomited.

Serum electrolytes were sodium, 140 mEq/L; potassium, 3.0 mEq/L; chloride, 107 mEq/L; bicarbonate, 16 mEq/L; blood urea nitrogen (BUN), 8 mg/dL; creatinine, 1 mg/dL; and glucose, 248

mg/dL. One liter of normal saline was administered by intravenous bolus and potassium chloride (40 mEq IV) was administered twice by infusion over 1 hour. Electrolytes repeated 3 hours after admission and subsequent to potassium repletion were sodium, 141 mEq/L; potassium, 2.8 mEq/L; chloride, 110 mEq/L; and bicarbonate, 17 mEq/L. The patient continued to have a sinus tachycardia with frequent PVCs, and her blood pressure decreased to 98/50 mm Hg. Two liters of lactated Ringer solution was administered by bolus, and her blood pressure increased to 108/56 mm Hg. Activated charcoal with sorbitol was again orally administered, this time without ensuing emesis. Approximately 4 hours after presentation and 6 hours after ingestion, a serum sample for a quantitative caffeine level was obtained. The treating institution lacked the capability to determine a quantitative caffeine level, and the blood sample was sent to a reference laboratory. Serum electrolytes were repeated at approximately 7 hours postingestion. Although the bicarbonate had increased to 20 mEq/L, the potassium was still 2.8

mEq/L. The patient again received potassium chloride (40 mEq IV) by infusion over 1 hour. The severity and persistence of hypotension and hypokalemia combined with a lack of intensive care capabilities necessitated transfer to the intensive care unit in a nearby children's hospital.

At the children's hospital, her vital signs improved and were blood pressure, 110/64 mm Hg; heart rate, 110 beats/min; respiratory rate, 18 breaths/min; and temperature, 99°F (37.2°C). Fifty grams of activated charcoal without sorbitol was administered. The patient experienced anxiety and agitation that responded to lorazepam (3 mg IV). She was awakened during the night to perform a physical examination and to receive another dose of activated charcoal orally. Otherwise, the patient remained sedated through the night. She awoke in the morning with a normal mental status and reported feeling unwell but much improved. Repeat electrolytes were normal except for a potassium of 3.1 mEq/L. A serum caffeine level at that time, approximately 18 hours postingestion, was 88 µg/mL. Caffeine levels were repeated twice that day, with results of 56 µg/mL and 40 µg/mL, at which time further assays were deemed unnecessary. Serum electrolytes repeated that evening and at all subsequent times were normal. The patient was discharged from intensive care and admitted to a psychiatric service. The 6-hour caffeine level drawn at the initial institution was later reported to be 149 µg/mL.

Methylxanthines, which include caffeine (1,3,7-trimethylxanthine), theobromine (3,7-dimethylxanthine), and theophylline (1,3-dimethylxanthine), are so named because they are methylated deriv-atives of xanthine (Fig. 39–1). Members of this group of plant-derived alkaloids have very similar pharmacologic properties and cause similar clinical effects. Methylxanthines are used ubiquitously throughout the world, most commonly in beverages imbibed for their stimulant, mood-elevating, and fatigue-abating effects. *Coffea arabica* and related species, from which coffee beans are obtained, are used to make coffee, a beverage rich in caffeine. Cocoa and chocolate are derived from the seeds of *Theobroma cacao*, which contains theobromine and, to a lesser extent, caffeine. *Thea sinensis*, a bush native to China but now cultivated worldwide, produces leaves from which various teas, rich in caffeine and containing small amounts of theophylline and theobromine, are brewed.

EPIDEMIOLOGY

From 1991 to 1999, the American Association of Poison Control Centers (AAPCC) reported a noteworthy downward trend of theophylline exposures from 6744 exposures in 1991 to 1641 exposures in 1999. The number of deaths reported from theophylline exposure has decreased progressively, from 38 in 1991 to 10 in 1999. The decrease in theophylline exposures presumably reflects decreased use of theophylline as a therapeutic agent. The number of caffeine exposures, 5639 in 1991 and 6264 in 1999, has essentially remained stable, reflecting steady use of caffeine, particularly caffeine in substances other than coffee, tea, and soft drinks. Deaths from caffeine exposure continue to be uncommon: The

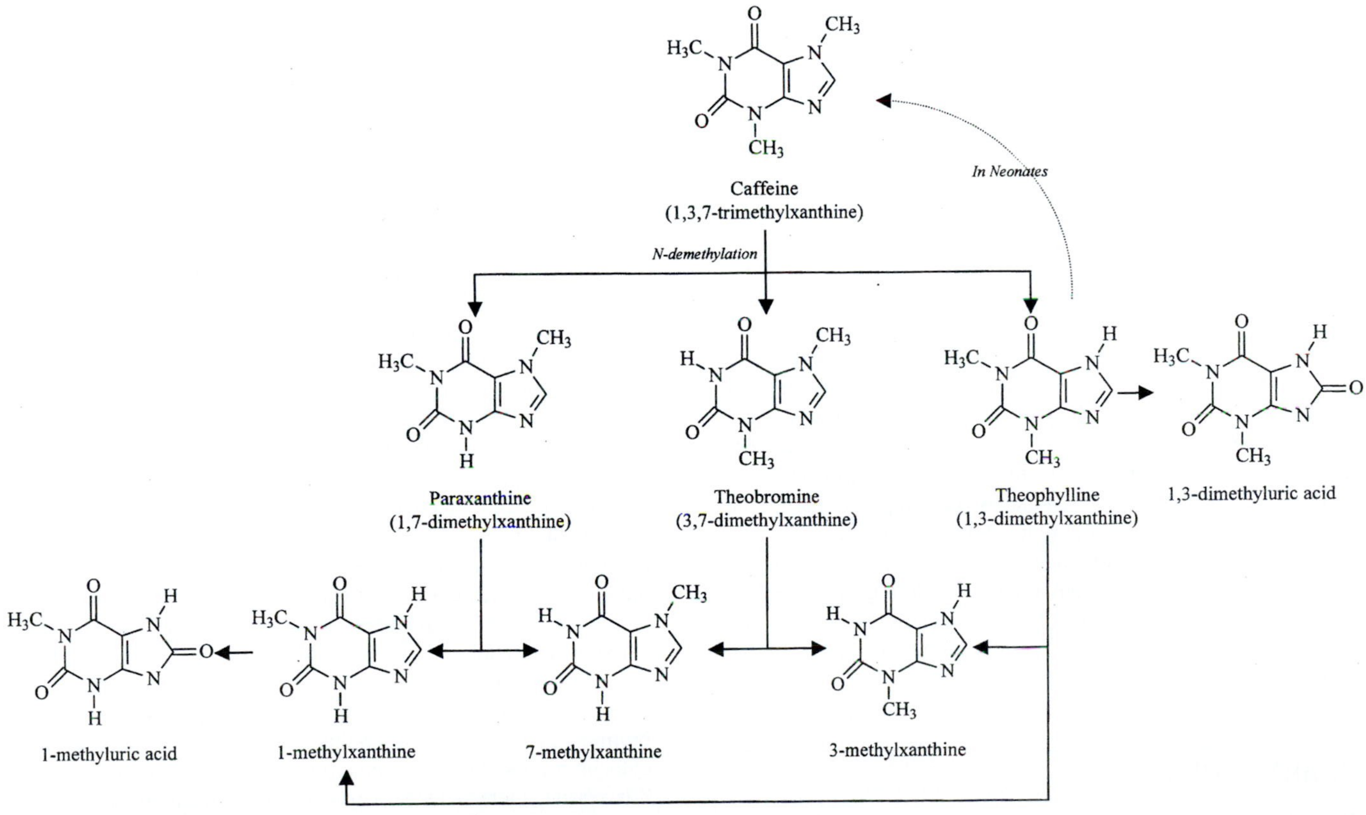

Figure 39-1.   Metabolism of caffeine and other methylxanthines by the hepatic P450 enzyme system.

maximal number of deaths associated with caffeine exposure in this time period was 3 per year (page XX and Chap. 116).

The overwhelming preponderance of caffeine consumed is in beverages, and a lesser portion in foods and tablets or capsules. Users typically seek the stimulant and psychoactive effects of caffeine. The use of guarana, a plant with very high caffeine content, for weight loss and athletic performance enhancement has increased dramatically in recent years. In particular, guarana or caffeine is frequently combined with ephedrine or ma huang, a dietary supplement product containing ephedrine. These combination pills are marketed for use as diet agents, anorectics, "energy" boosters, and athletic-performance-enhancement products. Despite the limited experience with overdose from these combination preparations, formulations containing caffeine/guarana combined with ephedrine/ ma huang cause illnesses such as myocardial infarctions and death.[77] Formulations containing phenylpropanolamine and caffeine, also once marketed as an anorexiant diet aid, were removed from US markets because of adverse drug events and a demonstrated lack of benefit from the inclusion of caffeine and a sympathomimetic agent for the purpose of appetite suppression.[80]

Medicinally, caffeine is used to treat neonatal apnea and bradycardia syndrome; as an analgesic adjuvant, particularly when combined with relatively mild analgesics such as acetaminophen, aspirin, and ibuprofen; and as an adjuvant treatment for migraine headache.

Theophylline, or its salt aminophylline, is used to treat varied respiratory conditions. Most prevalently, theophylline is used to treat obstructive airway disease, particularly asthma and chronic obstructive pulmonary disease. Although theophylline was once the mainstay of therapy for such diseases, more selective agents with fewer side effects, such as albuterol and other selective β_2-adrenergic agonists, are now more commonly utilized. However, because anti-inflammatory and other beneficial effects of theophylline were recently described, its role in the treatment of pulmonary disease may again expand.[100] In neonates, theophylline and aminophylline are used similarly to caffeine to treat neonatal apnea and bradycardia syndrome. The result of such treatment is increased respiratory rate, decreased apnea, increased cardiac chronotropy and inotropy, and increased cardiac output.[33]

Caffeine or theophylline toxicity result from iatrogenic events as well as self-administration, and acute or chronic toxicity may result from either drug or circumstance. Chronic toxicity from caffeine is most typically described as a result of the frequent self-administration of caffeine. A particular syndrome associated with chronic caffeine use consisting of headache, palpitations, tachycardia, insomnia, and delirium is termed *caffeinism*. Chronic theophylline toxicity results from the use of theophylline as a medicinal therapeutic agent. Neonates receiving caffeine therapy may develop either acute or chronic caffeine toxicity.[6,15]

Most reported cases of theobromine poisoning occur in animals and typically result from small animals ingesting cocoa or chocolate.[29,46,50,78,181] Humans may theoretically experience theobromine poisoning from ingestion of chocolate or cocoa, although evidence of such occurrence is lacking.

PHARMACOLOGY

Methylxanthines cause the release of endogenous catecholamines, resulting in stimulation of adrenergic receptors. The resulting adrenergic agonism plays a significant role in their therapeutic ef-

fects and in their untoward effects in cases of toxicity.[187] Levels of endogenous catecholamines are extremely elevated in patients with acute methylxanthine poisoning.[20]

Methylxanthines are also structural analogues of adenosine and function pharmacologically as adenosine antagonists. Adenosine is believed to modulate histamine release and to cause constriction of respiratory smooth muscle, which may explain the efficacy of adenosine antagonists in the treatment of bronchoconstriction. Additionally, adenosine antagonism results in release of norepinephrine, and, to a lesser extent, epinephrine.

At supertherapeutic doses, methylxanthines also inhibit phosphodiesterase, the enzyme responsible for degradation of intracellular cyclic AMP. This likely occurs as a result of the structural similarity of cyclic AMP and methylxanthines. Cyclic AMP is involved in the postsynaptic second messenger system of β-adrenergic stimulation. Thus, elevated cyclic AMP levels cause clinical effects similar to adrenergic stimulation including smooth muscle relaxation, peripheral vasodilation, myocardial stimulation, and central nervous system (CNS) excitation. Phosphodiesterase inhibition was long considered to be the primary therapeutic mechanism of the methylxanthines, but clinically significant elevations in cyclic AMP levels are not achieved until serum methylxanthine levels are well above the therapeutic range.

PHARMACOKINETICS AND TOXICOKINETICS

Caffeine

Caffeine is bioavailable by oral, intravenous, subcutaneous, intramuscular, and rectal routes of administration. Oral administration, which is by far the most common route of exposure, results in nearly 100% bioavailability of the drug. The presence of food in the gut does little to affect peak concentration. However, food in the gut does delay time until the peak serum concentration is reached, which is typically 30–60 minutes in the absence of food. Caffeine rapidly diffuses into the total body water and all tissues and readily crosses the blood-brain barrier and placenta. Caffeine is secreted in breast milk.[185] The volume of distribution is 0.6 L/kg, and 36% is protein bound.

Caffeine is metabolized via the cytochrome P450 system, primarily by the isozyme CYP1A2. The major pathway involves demethylation to 1,7-dimethylxanthine (paraxanthine) followed by hydroxylation, or repeated demethylation followed by hydroxylation. To a lesser extent caffeine is also metabolized to 3,7-dimethylxanthine (theobromine) and to 1,3-dimethylxanthine (theophylline). Neonates demethylate caffeine, producing theophylline, and also possess the unique ability to convert theophylline to caffeine by methylation.[2,10] By approximately 4–7 months of age, infants metabolize and eliminate caffeine in a manner similar to adults.[9] Less than 5% of caffeine is excreted in the urine unchanged. All patients metabolize some quantity of caffeine to active metabolites including theophylline and theobromine. The degree to which this occurs is dependent on the age, cytochrome P450 enzyme induction status, and other factors. For this reason, there may be a role for assessment of serum theophylline concentration in the management of patients with suspected caffeine overdose, but such role is not clearly defined and obviously limited.

The half-life of caffeine is highly variable and dependent on several factors. Generally speaking, younger patients, particularly infants, as well as patients with cytochrome P450 inhibition, such as pregnant patients and patients with cirrhosis, have longer caffeine half-lives than the 4.5-hour half-life in healthy, adult, nonsmoking patients.[34,45,47,178] Caffeine also exhibits Michaelis-Menten kinetics (Chap. 11).

Caffeine poisoning is a dose-dependent phenomenon. Unfortunately, the range of toxicity reported in different references varies greatly, and no definite conclusions can be drawn regarding serum levels and symptomatology in overdose. Therapeutic dosing in adults is 100–200 mg orally every 4 hours, and in neonates a typical loading dose is 20 mg/kg, with daily maintenance dosing of 5 mg/kg. Based on case reports and series, lethal dosing in adults is estimated at 150–200 mg/kg, and death was associated with serum levels above 80 μg/mL. Although numerous fatalities occur with serum levels under 200 μg/mL, survival of a patient with an acute caffeine overdose and a serum level over 400 μg/mL has been reported.[183] Infants survive toxicity with greater serum concentrations of caffeine than are tolerated by children and adults.

Theophylline

Theophylline, or its water-soluble ethylenediethylamine salt derivative aminophylline, is approximately 100% bioavailable by both the oral and intravenous routes. Many of the available oral preparations are sustained-release, designed to provide stable serum concentrations over a prolonged period of time with less frequent dosing. Peak absorption generally occurs 6–10 hours after ingestion of these products. However, following overdose of sustained-release preparations, the time to peak absorption may be twice as long as that of the intermediate-release preparations.

Like caffeine, theophylline rapidly diffuses into the total body water and all tissues, readily crosses the blood-brain barrier and placenta, and is secreted into breast milk.[13,102,179,199] Theophylline's volume of distribution is 0.5 L/kg, and 56% of it is protein bound.

Theophylline is metabolized via the cytochrome P450 system, primarily by the isozyme CYP1A2. The major pathway is demethylation to 3-methylxanthine, in addition to being demethylated or oxidized to other metabolites. Neonates have the unique ability to readily methylate and demethylate methylxanthines, and a portion of theophylline administered to neonates is methylated to form 1,3,7-trimethylxanthine (caffeine).[11,31,65] Less than 10% of theophylline is excreted in the urine unchanged.

Like caffeine, the half-life of theophylline is highly variable, and is dependent on several factors. In healthy, adult, nonsmoking patients, the half-life is 4.5 hours. Infants and the elderly, as well as patients with cytochrome P450 inhibition, pregnant patients, and patients with cirrhosis, have longer theophylline half-lives than do healthy children and adult nonsmoking patients.[59,87,119,177] Factors that induce cytochrome P450, such as cigarette smoking, or others that inhibit cytochrome P450, such as exposure to cimetidine, erythromycin, rifampin, and oral contraceptives, can significantly alter theophylline clearance.[73,95,96,103,118,134,135,152,189] Decreased theophylline or caffeine metabolism or reversal of enzyme induction predisposes to the development of chronic toxicity.

Like caffeine, theophylline exhibits Michaelis-Menten kinetics. At low doses, it is metabolized by first-order kinetics, and increases in dose result in concomitant increases in elimination.[151]

At higher doses and in overdose it undergoes zero-order elimination, and only a fixed amount of the drug can be eliminated in a given time because of saturation of metabolic enzymes.[149]

Therapeutic serum levels of theophylline are 10–15 μg/mL, and higher levels are considered toxic. Morbidity and mortality occur with relatively lower levels in chronic toxicity. Although morbidity and mortality are not always predictable based on serum levels, life-threatening toxicity, including seizures, ventricular dysrhythmias, and death, are associated with serum levels of 80–100 μg/mL in acute overdoses and serum levels of 40–60 μg/mL in chronic toxicity.

Theobromine

As is the case with the other methylxanthines, theobromine is well absorbed from the gut, and is 80% bioavailable when administered in solution. It is bioavailable orally, intravenously, and rectally. Theobromine has 21% protein binding, a volume of distribution of 0.62 L/kg, and a plasma half-life of 6–10 hours.[51,146] Theobromine undergoes hepatic metabolism by the CYP450 system similarly to caffeine and theophylline.[30] Like the other methylxanthines, theobromine is excreted in breast milk, and consumption of chocolate results in measurable concentrations in breast milk. Toxic concentrations of theobromine in animals are known, but comparable human data are lacking. A serum concentration of 133 μg/mL was reported in a lethal ingestion by a dog.[67]

PATHOPHYSIOLOGY

Caffeine, theobromine, and theophylline affect the same organ systems and cause qualitatively similar effects. For the purposes of this chapter, the adverse effects of all methylxanthines in acute overdose are considered to be similar. It should be noted, however, that there are distinct differences in the activity and effects of the various methylxanthines, particularly in therapeutic dose. The major clinical effects at both therapeutic doses and in overdose result from adenosine antagonism, release of endogenous norepinephrine and consequent β-adrenergic receptor stimulation, and phosphodiesterase inhibition. Toxicity affects the gastrointestinal, cardiovascular, central nervous, and musculoskeletal systems in addition to causing a constellation of metabolic derangements. Polypharmacy poisoning with methylxanthines and other agents that result in adrenergic stimulation, such as ephedrine, amphetamines, or cocaine, may be particularly severe.[48,190]

Theobromine toxicity is exceedingly rare. There are limited human data and most published cases are actually veterinary. Animals with theobromine poisoning may experience emesis, incontinence, restlessness, excitement, tachycardia, seizures, coma, and death. These characteristic symptoms, as well the pharmacologic similarity between theobromine and other methylxanthines, dictate that management principles for caffeine and theophylline be applied in cases of theobromine toxicity.

Gastrointestinal

In overdose, methylxanthines cause nausea and most significant acute overdoses result in severe and protracted emesis. Emesis occurs in 75% of cases of acute theophylline poisoning, whereas only 30% of cases of chronic poisoning are characterized by emesis.[169] This emesis is often quite severe and may be difficult to control despite the use of potent antiemetics. In particular, poisoning with sustained-release theophylline preparations may cause particularly severe emesis refractory to treatment.[4]

Methylxanthines cause an increase in gastric acid secretion and smooth-muscle relaxation. These factors contribute to the gastritis and esophagitis reported in chronic methylxanthine users.[42] Gastritis is noted in drinkers of decaffeinated coffee, so some adverse gastric effects associated with coffee drinking may be due to ingredients other than caffeine alone.

Cardiovascular

Methylxanthines are cardiac stimulants, and result in positive inotropy and chronotropy. Dysrhythmias, particularly tachydysrhythmias, are common in methylxanthine overdose. Considering the adenosine antagonist properties of methylxanthines, it is not surprising that supraventricular tachycardias (SVTs) commonly occur in overdose. Tachydysrhythmias, particularly ventricular extrasystoles, are uncommon following therapeutic doses, whereas they are common in overdose.[40,126,164] In the setting of acute poisoning, generally benign sinus tachycardia is nearly universal in patients without antecedent cardiac disease. In any patient, particularly those with underlying cardiac disease, a sinus tachycardia can degenerate to a more severe rhythm disturbance, which is the most common cause of fatality associated with methylxanthine poisoning. Supraventricular tachycardias, atrial fibrillation, atrial flutter, multifocal atrial tachycardia, ventricular tachycardia, and ventricular fibrillation may all result from methylxanthine toxicity.[18] Electrolyte disturbances, particularly hypokalemia, may be a contributing factor in the development of dysrhythmias. Dysrhythmias occur more commonly and at lower serum concentrations in cases of chronic poisoning. Consequential dysrhythmias occur in 35% of chronic theophylline poisonings, but in only 10% of acute poisonings.[173] These dysrhythmias occur at serum levels of 40–80 μg/mL in chronic theophylline overdoses and most commonly at serum levels greater than 80 μg/mL in acute overdose. Neonates born to mothers who consumed >500 mg/d of caffeine are more likely to have dysrhythmias as compared to cohorts born to mothers consuming less then 250 mg/d of caffeine.[74] Myocardial ischemia and myocardial infarction may result from acute caffeine or theophylline poisoning.[58,79]

At therapeutic doses, and initially in overdose, methylxanthines result in tachycardias and increased blood pressure, both by the effect of adenosine antagonism on the sinoatrial or atrioventricular node, and by causing the release of endogenous catecholamines. Tolerance to these pressor effects develops after several days of use and rapidly disappears after relatively brief periods of abstinence.

At elevated serum concentrations, methylxanthines will result in peripheral vasodilation, causing a characteristic widened pulse pressure. β_2-Adrenergic agonism is one major mechanism by which hypotension occurs. In cases of acute theophylline overdose, serum levels greater than 100 μg/mL are usually associated with severe hypotension.

In therapeutic doses, methylxanthines cause cerebral vasoconstriction, which is a desirable effect when caffeine is used to treat a migraine headache. However, in overdose, this effect likely exacerbates CNS toxicity by diminishing cerebral perfusion.[121] Methylxanthines cause renal vasodilation, which, in addition to the increased cardiac output, results in a mild diuresis.[136]

Pulmonary

Methylxanthines stimulate the CNS respiratory center, causing an increase in respiratory rate. For this reason, caffeine and theophylline are used to treat neonatal apnea syndromes. Caffeine and theophylline overdose may cause hyperventilation, respiratory alkalosis, respiratory failure, respiratory arrest, and acute lung injury.

Neuropsychiatric

The stimulant and psychoactive properties of methylxanthines, particularly caffeine, elevate mood and improve performance of manual tasks.[24,35,89,111] These stimulant effects are typically considered desirable, and are one reason caffeine is so widely used. CNS stimulation is an effect sought by users of coffee, tea, cocoa, and chocolate, but CNS stimulation resulting from therapeutic use of theophylline is generally considered to be an undesirable side effect. Caffeine is an effective analgesic adjuvant, possibly because of the stimulant properties of the drug.[90,91,125,127,160,165]

Agitation, insomnia, nervousness, and irritability are common following initial administration of methylxanthines, but tolerance to these effects develops quickly. Although at low doses methylxanthines improve cognitive performance and elevate mood, with increasing doses they result in adverse effects. Headache, anxiety, agitation, insomnia, tremor, irritability, hallucinations, and seizures may result from caffeine or theophylline poisoning. In adults, caffeine doses of 50–200 mg result in increased alertness, decreased drowsiness, and lessened fatigue, and caffeine doses of 200–500 mg produce adverse effects. Children tend to develop CNS symptoms at lower serum theophylline concentrations than do adults, and such excitation is a significant clinical disadvantage of theophylline use. Although not reported, theobromine is probably capable of causing similar CNS symptoms reported with caffeine and theophylline.

Seizures are a major complication of methylxanthine poisoning. The additional methyl group possessed by caffeine (1,3,7-trimethylxanthine) affords this agent greater CNS penetration relative to theophylline and theobromine, which are dimethylxanthines. Caffeine's ability to both promote and prolong seizures is well recognized, and caffeine has been used to prolong therapeutically induced seizures in electroconvulsive therapy (ECT).[98,174] Seizures resulting from methylxanthine overdose tend to be severe and recurrent, and may be refractory to treatment. Antagonism of adenosine, the endogenous neurotransmitter responsible for halting seizures, contributes to the profound seizures associated with methylxanthine overdose.[53,60,171,198]

When studied prospectively, chronic theophylline toxicity results in seizures in 14% of patients, whereas 5% of acutely poisoned patients experience seizures. Seizures are more likely to occur in cases of chronic overdose, and in such situations they occur at lower serum levels.[138] Patients at extremes of age, younger than 3 years and older than 60 years, are more likely to experience seizure with overdose.

Musculoskeletal

Methylxanthines increase intracellular calcium content and increase striated muscle contractility, secondarily decreasing muscle fatigue. They also increase muscle oxygen consumption and increase the basal metabolic rate. These effects are sought by users of methylxanthines to enhance or improve athletic performance or to lose weight.[8,17,41,54,69,70,116,130] Theobromine has the most potent activity on the muscles, more than 100 times that of caffeine, and theophylline has the least muscle-stimulating activity. All methylxanthines cause smooth-muscle relaxation.

Skeletal muscle excitation, which may include tremor, fasciculation, hypertonicity, myoclonus, or even rhabdomyolysis, can all occur with methylxanthine overdose.[104,117,142,154,192,196] Mechanisms by which rhabdomyolysis may result include increased muscle activity, particularly from seizures, and direct cytotoxicity from excessive sequestered intracytoplasmic calcium. Interestingly, there are multiple case reports of compartment syndrome resulting from theophylline overdose.[115,184] This phenomenon is not described as a result of caffeine or theobromine overdose.

Metabolic

Numerous metabolic derangements may result from acute methylxanthine toxicity, and are similar to other states of excess adrenergic agonism or increased metabolism.[75,76,159,170]

Transient hypokalemia resulting from β-adrenergic agonism occurs in 85% of patients with acute theophylline overdose, and typically the serum potassium falls to approximately 3 mEq/L.[5,167] Stimulation of Na^+/K^+ ATPase results in a shift of serum potassium to the intracellular compartment of skeletal muscle. This hypokalemia is only a shift of potassium from the extracellular to the intracellular compartment rather than a loss of potassium, and total body potassium stores are unchanged. The significance of hypokalemia in patients with methylxanthine overdose is unclear. Vomiting and renal losses contribute significantly to true total body hypokalemia. Hyperkalemia may result from overly aggressive repletion of potassium or as a result of rhabdomyolysis.

Metabolic acidosis with increased serum lactate levels is commonly noted as a complication of theophylline overdose.[23,108] Tachypnea and respiratory alkalosis secondary to stimulation of the respiratory center are common.

Hyperglycemia, with serum glucose of approximately 200 mg/dL, is common and occurs in 75% of acute theophylline overdoses. Hypophosphatemia, hypomagnesemia, hypocalcemia, hypercalcemia, and ketosis may also result from methylxanthine toxicity.[156]

Hyperthermia caused by increased metabolic activity and increased muscle activity may result from caffeine and theophylline overdose.

Leukocytosis, probably secondary to the high levels of circulating catecholamines, results from acute methylxanthine overdose. This phenomenon apparently lacks clinical significance.

In the absence of seizures or protracted emesis, chronic methylxanthine poisoning does not typically lead to metabolic derangements because such toxicity is an ongoing, compensated process.

Chronic Methylxanthine Toxicity

The major difference between acute and chronic toxicity is the duration of exposure to the drug. Patients with chronic toxicity may manifest subtle signs such as anorexia, nausea, palpitations, or emesis, although they may also present with seizures or dysrhythmias.

The patient chronically receiving theophylline or caffeine has higher total body stores, and may develop toxicity with a smaller amount of additional theophylline or caffeine. Chronic theophylline poisoning typically occurs in the setting of therapeutic use of theophylline and may occur with iatrogenic administration of caffeine or from frequent, chronic consumption of caffeinated products. Patients often manifest subtle signs of illness, such as anorexia, nausea, palpitations, or emesis. However, the initial presentation in these patients, even with levels in the 40–60 μg/mL range, may be a seizure. In children chronically overdosed with theophylline, the peak serum theophylline concentration may fail to identify those who will progress to life-threatening toxicity. In the absence of protracted emesis or seizures, the initial electrolytes and blood gases are expected to be normal in patients with chronic methylxanthine toxicity.

CHRONIC METHYLXANTHINE USE

An inconclusive link to cancer, heart disease, osteoporosis, hyperlipidemia, and hypercholesterolemia is associated with caffeine use.[57,61,72,110,131,150,193,194] Excessive consumption of caffeine-containing beverages can cause hypokalemia.[153]

A substantial debate centers on the psychiatric and cognitive effects of chronic theophylline use, particularly in children.[114] To date, evidence suggests that although theophylline may acutely result in excessive CNS stimulation and hyperactivity, chronic use of methylxanthines does not adversely affect children's cognitive development.[19,180]

CAFFEINISM

Caffeinism is a syndrome of chronic toxicity resulting from excessive caffeine consumption. It may involve anxiety, palpitations, tremulousness, tachycardia, diuresis, headache, and diarrhea.[188] Patients suffering caffeinism also experience withdrawal symptoms upon abstinence. The chronic toxicity from excessive caffeine use, caffeinism, is a distinctly different entity from caffeine withdrawal.

CAFFEINE WITHDRAWAL

Caffeine is habit-forming and a withdrawal syndrome, including headache, yawning, nausea, drowsiness, rhinorrhea, lethargy, irritability, nervousness, a disinclination to work, and depression, may result upon abstinence.[25,182] Caffeine withdrawal symptoms are described in neonates born to mothers with consequential caffeine use.[123] The onset of caffeine withdrawal symptoms begins 12–24 hours after cessation, and lasts up to 1 week.[71] In a double-blind trial, 52% of adults with moderate caffeine intake developed a withdrawal syndrome upon caffeine abstinence.[175]

REPRODUCTION

Massive doses of methylxanthines are teratogenic, but the doses of typical use are not associated with birth defects. Decreased fecundity and adverse fetal outcome are noted in animals with chronic exposure to methylxanthines.[62,66,122] Human studies of fertility, fetal loss, and fetal outcome produce divergent results, and the effects of methylxanthine use during gestation are unclear.[1,21,55,86,94,128,133]

DIAGNOSTIC TESTING

An electrocardiogram (ECG) and serum electrolytes, as well as a serum caffeine or theophylline level as appropriate, are indicated in cases of suspected methylxanthine toxicity.

Some degree of methylation and demethylation of methylxanthines may occur in patients of all ages, and methylxanthine poisoning may result in elevation in the serum level of other methylxanthine metabolites. Overdose of caffeine may cause a spuriously elevated serum measurement for theophylline.[56,93] The utility of a serum theophylline level in cases of caffeine toxicity is undemonstrated, and at this time, obtaining such levels should only be considered an academic exercise.

Theophylline levels, and to a lesser extent caffeine levels, may be used to guide management of poisoning with the respective agents. For these levels to be maximally useful it is important to know whether they reflect acute or chronic poisoning. In the setting of acute toxicity, serum methylxanthine levels should be obtained immediately and then serially every 1–2 hours until a downward trend is evident.

Acute poisoning by caffeine and theophylline is well described. Because toxicity is dose related, serum concentrations of caffeine and theophylline may be loosely applied as a correlate with toxicity.

Unfortunately, serum caffeine concentrations are usually readily available only in institutions in which neonates are therapeutically treated with caffeine. Serum theophylline concentration is a more readily available laboratory assay, and the greater clinical experience with theophylline in therapeutic dose and in overdose provides an established correlation between serum theophylline concentration and symptomatology.

Likewise, serum electrolytes, particularly potassium, should be monitored serially as long as the poisoned patient remains symptomatic and such values are in a range that may warrant treatment. Cardiac monitoring should continue until the patient is free of any dysrhythmia other than sinus tachycardia, the patient has a decreasing serum methylxanthine level, and the patient is not systemically ill. In patients with systemic illness, hyperthermia, or increased muscle tone, assessing serum creatine phosphokinase (CPK) and urinalysis to detect rhabdomyolysis are also indicated.

MANAGEMENT

General Principles and Gastrointestinal Decontamination

After assuring adequacy of airway, breathing, and circulation, supportive care and maintenance of vital signs within acceptable limits are the mainstay of therapy for methylxanthine overdose. Decisions regarding gastrointestinal decontamination including orogastric lavage, induction of emesis with syrup of ipecac, administration of activated charcoal, or whole-bowel irrigation depend on the dosage and type of preparation of theophylline or caffeine involved, time since exposure, and the patient's physical condition.

Emesis

Emesis with syrup of ipecac should only be rarely considered for minimally symptomatic patients whose ingestions occurred less than 1 hour previously. A simulated overdose controlled volunteer study with sustained-release theophylline was unable to demonstrate reduction of absorption of theophylline in patients treated with syrup of ipecac.[129] Seizures are possible with any significant methylxanthine poisoning, and emesis in a patient experiencing a seizure is an obvious danger. Because the benefits of emetics are undemonstrated and emesis interferes with administration of activated charcoal, syrup of ipecac is rarely indicated for methylxanthine poisoning.[3,63]

Orogastric Lavage

Orogastric lavage may be considered for patients with potentially toxic methylxanthine ingestions, particularly those who are ill enough to require endotracheal intubation. Orogastric lavage may not be effective in removing theophylline tablets, probably because of the large size of the tablets relative to the lumen of the orogastric tube.

Ingestion of sustained-release theophylline tablets is associated with the formation of bezoars that may be difficult to remove or dislodge.[26] Treatment in such cases has included endoscopic removal.[38]

Whole-Bowel Irrigation

Treatment of patients with significant ingestions of sustained-release pills may include whole-bowel irrigation (WBI) with a balanced electrolyte solution to enhance gastrointestinal elimination. (Antidotes in Depth: Whole-Bowel Irrigation) Polyethylene glycol solution used for WBI may displace theophylline already bound to charcoal.[83] This may be a particular problem in patients who have taken several doses of activated charcoal prior to WBI, in which desorption of methylxanthine from activated charcoal may result in a bolus of methylxanthine available for gastrointestinal absorption. Also, WBI is experimentally demonstrated to provide no additional benefit to activated charcoal in treatment of sustained-released theophylline ingestion.[37] Despite these data, WBI remains the preferred and recommended treatment of an ingestion of sustained-release theophylline.

Activated Charcoal

Activated charcoal plays an important role in the treatment of methylxanthine poisoning. Activated charcoal can bind methylxanthines present in the gastrointestinal (GI) tract prior to absorption of the methylxanthine, limiting the absorption of a given methylxanthine dose. Multiple-dose activated charcoal (MDAC) also plays a significant role in the management of methylxanthine toxicity. MDAC enhances elimination of theophylline by gut dialysis. Such enhanced elimination by gut dialysis is not demonstrated, experimentally or otherwise, for caffeine or theobromine toxicity. Because caffeine is to some extent metabolized to theophylline, MDAC in cases of caffeine poisoning would, at the very least, enhance elimination of theophylline metabolites. The pharmacologic similarity of the methylxanthines and the relative safety of MDAC therapy warrant the use of such treatment for any methylxanthine toxicity. MDAC is for the purpose of enhanced elimination and is discussed in depth later in this chapter.

Selecting a Method of Decontamination

The use of decontamination methods that involve more than minimal risk, specifically emesis with syrup of ipecac or orogastric lavage, should only occur after careful consideration of the indications. Acute ingestion occurring not more than 1 hour previously in a patient without CNS depression or contraindicating factors may be treated with syrup of ipecac, and potentially life-threatening acute ingestions may be treated with orogastric lavage.

Treatment of Gastrointestinal Toxicity

Phenothiazine antiemetics are relatively contraindicated in methylxanthine poisoning because they are typically ineffective and may lower the seizure threshold. Metoclopramide may be used, but a more potent antiemetic such as ondansetron or granisetron may be required.[44,147,157] Histamine (H_2) blockers or proton-pump inhibitors may be administered to any patient with hematemesis. Use of such agents should be reserved for cases in which they are certainly needed, because some H_2 blockers (cimetidine) may inhibit CYP450, delaying clearance of methylxanthines.

Treatment of Cardiovascular Toxicity

Hypotension should initially be treated by administration of an isotonic intravenous fluid, such as 0.9% sodium chloride or lactated Ringer solution, in bolus volumes of 20 mL/kg. If acceptable blood pressure cannot be maintained despite several fluid boluses, or if there are contraindications to fluid bolus, vasopressor therapy should be considered.

Methylxanthine toxicity typically results in excessive β-adrenergic agonism; therefore, administration of vasopressors with β-adrenergic agonist effects, such as epinephrine, dobutamine, or isoproterenol, are not preferred. A strictly α-adrenergic agonist such as phenylephrine is the first-line pressor of choice in such a situation, although norepinephrine is also acceptable (Table 39–1).

Hypotension may be refractory to treatment with intravenous fluid and pressor therapy, and in such cases the administration of a β-adrenergic antagonist may be warranted.[49] This approach may seem counterintuitive. Methylxanthine-induced hypotension is to a significant extent mediated by $β_2$-adrenergic vasodilation, and a nonselective β-adrenergic antagonist suppresses $β_2$-adrenergic stimulation. In addition, $β_1$-adrenergic antagonism treats tachycardia and any decreased cardiac output that may result from inefficient cardiac activity. In canines with aminophylline-induced tachycardia and hypotension, administration of esmolol results in a return to normal heart rate and blood pressure, and does not exacerbate hypotension.[63] Propranolol, esmolol, and metoprolol have been used successfully to treat methylxanthine-induced hypotension in humans.[27,144,161,186] It is more appropriate to use a β-adrenergic antagonist with a brief duration of action, such as esmolol or metoprolol, at least initially, in such circumstances. In the event of an adverse reaction or side effect such as hypotension or bronchospasm, the duration of such will be relatively brief. Any β-adrenergic antagonist therapy should ideally be preceded and accompanied by measurement of cardiac output and central venous blood pressure with a device such as a pulmonary artery catheter.[99]

In most other situations, adenosine or electrical cardioversion is the preferred treatment for SVT, but this is not so for SVT resulting from methylxanthine toxicity. Although adenosine or electrical cardioversion may be effective, neither is likely to be effective. Because of the adenosine antagonist effects of methylxanthines, administration of adenosine should not be expected to convert an SVT. However, even if adenosine is successfully used to convert an SVT, the effect is likely to be transient. Because methylxanthine toxicity has a global effect on the myocardium, cardioversion, which is effective in electrically "reorganizing" depolarization, is unlikely to work because this SVT does not result from a single locus of aberrant electrical activity.

Primary treatment for methylxanthine-induced SVT includes administration of benzodiazepines, which work to abate CNS stimulation and concomitant release of catecholamines. More focused pharmacologic therapy to treat SVT is through administration of a conduction-attenuating calcium channel blocker such as diltiazem.

In rat and dog models, treatment of acute theophylline toxicity with calcium channel blockers verapamil, diltiazem, or nifedipine results in decreased cardiac-related deaths and prevented dysrhythmias, hypotension, myocardial necrosis, and seizures.[91] In addition to the cardiovascular benefit of calcium channel blockers, they also afford some neurologic protection and prevention of seizure. In the nonasthmatic patient, methylxanthine-induced supraventricular tachycardia and other tachydysrhythmias may be treated by administration of β-adrenergic antagonist.

Correction of hypokalemia may be crucial in methylxanthine poisoning associated with ventricular dysrhythmias. Hypokalemia is a well-described consequence of excess adrenergic agonism, including poisoning from methylxanthines as well as sympathomimetic agents. In the absence of associated dysrhythmia, the clinical significance of such hypokalemia is unclear. Such hypokalemia has been experimentally demonstrated to respond to treatment with β-adrenergic antagonists.

Treatment of Central Nervous System Toxicity

Administration of a benzodiazepine such as diazepam or lorazepam is appropriate treatment for anxiety, agitation, or seizure. The seizures associated with methylxanthine toxicity are severe and often refractory to treatment. Seizures not controlled with 1 or 2 therapeutic doses of a benzodiazepine should be treated with a barbiturate such as pentobarbital or phenobarbital, or a suitable sedative-hypnotic such as propofol. No delay should occur before administering such medications. Unsuccessful treatment of methylxanthine-induced seizures with any particular agent should quickly be abandoned in favor of treatment with an additional or more efficacious anticonvulsant. The administration of barbiturates may result in or exacerbate hypotension. Treatment of any aforementioned problem with benzodiazepines, barbiturates, or other sedative-hypnotic may require repeated dosing until clinical effect is achieved.

Administration of phenobarbital to prevent seizures in theophylline-poisoned rabbits and mice increases survival by decreasing the incidence of seizures.[43,68] Patients at increased risk for seizures should be prophylactically administered a benzodiazepine such as lorazepam. These patients include those identified earlier in this chapter: patients older than 60 years or younger than 3 years of age, those with chronic overdose and a serum level of 40–60 μg/mL, and acutely overdosed patients with serum levels greater than 100 μg/mL.

Phenytoin and fosphenytoin are of no benefit in controlling methylxanthine-induced seizures and they have no role in such

TABLE 39–1.   Therapeutic Agents for Methylxanthine Poisoning

System	Indication	Therapeutic agent	Comments
Cardiovascular	Hypotension	Fluids	
		Vasopressors	
		Phenylephrine	
		Norepinephrine	
		β-Adrenergic antagonist	Relatively contraindicated in asthmatic patients
		Esmolol	
		Metoprolol	
		Propranolol	
	Supraventricular dysrhythmias	Calcium channel blocker	Dihyrdopyridine agents such as nifedipine and amlodipine are not indicated
		Diltiazem	
		Verapamil	
		β-Adrenergic antagonist	Relatively contraindicated in asthmatic patients
		Esmolol	
		Metoprolol	
		Propranolol	
	Ventricular dysrhythmias	Antidysrhythmic	
		Lidocaine	
		β-Adrenergic antagonist	Relatively contraindicated in asthmatic patients
		Esmolol	
		Metoprolol	
		Propranolol	
Gastrointestinal	Emesis	Antiemetic	
		Metoclopramide	
		Ondansetron	
		Granisetron	
	Hematemesis	Proton pump inhibitor	
		Omeprazole	
		Histamine H_2 antagonist	Cimetidine may decrease clearance of methylxanthines and prolong toxicity
		Ranitidine	
		Famotidine	
CNS	Anxiety Agitation	Benzodiazepine	
		Diazepam	
		Lorazepam	
	Seizure and seizure prophylaxis	Benzodiazepine	
		Diazepam	
		Lorazepam	
Metabolic	Metabolic acidosis	Sodium bicarbonate	
	Hypokalemia	Potassium chloride	
		β-Adrenergic antagonist	Not routinely recommended for this purpose; relatively contraindicated in asthmatic patients
		Esmolol	
		Metoprolol	
		Propranolol	

treatment.[82,120] Retrospective review of human cases demonstrated phenytoin to be ineffective in treating seizures in 21 of 22 cases.[88] In a rabbit model, phenytoin is ineffective in the treatment of seizures, results in the occurrence of seizures at an earlier time after overdose, and results in higher mortality when administered to theophylline-poisoned mice.[28]

Treatment of Metabolic Disorders

Patients with symptomatic hypokalemia, hyperkalemia, or hypocalcemia should be treated accordingly. Most cases of hyperkalemia are well tolerated, but any patient with symptomatic hypokalemia, particularly those associated with ECG changes of T waves or QTc prolongation, should be treated. The frequency of

ventricular dysrhythmias in methylxanthine poisoning, which may be the exacerbated by hypokalemia coupled with increased intrinsic catecholamine release, prompts the recommendation that otherwise asymptomatic hypokalemia below 2.7 mEq/L be treated.

Cautious administration of potassium to treat symptomatic hypokalemia may be indicated, but this is distinct from higher doses of potassium used in total body potassium repletion. In cases of hypokalemia secondary to β-adrenergic agonism, after the β-adrenergic agonism returns to baseline level an efflux of potassium from the intracellular compartment occurs. Concomitant rise of the serum potassium concentration occurs at that time. Overly aggressive attempts to correct hypokalemia may result in hyperkalemia after the β-adrenergic agonist effects abate. Acute methylxanthine-induced hypokalemia may be treated with potassium supplementation, but because of the nature of the problem—excess β-adrenergic agonism—potassium supplementation is typically ineffective.

Experimentally, administration of propranolol to theophylline-poisoned dogs prevented or partially reversed hypokalemia, hypophosphatemia, hyperglycemia, and metabolic acidosis, as well as hypotension.[97] Prevention or correction of the metabolic derangements associated with theophylline toxicity by administration of a β-adrenergic antagonist is congruent with the fact that these derangements, particularly hypokalemia, are the consequence of β-adrenergic agonism. The efficacy of β-adrenergic antagonists as therapy for hypokalemia resulting from acute methylxanthine poisoning in humans is unstudied. However, the pathophysiology of acute methylxanthine-induced hypokalemia and available animal data suggest that therapy with a β-adrenergic antagonist is probably the optimal treatment of such hypokalemia. As mentioned previously, this is relatively contraindicated in an asthmatic patient, and any such treatment should initially be with a short-acting β-adrenergic antagonist such as esmolol or metoprolol to afford greater safety in the event of untoward effects.

The importance of treating hypomagnesemia, hypophosphatemia, and hypocalcemia is not evident, and these disorders should be treated as they would for other patients experiencing them. As with hypokalemia, QTc prolongation is an absolute indication to treat these derangements.

Hyperglycemia, likely resulting from increased circulating catecholamines, is common. This hyperglycemia does not necessitate treatment with any type of hypoglycemic agent, both because it is a transient effect and because in other situations of hyperglycemia resulting from adrenergic agonism a rebound hypoglycemia may occur.

Treatment of Musculoskeletal Toxicity

The use of benzodiazepines is appropriate treatment for fasciculation, hypertonicity, myoclonus, or rhabdomyolysis. Rhabdomyolysis necessitates aggressive intravenous fluid therapy, possibly with sodium bicarbonate (Antidotes in Depth: Sodium Bicarbonate).

Enhanced Elimination

Fortunately, methylxanthine toxicity lends itself well to several methods of enhanced elimination, including gut dialysis with MDAC, charcoal hemoperfusion, and hemodialysis, as well as less used methods such as continuous arteriovenous hemoperfusion (CAVHP) and plasmapheresis.[14,105,113]

Infants with methylxanthine poisoning may be too ill, too unstable, or too small to be treated with hemodialysis or hemoperfusion. Both MDAC and exchange blood transfusion are effective methods of enhanced elimination in infants, and may be the preferred method of treatment in these patients.[16,81,92,139,143,166,168]

MDAC is extremely effective at enhancing elimination of theophylline.[22,64,112,137,140] Experimentally in dogs, rabbits, and human volunteers, activated charcoal administered after IV aminophylline administration results in increased systemic clearance and decreased half-life of theophylline.[32,85,101,124,145] The therapeutic effects of activated charcoal in such cases are much greater than simply limiting absorption of ingested methylxanthine. Activated charcoal, particularly MDAC, enables elimination of theophylline by way of gastrointestinal dialysis.[12] Gut dialysis works to eliminate a drug by virtue the drug diffusing across the gut mucosa. Activated charcoal in the gut lumen acts to adsorb that drug, after which it is eliminated in stool. The pharmacologic similarity of the methylxanthines suggests that MDAC may be effective in gut dialyzing caffeine or theobromine, and MDAC certainly will be effective in eliminating any theophylline generated from metabolism of caffeine or theobromine. The extreme efficacy of MDAC combined with the safety and ease with which this therapy can be administered make MDAC the mainstay of enhanced elimination in methylxanthine toxicity. Severe emesis associated with methylxanthine poisoning may result in intolerance of MDAC, and in case series, has been shown to necessitate abandonment of MDAC for definitive enhancement of methylxanthine elimination by charcoal hemoperfusion[162] (Antidotes in Depth: Activated Charcoal).

Charcoal hemoperfusion is the single most effective method of enhanced elimination of methylxanthines, decreasing theophylline's half-life to 2 hours, and increasing its clearance possibly up to 6-fold.[36,52,132,141,155,158,195] Variations of charcoal hemoperfusion, including albumin colloid hemoperfusion, resin hemoperfusion, and charcoal hemoperfusion, in series with hemodialysis are reported.[39,84,106,148,179]

Charcoal hemoperfusion in series with hemodialysis may be superior to either method alone, because it extends the life of the charcoal perfusion cartridge, increases overall methylxanthine extraction and clearance, and allows fluid and electrolyte abnormalities to be corrected. Charcoal hemoperfusion is typically less readily available and somewhat more complicated than hemodialysis, and this may influence selection between charcoal hemoperfusion and hemodialysis as therapeutic options. Combined hemodialysis and MDAC are an easily performed regimen that provides superior theophylline clearance to hemodialysis alone.

Although employed as an effective treatment modality, hemodialysis has always been less efficient than hemoperfusion in the extracorporeal removal of methylxanthines.[7,107,109,176] Traditionally, hemodialysis was not preferred because methylxanthine elimination rates by hemodialysis were much lower than that those achieved by charcoal hemoperfusion, and even lower than a much safer, easier, noninvasive method—MDAC.

Improvement of hemodialysis equipment allows blood flow rates as much as 2 times faster than in the recent past, and has tremendously increased the potential rates of methylxanthine clearance by hemodialysis. As a result, the difference in elimination achieved by hemoperfusion and hemodialysis is less. This fact, in combination with the ability of hemodialysis to correct fluid and electrolyte imbalances, the greater availability of hemodialysis, its greater technical ease, and its lower complication rates, has resulted in a paradigm shift from considering charcoal hemoperfusion to be the definitive treatment for significant methylxanthine toxicity to one in which charcoal hemoperfusion and hemodialysis are considered fairly equivalent treatment options[172] (Chap. 6).

In the treatment of methylxanthine poisoning, the specific indications for therapy to enhance elimination are not agreed upon. Several studies and clinical experience are the basis for the following suggested indications for extracorporeal elimination by charcoal hemoperfusion, hemodialysis, combined charcoal hemoperfusion/hemodialysis, or combined hemodialysis and MDAC.

Most cases of methylxanthine toxicity and overdoses occur with theophylline, and theophylline levels tend to be both readily available and correlate with toxicity. Therefore, many recommendations regarding hemoperfusion and/or hemodialysis for theophylline toxicity use serum theophylline concentration as a guideline. Serum levels may not be available in instances of caffeine poisoning and do not exist for theobromine poisoning. The clinical aspects of theophylline management guidelines can probably be generalized to all methylxanthine toxicities.

When indicated, charcoal hemoperfusion and/or hemodialysis should be initiated while the patient is still hemodynamically stable, or considered alternatively, before the patient becomes unstable. Charcoal hemoperfusion and/or hemodialysis therapy should be employed for chronic theophylline poisoning associated with a serum theophylline concentration above 40–60 μg/mL or with a deteriorating clinical status.

Our recommendation is that charcoal hemoperfusion and/or hemodialysis be performed any time a methylxanthine exposure results in a serum theophylline or caffeine concentration of greater than 90 μg/mL and symptoms, regardless of clinical stability (Table 39–2). Any methylxanthine exposure resulting in a serum theophylline or caffeine concentration greater than 40 μg/mL that is associated with ventricular dysrhythmias, seizures, hypotension unresponsive to fluids, or emesis unresponsive to antiemetics should also be treated with charcoal hemoperfusion and/or hemodialysis.

A patient who experiences a seizure or dysrythmias or who becomes extremely ill remains a candidate for extracorporeal drug removal. To the contrary, these events make administration of such therapy more critical to ensure survival of the patient.

TABLE 39–2. Indications for Charcoal Hemoperfusion and/or Hemodialysis

1. Theophylline or caffeine serum level >90 μg/mL
2. Acute theophylline or caffeine overdose with seizures or cardiovascular compromise
3. Chronic theophylline or caffeine serum level >40 μg/mL and
   A. Seizures or
   B. Hypotension unresponsive to intravenous fluid or
   C. Ventricular dysrhythmias

Treatment of Chronic Methylxanthine Toxicity

Treatment of chronic methylxanthine toxicity is determined by the patient's clinical status and by the efficacy of MDAC. The precise serum theophylline or caffeine concentration at which patients with chronic theophylline or caffeine toxicity should receive charcoal hemoperfusion or hemodialysis is controversial. For a hemodynamically stable patient without signs of life-threatening methylxanthine toxicity such as ventricular dysrhythmias or seizure, therapy with MDAC may be sufficient. If the serum theophylline or caffeine concentration does not decline following the administration of activated charcoal, or if the patient's clinical status deteriorates, charcoal hemoperfusion or hemodialysis is indicated.

Treatment of Acute-on-Chronic Methylxanthine Toxicity

Patients chronically receiving theophylline or caffeine who acutely overdose should be initially managed in the same manner as patients with acute overdose. The clinical presentation of such patients resembles that of acute poisoning, and the initial management issues of gastrointestinal decontamination are the same as for acute poisoning. Such issues include gastrointestinal decontamination, emesis and other gastrointestinal toxicity, and metabolic derangement.

Because total body stores of the methylxanthine are higher in patients who are chronically exposed, the threshold for toxicity may be reached at lower serum concentrations. After issues of gastrointestinal decontamination and control of emesis are addressed, acute-on-chronic methylxanthine poisoning is managed similarly to chronic poisoning. Seizure prophylaxis indications are the same as those for chronic methylxanthine poisoning, and enhanced elimination is indicated at the lower serum methylxanthine concentrations applied in chronic methylxanthine poisoning.

SUMMARY

Methylxanthines are ubiquitously used by cultures throughout the world. Toxicity results from both the use of medicinal and therapeutic agents, as well as from consumption of methylxanthine-containing foods and beverages. There are significant differences in the clinical presentation and management of patients with acute and chronic poisoning. Supportive care and treatment of gastrointestinal, cardiovascular, CNS, metabolic, and musculoskeletal toxicities are the mainstay of therapy. The unique properties of methylxanthines necessitate specific therapies for the gastrointestinal, cardiovascular, and CNS toxicities of methylxanthines. Methods of enhanced elimination, particularly extracorporeal elimination by charcoal hemoperfusion, hemodialysis, or charcoal hemoperfusion and hemodialysis in series, as well as gut dialysis with MDAC are effective treatments.

REFERENCES

1. Aaronson LS, Macnee CL: Tobacco, alcohol, and caffeine use during pregnancy. J Obstet Gynecol 1989;18:279–287.
2. Aldrigde A, Aranda JV, Neims AH: Caffeine metabolism in the newborn. Clin Pharmacol Ther 1979;25:447–453.
3. Amitai Y, Yeung A, Moye J, Lovejoy FH Jr: Repetitive oral activated charcoal and control of emesis in severe theophylline toxicity. Ann Intern Med 1986;105:386–387.
4. Amitai Y, Lovejoy FH Jr: Characteristics of vomiting associated with acute sustained-release theophylline poisoning: Implications for management with oral activated charcoal. Clin Toxicol 1987;25:539–554.
5. Amitai Y, Lovejoy FH Jr: Hypokalemia in acute theophylline poisoning. Am J Emerg Med 1988;6:214–218.
6. Anderson BJ, Gunn TR, Holford NH, Johnson R: Caffeine overdose in a premature infant: Clinical course and pharmacokinetics. Anaesth Intensive Care 1999;27:307–311.
7. Anderson JR, Poklis A, McQueen RC, et al: Effects of hemodialysis on theophylline kinetics. J Clin Pharmacol 1983;23:428–432.
8. Anselme F, Collomp K, Mercier B, Ahma'idi S, Prefault C: Caffeine increases maximal anaerobic power and blood lactate concentration. Eur J Appl Physiol 1992;65:188–191.
9. Aranda JV, Collinge JM, Zinman R, Watters G: Maturation of caffeine elimination in infancy. Arch Dis Child 1979;54:946–949.
10. Aranda JV, Cook CE, Gorman W, et al: Pharmacokinetic profile of caffeine in the premature newborn infant with apnea. J Pediatr 1979;94:663–668.
11. Aranda JV, Sitar DS, Parsons WD, et al: Pharmacokinetic aspects of theophylline in premature newborns. N Engl J Med 1976;295:413–416.

12. Arimori K, Nakano M: Transport of theophylline from blood to the intestinal lumen following IV administration to rats. J Pharmacobiodyn 1985;8:324–327.

13. Arwood LL, Dasta JF, Friedman C: Placental transfer of theophylline: Two case reports. Pediatrics 1979;63:844–846.

14. Bania TC, Hoffman RS, Howland MA, et al: Plasmapheresis for theophylline intoxication. Vet Hum Toxicol 1992;34:330.

15. Banner W, Czajka P: Acute caffeine overdose in the neonate. Am J Dis Child 1980;134:495–498.

16. Barazarte V, Rodriguez Z, Ceballos S, et al: Exchange transfusion in a case of severe theophylline poisoning. Vet Hum Toxicol 1992;34:524.

17. Bell DG, Jacobs I, Zamecnik J: Effects of caffeine, ephedrine, and their combination on time to exhaustion during high-intensity exercise. Eur J Appl Physiol 1998;77:427–433.

18. Bender PR, Brent J, Kulig K: Cardiac arrhythmias during theophylline toxicity. Chest 1991;100:884–886.

19. Bender BG, Ikl'e DN, DuHamel T, Tinkelman D: Neuropsychological and behavioral changes in asthmatic children treated with beclomethasone dipropionate versus theophylline. Pediatrics 1998;101:355–360.

20. Benowitz NL, Osterloh J, Goldschlager N, et al: Massive catecholamine release from caffeine poisoning. JAMA 1982;248:1097–1098.

21. Berger A: Effects of caffeine consumption on pregnancy outcome. A review. J Reprod Med 1988;33:945–956.

22. Berlinger GW, Spector R, Goldberg MJ, et al: Enhancement of theophylline clearance by oral activated charcoal. Clin Pharmacol Ther 1983;33:351–354.

23. Bernard S: Severe lactic acidosis following theophylline overdose. Ann Emerg Med 1991;20:1135–1137.

24. Bernstein GA, Carroll ME, Crosby RD, et al: Caffeine effects on learning, performance, and anxiety in normal school-age children. J Am Acad Child Adolesc Psychiatry 1994;33:407–415.

25. Bernstein GA, Carroll ME, Dean NW, et al: Caffeine withdrawal in normal school-age children. J Am Acad Child Adolesc Psychiatry 1998;37:858–865.

26. Bernstein G, Jehle D, Bernaski E, Braen GR: Failure of gastric emptying and charcoal administration in fatal sustained-release theophylline overdose: Pharmacobezoar formation. Ann Emerg Med 1992;21:1388–1390.

27. Biberstein MP, Ziegler MG, Ward DM: Use of β-blockade and hemoperfusion for acute theophylline poisoning. West J Med 1984;141:485–490.

28. Blake KV, Massey KL, Hendeles L, et al: Relative efficacy of phenytoin and phenobarbital for the prevention of theophylline-induced seizures in mice. Ann Emerg Med 1988;17:1024–1028.

29. Blakemore F, Shearer GD: The poisoning of livestock by cacao products. Vet Rec 1943;55:165.

30. Bonati M, Latini R, Sadurska B, et al: Kinetics and metabolism of theobromine in male rats. Toxicology 1984;30:327–341.

31. Bory C, Baltassat P, Porthault M, et al: Metabolism of theophylline to caffeine in premature newborn infants. J Pediatr 1979;94:988–993.

32. Brashear RE, Argonoff GR, Brier RA: Activated charcoal in theophylline intoxication. J Lab Clin Med 1985;106:242–245.

33. Brouard C, Moriette G, Murat I, et al: Comparative efficacy of theophylline and caffeine in the treatment of idiopathic apnea in premature infants. Am J Dis Child 1985;139:698–700.

34. Brown CR, Jacob P 3d, Wilson M, Benowitz NL: Changes in rate and pattern of caffeine metabolism after cigarette abstinence. Clin Pharmacol Ther 1988;43:488–491.

35. Bryant CA, Farmer A, Tiplady B, et al: Psychomotor performance: Investigating the dose-response relationship for caffeine and theophylline in elderly volunteers. Eur J Clin Pharmacol 1998;54:309–313.

36. Burgess E, Sargious P: Charcoal hemoperfusion for theophylline overdose: Case report and proposal for predicting treatment time. Pharmacotherapy 1995;15:621–624.

37. Burkhart K, Wuerz R, Donovan JW: Whole-bowel irrigation as adjunctive treatment for sustained-release theophylline poisoning. Ann Emerg Med 1992;21:1316–1320.

38. Cereda JM, Scott J, Quigley EMM: Endoscopic removal of pharmacobezoar of slow release theophylline. Br Med J 1986;293:1143.

39. Chang TMS, Espinosa-Melendez E, Francoeur TE, Eade NR: Albumin-collodion activated charcoal hemoperfusion in the treatment of severe theophylline intoxication in a three-year-old patient. Pediatrics 1980;65:811–814.

40. Chazan R, Karwat K, Tyminska K, et al: Cardiac arrhythmias as a result of intravenous infusions of theophylline in patients with airway obstruction. Int J Clin Pharmacol Therap 1995;32:170–175.

41. Cohen BS, Nelson AG, Prevost MC, et al: Effects of caffeine ingestion on endurance racing in heat and humidity. Eur J Appl Physiol 1996;73:358–363.

42. Cohen S, Booth G: Gastric acid secretion and lower esophageal sphincter pressure in response to coffee and caffeine. N Engl J Med 1975;293:897–899.

43. Czuczwar SJ, Janusz W, Wamil A, Kleinrok Z: Inhibition of aminophylline-induced convulsions in mice by antiepileptic drugs and other agents. Eur J Pharmacol 1987;144:309–315.

44. Daly D, Taylor JN: Ondansetron in theophylline overdose. Anaesth Intensive Care 1993;21:474–475.

45. Dalvi R. Acute and chronic toxicity of caffeine: A review. Vet Hum Toxicol 1986;28:144–150.

46. Decker RA, Meyers GH: Theobromine poisoning in a dog. J Am Vet Med Assoc 1972;161:198–199.

47. Denaro CP, Wilson M, Jacob P 3d, Benowitz NL: The effect of liver disease on urine caffeine metabolite ratios. Clin Pharmacol Ther 1996;59:624–635.

48. Derlet RW, Tseng JC, Albertson TE: Potentiation of cocaine and d-amphetamine toxicity with caffeine. Am J Emerg Med 1992;10:211–216.

49. Dettloff RW, Touchette MA, Zarowitz BJ: Vasopressor-resistant hypotension following a massive ingestion of theophylline. Ann Pharmacother 1993;27:781–784.

50. Drolet R, Arendt TD, Stowe CM: Cacao bean shell poisoning in a dog. J Am Vet Med Assoc 1984;185:902.

51. Drouillard DD, Vesell ES, Dvorchick BH: Studies of theobromine disposition in normal subjects. Clin Pharmacol Ther 1978;23:296–302.

52. Ehlers SM, Zaske DE, Sawchuk RJ: Massive theophylline overdose. Rapid elimination by charcoal hemoperfusion. JAMA 1978;240:474–475.

53. Eldridge FL, Paydarfar D, Scott SC, Dowell RT: Role of endogenous adenosine in recurrent generalized seizures. Exp Neurol 1989;103:179–185.

54. Falk B, Burstein R, Ashkenazi I, et al: The effect of caffeine ingestion on physical performance after prolonged exercise. Eur J Appl Physiol 1989;59:168–173.

55. Fernandes O, Sabharwal M, Smiley T, et al: Moderate to heavy caffeine consumption during pregnancy and relationship to spontaneous abortion and abnormal fetal growth: A meta-analysis. Reprod Toxicol 1998;12:435–444.

56. Fligner CL, Opheim KE: Caffeine and its dimethylxanthine metabolites in two cases of caffeine overdose: A cause of falsely elevated theophylline concentrations in serum. J Anal Toxicol 1988;12:339–343.

57. Folsom AR, McKenzie DR, Bisgard KM, et al: No association between caffeine intake and postmenopausal breast cancer incidence in the Iowa Women's Health Study. Am J Epidemiol 1993;138:380–383.

58. Forman J, Aizer A, Young CR: Myocardial infarction resulting from caffeine overdose in an anorectic woman. Ann Emerg Med 1997; 29:178–180.

59. Frederiksen MC, Ruo TI, Chow MJ, Atkinson AJ Jr: Theophylline pharmacokinetics in pregnancy. Clin Pharmacol Ther 1986;40: 321–328.

60. Fredholm BB: Theophylline action on adenosine receptors. Eur J Respir Dis 1980;18:29–36.

61. Fried RE, Levine DM, Kwiterovich MD, et al: The effects of filtered coffee consumption on plasma lipid levels. JAMA 1992;267: 811–815.

62. Friedman L, Weinberger MA, Farber TM, et al: Testicular atrophy and impaired spermatogenesis in rats fed high levels of methylxanthines, caffeine, theobromine or theophylline. J Environ Pathol Toxicol 1979;2:687–706.

63. Gaar GG, Banner W Jr, Laddu AR: The effects of esmolol on the hemodynamics of acute theophylline toxicity. Ann Emerg Med 1987; 16:1334–1339.

64. Gal P, Miller A, McCue JD: Oral activated charcoal to enhance theophylline elimination in an acute overdose. JAMA 1984;251: 3130–3131.

65. Giacoia G, Jusko WJ, Menke J, Koup JR: Theophylline pharmacokinetics in premature infants with apnea. J Pediatr 1976;89:829–832.

66. Gilbert SG, Rice DC: Somatic development of the infant monkey following in utero exposure to caffeine. Fundam Appl Toxicol 1991; 17:454–465.

67. Glauberg A, Blumenthal HP: Chocolate poisoning in the dog. J Am Animal Hosp Assoc 1983;19:246–248.

68. Goldberg MJ, Spector R, Miller G: Phenobarbital improves survival in theophylline-intoxicated rabbits. Clin Toxicol 1986;24:203–211.

69. Graham TE, Rush JW, van Soeren MH: Caffeine and exercise: Metabolism and performance. Can J Appl Physiol 1994;19:111–138.

70. Graham TE, Spriet LL: Metabolic, catecholamine, and endurance responses to caffeine during intense exercise. J Appl Physiol 1996; 81:1658–1663.

71. Griffiths RR, Woodson PP: Caffeine physical dependence: A review of human and laboratory animal studies. Psychopharmacology 1988; 94:437–451.

72. Grobbee DE, Rimm EB, Giovannucci E, et al: Coffee, caffeine, and cardiovascular disease in men. N Engl J Med 1990;323:1026–1032.

73. Grygiel JJ, Birkett DJ: Cigarette smoking and theophylline clearance and metabolism. Clin Pharmacol Ther 1981;30:491–496.

74. Hadeed A, Siegel S: Newborn cardiac arrhythmias associated with maternal caffeine use during pregnancy. Clin Pediatr 1993;32:45–47.

75. Hagley MT, Traeger SM, Schuckman H: Pronounced metabolic response to modest theophylline overdose. Ann Pharmacother 1994; 28:195–196.

76. Hall KW, Dobson KE, Dalton JG, et al: Metabolic abnormalities associated with intentional theophylline overdose. Ann Intern Med 1984;101:457–462.

77. Haller CA, Benowitz NL: Adverse cardiovascular and central nervous system events associated with dietary supplements containing ephedra alkaloids. N Engl J Med 2000;343:1833–1838.

78. Hanington E, Bell H: Suspected chocolate poisoning of calves. Vet Rec 1972;90:408–409.

79. Hantson P, Gautier P, Vekemans MC, et al: Acute myocardial infarction in a young woman: Possible relationship with sustained-release theophylline acute overdose? Intensive Care Med 1992;18:496–498.

80. Hayes AH: New drug status of OTC combination products containing caffeine, phenylpropanolamine, and ephedrine. Fed Reg 1982; 47:35344–35346.

81. Henry GC, Wax PM, Howland MA, et al: Exchange transfusion for the treatment of a theophylline overdose in a premature neonate. Vet Human Toxicol 1991;33:354.

82. Hoffman A, Pinto E, Gilhar D: Effect of pretreatment with anticonvulsants on theophylline-induced seizures in the rat. J Crit Care 1993;8:198–202.

83. Hoffman RS, Chiang WK, Howland MA, et al: Theophylline desorption from activated charcoal caused by whole-bowel irrigation solution. J Toxicol Clin Toxicol 1991;29:191–201.

84. Hootkins R Sr, Lerman MJ, Thompson JR: Sequential and simultaneous "in series" hemodialysis and hemoperfusion in the management of theophylline intoxication. J Am Soc Nephrol 1990;1: 923–926.

85. Huang JD: Kinetics of theophylline clearance in gastrointestinal dialysis with charcoal. J Pharm Sci 1987;76:525–527.

86. Infante-Rivard C, Fernandez A, Gauthier R, et al: Fetal loss associated with caffeine intake before and during pregnancy. JAMA 1993; 270:2940–2943.

87. Jackson SH, Johnston A, Woollard R, Turner P: The relationship between theophylline clearance and age in adult life. Eur J Clin Pharmacol 1989;36:29–34.

88. Jacobs MH, Senior RM: Theophylline toxicity due to impaired theophylline degradation. Am Rev Resp Dis 1974;110:342–345.

89. Jacobson BH, Thurman-Lacey SR: Effect of caffeine on motor performance by caffeine-naïve and familiar subjects. Percept Mot Skills 1992;74:151–157.

90. Jain AK, McMahon FG, Ryan JR, et al: Aspirin and aspirin-caffeine in postpartum pain relief. Clin Pharmacol Ther 1978;24:69–75.

91. Jain AK, McMahon FG, Ryan JR, Narcisse C: A double-blind study of ibuprofen 200 mg in combination with caffeine 100 mg, ibuprofen 400 mg, and placebo in episiotomy pain. Curr Ther Res 1988;43: 762–769.

92. Jain R, Tholl DA: Activated charcoal for theophylline toxicity in a premature infant on the second day of life. Dev Pharmacol Ther 1992;19: 106–110.

93. Jenny RW, Jackson KY: Two types of error found with the Seralyzer ARIS assay of theophylline. Clin Chem 1986;32:2122–2123.

94. Jensen TK, Henriksen TB, Hjollund NH, et al: Caffeine intake and fecundability: A follow-up study among 430 Danish couples planning their first pregnancy. Reprod Toxicol 1988;12:289–295.

95. Jusko WJ, Gardner MJ, Mangione A, et al: Factors affecting theophylline clearances: Age, tobacco, marijuana, cirrhosis, congestive heart failure, obesity, oral contraceptives, benzodiazepines, barbiturates, and ethanol. J Pharm Sci 1979;68:1358–1366.

96. Jusko WJ, Schentag JJ, Clark JH, et al: Enhanced biotransformation of theophylline in marijuana and tobacco smokers. Clin Pharmacol Ther 1978;24:405–410.

97. Kearney TE, Manoguerra AS, Curtis GP, et al: Theophylline toxicity and the beta-adrenergic system. Ann Intern Med 1985;102: 766–769.

98. Kelsey MC, Grossberg GT: Safety and efficacy of caffeine-augmented ECT in elderly depressives: A retrospective study. J Geriatr Psychiatry Neurol 1995;8:168–172.

99. Kempf J, Rusterholtz TH, Ber C, et al: Haemodynamic study as guideline for the use of beta blockers in acute theophylline poisoning. Intensive Care Med 1996;22:585–587.

100. Kraft M, Torvik JA, Trudeau JB, et al: J Allergy Clin Immunol 1996; 97:1242–1246.

101. Kulig KW, Bar-Or D, Rumack BH: Intravenous theophylline poisoning and multiple-dose charcoal in an animal model. Ann Emerg Med 1987;16:842–846.

102. Labovitz E, Spector S: Placental theophylline transfer in pregnant asthmatics. JAMA 1982;247:786–788.

103. Lalonde RL, Koob RA, McLean WM, Balsys AJ: The effects of cimetidine on theophylline pharmacokinetics at steady state. Chest 1983;2:221–224.

104. Laurence AS, Wight J, Forrest AR: Fatal theophylline poisoning with rhabdomyolysis. Anaesthesia 1992;47:82.

105. Laussen P, Shann F, Butt W, Tibbals J: Use of plasmapheresis in acute theophylline toxicity. Crit Care Med 1991;19:288–290.

106. Lawyer C, Aitchison J, Sutton J, Bennett W: Treatment of theophylline neurotoxicity with resin hemoperfusion. Ann Intern Med 1978; 38:516–517.

107. Lee CS, Marbury TC, Perrin JH, Fuller TJ: Hemodialysis of theophylline in uremic patients. J Clin Pharmacol 1979;19:219–226.
108. Leventhal LJ, Kochar G, Felman NH, et al: Lactic acidosis in theophylline overdose. Am J Emerg Med 1989;7:417–418.
109. Levy G, Gibson TP, Whitman W, Procknal J: Hemodialysis clearance of theophylline. JAMA 1977;237:1466–1467.
110. Lewis CE, Caan B, Funkhouser E, et al: Inconsistent associations of caffeine containing beverages with blood pressure and with lipoproteins. Am J Epidemiol 1993;138:502–507.
111. Lieberman HR, Wurtman RJ, Emde GG, Coviella IL: The effects of caffeine and aspirin on mood and performance. J Clin Psychopharmacol 1987;75:315–320.
112. Lim DT, Singh P, Nourtsis S, Delacruz R. Absorption inhibition and enhancement of elimination of sustained-release theophylline tablets by oral activated charcoal. Ann Emerg Med 1986;15: 1303–1307.
113. Lin JL, Jeng LB: Critical, acutely poisoned patients treated with continuous arteriovenous hemoperfusion in the emergency department. Ann Emerg Med 1995;25:75–80.
114. Lindgren S, Lokshin B, Stromquist A, et al: Does asthma or treatment with theophylline limit children's academic performance? N Engl J Med 1992;327:926–930.
115. Lloyd DM, Payne SP, Tomson CR, et al: Acute compartment syndrome secondary to theophylline overdose. Lancet 1990;336:312.
116. Lopes JM, Aubier M, Jardim J, et al: Effect of caffeine on skeletal muscle function before and after fatigue. J Appl Physiol 1983;54: 1303–1305.
117. MacDonald JB, Jones HM, Cowan RA: Rhabdomyolysis and acute renal failure after theophylline overdose. Lancet 1985;1:932–933.
118. Maddux MS, Leeds NH, Organek HW, et al: The effect of erythromycin on theophylline pharmacokinetics at steady state. Chest 1982;5:563–565.
119. Mangione A, Imhoff TE, Lee RV, et al: Pharmacokinetics of theophylline in hepatic disease. Chest 1978;73:616–622.
120. Marquis JF, Carruthers SG, Spence JD, et al: Phenytoin-theophylline interaction. N Engl J Med 1982;307:1189–1190.
121. Mathew RJ, Wilson WH: Caffeine induced changes in cerebral circulation. Stroke 1985;16:814–817.
122. Matsuoka R, Uno H, Tanaka H, Kerr CS, et al: Caffeine induces cardiac and other malformations in the rat. Am J Med Genet 1987;3: 433–443.
123. McGowan JD, Altman RE, Kanto WP: Neonatal withdrawal symptoms after chronic maternal ingestion of caffeine. South Med J 1988;81:1092–1094.
124. Mckinnon RS, Desmond PV, Harman PJ, et al: Studies on the mechanisms of action of activated charcoal on theophylline pharmacokinetics. J Pharm Pharmacol 1987;39:522–555.
125. McQuay HJ, Angell K, Carroll D, et al: Ibuprofen compared with ibuprofen plus caffeine after third molar surgery. Pain 1996;66: 247–251.
126. Mehta A, Jain AC, Mehta MC, Billie M: Caffeine and cardiac arrhythmias. An experimental study in dogs with review of literature. Acta Cardiol 1997;52:273–283.
127. Migliardi JR, Armellino JJ, Friedman M, et al: Caffeine as an analgesic adjuvant in tension headache. Clin Pharmacol Ther 1994;56: 576–586.
128. Mills JL, Holmes LB, Aarons JH, et al: Moderate caffeine use and the risk of spontaneous abortion and intrauterine growth retardation. JAMA 1993;269:593–597.
129. Minton NA, Glucksman E, Henry JA: Prevention of drug absorption in simulated theophylline overdose. Hum Exp Toxicol 1995;14: 170–174.
130. Morton AR, Scott CA, Fitch KD: The effects of theophylline on the physical performance and work capacity of well-trained athletes. J Allergy Clin Immunol 1989;83:55–61.
131. Myers MG, Basinski A: Coffee and coronary heart disease. Arch Intern Med 1992;152:1767–1772.

132. Nagesh RV, Murphy KA: Caffeine poisoning treated by hemoperfusion. Am J Kidney Dis 1988;4:316–318.
133. Nehlig A, Debry G: Potential teratogenic and neurodevelopmental consequences of coffee and caffeine exposure: A review on human and animal data. Neurotoxicol Teratol 1994;16:531–543.
134. Nicot G, Charmes JP, Lachatre G, et al: Theophylline toxicity risks and chronic renal failure. Int J Clin Pharmacol Ther Toxicol 1989; 27:398–401.
135. Nix DE, DiCicco RA, Miller AK, et al: The effect of low-dose cimetidine (200 mg twice daily) on the pharmacokinetics of theophylline. J Clin Pharmacol 1999;39:855–865.
136. Nobel PA, Light GS: Theophylline-induced diuresis in the neonate. J Pediatr 1977;90:825–826.
137. Ohning BL, Reed MD, Blumer JL. Continuous nasogastric administration of activated charcoal for the treatment of theophylline intoxication. Pediatr Pharmacol 1986;5:241–245.
138. Olson KR, Benowitz NL, Woo OF, Pond SM: Theophylline overdose: Acute single ingestion versus chronic repeated overmedication. Am J Emerg Med 1985;3:386–394.
139. Osborn HH, Henry G, Wax P, et al: Theophylline toxicity in a premature neonate—Elimination kinetics of exchange transfusion. J Toxicol 1993;31:639–644.
140. Park GD, Radomski L, Goldberg MJ, et al: Effects of size and frequency of oral doses of charcoal on theophylline clearance. Clin Pharmacol Ther 1983;34:663–666.
141. Park GD, Spector R, Roberts RJ, et al: Use of hemoperfusion for the treatment of theophylline toxicity. Am J Med 1983;74:961–966.
142. Parr MJA, Willatts SM: Fatal theophylline poisoning with rhabdomyolysis. Anaesthesia 1991;46:557–559.
143. Perrin C, Debruyne D, Lacotte J, et al: Treatment of caffeine intoxication by exchange transfusion in a newborn. Acta Paediatr Scand 1987;76:679–681.
144. Price KR, Fligner DJ: Treatment of caffeine toxicity with esmolol. Ann Emerg Med 1990;19:44–46.
145. Radomski L, Park GD, Goldberg MJ, et al: Model for theophylline overdose treatment with oral activated charcoal. Clin Pharmacol Ther 1984;35:402–408.
146. Resman BH, Blumenthal HP, Jusko WJ. Breast milk distribution of theobromine from chocolate. J Pediatrics 1977;91:477–480.
147. Roberts JR, Carney S, Boyle SM, Lee DC: Ondansetron quells drug-resistant emesis in theophylline poisoning. Am J Emerg Med 1993; 11:609–610.
148. Rongved G, Westlie L: Hemoperfusion/hemodialysis in the treatment of acute theophylline poisoning: Description of a fatal case. Int J Clin Pharmacol Ther Toxicol 1986;24:85–87.
149. Rosenberg J, Benowitz NL, Pond S: Pharmacokinetics of drug overdose. Clin Pharacokinet 1981;6:161–192.
150. Ross PC: Osteoporosis frequency, consequences and risk factors. Arch Intern Med 1996;156:1399–1411.
151. Rovei V, Chanoine F, Strolin Benedetti M: Pharmacokinetics of theophylline: A dose-range study. Br J Clin Pharmacol 1982;14: 769–778.
152. Roy AK, Cuda MP, Levine RA: Induction of theophylline toxicity and inhibition of clearance rates by ranitidine. Am J Med 1988; 85: 525–527.
153. Rudy DR, Lee S: Coffee and hypokalemia. J Fam Pract 1988;26: 679–680.
154. Rumpf DW, Wagner H, Criee CP, et al: Rhabdomyolysis after theophylline overdose. Lancet 1985;1:1451–1452.
155. Russo ME: Management of theophylline intoxication with charcoal-column hemoperfusion. N Engl J Med 1979;300:24–26.
156. Ryan T, Coughlan G, McGing P, Phelan D: Ketosis, a complication of theophylline toxicity. J Intern Med 1989;226:277–278.
157. Sage TA, Jones WN, Clark RF: Ondansetron in the treatment of intractable nausea associated with theophylline toxicity. Ann Pharmacother 1993;27:584–585.

158. Sahney S, Abarzua J, Sessums L: Hemoperfusion in theophylline neurotoxicity. Pediatrics 1983;71:615–619.

159. Sawyer WT, Caravati EM, Ellison MJ, Krueger KA: Hypokalemia, hyperglycemia, and acidosis after intentional theophylline overdose. Am J Emerg Med 1985;3:408–411.

160. Sawynok J, Yaksh TL: Caffeine as an analgesic adjuvant: A review of pharmacology and mechanisms of action. Pharmacol Rev 1993; 45:43–85.

161. Seneff M, Scott J, Friedman B, Smith M: Acute theophylline toxicity and the use of esmolol to reverse cardiovascular instability. Ann Emerg Med 1990;19:671–673.

162. Sessler CN, Glauser FL, Cooper KR: Treatment of theophylline toxicity with oral activated charcoal. Chest 1985;87:325–329.

163. Sessler CN: Poor tolerance of oral activated charcoal with theophylline overdose. Am J Emerg Med 1987;5:492–495.

164. Sessler CN, Cohen MD: Cardiac arrhythmias during theophylline toxicity: A prospective continuous electrocardiographic study. Chest 1990;98:672–678.

165. Schaftel BP, Fillman JM, Lane AC, et al: Caffeine as an analgesic adjuvant. Arch Intern Med 1991;151:733–737.

166. Shannon M, Amitai Y, Lovejoy FH Jr: Multiple-dose activated charcoal for theophylline poisoning in young infants. Pediatrics 1987; 80:368–370.

167. Shannon M, Lovejoy FH Jr: Hypokalemia after theophylline intoxication. The effects of acute vs chronic poisoning. Arch Intern Med 1989;149:2725–2729.

168. Shannon M, Wernovsky G, Morris C: Exchange transfusion in the treatment of severe theophylline poisoning. Pediatrics 1992;89: 145–147.

169. Shannon M: Predictors of major toxicity after theophylline overdose. Ann Intern Med 1993;119:1161–1167.

170. Shannon M: Hypokalemia, hyperglycemia and plasma catecholamine activity after severe theophylline intoxication. Clin Toxicol 1994;32:41–47.

171. Shannon MW, Maher TJ: Anticonvulsant effects of intracerebroventricular adenosine in theophylline-induced seizures. Ann Emerg Med 1995;26:723–724.

172. Shannon MW: Comparative efficacy of hemodialysis and hemoperfusion in severe theophylline intoxication. Acad Emerg Med 1997;4: 674–678.

173. Shannon M: Life-threatening events after theophylline overdose: A 10-year prospective analysis. Arch Intern Med 1999;159:989–994.

174. Shapira B, Lerer B, Gilboa D, et al: Facilitation of ECT by caffeine pretreatment. Am J Psychiatry 1987;144:1199–1202.

175. Silverman K, Evans SM, Strain EC, Griffiths RR: Withdrawal syndrome after the double-blind cessation of caffeine consumption. N Engl J Med 1992;327:1109–1114.

176. Slaughter RL, Green L, Kohli R: Hemodialysis clearance of theophylline. Ther Drug Monit 1982;4:191–193.

177. Staib AH, Schuppan D, Lissner R, et al: Pharmacokinetics and metabolism of theophylline in patients with liver disease. Int J Clin Pharm Ther Toxicol 1980;18:500–502.

178. Statland BE, Demas TJ: Serum caffeine half-lives. Healthy subjects vs. patients having alcoholic hepatic disease. Am J Clin Pathol 1980; 73:390–393.

179. Stegmayr BG: On-line hemodialysis and hemoperfusion in a girl intoxicated by theophylline. Acta Med Scand 1988;223:565–567.

180. Stein MA, Krasowski M, Leventhal BL, et al: Behavioral and cognitive effects of methylxanthines. A meta-analysis of theophylline and caffeine. Arch Pediatr Adolesc Med 1996;150:284–288.

181. Strachan ER, Bennett A: Theobromine poisoning in dogs. Vet Rec 1994;134:284.

182. Strain EC, Mumford GK, Silverman K, Griffiths RR: Caffeine dependence syndrome. JAMA 1994;272:1043–1048.

183. Tisdell R, Iacobucci M, Snodgrass WR: Caffeine poisoning in an adult—Survival with a serum concentration of 400 mg/L and need for adenosine agonist antidotes. Vet Human Toxicol 1986;28:492.

184. Titley OG, Williams N: Theophylline toxicity causing rhabdomyolysis and acute compartment syndrome. Intensive Care Med 1992;18: 129–130.

185. Tyrala EE, Dodson WE: Caffeine secretion into breast milk. Arch Dis Child 1979;54:787–800.

186. Vanden Hoek T, Murphy C, Aks S, et al: The use of esmolol to reverse unstable supraventricular tachycardia in a theophylline toxic patient. Vet Hum Toxicol 1991;33:390.

187. Vestal RE, Eiriksson CE Jr, Musser B, et al: Effect of intravenous aminophylline on plasma levels of catecholamines and related cardiovascular and metabolic responses in man. Circulation 1983;67: 162–171.

188. Victor BS, Lubetsky M, Greden JF: Somatic manifestations of caffeinism. J Clin Psychiatry 1981;42:185–188.

189. Vozeh S, Powell R, Riegelman S, et al: Changes in theophylline clearances during acute illness. JAMA 1978;240:1882–1884.

190. Weinberger M, Bronsky E, Bensch GW, et al: Interaction of ephedrine and theophylline. Clin Pharmacol Ther 1975;291: 151–153.

191. Whitehurst VE, Joseph X, Vick JA, et al: Reversal of acute theophylline toxicity by calcium channel blockers in dogs and rats. Toxicology 1996;110:113–121.

192. Wight JP, Laurence S, Holt S, Forrest AR: Rhabdomyolysis with hyperkalaemia after aminophylline overdose. Med Sci Law 1987;27: 103–105.

193. Willett WC, Stampfer MJ, Manson JE, et al: Coffee consumption and coronary heart disease in women. JAMA 1996;275:458–462.

194. Wilson PW, Garrison RJ, Kannel WB, et al: Is coffee consumption a contributor to cardiovascular disease? Arch Intern Med 1989;149: 1169–1172.

195. Woo OF, Pond SM, Benowitz NL, Olson KR: Benefit of hemoperfusion in acute theophylline intoxication. J Toxicol Clin Toxicol 1984; 22:411–424.

196. Wrenn KD, Oschner I: Rhabdomyolysis induced by caffeine overdose. Ann Emerg Med 1989;18:94–97.

197. Yeh TF, Pildes R: Transplacental aminophylline toxicity in a neonate. Lancet 1977;1:9–10.

198. Young D, Dragunow M: Status epilepticus may be caused by a loss of adenosine anticonvulsant mechanisms. Neuroscience 1994;58: 245–261.

199. Yurchak AM, Jusko WJ: Theophylline secretion into breast milk. Pediatrics 1976;57:518–520.

George M. Bosse

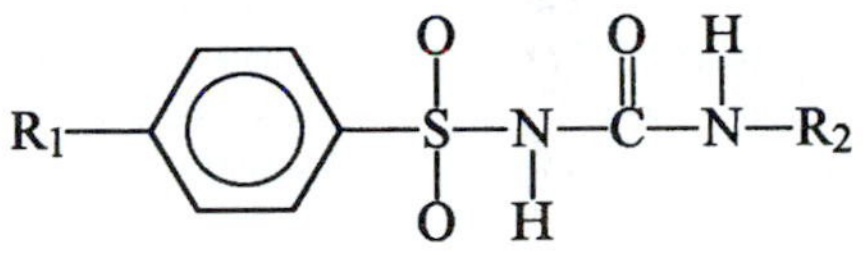

Sulfonylureas

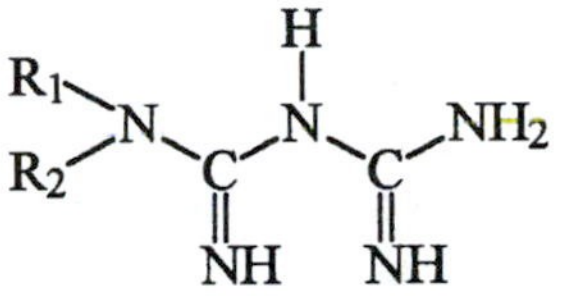

Biguanides

Glucose

MW	=	180 daltons
Normal range (blood)	=	60–110 mg/dL
	=	3.3–6.1 mmol/L

Values less than or equal to the action level necessitate clinical intervention. Values greater than this level may necessitate intervention based on the clinical characteristics of the patient.

Five police officers entered the Emergency Department (ED) with an obese, middle-aged man whose arms were handcuffed behind his back. He was extremely agitated, diffusely diaphoretic, bleeding from the mouth, and had several small lacerations and multiple contusions. His respirations were labored. The police stated that the man's family had called them after he had "gone berserk." When they arrived at the apartment, several pieces of furniture had been broken, and it took all five police officers to restrain the man. In a few minutes, the family arrived in the ED. They related that the patient had been despondent recently; they suspected he had been drinking. In addition, they reported, he was taking various unknown medications, "because he's been sick." Shortly after the handcuffs were removed to permit physical examination, the patient developed a focal seizure that began in his right hand and progressed to become a typical generalized tonic-clonic seizure lasting 2 minutes. Postictal vital signs were: blood pressure, 120/80 mm Hg; pulse, 120 beats/min; respiration, 24 breaths/min; and temperature, 36.8°C (98.4°F). The patient was lethargic but oriented. The remainder of the neurologic examination revealed a right hemiparesis, right conjugate gaze, right central facial paralysis, and right-sided plantar extension. The pupils were equal and reactive to light, and the fundi were unremarkable. He had no evidence of significant head trauma. His chest was clear to percussion and auscultation, and heart sounds were normal except for tachycardia. Multiple contusions were clearly visible on his extremities, but there were no overt fractures and there was no edema.

Within 5 minutes of empiric administration of 100 mL of $D_{50}W$ and 100 mg thiamine IV, the right-sided neurologic findings disappeared, the lethargy cleared, and the patient was sufficiently alert to relate a history. The patient stated that his private physician had placed him on chlorpropamide for "mild diabetes." Because his mother had died of diabetes, he thought he knew the type of complications he might expect. He became despondent, he said, because of his "inevitable fate" and began to drink. The alcohol, however, only led to more frequent episodes of despondency.

His pretreatment serum glucose was 18 mg/dL. Although the patient's blood sugar remained elevated in the ED, he was admitted to the hospital so that he could be observed, and if necessary treated, for recurrent hypoglycemia. An IV line was maintained for 24 hours until the patient began to eat regularly. No neurologic sequelae were observed. Diabetic education and alcoholism counseling were initiated during his 2-day hospitalization, which was uneventful. He was discharged to the care of his private physician and the chlorpropamide was discontinued.

Although various pharmacologic agents and medical conditions may cause hypoglycemia, the focus of this chapter is on the drugs used in the treatment of diabetes mellitus. This includes the various forms of insulin and several oral agents: the sulfonylureas, biguanides, α-glucosidase inhibitors, thiazolidinediones, and meglitinides. This chemically heterogeneous group of drugs has the potential to cause various unique toxic effects in addition to hypoglycemia.

Most patients with diabetes mellitus are classified as either insulin-dependent (IDDM) (Type 1) or noninsulin-dependent (NIDDM) (Type 2). This classification scheme for diabetes mellitus is not perfect. For example, patients with NIDDM may be managed with insulin therapy. Early in the course of IDDM, patients may enter a remission period during which insulin is not required.

In general, neurohormonal control of glucose production in healthy individuals maintains a serum glucose level in the range of 60–110 mg/dL. Hypoglycemia is the failure to maintain serum glucose above a level that does not cause signs or symptoms of glucose deficit. The glycemic threshold is the plasma glucose concentration below which clinical manifestations develop. This threshold level for symptoms to occur is quite variable. In one study, the mean glycemic threshold for hypoglycemic symptoms was 78 mg/dL in poorly controlled diabetics as compared to 53 mg/dL in nondiabetics.[11]

HISTORY AND EPIDEMIOLOGY

Insulin first became available for use in 1922.[7] Since its introduction, several forms with varying kinetic properties have become available. In an attempt to more closely simulate physiologic conditions, newer, designer insulins have been developed, including an ultrashort-acting preparation known as lispro.[49,97] Research into an oral form of insulin with resistance to the protein degradation effects of the gut is ongoing and of particular interest.[36] Emphasis on tighter diabetic control as a means of preventing microvascular effects of diabetes mellitus carries with it an increased risk of hypoglycemia.[22,23] Insulin-induced hypoglycemia may be used therapeutically in alternative medicine practices and psychiatrists use this therapy for patients with severe depression.

The hypoglycemic activity of a sulfonamide derivative used for typhoid fever in World War II was noted by the French physician Janbon.[51] This discovery was subsequently verified in animals. The sulfonylureas in use today are all chemical modifications of that original sulfonamide compound. In the mid-1960s, the first-generation sulfonylureas were widely used. The newer, second-generation agents differ from those early first-generation agents primarily in their potency. Although insulin is widely used, overdose with the sulfonylureas is more commonly reported than is insulin overdose, based on 10 years of data from the 1989 through 1998 reports of the American Association of Poison Control Centers Toxic Exposure Surveillance System (Chap. 116 and page 1752). However, insulin-induced hypoglycemia probably occurs more frequently than reported.

The biguanides metformin and phenformin were developed as derivatives of *Galega officinalis,* the French lilac which was recognized in medieval Europe as a treatment for diabetes mellitus.[4] Phenformin was used in the United States until 1977, when it was banned because of its association with life-threatening lactic acidosis (64 cases/100,000 patient-years). However, it is still available in certain countries, including Spain and Italy.[57] Travelers and immigrant patients who continue to receive medication from their native countries may still present here with phenformin-induced lactic acidosis. Metformin became available in the United States in 1995. Its use is also associated with lactic acidosis, but to a much lesser degree than with phenformin (only 3 cases/100,000 patient-years).[20]

Several newer agents have been introduced in the treatment of diabetes mellitus. Although overdose data are limited, some of these drugs have unique toxicity related to therapeutic use. These include the thiazolidinedione derivatives (troglitazone, rosiglitazone, pioglitazone), acarbose and miglitol (α-glucosidase inhibitors), and repaglinide and nateglinide (meglitinides).

Hypoglycemia and its secondary effects on the central nervous system are the most common adverse effects related to insulin and the sulfonylureas. Ethanol is also a common cause of hypoglycemia and is discussed in depth in Chapter 64. Although this classically occurs in alcoholics with decreased carbohydrate intake and depleted hepatic glycogen stores, other populations, such as children, are also particularly vulnerable to ethanol-induced hypoglycemia. Various other drugs, including β-adrenergic antagonists and salicylates, as well as various medical conditions, such as sepsis and insulin-secreting tumors, may cause hypoglycemia (see Table 40–1). Certain plant products may be implicated as well. Although not a particular problem in the United States, ingestion of the unripe fruit of the Ackee tree (*Blighia sapida*) in countries

TABLE 40–1.   Causes of Hypoglycemia

Endocrine Disorders	Rheumatoid arthritis
Addison disease	Graves disease
Glucagon deficiency	Burns
Panhypopituitarism	Diarrhea (childhood)
(Sheehan syndrome)	Leucine sensitivity
	Muscular activity (excessive)
Neoplasms	Postgastric surgery
Carcinomas (diverse	Pregnancy
extrapancreatic)	Protein calorie malnutrition
Hematologic	Septicemia
Insulinoma	Shock
Mesenchymal	Wasting syndrome
Multiple endocrine adenopathy	
type 1 (Werner syndrome)	**Exogenous**
	Ackee (hypoglycin)
Reactive Hypoglycemia	Alloxan
	β-Adrenergic antagonists
Hepatic Disease	Cocaine
Acute hepatic atrophy	Disopyramide
Alcoholism	Ethanol
Cirrhosis	Hypoglycemic agents (insulin,
Galactose or fructose intolerance	sulfonylureas)
Glycogen storage disease	Opioids
Neoplasia	Pentamidine
	Quinine
Renal Disease	Quinidine
Chronic hemodialysis	Ritodrine
Chronic renal insufficiency	Salicylates
	Streptozocin
Miscellaneous	Sulfonamides
Acquired immunodeficiency	Vacor
syndrome (AIDS)	Valproic acid
Anorexia nervosa	
Autoimmune disorders	**Artifactual**
SLE	Chronic myelogenous leukemia
	Polycythemia vera

where food is in short supply may result in significant hypoglycemia due to the compound hypoglycin.

PHARMACOLOGY

Insulin is synthesized in the β cells of the pancreas as a prohormone, which upon release is cleaved, resulting in a C-peptide and insulin itself, a double-chain molecule containing 51 amino acid residues. Glucose concentration plays a major role in the regulation of insulin release. The activation of insulin secretion by glucose is complex and not well understood. Likely steps in the triggering process include the activation of signal transduction pathways, ATP production via glucose metabolism, closure of adenosine triphosphate (ATP)-sensitive potassium channels, cellular depolarization, and calcium entry into the β cell. Insulin binds to specific receptors on cell surfaces in insulin-sensitive tissues, particularly liver, muscle, and adipose. The action of insulin on these tissues is complex and involves various phosphorylation and dephosphorylation reactions.[86] Chapter 26 has a detailed discussion of the endocrine principles of insulin and other antidiabetic agents. Figure 40–1 depicts the chemical structures of representative oral agents. The sulfonylureas stimulate the β cells of the pancreas to produce insulin; as such, they are ineffective in IDDM

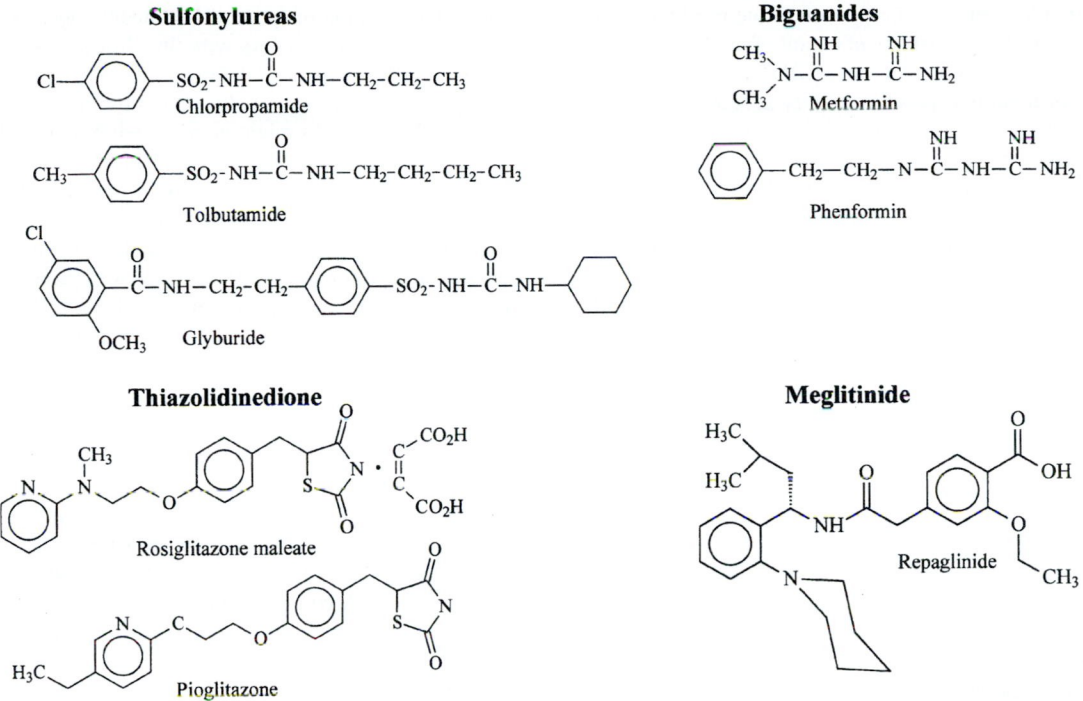

Figure 40–1. The chemical structures of representative oral antidiabetic and hypoglycemic agents.

where the patient is insulinopenic (Fig. 40–2). This stimulatory effect diminishes with chronic therapy. All the sulfonylureas have molecular mechanisms that involve binding to high-affinity receptors on the pancreatic β-cell membrane, with subsequent closure of potassium channels sensitive to adenosine triphosphate (K_{ATP} channels).[27,31,32] This inhibition of potassium ion efflux from pancreatic β cells causes membrane depolarization, calcium influx, and activation of the secretory machinery independent of glucose concentration. High-affinity sulfonylurea receptors are also present within pancreatic β cells and are postulated to be either on granular membranes or part of a regulatory exocytosis kinase. Binding to these receptors promotes exocytosis by direct interaction with secretory machinery not involving closure of the plasma membrane K_{ATP} channels.[27,31,32] Repaglinide is a new oral agent that is structurally different from the sulfonylureas. However, it also binds to ATP-sensitive potassium channels on β cells of the pancreas, resulting in increased insulin secretion.[61]

The linkage of two guanidine molecules forms the biguanides. In the process, an amino group is eliminated. Metformin, the only biguanide available in the United States, is an oral compound used in the treatment of NIDDM. Its glucose-lowering effect is caused by several underlying mechanisms. The most important mechanism appears to involve the inhibition of gluconeogenesis and subsequent decreased hepatic glucose output. Enhanced peripheral glucose uptake also plays a significant role. Other contributing factors include decreased fatty acid oxidation and increased intestinal use of glucose.[5,99] In skeletal muscle and adipose cells, metformin causes enhanced activity and translocation of glucose transporters. Although the details are unclear, the mechanism by which this occurs involves an interaction between metformin and

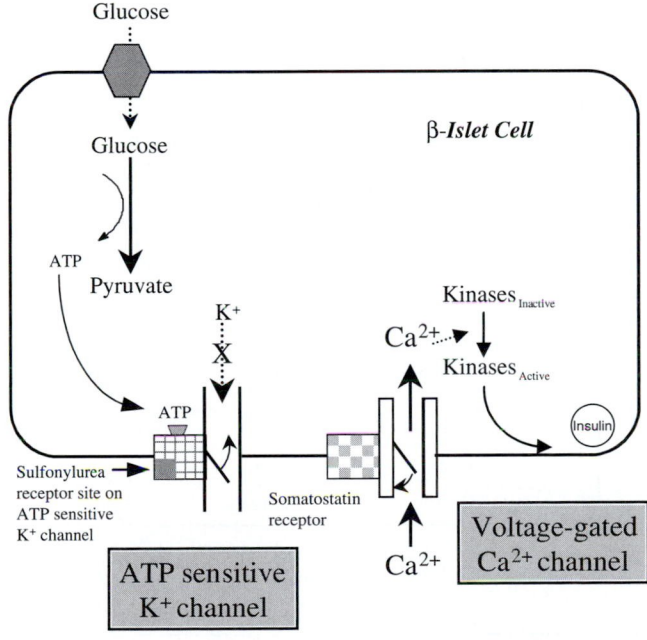

Figure 40–2. Under normal conditions, cells release insulin in response to an elevation of intracellular ATP levels. Sulfonylureas potentiate the effects of ATP at its "sensor" on the ligand gated K^+ channels and prevent efflux of K^+. The subsequent rise in intracellular potential opens voltage-gated Ca^{2+} channels, which sets in action a series of phosphorylation reactions culminating in fusion of the insulin-containing vesicle with the cell membrane and release of insulin.

tyrosine kinase on the intracellular portion of the insulin receptor. Figure 40–3 depicts the mechanism of action of metformin.

Insulin resistance is common in NIDDM. Resistance may occur because of abnormal β-cell secretory products, circulating insulin antagonists, and target tissue defects in insulin action.[66] The thiazolidinedione derivatives decrease insulin resistance by the potentiation of insulin sensitivity in the liver, adipose tissue, and skeletal muscle. Uptake of glucose into adipose tissue and skeletal muscle is enhanced, while hepatic glucose production is reduced.[13,41]

Acarbose and miglitol are oligosaccharides that inhibit α-glucosidase enzymes in the brush border of the small intestine, mainly glucoamylase, sucrase, and maltase. As a result, postprandial elevations in blood glucose levels after carbohydrate ingestion are blunted.[105] Delayed gastric emptying may be another mechanism for their antihyperglycemic effect.[76]

PHARMACOKINETICS AND TOXICOKINETICS

Some of the pharmacokinetic parameters of the hypoglycemic agents are outlined in Tables 40–2 and 40–3. Insulin is a peptide that is degraded in the gut and is therefore not active by the oral

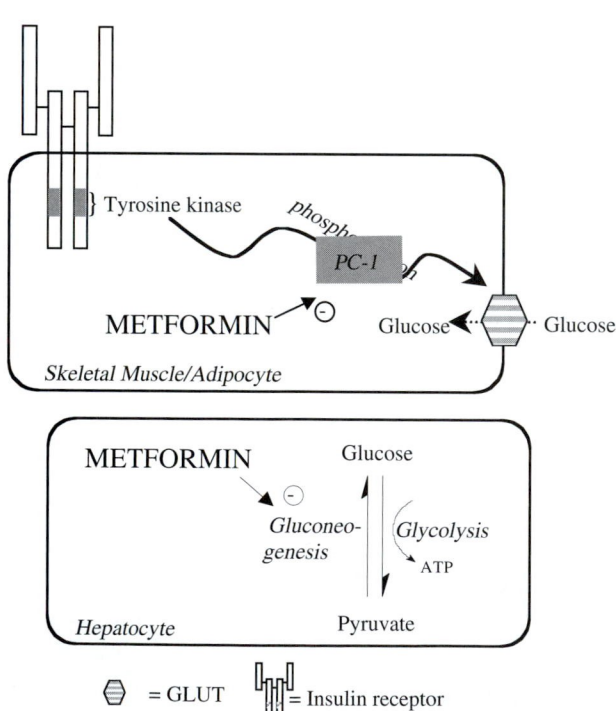

Figure 40–3. Under normal conditions, insulin binding to its receptor on myocytes and adipocytes activates tyrosine kinase, resulting in phosphorylation, and activation, of the membrane bound glucose transporter, GLUT. NIDDM is causally associated with an increased activity of PC-1, a glycoprotein that inhibits tyrosine kinase activity and thus reduces myocyte and adipocyte glucose uptake. Metformin reduces PC-1 activity in these cells, enhancing peripheral glucose utilization. In addition, gluconeogenesis in hepatic cells is reduced through interference with pyruvate carboxylase, the enzyme responsible for the conversion of pyruvate to oxaloacetate (Chap. 13).

route. The duration of action in therapeutic doses varies considerably from less than 5 hours with the ultrashort-acting lispro to as long as 36 hours with protamine zinc (NPH) and Ultralente insulin. Insulin overdose usually occurs by the subcutaneous or intramuscular route. As might be predicted based on the duration of action of some of the preparations, insulin overdose may result in prolonged hypoglycemia. However, this may also occur with short-acting forms because of some unusual toxicokinetic features. Insulin overdose of any type presents the potential for unusually delayed and profound hypoglycemia as well. Some of these unpredicted responses may be caused by a depot effect, and poor absorption may be further potentiated by the poor perfusion that can occur in hypoglycemia.[62,96] The clinical course after insulin overdose can also vary quite widely and is often unpredictable based on the dose injected. Delayed release of insulin from adipose tissue at the injection site(s) and in diabetics the presence of insulin antibodies may explain a victim's recovery in spite of massive overdoses.[80] As there are a finite number of insulin receptors, insulin overdoses of varying size are probably equivalent in terms of the degree of hypoglycemia but not its duration once receptor saturation occurs. A comparison can be made with the current treatment of diabetic ketoacidosis, in which lower doses of insulin are as effective as the higher doses used in the past.[48]

Many of the sulfonylureas have a long duration of action, and this may explain the unusually long period of hypoglycemia that may occur with therapeutic use and in the overdose setting. The first-generation sulfonylureas (acetohexamide, chlorpropamide, tolazamide, and tolbutamide) reduce hepatic clearance of insulin, and produce active hepatic metabolites. These agents are dependent on their effective urinary excretion to maintain euglycemia and avoid hypoglycemia. The second-generation sulfonylureas (glimepiride, glipizide, and glyburide) have half-lives that approach 24 hours and are associated with substantial fecal excretion of the parent drug. These agents are associated with frequent episodes of hypoglycemia (Table 40–2). The sulfonylureas, like insulin, may cause delayed onset of hypoglycemia in the overdose setting.[68,75] The reason for the potential delayed onset of effects with sulfonylureas is unclear and cannot be explained by known kinetic principles.

The kinetics of acarbose are notable for minimal systemic absorption and metabolism that occurs in the gut. As a result, serious systemic toxicity would not be expected.[81] Related symptoms are usually gastrointestinal in nature.

PATHOPHYSIOLOGY

Hypoglycemic agents are a diverse group of drugs, all of which, with the possible exception of metformin, the thiazolidinedioness and acarbose, may produce a nearly identical clinical condition of hypoglycemia. The etiologies of hypoglycemia are divided into three general categories:[29] physiologic or pathophysiologic conditions (Table 40–1), direct effects of various hypoglycemic agents (Tables 40–2 and 40–3), and the potentiation of hypoglycemic agents by interactions with other pharmacologic agents (Table 40–4). The most common cause of severe hypoglycemia resulting in an emergency department visit is excessive insulin use or insulin use that is relatively excessive for the caloric intake or exercise level of the individual.

Central nervous system symptoms predominate in hypoglycemia because the brain relies almost entirely on glucose as an

TABLE 40–2   Characteristics of Orally Administered Hypoglycemic Agents

Drug	Duration of Action (h)	Active Hepatic Metabolite	Active Urinary Excretory Product (% of dose)	Fecal Excretion (% of dose)	Frequency of Severe Hypoglycemia (other complications)
I. Sulfonylureas					
First generation					
Acetohexamide (Dymelor)	12–18	Hydroxyhexamide (+++)	Hydroxyhexamide (65%) Acetohexamide (2%)	Negligible	~1%
Chlorpropamide (Diabinese)	24–72	2-Hydroxychlorpropamide (+) 3-Hydroxychlorpropamide (+)	Chlorpropamide (20%) 2-Hydroxychlorpropamide (55%) 3-Hydroxychlorpropamide (2%)	Negligible	4–6%
Tolazamide (Tolinase)	16–24	Hydroxytolazamide (++)	Hydroxytolazamide (35%) Tolazamide (7%)	Negligible	~1%
Tolbutamide (Orinase)	6–12	Hydroxytolbutamide (+)	Hydroxytolbutamide (30%) Tolbutamide (2%)	Negligible	<1%
Second generation					
Glimepiride (Amaryl)	24	Cyclohexylhydroxy ethyl derivative (++)	Cyclohexylhydroxy methyl derivative (63%)	15%	1–2%
Glipizide (Glucotrol, Glucotrol XL)	16–24	None	Glipizide (3%)	12%	2–4%
Glyburide (Micronase, Glynase, DiaBeta)	18–24	4-Hydroxyglyburide (++)	4-Hydroxyglyburide (36%) Glyburide (3%)	50%	4–6%
II. Biguanides					
Metformin (Glucophage, Glucophage XR) Metformin/Glyburide (Glucovance)	1.3–4.5	None	Metformin (90%)	Neglibible	None (?) (lactic acidosis 0.03 cases/1000 patient years)
Phenformin	6–8	None	Phenformin (66%)	Negligible	Uncommon (lactic acidosis 0.64 cases/1000 patient years)
III. α-Glucosidase Inhibitors					
Acarbose (Precose)	2	None	4-Methyl pryogallol derivative (<2%)	None	None
Miglitol (Glyset)	2	None	100%	None	None
IV. Thiazolidinedione Derivatives					
Pioglitazone (Actos)	16–24	Hydroxyderivative Keto derivative	?<15–30%	70%	None
Rosiglitazone (Avandia)	12–24	None	None	23%	None
V. Meglitinides					
Nateglinide (Starlix)	2–4	Isoprene derivative (++) Hydroxylation metabolites (+)	~16% as parent	10%	<1%
Repaglinide (Prandin)	1–3	None	None	90%	4–6%

+ = Weakly active; ++ = moderately active; +++ = more active than parent drug. The durations of action for the oral agents are cited for therapeutic doses. These values increase for overdoses.

energy source. The brain cannot use free fatty acids for fuel because they do not cross the blood-brain barrier. However, during prolonged starvation, the brain is able to utilize ketones derived from free fatty acids. Other major organs such as the heart, liver, and skeletal muscle are able to use various fuel sources, particularly free fatty acids.[87]

The regulation of glucose control to near normal glucose values, the characteristics of each individual's awareness of hypoglycemia, and the individual counterregulatory mechanisms define the frequency and intensity of hypoglycemia.[85] The Diabetic Control and Complications Trial (DCCT) research group reported 62 episodes of blood glucose <50 mg/dL with central nervous system (CNS) manifestations requiring assistance for every 100 patient years on an intensive insulin therapy regimen. This was in comparison to a conventional therapy group which had 19 such episodes per 100 patient years.[22,23] In a review of 1418 medication-related cases of hypoglycemia, sulfonylureas (especially the long-acting agents chlorpropamide and glyburide) alone or with a second agent accounted for the largest percentage of cases: 63%.[84] Alcohol, propranolol, and salicylate, either alone or with another

TABLE 40–3. Characteristics of Routinely Used Forms of Insulin

Insulin	Duration of Action (h)	Metabolism
Ultrashort Acting		
Lispro (Humalog)	<5	Renal and hepatic metabolism
Short Acting		
Regular	5–8	Renal and hepatic metabolism
Semilente	12–16	Renal and hepatic metabolism
Intermediate Acting		
Lente	18–24	Renal and hepatic metabolism
Mixtard	24	
70% isophane		
30% regular		
NPH	18–24	
Long Acting		
Protamine zinc insulin (PZI)	24–36	Renal excretion
Ultralente	20–36	

hypoglycemic drug, accounted for another 19% of cases of hypoglycemia, and quinine, quinidine, pentamidine, ritodrine, and disopyramide were the most common of the less frequently associated agents. Conversely, hypoglycemia is reported in as many as 20% of patients using sulfonylureas.[42] Besides sulfonylurea use, advanced age and fasting are identified as major risk factors for hypoglycemia. Avoidance of sulfonylurea prescribing in elderly diabetics may occur because of the concern for hypoglycemia. However, a recent prospective placebo controlled study provides opposing evidence.[15] Fifty-two diabetic subjects (mean age, 65 years) underwent three separate 23-hour fasting sessions following therapy with placebo, glyburide, and glipizide. No hypoglycemia (defined as plasma glucose <60 mg/dL) occurred over the course of 156 fasting studies.

The autonomic nervous system regulates glucagon and insulin secretion, muscle glycogenolysis, adipose lipolysis, and hepatic glucose production. Propranolol and other β-adrenergic antagonists affect all these mechanisms and can result in hypoglycemia. In the presence of chronic renal failure, β-adrenergic antagonist-induced hypoglycemia is a particular risk.[35] This likely relates to

TABLE 40–4. Drugs or Toxins Known to React with Hypoglycemic Agents Resulting in Hypoglycemia

Angiotensin-converting enzyme (ACE) inhibitors	Monamine oxidase inhibitors
Allopurinol	Para-aminobenzoic acid
Anabolic steroids	Pentamidine
Beta-adrenergic antagonists	Phenylbutazone
Chloramphenicol	Probenecid
Clofibrate	Propoxyphene
Dicoumarol	Quinine
Disopyramide	Salicylates
Ethanol	Sulfinpyrazone
Haloperidol	Sulfonamide
Methotrexate	Trimethoprim-sulfamethoxazole

increased insulin half-life and reduced renal gluconeogenesis.[69] In addition, the clinical presentation of hypoglycemia in diabetics may be muted when β-adrenergic antagonists are used concurrently with hypoglycemic agents. Expected autonomic responses such as tachycardia, diaphoresis, and anxiety may not occur. Although this is assumed to be true, an adverse effect on hypoglycemic awareness could not be demonstrated in healthy volunteers given metoprolol, atenolol, and propranolol.[47]

Drug dispensing errors are often responsible for inadvertent hypoglycemia. Common medication errors associated with oral hypoglycemic agents attributable to pharmacists, physicians, or patients include the mistaken substitution of Orinase for Ornade, Tolinase for Tolectin, Diabinese for Diamox, chlorpropamide for chlorpromazine,[40,88] or acetohexamide for acetazolamide. The last pair are particularly problematic because their corresponding brand names are Dymelor and Diamox, respectively.[90]

Besides a decrease in glucose concentrations, the hypoglycemic agents are capable of producing a number of adverse effects, both in overdose and in therapeutic doses. The sulfonylureas, predominantly chlorpropamide, can cause a syndrome of inappropriate antidiuretic hormone secretion.[44] Concomitant use of sulfonylureas and ethanol can cause a disulfiram-ethanol reaction, as sulfonylureas inhibit aldehyde dehydrogenase.[73]

The biguanides are unique because of their association with the occurrence of lactic acidosis. Mechanisms for production of lactic acid with phenformin include interference with cellular aerobic metabolism and subsequent enhanced anaerobic metabolism. Phenformin also suppresses hepatic gluconeogenesis from pyruvate and causes a decrease in hepatocellular pH, resulting in decreased lactate consumption and hepatic lactate uptake. Metformin-associated lactic acidosis is about 20 times less common than that occurring with phenformin. Although the exact mechanism for metformin-associated lactic acidosis is not clear, the mechanism of phenformin-associated lactic acidosis is often extrapolated as an explanation. Lactic acidosis related to metformin use usually occurs in the presence of an underlying condition, particularly renal impairment,[18] which probably relates to increased tissue burden of metformin as a cause. Other associated factors include cardiorespiratory insufficiency, septicemia, liver disease, a history of lactic acidosis, advanced age, alcohol abuse, and the use of radiologic contrast media.[5,18] Iodinated contrast material may induce acute renal failure, leading to accumulation of metformin, and a subsequent risk for the development of lactic acidosis. In their 2001 data sheet, the manufacturers of metformin (Bristol-Myers Squibb) recommend that "Glucophage should be temporarily discontinued for 48 hours in patients following radiologic studies involving intravascular administration of iodinated contrast materials, because use of such products may result in acute alteration of renal function." Glucophage can be restarted 48 hours later when the serum creatinine is normal. Although lactic acidosis associated with the therapeutic use of metformin can occur without underlying risk factors, this appears to be uncommon.[18] Lactic acidosis has rarely been associated with acute intentional overdose.

CLINICAL MANIFESTATIONS

The presentations of patients with hypoglycemia are extremely variable. Any neuropsychiatric abnormality, whether persistent or transient, focal or generalized, must be considered a possible effect of hypoglycemia (Table 40–5). The cerebral cortex is usually most severely affected. Categorization of these findings are:[72]

- Delirium with subdued, confused, or manic behavior.
- Coma with multifocal brainstem abnormalities, including posturing and respiratory abnormalities, with preservation of the oculocephalic (doll's eyes) response, oculovestibular (cold-caloric) response, and pupillary responses.
- Focal neurologic deficits simulating a cerebrovascular accident (CVA) with or without the presence of coma. During a 12-month study period, 3 of 125 (2.4%) hypoglycemic patients presented with hemiplegia.[55] There are numerous reports[1,92] and series[83,104] of patients with focal neurologic deficits.
- Solitary or multiple seizures, with or without a significant post-ictal phase.

These neuropsychiatric symptoms are usually reversible if the hypoglycemia is corrected promptly. The morbidity resulting from undiagnosed hypoglycemia is related partly to the etiology and partly to the duration and severity of the hypoglycemia. Because the etiologies of hypoglycemia encompass both severe diseases such as fulminant hepatic failure and some benign problems such as a missed meal by an insulin-requiring diabetic, the literature is confusing with regard to outcome. For example, although a study of 125 ED cases of symptomatic hypoglycemia reported an 11% mortality rate,[55] only 1 death (0.8%) was attributed directly to hypoglycemia, and 4 survivors (3.2%) suffered from residual neurologic deficits. In a tertiary care medical center, 1.2% of all admitted patients had hypoglycemia (defined as a serum or plasma glucose level less than 50 mg/dL). The overall mortality was 27% for this group of 94 patients.[29] The longer and more profound the hypoglycemic episode, the more likely that permanent CNS damage will occur.[3] It cannot be overemphasized that there are no absolute criteria available from the physical examination or history to distinguish one form of metabolic coma from another. Moreover, the findings classically associated with hypoglycemia—tremor, sweating, tachycardia, confusion, coma, and convulsion—frequently may not occur (Table 40–5).[38]

Currently there is a great interest in the concept that patients may be unaware of hypoglycemia, particularly in those with well-controlled insulin-dependent diabetes mellitus. It appears that even in the presence of numerical hypoglycemia, those diabetic individuals with near normal glycosylated hemoglobin values maintain near normal glucose uptake by the brain, thereby preserving cerebral metabolism and limiting the response of counterregulatory hormones. The result of this limited response is unawareness of hypoglycemia.[10,11] The authors suggest that a threshold level is achieved below which the glucose concentration is inadequate, but this may be a level so close to that which causes serious neuroglycopenia that patients have limited opportunity for corrective action.[10]

Hypoglycemia may not occur until 18 hours after Lente insulin overdose,[62] and may persist for up to 6 days after Ultralente insulin overdose.[56] Survival after insulin overdose cannot be correlated directly with either the dose or preparation type, as some patients have died with doses estimated in the hundreds of units, whereas others have survived doses in the thousands of units.[80] Mortality and morbidity are more likely correlated with delay in recognition of the problem, duration of symptoms, onset of therapy, and type of complications, as opposed to the absolute degree of hypoglycemia or persistence of elevated insulin levels. A significant correlation exists between the amount of insulin injected and either the total amount of dextrose used for treatment or the duration of dextrose infusion.[96] In this retrospective study of insulin overdose, 7 of 17 cases (41%) developed recurrent hypoglycemia between 5 and 39 hours after overdose, despite oral feeding and intravenous glucose infusion ranging from 5 to 17 g of glucose per hour.

In a retrospective review of 40 sulfonylurea overdose cases, the time from ingestion to the onset of hypoglycemia, when known, was variable.[68] The longest delay was 21 hours after ingestion of glyburide, and 48 hours after ingestion of chlorpropamide. In a retrospective poison center review of 93 cases of sulfonylurea exposure in children, 25 patients (27%) developed hypoglycemia, in which the time of onset ranged from 0.5 to 16 hours, with a mean of 4.3 hours.[75] In a prospective poison center study of sulfonylurea exposure in children, 56 of 185 cases (30%) developed hypoglycemia, with a time of onset ranging from 1 to 21 hours and a mean of 5.3 hours.[93] Single-tablet ingestions of chlorpropamide (250 mg), glipizide (5 mg), and glyburide (2.5 mg) can result in hypoglycemia in young children[75]; the hypoglycemia may be delayed.[100]

Sinus tachycardia, atrial fibrillation, and ventricular premature contractions are the most common dysrhythmias associated with hypoglycemia.[50,65] An outpouring of catecholamines, hypoglycemia itself, transient electrolyte abnormalities, and underlying heart disease appear to be the most likely etiologies, as evidenced by the disappearance of these dysrhythmias with glucose repletion. Based on their mechanisms of action, both insulin and the sulfonylureas would be expected to promote the shift of potassium into cells, and hypokalemia after insulin overdose is well documented.[2,96] Other cardiovascular manifestations include angina and ischemia, which may be the sole manifestations of hypoglycemia.[26] Both are directly related to hypoglycemia.[8,71]

Hypothermia may occur in hypoglycemic patients.[30,46,98] If present, hypothermia is usually mild (32–35°C; 90–95°F), unless coexisting conditions are present, such as environmental exposure, infection, head injury, or hypothyroidism. In a study comparing two groups of comatose and stuporous patients, hypothermia was almost exclusively limited to the hypoglycemic patients; of these, 53% with demonstrated hypoglycemia showed hypothermia.[98] Hypoglycemic hypothermic patients who have grand mal seizures may have initially been even more hypothermic since a tempera-

TABLE 40–5.   Manifestations of Hypoglycemia

Caused by Catecholamine Release (Neurogenic, Autonomic)	Caused by Cerebral Glucose Deprivation (Neuroglycopenia)
Tremor, shivering	Blurred vision
Tachycardia, palpitations	Dysesthesias, paresthesias
Diaphoresis	Inability to concentrate
Pallor	Loss of coordination
Piloerection	Weakness
Anxiety	Somnolence, fatigue
Hypertension	Altered behavior pattern
Headache	Hypothermia
Dry mouth	Seizures
Hunger	Hemiplegia
Nausea	Coma
Angina	Death

ture elevation of several degrees Fahrenheit or Celsius is commonly noted for several hours after a major motor seizure.[103] The central hypothalamic response to hypoglycemia stimulated by the sympathetic nervous system may actually "overshoot" normal temperatures, resulting in hyperthermia.[19]

Case reports in 6 patients document the occurrence of severe lactic acidosis after metformin overdose.[59,67,101] In a larger poison center series of 65 adult overdose cases, 2 patients developed significant lactic acidosis, 1 of whom died.[94] One patient developed diffuse intravascular coagulation (DIC), and hypoglycemia occurred in 7 patients with concomitant insulin or sulfonylurea overdose. The remaining cases were described as having minimal toxicity. In a poison center series of 46 pediatric metformin exposures, lactic acidosis was not reported and no significant adverse effects were noted.[95] The dose ingested ranged from 250 mg to 16.6 g, with a mean of 1.8 g. However, many patients on metformin also take sulfonylureas, so hypoglycemia should be expected. Phenformin ingestion alone rarely causes hypoglycemia, both in overdose and with therapeutic use.[84]

Repaglinide, nateglinide, troglitazone, rosiglitazone, pioglitazone, and acarbose are newer agents for which overdose data are limited. Hypoglycemia should be anticipated after repaglinide and nateglinide ingestion.[61] Limited data suggest that the thiazolidinediones are less likely to cause hypoglycemia. Of these agents, there is more experience with the use of troglitazone. Its most prominent adverse effect is the development of liver toxicity with therapeutic doses, which may be severe and may require liver transplantation.[33,63] As a result, the FDA issued a directive for the withdrawal of this product from the US market in March 2000.

It appears unlikely that acarbose would cause hypoglycemia based on its mechanism of action of inhibition of α-glucosidase. The most common adverse effects associated with therapeutic use are gastrointestinal, including nausea, bloating, abdominal pain, flatulence, and diarrhea. Elevated aminotransferase levels were noted in clinical trials.[39] Most patients were asymptomatic and the aminotransferases returned to normal after discontinuation of the drug.

DIAGNOSTIC TESTING

Suspicion of possible hypoglycemia is particularly important in the patient with an abnormal neurologic examination. The most frequent reasons for failure to diagnose hypoglycemia and mismanaging patients are the erroneous conclusions that the patient is not hypoglycemic, but psychotic, epileptic, experiencing a CVA, or intoxicated because of an "odor of alcohol" on the breath (Chap. 64); compounding the problem of misdiagnosis is the erroneous assumption that a single bolus of 0.5–1 g/kg of 50% dextrose in water for an adult will always be sufficient.

Serum glucose levels are accurate, but treatment cannot be delayed pending the results. Glucose reagent strip testing can be performed at the bedside, and sensitivity for detecting hypoglycemia is excellent, but these tests are not perfect. In a comparison of reagent strips to plasma glucose determinations, 87% of the reagent strips were within 60 mg/dL of the actual glucose level.[82] This determination was accurate for plasma glucose levels less than 350 mg/dL. It is also important to remember that hypoglycemia is a clinical disorder, not a numerical disorder. Patients with poorly controlled diabetes in particular may become symptomatic at higher glucose levels than those without the disease.[11]

The threshold reagent strip level that should be used for the administration of hypertonic dextrose may be debated, but we would argue that based on the available data,[82] a cutoff of 120 mg/dL is appropriate. Bedside glucose testing is discussed in more detail in Antidotes in Depth: Dextrose.

Other than glucose determinations, various diagnostic studies may be indicated, depending on the clinical situation. Serum ethanol determination may be helpful in confirming a contributing or sole etiologic factor. Renal function tests may indicate the presence of renal impairment as a causative factor of hypoglycemia. This is a common scenario in insulin-dependent diabetics, as renal failure often occurs after patients have had diabetes mellitus for several years, and insulin half-life increases as renal function declines. Hepatic function tests may be a clue to liver disease as a cause of hypoglycemia, although this may also be evident on physical examination. Although seizures are clearly associated with hypoglycemia, other studies, such as electrolytes, calcium, magnesium, and computed tomographic scanning of the head, may be indicated if there is any doubt as to the etiology.

In known diabetics in whom overdose is not suspected, the clinician must search for a cause of hypoglycemia. Sometimes, it is as simple as a missed meal or an unusually strenuous exercise routine, but in many cases it may not be so clear. Numerous other medical conditions, as well as various drugs, may be involved (Table 40–1), and diagnostic testing will be tailored to each individual episode depending on the clinical suspicion. It is never acceptable to diagnose the etiology as "idiopathic."

Evaluation of Malicious, Surreptitious, or Unintentional Insulin Overdose

The physical examination may give helpful clues in the evaluation of a suspected malicious, surreptitious, or unintentional insulin overdose. A meticulous search may reveal a site that is erythematous, hemorrhagic, atypically boggy in nature, or even painful if the subcutaneous (or intramuscular) injection of insulin was particularly large.

An understanding of how the β cells of the pancreas secrete insulin in response to glucose levels in the blood is essential to understand the investigation of fasting hypoglycemia.[21] When the plasma glucose is less than 45 mg/dL, insulin secretion should be almost completely suppressed and therefore plasma insulin concentrations should be minimal or absent.[74] Moreover, insulin is secreted as proinsulin, which is cleaved in vivo to form insulin (a double-stranded peptide) and C-peptide, which are released into the blood in equimolar quantities. Insulin is biologically active, whereas proinsulin has limited activity, and C-peptide has no activity. Although insulin is normally cleared during hepatic transit, C-peptide is not; therefore C-peptide can be utilized as a quantitative marker of endogenous insulin secretion. Commercially available exogenous human insulin does not contain C-peptide fragments (Table 40–6). When plasma glucose concentration falls to hypoglycemic levels (usually <60 mg/dL), insulin secretion should fall to less then 6 μU/mL. Therefore, when hypoglycemia is caused by exogenous insulin administration, plasma C-peptide levels should be less than 0.2 nmol/L in the presence of insulin levels that are substantially higher than insulin levels resulting from an insulinoma. With insulinoma, insulin levels are generally greater than 6 μU/mL in the presence of hypoglycemia. Sulfonylurea ingestion and insulinomas will both result in elevated C-peptide and insulin levels, but in the face of uncertainty sulfonylurea

TABLE 40–6.   The Laboratory Assessment of Fasting Hypoglycemia

Clinical State	Insulin[a] (Plasma) (μU/mL)	C Peptide (Plasma) (nmol/L)	Proinsulin (pmol/L)	Anti-insulin Antibodies[c]
Normal	<6	<0.2	<5	—
Exogenous insulin	Very high	Low (suppressed)	Absent	Present[d]
Insulinoma	High	High	Present	Absent
Sulfonylurea ingestion[b]	High	High	Present	Absent
Autoimmune	Very high (artifact)	Low (or) high (artifact)	Present	Present
Decreased glucose production	Low	Low	Present	Absent
Neoplasia (non-β-cell)	Low	Low	Present	Absent

[a]Insulin levels are determined during fasting hypoglycemia at low levels of glucose, preferably <45 mg/dL of blood glucose.
[b]Sulfonylurea ingestion is diagnosed by detection of the drugs or their metabolites in plasma or urine.
[c]The anti-insulin antibodies produced spontaneously differ from those of treated (exposed to exogenous insulin) and those of untreated insulin-dependent diabetics.
[d]The presence of anti-insulin antibodies occurs less frequently in those exposed only to human insulin.

levels are readily available from reference laboratories. Animal insulin can be distinguished from human insulin by high-performance liquid chromatography.[34] However, this technique has limited use because of the virtually exclusive use of human insulin at present.

In summary, patients with chronic insulin-induced factitious or surreptitious hypoglycemia will have high insulin levels, the presence of insulin-binding antibodies,[28] and low C-peptide levels. Those who have taken sulfonylureas will have high insulin levels, absent insulin-binding antibodies, high C-peptide levels, and the presence of urinary sulfonylurea metabolites (Table 40–6). The issues of evidence collection that are appropriate to document malicious or surreptitious use of insulin successfully have been described[53] (Chap. 118).

MANAGEMENT

Treatment centers on the correction of hypoglycemia and the anticipation that hypoglycemia may recur in the overdose setting. Symptomatic patients with hypoglycemia require immediate treatment with 0.5–1 g/kg of concentrated intravenous dextrose in the form of $D_{50}W$ in adults, $D_{25}W$ in children, and $D_{10}W$ in neonates. Occasionally, patients require a larger dose to achieve an initial response. If hypoglycemia is suspected but not confirmed, such as in the absence of rapid reagent strip availability or when such readings are "borderline," glucose should still be administered rapidly.

The kinetics of intravenous administration of 25 g of 50% dextrose have been studied in healthy euglycemic volunteers.[6] Serum glucose levels rise rapidly to a mean of 244 mg/dL at 5 minutes and return to baseline at 30 minutes. Most similar studies on this topic have been done in healthy euglycemic volunteers, and there is no evidence that this is predictive of what time there will be a return to baseline in patients who have hypoglycemia of various etiologies. There is no mechanism to extrapolate back to pre-$D_{50}W$ levels. Although the use of concentrated dextrose has some theoretical risks, such as in the setting of cerebral ischemia, failure to rapidly correct hypoglycemia may lead to deleterious neurologic effects. Appropriate emergency and toxicologic uses of hypertonic dextrose are covered in detail in Antidotes in Depth: Dextrose. A dose of 100 mg of thiamine hydrochloride should be given as well in view of the substantial association of hypoglycemia with alcoholism and malnutrition.

Glucagon should not be considered except in the uncommon situation in which intravenous access cannot be obtained. Glucagon requires time to take effect and may be ineffective in patients with depleted glycogen stores, such as in the elderly, or those patients with alcoholism or neoplasms. Glucagon also stimulates insulin release by the pancreas, which may lead to prolonged hypoglycemia in settings such as sulfonylurea ingestion and insulinoma.[102]

Numerous articles have evaluated approaches for treating insulin reactions with carbohydrates in tablet, solution, or gel forms in a well-defined diabetic population.[14,89] None of these are appropriate gestures (other than as temporizing measures) for the undefined, possibly hypoglycemic patient. ED patients who have clinical symptoms of hypoglycemia run the risk of grave CNS complications unless treated quickly and adequately with glucose.

A common occurrence is that of a symptomatic hypoglycemic patient receiving treatment with intravenous dextrose in the prehospital setting, with subsequent refusal of transport to the hospital. Two recent studies address this issue. One is a retrospective review of 571 paramedic runs on patients with hypoglycemic signs and fingerstick glucose levels <80 mg/dL.[91] The conclusion of the authors is that out-of-hospital treatment of hypoglycemic diabetic patients is safe and effective even when transport is refused. Seventy-two percent of the 571 patients seen by paramedics refused care. Of 159 patients who were transported to the hospital, 40% were admitted. This very fact either suggests that paramedics can easily determine who does not need to be admitted to the hospital or demonstrates the tremendous risk associated with permitting self-discharge. The other study prospectively evaluates the short-term outcome of 132 hypoglycemic diabetic patients who refused transport.[60] The authors conclude that most such patients have good short-term outcome, although they do encourage transport because of the risk of recurrent hypoglycemia. In this study, 9 of 132 patients (7%) had recurrent hypoglycemia, and 29 of 132 (22%) were lost to followup. One patient died in each of the two studies, and neither article addresses associated ethanol use, which is a major cause of hypoglycemia. We encourage the further education of paramedics, emphasizing the importance of transporting hypoglycemic patients to emergency departments.

The benefits of emesis, lavage, and catharsis should be considered in managing a patient with an overdose of oral hypoglycemic agents. The extensive affinity between chlorpropamide, tolazamide, tolbutamide, glyburide, glipizide, and carbutamide and activated charcoal has been demonstrated in vitro.[45] The affinities ranged from 0.45 to 0.52 g/g activated charcoal at pH 7.5, and were higher at pH 4.9. Single-dose activated charcoal and possibly multiple-dose activated charcoal should theoretically be beneficial in the management of these overdoses. Patients who overdose on glipizide, an agent that has an enterohepatic circulation, may theoretically benefit from multiple-dose activated charcoal. In theory, multiple-dose activated charcoal and whole-bowel irrigation may be of benefit and should be considered after overdose of sustained-release oral agents. In patients who overdose on insulin, case reports describe the use of surgical excision of the injection site.[17,52,58] However, this has not been studied in a systematic fashion and therefore further data are necessary before recommending this approach.

Urinary alkalinization to a pH of 7–8 can reduce the half-life of chlorpropamide from 49 hours to approximately 13 hours. Urinary alkalinization is not useful for other oral agents.[64] Outcome studies have not been performed.

Maintaining Euglycemia after Initial Control

After the patient is awake and alert, further therapy depends on the agent involved and pancreatic islet cell function. A determination must be made as to whether the setting was unintentional versus intentional with suicidal or homicidal intent. One problem that occurs with dextrose administration is that individuals who can produce insulin through glucose-stimulated insulin release (nondiabetics and those with NIDDM) are at substantial risk of recurrent hypoglycemia. This can occur with insulin overdose and may be particularly problematic with sulfonylurea or meglitinide overdose, as these oral agents stimulate insulin release. Treatment with hypertonic dextrose solutions can be expected to result in dramatic yet transient increases in glucose concentrations, with a subsequent fall in serum glucose possibly to hypoglycemic levels again.

For diabetic patients who unintentionally inject an excessive amount of insulin, feeding should be initiated and 5% dextrose in water should be given intravenously and the rate of infusion adjusted to keep the patient relatively euglycemic (100–150 mg/dL). Overdose in the setting of suicidal or homicidal intent is likely to involve significant quantities of insulin and nondiabetics may be particularly prone to significant hypoglycemia because they lack insulin resistance. As with unintentional overdose, feeding should be started and glucose levels maintained in the 100–150 mg/dL range. However, a more concentrated dextrose infusion (10%) should be used.

Some patients may need more concentrated dextrose infusions, such as 20% dextrose in water augmented by repeated doses of 50% dextrose in water. Central venous lines should be used when an infusion of 20% dextrose is instituted, as the solution is a substantial venous irritant. The presence of glycosuria is not an adequate indicator of euglycemia; frequent serial blood glucose or reagent strip glucose levels should be obtained. The appropriate timing of glucose monitoring varies depending on the clinical situation. Mental status must be observed as well. As a rough guide, glucose monitoring every 1–2 hours after initial control is reasonable, with subsequent spacing of the intervals to once every 4–6 hours. Potassium and phosphate levels must also be monitored, as glucose administration may lead to hypokalemia and hypophosphatemia. The duration of sampling necessary will depend on the stability of the patient, the underlying metabolic disorders, the extent of overdose, and the rate of improvement. When the patient

begins to eat an adequate diet and the initial hypoglycemia is controlled, the serum glucose will rise and the concentration and rate of infusion may then be tapered. Many patients may actually develop significant hyperglycemia.

The therapeutic approach differs for patients who overdose on sulfonylureas or meglitinides. After initial control of hypoglycemia with concentrated dextrose, the patient should be fed. Intravenous access is necessary, but routine dextrose infusion should be avoided. As with insulin overdose, frequent monitoring of glucose levels and mental status is critical. We recommend early use of octreotide in this setting because of the significant risk of glucose-stimulated insulin release.

Octreotide, a semisynthetic long-acting analog of somatostatin with an intravenous half-life of 72 minutes, inhibits glucose-stimulated β-cell insulin release through receptors coupled to G proteins on β islet cells.[9] Somatostatin present in diverse tissues such as the hypothalamus, pancreas, and GI tract alters the secretion of growth hormone and thyroid-stimulating hormone, gastrointestinal secretions, and the endocrine pancreas (glucagon and insulin).[77,78] In normal subjects brought to hypoglycemia with glipizide, octreotide was compared to intravenous hypertonic dextrose and also to diazoxide and concomitant dextrose.[9] There were fewer episodes of recurrent hypoglycemia and overall dextrose requirements were lower than in the dextrose-alone and dextrose-plus-diazoxide groups. Several successful clinical experiences with octreotide have been reported with quinine-induced hypoglycemia resulting from malaria therapy,[70] with an insulinoma,[37] with nesidioblastosis of infancy,[24] with hypoglycemia related to therapeutic use of gliclazide,[12] and with a tolbutamide overdose.[9] It appears to be relatively free of serious side effects. The most likely adverse effects are injection-site discomfort (if administered subcutaneously), and gastrointestinal symptoms such as nausea, bloating, diarrhea, and constipation.[54] The suggested adult octreotide dose is 50 µg subcutaneously every 6–8 hours (Antidotes in Depth: Octreotide).

Diazoxide, a formely used parenteral antihypertensive agent, directly inhibits insulin secretion by opening K_{ATP} channels in β cells. Like octreotide, it may be effective in patients who have insulin-secreting tumors and for refractory sulfonylurea-induced hypoglycemia.[43,68] Unfortunately, diazoxide has more potential for adverse effects, particularly significant hypotension and its associated complications, and should only be considered if octreotide is ineffective. It should be given by slow intravenous infusion (300 mg over 30 minutes every 4 hours), in an attempt to limit hypotension. If diazoxide is used continuously, sodium retention may occur, and therefore a diuretic such as furosemide may need to be employed, particularly when the urine is alkalinized for a chlorpropamide overdose. Oral diazoxide can also be used at a dose of 200–300 mg every 4 hours, as indicated.

Admitting Patients to the Hospital

The decision to admit a patient may be difficult, but several guidelines may be followed. Admission is required for hypoglycemia related to ethanol, starvation, hepatic failure, and renal failure, as well as in hypoglycemia of unknown etiology. Patients on therapeutic doses of insulin require inpatient evaluation of recurrent and unexplained hypoglycemic episodes. All patients who present with hypoglycemia caused by a sulfonylurea or after unintentional overdose with long-acting insulin should be admitted. Hospitalization is recommended after unintentional overdose with ultrashort-, short-, or intermediate-acting insulin if hypoglycemia is persistent or recurs during a 4–6 hour observation period in the ED. Many factors may be responsible for unintentional insulin overdose, such as patient error because of impaired vision, syringe structure, and prescription error and hospital admission may be warranted. Admission is also indicated for any patient, regardless of serum glucose or symptoms, who intentionally overdoses on a sulfonylurea or any form of insulin, as delayed, profound, and protracted hypoglycemia may result. Although insulin overdose by the intravenous route might be expected to result in more immediate symptoms, admission is still recommended in asymptomatic patients, as experience with this scenario is limited. Those with possible self-induced factitious hypoglycemia should also be admitted. "Factitious" (intentionally self-induced) hypoglycemia is particularly prevalent among members of the medical profession. Administration of insulin to a nondiabetic child is a form of child abuse or an attempt at homicide.[25] Children who have been given an inappropriate dose of insulin, as well as any patient who may be a victim of attempted homicide, should be admitted.

Although severe hypoglycemia has not been reported with repaglinide, this is a new agent that is expected to behave like a sulfonylurea. Hospital admission after overdose is advisable, even in asymptomatic patients. Although hypoglycemia is unexpected after metformin, troglitazone, rosiglitazone, or pioglitazone overdose, experience is limited. Metformin overdose may result in lactic acidosis. In one case,[59] lactic acidosis was not diagnosed until 14 hours after metformin overdose. The patient had early symptoms of repeated vomiting at 1 hour postingestion. Until further data become available, asymptomatic patients who have overdosed on either metformin or the thiazolidinediones should probably be admitted for observation. Patients who overdose on acarbose would not be expected to have delayed or serious systemic toxicity and routine medical admission is unnecessary, although if the overdose is intentional psychiatric support is indicated.

Children who have unintentionally ingested as little as one sulfonylurea tablet should be admitted. Although this is controversial and some authors have suggested shorter observation periods,[16] and even home monitoring in some cases,[79] we feel that delayed effects of sulfonylurea ingestion in children are well documented in the literature[75,93,100] and convincing enough to support our position. It has been suggested, however, that asymptomatic children with single-tablet exposures to sulfonylureas be managed without prophylactic intravenous glucose, as this could contribute to delayed onset of hypoglycemia,[16] and we agree. Such patients are best managed by early feeding, frequent checks of glucose levels, and observation of mental status.

SUMMARY

Numerous drugs, chemicals, and medical conditions may cause hypoglycemia. Hypoglycemia is the predominant adverse effect related to therapeutic use and overdose of the agents used in the treatment of diabetes mellitus. Various clinical manifestations, particularly neurologic, may occur and can be confused with conditions such as ethanol intoxication, psychosis, epilepsy, and cerebrovascular accidents. The potential for delayed and prolonged hypoglycemia must be recognized in the overdose situation. Although several treatment options exist, rapid intravenous administration of glucose is the most important measure. Octreotide may be useful in patients with refractory hypoglycemia following sulfonylura or meglitinide overdose.

REFERENCES

1. Andrade R, Mathew V, Morgenstern MJ, et al: Hypoglycemic hemiplegic syndrome. Ann Emerg Med 1984;13:529–531.
2. Arem R, Zoghbi W: Insulin overdose in eight patients: Insulin pharmacokinetics and review of the literature. Medicine (Baltimore) 1985;64:323–332.
3. Arky RA, Veverbrants E, Abramson EA: Irreversible hypoglycemia. A complication of alcohol and insulin. JAMA 1968;206:575–578.
4. Bailey CJ, Day C: Traditional plant medicines as treatments for diabetes. Diabetes Care 1989;12:553–564.
5. Bailey CJ, Turner RC: Metformin. N Engl J Med 1996;334:574–579.
6. Balentine JR, Gaeta TJ, Kessler D, et al: Effect of 50 milliliters of 50% dextrose in water administration on the blood sugar of euglycemic volunteers. Acad Emerg Med 1998;5:691–694.
7. Banting FG, Best CH, Collip JB, et al: Pancreatic extracts in the treatment of diabetes mellitus: Preliminary report. CMAJ 1922;12:141–146.
8. Bowman CE, MacMahon DG, Mourant AJ: Hypoglycaemia and angina. Lancet 1985;1:639–640.
9. Boyle PJ, Justice K, Krentz AJ, et al: Octreotide reverses hyperinsulinemia and prevents hypoglycemia induced by sulfonylurea overdoses. J Clin Endocrinol Metab 1993;76:752–756.
10. Boyle PJ, Kempers SF, O'Connor AM, et al: Brain glucose uptake and unawareness of hypoglycemia in patients with insulin-dependent diabetes mellitus. N Engl J Med 1995;333:1726–1731.
11. Boyle PJ, Schwartz NS, Shah SD, et al: Plasma glucose concentrations at the onset of hypoglycemic symptoms in patients with poorly controlled diabetes and in nondiabetics. N Engl J Med 1988;318:1487–1492.
12. Braatvedt GD: Octreotide for the treatment of sulphonylurea induced hypoglycaemia in type 2 diabetes. N Z Med J 1997;110:189–190.
13. Bressler R, Johnson D: New pharmacological approaches to therapy of NIDDM. Diabetes Care 1992;15:792–805.
14. Brodows RG, Williams C, Amatruda JM: Treatment of insulin reactions in diabetics. JAMA 1984;252:3378–3381.
15. Burge MR, Schmitz-Florentino K, Fischette C, et al: A prospective trial of risk factors for sulfonylurea-induced hypoglycemia in Type 2 diabetes mellitus. JAMA 1998;279:137–143.
16. Burkhart KK: When does hypoglycemia develop after sulfonylurea ingestion? Ann Emerg Med 1998;31:771–772.
17. Campbell IW, Ratcliffe JG: Suicidal insulin overdose managed by excision of insulin injection site. Brit Med J Clin Res 1982;285:408–409.
18. Chan NN, Brain HP, Feher MD: Metformin-associated lactic acidosis: A rare or very rare clinical entity. Diabet Med 1999;16:273–281.
19. Chochinov R, Daughaday WH: Marked hyperthermia as a manifestation of hypoglycemia in long-standing diabetes mellitus. Diabetes 1975;24:859–860.
20. Crofford OB: Metformin. N Engl J Med 1995;333:588–589.
21. Cryer PE, Polonsky KS: Glucose homeostasis and hypoglycemia. In: Wilson JD, Foster DW, Kronenberg HM, Larsen PR, eds: Williams Textbook of Endocrinology, 9th ed. Philadelphia, WB Saunders, 1998, pp. 939–971.
22. DCCT Research Group: The effect of intensive treatment of diabetes on the development and progression of long-term complications in insulin-dependent diabetes mellitus. Am J Med 1991;90:450–459.
23. DCCT Research Group: The effect of intensive treatment of diabetes on the development and progression of long-term complications in insulin-dependent diabetes mellitus. N Engl J Med 1993;329:977–986.
24. Delemarre-van de Waal HA, Veldkamp EJ, Schrander-Stumpel CT: Long-term treatment of an infant with nesidioblastosis using a somatostatin analogue. N Engl J Med 1987;316:222–223.
25. Dine MS, McGovern ME: Intentional poisoning of children—An overlooked category of child abuse: Report of seven cases and review of the literature. Pediatrics 1982;70:32–35.

26. Duh E, Feinglos M: Hypoglycemia-induced angina pectoris in a patient with diabetes mellitus. Ann Intern Med 1994;121:945–946.

27. Eliasson L, Renstrom E, Ammala C, et al: PKC-dependent stimulation of exocytosis by sulfonylureas in pancreatic β cells. Science 1996;271:813–815.

28. Fineberg SE, Galloway JA, Fineberg NS, et al: Immunogenicity of recombinant DNA human insulin. Diabetologia 1983;25:465–469.

29. Fischer KF, Lees JA, Newman JH: Hypoglycemia in hospitalized patients. Causes and outcomes. N Engl J Med 1986;315:1245–1250.

30. Fitzgerald FT: Hypoglycemia and accidental hypothermia in an alcoholic population. West J Med 1980;133:105–107.

31. Gaines KL, Hamilton S, Boyd AE: Characterization of the sulfonylurea receptor on β cell membranes. J Biol Chem 1988;263:2589–2592.

32. Gerich JE: Oral hypoglycemic agents [published erratum appears in N Engl J Med 1990;322(1):71]. N Engl J Med 1989;321:1231–1245.

33. Gitlin N, Julie NL, Spurr CL, et al: Two cases of severe clinical and histologic hepatotoxicity associated with troglitazone. Ann Intern Med 1998;129:36–38.

34. Given BD, Ostrega DM, Polonsky KS, et al: Hypoglycemia due to surreptitious injection of insulin. Identification of insulin species by high-performance liquid chromatography. Diabetes Care 1991;14:544–547.

35. Grajower MM, Walter L, Albin J: Hypoglycemia in chronic hemodialysis patients: Association with propranolol use. Nephron 1980; 26:126–129.

36. Gura T: New lead found to a possible "insulin pill." Science 1999;284:886.

37. Hearn PR, Ahmed M, Woodhouse NJ: The use of SMS 201–995 (somatostatin analogue) in insulinomas. Additional case report and literature review. Horm Res 1988;29:211–213.

38. Hoffman JR, Schriger DL, Votey SR, et al: The empiric use of hypertonic dextrose in patients with altered mental status: A reappraisal. Ann Emerg Med 1992;21:20–24.

39. Hollander P: Safety profile of acarbose an alpha-glucosidase inhibitor. Drugs 1992;44(Suppl 3):47–53.

40. Huminer D, Dux S, Rosenfeld JB, et al: Inadvertent sulfonylurea-induced hypoglycemia. A dangerous but preventable condition. Arch Intern Med 1989;149:1890–1892.

41. Iwamoto Y, Kosaka K, Kuzuya T, et al: Effects of troglitazone: A new hypoglycemic agent in patients with NIDDM poorly controlled by diet therapy. Diabetes Care 1996;19:151–156.

42. Jennings AM, Wilson RM, Ward JD: Symptomatic hypoglycemia in NIDDM patients treated with oral hypoglycemic agents. Diabetes Care 1989;12:203–208.

43. Johnson SF, Shade DS, Peake GT: Chlorpropamide-induced hypoglycemia: Successful treatment with diazoxide. Am J Med 1977;63:799–804.

44. Kadowaki T, Hagura R, Kajinuma H, et al: Chlorpropamide-induced hyponatremia: Incidence and risk factors. Diabetes Care 1983;6:468–471.

45. Kannisto H, Neuvonen PJ: Adsorption of sulfonylureas onto activated charcoal in vitro. J Pharm Sci 1984;73:253–256.

46. Kedes LH, Field JB: Hypothermia: A clue to hypoglycemia. N Engl J Med 1964;271:785–787.

47. Kerr D, MacDonald IA, Heller SR, et al: Beta-adrenoceptor blockade and hypoglycaemia. A randomised double-blind placebo controlled comparison of metoprolol CR atenolol and propranolol LA in normal subjects. Brit J Clin Pharmacol 1990;29:685–693.

48. Kitabchi AE: Low-dose insulin therapy in diabetic ketoacidosis: Fact or fiction? Diabetes Metab Rev 1989;5:337–363.

49. Koivisto VA : The human insulin analogue insulin lispro. Ann Intern Med 1998;30:260–266.

50. Leak D, Starr P: The mechanism of arrhythmias during insulin-induced hypoglycemia. Am J Heart 1962;63:688–691.

51. Lebovitz HE: The oral hypoglcemic agents. In: Porte D Jr, Sherwin RS, eds: Ellenberg & Rifkin's Diabetes Mellitus, 5th ed. Stamford, CT, Appleton & Lange, 1997, pp. 761–788.

52. Levine DF, Bulstrode C: Managing suicidal insulin overdose. Brit Med J 1982;285:974–975.

53. Levy WJ, Gardner D, Moseley J, et al: Unusual problems for the physician in managing a hospital patient who received a malicious insulin overdose. Neurosurgery 1985;17:992–996.

54. Longnecker SM: Somatostatin and octreotide: Literature review and description of therapeutic activity in pancreatic neoplasia. Drug Intell Clin Pharm 1988;22:99–106.

55. Malouf R, Brust JC: Hypoglycemia: Causes, neurological manifestations, and outcome. Ann Neurol 1985;17:421–430.

56. Martin FI, Hansen N, Warne GL: Attempted suicide by insulin overdose in insulin-requiring diabetics. Med J Aust 1977;1:58–60.

57. Martindale W: Phenformin hydrochloride. In: Parfitt K, ed: Martindale: The Complete Drug Reference. London, Pharmaceutical Press, 1999, p. 331.

58. McIntyre AS, Woolf VJ, Burnham WR: Local excision of subcutaneous fat in the management of insulin overdose. Br J Surg 1986;73:538.

59. McLelland J: Recovery from metformin overdose. Diabet Med 1985;2:410–411.

60. Mechem CC, Kreshak AA, Barger J, et al: The short-term outcome of hypoglycemic diabetic patients who refuse ambulance transport after out-of-hospital therapy. Acad Emerg Med 1998;5:768–772.

61. Repaglinide for type 2 diabetes mellitus. Med Lett Drugs Ther 1998;40(1027):55–56.

62. Munck O, Quaade F: Suicide attempted with insulin. Dan Med Bull 1963;10:139–141.

63. Neuschwander-Tetri BA, Isley WL, Oki JC, et al: Troglitazone-induced hepatic failure leading to liver transplantation. A case report. Ann Intern Med 1998;129:38–41.

64. Neuvonen PJ, Karkkainen S: Effects of charcoal sodium bicarbonate and ammonium chloride on chlorpropamide kinetics. Clin Pharm Ther 1983;33:386–393.

65. Odeh M, Oliven A, Bassan H: Transient atrial fibrillation precipitated by hypoglycemia. Ann Emerg Med 1990;19:565–567.

66. Olefsky JM: Insulin resistance. In: Porte JD, Sherwin RS, eds: Ellenberg & Rifkin's Diabetes Mellitus, 5th ed. Stamford, CT, Appleton & Lange, 1997, pp. 513–552.

67. Palatnick W, Meatherall R, Tenenbein M: Severe lactic acidosis from acute metformin overdose [abstract]. J Toxicol Clin Toxicol 1999; 37:638–639.

68. Palatnick W, Meatherall RC, Tenenbein M: Clinical spectrum of sulfonylurea overdose and experience with diazoxide therapy. Arch Intern Med 1991;151:1859–1862.

69. Peitzman SJ, Agarwal BN: Spontaneous hypoglycemia in end-stage renal failure. Nephron 1977;19:131–139.

70. Phillips RE, Warrell DA, Looareesuwan S, et al: Effectiveness of SMS 201–995 a synthetic long-acting somatostatin analogue in treatment of quinine-induced hyperinsulinaemia. Lancet 1986;1: 713–716.

71. Pladziewicz DS, Nesto RW: Hypoglycemia-induced silent myocardial ischemia. Am J Cardiol 1989;63:1531–1532.

72. Plum F, Posner JB: The Diagnosis of Stupor and Coma, 3rd ed. Philadelphia, FA Davis, 1980.

73. Podgainy H, Bressler R: Biochemical basis of the sulfonylurea-induced Antabuse syndrome. Diabetes 1968;17:679–683.

74. Polonsky KS : A practical approach to fasting hypoglycemia. N Engl J Med 1992;326:1020–1021.

75. Quadrani DA, Spiller HA, Widder P: Five-year retrospective evaluation of sulfonylurea ingestion in children. J Toxicol Clin Toxicol 1996;34:267–270.

76. Ranganath L, Norris F, Morgan L, et al: Delayed gastric emptying occurs following acarbose administration and is a further mechanism for its anti-hyperglycaemic effect. Diabet Med 1998;15:120–124.

77. Reichlin S: Somatostatin. N Engl J Med 1983;309:1495–1501.

78. Reichlin S: Somatostatin (second of two parts). N Engl J Med 1983; 309:1556–1563.

79. Robertson WO: Sulfonylurea ingestions: Hospitalization not mandatory. J Toxicol Clin Toxicol 1997;35:115–118.

80. Samuels MH, Eckel RH: Massive insulin overdose: Detailed studies of free insulin levels and glucose requirements. J Toxicol Clin Toxicol 1989;27:157–168.

81. Scheen AJ, Lefebvre PJ: Oral antidiabetic agents. A guide to selection. Drugs 1998;55:225–236.

82. Scott PA, Wolf LR, Spadafora MP: Accuracy of reagent strips in detecting hypoglycemia in the emergency department. Ann Emerg Med 1998;32:305–309.

83. Seibert DG: Reversible decerebrate posturing secondary to hypoglycemia. Am J Med 1985;78:1036–1037.

84. Seltzer HS: Drug-induced hypoglycemia. A review of 1418 cases. Endocrinol Metab Clin North Am 1989;18:163–183.

85. Service FJ: Hypoglycemic disorders. N Engl J Med 1995;332: 1144–1152.

86. Sherwin RS: Diabetes Mellitus. In: Bennett JC, Plum F, eds: Cecil Textbook of Medicine, 20th ed. Philadelphia, WB Saunders, 1996, pp. 1258–1277.

87. Shulman GI, Barrett EJ, Sherwin RS: Integrated fuel metabolism. In: Porte JD, Sherwin RS, eds: Ellenberg & Rifkin's Diabetes Mellitus, 5th ed. Stamford, CT, Appleton & Lange, 1997, pp. 1–17.

88. Shumak SL, Corenblum B, Steiner G. Recurrent hypoglycemia secondary to drug-dispensing error. Arch Intern Med 1991;151: 1877–1878.

89. Slama G, Traynard PY, Desplanque N, et al: The search for an optimized treatment of hypoglycemia. Carbohydrates in tablets solution or gel for the correction of insulin reactions. Arch Intern Med 1990; 150:589–593.

90. Sledge ED, Broadstone VL: Hypoglycemia due to a pharmacy dispensing error. South Med J 1993;86:1272–1273.

91. Socransky SJ, Pirrallo RG, Rubin JM: Out-of-hospital treatment of hypoglycemia: Refusal of transport and patient outcome. Acad Emerg Med 1998;5:1080–1085.

92. Spiller HA, Schroeder SL, Ching DS: Hemiparesis and altered mental status in a child after glyburide ingestion. J Emerg Med 1998; 16:433–435.

93. Spiller HA, Villalobos D, Krenzelok EP, et al: Prospective multicenter study of sulfonylurea ingestion in children. J Pediatr 1997;131: 141–146.

94. Spiller HA, Weber J, Hofman M, et al: Multicenter case series of adult metformin ingestion [abstract]. J Toxicol Clin Toxicol 1999; 37:639.

95. Spiller HA, Weber J, Hofman M, et al: Multicenter case series of pediatric metformin ingestion [abstract]. J Toxicol Clin Toxicol 1999; 37:639–640.

96. Stapczynski JS, Haskell RJ: Duration of hypoglycemia and need for intravenous glucose following intentional overdoses of insulin. Ann Emerg Med 1984;13:505–511.

97. Stocks AE: Insulin lispro: Experience in a private practice setting. Med J Aust 1999;170:364–367.

98. Strauch BS, Felig P, Baxter JD, et al: Hypothermia in hypoglycemia. JAMA 1969;210:345–346.

99. Stumvoll M, Nurjhan N, Perriello G, et al: Metabolic effects of metformin in non-insulin-dependent diabetes mellitus. N Engl J Med 1995;333:550–554.

100. Szlatenyi CS, Capes KF, Wang RY: Delayed hypoglycemia in a child after ingestion of a single glipizide tablet. Ann Emerg Med 1998;31:773–776.

101. Teale KF, Devine A, Stewart H, et al: The management of metformin overdose. Anaesthesia 1998;53:698–701.

102. Thoma ME, Glauser J, Genuth S. Persistent hypoglycemia and hyperinsulinemia: Caution in using glucagon. Am J Emerg Med 1996; 14:99–101.

103. Wachtel TJ, Steele GH, Day JA: Natural history of fever following seizure. Arch Intern Med 1987;147:1153–1155.

104. Wallis WE, Donaldson I, Scott RS, et al: Hypoglycemia masquerading as cerebrovascular disease (hypoglycemic hemiplegia). Ann Neurol 1985;18:510–512.

105. Welborn TA. Acarbose an α-glucosidase inhibitor for non-insulin-dependent diabetes. Med J Aust 1998;168:76–78.

ANTIDOTES IN DEPTH

Dextrose
Kathleen A. Delaney

CH₂OH
H   O OH
H
OH H
OH   H
H   OH

Dextrose (D-glucose)

Glucose is the primary energy source for the human brain. Although the adult human brain can use alternate substrates, such as fatty acids, amino acids, and ketones, for metabolic energy, glucose is the only source of metabolic energy for the brain of the fetus and neonate.[66] Hypoglycemia causes neurologic effects that are clinically indistinguishable from those of a variety of toxic-metabolic and structural brain injuries, which include focal stroke syndromes, seizures, confusion, delirium, and coma.[3,16,22,35,47,57,69,76] Hypoglycemia also precipitates myocardial stress and is associated with angina, electrocardiogram (ECG) changes, and dysrhythmias.[23,38,46,49] Although in most cases these effects reverse following treatment of hypoglycemia, prolonged or severe hypoglycemia may result in permanent brain injury, myocardial infarction, and death.[24,32,59] The mortality rate of critically ill children who are hypoglycemic is significantly higher than children who are normoglycemic.[42]

The administration of 0.5–1 g/kg of concentrated intravenous dextrose immediately reverses the clinical effects of uncomplicated hypoglycemia when the duration of hypoglycemia is brief. (Table 40–7). Because of the myriad presentations of hypoglycemia, the difficulties inherent in its clinical diagnosis, and the serious consequences of failure to treat it, the empirical administration of hypertonic dextrose to all patients with mental status alteration has been a standard Emergency Department (ED) practice. Only clinically insignificant or very rare complications have been attributed to this practice. For example, the administration of dextrose by bolus or infusion causes mild hypophosphatemia.[43,53,55] Dextrose infusion has also been reported to precipitate hyperkalemia in insulin-dependent diabetics with type 4 renal tubular acidosis or hyporeninemic hypoaldosteronism.[26] There is a theoretical concern that the osmotic effects of hypertonic dextrose could precipitate pulmonary edema in patients with fragile cardiac function.[34] Rarely, the administration of hypertonic dextrose is associated with lactic acidosis in cancer patients with large tumor loads.[27] Concentrated dextrose solutions commonly cause phlebitis, and tissue necrosis is described following soft tissue infiltration of 50% dextrose.[20] Tissue infarction has also followed inadvertent intraarterial injection of 50% dextrose.[4] Seizures, hyperosmolar coma, and death have been attributed to the administration of inappropriately large boluses of 50% dextrose to

children.[58] Anecdotal reports of the precipitation of acute Wernicke encephalopathy by the administration of dextrose led to the inclusion of thiamine in the "coma cocktail" (Antidotes in Depth: Thiamine Hydrochloride). These potential complications of dextrose administration are easily accepted when contrasted with the risks posed by delay in the recognition and treatment of hypoglycemia. Serious problems associated with the administration of hypertonic dextrose are also caused by medication errors, such as the inadvertent substitution of a look-alike bolus of concentrated lidocaine or magnesium.[29]

CONCERNS REGARDING ELEVATED BLOOD GLUCOSE LEVELS IN THE PATIENT WITH CEREBRAL ISCHEMIA

Since the early 1980s a growing body of clinical and laboratory studies in the neuroscience literature suggests that preexisting hyperglycemia is either a marker for, or a cause of, more extensive brain injury in the presence of cerebral ischemia.[71] Clinical studies have shown that elevation of blood glucose was associated with more serious neurologic outcomes in patients with head injury or cerebrovascular accidents.[10,52] These descriptive clinical studies do not distinguish the primary effects of hyperglycemia from those of obvious associated conditions, such as hyperglycemia secondary to the intense sympathetic response accompanying more severe brain injury, or hyperglycemia as a marker of diabetes and its attendant severe cerebrovascular disease.[77] However, controlled laboratory investigations of ischemic brain injury in the presence of hyperglycemia induced prior to the ischemic insult consistently support the clinical observation that higher blood glucose levels are in fact associated with more extensive cerebral injury. Most such studies were conducted in animal models of global cerebral ischemia, using cardiac arrest or 4-vessel ligation, and in models of focal ischemia using 1- or 2-vessel ligation.[50] These animal models of ischemic injury demonstrated deleterious effects of preischemic hyperglycemia using a variety of outcome endpoints. Monkeys given 0.76 g/kg of dextrose followed by 17 minutes of global ischemia have significantly greater neurologic and histopathologic evidence of cerebral injury at 96 hours as compared with controls given saline instead of dextrose. Dextrose infusions resulted in increases in the blood glucose levels from a mean of 57 mg/dL to a mean of 244 mg/dL.[36] Hyperglycemic rats subjected to 12.5 minutes of forebrain ischemia by bilateral carotid ligation showed significant increases in pathologic injury compared to normoglycemic rats.[40] Infusion of 10% dextrose into cats prior to middle cerebral artery occlusion resulted in a 3-fold increase in the size of the resultant infarct measured at 2 weeks. Serum glucose levels increased from 90 mg/dL to 360 mg/dL following dextrose infusion in this study.[18] A dog model of cardiac arrest compared 6 animals maintained with a solution of 5% dextrose in lactated Ringer solution (D₅LR) with 6 animals treated with LR alone. Glucose levels were 335 mg/dL in the treated ani-

TABLE 40–7.   Dosing of Dextrose

Bolus

Adult
D$_{50}$W (50% = 0.5 g/mL)   0.5–1.0-g/kg bolus
Child
D$_{25}$W (25% = 0.25 g/mL);   0.5-g/kg bolus
    1:1 dilution of D$_{50}$W with sterile water
Infant
D$_{10}$W (10% = 0.1 g/mL);   0.5-g/kg bolus
    1:4 dilution of D$_{50}$W with sterile water

Infusion

Adults and Children
D$_{10}$W (10% = 0.1 g/mL)   Titrate infusion as
D$_5$W (5% = 0.05 g/mL)   indicated to
                                                     maintain serum
                                                     glucose in normal
                                                     range

mals and 129 mg/dL in the controls. At 24 hours all of the dextrose-infused animals were dead or had severe neurologic deficits, whereas all of the LR-treated animals walked and ate.[15] In rats subjected to 10 minutes of global ischemia none of the 6 made hyperglycemic prior to ischemia survived whereas 100% (10 of 10) of the normoglycemic animals survived.[60] The most severe injuries are evident when ischemia is incomplete or focal so that a small amount of blood flow is present, such as when collateral circulation is present near an area of focal infarction.[18,30,50,51] Hypoglycemia was deleterious in all models where it was studied.[18,30,33,60]

The biochemical impact of hyperglycemia in the setting of ischemia has been extensively investigated. Studies of global ischemia demonstrate rapid depletion of brain glucose, ATP, and phosphocreatine, followed by a rapid rise in the intracellular content of lactic acid, disruption of energy-dependent electrolyte gradients, activation of phospholipase by increased intracellular calcium, and generation of destructive free radicals.[61–63,68,71,74] The deleterious effect of hyperglycemia appears to be consistently associated with increased intraneuronal production of lactate, particularly in models of focal ischemia.[63,68,71] This was attributed to the continued availability of a trickle of glucose in the penumbra of ischemia, resulting in acidosis that extends the area of infarction.[3,50,62,81] The magnitude of intracellular lactic acid accumulation following the onset of ischemia is proportional to the blood glucose level.[30,48,54,73] Hyperglycemia is also associated with increased capillary permeability in ischemic tissue and delay in the resolution of intracellular calcium elevation during recovery from ischemia.[5,21] It may also interfere with membrane repair systems in injured cells by suppressing the synthesis of "heat shock" proteins.[14,74] The administration of insulin to control preischemic hyperglycemia decreases the extent of ischemic injury.[17,19,28,39,70,72] Insulin, a promoter of "heat shock" protein synthesis in ischemic cells, may have a protective effect that is independent of its effect on blood glucose.[18,28,39,65,67] In all studies hypoglycemia is clearly detrimental.[7] Recently, significant increases in the deposition of neutrophils were demonstrated in areas of focal brain injury associated with hyperglycemia, suggesting a role in injury production.[41] In contrast to the situation in adult models, hyperglycemia has not been shown to be detrimental in fetal and neonatal animal models of anoxia.[11,66]

CLINICAL IMPLICATIONS OF ANIMAL STUDIES OF HYPERGLYCEMIA AND CEREBRAL ISCHEMIA

The studies described above have led to calls for reassessment of the standard practice of routine inclusion of D$_{50}$W in the antidote cocktail for patients with altered mental status.[9] A thoughtful assessment recognizes that the possible detriment of raising blood glucose levels in a patient whose altered mental status or focal neurologic symptoms are caused by ischemia must be weighed against the risk of failure to treat hypoglycemia and the potential resultant neurologic injury. There is no question that the reversal of hypoglycemia is a sound clinical intervention in the patient who is hypoglycemic, regardless of the presence of cerebral ischemia, and that the failure to administer dextrose in a timely fashion to a patient with significant hypoglycemia may result in permanent neurologic injury.

Although they raise reasonable concerns, the applicability of the above studies to the empirical administration of dextrose in the emergency department is unclear. All of the studies utilize pretreatment models; that is, the serum glucose was raised prior to the induction of the ischemic insult. In addition, the blood glucose levels attained in some of these models were much higher than would be expected following the administration of a 0.5 g/kg dose of hypertonic dextrose to an adult. In a postinfarct scenario, the induction of transient hyperglycemia would not be expected to affect the area where irreversible infarction had occurred. However, in the patient with focal symptoms, the delivery of excessive amounts of glucose could be of greater concern. The retrospective clinical studies that show poorer outcomes in head-injured or stroke patients who are hyperglycemic do not distinguish the effects of hyperglycemia per se from hyperglycemia as a marker of a sympathetic response to a more severe neurologic insult, or hyperglycemia as a marker of the more severe cerebrovascular disease associated with diabetes. No studies evaluate the effects of a transient elevation of the blood glucose after the onset of ischemia that might occur during clinical practice.

THE RELIABILITY OF BEDSIDE BLOOD GLUCOSE DETERMINATIONS

These concerns would be easily resolved if bedside blood glucose determinations with reagent strips were as reliable as the chemistry laboratory. Several studies of commonly available reagent strips have failed to demonstrate 100% sensitivity for distinguishing normoglycemia from hypoglycemia.[12,13,25,37,44,56] The best published sensitivities for the detection of hypoglycemia by fingerstick using reagent strips range between 92% and 94%.[31,37] A recent study of reagent strip testing of venous blood identified 28 of 29 hypoglycemic patients (97% sensitivity).[56] In one study, 2 of 33 hypoglycemic patients (blood glucose <60 mg/dL) were not detected, but a 90-mg/dL cutoff would have detected 100% of numerically hypoglycemic patients.[37] The "safe" number at which no cases of symptomatic hypoglycemia are missed by reagent strip testing is a subject of debate because poorly controlled diabetics experience hypoglycemic symptoms at blood glucose levels that can be regarded as normoglycemic.[8] In an important study, the mean blood glucose level for symptomatic hypoglycemia in poorly controlled diabetics was 78 ± 5 mg/dL as compared to 53 ± 2 mg/dL in normal controls.[8] False-positive indications of hypoglycemia are more common than false-negatives, especially in patients with shock. A recent study of fingerstick capillary samples from 50 patients after cardiac arrest identified 8 patients as hypoglycemic, although only 3 of 8 were actually hypoglycemic when venous blood was analyzed. Furthermore, bedside testing missed one hypoglycemic patient. Reagent strip tests of venous blood correctly identified all numerically hypoglycemic patients.[64] In another study, 32% of hypotensive patients were incorrectly diagnosed as hypoglycemic by capillary blood glucose measurement. Again, the use of venous blood for reagent strip testing correctly classified all patients.[6] Based on these studies a reasonably conservative cutoff for the assurance of clinical normoglycemia in all patients would be a bedside reagent measurement of 120 mg/dL.

PHARMACOKINETICS OF DEXTROSE

Studies of the pharmacokinetics of dextrose are limited, making it difficult to predict the amount of dextrose required to effectively treat hypoglycemia. In one study the administration of 25 g (50 mL) of $D_{50}W$ to adults resulted in elevation of the blood glucose from 40 mg/dL to 350 mg/dL above baseline when measured at random times after administration.[1] In a human model of insulin-induced hypoglycemia, the oral administration of 20 g of dextrose raised serum blood glucose from 60 mg/dL to 120 mg/dL over 1 hour. Ten grams raised the level from 60 mg/dL to 100 mg/dL.[75]

A RATIONAL CLINICAL SOLUTION

An ideal clinical solution to the management of patients with altered mental status or focal neurologic symptoms would miss no cases of significant symptomatic hypoglycemia and would avoid the administration of dextrose to patients with brain ischemia. A realistic approach can be fashioned from our understanding of the reliability of reagent test strips and a risk-benefit assessment of the presenting problem. Infants and neonates should receive dextrose when clinically indicated without concern for the presence of associated ischemia or anoxia. The patient with coma or status epilepticus from hypoglycemia will benefit greatly from empiric treatment and will suffer the greatest deterioration if not treated. A patient who is comatose from a major cerebrovascular accident has a very limited chance for recovery and the administration of dextrose is unlikely to impact heavily on the prognosis. It is rational to administer $D_{50}W$ to patients in coma who do not have a measured blood glucose of at least 100 mg/dL on bedside reagent strip testing. Similarly, while confusion and delirium in the absence of focal neurologic findings can and do occur as a manifestation of structural brain injury, toxic-metabolic etiologies are more common in our experience. These patients should also receive dextrose if the bedside glucose test is not greater than 100 mg/dL. When a reliable bedside glucose determination cannot be done, all of these patients should receive $D_{50}W$ empirically. Fingerstick glucose samples are especially unreliable in the patient with hypotension or cardiac arrest; however, bedside reagent strip testing of venous blood appears to be more reliable.[6,56,64] Patients in shock or cardiac arrest should have reagent testing done on a *venous* blood sample (not a fingerstick sample) and should receive dextrose if they are numerically hypoglycemic. The administration

of dextrose to the patient in cardiac arrest who is normoglycemic by reagent strip testing should be considered if the patient is a diabetic.

Patients with focal deficits caused by ischemia constitute a population that would reasonably be expected to have the greatest theoretical benefit from the maintenance of normoglycemia. Although focal presentations of hypoglycemia are not rare, they are small relative to the numbers of patients with focal presentations who have suffered cerebrovascular accidents. In one study, 3% of patients with hypoglycemia presented with focal symptoms.[45] In the patient with a history of diabetes who is being treated with insulin or an oral hypoglycemic agent and who presents with focal symptoms, symptomatic hypoglycemia must be strongly considered when the reagent strip shows a blood glucose level less than 90 mg/dL.

The patient with a clear history and evidence of significant head injury antedated by normal activity (eg, crossing the street, struck by car) should not be treated unless the bedside test indicates hypoglycemia (<60 mg/dL). Diabetic patients, of course, may suffer unintentional injuries predisposed by hypoglycemic episodes. The treating physician must use his or her best judgment of the mechanism and evidence of injury, witness reports, available medical history, and results of bedside glucose determination to make a decision regarding administration of $D_{50}W$ to the head-injured trauma patient.

In summary, concerns regarding effects of elevated blood glucose on cerebral ischemia should not cause a physician to withhold dextrose in patients with neurologic impairment when symptomatic hypoglycemia cannot be excluded. Studies indicated that the currently available reagent strips reliably demonstrate the absence of significant hypoglycemia at readings of greater than 100 mg/dL. It is unlikely that profound neurologic impairment is caused by hypoglycemia when such levels are demonstrated. Patients with altered levels of consciousness who do not have capillary blood glucose levels greater than 100 mg/dL should receive $D_{50}W$. We also recommend empiric administration when reagent strip testing is not available. For alert patients with focal neurologic symptoms, a more cautious approach should recognize that poorly controlled diabetic patients had symptomatic hypoglycemia at serum blood glucose levels as high as 85 mg/dL.[8]

REFERENCES

1. Adler PM: Serum glucose changes after administration of 50% dextrose solution: Pre- and in-hospital calculations. Am J Emerg Med 1986;4:504–506.
2. Anderson RE, Tan WK, Martin HS, Meyer FB: Effects of glucose and PaO$_2$ modulation on cortical intracellular acidosis, NADH redox state, and infarction in the ischemic penumbra. Stroke 1999;30:160–170.
3. Andrade R, Mathew V, Morgenstern MJ, et al: Hypoglycemic hemiplegic syndrome. Ann Emerg Med 1984;13:529–531.
4. Arad I, Benady S: Gangrene following intraumbilical injection of hypertonic glucose. J Pediatr 1976;89:327–328.
5. Araki N, Greenberg JH, Sladky JT, et al: The effect of hyperglycemia on intracellular calcium in stroke. J Cereb Blood Flow Metab 1992;12:469–476.
6. Atkin SH, Dasmahapatra A, Jaker MA, et al: Fingerstick glucose determination in shock. Ann Intern Med 1991;114:1020–1024.
7. Auer RN: Insulin, blood glucose levels, and ischemic brain damage. Neurology 1998;51:S039–S043.
8. Boyle PJ, Schwartz NS, Shah SD, et al: Plasma glucose concentrations at the onset of hypoglycemic symptoms in patients with poorly

controlled diabetes and in nondiabetics. N Engl J Med 1988;318: 1487–1492.

9. Browning RG, Olson DW, Stueven HA, Mateer JR: 50% dextrose: Antidote or toxin? Ann Emerg Med 1990;19:683–687.

10. Candelise L, Landi G, Orazio E, et al: Prognostic significance of hyperglycemia in acute stroke. Arch Neurol 1985;42:661–733.

11. Chang YS, Park WS, Lee M, et al: Effect of hyperglycemia on brain cell membrane function and energy metabolism during hypoxia-ischemia in newborn piglets. Brain Res 1998;798:271–280.

12. Cheeley RD, Joyce SM: A clinical comparison of the performance of four blood glucose reagent strips. Am J Emerg Med 1990;8:11–15.

13. Chernow A, Diaz M, Cruess D, et al: Bedside blood glucose determinations in critical care medicine: A comparative analysis of two techniques. Crit Care Med 1982;10:463–465.

14. Combs DJ, Dempsey RJ, Donaldson D, et al: Hyperglycemia suppresses C-fos mRNA expression following cerebral ischemia in gerbils. J Cereb Blood Flow Metab 1992;12:169–172.

15. D'Alecy LG: Dextrose containing intravenous fluid impairs outcome and increases death after eight minutes of cardiac arrest and resuscitation in dogs. Surgery 1986;3:505–511.

16. DCCT Research Group: Epidemiology of severe hypoglycemia in the diabetes control and complications trial. Am J Med 1991;90: 450–459.

17. de Courten-Meyers GM, Kleinholz M, Wagner KR, et al: Normoglycemia (not hypoglycemia) optimizes outcome from middle cerebral artery occlusion. J Cereb Blood Flow Metab 1994;14:227–236.

18. de Courten-Myers G, Myers RE, Schoolfield L: Hyperglycemia enlarges infarct size in cerebrovascular occlusion in cats. Stroke 1988; 19:623–630.

19. de Courten-Myers GM, Wagner KR, Myers RE: Insulin reduction of cerebral infarction. J Neurosurg 1996;84:146–148.

20. DeLorenzo RA, Vista JP: Another hazard of hypertonic dextrose. Am J Emerg Med 1994;12:262–263.

21. Dietrich WD, Alonso O, Busto R: Moderate hyperglycemia worsens acute blood-brain barrier injury after forebrain ischemia in rats. Stroke 1993;24:111–116.

22. Duarte J, Perez A, Coria F, et al: Hypoglycemia presenting as acute tetraplegia [letter]. Stroke 1993;24:143.

23. Duh E, Feinglos M: Hypoglycemia-induced angina pectoris in a patient with diabetes mellitus. Ann Intern Med 1994;121:945–946.

24. Duvanel CB, Fawer CL, Cotting J, et al: Long-term effects of neonatal hypoglycemia on brain growth and psychomotor development in small-for-gestational-age preterm infants. J Pediatr 1999;134: 492–498.

25. Frantz ID, Medina G, Taeusch HW: Correlation of Dextrostix values with true glucose in the range less than 50 mg/dL. J Pediatr 1975; 87:417–420.

26. Goldfarb S, Cox M, Singer I, Goldberg M: Acute hyperkalemia induced by hyperglycemia: Hormonal mechanisms. Ann Intern Med 1976;84:426–432.

27. Goodgame JT, Pizzo P, Brennan MF: Iatrogenic lactic acidosis. Cancer 1978;42:800–803.

28. Hamilton MG, Tranmer BI, Auer RN: Insulin reduction of cerebral infarction due to transient focal ischemia. J Neurosurg 1995;82: 262–268.

29. Hoffman RS, Smilkstein MJ, Rubenstein F: An "AMP" by any other name: The hazards of intravenous magnesium dosing [letter]. JAMA 1989;261:557.

30. Ibayashi S: Cerebral blood flow and tissue metabolism in experimental cerebral ischemia of spontaneously hypertensive rats with hyper, normo- and hypoglycemia. Stroke 1986;17:261–266.

31. Jones JL, Ray VG, Gough JE, et al: Determination of prehospital blood glucose: A prospective, controlled study. J Emerg Med 1992; 10:679–682.

32. Kalimo H, Olsson Y: Effects of severe hypoglycemia on the human brain: Neuropathological case reports. Acta Neurol Scand 1980;62: 345–356.

33. Kim YB, Gidday JM, Gonzalez FR, et al: Effect of hypoglycemia on postischemic cortical blood flow, hypercapnic reactivity, and interstitial adenosine concentration. J Neurosurg 1994;81:877–884.

34. Kulling P, Lindholm M, Eklund J: Hemodynamic effects of hyperosmolal glucose infusion in the critically ill patient. Crit Care Med 1981;9:768–771.

35. Lala VR, Vedanarayana VV, Ganesh S, et al: Hypoglycemic hemiplegia in an adolescent with insulin-dependent diabetes mellitus: A case report and a review of the literature. J Emerg Med 1989;7: 233–236.

36. Lanier WL, Strangland KJ, Scheithauer BW, et al: The effects of dextrose infusion and head position on neurologic outcome after complete cerebral ischemia in primates: Examination of a model. Anesthesiology 1987;66:39–48.

37. Lavery RF, Allegra JR, Cody RP, et al: A prospective evaluation of glucose reagent test strips in the prehospital setting. Am J Emerg Med 1991;9:304–308.

38. Leak D, Starr P: The mechanism of arrhythmias during insulin-induced hypoglycemia. Am Heart J 1962;63:688–691.

39. LeMay DR, Gehua L, Zelenock GB, D'Alecy LG: Insulin administration protects neurologic function in cerebral ischemia in rats. Stroke 1988;19:1411–1419.

40. Lin B, Ginsberg MD, Busto R: Hyperglycemic exacerbation of neuronal damage following forebrain ischemia: Microglial, astrocytic and endothelial alterations. Acta Neuropathol 1998;96:610–620.

41. Lin B, Ginsberg MD, Busto R, Li L: Hyperglycemia triggers massive neutrophil deposition in brain following transient ischemia in rats. Neurosci Lett 2000;278:1–4.

42. Losek J: Hypoglycemia and the ABC's (sugar) of pediatric resuscitation. Ann Emerg Med 2000;35:43–46.

43. MacLeod DB, Montoya DR, Fick GH, Jessen KR: The effect of 25 grams IV glucose on serum inorganic phosphate levels. Ann Emerg Med 1994;23:524–528.

44. Maisels MJ, Lee CA: Chemstrip glucose test strips: Correlation with true glucose values less than 80 mg/dL. Crit Care Med 1983;11: 293–295.

45. Malouf R, Brust JM: Hypoglycemia: Causes, neurological manifestations, and outcome. Ann Neurol 1985;17:421–430.

46. Meinhold J, Heise T, Rave K, Heinemann L. Electrocardiographic changes during insulin-induced hypoglycemia in healthy subjects. Horm Metab Res 1998;30:694–697.

47. Montgomery BM, Pinner CA: Transient hypoglycemic hemiplegia. Arch Intern Med 1964;114:680–684.

48. Morikawa S, Inubushi T, Ishii H, Nakasu Y: Effects of blood sugar level on rat transient focal brain ischemia consecutively observed by diffusion-weighted EPI and (1) H echo planar spectroscopic imaging. Magn Reson Med 1999;42:895–902.

49. Odeh M, Oliven A, Bassan H: Transient atrial fibrillation precipitated by hypoglycemia. Ann Emerg Med 1990;19:565–567.

50. Plum F: What causes infarction in ischemic brain? The Robert Wartenberg Lecture. Neurology 1983;33:222–226.

51. Prado R, Ginsberg MD, Dietrich WD, et al: Hyperglycemia increases infarct size in collaterally perfused but not end-arterial vascular territories. J Cereb Blood Flow Metab 1988;8:186–191.

52. Pulsinelli WA, Levy DE, Sigsbee B, et al: Increased damage after ischemic stroke in patients with hyperglycemia with or without established diabetes mellitus. Am J Med 1983;74:540–544.

53. Rasmussen A: Hypophosphatemia during postoperative glucose infusion. Acta Chir Scand 1985;151:497–500.

54. Rehncrona S, Rosen I, Siesjo BK: Brain lactic acidosis and ischemic cell damage: 1. Biochemistry and neurophysiology. J Cereb Blood Flow Metabol 1981;1:297–309.

55. Rowlands BJ, Giddings AEB: Postoperative hypophosphataemia. Lancet 1976;3:1077–1078.

56. Scott PA, Wolf LR, Spadafora MP: Accuracy of reagent strips in detecting hypoglycemia in the Emergency Department. Ann Emerg Med 1998;32:305–309.

57. Seibert DG: Reversible decerebrate posturing secondary to hypoglycemia. Am J Med 1985;78:1036–1037.

58. Shah A, Stanhope R, Matthew D: Hazards of pharmacological tests of growth hormone secretion in childhood. Br Med J 1992;304:173–174.

59. Shorr RI, Ray WA, Daugherty JR, Griffin MR: Individual sulfonylureas and serious hypoglycemia in older people. J Am Geriatr Soc 1996;44:751–756.

60. Siemkowicz E, Hansen AJ: Clinical restitution following cerebral ischemia in hypo-, normo-, and hyperglycemic rats. Acta Neurol Scand 1978;58:1–8.

61. Siesjo BK: Basic mechanisms of traumatic brain damage. Ann Emerg Med 1993;22:959–969.

62. Siesjo BK: Cell damage in the brain: A speculative synthesis. J Cereb Blood Flow Metab 1981;1:155–183.

63. Swain JA, Anderson RV, Siegman MG: Low-flow cardiopulmonary bypass and cerebral protection: A summary of investigations. Ann Thorac Surg 1993;56: 1490–1492.

64. Thomas SH, Gough JE, Benson N, et al: Accuracy of fingerstick glucose determination in patients receiving CPR. South Med J 1994; 87:1072–1075.

65. Ting LP, Tu CL, Chou CK: Insulin-induced expression of human heat-shock protein hsp-70. J Biol Chem 1989;264:3404–3408.

66. Vannucci RC, Yager JY: Glucose, lactic acid, and perinatal hypoxic-ischemic brain damage. Pediatr Neurol 1992;8:3–12.

67. Voll CL, Auer RN: Insulin attenuates ischemic brain damage independent of its hypoglycemic effect. J Cereb Blood Flow Metab 1991;11: 1006–1014.

68. Wagner SR, Lanier WL: Metabolism of glucose, glycogen, and high-energy phosphates during complete cerebral ischemia. Anesthesiology 1994;81:1516–1526.

69. Wallis WE, Donaldson I, Scott RS, Wilson J: Hypoglycemia masquerading as cerebrovascular disease (hypoglycemic hemiplegia). Ann Neurol 1985;18:510–512.

70. Warner DS, Gionet TX, Todd MM, McAllister AM: Insulin-induced normoglycemia improves ischemic outcome in hyperglycemic rats. Stroke 1992;23:1775–1780.

71. Wass CT, Lanier WL: Glucose modulation of ischemic brain injury: Review and clinical recommendations. Mayo Clin Proc 1996;71: 801–812.

72. Wass CT, Scheithauer BW, Bronk J, et al: Insulin treatment of corticosteroid-associated hyperglycemia and its effect on outcome after forebrain ischemia in rats. Anesthesiology 1996;84:644–651.

73. Welsh FA, Ginsberg MD, Rieder W, et al: Deleterious effect of glucose pretreatment on recovery from diffuse cerebral ischemia in the cat: II. Regional metabolite levels. Stroke 1980;11:355–363.

74. White BC, Krause GS: Brain injury and repair mechanisms: The potential for pharmacologic therapy in closed head trauma. Ann Emerg Med 1993;22:970–979.

75. Wiethop BV, Cryer PE: Alanine and terbutaline in the treatment of hypoglycemia in IDDM. Diabetes Care 1993;16:1131–1136.

76. Winer JB, Fish DR, Sawyers D, Marsden CD: A movement disorder as a presenting feature of recurrent hypoglycemia. Mov Disord 1990; 5:176–177.

77. Woo E, Ma JTC, Robinson JD, et al: Hyperglycemia is a stress response in acute stroke. Stroke 1988;19:1359–1364.

ANTIDOTES IN DEPTH

OCTREOTIDE

Mary Ann Howland

Octreotide is a long-acting, synthetic octapeptide analogue of so-matostatin that inhibits pancreatic insulin secretion. It currently is considered secondary only to glucose for the treatment of refractory hypoglycemia induced by intentional and unintentional overdoses of oral hypoglycemic agents such as sulfonylureas, as well as for quinine.

HISTORY

"Somatostatin" is a collective term for shorter fragments (SRIF-28, SRIF-25, and SRIF-14) cleaved by tissue-specific enzymes from preprosomatostatin (116 amino acids) and prosomatostatin (92 amino acids).[10] Somatostatin is a protein that was discovered in 1973, during the search for growth hormone releasing factor.[6] In addition to its effects on growth hormone and insulin secretion, somatostatin, which is widely distributed in the body, has far-reaching effects as a central nervous system (CNS) neurotransmitter and as a modulator of hormonal release.[21] Somatostatin is very short acting. Octreotide was purposefully synthesized in 1982 at Sandoz Labs in a quest to develop a longer-acting analogue of somatostatin.[3] Octreotide is currently used therapeutically in the treatment of acromegaly, pituitary adenomas, pancreatic islet cell tumors, carcinoid tumors, esophageal varices, and secretory diarrhea.[21] Octreotide is also being investigated for its inhibitory effects on tumor cell proliferation. [21]

RECEPTOR AFFINITY

Somatostatin's effects are mediated by high-affinity binding to membrane receptors on target tissues. Five different somatostatin receptor subtypes (SSTR 1–5) that belong to a superfamily of G-protein-coupled receptors have been identified and assigned numbers according to their order of discovery.[10] Octreotide has high binding affinity for SSTR 2 and 5 subtypes, low affinity for SSTR 1 and 4 subtypes, and intermediate affinity for SSTR 3 subtype.[21] SSTR 2 is found in the pancreas, brain, and kidney, whereas SSTR 5 is found in the brain, heart, adrenal glands, placenta, small intestine, and skeletal muscle.[21,24]

EFFECTS ON INSULIN SECRETION AND OTHER HORMONES

Experiments utilizing a whole-cell patch clamp technique on a hamster β-cell line suggest that somatostatin inhibits insulin secretion by a G-protein-mediated decrease in calcium entry through voltage-dependent Ca^{++} channels[15] while demonstrating no evidence that somatostatin inhibited insulin release by promoting K^+ efflux through K^+ channels (Fig. 40–2).[26]

Experiments with somatostatin in healthy human volunteers and in an isolated perfused canine pancreas model demonstrate the ability of somatostatin to inhibit glucose-stimulated insulin release as well as its short duration of action.[1,12]

One study in human volunteers confirmed the ability of somatostatin to inhibit the increased insulin response to both glucose and glucagon.[12] An intravenous infusion of 1 g of tolbutamide over 2 minutes caused insulin levels to rise and serum glucose to drop sharply. However, treatment with somatostatin blocked these changes. Similarly, in the presence of somatostatin and tolbutamide, administration of IV glucagon caused a rise in glucose without the expected subsequent glucose-stimulated rise in insulin. These effects of somatostatin were short-lived. The prolonged effects of tolbutamide stimulated increasing insulin levels within 5 minutes after somatostatin was stopped; within 15 minutes the serum glucose fell and peak insulin levels were achieved within 25 minutes.

Studies in rats and monkeys, comparing octreotide to somatostatin, demonstrated that octreotide was 1.3 times as potent as somatostatin in inhibiting insulin secretion by 50%. In this model, octreotide was 45 times more potent in inhibiting growth hormone secretion and 11 times more potent in inhibiting glucagon release.[3]

The actions of octreotide on various hormones have been studied.[19] Using a hyperglycemic glucose clamp technique, administration of octreotide 30 ng/kg/min by continuous IV infusion demonstrated the ability of octreotide to suppress endogenous insulin secretion, growth hormone, and glucagon. Octreotide also blocked the counterregulatory response to the effects of 0.1 U/kg intravenous insulin by preventing an increase in glucagon and growth hormone. Moreover, epinephrine and norepinephrine concentrations nearly achieved control levels. In a subsequent study of octreotide on the responses of adrenocorticotropin (ACTH), cortisol, prolactin, luteinizing hormone (LH), and follicle-stimulating hormone (FSH) to insulin-induced hypoglycemia all remained intact, in contrast to growth hormone and thyroid-stimulating hormone (TSH), which were significantly inhibited.[22] A study of octreotide demonstrated rapid suppression of the rises in both growth hormone and insulin in response to arginine with a more persistent effect on growth hormone.[7]

PHARMACOKINETICS

The pharmacokinetics of intravenous and subcutaneous octreotide were studied in 8 healthy adult volunteers.[20] Subjects received 25, 50, 100, 200 µg IV octreotide over 3 minutes and 50, 100, 200, and 400 µg SC octreotide in random order. Following IV administration, the α distribution half-life averaged 12 minutes and the elimination half-life ranged from 72 ± 22 to 98 ± 37 minutes and was linear. The Vi (volume of distribution of the central compartment) was dose-dependent and increased from about 5.7 L at 25, 50, and 100 µg IV to 10 L at 200-µg IV doses.[20] The Vβ (volume of distribution determined by area) was 18 ± 6 to 30 ± 30 L and showed no dose dependency.[20] Renal elimination accounted for about 30% and was reduced in the elderly and in those with severe renal failure.[28]

After subcutaneous administration, bioavailability was 100% and the peak levels were achieved within 30 minutes with an absorption half-life of 5–12 minutes. The elimination half-life was $88–102 \pm 16$ minutes. Peak plasma concentrations ranged from 2.4 ng/mL at doses of 50 µg to 23.5 ng/mL at doses of 400 µg, approximately half of the intravenously administered level.[20]

The pharmacokinetics in patients with clinical conditions may differ from the healthy as exemplified by a lower peak concentration and higher steady-state Vd in patients with acromegaly.[28]

CLINICAL USE FOR INSULIN SUPPRESSION

Octreotide was studied in several clinical conditions such as the hyperinsulinemic condition associated with insulinomas and hypoglycemia of infancy.[2,13,17,31,30] In most instances octreotide suppressed insulin levels, and glucose levels rose. However, there are reports of worsening hypoglycemia when glucagon suppression outlasted insulin suppression.[4,9,11,29]

Octreotide is currently used for the treatment of drug-induced endogenous secretion of insulin. In two controlled studies in healthy volunteers, octreotide suppressed the release of insulin associated with quinine and glipizide therapy.[5,27] Several case reports and limited case series also demonstrated octreotide's effectiveness in the management of intentional and unintentional sulfonylurea overdoses.[5,14,16,18,23,25]

Life-threatening hypoglycemia is a well-recognized complication of the quinine treatment of *Plasmodium falciparum* malaria. In this setting, hypertonic dextrose and diazoxide are frequently inadequate therapy. In an investigation of the potential hypoglycemia-sparing effect of octreotide for quinine-induced hypoglycemia, healthy adults were given 50 µg/h of octreotide or placebo as a continuous IV infusion for 4 hours followed at the first hour by the infusion of 490 mg of quinine base.[27] In the control subjects, plasma insulin levels rose and plasma glucose levels fell significantly, whereas in the octreotide group, insulin levels fell and glucose levels remained constant. This effect of octreotide began within 30 minutes and persisted for 2 hours after the octreotide was stopped. Octreotide was successfully utilized to treat severe hypoglycemia in a woman receiving 600 mg of quinine dihydrochloride IV for malaria.[27]

The efficacy of octreotide was demonstrated in a subsequent study. Eight healthy volunteers were given 1.43 mg/kg of glipizide orally and randomized to receive either a variable dextrose infusion to remain euglycemic, diazoxide 300 mg IV over 30 minutes and repeated every 4 hours along with dextrose or octreotide 30 ng/kg/min IV continuously.[5] Following the administration of glipizide, hypoglycemia of 50 mg/dL was achieved within 30–165 minutes.[5] Insulin levels in the octreotide group were comparable to those in the glipizide group with resultant glucose levels slightly higher than the other groups. Four of the 8 patients in the octreotide group did not require supplemental dextrose. At the fifth hour of the protocol an IV bolus of 50 mL of 50% dextrose was given to study the response to hyperglycemia in the octreotide group. Approximately 6.5 hours were necessary for the plasma glucose to drop to 85 mg/dL, whereas it only took 3 hours in the dextrose and diazoxide groups.[5] Diazoxide infusion was associated with higher norepinephrine levels, whereas epinephrine levels were similar in all groups.[5] All agents were stopped at 13 hours and plasma glucose levels fell below 65 mg/dL within 1.5 hours in

subjects who received the dextrose and diazoxide, whereas the plasma glucose levels remained above 65 mg/dL in 6 of the 8 octreotide subjects for the 4-hour observation period. Without additional octreotide, hypoglycemia continued to recur for as long as 30 hours after the initial glipizide administration.

Several case studies and a case series of 9 patients support the efficacy of octreotide in overdoses of glipizide, glyburide, gliclazide and tolbutamide, whether intentional or unintentional, NIDDM or IDDM, and in a pediatric patient.[5,8,14,16,18,23,25] In these case reports, therapeutic doses have ranged considerably with the most frequent doses being 50–100 µg SC repeated every 8–12 hours in the adult patients.

ADVERSE REACTIONS

Octreotide is generally well tolerated but experience in the toxicologic setting is limited. Adverse reactions occurring with short-term administration are usually local or gastrointestinal in nature. Stinging at the site of injection occurs in approximately 7% of patients, but rarely lasts more than 15 minutes.[32] Healthy volunteers receiving octreotide noted no side effects at intravenous doses of 25 or 50 µg, or subcutaneous doses of 50 or 100 µg. At higher doses early transient nausea and later-appearing but longer-lasting diarrhea and abdominal pain frequently occur.[19,20] Healthy volunteers were given IV bolus doses of octreotide as high as 1000 µg and infusion doses of 30,000 µg over 20 minutes and 120,000 µg over 8 hours without serious side effects. Single doses in healthy volunteers resulted in decreased biliary contractility and bile secretion.[28] Long-term therapy lasting weeks to months results in biliary tract abnormalities.[28,32]

Other adverse effects reported with long-term administration of octreotide include hypothyroidism, cardiac conduction abnormalities, and worsening congestive heart failure (in at-risk patients with acromegaly); bradycardia; pancreatitis; cholecystitis; biliary obstruction; cholestatic hepatitis; altered fat absorption; and decreased vitamin B_{12} levels.[28] Anaphylactoid reactions were reported.[28]

Drug interactions are expected with agents that affect glucose regulation. In addition, octreotide may significantly decrease the oral absorption of cyclosporine.[28]

ADMINISTRATION

Both subcutaneous and intravenous administration are acceptable, although the usual route of administration is subcutaneous.[28] The administration sites should be rotated. For IV infusion, octreotide may be diluted in sterile normal saline or D_5W and infused over 15–30 minutes or by IV bolus over 3 minutes.[28] Rapid IV bolus may be indicated for carcinoid crisis.[28] Refrigeration of octreotide is recommended for prolonged storage although octreotide is stable at room temperature for 14 days when protected from light. Active warming of refrigerated octreotide is not recommended, although passive warming to room temperature prior to administration is suggested. A depot formula designed to last for 4 weeks is available (Sandostatin LAR Depot). Although useful in the case of patients with insulinomas, this duration of action would far exceed that of any oral hypoglycemic agent making it an inappropriate and unnecessary choice for the management of drug-induced hypoglycemia.

DOSING

There is no controlled trial evaluating the dose of octreotide in the overdose setting. A 50-μg SC dose of octreotide every 6 hours is suggested to treat adults. Several days of therapy may be required depending on the duration of action of the ingested agent. In children, a dose of 4–5 μg/kg/d SC divided every 6 hours, up to the adult dose, may be used for initial therapy. This pediatric dose is derived from the literature on treating persistent hyperinsulinemic hypoglycemia of infancy.[13] Further experience in the toxicologic setting should permit a better delineation of these dosing recommendations. Several days of therapy may be required depending on the duration of the offending agent. All patients must be carefully monitored for recurrent hypoglycemia during octreotide therapy and for perhaps 24 hours following termination of octreotide therapy before discharge. Octreotide is considered a category B drug (Table 105–1) and pregnant women must be carefully monitored for recurrent hypoglycemia. The use of octreotide should not diminish this vigilance.

AVAILABILITY

Octreotide acetate (Sandostatin) injection is available in ampules and multidose vials ranging in concentration from 50–1000 μg/mL.

SUMMARY

Octreotide appears to be useful in treating refractory hypoglycemia induced by agents such as sulfonylureas and quinine that cause the endogenous release of insulin. Octreotide is more effective than diazoxide in suppressing insulin and is much better tolerated. Although octreotide may result in gastrointestinal symptoms, diazoxide often causes sodium and water retention, tachycardia, and orthostatic hypotension.

REFERENCES

1. Alberti KGMM, Christensen NJ, Christensen S, et al: Inhibition of insulin secretion by somatostatin. Lancet 1973;2:1299–1301.
2. Alberts AS, Falkson G: Rapid reversal of life-threatening hypoglycemia with a somatostatin analogue (octreotide). S Afr Med J 1988;74:75–76.
3. Bauer W, Briner U, Doepfner W, et al: SMS 201–995: A very potent and selective octapeptide analogue of somatostatin with prolonged action. Life Sci 1982;31:1133–1140.
4. Boden G, Ryan IG, Shuman CR: Ineffectiveness of SMS 201–995 in severe hyperinsulinemia. Diabetes Care 1988;11:664–668.
5. Boyle PJ, Justice K, Krentz AJ, et al: Octreotide reverses hyperinsulinemia and prevents hypoglycemia induced by sulfonylurea overdoses. J Clin Endocrin 1993;76:752–756.
6. Bradeau P, Vale W, Burgus R, et al: Hypothalamic polypeptide that inhibits the secretion of immunoreactive pituitary growth hormone. Science 1973;179:77–79.
7. del Pozo E: Endocrine profile of a long-acting somatostatin derivative. Acta Endocrinologica 1986;111:433–439.
8. Braatvedt GD: Octreotide for the treatment of sulphonylurea-induced hypoglycemia in type 2 diabetes. N Z Med J 1997;110:189–190.
9. Brunner JE, Kruger DF, Basha MA, et al: Hypoglycemia after administration of somatostatin analog in metastatic carcinoid. Henry Ford Hosp Med J 1989;37:60–62.
10. Bruns C, Weckbecker G, Raulf F, et al: Molecular pharmacology of somatostatin-receptor subtypes. Ann N Y Acad Sci 1994;733: 138–146.
11. Gama R, Marks V, Wright J, Teale JD: Octreotide exacerbated fasting hypoglycemia in a patient with a proinsulinoma: The glucostatic importance of pancreatic glucagons. Clin Endocrin 1995;43:117–120.
12. Gerich J, Lorenzi M, Schneider V, Forsham P: Effect of somatostatin on plasma glucose and insulin to responses to glucagon and tolbutamide in man. J Clin Endocrinol Metab 1974;39:1057–1060.
13. Glaser B, Hirsch H, Landau H: Persistent hyperinsulinemic hypoglycemia of infancy: Long-term octreotide treatment without pancreatectomy. J Pediatr 1993;123:644–650.
14. Graudins A, Linden C, Ferm R: Diagnosis and treatment of sulfonylurea-induced hyperinsulinemic hypoglycemia. Am J Emerg Med 1997;15:95–96.
15. Hsu W, Xiang H, Rajan A, et al: Somatostatin inhibits insulin secretion by a G-protein-mediated decrease in Ca^{2+} entry through voltage dependent Ca^{2+} channels in the beta cell. J Biol Chem 1991;206: 837–843.
16. Hung O, Eng J, Ho J, et al: Octreotide as an antidote for refractory sulfonylurea hypoglycemia [abstract]. J Toxicol Clin Toxicol 1997; 35:540.
17. Kane C, Lindley K, Johnson P, et al: Therapy for persistent hyperinsulinemic hypoglycemia of infancy. J Clin Invest 1997;100: 1888–1893.
18. Krentz AJ, Boyle PJ, Justice KM, et al: Successful treatment of severe refractory sulfonylurea-induced hypoglycemia with octreotide. Diabetes Care 1993;16:184–186, 189–190.
19. Krentz AJ, Boyle PJ, Mavdonald LM, Schade DS: Octreotide: A long-acting inhibitor of endogenous hormone secretion for human metabolic investigations. Metabolism 1994;43:24–31.
20. Kutz K, Nuesch E, Rosenthaler J: Pharmacokinetics of SMS 201–995 in healthy subjects. Scand J Gastroenterol 1986;21(Suppl 119):65–72.
21. Lamberts SWJ, Vaanderlely AJ, DeHerder WW, Hofland LJ: Octreotide. N Engl J Med 1996;334:246–254.
22. Lightman SL, Fox P, Dunne MJ: The effects of SMS 201–995, a long-acting somatostatin analogue, on anterior pituitary function in healthy male volunteers. Scand J Gastroenterol 1986;21(Suppl 119):84–95.
23. McLaughlin SA, Crandall CS, McKinney PE: Octreotide: An antidote for sulfonylurea-induced hypoglycemia. Ann Emerg Med 2000;36: 133–138.
24. Moldovan S, Atiya A, Adrian T, et al: Somatostatin inhibits β-cell secretion via a subtype-2 somatostatin receptor in the isolated perfused human pancreas. J Surg Research 1995;59:85–90.
25. Mordel A, Sivilotti MLA, Old AC, Ferm RP: Octreotide for pediatric sulfonylurea poisoning [abstract]. J Toxicol Clin Toxicol 1998; 36:437.
26. Pace CS, Tarvin JT: Somatostatin: Mechanism of action in pancreatic islet cells beta cells. Diabetes 1981;30:836–842.
27. Philips RE, Looareesuwan S, Bloom SR, et al: Effectiveness of SMS 201–995, a synthetic, long-acting somatostatin analogue, in treatment of quinine-induced hyperinsulinemia. Lancet 1986;1:713–715.
28. Product information: Sandostatin octreotide acetate injection. East Hanover, NJ, Novartis Pharmaceuticals Corporation, 1999.
29. Stehouwer CDA, Lems WF, Fischer HRA, et al: Aggravation of hypoglycemia in insulinoma patients by the long-acting somatostatin analogue octreotide (Sandostatin). Acta Endocrinol 1989;121:34–40.
30. Thorton P, Alter C, Levitt-Katz L, et al: Short- and long-term use of octreotide in the treatment of congenital hyperinsulinism. J Pediatr 1993;123:637–643.
31. Verschoor L, Uitterlinden P, Lamberts J, del Pozo E: On the use of a new somatostatin analogue in the treatment of hypoglycemia in patients with insulinoma. Clin Endocrinol (Oxf) 1986;25:555–560.
32. Waas JAH, Popovic V, Chayvialle JA: Proceedings of the discussion, tolerability and safety of Sandostatin. Metabolism 1992;41(Suppl 2): 80–82.

CHAPTER 41

ANTICONVULSANTS

Suzanne Doyon

Drug	Therapeutic serum levels	
	mg/L	μmol/L
Carbamazepine	4–12	17–51
Ethosuximide	40–100	283–708
Felbamate	N/R	N/R
Gabapentin	2–15*	12–88
Lamotrigine	≤5*	≤19.5
Phenobarbital	15–40	65–172
Phenytoin	10–20	40–79
Valproic acid	50–120	347–833
Vigabatrin	N/R	N/R

*Proposed.
N/R = Not recommended.

A 45-year-old man with a past history of alcoholism, posttraumatic stress disorder, and bipolar mood disorder was brought to the Emergency Department (ED) after ingesting unknown amounts of valproic acid and gabapentin. He had recently become depressed and on the day of presentation he ingested all of his remaining tablets with alcohol.

On arrival in the ED, the patient was comatose with a blood pressure of 136/80 mm Hg, pulse of 110 beats/min, respiratory rate of 12 breaths/min, and a temperature of 37°C (98.6°F). The patient withdrew to deep pain in all 4 extremities. His head was atraumatic with 3-mm pupils that responded sluggishly to light. Gag reflex was absent. The examination of his lungs, heart, and abdomen was normal. There were no signs of track marks, cyanosis, or edema. Deep-tendon reflexes were symmetrically brisk and there was bilateral plantar extension.

The patient was endotracheally intubated and placed on a ventilator. A fingerstick for glucose was 70 mg/dL and 50 mL of 50% dextrose was administered intravenously with no change in his mental status. The electrocardiogram (ECG) revealed a sinus tachycardia with normal axis and intervals. A 40-French orogastric tube was inserted for lavage, and 75 g of activated charcoal was instilled through the lavage tube after the lavage fluid was clear.

Laboratory evaluation revealed a normal complete blood count (CBC), serum chemistry profile, liver enzymes, and ammonia level. The serum ethanol level was 391 mg/dL; APAP (serum acetaminophen) was negative. The initial plasma valproic acid level was 236 mg/L.

The patient was admitted to the intensive care unit (ICU). Four hours later, the repeat valproic acid level was 800 mg/L and the initial plasma gabapentin level was 19 mg/L. Multiple doses of activated charcoal were administered. Hemoperfusion was considered but not instituted. The third valproic acid level was 933 mg/L, approximately 6 hours after initial presentation. His mental status remained unchanged. Approximately 18 hours postingestion the valproic acid level decreased to 735 mg/L. The 28-hour valproic acid level was 481 mg/L and gabapentin level was 2.7 mg/L. The patient required additional sedation approximately 18 hours postadmission and developed a fever and a right-lower-lobe infiltrate. He remained intubated and mechanically ventilated. Two days later, his platelets dropped to 30,000/mm³ from 156,000/mm³ on admission. There were no overt signs of bleeding but an expanding hematoma developed at an arterial puncture site. He responded well to platelet transfusion. His liver enzymes remained normal throughout his hospital stay. He recovered uneventfully and his CBC normalized 3 days later. He was discharged without permanent sequelae and with psychiatric support and substance abuse counseling.

HISTORY AND EPIDEMIOLOGY

The prevalence of seizures in the United States is 3%. Historically, seizures have been treated by a variety of methods including barbituric acid compounds, bromides, ketogenic diets, fluid restriction, and surgical excision of scars or irritable cortical foci. The first truly effective therapy was introduced in 1857, when it was noted that administration of bromides sedated patients and significantly reduced their seizures. Phenobarbital was first used to treat seizures in 1912. Consequently, it was erroneously believed that sedation was an essential component of seizure therapy.

The search for nonsedating anticonvulsive agents led to the introduction of phenytoin in 1938.[92] Most of the anticonvulsive agents introduced subsequently, such as primidone, had chemical structures similar to that of phenobarbital.[6] After 1965, benzodiazepines, carbamazepine, and valproic acid were introduced, and widely gained use as anticonvulsants. These remained the only available agents until the most recent decade when numerous new anticonvulsants received approval for clinical use: gabapentin, felbamate, lamotrigine, levetiracetam, oxcarbazepine, tiagabine, topiramate, and vigabatrin.

The indications for the use of these anticonvulsant agents broadened and clinicians now use agents such as valproic acid, gabapentin, and lamotrigine to treat mood disorders. Valproic acid and gabapentin, are also used for the treatment of drug withdrawal syndromes. Some anticonvulsants are used in the treatment of diverse disorders, such as refractory pain syndromes like trigeminal neuralgia, bruxism, and migraine headache prophylaxis. There is also an emerging role for anticonvulsants in the treatment of social phobias.

In a review of more than 5000 patient suicides, anticonvulsants were implicated in 8.2% of cases, suggesting a fairly high rate of suicidal ideation among people who have access to these medications.[60] In the last decade, there has been a shift from predominantly carbamazepine and phenytoin exposures to valproic acid and second-generation anticonvulsants. The 1989 annual report from the American Association of Poison Control Centers and the National Data Collection Systems implicated carbamazepine in 44.1%, phenytoin in 42.7%, valproic acid in 10.1%, and other anticonvulsants in 2% of all anticonvulsant exposures. Carbamazepine was responsible for 50% of anticonvulsant deaths. The 1999 annual report implicated valproic acid in 37.5%, carbamazepine in 26.1%, phenytoin in 17.4%, and other anticonvulsants in 18.8% of all anticonvulsant exposures. Also, valproic acid is now responsible for 89% of anticonvulsant-related deaths (Chap. 116 and p. 1752).

This chapter reviews the toxicity and management of overdoses with anticonvulsants. The toxicities of benzodiazepines and barbiturates are discussed in Chapter 63 and are not reviewed in this chapter.

PHARMACOLOGY

A seizure is defined as the clinical manifestation of excessive neuronal activity within the cerebral cortex. It is accompanied by various degrees of motor, sensory, and cognitive dysfunction. Seizures result from abnormal sodium channel function, excessive calcium conductance, increased interaction between excitatory neurotransmitters, such as glutamate, and their receptors, or loss of inhibitory γ-aminobutyric acid (GABA) control.

Extensive research performed over the past decade serves to elucidate the mechanism of action of most of the major anticonvulsants. Suppression of high-frequency firing in neuronal pacemaker cells results in lowering of excitability and suppression of seizures. A number of different mechanisms of action may suppress high-frequency firing. They usually fall into one of four specific categories: voltage-dependent sodium channel blockade, calcium channel blockade, antiglutamatergic, and GABAergic effects. Frequently, more than one mechanism may account for a drug's anticonvulsive action.[135]

Phenytoin, carbamazepine, and valproic acid all inhibit inactivated time, voltage, and use-dependent sodium channels. More specifically they attach themselves to the batrachotoxin H-20 α-benzoate binding sites. After a depolarization-triggered sodium channel opening, the sodium channels are prevented from closing spontaneously by the anticonvulsant and are, therefore, unable to evoke another action potential.[83,91,147,148] At therapeutic concentrations the sodium channel blockade is selective. At toxic levels, the selectivity is lost and both spontaneous and high-frequency sodium channels are inhibited, and some GABA enhancement is

detected. Lamotrigine, felbamate, and the newer agents—topiramate, oxcarbazepine, zonisamide, and possibly gabapentin—all inhibit sodium channels as part of their mechanism of action.[145] Myocardial sodium channels may also be inhibited by all of these agents at very high levels, resulting in conduction abnormalities.[9]

GABA, synthesized from glutamate, is an inhibitory neurotransmitter whose accumulation is protective against seizures.[5] Increased intrasynaptic levels of GABA enhance $GABA_A$ receptor binding and membrane hyperpolarization through increased inward chloride movement.[91] This reduces neuronal excitability and raises the patient's seizure threshold. Gabapentin may increase the release of GABA from vesicles within the presynaptic neurons.[8,51] Vigabatrin irreversibly inhibits GABA transaminase, the enzyme primarily responsible for the metabolism of GABA.[46] Valproic acid has similar effects.[91] Tiagabine inhibits GABA reuptake thereby increasing the availability of GABA at the neuronal junction.[82]

The N-methyl-D-aspartate (NMDA) receptor is, clinically, the glutamate receptor of greatest importance with respect to the development of seizures. When activated by glutamate, the NMDA receptor activates a ligand-gated ion channel that permits entry of Na^+ and Ca^{++} into the neuronal cells. Suppression of the glutamate-NMDA interaction is protective against seizures.[91] Felbamate and possibly valproic acid are competitive glutamate antagonists.[54] Felbamate acts at the strychnine-insensitive glycine recognition site on the NMDA receptor.[90] Lamotrigine and phenytoin exert antiglutamate activity by inhibiting glutamate release, possibly by binding to presynaptic Na^+ channels.[47,85,135] Phenytoin's antiglutamatergic activity only occurs at very high doses. Topiramate binds to the kainate, not the NMDA, glutamate receptor subtype and blocks the Na^+ entry into the neuronal cell.[108] Figure 41–1 summarizes these findings.

Modulation of voltage-dependent calcium channels occurs with ethosuximide, gabapentin, and zonisamide.[45,105] And, finally, there is evidence that gabapentin may work by binding to a novel site in the cerebral cortex.[56]

PHENYTOIN/FOSPHENYTOIN

Phenytoin (5,5-diphenyl-2,4-imidazolidinedione), first discovered in 1938, is still a first-line anticonvulsive agent for most seizure disorders, except absence seizures.[86] However, currently available data suggest that phenytoin has no role in the treatment of most toxin-induced seizures, including the alcohol withdrawal syndrome.[4,20] Phenytoin is nonsedating in therapeutic doses and, therefore, is often preferred over the GABAergic anticonvulsants for the long-term management of epilepsy.

Fosphenytoin is a water-soluble phenytoin derivative introduced in 1997 that was developed to address the apparent shortcomings of parenteral phenytoin. Its clinical utility derives from

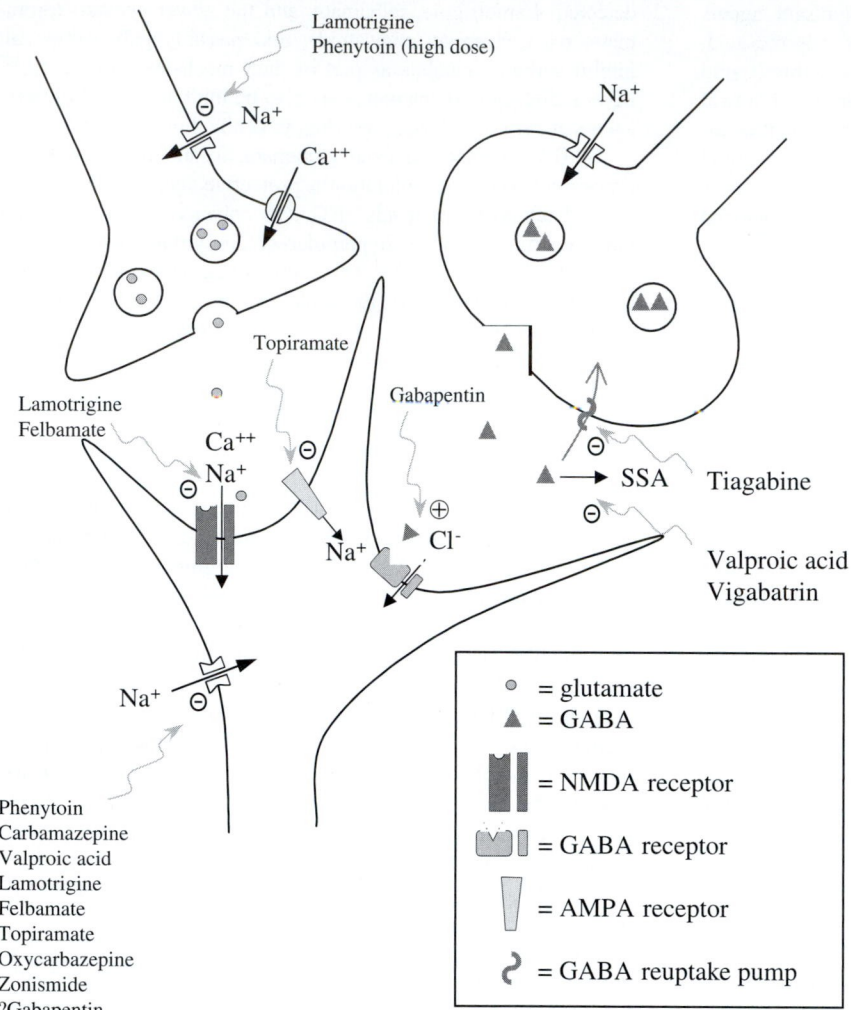

Figure 41–1. Mechanism of action of anticovulsants.

Pharmacokinetics and Toxicokinetics

Phenytoin is a weak acid (pK_a 8.3) that is highly protein-bound and is rapidly distributed to all tissues. Single-dose oral therapeutic loading using 18 mg/kg of phenytoin is well tolerated but is incomplete in 36% of patients at 8 hours.[103] In larger oral overdoses, gastrointestinal absorption can be delayed even more, especially following ingestion of sustained-release preparations.[19] Some authors also suggest that phenytoin may be subjected to continued absorption in the colon because of its lipophilic properties.[138] Phenytoin occasionally forms concretions in the gastrointestinal tract.[19] Once absorbed, it is extensively bound to albumin and only the unbound free fraction can cross biologic membranes and exert pharmacologic action. A significant fraction of phenytoin remains unbound in the neonate and uremic patient and other patients suffering from hypoalbuminemia.[50]

Less than 5% of a given dose of phenytoin is excreted unchanged in the urine. The remainder is metabolized in the endoplasmic reticulum of hepatocytes. The major phenytoin metabolite, a parahydroxylphenyl derivative, is inactive but is believed to be responsible for the hypersensitivity reaction associated with the administration of phenytoin.[72] The Michaelis-Menten model of saturable enzyme kinetics explains the relationship between phenytoin doses and plasma concentrations at steady state. At phenytoin concentrations below 10 mg/L, elimination is usually first order and elimination half-life ranges between 6 and 24 hours. At higher concentrations, zero-order elimination (ie, dose-dependent elimination) occurs as a result of saturation of the hydroxylation reaction and the apparent elimination half-life increases to 20–60 hours.[19,22] Therefore, phenytoin's apparent half-life of elimination is progressively prolonged as the plasma concentration increases[91] (Chap. 11).

Phenytoin is dissolved in propylene glycol when administered intravenously because it is poorly water soluble. It is inadequately absorbed when administered intramuscularly. The maximum rate of intravenous infusion of phenytoin is 50 mg/min; higher infusion rates are associated with significant hypotension and local irritation.

Fosphenytoin (1.5 mg fosphenytoin = 1 mg phenytoin) is a water-soluble phosphate ester prodrug of phenytoin. It is only available in a parenteral formulation that contains no ethanol or propylene glycol. Diluted instead with nontoxic, nonirritating additives, fosphenytoin has a pH of 8–9. Fosphenytoin is converted entirely to phenytoin by circulating phosphatases within 6–16 minutes of injection. The loading dose expressed in phenytoin equivalents is the same as phenytoin. Fosphenytoin can be infused at a maximal rate of 150 mg phenytoin-equivalents/min.[15]

Clinical Manifestations

Acute phenytoin toxicity produces predominantly neurologic dysfunction starting with the cerebellar and vestibular systems. In patients with normal albumin concentrations, phenytoin levels greater than 15 mg/L are typically associated with nystagmus, levels greater than 30 mg/L are associated with ataxia, and levels exceeding 50 mg/L are associated with lethargy, slurred speech, and pyramidal and extrapyramidal manifestations.[74,93] Patients with low albumin concentrations and consequently higher free serum concentrations of phenytoin can develop symptoms at lower levels because central nervous system (CNS) levels correlate best with free phenytoin levels.[11,50] Toxic phenytoin levels may produce seizures, but this event is extremely rare; when it occurs, it is usually in the setting of acute overdose in an epileptic patient on chronic therapy.[139] Young children and the elderly may present with atypical manifestations of toxicity. For example, phenytoin-induced chorea and opisthotonic posturing are reported following oral overdoses in children.[93]

There is no reported cardiotoxicity resulting from oral overdoses of phenytoin.[37,148] Intravenous phenytoin, however, impairs myocardial contractility, decreases peripheral vascular resistance, and depresses myocardial conduction. In a large case series, it was associated with a 3.5% incidence of hemodynamic complications.[35] Death has been reported.[49,120,144,150] These complications correlate with rate of administration and total dose and can be partially ascribed to the diluents used in the intravenous preparation of phenytoin: propylene glycol (40%) and ethanol (10%).[94] Propylene glycol in particular depresses myocardial tissue and decreases peripheral vascular resistance (Chap. 56). Fosphenytoin also seems to impair cardiac conduction and contractility. Two reports of large doses of fosphenytoin, 5–10 times in excess of the required dose, administered to young infants with status epilepticus, resulted in bradycardia, hypotension, and asystole.[76,116]

Intravenous phenytoin is commonly associated with local irritation. Extravasation may lead to skin necrosis, possibly necessitating surgical intervention.[23,35,70] The risk of fosphenytoin-induced skin necrosis is minimal because of its increased water solubility and decreased osmolarity.

Chronic high phenytoin levels may result in cerebello-vestibular symptoms, behavioral changes, and encephalopathy. Hyperactivity, confusion, lethargy, and hallucinations characterize behavioral changes.

Adverse Effects

Acute, dose-related adverse events associated with phenytoin therapy include nystagmus, ataxia, dizziness, diplopia, drowsiness, and involuntary movements. Phenytoin-induced involuntary movements are similar to the dyskinesias encountered during long-term antipsychotic drug therapy. All these adverse effects, including the involuntary movements, are completely reversible upon discontinuation of phenytoin therapy.

Adverse events related to long-term phenytoin therapy include gingival hyperplasia, facial coarsening, peripheral neuropathy, bone diseases, and vitamin deficiencies. Gingival hyperplasia is a dose-related effect that occurs in more than 40% of adult patients. Improving dental and gingival care usually prevents this problem. Chronic phenytoin therapy is associated with disturbances in collagen resulting in dysmorphic changes in the nose, lips, and brow. It is also associated with acne, hirsutism, and alopecia. Peripheral neuropathy is characterized by hyporeflexia and sensory deficits. The peripheral neuropathy is common during polydrug therapy and is irreversible. Phenytoin-induced megaloblastic anemia with folic acid deficiency occurs in less than 1% of patients and usually responds to folic acid therapy. Clinically apparent osteomalacia and osteoporosis can result from chronic phenytoin therapy. Phenytoin-induced hypovitaminosis D may contribute to this problem. Vitamin D and calcium supplementation are recommended to treat these problems.[115]

Idiosyncratic adverse events include hematologic disturbances and the hypersensitivity syndrome. Hematopoietic complications include leukopenia, thrombocytopenia, and, very rarely, aplastic anemia and agranulocytosis. The anticonvulsant hypersensitivity syndrome is discussed below. Patients with severe idiosyncratic adverse reactions to phenytoin should never be challenged with phenytoin again.

Diagnostic Testing

Serum phenytoin levels should be performed in all cases of phenytoin exposure. Because of unpredictable absorption, phenytoin levels should be repeated and monitored. Therapeutic levels are 10–20 mg/L. Patients with very high levels may take days or weeks before the levels fall to the therapeutic range.

Individual variations in protein-binding capacity may explain the variance that occurs in the relationship between serum concentration and clinical toxicity. Patients with impaired or decreased protein-binding capacity can theoretically develop symptoms at total phenytoin levels within the therapeutic range. Those at greatest risk include neonates, elderly, hypoalbuminemic, hyperbilirubinemic, and uremic patients, as well as patients on combination therapy with valproic acid, salicylates, sulfonamides, and tolbutamide, because these agents displace phenytoin from its albumin binding sites. In such patients, determination of the free phenytoin fraction is helpful. The free phenytoin fraction can be measured directly by a number of analytical methods, including serum ultrafiltration followed by gas chromatography or enzyme-multiplied immunoassay technique (EMIT).[11,50] Free phenytoin levels should not exceed 2.1 mg/L. Interestingly, CSF levels compare more favorably to free phenytoin than to total phenytoin.[11]

Equation 41–1 approximates the total phenytoin concentration that would be observed based on a given measured serum phenytoin concentration and measured albumin concentration.

$$\text{Phenytoin} = \frac{\text{measured phenytoin}}{(0.25 \times \text{measured albumin}) + 0.1}$$

(Eq. 41–1)

Management

The treatment of patients with acute or chronic phenytoin overdoses remains largely supportive and phenytoin-related deaths are rare, even after massive overdoses. Because the use of multiple-dose activated charcoal (MDAC) reduces the elimination half-life of intravenously administered phenytoin from 44.5 to 22.3 hours, it is recommended in cases where serial serum levels are increasing or persistently elevated although one study demonstrated no improvement in morbidity and mortality.[87] Aggressive lowering of the phenytoin serum level may be harmful to the epileptic patient and multiple doses of activated charcoal should be used cautiously in these patients.

Severe ataxia mandates that patients be followed carefully with serial neurologic examinations. Patients presenting with oral overdoses of phenytoin do not need routine cardiac monitoring.[37,148] Serial blood determinations are necessary because of the unpredictable absorption and delayed peak levels.

Stopping the phenytoin infusion for a few minutes and administering a bolus of 250–500 mL of 0.9% sodium chloride solution best treats propylene glycol–related hypotension. Restarting the infusion at half the initial rate is prudent.[35] Dyskinetic movements occurring during infusion of phenytoin are usually transient and resolve spontaneously in 30–60 minutes.

Prolonged periods of cardiopulmonary resuscitation (CPR) may be beneficial in cases of fosphenytoin or parenteral phenytoin-induced dysrhythmias, in order to allow the (newly converted) phenytoin to distribute into other tissues and the cardiotoxicity to resolve.[76, 117]

Given the extensive protein binding, hemodialysis and hemoperfusion are of little benefit in the management of phenytoin/fosphenytoin toxicity.[67,74] No specific antidote is available.

For a discussion of the management of extravasation see Chapter 8.

CARBAMAZEPINE

Introduced in 1947, carbamazepine, a carbamylated derivative of iminostilbene, is related structurally to the cyclic antidepressants. It is a potent anticonvulsant used in the treatment of seizures, for patients with chronic pain syndromes such as trigeminal neuralgia, for migraine headache prophylaxis, and for bipolar affective disorder. Like phenytoin, it is ineffective in the treatment of absence seizures. Carbamazepine is a first-line therapy for seizures and may be useful especially for pregnant women with epilepsy.[86] Carbamazepine is considered the best anticonvulsant by many and is only available for oral use.

Pharmacokinetics and Toxicokinetics

Carbamazepine is lipophilic with slow and unpredictable absorption following oral administration. Levels may take up to 24 hours to reach a peak, especially following a large overdose.[29,32,44] Carbamazepine also possesses weak anticholinergic properties and can depress gastrointestinal motility, delaying its own absorption. Hence, there is no simple relationship between the dose of carbamazepine and the plasma concentration. There is evidence supporting some degree of enterohepatic circulation following carbamazepine ingestions.[80] Carbamazepine distributes rapidly to all tissues.

It is metabolized primarily by the mixed function oxidase system. CYP 3A4 metabolism produces the pharmacologically active and quantifiable carbamazepine 10,11-epoxide metabolite. This metabolite is further degraded by epoxide hydrolase to carbamazepine-diol, a largely inactive compound.[69] The enzymes responsible for the degradation of carbamazepine are not considered saturable.[36] The elimination of carbamazepine increases over the first few weeks of therapy because of autoinduction, and the half-life on chronic therapy shortens substantially. Therefore, the dose must be increased gradually over a 2–4 week period to a final daily dose of 10–20 mg/kg for adults and 20–70 mg/kg for children. Children require a proportionally higher dose because they eliminate the drug more rapidly. During chronic therapy, the elimination half-life is on the order of 10–20 hours.[80] The elimination half-life is unpredictable and potentially longer after single acute overdoses.

Clinical Manifestations

Acute carbamazepine toxicity produces neurologic signs and symptoms in association with cardiovascular effects.

The initial neurologic disturbances include nystagmus, ataxia, and dysarthria. In patients with large overdoses, they are followed by lethargy and coma. Fluctuations in level of consciousness are common.[29,34,125,127] Carbamazepine toxicity leads to seizure development in nonepileptic patients and causes seizure deterioration in patients with epilepsy. In some cases, an increase in seizure frequency, unaccompanied by other neurologic symptoms, is the only presenting symptom of carbamazepine toxicity. Status epilepticus may also complicate acute carbamazepine toxicity.[130,146] The mechanism underlying carbamazepine-induced seizures are poorly understood.[57,105] In one case series, 55% of adult patients with carbamazepine levels greater than 40 mg/L developed seizures.[57] Children may experience seizures at slightly lower levels.[133]

Cardiovascular effects include sinus tachycardia, hypotension, and cardiac conduction abnormalities. Sinus tachycardia occurs in 35% of overdoses and is ascribed to the anticholinergic effects of the drug.[57] Hypotension is possible and may also be accompanied by myocardial suppression.[44,78] At high levels of carbamazepine, depression of phase 0, phase 2, and phase 4 of the action potential has been reported in cardiac muscle.[137] In a large case series of mostly adult patients with confirmed carbamazepine overdoses, there were a 15% incidence of QRS widening (>100 msec), a 50% incidence of QTc prolongation (>420 msec), and no cases of terminal axis deviation of the QRS in limb leads.[9] The reported ECG abnormalities can be delayed for as long as 20 hours and may occur with chronic therapy.[9,25,32,66,141]

The toxicity of carbamazepine in children differs slightly from that of adults. The pediatric population reportedly experiences a higher incidence of dystonic reactions, choreoathetosis, and seizures and has a lower incidence of electrocardiographic abnormalities.[12,14,63,132,133,140]

Chronic carbamazepine overdose can result in headaches, diplopia, or ataxia. At high serum concentrations of carbamazepine, vasopressin secretion can be stimulated, leading to hyponatremia (syndrome of inappropriate antidiuretic hormone, SIADH).[42,109] This effect is especially detrimental to young children, the elderly, and patients with impaired cardiac function.

Adverse Effects

Dose-related neuropsychiatric events include irritability, impaired concentration, and cognitive and memory impairment. Most symptoms can be controlled by more prudent dose escalation, reduction of the total dose, or usage of sustained-release preparations.

Idiosyncratic adverse events include rashes, hepatitis, drug-induced systemic lupus erythematosus (SLE) syndromes, and hematopoietic disorders. Benign maculopapular or morbilliform rashes occur in 5% of patients, usually in the initial weeks. Isolated mild elevations of the hepatic aminotransferases occur in 10% of individuals and are of little clinical importance. Drug-induced SLE is a serious disorder that can occur in the first 6 months and necessitates discontinuation. Idiosyncratic carbamazepine-induced leukopenia occurs in 10% of patients and is usually self-limited, although 2% of patients will require discontinuation of the drug.[55,119] Aplastic anemia is a serious, often fatal, disorder occurring in 0.5 per 100,000 treatment-years. The anticonvulsant hypersensitivity syndrome is discussed later in this chapter.

Diagnostic Testing

Serum carbamazepine levels should be performed in all cases of carbamazepine exposure. Because of erratic absorption, the levels should be repeated and closely monitored. Therapeutic levels are 4–12 mg/L. Patients receiving multiple anticonvulsants may not tolerate high levels of carbamazepine and should be maintained at 4–8 mg/L. Levels of ≥40 mg/L tend to be associated with increased incidence of coma, seizure, respiratory depression, and cardiotoxicity.[57] Although free carbamazepine levels are available in certain laboratories, they are rarely used in overdose settings.

The contribution of active metabolites to the toxicity of carbamazepine must not be overlooked. Patients receiving multiple anticonvulsants, especially combination therapy with valproic acid and lamotrigine, develop clinical toxicity with carbamazepine concentrations within the reference range and elevated levels of the circulating carbamazepine-10,11-epoxide metabolite. This finding is attributed to the additive inhibitory effects of valproic acid and lamotrigine on the enzyme epoxide hydrolase. The carbamazepine-10,11-epoxide levels in the 1–10 mg/L range are detected.[107] The carbamazepine/carbamazepine-epoxide ratio is usually above 1.7 and is approximately 5 in patients on monotherapy.[107]

Management

Multiple-dose activated charcoal has a definite therapeutic role in the management of patients with carbamazepine overdose, and is particularly helpful by reducing enterohepatic circulation.[99,142] Concretions of carbamazepine should be suspected when plasma levels rise or the occurrence of symptoms is delayed. Cardiac monitoring for occurrence of QRS or QTc abnormalities is recommended. Although not formally studied, sodium bicarbonate should be considered if the QRS duration exceeds 100 msec. Carbamazepine-induced seizures respond to benzodiazepines.

Because carbamazepine is poorly water soluble, hemodialysis is relatively ineffective. Hemoperfusion may be associated with a 20% reduction in serum carbamazepine levels and marginal clinical improvement.[44] Recently, some authors report success with the use of high-efficiency hemodialysis.[126] It must be emphasized that MDAC remains as effective as charcoal hemoperfusion, is much less invasive, and has comparable outcome.[142]

VALPROIC ACID

$$CH_3-CH_2-CH_2 \Big\backslash \atop CH_3-CH_2-CH_2 \Big/ CH-\overset{\displaystyle O}{\overset{\displaystyle \|}{C}}-OH$$

Valproic acid (di-*n*-propylacetic acid) (VPA), a simple branched-chain carboxylic acid, is used to treat a broad spectrum of seizure disorders from simple and complex absence seizures to complex partial and myoclonic seizures. It is also widely used as a mood stabilizer in the management of many psychiatric illnesses, especially bipolar affective disorders for which it is a first-line agent. Other therapeutic uses for VPA include migraine headache prophylaxis and the treatment of minor urinary incontinence following ileoanal anastomosis.

Pharmacokinetics and Toxicokinetics

VPA is available in soft, gelatin capsules, in syrup form, as enteric-coated and ER tablets, and in sprinkle capsules that may be added to food. An intravenous form is available as well, but intramuscular VPA is not well tolerated.

VPA is almost 100% absorbed from the gastrointestinal tract. Peak levels are reached in hours except for enteric-coated preparations, which delay complete absorption for up to 24 hours.[16,53] VPA is 90% protein-bound at therapeutic levels, but this percentage decreases as the VPA level increases.

VPA metabolism is complex. It is extensively metabolized (95%) by hepatocytes in a multistep process. First, VPA is conjugated by glucuronic acid. It is then oxidized in one of two ways: mitochondrial β-oxidation or microsomal ω oxidation. Nine different metabolites are isolated. The three β-oxidation metabolites are the major metabolites and ω- and ω_1-metabolites are relatively less important quantitatively.[33]

Mitochondrial β-oxidation of short-chain fatty acids such as VPA involves activation and linkage to coenzyme A (CoA) followed by transfer to carnitine or undergoes β-oxidation in the mitochondrial matrix. The first steps, the activation and linkage of VPA, occur on the outer mitochondrial membrane and are mediated by the ATP-dependent medium-chain acyl-CoA synthetase, resulting in the formation of valproylCoA. ValproylCoA is transferred to carnitine, resulting in the formation of valproylcarnitine, which is shuttled across the inner mitochondrial membrane to the mitochondrial matrix where it enters a slow, modified form of β-oxidation that yields 3-en-VPACoA. This metabolite is not cleaved thiolytically by any mitochondrial enzymes, but is rather very slowly hydrolyzed to CoA and 3-en-VPA, the major extracellular VPA metabolite that exerts negative feedback on the β-oxidation process. An understanding of VPA metabolism permits the study of its effect on the mitochondrial carnitine pool and β-oxidation[81] (Fig. 41–2).

VPA decreases carnitine stores through a number of different mechanisms. VPA increases carnitine excretion via formation of valproylcarnitine and valproylcarnitine also inhibits the carnitine

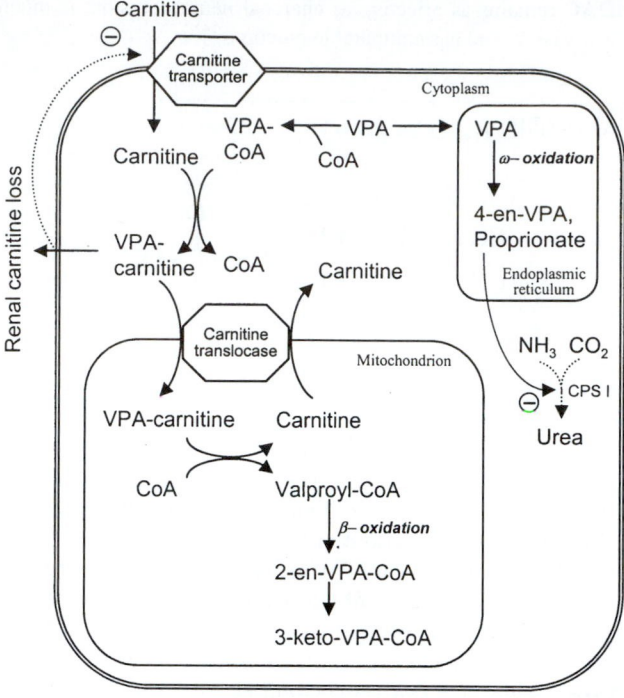

Figure 41–2. Valproic acid metabolism by the hepatocyte. Valproic acid, a short-chain fatty acid, is joined to coenzyme A (CoA) by acyltransferase I and subsequently transferred to carnitine. Valproylcarnitine is shuttled into the mitochondrion where, after transfer back to CoA by acyltransferase II, it undergoes β-oxidation yielding several metabolites. These metabolites sequester CoA, preventing its use in the β-oxidation of other fatty acids; this may lead to a Reyelike syndrome of hepatic steatosis. Alternatively, valproylcarnitine may diffuse from the cell and be renally eliminated, or it may inhibit cellular uptake of carnitine. In either case, the cellular depletion of carnitine shifts valproate metabolism toward microsomal ω-oxidation. This pathway forms 4-en-valproate, a putative hepatotoxin responsible for the severe hepatotoxicity associated with valproic acid. ω-Oxidation products also interfere with carbamoyl phosphate synthase I (CPS I), the initial step in the urea cycle resulting in hyperammonemia. Carnitine therapy steers metabolism toward β-oxidation.

transporter located on the plasma membrane preventing the transport of extracellular carnitine into the cell. The net result is depletion of intramitochondrial carnitine stores. Second, VPA metabolites trap the mitochondrial CoA. Depletion of the mitochondrial CoA pool then sequesters acyl carnitine, resulting in a further decrease in free mitochondrial carnitine stores. Mitochondrial CoA depletion may also negatively affect β-oxidation. Inhibition of β-oxidation decreases adenosine triphosphate (ATP) production and interferes with the ATP-dependent carnitine transporter located on the plasma membrane[110] (Fig. 41–2).

The predominant effect of carnitine depletion is impaired transport of long-chain fatty acids across the inner mitochondrial membrane and subsequent interruption of β-oxidation. Other effects include loss of acceptance of toxic acyl moieties from CoA, inhibition of α-ketoacid oxidation, accumulation of products of peroxisomal β-oxidation, and interruption of the carnitine-based esterification process that protects the urea cycle, the citric acid cycle, and the pathways of gluconeogenesis from toxic metabolites. Interruption of the urea cycle results in accumulation of ammonia. This finding is supported by the fact that there is a significant inverse correlation between plasma carnitine levels and blood ammonia values in patients on chronic VPA therapy.[101] Furthermore, interruption of β-oxidation will shift the metabolism of VPA predominantly toward ω-oxidation and excessive production of 4-en-VPA, a suspected hepatotoxin. VPA-induced hypocarnitinemia is associated with hyperammonemia. This is possible due to the inhibition by ω-oxidation metabolites of carbamoyl phosphate synthase I, a key urea cycle enzyme.

Clinical Manifestations

Mild overdoses of VPA result in a benign clinical course characterized by self-limited drowsiness. Coma and respiratory depression typically occur with overdoses greater than 30 mg/kg. Dysarthria, nystagmus, ataxia, and tremor do not occur. The neurotoxicity is less severe if the ingestion represents an acute overdose in a chronically treated patient.[64]

Metabolic complications following acute valproic acid overdoses include hypernatremia, hypocalcemia, metabolic acidosis, hypocarnitinemia, and hyperammonemia.[7,68] These metabolic disturbances are usually present at an early stage.[110]

Hyperammonemia (>60 μmol/L) occurs in 35–45% of patients on chronic VPA therapy.[26,101] It may also occur after acute overdose in patients on chronic therapy, but has not been reported after acute overdose in patients who are not on VPA therapy.[53,95,96]

Metabolic acidosis and elevation of serum lactate occur following acute massive VPA overdose and are not necessarily related to hypotension.[39,61] Severe metabolic acidosis resulting from massive VPA overdoses is a poor prognostic sign.[7,24,53,61,95,96,116]

Bone marrow suppression occurs 3–5 days following acute massive overdoses of VPA and is characterized by leukopenia, thrombocytopenia, and anemia.[7,24,116] These hematopoietic disturbances resolve spontaneously within a few days.

Pancreatitis and hepatic and renal failure are rare manifestations of acute toxicity.[7,24,68] Chronic valproic acid therapy may lead to hepatotoxicity secondary to the aforementioned metabolic aberration rather than to a hypersensitivity reaction. The clinical findings may vary from asymptomatic elevation of aminotransferases to fatal hepatitis.

Adverse Effects

Valproic acid–induced hepatotoxicity may be classified into 4 distinct subtypes: transient reversible elevation of aminotransferases, reversible hyperammonemia, toxic hepatitis, and a Reyelike syndrome.[26, 110] The mechanism for VPA-induced hepatotoxicity may be related to a relative imbalance between β- and ω-oxidation, and to VPA-induced carnitine deficiency. Transient reversible aminotransferase elevation responds to reduction in dosing, supplemental carnitine therapy, or discontinuation of VPA. Gastrointestinal symptoms, anorexia, and seizures may precede the development of fulminant hepatic failure. Fulminant hepatitis, when it occurs, is not consistently preceded by abnormalities in liver enzymes.[31,52,115] The prognosis is improved if therapy is discontinued promptly. The incidence of fatal idiosyncratic hepatotoxicity is 1/49,000 adults and 1/800 children.[110] Risk factors for valproic acid–induced fulminant hepatitis include age less than 2 years, the presence of neurologic or metabolic disorders, recent liver dysfunction, ketogenic diets, and polydrug therapy. The Reyelike syndrome is probably due to depletion of mitochondrial CoA. Other important adverse effects include tremors, pancreatitis, and alopecia.

Diagnostic Testing

Serum valproic acid levels should be performed in all cases of valproic acid exposure. The levels should be repeated every 2–3 hours and closely monitored. Therapeutic levels reside in the 50–100-mg/L range, although higher levels are used by some clinicians. Free valproic acid levels are available in certain laboratories, but their clinical relevance in the overdose setting remains unproven.

Some authors measure the blood carnitine levels and β- and ω-metabolites in the urine. Free blood carnitine levels ≤20 μM or a acylcarnitine/free carnitine ratio ≥0.4 is an index of carnitine deficiency. The latter is a more precise measurement of drug-induced hypocarnitinemia. All 9 VPA metabolites can be measured in the urine. 4-en-VPA may be elevated in patients with acute or chronic overdoses, indicating excessive ω-oxidation. 2-en-VPA may be low or absent from the urine of VPA-intoxicated patients secondary to VPA-induced inhibition of β-oxidation or carnitine depletion. 2-en-VPA levels increase 1–3 days following acute ingestion. This represents a shift from predominantly ω- to β-oxidation and normalization of hepatic functions.[61,96]

Serum ammonia levels are inversely correlated with carnitine levels in patients on chronic therapy. They should be monitored if the patient presents with an altered mental status following overdose with VPA.

Management

Supportive management is all that is required to ensure complete recovery in most patients with VPA overdoses. Appropriate airway intervention and maintenance of good renal output, as well as discontinuation of all medications likely to affect VPA metabolism, are usually sufficient.

Multiple-dose activated charcoal reduces the half-life of valproic acid from a mean of 12 hours to 4.8 hours and is recommended in patients with large acute overdoses and in instances where serum levels are continuously rising.[39] Although VPA is extensively protein-bound and theoretically not amenable to MDAC, the percentage of bound VPA decreases significantly (89% to 29%) as the plasma concentration increases.[39] Whole-bowel irrigation may be beneficial in the treatment of patients with large acute overdoses of enteric-coated preparations of VPA.[53]

In vitro studies suggest that naloxone may have GABA antagonistic properties and may inhibit the effects of VPA on GABA metabolism.[30,59] Two case reports describe rapid resolution of CNS symptoms in VPA-overdosed patients following the administration of naloxone.[3,136] These patients had minimally elevated VPA levels (<200 mg/L). Other reports, however, showed no effect in patients with much higher VPA levels (>1000 mg/L).[24,95] Clinical experience does not support the use of naloxone to reverse valproic acid–induced CNS depression.

The role of carnitine supplementation in VPA overdoses is not well defined. In spite of a lack of controlled studies, the Pediatric Neurology Advisory Committee indicated, in 1996, that carnitine supplementation should be administered to children with VPA overdoses.[28] Other authors are more precise and recommend prophylactic carnitine supplementation to children who have acutely

ingested more than 400 mg/kg of valproic acid.[61,96] Administration of prophylactic parenteral carnitine led to normalization of β- and ω-oxidation within 3 days in 2 children presenting after acute VPA ingestions, each with VPA levels above 1300 mg/L.[61,96] Caution is advised, however, in the interpretation of these reports. Hepatic failure following acute severe VPA overdose is a rarity. In fact, a review of all published cases of acute or acute-on-chronic overdoses with VPA levels above 1000 mg/L reveals only 1 case of mild, transient, and clinically irrelevant elevation in aminotransferases.[7] The absence of enzyme elevation following prophylactic carnitine therapy probably reflects the natural history of the overdoses and not the hepatoprotective effect of carnitine. Supplemental carnitine is strongly recommended, however, in certain pediatric subpopulations: pediatric patients younger than 2 years of age who are receiving VPA, especially those with complex neurologic disorders requiring more than 1 anticonvulsant; and pediatric patients with poor nutrition, or failure to thrive, or who are on ketogenic diets, which are commonly used to treat seizure patients. Supplemental carnitine is also probably beneficial to patients with VPA-induced hepatic dysfunction or hyperammonemia regardless of the chronicity of the exposure. There are few data to support the use of carnitine in patients with VPA-induced CNS depression. The delineation of the prophylactic and therapeutic role of carnitine in acute or chronic overdoses necessitates further study.

Carnitine should be administered in doses of 100 mg/kg/d to 2 g/d divided in 3 doses orally or 150–500 mg/kg/d divided in 3 doses intravenously.[110] It should be administered for a period of 3–4 days or until clinical improvement is noted. Carnitor (Sigma-Tau, Gaithersburg, MD) is available as an injection (200 mg/mL) and as a solution (100 mg/mL) for oral use. Carnitine is generally well tolerated and is primarily associated with gastrointestinal effects. Large doses can produce a fishy body odor.[48,110]

Hemodialysis and hemoperfusion increase clearance of valproic acid and, occasionally, produce some improvement in clinical outcome.[53,95] Extracorporeal removal of valproic acid should probably be reserved for patients with rapid deterioration, evidence of hepatic dysfunction, apparent continued absorption of the drug, and serum levels in excess of 1000 mg/L.

GABAPENTIN

Gabapentin is a chemically unique cyclohexane derivative of GABA and has become an approved adjunct medication in the treatment of partial seizures with and without secondarily generalized seizures in adults. It is currently also used as a treatment for posttraumatic stress disorder, behavioral disorders, mood disorders, bruxism, and a number of neurologic disturbances where it is used in doses exceeding 70 mg/kg.

Pharmacokinetics and Toxicokinetics

The bioavailability of gabapentin is approximately 60% at therapeutic dose ranges. It is not appreciably metabolized in humans and all its pharmacologic activity is attributed to the parent compound. Gabapentin is not bound to plasma proteins and is excreted entirely by the kidney. It is highly lipophilic and easily crosses the blood-brain barrier. Dosage adjustments must be made in patients with decreased renal function (creatinine clearance <60 mL/min). It is not metabolized and does not affect the mixed function oxidase system.

Clinical Manifestations

Sedation, ataxia, and slurred speech are observed following acute gabapentin overdose.[40,41,43] In a large case series, 76 acute, self-reported gabapentin overdoses were divided into 2 groups: single versus mixed drug ingestions. In the single group (n=20), 15% were treated at home and 85% were treated and released from the ED. No moderate, major effects or deaths occurred. In the second group (n=56), the clinical picture was comparable to that expected from the coingestant. Laboratory confirmation of the ingestion was not obtained in either group.[58] The clinical features of acute gabapentin toxicity compare favorably to the serious neurologic and cardiovascular toxicities that occur with phenytoin and carbamazepine overdoses.[40,41,43]

In one case report of chronic overdose in a patient with renal failure, tremulousness and cognitive deficits were noted. The serum level was 85 mg/dL. Symptoms were self-limited and resolved following a dose adjustment.[143]

A gabapentin withdrawal syndrome has recently been described.

Adverse Effects

Gabapentin can cause somnolence, dizziness, ataxia, fatigue, nystagmus, headache, and rhinitis. Most of these adverse events disappear with prolonged therapy.

Movement disorders, such as oculogyric crises, asterixis, and choreoathetoid movements, occasionally are associated with gabapentin therapy. All symptoms resolve upon discontinuation and without pharmacologic intervention.[18,62,111] Catatonia following abrupt withdrawal of gabapentin therapy is reported.[118]

In spite of these reports of gabapentin-related adverse events, available data support the relatively benign nature of this anticonvulsive agent.

Diagnostic Testing

A therapeutic plasma concentration for seizure control of 2–15 mg/L is recommended. Because gabapentin is not appreciably protein-bound, this range essentially represents free gabapentin. The preferred method for analysis for gabapentin is high-pressure liquid chromatography.

Management

The treatment of patients with gabapentin overdose is largely supportive. Activated charcoal may be useful. Patients with persistent neurologic symptoms need to be admitted to the hospital. There are no available data on the value of hemodialysis or hemoperfusion and no specific antidote exists for gabapentin overdose.

FELBAMATE

Felbamate is a phenyl dicarbamate derivative structurally similar to meprobamate, which received FDA approval in 1993, with indications similar to gabapentin and lamotrigine. Because of its potential for causing hepatic failure and aplastic anemia, the FDA recommends that felbamate be considered a therapy of last resort that is to be used only after written consent is obtained.[98]

Pharmacokinetics

Felbamate is rapidly absorbed from the gastrointestinal tract. Peak levels of therapeutic doses are reached within 1–4 hours. Felbamate has low plasma protein binding and no active metabolites, and 90% of a dose is excreted unchanged in the urine. Felbamate has a plasma elimination half-life in the range of 13–23 hours in adults. The recommended daily dose is 50 mg/kg/d in 3 or 4 divided doses.[54]

Clinical Manifestations

There are very few reports of acute felbamate overdoses. Mild lethargy and gastrointestinal symptoms characterized one report of acute felbamate toxicity where felbamate levels of 141 and 111 mg/L were measured, respectively, 4 and 7 hours postingestion. All symptoms resolved spontaneously over the next few hours and the patient was discharged. The hepatic aminotransferases and the blood counts remained within normal limits 4 hours postingestion and on followup 6 weeks later.[98]

Intubation was required in 1 report of acute valproic acid and felbamate ingestion with peak levels of 200 mg/L and 470 mg/L, respectively. It resulted in crystalluria and reversible acute renal failure and the patient made an uneventful recovery.[113]

In animal studies on its chronic neurotoxicity, felbamate compared favorably to phenytoin and carbamazepine, with a profile similar to that of valproic acid and a large therapeutic index.

Adverse Effects

Weight gain or loss, insomnia or somnolence, nausea, vomiting, pancreatitis, and psychosis following felbamate are documented.[104] Fulminant hepatic failure is associated with chronic felbamate therapy in case reports.[102] The number of cases reported greatly exceeds the expected incidence of hepatic failure. Felbamate-induced hepatic failure has a 20% mortality rate. Among individuals treated with felbamate the incidence of aplastic anemia is about 100-fold greater than expected. Felbamate-induced aplastic anemia is associated with a high mortality rate.[1]

Diagnostic Testing

Felbamate levels can be measured by high-performance liquid chromatography. Levels greater than 135 mg/L are potentially toxic.

Management

The treatment of felbamate toxicity is largely supportive. Activated charcoal may be useful. There are no data on the value of hemodialysis or hemoperfusion.

LAMOTRIGINE

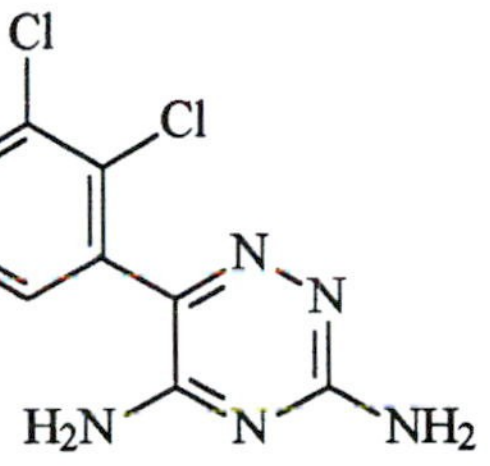

Lamotrigine is an anticonvulsant approved as an adjunctive medication for the treatment of partial seizures or in those adult patients with secondarily generalized seizures. An increasing body of literature also advocates the use of lamotrigine therapy in cases of refractory bipolar mood disorder. It is not structurally related to other anticonvulsants.[47]

Pharmacokinetics and Toxicokinetics

Lamotrigine's bioavailability is 98%. It is metabolized solely by glucuronidation to an inactive metabolite. It does not affect the cytochrome P450 system. Its elimination half-life is approximately 25 hours, but can be halved in the presence of phenytoin and carbamazepine and doubled in the presence of valproic acid. The mechanism for these interactions is not well elucidated. It is believed that phenytoin and carbamazepine can induce glucuronidation and increase elimination of lamotrigine. Valproic acid may compete with lamotrigine for the same step in the glucuronidation process and decrease the elimination of lamotrigine. A significantly reduced clearance of lamotrigine occurs in patients with Gilbert syndrome (a syndrome of defective glucuronidation). Lamotrigine does not affect the cytochrome P450 system or the metabolism of other drugs except when administered concomitantly with carbamazepine and valproic acid, where it is associated with accumulation of the carbamazepine epoxide metabolite.[47]

Clinical Manifestations

Overdoses with between 19 and 64 mg/kg of lamotrigine are reported. Signs and symptoms include lethargy, ataxia, nystagmus, slurred speech, seizures, and electrocardiographic abnormalities.

Rotational nystagmus, slurred speech, and ataxia developed in a patient with a lamotrigine level of 35.8 mg/L following an acute-on-chronic overdose. No electrocardiographic abnormalities occurred and the patient made an uneventful recovery.[100]

A previously healthy toddler developed seizures 50 minutes after an acute lamotrigine ingestion. The lamotrigine level, 2 hours postingestion, was 3.8 mg/L. Repeat levels were lower. Seizure activity did not recur and the ataxia and muscle weakness resolved over 48 hours.[13]

An adult who ingested 19.2 mg/kg of lamotrigine developed mild lethargy, vertical and horizontal nystagmus, and QRS prolon-

gation (112 msec). The reported peak serum level was 17.4 mg/L. Other explanations for the QRS prolongation were not sought.[17] The 2-N-methyl metabolite of lamotrigine causes QRS prolongation in animals and may accumulate in humans when glucuronidation is defective, although this finding has never been reported in humans.[13,38]

Chronic overdoses of lamotrigine result in multiorgan involvement, often sparing the CNS. Rashes, elevation in hepatic aminotransferases, and elevation of serum creatinine phosphokinase are documented in a single case. All abnormalities resolved upon withdrawal of the drug.[97]

Adverse Effects

The adverse effects associated with lamotrigine are usually mild and resolve with dosage reduction. The most frequently reported adverse events are dizziness, headache, diplopia, and ataxia. A rash develops in 10% of patients and usually responds to discontinuation of therapy. However, some patients may progress to Stevens-Johnson syndrome. At high risk are children ≤ 16 years old and those patients whose dose is rapidly titrated. Sudden deaths while on chronic lamotrigine therapy are reported. Most of these patients had a rapidly progressing illness with rhabdomyolysis, disseminated intravascular coagulation, and renal failure secondary to status epilepticus.[84,123] Lamotrigine can induce the anticonvulsant hypersensitivity syndrome.[123]

Diagnostic Testing

Lamotrigine levels can be measured by high-performance liquid chromatography. Levels greater than 5 mg/L are potentially toxic. The 2-N-methyl metabolite is detected in animals but has yet to be quantified in humans, even after large overdoses.[13]

Management

Orogastric lavage may be used in cases of large lamotrigine overdose. Ipecac-induced emesis is contraindicated because of the potential for seizures. Activated charcoal therapy should probably be administered. Signs and symptoms of lamotrigine overdose, including ECG changes, usually resolve over 48 hours without any specific therapy.[17,100] Until more is known about the cardiac toxicity of lamotrigine, close ECG monitoring for a period of 24 hours is recommended. If the initial QRS duration is longer than 100 msec, consideration should be given to the administration of hypertonic sodium bicarbonate, although this is not studied. Lamotrigine-induced seizures can be treated with benzodiazepines.[13] There are no data on the value of hemodialysis and hemoperfusion.

VIGABATRIN

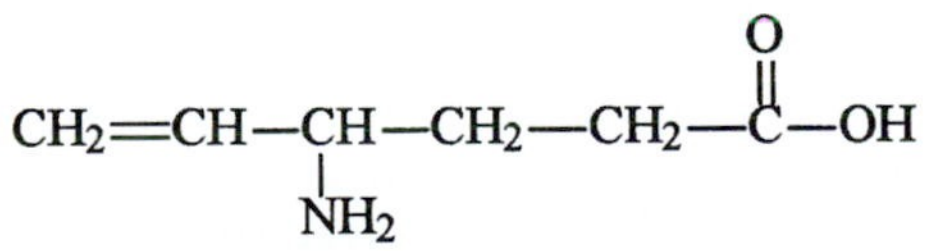

Vigabatrin, structurally similar to GABA, is a stereospecific irreversible inhibitor of GABA-transaminase. The R-enantiomer has virtually no effect, whereas the S-enantiomer inhibits the enzyme.[46]

Pharmacokinetics and Toxicokinetics

Although vigabatrin possesses a short elimination half-life, its duration of action is 24 hours. As for gabapentin, dosage adjustments are necessary in the patient with impaired renal function.[46] Experimental data in animals demonstrate that vigabatrin does not interact, potentiate, or increase serum levels of diazepam or other GABAergic agents.[114] It does not affect the mixed function oxidase system. Additional pharmacokinetic data are available in Table 41–1.

Clinical Manifestations

There are 4 case reports of acute vigabatrin overdose. Long-term psychosis developed in 1 patient who overdosed on 8–10 g of vigabatrin.[122] Coma occurred after a mixed ingestion including 30 g of vigabatrin.[89] One patient ingested a total of 60 g of vigabatrin and presented with severe agitation.[27]

Chronic toxicity may result in psychosis, which is usually mild and transient.[121,122,129] Chronic ingestion of 14 g/d for 3 days resulted in vertigo and tremor, and in an uneventful recovery.[89]

Adverse Effects

Several vigabatrin-induced adverse events are observed. Neuropathologic studies in rats, mice, and dogs find microvacuoles in the CNS white matter.[106] Studies in humans do not confirm this finding. However, vigabatrin therapy is associated with an increased incidence of depression (12%) and psychosis (2.5%) in a large case series.[79] This finding may be linked to the regional increases in dopamine metabolites found in the cerebrospinal fluid and the decreased selective dopamine receptor binding observed in the CNS following vigabatrin therapy. There is no simple biochemical relationship between vigabatrin therapy and psychosis, but the risk of developing psychosis is probably limited.

Diagnostic Testing

Vigabatrin levels can be measured by high-performance liquid chromatography. Plasma levels greater than 80 mg/L are potentially toxic.

Management

The treatment of vigabatrin toxicity is largely supportive. Severe delirium is best treated with intravenous benzodiazepines and, occasionally, administration of an antipsychotic.[27,122] Some cases of mild vigabatrin-induced psychosis resolve simply by withdrawal of the medication.[79]

TOPIRAMATE

Topiramate is approved as adjunctive therapy for adults with partial seizures. Although the precise mechanism of action is unclear, it can block sodium channels, enhance the action of GABA, and diminish the action of glutamate excitatory receptor stimulation.[108]

Pharmacokinetics and Toxicokinetics

The therapeutic dose of topiramate is 50–400 mg daily. Peak plasma levels are reached in about 2 hours. Seventy percent of the drug is eliminated unchanged in the urine. The plasma elimination half-life is about 22 hours.[65] Topiramate has a sulfamate moiety that can interfere with carbonic anhydrase enzyme activity.[127]

Clinical Manifestations

There are no reports of acute or chronic overdose in the literature. Large overdoses are predicted to cause neurologic impairment, cardiac conduction defects, metabolic acidosis, and electrolyte disturbances based on its mechanism of action.

TABLE 41–1.   Pharmacokinetics of Anticonvulsants

	Dose (mg/kg/d)	Time to Peak Plasma Level (h)	Therapeutic Serum Levels (mg/L)	Vd (L/kg)	Plasma Protein Binding (%)	Urinary Elimination Unchanged (%)	Active Metabolites	Plasma Elimination Half-Life (h)
Carbamazepine	5–70 children 5–30 adults	3–24 in overdose	4–12	0.8–1.8	75	1	CBZ 10, 11-epoxide	6–20 overdose 4.9–11.5 chronic
Felbamate	15–45 children 25–50 adults	4	17–134	0.75	25	40	None	20–23
Gabapentin	10–30 children 8–70 adults	3	1–2	0.8	0	100	None	5–7
Lamotrigine	5–15 children 3–7 adults	2.5	0.5–4.5	1.2	55	10	None	14–50
Phenytoin	3–8	5–24 in overdose	10–20	0.6	>90	<5	None	6–60
Topiramate	3–22 adults	1–4	14–27	0.5–0.8	15	60	None	20–30
Valproic acid	15–60	1–24 in overdose	50–120	0.1–0.2	>90*	<5	2-en-VPA 3-OHVPA 3-keto-VPA	6–18
Vigabatrin	14–57 adults	4	20–80	0.8	0	100	None	4–8

*Concentration dependent.
See references 8, 46, 47, 54, 71, 91, and 108.

Adverse Effects

Adverse effects noted with therapeutic regimens include lethargy, confusion, somnolence, dizziness, ataxia, diplopia, paresthesias, and weight loss.[112] Nephrolithiasis occurs in about 1–2% of patients, and may be the result of the interference with the carbonic anhydrase enzyme.

Diagnostic Testing

Topiramate levels are performed by gas chromatography. Therapeutic levels are between 4 and 27 mg/L.

Management

Overdose management should include basic GI decontamination with activated charcoal. Electrocardiographic monitoring for potential effects on the myocardial sodium channel is recommended as is monitoring of serum electrolytes and acid-base status.

OTHER ANTICONVULSANTS

Ethosuximide

Ethosuximide, which affects T calcium channels, has largely replaced trimethadione in the management of absence seizures. Its major metabolite, the hydroxyethyl derivative, is inactive. Acute toxicity presents with sedation and gastrointestinal symptoms. Adverse effects include behavioral disturbances, psychosis (especially in children), Stevens-Johnson syndrome, aplastic anemia, and drug-induced systemic lupus erythematosus.

Tiagabine

Tiagabine is a novel anticonvulsive agent with pro-GABA effects. The tiagabine dose range is 160–320 mg/d divided in 4 doses. It is rapidly absorbed after an oral dose, and quickly metabolized in the liver. Its elimination half-life is 4–13 hours. The elimination half-life is reduced by 50% in patients on enzyme-inducing anticonvulsive agents.[82] Therapeutic levels are 15–420 mg/L. Few adverse events are reported.[77] Development of severe CNS depression was reported following an acute overdose of tiagabine and phenytoin. The patient recovered uneventfully after 12 hours of supportive care.[75]

Oxcarbazepine

Oxcarbazepine recently received FDA approval for both adjunctive therapy and monotherapy in adults and adjunctive therapy in children. It is rapidly absorbed after an oral dose and is rapidly metabolized in the liver. Hepatic noncytochrome P450–related metabolism yields the 10-monohydroxy metabolite (MHD), which is responsible for the pharmacologic effects of the drug. Further metabolism of MHD by conjugation with glucuronic acid is increased in the presence of phenobarbital, phenytoin, and carbamazepine. The starting dose of oxcarbazepine is 300 mg bid, which can be increased to 2400 mg/d. Oxcarbazepine is known to induce CYP2C19 and inhibit CYP3A4/5, leading to potential serious drug interactions (Table 41–2). For example, it can increase phenytoin levels and decrease the effectiveness of oral contraceptives. Two significant differences between carbamazepine and oxcarbazepine should be noted. Oxcarbazepine is associated with a

TABLE 41–2. The Anticonvulsants and Cytochrome P450 System

	Metabolized by	Induces the Following	Inhibits the Following	References
Carbamazepine	1A2 2C8 2C9 3A4	2C9 3A subtype	None	69, 133
Felbamate	3A4/2E1	3A4	2C19	54
Phenobarbital	2C9 2C19	2C 3A	None	7
Phenytoin	2C9 2C19	2C subtype 3A subtype	None	73
Topiramate	None	β-Oxidation	2C19	65
Valproic acid	2A6 2C9 2C19		2C9	10

lower incidence of skin rash but is frequently associated with hyponatremia. Overdose management includes basic GI decontamination, administration of activated charcoal, and close cardiac, neurologic, and metabolic monitoring. ECG abnormalities, such as QRS prolongation, are expected following such an overdose, but have not been reported.[88]

Levetiracetam

Levetiracetam is the seventh drug recently approved by the FDA for adjunct therapy of partial seizures in adults. The exact mechanism of action is unknown. Levetiracetam is rapidly absorbed. It is not metabolized by the hepatic CYP450 system and is not protein bound. It is unlikely to cause any drug interactions. Among other anticonvulsants only gabapentin and vigabatrin share these characteristics. Dosage ranges from 1000 to 3000 mg/d in 2 divided doses. Lower doses are recommended for patients with renal insufficiency and for the elderly. Adverse effects include somnolence, asthenia, and psychiatric symptoms in 13% of patients. Polycythemia and leukocytosis are rarely reported and do not necessitate discontinuation of the drug. Overdose management should include basic GI decontamination, administration of activated charcoal therapy, and frequent cardiac and neurologic monitoring. Although levetiracetam-induced psychosis responds to withdrawal of therapy, symptoms may take up to 2 weeks to resolve[88] (Tables 41–3 and 41–4).

Anticonvulsant Hypersensitivity Syndrome

Ill-defined since it was first described in 1950, the anticonvulsant hypersensitivity syndrome (AHS) is a disorder that probably occurs in 1 of every 1000 to 10,000 exposures to anticonvulsants. AHS is traditionally associated with exposures to aromatic anticonvulsants such as phenytoin, carbamazepine, and phenobarbital. Recent literature supports the inclusion of the nonaromatic lamotrigine as a causative agent. The incidence remains the same regardless of gender and ethnic origin. The development of AHS may be under genetic control; first-degree relatives of patients with AHS have a 1:4 risk of developing this affliction.[72]

TABLE 41–3. **Drug Interactions**

	Increases Levels of	Decreases Levels of	Drug Toxicity Enhanced by	Drug Anticonvulsant Effect Decreased by
Carbamazepine	None known	Doxycycline, felbamate, haloperidol, lamotrigine, ?methadone, phenytoin, primidone, tiagabine, valproic acid, warfarin	Allopurinol, cimetidine, danazol, diltiazem, fluoxetine, fluvoxamine, gemfibrozil, INH, ketoconazole, lamotrigine, macrolides, nefazodone, nicotine, propoxyphene, protease inhibitors, verapamil	Benzodiazepines, carbamazepine, felbamate, isotretinoin, pheno-barbital, phenytoin, primidone, succinimides, valproic acid
Felbamate	Carbamazepine epoxide, phenytoin, valproic acid	Carbamazepine	Valproic acid, gabapentin	Carbamazepine, phenytoin
Gabapentin	Felbamate	None known	None known	Antacids
Lamotrigine	Carbamazepine	None known	Valproic acid	Antituberculous agents, carb-amazepine, phenytoin, phen-obarbital
Phenobarbital	Valproic acid metabolites	Carbamazepine, corticosteroids, doxycycline, estradiol, griseofulvin, lamotrigine, phenytoin, propranolol, quinidine, theophylline, valproic acid, warfarin	Acetazolamide, chloramphenicol, CNS depressants, dextro-propoxyphene, furosemide, methylphenidate, MAOIs, valproic acid	Ammonium chloride, antacids, folic acid, pyridoxine, warfarin
Phenytoin	N-acetyl-p-benzo quinoneimine (NAPQI), oral anticoagulants, phenobarbital, primidone	Amiodarone, carbamazepine, cardiac glycosides, contra-ceptives, corticosteroids, cyclosporine, disopyramide, dopamine, doxycycline, furosemide, haloperidol, influenza vaccine, levodopa, methadone, mexilitene, phenothiazines, quinidine, tiagabine, theophylline, tolbutamide, valproic acid	Allopurinol, amiodarone, chlor-amphenicol, chlorphenira-mine, clarithromycin, cloxa-cillin, cimetidine, disulfiram, ethosuximide, felbamate, fluconazole, fluoxetine, flu-voxamine, imipramine, INH, methylphenidate, metronidazole, miconazole, omeprazole, oral anticoagulants, phenylbutazone, sulfonamides, trimethoprim, tolbutamide, tolazamide, topiramate, valproic acid	Antacids, antineoplastic agents, carbamazepine, calcium, diazepam, diazoxide, ethanol (chronic), folic acid, influenza vaccine, loxapine, nitrofuran-toin, phenobarbital, phenylbu-tazone, pyridoxine, rifampin, salicylates, sulfisoxazole, sucralfate, theophylline, tolbutamide, valproate, vigabatrin
Topiramate	Phenytoin	Contraceptives	None known	Carbamazepine, phenytoin, val-proic acid
Valproic acid	Felbamate, lamotrigine, phenobarbital, primidone	Carbamazepine, tiagabine	Cimetidine, felbamate, ranitidine	Antacids, carbamazepine, chlorpromazine, felbamate, INH, methotrexate, phen-obarbital, phenytoin, prim-idone, salicylates
Vigabatrin	None known	Phenytoin	None known	None known

See references 2, 7, 8, 10, 46, 47, 54, 73, 114, and 134.

AHS occurs most frequently within the first 2 months of ther-apy and is not related to dose or serum concentration. The patho-physiology of AHS is related to the accumulation of toxic metabolites, notably the arene oxide metabolites, resulting from insufficient detoxification by the enzyme epoxide hydrolase. The arene oxides are capable of binding to macromolecules and caus-ing cellular necrosis. Interestingly, the same metabolite is believed to cause other serious dermatologic reactions such as Stevens-Johnson syndrome and toxic epidermal necrolysis. The pathophys-iology of lamotrigine-induced hypersensitivity syndrome remains largely unknown.[123]

AHS is defined by a triad of fever, rash, and internal organ in-volvement. The initial symptoms include fever, malaise, pharyngi-tis, and, occasionally, cervical adenopathy. A skin eruption usually follows, which is characterized by macular erythema and evolves into a papular rash primarily involving the trunk and then the extremities. Severely affected cases develop a Stevens-John-son syndrome or toxic epidermal necrolysis. Other dermatologic manifestations include pustule formation, facial edema, and con-junctivitis. The rash usually spares the other mucous membranes. Internal organ involvement usually occurs 1–2 weeks into the syn-drome. The liver is the most frequently affected organ, although involvement of the CNS (encephalitis), cardiac muscle (myocardi-tis), lungs (pneumonitis), renal system (nephritis), and thyroid (thyroiditis) is possible. Liver disturbances range from mild eleva-tion in aminotransferases to fulminant hepatic necrosis.

Prompt discontinuation of the offending agent is essential to prevent symptom progression. Patients with all but the mildest

TABLE 41–4. Adverse Events Associated with Anticonvulsants

	Predictable	Idiosyncratic
Carbamazepine	Diplopia	Agranulocytosis
	Hyponatremia	Aplastic anemia
	Hypocalcemia	Hepatotoxicity
	Orofacial dyskinesias	Photosensitivity
	Cardiac dysrhythmias	Stevens-Johnson syndrome
		Lupus syndrome
		Morbilliform rash
		Thrombocytopenia
		Pseudolymphoma
		Myocarditis
		Anticonvulsant hypersensitivity syndrome
Felbamate	Irritability	Fulminant hepatic failure
	Insomnia	Aplastic anemia
	Anorexia	
Gabapentin	Diplopia	Dystonic movements
	Ataxia	Asterixis
Lamotrigine	Tremor	Agranulocytosis
	Diplopia	Rash
	Ataxia	Erythema multiforme
		Stevens-Johnson syndrome
		Toxic epidermal necrolysis
		Anticonvulsant hypersensitivity syndrome
Phenytoin	Anorexia	Blood dyscrasias
	Aggression	Lupus syndrome
	Ataxia	Reduced IgA
	Cognitive impairment	Pseudolymphoma
	Depression	Peripheral neuropathy
	Nystagmus	Pseudotumour cerebri
	Neonatal hemorrhage	Rash
	Gingival hypertrophy	Stevens-Johnson syndrome
	Coarse facies	Dupuytren contractures
	Hirsutism	Hepatotoxicity
	Megaloblastic anemia	Teratogenicity
	Hyperglycemia	Gingival hyperplasia
	Hypocalcemia	Aplastic anemia
	Osteomalacia	Anticonvulsant hypersensitivity syndrome
	Hypothyroidism	
Topiramate	Diplopia	
	Weight loss	
	Paresthesias	
	Nephrolithiasis	
Valproic acid	Anorexia	Pancreatitis
	Tremor	Hepatotoxicity
	Alopecia	Thrombocytopenia
	Peripheral edema	Hyperammonemia
	Rash	Encephalopathy
	Weight gain	Teratogenicity
Vigabatrin	Weight gain	Psychosis
	Behavioral changes	

Most anticonvulsants cause dizziness, sedation, nausea, headache, and other mild gastrointestinal and central nervous system adverse effects.

syndrome should be admitted to the hospital. In severe cases, prednisone 1–2 mg/kg/d may be beneficial. This recommendation is based on a single case report.[21] The role of corticosteroids in mild cases remains controversial. If steroids are administered, gradual weaning is recommended because symptoms can reoccur after abrupt discontinuation. In one case study, 90% of patients with AHS showed in vitro cross-reactivity to a different aromatic

anticonvulsant.[130] Based on this evidence, avoidance of phenytoin, carbamazepine, phenobarbital, and potentially oxcarbazepine is recommended. Although there is no evidence of cross-reactivity to lamotrigine, it should probably be avoided as well. Benzodiazepines, valproic acid, gabapentin, topiramate, and vigabatrin are safer alternatives.[130]

SUMMARY

All anticonvulsant drugs produce CNS symptoms in overdose situations. Differentiation on the basis of clinical findings is difficult. Lethargy and sedation occur following overdoses with almost all of these anticonvulsants, but ataxia, slurred speech, and nystagmus occur predominantly with phenytoin and carbamazepine.

Coma is reported following overdoses with carbamazepine, phenytoin, and valproic acid, but is rare with the second-generation anticonvulsants. Seizures occur with carbamazepine, phenytoin, and lamotrigine overdoses.

Hemodynamic instability and abnormal electrocardiograms are rare findings. Carbamazepine, lamotrigine, and possibly topiramate can cause QRS prolongation. In sharp contrast to parenteral overdose of phenytoin, oral overdose with phenytoin is not associated with electrocardiographic or hemodynamic abnormalities.

Although not universally available, all anticonvulsants are quantifiable in the blood. Frequent and sequential levels are recommended in most cases because of unpredictable and erratic absorption patterns.

Anticonvulsants interact with numerous other drugs. Gabapentin, vigabatrin, and levetiracetam have the fewest drug interactions (Table 41–3). Gabapentin, vigabatrin, levetiracetam, and lamotrigine have no effect on the mixed function oxidase enzyme system.

Meticulous supportive care is required to achieve a good outcome after anticonvulsant drug poisoning. Administration of activated charcoal is generally recommended because of its safety and efficacy. Extracorporeal drug removal is rarely necessary and should be reserved for the severe overdose with hemodynamic instability and clinical deterioration.

Poisonings with the newer anticonvulsants are not frequently reported.

REFERENCES

1. Ahmad SR: Felbamate and aplastic anemia. Lancet 1994;344:465.
2. Albani F, Theodore WH, Washington P, et al: Effect of felbamate on plasma levels of carbamazepine and its metabolites. Epilepsia 1991;32;130–132.
3. Alberto G, Erickson T, Popiel R, et al: Central nervous system manifestations of a valproic acid overdose responsive to naloxone. Ann Emerg Med 1989;18:889–891.
4. Alldredge BK, Lowenstein DH, Simon RP: Placebo-controlled trial of intravenous diphenylhydantoin for short-term treatment of alcohol withdrawal seizures. Am J Med 1989;87:645–648.
5. Anderson GD: A mechanistic approach to antiepileptic drug interactions. Ann Pharmacother 1998;32:554–563.
6. Anderson GD: Phenobarbital: Chemistry and biotransformation. In: Levy RH, Mattson RH, Meldrum BS, eds: Antiepileptic Drugs, 4th ed. New York, Raven Press, 1995, pp. 371–400.
7. Anderson GO, Ritland S: Life-threatening intoxication with sodium valproate. J Toxicol Clin Toxicol 1995;33:279–284.

8. Andrews CO, Fischer JH: Gabapentin: A new agent for the management of epilepsy. Ann Pharmacother 1994;28:1188–1196.

9. Apfelbaum JD, Caravati EM, Kerns WP, et al: Cardiovascular effects of carbamazepine toxicity. Ann Emerg Med 1995;25:631–635.

10. Baille TA, Sheffels PR: Valproic acid: Chemistry and biotransformation. In: Levy RH, Mattson RH, Meldrum BS, eds: Antiepileptic Drugs, 4th ed. New York, Raven Press, 1995, pp. 589–604.

11. Booker HE, Darcey B: Serum concentrations of free diphenylhydantoin and their relationship to clinical intoxication. Epilepsia 1973;14:177–184.

12. Bradury AJ, Bentick B, Todd PJ: Dystonia associated with carbamazepine toxicity. Postgrad Med J 1982;58:525–526.

13. Briassoulis G, Kalabalikis P, Tamiolaki M: Lamotrigine childhood overdose. Pediatr Neurol 1998;19:239–242.

14. Bridge TA, Norton RL, Robertson WO: Pediatric carbamazepine overdoses. Pediatr Emerg Care 1994;10:260–263.

15. Browne TR, Kugler AR, Eldon MA: Pharmacology and pharmacokinetics of fosphenytoin. Neurology 1996;46:S3–S7.

16. Brubacher JR, Dahghani P, McKnight D: Delayed toxicity following ingestion of enteric-coated divalproex sodium (Epival). J Emerg Med 1999;17:463–467.

17. Buckley NA, Whyte IM, Dawson AH: Self-poisoning with lamotrigine. Lancet 1993;342:1552–1553.

18. Buetefisch CM, Gutierrez A, Gutmann L: Choreoathetotic movements: A possible side effect of gabapentin. Neurology 1996;46:851–852.

19. Chaikin P, Adir J: Unusual absorption profile of phenytoin in a massive overdose case. J Clin Pharmacol 1987;27:70–73.

20. Chance JF: Emergency department treatment of alcohol withdrawal seizures with phenytoin. Ann Emerg Med 1991;20:520–522.

21. Chopra S, Levell NJ, Cowley G, et al: Systemic corticosteroids in the phenytoin hypersensitivity syndrome. Br J Dermatol 1996;134:1109–1112.

22. Chua HC, Venketasubramanian N, Tjia H, et al: Elimination of phenytoin in toxic overdose. Clin Neurol Neurosurg 2000;102:6–8.

23. Comer JB: Extravasation from intravenous phenytoin. Intrav Ther Clin Nutr 1984;11:23–29.

24. Connacher AA, Macnab JP, Jung RT: Fatality due to massive overdose of sodium valproate. Scott Med J 1987;32:85–86.

25. Corday E, Enescu V, Vyden JK, et al: Antiarrhythmic properties of carbamazepine. Geriatrics 1971;26:78–81.

26. Coulter DL, Allen RJ: Secondary hyperammonemia: A possible mechanism for valproate encephalopathy. Lancet 1980;1:1310–1311.

27. Davie MB, Cook MJ, Ng C: Vigabatrin overdose [letter]. Med J Aust 1996;165:403.

28. DeVivo DC, Bohan TP, Coulter DL et al: L-Carnitine supplementation in childhood epilepsy: Current perspectives. Epilepsia 1998;39:1216–1225.

29. De Zeuw R, Westemberg H, Van der Kleijn E: An unusual case of carbamazepine poisoning with a near fatal relapse after two days. J Toxicol Clin Toxicol 1979;14:263–269.

30. Dingledine R, Iversen LL, Breuker E, et al: Naloxone as a GABA antagonist. Eur J Pharmacol 1978;47:19–27.

31. Dreifuss FE, Langer DH, Moline KA, et al: Valproic acid hepatic fatalities. Neurology 1989:39:201–207.

32. Drenck NE, Risbo A: Carbamazepine poisoning, a suprisingly severe case. Anesth Intens Care 1980;8:203–204.

33. Dupuis RE, Lichtman SN, Pollack GM: Acute valproic acid overdose. Clinical course and pharmacokinetic disposition of valproic acid and metabolites. Drug Saf 1990;5:65–71.

34. Durelli L, Massazza V, Cavallo R: Carbamazepine toxicity and poisoning. Incidence, clinical features and management. Med Toxicol Adv Drug Exp 1989;4:95–107.

35. Earnest MP, Marx JA, Drury LR: Complications of intravenous phenytoin for acute treatment of seizures. JAMA 1983;249:762–765.

36. Eichelbaum M, Ekbom K, Bertilsson L, et al: Plasma kinetics of carbamazepine and its epoxide metabolite in man after single and multiple doses. Eur J Clin Pharmacol 1975;8:337–341.

37. Evers ML, Ishar A, Agil A: Cardiac monitoring after phenytoin overdose. Heart Lung 1997;26:325–328.

38. Cada DJ, Civington TR, Generali JA, et al, eds: Drug Facts and Comparisons 2000. St Louis, MO: Wolters Kluwer, 2000, pp. 1029–1033.

39. Farrar HC, Harold DA, Reed MD: Acute valproic acid intoxication: Enhanced drug clearance with oral-activated charcoal. Crit Care Med 1993;21:299–301.

40. Fernandez MC, Walter FG, Peterson LR, et al: Gabapentin, valproic acid and ethanol intoxication: Elevated blood levels with mild clinical effects. J Toxicol Clin Toxicol 1996;34:437–439.

41. Fischer JH, Barr AN, Rogers SL, et al: Lack of serious toxicity following gabapentin overdose. Neurology 1994;44:982–983.

42. Gandelman MS: Review of carbamazepine-induced hyponatremia. Prog Neuropsychopharmacol Biol Psychiatry 1994;18:211–233.

43. Garofalo E, Koto E, Feuerstein T, Goedecke AG: Experience with gabapentin overdose: Five case studies [abstract]. Epilepsia 1993;34:157.

44. Gary NE, Byra WM, Eisinger RP: Carbamazepine poisoning: Treatment by hemoperfusion. Nephron 1981;27:202–203.

45. Gee NS, Brown JP, Dissanayake VU, et al. The novel anticonvulsant drug gabapentin (Neurontin) binds to the alpha-2-delta subunit of a calcium channel. J Biol Chem 1996;271:5768–5776.

46. Gidal BE, Privitera MD, Sheth RD, Gilman JT: Vigabatrin: A novel therapy for seizure disorders. Ann Pharmacother 1999;33:1277–1286.

47. Gilman JT: Lamotrigine: An antiepileptic agent for the treatment of partial seizures. Ann Pharmacother 1993;29:144–151.

48. Goa KL, Brogden RN: L-Carnitine. Drugs 1987;34:1–24.

49. Goldschlager AW, Karliner JS: Ventricular standstill after intravenous diphenylhydantoin. Am Heart J 1967;74:410–412.

50. Gordon MF, Gerstenblitt D: The use of free phenytoin levels in averting phenytoin toxicity. N Y State J Med 1990;90:469–470.

51. Gotz E, Feuerstein TJ, Lais A, et al: Effects of gabapentin on release of gamma-aminobutyric acid from slices of rat neostriatum. Arzneimittelforschung 1993;43:636–638.

52. Gram L, Bentson KD: Hepatic toxicity of antiepileptic drugs: A review. Acta Neurol Scand Suppl 1983:97:81–90.

53. Graudins A, Aaron CK: Delayed peak serum valproic acid in massive divalproex overdose: Treatment with charcoal hemoperfusion. J Toxicol Clin Toxicol 1996;34:335–341.

54. Graves NM: Felbamate. Ann Pharmacother 1993;27:1073–1081.

55. Hart RG, Easton JD: Carbamazepine and hematological monitoring. Ann Neurol 1982;11:309–312.

56. Hill DR, Suman-Chauhan N, Woodruff GN: Localization of (3H)gabapentin to a novel site in rat brain: Autoradiographic studies. Eur J Pharmacol 1993;244:303–309.

57. Hojer J, Malmlund HO, Berg A: Clinical features in 28 consecutive cases of laboratory confirmed massive poisoning with carbamazepine alone. J Toxicol Clin Toxicol 1993;31:449–458.

58. Hopkins U, Shepherd G, Klein-Schwartz W, Gorman S, Crouch B: Multicenter case series of gabapentin exposures [abstract]. J Toxicol Clin Toxicol 2000;38:575.

59. Hyden H, Cupello A, Palm A. Naloxone reverses the inhibition by valproate of GABA transport across dieter's neuronal plasma membrane. Ann Neurol 1987;21:64–68.

60. Isacsson G, Holmgren P, Druid H, Bergman U: Psychotropics and suicide prevention. Implication from toxicological screening of 5281 suicides in Sweden 1992–1994. Br J Psychiatry 1999;174:259–265.

61. Ishikura H, Matsuo N, Matsubara M, et al: Valproic acid overdose and L-carnitine therapy. J Anal Toxicol 1996;20:55–58.

62. Jacob PC, Chand RP, Omeima el-S: Asterixis induced by gabapentin. Clin Neuropharm 2000;23:53.

63. Jacome D: Carbamazepine-induced dystonia [letter]. JAMA 1979; 241:2263.

64. Jones AL, Proudfoot AT: Features and management of poisoning with modern drugs used to treat epilepsy. Q J Med 1998;91: 325–332.

65. Johannessen SI: Pharmacokinetics and interaction profile of topiramate. Review and comparison with other newer antiepileptic drugs. Epilepsia 1997;38:S18–S33.

66. Karsarkis EJ, Kuo CS, Berger R, et al: Carbamazepine-induced cardiac dysfunction. Characterization of two distinct clinical syndromes. Arch Intern Med 1992;152:186–191.

67. Kawasaki C, Nishi R, Vekihara S, et al: Charcoal hemoperfusion in the treatment of phenytoin overdose. Am J Kidney Dis 2000;35: 323–326.

68. Khoo SH, Layland MJ: Cerebral edema following acute sodium valproate overdose. J Toxicol Clin Toxicol 1992;30:209–214.

69. Kerr BM, Thummel KE, Wurden CJ, et al: Human liver carbamazepine metabolism. Role of CYP3A4 and CYP2C8 in 10,11-epoxide formation. Biochem Pharmacol 1994;47:1969–1079.

70. Kilarski DJ, Buchanan C, Von Behren L: Soft-tissue damage associated with intravenous phenytoin [letter]. N Engl J Med 1984;311: 1186–1187.

71. Klotz U, Antonin KH: Pharmacokinetics and bioavailability of sodium valproate. Clin Pharmacol Ther 1977;21:736–743.

72. Knowles SR, Shapiro LE, Shear NH: Anticonvulsant hypersensitivity syndrome: Incidence, prevention and management. Drug Saf 1999;21:489–501.

73. Kutt H: Phenytoin: Interactions with other drugs. Parts I and II. In: Levy RH, Mattson RH, Meldrum BS, eds: Antiepileptic Drugs, 4th ed. New York, Raven Press, 1995, pp. 315–344.

74. Larsen JR, Larsen LS: Clinical features and management of poisoning due to phenytoin. Med Toxicol Adv Drug Exp 1989;4:229–245.

75. Leach JP, Storalek I, Brodie MJ: Deliberate overdose with the novel anticonvulsant tiagabine. Seizure 1995;4:155–157.

76. Leiber BL, Snodgrass WR: Cardiac arrest following large intravenous fosphenytoin overdose in an infant [abstract]. J Toxicol Clin Toxicol 1998:36:473.

77. Leppik IE, Gram L, Deaton R, Sommerville KW: Safety of tiagabine: Summary of 53 trials. Epilepsy Res 1999;33:235–246.

78. Leslie PJ, Heyworth R, Prescott LF: Cardiac complications of carbamazepine intoxication: Treatment by haemoperfusion [letter]. Br Med J 1983;286:1018.

79. Levinson DF, Devinsky O: Psychiatric adverse events during vigabatrin therapy. Neurology 1999;53:1503–1511.

80. Levy RH, Pitlick WHJ, Troupin AS, et al: Pharmacokinetics of carbamazepine in normal man. Clin Pharmacol Ther 1975;17:657–668.

81. Li J, Norwood DL, Li-Feng M, Schulz H. Mitochondrial metabolism of valproic acid. Biochemistry 1991;30:388–394.

82. Luer MS, Rhoney DH: Tiagabine: A novel antiepileptic drug. Ann Pharmacother 1998;32:1173–1180.

83. Macdonald RL: Anticonvulsant drug actions on neurons in cell culture. J Neural Transm 1988;72:173–183.

84. Mackey FJ, Wilton GL, Pearce SN, et al: Safety of long-term lamotrigine in epilepsy. Epilepsia 1997;38:881–886.

85. Matsuo F: Lamotrigine. Epilepsia 1999;40:S30–S36.

86. Mattson RH, Cramer JA, Collins JF, et al: Comparison of carbamazepine, phenobarbital, phenytoin and primidone in partial and secondarily generalized tonic-clonic seizures. N Engl J Med 1985; 313:145–151.

87. Mauro LS, Mauro V, Brown D, et al: Enhancement of phenytoin elimination by multiple-dose activated charcoal. Ann Emerg Med 1987;16:1132–1135.

88. Anonymous: Two new drugs for epilepsy. Med Letter 2000;42: 33–35.

89. Merrell Dow Research Institute Clinical Investigator Bureau: Vigabatrin (GABA transaminase inhibitor). Merrell Dow Pharmaceuticals, 1988.

90. McCabe RT, Sofia RD, Layer RT, et al: Felbamate increases (3H)glycine binding in rat brain and section of human postmortem brain. J Pharmacol Exp Ther 1998;286:991–999.

91. McNamara JO: Drugs effective in the therapy of the epilepsies. In: Hardman JG, Limbird LE, Molinoff PB, Ruddon RW, eds: Goodman and Gilman's The Pharmacological Basis of Therapeutics, 9th ed. New York, McGraw-Hill, 1996, pp. 461–486.

92. Merritt HH, Putnam TJ: Sodium diphenylhydantoinate in treatment of convulsive disorders. JAMA 1938;111:1068–1073.

93. Mellick LB, Morgan JA, Mellick GA: Presentations of acute phenytoin overdose. Ann Emerg Med 1989;7:61–67.

94. Mixter CG, Moran JM, Austen WG: Cardiac and peripheral vascular effects of diphenylhydantoin sodium. Am J Cardiol 1966;17: 332–338.

95. Mortensen PB, Hansen HE, Pedersen B, et al: Acute valproate intoxication: Biochemical investigations and hemodialysis treatment. Int J Clin Pharmacol Ther Toxicol 1983;21:64–68.

96. Murakami K, Sugimoto T, Woo M, et al: Effect of L-carnitine supplementation on acute valproate intoxication. Epilepsia 1996;37: 687–689.

97. Mylonakis E, Vittorio CC, Hollick DA, et al: Lamotrigine overdose presenting as anticonvulsant hypersensitivity syndrome. Ann Pharmacother 1999;33:557–559.

98. Nagel TR, Schunk JE: Felbamate overdose: A case report and discussion of a new antiepileptic drug. Pediatr Emerg Care 1995;11: 369–371.

99. Neuvonen PJ, Elonen E: Effect of activated charcoal on absorption and elimination of phenobarbitone, carbamazepine and phenylbutazone in man. Eur J Clin Pharmacol 1980;17:51–57.

100. O'Donnell John, Bateman ND: Lamotrigine overdose in an adult. J Toxicol Clin Toxicol 2000;38:659–660.

101. Ohtani Y, Endo F, Matsuda I. Carnitine deficiency and hyperammonemia associated with valproic acid therapy. J Pediatr 1982;101: 782–785.

102. O'Neil MG, Perdun CS, Wilson MB, et al: Felbamate-associated fatal acute hepatic necrosis. Neurology 1996;46:1457–1459.

103. Osborn HH, Zistein J, Sparano R: Single-dose oral phenytoin loading. Ann Emerg Med 1987;16:407–412.

104. Palmer KJ, Mctavish D: Felbamate. A review of its pharmacodynamic and pharmacokinetic properties and therapeutic efficacy in epilepsy. Drugs 1993;32:130–132.

105. Perucca E, Gram L, Avanzini G, Dulac O: Antiepileptic drugs as a cause of worsening seizures. Epilepsia 1998;39:5–17.

106. Peyster RG, Sussman NM, Hershey BL, et al: Use of ex vivo magnetic resonance imaging to detect onset of vigabatrin-induced intramyelinic edema in canine brain. Epilepsia 1995;36:93–100.

107. Potter JM, Donnelly A. Carbamazepine-10,11-epoxide in therapeutic drug monitoring. Ther Drug Monit 1998;20:652–657.

108. Privitera MD: Topiramate: A new antiepileptic drug. Ann Pharmacother 1997;31:1164–1173.

109. Ramzy Y, Nastase C, Camille Y, et al: Carbamazepine, diuretics and hyponatremia: A possible interaction. J Clin Psychiatry 1987;48: 281–283.

110. Raskind JY, EI-Chaar GM: The role of carnitine supplementation during valproic acid therapy. Ann Pharmacother 2000;34: 630–638.

111. Reeves AL, So EL, Sharbrough FW, et al: Movement disorders associated with the use of gabapentin. Epilepsia 1996;37:988–990.

112. Reife RA, Lim P, Pledger G: Topiramate: Side effect profile in double-blind studies [abstract]. Epilepsia 1995;36:534.

113. Rengstroff DS, Milstone AP, Seger DL, et al: Felbamate overdose complicated by massive crystalluria and acute renal failure. J Toxicol Clin Toxicol 2000;38:666–667.

114. Richens A: Pharmacokinetic and pharmacodynamic drug interaction during treatment with vigabatrin. Acta Neurol Scand 1995;93 (Suppl):43–46.

115. Rogvi-Hansen B, Gram L: Adverse effects of established and new antiepileptic drugs: An attempted comparison. Pharmacol Ther 1993;68:425–434.

116. Roodhooft AM, Van Dam K, Haentjens D, et al: Acute sodium valproate intoxication: Occurrence of renal failure and treatment with haemoperfusion-haemodialysis. Eur J Pediatr 1990;149:363–364.

117. Rose R, Cisek J, Michell J: Fosphenytoin-induced bradyasystole arrest in an infant treated with charcoal hemofiltration [abstract]. J Toxicol Clin Toxicol 1998;36:473.

118. Rosebush PI, MacQueen GM, Mazurek MF: Catatonia following gabapentin withdrawal. J Clin Psychopharmacol 1999;19:188–189.

119. Rush JA, Beran RG: Leucopenia as an adverse reaction to carbamazepine therapy. Med J Aust 1984;140:426–428.

120. Russell MA, Bousvaros G: Fatal results from diphenylhydantoin administered intravenously. JAMA 1968;20:2118–2119.

121. Salke-Kellerman A, Baier H: Acute encephalopathy with vigabatrin [letter]. Lancet 1993;342:185.

122. Sander JW, Hart YM, Trimble MR, et al: Vigabatrin and psychosis. J Neurol Neurosurg Psychiatry 1991;54:435–439.

123. Schaub JEM, Williamson PJ, Barnes EW, Trewby PN: Multisystem adverse reaction to lamotrigine [letter]. Lancet 1994;344:481.

124. Schlienger RG, Knowles SR, Shear NH: Lamotrigine-associated anticonvulsant hypersensitivity syndrome. Neurology 1998;51:1172–1175.

125. Schmidt S, Schmitz-Buhl M: Signs and symptoms of carbamazepine overdose. J Neurol 1995;242:169–173.

126. Schuerer DJE, Brophy PD, Maxvold NJ, et al: High-efficiency dialysis for carbamazepine overdose. J Toxicol Clin Toxicol 2000;38:321–323.

127. Seymour JF: Carbamazepine overdose. Features of 33 cases. Drug Saf 1993;8:81–88.

128. Shank RP, Vaught JL, Raffa JL, et al: Topiramate: Investigation of the mechanism of topiramate's anticonvulsant activity. Epilepsia 1991;32:7–8.

129. Sharief MK, Sander JWA, Shorvon SD: Acute encephalopathy with vigabatrin [letter]. Lancet 1993;342:619.

130. Sharma P, Gupta RC, Bhardwaja B, et al: Status epilepticus and death following acute carbamazepine poisoning. J Assoc Physicians India 1992;40:561–562.

131. Shear N, Spielberg S: Anticonvulsant hypersensitivity syndrome, in vitro assessment of risk. J Clin Invest 1988;82:1826–1832.

132. Soman P, Jain S, Rajsekhar V, et al: Dystonia—A rare manifestation of carbamazepine toxicity. Postgrad Med J 1994;70:54–56.

133. Spiller HA, Krenzelok EP, Cookson E: Carbamazepine overdose: A prospective study of serum levels and toxicity. J Toxicol Clin Toxicol 1990;28:445–458.

134. Spina E, Pisani F, Perucca E: Clinically significant interactions with carbamazepine. An update. Clin Pharmacokinet 1996;31:198–214.

135. Stahl S: Four key neurotransmitter systems. In Stahl S, ed: Psychopharmacology of Antipsychotics, 1st ed. London, Martin Dunitz, 1999, pp. 4–13.

136. Steiman GS, Woerpel RW, Sherard ES: Treatment of accidental sodium valproate overdose with an opiate antagonist. Ann Neurol 1979;6:274.

137. Steiner C, Wit AL, Weiss MB, et al: The antiarrhythmic actions of carbamazepine. J Pharmacol Exp Ther 1970;173:323–335.

138. Stevenson CM, Kim J, Felischer D: Colonic absorption of antiepileptic agents. Epilepsia 1997;38:63–67.

139. Stilman N, Masdeu JC: Incidence of seizures with phenytoin toxicity. Neurology 1985;35:1769–1772.

140. Stremski ES, Brady W, Prasad K, et al: Pediatric carbamazepine intoxication. Ann Emerg Med 1995;25:624–630.

141. Sullivan JB, Rumack BH, Peterson RG: Acute carbamazepine toxicity resulting from overdose. Neurology 1981;31:621–624.

142. Vale JA: Carbamazepine overdose. J Toxicol Clin Toxicol 1992;30:481–482.

143. Verma A, St Clair EW, Radtke RA: A case of sustained massive gabapentin overdose without serious side effects. Ther Drug Monit 1999;21:615–617.

144. Voigt GC: Death following intravenous sodium diphenylhydantoin (Dilantin). Johns Hopkins Med J 1968;123:153–157.

145. Wamil AW, McLean MJ: Limitation by gabapentin of high-frequency action potential firing by mouse central neurons in cell culture. Epilepsy Res 1994;17:1–11.

146. Weaver DF, Camfield P, Fraser A: Massive carbamazepine overdose: Clinical and pharmacologic observation in five episodes. Neurology 1988;38:755–759.

147. Willow M, Gonoi R, Catterall WA: Voltage clamp analysis of the inhibitory actions of diphenylhydantoin and carbamazepine on voltage-sensitive sodium channels in neuroblastoma cells. Mol Pharmacol 1985;27:549–558.

148. Wyte CD, Berk WA: Severe oral phenytoin overdose does not cause cardiovascular morbidity. Ann Emerg Med 1991;20:508–512.

149. Yoari, Y, Selzer ME, Pincus JH: Phenytoin: Mechanisms of its anticonvulsant action. Ann Neurol 1986;20:171–184.

150. Zoneraich S, Zoneraich O, Seigel J: Sudden death following intravenous sodium diphenylhydantoin. Am Heart J 1976;91:375–377.

Mark Su / Robert S. Hoffman

A 66-year-old man presented to the Emergency Department (ED) with a complaint of lower abdominal pain of 24 hours duration that radiated to his left groin. The pain had increased in intensity and resulted in syncope. His past medical history was significant for atrial fibrillation, hypertension, congestive heart failure, colonic polyps, diverticulosis, cataracts, and sciatica. His medications included warfarin 2.5 mg daily, oxybutynin 2 mg twice daily, labetalol 300 mg three times daily, quinapril 40 mg daily, rofecoxib 25 mg daily, and zolpidem 10 mg as needed for sleep.

On physical examination, he was awake and alert, but ill appearing and pale. Vitals signs were blood pressure, 101/38 mm Hg; pulse, 92 beats/min; respiratory rate, 18 breaths/min; and temperature, 37°C (98.6°F); symptomatic orthostasis was present. Examination of the head, eyes, ears, nose, and throat were unremarkable. His chest was clear to auscultation bilaterally and heart examination revealed an irregularly irregular rate. The patient's abdomen was noted to be moderately distended and tender in the left upper-quadrant and left flank, with scrotal edema. Rectal examination and testing for occult blood were negative. The skin and extremities were normal with no evidence of petechiae or ecchymoses.

The patient was immediately placed on 100% oxygen via a non-rebreather mask and treated with intravenous normal saline via two large-bore catheters, and bloods were drawn for laboratory studies. Electrocardiogram demonstrated atrial fibrillation at a rate of 99 beats/min with no evidence of acute myocardial ischemia.

Initial laboratory studies showed a WBC (white blood cell) count of $14 \times 10^3/mm^3$; hemoglobin, 10.3 g/dL; hematocrit, 32.1%; and platelets, $317 \times 10^3/mm^3$. The initial prothrombin time (PT) was 66.7 seconds (international normalized ratio (INR) of 5.7), and activated partial thromboplastin time (PTT) was 81.4 seconds. Urinalysis revealed a specific gravity of 1.025, small bilirubin, trace ketones, 100 mg/dL protein, and no red blood cells.

After the patient's coagulopathy was discovered, the patient was given 10 mg of vitamin K_1 subcutaneously. He was also given 4 units of fresh-frozen plasma and then taken emergently for a non-contrast abdominal computed tomography (CT) scan of the abdomen, which revealed a large retroperitoneal hematoma extending from the inferior pole of the spleen into the pelvis (Fig. 42–1). On repeat abdominal CT scan with contrast 3 hours later, the retroperitoneal hematoma was noted to have increased in size.

The patient was admitted to the surgical intensive care unit where his repeat coagulation studies were significant for a PT of 27 seconds, INR of 2.3, and PTT of 56.2 seconds. His hematocrit decreased to 22.6% and he received an additional 6 units of fresh-frozen plasma and 6 units of packed red blood cells prior to surgery. Intraoperatively, a large hematoma with clots was evacuated and although no active bleeding was visualized at the time, the retroperitoneal blood was believed to originate from his psoas muscles. The patient had an uneventful course postoperatively and was discharged home 5 days later.

HISTORY AND EPIDEMIOLOGY

The origins and discovery of anticoagulants are extraordinary.[1,16,20,68,118] Currently, there are numerous clinical applications including the treatment of coronary artery disease, acute coronary syndromes, cerebrovascular events, deep venous thrombosis, and pulmonary embolism.

The discovery of modern-day oral anticoagulants originated following investigations of a hemorrhagic disorder in cattle in the early 20th century that resulted from the ingestion of spoiled sweet clover silage. The hemorrhagic agent identified as bishydroxy-coumarin was the precursor to its synthetic congener warfarin. This knowledge also led to the utilization of warfarin as a rodenticide. "Superwarfarins" were subsequently developed as rats developed genetic resistance to warfarin. These potent agents permitted either small, repetitive ingestions or single, larger ingestions to function successfully in rodent control.

A medical student initially attempting to study ether-soluble procoagulant agents serendipitously found that, over time, these apparent "procoagulants" actually prevented the normal coagulation of blood. The phospholipid anticoagulant responsible for this effect was later identified as an early form of heparin. Shortly thereafter, the water-soluble mucopolysaccharide termed *heparin* (because of its abundance in the liver) was discovered. *Unfractionated* heparin is a mixture of polysaccharide chains with varying molecular weights. Following the identification of the active pentasaccharide segment of heparin in the 1970s, multiple *low-molecular-weight* heparin variants were isolated.

As early as the late 19th century, human urine was noted to have proteolytic activity with a specificity for fibrin. A substance found to be an activator of endogenous plasminogen, leading to the consumption of fibrin, fibrinogen, and other coagulation proteins, was isolated and purified and given the name *urokinase*. Streptokinase, a protein produced by β-hemolytic streptococci, and tissue plasminogen activator (t-PA) and other synthetic thrombolytic agents were later discovered. Ancrod (a purified derivative of snake venom) and hirudin (a product of leeches), although known to exist for many years, have only recently gained attention as naturally occurring antithrombotic therapeutic agents.

The diversity of these anticoagulants has led to their ever-increasing use in many fields of medicine. Warfarin was the 21st most commonly prescribed drug in the United States in the year

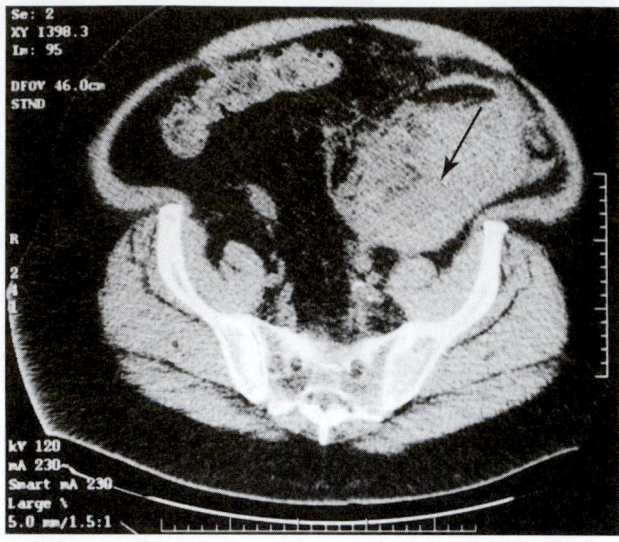

Figure 42–1. Abdominal CT scan illustrating a large left-sided retroperitoneal hematoma in a patient with an INR of 5.7 presenting with left flank pain radiating to the groin.

2000[169] reported to the American Association of Poison Control Centers. During the last decade, the annual number of cases of warfarin exposures has doubled, including 12 deaths. Additionally, the common problem of excessive warfarin effects leading to hemorrhage is poorly quantitated as an adverse drug reaction and frequently goes untabulated. Thus, as long as warfarin continues to be routinely prescribed, it is likely that the incidence of adverse drug events will only increase. Physicians must therefore be cognizant of the complications of warfarin and other anticoagulants, as well as their various therapeutic modalities, while balancing the potential for their risk and benefits.

BALANCE BETWEEN COAGULATION AND ANTICOAGULATION

An understanding of the normal function of the coagulation pathways is essential to appreciate the etiology of a coagulopathy. The critical steps of the coagulation cascade are summarized here. For additional detail, see Chapter 25 and several reviews.[59,115,139]

Coagulation consists of a series of events that prevent excess blood loss and that assist in the restoration of blood vessel integrity. Although the traditional understanding of the events that occur in the coagulation cascade,[45,103] as discussed below, adequately describes in vitro events, current comprehension emphasizes some distinct differences that occur in vivo.[59,115,139] Despite these differences, an understanding of the traditional model is most useful for interpreting the results of diagnostic tests of coagulation.

Within the cascade, coagulation factors exist as inert precursors and are transformed into enzymes when activated. Activation of the cascade occurs through one of two distinct pathways, the intrinsic and extrinsic systems (Fig. 42–2).[45,103] Once activated, these enzymes catalyze a series of reactions that ultimately con-

verge and lead to the generation of thrombin and the formation of a fibrin clot.

The intrinsic pathway is activated by the complexation of factor XII (Hageman factor) with high-molecular-weight kininogen (HMWK) and prekallikrein or vascular subendothelial collagen. This results in sequential activation of factor XII, active kallikrein, and active factors IX to XI and prothrombin II (Fig. 42–2). Prothrombin is converted to thrombin in the presence of factor V, calcium, and phospholipid. The integrity of this system is usually evaluated by determining the PTT.

In the extrinsic, or tissue factor–dependent, pathway, a complex is formed between factor VII, calcium, and tissue factor. A calcium and lipid-dependent complex is then created between factors VII and X. The factor VII–X complex subsequently converts prothrombin to thrombin, which promotes the formation of fibrin from fibrinogen (Fig. 42–2). The integrity of this pathway is usually assessed by determining the PT (or INR, described later).

Activation of factors IX and X provides the important link between the intrinsic and extrinsic coagulation pathways. Additional evidence that tissue factors can activate both factors IX and X suggests that there are more interrelations between the two pathways than originally thought.[127] Furthermore, cell surfaces facilitate the process of clotting. Platelets are also known to interact with proteins of the coagulation cascade through surface receptors for factors V, VIII, IX, and X.[61,154] As a final step, factor XIII assists in the cross-linking of fibrin to form a stable thrombus.

Antithrombin III, protein C, and protein S serve as inhibitors, maintaining the homeostasis that is required to prevent spontaneous clotting and keep blood fluid. Protein C, when aided by protein S, inactivates two plasma factors, V and VIII.[25,38,59] Antithrombin III complexes with all the serine protease coagulation factors except factor VII.[25,59,140]

Thrombolytic agents such as streptokinase, urokinase, anistreplase, recombinant tissue plasminogen activator (rt-PA) reteplase, and tenectoplase enhance the normal processes that lead to clot degradation.[115] Thrombosis is initiated when exposed endothelium or released tissue factor leads to platelet adherence and aggregation, the formation of thrombin, and cross-linking of fibrinogen to form fibrin strands.[59,115,139] This results in a hemostatic plug or thrombus formation. Thrombus formation, in turn, leads to generation of plasmin from plasminogen, which causes fibrinolysis and eventual dissolution of the hemostatic plug.[40,41] Thus, the fibrinolytic system may be thought of as a natural balance against unregulated coagulation. Thrombolytic therapy increases fibrinolytic activity by accelerating the conversion of plasminogen to plasmin, which actively degenerates fibrin.[15,40,41] Following the administration of thrombolytic agents, a consequential coagulopathy results, and fibrin degradation products are elevated secondary to the rapid turnover of clot.

DEVELOPMENT OF COAGULOPATHY

Impaired coagulation results from decreased production or enhanced consumption of coagulation factors, the presence of inhibitors of coagulation, activation of the thrombolytic system, or abnormalities in platelet number or function. For the purposes of this chapter, a discussion of platelet-related abnormalities is excluded. Some of this information is found in Chapter 25.

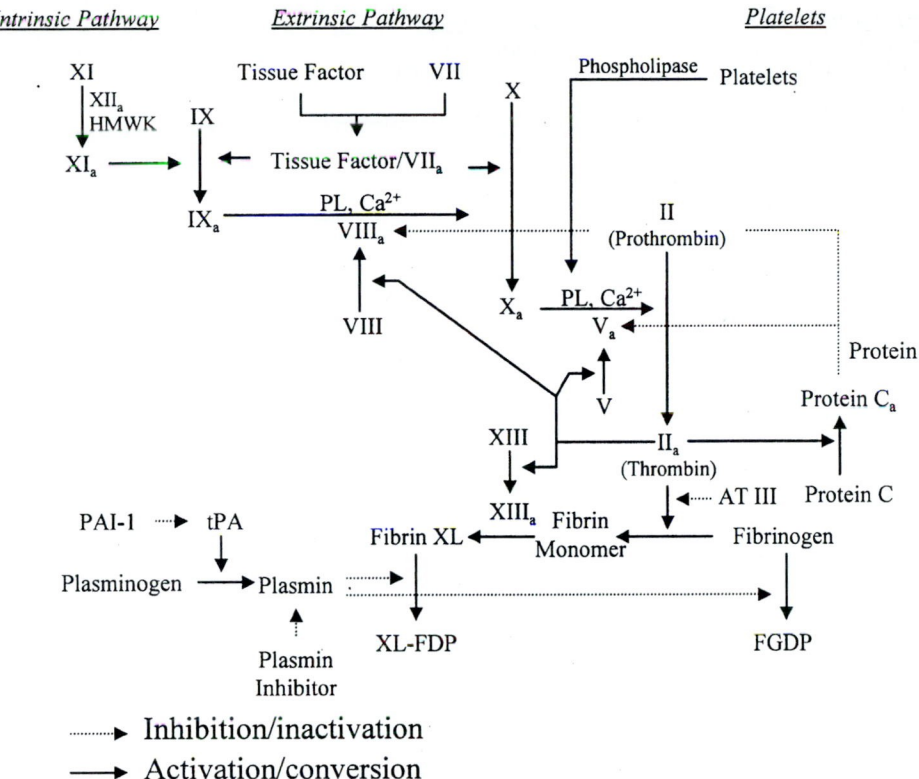

Intrinsic Pathway   *Extrinsic Pathway*   *Platelets*

Figure 42–2. The figure presents a schematic overview of the coagulation and fibrinolytic pathways and indicates where phospholipids on the platelet surface interact with the coagulation pathway intermediates. Inhibitory interactions produced by the venom proteins are shown by the side dashed lines; activation or conversion interactions are shown by the wide solid black lines. The narrow solid lines indicate the normal interactions of the coagulation and fibrinolytic proteins.

Decreased production of coagulation factors results from congenital and acquired etiologies. Although congenital disorders of factor V (Leiden), factor VIII (hemophilia), factor IX (Christmas factor), factor XI, and factor XII (Hageman factor) are all reported, their overall incidence is still quite low. Clinical conditions that result in acquired factor deficiencies are much more common and result from either a decrease in synthesis or activation. Factors II, V, VII, and X are entirely synthesized in the liver;[59,115,139] thus, hepatic dysfunction is a common cause of acquired coagulopathy. In addition, factors II, VII, IX, and X require postsynthetic activation by vitamin K,[157,163,164] such that vitamin K deficiency (from malnutrition, changes in gut flora, or malabsorption) or inhibition (from warfarin, as will be described) is capable of impairing coagulation.

Excessive consumption of coagulation factors usually results from massive activation of the coagulation cascade. Massive activation occurs during severe hemorrhage or disseminated intravascular coagulation. The latter results from infection (eg, gram-negative sepsis), conditions that introduce tissue factor into the blood (eg, neoplasms, snake envenomations), stagnant blood flow, and diffuse endothelial injury (eg, hyperthermia, aortic aneurysm, or dissection). The hallmark of a consumptive coagulopathy is a depressed level of fibrinogen with an elevation of fibrin-degradation products. This combination suggests the rapid turnover of fibrin in the coagulation process. In the other coagulopathic conditions, the failure to activate the coagulation cascade is associated with normal or high fibrin levels and low levels of fibrin-degradation products, because of limited clot formation.

Inhibitors of the coagulation cascade (circulating anticoagulants) are of two types: immunoglobulin and nonimmunoglobulin. Immunoglobulins, which are often antibodies to existing coagula-

tion factors, may occur without obvious cause, as part of a systemic autoimmune disorder, or as a result of repeated transfusions with exogenous factors (as occurs in hemophilia).[72,97,149] The clinical syndromes associated with antibody inhibitors are similar to those associated with deficiencies of the particular coagulation factors involved. Antibodies to factors V, VII to XI, and XIII are described.[20,149] Alternatively, nonimmunoglobulin neutralizers of coagulation occur in conditions associated with rapid white cell turnover.[20,70] These neutralizers are positively charged lysosomal proteins that compete with coagulation factors for negatively charged phospholipid membrane surfaces. Although they prolong in vitro coagulation times, they are rarely responsible for clinical coagulopathy because of the excess of phospholipid surface area available in vivo.[72,97]

ORAL ANTICOAGULANTS

Warfarin and "Warfarinlike" Anticoagulants

The short-acting oral anticoagulants may be divided into two groups: (a) hydroxycoumarins, including warfarin (Coumadin), panwarfin, warficide, coumachlor, coumafuryl, fumasol, prolin, ethyl biscoumacetate (Tromexan), phenprocoumon, dicumarol bishydroxycoumarin, and acenocoumarin (sintrom); and (b) indanediones, including pindone, pivalyn, diphacinone, diphenadione, phenindione, and anisindione. Regardless of the classification, the mechanism of action involves vitamin K inhibition. Vitamin K is a cofactor in the postribosomal synthesis of clotting factors II, VII, IX, and X (Fig. 42–3). The vitamin K–sensitive step involves the carboxylation in the liver of 10 or more glutamic acid residues at the

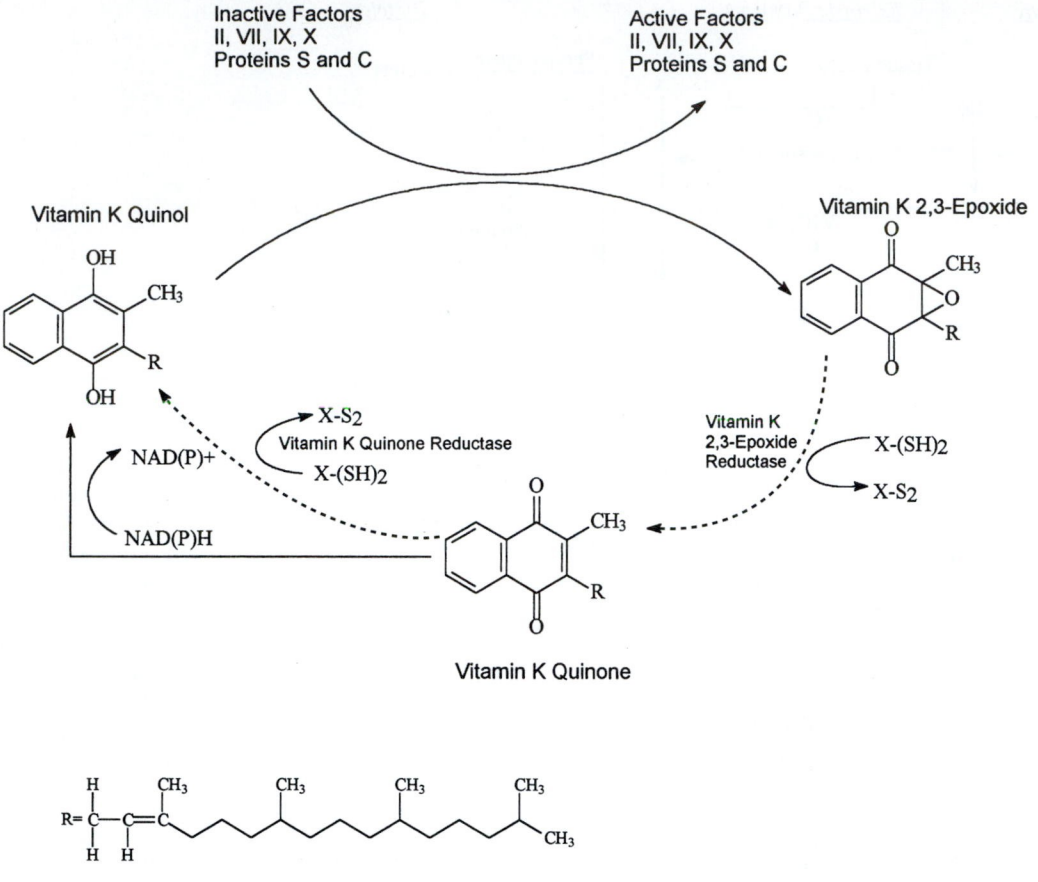

Figure 42–3. The vitamin K cycle. Dotted lines represent pathways that can be blocked with warfarin and warfarinlike anticoagulants. The aliphatic side chain (R) of vitamin K is shown below the metabolic pathway.

amino terminal end of the precursor proteins, to form a unique amino acid γ-carboxyglutamate.[49,157,163,164] These amino acids chelate calcium in vivo, which allows the binding of the four vitamin K–dependent clotting factors to phospholipid membranes during activation of the coagulation cascade.[180]

Vitamin K is not active until it is reduced from its quinone form to a quinol (or hydroquinone) form in hepatic microsomes. This reduction of vitamin K must precede the carboxylation of the precursor factors. The carboxylase activity is coupled to an epoxidase activity for vitamin K, whereby vitamin K is oxidized simultaneously to vitamin K 2,3-epoxide (Fig. 42–3).[163,180] This inactive form of the vitamin is converted to the active form by two successive reductions.[49,105,123] In the first step, an epoxide reductase (known as vitamin K 2,3-epoxide reductase) uses reduced nicotinamide adenine dinucleotide (NADH) as a cofactor to convert vitamin K 2,3-epoxide to a quinone form.[123,163] Subsequently, the quinone is reduced to the active vitamin K quinol form by vitamin K quinone reductase (Antidotes in Depth: Vitamin K).

Warfarin is a racemic mixture of R-warfarin and S-warfarin enantiomers. In rodents, S-warfarin is 3–6 times more potent than R-warfarin at producing hypoprothrombinemia.[28] In humans, S-warfarin may only be about 1.5 times as potent as R-warfarin.[29] Warfarin and all warfarinlike compounds inhibit the activity of vitamin K 2,3-epoxide reductase, as can be demonstrated by the observation of elevated levels of vitamin K 2,3-epoxide in

anticoagulated subjects.[37,183] Additional evidence suggests that the other enzyme system, vitamin K quinone reductase, is also inhibited by warfarin and its related compounds (Fig. 42–3).[49,52] This subsequently inhibits the formation of activated clotting factors.

Pharmacology of Warfarin. Orally ingested warfarin is virtually completely absorbed and peak plasma concentrations occur approximately 3 hours after drug administration.[162] Because only the free warfarin is therapeutically active, concurrent administration of drugs that alter the level of free warfarin (eg, by competing for binding to albumin or inhibiting warfarin metabolism) may markedly influence the anticoagulant effect.[12,57,162] Drugs that interfere with or potentiate warfarin's effects are listed in Table 42–1. Although vitamin K regeneration is inhibited almost immediately, the anticoagulant effect of warfarin (and other oral anticoagulant agents) is delayed until the existing stores of vitamin K are depleted and the active coagulation factors are removed from circulation. Because vitamin K turnover is rapid, this effect is dependent on factor half-life ($t_{1/2}$), with factor VII ($t_{1/2} \approx 5$ hours) depleted most rapidly.[57] For a prolongation of the PT to occur, factor levels must fall to about 25% of normal values. This suggests that, in most patients who are not originally anticoagulated, at least 15 hours (3 factor VII half-lives) are required before warfarin's effect is evident.[57]

TABLE 42–1. Common Drug Interactions with Warfarin Anticoagulation

Potentiation		Antagonism
Acetaminophen	Metronidazole	Antacids
Allopurinol	Nonsteroidal anti-	Antihistamines
Amiodarone	inflammatory agents	Barbiturates
Anabolic steroids	Omeprazole	Carbamazepine
Aspirin	Phenytoin	Cholestyramine
Carbenicillin	Propafenone	Colestipol
Clarithromycin	Propoxyphene	Corticosteroids
Cephalosporins	Quinidine	Griseofulvin
Chloral hydrate	Quinolones	Oral contraceptives
Cimetidine	Simvastatin	Phenytoin
Clofibrate	Sulfonylureas	Rifampin
Cyclic anti-	Tamoxifen	Vitamin K
depressants	Tetracycline	
Disulfiram	Thyroxine	
Erythromycin	Trimethoprim-	
Ethanol	sulfamethoxazole	
Fluconazole	Vitamin E	
Isoniazid		
Ketoconazole		

The half-life of warfarin in humans is 35 hours; thus, its duration of action may be up to 5 days.[28,57,162] On average, it takes approximately 6 days of warfarin administration to reach a steady-state anticoagulant effect.

Warfarin is metabolized by isoenzymes CYP1A2 and CYP3A4 of the hepatic microsomal P450 enzyme system. R-warfarin is metabolized by side-chain reduction to secondary alcohols that are subsequently excreted by the kidney, whereas S-warfarin is metabolized by hydroxylation to 7-hydroxy warfarin, which is excreted into the bile.[57,162] The elimination of S-warfarin is more rapid than that of R-warfarin.[28]

The therapeutic dose of warfarin is established for both adults and children. Typical adult recommendations are to give a dose of 5 mg/d for several days and then maintain the patient on 2–10 mg/d as determined by the INR.[105] Therapeutic dosing equivalents for the other oral anticoagulants are available.[105] For children, the suggested loading dose of warfarin is 0.1 mg/kg/d, followed by a daily maintenance dose that is 15–25% of the loading dose.[34] A 2-year prospective study in children demonstrated that the optimal daily dose of warfarin could be calculated using this formula[166]:

$$\text{Dose (mg / day)} = 0.07 \times \text{weight (kg)} + 0.54$$

Long-Acting Anticoagulants

Within the coumarin group are two 4-hydroxycoumarin derivatives—difenacoum and brodifacoum. These agents differ from warfarin by their longer, higher-molecular-weight polycyclic hydrocarbon side chain (Fig. 42–4). Together with a third agent, chlorophacinone, an indandione derivative, they are known as "superwarfarins," or long-acting anticoagulants.

Long-acting anticoagulants were designed to be effective rodenticides in warfarin-resistant rodents.[101] Their mechanism of action is identical to that of the traditional warfarinlike anticoagulants, as demonstrated by the measurement of increased levels of vitamin K 2,3-epoxide after long-acting anticoagulant administration.[26,27,30,98,130] The ability of these agents to perform as superior rodenticides is attributed to their high lipid solubility and concentration in the liver.[98,101,130] They also may saturate hepatic enzymes at very low levels, as demonstrated by zero-order elimination following overdose.[30] These issues make them about 100 times more potent than warfarin on a mole-for-mole basis.[98,101,130] In addition, they have a longer duration of action than the traditional warfarins.[98,101,130] For example, to obtain 100% lethality in a common house mouse, more than 21 days of feeding with a warfarin-containing rodenticide (0.025% anticoagulant by weight of bait) is required.[101] Similar efficacy can be achieved with a single day's ingestion of brodifacoum (0.005% anticoagulant by weight of bait).[101]

Many animals have been poisoned with long-acting anticoagulants, either secondary to the unintentional ingestion of rodenticides or intentionally for the purposes of investigation. In rats, the half-life of brodifacoum is reported to be 156 hours.[7] The half-life in dogs is reported to be between 6 and 120 days.[100,184] Horses intentionally poisoned with brodifacoum showed a half-life of 1.22 days.[22] The veterinary literature is replete with reports of fatalities and animals that remained anticoagulated in excess of 1 month.[116,160]

Many cases of intentional overdose of long-acting anticoagulants in humans are also described in the literature. Table 42–2

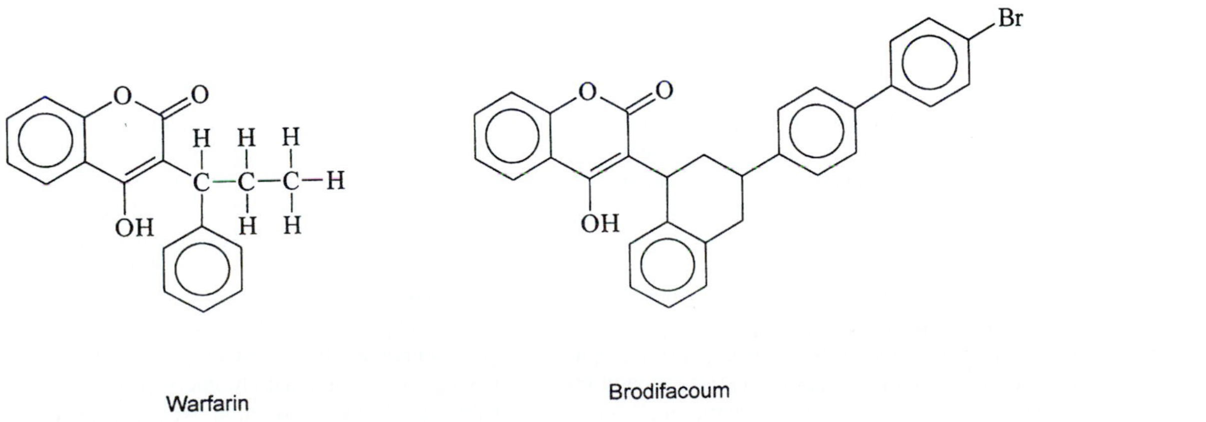

Figure 42–4. Structural comparison of prototypical short-acting (warfarin) and long-acting (brodifacoum) anticoagulants.

TABLE 42–2. Intentional Long-Acting Anticoagulant Overdoses

Reference	Age, Sex	Product	Complications	Initial PT ratio/INR	Duration of Coagulopathy
Babcock[5]	2	Brodifacoum	Purpura		9 mo
Barlow[9]	17F	Difenacoum	None	15	5 wk
Reingestion			GI bleeding		42 d
Barnett[10]	27F	Brodifacoum	Hemoptysis	7	—
Basehore[11]	Unknown	Brodifacoum	Epistaxis, hematuria, death	5	—
Berry[18]	57F	Brodifacoum	Wound bleeding		—
Bruno[30]	52M	Brodifacoum	Hematuria, oral bleeding	6	46 d
Burucoa[32]	20F	Chlorophacinone	Hematuria	8	49 d
	60F	Chlorophacinone	Hematuria, menorrhagia	7	25 d
	23M	Chlorophacinone	Oral bleeding	6	132 d
Butcher[33]	M	Difenacoum	Hematuria	6	10 wk
Casner[35]	61F	Brodifacoum	Ecchymoses, GI/vaginal bleeding		>14 wk
Chong[36]	20M	Brodifacoum	Oral bleeding, hematuria	2	8 mo
Corke[44]	26M	Brodifacoum	Hematuria, oral bleeding, mesenteric hematoma		>5 wk
Exner[51]	25F	Brodifacoum	Hemoptysis	7	>8 mo
Helmuth[73]	25M	Brodifacoum	CNS bleed, death	>6	—
Hoffman[77]	30M	Brodifacoum	Hematuria, GI bleeding	10	64 d
Hollinger[79]	38M	Brodifacoum	Hematuria	11	114 d
Hui[82]	76M	Brodifacoum	Hematuria, GI bleeding	>10	>3 mo
Jones[86]	17M	Brodifacoum	Hematuria	>10	55 d
Kruse[92]	25M	Brodifacoum	Upper GI bleeding	4	15 wk
Reingestion			Fatal CNS bleed		
Lipton[100]	31F	Brodifacoum	Abortion	6	300 d*
McCarthy[111]	41M	Difenacoum	Ecchymoses, hematuria, GI bleeding	>10	>7 mo*
Murdoch[119]	37F	Chlorophacinone	None	4	3 mo
Palmer[129]	15F	Brodifacoum	Pulmonary hemorrhage, death		—
Rauch[136]	26M	Brodifacoum	Calf hematoma, hematemesis	9	24 mo*
	37F	Brodifacoum	Ecchymoses	>8	6 mo
	42M	Brodifacoum	Hematuria, epistaxis	>4	>3 mo
Ross[141]	62M	Brodifacoum	Hematuria	4	3 mo
Routh[142]	29F	Brodifacoum	Death	9	—
Seidelman[147]	24M	Unconfirmed	None	>12	>37 d
Sheen[150]	39M	Brodifacoum	Hematuria	>12	>152 d
Swigar[165]	52M	Unconfirmed	Compartment syndrome		>82 d
Tecimer[167]	37M	Brodifacoum	Hematuria, occult GI bleeding	8	17 d
Wallace[175]	36M	Brodifacoum	Upper GI bleeding	10	—
Weitzel[178]	20F	Brodifacoum	Melena, menorrhagia, hematuria	>4	>11 mo
	25M	Brodifacoum	Epistaxis, compartment syndrome	>4	100 d
	37M	Brodifacoum	Hematuria	>5	>150 d

*Denotes possible repeat ingestion.

summarizes these cases. These patients' clinical courses are characterized by a severe coagulopathy that may last weeks to months, often accompanied by consequential blood loss. The most common sites of bleeding include the gastrointestinal and genitourinary tracts. Although initial parenteral vitamin K_1 doses as high as 400 mg have been used,[32] daily oral vitamin K_1 requirements may be in the range of 50–100 mg. Recent experience in both animals and humans suggests that parenteral vitamin K_1 therapy may not be required[30,184] (Antidotes in Depth: Vitamin K).

Patients with unintentional ingestions must be distinguished from those with intentional ingestions, because the former individuals demonstrate a low likelihood of producing coagulation abnormalities and rare morbidity or mortality. Actually, with a single, small ingestion of a superwarfarin rodenticide, prolongation of the PT or INR is unlikely. Clinically significant anticoagulation is even rarer. In the combined pediatric case series, prolongation of the PT occurred in only 8 of 142 children (5.6%) reported with single small ingestions of long-acting anticoagulants.[15,87,89,156] Only 1 child in this group was reported to have "abnormal prolonged bleeding," but this required no medical attention.[156] In a single case report, a 36-month-old child developed a coagulopathy manifested by epistaxis and hematuria with anticoagulation persisting for over 100 days after a presumed, but unwitnessed, single unintentional ingestion of brodifacoum.[170] Clinically significant coagulopathy can result, however, following small repeated ingestions. Two children reportedly became unintentionally poisoned by repeated ingestions of a long-acting anticoagulant. One child presented with a neck hematoma that compromised his airway; the other child presented with a hemarthrosis.[64] Similarly, a 7-year-old girl required multiple hospitalizations over a 20-month period following an unintentional chronic ingestion of brodifacoum.[177] Finally, a 24-month-old child who presented with unexplained bruising and a PT >125 seconds, was the victim of brodifacoum poisoning caused by a Munchausen syndrome by proxy.[6]

Following an acute unintentional exposure, most patients (usually children) are entirely asymptomatic and have a normal coagulation profile. Knowing that the risk of coagulopathy is low and that it will occur over days, most authors recommend nonintervention.[88,156] Despite the fact that significant toxicity from superwarfarins is rare, it should be recognized that the reported benign courses of pediatric exposures may be misleading. Multiple retrospective studies suggest that children with unintentional acute exposures do not require any followup coagulation studies.[31,117,132,151] This conclusion and approach to management are an unjustified attempt to decrease the cost of "unnecessary" coagulation studies. However, there are clearly insufficient data to justify this conclusion as many of these "exposed" children were never documented to have actually ingested long-acting anticoagulants (Chap. 116). We recommend that clinicians continue to manage these children as possible ingestions and that all children be followed up with daily INR studies for at least 48 hours.

Laboratory Assessment

Established screening tests are helpful for diagnosis. Four studies —PT(INR), PTT, thrombin time, and fibrinogen concentration— are available. Prothrombin time is calculated by adding standardized thromboplastin reagent (phospholipid and tissue factor) to a sample of the patient's citrated plasma (the citrate removes calcium). Calcium is then introduced and the time to clotting measured. The PT is unaffected by the presence or absence of factors VIII to XIII (with the exception of X), platelets, prekallikrein, and HMWK. An individual's PT was formerly expressed as a ratio (PT observed/PT control). Because both laboratory methodology and the source of the thromboplastin reagent used directly affect this ratio, the results generated suffered from significant variability. A new standard, the international normalized ratio (INR) was developed in an attempt to limit interlaboratory variability.[74,121] The INR is derived by raising the PT ratio to a power value known as the international sensitivity index (ISI): $(PT\ ratio)^{ISI}$. The ISI is a measure of responsiveness of the particular thromboplastin to warfarin. Although the use of the INR does not completely eliminate variability,[76,120] it does improve the potential for standardized interpretation and limits interinstitutional variations.

Partial thromboplastin time is measured by adding kaolin or celite to citrated plasma in order to activate the "contact" components of the intrinsic system. This mixture is then recalcified and the time to clotting observed. Some tests use phospholipids in the reagent to activate the remaining coagulation factors, thereby giving rise to the term *activated PTT* (aPTT). Because the PTT and aPTT are essentially interchangeable, the term PTT is used hereafter to represent the concept. The PTT is not affected by factors VII, XIII, or platelets.

The thrombin time, which is determined by adding exogenous thrombin to citrated plasma, evaluates the ability to convert fibrinogen to fibrin, and is thus unaffected by factors II, V, VII to XIII, platelets, prekallikrein, or HMWK. Finally, either a fibrinogen level or a determination of fibrin degradation products helps to distinguish between problems with clot formation and consumptive coagulopathy. An evaluation of the combination of normal and abnormal results of these tests determines the patient's abnormality (Table 42–3).

Inhibitors can be diagnosed by "mixing studies," because only a small percentage of the coagulation factor levels present in normal plasma are necessary to have a normal PTT. If the patient with

TABLE 42–3. Evaluation of Abnormal Coagulation Times

INR Normal, PTT Prolonged, Bleeding
Deficiencies of factors VIII, IX, XI
Von Willebrand disease
Heparin therapy (low dose)

INR Normal, PTT Prolonged, No Bleeding
Deficiencies of factor XII, prekallikrein, high-molecular-weight-kininogen
Inhibitor syndrome

INR Prolonged, PTT Normal
Deficiency of factor VII
Warfarin therapy (early)
Vitamin K deficiency (mild)
Liver disease (mild)

INR and PTT Prolonged, Thrombin Time Normal, Fibrinogen Normal
Deficiencies of factors II, V, IX, vitamin K (severe)
Warfarin therapy (late)

INR and PTT Prolonged, Thrombin Time Abnormal, Fibrinogen Normal
Heparin effect
Dysfibrinogenemia

INR and PTT Prolonged, Thrombin Time Abnormal, Fibrinogen Abnormal
Liver disease
Disseminated intravascular coagulation
Fibrinolytic therapy
Crotaline envenomation

an abnormal PTT suffers from even a severe factor deficiency, restoration of that factor activity to 50% of normal will completely normalize the PTT. Thus, the presence of an abnormal PTT that will not correct by incubation of the patient's plasma with an equal volume of normal plasma is diagnostic of an inhibitor of coagulation. More sophisticated studies can be used to identify specific coagulation factor deficiencies. The reader is referred to one of several standard references for a more detailed discussion of the approach to patients with abnormal coagulation studies.[2,70]

Although warfarin levels may be useful to confirm the diagnosis in unknown cases and to study drug kinetics,[67,122] the routine use of simple and inexpensive measures such as INR determination seems more appropriate.

Evaluation of Long-Acting Anticoagulants

For patients who have known ingestions of long-acting anticoagulants and are considered likely to develop a coagulopathy, baseline coagulation studies are not usually helpful, but they may provide information about chronic exposures. If the history is reliable and the patient is healthy, baseline studies can be avoided. Serial INRs at 24 and 48 hours should identify all patients at risk of coagulopathy.[156] These studies can be obtained while the patient remains in the home setting, depending on the social situation.

In contrast, all patients with intentional ingestions of long-acting anticoagulants should be presumed to be at risk for a severe coagulopathy. In fact, most patients do not seek medical care until bruising or bleeding is evident.[9,30,32,36,51,73,77,86,87,89,92,100,119,142,165] These events often occur many days after ingestion, which obviates the need for gastric decontamination unless there is a suggestion of repetitive ingestion. These patients should be managed as described below.

For patients who have a suspected long-acting anticoagulant overdose, daily or twice-daily INR evaluations should be adequate to identify most patients at risk for coagulopathy. Early detection (through coagulation factor analysis) may be preferred,[67] however, and levels of long-acting anticoagulants can now be measured.[54,94,122] Emphasis has been placed on determining a critical superwarfarin level below which anticoagulation does not occur,[32] and in one case report, brodifacoum was observed to follow zero-order elimination kinetics.[30] If this type of toxicokinetics is consistent in the analysis of other long-acting anticoagulants, these laboratory measurements may prove more reliable than the current empiric endpoints of therapy.

Clinical Manifestations

Typical warfarin-containing rodenticides contain only small concentrations of anticoagulant, such as 0.025% (or 25 mg of warfarin per 100 g of product). Using the data previously listed, a 10-kg child requires a dose of 1 mg of warfarin (4 g of rodenticide) and a daily dose of about 1.2 mg of warfarin (5 g of rodenticide) to remain anticoagulated. These quantities are far greater than those that occur in typical "tastes." Thus, single unintentional ingestions of warfarin-containing rodenticides pose virtually no threat to either normal or anticoagulated patients.[88] In contrast, intentional and large unintentional ingestions of pharmaceutical-grade anticoagulants have the potential to produce a coagulopathy and consequential bleeding. In one study describing 12 patients with surreptitious ingestion of oral anticoagulants, 9 were healthcare professionals.[124] These patients presented with typical manifestations of impaired coagulation: bruising, hematuria, hematochezia, and menorrhagia. Rare but life-threatening complications, such as hemorrhage into the neck with resultant airway compromise, are reported.[23]

Although intentional ingestions of warfarin-containing products are uncommon, adverse drug events resulting in excessive anticoagulation and bleeding occur frequently. The risk of hemorrhage during oral anticoagulant therapy depends upon a myriad of factors, including the intensity of anticoagulation, patient characteristics and comorbid conditions (ie, hypertension, renal insufficiency, malignancy, etc), length of anticoagulant therapy, and indications for anticoagulation (ie, cerebral vascular disease, prosthetic heart valves, atrial fibrillation, ischemic heart disease, and venous thromboembolism). The significance of each of these clinical conditions varies among different reports; however, most studies demonstrate that there is a greater incidence of bleeding complications with increasing INR,[39] increasing intensity (or variation) of coagulation, advanced age, a history of previous bleeding episodes while on therapeutic warfarin, drug interactions, impaired liver function, and dietary changes.[55,57,66,71,135,182] Clearly, the most serious complication of excessive anticoagulation is intracranial hemorrhage, reported to occur in as many as 2% of patients on long-term therapy.[57] This complication is associated with a fatality rate as high as 77%.[109]

Recently, an Outpatient Bleeding Risk Index was created and shown to be more accurate than physician's judgment in classifying patients according to the risk of major bleeding.[19] The index was based on 4 independent risk factors: age ≥65 years; history of cerebrovascular accident; history of gastrointestinal bleeding; and either history of recent myocardial infarction, hematocrit <30%, serum creatinine >1.5 mg/dL, or diabetes mellitus. The sum of the number of risk factors successfully predicted major bleeding at 48 months to be 3%, 12%, and 53% in low-risk (0 risk factors), intermediate-risk (1–2 risk factors), and high-risk (3–4 risk factors) patients, respectively. Physicians had little ability to accurately estimate the probability of bleeding and use of the Outpatient Bleeding Risk Index would therefore seem appropriate to improve awareness and treatment of these high-risk patients.

In a study of 32 patients who developed life-threatening hemorrhage while on warfarin therapy, most patients had multiple risk factors for hemorrhage, including excessive anticoagulation.[182] The gastrointestinal tract was identified as the source of bleeding in two-thirds of the patients.[182] Sixty-six percent of patients were given vitamin K$_1$, 50% were given FFP, and 7% were given both therapies.[182]

GENERAL MANAGEMENT

Gastrointestinal decontamination should be performed on patients who are believed to have potentially significant life-threatening ingestions, but for patients who present a few hours after ingestion, gastric decontamination with either orogastric lavage or syrup of ipecac-induced emesis is not indicated (Chap. 5). Although convincing data on the efficacy of either single- or multiple-dose activated charcoal (possible enterohepatic circulation) are lacking, at least a single dose should be administered unless it is contraindicated. Oral cholestyramine can also be used to enhance warfarin elimination,[137] but no studies are available that compare these two therapies or that evaluate the role of combined activated charcoal and cholestyramine therapy. Although phenobarbital also enhances elimination in animal models, it would be contraindicated in humans because of the decreased ability to reliably monitor the mental status of a patient who had the possibility of spontaneous intracranial hemorrhage. In addition to general supportive measures, the patient should be placed in a supportive medical and psychiatric environment that offers protection against external or self-induced trauma, and permits observation for the onset of coagulopathy.

Blood is required for any patient with a history of blood loss or active bleeding who is hemodynamically unstable, has impaired oxygen transport, or is expected to become unstable. Although a transfusion of packed red blood cells is ideal for replacing lost blood, it cannot correct a coagulopathy, and thus patients will continue to bleed. Whole blood contains not only the cellular elements the patient is losing, but the necessary coagulation factors to reverse the coagulopathy. Although transfusion of whole blood should be considered in severe cases, whole blood contains many components (platelets, white blood cells, and nonvitamin K–dependent factors) that might benefit other patients, and relatively small amounts of vitamin K–dependent factors. Thus, selective use of specific blood products is generally preferred. Packed red blood cells should be given to correct the anemia and fresh-frozen plasma (FFP) or other factor concentrates (cryoprecipitate, Konyne) to correct the coagulopathy. FFP is rich in active vitamin K–dependent coagulation factors and will reverse oral anticoagulant–induced coagulopathy in most patients. Multiple FFP transfusions may be required, however, because of the rapid degradation of coagulation factors in the absence of vitamin K. Although vitamin K administration is required to reverse the blockade of coagulation factor activation, it cannot be relied upon for the patient with acute and consequential hemorrhage (Antidotes in Depth: Vitamin K).

Treatment with vitamin K takes several hours to activate enough factors to reverse the patient's coagulopathy,[107,131] and this delay may potentially be fatal.

Antidotal Treatment

Several issues influence the decision to treat a patient with a suspected overdose of a warfarinlike anticoagulant. Answers to the following questions should always be considered: Does the ingestion involve a warfarin-containing rodenticide or a pharmaceutical preparation? Is the ingestion unintentional or intentional? Does the patient require maintenance of therapeutic anticoagulation?

Life-threatening hemorrhage should immediately be reversed with FFP and vitamin K_1. The amount of FFP to adequately replace the vitamin K–dependent clotting factors to a level of 25% is equivalent to approximately 10–25 mL/kg.[159] In most cases, this should be adequate to reverse any coagulopathy. However, the specific factor quantities and volume of each unit may be varied, leading to an unpredictable response.[106] A recent study comparing the efficacy of FFP and clotting factor concentrates in rapid reversal of anticoagulation showed that despite significant reduction in the INR, FFP had an extremely varied effect on factor IX repletion. Clotting factor concentrates not only significantly decreased the INR, but completely corrected it and factor IX replacement was much more consistent.[106]

Repetitive, large doses of vitamin K_1 (on the order of 60 mg/d) may be required in some patients.[23,67,124] If complete reversal of the PT prolongation occurs or is desirable (as in most cases of life-threatening bleeding) and the patient's underlying medical condition still requires some degree of anticoagulation, they can then receive controlled anticoagulation with heparin until the bleeding is controlled and they are otherwise stable. This approach was used in 25% of patients in one study.[182]

Vitamin K_1 is the preferred form of vitamin K because the other forms of vitamin K are ineffective[86,119,123,171] and potentially toxic.[8] Parenteral administration of vitamin K_1 (AquaMEPHYTON) is traditionally preferred as initial therapy by many authors, but success can be achieved with early oral therapy as well.[30] In most cases reviewed, the patient was switched to oral vitamin K_1 preparations for long-term care. Vitamin K_1 can be administered intramuscularly, subcutaneously, intradermally, or intravenously. Although intravenous therapy has the most rapid onset of action of all routes of delivery, its use as the sole therapeutic agent is still associated with a delay of several hours[107,131] and carries the added risk of anaphylactoid reactions.[138] The use of low doses and slow rates of administration reduces this risk,[153] but we generally prefer that vitamin K_1 be administered by other than the intravenous route (Antidotes in Depth: Vitamin K).

For patients with non-life-threatening hemorrhage, the clinician must consider whether anticoagulation is required for long-term care. In patients not requiring chronic anticoagulation, even small elevations of the PT may be treated (with vitamin K_1 alone) to prevent a deterioration in coagulation status and reduce the risk of bleeding. Because in most cases, coagulopathy persists only for several days, there may be a rationale for prophylactic vitamin K_1 administration in known warfarinlike anticoagulant ingestions in patients not requiring anticoagulation. In contrast to ingestions of warfarin, prophylactic vitamin K_1 should never be given to asymptomatic children with unintentional ingestions of long-acting anticoagulants, for several reasons: (a) if the child develops a coagulopathy it will last for weeks, and the one or two doses of vi-

tamin K_1 given will not prevent complications; (b) because a gradual decline in coagulation factors occurs over the first day of anticoagulation, no child would be expected to develop a life-threatening coagulopathy in a single day; and (c) after vitamin K_1 is administered, the onset of an INR abnormality will be delayed, which could impair the clinician's ability to diagnose any coagulation abnormality, or, more likely, require an unnecessarily prolonged observation period.

For patients requiring chronic anticoagulation, The American College of Chest Physicians has issued guideline for management of patients with elevated INR values[2] (Table 42–4). Moreover, a recent study investigated the use of a regression formula to calculate the amount of oral vitamin K_1 necessary to partially correct the INR without completely discontinuing the oral anticoagulant. If validated, it would be extremely useful prior to minor surgery or dental procedures in patients requiring chronic anticoagulation while theoretically decreasing the likelihood of thromboembolism.[179]

Treatment of Long-Acting Anticoagulant Overdoses

The goal of therapy is to reverse the coagulopathy and to replace lost blood. Patients should have large-bore venous access established at the first sign of bleeding and have a blood type and crossmatch available for packed red blood cells and FFP. FFP is the initial treatment of choice for patients with active blood loss. It should be infused as needed, based on clinical symptoms and sequential PT or INR determinations. Vitamin K_1 is required, however, for long-term control of the INR.

Long-acting anticoagulants are metabolized by the hepatic mixed-function oxidase system (cytochrome P450).[7,123] In a rat model, the duration of coagulopathy was shortened by administering phenobarbital, a CYP3A4 inducer.[7] Although a phenobarbital effect has never been systematically studied in humans, this approach was employed by several authors in isolated human cases of long-acting anticoagulant toxicity.[32,86,100,170,177] Although these

TABLE 42–4. American College of Chest Physicians Consensus Conference 2001 Guidelines for Management of Excessive INR with and without Bleeding in Patients Requiring Chronic Anticoagulation.[2]

INR	Recommendations
Below 5.0	Lower dose or omit next dose of warfarin
Between 5.0–9.0	*Low risk:*[a] Discontinue warfarin for several doses or *High risk:*[a] Omit next dose and give oral vitamin K_1 (1–2.5 mg)
	If cannot be treated with oral medication then give parenteral vitamin K_1 (0.5–1 mg)
Between 9.0–20.0	Higher dose of oral vitamin K_1 (3–5 mg)
Greater than 20.0 (or rapid reversal of anticoagulation needed)	Vitamin K_1 10 mg slow parenteral[b] infusion with fresh-frozen plasma or prothrombin complex concentrate; vitamin K_1 administration may need to be repeated q12 h

[a]Low and high risk are determined by assessing parameters associated with potential hemorrhage such as recent hemorrhage, alcohol abuse, hepatic or renal impairment, and use of aspirin or other nonsteroidal anti-inflammatory agents.
[b]Although parenteral infusion of vitamin K is recommended, we urge caution when this route of administration is used because there may not be an appreciable difference in onset of therapeutic effect and, although rare, severe anaphylactoid reactions may occur.

anecdotal reports suggest some improvement with phenobarbital therapy, the risks of producing sedation in a patient who might be prone to bleeding complications appear consequential.[77]

Patients should be followed until their coagulation studies remain normal while off therapy for several days. This usually requires daily or even twice-daily INR measurements until the INR is at the lower limit of the therapeutic range. Monitoring of serial INR measurements should allow for a gradual decrease in vitamin K_1 requirement over time. Periodic coagulation factor analysis, however, may provide an early clue to the resolution of toxicity.[77] The patient may require weeks to months of close observation for both psychiatric and medical reasons.

PARENTERAL ANTICOAGULANTS

Heparin

Conventional or unfractionated heparin is a heterogeneous group of molecules within the class of glycosaminoglycans.[85] The heparin precursor molecule is composed of long chains of mucopolysaccharides, a polypeptide, and carbohydrates. The main carbohydrate components of heparin molecules include uronic acids and amino sugars in polysaccharide chains. Heparin for pharmaceutical use is extracted from bovine lung tissue and porcine intestines.[146]

As a therapeutic agent, heparin inhibits thrombosis by accelerating the binding of the protease inhibitor antithrombin III to thrombin and other serine proteases involved in coagulation.[105,140] Thus, factors IX to XII, kallikrein, and thrombin are inhibited. Heparin also affects plasminogen activator inhibitor, protein C inhibitor, and other components of coagulation. Heparin's therapeutic effect is usually measured through the activated PTT. The activated blood coagulation time (ACT) may be more useful for monitoring large therapeutic doses or in the overdose situation.[94]

Low-molecular-weight heparins are 4000–6000-dalton fractions obtained from conventional (unfractionated) heparin.[58] As such, they share many of the pharmacologic and toxicologic properties of conventional heparin.[24] The major differences between low-molecular-weight heparins and conventional heparin are greater bioavailability, longer half-life, more predictable anticoagulation with fixed dosing, and targeted activity against activated factor X, and less against activated factor II.[24,58] As a result of this targeted factor X activity, low-molecular-weight heparins have minimal effect on the activated PTT, thereby eliminating either the need for or the utility of monitoring. As such, they are administered on a fixed-dose schedule.

Low-molecular-weight heparins have been investigated for prevention of thromboembolic disease after hip surgery and trauma, in patients with stroke or deep venous thrombosis, in pregnancy, and in other conditions where anticoagulation with heparin would otherwise be indicated. Although these drugs are presumed to have a minimal risk in pregnancy[113] because they do not cross the placenta,[56,161] they are not approved for treatment or prophylaxis of thromboembolic disease. Most studies demonstrate a lower incidence of embolization; however, there is still a trend toward increased bleeding.[17,65,99]

Pharmacology

Because of heparin's large size and negative charge, it is unable to cross cellular membranes. For this reason, heparin is usually recommended for anticoagulation in pregnant women. These factors also eliminate oral administration as a therapeutic route, and heparin must be administered by either deep subcutaneous injection or by continuous intravenous infusion. Following parenteral administration heparin remains in the intravascular compartment, in part bound to globulins, fibrinogen, and low-density lipoproteins, thus resulting in a volume of distribution of 0.06 L/kg in humans.[50,125] Heparin has a short duration of effect, as a result of its rapid metabolism in the liver by a heparinase and by the reticuloendothelial system.[105] Although the half-life of elimination is dose dependent and ranges from 1 to 2.5 hours,[105,110,125] the duration of anticoagulant effect is usually reported as 1–3 hours.[105] Dosing errors or drug interactions with thrombolytic agents, antiplatelet drugs, or nonsteroidal antiinflammatory drugs may increase the risk of hemorrhage.[71]

Clinical Manifestations

Intentional overdoses with heparin are rare.[67,108] Most reported cases involve unintentional poisoning in hospitalized infants.[60,63,108,145] One neonate received 8000 U (2666 U/kg) of heparin. Bleeding from injection sites and intra-abdominal hemorrhage occurred after 17 hours despite administration of a total of 25.4 mg of protamine sulfate, and the infant died.[60] Similarly, the inadvertent administration of 8620 U/kg of heparin over 4 hours to a neonate via an umbilical catheter resulted in excessive bleeding from all skin puncture sites.[63] Another 3 cases of toxicity in infants related to flushing an indwelling catheter with heparin instead of saline.[145] These infants received 500–50,000 U of heparin and presented with respiratory distress, hypotension, bleeding from puncture sites and umbilical stumps, and gross hematuria. Finally, following the unintentional intramuscular administration of 20,000 U of heparin to an 8-month-old girl, a hematoma formed, bleeding from injection sites began within 2 hours, and her hemoglobin fell to 5.5 g/dL. Capillary coagulation times remained abnormal for 31 hours.[128]

Although no overdoses of low-molecular-weight heparins are reported, similar adverse effects to unfractionated heparins have been reported to include epidural/spinal hematoma, intrahepatic hemorrhage,[80] abdominal wall hematomas,[3] psoas hematoma after lumbar plexus block,[90] and intracranial hemorrhage in patients with malignancy in the brain.[48] These complications were all reported in patients who received the low-molecular-weight enoxaparin.

Evaluation and Treatment

After stabilization of the airway, breathing, and circulation are assured, the physician should be prepared to replace blood loss and reverse the coagulopathy, if indicated. Because of the relatively short duration of action of heparin, observation alone may be indicated if significant bleeding has not occurred. For the patient requiring anticoagulation, serial PTT determinations will indicate when it is safe to resume therapy. If significant bleeding occurs, either removal of the heparin or reversal of its anticoagulant effect is indicated. Because heparin has a very small volume of distribution, it can be effectively removed by exchange transfusion.[145] Although this technique has been used successfully in neonates, it is not generally applicable to older children and adults.

When severe bleeding occurs, heparin may be effectively neutralized by protamine sulfate. Protamine is a low-molecular-weight protein found in the sperm and testes of salmon, which forms ionic bonds with heparin and renders it devoid of anticoagulant activity.[105] One milligram of protamine sulfate injected intravenously neutralizes 100 U of heparin.[105] The dose of protamine should be calculated from the dose of heparin administered and heparin's approximate half-life, such that the amount of protamine does not exceed the amount of heparin expected to be found intravascularly at the time of infusion. As with other foreign proteins, protamine administration is associated with numerous adverse effects. Because approximately 0.2% of patients receiving protamine experience anaphylaxis, a complication that carries a 30% mortality rate, most authors commonly recommend that protamine be reserved for patients with life-threatening hemorrhage[78] (Antidotes in Depth: Protamine).

Because of the severe adverse effects associated with protamine, current research is focusing on safer methods to reverse heparin anticoagulation. These experimental agents include heparinase,[114] designer protamine variants,[173,174] and platelet factor 4.[46]

If life-threatening bleeding occurs following low-molecular-weight heparin administration, patients should be treated supportively. The newer (safer) experimental protamine variants appear to be effective against low-molecular-weight heparins but as of yet are unavailable.[173,174]

NONBLEEDING COMPLICATIONS OF ANTICOAGULANTS

Warfarin therapy is associated with three nonhemorrhagic lesions of the skin: urticaria,[144] purple toe syndrome,[53] and warfarin skin necrosis.[42,91,95,112,172] Although skin necrosis was once thought to be a rare and idiosyncratic reaction,[91,95] more recent evidence suggests a link between this disorder and protein C deficiency.[95,172] Protein C is also dependent on vitamin K.[38] Patients who are homozygotes for protein C deficiency have an increased incidence of thrombosis and embolic events, such that they often require long-term anticoagulant therapy.[38] Because the half-life of protein C is shorter than that of many of the vitamin K–dependent coagulation factors, protein C levels fall rapidly during the first hours of warfarin therapy. In the protein C–deficient patient, protein C levels fall dramatically prior to a reduction in coagulation factors. This results in an imbalance that actually favors coagulation, and skin necrosis results.[112,172] Although warfarin skin necrosis is more common in patients with protein C deficiency, this disorder is also described in patients with protein S and antithrombin III deficiencies.[42] Unfortunately, these deficiencies are neither necessary nor sufficient to account for the incidence of warfarin necrosis.[42] If necrosis occurs, warfarin should be discontinued and heparin should be initiated to decrease thrombosis of postcapillary venules. Some patients may also require surgical debridement.[168] The purple toe syndrome, in contrast to warfarin-induced skin necrosis, is presumed to result from small atheroemboli that are no longer adherent to their plaques by clot.

An additional major nonhemorrhagic complication of warfarin therapy relates to its use in pregnant women. Most warfarin-induced fetal abnormalities occur during weeks 6 to 12 of gestation, but central nervous system (CNS) and ocular abnormalities can develop at any time during gestation.[69,158]

Heparin therapy is associated with a transient and mild heparin-induced thrombocytopenia (HIT) that occurs in about 25% of patients during the first few days of therapy. Although this syndrome results from heparin-induced platelet aggregation, a more severe form of thrombocytopenia occurs in 1–5% of patients between days 7 and 14 of therapy (Heparin-induced thrombocytopenia and thrombosis, or HITT).[5,104,105,185] Heparin stimulates platelets to release platelet factor 4, which subsequently complexes with heparin to provoke an IgG response. These antibodies against the heparin-platelet factor 4 complex activate platelets, leading to platelet-fibrin thrombotic events known as the white clot syndrome. Because low-molecular-weight heparins do not stimulate the release of platelet factor 4, their use is not associated with either severe thrombocytopenia or the white clot syndrome.[176] However, once HITT occurs, low-molecular-weight heparins are not recommended as alternative therapy. In patients previously treated with heparin these events can occur earlier than 7 days. Patients may present with either hemorrhagic or thromboembolic complications. Necrotizing skin lesions[134] and hyperkalemia from aldosterone suppression[126] are rarely reported in patients receiving heparin therapy.

Some additional complications of heparin use include osteoporosis, which mostly occurs in patients on long-term therapy with unfractionated heparin.[81] A small percentage of these patients may develop bone fractures if treated continuously for more than 3 months. Data for low-molecular-weight heparins are limited and the incidence of osteoporosis may be less as compared to unfractionated heparin.[81]

OTHER ANTICOAGULANTS
Snake Venoms

A detailed discussion of snake envenomations is found in Chapter 101; only a few specific issues are discussed here. Snake venoms may be composed of a vast number of complex proteins and peptides that interact with components of the human hemostatic system. Their functions may be thought of in general as being procoagulant, anticoagulant, fibrinolytic, vessel wall interactive, platelet active, or as protein inactivators. Additionally, they may more specifically also be classified based on their specific biologic activity and some of the various mechanisms include individual factor activating, inhibition of protein C and thrombin, fibrinogen degradation, platelet aggregation, and inhibitors of serine protease inhibitors (SERPINS). Currently, there are more than 100 different snake venoms that affect the hemostatic system;[83,84] Figure 42–2 provides an overview of their multiple interactions with the coagulation and fibrinolytic systems.[102]

Some of these venom proteins are used as therapeutic agents for human diseases. Ancrod, a purified derivative of the Malaysian pit viper, *Calloselasma rhodostoma*, is used in the treatment of deep-vein thrombosis, myocardial infarction, pulmonary embolus, and acute cerebrovascular thrombosis because of its defibrinogenating property.[13] In a multicenter study of 500 patients with acute or progressing ischemic neurologic events, ancrod showed a favorable benefit-risk as compared to placebo.[152] As expected, an increased risk of hemorrhage was observed; however, the risk appears to be less than that with thrombolytic agents.[152] Monitoring of fibrinogen levels is essential to avoid potential complications and no specific antidote exists. For envenomation of other snake venoms (such as from the Crotalidae family) that induce hemorrhage, antivenin treatment may be required.

Hirudin

Hirudin, a 65-amino-acid polypeptide produced by the salivary glands of the medicinal leech (*Hirudo medicinalis*), irreversibly blocks thrombin without the need for antithrombin III.[148] Unlike heparin, the small size of hirudin allows it to enter clots and inhibit clot-bound thrombin, offering the distinct advantage of restricting further thrombus formation. Hirudin demonstrates enhanced bioavailability and a longer half-life than unfractionated heparin. In addition, there are no known natural inhibitors of hirudin, such as platelet factor 4. Desirudin is a recombinant hirudin that is used in acute coronary syndromes, in the prevention of thromboembolic diseases, and in patients with heparin-induced thrombocytopenia.[21,143,148] Both of these compounds appear to be at least as effective as unfractionated heparin, and without increased bleeding or thrombocytopenia. However, in the GUSTO IIb study of patients with unstable angina/non-Q-wave myocardial infarction, there was an increase in the number of blood transfusions in patients who received desirudin as compared to those who received heparin.[62]

Thrombolytic Agents

The fibrinolytic system is designed to remove unwanted clots and leave those clots protecting sites of vascular injury intact. Plasminogen exists as a proenzyme and is converted to the active form, plasmin, by various plasminogen activators.[40,41] t-PA is released from the endothelium, and is under the inhibitory control of two inactivators known as tissue plasminogen activator inhibitors 1 and 2 (t-PAI-1 and t-PAI-2).[40,41,105,115] Plasmin's actions are non-specific in that it degrades not only fibrin clots but also some plasma proteins and coagulation factors.[105] Inhibition at the level of plasmin occurs through α_2-antiplasmin.

With their diverse indications in acute myocardial infarction, unstable angina, arterial and venous thrombosis and embolism, and cerebrovascular disease, the thrombolytic agents (streptokinase, urokinase, alteplase, reteplase, tenectaplase, and anistreplase) are used commonly.[14] The reader is referred to one of a number of reviews for specific indications and dosing regimens.[43,96,105,133,155,181] Although all agents enhance fibrinolysis, they differ in their specific sites of action and durations of effect. Alteplase (t-PA), reteplase, and tenectaplase are specific for clot (they do not increase fibrinolysis in the absence of a thrombus), whereas streptokinase, urokinase, and anistreplase are not clot-specific. Alteplase has the shortest half-life and duration of effect (5 minutes and 2 hours, respectively), and anistreplase has the longest (90 minutes and 18 hours, respectively).[133,155] Streptokinase has the additional risk of severe allergic reaction on rechallenge, limiting its use to once in a lifetime.

Newer thrombolytic drugs such as monteplase, lanoteplase, pamiteplase, and staphylokinase are being evaluated for therapeutic use. These agents have a longer half-life in plasma and may be administered via single or repeated bolus injections. Although they also have increased fibrin selectivity, no improvement in long-term mortality has been demonstrated.[4] Although the incidence of bleeding requiring transfusion may be as high as 7.7% following high-dose (150 mg) alteplase and 4.4% following low-dose alteplase,[43] the incidence of life-threatening hemorrhage is much lower.[181] The addition of heparin to the thrombolytic regimen increases the risk of bleeding. Reviews of multiple trials suggest that life-threatening events such as intracranial hemorrhage occur in 0.30–0.58% of patients receiving anistreplase, 0.42–0.73% of patients receiving alteplase, and 0.08–0.30% of patients receiving streptokinase.[181] The frequency of bleeding events is essentially equal regardless of the thrombolytic agent used even with the newer agents, with the exception of lanoteplase.[47] Currently, no agents exist to reverse thrombolysis, and prevention is best practiced with the use of weight-based doses of thrombolytic agents and heparin. Only supportive care is indicated for patients with bleeding complications.

SUMMARY

The ever-increasing frequency of anticoagulant therapeutic use is associated with complications and adverse outcomes. A complete understanding of the normal mechanisms of coagulation, anticoagulation, and thrombolysis combined with an understanding of the pharmacology of the agents and the patient's clinical needs allows the clinician to better choose among the complex therapies currently available.

REFERENCES

1. Ancalmo N, Ochsner J: Heparin, the miracle drug: A brief history of its discovery. J La State Med Soc 1990;142:22–24.
2. Ansell J, Hirsh J, Dalen J, et al: Managing oral anticoagulant therapy. Chest 2001;119:22S–38S.
3. Antonelli D, Fares L 2nd, Anene C: Enoxaparin associated with huge abdominal wall hematomas: A report of two cases. Am Surg 2000;66:797–800.
4. Assessment of the safety and efficacy of a new thrombolytic (ASSENT-II investigators): Single-bolus tenecteplase compared with front-loaded alteplase in acute myocardial infarction: The ASSENT-II double-blind randomized trial. Lancet 1999;354:716–722.
5. Aster RH: Heparin-induced thrombocytopenia and thrombosis. N Engl J Med 1995;332:1374–1376.
6. Babcock J, Hartman K, Pedersen A, et al: Rodenticide-induced coagulopathy in a young child. A case of Munchausen syndrome by proxy. Am J Pediatr Hematol Oncol 1993;15:126–130.
7. Bachmann KA, Sullivan TJ: Dispositional and pharmacodynamic characteristics of brodifacoum in warfarin-sensitive rats. Pharmacology 1983;27:281–288.
8. Badr M, Yoshihara H, Kauffman F, Thurman RA: Menadione causes selective toxicity to periportal regions of the liver lobule. Toxicol Lett 1987;35:241–246.
9. Barlow AM, Gay AL, Park BK: Difenacoum (Neosorexa) poisoning. Br Med J 1982;285:541.
10. Barnett VT, Bergmann F, Humphrey H, Chediak J: Diffuse alveolar hemorrhage secondary to superwarfarin ingestion. Chest 1992;102:1301–1302.
11. Basehore LM, Mowry JM: Death following ingestion of superwarfarin rodenticide: A case report. Vet Hum Toxicol 1987;29:459.
12. Becker RC: Seminars in thrombosis, thrombolysis, and vascular biology. Cardiology 1991;78:257–266.
13. Bell WR Jr: Defibrinogenating enzymes. Drugs 1997;54(Suppl 3):15–31.
14. Benedict CR, Mueller S, Anderson HV, Willerson JT: Thrombolytic therapy: A state of the art review. Hosp Pract 1991;27:61–72.
15. Bennett DL, Caravatti DM, Veltri JC: Long-acting anticoagulant ingestion: A prospective study [abstract]. Vet Hum Toxicol 1987;29:472.
16. Beretz A, Cazenave JD: Old and new natural products as the source of modern antithrombotic drugs. Planta Med 1991;57(7):S68–S72.

17. Bergqvist D, Benoni G, Bjorgell O, et al: Low-molecular-weight heparin (enoxaparin) as prophylaxis against venous thromboembolism after total hip replacement. N Engl J Med 1996;335: 696–700.

18. Berry RG, Morrison JA, Watts JW, et al: Surreptitious superwarfarin ingestion with brodifacoum. South Med J 2000;93:74–75.

19. Beyth RJ, Quinn LM, Landefeld S: Prospective evaluation of an index for predicting the risk of major bleeding in outpatients treated with warfarin. Am J Med 1998;105:91–99.

20. Bithell TC: Acquired coagulation disorders. In: Lee GR, Bithell TC, Foerster J, et al, eds: Wintrobe's Clinical Hematology, 9th ed. Philadelphia, Lea & Febiger, 1993, pp. 1473–1503.

21. Bittl JA, Strony J, Brinker JA: Treatment with bivalirudin (Hirulog) as compared to heparin during coronary angioplasty for unstable or postinfarction angina. N Engl J Med 1995;333:764–769.

22. Boermans HJ, Johnstone I, Black WD, Murphy M: Clinical signs, laboratory changes and toxicokinetics of brodifacoum in the horse. Can J Vet Res 1991;55:21–27.

23. Boster SR, Bergin JL: Upper airway obstruction complicating warfarin therapy: With a note on reversal of warfarin toxicity. Ann Emerg Med 1983;12:711–715.

24. Bounameaux H, Goldhaber SZ: Uses of low-molecular-weight heparin. Blood Rev 1995;9:213–219.

25. Bowen KJ, Vukeljia SJ: Hypercoagulable states: Their causes and management. Postgrad Med 1992;91:117–132.

26. Braithwaite GB: Vitamin K and brodifacoum. J Am Vet Med Assoc 1982;181:531–534.

27. Breckenridge A, Leck JB, Serlin MJ, Wilson A: Mechanisms of action of the anticoagulants warfarin, 2-chloro-3-phytylnaphthoquinone (CL-K), acenocoumarol, brodifacoum, and difenacoum in the rabbit. Br J Pharmacol 1978;64:339.

28. Breckenridge A, Orme M: Plasma half-lives and the pharmacological effect of the enantiomers of warfarin in rats. Life Sci 1972;11: 337–345.

29. Breckenridge A, Orme M, Wessling H, et al: Pharmacokinetics and pharmacodynamics of the enantiomers of warfarin in man. Clin Pharmacol Ther 1974;15:424–430.

30. Bruno GR, Howland MA, McMeeking A, Hoffman RS: Long-acting anticoagulant overdose: Brodifacoum kinetics and optimal vitamin K dosing. Ann Emerg Med 2000;36:262–267.

31. Burgess JL, Robertson WO: Washington's experience and recommendations re: Anticoagulant rodenticides. Vet Hum Toxicol 1995; 37:362–363.

32. Burucoa C, Mura P, Robert R, et al: Chlorophacinone intoxication a biological and toxicological study. J Toxicol Clin Toxicol 1989;27: 79–89.

33. Butcher GP, Shearer MH, MacNicoll AD, et al: Difenacoum poisoning as a cause of hematuria. Hum Exp Toxicol 1992;11:553–554.

34. Carpentieri U, Mghiem QX, Harris LC: Clinical experience with an oral anticoagulant in children. Arch Dis Child 1976;51:445–448.

35. Casner PR: Superfwarfarin toxicity. Am J Ther 1998;5:117–120.

36. Chong L, Chau WK, Ho CH: A case of "superwarfarin" poisoning. Scand J Haematol 1986;36:314–315.

37. Choonara BA, Scott AK, Haynes BP, et al: Vitamin K₁ metabolism in relation to pharmacodynamic response in anticoagulated patients. Br J Clin Pharmacol 1985;20:643–648.

38. Clouse LH, Comp PC: The regulation of hemostasis: The protein C system. N Engl J Med 1986;314:1298–1303.

39. Coccheri S, Gualtiero, P, Cosmi B: Oral anticoagulant therapy: Efficacy, safety, and the low-dose controversy. Haemostasis 1999;29: 150–165.

40. Collen D: On the regulation and control of fibrinolysis. Thromb Haemost 1980;43:77–89.

41. Collen D, Lijnen HR: Basic and clinical aspects of fibrinolysis and thrombosis. Blood 1991;78:3114–3124.

42. Comp PC: Coumarin-induced skin necrosis: Incidence, mechanisms, management and avoidance. Drug Saf 1993;8:128–135.

43. Conti RC: Brief overview of the endpoints of thrombolytic therapy. Am J Cardiol 1991;67:8E–10E.

44. Corke PJ: Superwarfarin (brodifacoum) poisoning. Anaesth Intens Care 1997;25:707–709.

45. Davie EW, Ratnoff OD: Waterfall sequence for intrinsic blood clotting. Science 1964;145:1310–1312.

46. Dehmer GJ, Fisher M, Tate DA, Teo S: Reversal of heparin anticoagulation by recombinant platelet factor 4 in humans. Circulation 1995;91:2188–2194.

47. den Heijer P, Vermeer F, Ambrosioni E, et al, on behalf of the InTIME-1 investigators: Evaluation of a weight-adjusted single-bolus plasminogen activator in patients with myocardial infarction. A double-blind, randomized angiographic trial of lanoteplase versus alteplase. Circulation 1998;98:2117–2125.

48. Dickinson LD, Miller L, Patel CP, Gupta SK: Enoxaparin increases the incidence of postoperative intracranial hemorrhage when initiated preoperatively for deep venous thrombosis prophylaxis with brain tumors. Neurosurgery 1998;43:1074–1081.

49. Dowd P, Ham S, Naganathan S, Hershline R: The mechanism of action of vitamin K. Annu Rev Nutr 1995;15:419–440.

50. Estes JW, Poulem PF: Pharmacokinetics of heparin. Thromb Diath Haemorrh 1974;33:26–37.

51. Exner DV, Brien WF, Murphy MJ: Superwarfarin ingestion. Can Med Assoc J 1992;146:34–35.

52. Fasco MJ, Hildebrandt EF, Suttie JW: Evidence that warfarin anticoagulant action involves two distinct reductase activities. J Biol Chem 1982;257:11210–11212.

53. Feder W, Auerbach R: Purple toes: An uncommon sequela of oral coumarin drug therapy. Ann Intern Med 1961;55:911–917.

54. Felice LJ, Chalermchaikit T, Murphy MJ: Multicomponent determination of 4-hydroxycoumarin anticoagulant rodenticides in blood serum by liquid chromatography with fluorescence detection. J Anal Toxicol 1991;15:126–129.

55. Fihn SD, Callahan CM, Marin DC, et al: The risk for and severity of bleeding complications in elderly patients treated with warfarin. The National Consortium of Anticoagulation. Ann Intern Med 1996;124: 970–979.

56. Forestier F, Daffos F, Capella-Pavlovsky M: Low-molecular-weight heparin (PH 10169) does not cross the placenta during the second trimester of pregnancy: Study by direct foetal blood sampling under ultrasound. Thromb Res 1984;34:557–560.

57. Freedman MD, Olatidoye AG: Clinically significant drug interactions with the oral anticoagulants. Drug Saf 1994;10:381–394.

58. Frydman A: Low-molecular-weight-heparins: An overview of pharmacodynamics, pharmacokinetics and metabolism in humans. Haemostasis 1996;26(Suppl 2):24–38.

59. Furie B, Furie BC: Molecular and cellular biology of blood coagulation. N Engl J Med 1992;326:800–806.

60. Galant SP: Accidental heparinization of a newborn infant. Am J Dis Child 1967;114:313–319.

61. Gilbert GE, Sims PJ, Wiedmer T, et al: Platelet derived microparticles express high affinity receptors for factor VIII. J Biol Chem 1991;266:17261–17268.

62. Global Use of Strategies to Open Occluded Coronary Arteries (GUSTO) IIb investigators: A comparison of recombinant hirudin with heparin for the treatment of acute coronary syndromes. N Engl J Med 1996;335:775–782.

63. Glueck HI, Light IJ, Flessa H, et al: Sodium heparin administration to a newborn infant. JAMA 1965;191:159–160.

64. Greeff MC, Mashile O, MacDougall LG: Superwarfarin (bromodialone) poisoning in two children resulting in prolonged anticoagulation. Lancet 1987;2:1269.

65. Green D, Hirsh J, Heit J, et al: Low-molecular-weight heparin: A critical analysis of clinical trials. Pharmacol Rev 1994;46:89–109.

66. Gurwitz JH, Avron J, Ross-Degnan D, et al: Aging and the anticoagulant response to warfarin therapy. Ann Intern Med 1992;116: 901–904.

67. Hackett LP, Ileet KF, Chester A: Plasma warfarin concentrations after a massive overdose. Med J Aust 1985;142:642–643.

68. Haines ST, Bussey HI: Thrombosis and pharmacology of antithrombotic agents. Ann Pharmacotherapy 1995;29:892–905.

69. Hall JG, Pauli RM, Wilson KM: Maternal and fetal sequelae of anticoagulation during pregnancy. Am J Med 1980;68:122–140.

70. Handin RI, Rosenberg RD: Hemorrhagic disorders. III: Disorders of primary and secondary hemostasis. In: Beck WS, ed: Hematology, 2nd ed. Cambridge, MA, MIT Press, 1977, pp. 547–567.

71. Harrington R, Ansell J: Risk-benefit assessment of anticoagulant therapy. Drug Saf 1991;6:54–69.

72. Harris EN, Gharavi AE, Asherson RA, Hugher GR: Antiphospholipid antibodies: A review. Eur J Rheumatol Inflamm 1984;7:5–8.

73. Helmuth RA, McCloskey OW, Doeden DJ, et al: Fatal ingestion of a brodifacoum-containing rodenticide. Lab Med 1989;20:25–27.

74. Hirsh J: Substandard monitoring of warfarin in North America. Arch Intern Med 1992;152:257–258.

75. Hirsh J, Dalen, JE, et al: Oral anticoagulants: Mechanism of action, clinical effectiveness, and optimal therapeutic range. Chest 1998; 114:445S–469S.

76. Hirsh J, Poller L: The international normalized ratio: A guide to understanding and correcting its problems. Arch Intern Med 1994;154: 282–288.

77. Hoffman RS, Smilkstein MJ, Goldfrank LR: Evaluation of coagulation factor abnormalities in long-acting anticoagulant overdose. J Toxicol Clin Toxicol 1988;26:233–248.

78. Holland CL, Singh AK, McMaster PRB, et al: Adverse reactions to protamine sulfate following cardiac surgery. Clin Cardiol 1984;7: 157–162.

79. Hollinger BR, Pastoor TP: Case management and plasma half-life in a case of brodifacoum poisoning. Arch Intern Med 1993;153: 1925–1928.

80. Houde JP, Steinberg G: Intrahepatic hemorrhage after use of low-molecular weight heparin for total hip arthroplasty. J Arthroplasty 1999;14:372–374.

81. Hovanessian HC: New-generation anticoagulants: The low-molecular-weight heparins. Ann Emerg Med 1999;34:768–779.

82. Hui CH, Lie A, Lam CK, Bourke C: "Superwarfarin" poisoning leading to prolonged coagulopathy. Forensic Sci Int 1996;78:13–18.

83. Iyaniwura TT: Snake venom constituents: Biochemistry and toxicology, part 1. Vet Hum Toxicol 1991;33:468–474.

84. Iyaniwura TT: Snake venom constituents: Biochemistry and toxicology, part 2. Vet Hum Toxicol 1991;33:475–480.

85. Jacques LB: The discovery of heparin. Semin Thromb Hemost 1978; 4:350–353.

86. Jones EC, Growe GH, Naiman SC: Prolonged anticoagulation in rat poisoning. JAMA 1984;252:3005–3007.

87. Katona B, Sigell LT, Wason S: Anticoagulant rodenticide poisoning [abstract]. Vet Hum Toxicol 1986;28:478.

88. Katona B, Wason S: Superwarfarin poisoning. J Emerg Med 1989; 7:627–631.

89. Katona B, Wason S: Anticoagulant rodenticide poisoning. Clin Toxicol Rev 1986;8:1–2.

90. Klein SM, D'Ercole F, Greenglass RA, Warner DS: Enoxaparin associated with psoas hematoma and lumbar plexopathy after lumbar plexus block. Anesthesiology 1997;87:1576–1579.

91. Koch-Weser J: Coumarin necrosis. Ann Intern Med 1968;68: 1365–1367.

92. Kruse JA, Carlson RW: Fatal rodenticide poisoning with brodifacoum. Ann Emerg Med 1992;21:333–336.

93. Kuijpers EA, den Hartigh J, Savelkoul TJ: A method for the simultaneous identification and quantitation of five superwarfarin rodenticides in human serum. J Anal Toxicol 1995;19:557–562.

94. Kunert M, Sorgenicht R, Scheuble L, et al: Value of activated blood coagulation time in monitoring anticoagulation during coronary angioplasty. Z Kardiol 1996;85:118–124.

95. Lacy JP, Godin RR: Warfarin induced necrosis of the skin. Ann Intern Med 1975;82:381–382.

96. Lawrence PF, Goodman GR: Thrombolytic therapy. Surg Clin North Am 1992;72:899–918.

97. Lechner K, Pabinger-Fasching I: Lupus anticoagulants and thrombosis: A study of 25 cases and review of the literature. Haemostasis 1985;15:254–262.

98. Leck JB, Park BK: A comparative study of the effect of warfarin and brodifacoum on the relationship between vitamin K_1 metabolism and clotting factor activity in warfarin-susceptible and warfarin-resistant rats. Biochem Pharmacol 1981;30:123–128.

99. Levine M, Gent M, Hirsh J, et al: A comparison of low-molecular-weight heparin administered primarily at home with unfractionated heparin administered in the hospital for proximal deep-vein thrombosis. N Engl J Med 1996;334:677–681.

100. Lipton RA, Klass EM: Human ingestion of a "superwarfarin" rodenticide resulting in a prolonged anticoagulant effect. JAMA 1984; 252:3004–3005.

101. Lund M: Comparative effect of the three rodenticides warfarin, difenacoum, and brodifacoum on eight rodent species in short feeding periods. J Hyg 1981;87:101–107.

102. Markland FS: Snake venoms and the hemostatic system. Toxicon 1998;36:1749–1800.

103. MacFarlane RG: An enzyme cascade in the blood clotting mechanism and its function as a biochemical amplifier. Nature 1964;202: 498–499.

104. MacLean JA, Moscicki R, Bloch KJ: Adverse reactions to heparin. Ann Allergy 1990;65:254–259.

105. Majerus PW, Broze GJ, Miletich JP, Tollefsen DM: Anticoagulant, thrombolytic, and antiplatelet drugs. In: Hardman JG, Limbird LE, Molinoff PB, Ruddon RW, eds: Goodman and Gilman's The Pharmacological Basis of Therapeutics, 9th ed. New York, McGraw-Hill, 1996, pp. 1341–1359.

106. Makris M, Greaves M, Phillips WS, et al: Emergency oral anticoagulant reversal: The relative efficacy of infusions of fresh frozen plasma and clotting factor concentrate on correction of the coagulopathy. Thromb Haemost 1997;77:477–480.

107. Marcus AJ: Hemorrhagic disorders: Abnormalities of platelet and vascular function. In: Wyngaarden JB, Smith LH, eds: Cecil Textbook of Medicine, 18th ed. Philadelphia, WB Saunders, 1988, pp. 1042–1051.

108. Martin CMM, Engstrom PF, Barrett O: Surreptitious self-administration of heparin. JAMA 1970;212:475–476.

109. Mathiesen T, Benediktsdottir K, Johnsson H, Lindqvist M: Intracranial traumatic and nontraumatic haemorrhagic complications of warfarin treatment. Acta Neurol Scand 1995;91:208–214.

110. McAvoy TJ: Pharmacokinetic modeling of heparin and its clinical implications. J Pharmacokinet Biopharm 1979;7:331–354.

111. McCarthy PT, Cox AD, Harrington DJ, et al: Covert poisoning with difenacoum: Clinical and toxicological observations. Hum Exp Toxicol 1997;16:166–170.

112. McGhee WG, Klotz TA, Epstein DJ, et al: Coumarin necrosis associated with hereditary protein C deficiency. Ann Intern Med 1984; 101:59–60.

113. Melissari E, Parker CJ, Wilson NV, et al: Use of low-molecular-weight heparin in pregnancy. Thromb Haemost 1992;68:652–656.

114. Michelsen LG, Kikura M, Levy JH, et al: Heparinase I (neutralase) reversal of systemic anticoagulation. Anesthesiology 1996;85: 339–346.

115. Mosher DF: Blood coagulation and fibrinolysis: An overview. Clin Cardiol 1990;13:5–11.

116. Mount ME: Diagnosis and therapy of anticoagulant rodenticide intoxications. Vet Clin North Am 1988;18:115–130.

117. Mullins ME, Brands CL, Daya, MR: Unintentional pediatric superwarfarin exposures: Do we really need a prothrombin time? Pediatrics 2000;105:402–404.

118. Mueller RL: History of drugs for thrombotic disease: Discovery, development, and directions for the future. Circulation 1994;89:432–450.

119. Murdoch DA: Prolonged anticoagulation in chlorophacinone poisoning. Lancet 1983;1:355–356.

120. Ng VL, Lewin J, Corash L, Gottfried EL: Failure of the International Normalized Ratio to generate consistent results within a local medical community. Am J Clin Pathol 1993;99:689–694.

121. Nichols WL, Bowie EJW: Standardization of the prothrombin time for monitoring orally administered anticoagulant therapy with use of the international normalized ratio system. Mayo Clin Proc 1993;68:897–898.

122. O'Bryan SM, Constable DJ: Quantification of brodifacoum in plasma and liver tissue by HPLC. J Anal Toxicol 1991;15:144–147.

123. O'Reilly RA: Vitamin K antagonists. In: Colman RW, Hirsh J, Marder VJ, Salzman EW, eds: Hemostasis and Thrombosis. Philadelphia, Lippincott, 1987, pp. 846–860.

124. O'Reilly RA, Aggeler PM: Surreptitious ingestion of coumarin anticoagulant drugs. Ann Intern Med 1966;64:1034–1041.

125. Olsson P, Lagergren H, Ek S: The elimination from plasma of intravenous heparin. Acta Med Scand 1963;173:619–630.

126. Oster JR, Singer I, Fishman LM: Heparin-induced aldosterone suppression and hyperkalemia. Am J Med 1995;98:575–586.

127. Osterud B, Rapaport SI: Activation of factor IX by the reaction product of tissue factor and factor VII: Additional pathway for initiating blood coagulation. Proc Natl Acad Sci U S A 1977;74:5260–5264.

128. Pachman DJ: Accidental heparin poisoning in an infant. Am J Dis Child 1965;110:210–212.

129. Palmer RB, Alakija P, Cde Baka JE, Nolte KB: Fatal brodifacoum rodenticide poisoning: Autopsy and toxicologic findings. J Forensic Sci 1999;44:851–855.

130. Park BK, Leck JB: A comparison of vitamin K antagonism by warfarin, difenacoum, and brodifacoum in the rabbit. Biochem Pharmacol 1982;31:3535–3639.

131. Park BK, Scott AK, Wilson AC, et al: Plasma disposition of vitamin K_1 in relation to anticoagulant poisoning. Br J Clin Pharmacol 1984;18:655–661.

132. Parsons BJ, Day LM, Ozanne-Smith J, Dobbin M: Rodenticide poisoning among children. Aust N Z J Public Health 1996;20:488–492.

133. Paspa PA, Movahed A: Thrombolytic therapy in acute myocardial infarction. Am Fam Physician 1992;45:640–647.

134. Platell CFE, Tan EGC: Hypersensitivity reactions to heparin: Delayed onset thrombocytopenia and necrotizing skin lesions. Aust N Z J Surg 1986;56:621–623.

135. Raskob GE, Pineo GF, Hull RD: The technique of administering oral anticoagulant therapy. J Crit Illness 1991;6:923–930.

136. Rauch AE, Weininger R, Pasquale D, et al: Superwarfarin poisoning: A significant public health problem. J Community Health 1994;19:55–65.

137. Renowden S, Westmoreland D, White JP, Routledge PA: Oral cholestyramine increases the elimination of warfarin after overdose. Br Med J 1985;291:513–514.

138. Rich EC, Prage CW: Severe complications of intravenous phytonadione therapy. Postgrad Med 1982;72:303–306.

139. Roberts HR, Lozier JN: New perspectives on the coagulation cascade. Hosp Pract 1992;27:97–112.

140. Rosenberg RD: Actions and interactions of antithrombin and heparin. N Engl J Med 1975;292:146–151.

141. Ross GS, Zacharski LR, Robert D, Rabin DL: An acquired hemorrhagic disorder from long-acting rodenticide ingestion. Arch Intern Med 1992;151:411–412.

142. Routh CR, Triplett DA, Murphy MJ, et al: Superwarfarin ingestion and detection. Am J Hematol 1991;36:50–54.

143. Schiele F, Vuillemenot A, Mouhat T, et al: Anticoagulant therapy with recombinant hirudin in patients with thrombocytopenia induced by heparin. Presse Med 1996;25:757–760.

144. Schiff BL, Kern AB: Cutaneous reactions to anticoagulants. Arch Dermatol 1968;98:136–137.

145. Schreiner RL, Wynn RJ, McNulty C: Accidental heparin toxicity in the newborn intensive care unit. J Pediatr 1978;92:115–116.

146. Schwartz BS: Heparin: What is it? How does it work? Clin Cardiol 1990;13:12–15.

147. Seidelmann S, Kubic V, Burton E, Schmitz L: Combined superwarfain and ethylene glycol ingestion: A unique case report with misleading clinical history. Am J Clin Pathol 1995;104:663–666.

148. Serruys PW, Herrman JR, Simon R: A comparison of hirudin with heparin in the prevention of restenosis after coronary angioplasty. N Engl J Med 1995;333:757–763.

149. Shapiro SS: Acquired anticoagulants. In: Williams WJ, Beutler E, Erslev AJ, Rundles RW, eds: Hematology, 2nd ed. New York, McGraw-Hill, 1973, pp. 1447–1454.

150. Sheen SR, Spiller HA, Grossman D: Symptomatic brodifacoum ingestion requiring high-dose phytonadione therapy. Vet Hum Toxicol 1994;36:216–217.

151. Shepard G, Klein-Schwartz W, Anderson B: Acute pediatric brodifacoum ingestions [abstract]. J Toxicol Clin Toxicol 1998;36:464.

152. Sherman DG, Atkinson RP, Chippendale T, et al: Intravenous ancrod for treatment of acute ischemic stroke: The stat study: A randomized controlled trial. JAMA 2000;283:2395–2403.

153. Shields RC, McBane RD, Kuiper JD, Li H, Herr JA: Efficacy and safety of intravenous phytonadione (vitamin K_1) in patients on long-term oral anticoagulant therapy. Mayo Clin Proc 2001;76:260–266.

154. Sims PJ, Faioni EM, Wiedmer T, Shattil SJ: Complement proteins CX5b–9 cause release of membrane vesicles from the platelet surface that are enriched in the membrane receptor for coagulation factor Va and express prothrombinase activity. J Biol Chem 1988;263:18205–18212.

155. Smitherman TC: Considerations affecting selection of thrombolytic agents. Mol Biol Med 1991;8:207–218.

156. Smolinske SC, Scherger DL, Kearns PS, et al: Superwarfarin poisoning in children: A prospective study. Pediatrics 1989;84:490–494.

157. Stenflo J, Suttie JW: Vitamin K-dependent formation of the γ-carboxyglutamic acid. Annu Rev Biochem 1977;46:157–172.

158. Stevenson RE, Burton AM, Ferlauto GJ, et al: Hazards of oral anticoagulants during pregnancy. JAMA 1980;243:1549–1551.

159. Storer DL: Blood and blood component therapy. In: Rosen P, Barkin R, et al, eds: Emergency Medicine Concepts and Clinical Practice, 4th ed., Vol 1. St Louis, Mosby, 1998, pp. 124–137.

160. Stowe CM, Metz AL, Arendt TD, Schulman J: Apparent brodifacoum poisoning in a dog. J Am Vet Med Assoc 1983;182:817–818.

161. Sturridge F, de Swiet M, Letsky E: The use of low-molecular-weight heparin for thromboprophylaxis in pregnancy. Br J Obstet Gyn 1994;101:69–71.

162. Sutcliffe FA, MacNicoll AD, Gibson GG: Aspects of anticoagulant action: A review of the pharmacology, metabolism and toxicology of warfarin and congeners. Drug Metabol Drug Interact 1987;5:225–271.

163. Suttie JW: Warfarin and vitamin K. Clin Cardiol 1990;13:16–18.

164. Suttie JW, Jackson CM: Prothrombin structure, activation, and biosynthesis. Physiol Rev 1977;57:1–70.

165. Swigar ME, Clemow LP, Saidi P, Kim HC: Superwarfarin ingestion: A new problem in covert anticoagulant overdose. Gen Hosp Psychiatry 1990;12:309–312.

166. Tait RC: Oral anticoagulation in paediatric patients: Dose requirements and complications. Arch Dis Child 1996;74:228–231.

167. Tecimer C, Yam LT: Surreptitious superwarfarin poisoning with brodifacoum. South Med J 1997;10:1053–1055.

168. Thomas JG, Beeson MS: Warfarin-induced skin necrosis. Am J Emerg Med 1998;16:541–543.

169. Top 200 Drugs. 2000 Drug Topics Red Book. Montvale, NJ, Medical Economics, 2000.

170. Travis SF, Warfield W, Breenbaum BH, et al: Spontaneous hemorrhage associated with accidental brodifacoum poisoning in a child. J Pediatr 1993;122:982–984.

171. Udall JA: Don't use the wrong vitamin K. West J Med 1970;112:65–67.

172. Vigano D'Angelo S, Comp PC, Esmon CT, et al: Relationship between protein C antigen and anticoagulant activity during oral anticoagulation and in selected disease states. J Clin Invest 1984;77:416–425.

173. Wakefield TW, Andrews PC, Wroblеski SK, et al: Effective and less toxic reversal of low-molecular-weight heparin anticoagulation by a designer variant of protamine. J Vasc Surg 1995;21:839–849.

174. Wakefield TW, Andrews PC, Wroblеski SK, et al: A protamine variant for nontoxic and effective reversal of conventional heparin and low-molecular-weight heparin anticoagulation. J Surg Res 1995;63:280–286.

175. Wallace S, Paull P, Worsnop C, Mashford ML: Covert self-poisoning with brodifacoum, a "superwarfarin." Aust N Z J Med 1990;20:713–715.

176. Warkentin TE, Levine MN, Hirsh J, et al: Heparin-induced thrombocytopenia in patients treated with low-molecular-weight heparin or unfractionated heparin. N Engl J Med 1995;332:1330–1335.

177. Watts RG, Castleberry RP, Sadowski JA: Accidental poisoning with a superwarfarin compound (brodifacoum) in a child. Pediatrics 1990;86:883–887.

178. Weitzel JN, Sadowski JA, Furie BC, et al: Surreptitious ingestion of a long-acting vitamin K antagonist/rodenticide, brodifacoum: Clinical and metabolic studies in three cases. Blood 1990;76:2555–2559.

179. Weintzen TH, O'Reilly RA, Kearns PJ: Prospective evaluation of anticoagulant reversal with oral vitamin K_1 while continuing warfarin therapy unchanged. Chest 1998;114:1546–1550.

180. Wessler S, Gitel SN: Warfarin: From bedside to bench. N Engl J Med 1984;311:645–652.

181. White HD: Comparative safety of thrombolytic agents. Am J Cardiol 1991;67:30E–37E.

182. White RH, McKittrick T, Takakuwa J, et al: Management and prognosis of life-threatening bleeding during warfarin therapy. National Consortium of Clinical Anticoagulation. Arch Intern Med 1996;156:1197–1201.

183. Whitlon DS, Sadowski JA, Suttie JW: Mechanisms of coumarin action: Significance of vitamin K epoxide reductase inhibition. Biochemistry 1978;17:1371–1377.

184. Woody BJ, Murphy MJ, Ray AC, Green RA: Coagulopathic effects and therapy of brodifacoum toxicosis in dogs. J Vet Intern Med 1992;6:23–28.

185. Young MA, Ehrenpreis ED, Ehrenpreis M, et al: Heparin-associated thrombocytopenia and thrombosis syndrome in a rehabilitation patient. Arch Phys Med Rehabil 1989;70:468–470.

ANTIDOTES IN DEPTH

Vitamin K$_1$
Mary Ann Howland

Vitamin K$_1$

Vitamin K$_1$ (phytonadione) is indicated for the reversal of elevated prothrombin times and international normalized ratios (INRs) in patients with xenobiotic-induced vitamin K deficiency states. Vitamin K deficiency states are typically induced following the therapeutic administration of warfarin or following the ingestion of warfarin or the long-acting anticoagulant rodenticides (LAARs) such as brodifacoum. The optimal dosage regimen of vitamin K$_1$ to treat patients who overdose on either is not adequately studied. Oral administration of large doses of vitamin K$_1$ is used safely and successfully. Intravenous administration of vitamin K$_1$ is associated with anaphylactoid reactions and should be avoided if possible. Subcutaneous administration is an acceptable route as initial therapy and when oral administration is not feasible.

HISTORY

It was noted in 1929 that chickens fed a poor diet developed spontaneous bleeding. In 1935, Dam and coworkers discovered that incorporating a fat-soluble substance in the chickens' diet could correct the bleeding. They named this substance a "koagulation factor," vitamin K.[15,24]

CHEMISTRY OF THE NATURAL VITAMINS K$_1$ AND K$_2$

Vitamin K, an essential fat-soluble vitamin, is actually a broad term that encompasses at least two distinct natural forms. Vitamin K$_1$ (phytonadione, phylloquinone) is the only form synthesized by plants and algae. Vitamin K$_2$ (menaquinones) is actually a series of compounds with the same 2-methyl-1,4-naphthoquinone ring structure as phylloquinone but with a variable number (1–13) of repeating 5 carbon units on the side chain. Bacteria synthesize the menaquinones. Most of the vitamin K ingested in the diet is phylloquinone.

PHARMACOLOGY

Activation of the coagulation factors II, VII, IX, and X requires γ-carboxylation of the glutamate residues, a vitamin K–dependent process. Only the reduced (quinol, hydroquinone) form of vitamin K manifests biologic activity (Fig. 42–3). The quinone form of vitamin K can be activated to the quinol form directly by an NADPH-dependent pathway that is relatively insensitive to warfarin.[24,28] During the carboxylation step, the K quinol form is converted to an epoxide. This 2,3-epoxide is reduced and recycled to the active K quinol in a two-step process that is inhibited by warfarin. An in-depth model of the chemical basis of this reaction was recently proposed.[7]

DAILY REQUIREMENT

The human daily requirement for vitamin K is small; the Food and Nutrition Board set the recommended daily allowance at 1 μg/kg/d of phylloquinone for adults, although 10 times that amount is required for infants to maintain normal hemostasis. This value is determined to meet the coagulation function.[23] Extrahepatic enzymatic reactions that are vitamin K–dependent relate to carboxylation of proteins in the bone, kidney, placenta, lung, pancreas, and spleen, and include the synthesis of osteocalcin, matrix Gla protein, plaque Gla protein, and one or more renal Gla proteins.[23,24,28]

VITAMIN K DEFICIENCY AND MONITORING

Vitamin K deficiency can result from inadequate intake, malabsorption, or interference with the vitamin K cycle. Malnourishment and any condition in which bile salts or fatty acids are inadequate, such as extrahepatic cholestasis or severe pancreatic insufficiency, can lead to vitamin K deficiency. Newborns are at risk for hemorrhage because: (a) phylloquinone does not readily cross the placenta; (b) breast milk contains less phylloquinone than vitamin K–fortified formula; (c) fetal hepatic stores of phylloquinone are low; and (d) maternal anticonvulsant therapy may lead to increased vitamin K metabolism.[24,28] Although menaquinones are produced in the colon by bacteria, it is unlikely that enteric production contributes significantly to vitamin K stores or that eradication of the bacteria with antibiotics, without a coexistent dietary deficiency of vitamin K, results in deficiency.[24] Determination of vitamin K deficiency is usually established on the basis of a prolonged prothrombin time (PT) or INR, an indirect measure. Measurement of the vitamin K–dependent factors, II, VII, IX, and X, appears to be an effective way to determine the adequacy of vitamin K_1 dosing.[12] Serial measurements of factor VII, the factor with the shortest half-life, allows for the early detection of inadequate vitamin K_1 in the diet or a therapeutic regimen.[5] Direct measurement of serum vitamin K plasma levels is done by high-performance liquid chromatography (HPLC) analysis. The human plasma vitamin K concentration required for adequate production of activated clotting factors in the presence of LAAR is still unclear. One study in a patient who overdosed on brodifacoum suggested that a plasma vitamin K concentration of 0.2–0.4 µg/mL as opposed to the 1 µg/mL reported in rabbits was sufficient.[5,19]

MECHANISM OF ACTION FOR XENOBIOTIC-INDUCED VITAMIN K–DEFICIENT STATES

Oral anticoagulants are vitamin K antagonists that interfere with the vitamin K cycle, causing the accumulation of vitamin K 2,3-epoxide, an inactive metabolite. Warfarin is a strong irreversible inhibitor of the dithiol-dependent vitamin K reductases (epoxide reductase and quinone reductase), which maintain vitamin K in its active (quinol, hydroquinone) form.[2] The superwarfarins are even more potent vitamin K reductase inhibitors. Without exogenous interference vitamin K is recycled and only 1 µg/kg in the adult is required to maintain adequate coagulation. Nicotinamide adenine dinucleotide phosphate (NADPH)-dependent quinone reductase is a warfarin-insensitive enzyme capable of reducing vitamin K_1 to its active hydroquinone form, but it is incapable of regenerating vitamin K from vitamin K epoxide following carboxylation of the coagulation factor[2] (Fig. 42–3). It is presumed that additional vitamin K_1 must be administered to supply this active cofactor for each and every carboxylation step.[5] The minimum vitamin K_1 requirement in the presence of LAAR is unknown. Other compounds have varying degrees of vitamin K antagonistic activity and include the *N*-methyl-thiotetrazole side chain containing antibiotics (moxalactam, cefamandole) and salicylates.[24]

PHARMACOKINETICS OF DIETARY VITAMIN K

Dietary vitamin K in the form of phylloquinone and menaquinones is solubilized with the bile salts, free fatty acids, and monoglycerides to enhance absorption. Vitamin K, bound to chylomicrons, enters the circulation via the lymphatic system and then is taken up by the liver.[24] Plasma vitamin K is primarily in the form of phylloquinone, whereas liver stores are 90% menaquinones and 10% phylloquinone.[24] Following 3 days of low vitamin K intake, a group of surgical patients showed a 4-fold lowering of liver vitamin K concentrations.[27] Rats given a vitamin K–deficient diet developed severe bleeding within 2–3 weeks.

AVAILABILITY OF DIFFERENT FORMS OF VITAMIN K

Table 42–5 lists the currently marketed vitamin K products. Vitamin K_1 (phylloquinone, phytonadione) is the only vitamin K preparation that should be used to reverse anticoagulant-induced vitamin K deficiency or to treat infants, pregnant women, or patients with glucose 6-phosphate dehydrogenase (G6PD) deficiency. Vitamin K_1 is superior to other no longer commercially available vitamin K preparations because it is more active, thus requiring comparatively smaller doses, and because it works more rapidly (6 vs. 12 hours).[10,26]

Vitamins K_3 (menadione) and K_4 (menadiol sodium diphosphate) may produce hemolysis, hyperbilirubinemia, and kernicterus in neonates and hemolysis in G6PD-deficient patients. The only advantage of menadione and menadiol sodium diphosphate is that these preparations are absorbed directly from the intestine by a passive process that does not require the presence of bile salts. Therefore, these agents may be advantageous for patients with cholestasis or severe pancreatic insufficiency. They are neither interchangeable with vitamin K_1, nor a substitute for vitamin K_1, when anticoagulants such as warfarin or LAAR are re-

TABLE 42–5.   Vitamin K Products

	Commercial Preparation	Route of Administration	Strength	Comments
Vitamin K_1 (phylloquinone, phytonadione)	Mephyton AquaMEPHYTON	Oral SC, IM, IV	5 mg 2 mg/mL 10 mg/mL	Best for anticoagulant-induced prolonged prothrombin time. Oral route preferred; divided doses may be necessary for large requirements; IV reserved for life-threatening situations. Must be carefully diluted and slowly infused (IV) to avoid anaphylactoid reactions; SC for small doses; IM should be avoided; may be used for infants, pregnant women, G6PD deficiency; oral absorption requires presence of bile salts.

sponsible for coagulation deficits. For a patient deficient in bile salts who requires vitamin K_1, exogenous bile salts (ie, ox bile extract 300 mg or dehydrocholic acid 500 mg) should be given with each dose of vitamin K_1.[20]

PHARMACOKINETICS AND PHARMACODYNAMICS OF VITAMIN K_1

There are only a limited number of pharmacokinetic studies of vitamin K_1.[5,11,19,30] One study evaluated the pharmacokinetics of vitamin K_1 in healthy volunteers, brodifacoum-anticoagulated rabbits, and a patient poisoned with brodifacoum.[19] In the volunteers and the poisoned patient, a 10-mg IV dose of vitamin K_1 had a half-life of 1.7 hours. After oral administration of doses of 10 and 50 mg of vitamin K_1, peaks of 100–400 ng/mL and 200–2000 ng/mL, respectively, occurred at 3–5 hours. Bioavailability varied significantly between patients (10–65%) for both doses and in individual patients with the 50-mg dose. Oral vitamin K_1 (phytonadione, phylloquinone) is absorbed in an energy-dependent saturable process in the proximal small intestine, and this likely contributes to the variability.[19] In maximally brodifacoum-anticoagulated rabbits, IV vitamin K_1 (10 mg/kg) increased prothrombin complex activity (PCA) from 14 to 50% by 4 hours and to 100% by 9 hours, after which it declined with a half-life of 6 hours. The minimum effective concentration of vitamin K_1 was approximately 1 μg/mL. High doses of oral vitamin K_1 were used to treat a patient anticoagulated with brodifacoum.[5] In this patient, a serum vitamin K_1 concentration as low as 200 ng/mL (0.2 μg/mL) was effective in maintaining a normal coagulation profile.[5] The pharmacokinetics of oral and IM vitamin K_1 were compared in 8 healthy female volunteers. Baseline plasma vitamin K levels were 0.23 ng/mL. Following the oral administration of 5 mg of vitamin K, peak plasma levels of 90 ng/mL were achieved between 4 and 6 hours. These levels dropped to a steady state of 3.8 ng/mL and exhibited a half-life of about 4 hours. The pharmacokinetics were distinctly different after IM administration and quite variable. IM administration of 5 mg of vitamin K, resulted in peak plasma levels of only 50 ng/mL with delays from 2 to 30 hours following administration and with the maintenance of a plateau for about 30 hours.[11]

ROUTES OF ADMINISTRATION AND ADVERSE EFFECTS

Although vitamin K_1 may be administered orally, subcutaneously, intramuscularly, or intravenously, the oral route is preferred when possible for maintenance therapy. When administered orally, vitamin K_1 is virtually free of adverse effects, except for overcorrection of the INR in the setting of a patient who requires maintenance anticoagulation. Subcutaneous administration is limited to about 5 mL, which is the amount that can be physically injected at any one administration site. The intramuscular route is best avoided in patients who are anticoagulated and at risk for hematoma formation. The only preparation available for intravenous administration is AquaMEPHYTON, which is associated with rare anaphylactoid reactions. This preparation is not available in solution but as an aqueous colloidal suspension of a polyoxyethylated fatty acid–derivative dextrose and benzyl alcohol. AquaMEPHYTON is for-

mulated as a colloidal suspension because of the vitamin's lipid solubility. Intravenous administration has resulted in death secondary to anaphylactoid reactions, probably as a result of the preparation's colloidal formulation.[3,6,16] More than 57 anaphylactoid reactions have been reported, even when properly diluted and administered slowly.[18]

ONSET OF EFFECT

The time necessary for PT or INR to return to a safe or normal range is very variable and depends on the rate of absorption of vitamin K_1, the plasma concentration achieved, and the time necessary for the synthesis of activated clotting factors. A decrease in the INR can often be seen within several hours, while it may take 8–24 hours to reach target values.[4,9,17,21] Maintenance of a normal PT or INR depends on the half-life of the vitamin K_1, maintenance of an effective plasma concentration, and the half-life of the anticoagulant involved. The IV route is only slightly faster than the oral route in restoring the INR to a safe range.[11] The subcutaneous route has never been studied in the management of overdoses nor has it ever been compared to the oral route even in the therapeutic setting. One study compared subcutaneous (SC) to IV for patients chronically on warfarin with markedly elevated INRs.[17] The warfarin dose was stopped in each group. SC doses of vitamin K_1 were slightly less effective than IV doses at 24 hours, but there were no differences between the 2 regimens at 72 hours.[17] It is presumed that the SC route is more rapidly effective than the oral route and is appropriate for initial administration. If the oral route is not feasible and the dose requirements exceed the 5 mL of SC administration (ie, >50 mg), then the IV route may be used for an initial dose.

DOSING AND ADMINISTRATION

The optimal dosage regimen for vitamin K_1 remains unclear. Variables include the vitamin K_1 pharmacokinetics, as well as the amount and type of anticoagulant ingested.[22] Reported cases of LAAR poisoning have required as much as 50–250 mg of vitamin K_1 daily for weeks to months.[1,5,8,13,14,25,29] A reasonable starting approach for a patient who has overdosed on warfarin or LAAR is 25–50 mg of vitamin K_1, orally 3–4 times a day for 1–2 days. This oral dose may be preceded by a SC dose of 10–25 mg of vitamin K_1 if desired. The INR should be monitored and the vitamin K_1 dose adjusted accordingly. Once the INR is <2, a downward titration in the dose of vitamin K_1 can be made on the basis of factor VII analysis. For a patient who has overdosed on an LAAR, treatment for many months may be required.[25] For an ingestion of brodifacoum, serial serum levels of brodifacoum may be helpful in determining the ultimate duration of treatment.[5]

IV administration of vitamin K_1 should be reserved for life-threatening situations when oral and SC administration are not feasible. Under these circumstances these patients will also probably be receiving blood and will necessitate blood products such as fresh-frozen plasma. A starting dose of 10–25 mg of vitamin K_1 is reasonable. To minimize the risk of an anaphylactoid reaction, the preparation should be diluted with preservative-free 5% dextrose, 0.9% sodium chloride, or 5% dextrose in 0.9% sodium chloride, and administered slowly, at a rate not to exceed 1 mg/min in adults. Preparations should be made for treating an anaphylactoid reaction should it occur.

Because the duration of action of vitamin K_1 is short-lived, the dose must be repeated 2–4 times daily. The onset of the effect of vitamin K_1 is not immediate, regardless of the route of administration. The risks of anaphylactoid reaction from the IV administration of vitamin K_1 and hematoma formation from IM administration are substantial concerns.

Vitamin K_1 is available orally as a 5-mg tablet, requiring the patient to initially consume 5–10 tablets every 6–8 hours.

REFERENCES

1. Babcock J, Hartman K, Pedersen A, et al: Rodenticide induced coagulopathy in a young child. Am J Ped Hematol Oncol 1993;15:126–130.
2. Baglin T: Management of warfarin (Coumadin) overdose. Blood Rev 1998;12:91–98.
3. Barash P, Kitahata LM, Mandel S: Acute cardiovascular collapse after intravenous phytonadione. Anesth Analg 1976;55:304–306.
4. Brophy M, Fiore L, Deykin D: Low-dose vitamin K therapy in excessively anticoagulated patients: A dose finding study. J Thrombosis Thrombolysis 1997;4:289–292.
5. Bruno GR, Howland MA, McMeeking A, Hoffman RS: Long-acting anticoagulant overdose: Brodifacoum kinetics and optimal vitamin K_1 dosing. Ann Emerg Med 2000;36:262–267.
6. De la Rubia J, Grau E, Montserrat I, et al: Anaphylactic shock and vitamin K_1. Ann Intern Med 1989;110:943.
7. Dowd P, Ham SW, Naganathan S, et al: The mechanism of action of Vitamin K. Annu Rev Nutr 1995;15:419–440.
8. Exner DV, Brien WF, Murphy MJ: Superwarfarin ingestion. Can Med J 1992;146:34–35.
9. Fetrow CW, Overlock T, Leff L: Antagonism of warfarin induced hypoprothrombinemia with use of low-dose subcutaneous vitamin K_1. J Clin Pharmacol 1997;37:751–757.
10. Gamble JR, Dennis EW, Coon WW, et al: Clinical comparison of vitamin K_1 and water-soluble vitamin K. Arch Intern Med 1955;5:52–58.
11. Hagstrom JN, Bovill EG, Soll R, et al: The pharmacokinetics and lipoprotein fraction distribution of intramuscular versus oral vitamin K_1 supplementation in women of childbearing age: Effects on hemostasis. Thromb Haemost 1995;74:1486–1490.
12. Hoffman R, Smilkstein M, Goldfrank L: Evaluation of coagulation factor abnormalities in long-acting anticoagulant overdose. J Toxicol Clin Toxicol 1998;26:233–248.
13. Hollinger B, Pastoor T: Case management and plasma half-life in a case of brodifacoum poisoning. Arch Intern Med 1993;153:1925–1928.
14. La Rosa F, Clarke S, Lefkowitz J: Brodifacoum intoxication with marijuana smoking. Arch Pathol Lab Med 1997;121:67–69.
15. Marcus R, Coulston AM: Water-soluble vitamins: The vitamin B complex and ascorbic acid. In: Gilman AG, Rall TW, Nies AS, Taylor P, eds: Goodman and Gilman's The Pharmacological Basis of Therapeutics, 8th ed. New York, Pergamon, 1990, pp. 1563–1566.
16. Mattea E, Quinn K: Adverse reactions after intravenous phytonadione administration. Hosp Pharm 1981;16:230–235.
17. Nee R, Doppenschmidt, Donovan D, Andrews T: Intravenous versus subcutaneous vitamin K1 in reversing excessive oral anticoagulation. Am J Cardiol 1999;83:286–288.
18. O'Reilly R, Kearns P: Intravenous vitamin K_1 injections: Dangerous prophylaxis. Arch Intern Med 1995;155:2127–2128.
19. Park BK, Scott AK, Wilson AC, et al: Plasma disposition of vitamin K_1 in relation to anticoagulant poisoning. Br J Clin Pharmacol 1984;18:655–662.
20. Phytonadione. In: AHFS Drug Information, ed. American Society of Health System Pharmacists. Bethesda, MD, 2000, pp. 3343–3346.
21. Raj G, Kumar R, Mckinney P: Time course of reversal of anticoagulant effect of warfarin by intravenous and subcutaneous phytonadione. Arch Intern Med 1999;159:2721–2724.
22. Routh CR, Triplett DA, Murphy MJ, et al: Superwarfarin ingestion and detection. Am J Hematol 1991;36:50–54.
23. Shearer MJ: Vitamin K. Lancet 1995;345:229–233.
24. Shearer MJ: Vitamin K metabolism and nutrition. Blood Rev 1992;6:92–104.
25. Sheen S, Spiller H: Symptomatic brodifacoum ingestion requiring high-dose phytonadione therapy. Vet Hum Toxicol 1994;36:216–217.
26. Udall JA: Don't use the wrong vitamin K. West J Med 1970;112:65–67.
27. Usuri Y, Taminura M, Nishimura, N, et al: Vitamin K concentrations in the plasma and liver of surgical patients. Am J Clin Nutr 1990;51:846–852.
28. Vermeer C, Hamulyak K: Pathophysiology of vitamin K deficiency and oral anticoagulants. Thromb Haemost 1991;66:153–159.
29. Weitzel J, Sadowski J, Furie BC, et al: Surreptitious ingestion of a long-acting vitamin K antagonist/rodenticide, brodifacoum: Clinical and metabolic studies of three cases. Blood 1990;76:2555–2559.
30. Winn MJ, Cholerton S, Park BK: An investigation of the pharmacological response to vitamin K_1 in the rabbit. Br J Pharmacol 1988;94:1077–1084.

ANTIDOTES IN DEPTH

Protamine

Mary Ann Howland

Protamine is a rapidly acting antidote utilized for heparin overdoses. The antidotal property of protamine was recognized in the late 1930s and it was approved for use as an antidote for heparin overdose in 1968.[41] However, the largest body of literature pertaining to protamine originates from its use in neutralizing heparin following cardiopulmonary bypass and dialysis procedures.

CHEMISTRY

The protamines are a group of simple basic cationic proteins found in fish sperm. Commercially available protamine sulfate is derived from the sperm of mature testes of salmon and related species. On hydrolysis it yields basic amino acids, particularly arginine, proline, serine, and valine, but not tyrosine and tryptophan. The effects of protamine sulfate appear to be comparable to those of protamine chloride.[34]

MECHANISM OF ACTION

Heparin is a large electronegative substance that is rapidly complexed by the electropositive protamine, forming an inactive salt. Heparin binds to antithrombin III (AT III), altering its stereochemistry and thereby catalyzing the subsequent inactivation of thrombin and other clotting factors. Immunoelectrophoresis demonstrates that due to its net positive charge, protamine has a greater affinity for heparin than AT III, thereby producing a dissociation of the heparin-AT III complex in favor of a protamine-heparin complex.[42]

ADVERSE EFFECTS, RISK FACTORS, AND SAFETY ISSUES

Since the advent of cardiopulmonary bypass surgery, protamine has been routinely employed in the neutralization of heparin at the completion of the procedure. More than 2 million patients are exposed to protamine each year. Nearly 100 deaths have been attributed to the use of protamine under these circumstances. It is largely in this setting that the adverse effects of protamine are also documented and studied.[22,23,36] It is often difficult to separate the adverse effects caused by protamine from those of the protamine-heparin complex and those actually related to heparin. Adverse effects associated with protamine include both rate- and non-rate-related hypotension,[12–15,17,26,29,46,49] anaphylactic[25] and anaphylactoid reactions,[28,38,40] bradycardia,[1] thrombocytopenia,[55] leukopenia, decreased oxygen consumption,[52,54] acute lung injury,[3,51] pulmonary hypertension,[5] and anticoagulant effects.[2]

The mechanisms for these adverse effects are multifactorial. The strong net-positive charge of protamine may be responsible for some of the adverse effects and probably directly injures a variety of organelles, including platelets.[7,56] The protamine-heparin complex activates the arachidonic acid pathway and the production of thromboxane is at least partly responsible for some of the hemodynamic changes, including pulmonary hypertension.[5,9,21,39,56] Pretreatment with indomethacin limits these effects.[9,21,39,56] Free protamine or protamine complexed with heparin can convert L-arginine to endothelium-derived relaxing factor (nitric oxide), which, in turn, causes vasodilation and inhibits platelet aggregation and adhesion.[43] Protamine administered in the absence of heparin or in an amount exceeding that necessary for heparin neutralization can act as an anticoagulant and may inhibit platelet function with a resultant weaker clot.[4,27] This anticoagulant effect may result from effects on factor VII and/or AT III. Protamine in excess of heparin can enter the myocardium and decrease cyclic adenosine monophosphate (cAMP), causing myocardial depression.[5] Protamine and protamine-heparin complexes can activate the classic complement pathway and contribute to vasoactive events.[5,44] Protamine stimulates mast cells in the human heart and skin to release histamine.[5]

Risk factors for protamine-induced adverse reactions include prior exposure (eg, during a previous surgery), vasectomy, history of nonprotamine medication allergy, rapid rate of infusion, or a history of allergy to fish.[44] Diabetic patients receiving daily subcutaneous injections of a protamine-containing insulin (neutral protamine Hagedorn, or NPH) have a 40–50% increased risk of adverse reactions.[16,19,25,33,49] One prospective study reported a 0.06% incidence of anaphylactic reactions to protamine in all patients undergoing coronary artery bypass, but a 2% incidence in diabetics using NPH insulin.[5] The resultant elevation of histamine levels, the activation of complement, and elevated IgE, IgA, and IgG levels are also suggested as mechanisms for the adverse effects.[35,50,57,58] Occasionally, patients manifesting a protamine allergy are presumed to have insulin allergy.[32] In diabetic patients receiving protamine insulin injections, the presence of serum antiprotamine IgE antibody is a significant risk factor for acute protamine reactions. Only patients with previous exposure to protamine insulin injections had serum antiprotamine IgE antibodies. However, in the group without previous protamine insulin exposure, antiprotamine IgG antibody was noted as a risk factor for protamine reactions.[58] Either naturally occurring cross-reacting antibodies, or perhaps previously unrecognized protamine exposure, was responsible for the generation of these IgG antibodies.

ALTERNATIVES TO PROTAMINE IN PATIENTS AT HIGH RISK FOR AN ADVERSE DRUG REACTION

There are limited options for the reversal of heparin in patients who have previously experienced clinical anaphylaxis following protamine therapy, or in patients who are expected to be at high risk for a protamine reaction. Clotting factors may be replaced, or exchange transfusion instituted in neonates, and protamine avoided, or protamine may be used while preparing to treat ana-phylaxis expectantly. Several alternatives are under investigation and include the placement of heparin removal devices in the extra-corporeal circuit, as well as the use of hexadimethrine, methylene blue, platelet factor 4, and heparinase as antidotes.[5,31] Pretreatment with antihistamines and corticosteroids may be sufficient for im-mune-mediated mechanisms, but will probably not be beneficial for pulmonary vasoconstriction and non-immune-mediated ana-phylactoid reactions.[24]

DOSING IN CARDIOPULMONARY BYPASS

Protamine is most frequently used at the end of cardiopulmonary bypass operations to reverse the effects of heparin. There are many regimens used for protamine dosing, including: (a) giving an arbi-trary amount of protamine (eg, 0.2 mg/kg); (b) giving protamine in a ratio of 0.6–1.5:1 times the initial heparin dose, resulting in an activated coagulation time (ACT) of about 480 seconds; and (c) giving protamine in a ratio of 0.75–2.1:1 times the total opera-tive heparin dose.[59] Two new methods of calculating the prota-mine dose to improve accuracy and avoid excess protamine have been proposed.[27,59] One advocates an initial protamine dose based on ACT, with subsequent doses based on the ratio of the change in thrombin time to the heparin-neutralized thrombin time. If this ratio is greater than 12 seconds, then 10-mg incremental protamine doses should be administered.[27] The other uses a nomogram based on heparin activity in mg/kg versus ACT.[59] Both methods demon-strate efficacy with 2-mg/kg doses of protamine, about one-half of the dose previously used. With these approaches, the ACT re-sponded to protamine within 5 minutes, decreasing in value from between 550 to 700 seconds to a control of 150 seconds. Other re-ports discuss a variety of monitoring methods and dosing in this setting.[10,20,47]

HEPARIN REBOUND AND REDOSING OF PROTAMINE

A heparin rebound effect was noted after cardiopulmonary bypass. This anticoagulant effect recurs, and is attributed to the presence of detectable circulating heparin several hours after apparently ad-equate heparin neutralization with protamine. The incidence of heparin rebound and the need for additional protamine (range, 4–42%) varies, depending on the neutralization protocol.[18,37,45] It is likely that larger heparin doses may prolong the clearance of heparin, contributing to higher than expected heparin levels.[45] When 300-U/kg body weight doses of heparin were reversed at the end of cardiopulmonary bypass with 3 mg/kg of protamine, a 14% incidence of small but detectable concentrations of circulating heparin was noted at 2 hours, which lasted less than 1 hour in all but one case.[37] The prothrombin time was prolonged and thrombo-cytopenia was noted, but there was no increase in blood loss.

DOSING CONSIDERATIONS

Approximately 1 mg of protamine will neutralize about 100 U (1 mg) of heparin. A limited number of studies suggest incomplete neutralization by protamine of enoxaparin, dalteparin, and tinzapa-rin low-molecular-weight heparins.[11] A number of tests can directly measure heparin levels or indirectly measure heparin's effect on the clotting cascade.[6,8,10] These tests may be helpful in determining the appropriate dose of protamine. Because excessive protamine can act as an anticoagulant, the dose chosen should always be an underesti-mation of that which is needed. In the case of unintentional over-dose, the half-life of heparin should be considered, because half of the administered dose of heparin is eliminated within 60–90 min-utes. In the case of an unintentional overdose without bleeding, the short half-life of heparin and the potential risks of protamine admin-istration usually argue for a conservative approach of patient obser-vation, rather than protamine reversal of anticoagulation. If protamine use is necessary to treat active bleeding, the dose must be administered intravenously over 15 minutes to limit rate-related hy-potension.[30,53]

DOSING IN THE OVERDOSE SETTING

When faced with a patient believed to have received an overdose of an unknown quantity of heparin, the decision to use protamine should be made when the setting is correct and a prolonged partial thromboplastin time (PTT) and persistent bleeding are present. In each circumstance, the potential risks of protamine use (especially in those who have had a prior life-threatening reaction to prota-mine as well as in a diabetic receiving a protamine-containing in-sulin) and the risks of continued heparin anticoagulation should be evaluated. A baseline ACT, thrombin time, heparin-neutralized thrombin time, heparin activity, platelets, PT/PTT, hemoglobin, and hematocrit should be obtained. Because of the routine nature of heparin reversal following cardiopulmonary bypass, consulta-tion with members of the bypass team may be helpful. An empiric dose of protamine may be suggested by the baseline ACT: (a) an ACT of 150 seconds necessitates no protamine; (b) an ACT of 200–300 seconds necessitates 0.6 mg/kg; and (c) an ACT of 300–400 seconds necessitates 1.2 mg/kg. These doses have not been tested outside the operating room. The ACT should be re-peated 5–15 minutes following the protamine dose and in 2–8 hours (to evaluate the potential for heparin rebound) and further dosing should be based on these values.

When the ACT is not available, 25–50 mg of protamine can be administered to an adult and adjusted accordingly. Repeat dosing in several hours may be necessary if heparin rebound occurs. The dose should be administered intravenously slowly over 15 minutes with resuscitative equipment immediately available. Neonates should not receive protamine that has been reconstituted with bac-teriostatic water containing benzyl alcohol.

AVAILABILITY

Protamine is available either as a parenteral solution ready for in-jection or as a powder to be reconstituted with 5 mL of sterile or bacteriostatic water for injection. When the vials containing 50 mg of protamine are used, they should be shaken vigorously after the water is added. The final solution of either preparation contains 10 mg of protamine per mL.

REFERENCES

1. Alvarez J, Alvarez L, Escudero C, Olivares JLC: Sinus node function and protamine sulfate. J Cardiothorac Anesth 1989;3:44–51.

2. Andersen MN, Mendelow M, Alfano GA: Experimental studies of heparin-protamine activity with special reference to protamine inhibition of clotting. Surgery 1959;46:1060–1068.

3. Brooks JC: Noncardiogenic pulmonary edema immediately following rapid protamine administration. Ann Pharmacother 1999;33:927–930.

4. Carr ME, Carr, SL: At high heparin concentrations, protamine concentrations which reverse heparin anticoagulant effects are insufficient to reverse heparin antiplatelet effects. Thromb Res 1994;75:617–630.

5. Carr JA, Silverman N: The heparin-protamine interaction. A review. J Cardiovasc Surg (Torino) 1999;40:659–666.

6. Castellani WJ, Hodges ED, Bode AP: Effect of protamine sulfate on the ACA heparin assay. Clin Chem 1991;37:1119–1120.

7. Chang SW, Westcott JY, Henson JE, Voelkel NF: Pulmonary vascular injury by polycations in perfused rat lungs. J Appl Physiol 1987;62:1932–1943.

8. Chen W, Yang V: Versatile non-clotting based heparin assay requiring no instrumentation. Clin Chem 1991;37:832–837.

9. Conzen PF, Habazettl H, Gutmann R, et al: Thromboxane mediation of pulmonary hemodynamic responses after neutralization of heparin by protamine in pigs. Anesth Analg 1989;68:25–31.

10. Despotis GJ, Gravlee G, Filos K, Levy J: Anticoagulation monitoring during cardiac surgery: A review of current and emerging techniques. Anesthesiology 1999;91:1122–1151.

11. Dietrich CP, Shinjo SK, Moraes FA, et al: Structural features and bleeding activity of commercial low-molecular-weight heparins: Neutralization by ATP and protamine. Semin Thromb Hemost 1999;3:43–50.

12. Fadali MA, Ledbetter M, Papacostas CA, et al: Mechanism responsible for the cardiovascular depressant effect of protamine sulfate. Ann Surg 1974;180:232–235.

13. Fadali MA, Papacostas CA, Duke JJ, et al: Cardiovascular depressant effect of protamine sulfate. Thorax 1976;31:320–323.

14. Frater RMW, Oka Y, Hong Y, et al: Protamine-induced circulatory changes. J Thorac Cardiovasc Surg 1984;87:687–692.

15. Goldman BS, Joison J, Austen WG: Cardiovascular effects of protamine sulfate. Ann Thorac Cardiovasc Surg 1969;7:459–471.

16. Gottschlich GM, Gravlee GP, Georgitis JW: Adverse reactions to protamine sulfate during cardiac surgery in diabetic and nondiabetic patients. Ann Allergy 1988;61:277–281.

17. Gourin A, Streisand RL, Greineder JK, Stuckey JH: Protamine sulfate administration and the cardiovascular system. J Thorac Cardiovasc Surg 1971;62:193–204.

18. Gundry SR, Drongowski RA, Klein MD, et al: Postoperative bleeding in cardiovascular surgery: Does heparin rebound really exist? Am Surg 1989;55:162–165.

19. Gupta SK, Veith FJ, Wengerter KR, et al: Anaphylactoid reactions to protamine: An often lethal complication in insulin-dependent diabetic patients undergoing vascular surgery. J Vasc Surg 1989;9:342–350.

20. Hall RI: Protamine dosing—The quandary continues. Can J Anaesth 1998;45:1–5.

21. Hobbhahn J, Conzen PF, Zenker B, et al: Beneficial effect of cyclooxygenase inhibition on adverse hemodynamic responses after protamine. Anesth Analg 1988;67:253–260.

22. Holland CL, Singh AK, McMaster PRB, Fang W: Adverse reactions to protamine sulfate following cardiac surgery. Clin Cardiol 1984;7:157–162.

23. Horrow JC: Protamine: A review of its toxicity. Anesth Analg 1985;64:348–361.

24. Hughes C, Haddock M: Protamine reaction in a patient undergoing coronary artery bypass grafting. Clin Forum Nurse Anesth 1995;6:172–176.

25. Jackson DR: Sustained hypotension secondary to protamine sulfate. Angiology 1970;21:295–298.

26. Jastrebski MK, Sykes MK, Woods DG: Cardiorespiratory effects of protamine after cardiopulmonary bypass in man. Thorax 1974;20:534–538.

27. Jobes DR, Aitken GL, Shaffer GW: Increased accuracy and precision of heparin and protamine dosing reduces blood loss and transfusion in patients undergoing primary cardiac operations. J Thorac Cardiovasc Surg 1995;110:36–45.

28. Kambam JR, Merrill WH, Smith BE: Histamine₂ receptor blocker in the treatment of protamine-related anaphylactoid reactions: Two case reports. Can J Anaesth 1989;36:463–465.

29. Katz NM, Kim YD, Siegelman R, et al: Hemodynamics of protamine administration. J Thorac Cardiovasc Surg 1987;94:881–886.

30. Kien ND, Quam DD, Reitan JA, White DA: Mechanism of hypotension following rapid infusion of protamine sulfate in anesthetized dogs. J Cardiothorac Vasc Anesth 1992;6:143–147.

31. Kikura M, Lee MK, Levy JH: Heparin neutralization with methylene blue, hexadimethrine, or vancomycin after cardiopulmonary bypass. Anesth Analg 1996;83:223–227.

32. Kim R: Anaphylaxis to protamine masquerading as an insulin allergy. Del Med J 1993;65:17–23.

33. Kimmel SE, Sekers MA, Berlin JA, et al: Risk factors for clinically important adverse events after protamine administration following cardiopulmonary bypass. J Am Coll Cardiol 1998;32:1916–1922.

34. Kuitunen AH, Salmenpera MT, Heinonen J, et al: Heparin rebound: A comparative study of protamine chloride and protamine sulfate in patients undergoing coronary artery bypass surgery. J Cardiothorac Vasc Anesth 1991;5:221–226.

35. Lakin JD, Blocker TJ, Strong DM, Yocum MW: Anaphylaxis to protamine sulfate mediated by a complement dependent IgG antibody. J Allergy Clin Immunol 1978;61:102–107.

36. Lindblad B: Protamine sulphate: A review of its effects—Hypersensitivity and toxicity. Eur J Vasc Surg 1989;3:195–201.

37. Martin P, Horkay F, Gupta NK, et al: Heparin rebound phenomenon: Much ado about nothing. Blood Coagul Fibrinolysis 1992;3:187–191.

38. Moorthy SS, Pond W, Rowland RG: Severe circulatory shock following protamine (an anaphylactoid reaction). Anesth Analg 1980;59:77–78.

39. Morel DR, Zapol WM, Thomas SJ, et al: C5a and thromboxane generation associated with pulmonary vaso- and broncho-constriction during protamine reversal of heparin. Anesthesiology 1987;66:597–604.

40. Neidhart PP, Meier B, Polla BS, et al: Fatal anaphylactoid response to protamine after percutaneous transluminal coronary angioplasty. Eur Heart J 1992;13:856–858.

41. New Drug Application. Washington DC, Food and Drug Administration, 1968; 6460, log 775.

42. Okajirna Y, Kanayama S, Maeda Y, et al: Studies on the neutralizing mechanism of antithrombin activity of heparin by protamine. Thromb Res 1981;24:21–29.

43. Pearson PJ, Evora PRB, Ayrancioglu K, Schaff HV: Protamine releases endothelium-derived relaxing factor from systemic arteries. Anesth Prog 1991;38:99–100.

44. Porsche R, Brenner ZR: Allergy to protamine sulfate. Heart Lung 1999;28:418–428.

45. Raul TK, Crow MJ, Rajah SM, et al: Heparin administration during extracorporeal circulation: Heparin rebound and postoperative bleeding. J Thorac Cardiovasc Surg 1979;78:95–102.

46. Shapira N, Schaff HV, Piehler JM, et al: Cardiovascular effects of protamine sulfate in man. J Thorac Cardiovasc Surg 1982;84:505–514.

47. Shore-Lesserson L, Reich DL, DePerio M: Heparin and protamine titration do not improve haemostasis in cardiac surgical patients. Can J Anaesth 1998;45:10–18.

48. Stefaniszyn HJ, Novick RJ, Salerno TA: Toward a better understanding of the hemodynamic effects of protamine and heparin interaction. J Thorac Cardiovasc Surg 1984;87:678–686.

49. Stewart WJ, McSweeney SM, Kellett MA, et al: Increased risk of severe protamine reactions in NPH insulin-dependent diabetics undergoing cardiac catheterization. Circulation 1984;70:788–792.

50. Stoelting RK, Henry DD, Verburg KM: Hemodynamic changes and circulating histamine concentrations following protamine administration to patients and dogs. Can Anaesth Soc J 1984;31:534–540.

51. Urdaneta F, Lobato EB, Kirby RR, Horrow JC: Noncardiogenic pulmonary edema associated with protamine administration during coronary artery bypass graft surgery. J Clin Anesth 1999;11:675–681.

52. Wakefield TW, Bies LE, Wrobleski SK, et al: Impaired myocardial function and oxygen utilization due to protamine sulfate in an isolated rabbit heart preparation. Ann Surg 1990;212:387–393.

53. Wakefield TW, Mantler CB, Wrobleski SK, et al: Effects of differing rates of protamine reversal of heparin anticoagulation. Surgery 1996; 119:123–128.

54. Wakefield TW, Ucros I, Kresowik TF, et al: Decreased oxygen consumption as a toxic manifestation of protamine sulfate reversal of heparin anticoagulation. J Vasc Surg 1989;9:772–777.

55. Wakefield TW, Wrobleski SK, Nichol BJ, et al: Heparin-mediated reduction of the toxic effects of protamine sulfate on rabbit myocardium. J Vasc Surg 1992;16:47–53.

56. Wakefield TW, Wrobleski BS, Wirthlin DJ, et al: Increased prostacyclin and adverse hemodynamic responses to protamine sulfate in an experimental canine model. J Surg Res 1991;50:449–456.

57. Weiss ME, Chatham F, Kagey Sobotka A, Adkinson NF: Serial immunological investigations in a patient who had a life-threatening reaction to intravenous protamine. Clin Exp Allergy 1990;20:713–720.

58. Weiss ME, Nyhan D, Zhikang P, et al: Association of protamine IgE and IgG antibodies with life-threatening reactions to intravenous protamine. N Engl J Med 1989;320:886–892.

59. Wright SJ, Murray WB, Hampton WA, et al: Calculating the protamine-heparin reversal ratio: A pilot study investigating a new method. J Cardiothorac Vasc Anesth 1993;7:416–421.

Edward W. Boyer

A 15-year-old girl who recently emigrated from Vietnam began to seize while in class at school. Paramedics were called, and the patient suffered two additional seizures during transport to the Emergency Department (ED). Upon presentation she had a blood pressure of 122/50 mm Hg; a pulse of 107 beats/min; 22 breaths/min; and a temperature of 99.4°F (37.4°C). Physical examination revealed an obtunded young female who had no signs of head trauma. Her pupils were 3 mm and sluggishly reactive. Her oropharynx showed no signs of trauma. Her lungs were clear, and she was tachycardic with no murmur, rub, or gallop appreciated on cardiac examination. Her abdomen was soft with normal bowel sounds. Her skin was warm, dry, and well perfused. There was an abrasion on her left forearm, but there was no other extremity injury. She was minimally responsive to painful stimuli in all extremities.

An intravenous catheter was established and she was placed on 100% oxygen nonrebreathing facemask. Pulse oximetry demonstrated an oxygen saturation of 100%. Her serum glucose by fingerstick was normal. She received 8 mg IV lorazepam in the ED but had an additional seizure. Family members said that the patient had started taking medicine for a "lung problem" that was identified when she emigrated. On the basis of this information, she received 5 g of intravenous pyridoxine. Seizure activity ceased. A nasogastric tube was inserted and, after verification of placement, 50 g activated charcoal was instilled.

Laboratory values were a white blood cell count of 13,600/mm^3; hemoglobin, 12.9 g/dL; platelets, 287 × 10^3/mm^3; sodium, 142 mEq/L; potassium, 3.7 mEq/L; chloride, 103 mEq/L; bicarbonate, 7 mEq/L; blood urea nitrogen (BUN), 7 mg/dL; creatinine, 0.6 mg/dL; serum glucose, 97 mg/dL; and anion gap, 29 mEq/L. Arterial blood gas was pH 7.19; Pco$_2$, 33 mm Hg; Po$_2$, 105 mm Hg; and 98% oxygen saturation. Creatinine phosphokinase was 1067 U/L. Cerebrospinal fluid (CSF) showed 4 RBC (red blood cells) per mm^3 and 33 WBC (white blood cells) per mm^3. Cerebrospinal glucose was 76 mg/dL and protein was 27 mg/dL.

She was admitted to the Intensive Care Unit (ICU), and her level of consciousness did not improve over the next 6 hours. An EEG (electroencephalogram) that was performed because of persistent depression of consciousness was normal. The Toxicology Service was consulted; it recommended that the patient be given an additional 5 g of intravenous pyridoxine. The patient's level of consciousness improved over the next 15 minutes, at which point she revealed that she ingested approximately 8 g of isoniazid in a suicide attempt. A CT scan and MRI of the brain were normal. The remainder of her hospitalization was uneventful. Titers for herpes simplex virus, equine encephalitis virus, and West Nile virus were negative, as were blood cultures. She was discharged from medical care and transferred to a psychiatric facility.

HISTORY AND EPIDEMIOLOGY

The global burden of tuberculosis is enormous. Approximately 1.86 billion people are infected with *Mycobacterium tuberculosis;* 7.96 million new cases are diagnosed each year. An estimated 1.87 million persons worldwide die from the infection annually.[37] After the introduction of isoniazid (INH) into clinical practice in 1952, the number of reported United States cases of tuberculosis steadily decreased over a 30-year period. From 1985 to 1991, however, reported tuberculosis cases increased by 18%. This increase was a result of, among other factors, the human immunodeficiency virus (HIV) epidemic, homelessness, deterioration in the healthcare infrastructure, and increased numbers of cases among foreign-born persons. At the same time, the emergence of multidrug-resistant tuberculosis became a serious health concern. One-third of newly diagnosed cases are resistant to INH and one-fifth are resistant to both INH and rifampin, the two most effective drugs for treating tuberculosis. Because of these dramatic increases, containment strategies such as aggressive case identification and directly observed therapy were initiated to slow the spread of the infection.[22,45,59] Consequently, the number of reported cases in the United States in 1998 decreased by 31% from the peak incidence reported in 1992. Populations that remain at risk for tuberculosis are HIV-positive patients, the homeless, intravenous drug users, healthcare workers, prisoners, prison workers, and Native Americans. In addition, the tuberculosis rate in foreign-born persons was 4–6 times higher than for US-born people. The birth countries generating the highest number of US tuberculosis cases were Mexico, the Philippines, and Vietnam.[21,23–25,59]

The emergence of multidrug-resistant tuberculosis has forced the use of multidrug regimens and the rapid application of newer antibiotics, as well as the reintroduction of older antituberculous agents. This likely results in an increased incidence of adverse drug effects. For example, multidrug antituberculous regimens are associated with a 15% incidence of an adverse event.[3] Hepatotoxicity, peripheral neuropathy, and ocular neuropathy are common, often irreversible, and potentially fatal. Moreover, many of those receiving antituberculous therapy are chronically ill and are therefore at increased risk for intentional overdose. Fortunately, poisoning from antituberculous agents is often responsive to treatment if identified. This chapter describes the toxicity of antituberculous agents, their manifestations, and their management.

ISONIAZID

Pharmacology

Isoniazid (INH, or isonicotinic hydrazide) is structurally related to nicotinic acid (niacin, or vitamin B_3), nicotinamide-adenosine dinucleotide (NAD), and pyridoxine (vitamin B_6) (Fig. 43–1). The pyridine ring is essential for antituberculous activity. The mechanism of action of INH involves an interaction with InhA, a mycobacterial enzyme that functions as an enoyl-acyl carrier protein (enoyl-ACP) reductase.[86,87] Enoyl-ACP reductases catalyze the nicotinamide adenine dinucleotide (NADH)-dependent reduction of the double bonds in the growing fatty acid chain linked to acyl carrier proteins. InhA is required for the synthesis of very-long-chain lipids known as mycolic acids (containing between 40 and 60 carbons) that are important components of mycobacterial cell walls.

Isonicotinic hydrazide itself does not directly interact with the InhA enzyme. Instead, INH is a prodrug that undergoes metabolic activation by a catalase-reductase known as KatG to produce a highly reactive intermediate.[86,123] This activated form of INH is either an anion or radical that is stabilized by the pyridine ring. The INH-derived species enters the binding site of InhA where it reacts with NADH. The covalently linked INH-NADH complex remains bound to the active site of InhA, irreversibly inhibiting the enzyme.[74,88]

Pharmacokinetics and Toxicokinetics

When therapeutic doses of 5–15 mg/kg are administered orally, INH is rapidly absorbed, reaching peak plasma concentrations within 2 hours.[56,81,84] Isonicotinic hydrazide diffuses into all body fluids with a volume of distribution of approximately 0.6 L/kg and has negligible binding to serum proteins. After the drug penetrates infected tissue, it persists in quantities well above those required for bacteriostasis.

Metabolism of INH occurs via a cytochrome P450–mediated process, with approximately 75–95% of INH renally eliminated as hepatic metabolites within 24 hours of administration.[71] The primary metabolic pathway for INH is via N-acetylation, which occurs primarily in hepatocytes and gut mucosa. N-Acetyltransferase, the enzyme responsible for this conversion, exhibits Michaelis-Menten kinetics, although the activity of any individual's enzyme is controlled by an autosomal dominant inheritance pattern. Phenotypically, patients with the polymorphic forms of N-acetyltransferase are distinguishable as slow and fast acetyla-

tors. The isoforms are distinguishable by these characteristics: (a) Slow acetylators have less presystemic clearance, or first-pass effect, than do fast acetylators; (b) fast acetylators metabolize INH 5–6 times faster than slow acetylators; and (c) plasma INH concentrations are 30–50% lower in fast acetylators than in slow acetylators. The elimination half-life of INH is approximately 70 minutes and 180 minutes in fast and slow acetylators, respectively. The slow acetylation isoenzyme is found in 50–60% of American whites and African-Americans, whereas the fast acetylator isoenzymes are found in 90% of Asians and Inuits.[38] Twenty-seven percent of INH is excreted unchanged in slow acetylators, as compared with 11% in fast acetylators. The clearance of INH averages approximately 46 mL/min.[11,117] INH is transformed either via a stepwise process to acetylhydrazine and isonicotinic acid, or directly to hydrazine. In the first instance, INH is initially acetylated to acetylisoniazid and then hydrolyzed to acetylhydrazine. This intermediate may then be oxidized by hepatic microsomes to reactive intermediates that damage hepatocytes.[114] Figure 43–2 illustrates the metabolism of INH.

Mechanism of Toxicity

Isonicotinic hydrazide alters pyridoxine metabolism to create a functional deficiency of pyridoxine by at least two mechanisms (Fig. 43–3). First, INH metabolites inhibits pyridoxine phosphokinase, the enzyme that converts pyridoxine to its active form, pyridoxal-5′-phosphate.[27,55,69] Second, INH reacts with pyridoxal phosphate to produce an inactive hydrazone complex that is renally excreted.[69,117] Urinary excretion of pyridoxine and its metabolites increases with increasing INH dosage, reflecting the effect of INH on pyridoxine metabolism. The consequences of pyridoxine depletion include impaired activity of pyridoxine-dependent enzyme systems, as well as a decrease in catecholamine synthesis. In addition, INH either replaces nicotinic acid in the synthesis of NAD or reacts with NAD to form inactive hydrazones. Isonicotinic hydrazide disrupts cellular reduction/oxidation capabilities through both of these mechanisms.

Isonicotinic hydrazide interferes with the synthesis and metabolism of γ-amino butyric acid (GABA), the primary inhibitory neurotransmitter in the central nervous system. Two pyridoxine-dependent enzymes control GABA metabolism: glutamic acid decarboxylase (GAD) and GABA aminotransferase. The former catalyzes GABA synthesis, while the latter degrades the neurotransmitter. The inhibitory effects of INH are greater on GAD, which leads to decreased GABA concentrations.[7,119] Depletion of GABA is thought to be the etiology of INH-induced seizures.

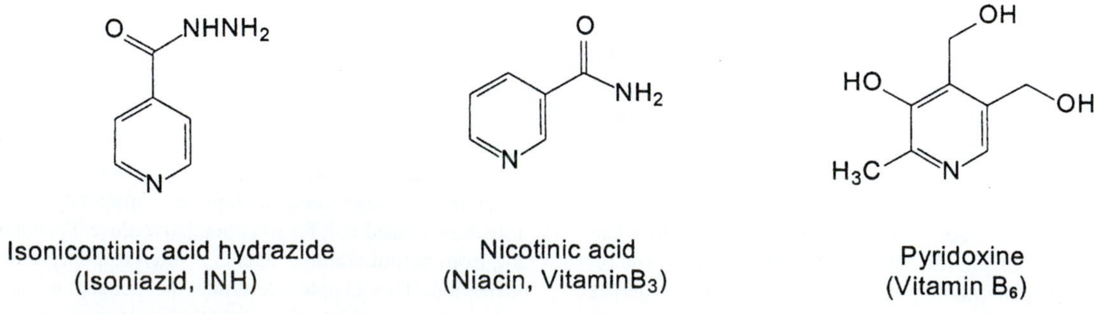

Isonicotinic acid hydrazide
(Isoniazid, INH)

Nicotinic acid
(Niacin, VitaminB$_3$)

Pyridoxine
(Vitamin B$_6$)

Figure 43–1. INH and related compounds.

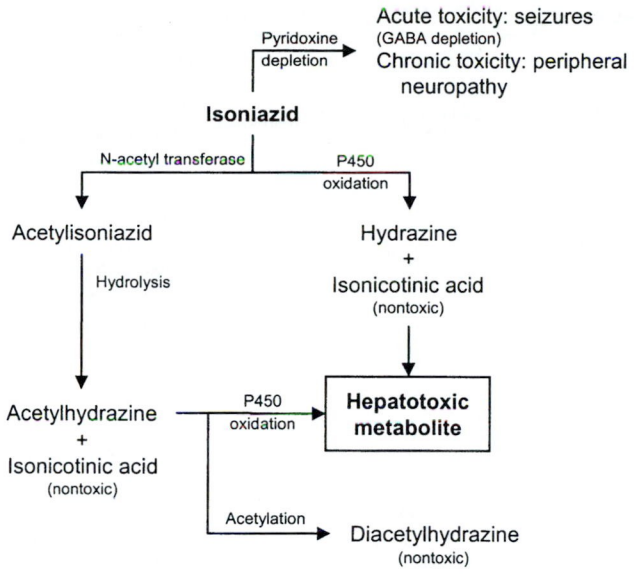

Figure 43–2. Metabolism of INH. Acetylator status is determined by polymorphism in N-acetyl transferase.

Monomethylhydrazine, a metabolite produced from gyromitrin isolated from the *Gyromitra* species ("false morel") mushroom, has a similar mechanism of action (Chap. 76).

Isonicotinic hydrazide crosses the placenta to enter the fetal compartment, reaching umbilical cord blood concentrations comparable to maternal levels.[13] INH does not appear to be a human teratogen, although fetal deformities following acute overdose of INH are reported.[65,117] Administration of INH to pregnant women was not associated with cancer in their offspring. Isonicotinic hydrazide readily enters breast milk, but breast-feeding during therapy is considered acceptable.[93,117]

Interactions with Other Drugs and Foods

Of patients receiving the drug, INH has an overall incidence of drug-drug interactions of 5.4%.[71,97] INH potentially inhibits several cytochrome P450–mediated transformations, particularly demethylation, oxidation, and hydroxylation (Chap. 11). Clinically relevant adverse effects have been documented with

theophylline (CYP1A2), phenytoin (CYP2C9/CYP2C19), Coumadin (CYP2C9/CYP2C19), valproate, and carbamazepine (CYP3A4).[54,97] Furthermore, therapeutically dosed INH interacts with CYP2E1 in at least two ways: INH induces CYP2E1, and then inhibits it. The binding of INH to CYP2E1 simultaneously decreases the metabolism of its substrate as well as inhibits the degradation of CYP2E1 itself. CYP2E1 is therefore stabilized, leading to increased cellular concentrations of the enzyme. After INH diffuses from the CYP2E1 active site, greater-than-normal amounts of cytochrome become available to metabolize potential substrates.[97] CYP2E1 catalyzes the formation of NAPQI (*N*-acetyl-*p*-benzoquinoneimine), the acetaminophen metabolite responsible for toxicity.[26] Consequently, INH use may increase the likelihood of acetaminophen-induced hepatotoxicity.[26]

Isonicotinic hydrazide has numerous food interactions. Carbohydrate meals ingested concurrently with INH lower serum drug concentrations by 34%.[72] Isonicotinic hydrazide is a weak monoamine oxidase inhibitor, and tyramine reactions to both foods and meperidine are reported in patients taking INH. Clinical effects include flushing, tachycardia, and hypertension.[32,42,64,107] Furthermore, INH inhibits the enzyme histaminase, leading to exacerbated reactions following the ingestion of histamine in scombrotoxic fish.[4,52,54,97] Table 43–1 summarizes additional INH drug and food interactions.

Clinical Manifestations of INH Toxicity

Acute Toxicity. Patients with severe, acute toxicity from INH present with the triad of seizures refractory to conventional therapy, severe metabolic acidosis, and coma. These clinical manifestations may appear as soon as 30 minutes following ingestion.[50,54,113] The case fatality rate of a single acute ingestion approaches 20%.[15,18] Although vomiting, slurred speech, dizziness, and tachycardia may represent early manifestations of toxicity, seizures may be the initial sign of acute overdose.[68] Seizures may occur following the ingestion of greater than 20 mg/kg of INH, and invariably occur with ingestions greater than 35–40 mg/kg. Patients with underlying seizure disorders, however, may develop seizures at lower doses.[15] Hyperreflexia or areflexia may herald INH-induced seizures. Patients may exhibit improvement in consciousness between seizures.[31,78]

A second feature of acute INH toxicity is severe anion gap metabolic acidosis associated with a high serum lactate. Typically, serum pH ranges between 6.80 and 7.30, although survival in the

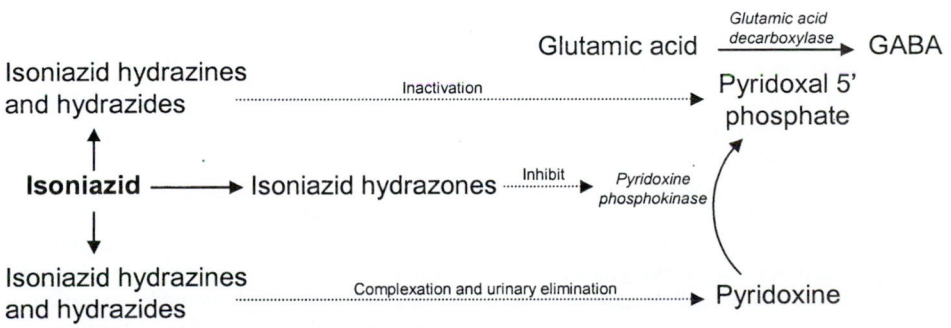

Figure 43–3. The effect of isoniazid on gamma-aminobutyric acid (GABA) synthesis.

TABLE 43–1. Adverse Reactions and Drug Interactions of Antituberculous Agents

Drug	Major Adverse Reactions	Drug Interactions-Clinical Effect	Monitoring	Comments
INH	Acute: Seizures, acidosis, coma, hyperthermia, oliguria, anuria Chronic: Elevation of liver enzymes, hepatitis, autoimmune disease (arthritis, anemia, hemolysis, eosinophilia), peripheral neuropathy, optic neuritis, vitamin B_6 deficiency (pellagra)	Rifampin, PZA, EtOH: Hepatic necrosis Acetaminophen: Hepatic necrosis Coumadin: Increased prothrombin time Theophylline: tachycardia, vomiting, seizures, acidosis Phenytoin: Increased phenytoin levels Carbamazepine: Altered mental status Meperidine: Hypertension Lactose: Decreased INH absorption Antacids: Decreased INH absorption Red wine/soft cheese: Tyramine reaction Fish (scombroid): Flushing, pruritis	Liver enzymes, ANA, CBC	HIV enteropathy may decrease absorption; INH should not be given with lactose-containing drug formulations because lactose can form hydrazones and lower INH concentrations
Rifampin	Acute: Diarrhea, periorbital edema Chronic: Hepatitis, reddish discoloration of body fluids	Protease inhibitors: Decreased serum concentration of protease inhibitor Delavirdine: Increased HIV resistance Cyclosporine: Graft rejection Coumadin: Decreased INR Oral contraceptives: Ineffective contraception Methadone: Opiate withdrawal Phenytoin: Higher frequency of seizures Theophylline: Decreased theophylline levels Verapamil: Decreased cardiovascular effect	If administered with HIV antiretroviral agents, viral titers should be followed. Liver enzymes; should monitor serum levels of drugs (ie, phenytoin, cyclosporine) or clinical markers of efficacy (ie, coagulation times)	Interactions of rifampin with several HIV medications are very poorly described; changes in dosing or dosing interval for both rifampin and antiretroviral drugs may be required; has teratogenic effects
Ethambutol	Chronic: Optic neuritis, loss of red-green discrimination, loss of peripheral vision		Visual acuity, color discrimination	Contraindicated in children too young for formal ophthalmologic examination
Pyrazinamide	Chronic: Hepatitis, decreased urate excretion	INH: Increased rates of hepatotoxicity (when extended courses or high dose pyrazinamide used)	Liver enzymes	Courses of therapy of 2 months or less recommended
Cycloserine	Chronic: Depression, paranoia, seizures, megaloblastic anemia	INH: Increased frequency of seizures	CBC, psychiatric monitoring	
Ethionamide	Chronic: Orthostatic hypotension, depression	Cycloserine: May increase CNS effects	Follow clinical signs of orthostasis	
Para-amino-salicylic acid	Chronic: Malaise, GI upset, elevated liver enzymes, hypersensitivity reactions, thrombocytopenia		Liver enzymes, CBC	
Capreomycin	Chronic: Hearing loss, tinnitus, proteinuria, sterile abscess at IM injection sites		Audiometry, renal function tests	

setting of an arterial pH 6.49 was reported.[50] Because paralyzed animals poisoned with INH do not develop lactic acidemia, muscular activity is thought to be the etiology of the acidosis.[27,79] Although not borne out in clinical practice, the acidosis from INH-induced seizures has been described as resolving more slowly than the lactic acidemia from typical seizures, the mechanism for which may be the formation of NAD hydrazones that prevent the transformation of lactate to pyruvate.[27,118] Alternate explanations of INH-associated acidosis include the generation of acidic INH metabolites and enhanced fatty acid oxidation leading to increased serum ketoacids.[79,117]

Protracted coma is the third component of acute INH toxicity. Coma may last as long as 24–36 hours and persist beyond the ter-mination of seizure activity and the resolution of acidosis. The cause of coma is unknown.[50]

Additional effects from acute INH intoxication include renal failure, hyperglycemia, glycosuria, and ketonuria along with hypotension and hyperpyrexia.[6,19,117]

Chronic Toxicity. Because of its many biochemical mechanisms, chronic, therapeutic INH use is associated with a variety of adverse effects. Most concerning of these is hepatocellular dysfunction. Although asymptomatic elevation of liver enzymes is common in the early stages of treatment, laboratory testing may reveal the onset of hepatitis up to 1 year after starting INH therapy. Following several deaths among patients receiving INH prophylaxis, the United States Public Health Service, in 1978, reported the incidence of clinically evident hepatitis as 1% of those taking INH; of that subgroup, 10% died, for an overall mortality of 0.1%.[17,62] Research performed since the resurgence of tuberculosis (TB), however, identified a considerably lower rate of hepatotoxicity. Clinically relevant hepatitis occurred in only 11 patients in a population of 11,141 persons receiving INH, an incidence of 0.1%.[77] Additional studies suggest that the death rate because of INH hepatotoxicity is 0.001% (2 of 202,497 treated patients).[91] The decrease in mortality from INH-associated hepatitis may be a result of improved surveillance protocols allowing for earlier removal of drugs or decision analysis concerning continued use of INH.

INH-induced hepatitis can arise via two pathways.[35] The first involves an autoimmune mechanism resulting in hepatic injury that is thought to be idiopathic.[9,106,117,122] The association of INH hepatitis with lupus erythematosus, hemolytic anemia, thrombocytopenia, arthritis, vasculitis, and polyserositis supports an immunologic process.[9,106,117,122] However, symptoms commonly found in autoimmune disorders such as fever, rash, and eosinophilia are usually absent, and rechallenge with INH often fails to provoke recurrence of hepatocellular injury.[35] The second, more likely mechanism involves direct hepatic injury by INH or its metabolites. The metabolite believed responsible for hepatic injury is acetylhydrazine, which arises from the acetylation of INH followed by its hydrolysis.[75] Hepatotoxicity is associated with chronic overdosage, increasing age, comorbid conditions such as malnutrition, and combinations of antituberculous drugs that may serve as P450 inducers. Frank hepatic failure often occurs if INH therapy is continued after onset of hepatocellular injury.[35,36,40,49,73,101,102] The incidence of hepatitis is 2–4 times higher in pregnant women than in nonpregnant women.[41]

Peripheral neuropathy or optic neuritis may also accompany chronic INH use. Peripheral neuropathy, the most common complication of INH therapy, presents as a stocking-glove distribution that progresses proximally. Although primarily sensory in nature, myalgias and weakness may occur.[103] Peripheral neuropathy is caused only by the parent drug and is generally observed in severely malnourished, alcoholic, uremic, or diabetic patients; it is also associated with slow acetylator status, an effect which leads to increased INH levels in patients.[44] Neurotoxicity is probably caused by pyridoxine deficiency aggravated by the formation of pyridoxine-INH hydrazones.[38] Optic neuritis presents as decreased visual acuity; visual field testing may reveal central scotomata.[46,54] Isonicotinic hydrazide is also associated with central CNS toxicity with findings of ataxia, psychosis, hallucinosis, and coma.[1,10,43,90]

Diagnostic Testing

Acute INH toxicity is a clinical diagnosis that may be confirmed by measuring serum INH levels.[96] Isonicotinic hydrazide toxicity has been defined as a serum INH concentration (a) greater than 10 mg/L at 1 hour after ingestion, (b) greater than 3.2 mg/L 2 hours after ingestion, or (c) greater than 0.2 mg/L 6 hours after the ingestion.[78] Because rapid serum INH concentration measurements are not commonly available, clinicians cannot rely upon serum concentrations to confirm the diagnosis or begin therapy. Because of the risk of hepatitis associated with chronic INH use, hepatic aminotransferases should be regularly monitored once therapy is started.

Management

Acute Toxicity.

The initial management of a patient with INH toxicity requires termination of seizures; stabilization and correction of vital signs with maintenance of a patent airway; cardiovascular support with intravenous fluids; and administration of sodium bicarbonate to treat severe acidemia. Orogastric lavage may be indicated for patients presenting soon after the ingestion of large amounts of INH. Activated charcoal should be administered for gastrointestinal decontamination.[100] Emetics are contraindicated because of the underlying risk of seizures. Delayed absorption of INH has not been observed, suggesting that late gastrointestinal decontamination with charcoal is ineffective in preventing toxicity.[95]

The antidote for INH-induced neurologic dysfunction is pyridoxine. Pyridoxine rapidly terminates seizures, independently corrects metabolic acidosis, and reverses coma. The efficacy of pyridoxine is correlated with the administered dose; one study identified recurrent seizures in 60% of patients who received no pyridoxine, in 47% of those who received 10% of the ideal pyridoxine dose, and in no patients that received the full dose of pyridoxine.[116] To treat acute toxicity, the pyridoxine dose in grams should probably equal the amount of INH ingested in grams. Unknown quantities of ingested INH warrant initial empiric treatment with a pyridoxine dose of no more than 5 g (pediatric dose: 70 mg/kg to a maximum of 5 g). Pyridoxine should be administered at a rate of 1 g every 2–3 minutes. Seizures that persist beyond administration of the initial 5-g dose should be treated by administration of an additional 5 g pyridoxine.[8]

Hospital pharmacies may stock insufficient quantities of pyridoxine to treat even a single large INH ingestion.[94] In the event that intravenous formulations are unavailable in sufficient quantities, pyridoxine tablets may be crushed and administered via nasogastric tube.[94]

Conventional anticonvulsants demonstrate variable effectiveness against INH-induced seizures. Benzodiazepines may be used to potentiate the antidotal effect of suboptimal doses of pyridoxine if gram-for-gram replacement doses are unavailable. The benzodiazepines act synergistically with pyridoxine as well as possess inherent GABA-agonist activity, but as single agents they may be ineffective in the treatment of acute INH poisoning.[28,29,54,116] Phenytoin has no intrinsic GABAergic effect and is not recommended as therapy for INH overdose.[54,78,89] Barbiturates, which have potent GABA-agonist activity, are expected to be as effective as the benzodiazepines, although the risk of complications is greater with this class of anticonvulsant.

Hemodialysis has been used to enhance elimination of INH in acute overdose, with clearance rates as high as 120 mL/min. Hemodialysis is rarely indicated and is usually reserved for patients who develop INH-induced renal failure.[19,117]

Asymptomatic patients who present to the ED within 2 hours of ingestion of toxic amounts of INH should receive prophylactic administration of 5 g pyridoxine. This recommendation is based on the observation that INH reaches its peak serum concentration within 2 hours of ingestion of therapeutic doses. Asymptomatic patients may be observed for a 6-hour period for signs of toxicity. Acute toxicity is unlikely to appear more than 6 hours beyond ingestion.

Chronic Toxicity.

Hepatitis (aminotransferase concentrations twice normal) resulting from therapeutic INH administration mandates termination of therapy; malnourished patients may require nutritional support. After liver injury has resolved, INH may be restarted if liver enzymes are closely monitored.[35,102] Pyridoxine does not reverse hepatic injury; consequently, surveillance for and recognition of hepatocellular injury remains vital. Cases of hepatitis refractory to medical therapy may require liver transplantation.[39,51]

Neurologic toxicity, including peripheral neuropathies, cerebellar findings, and psychosis, is commonly treated with as much as 50 mg/d of pyridoxine, although doses as low as 6 mg/d appear to be effective.[1,10,90,108] Because of its effectiveness, pyridoxine is almost always used concomitantly with INH therapy.

RIFAMYCINS

Rifampin

Pharmacology

Rifamycins are a class of semisynthetic macrocyclic antibiotics derived from *Streptomyces mediterranei*. The drugs included in this class are rifampin, rifabutin, and rifapentine, of which the first two receive the greatest clinical use.[67] Rifampin and RNA polymerase form a stable complex that inhibits the initial steps in RNA chain polymerization. Disruption of RNA synthesis interrupts protein synthesis, leading to cell death. While mycobacterial RNA polymerase is susceptible to rifampin, eukaryotic RNA polymerase is not.[71]

Pharmacokinetics and Toxicokinetics

When administered orally, rifampin reaches peak plasma concentrations in 2–4 hours; foods, but not antacids, interfere with absorption.[83] Rifampin is secreted into the bile and undergoes enterohepatic recirculation. Although the recirculating antibiotic is deacetylated, the metabolite retains antimicrobial activity. The half-life of rifampin, normally between 1.5 and 5 hours, increases in the setting of hepatic dysfunction. After therapy is started, however, rifampin induces its own metabolism to lower its half-life by approximately 40%. Rifampin is approximately 75% protein-bound, but distributes widely into body compartments. It imparts a reddish color to all body fluids, including the CSF, leading to confusion with xanthochromia from subarachnoid hemorrhage.[54,71] The reddish discoloration of the skin may be removed by washing.[71] This property distinguishes rifampin from the "red man syndrome" associated with vancomycin, in which extreme flushing produces intense skin discoloration (Chap. 46).[60]

Rifampin therapy carries greater teratogenic risk than other antituberculous therapies, with an incidence of malformation of 4.4%. Anencephaly, hydrocephalus, and congenital limb abnormality and dislocations are reported.[14,110] Rifampin is associated with hemorrhagic disease of the newborn.[14] The antibiotic is compatible with breast-feeding as only minute amounts of rifampin are secreted into breast milk.[109]

Drug-Drug Interactions

Rifamycins are potent inducers of cytochrome P450 oxidative enzymes, which result in numerous significant drug interactions (Chap. 11). Of the rifamycins, rifampin has greater activity in inducing CYP3A4 than rifapentine; rifabutin has the least inductive activity of the class.[67] In addition, rifampin is thought to induce CYP1A2, CYP2C8, and CYP2C9.[47,112] Concomitant administration of rifampin thus affects the metabolism of an array of drugs such as Coumadin, cyclosporine, phenytoin, opioids, and oral contraceptives.[47,98,112] Enzyme induction by rifampin may therefore be responsible for a variety of processes, including insufficient anticoagulation in patients receiving Coumadin, acute graft rejection in transplant patients, graft-versus-host disease, difficulty controlling phenytoin levels, methadone withdrawal, and unplanned pregnancy. Effects arising from CYP3A4 induction begin within 5–6 days after rifampin is started, and persist for up to 7 days after therapy is stopped.[71]

The cytochrome isoforms induced by rifampin also control the metabolism of drugs used in the treatment of HIV. Rifampin decreases the concentration of available protease inhibitors by 35–92%.[16] The antiviral effect of protease inhibitors correlates best with their trough concentration.[111] Lower trough concentrations increase the frequency of drug-resistant mutations in the protease gene and lead to the outgrowth of drug-resistant HIV strains. The reduction of serum concentrations of protease inhibitors is of such magnitude that it may not be overcome by increasing the dose of protease inhibitor. Coadministration of rifampin with protease inhibitors may therefore lead to loss of HIV suppression and to the emergence of resistant HIV strains.[16]

Rifampin decreases the serum concentrations of nucleoside reverse transcriptase inhibitors such as zidovudine. The efficacy of zidovudine and congeners is not related to the serum concentration of drug, but is, instead, related to the intracellular concentration of the active metabolite, a triphosphate derivative. Even though rifampin decreases zidovudine concentrations by 47%, active metabolite is present within cells in sufficient levels for activity. Rifampin, therefore, has minimal effect on the efficacy of nucleoside reverse transcriptase inhibitors. Table 43–1 lists the drug interactions of rifampin.

Rifampin suppresses the transformation of antigen-stimulated lymphocytes as well as normal T-cell function, leading to decreased hypersensitivity to tuberculin. Rifampin also causes immunosuppression in animal models, an effect that may be caused by decreased protein synthesis in immune system cells. The clinical importance of this effect is uncertain.[71]

Clinical Manifestations

Acute Toxicity.   Rifamycin overdose infrequently produces serious effects. Nonetheless, 3 deaths from rifampin and rifampicin are reported, with 1 death the result of pulmonary edema.[12,58,85] The most common side effects of acute rifampin overdose are gastrointestinal symptoms consisting of epigastric pain, nausea, vomiting, and diarrhea. The presence of diarrhea distinguishes rifampin ingestion from other antimycobacterial agents.[35] Other effects include flushing, angioedema, and obtundation; children who received an overdose of rifampin developed facial or periorbital edema. Anterior uveitis is occasionally observed, as are neurologic effects consisting of generalized numbness, extremity pain, ataxia, and muscular weakness.[48,71]

Chronic Toxicity. When rifampin was originally introduced as an antituberculous agent, hepatitis was more frequently observed in patients taking combination therapy of rifampin and INH than in those taking INH alone. These results arise from rifampin's ability to induce cytochromes responsible for INH hepatotoxicity and are not commonly a result of direct hepatic injury that is caused by rifampin itself. Liver injury, when attributable to rifampin alone, is predominantly cholestatic, prompting suggestions that clinical surveillance for hepatic injury may be preferable over regular biochemical monitoring.[35,80] Rifampin alters the metabolism of other substances, such as INH and acetaminophen, to augment their hepatotoxicity.[35,76] Although more prevalent in combined regimens, adverse effects are uncommon; the increased efficacy of multidrug regimens generally outweighs the risks associated with their use. A recent report underscores the risks of the 9-month isoniazid, 2-month rifampin, and pyrazinamide regimen which has resulted in two cases of fatal and severe hepatitis following treatment for latent tuberculosis.[124]

An influenzalike syndrome that may result from hypersensitivity reactions is associated with rifampin therapy. The syndrome, which occurs in 20% of patients receiving high doses, includes fever, chills, myalgias, and nonproductive cough. Eosinophilia, hemolytic anemia, thrombocytopenia, and interstitial nephritis may develop in severe cases.[71] Intermittent dosing of rifampin is also a risk factor for renal failure, the mechanism for which is unknown. Renal failure is rarely oliguric and is usually self-limited; patients usually recover with supportive care, although rechallenge with rifampin should be undertaken only with caution.[80]

The concomitant administration of rifampin and protease inhibitors results in increased rates of arthralgias, uveitis, leukopenia, and skin discoloration. Identical side effects occurred during the simultaneous administration of rifampin and CYP3A4 inhibitors such as clarithromycin, suggesting that toxic effects arise from elevated serum rifampin concentrations.[16] Current recommendations are that rifampin dosing be decreased when administered with nelfinavir, indinavir, and amprenavir. The administration of rifampin with ritonavir is not recommended.[16,20]

Therapeutic Testing and Management

Management of patients with acute rifampin overdose is primarily supportive. Stabilization of vital signs and administration of charcoal are usually adequate, although clinicians should remain vigilant for coingestants. For chronic toxicity, recognition of interactions between rifampin and other drugs is critical. Hepatic function should be monitored because of rifampin's ability to augment the hepatotoxicity of other pharmaceutics. Treatment for hepatic injury involves withholding rifampin therapy and reassessing the appropriateness of other drugs administered to the patient. Supportive care for hepatotoxicity may be required. Influenzalike symptoms and renal failure secondary to rifampin may respond to decreasing the interval between administration of the drug.[80] Although rifampin interacts with protease inhibitors, the utility of

therapeutic drug monitoring is uncertain because the correlation of clinical events with serum concentrations of rifampin and antiretroviral drugs is unknown.[16]

ETHAMBUTOL

$$H-\underset{\underset{C_2H_5}{|}}{\overset{\overset{CH_2OH}{|}}{C}}-\underset{\underset{H}{|}}{\overset{\overset{H}{|}}{N}}-\underset{\underset{H}{|}}{\overset{\overset{H}{|}}{C}}-\underset{\underset{H}{|}}{\overset{\overset{H}{|}}{C}}-\underset{\underset{H}{|}}{\overset{\overset{H}{|}}{N}}-\underset{\underset{CH_2OH}{|}}{\overset{\overset{C_2H_5}{|}}{C}}-H$$

Pharmacology and Pharmacokinetics

Ethambutol, an antibiotic to which almost all strains of *M. tuberculosis* are sensitive, has no effect on other bacteria. Ethambutol binds to arabinosyltransferases, which are enzymes that incorporate glycan subunits into cell wall polymers known as arabinogalactan and lipoarabinomannan.[66] Only the D(+)− isomer is used therapeutically, but both enantiomers are bacteriocidal.[54] The drug is active only in growing cells, where bacteriostatic effects appear approximately 24 hours after ethambutol is incorporated by mycobacteria.[71]

Maximum serum concentrations are reached within 4 hours of oral administration and are proportional to the dose. Both foods and antacids decrease absorption.[16] Ethambutol is approximately 20–30% protein bound and has a half-life of between 4 and 6 hours.[63,71] Three-fourths of a standard dose is excreted unchanged into the urine by a combination of glomerular filtration and tubular secretion. Consequently, ethambutol accumulates in patients with renal failure, making adjustments in dosing necessary.[71]

Ethambutol is considered safe for use during pregnancy as a first-line agent. Although a 2.2% incidence of congenital abnormalities was identified in women undergoing ethambutol therapy, no consistent pattern of abnormalities occurred in their offspring.[14] Even though ethambutol is excreted into breast milk in approximately a 1:1 ratio with serum, it is compatible with breastfeeding.[14]

Clinical Manifestations of Toxicity and the Management of Toxicity

Acute overdosage of ethambutol is generally well tolerated, although death is reported.[58] More commonly, nausea, abdominal pain, confusion, visual hallucinations, and optic neuropathy occur following acute ingestions of greater than 10 g.[34] Hemodialysis is rarely used as treatment for multidrug ingestions including ethambutol.[34] Although stabilization of vital signs and gastric decontamination consisting of activated charcoal remain the hallmarks of therapy, clinicians must remain vigilant for coingestants.

While peripheral neuropathy and asymptomatic hyperuricemia occur with chronic therapy, the most significant effect of ethambutol is dose-related optic or retrobulbar neuritis, which may be unilateral or bilateral.[57,104] Approximately 15% of patients receiving 50 mg/kg/d, 5% of patients receiving 25 mg/kg/d, and fewer than 1% of those receiving 15 mg/kg/d developed optic neuritis.[80] Patients may develop subclinical ocular disease within 30 days of starting ethambutol.[120] If clinically apparent, patients may complain of loss of red/green discrimination, decreased visual acuity, and loss of peripheral vision. The loss of peripheral vision and color discrimination seen in those with optic neuropathy from ethambutol distinguishes this condition from optic neuropathy secondary to INH.[54,80]

Management of chronic toxicity from ethambutol involves cessation of therapy, although improvement may be hastened by treatment with hydroxocobalamin.[54] Recovery is less likely in older patients, is related to the degree of visual impairment, and requires terminating ethambutol therapy.[115]

Optic neuritis may be related to derangements in mitochondrial copper or zinc metabolism; ethambutol chelates both metals.[30] The visual abnormalities induced by ethambutol have clinical features similar to a hereditary condition known as Leber optic neuropathy. In this disorder, the mechanism of visual loss is defective mitochondrial metabolism of copper.[61] Ethambutol is suspected of mimicking this condition by binding intracellular copper, altering mitochondrial function and producing neuronal injury.[53,61] Alternatively, optic neuritis may be related to zinc metabolism. Ethambutol chelates intracellular zinc to induce reversible vacuolar degeneration in retinal cultures. Progressive degeneration leads to irreversible neuronal destruction.[121] The clinical effect of this injury is a shift in the threshold for wavelength discrimination without changing the absolute sensitivity of the cone system, which patients discern as loss of red-green discrimination.[105]

Diagnostic Testing

All patients should receive neuro-ophthalmic testing prior to ethambutol therapy. The use of visual-evoked potentials is especially useful in identifying subclinical optic nerve disease. Furthermore, patients should receive regular visual acuity exams, and clinicians should encourage patients to report any subjective symptoms related to vision. The use of ethambutol may be relatively contraindicated in children who are unable to comply with an ophthalmic examination.[54,80]

PYRAZINAMIDE

Pharmacology and Pharmacokinetics

Pyrazinamide (PZA) is a structural analogue of nicotinamide whose mechanism of action is similar to that of INH. Like INH, PZA is a prodrug. Pyrazinamide requires deamidation by an endogenous bacterial enzyme, pyrazinamidase, to pyrazinoic acid, the active form of the drug. The precise cellular functions inhibited by pyrazinoic acid have not been defined, but an acid pH is required for activity. Pyrazinamide is active against both active and dormant bacteria.[5] Pyrazinamide is used in antituberculosis regimens as a means of shortening the course of therapy. If PZA is administered during the first 2 months of treatment with INH and rifampin, a course of chemotherapy may be shortened to only 6 months, the shortest effective regimen.[82] After oral administration, PZA is rapidly absorbed, with maximum concentrations occurring within 1 hour of administration. Its volume of distribution is 0.7 L/kg and PZA remains approximately 10% protein bound in the plasma. Pyrazinamide is metabolized to pyrazinoic acid and 5-hydroxypyrazinoic acid, which are then renally excreted. The drug has a half-life of approximately 9 hours.[71]

When introduced in the 1950s, PZA was administered in doses of 40–50 mg/kg for extended periods. The dosages caused cytolytic hepatitis, with clinical manifestations of highly elevated transaminase and bilirubin concentrations. Among patients taking high-dose PZA, elevations in transaminases were identified in 20% and symptomatic hepatitis in 10%. A small number of the latter population succumbed after a fulminant course. As a result of these findings, PZA was believed to be highly hepatotoxic and its use was discouraged. The resurgence of multidrug-resistant mycobacteria, however, has forced clinicians to reassess the role of PZA. Modern dosing regimens of 30 mg/kg for brief courses of 2 months produce infrequent hepatic injury, with some studies suggesting that addition of PZA to multidrug TB regimens confers no additional risk for hepatotoxicity.[35,80,82] A recent report of PZA, rifampin, and INH therapy resulting in fatal and severe hepatitis is of great concern.[124] Pyrazinamide administration for short courses is not associated with hepatitis in children.[92]

Pyrazinamide is rarely used in pregnancy because the risk of birth defects is poorly defined. Animal studies suggest that PZA has no teratogenic potential at therapeutic doses.[2] Pyrazinamide has minimal excretion into breast milk, and is presumed safe for breast-feeding.[14]

Clinical Manifestations and Management

Proper dosing of PZA and short courses of therapy are the most important factors in preventing toxicity. At doses higher than 30 mg/kg/d and at durations greater than 2 months, PZA is associated with cytolytic hepatitis characterized by highly elevated aminotransferases and bilirubin concentrations. Treatment for hepatotoxicity involves cessation of PZA therapy in conjunction with supportive care.[35] Pyrazinamide inhibits the renal excretion of uric acid, and hyperuricemia is observed. Greater than 90% of children treated with short courses developed elevated uric acid concentrations.[92] While most patients regardless of age remain asymptomatic and do not develop symptoms of gout, polyarthralgias responsive to probenecid or allopurinol may be observed.[82] Cutaneous hypersensitivity responsive to antihistamines has been rarely described.[99] Toxic effects from acute overdose of pyrazinamide have not been reported.

CYCLOSERINE

Cycloserine is used in conjunction with other tuberculostatic agents when treatment with primary agents (INH, rifampin, ethambutol, and streptomycin) has failed. Cycloserine, a structural analogue of alanine, inhibits reactions in which D-alanine is required for cell wall biosynthesis. After oral doses, 70–90% of the drug is absorbed. Peak concentrations of the drug are reached in 3–4 hours. Cycloserine is distributed throughout all tissues and body fluids. No appreciable blood-brain barrier exists, because CSF concentrations are approximately equal to those in the serum.

Very little of the antibiotic is metabolized, and the drug is excreted unchanged in the urine.[71]

Toxicity, occurring in as many as 50% of patients taking cycloserine, is dose dependent. Neurologic effects consist of somnolence, headache, tremor, dysarthria, vertigo, confusion, irritability, and seizures. Psychiatric manifestations include paranoid reactions, depression, and suicidal ideation. These effects are thought to be caused by agonism of glycine B receptors by cycloserine. Cycloserine is contraindicated in patients with a history of either seizures or depression. If used, cycloserine should be introduced slowly to avoid CNS toxicity.[54,80,82] Toxicity is potentiated by alcohol, usually appears within the first 2 weeks of therapy, and ceases upon termination of the drug. Because cycloserine is renally excreted, patients with renal failure may be predisposed to toxicity; it is removed by hemodialysis. Although no teratogenic effects were noted in 3 women exposed to cycloserine during the first trimester, cycloserine is not recommended for use during pregnancy. Cord blood concentrations are approximately 70% of serum levels, and no adverse effects were seen in breast-fed infants. Consequently, cycloserine is considered to be compatible with breast-feeding.[14]

OTHER ANTIMYCOBACTERIAL AGENTS

Ethionamide

Aminosalicylic acid

Ethionamide, a congener of INH, is thought to have a similar mechanism of action to INH. Oral doses yield peak serum concentrations within approximately 3 hours of administration. The half-life of the drug is approximately 2 hours. Toxic effects include orthostatic hypotension, depression, and drowsiness. Rash, purpura, and gynecomastia are observed, as are tremor, paresthesias, and olfactory disturbances. Approximately 5% of patients receiving ethionamide develop hepatitis. Treatment for toxicity involves withholding ethionamide therapy, although patients should be given pyridoxine concomitantly with ethionamide.[71] Birth defects were observed in 7 of 23 infants antenatally exposed to ethionamide, although a consistent pattern of anomalies was lacking. Data regarding the safety of ethionamide are lacking.[14] Reports of toxicity from ethionamide overdose are absent from the English literature.[33]

Para-aminosalicylic acid (PAS) is thought to inhibit enzymes responsible for folate biosynthesis in mycobacteria but not other organisms. PAS is readily absorbed from the gut, and is rapidly distributed into all tissues, especially the pleural fluid and caseous material. PAS has a brief half-life, and is renally excreted. Adverse effects associated with PAS use include gastrointestinal

upset, sore throat, and malaise. Between 5 and 10% of patients receiving PAS develop hypersensitivity reactions characterized by high fever, rash, and arthralgias. Finally, hematologic abnormalities of agranulocytosis, leukopenia, eosinophilia, thrombocytopenia, and acute hemolytic anemia have been observed.[71] In renal failure and acute overdose, PAS may be removed by hemodialysis.[70] Adverse effects associated with chronic therapy may be treated with withdrawal of the drug. Data regarding the safety of PAS in pregnancy and breast-feeding are lacking.[14]

Capreomycin is a cyclic polypeptide with an unknown mechanism of action. Because of poor absorption after oral dosing, capreomycin must be administered intramuscularly. Toxicity associated with capreomycin use includes hearing loss, tinnitus, proteinuria, and electrolyte disturbances, although severe renal failure is rare. Eosinophilia, leukocytosis, and rashes have been described. Pain and sterile abscesses at the site of capreomycin injection have been reported.[71] Data regarding the safety of capreomycin in pregnancy and breast-feeding are lacking.[14]

SUMMARY

Antituberculous agents continue to represent a significant toxicologic threat. Patients acutely poisoned with INH require immediate and appropriate action to reverse seizures, acidosis, and coma. As an antidote to INH overdose, pyridoxine is effective therapy, although its action may be augmented by the use benzodiazepines. Although less common than previously believed, hepatocellular injury manifested from therapeutic dosing of INH nonetheless requires surveillance to prevent fulminant hepatic failure.

Other antituberculous agents possess significant adverse effects. In particular, rifampin has numerous drug-drug interactions, including several with anti-HIV therapies. Because antituberculous therapies are common in the HIV population, potential interactions between rifampin and antiretroviral agents force clinicians to remain vigilant for unanticipated adverse effects. Patients receiving ethambutol, pyrazinamide, and other antituberculous agents benefit from surveillance for specific effects such as decreased visual acuity, hepatic injury, and psychiatric manifestations. Despite the toxicity of this class of drugs, poisoning is often responsive to intervention if recognized and treated appropriately.

REFERENCES

1. Alao A, Yolles J: Isoniazid-induced psychosis. Ann Pharmacother 1998;32:889–890.
2. Al-Haggag M, Al Haider A, Islam M: Evaluation of the teratogenic potential of pyrazinamide in Wistar rats. Ups J Med Sci 1999;104:259–270.
3. Aziz S, Hassan R, Fairoz S, Hassan K: Hepatotoxicity to different antituberculosis drug combinations. J Pakistan Med Assoc 1990;40:290–294.
4. Baciewicz AW, Self TH: Isoniazid interactions. South Med J 1985;78:714–718.
5. Barry C: New horizons in the treatment of tuberculosis. Biochem Pharmacol 1997;54:1165–1172.
6. Bear E, Hoffman P, Siegel S, Randall R: Suicidal ingestion of isoniazid: An uncommon cause of metabolic acidosis and seizures. South Med J 1976;69:31–32.
7. Biggs CS, Pearce BR, Fowler LJ, Whitton PS: Effect of isonicotinic acid hydrazide on extracellular amino acids and convulsions in the

rat: Reversal of neurochemical and behavioural deficits by sodium valproate. J Neurochem 1994;63:2197–2201.

8. Blanchard PD, Yao JDC, McAlpine DE, et al: Isoniazid overdose in the Cambodian population of Olmstead County, Minnesota. JAMA 1986;256:3131–3133.

9. Blowey D, Johnson D, Verjee Z: Isoniazid-associated rhabdomyolysis. Am J Emerg Med 1995;13:543–544.

10. Blumberg E, Gil R: Cerebellar syndrome caused by isoniazid. Ann Pharmacother 1990;24:829–831.

11. Boxenbaum HC, Riegelman S: Pharmacokinetics of isoniazid and some metabolites in man. J Pharmacokinet Biopharm 1976;4:287–325.

12. Broadwell R, Broadwell S, Comer P: Suicide by rifampin overdose. JAMA 1978;240:2283–2284.

13. Bromberg Y, Salzberger M, Bruderman I: Placental transfer of isonicotinic acid hydrazide. Gynecology 1955;140:141–145.

14. Brost B, Newman R: The maternal and fetal effects of tuberculosis therapy. Obstet Gynecol Clin North Am 1997;24:659–673.

15. Brown C: Acute isoniazid poisoning. Am Rev Resp Dis 1972;105:206–216.

16. Burman W, Gallicano K, Peloquin C: Therapeutic implications of drug interactions in the treatment of human immunodeficiency virus-related tuberculosis. Clin Infect Dis 1999;28:419–430.

17. Byrd R, Nelson R, Elliott R: Isoniazid toxicity: A prospective study in secondary complications. JAMA 1972;220:1471–1473.

18. Cameron W: Isoniazid overdose. Can Med Assoc J 1978;118:1413–1415.

19. Cash J, Zawada E: Isoniazid overdose: Successful treatment with pyridoxine and hemodialysis. West J Med 1991;155:644–646.

20. Cato A, Cavanaugh J, Shi H, et al: The effect of multiple doses of ritonavir on the pharmacokinetics of rifambutin. Clin Pharmacol Ther 1998;63:414–421.

21. Centers for Disease Control: Approaches to improving adherence to antituberculosis therapy. MMWR Morb Mortal Wkly Rep 1993;42:74–75.

22. Centers for Disease Control: Initial therapy for tuberculosis in the era of multidrug resistance: Recommendations of the Advisory Council for the Elimination of Tuberculosis. JAMA 1993;270:694–698.

23. Centers for Disease Control: Probable transmission of multidrug-resistant tuberculosis in correctional facility—California. MMWR Morb Mortal Wkly Rep 1993;42:48–51.

24. Centers for Disease Control: Progress toward the elimination of tuberculosis—United States, 1998. MMWR Morb Mortal Wkly Rep 1999;48:732–734.

25. Centers for Disease Control: Tuberculosis transmission in a state correctional institution—California, 1990–1991. MMWR Morb Mortal Wkly Rep 1993;41:927–929.

26. Chien J, Peter R, Nolan C, et al: Influence of polymorphic N-acetyltransferase phenotype on the inhibition and induction of acetaminophen bioactivation with long-term isoniazid. Clin Pharmacol Ther 1997;61:24–34.

27. Chin L, Sievers ML, Herrier HE, et al: Convulsions as the etiology of lactic acidosis in acute isoniazid toxicity in dogs. Toxicol Appl Pharmacol 1979;49:377–384.

28. Chin L, Sievers ML, Laird HE, et al: Evaluation of diazepam and pyridoxine as antidotes to isoniazid intoxication in rats and dogs. Toxicol Appl Pharmacol 1978;45:713–722.

29. Chin L, Sievers ML, Laird HE, et al: Potentiation of pyridoxine by depressants and anticonvulsants in the treatment of acute isoniazid intoxication in dogs. Toxicol Appl Pharmacol 1981;58:504–509.

30. Cole A, May P, Williams D: Metal binding by pharmaceuticals. Part 1. Copper (II) and zinc (II) interactions following ethambutol administration. Agents Actions 1981;11:296–305.

31. Coyer J, Nicholson DP: Isoniazid-induced convulsions. South Med J 1976;69:294–297.

32. DiMartini A: Isoniazid, tricyclics and the "cheese reaction." Int Clin Psychopharmacol 1995;10:197–198.

33. Dolgikh-Litt N: Attempted of suicide with ethionamide. Klin Med 1967;45:148–150.

34. Ducobu J, Dupont P, Laurent M: Acute isoniazid/ethambutol/rifampin overdosage. Lancet 1982;1:632.

35. Durand F, Jebrak G, Pessayre D, Fournier M, Bernuau J: Hepatotoxicity of antitubercular treatments: Rationale for monitoring liver status. Drug Saf 1996;15:394–405.

36. Durand F, Pessayre D, Fournier M, et al: Antituberculous therapy and acute liver failure. Lancet 1995;345:1170.

37. Dye C, Scheele S, Dolin P, Pathania V, Raviglione MC: Consensus statement. Global burden of tuberculosis: Estimated incidence, prevalence, and mortality by country. WHO Global Surveillance and Monitoring Project. JAMA 1999;282:677–686.

38. Ellard G: The potential clinical significance of the isoniazid acetylator phenotype in the treatment of pulmonary tuberculosis. Tubercle 1984;65:211–227.

39. Farrell FJ, Keeffe EB, Man KM, Imperial JC, Esquivel CO: Treatment of hepatic failure secondary to isoniazid hepatitis with liver transplantation. Dig Dis Sci 1994;39:2255–2259.

40. Farrell G: Drug-induced acute hepatitis. In: Farrell G, ed. Drug-Induced Liver Disease. Edinburgh, Churchill Livingstone, 1994, pp. 247–299.

41. Franks A, Binkin N, Snider D: Isoniazid hepatitis in pregnant and postpartum Hispanic patients. Pub Health Rep 1989;104:151–155.

42. Gannon R, Pearsall W, Rowley R: Isoniazid, meperidine, and hypotension. Ann Intern Med 1983;99:415.

43. Gnam W, Flint A, Goldbloom D: Isoniazid-induced hallucinosis: Response to pyridoxine. Psychosomatics 1993;34:537–539.

44. Goel U, Baja S, Gupta O, Dwiedi N: Isoniazid-induced neuropathy in slow versus rapid acetylators. J Assoc Physicians India 1992;40:671–672.

45. Goldberger M: Treatment of tuberculosis: Current status and future promise. Semin Resp Crit Care Med 1997;18:439–448.

46. Gonzalez-Gay MA, Sanchez-Andrade A, Aguero JJ, et al: Optic neuritis following treatment with isoniazid in a hemodialyzed patient. Nephron 1993;63:360.

47. Grange J, Winstanley P, Davies P: Clinically significant drug interactions with antituberculosis agents. Drug Saf 1994;11:242–251.

48. Griffith D, Brown B, Girard W, Wallace R: Adverse events associated with high-dose rifabutin in macrolide-containing regimens for treatment of Mycobacterium avium complex lung disease. Clin Infect Dis 1995;21:594–598.

49. Gurumurthy P, Krishnamurthy M, Nazareth O: Lack of relationship between hepatic toxicity and acetylator phenotype in South Indian patients during treatment with isoniazid for tuberculosis. Am Rev Resp Dis 1984;129:58–61.

50. Hankinns DG, Saxena K, Faville RJ, et al: Profound acidosis caused by isoniazid ingestion. Am J Emerg Med 1987;5:165–166.

51. Hasagawa T, Reyes J, Nour B, et al: Successful liver transplantation for isoniazid-induced hepatic failure—A case report. Transplant 1994;57:1274–1277.

52. Hauser M, Baier H: Interactions of isoniazid with foods. Clin Pharmacokinet 1982;16:617–618.

53. Heng J, Vorwerk C, Lessell E, Zurakowski D, Levin L, Dreyer E: Ethambutol is toxic to retinal ganglion cells via an excitotoxic pathway. Invest Ophthalmol Vis Sci 1999;40:190–196.

54. Holdiness MR: Neurological manifestations and toxicities of the antituberculosis drugs—A review. Med Toxicol 1987;2:33–51.

55. Holtz P, Palm D: Pharmacological aspects of vitamin B-6. Pharmacol Rev 1964;16:113–178.

56. Hurwitz A, Schlozman DL: Effects of antacids on gastrointestinal absorption of isoniazid in rat and man. Am Rev Respir Dis 1974;109:41–47.

57. Jaanus S: Ocular side effects of selected systemic drugs. Optom Clin 1992;2:73–96.

58. Jack D, Knepil J, McLay W, Fergie R: Fatal rifampicin-ethambutol overdose. Lancet 1978;2:1107–1108.

59. Jasmer RM, Hahn JA, Small PM, et al: A molecular epidemiologic analysis of tuberculosis trends in San Francisco, 1991–1997. Ann Intern Med 1999;130:971–978.

60. Kapusnik-Uner, Sande M, Chambers H: Antimicrobial agents: Tetracyclines, chloramphenicol, erythromycin, and miscellaneous antibacterial agents. In: Hardman JG, Limbird LE, Molinoff PB, Ruddon RW, Gilman AG, eds: Goodman and Gilman's The Pharmacological Basis of Therapeutics, 9th ed. New York, McGraw-Hill, 1996, pp. 1123–1154.

61. Kozak S, Inderlied C, Hsu H, Keller K, Sadun A: The role of copper on ethambutol's antimicrobial action and implications for ethambutol-induced optic neuropathy. Diagn Microbiol Infect Dis 1998;30:83–87.

62. Kozanoff D, Snider D, Caras G: Isoniazid hepatitis: A US Public Health Service Cooperative Surveillance Study. Am Rev Resp Dis 1978;117:991–1001.

63. Lee C, Gambertoglio J, Brater D, Benet L: Kinetics of oral ethambutol in the normal subject. Clin Pharmacol Ther 1977;22:615–621.

64. Lejonc J, Schaeffer A, Brochard P, Portos J: Paroxystic hypertension after ingestion of gruyere cheese during isoniazid treatment: A report of two cases. Ann Med Interne (Paris) 1980;131:346–348.

65. Lenke R, Turkel S, Monsen R: Severe fetal deformities associated with ingestion of excessive isoniazid in early pregnancy. Acta Obst Gynecol Scand 1985;64:281–282.

66. Lety M, Nair S, Berche P, Escuyer V: A single point mutation in the embB gene is responsible for resistance to ethambutol in *Mycobacterium smegmatis*. Antimicrob Agents Chemother 1997;41:2629–2633.

67. Li A, Reith M, Rasmussen A, et al: Primary human hepatocytes as a tool for the evaluation of structure-activity relationship in cytochrome P450 induction potential of xenobiotics: Evaluation of rifampin, rifapentine, and rifabutin. Chem Biol Interact 1997;107: 17–30.

68. Lopez-Samblas A, Tsiligiannis T: Isoniazid intoxication in three adolescent patients. Hosp Pharm 1991;26:119–121.

69. Mailler J, Robinson A, Percy AKL: Acute isoniazid poisoning in childhood. Am J Dis Child 1980;134:290–292.

70. Malone R, Fish D, Spiegel D, Childs M, Peloquin C: The effect of hemodialysis on cycloserine, ethionamide, para-aminosalicylic acid, and clofazimine. Chest 1999;116:984–990.

71. Mandell G, Petri W. Antimicrobial agents: Drugs used in the chemotherapy of tuberculosis, *Mycobacterium avium* complex and leprosy. In: Hardman JG, Limbird LE, Molinoff PB, Ruddon RW, Gilman AG, eds: Goodman and Gilman's The Pharmacological Basis of Therapeutics, 9th ed. New York, McGraw-Hill, 1996, pp. 1155–1174.

72. Mannisto P, Mantyla R, Klinge R: Influence of various diets on the bioavailability of isoniazid. J Antimicrob Chemotherap 1982;10:427–434.

73. Martinez-Roig A, Cami J, Llorens-Terol J: Acetylation phenotype and hepatotoxicity in the treatment of tuberculosis in children. Pediatrics 1986;77:912–915.

74. Mdluli K, Slayden R, Zhu Y, et al: Inhibition of a *Mycobacterium tuberculosis* beta-ketoacyl ACP synthetase by isoniazid. Science 1998;280:1607–1610.

75. Nelson S, Mitchell J, Timbrell J, Snodgrass W: Isoniazid activation of metabolites to toxic intermediates in man and rat. Science 1975;193:901–903.

76. Nicod L, Villon C, Regnier A, Jacqueson A, Richert L: Rifampicin and isoniazid increase acetaminophen and isoniazid cytotoxicity in human HapG2 hepatoma cells. Hum Exp Toxicol 1997;16: 28–34.

77. Nolan C, Goldberg S, Buskin S: Hepatotoxicity associated with isoniazid preventive therapy: A 7-year survey from a public health tuberculosis clinic. JAMA 1999;281:1014–1081.

78. Orlowski JP, Paganini EP, Pippenger CE: Treatment of a potentially lethal dose of isoniazid ingestion. Ann Emerg Med 1988;17:73–76.

79. Pahl MV, Vaziri ND, Ness R, et al: Association of beta-hydroxybutyric acidosis with isoniazid intoxication. J Toxicol Clin Toxicol 1984;22:167–176.

80. Patel A, McKeon: Avoidance and management of adverse reactions to antituberculosis drugs. Drug Saf 1995;12:1–25.

81. Paulsen O, Hoglund P, Nilsson LG, Gredeby H: No interaction between H2 blockers and isoniazid. Eur J Respir Dis 1986;68: 286–290.

82. Peloquin C: Pharmacology of antimycobacterial drugs. Med Clin North Am 1993;77:1253–1262.

83. Peloquin C, Namdar R, Singleton M, Nix D: Pharmacokinetics of rifampin under fasting conditions, with food, and with antacids. Chest 1999;115:12–18.

84. Peloquin CA, Namdar R, Dodge AA, Nix DE: Pharmacokinetics of isoniazid under fasting conditions, with food, and with antacids. Int J Tuberc Lung Dis 1999;3:703–710.

85. Plomp T, Battista H, Unterdorfer H: A case of fatal poisoning by rifampicin. Arch Toxicol 1981;48:245–248.

86. Quemard A, Dessen A, Sugantino M, Jacobs W, Sacchettini J, Blanchard J: Binding of catalase-peroxidase activated isoniazid to wild-type and mutant *Mycobacterium tuberculosis* enoyl-ACP reductases. J Am Chem Soc 1996;118:1561–1562.

87. Quemard A, Sacchettini J, Dessen A, et al: Enzymatic characterization of the target for isoniazid in *Mycobacterium tuberculosis*. Biochem 1995;34:8235–8241.

88. Rozwarski D, Grant G, Barton D, Jacobs W, Casshettini J: Modification of the NADH of the isoniazid target (InhA) from *Mycobacterium tuberculosis*. Science 1998;279:98–101.

89. Saad S, el Masry A, Scott P: Influence of certain anticonvulsants on the concentration of GABA in the cerebral hemispheres of mice. J Am Chem Soc 1954;76:300–304.

90. Salkind A, Hewitt C: Coma from long-term overingestion of isoniazid. Arch Intern Med 1997;157:2518–2520.

91. Salpeter SR: Fatal isoniazid-induced hepatitis—Its risk during chemoprophylaxis. West J Med 1993;159:560–564.

92. Sanchez-Albisua I, Vidal L, Joya-Verde F, Castillo F, De Jose I, Garcia-Hortelano J: Tolerance of pyrazinamide in short course chemotherapy for pulmonary tuberculosis in children. Pediatr Infect Dis J 1997;16:760–763.

93. Sanders B, Draper G: Childhood cancer and drugs in pregnancy. Br Med J 1979;1:717–718.

94. Santucci K, Shah B, Linakis J: Acute isoniazid exposures and antidote availability. Pediatr Emerg Care 1999;15:99–101.

95. Scolding N, Ward M, Hutchings A, Routledge P: Charcoal and isoniazid pharmacokinetics. Hum Toxicol 1986;5:285–286.

96. Scott E, Wright R: Fluorimetric determination of INH in serum. J Lab Clin Med 1967;70:355–360.

97. Self T, Chrisman C, Baciewicz A, Bronze M: Isoniazid drug and food interactions. Am J Med Sci 1999;317:304–311.

98. Shenfield G: Oral contraceptives. Are drug interactions of clinical significance? Drug Saf 1993;9:211–237.

99. Shorr A, Trotta R: PZA hypersensitivity. Chest 1996;109:855–856.

100. Siefkin A, Albertson T, Corbett M: Isoniazid overdose: Pharmacokinetics and effects of oral charcoal in treatment. Hum Toxicol 1987;6:497–501.

101. Singh J, Arora A, Garg P, Thakur V, Pande J, Tandon R: Antituberculosis treatment induced hepatotoxicity: Role of predictive factors. Postgrad Med J 1995;71:359–362.

102. Singh J, Garg P, Tandon R: Hepatotoxicity due to antituberculosis therapy: Clinical profile and reintroduction of therapy. J Clin Gastroenterol 1996;22:211–214.

103. Siskind MS, Thienemann D, Kirlin L: Isoniazid-induced neurotoxicity in chronic dialysis patients: Report of three cases and a review of the literature. Nephron 1993;64:303–306.

104. Sivakumaran P, Marschner J, Martin P: Ocular toxicity from ethambutol: A review of four cases and recommended precautions. N Z Med J 1998;111:428–430.

105. Sjoerdsma T, Kamermans M, Spekreijse H: Modulating wavelength discrimination in goldfish with ethambutol and stimulus intensity. Vision Res 1996;36:3519–3525.

106. Skaer NL: Medication-induced systemic lupus erythematosus. Clin Ther 1992;14:496–505.

107. Smith C, Durack D: Isoniazid and reaction to cheese. Ann Intern Med 1979;88:520–521.

108. Snider D: Pyridoxine supplementation during isoniazid therapy. Tubercle 1980;61:191–196.

109. Snider D, Pwell K: Should women taking antituberculosis drugs breast-feed? Arch Intern Med 1984;144:589–590.

110. Steen J, Stainton-Ellis D: Rifampicin in pregnancy. Lancet 1977;2: 604–605.

111. Stein D, Fish D, Bilello J, Preston S, Martineau G, Drusano G: A 24-week open-label Phase I/II evaluation of the HIV protease inhibitor MK-639 (indinavir). AIDS 1996;10:485–492.

112. Strayhorn V, Baciewicz A, Self T: Update in rifampin drug interactions, III. Arch Intern Med 1997;157:2453–2457.

113. Terman DS, Teitelbaum DT: Isoniazid self-poisoning. Neurology 1970;20:299–304.

114. Timbrell J, Mitchell J, Snodgrass W: Isoniazid hepatotoxicity: The relationship between covalent binding and metabolism in vivo. J Pharmacol Exp Ther 1980;213:364–369.

115. Tsai R, Lee Y: Reversibility of ethambutol optic neuropathy. J Ocul Pharmacol Ther 1997;13:473–477.

116. Wason S, Lacouture PG, Lovejoy F: Single high-dose pyridoxine treatment for isoniazid overdose. JAMA 1981;246:1102–1104.

117. Weber WW, Hein DW: Clinical pharmacokinetics of isoniazid. Clin Pharmacol 1979;4:401–422.

118. Whitefield C, Klein R: Isoniazid overdose: Report of 40 patients with a critical analysis of treatment and suggestions for prevention. Am Rev Resp Dis 1971;103:887–893.

119. Wood JD, Paesker SJ: The effect on GABA metabolism in brain of isonicotinic acid hydrazide and pyridoxine as a function of time after administration. J Neurochem 1972;19:1527–1537.

120. Yiannidas C, Walsh J, McLeod J: Visual evoked potentials in the detection of subclinical optic toxic effects secondary to ethambutol. Arch Neurol 1983;40:645–648.

121. Yoon Y, Jung K, Sadun A, Shin H, Koh J: Ethambutol-induced vacuolar changes and neuronal loss in rat retinal cell culture: Mediation by endogenous zinc. Toxicol Appl Pharmacol 2000;162:107–114.

122. Yung RL, Richardson BC: Drug-induced lupus. Rheum Dis Clin North Am 1994;20:61–84.

123. Zabinski R, Blanchard J: Activation of INH by KatG. J Am Chem Soc 1997;1999:2331–2332.

124. Centers for Disease Control. Fatal and severe hepatitis associated with rifampin and pyrazinamide for the treatment of latent tuberculosis infection—New York and Georgia, 2000. MMWR Morb Mortal Wkly Rep 2001;50:289–291.

ANTIDOTES IN DEPTH

Pyridoxine
Mary Ann Howland

H_3C ... N ... H

HO ... CH_2OH

CH_2OH

Vitamin B$_6$
(pyridoxine)

Pyridoxine is administered as an antidote for isonicotinic acid hydrazide (isoniazid, INH), monomethylhydrazine, and perhaps ethylene glycol overdoses. The first two overdoses result in seizures caused by the competitive inhibition of pyridoxal-5-phosphate (PLP), and pyridoxine may overcome this inhibition. The administration of pyridoxine may enhance a less toxic pathway of ethylene glycol metabolism.[3]

HISTORY

A deficiency syndrome was first identified in 1926; it was mistakenly attributed to vitamin B_2.[22] Ten years later, the active compound was isolated and named vitamin B_6.[22]

CHEMISTRY

The active form of pyridoxine, also known as vitamin B_6, is the phosphate ester of pyridoxine (vitamin B_6; PLP).[22] Pyridoxine, an alcohol, pyridoxal, an aldehyde, and pyridoxamine, an aminomethyl form, are all naturally occurring related compounds that are metabolized by the body to the active PLP.[22] Pyridoxine was chosen by the Council on Pharmacy and Chemistry to represent vitamin B_6.[22] Pyridoxine hydrochloride was chosen as the commercial preparation because of its stability.[38]

PHARMACOLOGY

PLP is an important cofactor in more than 100 enzymatic reactions, including decarboxylation and transamination of amino acids, and the metabolism of tryptophan to 5-hydroxytryptamine and methionine to cysteine.[17,22] Iatrogenic pyridoxine deficiency in animals produces seizures associated with reduced brain levels of PLP, glutamic acid decarboxylase, and γ-aminobutyric acid (GABA).[12]

PHARMACOKINETICS

Pyridoxine is not protein bound, has a volume of distribution of 0.6 L/kg, and easily crosses cell membranes; in contrast PLP is nearly entirely plasma protein bound.[38] Pyridoxine is rapidly metabolized at extrahepatic sites to pyridoxal, PLP, and 4-pyridoxic acid, with only 7% excreted unchanged in the urine.[38] After intravenous infusion of 100 mg of pyridoxine over 6 hours, PLP concentration increases in plasma from a baseline of 183 nmol/L to a peak of 892 nmol/L at 3 hours after the end of the infusion. In erythrocytes, the PLP level rose from 88 nmol/L to a peak of 1646 nmol/L at 4 hours into the infusion.[38] Pyridoxal rose from 37 nmol/L to 2183 nmol/L in plasma and 5593 nmol/L in erythrocytes, with peak levels achieved at the end of the infusion.[38] Oral pyridoxine in doses of 600 mg is 50% absorbed within 20 minutes by a first-order process.[37] Peak plasma concentrations of pyridoxine, PLP, and pyridoxal were 25,053, 945, and 8682 nmol/L at 1.3, 2.3, and 3.3 hours, respectively, following the oral ingestion of 600 mg of pyridoxine.[37] The concentration of PLP appears to be tightly controlled in the plasma and related to alkaline phosphatase activity. Oral doses of pyridoxine from 10–800 mg result in PLP concentrations of 518–732 nmol/L 4 hours after ingestion.[37] Chronic alcoholics have lower baseline PLP plasma levels, as acetaldehyde enhances the degradation of PLP in erythrocytes through stimulation of an erythrocyte membrane-bound phosphatase that hydrolyzes phosphate-containing B_6 compounds.[21]

MECHANISM OF HYDRAZIDE- AND HYDRAZINE-INDUCED SEIZURES

The antidotal role of pyridoxine in the management of isonicotinic acid hydrazide (isoniazid; INH) and monomethylhydrazine (MMH) poisoning is based on these drugs' interference with the normal utilization and function of pyridoxine as a coenzyme. INH produces a syndrome resembling cerebral vitamin B_6 deficiency, which results in seizures. Specifically, INH and other hydrazides and hydrazines inhibit the enzyme pyridoxine phosphokinase that converts pyridoxine to its active form, PLP.[17] In addition, hydrazides directly combine with PLP, causing inactivation through the production of hydrazones that are rapidly excreted by the kidney.[17] PLP is a coenzyme for L-glutamic acid decarboxylase that permits the synthesis of GABA from L-glutamic acid. Animal studies suggest that the interference with PLP by INH disrupts the formation of GABA, an inhibitory neurotransmitter.[17,35] The decreased GABA formation may reduce the cerebral inhibition, which may contribute in part to the seizures resulting from INH and MMH exposure.[30]

ANIMAL STUDIES

In a dog model of INH-induced toxicity, pyridoxine reduced the severity of seizures and the time to seizure and prevented the mortality of a previously lethal dose of INH in a dose-dependent fashion.[9,10] Lower molar ratios prevented deaths and higher molar ratios prevented deaths and seizures.[10] When used as single agents phenobarbital, pentobarbital, phenytoin, ethanol, and diazepam were ineffective in controlling seizures and mortality, but when combined with pyridoxine each one protected the animals from seizures and death.[9] These same authors were unable to demonstrate a benefit with pyridoxine in a rat model, apparently because of dosing constraints.[10] Small-animal experiments have documented the effectiveness of pyridoxine against MMH-induced seizures when used alone[17] or in combination with diazepam.[14] Anticonvulsant efficacy has also been noted in cat[29] and monkey[31] models.

Rat studies with 1,1-dimethylhydrazine (UDMH) given IP also demonstrate the protective effects of pyridoxine given IP 90 minutes later.[11] Doses of 10, 20, or 50 mg/kg of pyridoxine prevented seizures and death secondary to 20 mg/kg compared to 94% mortality and 100% seizing without pyridoxine.[11] When rats were administered 100 mg/kg IP UDMH and 15 mg/kg pyridoxine IV 20 minutes later, 17% died at 24 hours, as compared to a 100% mortality without pyridoxine.[11] A higher dose of pyridoxine would probably have been completely protective.

HUMAN DATA

Clinical experience with the use of pyridoxine for INH overdose in humans demonstrates favorable results.[2,8] Rapid seizure control with no morbidity or mortality was achieved when the ratio in grams of pyridoxine administered to INH ingested ranged from 0.14 to 1.3, although in practice, most patients receive approximately gram-for-gram amounts. In 5 patients, the use of gram-for-gram amounts of pyridoxine resulted in the complete control of seizures and a resolution of the metabolic acidosis.[34] In 8 patients with intentional INH overdoses, basic poison management, intensive supportive care, and a mean dose of 5 g of pyridoxine IV resulted in no fatalities.[5] Seizures were controlled in a 22-month-old boy given 100 mg of IV pyridoxine, after an estimated INH ingestion of 5 g,[30] although variable results are reported when relatively small doses of pyridoxine are used.[23] Seizure activity is reported in 2 patients following the ingestion of INH-pyridoxine combination tablets, although the actual amount of pyridoxine ingested was not noted.[32]

In addition to controlling seizures, the administration of pyridoxine also appears to restore consciousness. Two patients, who had experienced seizures after INH overdoses and were obtunded for as long as 72 hours after the apparent resolution of the seizures, were reported to awaken immediately after 3–10 g of IV pyridoxine was administered.[7] A third patient who was lethargic awakened with IV pyridoxine. This work suggests that mental status abnormalities associated with INH overdose, and conceivably hydrazine overdoses, may be responsive to pyridoxine and also may require repetitive dosing.[8,34] These papers indicate that patients treated with large doses of pyridoxine awaken more rapidly even after experiencing sustained seizure activity or status epilepticus.

MMH poisoning may be encountered in a variety of clinical situations. In the aerospace industry, where MMH is used as a rocket propellant, percutaneous or inhalational poisoning may occur. Ingestion of the false morel mushroom, *Gyromitra esculenta*, can theoretically also produce toxicity when its major toxic

compound, known as gyromitrin, a volatile, water-soluble toxin, is metabolized to MMH. *G. esculenta* is usually toxic if eaten raw (Chap. 76).

The neurologic effects of MMH poisoning are similar to those of INH toxicity and include seizures and respiratory failure, and severe liver damage similar to INH-induced hepatotoxicity is also described.[13] There is no evidence that MMH-induced hepatotoxicity can be treated by administration of pyridoxine.[6]

A patient who was exposed to hydrazine became comatose 14 hours later and remained comatose for 60 hours until 25 mg/kg of pyridoxine aroused him.[18] Another case report describes improvement in the mental status and supposedly the liver function tests of a confused, lethargic, and restless man who had ingested a mouthful of hydrazine and was treated with 10-g dose of pyridoxine.[16] This improvement developed over 24 hours and may have been unrelated to pyridoxine therapy. A severe sensory peripheral neuropathy lasting for 6 months developed 1 week following the overdose and was most likely due to the hydrazine ingestion and not the pyridoxine.

ETHYLENE GLYCOL

PLP is a cofactor in the conversion of glycolic acid to nonoxalate compounds (Chap. 66). Patients poisoned with ethylene glycol may receive 100 mg/d of pyridoxine IV in an attempt to shunt metabolism preferentially away from the production of oxalic acid. This approach was suggested by an animal model[3] and by the study of primary hyperoxaluria,[15] but has not been conclusively demonstrated in cases of human ethylene glycol poisoning.[25]

SAFETY ISSUES

Pyridoxine is clearly neurotoxic to animals and humans when administered chronically in supraphysiologic doses.[19,20] Delayed peripheral neurotoxicity occurred in patients taking large daily doses of 200 mg to 6 g of pyridoxine for 1 month.[24,27,28] Healthy volunteers administered 1 or 3 g/d developed a small- and large-fiber distal axonopathy with sensory findings and quantitative sensory threshold abnormalities occurring after 1.5 months in the high-dose and 4.5 months in the low-dose patients. Once symptoms occurred, the pyridoxine was immediately stopped, but symptoms progressed for 2–3 weeks, leading to speculation that it took time for the reversal of neuronal metabolic manifestations.[4]

Pyridoxine may also induce a sensory neuropathy when massive doses are administered either as a single dose or over several days.[1,20,33] Ataxia has occurred (with subsequent resolution) in dogs receiving 1 g/kg of pyridoxine.[33] Larger doses of pyridoxine produce incoordination, ataxia, seizures, and death.[33] Death after pyridoxine administration was sometimes delayed for 2–3 days.[33] Two patients treated with 2 g/kg of IV pyridoxine (132 and 183 g, respectively) over 3 days developed severe and crippling sensory neuropathies.[1] One year later, both patients were unable to walk. Inadequate information is available to determine the maximal single acute nontoxic dose in humans; however, there appears to be a wide margin of safety. Doses of pyridoxine ranging from 70 to 375 mg/kg or doses equivalent to the milligram-per-kilogram historical dose of ingested INH have been administered without adverse effects.[34]

DOSING

Considering all of the available data, a safe and effective pyridoxine regimen for INH overdoses in adults is 1 g of pyridoxine for each gram of INH ingested, to a maximum of 5 g or 70 mg/kg when the history is uncertain. Initial doses of pyridoxine in children probably should not exceed 70 mg/kg.[34] These doses are sufficient in the majority of patients. The best way to administer pyridoxine in a patient after an INH overdose has not been established. For a patient who is actively seizing, pyridoxine may be given by slow IV infusion at approximately 0.5 g/min until the seizures stop or the maximum dose has been reached. When the seizures stop, the remainder of the dose should be infused over 4–6 hours to maintain pyridoxine availability while the INH is being eliminated. The dose should be repeated if seizures persist or recur or if the patient exhibits mental status depression. In the event of inadequate availability of intravenous pyridoxine, pyridoxine should be administered orally.[26] For MMH poisoning, there is no established dose. Using the same dosage regimen as for INH is theoretically reasonable, but has never been tested in humans. A benzodiazepine should be used with pyridoxine in an attempt to achieve synergistic control of seizures. Pyridoxine should not be the sole agent used for INH or MMH poisoning. If the seizures do not respond to both of these measures, they can be repeated, followed by intravenous agents such as propofol, pentobarbital, or phenobarbital, and, if necessary, neuromuscular blockade and general anesthesia. When neuromuscular blockade is achieved without extinguishing the central nervous system (CNS) seizure activity, irreversible neuronal damage may result. Although metabolic acidosis is probably a result of the seizures and should therefore resolve once the underlying condition is controlled, severe or refractory metabolic acidosis may require appropriate quantities of sodium bicarbonate.

AVAILABILITY

Pyridoxine HCl is available parenterally at a concentration of 100 mg/mL in 1-mL ampules from various manufacturers.

REFERENCES

1. Albin R, Albers J, Greenberg H, et al: Acute sensory neuropathy-neuronopathy from pyridoxine overdose. Neurology 1987;37:1729–1732.
2. Alvarez EG, Guntupalli KK: Isoniazid overdose: Four case reports and review of the literature. Intensive Care Med 1995;21:641–644.
3. Beasley UR, Buck WB: Acute ethylene glycol toxicosis: A review. Vet Hum Toxicol 1980;22:255–263.
4. Berger AR, Schaumberg HH, Schroeder C, et al: Dose response, coasting, and differential fiber vulnerability in human toxic neuropathy: A prospective study of pyridoxine neurotoxicity. Neurology 1992;42:1367–1370.
5. Blanchard P, Yao J, McAlpine D, et al: Isoniazid overdose in the Cambodian population of Olmsted County, Minnesota. JAMA 1986; 256:3131–3133.
6. Braun R, Greeff U, Netter KJ: Liver injury by the false morel poison gyromitrin. Toxicology 1979;12:155–163.
7. Brent J, Vo N, Kulig K, Rumack BH: Reversal of prolonged isoniazid-induced coma by pyridoxine. Arch Intern Med 1990;150: 1751–1753.
8. Brown CV: Acute isoniazid poisoning. Am Rev Respir Dis 1972; 105:206–216.
9. Chin L, Sievers ML, Herrier RN, et al: Potentiation of pyridoxine by depressants and anticonvulsants in the treatment of acute isoniazid intoxication in dogs. Toxicol Appl Pharmacol 1981;58:504–509.
10. Chin L, Sievers ML, Laird HE, et al: Evaluation of diazepam and pyridoxine as antidotes to isoniazid intoxication in rats and dogs. Toxicol Appl Pharmacol 1978;45:713–722.
11. Cornish HH: The role of B6 in toxicity of hydrazines. Ann N Y Acad Sci 1969;166:136–145.
12. Dakshinamurti K, Paulose CS, Viswanathan M, et al: Neurobiology of pyridoxine. Ann N Y Acad Sci 1990;585:128–144.
13. Franke S, Freimuth U, List PH: Uber die Giftigkeit der fruhjahrslorchel Gyromitra (Helvella) esculenta. Fr Arch Toxicol 1967;22: 293–332.
14. George ME, Pinkerton MK, Bach KC: Therapeutics of monomethylhydrazine intoxication. Toxicol Appl Pharmacol 1982;63:201–208.
15. Gibbs DA, Watts RWE: The action of pyridoxine in primary hyperoxaluria. Clin Sci 1970;38:277–286.
16. Harati Y, Niakan E: Hydrazine toxicity, pyridoxine therapy and peripheral neuropathy. Ann Intern Med 1986;104:728–729.
17. Holtz P, Palm D: Pharmacological aspects of vitamin B6. Pharmacol Rev 1964;16:113–178.
18. Kirlin JK: Treatment of hydrazine induced coma with pyridoxine. N Engl J Med 1976;294:938–939.
19. Krinke G, Schaumberg IIH, Spencer PS, et al: Pyridoxine megavitaminosis produces degeneration of peripheral sensory neurons (sensory neuropathy) in the dog. Neurotox 1980;2:13–24.
20. Krinke G, Naylor DC, Skorpil V: Pyridoxine megavitaminosis: An analysis of the early changes induced with massive doses of vitamin B6 in rat primary sensory neurons. J Neuropath Exp Neurol 1985;44: 117–129.
21. Lumeng L, Li T: Vitamin B6 metabolism in chronic alcohol abuse. J Clin Invest 1974;53:693–704.
22. Marcus R, Coulston AM: Water-soluble vitamins. In: Hardman JG, Limbird LE, Molinoff PB, Ruddon RW, eds: Goodman and Gilman's The Pharmacological Basis of Therapeutics, 9th ed. New York, McGraw-Hill, 1996, pp. 1561–1563.
23. Miller J, Robinson A, Percy AK: Acute isoniazid poisoning in childhood. Am J Dis Child 1980;134:290–292.
24. Parry G, Bredesen D: Sensory neuropathy with low dose pyridoxine. Neurology 1985;35:1466–1468.
25. Parry MF, Wallach R: Ethylene glycol poisoning. Am J Med 1974; 57:143–150.
26. Scharman EJ, Rosencrance JG: Isoniazid toxicity: A survey of pyridoxine availability. Am J Emerg Med 1994;12:386–388.
27. Schaumburg H: Sensory neuropathy from pyridoxine abuse. N Engl J Med 1984;310:198.
28. Schaumburg H, Kaplan J, Windebank A, et al: Sensory neuropathy from pyridoxine abuse: A new megavitamin syndrome. N Engl J Med 1983;309:445–448.
29. Shouse MN: Acute effects of pyridoxine hydrochloride on monomethylhydrazine seizure latency and amygdaloid kindled seizure thresholds in cats. Exp Neurol 1982;75:79–88.
30. Starke H, Williams S: Acute poisoning from overdose of isoniazid: A case report. Lancet 1963;83:406–408.
31. Sterman MB, Kovalesky RA: Anticonvulsant effects of restraint and pyridoxine on hydrazine seizures in the monkey. Exp Neurol 1979; 65:78–86.
32. Terman DS, Teitelbaum DT: Isoniazid self-poisoning. Neurology 1970;20:299–304.
33. Unna IC: Studies of the toxicity and pharmacology of vitamin B6 (2-methyl, 3-hydroxy-4, 5-bis-pyridine). Pharmacol Exp Ther 1940; 70:400–407.
34. Wason S, Lacouture PG, Lovejoy FH: Single high-dose pyridoxine treatment for isoniazid overdose. JAMA 1981;246:1102–1104.

35. Wood JD, Peesker SJ: The effect on GABA metabolism of isonicotinic acid hydrazide and pyridoxine as a function of time after administration. J Neurochem 1972;19:1527–1537.

36. Wood JD, Peesker SJ: A correlation between changes in GABA metabolism and isonicotinic acid. Hydrazide-induced seizures. Brain Res 1972;45:489–498.

37. Zempleni J: Pharmacokinetics of vitamin B6 supplements in humans. J Am Coll Nutr 1995;14:579–586.

38. Zempleni J, Kubler W: The utilization of intravenously infused pyridoxine in humans. Clin Chim Acta 1994;229:27–36.

CHAPTER 44 ANTIMALARIAL AGENTS

G. Randall Bond

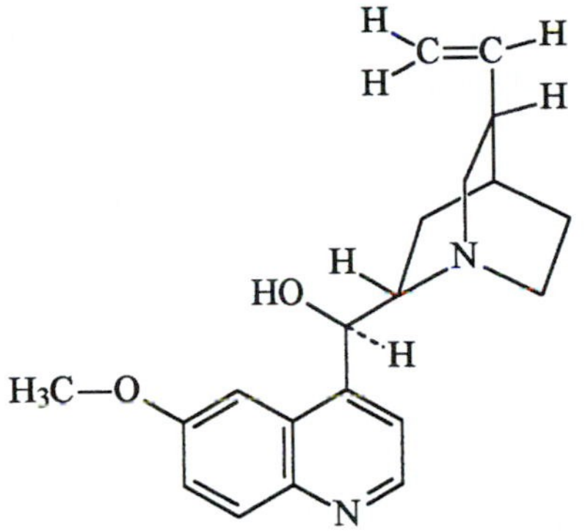

Quinine

Quinine

MW	=	324.41 daltons
Cinchonism	=	8–15 µg/mL
(serum levels)	=	24.7–46.02 µmol/L
Visual Toxicity		
Early	=	> 15 µg/mL
		> 46.2 µmol/L
Late	=	> 10 µg/mL
		> 30.8 µmol/L

Values greater than or equal to the action level necessitate clinical intervention. Values less than this level may necessitate intervention based on the clinical condition of the patient.

A 30-year-old man stumbled into Emergency Department (ED) appearing to be intoxicated and agitated. However, he was quite coherent. He complained of inability to see, difficulty in hearing, with a continuous ringing in his ears, and the sensation of "a train rushing through his head."

He stated that he had taken "a bunch of pills," drunk some wine, and went off to sleep about 7 hours before coming to the ED. On awakening approximately 6 hours later, he was unable to keep his balance.

His mother related an extensive family, medical, and social history: The patient was an asthmatic taking many drugs. In addition, he took "water pills," later identified as furosemide, to control hypertension. The patient, she said, took aspirin "for arthritis," and "some other pills for malaria." She insisted that he used no illicit drugs and seldom drank, but did smoke 2 packs of cigarettes per day. She further noted that he had been extremely depressed recently, after his loss of unemployment benefits. In addition, he had had a quarrel on the day of admission.

Physical examination revealed a well-developed, talkative, anxious man, with blood pressure, 100/40 mm Hg; pulse, 100 beats/min; respiration, 18 breaths/min; and temperature, 97.2°F (36.2°C). The skin was warm, dry, anicteric, and without pallor or cyanosis.

Ophthalmic examination revealed fixed, widely dilated pupils (OD 7 mm, OS 8 mm) unresponsive to light and accommodation. Assessment of visual acuity demonstrated some perception of distant shadows but no perception of close objects. The fundi were easily visualized. The optic discs were pale and flat. There was severe arteriolar constriction starting at the disc border with thread-like vessels. The veins appeared normal in diameter. The arteriovenous ratio was 1:7. Extraocular movements were intact.

Examination of the ears revealed normal tympanic membranes. The patient was able to hear a tuning fork on each side, but could not hear the ticking of a watch. The remainder of the examination was normal except for a systolic ejection murmur.

Blood samples were drawn and an electrocardiogram (ECG) was obtained. An IV line was established with 5% dextrose in water (D_5W), and 1 g/kg body weight of activated charcoal and 50 g of sorbitol were given orally.

The initial laboratory data revealed a hematocrit of 37.6%; hemoglobin, 12.1 g/dL; and white blood cell count (WBC), 8600/mm^3 with 80% polymorphonuclear cells, 18% lymphocytes, 1% monocytes, and 1% eosinophils. The platelet count and international normalized ratio (INR) were normal.

The electrolyte analysis revealed sodium, 143 mEq/L; potassium, 4.4 mEq/L; chloride, 106 mEq/L; bicarbonate, 29 mEq/L; blood urea nitrogen (BUN), 9 mg/dL; and glucose, 65 mg/dL. The creatine phosphokinase (10,250 IU/L), lactic dehydrogenase (700 IU/L), and aspartate aminotransferase (75 IU/L) were all elevated. The urinalysis was normal with a negative urine ferric chloride test for salicylates. The ECG showed a normal sinus rhythm at 96 beats/min, an axis of 90°, and inverted T waves in leads II, III, and aVF. Peaked T waves were present in V_2 to V_4. The QRS and QTc intervals were both normal. The chest radiograph was normal. The patient was admitted to the intensive care unit.

Without any additional specific therapy the ophthalmic and auditory symptoms rapidly abated. Ophthalmic findings returned to normal. The fundi showed normal vasculature and color within 24 hours. Blood pressure returned to normal by the second day. The abnormal auditory and visual findings entirely resolved within 48 hours. The patient's mother subsequently revealed that he had taken ten 300-mg quinine tablets, originally intended for the treatment of the *Plasmodium falciparum* malaria.

The malaria parasite has caused untold grief throughout human history. Today, 40% of humanity lives in areas of endemic malaria. One-half billion people suffer infection and 2 million die each year.[62] Included in those at risk are 50,000,000 travelers from industrialized countries who visit the developing world each year. In spite of prophylactic medications, 30,000 will acquire malaria (Table 44–1).[76] The battle against malaria and its vectors is also responsible for much of the DDT used in the developing world in the mid-20th century and currently (Chap. 89).

HISTORY AND EPIDEMIOLOGY

The bark of the cinchona tree, the first effective remedy for malaria, was introduced to Europeans more than 350 years ago.[86] The toxicity of the active ingredient, quinine, was noted from the beginning. In this century, the need to fight wars in malaria-infested areas and the toxicity of quinine led to pharmaceutical advances, funded by the military during WWII (chloroquine, proguanil, amodiaquine, pyrimethamine) and the Vietnam conflict (mefloquine, halofantrine).[86,87] Chloroquine, hydroxychloroquine, primaquine, amodiaquine, mefloquine, and halofantrine are related to quinine, but have different patterns of toxicity. Other agents include the folate inhibitors proguanil and pyrimethamine; which are frequently utilized in combination with the sulfonamide, sulfadoxine, or the sulfone, dapsone, and other antibiotics; such as the tetracyclines, clindamycin, and azithromycin (Chap. 46).

As each new agent has been introduced, resistance has developed, particularly in Oceania, Southeast Asia, and Africa.[86,87] In some places, quinine has again become the first-line therapy for severe malaria.[87] In the last two decades, the search for active agents has returned to a natural product, the Chinese herb qinghaosu.[49,93] Artemisinin, the active ingredient, is widely used in areas with multidrug-resistant malaria.[93] With increased leisure travel, a greater number of North Americans are taking ever more toxic prophylactic agents. Some return with unused medications.

Those who acquire malaria abroad may return with medications unavailable in the United States.

QUININE

In addition to its use as an antimalarial, quinine is also available in small amounts in tonic water. It has been used for muscle cramps and, because of its extremely bitter taste (like heroin), as an adulterant in drugs of abuse.

Pharmacokinetics and Toxicodynamics

Quinine is rapidly and relatively completely absorbed orally (Table 44–2). Peak plasma levels are achieved within 3 hours, and 85 to 95% of quinine is protein bound, primarily to human serum albumin and α_1 acid glycoprotein.[81,90] The apparent volume of distribution is 1.8 L/kg. Peak myocardial concentrations are achieved at 3 to 6 hours. The average therapeutic plasma half-life of quinine is 9 to 15 hours. In overdose, the elimination half-life is approximately 25 to 26 hours.[7] The liver, kidneys, and muscles metabolize 80% of the ingested dose. Approximately 20% is excreted unaltered in urine. Quinine passes transplacentally as well as via breast milk.

In pregnant women, high doses of cinchona alkaloids exhibit oxytocic activity that may induce abortion or premature labor. For this reason, despite its known dangers, quinine was once used commonly as an abortifacient (Chap. 30).[60]

Quinine and quinidine are optical isomers and share similar pharmacologic effects as antidysrhythmics and antimalarials. Because of the tissue toxicity of quinine, intravenous quinidine is used in the United States when a parenteral form is needed to treat severe or resistant malaria. Quinine has direct irritant properties on

TABLE 44–1.   Common Doses of Antimalarial Drugs Used Worldwide

Drug	Prophylactic Dose (Adult)	Upper Dose Range, Treatment (Adult)
Quinine sulfate	Not used	650 mg tid × 6–12 days
Chloroquine phosphate	500 mg/wk as single dose	1000 mg stat then 500 mg at 6 hours, 24 hours, and 48 hours
Hydroxychloroquine sulfate	400 mg/wk as single dose	Rarely used
Primaquine phosphate	30 mg/d × 14 days after leaving *P. vivax* or *P. ovale* area	15 mg/d × 14–21 days
Halofantrine	Not used	500 mg po q6h × 3 doses, repeat in 7 days
Mefloquine	250 mg/wk as single dose	750 mg stat, then 500 mg q6–8h × 3–5 days
Pyrimethamine/sulfadoxine	Not used	75 mg & 1500 mg as single dose
Pyrimethamine/dapsone*	12.5 mg & 100 mg/wk single dose	Rarely used
Artemisinin	Not used	25 mg/kg po on day 1 then 12.5 mg/kg on days 2** and 3
Artesunate	Not used	5 mg/kg po on day 1 then 2.5 mg/kg on days 2** and 3
Artemether	Not used	3.2 mg/kg IM on day 1 then 1.6 mg/kg/d until po treatment tolerated
Doxycycline	100 mg/d	100 mg bid^
Proguanil	100 mg once per day§	Rarely used
Atovaquone	250 mg once per day#	Rarely used

*with chloroquine; ** often with mefloquine 15 mg/kg; ^with quinine sulfate for chloroquine-resistant cases; §usually with chloroquine or atovaquone; #usually with proguanil.

TABLE 44–2. Pharmacokinetic Properties of Antimalarial Agents

	Quinine	Chloroquine	Mefloquine	Halofantrine	Pyrimethamine	Dapsone
Bioavailability (%)	76	80	>85	Low, varies	>95	90
Time to peak (oral)	1–3h	2–5h	3.8h	4–7h	2–6h	3–6h
Plasma bound (%)	93	50–65	98	—	87	70–80
Volume of distribution (L/kg)	1.8–4.6	>100	15–40	>100	3	0.5–1
Half-life	9–15h	40–55d	15–27d	1–5d	3–4d	21–30h
Urinary excretion (20%)	20	50	<1	—	16–32	20

For additional information, see references 15, 25, 37, 43, 45, 63, and 86.

the GI tract and stimulates the nausea center in the brainstem.[86] Much of the cardiac and endocrine toxicity of quinine can be attributed to its effect on sodium and potassium channels.

Pathophysiology

As with quinidine, the anti- and prodysrhythmic effects of quinine result from its inhibiting effect on two classes of cardiac ion channel—the sodium channel and various potassium channels (Chaps. 21 and 52).[29] With sodium channel blockade, the result is a negative inotropic effect, slowed rate of depolarization, slowed conduction, and increased action potential duration. Inhibition of the rapid inward sodium current is increased at higher heart rates, leading to rate-dependent widening of the QRS complex. Inhibition of the potassium channels results in suppression of the repolarizing delayed rectifier potassium current, particularly the rapidly activating component. This increase in the effective refractory period is rate dependent, with greater repolarization delay at slower heart rates. This repolarization delay predisposes to the unique ventricular tachycardia torsades de pointes. The result is risk for syncope and sudden death. In addition, syncope may be the result of vasodilation from the α-blocking effect of quinine.

The mechanism of quinine-induced inhibition of hearing appears to be multifactorial.[87] Microstructural lengthening of the outer hair cells of the cochlea and organ of Corti is noted.[2,32] Vasoconstriction and local prostaglandin inhibition within the organ of Corti may contribute to the inhibition of hearing.[87] Inhibition of the potassium channel may also be responsible for hearing loss and vertigo. Deafness associated with the long QT syndrome (Jervell and Lange-Nielson syndrome) is caused by the homozygous absence of gene products that form part of some potassium channels, including those in the inner ear (Chap. 28).[84]

Quinine also inhibits the ATP-sensitive potassium channels of the pancreatic β cells resulting in the release of insulin similar to the action of sulfonylureas (Chap. 40).[20] Mild hyperinsulinism may occur, but hypoglycemia is unusual following oral quinine overdose.[12,14,46,95] The significance of quinine-induced hyperinsulinism may be limited to patients receiving high-dose IV quinine and to those patients with other metabolic stresses such as concurrent malaria, malnutrition, or alcohol consumption.[14,46,66,67]

The ophthalmic toxicity of quinine is most likely a direct retinal toxic effect, and not the consequence of retinal vasospasm as was once postulated.[28,33] Electroretinographic studies demonstrate a rapid and direct effect on the retina (decreased potentials) within minutes after doses of quinine.[28] These early retinographic changes, as well as histologic lesions in photoreceptor and ganglion cell layers, provide evidence of direct damage.[28] Changes in

the electro-oculogram, suggesting changes in the retinal pigment epithelium, parallel changes in visual acuity. In contrast, no electrophysiologic, angiographic, or morphologic experimental evidence for retinal ischemia has been found.[28,33] Quinine may also antagonize cholinergic neurotransmission in the inner synaptic layer.

Clinical Manifestations

For quinine in particular, there is a small margin between therapeutic and toxic dosing. Patients receiving therapeutic doses often experience a syndrome known as "cinchonism." Common features include nausea, vomiting, decreased hearing acuity, tinnitus, and headache.[37,49,64] Tachycardia is often noted. Diarrhea and abdominal pain are less frequently observed. The skin may be warm and flushed. As serum concentrations rise, visual disturbances, including blindness, are common.[37,49,64] Patients experience vertigo, syncope, ventricular dysrhythmias (including torsades de pointes), and hypoglycemia.[37,49,64,86]

The average oral lethal dose of quinine is 8 g, although a dose as small as 1.5 g has been reported to cause death.[26,37] Delirium, coma, and seizures are also uncommon, usually occur only after severe overdoses, and may be associated with myocardial depression.[12]

Cardiovascular manifestations are related to myocardial drug levels and are similar to those of quinidine.[11] They manifest on the ECG as a prolonged PR interval, QRS complex, QT interval, and as ST depression with or without T-wave inversion.[11] Patients may develop complete heart block, markedly prolonged QRS complexes, or dysrhythmias.[11] Patients on high doses of quinine must be monitored for torsades de pointes, ventricular tachycardia, and ventricular fibrillation. Quinine toxicity can also result in significant hypotension, because of vasodilation and probably a concomitant decrease in myocardial contractility.

Ophthalmic presentations include blurred vision, visual field constriction, tunnel vision, diplopia, altered color perception, mydriasis, photophobia, scotomata, and sometimes complete blindness due to the direct toxicity.[12,22,28] Onset of blindness is invariably delayed and usually follows the onset of other manifestations by at least 6 hours. The pupillary dilation that occurs is usually nonreactive and correlates with the severity of visual loss. Vermiform motion or tonic pupil with denervation supersensitivity has been reported.[26] Funduscopic examination may be normal, but usually demonstrates extreme arteriolar constriction associated with optic disc and retinal edema. Normal arteriolar caliber may be present, but funduscopic manifestations such as vessel attenuation and disc pallor may develop as clinical improvement occurs.

Improvement in vision may occur rapidly, but is usually slow, occurring over a period of months after a severe exposure. Initially, improvement occurs centrally and is followed later by improvement in peripheral vision. The pupils may remain dilated even after return to normal vision.[26] Those with the greatest exposure may develop optic atrophy.

Eighth-nerve dysfunction results in tinnitus and deafness. This causes a rapid decrease in auditory acuity with a flattening of audiograms. The decreased acuity is not usually clinically apparent, although the patient recognizes tinnitus.[74] These findings usually resolve within 48–72 hours, and permanent hearing impairment is unlikely.

Although mild hyperinsulinemia may occur, hypoglycemia is rare following oral quinine overdose.[12,14,46,95] Hypoglycemia with elevated plasma insulin levels following therapeutic dosing has been noted in a patient with severe congestive heart failure,[46] and in a healthy patient who had consumed a large quantity of whiskey.[46] It also has occurred in a healthy patient following overdose.[92]

A number of hypersensitivity reactions are described. These are the result of antiquinine or antiquinine/hapten antibodies cross-reacting with a variety of membrane glycoproteins.[43,78] Asthma sometimes occurs. Dermatologic manifestations include photosensitivity dermatitis, lichen planus, and angioedema.[24] Hematologic manifestations of hypersensitivity are rare, but include thrombocytopenia (Chap. 25), agranulocytosis, microangiopathic hemolysis, and diffuse intravascular coagulation (DIC), which can lead to jaundice, hemoglobinuria, and renal failure.[43,78] Hepatitis is a rare hypersensitivity reaction.[23]

Hemolysis may also occur in those with glucose-6-phosphate dehydrogenase deficiency.

Diagnostic Testing

Urine thin-layer chromatography is sensitive enough to confirm the presence of quinine even following the ingestion of tonic water.[95] However, this test may have difficulty differentiating between quinine and quinidine if the latter is a clinical possibility.

Immunoassay techniques are the most reliable, but quantitative serum testing is not rapidly or widely available. Quinidine immunoassays cannot be substituted. In any case, no specific serum drug level determines a unique management intervention. However, plasma quinine concentrations are higher in individuals who develop severe toxicity, including blindness. If available, they can be used as a predictor of blindness.[7] After absorption and distribution, plasma quinine levels greater than 10 μg/mL are associated with temporary blindness, and levels of 15 μg/mL are associated with increased risk of permanent visual damage,[10] dysrhythmias, and death.[22,37] Similar levels in individuals who are severely ill with malaria do not result in as severe toxicity because of the increase in α_1-acid glycoprotein and consequent reduction in free fraction of quinine present.[77,81]

Management

Even if the patient has not already vomited on his or her own, emetic agents should not be used, as seizures, dysrhythmias, and hypotension may also develop rapidly. Because activated charcoal is so effective at adsorbing quinine, orogastric lavage should only be performed for patients with recent and substantial ingestions and no spontaneous emesis. Otherwise, standard overdose management is indicated, which includes activated charcoal (1 g/kg), catharsis, and supportive techniques such as oxygen, cardiac monitoring, an IV line with 0.9% sodium chloride, and dextrose support as needed. Because toxic manifestations are serum concentration dependent, measures to enhance elimination may be effective in preventing or reducing the toxic manifestations.

Cardiac. The cardiotoxic manifestations of quinine make the choice of serum alkalinization a logical therapeutic intervention. In a case report of a patient with quinine overdose, alkalinization with sodium bicarbonate was dramatically effective in narrowing the QRS complex, but torsades de pointes nevertheless ensued, perhaps because of hypokalemia combined with quinine-induced potassium channel blockade.[10] It was responsive only to an overdrive pacemaker.[10] Sodium bicarbonate should only be given if there is a clear indication. Prolonged QRS or heart block should be treated with sodium bicarbonate alkalinization to achieve a serum pH of 7.45–7.50, as would be done in the presence of a patient with a serious cyclic antidepressant overdose (Antidotes in Depth: Sodium Bicarbonate). Hypertonic sodium bicarbonate may result in hypokalemia, potentially exacerbating the effect of potassium channel blockade. The QTc should be carefully monitored for prolongation. Intervention for torsades de pointes, including magnesium administration, potassium supplementation, and overdrive pacing, may be necessary (Chap. 21).

Class IA, IC, or III antidysrhythmic agents, those with sodium channel and/or potassium channel blocking activity, should not be used to treat a quinine-, quinidine-, or chloroquine-overdosed patient because they may exacerbate the toxin-related conduction disturbances or dysrhythmias. Type IB agents may be useful (Chap. 21).

Extracorporeal membrane oxygenation (ECMO) was used in one case of severe quinidine poisoning with bradydysrhythmia and refractory hypotension.[85] It stabilized the cardiovascular system while a quinidine/charcoal bezoar was removed, and the patient metabolized the remaining quinidine. A similar approach should be considered for intractable quinine toxicity.

Ophthalmic. Funduscopic examination, visual field examination, and color testing may be appropriate bedside diagnostic studies. Electroretinography, electro-oculogram, visual-evoked potentials, and dark adaptation may be helpful in assessing the injury, but require equipment that is not portable. Because the mechanism of ocular toxicity is most likely caused by a directly acting retinal toxin and not by retinal artery vasospasm, techniques to improve retinal arterial flow, including stellate ganglion blockade and vasodilators, have not resulted in improvement. Hyperbaric oxygen (HBO) was used in 3 patients who recovered vision, but the role of HBO in that recovery was not established.[28,96] There is no specific, effective treatment for quinine retinal toxicity.[28,30]

Hypoglycemia. Significant quinine-induced hyperinsulinism is rare except in patients receiving high-dose IV quinine and those with other metabolic stresses such as concurrent malaria, malnutrition, or alcohol consumption.[14,46,66,67] Serum glucose should be supported with an adequate infusion of dextrose. Serum potassium and the QTc interval should be monitored during correction and maintenance. Diazoxide has not been helpful in raising serum glucose.[66] Octreotide, a somatostatin analogue that blocks insulin secretion, was used intravenously in a dose of 50 μg/h to correct quinine-induced hyperinsulinemia in adult malaria victims.[66,67] In volunteers, quinine-induced hyperinsulinemia was suppressed within 15 minutes following a 100-μg intramuscular dose of octreotide (Antidotes in Depth: Octreotide).[67]

Enhanced Elimination

The effect of multiple-dose activated charcoal (MDAC) on quinine elimination was studied in an experimental human model as well as in symptomatic patients.[48,69] In these patients, MDAC decreased quinine half-life from approximately 8 hours to about 4.5 hours, and increased clearance by 56%.[69] Numerous authors have shown that activated charcoal decreases quinine half-life.[7,48,69] It is unclear whether the reduction in half-life improves clinical outcome. Nevertheless, because ophthalmic, CNS, and cardiovascular toxicity are related to serum concentration, it is prudent to reduce levels as quickly as practicable. Activated charcoal should be administered every 2–4 hours.

There is conflicting evidence about a benefit of urinary acidification in enhancing clearance.[7,77] However, because of the increased potential for cardiotoxicity associated with acidification, this technique is not recommended. Forced diuresis is likewise unhelpful. In one study, the mean half-life of quinine in the forced acid diuresis group was 25.1 hours, as compared with 26.5 hours in the control group.[7]

Because quinine has a relatively large volume of distribution and is highly protein bound to plasma albumin and α_1-acid glycoprotein, peritoneal dialysis, hemoperfusion, hemodialysis, and exchange transfusion have a limited effect on drug removal.[7,12,53,59,77,86] Although the blood compartment can be cleared with the last three of these techniques, total body clearance is only marginally altered. After the rapid tissue distribution occurs, there is little impact on the total body burden because of the relatively large volume of distribution and the very extensive protein binding.

CHLOROQUINE, HYDROXYCHLOROQUINE, AND AMODIAQUINE

Chloroquine

The structurally related compounds chloroquine and amodiaquine were once used extensively for malaria prophylaxis. With growing resistance they are used in fewer regions. Amodiaquine is now rarely used because of a higher incidence of unacceptable side effects. Hydroxychloroquine is similar to chloroquine in therapeutic, pharmacokinetic, and toxicologic properties.[25,53] The side-effect profile is slightly different, favoring chloroquine for malarial pro-

phylaxis and hydroxychloroquine for use as an anti-inflammatory agent.[49,86]

Pharmacokinetics and Toxicodynamics

Chloroquine is rapidly and completely absorbed (Table 44–2). Chloroquine is highly bound to many different tissues, particularly kidney, liver, and lung.[32] Consequently, it has a very large apparent volume of distribution of 61 L/kg.[86] As such, serum values reflect a small part of total chloroquine load. Chloroquine is eliminated in the urine, up to 70% as the parent molecule and the remainder as metabolites.[45,53] An exceedingly long half-life averaging 41 days was reported.[53] Hydroxychloroquine has a similarly rapid absorption and a half-life of 40 days in routine use.[39] However, half-life in overdose is 15–30 hours.[39]

Pathophysiology

Like quinine, chloroquine has a small toxic-to-therapeutic margin. Severe chloroquine poisoning is usually associated with ingestions of 5 g or more, or with serum concentrations exceeding 5 μg/mL. The cardiovascular effects of chloroquine and hydroxychloroquine are similar to those of quinine, but other features, including cinchonism, are uncommon. These agents have low toxicity when used in therapeutic doses. Because of this, chloroquine remains the first-line drug for malaria prophylaxis and treatment in areas of *Plasmodium* sensitivity. Visual changes are not described with prophylactic doses but occur rarely with daily dosing of chloroquine or hydroxychloroquine for arthritis. The mechanism involves binding to melanin granules in the pigmented epithelial layer of the retina.[49] A related process with skin melanin is responsible for pruritus noted frequently in Africans (8–20%).[49]

Amodiaquine metabolism produces a quinone imine metabolite that can link with a hapten to induce a hypersensitivity reaction in some hosts.[14] This has led to reduced use as a prophylactic agent, particularly among Western travelers. Nonetheless, the drug is still used in some tropical countries for treatment of acute and chronic malaria.

Clinical Manifestations

Chloroquine is rapidly absorbed from the gastrointestinal (GI) tract. Symptoms are usually noted within 1–3 hours.[72] The range of symptoms associated with chloroquine toxicity is quite similar to quinine, but the frequencies of various manifestations differ. Nausea, vomiting, diarrhea, and abdominal pain are less common than with quinine.[37,49] Apnea, hypotension, and cardiovascular compromise can be precipitous.[37] The neurologic manifestations include CNS depression, dizziness, headache, and convulsions.[37] Electrocardiographic abnormalities include QRS prolongation, AV block, ST-T depression, increased U waves, and QT interval prolongation, but these are less frequent than with quinine.[37] Significant hypokalemia is invariably associated with the cardiac manifestations.[16,37] Hypokalemia results from direct chloroquine-induced intracellular shifts and is exacerbated by epinephrine therapy. Hypotension is a more prominent feature than with quinine.[37] Respiratory depression often occurs.

The ophthalmic manifestations are infrequent in acute toxicity, usually less consequential, and transient in nature.[37,49] More severe and irreversible vision and hearing changes are described in association with use of chloroquine and hydroxychloroquine as anti-inflammatory agents.[49] Myopathy, neuropathy, and cardiomyopathy are described in this context as well.[5,91] Dermatologic findings and hypersensitivity reactions similar to those associated with quinine are described.[21] Red blood cell (RBC) oxidant stress from chloroquine may result in hemolysis in patients with G6PD deficiency (Chap. 25).

Acute hydroxychloroquine toxicity is similar to chloroquine toxicity.[39,54] Side effects in routine dosing include nausea and abdominal pain, hemolysis in G6PD-deficient patients, and, rarely, retinal damage, sensineuronal deafness, and hypoglycemia.[9,38,80] Hypersensitivity reactions, including myocarditis and hepatitis, are described.[27,52]

One report of amodiaquine toxicity suggests that neurologic toxicity including involuntary movements, muscle stiffness, dysarthria, syncope, and seizures may occur.[37] Amodiaquine is associated with a hypersensitivity hepatitis and neutropenia in prophylactic use, but not therapeutic use.[14] There is no overdose experience reported.

Management

Early, aggressive management of severe chloroquine toxicity decreased the fatality rate in one study from 91% to 9%.[72] The protocol involves the use of epinephrine for chloroquine-related vasodilation and myocardial depression and diazepam for possible direct cardiovascular effect and for sedation to minimize CNS-based cardiac excitation.[73] The use of epinephrine and diazepam is reported to be successful in reversing severe cardiovascular toxicity.[8,34,39,56,94]

Patients should receive early endotracheal intubation and mechanical ventilation if warranted. An adequate FIO_2 tidal volume, and ventilatory rate should be assured. Orogastric lavage should be performed for patients evaluated with recent and substantial ingestions and no spontaneous emesis. Activated charcoal should be administered. During decontamination, 2 mg/kg of IV diazepam is given over 30 minutes and then 1–2 mg/kg/d for 2–4 days. Simultaneously, epinephrine (0.25 µg/kg/min) should be given IV with D_5W, adjusted incrementally until a systolic blood pressure over 100 mm Hg is achieved. Even after this initial therapy, some patients may manifest transient cardiovascular compromise and require additional epinephrine and other catecholamines.[72] Serum potassium levels should be monitored and potassium supplementation administered, but aggressive replacement therapy is not encouraged because hypokalemia represents intracellular shift, not total body potassium depletion.[16,37,39]

Because chloroquine has a high volume of distribution, significant protein binding, and a long terminal elimination half-life, enhanced elimination procedures have not been beneficial.

PRIMAQUINE

Pharmacokinetics and Toxicodynamics

Primaquine causes RBC oxidant stress. Subclinical methemoglobinemia is common. Methemoglobinemia and hemolysis can occur in normal individuals given high doses.[49] The primary toxicity of primaquine in therapeutic use has been hemolysis in G6PD-deficient individuals.[19] It is contraindicated in pregnant women because the fetal G6PD status is unknown. Reversible bone marrow suppression can occur.

Clinical Manifestations

Overdose with primaquine occurs rarely. Nausea, headache, and abdominal cramps are described. A case of extreme, iatrogenic overdose (1260 mg followed by 15 mg/d × 5 days) resulted in hallucinations, abdominal cramps, nausea, jaundice, hepatitis, and black urine.[47] Bilirubin peaked at 7.4 mg/dL. Aminotransferases peaked at AST 3309 IU/L and ALT 2654 IU/L. Renal function, hemoglobin, and white blood cell count were not reported. Resolution occurred over 1 month.

Management

In the event of overdose, therapy should be directed at minimizing absorption with appropriate decontamination, reversing significant methemoglobinemia with methylene blue (Chap. 94 and Antidotes in Depth: Methylene Blue), supporting adequate circulating red cell mass with transfusion if necessary, and preventing hemoglobin-induced renal injury by maintaining adequate urine output and alkalinizing the urine to a pH greater than 6 if necessary (Chap. 6 and Antidotes in Depth: Sodium Bicarbonate and Activated Charcoal).

MEFLOQUINE

Pharmacokinetics and Toxicodynamics

Mefloquine is slowly absorbed (Table 44–2).[79] Absorption is enhanced with food. There is extensive protein binding and a very large volume of distribution (22 L/kg).[43,79] Hepatic metabolism results in an inactive metabolite, with a terminal elimination half-life of 18 days, but significant interindividual variation occurs.[79] Because it has such a long half-life, it may take several weeks to achieve steady state, delaying the onset of toxic manifestations.

Clinical Manifestations

Common effects include nausea, vomiting, and diarrhea.[63] These effects are noted in patients, particularly children, with high therapeutic dosing, and are expected in acute overdose.[93]

Mefloquine has a mild cardiodepressant effect—less than that of quinine or quinidine. This has not been significant in prophylactic dosing or with therapeutic administration. With prophylactic use, neither the PR interval nor the QRS complex is prolonged, but the QT interval may be prolonged.[21,49] Clinically insignificant bradycardia is common.[49,63] Reports of torsades de pointes are rare, but the increase in QTc and risk of torsades de pointes are increased when mefloquine is used with quinine, chloroquine, or most particularly, with halofantrine.[49,62,63] Risk would also be increased with acute overdose. The long half-life of mefloquine, about 18 days, means that particular care must be taken with therapeutic use of these agents when breakthrough malaria occurs during mefloquine prophylaxis or within 28 days of mefloquine therapy. Given the lack of alternatives for severe malaria, quinine is often used.

During prophylactic use, many patients experience insomnia and an alteration in dreams and complain of dizziness, headache, and vertigo.[79] In only 2–10% of those experiencing these effects are they significant enough to cause the traveler to "feel sick" or to change normal activities.[36] Intolerance occurs more commonly in women.[6,65] Seizures occur very rarely in prophylaxis and therapeutic use.[68,75] In many of these cases, there is a history of previous seizures, seizures in a first-degree relative, or other risk factors. Other neuropsychiatric symptoms, including dysphoria, "clouded" consciousness, toxic encephalopathy, anxiety, depression, giddiness, and an agitated delirium with psychosis, comprise the bulk of serious adverse event reports. These effects may be related to the serum or CNS concentration. The frequency of hallucinations and delirium rises from about 1:10,000 with prophylaxis to as high as 1:250 with therapeutic dosing.[19] Because mefloquine has a very long half-life, the onset of CNS toxicity often begins after several weeks of prophylaxis as concentrations rise. Serious CNS symptoms may be delayed 2–3 weeks after treatment.[51,75] In at least one severe case, the neuropsychiatric manifestations of mefloquine were reversed with physostigmine, suggesting a central anticholinergic etiology.[83] Risk of CNS toxicity is increased by administration of quinine or chloroquine with or after mefloquine.

The effect of mefloquine on the pancreatic potassium channel is much less than that of quinine, resulting in only a mild increase in insulin secretion.[20,21] Symptomatic hypoglycemia has not been reported as an effect of mefloquine alone in healthy individuals, but has occurred with coadministration of alcohol and in a severely malnourished patient with AIDS.[4,21,49] In overdose, particularly with alcohol or recent starvation, this effect may be significant.

Two cases of prolonged, daily mefloquine overdosing (pharmacy error substituting mefloquine for terbinafine) are reported.[47] Symptoms included confusion, agitation, ataxia, dizziness, speech difficulties, and high-frequency hearing loss in one case, and nausea, fatigue, weakness, depression, disorientation, and paresthesia in the other. In the first case, resolution, except residual hearing loss occurred over 1 year. In the second case, symptoms persisted 1 year later.

In another case of a therapeutic error, a man took 5.25 g over 6 days.[13] Symptoms included weakness, myalgia, vertigo, visual accommodation difficulties, mild hypotension (90/50 mm Hg), tachycardia (120/min) with occasional ventricular premature complexes, minimal increase in liver function test, and prolonged INR. His symptoms resolved over 5 days except the weakness, which resolved over 2 months. The INR corrected over 2 weeks. In this case, cardiovascular symptoms were more significant than were neurologic symptoms.

Rare events reported with prophylaxis include urticaria, alopecia, erythema multiforme, toxic epidermal necrolysis, myalgias, mouth ulcers, neutropenia, and thrombocytopenia.[55,63,79] These are most likely hypersensitivity reactions. It is unclear which, if any, would be significant following an acute large dose ingestion.

Management

In overdose, supportive care is the primary therapy. Decontamination with activated charcoal is indicated if the patient presents soon after the ingestion. Specific monitoring for ECG abnormalities, hypoglycemia, and liver injury should occur. Patients should be followed for CNS and cranial nerve complications. Physostigmine may be considered if central anticholinergic syndrome is present (Chap. 35 and Antidotes in Depth: Physostigmine).[83]

In two renal-failure patients taking prophylactic mefloquine, hemodialysis did not remove mefloquine.[18] Given the large volume of distribution and high degree of protein binding of mefloquine, hemodialysis is unlikely to be effective.

HALOFANTRINE

Pharmacokinetics and Toxicodynamics

Halofantrine is slowly and incompletely absorbed (Table 44–2).[15,37] It is metabolized to an active metabolite, N-desbutylhalofantrine.[15] Its half-life is 1–6 days.[15,37] Prolongation of the QT interval is proportional to the dose and serum halofantrine concentration.[44,58,88] Fifty percent of children receiving a therapeutic course of halofantrine will have a QTc >440 msec.[82] Given the long half-life of mefloquine, a drug that also prolongs the QT interval, the use of halofantrine is contraindicated within 4 weeks of mefloquine use.

Clinical Manifestations

The primary toxicity in therapeutic and supertherapeutic doses is torsades de pointes and ventricular fibrillation associated with prolongation of the QTc.[17,31,62,88] Palpitations, hypotension, and syncope may occur. Because the QTc duration is related to serum concentration, dysrhythmias would be expected in overdose.[62] Dysrhythmias are also likely in the context of combined overdose or combined/serial therapeutic use with other drugs that cause QTc prolongation, particularly mefloquine.[44]

Other side effects, including nausea, vomiting, diarrhea, abdominal cramping, headache, and lightheadedness, which are frequently seen in therapeutic use, are expected in overdose.[49] Less frequently described side effects—pruritus, myalgias, and rigors—may occur. In a very few patients, seizures, minimal liver enzyme elevation, and hemolysis are described.[49,58,89] Whether these manifestations are related to halofantrine or to the underlying malaria is not clear.

Management

Management of halofantrine overdose should focus on decontamination as for quinine, supportive care, and monitoring for QTc prolongation and associated dysrhythmias. Treatment of prolonged QTc and torsades de pointes is discussed above under quinine (Chap. 21).

PROGUANIL, PYRIMETHAMINE, SULFADOXINE, AND DAPSONE

Pharmacokinetics and Toxicodynamics

These four agents all interfere with folate metabolism and are usually used in combination with each other. Proguanil (chlorguanide) may be used alone, but is often used with dapsone, chloroquine, or the antiparasitic atovaquone for prophylaxis. Pyrimethamine is used in combination with sulfadoxine (Fansidar) or with dapsone (Maloprim). Genetic polymorphism is described in the metabolism of proguanil and dapsone.[40,71] This may be the cause of the significant hypersensitivity reactions noted with dapsone.[71]

Clinical Manifestations

Information on proguanil overdose is limited. Proguanil's side effects during prophylaxis include nausea, diarrhea, and mouth ulcers.[49] Because of folate interference, megaloblastic anemia is a rare complication. Folate supplementation may be required in pregnancy and renal failure.[19] Rarely, neutropenia, thrombocytopenia, rash, and alopecia are also noted.[19] In a single case report, hypersensitivity hepatitis was described.[19]

Dapsone and the sulfonamides have a long history of causing idiosyncratic reactions including neutropenia, thrombocytopenia, eosinophilic pneumonia, aplastic anemia, neuropathy, and hepatitis.[49] The rare occurrence of life-threatening erythema multiforme major associated with pyrimethamine/sulfadoxine prophylaxis has limited the use of this combination for prophylaxis.

Acute ingestion of dapsone may result in nausea, vomiting, and abdominal pain.[37] Following overdose, dapsone produces RBC oxidant stress leading to methemoglobinemia and, to a much lesser extent, sulfhemoglobinemia (Chap. 94).[50] The onset may be both immediate and delayed hemolysis.[97] Other symptoms, particularly cardiac and neurologic symptoms, resulting from end-organ hypoxia, may occur.[37] In addition, in overdose, hepatitis and neuropathy are also described.

Overdose of pyrimethamine alone is rare. In children, it results in nausea, vomiting, rapid onset of seizures, fever, and tachycardia.[1,37] Blindness, deafness, and mental retardation have followed.[1,37] Chronic high-dose use may be associated with a megaloblastic anemia requiring folate replacement (Chap. 25 and Antidotes in Depth: Folic Acid and Leucovorin).[1]

Management

Folate supplementation should be considered after overdose of proguanil or pyrimethamine (Antidotes in Depth: Folic Acid and Leucovorin). Other efforts should include supportive care.

Following dapsone ingestion, significant methemoglobinemia should be treated with methylene blue (Chap. 94 and Antidotes in Depth: Methylene Blue). Sulfhemoglobinemia is irreversible, but constitutes an insignificant portion of total hemoglobin. Both hemodialysis and repeat dose activated charcoal are associated with enhanced elimination of dapsone during therapy.[61,97] Multidose activated charcoal is recommended in the treatment of dapsone overdose.[3] Required support may include RBC transfusion and urinary alkalinization if hemolysis is extensive (Antidotes in Depth: Sodium Bicarbonate).

ARTEMISININ DERIVATIVES: ARTEMETHER, ARTEETHER, AND ARTESUNATE

Artemisinin and its derivatives—artemether, arteether, and artesunate—come from the Chinese herb qinghaosu. They were introduced in the 1980s in China for the treatment of malaria. Millions of doses of artemisinin derivatives have been used in Asia and Africa.

Clinical Manifestations

Low-frequency side effects include nausea, vomiting, abdominal pain, diarrhea, and dizziness. In animals, damage to brainstem nuclei is consistently produced following prolonged, high-dose administration. Rare reports of CNS side effects during therapeutic use suggest the possibility of CNS depression, seizures, or cerebellar symptoms following intentional self-poisoning. In children with cerebral malaria, a higher incidence of seizures and a delay to recovery from coma were noted in a comparison with quinine.[11]

No neurologic difference was noted in long-term follow up. In an artemether/quinine comparative trial of adults with severe malaria, recovery from coma was also prolonged in the artemether group.[35] A small number (<1%) of patients receiving an artemisinin derivative in a third study experienced transient cerebellar signs.[57] Most recovered within days. One patient in that study and one in another report suffered prolonged symptoms—1 month and 4 months, respectively—but both ultimately recovered.[57,70] Attribution of these symptoms to artemisinin compounds as opposed to other drugs and malaria is debated.

In patients receiving serial ECGs, a small, but statistically significant fall in heart rate is noted coincident with peak drug levels.[57] In one therapeutic trial, 7% of adult patients receiving artemether had an asymptomatic QTc prolongation of at least 25%.[35]

Hypoglycemia and changes in the QRS have not been noted.

Management

Overdose patients should be managed with supportive measures and expectant observation including cardiovascular monitoring. CNS manifestations are the most likely.

SUMMARY

A variety of agents are used in the prevention and treatment of malaria. The optimal choices, and consequently the most widely available agents, are changing rapidly with shifting patterns of parasite resistance. Most of these agents have significant toxicity in acute overdose. Although many are related to quinine, even within this group, the pattern of predominant symptoms varies. Effects seen in the low doses associated with prophylaxis and therapy include nausea, vomiting, headache, and confusion. Autoimmune-mediated idiosyncratic reactions are described with most of the antimalarials. In overdose, cardiovascular, neurologic, and hematologic symptoms predominate. Dysrhythmias are the most life-threatening. They result from the sodium channel blockade effects, potassium channel blockade, and myocardial depression. Coma, seizures, and neurologic injury, especially to the special senses, occur. Primaquine and dapsone produce significant oxidant stress resulting in methemoglobinemia. Little is known of the acute toxicity of the newest agent, artemisinin.

Decontamination, including the administration of activated charcoal, is recommended. Agent-specific symptoms should be anticipated, and specific management strategies should be followed. These have resulted in improved outcome, particularly for chloroquine poisoning. Multidose activated charcoal is particularly important following quinine and dapsone ingestions.

REFERENCES

1. Akinyanju O, Goddell JC, Ahmed I: Pyrimethamine poisoning. Lancet 1973;4:147–148.
2. Alvan G, Karlsson KK, Villen T: Reversible hearing impairment related to quinine blood concentrations in guinea pigs. Life Sci 1989; 45:751–755.
3. American Academy of Clinical Toxicology, European Association of Poisons Centres and Clinical Toxicologists: Position statement and practice guidelines on the use of multi-dose activated charcoal in the treatment of acute poisoning. J Toxicol Clin Toxicol 1999;37: 731–751.

4. Assan R, Perronne C, Chotard L, et al: Mefloquine-associated hypoglycemia in a cachectic AIDS patient. Diabete Metab (Paris) 1995; 21:54–57.

5. Baguet JP, Tremel F, Fabre M: Chloroquine cardiomyopathy with conduction disorders. Heart 1999;81:221–223.

6. Barrett PJ, Emmins PD, Clarke PD, Bradley DJ: Comparison of adverse events associated with the use of mefloquine and combination chloroquine and proguanil as antimalarial prophylaxis: Postal and telephone survey of travelers. BMJ 1996;313:525–528.

7. Bateman DN, Blain PG, Woodhouse KW, et al: Pharmacokinetics and clinical toxicity of quinine overdose: Lack of efficacy of techniques intended to enhance elimination. Q J Med 1985;54:125–131.

8. Bauer P, Bruno M, Weber M, et al: Full recovery after a chloroquine suicide attempt. J Toxicol Clin Toxicol 1991;29:23–30.

9. Block JA: Hydroxychloroquine and retinal safety [commentary]. Lancet 1998;351:1388.

10. Bodenhamer JE, Smilkstein MJ: Delayed cardiotoxicity following quinine overdose: A case report. J Emerg Med 1993;11:279–285.

11. Boele van Hensbroek M, Onyiorah E, Jaffar E, et al: A trial of artemether or quinine in children with cerebral malaria. N Engl J Med 1996;335:65–75.

12. Boland ME, Roper SMB, Henry JA: Complications of quinine poisoning. Lancet 1985;384–385.

13. Bourgeade A, Tonin V, Keudjian F, et al: Intoxication accidentale a la mefloquine [letter]. Presse Medicale 1990;19:1903.

14. Breckenridge AM, Winstanley PA: Clinical pharmacology and malaria. Ann Trop Med Parasitol 1997;91:727–733.

15. Bryson HM, Goa KL: Halofantrine: A review of its antimalarial activity, pharmacokinetic properties and therapeutic potential. Drugs 1992; 43:236–258.

16. Clemessey JL, Favier C, Borron SW, et al: Hypokalemia related to acute chloroquine ingestion. Lancet 1995;346:877–880.

17. Costot A, Rapoport P, Le Coz P: Prolonged QT interval with halofantrine [letter]. Lancet 1993;341:1541.

18. Crevoisier C, Joseph I, Fischer M, Graf H: Influence of hemodialysis on plasma concentration-time profiles of mefloquine in two patients with end stage renal disease: A prophylactic drug monitoring study. Antimicrob Agents Chemother 1995;39:1892–1895.

19. Davis TME: Adverse effects of antimalarial prophylactic drugs: An important consideration in the risk-benefit equation. Ann Pharmacother 1998;22:1104–1106.

20. Davis TME: Antimalarial drugs and glucose metabolism. Br J Clin Pharmacol 1997;44:1–7.

21. Davis TME, Dembo LG, Kaye-Eddie SA, et al: Neurological, cardiovascular, and metabolic effects of mefloquine in healthy volunteers: A double-blind placebo controlled trial. Br J Clin Pharmacol 1996; 42:415–421.

22. Dyson EH, Proudfoot AT, Bateman DN: Quinine amblyopia: Is current management appropriate? J Toxicol Clin Toxicol 1985;23: 571–578.

23. Farver DK, Lavin MN: Quinine-induced hepatotoxicity. Ann Pharmacother 1999;33:32–34.

24. Freedberg IM, Eisen AZ, Wolff K, et al: Fitzpatrick's Dermatology in General Medicine, 5th ed. New York, McGraw-Hill, 1999.

25. Furst DE: Pharmacokinetics of hydroxychloroquine and chloroquine during treatment of rheumatic diseases. Lupus 1996;5:S11–S15.

26. Gangitano JL, Keltner JL: Abnormalities of the pupil and visual-evoked potential in quinine amblyopia. Am J Ophthalmol 1980;89: 425–430.

27. Getz MA, Subramian R, Logeman R, Bellantyne F: Acute necrotizing eosinophilic myocarditis as a manifestation of severe hypersensitivity myocarditis. Ann Intern Med 1991;115:201–202.

28. Grant WM, Schuman JS: Quinine Sulfate in Toxicology of the Eye, Volume II: Effects on the Eyes and Visual System from Chemicals, Drugs, Metals and Minerals, Plants, Toxins and Venoms, 4th ed. Springfield, IL, Charles C. Thomas, 1993, pp. 1225–1233.

29. Grace AA, Camm AJ: Quinidine. N Engl J Med 1998; 338:35–45.

30. Guly U, Driscoll P: The management of quinine induced blindness. Arch Emerg Med 1992;9:317–322.

31. Gundersen SG, Rostrup M, von der Lippe E, et al: Halofantrine-associated ventricular fibrillation in a young woman with no predisposing QTc prolongation. Scand J Infect Dis 1997;29:207–208.

32. Gustafsson LI, Walker O, Alvan G, et al: Disposition of chloroquine in man after single intravenous and oral doses. Br J Clin Pharmacol 1983;15:471–479.

33. Hall A, Williams S, Rajkumar K, Galloway R: Quinine-induced blindness. Br J Ophthalmol 1997;81:1–4.

34. Havens PL, Splaingard ML, Bousounis D, et al: Survival after chloroquine ingestion in a child. J Toxicol Clin Toxicol 1988;26: 381–388.

35. Hein TT, Day NPJ, Phu NH, et al: A controlled trial of artemether or quinine in Vietnamese adults with severe falciparum malaria. N Engl J Med 1996;335:76–83.

36. Ingram RJH, Ellis-Pegler RB: Malaria, mefloquine and the mind. N Z Med J 1997;110:137–138.

37. Jaeger A, Sauder P, Kopferschmitt J, Flesch F: Clinical features and management of poisoning due to antimalarial drugs. Med Toxicol 1987;2:242–273.

38. Johansen PB, Gran JT: Ototoxicity due to hydroxychloroquine: Report of two cases. Exper Rheumatol 1998;16:472–474.

39. Jordan P, Brookes JG, Nickolic G, LeCouteur DG: Hydroxychloroquine overdose, toxicokinetics and management. J Toxicol Clin Toxicol 1999;37:861–864.

40. Kaneko A, Bergqvist Y, Taleo G, et al: Proguanil disposition and toxicity in malaria patients from Vanuatu with high frequencies of CYP2C19 mutations. Pharmacogenetics 1999;9:317–326.

41. Karlsson KK, Flock A: Quinine causes isolated outer hair cells to change length. Neurosci Lett 1990;116:101–105.

42. Kedia RK, Wright AJ: Quinine-mediated disseminated intravascular coagulation. Postgrad Med J 1999;75:429–430.

43. Karbwang J, White NJ: Clinical pharmacokinetics of mefloquine. Clin Pharmacokinet 1990;19:264–279.

44. Karbwang J, Na Bangchang K, Bunnag D, et al: Cardiac effect of halofantrine [letter]. Lancet 1993;342:501.

45. Krishna S, White NJ: Pharmacokinetics of quinine, chloroquine and amodiaquine: Clinical implications. Clin Pharmacokinet 1996;30: 263–299.

46. Limburg PJ. Katz H, Grant CS, Service FJ: Quinine-induced hypoglycemia. Ann Intern Med 1993;119:218–219.

47. Lobel Ho, Coyne PE, Rosenthal PJ: Drug overdoses with antimalarial agents: Prescribing and dispensing errors [letter]. JAMA 1998;280: 1483.

48. Lockey D, Bateman DN: Effect of oral activated charcoal on quinine elimination. Br J Clin Pharmacol 1989;27:92–94.

49. Luzzi GA, Peto TWA: Adverse effects of antimalarials. Drug Saf 1993;8:295–311.

50. MacDonald RD, McGuigan MA: Acute dapsone intoxication: A pediatric case report. Pediatr Emerg Care 1997;13:127–129.

51. Mai N, Day N, Van Chuong L, et al: Post-malaria neurological syndrome. Lancet 1996;348:917–921.

52. Makin AJ, Wendon J, Fitt S, et al: Fulminant hepatic failure secondary to hydroxychloroquine. Gut 1994;35:569–571.

53. Markham TN, Dodson VN, Eckberg DL: Peritoneal dialysis in quinine sulfate intoxication. JAMA 1967;202:1102–1103.

54. Marquart K, Albertson T: A life-threatening hydroxychloroquine overdose [abstract]. J Toxicol Clin Toxicol 1999;37:630.

55. McBride SR, Lawrence CM, Pape SA, Reid CA: Fatal toxic epidermal necrolysis associated with mefloquine antimalarial prophylaxis. Lancet 1997;349:101.

56. Meeran K, Jacobs MG, Scott J, et al: Chloroquine poisoning. Rapidly fatal without treatment. BMJ 1993;307:49–50.

57. Miller LG, Panosian CB: Ataxia and slurred speech after artesunate treatment for falciparum malaria [letter]. N Engl J Med 1997;336: 1328.

58. Monlun E, Le Metayer P, Szwandt S, et al: Cardiac complications of halofantrine: A prospective study of 20 patients. Trans R Soc Trop Med Hyg 1995;89:430–433.

59. Morgan MD, Rainford DJ, Pusey CD, et al: The treatment of quinine poisoning with charcoal hemoperfusion. Postgrad Med J 1983;59:365–367.

60. Netland K, Martinez J: Abortifacients: Toxidromes, ancient to modern—A case series and review of the literature. Acad Emerg Med 2000;7:824–829.

61. Neuvonen PJ, Elonen E, Haapenen EJ: Acute dapsone poisoning: Clinical findings and effect of oral activated charcoal and haemodialysis on dapsone elimination. Acta Med Scand 1983;214:215–220.

62. Nosten F, ter Kuile FO, Luxemburger C, et al: Cardiac effects of antimalarial treatment with halofantrine. Lancet 1993;341:1054–1056.

63. Nosten F, Price RN: New antimalarials: A risk-benefit analysis. Drug Saf 1995;12:264–272.

64. Okitolonda W, Delacollette C, Malengreau M, Henquin JC: High incidence of hypoglycemia in African patients treated with intravenous quinine for severe malaria. Br Med J 1987;295:716–718.

65. Phillips M: Women may be more susceptible to adverse effects [letter]. BMJ 1996;313:1552–1553.

66. Phillips RE, Looareesuwan S, Bloom SR, et al: Effectiveness of SMS 201–995, a synthetic long-acting somatostatin analogue, in treatment of quinine-induced hyperinsulinemia. Lancet 1986;i:713–716.

67. Phillips RE, Looareesuwan S, Molyneux ME, et al: Hypoglycemia and counterregulatory hormone responses in severe falciparum malaria: Treatment with Sandostatin. Q J Med 1993;86:233–240.

68. Pous E, Gascon J, Obach J, Corachan M: Mefloquine-induced grand mal seizure during malaria chemoprophylaxis in a non-epileptic subject. Trans R Soc Trop Med Hyg 1995;89:434.

69. Prescott LF, Hamilton AR, Heyworth R: Treatment of quinine overdose with repeated oral charcoal. Br J Clin Pharmacol 1989;27:95–97.

70. Price R, van Vugt M, Phaipun L, et al: Adverse effects in patients with acute falciparum malaria treated with artemisinin derivatives. Am J Trop Med Hyg 1999;60:547–555.

71. Reilly TP, Woster PM, Swensson CK: Methemoglobin formation by hydroxylamine metabolites of sulfamethoxazole and dapsone: Implications for differences in adverse drug reactions. J Pharmacol Exper Therap 1999;288:951–959.

72. Riou B, Barriot P, Rimailho A, Baud FJ: Treatment of severe chloroquine poisoning. N Engl J Med 1988;318:1–7.

73. Riou B, Rimailho A, Galliot M, et al: Protective cardiovascular effects of diazepam in experimental acute chloroquine poisoning. Intensive Care Med 1988;14:610–616.

74. Roche RJ, Silamut K, Pukrittayakamee S, et al: Quinine induces reversible high tone hearing loss. Br J Clin Pharmacol 1990;29:780–782.

75. Rouviex B, Bricaire F, Michon C, et al: Mefloquine and an acute brain syndrome. Ann Intern Med 1989;110:577–578.

76. Ryan ET, Kain KC: Health advice and immunizations for travelers. N Engl J Med 2000;342:1716–1725.

77. Sabto J, Pierce RM, West RH, Gurr FW: Haemodialysis, peritoneal dialysis, plasmapheresis and forced diuresis for the treatment of quinine overdose. Clin Nephrol 1981;16:264–268.

78. Schattner A: Quinine hypersensitivity simulating sepsis. Am J Med 1998;104:488–490.

79. Schlagenhauf P: Mefloquine for malaria prophylaxis: A review. J Travel Med 1999;6:122–133.

80. Shojania K, Koehler BE, Elliot T: Hypoglycemia induced by hydroxychloroquine in a Type II diabetic treated for polyarthritis. J Rheumatol 1999;26:195–196.

81. Sialmut K, Molunto P, Ho M, et al: α_1-Acid glycoprotein (orosomucoid) and plasma protein binding of quinine in falciparum malaria. Br J Clin Pharmacol 1991;32:311–315.

82. Sowunmi A, Fehintola FA, Ogundahansi AT, et al: Comparative cardiac effects of halofantrine and chloroquine plus chlorpheniramine in children with acute uncomplicated falciparum malaria. Trans R Soc Trop Med Hyg 1999;93:78–83.

83. Speich R, Haller A: Central anticholinergic syndrome with the antimalarial drug mefloquine. N Engl J Med 1994;331:57–58.

84. Splawski I, Timothy KW, Vincent GM, Atkinson DL, Keating MT: Molecular basis of the long-QT syndrome associated with deafness. N Engl J Med 1997;336:1562–1567.

85. Tecklenburg FW, Thomas NJ, Webb SA, Case C, Habib DM: Pediatric ECMO for severe quinidine cardiotoxicity. Pediatr Emerg Care 1997;13:111–113.

86. Tracy JW, Webster LT: Drugs used in the chemotherapy of protozoal infection: Malaria. In: Hardman JG, Limbird LE, Molinoff PB, et al, eds: Goodman and Gilman's The Pharmacological Basis of Therapeutics, 9th ed. New York, McGraw-Hill, 1996, pp. 965–985.

87. Tange RA: Ototoxicity. Adverse Drug React Toxicol Rev 1998;17:75–89.

88. Touze JE, Keundjian BA, Viguier PIA, et al: Electrocardiographic changes and halofantrine plasma level during acute falciparum malaria. Am J Trop Med Hyg 1996;54:225–228.

89. Vachon F, Fajac I, Gachot B, et al: Halofantrine and acute intravascular haemolysis. Lancet 1992;340:909–910.

90. Wanwimolruk S, Denton JR: Plasma protein binding of quinine: Binding to human serum albumin, α_1-acid glycoprotein and plasma from patients with malaria. J Pharm Pharmacol 1992;44:806–811.

91. Wasay M, Wolfe GI, Herrold JM, et al: Chloroquine myopathy and neuropathy with elevated CSF protein. Neurology 1998;51:1226–1227.

92. Wenstone R, Bell M, Mostafa SM: Fatal adult respiratory distress syndrome after quinine overdose [letter]. Lancet 1989;1:1143–1144.

93. White NJ: The treatment of malaria. N Engl J Med 1996;335:800–806.

94. Wilkinson R, Mahatane J, Wade P, Pasvol G: Chloroquine poisoning [letter]. BMJ 1993;307:504.

95. Wolf LR, Otten EJ, Spadafora MP: Cinchonism: Two case reports and review of acute quinine toxicity and treatment. J Emerg Med 1992;10:295–301.

96. Wolff RS, Wirtschafter D, Adkinson C: Ocular quinine toxicity treated with hyperbaric oxygen. Undersea Hyperb Med 1997;24:131–134.

97. Woodhouse KW, Henderson DB, Peaston RT, et al: Acute dapsone poisoning: Clinical features and pharmacokinetic studies. Hum Toxicol 1983;3:507–510.

CHAPTER 45   ANTIMIGRAINE AGENTS

Jason Chu / Neal A. Lewin

A 33-year-old man presented to the Emergency Department (ED) with substernal chest pain. His past medical history was remarkable for 2 weeks of daily headaches. He had visited his personal physician, who prescribed Fiorinal (caffeine 50 mg, aspirin 300 mg, and butalbital 50 mg) for migraine headaches. After failing a trial of Fiorinal, the patient was started on Cafergot (ergotamine tartrate 1 mg and caffeine 100 mg). He was specifically instructed to take no more than 6 Cafergot tablets per day and no more than 10 tablets per week. For the first 5 days he took 4 tablets each day, which relieved his headache. On day 6 he took 4 tablets in the morning, but the headache returned in the afternoon and he took an additional 10 tablets. A total of 34 tablets (34 mg of ergotamine) were consumed within 6 days. Within 10 minutes of taking the 10 tablets he noted tingling in his forehead and the onset of substernal pressure.

The emergency medical service was called within half an hour of the onset of his chest pain. The patient vomited once in the ambulance. On arrival in the ED he still had substernal pressure. His vital signs were blood pressure, 150/90 mm Hg; pulse, 100 beats/min; respirations, 20 breaths/min; and rectal temperature, 98.6°F (37°C). His head was without signs of trauma. His pupils were equal, round (at 3–4 mm), and reactive to light, and extraocular movements were intact. Funduscopic examination showed no evidence of increased intracranial pressure or hemorrhage. His neck was supple and there was no thyromegaly or carotid bruits. The chest was clear to auscultation and percussion. Heart sounds were normal. His abdomen was soft, nontender, and without organomegaly. Stool was negative for occult blood. Pulses were strong and symmetric, and there were no signs of clubbing, cyanosis, edema, or ulcerations on the extremities. There were no focal neurologic findings. One inch of 2% nitropaste (nitroglycerin paste) was immediately applied to the chest and an electrocardiogram (ECG) was performed, which showed ST segment elevations in precordial leads V_2 to V_5 interpreted as early repolarization abnormalities, with biphasic T waves in leads III and aVF (Fig. 45–1). Intravenous nitroglycerin was started and the pain resolved. Subsequent ECGs showed inversion of the T waves in leads III and aVF, consistent with inferior myocardial injury (Fig. 45–2). Cardiac isoenzymes were nondiagnostic. A cardiac pyrophosphate scan was consistent with anteroseptal and inferior myocardial infarction.

Migraine is a neurovascular disorder with multiple manifestations that include headache and neurologic symptoms. The International Headache Society has established diagnostic criteria for the various types of migraine.[22] The pathophysiology of migraines is complex and not fully understood, but it does involve activation of the trigeminovascular system. Current theories postulate that headache pain begins with cerebral blood vessel dilation and activation of trigeminal sensory neurons on the vessels. Pain impulses are relayed to the trigeminal nucleus in the lower brainstem and upper cervical spinal cord, then to the thalamus and higher cortical areas. Vasoactive neuropeptides are released and exacerbate the vasodilation and pain cycle. Calcitonin-gene-related peptide (CGRP) from trigeminal Aδ-fibers produces dural vasodilation, while substance P and neurokinin A from trigeminal C-fibers increase dural vessel permeability.[13,20] Headache therapy would ideally target these processes.

Treatment of migraines can be divided into avoidance of migraine triggers, prophylactic therapy, and acute management. Medications used include aspirin, acetaminophen, nonsteroidal anti-inflammatory drugs (NSAIDs), antiemetics, opioids, ergots, triptans, β-adrenergic antagonists, calcium channel blockers, anticonvulsants, serotonin reuptake inhibitors, monoamine oxidase inhibitors, and tricyclic antidepressants. Toxicity of all of these medications is discussed in depth elsewhere in the text. Ergots were formerly the mainstay of therapy for acute migraines, but with the advent of sumatriptan, the triptans rapidly replaced the ergots.

ERGOT ALKALOIDS

History and Epidemiology

Ergot is the product of *Claviceps purpurea*, a fungus that contaminates rye and other grains. The spores of the fungus are both windborne and transported by insects to young rye, where they germinate into hyphal filaments. When these spores germinate, they destroy the grain and harden into a curved body called the sclerotium, which is a major commercial source of ergot alkaloids.[46] This fungus can elaborate diverse substances, including ergotamine, histamine, tyramine, isomylamine, acetylcholine, and acetaldehyde.

In 600 BC, an Assyrian tablet made mention of contamination of grain believed to be *Claviceps purpurea*. In approximately 400 BC, contaminated grass that killed pregnant women was described. In the Middle Ages, epidemics causing gangrene of the extremities, with mummification of limbs, were depicted in the literature. The disease was called holy fire or St. Anthony's fire, because of the blackened limbs resembling the charring from fire and the burning sensation expressed by its victims. It is postulated that improvement occurred when victims went to visit the shrine of St. Anthony as a result of a diet free of contaminated grain.[21] Abortion and seizures were also reported with this poisoning. As early as 1582, midwives used ergot to assist in the childbirth process.

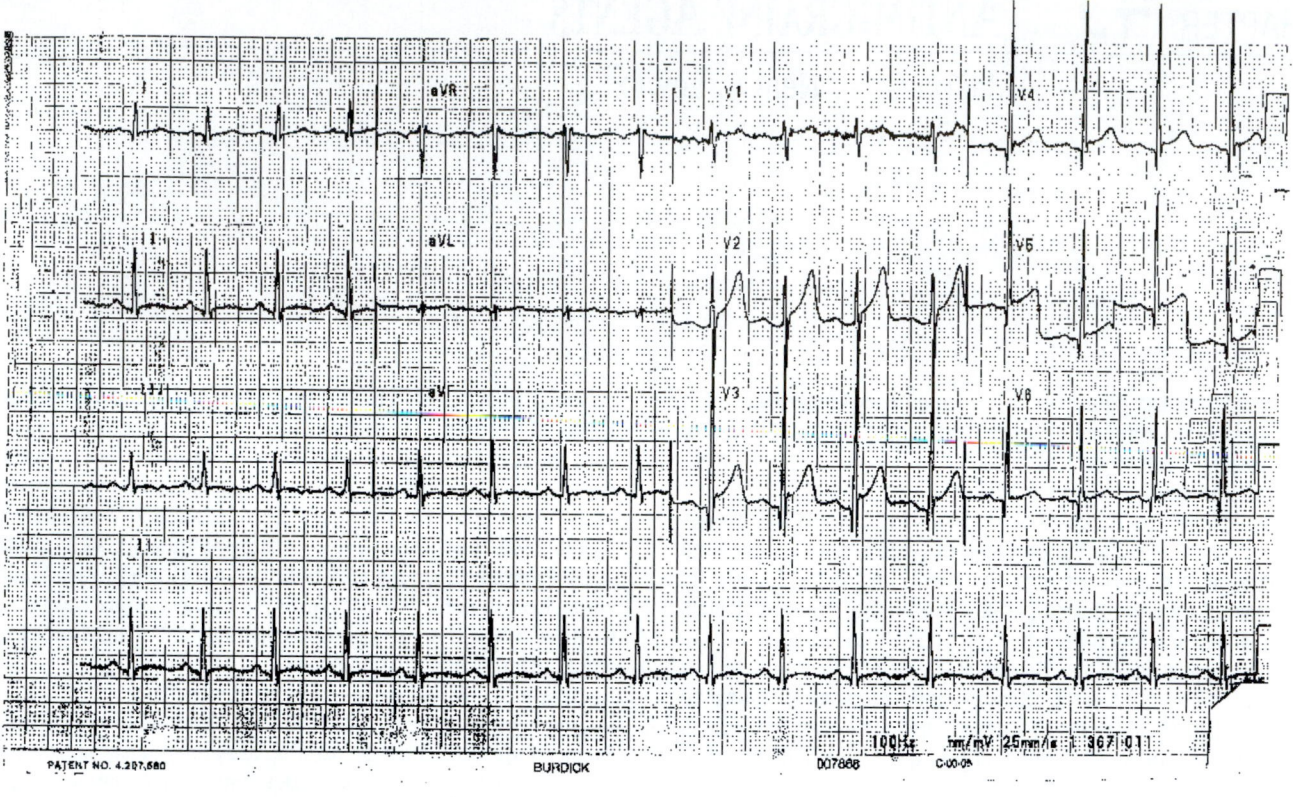

Figure 45–1. This 12-lead electrocardiogram (ECG) was obtained in the patient after the application of 2% nitropaste. The ECG shows ST segment elevation in the precordial leads (V_2 to V_5) interpreted as early repolarization, and biphasic T waves in leads III and aVF.

Desgranges was the first physician to use ergot for obstetric care in 1818. In 1824, Hosack reported that the ergot could be used for the control of postpartum hemorrhage, but that its routine use during labor was to be avoided because of the drug's toxicity.[46] Ergot's clinical use since 1950 has been almost entirely limited to the treatment of vascular headaches. Ergonovine, another ergot derivative, is used in obstetric care for its stimulant effect on uterine smooth muscle. It is also employed during cardiac catheterizations to induce coronary artery spasm and assist in the diagnosis of Prinzmetal angina. Methylergonovine is used for postpartum uterine atony and hemorrhage. Ergots have also been used as a putative cognition enhancer,[59] in the management of orthostatic hypotension,[55] and to prevent the secretion of prolactin.[48]

Presently, epidemics of ergotism in the United States are prevented by government inspections of grain fields. If a grain field contains more than 0.3% infected grain, it is rejected for commercial sale; there have been years in which as much as 36% of grain was rejected.[17] Ergot toxicity remains a problem elsewhere in the world, however, especially in animals.[29,45]

Pharmacology and Pharmacokinetics

The ergot alkaloids can be divided into three groups: amino acid alkaloids, dihydrogenated amino acid alkaloids, and amine alkaloids. All ergot alkaloids are derivatives of the tetracyclic compound 6-methylergoline (Fig. 45–3).

The amino acid alkaloid group, or ergopeptines, includes ergotamine, ergocristine, ergosine, ergocornine, and bromocriptine.

The dihydrogenated group includes dihydroergotamine, dihydroergocristine, dihydroergosine, and dihydroergocornine. The amine alkaloids include ergonovine, ergometrine, ergobasine, and methysergide. The pharmacokinetics of the ergot alkaloids are well defined from controlled human volunteer studies, whereas the toxicokinetics are unknown. Almost all of the ergots are poorly absorbed orally and there is considerable first-pass hepatic metabolism, resulting in highly variable bioavailability. Intramuscular absorption is unpredictable and actions are often delayed.[41] The effective oral dose is approximately 10 times the intramuscular dose.[41] Ergotamine suppositories increase bioavailability 20 times compared to orally administered doses.[25,52] Peak plasma levels with most ergot alkaloids occur within 30–120 minutes.[41] The volume of distribution is approximately 2 L/kg, and the half-life varies from 1.4–6.2 hours.

The pharmacologic effects of the ergot alkaloids are complex and can be mutually antagonistic.[46] The actions of the ergot alkaloids can be subdivided into central and peripheral effects. In the central nervous system (CNS), ergotamine is believed to have a sympatholytic effect, stimulating and potentiating serotonergic (tryptaminergic) receptors and interfering with neuronal serotonin reuptake (Table 45–1).[48] The ergot alkaloids interact with all known $5-HT_1$ and $5-HT_2$ receptors.[46] The result is increased intrasynaptic serotonin activity in the median raphe neurons of the brainstem.[49] Because serotonin is an inhibitory CNS neurotransmitter, ergotamine is thought to decrease the neuronal firing rate and stabilize the cerebrovascular smooth musculature. The stabilization of the cerebrovascular beds by the ergot alkaloids makes

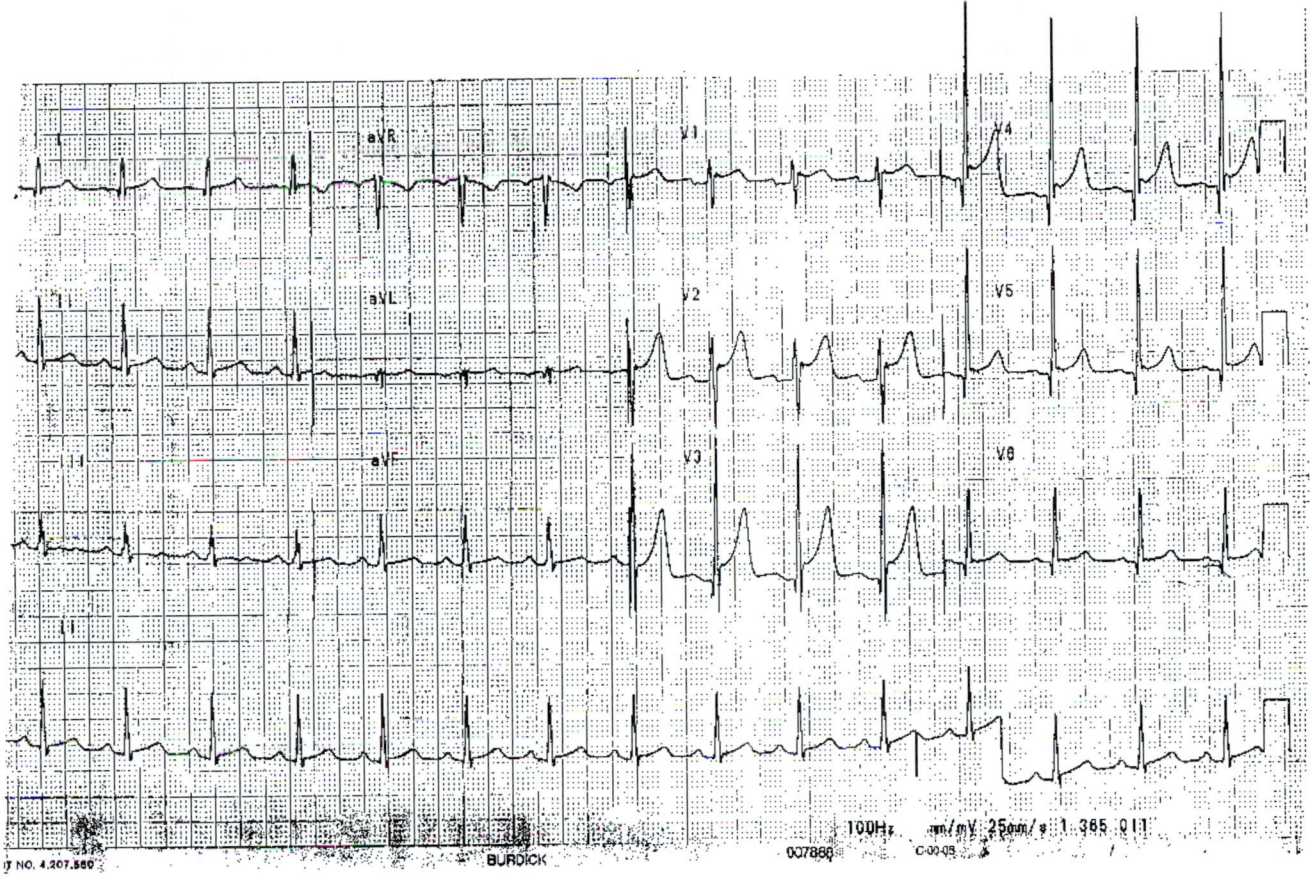

Figure 45–2. A subsequent 12-lead electrocardiogram (ECG) from the patient taken after the initiation of IV nitroglycerin therapy. The ECG now demonstrates and normalization of the T wave in aVF.

them useful drugs for the treatment of migraine headaches, which are characterized by cerebrovascular hyperreactivity.

Peripherally, ergotamine acts as a partial α-adrenergic agonist or as an antagonist at adrenergic, dopaminergic, and serotonergic (tryptaminergic) receptors.[46] Table 45–2 summarizes the pharmacologic actions of selected ergot alkaloids currently used in clinical medicine. The spectrum of effects depends on dosage, host response, and physiologic conditions. The usual clinical effect at therapeutic doses is vasoconstriction. There may be an additional vasoconstrictive effect caused by the direct action of ergotamine on the media of the arterioles.[48]

The difference between the effects of therapeutic and toxic doses, both peripherally and centrally, is that in the peripheral vessels, therapeutic doses of ergotamine produce mild vasoconstriction. The effect is directly dose related; therefore, at toxic doses, extreme vasoconstriction produces the characteristic ischemic changes that occur in ergotism.

The cerebrovascular effects of ergot alkaloids are not as clearly understood. In migraine treatment, for example, therapeutic doses of ergotamine produce a mild vasoconstriction via α-adrenergic agonism, especially in intracranial vessels that are already dilated during a migraine attack. This vasoconstriction is considered the basis for the ergot's ability to terminate a migraine headache. There is very little definitive information, however, regarding toxic doses of the ergot alkaloids on the cerebrovasculature.

Cephalic vasodilation may occur, but the mechanism for this effect is unknown. One hypothesis is that toxic doses of the drug initially produce vasoconstriction and ischemia, just as in the periphery, but as the cerebrovasculature cannot tolerate hypoxia and hypercapnia, rapid vasodilation then ensues to improve local perfusion. α-Adrenergic receptors in the CNS function differently from those in the periphery, and it may be that CNS vascular tone cannot be maintained in the setting of local tissue hypoxia.

Clinical Manifestations

Ergotism, a toxicologic syndrome resulting from excessive use of ergot alkaloids, is characterized by intense burning of the extremities, hemorrhagic vesiculations, pruritus, formications, nausea, vomiting, and gangrene (Table 45–1). Headache, fixed miosis, hallucinations, delirium, cerebrovascular ischemia, and convulsions are also associated with this condition, which has been called "convulsive" ergotism.[21] Chronic ergotism usually presents with peripheral ischemia of the lower extremities, although ischemia of cerebral, mesenteric, coronary, and renal vascular beds is well documented.[2,14,15,49,50]

Ergotaminism is a syndrome caused specifically by ergotamine use. Symptoms of vascular insufficiency such as cold extremities, extremity pain at rest, numbness, cyanosis, and intermittent claudication are most commonly reported.[21] Central nervous system

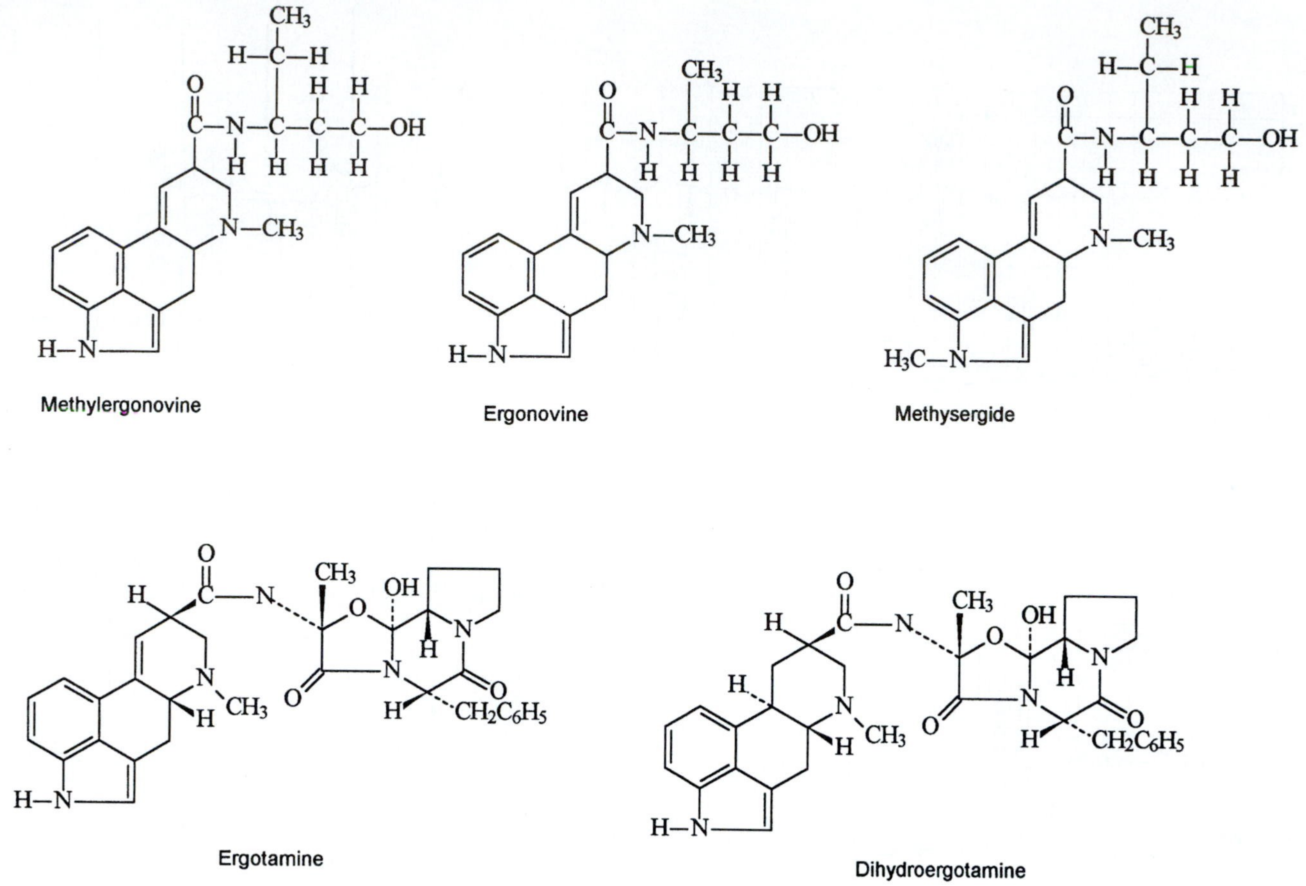

Figure 45–3. Chemical structures of ergot derivatives.

manifestations are rarely seen in ergotaminism. Many published cases describe ingestions of combination therapeutic preparations containing an ergot alkaloid and caffeine. In an acute overdose—although restlessness, nausea, vomiting, or agitation develop within 4 hours—peripheral vasospasm may not be obvious for 24 hours.

The toxic vascular effects ascribed to ergot alkaloids are complex and sometimes conflicting (Table 45–2). Subintimal and medial fibrosis, vasospasm, and arteriolar and venous thrombi (in general, stasis related) are all reported.[34] Angiography can demonstrate distal, segmental vessel spasm with increased collateralization in patients with chronic ergotism. The coronary, renal,

cerebral, ophthalmic, and mesenteric vasculature,[51] as well as the vessels of the extremities, may also be affected.[53] Neuropathic changes may be secondary to ischemia of the vasa nervorum injury.

Bradycardia is a characteristic effect of the ergot alkaloids. Bradycardia is believed to be a reflex baroreceptor–mediated phenomenon associated with vasoconstriction, but a reduction in sympathetic tone, direct myocardial depression, and increased vagal activity may also be factors.[46]

Myocardial valvular abnormalities are reported with ergot alkaloid use and abuse. Ergotamine and methysergide both cause mitral and aortic valve leaflet thickening and immobility resulting in valvular regurgitation.[16,50] This is similar to the valve abnormalities acquired following the use of fenfluramine, dexfenfluramine, and phentermine[7,60] (Chap. 38).

Methysergide, an amine alkaloid, has potent vasoconstrictive characteristics and is a serotonin antagonist that is used to prevent migraine headaches.[18] Methysergide use is limited because of its well-described adverse effects of retroperitoneal fibrosis,[50] as well as pleuropericardial, endocardial, and endovascular fibrosis.[40,50]

Treatment

The treatment for ergot alkaloid toxicity depends on the nature of the clinical findings (Table 45–3). Shortly after an acute oral overdose, if vomiting is not present, basic management should include

TABLE 45–1. Clinical Manifestations of Ergotism

Central Effects	Peripheral Effects
Agitation	Bradycardia
Cerebrovascular ischemia	
Hallucinations	**Ischemic Effects**
Headaches	Angina
Miosis (fixed)	Gangrene
Nausea	Hemorrhagic vesiculations and bullae
Seizures	Mesenteric infarction
Twitching (facial)	Myocardial infarction
Vomiting	Renal infarction

TABLE 45–2. **Ergotamine Compounds**

Compound	Interactions with Tryptaminergic (Serotonergic) Receptors	Interactions with Dopaminergic Receptors	Interactions with α-Adrenergic Receptors
Ergotamine (amino acid alkaloid)	Vasculature: Partial agonist Smooth muscles: Nonselective antagonist CNS: Poor agonist/antagonist	CNS: Emetic (potent)	Vasculature: Partial agonist/antagonist Smooth muscles: Partial agonist/antagonist CNS: Antagonist PNS: Antagonist
Bromocriptine (amino acid alkaloid)	Weak antagonist	CNS: Partial agonist/antagonist; inhibits prolactin secretion; emetic (mild)	Vasculature: Antagonist
Dihydroergotamine (dihydrogenated group)	Smooth muscles: Partial agonist/antagonist CNS: Agonist lateral geniculate nucleus	CNS: Emetic (mild) Sympathetic ganglia: Antagonism	Vasculature: Partial agonist: veins; antagonist: arteries Smooth muscles: Antagonism CNS/PNS: Antagonism
Ergonovine and methyl ergonovine (amine alkaloid)	Smooth muscles: Potent antagonist Vasculature: Agonist in umbilical and placental vessels CNS: Partial antagonist/agonist	CNS: Emesic (mild); inhibits prolactin (weak); partial agonist/antagonist Vasculature: Weak antagonist	Vasculature: Partial agonists
Methysergide (amine alkaloid)	Vasculature: Partial agonist CNS: Potent antagonist	None	None

Adapted, with permission, from Peroutka SJ: Drugs effective in the therapy of migraine. In: Hardman JG, Limbird LE, Molinoff PB, et al, eds: Goodman and Gilman's The Pharmacological Basis of Therapeutics, 9th ed. New York, McGraw-Hill, 1996, pp. 491–496.

multiple-dose activated charcoal with a single dose of sorbitol. If emesis is present, metoclopramide or 5-HT$_3$ antagonists, such as ondansetron, can be used as an antiemetic to facilitate the administration of activated charcoal. Ipecac-induced emesis or orogastric lavage should be used rarely, if at all, because vomiting is a common early occurrence of acute ergot alkaloid toxicity. In mild cases, characterized by minimal pain of the extremities, supportive measures such as hydration and analgesia are all that is needed. In more serious cases, severe peripheral vasoconstriction may produce ischemic changes including angina, myocardial infarction, cerebral ischemia, intermittent claudication, and mesenteric ischemia. Intravenous vasodilators, such as sodium nitroprusside,[2,4,39] nitroglycerin,[24] and phentolamine, are indicated to reverse the ischemia. Prazosin,[6] captopril,[61] and nifedipine[9] have also been used to achieve peripheral vasodilation, and may be ap-

TABLE 45–3. **Treatment of Ergotism**

Acute
  Basic Management
    Syrup of ipecac or orogastric lavage—often will not be necessary due to spontaneous emesis
    Multiple-dose activated charcoal and sorbitol or magnesium sulfate cathartic
  Advanced Management
    Hypertension or cerebral, mesenteric, or cardiac ischemia: IV nitroglycerin, nitroprusside, or phentolamine titrated to adequate blood pressure and perfusion
    Mild peripheral vascular ischemia with adequate perfusion: Oral prazosin, captopril, or nifedipine titrated to adequate perfusion
    Seizures and hallucinations: Diazepam, lorazepam titrated until seizures and hallucinations cease
    Hypercoagulable conditions: Heparin or dextran titrated until anticoagulated; thrombolytic therapy?
Chronic
  Withdraw drug
  Surgery if gangrene is advanced or to remove a clot

propriate with less severe vasospasm, manifested by dysesthesias and minimal ischemic pain of the digits, where immediate reversal may not yet be imperative.

Although sympathetic block, epidural block, or sympathectomy—all of which have been used in past—may relieve vasoconstriction mediated via the CNS, these modalities are not expected to antagonize the direct action of the ergot alkaloids on arteriolar smooth muscle.[2] Heparinization, corticosteroids, or low-molecular-weight dextran may be used to prevent sludging and subsequent clot formation. The use of thrombolytic agents in this setting has not been evaluated but may have some theoretical utility. Arteriotomy may be necessary to remove large clots. Hyperbaric oxygen may correct local tissue hypoxia.

SUMMARY

Although epidemic ergotism is no longer a concern in this country because testing of grain by the government exists, ergot poisoning both by unintentional and intentional ingestions continues to be reported. Knowledge of these agents' complex pharmacologic and physiologic actions and use of appropriate pharmacologic antidotes enable the clinician to minimize the morbidity and mortality previously associated with ergot alkaloids.

TRIPTANS

In the latter part of the 20th century, it was known that cerebral blood flow and serotonin abnormalities played a role in the pathogenesis of migraines. Based on this understanding, in 1974 investigation began on new compounds with vasoconstrictive effects via 5-HT receptors. The first compound found was 5-carboxamidotryptamine (5-CT). When applied to an isolated dog saphenous vein, 5-CT caused potent constriction and induced significant hypotension in vivo. The next compound developed, AH25086

[(3–2-aminoethyl)-*N*-methyl-1-H-indole-5-acetamide], also constricted dog saphenous veins but had more 5-HT receptor selectivity. It was effective against acute migraine in human volunteers, but further research was stopped because it was deemed less suitable for development in humans.[47] In 1984, sumatriptan was synthesized and its clinical success led to the rapid development of other triptans such as naratriptan, zolmitriptan, rizatriptan, and eletriptan (Fig. 45–4).

Pharmacology

The triptans are all primarily 5-HT$_{1B}$ and 5-HT$_{1D}$ receptor agonists and have less activity at 5-HT$_{1A}$ and 5-HT$_{1E}$ receptors[17] (Chap. 10). In the CNS, 5-HT$_{1B}$ receptors are located on cerebral vessels.[19] Stimulation of these receptors results in cerebral vasospasm.[10] This effect reverses the abnormal cerebral vasodilation and decreases the trigeminal sensory nerve activity associated with migraines. In contrast, the 5-HT$_{1D}$ receptors are located presynaptically on trigeminal neurons, and act as "autoreceptors" to decrease neurotransmitter release from central trigeminal nerve terminals.[27] The triptans also inhibit dural neurogenic inflamma-

tion by preventing the release of vasodilating neuropeptides from peripheral trigeminal nerves.[37,54] Peripherally, triptans cause vasospasm systemically through the 5-HT$_{1B}$ receptor.[12,31]

The available triptans have limited pharmacologic differences. Sumatriptan has an oral bioavailability of only 14% (range, 10–26%) because of extensive first-pass hepatic metabolism. Peak plasma levels are achieved by 1.5 hours (range, 0.5–4.5 hours).[17] An intranasal formulation is available, but the bioavailability is also only 17%.[52] Subcutaneous administration results in a much higher bioavailability (96%) and faster peak plasma levels at 10 minutes. Sumatriptan is, therefore, preferentially given by this route. The volume of distribution is 2.4–3.3 L/kg, and the half-life is approximately 2 hours. The newer triptans differ substantially from sumatriptan with regard to oral bioavailability—zolmitriptan, 40–49%; naratriptan, 63–74%; rizatriptan, 40–45%[11]—and with regard to their potency. All the triptans are hepatically metabolized.

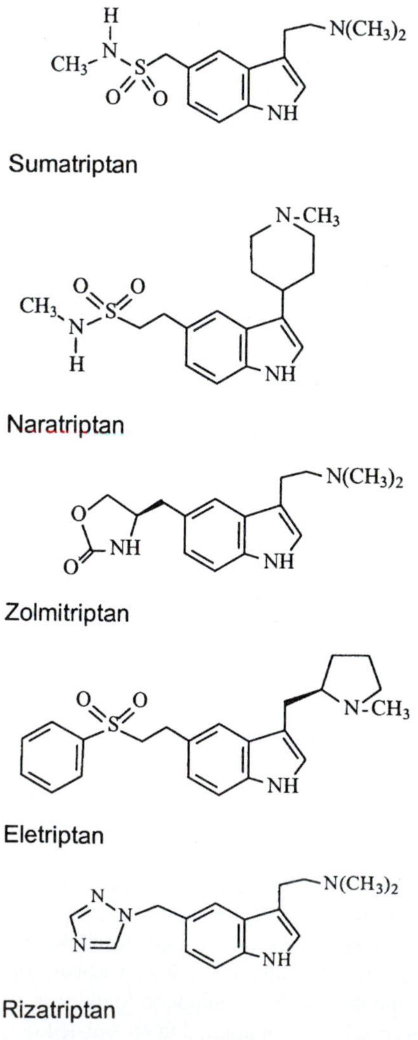

Clinical Manifestations

With appropriate therapeutic use, the adverse effects associated with the triptans are limited. The most common effects are nausea, vomiting, and taste disturbances followed by a feeling of heaviness or pressure in various body parts, warmth, and paresthesias.[11,46] The most consequential adverse effects are related to vasospasm. Chest pressure symptoms are reported in up to 15% of sumatriptan users.[3,42] Therapeutic sumatriptan use is also associated with myocardial infarction, dysrhythmias, and ischemic colitis.[1,8,28,33,36,38,43] Although cephalic vasospasm is the desired effect with sumatriptan, there are reports of adverse neurologic events ranging from transient hemiparesis to strokes and spinal cord infarction.[5,26,30,35,58] Although these complications have not been reported with the other triptans, they have only been recently become clinically available. All the triptans show some degree of coronary artery constriction in in vitro studies.[32,57]

Animal studies on acute toxicity showed a wide margin of safety with oral sumatriptan. Subcutaneous administration of 2 g/kg of sumatriptan to Sprague-Dawley rats was lethal. Death was preceded by erythema, inactivity, and tremor.[23] Dogs survived 20 mg/kg and 100 mg/kg subcutaneous doses, but developed hind limb paralysis, erythema, tremor, salivation, and loss of vocalization.[23] Reactions in other animals include convulsions, inactivity, reduced respiratory rate, cyanosis, ptosis, ataxia, mydriasis, salivation, and lacrimation.[23,56] Dogs given oral sumatriptan at 2 mg/kg developed corneal opacities and corneal epithelium defects.[44,56]

There are no published reports of human overdose with triptans. During clinical trials, a 33-year-old woman developed confusion, drowsiness, right-sided tingling, blurred vision, and possibly hallucinations after 600 mg of oral sumatriptan (approximately 30 times the usual therapeutic dose). She was treated with activated charcoal, sorbitol, and intravenous fluids, and recovered completely.[56]

Treatment

Treatment of triptan-induced vasospasm is dependent on the route of exposure and the organ system affected. Sumatriptan is marketed in oral, intranasal, and subcutaneous formulations. Decontamination is not feasible in subcutaneous exposures, but can be effective in oral overdose settings. The newer triptans are all oral preparations; therefore, basic GI decontamination should be performed with activated charcoal and a cathartic. Because vomiting

Figure 45–4. Chemical structures of the triptans.

is not as prominent with triptan exposure as with exposure to the ergot alkaloids, gastric emptying procedures such as ipecac and orogastric lavage may be considered early, but only following massive exposure.

In the setting of triptan-induced end-organ ischemia, intravenous vasodilators, such as sodium nitroprusside, nitroglycerin, or phentolamine, may be used. Prior cases of sumatriptan-associated myocardial infarction were treated with aspirin, heparinization, and intravenous nitroglycerin.[43] Thrombolytic therapy has not been investigated in this setting.

SUMMARY

The introduction of the triptans has decreased the use of ergot alkaloids for treatment of migraine. Triptan toxicity is presently infrequent, but has consequential complications. The clinician should be aware of the pharmacologic effects of these agents in order to anticipate and to minimize the adverse effects of exposure.

REFERENCES

1. Abbrescia VD, Pearlstein L, Kotler M: Sumatriptan-associated myocardial infarction: Report of a case with attention to potential risk factors. J Am Osteopath Assoc 1997;97:162–164.
2. Anderson PK, Christensen KN, Hole P, et al: Sodium nitroprusside and epidural blockage in treatment of ergotism. N Engl J Med 1977; 296:1271–1273.
3. Brown EG, Endersby CA, Smith RN, et al: The safety and tolerability of sumatriptan: An overview. Eur Neurol 1991;31:339–344.
4. Carliner NH, Denune DP, Finch CS, Goldberg LI: Sodium nitroprusside treatment of ergotamine-induced peripheral ischemia. JAMA 1974;227:308–309.
5. Cavazos JE, Caress JB, Chilukuri VR, et al: Sumatriptan-induced stroke in sagittal sinus thrombosis. Lancet 1994;343:1105–1106.
6. Cobaugh DS: Prazosin treatment of ergotamine induced peripheral ischemia. JAMA 1980;244:1360.
7. Connolly HM, Crary JL, McGoon MD, et al. Valvular heart disease associated with fenfluramine-phentermine. N Engl J Med 1997;337: 581–588.
8. Curtain T, Brooks AP, Roberts J: Cardiorespiratory distress after sumatriptan given by injection. BMJ 1992;305:713–714.
9. Dagher FJ, Paris SO: Severe unilateral ischemia of the lower extremity caused by ergotamine. Surgery 1985;97:369–373.
10. Dechant KL, Clissold SP: Sumatriptan: A review of its pharmacodynamic and pharmacokinetic properties, and therapeutic efficacy in the acute treatment of migraine and cluster headache. Drugs 1992;43:776–798.
11. Deleu D, Hanssens Y: Current and emerging second-generation triptans in acute migraine therapy: A comparative review. J Clin Pharmacol 2000;40:687–700.
12. Dixon RM, Meire HB, Evans, et al: Peripheral vascular effects and pharmacokinetics of the antimigraine compound, zolmitriptan, in combination with oral ergotamine in healthy volunteers. Cephalagia 1997;17:639–646.
13. Ferrari MD: Migraine. Lancet 1998;251:1043–1051.
14. Finchan RW, Perdue Z, Dunn VD: Bilateral focal cortical atrophy and chronic ergotamine abuse. Neurology 1985;35:720–722.
15. Fisher PE, Silk DBA, Menzies-Gow N, Dingle M: Ergotamine abuse and extra-hepatic portal hypertension. Postgrad Med J 1988;61: 461–463.
16. Flaherty KR, Bates JR: Mitral regurgitation caused by chronic ergotamine use. Am Heart J 1996;131:603–606.
17. Fowler PA, Lacey LF, Thomas M, et al: The clinical pharmacology, pharmacokinetics and metabolism of sumatriptan. Eur Neurol 1991; 31:291–294.
18. Graham JR: Methysergide for prevention of headache. N Engl J Med 1964;270:67–72.
19. Hamel E: The biology of serotonin receptors: Focus on migraine pathophysiology and treatment. Can J Neurol Sci 1999;26(Suppl 3): S2–S6.
20. Hargreaves RJ, Shepheard SL. Pathophysiology of migraine—New insights: Can J Neurol Sci 1999;26(Suppl 3):S12–S19.
21. Harrison TS: Ergotaminism. JACEP 1978;7:162–169.
22. Headache Classification Committee of the International Headache Society: Classification and diagnostic criteria for headache disorders, cranial neuralgias and facial pain. Cephalgia 1988;8(Suppl 7):1–96.
23. Humphrey PP, Feniuk W, Marriott AS, et al: Preclinical studies on the anti-migraine drug, sumatriptan. Eur Neurol 1991;31:282–290.
24. Husum B, Metz P, Rasmussen JP, et al: Nitroglycerin infusion for ergotism. Lancet 1979;2:794–795.
25. Ibraheem JJ, Paalzow L, Tfelt-Hansen P: Kinetics of ergotamine after intravenous and intramuscular administration of migraine sufferers. Eur J Clin Pharmacol 1982;23:235–240.
26. Jayamaha JEL, Street MK: Fatal cerebellar infarction in a migraine sufferer whilst receiving sumatriptan. Intensive Care Med 1995;21: 82–83.
27. Kaube H, Hoskin KL, Goadsby PJ: Inhibition by sumatriptan of central trigeminal neurons only after blood-brain barrier disruption. Br J Pharmacol 1993;109:788–792.
28. Knudsen JF, Friedman B, Chen M, et al: Ischemic colitis and sumatriptan use. Arch Intern Med 1998;158:1946–1948.
29. Lopez TA, Campero CM, Chayer R, et al: Ergotism and photosensitization in swine produced by the combined ingestion of Claviceps purpurea sclerotia and Ammi majus seeds. J Vet Diagn Invest 1997; 9:68–71.
30. Luman W, Gray RS: Adverse reactions associated with sumatriptan. Lancet 1993;341:1091–1092.
31. MacIntyre PD, Bhargava B, Hogg KJ, et al: Effect of subcutaneous sumatriptan, a selective 5-HT$_1$ agonist, on the systemic, pulmonary, and coronary circulation. Circulation 1993;87:401–405.
32. MaassenVanDenBrink A, Reekers M, Bax WA, et al: Coronary side-effect potential of current and prospective antimigraine drugs. Circulation 1998;98:25–30.
33. Main ML, Ramaswamy K, Andrews TC: Cardiac arrest and myocardial infarction immediately after sumatriptan injection. Ann Intern Med 1998;128:874.
34. Merhoff GC, Porter JM: Ergot intoxication: Historical review and description of unusual clinical manifestations. Ann Surg 1974;180: 733–779.
35. Meschia JF, Malkoff MD, Biller J: Reversible segmental cerebral arterial vasospasm and cerebral infarction: Possible association with excessive use of sumatriptan and Midrin. Arch Neurol 1998;55: 712–714.
36. Mueller L, Gallagher M, Ciervo CA: Vasospasm-induced myocardial infarction with sumatriptan. Headache 1996;36:329–331.
37. Moskowitz MA: Neurogenic versus vascular mechanisms of sumatriptan and ergot alkaloids in migraine. Trends Pharmacol Sci 1992; 13:307–312.
38. O'Conor P, Gladstone P: Oral sumatriptan associated transmural myocardial infarction. Neurology 1995;45:2274–2276.
39. O'Dell CW, Davis GB, Johnson AD, et al: Sodium nitroprusside in the treatment of ergotism. Radiology 1977;124:73–74.
40. Orlando RC, Moyer P, Barnett TB: Methysergide therapy and constrictive pericarditis. Ann Intern Med 1978;88:213–214.
41. Orton DA, Richardson RJ: Ergotamine absorption and toxicity. Postgrad Med J 1982;58:6–11.
42. Ottervanger JP, van Witsen TB, Valkenberg HA, et al: Postmarketing study of cardiovascular adverse reactions associated with sumatriptan. BMJ 1993;307:1185.

43. Ottervanger JP, Paalman HJA, Boxma GL, et al: Transmural myocardial infarction with sumatriptan. Lancet 1993;341:861–862.

44. Owen K, Hartley K, Tucker ML, et al: The preclinical toxicological evaluation of sumatriptan. Hum Exp Toxicol 1995;14:959–973.

45. Peet RL, McCarthy MR, Barbetti MJ: Hyperthermia and death in feedlot cattle associated with the ingestion of Claviceps purpurea. Aust Vet J 1991;68:121.

46. Peroutka SJ: Drugs effective in the therapy of migraine. In: Hardman JG, Limbird LE, Molinoff PB, et al, eds: Goodman and Gilman's The Pharmacological Basis of Therapeutics, 9th ed. New York, McGraw-Hill, 1996, pp. 491–496.

47. Peroutka SJ: Sumatriptan in acute migraine: Pharmacology and review of world experience. Headache 1990;(Suppl 2):554–559.

48. Graves CR: Agents that cause contraction or relaxation of the uterus. In: Hardman JG, Limbird LE, Molinoff PB, et al, eds: Goodman and Gilman's The Pharmacological Basis of Therapeutics, 9th ed. New York, McGraw-Hill, 1996, pp. 939–949.

49. Raskin N, Appenzeller O: Migraine pathogenesis. In: Raskin N, Appenzeller O, eds: Major Problems in Internal Medicine, vol. 19. Philadelphia, WB Saunders, 1980, pp. 84–104.

50. Redfield MM, Nicholson WJ, Edwards WD, Tajik AJ: Valve disease associated with ergot alkaloid use: Echocardiographic and pathologic correlations. Ann Intern Med 1992;117:50–52.

51. Rogers PA, Mansberger JA: Gastrointestinal vascular ischemia caused by ergotamine. South Med J 1989;82:1058–1059.

52. Sanders SW, Haering N, Mosberg H, Jaegger H: Pharmacokinetics of ergotamine in healthy volunteers following oral and rectal dosing. Eur J Clin Pharmacol 1986;30:331–334.

53. Senta HJ, Lieberman AN, Pinto R: Cerebral manifestations of ergotism: Report of a case and review of the literature. Stroke 1976;7: 88–92.

54. Shepheard SL, Williamson DJ, Beer MS, et al: Differential effects of 5-HT$_{1B/1D}$ receptor agonists on neurogenic dural plasma extravasation and vasodilation in anaesthetized rats. Neuropharmacology 1997;36: 525–533.

55. Stumpf JL, Mitrzyk B: Management of orthostatic hypotension. Am J Hosp Pharm 1994;51:618–660.

56. Sumatriptan: Product information and personal communication. Glaxo Wellcome, Inc.

57. Van den Broek RWM, MaassenVanDenBrink A, de Vries R, et al: Pharmacological analysis of contractile effects of eletriptan and sumatriptan on human isolated blood vessels. Eur J Pharmacol 2000;407: 165–173.

58. Vijayan N, Peacock JH: Spinal cord infarction during use of zolmitriptan: A case report. Headache 2000;40:57–60.

59. Wadsworth AN, Chrisp P: Co-dergocrine mesylate. A review of its pharmacodynamic and pharmacokinetic properties and therapeutic use in age-related cognitive decline. Drugs Aging 1992;2:153–173.

60. Weissman NJ, Tighe JF, Gottdiener JS, et al: An assessment of heart valve abnormalities in obese patients taking dexfenfluramine, sustained release dexfenfluramine, or placebo. N Engl J Med 1998; 339: 725–732.

61. Zimran A, Ofek B, Hershko C, et al: Treatment with captopril for peripheral ischemia induced by ergotamine. Br Med J 1984;288:364.

A 16-year-old female was brought to the Emergency Department (ED) after an intentional ingestion of her "strep throat" prescription. She had vomited twice and had a headache, but otherwise had no complaints. She was alert and oriented with vital signs of heart rate, 80 beats/min; blood pressure, 110/60 m'm Hg; respiratory rate, 16 breaths/min; and temperature (rectal), 37°C (98.6°F). The remainder of the physical examination was noncontributory and an initial electrocardiogram (ECG) was normal with a QRS complex duration of 80 msec. Activated charcoal (1 g/kg) was administered orally. All laboratory reports were normal and an acetaminophen level drawn 4 hours after exposure was negative. The patient was able to tolerate feeding after 4 hours. The prescription bottle was obtained by her parents and contained clarithromycin (Biaxin) 500-mg tablets, 14 of which were missing.

HISTORY AND EPIDEMIOLOGY

The majority of the adverse effects related to antibiotics occur as a result of iatrogenic complications rather than intentional overdose. The origins of these complications are diverse and include dosing and decision errors, allergic reactions, adverse drug reactions, and drug interactions. This chapter focuses on each of these adverse drug effects as they relate to the specific antibiotics. Overdose data will also be presented, if available.

Prevention in the form of process improvements and continued vigilance is required to minimize adverse effects. As dosing errors are commonly noted in neonates and infants treated with intravenous antibiotics, careful and constant diligence on the part of all healthcare providers is required to minimize such errors. Antibiotics have a higher risk for anaphylactic reactions than other medications. The reason for this is unclear, but it may be a result of the high frequency of use and the high incidence of repeated interrupted exposures caused by prescriptive use and environmental contamination. A complete and clear allergy history is essential to minimize these reactions in patients being considered for antibiotic therapy.

Many of the adverse effects of antibiotics are difficult to predict even when given patient- and population-specific parameters. In some cases, a diluent or chemical constituent of the drug is responsible for the adverse effect, as recognized with the use of procaine penicillin G.

Antibiotics are involved in many of the common and severe drug interactions primarily through the inhibition of metabolic enzymes. Patients being considered for antibiotic therapy should be carefully assessed for the existence of concomitant drug therapy that will interact with the chosen antibiotic. Drug interactions related to antibiotics are discussed in numerous chapters throughout this text.

PHARMACOLOGY AND TOXICOLOGY

Antibiotic pharmacology is aimed at the destruction of invasive microorganisms through the inhibition of cell cycle reproduction or by directly altering a microorganism's critical function. Table 46–1 lists antibiotics and their associated mechanisms of antimicrobial activity. Often the mechanisms for toxicologic effects following acute overdose differ from the therapeutic mechanisms. Table 46–1 also lists the toxicologic effects and related mechanisms. Table 46–2 lists the pharmacokinetics of each class of drugs.

ANTIBACTERIALS

Aminoglycosides

Gentamicin C: $R_1 = R_2 = CH_3$
Gentamicin C$_2$: $R_1 = CH_3$, $R_2 = H$
Gentamicin C$_{1a}$: $R_1 = R_2 = H$

Aminoglycoside antibiotics that are in current use include amikacin, gentamicin, kanamycin, neomycin, netilmicin, streptomycin, and tobramycin.

TABLE 46–1.   Antibiotic and Antifungal Pharmacology

	Pharmacology of Antibiotic Effect	Acute Overdose Effect and Related Pharmacology, If Known	Chronic Administration Adverse Effect and Related Pharmacology, If Known
Antibiotic			
Aminoglycosides	Inhibit 30s ribosomal subunit	*Neuromuscular blockade*—inhibit the release of acetylcholine from presynaptic nerve terminals and antagonist at acetycholine receptors	*Renal toxicity/ototoxicity*—form an iron complex that inhibits mitochondrial respiration and causes lipid peroxidation
Penicillins, cephalosporins, and other β-lactams	Inhibit cell wall mucopeptide synthesis	*Seizures*—agonist at picrotoxin binding site causing GABA antagonism	*Hypersensitivity*—immune *Other*—see text
Chloramphenicol	Inhibits 50s ribosomal subunit and inhibits protein synthesis in rapidly dividing cells	Inhibits 50s ribosomal subunit and inhibits protein synthesis in rapidly dividing cells	Inhibits 50s ribosomal subunit and inhibits protein synthesis in rapidly dividing cells
Fluoroquinolones	Inhibit DNA topoisomerase and DNA gyrase	Not entirely known; bind to cations, particularly magnesium	Not entirely known, bind to cations, particularly magnesium
Macrolides	Inhibit 50s ribosomal subunit in multiplying cells	*Wide QT*—block delayed rectifier potassium channel	Not entirely known, cytotoxic effect
Sulfonamides	Inhibit para-amino benzoic acid and/or para-amino glutamic acid in the synthesis of folic acid	None clinically relevant	*Hypersensitivity*—metabolite is hapten generating *Hemolysis/methemoglobinemia*—exposure to ultraviolet B causes free radical formation, which results in an oxidant stress
Tetracycline	Inhibits 30s and 50s ribosomal subunits; binds to aminoacyl transfer RNA	None clinically relevant	Unknown
Vancomycin	Inhibits glycopeptidase polymerase in cell wall synthesis	*"Red-man syndrome"*— anaphylactoid	Unknown
Antifungal			
Amphotericin B	Binds with ergosterol on cytoplasmic membrane to cause pores to facilitate organelle leak	Assumed same as mechanism of action	Nephrotoxicity—vehicle deoxycholate may be involved, nephrocalcinosis
Triazoles and imidazoles	Increase permeability of cell membranes	None clinically relevant	None clinically relevant

Acute Overdose.   Because they are only available in parenteral forms, acute overdoses of aminoglycoside antibiotics are almost exclusively the result of dosing errors, especially in neonates. Fortunately, these overdoses are rarely life-threatening, and most patients can be safely managed with minimal intervention.[72,99,117] Large intravenous doses are found to be safe when studied for use in single daily doses. A multiple meta-analysis studying four previous meta-analyses examined the efficacy and toxicity of once-daily aminoglycoside dosing studies and failed to find an increase in adverse effects including nephrotoxicity, ototoxicity, or vestibular toxicity despite these relatively large doses of aminoglycosides.[5]

TABLE 46–2.   Antibiotic and Antifungal Pharmacokinetics

	Absorption	Volume of Distribution (L/kg)	Elimination Route	Half-Life (h)
Antibiotic				
Aminoglycosides	Parenteral	0.25	Renal	2–3
Penicillins, cephalosporins, and other β-lactams	Oral, parenteral	Variable	Renal	Variable
Chloramphenicol	Oral, parenteral, otic	0.5–1.0	Hepatic 90%, renal 10%	1.6–3.3
Fluoroquinolones	Oral, parenteral	Variable	Renal	3–5
Macrolides	Oral, parenteral	Variable	Hepatic	Variable
Sulfonamides	Oral, parenteral	Variable	Hepatic	Variable
Tetracyclines	Oral	Variable	Hepatic	6–26
Vancomycin	Parenteral	0.2–1.25	Renal	4–6
Antifungal				
Amphotericin B	Parenteral	4.0	Hepatic	360
Triazoles and imidazoles	Oral	Variable	Hepatic	Variable

Rarely, acute overdose results in toxic effects. In a case report of a massive gentamicin overdose, vestibular dysfunction and hearing loss occurred.[134] Also, aminoglycosides may infrequently exacerbate neuromuscular blockade corresponding with high-peak serum aminoglycoside levels (Chap. 54).[163,234] These effects relate to the fact that aminoglycosides inhibit the release of acetylcholine from presynaptic nerve terminals and block acetylcholine receptors.[2,90] Risk factors for enhanced neuromuscular blockade include patients with abnormal neuromuscular junction function, such as those with myasthenia gravis and botulism and patients receiving concomitant neuromuscular blocking drugs.[2]

Adverse Effects After Therapeutic Use. Adverse effects, including nephrotoxicity and ototoxicity, correlate more closely with elevated trough serum concentrations of aminoglycosides.[2,68,104,141,145] The mechanism of nephrotoxicity and ototoxicity is inconclusive, but appears to include the ability of the aminoglycoside to reach these organs, to be sequestered, and to form reactive oxygen species with iron. Mitochondrial respiration is inhibited, lipid peroxidation occurs, and stimulation of glutamate activated N-methyl-D-aspartate (NMDA) receptors may play a role.[91,193,202,230] The incidence of nephrotoxicity with aminoglycoside therapy is estimated at 5–10%.[9] Although the aminoglycosides are almost completely excreted prior to biotransformation in the kidney, a small fraction of filtered aminoglycoside is transported by absorptive endocytosis across the apical membrane of proximal tubular cells and becomes sequestered within lysosomes. Toxicity results as the aminoglycoside binds to and destroys phospholipids contained on brush border membranes in the proximal renal tubule.[9]

Clinically, acute tubular necrosis occurs after 7–10 days of standard dose therapy. Laboratory abnormalities include granular casts, proteinuria, elevated urinary sodium, and increased fractional excretion of sodium. Usually the renal dysfunction is reversible; however, irreversible toxicity is reported.[8] Functional renal injury occurs days prior to elevations in serum creatinine, and for this reason, a delay in diagnosis is common.[194] Risk factors for the development of nephrotoxicity include increasing age, renal dysfunction, female sex, previous aminoglycoside therapy, liver dysfunction, large total dose, long duration of therapy, frequent doses, high trough levels, presence of other nephrotoxic drugs, and the presence of shock.[9,147,172] Because the uptake of aminoglycosides into organs causing toxicity is saturable, large doses once daily are less problematic than several lesser doses given in a single day.

Ototoxicity can occur after prolonged exposure to aminoglycosides. Both cochlear and vestibular dysfunction are correlated with high aminoglycoside trough concentrations.[33,146] Because aminoglycosides bioaccumulate in the endolymph and perilymph spaces, they have prolonged contact time with sensory hair cells. Type I hair cells appear to be more susceptible than type II hair cells, although both are affected.[116]

Vestibular toxicity, caused by destruction of sensory receptor portions of the inner ear or destruction of hair cells in the utricle and saccule, occurs in 0.4–6% of patients.[146] Symptoms include vertigo or tinnitus. The relative risks of various aminoglycosides to cause vestibular versus cochlear dysfunction are detailed in Table 46–3.

Full-tone audiometric testing may first show high-frequency hearing loss, which may subsequently progress. Given the inability of hair cells to regenerate, all hearing loss that develops is per-manent. Electronystagmography is the diagnostic tool of choice for vestibular dysfunction, and up to 50% of patients with early findings of vestibular dysfunction may have improvement after discontinuation of the drug.[66] Simultaneous administration of other drugs capable of causing ototoxicity enhances ototoxicity of aminoglycoside antibiotics (Chap. 28).[27,116,217]

Treatments for both nephrotoxicity and ototoxicity caused by the aminoglycoside antibiotics include withdrawal of the offending agent and supportive care. Experimental treatments in animal models include the use of deferoxamine, glutathione, and NMDA receptor antagonists in an attempt to chelate and/or detoxify a reactive intermediate.[158,214] The antibiotic ticarcillin forms a complex with aminoglycosides to inactivate both antimicrobial efficacy and toxicity. In animals given tobramycin with and without concurrent ticarcillin, ticarcillin provided protection against tobramycin-induced renal toxicity.[64] In humans, ticarcillin removes 50% more aminoglycoside in 48 hours than two hemodialysis sessions.[193] Ticarcillin therapy is of limited value because in most instances, the aminoglycoside has decreased to a much lower serum concentration before any therapeutic measures can be employed. The use of ticarcillin should be considered only in patients with either demonstrated toxicity or renal failure in which the risks of toxicity are significant.

Less common adverse effects associated with chronic aminoglycoside use include electrolyte abnormalities, allergic reactions, hepatotoxicity, anemia, granulocytopenia, thrombocytopenia, eosinophilia, retinal toxicity, reproductive dysfunction, tetany, and toxic psychosis.[49,52,108,122,210,223] When aminoglycosides are administered at high doses or during once-daily dosing, sepsislike reactions can occur.[7] This is likely a result of an increased dose of endotoxin contaminants derived from the fungus that are delivered to the patient during the infusion.

Penicillins

Penicillin nucleus

There are several penicillins available in the United States. They are natural or semisynthetic derivatives from the fungus *Penicillium*. Penicillins are β-lactam antibiotics that contain a 6-aminopenicillanic acid nucleus composed of a β-lactam ring fused

TABLE 46–3. Predominant Aminoglycoside Toxicity

Cochlear	Cochlear and Vestibular	Vestibular	Renal
Kanamycin	Gentamicin	Streptomycin	Amikacin
Neomycin	Tobramycin		Gentamicin
Amikacin			Kanamycin
			Neomycin
			Streptomycin
			Tobramycin

to a 5-member thiazolidine ring. Currently available penicillins include penicillin G, penicillin V, cloxacillin, nafcillin, dicloxacillin, oxacillin, amoxicillin, bacampicillin, ampicillin, piperacillin, carbenicillin, ticarcillin, and mezlocillin. Table 46–1 lists the pharmacologic mechanism of penicillins and Table 46–2 lists their pharmacokinetic properties.

Acute Overdose. Acute oral overdoses of penicillin-containing drugs are usually not life-threatening, and most patients can be safely and effectively managed in the home by poison center staff unless psychological or social reasons necessitate hospital evaluation. The most frequent complaints following acute overdose are nausea, vomiting, and diarrhea. Rarely, hyperkalemia resulting in electrocardiographic abnormalities occurs after rapid intravenous doses of potassium penicillin G are administered to patients with renal failure.

Seizures occur in humans given large intravenous or intraventricular doses of penicillins.[26,110,119,202] Doses of penicillin required to produce seizures are high, usually greater than 50 million units intravenously.[200] In animals, seizures develop when high doses are administered parenterally, or when penicillin is administered via intraventricular or intracisternal injection.[88] Penicillin-induced seizures appear to be mediated through an interaction with the picrotoxin-binding site on the neuronal chloride channel near the γ-amino butyric acid (GABA) site (Chap. 10). When this binding site is activated, an allosteric change prevents GABA from binding to its receptor, resulting in a relative lack of inhibitory tone.[53] Penicillin analogues (such as imipenem) also cause seizures in both animal models and humans, presumably through a similar mechanism.[202] Treatment of patients who develop penicillin-induced seizures include GABA agonists such as benzodiazepines and barbiturates, if needed. Rarely, intraventricular overdoses require cerebral spinal fluid exchange to attenuate seizure activity.[119]

Adverse Effects After Therapeutic Use. Penicillin class antibiotics are associated with a myriad of adverse effects after therapeutic use, the most common of which are allergic reactions. They are commonly implicated in immune-related reactions such as bone marrow suppression, interstitial nephritis, and vasculitis.[75,150,151,213] Rare effects include pemphigus after penicillin use and corneal damage after the use of methicillin.[18,238]

Acute Allergy. Penicillins are the agents most commonly implicated in the development of acute anaphylactic reactions (Chap. 15). The incidence of hypersensitivity after penicillin use is 5% overall, with 1% of penicillin reactions resulting in anaphylaxis. The risk for a fatal hypersensitivity reaction after penicillin administration is 2/100,000 (0.002%).[229] All routes of penicillin administration can result in anaphylaxis; however, it is most common after intravenous administration. The anaphylactic syndrome is caused by local and systemic release of endogenous vasoactive substances including leukotrienes C_4 and D_4, histamine, eosinophilic chemotactic factor, and other vasoactive substances, such as bradykinin, kallikrein, prostaglandin D_2, and platelet-activating factor (Table 46–4; Chap. 15). Type 1 hypersensitivity, or anaphylaxis, results after prior exposure to the antigen produces IgE, which is bound to mast cells and basophilic surfaces. With secondary exposure, the antigen combines with the antibody and results in mast cell and basophil degranulation.

TABLE 46–4. Classification of Anaphylactic Reactions

Grade	Classification Description
I	Large local contiguous reaction (>15 cm)
II	Pruritus (urticaria), generalized
III	Asthma, angioedema, nausea, vomiting
IV	Airway (asthma, tongue swelling, dysphagia, respiratory distress, laryngeal edema)
	Cardiovascular (hypotension, may progress to cardiovascular collapse)

Treatment is supportive with careful attention to airway, breathing, and circulation. If the penicillin was ingested orally, the patient may theoretically benefit from activated charcoal 1 g/kg orally. Initial drug therapy includes epinephrine at 0.01 mL/kg (up to 0.5 mL) of 1:1000 dilution SC every 10–20 minutes. Epinephrine, through β-receptor stimulation, results in bronchodilation and increased cardiac output. In addition, its α-receptor stimulation results in increased peripheral vascular tone. Oxygen and inhaled β$_2$-adrenergic agonists are warranted in severe cases, as are corticosteroids and H$_1$-receptor antagonists.

H$_2$-Receptor antagonism as a treatment for anaphylaxis is controversial. H$_2$-Receptors, when stimulated in the peripheral vasculature, cause vasodilation; in the heart, cause positive inotropy, positive chronotropy, and coronary vasodilation; and in the lung, cause increased mucus production.[188] Theoretically, H$_2$-receptor antagonists can lead to a decrease in myocardial activity at a time when H$_1$-receptor stimulation is causing hypotension, coronary vasoconstriction, and bronchospasm. In vitro and animal models demonstrate decreases in coronary circulation and decreases in the overall anaphylactic response following H$_1$ blockers.[15,20] In humans, cimetidine and ranitidine are useful for the treatment of pruritus and flushing after acute allergic skin reactions.[130,143] Cimetidine, used following anaphylaxis, may result in clinical improvement, particularly hypotension and tachycardia.[57,239] However, in one case, chronic ranitidine administration was postulated to result in heart block after an anaphylactic response to latex.[166] Treatment using H$_2$-receptor antagonists should only be considered when other therapies have failed and the patient is adequately H$_1$-receptor blocked.

Aminophylline, although mentioned in some references for the treatment of anaphylaxis, is not adequately studied and should not be routinely employed. Lastly, glucagon may be of some benefit, particularly in patients who are maintained on β-adrenergic antagonists.

Dosing of specific therapy, along with information on side effects, is found in Chapter 15.

Amoxicillin/Clavulanic Acid and Hepatitis. Intrahepatic cholestatic hepatitis occurs after treatment with amoxicillin/clavulanate.[40,129,155,177,208] The incidence of hepatotoxicity that typically occurs 1–6 weeks after initiation of therapy is estimated at 1.1–2.7/100,000 prescriptions.[74] The mechanism of hepatotoxicity is not clear, but may include toxicity of clavulanate or one of its metabolites. Treatment is supportive with symptoms typically resolving after the discontinuation of therapy. However, prolonged hepatitis, ductopenia, and pancreatitis may rarely occur.[40,177]

Penicillin G. The most common adverse effects occurring after administration of intramuscular procaine penicillin G are the Hoigne syndrome and the Jarisch-Herxheimer reaction.[11,50,98,106,139,207,245] Both occur after the administration of large intramuscular or intravenous doses of penicillin G.[73,84] Hoigne syndrome is characterized by extreme apprehension and fear, illusions, or hallucinations; changes in auditory and visual perception; tachycardia; systolic hypertension; and, occasionally, seizures that begin within minutes of injection.[228] These effects occur in the absence of signs or symptoms of anaphylaxis. The cause of this syndrome is unknown. Procaine is implicated as the causative agent because of this syndrome's similarity to events that occur after the administration of other pharmacologically similar local anesthetics.[190,201,225]

Hoigne syndrome is 6 times more common in males than females.[206] The reason for this increased prevalence is unclear, but autosomal dominance and influences of prostaglandin and thromboxane A_2 activity in this population may be responsible.[11]

The Jarisch-Herxheimer reaction is a self-limited reaction that develops within a few hours of treatment of early syphilis. Symptoms include myalgias, chills, headache, rash, and fever. Symptoms spontaneously resolve within 18–24 hours, even with continued antibiotic therapy.[144,184] The pathogenesis of this reaction is unclear, but some authors hypothesize that the reaction is caused by an acute antigen response to lysed bacteria. Similar reactions are reported after treatment of other spirochetal and bacterial infections such as Lyme disease.[30]

Cephalosporins

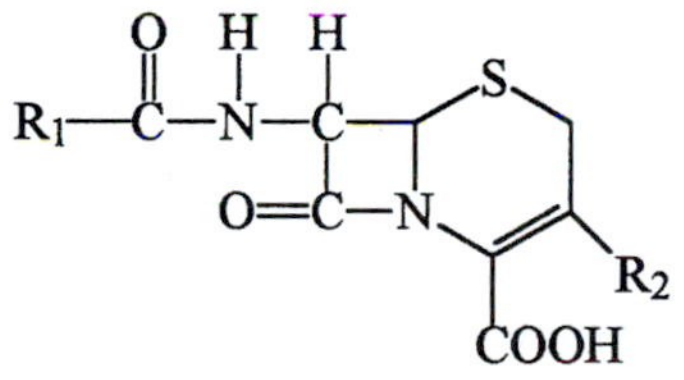

Cephem nucleus

Cephalosporins are semisynthetic derivatives of cephalosporin C produced by the fungus *Acremonium,* previously called *Cephalosporium.* Cephalosporins have a similar ring structure to penicillins. Cephalosporins are generally divided into first, second, third, and fourth generations based on their antimicrobial spectrum. First-generation cephalosporins include cefadroxil, cefazolin, cephalexin, cephapirin, and cephadrine. Second-generation cephalosporins include cefaclor, cefamandole, cefonicid, cefotetan, cefoxitin, cefprozil, and cefuroxime. Third-generation cephalosporins include cefdinir, ceftazidime, cefixime, ceftibuten, cefoperazone, ceftizoxime, cefotaxime, ceftriaxone, and cefpodoxime. Finally, of the fourth-generation cephalosporins, cefepime is the first to be marketed.

Acute Overdose. Effects occurring after acute overdose of cephalosporins resemble those occurring after penicillin exposure. Some cephalosporins have similar epileptogenic potential to penicillin in the animal model.[77,231] Management guidelines for cephalosporin overdose are similar to those of penicillin overdose. Table 46–1 lists the pharmacologic mechanism of cephalosporins and Table 46–2 lists their pharmacokinetic properties.

Adverse Effects After Therapeutic Use. Cephalosporins are also capable of causing an immune-mediated acute hemolytic crisis.[21,63] Cefaclor is the most common cephalosporin reported to cause serum sickness, although it can occur with other cephalosporins.[114,133] Also, like penicillins, cephalosporins are associated with chronic toxicity, including interstitial nephritis and hepatitis with first-generation agents.[150,151,237]

Cross-Hypersensitivity. The cephalosporins contain a 6-member dihydrithiazine ring instead of the 5-member thiazolidine penicillin ring. The incidence of allergy after cephalosporin use is approximately 4% in the general population and 8% in those with prior penicillin allergy. The incidence of anaphylaxis to cephalosporins is less than 0.02%, with an increase to less than 0.04% in those patients with previous penicillin allergy. Cross-reactivity may be greater with agents that are structurally similar to penicillin or that are contaminated by penicillin.[6] Antibody binding after cephalosporin exposure occurs at the determinants located on the side chain groups of the cephalosporin.[13] These determinants are quite distinct between cephalosporins, which causes the pattern of cross-hypersensitivity between cephalosporins to be much less well defined than between the penicillins. Caution should be used when considering cephalosporins in penicillin- or cephalosporin-allergic patients; however, if a risk-benefit analysis demonstrates a clear benefit to the patient without equivalent alternatives, the cephalosporin should be given.

nMTT Side Chain Effects. Cephalosporins containing an *N*-methylthiotetrazole (nMTT) side chain (moxalactam, cefazolin, cefoperazone, cefmetazole, cefamandole, cefotetan) have toxic effects unique to their group structure. These cephalosporins are metabolized spontaneously and release free nMTT, which is responsible for their effects (Fig. 46–1).[140]

Free nMTT inhibits the enzyme aldehyde dehydrogenase similarly to disulfiram, and in conjunction with ethanol can cause a disulfiramlike reaction (Chap. 65).[31] Patients report flushing, nausea, and vomiting after even small doses of ethanol as a result of the accumulation of acetaldehyde. Those experiencing more severe manifestations may present with hypotension and shock. Treatment is supportive, with careful attention to hemodynamic

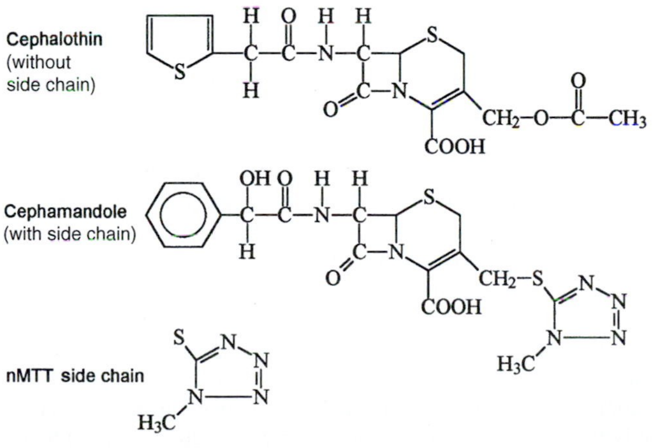

Figure 46–1. Characteristic structures of cephalosporins emphasizing the nMTT side chain.

status. Activated charcoal may be useful if the cephalosporin is recently ingested or has enterohepatic recirculation (ie, cefazolin).

The nMTT side chain is also associated with hypoprothrombinemia, although a causal relationship is controversial.[85] It is thought that nMTT depletes vitamin K–dependent clotting factors by inhibition of vitamin K epoxide reductase.[160] Treatment of patients suspected of hypoprothrombinemia caused by these cephalosporins consists of fresh-frozen plasma, if bleeding is evident, and vitamin K_1 in doses required to resynthesize vitamin K cofactors (Chap. 42).

The amount of nMTT formed per dose of cephalosporin is variable among the cephalosporins. In a study involving healthy humans, cefoperazone produced the greatest amount of nMTT, followed by cefotetan and cefmetazole.[236]

Other β-Lactam Antibiotics

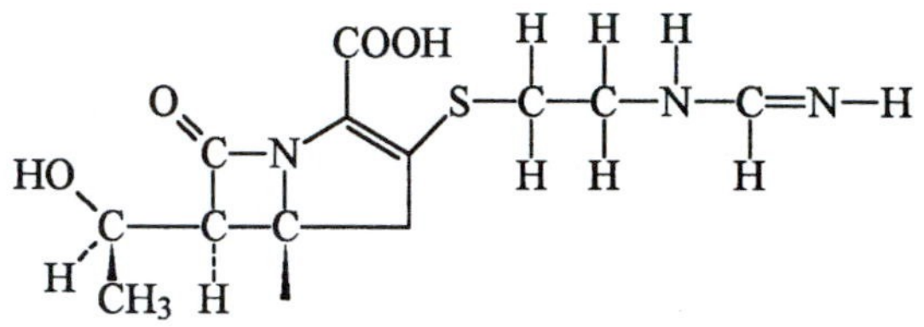

Imipenem

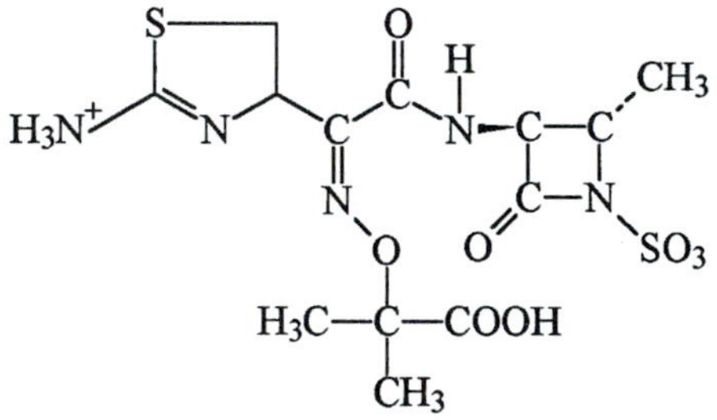

Aztreonam

Included in this group are monobactams such as aztreonam and carbapenems such as imipenem and meropenem. Table 46–1 lists the pharmacologic mechanism of these drugs, and Table 46–2 lists their pharmacokinetic properties.

Acute Overdose.   Effects occurring after acute overdose of other β-lactam antibiotics resemble those occurring following penicillin exposure. Imipenem has clear epileptogenic potential (Adverse Effects After Therapeutic Use). Management guidelines for other β-lactam overdoses are similar to those of penicillin overdoses.

Adverse Effects After Therapeutic Use.   Imipenem, a member of the class of carbapenem compounds, can cause seizures in therapeutic doses.[37,113,125,165,212] The risk factors for seizures include central nervous system disease, prior seizure disorders, or abnormal renal function.[167] The mechanism for seizures appears to be GABA antagonism (similar to the penicillins) in conjunction with enhanced activity of excitatory amino acids. In mice, the addition of both excitatory amino acid antagonists and GABA agonists increases the threshold required to provoke carbapenem-induced seizure activity.[55] In animals, the C-2 side chain of imipenem provoked seizure

activity, providing a structural relationship between imipenem and the development of seizures.[218] Treatment for patients with seizures after imipenem use is supportive. GABA agonists such as benzodiazepines or barbiturates should be used if pharmacologic therapy is required for termination of seizure activity.

Cross-Hypersensitivity.   Aztreonam is a monobactam that does not contain the antigenic components required for cross-allergy with penicillins. Therefore, generalized cross-allergenicity is not expected.[191] However, aztreonam cross-reacts in vitro with ceftriaxone, thought to be the result of the similarity in their side chain structure.[170] Cross-allergenicity has also been noted between imipenem and penicillin, although the incidence has yet to be determined.

Chloramphenicol

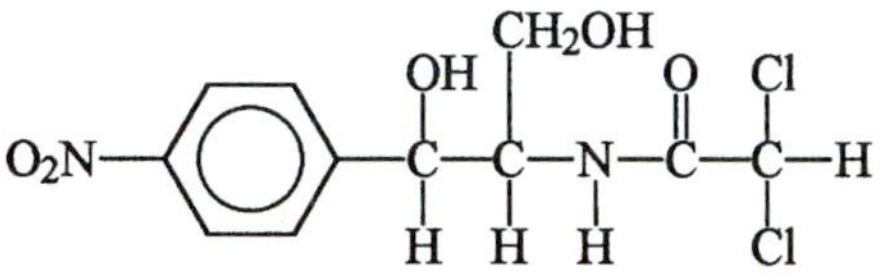

Chloramphenicol

Chloramphenicol was originally derived from *Streptomyces venezuelae* and is now produced synthetically. Antimicrobial activity exists against many gram-positive and gram-negative aerobes and anaerobes. Table 46–1 lists the pharmacologic mechanism of chloramphenicol, and Table 46–2 lists its pharmacokinetic properties.

Acute Overdose.   Acute overdose of chloramphenicol commonly causes nausea and vomiting. Effects are caused by its ability to inhibit protein synthesis in rapidly proliferating cells. Metabolic acidosis occurs due to the inhibition of mitochondrial enzymes, oxidative phosphorylation, and mitochondrial biogenesis.[70] Infrequently, sudden cardiovascular collapse may occur 5–12 hours after acute overdoses. In case series, cardiovascular compromise was more frequent in patients with elevated serum concentrations (>50 μg/mL).[70,115,148,168,222] Because levels are not readily available, all poisoned patients should receive close observation for at least 12 hours after exposure. Orogastric lavage may be useful for recent ingestions in which the patient has not vomited, and activated charcoal 1 g/kg should be given orally.

Extracorporeal means of eliminating chloramphenicol are not usually required because of its rapid metabolism (Table 46–2). However, it may be of benefit in patients with large overdoses, or in patients with severe hepatic or renal dysfunction. Both hemodialysis and charcoal hemoperfusion decrease elevated plasma chloramphenicol levels.[69,142,209] Exchange transfusion also lowers chloramphenicol serum concentrations in neonates.[115,216] Surviving patients should be closely monitored for signs of bone marrow suppression.

Adverse Effects After Therapeutic Use.   Chronic toxicity of chloramphenicol is similar to that seen after acute poisoning. A classic description of the chronic toxicity of chloramphenicol is the "gray baby syndrome."[69,70,142,216] Children with this syndrome exhibit vomiting, anorexia, respiratory distress, abdominal distension, green stools, lethargy, cyanosis, ashen color, metabolic acidosis, hypotension, and cardiovascular collapse. The majority (90%) of a dose of chloramphenicol is metabolized via glucuronyl transferase forming a glucuronide conjugate. The remainder is excreted renally unchanged. Infants, in particular, are predisposed to the gray baby syndrome because they have a limited capacity to conjugate chloramphenicol and to excrete unconjugated chloramphenicol in the urine.[80,235]

Dose-dependent bone marrow depression occurs with high serum concentrations of chloramphenicol.[102,103,199] Clinical manifestations usually occur after several weeks of therapy and include anemia, thrombocytopenia, and leukopenia. Bone marrow suppression is reversible with discontinuation of therapy. Chloramphenicol causes bone marrow suppression by inhibiting protein synthesis in the mitochondria of marrow cell lines.[152,153]

Rarely, aplastic anemia occurs after topical application.[1] The development of aplastic anemia after chloramphenicol use is not dose related and generally occurs in susceptible patients within 5 months of treatment (Chap. 25).[61,242] Although the exact mechanism is unknown, it is theorized that the *p*-nitrosulfathiazole group on chloramphenicol inhibits DNA synthesis in marrow stem cells.[241]

Other adverse effects associated with chloramphenicol include peripheral neuropathy;[112,174] neurologic abnormalities, including confusion and delirium;[127] optic neuritis;[46,112] nonlymphocytic leukemia;[205] and contact dermatitis.[120]

Fluoroquinolones

Quinolone nucleus

The fluoroquinolones are a structurally similar, synthetically derived group of antibiotics that may exhibit a diverse spectrum of activity. The fluoroquinolones include balofloxacin, ciprofloxacin, clinafloxacin, enoxacin, fleroxacin, gatifloxacin, gemifloxacin, grepafloxacin, levofloxacin, lomefloxacin, moxifloxacin, nadifloxacin, nalidixic acid, norfloxacin, ofloxacin, pefloxacin, rufloxacin, sparfloxacin, temafloxacin, tosufloxacin, and trovafloxacin. Table 46–1 lists the pharmacologic mechanism of fluoroquinolones, and Table 46–2 lists their pharmacokinetic properties.

Acute Overdose. Like other antimicrobials, the fluoroquinolones are rarely life-threatening after acute overdose, and most patients can be safely managed with minimal intervention.[10] Rarely, acute overdose of a fluoroquinolone results in renal failure or seizures.[48]

The mechanism of renal failure after fluoroquinolone exposure is controversial. In animals, ciprofloxacin and norfloxacin cause pathologic changes in the kidney, especially in the setting of neutral or alkaline urine.[195] In humans, renal failure is reported after both acute and chronic exposure to fluoroquinolones. A hypersensitivity reaction is postulated to explain pathologic changes con-

sistent with interstitial nephritis.[101,150,151,179,240] Treatment is supportive with discontinuation of the fluoroquinolone. Improvement in renal function is usually noticed within several days.

Seizures are reported with ciprofloxacin and may be a result of the inhibition of GABA.[211,224] Others postulate that the ability of fluoroquinolones to bind efficiently to cations, particularly magnesium, results in seizure activity. This hypothesis is related to magnesium's inhibitory role at the excitatory NMDA-gated ion channel (Chap. 10).[56,196] Treatment is supportive, using benzodiazepines and, if necessary, barbiturates to increase GABAergic activity.

Adverse Effects After Therapeutic Use. Several fluoroquinolones are substrates and/or inhibitors of cytochrome P450 isoenzymes. This can result in drug interactions, especially important with drugs that have a narrow therapeutic index. See Chapter 11 for clinical implications.

Serious adverse effects related to fluoroquinolone use consist of central nervous system toxicity as discussed, cardiovascular toxicity, hepatotoxicity, and articular/tendon toxicity.

Fluoroquinolones cause prolongation of the QTc complex duration that may cause torsades de pointes.[54,109,189] Although the mechanism of this effect is unclear, sequestering of magnesium resulting in clinical hypomagnesemia is postulated.[196] Treatment of patients presenting with widening of the QTc interval duration is supportive with careful attention to magnesium supplementation if necessary.

The fluoroquinolones rarely result in potentially fatal hepatotoxicity.[41,42,71,81,92,123,135,181] This adverse effect is most notable with trovafloxacin, although the reason for an increased risk with this particular fluoroquinolone is not clear. As a result, trovafloxacin (Trovan) is now reserved only for the treatment of patients with life-threatening infections in whom the benefits are thought to outweigh the risks. In addition, the manufacturer has initiated a limited distribution system that allows drug shipment only to pharmacies within inpatient healthcare facilities.

Fluoroquinolones should be used with caution in children and pregnant women because of their potential adverse effects on developing cartilage and bone. Damage to articular cartilage is demonstrated in young dogs and rats although it was variable with different fluoroquinolones.[34,220] There are very limited data in humans; however, children given ciprofloxacin on a compassionate basis developed complaints of swollen, painful, and stiff joints after 3 weeks of therapy.[111] All signs and symptoms abated within 2 weeks of discontinuation of therapy. However, 29 additional children treated with ofloxacin or ciprofloxacin showed no differences with respect to cartilage thickness, cartilage structure, edema, cartilage-bone borderline, or synovial fluid. Women who received quinolones during pregnancy had larger babies and more caesarean deliveries because of fetal distress than did controls.[17] However, there were no congenital malformations, delay to developmental milestones, or musculoskeletal abnormalities found.

Fluoroquinolones are also implicated as a cause of tendon rupture, which is reported to occur for up to 120 days after the start of treatment and even after the discontinuation of therapy.[169] The fluoroquinolone should be discontinued in patients, particularly athletes who complain of symptoms consistent with painful and swollen tendons.

Other adverse effects include acute psychosis, rash, tinnitus, eosinophilia, serum sickness, and, commonly, photosensitivity.[32,86,215,149]

Macrolides

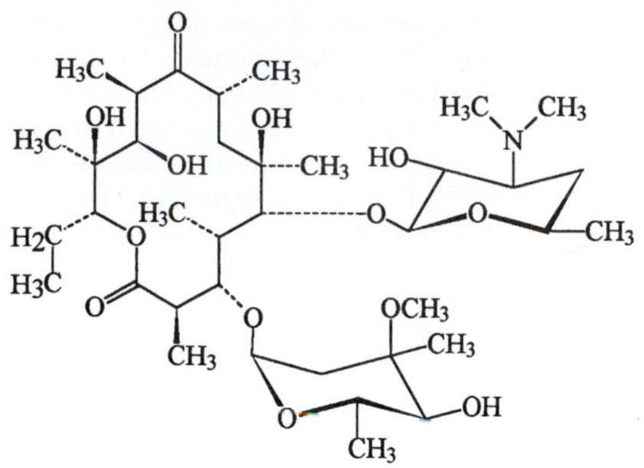

Erythromycin

The macrolide antibiotics include various forms of erythromycin (base, estolate, ethylsuccinate, gluceptate, lactobionate, stearate), azithromycin, clarithromycin, troleandomycin, and dirithromycin. Table 46–1 lists the pharmacologic mechanism of macrolides, and Table 46–2 lists their pharmacokinetic properties.

Acute Overdose. Acute oral overdoses of macrolide antibiotics are usually not life-threatening and symptoms are generally confined to the gastrointestinal tract. Treatment is similar to acute oral penicillin overdoses. Erythromycin lactobionate causes QT prolongation and torsades de pointes after intravenous use.[161] In vitro models demonstrate erythromycin's ability to slow repolarization in a concentration-dependent manner.[156] The cause for widened QT was once thought to result from hypokalemia-induced promotion of intracellular efflux of potassium.[175] Current data, however, demonstrate that the QT prolongation results from blockade of delayed rectifier potassium currents (Chap. 21).[183] QTc prolongation and torsades de pointes are common after intravenous erythromycin lactobionate.[161] More pronounced widening occurs in patients with underlying heart disease and correlates with the infusion rate.[89] Epidemiologic studies associate an increased incidence of ventricular dysrhythmias in females treated with erythromycin.[59] The implications of this finding are unknown.

Adverse Events After Therapeutic Use

Drug Interactions. Erythromycin is the prototypical macrolide and as such has received the most attention with respect to potential and documented drug interactions. Clarithromycin, erythromycin, and troleandomycin are all potent inhibitors of the cytochrome CYP3A4 enzyme system, whereas azithromycin provides little to no inhibition.[51] Erythromycin inhibits P450 after metabolism to a nitroso intermediate, which then forms an inactive complex with the iron (II) of cytochrome P450. Chapter 11 lists some substrates for the CYP3A4 system. Clinically significant interactions occur with erythromycin and astemizole, carbamazepine, cisapride, and terfenadine.[35,83,95,100,173] Inhibition of terfenadine, astemizole, and cisapride metabolism results in increased concentrations of the parent drug, all of which are capable of causing a widening of the QTc interval and torsades de pointes.[24,164] Cases of carbamazepine toxicity are documented with erythromycin use.[95] Erythromycin also inhibits CYP1A2,

producing clinically significant interactions with clozapine, theophylline, and warfarin.[180]

Macrolides may also interact with the absorption and renal excretion of drugs that are amenable to intestinal *p*-glycoprotein excretion, or interfere with normal gut flora responsible for metabolism. This may be part of the underlying mechanism of cases of macrolide-induced digoxin toxicity[159] (Chap. 48).

End-Organ Effects. The most common toxic effect of macrolides after chronic use is hepatitis, which may be immune mediated.[38] Erythromycin estolate is the agent most frequently implicated in causing cholestatic hepatitis.[79,107]

Large doses of macrolide antibiotics are also associated with high-frequency sensorineural hearing loss.[28,198] A review of 11 patients who experienced hearing loss following erythromycin therapy showed that the therapy employed a dose greater than 4 g/d or that the patient had prior renal impairment as a potential risk factor.[185] The hearing loss was reversible in all 11 cases after dosage reduction or discontinuation. A similar case-control study found that 5 of 30 patients treated with erythromycin therapy experienced ototoxicity, while none of the 15 controls had any manifestations.[219] Ototoxicity occurred only with doses of 4 g/d or more, and was found to correlate with higher serum concentrations. Ototoxicity resolved in all patients 6–14 days after discontinuation of therapy. However, there are rare case reports in which ototoxicity did not resolve following discontinuation of therapy.[62,126] There are insufficient data concerning the ototoxic potential of the other macrolide antibiotics.

Other, rare toxic effects associated with macrolides include cataracts after clarithromycin use in animals and acute pancreatitis in humans.[65,227,172]

Sulfonamides

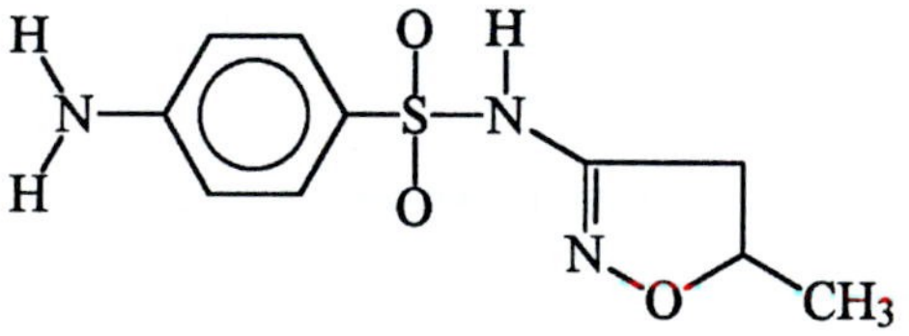

Sulfamethoxazole

Sulfonamides are antibiotics that antagonize *p*-aminobenzoic acid or *p*-aminobenzyl glutamic acid, which are required for the biosynthesis of folic acid. Table 46–1 lists the pharmacologic mechanism of sulfonamides, and Table 46–2 lists their pharmacokinetic properties.

Acute Overdose. Acute oral overdoses of sulfonamides are usually not life-threatening and symptoms are generally confined to nausea, although allergy and methemoglobinemia are rarely seen. Treatment is similar to acute oral penicillin overdoses.

Adverse Effects After Therapeutic Use. The most common adverse effects associated with chronic therapy with sulfonamides are nausea and cutaneous hypersensitivity reactions. Hypersensitivity reactions are thought to be caused by the formation of hapten sulfamethoxazole metabolites, *N*-hydroxy-sulfamethoxazole-NHOH and nitroso-sulfamethoxazole-NO. The degree of hapten binding is mitigated in vitro by cysteine and glutathione.[154] The incidence of adverse reactions to sulfonamides, including allergy, is increased in the HIV-positive population and is positively correlated to the number of opportunistic infections that the patient has had despite similar CD4 counts among the groups.[124] This may be caused by a decrease in the mechanisms available for detoxification of free radical formation as cysteine and glutathione levels are low in these patients.[233] It is unknown whether supplementation with a glutathione precursor such *N*-acetylcysteine will reduce the incidence of these reactions. One study using 800 mg of *N*-acetylcysteine daily found no difference in the incidence of adverse effects between the groups.[3]

Methemoglobinemia and hemolysis also rarely occur.[60,132] The mechanism for adverse reactions is not entirely clear. However, when sulfamethoxazole is exposed to ultraviolet B (UVB) radiation in vitro, free radicals are formed that can participate in the development of tissue peroxidation and hemolysis.[244] This finding may be of particular importance in treating patients with G6PD deficiency caused by a decrease in reducing capabilities.[4]

The sulfonamides are associated with many chronic adverse effects. Bone marrow suppression is rare, but an increased incidence occurs in patients with folic acid or vitamin B_{12} deficiency, and in children, pregnant women, alcoholics, dialysis patients, and immunocompromised patients, as well as in those patients those receiving other folate antagonists. Other adverse effects include hypersensitivity pneumonitis, stomatitis, aseptic meningitis, hepatotoxicity, renal toxicity, and central nervous system toxicity.[22]

Tetracyclines

Tetracycline

Tetracyclines are derivatives of *Streptomyces* cultures. Currently available tetracyclines include demeclocycline, doxycycline, methacycline, minocycline, oxytetracycline, and tetracycline. Table 46–1 lists the pharmacologic mechanism of tetracyclines, and Table 46–2 lists their pharmacokinetic properties.

Acute Overdose. Significant toxicity after acute overdose of tetracyclines is unlikely. Gastrointestinal effects consisting of nausea, vomiting, and epigastric pain have been reported.[29]

Adverse Effects After Therapeutic Use. Tetracycline should not be used in children during the first 6–8 years of life or in pregnant women after the 12th week of pregnancy because of the risk of development of secondary tooth discoloration in the child or in the offspring.

Other chronic effects associated with the tetracyclines include nephrotoxicity, hepatotoxicity, and skin hyperpigmentation in sun-exposed areas and hypersensitivity reactions.[38,82,105,221] More severe hypersensitivity reactions, drug-induced lupus, and pneumonitis are reported after minocycline use, as are cases of necrotizing vasculitis of the skin and uterine cervix, and lymphadenopathy with eosinophilia.[137,197,204] Demeclocycline is reported in a single case to cause nephrogenic diabetes insipidus.[39] Outdated older formulations, but not newer formulations, of tetracycline are reported to cause hypouricemia, hypokalemia, and a proximal and distal renal tubular acidosis.[44]

Vancomycin

Vancomycin is obtained from cultures of *Nocardia orientalis* and is a tricyclic glycopeptide. Vancomycin is biologically active against numerous gram-positive organisms. Table 46–1 lists the pharmacologic mechanism of vancomycin, and Table 46–2 lists its pharmacokinetic properties.

Acute Overdose. Acute oral overdoses of vancomycin rarely cause significant toxicity and most cases can be treated with supportive care alone. Multiple-dose activated charcoal therapy decreases the half-life of vancomycin and can be considered in patients with large overdoses when the patient is expected to have a long clearance time.[121]

Adverse Effects After Therapeutic Use. Patients who receive intravenous vancomycin may develop the "red man syndrome," which is a glycopeptide-induced anaphylactoid reaction.[76] Symptoms include chest pain, dyspnea, pruritus, urticaria, flushing, and angioedema.[182] Signs and symptoms spontaneously resolve, typically within 15 minutes. Other symptoms attributable to "red man syndrome" may include hypotension, cardiovascular collapse, and seizures.[12,157]

The incidence, signs, and symptoms of red man syndrome are variable. The incidence of red man syndrome appears to be related to the rate of infusion. The incidence is 14% (11/76) when 1 g is given over 10 minutes versus 3.4% when given over 1 hour.[157,162] A trial in healthy humans studied the relationship between intradermal skin hypersensitivity and the development of red man syndrome. Each of the 11 subjects underwent skin testing followed 1 week later by an intravenous dose of vancomycin 15 mg/kg over 60 minutes. Following intravenous vancomycin, all subjects developed dermal flare responses and erythema, and 10 of 11 subjects developed pruritus within 20–45 minutes. After the infusion was terminated, symptoms resolved within 60 minutes.[171]

The signs and symptoms of the red man syndrome are related to the rise and fall of histamine concentrations.[94,128] Tachyphylaxis occurs in patients given multiple doses.[93,232] Animal models demonstrated a direct myocardial depressant and vasodilatory effect of vancomycin.[47] More serious reactions result when vancomycin is given via intravenous bolus, further supporting a rate-related anaphylactoid mechanism.[19]

Patients most often experience red man syndrome after vancomycin is administered intravenously. In rare cases, oral administration of vancomycin can also result in the syndrome.[16] Treatment includes increasing the dilution of vancomycin and a slower intravenous administration. Antihistamines may be useful as pretreatment, especially prior to the first dose.[176] A placebo-controlled trial in adult patients studied the incidence of these symptoms in patients given 1 g of vancomycin over 1 hour, as well as the effect of diphenhydramine in the prevention of the syndrome.[232] There was a 47% incidence of reaction without diphenhydramine and a 0% incidence with diphenhydramine.

Chronic use of vancomycin may cause reversible nephrotoxicity, particularly in patients with prolonged excessive steady-state serum levels.[8,178] Concomitant administration of aminoglycoside antibiotics may increase the risk of nephrotoxicity.[186] Vancomycin also rarely causes thrombocytopenia and neutropenia.[43,58]

ANTIFUNGALS

Numerous antifungals are available. Toxicity related to the use of antifungal agents is variable and is based generally upon their mechanism of action.

Amphotericin B

Amphotericin B is a potent antifungal derived from *Streptomyces nodosus*. Amphotericin B is generally fungistatic against fungi that contain sterols in their cell membrane. Table 46–1 lists the pharmacologic mechanism of amphotericin B, and Table 46–2 lists its pharmacokinetic properties.

Acute Overdose. There are several case reports of amphotericin B overdose in infants and children. Significant clinical findings include hypokalemia, aspartate aminotransferase elevations, and cardiac complications including dysrhythmias and cardiac arrest after being given 5–15 mg/kg of amphotericin B.[45,118]

Exchange transfusion may be useful in neonates and infants and should be considered after large intravenous exposures.[25] In adults, extracorporeal elimination is not expected to be useful because of the drug's low water solubility and high blood-protein binding.

Adverse Effects After Therapeutic Use. Infusion of amphotericin B results in fever, rigors, headache, nausea, vomiting, hypotension, tachycardia, and dyspnea.[138] Pretreatment with acetaminophen, diphenhydramine, ibuprofen, and hydrocortisone is helpful in alleviating the febrile symptoms along with slower rates of infusion and lower total daily doses.[78,226] Doses greater than 1 mg/kg/d and rapid administration of drug in less than 1 hour are not recommended. Infusion concentrations of amphotericin B greater than 0.1 mg/mL can result in localized phlebitis. Slower infusion rates, hot packs, and frequent line flushing with dextrose in water may also help to alleviate symptoms.

Eighty percent of patients exposed to amphotericin B will sustain some degree of renal insufficiency (Chap. 23).[36] Azotemia is caused by distal renal tubule damage, which causes renal artery vasoconstriction. Studies in animals show depressed renal blood flow and glomerular filtration rate, and increased renal vascular resistance. It is unclear why this occurs, but at this time, renal nerves, angiotensin II, endothelium-derived relaxing factor, and tubuloglomerular feedback are excluded.[187,192] The toxic effects associated with amphotericin B may be caused by the vehicle, deoxycholate.[243] After large total doses of amphotericin B, residual decreases in glomerular filtration rate may occur even after discontinuation of therapy. This is hypothesized to be the result of nephrocalcinosis. Potassium and magnesium wasting, proteinuria, decreased renal concentrating ability, renal tubular acidosis, and hematuria also occur.[14,138] Strategies to reduce renal toxicity after amphotericin B include intravenous saline or magnesium and potassium supplementation.[23,67,96]

Lipid and colloidal formulations of amphotericin B attenuate the adverse effects associated with amphotericin B.[87] Here the amphotericin B is complexed with either a lipid or cholesteryl sulfate. Upon contact with a fungus, lipases are released to free the complexed amphotericin B, resulting in focused cell death.[97]

Other adverse effects reported after treatment with amphotericin B include normochromic, normocytic anemia; decreased erythropoietin release; respiratory insufficiency with infiltrates; and, rarely, dysrhythmias, tinnitus, thrombocytopenia, peripheral neuropathy, and leukopenia.[131,136,138]

Triazole and Imidazoles

Fluconazole

TABLE 46–5. Consequential Organ System Manifestations Associated with Antibiotics and Antifungals

Drug	Organ System Toxicity	Signs, Symptoms, Laboratory
Antibiotics		
Bacitracin	Immune	Hypersensitivity reactions
Clindamycin	Immune	Hypersensitivity reactions
	Gastrointestinal	Nausea, vomiting, diarrhea
	Nervous	Dizziness, headache, vertigo
Colistimethate (colistin sulfate)	Renal	Decreased function, acute tubular necrosis
	Nervous	Peripheral paresthesias, confusion, coma, seizures, neuromuscular blockade
Griseofulvin	Renal	Proteinuria, nephrosis
	Hepatic	Increased liver enzymes
	Gastrointestinal	Nausea, vomiting, diarrhea
	Immune	Granulocytopenia
	Other	Disulfiram reactions, increased porphyrins
Lincomycin	Gastrointestinal	Nausea, vomiting, diarrhea
	Immune	Hypersensitivity reactions
Metronidazole	Neurologic	Peripheral neuropathy, seizures
	Gastrointestinal	Nausea, vomiting
	Other	Disulfiram reactions
Nitrofurazone	Immune	Hypersensitivity reactions
	Other	Ointment contains polyethylene glycols (renal dysfunction)
Nitrofurantoin	Gastrointestinal	Nausea, vomiting, diarrhea
	Hepatic	Jaundice
	Immune	Rash; acute and chronic pulmonary hypersensitivity
	Neurologic	Peripheral neuropathy
Novobiocin	Immune	Skin rash
	Gastrointestinal	Nausea, vomiting, diarrhea
	Hematologic	Pancytopenia, hemolytic anemia
Polymyxin B sulfate	Neurologic	Muscle weakness, seizures
	Renal	Azotemia, proteinuria
Selenium sulfide	Cutaneous	Contact dermatitis
	Other	Selenium: hair loss (rare)
Silver sulfadiazine	Cutaneous	Contact dermatitis
	Hematologic	Anemia, aplastic anemia
Spectinomycin	Immune	Rash (rare)
Antifungals		
Benzoic acid	Gastrointestinal	Nausea, vomiting, diarrhea
Carbol-fuchsin solution (phenol/resorcinol/fuchsin)	Gastrointestinal	Nausea, vomiting, diarrhea
Gentian violet	Gastrointestinal	Nausea, vomiting, diarrhea
	Immune	Rarely rash
Nystatin	Gastrointestinal	Nausea, vomiting, diarrhea
Pradimicins (investigational)	Unknown	Unknown
Salicylic acid	Gastrointestinal and dermal	Higher concentrations are caustic
Undecylenic acid and undeclyenate salt	Gastrointestinal	Nausea, vomiting, diarrhea

Common triazole antifungals include fluconazole and itraconazole. Common imidazoles include clotrimazole, econazole, ketoconazole, and miconazole. Severe toxicity is not expected in the overdose setting. The majority of toxic effects seen after the use of these drugs result from their drug interactions. Fluconazole, itraconazole, ketoconazole, and miconazole competitively inhibit CYP3A4, the enzyme system responsible for the metabolism of many drugs. Clinically significant interactions are reported with many of the drugs listed in Chapter 11. Table 46–5 lists other organ system manifestations associated with antifungal agents and other antibiotics.

SUMMARY

Adverse effects attributable to antibiotics are largely related to chronic administration, although rarely, acute toxicity does occur. Acute toxic effects of antibiotics are more common after large intravenous administration, drug interactions, or iatrogenic overdose. Careful vigilance on the part of the healthcare provider will prevent the majority of acute toxic manifestations following antibiotic use.

REFERENCES

1. Abrams SM, Degnan TJ, Vinciguerra V: Marrow aplasia following topical application of chloramphenicol eye ointment. Arch Intern Med 1980;140:576–577.
2. Adams SL, Mathews J, Grammer LC: Drugs that may exacerbate myasthenia gravis. Ann Emerg Med 1984;13:532–538.
3. Akerlund B, Tynell E, Bratt G, et al: N-Acetylcysteine treatment and the rise of toxic reactions to trimethoprim-sulfamethoxazole in primary pneumocystis carinii prophylaxis in HIV-infected patients. J Infect 1997;35:143–147.
4. Ali NA, Al-Naama LM, Khalid LO: Haemolytic potential of three chemotherapeutic agents and aspirin in glucose-6-phosphate dehydrogenase deficiency. East Mediterr Health J 1999;5(3):457–464.
5. Ali MZ, Goetz MB: A meta-analysis of the relative efficacy and toxicity of single daily dosing versus multiple daily dosing of aminoglycosides. Clin Infect Dis 1997;24:796–809.
6. Anne S, Reisman RE: Risk of administering cephalosporin antibiotics to patients with history of penicillin allergy. Ann Allergy Asthma Immunol 1995;74:167–170.
7. Anonymous: Endotoxin-like reactions associated with intravenous gentamicin—California, 1998. MMWR Morb Mortal Wkly Rep 1998;47(41):877–80.
8. Appel GB, Given DB, Levine LR, et al: Vancomycin and the kidney. Am J Kidney Dis 1986;8:75–80.
9. Appel GB: Aminoglycoside nephrotoxicity. Am J Med 1990;88 (Suppl 3C):16S–20S.
10. Arcieri GM, Becker N, Esposito B, et al: Safety of intravenous ciprofloxacin. Am J Med 1989;87(Suppl 5A):92S–97S.
11. Backon J: Hoigne's syndrome: Relevance of anomalous dominance and prostaglandins [letter]. Am J Dis Child 1986;140:1091–1092.
12. Bailie GR, Yu R, Morton R, Waldek S: Vancomycin, red neck syndrome and fits. Lancet 1985;2:279–280.
13. Balso BA, Pham NH: Invited review: Structure-activity studies on drug-induced anaphylactic reactions. Chem Res Toxicol 1994;7:703–721.
14. Barton CH, Pahl M, Vaziri ND: Renal magnesium wasting associated with amphotericin B therapy. Am J Med 1984;77:471–474.
15. Baumann G, Loher U, Felix SB, et al: Deleterious effects of cimetidine in the presence of histamine on coronary circulation. Res Exp Med 1982;180:209–213.

16. Bergeron L, Boucher FD: Possible red-man syndrome associated with systemic absorption of oral vancomycin in a child with normal renal function. Ann Pharmacother 1994;28:581–584.

17. Berkovitch M, Pastuszak A, Gazarian M, et al: Safety of the new quinolones in pregnancy. Obstet Gynecol 1994;84:535–538.

18. Berry M, Gurung A, Easty DL: Toxicity of antibiotics and antifungals on cultured human corneal cells: Effect of mixing, exposure and concentration. Eye 1995;9:110–115.

19. Best CJ, Ewart M, Sumner E: Perioperative complications following the use of vancomycin during anaesthesia: Two clinical reports. Br J Anaesth 1989;62:567–577.

20. Blandana P, Brunelleschi S, Fantozzi R, et al: The antianaphylactic action of histamine H2-receptor agonists in the guinea pig isolated heart. Br J Pharmacol 1987;90:459–466.

21. Borgna-Pignatti C: Fatal ceftriaxone-induced hemolysis in a child with acquired immunodeficiency syndrome. Pediatr Infect Dis J 1995;14:1116–1117.

22. Bovino JA, Marcus DF: The mechanism of transient myopia induced by sulfonamide therapy. Am J Ophthalmol 1982;94:99–102.

23. Branch RA: Prevention of amphotericin B-induced renal impairment. Arch Intern Med 1988;148:2389–2394.

24. Brandriss MW, Richardson WS, Barold SS: Erythromycin-induced QT prolongation and polymorphic ventricular tachycardia (torsades de pointes): Case report and review. Clin Infect Dis 1994;18:995–998.

25. Brent J, Hunt M, Kulig K, Rumack B: Amphotericin B overdoses in infants: Is there a role for exchange transfusion? Vet Hum Toxicol 1990;32:124–125.

26. Brozanski BS, Scher MS, Albright AL: Intraventricular nafcillin-induced seizures in a neonate. Pediatr Neurol 1988;4:188–190.

27. Brummett RE, Traynor J, Brown R, Himes D: Cochlear damage resulting from kanamycin and furosemide. Acta Otolaryngol (Stockh) 1975;80:86–92.

28. Brummett RE: Ototoxic liability of erythromycin and analogues. Otolaryngol Clin North Am 1993;26:811–819.

29. Bryant SG, Fisher S, Kluge RM: Increased frequency of doxycycline side effects. Pharmacotherapy 1987;7:125–129.

30. Bryceson ADM: Clinical pathology of the Jarisch-Herxheimer reaction. J Infect Dis 1976;133:696–704.

31. Buening MK, Wold JS, Israel KS, Kammer RB: Disulfiram-like reaction to beta-lactams. JAMA 1980;245:2027–2028.

32. Burdge DR, Nakielna EM, Rabin HR: Photosensitivity associated with ciprofloxacin use in adult patients with cystic fibrosis [letter]. Antimicrob Agents Chemother 1995;39:793.

33. Buring JE, Evans DA, Mayrent SL, et al: Randomized trials of aminoglycoside antibiotics: Quantitative overview. Rev Infect Dis 1988;10:951–957.

34. Burkhardt JE, Hill MA, Lamar CH, et al: Effects of difloxacin on the metabolism of glycosaminoglycans and collagen in organ cultures of articular cartilage. Fundam Appl Toxicol 1993;20:257–263.

35. Bussey HI, Knodel LC, Boyle DA: Warfarin-erythromycin interaction. Arch Intern Med 1985;145:1736–1737.

36. Butler WT, Bennett JE, Hill GJ, et al: Electrocardiographic and electrolyte abnormalities caused by amphotericin B in dog and man. Proc Soc Exp Biol Med 1964;116:857–863.

37. Calandra GB, Wang C, Aziz M, Brown KR: The safety profile of imipenem/cilastatin: Worldwide experience base on 3,470 patients. J Antimicrob Chemother 1986;18(Suppl E):193–202.

38. Carson JL, Strom BL, Duff A, et al: Acute liver disease associated with erythromycins, sulfonamides, and tetracyclines. Ann Intern Med 1993;119:576–583.

39. Castell DO, Sparks HA: Nephrogenic diabetes insipidus due to demethylchlortetracycline hydrochloride. JAMA 1965;193:237.

40. Chawla A, Kahn E, Yunis EJ, Daum F: Rapidly progressive cholestasis: An unusual reaction to amoxicillin/clavulanic acid therapy in a child. J Pediatr 2000;136:121–123.

41. Chen JH, Wiener L, Distenfeld A: Immunologic thrombocytopenia. N Y State J Med 1980;80:1134–1135.

42. Chen HJ, Bloch KL, Maclean JA: Acute eosinophilic hepatitis from trovafloxacin [letter]. N Engl J Med 2000;342:359–360.

43. Christie DJ, Van Buren N, Lennon SS, et al: Vancomycin-dependent antibodies associated with thrombocytopenia and refractoriness to platelet transfusion in patients with leukemia. Blood 1990;75:518–525.

44. Chusil S, Tungsanga K, Wathanavaha A, Pansin P: Hypouricemia, hypokalemia, proximal and distal tubular acidification defect following administration of outdated tetracycline: A case report. J Med Assoc Thai 1994;77:98–102.

45. Cleary JD, Hayman J, Sherwood J, et al: Amphotericin B overdose in pediatric patients with associated cardiac arrest. Ann Pharmacother 1993;27:715–719.

46. Cocke JG, Brown RE, Geppert LJ: Optic neuritis with prolonged use of chloramphenicol. J Pediatr 1966;68:27–31.

47. Cohen LS, Wechsler AS, Mitchell JH, Glick G: Depression of cardiac function by streptomycin and other antimicrobial agents. Am J Cardiol 1970;26:505–511.

48. Connor JP, Curry JM, Selby TL, Perlmutter AD: Acute renal failure secondary to ciprofloxacin use. J Urol 1994;154:975–976.

49. Covinsky JO: Aminoglycoside-induced electrolyte imbalance. Hosp Ther 1986;5:17–29.

50. Cummings JL, Barritt CF, Horan M: Delusions induced by procaine penicillin: Case report and review of the syndrome. Int J Psychiatry Med 1986–1987;16:163–168.

51. Danan G, Descatoire V, Pessayre D: Self-induction of erythromycin by its own transformation into a metabolite forming an inactive complex with reduced cytochrome P-450. J Pharmacol Exp Ther 1989;250:746–751.

52. Danisovicova A, Brezina M, Belan S, et al: Magnetic resonance imaging in children receiving quinolones: No evidence of quinolone-induced arthropathy. A multicenter survey. Chemotherapy 1994;40:209–214.

53. De Boer T, Stoof JC, Van Duyn H: Effect of penicillin on neurotransmitter release from rat cortical tissue. Brain Res 1980;192:296–300.

54. Demolis JL, Charransol A, Funck-Brentano C, Jaillon P: Effects of a single oral dose of sparfloxacin on ventricular repolarization in healthy volunteers. Br J Clin Pharmacol 1996;41:499–503.

55. De Sarro A, Ammendola D, De Sarro G: Effects of some quinolones on imipenem-induced seizures in DBA/2 mice. Gen Pharmacol 1994;25:369–379.

56. De Sarro G, Nava F, Calapai G, et al: Effects of some excitatory amino acid antagonists and drugs enhancing gamma-amino butyric acid neurotransmission on pefloxacin-induced seizures in DBA/2 mice. Antimicrob Agents Chemother 1997;41:427–434.

57. DeSoto H: Cimetidine in anaphylactic shock refractory to standard therapy. Anesth Analg 1989;69:260–269.

58. Domen RE, Horowitz S: Vancomycin-induced neutropenia associated with anti-granulocyte antibodies. Immunohematology 1990;6:41–43.

59. Drici MD, Knollmann BC, Wang WX, Woosley RL: Cardiac actions of erythromycin: Influence of female sex. JAMA 1998;280:1774–1776.

60. Dunn RJ: Massive sulfasalazine and paracetamol ingestion causing acidosis, hyperglycemia, coagulopathy and methemoglobinemia. J Toxicol Clin Toxicol 1998;36:239–242.

61. Durosinmi MA, Ajayi AA: A prospective study of chloramphenicol-induced aplastic anaemia in Nigerians. Trop Geographic Med 1993;45:159–161.

62. Dylewski J: Irreversible sensorineural hearing loss due to erythromycin. Can Med Assoc J 1988;139:230–231.

63. Ehmann WC: Cephalosporin-induced hemolysis: A case report and review of the literature. Am J Hematol 1992;40:121–125.

64. English J, Gilbert DN, Kohlhepp S, et al: Attenuation of experimental tobramycin nephrotoxicity by ticarcillin. Antimicrob Agents Chemother 1985;27:897–902.

65. Fang CC, Wang HP, Lin JT: Erythromycin-induced acute pancreatitis. J Toxicol Clin Toxicol 1996;34:93–95.

66. Fee WE: Aminoglycoside ototoxicity in the human. Laryngoscope 1980;90(Suppl 24):1–19.

67. Fisher MA, Talbot GH, Maislin G, et al: Risk factors for amphotericin B associated nephrotoxicity. Am J Med 1989;87:547–552.

68. French MA, Cerra FB, Plaut ME, Schentag JJ: Amikacin and gentamicin accumulation pharmacokinetics and nephrotoxicity in critically ill patients. Antimicrob Agents Chemother 1981;19:147–152.

69. Freundlich M, Cynamon H, Tames A, et al: Management of chloramphenicol intoxication in infancy by charcoal hemoperfusion. J Pediatr 1983;103:485–487.

70. Fripp RR, Carter MC, Werner JC: Cardiac function and acute chloramphenicol toxicity. J Pediatr 1983;103:487–490.

71. Fuchs S, Simon Z, Brezis M: Fatal hepatic failure associated with ciprofloxacin [letter]. Lancet 1994;343:738–739.

72. Fuguay D, Koup J, Smith AL: Management of neonatal gentamicin overdose. J Pediatr 1981;99:473–476.

73. Galpin JE, Chow AW, Yoshikawa TT, Guze LB: Pseudoanaphylactic reactions for inadvertent infusion of procaine penicillin G. Ann Intern Med 1974;81:358–359.

74. Garica RLA, Stricker BH, Zimmerman HJ: Risk of acute liver injury associated with the combination of amoxicillin and clavulanic acid. Arch Intern Med 1996;156:1327–1332.

75. Garratty G: Immune cytopenia associated with antibiotics. Transfus Med Rev 1993;7:255–267.

76. Garrelts JC, Peterie JD: Vancomycin and the "red man's syndrome" [letter]. N Engl J Med 1985;312:245.

77. Gerald MD, Massey J, Spadoro DC: Comparative convulsant activity of various penicillins after intracerebral injection in mice. Pharmacology 1973;25:104–106.

78. Gigliotti F, Shenep JL, Lott L, et al: Induction of prostaglandin synthesis as the mechanism responsible for the chills and fever produced by infusing amphotericin B. J Infect Dis 1987;156:784–789.

79. Gilbert FI Jr: Cholestatic hepatitis caused by esters of erythromycin and oleandomycin 1962 (classical article). Hawaii Med J 1995;54:603–605.

80. Glazko AJ: Identification of chloramphenicol metabolites and some factors affecting metabolic disposition. Antimicrob Agents Chemother 1966;6:655–665.

81. Gonzolez CP, Huidobro ML, Zabala AP, Vicente EM: Fatal subfulminant hepatic failure with ofloxacin [letter]. Am J Gastroenterol 2000;95:1606.

82. Gordon G, Sparano BM, Iatripoulos MJ: Hyperpigmentation of the skin associated with minocycline therapy. Arch Dermatol 1985;121:618–623.

83. Goss JE, Ramo BW, Blake K: Torsades de pointes associated with astemizole (Hismanal) therapy [letter]. Arch Intern Med 1993;153:2705.

84. Green RL, Lewis JE, Kraus ST, et al: Elevated plasma procaine concentration after administration of procaine penicillin G. N Engl J Med 1979;291:223–226.

85. Goss TF, Walawander CA, Grasela TH, et al: Prospective evaluation of risk factors for antibiotic-associated bleeding in critically ill patients. Pharmacotherapy 1992;12:283–291.

86. Guharoy SR: Serum sickness secondary to ciprofloxacin use. Vet Hum Toxicol 1994;36:540–541.

87. Gurwith M, Mamelok R, Pietrelli L, DuMond C: Renal sparing by amphotericin B colloidal dispersion: Clinical experience in 572 patients. Chemotherapy 1999;45(Suppl 1):39–47.

88. Gutnick MJ, Van Duijn H, Citri N: Relative convulsant potencies of structural analogs of penicillin. Brain Res 1976;114:139–143.

89. Haefeli WE, Schoenberger RA, Weiss PH, Ritz R: Possible risk for cardiac arrhythmias related to intravenous erythromycin. Intensive Care Med 1992;18:469–473.

90. Hall DR, McGibbin DH, Evans CC, et al: Gentamycin, tubocurarine, lignocaine, and neuromuscular blockade. Br J Anaesth 1972;44:1329–1331.

91. Harvey SC, Li X, Skolnick P, Kirst HA: The antibacterial and NMDA receptor activating properties of aminoglycosides are dissociable. Eur J Pharmacol 2000;387:1–7.

92. Hautekeete ML, Kockx MM, Naegels S, et al: Cholestatic hepatitis related to quinolones: A report of two cases. J Hepatol 1995;23:759–760.

93. Healy DP, Polk RE, Garson ML, et al: Comparison of steady-state pharmacokinetics of two dosage regimens of vancomycin in normal volunteers. Antimicrob Agents Chemother 1987;31:393–397.

94. Healy DP, Sahai JV, Fuller SH, Polk RE. Vancomycin-induced histamine release and "red mans syndrome": Comparison of 1- and 2-hour infusions. Antimicrob Agents Chemother 1990;34:550–554.

95. Hedrick R, Williams F, Morin R, et al: Carbamazepine-erythromycin interaction leading to carbamazepine toxicity in four epileptic children. Ther Drug Monit 1983;5:405–407.

96. Heidemann HT, Gerkens JF, Spickard WA, et al: Amphotericin B nephrotoxicity in humans decreased by salt repletion. Am J Med 1983;75:476–481.

97. Hiemenz JW, Walsh TJ: Lipid formulation of amphotericin B: Recent progress and future directions. Clin Infect Dis 1996;22:S133–S144.

98. Heye N, Dunne JW: Jarisch-Herxheimer reaction in a patient with neurosyphilis: Non-convulsive status epilepticus [letter]? J Neurol Neurosurg Psychiatry 1995;58:521.

99. Ho PW, Pien FD, Koninami N: Massive amikacin overdose. Ann Intern Med 1979;91:227–228.

100. Honig PK, Woolsley RL, Zamani K, et al: Changes in the pharmacokinetics and electrocardiographic pharmacodynamics of terfenadine with concomitant administration of erythromycin. Clin Pharmacol Ther 1992;52:231–238.

101. Hootkins R, Fenves AZ, Stephens MK: Acute renal failure secondary to oral ciprofloxacin therapy: A presentation of three cases and a review of the literature. Clin Nephrol 1989;32:75–78.

102. Hughes DW: Studies on chloramphenicol II. Possible determinants and progress of hemopoietic toxicity during chloramphenicol therapy. Med J Aust 1973;2:1142–1146.

103. Hughes DW: Studies on chloramphenicol I. Assessment of hemopoietic toxicity. Med J Aust 1968;2:436–438.

104. Humes HD: Aminoglycoside nephrotoxicity. Kidney Int 1988;33:900–901.

105. Hunt CM, Washington K: Tetracycline-induced bile duct paucity and prolonged cholestasis. Gastroenterology 1994;107:1844–1847.

106. Ilechukwu STC: Acute psychotic reactions and stress response syndromes following intramuscular aqueous procaine penicillin. Br J Psychiatry 1990;156:554–559.

107. Inman WH, Rawson NS: Erythromycin estolate and jaundice. Br Med J 1983;286:1954–1955.

108. Jackson TL, Williamson TH: Amikacin retinal toxicity [letter]. Br J Ophthalmol 1999;83:1199–1200.

109. Jaillon P, Morganroth J, Brumpt I, Talbot G: Overview of the electrocardiographic and cardiovascular safety data for sparfloxacin. Sparfloxacin safety group. J Antimicrob Chemother 1996;37(Suppl A):161–167.

110. Jalbert EO: Seizures after penicillin administration [letter]. Am J Dis Child 1985;139:1075.

111. Jawad ASM: Cystic fibrosis and drug induced arthropathy. Br J Rheumatol 1989;28:179–180.

112. Joy RJT, Scalettar R, Sodee DB: Optic and peripheral neuritis. Probable effect of prolonged chloramphenicol therapy. JAMA 1960;173:1731–1734.

113. Kaloyanides GJ: Renal pharmacology of aminoglycoside antibiotics. In: Bianchi C, Bertelli A, Duarte CG, eds: Contributions to Nephrology 42, Drug-Induced Nephrotoxicity. Basel, Karger, 1984, pp. 148–167.

114. Kearns OL, Wheeler JO, Childress SH, Letzig LU: Serum sickness-like reactions to cefaclor: Role of hepatic metabolism and individual susceptibility. J Pediatr 1994;125:805–811.

115. Kessler DL, Smith AL, Woodrum DE: Chloramphenicol toxicity in a neonate treated with exchange transfusion. J Pediatr 1980;96: 140–141.

116. Koegel L: Ototoxicity: A contemporary review of aminoglycosides, loop diuretics, acetylsalicylic acid, quinine, erythromycin, and cisplatinum. Am J Otol 1985;6:190–199.

117. Koren G, Barzilay Z, Greenwald M: Tenfold errors in administration of drug doses: A neglected iatrogenic disease in pediatrics. Pediatrics 1986;77:848–849.

118. Koren G, Lau A, Kenyon CF, et al: Clinical course and pharmacokinetics following a massive overdose of amphotericin B in a neonate. J Toxicol Clin Toxicol 1990;28:371–378.

119. Kristof RA, Clusmann H, Koehler W, et al: Treatment of accidental high-dose intraventricular mezlocillin application by cerebrospinal fluid exchange. J Neurol Neurosurg Psychiatry 1998;64:379–381.

120. Kubo Y, Nonaka S, Yoshida H: Contact sensitivity to chloramphenicol. Contact Dermatitis 1987;17:245–247.

121. Kucukguclu S, Tuncok Y, Ozkan H, et al: Multiple-dose activated charcoal in an accidental vancomycin overdose. J Toxicol Clin Toxicol 1996;34:83–87.

122. Kumar A, Dada T: Preretinal hemorrhages: An unusual manifestation of intravitreal amikacin toxicity. Aust N Z J Ophthalmol 1999; 27:435–436.

123. Labowitz JK, Silverman WB: Cholestatic jaundice induced by ciprofloxacin. Dig Dis Sci 1997;42:192–194.

124. Lehmann DF, Liu A, Newman N, Blair DC: The association of opportunistic infections with the occurrence of trimethoprim/sulfamethoxazole hypersensitivity in patients infected with human immunodeficiency virus. J Clin Pharmacol 1999;39:533–537.

125. Leo RJ, Ballow CH: Seizure activity associated with imipenem use: Clinical case reports and review of the literature. Ann Pharmacother 1991;25:351–354.

126. Levin G, Behrenth E: Irreversible ototoxic effect of erythromycin. Scand Audiol 1986;15:41–42.

127. Levine PH, Regelson W, Holland JF: Chloramphenicol-associated encephalopathy. Clin Pharmacol Ther 1970;11:194–199.

128. Levy JH, Kettlekamp N, Goertz P, et al: Histamine release by vancomycin: A mechanism for hypotension in man. Anaesthesia 1987;67:122–125.

129. Limauro DL, Chan-Tompkins NH, Carter RW, et al: Amoxicillin/clavulanate-associated hepatic failure with progression to Stevens-Johnson syndrome. Ann Pharmacother 1999;33:560–564.

130. Lin RY, Curry A, Pesola GR, et al: Improved outcomes in patients with acute allergic syndromes who are treated with combined H1 and H2 antagonists. Ann Emerg Med 2000;36:462–468.

131. Lin AC, Goldwasser E, Bernard EM, et al: Amphotericin B blunts erythropoietin response to anemia. J Infect Dis 1990;161:348–351.

132. Lopez A, Bernado B, Lopez-Herce J, et al: Methaemoglobinaemia secondary to treatment with trimethoprim and sulfamethoxazole associated with inhaled nitric oxide [letter]. Acta Paediatrica 1999;88: 915–916.

133. Lowery N, Kearns GL, Young RA, Wheeler JG: Serum sickness-like reactions associated with cefprozil therapy. J Pediatr 1994;125: 325–328.

134. Lu CMC, James SH, Lien YHH: Acute massive gentamicin intoxication in a patient with end-stage renal disease. Am J Kidney Dis 1996;28:767–771.

135. Lucena MI, Andrake RJ, Rodrigo L, et al: Trovafloxacin-induced acute hepatitis. Clin Infect Dis 2000;30:400–401.

136. MacGregor RR, Bennett JE, Erslev AJ: Erythropoietin concentration in amphotericin B induced anemia. Antimicrob Agents Chemother 1978;14:270–273.

137. MacNeil M, Haase DA, Tremaine R, Marrie TJ: Fever, lymphadenopathy, eosinophilia, lymphocytosis, hepatitis and dermatitis: A severe adverse reaction to minocycline. J Am Acad Dermatol 1997;36:347–350.

138. Maddux MS, Barriere SL: A review of complications of amphotericin therapy: Recommendations for prevention and management. DICP 1980;14:177–180.

139. Malone JD, Lebar RD, Hilder R: Procaine-induced seizures after intramuscular procaine penicillin G. Mil Med 1988;153:191–192.

140. Matsubara T, Otsubo S, Ogawa A, et al: Effects of beta-lactam antibiotics and N-methyltetrazolethiol on the alcohol-metabolizing system in rats. Jpn J Pharmacol 1987;45:303–315.

141. Mattle H, Craig WA, Pechere PC: Determinants of efficacy and toxicity of aminoglycosides. J Antimicrob Chemother 1989;24:281–293.

142. Mauer SM, Chavers BM, Kjellstrand CM: Treatment of an infant with severe chloramphenicol intoxication using charcoal-column hemoperfusion. J Pediatr 1980;96:136–139.

143. Mayumi H, Kimura S, Asano M, et al: Intravenous cimetidine as an effective treatment for systemic anaphylaxis and acute allergic skin reactions. Ann Allergy 1987;58:447–450.

144. Meislin HW, Bremer JC: Jarisch-Herxheimer reaction case report. JACEP 1976;5:779–781.

145. Moore RD, Lietman PS, Smith CR: Clinical response to aminoglycoside therapy: Importance of the ratio of peak concentration to minimal inhibitory concentration. J Infect Dis 1987;155:93–99.

146. Moore RD, Smith CR, Lietman PS: Risk factors for the development of auditory toxicity in patients receiving aminoglycosides. J Infect Dis 1984;149:23–30.

147. Moore RD, Smith CR, Lipsky JJ, et al: Risk factors for nephrotoxicity in patients treated with aminoglycosides. Ann Intern Med 1984; 100:352–357.

148. Mulhall A, deLouvois J, Hurley R: Chloramphenicol toxicity in neonates: Its incidence and prevention. Br Med J 1983;287: 1424–1427.

149. Mulhall JP, Bergmann LS: Ciprofloxacin-induced acute psychosis. Urology 1995;46:102–103.

150. Murray KM, Keane WR: Review of drug-induced acute interstitial nephritis. Pharmacotherapy 1992;12:462–467.

151. Murray KM, Wilson MG: Suspected ciprofloxacin-induced interstitial nephritis. DICP 1990;24:379–380.

152. Nahtha MC: Lack of predictability of chloramphenicol toxicity in pediatric patients. J Clin Pharmacol Ther 1989;14:297–303.

153. Nahtha MC: Serum concentrations and adverse effects of chloramphenicol in pediatric patients. Chemotherapy 1987;33:322–327.

154. Naisbitt DJ, Hough SJ, Gill HJ, et al: Cellular deposition of sulphamethoxazole and its metabolites: Implications for hypersensitivity. Br J Pharmacol 1999;126:1393–1407.

155. Nathani MG, Mutchnick MG, Tynes DJ, Ehrinpreis MN: An unusual case of amoxicillin/clavulanic acid-related hepatotoxicity. Am J Gastroenterol 1998;93:1363–1365.

156. Nattel S, Ranger S, Talajic M, et al: Erythromycin-induced prolonged QT syndrome: Concordance with quinidine and underlying cellular electrophysiologic mechanism. Am J Med 1990;89: 235–238.

157. Newfield P, Roizen MF: Hazards of rapid administration of vancomycin. Ann Intern Med 1979;91:58.

158. Nishidi I, Takumida M: Attenuation of aminoglycoside ototoxicity by glutathione. ORL J Otorhinolaryngol Relat Spec 1996;58:68–73.

159. Nordt SP, Williams SR, Manoguerra AS, Clark RF: Clarithromycin induced digoxin toxicity. J Accident Emerg Med 1998;15:194–195.

160. Obata H, Lizuka B, Uchida K: Pathogenesis of hypoprothrombinemia induced by antibiotics. J Nutr Sci Vitaminol (Tokyo) 1992; S13–S15:421–424.

161. Oberg KC, Bauman JL: QT prolongation and torsades de pointes due to erythromycin lactobionate. Pharmacotherapy 1995;15:687–692.

162. O'Sullivan TL, Ruffing MJ, Lamp KC, et al: Prospective evaluation of red man syndrome in patients receiving vancomycin. J Infect Dis 1993;168:773–776.

163. Paradelis AG: Aminoglycoside antibiotics and neuromuscular blockade. J Antimicrob Chemother 1979;5:737–738.

164. Paris DG, Parente TF, Bruschetta HR, et al: Torsades de pointes induced by erythromycin and terfenadine. Am J Emerg Med 1994; 12:636–638.

165. Park SY, Parker RH: Review of imipenem. Infect Control 1986; 7:333–337.

166. Patterson LJ, Milne B: Latex anaphylaxis causing heart block: Role of ranitidine. Can J Anesth 1999;46:776–778.

167. Pestotnik SL, Classen DC, Evans RS, et al: Prospective surveillance of imipenem/cilastatin use and associated seizures using a hospital information system. Ann Pharmacother 1993;27:497–501.

168. Phelps SJ, Tsiu W, Barrett FF, et al: Chloramphenicol-induced cardiovascular collapse in an anephric patient. Pediatr Infect Dis J 1987; 6:285–288.

169. Picrfitte C, Gillet P, Royer RJ: More on fluoroquinolone antibiotics and tendon rupture [letter]. N Engl J Med 1995;332(3):193.

170. Pimiento PA, Martinez GM, Mena MA, et al: Aztreonam and ceftazidime: Evidence of in vivo cross allergenicity. Allergy 1998;53: 624–625.

171. Polk RE, Israel D, Wang J, et al: Vancomycin skin tests and prediction of "red man syndrome" in healthy volunteers. Antimicrob Agents Chemother 1993;37:2139–2143.

172. Prazic M, Salaj B, Sunotic R: Familial sensitivity to streptomycin. J Laryngol Otol 1964;78:1037–1043.

173. Ptachainski RJ, Carpenter BJ, Burckart GJ, et al: Effect of erythromycin on cyclosporine levels [letter]. N Engl J Med 1985;313: 1416–1417.

174. Ramilo O, Kinane BT, McCracken GH: Chloramphenicol neurotoxicity. Pediatr Infect Dis J 1988;7:358–359.

175. Regan TJ, Khan MI, Olde IHA, Passannant AJ: Antibiotic effect on myocardial K transport and the production of ventricular tachycardia [abstract]. J Clin Invest 1969;48:66A.

176. Renz CL, Thurn JD, Finn HA, et al: Antihistamine prophylaxis permits rapid vancomycin infusion. Crit Care Med 1999;27:1732–1737.

177. Richardet JP, Mallat A, Zafrani ES, et al: Prolonged cholestasis with ductopenia after administration of amoxicillin/clavulanic acid. Dig Dis Sci 1999;44:1997–2000.

178. Riley HD Jr: Vancomycin and novobiocin. Med Clin North Am 1970;54:1277–1289.

179. Rippelmeyer DJ, Synhavsky A: Ciprofloxacin and allergic interstitial nephritis [letter]. Ann Intern Med 1988;109:170.

180. Rockwood RP, Embardo LS: Theophylline, ciprofloxacin, erythromycin: A potentially harmful regimen [letter]. Ann Pharmacother 1993;27:651–652.

181. Romero-Gomez M, Suarez GE, Fernandez MC: Norfloxacin-induced acute cholestatic hepatitis in a patient with alcoholic liver cirrhosis [letter]. Am J Gastroenterol 1999;94:2324–2325.

182. Rothenberg HJ: Anaphylactoid reaction to vancomycin. JAMA 1959;171:1101–1102.

183. Rubart M, Pressler ML, Pride HP, Zipes DP: Electrophysiological mechanisms in a canine model of erythromycin-associated long QT syndrome. Circulation 1993;88(pt 1):1832–1844.

184. Rudolph AH, Prince EV: Penicillin reactions among patients in venereal disease clinics: A national survey. JAMA 1973;223: 499–501.

185. Sacristan JA, Soto JA, deCos MA: Erythromycin-induced hypoacusis: 11 new cases and literature review. Ann Pharmacother 1993;27: 950–955.

186. Rybak MJ, Boike SC: Additive toxicity in patients receiving vancomycin and aminoglycosides [letter]. Clin Pharm 1983;2:508.

187. Sabra R, Takahashi K, Branch RA, Badr KF: Mechanisms of amphotericin B-induced reduction of glomerular filtration rate: A micropuncture study. J Pharmacol Exp Ther 1990;253:34–37.

188. Sage DJ: Management of acute anaphylactoid reactions. Int Anesthesiol Clin 1985;23(3):175–86.

189. Samaha FF: QTC interval prolongation and polymorphic ventricular tachycardia in association with levofloxacin [letter]. Am J Med 1999;107:528–529.

190. Saraway SM, Marke J, Steinberg M, et al: Doom anxiety and delirium in lidocaine toxicity. Am J Psychiatry 1987;144:159–163.

191. Saxon A, Swabb EA, Adkinson NF Jr: Investigation into the immunologic cross-reactivity of aztreonam with other beta lactam antibiotics. Am J Med 1985;78(Suppl A):19–26.

192. Sayawa BP, Weihprecht H, Cambell WR, et al: Direct vasoconstriction as a possible cause for amphotericin B-induced nephrotoxicity in rats. J Clin Invest 1991;87:2079–2107.

193. Schacht J: Biochemistry and pharmacology of aminoglycoside-induced hearing loss. Acta Physiol Pharmacol Ther Latinoam 1999; 49:251–256.

194. Schentag JJ, Plaut ME: Patterns of beta-2-microglobulin excretion in patients treated with aminoglycosides. Kidney Int 1980;16:654–661.

195. Schluter G: Ciprofloxacin: Review of potential toxicologic effects. Am J Med 1987;82(Suppl 4A):91–93.

196. Schmuck G, Schurmann A, Schluter G: Determination of the excitatory potencies of fluoroquinolones in the central nervous system by an in vitro model. Antimicrob Agents Chemother 1998;42: 1831–1836.

197. Schrodt BJ, Kulp-Shorten CL, Callen JP: Necrotizing vasculitis of the skin and uterine cervix associated with minocycline therapy for acne vulgaris. South Med J 1999;92:502–504.

198. Schweitzer VG, Olson NR: Ototoxic effect of erythromycin therapy. Arch Otolaryngol 1984;110:258–260.

199. Scott JL, Finegold SM, Belkins GA, et al: A controlled double-blind study of the hematologic toxicity of chloramphenicol. N Engl J Med 1965;272:1137.

200. Seamans KB, Gloor P, Dobell RAR, Wyant JD: Penicillin-induced seizures during cardiopulmonary bypass: A clinical and electroencephalographic study. N Engl J Med 1968;278:861–868.

201. Seldon R, Sasahara AA: Central nervous system toxicity induced by lidocaine. JAMA 1967;202:908–909.

202. Serdaru M, Diquet B, Lhermitte F: Generalized seizures after ampicillin [letter]. Lancet 1982;2:617–618.

203. Sha SH, Schacht J: Are aminoglycoside antibiotics excitotoxic? Neuroreport 1998;9:3893–3895.

204. Shapiro LE, Knowles SR, Shear: Comparative safety of tetracycline, minocycline and doxycycline. Arch Dermatol 1997;133:1224–1230.

205. Shu XO, Gao YT, Linet MS, et al: Chloramphenicol use and childhood leukaemia in Shanghai. Lancet 1987;2:934–937.

206. Silber T, D'Angelio L: Doom, anxiety, and Hoigne's syndrome [letter]. Am J Psychiatry 1987;144:1365.

207. Silber TJ, D'Angelio LJ: Panic attack following injection of aqueous procaine penicillin G (Hoigne's syndrome). J Pediatr 1985;107: 314–315.

208. Silvian C, Levillain P, Labat-Labourdette J, Beauchant M: Granulomatous hepatitis due to a combination of amoxicillin and clavulanic acid. Dig Dis Sci 1992;37:150–152.

209. Slaughter RL, Cerra FB, Koup JR: Effect of hemodialysis on total body clearance of chloramphenicol. Am J Hosp Pharm 1980;37(8): 1083–1086.

210. Slayton W, Anstine D, Lakhdir F, et al: Tetany in a child with AIDS receiving intravenous tobramycin. South Med J 1996;89:1108–1110.

211. Slavich IL, Gleffe RF, Haas EJ: Grand mal epileptic seizures during ciprofloxacin therapy. JAMA 1989;261:558–559.

212. Solomkin JS, Fant WK, Rivera JU, Alexander JW: Randomized clinical trial of imipenem/cilastatin versus gentamycin and clindamycin in mixed flora infections. Am J Med 1985;78(Suppl 6A):85–91.

213. Somer T, Finegold SM: Vasculitis associated with infections, immunization, and antimicrobial drugs. Clin Infect Dis 1995;20:1010–1036.

214. Song BB, Sha SH, Schacht J: Iron chelators protect from aminoglycoside-induced cochleo- and vestibulo-toxicity. Free Radic Biol Med 1998;25:189–195.

215. Stahlmann R, Lode H: Toxicity of quinolones. Drugs 1999;58(Suppl 2):37–42.

216. Stevens DC, Kleiman MB, Lietman PS, et al: Exchange transfusion in acute chloramphenicol toxicity. J Pediatr 1981;99:651–653.

217. Stupp H, Kupper K, Lagler F, et al: Inner ear concentrations and ototoxicity of different antibiotics in local and systemic application. Audiology 1973;12:350–363.

218. Sunagawa M, Matsumura H, Sumita Y, Nouda H: Structural features resulting in convulsive activity of carbapenem compounds: Effect of C-2 side chain. J Antibiot (Tokyo) 1995;48:408–416.

219. Swanson DJ, Sung RJ, Fine MJ, et al: Erythromycin ototoxicity: Prospective assessment with serum concentrations and audiograms in a study of patients with pneumonia. Am J Med 1992;92:61–68.

220. Takada S, Kato M, Takayama S: Comparison of lesions induced by intra-articular injections of quinolones and compounds damaging cartilage components in rat femoral condyles. J Toxicol Environ Health 1994;42:73–88.

221. Teitelbaum JE, Perez-Atayde AR, Cohen M, et al: Minocycline-related autoimmune hepatitis: case series and literature review. Arch Pediatr Adolesc Med 1998;152:1132–1136.

222. Thompson WL, Anderson SE Jr, Lipsky JJ, et al: Overdose of chloramphenicol. JAMA 1975;234:149–150.

223. Timmermans L: Influence of antibiotics on spermatogenesis. J Urol 1974;112:348–349.

224. Tsuji A, Sato H, Kume Y, et al: Inhibitory effects of quinolone antibacterial agents on gamma-aminobutyric acid binding to receptor sites in rat brain membranes. Antimicrob Agents Chemother 1988;32:190–194.

225. Turner WM: Lidocaine and psychotic reactions. Ann Intern Med 1982;97:149–150.

226. Tynes BS, Utz JP, Bennett JE, et al: Reducing amphotericin B reactions. Am Rev Resp Dis 1963;87:264–268.

227. Unal M, Peyman GA, Liang C, et al: Ocular toxicity of intravitreal clarithromycin. Retina 1999;19:442–446.

228. Utley PM, Lucas JB, Billings TE: Acute psychotic reactions to aqueous procaine penicillin. South Med J 1966;59:1271–1274.

229. Van Arsdel PP Jr: The risk of penicillin reactions. Ann Intern Med 1968;69:1071–1073.

230. Walker PD, Barri Y, Shah SV: Oxidant mechanisms in gentamycin nephrotoxicity. Ren Fail 1999;21:433–442.

231. Wallace KL: Antibiotic-induced convulsions. Med Toxicol 1997;13:741–762.

232. Wallace MR, Mascola JR, Oldfield EC 3rd: Red man syndrome: Incidence, etiology and prophylaxis. J Infect Dis 1991;164:1180–1185.

233. Walmsley SL, Winn LM, Harrison ML, et al: Oxidative stress and thiol depletion in plasma and peripheral blood lymphocytes from HIV-infected patients: Toxicological and pathological implications. AIDS 1997;11:1689–1697.

234. Warner WA, Sanders E: Neuromuscular blockade associated with gentamycin therapy. JAMA 1971;215:1153–1154.

235. Weisberger AS, Wessler S, Avioli LV: Mechanisms of action of chloramphenicol. JAMA 1969;209:97–103.

236. Welage LS, Borin MT, Wilton JH, et al: Comparative evaluation of the pharmacokinetics of N-methylthiotetrazole following administration of cefoperazone, cefotetan and cefmetazole. Antimicrob Agents Chemother 1990;34:2369–2374.

237. Westphal JF, Vetter D, Brogard JM: Hepatic side-effects of antibiotics. J Antimicrob Chemother 1994;33:387–401.

238. Wolf R, Brenner DS: An active amide group in the molecule of drugs that induce pemphigus: A casual or causal relationship? Dermatology 1994;189:1–4.

239. Yarbrough JA Moffitt JE, Brown DA, Stafford C: Cimetidine in the treatment of refractory anaphylaxis. Ann Allergy 1989;63:235–238.

240. Ying LS, Johnson CA: Ciprofloxacin-induced interstitial nephritis. Clin Pharm 1989;8:518–521.

241. Yunis AA: Chloramphenicol toxicity: 25 years of research. Am J Med 1989;87:3–44N–3–48N.

242. Yunis AA: Chloramphenicol-induced bone marrow suppression. Semin Hematol 1973;10:255–234.

243. Zager RA, Bredl CR, Schimpf BA: Direct amphotericin B-mediated tubular toxicity: Assessments of selected cytoprotective agents. Kidney Int 1992;42:1588–1594.

244. Zhou W, Moore DE: Photosensitizing activity of the anti-bacterial drugs sulfamethoxazole and trimentoprim. J Photochem Photobiol 1997;39:63–72.

245. Zifko U, Wimberger D, Volc B, Grisold W: Jarisch-Herxheimer reaction in a patient with neurosyphilis. J Neurol Neurosurg Psychiatry 1994;57:865–867.

CHAPTER *47* ANTINEOPLASTIC AGENTS

Richard Y. Wang / Paul Calabresi

A 70-year-old female was brought to the Emergency Department (ED) from an extended-care facility because of the sudden onset of epistaxis. Vital signs were blood pressure, 120/70 mm Hg; pulse, 100 beats/min; respiratory rate, 18 breaths/min; and temperature, 37°C (98.6°F). The patient stated that for the last 2 days she had dysphagia, progressive weakness, and intermittent shakes. The patient had a past medical history of rheumatoid arthritis and pulmonary emboli. The patient's medications include methotrexate (MTX) and Coumadin, which were both started in the last month for her underlying medical disorders. An anterior nasal packing was placed to stop the bleeding. Further examination of the oropharynx demonstrated several ulcers. The skin showed ecchymoses. Chest and abdominal findings were unremarkable. A large-bore IV line was established, and blood was drawn for complete blood count (CBC) with platelets, prothrombin time (PT), partial thromboplastin time (PTT), electrolytes, blood urea nitrogen (BUN), and creatinine. Blood was also sent for an MTX level and a type and cross-match. The CBC showed hemoglobin, 8 g/dL; white cell count, 2000/mm^3 (81% neutrophils, 13% lymphocytes, 1% monocytes, 5% eosinophils); platelet count, 3000/mm^3; prothrombin time, 16.5 seconds; and international normalized ratio (INR), 2.0. PTT and renal function were normal. The extended-care facility was contacted, and it was discovered that the patient was inadvertently administered methotrexate 2.5 mg qd instead of once a week for 1 month.

The patient was transfused with packed red blood cells, platelets, and fresh-frozen plasma. Prophylactic broad-spectrum antibiotics were initiated. Leucovorin 10 mg/m^2 was started and administered every 4 hours IV. The serum MTX was determined later to be zero, and leucovorin therapy was discontinued. The white blood cell count (WBC) was lowest on day 3 of hospitalization and rose thereafter.

Overdoses of antineoplastic medications are infrequent; however, they are of greater consequence than many other medications because of their narrow therapeutic margin.[160,217] From 1987 to 1999, 85% of the annual exposures to these agents that were reported to the American Association of Poison Control Centers Toxic Exposure Surveillance System (AAPCC TESS) were unintentional (Chap. 116 and page 1752) Twenty percent of all reported exposures resulted in moderate or severe symptoms.

A review of the 2819 orders for cytotoxic agents at a pharmacy satellite showed that 93 orders (3%) contained at least 1 error in the dosage regimen and 442 (16%) contained at least 1 error in the instructions for drug preparation.[87] Three of the errors in dosage regimen were classified as potentially lethal, 13 as serious, 5 as significant, and 72 as minor. Two of the potentially lethal overdoses of cisplatin were a result of errors in duration of administration (100 mg/m^2 for 3–4 consecutive days instead of for a single day). Lack of healthcare-provider familiarity with the agent and its dosing was a major cause of these events. In another study evaluating drug errors, 49% occurred at the ordering/prescribing stage. This was most commonly caused by physicians who lacked knowledge of the drug and of the intended patient.[155] Other areas in which errors occurred were during transcription and nurse administration. As more antineoplastic agents become available and their indications broaden, exposures will increase in number and frequency. In the last 10 years, the annual number of exposures reported to the AAPCC TESS increased 4-fold (Chap. 116 and page 1752).

Most antineoplastic agents can be grouped into one of these four categories: alkylating agents, antimetabolites, antimitotics, and antibiotics (Table 47–1). The antimetabolites are grouped by the substrates with which they interfere. They include pyrimidine, purine, and folic acid antagonists. Methotrexate is a folate antagonist, and other agents with similar but lesser toxicity include trimethoprim and pyrimethamine. The antimitotics include the plant alkaloids (eg, vinca, taxanes, and epipodophyllotoxins). These agents exert toxic effects by interrupting microtubule assembly. The antibiotic agents are isolated from bacteria and comprise the anthracyclines bleomycin, mitomycin, and dactinomycin. The alkylating agents are more commonly used than their counterparts and cause covalent binding to nucleic acids, which inhibits DNA activity. These agents include the nitrogen mustards, platinoids, and nitrosoureas. The antimetabolites and the alkylating agents are cell-cycle active, meaning they only affect cells undergoing cell division. Some agents are phase specific; that is, they affect the cell only at a period during cell division. Vincristine is M (mitotic)-phase specific and cytarabine is S (DNA replication)-phase specific. Because the majority of the cases of antineoplastic agent overdoses involve the mustards, cisplatin, methotrexate, vincristine, and mitoxantrone (related to the anthracyclines), this discussion focuses on these agents.

METHOTREXATE

Pharmacology

TABLE 47–1. **Classification of Antineoplastic Agents and Their Effects**

Class	Agent	Adverse Effects	Overdose
Alkylating	Busulphan	Hyperpigmentation, pulmonary fibrosis, hyperuricemia	
	Dacarbazine	Hypotension, transaminitis, flulike syndrome	
	Melphalan	Pulmonary fibrosis	
	Mustards		
	Chlorambucil, Cyclophosphamide, Ifosfamide, Mechlorethamine	Hemmorrhagic cystitis, encephalopathy, pulmonary fibrosis	Seizures, myocardial necrosis
	Nitrosoureas		
	Carmustine, Lomustine, Semustine	Pulmonary fibrosis, transaminitis, renal insufficiency	
	Platinoids		
	Cisplatin	Renal failure, peripheral neuropathy, hypomagnesemia, hypocalcemia, hyponatremia, ototoxicity	Seizures, encephalopathy, ototoxicity, retinal toxicity
	Carboplatin, Iproplatin	Myelosuppression, hypomagnesemia, hypocalcemia, hyponatremia	
	Procarbazine	MAOI activity	
	Thiotepa		
Antimetabolite	Hydroxyurea		
	Methotrexate	Mucositis, nausea, diarrhea, transaminitis	Mucositis, myelosuppression, renal failure
	Purine Analogues		
	Chlordeoxyadenosine		
	Fludarabine	Encephalopathy, muscle weakness	
	Mercaptopurine	Hyperuricemia, pancreatitis, cholestasis	
	Pentostatin	Transaminitis	
	Thioguanine	Hyperuricemia	
	Pyrimidine Analogues		
	Cytarabine	Acute lung injury, neuropathy, cerebellar ataxia	
	Fluorouracil	Cardiogenic shock, cardiomyopathy, neuropathy, cerebellar ataxia	
Antimitotic	Epipodophyllotoxin		
	Etoposide, Teniposide	CHF, hypotension	
	Paclitaxel	GI perforation, peripheral neuropathy, dysrhythmias	
	Vinca Alkaloids		
	Vinblastine, Vincristine, Vindesine	Peripheral neuropathy	Encephalopathy, seizures, autonomic instability, SIADH, paralytic ileus, myelosuppression
Antibiotics	Anthracyclines		
	Daunorubicin, Doxorubicin, Epirubicin, Idarubicin	Congestive cardiomyopathy	Dysrhythmias, CHF
	Bleomycin	Pulmonary fibrosis	
	Dactinomycin	Transaminitis	
	Mithramycin	Skin flushing	
	Mitomycin C	Hemolytic uremic syndrome	
	Mitoxantrone	Congestive cardiomyopathy	
Enzyme	L-Asparaginase	Hypersensitivity, pancreatitis	

MTX is an important therapy for a variety of cancers, such as non-Hodgkin lymphoma, lymphocytic leukemia, breast cancer, and small-cell lung carcinoma. Its immunosuppressive activity allows it to also be used for rheumatoid arthritis, organ transplantation, psoriasis, trophoblastic diseases, and therapeutic abortion.[50,131] MTX's therapeutic and toxic effects are based on its ability to limit DNA and RNA synthesis by inhibiting dihydrofolate reductase (DHFR) and thymidylate synthetase (Fig. 47–1). DHFR reduces folic acid to tetrahydrofolate (FH_4), which serves as an essential cofactor in the synthesis of purine nucleotides. These reduced folates are required by thymidylate synthetase to serve as methyl donors in the formation of thymidylate as well. Thymidylate is then used for DNA synthesis. MTX is a structural analogue of folate and competitively inhibits DHFR by binding to this substrate's site of action. This stops reduced folate production, which is necessary for nucleotide formation and DNA/RNA synthesis. Administration of the reduced folate (folinic acid or leucovorin) allows for continual purine synthesis despite a blocked DHFR.

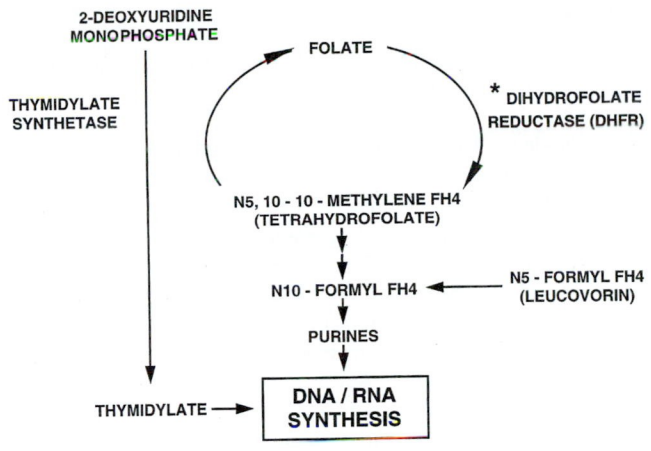

Figure 47–1. Mechanism of methotrexate (MTX) toxicity. MTX inhibits DHFR activity, which is necessary for DNA and RNA synthesis. Leucovorin bypasses blockade to allow for continued synthesis.

Leucovorin is used as an antidote or rescue agent to limit the toxic effects of high-dose methotrexate therapy.

The bioavailability of methotrexate appears to be limited by a saturable intestinal absorption mechanism. At doses less than 30 mg/m², the absorption is 90%; at doses greater than 80 mg/m², the absorption is less than 10–20%.[35] The weekly adult dose used for the treatment of psoriasis and rheumatoid arthritis is low (ie, 7.5–15 mg) and can be administered orally. The dose used to induce abortion is higher (50 mg/m² or 1 mg/kg) and must be administered parenterally to achieve effective drug concentrations. MTX dosing regimens for chemotherapy are variable, but can be generally classified as low dose—30–40 mg/m² IV every 1–3 weeks; moderate dose—250–500 mg/m² IV infusion every 2–3 weeks; and high dose—greater than 1000 mg/m² (or 20 mg/kg) infusion every 2–3 weeks. Conventional doses of up to 100 mg/m² can be administered without leucovorin rescue. Doses of 1000 mg/m² are considered potentially lethal. Much higher doses (eg, 2–3 g/m²) can be given when MTX is followed by leucovorin in order to prevent life-threatening toxicity. Mortality from high-dose MTX is about 6%, and occurs primarily when patients' MTX levels are not monitored.[84,239,259] Neurotoxicity may occur with high-dose therapy; however, the process reverses upon discontinuation of MTX treatment. The mechanisms remain unclear, but may be the result of direct toxicity to neuronal glial and endothelial cells and decreased neurotransmitter synthesis.[2]

MTX has a triphasic plasma clearance. The initial plasma distribution half-life is short—0.75 hours. The second half-life is 2–3.4 hours and represents renal clearance of the drug. The third phase has a half-life of about 8–10.4 hours and represents tissue redistribution into the plasma. This phase can be prolonged in the setting of renal failure and is associated with bone marrow and gastrointestinal (GI) toxicity. The kidneys eliminate 50–80% of MTX unchanged. At high doses, drug and insoluble drug metabolites—7-hydroxy methotrexate and 2,4-diamino-10-methyl pteroic acid—accumulate and may precipitate in the renal tubules, causing reversible acute tubular necrosis. MTX is one-tenth as soluble at a pH of 5.5 as it is at a pH of 7.5.[35,219] The serum concentration threshold for nephrotoxicity is 2.2 mmol/L at a urine pH of 5.5, and 22 mmol/L at a urine pH of 6.9. Acute renal failure may result

from drug precipitation in the renal tubule, and is most common in patients who are inadequately hydrated or not alkalinized.[3,90,133] The majority (90%) of MTX is excreted unchanged in the urine, within 48 hours, by both glomerular filtration and active tubular secretion. Folic acid blocks MTX renal reabsorption and can enhance drug elimination during leucovorin rescue.[117] A small amount of MTX is metabolized intracellularly to polyglutamate derivatives, which inhibit DHFR and are believed to be responsible for MTX's persistent cytotoxic effect.

Toxicity of MTX is dependent more on the duration of concentration than the dose itself. Thus, greater toxicity is expected from a 7 g IV dose administered over 48 hours than from a 20 g dose administered over 24 hours.[98] Patients with a plasma MTX concentration greater than 1.0 μmol/L at 48 hours posttreatment are considered at risk for bone marrow and gastrointestinal mucosal toxicity.[239] Risk factors for MTX toxicity are impaired renal function (primary route of drug elimination), third compartment spacing (eg, ascites, pleural effusions), use of nonsteroidal anti-inflammatory drugs (NSAIDs), age, folate deficiency, and concurrent infection.[239]

Clinical Manifestations

In the course of MTX therapy, a variety of disorders may occur, resulting from either increased patient susceptibility to toxicity or an excessive administration. The clinical manifestations of MTX toxicity include stomatitis, esophagitis, renal failure, and myelosuppression. Hepatitis and central neurologic system dysfunction may appear as well. In a group of 23 patients who received 45 courses of high-dose MTX therapy, the commonly observed signs included increased AST/ALT (81%), nausea and vomiting (66%), mucositis (33%), dermatitis (18%), leukopenia (11%), thrombocytopenia (9%), and creatinine elevation (7%).[204]

Nausea and vomiting, considered rare after low-dose therapy, typically begin 2–4 hours after high-dose therapy and last for about 6–12 hours. Mucositis, characterized by mouth soreness, stomatitis, or diarrhea, usually occurs 1–2 weeks after therapy and can last for 4–7 days. Other gastrointestinal symptoms resulting from MTX therapy include pharyngitis, anorexia, gastrointestinal hemorrhage, and toxic megacolon.[15] Hepatotoxicity, as described by increased AST (<1000), ALT (<1000), and hyperbilirubinemia, can be observed with both acute and chronic therapy.[172,185] It is usually associated with high-dosage regimens. Laboratory abnormalities improve within 1–2 weeks of discontinuation of MTX. The mechanism is not completely understood, but toxicity is attributed to reduced liver folate stores.[18] Factors associated with hepatotoxicity are sustained high plasma levels, cumulative dosages, chronic therapy, and host factors such as increase in age, obesity, diabetes, and alcoholism.[263]

Pancytopenia usually occurs within the first 2 weeks after an acute exposure. The CBC should be monitored on days 7, 10, and 14 because life-threatening complications, such as bleeding disorders and overwhelming sepsis, may occur.[152] There are several reports demonstrating the occurrence of pancytopenia in individuals receiving chronic low-dose MTX therapy for rheumatoid arthritis and psoriasis.[72,145,172,209] Leucovorin therapy may be beneficial in these instances, and has been recommended for treatment until the pancytopenia resolves and MTX is no longer detected in the serum.[166]

When used in small IV doses of 40–60 mg/m², MTX is not associated with appreciable nephrotoxicity. However, at doses greater than 5000 mg/m^2 (100 mg/kg), several investigators have reported severe kidney damage, with oliguria, azotemia, and fatal renal failure.[34] The renal function can normalize over time. Patients at risk for nephrotoxicity include the elderly, those with underlying renal disease (glomerular filtration rate [GFR] less than 50 mL/min), and those who receive concurrent drug therapy that can delay MTX excretion. This includes agents that reduce renal blood flow (eg, NSAIDs), that are nephrotoxic (eg, cisplatin, aminoglycoside), or that are weak organic acids (eg, salicylate, piperacillin).[125,239]

The neurologic complications associated with either high-dose systemic MTX therapy or intrathecal administration are the most consequential manifestations. The incidence of neurologic toxicity from high-dose MTX therapy is about 5–15%.[134] The manifestations usually occur from hours to days after the initiation of therapy and include hemiparesis, paraparesis, tetraparesis, seizures, and dysreflexia.[82,171,261] These events are reversible to varying degrees. Those that occur within several hours (usually within 12 hours) of therapy are attributed to chemical arachnoiditis from increased central nervous system MTX concentration. The clinical findings include meningismus, pleocytosis, and increased cerebrospinal fluid (CSF) protein concentration. The CSF may be assayed for MTX to confirm the exposure. The CSF MTX concentration is about 0.1 µmol/L and lasts for 48 hours after an IV MTX dose of 1500 mg/m^2, and 100 µmol/L for the peak therapeutic concentration for a 12 mg intrathecal MTX dose.[190] Magnetic resonance imaging (MRI) of the brain may demonstrate a high signal throughout the pachymeningeal region, which is consistent with a chemical meningitis.[91]

The onset of behavioral disorders and progressive dementia from months to years after treatment is associated with leukoencephalopathy, which is irreversible.[7] CSF analysis and computerized tomography of the brain may be normal or show demyelination of white matter (especially in the anterior and frontal lobes).[7] T2-weighted MRI scans of the brain of patients with leukoencephalopathy shows hyperintense lesions in the white matter area.[91] This is a similar finding in patients presenting with subacute neurologic symptoms following MTX therapy.[171] Patients presenting with meningismus or altered mental status following MTX therapy require an initial computed tomography (CT) scan of the brain and then CSF analysis for infection.[143] Leucovorin does not appear to limit or prevent MTX-induced neuropathy.

Management

In the event of an oral overdose of methotrexate, the initial concern should be gastrointestinal decontamination. Activated charcoal adsorbs methotrexate and should be administered as soon as possible to limit drug absorption.[92] The administration of multiple-dose activated charcoal and cholestyramine[82] can significantly decrease the elimination half-life of methotrexate by interrupting enterohepatic circulation.[92,104] This is of most benefit to patients with diminished renal creatinine clearance.

Adequate hydration with saline diuresis is also important to prevent renal failure in patients who receive inadvertent high doses. To prevent precipitation of drug and drug metabolites in the renal tubules, the urine should be alkalinized with sodium bicarbonate (to pH 7–8) as well.

Antidotes

Folinic acid (leucovorin, N-5-formyl-tetrahydrofolate) rescue therapy has allowed higher doses of methotrexate to be administered therapeutically, as leucovorin limits bone marrow and gastrointestinal toxicity. The effectiveness of leucovorin depends on the timing of administration and the dose (Fig. 47–2). Leucovorin is most beneficial when administered within 1 hour of exposure, but should still be given to patients as soon as possible after an excessive exposure, because the only complications associated with leucovorin administration are drug interactions[206] and hypersensitivity reactions.[119] Routine doses of leucovorin (eg, 15–25 mg/m^2) used for rescue therapy are inadequate for overdose situations[144] (Antidotes in Depth: Folinic Acid).

The initial leucovorin dose to be administered should achieve a plasma concentration equal to or greater than that of the MTX. In this manner, the reduced folate antidote can successfully compete with MTX for active transport sites on the cell membrane, displace MTX from its intracellular binding site, and, most importantly, restore reduced folate stores.[132,200] The lower doses of leucovorin used during MTX therapy are an attempt to protect normal body cells but not tumor cells. Under therapeutic circumstances it is recommended to delay leucovorin rescue as long as possible, administer the minimal effective dose, and discontinue therapy as soon as it is no longer necessary.[34]

Serum MTX levels should be monitored at 12, 24, and 48 hours postexposure so that leucovorin therapy can be adjusted ac-

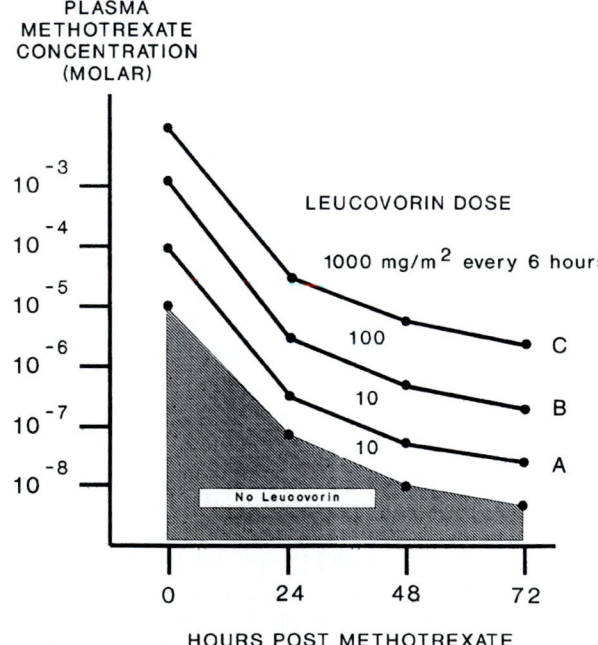

Figure 47–2. Leucovorin rescue nomogram for methotrexate toxicity. Shaded area = MTX levels observed after doses <60 mg/m^2; leucovorin is usually not required. Up to curve B requires 10 mg/m^2 of leucovorin per dose every 6 hours until the MTX level is $<1 \times 10^7$ M. Up to curve C requires 100 mg/m^2 per dose. *(Reprinted, with permission, from Young LY, Koda-Kimble MA, eds: Applied Therapeutics: The Clinical Use of Drugs, 4th ed. Vancouver, WA, Applied Therapeutics, Inc., 1988.)*

cordingly (Fig. 47–2). Generally, leucovorin therapy is continued if the plasma MTX level is above 1.0 μmol/L at 48 hours postexposure,[239] and maintained until the level is below 0.1 μmol/L in patients undergoing chemotherapy.[248] However, for patients without cancer, the leucovorin therapy should be continued until the MTX level is less than 0.01 μmol/L because DNA synthesis is impaired above this value.[51] In severe cases, leucovorin therapy should be considered until marrow recovery, even if serum MTX is no longer detectable. This is because intracellular MTX activity may still be ongoing and folinic acid would be of benefit. It should be noted that trimethoprim, a folate antagonist, can interfere with certain MTX assays (radioenzymatic, enzyme inhibition).[21] Spectrophotofluorimetric analysis may misinterpret folinic acid for MTX and should not be used as the analytic method during leucovorin therapy.[146]

Thymidine has also been used to rescue cells from the cytotoxic effects of MTX by what is called "thymidylate salvage."[80,243] Thymidine can be converted to thymidine triphosphate by thymidine kinase, which is not inhibited by MTX, thus allowing for DNA synthesis. Thymidine rescue has limited application as it does not appear to be as effective as leucovorin.[177,243] It is currently available under an investigational protocol (NCI 92-C-0134, prpl@mail.cc.nih.gov, Tel. 800-411-1222 or 301-496-5725, Fax 301-480-9793) for use by patients with high serum MTX concentration, severe manifestations of toxicity (ie, mucositis, thrombocytopenia, neutropenia, and hepatic insufficiency), and renal insufficiency. The investigational dose for thymidine is 8 g/m²/d IV, and this treatment is used in conjunction with leucovorin and carboxypeptidase.

Carboxypeptidase G2 (CPDG2) is a rescue agent that inactivates MTX by cleaving its terminal glutamate group.[275] It is a recombinant bacterial (*Pseudomonas*) enzyme that is well tolerated by patients undergoing high-dose MTX therapy.[66,266,267,275] Upon its administration, serum MTX concentration decreases rapidly (ie, within 1 hour). Hypersensitivity reactions may occur because of this agent's bacterial origin. CPDG2 is available for compassionate use by patients with high serum MTX concentration (at least 10 μmol/L and more than 42 hours after initiation of MTX therapy) or under investigational protocol (NCI 92-C-0134; see above) with thymidine from the National Cancer Institute. Leucovorin and thymidine treatments are continued during CPDG2 use because this enzyme does not enter the cell where toxicity is ongoing. The investigational dose for CPDG2 is 50 U/kg IV and repeat administration may be necessary if the MTX concentration remains greater than 1 μmol/L. It is essential that the high-performance liquid chromatography (HPLC) technique be used to assay for MTX concentration after CPDG2 therapy because the enzymatic byproducts of MTX yield falsely elevated values with the routine enzyme immunosorbent assay method.[275]

Extracorporeal Elimination

There are several reports of the use of hemodialysis and/or hemoperfusion for patients with MTX toxicity. Although the volume of distribution (0.6–0.9 L/kg) and protein binding (50%) suggest that methotrexate is dialyzable, clinical evidence suggests otherwise.[235] In one report, less than 10% of an initial 0.7 g of methotrexate was cleared in 12 sessions of hemodialysis.[245] The measured clearance was only 38 mL/min, which can be compared to 5 mL/min for peritoneal dialysis,[110] 0.28–24 mL/min for continuous venovenous

hemodiafiltration,[135,144] and 180 mL/min for normal renal clearance.[161] Using plasma exchange transfusion to remove MTX is not recommended because the redistribution of drug from tissue stores limits the efficacy of this procedure.[24,144,245]

Charcoal hemoperfusion removed more than 50% of methotrexate in 4 patients with impaired renal MTX clearance during high-dose MTX therapy.[71] This was felt to have prevented severe skin and mucosal toxicity. Sequential hemodialysis and hemoperfusion were used for a patient with substantial MTX toxicity.[104] These procedures decreased the half-life of elimination from 45 hours to 7.6 hours. In experimental animals, hemoperfusion significantly reduced the terminal half-life of methotrexate. In anephric dogs, hemoperfusion decreased the half-life from more than 20 hours to 1.3 hours.[124] Thus, hemoperfusion is recommended over hemodialysis.

In vitro studies indicate that the toxic effects of 100 μmol/L of MTX cannot be reversed by 1000 μmol/L of leucovorin.[200] This suggests the need for hemoperfusion to lower persistent MTX plasma concentrations of greater than 100 μmol/L.[205] It is important to perform hemoperfusion early, prior to distribution into tissues. Rebound in MTX levels from tissues may be expected after hemodialysis, which can begin at 2 hours postdialysis and plateau at 16 hours.[97,110,262] If hemoperfusion is not available and the patient is in renal failure and has a plasma MTX concentration greater than 8 μmol/L, hemodialysis may be considered until more definitive treatment is available (eg, enzymatic cleavage).[71]

Acute intermittent hemodialysis with a high-flux dialyzer membrane (Fresenius F-80, Fresenius Inc., Walnut Creek, GA) yielded an effective mean plasma MTX clearance of 92 mL/min in 6 patients with renal failure, resulting from either chronic disease or high-dose MTX therapy.[262] These patients received high-dose MTX therapy and had a predialysis plasma MTX concentration ranging from 1.45 to 1813 μmol/L. The time of dialysis initiation after MTX treatment was from 1 hour to 6 days in this patient population. A plasma MTX concentration of 0.3 μmol/L was used as an endpoint for dialysis. The reported plasma MTX clearance by this technique closely approximates normal renal MTX clearance and should be considered if it is available.

Other treatment options, including leucovorin and urinary alkalinization, should be continued during extracorporeal MTX removal. Folic acid is water soluble and can be removed by hemodialysis.[62,226,230] This is probably also applicable for leucovorin, and replacement doses of leucovorin postdialysis should be considered.

Granulocyte Colony-Stimulating Factor

The decision for using granulocyte colony-stimulating factor (G-CSF) in patients with agranulocytosis depends on the severity of neutropenia and anticipated speed of recovery. Granulocyte-macrophage colony-stimulating factor (GM-CSF) was used in a patient with a chronic MTX overdose and pancytopenia.[235] The patient had a serum MTX concentration of 1.25 μmol/L upon admission and was in renal failure. Bone marrow biopsy showed promyelocytes, but no mature white cells and a marked reduction of megakaryocytes. Because of deteriorating conditions, GM-CSF (125 μg/m²/d) was administered when the MTX level fell below the reference limit for toxicity. Seven days after the initiation of GM-CSF, the WBC count rose and reached normal values within 10 days. Thus, if promyelocytes and myelocytes are present in the bone marrow, neutrophil recovery will occur spontaneously in 4–7 days following the withdrawal of the offending agent.[89] However, when granulopoiesis is completely absent, neutrophil recovery cannot be expected for at least 14 days. Using G-CSF or GM-CSF can accelerate neutrophil recovery. When myeloid precursors are present in the bone marrow, G-CSF can accelerate neutrophil recovery in 1–4 days. If myeloid precursors are absent, neutrophil recovery with G-CSF may take longer, but can be expected to occur sooner than without GCSF therapy. Serum levels of the antineoplastic agent should be below detection before institution of G-CSF; otherwise, no benefit may be expected. The initial dose is 5 μg/kg/d IV or SC and it is continued beyond the expected WBC nadir. This is usually a 2-week course; however, it can be prolonged with lomustine overdoses.[1,247] The dose may be adjusted depending on the patient's WBC response. Therapy can be discontinued when the postnadir absolute neutrophil count is greater than 10,000 cells/mm³.

GM-CSF may produce a transient beneficial response in the WBC in patients with aplastic anemia.[53] However, when the anemia was severe, the GM-CSF therapy was not effective. Another hematopoietic growth factor is erythropoietin (EPO), which is approved for use in patients with anemia associated with cancer chemotherapy treatment.[99]

VINCRISTINE

Pharmacology

Vinblastine: R₁ = CH₃
Vincristine: R₁ = CHO

Vincristine and vinblastine are derived from the periwinkle plant (*Catharanthus roseus*) and used for the treatment of leukemias, lymphomas, and certain solid tumors. Their mechanism of activity is similar to that of colchicine, podophyllotoxin, and the taxoids (eg, paclitaxel, docetaxel).[67,76] These agents disrupt microtubule assembly by either preventing their formation or depolymerization, which is necessary for routine cell maintenance. Microtubules are responsible for several basic cellular functions including cell division, axonal transport of organelles, and cellular movement. Mitotic metaphase arrest is commonly observed because of the inability to form spindle fibers from the microtubules. Cell death quickly ensues as a result of the interruption of these homeostatic functions, accounting for the clinical manifestations.

The vinca alkaloids are primarily eliminated through the liver and have a terminal plasma half-life of about 24 hours.[184] The typical dose for vincristine is 1–1.4 mg/m². Patients with hepatic dysfunction are susceptible to toxicity.

Vincristine overdose is the most frequently reported antineoplastic overdose in the literature. This is because there are four different ways to misdose this agent, including confusing it with vinblastine, misinterpreting the dose, administering by the wrong route, and confusing two different-strength vials. The normal dose for vincristine is 0.06 mg/kg, and a single dose is not to exceed 2.0 mg for an adult or child.

Clinical Manifestations

Despite their similarity in structure, vincristine and vinblastine differ in clinical toxicity. Vincristine produces less bone marrow suppression and more neurotoxicity than vinblastine. During the therapeutic use of vincristine, myelosuppression occurs in only 5–10% of patients.[114] However, this effect is common in the overdose setting and the need for replacement blood products and concern for overwhelming infection is apparent.[165] The fall in cell counts begins within the first week and may last for up to 3 weeks. Other manifestations of acute vincristine toxicity are mucositis, CNS disorders, and the syndrome of inappropriate antidiuretic hormone (SIADH).

CNS disorders are varied and unusual during therapeutic vincristine therapy because of the agent's poor penetrance of the blood-brain barrier.[129] They are, however, more common when there is delayed drug elimination, damage to the blood brain-barrier, overdose, or inadvertent intrathecal administration. Generalized seizures from toxicity or secondary effects may occur from 1–7 days after drug exposure.[120,138,142,240] Treatment with benzodiazepines and phenobarbital is usually successful, and phenytoin was used successfully in a patient with barbiturate hypersensitivity.[142] Other manifestations are depression, agitation, insomnia, and hallucinations. Vincristine stimulation of the hypothalamus may be responsible for the fevers and SIADH noted in overdosed patients.[210] The fevers begin 24 hours after exposure and last 6–96 hours. Serum electrolytes need to be monitored, typically for 10 days.

Autonomic dysfunction is observed, and it commonly includes bowel ileus, constipation, and abdominal pain. Atony of the bladder, hypertension, and hypotension can occur as well.[142]

Ascending peripheral neuropathies occur during vincristine therapy and can be limited by keeping the total for a single dose below 2 mg.[231] Neuropathy may appear after an overdose, starting at about 2 weeks and lasting for 6–7 weeks. Paresthesias, neuritic pain, ataxia, bone pain, wrist drop, foot drop, cranial nerve involvement (III–VII and X), and diminished reflexes can be observed.[264] The incidence of paresthesia increases with dose and is reported to be 56% in patients treated at doses between 12.5 and 25 μg/kg.[114] At a dose of 75 μg/kg, the incidence of patients with a sensory disorder increased by 6-fold. The loss of reflexes, the earliest and most consistent sign of vincristine neuropathy, is maximal at 17 days after a single massive dose. Muscular weakness is a limiting point in therapy, and typically involves the distal dorsiflexors of the extremities, although laryngeal involvement is also reported.[158,218] These severe neurologic symptoms may be reversed by either withholding therapy or reducing dosage upon manifestation of these findings.[158] The mechanism of toxicity is not well understood, but appears to be related to inhibition of microtubular synthesis, which leads to axonal degeneration.[102,186] A brain biopsy of a patient suffering a vincristine-related death showed neurotubular dissociation, which is characteristic of vincristine damage in experimental animals.[40,55] Unlike the vinca alkaloids, taxoid-induced peripheral neuropathy is predominantly sensory and resolves faster upon discontinuation of the offending agent.[163] This is because of the varied effects on microtubule assembly by these agents. Nerve conduction studies and the Achilles tendon reflex are useful in monitoring patients for toxicity after exposure.

Vincristine-induced myocardial infarctions are reported but their cause is not understood.[168,232,241,272] It may be related to vinca alkaloid–induced platelet aggregation, coronary artery spasm, or increased sensitivity of myocardium to hypoxia.

Management

Patients receiving an inadvertent amount of an IV dose of vincristine are to be admitted to a cardiac-monitored bed and observed for 24–72 hours.[167] Seizures, dysrhythmias, and alterations in blood pressure can be expectantly managed, although prophylactic phenobarbital and benzodiazepine were used to prevent seizures in two patients.[52,148] Calcium channel blocking agents (nifedipine and amlodipine) were used to control hypertension in a patient with vincristine overdose.[52] Blood counts must be monitored daily, and GCSF may be used to treat neutropenia.[52,165,240]

If patients remain asymptomatic, they can be discharged with followup for bone marrow suppression and SIADH; otherwise, depending upon the patients' clinical condition, continual observation for progression of neurologic symptoms is warranted.[26] The symptoms of acute toxicity usually last for 3–7 days, and the neurologic sequelae may last for months with some resolution.

In the early 1960s, some investigations suggested that glutamic acid might reduce the incidence of vinblastine-induced myelosuppression.[14,64,139,251] Further investigations led to a controlled study, in which patients receiving vincristine therapy were given glutamic acid as 500 mg orally 3 times a day.[130] It was observed that there was a decreased incidence in loss of Achilles tendon reflex and delayed onset of paresthesias in the glutamic acid–treated group. However, the frequency of hematologic and gastrointestinal effects from vincristine was not significantly different between the two treatment groups. There were no reported adverse effects with glutamic acid in this investigation. Animal studies involving the administration of glutamic and aspartic acid to mice poisoned with either vinblastine or vincristine demonstrate increased survival and decreased sensorimotor peripheral neuropathy.[39,64,128] The mechanisms of these observed effects with glutamic acid are not clear. One possibility is that glutamic acid may competitively inhibit a common cellular transport mechanism for vincristine.[36,61] Another possibility would be that glutamic acid may assist in the stabilization of tubulin and promote its polymerization into microtubules, thus improving peripheral neuropathy.[41,109] Finally, exogenous glutamic acid may improve cellular metabolism by overcoming its inhibition by these agents in the Krebs cycle.[75,207] Although the role of glutamic acid for acute toxicity needs further study, it is probably not harmful and should be considered. Glutamic acid may be initiated as 500 mg orally 3 times a day and continued until the serum drug concentration is below toxicity.[130]

Leucovorin may shorten the course of vincristine-induced peripheral neuropathy[106] and myelosuppression.[148] The mechanism is attributed to leucovorin's ability to overcome a vincristine-mediated block of dihydrofolate reductase and thymidine synthetase.[106] However, neither leucovorin[23,126,246] nor pyridoxine[127] has been shown to be definitely effective. An initial experimental investigation evaluating the efficacy of antibody therapy to limit vinca alkaloid toxicity shows promise.[107]

Enhanced Elimination

Vincristine is rapidly distributed to tissue stores and highly bound to proteins and red cells.[48] Elimination is via the hepatobiliary system.[48] In more than 50% of children given this agent IV, their plasma levels were not detected 4 hours after administration.[181] Such characteristics favor early intervention and methods other than hemodialysis. Double-volume exchange transfusion was performed at 6 hours postexposure in 3 children who were overdosed with 7.5 mg/m^2 of vincristine IV.[148] Of the two survivors, their respective postexchange serum vincristine concentrations were 57 and 71% lower than their preexchange concentrations. The amount of vincristine removed was not determined. Although these patients developed peripheral neuropathies, myelosuppression, and autonomic instability, the author noted that the duration of illness was shorter than previously reported.

Plasmapheresis was attempted with vinca alkaloid overdoses.[165,198] In an 18-year-old patient who received two 8-mg IV doses of vincristine at 12-hour intervals, the procedure was performed 6 hours after the second dose and 1.5 times the plasma volume was pheresed.[198] Postpheresis serum vincristine concentration was 23% lower than the starting concentration. The patient survived with myelosuppression, neurotoxicity, and SIADH. Thus, based on the pharmacodynamic profile of vincristine and these two reports, exchange transfusion in the child would be the preferred method of enhanced elimination upon early arrival and plasmapheresis in the adult.

ANTHRACYCLINES

Pharmacology

Doxorubicin

The antineoplastic agents derived from the bacterium *Streptomyces* are dactinomycin, daunorubicin, doxorubicin, bleomycin, mitomycin, and plicamycin. Only plicamycin crosses the blood-brain barrier. The terminal elimination half-life for doxorubicin is about 30 hours.[103] Doxorubicin and daunorubicin are both eliminated by the liver and patients with hepatic dysfunction should have their dosage decreased. Delayed drug elimination contributes to increased drug area-under-the-time-versus-concentration-curve (AUC) and peak serum concentration, which are associated with myelosuppression and cardiac toxicity, respectively[159] These agents are metabolized to active metabolites, which have lesser degrees of activity than their parent compounds. A typical dose schedule for daunorubicin is 30–60 mg/m^2 daily for 3 days. For doxorubicin, this is 45–60 mg/m^2 every 18–21 days. Daunorubicin and doxorubicin share many common indications for cancer therapy, but they differ by doxorubicin's use in solid tumors (eg, breast carcinoma).

The red anthracycline antibiotics—dactinomycin and doxorubicin—are best known for their associated cardiotoxicity, which limits their therapeutic use. The mechanism responsible for their therapeutic effects is different from that which causes cardiotoxicity.[244] The mechanism of therapeutic action of the anthracyclines is attributed to DNA intercalation[215] and activation of topoisomerase II,[244] which is an enzyme that promotes DNA strand breakage and resealing. The mechanism of cardiac toxicity is believed to result from the formation of free radicals.[182] Doxorubicin and dactinomycin are quinone derivatives and can be reduced to free radicals. These metabolites are extremely cytotoxic through the promotion of lipid peroxidation. Paraquat and bleomycin have similar mechanisms of toxicity. The limited efficacy of free radical scavengers (α-tocopherol, N-acetylcysteine) for anthracycline cardiotoxicity have led to the evaluation of other toxic mechanisms.[183] From this, the importance of iron as a cofactor for these radical-producing reactions was realized. The anthracyclines have a high affinity for metal ions. Doxorubicin has an iron (Fe^{3+})-binding constant of 10,[41] which is comparable to deferoxamine.[95] The heart's increased susceptibility to free radicals is attributed to its lack of sufficient enzyme activity responsible for free radical scavenging.[73]

Newer agents with less cardiotoxicity are aclarubicin, epirubicin, idarubicin, and mitoxantrone. The potential therapeutic benefits and questionable degree of lesser toxicity of aclarubicin and epirubicin limit their current use.

Clinical Manifestations

The cardiotoxic manifestations can be divided into acute and chronic categories. The acute form of toxicity consists of dysrhythmias, ST and T-wave changes on the electrocardiograph, diminished ejection fraction that usually resolves over 24 hours, and sudden death.[42,236,271] Abnormal findings on the ECG are present in 41% of patients receiving doxorubicin.[12,111,157,236,260,274,277] These are neither dose related nor associated with the development of cardiomyopathy. Acute pericarditis and myocarditis resulting in conduction defects and congestive heart failure are also reported.[42] Animal studies with doxorubicin demonstrate beneficial effects of adrenergic antagonists for toxicity because of elevated levels of catecholamines,[43] although the use of β-adrenergic antagonists in the potential setting of diminished cardiac output needs to be considered.

Significant cardiotoxicity results from elevated peak serum drug levels and accounts for the continuous and periodic infusions practiced in therapy. In cumulative doses, the anthracycline antibiotics cause a cardiomyopathy that results in congestive heart failure. The condition is irreversible and is associated with a 48%

mortality.[201] This drug-induced congestive heart failure (CHF) is associated with pathognomonic changes on electron microscopy that can distinguish it from infectious and ischemic etiologies. These histologic changes include reduced number of myocardial fibrils, and mitochondrial and cellular degeneration.[32] The potential mechanisms for cardiac failure include free radical damage and impaired intracellular calcium homeostasis.[196] The incidence of chronic cardiotoxicity for doxorubicin is between 1 and 10% when the cumulative dose is less than 450 mg/m^2, and becomes greater than 20% when more than 550 mg/m^2 (comparable to dactinomycin, 950 mg/m^2) is administered.[258] At a cumulative dose of 720 mg/m^2 for epirubicin, the incidence of cardiac dysfunction was reported to be 19%.[178]

The best way of monitoring cardiac function during therapy is by measuring left ventricular ejection fraction by radionuclide cineradiography.[6] Therapy should be discontinued when the ejection fraction falls below 50%. Two-dimensional echocardiography can demonstrate left-ventricular wall thickening and fractional shortening from anthracycline overexposure. Newer techniques used to assess subclinical cardiac muscle pathology from these agents include cardiac-specific contractile protein troponin-T and troponin-I,[162] and radionuclide-tagged monoclonal antibody imaging.[49] Further studies are necessary to determine their role in clinical management.

Some of the factors associated with an increased risk for cardiotoxicity include mediastinal irradiation; preexisting cardiac disease; children (especially females); age more than 70 years; and the concomitant use of cyclophosphamide, paclitaxel, and other anthracycline agents.[42] Fatalities are been reported with minimum doses of 150–333 mg/m^2, and occur within 1–16 days after exposure.[63]

Myelosuppression and mucositis are other effects associated with the use of the anthracycline agents. They typically occur in 1–2 weeks and patients recover.[25] The white cells are affected more than either the red cells or platelets. Patients with diminished drug clearance (eg, liver failure) are at risk for the development of these findings.

Mitoxantrone is recognized to be less toxic than doxorubicin and daunorubicin. Major organs of toxicity remain the heart, bone marrow, and gut. Gastrointestinal effects are less severe and frequent with mitoxantrone than doxorubicin.[229] Four cases of mitoxantrone overdose are reported in the literature.[108,229] Common to these events is a 10-fold error in dosing (100 mg/m^2 instead of 10 mg/m^2), early onset of nausea with vomiting, and myelosuppression with fever. Acute decreased cardiac contractility was observed by echocardiography in 1 patient who was asymptomatic.[108] Otherwise, no patient developed dysrhythmias, congestive failure, ECG changes, or elevated creatine phosphokinase levels early after exposure. Three patients developed fatal CHF from 1–4 months later.[229]

Management

There are no specific antidotes for this class of agents; thus, management is largely supportive. Monitoring for cardiotoxicity and pancytopenia is necessary. A baseline chest radiograph, electrocardiogram, and left-ventricular ejection fraction (at rest and/or with stress) are required. Endomyocardial biopsy and cardiac catheterization can assist in distinguishing variable causes of cardiac dysfunction. Left-ventricular function is the best predictor for cardiomyopathy.[86,222] A 10% absolute decrease in the left-ventricular ejection fraction (LVEF) or a drop in LVEF of 50% from baseline is a significant finding for the discontinuation of further anthracycline therapy.[222] Although digoxin and furosemide should be used to manage acute CHF, a variable response can be expected.[229]

A variety of cardioprotectants have been evaluated for doxorubicin therapy. Further clinical investigations are necessary to define their beneficial role in the treatment of patients with overexposures. Digoxin and low-dose verapamil benefit patients treated with doxorubicin.[94,265] At higher doses of verapamil, hypotension and heart block were observed and limited further use.[192,238] Dexrazoxane (ICRF-187), an iron chelator, limited the cardiotoxic effects of doxorubicin in a randomly controlled human trial.[233] In comparison with the controls, the treatment group had smaller decreases in the left ejection fraction per dose of doxorubicin and fewer histologic changes on cardiac biopsy, and more patients tolerated doses greater than 600 mg/m^2. The use of dexrazoxane in this study also had a slight increase in myelosuppression. The current role of this chelator is in limiting cardiotoxicity in patients receiving greater than 300 mg/m^2 of doxorubicin.[224] It is administered 30 minutes before doxorubicin in a 10:1 ratio. Dexrazoxane was shown to increase the systemic clearance of epirubicin in a clinical trial, which would be an important benefit to patients with increased exposure.[22] Further investigations are required to determine the use of dexrazoxane in overdose exposures and with other anthracycline agents.[5,178] Monohydroxyethylrutoside is a semisynthetic flavonoid that is being evaluated as an alternative cardioprotectant agent. The beneficial properties of the flavonoids include iron chelation and the scavenging of free radicals. In experimental models, monohydroxyethylrutoside was shown to decrease doxorubicin-induced cardiotoxicity as measured by ST segment elevation on the ECG[252] and left-ventricular function.[121] Clinical trials are lacking with this agent.

Enhanced Elimination

The anthracycline agents are highly protein bound and have a large volume of distribution, which makes them unlikely candidates for hemodialysis. However, the early institution of hemoperfusion may enhance elimination. In an animal model, plasma doxorubicin clearance could be enhanced up to 20-fold with hemoperfusion.[269] Factors determining this were duration of therapy, rate of flow, and the use of a 2% acrylic hydrogel-coated cartridge. Three patients with a doxorubicin overdose were treated with hemoperfusion, 1 with an Amberlite cartridge, and all had a rapid reduction in their serum levels.[63] One survived a 10-fold error in dosing. In a patient with a mitoxantrone overdose of 98 mg IV, hemoperfusion was begun within hours and only 0.287 and 0.236 mg of drug was removed in two trials.[108]

NITROGEN MUSTARDS
Pharmacology

Mechlorethamine

The nitrogen mustard agents are cyclophosphamide, ifosfamide, chlorambucil, mechlorethamine, and melphalan. Their indicated uses include immunosuppression (eg, controlling graft-versus-host rejection, collagen vascular diseases) and chemotherapy. The tumoricidal activity of these agents is the result of the formation of reactive intermediates that bind to nucleophilic moieties on the DNA chain, which inactivates DNA synthesis. Unlike the other agents, cyclophosphamide and ifosfamide require mixed function oxidation to achieve their alkylating properties. Mechlorethamine is the original compound from which all of the others were derived. It is highly reactive when it comes in contact with water and undergoes rapid chemical transformation. Local reactions caused by mechlorethamine spillage (eg, extravasation) include tissue injury and thrombophlebitis (Chap. 100). Nonenzymatic hydrolysis is the major route by which these agents are metabolized, thus accounting for their relatively short elimination half-lives (ie, less than 3 hours).[30] Cyclophosphamide, ifosfamide, and chlorambucil have active metabolites, which prolongs their alkylating activity after administration.[140]

Clinical Manifestations

Chlorambucil and ifosfamide can produce altered mental status and seizures from therapeutic use or from an overdose.[46] Both compounds undergo *N*-dechloroethylation to produce chloroacetaldehyde, which is purported to be a nervous system toxin.[101] Encephalopathy occurs in 9% of patients receiving 5 g/m^2 of ifosfamide, and is more frequent with oral versus IV administration because of the first-pass effect and increased chloroacetaldehyde production.[173] Seizures are more commonly associated with chlorambucil. Acute overdoses reported in the literature are all from the oral route, and range in dosing from 1.5–6.8 mg/kg (therapeutic is 0.1–0.2 mg/kg).[9,47] The seizures occur within 6 hours, may appear as generalized tonic-clonic activity or staring spells, and can last for 24 hours. However, in one instance in which therapeutic dosing was increased, seizures occurred 17 hours later. This delay may be attributed to a lower serum concentration or a slower time to peak than in the overdose setting. A similar reasoning would explain why a patient with a chronic overdose of 4.1 mg/kg over 5 days did not sustain CNS toxicity.[79] Patients with increased likelihood to seize are those with underlying seizure disorders or with nephrotic syndrome, which can alter pharmacokinetics.[216] Electroencephalograms (EEGs) demonstrated multiple paroxysms of bilaterally symmetric 2–3-Hz spikes and slow high-voltage rhythmic slowing that progressed to slower bursts of rhythmic spike and wave discharge in a child with an acute overdose.[47] Myelosuppression occurs in patients with both acute and chronic overdoses, and can present as late as 41 days postexposure. Recovery is expected within 1 week of the nadir, and GCSF treatment may be necessary.[137]

Cyclophosphamide and its analogue ifosfamide are known for inducing hemorrhagic cystitis from their irritating metabolite, acrolein. This occurs in about 5–10% of patients who receive therapy.[45,60] The incidence of cystitis does not appear to be related to the total dose and route administered, age, or gender. The course is usually self-limiting, although blood transfusions may be required. Free water retention is observed in patients receiving greater than 50 mg/kg of cyclophosphamide.[68] This effect is attributed to the activity of the alkylating metabolite on the renal tubule and is observed at 6–8 hours after drug administration. The patient experiences decreased urinary output, increased urine osmolality, and decreased serum osmolality. This is self-limiting, lasting for about 12–16 hours. Treatment with furosemide during this period can prevent free water loading in the patient.

In the overdose setting, cyclophosphamide can cause dysrhythmias, myocardial necrosis, and death. ECG changes are noted at doses of 120 mg/kg and heart failure and myocarditis at doses greater than 150 mg/kg.[11,179] An error in writing an order led to the death of 1 patient and irreversible cardiac damage in another patient from cyclophosphamide overdose. These 2 patients received 6520 mg of the agent daily for 4 consecutive days, when the amount was to be divided over 4 days.[212] The onset of heart failure can be sudden, and patients older than 50 years of age, and those with prior treatment with anthracyclines, are at greatest risk for cardiac toxicity.[237]

Management

Recommendations for an acute chlorambucil exposure include routine gastrointestinal decontamination, a 6-hour observation, a baseline CBC and liver function test (LFT), and a followup CBC weekly for 4 weeks.[253] Ifosfamide-induced encephalopathy can be managed with methylene blue (50 mg IV as a 1% solution), although the mechanism is unknown.[150,276] Seizures were reported to be more effectively managed with barbiturates and benzodiazepines than with phenytoin.[9,33,270]

When gross hematuria from cyclophosphamide or ifosfamide therapy persists, treatments reported to be effective in the literature may be considered. These include electrocauterization, systemic vasopressin,[202] and intravesical administration of silver nitrate,[149] formalin,[88,225] prostaglandin F_2 α,[228] and hydrostatic pressure.[115] Some of the preventive therapies that seem to reduce this occurrence include adequate hydration for dilution effect, frequent bladder emptying, IV administration of sodium 2-mercaptoethanesulfonate (MESNA), and intravesical N-acetylcysteine.[45] The thiol group of N-acetylcysteine is believed to directly interact with acrolein to limit its irritating effect on the bladder epithelium. MESNA is believed to work by inactivating acrolein to an inert thioether.[116] The IV dose of MESNA is 20% of the cyclophosphamide or ifosfamide amount (wt/wt) and administered during therapy and again at 4 and 8 hours. MESNA is used during standard-dose therapy for ifosfamide and high-dose therapy for cyclophosphamide.

Patients with increased exposures to cyclophosphamide require baseline ECGs and echocardiograms. Intravenous fluid restriction, digoxin, and furosemide were successfully used to treat a patient with cyclophosphamide-induced congestive cardiomyopathy.[257]

PLATINOIDS
Pharmacology

Cisplatin   Carboplatin

The cytotoxic effects of the platinum-containing compounds were first recognized in 1965; since then, many types have been derived. The ones of clinical significance are cisplatin, carboplatin, and oxaliplatin.[180] These agents were designed to reduce the incidence of nephrotoxicity and to counter drug resistance. Differences in chemical structure exist among these agents as well. Most notably, cisplatin is an inorganic and carboplatin an organic compound. Similarities exist in their mechanism of toxicity, which is the binding of platinum to DNA to incapacitate DNA function. These agents are eliminated from the body primarily in the urine and at varying rates. The amount eliminated at 24 hours is 25% for cisplatin and 90% for carboplatin. Patients with decreased creatinine clearance (less than 30 mg/m^2) will have prolonged elimination half-lives of platinoids.[81]

Clinical Manifestations

The more common manifestations of toxicity with cisplatin during therapy are renal dysfunction, auditory impairment, and peripheral sensory neuropathy. The other antineoplastic agents recognized to cause a peripheral neuropathy are the vinca alkaloids and the taxoids. Oxaliplatin-induced neuropathy is triggered or enhanced by exposure to cold and can subside over several months.[85] Myelosuppression is a dose-limiting factor for carboplatin and iproplatin, which does not occur with cisplatin. At a carboplatin dose of 800 mg/m^2, 25% of patients develop marrow toxicity.[193] The marrow effects are delayed, with nadir occurring 3–5 weeks after the start of therapy. Patients developing an anemia within the first week of cisplatin therapy should be evaluated for hemolytic anemia.[57]

The sources of error associated with cisplatin overdoses are frequency of administration (total dose versus over a period of time), mistaking it for carboplatin, and writing the wrong dose.[58,199] Manifestations in the overdose setting involve neurologic, visual, hearing, bone marrow, pancreatic, and renal disorders.[227] The most common renal disorder is renal failure, which is dose-related and begins at 50 mg/m^2. The result is irreversible distal tubular necrosis.[211,220] Cell death may be from intracellular glutathione depletion.[65,70,100] The presence of urinary alanine aminopeptidase and N-acetyl-β-D-glucosaminidase may be used as early indicators of renal tubular damage.[65,70,100] Saline-induced diuresis can limit renal toxicity. At doses greater than 200 mg/m^2, the development of seizures, encephalopathy, and irreversible peripheral sensory neuropathy is of concern.[27,59,113,193,194] Pathologic evaluation demonstrates axonal degeneration and damage to the dorsal root ganglion. At this dose, visual impairment may occur within the first week of exposure.[56,170,268] This can include temporary visual loss with permanent loss of color discrimination. Physical examination of the anterior chamber and fundus of the eye will be normal; however, an electroretinogram will be abnormal with a negative-type response. Some other ocular disorders are papilledema and retrobulbar neuritis. High-frequency (greater than 2000 Hz) hearing loss is evident 2–3 days after exposure to doses greater than 500 mg/m^2.[54]

Management

Renal protection and enhanced elimination of platinum are the two primary goals in the management of a cisplatin overdose. Expectant management for myelosuppression and neurotoxicity can follow. Sodium chloride diuresis both promotes the inactive anionic state of cisplatin and decreases the urine platinum concentration to limit nephrotoxicity during therapy.[8,256] Hydration with 0.9%

NaCl and an osmotic diuretic (eg, mannitol) should be administered to achieve a high urine output (eg, 1–3 mL/kg/h) for 6–24 hours postexposure. In the setting of nonoliguric renal failure, careful hydration is recommended to maintain urinary output, because platinum renal excretion is directly related to urinary flow and independent of creatinine clearance.[56] Aside from the serum BUN and creatinine, assessment of renal function can include the glomerular filtration, filtration fraction, and renal plasma flow.[105,175,176,187]

Amifostine and sodium thiosulfate are effective nephroprotectants. Amifostine's role is more preventative and its mechanisms are attributed to free radical scavenging, prevention of cisplatin-DNA adduct formation, and facilitation of DNA repair.[147] Sodium thiosulfate is effective postexposure. Thiosulfate remains in the extracellular space to bind free platinum to limit cellular damage. Little or no renal toxicity was seen in patients receiving as much as 270 mg/m^2 of cisplatin when thiosulfate was given as an IV bolus of 4 g/m^2 with an infusion of 12 g/m^2 over 6 hours.[112,197] Thiosulfate may offer the additional benefit of limiting neurotoxicity and should be administered to all patients after an overdose.[169,254] Diethyldithiocarbamate (DDTC) demonstrated efficacy as a nephroprotectant in animal models; however, it failed to do so in clinical trials.[93] The use of thiosulfate is limited by the time in which it needs to be administered after exposure (ie, 1–2 hours). Although N-acetylcysteine was effective as a nephroprotectant in an experimental cisplatin model, clinical trials are required to determine its role in therapy.[227]

Plasmapheresis and hemodialysis have been attempted in patients with cisplatin overdoses, and owing to this agent's high protein binding, hemodialysis was ineffective.[44] However, in patients with renal failure, dialysis may benefit. Plasmapheresis was performed in 2 adults and there was a fall in blood platinum levels with clinical improvement. The first patient received an overdose of 280 mg/m^2 and was plasmapheresed on day 12 of exposure.[56] After 3 daily treatments, the serum platinum level decreased from 2900 to 200 ng/mL and the patient had noticeable improvement in gastrointestinal and visual symptoms. On day 20, the serum platinum level rebounded to 700 ng/mL and the symptoms worsened. Further plasmapheresis lowered the level to 290 ng/mL by day 27 and symptoms improved. The other patient received 300 mg/m^2 of cisplatin and received 4 daily treatments of plasmapheresis starting on day 6 postexposure.[141] The plasma platinum level declined from 2979 to 430 ng/mL and the patient became more awake and less nauseous. On day 11, platinum levels rebounded to 834 ng/mL and fell to 279 ng/mL upon reinstitution of plasmapheresis. The amount of platinum removed by three trials was 4622 μg. The author of the paper contends that plasmapheresis prevented the need for hemodialysis for renal failure. Thus, plasmapheresis appears to be effective in cisplatin overdose and should be instituted immediately after exposure. Patients who remain symptomatic days later may benefit as well.

INTRATHECAL OVERDOSE

Intrathecal overdoses with vincristine, methotrexate, doxorubicin, daunorubicin, and cytarabine are reported in the literature.[151] Common sources of error are confusing the IV for the intrathecal agent and misidentifying the strength of the solution vial in the preparation of the medication. These events are stressful because of the disastrous consequences they bring and the immediacy with which the agent must be removed from the thecal space. Removal of as much of the agent as possible is the patient's only chance of having an acceptable prognosis.

Upon recognition of the occurrence, the patient needs to be placed in a gravity-dependent position to prevent upward flow of the agent towards the cisterna magnum. The upright position significantly delays the flow of an intralumbar administered agent to the cerebral ventricles when compared to lying flat or being in the Trendelenburg position.[78] The lumbar puncture site needs to be maintained or reestablished so that as much of the CSF can be drained as possible. With an intrathecal MTX model, if 20 mL of CSF is removed within 30 minutes of administration, then 94% of the agent given is retrieved.[4] However, by removing the same volume at 3 hours, only 10% of the agent is recovered. CSF drainage can be accomplished in short time intervals, considering that CSF production is 30 mL/h. CSF exchange should be accomplished by lavaging the intrathecal space with lactated Ringer solution. An equal volume of the CSF space should be used in each pass, and 2–3 passes should be performed. The volume of CSF in a child older than 3 years approaches that of an adult (ie, 120 mL). For large and significant exposures, CSF perfusion must follow. This is performed by passing solution through a ventriculostomy and out a lumbar drainage catheter. Lactated Ringer solution with 15–25 mL of fresh-frozen plasma added per liter of crystalloid is infused at 150 mL/h for 18–24 hours.[77,273] The ventriculostomy and lumbar drain can then be removed. The thecal effluent can be collected to determine the amount of agent recovered. Depending on the antineoplastic agent involved, additional measures may be necessary.

Intrathecal vincristine overdoses are devastating. Only 2 of 13 patients reported in the literature survived.[77,273] There is no indication for the intrathecal administration of vincristine or vinblastine. This mishap is usually the result of confusing vincristine with the other medications (eg, cytarabine, MTX) that are commonly dispensed for intrathecal use. Death follows a characteristic course, consisting of back pain, meningismus, lower limb weakness, urinary difficulty, loss of deep tendon reflexes, encephalopathy, and then respiratory failure. Alteration in mental status appeared earlier when vincristine was administered intraventricularly.[174] Pathologic changes are most notable in the cerebellum, the brainstem, and the anterior horns of the spinal cord.[17] There are only 2 reported survivors from intrathecal vincristine, and it is believed that their success was because CSF evacuation of the agent was instituted within minutes as described above.[77,273] The amount of vincristine recovered in one case was 95% of the 2 mg of vincristine that had been administered.[77] Additional therapies provided in these cases were glutamic acid (10 g IV over 24 hours, then 500 mg po 3 times a day),[130] folinic acid (25 mg IV every 6 hours), and pyridoxine (50 mg IV every 8 hours). These agents were continued for 1 week or until the neurologic symptoms stabilized. Dexamethasone (4 mg/m^2 IV every 6 hours) may be given for meningeal inflammation. The role for these agents is unclear, but because of the seriousness of the situation, aggressive therapy should be offered.

Intrathecal overdoses of MTX commonly occur because a more concentrated solution vial is mistaken for one that is less concentrated.[234,156] Overdoses reported in the literature range as high as 650 mg and death is associated with amounts greater than 500 mg.[234] The therapeutic intrathecal MTX dose according to age is 6 mg for a patient younger than 1 year old; 8 mg for a patient between the ages of 1 and 2 years; 10 mg for a patient between the ages of 2 and 3 years; and 12 mg for a patient older than 3 years of age.[35] The neurotoxicity associated with these events includes chemical arachnoiditis, ascending neuropathy, encephalopathy, and seizures. The seizures can be treated with phenobarbital and benzodiazepines.[156,208] The most common form of toxicity is chemical arachnoiditis, which is associated with the acute onset of fever, back pain, dizziness, neck stiffness, vomiting, and headaches that can last for hours.[118] The CSF in these cases demonstrated elevated intracranial pressure, pleocytosis, and elevated protein levels.

Unlike intrathecal vincristine overdoses, the prognosis for an intrathecal MTX exposure is more favorable because of the agent's different mechanism of action and the availability of rescue therapy. Two deaths have been reported with intrathecal MTX overdose and they received amounts greater than 500 mg.[83,234] CSF removal of MTX is still crucial, and for amounts less than 100 mg CSF, drainage may be adequate if performed within 30–60 minutes of administration.[136,190] When a longer period of time has elapsed, or a larger amount is involved, CSF exchange is necessary, and possibly CSF perfusion as well. At amounts greater than 500 mg, CSF perfusion must follow because drainage and exchange cannot remove enough MTX to prevent significant toxicity. CSF decontamination should continue until the final MTX concentration is about 100 µmol/L, which is a peak therapeutic level for a 12 mg intrathecal MTX dose.[190] Large amounts of MTX administered intrathecally pass into the systemic circulation, which poses a threat to the bone marrow. Although there are no reports of myelosuppression resulting from such an event, IV leucovorin is indicated. High-dose leucovorin rescue is to be started upon recognition of the overdose. The following IV regimen was used in a patient who received 600 mg and survived: 1000 mg/m^2, followed by 100 mg/m^2 every 3 hours until the plasma MTX was less than 0.1 µmol/L.[190] Leucovorin is not to be administered intrathecally because seizures with resultant death can occur, and the etiology of MTX-induced neurotoxicity is chemical irritation, not folate inhibition.[136] Additional therapies are hydration and urinary alkalinization to prevent renal toxicity, and IV dexamethasone to lessen meningeal inflammation. Enzymatic agents that inactivate MTX are a new and promising form of rescue therapy for intrathecal overdoses. Carboxypeptidase G2 (CPDG2) dramatically shortens the MTX CSF half-life in a patient with a 600-mg intrathecal overdose.[190] The patient received the carboxypeptidase agent intrathecally, following CSF decontamination, and survived. CPDG2 is currently available for patients with intrathecal MTX overdose by investigational protocol at the National Cancer Institute (Protocol number 92-C-0137, Tel. 800-411-1222 or 301-496-5725, Fax 301-480-9793, email: prpl@mail.cc.nih.gov). Enzymatic cleavage may obviate the future need for CSF perfusion in large overdoses.

ANTINEOPLASTIC EXTRAVASATIONS

Extravasational injuries are among the most consequential local toxic events. When an antineoplastic agent leaks from the blood vessel into the surrounding tissue, significant necrosis of skin, muscles, and tendons can occur with resultant loss of function. The initial manifestations may include swelling, pain, and a burning sensation that can last for hours. Days later, the area becomes erythematous and indurated and can either resolve or proceed to ulceration and necrosis.[213] Sometimes, these early findings may be difficult to distinguish from other forms of local drug toxicity, such as irritation and hypersensitivity. Either the agent or its vehicle (ethanol, propylene glycol) can cause local irritation. The agents associated with local irritation include fluorouracil, carmustine, bisantrene, cisplatin, and dacarbazine. The local irritation and hypersensitivity manifestations are self-limiting and typified by an immediate onset of a burning sensation, pruritus, erythema, and a flare reaction of the vein in which the agent is being infused. Pretreatment with an antihistamine usually prevents some of the hypersensitivity manifestations upon subsequent administrations.[255] Agents reported to cause hypersensitivity reactions include daunorubicin, doxorubicin, idarubicin, and mitoxantrone. This event is typified by the presence of pruritus. Nevertheless, when local reactions cannot be differentiated, it is always best to presume extravasation and manage the situation accordingly.

The occurrence of these inadvertent events appears to be about 50 times more frequent in the hands of the inexperienced clinician.[122] There are several factors that are associated with extravasational injuries from peripheral intravenous lines, including (a) patients with poor vessel integrity and blood flow, such as the elderly, those who undergo numerous venipunctures, and radiation therapy to the site; (b) limited venous and lymphatic drainage caused by either obstruction or surgical resection; and (c) use of sites over joints, which increases the risk of dislodgments because of movement.[123,213] Extravasational injuries from implanted ports in central venous vessels can occur from inadequate placement of the needle, needle dislodgment, fibrin sheath formation around the catheter, perforation of the superior vena cava, and fracture of the catheter.[221] When extravasation from a port is suspected, a CT scan of the chest with a contrast dye study is necessary for evaluation, if radiographic studies are not diagnostic.[10]

The factors associated with a poor outcome from extravasational injuries include (a) areas of the body with little subcutaneous tissue, such as the dorsum of the hand, volar surface of the wrist, and antecubital fossa, where healing is poor and vital structures are more likely to be involved; (b) concentration of extravasant; (c) increased volume and duration of contact with tissue; and (d) the type of agent.[213,214] The vesicant agents appear to result in more significant local tissue destruction. These include doxorubicin, daunorubicin, dactinomycin, epirubicin, idarubicin, mechlorethamine, mitomycin, and the vinca alkaloids. Mitomycin infusions can cause dermal ulcerations at venipuncture sites, remote from the location of administration.[195] The anthracycline antibiotics are associated with a higher incidence of significant injuries and delayed healing, which may be a result of their slow release from bound tissue into surrounding viable tissue. Doxorubicin extravasation is associated with local tissue necrosis in approximately 25% of cases. The extravasational injuries from taxanes appear similar to the vesicant agents, but milder in response and later in days to presentation.[16,203] The best form of therapy for these injuries is one of prevention. Specialized nursing care and the use of indwelling central venous catheters have limited the extent of these injuries.

Management

The treatment for extravasational injuries is somewhat controversial, varying from conservative care to early surgical débridement and the use of selective antidotes.[223] This uncertainty is because of the limited number of clinical cases available for study, and the discordance between animal studies and clinical findings. However, there are some recommended general management guidelines for an extravasation (Table 47–2).[28,38]

Once extravasation of an agent is suspected, the infusion should be immediately halted. A physician should be notified and the agent, its concentration, and the approximate amount infused should be noted. The venous access should be maintained so that aspiration of as much of the infusate as possible can be performed and antidote can be administered, if indicated. Injection of normal saline into the catheter to dilute the extravasant may be beneficial.[223] The intermittent local application of ice (20 minutes 4 times a day) and elevation of the extremity should be done for 24–48 hours, so as to limit further progression of the agent. Cooling the area is believed to prevent cell injury by reducing the amount of drug absorbed by the tissue and lowering the cellular metabolic rate. It was demonstrated that with just cold application and strict elevation, only 13 (11%) of 119 patients required surgical intervention for their injuries.[153] In the past, heat was recommended to disperse the agent, but investigations with mice demonstrated that this practice increases the area of skin ulceration.[74,153] However, dry, warm compresses are still recommended for the vinca alkaloids and etoposide to promote systemic uptake.[28] This is combined with the local infiltration with hyaluronidase to enhance absorption (Table 47–2). The wound should be observed closely for the first 7 days, and a surgeon consulted if either pain persists or evidence of ulceration appears.[213] However, in severe extravasations—where there is a high incidence of necrosis due to the type of drug (doxorubicin), the volume or concentration, and any area in which there may be significant long-term morbidity (over joints)—early surgical consultation would be warranted. If tissue ulceration occurs, initial

management can be with antiseptic dressings. After the area of necrotic skin has evolved to the point where it can be clearly delineated from surviving tissue, surgical débridement may be beneficial to limit secondary infection. The use of intravenous fluorescein can aid in identifying viable tissue.[13]

Antidotal therapy should be considered when the extravasant is known to respond poorly to conservative care. The vesicant-type agents are associated with a significantly worse outcome, and when the exposure is large, a more aggressive approach should be initiated. Otherwise, conservative management may be the accepted form of care. The specific antidotal treatments can be divided into several categories based upon their mechanism of action, one of which is the reduction of the inflammatory response through the application of steroids. Hydrocortisone has been used in varying concentrations (50–200 mg) as either subcutaneous or intradermal injections for doxorubicin and the vinca alkaloids.[19,122,154,250] Steroids may have only a limited role in doxorubicin-induced lesions because inflammatory cells are not found in predominance at the wound site.[31] The addition of steroids to doxorubicin infusions, so as to limit morbidity if extravasation should occur, is not recommended because the drugs are chemically incompatible.[249] Another approach is to inactivate the agents by affecting the pH of the environment. The administration of 5 mL of 8.4% sodium bicarbonate through the same IV line has been advocated to decrease the DNA binding of doxorubicin.[20] The use of bicarbonate should be cautious because its hyperosmolarity can cause tissue necrosis.[96] Sodium thiosulfate is recommended for mechlorethamine extravasations, and is believed to work by inactivating the agent by reacting with the active ethylenimmonium ring.[123,191] The site is infiltrated with sterile sodium thiosulfate solution and then ice compresses are applied intermittently for 6–12 hours.[28] Finally, there are agents, such as dimethyl sulfoxide (DMSO), that scavenge the free radicals that are believed to cause tissue damage from doxorubicin. Dimethyl sulfoxide is beneficial for anthracycline extravasations in both animal and human clinical trials.[29,69,154,189,191,242] The concentration of DMSO used ranged from 55 to 99% and was applied topically with intermittent cool compresses.[28,154,188] Some of the other beneficial properties of DMSO are its anti-inflammatory, analgesic, and vasodilatory effects, and its ability to promote systemic absorption of drug at local sites.[164] The use of other free radical scavengers (eg, α-tocopherol) for extravasations of antimitotic agents requires further clinical investigation.[37] Although the overall incidence of extravasations with antineoplastic agents is small, the associated morbidity from any one event may be significant. The best form of therapy is one of prevention.

TABLE 47–2. Management of Extravasational Injuries

Agent	Therapy	Mechanism
Anthracyclines	Dimethyl sulfoxide (DMSO)—Applied topically and allowed to dry. Every 6–8 hours for 3–10 days.	Free radical scavenger.
	Apply cool compresses for 1 hour, every 8 hours for 3 days.	Localizes area of involvement.
Mechlorethamine	Sodium thiosulfate—Prepare a sterile 0.17 M solution by mixing 4 mL thiosulfate 10% weight/volume with 6 mL water for injection. Infiltrate the site of extravasation.	
Mitomycin	DMSO	
Vinca alkaloids and epipodophyllotoxins	Hyaluronidase—Reconstitute with normal saline (15 U/mL) and inject, intradermally or subcutaneously, 150–900 U into the site.	Degrades hyaluronic acid to enhance systemic absorption.
	Dry, warm compresses only.	To promote systemic absorption.

Adapted with permission from Bertelli G: Prevention and management of extravasation of cytotoxic drugs. Drug Saf 1995;12:245–255.

SUMMARY

The antineoplastic agents are a unique class of drugs because their cellular toxic effects are desired for therapeutic use. Medicine is challenged to carefully balance this measure so that native cells, and thus the patient, are not harmed. Over the years, the number of human antineoplastic drug exposures reported to the AAPCC TESS has remained small; however, the consequences of toxicity to the patient were great. The majority of these occurrences were iatrogenic, involving misreading of the product label and errors in dosing and transcription of orders. A key element was the lack of familiarity of the healthcare provider with the use of these select agents. The number of antineoplastic agents and their indicated use have increased over the years and will continue in this fashion into the future, increasing the chance for medical error and patient toxicity. The clinical manifestations of toxicity can develop in various organ systems and are primarily determined by the agent's mechanism of action, route of administration, and duration of exposure. The gut epithelium and bone marrow are extremely susceptible to toxicity because of their high mitotic activity. They are important because their failure will lead to overwhelming sepsis and death. Treatment remains primarily supportive in nature. New additions in this area include carboxypeptidase, the antidote for MTX, and GCSF to limit the severity of neutropenia. Further work is necessary to define the role of erythropoietin in exposures resulting in anemia. Although cytoprotectants will continue to be developed, they cannot be relied on to rescue patients from exposures because their number will be few in comparison to the quantity of available antineoplastic agents, and their effectiveness limited to pretreatment. Thus, the best treatment is one of prevention, which can be accomplished by maintaining a heightened awareness when working with these agents, educating the patient and healthcare provider regarding their use, and providing increased skilled care.

REFERENCES

1. Abele M, Leonhardt M, Dichgans J, Weller M: CCNU overdose during PCV chemotherapy for anaplastic astrocytoma. J Neurol 1998; 245:236–238.

2. Abelson HT: Methotrexate and central nervous system toxicity. Cancer Treat Rep 1978;62:1999–2001.

3. Abelson HT, Fosburg MT, Beardsley P, et al: Methotrexate-induced renal impairment: Clinical studies and rescue from systemic toxicity with high dose leucovorin and thymidine. J Clin Oncol 1983;1: 208–216.

4. Addiego JE, Ridgway D, Bleyer WA: The acute management of intrathecal methotrexate overdose: Pharmacologic rationale and guidelines. J Pediatr 1981;98:825–828.

5. Alderton PM, Gross J, Green MD: Comparative study of doxorubicin, mitoxantrone, and epirubicin in combination with ICRF-187 (ADR-529) in a chronic cardiotoxicity animal model. Cancer Res 1992;52:194–201.

6. Alexander J, Dainiak N, Berger HJ, et al: Serial assessment of doxorubicin cardiotoxicity with quantitative radionuclide angiocardiography. N Engl J Med 1979;300:278–283.

7. Allen JC, Rosen G, Mehta BM, Horten B: Leukoencephalopathy following high-dose IV methotrexate chemotherapy with leucovorin rescue. Cancer Treat Rep 1980;64:1261–1273.

8. Al-Sarraf M, Fletcher W, Oishi N, et al: Cisplatin hydration with and without mannitol diuresis in refractory disseminated malignant melanoma. Cancer Treat Rep 1982;66:31–35.

9. Ammenti A, Reitter B, Muller-Wiefel DE: Chlorambucil neurotoxicity: Report of two cases. Helvetic Paediatr Acta 1980;35:281–287.

10. Anderson CM, Walters RS, Hortobagyi GN: Mediastinitis related to probable central vinblastine extravasation in a woman undergoing adjuvant chemotherapy for early breast cancer. Am J Clin Oncol 1996;19:566–568.

11. Appelbaum FR, Strauchen JA, Gram RG: Acute lethal carditis caused by high-dose combination chemotherapy. Lancet 1976;31: 58–62.

12. Arena E, D'Alessandro N, Dusonchet L, et al: Influence of pharmacokinetic variations on the pharmacologic properties of adriamycin. In: Carter SK, DiMarco A, Ghione M, et al, eds: International Symposium on Adriamycin. Berlin, Springer-Verlag, 1972, pp. 96–116.

13. Argenta LC, Manders EK: Mitomycin C extravasation injuries. Cancer 1983;51:1080–1082.

14. Armstrong JG, Dyke RW, Forts PJ, et al: Hodgkin's disease, carcinoma of the breast, and other tumors treated with vinblastine sulfate. Cancer Chemother Rep 1962;18:49–51.

15. Atherton LD, Leib ES, Kaye MD: Toxic megacolon associated with methotrexate therapy. Gastroenterology 1984;86:1583–1585.

16. Bailey WL, Crump RM. Taxol extravasation: A case report. Can Oncol Nurs J 1997;7:96–99.

17. Bain PG, Lantos PL, Djurovic V, West I: Intrathecal vincristine: A fatal chemotherapeutic error with devastating central nervous system effects. J Neurol 1991;238:230–234.

18. Barak AJ, Tuma DJ, Beckenhauer HC: Methotrexate hepatotoxicity. J Am Coll Nutr 1984;3:93–96.

19. Barlock AL, Howsen DM, Hubbard SM: Nursing management of Adriamycin extravasation. Am J Nurs 1979;79:94–96.

20. Bartowski-Dodds L, Daniels JR: Use of sodium bicarbonate as a means of ameliorating doxorubicin-induced dermal necrosis in rats. Cancer Chemother Pharmacol 1980;4:179–181.

21. Baselt RC: Disposition of Toxic Drugs and Chemicals in Man. Davis, CA, Biomedical Publications, 1982.

22. Basser RK, Sobol MM, Duggan G, et al. Comparative study of the pharmacokinetics and toxicity of high-dose epirubicin with or without dexrazoxane in patients with advanced malignancy. J Clin Oncol 1994;12:1659–1666.

23. Beer M, Cavalli F, Martz G: Vincristine overdose: Treatment with and without leucovorin rescue. Cancer Treat Rep 1983;67:746–747.

24. Benezet S, Chatelut E, Bagheri H, et al: Inefficacy of exchange-transfusion in case of a methotrexate poisoning. Bull Cancer 1997; 84:788–790.

25. Benjamin RS, Wiernik PH, Bachur NR: Adriamycin chemotherapy—Efficacy, safety, and pharmacologic basis of an intermittent single high-dosage schedule. Cancer 1974;33:19–27.

26. Berenson MP: Recovery after inadvertent massive overdosage of vincristine. Cancer Chemother Rep 1971;55:525–526.

27. Berman IF, Mann MP: Seizures and transient cortical blindness associated with cisplatinum diamminedichloride therapy in a thirty-year-old man. Cancer 1980;45:764–766.

28. Bertelli G: Prevention and management of extravasation of cytotoxic drugs. Drug Saf 1995;12:245–255.

29. Bertelli G, Gozza A, Forno GB, et al: Topical dimethylsulfoxide for the prevention of soft tissue injury after extravasation of vesicant cytotoxic drugs: A prospective clinical study. J Clin Oncol 1995;13: 2851–2855.

30. Betcher DL, Burnham N: Melphalan. J Pediatr Oncol Nurs 1990;7: 35–36.

31. Bhawan J, Petry J, Pybak ME: Histologic changes induced in skin by extravasation of doxorubicin. J Cutan Pathol 1989;16:158–163.

32. Billingham ME, Mason GW, Bristow MT, Daniels JR: Anthracycline cardiomyopathy monitored by morphologic changes. Cancer Treat Rep 1978;62:865–872.

33. Blank DQ, Nanji AA, Schreiber DH: Acute renal failure and seizures associated with chlorambucil overdose. J Toxicol Clin Toxicol 1983; 20:361–365.

34. Bleyer WA: New vistas for leucovorin in cancer chemotherapy. Cancer 1989;63:995–1007.

35. Bleyer WA: The clinical pharmacology of methotrexate. Cancer 1978;41:36–51.

36. Bleyer WA, Frisby SA, Oliverio VT: Uptake and binding of vincristine by murine leukemia cells. Biochem Pharmacol 1975;24: 633–639.

37. Bonnetblanc JM, Bordessoule D, Fayol J, Amici JM: Treatment of accidental extravasation of antitumor agents with dimethylsulfoxide and alpha-tocopherol. Ann Dermatol Venereol 1996;123:640–643.

38. Boyle D, Engelking C: Vesicant extravasation: Myths and realities. Oncol Nurs Forum 1995;22:57–67.

39. Boyle FM, Wheeler HR, Shenfield GM: Glutamate ameliorates experimental vincristine neuropathy. J Pharmacol Exp Ther 1996;279: 410–415.

40. Bradley WG, Lassman LP, Pearce GW, Walton JN: The neuromyopathy of vincristine in man: Clinical electrophysiological and pathological studies. J Neurol Sci 1970;10:107–131.

41. Brady ST: Basic properties of fast axonal transport and the role of fast axonal transport in axonal growth. In: Elam JS, ed: Axonal Transport in Neuronal Growth and Regeneration. New York, Plenum, 1984, pp. 13–27.

42. Bristow MR: Toxic cardiomyopathy due to doxorubicin. Hosp Pract 1982;17:101–111.

43. Bristow MR, Minobe WA, Billingham BE, et al: Anthracycline associated cardiac and renal damage in rabbits. Lab Invest 1981;45: 1579–1681.

44. Brivet F, Pavlovitch JM, Gouyette A, et al: Inefficiency of early prophylactic hemodialysis in cis-platinum overdose. Cancer Chemother Pharmacol 1986;18:183–184.

45. Brock N, Pohl J: Prevention of urotoxic side effects by regional detoxification with increased selectivity of oxazaphosphorine cytostatics. IARC Sci Publ 1986;78:269–279.

46. Brock N, Stekar J, Pohl J, et al: Acrolein, the causative factor of nontoxic side effects of cyclophosphamide, ifosfamide, trofosfamide and sufosfamide. Arzneimittelforschung 1979;29:659–661.

47. Byrne TN, Moseley TA, Finer MA: Myoclonic seizures following chlorambucil overdose. Ann Neurol 1981;9:191–194.

48. Calabresi P, Chabner BA: Antineoplastic agents. In: Goodman LS, Limbird LE, Milinoff PB, Gilman AG, Rall TW, eds: The Pharmacological Basis of Therapeutics, 9th ed. New York, McGraw-Hill, 1996, p. 1224–1287.

49. Carrio I, Lopez-Pousa A, Estorch M, et al: Detection of doxorubicin cardiotoxicity in patients with sarcomas by indium-111-antimyosin monoclonal antibody studies. J Nucl Med 1993;34:1503–1507.

50. Chabner BA, Allegre CG, Curt GA, et al: Polyglutamation of methotrexate. Is methotrexate a pro-drug? J Clin Invest 1985;76: 907–912.

51. Chabner BA, Young RC: Threshold methotrexate concentration for in vivo inhibition of DNA synthesis in normal and tumorous target tissues. J Clin Invest 1973;52:1804–1811.

52. Chae L, Moon HS, Kim SC: Overdose of vincristine: Experience with a patient. J Korean Med Sci 1998;13:334–348.

53. Champlin RE, Nimer SD, Ireland P, et al: Treatment of refractory aplastic anemia with recombinant human granulocyte-macrophage-colony-stimulating factor. Blood 1989;15(73):694–699.

54. Chiuten D, Vogl SE, Kaplan BH, Greenwald R: Is there a cumulative or delayed toxicity from cis-diamminedichloroplatinum? Proc Am Assoc Cancer Res 1981;22:163–164.

55. Cho ED, Lowndes HE, Goldstein BD: Neurotoxicology of vincristine in the cat. Arch Toxicol 1983;52:83–90.

56. Chu G, Mantin R, Shen YM: Massive cisplatin overdose by accidental substitution for carboplatin. Cancer 1993;73:3707–3714.

57. Cinollo G, Dini G, Lanino E, et al: Positive direct antiglobulin test in a pediatric patient following high-dose cisplatin. Cancer Chemother Pharmacol 1988;21:85–86.

58. Cohen MR: Medication errors. Cisplatin death. Nursing 1998;28:18.

59. Cohen RJ, Cuneo RA: Transient left homonymous hemianopsia and encephalopathy following treatment of testicular carcinoma with cisplatin, vinblastine and bleomycin. J Clin Oncol 1983;1:392–393.

60. Cox PJ: Cyclophosphamide cystitis—Identification of acrolein as the causative agent. Biochem Pharmacol 1979;28:2045–2049.

61. Creasey WA, Bensch KB, Malawista SE: Colchicine, vinblastine and griseofulvin pharmacological studies with human leukocytes. Biochem Pharmacol 1971;20:1579–1588.

62. Cunningham J, Sharman BL, Goodwin FJ, et al: Do patients receiving hemodialysis need folic acid supplements? Br Med J 1981;282: 1582–1585.

63. Curran CF: Acute doxorubicin overdoses [letter]. Ann Intern Med 1991;115:913.

64. Cutts HJ: Effects of other agents on the biologic responses to vincaleukoblastine. Biochem Pharmacol 1964;13:421–430.

65. Daugaard G, Abildgarrd U, Holstein-Rathlou N, et al: Renal tubular function in patients treated with high-dose cisplatin. Clin Pharmacol Ther 1988;44:164–172.

66. DeAngelis LM, Tong WP, Lin S, Fleisher M, Bertino JR: Carboxypeptidase G2 rescue after high-dose methotrexate. J Clin Oncol 1996;14:2145–2149.

67. Deconti RC, Creasey WA: Clinical aspects of the dimeric Catharanthus alkaloids. In: Taylor WI, Farnsworth NR, eds: The Catharanthus Alkaloids: Botany, Chemistry, Pharmacology and Clinical Use. New York, Marcel Dekker, 1975, pp. 237–278.

68. DeFronzo RA, Braine H, Colvin M, Davis PJ. Water intoxication in man after cyclophosphamide therapy. Time course and relation to drug activation. Ann Intern Med 1973;78:861–869.

69. Desao MH, Teres D: Prevention of doxorubicin-induced skin ulcers in the rat and pig with dimethyl sulfoxide. Cancer Treat Rep 1982; 66:1371–1374.

70. Diener U, Knoll E, Langer G, et al: Urinary excretion of N-acetyl-β-D-glucosaminidase and alanine aminopeptidase in patients receiving amikacin or cisplatin. Clin Chim Acta 1981;112:149–157.

71. Djerassi I, Ciesielka W, Kim JS: Removal of methotrexate by filtration adsorption using charcoal filters or by hemodialysis. Cancer Treat Rep 1977;61:751–752.

72. Doolittle GC, Simpson KM, Lindsley HB: Methotrexate associated, early onset pancytopenia in rheumatoid arthritis. Arch Intern Med 1989;149:1430–1431.

73. Doroshow JH, Locker GY, Myers CE: The enzymatic defenses of the heart against reactive oxygen metabolites. J Clin Invest 1980; 65:128–135.

74. Dorr RT, Alberts DS, Stone A: Cold protection and heat enhancement of doxorubicin skin toxicity in the mouse. Cancer Treat Rep 1985;69:431–437.

75. Dorr RT, Fritz WL: Cancer Chemotherapy Handbook. New York, Elsevier, 1980, pp. 677–684.

76. Dustin P: Micorotubule poisons. In: Justin P, ed: Microtubules. Berlin, Springer-Verlag, 1984, pp. 167–225.

77. Dyke RW: Vincristine must not be administered intrathecally [letter]. JAMA 1982;248:171.

78. Echelberger CK, Ricccardi R, Bleyer A, et al: Influence of body position on ventricular cerebrospinal fluid methotrexate concentration following intralumbar administration. Proc Am Assoc Cancer Res Am Soc Clin Oncol, March 1981, p. 365, Abstract C-131.

79. Enck RE, Bennett JM: Inadvertent chlorambucil overdose in adult. N Y State J Med 1977;77:1480–1485.

80. Ensminger WD, Frei E: The prevention of methotrexate toxicity thymidine infusions in humans. Cancer Res 1977;37:1857–1863.

81. Egorin MJ, Van Echo DA, Tipping SJ, et al: Pharmacokinetics and dosage reduction of cis-diammine (1,1-cyclobutanedicarboxylato) platinum in patients with impaired renal function. Cancer Res 1984; 44:5432–5438.

82. Erttmann R, Landbeck G: Effect of oral cholestyramine on the elimination of high-dose methotrexate. J Cancer Res Clin Oncol 1985; 110:48–50.

83. Ettinger LJ: Pharmacokinetics and biochemical effects of a fatal intrathecal methotrexate overdose. Cancer 1982;50:444–450.

84. Evans WE, Pratt CB, Taylor RH, et al: Pharmacokinetic monitoring of high-dose methotrexate: Early recognition of high risk patients. Cancer Chemother Pharmacol 1979;3:161–166.

85. Extra JM, Marty M, Brienza S, Misset JL: Pharmacokinetics and safety profile of oxaliplatin. Semin Oncol 1998;25(2 Suppl 5): 13–22.

86. Fantine EO, Garnier-Suillerot G: Interaction of 5-amino daunorubicin with Fe II and with cardiolipin-containing vesicles. Biochim Biophys Acta 1986;856:130–136.

87. Favier M, de Carzanove F, Saint-Martin F, et al: Preventing medication errors in antineoplastic therapy [letter]. Am J Hosp Pharm 1984;51:832–833.

88. Firlit CF: Intractable hemorrhagic cystitis secondary to extensive carcinomatosis: Management with formalin solution. J Urol 1973; 110:57–58.

89. Fleischman RA: Clinical use of hematopoietic growth factors. Am J Med Sci 1993;11:248–273.

90. Fox RM: Methotrexate nephrotoxicity. Clin Exp Pharmacol Physiol 1977;5:43–45.

91. Fukushima T, Sumazaki R, Koike K, et al: A magnetic resonance abnormality correlating with permeability of the blood-brain barrier in a child with chemical meningitis during central nervous system prophylaxis for acute leukemia. Ann Hematol 1999;78:564–567.

92. Gadgil SD, Damle SR, Advani SH, Vaidya AB: Effect of activated charcoal on the pharmacokinetics of high dose methotrexate. Cancer Treat Rep 1982;66:1169–1171.

93. Gandara DR, Nahhas WA, Adelson MD, et al: Randomized placebo-controlled multicenter evaluation of diethyldithiocarbamate for chemoprotection against cisplatin-induced toxicity. J Clin Oncol 1995;13:490–496.

94. Garbrecht M, Mullerlie U: Verapamil in the prevention of Adriamycin-induced cardiomyopathy. Klin Wochenschr 1986;64: 132–134.

95. Garnier-Suillerot A: Metal anthracycline and anthracenedione complexes as a new class of anticancer agents. In: Lown JW, ed: Anthracycline and Anthracenedione-Based Anticancer Agents. Amsterdam, Elsevier, 1988, pp. 129–157.

96. Gaze NR: Tissue necrosis caused by commonly used intravenous infusions. Lancet 1978;2:417–419.

97. Gibson TP, Reisch SD, Krumlousky FA, et al: Hemoperfusion for methotrexate removal. Clin Pharmacol Ther 1978;23:351–355.

98. Goldie JH, Price LA, Harrap KR: Methotrexate toxicity: Correlation with duration of administration, plasma levels, dose and excretion pattern. Eur J Cancer 1072;8:409–414.

99. Goodnough LT, Anderson KC, Kurtz S, et al: Indications and guidelines for the use of hematopoietic growth factors. Transfusion 1993; 33:944–959.

100. Goren MP, Wright RK, Horowitz ME: Cumulative renal tubular damage associated with cisplatin nephrotoxicity. Cancer Chemother Pharmacol 1986;18:69–73.

101. Goren MP, Wright RK, Pratt CP, Pell FE: Dechlorethylation of ifosfamide and neurotoxicity. Lancet 1986;2:1219–1220.

102. Green LS, Donoso JA, Heller-Bettinger IE, Samson FE: Axonal transport of disturbances in vincristine-induced peripheral neuropathy. Ann Neurol 1977;12:255–262.

103. Greene RF, Collins JM, Jenkins JF, Speyer JL, Myers CE: Plasma pharmacokinetics of Adriamycin and adriamycinol: Implications for the design of in vitro experiments and treatment protocols. Cancer Res 1983;43(7):3417–3421.

104. Grimes DJ, Bowles MR, Buttsworth JA, et al: Survival after unexpected high serum methotrexate concentrations in a patient with osteogenic sarcoma. Drug Saf 1990;5:447–454.

105. Groth S, Nielsen H, Sorensen JB, et al: Acute and long-term nephrotoxicity of cisplatinum in man. Cancer Chemother Pharmacol 1986; 17:191–196.

106. Grush OC, Morgan SK: Folinic acid rescue for vincristine toxicity. Clin Toxicol 1979;14:71–78.

107. Gutowski MC, Fix DV, Corvalan JR, Johnson DA: Reduction of toxicity of a vinca alkaloid by an anti-vinca alkaloid antibody. Cancer Invest 1995;13:370–374.

108. Hachimi-Idrissi S, Schots R, DeWolf D, et al: Reversible cardiopathy after accidental overdose of mitoxantrone. Pediatr Hematol Oncol 1993;10:35–40.

109. Hamel E, Lin CM: Glutamate induced polymerization of tubulin: Characteristics of the reaction and application to the large-scale purification of tubulin. Arch Biochem Biophys 1981;209:29–40.

110. Hande KR, Balow JE, Drake JC, et al: Methotrexate and hemodialysis. Ann Intern Med 1977;87:495–596.

111. Herman EH, Matre RM, Lee IP, et al: A comparison of the cardiovascular actions of daunomycin, Adriamycin and N-acetyl-daunomycin in hamsters and monkeys. Pharmacology 1971;6:230–241.

112. Hirosawa A, Niitani H, Hayashibara K, Tsuboi E: Effects of sodium thiosulfate in combination therapy of cis-dichlorodiammineplatinum and vindesine. Cancer Chemother Pharmacol 1989;23:255–258.

113. Hitchings RN, Thompson DB: Encephalopathy following cisplatin, bleomycin and vinblastine therapy for non-seminomatous germ cell tumor of testis. Aust N Z J Med 1988;18:67–68.

114. Holland JF: Vincristine treatment of advanced cancer: A cooperative study of 392 cases. Cancer Res 1973;33:1258–1265.

115. Holstein P, Jacobsen K, Pedersen JF, Sorensen JS: Intravesical hydrostatic pressure treatment: New method for control of bleeding from the bladder mucosa. J Urol 1973;109:234–236.

116. Hows JM, Mehta AM, Ward L, et al: Comparison of mensa with forced diuresis to prevent cyclophosphamide induced hemorrhage cystitis in marrow transplantation: A prospective randomized study. Br J Cancer 1984;50:753–756.

117. Huang KC, Wenczak BA, Liu YK: Renal tubular transport of methotrexate in the rhesus monkey and dog. Cancer Res 1979; 39:4843–4848.

118. Hughes PJ, Lane RJM: Acute cerebral edema induced by methotrexate. BMJ 1989;289:1315.

119. Hunter R, Barnes J, Oakeley JF, Mattews DM: Toxicity of folic acid given in pharmacological doses to healthy volunteers. Lancet 1970; 1:61–63.

120. Hurwitz RL, Mahoney DH, Armstrong DL, Browder TM: Reversible encephalopathy and seizures as a result of conventional vincristine administration. Med Pediatr Oncol 1988;16:216–219.

121. Husken BC, de Jong J, Beekman B, et al: Modulation of the in vitro cardiotoxicity of doxorubicin by flavonoids. Cancer Chemother Pharmacol 1995;37:55–62.

122. Ignoffo RJ: Neoplastic disorders. In: Young LY, Koda Kimble MA, eds: Applied Therapeutics: The Clinical Use of Drugs. Vancouver, WA Applied Therapeutics, 1988, pp. 1197–1201.

123. Ignoffo RJ, Friedman MA: Therapy of local toxicities caused by extravasation of cancer chemotherapeutic drugs. Cancer Treat Res 1980;7:17–27.

124. Isacoff WH: Effects of extracorporeal charcoal hemoperfusion on plasma methotrexate [abstract]. Proc Am Assoc Cancer Res 1977; 18:145.

125. Iven H, Brasch H: The effects of antibiotics and uricosuric drugs on the renal elimination of methotrexate and 7-hydroxy methotrexate in rabbits. Cancer Chemother Pharmacol 1988;21:337–342.

126. Jackson DV, McMahan RA, Pope EK, et al: Clinical trial of folinic acid to reduce vincristine neurotoxicity. Cancer Chemother Pharmacol 1986;17:281–284.

127. Jackson DV, Pope EK, McMahan RA, et al: Clinical trial of pyridoxine to reduce vincristine neurotoxicity. J Neurol Oncol 1986;4: 37–41.

128. Jackson DV, Pope EK, Case LD, et al: Improved tolerance of vincristine by glutamic acid. A preliminary report. J Neurooncol 1984; 2:219–222.

129. Jackson DV, Rosenbaum DL, Carlisle LJ, et al: Glutamic acid modification of vincristine toxicity. Cancer Biochem Biophys 1984;7: 245–252.

130. Jackson DV, Wells HB, Atkins JN, et al: Amelioration of vincristine neurotoxicity by glutamic acid. Am J Med 1988;84:1016–1022.

131. Jackson RC: Biological effects of folic acid antagonists with antineoplastic activity. Pharmacol Ther 1984;25:61–82.

132. Jackson RC, Grindey GB: The biochemical basis for methotrexate cytotoxicity. In: Sirotnak FM, ed: Folate Antagonists as Therapeutic Agents, Vol. 1. Orlando, FL, Academic Press, 1984, pp. 289–315.

133. Jacobs SA, Stoller RG, Chabner BA, Johns DG: 7-Hydroxy methotrexate as a urinary metabolite in human subjects and rhesus

monkeys receiving high-dose methotrexate. J Clin Invest 1978;57: 534–538.

134. Jaffe N, Takaue Y, Anzai T, Robertson RR: Transient neurologic disturbances induced by high-dose methotrexate treatment. Cancer 1985;56:1356–1360.

135. Jambou P, Levraut J, Favier C, et al: Removal of methotrexate by continuous venovenous hemodiafiltration. Contrib Nephrol 1995; 116:48–52.

136. Jardine LF, Ingram LC, Bleyer WA: Intrathecal leucovorin after intrathecal methotrexate overdose. J Pediatr Hematol Oncol 1996;18: 302–304.

137. Jirillo A, Gioga G, Bonciarelli G, Dalla Valle G: Accidental overdose of melphalan per os in a 69-year-old woman treated for advanced endometrial carcinoma. Tumori 1998;84:611.

138. Johnson FL, Bernstein ID, Hartman JR: Seizures associated with vincristine sulfate therapy. J Pediatr 1973;82:699–702.

139. Johnson IS, Wright HF, Svoboda GH, et al: Antitumor principles derived from vinca rosea linn, I. Vincaleukoblastine and leurosine. Cancer Res 1960;20:1016–1022.

140. Juma FD, Rogers HJ, Trounce JR. The pharmacokinetics of cyclophosphamide, phosphoramide mustard and nor-nitrogen mustard studied by gas chromatography in patients receiving cyclophosphamide therapy. Br J Clin Pharmacol 1980;10:327–335.

141. Jung HK, Lee J, Lee SN: A case of massive cisplatin overdose managed by plasmapheresis. Korean J Intern Med 1995;10: 150–154.

142. Kaufman IA, Kung FH, Koenig HM, Giammona ST: Overdosage with vincristine. J Pediatr 1976;89:671–674.

143. Kelkar R, Gordon SM, Giri N, et al: Epidemic iatrogenic *Acinetobacter spp.* meningitis following administration of intrathecal methotrexate. J Hosp Infect 1989;14:233–243.

144. Kepka L, De Lassence A, Ribrag V, et al: Successful rescue in a patient with high-dose methotrexate-induced nephrotoxicity and acute renal failure. Leuk Lymphoma 1998;29:205–209.

145. Kevat SG, McCarthy PJ, Hill WR, Ahern MJ: Pancytopenia induced by low-dose methotrexate for rheumatoid arthritis. Aust N Z J Med 1988;18:697–700.

146. Kinkade JM, Volger WR, Dayton PG: Plasma levels of methotrexate in cancer patients as studied by an improved spectrophotofluorimetric method. Biochem Med 1974;10:337–350.

147. Korst AE, van der Sterre ML, Eeltink CM, et al: Pharmacokinetics of carboplatin with and without amifostine in patients with solid tumors. Clin Cancer Res 1997;3:697–703.

148. Kosmidos HV, Bouhoutsou DO, Varvoutsi MC, et al: Vincristine overdose: Experience with 3 patients. Pediatr Hematol Oncol 1991; 8:171–178.

149. Kumar APN, Wrenn EL, Conrad L, et al: Silver nitrate irrigation to control bladder hemorrhage in children receiving cancer therapy. J Urol 1976;166:85–86.

150. Kupfer A, Aeschlimann C, Wermuth B, Cerny T: Prophylaxis and reversal of ifosfamide encephalopathy with methylene-blue. Lancet 1994;26:763–764.

151. Lafolie P, Liliemark J, Bjork O, et al: Exchange of cerebrospinal fluid in accidental intrathecal overdose of cytarabine. Med Toxicol Adverse Drug Exp. 1988;3:248–252.

152. Langlsow A: Nursing and the law. Deadly doses of methotrexate. Aust Nurs J 1995;2:32–34.

153. Larson DL: Treatment of tissue extravasation by antitumor agents. Cancer 1982;49:1796–1799.

154. Lawrence HJ, Goodnight SH: Dimethyl sulfoxide and extravasation of anthracycline agents [letter]. Ann Intern Med 1983;98:1026.

155. Leape LL, Bates DW, Culler DJ, et al: Systems analysis of adverse drug events. JAMA 1995;274:35–43.

156. Lee AC, Wong KW, Fong KW, So KT: Intrathecal methotrexate overdose. Acta Paediatr 1997;86:434–437.

157. LeFrak EA, Pitha J, Rosentheim S, Gottlieb JA: A clinicopathologic analysis of Adriamycin cardiotoxicity. Cancer 1973;32:302–314.

158. Legha SS: Vincristine neurotoxicity, pathophysiology and management. Med Toxicol 1986;1:421–427.

159. Legha SS, Benjamin RS, Mackay B, et al: Reduction of doxorubicin cardiotoxicity by prolonged continuous intravenous infusion. Ann Intern Med 1982;96:133–139.

160. Lesar TS, Briceland L, Stein D: Factors related to errors in medication prescribing. JAMA 1997;227:312–317.

161. Liegler DG, Henderson ES, Hahn MA, Oliverio VT: The effect of organic acids on renal clearance of methotrexate in man. Clin Pharmacol Ther 1969;10:849–857.

162. Lipshultz SE, Rifai N, Sallan SE, et al: Predictive value of cardiac troponin T in pediatric patients at risk for myocardial injury. Circulation 97:96:2641–2648.

163. Lipton RB, Apfel SC, Dutcher JP, et al. Taxol produces a predominantly sensory neuropathy. Neurology 1989;39:368–373.

164. Lopez AM, Wallace L, Dorr RT, et al: Topical DMSO treatment for pegylated liposomal doxorubicin-induced palmar-plantar erythrodysesthesia. Cancer Chemother Pharmacol 1999;44:303–306.

165. Lotz JP, Chapiro J, Voinea A, et al: Overdosage of vinorelbine in a woman with metastatic non-small-cell lung carcinoma. Ann Oncol 1997:7:714–715.

166. MacKinnon SK, Starkebaum G, Wilkens RF: Pancytopenia associated with low-dose pulse methotrexate in the treatment of rheumatoid arthritis. Semin Arthritis Rheum 1985;15:119–126.

167. Maeda K, Ueda M, Ohtaka H, et al: A massive dose of vincristine. Jpn J Clin Oncol 1987;7:247–253.

168. Mandel EM, Lewinski U, Djaldetti M: Vincristine-induced myocardial infarction. Cancer 1975;36:1979–1982.

169. Markman M, Cleary S: High-dose intracavitary cisplatin with intravenous thiosulfate. Low incidence of serious neurotoxicity. Cancer 1985;56:2364–2368.

170. Marmor MF: Negative type electroretinogram from cisplatin toxicity. Doc Ophthalmol 1993;84:237–246.

171. Massenkeil G, Spath-Schwalbe E, Flath B, et al: Transient tetraparesis after intrathecal and high-dose systemic methotrexate. Ann Hematol 1998;77:239–242.

172. McIntosh S, Davis DL, O'Brian RT, Pearson HA: Methotrexate hepatotoxicity in children with leukemia. J Pediatr 1977;90: 1019–1021.

173. Meanwell CA, Blake AE, Kelly KA, et al: Prediction of ifosfamide mesna associated encephalopathy. Eur J Cancer Clin Oncol 1986;22: 815–819.

174. Meggs WJ, Hoffman RS: Intraventricular vincristine fatality [abstract]. J Toxicol Clin Toxicol 1996;34:575.

175. Meijer S, Mulder NH, Sleiffer DT, et al: Influence of combination chemotherapy with cis-diamminedichloroplatinum on renal function: Long-term effects. Oncology 1983;40:170–173.

176. Meijer S, Sleijfer DT, Mulder NH, et al: Some effects of combination chemotherapy with cisplatinum on renal function in patients with nonseminomatous testicular carcinoma. Cancer 1983;51: 2035–2040.

177. Meyer WH, Houghton JA, Houghton PJ: Hypoxanthine: Guanine phosphoribosyltransferase activity in primary human osteosarcomas. A rationale for therapy with methotrexate-thymidine rescue? J Clin Oncol 1987;5:657–661.

178. Michelotti A, Venturini M, Tibaldi C, et al: Single agent epirubicin as first line chemotherapy for metastatic breast cancer patients. Breast Cancer Res Treat 2000;59:133–139.

179. Mills BA, Roberts RW: Cyclophosphamide-induced cardiomyopathy: A report of two cases and review of the English literature. Cancer 1979;43:2223–2226.

180. Misset JL: Oxaliplatin in practice. Br J Cancer 1998;77(Suppl 4):4–7.

181. Moraska L, Rainisio C, Masera G: Duration of cytotoxicity activity of vincristine in the blood of leukemia in children. Rur J Cancer 1969;5:79–84.

182. Myers CE: Role of iron in anthracycline action. In: Hacker MP, Lazo JS, Tritton TR, eds: Organ Directed Toxicities of Anticancer Drugs. Boston, Martinus Nijhoff, 1988, pp. 17–30.

183. Myers CE, Bonow R, Palmeri S, et al: Prevention of doxorubicin cardiomyopathy by *N*-acetylcysteine. Semin Oncol 1983;10:53–55.

184. Nelson RL: The comparative clinical pharmacology and pharmacokinetics of vindesine, vincristine, and vinblastine in human patients with cancer. Med Pediatr Oncol 1982;10:115–127.

185. Nesbit M, Kririt W, Heyn R, Sharp H: Acute and chronic methotrexate on hepatic, pulmonary, and skeletal systems. Cancer 1976;27:1048–1057.

186. Ochs S, Worth R: Comparison of the block of fast axoplasmic transport in mammalian nerve by vincristine, vinblastine, and desacetyl vinblastine amide sulfate (DVA). Proc Am Assoc Cancer Res 1975;16:70–75.

187. Offerman JJ, Meijer S, Sleijfer DT, et al: Acute effects of cis-diamminedichloroplatinum on renal function. Cancer Chemother Pharmacol 1984;12:36–38.

188. Olver IN, Aisner J, Hament A, et al: A prospective study of topical dimethyl sulfoxide for treating anthracycline extravasation. J Clin Oncol 1988;6:1732–1735.

189. Olver IN, Schwartz MA: The use of dimethyl sulfoxide in limiting tissue damage caused by extravasation of doxorubicin. Cancer Treat Rep 1983;67:407–408.

190. O'Marcaigh AS, Johnson MC, Smithson WA, et al: Successful treatment of intrathecal methotrexate overdose by using ventriculolumbar perfusion and intrathecal instillation of carboxypeptidase G2. Mayo Clin Proc 1996;71:161–165.

191. Owen OE, Dellatorre DL, Van Scott EJ, Cohen MR: Accidental intramuscular injection of mechlorethamine. Cancer 1980;45: 2225–2226.

192. Ozols RF, Cunnion RE, Klecker RW, et al: Verapamil and adriamycin in the treatment of drug-resistant ovarian cancer patients. J Clin Oncol 1987;5:641–664.

193. Ozols RF, Ostchega Y, Curt G, Young RC: High dose carboplatin in refractory ovarian cancer patients. J Clin Oncol 1987;5:197–201.

194. Panici PB, Greggi S, Scambia G, et al: High-dose cisplatin-induced neurotoxicity in primary advanced ovarian cancer patients. Cancer Treat Rep 1987;71:669–670.

195. Patel JS, Krusa M: Distant and delayed mitomycin C extravasation. Pharmacotherapy 1999;19:1002–1005.

196. Pessah IN, Durie EL, Schiedt MJ, Zimanyi I: Anthraquinone-sensitized Ca^{2+} release channel from rat cardiac sarcoplasmic reticulum: Possible receptor-mediated mechanism of doxorubicin cardiomyopathy. Mol Pharmacol 1990;37:503–514.

197. Pfeifle CE, Howell SB, Felthouse RD, et al: High-dose cisplatin with sodium thiosulfate protection. J Clin Oncol 1985;3:237–244.

198. Pierga JY, Beuzeboc P, Dorval T, et al: Favorable outcome after plasmapheresis for vincristine overdose [letter]. Lancet 1992;640:185.

199. Pike IM, Arbus MH: Cisplatin overdosage [letter]. J Clin Oncol 1992;10:1503–1504.

200. Pinedo HM, Zaharko DS, Bull JM: The reversal of methotrexate cytotoxicity to mouse bone marrow cells by leucovorin and nucleoside. Cancer Res 1976;336:4418–4424.

201. Pratt CB, Ransom JL, Evans WE: Age-related Adriamycin cardiotoxicity in children. Cancer Treat Rep 1978;62:1381–1385.

202. Pyeritz RE, Droller MJ, Bender WL, Saral R: An approach to the control of massive hemorrhage in cyclophosphamide induced cystitis by intravenous vasopressin: A case report. J Urol 1978;120:253–254.

203. Raley J, Geisler JP, Buekers TE, Sorosky JI: Docetaxel extravasation causing significant delayed tissue injury. Gynecol Oncol 2000;78:259–260.

204. Reggev A, Djerassi I: The safety of administration of massive doses of methotrexate (50 g) with equimolar citrovorum factor rescue in adult patients. Cancer 1988;61:2423–2428.

205. Relling MV, Srapleton FB, Ochs J, et al: Removal of methotrexate, leucovorin, and their metabolites by combined hemodialysis and hemoperfusion. Cancer 1988;62:884–888.

206. Reynolds EH: Mental effects of anticonvulsants and folic acid metabolism. Brain 1968;91:197–214.

207. Reynolds JEF: Vinblastine. In: Reynolds JEF, ed: Martindale: The Extra Pharmacopoeia. England, The Pharmaceutical Press, 1989, pp. 655–657.

208. Riva L, Conter V, Rizzari C, et al: Successful treatment of intrathecal methotrexate overdose with folinic acid rescue: A case report. Acta Paediatr 1999;88:780–782.

209. Roenigk H, Maibach HI, Weinstein GP: Methotrexate therapy for psoriasis. Guidelines revisions. Arch Dermatol 1973;108:35.

210. Rosenthal S, Kaufman S: Vincristine neuropathy. Ann Intern Med 1974;81:733–737.

211. Rossof RH, Slayton RE, Perlia CP: Preliminary clinical experience with cis-diamminedichloroplatinum. Cancer 1972;30:1451–1456.

212. Roush W: Dana-Farber death sends a warning to research hospitals. Science 1995;269:295–306.

213. Rudolph R, Larson DL: Etiology and treatment of chemotherapeutic agent extravasation injuries: A review. J Clin Oncol 1987;5:1116–1126.

214. Rudolph R, Suzuki M, Luca JK: Experimental skin necrosis produced by Adriamycin. Cancer Treat Rep 1979;63:529–537.

215. Rusconi A, Calendi E: Action of daunomycin on nucleic acid metabolism in HeLa cells. Biochem Biphys Acta 1996;119:413–415.

216. Salloum E, Khan KK, Cooper DL: Chlorambucil-induced seizures. Cancer 1997;1;79:1009–1013.

217. San Angel F: Current controversies in chemotherapy administration. J Intraven Nurs 1995;18:16–23.

218. Sandler SG, Tobin W, Henderson ES: Vincristine induced neuropathy: A clinical study of fifty leukemic patients. Neurology 1969;19:367–374.

219. Sasaki K, Tanaka J, Fujimoto T: Theoretically required urinary flow during high dose methotrexate infusion. Cancer Chemother Pharmacol 1984;13:9–14.

220. Schilsky RL: Renal and metabolic toxicities of cancer chemotherapy. Semin Oncol 1982;9:75–83.

221. Schulmeister L, Camp-Sorrell D: Chemotherapy extravasation from implanted ports. Oncol Nurs Forum 2000;27:531–538; quiz 539–540.

222. Schwartz RG, McKenzie WB, Alexander J, et al: Congestive heart failure and left ventricular dysfunction complication doxorubicin therapy. Am J Med 1987;82:1110–1118.

223. Scuderi N, Onesti MG: Antitumor agents: Extravasation, management, and surgical treatment. Ann Plast Surg 1994;32:39–44.

224. Seymour L, Bramwell V, Moran LA. Use of dexrazoxane as a cardioprotectant in patients receiving doxorubicin or epirubicin chemotherapy for the treatment of cancer. The Provincial Systemic Treatment Disease Site Group. Cancer Prev Control 1999;3:145–159.

225. Shah BC, Albert DJ: Intravesical instillation of formalin for the management of intractable hematuria. J Urol 1973;110:519–520.

226. Sharman VL, Cunningham J, Goodwin JF, et al: Do patients receiving regular hemodialysis need folic acid supplements? Br Med J 1982;285:96–97.

227. Sheikh-Hamad D, Timmins K, Jalali Z. Cisplatin-induced renal toxicity: Possible reversal by *N*-acetylcysteine treatment. J Am Soc Nephrol 1997;8:1640–1644.

228. Shurafa M, Shumaker E, Cronin S: Prostaglandin F_2-alpha bladder irritation for control of intractable cyclophosphamide induced hemorrhagic cystitis. J Urol 1987;137:1230–1231.

229. Siegert W, Hiddemann W, Koppensteiner R, et al: Accidental overdose of mitoxantrone in three patients. Med Oncol Tumor Pharmacother 1989;6:275–278.

230. Skoutakis VA, Acchiardo DR, Meyer MC, Hatch FE: Folic acid dosage for chronic hemodialysis patients. Clin Pharmacol Ther 1975;18:200–204.

231. Slimowitz R: Thoughts on a medical disaster. Am J Health Syst Pharm 1995;52:1464–1465.

232. Somers G, Abramow M, Witter M, Naets JP: Myocardial infarction: A complication of vincristine treatment [letter]? Lancet 1976;2:690.

233. Speyer J, Green MD, Kramer E, et al: Protective effect of the bispiperazinedione ICRF-187 against doxorubicin induced cardiac toxicity in women with advanced breast cancer. N Engl J Med 1988;319:745–752.

234. Spiegel RJ, Cooper PR, Blum RH, et al: Treatment of massive intrathecal methotrexate overdose by ventriculolumbar perfusion. N Engl J Med 1984;311:386–388.

235. Steger GG, Mader RM, Gnant MFX, et al: GM-CSF in the treatment of a patient with severe methotrexate intoxication. J Intern Med 1993;233:499–502.

236. Steinberg JS, Cohen AJ, Wasserman AG, et al: Acute arrhythmogenicity of doxorubicin administration. Cancer 1987;60:1213–1218.

237. Steinherz LJ, Steinherz PG, Mangiacasale D, et al: Cardiac changes with cyclophosphamide. Med Pediatr Oncol 1981;9:417–422.

238. Stephens LC, Wang YM, Schultheiss TE, Jarkdine JN: Enhanced cardiotoxicity in rabbits treated with verapamil and Adriamycin. Oncology 1987;44:302–306.

239. Stoller RG, Hande KR, Jacobs SA, et al: Use of plasma pharmacokinetics to predict and prevent methotrexate toxicity. N Engl J Med 1977;297:630–633.

240. Stones DK: Vincristine overdosage in paediatric patients. Med Pediatr Oncol 1998;30:193.

241. Subar M, Muggia FM: Apparent myocardial ischemia associated with vinblastine administration. Cancer Treat Rep 1986;70:690–691.

242. Svingen BA, Powis G, Appel PL, Scott M: Protection against Adriamycin-induced skin necrosis in the rat by dimethyl sulfoxide and alpha-tocopherol. Cancer Res 1979;41:3395–3399.

243. Tattersall MHN, Brown B, Frei E: The reversal of methotrexate toxicity by thymidine with maintenance of antitumor effects. Nature 1981;253:198–200.

244. Tewey KM, Chen GL, Nelson EM, Liu IF: Interactive anticancer drugs interfere with the breakage reunion reaction of mammalian DNA topoisomerase II. J Biol Chem 1984;259:9182–9187.

245. Thierry FX, Vernier I, Dueymes HM, et al: Acute renal failure after high dose methotrexate therapy. Nephron 1989;51:416–417.

246. Thomas LL, Brasst PC, Somers R, Goudsmit R: Massive vincristine overdose: Failure of leucovorin to reduce toxicity. Cancer Treat Rep 1982;66:1967–1969.

247. Trent KC, Myers L, Moreb J: Multiorgan failure associated with lomustine overdose. Ann Pharmacother 1995;29:384–386.

248. Treon SP, Chabner BA: Concepts in use of high dose methotrexate therapy. Clin Chem 1996;42:1322–1329.

249. Trissel LA: Handbook of Injectable Drugs. Bethesda, MD, American Society of Hospital Pharmacists, 1988.

250. Tsavaris NB, Karagiaouris P, Tzannou I: Conservative approach to the treatment of chemotherapy-induced extravasation. J Dermatol Surg Oncol 1990;16:519–522.

251. Vaitkevicius VK, Talley RW, Tucker JL, et al: Cytological and clinical observations during vincaleukoblastine therapy of disseminated cancer. Cancer 1962;15:294–297.

252. van Acker FA, van Acker SA, Kramer K, et al: 7-Monohydroxyethylrutoside protects against chronic doxorubicin-induced cardiotoxicity when administered only once per week. Clin Cancer Res 2000;6:1337–1341.

253. Vandenberg SA, Julig K, Spoerke DG, et al: Chlorambucil overdose: Accidental ingestion of an antineoplastic drug. J Emerg Med 1988;6:495–508.

254. van Rijswijk RE, Hoekman K, Burger CW, et al: Experience with intraperitoneal cisplatin and etoposide and i.v. sodium thiosulphate protection in ovarian cancer patients with either pathologically complete response or minimal residual disease. Ann Oncol 1997;8:1235–1241.

255. Vogelzang NJ: "Adriamycin flare": A skin reaction resembling extravasation. Cancer Treat Rep 1979;63:2067–2069.

256. Vogl SE, Zaravinos T, Kaplan BH: Toxicity of cis-diamminedichloroplatinum given in a two-hour outpatient regimen of diuresis and hydration. Cancer 1980;45:11–15.

257. von Bernuth G, Adam D, Hofstetter R, et al: Cyclophosphamide cardiotoxicity. Eur J Pediatr 1980; 134:87–90.

258. Von Hoff DD, Layard MY, Basa P, et al: Risk factors for doxorubicin induced congestive heart failure. Ann Intern Med 1979;91:710–717.

259. Von Hoff DD, Penta JS, Helman LG, Slavik M: Incidence of drug-related deaths secondary to high-dose methotrexate and citrovorum factor administration. Cancer Treat Rep 1977;61:745–748.

260. Von Hoff DD, Rozencweig M, Picat M: The cardiotoxicity of anticancer agents. Semin Oncol 1982;9:23–33.

261. Walker RW, Allen JC, Rosen G, Caparros B: Transient cerebral dysfunction secondary to high dose methotrexate. J Clin Oncol 1986;4:1845–1850.

262. Wall SM, Johansen MJ, Molony DA, et al: Effective clearance of methotrexate using high-flux hemodialysis membranes. Am J Kidney Dis 1996;28:846–854.

263. Weinstein GO: Methotrexate. Ann Intern Med 1988;86:199–204.

264. Weiss HD, Walker MD, Wiernick PH: Neurotoxicity of commonly used antineoplastic agents. N Engl J Med 1974;29:75–81.

265. Whittaker JA, Al-Ismail SA: Effect of digoxin and vitamin E in preventing cardiac damage caused by doxorubicin in acute myeloid leukemia. Br Med J 1984;288:283–284.

266. Widemann BC, Balis FM, Murphy RF, et al: Carboxypeptidase-G2, thymidine, and leucovorin rescue in cancer patients with methotrexate-induced renal dysfunction. J Clin Oncol 1997;15:2125–2134.

267. Widemann BC, Hetherington ML, Murphy RF, et al: Carboxypeptidase-G2 rescue in a patient with high-dose methotrexate-induced nephrotoxicity. Cancer 1995;1;76:521–526.

268. Wilding G, Caruso R, Lawrence TS, et al: Retinal toxicity after high-dose cisplatin therapy. J Clin Oncol 1985;3:1683–1689.

269. Winchester JF, Rahman A, Tilstone WJ, et al: Will hemoperfusion be useful for cancer chemotherapeutic drug removal? Clin Toxicol 1980;17:557–569.

270. Wolfson S, Olney MB: Accidental ingestion of a toxic dose of chlorambucil. Report of a case in a child. JAMA 1957;165:239–240.

271. Wortman JR, Lucas VS, Schuster E, et al: Sudden death during doxorubicin administration. Cancer 1979;44:1588–1590.

272. Yancey RS, Talpaz M: Vindesine-associated angina and ECG changes. Cancer Treat Rep 1982;66:587–589.

273. Zaragoza MR, Ritchey ML, Walter A: Neurologic consequences of accidental intrathecal vincristine: A case report. Med Pediatr Oncol 1995;24:61–62.

274. Zbinden G, Brandle E: Toxicologic screening of daunorubicin, NSC-82151, Adriamycin, NSC-123127 and their derivatives in rats. Cancer Chemother Rep 1975;59:707–715.

275. Zoubek A, Zaunschirm HA, Lion T, et al: Successful carboxypeptidase G2 rescue in delayed methotrexate elimination due to renal failure. Pediatr Hematol Oncol 1995;12:471–477.

276. Zulian GB, Tullen E, Maton B: Methylene blue for ifosfamide associated encephalopathy. N Engl J Med 1996;332:1239–1240.

277. Zweier JL: Iron-mediated formation of an oxidized adriamycin free radical. Biochim Biophys Acta 1985;839:209–213.

Jason B. Hack / Neal A. Lewin

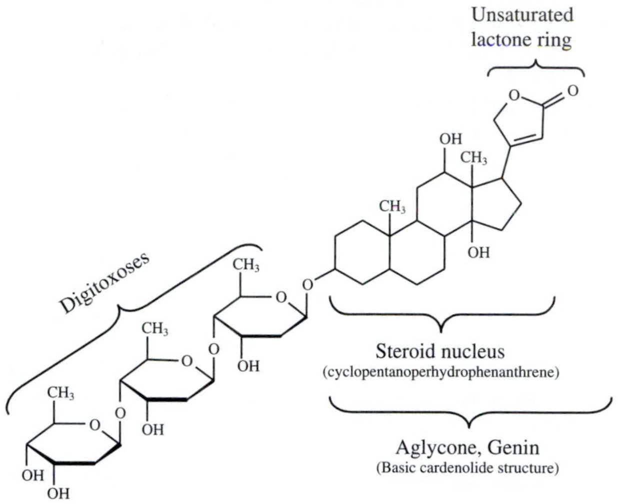

Unsaturated lactone ring

Digitoxoses

OH
CH₃

CH₃

CH₃

CH₃
O
OH

CH₃
O O
OH

CH₃
O O
OH

OH
OH

OH

OH

CH₃

OH

Steroid nucleus
(cyclopentanoperhydrophenanthrene)

Aglycone, Genin
(Basic cardenolide structure)

Digoxin		
MW:	=	780 daltons
Action Levels		
Serum Digoxin	=	> 2 ng/mL
	=	≥ 10 ng/mL 6h postingestion
	=	≥ 15 ng/mL at any time
Serum Digitoxin	=	> 4 ng/mL
	=	> 150 ng/mL (serious)
Ingestion	=	> 4 mg digoxin in child
	=	> 10 mg digoxin in adult
Serum K⁺ level	=	≥ 5.0 mEq/L (acute)

Values greater than or equal to the action level necessitate clinical intervention. Values less than this level may necessitate intervention based on the clinical condition of the patient.

A 92-year-old woman was brought to the hospital by her grandson. The grandson stated that she had lost her appetite for several days, refused her medications for 2 days, and had begun to vomit on the day of admission. The woman complained of being weak and having no appetite because of her constant nausea. Her grandson reported that 5 days prior to admission, she had initiated a course of clarithromycin for sinusitis, and her past medical history was significant for congestive heart failure and hypertension. Her medications included digoxin, furosemide, and enteric-coated aspirin.

On presentation to the Emergency Department (ED) the patient was not in acute distress, laying quietly on the bed, alert and oriented to place and person. Her vital signs were blood pressure, 140/95 mm Hg; pulse, 50 beats/min and regular; respiratory rate, 16 breaths/min; and rectal temperature, 98.8°F (37.1°C). The woman weighed 55 kg. Her neck was supple; she had no jugular venous distension or carotid bruits. Lung examination revealed bibasilar rales. Heart examination revealed a normal S_1 and S_2 with an S_3 gallop, but no murmurs were heard. Abdominal examination revealed increased bowel sounds, with no other abnormal findings. Examination of the patient's extremities revealed 1+ pitting edema without clubbing, or cyanosis, and all pulses were 2+. Neurologic examination was nonfocal.

The patient was attached to a cardiac monitor with continuous pulse oximetry. An IV line was inserted, and blood samples were obtained for complete blood count (CBC); electrolytes, including calcium and magnesium; blood urea nitrogen (BUN); creatinine; glucose; liver enzymes; amylase and lipase; digoxin; and salicylate levels. An initial rhythm strip and 12-lead electrocardiogram (ECG) revealed high-degree heart block with a ventricular rate of 30–50 beats/min (Fig. 48–1), which then converted into atrial flutter with variable block, and a ventricular response rate of 30–40 beats/min (Fig. 48–2). Transcutaneous pacer pads were placed on standby, and 5 vials of Digibind (digoxin-specific Fab) were requested. Stat

laboratory results returned: serum sodium, 142 mEq/L; chloride, 114 mEq/L; potassium, 3.6 mEq/L; bicarbonate, 24 mEq/L; BUN, 12 mg/dL; creatinine, 1.4 mg/dL; glucose, 98 mg/dL; calcium, 9.8 mg/dL, magnesium, 2.0 mEq/L. Liver enzymes, amylase, and lipase were normal. Hematocrit was 37.8%. A serum digoxin level was pending.

Fifteen minutes after the examination was completed, the patient vomited. Although her heart rate decreased to 30 beats/min, her blood pressure remained at 130/80 mm Hg. Atropine 1 mg IV was administered for the bradycardia with no response, and 5 vials of Digibind were administered IV. Within 20 minutes of the infusion of Digibind, her heart rate had increased to 86 beats/min. The initial digoxin level was 3.8 ng/mL.

HISTORY AND EPIDEMIOLOGY

Although there is evidence in the *Ebers Papyrus* (Papyrus Smith) that the Egyptians used plants containing cardiac glycosides at least 3000 years ago, it was not until William Withering wrote the first organized account about the effects of the foxglove plant in 1785 that its use was more widely accepted into the Western apothecary. The discussion and case reports of the 163 patients for whom Withering prescribed foxglove and his correspondence with other physicians on the subject, comprise the first work related to the medical use of cardiac glycosides. Foxglove was initially used as a diuretic and for the treatment of "dropsy," and Withering eloquently described its "power over the motion of the heart, to a degree yet unobserved in any other medicine."[95]

Subsequent to these reports, cardiac glycosides became the mainstay of treatment for chronic heart failure, and for the control the ventricular response rate in atrial tachydysrhythmias. Because of the widespread use of cardiac glycosides, both acute and

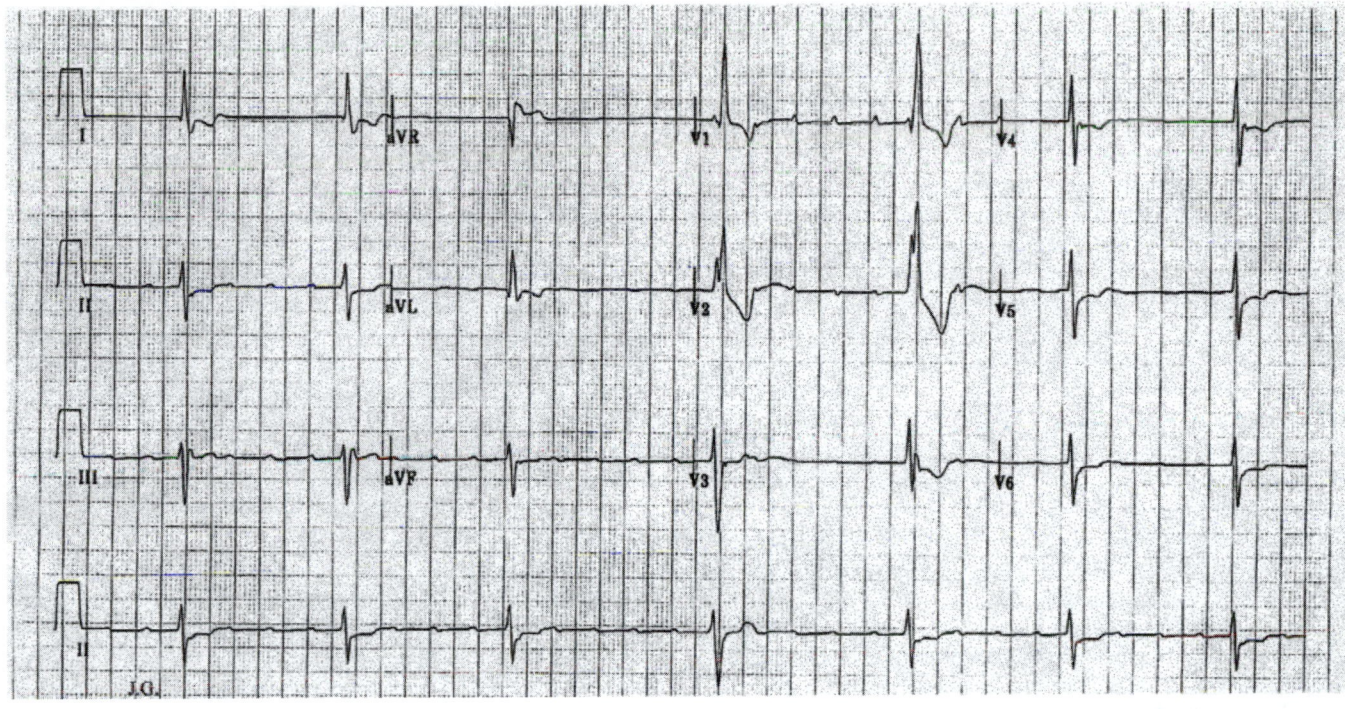

Figure 48–1.   High-degree heart block with a ventricular rate of 30–50 beats/min.

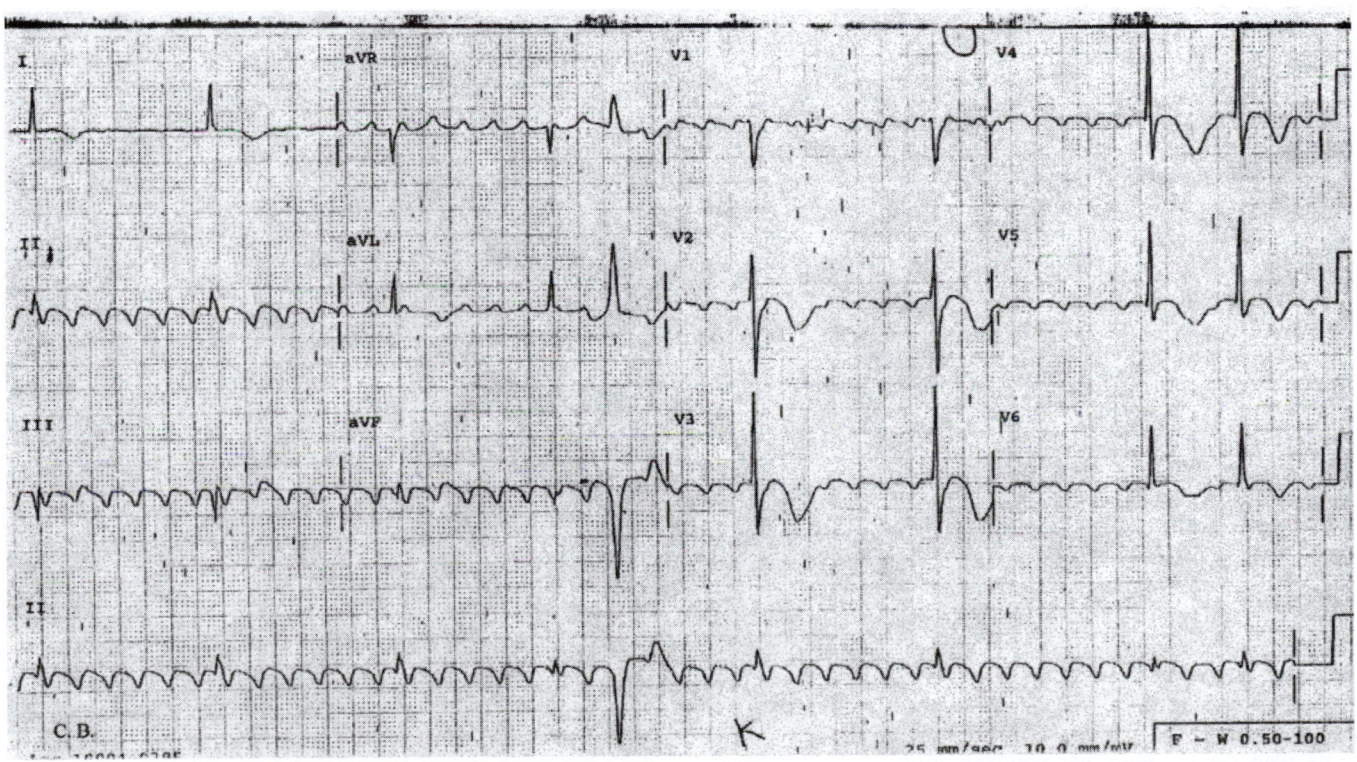

Figure 48–2.   The patient in Figure 48–1 subsequently converted into atrial flutter with variable block and a ventricular rate of 30–40 beats/min.

chronic toxicity has remained an important problem.[62] According to the American Association of Poison Control Centers data, between the years 1995 and 1999 there were approximately 18,000 exposures to cardiac glycoside-containing products resulting in over 70 deaths. In 1999 it was noted that 75% of the deaths were a result of "therapeutic errors" (Chap. 116 and page 1752).

Poisoning is typically encountered in the very young or the very old. In children most acute overdoses result from dosing errors, usually a decimal point error resulting in 10 times the appropriate dose, or inadvertent ingestions. Older patients more often have acute exposures related to intentional ingestion of the drug. Adults are also at risk for acute toxicity complicating a chronic regimen related to changes in chronic dosing or an alteration in the absorption or elimination kinetics, which results in an increased serum concentration of the drug. This may be caused by drug-drug interactions that change cardiac glycoside clearance in the liver or kidney, or from altered protein binding, or from coingested medications that increase the bioavailability. The most commonly prescribed cardiac glycoside in the United States is digoxin; other, less commonly used preparations are digitoxin, ouabain, lanatoside C, deslanoside, and gitalin.

Cardiac glycoside poisoning also results from specific plant or animal ingestions. Documented sources of plant toxicities include oleander, foxglove, lily of the valley, dogbane, Siberian ginseng, and red squill; foods skewered and cooked with cardiac glycoside–containing plants and teas containing seeds of these plants; drinking contaminated water; and contaminated herbal products (Chap. 77).[12,36,59,67,73,87] Cardiac glycoside poisoning also results from ingestion, instead of topical application, of a purported aphrodisiac derived from the dried secretion of the *Bufo* toad containing certain cardioactive bufadienolide-class agents.[8,9,11]

PHARMACOLOGY

Cardiac glycosides all contain an aglycone or "genin" nucleus structure with a steroid core and an unsaturated lactone ring attached at C-17 and several sugars attached to C-3. Cardenolides are plant-derived aglycone structures with a 5-member unsaturated lactone ring. The bufadienolide group of cardioactive steroid molecules are mainly animal derived (with notable exceptions such as scillaren from red squill) and have a 6-member unsaturated lactone ring. Digoxigenin needs sugar residues to become a glycoside. Digoxin, which is the most widely prescribed cardiac glycoside in the United States, may be thought of as the model molecule for cardenolides. Digitoxin aglycone differs from digoxin aglycone by the lack of a hydroxyl group on C-12, and ouabain differs by both the absence of a hydroxyl group on C-12 and the addition of hydroxyl groups on C-1, 5, 10, and 11. These plant-derived aglycone molecules are linked to one or more hydrophilic sugar (digitoxoses) residues at C-3, which confer increased water solubility and enhanced ability to enter cells, to compose a cardiac glycoside. The cardioactive components in toad venom are genins, and lack sugar moieties.

The clinical manifestations following the ingestion of cardiac glycoside-containing plants or toad venom are clinically indistinguishable from those following the ingestion of digoxin. Those patients with cardiac glycoside poisoning from plant or animal ingestion may differ from pharmaceutic digoxin ingestions by a low or nonexistent digoxin level (depending on the digoxin assay),

despite the persistence of toxicity and the need for large doses of digoxin-specific antibody fragments (Chaps. 77 and 78.)

Mechanisms of Action and Pathophysiology

Electrophysiologic Effects on Inotropy. The cardiac glycosides increase the force of contraction of the heart (positive inotropic effect) because of an increase of cytosolic Ca^{2+} during systole. Both Na^+ and Ca^{2+} ions enter and exit cardiac muscle cells during each cycle of depolarization, contraction, and repolarization. Sodium entry heralds the start of the action potential (phase 0) and carries the inward, depolarizing positive charge. Calcium enters the cardiac myocyte through L-type calcium channels during the plateau phase of depolarization, which subsequently triggers the release of more calcium into the cytosol from the sarcoplasmic reticulum. During repolarization and relaxation (diastole), calcium is pumped back into the sarcoplasmic reticulum by a local Ca^{2+}-ATPase and is removed from the cytoplasm by an Na^+-Ca^{2+} antiporter and a sarcolemmal Ca^{2+}-ATPase[58] (Fig. 48–3).

All cardiac glycosides inhibit active transport of Na^+ and K^+ across cell membranes by binding to a specific site on the extracytoplasmic face of the α subunit of the membrane Na^+-K^+-ATPase preventing its normal function. This Na^+-Ca^{2+} exchanger derives its power not from ATP but rather from the Na^+ gradient generated by the Na^+- K^+ transport mechanism.[18] The amount of intracellular Na^+ determines how much Ca^{2+} is extruded from the cell. The cardiac glycosides bind to sarcolemmal Na^+-K^+-ATPase, and inhibit cellular Na^+ pump activity, which decreases Na^+ extrusion and increases Na^+ in the cytosol, thereby decreasing the transmembrane Na^+ gradient preventing extrusion of intracellular Ca^{2+} during repolarization. Small changes in intracellular Na^+ concentration yield large increases in cardiac muscle shortening. Other proposed mechanisms under investigation for cardiac glycosides increasing cytosolic Ca^{2+} include an interaction with the L-type calcium channels, and interactions with the Ca^{2+}-triggered calcium release from myocardial sarcoplasmic reticulum.[41]

Effects on Cardiac Conduction. At therapeutic levels, cardiac glycosides increase inotropy, increase automaticity, and shorten the repolarization intervals of the atria and ventricles (Table 48–1). There is a concurrent decrease in the rate of conduction through the SA and AV nodes with direct depression of this tissue and an indirect effect through an increase in vagally mediated parasympathetic tone. These changes in repolarization are reflected on the ECG by a decrease in ventricular response rate to suprajunctional rhythms, QT segment shortening, and ST segment and T-wave forces opposite in direction to the major QRS forces. That last effect results in the characteristic scooping of the ST segments (referred to as "digitalis effect"). Excessive increases in intracellular Ca^{2+} caused by excessive cardiac glycoside levels result in transient late depolarizations (delayed afterdepolarizations), which may initiate contractions.[17,42]

Effects of Cardiac Glycosides on the Autonomic Nervous System. Digitalis affects the parasympathetic system by increasing the release of acetylcholine from vagal fibers,[55,86] possibly through augmentation of intracellular calcium. Cardiac glycosides affect the sympathetic system by increasing efferent sympathetic discharge,[63,82] which, in turn, may exacerbate myocardial intracellular hypercalcemia.

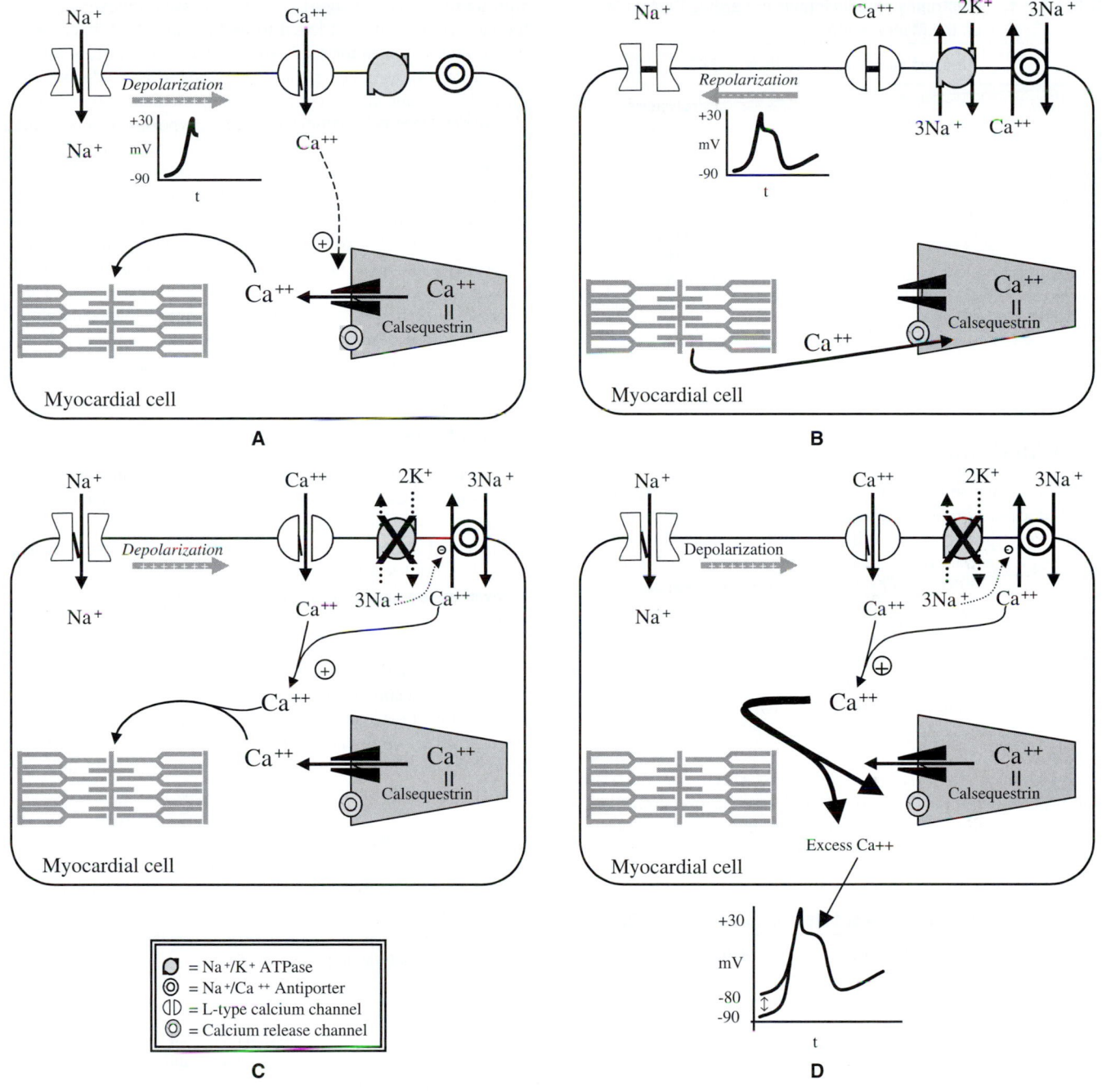

Figure 48–3. A. *Normal Depolarization.* Depolarization occurs following the opening of fast Na$^+$ channels; the rise in intracellular potential opens voltage-dependent Ca^{2+} channels; the influx of Ca^{2+} induces the massive release of Ca^{2+} from the sarcoplasmic reticulum, producing contraction. **B.** *Normal Repolarization.* Repolarization begins with active expulsion of Na$^+$ ions in exchange for K$^+$ using an ATPase. This electrogenic (3 for 2) pump creates an Na$^+$ gradient that is used to expel Ca^{2+} via an antiporter. The sarcoplasmic reticulum resequesters its Ca^{2+} load via a separate ATPase. **C.** *Pharmacologic Cardiac Glycoside.* Digitalis inhibition of the Na$^+$/K$^+$ ATPase raises the intracellular Na$^+$ content, preventing the antiporter from expelling Ca^{2+} in exchange for Na$^+$. The net result is an elevated intracellular Ca^{2+}, resulting in enhanced inotropy. **D.** *Toxic Cardiac Glycoside.* Excessive elevation of the intracellular Ca^{2+} elevates the resting potential, producing myocardial sensitization, and predisposes to dysrhythmias. The addition of exogenous Ca^{2+} may overwhelm the capacity of the sarcoplasmic reticulum to sequester this ion, resulting in systolic arrest.

TABLE 48–1. Electrophysiologic Effects of Cardiac Glycoside on the Myocardium

	Atria and Ventricles	AV Node	ECG
Excitability	↑	—	Extrasystoles, tachydys-rhythmias
Automaticity	↑	—	Extrasystoles, tachydys-rhythmias
Conduction velocity	↓	↓	↑ PR interval, AV block
Refractoriness	↓	↑	↑ PR interval, AV block, decreased QTc interval

PHARMACOKINETICS

Whether an ingestion of cardiac glycosides will result in a toxic effect depends upon the preparation, mode of administration, amount absorbed, volume of distribution, route of administration, and drug-drug interactions, together with the pathophysiologic characteristics of the host (Table 48–2). Correlation between clinical effects and toxic serum levels are based on steady-state levels; measurement of a level before 6 hours after an ingestion gives misleadingly high levels, which reflect a biphasic distribution. After therapeutic dosing, the intravascular distribution and elimination of digoxin are best described by a two-compartment system with the first (the α phase) a 30-minute half-life and exponential decline because of rapid distribution from the blood volume to peripheral tissues. This phase is followed by an elimination phase (the β phase) with a half-life of 36–48 hours for total body clearance, which is achieved primarily by the kidneys (70% in a person

TABLE 48–2. Pharmacology of Selected Cardiac Glycosides

Onset of Action	Digoxin	Digitoxin
Oral	1.5–6 h	3–6 h
IV	5–30 min	30 min–2 h
Maximal effect		
Oral	4–6 h	6–12 h
IV	1.5–3 h	4–8 h
Intestinal absorption	40–90% (mean 75%)	>95%
Plasma protein binding	25%	97%
Volume of distribution	6–7 L/kg (adults) 16 L/kg (infants) 10 L/kg (neonates) 4–5 L/kg (adults with renal failure)	0.6 L/kg (adults)
Elimination half-life	1.6 days	6–7 days
Route of elimination	Renal (60–80%), with limited hepatic metabolism	Hepatic metabolism (80%)
Enterohepatic circulation	7%	26%

with normal renal function).[13] After a massive digoxin ingestion the half-life may be shortened to as little as 13–15 hours. With therapeutic administration of cardiac glycosides, factors such as age, hypothyroidism, hepatic and renal disease associated with decreased creatinine clearance, hypokalemia, hypernatremia, alkalosis, hypercalcemia, hypomagnesemia, hypoxemia, myocardial disease, and cor pulmonale can all result in toxicity unless dosage and frequency regimens of the drug are appropriately adjusted. Drug interactions between digoxin and quinidine, verapamil, diltiazem, amiodarone, and spironolactone are common.[15,31,49,68] In approximately 10–15% of the population, a significant amount of digoxin is inactivated in the gut by enteric bacterium, primarily *Eubacterium lentum*, and the reversal of this inactivation by erythromycin or tetracycline may result in increased bioavailability.[53] Indeed, the use of certain antibiotics may produce as much as a 2-fold increase in serum cardiac glycoside concentration, potentially leading to toxicity.[68]

Clinical Manifestations

"The Foxglove when given in very large and quickly-repeated doses, occasions sickness, vomiting, purging, giddiness, confused vision, objects appearing green or yellow; increased secretion of urine, with frequent motion to part with it, and sometimes inability to retain it; slow pulse, even as low as 35 in a minute, cold sweats, convulsions, syncope, death."[95]

In general, adults and children with cardiac glycoside poisoning present in a similar manner depending upon whether the exposure is acute or chronic. Both groups may present with either acute or chronic poisoning and while clinical manifestations differ, the types of poisoning are treated in similar manners. The following descriptions apply to both clinical situations.

Noncardiac Toxicity

Acute Toxicity. An asymptomatic period of several minutes to several hours may follow a single orally administered toxic dose of cardiac glycoside. The first symptom is typically nausea, vomiting, or abdominal pain. Central nervous system effects of acute toxicity may include lethargy, confusion, and weakness that are not caused by hemodynamic changes.[12]

Chronic Toxicity. Chronic toxicity is often difficult to diagnose secondary to its insidious development and protean manifestations. Symptoms may include those that occur with acute poisonings; however, they are often less obvious. Gastrointestinal symptoms include, anorexia, nausea, vomiting, abdominal pain, and weight loss. Neuropsychiatric disorders include delirium, confusion, disorientation, drowsiness, headache, hallucinations, or, rarely, convulsions.[12,25,26] Visual disturbances include transient amblyopia, photophobia, blurring, scotomata, photopsia, decreased visual activity, and aberrations of color vision (chromatopsia), such as yellow halos (xanthopsia) around lights.[50]

Electrolyte Abnormalities. Elevated serum potassium levels frequently occur in patients with acute cardiac glycoside poisoning.[42,45] Hyperkalemia in acute cardiac glycoside poisoning has important prognostic implications, as the serum potassium concentration is a better predictor of lethality than either the initial ECG changes or the serum cardiac glycoside concentration.[4,5] In a study of 91 acutely digitalis-poisoned (digitoxin) patients conducted before digoxin-specific Fab was available, approximately 50% of the patients with serum potassium levels of 5.0–5.5 mEq/L died. Although a serum potassium level lower than 5.0 mEq was associated with no deaths, all of the 10 patients with serum potassium levels above 5.5 mEq died.[4] This hyperkalemia causes further depolarization of myocardial conduction tissue, in particular increasing AV nodal block, thereby exacerbating cardiac glycoside–induced bradydysrhythmias and conduction delays.[42] However, correction of hyperkalemia does not increase patient survival,[4] as it is a marker of, and not the cause of, the morbidity and mortality associated with cardiac glycoside poisoning. Elevation of the serum potassium concentration after toxic as well as therapeutic administration of cardiac glycoside is a result of (a) the release of potassium from many tissues, including the liver; (b) cardiac glycoside inhibition of potassium uptake by skeletal muscle; and (c) cardiac glycoside inhibition of the cardiac Na^+-K^+-ATPase pump. The interrelationships between intracellular and extracellular potassium and cardiac glycoside therapy are complex and not clearly understood.

Hypokalemia resulting from a variety of mechanisms, such as the use of loop diuretics, poor dietary intake, diarrhea, and the administration of potassium binding resins, enhances the effects of cardiac glycosides on the myocardium and is associated with dysrhythmias at lower cardiac glycoside levels. Hypokalemia itself inhibits Na^+-K^+-ATPase activity and contributes to the pump inhibition induced by cardiac glycosides, enhances myocardial automaticity, and therefore increases myocardial susceptibility to cardiac glycoside–related dysrhythmias. This may be partly a result of decreased competitive inhibition between the cardiac glycoside and potassium at the Na^+-K^+-ATPase exchanger.[71] Severe hypokalemia (<2.5 mEq/L) reduces the rate of sodium pump function, slowing the pump and exacerbating concomitant sodium pump inhibition because of cardiac glycosides.[42] Chronic hypokalemia reduces the number of Na^+-K^+-ATPase units in skeletal muscle, thereby potentially decreasing the volume of drug distribution.[2,45]

Cardiac Toxicity. The alterations in cardiac rate and rhythm occurring with cardiac glycoside toxicity may produce almost every known type of dysrhythmia with the exception of the rapidly conducted supraventricular tachydysrhythmias. In 10–15% of cases, the appearance of an ectopic ventricular rhythm is the first sign of toxicity and this is the most frequent rhythm disturbance noted.[70] Although no dysrhythmia is diagnostic of cardiac glycoside toxicity (with perhaps the exception of bidirectional ventricular tachycardia), toxicity should be suspected when there is evidence of increased automaticity in combination with depressed conduction through the SA and AV nodes.[42] These dysrhythmias result from the complex electrophysiologic influences on the heart and the direct, vagotonic, and antiadrenergic actions of these cardiac glycosides. The effects of digoxin vary with the dose and differ depending on the type of cardiac tissue involved. The atrial and ventricular myocardial tissues exhibit increased automaticity and excitability, resulting in extrasystoles and tachydysrhythmias. Conduction velocity is reduced in both the conducting system and nodal tissue, resulting in an increased PR interval and AV nodal block accompanied by a decreased QT interval. Indeed, AV junctional blocks of varying degrees, associated with increased ventricular automaticity, are the most common manifestations, occurring in 30–40%, of patients with cardiac glycoside toxicity.[56]

Atrioventricular dissociation may result from suppression of the dominant pacemaker with escape of a subsidiary pacemaker or from inappropriate acceleration of a ventricular pacemaker. Hypotension, shock, and cardiovascular collapse can ensue. Table 48–1 summarizes these phenomena.

Acute Toxicity. The initial electrophysiologic manifestations of digitalis are usually mediated indirectly by increased vagal tone resulting in bradydysrhythmias. In the initial phase of acute poisoning, depression of SA or AV nodal function may be reversed by atropine. Cardiac dysrhythmias—nonparoxysmal atrial tachydysrhythmias with block,[54] atrial flutter, and fibrillation with block; conduction system dysfunction including nonparoxysmal junctional tachycardia,[42] high-degree AV block, occasionally with depression of the atrial pacemakers resulting in SA arrest, and sinus exit block; and ventricular ectopies including premature extrasystoles, ventricular salvoes, ventricular bigeminy, ventricular flutter and fibrillation, and bidirectional ventricular tachycardia—are caused by enhanced automaticity, reentry, or both (Table 48–1).[70] Bidirectional ventricular tachycardia is particularly characteristic of severe cardiac glycoside toxicity and results from alterations of intraventricular conduction, junctional tachycardia with aberrant intraventricular conduction, or, on rare occasions, alternating ventricular pacemakers.

Chronic Toxicity. Bradydysrhythmias that appear late in acute poisonings or those resulting from chronic toxicities occur by direct actions of the drug on the heart and often are minimally responsive, or cannot be corrected by the administration of atropine. The rhythms seen include all of those encountered after acute poisonings.

Diagnostic Testing

Properly obtained and interpreted serum digoxin concentrations significantly aid in the management of cardiac glycoside poisoning. Serum cardiac glycoside levels must be interpreted in relation to other metabolic abnormalities and medications, including hypokalemia; hypomagnesemia; hypercalcemia; hypernatremia; alkalosis; hypothyroidism; hypoxemia; catecholamines; and the use of calcium channel blockers, quinidine, amiodarone, or diuretics.

Although cardiac glycoside poisonings are multifactorial, being the result of interactions of the many diverse factors previously mentioned, there is a significant correlation between the clinical condition and the serum digoxin or digitoxin concentration. In general, patients with cardiac glycoside toxicity have mean serum concentrations above 2 ng/mL measured at least 6 hours postingestion for digoxin and above 40 ng/mL for digitoxin.[41] The significance of these concentrations depends on when the value is obtained in relation to an acute ingestion and the distribution phase of the drug. A value of 15 ng/mL of digoxin is, therefore, more ominous 6 hours after an ingestion than 1 hour after an ingestion. Because there are multiple determinants of digoxin poisoning and there is an overlap in serum digoxin concentrations between toxic and nontoxic patients, it may be inaccurate to use the therapeutic range of digoxin of 0.5–2.0 ng/mL as the sole indicator of toxicity, as this can be misleading, and must be correlated with the clinical presentation.[76]

In most hospitals, "digoxin levels" are ordered to evaluate therapeutic or toxic levels of digoxin and also for digitoxin, if digitoxin levels are unavailable. The polyvalent assays typically used in most institutions frequently but unpredictably cross-react with other plant or animal cardiac glycosides. Only digoxin is accurately detected by monoclonal digoxin immunoassay. Thus an elevated "digoxin level" in the correct clinical setting may qualitatively assist in making a presumptive diagnosis of a nondigoxin cardiac glycoside poisoning (Chaps. 77 and 78). Serum levels of digoxin are measured in one of two ways: free digoxin and total digoxin. The most common method of quantifying total digoxin in the serum is by fluorescence polarization immunoassay (FPIA). Under normal circumstances, measuring total digoxin in the serum is sufficient. However, after the use of digoxin-specific Fab, which draws cardiac glycoside from the tissues into the intravascular space, there is a large elevation in total cardiac glycoside levels as measured by total digoxin immunoassay techniques. Paradoxically, excess digoxin antibody may cause a false elevation in "digoxin concentration" (Chap. 7). Other methods, such as treating the serum with Fab denaturing agents, utilizing ultrafiltration techniques to remove digoxin-Fab complexes, or equilibrium dialysis techniques, allow the quantification of free digoxin in the serum.[23]

ENDOGENOUS DIGOXINLIKE IMMUNOREACTIVE SUBSTANCE

Some patients who are not receiving a cardiac glycoside may also have a false-positive digoxin assay as a result of an endogenous substance that is structurally and functionally similar to the prescribed cardiac glycosides.[30] This finding is described in pregnancy,[20,28,35] in neonates,[88] and in patients with renal insufficiency,[10,27,37] liver disease,[60] subarachnoid hemorrhage,[94] congestive heart failure,[29,77] insulin-dependent diabetes,[22] stress,[26,89] acromegaly,[16] and hypothermia,[88] which are all states of increased inotropic need or reduced renal clearance. Endogenous substances, for example bilirubin[60] (and exogenous substances, such as spironolactone[78]), may cross-react with the digoxin assay and cause a false-positive result. An endogenous sodium pump inhibiting dihydropyrone-substituted steroid has been isolated from human placenta and structurally is a bufenolide. It differs from the toad bufadienolides solely by a single double-bond pyrone ring. Because bufenolides are not found in plants or humans, a synthetic pathway to produce dihydropyrone-substituted steroids in humans may be responsible for this endogenous digoxinlike immunoreactive substance (DLIS). Further research is necessary to confirm this pathway.[35] The use of ultrafiltration techniques while altering incubation time and temperature at which the digoxin assay is performed can eliminate the contribution of DLIS.[21] The clinician suspecting this problem should consult the laboratory. Clinical observations indicate that the serum digoxin level contributed by endogenous digoxinlike immunoreactive substances is usually less than 2 ng/mL.

THERAPY

Management Overview

Initial treatment of a patient with acute digitalis poisoning includes providing general supportive care, discontinuing cardiac glycoside therapy, preventing further exposure, preventing further gastrointestinal (GI) absorption, monitoring for dysrhythmias, de-

termining electrolyte and digoxin levels, administering digoxin-specific antibodies, and treating specific complications such as dysrhythmias and electrolyte abnormalities.

Gastrointestinal Decontamination

Initial therapy should be directed toward prevention of further GI absorption. Emesis or lavage, may be considered; however, efficacy is limited secondary to rapid absorption from the gut, and the emetic effects of the drug itself. Patients with chronic ingestions do not usually benefit from these GI decontamination techniques. Because many cardiac glycosides such as digitoxin and digoxin are recirculated enterohepatically and enteroenterically, late as well as repeated activated charcoal administration (1 g/kg body weight every 2–4 hours) may be beneficial.[13,48,51,64,92] Steroid-binding resins, such as cholestyramine and colestipol,[34] like activated charcoal, can block reabsorption of cardiac glycoside from the GI tract and reduce the serum half-life by interrupting both enteroenteric and enterohepatic circulation.

Advanced Management

"If inadvertently the doses of the Foxglove should be prescribed too largely, exhibited too rapidly, or urged too great a length; the knowledge of a remedy to counteract its effects would be a desirable thing"[95]

Digoxin-Specific Antibody Fragments. The standard of care for patients with life-threatening cardiac glycoside toxicity is the use of digoxin-specific antibodies.[1,21,23,65,67,73,80,84,96] Purified digoxin-specific Fab causes a sharp decrease in free digoxin levels, a concomitant, but clinically unimportant massive increase in total serum digoxin, an increase in renal clearance of cardiac glycoside, and a decrease of serum potassium.[1] Digoxin-specific Fab represents a significant advance when life-threatening digoxin or digitoxin toxicity is present. The administration of digoxin-specific Fab is financially beneficial for both the hospital and the patient. While the drug itself is expensive, its expense is far outweighed by obviating the need, risk, and expense of long-term ICU stays, and of repetitive evaluation of potassium and digoxin levels. Table 48–3 lists the indications for administering digoxin-specific Fab. Extensive discussion is found in Antidotes in Depth: Digoxin-Specific Antibody Fragments (Fab).

Additional Cardiac Therapies. In the event that digoxin-specific fragments are not immediately available, the secondary drugs for the management of ventricular irritability include phenytoin and lidocaine. These drugs depress the enhanced ventricular automaticity without significantly slowing and perhaps enhancing AV nodal conduction.[72] In fact, phenytoin may reverse digitalis-induced prolongation of AV nodal conduction. Phenytoin dissociates the inotropic and dysrhythmic actions of digitalis, thus suppressing digitalis-induced tachydysrhythmia without diminishing the contractile effects. In addition, phenytoin can terminate supraventricular dysrhythmias induced by digitalis more effectively than lidocaine.[72] Atrial fibrillation and flutter typically do not respond to phenytoin or lidocaine. When used, phenytoin should be infused slowly intravenously (≤50 mg/min) until control of the dysrhythmias is achieved or a maximum of 1000 mg has been given in an adult or 15–20 mg/kg in a child. Fosphenytoin offers several theoretical advantages over phenytoin in avoiding drug effects associated with rate of administration, but has not

TABLE 48–3. **Indications for Administration of Digoxin-Specific Antibody Fragments**

Any potentially digoxin-related life-threatening dysrhythmia
Potassium concentration >5.0 mEq/L in setting of acute digoxin poisoning
Chronic digoxin poisoning with dysrhythmias, significant gastrointestinal symptoms, or acute onset of significantly altered mental status, or renal insufficiency
Serum digoxin concentration ≥15 ng/mL at any time, or ≥10 ng/mL 6 h postingestion
Ingestion of 10 mg in adult
Ingestion of 4 mg in a child
To aid in treatment of suspected cardiac glycoside poisoning without a confirmatory level
Poisoning by nondigoxin cardiac glycoside

Digoxin Fab Dosing: (Round up vial calculation)

$$\text{No. of vials} = \frac{\text{Digoxin serum concentration (ng/mL)} \times \text{Pt Wt (kg)}}{100}$$

$$\text{No. of vials} = \frac{\text{Amount ingested (mg)}}{0.5 \text{ (mg/vial)}}$$

Empiric therapy for acute poisoning:
  10–20 vials (adult or pediatric)
Empiric therapy for chronic poisoning:
  3–6 vials (adult)
  1–2 vials (pediatric)

been evaluated in this setting. Maintenance oral doses of phenytoin 300–400 mg/d in an adult and 6–10 mg/kg/d in a child should be continued until digoxin toxicity is resolved. Lidocaine is given as a 1.0–1.5 mg/kg IV bolus followed by continuous infusion at 1–4 mg/min in an adult, or given as a 1.0–1.5 mg/kg IV bolus followed by 30–50 µg/kg/min in a child, as required to control the rhythm disturbance. Fifteen minutes after the initial bolus, an additional 1 mg/kg IV bolus should be administered in an adult and child (Chap. 52).

In general, class IA antidysrhythmic agents are contraindicated in the setting of cardiac glycoside poisoning because they may induce or worsen AV nodal block and decrease His-Purkinje conduction. IA antidysrhythmic agents may also induce ventricular dysrhythmias (prodysrhythmogenic effects).

In patients with severe supraventricular bradydysrhythmias or high degrees of AV block, atropine 0.5 mg should be administered intravenously to an adult, or 0.02 mg/kg with a minimum of 0.1 mg to a child. Atropine should be titrated to block the vagotonic effects of the cardiac glycoside. The dose may be repeated at 5-minute intervals if necessary. Therapeutic success is unpredictable because the depressant actions of digitalis are mediated only in part through the vagus nerve. The use of isoproterenol should be avoided in digitalis-induced conduction disturbances, as there may be an increased incidence of ventricular ectopic activity in the presence of toxic levels of digitalis.

Pacemakers and Cardioversion

External or transvenous pacemakers have limited indication since the availability of digoxin-specific Fab. In one retrospective study over a 6-year period, 92 digitalis-poisoned patients were studied.[85]

Fifty-one patients were treated with cardiac pacing and/or digoxin-specific Fab, and the overall mortality rate was 13%. Prevention of life-threatening dysrhythmias failed in 8% of patients treated with immunotherapy and in 23% of patients treated with pacemakers. The main reason for failure of digoxin-specific Fab was pacing-induced dysrhythmias and delayed or insufficient administration of digoxin-specific Fab. Iatrogenic complications of pacing occurred in 36% of patients. Thus, overdrive suppression with a temporary transvenous pacemaker should not be used to abolish ventricular tachydysrhythmias in the presence of cardiac glycoside poisoning.[5,85] The authors concluded that the pacemaker has limited utility in cardiac glycoside toxicity and encouraged early use of digoxin-specific Fab as first-line therapy.[85]

Transthoracic electrical cardioversion for atrial tachydysrhythmias in the setting of digoxin toxicity is both clinically and experimentally associated with the development of potentially lethal ventricular dysrhythmias. The dysrhythmias induced were similar to digoxin toxic rhythms, and seemed to be related to the degree of cardiac glycoside poisoning, and the amount of administered current.[74] In cardiac glycoside–toxic patients with unstable rhythms such as ventricular tachycardia or ventricular fibrillation, cardioversion and defibrillation, respectively, are indicated.

Electrolyte Therapy

Potassium. Hypokalemia and hyperkalemia can exacerbate digitalis cardiotoxicity. When hypokalemia is noted in conjunction with tachydysrhythmias or bradydysrhythmias, potassium replacement should be given, with close monitoring of serum potassium, because iatrogenic hyperkalemia is detrimental and avoidable.

In the presence of acute cardiac glycoside toxicity when potassium exceeds 5.0 mEq/L, digoxin-specific antibodies are probably indicated. Most investigators agree that when marked hyperkalemia develops in conjunction with ECG evidence of potassium toxicity and if digoxin-specific Fab is not available immediately, an attempt should be made to lower the serum potassium with IV insulin, dextrose, sodium bicarbonate, and oral administration of ion-exchange resins such as sodium polystyrene sulfonate. Caution should be used in the subsequent administration of Fab because the reinstitution of the exchange of Na^+ for K^+ causes hypokalemia which may be profound.

In most hyperkalemic patients calcium chloride is beneficial, but in the presence of digitalis poisoning calcium may be disastrous, as intracellular hypercalcemia is already present. A number of experimental studies cite the additive or synergistic actions of calcium and cardiac glycosides on the heart, resulting in increasing dysrhythmias,[24,61,79] cardiac dysfunction[43] (eg, hypercontractility, hypocontractility), and cardiac arrest.[52,79,90] Furthermore, 3 case reports[7,46] of deaths in cardiac glycoside–poisoned patients following calcium administration support the withholding of bolus calcium administration in the setting of hyperkalemia caused by this specific etiology. The purported mechanism is augmented intracellular cytoplasmic calcium resulting from an increased transmembrane concentration gradient further inhibiting calcium extrusion through the Na^+-Ca^{++} exchange and/or increased intracytoplasmic stores.[41] This additional cytoplasmic calcium may result in altered contraction of myofibril organelles,[43] altered ion exchange affecting intracellular electronegativity (resting potential and Phase 4) allowing afterdepolarizations to reach firing threshold,[33,41,61] altered function of the sarcoplasmic reticulum,[43,71] or increased calcium interfering with myocardial mitochondrial function.[43] Although some investigators suspect that the rate of administration of the calcium may be a factor in the subsequent cardiac toxicity,[61,52] calcium administration should be avoided as there are better, safer alternative treatments available for cardiac glycoside-induced hyperkalemia (digoxin-specific Fab, insulin, sodium bicarbonate). Intractable ventricular fibrillation, ventricular tachycardia, or even a systolic arrest (the so-called "stone heart") could ensue if additional calcium is administered, although the literature is unclear whether this effect is additive or synergistic.[7,24,46,61,79]

Magnesium. Hypomagnesemia may also occur in cardiac glycoside-poisoned patients secondary to the contributory factors mentioned with hypokalemia (eg, diuretic use, congestive heart failure). Concomitant hypomagnesemia may result in refractory hypokalemia despite potassium replacement. The theoretical benefits of magnesium therapy include transient inward calcium current blockade, antagonism of calcium at intracellular binding sites, decreased cardiac glycoside-related ventricular irritability, and blockade of potassium egress from cardiac glycoside-poisoned cells.[3,19,38,66,75,83,93]

Hypomagnesemia increases myocardial digoxin uptake and decreases cellular Na^+-K^+-ATPase activity. Patients with hypomagnesemia, hypokalemia, or both may become cardiotoxic even with therapeutic digitalis levels.[93]

The successful use of intravenous magnesium sulfate in the treatment of ventricular tachydysrhythmias caused by digoxin toxicity, even in the presence of elevated serum magnesium levels, is reported.[44] The mechanism of efficacy of magnesium may be its ability to suppress early afterdepolarizations and its indirect antagonism of digoxin at the sarcolemma Na^+-K^+-ATPase pump. However, this treatment is only temporizing until digoxin-specific Fab is available for definitive therapy, and is not advocated as first-line therapy. The precise dosing of magnesium sulfate in digitalis-poisoned patients is not established.[3,19,38,44,66,75,93] A common regimen uses 2 g of magnesium sulfate IV over 20 minutes in an adult, or 25–50 mg/kg/dose to a maximum of 2 g in a child. Following stabilization, a patient with severe hypomagnesemia may require a magnesium infusion of 1–2 g/h in an adult or 25–50 mg/kg/h to a maximum of 2 g in a child with serial monitoring of serum magnesium levels, telemetry, respiratory rate (observing for bradypnea), deep-tendon reflexes (observing for hyporeflexia), and monitoring of blood pressure. Magnesium is contraindicated in the setting of bradycardia or atrioventricular block.

Extracorporal Removal. Forced diuresis,[47] hemoperfusion,[57,91] and hemodialysis[91] are ineffective in enhancing the elimination of digoxin because of its large volume of distribution (4–10 L/kg), which makes it relatively inaccessible to these techniques. Because of its high affinity for tissue proteins, approximately 10–50 times less digoxin is found in the serum than is found at the tissue level, and of that amount approximately 20–40% is protein-bound.[39]

SUMMARY

Cardiac glycosides have a narrow therapeutic index. Signs and symptoms of cardiac glycoside toxicity range from subtle to profound. Both cardiac and noncardiac effects follow cardiac glycoside poisoning. A systematic approach toward treating patients utilizing basic supportive and decontamination management techniques, supplemented by the early administration of immunotherapy, can significantly reduce morbidity and mortality in these high-risk patients.

ACKNOWLEDGMENTS

Mary Ann Howland, PharmD, and Robert H. Kirstein, MD, contributed to this chapter in a previous edition.

REFERENCES

1. Banner W, Bach P, Burk B, et al: Influence of assay methods on serum concentrations of digoxin during Fab fragment treatments. J Toxicol Clin Toxicol 1992;30:259–267.
2. Bayer MJ: Recognition and management of digitalis intoxication: Implications for emergency medicine. Am J Emerg Med 1991;9(Suppl 1):29–32.
3. Beller GA, Hood WB, Smith TW, et al: Correlation of serum magnesium level and cardiac digitalis intoxication. Am J Cardiol 1974;33:225–229.
4. Bismuth C, Gaultier M, Conso F, Efthymiou ML: Hyperkalemia in acute digitalis poisoning: Prognostic significance and therapeutic implications. Clin Toxicol 1973;6:153–162.
5. Bismuth C, Motte G, Conso F, Chauvin M: Acute digitoxin intoxication treated by intracardiac pacemaker: Experience in sixty-eight patients. Clin Toxicol 1977;10:443–456.
6. Blaustein MP: Physiologic effects of endogenous ouabain: Control of intracellular Ca^{2+} stores and cell responsiveness. Am J Physiol 1993;264:C1367–C1387.
7. Bower JO, Mengle HAK: The additive effect of calcium and digitalis. JAMA 1936;106:1151–1153.
8. Brubacher JR, Hoffman RS, Bania T, et al: Deaths associated with a purported aphrodisiac. New York City, February 1993–May 1995. MMWR Morb Mortal Wkly Rep 1995;44:853–855.
9. Brubacher JR, Ravikumar PR, Bania T, et al: Treatment of toad venom poisoning with digoxin-specific Fab fragments. Chest 1996;110:1282–1288.
10. Carver JL, Valdes R: Anomalous serum digoxin concentrations in uremia. Ann Intern Med 1983;98:483–484.
11. Chern MS, Ray CY, Wu DL: Biological intoxication due to digitalis-like substance after ingestion of cooked toad soup. Am J Cardiol 1991;67:443–444.
12. Cooke D: The use of central nervous system manifestations in the early detection of digitalis toxicity. Heart Lung 1993;22:477–481.
13. Critchley JA, Critchley LA: Digoxin toxicity in chronic renal failure: Treatment by multiple-dose activated charcoal intestinal dialysis. Hum Exp Toxicol 1997;16:733–735.
14. Cummins RO, Haulman J, Quan L: Near-fatal yew berry intoxication treated with external cardiac pacing and digoxin-specific Fab antibody fragments. Ann Emerg Med 1990;19:38–43.
15. Doering W: Quinidine-digoxin interaction: Pharmacokinetics, underlying mechanism and clinical implications. N Engl J Med 1979;301:400–404.
16. Doolittle MH, Lincoln K, Graves SW: Unexplained increase in serum digoxin: A case report. Clin Chem 1994;40:487–492.
17. Eisner DA, Lederer WJ, Vaughan-Jones RD: The quantitative relationship between twitch tension and intracellular sodium activity in sheep cardiac Purkinje fibres. J Physiol 1984;355:251–266.
18. Eisner DA, Smith TW: The Na-K pump and its effect in cardiac muscle. In: Fozzard HA, ed: The Heart and Cardiovascular System, 2nd ed. New York, Raven Press, 1991, pp. 863–902.
19. French JH, Thomas RG, Siskind AP, et al: Magnesium therapy in massive digoxin intoxication. Ann Emerg Med 1984;13:562–566.

20. Friedman HS, Abramowitz I, Nguyen T, et al: Urinary digoxin-like immunoreactive substance in pregnancy. Am J Med 1987;83: 261–264.

21. George S, Brathwaite RA, Hughes EA: Digoxin measurements following plasma ultrafiltration in two patients with digoxin toxicity treated with specific Fab fragments. Ann Clin Biochem 1994;31: 380–381.

22. Giampietro O, Clerico A, Gregori G, et al: Increased urinary excretion of digoxin-like immunoreactive substance by insulin-dependent diabetic patients: A linkage with hypertension? Clin Chem 1988;34: 2418–2422.

23. Gibb T, Adams PC, Parnham AJ, Jennings K: Plasma digoxin: Assay anomalies in Fab-treated patients. Br J Clin Pharmacol 1983;16: 445–447.

24. Gold H, Edwards DJ: The effects of ouabain on heart in the presence of hypercalcemia. Am Heart J 1927;3:45–50.

25. Gorelick DA, Kussin SZ, Kahn I: Paranoid delusions and auditory hallucinations associated with digoxin intoxication. J Nerv Ment Dis 1978;166:817–819.

26. Graves SW, Adler G, Stuenkel C, et al: Increases in plasma digitalis-induced hypoglycemia. Neuroendocrinology 1989; 49:586–591.

27. Graves SW, Brown BA, Valdes R: Digoxin-like substances measured in patients with renal impairment. Ann Intern Med 1983;99: 604–608.

28. Graves SW, Valdes R, Brown BA, et al: Endogenous immunoreactive digoxin-like substance in human pregnancies. J Clin Endocrinol Metab 1984;58:748–751.

29. Graves SW: Endogenous digitalis-like factors. Crit Rev Clin Lab Sci 1986;23:177–200.

30. Haddy FJ: Endogenous digitalis-like factor or factors [letter]. N Engl J Med 1987;316:621–622.

31. Hager WD, Fenster P, Mayersohn M, et al: Digoxin-quinidine interaction: Pharmacokinetic evaluation. N Engl J Med 1979;300: 1238–1241.

32. Hastreiter AR, John EG, van der Horst RL: Digitalis, digitalis antibodies, digitalis-like immunoreactive substances, and sodium homeostasis: A review. Clin Perinatol 1988;15:491–522.

33. Hauptman PJ, Kelly RA: Digitalis. Circulation 1999;99:1265–1270.

34. Henderson RP, Solomon CP: Use of cholestyramine in the treatment of digoxin intoxication. Arch Intern Med 1988;148:745–746.

35. Hilton PJ, White G, Lord A, et al: An inhibitor of the sodium pump obtained from human placenta. Lancet 1996;348:303–305.

36. Hollman A: Plants and cardiac glycosides. Br Heart J 1985;54: 258–261.

37. Isensee L, Solomon RJ, Weinberg MS, et al: Digoxin levels in dialysis patients. Hosp Physician 1988;24:50–52.

38. Karkal SS, Ordog G, Wasserberg J: Digitalis intoxication: Dealing rapidly and effectively with a complex cardiac toxidrome. Emerg Med Rep 1991;12:29–44.

39. Katzung BG, Parmley WM: Cardiac glycosides & other drugs used in congestive heart failure. In: Katzung BG, ed: Basic & Clinical Pharmacology, 7th ed. Stamford, CT, Appleton & Lange, 1998, pp. 197–215.

40. Kelly RA, Smith TW: Endogenous cardiac glycosides. Adv Pharmacol 1994;25:263–288.

41. Kelly RA, Smith TW: Pharmacological treatment of heart failure. In: Hardman JG, Limbird LE, Molinoff PB, Ruddon RW, eds: Goodman and Gilman's The Pharmacological Basis of Therapeutics, 9th ed. New York, McGraw-Hill, 1996, pp. 809–838.

42. Kelly RA, Smith TW: Recognition and management of digitalis toxicity. Am J Cardiol 1992;69:108–109.

43. Khatter JC, Agbanyo M, Navaratnam S, Nero B, et al: Digitalis cardiotoxicity: Cellular calcium overload as a possible mechanism. Basic Res Cardiol 1989;84:553–563.

44. Kinlay S, Buckley N: Magnesium sulfate in the treatment of ventricular arrhythmias due to digoxin toxicity. J Toxicol Clin Toxicol 1995; 33:55–59.

45. Klausen T, Kjeldsen K, Norgaard A: Effects of denervation on sodium, potassium and [3H] ouabain binding in muscles of normal and potassium depleted rats. J Physiol 1983;345:123–124.

46. Kne T, Brokaw M, Wax P: Fatality from calcium chloride in a chronic digoxin toxic patient. J Toxicol Clin Toxicol 1997;5:505.

47. Koren G, Klein J: Enhancement of digoxin clearance by mannitol diuresis: In vivo studies and their clinical implications. Vet Hum Toxicol 1988;30:25–27.

48. Lalonde RL, Deshpande R, Hamilton PP, et al: Acceleration of digoxin clearance by activated charcoal. Clin Pharmacol Ther 1985; 37:367–371.

49. Leahy EB Jr, Reiffel JA, Drusin RE, et al: Interaction between quinidine and digoxin. JAMA 1978;240:533–534.

50. Lee TC: Van Gogh's vision. JAMA 1981;245:727–729.

51. Levy G: Gastrointestinal clearance of drugs with activated charcoal. N Engl J Med 1982;307:676–678.

52. Lieberman AL: Studies on calcium VI. Some interrelationships of the cardiac activities of calcium gluconate and scillaren-B. J Pharmacol Exp Ther 1933;47:183–192.

53. Lindenbaum J, Rund DG, Butler VP: Inactivation of digoxin by the gut flora: Reversal by antibiotic therapy. N Engl J Med 1981;305: 789–794.

54. Lown B, Byatt NF, Levine HD: Paroxysmal atrial tachycardia with block. Circulation 1960;21:129–143.

55. Madan BR, Khanna NK, Soni RK: Effect of some arrhythmogenic agents upon the acetylcholine content of the rabbit atria. J Pharm Pharmacol 1970;22:621–622.

56. Mahdyoon H, Battilana G, Rosman H, et al: The evolving pattern of digoxin intoxication: Observations at a large urban hospital from 1980 to 1988. Am Heart J 1990;120:1189–1194.

57. Marbury T, Mahoney J, Juncos L, et al: Advanced digoxin toxicity in renal failure: Treatment with charcoal hemoperfusion. South Med J 1979;72:279–282.

58. McGary SJ, Williams AJ: Digoxin activates sarcoplasmic reticulum Ca^{2+} release channels: A possible role in cardiac inotropy. Br J Pharmacol 1993;108:1043–1050.

59. McRae S: Elevated serum digoxin levels in a patient taking digoxin and Siberian ginseng. Can Med Assoc J 1996;155:292–295.

60. Nanji AA, Greenway DC: Falsely raised plasma digoxin concentrations in liver disease. Br Med J 1985;290:432–433.

61. Nola GT, Pope S, Harrison DC: Assessment of the synergistic relationship between serum calcium and digitalis. Am Heart J 1970;79: 499–507.

62. Ordog GJ, Benaron S, Bhasin V, et al: Serum digoxin levels and mortality in 5,100 patients. Ann Emerg Med 1987;16:32–39.

63. Pace DG, Gillis RA: Neuroexcitatory effects of digoxin in the cat. J Pharmacol Exp Ther 1976;199:583–600.

64. Pond S, Jacos M, Marks J, et al: Treatment of digitoxin overdose with oral activated charcoal. Lancet 1981;2:1177–1178.

65. Rabetory GM, Price CA, Findlay JWA, et al: Treatment of digoxin intoxication in a renal failure patient with digoxin-specific antibody fragments and plasmapheresis. Am J Nephrol 1990;10:518–521.

66. Reisdorff EJ, Clark MR, Walter BL: Acute digitalis poisoning: The role of intravenous magnesium sulfate. J Emerg Med 1986;4: 463–469.

67. Rich SA, Libera JM, Locke RJ: Treatment of foxglove extract poisoning with digoxin-specific Fab fragments. Ann Emerg Med 1993;22: 1904–1907.

68. Rodin SM, Johnson BF: Pharmacokinetic interactions with digoxin. Clin Pharmacokinetic 1988;15:227–244.

69. Rose AM, Valdes R: Understanding the sodium pump and its relevance to disease. Clin Chem 1994;40:1674–1685.

70. Rosen MR, Wit AL, Hoffman BF: Cardiac antiarrhythmic and toxic effects of digitalis. Am Heart J 1975;89:391–399.

71. Rosen MR: Cellular electrophysiology of digitalis toxicity. J Am Coll Cardiol 1985;2:22A–34A.

72. Rumack BH, Wolfe RR, Gilfinch H: Diphenylhydantoin treatment of massive digoxin overdose. Br Heart J 1974;36:405–408.

73. Safadi R, Levy T, Amitai Y, et al: Beneficial effect of digoxin-specific Fab antibody fragments in oleander intoxication. Arch Intern Med 1995;155:2121–2125.

74. Sarubbi B, Ducceschi V, D'Antonello A, et al: Atrial fibrillation: What are the effects of drug therapy on the effectiveness and complications of electrical cardioversion? Can J Cardiol 1998;14: 1267–1273.

75. Seller RH: The role of magnesium in digitalis toxicity. Am Heart J 1971;82:551–556.

76. Selzer A: Role of serum digoxin assay in patient management. J Am Coll Cardiol 1985;5:106A–110A.

77. Shilo LM, Adawi A, Solomon G, Shenkman L: Endogenous digoxin-like immunoreactivity in congestive heart failure. Br Med J 1987; 295:415–416.

78. Silber B, Sheiner LB, Powers JL, et al: Spironolactone-associated digoxin radioimmunoassay interference. Clin Chem 1979;25:48–54.

79. Smith PK, Winkler AW, Hoff HE: Calcium and digitalis synergism: The toxicity of calcium salts injected intravenously into digitalized animals. Arch Intern Med 1939;64:322–328.

80. Smith TW, Haber E, Yeatman L, et al: Reversal of advanced digoxin intoxication with Fab fragments of digoxin-specific antibodies. N Engl J Med 1976;294:797–800.

81. Smith TW: Digitalis. N Engl J Med 1988;318:358–365.

82. Somberg JC, Bounous H, Levitt B: The antiarrhythmic effects of quinidine and propranolol in the ouabain-intoxicated spinally transected cat. Eur J Pharmacol 1979;54:161–166.

83. Spechter MJ, Schweizer E, Goldman RH: Studies on magnesium's mechanism of action in digitalis-induced arrhythmias. Circulation 1975;52:1001–1005.

84. Sullivan JB: Immunotherapy in the poisoned patient. Med Toxicol 1986;1:47–60.

85. Taboulet P, Baud FJ, Bismuth C, et al: Acute digitalis intoxication: Is pacing still appropriate? J Toxicol Clin Toxicol 1993;31:261–273.

86. Torsti P: Acetylcholine content and cholinesterase activities in the rabbit heart in experimental heart failure and the effect of g-strophanthin treatment on them. Ann Med Exp Biol Fenn 1959;37(Suppl 4): 4–9.

87. Tuncok Y, Kozan O, Cavdar C, et al: Urginea maritima (squill) toxicity. J Toxicol Clin Toxicol 1995;33:83–86.

88. Valdes R, Graves SW, Brown BA, et al: Endogenous substances in newborn infants causing false-positive digoxin measurements. J Pediatr 1983;102:947–950.

89. Valdes R, Hagberg JM, Vaughn TE, et al: Endogenous digoxin-like immunoreactivity in blood is increased during prolonged strenuous exercise. Life Sci 1988;42:103–110.

90. Wagner J, Salzer WW: Calcium-dependent toxic effects of digoxin in isolated myocardial preparations. Arch Int Pharmacodyn 1976;223: 4–14.

91. Warren SE, Fanestil DD: Digoxin overdose: Limitations of hemoperfusion-hemodialysis treatment. JAMA 1979;242:2100–2101.

92. Watson WA: Factors influencing the clinical efficacy of activated charcoal. Drug Intell Clin Pharm 1987;21:160–166.

93. Whang R, Aikawa J: Magnesium deficiency and refractoriness to potassium repletion. J Chron Dis 1977;30:65–68.

94. Wildicks EFM, Vermeulen M, van Brummelen P, et al: Digoxin-like immunoreactive substance in patients with aneurysmal subarachnoid hemorrhage. Br Med J 1987;294:729–732.

95. Withering W: An account of the foxglove and some of its medical uses: With practical remarks on dropsy and other diseases. Med Classics 1937;2:295–443.

96. Woolf AD, Wenger T, Smith TW, et al: The use of digoxin-specific Fab fragments for severe digitalis intoxication in children. N Engl J Med 1992;326:1739–1744.

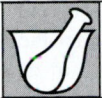

ANTIDOTES IN DEPTH

Digoxin-Specific Antibody Fragments (Fab)

Mary Ann Howland

Digoxin-specific antibody fragments (Fab) are indicated for the management of patients with toxicity related to digoxin, digitoxin, and all natural cardiac glycosides, including oleander, squill, and toad venom. Digoxin-specific antibody fragments have an excellent record of efficacy and safety, and should be administered early in established and suspected digoxin and digoxinlike cardiac steroid poisoning.

HISTORY

The production of antibody fragments to treat patients poisoned with digoxin was initiated subsequent to the development of digoxin antibodies for measuring serum digoxin concentrations by radioimmunoassay (RIA).[10] The RIA technique permitted the correlation between serum digoxin concentrations and clinical digoxin toxicity. One of the earliest prospective studies of patients receiving therapeutic digoxin demonstrated that toxic patients had statistically significantly higher mean serum digoxin concentrations (2.3 ± 1.6 ng/mL) than nontoxic patients (1.0 ± 0.5 ng/mL), although considerable overlap was present (29% of the toxic group had levels less than 1.7 ng/mL and 15% of the nontoxic group had levels greater than 1.7 ng/mL).[3] Subsequent studies reaffirmed the benefits of appropriate monitoring of serum digoxin concentrations.[16,17,46]

Butler and Chen suggested that purified digoxin antibodies with a high affinity and specificity should be developed to treat digoxin toxicity in humans.[10] The digoxin molecule alone, with a molecular weight of 780 daltons, would be too small to be immunogenic. But digoxin could function as a hapten when joined to an immunogenic protein carrier such as serum albumin. These investigators immunized sheep with this conjugate to generate antibodies. The immunized sheep subsequently produced a mixture of antibodies that included antialbumin antibodies and antidigoxin antibodies. The antibodies were separated and highly purified to retain the digoxin antibodies while removing the antibodies to the albumin and all other extraneous proteins. The antibodies developed have a high affinity for digoxin and sufficient cross-reactivity with digitoxin to be clinically useful for the treatment of poisoning from either agent. Moreover, the specificity is so significant that endogenous steroids, which resemble digoxin structurally, are not affected by antibody administration.

In vitro studies followed by in vivo studies in animals demonstrated biologic activity of these antibodies.[12,15,57,58] Investigations proceeded and contributed significantly to understanding of the pharmacodynamics and pharmacokinetics of the antibodies.[11,39,65] Intact IgG antidigoxin antibodies reversed digoxin toxicity in dogs. Unfortunately, the urinary excretion of digoxin was delayed, and free digoxin was released later after antibody degradation occurred. Furthermore, concern for hypersensitivity reactions also existed. To make these antibodies safe and effective in humans, the whole IgG antidigoxin antibodies were cleaved with papain, yielding 2 antigen-binding Fab with a molecular weight of 50,000 daltons each and 1 Fc.[11] Because the Fc does not bind antigen, but it does increase the potential for hypersensitivity reactions, it was eliminated. The advantages of the digoxin-specific Fab when compared to the whole IgG antibodies include larger volume of distribution, more rapid onset of action, smaller risk of adverse immunologic effects, and more rapid elimination.[11,39,41] Ultimately, the commercial product (Digibind) is a relatively pure Fab product that is very safe and extremely effective. Other commercial products are now available abroad and may be available in the United States shortly.

MECHANISM OF ACTION OF DIGOXIN-SPECIFIC ANTIBODIES

Immediately following IV administration, Fab digoxin-specific antibodies bind intravascular free digoxin. They then diffuse into the interstitial space, binding free digoxin there. This accounts for the 3-fold larger apparent volume of distribution (V_d) at steady state.[68] A concentration gradient is then established, which facilitates movement of the free intracellular digoxin and digoxin that is dissociated from its binding sites (the external surface of Na^+-K^+-ATPase enzyme) in the heart, into the interstitial or intravascular spaces. The binding affinity of Digibind for digoxin is about 10^9–10^{11}, which is greater than the affinity of digoxin for the Na^+-K^+-ATPase pump receptor. Intravascular concentrations of inactive, antibody-bound digoxin rise substantially. The elimination kinetics of the Fab-bound digoxin are dependent on the patient's renal function and capacity for renal and nonrenal elimination.

EFFICACY OF DIGOXIN-SPECIFIC ANTIBODIES

One hundred twenty-five patients with a median age of 65 years (all ≥16 years) and 25 patients with a median age of 3 years were treated.[1] Forty-nine percent of cases involved a single unintentional or suicidal overdose, and the remainder involved patients on chronic digitalis therapy. Of the 150 patients treated, 148 were evaluated for cardiovascular manifestations of toxicity: 79 patients (55%) had high-grade AV block, 68 (46%) had refractory ventricular tachycardia, 49 (33%) had ventricular fibrillation, and 56 (37%) had hyperkalemia. Ninety percent of patients had a response to digoxin-specific Fab within minutes to several hours of Digibind administration. Complete resolution of all signs and symptoms of digoxin toxicity occurred in 80% of cases. A partial response was observed in 10% of patients, and of the 15 patients who did not respond, 14 were moribund or actually found not to be digoxin toxic. The spectacular success of digoxin-specific Fab for patients with digoxin toxicity is demonstrated by the fact that of the 56 patients who had cardiac arrest caused by digoxin, 54% survived hospitalization, as compared with 100% mortality before the advent of these fragments.[1,5] Newborns, infants, and children have all been successfully treated with Digibind.[4,32,59] Pediatric patients with cardiac abnormalities who develop chronic digoxin toxicity require small doses of Fab because the total body burden of digoxin is small, whereas children with acute overdoses require Fab doses based on the amount of digoxin ingested, in a manner similar to adults.

PHARMACOKINETICS AND PHARMACODYNAMICS

In 1976, Smith and associates described the first clinical use of digoxin-specific antibody fragments in a human.[56] Within 1 hour of administration, free (unbound and active) digoxin dropped to an undetectable level. It did not rise until 9 hours later, and the free digoxin reached a peak of only 2 ng/mL at 16 hours and remained at approximately 1.5 ng/mL for the next 40 hours.[64] Total (free plus bound) digoxin, which was 17.6 ng/mL before digoxin-specific antibody fragments were given, rose to 226 ng/mL 1 hour after the start of the infusion, remained there for 11 hours, and then fell over the next 44 hours, with a half-life of 20 hours.[64] Fab concentrations peaked at the end of the infusion and then apparently exhibited a biphasic or triphasic decline, probably reflecting distribution into different compartments as well as excretion and catabolism. An analysis of renal elimination based on an incomplete collection suggested that digoxin was excreted only in the bound form during the first 6 hours, but by 30 hours after Fab administration all digoxin was free digoxin. However, the amount of free digoxin is dependent on the dose of Fab as compared to the total body load of digoxin.

The pharmacokinetics of Fab were evaluated in two different studies of 33 adult patients (total) who had attempted suicide.[52,56] The distribution half-life was 1.1–1.5 hours. Data from 11 patients in the first study were used to calculate a median total body digoxin-specific Fab clearance of 24.5 mL/min, of which 13.6 mL/min was renal clearance. The second study demonstrated a total body clearance of 18 mL/min, which was directly related to creatinine clearance and age.[52] The apparent distribution volume for the Fab in the first study varied from 25.4 to 54 L, depending on when the calculation was made, and averaged 20 L in the second study.[52,56] In the first 11 patients, the dose was 400–480 mg (10–12 vials), infused over 0.5–5 hours. In the last 6 patients, 160 mg (4 vials) was given as a loading dose over 15 minutes, followed by an additional 160 mg given over 7 hours. If the Fab is given so rapidly that elimination occurs before redistribution of digoxin from the binding sites, the total amount of Fab actually bound to digoxin is less than the predicted or the optimal amount, and digoxin levels may once again increase. In the first 11 patients, the ratio of bound to unbound digoxin-specific Fab was about 50%, free digoxin concentrations appeared earlier, and maximum levels were higher than in the subsequent 6 patients. In those 6 patients who received a loading dose followed by a maintenance infusion, the amount of bound Fab was 70%, indicating a more effective access of Fab to digoxin. Free digoxin levels reappeared at 12–24 hours and maximum levels averaged only 2.2 ng/mL (0–4.4 ng/mL).[56]

A pharmacokinetic study in a rat model using a monoclonal Fab that cross-reacted well with digoxin and active digoxin metabolites evaluated the effects of dose and timing on efficacy.[53] Administration of Fab was more effective prior to complete distribution of digoxin. Postdistribution, increasing the dose of Fab improved efficacy as measured by comparing the area-under-the-time-versus-concentration-curve (AUC) of digoxin to that of the Fab-digoxin complex.[53]

These findings[53,56] suggest some important points. It is more logical to give a loading dose of Fab followed by a maintenance infusion to optimize the binding of digoxin to Fab. The loading dose immediately captures digoxin already in the vascular space and digoxin that can be rapidly redistributed to the vascular space. The maintenance dose provides enough Fab to bind any digoxin that redistributes from the tissues into the serum. It appears that in acute intentional overdose, 4–6 vials given as a loading dose, followed by 0.5 mg/min for 8 hours, and then followed by 0.1 mg/min for about 6 hours should be safe, effective, and efficient.[56] More patients should be studied and the protocol validated before this approach can be generally adopted or recommended. The other important issue raised by these authors is that the apparent volume of distribution (V_d) of Fab suggests that the molecule does enter the cells in spite of a molecular weight of 50,000 daltons.[56]

Additional pharmacokinetic studies indicate that in renal failure, the half-life of Fab is prolonged 10-fold with no change in the apparent V_d.[68] Fab serum concentrations remain detectable for 2–3 weeks. Total digoxin serum concentrations generally follow Fab. There is no evidence for dissociation of digoxin-Fab over time.[74] However, there is a rebound in free digoxin levels that appears later, up to 130 hours following administration, in patients with renal dysfunction, as compared to 12–24 hours in patients with normal renal function.[14,18,21,34,43,44,60,62,69,70,74] This rebound is presumed secondary to changes associated with digoxin redistribution to vascular space in the absence of any Fab. The rebound is delayed in patients with renal dysfunction presumably secondary to prolonged distribution and elimination phases.

SAFETY OF DIGOXIN-SPECIFIC ANTIBODY FRAGMENTS

Digoxin-specific antibody fragments are effective, as well as very safe. In the multicenter study of 150 patients, the only acute clinical manifestations were hypokalemia in 6 patients (4%), worsening of congestive heart failure in 4 patients (3%), and transient apnea in a several-hours-old neonate.[1] There were no other reactions reported in any of the patients in this series, although vigilance should continue with regard to concern for allergic reactions and serum sickness. In a postmarketing surveillance study of Digibind that included 451 patients, however, 2 patients with a prior history of allergy to antibiotics reportedly developed rashes.[49] One of these patients developed a total body rash, facial swelling, and a flush during the infusion. The other experienced a pruritic rash. Two other adverse reactions (thrombocytopenia and shaking chills) were probably unrelated to the use of Digibind.[49] One patient received Digibind on 3 separate occasions over the course of 1 year for multiple suicide attempts with no adverse effects.[7]

INDICATIONS FOR DIGOXIN-SPECIFIC FAB

To define the indications for digoxin-specific Fab, the signs and symptoms of digoxin toxicity must be recognized.[19,63] In general, the manifestations of digoxin toxicity are exaggerations of the pharmacologic effects or alterations of these effects caused by ingestion of a single large dose (suicidal or unintentional) or accumulation from chronic dosing, the presence or absence of cardiac pathology, or the patient's age.[19,63] Pediatric patients with normal cardiac function generally tolerate higher μg/kg dosages of digoxin than do adults. Potassium concentrations in these children tend to remain in the therapeutic range except in extreme circumstances. Serum potassium concentrations result from a balance between the degree and extent of inhibition of the Na⁺-K⁺-ATPase pump and the patient's renal function.[19,63] Both adults and children with diseased hearts become digoxin toxic at lower levels of toxic exposure than their respective healthy counterparts. In the chronically exposed patient, the magnitude of Na⁺-K⁺-ATPase enzyme inhibition in the heart and throughout the body is less extensive prior to the development of symptoms. Many patients who chronically receive digoxin also receive diuretics, which may contribute to smaller rises in serum potassium levels in these patients. Adult patients who ingest a large, single dose of digoxin or digitoxin have extensive Na⁺-K⁺-ATPase inhibition, and, consequently, have significant elevations in potassium. When hyperkalemia occurred, before the advent of digoxin-specific Fab, rises in potassium above 5.0 or 5.5 mEq/L indicated a 50 or 100% probability of death, respectively.[5]

Digoxin-specific antibody fragments are indicated for potentially life-threatening digoxin or digitoxin toxicity.[48] Patients with progressive bradydysrhythmias, including severe sinus bradycardia or second- or third-degree heart block unresponsive to atropine, and those patients with severe ventricular dysrhythmias, including ventricular tachycardia or ventricular fibrillation, should be treated with digoxin-specific antibody fragments. A ventricular tachycardia with a fascicular block is likely to be a digoxin-toxic rhythm.[40] Any patient with a potassium concentration exceeding 5 mEq/L should also be treated. Acute ingestions greater than 4 mg in a healthy child, or 10 mg in a healthy adult, probably require antibody treatment. Serum digoxin concentrations do not correlate with myocardial concentrations and are not stable until tissue distribution occurs within about 4–6 hours. This time delay is required for digoxin to distribute from the serum to the heart. Serum concentrations of ≥15 ng/mL in an acute ingestion will probably require digoxin-specific antibody fragments and are an indication for treatment. Because the elderly appear at greatest risk of lethality, the threshold for treating those older than 60 should be lowered.[6] Before the advent of digoxin-specific antibody fragments mortality in patients older than 60 years of age was 58%, as compared to 8% in those younger than 40 years of age, and to 34% in those between the ages of 40 and 50 years of age.[6] A rapid progression of clinical signs and symptoms, such as cardiac and gastrointestinal effects and a rising potassium level in the presence of an acute overdose, suggests a potentially life-threatening ingestion and the need for digoxin antibodies.

In a patient with an unknown ingestion who is clinically ill with characteristics suggestive of intoxication by digoxin, a calcium channel blocking agent, or a β-adrenergic antagonist, digoxin antibodies should be administered early in management, and always prior to calcium use. If digoxin is involved, its effects can be reversed, obviating the need to administer calcium and avoiding the danger of giving calcium to a digoxin-toxic patient. Digoxin toxicity causes intracellular myocardial hypercalcemia, and the administration of exogenous calcium may further exacerbate conduction abnormalities.

When it is difficult to distinguish clinically between digoxin intoxication and intrinsic cardiac disease, the administration of digoxin antibodies can help establish the diagnosis.

TIME OF ONSET OF RESPONSE TO DIGOXIN-SPECIFIC FAB

In the multicenter study of 150 patients, the mean time to initial response from the completion of the digoxin antibody infusion (accomplished over 15 minutes to 2 hours) was 19 minutes (range, 0–60 minutes), and the time to complete response was 88 minutes (range, 30–360 minutes).[15] Time to response was not affected by age, concurrent cardiac disease, or presence of chronic or acute ingestion.[1]

DOSING OF DIGOXIN-SPECIFIC FAB

The dose of antibodies depends on the total body load (TBL) of digoxin. Estimates of TBL can be made in three ways: (a) estimate the quantity of digoxin acutely ingested and assume 80% bioavailability (X mg ingested × 0.8 = TBL); (b) obtain a serum digoxin concentration, and using a pharmacokinetic formula, incorporate the apparent V_d of digoxin and the patient's body weight (in kg); or (c) use an empiric dose based on the average requirements for an acute or chronic overdose in an adult or child. Sample calculations for each of these methods are shown in Tables 48–4 to 48–6. Each vial of Digibind contains 38 mg of purified digoxin-specific antibody fragments, which will bind approximately 0.5 mg of digoxin or digitoxin. If the quantity of ingestion cannot be reliably estimated, it may be safest to use the largest calculated estimate. Alternatively, the clinician should be prepared to increase dosing should resolution be incomplete. Inaccurate estimations can occur if the history is faulty; if serum digoxin concentration is determined during the acute phase of distribution (overestimating requirements); and because the volume of distribution of 5 L/kg is merely a population estimate that varies considerably in individuals and in certain disease states, such as the decreases that occur in patients with renal disease and hypothyroidism.[75]

Administration

According to the manufacturer, Digibind should be administered IV over 30 minutes via a 0.22-micron membrane filter.[48] The 38-

---

TABLE 48–4. Sample Calculation Based on History of Acute Digoxin Ingestion

Adult
Weight: 70 kg
Ingestion: Fifty 0.25-mg digoxin tablets
Calculation:
0.25 mg × 50 = 12.5 mg ingested dose
12.5 mg × 0.80 (80% bioavailability) = 10.0 mg (absorbed dose)

$$\frac{10.0 \text{ mg}}{0.5 \text{ mg}} = 20 \text{ vials}$$

Child
Weight: 10 kg
Ingestion: Fifty 0.25-mg digoxin tablets
Calculation: Same as for adult. Child will require 20 vials

TABLE 48–5. Sample Calculations Based on the Serum Digoxin Concentration

Adult
Weight: 70 kg
Serum digoxin concentration = 10 ng/mL
Volume of distribution = 5 L/kg
Calculation[a]:

$$\text{No. of vials} = \frac{\text{Total body load (mg)}}{0.5 \text{ mg / vial}}$$

$$= \frac{\text{Digoxin serum concentration} \times V_d \times \text{Pt Wt (kg)}}{1000 \times 0.5 \text{ mg / vial}}$$

$$\text{No. of vials} = \frac{10 \text{ ng / mL} \times 5 \text{ L / kg} \times 70 \text{ kg}}{1000 \times 0.5 \text{ mg / vial}} \quad \text{(Round up)}$$

No. of vials = 7

Child
Weight: 10 kg
Serum digoxin concentration: 10 ng/mL
Volume of distribution: 5 L/kg
Calculation[a]:

$$\text{No. of vials} = \frac{10 \text{ ng / mL} \times 5 \text{ L / kg} \times 10 \text{ kg}}{1000 \times 0.5 \text{ mg / vial}} \quad \text{(Round up)}$$

No. of vials = 1

Quick Estimation (for Adults and Children)

$$\text{No. of vials} = \frac{\text{Digoxin serum concentration (ng / mL)} \times \text{Pt Wt (kg)}}{100}$$

[a]1000 is a conversion factor to change ng/mL to mg/L.

mg vial must be reconstituted with 4 mL of sterile water for IV injection, furnishing an isoosmotic solution. This preparation can be further diluted with sterile isotonic saline (for small infants, addition of 34 mL to the 4 mL (for 38 mL total achieves 1 mg/mL). After it is reconstituted, it should be used immediately, or if refrigerated, it should be used within 4 hours.[48] In the critically ill, Digibind maybe given by IV bolus.

Availability

Digoxin-specific antibody fragments are available as Digbind (Digoxin Immune Fab—Ovine). Vials contain 38 mg of purified lyophilized digoxin-specific Fab fragments and each vial binds 0.5

TABLE 48–6. Empiric Dosing Recommendations

Acute Ingestion	
Adult: 10–20 vials	
Child[a]: 10–20 vials	
Chronic Toxicity	
Adult: 3–6 vials	
Child[b]: 1–2 vials	

[a]Monitor for volume overload in children.
[b]Package insert contains table for infants and children, with corresponding serum concentrations.

mg of digoxin or digitoxin. A new product called DigiTab is currently undergoing FDA review.

MEASUREMENT OF DIGOXIN SERUM CONCENTRATION AFTER FAB ADMINISTRATION

Many laboratories are not equipped to determine free serum digoxin concentrations. Therefore, after digoxin-specific antibody fragments are administered, serum digoxin concentrations are no longer clinically useful, because they represent free plus bound digoxin.[2,24,29,37,66] The type of test employed can either result in falsely high or falsely low serum concentrations, depending on which phase (solid or supernatant) is sampled.[28] If the correct dose of Fab is administered, the free serum digoxin concentrations should be near zero. Free digoxin concentrations begin to reappear 5–24 hours or longer after Fab administration, depending on the antibody dose, infusion technique, and the patient's renal function. Newer commercial methods employing ultrafiltration or immunoassays make free digoxin measurements easier to perform and, therefore, more clinically useful, but they remain associated with errors in the underestimation or overestimation of the free digoxin level.[23,30,45,51,67,71] Free digoxin concentrations are particularly useful in patients with severe renal dysfunction. Independent of the availability of these data, the patient's cardiac status must be carefully monitored for signs of recurrent toxicity.

Other pitfalls in the measurement and utility of serum digoxin concentrations include endogenous and exogenous factors. Endogenous digoxinlike immunoreactive substances (DLIS) have been described in infants, in women in the third trimester of pregnancy, and in patients with renal and hepatic failure.[22,25,26,31,33,42,72,73] When endogenous DLIS are free or weakly bound, as in these circumstances, they are measurable by the typical RIA and can account for factitiously high reported serum digoxin concentrations in the absence of digoxin treatment. The role of endogenous DLIS in the body has not been fully elucidated, but it does have an effect on both the sodium potassium ATPase pump and the digoxin glycoside receptor site.[26] Endogenous DLIS are implicated as a causative factor in hypertension and renal disease. Exogenous factors relate primarily to measurement techniques and interpretation.[35] Digoxin is metabolized to compounds with varying levels of cardioactivity.[38] Some metabolites cross-react and are measured by RIA, while others are not. The in vivo production of these metabolites varies in patients, and may depend on intestinal metabolism by gut flora as well as renal and liver clearance.

EXTRACORPOREAL REMOVAL

Hemodialysis and activated charcoal hemoperfusion have no role in the management of digoxin poisoning. Even in the absence of Fab, these procedures are not indicated because both the molecular weight and volume of distribution of digoxin are too large to make either approach useful. Digoxin-specific antibody fragments are effective even in anephric patients, although toxic symptoms may recur 7–14 days later, possibly indicating the need for another dose of Fab. Hemoperfusion through columns with antidigoxin antibodies bound to agarose polyacrolein microsphere beads has been accomplished, but the availability of Fab in the United States has supplanted this modality.[41,55] The principles that make activated charcoal hemoperfusion less than ideal (V_d of digoxin, extracorporeal access, anticoagulation) also apply to the antidigoxin antibody columns. Continuous arteriovenous hemofiltration in an experimental model has failed to remove the digoxin-Fab complex.[50]

ROLE OF DIGOXIN-SPECIFIC ANTIBODY FRAGMENTS IN POISONING WITH OTHER CARDIAC GLYCOSIDES

Digoxin-specific antibody fragments were designed to have high-affinity binding for digoxin and digitoxin. There are structural similarities, however, between all cardiac glycosides. In fact, RIA-determined digoxin levels have been reported in patients following intoxication with nondigoxin cardiac glycosides,[27,47,61] suggesting that cross-reactivity exists between digoxin-specific antibodies and other cardiac glycosides. Thus, Digibind may have some efficacy in all natural cardiac glycoside poisonings including oleander, squill, and toad venom.[8,9,13,20,54] The successful reversal by Digibind of cardiotoxicity resulting from ingestion of *Nerium oleander* was reported.[61] This patient responded to 5 vials (200 mg) of Fab, but larger doses may be required in other cardiac glycoside poisonings because of the lower-affinity binding of Digibind for these toxins. Treatment decisions should be based on empirical grounds, with initial therapy consisting of 10–20 vials. Subsequent doses can be based on clinical response.

REFERENCES

1. Antman EM, Wenger TL, Butler VP, et al: Treatment of 150 cases of life-threatening digitalis intoxication with digoxin specific Fab antibody fragments: Final report of multicenter study. Circulation 1990; 81:1744–1752.
2. Argyle JC: Effect of digoxin antibodies on TDX digoxin assay. Clin Chem 1986;32:1616–1617.
3. Beller GA, Smith TW, Abelmann WH, et al: Digitalis intoxication: A prospective clinical study with serum level correlations. N Engl J Med 1971;284:989–997.
4. Berkovitch M, Akilesh MR, Gerace R, et al: Acute digoxin overdose in a newborn with renal failure: Use of digoxin immune Fab and peritoneal dialysis. Ther Drug Monit 1994;16:531–533.
5. Bismuth C, Gaultier M, Conso F, et al: Hyperkalemia in acute digitalis poisoning: Prognostic significance and therapeutic implications. Clin Toxicol 1973;6:153–162.
6. Borron S, Bismuth C, Muszynski J: Advances in the management of digoxin toxicity in the older patient. Drugs Aging 1997;10:18–33.
7. Bosse GM, Pope TM: Recurrent digoxin overdose and treatment with digoxin-specific Fab antibody fragments. J Emerg Med 1994;12: 179–185.
8. Brubacher J, Lachmanen D, Ravikumar PR, Hoffman RS: Efficacy of digoxin specific Fab fragments (Digibind) in the treatment of toad venom poisoning. Toxicon 1999;37:931–942.
9. Brubacher J, Ravikumar P, Bania T, et al: Treatment of toad venom poisoning with digoxin-specific Fab fragments. Chest 1996;110: 1282–1288.
10. Butler VP, Chen J: Digoxin specific antibodies. Proc Natl Acad Sci U S A 1967;57:71–78.
11. Butler VP, Schmidt DH, Smith TW, et al: Effects of sheep digoxin: Specific antibodies and their Fab fragments on digoxin pharmacokinetics in dogs. J Clin Invest 1977;59:345–359.
12. Butler VP, Smith TW, Schmidt DH, et al: Immunological reversal of the effects of digoxin. Fed Proc 1977;36:2235–2241.
13. Cheung K, Urech R, Taylor L, et al: Plant cardiac glycosides and digoxin Fab antibody. J Pediatr Child Health 1991;27:312–313.
14. Colucci R, Choses M, Kluger J, et al: The pharmacokinetics of digoxin immune Fab, total digoxin and free digoxin in patients with renal impairment [abstract]. Pharmacotherapy 1989;9:175.
15. Curd J, Smith TW, Jaton J, et al: The isolation of digoxin specific antibody and its use in reversing the effects of digoxin. Proc Natl Acad Sci U S A 1971;68:2401–2406.
16. D'Angio RG, Stevenson JG, Lively BT, et al: Therapeutic drug monitoring: Improved performance through educational intervention. Ther Drug Monit 1990;12:173–181.
17. Duhme DW, Greenblatt DJ, Kock-Weser J: Reduction of digoxin toxicity associated with measurement of serum levels: A report from the Boston Collaborative Drug Surveillance Program. Ann Intern Med 1974;80:516–519.
18. Durham G, Califf RM: Digoxin toxicity in renal insufficiency treated with digoxin immune Fab. Prim Cardiol 1988;1:31–34.
19. Eagle KA, Haber E, DeSanctis RW, et al, eds: The Practice of Cardiology, 2nd ed. Boston, Little, Brown, 1989.
20. Eddleston M, Rajapakse S, Rajakanthan, et al: Anti-digoxin Fab fragments in cardiotoxicity induced by ingestion of yellow oleander: A randomized controlled trial. Lancet 2000;355:967–972.
21. Erdmann E, Mair W, Knedel M, et al: Digitalis intoxication and treatment with digoxin antibody fragments in renal failure. Klin Wochenschr 1989;67:16–19.
22. Frisolone J, Sylvia LM, Gelwan J, et al: False-positive serum digoxin concentrations determined by three digoxin assays on patients with liver disease. Clin Pharm 1988;7:444–449.
23. George S, Braithwaite RA, Hughes EA: Digoxin measurements following plasma ultrafiltration in two patients with digoxin toxicity treated with specific Fab fragments. Ann Clin Biochem 1994;31: 380–381.
24. Gibb I, Adams PC, Parnham AJ, et al: Plasma digoxin: Assay anomalies in Fab treated patients. Br J Clin Pharmacol 1983;16:445–447.
25. Graves SW, Brown B, Valdes R: An endogenous digoxin like substance in patients with renal impairment. Ann Intern Med 1983;99: 604–608.
26. Hastreiter AR, John EG, Nander Hoist RL: Digitalis, digitalis antibodies, digitalis-like immunoreactive substances, and sodium homeostasis: A review. Clin Perinatol 1988;15:491–522.
27. Haynes BE, Bessen HA, Wightman WD, et al: Oleander tea: Herbal draught of death. Ann Emerg Med 1985;14:350–353.
28. Honda SAA, Rios CN, Murakami L, et al: Problems in determining levels of free digoxin in patients treated with digoxin immune Fab. J Clin Lab Anal 1995;9:407–412.
29. Hursting MJ, Raisys VA, Opheim KE, et al: Determination of free digoxin concentrations in serum for monitoring Fab treatment of digoxin overdose. Clin Chem 1987;33:1652–1655.
30. Jortani S, Pinar A, Johnson N, Valdes R: Validity of unbound digoxin measurements by immunoassays in presence of antidote (Digibind). Clin Chim Acta 1999;283:159–169.
31. Karboski JA, Godley PJ, Frohna PA, et al: Marked digoxin like immunoreactive factor interference with an enzyme immunoassay. Drug Intell Clin Pharm 1988;2:703–705.
32. Kaufman J, Leikin J, Kendzierski D, Polin K: Use of digoxin Fab immune fragments in a seven-day-old infant. Pediatr Emerg Care 1990;6:118–121.
33. Kelly RA, O'Hara DS, Canessa MG, et al: Characterization of digitalis like factors in human plasma. J Biol Chem 1905;260: 11396–11405.
34. Koren G, Deatie D, Soldin S: Agonal elevation in serum digoxin concentrations in infants and children long after cessation of therapy. Crit Care Med 1988;16:793–795.
35. Koren G, Parker R: Interpretation of excessive serum concentrations of digoxin in children. Am J Cardiol 1985;55:1210–1214.

36. Lechat P, Mudgett-Hunter M, Margolies M, et al: Reversal of lethal digoxin toxicity in guinea pigs using monoclonal antibodies and Fab fragments. J Pharmacol Exp Ther 1984;229:210–215.

37. Lemon M, Andrews DJ, Binks AM, et al: Concentrations of free serum digoxin after treatment with antibody fragments. Br Med J 1987;295:1520–1521.

38. Lindenbaum J, Rund D, Butler VP, et al: Inactivation of digoxin by the gut flora: Reversal by antibiotic therapy. N Engl J Med 1981; 305:789–794.

39. Lloyd BL, Smith TW: Contrasting rates of reversal of digoxin toxicity by digoxin: Specific IgG and Fab fragments. Circulation 1978;58: 280–283.

40. Marchlinski FE, Hook BG, Callans DJ: Which cardiac disturbances should be treated with digoxin immune Fab (ovine) antibody? Am J Emerg Med 1991;9:24–34.

41. Marcus L, Margel S, Savin H, et al: Therapy of digoxin intoxication in dogs by specific hemoperfusion through agarose polyacrolein microsphere beads: Antidigoxin antibodies. Am Heart J 1985;110: 30–39.

42. Naomi S, Graves S, Lazarus M, et al: Variation in apparent serum digitalis-like factor levels with different digoxin antibodies: The "immunochemical fingerprint." Am J Hypertens 1991;4:795–800.

43. Nollet H, Verhaaren H, Stroobandt R, et al: Delayed elimination of digoxin antidotum determined by RIA. J Clin Pharmacol 1989;29: 41–45.

44. Nuwayhid N, Johnson G: Digoxin elimination in a functionally anephric patient after digoxin specific Fab fragment therapy. Ther Drug Monit 1989;11:680–685.

45. Ocal I, Green T: Serum digoxin in the presence of Digibind: Determination of digoxin by the Abbott AxSYM and Baxter Stratus II immunoassays by direct analysis without pretreatment of serum samples. Clin Chem 1998;44:1947–1950.

46. Ordog GJ, Benaron S, Bhasin V: Serum digoxin levels and mortality in 5100 patients. Ann Emerg Med 1987;16:32–39.

47. Osterloh J, Herold S, Pond S: Oleander interference in the digoxin radioimmunoassay in a fatal ingestion. JAMA 1982;247:1596–1597.

48. Physicians Desk Reference, 55th ed. Oradell, NJ, Medical Economics, 2001, pp. 1372–1373.

49. Postmarketing Surveillance Study of Digibind: Interim Report to Contributors. Research Triangle Park, NC, Burroughs Wellcome, July 1986–July 1987.

50. Quaife EJ, Banner W, Vernon D, et al: Failure of CAVH to remove digoxin Fab complex in piglets. J Toxicol Clin Toxicol 1990;28: 61–68.

51. Rainey P: Digibind and free digoxin. Clin Chem 1999;5:719–721.

52. Renard C, Grene-Lerouge N, Beau N, et al: Pharmacokinetics of digoxin-specific Fab: Effects of decreased renal function and age. Br J Clin Pharmacol 1997;44:135–138.

53. Renard C, Weinling E, Pau B, Schermann JM: Time and dose-dependent digoxin redistribution by digoxin-specific antigen binding fragments in a rat model. Toxicology 1999;137:117–127.

54. Safadi R, Levy I, Amitai Y, Caraco Y: Beneficial effect of digoxin-specific Fab antibody fragments in oleander intoxication. Arch Intern Med 1995;155:2121–2125.

55. Savin H, Marcus L, Margel S, et al: Treatment of adverse digitalis effect by hemoperfusion through columns with antidigoxin antibodies bound to agarose polyacrolein microsphere beads. Am Heart J 1987; 113:1078–1084.

56. Schaumann W, Kaufmann B, Neubert P, et al: Kinetics of the Fab fragments of digoxin antibodies and of bound digoxin in patients with severe digoxin intoxication. Eur J Clin Pharmacol 1986;30:527–533.

57. Schmidt DH, Butler VP: Immunological protection against digoxin toxicity. J Clin Invest 1971;50:866–871.

58. Schmidt DH, Butler VP: Reversal of digoxin toxicity with specific antibodies. J Clin Invest 1971;50:1738–1744.

59. Schmitt K, Tulzer G, Hackel F, et al: Massive digitoxin intoxication treated with digoxin-specific antibodies in a child. Pediatr Cardiol 1994;15:48–49.

60. Sherron PA, Gelband H: Reversal of digoxin toxicity with Fab fragments in a pediatric patient with acute renal failure. Paper presented at Management of Digitalis Toxicity: The Role of Digibind, San Francisco, July 26–28, 1985. Burroughs Wellcome, sponsor.

61. Shumaik GM, Wu AU, Ping AC: Oleander poisoning: Treatment with digoxin-specific Fab antibody fragments. Ann Emerg Med 1988;17: 732–735.

62. Sinclair AJ, Hewick DS, Johnston PC, et al: Kinetics of digoxin and anti-digoxin antibody fragments during treatment of digoxin toxicity. Br J Clin Pharmacol 1989;28:352–356.

63. Smith TW: New advances in the assessment and treatment of digitalis toxicity. J Clin Pharmacol 1985;25:522–528.

64. Smith TW, Haber E, Yeatman L, et al: Reversal of advanced digoxin intoxication with Fab fragments of digoxin specific antibodies. N Engl J Med 1976;294:797–800.

65. Smith TW, Lloyd BL, Spicer N, et al: Immunogenicity and kinetics of distribution and elimination of sheep digoxin specific IgG and Fab fragments in the rabbit and baboon. Clin Exp Immunol 1979;36: 384–396.

66. Soldin S: Digoxin: Issues and controversies. Clin Chem 1986;32: 5–12.

67. Ujhelyi MR, Colucci RD, Cummings DM, et al: Monitoring serum digoxin concentrations during digoxin immune Fab therapy. Ann Pharmacother 1991;25:1047–1049.

68. Ujhelyi MR, Robert S: Pharmacokinetic aspects of digoxin-specific Fab therapy in the management of digitalis toxicity. Clin Pharmacokinet 1995;28:483–493.

69. Ujhelyi MR, Robert S, Cummings DM, et al: Disposition of digoxin immune Fab in patients with kidney failure. Clin Pharmacol Ther 1993;54:388–394.

70. Ujhelyi MR, Robert S, Cummings DM, et al: Influence of digoxin immune Fab therapy and renal dysfunction on the disposition of total and free digoxin. Ann Intern Med 1993;119:273–277.

71. Valdes R, Jortani S: Monitoring of unbound digoxin in patients treated with antidigoxin antigen-binding fragments: A model for the future? Clin Chem 1998;44:1883–1885.

72. Vasdev S, Johnson E, Longerich L, et al: Plasma endogenous digitalis-like factors in healthy individuals and in dialysis dependent and kidney transplant patients. Clin Nephrol 1987;27:169–174.

73. Vinge E, Ekman R: Partial characterization of endogenous digoxin-like substance in human urine. Ther Drug Monit 1988;10:8–15.

74. Wenger TL: Experience with digoxin immune Fab (ovine) in patients with renal impairment. Am J Emerg Med 1991;9:21–23.

75. Winter ME: Digoxin. In: Koda-Kimble MA, Young LY, eds: Basic Clinical Pharmacokinetics, 3rd ed. Vancouver, WA, Applied Therapeutics, 1994, pp. 198–235.

CHAPTER 49 β-ADRENERGIC ANTAGONISTS

Jeffrey R. Brubacher

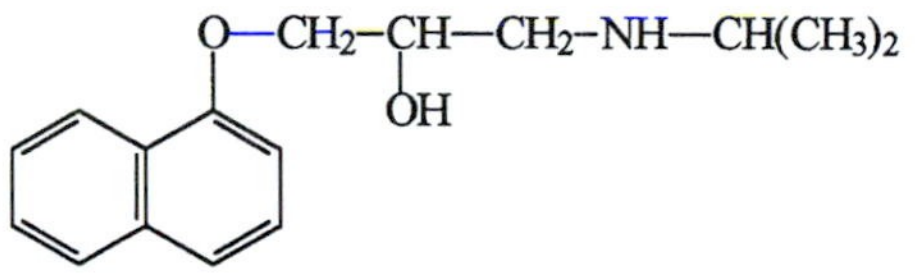

Propranolol

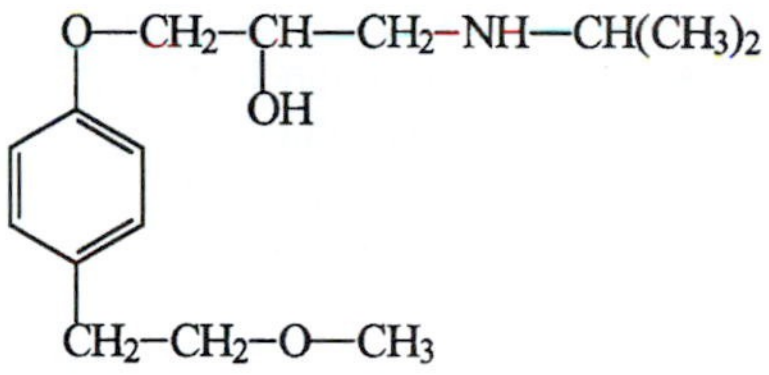

Metoprolol

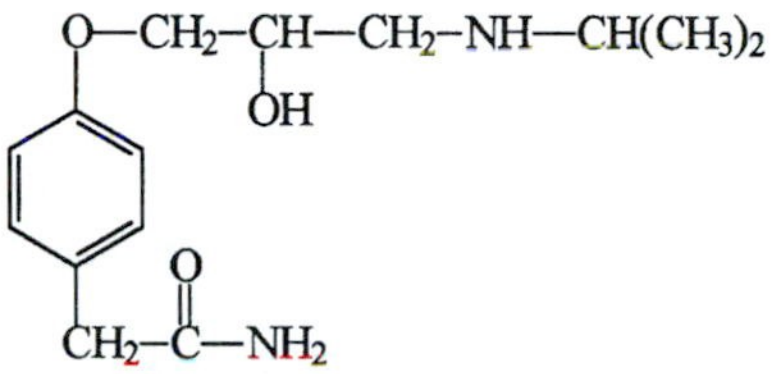

Atenolol

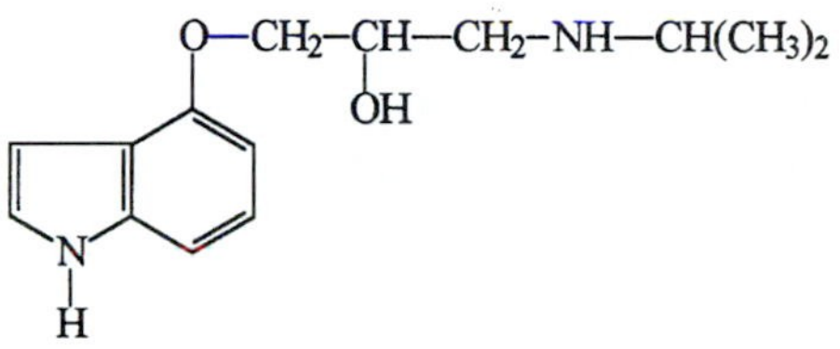

Pindolol

A 64-year-old man was brought to the emergency department by ambulance after being found comatose by his family. The emergency medical personnel found him hypoventilating with respirations of 10 breaths/min, a pulse of 45 beats/min, and a blood pressure of 80 mm Hg by palpation. They intubated him and gave him 2 mg naloxone, 1 mg atropine, and a 500-mL bolus of 0.9% NaCl. During transport, the patient had a generalized seizure that responded to 5 mg of intravenous diazepam. On arrival in the emergency department the patient was intubated, ventilated, and comatose with the following vital signs: blood pressure, 85 mm Hg by palpation; pulse, 50 beats/min; and temperature 36°C (96.8°F). On 100% oxygen the patient's oxygen saturation by pulse oximetry was 99% and his fingerstick blood glucose was 80 mg/dL. Physical examination showed that the pupils were 6 mm and reactive and the skin was cool. There were scattered basilar crackles. Heart sounds were normal with no murmurs. Bowel sounds were decreased. The patient was given 100 mg thiamine IV, 50 mL 50% dextrose IV, and 2 mg naloxone IV with no response. One of the medical staff was sent to interview the family.

Blood was obtained for laboratory analysis and sent for a complete blood count, electrolytes, glucose, renal function, and creatine phosphokinase. Arterial blood was sent for blood gas analysis. A 12-lead electrocardiogram showed sinus bradycardia with a PR interval of 280 msec and a QRS duration of 140 msec. During the next several minutes the patient's vital signs deteriorated. His blood pressure decreased to 75 mm Hg and his pulse decreased to 40 beats/min. He was given an additional 2 mg of atropine and another 500 mL of 0.9% NaCl with little change in blood pressure or heart rate. External cardiac pacing was instituted with an increase in the pulse to 70 beats/min. The blood pressure fell to 60 mm Hg with pacing and this intervention was discontinued. A central venous line

was placed and dopamine was started. There was no response to a dopamine infusion at 20 µg/kg/min.

Further history was obtained from the patient's son. The patient was previously healthy except for a history of depression and hypertension. The patient stopped taking antidepressants several months ago. He was currently taking only an antihypertensive medication, and no one else in the family took any pills. The family stated that the patient was more depressed in the last 2 weeks with apathy, decreased appetite, and inability to sleep. On the day of admission, however, he seemed better. He ate breakfast, took a shower, and went for a walk before he returned home to take a nap before lunch. The patient was well prior to taking his nap but 2 hours later, when the family could not arouse him for lunch, they called the ambulance. A family member was requested to return home and bring all medication bottles to the emergency department. A call was placed to the patient's family physician.

Given the possibility of an overdose, blood was analyzed for acetaminophen. The history of depression, seizures, hypotension, and widened QRS interval suggested a tricyclic antidepressant overdose and the patient was given 100 mEq of hypertonic sodium bicarbonate. There was no change in the patient's vital signs following this and a repeat electrocardiogram was essentially unchanged except that the QRS interval had decreased to 130 msec from 140 msec. A bicarbonate infusion was started. Because of the possibility of a calcium-channel-blocking medication, the patient was given 1 g of calcium chloride intravenously. Following this, his blood pressure increased to 75 mm Hg and the pulse remained at 40 beats/min.

The family physician returned the call and stated that propranolol had just been prescribed for hypertension 2 weeks earlier. One of the patient's daughters returned with all the medication bottles that she could find. Several bottles of vitamins and over-the-counter analgesics were almost full; however, the propranolol bottle was empty; an estimated 5 g of propranolol was missing.

With this additional information, the patient was given intravenous glucagon. After a total of 5 mg of glucagon given over a 10-minute period, the patient improved. His blood pressure increased to 105/60 mm Hg and his pulse increased to 55 beats/min. A glucagon infusion at 5 mg/h was started and the patient was admitted to the intensive care unit. Laboratory analysis was negative for acetaminophen. The electrolytes, glucose, renal function, complete blood count, and arterial blood gases were all within normal limits except for a mild anion gap metabolic acidosis, which resolved on repeat analysis performed after the patient's vital signs normalized.

By the next day, the patient had regained consciousness and was able to maintain his blood pressure after the glucagon infusion was stopped. He was extubated and stated that he had taken an overdose of propranolol in a suicide attempt. The patient was assessed by a psychiatrist who suggested that his depression was exacerbated by the propranolol. Propranolol was discontinued and his antidepressants were restarted. The patient was started on a calcium channel blocker for hypertension and briefly admitted to the psychiatric service. On followup examination 1 month later, the patient was doing well with no complaints. He no longer felt depressed, and his blood pressure was well controlled.

β-Adrenergic antagonists have been available for clinical use for four decades. They are commonly used in the treatment of cardiovascular disease: hypertension, coronary artery disease, and tachydysrhythmias. Additional indications for β-adrenergic antagonists include congestive heart failure, migraine headaches, tremor, panic attacks, and hyperthyroidism. Ophthalmic preparations containing β-adrenergic antagonists are also used in the treatment of glaucoma.[51] When taken in overdose, β-adrenergic antagonists cause hypotension and bradycardia. The clinical course is often benign, although patients with any compromise in cardiac status and those who have taken a cardioactive coingestant are at risk for cardiovascular collapse and death.

HISTORY

In 1948, Raymond Alquist postulated that the cardiovascular actions of epinephrine, hypertension and tachycardia, were best explained by the existence of two distinct sets of receptors that he generically named α and β receptors.[5] Contemporary "antiepinephrine" drugs such as phenoxybenzamine reversed the hypertension but not the tachycardia associated with epinephrine. According to Alquist's theory, these drugs acted at the α receptors, whereas the β receptors mediated catecholamine-induced tachycardia. The British pharmacist Sir James Black was influenced by Alquist's work and recognized the potential clinical benefit of a β-adrenergic antagonist. In 1958, Black synthesized the first β-adrenergic antagonist, pronethalol. This drug was briefly marketed as Alderlin, named after Alderly Park, the research headquarters of ICI Pharmaceuticals. Pronethalol was discontinued because it produced thymic tumors in mice. Propranolol was soon developed and marketed as Inderal (an anagram of Alderlin) in the United Kingdom in 1964,[16,131] and in the United States in 1973. Prior to the introduction of β-adrenergic antagonists, the management of angina was limited to agents such as nitrates that increased myocardial oxygen delivery by vasodilation of the coronary arteries. Propranolol gave clinicians the ability to decrease myocardial oxygen requirements. This new approach decreased morbidity and mortality in angina sufferers.[69] New drugs soon followed, and by 1979, there were 10 β-adrenergic antagonists available in the United States.[31] Unfortunately, it soon became apparent that these agents were dangerous when taken in overdose, and by 1979, cases of severe toxicity and death from β-adrenergic overdose were reported.[31]

EPIDEMIOLOGY

Intentional β-adrenergic antagonist overdose, although relatively uncommon, continues to account for a number of deaths annually. From 1985 to 1995, there were 52,156 β-adrenergic antagonist exposures reported to the toxic exposure surveillance system of the American Association of Poison Control Centers (Chap. 116 and p. 1752). These exposures accounted for 164 deaths with β-adrenergic antagonists implicated as the primary cause of death in 38 cases. The other fatalities could not be clearly ascribed to β-adrenergic antagonists because of coingestants with cardioactive drugs such as calcium channel blockers or because of other factors. Children younger than 6 years of age accounted for 19,388 exposures but no fatalities. The youngest fatality reported in this age group was 7 years old. More than half of the patients who died developed cardiac arrest only after arriving at a healthcare facility.[84] In England and Wales, β-adrenergic antagonist toxicity accounted for just over 20 deaths annually during the period from 1975 to 1984.

Several authors report that, as compared to the other β-adrenergic antagonists, propranolol accounts for a disproportionate number of cases of self-poisoning[22,112] and deaths.[68,84] This may be explained by the fact that propranolol is frequently prescribed for patients with diagnoses such as anxiety, stress, and migraine who may be more prone to suicide attempts.[112] Propranolol is also more toxic because of its lipophilic and membrane-stabilizing properties.[44,112]

PHARMACOLOGY

Myocyte Calcium Flow and Contractility

Myocyte contraction occurs when actin and myosin filaments interact and slide past each other. At rest, the troponin-tropomyosin complex blocks this interaction. Excitation triggers a series of events that increase cytoplasmic calcium concentrations. Calcium binds to troponin C causing movement of the troponin-tropomyosin complex. This permits actin-myosin linkage and results in sliding of myosin and actin chains relative to each other and ultimately in muscle contraction.[2,9,120]

Low intracellular calcium concentrations are maintained by pumps that actively remove calcium from the cytoplasm.[108,111] Voltage-sensitive slow calcium channels open in response to depolarization and allow calcium to flow into the myocyte. This triggers the opening of calcium release channels in the sarcoplasmic reticulum, a phenomenon known as calcium-induced calcium release.[39,152] More calcium causes stronger actin-myosin interaction and greater contractility. Actin-myosin interaction is also modulated by troponin phosphorylation, ischemia, intracellular pH, and myofilament stretch[9,120] (Fig. 49–1A).

Relaxation occurs when calcium is released from troponin and removed from the cytoplasm. Most calcium is pumped back into the sarcoplasmic reticulum by the sarcoplasmic calcium pump. This pump is modulated by β-adrenergic stimulation as discussed below. Calcium is also removed by an active cytoplasmic membrane calcium pump and by the calcium-sodium transporter, which exchanges 1 molecule of calcium for 3 molecules of sodium (Fig. 49–1B).[9,13]

β-Adrenergic Receptors

β-Adrenergic receptors are divided into $β_1$, $β_2$, and $β_3$ subtypes. $β_1$-Adrenergic receptors are coupled to G_s proteins, which activate adenylate cyclase when the receptor is stimulated. This increases intracellular production of cyclic adenosine monophosphate (cAMP), which binds to and activates protein kinase A and other cAMP-dependent protein kinases.[75] Protein kinase A, in turn, phosphorylates important myocyte proteins including phospholamban, the voltage-sensitive calcium channels, and troponin.[42,138] Calcium channel phosphorylation increases contractility by increasing the influx of calcium during each cell depolarization.[113,129] Phosphorylation of phospholamban increases the activity of the sarcoplasmic calcium ATPase and thus enhances contractility by increasing sarcoplasmic calcium stores.[24,138] This also results in a more rapid removal of cytoplasmic calcium during diastole, and aids in myocyte relaxation. Troponin phosphorylation facilitates calcium unbinding and decreases contractility, but improves cardiac performance by enhancing myocyte relaxation[2,9,77,138] (Fig. 49–2).

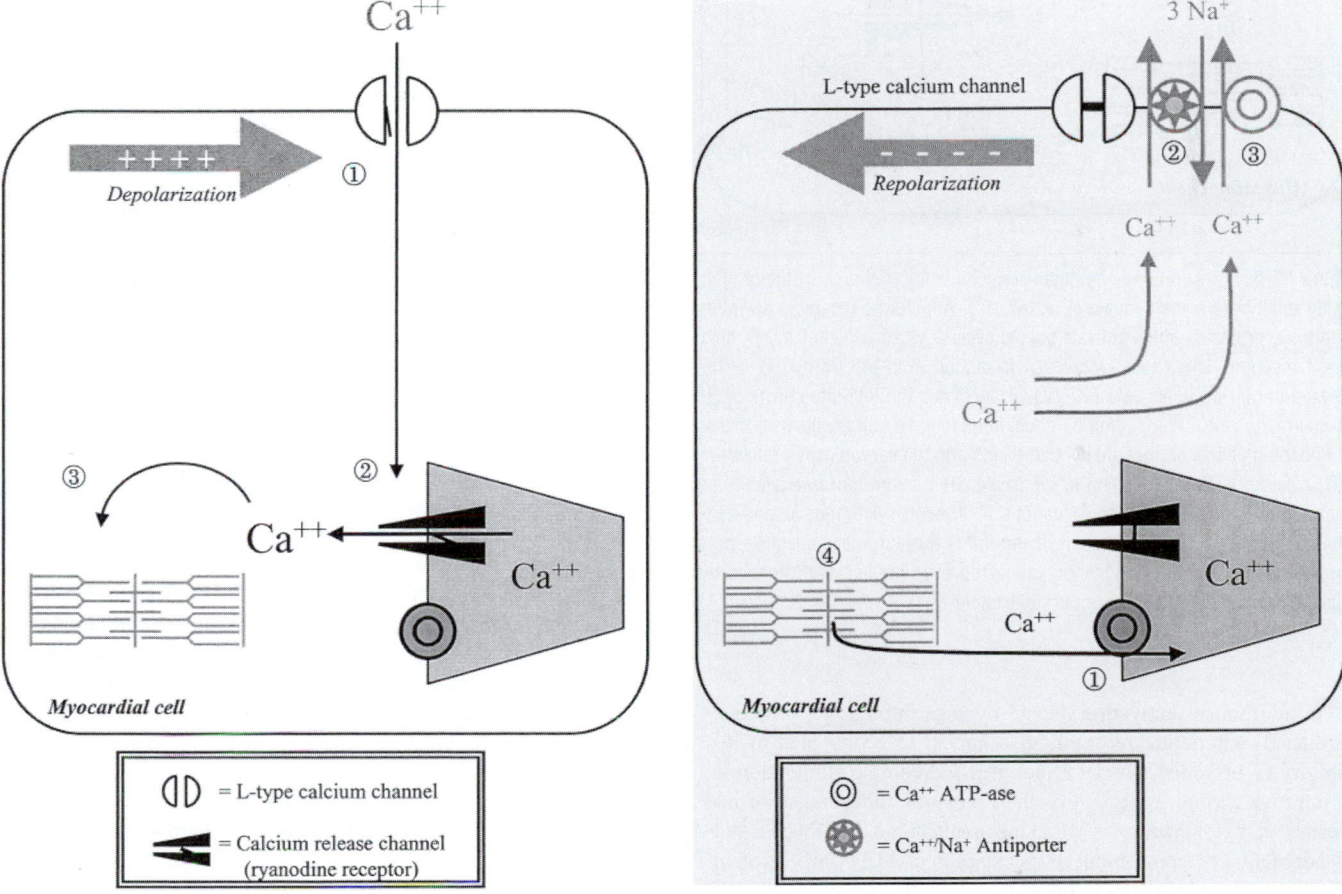

Figure 49–1. **A.** Fluctuations in calcium levels couple myocyte depolarization with contraction and myocyte repolarization with relaxation. ① Depolarization causes voltage-sensitive calcium channels to open and calcium to flow down its concentration gradient into the myocyte. ② This calcium current triggers the opening of calcium release channels (ryanodine receptor) in the sarcoplasmic reticulum (SR) and calcium pours out. The amount of calcium released from the SR is proportional to the initial inward calcium current and to the amount of calcium stored in the SR. ③ At rest, actin-myosin interaction is prevented by troponin. When calcium binds to troponin, this inhibition is removed, actin and myosin slide relative to each other, and the cell contracts. **B.** Following contraction, calcium is actively removed from the myocyte to allow relaxation. ① Most calcium is actively pumped into the SR where it is bound to calsequestrin. Calcium stored in the SR is thus available for release during subsequent depolarizations. The sarcoplasmic calcium ATPase is inhibited by phospholamban (Fig. 49–2). ② The calcium sodium antiporter couples the flow of 3 molecules of sodium in one direction to that of a single molecule of calcium in the opposite direction. This transporter is passively driven by electrochemical gradients which usually favor the inward flow of sodium coupled to the extrusion of calcium. Extrusion of calcium is therefore inhibited by high intracellular sodium or extracellular calcium concentrations and by cell depolarization. Under these conditions, the pump may "run in reverse." ③ Some calcium is actively pumped from the cell by calcium ATPase. ④ As myocyte calcium concentrations fall, calcium is released from troponin and the myocyte relaxes.

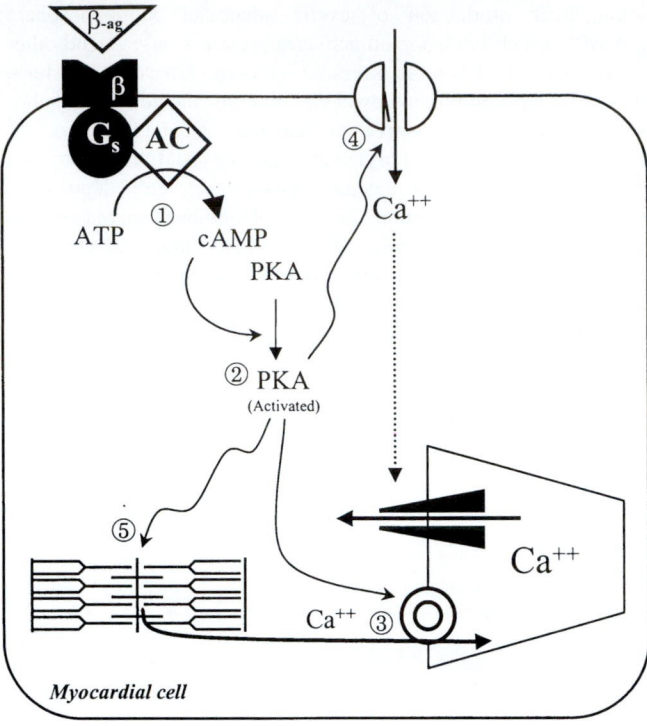

Figure 49–2. β-Adrenergic agonists are positive inotropes by virtue of their ability to activate protein kinase A (PKA). ① β-Adrenergic receptors are coupled to G_s proteins, which activate adenyl cyclase when catecholamines bind to the receptor. This causes increased formation of cAMP from ATP. ② Increased cAMP levels activate PKA, which mediates the ultimate effects of β-adrenergic receptor stimulation by phosphorylating key intracellular proteins. ③ Phosphorylation of phospholamban disinhibits the sarcoplasmic reticulum (SR) calcium ATPase, resulting in increased SR calcium stores available for release during subsequent depolarizations. ④ Phosphorylation of voltage-sensitive calcium channels increases calcium influx through these channels during systole. ⑤ Troponin phosphorylation improves cardiac performance by facilitating unbinding of calcium during diastole.

In addition to activating adenyl cyclase through G_S proteins, cardiac $β_2$-adrenergic receptors also appear to be coupled to inhibitory G_I proteins. The net effect of $β_2$-adrenergic stimulation is to improve cardiac contractility and relaxation independent of increases in cytoplasmic cAMP. One explanation for this is that $β_2$-adrenergic receptor–induced increases in cAMP (via G_S protein stimulation) are localized to the cell membrane, where they result in phosphorylation and improved function of slow calcium channels. The G_I protein-linked receptor inhibits adenyl cyclase elsewhere in the cytoplasm and prevents the global increase in cAMP that occurs with $β_1$-adrenergic activation. $β_2$-Adrenergic receptor stimulation may also improve contractility by increasing cytoplasmic pH independent of G protein activation.[132,154]

The pharmacology of the $β_3$-adrenergic receptor differs substantially from that of the other β receptors. Whereas isoproterenol is an agonist at all three β-adrenergic receptors, classic β-adrenergic antagonists actually act as agonists at the $β_3$ receptor.[135] The role of the $β_3$-adrenergic receptor in man is incompletely understood. This receptor is found on human adipocytes where it plays a role in thermogenesis and lipolysis,[27] and is also found in human

hearts,[34,35] where it appears to be a mediator of negative inotropy.[34]

Effects of β-Adrenergic Receptor Activation

β-Adrenergic stimulation modulates the function of the heart, vasculature, lungs, and numerous other organs, and causes complex metabolic effects. The most prevalent subtype in the heart is the $β_1$-adrenergic receptor. The relative density of cardiac $β_2$-adrenergic receptors increases in persons with heart failure.[132] $β_1$-Adrenergic stimulation of the heart results in increased contractility, increased conduction velocity, and increased automaticity. Peripheral vascular resistance is largely controlled by arteriolar muscle tone. α-Adrenergic stimulation causes arteriolar constriction in contrast to $β_2$-adrenergic receptors, which mediate arteriolar dilation.

In the lungs, $β_2$-adrenergic receptor stimulation results in bronchodilation and decreased respiratory secretions. β-Adrenergic agonists have important endocrine and metabolic effects. Renin secretion is increased by $β_1$-adrenergic stimulation. Insulin secretion is increased by $β_2$-adrenergic receptor stimulation, but is decreased by $α_2$-adrenergic receptor stimulation so that the net effect of epinephrine is to decrease insulin levels. $β_2$-Adrenergic receptor stimulation causes increased glucose secondary to increased hepatic gluconeogenesis, and skeletal muscle and hepatic glycogenolysis. Skeletal muscle potassium uptake is increased by $β_2$ stimulation, resulting in hypokalemia. Gut motility is decreased by both $β_1$- and $β_2$-adrenergic stimulation. β-Adrenergic agonists act at fat cells to cause lipolysis and thermogenesis.[51]

Action of β-Adrenergic Antagonists

β-Adrenergic antagonists competitively antagonize the effects of catecholamines at the β-adrenergic receptor. This causes decreased chronotropy and contractility, which is manifested clinically as lowered heart rate and blood pressure. These effects are more important in times of exertion, stress, or illness, when sympathetic tone is increased. The antihypertensive effect of β-adrenergic antagonists is counteracted by a reflex increase in peripheral vascular resistance. This effect is augmented by the $β_2$-adrenergic antagonism of nonselective β-adrenergic antagonists. With long-term use of β-adrenergic antagonists there is a fall in peripheral vascular resistance. The mechanism for this effect is poorly understood.[51]

Several adverse effects are related to $β_2$-adrenergic antagonism. β-Adrenergic antagonists cause bradycardia and hypotension which may be severe in patients with cardiac conduction defects and in those who take calcium channel blockers or other medications that impair cardiac conduction. Although β-adrenergic antagonists slow the progression of congestive heart failure and have become a standard of care for mild heart failure,[1] they acutely exacerbate symptoms in some patients with congestive heart failure. Rarely, β-Adrenergic antagonists will worsen peripheral vascular disease. Patients with reactive airways disease may suffer severe bronchospasm after using β-adrenergic antagonists because of loss of $β_2$-mediated bronchodilation. Catecholamines inhibit mast cell degranulation through a $β_2$-adrenergic mechanism, and interference with this may predispose to life-threatening anaphylactic reactions in atopic individuals.[55] Patients taking β-adrenergic antagonists who develop allergic reactions should be monitored more closely than other patients are monitored and allergy testing should be avoided in these patients. Although β_2-adrenergic stimulation augments insulin release, β-adrenergic antagonists rarely lower insulin levels. β_2-Adrenergic antagonists interfere with glycogenolysis and gluconeogenesis, resulting in impaired ability to recover from hypoglycemia. Furthermore, β-adrenergic antagonism may mask the sympathetic discharge that serves to warn of hypoglycemia. This combination of effects frequently proves dangerous for diabetic patients at risk for hypoglycemic episodes. The β_1-adrenergic-selective agents may be safer in patients with reactive airways or diabetes mellitus. Because β_2-adrenergic antagonism interferes with peripheral vasodilation, the β_1-adrenergic-selective agents may also be more effective antihypertensive agents. It is important to realize that β_1-adrenergic selectivity is incomplete, and that adverse reactions secondary to β_2-adrenergic antagonism may occur with the β_1-adrenergic-selective agents. This is especially likely to be the case when higher doses are used.[11,51,78,126]

Intrinsic sympathomimetic activity (ISA) describes the properties of β-adrenergic antagonists that are actually partial agonists at the β-adrenergic receptors. This property is unrelated to β_1-adrenergic selectivity. Like other β-adrenergic antagonists, these agents are antihypertensives and prevent exercise-induced tachycardia. These agents may avoid the severe decrease in resting heart rate that occurs with β-adrenergic antagonism in susceptible patients, but their clinical benefit is not demonstrated in controlled trials.[28] Table 49–1 lists the important agents with ISA.

Three of the β-adrenergic antagonists are also vasodilators. Carvedilol and labetalol are α-adrenergic antagonists, and nebivolol causes vasodilation by increasing nitric oxide release.[89]

Vasodilation may prove beneficial in patients with congestive heart failure and may make these agents more effective antihypertensives. Because labetalol is 5- to 10-fold more potent as a β-adrenergic antagonist than as an α antagonist, it remains contraindicated in situations such as pheochromocytoma or cocaine toxicity, where β-adrenergic antagonism could result in an "unopposed α" adrenergic effect.[37,51]

Sotalol is unique in that it prolongs action potential duration and increases the refractory period by blocking delayed rectifier potassium channels.[52] These actions make sotalol an effective class III antidysrhythmic agent; unfortunately, these actions also predispose patients to the development of polymorphic ventricular tachycardia (torsades de pointes) (see "Clinical Manifestations").

PHARMACOKINETICS

β-Adrenergic antagonists differ in their lipophilicity, oral bioavailability, first-pass metabolism, protein binding, β_1-adrenergic selectivity, and intrinsic sympathomimetic activity (Table 49–1).

Lipid solubility is a measure of the ability of a drug to partition into fat. Highly lipid-soluble agents cross lipid membranes rapidly and concentrate in adipose tissue. These properties allow rapid entry into the central nervous system (CNS), and typically result in large volumes of distribution. Lipid solubility enhances intestinal absorption by allowing rapid transit across lipid membranes but because compounds must enter an aqueous phase in the intestines before being absorbed, excessive lipid solubility may actually impede absorption. Highly lipid-soluble and highly pro-

TABLE 49–1.   Pharmacologic Properties of the β-Adrenergic Antagonists

	Adrenergic Blocking Activity	Partial Agonist Activity (ISA)	Membrane-Stabilizing Activity	Lipid Solubility	Protein Binding	Oral Bio-availability	Half-Life (hours)	Metabolism	Volume of Distribution (L/kg)
Acebutolol	β_1	Yes	Yes	Low	25%	40%	2–4	Hepatic/renal	1.2
Atenolol	β_1	No	No	Low	<5%	50%	5–8	Renal	1
Betaxolol	β_1	No	Yes	Low	50%	90%	14–22	Hepatic/renal	5–10
Bisoprolol	β_1	No	No	Low	30%	80%	9–12	Hepatic/renal	?
Carteolol	β_1, β_2	Yes	No	Low	30%	85%	6	Renal	?
Carvedilol	α_1, β_1, β_2	No		High	~98%	25–35%	7–10	Hepatic	115
Esmolol	β_1	No	No	Low	50%	N/A	~8 minutes	RBC esterases	2
Labetalol	α_1, β_1, β_2	No	Low	Moderate	50%	20%	4–6	Hepatic	9
Metoprolol*	β_1	No	Low	Moderate	10%	40%	3–4	Hepatic	4
Nadolol	β_1, β_2	No	No	Low	20%	35%	10–20	Renal	2
Nebivolol	β_1	No		High	98%	12–96%	10–32	Hepatic	10–40
Oxprenolol	β_1, β_2	Yes	Yes	High	80%	20–70%	1–2	Hepatic	1.3
Penbutolol	β_1, β_2	Yes	No	High	90%	~100%	5	Hepatic/renal	?
Pindolol	β_1, β_2	Yes	Low	Moderate	50%	75%	3–4	Hepatic/renal	2
Propranolol*	β_1, β_2	No	Yes	High	90%	25%	3–5	Hepatic	4
Sotalol	β_1, β_2	No	No	Low	0%	90%	~12	Renal	2
Timolol	β_1, β_2	No	No	Moderate	60%	75%	3–5	Hepatic/renal	2

*Long acting preparation available. Data from references 44, 51, 89, and 98.

tein-bound agents are poorly excreted by the kidneys and require hepatic biotransformation before they can be eliminated. These drugs tend to accumulate in patients with liver failure.[51,98,104,140] Propranolol is the most lipid-soluble of the β-adrenergic antagonists.

Highly water-soluble compounds cross lipid membranes slowly and distribute in total body water. These compounds are generally slowly absorbed, poorly protein bound, renally eliminated, and slow to enter the CNS. They tend to accumulate in patients with renal failure, and generally have less CNS toxicity. Esmolol, although water-soluble, is rapidly eliminated by red blood cell esterases and does not accumulate in renal failure.[114] Atenolol is the most water-soluble β-adrenergic antagonist.

Bioavailability reflects both the degree of absorption and the amount of first-pass metabolism. Compounds with extensive first-pass hepatic metabolism or poor absorption will have low bioavailability. β-Adrenergic antagonist bioavailability ranges from approximately 25% for propranolol to almost 100% for pindolol. Propranolol and other lipophilic agents with extensive first-pass hepatic metabolism have increased bioavailability in overdose when hepatic enzymes become saturated.

The half-life of β-adrenergic antagonists ranges from 8 minutes for esmolol to 32 hours with nebivolol. Most agents have half-lives in the range of 2–8 hours. Sustained-release formulations, which prolong the clinical effect without changing the half-life, are available for some β-adrenergic antagonists.

Protein binding ranges from essentially none with sotalol to 90% with propranolol and penbutolol and to almost 100% with nebivolol. The volume of distribution of most β-adrenergic antagonists is in the range of 2–4 L/kg. Atenolol, being the most water-soluble, has the lowest volume of distribution (approximately 1 L/kg) and carvedilol has the largest volume of distribution ($\approx$115 L/kg).[51]

PATHOPHYSIOLOGY

β-Adrenergic antagonists competitively antagonize the action of catecholamines at cardiac and peripheral β-adrenergic receptors. This, at least partially, explains the bradycardia and impaired contractility that occur with β-adrenergic antagonist toxicity. The effects of peripheral β-adrenergic antagonism are less prominent in overdose, but may explain the hypoglycemia, mild hyperkalemia, and respiratory impairment which sometimes occur. β-Adrenergic antagonists may also cause toxic effects independent of their action at catecholamine receptors. In catecholamine-depleted, spontaneously beating isolated rat hearts, propranolol decreased heart rate and contractility. Timolol and sotalol cause similar, but less dramatic, results.[153] Surprisingly, the decreases in heart rate and contractility are similar in catecholamine-depleted and nondepleted hearts.[71] It may be concluded that β-adrenergic antagonists cause myocardial depression by an action independent of catecholamine antagonism. A membrane-depressant effect may explain some of the cardiac-depressant effects of propranolol, but not of other β-adrenergic antagonists such as timolol or sotalol.[71] Although this effect is assumed to be similar to that of quinidine, it is controversial.[81] Other investigators provide evidence that β-adrenergic antagonists may cause myocardial hyperpolarization. Lowering extracellular potassium or raising extracellular sodium concentrations partially reverses propranolol and atenolol toxicity in isolated hearts. Thus, these agents may interfere with calcium

intake into intracellular organelles. This increased cytosolic calcium, in turn, would increase the activity of calcium-sensitive outward potassium channels, ultimately resulting in hyperpolarization.[58]

Although cardiovascular effects are most prominent in overdose, β-adrenergic antagonists also cause respiratory depression.[72] This effect is centrally mediated and appears to be an important cause of death in spontaneously breathing animal models of β-adrenergic antagonism toxicity.[73] There is evidence that propranolol may interfere with synaptic transmission and this may explain some of the CNS effects noted in propranolol overdose.[38]

CLINICAL MANIFESTATIONS

β-Adrenergic antagonist overdose is often quite benign, with about one-third of patients remaining asymptomatic.[26,140] This is partially explained by the fact that β-adrenergic antagonism is often well tolerated in healthy persons who do not rely on sympathetic stimulation to maintain cardiac output. On the other hand, persons with congestive heart failure, sick sinus syndrome, or impaired arteriovenous (AV) conduction may rely on sympathetic stimulation to maintain heart rate or cardiac output, and β-adrenergic antagonists may be harmful in these persons. In addition, β-adrenergic antagonists severely impair the heart's ability to respond to peripheral vasodilation, bradycardia, or decreased contractility caused by other toxins. Therefore, even relatively benign toxins may cause catastrophic toxicity when coingested with β-adrenergic antagonists.[32] The most important predictor of toxicity in β-adrenergic antagonist overdose is likely to be a cardioactive coingestant.[80] However, severe toxicity and death may still occur in healthy persons who have ingested β-adrenergic antagonists alone.[31,112,130] This may be explained by an increased susceptibility of certain persons to β antagonism or by special properties that increase the toxicity of certain β-adrenergic antagonists (see below). In patients without a coingestant, toxicity is most likely to occur in those who ingest a β-adrenergic antagonist with membrane-stabilizing activity.[80]

Patients with symptomatic β-adrenergic antagonist overdose will be hypotensive and bradycardic. Decreased sinoatrial (SA) node function results in sinus bradycardia, sinus pauses, or sinus arrest. Impaired atrioventricular conduction manifested as prolonged PR interval or high-grade AV block rarely occurs. Prolonged QRS and QT intervals may occur and severe poisonings may result in asystole. Congestive heart failure often complicates β-adrenergic antagonist overdose. Delirium, coma, and seizures occur most commonly in the setting of severe hypotension, but may also occur with normal blood pressure, especially with exposure to the more lipophilic agents.[31,112] Respiratory depression and apnea may have an additional role.[6] In a review of reported cases, 18% of patients with propranolol toxicity and 6% of those with atenolol toxicity had a respiratory rate less than 12.[112] Respiratory depression following β-adrenergic antagonist overdose typically occurs in patients who are hypotensive and comatose, but is also reported in awake patients.[93] Hypoglycemia, although relatively common in children after β-adrenergic antagonist poisoning,[46] is uncommon in acutely poisoned adults. In a series of 15 cases of β-adrenergic antagonist overdose, none of the 13 adults were hypoglycemic whereas both of the 2 children had symptomatic hypoglycemia.[31] Bronchospasm is relatively uncommon following β-adrenergic antagonist overdose and appears to occur only in susceptible patients. In the series mentioned above, only 2 of the 15 patients developed bronchospasm,[31] and in a recent review of 39 cases of symptomatic adults with β-adrenergic antagonist overdose, only 1 patient developed bronchospasm.[86] Clinical use of β-adrenergic antagonists slightly increases serum potassium;[88] however, significant hyperkalemia rarely complicates acute overdose.

Toxicity generally occurs early following β-adrenergic antagonist ingestion. Propranolol overdose, in particular, may be complicated by the rapid development of seizures, coma, and dysrhythmias. In a retrospective review of published reports of adult β-adrenergic antagonist overdose, there were 39 symptomatic patients with well-documented time from ingestion to symptom onset. Only one of these patients had ingested a sustained-release product. Thirty-one patients were symptomatic at 2 hours, 30 at 4 hours, and all developed symptoms within the first 6 hours. The authors concluded that there are no well-documented reports of toxicity delayed more than 6 hours after β-adrenergic antagonist overdose.[86] The authors of an Australian series also noted that, in their 58 patients with β-adrenergic antagonist overdose, all major symptoms began within 6 hours of ingestion.[112] These observations do not apply to sotalol overdoses, which are well known to cause delayed toxicity. All the authors caution against applying these observations to sustained-release products.

PROPERTIES THAT MODIFY TOXICITY

Membrane-Stabilizing Effects

β-Adrenergic antagonists that inhibit fast sodium channels are said to possess membrane-stabilizing activity. Propranolol possesses the most membrane-stabilizing activity of this class, and propranolol poisoning is characterized by coma, seizures, hypotension, bradycardia, impaired atrioventricular conduction, and widened QRS interval; ventricular tachydysrhythmias may also occur.[3,84] Hypotension may be out of proportion to bradycardia, and deaths from propranolol overdose are frequently reported.[31,44,84] Acebutolol, betaxolol, and oxprenolol also possess significant membrane-stabilizing activity and have caused fatalities when taken in overdose (Table 49–1).[14,44,61,98,104]

Lipid Solubility

Lipid solubility is another important modifier of β-adrenergic antagonist toxicity. In overdose, the more lipophilic β-adrenergic antagonists may cause delirium, coma, and seizures, even in the absence of hypotension.[31,112] Atenolol is the least lipid-soluble of the β-adrenergic antagonists and also appears to be one of the safer β-adrenergic antagonists when taken in overdose.[44] In fact, in one series of β-adrenergic antagonist overdoses none of 18 patients with atenolol overdose had seizures, compared with 8 of 28 patients with propranolol overdose.[112] Nevertheless, atenolol overdose may result in severe toxicity and death.[84,100,133]

Intrinsic Sympathomimetic Activity

Acebutolol, oxprenolol, penbutolol, and pindolol act as partial agonists at β-adrenergic receptors and are said to have intrinsic sympathomimetic activity. In theory, ISA should make these drugs safer than the other β-adrenergic antagonists; however, there is little experience with overdose of these agents. Sympathetic stim-

ulation with tachycardia or hypertension often predominates in pindolol overdose and this agent does appear to be relatively safe in overdose.[31,68,105] In addition to ISA, acebutolol and oxprenolol have significant membrane-stabilizing activity, making them dangerous in overdose, and deaths as a result of acute toxicity from these agents are reported.[31,44,104] Penbutolol overdose has not yet been reported.

β₁ Selectivity

Cardioselective agents may be safer in clinical practice because they are less likely to cause bronchospasm and the other undesirable effects of β₂-adrenergic antagonism. In overdose, cardioselectivity is largely lost and deaths are reported from all of the β₁-adrenergic-selective agents, including acebutolol,[44] atenolol,[84] betaxolol,[14] and metoprolol.[117,130]

Potassium Channel Blockade

Sotalol is a nonselective β-adrenergic antagonist with low lipophilicity, no membrane-stabilizing effect, and no ISA. Sotalol is unique among β adrenergic antagonists because of its ability to block the delayed rectifier potassium current responsible for repolarization. This prolongs the action potential duration and is manifested on the electrocardiogram by a prolonged QT interval.[52] The prolonged QT interval predisposes to torsades de pointes, and ventricular dysrhythmias may complicate the therapeutic use of sotalol.[67] Torsades de pointes, is most common in patients taking sotalol therapeutically who also use other agents that prolong the QT interval or who have predisposing factors such as renal failure, hypokalemia, hypomagnesemia, or bradycardia.[23,52] Some authors suggest that QT dispersion is a better predictor of sotalol-induced torsades de pointes than is QT prolongation alone. A difference between the longest and shortest QT interval on the 12-lead ECG of over 100 msec indicates an increased risk of torsades de pointes.[23]

Sotalol overdoses also are frequently complicated by QT prolongation and ventricular dysrhythmias, especially torsades de pointes.[12] In 6 patients with sotalol overdose, the average QT interval was 172% of normal, and 5 patients had ventricular dysrhythmias, including multifocal ventricular extrasystoles, ventricular tachycardia, and ventricular fibrillation.[97] Sotalol overdose may also be complicated by hypotension, bradycardia, and asystole,[4,97] and fatalities are well documented.[92,99]

Sotalol overdose may cause delayed and prolonged toxicity, although electrocardiographic changes occur early. In a series of 6 patients with sotalol overdose, all had prolonged QT interval noted on the initial electrocardiogram taken 30 minutes to 4.5 hours after ingestion. The greatest QT prolongation occurred 4–15 hours after ingestion, and the risk of ventricular dysrhythmias was highest between 4 and 20 hours. All 4 patients who developed ventricular tachycardia did so after 4 hours, and in 2 patients, ventricular dysrhythmias first occurred 9 hours after ingestion. One patient continued to have ventricular dysrhythmias at 48 hours, and abnormally prolonged QT intervals were noted as long as 100 hours after ingestion. In this series, average sotalol half-life was 13 hours and the average time until normalization of the QT interval was 82 hours.[97]

Acebutolol also prolongs the QT interval, presumably secondary to blockade of outward potassium channels.[87] This effect may partially explain the ventricular tachydysrhythmias that occur with severe acebutolol toxicity.[25,84,87]

Vasodilation

Labetalol and carvedilol are nonselective β-adrenergic antagonists that also possess α-adrenergic antagonist activity, making them vasodilators. Overdose with these agents is seldom reported, but appears to cause similar effects as other β-adrenergic antagonists, with hypotension and bradycardia prominent. $α_1$-Adrenergic antagonism would theoretically act in synergy with β-adrenergic antagonism to increase toxicity. Conversely, the low membrane-stabilizing effect of these agents may make them relatively safe in overdose. Renal failure has complicated labetalol overdose.[64,127] Experience with carvedilol overdose is extremely limited. One patient developed hypotension responsive to dopamine without significant bradycardia and had a benign course.[40] Nebivolol is a selective $β_1$-adrenergic antagonist, which does not act at the α receptor but causes vasodilation by release of nitric oxide.[89] In a single case report from Germany, nebivolol overdose was complicated by bradycardia, lethargy, and hypoglycemia. The patient received standard treatment and had a benign outcome.[43]

Other Preparations

There has been very little experience with overdoses of the sustained-release β-adrenergic antagonists, but it is reasonable to expect that overdose with these agents will result in both delayed onset and prolonged duration of toxicity. Therapeutic use of ophthalmic solutions containing β-adrenergic antagonists may cause adverse effects such as bradycardia, heart failure, bronchospasm, and depression,[17,147] but acute overdose of these agents has not been reported. Combined overdoses with calcium channel blockers and β-adrenergic antagonists are likely to be very difficult to manage because of synergistic toxicity. An extended-release tablet containing a combination of the calcium channel blocker felodipine and metoprolol is being studied as an antihypertensive medication.[41,53] This medication would be expected to be quite dangerous in overdose.

DIFFERENTIAL DIAGNOSIS OF BRADYCARDIA

Bradycardia may result from numerous toxic exposures and medical conditions. The three most common causes of drug-induced bradycardia are calcium channel blockers (Chap. 50), β-adrenergic antagonists, and digoxin (Chap. 48). Other important toxicologic causes of bradycardia include $α_1$-adrenergic agonists, such as phenylpropanolamine (Chap. 38); $α_2$-adrenergic agonists, such as clonidine and other imidazolines (Chap. 51); cholinergic agents, such as carbamates and organic phosphorus compounds (Chap. 88); sodium channel blockers (Chap. 52); opioids (Chap. 62); and most sedative hypnotics such as the barbiturates (Chap. 63). Many patients with toxicologic causes of bradycardia present with a recognizable toxidrome. Medical causes of bradycardia include hyperkalemia, hypothermia, myocardial infarction, sick sinus syndrome, vasovagal episodes, intracranial hypertension, hypothyroidism and benign physiologic bradycardia in resting athletes. The differential diagnosis of bradycardia is summarized in Table 49–2 and discussed in detail in Chapter 21.

β-Adrenergic antagonist toxicity typically results in bradycardia and hypotension with depressed mental status, mild hypoglycemia, and slight hyperkalemia (see "Clinical Manifestations").

TABLE 49–2. Drug-Induced Bradycardia

Drug	Clinical Characteristics	Electrocardiogram
β-Adrenergic antagonists	Depressed mental status, hypotension, slight hyperkalemia, hypoglycemia, respiratory depression	Prolonged PR QRS narrow or wide
Calcium channel blockers	Preservation of mental status, hypotension, hyperglycemia	Prolonged PR QRS narrow or wide
Digoxin/cardiac glycosides	Prominent vomiting, hyperkalemia, BP preserved, mental status preserved	Prolonged PR, ST changes, atrial and ventricular dysrhythmias
Sodium channel blockers	Altered mental status, seizures, hypotension	Wide QRS
Cholinergics	Cholinergic toxidrome: SLUDGE	Sinus bradycardia
α-Adrenergic agonists (phenylpropanolamine)	Hypertension, intracranial hemorrhage	Sinus bradycardia
$α_2$-Adrenergic agonists (clonidine)	Opioid toxidrome: miosis, respiratory depression, sedation	Sinus bradycardia
Opioids	Opioid toxidrome: miosis, respiratory depression, sedation	Sinus bradycardia
Sedative hypnotics	Sedation, +/– miosis, +/– respiratory depression	Sinus bradycardia or tachycardia
γ-Hydroxybutyrate	Sedation, vomiting	Sinus bradycardia

Calcium channel blocker toxicity invariably causes hypotension but may result in bradycardia, normal heart rate, or even reactive tachycardia depending on which agent is ingested. Calcium channel blocker overdose is often characterized by preservation of mental status in the setting of marked hypotension. The ECG may show a prolonged PR with normal QRS interval. In contrast to the case with β-adrenergic antagonists, patients with calcium channel blocker overdose may be hyperglycemic.[50,106] The presence of profound hypotension with preserved mental status and hyperglycemia may differentiate a patient with calcium channel blocker toxicity from one with β-adrenergic antagonist toxicity; however, the two conditions are easily confused clinically. Fortunately, the therapy for these two poisonings is similar.

Acute digoxin toxicity is invariably associated with vomiting. Patients may be bradycardic secondary to increased vagal tone, but may also develop ventricular tachydysrhythmias. Typically, blood pressure is preserved despite significant bradycardia. Patients with digoxin toxicity usually maintain a normal mental status. Hyperkalemia is an important marker of acute digoxin toxicity. Digoxin results in typical electrocardiographic findings that reflect impaired AV conduction, repolarization changes ("digoxin effect"), and ventricular irritability. Acute digoxin toxicity is differentiated from β-adrenergic antagonist toxicity by the presence of vomiting, bradycardia with preserved blood pressure, characteristic ECG changes, and prominent hyperkalemia.

Sodium channel blocker toxicity results in hypotension, seizures, and depressed mental status. Most cases of sodium channel blocker toxicity are associated with tachycardia, but bradycardia may occur. The electrocardiogram is characterized by a markedly widened QRS interval that narrows with administration of hypertonic sodium bicarbonate. β-Adrenergic antagonists with membrane-stabilizing effect, such as propranolol, may also prolong the QRS interval.

α-Adrenergic agonists cause marked hypertension and a reactive bradycardia. Patients often complain of headaches, and the clinical course may be complicated by intracranial hemorrhage or cerebral edema. Cholinergic toxicity causes an easily recognized symptom complex characterized by vomiting, diarrhea, salivation, lacrimation, urinary incontinence, fasciculations, muscle paralysis, seizures, coma, and hypoxia. Patients may be bradycardic as a result of muscarinic stimulation, or may be tachycardic secondary to hypoxia and nicotinic stimulation. Opioids, α_2 agonists, and certain sedative hypnotics result in marked sedation, respiratory depression, miosis, and only moderate physiologic bradycardia. Toxicity from these agents is usually easily differentiated from that caused by β-adrenergic antagonists.

γ-Hydroxybutyrate (GHB) is a sedative that has recently gained popularity as a drug of abuse. GHB overdose is characterized by profound depression of consciousness of several hours duration. Vomiting and mild respiratory depression are common, but aspiration seems to be rare and intubation is not always necessary. Mild bradycardia occurs in about one-third of patients. Hypotension occurs in about 10% of cases, usually when GHB is taken with a coingestant such as ethanol. Seizurelike activity is sometimes reported. The combination of severely depressed consciousness with relatively mild bradycardia should make GHB and other sedative hypnotic poisoning easy to differentiate from β-adrenergic antagonist toxicity.[21,76] The medical causes of bradycardia are distinguished from β-adrenergic antagonist toxicity by history, physical examination, the electrocardiogram, and simple laboratory tests (Chap. 21).

DIAGNOSTIC TESTING

All patients suspected of ingesting an overdose of a β-adrenergic antagonist should be attached to a cardiac monitor and have a 12-lead electrocardiogram. Serum glucose should be measured regardless of mental status because β-adrenergic antagonists can cause hypoglycemia. If the patient appears to be in congestive heart failure, a chest radiograph and measurement of oxygen saturation should be obtained. For patients with bradycardia of uncertain etiology, measurement of potassium, renal function, cardiac enzymes, and digoxin levels may prove helpful. Serum levels of β-adrenergic antagonists are not readily available for routine clinical use but may prove helpful in making a diagnosis in selected cases.

MANAGEMENT

The initial management of the critically ill patient who ingests β-adrenergic antagonists is similar to that of other acutely ill patients. Airway and ventilation should be maintained with endotracheal intubation if necessary. Because laryngoscopy may induce a vagal response, it is reasonable to give atropine prior to intubation of the bradycardic patient. The initial treatment of bradycardia and hypotension consists of atropine and fluids. These measures will likely be insufficient in patients with severe toxicity, but may suffice in patients with mild poisoning or other etiologies. It is important to have an organized approach to the care of these patients (Table 49–3 and below under "Specific Management").

Gastrointestinal decontamination is warranted for all persons who have ingested significant amounts of a β-adrenergic antagonist. Induction of emesis with ipecac is contraindicated because of the potential for catastrophic deterioration of mental status and vital signs, and because vomiting increases vagal stimulation and may worsen bradycardia.[128] Orogastric lavage is recommended for patients with significant symptoms, such as seizures, significant hypotension, or bradycardia, if the drug is still expected to be in the stomach, and for all patients who present within 1 hour of ingesting large amounts of propranolol or one of the other more toxic β-adrenergic antagonists (acebutolol, betaxolol, metoprolol, oxprenolol, and sotalol). Orogastric lavage also causes vagal stimulation and carries the risk of worsening bradycardia so it is reasonable to pretreat bradycardic patients with standard doses of atropine and to have atropine available at the bedside for all other persons. We recommend activated charcoal alone for persons with minor symptoms following an overdose with one of the more water-soluble β-adrenergic antagonists such as atenolol, and for those who present later than 1 hour following ingestion. Whole-bowel irrigation with polyethylene glycol should be considered in patients who have ingested sustained-release preparations (Antidotes in Depth: Whole-Bowel Irrigation).

Seizures associated with cardiovascular collapse are treated by attempting to restore circulation. Seizures in the patient with relatively normal vital signs should be treated with benzodiazepines followed by barbiturates if benzodiazepines fail. Refractory seizures are rare in β-adrenergic antagonist overdose. Consideration should be given for the administration of glucose, thiamine, and naloxone in the lethargic or comatose patient. Naloxone may be effective for patients who are comatose following a mixed drug overdose where opioid or clonidine ingestion is suspected, but will not reverse coma in patients with pure β-adrenergic antagonist overdose.

Mechanism of Inotropic Action

Before discussing their clinical use, it is helpful to understand how inotropes act. As discussed earlier, β-adrenergic agonists have a positive inotropic effect mediated by cAMP and protein kinase A. Other inotropes whose effects are mediated by cAMP include glucagon, phosphodiesterase inhibitors, and the experimental agent forskolin. Glucagon receptors, like β-adrenergic receptors, are coupled to G_S proteins and glucagon binding increases adenyl cyclase activity independent of β-adrenergic receptor binding.[155] Humans have cardiac glucagon receptors identical to those found in the pancreas[149] and it is probable that the positive inotropic action of glucagon is a result of increased adenyl cyclase activity causing increased myocyte cAMP levels. The inotropic effect of glucagon is enhanced by its ability to inhibit phosphodiesterase and thereby prevent cAMP breakdown.[91] Forskolin and its derivatives directly activate adenyl cyclase and are often used experimentally for this purpose. Phosphodiesterase inhibitors, such as amrinone (inamrinone), milrinone, and enoximone, inhibit the breakdown of cAMP by phosphodiesterase, thereby increasing cAMP levels.

Cardiac contractility can be increased by increasing calcium influx using calcium channel openers[146] or by inhibiting calcium ex-

TABLE 49–3.   Management of β-Adrenergic Antagonist Poisoning

The following categories of toxicity are to be used as a guide only. Some patients may tolerate bradycardia and hypotension poorly and require more aggressive treatment. Clinical judgement is required see Antidotes in Depth for pediatric doses

Asymptomatic
   1. Activated charcoal.
   2. Consider orogastric lavage within the first hour postingestion.
   3. Consider whole-bowel irrigation with polyethylene glycol electrolyte lavage solution for management of ingested sustained-release preparations

Mild Toxicity
   Mild hypotension (BP <100 systolic) or bradycardia (HR <60) without hypoperfusion
   1. All of the above plus:
   2. Atropine 1 mg for bradycardia
   3. Fluid boluses (20–40 mL/kg of 0.9% NaCl) for hypotension (monitor closely to avoid pulmonary edema)

Moderate Toxicity
   Failure of the above therapy, or
       severe bradycardia (HR <40), or hypotension (BP <80), or
       clinical evidence of hypoperfusion: for example, congestive heart failure or
       decreased consciousness
   1. All of the above plus:
   2. Monitor ventilation and intubate if necessary
   3. Glucagon: 3–5 mg IV over 1–2 minutes (may give up to 10 mg) then 2–5 mg/h (up to 10 mg/h)
   4. More atropine up to 3 mg for bradycardia
   5. Calcium salts for hypotension: 1–3 grams calcium chloride slow IV push (alternatively, 3–9 g calcium gluconate)
   6. High-dose insulin: regular insulin 0.5–1.0 U/kg/h intravenously with dextrose 1 g/kg/h (eg, 10 mL/kg/h of 10% dextrose or 2 mL/kg/h of 50% dextrose); glucose should be monitored every 30 minutes and the infusion tapered or increased as required

Severe Toxicity
   Failure of the above therapy, or
       evidence of severe hypoperfusion such as cardiogenic shock or coma
   1. All of the above plus:
   2. Increase glucagon infusion to 10 mg/h
   3. Intra-arterial and pulmonary artery pressure monitoring and frequent reassessment
   4. Catecholamine infusion: *Very high doses of the following are typically required; invasive hemodynamic monitoring is recommended*
       (a) Isoproterenol (β_1, β_2 agonist—caution for β_2-mediated vasodilation);
           start at 0.1 μg/kg/min; titrate rapidly to effect
       (b) Epinephrine (α, β agonist—caution for "unopposed α" effect);
           start at 0.02 μg/kg/min; titrate rapidly to effect
       (c) Dobutamine (β_1 agonist—theoretically useful but limited experience);
           start at 2.5 μg/kg/min; titrate rapidly to effect;
       (d) Norepinephrine (α, β_1 agonist—caution for "unopposed α" effects);
           start at 0.1 μg/kg/min; titrate rapidly to effect;
   5. Phosphodiesterase inhibitors:
       (a) Milrinone: 50 μg/kg IV bolus over 2 min, then 0.25–1.0 μg/kg/min
       (b) Amrinone (inamrinone): 0.75 mg/kg IV bolus over 2 min (may repeat in 30 min), then 2–20 μg/kg/min
   6. Ventricular pacing: *This often increases heart rate without improving cardiac output*
   7. Intra-aortic balloon pump or extracorporeal circulation

trusion via the sodium-calcium exchange pump. Inhibition of the sodium-calcium exchange pump provides higher calcium concentrations throughout the cardiac cycle and allows greater time for the sarcoplasmic pump to move calcium into the sarcoplasmic reticulum. The sodium-calcium exchange pump is driven by electrochemical gradients, and calcium extrusion requires low intracellular sodium and a negative intracellular charge. Agents that increase intracellular sodium will thus act as positive inotropes by

inhibiting calcium extrusion. This is the basis for the positive inotropic action of experimental sodium channel openers,[95,96,107,137] as well as of digoxin and other cardioactive steroids that increase intracellular sodium by inhibition of the sodium-potassium ATPase. The sodium-calcium exchange pump is inhibited by the high intracellular potential that occurs during myocyte depolarization, so agents that prolong the action potential duration (APD) also inhibit the extrusion of calcium. Increased APD further increases intracellular calcium concentrations by prolonging the time that voltage-sensitive calcium channels are open. This mechanism partially explains the inotropic action of 4-aminopyridine, which prolongs the APD by blocking outward potassium channels.[9,10,48,139] A secondary effect of 4-aminopyridine is to induce an intracellular alkalosis, which also increases contractility, as discussed below.[124]

All of the inotropes discussed so far act by increasing intracellular calcium. Unfortunately, intracellular calcium loading predisposes to ventricular dysrhythmias and all of the preceding agents are dysrhythmogenic.[110,137] A different approach to improving cardiac function is to sensitize the contractile proteins to calcium.[146] Alkalosis augments the sensitivity of the contractile proteins to calcium. Agents such as angiotensin II and endothelin are believed to exert their inotropic effect by increasing intracellular pH. Novel agents that directly sensitize the contractile proteins to calcium also increase contractility, but without increasing intracellular calcium. These agents have a lower risk of inducing ventricular dysrhythmias, but they impede diastolic relaxation by slowing calcium dissociation from troponin[109] (Fig. 49–3).

Specific Management

Patients who fail to respond to atropine and fluids require management with the inotropic agents discussed below. When time permits, it is preferable to introduce new medications sequentially so that the effects of each may be assessed. We recommend glucagon followed by calcium, high-dose insulin, a catecholamine pressor, and, if this fails, a phosphodiesterase inhibitor. In the critically ill patient, there may not be enough time for this approach, and multiple treatments may be started simultaneously. It is often difficult to differentiate clinically between β-adrenergic antagonist and calcium channel blocker toxicity, and it is fortunate that the therapies for these ingestions are similar (Chap. 50).

Glucagon.   With almost 30 years of clinical use for β-adrenergic antagonist overdose,[66] glucagon is recognized as a treatment of choice for severe β-adrenergic antagonist toxicity.[103,140,151] Several animal models show the effectiveness of glucagon in treating β-adrenergic antagonist toxicity,[36,65] and a recent case series suggests that glucagon may also be effective in correcting symptomatic bradycardia and hypotension secondary to therapeutic β-adrenergic antagonist use.[85] Glucagon is a vasodilator and in animal models of propranolol poisoning it is more effective in restoring contractility, cardiac output, and heart rate than in restoring blood pressure.[82] The initial adult dose of glucagon for β-adrenergic antagonist toxicity is 3–5 mg given slowly over 1–2 minutes. The initial pediatric dose is 50 μg/kg. Normal saline (0.9% NaCl) or 5% dextrose is recommended as a diluent for doses of glucagon exceeding 2 mg because the packaged diluent contains 0.2% (2 mg/ mL) phenol. If there is no response to the initial dose, higher doses up to a total of 10 mg may be used. Once a response occurs, a glucagon infusion is started. Most authors recommend using an infusion of 2–5 mg/h, although many authorities recommend glucagon infusions as high as 10 mg/h. We suggest that the glucagon infusion be started at the "response dose" per hour. Thus, for example, if the patient receives 7 mg of glucagon before a response occurs, the glucagon infusion should be started at 7 mg/h. When a full dose of glucagon fails to restore blood pressure and heart rate, and the diagnosis of β-adrenergic antagonist toxicity is probable, we would still recommend starting an infusion of glucagon at 10 mg/h. Side effects of glucagon in this setting in-

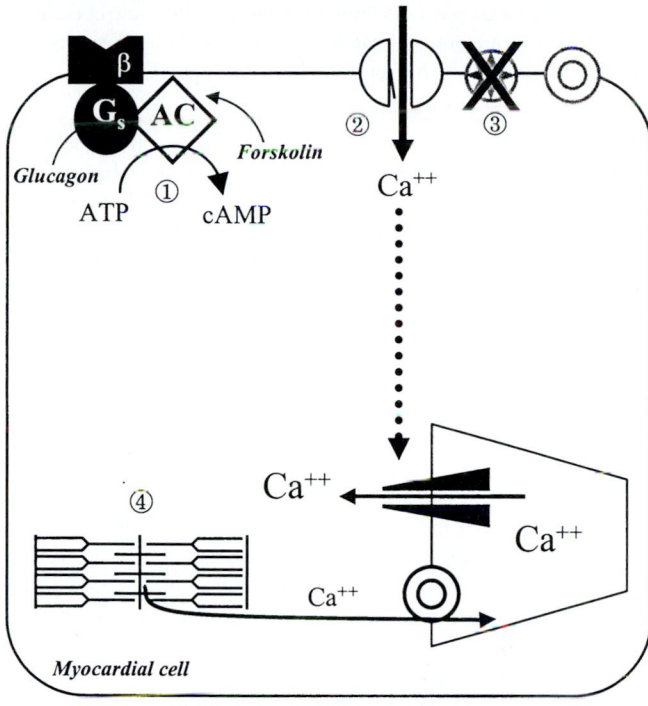

Figure 49–3.   Positive inotropes improve cardiac function by a number of mechanisms that usually result in increased intracellular calcium.
① Agents that increase cAMP: Glucagon receptors and β-adrenergic receptors are coupled to G_s proteins so that receptor binding increases cAMP by activation of adenyl cyclase. Phosphodiesterase inhibitors increase cAMP by inhibiting it's breakdown. Forskolin increases cAMP by directly activating adenyl cyclase.
② Calcium channel openers increase calcium influx during cell depolarization and result in higher intracellular calcium stores.
③ Agents that inhibit extrusion of calcium via the sodium-calcium exchange pump: Digoxin and sodium channel openers that increase intracellular sodium and agents such as 4-aminopyridine that prolong the action potential duration alter the electrochemical gradients that usually favor removal of calcium.
④ Agents that increase the sensitivity of the contractile elements to calcium: Angiotensin II and endothelin do this by inducing an intracellular alkalosis. Experimental drugs that directly increase the sensitivity of troponin to calcium are being investigated.

clude vomiting, hyperglycemia, and mild hypocalcemia,[54] and these should be treated appropriately if they develop (Antidotes in Depth: Glucagon).

Calcium.   Calcium salts effectively treat hypotension from calcium channel blocker overdose and are also effective in restoring blood pressure but not heart rate in animal models of β-adrenergic antagonist toxicity.[71,79] Calcium chloride successfully reverses hypotension in patients with β-adrenergic antagonist overdose[18,100] and in combined calcium channel blocker and β-adrenergic antagonist toxicity.[45] The adult starting dose of calcium chloride is 1 g of the 10% solution given as a slow intravenous push. We recommend using up to 3 g of calcium chloride. The initial pediatric dose of calcium chloride is 20 mg/kg up to 1 g and up to 60 mg/kg may be given. Calcium gluconate is less irritating and may be preferable if venous access is tenuous. Calcium gluconate contains one-third as much elemental calcium as the chloride salt, so doses must be proportionately higher (Antidotes in Depth: Calcium).

Insulin. Recent evidence suggests that high-dose insulin combined with sufficient glucose to maintain euglycemia is beneficial in β-adrenergic antagonist poisoning. In a canine model of propranolol toxicity, all 6 animals treated with insulin and glucose survived as compared to 4 of 6 animals in the glucagon group, 1 of 6 animals in the epinephrine group, and no survivors in the sham treatment group. The authors speculate that insulin may increase survival by increasing myocardial glucose utilization or by altering myocardial calcium handling.[60] High-dose insulin is also effective in animal models of verapamil toxicity.[62] Insulin infusions averaging 0.5 U/kg/h combined with 1 g/kg/h of glucose proved effective in a series of 5 patients with severe calcium channel blocker toxicity. In that series, one patient who ingested atenolol and amlodipine also had a beneficial response to high-dose insulin.[156] High-dose insulin is simple to use, relatively safe (as long as glucose is monitored), and does not require invasive monitoring. For these reasons and despite limited clinical experience for this indication, we recommend using insulin and glucose infusions for β-adrenergic antagonist toxicity unresponsive to fluids, atropine, and glucagon. We recommend an insulin infusion of 0.5 U/kg/h to be continued until the patient's status stabilizes and pressors are discontinued. Glucose should be given at an initial rate of 1 g/kg/h, monitored every 30 minutes for the first 4 hours, and titrated to maintain euglycemia. Unfortunately, the response to insulin is typically delayed for 15–60 minutes so it will probably be necessary to start a catecholamine infusion before the full effects of insulin are apparent. The effects of insulin will last for hours after the infusion stops so abrupt deterioration is unlikely to occur. It is important to continue monitoring glucose for several hours after insulin is discontinued.

Catecholamines. Patients who do not respond to the preceding usually require a catecholamine infusion. The choice of catecholamine is somewhat controversial. Theoretically, the β agonist isoproterenol is the ideal agent. Unfortunately, this therapy has several potential drawbacks that limit its efficacy. In the presence of β-adrenergic antagonism, extraordinarily high doses of isoproterenol and other catecholamines are frequently required.[104,115,140,145] In fact, one author suggests that catecholamine infusion rates up to 10,000 times the usual effective rate may be required.[22] Case reports document isoproterenol infusions of 800 μg/min, dobutamine infusions of 500 μg/min, 6 mg of epinephrine given over 1 hour, and dopamine infusions of 4800 μg/min.[104] At these high doses the β2-adrenergic effects of isoproterenol cause peripheral vasodilation and may cause consequential hypotension.[116] Furthermore, isoproterenol is very dysrhythmogenic and is thus potentially harmful in calcium channel blocker overdose and other causes of hypotension and bradycardia. Nevertheless, in some animal models, isoproterenol is the most effective catecholamine and is even more effective than glucagon in reversing β-adrenergic antagonist toxicity.[136,150] Clinical experience, however, has not shown this to be the case. In a review of reported cases, glucagon increased heart rate 67% of the time and blood pressure 50% of the time. In contrast, isoproterenol was effective in increasing heart rate only 11% of the time and blood pressure only 22% of the time; epinephrine was more effective than isoproterenol.[151]

The selective β1 agonist prenalterol may avoid some of the problems associated with isoproterenol and has been used successfully to treat β-adrenergic antagonist overdose.[29,68] This agent is expected to be especially effective following overdose of the cardioselective β-adrenergic antagonists.[29] Prenalterol is not readily available for clinical use in North America and has limited therapeutic potential as its relatively long half life (≈2 hours) makes titration difficult.[118] Dobutamine is a β-adrenergic agonist with relatively little effect on vascular resistance that may be useful in this setting. However, experience is limited and dobutamine is not always effective in patients with β-adrenergic antagonist overdose, perhaps because of inadequate dosing.[104,125] In the setting of β-adrenergic antagonism, catecholamines with substantial α-adrenergic agonist properties may increase peripheral vascular resistance without improving contractility, resulting in acute cardiac failure. Severe hypertension because of lack of β2-adrenergic-mediated vasodilation is another potential adverse reaction from this so called "unopposed α" adrenergic effect.[33] Because of these potential problems, we recommend that the use of catecholamines be guided by invasive or echocardiographic monitoring of cardiac performance whenever possible. Catecholamine infusions should be started at the usual rates and then increased rapidly until a clinical effect is obtained. If advanced monitoring is impossible and the diagnosis of β-adrenergic antagonist overdose is fairly certain, it is reasonable to begin an isoproterenol or epinephrine infusion with careful monitoring of the patient's blood pressure and clinical status. The infusion should be stopped immediately if the patient either becomes more hypotensive or develops congestive heart failure.

Phosphodiesterase Inhibitors. The phosphodiesterase inhibitors (PDIs) amrinone (inamrinone), milrinone, and enoximone are theoretically beneficial in β-adrenergic antagonist overdose because they increase cAMP independent of β-receptor stimulation. PDIs are able to increase inotropy in the presence of β-adrenergic antagonism both in animal models[74] and in humans.[144] Although these agents appear to be as effective as glucagon in animal models of β-adrenergic antagonist toxicity,[82,123] controlled dog models are unable to demonstrate an additional benefit of these agents over glucagon.[83,122] PDIs have been used clinically to treat β-adrenergic antagonist poisoning in selected patients who fail glucagon therapy.[49,63] Therapy with PDIs is often limited by hypotension secondary to peripheral vasodilation. Furthermore, these agents are difficult to titrate because of relatively long half-lives (30–60 minutes for milrinone, 2–4 hours for amrinone (inamrinone), and approximately 2 hours for enoximone).[56,94] For these reasons, the PDIs should generally be considered only for patients who have arterial and pulmonary artery pressure monitoring.

Ventricular Pacing. Ventricular pacing is not a particularly useful intervention in patients with β-adrenergic antagonist toxicity, but it will increase the heart rate in some patients.[57] Unfortunately, there will frequently be failure to capture, or pacing may increase the heart rate with no increase in cardiac output or blood pressure.[3,68,70,140] In fact, some authors noticed that ventricular pacing occasionally decreases blood pressure, perhaps secondary to loss of atrial contraction or impaired ventricular relaxation.[140]

Extracorporeal Removal. Extracorporeal removal is ineffective for the lipid-soluble β-adrenergic antagonists because of their large volumes of distribution. Hemodialysis may remove water-soluble β-adrenergic antagonists such as atenolol[121] and acebutolol.[119] Hemodialysis is technically difficult in these patients because of hypotension and bradycardia. Thus, hemodialysis is rarely indicated in patients with β-adrenergic antagonist overdose, but may be considered in selected cases.

Mechanical Life Support.   It is important to remember that the patient with severe hypotension from an acute overdose typically recovers without sequelae if ventilation and circulation can be maintained until the toxin is eliminated. When the preceding medical treatment fails in patients with severe β-adrenergic antagonist overdose, it is appropriate to consider the use of an intra-aortic balloon pump or extracorporeal circulation. Several case reports describe remarkable recoveries following the use of these therapies for refractory β-adrenergic antagonist toxicity[70,90] or combined β-adrenergic antagonist and calcium channel blocker overdose.[30]

Special Circumstances

The preceding discussion applies to the generic management of β-adrenergic antagonists. Certain β-adrenergic antagonists have unique properties that modify their toxicity. The management considerations for these unique agents are discussed below.

Sotalol.   Sotalol toxicity may result in a prolonged QT interval and ventricular dysrhythmias, including torsades de pointes, in addition to bradycardia and hypotension. Sotalol-induced bradycardia and hypotension should be managed as are other β-adrenergic antagonists. Specific management of patients with sotalol overdose includes correction of hypokalemia and hypomagnesemia. Overdrive pacing and magnesium infusions may be effective for sotalol-induced ventricular dysrhythmias.[7,142] Lidocaine is also effective for sotalol-induced torsades de pointes.[8] In the future, potassium channel openers such as the cardioprotective drug nicorandil may prove effective for sotalol-induced torsades de pointes.[141,148]

Peripheral Vasodilating Effect.   Treatment of patients who have overdosed with labetalol, carvedilol, or nebivolol is similar to the treatment for patients who ingest other β-adrenergic antagonists. If vasodilation from α_1 antagonism is a prominent feature, then high doses of pressors with α-adrenergic agonist properties may be required.[47] Conversely, if β-adrenergic antagonism is prominent, then agents that act to increase intracellular cAMP may be needed.[63]

Membrane-Stabilizing Effects.   Acebutolol, propranolol, and the other β-adrenergic antagonists with membrane-stabilizing activity are particularly toxic and responsible for a disproportionate number of deaths. It might be expected that hypertonic sodium bicarbonate would be beneficial in treating the ventricular dysrhythmias seen with these agents. Unfortunately, there is limited experience with the use of bicarbonate in this situation and the experimental data are mixed. Bicarbonate was not beneficial in a canine model of propranolol toxicity, although there was a trend toward QRS interval narrowing in the bicarbonate group.[81] In models with propranolol-poisoned isolated rat hearts, however, hypertonic sodium proved beneficial.[58,59] Perhaps most compelling is that bicarbonate appeared to reverse ventricular tachycardia in a human case of acebutolol poisoning.[25] Because

bicarbonate is a relatively safe and simple intervention, we recommend that it be used in addition to standard therapy for β-adrenergic antagonist–poisoned patients with QRS widening, ventricular dysrhythmias, or severe hypotension. The usual dose of hypertonic bicarbonate is 1–2 mEq/kg given as an intravenous bolus. This may be followed by an infusion or repeated boluses may be given as needed. Care should be taken to avoid severe alkalosis or hypokalemia (Antidotes in Depth: Bicarbonate).

Observation.   All patients who have bradycardia, hypotension, abnormal ECGs, or CNS toxicity following a β-adrenergic antagonist overdose should be observed in an intensive care setting until these findings resolve. Toxicity from regular-release β-adrenergic antagonist poisoning almost always occurs within the first 6 hours.[80,86,112] Therefore, patients without any findings of toxicity following an overdose of a regular-release β-adrenergic antagonist may be discharged from medical care after an observation time of 6–8 hours if they remain asymptomatic with normal vital signs and normal electrocardiograms. Ingestion of extended-release preparations may cause delayed toxicity, and such patients should be observed for 24 hours in an intensive care unit. Patients who may have delayed absorption because of a mixed overdose, or because of underlying gastrointestinal disease, may also require longer observation. Sotalol toxicity may also be delayed with ventricular dysrhythmias first occurring as late as 9 hours after ingestion.[97] We recommend that all patients with sotalol overdoses be monitored for at least 12 hours. Patients who remain stable without QT prolongation may then be discharged from a monitored setting.

Experimental Treatment

In the future, novel medications may prove beneficial in β-adrenergic antagonist overdose. Forskolin is a drug derived from the root of *Coleus forskalii,* which is used as a tonic in traditional East Indian medicine. Forskolin is known to directly activate adenyl cyclase independently of the β receptor, and is often used experimentally for this purpose. There is limited experience with the use of forskolin in Western medicine, but it is being investigated for the treatment of psychiatric disorders and asthma,[11,15] and it does improve the performance of human myocardium.[19,20,102,143] By directly increasing cAMP production, forskolin may prove beneficial in the management of β-adrenergic antagonist poisoning. The potassium channel blocker 4-aminopyridine increases intracellular calcium stores and may counteract some of the adverse effects of β-adrenergic antagonist toxicity. Currently, 4-aminopyridine is used in patients with multiple sclerosis. Overdose with 4-aminopyridine is complicated by neurologic symptoms ranging from paresthesias to seizures.[101,134] Calcium channel openers, sodium channel openers, and calcium sensitizers may also prove useful for β-adrenergic antagonist toxicity, but their role is strictly experimental at this time.

SUMMARY

β-Adrenergic antagonists are commonly used to treat hypertension, angina, tachydysrhythmias, tremor, migraines, and panic attack. Overdoses of β-adrenergic antagonists are relatively uncommon but continue to cause deaths in the United States and around the world. Patients who develop symptoms after ingesting regular-release β-adrenergic antagonists do so within the first 6 hours. Sotalol ingestions are an exception to this and may cause delayed and prolonged toxicity. Extended-release formulations may also result in delayed toxicity and require 24 hours observation. Patients with β-adrenergic antagonist overdose, when symptomatic, typically develop bradycardia and hypotension. Propranolol and other β-adrenergic antagonists with membrane-stabilizing properties and high lipid solubility are the most toxic in overdose. These drugs cause prolongation of the QRS interval, severe hypotension, coma, seizures, and apnea. Hypoglycemia is rare in adults following β-adrenergic antagonist ingestions, but it may complicate overdose in children. Bronchospasm may occur in acute β-adrenergic antagonist toxicity in susceptible persons. Sotalol is unique in its ability to prolong the QT interval and sotalol toxicity often results in refractory ventricular dysrhythmias, which may respond to overdrive pacing or to magnesium infusions. In addition to supportive care, the most important therapy for β-adrenergic antagonist toxicity is glucagon. High doses of insulin together with glucose provide a promising new treatment modality. Catecholamine infusions may also be helpful but should be closely monitored; large doses are typically required. Patients who fail treatment with glucagon, insulin, and catecholamines are critically ill and may respond to phosphodiesterase inhibitors or to mechanical support of circulation. Fortunately, most patients respond to simpler measures and this aggressive therapy is rarely required.

REFERENCES

1. Abraham W. β-Blockers: The new standard of therapy for mild congestive heart failure. Arch Intern Med 2000;160:1237–1247.
2. Adelstein RS, Eisenberg E: Regulation and kinetics of the actin-myosin-ATP interaction. Ann Rev Biochem 1980;49:921–956.
3. Agura ED, Wexler LF: Massive propranolol overdose. Am J Med 1986;80:755–757.
4. Alderfliegel F, Leeman M, Demaeyer P, Kahn RJ: Sotalol poisoning associated with asystole. Intensive Care Med 1993;19:57–58.
5. Alquist RP: A study of the adrenotropic receptors. Am J Physiol 1948;153:586–600.
6. Annane D: Beta-adrenergic mediation of the central control of respiration: Myth or reality. J Toxicol Clin Exp 1991;11:325–336.
7. Arstall MA, Hii JT, Lehman RG, Horowitz JD: Sotalol-induced torsade de pointes: Management with magnesium infusion. Postgrad Med J 1992;68:289–290.
8. Assimes T, Malcolm I: Torsades de pointes with sotalol overdose successfully treated with lidocaine. Can J Cardiol 1998;14:753–756.
9. Barry WH, Bridge JHB: Intracellular calcium homeostasis in cardiac myocytes. Circulation 1993;87:1806–1815.
10. Basavappa S, Romano-Silva MA, Mangel AW, et al: Inhibition of K⁺ channel activity by 4-AP stimulates N-type Ca⁺ channels in CHP-100 cells. Neuroreport 1994;5:1256–1258.
11. Bauer K, Dietersdorfer F, Sertl K, Kaik B, Kaik G: Pharmacodynamic effects of inhaled dry powder formulations of fenoterol and colforsin in asthma. Clin Pharmacol Ther 1993;53:76–83.
12. Beattie JM: Sotalol-induced torsade de pointes. Scott Med J 1984;29:240–244.
13. Ber DM: Calcium fluxes involved in the control of cardiac myocyte contraction. Circ Res 2000;87:275–281.
14. Berthault F, Kintz P, Tracqui A, Mangin P: A fatal case of betaxolol poisoning. J Anal Toxicol 1997;21:228–231.
15. Berudsky Y, Kotler M, Shifrin M, Belmaker RH: A preliminary study of possible psychoactive effects of intravenous forskolin on depressed and schizophrenic patients. J Neural Transm 1996;103:1463–1467.
16. Black JW, Duncan WA, Shanks RG: Comparison of some properties of pronethalol and propranolol. Br J Pharmacol 1997;120(Suppl 4):285–299.
17. Bourgeois JA: Depression and topical ophthalmic beta-adrenergic blockade. J Am Optom Assoc 1991;62:403–406.
18. Brimacombe JR, Scully M, Swainston R: Propranolol overdose—A dramatic response to calcium chloride. Med J Aust 1991;155:267–268.
19. Bristow MR, Ginsburg R, Strosberg A, Montgomery W, Minobe W: Pharmacology and inotropic potential of forskolin in the human heart. J Clin Invest 1984;74:212–213.
20. Buschmans E, Hearse DJ, Manning AS: Forskolin: Effects on cyclic AMP and contractile function in the isolated rat and guinea pig heart. Can J Cardiol 1985;1:385–394.
21. Chin RL, Sporer KA, Cullison B, Dyer JE, Wu TD: Clinical course of γ-hydroxybutyrate overdose. Ann Emerg Med 1998;31:716–722.
22. Critchley JA, Ungar A: The management of acute poisoning due to beta adrenoreceptor antagonists. Med Toxicol 1989;4:32–45.
23. Dancey D, Wulffhart Z, McEwen P: Sotalol-induced torsades de pointes in patients with renal failure. Can J Cardiol 1997;13:55–58.
24. Davis BA, Edes I, Gupta RC, et al: The role of phospholamban in the regulation of calcium transport by cardiac sarcoplasmic reticulum. Mol Cell Pharmacol 1990;99:83–88.
25. Donovan KD, Gerace RV, Dreyer JF: Acebutolol-induced ventricular tachycardia reversed with sodium bicarbonate. J Toxicol Clin Toxicol 1999;37:481–484.
26. Elkharrat D, Bismuth C, Davy JM: Le blocage des beta-recepteurs: Phenomene auto-limite exploquant la benignite des intoxictiona aigues par les beta-bloquantes. Mortalite nulle a la clinique toxicologique de Fernand-Widal sur quarante cas. Sem Hop 1982;58:1073–1076.
27. Enocksson S, Shimizu M, Lonnqvist F, et al: Demonstration of an in vivo functional beta 3-adrenoceptor in man. J Clin Invest 1995;95:2239–2245.
28. Fitzgerald JD: Do partial agonist beta-blockers have improved clinical utility? Cardiovasc Drugs Ther 1993;7:303–310.
29. Freestone S, Thomas HM, Bharma RK, et al: Severe atenolol poisoning: Treatment with prenalterol. Hum Toxicol 1986;5:343–345.
30. Frierson J, Bailly D, Shultz T, et al: Refractory cardiogenic shock and complete heart block after unsuspected verapamil-SR and atenolol overdose. Clin Cardiol 1991;14:933–935.
31. Frishman W, Jacob H, Eisenberg E, et al: Clinical pharmacology of the new beta-adrenergic blocking drugs. Part 8: Self-poisoning with beta-adrenoreceptor blocking agents: Recognition and management. Am Heart J 1979;98:798–811.
32. Frithz G. Toxic effects of propranolol on the heart. Br Med J 1976;1:769–770.
33. Gandy W: Severe epinephrine-propranolol interaction. Ann Emerg Med 1989;18:98–99.
34. Gautier C, Lablais V, Kobzic L, et al: The negative inotropic effect of β3-adrenoreceptor stimulation is mediated by activation of a nitric oxide synthase pathway in human ventricle. J Clin Invest 1998;102:1377–1384.
35. Gautier C, Tavernier G, Charpentier F, Langin D, LeMarec H: Functional β3-adrenoreceptor in the human heart. J Clin Invest 1996;98:556–562.
36. Glick G, Parmley W, Weschler A, et al: Glucagon: Its enhancement of cardiac performance in the cat and dog and persistence of its inotropic action despite beta receptor blockade with propranolol. Circ Res 1968;22:789–799.
37. Gold EH, Chang W, Cohen M, et al: Synthesis and comparison of some cardiovascular properties of the stereoisomers of labetalol. J Med Chem 1982;25:1363–1370.
38. Gopalaswamy UV, Satav JG, Katyare SS, Bhattacharya RK: Effect of propranolol on rat brain synaptosomal Na⁺-K⁺-ATPase and Ca2⁺-ATPase. Chem Biol Interact 1997;103:51–58.

39. Gyorke I, Gyorke S: Regulation of cardiac ryanodine receptor channel by luminal Ca^{2+} involves luminal calcium sensing sites. Biophys J 1998;75:2801–2810.

40. Hanston P, Lambermont JY, Simoens G, Mathieu P: Carvedilol overdose. Acta Cardiol 1997;52:369–371.

41. Haria M, Plosker GL, Markham A: Felodipine/metoprolol: A review of the fixed-dose controlled-release formulation in the management of essential hypertension. Drugs 2000;59:141–157.

42. Hartzell HC, Hirayama Y, Petit-Jacques J: Effects of protein phosphatase and kinase inhibitors on the cardiac L-type calcium current suggests two sites are phosphorylated by protein kinase A and another protein kinase. J Gen Physiol 1995;106:393–414.

43. Heinroth KM, Walper R, Busch I, Winkler M, Prondzinsky R: Acute beta$_1$-selective blocker nebivolol poisoning in attempted suicide. Dtsch Med Wochenschr 1999;124:1230–1234.

44. Henry JA, Cassidy SL: Membrane stabilizing activity: A major cause of fatal poisoning. Lancet 1986;8495:1414–1417.

45. Henry M, Kay MM, Viccellio P: Cardiogenic shock associated with calcium channel blockers and beta blockers: Reversal with calcium chloride. Am J Emerg Med 1985;3:334–336.

46. Hesse B, Pederson JT: Hypoglycemia after propranolol in children. Acta Med Scand 1973;193:551–552.

47. Hicks PR, Rankin AP: Massive adrenaline doses in labetalol poisoning. Anaesth Intensive Care 1991;19:447–449.

48. Hilgemann DW: Extracellular calcium transients and action potential configuration changes related to post-stimulatory potentiation in rabbit atrium. J Gen Physiol 1986;87:675–706.

49. Hoeper MM, Boeker KH: Overdose of metoprolol treated with enoximone. N Engl J Med 1996;335:1538.

50. Hofer CA, Smith JK, Tenholder MF: Verapamil intoxication: A literature review of overdoses and discussion of therapeutic options. Am J Med 1993;95:431–438.

51. Hoffman BB, Lefkowitz RJ: Catecholamines, sympathomimetic drugs, and adrenergic receptor antagonists. In: Hardman JG, Limbird LE, Molinoff PB, et al eds: Goodman & Gilman's The Pharmacological Basis of Therapeutics, 9th ed. New York, McGraw-Hill, 1996, pp. 199–248.

52. Hohnloser SH, Woosley RL: Sotalol. N Engl J Med 1994; 331: 31–38.

53. Hosie J, Dahlof B, Klein G: The long-term antihypertensive efficacy and safety of a new felodipine-metoprolol combination tablet. Blood Press 1993;(Suppl 1):46–50.

54. Illingworth R: Glucagon for beta-blocker poisoning. Lancet 1980; 8185:86.

55. Javeed N, Javeed H, Javeed S, Moussa G, Wong P, Rezai F: Refractory anaphylactic shock potentiated by beta-blockers. Catheter Cardiovasc Diagn 1996;39:383–384.

56. Kelly RA, Smith TW: Pharmacologic treatment of heart failure. In: Hardman JG, Limbird LE, Molinoff PB, et al eds: Goodman & Gilman's The Pharmacological Basis of Therapeutics, 9th ed. New York, McGraw-Hill, 1996, pp. 809–838.

57. Kenyon CJ, Aldonger GE, Joshipura P, Zaid GJ: Successful resuscitation using external cardiac pacing in beta-adrenergic antagonist-induced bradyasystolic arrest. Ann Emerg Med 1988;17:711–713.

58. Kerns W, Ransom M, Tomaszewski C, Kline J, Raymond R: The effects of extracellular ions on β-blocker cardiotoxicity. Toxicol Appl Pharmacol 1996;137:1–7.

59. Kerns W, Ransom M, Tomaszewski C, Raymond R: The effect of hypertonic sodium and dantrolene on propranolol toxicity. Acad Emerg Med 1997;4:545–551.

60. Kerns W, Schroeder D, Williams C, Tomaszewski C, Raymond R: Insulin improves survival in a canine model of acute β-blocker toxicity. Ann Emerg Med 1997;29:748–757.

61. Khan A, Muscat-Baron JM: Fatal oxprenolol poisoning. Br Med J 1977;6060:552.

62. Kline JA, Tomaszewski CA, Schroeder JD, Leonova ED, Raymond RM: Insulin is a superior antidote for cardiovascular toxicity induced by verapamil in anesthetized dogs. J Pharmacol Exp Ther 1993;267: 744–750.

63. Kollef MH: Labetalol overdose successfully treated with amrinone (inamrinone) and alpha receptor agonists. Chest 1994;105:626–627.

64. Korzets A, Danby P, Edmunds ME, et al: Acute renal failure associated with a labetalol overdose. Postgrad Med J 1990;66:66–67.

65. Kosinski E, Malindzak G: Glucagon and isoproterenol in reversing propranolol toxicity. Arch Intern Med 1973;132:840–843.

66. Kosinski EJ, Stein N, Malindzak GS, Boone E: Glucagon and propranolol (Inderal) toxicity. N Engl J Med 1971;285:1325.

67. Krapf R, Gertsch M: Torsade de pointes induced by sotalol despite therapeutic plasma sotalol concentrations. Br Med J 1985;290: 1784–1785.

68. Kulling P, Eleborg L, Persson H: β-Adrenoreceptor blocker intoxication: Epidemiological data. Prenalterol as an alternative in the treatment of cardiac dysfunction. Hum Toxicol 1983;2:175–181.

69. Lambert DM: Effect of propranolol on mortality in patients with angina. Postgrad Med 1976;52(Suppl 4):57–60.

70. Lane AS, Woodward AC, Goldman MR: Massive propranolol overdose poorly responsive to pharmacologic therapy: Use of the intraaortic balloon pump. Ann Emerg Med 1987;16:1381–1383.

71. Langemeijer J, De Wildt D, De Groot G, et al: Calcium interferes with the cardiodepressive effects of beta-blocker overdose in isolated rat hearts. J Toxicol Clin Toxicol 1986;24:111–133.

72. Langemeijer J, De Wildt D, De Groot G, et al: Respiratory arrest as main determinant of toxicity due to overdose with different β-blockers in rats. Acta Pharmacol Toxicol 1985;57:352–356.

73. Langemeijer JJM, De Wildt D, De Groot G, et al: Centrally induced respiratory arrest: Main cause of death in β-adrenoreceptor antagonist intoxication. Hum Toxicol 1986;5:65.

74. Lee KC, Canniff PC, Hamel DW, et al: Cardiovascular and renal effects of milrinone in β-adrenoreceptor blocked and non-blocked anaesthetized dogs. Drugs Exp Clin Res 1991;18:145–158.

75. Levitzki A, Marbach I, Bar-Sinai A: The signal transduction between beta receptors and adenyl cyclase. Life Sci 1993;52: 2093–2100.

76. Li J, Stokes SA, Woeckener A: A tale of novel intoxication: γ-Hydroxybutyrate overdose. Ann Emerg Med 1998;31:723–728.

77. Li L, DeSantiago J, Chu G, Kranias EC, Bers DM: Phosphorylation of phospholamban and troponin I in β-adrenergic-induced acceleration of cardiac relaxation. Am J Physiol Heart Circ Physiol 2000; 278:H769–H779.

78. Lofdahl CG, Svedmyr N: Cardioselectivity of atenolol and metoprolol. A study in asthmatic patients. Eur J Resp Dis 1981;62:396–404.

79. Love JN, Hanfling D, Howell JM: Hemodynamic effects of calcium chloride in a canine model of acute propranolol intoxication. Ann Emerg Med 1996;28:1–6.

80. Love JN, Howell JM, Litovic TL, Klein-Schwartz W: Acute beta-blocker overdose: Factors associated with the development of cardiovascular morbidity. J Toxicol Clin Toxicol 2000;38:275–281.

81. Love JN, Howell JM, Newsome JT, et al: The effect of bicarbonate on propranolol-induced cardiovascular toxicity in a canine model. J Toxicol Clin Toxicol 2000;38:421–428.

82. Love JN, Leasure JA, Mundt DJ, et al: A comparison of amrinone (inamrinone) and glucagon therapy for cardiovascular depression associated with propranolol toxicity in a canine model. J Toxicol Clin Toxicol 1992;30:399–412.

83. Love JN, Leasure JA, Mundt DJ: A comparison of combined amrinone (inamrinone) and glucagon therapy to glucagon alone for cardiovascular depression associated with propranolol toxicity in a canine model. Am J Emerg Med 1993;11:360–363.

84. Love JN, Litovitz TL, Howell JM, Clancy C: Characterization of fatal beta-blocker ingestion: A review of the American Association of Poison Control Centers data from 1985 to 1995. J Toxicol Clin Toxicol 1997;35:353–359.

85. Love JN, Sachdeva DK, Bessman ES, Curits LA, Howell JM: A potential role for glucagon in the treatment of drug-induced symptomatic bradycardia. Chest 1998;114:323–326.

86. Love JN: Beta-blocker toxicity after overdose: When do symptoms develop in adults? J Emerg Med 1994;12:799–802.

87. Love JN: Acebutolol overdose resulting in fatalities. J Emerg Med 1999;18:341–344.

88. Lundborg P: The effect of adrenergic blockade on potassium concentrations in different conditions. Acta Med Scand 1983;672:121–126.

89. Mangrella M, Rossi F, Fici F, Rossi F: Pharmacology of nebivolol. Pharmacol Res 1998;38:419–431.

90. McVey FK, Corke CF: Extracorporeal circulation in the management of massive propranolol overdose. Anaesthesia 1991;46:744–746.

91. Mery PF, Brechler V, Pavoine C, et al: Glucagon stimulates the cardiac Ca^{2+} current by activation of adenyl cyclase and inhibition of phosphodiesterase. Nature 1990;345:158–161.

92. Montagna M, Groppi A: Fatal sotalol poisoning. Arch Toxicol 1980;43:221–226.

93. Montgomery AB, Stager MA, Schoene RB: Marked suppression of respiration while awake following massive ingestion of atenolol. Chest 1985;88:920–921.

94. Morita S, Sawai Y, Heeg JF, Koike Y: Pharmacokinetics of enoximone after various intravenous administrations to healthy volunteers. J Pharm Sci 1995;84:152–157.

95. Muller-Ehmsen J, Brixius K, Schwinger RH: Positive inotropic effects of the novel Na^+ channel modulator BDF 9198 in human nonfailing and failing myocardium. J Clin Pharmacol 1998;31:684–689.

96. Muller-Ehmsen J, Frank K, Brixius K, Schwinger RH: Increase in force of contraction by activation of the Na^+/Ca^{2+} exchanger in human myocardium. Br J Clin Pharmacol 1997;43:399–405.

97. Neuvonen PJ, Elonen E, Vuorenmaa T, et al: Prolonged QT interval and severe tachyarrhythmias, common features of sotalol intoxication. Eur J Clin Pharmacol 1981;20:85–89.

98. Olin BR, Blasing S, Bastean JN, et al: Beta-adrenergic blocking agents. In: Kastrup EK, et al, ed. Drug Facts and Comparisons. St. Louis, Wolters Kluwer, 2000, pp. 467–486.

99. Perrot D, Bui-Xuan B, Lang J, et al: A case of sotalol poisoning with fatal outcome. J Toxicol Clin Toxicol 1988;26:389–396.

100. Pertoldi F, D'Orlando L, Mercante WP: Electromechanical dissociation 48 hours after atenolol overdose: Usefulness of calcium chloride. Ann Emerg Med 1998;31:777–781.

101. Pickett TA, Enns R: Atypical presentation of 4-aminopyridine overdose. Ann Emerg Med 1996;27:382–385.

102. Pieske B, Trost S, Schutt K, et al: Influence of forskolin on the force-frequency behaviour in failing and end stage failing human myocardium. Basic Res Cardiol 1998;93(Suppl 1):66–75.

103. Pollack CV: Utility of glucagon in the emergency department. J Emerg Med 1993;11:195–205.

104. Pritchard BN, Battersby LA, Cruikshank JM: Overdosage with β-adrenergic blocking agents. Adverse Drug React Acute Poisoning Rev 1984;3:91–111.

105. Pritchard BN, Thorpe P: Pindolol in hypertension. Med J Aust 1971;58:1242.

106. Proano L, Chiang WK, Wang RY: Calcium channel blocker overdose. Am J Emerg Med 1995;13:444–450.

107. Raap A, Armah B, Stenzel W, Schloos J, Blechacz W: Investigations of action of the positive inotropic action of BDF 9148: Comparison with DPI 210–106 and the enantiomers. J Cardiovasc Pharmacol 1997;29:164–173.

108. Rasmussen H: The calcium messenger system. N Engl J Med 1986;314:1094–1102.

109. Ravens U, Flub MO, Li Q, et al: Stereoselectivity of actions of the calcium sensitiver [+]−EMD 60263 and its enantiomer [−]−EMD 60264. Arch Pharmacol 1997;355:733–742.

110. Ravens U, Himmell HM: Drugs preventing Na^+ and Ca^{2+} overload. Pharmacol Res 1999;39:167–174.

111. Reiter M: Calcium mobilization and cardiac inotropic mechanisms. Pharmacol Rev 1988;40:189–217.

112. Reith DM, Dawson AH, Epid D, et al: Relative toxicity of beta blockers in overdose. J Toxicol Clin Toxicol 1996;34:273–278.

113. Reuter H, Porzig H: Beta-adrenergic actions on cardiac cell membranes. Adv Myocardiol 1982;3:87–93.

114. Reynolds RD, Gorczynske RJ, Quon CY: Pharmacology and pharmacokinetics of esmolol. J Clin Pharmacol 1986;26:A3–A14.

115. Richards DA, Prichard BN, Boakes AJ, et al: Pharmacologic basis for antihypertensive effects of intravenous labetalol. Br Heart J 1977;39:99–106.

116. Richards DA, Prichard BN: Self-poisoning with β-blockers. Br Med J 1978;6127:1623–1624.

117. Riker CD, Wright RK, Matusiak W, et al: Massive metoprolol ingestion associated with a fatality: A case report. J Forensic Sci 1987;32:1447–1452.

118. Ronn O, Graffner C, Johnsson G, et al: Haemodynamic effects and pharmacokinetics of a new selective $beta_1$-adrenoreceptor agonist, prenalterol, and its interaction with metoprolol in man. Eur J Clin Pharmacol 1979;15:9–13.

119. Rooney M, Massey KL, Jamali F, et al: Acebutolol overdose treated with hemodialysis and extracorporeal membrane oxygenation. J Clin Pharmacol 1996;36:760–763.

120. Ruegg JC: Cardiac contractility: How calcium activates the myofilaments. Naturwissenschaften 1998;85:575–582.

121. Saitz R, Williams BW, Farber HW: Atenolol-induced cardiovascular collapse treated with hemodialysis. Crit Care Med 1991;19:116–119.

122. Sato S, Tsuji MH, Okubo N, et al: Combined use of glucagon and milrinone may not be preferable for severe propranolol poisoning in the canine model. J Toxicol Clin Toxicol 1995;33:337–343.

123. Sato S, Tsuji MH, Okubo N, et al: Milrinone versus glucagon: Comparative hemodynamic effects in canine propranolol poisoning. J Toxicol Clin Toxicol 1994;32:277–289.

124. Shahid M, Rogers IW: The inotropic effect of 4-aminopyridine and pH changes in rabbit papillary muscle. J Pharm Pharmacol 1989;49:601–606.

125. Shore ET, Cepin D, Davidson MJ: Metoprolol overdose. Ann Emerg Med 1981;10:524–527.

126. Singh BN, Nisbet HD, Harris EA, et al: A comparison of the actions of ICI66082 and propranolol on cardiac and peripheral beta receptors. Eur J Pharmacol 1975;34:75–86.

127. Smit AJ, Mulder PO, de Jong PE, et al: Acute renal failure after overdose of labetalol. Br Med J 1986;293:1142–1143.

128. Soni N, Baines D, Pearson IY: Cardiovascular collapse and propranolol overdose. Med J Aust 1983;2:629–630.

129. Sperelakis N, Xiong Z, Haddad G, et al: Regulation of slow calcium channels of myocardial cells and vascular smooth muscle by cyclic nucleotides and phosphorylation. Mol Cell Biochem 1994;140:103–117.

130. Stajic M, Granger RH, Beyer JC: Fatal metoprolol overdose. J Anal Toxicol 1984;8:228–230.

131. Stapleton MP: Sir James Black and propranolol: The role of the basic sciences in the history of cardiovascular pharmacology. Tex Heart Inst J 1997;24:236–242.

132. Steinberg SF: The molecular basis for distinct β-adrenergic receptor subtype actions in cardiomyocytes. Circ Res 1999;85:1101–1111.

133. Stinson J, Walsh M, Feely J: Ventricular asystole and overdose with atenolol. BMJ 1992;305:693.

134. Stork CM, Hoffman RS: Characterization of 4-aminopyridine in overdose. J Toxicol Clin Toxicol 1994;32:583–587.

135. Strosberg AD: Structure, function, and regulation of the three beta-adrenergic receptors. Obes Res 1995;3(Suppl 4):501S–505S.

136. Strubelt O: Evaluation of antidotes against the acute cardiovascular toxicity of propranolol. Toxicology 1984;31:261–270.

137. Stump GL, Wallace AA, Gilberto DB, Gehret JR, Lynch JJ: Arrhythmogenic potential of positive inotropic agents. Basic Res Cardiol 2000;95:186–198.

138. Sulakhe PV, Vo XT: Regulation of phospholamban and troponin-I phosphorylation in the intact rat cardiomyocytes by adrenergic and

cholinergic stimuli: Roles of cyclic nucleotides, calcium, protein kinases and phosphatases and depolarization. Mol Cell Biochem 1995;149/150:103–126.

139. Szigligeti P, Pankucsi C, Banyasz T, et al: Action potential duration and force-frequency relationship in isolated rabbit, guinea pig and rat cardiac muscle. J Compar Physiol 1996;166:150–155.

140. Taboulet P, Cariou A, Berdeaux A, et al: Pathophysiology and management of self-poisoning with β-blockers. J Toxicol Clin Toxicol 1993;31:531–551.

141. Takahashi N, Ito M, Saikawa T, et al: Clinical suppression of bradycardia-dependent premature ventricular contractions by the potassium channel opener nicorandil. Heart 1998;79:64–68.

142. Totterman KJ, Turto H, Pellinen T: Overdrive pacing as treatment of sotalol-induced ventricular tachydysrhythmias (torsades de pointes). Acta Med Scand 1982;668:28–33.

143. Toya Y, Schwencke C, Ishikawa Y: Forskolin derivatives with increased selectivity for cardiac adenyl cyclase. J Mol Cell Cardiol 1998;30:97–108.

144. Travill CM, Pugh S, Noble MIM: The inotropic and hemodynamic effects of intravenous milrinone when reflex adrenergic stimulation is suppressed by beta-adrenergic blockade. Clin Ther 1994;16:783–792.

145. Tynan RF, Fisher M, Ibels LS: Self-poisoning with propranolol. Med J Aust 1981;1:82–83.

146. Varro A, Papp JG: Classification of positive inotropic actions based on electrophysiologic characteristics: Where should calcium sensitizers be placed? J Cardiovasc Pharmacol 1995;26(Suppl 1):S32–S44.

147. Vinti H, Chichmanian RM, Fournier JP, et al: Systemic complications of beta-blocking eyedrops. Apropos of 6 cases. Rev Med Interne 1989;10:41–44.

148. Watanabe O, Okumura T, Takeda H, et al: Nicorandil, a potassium channel opener, abolished torsades de pointes in a patient with complete atrioventricular block. Pacing Clin Electrophysiol 1999;22:686–688.

149. Wei J, Mojsoc S: Tissue-specific expression of the human receptor for glucagon-like peptide-1: Brain, heart and pancreatic forms have the same deduced amino acid sequences. FEBS Lett 1995;358:219–224.

150. Wei J, Spotnitz H, Spotnitz W, et al: Pharmacologic antagonism of propranolol in dogs. J Thorac Cardiovasc Surg 1984;87:732–742.

151. Weinstein RS: Recognition and management of poisoning with beta-adrenergic blocking agents. Ann Emerg Med 1984;13:1123–1131.

152. Wier WG, Balke CW: Ca^{2+} release mechanisms, Ca^{2+} sparks, and local control of excitation-contraction coupling in normal heart muscle. Circ Res 1999;85:770–776.

153. Wildt D, Sangster B, Langemeijer J, De Groot G: Different toxicologic profiles for various beta-blocking agents in cardiac function in isolated rat hearts. J Toxicol Clin Toxicol 1984;22:115–132.

154. Xiao RP, Heping YY, Kuschel M, Lakatta EG: Recent advances in cardiac β2-adrenergic signal transduction. Circ Res 1999;85:1092–1100.

155. Yagami T: Differential coupling of glucagon and beta-adrenergic receptors with the small and large forms of the stimulatory G protein. Mol Pharmacol 1995;48:849–854.

156. Yuan TH, Kerns WP, Tomaszewski CA, Ford MD, Kline JA: Insulin-glucose as adjunctive therapy for severe calcium channel antagonist poisoning. J Toxicol Clin Toxicol 1999;37:463–474.

ANTIDOTES IN DEPTH

Glucagon
Mary Ann Howland

Glucagon is a polypeptide counterregulatory hormone with a molecular weight of 3500 daltons, secreted by the α cells of the pancreas. Its traditional role has been to reverse life-threatening hypoglycemia in diabetic patients, who are unable to ingest glucose. In clinical toxicology, glucagon is used as an adjunct in the management of β-adrenergic antagonist and calcium channel blocker overdoses. Stimulation of glucagon receptors in the liver and adipose tissue increases cyclic adenosine monophosphate (cAMP) synthesis, resulting in glycogenolysis, gluconeogenesis, and ketogenesis.[25] Stimulation of glucagon receptors in the heart also increases cAMP levels and produces an increase in inotropy and chronotropy.[9,23,24,32,37] Other properties of glucagon include relaxation of smooth muscle in the lower esophageal sphincter, stomach, small and large intestines, common bile duct, and ureters.[16,18,23]

ROLE IN HYPOGLYCEMIA

Glucagon was formerly proposed to be part of the initial treatment for all comatose patients.[40] The theoretical rationale for this approach is only partially sound: Hypoglycemic patients may present in coma or with an altered mental status and hypoglycemia can be present concomitantly with a drug overdose. Immediately restoring the patient's blood glucose level may be lifesaving. Glucagon, however, requires time to act and may be ineffective in a patient with depleted glycogen stores. The intravenous administration of 0.5–1.0 g/kg of 50% dextrose in adults rapidly reverses hypoglycemia and does not rely on glycogen stores for its effect. Intravenous dextrose, therefore, is preferred over glucagon as the initial substrate to be given to all patients with an altered mental status presumed to be related to hypoglycemia (Antidotes in Depth: Dextrose). Glucagon retains a role as a temporizing measure, until medical help can be obtained, in settings such as in the home where IV dextrose is not an option.

CARDIOVASCULAR EFFECTS

Mechanism of Action

Investigations into the mechanism of action of glucagon on the heart have been performed on cardiac tissue obtained from patients during surgical procedures and in a variety of in vivo and ex vivo animal studies. The results are species specific and dependent on the presence or absence of congestive heart failure. The inotropic action of glucagon appears to be related to an increase in cardiac cAMP levels.[9,24,32] The positive inotropic[2,13,30,37] and chronotropic[2,13,22,30,37,54] actions of glucagon are very similar to those of the β-adrenergic agonists except that they are not blocked by β-adrenergic antagonists.[56] Glucagon was not dysrhythmogenic in some early studies, but in several canine experiments, glucagon was associated with ventricular tachycardia.[21,26,31,34] The effects of

glucagon are markedly diminished as the severity and chronicity of congestive heart failure increases.

Administration of ^{125}I-labeled glucagon in the cat demonstrated the presence of a specific glucagon receptor and binding was closely correlated with activation of cardiac adenylate cyclase.[25] This experiment demonstrated a large number of glucagon binding sites, with as few as 10% of the binding sites occupied at near maximal stimulation of adenylate cyclase. Glucagon receptors have been identified on the human heart and brain, and resemble those on the pancreas.[51] The binding of glucagon to its receptor results in coupling with two isoforms of the G_s protein, catalyzing the exchange of guanosine triphosphate (GTP) for guanosine diphosphate (GDP) on the α subunit of the G_s protein.[18,41,56] One isoform is coupled to β agonists, while both isoforms are coupled to glucagon.[56] The GTP-G_s units then stimulate adenylate cyclase to convert ATP to cAMP.[24,32] In the rat ventricular myocyte, stimulation of adenylate cyclase enhances cAMP phosphorylation of L-type Ca^{2+} channels.[35] These effects are antagonized by acetylcholine.[35]

Evidence now suggests an additional mechanism of action for glucagon independent of cAMP and dependent on arachidonic acid.[47] Cardiac tissue metabolizes glucagon, liberating miniglucagon, an apparently active smaller terminal fragment.[47,53] Mini-glucagon stimulates phospholipase A_2 in chick ventricular myocytes, releasing arachidonic acid. Arachidonic acid then acts to increase cardiac contractility through an effect on calcium. The effect of arachidonic acid, and therefore of mini-glucagon, is synergistic with the effect of glucagon and cAMP.[46]

COMBINED EFFECTS WITH PHOSPHODIESTERASE INHIBITORS AND CALCIUM

Strategies for enhancing the beneficial effects of glucagon have involved combining it with the phosphodiesterase inhibitor amrinone (inamrinone) and its derivative milrinone. In a canine model, both amrinone (inamrinone) and milrinone alone were comparable to glucagon,[28,45] but the combination of amrinone and glucagon resulted in a decrease in mean arterial pressure whereas a tachycardia occurred when milrinone was used with glucagon.[27,44] The relationship between calcium and the chronotropic effects of glucagon was demonstrated in rats.[5] The maximal chronotropic effects of glucagon are dependent on a normal circulating ionized calcium. Both hypocalcemia and hypercalcemia blunt the maximal chronotropic response.[4,5]

VOLUNTEER STUDIES

The cardiovascular effects of glucagon were extensively studied in 21 patients with heart failure who were given varied doses and durations of infusion.[38] In 11 patients who received 3–5 mg via IV bolus, increases in the force of contraction as measured by maximum dP/dT, heart rate, cardiac index, blood pressure, and stroke work were all demonstrated. There was no change in systemic vascular resistance, left-ventricular end-diastolic pressure (LVEDP), or stroke index. Additionally, glucose increased by 50% and the potassium level fell. Another study in 9 patients demonstrated a 30% increase in coronary blood flow following a 50-μg/kg IV dose.[34] Patients who received 1 mg via IV bolus also had an increase in cardiac index, but systemic vascular resistance fell, probably secondary to splanchnic and hepatic vascular smooth muscle relaxation. Patients who received an infusion of 2–3 mg/min for 10–15 minutes responded similarly to those who received the 3–5-mg IV boluses, but the latter experienced significant dose-limiting nausea and vomiting.

ROLE IN OVERDOSES WITH β-ADRENERGIC ANTAGONISTS

Overdoses with β-adrenergic antagonists are particularly dangerous and are manifested by hypotension, bradycardia, prolonged atrioventricular conduction times, depressed cardiac output, and cardiac failure, in addition to alterations in consciousness, seizures, and, rarely, hypoglycemia.[1,7,10,12,17,52] Management is often complicated and many agents have been used with variable success, including atropine, isoproterenol, epinephrine, norepinephrine, dopamine, dobutamine, or combinations thereof.[11] Animal studies document the ability of glucagon to either reverse cardiac toxicity or to improve survival.[28,45] Glucagon has successfully reversed bradydysrhythmias and hypotension in patients unresponsive to the aforementioned drugs, and should be administered early in the management of patients with severe overdoses.[7,10,22,43,50] By increasing myocardial cAMP levels independent of the β receptor,[24,32] glucagon is able to increase the inotropic[2,13,30,37] and the chronotropic[2,13,22,30,37,54] activity of the heart.

ROLE IN CALCIUM CHANNEL BLOCKER OVERDOSE

Calcium channel blocker overdoses produce a constellation of clinical findings similar to those recognized with β-adrenergic antagonist overdoses, including hypotension, bradycardia, heart block, and myocardial depression. Animal studies[20,42,48,49,58,59] demonstrate the ability of glucagon to reverse the myocardial depression produced by nifedipine, diltiazem, and verapamil. Several human case reports,[8,33,36] including one where amrinone was used in addition to glucagon therapy, also show this benefit.[55]

PHARMACOKINETICS AND PHARMACODYNAMICS

Glucagon has a volume of distribution of 0.25 L/kg. The elimination half-life is 8–18 minutes. The plasma, liver, and kidney extensively metabolize glucagon.

The effects of glucagon on the heart in human volunteers begin within 1–3 minutes, are maximal within 5–7 minutes, and last up to 10–15 minutes after a single IV bolus.[37]

Tachyphylaxis or desensitization may occur with continual dosing. Guinea pig hearts exposed to glucagon for varying lengths of time demonstrated a decrease in the amount of cAMP generated.[57] Calcium or isoproterenol administration was subsequently

unaffected and cAMP rose following glucagon administration. The author suggested uncoupling from the glucagon receptor as a plausible explanation.[57] β-Adrenergic agonists are also known to exhibit desensitization.[53,60] A canine experiment also demonstrated a transient effect of glucagon on contractility and on the resultant hyperglycemia, also suggesting tachyphylaxis.[21]

ADVERSE EFFECTS AND SAFETY ISSUES

Side effects associated with glucagon include a dose-dependent nausea and vomiting,[31] hyperglycemia, hypokalemia, gastric hypotonicity, and rarely allergic manifestations. Although commercial glucagon was previously derived from beef or pork pancreas, today commercial glucagon is prepared by recombinant DNA. No glucagon-specific antibodies were detected following glucagon administration.[14] In patients with insulinoma glucagon may worsen hypoglycemia, after an initial hyperglycemic response, as a result of a feedback mechanism. Glucagon may increase the release of catecholamines in a patient with a pheochromocytoma, resulting in a hypertensive crisis. Phentolamine can be used to manage this hypertensive reaction.[14]

DOSING

An initial IV bolus of 50 μg/kg infused over 1–2 minutes is recommended (3–5 mg in a 70-kg person).[12] Higher doses may be necessary if the initial bolus is ineffective, and up to 10 mg may be utilized in an adult.[19] In many cases, the bolus dose should be followed by a continuous infusion of 2–5 mg/h (up to 10 mg/h), in 5% dextrose in water, which can then be tapered as the patient improves.[1,17,19,39,43,52]

AVAILABILITY

Glucagon is available as a 1-mg (1-unit) lyophilized powder for injection with an accompanying 1 mL of diluent. The diluent contains 12 mg/mL of glycerin, water for injection, and hydrochloric acid if needed for pH adjustment. Older formulations, which should no longer be used, contained 2 mg of phenol/mL as a preservative in the diluent. As a precaution against phenol toxicity, the manufacturer had recommended reconstituting the glucagon with sterile water for injection, rather than the accompanying phenol-containing diluent, when glucagon doses exceeded 2 mg.[3,15]

The availability of an adequate supply of glucagon in the ED (at least 20 1-mg vials) with another 30 mg in the pharmacy should be ensured.[6,29]

SUMMARY

Glucagon produces positive inotropic and chronotropic effects despite β-adrenergic and calcium channel antagonism. Glucagon is beneficial in the treatment of patients with severe overdoses of β-adrenergic antagonists and calcium channel blockers. The effects of glucagon may not persist and other therapies such as insulin and glucose should also be considered (Chaps. 49 and 50). The benign character of an IV bolus of glucagon in the patient with a serious overdose of a β-adrenergic antagonist or calcium channel blocker should lead the clinician to use glucagon early in patient management.

REFERENCES

1. Agura E, Wexler L, Witzburg R: Massive propranolol overdose. Am J Med 1986;80:755–757.
2. Benvenisty A, Spotnitz H, Rose EA, et al: Antagonism of chronic canine beta-adrenergic blockage with dopamine, isoproterenol, dobutamine, and glucagon. Surg Forum 1979;30:187–188.
3. Brancato DJ: Recognizing potential toxicity of phenol. Vet Hum Toxicol 1982;24:29–30.
4. Chernow B, Reed L, Geelhoed G, et al: Glucagon endocrine effects and calcium involvement in cardiovascular actions in dogs. Circ Shock 1986;19:393–407.
5. Chernow B, Zaloga G, Malcolm D, et al: Glucagon's chronotropic action is calcium dependent. J Pharm Exp Ther 1987;241:833–837.
6. Dart RC, Goldfrank LR, Chyka PA: Combined evidence-based literature analysis and consensus guidelines for stocking of emergency antidotes in the United States. Ann Emerg Med 2000;36:126–132.
7. Ehgartner GR, Zelinka MA: Hemodynamic instability following intentional nadolol overdose. Arch Intern Med 1988;148:801–802.
8. Fant JS, James LP, Fiser RT, Kearns GL: The use of glucagon in nifedipine poisoning complicated by clonidine ingestion. Pediatr Emerg Care 1997;13:417–419.
9. Farah A: Glucagon and the circulation. Pharm Rev 1983;35:181–217.
10. Fernandes CMB, Daya MR: Sotalol-induced bradycardia reversed by glucagon. Can Fam Physician 1995;41:659–665.
11. Frishman W: Beta-adrenoceptor antagonists: New drugs and new indications. N Engl J Med 1980;305:500–506.
12. Frishman W, Jacob H, Eisenberg E, Ribner H: Clinical pharmacology of the new beta-adrenergic blocking drugs. Part 8. Self-poisoning with beta-adrenoceptor blocking agents: Recognition and management. Am Heart J 1979;98:798–811.
13. Glick G, Parmley W, Wechsler AS, Sonnenblick EH: Glucagon. Circ Res 1968;22:798–799.
14. Glucagon. Package Insert. Eli Lilly, 1999.
15. Golightly L, Smolinske S, Bennett M, et al: Pharmaceutical excipients. Med Toxicol 1988;3:128–165.
16. Hall-Boyer K, Zaloga G, Chernow B: Glucagon: Hormone or therapeutic agent. Crit Care Med 1984;12:584–589.
17. Heath A: β-Adrenoreceptor blocker toxicity: Clinical features and therapy. Am J Emerg Med 1984;2:518–526.
18. Homcy CJ: The β-adrenergic signaling pathway in the heart. Hosp Pract 1991;26:43–50.
19. Illingworth RN: Glucagon for beta-blocker poisoning. Practitioner 1979;223:683–685.
20. Jolly S, Kipnis J, Lucchesi B: Cardiovascular depression by verapamil: Reversal by glucagon and interactions with propanolol. Pharmacology 1987;35:249–255.
21. Kerns W II, Schroeder D, Williams C, et al: Insulin improves survival in a canine model of acute β-blocker toxicity. Ann Emerg Med 1997;29:748–757.
22. Kosinski EJ, Malidzak GS: Glucagon and isoproterenol in reversing propanolol toxicity. Arch Intern Med 1973;132:840–843.
23. Larner J: Insulin and oral hypoglycemic drugs: Glucagon. In: Gilman AG, Goodman LS, Gilman A, eds: The Pharmacologic Basis of Therapeutics, 6th ed. New York, Macmillan, 1980, pp. 1497–1523.
24. Levey G, Epstein S: Activation of adenyl cyclase by glucagon in cat and human heart. Circ Res 1969;24:151–156.
25. Levey GS, Fletcher MA, Klein I, et al: Characterisation of I-glucagon binding in a solubilized preparation of cat myocardial adenylate cyclase. J Biol Chem 1974;249:2665–2673.
26. Lipski JI, Kaminsky D, Donoso E, Friedberg CK: Electrophysiological effects of glucagon on the normal canine heart. Am J Physiol 1972;222:1107–1112.
27. Love JN, Leasure JA, Mundt DJ: A comparison of combined amrinone and glucagon therapy to glucagon alone for cardiovascular depression associated with propranolol toxicity in a canine model. Am J Emerg Med 1993;11:360–363.
28. Love JN, Leasure JA, Mundt DJ, Janz TG: A comparison of amrinone and glucagon therapy for cardiovascular depression associated with propanolol toxicity in a canine model. J Toxicol Clin Toxicol 1992;30:399–412.
29. Love JN, Tandy TK: β-Adrenoreceptor antagonist toxicity: A survey of glucagon availability [letter]. Ann Emerg Med 1993;22:151–152.
30. Lucchesi B: Cardiac actions of glucagon. Circ Res 1968;22:777–787.
31. Lvoff R, Wilcken D: Glucagon in heart failure and in cardiogenic shock—Experience in 50 patients. Circulation 1972;45:534–542.
32. MacLeod K, Rodgers R, McNeil J: Characterization of glucagon-induced changes in rate, contractility, and cyclic AMP levels in isolated cardiac preparations of the rat and guinea pig. J Pharmacol Exp Ther 1981;217:798–804.
33. Mahr NC, Valdes A, Lamas G: Use of glucagon for acute intravenous diltiazem toxicity. Am J Cardiol 1997;79:1570–1571.
34. Manchester JH, Parmley WW, Matloff JM, et al: Effects of glucagon on myocardial oxygen consumption and coronary blood flow in man and in dog. Circulation 1970;41:579–588.
35. Méry PF, Brechler V, Pavoine C, et al: Glucagon stimulates the cardiac Ca²⁺ current by activation of adenyl cyclase and inhibition of phosphodiesterase [letter]. Nature 1990;345:158–161.
36. Mullen JT, Walter FG, Ekins BR, Khasigian PA: Amelioration of nifedipine poisoning associated with glucagon therapy. Vet Hum Toxicol 1991;33:358.
37. Parmley WW: The role of glucagon in cardiac therapy. N Engl J Med 1971;285:801–802.
38. Parmley W, Glick G, Sonnenblick E: Cardiovascular effects of glucagon in man. N Engl J Med 1968;279:12–17.
39. Peterson C, Leeder S, Sterner S: Glucagon therapy for beta-blocker overdose. Drug Intell Clin Pharm 1984;18:394–398.
40. Rappolt R, Inaba D, Gay G: NAGD regime (Naloxone [Narcan], activated charcoal, glucagon, doxapram [Dopram]) for the coma of drug related overdoses. Clin Toxicol 1980;16:395–396.
41. Rodell M: The role of hormone receptors and GTP-regulatory proteins in membrane transduction. Nature 1980;284:17–22.
42. Sabatier J, Pouyet T, Shelvey G, Cavero I: Antagonistic effects of epinephrine, glucagon and methylatropine but not calcium chloride against atrioventricular conduction of disturbances produced by high doses of diltiazem, in conscious dogs. Fundam Clin Pharmacol 1991;5:93–106.
43. Salzberg M, Gallagher EJ: Propranolol overdose. Ann Emerg Med 1980;9:26–27.
44. Sato S, Tsuhi MH, Okubo N, et al: Combined use of glucagon and milrinone may not be preferable for severe propanolol poisoning in the canine model. J Toxicol Clin Toxicol 1995;33:337–342.
45. Sato S, Tsuhi MH, Okubo N, et al: Milrinone versus glucagon: Comparative effects in canine propranolol poisoning. J Toxicol Clin Toxicol 1994;32:277–289.
46. Sauvadet A, Rohn T, Pecker F, Pavione C: Synergistic actions of glucagons and miniglucagon on Ca²⁺ mobilization in cardiac cells. Cir Res 1996;78:102–109.
47. Sauvadet A, Rohn T, Pecker F, Pavione C: Arachidonic acid drives mini-glucagon action in cardiac cells. J Biol Chem 1997;272:12437–12445.
48. Stone CK, May WA, Carroll R: Treatment of verapamil overdose with glucagon. Ann Emerg Med 1995;25:369–374.
49. Stone CK, Thomas SH, Koury SI, Low RB: Glucagon and phenylephrine combination vs glucagon alone in experimental verapamil overdose. Acad Emerg Med 1996;3:120–125.

50. Ward DE, Jones B: Glucagon and beta-blocker toxicity. Br Med J 1976;2:151.

51. Wei Y, Mojsov S: Tissue-specific expression of the human receptor for glucagon-like peptide-I: Brain, heart and pancreatic forms have the same deduced amino acid sequences. FEBS Lett 1995;358: 219–224.

52. Weinstein R: Recognition and management of poisoning with beta-blocking agents. Ann Emerg Med 1984;13:1123–1131.

53. White CM: A review of potential cardiovascular uses of intravenous glucagon administration. J Clin Pharmacol 1999;39:442–447.

54. Whitehouse F, James T: Chronotropic action of glucagon on the sinus node. Proc Soc Exp Biol Med 1966;122:823–826.

55. Wolf LR, Spadafora MP, Otten EJ: Use of amrinone and glucagon in a case of calcium channel blocker overdose. Ann Emerg Med 1993; 22:1225–1228.

56. Yagami T: Differential coupling of glucagon and β-adrenergic receptors with the small and large forms of the stimulatory G protein. Mol Pharmacol 1995;48:849–854.

57. Yao L, Macleod KM, McNeill JH: Glucagon-induced desensitization: Correlation between cyclic AMP levels and contractile force. Euro J Pharmacol 1982;9:147–150.

58. Zaloga G, Malcolm D, Holaday J, et al: Glucagon reverses the hypotension and bradycardia of verapamil overdose in rats. Crit Care Med 1985;13:273.

59. Zaritsky A, Morowitz M, Chernow B: Glucagon antagonism of calcium blocker-induced myocardial dysfunction. Crit Care Med 1988; 16:246–251.

60. Zeiders JL, Seidler FJ, Iaccarino G, et al: Ontogeny of cardiac beta-adrenoceptor desensitization mechanisms: Agonist treatment enhances receptor/G-protein transduction rather than eliciting uncoupling. J Mol Cell Cardiol 1999;31:413–423.

Francis De Roos

A 47-year-old female with a history of insulin-dependent diabetes, coronary artery disease, and depression presented to the hospital with multiple nonspecific complains including "not feeling well," dyspnea, weakness in the legs, and lightheadedness. Physical examination revealed a morbidly obese female in no distress whose initial vital signs were blood pressure, 120/70 mm Hg; heart rate, 100 beats/min; respiratory rate, 18 breaths/min; temperature, 98.9°F (37.2°C). The lung fields were clear to auscultation and cardiac examination revealed normal S_1 and S_2, and an S_4 gallop, but no murmurs or rubs. Her abdomen was obese with active bowel sounds and no tenderness. Neurologic assessment revealed an alert and oriented female with no gross focal deficits.

Because of the nonspecific complaints in a patient with significant medical conditions, a broad diagnostic evaluation was begun which included a rapid glucose check, a urinalysis, electrolytes, renal function testing, liver enzymes, complete blood count, and an electrocardiogram (ECG). The ECG demonstrated a sinus rhythm at 100 beats/min with normal PR and QRS intervals, left atrial enlargement, and evidence of an old anterior wall myocardial infarction (Fig. 50–1). There was no change from previous ECGs.

Approximately 4 hours into her evaluation and hospital stay, the patient complained about lightheadedness and weakness. Repeat physical examination revealed a slightly lethargic but arousable and cooperative female. Blood pressure was now 70/30 mm Hg and her heart rate was 90 beats/min and regular. A repeat ECG revealed normal sinus rhythm and first-degree heart block with a PR interval of 24 msec (Fig. 50–2). At this time she confided to the physician that the true reason for her visit was that she was suicidal and that she ingested 20 diltiazem (90 mg) tablets in a suicide attempt just prior to coming to the hospital.

Initial therapy included boluses of normal saline, calcium chloride (2 g), glucagon (1 mg), and infusions of dopamine and isopro-

terenol, which resulted in transient improvement in systolic blood pressure from 70 to 98 mm Hg. One hour after her initial hypotensive episode, the patient suffered a cardiac arrest with an idioventricular rhythm of 65 beats/min and no measurable blood pressure (Fig. 50–3). With aggressive therapy, including cardiopulmonary resuscitation (CPR), endotracheal intubation, atropine (3 mg), large infusions of dopamine and isoproterenol, and a glucagon bolus (5 mg), the systolic blood pressure returned to between 40 and 65 mm Hg with a heart rate of 50–60 beats/min. Over the next 3 hours multiple pharmacologic agents, including repeat boluses of calcium chloride and continuous infusions of glucagon (5 mg/h), amrinone (200 mg bolus then 800 mg/h), and phenylephrine, were initiated without improvement in blood pressure. During this period the patient's serum glucose rose from 250 mg/dL to 800 mg/dL and an insulin infusion was begun.

Because there was only limited improvement after multiple pharmacologic agents, a transcutaneous pacer was applied but was unable to capture and a transvenous right ventricular pacemaker was then placed with intermittent capture at 70 beats/min, but the systolic blood pressure remained below 80 mm Hg. An intra-aortic balloon pump was placed and within 15 minutes the blood pressure improved to 100/50 mm Hg. The patient was maintained on the intra-aortic balloon pump (IABP) and transvenous pacemaker, and slowly weaned off the multiple inotropic agents and vasopressors over the next 24 hours. After a complicated 3-week hospitalization the patient was discharged to an inpatient psychiatric facility with complete neurologic recovery.

Calcium channel blockers (CCBs) were first used experimentally in the 1960s and their use has steadily risen to where they are now the most frequently prescribed cardiovascular drugs.[44] Mir-

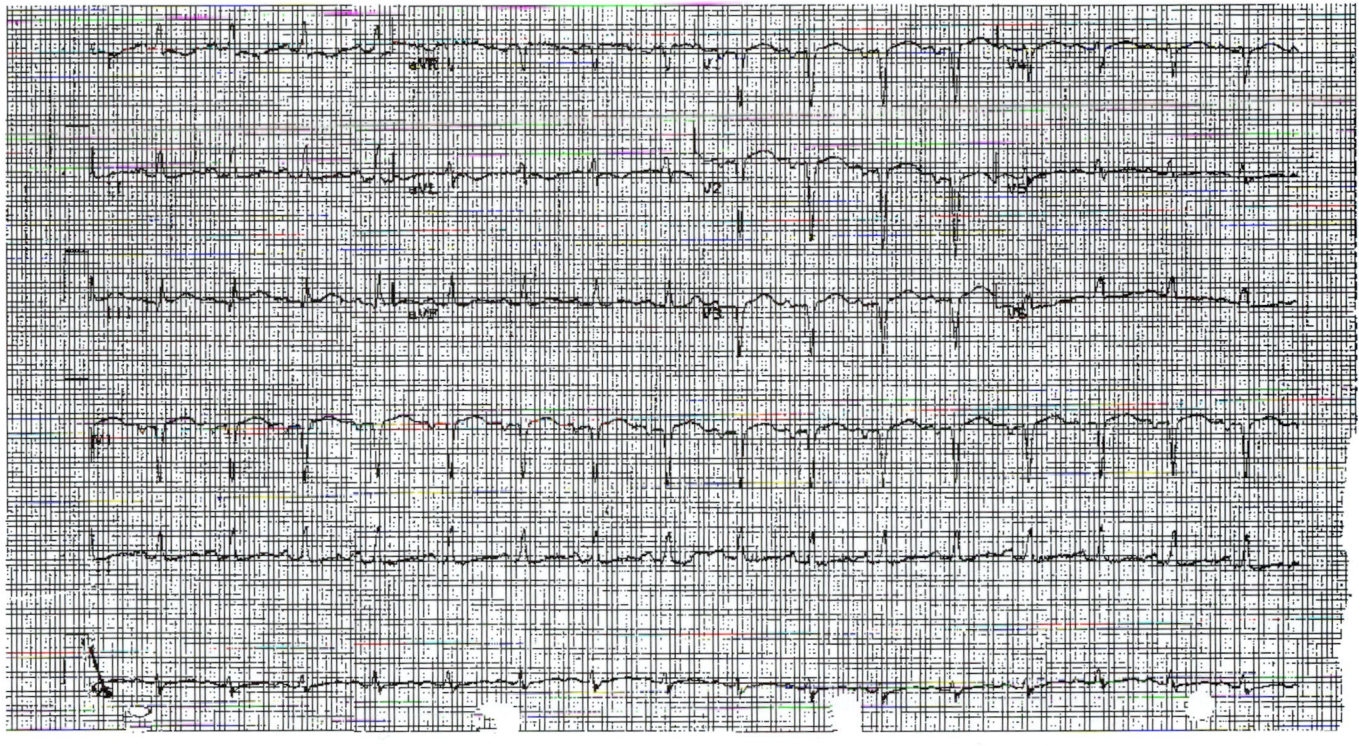

Figure 50–1. This 12-lead electrocardiogram taken 2 hours postingestion of 1800 mg of sustained-release diltiazem demonstrates a sinus tachycardia at 100 beats/min with a normal QRS axis, normal intervals, left atrial enlargement, and an old anterior wall myocardial infarction.

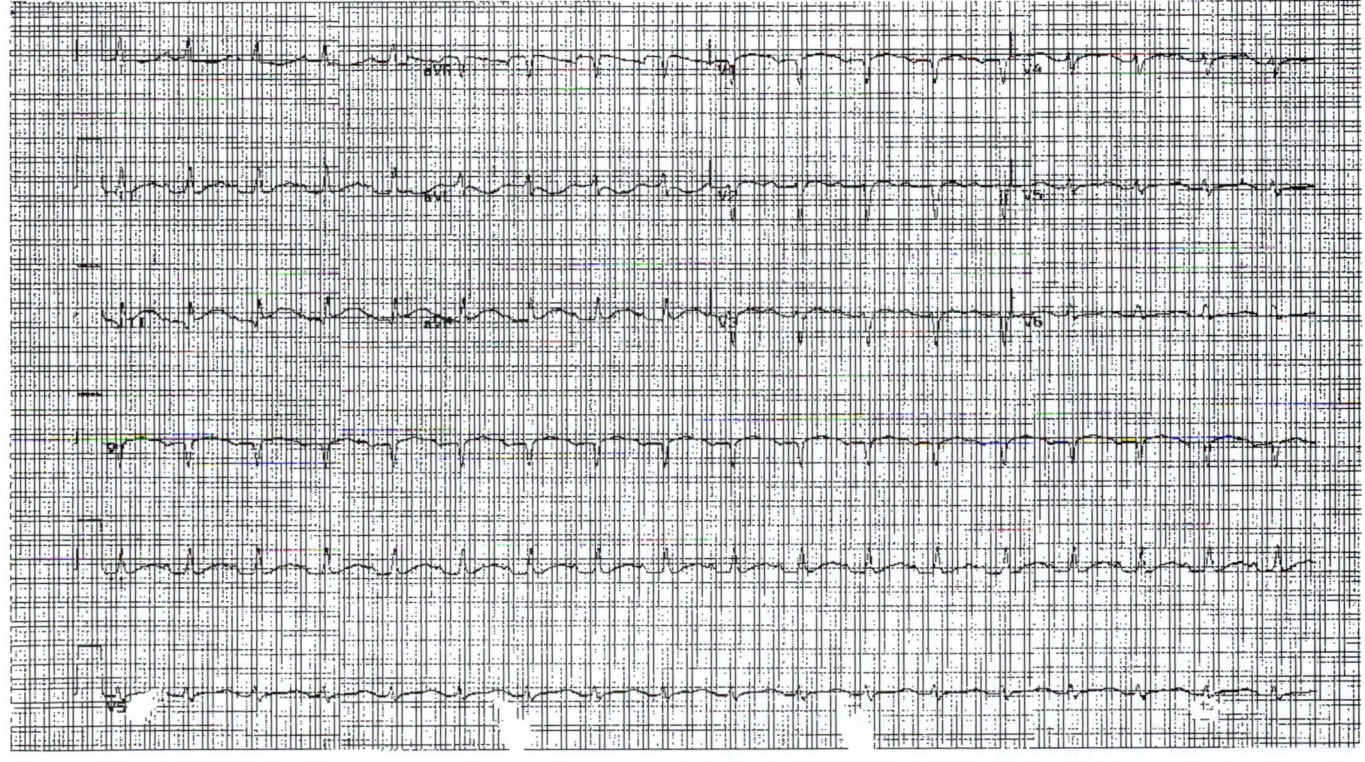

Figure 50–2. This 12-lead electrocardiogram taken 6 hours postingestion of 1800 mg of sustained-release diltiazem demonstrates first-degree heart block with a PR interval of 0.26 msec and no other changes as compared to the patient's previous electrocardiogram (Fig. 50–1).

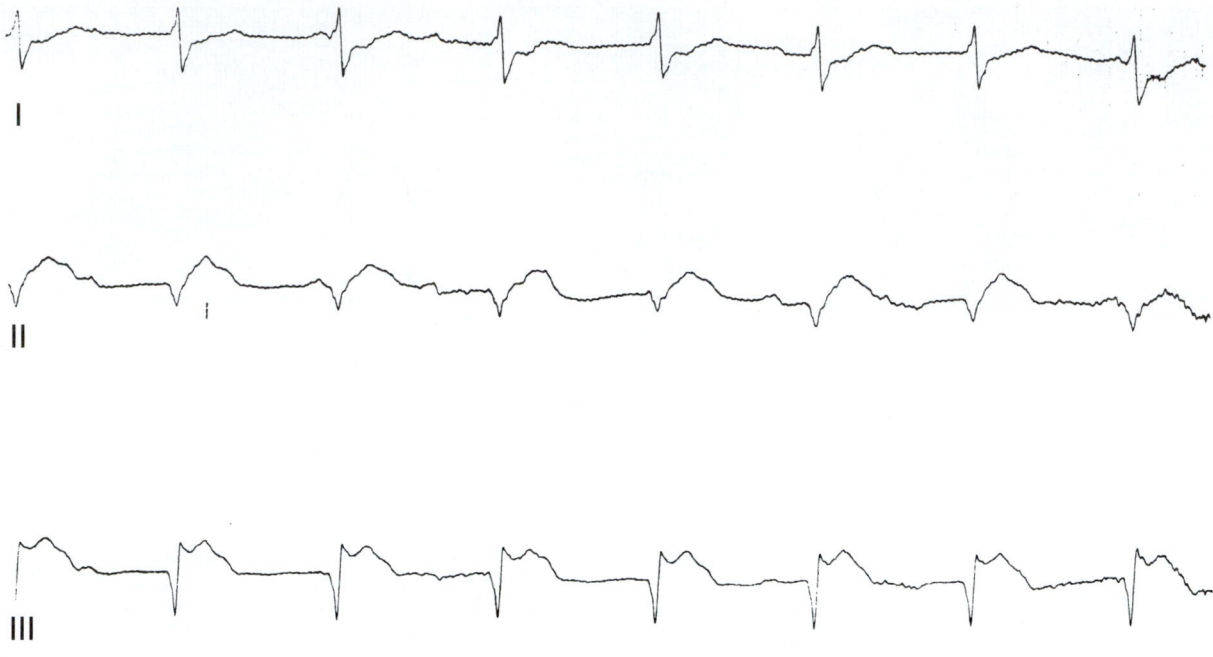

Figure 50–3. This 3-lead rhythm strip was obtained 9 hours postingestion of 1800 mg of sustained-release diltiazem, shortly after the patient became obtunded, hypotensive, and bradycardic. The electrocardiogram demonstrates a junctional bradycardia at 65 beats/min with widened QRS interval of 0.13 msec and possible inferior ischemia.

roring this widespread use, poisonings involving CCBs have also risen. Their combination of compliance-improving sustained-release formulations and potent hemodynamic effects makes poisoning with these agents extremely challenging. The hallmarks of toxicity include hypotension from vasodilation and impaired myocardial contractility, and bradydysrhythmias. In severely poisoned patients, no therapeutic intervention is demonstrated to be consistently effective. Management decisions must be made on an individual patient basis with careful assessment of the physiologic response to each treatment.

EPIDEMIOLOGY

CCBs were first introduced into the US pharmaceutical markets in the late 1970s. Currently there are 9 CCB agents available in either regular and/or sustained-release formulations (Table 50–1). They are used for a wide variety of medical conditions including hypertension, stable angina, dysrhythmias, migraine headaches, Raynaud phenomenon, and subarachnoid hemorrhage.

As the utility of CCBs expands, more and more poisonings occur. In 1986, there were just over 1200 exposures and 7 deaths associated with CCB exposures reported to the American Association of Poison Control Centers (AAPCC). In 1999, those figures increased to more than 8800 exposures, including more than 1100 exposures characterized by moderate to major toxicity, and 61 deaths (see page 1752 and Chap. 116). As a class of drugs, only cyclic antidepressants, opioids, cocaine, and benzodiazepines were associated with more deaths reported to the AAPCC (Chap. 116). This significant rise in fatalities is most likely the result of the increased use of these drugs, although the introduction of sustained-release preparations in 1988 may also play a role.

PHARMACOKINETICS AND TOXICOKINETICS

All CCBs are well absorbed orally and undergo hepatic oxidative metabolism predominantly via the CYP3A subgroup of the cytochrome P450 enzyme system.[42,58,113] Norverapamil, formed by *N*-demethylation, is the only active metabolite and retains 20% of the activity of the parent compound.[75] Diltiazem is predominantly deacetylated into minimally active deacetyldiltiazem, which is then eliminated via the biliary tract.[58] In overdose, these hepatic enzymes become saturated, reducing the potential control of the first-pass effect and increasing the quantity of active drug absorbed systemically. This saturation of drug metabolism contributes to the prolongation of various CCB half-lives that have been reported to be associated with overdose.[17,20,40,41,136] All CCBs are highly protein bound.[83,112] Volumes of distribution are large

TABLE 50–1.   Classification of Calcium Channel Blockers Available in the United States

Class	Specific Compounds
Phenylalkylamine	Verapamil (Calan, Isoptin, Verelan)
Benzothiazepine	Diltiazem (Cardizem, Dilacor, Tiazac)
Dihydropyridines	Nifedipine (Adalat, Procardia)
	Isradipine (DynaCirc)
	Amlodipine (Norvasc)
	Felodipine (Plendil)
	Nimodipine (Nimotop)
	Nisoldipine (Sular)
	Nicardipine (Cardene)
Diarylaminopropylamine ether	Bepridil (Vascor)
T channel blocker	None (mibefradil withdrawn)

for verapamil (5.5 L/kg)[113] and diltiazem (5.3 L/kg),[112] and somewhat smaller for nifedipine (0.8 L/kg).[89] Although not well studied, the substantial protein binding and the large volumes of distribution make it unlikely that extracorporeal drug removal with hemodialysis or hemoperfusion would be of any value in overdose. Several case reports offer clinical support for this conclusion.[139,141,158]

One interesting aspect of the pharmacology of CCBs is their potential for drug-drug interactions. The CYP3A isoenzyme group of the cytochrome P450 metabolizes most CCBs and is also responsible for the initial oxidation of numerous other drugs. Verapamil and diltiazem specifically compete for this isoenzyme pathway and can decrease the clearance of many agents including carbamazepine, cisapride, quinidine, various 3-hydroxy-3-methylglutaryl coenzyme A (HMG-CoA) reductase inhibitors, cyclosporine, tacrolimus, most HIV-protease inhibitors, and theophylline.[1,130] In June 1998, mibefradil, a uniquely structured CCB, was voluntarily withdrawn from the market following several reports of serious adverse drug interactions due in part to its potent inhibition of the CYP3A isoenzyme system.[8,100] While other inhibitors of this isoenzyme system, such as cimetidine, fluoxetine, some antifungals, macrolide antibiotics, and even grapefruit juice, may raise serum concentrations of several CCBs, its clinical significance remains unclear.[1]

In addition to affecting CYP3A, verapamil and diltiazem also inhibit *p*-glycoprotein-mediated drug transport into peripheral tissues. This inhibition results in elevated serum concentrations of drugs such as cyclosporine and digoxin, which utilize this transport system.[32,69] Unlike diltiazem and verapamil, nifedipine and the other dihydropyridines do not appear to affect the clearance of other agents via CYP3A or *p*-glycoprotein-mediated transport.[2]

PATHOPHYSIOLOGY

To understand the physiologic effects of CCBs and to develop a rational pharmacologic approach to overdose therapy, it is important to understand the role of calcium in normal muscle function (Fig. 50–4). Calcium plays an integral part in excitation-contraction coupling and in myocardial conduction. Initially, calcium is driven intracellularly down large concentration and electrical gradients through calcium-specific voltage-sensitive channels. These channels, specifically identified as L-type calcium channels, are located in the plasma membrane of all types of muscle cells[77] and are composed of homologous protein subunits also found in some sodium and potassium channels.[81] The α_{1c} subunit is the pore-forming portion of this channel and is where all CCBs bind to prevent calcium transport.[60] There are many other types of calcium channels, including N, P, T, Q, and R types, that can be found either intracellularly on the sarcoplasmic reticulum or on cell plasma membranes, particularly in neuronal and secretory tissue.[143] They may be stimulated by cellular stretch (stretch-operated), specific neurohormonal binding (receptor-operated), or voltage changes (voltage-sensitive).[134] Skeletal muscle depends exclusively upon intracellular calcium stores for excitation contraction coupling so intracellular influx of calcium has little physiologic consequence. In cardiac and smooth-muscle cells, however, this influx is critical.

In smooth muscle, the rapid influx of calcium binds calmodulin, and the resulting complex stimulates myosin light-chain kinase activity.[3] The myosin light-chain kinase phosphorylates and

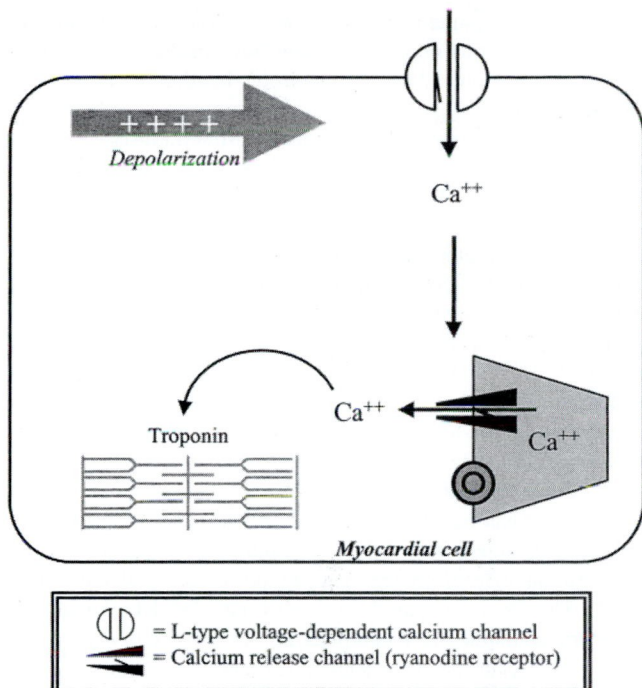

Figure 50–4. The role of calcium in contractile function of myocardial cells. Calcium channel blockers reduce ion influx through the L-type calcium channel and thus reduce contractility. Mechanisms to increase intracellular calcium include recruitment of new or dormant calcium channels by increasing cAMP either by stimulating its formation by adenyl cyclase (AC), with catecholamines or glucagon (see text), or by inhibiting its degradation with amrinone. Increasing the concentration gradient of calcium across the cellular membrane to futher its influx may improve contractility. The mechanism by which insulin therapy enhances inotropy is undefined. PDE; Phophodiesterase, PKA; Protein kinase A.

thus activates myosin, which subsequently binds actin, causing a contraction to occur.[78,121] In myocardial cells, this slow calcium influx creates the plateau phase (phase 2) of the action potential.[118] The calcium then acts as a second messenger by binding to and opening a receptor-operated calcium channel on the sarcoplasmic reticulum, which releases calcium from the vast stores of the sarcoplasmic reticulum into the cytosol.[70,71] This is often termed calcium-induced calcium release.[37,171] Calcium then binds troponin C, which causes a conformational change that displaces troponin and tropomyosin from the actin. This allows actin and myosin to bind, resulting in a contraction[80] (Chaps. 21 and 49).

In addition to its role in myocardial contractility, calcium influx is also important in myocardial conduction. Calcium influx plays an important role in the spontaneous depolarization (phase 4) of the action potential in the sinoatrial (SA) node.[118] This slow calcium influx also allows normal propagation of electrical impulses via the specialized myocardial conduction tissues, particularly the atrioventricular (AV) node.[137]

All commercially available CCBs exert their physiologic effects by antagonizing L-type voltage-sensitive slow calcium channels.[79] This impairs calcium influx into muscle cells, particularly the myocardial and smooth muscle, which are dependent on this influx for normal function. In the vascular smooth muscle, the cytosolic calcium concentration maintains basal tone and any influx of calcium results in relaxation and arterial vasodilation.[74] In the myocardium this impaired calcium flow results in a decreased force of contraction and negative inotropy. In addition, the SA and AV nodal tissues are inhibited, which produces a reduction in heart rate and intracardiac conduction.[114] Mibefradil is also a potent antagonist of calcium T channels; however, it is unclear what, if any, physiologic effects this antagonism produced.

The CCBs currently available in the United States are classified into four structural groups (Table 50–1). Each group binds a slightly different region of the α_{1c} subunit of the calcium channel and thus has different affinities for the various L-type calcium channels both in the myocardium and the vascular smooth muscle.[105,116,117,155] Verapamil, a phenylalkylamine, has the most profound inhibitory effects on the SA and AV nodal tissue, whereas diltiazem, a benzothiazepine, has only moderate myocardial conduction effects.[82,116,117] In contrast, nifedipine, the prototypical dihydropyridine, has little affinity for myocardial calcium channels but has the greatest pharmacologic effect on the peripheral vascular smooth-muscle.[82,116,155] Both verapamil and diltiazem have similar effects on vascular smooth-muscle calcium channels.[105] Therefore, verapamil is the most potent at decreasing heart rate, cardiac output, and blood pressure, while nifedipine produces the greatest decrease in systemic vascular resistance. Because nifedipine and all the dihydropyridines have little myocardial effect at therapeutic levels, the baroreceptor reflex remains intact and an actual slight increase in heart rate and cardiac output may occur.[155] Isradipine is the only dihydropyridine whose inhibitory effect on the SA node is significant enough to blunt any reflex tachycardia.[43]

Bepridil is unique because in addition to its calcium channel blocking effects, it is a potent fast sodium channel and potassium channel antagonist.[63] This impairs both myocardial contractility and conduction and results in prolongation of the AV nodal effective refractory period, the action potential itself, and myocardial repolarization.[63] Bepridil induces a prolongation of the QTc interval and may precipitate malignant ventricular dysrhythmias including torsades de pointes.[7,63] This dysrhythmogenic effect is potentiated in the setting of hypokalemia.

These receptor-binding differences among the CCB classes determine the potential therapeutic role of each. Verapamil and diltiazem are used in the management of hypertension, to reduce myocardial oxygen demand, to achieve rate control in atrial flutter or fibrillation, and for supraventricular reentry tachycardias.[2] Dihydropyridines are typically used to treat diseases with increased peripheral vascular tone such as hypertension, Raynaud phenomenon, Prinzmetal angina, esophageal spasm, vascular headaches, and postsubarachnoid hemorrhage vasospasm.[4,22,48,148] Bepridil is classified and used as an antidysrhythmic but because of its dysrhythmogenic potential, its use is limited only to patients who are refractory to all other therapy.[63]

CLINICAL MANIFESTATIONS

The life-threatening toxicity of CCBs is manifested largely within the cardiovascular system and is an extension of their therapeutic effects. Myocardial depression and peripheral vasodilation occur, producing bradycardia and hypotension.[142] Myocardial conduction may be impaired, producing AV conduction abnormalities, idioventricular rhythms, and complete heart block.[12,39,65,72,101,107,122,129]

Junctional escape rhythms are frequently noted in patients with significant poisonings.[27] The negative inotropic effects may be so profound, particularly with verapamil, that ventricular contraction may be completely inhibited.[13,54] Patients may present initially asymptomatic but deteriorate rapidly into severe cardiogenic shock.[61,147,165]

Hypotension is the most common physical finding following an overdose.[132,133] The signs and symptoms represent the degree of cardiovascular compromise and hypoperfusion of the patient's central nervous system. Early or mild symptoms include dizziness, fatigue, and lightheadedness while more severely poisoned patients may manifest lethargy, syncope, altered mental status, coma, and death.[28,56,61,65,95,122,138] Cases of seizures,[56,65,110,124,152] strokes,[140,145,167] ischemic bowel,[51,52,151,166] and renal failure[107,129] occurring in the setting of cardiogenic shock as a result of CCB poisonings are also reported. Severe CNS depression is distinctly uncommon, and if respiratory depression or coma is present without severe hypotension, coingestants or other causes of altered mental status must be considered. Gastrointestinal symptoms of nausea and vomiting are also uncommon.[67]

Although receptor selectivity is lost in overdose and all CCBs can produce severe bradycardia, hypotension, and death,[142] there are some subtle variations in presentation depending upon the agent. The CCBs with the most significant myocardial effects, verapamil and, to a lesser extent, diltiazem, are associated with more negative inotropic and chronotropic effects.[125,128] In a prospective, poison control center–based study, AV nodal block occurred much more frequently in the setting of verapamil poisoning.[132] In contrast, nifedipine, because of its limited myocardial binding, may produce tachycardia or a "normal" heart rate initially, with bradycardia developing only in patients with more substantial ingestions.[25,59,166,170] Deaths associated with dihydropyridines do occur, but they are uncommon.[95,125]

Numerous reports document hyperglycemia in patients with severe CCB poisoning.[16,28,35,56,65,107,115,129,152,165] Insulin release from the β islet cells in the pancreas is dependent on calcium influx via a slow calcium channel.[102,109] In CCB overdose, selectivity is lost and this channel is also antagonized. This impairs normal calcium influx and insulin release is reduced.[29] The hyperglycemic effect may be exacerbated in a diabetic patient or if glucagon is used as inotropic therapy[159] (Chap. 40).

Acute lung injury is also associated with CCB poisoning.[16,19,47,59,67,103] While the mechanism is unknown, it is postulated that there is precapillary vasodilation causing an increase in transcapillary hydrostatic pressure.[68] The elevated pressure gradient results in increased pulmonary capillary transudates and ultimately interstitial edema.

Several factors, including the agent involved, the dose ingested, the product formulation, and the patient's underlying cardiovascular health, may play a role in the ultimate degree of toxicity. Coingestion with other agents with cardiovascular activity, such as β-adrenergic antagonists digoxin, potentiates conduction abnormalities.[21,45,76,96,177]

The product formulation immediate or regular release vs. sustained-release) affects the onset of symptoms and duration of toxicity. With regular-release formulations, toxicity is often present within 2–3 hours of ingestion.[133] With sustained-release products, however, initial signs or symptoms may be delayed for 6–8 hours, and delays of up to 15 hours have been reported.[133,150,161] In addition, with sustained-release ingestions, the drug's apparent half-life is prolonged and toxicity may last longer than 48 hours.[10,12,99]

Comorbidity and age are two factors that negatively impact on both morbidity and mortality in CCB poisonings. Elderly patients and those with underlying cardiovascular disease, such as congestive heart failure, are much more sensitive to the myocardial depressant effects of CCBs.[25,111] Even with presumed therapeutic dosing these individuals may develop symptoms of mild hypoperfusion, such as dizziness and fatigue, much more frequently.[55,66,72,120]

DIAGNOSTIC TESTING

All patients with a suspected CCB ingestion should be attached to a cardiac monitor and have a 12-lead ECG performed to assess for any PR prolongation or bradydysrhythmias. Careful assessment of the degree of hypoperfusion, if any, may include a chest radiograph, oxygen saturation, and diagnostic testing for metabolic acidosis. Assays for various CCB serum concentrations are not routinely available and are not used to manage patients following overdose. If a patient presents with bradydysrhythmias of unclear origin, assessment of electrolytes, particularly potassium and magnesium, renal function, and a digoxin level may be helpful, although obtaining an accurate history often provides the most valuable clues. If hyperkalemia is present, careful consideration of cardiac glycoside poisoning should be made. Because calcium channel antagonist poisoning can impair insulin secretion from the pancreas, hyperglycemia may be present.

MANAGEMENT

Any patient with a suspected CCB ingestion should be immediately evaluated even if initial vital signs are normal and there are no symptoms. Intravenous access and continuous electrocardiographic monitoring should be initiated. A 12-lead ECG demonstrating the rhythm and intervals should be obtained and repeated every 1–2 hours for the first 8 hours, and if the patient's condition normalizes, at longer intervals subsequently. Initial treatment should begin with adequate oxygenation and airway protection, and aggressive gastrointestinal decontamination. If the patient is hypotensive and there is no evidence of congestive heart failure, an initial fluid bolus of 10–20 mL/kg of crystalloid should be given and repeated as needed.

Gastrointestinal decontamination is a critical intervention. Syrup of ipecac should be avoided because CCB-poisoned patients can rapidly deteriorate and become severely hypotensive. Orogastric lavage should be considered for all patients who present to have within 1–2 hours of the ingestion, those who are presumed to have large ingestions, and those who are critically ill. Whereas the effects of orogastric lavage in an overdose involving a sustained-release CCB have not been studied, and while most of these formulations tend to be large and poorly soluble, because of the significant danger in overdose, orogastric lavage should still be strongly considered. When performing orogastric lavage in a CCB-poisoned patient, remember that this procedure may increase vasomotor tone and potentially exacerbate any bradydysrhythmias.[160] All patients with CCB ingestions should receive 1 g/kg of activated charcoal orally. Multiple doses (0.5 g/kg) of activated charcoal (MDAC) without a cathartic should be administered to all patients with sustained-release pill ingestions or signs of continuing toxicity. Although data are limited, there is no evidence that MDAC increases CCB clearance from the serum.[136,157]

Rather, its efficacy may be a result of the continuous presence of activated charcoal throughout the gastrointestinal tract, which adsorbs any active drug from its slow-release formulation. Whole-bowel irrigation (WBI) with polyethylene glycol solution (1–2 L/h via nasogastric tube in adults; up to 500 mL/h in children) should be initiated for patients who ingest sustained-release products.[18,156] WBI may be the most effective means of gastrointestinal decontamination for sustained-release products.[87] Dosing should be continued until the rectal effluent is clear.

The importance of early initiation of MDAC and WBI, even for well-appearing patients, and particularly for children with a history of sustained-release CCB ingestion, cannot be overemphasized. It is imperative to minimize any absorption and to prevent delayed cardiovascular toxicity, which can be profound and difficult to reverse. Several reports describe patients who presented with mild signs of poisoning, in whom gastrointestinal decontamination was not performed aggressively and who subsequently displayed severe toxicity.[150,161]

Pharmacotherapy should focus upon maintenance or improvement of both cardiac output and peripheral vascular tone.[85] Although many agents, including atropine, calcium, insulin, glucagon, isoproterenol, dopamine, epinephrine, norepinephrine, and phosphodiesterase inhibitors, have been used with reported success in CCB-poisoned patients, no single agent has consistently demonstrated total efficacy.[65,125,128,132,133] Little prospective or basic science research specifically evaluates effective treatment modalities.

Although therapy should begin with crystalloids and atropine, the more critically poisoned patients will not respond and inotropics and vasopressors will be needed. Although it would be ideal to initiate each agent individually and to monitor the patient's hemodynamic response, in the most critically ill patients, multiple therapies should be administered simultaneously. A reasonable treatment sequence includes calcium followed by a catecholamine such as norepinephrine, high-dose insulin infusion, glucagon, and a phosphodiesterase inhibitor. The evidence and use of each of these drugs are discussed below.

Atropine

Atropine is considered to be the drug of choice for patients with symptomatic bradycardia. In an early dog model of verapamil poisoning, atropine improved heart rate and cardiac output.[46] In one prospective study, 2 of 8 bradycardic CCB-poisoned patients had an improvement in heart rate.[132] Clinical experience, however, demonstrates atropine to be largely ineffective in improving bradycardias in severe CCB-poisoned patients.[28,35,71,128,138,147,167] Initial treatment with calcium may improve the efficacy of atropine.[34,67,73] Given its availability, efficacy in mild poisonings, and safety profile, atropine should still be considered as initial therapy in patients with symptomatic bradycardia. Dosing should begin with 0.5–1.0 mg (0.02 mg/kg in children) IV every 2 or 3 minutes up to a maximum dose of 3 mg in all patients with symptomatic bradycardia. However, because of its limited efficacy in severely poisoned patients, treatment failures with this agent should be anticipated. In addition, it may be reasonable to withhold atropine from patients in whom whole-bowel irrigation is needed in order to avoid decreasing bowel motility.

Calcium

Pharmacologically, calcium appears to be a logical agent to treat patients with CCB poisoning. Pretreatment with intravenous calcium prior to verapamil use for supraventricular tachydysrhythmias prevents hypotension without diminishing the antidysrhythmic effects.[31,146,168] This is also observed in the overdose setting in which calcium tends to improve blood pressure more than it does the heart rate. Although the mechanism is unclear, boluses of calcium increase the extracellular calcium concentration and increase the intracellular concentration gradient. This may drive calcium intracellularly through unblocked calcium channels. Calcium salts are beneficial in experimental models of CCB poisoning.[34,46,54] Improvement in inotropy and blood pressure in verapamil-poisoned dogs was demonstrated after increasing the serum calcium by 2 mEq/L with an intravenous infusion of 10% calcium chloride at 3 mg/kg/min (Antidotes in Depth: Calcium).[54]

Calcium reverses the negative inotropy, impaired conduction, and hypotension in many humans poisoned with CCBs.[19,26,36,53,57,59,101,104,106,119,120,126,132,169,172] Unfortunately, this effect is often short-lived and more significantly poisoned patients may not improve with calcium salt administration.[24,28,35,40,47,50,61,71,136,141] Some authors feel that these failures may represent inadequate dosing.[18,67] However, the exact dosing of calcium salts remains unclear. Reasonable recommendations for poisoned adults include an initial intravenous bolus of approximately 13–25 mEq of calcium (10–20 mL of 10% calcium chloride or 30–60 mL of 10% calcium gluconate) followed by either repeat boluses every 15–20 minutes for 3 or 4 doses, or a continuous infusion of 0.5 mEq/kg/h of calcium (0.2–0.4 mL/kg/h of 10% calcium chloride or 0.6–1.2 mL of 10% calcium gluconate).[85,86,125] Careful selection of the calcium salt used is critical for dosing. While there is no difference in efficacy of calcium chloride or calcium gluconate, 1 g of calcium chloride contains 13.4 mEq of calcium, which is more than 3 times the 4.3 mEq found in 1 g of calcium gluconate. Therefore, in order to administer equal doses of calcium, one must administer 3 times the volume of standard calcium gluconate. If repeat dosing or continuous infusions are used, the serum calcium and phosphorous should be closely monitored to prevent hypercalcemia and hypophosphatemia. These concerns are not unfounded and may in fact significantly limit calcium therapy.[95] Other adverse effects of intravenous calcium include nausea, vomiting, flushing, constipation, confusion, and angina.[86] If there is any suspicion that a cardiac glycoside such as digoxin is involved in an overdose, calcium should be avoided until after digoxin-specific Fab therapy, because it may further elevate the intracellular calcium and worsen digoxin toxicity[15] (Chap. 48).

Catecholamines

Catecholamines and sympathomimetics are the next line of therapy in the treatment CCB poisoning. Numerous case reports describe the success or failure of a wide variety of vasopressors including epinephrine (success[9,24]; failure[56,107]), norepinephrine (success;[65,115] failure[107,110]), dopamine (success[10,36,167]; failure[9,24,33,50,56,107,115165]), isoproterenol (success[49,107,122,129,158]; failure[9,24,56,165]), and dobutamine (success[129]; failure[28,33,107]). Experimentally, no single agent is consistently effective.[46,92] This is not surprising given the significant variability in both the CCBs and the patients involved. Mechanistically, however, either stimulation of β_1-adrenergic receptors on the myocardium or α_1-adrenergic receptors on the peripheral vascular smooth muscle would appear to be the desirable, but which depends upon the etiology of the hypotension.

β-Adrenergic agonists activate adenylate cyclase via G_s protein.[144] This results in formation of cyclic adenosine monophosphate (cAMP), which then stimulates protein kinase A to phosphorylate the α_1 subunit of various calcium channels[149] (Fig. 50–5). It is unclear whether this phosphorylation allows calcium channels to remain open longer,[25,135] or if it opens dormant channels within the plasma membrane.[19,86] In addition, protein kinase A also phosphorylates phospholamban, which improves calcium release from troponin after contraction.[154] In the myocardium, this multifactorial increase in intracellular calcium results in improved chronotropy, dromotropy, and inotropy (Chap. 49).

In the peripheral vascular smooth muscle, α_1-adrenergic receptor agonists activate receptor-operated calcium channels. This opening of nonpoisoned calcium channels allows calcium influx[135] (see Fig. 50–6), which makes α_1-adrenergic agonists such as norepinephrine and phenylephrine logical choices if the hypotension is primarily the result of peripheral vasodilation.

Based upon these pharmacologic mechanisms, norepinephrine appears to be an appropriate initial catecholamine to use in hypotensive CCB-poisoned patients. Its significant β_1-adrenergic activity reverses the myocardial depressant effects, while its α_1-adrenergic effects increase peripheral vascular resistance. There is some theoretical concern about using pure β-adrenergic receptor agonists, such as isoproterenol and, to a lesser extent, dobutamine, because β_2-induced peripheral vasodilation may worsen hypotension, particularly at high doses.

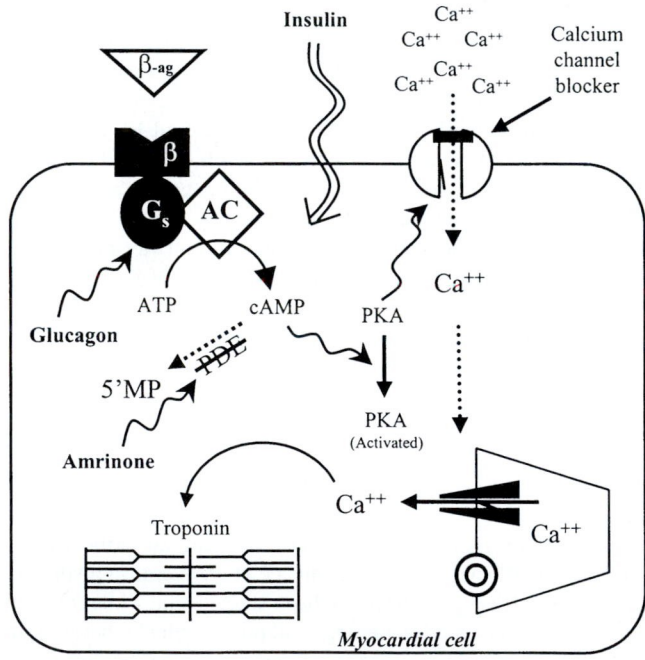

Figure 50–5. Calcium's role in contractile function of vascular smooth muscle cells and potential therapeutic options in severe calcium channel blocker poisoning. Calcium's entry via voltage-sensitive channels initiates a cascade of events resulting in actin-myosin coupling and contraction; this is inhibited by calcium channel blockers. Mechanisms to increase intracellular calcium include activation of receptor operated calcium channels with α_1 adrenergic agonists or increasing the calcium ion gradient across the cellular membrane to further its influx.

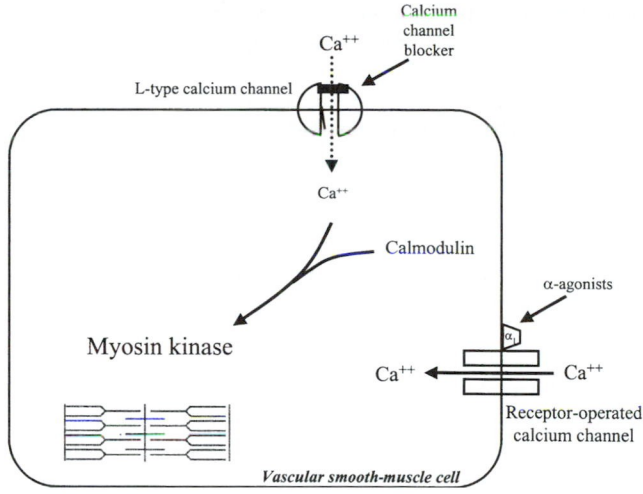

Figure 50–6. Vascular toxicity of calcium channel blockers and antidotal therapies. Calcium's entry via voltage-sensitive channels initiates a cascade of events resulting in actin-myosin coupling and contraction; this is inhibited by calcium channel blockers. Mechanisms to increase intracellular calcium include activation of receptor-operated calcium channels with α_1-adrenergic agonists or increasing the calcium ion gradient across the cellular membrane to further its influx.

Dopamine is predominantly an indirect-acting pressor that acts by stimulating the release of norepinephrine from the distal nerve terminal and not by direct α- and β-adrenergic receptor stimulation.[62] This may limit its effectiveness in severely stressed patients who may have mild catecholamine depletion.[165] Published clinical experience of severe CCB poisonings supports these concerns.[9,24,33,49,56,107,115,165] Improvement in blood pressure may be noted with dopamine at high dosing when the drug has additional direct α- and β-adrenergic effects.[62]

The choice of a sympathomimetic agent is based on numerous factors, including the pharmacologic profile of each drug, the patient's underlying physiologic condition, and the physician's familiarity and comfort with the agent. If one sympathomimetic agent is unsuccessful, invasive cardiovascular monitoring, such as a pulmonary artery catheterization, may be helpful in assessing whether the myocardial depressant or peripheral vasodilatory effects are responsible for the hypotension.[128]

Insulin

The most exciting new development in the treatment of patients who were severely poisoned with CCBs is the successful use of high-dose insulin and euglycemic therapy. It has been long known that insulin has positive inotropic effects.[38] While some indirect evidence suggests that increased calcium entry may be involved,[38,97] there is growing support for the hypothesis that improved myocardial utilization of carbohydrates is responsible for clinical improvement (Chap. 59).[93] Verapamil poisoning alters the normal metabolism of myocardial cells of primarily fatty acids and forces them to become carbohydrate dependent.[91,92,94] At the same time, CCBs impede the ability of myocardial tissues to use these carbohydrates by inhibiting calcium-mediated insulin secretion from the β islet cells in the pancreas,[29] and by somehow increasing myocardial resistance to insulin.[93] In a canine model of

verapamil toxicity, high-dose insulin in conjunction with continuous dextrose infusion to maintain euglycemia improved survival when compared to calcium, epinephrine, or glucagon.[90,94] A possible explanation is that epinephrine and glucagon increase myocardial contractility at the expense of increased myocardial oxygen consumption, whereas insulin improves overall myocardial efficiency. The use of insulin is particularly interesting because severe CCB toxicity often produces significant hyperglycemia and insulin infusions are often initiated.[35,152] Whether this is a nonspecific effect of insulin therapy in critically ill patients or a specific effect for calcium channel blocker poisoning is currently being investigated.[163]

In a case series of 4 verapamil-poisoned patients, adjuvant high-dose insulin therapy improved the cardiac function and blood pressure.[176] Notably, there was little effect on heart rate in any of these patients. One patient had an improvement in ejection fraction from 10% to 50%.[176]

Although there is limited clinical experience with the use of insulin/glucose therapy, because of the convincing animal evidence, the relative lack of other demonstrably effective therapeutics, and the seriousness and potentially fatal nature of CCB poisoning, we recommend high-dose insulin/glucose therapy early in the treatment of patients manifesting CCB toxicity. Based on the canine data and the case series, after an initial insulin bolus of 0.1 U/kg, a reasonable starting rate for the insulin infusion is 0.2–0.3 U/kg/h, which can be increased if there is no hemodynamic response in 60 minutes.[176] Remember, this increase should be done in a stepwise manner with concomitant increases in the dextrose infusion to maintain euglycemic control. After an initial bolus of 25–50 g of dextrose (0.5–1 g/kg) a reasonable starting rate for the dextrose infusion is 0.5 g/kg/h.[176] Serum glucose levels should be closely monitored throughout therapy, particularly during the first few hours, and should be continued for several hours after discontinuation of the insulin infusion. Because the hemodynamic effects of insulin are mediated via alterations in myocardial metabolism, the hemodynamic response is typically delayed for 30–60 minutes, necessitating the simultaneous use of catecholamines in profoundly hypotensive patients.

Glucagon

Glucagon is an endogenous polypeptide hormone secreted by the pancreatic α cells in response to hypoglycemia and catecholamines. In addition, it has significant inotropic and chronotropic effects.[23,123] Glucagon is the drug of choice for β-adrenergic antagonist poisoning (Chap. 49) because of its ability to bypass the β-adrenergic receptor and activate adenylate cyclase via a G_s protein in the myocardium.[174] Thus glucagon is unique in that it is functionally a "pure" β_1 agonist with no peripheral vasodilatory effects. However, in CCB poisoning, because the cellular lesion is "downstream" from adenylate cyclase, this alternative activation, other than its β_1 selectivity, offers no pharmacologic advantage over more traditional β-adrenergic agonist agents (see Fig. 50–4).

Cases of CCB-poisoned patients who failed to respond to fluids, calcium, or dopamine and dobutamine, but who had significant increases in both heart rate and blood pressure after glucagon administration, are reported.[33,164] However, other much more severely poisoned patients demonstrated no hemodynamic benefit with glucagon therapy.[9,24,56] Several animal models demonstrated the efficacy of glucagon in improving CCB-induced myocardial depression.[76,153,178,179] Unfortunately, none of these studies compared other therapies, including calcium, insulin, or catecholamines, with glucagon. Although the data are limited, given its experimental and anecdotal efficacy, glucagon should be considered in the management of refractory hypotension in patients with CCB poisoning. Dosing for glucagon is not well established. An initial dose of 2–5 mg intravenously over 30–60 seconds is reasonable in adults followed by retreatment in 5 minutes with 4–10 mg if there is no response. The initial pediatric dose is 50 µg/kg. Because of the short half-life of glucagon, a maintenance infusion should be initiated once a desired effect is achieved. Maintenance infusion dosing should begin at the "response dose" of glucagon per hour. For example, if an initial dose of 4 mg of glucagon effectively improved blood pressure, then the infusion should be started at 4 mg/h (Antidotes in Depth: Glucagon). Adverse effects include vomiting and hyperglycemia, particularly in diabetics or during continuous infusion.[159] Although the most common glucagon formulation currently available is a recombinant product, it is important to remember that older formulations also come with a 0.2% phenol diluent for intramuscular administration that should never be used intravenously.

Phosphodiesterase Inhibitors

Another class of agents that have demonstrated utility in CCB poisoning are amrinone, milrinone, and enoximone. These agents inhibit the breakdown of cAMP by phosphodiesterase and increase cAMP levels. These noncatecholamine inotropic agents do not disproportionately increase myocardial oxygen demand and have been traditionally used for congestive heart failure.[11,14] They specifically inhibit phosphodiesterase III, the enzyme responsible for cAMP breakdown found in cardiac and vascular tissue[30] (Fig. 50–4). This inhibition results in increased cAMP, increased intracellular calcium, and improved inotropy. Amrinone improved myocardial contractility in 2 canine models of verapamil poisoning.[5,108] In addition, amrinone is clinically successful in patients with CCB poisoning when used in combination with another inotropic agent such as isoproterenol or glucagon.[50,173] This "two-pronged" approach to increase myocardial cAMP levels—by stimulating formation and by inhibiting breakdown—makes pharmacologic sense. However, because amrinone nonselectively inhibits phosphodiesterase III, cAMP is also increased in the vascular smooth muscle. This causes smooth-muscle relaxation, peripheral vasodilation, and, often, hypotension.[88] Therefore amrinone should be used only as a second-line agent in combination with another inotropic agent, and in patients with invasive hemodynamic monitoring. Dosing of amrinone in CCB poisoning is not well defined. Based on traditional dosing for congestive heart failure, the experimental data, and the case reports, an initial bolus of 1 mg/kg over 2 minutes followed by a continuous infusion of 5–20 µg/kg/min is appropriate.[5,30,49,50,173]

Experimental Pharmaceutical Agents

Currently, there are several experimental agents that may be effective in treatment of severe hypotension and bradycardia in CCB-poisoned patients. 4-Aminopyridine has been used for many years as an antagonist to nondepolarizing neuromuscular blocking agents in Bulgaria.[6] It indirectly increases the calcium influx by blocking voltage-sensitive potassium channels in excitable membranes. This blockade of the outward potassium-rectifying current causes a prolonged depolarization at the nerve terminal, allowing

for greater calcium influx, and, ultimately, increasing neurotransmitter release.[46,175] In addition, 4-aminopyridine directly increases both skeletal and cardiac muscle contractility.[6] The net effect on the cardiovascular system is an increase in myocardial contractility and in peripheral vascular resistance. Several animal models of severe verapamil poisoning report improvements in hemodynamic status, as well as survival in animals receiving 4-aminopyridine.[6,46] 4-Aminopyridine was used in 1 patient who was poisoned with verapamil because of a therapeutic error, although other interventions including calcium and isoproterenol infusions were also administered.[158] Unfortunately, 4-aminopyridine has a narrow therapeutic index and its most notable toxicity is seizures, which has limited its utility. Two closely related and much more potent compounds, 3,4-diaminopyridine and Bay K 8664, have had similar experimental success at improving the hemodynamics in verapamil poisoning models but are limited by their significant toxicity, which includes muscle fasciculations, severe hypertension, and coronary artery vasospasm.[61,98,127]

Another drug used experimentally in CCB poisoning is digoxin. Cardiac glycosides inhibit the sodium/potassium/ATPase, which increases the intracellular sodium concentration and decreases the transmembrane sodium concentration gradient. This concentration gradient is the driving force for the sodium/calcium exchanger in the cell membrane. When it is decreased, less calcium can exit the cell in exchange for sodium during cellular repolarization.[84] In a canine model of mild/moderate verapamil poisoning, digoxin, in conjunction with atropine to block the vagally mediated inhibitory effects of digoxin on heart rate and AV nodal conduction, improved both myocardial dromatropy and inotropy, while increasing peripheral vascular resistance.[131] However, because digoxin takes a significant amount of time to distribute into tissue and because of its limited efficacy and the lack of safety data, much more work is required before digoxin should be administered to patients with CCB poisoning.

Adjunctive Hemodynamic Support

Many of the most severely poisoned patients may not respond to any pharmacologic intervention.[56] Transthoracic or intravenous cardiac pacing may be required to improve heart rate as demonstrated by several case reports.[36,147,165] However, in a prospective cohort of CCB poisonings, 2 of 4 patients with significant bradycardia requiring electrical pacing had no electrical capture.[132] In addition, even if electrical pacing is effective in increasing the heart rate, blood pressure often remains unchanged.[20,61,65,122]

Intra-aortic balloon counterpulsation is another invasive supportive option. A large balloon is inserted into the femoral artery, and it expands during diastole and deflates just before systole. This supports the diastolic pressure to the coronary and carotid arteries during inflation and acts as a vacuum that effectively reduces afterload when the balloon collapses.[162] Intra-aortic balloon counterpulsation was used successfully to improve cardiac output and blood pressure in a patient with a mixed verapamil and atenolol overdose.[45] The synchronized inflation and deflation are dependent on a regular cardiac electrical activity, so cardiac pacing is often required in addition to the intra-aortic balloon. It is important to understand that overdosed patients who may be candidates for intra-aortic balloon counterpulsation support have a much better prognosis than other patients with severe left-ventricular failure from ischemic heart disease in whom this technology is traditionally used. Between 24 and 48 hours of assisted cardiac output allows metabolism and elimination of the CCBs and a return of baseline myocardial function.

Although much more invasive and technologically demanding, emergent open and percutaneous cardiopulmonary bypass is also used to support patients with severe CCB poisoning.[56,64] The major limitation of all these technologies is that they are available only at tertiary care facilities.

DISPOSITION

Every patient who manifests any signs or symptoms of toxicity should be admitted to an intensive care setting. Because of the potential for delayed toxicity, all patients ingesting sustained-release products should be admitted for 24 hours to a monitored setting even if asymptomatic. This is particularly important for small children in whom even a few tablets may produce significant toxicity.[56,124] All admitted patients should be treated with multiple doses of activated charcoal, and whole-bowel irrigation should be strongly considered in any ingestion involving sustained-release products. Only patients with a precise history of an "immediate-release" preparation ingestion who have received adequate gastrointestinal decontamination, who have normal unchanged serial ECGs over 6–8 hours, and who are asymptomatic can be medically "cleared."

SUMMARY

Calcium channel blockers are commonly used to treat hypertension, stable and vasospastic angina, dysrhythmias, migraine headaches, Raynaud phenomenon, and subarachnoid hemorrhage. Because of their increasing frequency of use, CCB exposures continue to rise, resulting in numerous deaths from poisoning annually. Hallmarks of toxicity include bradydysrhythmias and hypotension, which are extensions of the pharmacologic effects of these agents. Although most patients develop symptoms of hypoperfusion such as lightheadedness, nausea, or fatigue within hours of a significant ingestion, sustained-release formulations may result in significant delays in any hemodynamic consequences, and will certainly prolong toxicity. Because of the significant lethality of large ingestions of sustained-release CCBs, it is imperative to make gastrointestinal decontamination with whole-bowel irrigation a top priority. Aggressive decontamination of patients with exposures to sustained-release products should begin as soon as possible and should not be delayed by waiting for signs of toxicity. Once hemodynamic toxicity develops, supportive care together with pharmacologic treatment with calcium boluses followed by high-dose insulin and glucose infusions should be initiated. Traditional catecholamines are also typically needed, but their use alone may not be sufficient for the most critically poisoned patients. Other therapeutic options include glucagon and phosphodiesterase inhibitors. Patients who fail to respond to all pharmaceutical interventions should be considered candidates for extracorporeal mechanical support, whenever available.

REFERENCES

1. Abernethy DR: Grapefruits and drugs: When is statistically significant clinically significant? J Clin Invest 1997;99:2297–2298.

2. Abernethy DR, Schwartz JB: Calcium-antagonist drugs. N Engl J Med 1999;341:1447–1457.

3. Adelstein RS, Sellers JR, Conti MA, et al: Regulation of smooth-muscle contractile proteins by calmodulin and cyclic AMP. Fed Proc 1982;41:2873–2878.

4. Allen GS: Role of calcium antagonists in cerebral arterial spasm. Am J Cardiol 1985;55:149B–153B.

5. Alousi AA, Canter JM, Fort DJ: The beneficial effect of amrinone on acute drug-induced heart failure in the anaesthetised dog. Cardiovasc Res 1985;19:483–494.

6. Agoston S, Maestrone E, van Hezik EJ, et al: Effective treatment of verapamil intoxication with 4-aminopyridine in the cat. J Clin Invest 1984;73:1291–1296.

7. Anonymous: Studies of bepridil in use against arrhythmias halted. Clin Pharm 1985;4:614.

8. Anonymous: Roche Laboratories announces withdrawal of Posicor from the market. FDA Talk Paper (T98–33), June 8, 1998.

9. Anthony T, Jastremski M, Elliot W, et al: Charcoal hemoperfusion for the treatment of a combined diltiazem and metoprolol overdose. Ann Emerg Med 1986;15:1344–1348.

10. Ashraf M, Chaudhary K, Nelson J, Thompson W: Massive overdose of sustained-release verapamil: A case report and review of literature. Am J Med Sci 1995;310:258–263.

11. Baim DS: Effect of phosphodiesterase inhibition on myocardial oxygen consumption and coronary blood flow. Am J Cardiol 1989;63:23A–26A.

12. Barrow PM, Houston PL, Wong DT: Overdose of sustained-release verapamil. Br J Anaesth 1994;72:361–365.

13. Beniam ME: Asystole after verapamil. Br Med J 1972;2:169–170.

14. Benotti JR, Grossman W, Braunwald E, Carabello BA: Effect of amrinone on myocardial energy metabolism and hemodynamics in patients with severe congestive heart failure due to coronary artery disease. Circulation 1980;62:28–35.

15. Bower JO, Mengle HAK: The additive effects of calcium and digitalis: A warning with a report of two deaths. JAMA 1936;106:1151–1153.

16. Brass BJ, Winchester-Penny S, Lipper BL: Massive verapamil overdose complicated by noncardiogenic pulmonary edema. Am J Emerg Med 1996;14:459–461.

17. Buckley CD, Aronson JK: Prolonged half-life of verapamil in a case of overdose: Implications for therapy. Br J Clin Pharmacol 1995;39:680–683.

18. Buckley N, Dawson AH, Howarth D, Whyte IM: Slow-release verapamil poisoning. Use of polyethylene glycol whole-bowel lavage and high-dose calcium. Med J Aus 1993;158:202–204.

19. Buckley NA, Whyte IM, Dawson AH: Overdose with calcium channel blockers. BMJ 1994;308:1639.

20. Braunwald E: Mechanism of action of calcium channel-blocking agents. N Engl J Med 1982;307:1618–1627.

21. Carruthers SG, Freeman DJ, Gailey DG: Synergistic adverse hemodynamic interaction between oral verapamil and propranolol. Clin Pharmacol Ther 1989;46:469–477.

22. Castell DO: Calcium-channel blocking agents for gastrointestinal disorders. Am J Cardiol 1985;55:210B–213B.

23. Chernow B, Zagola GP, Malcolm D, et al: Glucagon's chronotropic action is calcium dependent. J Pharmacol Exp Ther 1987;241:833–837.

24. Chimienti M, Previtali M, Medici A, Piccinini M: Acute verapamil poisoning: Successful treatment with epinephrine. Clin Cardiol 1982;5:219–222.

25. Clifton DG, Booth DC, Hobbs S, et al: Negative inotropic effect of intravenous nifedipine in coronary artery disease. Relation to plasma levels. Am Heart J 1990;119:283–290.

26. Coaldrake LA: Verapamil overdose. Anaesth Intensive Care 1984;12:174–175.

27. Connolly DL, Nettleton MA, Bastow MD: Massive diltiazem overdose. Am J Cardiol 1993;72:742–743.

28. Crump BJ, Holt DW, Vale JA: Lack of response to intravenous calcium in severe verapamil poisoning. Lancet 1982;2:939–940.

29. Devis G, Somers G, Van Obberghen E, Malaisse WJ: Calcium antagonists and islet function. I. Inhibition of insulin release by verapamil. Diabetes 1975;24:547–551.

30. DiBianco R: Acute positive inotropic interventions: The phosphodiesterase inhibitors. Am Heart J 1991;121:1871–1876.

31. Dolan DL: Intravenous calcium before verapamil to prevent hypotension. Ann Emerg Med 1991;20:588–589.

32. Doppenschmitt S, Langguth P, Regardh CG, et al: Characterization of binding properties to human p-glycoprotein: Development of a [3H] verapamil radioligand-binding assay. J Pharmacol Exp Ther 1999;288:348–357.

33. Doyon S, Roberts JR: The use of glucagon in a case of calcium channel blocker overdose. Ann Emerg Med 1993;22:1229–1233.

34. Eccleston DS, Dosen P, Smith AJ: A rat model for calcium channel antagonist toxicity in man. Clin Exp Pharmacol Physiol 1991, 18(suppl):15.

35. Enyeart JJ, Price WA, Hoffman DA, Woods L: Profound hyperglycemia and metabolic acidosis after verapamil overdose. J Am Coll Cardiol 1983;2:1228–1231.

36. Erickson FC, Ling LJ, Grande GA, Anderson DL: Diltiazem overdose: Case report and review. J Emerg Med 1991;9:357–366.

37. Fabiato A: Calcium-induced release of calcium from the cardiac sarcoplasmic reticulum. Am J Physiol 1983;245:C1–C14.

38. Farah AE, Alousi AA: The actions of insulin on cardiac contractility. Life Sci 1981;29:975–1000.

39. Fauville JP, Hantson P, Honore P, et al: Severe diltiazem poisoning with intestinal pseudo-obstruction: Case report and toxicological data. J Toxicol Clin Toxicol 1995;33:273–277.

40. Ferner RE, Monkman S, Riley J, et al: Pharmacokinetic and toxic effects of nifedipine in massive overdose. Hum Exp Toxicol 1990; 9:309–311.

41. Ferner RE, Odemuyiwa O, Field AB, et al: Pharmacokinetics and toxic effects of diltiazem in massive overdose. Hum Toxicol 1989; 8:497–499.

42. Foster TS, Hamann SR, Richards VR, et al: Nifedipine kinetics and bioavailability after single intravenous and oral doses in normal subjects. J Clin Pharm 1983;23:161–170.

43. Freedman DD, Waters DD: "Second-generation" dihydropyridine calcium antagonists. Greater vascular selectivity and some unique applications. Drugs 1987;34:578–598.

44. Freher M, Challapalli S, Pinto JV, et al: Current status of calcium channel blockers in patients with cardiovascular disease. Curr Probl Cardiol 1999;24:236–240.

45. Frierson J, Bailly D, Shultz T, et al: Refractory cardiogenic shock and complete heart block after unsuspected verapamil-SR and atenolol overdose. Clin Cardiol 1991;14:933–935.

46. Gay R, Angeo S, Lee R, et al: Treatment of verapamil toxicity in intact dogs. J Clin Invest 1986;77:1805–1811.

47. Gelbke HP, Schlicht HG, Schmidt G: Fatal poisoning with verapamil. Arch Toxicol 1980;37:89–94.

48. Gelmers HJ. Calcium-channel blockers in the treatment of migraine. Am J Cardiol 1985;55:139B–143B.

49. Goenen M, Col J, Compere A, Bonte J: Treatment of severe verapamil poisoning with combined amrinone-isoproterenol therapy. Am J Cardiol 1986;58:1142–1143.

50. Goenen M, Pedemonte O, Baele P, Col J: Amrinone in the management of low cardiac output after open-heart surgery. Am J Cardiol 1985;56:33B–38B.

51. Goglin WK, Elliott BM, Deppe SA: Nifedipine-induced hypotension and mesenteric ischemia. South Med J 1989;82:274–275.

52. Gutierrez H, Jorgensen M. Colonic ischemia after verapamil overdose. Ann Intern Med 1996;124:535.

53. Haddad LM: Resuscitation after nifedipine overdose exclusively with intravenous calcium chloride. Am J Emerg Med 1996;14: 602–603.

54. Hariman RJ, Mangiardi LM, McAllister RG, et al: Reversal of the cardiovascular effects of verapamil by calcium and sodium: Differences between electrophysiologic and hemodynamic responses. Circulation 1979;59:797–804.

55. Hattori VT, Mandel WJ, Peter T: Calcium for myocardial depression from verapamil. N Engl J Med 1982;306:238.

56. Hendren WC, Schreiber RS, Garretson LK: Extracorporeal bypass for the treatment of verapamil poisoning. Ann Emerg Med 1989; 18:984–987.

57. Henry M, Kay MM, Viccellio P: Cardiogenic shock associated with calcium channel and beta blockers. Reversal with intravenous calcium chloride. Am J Emerg Med 1985;3:334–336.

58. Hermann PH, Rodger SD, Remones G, et al: Pharmacokinetics of diltiazem after intravenous and oral administration. Eur J Clin Pharmacol 1983;24:349–352.

59. Herrington DM, Insley BM, Weinman GG: Nifedipine overdose. Am J Med 1986;81:344–346.

60. Hockermon GH, Peterson BZ, Johnson BD, Catterall WA: Molecular determinants of drug binding and action on L-type calcium channels. Annu Rev Pharmacol Toxicol 1997;37:361–369.

61. Hofer CA, Smith JK, Tenholder MF: Verapamil intoxication: A literature review of overdoses and discussion of therapeutic options. Am J Med 1993;95:431–438.

62. Hoffman BB, Lefkowitz RJ: Catecholamines, sympathomimetic drugs, and adrenergic receptor antagonists. In: Hardman JG, Limbird LE, Molinoff PB, Ruddon RW, eds: Goodman and Gilman's The Pharmacological Basis of Therapeutics, 9th ed. New York, McGraw-Hill, 1996, pp. 199–248.

63. Hollingshead LM, Faulds D, Fitton A: Bepridil. A review of its pharmacological properties and therapeutic use in stable angina pectoris. Drugs 1992;44:835–837.

64. Holzer M, Sterz F, Schoerkhuber W, et al: Successful resuscitation of a verapamil-intoxicated patient with percutaneous cardiopulmonary bypass. Crit Care Med 1999;27:2818–2823.

65. Horowitz BZ, Rhee KJ: Massive verapamil ingestion: A report of two cases and a review of the literature. Am J Emerg Med 1989;7: 624–631.

66. Hossack KF: Conduction abnormalities due to diltiazem. N Engl J Med 1982;307:953–954.

67. Howarth DM, Dawson AH, Smith AJ, et al: Calcium channel blocking drug overdose: An Australian series. Hum Exp Tox 1994;13: 161–166.

68. Humbert VH, Munn NJ, Hawkins RF: Noncardiogenic pulmonary edema complicating massive diltiazem overdose. Chest 1991;99: 258–260.

69. Hunter J, Hirst BH: Intestinal secretion of drugs: The role of P-glycoprotein, and related drug efflux systems in limiting oral drug absorption. Adv Drug Deliv Rev 1997;25:129–157.

70. Ikemoto N: Structure and function of the calcium pump protein of sarcoplasmic reticulum. Ann Rev Physiol 1982;44:297–317.

71. Immonen P, Linkola A, Waris E: Three cases of severe verapamil poisoning. Int J Cardiol 1981;1:101–105.

72. Ishikawa T, Imamura T, Koiwaya Y, Tanaka K: Atrioventricular dissociation and sinus arrest induced by oral diltiazem. N Engl J Med 1983;309:1124–1125.

73. Jakubowski AT, Mizgala HF: Effect of diltiazem overdose. Am J Cardiol 1987;60:932–933.

74. Johns A, Leijten P, Yamamoto H, et al: Calcium regulation in vascular smooth muscle contractility. Am J Cardiol 1987;59:18A–23A.

75. Johnson KE, Balderston SM, Pieper JA, et al: Electrophysiologic effects of verapamil metabolites in the isolated heart. J Cardiovasc Pharmacol 1991;17:830–837.

76. Jolly SR, Kipnis JN, Lucchesi BR: Cardiovascular depression by verapamil: Reversal by glucagon and interactions with propranolol. Pharmacology 1987;35:249–255.

77. Katz A: Contractile proteins of the heart. Physiol Rev 1970;50: 63–167.

78. Katz AM. Basic cellular mechanisms of action of the calcium-channel blockers. Am J Cardiol 1985;55:2B–9B.

79. Katz AM: Cardiac ion channels. N Engl J Med 1993;328:1244–1251.

80. Katz AM: Calcium channel diversity in the cardiovascular system. J Am Coll Cardiol 1996;28:522–529.

81. Katz AM, Hager DW, Messineo FC, Pappano AJ: Cellular actions and pharmacology of calcium-channel blockers. Am J Emerg Med 1985;3:1–9.

82. Kawai C, Konishi T, Matsuyama E, Okazaki H: Comparative effects of three calcium antagonists, diltiazem, verapamil, and nifedipine, on the sinoatrial and atrioventricular nodes. Circulation 1981;63:1035–1042.

83. Keefe DL, Yee YG, Kates RE: Verapamil protein binding in patients and normal subjects. Clin Pharmacol Ther 1981;29:21–26.

84. Kelly RA, Smith TW: Pharmacological treatment of heart failure. In: Hardman JG, Limbird LE, Molinoff PB, Ruddon RW, eds: Goodman and Gilman's The Pharmacological Basis of Therapeutics, 9th ed. New York, McGraw-Hill, 1996, pp. 809–838.

85. Kenny J: Treating overdose with calcium channel blockers. BMJ 1994;308:992–993.

86. Kerns W, Kline J, Ford MD: β-Blocker and calcium channel blocker toxicity. Emerg Med Clin North Am 1994;12:365–390.

87. Kirshenbaum LA, Mathews SC, Sitar DS, Tenenbein M: Whole-bowel irrigation versus activated charcoal in sorbitol for the ingestion of modified-release pharmaceuticals. Clin Pharmacol Ther 1989;46:264–271.

88. Kissling G, Brilla C, Vagt M, et al: Haemodynamic effects of amrinone in the anaesthetized pig. Eur Heart J 1991;9:800–810.

89. Kleinbloesem CH, van Brummelen P, van de Linde JA, Voogd PJ, Breimer DD: Nifedipine: Kinetics and dynamics in healthy subjects. Clin Pharmacol Ther 1984;35:742–749.

90. Kline JA, Leonova E, Raymond RM: Beneficial myocardial metabolic effects of insulin during verapamil toxicity in the anesthetized canine. Crit Care Med 1995;23:1251–1263.

91. Kline JA, Leonova E, Williams TC, et al: Myocardial metabolism during graded intraportal verapamil infusion in awake dogs. J Cardiovasc Pharmacol 1996;27:719–726.

92. Kline JA, Raymond RM, Leonova E, et al: Insulin improves heart function and metabolism during non-ischemic cardiogenic shock in awake canines. Cardiovasc Res 1997;34:289–298.

93. Kline JA, Raymond RM, Schroeder JD, Watts JA: The diabetogenic effects of acute verapamil poisoning. Toxicol Appl Pharmacol 1997;145:357–362.

94. Kline JA, Tomaszewski CA, Schroeder JD, Raymond RM: Insulin is a superior antidote for cardiovascular toxicity induced by verapamil in the anesthetized canine. J Pharm Exp Ther 1993;267:744–750.

95. Koch AR, Vogelaers DP, Decruyenaere JM, Callens B, Verstraete A, Buylaert WA: Fatal intoxication with amlodipine. J Toxicol Clin Toxicol 1995;33:253–256.

96. Kones RJ, Phillips JH: Insulin: Fundamental mechanism of action and the heart. Cardiology 1973;60:280–303.

97. Korstanje C, Honkman FAM, van Kemenade JE: Bay K 8644, a calcium entry promoter as an antidote in verapamil intoxication in rabits. Arch Int Pharmacodyn 1987;287:109–119.

98. Kounis N: Asystole after verapamil and digoxin. J Clin Pract 1980;43:57–58.

99. Kozlowski JH, Kozlowski JA, Schuller D: Poisoning with sustained-release verapamil. Am J Med 1988;85:127.

100. Krayenbuhl JC, Vozeh S, Kondo-Oestreicher M, Dayer P: Drug-drug interactions of new active substances: Mibefradil example. Eur J Clin Pharmacol 1999;55(8):559–565.

101. Kuo MJ, Tseng YZ, Chen TF, Fong DE: Verapamil overdose and severe hypocalcemia. J Toxicol Clin Toxicol 1992;30:309–311.

102. Lebrun P, Malaisse WJ, Herchuelz A: Nutrient-induced intracellular calcium movement in rat pancreatic β-cell. Am J Physiol 1982;243:E196–E205.

103. Leesar MA, Martyn R, Talley JD, Frumin H: Noncardiogenic pulmonary edema complicating massive verapamil overdose. Chest 1994;105:606–607.

104. Lipman J, Jardin I, Roos C, et al: Intravenous calcium chloride as an antidote to verapamil-induced hypotension. Intensive Care Med 1982;8:55–57.

105. Low R, Takeda P, Mason DT, DeMaria AN: The effects of calcium channel blocking agents on cardiovascular function. Am J Cardiol 1982;49:547–553.

106. Luscher TF, Noll G, Sturmer T, Huser B, Wenk M: Calcium gluconate in severe verapamil intoxication. N Engl J Med 1994;330:718–720.

107. MacDonald D, Alguire PC: Case report: Fatal overdose with sustained-release verapamil. Am J Med Sci 1992;303:115–117.

108. Malaisse WJ: Role of calcium in insulin secretion. Isr J Med Sci 1972;8:224–251.

109. Makela HMV, Kapur PA: Amrinone and verapamil-propranolol induced cardiac depression during isoflurane anesthesia in dogs. Anesthesiology 1987;66:792–797.

110. Malcolm N, Callegari P, Goldberg P, et al: Massive diltiazem overdosage: Clinical and pharmacokinetic observations. Drug Intell Clin Pharmacol 1993;20:888.

111. Materne P, Legrand V, Vandormael M, Collignon P, Kulbertus HE: Hemodynamic effects of intravenous diltiazem with impaired left ventricular function. Am J Cardiol 1984;54:733–737.

112. McAllister RG, Hamann SR, Blouin RA: Pharmacokinetics of calcium-entry blockers. Am J Cardiol 1985;55:30B–40B.

113. McAllister RG, Kirsten EB: The pharmacology of verapamil: IV. Kinetic and dynamic effects after single intravenous and oral doses. Clin Pharm Therap 1982;31:418–426.

114. McCall D: Excitation-contraction coupling in cardiac and vascular smooth muscle. Modification by calcium-entry blockade. Circulation 1987;75(Suppl V):V3–V64.

115. McMillan R: Management of acute severe verapamil intoxication. J Emerg Med 1988;6:193–196.

116. Millard RW, Lathrop DA, Grupp G, Ashraf M, Grupp IL, Schwartz A: Differential cardiovascular effects of calcium channel blocking agents: Potential mechanisms. Am J Cardiol 1982;49:246–251.

117. Mitchell BL, Schroeder JS, Mason JW: Comparative clinical electrophysiologic effects of diltiazem, verapamil, and nifedipine: A review. Am J Cardiol 1982;49:629–635.

118. Morad M, Tung L: Ionic events responsible for the cardiac resting and action potential. Am J Cardiol 1982;49:584–594.

119. Moroni F, Mannaioni PF, Dolara A, Ciaccheri M: Calcium gluconate and hypertonic sodium chloride in a case of massive verapamil poisoning. Clin Toxicol 1980;17:395–400.

120. Morris DL, Goldschlager N: Calcium infusion for reversal of adverse effects of intravenous verapamil. JAMA 1981;249:3212–3213.

121. Murphy RA, Askoy MO, Dillon PF, Gerthoffer WT, Kamm KE: Myosin phosphorylation and the crossbridge cycle in arterial smooth muscle. Fed Proc 1983;42:51–56.

122. Orr GM, Bodansky HJ, Dymond DS, Taylor M: Fatal verapamil overdose. Lancet 1982;2:1218–1219.

123. Parmley WW: The role of glucagon in cardiac therapy. N Engl J Med 1971;285:801–802.

124. Passal DB, Crespin FH: Verapamil poisoning in an infant. Pediatrics 1984;73:543–545.

125. Pearigen PD, Benowitz NL: Poisoning due to calcium antagonists. Drug Saf 1991;6:408–430.

126. Perkins CM: Serious verapamil poisoning: Treatment with intravenous calcium gluconate. Br Med J 1978;2:1127.

127. Plewa MC, Martin TG, Menegazzi JJ, Seaberg DC, Wolfson AB: Hemodynamic effects of 3,4-diaminopyridine in a swine model of verapamil toxicity. Ann Emerg Med 1994;23:499–507.

128. Proano L, Chiang WK, Wang RY: Calcium channel blocker overdose. Am J Emerg Med 1995;13:444–450.

129. Quezado Z, Lippmann M, Wertheimer J: Severe cardiac, respiratory, and metabolic complications of massive verapamil overdose. Crit Care Med 1991;19:436–438.

130. Quinn DI, Day RO: Drug interactions of clinical importance. Drug Saf 1995;12:393–452.

131. Ramo MP, Grupp I, Pesola MK, et al: Cardiac glycosides in the treatment of experimental overdose with calcium-blocking agents. Res Exp Med 1992;192:335–343.

132. Ramoska EA, Spiller HA, Myers A. Calcium channel blocker toxicity. Ann Emerg Med 1990;19:649–653.

133. Ramoska EA, Spiller HA, Winter M, Borys D: A one-year evaluation of calcium channel blocker overdoses: Toxicity and treatment. Ann Emerg Med 1993;22:196–200.

134. Rasmussen H: The calcium messenger system. N Engl J Med 1986; 314:1094–1102.

135. Reuter H, Stevens CF, Tsien RW, Yellen G: Properties of single calcium channels in cardiac cell culture. Nature 1982;297:501–504.

136. Roberts D, Honcharik N, Sitar DS, Tenenbein M: Diltiazem overdose: Pharmacokinetics of diltiazem and its metabolites and effect of multiple dose charcoal therapy. J Toxicol Clin Toxicol 1991;29: 45–52.

137. Roden DM, George AL: The cardiac ion channels: Relevance to management of arrhythmias. Annu Rev Med 1996;47:135–148.

138. Roper TA, Sykes R, Gray C: Fatal diltiazem overdose: Report of four cases and review of the literature. Postgrad Med J 1993; 69: 474–476.

139. Rosansky SJ: Verapamil toxicity—Treatment with hemoperfusion. Ann Intern Med 1991;114:340–341.

140. Samniah N, Schlaeffer F: Cerebral infarction associated with oral verapamil overdose. J Toxicol Clin Toxicol 1988;26:365–369.

141. Schiffl H, Ziupa J, Schollmeyer P: Clinical features and management of nifedipine overdosage in a patient with renal insufficiency. J Toxicol Clin Toxicol 1984;22:387–395.

142. Schoffstall JM, Spivey WH, Gambone LM, Shaw RP, Sit SP: Effects of calcium channel blocker overdose-induced toxicity in the conscious dog. Ann Emerg Med 1991;20:1104–1108.

143. Schwartz A: Molecular and cellular aspects of calcium channel antagonism. Am J Cardiol 1992;70:6F–8F.

144. Scott RH, Dolphin AC: Activation of a G protein promotes against responses to calcium channel ligands. Nature 1987;330:760–762.

145. Shah AR, Passalacqua BR: Case report: Sustained-released verapamil overdose causing stroke: An unusual complication. Am J Med Sci 1992;304:257–359.

146. Singh NA: Intravenous calcium and verapamil—When the combination may be indicated. Int J Cardiol 1983;4:281–284.

147. Snover SW, Bocchino V: Massive diltiazem overdose. Ann Emerg Med 1986;15:1221–1224.

148. Sorkin EM, Clissold SP, Brogden RN: Nifedipine: A review of its pharmacodynamic and pharmacokinetic properties and therapeutic efficacy in ischaemic heart disease, hypertension, and related cardiovascular disorders. Drugs 1985;30:182–274.

149. Sperelakis N: Cyclic AMP and phosphorylation in regulation of calcium influx into myocardial cells and blockade by calcium antagonist drugs. Am Heart J 1984;107:347–357.

150. Spiller HA, Meyers A, Ziemba T, Riley M: Delayed onset of cardiac arrhythmias from sustained-release verapamil. Ann Emerg Med 1991;20:201–203.

151. Sporer KA, Manning JJ: Massive ingestion of sustained-release verapamil with a concretion and bowel infarction. Ann Emerg Med 1993;22:603–605.

152. Spurlock BW, Virani NA, Henry CA: Verapamil overdose. West J Med 1991;154:208–211.

153. Stone CK, May WA, Carroll R: Treatment of verapamil overdose with glucagon in dogs. Ann Emerg Med 1995;25:369–374.

154. Sulakhe MV, Vox T: Regulation of phospholamban and troponin 1 phosphorylation in the intact rat cardiomyocytes by adrenergic and cholinergic stimuli: Roles of cyclic nucleotides, calcium, protein kinases, and phosphatases and depolarization. Mol Cell Biochem 1995;149–150:103–126.

155. Taira N: Differences in cardiovascular profile among calcium antagonists. Am J Cardiol 1987;59:24B–29B.

156. Tenenbein M, Cohen S, Sitar DS: Whole-bowel irrigation as a decontamination procedure after acute drug overdose. Arch Intern Med 1987;147:905–907.

157. Tenenbein M, Honcharik N, Roberts D, Sitar DS: Pharmacokinetics of massive diltiazem overdose and effects of multiple dose charcoal therapy [abstract]. Vet Human Tox 1989;31:335.

158. ter Wee PM, Kremer Hovinga TK, Uges DRA, van der Geest S: 4-Aminopyridine and haemodialysis in the treatment of verapamil intoxication. Hum Toxicol 1985;4:327–329.

159. Thomas SH, Stone K, May WA: Exacerbation of verapamil-induced hyperglycemia with glucagon. Am J Emerg Med 1995;13:27–29.

160. Thompson AM, Robbins, JP, Prescott JL: Changes in cardiorespiratory function during gastric lavage for drug overdose. Hum Toxicol 1987;6:215–218.

161. Tom PA, Morrow CT, Kelen GD: Delayed hypotension after overdose of sustained release verapamil. J Emerg Med 1994;12:621–625.

162. Underwood MJ, Firmin RK, Graham TR. Current concepts in the use of intra-aortic balloon counterpulsation. Br J Hosp Med 1993;50: 391–397.

163. Van den Berghe G, Wouters P, Weekers F, et al: Intensive insulin therapy in critically ill patients. N Engl J Med 2001;345:1359–1367.

164. Walter FG, Frye G, Mullen JT, Ekins BR, Khasigian PA: Amelioration of nifedipine poisoning associated with glucagon therapy. Ann Emerg Med 1993;22:1234–1237.

165. Watling SM, Crain JL, Edwards TD, Stiller RA: Verapamil overdose: Case report and review of the literature. Ann Pharmacother 1992;26:1373–1377.

166. Wax P: Intestinal infarction due to nifedipine overdose. J Toxicol Clin Toxicol 1995;33:725–728.

167. Welch RD, Todd K: Nifedipine overdose accompanied by ethanol intoxication in a patient with congenital heart disease. J Emerg Med 1990;8:169–172.

168. Wells TG, Graham CJ, Moss MM, Kearns GL: Nifedipine poisoning in a child. Pediatrics 1990;86:91–94.

169. Weiss AT, Lewis BS, Halon DA, Hasin Y, Gotsman M: The use of calcium with verapamil in the management of supraventricular tachyarrhythmias. Int J Cardiol 1983;4:275–280.

170. Whitebloom D, Fitzharris J: Nifedipine overdose. Clin Cardiol 1988; 11:505–506.

171. Winegrad S: Calcium release from cardiac sarcoplasmic reticulum. Ann Rev Physiol 1982;44:451–462.

172. Woie L, Storstein L: Successful treatment of suicidal verapamil poisoning with calcium gluconate. Eur Heart J 1981;2:239–242.

173. Wolf LR, Spadafora MP, Otten EJ: Use of amrinone and glucagon in a case of calcium channel blocker overdose. Ann Emerg Med 1993; 22:1225–1228.

174. Yagami T: Differential coupling of glucagon and beta-adrenergic receptors with the small and large forms of the stimulatory G protein. Mol Pharmacol 1995;48:849–854.

175. Yeh JZ, Oxford GS, Wu CH: Interactions of aminopyridines with potassium channels of squid axon membranes. Biophys J 1976;16: 77–81.

176. Yuan TH, Kerns WP, Tomaszewski CA, et al: Insulin-glucose as adjunctive therapy for severe calcium channel antagonist poisoning. J Toxicol Clin Toxicol 1999;37:463–474.

177. Yust I, Hoffman M, Aronson RJ: Life-threatening bradycardic reactions due to beta blocker-diltiazem interactions. Isr J Med Sci 1992;28:292–294.

178. Zaloga GP, Malcolm D, Holaday J, Chernow B: Glucagon reverses the hypotension and bradycardia of verapamil overdose in rats [abstract]. Vet Hum Toxicol 1985;13:273.

179. Zaritsky AL, Horowitz M, Chernow B: Glucagon antagonism of calcium channel blocker-induced myocardial dysfunction. Crit Care Med 1988;16:246–251.

CHAPTER 51

MISCELLANEOUS ANTIHYPERTENSIVES

Francis De Roos

Clonidine   Methyldopa   Guanabenz

Case 1 A 2-year-old male was brought to the emergency department lethargic and difficult to arouse. The patient had no significant medical history, but shortly before this event he was playing with a bottle of clonidine tablets. Physical examination revealed a lethargic but well-developed child whose initial vital signs were blood pressure, 110/70 mm Hg; heart rate, 55 beats/min at rest and 80 beats/min with stimulation; respiratory rate, 16–20 breaths/min with intermittent deep, sighing respirations; and temperature, 36.6°C (97.9°F). The head and neck examination was significant for 2-mm pupils that were slightly reactive to light. Lung and abdominal examinations were normal. Heart examination was notable for a regular bradycardia. Neurologic evaluation revealed a somnolent male with poor muscle tone and slight hyporeflexia. The gag reflex was intact. Of note, the patient became much more active, and at times agitated, with tactile stimulation, and he had strong purposeful movements when intravenous access was initiated.

Supplemental oxygen and intravenous doses of naloxone at 0.5 mg initially followed by a second dose of 1.5 mg were administered without clinical response. Activated charcoal (12.5 g) was given via nasogastric tube. An electrocardiogram (ECG) revealed sinus bradycardia at a rate of 60 beats/min with no conduction abnormalities. Laboratory tests included an arterial blood gas of pH 7.36, P_{CO_2} of 42 mm Hg, and P_{O_2} of 113 mm Hg. The patient was admitted to the pediatric intensive care unit for close observation and cardiac monitoring. Over the next 16 hours the patient's blood pressure remained stable, his heart rate increased to 90 beats/min, and his mental status returned to normal.

As our understanding of the medical complications of chronic hypertension has grown together with our understanding of how controlling this silent killer improves long-term morbidity and mortality, the list of available antihypertensive drugs has become extensive. Two of the most commonly used classes of antihypertensives, β-adrenergic antagonists and calcium channel blockers, were discussed in Chaps. 49 and 50, but numerous other agents are also marketed in the United States to control chronic hypertension and are discussed here.

Although overdoses involving these agents are rarely reported either because of limited use (e.g., the older agents such as reserpine, trimethaphan, and methyldopa) or limited toxicity (such as diuretics and angiotensin-converting enzyme inhibitors), poisoning does occur. Most of the adverse effects and toxicity in overdose are exaggerated pharmacologic effects. This chapter explores a variety of antihypertensive agents, their pharmacologic effects, their clinical effects in overdose, and overdose management recommendations.

CLONIDINE AND OTHER CENTRALLY ACTING ANTIHYPERTENSIVE AGENTS

Clonidine is an imidazoline compound that was synthesized in the early 1960s. Because of its potent α_2-adrenergic agonist effects, it was initially studied as a potential topical nasal decongestant. However, hypotension was a common side effect, which redirected its consideration for other therapeutic applications.[80] Clonidine is the best understood and the most commonly used of all the centrally acting antihypertensive agents. The other agents include methyldopa, guanfacine, and guanabenz. Whereas these drugs differ chemically and structurally, they all decrease blood pressure in a similar manner by reducing the sympathetic outflow from the central nervous system. Other imidazoline compounds, oxymetazoline and tetrahydrozoline, which are used as ocular topical vasoconstrictors and decongestants, produce similar systemic effects when ingested (Chap. 35).

Over the past 20 years, the increased efficacy and improved side-effect profiles of the newer antihypertensives have diminished the use of the α_2-adrenergic agonists in routine hypertension management. However, a variety of new applications for clonidine have been promoted, including migraine headache prophylaxis, attention deficit/hyperactivity disorder management, and management of opioid, ethanol, and nicotine withdrawal.[62,63,84,86,96] Although clonidine is a relatively uncommon exposure, it causes significant toxicity, particularly in children. One report from 2 large pediatric hospitals identified 47 children requiring hospitalization for clonidine ingestions over a 5-year period.[207]

Pharmacology and Pharmacokinetics

Clonidine is well absorbed from the gastrointestinal tract (approximately 75%) with an onset of action of 30–60 minutes and a peak effect at 2–3 hours, lasting as long as 8 hours.[43] It is widely distributed to all tissues including the brain, with 20–40% protein binding, and with an apparent volume of distribution of 3.2–5.6 L/kg.[118] Clonidine is predominantly eliminated unchanged via the kidneys.[118]

Guanfacine and guanabenz are structurally and pharmacologically very similar. They are well absorbed orally, achieving peak levels within 3–5 hours, and have large volumes of distribution (4–6 L/kg for guanfacine, 7–17 L/kg for guanabenz).[83,184] Guanabenz is metabolized predominantly in the liver and undergoes extensive first-pass effect, whereas guanfacine is eliminated equally by the liver and kidney.[83,184] Neither drug has significant active metabolites.

While clonidine, guanabenz, and guanfacine are all active agents with direct α_2-adrenergic agonist effects, methyldopa is a prodrug. It enters the central nervous system (CNS), probably by an active transport mechanism, before it is converted into its pharmacologically active degradation products.[18] α-Methylnorepinephrine is the most significant of the metabolites, although α-methyldopamine and α-methylepinephrine may also be important.[53,75,166] These metabolites are direct α_2-adrenergic agonists and exert their hypotensive effect in the same manner as the other centrally acting antihypertensives. Approximately 50% of an oral dose of methyldopa is absorbed, and peak serum levels are achieved in 2–3 hours.[135] However, because methyldopa must be metabolized into its active form, these serum levels have little correlation with its clinical effects. Methyldopa has a small volume of distribution (0.24 L/kg) with little protein binding (15%).[135] It is eliminated in the urine, both as parent compound and after hepatic sulfation.[141]

Clonidine is available in both oral and patch forms. The patch, referred to as the clonidine transdermal therapeutic system (TTS), allows slow, continuous delivery of drug over a prolonged period of time, typically 1 week. Similar delivery systems are effective in management of chronic pain with fentanyl and in the cessation of smoking tobacco with nicotine. This formulation, however, offers new challenges to the medical toxicologist. Each patch contains significantly more drug than is delivered. The patch that delivers 0.1 mg/d of clonidine contains 2.5 mg total, while the 0.3-mg/d product contains 7.5 mg.[25] Even after 1 week of use, between 35% and 50%, and in some instances, as much as 70%, of the drug remains in the patch.[25,73] Puncturing the outer membrane layer or backing opens the drug reservoir and allows significant drug to be released rapidly. In addition, many patients may not perceive this TTS as a medication and discard it in open wastebaskets. This is an invitation for toddlers, who often are fascinated with stickers and other adhesive objects, to remove an improperly disposed of patch and apply, chew, taste, or ingest it. Numerous reports of significant toxicity from dermal exposure, mouthing, or ingesting one clonidine patch emphasize this point.[25,33,70,73,76,99,161]

Pathophysiology

Clonidine and the other centrally acting antihypertensives exert their hypotensive effects primarily via stimulation of α-adrenergic receptors in the brain.[100,154] This central α-adrenergic receptor agonism enhances the activity of inhibitory neurons in the vasoregulatory regions of the CNS, notably the nucleus tractus solitarius in the medulla, resulting in decreased sympathetic outflow from the intermediolateral cell columns of the thoracolumbar spinal tracts into the periphery.[1,198] This sympathetic attenuation reduces heart rate, vascular tone, and ultimately arterial blood pressure.[155,210]

One area of controversy is the precise cellular location of the α-adrenergic receptors that are activated by clonidine. Although compelling arguments are published favoring both presynaptic and postsynaptic effects, it appears that they are in fact, postsynaptic.[117,199] When the central presynaptic pathways and receptors are destroyed or inactivated with various compounds, there is little influence on the hypotensive effects of clonidine.[100] Therefore, it appears that these α_2-adrenergic receptors are located postsynaptically.

In therapeutic oral dosing, clonidine and the other centrally acting antihypertensives have little effect on the peripheral α receptors, the peripheral sympathetic nervous system, or the normal circulatory responses seen with exercise or with Valsalva maneuvers.[134,145] In overdose or with intravenous administration, peripheral α-adrenergic stimulation can occur, causing increased norepinephrine release, thus producing vasoconstriction and hypertension.[31,137] This hypertension is short-lived, however, as the potent centrally mediated sympathetic inhibition of clonidine becomes overwhelming and hypotension ensues.[4,41,110,122] In addition, other imidazoline compounds, including oxymetazoline and tetrahydrozoline, which are used topically in the eye as vasoconstrictors, produce similar systemic toxicity when ingested[78] (Chap. 35).

Recently, imidazoline-specific binding sites have been identified in the ventrolateral medulla of the brain and in other tissues.[191] Direct stimulation of these receptors appears to lower blood pressure independently of central α_2-adrenergic effects.[19] In addition, a class of endogenous compounds, termed clonidine-displacing substances, has been found.[162] Although their significance is not yet known, these may become targets of new antihypertensive drug therapy.[80]

Clinical Manifestations

The signs and symptoms of poisoning with any centrally acting antihypertensive are variable but reflect an exaggeration of their pharmacologic action. Although the majority of the published cases involve clonidine, all these agents produce similar toxicity especially to the CNS and cardiovascular system. Common signs include CNS depression, bradycardia, hypotension, and, occasionally, hypothermia.[6,152,178,195] Most patients who ingest clonidine or the other similarly acting agents manifest symptoms rapidly, typically within 30–90 minutes.[207] The exception may be methyldopa, which requires metabolism before it is active. This may delay toxicity until several hours postingestion.[178,212]

CNS depression is the most frequent complication and can vary from mild lethargy to somnolence, stupor, or coma.[33,68,121,122,131,133,139,144,160] In addition, severely obtunded patients may suffer from decreased ventilatory effort and hypoxia.[4] Respirations may be slow and shallow with intermittent deep sighing breaths. Various terms have been used to describe this phenomenon including shallow, gasping, or Cheyne-Stokes respirations or periodic apnea.[6,10,99,122,123] This hypoventilation is typically responsive to tactile stimuli alone although endotracheal intubation may be required in severe cases.[4,6,77,99,131] The associated CNS depression typically resolves over 12–36 hours[10,74,144] although prolonged coma may rarely occur.[151] Other manifestations of CNS depression include hypotonia, hyporeflexia, and irritability.[31,122,186] The cranial nerve examination often demonstrates miotic pupils that may remain reactive to light.[4,6,147,189] Two unusual case reports describe seizures in the setting of clonidine poisoning.[87,119] The mechanism for producing these seizures is unclear.

Hypothermia is associated with overdoses involving centrally acting antihypertensives.[6,122,123,152] The hypothermia is thought to be due to α-adrenergic effects within the thermoregulatory center, although others suggest that these agents activate central serotonergic pathways which alter normal thermoregulation.[111,130] While this phenomenon may last several hours, it rarely requires treatment and responds well to passive rewarming.[31,152]

Sinus bradycardia may occur in up to 50% of ingestions.[186,207] Although sinus bradycardia is usually associated with hypotension, it may be an isolated finding. The exact mechanism responsible for it is not clearly defined, but plausible explanations include an exaggerated centrally mediated sympatholytic effect, a centrally mediated increase in vagal tone, or a direct stimulation of α₂-adrenergic receptors on the myocardium.[38,106,200,208]

Other conduction abnormalities, including first-degree heart block, Wenckebach and 2:1 second-degree atrioventricular block, and complete heart block, are described both from overdose as well as therapeutic dosing.[65,98,144,173,174,196,208] It appears that patients who have underlying sinus node dysfunction, concurrent sympatholytic drug therapy or renal insufficiency, and the very young are at greatest risk of developing sinus bradycardia and conduction delays.[23,186,192]

Hypotension is another hemodynamic manifestation of central antihypertensive toxicity,[6,25,131,144,186,207] which typically occurs within the first few hours after the exposure and represents profound inhibition of central sympathetic outflow.[55] Paradoxically, severe hypertension may be noted early in dosing or in massive overdoses.[4,41,87,110,122] This is the result of nonspecific peripheral α-adrenergic agonism resulting in norepinephrine release and vasoconstriction. Typically, the hypertensive effect is short-lived as the central sympatholytic effects become overwhelming.[87] However, in massive ingestions it can be protracted, requiring pharmacologic intervention.[4,41,122,186]

There is no clear association between the amount of any centrally acting antihypertensive ingested and the clinical manifestations. In children, clonidine ingestions as small as 0.2 mg have resulted in clinically severe poisoning.[144] Fatalities from any of these agents are extremely rare, with only a few published reports.[115,178]

In addition to the common clinical findings in overdose, these centrally acting antihypertensive agents also produce similar adverse effects with therapeutic dosing. Symptoms include drowsiness, depression, lightheadedness, dry mucous membranes, constipation, and sexual dysfunction.[49] In rare instances, hallucinations are reported,[21] and transdermal clonidine patch therapy may result in skin depigmentation.[42] While there was some concern about an association between patients with attention deficit hyperactivity disorder (ADHD) being treated with combination clonidine-methylphenidate therapy and sudden death, several well-designed studies, including an investigation by the Food and Drug Administration, concluded that there was inadequate evidence to confirm this association.[51,158]

Methyldopa has been associated with the highest incidence of adverse effects with therapeutic dosing, which explains its limited clinical use.[212] It is associated with a 10% incidence of a positive direct Coombs test; fatal hemolytic anemia is also reported.[26,209] Additionally, elevations in hepatic aminotransferases and clinical hepatitis are reported.[47,167]

Abrupt cessation of central antihypertensive therapy may result in withdrawal, which is characterized by excessive sympathetic activity. Symptoms include agitation, insomnia, tremor, palpitations, and hypertension, and present between 16 and 48 hours after cessation of therapy.[72,163,188] Ventricular tachycardia and myocardial infarction are associated with clonidine withdrawal.[16,136,153] The frequency and severity of symptoms appear to be greater in patients treated with higher doses for several months and in those with the most severe pretreatment hypertension.[163] However, cases occur even when the drug dosing is gradually reduced.[24,201] While these phenomena are associated with all centrally acting α₂-agonists, they appear to be most prominent from the shorter-acting agents such as clonidine and guanbenz.[6,22,159,211] The mechanism for these hyperadrenergic phenomena appear to involve an increase in CNS noradrenergic activity in the setting of decreased α₂-receptor sensitivity.[48] Reasonable treatment strategies include intravenous clonidine therapy followed by a closely monitored tapering of the dosing over several weeks or benzodiazepines. Animal and human data suggest that β-adrenergic antagonists, including labetalol, are harmful in the setting of clonidine withdrawal and their use is contraindicated.[9,94]

Diagnostic Testing

Clonidine and other centrally acting antihypertensives are not routinely included in typical serum or urine toxicologic assays. In addition, there is no evidence that quantitative serum clonidine levels correlate with clinical toxicity.[99] Therefore, management decisions should be based upon clinical parameters. No electrolyte or hematologic abnormalities are associated with this exposure. Because of the potential for bradydysrhythmias and hypoventilation, a 12-lead ECG and continuous cardiac and pulse oximetry monitoring are strongly recommended during the assessment.

Management

Appropriate therapy begins with particular focus on the patient's respiratory and hemodynamic status. Administration of activated charcoal is the primary mode of gastrointestinal decontamination. Emesis induced by syrup of ipecac is contraindicated because of the possibility for rapid deterioration in mental status. Orogastric lavage has limited utility because these agents are rapidly absorbed and patients often present following the onset of symptoms and respond well to supportive care. In cases involving clonidine patch ingestions, whole-bowel irrigation appears to be an effective intervention.[76]

All patients with CNS depression should be routinely evaluated for hypoxia and hypoglycemia. Respiratory compromise, including apnea, often responds well to simple auditory or tactile stimulation.[4,6,77,99] Significant arousal during preparation for intubation precluding any need for mechanical ventilation has been reported.[4] Endotracheal intubation may be required, however, for the most severely poisoned patients.

Naloxone was probably first used in clonidine poisoning because of the similarity in its clinical findings to opioid toxicity, namely CNS and respiratory depression and miosis. Although the interaction between clonidine and opioid receptors is poorly understood, several clonidine-poisoned patients have had significant arousal after naloxone administration, as well as increased respiratory effort, heart rate, and blood pressure.[10,103,138,140,189] Because of the short duration of effects from naloxone (20–60 minutes), redosing or a continuous naloxone infusion may be required. As with some synthetic opioids, such as propoxyphene and fentanyl, clinical improvement may occur only after high doses of naloxone (4–10 mg).[99] Some patients may have no response regardless of dosing.[11,121,207] Because of the paucity of clinical experience, it is unclear how efficacious naloxone may be in overdoses involving other α-adrenergic agents. In one adult with severe guanabenz poisoning, 7 mg of naloxone failed to improve her clinical status.[152] Rarely, naloxone administration in the setting of clonidine overdose may precipitate significant hypertension, so continuous hemodynamic monitoring is indicated.[99,207]

Bradycardia following a centrally acting α-adrenergic agonist ingestion may be mild and usually does not require any therapy if adequate peripheral perfusion exists. If the bradycardia is severe, however, standard doses of atropine are effective, but redosing may be required.[4,6,121,186] If bradycardia is associated with severe hypotension, dopamine may increase both heart rate and blood pressure.[6,66,121] Isolated hypotension should initially be treated with intravenous boluses of crystalloid. If ineffective, pressor support with a dopamine infusion is usually beneficial.[4,6,25]

Other authors recommend the use of α-adrenergic antagonists such as tolazoline as specific antidotes for patients with α-adrenergic agonist overdoses. Although some patients have had significant hemodynamic improvements,[131,144,172] tolazoline administration was ineffective in other patients.[4,186] An adult dose is 5–10 mg intravenous infusion every 15 minutes up to a total maximum of 40 mg.[31] Given that tolazoline treatment is variably successful and that most physicians are unfamiliar with this agent, it cannot be recommended in the primary management strategy for centrally acting antihypertensive poisoning. It should be considered only after tactile stimulation, naloxone, atropine, intravenous fluids, and dopamine have failed.

If the patient presents early or after a massive overdose, paradoxical hypertension may occur. It is typically self-limited and is routinely followed by profound hypotension. If severe or prolonged, then treatment with a short-acting antihypertensive such as sodium nitroprusside is appropriate.[122] Although oral nifedipine has been used,[41] its lack of titratability and its unpredictable efficacy make its use inappropriate.

OTHER SYMPATHOLYTIC ANTIHYPERTENSIVE AGENTS

In addition to the centrally acting α₂-adrenergic agonists such as clonidine, there are several other agents that exert their antihypertensive effect by decreasing the effects of the sympathetic nervous system. Often termed sympatholytics, they can be classified as either ganglionic-blocking agents, peripheral neuron-blocking agents, or α₁-adrenergic antagonists, depending on their mechanism of action. These agents are rarely used clinically and little is known about their effects in overdose.

Ganglionic-Blocking Agents

Ganglionic-blocking agents, such as trimethaphan, are extremely potent antihypertensive agents. They inhibit impulse transmission

down the postganglionic sympathetic, as well as parasympathetic, nerves, decreasing vascular tone, cardiac output, and blood pressure. These agents were used more frequently in the 1950s and 1960s in Europe, but because of their significant side effects, they were quickly replaced by other agents. These side effects stem from the unpredictable degree of sympathetic, as well as additional parasympathetic, blockade, and include paralytic ileus, constipation, urinary retention, impotence, dry mouth, and blurred vision.[141] Trimethaphan is the only ganglionic blocker available in the United States and it is administered intravenously. While there are no reported cases of intentional overdose reported, there are cases of cardiopulmonary arrest associated with administration of continuous doses or of a 10-fold pediatric dosing error of trimethaphan to treat a severe hypertensive crisis.[36,71] In overdose, the exaggerated hypotension should respond well to intravenous crystalloid boluses and a direct-acting vasopressor such as norepinephrine.

Peripheral Adrenergic Neuron-Blocking Agents

Guanethidine

These agents exert their sympatholytic action by decreasing norepinephrine release from the distal nerve terminals. Guanethidine and guanadrel interfere with the action potential triggering the release of norepinephrine,[176] while reserpine depletes norepinephrine and other catecholamines from the nerve end terminals, probably by direct binding and inactivation of catecholamine storage vesicles.[60] Adverse effects of these agents again limit their clinical utility. These effects include a high incidence of orthostatic and exercise-induced hypotension, diarrhea, increased gastric secretions, and impotence.[141] In addition, the hypotensive effects may be prolonged for as long as 1 week.[95,177] Because of its ability to cross the blood-brain barrier, reserpine may also deplete central catecholamines and produce drowsiness, extrapyramidal symptoms, hallucinations, or depression.[116] In overdose, an extension of the pharmacologic effects would be expected. Severe orthostatic hypotension should be anticipated and treated with intravenous crystalloid boluses and a direct-acting vasopressor. If reserpine is involved, significant CNS depression should be anticipated.[116]

Peripheral α₁-Adrenergic Antagonists

The fourth group of sympatholytic agents is the selective α₁-adrenergic antagonists, which include prazosin, terazosin, and doxazosin. The α₁ receptor is a postsynaptic receptor primarily located on vascular smooth muscle, although it is also found in the eye and in the gastrointestinal and genitourinary tracts.[34] In fact, this class of drugs provides first-line pharmacologic therapy for patients with urinary dysfunction secondary to benign prostatic hyperplasia. These drugs produce arterial smooth-muscle relaxation, vasodilation, and lowering of the blood pressure. Although better tolerated than ganglionic blockers and peripheral adrenergic neuron blockers, these agents may still produce significant symptoms of postural hypotension including lightheadedness, near syncope, and palpitations, particularly after the first dose or if the dosing is rapidly increased.[15] In overdose, hypotension and CNS depression ranging from lethargy to coma are reported.[109,113,125,171] In addition, priapism may occur.[113,164] Treatment with supportive care including intravenous fluid boluses and vasopressors such as dopamine was effective in the few overdose cases reported.[109,113,125]

DIRECT VASODILATORS

Nitroprusside

The direct vasodilators include hydralazine, minoxidil, diazoxide, and sodium nitroprusside. These drugs produce vascular smooth-muscle relaxation independent of innervation or known pharmacologic receptors.[44,101,102] This direct vasodilatory effect is related to alterations in smooth-muscle intracellular calcium ion homeostasis, most likely via cyclic guanosine monophosphate. Minoxidil exerts its vasodilatory effects by opening potassium channels and hyperpolarizing the smooth-muscle cell, making it less responsive to adrenergic effects.[107] As this vasodilation occurs, the baroreceptor reflexes, which remain intact, produce an increased sympathetic outflow to the myocardium, resulting in an increase in heart rate and contractile force. Typically, these agents are utilized in patients with severe, refractory hypertension and in conjunction with a β-adrenergic antagonist to diminish the reflex tachycardia. Hydralazine, minoxidil, and diazoxide are effective orally, whereas sodium nitroprusside is only used intravenously. Minoxidil is also used topically to promote hair growth in patients with male pattern baldness, and significant overdoses have occurred with this formulation.[129] Diazoxide, although previously used to rapidly reduce blood pressure in hypertensive emergencies, is rarely used for this indication now because of its poor titratability and its variable, and occasionally profound, hypotensive effect.[101]

Adverse effects associated with daily hydralazine use include several immunologic phenomena such as hemolytic anemia, vasculitis, acute glomerulonephritis, and most notably a lupuslike syndrome.[156] Minoxidil may cause electrocardiographic changes, both in therapeutic doses and in overdose, including sinus tachycardia, ST segment depressions, and T-wave inversions.[69,157,182] The significance of these changes is unknown; they typically resolve with either continued therapy or after other toxic manifestations resolve.[69,182]

In overdose, the toxic manifestations of these agents are an extension of their pharmacologic action. Symptoms may include lightheadedness, syncope, palpitations, and nausea.[3,120] Signs may be isolated to tachycardia alone,[88,157,182] or may include flushing or alterations in mental status depending upon the degree of hypotension.[129] Based on American Association of Poison Control Centers

annual poison data, it appears that in recent years, the majority of reported exposures to this class of agents involve the topical form of minoxidil[50] (see page 1752 and Chap. 116).

After appropriate gastrointestinal decontamination, routine supportive care with special consideration to maintaining adequate mean arterial pressure should be provided. If intravenous fluid boluses are insufficient, a peripherally acting vasopressor, such as norepinephrine or neosynephrine, is an appropriate next therapy. Catecholamines, such as dopamine and epinephrine, should be avoided to prevent an exaggerated myocardial response and tachycardia.

Sodium nitroprusside exerts its vasodilatory effects after being metabolized in the erythrocyte and then releasing the vasodilator nitric oxide, and 5 atoms of cyanide. Patients who have renal insufficiency, low thiosulfate stores (infant, malnourished, critically ill), or who are maintained on infusion rates greater than 3–4 mg/kg/min are at risk of developing cyanide toxicity.[35] Signs and symptoms of cyanide toxicity include an alteration in mental status, anion gap metabolic acidosis, and in late stages, hemodynamic instability. (For a complete discussion of cyanide see Chap. 98.)

DIURETICS

Antihypertensive diuretic agents can be divided into three main groups: (a) the thiazides and related compounds, including hydrochlorothiazide and chlorthalidone; (b) the loop diuretics, including furosemide, bumetanide, and ethacrynic acid; and (c) the potassium-sparing diuretics, including amiloride, triamterene, and spironolactone. Two other groups of diuretics—the carbonic anhydrase inhibitors, such as acetazolamide, and the osmotic diuretics, such as mannitol—are not used as antihypertensive agents.

The thiazides are a broad class of diuretics that share both a core benzothiadiazine structure and a similar function. Their diuretic effect involves inhibition of sodium and chloride reabsorption in the distal convoluted tubule. Loop diuretics, in contrast, inhibit the coupled transport of sodium, potassium, and chloride in the thick ascending limb of the loop of Henle. Although their exact antihypertensive mechanism is unclear, an increased urinary excretion of sodium, potassium, and magnesium results from their use. Potassium-sparing diuretics act either as aldosterone antagonists, such as spironolactone, or as renal epithelial sodium channel antagonists, such as triamterene, in the late distal tubule and collecting duct.[91]

The major toxicity associated with these agents is metabolic and occurs during chronic therapy or overuse.[206] Hyponatremia develops within 2 weeks of initiation of therapy in more than two-thirds of susceptible patients.[183] Patients who are elderly, female, malnourished, or using thiazides are at greatest risk.[8] With severe hyponatremia (<120 mEq/L) symptoms may include headache, nausea, vomiting, confusion, seizures, or coma. Pontine demyelination has been reported during correction of severe hyponatremia secondary to diuretic abuse[32] (Chap. 24).

Other electrolyte abnormalities associated with diuretic use include hypokalemia and hypomagnesemia, which raise the concern of precipitating ventricular dysrhythmias and sudden death. Diuretic use is an extremely controversial topic, with several excellent studies providing conflicting results.[17,54,148,179,180] Although it is unclear how great a risk, if any, diuretic use may be, it remains prudent to monitor and correct the patient's potassium levels.[82,179,205] This is particularly important for elderly patients, and for those patients who concomitantly use digoxin, in which setting hypokalemia is clearly associated with dysrhythmias.[20,187] Potassium-sparing diuretics may cause hyperkalemia, particularly in the presence of renal insufficiency.

Several unusual reactions are associated with diuretic use, including pancreatitis, cholecystitis, and hematologic abnormalities such as hypercoagulability, thrombocytopenia, and hemolytic anemia.[45,46,168,170,194,204] Impotence remains an underappreciated adverse effect of these agents.

Despite the widespread use of these agents, acute overdoses are distinctly rare.[112] Major signs and symptoms of acute overdose include gastrointestinal distress, brisk diuresis, possible hypovolemia, electrolyte abnormalities, and altered mental status.[112] Typically, the diuresis is short-lived because of the limited duration of effect and the rapid clearance of the majority of diuretics. Assessment should focus on fluid and electrolyte status, which should be corrected as needed. If hyperkalemia is unexpectedly discovered, consider an ingestion of a potassium-sparing agent or, more likely, an overdose of potassium supplements, which are frequently prescribed in conjunction with thiazides.[85,89] Altered mental status including coma may result from diuretic overdosage without evidence of any fluid or electrolyte abnormalities.[14,112,169] Postulated mechanisms include a direct drug effect or induction of transient cerebral ischemia.[142]

Case 2 A 56-year-old male complained of progressive lip and tongue swelling. The patient had a history of noninsulin-dependent diabetes mellitus and hypertension. His medications included aspirin, glyburide, and hydrochlorothiazide, and 3 weeks earlier he began a second antihypertensive agent. Physical examination revealed a well-appearing male in mild distress with obvious swelling of lips, face, and tongue. Initial vital signs were blood pressure, 154/88 mm Hg; heart rate, 90 beats/min; respiratory rate, 18 breaths/min; and temperature, 36.6°C (97.8°F). Head and neck examination was remarkable for marked swelling of lips, slight protrusion of tongue forcing the mouth open at rest, and left cheek swelling. Lung examination revealed no wheezes or rhonchi with good air movement. No stridor was noted, although his voice was muffled. Heart, abdominal, and neurologic examinations were unremarkable. A diagnosis of angiotensin-converting enzyme inhibitor–induced angioedema was made and a nasopharyngeal airway was immediately placed. Diphenhydramine (50 mg IV) and methylprednisolone (125 mg IV) were administered without significant improvement. Although the patient's upper airway was patent, the rapidity of the onset of such significant oropharyngeal swelling threatened his respiratory status. Topical anesthetics and systemic anxiolytics were used, and direct fiberoptic nasopharyngeal intubation was performed. The patient remained intubated for 36 hours. After the swelling had decreased, the patient tolerated extubation without difficulty. He was discharged from the hospital with specific instructions to discontinue his new antihypertensive, enalapril, and instead to substitute a replacement antihypertensive, verapamil.

ANGIOTENSIN-CONVERTING ENZYME INHIBITORS

Angiotensin-converting enzyme (ACE) inhibitors are among the most widely prescribed antihypertensive drugs. At the time of this writing there were 10 ACE inhibitors approved by the US Food and Drug Administration for the treatment of hypertension (Table 51–1). In general, these agents are well absorbed from the gastrointestinal tract, reaching peak serum levels within 1–4 hours. Enalapril and ramipril are prodrugs and require hepatic metabolism to produce their active forms. These agents are primarily eliminated via the kidneys.

All ACE inhibitors have a common core structure of a 2-methyl propanolol-L-proline moiety.[58] This structure binds directly to the active site of the angiotensin-converting enzyme, which is found in the lung and vascular endothelium. Binding blocks the conversion of angiotensin I to angiotensin II. Because angiotensin II is a potent vasoconstrictor and stimulant of aldosterone secretion, vasodilation, decreased peripheral vascular resistance, decreased blood pressure, increased cardiac output, and a relative increase in renal, cerebral, and coronary blood flow occur.[58] This hypotensive response may be severe in select patients after their initial dose, resulting in syncope and cardiac ischemia.[29,79] Patients with renovascular-induced hypertension and those who are mildly hypovolemic from concomitant diuretic use appear to be at greatest risk.[79] Overall, however, these agents are well tolerated and have a very low incidence of side effects. Some reported adverse effects include rash, dysgeusia, neutropenia, hyperkalemia, chronic cough, and angioedema.[40,58,190] Because of their interference with the renin-angiotensin system, ACE inhibitors are potential teratogens and should never be used by pregnant patients.[13]

ACE Inhibitor–Induced Angioedema

Angioedema is an inflammatory reaction in which there is increased capillary blood flow and permeability, resulting in an increase in interstitial fluid. If this process is confined to the

---

TABLE 51–1. Classification of Antihypertensive Agents Available in the United States

β-Adrenergic antagonists (Chap. 49)
Calcium channel blockers (Chap. 50)
Sympatholytics
    Central acting agents: α_2-adrenergic agonists
        Methyldopa, clonidine, guanabenz, guanfacine
    Ganglionic-blocking agents
        Trimethaphan
    Peripheral adrenergic neuron blocking agents
        Guanethidine, guanadrel, metyrosine, reserpine
    Peripheral α_1-adrenergic antagonists
        Prazosin, terazosin, doxazosin
Diuretics
    Thiazide
        Chlorothiazide, hydrochlorothiazide, chlorthalidone, indapamide, metolazone
    Loop diuretics
        Furosemide, bumetanide, ethacrynic acid, torsemide
    Potassium sparing
        Amiloride, spironolactone, triamterene
Vasodilators
    Hydralazine, minoxidil, diazoxide, nitroprusside
ACE inhibitors
    Captopril, benazepril, enalapril, fosinopril, lisinopril, moexipril, perindopril, quinapril, ramipril, trandolapril
Angiotensin II receptor antagonists
    Candesartan cilexetil, eprosartan, irbesartan, losartan, telmisartan, valsartan

superficial dermis, urticaria develops, whereas if the deeper layers of the dermis or subcutaneous tissue are involved, angioedema results. Angioedema most commonly involves the periorbital, perioral, or oropharyngeal tissues.[165] This swelling may progress rapidly over minutes and result in complete airway obstruction and death.[57,61,175] The pathogenesis of acquired angioedema involves multiple vasoactive substances including histamine, prostaglandin D_2, leukotrienes, and bradykinin. Angiotensin-converting enzyme not only converts angiotensin I to angiotensin II, but also metabolizes bradykinin and substance P into inactive products (Fig. 51–1). Thus, ACE inhibition results in elevations in bradykinin levels, which appears to be the primary cause of ACE inhibitor–induced angioedema, as well as of cough.[5,90] There is no evidence that this is an IgE-mediated phenomenon.[5]

Although the literature is replete with ACE inhibitor–induced angioedema, the overall incidence is only approximately 0.1%.[52,90,93,181] One-third of these reactions occur within hours of the first dose and another one-third within the first week.[181] It is important to remember that in the additional one-third of cases angioedema may occur at any time during therapy, even after years of therapy.[28] Patients with a history of idiopathic angioedema, and possibly atopy, may be at greater risk.[146] There does not appear to be any dose-response relationship.

Treatment varies depending upon the severity and rapidity of the swelling. Because of the propensity to involve the tongue, face, and oropharynx, the airway must remain the primary focus of management. A nasopharyngeal airway is often helpful. If there is any potential for, or suggestion of, airway compromise, endotracheal intubation should be performed. Severe tongue and oropharyngeal swelling may make orotracheal or nasotracheal intubation extremely difficult, if not impossible. If this occurs, fiberoptic nasal intubation may be an attractive option, provided the resources are available. Other techniques, including retrograde intubation over a guidewire previously passed through the cricothyroid membrane and emergent cricothyrotomy, should also be considered.[165]

Pharmacologic therapy for ACE inhibitor–induced angioedema should include standard agents used for anaphylaxis such as subcutaneous epinephrine, intravenous diphenhydramine, and corticosteroids. However, because this is not an antibody-mediated allergic phenomenon, these interventions may be ineffective.

All patients with mild or quickly resolving angioedema should be observed for several hours to assure that the swelling does not progress or return. Outpatient therapy with a short course of oral antihistamines and corticosteroids is appropriate. Such patients should be instructed to discontinue ACE inhibitor therapy permanently and to consult their primary physicians about other antihypertensive options. Because this is related to the mechanism of action of the drug and is not an allergic adverse effect, the use of any other ACE inhibitors is contraindicated.

ACE Inhibitor Overdose

The toxicity of ACE inhibitors in overdose appears to be limited.[30,81,114,185] Although several reports of overdoses involving ACE inhibitors have been published, the majority of the cases reported manifested toxicity of a coingestant.[37,67,92,193,205] Hypotension may occur in select patients,[12,105] but deaths are rarely reported in isolated ACE inhibitor ingestions.[149,203] Other patients may remain asymptomatic despite high serum drug levels.[108] Two studies suggest that unintentional pediatric exposures to adult therapeutic doses rarely produce any clinical effects.[81,185]

Treatment should focus on supportive care and on identifying any coingestants that may be more toxic, particularly other antihypertensives such as β-adrenergic antagonists and calcium channel blockers. Activated charcoal alone is sufficient gastrointestinal decontamination in most cases. Intravenous crystalloid boluses are often effective in correcting hypotension, although in rare cases, catecholamines may be required.[7]

Naloxone may also be effective in reversing the hypotensive effects of ACE inhibitors. ACE inhibitors may inhibit the metabo-

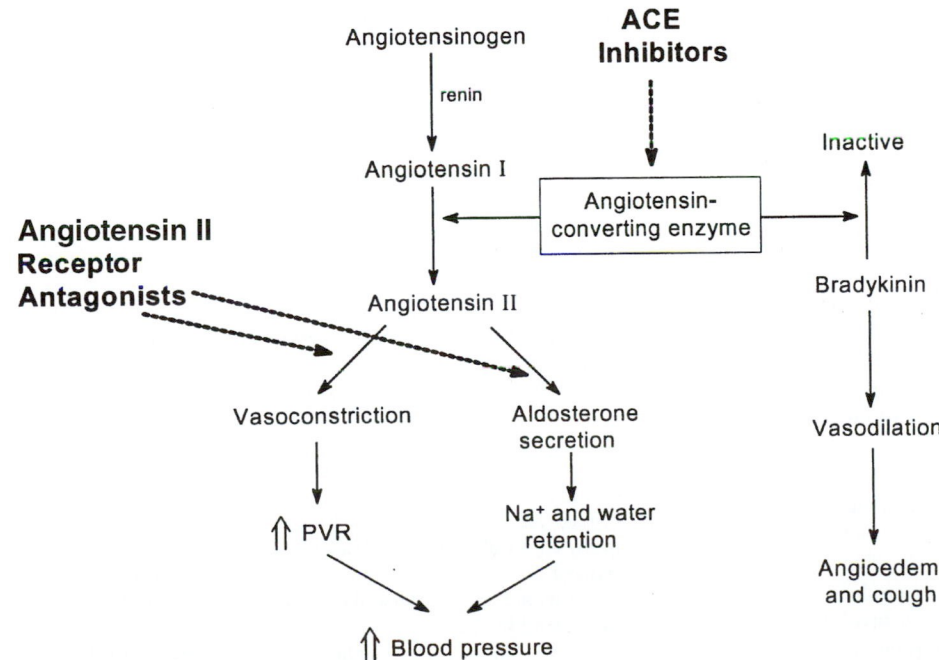

Figure 51–1. An overview of the normal function of angiotensin II and the mechanisms of action of angiotensin-converting enzyme inhibitors and the angiotensin II receptor antagonists. PVR = peripheral vascular resistance.

lism of enkephalins and may potentiate their opioid effects, which include lowering blood pressure.[39,132] In a controlled human volunteer study, continuous naloxone infusion effectively blunted the hypotensive response of captopril.[2] In one case report, naloxone appeared to be effective in reversing symptomatic hypotension secondary to a captopril overdose.[202] In another published case, naloxone was ineffective.[12] Although its role in the setting of ACE inhibitor overdose remains unclear, naloxone may obviate the need for large quantities of crystalloid or vasopressors and should therefore be utilized.

ANGIOTENSIN II RECEPTOR ANTAGONISTS

In 1995, a new class of antihypertensives named the angiotensin II receptor antagonists became available, and six members of this class are currently marketed in the United States. These drugs are rapidly absorbed in the gastrointestinal tract, reaching peak serum levels in 1–4 hours and they are either eliminated unchanged in the feces, or, after undergoing hepatic metabolism via the mixed function oxidase system, are eliminated in the bile.[124,126–128,143]

Although these agents are similar to ACE inhibitors in that they decrease the effects of angiotensin II, rather than decreasing the formation of angiotensin II, drugs antagonize angiotensin II at the type 1 angiotensin (AT-1) receptor[97] (Fig. 51–1). This allows the drugs to inhibit the vasoconstrictive and aldosterone promoting effects of angiotensin II without interfering with bradykinin degradation,[124] significantly reducing the adverse effects of cough and angioedema seen with ACE inhibitor therapy.[104,150] However, rare cases of angioedema associated with angiotensin II receptor antagonist therapy have been reported.[27,197] Although it is clear that these agents have an improved adverse effect profile because they do not affect bradykinin metabolism, there is a potential concern that this may make them less effective antihypertensives, or may limit, or even eliminate, the renal and cardioprotective effects associated with ACE inhibitors.[56]

Like ACE inhibitors, angiotensin II receptor antagonists should never be used by pregnant patients because of their teratogenic potential.[13] In addition, approximately 0.5–1% of patients develop first-dose orthostatic hypotension.[64]

There are no published reports of overdoses involving these agents but hypotension should be anticipated and treated with intravenous crystalloid therapy and traditional catecholamines.

SUMMARY

Numerous medications are currently marketed for the treatment of chronic hypertension, including centrally acting agents, other sympatholytics, direct vasodilators, diuretics, ACE inhibitors, and angiotensin II receptor antagonists. Although none are typically associated with severe poisonings either because of limited use, as with many of the sympatholytics and direct vasodilators, or because of limited toxicity, as with diuretics, ACE inhibitors, and angiotensin II receptor antagonists, severe poisonings have and will probably continue to occur. While centrally acting agents, such as the α_2 agonist clonidine, may produce significant CNS depression and bradycardia, most of these agents produce hypotension in overdose. Management of ingestions involving these antihypertensive agents should focus on appropriate gastrointesti-

nal decontamination, typically, oral activated charcoal, and hemodynamic monitoring and support with intravenous crystalloids and catecholamines. Naloxone may be used in clonidine- and ACE inhibitor–poisoned patients, but its efficacy is variable.

REFERENCES

1. Abrams WB: In summary: Satellite symposium on central α-adrenergic blood pressure regulating mechanisms. Hypertension 1984;6 (Suppl II):87–93.
2. Ajayi AA, Campbell BC, Rubin PC, Reid JL: Effect of naloxone on the actions of captopril. Clin Pharmacol Ther 1985;38:560–565.
3. Allon M, Hall WD, Macon EJ: Prolonged hypotension after initial minoxidil dose. Arch Intern Med 1986;146:2075–2076.
4. Anderson FJ, Hart GR, Crumpler CP, Lerman MJ: Clonidine overdose: Report of six cases and review of the literature. Ann Emerg Med 1981;10:107–112.
5. Anderson MW, deShazo RD: Studies of the mechanism of ACE inhibitor-associated angioedema: The effect of an ACE inhibitor on cutaneous responses to bradykinin, codeine, and histamine. J Allergy Clin Immunol 1990;85:856–858.
6. Artman M, Boerth RC: Clonidine poisoning. Am J Dis Child 1983; 137:171–174.
7. Augenstein WL, Kulig KW, Rumack BH: Captopril overdose resulting in hypotension. JAMA 1988;259:3302–3305.
8. Baglin A, Boulard JC, Hanslink T, Prinseau J: Metabolic adverse reactions to diuretics. Drug Saf 1995;12:161–167.
9. Bailey RR, Neale TJ: Rapid clonidine withdrawal with blood pressure overshoot exaggerated by beta-blockade. Br Med J 1976;1: 942–943.
10. Bamshad MJ, Wasserman GS: Pediatric clonidine intoxications. Vet Hum Toxicol 1990;32:220–223.
11. Banner WJR, Lund ME, Clawson L: Failure of naloxone to reverse clonidine toxic effect. Am J Dis Child 1983;137:1170–1171.
12. Barr CS, Payne R, Newton RW: Profound prolonged hypotension following captopril overdose. Postrgrad Med J 1991;67:953–954.
13. Barr M Jr: Teratogen update: Angiotensin-converting enzyme inhibitors. Teratology 1994;50:399–409.
14. Bass JW, Beisel WR: Coma due to acute chlorothiazide intoxication. Am J Dis Child 1973;106:620–623.
15. Bendall MJ, Baloch KH, Wilson PB: Side effects due to treatment of hypertension with prazosin. Br Med J 1975;2:727–729.
16. Berge KH, Lanier WL: Myocardial infarction accompanying acute clonidine withdrawal in a patient without a history of ischemic coronary artery disease. Anesth Analg 1991;72:259–261.
17. Bigger TJ: Diuretic therapy, hypertension, and cardiac arrest. N Engl J Med 1994;330:1899–1900.
18. Bobik A, Jennings G, Jackman G, et al: Evidence for a predominantly central hypotensive effect of alpha-methyldopa in humans. Hypertension 1986;8:16–23.
19. Bousquet P, Feldman J, Tibirica E, et al: A new concept in central regulation of the arterial blood pressure. Am J Hypertens 1992;4: 47S–50S.
20. Brater DC, Morrelli HF: Digoxin toxicity in patients with normokalaemic potassium depletion. Clin Pharmacol Ther 1978;22: 21–33.
21. Brown MJ: Clonidine hallucinations. Ann Intern Med 1980;93: 456–457.
22. Burden AC, Alexander CPT: Rebound hypertension after acute methyldopa withdrawal. Br Med J 1976;2:1056–1057.
23. Byrd BF III, Collins HW, Primm RK: Risk factors for severe bradycardia during oral clonidine therapy for hypertension. Arch Intern Med 1988;148:729–733.
24. Cairns SA, Marshall AJ: Clonidine withdrawal. Lancet 1976;1:368.

25. Caravati EM, Bennett DL: Clonidine transdermal patch poisoning. Ann Emerg Med 1988;17:175–176.

26. Carstairs KC, Brechenridge A, Dollery CT, Worlledge SM: Incidence of a positive direct Coombs test in patients on alpha-methyldopa. Lancet 1966;2:133–135.

27. Cha YJ, Pearson VE: Angioedema due to losartan. Ann Pharmacother 1999;33:936–938.

28. Chin HL, Buchan DA: Severe angioedema after long-term use of an angiotensin-converting enzyme inhibitor. Ann Intern Med 1990;112:312–313.

29. Cleland JGF, Dargie HJ, McAlpine, et al: Severe hypotension after first dose of enalapril in heart failure. Br Med J 1985;291:1309–1312.

30. Cobaugh DJ, Everson GW, Normann SA, et al: Angiotensin-converting enzyme inhibitor overdoses: A multi-centre study. Vet Hum Toxicol 1990;32:352.

31. Conner CS, Watanabe AS: Clonidine overdose: A review. Am J Hosp Pharm 1979;36:906–911.

32. Copeland PM: Diuretic abuse and central pontine myelinolysis. Psychother Psychosom 1989;52:101–105.

33. Corneli HM, Banner WW, Vernon DD, Swenson PH: Toddler eats clonidine patch and nearly quits smoking for life. JAMA 1989;261:42.

34. Cubeddu LX: New alpha-1-adrenergic receptor antagonists for the treatment of hypertension: Role of vascular alpha receptors in the control of peripheral resistance. Am Heart J 1988;116:133–162.

35. Curry SC, Arnold-Capell P: Nitroprusside, nitroglycerin, and angiotensin-converting enzyme inhibitors. Crit Care Clin 1991;7:555–581.

36. Dale RC, Schroeder ET: Respiratory paralysis during treatment of hypertension with trimethaphan camsylate. Arch Intern Med 1976;126:816–818.

37. Dawson AH, Harvey D, Smith AJ, et al: Lisinopril overdose. Lancet 1990;335:487–488.

38. De Jonge A, Timmermans PB, van Zwieten PA: Qualitative aspects of α-adrenergic effects induced by clonidine-like imidazolines: II. Central and peripheral bradycardia activities. J Pharmacol Exp Ther 1982;222:712–719.

39. Di Nicolantonia R, Hutchinson JS, Takata Y, Veroni M: Captopril potentiates the vasodepressor action of metenkephalin in anaesthetised dogs. Br J Pharmacol 1983;80:405–408.

40. DiBianco R: Adverse reactions with angiotensin converting enzyme (ACE) inhibitors. Med Toxicol 1986;1:122–141.

41. Dire DJ, Kuhns DW: The use of sublingual nifedipine in a patient with a clonidine overdose. J Emerg Med 1988;6:125–128.

42. Doe N, Seth S, Hebert LA: Skin depigmentation related to transdermal clonidine therapy. Arch Intern Med 1995;155:2129.

43. Dollery CT, Davies DS, Draffan GH, et al: Clinical pharmacology and pharmacokinetics of clonidine. Clin Pharmacol Ther 1976;19:11–17.

44. DuCharme DW, Freyburger WA, Graham BE, Carlson RG: Pharmacologic properties of minoxidil: A new hypertensive agent. J Pharmacol Exp Ther 1973;184:662–670.

45. Eckhauser ML, Dokler MA, Imbembo AL: Diuretic-associated pancreatitis: A collective review and illustrative cases. Am J Gastroenterol 1987;82:865–870.

46. Eisner EV, Crowell EB: Hydrochlorothiazide-dependent thrombocytopenia due to IgM antibodies. JAMA 1971;215:480–482.

47. Elkington SG, Schreiber WM, Conn HO: Hepatic injury caused by L-alpha-methyldopa. Circulation 1969;40:589–590.

48. Engberg G, Elam M, Svensson TH: Clonidine withdrawal: Activation of brain noradrenergic neurons with specifically reduced alpha-2-receptor sensitivity. Life Sci 1982;30:235–243.

49. Engelman K: Side effects of sympatholytic antihypertensive drugs. Hypertension 1988;11(Suppl II):30–33.

50. Farrell SE, Epstein SK: Overdose of Rogaine Extra Strength for Men topical minoxidil preparation. J Toxicol Clin Toxicol 1999;37:781–783.

51. Fenichel RR: Post-marketing surveillance identifies three case of sudden death in children during treatment with clonidine and methylphenidate. J Child Adolesc Psychopharmacol 1995;5:157–166.

52. Finley CJ, Silverman MA, Nunez AE: Angiotensin-converting enzyme inhibitor-induced angioedema: Still unrecognized. Am J Emerg Med 1992;10:550–552.

53. Freed CR, Quintero E, Murphy RC: Hypotension and hypothalamic amine metabolism after long-term alpha-methyldopa infusions. Life Sci 1978;23:313–322.

54. Freis ED: Adverse effects of diuretics. Drug Saf 1992;7:364–373.

55. Frohlich ED, Messerli FH, Pegram BL, Kardon MB: Hemodynamic and cardiac effects of centrally acting antihypertensive drugs. Hypertension 1984;6(Suppl II):76–81.

56. Gainer JV, Morrow JD, Loveland A, et al: Effect of bradykinin-receptor blockade on the response to angiotensin-converting-enzyme inhibitor in normotensive and hypertensive subjects. N Engl J Med 1998;339:1285–1292.

57. Gannon TH, Eby Tl: Angiocdema for angiotensin-converting enzyme inhibitors: A cause of upper airway obstruction. Laryngoscope 1990;100:1156–1160.

58. Gavras H, Gavras I: Angiotensin-converting enzyme inhibitors. Properties and side effects. Hypertension 1988;11(Suppl II):37–41.

59. Geyskes GG, Boer P, Dorhout MEJ: Clonidine withdrawal: Mechanism and frequency of rebound hypertension. Br J Clin Pharmacol 1979;7:55–62.

60. Giachetti A, Shore PA: The reserpine receptor. Life Sci 1978;23:89–92.

61. Giannoccaro PJ, Wallace GJ, Higginson LAJ, et al: Fatal angioedema associated with enalapril. Can J Cardiol 1989;5:335–336.

62. Glassman AH, Steiner F, Walsh BT, et al: Heavy smokers, smoking cessation, and clonidine. JAMA 1988;259:2863–2866.

63. Gold MS, Pottash AC, Sweeney DR, Kleber HD: Opiate withdrawal using clonidine. A safe, effective and rapid nonopiate treatment. JAMA 1980;243:343–346.

64. Goldberg AJ, Dunlay MC, Sweet CS: Safety and tolerability of losartan potassium, an angiotensin II receptor antagonist, compared with hydrochlorothiazide, atenolol, felodipine ER, and angiotensin-converting enzyme inhibitors for the treatment of systemic hypertension. Am J Cardiol 1995;75:793–795.

65. Golusinski CL, Blount BW: Clonidine-induced bradycardia. J Fam Pract 1995;41:399–401.

66. Grabert B: Clonidine: Recurrent apnea following overdose. DICP 1979;13:1778–1780.

67. Graham SR, Day RO, Hardy M: Captorpril overdose. Med J Aust 1989;151:111.

68. Hall AH, Smolinske SC, Kulig KW, Rumack BH: Guanabenz overdose. Ann Intern Med 1985;102:787–788.

69. Hall D, Charocopos F, Froer K-L, Rudolph W: ECG changes during long-term minoxidil therapy for severe hypertension. Arch Intern Med 1979;139:790–794.

70. Hamblin JE, Martin CA: Transdermal patch poisoning. Pediatrics 1987;79:161.

71. Hammer GB: Ultra-high dose trimethaphan in an infant with severe hypertension. Clin Toxicol 1996;34:227–229.

72. Hansson L: Clinical aspects of blood pressure crisis due to withdrawal of centrally acting antihypertensive drugs. Br J Clin Pharmacol 1983;15:485–490.

73. Harris JM: Clonidine patch toxicity. DICP 1990;24:1191–1194.

74. Heidemann SM, Sarnaik AP: Clonidine poisoning in children. Crit Care Med 1990;18:618–620.

75. Henning M, Rubenson A: Evidence that the hypotensive action of alpha-methyl-DOPA is mediated by central actions of methylnoradrenaline. J Pharm Pharmacol 1971;23:407–411.

76. Henretig F, Wiley J, Brown L: Clonidine patch toxicity: The proof is in the poop [abstract]. J Toxicol Clin Toxicol 1995;33:520.

77. Henretig F. Clonidine and central acting antihypertensives. In: Ford M, Delaney DA, Ling L, Erickson T, eds: Clincal Toxicology. Philadelphia, WB Saunders, 2001, pp. 391–396.

78. Higgins GL, Campbell B, Wallace K, et al: Pediatric poisoning from over-the-counter imidazoline-containing products. Ann Emerg Med 1991;20:655–658.

79. Hodsman GP, Isles CG, Murray GD, et al: Factors related to first-dose hypotensive effect of captopril: Prediction and treatment. Br Med J 1993;286:832–834.

80. Hoffman BB, Lefkowitz RJ: Catecholamines, sympathomimetic drugs, and adrenoceptor antagonists. In: Hardman JG, Limbird LE, Molinoff PB, Ruddon RW, eds: Goodman and Gilman's The Pharmacological Basis of Therapeutics, 9th ed. New York, McGraw-Hill, 1996, pp. 199–248.

81. Hogue-Murray K, Horowitz R, Dart RC: Outcome of ACE inhibitor ingestion in children under the age of six years [abstract]. J Toxicol Clin Toxicol 1995;33:509.

82. Holland OB, Nixon JV, Kuhnet L: Diuretic induced ventricular ectopic activity. Am J Med 1981;70:762–765.

83. Holmes B, Brogden RN, Heel RC: Guanabenz. A review of its pharmacodynamic properties and therapeutic efficacy in hypertension. Drugs 1983;26:212–229.

84. Hughes PL, Morse RM: Use of clonidine in a mixed drug detoxification regimen: Possibility of masking of clinical signs of sedative withdrawal. Mayo Clin Proc 1985;60:47–49.

85. Hume L, Forfar JC: Hyperkalaemia and overdose of antihypertensive agents. Lancet 1977;2:1182.

86. Hunt RD, Minderaa RB, Cohen DJ: Clonidine benefits children with attention deficit disorder and hyperactivity: Report of a double-blind placebo-crossover therapeutic trial. J Am Acad Child Psychiatry 1985;24:617–629.

87. Hunyor SN, Bradstock K, Somerville PJ, Lucas N: Clonidine overdose. Br Med J 1975;4:23.

88. Iles C, Mackay A, Barton PJM, Mitchell I: Accidental overdose of minoxidil in a child. Lancet 1981;1:97.

89. Illingworth RN, Proudfoot AT: Rapid poisoning with slow-release potassium. Br Med J 1980;2:485–486.

90. Israili ZH, Hall WD: Cough and angioneurotic edema associated with angiotensin-converting enzyme inhibitor therapy. Ann Intern Med 1992;117:234–242.

91. Jackson EK: Diuretics. In: Hardman JG, Limbird LE, Molinoff PB, Ruddon RW, eds: Goodman and Gilman's The Pharmacological Basis of Therapeutics, 9th ed. New York, McGraw-Hill, 1996, pp. 199–248.

92. Jackson T, Corke C, Agar J: Enalapril overdosage treated with angiotensin infusion. Lancet 1993;341:703.

93. Jett KG: Captopril-induced angioedema. Ann Emerg Med 1984;13:489–490.

94. Jonkman FA, Man PW, Breurkes R, van Zwieten PA: Beta-2-adrenoceptor antagonists intensify clonidine withdrawal syndrome in conscious rats. J Cardiovasc Pharmacol 1989;14:886–891.

95. Kalmanovitch DV, Hardwick PB: Hypotension after guanethidine block. Anaesthesia 1988;43:256.

96. Kallanranta T, Hakkarainen H, Kokkanen E, et al: Clonidine in migraine prophylaxis. Headache 1977;17:169–172.

97. Kang PM, Landau AJ, Eberhardt RT, Frishman WH: Angiotensin II receptor antagonists: A new approach to blockade of the renin-angiotensin system. Am Heart J 1994;127:1388–1401.

98. Kibler LE, Gazes PC: Effect of clonidine on atrioventricular conduction. JAMA 1977;238:1930–1932.

99. Knapp JF, Fowler MA, Wheeler CA, Wasserman GS: Case 01–1995: A two-year-old female with alteration of consciousness. Ped Emerg Care 1995;11:62–65.

100. Kobinger W: Central α-adrenergic systems as target for hypotensive drugs. Rev Physiol Biochem Pharmacol 1978;81:39–75.

101. Koch-Weser J: Diazoxide. N Engl J Med 1976;294:1271–1274.

102. Koch-Weser J: Hydralazine. N Engl J Med 1976;295:320–323.

103. Kulig K, Duffy J, Rumack BH, et al: Naloxone for treatment of clonidine overdose. JAMA 1982;247:1697.

104. Lacourciere Y, Lefebvre J, Nakhle G, et al: Association between cough and angiotensin-converting enzyme inhibitors versus angiotensin II antagonists: The design of a prospective, controlled study. J Hypertens 1994;12:S49–S53.

105. Lau CP: Attempted suicide with enalapril. N Engl J Med 1986;315:197.

106. Laubie M, Schmitt H, Drouillat M: Action of clonidine on the baroreceptor pathway and medullary sites mediating vagal bradycardia. Eur J Pharmacol 1976;38:293–303.

107. Leblanc N, Wilde DW, Keef KD: Electrophysiological mechanisms of minoxidil sulfate-induced vasodilation of rabbit portal vein. Circ Res 1989;65:1102–1111.

108. Lechleitner P: Uneventful self-poisoning with a very high dose of captopril. Toxicology 1990;64:325–329.

109. Lenz K, Druml W, Kleinbergeer G, et al: Acute intoxication with prazosin. A case report. Hum Toxicol 1985;4:53–56.

110. Levine RH, Stauch BS: Hypertensive responses to methyldopa. N Engl J Med 1966;257:946–948.

111. Lin MT, Chandra A, Ko WC, Chen YM: Serotonergic mechanisms of clonidine-induced hypothermia in rats. Neuropharmacology 1981;20:15–21.

112. Lip GYH, Ferner RE: Poisoning with anti-hypertensive drugs: Diuretics and potassium supplements. J Hum Hypertens 1995;9:295–301.

113. Lip GYH, Ferner RE: Poisoning with anti-hypertensive drugs: Alpha-adrenoreceptor antagonists. J Hum Hypertens 1995;9:523–526.

114. Lip GYH, Ferner RE: Poisoning with anti-hypertensive drugs: Angiotensin converting enzme inhibitors. J Hum Hypertens 1995;9:711–715.

115. Litovitz TL, Schmitz BF, Holm KC: 1988 Annual Report of the American Association of Poison Control Centers National Data Collection System. Am J Emerg Med 1989;7:495–545.

116. Loggie JMH, Saito H, Kahn I, Femmer A, Gaffmeu TE: Accidental reserpine poisoning: Clinical and metabolic effects. Clin Pharmacol Ther 1967;8:692–695.

117. Lowenstein JS: Clonidine. Ann Intern Med 1980;92:74–77.

118. Lowenthal DT: Pharmacokinetics of clonidine. J Cardiovasc Pharmacol 1980;2(Suppl):529–537.

119. MacFaul R, Miller G: Clonidine poisoning in children. Lancet 1979;1:1266–1267.

120. MacMillan AR, Warshawski FJ, Steinberg RA: Minoxidil overdose. Chest 1993;103:1290–1291.

121. Maggi JC, Iskra MK, Nussbaum E: Severe clonidine overdose in children requiring critical care. Clin Pediatr 1986;25:453–455.

122. Marruecos L, Roglan A, Frati ME, Artigas A: Clonidine overdose. Crit Care Med 1983;11:959–960.

123. Mathew PM, Addy DP, Wright N. Clonidine overdose in children. Clin Toxicol 1981;18:169–173.

124. Mazzolai L, Burnier M: Comparative safety and tolerability of angiotensin II receptor antagonists. Drug Saf 1999;21:23–33.

125. McClean WJ: Prazosin overdose. Med J Aust 1976;1:592.

126. McClellan KJ, Balfour JA: Eprosartan. Drugs 1997;55:713–720.

127. McClellan KJ, Goa KL: Candesartan cilexetil. A review of its use in essential hypertension. Drugs 1998;56:847–869.

128. McClellan KJ, Markham A: Telmisartan. Drugs 1998;56:1039–1046.

129. McCormick MA, Forman MH, Manoguerra AS: Severe toxicity from ingestion of a topical minoxidil preparation. Am J Emerg Med 1989;7:419–421.

130. McLennan PL: The hypothermic effect of clonidine and other imidazolines in relation to their ability to enter the central nervous system in mice. Eur J Pharmacol 1981;69:477–482.

131. Mendoza JE, Medalie M: Clonidine poisoning with marked hypotension in a 2½-year-old child. Clin Pediatr 1079;18:123–127.

132. Millar JA, Sturani A, Rubin PC, Reid JL: Attenuation of the antihypertensive effect of captopril by the opioid receptor antagonist naloxone. Clin Exp Pharmacol Physiol 1983;10:253–259.

133. Moore MA, Philips P: Clonidine overdose. Lancet 1976;2:694.

134. Muir AL, Burton JL, Lawrie DM: Circulatory effects at rest and exercise of clonidine, an imidazoline derivative with hypotensive properties. Lancet 1969;2:181–185.

135. Myhre E, Rugstad HE, Hansen T: Clinical pharmacokinetics of methyldopa. Clin Pharmacokinet 1982;7:221–223.

136. Nakagawa S, Yamamoto Y, Koiwaya Y: Ventricular tachycardia induced by clonidine withdrawal. Br Heart J 1985;53:654–658.

137. Nayler WG, Price JM, Swann JB, et al: Effect of the hypotensive drug ST 155 (Catapres) on the heart and peripheral circulation. J Pharmacol Exp Ther 1968;164:45–59.

138. Neimann JT, Getzug T, Murphy W: Reversal of clonidine toxicity by naloxone. Ann Emerg Med 1986;15:1229–1231.

139. Neuvonen PJ, Vilska J, Keranen A: Severe poisoning in a child caused by small dose of clonidine. Clin Toxicol 1978;14:369–374.

140. North DS, Wieland MJ, Peterson CD, Krenzelok EP: Naloxone administration in clonidine overdosage. Ann Emerg Med 1981;10:397.

141. Oates JA: Antihypertensive agents and the drug therapy of hypertension. In: Hardman JG, Limbird LE, Molinoff PB, Ruddon RW, eds: Goodman and Gilman's The Pharmacological Basis of Therapeutics, 9th ed. New York, McGraw-Hill, 1996, pp. 199–248.

142. O'Doherty NJ: Thiazides and cerebral ischaemia. Lancet 1965;2:1297.

143. Ohtawa M, Takayama F, Saitoh K, et al. Pharmacokinetics and biochemical efficacy after single and multiple oral administration of losartan, an orally active nonpeptide angiotensin II receptor antagonist, in humans. Br J Clin Pharmacol 1993;35:290–297.

144. Olsson JM, Pruitt AW: Management of clonidine ingestion in children. J Pediatr 1983;103:646–650.

145. Onesti G, Schwartz AB, Kim KE, et al: Pharmacodynamic effects of a new antihypertensive drug. Catapres (ST-155). Circulation 1969;34:219–228.

146. Orfan N, Patterson R, Dykewicz MS: Severe angioedema related to ACE inhibitor in patients with a history of idiopathic angioedema. JAMA 1990;264:1287–1290.

147. Pai GS, Lipsitz DJ: Clonidine poisoning. Pediatrics 1976;58:749–750.

148. Papademetriou V, Burris JF, Notargiacomo A, et al: Thiazide therapy is not a cause of arrhythmia in patients with systemic hypertension. Arch Intern Med 1988;148:1272–1276.

149. Park H, Purnell GV, Mirchandani HG: Suicide by captopril overdose. J Toxicol Clin Toxicol 1990;28:379–382.

150. Paster RZ, Snaely DB, Sweet AR, et al: Use of losartan in the treatment of hypertensive patients with a history of cough induced by angiotensin-converting enzyme inhibitors. Clin Ther 1998;20:978–989.

151. Patnode RE, Brouhard BH, Travis LB, et al. Prolonged clonidine overdosage in a child. J Pediatr 1977;90:849–850.

152. Perrone J, Hoffman RS, Jones B, Hollander JE: Guanabenz-induced hypothermia in a poisoned elderly female. J Toxicol Clin Toxicol 1994;32:445–449.

153. Peters RW, Hamilton BP, Hamilton J, et al: Cardiac arrhythmias after abrupt clonidine withdrawal. Clin Pharmacol Ther 1983;34:435–439.

154. Pettinger WA: Clonidine, a new antihypertensive drug. N Engl J Med 1975;293:1179–1180.

155. Pettinger WA: Pharmacology of clonidine. J Cardiovasc Phamacol 1980;2:521–528.

156. Pettinger WA, Mitchell HC: Side effects of vasodilator therapy. Hypertension 1988;11(Suppl II):34–36.

157. Poff SW, Rose SR: Minoxidil overdose with ECG changes: Case report and review. Am J Emerg Med 1992;10:53–57.

158. Popper CW. Combined methylphenidate and clonidine: News reports about sudden death. J Child Adolesc Psychopharmacol 1995;5:155–166.

159. Ram VCS, Holland B, Fairchild C, Gomez-Sanchez CE: Withdrawal syndrome following cessation of guanabenz therapy. J Clin Pharmacol 1979;19:148–150.

160. Raper JH, Shinar C, Finkelstein S: Clonidine patch ingestion in an adult. Ann Pharmacother 1993;27:719–722.

161. Reed MT, Hamburg EL: Person to person transfer of transdermal drug-delivery systems: A case report. N Engl J Med 1986;314:1120–1121.

162. Regunathan S, Reis DJ: Imidazoline receptors and their endogenous ligands. Ann Rev Pharm Toxicol 1996;36:511–544.

163. Reid JL, Campbell BC, Hamilton CA: Withdrawal reactions following cessation of central α-adrenergic receptor agonists. Hypertension 1984;6(Suppl II):71–75.

164. Robbins DN, Crawford ED, Lackner LH: Priapism secondary to prazosin overdose. J Urol 1983;130:975.

165. Roberts JR, Wuerz RC: Clinical characteristics of angiotensin-converting enzyme inhibitor-induced angioedema. Ann Emerg Med 1991;20:555–558.

166. Robertson D, Tung C, Goldberg MR, et al: Antihypertensive metabolites of α-methyldopa. Hypertension 1984;6(Suppl II):45–50.

167. Rodman JS, Deutsch DJ, Gutman SI: Methyldopa hepatitis. A report of six cases and review of the literature. Am J Med 1976;60:941–948.

168. Rosenberg L, Shapiro S, Slone D, et al: Thiazides and acute cholecystitis. N Engl J Med 1980;303:546–548.

169. Rougraff ME: Chlorothiazide overdosage effects in two-year-old child. PA Med J 1959;62:694.

170. Rubinstein I: Fatal thrombosis of left internal carotid artery following diuretic abuse. Ann Emerg Med 1985;14:275.

171. Rygnestad TK, Dale O: Self-poisoning with prazosin. Acta Med Scand 1983;213:157–158.

172. Schieber RA, Kaufman ND: Use of tolazoline in massive clonidine poisoning. Am J Dis Child 1981;135:77–78.

173. Scheinman MM, Strauss HC, Evans GT, et al: Adverse effects of sympatholytic agents in patients with hypertension and sinus node dysfunction. Am J Med 1978;64:1013–1020.

174. Schwartz E, Friedman E, Mouallem M, Farfel Z: Sinus arrest associated with clonidine therapy. Clin Cardiol 1987;11:53–54.

175. Self F, Bates GHEM, Drake-Lee A: Severe angioneurotic oedema causing acute airway obstruction. J R Soc Med 1988;81:544–545.

176. Shand DG, Morgan DH, Oates JA: The release of guanethidine and bethanidine by splenic nerve stimulation; A quantitative evaluation showing dissociation from adrenergic blockade. J Pharmacol Exp Ther 1973;184:73–80.

177. Sharpe E, Milaszkiewicz R, Carli R: A case of prolonged hypotension following intravenous guanethidine blockade. Anaesthesia 1987;42:1081–1084.

178. Shnaps Y, Almog S, Halkin H, Tirosh M: Methyldopa poisoning. Clin Toxicol 1982;19:501–503.

179. Siegel D, Hulley SB, Black DM, et al: Diuretics, serum and intracellular electrolyte levels, and ventricular arrhythmias in hypertensive men. JAMA 1992;267:1083–1089.

180. Siscovick DS, Raghunathan TE, Psaty BM, et al: Diuretic therapy for hypertension and the risk of primary cardiac arrest. N Engl J Med 1994;330:1852–1857.

181. Slater EE, Merril DD, Guess HA, et al: Clinical profile of angioedema associated with angiotensin-converting enzyme inhibition. JAMA 1988;260:967–970.

182. Smith BA, Ferguson DB: Acute hydralazine overdose: Marked ECG abnormalities in a young adult. Ann Emerg Med 1992;21:326–330.

183. Sonnenblick M, Friedlander Y, Rosin AJ: Diuretic-induced hyponatremia. Reproducibility by single-dose rechallenge and an analysis of pathogenesis. Chest 1993;103:601–606.

184. Sorkin EM, Heel RC: Guanfacine. A review of its pharmacodynamic and pharmacokinetic properties and therapeutic efficacy in the treatment of hypertension. Drugs 1986;31:301–336.

185. Spiller HA, Udicious TM, Muir S: Angiotensin-converting enzyme inhibitor ingestion in children. J Toxicol Clin Toxicol 1989;27:345–353.

186. Stein B, Volans GN: Dixarit overdose: The problem of attractive tablets. Br Med J 1978;2:667–668.

187. Steiners E: Diuretics, digitalis, and arrhythmias. Acta Med Scand 1981;647(Suppl):75–78.

188. Stelzer FP, Stubenbord JJ, Sreenivasan V, Venuto RC: Late toxicity of clonidine withdrawal. N Engl J Med 1976;294:1182.

189. Tenenbein M: Naloxone in clonidine toxicity. Am J Dis Child 1984;138:1084–1085.

190. Textor SC, Bravo EL, Fouad FM, Tarazi RC: Hyperkalemia in azotemic patients during angiotensin-converting enzyme inhibition and aldosterone reduction with captopril. Am J Med 1982;73:719–725.

191. Tibirica E, Feldman J, Mermet C, et al: An imidazoline-specific mechanism for the hypotensive effect of clonidine: A study with yohimbine and idazoxan. J Pharmacol Exp Ther 1991;256:606–613.

192. Thormann J, Neuss H, Schlepper M, Mitrovic V: Effects of clonidine on sinus node function in man. Chest 1981;80:201–206.

193. Tovar JL, Bujons I, Ruiz JC, et al: Treatment of severe combined overdose of calcium antagonists and converting enzyme inhibitors with angiotensin II. Nephron 1997;77:239.

194. Van der Linden W, Ritter B, Edlund G: Acute cholecystitis and thiazides. Br Med J 1984;289:654–655.

195. Van Dyke MW, Bonace AL, Ellenhorn MJ: Guanfacine overdose in a pediatric patient. Vet Hum Toxicol 1990;32:46–47.

196. van Etta L, Burchell H: Severe bradycardia with clonidine. JAMA 1978;240:2047.

197. van Rijnsoever EW, Kwee-Zuiderwijk WJ, Feenstra J: Angioneurotic edema attributed to the use of losartan. Arch Intern Med 1998;158:2063–2065.

198. van Zweiten PA: Antihypertensive drugs with a central action. Prog Pharmacol 1975;1:1–66.

199. van Zwieten PA: The pharmacology of centrally acting hypotensive drugs. Br J Clin Pharmacol 1980;10:135S–138S.

200. van Zwieten PA, Thoolen MJMC, Timmermans PBMWM: The hypotensive activity and side effects of methyldopa, clonidine, and guanfacine. Hypertension 1984;6(Suppl II):28–33.

201. Vanholder R, Carpentier J, Schurgers M, Clement DL: Rebound phenomenon during gradual withdrawal of clonidine. Br Med J 1977;1:1138.

202. Varon J, Duncan SR: Naloxone reversal of hypotension due to captopril overdose. Ann Emerg Med 1991;20:1125–1127.

203. Varughese A, Taylor AA, Neslon EB: Consequences of angiotensin-converting enzyme inhibitor overdose. Am J Hypertens 1989;2:355–357.

204. Vila JM, Blum L, Dosik H: Thiazide-induced immune hemolytic anemia. JAMA 1976;236:1723–1724.

205. Waeber B, Nussberger J, Brunner HR. Self-poisoning with enalapril. Br Med J 1984;288:287–288.

206. Weinberger MH: Diuretics and their side effects. Hypertension 1988;11(Suppl II):16–20.

207. Wiley JF, Wiley CC, Torrey SB, Henretig FM: Clonidine poisoning in young children. J Pediatr 1990;116:654–658.

208. Williams PL, Krafcik JM, Potter BB, et al: Cardiac toxicity of clonidine. Chest 1977;72:784–785.

209. Worlledge SM, Carstairs KC, Dacie JV: Autoimmune hemolytic anaemia associated with α-methyldopa therapy. Lancet 1966;2:135–139.

210. Yeh BK, Natel A, Goldberg LI: Antihypertensive effect of clonidine. Arch Intern Med 1971;127:233–237.

211. Zamboulis C, Reid JL: Withdrawal of guanfacine after long-term treatment in essential hypertension. Eur J Clin Phamacol 1981;19:19–24.

212. Zarifis J, Lip GYH, Ferner RE: Poisoning with anti-hypertensive drugs: Methyldopa and clonidine. J Hum Hypertens 1995;9:787–790.

Neal A. Lewin / Lewis S. Nelson

A 78-year-old woman was brought to the Emergency Department (ED) complaining of nausea. She had a history of "heart trouble" and reported taking a "water pill" for high blood pressure. On closer questioning, she described four episodes of syncope over the previous 9 days.

Her vital signs were blood pressure, 130/90 mm Hg; irregular pulse at 100 beats/min; respirations, 20 breaths/min; and temperature, 37°C (98.6°F). The patient was moderately obese, slightly diaphoretic, and in moderate distress. There was no cyanosis or peripheral edema. Her lungs were clear. The left ventricular apex impulse was in the sixth intercostal space, midway between the midclavicular and anterior axillary line. Auscultation of the heart revealed an irregular rhythm without murmurs. Her abdomen was soft, nontender, and without organomegaly, and her neurologic examination was within normal limits.

An ECG revealed a sinus rhythm of 70 beats/min with runs of a wide complex dysrhythmia at a rate of 160 beats/min. An intravenous (IV) line was inserted and blood was sent for analysis. The patient was given a 100-mg bolus of lidocaine followed by an infusion at a rate of 2 mg/min. (At the time of this case, IV infusion pump devices were not routinely used in Emergency Departments.) A second IV line with 0.9% NaCl was placed in the other arm for the administration of fluids. A repeat electrocardiogram (ECG) showed sinus rhythm without evidence of ectopy.

Over the next hour, the urine output by Foley catheter was noted to be only 10 mL and the rate of her saline infusion was ordered increased. Inadvertently, the lidocaine infusion was run "wide open" and the patient received 600 mg of lidocaine (150 mL of solution) over a 10-minute period. She rapidly became hypotensive with a palpable blood pressure of 70 mm Hg followed by status epilepticus and then cardiorespiratory arrest. Cardiopulmonary resuscitation (CPR) was initiated, during the course of which the patient was given 1 mg of epinephrine intravenously without effect. While a transvenous pacemaker was being inserted, a sinus rhythm of 70 beats/min returned spontaneously and the blood pressure rose to 120/80 mm Hg. The patient was admitted to the intensive care unit (ICU).

The patient's mental status returned to normal 7 hours after her cardiac arrest, during which time her initial laboratory data were returned and were normal. As she continued to have intermittent multifocal ventricular extrasystoles, a lidocaine infusion was reinstituted using an infusion pump. Because the lidocaine infusion at a rate of 4 mg/min did not control her dysrhythmia, 400 mg of procainamide was slowly administered intravenously and the ectopy resolved. Serial ECGs and cardiac enzyme studies did not demonstrate any evidence of a myocardial infarction. Oral doses of pro-cainamide were instituted and the patient was discharged home from the hospital.

The term *dysrhythmia* encompasses an array of abnormal cardiac rhythms that range in clinical significance from merely annoying to instantly life-threatening. Antidysrhythmics include all agents that are used to treat any of the various dysrhythmias. Although most antidysrhythmic agents find their only utility in the relief of serious dysrhythmias, many have other important clinical effects and are antidysrhythmic only secondarily. Examples include the use of lidocaine for local anesthesia or phenytoin for seizure control.

The importance of dysrhythmia management in the modern practice of medicine cannot be overstated, as these are among the most common causes of preventable sudden cardiac death. However, despite an incomplete understanding of the underlying mechanisms of dysrhythmia formation, an abundance of antidysrhythmic agents have been developed, each attempting to alter specific electrophysiologic components of the cardiac impulse generating or conducting system. In addition to the predictable, mechanism-based adverse effect of each agent, unique and often unanticipated effects also occur.[99] Experience with overdose of any of these agents is limited, and management is generally based on the underlying pharmacologic principles, existing case reports, and experimental literature.

HISTORY AND EPIDEMIOLOGY

Until recently, antidysrhythmic agents were considered among the most rational of the available cardiac medications. This well-earned reputation related to their high efficacy at reducing the incidence of malignant dysrhythmias. Similarly, they are effective at controlling nuisance rhythm disorders. However, this approach changed dramatically in the recent past, both with the rise of mechanical interventions such as ablation therapy and implantable defibrillators, and with the reporting of the Cardiac Arrhythmia Suppression Trial (CAST).[20] This trial assessed the ability of three antidysrhythmic agents to suppress asymptomatic ventricular dysrhythmias known to be harbingers of malignant dysrhythmias. This study was discontinued prematurely in April 1989, when it was noted that encainide and flecainide, two of the examined agents, not only failed to prevent sudden death, but they actually increased overall mortality. The CAST II trial continued to evaluate the remaining agent, moricizine, but ultimately this agent met a similar fate.[21] It has since become clear that the enhanced mortality associated with many antidysrhythmic agents is a result of their prodysrhythmogenic effects, and that virtually all agents of this group carry such risk.

This chapter focuses on the agents that serve their primary clinical role as antidysrhythmic agents and, with the exception of lidocaine, have little other medicinal function. A more detailed description of the various dysrhythmias and a discussion of their genesis is found in Chapter 21. The toxicities from β-adrenergic antagonists and calcium channel blockers are discussed separately in Chapters 49 and 50.

CLASSIFICATION OF ANTIDYSRHYTHMIC AGENTS

Antidysrhythmic agents modify impulse generation and conduction by interacting with various membrane sodium, potassium, and calcium ion channels. Generally, antidysrhythmic agents alter electrophysiologic effects either through blockade of the channel pore or by modification of its gating mechanism (described in Fig. 52–1).[57] Unfortunately, given the exceedingly complex mechanisms of action of the antidysrhythmic drugs, the descriptive terms used to explain their molecular selectivities are not always completely accurate. For example, the description of an antidysrhythmic agent as a "channel blocker" or a "channel opener," although

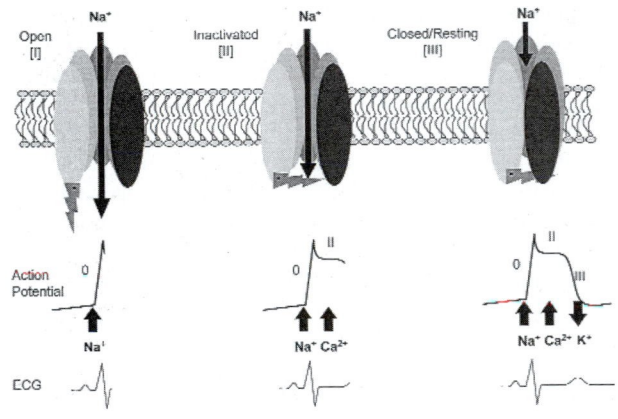

Figure 52–1. Sodium channel blockade. Upon appropriate signal, sodium channel activation occurs, in which the sodium channel coverts from the resting [III] state to the open state [I]. This allows sodium ion influx to initiate phase 0 of the action potential, or cellular depolarization. The sodium channels subsequently assume the inactivated state by closure of an inactivation gate; this is a voltage-dependent phenomena and occurs concomitantly with, although more slowly than, channel activation. Cellular depolarization is maintained for a period of time by other ion channels that form the plateau of the action potential. Prior to reactivating, sodium channels must convert back to the resting state, which also occurs in a voltage-dependent fashion. Many antidysrhythmic agents stabilize the inactivated state of the channel and, by slowing conversion to the resting state, prevent its reopening, reducing the excitability of the cell. As this is a population phenomena, there are dose-dependent effects on channel blockade; thus, more drug interferes with more channels. Interestingly, certain toxins, such as ciguatoxin and aconitine, stabilize the open state of the sodium channel and produce persistent depolarization.

representative of a specific action of that drug, is often incomplete because many of these agents are active at other channels or on other cells. Nonspecific effects on a plasma membrane ion channel may modify several different proteins within the bilayer, not just the anticipated target.

The Vaughan Williams (VW) classification of antidysrhythmic agents by electrophysiologic properties emphasizes the connection between the basic electrophysiologic actions and the antidysrhythmic effects.[120,121] Although initially proposed as a descriptive model for electrophysiologic actions and not for clinical effects, the VW classification is commonly invoked as a user-friendly guide to clinical therapy. In 1991, a competing system known as "the Sicilian Gambit"[127] was constructed by a task force of European cardiologists based on the mechanisms by which antidysrhythmic drugs modify dysrhythmogenic mechanisms. Although perhaps more contemporary in theory, this latter classification system is complex and is therefore not widely implemented. An even more rational, and unusable, classification would match the electrophysiologic effects of the antidysrhythmic agents with their molecular interactions on different regions of the various ion channels, such as channel gating and pore conductance.[57]

This discussion of antidysrhythmic agents utilizes the Vaughan Williams classification, while recognizing the shortcomings delineated above.[118]

CLASS I ANTIDYSRHYTHMICS

All antidysrhythmic agents in VW Class I (A, B, and C) alter Na^+ conductance through cardiac voltage-gated, fast inward Na^+ channels (see Table 52–1). These agents bind to the Na^+ channels and slow their recovery from the open or inactivated state to the resting state (Fig. 52–2). This conversion must occur before the channel can reopen and participate in another depolarization. Thus, when drug is bound to a proportion of the available Na^+ channels, fewer are capable of reactivation upon the arrival of the next depolarizing impulse. As a result, by reducing the excitability of the myocardium, abnormal rhythms are both prevented and terminated.[63]

Blockade of these sodium channels slows the rise of phase 0 of the cellular action potential, which correlates with a reduction in the rate of depolarization of the myocardial cell (or V_{max}). Similarly, conduction through the myocardium is slowed, producing a measurable prolongation of the QRS complex on the surface electrocardiogram. Correspondingly, slowed intramyocardial conduction is associated with reduced contractility, manifesting as negative inotropy. Myocardial depression is also a result of the reduced availability of intracellular Na^+ to participate in Na^+/Ca^{2+} exchange. This latter effect causes a fall in the intracellular Ca^{2+} concentrations, normal levels of which are required for adequate contractility.

It is now clear that the differences between Class I agents are directly related to their pharmacologic relationships with the Na^+ channel. Type IB agents have their highest affinity for Na^+ channels that are in the inactivated state. This occurs at the end of depolarization, during early repolarization, and during periods of myocardial ischemia, all situations in which the myocardium is partially depolarized. These agents also have rapid "on-off" binding kinetics and are thus bound only briefly, during late systole, the period during which the Na^+ channels are predominantly in the inactivated form. They are essentially unbound during diastole,

TABLE 52–1. Antidysrhythmic Agents: Pharmacology, Pharmacokinetics and Adverse Effects

Drug	Route	Primary Route of Elimination	VW Class	Channel/Receptor Effects*	Adverse Effects and Complicating Factors	V_d (L/kg)	Protein Binding (%)	$t_{1/2}$ in Healthy Patients
Disopyramide (Norpace)	PO	Liver: mono-*N*-dealkylated Kidney: unchanged 50%	IA	Na+, K+	Congestive heart failure, negative inotropic effects, anticholinergic, torsades de pointes, heart block, hypoglycemia	0.59 ± 0.15	35–95	Parent: 6–8 h Metabolite: 3–4 h
Procainamide (Pronestyl)	IV, PO	Kidney: unchanged 50–60% Liver: NAPA (active)	IA	Na+, K+	Hypotension, QRS widening, fever, SLE-like syndrome, torsades de pointes	1.9 ± 0.3	16 ± 9	Parent: 2–4 h Metabolite: 6–10 h
Quinidine	PO	Liver: several metabolites (?activity) Kidney: unchanged 10–30%	IA	Na+, K+, Ca2+	Heart block, severe sinus node dysfunction, prolonged QT syndrome, hypotension, cinchonism, torsades de pointes, thrombocytopenia, ↑ digoxin levels, hypoglycemia	2.7 ± 1.2	87 ± 3	Parent: 3–19 h
Lidocaine (Xylocaine)	SQ, IV PO	Liver: MEGX (active)	IB	Na+	Fatigue, agitation, paresthesias, seizures, hallucinations, rarely bundle-branch block; Vd reduced by CHF and increased in liver failure	1.1 ± 0.4	70 ± 5	Parent: ~2 h MEGX: 2 h GX: 1 h
Mexiletine (Mexitil)	IV, PO	Liver Kidney: unchanged <10%	IB	Na+	See lidocaine	4.9 ± 0.5	63 ± 3	12–13 h
Phenytoin (Dilantin)	IV, PO	Liver	IB	Na+	Hypotension and asystole related to IV infusion, nystagmus, ataxia	0.64 ± 0.04	89 ± 23	
Tocainide (Tonocard)	IV, PO	Kidney, Liver	IB	Na+	See lidocaine; aplastic anemia, interstitial pneumonia	3.0 ± 0.2	10 ± 15	9–12 h
Flecainide (Tambocor)	IV, PO	Liver 75% Kidney 25%	IC	Na+, Ca2+, K+	Negative inotropic effects, bradycardia, heart block, ventricular fibrillation, ventricular tachycardia, neutropenia	4.9 ± 0.4	61 ± 10	12–27 h
Propafenone (Rhythmol)	IV, PO	Liver	IC	Na+, K+	Asthma, congestive heart failure, hypoglycemia, AV block, QRS prolongation, bradycardia, ventricular fibrillation, ventricular tachycardia	3.6 ± 2.1	85–95	2–32 h
Moricizine (Ethmozine)	PO	Liver, Kidney	IB?	Na+	Bradycardia, CHF, ventricular fibrillation, ventricular tachycardia	?	95	6–13 h
β-Adrenergic antagonists	IV, PO	Liver	II		Congestive heart failure, asthma, hypoglycemia, Raynaud disease			
Amiodarone (Cordarone)	IV, PO	Liver: desethylamiodarone	III	Na+, K+, Ca2+	Negative inotropic effects, pulmonary fibrosis, corneal microdeposits, thyroid abnormalities, photosensitivity, ↑ digoxin, warfarin effects	66 ± 44	99.98 ± 0.01	2 mo
Bretylium (Bretylol)	IV, IM	Kidney	III	K+	Hypertension followed by hypotension, nausea, and vomiting	5.9 ± 0.8	(0–8)	
Dofetilide (Tikosyn)	IV, PO	Kidney	III	K+	Torsades de pointes	3.6 ± 0.8	64	
Ibutilide (Corvert)	IV	Kidney	III	K+, Na+ (opener)	Torsades de pointes, heart block	11	40	2–12 h
Calcium channel blockers (various)	IV, PO	Liver	IV	Ca2+	Asystole (if used IV with IV β-adrenergic antagonists), AV block, hypotension, congestive heart failure, constipation, ↑ digoxin levels			
Adenosine (Adenocard)		All cells (adenosine deaminase)	None	Adenosine (agonist)	Transient asystole <5 sec, chest pain, dyspnea, atrial fibrillation, ↓ BP, ↑ effects potentiated by dipyridamole and in heart transplant patients, ↑ dose needed with methylxanthine use			8 sec

V_d = volume distribution; VW class=Vaughan Williams class.
*Blocker or antagonist unless specified.

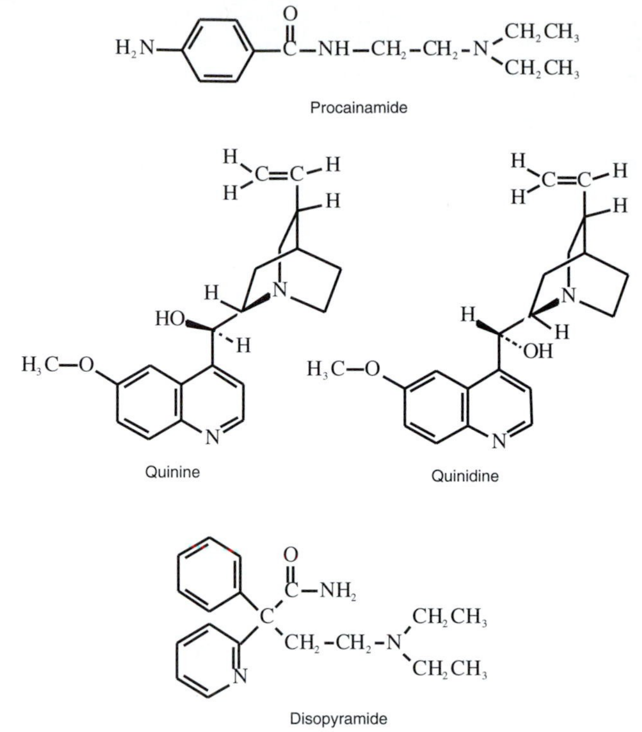

myocardial potassium channels. Class IB agents do not alter refractoriness or the QTc. In fact, Class IB agents often reduce the action potential duration and thereby shorten refractoriness. Further discussion of potassium channel blockade is found in Chapter 21 and below in the discussion of Class III antidysrhythmic agents.

Class IA Antidysrhythmic Agents: Procainamide, Quinidine, and Disopyramide

Procainamide. Procainamide (Fig. 52-2) may be used to suppress either atrial or ventricular tachydysrhythmias. Although absorption from the GI tract is rapid and relatively complete following a therapeutic dose (75–95%), it may be delayed in overdose situations. A sustained-release preparation is available as well. Importantly, procainamide undergoes hepatic biotransformation by acetylation to N-acetylprocainamide (NAPA),[29] the rate of which is genetically determined. Although NAPA lacks the Na+ channel–blocking activity of procainamide, it prolongs the action potential duration through K+ channel blockade and is an investigational Class III antidysrhythmic agent. Both procainamide and NAPA are renally eliminated and may accumulate in patients with renal insufficiency.[32,34]

Rapid intravenous dosing of procainamide is dangerous because it distributes into an initial volume of distribution that is smaller than its final volume of distribution. Because this initial compartment includes the heart, myocardial effects may be unexpectedly pronounced. Thus, to prevent toxicity during drug infusion, the intravenous loading dose should be administered by slow infusion with electrocardiogram monitoring. Although the chronic use of procainamide is commonly accompanied by the development of antinuclear antibodies or drug-induced lupus,[48] this syndrome is not associated with acute poisoning. Other reported adverse effects include myopathic pain, thrombocytopenia, and agranulocytosis.

Both procainamide and NAPA serum concentrations should be determined both in monitoring therapeutic serum levels (5–20 µg/mL) and in patients with procainamide overdose. Because the elimination half-life of procainamide is 3–4 hours, which is substantially shorter than that of NAPA (6–10 hours), chronic overdosing typically results in NAPA toxicity. In this situation, the QTc interval, a reflection of K+ channel blockade, correlates directly, and blood pressure correlates inversely, with the degree of poisoning. Severe effects usually do not occur until total (procainamide plus NAPA) serum concentrations are greater than 60 µg/mL.[4]

Quinidine. Quinidine (Fig. 52-2), the d-isomer of quinine, is derived from the bark of the cinchona tree.[73] Because it is a weak base, it is formulated as the sulfate, gluconate, or other salt. It is used for the management of atrial or ventricular dysrhythmias. Quinidine undergoes hydroxylation by the liver, and its metabolites, both active and inactive, are renally eliminated. Thus, the drug's elimination t½ of approximately 6–8 hours is prolonged by both liver disease (to >50 hours) and renal failure (to 9–12 hours).

Quinidine has substantial acute cardiotoxicity following overdose that includes intraventricular conduction abnormalities and increased QTc duration. "Quinidine syncope," in which patients on therapeutic doses of quinidine experience paroxysmal, transient loss of consciousness, is most frequently a result of torsades de

the major portion of the cardiac cycle at normal heart rates. However, the degree of binding increases as the heart rate accelerates because the duration of diastole decreases and the relative proportion of time spent in systole increases; this is termed *use dependence* (Chap. 21). Because they do not bind to activated sodium channels, Class IB agents do not affect the rate of rise of phase 0 of the action potential, or V_{max}, and have no effect on the electrocardiogram in conventional doses.[120] Alternatively, the Class IA and IC agents either prefer activated Na+ channels or they[99,120] release from the Na+ channels very slowly, and are thus bound throughout most, if not all, of the cardiac cycle. This prolonged channel blockade and reduced channel reactivation results in greater pharmacologic effects, and toxicity, even at slow heart rates. Thus, these agents reduce V_{max} and prolong the QRS complex on the electrocardiogram. Class IA agents fall intermediate between the other two subclasses. It is important to note that the original subdivision of Class I drugs was based on clinical observations, not current pharmacologic awareness, accounting for the somewhat illogical ordering of the Class I subdivisions.[120]

Although by the VW classification Class I agents are considered primarily sodium channel blockers, many of the represented agents, particularly those in Class IA, have important effects on cardiac potassium channels. These channels are critical to maintenance of the cardiac action potential and repolarization of the myocardial cell. Slowing of potassium efflux thus prolongs the duration of the action potential and accounts for the persistence of refractoriness, or the time during which the cell is incapable of repolarization. Through blockade of myocardial potassium channels the Class I agents produce QT prolongation on the surface electrocardiogram, predisposing to the triggering of polymorphic ventricular tachycardia.[51] Because they have no effect on

Figure 52-2. Structures of Class IA antidysrhythmic agents and quinine.

Disopyramide

Quinidine

Quinine

Procainamide

pointes.[53,113,123] Many of the ECG changes mimic those of hypokalemia.

Quinidine shares many pharmacologic properties with quinine (Chap. 44). Therefore, it is not surprising that patients may occasionally suffer from cinchonism following either chronic or acute overdose. This syndrome includes abdominal symptoms, tinnitus, and altered mental status. Quinidine also produces peripheral and cardiac antimuscarinic effects. Through these vagolytic effects, conduction via the AV node is enhanced. Thus, quinidine may actually exacerbate the ventricular response to atrial fibrillation, explaining the need for rate control prior to chemical cardioversion of this rhythm.[101] Furthermore, as with quinine, quinidine-induced blockade of K^+ channels in pancreatic islet cells may cause uncontrolled insulin release and hypoglycemia.[124]

Serum quinidine concentrations greater than 14 μg/mL are associated with cardiotoxicity,[61] as evidenced by a 50% increase in either the QRS or QTc interval. However, in contradistinction to procainamide, quinidine is associated with an increased QTc at both subtherapeutic and therapeutic serum concentrations.[51]

Disopyramide. Disopyramide (Fig. 52–2) is more likely than the other Class IA antidysrhythmic agents to produce negative inotropy and congestive heart failure. This effect may be noted in patients with therapeutic dosing,[95] and in those who overdose. This propensity may relate in part to disopyramide's ability to block myocardial calcium channels.[82,120] Disopyramide, through its mono-N-dealkylated metabolite, produces the most pronounced anticholinergic effects of the class.[82]

Electrophysiologic abnormalities similar to those associated with poisoning from other Class IA drugs can occur. These include atrioventricular and intraventricular conduction abnormalities, torsades de pointes, and other ventricular dysrhythmias. Disopyramide is also the most likely Class IA agent to cause hyperinsulinemic hypoglycemia through its antagonism of K^+ channels in the pancreatic islet cells.[17]

Patients who overdose on disopyramide frequently develop classic anticholinergic manifestations, including mydriasis, urinary retention, and gastrointestinal stasis. Lethargy, confusion, or hallucinations may be prominent.

Management. Management of patients following overdoses of a Class IA antidysrhythmic agent centers on assessment and correction of cardiovascular dysfunction. Following airway evaluation and intravenous line placement, the 12-lead ECG and continuous electrocardiographic monitoring are of paramount importance. For patients with severe cardiovascular manifestations of poisoning, a pulmonary artery catheter is useful to guide therapy. Appropriate gastrointestinal decontamination is recommended when the patient is stabilized and should include whole-bowel irrigation if a sustained-release preparation is involved.

For patients with widening of the QRS complex, bolus administration of intravenous hypertonic sodium bicarbonate is indicated. Depolarization is accelerated and the QRS complex duration is reduced by enhancing rapid sodium ion influx through the myocardial sodium channels.[109,122] However, hypokalemia from the use of sodium bicarbonate may further prolong the QT interval, requiring careful monitoring of the serum K^+ and ECG. Class IA antidysrhythmic agent–induced hypotension is treated primarily with rapid saline infusion in order to expand the patient's intravascular volume and to simultaneously increase myocardial contractility (ie, enhanced Starling force). Hypotension in the set-

ting of QRS complex duration prolongation may respond favorably to hypertonic sodium bicarbonate, which enhances inotropy by both accelerating depolarization and raising intravascular volume. Dopamine, dobutamine, isoproterenol, norepinephrine, and intra-aortic balloon pump insertion may also be required, but their use has not been systematically evaluated. Because disopyramide also blocks calcium channels, calcium chloride administration has reportedly been beneficial,[1] although evidence to support this antidotal effect is lacking. The use of glucagon and bretylium effectively reversed myocardial depression in canine models, but it has not been evaluated in humans.

Patients with ventricular dysrhythmias occurring in the setting of Class IA antidysrhythmic agent poisoning are usually treated with hypertonic sodium bicarbonate or lidocaine. Sodium bicarbonate enhances conduction through the myocardium promoting spontaneous termination of the ventricular dysrhythmia. Although it may seem counterintuitive to administer another Class I antidysrhythmic agent to a patient already poisoned by a Class I antidysrhythmic agent, there is sound theoretical and experimental literature to support the practice. That is, because lidocaine is a Class IB agent with rapid on-off receptor kinetics, it may displace the "slower" Class IA agent from the sodium channel, effectively reducing channel blockade. Magnesium sulfate and overdrive pacing may be helpful in treating torsades de pointes, should the dysrhythmia not spontaneously terminate.[117] Drugs that must be avoided in treating patients with dysrhythmias associated with Class IA poisoning include other Class IA and IC agents as well as the β-adrenergic antagonists and calcium channel blockers, all of which may exacerbate conduction abnormalities.

The roles of charcoal hemoperfusion, hemofiltration, and continuous arteriovenous hemodialtration are inadequately defined, but may be most beneficial for removing NAPA.[4,14,56] There is no clinical evidence to support the use of hemodialysis or hemoperfusion for quinidine or disopyramide poisoning.

Class IB Antidysrhythmic Agents: Lidocaine, Tocainide, Mexiletine, and Moricizine

Lidocaine. Lidocaine (Fig. 52–3), known internationally as lignocaine, is an aminoacyl amide that is a synthetic derivative of cocaine. Its predominant clinical uses are as an antidysrhythmic agent and, for mechanistically similar reasons, as a local anesthetic agent.[6,47,82,96,103] Lidocaine is effective in controlling ventricular dysrhythmias resulting from increased automaticity and reentry. Lidocaine may prevent reentry by preferentially suppressing conduction in compromised tissue.[33,74] Following an intravenous bolus, lidocaine initially enters the central nervous system but quickly redistributes into the peripheral tissue with a distribution half-life of approximately 8 minutes.[9,13,46] Lidocaine is 95% dealkylated by hepatic CYP3A4 to an active metabolite, monoethylglycylxylidide (MEGX) and, subsequently, to the inactive glycine xylidide (GX). GX is further metabolized to monoethyl-glycine and xylidide.[112] MEGX, although less potent as a Na^+ channel blocker than the parent drug,[8] may bioaccumulate because of its substantially longer half-life.[99]

Patients with lidocaine poisoning develop both central nervous system and cardiovascular effects. Acute, massive lidocaine poisoning, as occurs following infusion pump malfunction or incorrect dose calculation, typically produces central nervous system dysfunction, particularly seizures, as its initial manifestation.[35,39,94] This may relate to preferential suppression of inhibitory neurons or be a result of the initial distribution of the drug into the brain.[96] Concomitant respiratory arrest generally occurs, probably for similar reasons. Shortly following the central nervous system effects, depression in the intrinsic cardiac pacemakers leads to sinus arrest, AV block, hypotension, and/or cardiac arrest.[5] If the patient is supported through this period, the drug distributes from the heart and cardiac function recurs.

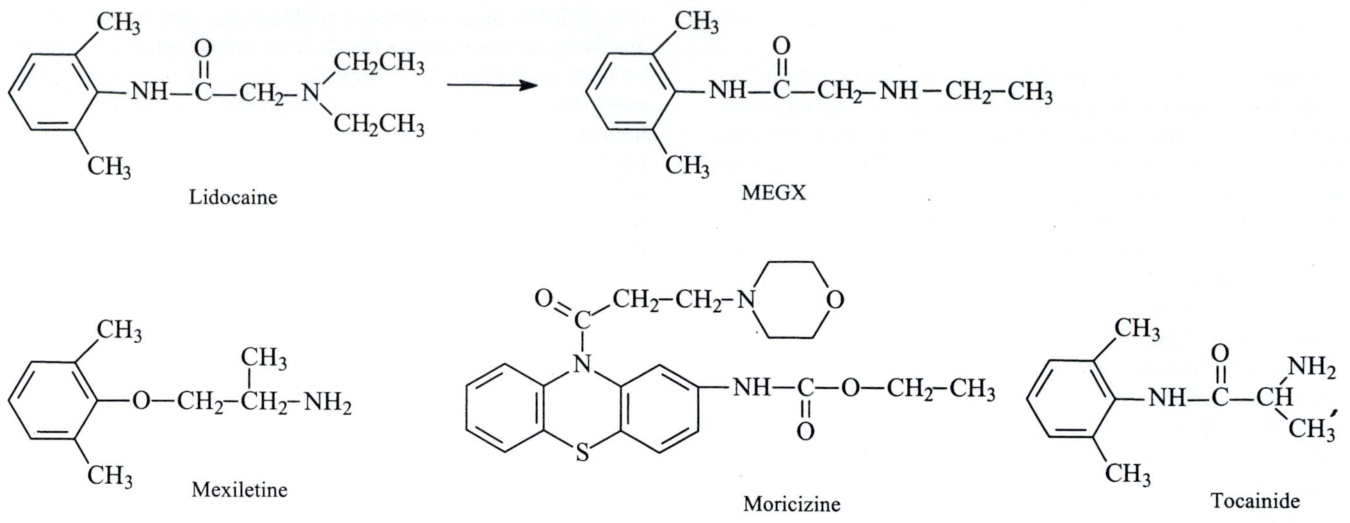

Nonmassive acute lidocaine poisoning has a variety of causes, most of which relate to excessive or inappropriate therapeutic dosing. Common settings include intravenous administration when the intended route was subcutaneous, inadvertent excessive subcutaneous administration during laceration repair, or medication errors. The high frequency of lidocaine-related medication errors relates in part to its availability in multiple different diverse "amps" designed for varying indications including resuscitation, preparation of infusions,[58] and local anesthesia.[62] With the reduced emphasis on lidocaine in the newest Advanced Cardiac Life Support (ACLS) protocols, one important setting for acute lidocaine poisoning may be eliminated. The typical CNS manifestations of nonmassive acute lidocaine poisoning include drowsiness, weakness, a sensation of "drifting away," euphoria, dysphoria, diplopia, decreased hearing, paresthesias, muscle fasciculations, and convulsions. The more severe of these effects develop when blood lidocaine concentrations exceed 5 μg/mL and are often preceded by paresthesias or somnolence. Either of these symptoms should therefore prompt the clinician to examine the patient's medication administration history or drug-infusion rate. In neonates, apnea, hypotonia, and seizures are reported to result from lidocaine toxicity.[65] Apnea and seizures may also occur in adults, as occurred following the unintentional subdural administration of lidocaine during regional anesthesia.[80]

When lidocaine is absorbed from the oral or nongastrointestinal mucosal surfaces, hepatic metabolism is bypassed resulting in enhanced systemic bioavailability of the parent compound.[6,81] Seizures are reported with topical tracheal application of lidocaine used for bronchoscopy,[12,128] as well as intraureteral application during ureteroscopic stone extraction.[92] Five deaths related to tumescent liposuction are reported. In this technique, a large vol-

ume of dilute lidocaine is used to distend subcutaneous fat prior to liposuction.[97] Three patients died as a consequence of hypotension and bradycardia; postmortem blood lidocaine concentrations in two of these patients were 5.2 μg/mL and 2 μg/mL. Because death typically occurred several hours following the procedure, it is likely that MEGX and other metabolites were more consequential than the parent compound.[93] Interestingly, proponents of this procedure suggest that lidocaine doses up to a maximum of 55 mg/kg are safe, whereas the conventional recommended limit for subcutaneous lidocaine with epinephrine is 5–7 mg/kg. Of concern, the recommendation in liposuction procedures does not take into account the ability of lidocaine to saturate the CYP3A4 hepatic microsomal enzyme. When saturation occurs, elimination lags behind absorption and lidocaine toxicity may result.

Chronic lidocaine poisoning most commonly occurs as a therapeutic misadventure in a critical care unit. Hepatic blood flow and hepatic function influence the rate of lidocaine degradation and only a small percentage is excreted unchanged by the kidney. Consequently, poisoning following appropriate therapeutic dosing is most likely to occur in patients with congestive heart failure, shock, liver disease, or concomitant drug therapy with CYP3A4 inhibitors such as cimetidine.[52,115] Adverse reactions to lidocaine also appears to increase with advancing age, decreasing body weight, and increasing infusion rate.[28,30,94] Lidocaine poisoning occurs in 6–15% of patients receiving infusions at 3 mg/min.[46,105] In part for this reason, lidocaine is no longer used routinely to prevent dysrhythmias in the immediate postmyocardial infarction period.[49]

Note that when used as an antidysrhythmic agent, lidocaine must be administered parenterally to avoid the extensive first-pass hepatic metabolism associated with oral ingestion.[13] However, numerous publications unequivocally demonstrate the toxicity associated with orally administered lidocaine.[47,103] Following gastrointestinal tract absorption only one-third of the drug is bioavailable. However, because the primary metabolite, MEGX, is nearly as toxic as lidocaine itself, substantial toxicity may still occur following ingestion. Because of their small size and the relatively high concentration of viscous lidocaine (typically 4%), chil-

Figure 52-3. Structures of Class IB antidysrhythmic agents: Lidocaine (and metabolite MEGX), tocainide, mexiletine, and moricizine.

dren seem overrepresented in reports of oral lidocaine poisoning. As little as 15 mL of 2% viscous lidocaine in a 3-year-old child (estimate, 300 mg or 21.4 mg/kg/dose) may cause seizures.[47,103]

Tocainide. Tocainide (Fig. 52-3) is indicated for the treatment of ventricular dysrhythmias and is only available for oral administration. Although a lidocaine analogue, it does not undergo first-pass metabolism and is therefore almost 100% orally bioavailable.[67] Tocainide has pharmacologic effects that are nearly identical to lidocaine.[45,66,102] Both renal failure and congestive heart failure prolong its half-life considerably.[67] The few overdoses reported with tocainide are associated with CNS and cardiovascular complications similar to those that occur with lidocaine overdose.[7,23,36] Therapeutic dosing is rarely associated with blood dyscrasias, which has limited its widespread use.

Mexiletine. Mexiletine (Fig. 52-3), originally developed as an anorectic agent, was found to have antidysrhythmic, local anesthetic, and anticonvulsant activity.[18,19] It is currently available in oral form for the management of ventricular dysrhythmias. Its chemical structure and electrophysiologic properties are similar to those of lidocaine. Mexiletine, a base, is absorbed in the small intestine; therefore, its absorption is increased when the gastric contents are alkalinized. Congestive heart failure and cirrhosis, as well as therapy with cimetidine, isoniazid, and disulfiram, decrease the clearance of mexiletine.[65] Its metabolism, predominantly through CYP2D6, is accelerated by concomitant use of phenobarbital, rifampin, and phenytoin.[65]

Adverse therapeutic effects are primarily neurologic and are similar to those that occur with lidocaine. The few reported cases of mexiletine overdose describe prominent cardiovascular effects such as complete heart block, torsades de pointes, and asystole.[24,40,54] Neurotoxicity resulting from overdose includes self-limited seizures, generally in the setting of cardiotoxicity. Moreover, a single case report described a patient with mexiletine poisoning who experienced status epilepticus without any hemodynamic or electrocardiographic abnormalities.[88] The use of other IB antidysrhythmics such as lidocaine or tocainide may potentiate the neurotoxicity of mexiletine.

Moricizine. Moricizine (Fig. 52-3) is a phenothiazine derivative that possesses qualities of Class I agents in general, but is difficult to specifically subclassify. It depresses Na$^+$ current in a manner consistent with the other Class IA agents,[119] but has other properties that more appropriately place the drug in Class IB or IC. It is historically discussed as a Class IB agent, as it is here. The parent drug undergoes extensive and rapid metabolism. Dose-related increases in PR and QRS intervals are expected, as well as hemiblocks, bundle-branch blocks, and sustained ventricular tachydysrhythmias. Experience with this drug during the CAST II trial in the setting of myocardial infarction suggests that it is prodysrhythmic.[21] However, clinical experience with overdose of this drug is limited but is expected to be similar to other Class I antidysrhythmic agents. The manufacturer reports two lethalities related to overdose of the drug. These patients manifested respiratory failure, congestive heart failure, and ventricular dysrhythmia, which are similar to the effects noted in experimental studies.[37]

Treatment. The focus of the initial management for intravenous lidocaine-induced cardiac arrest is continuous cardiopulmonary resuscitation to allow lidocaine to redistribute from the heart. Out-side of this setting, management of hemodynamic compromise includes fluid replacement and other conventional strategies. Resistant hypotension may require dopamine or norepinephrine administration or insertion of an intra-aortic balloon assist pump.[42] Bradydysrhythmias typically do not respond to atropine, requiring the administration of dopamine, norepinephrine, or isoproterenol. External pacing or insertion of a transvenous pacemaker may be useful,[89] but the myocardium is often refractory to electrical capture. Lidocaine-induced seizures, or those related to lidocaine analogues, are generally brief in nature and do not require specific therapy. For patients requiring treatment, an intravenous benzodiazepine generally suffices; rarely, a barbiturate may be required.

Following oral poisoning by a Class IB agent, administration of activated charcoal is appropriate. The use of whole-bowel irrigation with a polyethylene glycol solution is undefined.[3] Enhanced elimination techniques are limited following intravenous poisoning because of the rapid time course of poisoning. Cardiopulmonary bypass, which does not directly enhance elimination, maintains hepatic perfusion, thereby allowing the lidocaine to be metabolized.[42,89] Hemoperfusion may rarely be warranted following lidocaine overdose if liver failure or circulatory collapse does not allow for other treatment modalities to be used. Hemoperfusion or hemodialysis may increase the clearance of tocainide but its indications remain unclear.[125] Mexiletine's extensive distribution and its rapid metabolism make it a poor candidate for extracorporeal drug removal.

Class IC Antidysrhythmic Agents: Flecainide and Propafenone

Flecainide. Flecainide, a fluorobenzamide derivative of procainamide, is used orally to treat both supraventricular and ventricular dysrhythmias.[2,90] Seventy percent of flecainide is metabolized hepatically by CYP2D6 to two major metabolites, one active and the other inactive; the remaining 30% is excreted renally. Thus, renal insufficiency, metabolic drug interactions, and congestive heart failure all decrease its clearance. Additionally, alkaluria reduces its clearance, presumably through enhanced tubular reuptake of nonionized drug. Patients using therapeutic doses may develop left ventricular dysfunction with worsening congestive heart failure. This is presumably due to flecainide's negative inotropic effect, which itself may relate to its antagonistic effects on calcium channels. Furthermore, sudden dysrhythmic death may occur, particularly in patients with underlying ischemic heart disease.[126]

Reported overdose experience is limited to case reports that uniformly involve polysubstance overdose. A 50% increase in QRS duration, a 30% prolongation of the PR interval, or a 15% increase in the QTc interval is consistent with flecainide toxicity.[83,90] The expected electrophysiologic consequences of these electrophysiologic disturbances include bradycardia, premature ventricular contractions, and ventricular tachydysrhythmias, including fibrillation.[22,108] The combination of marked QRS and PR interval changes associated with minimal QTc prolongation is characteristic of flecainide toxicity and contrasts with those described with other antidysrhythmic agents.

Propafenone. Propafenone bears a structural resemblance to propranolol,[43] and, not unexpectedly, has qualitatively, but not quantitatively, similar electrophysiologic properties.[25,79] Propafenone blocks fast inward sodium channels, is a weak β-adrenergic antagonist, and is an L-type calcium channel blocker.[110] Bioavailability is low as a result of first-pass metabolism by CYP-2D6 to 5-OH-propafenone, the primary active metabolite.[111] Accumulation of parent compound in patients with the slow metabolizer pharmacogenetic variant of CYP2D6 may cause excessive β-adrenergic antagonism.[70,71] The activity of a second metabolite, N-depropylpropafenone, is unknown.[111] Not unexpectedly, propafenone overdose produces sinus bradycardia, as well as ventricular dysrhythmias and negative inotropy.[87]

Acute overdose experience includes a 2-year-old child who reportedly ingested 1800 mg and developed a wide complex tachycardia, right bundle-branch block, first-degree AV block, and prolongation of the QT interval, as well as a generalized seizure.[78] The administration of phenytoin was associated with a simultaneous prolongation of the QRS interval, which initially responded to sodium bicarbonate, but the patient subsequently developed bradyasystolic arrest. Massive overdose in a young suicidal adult was linked to the development of a mild cardiomyopathy and a left bundle-branch block.[59] It is unclear if this was a result of the overdose, the epinephrine infusion used to manage the overdose, or if it was unrelated.

Treatment.   Initial stabilization should include standard management strategies for hypotension and seizures. Additionally, therapy for hypotension, and for the electrocardiographic manifestations of Class IC poisoning, includes intravenous hypertonic sodium bicarbonate to overcome the Na^+ channel blockade.[84] An animal study documents the beneficial effects of hypertonic sodium bicarbonate on flecainide-induced ventricular dysrhythmias,[60] and three reports of human overdose verify QRS narrowing in response to sodium bicarbonate administration.[15,75,43] Although sodium loading with hypertonic saline may be similarly effective, it remains unproved. Following overdose with tricyclic antidepressants, the renal elimination of flecainide is reduced by urinary alkalinization suggesting that sodium chloride, in equimolar doses, may ultimately prove superior to sodium bicarbonate.[84] The administration of other Class IA or IC antidysrhythmic agents is clearly contraindicated because of their additive blockade of the Na^+ channel. The efficacy of an external or internal pacemaker may be limited because of the drug-induced increased electrical pacing threshold of the ventricle.[108] Heroic therapy with cardiopulmonary bypass for flecainide overdose is reported,[22,26] and should be considered if readily available.

Extracorporeal removal is not expected to be beneficial for patients with flecainide poisoning, and in fact has been unsuccessful. However, although hemodialysis was successful at removing drug following propafenone overdose, additional studies are needed to determine its clinical benefit.[16]

CLASS III ANTIDYSRHYTHMIC AGENTS: AMIODARONE, BRETYLIUM, DOFETILIDE, AND IBUTILIDE

The Class III antidysrhythmic agents (Fig. 52-4) prevent and terminate reentrant dysrhythmias by prolonging the action potential duration and effective refractory period without slowing conduction velocity during phase 0 or 1 of the action potential. This drug-induced effect on the action potential is generally caused by blockade of the rapidly activating component of the delayed rectifier potassium current, which is responsible for repolarization. The Class III antidysrhythmic agents in use today prolong repolarization of both the atria and ventricles.[104] Thus, common electrocardiographic effects of the Class III agents at therapeutic doses are prolongation of the PR and QTc intervals and abnormal T and U waves. A detailed discussion of the pharmacologic mechanisms of this class can be found in Chapter 21. A discussion of sotalol can be found in Chapters 21 and 49.

Amiodarone

Amiodarone (Fig. 52-4) is an iodinated benzofuran derivative that is structurally similar to both thyroxine and procainamide. A recent study revealed that treatment with amiodarone of patients with out-of-hospital cardiac arrests caused by refractory ventricular dysrhythmias resulted in a higher rate of survival to hospital admission.[64] Furthermore, the newest revision of the ACLS guidelines places tremendous emphasis on the early intravenous administration of amiodarone. These, and perhaps other, studies will presumably lead to the increased use of this drug in patients with malignant dysrhythmias along with both its misuse and associated adverse effects.

Although it has multiple pharmacologic effects, its efficacy as an antidysrhythmic agent is presumably a result of its Class III effects. It also has weak α- and β-adrenergic antagonist activity and can block both calcium channels and inactivated sodium channels.[50] Amiodarone is slowly absorbed by the oral route and concentrates in the liver, lung, and adipose tissue. Steady-state pharmacokinetics may not occur for more than a month, and the elimination half-life is extremely long.

The electrocardiographic effects of amiodarone differ based on the route of drug administration. Therapeutic oral doses prolong PR and QTc intervals but not the QRS complex. Intravenous dosing may produce a prolongation of the PR interval, but has few other electrocardiographic manifestations. The differences may be because of the drug's active metabolite, desethylamiodarone, or because of the agent's vehicle, polysorbate 80. Ventricular dysrhythmias and sinus bradycardia are the most serious cardiac com-

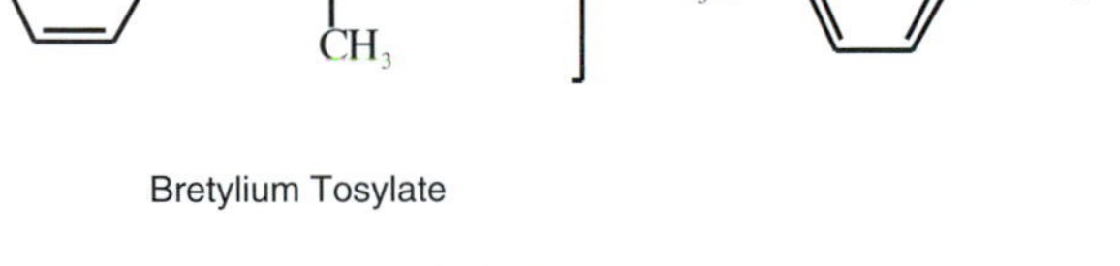

Bretylium Tosylate

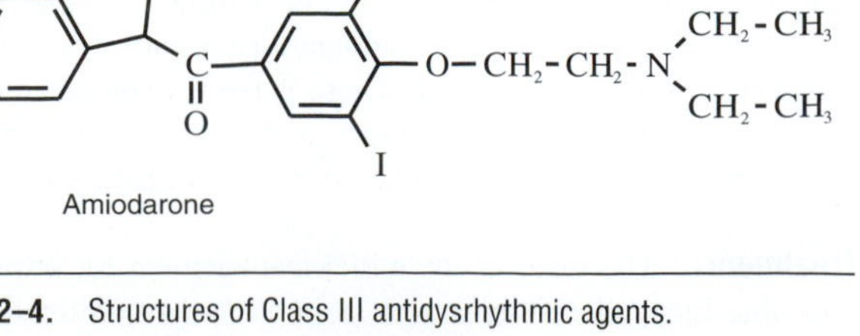

H_3C—⟨SO$_3^-$⟩ · [Br, CH_2—$N^+(CH_3)_2$—CH_2CH_3]

Amiodarone

CH_3; O (furan); C=O; I; I; O—CH_2—CH_2—$N(CH_2$—$CH_3)(CH_2$—$CH_3)$

Figure 52-4.   Structures of Class III antidysrhythmic agents.

plications of therapeutic doses of amiodarone.[77,106] Monomorphic and polymorphic ventricular tachycardias resistant to cardioversion and pharmacologic interventions are uncommon, but reported.[11,69] Important consequences of drug interactions include elevated digoxin levels, enhanced effectiveness of warfarin anticoagulation, and elevated cyclosporine levels, such as in patients with heart transplants.

Excessive intravenous dosing decreases myocardial contractility and peripheral vascular resistance and results in hypotension. Bradycardia is also common. The complications associated with long-term therapy do not occur following short-term intravenous use. Chronic therapy with oral amiodarone is associated with substantial pulmonary, thyroid, corneal, hepatic, and cutaneous toxicity.[76] Many of these effects appear to be dose related, but because of the wide range of bioavailabilities and metabolic patterns among different patients, as well as the overlap between therapeutic and toxic serum concentrations, therapeutic drug monitoring is of limited benefit. Pulmonary toxicity, the most consequential extracardiac adverse effect, may develop within days of initiating therapy but typically occurs following years of therapy. It is more common in patients with preexisting lung disease. Manifestations include dyspnea, cough, hemoptysis, rales, hypoxia, and radiographic changes.[98] Lung biopsy typically reveals interstitial pneumonitis with many macrophages and a characteristic finely vacuolated foamy cytoplasm. Thyroid dysfunction, either hypo- or hyper-, which occurs in about 4% of patients, is a predictable adverse effect because nearly 40% of the molecular weight of the drug is iodine. Hypothyroidism may be caused by noncompetitive inhibition by desethylamiodarone of thyroid hormone's binding to nuclear receptors.[68] Corneal microdeposits are extremely common during chronic therapy and may lead to vision loss. Abnormal elevation of hepatic enzymes occurs in more than 30% of those on therapy, and the hepatotoxicity may be associated with progression to cirrhosis. Slate gray or bluish discoloration of the skin is common particularly in sun-exposed portions of the body.

Bretylium Tosylate

Bretylium tosylate (Fig. 52–4), a quaternary benzylammonium compound, is frequently used to treat resistant ventricular dysrhythmias, including those that occur following myocardial infarction. Its removal from the ACLS guidelines and subsequent unavailability will reduce the risk for inadvertent iatrogenic drug overdose. Bretylium is concentrated in adrenergic neurons, where it initially releases and later inhibits the release of norepinephrine by adrenergic nerve endings.[100] Expectedly, administration is associated with transient hypertension initially followed later by hypotension.[10]

Dofetilide

Dofetilide is a newer Class III antidysrhythmic agent that is FDA approved for conversion of atrial fibrillation or atrial flutter to a normal sinus rhythm. Dofetilide increases the effective refractory period more substantially in atrial tissue than in ventricular fibers, accounting for this clinical indication. Still, it may also be of use in the treatment and prevention of paroxysmal supraventricular tachycardia and prevention of ventricular tachycardia. Unlike many of the other antidysrhythmics, it may reduce morbidity of patients with congestive heart failure. This is supported by experimental models in which increased myocardial contractility occurs.[114] Furthermore, it has no known effect on calcium, potassium, or sodium channels nor does it also result in β-adrenergic antagonism.[55] Dofetilide increases the QTc intervals, but does not change either the PR or QRS intervals in humans. Heart rate and blood pressure are also not appreciably affected.[107]

Although limited data are available, the expected and reported adverse cardiac events include ventricular tachycardia, particularly torsades de pointes. The approximate incidence of torsades de pointes in patients receiving high therapeutic doses of the drug is 3%.[38]

Overdose data reported by the manufacturer include two cases. One patient reportedly ingested 28 capsules and experienced no events, whereas a second patient inadvertently received 2 supratherapeutic doses 1 hour apart and experienced fatal ventricular fibrillation after the second dose.[116]

Ibutilide

Ibutilide, a methanesulphonamide derivative, is an antidysrhythmic with predominant Class III activity. It was recently marketed for the rapid conversion of atrial fibrillation and flutter to normal sinus rhythm. Because of ibutilide's extensive first-pass metabolism it can only be administered parenterally. Its metabolic pathways are not well understood, but they do not involve the cytochrome P450 isoenzymes CYP3A4 or CYP2D6. Pharmacokinetic data thus far do not indicate that age, sex, hepatic, or renal dysfunction would necessitate adjustment of ibutilide's recommended dosage. In addition to its effects on the delayed rectifier current, ibutilide, at nanomolar concentrations, activates a slow inward sodium current that is unaffected by potassium channel blockers.[86]

Ibutilide can increase the QTc interval and cause torsades de pointes, especially in patients with congenital long-QT syndrome (see Chap. 21). Although ibutilide can enhance the efficacy of transthoracic cardioversion for atrial fibrillation, its use in patients with ejection fractions below 20% is associated with a increased incidence of sustained polymorphic ventricular tachycardia.[91] Although acute renal failure, including biopsy-identified crystals consistent with other sulfonamide derivatives, is reported in association with ibutilide cardioversion, a causal relationship is not yet definitive.[41] Acute overdose information, only available in limited form through the manufacturer, suggests that ventricular dysrhythmias and high-degree AV conduction abnormalities should be expected.[27]

Treatment

Treatment experience with Class III agent overdose is limited. Torsades de pointes induced by amiodarone was successfully treated with isoproterenol and overdrive pacing.[106] Administration of Class IB antidysrhythmic agents or propranolol for the control of monomorphic ventricular tachycardia, while reported, cannot be recommended on theoretical grounds. Because the hypotension following bretylium is caused by inhibition of norepinephrine uptake and not by myocardial depression, intravenous fluids may effectively raise the blood pressure. The use of dopamine should be avoided following bretylium because it may result in uncontrollable hypertension.

Hemodialysis is not expected to be beneficial in general either because of extensive protein binding or because of large volumes of distribution. Multiple-dose activated charcoal and charcoal heimoperfusion may be of help if used immediately following overdose, but these approaches have not been studied in humans.

UNCLASSIFIED: ADENOSINE

Adenosine, a nucleoside found in all cells, is released from myocardial cells under physiologic and pathophysiologic conditions. It is administered as a rapid IV bolus to terminate reentrant supraventricular tachycardia.[31,85] The effects of adenosine are mediated by its interaction with specific G protein–coupled adenosine (A_1) receptors that activate acetylcholine-sensitive outward K^+ current in the atrium, sinus nodes, and AV nodes. The resultant hyperpolarization reduces the rate of cellular firing. Adenosine also reduces the Ca^{2+} currents and its antidysrhythmic activity results from its effect in increasing AV nodal refractoriness and inhibiting delayed afterdepolarizations (DADs) elicited by sympathetic stimulation.[72]

Adverse effects of adenosine administration are very common and include transient asystole, dyspnea, chest tightness, flushing, hypotension, and atrial fibrillation.[31] Although bronchospasm occurs following intrapulmonary administration, it is not reported following intravenous use. Fortunately, most of the adverse effects of adenosine are transitory because of its rapid metabolism to inosine by both extracellular and intracellular deaminases. Overdose of adenosine is not reported, but its clinical effects are potentiated by dipyridamole, an adenosine uptake inhibitor, and in cardiac transplant recipients, who develop denervation hypersensitivity. Methylxanthines may produce adenosine receptor blockade, and in this setting (Chap. 39), larger-than-usual doses of adenosine are required to produce an antidysrhythmic effect. Treatment would likely be supportive due to the rapid elimination of the drug.

SUMMARY

There are many antidysrhythmic agents presently in clinical use. In the overdose setting, the Class IA, B, and C drugs are associated with sodium channel blockade, which can cause profound cardiac dysrhythmias and morbidity if not treated judiciously. Most of the Class III antidysrhythmic agents in overdose can also cause malignant dysrhythmias, as well as severe multisystem derangements. It is only by understanding the pharmacokinetics and toxicokinetics of these agents that proper management can be accomplished.

ACKNOWLEDGMENTS

Mary Ann Howland, PharmD, and Harold Osborn, MD, contributed to this chapter in a previous edition.

REFERENCES

1. Accomero F, Pellanda A, Ruffini C, et al: Prolonged cardiopulmonary resuscitation during acute disopyramide poisoning. Vet Hum Toxicol 1993;35:231–232.
2. Anderson JL, Stewart JR, Perry BA, et al: Oral flecainide acetate for the treatment of ventricular arrhythmias. N Engl J Med 1981;305:473–477.
3. Arimori K, Deshimaru M, Furukawa E, Nakano M: Adsorption of mexiletine on to activated charcoal in Macrogel-electrolyte solution. Chem Pharm Bull (Tokyo) 1993;41:766–782.
4. Atkinson AJ, Krumlovsky FA, Huang CM, et al: Hemodialysis for severe procainamide toxicity: Clinical and pharmacokinetic observations. Clin Pharmacol Ther 1976;20:585–592.
5. Badui E, Garcia-Rubi D, Estañ B: Inadvertent massive lidocaine overdose causing temporary complete heart block in myocardial infarction. Am Heart J 1981;102:801–803.
6. Bailey DN: Percutaneous absorption of lidocaine hydrochloride in vivo. J Toxicol Cut Ocular Toxicol 1987;6:233–236.
7. Barnfield C, Kemmenoe AV: A sudden death due to tocainide overdose. Hum Toxicol 1986;5:337–340.
8. Bennett PB, Woolsey RL, Hondeghem LM: Competition between lidocaine and one of its metabolites, glycylxylidide, for cardiac sodium channels. Circulation 1988;78:692–700.
9. Benowitz NL, Forsyth RP, Melmon KL, Rowland M: Lidocaine disposition kinetics in monkey and man. 1. Prediction by a perfusion model. Clin Pharmacol Ther 1974;16:87–98.
10. Bodner T, Nowak R, Tomlanovich MC: Massive intravenous bolus bretylium tosylate. Ann Emerg Med 1980;9:630–633.
11. Bonati M, D'Arranno V, Galletti F: Acute overdose of amiodarone in a suicide attempt. J Toxicol Clin Toxicol 1983;20:181–186.
12. Boster SR, Danzl DF: Translaryngeal absorption of lidocaine. Ann Emerg Med 1982;11:461–465.
13. Boyes RN, Scott DB, Jebson PJ, et al: Pharmacokinetics of lidocaine in man. Clin Pharmacol Ther 1971;12:105–116.
14. Braden G, Fitzgibbons JP, Germain MJ, et al: Hemoperfusion for treatment of N-acetylprocainamide intoxication. Ann Intern Med 1986;105:64–65.
15. Brazil E, Bodiwala GG, Bouch DC: Fatal flecainide intoxication. Acad Emerg Med 1998;15:423–425.
16. Burgess ED, Duff HJ: Brief reports: Hemodialysis removal of propafenone. Pharmacotherapy 1989;9:331–333.
17. Cacoub P, Deray G, Baumelou A, et al: Disopyramide-induced hypoglycemia: Case report and review of the literature. Fundam Clin Pharmacol 1989;3:527–535.
18. Campbell NPS, Zaidi SA, Adgey AA, et al: Observations on hemodynamic effects of mexiletine. Br Heart J 1979;41:182–186.
19. Campbell RW: Mexiletine. N Engl J Med 1987;316:29–34.
20. The CAST Investigators: Preliminary report: Effect of encainide and flecainide on mortality in a randomized trial of arrhythmia suppression after myocardial infarction. N Engl J Med 1989;32:406–412.
21. The CAST II Investigators: Effects of the antiarrhythmic agent moricizine on survival after myocardial infarction. N Engl J Med 1991;327:227–233.
22. Chung PKC, Tuso P: The electrocardiographic changes in a case of flecainide overdose. Conn Med 1990;54:183–185.
23. Clark CWF, El-Mahdi EO: Fatal oral tocainide overdosage. Br Med J 1984;288:760.
24. Cocco G, Strozzi C, Chu D, Pansini R: Torsade de pointes as a manifestation of mexiletine toxicity. Am Heart J 1980;100:878–880.
25. Connolly SJ, Kates RE, Lebsack CS, et al: Clinical pharmacology of propafenone. Circulation 1983;68:589–596.
26. Corkeron MA, Van Heerden PV, Newman LD: Extracorporeal circulatory support in near fatal flecainide overdose. Anaesth Intensive Care 1999;27:405–408.
27. Corvert (ibutilide) package insert. Pharmacia & Upjohn, Kalamazoo, MI, 2000.
28. Cusson J, Rattel S, Matthew C, et al: Age-dependent lidocaine disposition in patients with acute myocardial infarction. Clin Pharmacol Ther 1985;37:381–386.
29. Dangman KH, Hoffman BF: In vivo and in vitro antiarrhythmic and arrhythmogenic effects of N-acetylprocainamide. J Pharmacol Exp Ther 1981;217:851–862.
30. Davison R, Parker M, Atkinson AJ Jr: Excessive serum lidocaine levels during maintenance infusions: Mechanisms and prevention. Am Heart J 1982;104:203–207.

31. DiMarco JP, Sellers TD, Lerman BB, et al: Diagnostic and therapeutic use of adenosine in patients with supraventricular tachyarrhythmias. J Am Coll Cardiol 1985;6:417-425.

32. Domoto D, Brown WW, Briggensmith P: Removal of toxic levels of N-acetylprocainamide with continuous arteriovenous hemofiltration or continuous arteriovenous hemodiafiltration. Ann Intern Med 1987;106:550-552.

33. Dorian P, Fain ES, Davy JM, Winkle RA: Lidocaine causes a reversible, concentration-dependent increase in defibrillation energy requirements. J Am Coll Cardiol 1986;8:327-332.

34. Drayer DE, Lowenthal DT, Woosley RL, et al: Accumulation of N-acetylprocainamide, a metabolite of procainamide, in patients with impaired renal function. Clin Pharmacol Ther 1977;22:63-69.

35. Edgren B, Tilelli J, Gehrz R: Intravenous lidocaine overdosage in a child. J Toxicol Clin Toxicol 1986;24:51-58.

36. Engler RL, Le Winter M: Tocainide-induced ventricular fibrillation. Am Heart J 1981;101:494-496.

37. Ethmozine (moricizine) package insert. Roberts Pharmaceutical Corp, Eatontown, NJ.

38. Falk RH, Pollak A, Singh S, et al: Intravenous dofetilide, a class III antiarrhythmic agent, for the termination of sustained atrial fibrillation or flutter. J Am Coll Cardiol 1997;29:385-390.

39. Finkelstein F, Kreeft J: Massive lidocaine poisoning. N Engl J Med 1979;301:50.

40. Frank SE, Snyder JT: Survival following severe overdose with mexiletine, nifedipine and nitroglycerine. Am J Emerg Med 1991;9:43-46.

41. Franz M, Geppert A, Kain R, et al: Acute renal failure after ibutilide. Lancet 1999;353:467.

42. Freedman MD, Gal J, Freed CR: Extracorporeal pump assistance: Novel treatment for acute lidocaine poisoning. Eur J Clin Pharmacol 1982;22:129-135.

43. Funk-Brentano C, Kroemer HK, Lee JT: Drug therapy: Propafenone. N Engl J Med 1990;322:518-525.

44. Goldman MJ, Mowry JB, Kirk MA: Sodium bicarbonate to correct widened QRS in a case of flecainide overdose. J Emerg Med 1997;15:183-186.

45. Graffner C, Conradson TB, Hofvendahl S, et al: Tocainide kinetics after intravenous and oral administration in healthy subjects and in patients with acute myocardial infarction. Clin Pharmacol Ther 1980;27:64-71.

46. Greenblatt DJ, Bolognini V, Koch-Weser J, et al: Pharmacokinetic approach to the clinical use of lidocaine intravenously. JAMA 1976;236:273-277.

47. Hess GP, Walson PD: Seizures secondary to oral viscous lidocaine. Ann Emerg Med 1988;17:725-727.

48. Heyman MR, Flores RH, Edelman BB, Carliner NH. Procainamide-induced lupus anticoagulant. South Med J 1988;81:934-936.

49. Hine LK, Laird N, Hewitt P, Chalmers TC: Meta-analytic evidence against prophylactic use of lidocaine in acute myocardial infarction. Arch Intern Med 1989;149:2694-2698.

50. Hondeghem LM, Mason JW, Katzung BG: Block of inactivated sodium channels and of depolarization-induced automaticity in guinea pig papillary muscle by amiodarone. Circ Res 1984;55:277-285.

51. Jackman WM, Friday KJ, Anderson JL, et al: The long QT syndromes: A critical review, new clinical observations and a unifying hypothesis. Prog Cardiovasc Dis 1988;31:115-172.

52. Jackson JE, Bentley JB, Glass SJ, et al: Effects of histamine-2 receptor blockade on lidocaine kinetics. Clin Pharmacol Ther 1985;37:544-548.

53. Jenzer HJ, Hagemeijer F: Quinidine syncope: Torsades de pointes with low quinidine plasma concentrations. Eur J Cardiol 1976;4:447-451.

54. Jequier P, Jones R, Mackintosh A: Fatal mexiletine overdose [letter]. Lancet 1976;1:429.

55. Kalus JS, Mauro VF: Dofetilide: A Class III-specific antiarrhythmic agent. Ann Pharmacother 2000;34:44-56.

56. Kar PM, Kellner K, Ing T, et al: Combined high-efficiency hemodialysis and charcoal hemoperfusion in severe N-acetylprocainamide intoxication. Am J Kidney Dis 1992;4:403-406.

57. Katz AM: Selectivity and toxicity of antiarrhythmic drugs: Molecular interactions with ion channels. Am J Med 1998;179-195.

58. Kempden PM: Lethal/toxic injection of 20% lidocaine: A well-known complication of an unnecessary preparation? Anesthesiology 1986;65:564-565.

59. Kerns W, English B, Ford M: Propafenone overdose. Ann Emerg Med 1994;24:98-103.

60. Keyler DE, Pentel PR: Hypertonic sodium bicarbonate partially reverses QRS prolongation due to flecainide in rats. Life Sci 1989;45:101-107.

61. Kim SY, Benowitz NL: Poisoning due to class Ia antiarrhythmic drugs, quinidine, procainamide and disopyramide. Drug Saf 1990;5:393-420.

62. Kim WY, Pomerance JJ, Miller AA: Lidocaine intoxication in a newborn following local anesthesia for episiotomy. Pediatrics 1979;64:643-645.

63. Kolecki PF, Curry SC: Poisoning by sodium channel blocking agents. Crit Care Clin 1997;13:829-848.

64. Kudenchuk PJ, Cobb LA, Copass MK, et al: Amiodarone for resuscitation after out-of-hospital cardiac arrest due to ventricular fibrillation. N Engl J Med 1999;341:871-878.

65. Kuhn P, Klicpera M, Kroiss A, et al: Antiarrhythmic and hemodynamic effects of mexiletine. Postgrad Med J 1977;53(Suppl 1):81-84.

66. Kvatiek SP, Morganroth J, Horowitz LN: Tocainide: A new oral antiarrhythmic agent. Ann Intern Med 1985;103:387-391.

67. Lalka D, Meyer MB, Duce BR, et al: Kinetics of the oral antiarrhythmic lidocaine congener, tocainide. Clin Pharmacol Ther 1976;19:757-766.

68. Latham KR, Sellitti DF, Goldstein RE: Interaction of amiodarone and desethylamiodarone with solubilized nuclear thyroid hormone receptors. J Am Coll Cardiol 1987;9:872-876.

69. Lazzara R: Amiodarone and torsade de pointes. Ann Intern Med 1989;549-551.

70. Lee JT, Kroemer HK, Silberstein DJ, et al: The role of genetically determined polymorphic drug metabolism in the beta-blockade produced by propafenone. N Engl J Med 1990;322:1764-1768.

71. Lee JT, Lineberry MD, Funck-Brentano C, et al: Propafenone-induced β-blockade in extensive and poor metabolizer subjects. Circulation 1988;78(Suppl II):499.

72. Lerman BB, Belardinelli L: Cardiac electrophysiology of adenosine: Basic and clinical concepts. Circulation 1991;83:1499-1509.

73. Levy S, Azoulay S: Stories about the origin of quinine and quinidine. J Cardiovasc Electrophysiol 1994;5:635-636.

74. Lie KI, Wellens HJ, van Capelle FJ, Durrer D: Lidocaine in the prevention of primary ventricular fibrillation: A double-blind, randomized study of 212 consecutive patients. N Engl J Med 1974;29:1324-1326.

75. Lovecchio F, Berlin R, Brubacher JR, et al: Hypertonic sodium bicarbonate in an acute flecainide overdose. Am J Emerg Med 1998;16:534-537.

76. Mason JW: Amiodarone. N Engl J Med 1987;316:455-466.

77. McGovern B, Garan H, Kelly E, Ruskin J: Adverse reactions during treatment with amiodarone hydrochloride. Br Med J 1983;287:175-180.

78. McHugh TP, Perina DG: Propafenone ingestion. Ann Emerg Med 1987;16:437-440.

79. McLeod AA, Stiles GL, Spand DG: Demonstration of beta adrenoreceptor blockade by propafenone hydrochloride. Clinical, pharmacologic, radioligand binding and adenyl cyclase activation studies. J Pharmacol Exp Ther 1983;228:461-466.

80. Mizuyama K, Dohi SD: An accidental subdural injection of a local anaesthetic resulting in respiratory depression. Anaesth 1993;40:83-84.

81. Mofenson HC, Caraccio TR, Miller H, et al: Lidocaine toxicity from topical mucosal application. Clin Pediatr 1983;22:190-192.

82. Morady F, Scheinman MM, Desai J: Disopyramide. Ann Intern Med 1982;96:337-343.

83. Horowitz LN, Morganroth J, Horowitz J: Flecainide: Its proarrhythmic effect and expected changes on the surface electrocardiogram. J Am Coll Cardiol 1984;53:89B-94B.

84. Muhiddin KA, Johnston A, Turner P: The influence of urinary pH on flecainide excretion and its serum pharmacokinetics. Br J Clin Pharm 1984;17:447-451.

85. Munoz A, Leenhardt A, Sassine A, et al: Therapeutic use of adenosine for terminating spontaneous paroxysmal supraventricular tachycardia. Eur Heart J 1984;5:735-738.

86. Murray KT: Ibutilide. Circulation 1998;97:493-497.

87. Nathan AW, Bexton RS, Hellestrand KJ, et al: Fatal ventricular tachycardia in association with propafenone, a new class IC antiarrhythmic agent. Postgrad Med J 1984;60:155-156.

88. Nelson L, Hoffman R: Mexiletine overdose producing status epilepticus without cardiovascular abnormalities. J Toxicol Clin Toxicol 1994;32:731-736.

89. Noble J, Kennedy DJ, Lattimer RD, et al: Massive lignocaine overdose during cardiopulmonary bypass, successful treatment with cardiac pacing. Br J Anesth 1984;56:1439-1441.

90. Olsson SB, Edvardsson N: Clinical electrophysiologic study of antiarrhythmic properties of flecainide: Acute intraventricular delayed conduction and prolonged repolarization with programmed stimulation. Am Heart J 1981;102:864-871.

91. Oral H, Souza JJ, Michand GF: Facilitating transthoracic cardioversion of atrial fibrillation with ibutilide pretreatment. N Engl J Med 1999;340:1849-1854.

92. Pantuck A, Goldsmith JW, Kuriyan JB, Weiss RE: Seizures after ureteral stone manipulation with lidocaine. J Urol 1997;157:2248.

93. Peat MA, Deyman ME, Crouch DJ, et al: Concentrations of lidocaine and monoethylglycylxylidide (MEGX) in lidocaine-associated deaths. J Forensic Sci 1985;30:1048-1057.

94. Pfeifer HJ, Greenblatt DJ, Koch-Weser J: Clinical use and toxicity of intravenous lidocaine. A report from the Boston Collaborative Drug Surveillance Program. Am Heart J 1976;92:168-173.

95. Podrid PJ, Schoenberger A, Lown B: Congestive heart failure caused by oral disopyramide. N Engl J Med 1980;302:614-618.

96. Pokis A, Mackell MA, Tucker EF: Tissue distribution of lidocaine after fatal accidental injection. J Forensic Sci 1984;29:1129-1236.

97. Rao R, Ely SF, Hoffman RS: Deaths related to liposuction. N Engl J Med 1999;340:1471-1475.

98. Ravishankar R, Samuels LF, Kaufman MS: Amiodarone-associated hemoptysis. Am J Med Sci 1998;316:390-392.

99. Roden DM: Risks and benefits of antiarrhythmic drug therapy. N Engl J Med 1994;331:785-791.

100. Roden DM: Current status of class III antiarrhythmic drug therapy. Am J Cardiol 1993;72:44B-49B.

101. Roden DM, Hoffman BF: Action potential prolongation and induction of abnormal automaticity by low quinidine concentrations in canine Purkinje fibers. Relationship to potassium and cycle length. Circ Res 1985;56:857-867.

102. Roden DM, Woolsey RL: Tocainide. N Engl J Med 1986;315:41-45.

103. Rothstein P, Dornbusch J, Shaywitz B: Prolonged seizures associated with the use of viscous lidocaine. J Pediatr 1982;101:461-463.

104. Sager PT: New advances in Class III antiarrhythmic drug therapy. Curr Opin Cardiol 2000;15:41-53.

105. Sawyer DR, Ludden TM, Crawford MH: Lidocaine infusions with cardiac arrhythmias: Unpredictability of plasma concentrations. Arch Intern Med 1981;141:43-45.

106. Sclarovsky S, Lewin RF, Kracoff O, et al: Amiodarone-induced polymorphous ventricular tachycardia. Am Heart J 1983;105:6-12.

107. Sedgewick ML, Rasmussen HS, Cobbe SM: Clinical and electrophysiologic effects of intravenous dofetilide (UK-68,798)—A new Class III antiarrhythmic drug in patients with angina pectoris. Am J Cardiol 1992;69:513-517.

108. Sellers TD, DiMarco JP: Sinusoidal ventricular tachycardia associated with flecainide acetate. Chest 1984;85:647-649.

109. Shub C, Gan GT: Management of acute quinidine intoxication. Chest 1978;73:173-178.

110. Siddoway LA, Roden DM, Woosley RE: Clinical pharmacology of propafenone: Pharmacokinetics, metabolism and concentration-response relations. Am J Cardiol 1984;54:9D-12D.

111. Siddoway LA, Thompson KA, McAllister CB, et al: Polymorphism of propafenone metabolism and disposition in man: Clinical and pharmacokinetic consequences. Circulation 1987;75:785-791.

112. Strong JM, Mayfield DE, Atkinson AJ Jr, et al: Pharmacological activity, metabolism and pharmacokinetics of glycine xylidide. Clin Pharmacol Ther 1975;17:184-194.

113. Swiryn S, Kim SS: Quinidine induced syncope. Arch Intern Med 1983;143:314-316.

114. Tande PM, Bjornstad H, Yang T, Refsum H: Rate-dependent Class III antiarrhythmic action, negative chronotropy, and positive inotropy of a novel Ik blocking drug UK-668,798: Potent in guinea pig but not effective in rat myocardium. J Cardiovasc Pharmacol 1990;16:401-410.

115. Thomson PD, Rowland M, Melmon KL: The influence of heart failure, liver disease, and renal failure on the disposition of lidocaine in man. Am Heart J 1971;82:417-421.

116. Tikosyn (dofetilide) package information. Pfizer Laboratories.

117. Tzivoni D, Banai S, Schuger C, et al: Treatment of torsades de pointes with magnesium sulfate. Circulation 1988;77:392-397.

118. Vaughan Williams EM: Classifying antiarrhythmic actions: By facts or speculation. J Clin Pharmacol 1992;32:964-977.

119. Vaughan Williams EM: Classification of the antiarrhythmic action of moricizine. J Clin Pharmacol 1991;31:216-221.

120. Vaughan Williams EM: Significance of classifying antiarrhythmic actions since the Cardiac Arrhythmia Suppression Trial. J Clin Pharmacol 1991;31:123-135.

121. Vaughan Williams EM: Classification of antiarrhythmic drugs. Pharmacol Ther [B] 1975;1:115-138.

122. Wasserman F, Brodsky L, Dick MM, et al: Successful treatment of quinidine and procainamide intoxication. N Engl J Med 1958;259:797-802.

123. Wetherbee DG, Holzman D, Brown MG: Ventricular tachycardia following the administration of quinidine. Am Heart J 1951;42:89-96.

124. White NJ, Warrell DA, Chanthavanich P, et al: Severe hypoglycemia and hyperinsulinemia in falciparum malaria. N Engl J Med 1983;309:61-66.

125. Wieger U, Hanrath P, Kuck KH: Pharmacokinetics of tocainide in patients with renal dysfunction and during hemodialysis. Eur J Clin Pharmacol 1983;24:503-507.

126. Winkelmann BR, Leinberger H: Life-threatening flecainide toxicity: A pharmacodynamic approach. Ann Intern Med 1987;106:807-814.

127. Working Group on Arrhythmias of the European Society of Cardiology: The Sicilian Gambit. Circulation 1991;84:1831-1851.

128. Wu FL, Razzaghi A, Souney PF: Seizure after lidocaine for bronchoscopy: Case report and review of the use of lidocaine. Airway Pharmacotherapy 1993;3:72-78.

Brian Kaufman

A 40-year-old dentist was found unresponsive in his procedure room by his office staff. The paramedics noted that the mask he had on his face was attached to a supply of nitrous oxide and oxygen. The oxygen tank was empty. His blood pressure was 140/90 mm Hg; his pulse was 120 beats/min; and his respiratory rate was 22 breaths/min and regular. In the Emergency Department (ED), his oxygen saturation by pulse oximetry was 63%. His pupils were dilated and minimally reactive. He remained unresponsive to painful stimulation. His blood glucose was 110 mg/dL. His serum electrolytes and complete blood count were normal. A CT scan of the head was normal. A presumptive diagnosis of anoxic encephalopathy secondary to unintentional inhalation of pure nitrous oxide was made. Neurologic improvement did not occur.

General anesthesia occurs as a result of reversible changes in neurologic function caused by drugs that modulate synaptic neurotransmission. The elements of general anesthesia include amnesia, analgesia, inhibition of noxious reflexes, and skeletal muscle relaxation.

Reversible changes in neurologic function cause loss of perception and reaction to pain, unawareness of immediate events, and loss of memory of those events. The exact mechanism by which the inhaled (volatile) anesthetics produce general anesthesia remains uncertain, but there are experimental data to support several theories. The pharmacologic mechanisms for general anesthesia include the physical-chemical behavior of volatile hydrocarbons within the hydrophobic regions of biologic membrane lipids and proteins.

Because a wide range of chemically distinct compounds can produce anesthesia, it is unlikely that a unique receptor exists for the inhaled anesthetic drugs; it is more likely that the volatile agents probably cause general anesthesia by modulating synaptic function from within cell membranes.

HISTORY

Modern anesthetic practice is often stated to have begun on Friday, October 16, 1846, at the Massachusetts General Hospital when a dentist, William Morton, gave the first public demonstration of the ability of inhaled ether vapor to alleviate the pain of surgery. Following this feat, John C. Warren, the chief of surgery, remarked to the assembled gallery, "Gentleman, this is no humbug." Oliver Wendell Holmes then chose the Greek-related noun anesthesia (without feeling) to characterize the process.

The earliest description of the use of an inhalational agent was by Paracelsus, a Swiss physician and alchemist who prepared a mixture of ether, alcohol, and water called sweet oil of vitriol. He described how he fed this preparation to hens who fell into a deep sleep from which they recovered unharmed. In 1735, Wilhelm Froben gave this substance its modern name of ether. Ether was used topically, particularly by the intranasal route, as a treatment of headache, nervous diseases, and fits.

Observations on the physiology of the circulation and respiration eventually led to an understanding of the effects of inhalation gases and vapors. In the last decade of the 18th century, centers for the pneumatic treatment of disease were established in Birmingham and Bristol, England. Experiments were conducted at these institutions with the use of ether inhaled via a funnel and with nitrous oxide. Humphry Davy's description of his own pleasurable and exhilarating experience when he inhaled the "laughing" gas led to many of his colleagues and friends inhaling nitrous oxide to experience its inebriating effects. Davy also described how the inhalation of nitrous oxide relieved headache and the pain of an erupting molar tooth. Although recognizing the analgesic properties of nitrous oxide and its possible application for surgery, he failed to pursue the idea.

The public soon took up the use of nitrous oxide in the form of nitrous oxide frolics. Audiences to itinerant medicine shows would volunteer to experience the exhilarating effects of nitrous oxide inhalation. At one such show in 1844, at Hartford Connecticut, a man under the influence of nitrous oxide injured his leg but did not feel any pain. Dr. Horace Wells, a dentist in the audience that day, inhaled nitrous oxide the following day and had his partner painlessly remove a troublesome tooth. A subsequent public demonstration of the use of nitrous oxide for dental extraction went poorly, impeding the general acceptance of this agent as a surgical anesthetic, and led to the subsequent initial acceptance of ether as a general anesthetic agent.

In Great Britain in 1847, James Simpson, an obstetrician, first utilized ether to relieve the pain of labor. He subsequently adopted chloroform for this purpose because of its more pleasant odor and more rapid induction and emergence. The clergy and other physicians opposed the concept of relieving pain during childbirth, but the method was ultimately accepted after Queen Victoria gave birth to Prince Leopold with chloroform given by John Snow.

Over the next century, several volatile anesthetic agents were introduced, including ethyl chloride (1848), divinyl ether (1933), trichloroethylene (1934), and ethyl vinyl ether (1947). All of these agents had significant safety problems associated with their use including the combustibility of most of these agents and direct organ toxicity.

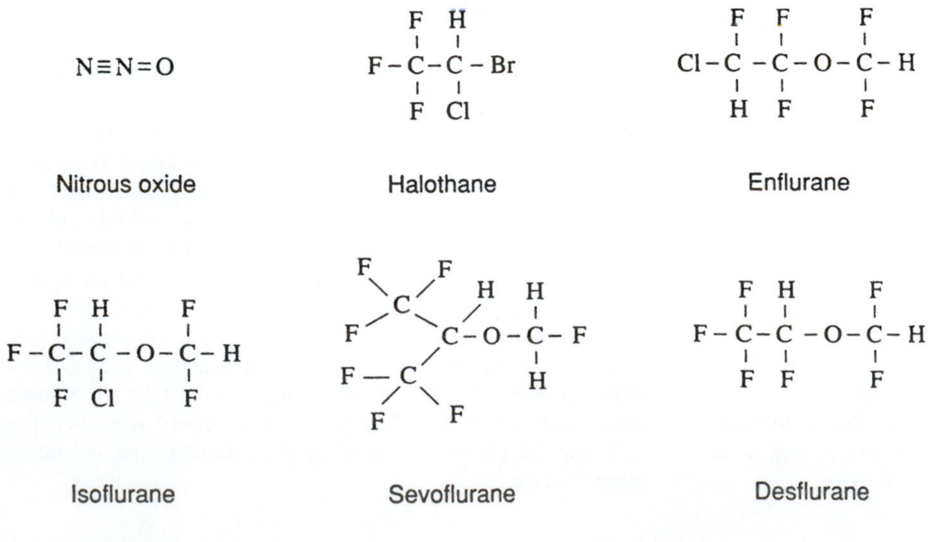

Figure 53-1. The inhalational anesthetics.

Advances in fluorine chemistry associated with nuclear research in the 1940s, which led to the cost-effective incorporation of fluorine into molecules, were pivotal in the development of modern anesthetics. Fluroxene was the first of the new fluorinated anesthetics to be widely used clinically. However, this agent was flammable and hepatotoxic. It was largely replaced by the nonflammable halothane, which was synthesized in 1951 and introduced into clinical practice in 1956. Methoxyflurane was evaluated in humans in 1960, but is no longer used because of nephrotoxicity and hepatotoxicity. Other halogenated hydrocarbons with improved clinical properties have subsequently been introduced, including enflurane, isoflurane, desflurane, and sevoflurane (Fig. 53-1).

PHARMACOKINETICS

The potency of the various inhaled anesthetic drugs is correlated with their physicochemical properties. The dominant theories of the molecular mechanisms by which volatile agents affect membrane function are based on the lipid solubility of the drugs and experimental demonstration of pressure reversal of anesthesia. The anesthetic potency of volatile agents correlates directly with the relative lipid solubility of each drug. This suggests that the primary molecular actions of anesthetics occur in the lipid portion of cell membranes known as the Meyer-Overton lipid solubility theory. Potential membrane regions for anesthetic action include the hydrophobic areas of proteins and protein–lipid interface regions, as well as the phospholipid matrix. Because high pressures (100–200 atmospheres) can reverse the anesthetic effects of several drugs, this suggests that the drugs could be causing anesthesia by increasing membrane volume at normal atmospheric pressure known as the volume expansion theory.

Because the inhaled anesthetics enter the body through the lungs, the factors that influence their absorption by blood and distribution to other tissues include the solubility of the drug in blood, blood flow through the lungs, and distribution to the various organs, solubility of the anesthetic in tissue, and the mass of the tissue. The goal of inhalation anesthesia is to develop and maintain a satisfactory partial pressure of anesthetic in the brain, the primary site of action.

The pharmacokinetics of anesthetics can be linked to their pharmacodynamics by consideration of anesthetic potency. The linkage exists because the desired alveolar concentration is what one strives to achieve and maintain during anesthesia. For the inhaled drugs, potency is commonly referred to as the minimum alveolar concentration (MAC) of the anesthetic. This is the alveolar concentration at 1 atmosphere that prevents movement in 50% of subjects in response to a painful stimulus. MAC is used when comparing the effects of equipotent doses of anesthetics on various organ functions.

NITROUS OXIDE

Nitrous oxide is the most commonly used inhalational anesthetic in the world. Its advantages include a mild odor, absence of airway irritation, rapid induction and emergence from anesthesia, potent analgesia, and minimal respiratory and circulatory effects. When administered in a modern operating room using current standards of monitoring to prevent unintentional hypoxia, it is a remarkably safe agent. Unfortunately, nitrous oxide also has a potential for abuse, particularly among hospital and dental personnel.[24] Death and permanent brain damage are reported. However, these do not result from direct toxic effects; instead, they are secondary to asphyxia, such as from inhalation of insufficient oxygen, or from use of high concentrations of the gas in a poorly ventilated room.[12] If a patient who is exposed to nitrous oxide fails to regain consciousness within several minutes after breathing fresh air or oxygen, other etiologies for the altered mental status such as hypoxic encephalopathy or concomitant ingestion of a central nervous system (CNS)–depressant drug should be suspected.

Deaths may occur when patients receive commercially prepared nitrous oxide from tanks contaminated with impurities such as nitric oxide or nitrogen dioxide, and pulmonary toxicity was described when similar contaminants were produced by individual preparation of nitrous oxide by the combustion of ammonium nitrate fertilizer.[28]

Injury can also result from the physical properties of this agent. Nitrous oxide is 35 times more soluble in blood than is nitrogen. When it is inhaled, any compliant air-containing space, such as bowel, will increase in size, while noncompliant spaces, such as disorder improved slowly when the patients abstained from further nitrous oxide abuse. As discussed, this neuropathy is clinically indistinguishable from subacute combined degeneration of the spinal cord associated with pernicious anemia. The syndrome of nitrous oxide neuropathy is characterized by sensorimotor polyneuropathy, often combined with signs of posterior and lateral spinal cord involvement. Signs and symptoms include numbness and paresthesias in the extremities, weakness, and truncal ataxia. Neurologic changes develop only after several months of frequent exposure to nitrous oxide. Those at risk include individuals who chronically abuse the gas as well as those who are occupationally exposed to grossly contaminated environments for prolonged periods.[4] This is a very unlikely scenario in the modern operating room, where inhalational anesthetics are scavenged, but it may occur in poorly ventilated dental offices, where personnel are exposed to greater than 1000 parts per million (ppm) of nitrous oxide. This problem is probably markedly underdiagnosed, because the neurologic changes that occur in mild cases mimic other more common neurologic conditions.[7]

Chronic Exposure to Trace Levels of Nitrous Oxide

Dentists and dental assistants are often exposed to greater concentrations of waste anesthetic gases than individuals working in well-vented operating rooms. Animal studies demonstrate that methionine synthase may be inactivated by exposure to greater than 1000 ppm nitrous oxide, a level often exceeded in dental procedure rooms. An epidemiologic survey of dentists compared 15,000 who used and 15,000 who did not use nitrous oxide in their practices.[7] A 1.2–1.8-fold increase in liver, kidney, and neurologic disease was found in the dentists and their chair-side assistants who were chronically exposed to trace levels of nitrous oxide. For those with heavy office use of nitrous oxide, there was a 4-fold increase in the incidence of neurologic complaints as compared to the nonexposed group. Female dental assistants who were exposed to nitrous oxide also had a 2–3-fold increase in spontaneous abortion rates, reduced fertility, and a higher rate of congenital abnormalities in their offspring.

Treatment

General. Removal of the acutely affected person from the toxic environment should be the initial intervention. Individuals who

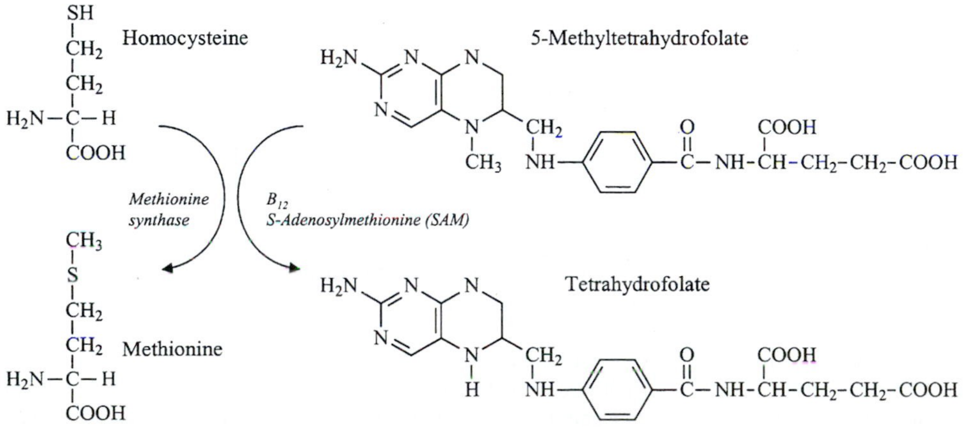

the eustachian tubes, will exhibit an increase in pressure. These effects occur because nitrous oxide diffuses along the concentration gradient from the blood into a closed space much more rapidly than nitrogen can be transferred in the opposite direction. Clinical consequences include rapid progression of a pneumothorax to tension pneumothorax, tympanic membrane rupture with hearing loss, bowel distention, and tracheal or laryngeal trauma caused by increased endotracheal cuff pressure.

Hematologic Effects

Bone marrow depression was first recognized as a complication of long-term nitrous oxide exposure in the 1950s, when the gas was used to sedate intubated patients with severe tetanus.[23] Leukopenia with hypoplastic bone marrow and megaloblastic erythropoiesis developed 3–5 days after initial exposure, followed by thrombocytopenia. Bone marrow recovery usually occurs within 4 days after the agent is discontinued. Healthy patients undergoing routine surgical procedures demonstrate mild megaloblastic bone marrow changes after 12 hours of exposure to 50% nitrous oxide and marked changes after 24 hours.[32] Critically ill patients may be more sensitive to the effects of nitrous oxide on the bone marrow, because megaloblastic changes are described after as little as 1 hour of exposure.[3]

The hematologic effects of exposure to nitrous oxide strongly resemble the biochemical characteristics of pernicious anemia.[2,30] Vitamin B_{12}, or cyanocobalamin, is a bound coenzyme of cytoplasmic methionine synthase. The cobalt moiety in the enzyme functions as a methyl carrier in its transfer from 5-methyltetrahydrofolate to homocysteine to form methionine (Fig. 53–2). Nitrous oxide oxidizes the cobalt, converting vitamin B_{12} from the active monovalent form (cob(I)alamin) to an inactive bivalent form (cob(II)alamin), which irreversibly inhibits methionine synthase.[30] The metabolic consequences of this block are quite significant, because methionine and tetrahydrofolate are required for both DNA synthesis and for production of myelin. This interference is responsible for the development of bone marrow depression and polyneuropathy resembling those that occur in pernicious anemia.[30]

Neurologic Effects

Disabling polyneuropathy in healthcare workers who habitually abused nitrous oxide was first described in 1978.[24] The neurologic

Figure 53–2. The hematologic effects of exposure to nitrous oxide resemble those characteristic of pernicious anemia and are related to oxidation and inactivation of vitamin B_{12}. The irreversible blockade of the methionine synthase is consequential with regard to DNA synthesis and myelin production.

have developed toxicity from abuse of the gas should be educated about the relationship between their recreational activities and their clinical findings.

Specific. Vitamin B_{12} may help patients with a masked vitamin B_{12} deficiency who develop megaloblastic anemia and neurologic dysfunction after brief exposure to nitrous oxide, but it is not beneficial in patients who have toxicity resulting from more chronic exposure.[34] The reason for the ineffectiveness of vitamin B_{12} in this situation is uncertain.

The bone marrow abnormalities associated with nitrous oxide toxicity may be reversed by the administration of a single 30-mg intravenous dose of folinic acid (the active form of folate)[31] (Antidotes in Depth: Folic Acid and Leucovorin). A methionine-supplemented diet also greatly reduced the demyelination and neurologic damage induced in monkeys by chronic exposure to 15% nitrous oxide.[35]

HALOGENATED HYDROCARBONS

The inhaled anesthetics were initially considered to be biochemically inert drugs with therapeutic efficacy. Initial reports of toxicity following their administration were poorly explained and attributed to direct effects of the drugs on susceptible organs. It is now clear that the inhalational anesthetics are not inert but are metabolized in vivo, and that their metabolites are responsible for acute and chronic toxicity.

Halothane Hepatitis

Two distinct types of hepatotoxicity are associated with the use of halothane. The first is a mild dysfunction that develops in approximately 20% of exposed patients. Patients are often asymptomatic, but exhibit modest elevations of serum aminotransferase levels within a few days of anesthetic exposure. Recovery is complete.[29] The second is a life-threatening hepatitis that occurs in approximately 1 in 10,000 exposed patients, and which produces fatal massive hepatic necrosis in 1 of 35,000 patients.[38] The histologic findings of massive hepatocellular necrosis are indistinguishable from those of viral hepatitis.[42] Differentiating halothane hepatitis from viral or other toxic hepatitis that becomes clinically evident in the postoperative period is difficult without positive serologic studies. Jaundice, common following anesthesia and surgery, is usually due to factors such as preexisting liver disease, blood transfusion, sepsis, or other causes of hepatitis. Halothane hepatitis is thus a diagnosis of exclusion.

Factors that may increase the risk of developing hepatotoxicity from halothane include multiple exposures, obesity, female gender, age, and ethnic origin.

Several studies report an association between multiple exposures to halothane and subsequent development of hepatitis.[41,45] In one study, 95% of cases of halothane hepatitis followed multiple exposures, and 55% followed halothane reexposure within 4 weeks.[45] Under these circumstances, the liver dysfunction is usually more severe and the latency before clinical presentation is usually shorter than when the syndrome develops following initial exposure to halothane.[41]

Obesity is implicated in several reports as a risk factor for hepatotoxicity following prolonged exposure.[43] Increased fat stores may act as a "reservoir" for this agent, with slow and prolonged release into the circulation, and subsequent increase in production of potentially hepatotoxic metabolites.

Most cases of halothane hepatitis occur in middle-aged patients. Females reportedly have a 2-fold increase in risk of developing the syndrome.[20] Genetic factors may also play a role in some patients, as there is a report of this syndrome in three pairs of related women of Mexican-Indian or Mexican-Spanish ancestry.[19]

Mechanism of Toxicity. Halothane is the most extensively metabolized inhalational anesthetic. Approximately 20% of the absorbed drug undergoes oxidative metabolism, principally by cytochrome P450 in the liver, to trifluoroacetic acid. Reduction to trifluorochloroethane and difluorochloroethylene (Fig. 53–3) is a minor route of halothane metabolism that requires the absence of oxygen and the presence of an electron donor. These volatile metabolites are free radicals, which may directly produce acute hepatic toxicity by irreversibly binding to and destroying intracellular structures in the hepatocyte. Alternatively, by acting as haptens they may trigger an immune-mediated hypersensitivity response.[33,44] The high percentage of patients with halothane hepatitis who had recent prior exposure to the drug is most consistent with the latter mechanism.[20]

Enflurane, used extensively in North America since 1966, is weakly associated with hepatotoxicity. Some authorities believe that the evidence does not support the existence of enflurane-induced hepatic necrosis.[13,15,37] Isoflurane, desflurane, and sevoflurane all appear to have low hepatotoxic potential.

Nephrotoxicity

The kidneys are the only other organ at risk of toxicity from modern inhalational anesthetics. Methoxyflurane is an anesthetic introduced in 1962. In 1966, it was linked to the development of vasopressin-resistant polyuric renal insufficiency (nephrogenic diabetes insipidus) in 16 of 94 patients receiving prolonged methoxyflurane anesthesia for abdominal surgery[10] (Chap. 24). Polyuria was associated with a negative fluid balance; dehydration; elevation of serum sodium, osmolality, and urea nitrogen concentrations; and a fixed urinary osmolality close to that of serum. Renal abnormalities lasted from 10–20 days in most patients, but persisted in 3 patients for more than 1 year. Subsequent studies demonstrated that the renal toxicity was caused by inorganic fluoride (F) released during biotransformation of methoxyflurane.[40] The risk of toxicity was highly correlated with both the total dose of methoxyflurane (concentration × duration) and the peak serum (F) concentration.[9,27] The nephrotoxic serum fluoride concentration is 50–60 μmol/L.[9] Factors that enhance biotransformation (obesity, enzyme induction) increased the risk of toxicity. Although the precise mechanism by which fluoride produces its toxic effect on the kidney is not clear, one hypothesis is that fluoride inhibits adenylate cyclase and thereby interferes with the normal action of antidiuretic hormone on the distal convoluted tubules.

Although methoxyflurane is no longer used, lessons learned regarding its toxicity are applied when evaluating the nephrotoxic potential of other fluorinated anesthetics. Of the currently used agents (halothane, isoflurane, enflurane, desflurane, sevoflurane), only enflurane and sevoflurane undergo biotransformation by defluorination. This occasionally results in sufficient serum fluoride concentrations to produce transient decreases in urine concentrating ability. However, clinically evident renal impairment almost never occurs with the use of either agent.[22]

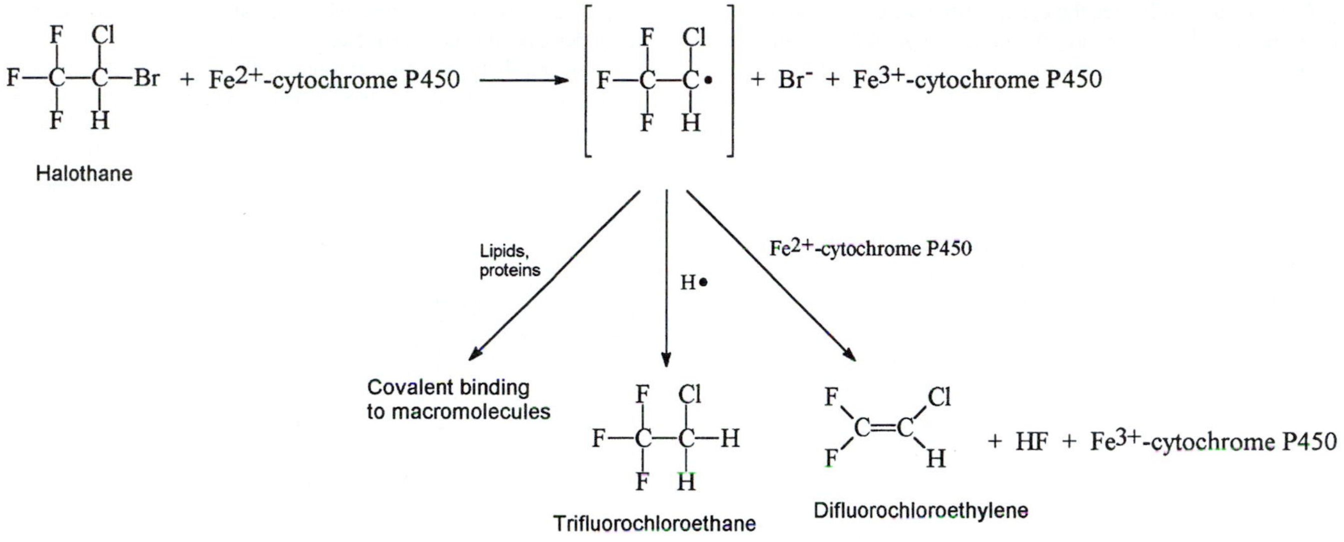

Pharmacokinetics

Chronic use of isoniazid induces CYP2E1, the enzyme responsible for the metabolism of enflurane. This induction results in elevated serum fluoride levels in approximately 50% of the isoniazid-treated patients who receive an enflurane anesthetic.[27] The fluoride concentrations, however, are neither high enough nor sustained long enough to produce clinically significant renal dysfunction. Nonetheless, it would seem prudent to avoid prolonged use of enflurane in patients taking isoniazid or other agents, such as ethanol, phenobarbital, and phenytoin, which elevate the hepatic activity of cytochrome CYP2E1 (Chap. 11).

Unusually high serum fluoride concentrations are also reported in morbidly obese patients anesthetized with enflurane.[8] This finding may be related to this group's large storage capacity for fat-soluble drugs. Although prolonged postoperative release and metabolism of enflurane may occur, renal dysfunction is not reported with the use of enflurane in this patient population.

Sevoflurane reacts with the alkali within carbon dioxide absorbers to produce several degradation products including a vinyl ether called compound A ($CF_2C(CF_3)OCH_2F$), which is nephrotoxic in rats.[21] The site of compound A–induced nephrotoxicity in the rat is the renal tubule, especially at the corticomedullary junction.[21] The extent of this nephrotoxicity is determined by both the concentration of compound A and the duration of exposure.

Technical Issues. Extensive clinical experience with sevoflurane involving several million patients and 4000 closely studied volunteers failed to demonstrate nephrotoxicity. A high fresh-gas flow rate dilutes the concentration of compound A. Concern that higher compound A concentrations generated when a low fresh-gas flow rate (eg, <2 L/min) is used in a closed circuit led to the current sevoflurane package labeling that warns the anesthetist that fresh-gas flow rates below 2 L/min in a circle absorber system are not recommended.

There has been some controversy regarding the safety of low-flow sevoflurane anesthesia. Although there are no clinical reports of sevoflurane-induced nephrotoxicity as measured by changes in blood urea nitrogen (BUN), serum creatinine, or creatinine clearance, there are clinical data demonstrating transient nephrotoxicity when more subtle measurements of both glomerular and tubular function are used.[14,18] For example, when young healthy patients without underlying renal disease were anesthetized with low-flow sevoflurane for a mean of 6.7 hours, transient but statistically significant increases in urinary glucose and protein excretion were documented but without any changes in BUN, creatinine, or creatinine clearance.[18] The clinical significance (if any) of such transient abnormalities in renal function is uncertain. It seems prudent that low-flow sevoflurane should not be used in patients with preexisting renal disease until clinical data become available documenting the safety of this practice.

INHALATIONAL ANESTHETIC–RELATED CARBON MONOXIDE POISONING

Pharmacology

Desflurane, enflurane, and isoflurane contain a difluoromethoxy moiety and can be degraded to carbon monoxide (CO). This occasionally results in patient exposure to toxic CO concentrations, and in rare instances, to severe CO poisoning.[6] The true incidence of CO exposure during clinical anesthesia is unknown and no adequate means to detect intraoperative exposure exists at this time.

Carbon monoxide production is inversely proportional to the water content of CO_2 absorbents. Soda lime and Baralyme, the two most frequently used CO_2 absorbents, are sold wet (13–15% water by weight), but wet absorbents may dry with high gas-inflow rates. Higher levels of CO are most apt to be present during the first case following a weekend because of drying of the CO_2 absorbent from a continuous inflow of dry oxygen over the weekend.[16]

Figure 53-3. The reductive metabolism of halothane results in the formation of trifluorochloroethane and difluorochloroethylene.

Other factors influence the concentration of CO that may result from anesthetic degradation, including temperature (higher temperature increase CO formation), type of absorbent, choice of anesthetic, and concentration of the anesthetic. Strong alkalis, such as potassium and sodium hydroxide, initiate the reaction that forms CO. Baralyme, which contains potassium hydroxide, forms more CO than does soda lime, which contains a combination of both.

In one experiment, Baralyme in an anesthetic circuit was exposed to 48 hours of dry gas flowing at 10 L/min. Nine swine were then anesthetized with desflurane. Three of the animals died of cardiac arrest within 20 minutes, and the other 6 were successfully resuscitated with intravenous epinephrine and discontinuation of the desflurane.[17] Extremely high concentrations of CO (mean peak concentration of 37,000 ppm) were detected in the circuit within 15 minutes of initiating desflurane anesthesia. All the animals had a carboxyhemoglobin concentration > 80% with a concentration of > 90% in 7 of the swine. Lower CO concentrations were detected when the CO_2 absorbent was exposed to only 24 hours of dry gas and when soda lime was substituted for Baralyme.

Technical Issues

Clinical monitors in routine use in the operating room cannot detect CO. Mass spectrometry (available in some operating rooms) cannot directly detect CO because its molecular weight is equivalent to that of nitrogen, a gas usually present in much greater amounts. In addition, detection of CO by fragmentation products is not possible by mass spectrometry because CO_2 is present in greater amounts and has similar fragmentation products. However, the presence of CO should be suspected if the mass spectrometer shows the presence of enflurane when this agent is not being administered.

Trifluoromethane is produced by the degradation of isoflurane and desflurane and is responsible for the false readings for enflurane.[49] The simultaneous production of trifluoromethane and CO during chemical decomposition of isoflurane and desflurane allows the false reading of the former as enflurane by mass spectrometry to serve as a gross CO monitor, and allows for interventions to prevent further CO production and enhance its elimination. The overall incidence of CO exposure from anesthetic degradation was 6 of 1372 (0.44%) of first cases of the day in which either isoflurane or desflurane was administered.[49] Mass spectrometry is a useful monitor for indirect detection of CO poisoning in the clinical arena.[48]

Although no case reports document patient morbidity or mortality from intraoperative CO exposures, carboxyhemoglobin levels reportedly as high as 36% can cause morbidity and mortality in patients with concurrent disease.[6] Unfortunately, the diagnosis of CO poisoning during anesthesia is difficult as the main clinical features of toxicity are masked by anesthesia, and there are no routinely available means to identify CO within the breathing circuit, nor to detect when the CO_2 absorbent has been desiccated. Delayed neurologic sequelae from intraoperative CO poisoning will be likely missed on the anesthesiologist's postoperative patient evaluation.[47]

The product labels of desflurane and isoflurane were recently altered to include a precaution that when a practitioner suspects that the CO_2 absorbent may be desiccated, it should be replaced. However, the problem associated with this warning is that a reli-

able method for determining when the absorbent is fully or partially desiccated is not available.

If an anesthetic machine is found with the fresh-gas flow on at the beginning of the day, it would be reasonable to replace the absorbent. Changing from the use of Baralyme to soda lime should also be considered as a protective measure. Newer CO_2 absorbents that are less likely to degrade anesthetics are being evaluated but are not yet available in the United States.

ABUSE OF HALOGENATED VOLATILE ANESTHETICS

Fatal or life-threatening complications occur when halogenated inhalational anesthetics are used for nonanesthetic purposes (suicide attempts, mood elevation, topical treatment of herpes simplex labialis). When ingested, halothane usually produces a gastroenteritis with vomiting, followed by depression of consciousness, hypotension, shallow breathing, bradycardia with extrasystoles, and pulmonary edema. Coma usually resolves within 72 hours.[11,46] The diagnosis should be suspected when these features occur in a patient with the odor (sweet/fruity) of halothane on his or her breath. Supportive care, including endotracheal intubation and nasogastric lavage, should be provided. Full recovery can occur without permanent organ injury.

Intravenous injections of halothane may occur as a suicide attempt or unintentionally during induction of anesthesia. Following IV injection a young patient was found unconscious and hypotensive with pulmonary edema. She was not successfully resuscitated.[5] A 16-year-old girl received an unintentional IV injection of 2.5 mL of halothane during induction of anesthesia.[39] She became unconscious and apneic within 30 seconds, but began to awaken within 2-3 minutes. Four hours later she developed respiratory distress from pulmonary edema but subsequently made a full recovery. Transient coma and apnea are probably secondary to a bolus of halothane reaching the brain on its first pass through the bloodstream. Redistribution then occurs, explaining the rapid awakening. The pulmonary edema that develops following injection of halothane may result from a direct toxic effect of high concentrations of this hydrocarbon drug on the pulmonary vascular bed. Following injection, the agent likely travels as a bolus during the first passage through the pulmonary circulation because of its poor solubility in blood.

Hospital personnel are involved in most reported cases of halothane abuse by inhalation.[36] Inhalation of halothane produces a pleasurable sensation similar to that described with glue sniffing. Death may result from upper airway obstruction following loss of consciousness or from dysrhythmias. Death also occurred in a student nurse anesthetist who applied a full 250-mL bottle of enflurane over 3 hours to "cold sores" on her lower lip.[25]

SUMMARY

Inhalational anesthetics remain popular choices for maintenance of general anesthesia. They have an advantage over intravenous agents in that the drug level within the body can be increased or decreased at will. Toxicity may result with the use of these agents through a variety of mechanisms including excessive physiologic drug effect, direct drug effects on metabolic pathways, and toxic effects of drug metabolites. Although life-threatening adverse reactions occur infrequently, physicians who use these agents should have knowledge of their pharmacology and potential toxicity.

REFERENCES

1. Abernathy D, Greenblatt D: Pharmacokinetics of drugs in obesity. Clin Pharmacokinet 1982;7:108–124.

2. Amess J, Burman J, Rees G, et al: Megaloblastic haemopoiesis in patients receiving nitrous oxide. Lancet 1978;2:339–342.

3. Amos R, Amess J, Hinds C, Mollin D: Incidence and pathogenesis of acute megaloblastic bone marrow change in patients receiving intensive care. Lancet 1982;2:835–839.

4. Baird P: Occupational exposure to nitrous oxide—Not a laughing matter. N Engl J Med 1992;327:1026–1027.

5. Berman P, Tattersall M: Self-poisoning with intravenous halothane [letter]. Lancet 1982;1:340.

6. Berry PD, Sessler DI, Larson MD: Severe carbon monoxide poisoning during desflurane anesthesia. Anesthesiology 1999;90:613–616.

7. Brodsky J, Cohen E, Brown B, et al: Exposure to nitrous oxide and neurologic disease among dental professionals. Anesth Analg 1981;60:297–301.

8. Cousins M, Greenstein L, Hitt B, Mazze R: Metabolism and renal effects of enflurane in man. Anesthesiology 1976;44:44–53.

9. Cousins M, Mazze R: Methoxyflurane nephrotoxicity: A study of dose-response in man. JAMA 1973;225:1611–1616.

10. Crandell W, Pappas S, MacDonald A: Nephrotoxicity associated with methoxyflurane anesthesia. Anesthesiology 1966;27:591–607.

11. Curelaru I, Stanciu S, Nicolau V, et al: A case of recovery from coma produced by the ingestion of 250 mL of halothane. Br J Anaesth 1968;40:283–288.

12. Di Maio V, Garriot J: Four deaths resulting from abuse of nitrous oxide. J Forensic Sci 1978;23:169–172.

13. Dykes M: Is enflurane hepatotoxic? Anesthesiology 1984;61:235–237.

14. Eger EI, Gong D, Koblin DD, et al: Dose-related biochemical markers of renal injury after sevoflurane versus desflurane anesthesia in volunteers. Anesth Analg 1997;85:1154–1163.

15. Eger E, Smuckler E, Ferrell L, et al: Is enflurane hepatotoxic? Anesth Analg 1986;65:21–30.

16. Fang ZX, Eger EI, Laster MJ, et al: Carbon monoxide production from degradation of desflurane, enflurane, isoflurane, halothane, and sevoflurane by soda lime and Baralyme. Anesth Analg 1995;80:1187–1193.

17. Frink EJ, Nogami WM, Morgan SE, Salmon RC: High carboxyhemoglobin concentrations occur in swine during desflurane anesthesia in the presence of partially dried carbon dioxide absorbents. Anesthesiology 1997;87:308–316.

18. Higuchi H, Sumita S, Wada H, et al: Effects of sevoflurane and isoflurane on renal function and on possible markers of nephrotoxicity. Anesthesiology 1998;89:307–322.

19. Hoff R, Bunker J, Goodman H: Halothane hepatitis in three pairs of closely related women. N Engl J Med 1981;304:1023–1024.

20. Inman W, Mushlin W: Jaundice after repeat exposure to halothane: A further analysis of reports to the committee on safety of medicines. Br Med J 1978;2:1455–1456.

21. Kandel L, Laster MJ, Eger EI, et al: Nephrotoxicity in rats undergoing a one-hour exposure to compound A. Anesth Analg 1995;81:559–563.

22. Kobayashi Y, Ochiai R, Takeda J, et al: Serum and urinary inorganic fluoride concentrations after prolonged inhalation of sevoflurane in man. Anesth Analg 1992;74:753–757.

23. Lassen H, Henriksen E, Neukirch F, Kristensen H: Treatment of tetanus: Severe bone marrow depression after prolonged nitrous-oxide anaesthesia. Lancet 1956;1:527–530.

24. Layzer R, Fishman R, Schafer J: Neuropathy following abuse of nitrous oxide. Neurology 1978;28:504–506.

25. Lingenfelter R: Fatal misuse of enflurane. Anesthesiology 1981;55:603.

26. Mazze RI, Jamison R: The renal effects of sevoflurane [editorial]. Anesthesiology 1995;83:443–445.

27. Mazze R, Woodruff R, Heerdt M: Isoniazid-induced enflurane defluorination in humans. Anesthesiology 1982;57:5–8.

28. Messina F, Wynne J: Homemade nitrous oxide: No laughing matter. Ann Intern Med 1982;96:333–334.

29. Neuberger J, Williams R: Halothane hepatitis. Digest Dis 1988;6:52–64.

30. Nunn J: Clinical aspects of the interaction between nitrous oxide and vitamin B12. Br J Anaesth 1987;59:3–13.

31. Nunn J, Chanarin I, Tanner A, Owen E: Megaloblastic bone marrow changes after repeated nitrous oxide anaesthesia. Br J Anaesth 1986;58:1469–1470.

32. O'Sullivan H, Jennings F, Ward K, et al: Human bone marrow biochemical function and megaloblastic hematopoiesis after nitrous oxide anesthesia. Anesthesiology 1981;55:645–649.

33. Pohl L, Gillette JR: A perspective on halothane-induced hepatotoxicity. Anesth Analg 1982;61:809–811.

34. Schilling R: Is nitrous oxide a dangerous anesthetic for vitamin B12 deficient subjects? JAMA 1986;255:1605–1606.

35. Scott J, Dinn J, Wilson P, Weir D: Pathogenesis of subacute combined degeneration: A result of methyl group deficiency. Lancet 1981;2:334–337.

36. Spencer J, Raasch F, Trefny F: Halothane abuse in hospital personnel. JAMA 1976;235:1034–1035.

37. Stock J, Strunin L: Unexplained hepatitis following halothane. Anesthesiology 1985;63:424–439.

38. Subcommittee on the National Halothane Study of the Committee on Anesthesia National Academy of Sciences—National Research Council: Summary of the national halothane study: Possible association between halothane anesthesia and postoperative hepatic necrosis. JAMA 1966;197:121–134.

39. Suton J, Harrison G, Hickie J: Accidental intravenous injection of halothane: Case report. Br J Anaesth 1971;43:513–520.

40. Taves D, Fry B, Freeman R, Gillies A: Toxicity following methoxyflurane anesthesia. II. Fluoride concentrations and nephrotoxicity. JAMA 1970;214:91–95.

41. Touloukian J, Kaplowitz N: Halothane-induced hepatic disease. Semin Liver Dis 1981;1:134–142.

42. Uzunalimoglu B, Yardley J, Boitnott J: The liver in mild halothane hepatitis: Light and electron microscopic findings with special reference to the mononuclear cell infiltrate. Am J Pathol 1970;61:457–478.

43. Vaughn R: Biochemical and biotransformation alterations in obesity. Contemp Anesth Pract 1982;5:55–70.

44. Vergani D, Tsantoulas D, Eddleston A, et al: Sensitization to halothane-altered liver components in severe hepatic necrosis after halothane anesthesia. Lancet 1978;2:801–803.

45. Walton B, Simpson B, Strunin L, et al: Unexplained hepatitis following halothane anesthesia. Lancet 1978;2:801–803.

46. Wig J, Chakravarty S, Krishnamurthy K, Mehta D: Coma following ingestion of halothane: Its successful management. Anaesthesia 1983;38:552–555.

47. Woehick HJ, Dunning M, Connolly LA: Reduction in the incidence of carbon monoxide exposures in humans undergoing general anesthesia. Anesthesiology 1997;87:228–234.

48. Woehick HJ, Dunning M, Gandhi S, et al: Indirect detection of intraoperative carbon monoxide exposure by mass spectrometry during isoflurane anesthesia. Anesthesiology 1995;83:213–217.

49. Woehick HJ, Dunning M, Nithipatikom K, et al: Mass spectrometry provides warning of carbon monoxide exposure via trifluoromethane. Anesthesiology 1996;84:1489–1493.

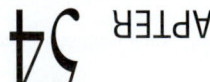
Kenneth M. Sutin / Brian Kaufman

A 25-year-old, 80-kg man with a 5-year history of steroid-dependent asthma presented to the Emergency Department (ED) complaining of acute shortness of breath. Physical examination revealed tachypnea (respiratory rate, 40 breaths/min) and diffuse wheezing. He was treated with intravenous fluids, nebulized albuterol, and methylprednisolone IV. Despite therapy, he remained in respiratory distress. An arterial blood gas determination while the patient was receiving 60% O_2 by facemask revealed a pH of 7.25, a $Paco_2$ of 65 mm Hg, and a Pao_2 of 70 mm Hg.

The patient was intubated and placed on mechanical ventilatory support. Initial pharmacologic therapy consisted of methylprednisolone 100 mg IV every 6 hours, nebulized bronchodilators, and IV antibiotics (ceftizoxime and erythromycin). Chest auscultation revealed equal but distant breath sounds bilaterally. A chest roentgenogram was normal except for diffuse hyperinflation. The patient's blood pressure decreased from 120/90 to 80/40 mm Hg. The respiratory rate was 35 breaths/min on synchronous intermittent mandatory ventilation at a rate of 20. The peak airway pressure was 65 cm H_2O. Evaluation of the expiratory flow waveform revealed the presence of auto-PEEP (positive end-expiratory pressure; air-trapping). Attempts to relieve this by prolonging the expiratory time were unsuccessful. Fentanyl and then lorazepam were infused to decrease the patient's dyspnea and allow for more complete exhalation. Although the patient's respiratory rate decreased to 15 breaths/min, the measured auto-PEEP was 15 cm H_2O. A 40-mg bolus of atracurium was given, followed by continuous infusion at 10–15 mg/h, adjusted to suppress spontaneous ventilatory efforts and to maintain 1–2 of 4 twitches on a train-of-four stimulus. The respiratory rate was decreased to 10 breaths/min and the inspiratory to expiratory ratio was reset to 1:3; with this treatment the level of auto-PEEP fell to 3 cm H_2O and the peak airway pressure decreased to 45 cm H_2O.

Sedation, paralysis, and bronchodilatory therapy were maintained for 7 days. Before attempting to wean him from mechanical ventilation, residual muscle relaxation was allowed to wear off. Reversal agents were not given because of concern that a cholinesterase inhibitor might exacerbate his bronchospasm.

Twenty-four hours after atracurium was discontinued, the patient was awake and alert, and able to move his eyes, tongue, and head. Train-of-four stimulation demonstrated 4 equal twitches without evidence of fade. His trachea was extubated. Initially, he noted difficulty holding his head up. Examination the next day revealed quadriparesis with absent deep-tendon reflexes. Sensory examination was normal. The maximum negative inspiratory force (NIF) was −15 cm H_2O (normal −60 to −90). His trachea was reintubated. Subsequently, during brief attempts to wean from mechanical ventilation with pressure support of 15 cm H_2O, he rapidly became dysp-

neic. The blood urea nitrogen (BUN), creatinine, and liver chemistry concentrations remained normal. The plasma creatine phosphokinase (CPK) peaked at 3172 U/L 2 days after the infusion was discontinued.

Over the next few days, attempts at weaning proved unsuccessful because of profound respiratory muscle weakness. Nerve conduction velocities were normal. Electromyography (EMG) demonstrated early evidence of motor denervation, with a decreased compound motor action potential and no evidence of neuromuscular block. A percutaneous needle quadriceps muscle biopsy revealed muscle atrophy and electron microscopy revealed loss of thick filaments in type 2 fibers. There was a slow but complete recovery of muscle strength over the subsequent 3 months.

Failure to wean or quadriparesis in the critically ill patient has multiple possible causes. In one study, myopathy was three times more likely than neuropathy to be the cause of acquired weakness in critically ill patients.[85] Because of the pattern of respiratory muscle weakness, diffuse motor weakness, preserved sensory function, increased CPK, and muscle biopsy results, a diagnosis of thick filament myopathy following the use of a neuromuscular blocking agent (NMB) was made. The etiology was likely multifactorial, and associated with NMBs, corticosteroids, and sepsis.[66] Normal nerve conduction velocities exclude the diagnosis of critical illness polyneuropathy. In some instances, progressive weakness and acute respiratory failure develop following a course of NMBs, critical illness, and ICU discharge.[87]

The purpose of neuromuscular blockers is to reversibly inhibit transmission at the skeletal neuromuscular junction (NMJ). The term *neuromuscular blocker* (NMB) is used instead of muscle relaxant to avoid confusion with drugs such as baclofen that are used to treat muscle spasms. Common indications for NMBs are to facilitate rapid-sequence tracheal intubation, to treat laryngospasm, and to maintain muscle paralysis during surgery and electroconvulsive therapy. The short-term use of muscle relaxants is only rarely a cause of a life-threatening reaction (eg, succinylcholine-related hyperkalemia, malignant hyperthermia, or anaphylaxis). These drugs are increasingly used outside the operating room and for prolonged periods, resulting in a new set of adverse side effects. The complications associated with NMB agents can be divided into those relating to care of a patient who is therapeutically paralyzed (eg, impaired ability to monitor neurologic function, unintentional patient awareness,[123] and chronic immobility) and those caused by specific untoward effects of the drug itself. The NMB drugs do not affect consciousness. Fortunately, the pupillary light reflex, an important indicator of midbrain function, is preserved in healthy subjects in the presence of vecuronium or pancuronium,[55] and presumably in the presence of other nondepolarizing NMBs (NDNMBs). However, the light reflex is depressed by sedatives, opioids, and inhalational general anesthetics. Misconceptions about the effects of NMB drugs are also common. In a 1989 survey, 10% of intensive care unit (ICU) nurses and 5% of physician house staff believed that pancuronium relieved pain, while 70% of ICU nurses and 50% of house staff believed that this agent relieved anxiety.[97] Standard methods for analysis of blood and tissue drug and metabolite levels employ gas or liquid chromatography coupled with mass spectrometry or high-pressure liquid chromatography.

In the largest study of its kind, involving 11,785 patients,[130] the incidence of explicit awareness or awake paralysis during general anesthesia was 0.18% when NMB, were used, and 0.10% when they were not used. Surprisingly, the rate of awareness was not affected by giving a benzodiazepine prior to anesthesia. More importantly, none of the nonparalyzed patients experienced anxiety during the interval of wakefulness or during the postoperative period, whereas 78% of the paralyzed patients experienced these symptoms.

HISTORY AND EPIDEMIOLOGY

Of all the NMBs, tubocurarine perhaps has the most exotic history.[155] Curare is a South American arrow poison derived from the *Strychnos* plant. It was used to paralyze hunted animals. Fortunately, for the people who used this toxin, ingestion does not cause paralysis. Claude Bernard used curare to study neuromuscular transmission. Curare was first used medically by Hunter in 1878 to treat tetanus, and later by West to reduce the muscular rigidity of hemiplegia. The most potent of the curare alkaloids, the toxiferines, are derived from the bark of the ligneous vine, *Strychnos toxifera*. The recent history of succinylcholine has been cloaked in legal mystery and intrigue as described by F. Lee Bailey in *The Defense Never Rests*. He describes an anesthesiologist, Dr. Carl Coppolino, who was accused of murdering his wife in 1965 by lethal injection of succinylcholine. His wife's autopsy revealed an abnormally high level of succinylcholine metabolites, succinic acid and choline, in the brain and liver. The evidence was deemed admissible even though prior to this case, the test was never validated. This set forth the legal precedent known as the Coppolino criteria, which states that a test can be used even if it is new and not in general use, provided that it is properly validated.[24]

MECHANISM OF NEUROMUSCULAR BLOCKER ACTION

The nicotinic cholinergic receptor at the skeletal muscle is a pentameric protein structure which exists in two primary forms, as either a mature receptor normally found at the NMJ ($\alpha\beta\delta\alpha\epsilon$) or as an embryonic (immature) receptor which can be found on muscle at extrajunctional sites ($\alpha\beta\delta\alpha\gamma$). All NMBs possess at least one positively charged quaternary ammonium group that can competitively bind the nicotinic ACH receptor. To understand neuromuscular block, it is helpful to explain normal neuromuscular transmission (Fig. 54–1).

There are two types of NMB: depolarizing and nondepolarizing. Succinylcholine, the only depolarizing NMB (DNMB) cur-

rently used, is similar structurally to ACH. It activates the ACH receptors, producing persistent localized depolarization of the muscle membrane, similar to the effect of ACH. The duration of the effect is longer than ACH because succinylcholine is relatively resistant to hydrolysis by true (junctional) acetylcholinesterase. Prolonged depolarization of the junctional muscle membrane renders it unexcitable to subsequent cycles of ACH release from the nerve terminal (called phase I block).

The NDNMBs cause skeletal muscle paralysis by competitively inhibiting the effects of ACH; one molecule of an NDNMB bound to a single α receptor competitively inhibits channel activation by ACH. The NDNMBs are classified by duration of action as either ultrashort, short, intermediate, or long. They are also classified by chemical structure as either synthetic benzylisoquinolinium drugs or the aminosteroids, which are comprised of the natural plant alkaloids and their congeners (Table 54–1). The NDNMBs do not block voltage-gated channels on the muscle membrane so direct electrical stimulation of muscle contraction is still possible.

There are different ACH receptors on the pre- and postjunctional membranes. The muscle paralysis produced by NMBs is primarily caused by inhibition of postjunctional receptors on the muscle. However, these agents also block prejunctional nicotinic receptors, inhibiting ACH-stimulated ACH production and release.[127] This effect reduces the available pool of ACH, enhances the postjunctional block, and also accounts for the decrease in tension ("fade") observed following train-of-four or tetanic stimulation during partial NDNMB block.[16]

The NMBs are highly water soluble and are relatively insoluble in lipid. Thus, NMBs do not rapidly cross lipid membranes (eg, blood-brain barrier, placenta) and are distributed mostly in the extracellular space. This explains why NMBs are devoid of central nervous system (CNS) affects.

Except for atracurium, which is a mixture of pharmacologically dissimilar isomers, the speed of onset of an NMB is inversely related to its molar drug potency (ie, ED_{95} in $\mu mol/kg$).[78,79] In other words, the fewer molecules per kilogram of tissue it takes to induce a given degree of ACH receptor occupancy, the more affinity the drug possess for that receptor. In general, small, fast-contracting muscles (eg, periorbital muscles) are more susceptible to block than are larger slower muscles (eg, diaphragm). Initially there is weakness of the small muscles of the hands, toes, and eyes, and then of the face and neck; this is followed by the extremities, and finally by the intercostals and the diaphragm. Following a large bolus of NDNMB, paralysis of the diaphragm is coincident with paralysis of the adductor pollicis and laryngeal muscles. Drug onset occurs quickly because of high perfusion of the NMJ and rapid drug diffusion into the NMJ.[31] Recovery is fastest for the diaphragm, intermediate for the larynx, and slowest for the adductor pollicis.[31] Termination of NMB effect is caused by drug elimination and/or metabolism.

NONSPECIFIC COMPLICATIONS COMMON TO NEUROMUSCULAR BLOCKERS

Histamine Release

The benzylisoquinolinium muscle relaxants (Table 54–1) produce direct, nonimmunologic (not related to IgE), dose- and rate-related histamine release from tissue mast cells. Histamine release causes

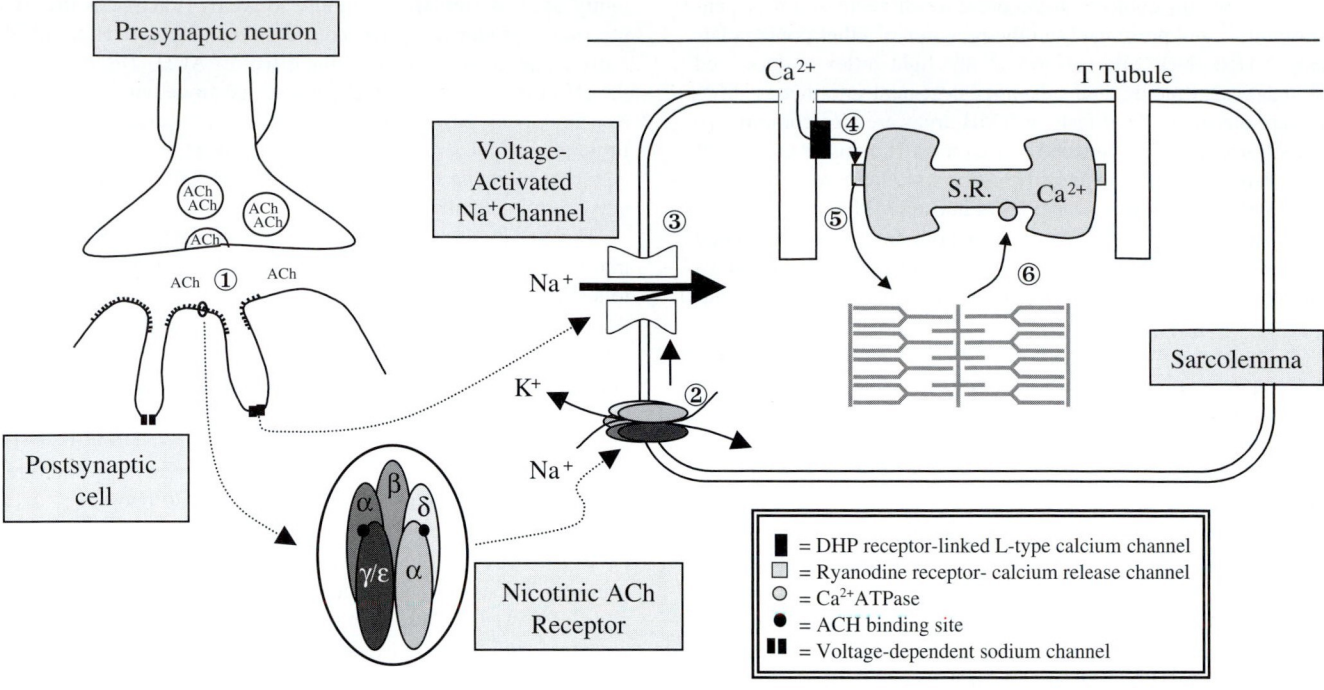

Figure 54–1. Excitation-contraction coupling in normal neuromuscular transmission. At the neuromuscular junction (NMJ), ACH released from the presynaptic nerve terminal crosses the 50-nm synaptic cleft to reach the nicotinic ACH receptor (①). There are two types of receptors, a mature receptor ($\alpha\beta\delta\alpha\varepsilon$) found at the normal adult NMJ, and an embryonic or immature receptor ($\alpha\beta\delta\alpha\gamma$) found on the muscle at extrajunctional sites (②). Proliferation of the immature receptor occurs during normal embryonic development and during certain pathologic states, such as motor nerve injury. There are two negatively charged sites on the receptor that can bind ACH: one at the α-γ interface and one at the α-δ interface. All NMBs possess at least one positively charged quaternary ammonium group that can competitively bind the ACH binding site. When both of the receptor sites are simultaneously occupied by ACH, the ACH-gated channel opens and the channel becomes nonselectively permeable to monovalent cations, resulting in an influx of Na^+ and an efflux of K^+. This then produces a local membrane depolarization (end-plate potential), which, in turn, opens voltage-activated Na^+ channels (③). If the depolarization is of sufficient amplitude, this results in a muscle action potential (MAP), which is propagated along the muscle membrane and down the transverse (T) tubules. In the T tubule, the MAP triggers opening of voltage-activated calcium channels (④, the dihyropyridine-sensitive L-type calcium channel). Calcium enters the cell and activates the ryanodine receptor/channel (⑤, RYR-1) on the sarcoplasmic reticulum (SR); this causes release of calcium from the terminal cisternae of the SR. The calcium then interacts with the troponin/tropomyosin complex to produce muscular contraction. This effect is terminated by active ATPase-driven reuptake of calcium into the longitudinal SR (⑥). The activity of the RYR-1 channel is affected by Ca^{2+}, Mg^{2+}, and anesthetic drugs, such as inhalation agents, which accelerate Ca^{2+} release in persons susceptible to malignant hyperthermia (MH).[124] In porcine MH an $ARG^{615} \rightarrow$ Cys mutation in the RYR-1 receptor has been found. A corresponding mutation in humans, however, has been observed in only 1:20 humans who are MH susceptible.

venous and arterial dilation, hypotension, tachycardia, bronchospasm, facial and upper body erythema, and increased bronchial secretions. This reaction is usually mild and clinically insignificant.[5] The approximate rank order for histamine release is tubocurarine > metocurine > atracurium, gallamine, and mivacurium > succinylcholine.[44] Pancuronium, rocuronium, vecuronium, cisatracurium, and pipecuronium do not induce histamine release. Hypersensitivity to NMB drugs may be more common and more severe in patients with asthma or other allergic diseases, possibly as a result of hypersensitivity to histamine.[44] Prophylaxis with both H_1 and H_2 blockers may be needed to inhibit the systemic effects of histamine release, because antagonism of only one receptor population may be insufficient.[98] Although the aminosteroid relaxants do not typically cause histamine release, unexplained episodes of hypotension and flushing have been reported; these are likely caused by noncompetitive inhibition of histamine *N*-methyl transferase (HNMT), which is the primary enzyme responsible for histamine degradation in humans.[54]

Anaphylaxis

Life-threatening anesthetic drug–related anaphylactoid (or anaphylactic) reaction occurs probably in less than 1 in 10,000 cases. Succinylcholine is the agent most often implicated in anaphylactic reactions (associated with IgE) during general anesthesia.[112] This agent was used in 283 (48%) of 590 severe anaphylactoid reactions associated with the use of NMB.[152] Surprisingly, in 20 of 28 patients with succinylcholine anaphylaxis, immediate circulatory collapse was the *only* manifestation; other signs, such as wheezing and skin rash, were notably absent.[158] In addition, more than 50% of these patients had sensitivities to other muscle relaxants. Succinylcholine anaphylaxis is 8 times more common in women than in men. Anaphylaxis with NDNMB is rare, but can occur even with some of the newer agents, such as atracurium and cisatracurium,[23] and there is even one report of a family history of anaphylaxis with NDNMB.[38] Pancuronium is the agent least associated with serious allergic reactions.[152]

TABLE 54–1. Pharmacology of Selected NMB Drugs.

	Class (1)	Duration	Initial Dose (mg/kg) (2,3)	Onset (min) (3)	Clinical Duration (min) (5)	Recovery Index 25–75% (min) (6)
Succinylcholine	Depolarizer	Ultrashort	1.0	1–1.5	7–12	2–4
Rapacuronium	Aminosteroid	Short	1.5	1–1.5	15–25	5–10
Mivacurium	Benzylisoquinolinium	Short	0.25	2–4	15–20	6–12
Vecuronium	Aminosteroid	Intermediate	0.1	3–4	20–40	10–15
Rocuronium	Aminosteroid	Intermediate	0.6–1.0	1.5–3	30–40	10–15
Atracurium	Benzylisoquinolinium	Intermediate	0.4–0.5	3–4	25–35	11
Cisatracurium	Benzylisoquinolinium	Intermediate	0.15–2.0	4–6	35–50	10–15
Pancuronium	Aminosteroid	Long	0.1	3–5	60–100	30–45
Pipecuronium	Aminosteroid	Long	0.14	3–5	90–120	30–45
Doxacurium	Benzylisoquinolinium	Long	0.05–0.07	5–7	90–120	30–45
Metocurine	Benzylisoquinolinium	Long	0.35–0.4	3–5	60–90	82
Tubocurarine	Benzylisoquinolinium	Long	0.2–0.3	3–5	60–90	48

	% Renal Excretion (7)	% Biliary Excretion (8)	Effect of Renal Failure	Effect of Hepatic Failure	Active Metabolite	Histamine Release	Effect on HR	Prolonged Block Reported
Succinylcholine	<10	Minimal	Minimal	Minimal ↑	? Succinic acid	Minimal	Rare severe bradycardia	Phase II block, atypical ACHase
Rapacuronium	10	<5	↑ Duration, esp metabolite		3-OH-rapacu-ronium		No	No (presumed)
Mivacurium	<10		↑ Duration	↑ Duration	No	Minimal	No	Atypical ACHase
Vecuronium	20–40	40–70	↑ Duration drug & metabolites	↑ Duration drug & metabolites	3-desacetyl-vecuronium	No	No	Yes
Rocuronium	10–25	50–70	Minimal ↑ duration	↑ Duration	No	No	Tachycardia at high dose	Yes
Atracurium	5–10		No effect	Minimal to none	No, but laudanosine	Minimal	No	Yes
Cisatracurium	10–20		No effect or minimal ↑	No effect	No, but laudanosine	No	No	Yes
Pancuronium	50–70	5–15	↑ To ↑↑ duration, esp metabolite	Mild ↑	3-OH-pancuronium	No	Tachycardia	Yes
Pipecuronium	38	Minimal	↑↑ Duration esp metabolite	Minimal ↑	No	No	No	No
Doxacurium	50–70	Minimal	↑↑ Duration	Minimal ↑	?	No	No	Yes
Metocurine	40–50	Minimal	↑ Duration	No effect	No	Moderate	Tachycardia	Yes
Tubocurarine	40–50	10	↑ Duration	Minimal ↑	No	Marked	Tachycardia	No

Adapted from: Atherton DP, Hunter JM: Clinical pharmacokinetics of the newer neuromuscular blocking drugs. Clin Pharmacokinet 1999;36:169–189; Coursin D, Prielipp R: Use of neuromuscular blocking drugs in the critically ill patient. Crit Care Clin N Am 1995;11:957–981; Donati F: Neuromuscular blocking drugs for the new millenium: Current practice, future trends—Comparative pharmacology of neuromuscular blocking drugs. Anesth Analg 2000;90:S2–S6; Hunter J: New neuromuscular blocking drugs. N Engl J Med 1995;332:1691–1699; and Mirakhur RK, McCourt KC, Kumar N: Use of intermediate acting muscle relaxants by infusion: The future. Acta Anaesthesiol Belg 1997;48:29–34.
Tubocurarine (Curare), metocurine (Metubine), atracurium (Tracrium), doxacurium (Nuromax), mivacurium (Mivacron), cisatracurium (Nimbex), pancuronium (Pavulon), vecuronium (Norcuron), pipecuronium (Arduan), rocuronium (Zemuron), rapacuronium (Raplon).
1. Nondepolarizers are classified as either benzylisoquinolinium or aminosteroid drugs.
2. Cisatracurium and rapacuronium are labeled as mg of base per mL, and for other drugs they are labeled and packaged as mg of salt per mL.
3. Typical initial dose is approximately 2 x ED95 (mg/kg).
4. Onset = time from bolus to 100% block.
5. Clinical duration = time from drug injection until recovery of 25% of single twitch height.
6. Recovery index = time between 25% and 75% twitch recovery.
7. % Renal excretion in first 24 h of unchanged drug.
8. % Biliary excretion in first 24 h of unchanged drug.

Autonomic Side Effects

In clinical doses, some NMBs have potentially serious dose- and rate-related effects on nicotinic and muscarinic receptors. Gallamine is now infrequently used because it produces substantial vagal block and tachycardia. As detailed below, pancuronium in-creases heart rate and blood pressure because of vagal block[132] and sympathetic stimulation.[136] These effects may be beneficial be-cause they may counteract the bradycardia and mild hypotension caused by high doses of opioids. However, this sympathetic stimu-lation may be hazardous when pancuronium is combined with halothane (which sensitizes the myocardium to catecholamine-induced dysrhythmias) and a tricyclic antidepressant.[41] Vecuronium has no chronotropic effect. This may be partly responsible for the rare bradydysrhythmias and cardiac arrests that have been observed after concurrent administration of high-dose opioids.[69] Succinylcholine stimulates cardiac muscarinic receptors, and may produce cardiac dysrhythmias including bradycardia, junctional rhythms, ventricular dysrhythmias, and cardiac arrest. Tubocurarine, and to a lesser extent metocurine, produces autonomic block at clinical doses, which may impair the sympathetic response to surgical stress or hypotension.[17]

Interactions of Muscle Relaxants and Pathologic States

Many medications and normal or pathologic physiologic states may alter the effects of NMBs (Table 54–2). It is especially important to be aware of conditions that are associated with an increased risk for hyperkalemia, rhabdomyolysis, and malignant hyperthermia.[36] Medications or diseases may affect the neuromuscular system at any level from the central nervous system (CNS) to the muscle itself.[120,150] For example, potent inhalation anesthetics depress CNS activity, lithium can inhibit presynaptic synthesis of ACH, local anesthetics inhibit action potential propagation at the nerve terminal, and dantrolene inhibits calcium release from muscle sarcoplasmic reticulum. All of these drugs augment the effects of NMBs.

In most neuromuscular diseases, such as Guillan-Barré syndrome or myasthenia gravis, there is increased sensitivity to the effect of NDNMBs.[4] However, in persons with myasthenia gravis, there is resistance to the effect of succinylcholine. Many systemic pathologic states will potentiate duration or intensity of NDNMBs, such as respiratory acidosis, hypokalemia, hypocalcemia, hypermagnesemia, hypophosphatemia, hypothermia, shock, and liver or kidney failure.[125] In acute sepsis, there may be resistance to the effect of NDNMBs.[114]

PHARMACOLOGY AND TOXICITY OF SUCCINYLCHOLINE

Succinylcholine (succinic acid-bischoline chloride, succinyldicholine, diacetylcholine, suxamethonium)[36] is a bis-quaternary ammonium ion, composed of two ACH molecules attached by their acetate groups. Following a typical IV induction dose (1 mg/kg), typical blood levels reach 62 μg/mL,[117] and intubating conditions are obtained in less than 60 seconds; paralysis usually lasts 3–5 minutes.

After an IV bolus of succinylcholine, plasma concentration rises and then rapidly declines as a result of redistribution into the extracellular fluid and neuromuscular junction; later, the concentration gradient reverses as a result of rapid plasma hydrolysis, and the concentration gradient is from the NMJ into the plasma.[51] Succinylcholine is hydrolyzed mostly by plasma cholinesterase (ACHase) and to a slight extent by alkaline hydrolysis. Hydrolysis is a two-step reaction to succinylmonocholine and choline, and then to succinic acid and choline (both of which are products of intermediary metabolism). The first-step reaction is about 6 times faster then the second.

Succinylcholine can be detected in the blood by gas chromatography and mass spectrometry.[142] Historically, detection of

the parent compound has proven difficult because of its rapid hydrolysis; however, techniques are described to detect parent compound in tissue even after embalming.[53] Succinylcholine can also be detected in the urine or at the site of prior intramuscular (IM) injection.

Plasma cholinesterase is also involved in the metabolism of mivacurium, heroin, cocaine, methylprednisolone, and ester local anesthetics (tetracaine, chloroprocaine, and procaine)[29] (Chap. 55). True ACHase is relatively specific to the substrate acetylcholine (ACH); it is found at the neuromuscular junction and in all excitable tissues and it does not catalyze the hydrolysis of succinylcholine.

The effect of succinylcholine may last for several hours if it cannot be degraded because of decreased plasma cholinesterase, abnormal cholinesterase activity (caused by genetic variance or drug inhibition), or a phase II block (see below). Plasma cholinesterase deficiency can be caused by hepatic disease, malnutrition, pregnancy, and fluoride accumulation.[71] On the other hand, partial enzyme deficiency of up to 70% of normal will no more than double the effective duration of succinylcholine.

The most commonly occurring atypical plasma cholinesterase variant (atypical type) can be assayed by its resistance to inhibition by the local anesthetic dibucaine, although there are different genetically aberrant plasma cholinesterases.[121] A history of a previously uneventful exposure to succinylcholine excludes the possibility of atypical plasma cholinesterase, except in case of hepatic transplantation. Dibucaine inhibits the ability of normal plasma cholinesterase to hydrolyze benzoylcholine by >70% (ie, dibucaine number >70%), heterozygous atypical variant enzyme by 40–60%, and homozygous atypical variant enzyme by ≤30%. Fresh-frozen plasma or plasma cholinesterase concentrates can be infused to hasten recovery in the case of genetic enzyme defect or acquired deficiency, but the simplest treatment is to keep the patient sedated, intubated, and ventilated until the block spontaneously reverses. In addition, blood samples should be drawn for measurement of cholinesterase level and activity. If the enzyme is deficient, inhibited, or unable to hydrolyze substrate, succinylcholine elimination proceeds by alkaline hydrolysis.[52] Phase II block may occur when large doses of succinylcholine are given over a short time (2–8 mg/kg IV); drug effect is prolonged and is similar to that of a nondepolarizing agent. A phase II block can be partially reversed by neostigmine.

Potentially life-threatening complications associated with succinylcholine are anaphylaxis; hyperkalemia in patients with neuropathy or myopathy; malignant hyperthermia in susceptible patients; and bradycardia from muscarinic stimulation, which occasionally occurs in children during anesthetic induction, especially following large or repeated doses in patients who have not been premedicated with atropine.

Succinylcholine 1 mg/kg IV typically causes serum [K$^+$] to increase by 0.5 mEq/L in normal individuals and in persons with renal failure. Severe hyperkalemia following succinylcholine is associated with increased extrajunctional muscle ACH receptors as a result of head or spinal cord injury, stroke, neuropathy, critical illness neuropathy or myopathy, muscular dystrophy, thermal burn or cold injury, crush injury, prolonged immobility, and malignant hyperthermia, or following prolonged use of NDNMBs. Susceptibility to hyperkalemia begins 4–7 days after neurologic injury, and it may persist indefinitely. In a study of ICU clinical directors in the United Kingdom, 68% of the respondents indi-

TABLE 54–2. **Prior Administration of Many Drugs Will Affect the Subsequent Response to Succinylcholine or NDNMB**

Drug	Response to Succinylcholine	Response to Nondepolarizer	Comments
Aminoglycosides (eg, amikacin, gentamicin)	Potentiation	Potentiation	Decrease ACH release and decrease postjunctional response to ACH. Some intrinsic neuromuscular blocking property and potentiate nondepolarizers. Partially reversible with calcium supplementation. Effect of neostigmine unpredictable.
Botulinum toxin, cosmetic		Early potentiation, delayed resistance	Single case report: Acutely, subclinical systemic denervation leads to vecuronium hypersensitivity. Subsequent NMJ remodelling, and ACH receptor upregulation leads to vecuronium resistance.
Calcium channel blockers: nifedipine and verapamil	Potentiation	Potentiation	Cause calcium channel block pre- and postjunctionally. Verapamil has local anestheticlike effect on nerve. May inhibit block reversal by cholinesterase inhibitor.
Carbamazepine	?	Resistant, shortened duration	Chronic therapy causes resistance to NDNMBs, except for mivacurium and atracurium.
Dantrolene	?	Potentiation	Blocks excitation-contraction coupling by blocking ryanodine calcium channel in sarcoplasmic reticulum of sketetal muscle.
Digoxin: cardiac glycosides	More prone to cardiac dysrhythmias	Pancuronium increases catecholamines and may cause dysrhythmias	
Edrophonium, neostigmine, physostigmine, pyridostigmine	Prolong succinylcholine	Inhibition	Inhibit plasma cholinesterase in dose-dependent manner. Succinylcholine 1–1.5 mg/kg lasts 35–180 min when given within 90 min after neostigmine.
Esmolol	? Mild prolongation	Slows onset of rocuronium and mivacurium	Inhibits plasma cholinesterase, slows degradation of mivacurium.
Furosemide <10 μg/kg 1–4 mg/kg	Potentiation Inhibition	Potentiation Inhibition	Biphasic dose-response in cats; protein-kinase inhibition at low doses and phosphodiesterase inhibition at high doses. Diuretic-related hypokalemia potentiates pancuronium in cats.
Glucocorticoids	Complex effects, ? mild prolongation of pancuronium	Inhibition	Chronic steroids induce resistance to pancuronium and decrease plasma cholinesterase activity by 50%. Steroids +/− NDNMBs given alone associated with myopathies.
Inhalational anesthetics: isoflurane, halothane, desflurane, sevoflurane	Potentiation	Potentiation	Decrease CNS neural activity and potentiates NMB in dose-dependent fashion (postsynaptic and muscle effects). Halothane and enflurane facilitate establishment of succinylcholine phase II block.
Lidocaine	Potentiation	Low-dose lidocaine potentiates block; high-dose lidocaine inhibits nerve terminals and blocks ACH binding site at postsynaptic membrane	The fast Na channel blockers decrease action potential propagation, ACH release, postsynaptic membrane sensitivity, and muscle excitability. Weak inhibitor of plasma cholinesterase.
Lithium carbonate	Prolongation of onset and duration	Prolongation of effect of pancuronium	Inhibits synthesis and release of ACH. Lithium alone may cause myasthenic reaction.
Magnesium	Potentiation, may block fasciculations	Potentiation, may also prolongs block	Decreases prejunctional ACH release, postjunctional membrane sensitivity, and muscle excitability.
Organic phosphorus, agents and carbamates	Potentiation		Irreversible plasma cholinesterase inhibitors. May decrease enzyme activity 100%.
Pancuronium	"Precurarization" with NDNMBs prolongs the onset and decreases side effects of succinylcholine; tubocurarine decreases and pancuronium increases block duration	Chronic NDNMBs induce resistance to their effect; mixing different NDNMBs may cause greater than additive effects, especially combining pancuronium with tubocurarine or metocurine	Pancuronium, and to a lesser extent vecuronium, inhibits plasma cholinesterase and prolongs mivacurium and succinylcholine block. Heterozygote for atypical cholinesterase may develop phase II block when given succinylcholine and pancuronium.
Phenelzine (MAO inhibitor)	Prolongation		Decreases plasma cholinesterase activity.
Phenytoin	?	Resistant, shortened duration	Acutely, potentiates NDNMB paralysis. Following chronic use, with the exception of mivacurium and atracurium, phenytoin induces resistance to NDNMBs and increases drug metabolism. This increases the initial dose and decreases the repeat dosing interval.

(continued)

TABLE 54–2. Prior Administration of Many Drugs Will Effect the Subsequent Response to Succinylcholine or NDNMB (continued)

Drug	Response to Succinylcholine	Response to Nondepolarizer	Comments
Propranolol	Potentiation in cat, effect in humans uncertain	Potentiation	Given alone may unmask myasthenic syndrome. Blocks ACH binding at postsynaptic membrane. Block reversal with cholinesterase inhibitor may cause bradycardia in patient on high-dose β-adrenergic antagonist.
Succinylcholine	Self-taming dose of succinylcholine may be used to limit muscular fasciculations	Tubocurarine, pancuronium, and vecuronium slightly prolonged by prior succinylcholine	
Theophylline		Inhibition	Pancuronium and theophylline can increase cardiac dysrhythmias.
Tricyclic antidepressants (TCA)		Pancuronium and TCA may cause cardiac dysrhythmias due to sympathetic effects	

Adapted from: Fiacchino F, Grandi L, Soliveri P, et al: Sensitivity to vecuronium after botulinum toxin administration. J Neurosurg Anesthesiol 1997;9:149–153; Ostergaard D, Engbaek J, Viby-Mogensen J: Adverse reactions and interactions of the neuromuscular blocking drugs. Med Toxicol Adverse Drug Exp 1989;4:351–368; and Viby-Mogensen J: Interaction of other drugs with muscle relaxants. In: Katz R, ed: Muscle Relaxants: Basic and Clinical Aspects. New York, Grune & Stratton, 1985, pp. 233–256.

cated that they would use succinylcholine to intubate an ICU patient with a history of sepsis, failure to wean and a prior difficult laryngoscopy.[65] However, in the chronic ICU patient, succinylcholine should be avoided when there is prolonged immobility or a possibility of myopathy or neuropathy because of the risk of inducing hyperkalemia, dysrhythmias, and cardiac arrest.[11] Severe hyperkalemia is not prevented by a small subparalyzing (defasciculating) dose of an NDNMB that is sufficient to prevent succinylcholine-induced muscle fasciculations.

Rarely, severe, or even fatal, hyperkalemia has been reported in a few patients who received succinylcholine immediately following exsanguinating hemorrhage or massive trauma. The mechanism for this is not the same as that following neurologic injury, because there is inadequate time for the proliferation of extrajunctional ACH receptors. Recently, it was reported that the tricarboxylic acid cycle intermediate, succinic acid (also a metabolite of succinylcholine), facilitates activation of voltage-gated sodium channels in a dose-dependent fashion.[58] Theoretically, succinic acid accumulates as a result of cell breakdown and anaerobic metabolism in hemorrhagic shock, and can augment the potassium-releasing effect of succinylcholine. Also, succinic acid formed by the degradation of succinylcholine may by an unclear mechanism be associated with masseter muscle rigidity (MMR), which can occur despite full neuromuscular block.

Severe hyperkalemia rarely occurs in the absence of a suggestive clinical history, which makes these conditions readily apparent, with one important exception. There are a few reports of acute rhabdomyolysis, hyperkalemic cardiac arrest, and death in apparently healthy children who were subsequently diagnosed with myopathy. Since March 1995, a warning appears in the succinylcholine package insert stating that succinylcholine should be avoided in elective situations in children, especially children younger than 8 years of age, because of a small risk of undiagnosed skeletal muscle myopathy, especially Duchenne muscular dystrophy.

Although this warning is controversial,[73] it seems prudent to use succinylcholine in children only when truly essential (eg, emergency airway management or laryngospasm). Sudden cardiac arrest that occurs immediately following succinylcholine is pre-

sumed to be caused by hyperkalemia, and immediate resuscitation should include calcium salts and measures to lower serum potassium. If there is coexisting fever, muscle rigidity, hyperlactemia, or metabolic and respiratory acidosis, dantrolene should also be given.

Cardiac dysrhythmias, including bradycardia, junctional rhythms, and ventricular dysrhythmias, occur infrequently after succinylcholine. The mechanism is most likely stimulation of cardiac muscarinic receptors, which can be prevented by pretreatment with atropine 15–20 μg/kg IV.

Especially under light anesthesia, succinylcholine (1 mg/kg IV) can increase cerebral blood flow, cortical electrical activity, intracranial pressure (ICP),[81] and intraocular pressure (IOP). When they occur, these effects are usually modest and can be blunted by deepening anesthesia (eg, IV opioid or lidocaine), or by prior administration of a small dose of an NDNMB. Even when it occurs, the increase in ICP is typically 10 mm Hg and lasts for 1–2 minutes. Surprisingly, this transient elevation in ICP is not observed in severely head-injured patients more than 3 days following injury.[81] Succinylcholine increases intragastric pressure; however, because lower esophageal sphincter pressure also increases, the gastric barrier pressure gradient (high pressure zone-intragastric pressure) actually increases following succinylcholine. Succinylcholine (1 mg/kg) causes muscle fasciculations that can be inhibited by giving tubocurarine 0.05 mg/kg or a small (defasciculating) dose of another NDNMB 3 minutes before succinylcholine. Pretreatment with an NDNMB partially antagonizes the succinylcholine block. Myalgias occur in one-half of patients after succinylcholine, and the severity is not correlated with CPK elevation or severity of fasciculations. Muscle fasciculations and incidence of myalgias are decreased by 30% with prior administration of a small, defasciculating dose of an NDNMB (eg, tubocurarine 0.05 mg/kg; or rocuronium 0.06 mg/kg). Masseter muscle rigidity may occur in as many as 1% of pediatric patients induced with halothane and succinylcholine, and it may precede malignant hyperthermia, especially if generalized muscle spasms occur. When given to a person with myotonic dystrophy or myotonia congenita, succinylcholine can induce severe myoclonic spasms, which can make ventilation and/or intubation impossible.

PHARMACOLOGY AND TOXICITY OF NONDEPOLARIZING NEUROMUSCULAR BLOCKING DRUGS

Extensive details with regard to the pharmacology and toxicity of these drugs are found in Table 54–1.

d-Tubocurarine is a monoquaternary ammonium and its *d*-isomer is the most potent component. It undergoes minimal metabolism and is eliminated in the urine. Renal failure prolongs neuromuscular block.[108] Tubocurarine produces autonomic block at clinical doses; this can impair the sympathetic response to surgical stress or hypotension.[17]

Metocurine is produced by methylation of tubocurarine, and is twice as potent. Like tubocurarine, it is minimally metabolized and is excreted primarily in the urine.[104] Elimination is also impaired in patients with renal insufficiency. The drug is prepared as the iodide, and may cause hypersensitivity in patients with seafood or shellfish allergy.

Doxacurium is a highly potent, long-acting NMB that does not significantly alter heart rate or blood pressure.[6] It is minimally hydrolyzed by plasma cholinesterase, and is eliminated mostly in the urine. Drug elimination and pharmacologic effect are significantly prolonged in renal but not hepatic insufficiency.

Mivacurium is short-acting drug composed of an unequal mixture of the three stereoisomers *trans-trans* (57% w/w), *cis-trans* (36%), and *cis-cis* (6%); the two more abundant are equipotent. They are rapidly hydrolyzed by plasma cholinesterase at a rate about 75% that of succinylcholine.[131] The *cis-cis* isomer is metabolized more slowly, but, fortunately, it also has about one-tenth the neuromuscular blocking activity of the two other isomers, so that accumulation of this isomer does not appear to cause prolonged drug effect. Mivacurium is a short-acting drug and recovery is twice as fast as that observed following atracurium. Prolonged block has been observed in persons with cholinesterase deficiency. In patients with atypical cholinesterase, the duration of effect is increased to 10–40 minutes in heterozygotes and up to 3–4 hours in homozygotes.[131] When mivacurium is given after an induction dose of pancuronium,[19] atracurium,[70] or cisatracurium,[70] its duration is more than doubled, probably because of a pharmacodynamic interaction.

Atracurium has four asymmetric sites, and this results in 10 different isomers, each with its own unique pharmacokinetic and pharmacodynamic profile. Atracurium is rapidly metabolized by spontaneous (nonenzymatic) Hofmann degradation (at a rate determined by temperature and pH) and by ester hydrolysis. The latter is catalyzed by nonspecific plasma esterases, distinct from the plasma cholinesterase that hydrolyzes succinylcholine. Drug elimination is independent of renal and hepatic function; however, it is prolonged during hypothermia or acidemia. Less than 10% of an administered dose of atracurium is eliminated unchanged in the urine or bile. None of the metabolites has NMB activity.

Each atracurium molecule when metabolized generates two molecules of laudanosine and an acrylate moiety, neither of which possesses neuromuscular blocking activity.[116] Laudanosine is excreted in the urine and bile, and its elimination is prolonged with renal insufficiency, biliary obstruction, or cirrhosis.[122] Laudanosine crosses the blood-brain barrier[39] and at high plasma concentrations, causes neuroexcitation and seizures in mice, rats, and dogs.[22] In humans, the toxic plasma laudanosine concentration is

unknown and seizures directly attributable to atracurium have not been observed (even following prolonged drug infusion in the ICU).[157] Unintentional overdose in a neonate was associated with flushing, hypotension, bronchospasm, and tachycardia, probably because of histamine release.[37]

Cisatracurium is a purified form of the 1R-*cis,* 1′R-*cis* isomer of atracurium (one of the 10 isomers), which retains the advantage of organ-independent elimination. It is eliminated from the plasma by pH- and temperature-dependent Hofmann degradation, but it undergoes only minimal plasma ester hydrolysis. Cisatracurium is an improvement over the parent drug; it is 3 times more potent and at clinically relevant doses does not produce histamine release or significant cardiovascular[94,134] or cerebrovascular effects.[135] Cisatracurium degrades to form laudanosine and a monoquaternary acrylate. The latter product is metabolized by nonspecific esterases in the plasma and liberates a second laudanosine molecule. Cisatracurium has a slower onset and is associated with lower plasma laudanosine levels than atracurium.[40] Drug elimination is not altered by liver or kidney failure, or following prolonged infusions in ICU patients.[68]

Pancuronium is a synthetic bisquaternary aminosteroid drug that is the prototype agent in its class. About 60% of the drug is excreted unchanged in the urine and 10–20% is metabolized. Because all aminosteroid drugs undergo some degree of deacetylation in the liver (especially pancuronium and vecuronium), clearance may be slowed and its effect prolonged in hepatic insufficiency. Drug effect is also prolonged in renal failure. Some of its metabolites are excreted in the urine and bile. The 3-OH-pancuronium metabolite retains 50% of the NMB activity of the parent drug[107] and accumulates in patients with renal failure.[148] Because the aminosteroid drugs undergo substantial biliary excretion (rocuronium > vecuronium > pancuronium > pipecuronium), their clearance is prolonged when this function is impaired.[67] Pancuronium is the only commonly used NMB drug that increases heart rate and arterial blood pressure; this is attributed to selective cardiac antimuscarinic (atropinelike) action,[132] indirect norepinephrine-releasing effect on postganglionic fibers, and block of presynaptic muscarinic receptors at the sympathetic nerve terminals.[136] In patients under general anesthesia, pancuronium 0.08–0.1 mg/kg IV causes an increase in heart rate, blood pressure, and cardiac output.[145] Combining pancuronium with halothane in patients on chronic tricyclic antidepressant therapy is associated with tachycardia and ventricular dysrhythmias.[41] At clinically relevant doses, pancuronium inhibits normal plasma cholinesterase and, to a lesser extent, atypical plasma cholinesterase, and slows the metabolism of drugs inactivated by this enzyme: succinylcholine, mivacurium, and procaine.[17]

Vecuronium is derived from pancuronium (it lacks one methyl group) and its potency is similar. The structural alteration eliminates the tachycardia and hypertension observed following pancuronium. Vecuronium does not cause clinically significant cardiovascular or autonomic side effects.[110] Approximately 10–25% of the agent is excreted in the urine within 24 hours. The drug is rapidly taken up by the liver and excreted in the bile.[8] In patients with cholestasis[89] or cirrhosis,[88] slowed elimination may prolong the effect of vecuronium. About one-third of the parent drug is hepatically metabolized to 3-desacetyl-, 17-desacetyl-, and 3,17-desacetylvecuronium; the last two metabolites have minimal activity. Overall, about 12% of vecuronium is converted to 3-desacetylvecuronium, which has 70–80% of the neuromuscular blocking potency of the parent compound.[20] This metabolite can accumulate during repeated dosing,[156] especially in renal failure. Neither vecuronium nor the 3-desacetyl metabolite is removed by hemodialysis.[138] Persistent paralysis was observed in 7 of 16 critically ill patients paralyzed with vecuronium for at least 2 days.[137] Paralysis lasted from 6 hours to >7 days, and was associated with elevated blood levels of 3-desacetylvecuronium, creatinine clearance <30 mL/min, metabolic acidosis, female gender, and elevated plasma magnesium.[137]

Because vecuronium is devoid of cardiovascular side effects, it is ideal for patients with cardiac disease. Rarely, when used in combination with fentanyl, sufentanil, etomidate, or propofol, especially when there is high vagal tone and if there is no concurrent painful stimulation, severe bradycardia, and even asystole, may occur.[69,76] Subparalyzing doses of vecuronium also blunt hypoxic ventilatory drive, probably because of an effect on the carotid body. In humans, when there was a partial residual vecuronium block, the ventilatory response to hypercapnia was normal; however, the response to isocapnic hypoxia was markedly depressed.[42]

Pipecuronium is an analogue of pancuronium with minimal hemodynamic and autonomic effects. It produces a block of long duration, similar to that of pancuronium. Parent drug is primarily eliminated by the kidney. The hepatic 3-desacetyl metabolite does not have pharmacologic activity and it is excreted in the urine.

Rocuronium is an aminosteroid drug that produces rapid-onset intubating conditions. When fast onset is necessary and succinylcholine is contraindicated, rocuronium may be substituted.[1] Rocuronium is eliminated mostly in the liver and bile and, to a lesser extent, by the kidneys. The drug is minimally metabolized by the liver, and the 17-desacetylrocuronium metabolite has one-twentieth the potency of the parent compound. Hepatic dysfunction increases the volume of distribution and elimination half-life, but does not affect the plasma clearance.[102] This may result in prolonged drug effect, especially following prolonged administration in patients with liver disease. Its effect is not prolonged by renal insufficiency. Rocuronium is associated with a slight increase in heart rate and stroke volume but does not produce histamine release.[105]

Rapacuronium is the newest aminosteroid drug designed for fast drug onset, and it can also be used in place of succinylcholine.[143] The drug is hydrolyzed by unidentified esterases, which are independent of the hepatic P450 system and plasma cholinesterase. The primary metabolite, 3-OH-rapacuronium, is 2.5 times more potent than the parent compound and it is cleared primarily by the kidneys. For this reason, the drug should not be given for more than 1 hour as an intermittent bolus or as an infusion,[133] especially in renal failure.[146] In premarket studies, rapacuronium caused dose-related histamine release, which was not associated with hemodynamic changes.[95] The package insert indicates a 3.2% incidence of bronchospasm. In March 2001, the drug was voluntarily withdrawn from the market because of several cases of severe bronchospasm, including a few unexplained fatalities.

MONITORING THE EFFECT OF NEUROMUSCULAR BLOCK

A portable nerve stimulator or visual evaluation of limb motion or respiratory efforts is the usual means of evaluating neuromuscular function; however, the nerve stimulator is considerably more reli-

able and should be used routinely when caring for any patient receiving an NMB.[149] Surprisingly, in a survey of ICUs,[59] neuromuscular monitoring was employed in only 21%, and was used routinely only 4% of the time. Even when a nerve stimulator is used to titrate the rate of NMB infusion, this does not guarantee that prolonged paralysis will not occur;[103,106] however, it may decrease the incidence of overdosage,[113] shorten the time to full recovery of muscle function,[28] and perhaps reduce the incidence of prolonged paralysis.[64]

The most common test of the extent of neuromuscular block is to deliver four supramaximal electrical impulses at 2 Hz (train-of-four, TOF) to the ulnar nerve at the wrist. Resultant movement of the adductor pollicis muscle is assessed by manual or visual inspection (typically), or by transduction of the electromyogram or twitch force. When the ratio of the force generated by the fourth twitch is ≥70% of the first (ie, TOF ratio ≥0.7), most subjects are able to protrude their tongue, open their eyes, grasp their hands, and maintain a sustained head lift.[18] With a TOF ratio ≤0.7, subjects usually experience weakness, diminished negative inspiratory force and vital capacity, and weakness of upper airway muscles.

Historically, a TOF ≥0.7 has been considered safe for tracheal extubation because it is associated with a sustained ability to maintain spontaneous airway and ventilation. It was recently emphasized that this does not represent a return of normal muscle function. At a TOF = 0.7–0.75, subjects experience significant signs and symptoms of residual weakness including subjective muscular weakness, inability to independently sit up, diplopia, problems with visual tracking, paralysis of facial muscles, and decreased grip strength.[80] At a TOF = 0.7, there is pharyngeal dysfunction and diminished upper esophageal resting muscle tone, which may increase the chance of vomiting and aspiration.[43] Adequate reversal of NMBs is important; in a prospective randomized study, inadequate NMB reversal was associated with an increase in postoperative pulmonary complications (ie, pneumonia or atelectasis).[9]

REVERSAL OF NONDEPOLARIZING NEUROMUSCULAR BLOCKING AGENTS AND ASSOCIATED COMPLICATIONS

Reversal of NMB block depends on drug redistribution, degradation, metabolism, and/or elimination. Neuromuscular block by NDNMBs can be pharmacologically reversed by ACHase inhibitors—drugs that inhibit junctional cholinesterase at nicotinic and muscarinic receptors (Table 54–3). The commonly used ACHase inhibitors are neostigmine, pyridostigmine, and edrophonium. Neostigmine and pyridostigmine, but not edrophonium, also inhibit plasma cholinesterase. The resultant increase in ACH concentration at the NMJ competitively reverses the effects of an NDNMB.

The goal of NMB reversal is to maximize the nicotinic (neuromuscular junctional) effect while minimizing muscarinic (ganglionic) side effects. This is accomplished by coadministering an antimuscarinic agent. The ACHase inhibitors are given in combination with the antimuscarinic agents glycopyrrolate or atropine. Because an increase or decrease in muscarinic effect leads to bradycardia or tachycardia, it is best to combine drugs with similar rates of onset. The rapid-acting agents edrophonium and atropine

TABLE 54–3. Pharmacology of Intravenous Neuromuscular Block Reversal Agents

CHOLINESTERASE INHIBITORS

	Neostigmine	Pyridostigmine	Edrophonium
Structure	Quaternary ammonium	Quaternary ammonium	Quaternary ammonium
Initial dose (mg/kg)	0.040–0.080	0.2–0.4	0.5–1.0
Onset (min)	7–11	10–16	1–2
Duration (min)	60–120	60–120	60–120
Recommended antimuscarinic	Glycopyrrolate	Glycopyrrolate	Atropine

ANTIMUSCARINICS

	Glycopyrrolate	Atropine
Structure	Quaternary ammonium	Tertiary amine
Initial dose (mg/kg)	0.01–0.02	0.02–0.03
Onset (min)	2–3	1
Duration (min)	30–60	30–60
Elimination	Renal	Renal
Crosses Blood-brain barrier	No	Yes

Adapted from: Bevan D, Donati F, Kopman A: Reversal of neuromuscular blockade. Anesthesiology 1992;77:785–805; and Cronnelly R: Muscle relaxant antagonists. In: Katz R, ed: Muscle Relaxants: Basic and Clinical Aspects. New York, Grune & Stratton, 1985, pp. 197–212.

are generally administered together, as are the slower-acting neostigmine or pyridostigmine and glycopyrrolate. ACHase inhibitors are eliminated primarily by renal excretion. In addition to their effects at the NMJ, acetylcholinesterase inhibitors inhibit plasma cholinesterase, and for this reason prolong the effects of drugs metabolized by this enzyme, such as succinylcholine and ester local anesthetics.

It should be possible in most situations to limit the incidence of postextubation complications in patients who have received an NMB, if standard criteria for extubation are rigidly adhered to. It should be noted that an overdose of an ACHase inhibitor may actually cause muscular weakness.[2] Administration of neostigmine in the presence of preexisting respiratory acidosis inhibits its effects; acidosis should be corrected by improving ventilation before administering the reversal agent.

The most common and troublesome clinical side effect of ACHase inhibition is bradycardia, which is usually prevented by coadministration of an antimuscarinic drug.[27] Bradydysrhythmia may be severe and lead to nodal or idioventricular rhythm, to complete heart block, or even to asystole.[96] These problems may be more common in patients with preexisting bradycardia or in those patients receiving chronic β-adrenergic antagonist therapy, and are not necessarily prevented by prior administration of atropine.[144] Other side effects that may result from excess ACHase inhibition are hypersalivation, bronchospasm, increased bronchial secretions, abdominal cramping and intestinal hyperperistaltic activity, miosis, ocular tearing, and increased bladder tone. Side effects of excess antimuscarinic effect include tachycardia, bronchodilation, pupillary dilatation, and increased intraocular pres-

sure. Following general anesthesia, use of anticholinesterases may increase the incidence of nausea, vomiting, and abdominal cramps.[75] Since atropine crosses the blood-brain barrier, it can produce central anticholinergic syndrome.

PERSISTENT WEAKNESS ASSOCIATED WITH NEUROMUSCULAR BLOCKERS

Weakness in critically ill patients is a common event; its etiology is multifactorial and it probably occurs in most patients with severe sepsis and/or multiple organ failure to a variable degree (Table 54–4). It occurs in about one-third of patients with status asthmaticus, possibly associated with use of glucocorticoids and NDNMBs and concomitant sepsis.[34] In patients undergoing liver transplantation, the incidence of myopathy was 7%,[21] and it is close to 100% following retransplantation. It is not surprising that severe illness is associated with injury to the neuromuscular system; systemic inflammatory response (SIRS), sepsis, multiple organ failure, glucocorticoids, toxic drug therapy, thermal injury, and electrolyte, endocrine, and nutritional disorders can have a contributory role. The first report of steroid myopathy appeared in 1977. An association was suggested between use of high-dose glucocorticoids (for asthma) and respiratory muscle weakness and quadriplegia.[99] It is interesting to note that this patient also received intermittent doses of pancuronium. The association between glucocorticoids and NDNMBs with severe myopathy has been observed for several years.[60] A possible explanation is that denervated skeletal muscle has an increased number of cytosolic glucocorticoid receptors;[35] glucocorticoids, in turn, promote muscular atrophy (especially in type II fibers) and induce selective myosin loss.[128]

Prolonged peripheral weakness (ie, not caused by central nervous system disorders) is a result of disorders of nerve, NMJ, and muscle, either alone or in combination. Reflecting a combination of the above, critical illness polyneuromyopathy (CIP)[87] was recently described. All of the following can cause peripheral weakness: (a) residual NMB effect because of inadequate reversal; (b) accumulation of the parent drug; (c) accumulation of an active metabolite (3-OH-pancuronium, 3-desacetylvecuronium), especially in the presence of renal or hepatic dysfunction;[137,148] (d) other causes of muscular weakness, such as hypothermia, hypophosphatemia, hypokalemia, hypermagnesemia, burn injury, and malnutrition; (e) peripheral neuropathy; (f) neuromuscular junction disorders or drug effect (eg, clindamycin); and (g) concomitant organ pathology in critically ill patients (eg, rhabdomyolysis). The evaluation of weakness in the ICU patient is reviewed elsewhere.[13]

Prolonged pharmacologic paralysis with an NDNMB mimics the effect of nerve injury. Both disrupt normal activity at the myoneural junction. In response, the muscle synthesizes embryonic ACH receptors (αβδαγ) that are dispersed over the entire muscle membrane, instead of localizing at the NMJ. There is also upregulation of these extrajunctional receptors, as well as muscle atrophy, subjective weakness, resistance to NDNMBs,[62] and hypersensitivity to DNMBs.[56] Resistance to the effect of NDNMB drugs can occur within the first few days after starting an NDNMB drug infusion, necessitating an increase in the rate of drug administration.[157] In ICU patients needing ventilation for more than 3 days, those with a high vecuronium requirement have more junc-

TABLE 54–4. Acute Neuromuscular Pathology Associated with Critical Illness and/or NDNMBs

Condition	Associated with Use of NDNMB	Incidence	Clinical Features	Creatine Phosphokinase (CPK)	Electromyogram (EMG) & Nerve Conduction Velocity (NCV)	Muscle Biopsy
Polyneuropathy						
Critical illness polyneuropathy (CIP)[15,92,159]	No	Common	Respiratory failure and symmetric quadriparesis (LE > UE) and associated with sepsis, SIRS, MOF, and aminoglycosides, but not NDNMBs.	Normal	Primary motor axonal polyneuropathy with decreased motor NCV, typically motor > sensory	Denervation atrophy, absence of inflammation, normal CSF
Acute motor polyneuropathy (AMP)[93,118,119]	Yes	Common	Similar to CIP except occurs in association with NDNMB. Associated with sepsis and MOF.	Normal	Primary axonal polyneuropathy, typically motor > sensory	Denervation atrophy, absence of inflammation, normal CSF
Hopkins syndrome[63,139] (poliomyelitislike syndrome in asthma)	No	Rare	Pediatric patient with asthma on steroids. Fever, flaccid paralysis of single arm or leg, possibly due to neuropathic nonpolio virus.	Normal	Evidence of anterior horn cell disease	No myonecrosis
Neuromuscular Transmission Defect						
Residual neuromuscular block[137,148]	Yes	Common	Flaccid Quadriplegia and respiratory failure. Associated with prolonged use of NDNMBs. Risk factors: active metabolites of vecuronium, pancuronium, or rapacuronium, and other drugs that potentiate weakness. Delayed drug clearance in MOF.	Normal	Abnormal muscle response to repetitive nerve stimulation	Normal
Myopathy						
Disuse myopathy[83] (cachectic myopathy)	Yes/No	Common	Catabolic state and immobility typically >7 days. Diffuse muscle wasting, reduced muscle mass.	Normal	Myopathic EMG changes and normal NCV	Normal or uniformly atrophic type 2 myofibers without patchy necrosis
Critical illness myopathy (CIM),[86] includes thick filament myopathy (TFM, aka steroid or asthma myopathy)[74,77] and acute myopathy of intensive care (AMIC)[7,34,84,99]	Yes/No	Common	Diffuse symmetric quadriparesis, respiratory failure, and weak neck flexors and facial muscles. Critically ill patient associated with sepsis/MOF, organ transplantation, renal failure, severe asthma, respiratory failure, aminoglycosides, and glucocorticoids.	Mild-moderate increase in 50%, typically <6000 IU	Myopathic changes including low amplitude or absent compound muscle action potentials, defibrillation potentials and positive sharp waves by needle EMG, normal NCV; normal sensory nerve action potentials. Intact NMJ function.[86]	Diffuse focal myonecrosis and vacuolization, myofibrolysis, myofibrillar disorganization. Preferential loss of thick filaments especially in type 2 fibers.
Acute necrotizing myopathy of intensive care (ANMIC)[126,160]	Yes	Rare	Flaccid quadriplegia and myoglobinuria, preserved sensation. Associated with sepsis, severe asthma, glucocorticoids, and NDNMBs (especially vecuronium). Renal failure commonly caused by rhabdomyolysis.	Very high, >10,000 IU	Myopathic EMG changes; normal NCV	Panfascicular necrotizing myopathy involving type 1 and 2 fibers, vacuolation and macrophage invasion, myosin loss, normal mitochondria

Adapted from: Bolton C: Sepsis and the systemic inflammatory response syndrome: Neuromuscular manifestations. Crit Care Med 1996;24:1408–1415; Hund E: Myopathy in critically ill patients. Crit Care Med 1999;27:2544–2547; Lacomis D, Giuliani MJ, Van Cott A, Kramer DJ: Acute myopathy of intensive care: Clinical, electromyographic, and pathological aspects. Ann Neurol 1996;40:645–654; and Nates JL, Cooper DJ, Day B, Tuxen DV: Acute weakness syndromes in critically ill patients.—A reappraisal. Anaesth Intensive Care 1997;25:502–513.
MOF = multiple organ failure; CSF = cerebral spinal fluid; SIRS = systemic inflammatory response; LE = lower extremity; UE = upper extremity.

tional ACH receptors than patients who have a lower drug requirement.[32] These alterations are assumed to result from absent muscle stimulation; however, this phenomenon has also been observed when subparalyzing doses of NMBs are used, suggesting that up-regulation may be a primary effect of the agent itself.[90] In fact, prolonged deep sedation without chemical paralysis can induce resistance to an NDNMB, presumably because of up-regulation of immature ACH receptors.[57]

The first reports of persistent weakness following NDNMB use appeared in 1985; severe reversible quadriplegia, muscular atrophy, and areflexia were described in 12 of 60 patients who received 4 mg of pancuronium every 3–4 hours for more than 6 days.[119] In all patients, biopsy revealed myopathic changes, while EMG was consistent with axonal degeneration. In a prospective study of 25 severe asthmatics who received corticosteroids, 22 of whom also received vecuronium, an elevation of CPK was observed in 76% and clinical myopathy was observed in 36%.[34] Patients with either abnormality had received a significantly higher dose of vecuronium and required more prolonged mechanical ventilation. There are other reports of weakness in 20–30% of patients receiving NMBs for as little as 48–72 hours, in 58% of critically ill patients ventilated for more than 7 days,[93] and in 70% of patients with sepsis and multiple organ failure.[12] In the ICU setting, weakness associated with NDNMB toxicity usually presents as failure to wean from mechanical ventilation. Prolonged weakness is associated with an increased mortality, and is probably a result of the severity of the underlying medical condition. Recovery in survivors may take up to 6 months and may be incomplete. Because myopathy can recur, it is helpful to determine the cause of prolonged weakness, especially in asthmatic patients, so that intravenous glucocorticoids can be avoided in the future whenever possible.

It is estimated that CIP occurs in 58–82% of critically ill patients with SIRS or sepsis and multiple organ failure,[93] and that the occurrence is unrelated to use of NDNMBs. The incidence of CIP is, however, related to the severity of multiple organ dysfunction syndrome (MODS),[92] and CIP is associated with an increase in ICU mortality (19% without CIP vs 48% with CIP, $p<0.05$[93]). Ultimately, 50% of patients with CIP make a complete recovery.[91]

It has been suggested that the term critical illness myopathy (CIM) supersede the disorders referred to as thick filament (or steroid) myopathy (TFM) and acute myopathy of intensive care (AMIC).[86] CIM is a common disorder, associated with sepsis, multiple organ failure, renal failure, hyperglycemia, hepatic transplantation, severe asthma, and high-dose glucocorticoids. Biopsy demonstrates loss of thick (myosin) filaments in type 2 fibers. Although sensory nerve action potentials are preserved, EMG reveals low-amplitude motor-unit potentials that are of short duration and that can be polyphasic. CPK is mildly elevated in about 50% of patients, about 2–5 days after start of therapy, and normalizes by day 16.[34]

A rare finding in patients receiving NDNMBs is acute necrotizing myopathy of intensive care (ANM-IC). This syndrome is associated with sepsis, severe myonecrosis, myoglobinuric renal failure, and death caused by multiple organ failure. The electrophysiologic signs of myopathy include low-amplitude motor response and normal to slightly abnormal spontaneous muscle activity.[160] It has been proposed that this syndrome may be caused when a "priming" factor (high dose of systemic glucocorticoids, myotropic infection, or sepsis) is combined with a "triggering" agent (an NDNMB).[126] Infection with certain myopathic agents,

such as influenza A or B, *Staphylococcus aureus* with toxic shock syndrome, *Escherichia coli*, *Legionella spp.*, *Mycoplasma pneumoniae*, and *Neisseria meningitidis*, might also predispose to myonecrosis and function as a priming factor. Early recognition of myonecrosis manifested by an increase in CPK, should prompt an immediate discontinuation of the NDNMB triggering agent and this may improve chances for survival.[126] Certainly, CPK should be monitored routinely in all patients receiving NMB's.[141]

Patients receiving NMBs should be reassessed on a daily basis to make sure that it is essential to continue NMBs. Monitoring of neuromuscular function should include daily testing of CPK and monitoring TOF q4–6h with a portable nerve stimulator and the dose of the agent adjusted to maintain 1–2 twitches of the TOF.[140] When an NMB must be used, it is beneficial to discontinue the NMB, sedation, and narcosis for a brief interval each day, a "drug holiday," to permit neurologic assessment and to prevent drug overdosing. This decreases the duration of mechanical ventilation and length of stay in the ICU.[82] Even when NMBs are avoided, there is a substantial risk of pathologic residual weakness associated with critical illness. Furthermore, unless NMBs are altogether avoided, it is impossible to always prevent the adverse effects of these drugs, including prolonged weakness. Before starting an NMB, always first try to optimize sedation and analgesia. Finally, it is unclear whether the pathophysiology of toxicity syndromes observed following exposure to organic phosphorus compounds (intermediate syndrome or organic phosphorus–induced delayed neuropathy) and neuromuscular blockers are related; it is clear that prolonged drug-induced alteration of normal neuromuscular transmission can have sustained adverse effects.

MALIGNANT HYPERTHERMIA

Malignant hyperthermia is a heterogeneous syndrome that typically affects individuals who are otherwise healthy, although there is an association with certain myopathic diseases (Table 54–5). Malignant hyperthermia usually occurs in the operating room shortly after initial exposure to anesthetic agents, but it can also occur after many hours of anesthesia,[111] and as long as 12 hours after surgery. In addition, recurrence can occur 24–36 hours after an initial episode.

Malignant hyperthermia is caused inconsistently by exposure to certain anesthetic agents that trigger abnormal calcium release from the sarcoplasmic reticulum (SR) into the cytoplasm. The disorder is associated with a defect of a skeletal muscle regulatory/receptor protein, and inheritance is autosomal dominant with variable penetrance.[101] The incidence of malignant hyperthermia is about 1:15,000 in children and 1:50,000 in adults. Drugs typically associated with triggering an attack of malignant hyperthermia are succinylcholine and the potent volatile inhalational anesthetics (the prototype agent is halothane). Diseases associated with malignant hyperthermia include Duchenne muscular dystrophy, central core disease, King-Denborough syndrome, myotonia, and osteogenesis imperfecta. Drugs that may be safely administered to individuals considered susceptible to malignant hyperthermia include NDNMBs, nitrous oxide, propofol, ketamine, etomidate, benzodiazepines, barbiturates, opioids, and local anesthetics.

The immediate systemic manifestations of malignant hyperthermia are a result of hypermetabolism following uncontrolled calcium release from the terminal cisternae of the sarcoplasmic reticulum. Calcium release produces skeletal muscle contrac-

TABLE 54–5.   Suggested Therapy for Malignant Hyperthermia Emergency

Acute Phase Treatment of Malignant Hyperthermia
1. Stop triggering agents: volatile inhalational anesthetics and succinylcholine.
2. Hyperventilate with 100% O_2.
3. Administer dantrolene sodium 2–3 mg/kg initial bolus rapidly with increments up to 10 mg/kg total. Continue to administer dantrolene until signs of MH (eg, tachycardia, rigidity, increased end-tidal CO_2, and temperature elevation) are controlled. Occasionally, a total dose greater than 10 mg/kg may be needed. Each vial of dantrolene contains 20 mg of dantrolene and 3 g mannitol. Each vial should be mixed with 50 mL of sterile distilled water for injection USP without a bacteriostatic agent. Dissolution of the lyophilized solution in water is slow and requires thorough mixing.
4. Administer sodium bicarbonate to correct metabolic acidosis as guided by blood gas analysis. In the absence of blood gas analysis, monitor end-tidal CO_2 and 1–2 mEq/kg should be administered.
5. Simultaneous with the above, actively cool the hyperthermic patient.
    • Cool patient. Immersion in ice-water slurry is fastest. Also, peritoneal or gastric lavage is useful.
    • Surface cool with ice and hypothermia blanket.
    • Monitor core temperature closely because overvigorous treatment may lead to hypothermia.
6. Dysrhythmias will usually respond to treatment of acidosis and hyperkalemia. If they persist or are life-threatening, standard antidysrhythmic agents may be used. Dysrhythmias should not be treated with calcium channel blockers (especially verapamil) because they may cause hyperkalemia and cardiovascular collapse.
7. Monitor end-tidal CO_2, arterial, and mixed venous blood gases, serum potassium, calcium, clotting studies, and urine output.
8. Hyperkalemia is common and should be treated with hyperventilation, sodium bicarbonate, intravenous glucose, and insulin. Life-threatening hyperkalemia may also be treated with calcium administration. Hypokalemia should be treated with great caution as potassium may trigger MH.
9. Ensure adequate urine output by hydration and/or administration of mannitol or furosemide. Consider central venous or PA monitoring.
10. Sudden unexpected cardiac arrest in children: Children younger than about 10 years of age who experience sudden cardiac arrest after succinylcholine in the absence of hypoxemia and anesthetic overdose should be treated for acute hyperkalemia first. In this situation, calcium chloride should be administered along with other means to reduce serum potassium. They should be presumed to have subclinical muscular dystrophy. A neurologist should be consulted.

Postacute Phase Treatment of Malignant Hyperthermia
1. Observe the patient in an ICU setting for at least 24 hours because recrudescence of MH may occur, particularly following a fulminant case resistant to treatment.
2. Administer dantrolene 1 mg/kg IV q6h for 24–48 hours following the episode. After that, oral dantrolene 1 mg/kg q6h may be used for 24 hours as necessary.
3. Follow arterial blood gases, CPK, potassium, calcium, urine and serum myoglobin, INR, PTT, and platelet count, and core body temperature until such time as they return to normal values (eg, q6h). Central temperature (eg, rectal, esophageal) should be continuously monitored until stable.
4. Counsel the patient and family regarding MH and further precautions.
    • Refer the patient to MHAUS. For nonemergency or patient referral calls, and to also reach MHAUS: 607-674-7901, 800-98-MHAUS, 39 East State Street, Sherburne, NY 13460. Fax-On-Demand at 800-440-9990.
    • Fill out an Adverse Metabolic Reaction to Anesthesia (AMRA) report available through the North American Malignant Hyperthermia Registry: 717-531-6936.
    • Alert family members to the possible dangers of MH and anesthesia.
5. Get an MH medical ID for the patient, and have them wear it at all times.

---

1. For emergency consultation to help with patient management (http://www.mhaus.org/hotline.html) call the MH Emergency Hotline:
    • Inside US or Canada call: 800-MH-HYPER (800-644-9737).
    • Outside the United States and Canada call: 0011 (315) 428-7924.
2. CAUTION: The guideline above may not apply to every patient and must of necessity be altered according to specific patient needs.
3. Also contact MHAUS at http://www.mhaus.org/.

---

tions. Continuous calcium reuptake by sarcoplasmic $Ca^{2+}ATPase$ causes depletion of cellular ATP, hypermetabolism, excess heat production, hyperthermia, increased O_2 consumption and CO_2 production, venous O_2 desaturation and hypercarbia, anaerobic metabolism, and lactic acid generation, and can cause cardiac dysrhythmias, hyperkalemia, rhabdomyolysis, and disseminated intravascular coagulopathy.[61] Tachycardia and initial hypertension or labile blood pressure are common. Elevation of venous, arterial, and exhaled CO_2 is among the earliest findings. The extreme elevation of metabolic rate causes severe mixed venous oxygen desaturation (far below the normal of 75%). Early septic shock is also associated with hypermetabolism, increased cardiac output, and fever, but typically the mixed venous O_2 saturation is >75%. The differential diagnosis of malignant hyperthermia also includes neuroleptic malignant syndrome, thyroid storm, baclofen withdrawal, drug overdose (eg, salicylate, amphetamine, cocaine and antimuscarinic), unintentional intraoperative patient overheating, heat stroke, transfusion reaction, and serotonin syndrome. Rare malignant hyperthermia–triggering agents/events include IV potassium salts (which depolarize the muscle membrane), severe exercise in a hot climate, antipsychotic drugs (eg, phenothiazines), and infection.[30,72] It is unlikely that these three cause true malignant hyperthermia. However, there are cases in which patients with hypermetabolism and rhabdomyolysis respond to dantrolene; this does not mean that these patients have malignant hyperthermia.

Potassium release from muscle cells may also cause life-threatening hyperkalemia during the acute reaction. Subsequently, rhabdomyolysis can occur, causing renal damage. Signs of malignant hyperthermia include tachycardia, tachypnea, skeletal muscle and jaw muscle rigidity, fever, and increased CO_2 production. In contrast to what its name suggests, although hyperthermia is a typical finding, it is not a universal finding; moreover, when it occurs, it is often a late finding.

In humans, several different chromosomal and protein defects have been causally associated with malignant hyperthermia, which may account for the heterogeneity of the inheritance and clinical presentation. Of practical importance, the existence of multiple mutations means that genetic testing is unlikely to prove useful in detecting all susceptible individuals. One possible defect involves an abnormal ryanodine-1 receptor (RYR-1, chromosome 19q13.1) that regulates intracellular calcium release in both fast- and slow-twitch skeletal muscle (Fig. 54–1).[100,101] According to this theory, a malignant hyperthermia–triggering agent keeps the RYR-1 channel open, leading to accelerated sarcoplasmic calcium release. A mutation of the ryanodine receptor may be necessary in some cases, but it may not be sufficient, and ryanodine receptor defects are observed in less than 50% of malignant hyperthermia–susceptible persons.[49] The association of defects in skeletal muscle sodium channels with certain myotonic disorders has led to research into the role of this channel in the genesis of malignant hyperthermia.[49] Also, malignant hyperthermia–susceptible persons and swine manifest increased skeletal muscle fatty acid production, and fatty acids augment halothane–induced sarcoplasmic calcium release.[46–48] Although it is not yet possible to define one pathogenic mechanism, any unitary hypothesis must account for the above observations.

By partially blocking the release of calcium from skeletal muscle sarcoplasmic reticulum, dantrolene rapidly reverses the signs and symptoms of hypermetabolism: fever, mottled skin, dysrhythmias, muscle rigidity, tachycardia, metabolic acidosis, and hypercapnia. Before the discovery of dantrolene, the mortality rate from malignant hyperthermia was 70%. Death from malignant hyperthermia resulted from cardiac arrest, dysrhythmias, brain damage, hemorrhage, or multiple organ failure. When acute malignant hyperthermia is treated immediately with dantrolene, volume resuscitation, active cooling, control of hyperkalemia, and supportive care, the mortality from acute malignant hyperthermia is under 5%. Therefore, the most important aspects of therapy are rapid initial diagnosis and immediate therapy (within minutes) with dantrolene. Even if delayed for hours or days, dantrolene may still improve survival following acute malignant hyperthermia. In acute malignant hyperthermia, significant dysrhythmias may be treated with standard antidysrhythmic agents; however, calcium entry blockers should *not* be given with dantrolene as they may precipitate hyperkalemia and severe cardiac depression.[129]

Persons who have had a possible episode of malignant hyperthermia, or who have a positive family history, may be considered for muscle biopsy and muscle testing; the fresh tissue specimen is placed in a tissue bath perfused with Krebs solution and then halothane or caffeine is added. According to the North America Malignant Hyperthermia Group, a positive muscle contraction in response to either halothane or caffeine is considered an indication of malignant hyperthermia susceptibility.

Dantrolene Sodium

Dantrolene is a hydantoin derivative, structurally similar to local anesthetics and anticonvulsants, but possessing none of their properties.[151] It is likely that dantrolene acts at the skeletal muscle ryanodine receptor, limiting its activation. Dantrolene does not affect nerve conduction or the neuromuscular junction and has minimal effect on cardiac and smooth muscle.[147]

Indications. Dantrolene is used to treat the hyperpyretic syndromes of peripheral etiology: malignant hyperthermia, baclofen withdrawal, and thyrotoxicosis. It may be used prophylactically prior to general anesthesia in patients with known malignant hyperthermia susceptibility—those with a previous episode of malignant hyperthermia after general anesthetic or in persons determined to be malignant hyperthermia susceptible. Dantrolene may also be considered for the patient with severe hyperpyrexia, when the diagnosis of malignant hyperthermia cannot be excluded with certainty, especially when there is coexisting metabolic acidosis, coagulopathy, or rhabdomyolysis.[30] Dantrolene has also been used to treat muscular spasticity; however, long-term administration is associated with hepatic and other toxicities.[151] If following initial dantrolene treatment the patient has a painful extremity or the CPK remains elevated, it is important to evaluate the patient for a possible compartment syndrome.

Pharmacology of Dantrolene. Dantrolene is supplied as a sterile lyophilized solution in a 70-mL vial that contains 20 mg of dantrolene sodium and 3000 mg of mannitol; following reconstitution with 60 mL of sterile water for injection USP (without a bacteriostatic agent), it has a pH of about 9.5. Dantrolene is lipophilic and relatively insoluble in water. In plasma, it is reversibly bound to plasma proteins, especially albumin. Dantrolene is metabolized in the liver to 5-hydroxydantrolene, and up to 25% is excreted in the urine as the hydroxy metabolite. The metabolite is less than half as potent as the parent drug. The elimination half-life is 6–9 hours for dantrolene and 15.5 hours for its metabolite.

Dosage. The initial dose of dantrolene for treatment of acute malignant hyperthermia is 2–3 mg/kg IV as a bolus; it is repeated every 15 minutes until the signs of hypermetabolism are reversed, or until a total dose of about 10 mg/kg has been administered. Following initial treatment, at least 1 mg/kg should be given every 4 hours for 48 hours to prevent recrudescence of the syndrome. For prophylaxis of malignant hyperthermia, 2.5 mg/kg of dantrolene is given IV 30 minutes prior to anesthesia or planned exposure. Oral prophylaxis can be given, but its absorption is less predictable.[50]

Side Effects and Toxicity. Because of its alkaline pH, dantrolene can cause venous irritation and thrombophlebitis. When given to healthy persons, or for malignant hyperthermia prophylaxis,[153] dantrolene causes skeletal muscle and diaphragm weakness, but not muscle paralysis.[154] In healthy volunteers, dantrolene 2.5 mg/kg does not depress peak expiratory flow rate or vital capacity, or alter end-tidal CO_2 or respiratory rate.[50]

SUMMARY

Problems associated with NMB drugs include predictable adverse effects, some of which may be life-threatening, interactions with other drugs and the patient's pathophysiology, and idiosyncratic and anaphylactic reactions. There is a predictable dose- and rate-related histamine release in the drugs belonging to the benzyliso-quinolinium family. True anaphylaxis caused by NMBs is most often caused by succinylcholine, and immediate circulatory collapse can be the initial and only presentation. Autonomic side effects include a predictable tachycardia caused by a vagolytic effect of pancuronium. The most important, and usually predictable, severe complications associated with succinylcholine are hyperkalemia, rhabdomyolysis, and malignant hyperthermia. Succinylcholine effect is predictably prolonged by rare congenital abnormalities of plasma cholinesterase or enzyme inhibition (eg, organic phosphorus eye drops). In most diseases affecting nerve, NMJ, or muscle, the effect of NDNMBs is enhanced. The effect of an NDNMB can be prolonged by residual neuromuscular block caused by slowed drug metabolism or accumulation of an active metabolite following either short-term (3-OH-rapacuronium) or long-term drug infusion (3-OH-pancuronium, 3-desacetylvecuronium). The effect of an NDNMB can also be prolonged by certain idiosyncratic reactions (acute motor polyneuropathy, critical illness myopathy, acute necrotizing myopathy of intensive care) that produce myopathy and/or neuropathy, typically following prolonged infusion of an NDNMB in a critically ill patient. Malignant hyperthermia is a true emergency with 95% survival, provided that dantrolene therapy is immediately instituted, which blocks calcium release from the muscle SR. Malignant hyperthermia is not a subtle diagnosis; hyperthermia is a late finding, whereas muscle fasciculations, cyanosis, signs of hypermetabolism, arterial and venous oxygen desaturation, and hyperlactemia are prominent early findings.

ACKNOWLEDGMENTS

The authors appreciate the thoughtful comments of Dr. Aaron F. Kopman, Department of Anesthesiology, St. Vincent's Hospital, New York City, and of Dr. David Lacomis, Department of Neurology, University of Pittsburgh.

REFERENCES

1. Andrews JI, Kumar N, van den Brom RH, et al: A large simple randomized trial of rocuronium versus succinylcholine in rapid-sequence induction of anaesthesia along with propofol. Acta Anaesthesiol Scand 1999;43:4–8.
2. Aracava Y, Deshpande S, Rickett D, et al: The molecular basis of anticholinesterase actions on nicotinic and glutaminergic synapses. Ann N Y Acad Sci 1987;505:226–255.
3. Atherton DP, Hunter JM: Clinical pharmacokinetics of the newer neuromuscular blocking drugs. Clin Pharmacokinet 1999;36:169–189.
4. Azar I: The response of patients with neuromuscular disorders to muscle relaxants: A review. Anesthesiology 1984;61:173–187.
5. Basta S: Modulation of histamine release by neuromuscular blocking drugs. Curr Opin Anaesth 1992;5:572–576.
6. Basta S, Savarese J, Ali H, et al: Clinical pharmacology of doxacurium chloride: A new long-acting non-depolarizing muscle relaxant. Anesthesiology 1988;69:478–486.
7. Behbehani NA, Al Mane F, Dyachkova Y, et al: Myopathy following mechanical ventilation for acute severe asthma: The role of muscle relaxants and corticosteroids. Chest 1999;115:1627–1631.
8. Bencini A, Scaf A, Sohn Y, et al: Hepatobiliary disposition of vecuronium bromide in man. Br J Anaesth 1986;58:988–995.
9. Berg H, Roed J, Viby Mogensen J, et al: Residual neuromuscular block is a risk factor for postoperative pulmonary complications. A prospective, randomized, and blinded study of postoperative pulmonary complications after atracurium, vecuronium and pancuronium. Acta Anaesthesiol Scand 1997;41:1095–1103.
10. Bevan D, Donati F, Kopman A: Reversal of neuromuscular blockade. Anesthesiology 1992;77:785–805.
11. Biccard BM, Grant IS, Wright DJ, et al: Suxamethonium and critical illness polyneuropathy. Anaesth Intensive Care 1998;26:590–591.
12. Bolton C: Neuromuscular complications of sepsis. Intensive Care Med 1993;19:S58–S63.
13. Bolton C: Neuromuscular conditions in the intensive care unit. Intensive Care Med 1996;22:841–843.
14. Bolton C: Sepsis and the systemic inflammatory response syndrome: Neuromuscular manifestations. Crit Care Med 1996;24:1408–1415.
15. Bolton C, Gilbert J, Hahn A, Sibbald W: Polyneuropathy in critically ill patients. J Neurol Neurosurg Psych 1984;47:1223–1231.
16. Bowman W: Prejunctional and postjunctional cholinoreceptors at the neuromuscular junction. Anesth Analg 1980;59:935–943.
17. Bowman W: Nonrelaxant properties of neuromuscular blocking drugs. Br J Anaesth 1982;54:147–160.
18. Brand J, Cullen D, Wilson N, Ali H: Spontaneous recovery from nondepolarizing neuromuscular blockade: Correlation between clinical and evoked responses. Anesth Analg 1977;56:55–58.
19. Brandom B, Meretoja O, Taivainem T, Wirtavuori K: Accelerated onset and delayed recovery of neuromuscular block induced by mivacurium preceded by pancuronium in children. Anesth Analg 1993;76:998–1003.
20. Caldwell J, Szenohradszky J, Segredo V, et al: The pharmacodynamics and pharmacokinetics of the metabolite 3-desacetylvecuronium (ORG 7268) and its parent compound, vecuronium, in human volunteers. J Pharmacol Exp Ther 1994;270:1216–1222.
21. Campellone JV, Lacomis D, Kramer DJ, et al: Acute myopathy after liver transplantation. Neurology 1998;50:46–53.
22. Chapple D, Miller A, Ward J, Wheatley P: Cardiovascular and neurological effects of laudanosine: Studies in mice and rats, and in conscious and anaesthetized dogs. Br J Anaesth 1987;59:218–225.
23. Clendenen SR, Harper JV, Wharen RE Jr, Guarderas JC: Anaphylactic reaction after cisatracurium. Anesthesiology 1997;87:690–692.
24. Conrad E: Landmarks and hallmarks in scientific evidence. J Forensic Sci 1971;16:465–470.
25. Coursin D, Prielipp R: Use of neuromuscular blocking drugs in the critically ill patient. Crit Care Clin N Am 1995;11:957–981.
26. Cronnelly R: Muscle relaxant antagonists. In: Katz R, ed: Muscle Relaxants: Basic and Clinical Aspects. New York, Grune & Stratton, 1985, pp. 197–212.
27. Cronnelly R, Morris R: Antagonism of neuromuscular blockade. Br J Anaesth 1982;54:183–194.
28. Darrah W, Johnston J, Mirakhur R: Vecuronium infusions for prolonged muscle relaxation in the intensive care unit. Crit Care Med 1989;17:1297–1300.
29. Davis L, Britten JJ, Morgan M: Cholinesterase. Its significance in anaesthetic practice. Anaesthesia 1997;52:244–260.
30. Denborough M: Malignant hyperthermia. Lancet 1998;352:1131–1136.
31. Dhonneur G, Kirov K, Slavov V, Duvaldestin P: Effects of an intubating dose of succinylcholine and rocuronium on the larynx and diaphragm: An electromyographic study in humans. Anesthesiology 1999;90:951–955.
32. Dodson B, Kelly B, Braswell L, Cohen N: Changes in acetylcholine receptor number in muscle from critically ill patients receiving mus-

cle relaxants: An investigation of the molecular mechanism of prolonged paralysis. Crit Care Med 1995;23:815–821.

33. Donati F: Neuromuscular blocking drugs for the new millennium: Current practice, future trends—Comparative pharmacology of neuromuscular blocking drugs. Anesth Analg 2000;90:S2–S6.

34. Douglass J, Tuxen D, Horne M, et al: Myopathy in severe asthma. Am Rev Respir Dis 1992;146:517–519.

35. Dubois D, Almon R: A possible role for glucocorticoids in denervation atrophy. Muscle Nerve 1981;4:370–373.

36. Durant N, Katz R: Suxamethonium. Br J Anaesth 1982;54:195–208.

37. Durcan J, Carter JA: Overdose of atracurium. Anaesthesia 1986; 41:767.

38. Duvaldestin P, Wigdorowicz C, Gabriel I: Anaphylactic shock to neuromuscular blocking agent: A familial history. Anesthesiology 1999;90:1211–1212.

39. Eddleston J, Harper N, Pollard B, et al: Concentrations of atracurium and laudanosine in cerebrospinal fluid and plasma during intracranial surgery. Br J Anaesth 1989;63:525–530.

40. Eddleston J, Harper N, Ward J, Weatley P: Cardiovascular and neurological effects of laudanosine. Br J Anaesth 1987;59:218–225.

41. Edwards R, Miller R, Roizen M, et al: Cardiac responses to imipramine and pancuronium during anesthesia with halothane and enflurane. Anesthesiology 1979;50:421–425.

42. Eriksson L, Sato M, Severinghaus J: Effect of a vecuronium-induced partial neuromuscular block on hypoxic ventilatory response. Anesthesiology 1993;78:693–699.

43. Eriksson LI, Sundman E, Olsson R, et al: Functional assessment of the pharynx at rest and during swallowing in partially paralyzed humans: Simultaneous videomanometry and mechanomyography of awake human volunteers. Anesthesiology 1997;87:1035–1043.

44. Ertama P: Histamine liberation in surgical patients following administration of neuromuscular blocking drugs. Ann Clin Res 1982;14: 15–26.

45. Fiacchino F, Grandi L, Soliveri P, et al: Sensitivity to vecuronium after botulinum toxin administration. J Neurosurg Anesthesiol 1997; 9:149–153.

46. Fletcher JE, Mayerberger S, Tripolitis L, et al: Fatty acids markedly lower the threshold for halothane-induced calcium release from the terminal cisternae in human and porcine normal and malignant hyperthermia susceptible skeletal muscle. Life Sci 1991;49:1651–1657.

47. Fletcher JE, Tripolitis L, Erwin K, et al: Fatty acids modulate calcium-induced calcium release from skeletal muscle heavy sarcoplasmic reticulum fractions: Implications for malignant hyperthermia. Biochem Cell Biol 1990;68:1195–1201.

48. Fletcher JE, Welter VE: Enhancement of halothane action at the ryanodine receptor by unsaturated fatty acids. Adv Pharmacol 1994; 31:323–331.

49. Fletcher JE, Wieland SJ, Karan SM, et al: Sodium channel in human malignant hyperthermia. Anesthesiology 1997;86:1023–1032.

50. Flewellen E, Nelson T, Jones W, et al: Dantrolene dose response in awake man: Implications for management of malignant hyperthermia. Anesthesiology 1983;59:275–280.

51. Foldes F: Distribution and biotransformation of succinylcholine. Int Anesth Clin 1975;13:101–115.

52. Foldes F, Rendell-Baker L, Birch J: Causes and prevention of prolonged apnea with succinylcholine. Anesth Analg 1956;35:609–615.

53. Forney RB Jr, Carroll FT, Nordgren IK, et al: Extraction, identification and quantitation of succinylcholine in embalmed tissue. J Anal Toxicol 1982;6:115–119.

54. Futo J, Kupferberg J, Moss J: Inhibition of histamine n-methyltransferase (HNMT) in vitro by neuromuscular relaxants. Biochem Pharmacol 1990;39:415–420.

55. Gray AT, Krejci ST, Larson MD: Neuromuscular blocking drugs do not alter the pupillary light reflex of anesthetized humans. Arch Neurol 1997;54:579–584.

56. Gronert G: Disuse atrophy with resistance to pancuronium. Anesthesiology 1981;55:547–549.

57. Gronert GA, Fung DL, Haskins SC, Steffey EP: Deep sedation and mechanical ventilation without paralysis for 3 weeks in normal beagles: Exaggerated resistance to metocurine in gastrocnemius muscle. Anesthesiology 1999;90:1741–1745.

58. Haesler G, Petzold J, Hecker H, et al: Succinylcholine metabolite succinic acid alters steady state activation in muscle sodium channels. Anesthesiology 2000;92:1385–1391.

59. Hansen-Flaschen J, Brazinsky S, Basile C, Lanken P: Use of sedating drugs and neuromuscular blocking agents in patients requiring mechanical ventilation for respiratory failure: A national survey. JAMA 1991;266:2870–2875.

60. Hansen-Flaschen J, Cowen J, Raps E: Neuromuscular blockade in the intensive care unit: More than we bargained for. Am Rev Respir Dis 1993;147:234–236.

61. Heffron J: Malignant hyperthermia: Biochemical aspects of the acute episode. Br J Anaesth 1988;60:274–278.

62. Hogue C, Ward J, Itani M, Martyn J: Tolerance and upregulation of acetylcholine receptors follow chronic infusion of *d*-tubocurarine. J Appl Physiol 1992;72:1326–1331.

63. Hopkins IJ, Shield LK: Poliomyelitis-like illness associated with asthma in childhood [letter]. Lancet 1974;1:760.

64. Hoyt JW: Persistent paralysis in critically ill patients after the use of neuromuscular blocking agents. New Hori 1994;2:48–55.

65. Hughes M, Grant IS, Biccard B, Nimmo G: Suxamethonium and critical illness polyneuropathy. Anaesth Intensive Care 1999;27: 636–638.

66. Hund E: Myopathy in critically ill patients. Crit Care Med 1999; 27:2544–2547.

67. Hunter J: New neuromuscular blocking drugs. N Engl J Med 1995; 332:1691–1699.

68. Hunter J, De Wolf A: The pharmacodynamics and pharmacokinetics of cisatracurium in patients with renal or hepatic failure. Curr Opin Anesthesiol 1996;9:S40–S44.

69. Inoue K, El-Banayosy A, Stolarski L, Reichelt W: Vecuronium induced bradycardia following induction of anaesthesia with etomidate or thiopentone, with or without fentanyl. Br J Anaesth 1988;60: 10–17.

70. Jalkanen L, Rautoma P, Taivainen T, Meretoja OA: The pharmacodynamics of mivacurium preceded by atracurium or cisatracurium in children. Anesth Analg 1998;86:62–65.

71. Kambam J, Parris W, Naukam R, et al: In vitro effects of fluoride and bromide on pseudocholinesterase and acetylcholinesterase activities. Can J Anaesth 1990;37:916–919.

72. Kasamatsu Y, Osada M, Ashida K, et al: Rhabdomyolysis after infection and taking a cold medicine in a patient who was susceptible to malignant hyperthermia. Intern Med 1998;37:169–173.

73. Kent R: Revised label regarding use of succinylcholine in children and adolescents: II, in reply. Anesthesiology 1994;80:244–245.

74. Khaleeli A, Edwards R, Gohil K, et al: Corticosteroid myopathy: A clinical and pathological study. Clin Endocrinol (Oxf) 1983;18: 155–166.

75. King M, Milazkiewicz R, Carli F, Deacock A: Influence of neostigmine on postoperative vomiting. Br J Anaesth 1988;61:403–406.

76. Kirkwood I, Duckworth R: An unusual case of sinus arrest. Br J Anaesth 1983;55:1273.

77. Knox AJ, Mascie Taylor BH, Muers MF: Acute hydrocortisone myopathy in acute severe asthma. Thorax 1986;41:411–412.

78. Kopman AF, Klewicka MM, Kopman DJ, Neuman GG: Molar potency is predictive of the speed of onset of neuromuscular block for agents of intermediate, short, and ultrashort duration. Anesthesiology 1999;90:425–431.

79. Kopman AF, Klewicka MM, Neuman GG: Molar potency is not predictive of the speed of onset of atracurium. Anesth Analg 1999; 89:1046–1049.

80. Kopman AF, Yee PS, Neuman GG: Relationship of the train-of-four fade ratio to clinical signs and symptoms of residual paralysis in awake volunteers. Anesthesiology 1997;86:765–771.

81. Kovarik W, Mayberg T, Lam A, et al: Succinylcholine does not change intracranial pressure, cerebral blood flow velocity, or the electroencephalogram in patients with head injury. Anesth Analg 1994;78:469–473.

82. Kress JP, Pohlman AS, O'Connor MF, Hall JB: Daily interruption of sedative infusions in critically ill patients undergoing mechanical ventilation. N Engl J Med 2000;342:1471–1477.

83. Kupfer Y, Okrent D, Twersky R, Tessler S: Disuse atrophy in a ventilated patient with status asthmaticus receiving neuromuscular blockade. Crit Care Med 1987;15:795–796.

84. Lacomis D, Giuliani MJ, Van Cott A, Kramer DJ: Acute myopathy of intensive care: Clinical, electromyographic, and pathological aspects. Ann Neurol 1996;40:645–654.

85. Lacomis D, Petrella JT, Giuliani MJ: Causes of neuromuscular weakness in the intensive care unit: A study of ninety-two patients. Muscle Nerve 1998;21:610–617.

86. Lacomis D, Zochodne DW, Bird SJ: Critical illness myopathy: What's in a name? Muscle Nerve 2000;23:1785–1788.

87. Latronico N, Guarneri B, Alongi S, et al: Acute neuromuscular respiratory failure after ICU discharge. Report of five patients. Intensive Care Med 1999;25:1302–1306.

88. Lebrault C, Berger J, D'Hollander A, et al: Pharmacokinetics and pharmacodynamics of vecuronium (ORG NC 45) in patients with cirrhosis. Anesthesiology 1985;62:601–605.

89. Lebrault C, Duvaldestin P, Henzel D, et al: Pharmacokinetics and pharmacodynamics of vecuronium in patients with cholestasis. Br J Anaesth 1986;58:983–987.

90. Lee C: Intensive care unit neuromuscular syndrome? Anesthesiology 1995;83:237–240.

91. Leijten F, De Weerd A: Critical illness polyneuropathy: A review of the literature, definition and pathophysiology. Clin Neurol Neurosurg 1994;96:10–19.

92. Leijten F, De Weered A, De Ridder V, et al: Critical illness polyneuropathy in multiple organ dysfunction syndrome and weaning from the ventilator. Intensive Care Med 1996;22:856–861.

93. Leijten F, Harinck-de Weerd J, Poortvliet D, de Weerd A: The role of polyneuropathy in motor convalescence after prolonged mechanical ventilation. JAMA 1995;274:1221–1225.

94. Lepage J-Y, Malinovsky J-M, Malinge M, et al: Pharmacodynamic dose-response and safety study of cisatracurium (51W89) in adult surgical patients during N_2O-O_2-opioid anesthesia. Anesth Analg 1996;83:823–829.

95. Levy JH, Pitts M, Thanopoulos A, et al: The effects of rapacuronium on histamine release and hemodynamics in adult patients undergoing general anesthesia. Anesth Analg 1999;89:290–295.

96. Lonsdale M, Stuart J: Complete heart block following glycopyrronium/neostigmine mixture. Anaesthesia 1989;44:448–449.

97. Loper K, Butler S, Nessly M, Wild L: Paralyzed with pain: The need for education. Pain 1989;37:315–316.

98. Lorenz W, Ennis M, Doenicke A, Dick W: Perioperative uses of histamine antagonists. J Clin Anesth 1990;2:345–360.

99. MacFarlane IA, Rosenthal FD: Severe myopathy after status asthmaticus. Lancet 1977;2:615.

100. MacLennan D, Duff C, Zorzato F, et al: Ryanodine receptor gene is a candidate for predisposition to malignant hyperthermia. Nature 1990;343:559–561.

101. MacLennan D, Phillips M: Malignant hyperthermia. Science 1992;257:789–794.

102. Magorian T, Wood P, Caldwell J, et al: The pharmacokinetics and neuromuscular effects of rocuronium bromide in patients with liver disease. Anesth Analg 1995;80:754–759.

103. Marik P: Doxacurium-corticosteroid acute myopathy: Another piece to the puzzle. Crit Care Med 1996;24:1266–1267.

104. Matteo R, Brotherton W, Nishitateno K: Pharmacodynamics and pharmacokinetics of metocurine in humans: Comparison to *d*-tubocurarine. Anesthesiology 1982;57:183–190.

105. McCoy E, Maddineni V, Elliott P, et al: Hemodynamic effects of rocuronium during fentanyl anaesthesia: Comparison with vecuronium. Can J Anaesth 1993;40:703–708.

106. Meyer K, Prielipp R, Grossman J, Coursin D: Prolonged weakness after infusion of atracurium in two intensive care unit patients. Anesth Analg 1994;78:772–774.

107. Miller R, Agoston S, Booij L, et al: The comparative potency and pharmacokinetics of pancuronium, and its metabolites in anesthetized man. J Pharmacol Exp Ther 1978;207:539–543.

108. Miller R, Matteo R, Benet L, Sohn Y: The pharmacokinetics of *d*-tubocurarine in man with and without renal failure. J Pharmacol Exp Ther 1977;202:1–207.

109. Mirakhur RK, McCourt KC, Kumar N: Use of intermediate acting muscle relaxants by infusion: The future. Acta Anaesthesiol Belg 1997;48:29–34.

110. Morris R, Cahalan M, Miller R, et al: The cardiovascular effects of vecuronium (ORG NC45) and pancuronium in patients undergoing coronary artery bypass grafting. Anesthesiology 1983;58:438–440.

111. Morrison AG, Serpell MG: Malignant hyperthermia during prolonged surgery for tumour resection. Eur J Anaesthesiol 1998;15:114–117.

112. Moss J: Muscle relaxants and histamine release. Acta Anaesthesiol Scand 1995;39:7–12.

113. Murray M, Coursin D, Scuderi P, et al: Double-blind, randomized, multicenter study of doxacurium vs pancuronium in intensive care unit patients who require neuromuscular-blocking agents. Crit Care Med 1995;23:450–458.

114. Narimatsu E, Nakayama Y, Sumita S, et al: Sepsis attenuates the intensity of the neuromuscular blocking effect of *d*-tubocurarine and the antagonistic actions of neostigmine and edrophonium accompanying depression of muscle contractility of the diaphragm. Acta Anaesthesiol Scand 1999;43:196–201.

115. Nates JL, Cooper DJ, Day B, Tuxen DV: Acute weakness syndromes in critically ill patients—A reappraisal. Anaesth Intensive Care 1997;25:502–513.

116. Nigrovic V, Fox J: Atracurium decay and the formation of laudanosine in humans. Anesthesiology 1991;74:446–454.

117. Nordgren IK, Forney RB Jr, Carroll FT, et al: Analysis of succinylcholine in tissues and body fluids by ion-pair extraction and gas chromatography-mass spectrometry. Arch Toxicol Suppl 1983;6: 339–350.

118. Op De Coul A, Verheul G, Leyten A: Critical illness polyneuropathy after artificial respiration. Clin Neurol Neurosurg 1991;93:27–33.

119. Op de Coul AA, Lambregts PC, Koeman J, et al: Neuromuscular complications in patients given Pavulon (pancuronium bromide) during artificial ventilation. Clin Neurol Neurosurg 1985;87:17–22.

120. Ostergaard D, Engbaek J, Viby-Mogensen J: Adverse reactions and interactions of the neuromuscular blocking drugs. Med Toxicol Adverse Drug Exp 1989;4:351–368.

121. Pantuck E: Plasma cholinesterase: Gene and variations. Anesth Analg 1993;77:380–386.

122. Parker C, Jones J, Hunter J: Disposition of infusions of atracurium and its metabolite, laudanosine, in patients in renal and respiratory failure in an ICU. Br J Anaesth 1988;61:531–540.

123. Parker M, Schubert W, Shelhamer J, Parrillo J: Perceptions of a critically ill patient experiencing therapeutic paralysis in an ICU. Crit Care Med 1984;12:69–71.

124. Pessah IN, Lynch Cr, Gronert GA: Complex pharmacology of malignant hyperthermia. Anesthesiology 1996;84:1275–1279.

125. Prielipp R, Coursin D: Applied pharmacology of common neuromuscular blocking agents in critical care. New Horiz 1994;2:34–47.

126. Ramsay D, Zochodne D, Robertson D, et al: A syndrome of acute severe muscle necrosis in intensive care unit patients. J Neuropath Exp Neurol 1993;52:387–398.

127. Riker W: Pre-junctional effects of neuromuscular blocking and facilitatory drugs. In: Katz R, ed: Muscle Relaxants. Amsterdam, North-Holland, 1975, pp. 59–102.

128. Rouleau G, Karpati G, Carpenter S, et al: Glucocorticoid excess induces preferential depletion of myosin in denervated skeletal muscle fibers. Muscle Nerve 1987;10:428–438.

129. Saltzman L, Kates R, Corke B, et al: Hyperkalemia and cardiovascular collapse after verapamil and dantrolene administration in swine. Anesth Analg 1984;63:473–478.

130. Sandin RH, Enlund G, Samuelsson P, Lennmarken C: Awareness during general anesthesia. Lancet 2000;355:707–711.

131. Savarese J, Lien C, Belmont M, Rubin L: The clinical and basic pharmacology of mivacurium: A short-acting nondepolarizing benzylisoquinolinium diester neuromuscular blocking drug. Acta Anaesthesiol Scand 1995;39:18–22.

132. Saxena P, Bonta I: Mechanism of selective cardiac vagolytic action of pancuronium bromide. Specific blockade of cardiac muscarinic receptors. Eur J Pharmacol 1970;3:332–341.

133. Schiere S, Proost JH, Schuringa M, Wierda JM: Pharmacokinetics and pharmacokinetic-dynamic relationship between rapacuronium (Org 9487) and its 3-desacetyl metabolite (Org 9488). Anesth Analg 1999;88:640–647.

134. Schmith V, Phillips L, Kisor D, et al: Pharmacokinetics/pharmacodynamics of cisatracurium in healthy adult patients. Curr Opin Anesthesiol 1996;9:S9–S15.

135. Schramm WM, Papousek A, Michalek Sauberer A, et al: The cerebral and cardiovascular effects of cisatracurium and atracurium in neurosurgical patients. Anesth Analg 1998;86:123–127.

136. Segarra Domenech J, Carlos Garcia R, Rodrigues Sasiain J, et al: Pancuronium bromide: An indirect sympathomimetic agent. Br J Anaesth 1976;48:1143–1148.

137. Segredo V, Caldwell J, Matthay M, et al: Persistent paralysis in critically ill patients after long-term administration of vecuronium. N Engl J Med 1992;327:524–528.

138. Segredo V, Shin Y, Sharma M, et al: Pharmacokinetics, neuromuscular effects, and biodisposition of 3-desacetylvecuronium (Org 7268) in cats. Anesthesiology 1991;74:1052–1059.

139. Shahar EM, Hwang PA, Niesen CE, Murphy EG: Poliomyelitis-like paralysis during recovery from acute bronchial asthma: Possible etiology and risk factors. Pediatrics 1991;88:276–279.

140. Shapiro B, Warren J, Egol A, et al: Practice parameters for sustained neuromuscular blockade in the adult critically ill patient: An executive summary. Crit Care Med 1995;23:1601–1605.

141. Shapiro J, Condos R, Cole R: Myopathy in status asthmaticus: Relation to neuromuscular blockade and corticosteroid administration. J Intensive Care Med 1993;8:144–152.

142. Somogyi G, Varga M, Prokai L, et al: Drug identification problems in two suicides with neuromuscular blocking agents. Forensic Sci Int 1989;43:257–266.

143. Sparr HJ, Mellinghoff H, Blobner M, Nˆldge Schomburg G: Comparison of intubating conditions after rapacuronium (Org 9487) and succinylcholine following rapid sequence induction in adult patients. Br J Anaesth 1999;82:537–541.

144. Sprague D: Severe bradycardia after neostigmine in a patient taking neostigmine to control paroxysmal atrial tachycardia. Anesthesiology 1975;42:208–210.

145. Stoelting R: The hemodynamic effects of pancuronium and *d*-tubocurarine in anesthetized patients. Anesthesiology 1976;36:612–615.

146. Szenohradszky J, Caldwell JE, Wright PM, et al: Influence of renal failure on the pharmacokinetics and neuromuscular effects of a single dose of rapacuronium bromide. Anesthesiology 1999;90:24–35.

147. Van Winkle W: Calcium release from skeletal muscle sarcoplasmic reticulum: Site of action of dantrolene sodium? Science 1976;193:1130–1131.

148. Vandenbrom R, Wierda J: Pancuronium bromide in the intensive care unit. A case of overdose. Anesthesiology 1988;69:996–997.

149. Viby-Mogensen J: Clinical assessment of neuromuscular transmission. Br J Anaesth 1982;54:209–223.

150. Viby-Mogensen J: Interaction of other drugs with muscle relaxants. In: Katz R, ed: Muscle Relaxants: Basic and Clinical Aspects. New York, Grune & Stratton, 1985, pp. 233–256.

151. Ward A, Chaffman M, Sorkin E: Dantrolene: A review of its pharmacodynamic and pharmacokinetic properties and therapeutic use in malignant hyperthermia, and neuroleptic malignant syndrome and an update of its use in muscle spasticity. Drugs 1986;32:130–168.

152. Watkins J: Adverse reaction to neuromuscular blockers: Frequency, investigation, and epidemiology. Acta Anaesthesiol Scand 1994;38:6–10.

153. Watson CB, Reierson N, Norfleet EA: Clinically significant muscle weakness induced by oral dantrolene sodium prophylaxis for malignant hyperthermia. Anesthesiology 1986;65:312–314.

154. Wedel D, Quilan J, Iaizzo P: Clinical effects of intravenously administered dantrolene. Mayo Clin Proc 1995;70:241–246.

155. West R: Curare in man. Proc R Soc Med 1932;25:1107–1116.

156. Wright P, Hart P, Lau M, et al: Cumulative characteristics of atracurium and vecuronium: A simultaneous clinical and pharmacokinetic study. Anesthesiology 1994;81:59–68.

157. Yate P, Flynn P, Arnold R, et al: Clinical experience and plasma laudanosine concentrations during the infusion of atracurium in the intensive therapy unit. Br J Anaesth 1987;59:211–217.

158. Youngman P, Taylor K, Wilson J: Anaphylactoid reactions to neuromuscular blocking agents: A commonly undiagnosed condition? Lancet 1983;2:597–599.

159. Zochodne D, Bolton C, Wells G, et al: Critical illness polyneuropathy: A complication of sepsis and multiple organ failure. Brain 1987;110:819–842.

160. Zochodne D, Ramsay D, Saly V: Acute necrotizing myopathy of intensive care: Electrophysiologic studies. Muscle Nerve 1994;17:285–292.

CHAPTER 55 LOCAL ANESTHETICS

Brian Kaufman / Staffan Wahlander

A 30-year-old female presented to the Emergency Department (ED) 4 hours after a laser epilation treatment. In preparation for the procedure, 150 g of EMLA (eutectic mixture of local anesthetics) cream (5 tubes) had been applied to her lower extremities under occlusive dressings. One hour later, she began to experience lightheadedness, dyspnea, tongue numbness, and muscular twitching. Her only medications were sertraline and an oral contraceptive. On physical examination she was alert and in mild respiratory distress with perioral/acral cyanosis, which did not resolve with supplemental oxygen. Her vital signs were blood pressure, 130/80 mm Hg; heart rate, 120 beats/min; respiratory rate, 20 breaths/min; and temperature 98.6°F (37°C). Her height was 5′4″, and she weighed 74 kg. Her lungs were clear and her heart sounds were normal. Her abdomen was soft and nontender with normal bowel sounds. Bilateral pretibial first-degree burns were still present from a prior laser treatment 1 week earlier. The remainder of her physical examination was normal. Her pulse oximeter revealed an 84% saturation while she was breathing 100% oxygen. An arterial blood gas (ABG) obtained on 100% oxygen was pH, 7.45; Pco_2, 36 mm Hg; and Po_2, 385 mm Hg; her methemoglobin was 20% by cooximeter. The patient received methylene blue, 50 mg IV, over 5 minutes and improved within 1 hour. A repeat methemoglobin level was 2.7%. Her lidocaine level, drawn several hours after initial placement of the EMLA cream, was 0.68 µg/mL, confirming systemic absorption from the EMLA cream. The patient subsequently improved and was discharged.[36]

Local anesthetics are drugs that block neural transmission along an axon in a predictable and reversible manner. The anesthesia that is produced is selective to the chosen body part in contrast to the unselective effects of a general anesthetic. Local anesthetics do not need the circulation as an intermediate carrier and are not usually transported to distant organs; therefore, the actions of local anesthetics are largely confined to the structures with which they come into direct contact. Local anesthetics may provide analgesia in various parts of the body by topical application, injection in the vicinity of peripheral nerve endings and major nerve trunks, or via instillation within the epidural or subarachnoid spaces. The various local anesthetic agents differ in their potency, duration of action, and degree of effects on sensory and motor fibers. Toxicity may be local or systemic, and when systemic typically involves the central nervous system (CNS) and cardiovascular systems.

HISTORY

Until the 1880s, the only drugs that were available to relieve pain were centrally acting depressants that blunted the perception of pain rather than attacking the root cause (eg, alcohol and opioids). The coca shrub (*Erythroxylon coca*) was brought back to Europe from Peru by Karl Von Scherzer, an Austrian explorer, in the mid-1800s. Some of the coca leaves were analyzed by a chemist, Albert Niemann, who, in 1860, successfully isolated and named the alkaloid (cocaine) derived from the erythroxyline extract. Although Niemann made the observation that cocaine crystals numbed his tongue, it was not until 1868 that Peruvian army surgeon Moreno y Mayz made the initial suggestion that cocaine might have medical applications as a local anesthetic. Sigmund Freud was interested in the analeptic actions of cocaine, which he hoped would help cure morphine addiction. Freud obtained a supply of cocaine from the manufacturing firm Merck and shared the supply with his good friend Carl Koller, who was a junior intern in the Ophthalmological Clinic at the University of Vienna. After dissolving coca powder in distilled water, Koller instilled the solution in the conjunctival sacs of a frog, a rabbit, and a dog, and was then able to touch their cornea without any evidence of reflex action. He then experimented on his own eye and that of his laboratory assistant, and demonstrated that the eye became insensitive to touch and injury within a minute. In 1884, Koller performed an operation for glaucoma with topical cocaine anesthesia, and 4 days later his findings were presented at the Congress of Ophthalmology in Heidelberg. Dr. Henry Noyes, an American who attended the Heidelberg meeting, reported the discovery in a letter to the *New York Medical Record,* and news of the discovery spread rapidly. Within 1 year, cocaine was in worldwide use as a pain-relieving drug for surgery of the eye, and was being tested on other mucous membranes, such as the upper airway.

After the 1884 publication of Dr. Noyes' letter, several surgeons investigated the direct injection of cocaine into tissues. Halsted, a year after Koller's discovery, reported on more than 1000 cases in which cocaine infiltration anesthesia was used at the Johns Hopkins Hospital.[37] Human spinal anesthesia and the associated spinal headache were reported by Bier in 1899.

Although the clinical benefits of cocaine anesthesia were great, so were its toxic and addictive potential. At least 13 deaths were reported in the first 7 years following its introduction, and within 10 years following its introduction as a regional anesthetic, reviews of "cocaine poisoning" appeared in the literature.[58,74] The toxicity of cocaine, coupled with its tremendous advantages for surgery, led to a search for less toxic substitutes. After the elucidation of cocaine's chemical structure (the benzoic acid methyl ester of the alkaloid ecgonine) in 1895, the hunt narrowed to benzoic acid esters. Synthetic compounds with local anesthetic activity were introduced but were either very toxic or irritating or had an impractical brief clinical effectiveness. In 1904, Einhorn synthesized procaine but its short duration of action limited its clinical utility, and research focused on synthesis of drugs with more prolonged duration of action.

The potent, long-acting local anesthetics dibucaine and tetracaine were synthesized in 1925 and 1928, respectively, and were introduced into clinical practice. However, these anesthetics could not be used safely for regional anesthetic techniques in which large volumes of drug were required because of systemic toxicity. These drugs were very useful, however, for spinal anesthesia.

Lofgren synthesized lidocaine from a series of aniline derivatives in 1943. Lidocaine, an amino amide, was a stable local anesthetic that combined high tissue penetrance with acceptably low systemic toxicity. Additionally, the metabolites of lidocaine did not include para-aminobenzoic acid, which was the reported cause of allergic reactions to amino ester derivatives. Lidocaine was introduced clinically in 1944. Subsequent to lidocaine's release, several amino amide compounds were synthesized and introduced into clinical practice, including mepivacaine in 1956, prilocaine in 1959, bupivacaine in 1963, etidocaine in 1971, and ropivacaine, synthesized in 1957 and released for use in the mid-1990s.

EPIDEMIOLOGY

Poisoning from topical benzocaine is common because of the large number of over-the-counter products available for teething and hemorrhoids. Fortunately, toxic effects following exposure are typically mild, and death occurs rarely. Toxicity usually occurs as a therapeutic misadventure, but child abuse or neglect should be considered if the patient is younger than 2 years of age, and suicide should be considered in older children or adults.

Considering the large number of local anesthetics administered, the frequency of clinically significant toxic reactions is quite low and usually iatrogenic. Most poisonings result from inadvertent injection of a therapeutic dose into a blood vessel, repeated use of a therapeutic dose, or unintentional administration of a toxic dose. Advanced age and liver disease increase the likelihood of toxicity.

In a large series of patients receiving bupivacaine, systemic toxicity occurred in only 15 of 11,080 nerve blocks.[65] Of these patients, 80% convulsed, whereas 20% had milder symptoms. However, during the late 1970s and early 1980s, a series of cases were described in which the use of bupivacaine, particularly in 0.75% concentration, was associated with the development of severe cardiovascular depression, ventricular dysrhythmias, and even death. Pregnant women were disproportionately affected. Some of these cases required prolonged and difficult resuscitation.[81] In 1983, 49 incidents of cardiac arrest or ventricular tachycardia occurring over a 10-year period were presented to the US Food and Drug Administration's Anesthetic and Life Support Advisory Committee. Of these cases, 0.75% bupivacaine was used in 27 obstetric patients with 10 deaths, and 0.5% bupivacaine was used in 8 obstetric patients with 6 deaths. In nonobstetric patients, there were only 14 patients, of whom 5 died. The overall mortality was 21/49 (43%). Partly as a result of these reports, in 1984, the US Food and Drug Administration withdrew approval of bupivacaine 0.75% for obstetric anesthesia.[81]

PHARMACOLOGY

Chemical Structure

The basic molecular structure of local anesthetics has three major components. A lipophilic, aromatic ring structure connected by a short alkyl, intermediate chain that contains either an amide or ester bound to a hydrophilic tertiary amine. The tertiary amine is a base (proton acceptor) and is partially protonated in the physiologic pH range. Clinically useful local anesthetics fall into one of two chemically distinct groups: (a) amino esters, which possess an ester link between the aromatic portion and the hydrophilic amine (eg, procaine, chloroprocaine, tetracaine, and cocaine), or (b) amino amides, which possess an amide link, (eg, lidocaine, mepivacaine, prilocaine, bupivacaine, etidocaine, and ropivacaine) (Table 55–1 and Fig. 55–1).

Mode of Action

Local anesthetics exert their main analgesic effect by inhibiting neuronal membrane conductance of sodium ions, thereby blocking impulse conduction. Local anesthetics function by reversibly binding to specific protein receptors within the sodium channel. Once bound, the anesthetic impedes sodium influx and blocks depolarization, creating a conduction block. The smaller-diameter nerve fibers carrying pain and temperature sensation are blocked before the larger fibers responsible for touch, motor function, and proprioception.[20]

These effects also occur in other conductive tissues, such as the heart and brain, which are the main target organs when systemic reactions to local anesthetics develop. It was initially believed that sodium channel blockade was the sole cause of systemic toxic reactions. However, the mechanisms of toxic effects are more complex, especially in the heart, and can occur at lower systemic concentrations than previously thought.[60] There is also growing evidence that local anesthetics can directly affect many other organ systems and functions, such as the coagulation, immune, and respiratory systems, at concentrations much lower than those required to achieve sodium channel blockade.[14,42,43]

Physicochemical Properties

The primary determinant of a local anesthetic's onset of action is its pK_a. All of the local anesthetics are weak bases, with a pK_a between 7.6 and 9.1. At physiologic pH (7.4) agents with a lower pK_a have relatively more uncharged molecules free to cross the

TABLE 55–1.   Classification of Local Anesthetics

Amino Esters	Amino Amides
Procaine	Lidocaine
Chloroprocaine	Mepivacaine
Tetracaine	Prilocaine
Cocaine	Etidocaine
Benzocaine	Ropivacaine

Generic/Proprietary Name	Chemical Structure
Benzocaine (Hurricaine)	
Procaine (Novocaine)	
Dibucaine (Nupercaine)	
Lidocaine (Xylocaine)	
Bupivacaine (Marcaine)	

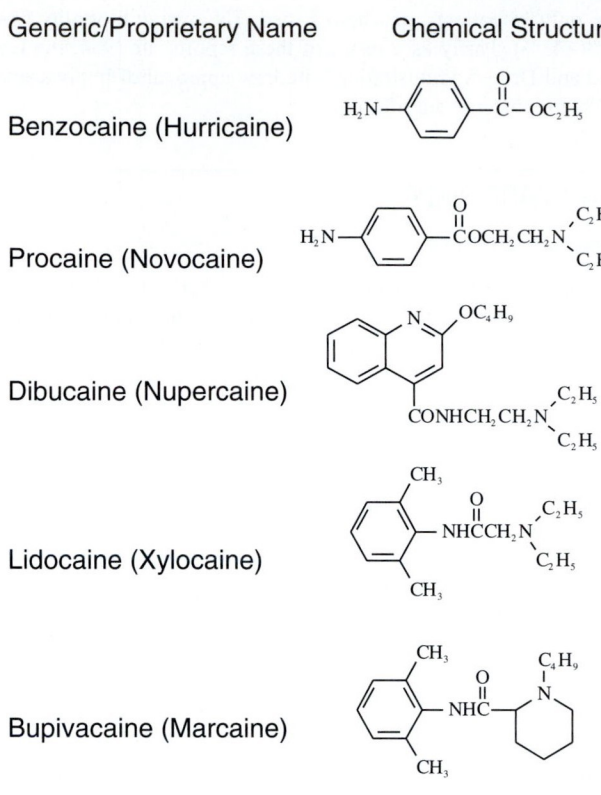

Figure 55–1. Representative local anesthetic agents in common clinical use.

nerve cell membrane, producing a faster onset of action than agents with a higher pK_a. Onset of action is also influenced by the total dose of local anesthetic administered.

Local anesthetic potency is determined by the drug's lipid solubility. The aromatic side of the anesthetic therefore determines potency. The hydrophilic amine is most involved in occupation of the sodium channel. The length of the intermediate chain is a determinant of local anesthetic activity, with 3–7 carbon-equivalents providing maximal activity.[20] Shorter or longer intermediate chain length is associated with rapid loss of local anesthetic action, suggesting that a critical length of separation of the aromatic group from the tertiary amine is required for sodium channel blockade to occur.

The degree of protein binding influences the duration of action of a local anesthetic. Agents with greater protein binding remain associated with the neural membrane for a longer time interval and therefore have a longer duration of action.[20]

Clinical Pharmacology

Systemic toxicity in humans usually presents with CNS symptoms. Animal studies and clinical observations demonstrate that lidocaine CNS toxicity develops at a lower plasma concentration than is needed to produce cardiac toxicity.[24] Local anesthetic–induced cardiac toxicity occurs less frequently than does CNS toxicity, but is more serious and more difficult to manage. It is possible that the reported low frequency of cardiac side effects at least partially reflects difficulty in detection. An experimental study in

pigs, attempting to identify early warning signs of bupivacaine-induced cardiac toxicity, compared bupivacaine-induced changes in cardiac output, heart rate, blood pressure, and electrocardiogram (ECG).[73] A 40% reduction in cardiac output was not associated with any significant change in blood pressure or heart rate. The ECG, on the other hand, showed a decrease in R-wave amplitude and a widening of the QRS complex. The R-wave depression changed gradually, correlating with the depression of the cardiac output. The observed electrophysiologic disturbances increase the likelihood of reentrant tachycardia, which may be either ventricular or supraventricular with aberrant conduction. Blood pressure may be maintained by a direct vasoconstrictive effect of bupivacaine on the peripheral circulation, which is dependent upon the plasma concentration of the drug.[15]

The mechanism and risk for cardiotoxicity are not exactly the same for the different local anesthetics. This difference in risk for cardiotoxicity is partially explained by different effects on the sodium channel. Local anesthetics depress the maximum rate of increase of the cardiac action potential (V_{max}) by blocking cardiac sodium channels. Lidocaine binds to both open and inactive channels and dissociates from the channels rapidly after an action potential. Bupivacaine, on the other hand, binds only to inactivated channels and dissociates much more slowly.[18] Additionally, several local anesthetics have an asymmetrically substituted carbon and their binding to sodium channels is stereospecific.[49] For example, the bupivacaine levo(S−)-enantiomer is significantly less cardiotoxic than the dextro(R+)-enantiomer.[4,60] Consequently, bupivacaine, a racemic mixture of both enantiomers, is more cardiotoxic than levobupivacaine, which contains only the levo-enantiomer.[35] Ropivacaine is a pure enantiomer and is less cardiotoxic than bupivacaine but is also slightly less potent as an analgesic.[75,76] The stereospecific effect on the sodium channels seems to differ between the heart and the peripheral nerves, however, because the local anesthetic potency of levobupivacaine is the same, or perhaps even greater than that of bupivacaine[27,71] (Chap. 52).

Interference with membrane ion conduction can explain the dysrhythmogenic properties of local anesthetics as well. Some agents, notably bupivacaine, also cause severe myocardial depression. Lipophilic local anesthetics directly impair mitochondrial energy transduction via two mechanisms: (a) uncoupling of oxygen consumption and adenosine triphosphate (ATP) synthesis and (b) inhibition of complex 1 in the respiratory chain.[92] This effect is related to the lipophilic properties of the drug rather than to stereospecific effects on ion channels; lidocaine has no effect on mitochondrial respiration and ropivacaine has less effect compared to bupivacaine.[100] There is no difference between the two bupivacaine enantiomers. These effects occur with higher concentrations of the drug as can happen after unintentional intravascular injection.

Low-dose bupivacaine-induced cardiotoxic effects are described in humans under certain circumstances, and at levels that are not associated with seizure activity in pigs.[99] Severe cardiac toxicity has been described after injection of a small subcutaneous dose of bupivacaine in a patient with secondary carnitine deficiency.[99] Myocytes are highly dependent on oxidation of fatty acids for energy turnover. It has been proposed that interference with this mechanism through bupivacaine-induced inhibition of carnitine-acylcarnitine translocase contributes to the cardiotoxicity of lipophilic local anesthetics[99] (Chap. 41 and Fig. 41–2). Bupivacaine may also produce dysrhythmias by blockage of GABAergic neurons that tonically inhibit the autonomic nervous system.[39] In addition to its other effects on the heart, bupivacaine may induce a marked decrease in cardiac contractility by alteration of Ca^{2+} release from sarcoplasmic reticulum.[54]

Local anesthetics have complex effects on target organs other than peripheral nerves and not all of these actions are detrimental. Lidocaine, for example, ameliorates anoxic/ischemic injury in neurons, partially mediated by inhibition of ischemia-induced increases in intracellular calcium, and there is interest in the potential use of local anesthetics as modulators of the inflammatory response.[42]

TOXICOKINETICS

When considering the pharmacokinetics of local anesthetics, a distinction should be made between local disposition (distribution and elimination) and systemic disposition. Local distribution is influenced by several factors including spread of the local anesthetic by bulk flow, diffusion, transport via local blood vessels, and binding to local tissues. Local elimination occurs through systemic absorption and transfer into the general circulation and by local hydrolysis of amino ester anesthetics. Systemic absorption decreases the amount of local anesthetic that is available for anesthetic effect and thereby limits the duration of the block. Systemic absorption is dependent on the avidity of binding of local anesthetics to tissues near the site of injection and on local perfusion. Both of these factors vary with the site of injection.

Local anesthetics, being lipophilic drugs, readily cross cell membranes, the blood-brain barrier, and the placenta. Therefore, tissue distribution is highly dependent on tissue perfusion. After entry into the venous circulation, local anesthetics pass through the lungs where significant uptake may occur, thereby lowering peak arterial blood concentrations. Part of the reason that most local anesthetic–induced seizures result from unintentional intravascular injection rather than absorptive uptake is that the lung uptake of these drugs appears to exceed 90% of the drug. Therefore, the lung may serve as a buffer to systemic toxicity.[51]

The two classes of local anesthetic agents undergo metabolism by different routes (Chap. 67). The amino esters are rapidly metabolized by plasma cholinesterase to the major metabolite para-aminobenzoic acid (PABA). The amino amides are metabolized more slowly in the liver to a variety of metabolites unrelated to PABA.[19] Patients with atypical plasma cholinesterase are at increased risk for systemic toxicity from amino ester local anesthetics. Factors that decrease hepatic blood flow or that impair hepatic function increase the risk of toxic reactions to the amino amides and make management of serious reactions more difficult. The patient's age may influence the rate of metabolism of local anesthetics. The lidocaine half-life following intravenous administration averaged 80 minutes in volunteers aged 22–26 years of age, whereas the half-life was 138 minutes in those aged 61–71 years of age.[70] Newborn infants with immature hepatic enzyme systems also have prolonged elimination of amino amides, which has been associated with seizures when high continuous infusion rates are used.[1,61]

Lidocaine elimination is reduced by coadministration of drugs that reduce hepatic blood flow. Decreased lidocaine extraction occurs with cimetidine and propranolol.[82] Administration of one local anesthetic increases the free plasma fraction of another agent by displacement from protein-binding sites.[44]

CLINICAL APPLICATIONS

Local anesthetics are utilized to provide regional anesthesia. On the basis of anatomic considerations, regional anesthesia can be divided into infiltrative anesthesia, intravenous regional anesthesia, peripheral nerve blockade, central neural blockade, topical anesthesia, and tumescent anesthesia.

Infiltrative anesthesia refers to the intradermal or subcutaneous administration of a local anesthetic, which blocks the ends of the peripheral nerves. The dosage required for adequate anesthesia depends on the size of the area to be anesthetized and the expected duration of the surgical procedure. If a large area needs to be anesthetized, the concentration of the anesthetic should be decreased within its clinically effective range so that the maximum safe dose of the anesthetic is not exceeded (eg, 5 mg/kg for lidocaine), thereby minimizing the risk for systemic toxicity. The onset of action is almost immediate with all agents.

Intravenous regional anesthesia involves intravenous administration of a local anesthetic into a tourniquet-occluded limb (Bier block). The local anesthetic diffuses from the peripheral veins to axons and nerve endings, producing nerve blockade. Lidocaine is the only local anesthetic approved for this technique in the United States, with a typical dose of 3 mg/kg of 0.5% preservative-free solution for an upper extremity block. Other drugs have been used successfully.[38] Systemic toxicity may ensue if the tourniquet is prematurely deflated while significant amounts of anesthetic remain within the peripheral veins. The use of bupivacaine for intravenous regional anesthesia is contraindicated due to reports of cardiovascular collapse following sudden, unintentional cuff release.[2]

Regional anesthetic procedures involving nerves of the peripheral nervous system are called peripheral nerve blocks. Peripheral nerve blocks can be divided into minor and major nerve blocks. Minor nerve blocks are procedures involving single nerves, whereas major nerve blocks involve the blocking of two or more distinct nerves or a nerve plexus (eg, brachial plexus block). Toxicity from minor nerve blocks is unusual because only small volumes of local anesthetic are injected. Much larger volumes of local anesthetic are used for the major nerve blocks, increasing the risk of overdosage. Additionally, because the injection is usually much deeper than with the minor nerve blocks, the possibility of an inadvertent intravascular injection is increased. Occasionally, toxic reactions follow administration of relatively small doses. This may occur, for example, with injections in the head or neck region when the local anesthetic gains access to the brain via alternative routes such as direct injection into the carotid or vertebral arteries, or by retrograde spread along nerves or veins.[47] Intrapleural regional anesthesia is a variant of a peripheral nerve block, which involves administration of local anesthetic solution into the pleural space using a catheter designed for epidural anesthesia. Large volumes of local anesthetic are administered with this technique which may result in extremely high plasma concentrations of anesthetic and risk for systemic toxicity.[80]

Central neural blockade will occur with introduction of local anesthetics into the epidural or subarachnoid space. Solutions injected into the epidural space will spread in all directions because there are no barriers to bulk flow. Suggested sites of action of local anesthetics administered into the epidural space include the paravertebral nerve trunks, the dorsal root ganglia, the spinal nerve roots, and the spinal cord. Systemic toxicity may develop from inadvertent intravascular injection.

Spinal anesthesia involves the injection of a small amount of a local anesthetic into the subarachnoid space. Because only a small amount of anesthetic is used, the risk for systemic toxicity is minimal; however, adverse reactions can occur because of overdosage (eg, total spinal anesthesia) with respiratory and cardiovascular compromise.

Topical anesthetics generally provide effective but short-duration analgesia when applied to mucous membranes or abraded skin. Absorption is very rapid and plasma concentrations can be reached comparable with those after direct intravenous placement. Topical anesthesia through cut skin may be provided by a mixture of tetracaine, epinephrine (adrenaline), and cocaine, known as TAC. TAC is a popular mixture for use in pediatric emergency rooms for liquid application into lacerations requiring suturing. TAC is usually supplied as tetracaine 0.5%, epinephrine 1:2000, and cocaine 11.8%. The generally recommended safe maximum dose is 3–4 mL for adults and 0.05 mL/kg for children. TAC should not come into contact with mucous membranes, the eye, or denuded or burned skin as rapid absorption through these surfaces can produce severe systemic toxicity and death.[21,95] A fatality related to TAC following its application to a nasal laceration with presumed dripping into the mouth and subsequent rapid mucosal absorption has been described.[8] TAC may also produce toxicity in the healthcare provider applying the mixture. Whenever a topical local anesthetic is applied to a large wound (eg, partial-thickness or full-thickness burns) or to deep skin abrasions, the potential exists for systemic toxicity. Definitive recommendations do not exist for maximal safe doses of topical agents applied to such wounds.

Local anesthetics are usually unable to penetrate intact skin in sufficient quantities to produce reliable anesthesia. Efficient skin penetration requires the combination of a high water content and a high concentration of the water-insoluble base form of the local anesthetic. This combination of properties has been achieved by mixing lidocaine and prilocaine in their base forms in a 1:1 ratio (EMLA).[11] EMLA 5% cream contains 25 mg of lidocaine and 25 mg of prilocaine per mL. Application for at least 45 minutes is required to achieve adequate dermal analgesia. Local anesthetic uptake continues for several hours during application. EMLA patches are also available over-the-counter in some countries. Both methemoglobinemia and systemic lidocaine toxicity have occurred with use of EMLA, although these toxicities occur rarely as in general the dose of the drugs is small.[36]

Tumescent anesthesia is a technique commonly employed by plastic surgeons for liposuction procedures. Large volumes of dilute local anesthetic in combination with epinephrine are injected subcutaneously. Total doses of up to 55 mg/kg have been reported to produce "safe" plasma concentrations. However, plasma concentrations can rise for up to 23 hours after injection.[12,78,87] Although good outcomes have been reported in large series, systemic toxicity has been described and may have contributed to the deaths of at least two patients.[17,78]

CLINICAL MANIFESTATIONS OF TOXICITY

Toxic Reactions

Regional Side Effects and Tissue Toxicity. All local anesthetics at some concentration are directly cytotoxic to nerve cells; however, in clinical dosage these drugs rarely produce localized nerve damage.[48,69] When nerve damage has occurred, it has been attributed to the use of excessively concentrated solutions or to inappropriate formulations. Several reports of cauda equina syndrome are associated with the use of hyperbaric 5% lidocaine solutions for spinal anesthesia. Hyperbaric solutions are those more dense than cerebrospinal fluid (CSF). This neurotoxicity appears to be a phenomena that especially occurs when the anesthetic is injected through narrow-bore needles or through continuous spinal catheters, which can result in very high local concentrations of the anesthetic that might pool around the sacral roots because of inadequate mixing.[83] The mechanism of this neurotoxic effect is unknown. Because an equally effective block can be achieved with injection of larger volumes of less concentrated drug, it is prudent to avoid use of 5% lidocaine.

Severe neurotoxic reactions have occurred following massive subarachnoid injection of chloroprocaine during attempted epidural anesthesia.[79] The neurotoxicity appears to have been associated with the use of the antioxidant sodium bisulfite and the low pH of the commercial solution, rather than with the use of the anesthetic per se.[98] Neural damage has not been reported since chloroprocaine was reformulated without bisulfite.

Skeletal muscle changes are observed following intramuscular injection of local anesthetics, especially with the more potent, longer-acting agents. The effect is reversible and muscle regeneration is complete within 2 weeks following injection of local anesthetics.[6]

Systemic Side Effects and Toxicity

Allergic Reactions. Allergic reactions to local anesthetics are extremely rare. Less than 1% of all adverse drug reactions caused by local anesthetics are caused by true IgE-mediated allergic reactions.[34] The amino esters are responsible for the majority of such cases. When hydrolyzed, the amino ester local anesthetics produce PABA, a known allergen. Cross-sensitivity to other amino ester anesthetics is common. Some multidose commercial preparations of amino amides may contain the preservative methylparaben, which is chemically related to PABA and is the most likely cause of the much rarer allergic reaction to amino amides. Thus, preservative-free amino amides, including lidocaine, can be used safely in patients who have reactions to drug preparations containing methylparaben, unless the patient is specifically sensitive to lidocaine. If a history of prior allergic reaction to a particular agent is obtained from a patient requiring a local anesthetic, a drug from the opposite class can be chosen as there is no cross-reactivity between the amides and esters.

Toxic Effects of Epinephrine. All local anesthetic agents, except cocaine, cause peripheral vasodilation by direct relaxation of vascular smooth muscle. The vasodilation enhances the vascular absorption of the local anesthetic. The addition of epinephrine (5 μg/mL or 1:200,000) to the local anesthetic solution decreases the rate of vascular absorption, thereby improving the depth and prolonging the duration of drug action. An epinephrine/local anesthetic mixture also decreases bleeding into the surgical field and serves as a marker for inadvertent intravascular injection when a test dose of the mixture is injected through a needle or catheter.[63]

There are significant drawbacks to the use of epinephrine, however, including the development of uncomfortable side effects such as palpitations and tremors, severe local tissue ischemia, and gangrene (eg, if used in the digits), and life-threatening systemic side effects in susceptible patients (eg, myocardial ischemia, hypertensive crisis). Inadvertent intravascular injection of local anesthetics mixed with epinephrine can have fatal consequences.[55]

Methemoglobinemia.   Methemoglobinemia is reported frequently as a side effect of topical and oropharyngeal benzocaine use, and occasionally with use of lidocaine, tetracaine, or prilocaine. Benzocaine is metabolized to aniline and then further metabolized to phenylhydroxylamine and nitrobenzene, which are capable of oxidizing hemoglobin to methemoglobin (Chap. 94).

Prilocaine is an amino ester local anesthetic primarily used in obstetric anesthesia because of its rapid onset of action and low systemic toxicity in both mother and fetus. Use of large doses of prilocaine can lead to the development of methemoglobinemia.[41,53] Prilocaine is an aniline derivative that, when metabolized in the liver, produces *ortho*-toluidine, which may oxidize hemoglobin to methemoglobin.[41] A direct relationship exists between the amount of epidural prilocaine administered and the incidence of methemoglobinemia. A dose greater than approximately 8 mg/kg is generally necessary to produce symptoms, which may not become apparent until several hours after epidural administration of the drug. If necessary, the patient should be treated with intravenous methylene blue (Chap. 94 and Antidotes in Depth: Methylene Blue). Standard doses of EMLA cream in term neonates being circumcised is associated with minimal production of methemoglobin, but risks may be increased in the neonate with metabolic disorders.[93]

Other Reactions.   The most common adverse reactions to local anesthetic agents are vasovagal reactions, and most "allergic reactions" attributed to local anesthetics by patients probably are vasovagal in origin.[96]

Central Nervous System Toxicity.   A gradually increasing blood level of lidocaine produces a common pattern of symptoms and signs. In the awake patient, the initial symptoms are subjective and include tinnitus, lightheadedness, circumoral numbness, disorientation, confusion, auditory and visual disturbances, and lethargy. Subjective side effects occur at plasma levels between 3 and 6 μg/mL. Significant psychologic effects of local anesthetics have also been reported. Near-death experiences and delusions of actual death have been described as specific symptoms of local anesthetic toxicity.[56] Thus, appearance of psychologic symptoms during administration of local anesthetics should not be discarded as unrelated nervous reactions by the patient or effects of sedatives given as premedication, but rather as an early sign of CNS toxicity.

Objective signs then develop, which are usually excitatory, including shivering, tremors, and ultimately general tonic-clonic seizures. Objective CNS toxicity is usually evident at levels between 5 and 9 μg/mL. Seizures may occur at levels above 10 μg/mL and higher levels produce coma, apnea, and cardiovascular collapse. The excitatory phase has a wide range of intensity and duration depending on the chemical properties of the local anesthetic. With the highly lipophilic, highly protein-bound drugs, the excitement phase is brief and mild. Toxicity from a large intravenous bolus of bupivacaine can even present without any CNS excitement and with bradycardia, cyanosis, and coma as the first signs.[85] Rapid intravascular injection of lidocaine may produce a brief excitatory phase, followed by generalized CNS depression with respiratory arrest. Seizures may follow even a small dose injected into the vertebral or carotid artery (as may occur during stellate ganglion block).[47] A relative overdose produces a slower onset of symptoms (usually within 5–15 minutes of drug injection), with irritability progressing into seizures.

The mechanism of the initial CNS excitation involves a selective block of cortical cerebral inhibitory pathways in the amygdala.[94,97] The resulting increase in unopposed excitatory activity leads to seizures. As the blood level rises further, both inhibitory and excitatory neurons are blocked and generalized CNS depression ensues.

The brain and heart are the primary target organs for systemic toxicity because of their rich perfusion, moderate tissue-blood partition coefficients, and lack of diffusion limitations.

There is a linear relationship between local anesthetic potency and CNS toxicity; however, several other factors influence the CNS effects, including the rate of injection (rapid infusion results in a higher blood level and a smaller dose necessary to produce toxicity), drug interactions (sedatives raise the threshold to local anesthetic–induced seizures), and acid-base status with acidosis increasing toxicity.[23] CNS-depressant drugs often modify the clinical presentation of a systemic toxic reaction. In general, CNS-depressant drugs minimize the signs and symptoms of CNS excitation, whereas flumazenil increases the sensitivity of the CNS to amino amide local anesthetics.[10]

Systemic toxicity for all local anesthetics correlates with plasma concentrations. The factors that determine the blood level include (a) dose of the drug; (b) rate of administration; (c) site of injection (absorption occurs more rapidly and completely from vascular areas such as with neck blocks and intercostal blocks); (d) presence or absence of a vasoconstrictor; and (e) drug-specific factors such as the degree of tissue protein binding, fat solubility, and pK_a of the drug.[64]

Intravenous infusion studies in volunteers demonstrated an inverse relationship between the anesthetic potency of various local anesthetics and the dosage required to induce signs of CNS toxicity.[89] A similar relationship exists between the convulsive blood level of various local anesthetics and their relative anesthetic potency. In humans, seizures have been reported at venous blood levels of approximately 2–4 μg/mL for bupivacaine and etidocaine, whereas concentrations in excess of 10 μg/mL are usually required for production of seizures when the less potent agents such as lidocaine are administered.

Although a general relationship exists between local anesthetic blood levels and risk of CNS toxicity, several factors limit the ability to monitor drug blood levels as a way to accurately predict the risk of toxicity. The rapidity with which a particular blood level is achieved influences the toxicity of the anesthetic. Volunteers could tolerate an average dose of 236 mg of etidocaine and a venous blood level of 3 μg/mL before the onset of CNS symptoms when the anesthetic was infused at a rate of 10 mg/min, but when the infusion rate was increased to 20 mg/min, the same individuals could only tolerate an average of 161 mg of the drug, which produced a venous blood level of approximately 2 μg/mL.[88] Other factors that can markedly affect the CNS activity of local anesthetics include the P_{CO_2}. The convulsive threshold of various local anesthetics is inversely related to the arterial P_{CO_2}.[25,28,29] Hypercarbia may lower seizure threshold by several mechanisms: (a) increased cerebral blood flow, which increases drug delivery to the CNS; (b) increased conversion of the drug base to the active cation in the presence of decreased intracellular pH; and (c) decreased plasma protein binding, which increases the amount of free drug available for diffusion into the brain.[13,25,28,29] Metabolic acidosis also decreases the plasma protein binding of local anesthetics, increasing the amount of free drug available to diffuse into the CNS. Diseases that decrease serum proteins also decrease the amount of protein binding and potentially magnify the toxicity of a given injected dose.

Recommendations have been published regarding maximal local anesthetic doses in an effort to minimize the risk for a systemic toxic reaction.[91] These maximal recommended doses are developed to prevent injection of excessive drug. However, because most episodes of systemic toxicity from local anesthetics occur secondary to unintentional intravascular injection, rather than from overdosage, limiting the maximal dose is irrelevant for preventing most toxic systemic reactions.[90]

Toxicity is also related to the metabolism for a given local anesthetic. The rapidity of elimination from the plasma determines the total dose delivered to the CNS. The amino esters are rapidly hydrolyzed in the plasma and eliminated, explaining their low potential for systemic toxicity. However, the amino amides have a much greater potential for producing systemic toxicity because termination of the therapeutic effect of these drugs is through redistribution and slower metabolic inactivation.[31] Another factor that creates difficulty in specifying the minimal toxic plasma level of lidocaine results from the fact that its N-dealkylated metabolites are pharmacologically active. These factors make it difficult to establish safe doses of local anesthetics (Fig. 55–2.). Table 55–2 summarizes the estimates of toxic doses of various local anesthetics.

Cardiovascular Toxicity. Local anesthetics have the potential for producing significant cardiovascular side effects. Although decreased blood pressure secondary to sympathetic nerve block is common after epidural and spinal analgesia, this is not a toxic drug effect, and treatment is relatively straightforward if the patient is properly monitored. True cardiotoxic effects of local anesthetics, on the other hand, include significant depression of cardiac output, dysrhythmias, and cardiac arrest. All local anesthetics are cardiotoxic at higher doses, but they differ in the exact mechanisms and in the potency for this side effect.

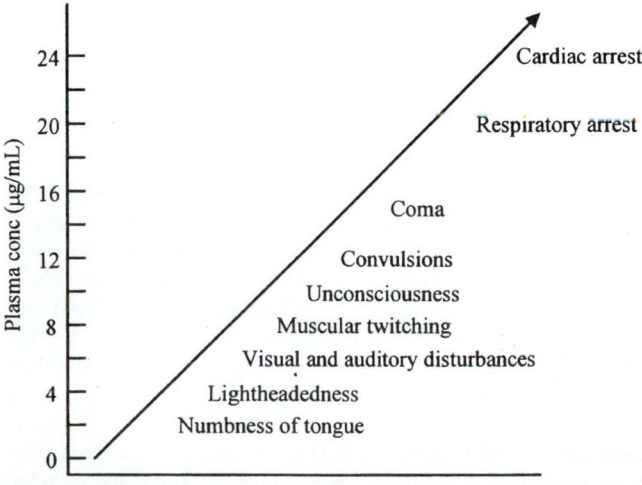

Figure 55–2. Relationship of signs and symptoms of lidocaine toxicity to its plasma concentrations.

TABLE 55–2. Toxic Doses of Local Anesthetics

Local Anesthetic	Minimum IV Toxic Dose of Local Anesthetic in Humans (mg/kg)
Procaine	19.2
Chloroprocaine	22.8
Tetracaine	2.5
Lidocaine	6.4
Mepivacaine	9.8
Bupivacaine	1.6
Etidocaine	3.4

Adapted, with permission, from Durrani Z, Winnie AP: Brainstem toxicity with reversible locked-in syndrome after intrascalene brachial plexus block. Anesth Analg 1991;72:249–252.

There are several mechanisms for local anesthetic–induced cardiac toxicity: (a) inhibition of sodium, potassium, and calcium channels; (b) central nervous system effects; and (c) direct inhibition of myocardial metabolism.[16,18,54,100] Blockade of fast sodium channels depresses myocardial automaticity, slows cardiac conduction, and depresses the rate of spontaneous depolarization, thereby increasing both PR interval and QRS duration. At progressively higher plasma drug levels, hypotension, sinus arrest with junctional rhythm, and, eventually, cardiac arrest occur.[3] Asystole has been described in patients who received unintentional intravenous bolus injections of 800–1000 mg of lidocaine.[3,30] Cardiovascular toxicity is the most feared complication of bupivacaine administration and usually occurs following a sudden increase in the plasma concentration, as in unintentional intravascular injection. Cardiovascular toxicity is rare in other circumstances, because a large dose of the drug is necessary to produce this effect, and also because CNS toxicity precedes cardiovascular events, thus providing a warning. Cardiac toxicity is not usually observed in humans with the use of lidocaine until the plasma lidocaine level greatly exceeds 10 μg/mL, unless the patient is also receiving medications that depress sinus and AV nodal conduction (calcium channel or β-adrenergic antagonists).

Bupivacaine is significantly more cardiotoxic than most other local anesthetics in common clinical use, such as lidocaine, ropivacaine, and even levobupivacaine. Animal studies have compared the dosage or plasma levels of local anesthetics required to produce irreversible circulatory collapse to those necessary to produce seizures.[67,68] This cardiovascular collapse/central nervous system toxicity ratio (CC/CNS) is approximately 7 for lidocaine; therefore, CNS toxicity should become evident well before potentially cardiotoxic levels are reached. In contrast, the CC/CNS ratio for bupivacaine is 3.7. The electrophysiologic toxicity of bupivacaine is approximately 16 times greater than that of lidocaine.[81]

The earliest signs of cardiac toxicity are ECG changes. The slowing of the action potential in the cardiac conduction system prolongs the PR, QRS, and QT intervals.

Subsequent cardiac events induced by bupivacaine include cardiovascular collapse, bradycardia, atrioventricular and intraventricular blocks, and ventricular dysrhythmias that are often refractory to treatment and may be fatal. Bupivacaine may cause significant reductions in cardiac output even while blood pressure is maintained, as the drug can produce a direct vasoconstrictive effect on the peripheral vasculature, which is dependent upon the plasma concentration of the drug.[15]

Acid-base and electrolyte status influence the cardiac toxicity of a given agent, because all of the depressant properties are potentiated by acidosis, hypoxia, or hypercarbia.[9] Table 55–3 summarizes the differential diagnosis of local anesthetic reactions.

LABORATORY

An ECG should be obtained to detect dysrhythmias and conduction disturbances. Serum electrolytes, blood urea nitrogen (BUN), and creatinine should be obtained to help assess the cause of cardiac dysrhythmias. Methemoglobin level should be obtained in symptomatic patients with cyanosis or when a SaO_2 of approximately 85% is obtained by pulse oximeter. Rapid sensitive assays are available for measuring concentrations of lidocaine and its monoethylglycylxylidide (MEGX) metabolite. When properly interpreted, the results of these assays can be used to decrease lidocaine's toxicity as well as to identify lidocaine toxicity in the nontherapeutic setting. Assays for determination of plasma levels of the other agents are not routinely available. Treatment should never be delayed waiting for the results of drug levels.

TREATMENT

Treatment of Local Anesthetic CNS Toxicity

At the first sign of possible CNS toxicity, administration of the agent must be discontinued. One hundred percent oxygen should be supplied immediately and ventilation should be supported if necessary. Minor symptoms usually do not require treatment provided that adequate respiratory and cardiovascular function is maintained. The patient must be followed closely so that progression to more severe effects can be detected quickly.

Although most seizures caused by local anesthetics are self-limited, they should be treated quickly because the hypoxia and respiratory and metabolic acidosis produced by prolonged convulsions may increase both CNS and cardiovascular toxicity.[66,68] Barbiturates and benzodiazepines have been used for treatment of local anesthetic–induced seizures. An induction dose of thiopental can rapidly terminate a seizure and acts more quickly than benzodiazepines, but any of these agents can exacerbate circulatory and respiratory depression.[23,62] Propofol 1 mg/kg IV was as effective as thiopental 2 mg/kg IV in stopping bupivacaine-induced seizures in rats and has been used successfully in a patient with uncontrolled muscle twitching secondary to local anesthetic toxicity.[7,40] Propofol, however, can cause significant bradydysrhythmias and even asystole, especially when it is used together with other drugs that cause bradycardia. It is not known whether propofol interacts with local anesthetics to enhance their bradydysrhythmic effects,

and it is not possible to generally recommend propofol over barbiturates and benzodiazepines for treatment of local anesthetic CNS toxicity. Intubation is not mandatory and the decision whether to intubate or not must be individualized.

Neuromuscular blocking agents have been proposed as adjunctive treatment for local anesthetic–induced seizures. They block muscular activity and thereby decrease oxygen demand from the skeletal muscles and lactic acid production. Neuromuscular blocking agents, however, should never be used to treat seizures per se because they have no effect on seizure activity in the CNS and can make clinical diagnosis of ongoing seizures problematic by abolishing muscle contractions. To avoid this potentially lethal complication, chemical paralysis should only be used to facilitate endotracheal intubation if needed. It is desirable that short-acting agents be used because their use allows subsequent repeated neurologic assessments. Succinylcholine may not be the ideal drug because of its significant side effects, including hyperkalemia and dysrhythmias. Newer short-acting agents with less potential for cardiac side effects should be considered.

The cardiovascular system must be monitored closely because when severe systemic toxicity occurs, cardiovascular depression may go unnoticed while the seizures are being treated. Because local anesthetic–induced myocardial depression can occur even with preserved blood pressure, it is important to be aware of early signs of cardiac toxicity, including ECG changes.

If toxicity has resulted from an oral ingestion, activated charcoal and orogastric lavage are unproved therapeutic considerations. Induction of emesis is contraindicated even after oral administration because of the risk of seizures and aspiration. Contaminated mucous membranes should be washed off. Hemodialysis is probably not useful; hemoperfusion might be useful for severe lidocaine toxicity but would be difficult to perform if significant cardiovascular depression is present.

Treatment of Local Anesthetic Cardiac Toxicity

Treatment of cardiovascular complications of local anesthetics is complicated by the fact that the effects of local anesthetics on the heart are so complex. Initial therapy should focus on correcting the physiologic derangements that may potentiate the cardiac toxicity of local anesthetics, including hypoxemia, acidosis, and hyperkalemia.[9,84] Prompt support of ventilation and circulation will limit hypoxia and acidosis. Early recognition of potential cardiac toxicity is critical if a good outcome is to be achieved, because cardiac toxicity that goes unrecognized for any interval is more difficult to resuscitate.[5] If a potentially massive intravascular local anesthetic injection is suspected, maximizing oxygenation of the patient before cardiovascular collapse occurs is critical.

Hypotension results from both peripheral vasodilation and myocardial depression and should be treated with α- and β-adrenergic agonists. Atropine should be used to treat bradycardia. The effectiveness of epinephrine in reversing local anesthetic–induced cardiac depression has been inconsistent in various animal models. The dysrhythmic effects of epinephrine are of particular concern. Amrinone, a phosphodiesterase III inhibitor, was evaluated for the treatment of bupivacaine-induced cardiac toxicity.[33,50] Anesthetized pigs with cardiovascular collapse induced by bupivacaine infusion survived when treated with amrinone; all of the control animals died of irreversible cardiac arrest.[50] Amrinone may also be a good choice for reversal of bupivacaine-induced cardiac depression during inhalation anesthesia.[86]

TABLE 55–3.   Types of Local Anesthetic Reactions

Etiology	Major Clinical Features
Local anesthetic toxicity	
Intravascular injection	Immediate seizure and/or cardiac toxicity
Reaction to catecholamine	Tachycardia, hypertension, headache
Vasovagal reaction	Rapid onset and recovery, bradycardia, hypotension, pallor
Allergic reaction	Anaphylaxis
High spinal or epidural block	Bradycardia, hypotension, respiratory distress, respiratory arrest

Bupivacaine-induced dysrhythmias are often refractory to cardioversion, defibrillation, and pharmacologic treatment. Lidocaine, phenytoin, magnesium, bretylium, amiodarone, calcium channel blockers, and combined therapy with clonidine and dobutamine have all been used in animal models, with variable results.[26,57,59] Therapy for bupivacaine toxicity should be directed toward dissociating bupivacaine from the myocardial sodium channel and thereby reversing the effects of the drug on cardiac conduction. Lidocaine competes with bupivacaine for cardiac sodium channels, and at high doses may displace it. Anecdotal reports suggest that lidocaine has occasionally helped in this application.[22] However, concern persists about additive CNS effects when lidocaine is used to treat bupivacaine cardiac toxicity.

Bretylium has been used successfully in some, but not all, animal models of bupivacaine cardiac toxicity.[45,46] The use of bretylium has several theoretical advantages for the treatment of this complication: (a) it does not slow conduction; (b) it does not exhibit CNS toxicity, unlike lidocaine, whose CNS effects are additive to those of bupivacaine; and (c) it produces norepinephrine release, which can help overcome some of the depressant effects of bupivacaine on cardiac output, stroke volume, and heart rate.[45] However, its α-blocking effects may worsen hypotension. The benefits of this drug need to be established in humans. This is unlikely to occur as bretylium is no longer available for clinical use.

Successful treatment of bupivacaine-induced cardiac dysrhythmias with phenytoin has been described in two full-term newborns after other therapies, including bretylium, had failed.[59] Phenytoin has direct cardiac effects similar to lidocaine, but it also blocks cardiac calcium channels and modulates the autonomic control centers in the brain.

With toxicity from the longer-acting, highly lipid-soluble, protein-bound amide local anesthetics (bupivacaine and etidocaine), if the patient does not respond promptly to therapy, cardiopulmonary resuscitation can be expected to be difficult and prolonged (1–2 hours) before the depression of the cardiac conduction system spontaneously reverses as a result of redistribution and metabolism of these drugs.[2,77] Vital organ perfusion is seriously compromised during cardiopulmonary resuscitation despite optimal chest compression. The significance of this problem increases with the duration of resuscitation; therefore, rapid initiation of cardiopulmonary bypass should be considered, if practical; its use has resulted in a successful outcome in some cases of lidocaine and bupivacaine overdose.[32,52] Cardiopulmonary bypass provides circulatory support that is far superior to closed chest cardiac massage. The improved perfusion prevents tissue hypoxia and the development of metabolic acidosis and, in turn, decreases the binding of local anesthetics to myocardial sodium channel receptors. Hepatic blood flow is also better maintained, enhancing local anesthetic metabolism, and increased myocardial blood flow helps redistribute local anesthetics out of the myocardium.[52]

Cardiac pacing was used successfully for treatment of cardiac arrest following unintentional administration of a 2-g bolus of lidocaine into a cardiopulmonary bypass circuit as the patient was being removed from bypass.[72] Pharmacologic therapy was unsuccessful and bypass had to be resumed. Forty-five minutes after the injection, atrioventricular pacing restored perfusion and permitted discontinuation of bypass.

The use of sodium bicarbonate early in resuscitation to prevent acidosis-mediated potentiation of cardiac toxicity may have had a beneficial effect in some cases.[22] High-dose sodium administration (1.8% saline) has also been suggested as a possibly useful therapeutic intervention.

SUMMARY

Local anesthetics are frequently used drugs that provide surgical analgesia and acute and chronic pain relief. Lidocaine is also frequently used to treat ventricular dysrhythmias. The local anesthetics analgesic effect is primarily caused by inhibition of neural conductance secondary to blockade of sodium channels. Systemic toxicity, which primarily effects the heart and brain, is also related to sodium channel blockade. Severe systemic toxicity usually occurs secondary to inadvertent intravascular injection. In most cases in which systemic toxicity occurs, CNS manifestations precede cardiovascular events. If cardiovascular collapse and cardiac arrest occur resuscitation may be difficult and prolonged. Cardiopulmonary bypass may be useful as it provides cardiovascular support and improves hepatic blood flow, thereby increasing local anesthetic metabolism.

REFERENCES

1. Agarwal R, Gutlove D, Lockhart C: Seizures occurring in pediatric patients receiving continuous infusion of bupivacaine. Anesth Analg 1992;75:284–286.
2. Albright G: Cardiac arrest following regional anesthesia with etidocaine or bupivacaine. Anesthesiology 1979;51:285–287.
3. Babui E, Garcia-Rubi D, Estanol B: Inadvertent massive lidocaine overdose causing temporary complete heart block in myocardial infarction. Am Heart J 1981;102:801–803.
4. Bardsley H, Gristwood R, Baker H, et al: A comparison of the cardiovascular effects of levobupivacaine and rac-bupivacaine following intravenous administration to healthy volunteers. Br J Clin Pharmacol 1998;46:245–249.
5. Batra MS, Bridenbaugh LD, Caldwell RD, Hecker BR: Bupivacaine cardiotoxicity in a pregnant patient with mitral valve prolapse: An example of an improperly administered epidural block. Anesthesiology 1984;60:170–171.
6. Benoit P, Belt WD: Some effects of local anesthetic agents on skeletal muscle. Exp Neurol 1972;34:264–278.
7. Bishop D, Johnstone R: Lidocaine toxicity treated with low-dose propofol. Anesthesiology 1993;78:788–789.
8. Bonadio W: TAC: A review. Pediatr Emerg Care 1989;5:128–130.
9. Bosnjak Z, Stowe D, Kampine J: Comparison of lidocaine and bupivacaine depression of sinoatrial node activity during hypoxia and acidosis in adult and neonatal guinea pigs. Anesth Analg 1986; 65:911–917.
10. Bruguerolle B, Emperaire N: Local anesthetic-induced toxicity may be modified by low-dose flumazenil. Life Sci 1992;50:185–187.
11. Buckley MM, Benfield P. Eutectic lidocaine/prilocaine cream: A review of the topical anaesthetic/analgesic efficacy of a eutectic mixture of local anaesthetics (EMLA). Drugs 1993;46:126–151.
12. Burk RW, Guzman-Stein G, Vasconez LO: Tumescent anesthesia with a lidocaine dose of 55 mg/kg is safe for liposuction. Dermatol Surg 1996;22:921–927.
13. Burney R, DiFazio C, Foster J: Effects of pH on protein binding of lidocaine. Anesth Analg 1978;57:478–480.
14. Butterworth JF, Strichartz G: Molecular mechanisms of local anesthesia: A review. Anesthesiology 1990;72:711–734.
15. Chang KS, Morrow DR, Kuzume K, et al: Bupivacaine inhibits baroreflex control of heart rate in conscious rats. Anesthesiology 2000;92:197–207.
16. Chazotte B, Vanderkooi G: Multiple sites of inhibition of mitochondrial electron transport by local anesthetics. Biochim Biophys Acta 1981;63:153–161.

17. Choi RH, Birknes JK, Popitz-Bergez FA, et al: Safety of tumescent liposuction in 15,336 patients: National survey results. Dermatol Surg 1995;21:459–462.

18. Clarkson C, Hondeghem LM: Mechanism for bupivacaine depression of cardiac conduction: Fast block of sodium channels during the action potential with slow recovery from block during diastole. Anesthesiology 1985;62:396–405.

19. Covino BG: New developments in the field of local anesthetics and the scientific basis for their clinical use. Acta Anaesth Scand 1982; 26:242–249.

20. Covino BG: Pharmacology of local anesthetic agents. Br J Anaesth 1986;58:701–716.

21. Dailey RH: Fatality secondary to misuse of TAC solution. Ann Emerg Med 1988;17:159–160.

22. Davis N, de Jong R: Successful resuscitation following massive bupivacaine overdose. Anesth Analg 1982;61:62–64.

23. de Jong R, Heavner J: Local anesthetic seizure prevention: Diazepam versus pentobarbital. Anesthesiology 1972;36:449–457.

24. de Jong R, Ronfeld R, DeRosa R: Cardiovascular effects of convulsant and supraconvulsant doses of amide local anesthetics. Anesth Analg 1982;61:3–9.

25. de Jong R, Wagman I, Prince D: Effect of carbon dioxide on the cortical seizure threshold to lidocaine. Exp Neurol 1967;17:221–232.

26. de la Coussaye J, Bassoul B, Brugada J, et al: Reversal of electrophysiologic and hemodynamic effects induced by high-dose of bupivacaine by the combination of clonidine and dobutamine in anesthetized dogs. Anesth Analg 1992;74:703–711.

27. Dyhre H, Lang M, Wallin R, el al: The duration of action of bupivacaine, levobupivacaine, ropivacaine, and pethidine in peripheral nerve block in the rat. Acta Anaesthesiol Scand 1997;41:1345–1352.

28. Englesson S: The influence of acid-base changes on central nervous system toxicity of local anesthetic agents. I. An experimental study in cats. Acta Anaesthesiol Scand 1974;18:79–87.

29. Englesson S: The influence of acid-base changes on central nervous system toxicity of local anesthetic agents: II. Acta Anaesthesiol Scand 1974;18:88–103.

30. Finkelstein F, Kreeft J: Massive lidocaine poisoning. N Engl J Med 1979;301:50.

31. Foldes FF, Davidson GM, Duncalf D, Kuwabara S: The intravenous toxicity of local anesthetic agents in man. Clin Pharm Ther 1965; 6:328–335.

32. Freedman M, Gal J, Freed C: Extracorporeal pump assistance—Novel treatment for acute lidocaine poisoning. Eur J Clin Pharmacol 1982; 22:129–135.

33. Fujita Y: Amrinone reverses bupivacaine-induced regional myocardial dysfunction. Acta Anaesthesiol Scand 1996;40:47–52.

34. Giovannitti JA, Bennett CR: Assessment of allergy to local anesthetics. J Am Dent Assoc 1979;98:701–706.

35. Graf BM, Martin E, Bosnjak ZJ, et al: Stereospecific effect of bupivacaine isomers on atrioventricular conduction in the isolated perfused guinea pig heart. Anesthesiology 1997;86:410–419.

36. Hahn I, Hoffman RS, Nelson LS: EMLA-induced methemoglobinemia (metHb) and lidocaine toxicity. J Toxicol Clin Toxicol 1999; 37:A621.

37. Halsted WS: Practical comments on the use and abuse of cocaine; suggested by its invariably successful employment in more than a thousand minor surgical operations. N Y Med J 1885;42:294.

38. Harris W, Slater E, Bell H: Regional anesthesia by the intravenous route. JAMA 1965;194:1273–1276.

39. Heavner JE: Cardiac dysrhythmias induced by infusion of local anesthetics into the lateral ventricle of cats. Anesth Analg 1986; 65:133–138.

40. Heavner J, Arthur J, Zou J, et al: Comparison of propofol with thiopentone for treatment of bupivacaine-induced seizures in rats. Br J Anaesth 1993;71:715–719.

41. Hjelm M, Holmdahl M: Biochemical effects of aromatic amines II. Cyanosis methemoglobinemia and Heinz-body formation induced by a local anaesthetic agent (prilocaine). Acta Anaesthesiol Scand 1965;2:99–120.

42. Hollmann MW, Durieux ME: Local anesthetics and the inflammatory response: A new therapeutic indication? Anesthesiology 2000; 93:858–875.

43. Hollmann MW, Fisher LG, Byforf AM, et al: Local anesthetic inhibition of m1 muscarinic acetylcholine signaling. Anesthesiology 2000;93:497–509.

44. Jorfeldt L, Lewis DH, Lofstrom JB, Post C: Lung uptake of lidocaine in man as influenced by anaesthesia, mepivacaine infusion or lung insufficiency. Acta Anaesth Scand 1983;27:5–9.

45. Kasten G, Martin S: Bupivacaine cardiovascular toxicity: Comparison of treatment with bretylium and lidocaine. Anesth Analg 1985; 64:911–916.

46. Kasten G, Martin S: Successful cardiovascular resuscitation after massive intravenous bupivacaine overdosage in anesthetized dogs. Anesth Analg 1985;64:491–497.

47. Kozody R, Ready L, Barsa J, Murphy T: Dose requirements of local anesthetic to produce grand mal seizure during stellate ganglion block. Can Anaesth Soc J 1982;29:489–491.

48. Lambert L, Lambert D, Strichartz G: Irreversible conduction block in isolated nerve by high concentrations of local anesthetics. Anesthesiology 1994;80:1082–1093.

49. Lee-Son S, Wang GK, Concus A, et al: Stereoselective inhibition of neuronal sodium channels by local anesthetics: Evidence for two sites of action? Anesthesiology 1992;77:324–335.

50. Lindgren L, Randell T, Suzuki N, et al: The effect of amrinone on recovery from severe bupivacaine intoxication in pigs. Anesthesiology 1992;77:309–315.

51. Lofstrom JB: Physiologic disposition of local anesthetics. Reg Anesth 1982;7:33–38.

52. Long W, Rosenblum S, Grady I: Successful resuscitation of bupivacaine-induced cardiac arrest using cardiopulmonary bypass. Anesth Analg 1989;69:403–406.

53. Lund P, Cwik J: Propitocaine (Eitanest) and methemoglobinemia. Anesthesiology 1965;26:569–571.

54. Lynch C III. Depression of myocardial contractility in vitro by bupivacaine, etidocaine, and lidocaine. Anesth Analg 1986;65: 551–559.

55. Mallampati SR, Liu PL, Knapp RM: Convulsions and ventricular tachycardia from bupivacaine with epinephrine: Successful resuscitation. Anesth Analg 1984;63:856–859.

56. Marsch SCU, Schaefer HG, Castelli I: Unusual psychological manifestation of systemic local anesthetic toxicity. Anesthesiology 1998; 88:531–533.

57. Matsuda F, Kinney W, Wright W, Kambam J: Nicardipine reduces the cardio-respiratory toxicity of intravenously administered bupivacaine in rats. Can J Anaesth 1990;37:920–923.

58. Mattison JB: Cocaine poisoning. Med Surg Rep 1891;60:645–650.

59. Maxwell L, Martin L, Yaster M: Bupivacaine-induced cardiac toxicity in neonates: Successful treatment with intravenous phenytoin. Anesthesiology 1994;80:682–686.

60. Mazoit JX, Decaux A, Bouaziz H, et al: Comparative ventricular electrophysiologic effect of racemic bupivacaine, levobupivacaine, and ropivacaine on the isolated rabbit heart. Anesthesiology 2000; 92:784–792.

61. McCloskey J, Haun S, Deshpande J: Bupivacaine toxicity secondary to continuous caudal epidural infusion in children. Anesth Analg 1992;75:287–290.

62. Moore D, Balfour R, Fitzgibbons D: Convulsive arterial plasma levels of bupivacaine and the response to diazepam therapy. Anesthesiology 1979;50:454–456.

63. Moore DC, Batra M: The components of an effective test dose prior to epidural block. Anesthesiology 1981;55:693–696.

64. Moore DC, Bridenbaugh LD, Thompson GE, et al: Factors determining dosages of amide-type local anesthetic drugs. Anesthesiology 1977;47:263–268.

65. Moore DC, Bridenbaugh LD, Thompson GE, et al: Bupivacaine: A review of 11,080 cases. Anesth Analg 1978;57:42–53.

66. Morishima H, Corvino B: Toxicity and distribution of lidocaine in nonasphyxiated and asphyxiated baboon fetuses. Anesthesiology 1981;54:182–186.

67. Morishima H, Pederson H, Finster M, et al: Bupivacaine toxicity in pregnant and nonpregnant ewes. Anesthesiology 1985;63:134–139.

68. Morishima H, Pederson H, Finster M, et al: Toxicity of lidocaine in adult, newborn, and fetal sheep. Anesthesiology 1981;55:57–61.

69. Myers RR, Kalichman MW, Reisner LS, et al: Neurotoxicity of local anesthetics: Altered perineural permeability, edema, and nerve fiber injury. Anesthesiology 1986;64:29–35.

70. Nation R, Triggs E, Selig M: Lignocaine kinetics in cardiac and aged subjects. Br J Clin Pharmacol 1977;4:439–445.

71. Nau C, Vogel W, Hempelmann G, et al: Stereoselectivity of bupivacaine in local anesthetic-sensitive ion channels of peripheral nerve. Anesthesiology 1999;91:786–795.

72. Noble J, Kennedy D, Latimer R, et al: Massive lignocaine overdose during cardiopulmonary bypass: Successful treatment with cardiac pacing. Br J Anaesth 1984;56:1439–1441.

73. Nystrom EUM, Heavner JE, Buffington CW: Blood pressure is maintained despite profound myocardial depression during acute bupivacaine overdose in pigs. Anesth Analg 1999;88:1143–1148.

74. Peterson RC: History of cocaine. NIDA Res Monogr 1977;13:17–34.

75. Pitkanen M, Feldman HS, Arthur GR, et al: Chronotropic and inotropic effects of ropivacaine, bupivacaine, and lidocaine in the spontaneously beating and electrically paced isolated perfused rabbit heart. Reg Anesth Pain Med 1992;17:183–192.

76. Polley LS, Columb MO, Naughton NN, et al: Relative analgesic potencies of ropivacaine and bupivacaine for epidural analgesia in labor: Implications for therapeutic indexes. Anesthesiology 1999;90:944–950.

77. Prentiss J: Cardiac arrest following caudal anesthesia. Anesthesiology 1979;50:51–53.

78. Rao RB, Ely SF, Hoffman RS: Deaths related to liposuction. N Engl J Med 1999;340:1471–1475.

79. Reisner LS, Hochman BN, Plumer MH: Persistent neurologic deficit and adhesive arachnoiditis following intrathecal 2-chloroprocaine injection. Anesth Analg 1980;59:452–454.

80. Reistad F, Stromskag K: Intrapleural catheter in the management of postoperative pain: A preliminary report. Reg Anesth 1986;11:89–91.

81. Reiz S, Nath S: Cardiotoxicity of local anesthetic agents. Br J Anaesth 1986;58:736–746.

82. Reynolds F: Adverse effects of local anaesthetics. Br J Anaesth 1987;59:78–95.

83. Rigler M, Drasner K, Krejcie T, et al: Cauda equina syndrome after continuous spinal anesthesia. Anesth Analg 1991;72:275–281.

84. Rosen M, Thigpen J, Schnider S, et al: Bupivacaine-induced cardiotoxicity in hypoxic and acidotic sheep. Anesth Analg 1985;64:1089–1096.

85. Rosenberg PH, Kalso EA, Tuominen MK, Linden HB: Acute bupivacaine toxicity as a result of venous leakage under the tourniquet cuff during a Bier block. Anesthesiology 1983;58:95–98.

86. Saitoh K, Hirabayashi Y, Shimizu R, Fukuda H: Amrinone is superior to epinephrine in reversing bupivacaine-induced cardiovascular depression in sevoflurane-anesthetized cats. Anesthesiology 1995;83:127–133.

87. Samdal F, Amland PF, Bugge JF: Plasma lidocaine levels during suction-assisted lipectomy using large doses of dilute lidocaine with epinephrine. Plastic Reconstr Surg 1994;93:1217–1223.

88. Scott DB: Evaluation of the toxicity of local anaesthetic agents in man. Br J Anaesth 1975;47:56–61.

89. Scott DB: Toxicity caused by local anaesthetic drugs. Br J Anaesth 1981;53:553–554.

90. Scott DB: "Maximal recommended doses" of local anaesthetic drugs. Br J Anaesth 1989;63:373–374.

91. Strichartz GR, Berde CB: Local anesthetics. In: Miller RD, ed: Anesthesia, 4th ed. New York, Churchill Livingstone, 1994, pp. 489–521.

92. Sztark F, Malgat M, Dabadie P, et al: Comparison of the effects of bupivacaine and ropivacaine on heart cell mitochondrial bioenergetics. Anesthesiology 1998;88:1340–1349.

93. Taddio A, Stevens B, Craig K, et al: Efficacy and safety of lidocaine-prilocaine cream for pain during circumcision. N Engl J Med 1997;336:1197–1201.

94. Tanaka K, Yamasaki M: Blocking of cortical inhibitory synapses by intravenous lidocaine. Nature 1966;209:207–208.

95. Tipton GA, DeWitt GW, Eisenstein SJ: Topical TAC (tetracaine, adrenaline, cocaine) solution for local anesthesia in children: Prescribing inconsistency and acute toxicity. South Med J 1989;82:1344–1346.

96. Verrill PJ: Adverse reactions to local anesthetics and vasoconstrictor drugs. Practitioner 1975;214:380–387.

97. Wagman IH, de Jong RH, Prince DA: Effects of lidocaine on the central nervous system. Anesthesiology 1967;28:155–172.

98. Wang BC, Hillman DE, Spielholz NI, et al: Chronic neurologic deficits and Nesacaine: An effect of the anesthetic 2-chloroprocaine or the antioxidant sodium bisulfite? Anesth Analg 1984;63:445–447.

99. Weinberg GL, Laurito C, Geldner P, et al: Malignant ventricular dysrhythmias in a patient with isovaleric acidemia receiving general and local anesthesia for suction lipectomy. J Clin Anesth 1997;9:668–670.

100. Weinberg GL, Palmer JW, VadeBoncourer TR, et al: Bupivacaine inhibits exchange in cardiac mitochondria. Anesthesiology 2000;92:523–528.

CHAPTER 56 PHARMACEUTICAL ADDITIVES

Sean P. Nordt / Lisa E. Vivero

A 32-year-old man presented to the Emergency Department (ED) after being found at a motel. When paramedics arrived on the scene, the patient was confused and inarticulate. The patient's tongue was bleeding, and he had urinary incontinence, suggestive of a seizure. In the ED the patient had a blood pressure of 152/80 mm Hg, a pulse of 101 beats/min, respirations of 20 breaths/min, and a temperature of 97.4°F (36.3°C). Physical examination revealed abrasions on the left side of the face; his pupils were 6 mm, equal and reactive to light; his lungs were clear to auscultation; and his abdomen was soft and nontender. A 12-lead electrocardiogram showed a sinus tachycardia, a rate of 102 beats/min, a PR interval of 200 msec, a QRS interval of 108 msec, and a corrected QT interval of 450 msec. An old ED chart revealed that the patient had suffered a gunshot wound to the head and subsequently had developed a seizure disorder.

A loading dose of 1 g of fosphenytoin was given intravenously over 5 minutes. Immediately following the fosphenytoin, the patient became hypotensive with a blood pressure of 85/50 mm Hg. His heart rate decreased to 52 beats/min, and his QRS interval widened to 140 msec. Atropine was given, resulting in an increase in heart rate to 82 beats/min. Wide open intravenous 0.9% sodium chloride was administered, which restored his blood pressure. Several minutes later the patient's QRS narrowed to 100 msec without other intervention. Subsequently, it was realized that the nurse had inadvertently drawn up phenytoin instead of fosphenytoin. The patient had an adverse reaction to the rapid infusion of phenytoin, which contains 400 mg/mL of propylene glycol.

During the last century there were several outbreaks of toxicity associated with pharmaceutical additives (Chap. 1). The Massengill sulfanilamide disaster in 1937 is the most notorious of these epidemics. Diethylene glycol, an excellent solvent that is also nephrotoxic, was substituted for the additives propylene glycol and glycerin due to its lower cost in the liquid formulation of a new sulfanilamide antibiotic.[21,45,52] As a result, 105 people died from acute renal failure.[21] More recently, outbreaks of acute renal failure occurred when diethylene glycol was used to solubilize acetaminophen in South Africa, Bangladesh, Nigeria, and Haiti.[14,41,54,83] One study identified diethylene glycol as the sole diluent in 19 of 69 foreign acetaminophen elixirs tested.[54]

In December 1983, E-Ferol, a new parenteral vitamin E formulation, was put on the market. It contained 25 U/mL of α-tocopherol acetate, 9% polysorbate 80, 1% polysorbate 20, and water for injection. At the time, no premarketing testing was required for new formulations of an already approved agent. Several months after its release a fatal syndrome in low-birth-weight infants, characterized by thrombocytopenia, renal dysfunction, cholestasis, hepatomegaly, and ascites, was described.[1,72] Thirty-eight deaths and 43 cases of severe symptoms were attributed to E-Ferol. Vitamin E was thought to be the cause and E-Ferol was recalled from the market 4 months after its release. It is now believed that the polysorbate emulsifiers were responsible.

Most recently there was concern over potential mercury toxicity from the preservative thimerosal, a mercury derivative that has been in use for 70 years. The FDA recently determined that some infants receiving routine vaccinations may be exposed to mercury levels exceeding recommended guidelines. Although there are a few reports of toxicity from large oral and injectable thimerosal dosages, no evidence has yet shown toxicity to result from routine vaccination. Potential concerns of toxicity have spurred ongoing efforts to eliminate thimerosal from vaccines wherever possible.

Although these additive-related occurrences are rare relative to the frequency of pharmaceutical additive use, they illustrate the potential of pharmaceutical additive toxicity.

Pharmaceutical agents are labeled specifically to focus attention on the active ingredient(s) of a product, thus giving the impression that additive ingredients are not important. Additives, or excipients as they are more properly termed, are necessary to act as vehicles, to add color, to improve taste, to provide consistency, to enhance stability and solubility, and to impart antibacterial and antifungal properties to medicinal formulations. Although these additives are considered to be inactive or inert ingredients, this is not always the case. While it is true that most cases of excipient toxicity involve exposure to large quantities, or prolonged or improper use, these adverse events are nonetheless related to excipient pharmacologic or toxicologic properties.

Prior to selecting specific additives and the quantity of each necessary for a drug formulation, the drug manufacturer must consider several factors, including the active ingredient's physical form, its solubility and stability, the desired final dosage form and route of administration, and compatibility with the dispensing container materials. The same active ingredient may require different excipients to impart different pharmacokinetic characteristics to different dosage forms, such as in long-acting and immediate-release formulations. Similarly, multiple-dose injection vials containing the same active ingredients as single-dose vials specifically require the addition of a bacteriostatic agent not necessary for single-dose vials.

Unlike active ingredients, there is no specific FDA approval system for pharmaceutical excipients. As such, the FDA determines the amount and type of data necessary to support the use of a specific excipient on a case-by-case basis. Under current practice, only excipients that were previously permitted for use in foods or pharmaceuticals are defined as generally recognized as safe (GRAS), or "GRAS listed." All components of a pharmaceutical product, including excipients, must be produced in accordance with current good manufacturing practice standards to assure purity. Recently, the Safety Committee of the International Pharmaceutical Excipients Council developed guidelines for the toxicologic testing of new excipients.[106]

Because of patent protection laws, it was not until very recently that manufacturers were required to provide a list of inactive ingredients contained in all pharmaceutical products. While it is becoming easier to identify pharmaceutical additives in products, information on their effects and the mechanisms by which they cause adverse responses are often unknown or difficult to obtain. This chapter summarizes the available literature on commonly used additives associated with direct toxicities. Data on pharmacokinetics and mechanism of toxicity are presented where data are available. Many additives are associated with hypersensitivity reactions, including anaphylaxis. Immunologic toxicities are not discussed; however, excipients should always be considered as possible causative agents in patients developing hypersensitivity reactions (Table 56–1).

BENZALKONIUM CHLORIDE

Benzalkonium chloride (BAK) or alkyldimethyl (phenylmethyl) ammonium chloride is a quaternary ammonium cationic surfactant composed of a mixture of alkyl benzyl dimethyl ammonium chlorides. Although it is the most widely used ophthalmic preservative in the United States, it is also considered the most cytotoxic[61,65] (Table 56–2). Benzalkonium chloride possesses activity against gram-positive and gram-negative bacteria, as well as against some

TABLE 56–1. Toxicity by Organ System of Common Pharmaceutical Excepients

Cardiovascular	Neurologic
Chlorobutanol	Benzyl alcohol
Propylene glycol	Chlorbutanol
Fluid and Electrolyte	Polyethylene glycol
Phenol	Propylene glycol
Polyethylene glycol	Thimerosal
Propylene glycol	Ophthalmic
Sorbitol	Benzalkonium chloride
Gastrointestinal	Chlorobutanol
Sorbitol	Renal
	Diethylene glycol
	Polyethylene glycol

TABLE 56–2. Benzalkonium Chloride Concentration in Common Ophthalmic Medications

Medication	%
Artificial tears (various)	0.005–0.01
Acular (ketorolac)	0.01
Betagan (levobunolol)	0.004
Betoptic (betaxolol)	0.01
Ciloxan (ciprofloxacin)	0.006
Cyclogyl (cyclopentolate)	0.01
Decadron (dexamethasone)	0.02
Garamycin (gentamicin)	0.01
Glaucon (epinephrine)	0.01
Isopto Carpine (pilocarpine)	0.01
Mydriacil (tropicamide)	0.01
Neosynephrine (phenylephrine)	0.01
Ocuflox (ofloxacin)	0.005
Ocupres (cartelol)	0.005
Polytrim (polymyxin B sulfate/trimethoprim)	0.004
Timoptic (timolol)	0.01
Tobrex (tobramycin)	0.01
Visine (tetrahydrozoline)	0.01

viruses, fungi, and protozoa. Because of its rapid onset of action, good tissue penetration, and long duration of action, BAK is preferred over other preservatives. The concentration of BAK in ophthalmic medications usually ranges from 0.004–0.01%.[65] Ingestion of strong BAK solutions (greater than 0.1%) may be caustic (Chap. 84).

Ophthalmic Toxicity

In an in vitro experiment, corneal epithelial cells harvested from human cadavers within 12 hours of death were exposed to a medium containing 0.01% BAK. Benzalkonium chloride's surfactant properties result in the dissolution of the intercellular matrix and loss of superficial layers of epithelial tissue. Immediately following exposure to the medium, mitotic activity ceased. Within 2 hours, degenerative changes to corneal epithelium were noted. No recovery of cytokinesis or mitosis occurred 24 hours after exposure to BAK.[104] Patients with a compromised corneal epithelium may be at increased risk to the adverse corneal effects of BAK.[104]

Two case reports demonstrate the potential toxicity of BAK and the difficulty in recognition of this potential problem. A 36-year-old woman complained of decreased vision when she inadvertently switched from Lensrins, a contact lens cleaning solution, to Dacriose, an isotonic boric acid solution preserved with BAK. After 3 days, she had inflammation, pain, and decreased visual acuity. Examination of the cornea revealed many superficial punctate erosions of the epithelium. An in vitro experiment identified significant binding of BAK to soft contact lenses.[44]

A 56-year-old man diagnosed with keratoconjunctivitis sicca was treated with topical antibiotics and artificial tears containing BAK. Following 1 year of continual use, the patient developed intractable pain, photophobia, and extensive breakdown of the corneal epithelium; however, neither of the BAK-containing products was suspected. The patient continued to use the artificial tears solution for an additional 9 years despite continued pain and decreasing visual acuity. The artificial tears solution was then replaced with a preservative-free saline solution with a dramatic resolution of pain, photophobia, and corneal changes.[65]

Nasopharyngeal and Oropharyngeal Toxicity

Benzalkonium chloride may decrease the viscosity of the normal protective mucous lining of the naso- and oropharynx resulting in cytotoxicity. In an in vitro experiment, human adenoidal tissue was exposed to oxymetalozine preserved with BAK at various concentrations. A dose- and time-dependent effect was demonstrated on epithelial cell morphology, with the highest concentrations resulting in irregular and broken epithelial cells within 36 hours. The number of beating ciliary bodies also decreased as the duration and the concentrations increased.[10]

An in vivo experiment was performed in rats comparing three nasal steroid sprays, beclomethasone diprorionate and flunisolide preserved with BAK, 0.031%, and 0.022%, respectively, and budenoside aqueous nasal spray without BAK. Sodium chloride 0.9% was used as a control. Each rat received one of the three nasal steroids in their right nostril and 0.9% sodium chloride in their left nostril twice daily for 21 days. No histologic differences occurred in either the preservative-free steroid or the control tissues. Nasal tissue exposed to the steroid sprays with BAK demonstrated squamous cell metaplasia, and a decrease in the number of goblet cells, cilia, and mucus.[11] Similar results were found when concentrations of 0.01%, 0.05%, and 0.10% BAK were applied to the nasal cavities of rats every hour for 8 hours. Epithelial desquamation, inflammation, and edema occurred in the two higher-concentration groups. No lesions developed in the nasal cavities of the rats receiving 0.01% BAK.[63]

BENZYL ALCOHOL

Benzyl alcohol (benzene methanol) is a colorless, oily liquid with a faint aromatic odor that is most commonly added to pharmaceuticals as a bacteriostatic agent (Table 56–3). In 1982, a "gasping" syndrome was first described in low-birth-weight neonates in intensive care units.[17,47] Children with this syndrome displayed hypotonia, progressive metabolic acidosis, bradycardia, gasping respirations, seizures, hypotension, cardiovascular collapse, and death.[17,47] The onset of symptoms typically occurred within the first 2 weeks of life.[70] All the infants had received either bacteriostatic water or sodium chloride containing 0.9% benzyl alcohol to flush intravenous catheters or in parenteral medications reconstituted with bacteriostatic water or saline.[17,47] The syndrome only occurred in infants who had received greater than 99 mg/kg of benzyl alcohol (range, 99–234 mg/kg).[47] The World Health Organization (WHO) estimates the acceptable daily intake of benzyl alcohol to be not more than 5 mg/kg body weight.[19]

TABLE 56–3. Benzyl Alcohol Concentration in Common Medications

Medication	%	mL/Avg Dose*
Bacteriostatic water for injection	1.5	—
Bacteriostatic saline for injection	1.5	—
Bactrim, septra (trimethoprim/ sulfamethoxazole)	1.0	0.61[†]
Bumex (bumetanide)	1.0	0.03
Compazine (prochlorperazine)	0.75	0.01
Cordarone (amiodarone)	2.0	0.42[†]
Lasix (furosemide)	0.9	0.04
Librium (chlordiazepoxide)	1.5	0.03
Methotrexate	0.9	0.01
Norcuron (vecuronium)	0.9	0.01
Pronestyl (procainamide)	0.9	0.06[†]
Tracrium (atracurium)	0.9	0.03
Valium (diazepam)	1.5	0.03
Vasotec (enalapril)	0.9	0.01
Vepesid (etoposide)	3.0	0.14
Versed (midazolam)	1.0	0.01
Vistaril (hydroxyzine)	0.9	0.01

*Based on dosage for a 70-kg person.
[†]Based on a 24-hour dosage.

Pharmacokinetics

In adults, benzyl alcohol is oxidized to benzoic acid, conjugated in the liver with glycine, and excreted in the urine as hippuric acid. The immature metabolic capacities of infants diminish their ability to metabolize and excrete benzyl alcohol.[47] Preterm babies have a greater ability to metabolize benzyl alcohol to benzoic acid than do term babies, but are unable to convert benzoic acid to hippuric acid, possibly because of glycine deficiency. This results in the accumulation of benzoic acid[64] (Fig. 56–1). A fatal case of metabolic acidosis was reported in a 5-year-old girl who had received 2.4 mg/kg/h diazepam preserved with benzyl alcohol for 36 hours to control status epilepticus. Elevated benzoic acid levels were identified in serum and urine samples. The estimated daily dosage of benzyl alcohol was 180 mg/kg.[47,66]

Hematologic Toxicity

An in vitro hemolytic effect was reported in red blood cells preserved with 1.5% benzyl alcohol.[74] Although the consequence of this in vitro phenomenon has not been elucidated in humans, it may have a role in the increased frequency of intraventricular hemorrhages and mortality reported in low-birth-weight infants (less than 1000 g) who received flush solutions preserved with benzyl alcohol.[57] An increased incidence of developmental delay and cerebral palsy was also noted in the same patient population.[8]

Neurologic Toxicity

Amplitudes of action potentials were measured in rats exposed to 0.9% or 1.5% benzyl alcohol in either 0.9% sodium chloride or distilled water. Rats were exposed to benzyl alcohol either acutely (less than 1 minute) or chronically (for 7 days). Acutely, benzyl alcohol inhibited action potentials. This was attributed to the local anesthetic effects of benzyl alcohol. Nerve function was 50–90% restored after rinsing the nerves with 0.9% sodium chloride. Fur-

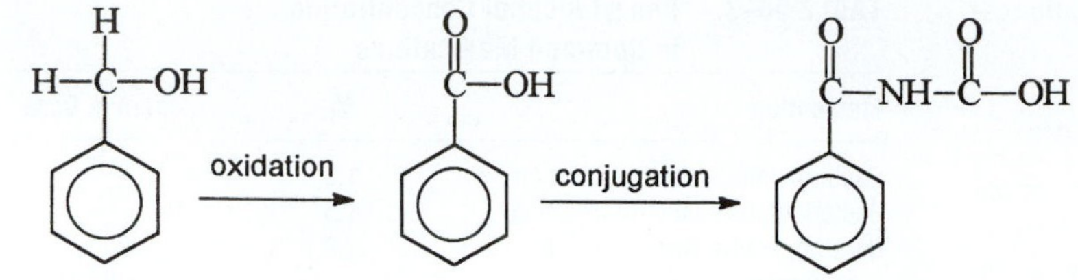

Benzyl alcohol → oxidation → Benzoic acid → conjugation → Hippuric acid

Figure 56–1. The oxidative metabolism of benzyl alcohol.

thermore, chronic exposure to benzyl alcohol 0.9% showed scattered areas of demyelinization and early remyelinization, whereas nerve roots exposed to 1.5% benzyl alcohol showed widespread areas of demyelinization and fatty degeneration of nerve fibers.[53] There are several reports of transient paraplegia following the intrathecal or epidural administration of antineoplastic or analgesic agents containing benzyl alcohol as the preservative.[6,30,53,91] While it is unknown whether these effects are transient, not necessitating therapy, resolution of symptoms occurred with cerebrospinal fluid exchange.[53]

CHLOROBUTANOL

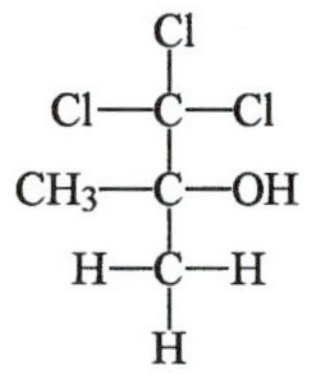

Chlorobutanol or chlorbutol (1,1,1-trichloro-2-methyl-2-propanol) is available as volatile, white crystals with an odor of camphor. Chlorobutanol has antibacterial and antifungal properties and is widely used as a preservative in injectable, ophthalmic, otic, and cosmetic preparations at concentrations up to 0.5% (Table 56–4). Chlorobutanol also has mild sedative and local anesthetic properties and is used therapeutically. The lethal human chlorobutanol dose is estimated to be 50–500 mg/kg.[80]

Central Nervous System Depression

Chlorobutanol has a chemical structure similar to trichloroethanol (Fig. 63–1), the active metabolite of chloral hydrate. Therefore, it has been suggested, without evidence, that chlorobutanol may have pharmacologic properties similar to those of chloral hydrate. Chlorobutanol central nervous system depression is demonstrated in a case report of a 40-year-old alcoholic male who chronically abused chlorobutanol in Seducaps, a nonprescription hypnotic available in Australia and several other countries. He was noted to have dysarthria, slurred speech, and occasional episodes of irregular myoclonic movements. The speech abnormality resolved over 4 weeks as plasma chlorobutanol levels declined. No drugs other than chlorobutanol were detected in the patient's urine or plasma.[13]

An additive central nervous system depressant effect from chlorobutanol was suggested in a 19-year-old woman treated with high doses of morphine preserved with chlorobutanol. She received approximately 90 mg/h of chlorobutanol for several days,

far in excess of the recommended dosage of 150 mg/d. Her peak plasma chlorobutanol concentration was 83 µg/mL, a level similar to that previously reported to result in somnolence.[13,35]

Cardiovascular Toxicity

In patients undergoing elective coronary artery bypass graft surgery, a clinically important decrease in arterial blood pressure (15.4 vs 1.3 mm Hg, $p = 0.01$) was reported when heparin preserved with 0.5% chlorobutanol was compared to preservative-free heparin. No effect on heart rate or central venous pressure was noted in this study.[15] Chlorobutanol is a halogenated hydrocarbon and therefore may theoretically sensitize the myocardium to catecholamines, although no cases of ventricular dysrhythmias are described in the literature to date.

Ophthalmic Toxicity

Although animal studies suggest toxic effects of chlorobutanol to the eye, it is a commonly used preservative in ophthalmic preparations. Chlorobutanol increases the permeability of cells by impairing cell membrane structure.[104] An in vitro experiment utilizing corneal epithelial cells harvested from human cadavers within 12 hours of death demonstrated arrested mitotic activity following chlorobutanol exposure.[104] However, in another study, although chlorobutanol was shown to be cytotoxic, it had less toxicity than other commonly used ophthalmic preservatives such as benzalkonium chloride.[82] Considering its widespread use, there have been few clinical reports of adverse ophthalmic effects.

PARABENS

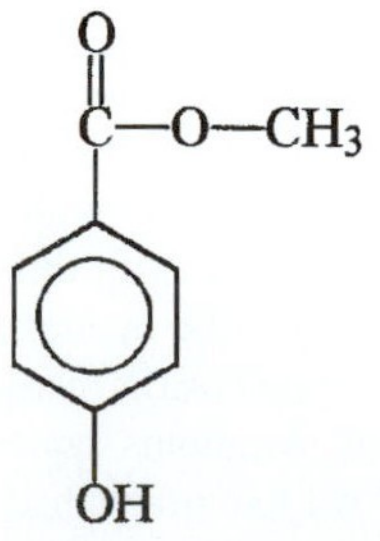

Methylparaben

The parabens or parahydroxybenzoic acids are a group of compounds widely employed as preservatives because of their bacteriostatic, fungistatic, and antioxidant properties[92] (Table 56–5). Parabens are often used in combination, because the presence of two or more parabens results in synergistic action.[67] The two most

TABLE 56–4. Chlorobutanol Concentrations in Common Medications

Medication	%	mg/Dose
Adrenalin chloride (epinephrine) injection	0.5	5
Chloroptic (chloramphenicol) ophthalmic solution	0.5	—
Dolophine (methadone) injection	0.5	10
Epinephrine ophthalmic solution	0.5	—
Novocain (procaine) injection	0.25	87
Phospholine iodine (echothiophate iodide) ophth. sol.	0.55	—
Rhinall (phenylephrine) nasal spray	0.14	—
Tobrex (tobramycin) ophthalmic ointment	0.5	—

commonly employed parabens are the methyl and propyl esters.[92] A survey conducted by the Food and Drug Administration identified the parabens as the second most commonly found ingredients in cosmetic formulations, with water being the most common.[67] Food and prescription medications containing greater than 0.1% parabens must be labeled as such, whereas over-the-counter preparations and cosmetics do not have this labeling requirement.[92] In the United States, the concentration of parabens usually ranges from 0.1% to 0.3%; however, Aureomycin and Achromycin far exceed these concentrations as each contains methyl paraben 2.4% and propyl paraben 0.6%. In Europe, parabens are used topically in a concentration of 5% as antifungal agents. An in vitro study demonstrated that the addition of 2-hydroxy propyl-β-cyclodextrin, used to solubilize methyl paraben, decreased the percutaneous absorption and promoted the bioconversion of methyl paraben to a less toxic metabolite, *p*-hydroxybenzoic acid, in the epidermis.[103] The potential for these pharmacokinetic effects to decrease toxicity was not studied. The WHO has set an estimated maximum acceptable daily intake at 10 mg/kg body weight for methyl and propyl parabens.[87]

Effects on Bilirubin Protein Binding

Gentamicin injection preserved with methyl and propyl paraben displaces bilirubin from albumin binding sites at serum concentrations ranging from 3 to 15 μg/mL.[33] An in vitro experiment demonstrated bilirubin displacement by methyl paraben 0.2 mg/mL in serum obtained from 28 hyperbilirubinemic newborns, while gentamicin alone had no effect on bilirubin displacement.[68]

TABLE 56–5. Paraben Concentration in Common Medications

Medication	%	mg/Dose
Aldomet (methyldopa) injection	0.17	8
Brofed (pseudoephedrine/brompheniramine) elixir	0.2	20
Haldol (haloperidol) injection	0.2	2
Inapsine (droperidol) injection	0.2	2
Isopto cetamide (sulfacetamide) ophthalmic soln	0.06	—
Narcan (naloxone) injection	0.2	2
Oncovin (vincristine) injection	0.15	4
Prolixin HCl (fluphenazine) injection	0.11	1
Prostigmin (neostigmine) injection	0.2	2
Romazicon (flumazenil) injection	0.2	4
Trandate (labetalol) injection	0.09	4
Xylocaine (lidocaine) injection	0.1	—
Zofran (ondansetron) injection	0.14	3

Spermicidal Activity

The in vitro spermicidal activity of methyl, ethyl, propyl, and butyl paraben was studied in human semen specimens. All the parabens possessed significant spermicidal activity in concentrations ranging from 1 to 8 mg/mL, leading to suggestions that the parabens be investigated as vaginal contraceptives.[98] Possible interferences with conception and potential for adverse effects on fertility were not investigated. The impact of routine topical application of cosmetics and medications, particularly to women, as well as the ingestion of foods containing parabens is not fully elucidated.[67] Because of the widespread exposure of humans to these agents, it is felt that the parabens have a relatively low order of toxicity, although they are associated with a higher incidence of allergic reactions than are other pharmaceutical additives.[92]

PHENOL

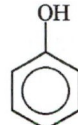

Phenol (carbolic acid, hydroxybenzene, phenylic acid, phenylic alcohol) is a commonly used preservative in injectable medications (Table 56–6). Phenol is a colorless to light pink, caustic liquid, with a characteristic odor. When exposed to air and light, phenol turns a red or brown color.[29] Phenol exerts antimicrobial activity against a wide variety of microorganisms such as gram-negative and gram-positive bacteria, mycobacteria, and some fungi and viruses.[29] Phenol is well absorbed from the gastrointestinal tract, skin, and mucous membranes, and is excreted in the urine as phenylglucuronide and phenyl sulfate metabolites.[29] Although there are numerous reports of phenol toxicity following intentional ingestions or unintentional dermal exposures (Chap. 84), adverse reactions to its use as a pharmaceutical excipient are uncommon, most likely because of the small quantities used.[29]

Commercially available glucagon is a lyophilized powder containing either 1 mg or 10 mg of glucagon. The diluent included with the packaging formerly contained phenol. According to the manufacturer, phenol was used to prolong the shelf life of the glucagon solution (personal communication, Lily Pharmaceuticals). The diluent contained 1 mL or 10 mL of sterile water preserved with 0.2% phenol and 1.6% glycerin. Reconstituted glucagon would subsequently contain 2 mg of phenol per mL. Glucagon in doses of 0.5–1 mg is employed in the treatment of hypoglycemia. High doses of glucagon is used in the treatment of se-

TABLE 56–6. Phenol Concentration in Common Medications

Medication	%	mg/Dose
Antivenom (Crotalidae)	0.25	25 (per vial)
Antivenom (*Micrurus fulvius*)	0.25	25 (per vial)
Pneumovax 23 (pneumococcal) vaccine	0.25	1.25
Prostigmin (neostigmine) injection	0.45	4.5
Quinidine gluconate injection	0.25	18.75
SusPhrine (epinephrine) injection	0.10	0.3

vere β-adrenergic antagonist and calcium channel blockade poisonings. There was a concern of systemic phenol toxicity following the administration of such high dosages of glucagon when reconstituted with the enclosed diluent.[29,75] It is recommended that the total intravenous phenol dosage in humans not exceed 50 mg in a 10-hour period.[16] Therefore, it was recommended that glucagon should be reconstituted with either 0.9% sodium chloride, 5% dextrose in water, or sterile water for injection when the dose exceeded 10 mg.[29,75] The diluent is enclosed for reconstitution for intramuscular administration when intravenous access is unavailable. Currently, glucagon does not contain phenol.[20] However, it is possible that some generic manufacturers may still include phenol in their diluents.

Cutaneous Absorption

Toxic effects following the topical administration of a phenol-containing product were reported in a 6-month-old child. Drowsiness, respiratory depression, and blue-colored urine were noted after repeated applications of magenta paint (also known as Castellani paint). Magenta paint contains 4% phenol, magenta, boric acid, resorcinol, acetone, and methylated spirit, and was widely employed in the treatment of seborrheic dermatitis in infants. Suspicion of systemic phenol toxicity led to the evaluation of urine samples from 16 children treated with topical magenta paint for the presence of phenol. Phenol was detected in the urine of four children, all of whom had approximately 11–15% of their body surface area painted twice daily for 48 hours.[88] Multifocal premature ventricular complexes were observed in a 10-year-old boy following the application of a chemical peeling solution containing 40% phenol. No phenol levels were obtained to confirm systemic absorption, and it is unclear what role the other components of the solution may have contributed to the cardiac effects.[108]

POLYETHYLENE GLYCOL

Polyethylene glycols (Carbowaxes) include several compounds with varying molecular weights (MWs) (150–10,000 MW).[9] Although regarded as relatively nontoxic, toxicity associated with polyethylene glycols (PEGs) includes renal failure, hyperosmolarity, and metabolic acidosis. Polyethylene glycols are mixtures that usually have a corresponding number denoting their average molecular weight. Polyethylene glycols are stable, hydrophilic substances, making them useful excipients in pharmaceuticals (Table 56–7) and cosmetics. At room temperature, PEGs with molecular weights less than 600 are clear, viscous liquids with a slight characteristic odor and bitter taste. Those PEGs with molecular weights greater than 1000 are solid and range in consistency from pastes to waxy flakes.[86] Oral ingestion of lower-molecular-weight

TABLE 56–7. Polyethylene Glycol (PEG) Content of Selected Medications*

Chloroptic (chloramphenicol) ointment	PEG 300
Decadron (dexamethasone) ophthalmic ointment	PEG 400
DepoProvera (medroxyprogesterone)	PEG 3350
Furacin (nitrofurazone) ointment	PEG Base
Polyethylene glycol electrolyte solution	PEG 3350
VePesid (etoposide) injection	PEG 300

*The number following PEG refers to the mean molecular weight of the constituent compounds.

PEGs, such as diethylene glycol and triethylene glycol, are associated with greater toxicity than PEGs with molecular weights above 6000.[95,96]

Commercially available products such as GoLytely and CoLyte are solutions of PEG 3350 combined with electrolytes (PEG-ELS). They are routinely employed to cleanse the bowel prior to surgery with minimal net water and electrolyte shifts. In addition, they are also used to decontaminate the gut following poisonings with sustained-release products or iron (Chap. 5). Polyethylene glycols combined with electrolytes are considered relatively nontoxic, even after massive quantities have been ingested. This is demonstrated by a case report in which a 33-month-old child received a total of 44.3 L PEG-ELS over 5 days following iron poisoning without any adverse effects.[60] In contrast, an 8-year-old female developed acute lung injury following the administration of 1 L of PEG-ELS. It is probable that this complication resulted from aspiration of the solution during several episodes of vomiting.[84]

Pharmacokinetics

When taken orally, lower-molecular-weight PEGs may be absorbed from the gastrointestinal tract, whereas higher-molecular-weight PEGs are not. The low-molecular-weight PEGs may be partially metabolized by alcohol dehydrogenase to hydroxyacid and diacid metabolites; however, they are mainly excreted unchanged in the urine.[86]

Nephrotoxicity

When rats fed various PEGs (200, 300, and 400) in their drinking water for 90 days were studied, a solution of 8% PEG 200 produced renal tubular necrosis in all the animals, followed by death within 15 days; however, a 4% PEG 200 solution resulted in only two of nine rats dying within 80 days. A 16% PEG 400 solution killed all animals within 13 days; however, both 8% and 4% PEG 400 solutions had no observable effect except for a decrease in kidney weights when compared to control animals.[97] Acute renal failure occurred in a 65-year-old male following his ingestion of the contents of a Lava Lamp in a suicide attempt. The lamp contained 13% PEG 200 in addition to water, paraffin, kerosene, and wax. Forty-eight hours after admission, the patient became oliguric with an anion gap metabolic acidosis and acute renal failure.[39] While his initial acute renal failure was probably multifactorial, he was discharged 3 months later with residual kidney dysfunction attributed to the PEG component of the lamp contents causing acute tubular necrosis.

Acute tubular necrosis was noted on autopsy of nine burn patients treated with a topical antibiotic cream in a PEG base. These effects were reproduced with the topical application of PEG for 7 days to rabbits with full-thickness skin defects.[101]

Neurotoxicity

There are reports of neurologic complications following intrathecal steroidal injections containing 3% PEG as a vehicle.[12] In an in vitro experiment, myelinated and unmyelinated rabbit nerves were exposed to concentrations of PEG 3350 ranging from 3% to 40% for 1 hour. Three percent and 10% PEG had no effect on either nerve conduction or the amplitude of action potentials. Twenty percent and 30% PEG markedly slowed nerve conduction and had varying effects on the amplitudes of action potentials. Forty percent PEG completely abolished action potentials.[9] This impairment of nerve conduction may be related to the osmotic effects of PEG.[9]

Fluid and Electrolyte Disturbances

Serum hyperosmolarity was reported in patients with burn surface areas ranging from 20% to 56%, following the application of Furacin, a topical dressing containing 63% PEG 300 and 32% PEG 1000.[18] Polyethylene glycol appears to produce a greater osmotic effect than can be accounted for by the number of PEG molecules in solution.[93]

Acid-Base Disturbances

Polyethylene glycol is oxidized by alcohol dehydrogenase to hydroxyacid and diacid metabolites, possibly contributing to metabolic acidosis.[56] Two cases of metabolic acidosis were reported following intravenous administration of nitrofurantoin mixed with polyethylene glycol (PEG 300).[102] Similarly, an increased anion gap was reported in three patients being treated with a topical PEG-based burn cream.[18]

PROPYLENE GLYCOL

Propylene glycol (PG), or 1,2-propanediol, is a clear, colorless, odorless, sweet viscous liquid. Propylene glycol is widely employed as a preservative and solvent in numerous pharmaceuticals (Table 56–8). The WHO has set the daily allowable dosage of PG at a maximum of 25 mg/kg.[34] Recently, the manufacturer of amprenavir (Agenerase) oral solution changed the product information to include a black-boxed warning regarding the high

TABLE 56–8. Propylene Glycol Concentration in Common Medications

Medication	%	g/Avg Dose*
Agenerase (amprenavir) oral solution	55	57.75
Ativan (lorazepam) injection	80	0.64
Bactrim, septra injection (trimethoprim/ sulfamethoxazole)	40	10.0[†]
Brevibloc (esmolol) injection	25	2.50[†]
Dilantin (phenytoin) injection	40	4.80
Lanoxin (digoxin) injection	40	0.40
Librium (chlordiazepoxide) injection	20	0.08
Luminal (phenobarbital sodium) injection	70	0.70
MVI-12 (multivitamins) injection	30	0.45
Tridil (nitroglycerin) injection	30	0.30[†]
Valium (diazepam) injection	40	0.4

*Based on dosage for a 70-kg person.
[†]Based on 24-hour dosage.

concentration of PG in this product.[90] No adverse reports have been attributed to amprenavir solution's PG content. (Personal communication, January 4, 2001 15:10 EST, Barbara I. Gary, R.N.C., Senior Customer Response Representative, III, Customer Response Center, Glaxo Wellcome Inc.)

Pharmacokinetics

Propylene glycol is rapidly absorbed from the gastrointestinal (GI) tract following oral administration and has a volume of distribution of approximately 0.6 L/kg.[71,99] When applied to intact epidermis, the absorption of PG is minimal. Percutaneous absorption may occur following application to damaged skin (eg, extensive burn surface areas). Propylene glycol is hepatically metabolized to lactic acid by alcohol dehydrogenase and is then further broken down to pyruvic acid, carbon dioxide, and water.[78] The terminal half-life is reported to be between 1.4 and 5.6 hours in adults, and as long as 16.9 hours in neonates.[36,99] Twelve percent to 45% of PG is excreted unchanged in the urine.[36]

Cardiovascular Toxicity

Intravenous preparations of phenytoin contain 40% PG to facilitate the solubility of phenytoin. Nine years after intravenous phenytoin became available, three deaths were attributed to the rapid administration of phenytoin used for the treatment of cardiac dysrhythmias.[46,105] Several years later, PG was identified as the cardiotoxin. Rapidly infusing PG results in hypotension, apnea, bradycardia, widening of the QRS interval, increased T waves with occasional inversions, and transient ST elevations. Conversely, when PG is infused slowly only minimal hypotension and ECG changes result. Bradycardia and depression of atrial conduction were not observed in cats pretreated with atropine, or in vagotomy following rapid intravenous infusion of PG, suggesting that these effects are vagally mediated. QRS widening was noted in these same pretreated cats, suggesting an additive direct cardiotoxic effect of PG.[69] Similar results were reported in calves pretreated with atropine that received oxytetracycline in a PG vehicle.[49]

Neurotoxicity

Smaller infants appear to have a decreased ability to clear PG when compared to older children and adults.[69] An increased frequency of seizures was reported in low-birth-weight infants who received greater than 10 mL/d of a parenteral multivitamin preparation containing 300 mg of PG/mL.[69] Seizures developed in an 11-year-old boy receiving long-term oral therapy with vitamin D dissolved in PG; seizures abated after the product was discontinued.[4] Propylene glycol is an alcohol and may possess some inebriating properties similar to ethanol.[57] Central nervous system depression was reported following an intentional oral ingestion of a PG-containing product.[71]

Ototoxicity

Many otic solutions and suspensions contain PG as part of their vehicles. Experimentally, concentrations of PG greater than 10% when instilled into the middle ears of guinea pigs resulted in cochlear hair cell loss and irreversible deafness.[77] A similar experiment found 10% PG produced no negative effects, while 90% PG did impair cochlear function; there was no greater increase in hair cell loss than in controls.[107] Topical otic solutions containing high concentrations of PG are contraindicated in patients with perforated tympanic membranes.[108]

Fluid and Electrolyte Disturbances

There are numerous reports of PG-induced serum hyperosmorality following the topical administration of silver sulfadiazine.[7,42,62] Systemic absorption of PG resulting in hyperosmorality occurred with topical application of silver sulfadiazine cream in 15 burn patients with burns over more than 35% of their body surface area.[62] Parenteral administration of medications containing a PG vehicle has also resulted in hyperosmorality. This occurred in four premature infants younger than 2 weeks of age receiving injectable multivitamins containing PG.[48] A correlation between decreased renal function and serum hyperosmorality was demonstrated. A significantly increased osmolar gap occurred in patients who had a calculated creatinine clearance of less than 30 mL/min and received intravenous nitroglycerin containing a PG vehicle.

Acid-Base Disturbances

Metabolic acidosis is also reported in patients receiving PG. The metabolic acidosis probably results from increased production of lactate, a metabolic by-product of PG.[22] Acute toxicity of propylene glycol in human proximal tubule cells was evaluated in an in vitro experiment that assessed lactate dehydrogenase and creatinine release as indicators of tubular toxicity. A concentration- and time-dependent effect associated with PG exposure suggested a direct toxic effect on proximal tubule cells.[79] Human proximal tubule cells exposed to concentrations of PG of 10, 25, and 50 mM for up to 6 days demonstrated a dose-dependent toxicity response. The highest degree of proximal tubule damage resulted from exposure to 50 mM, while the 10-mM group showed no significant differences from controls. These authors suggest that the chronic administration of PG in drug vehicle may contribute to proximal tubule damage and subsequent decreased renal function. However, the concentrations required to produce the proximal tubule damage would rarely exist except when very high doses of PG were administered. Caution should be utilized when prolonged administration of a PG-containing medication is necessary in the presence of impaired metabolic and/or renal function, which might result in the accumulation of PG.[78]

Thrombophlebitis

An increased frequency of thrombophlebitis occurred in patients who received intravenous diazepam in a PG solvent compared with diazepam suspended in another solvent, Cremophor-EL (polyethoxylated castor oil). Sixty-two percent of the PG-treated patients had evidence of thrombophlebitis 14 days after administration as compared to only 3.4% of the Cremophor-EL patients. Pain on injection was also greater in intensity in the PG patients than in those receiving the other preparation, 65% and 8.5%, respectively.[73] However, because Cremophor-EL is associated with several cases of anaphylaxis, it is not used.[37,38]

Drug Interactions

Propylene glycol may cause a transient inhibition of function of heparin by a mechanism similar to protamine.[27] Higher doses of heparin are sometimes required when used concomitantly with ni-

troglycerin containing propylene glycol as a diluent. However, further study has demonstrated that heparin resistance seems to occur in patients receiving nitroglycerin whether or not the product contains propylene glycol.[50]

SORBITOL

$$
\begin{array}{c}
CH_2OH \\
| \\
HC-OH \\
| \\
HO-CH \\
| \\
HC-OH \\
| \\
HC-OH \\
| \\
CH_2OH
\end{array}
$$

Sorbitol (D-glucitol) is widely used in the pharmaceutical industry as a sweetening agent, moistening agent, and a diluent (Table 56–9). It is particularly useful in chewable tablets because of its pleasant taste. In addition, it is widely used by the food industry in chewing gums, dietetic candies, foods, and enteral nutrition formulations. Sorbitol is about 50–60% as sweet as sucrose.[81] Sorbitol is not readily fermented by oral microorganisms and is generally considered noncariogenic.[81]

Sorbitol occurs naturally in the ripe berries of many fruits, trees, and plants, and was first isolated in 1872, from the berries of the mountain ash (*Sorbus aucuparia*). Sorbitol has a caloric value of 4 Kcal/g and is better tolerated by diabetics than sucrose; however, it is not considered unconditionally safe for diabetics.[81] Sorbitol is absorbed more slowly from the gastrointestinal tract than sucrose and is metabolized in the liver to fructose or glucose.[81] There is a concern of potentially fatal toxicity for fructose-intolerant individuals receiving sorbitol-containing agents.[43] There are several reports of patients with hereditary fructose intolerance dying following the parenteral infusion of sorbitol solutions.[28,94]

Gastrointestinal Toxicity

In large dosages, sorbitol can cause abdominal cramping, bloating, flatulence, vomiting, and diarrhea. Sorbitol appears to exert its cathartic effects by its osmotic properties, resulting in fluid shifts within the gastrointestinal tract. In a human volunteer study, 42 healthy adults ingested 10 g of a sorbitol solution. Sorbitol intolerance was detected in up to 55% of subjects.[58] Sorbitol is found in a great number of commonly used medications. Diarrhea resulting from sorbitol-containing medications is common and often over-

TABLE 56–9. Common Medications Containing Sorbitol

Medication	%	g/Dose
Brofed elixir	20	2
Calcium carbonate suspension	28	1.4
Fer-In-Sol drops	31	0.2
Symmetrel syrup	64	6.4
Triaminic syrup	7	0.7

looked as a possible etiology.[25,55] Sorbitol should be considered as a possible causative agent in patients experiencing gastrointestinal effects while receiving sorbitol-containing medications.[55] Ingestion of large quantities of sorbitol (greater than 20 g/d in adults) is not recommended[81] (Antidotes in Depth: Cathartics).

THIMEROSAL

Thimerosal (Merthiolate, Mercurothiolate) or sodium ethylmercuric thiosalicylate is an organic mercury compound that contains approximately 49% mercury by weight.[89] Thimerosal has a wide spectrum of antibacterial activity at concentrations ranging from 0.02% to 0.1%; however, higher concentrations are sometimes used.[76] Thimerosal has been widely used since the 1930s as a contact lens disinfectant and as a preservative in numerous biologics and vaccines, particularly those in multidose containers (Table 56–10). At doses much higher than those found in vaccines, thimerosal is associated with neurotoxicity and nephrotoxicity. In July 1999, the US Public Health Service (USPHS) and the American Academy of Pediatrics (AAP) issued a joint statement concerning the use of thimerosal in vaccines, prompting recommendations and expedited measures for the removal of thimerosal from vaccines.[3,23]

As part of the FDA Modernization Act of 1997, a review of thimerosal-containing vaccines revealed that infants receiving several thimerosal-containing vaccines over the first 6 months of life might exceed recommended federal guidelines for daily exposure limits of methylmercury (up to 187.5 μg Hg total).[3,24] Maximum recommended allowable daily exposures range from 0.1 μg Hg/kg (EPA) to 0.47 μg Hg/kg.[26] Although there is no evidence of adverse effects following recommended vaccination schedules, the actual risk that intermittent, cumulative thimerosal exposure poses to infants is unknown.[24]

Most recently, the Centers for Disease Control and Prevention (CDC) conducted preliminary screening of large databases that link vaccination and International Classification of Disease code (ICD-9) information from managed care organizations. A dataset from two organizations showed no association between exposure to thimerosal-containing vaccines and 12 of the 17 renal and neurologic ICD-9 codes examined; however, an inconclusive correlation was observed with the remaining 5 ICD-9 codes (language delays, speech delays attention deficit disorder, unspecified developmental delays, and tics). Premature infants did not appear to be at greater risk for these codes. Similarly, preliminary data from a third managed care organization showed no association between speech and language delays and attention deficit disorder. Unspecified developmental delays and tics were not analyzed. Further investigations of these data are planned.[2]

Despite the great progress made in the production and FDA approval of thimerosal preservative–free pediatric vaccines, there may be occasions when only a thimerosal-containing vaccine is available.[2]

Mercurial Toxicity

Oral Administration. A case report from Germany described a 44-year-old man who ingested 5 g (83 mg/kg) of thimerosal in a suicide attempt; within 15 minutes he began vomiting spontaneously. Gastric lavage was performed and chelation therapy begun with 300 mg of dimercaptopropane sulfonate (DMPS) instilled through a nasogastric tube into the stomach. Gastroscopy revealed a grade 2 hemorrhagic gastritis. Polyuric acute renal failure was noted on the day of admission and persisted for 40 days. Four days after admission the patient developed a fever and a maculopapular exanthem attributed to thimerosal. The patient also developed an autonomic and ascending peripheral polyneuropathy that persisted for 13 days. Chelation therapy was continued for a total of 50 days with DMPS followed by dimercaptosuccinic acid (DMSA). Elevated blood and urine mercury levels persisted for more than 140 days. The patient was discharged 148 days following the ingestion with only sensory defects in his toes. No other neurologic sequelae were noted.[85]

Oral absorption of thimerosal resulted in the fatal poisoning of an 18-month-old girl from the intraotic instillation of a solution containing 0.1% thimerosal and 0.14% sodium borate. Tympanostomy tubes, placed 1 year previously, allowed for the majority of the irrigation solution to flow through the auditory tube into the nasopharynx and subsequently to be swallowed and absorbed through the gastrointestinal tract. A total of 1.2 L of solution (500 mg mercury) was instilled over a 4-week period resulting in severe mercury poisoning. Chelation therapy with N-acetyl-D-penicillamine was initiated on day 51. Despite increased urinary mercury concentrations following the N-acetyl-D-penicillamine, her neurologic function and blood mercury levels remained unchanged. The child died 3 months after admission. An autopsy was not performed.[89]

Intramuscular Administration. A recent study evaluated 15 preterm (weight ≤ 1 kg) and 5 term (weight ≥ 3.5 kg) neonate blood mercury levels before and 48–72 hours after intramuscular injection of a hepatitis B vaccine containing thimerosal 0.005% (12.5

TABLE 56–10. Thimerosol Concentration in Common Medications

Medication	%	mg/Dose*
Antivenom (Crotalidae)	0.005	0.5 (per vial)
Antivenom (*Lactrodectus mactans*)	0.01	0.25 (per vial)
Antivenom (*Micrurus fulvius*)	0.005	0.5 (per vial)
Diphtheria & tetanus toxoids (various)	0.01	0.05
Engerix-B (hepatitis B vaccine)	0.005	0.025
Fluzone (influenza virus vaccine)	0.01	0.05
H-BIG (hepatitis B immune globulin)	0.01	0.05
Hib TITER (*Haemophilus* b conjugate vaccine)	0.01	0.05
Neosporin (triple antibiotic) ophthalmic sol.	0.001	—
Ocufren (flurbiprofen) ophthalmic sol.	0.005	—
Pnu-Imune 23 (pneumococcal vaccine)	0.01	0.05
Rabies immune globulin	0.012	1.2
Sulf-10 (sulfacetamide) ophthalmic solution	0.01	—
Varicella-zoster immune globulin	0.01	0.25

*Based on a 70-kg person.

μg of mercury) within the first week of life. Mean blood mercury levels were similar at baseline for both groups. Preterm neonates had a mean postvaccination blood mercury level 3 times greater than term neonates (7.36 μg/L vs 2.24 μg/L). Nine of the preterm neonates had blood mercury levels greater than 2.9 μg/L.[100] A retrospective National Institute of Health study showed blood mercury levels of term infants exposed to thimerosal-containing vaccines are similar to background blood mercury levels (less than 2 μg/L).[2]

Urine mercury levels of 26 patients with hypogammaglobulinemia who received weekly intramuscular IgG replacement therapy preserved with 0.01% thimerosal were studied. The dosages of IgG ranged from 25 to 50 mg/kg, containing 0.6–1.2 mg of mercury per dose.[51] The total estimated dose of mercury administered ranged from 4 to 734 mg over a period of 6 months to 17 years. Elevated urine mercury levels were determined in 19 patients; however, no patients had clinical evidence of chronic mercury toxicity.[51]

Six cases of severe mercury poisoning resulting in four deaths were reported from Africa following the intramuscular administration of chloramphenicol preserved with thimerosal. A manufacturing error produced vials containing 510 mg of thimerosal instead of 0.51 mg per vial. All six patients had extensive tissue necrosis at the site of injection. Fever, altered mental status, slurred speech, and ataxia were also noted. Autopsy showed evidence of widespread degeneration and necrosis of the renal tubules. Elevated mercury concentrations were found in the injection site tissues, and in the kidneys, livers, and brains.[5]

Topical Administration. Thirteen infants were exposed to 9–48 topical applications of a thimerosal tincture 0.1% for the treatment of exomphalos. Analysis for elevated mercury levels was performed in 10 of 13 infants who died unexpectantly. Mercury concentrations were determined in various tissues from six of the infants. Mean tissue concentrations in fresh samples of liver, kidney, spleen, and heart ranged from 5152 to 11,330 ppb, suggesting percutaneous absorption from these repeated topical applications.[40]

Ophthalmic Administration. Mercury concentrations of the aqueous humor and excised corneal tissues of nine patients undergoing keratoplasty were measured after application to one eye of a contact lens that was stored in a contact lens solution containing thimerosal. After 4 hours the lens was removed and mercury concentrations were determined. Elevated levels of mercury were determined in both aqueous humor (range, 20–46 ng/mL) and corneal tissues (range, 0.6–14 ng per tissue) as compared to the control eyes. Only residual amounts of mercury remained on the contact lenses after 4 hours of wear. The authors noted that although the aqueous humor concentrations were in the same range as those measured in 10 patients with symptomatic mercury poisoning (11–104 ng/mL),[109] adverse effects were not seen.

A possible drug interaction between orally administered tetracyclines and thimerosal was reported to result in acute, varying degrees of eye irritation in contact lens wearers using thimerosal-containing contact lens solutions who started treatment with tetracycline.[32]

Cutaneous Effects. A chemical interaction between thimerosal and aluminum electrodes caused skin burns in a woman following a surgical procedure. The thimerosal was applied topically as a 1:1000 thimerosal solution in 50% alcohol. Thimerosal acted as a catalyst that rapidly oxidized the aluminum electrode, generating heat and causing a subsequent thermal injury.[59]

SUMMARY

Pharmaceutical excipient benefits include improved drug solubility, stability and palatability, the ability to make available various dosage forms, the provision of products with long-term storage, and the availability of multiple-dose packaging. Excipients are often termed "inert," implying that they possess no pharmacologic or toxicologic properties of their own. While excipients are essential and efficacious, they may also be responsible for severe, and sometimes fatal, adverse effects.

The toxicity of pharmaceutical excipients should be considered for patients requiring high dosages or prolonged administration of any medication containing excipients, particularly those additives known to have toxicities. Individuals with decreased renal or hepatic functions or patients at the extremes of age may be at an increased risk of accumulating excipients. Under circumstances in which there is no option but to continue treating a patient with a particular therapeutic agent, switching to a preservative-free product, or to another brand without the offending excipient, may obviate the need for discontinuation of an effective agent. In addition to inherent toxicities, many excipients may also be responsible for allergic reactions. Their prevalence in numerous pharmaceuticals, cosmetics, and foods may allow for sensitization. However, in the majority of cases, pharmaceutical excipients are safe and effective, and their benefits far exceed their potential for adverse effects when administered properly.

REFERENCES

1. Alade SL, Brown RE, Paquet A: Polysorbate 80 and E-Ferol toxicity. Pediatrics 1986;77:593–597.
2. American Academy of Family Physicians, American Academy of Pediatrics, Advisory Committee on Immunization Practices, United States Public Health Service. Joint statement concerning removal of thimerosal from vaccines. Approved on June 22, 2000. URL: http://www.cdc.gov/nip/vacsafe/concerns/thimerosal/joint_statement_00.htm.
3. American Academy of Pediatrics Committee on Infectious Diseases and Committee on Environmental Health. Thimerosal in vaccines—An interim report to clinicians (RE9935). Pediatrics 1999;104:570–574.
4. Arulanantham K, Genel M: Central nervous system toxicity associated with ingestion of propylene glycol. J Pediatr 1978;93:515–516.
5. Axton JH: Six cases of poisoning after parenteral organic mercurial compound (Merthiolate). Postgrad Med J 1972;48:417–421.
6. Bagshawe KD, Magrath IT, Golding PR: Intrathecal methotrexate. Lancet 1969;2:1258.
7. Bekeris L, Baker C, Fenton J, et al: Propylene glycol as a cause of an elevated serum osmolality. Am J Clin Pathol 1979;72:633–636.
8. Benda GI, Hiller JL, Reynolds JW: Benzyl alcohol toxicity: Impact on neurologic handicaps among surviving very-low-birth-weight infants. Pediatrics 1986;77:507–512.
9. Benzon HT, Gissen AJ, Strichartz GR, et al: The effect of polyethylene glycol on mammalian nerve impulses. Anesth Analg 1987;66:553–559.
10. Berg ØH, Henriksen RN, Steisvåg SK: The effect of a benzalkonium chloride-containing nasal spray on human respiratory mucosa in vitro as a function of concentration and time of action. Pharmacol Toxicol 1995;76:245–249.

11. Berg ØH, Lie K, Steisvåg SK: The effects of topical nasal steroids on rat respiratory mucosa in vivo, with special reference to benzalkonium chloride. Allergy 1997;52:627–632.

12. Bernat JL: Intraspinal steroid therapy. Neurology 1981;31:168–171.

13. Borody T, Chinwah PM, Graham GG, et al: Chlorobutanol toxicity and dependence. Med J Aust 1979;1:288.

14. Bowie MD, McKenzie D: Diethylene glycol poisoning in children. S Afr Med J 1972;46:931–934.

15. Bowler GM, Galloway DW, Mieklejohn BH: Sharp fall in blood pressure after injection of heparin containing chlorbutol. Lancet 1986;1:848–849.

16. Brancato DJ: Recognizing potential toxicity of phenol. Vet Hum Toxicol 1982;24:29–30.

17. Brown WJ, Buist WJ, Cory Gipson HT, et al: Fatal benzyl alcohol poisoning in an neonatal intensive care unit [letter]. Lancet 1982;1: 1250.

18. Bruns DE, Herold DA, Rodheaver GT, et al: Polyethylene glycol intoxication in burn patients. Burns 1982;9:49–52.

19. Brunson EL: Benzyl alcohol. In: Kibbe AH, ed: Handbook of Pharmaceutical Excipients, 3rd ed. Washington, DC, American Pharmaceutical Association, 2000, pp. 41–43.

20. Burda AM, Kapustka CA J: Reformulated glucagon diluent phenol-free [letter]. J Toxicol Clin Toxicol 1999;37:1:127.

21. Calvery HO, Klumpp TG: The toxicity for human beings of diethylene glycol with sulfanilamide. South Med J 1939;32:1105–1109.

22. Cate JC, Hedrick R: Propylene glycol intoxication and lactic acidosis [letter]. N Engl J Med 1980;303:1237.

23. Centers for Disease Control and Prevention. Recommendations regarding the use of vaccines that contain thimerosal as preservative. MMWR Morb Mortal Wkly Rep 1999;48:996–998.

24. Centers for Disease Control and Prevention. Thimerosal in vaccines: A joint statement of the American Academy of Pediatrics and the Public Health Service. MMWR Morb Mortal Wkly Rep 1999; 48:563–565.

25. Chassany O, Michaux A, Bergmann JF: Drug-induced diarrheoea. Drug Saf 2000;22:53–72.

26. Clements CJ, Ball LK, Ball R, et al: Thiomersal in vaccines. Lancet 2000;355:1279–1280.

27. Col J, Col-Debeys C, Lavenne-Pardogne E, et al: Propylene glycol-induced heparin resistance during nitroglycerin infusion. Am Heart J 1985;110:171–173.

28. Collins J: Time for fructose solutions to go. Lancet 1993;341:600.

29. Conway V, Mulski M: Phenol. In: Kibbe AH, ed: Handbook of Pharmaceutical Excipients, 3rd ed. Washington, DC, American Pharmaceutical Association, 2000, pp. 367–369.

30. Craig DB, Habib GG: Flaccid paraparesis following obstetrical epidural anesthesia: Possible role of benzyl alcohol. Anesth Analg 1977;56:219–221.

31. Cronk JD: Phenol with glucagon in cardiotherapy. N Engl J Med 1971;284:219–220.

32. Crook TG, Freeman JJ: Reactions induced by the concurrent use of thimerosal and tetracycline. Am J Optom Physiol Optics 1983;60: 759–761.

33. Cukier JO, Seungdamrong S, Odell JL, et al: The displacement of albumin bound bilirubin by gentamicin. Pediatr Res 1974;8:399.

34. Dandiker Y: Propylene glycol. In: Kibbe AH, ed: Handbook of Pharmaceutical Excipients, 3rd ed. Washington, DC, American Pharmaceutical Association, 2000, pp. 442–444.

35. DeChristoforro R, Corden BJ, Hood JC, et al: High-dose morphine complicated by chlorobutanol-somnolence. Ann Intern Med 1983; 98:335–336.

36. Demey HE, Daelemans RA, Verpooten GA, et al: Propylene glycol-induced side effects during intravenous nitroglycerin therapy. Intensive Care Med 1988;14:221–226.

37. Doenicke A, Lorenz W, Beigl R, et al: Histamine release after intravenous application of short acting hypnotics. Br J Anaesth 1973; 45:1097–1104.

38. Dundee JW: Hypersensitivity to intravenous anaesthetic agents. Br J Anaesth 1976;48:57–58.

39. Erickson TB, Aks SE, Zabaneh R, et al: Acute renal toxicity after ingestion of lava light liquid. Ann Emerg Med 1996;27:781–784.

40. Fagan DG, Pritchard JS, Clarkson TW, et al: Organ mercury levels in infant with omphaloceles treated with organic mercurial antiseptic. Arch Dis Child 197;52:962–964.

41. Fatalities associated with ingestion of diethylene glycol-contaminated glycerin used to manufacture acetaminophen syrup—Haiti, November 1995–June 1996. MMWR Morb Mortal Wkly Rep 1996; 45:649–650.

42. Fligner CL, Jack R, Twiggs GA, et al: Hyperosmolality induced by propylene glycol, a complication of silver sulfadiazine therapy. JAMA 1985;253:1606–1609.

43. Florence AT, Salole EG, eds: Formulation Factors in Adverse Reactions. London, Wright, 1990, p. 11.

44. Gassett AR: Benzalkonium chloride toxicity to the human cornea. Am J Ophthamol 1977;84:169–171.

45. Geiling EM, Cannon PR: Pathologic effects of elixir of sulfanilamide (diethylene glycol) poisoning. JAMA 1938;111:919–926.

46. Gellerman GL, Martinez C: Fatal ventricular fibrillation following intravenous sodium diphenylhydantoin therapy. JAMA 1967;200: 337–338.

47. Gershanik J, Boecler B, Ensley H, et al: The gasping syndrome and benzyl alcohol poisoning. N Engl J Med 1982:1384–1388.

48. Glasgow AM, Boeckx RL, Miller MK, et al: Hyperosmolality in small infants due to propylene glycol. Pediatrics 1983;72:353–355.

49. Gross DR, Kitzman JV, Adams HR: Cardiovascular effects of intravenous administration of propylene glycol and oxytetracycline in propylene glycol in calves. Am J Vet Res 1979;40:783–791.

50. Habbab MA, Haft JI: Heparin resistance induced by intravenous nitroglycerin. Arch Intern Med 1987;147:857–860.

51. Haeney MR, Carter GF, Yeoman WB, et al: Long-term parenteral exposure to mercury in patients with hypogammaglobulinaemia. Br Med J 1979;2:12–14.

52. Hagebusch OE: Necropsies of four patients following administration of elixir sulfanilamide-massengill. JAMA 1937;109:1537–1539.

53. Hahn AF, Feasby TE, Gilbert JJ: Paraparesis following intrathecal chemotherapy. Neurology 1983;33:1032–1038.

54. Hanif M, Mobarak MR, Ronan A: Fatal renal failure by diethylene glycol in paracetamol elixir: The Bangladesh epidemic. BMJ 1995; 311:88–91.

55. Henley E: Sorbitol-based elixirs, diarrhea and enteral tube feeding. Am Fam Physician. 1997;1;55:2084–2086.

56. Herold DA, Keil K, Bruns DE: Oxidation of polyethylene glycols by alcohol dehydrogenase. Biochem Pharmacol 1989;38:73–76.

57. Hiller JL, Benda GI, Rahatzad M, et al: Benzyl alcohol toxicity: Impact on mortality and intraventricular hemorrhage among very-low-birth-weight infants. Pediatrics 1986;77:500–506.

58. Jain NK, Patel VP, Pitchumoni CS: Sorbitol intolerance in adults. Am J Gastroenterol 1985;80:678–681.

59. Jones HT: Danger of skin burns from thimersal. Br Med J 1972;2: 504–505.

60. Kaczorowski JM, Wax PM: Five days of whole-bowel irrigation in a case of pediatric iron ingestion. Ann Emerg Med 1996;27: 258–263.

61. Kibbe AH: Benzalkonium chloride. In: Kibbe AH, ed: Handbook of Pharmaceutical Excipients, 3rd ed. Washington, DC, American Pharmaceutical Association, 2000, pp. 33–35.

62. Kulick MI, Lewis NS, Bansal V, et al: Hyperosmolality in the burn patient: Analysis of an osmolal discrepancy. J Trauma 1980;20: 223–228.

63. Kuoyama Y, Suzuki K, Hara T: Nasal lesion induced by intranasal administration of benzalkonium chloride in rats. J Toxicol Sci 1997; 22:153–160.

64. LeBel M, Ferron L, Masson M, et al: Benzyl alcohol metabolism and elimination in neonates. Dev Pharmacol Ther 1988;11:347–356.

65. Lemp MA, Zimmerman LE: Toxic endothelial degeneration in ocular surface disease treated with topical medications containing benzalkonium chloride. Am J Ophthamol 1988;105:670–673.

66. Lopez-Herce J, Bonet C, Meana A, Albajara L: Benzyl alcohol poisoning following diazepam intravenous infusion [letter]. Ann Pharmacother 1995;29:632.

67. Lorenzetti OJ, Wernet TC: Topical parabens: Benefits and risks. Dermatologica 1977;154:244–250.

68. Loria CJ, Echeverria P, Smith AL: Effect of antibiotic formulations in serum protein: Bilirubin interaction of newborn infants. J Pediatr 1976;89:479–482.

69. Louis S, Kutt H, McDowell F: The cardiovascular changes caused by intravenous Dilantin and its solvent. Am Heart J 1967;74:523–529.

70. MacDonald MG, Getson PR, Glasgow AM, et al: Propylene glycol: Increased incidence of seizures in low-birth-weight infants. Pediatrics 1987;79:622–625.

71. Martin G, Finberg L: Propylene glycol: A potentially toxic vehicle in liquid dosage form. J Pediatr 1970;77:877–878.

72. Martone WJ, Williams WW, Mortensen ML, et al: Illness with fatalities in premature infants: Association with intravenous vitamin E preparation, E-Ferol. Pediatrics 1986;78:591–600.

73. Mattila MA, Ruoppi M, Korhonen HM, et al: Prevention of diazepam-induced thrombophlebitis with Cremophor as a solvent. Br J Anaesth 1979;51:891–894.

74. McOrmond P, Gulck B, Duggan HE, et al: Hemolytic effect of benzyl alcohol. Drug Intell Clin Pharm 1980;14:549.

75. Mofenson HC, Caraccio TR, Laudano J: Glucagon for propranolol overdose. JAMA 1986;255:2025–2026.

76. Möller H: Merthiolate allergy: A nationwide iatrogenic sensitization. Acta Derm Venereol 1977;57:509–517.

77. Morizono T, Johnstomne BM: Ototoxicity of chloramphenicol ear drops with propylene glycol as solvent. Med J Aust 1975;2:634–638.

78. Morshed KM, Jain SK, McMartin KE: Propylene glycol-mediated injury in a primary cell culture of human proximal tubule cells. Toxicol Sci 1998;46:410–417.

79. Morshed KM, Jain SK, McMartin KE: Acute toxicity of propylene glycol: An assessment using cultured proximal tubule cells of human origin. Fundam Appl Toxicol 1994;23:38–43.

80. Nash RA: Chlorbutanol. In: Kibbe AH, ed: Handbook of Pharmaceutical Excipients, 3rd ed. Washington, DC, American Pharmaceutical Association, 2000, pp. 126–128.

81. Nash RA: Sorbitol. In: Kibbe AH, ed: Handbook of Pharmaceutical Excipients, 3rd ed. Washington, DC, American Pharmaceutical Association, 2000, pp. 515–518.

82. Neville R, Dennis, P, Sens D, et al: Preservative cytotoxicity to cultured corneal epithelial cells. Curr Eye Res 1986;5:367–372.

83. Okuonghae HO, Ighogboja IS, Lawson JO, et al: Diethylene glycol poisoning in Nigerian children. Ann Trop Paediatr 1992;12:235–238.

84. Paap CM, Ehlirch R: Acute pulmonary edema after polyethylene glycol intestinal lavage in a child. Ann Pharmacother 1993;27:1044–1047.

85. Pfab R, Mückter H, Roider G, et al: Clinical course of severe poisoning with thimerosal. J Toxicol Clin Toxicol 1996;34:453–460.

86. Price JC: Polyethylene glycol. In: Kibbe AH, ed: Handbook of Pharmaceutical Excipients, 3rd ed. Washington, DC, American Pharmaceutical Association, 2000, pp. 392–398.

87. Rieger MM: Methylparaben. In: Kibbe AH, ed: Handbook of Pharmaceutical Excipients, 3rd ed. Washington, DC, American Pharmaceutical Association, 2000, pp. 340–344.

88. Rogers SC, Burrows D, Neill D: Percutaneous absorption of phenol and methyl alcohol in magenta paint BPC. Br J Dermatol 1978;98:559–560.

89. Rohyans J, Walson PD, Wood GA, et al: Mercury toxicity following Merthiolate ear irrigations. J Pediatr 1984;104:311–313.

90. Rubin M. Dear Health Care Professional Letter. Agenerase. Glaxo Wellcome, May 2000.

91. Saiki JH, Thompson S, Smith F, et al: Paraplegia following intrathecal chemotherapy. Cancer 1972;29:370–374.

92. Schamberg IL: Allergic contact dermatitis to methyl and propyl paraben. Arch Dermatol 1967;95:626–328.

93. Schiller LR, Emmett M, Santa CA, et al: Osmotic effects of polyethylene glycol. Gastroenterology 1988;94:933–941.

94. Schulte MJ, Lenz W: Fatal sorbitol infusion in patient with fructose-sorbitol intolerance. Lancet 1977;2:188.

95. Smyth HF, Carpenter CP, Shaffer CB: The toxicity of high-molecular-weight polyethylene glycols; Chronic oral and parenteral administration. J Am Pharm Assoc (Wash) 1947;36:157–160.

96. Smyth HF, Carpenter CP, Weil CS: The chronic oral toxicity of the polyethylene glycols. J Am Pharm Assoc (Wash) 1955;44;27–30.

97. Smyth HF, Carpenter CP, Weil CS: The toxicology of the polyethylene glycols. J Am Pharm Assoc (Wash) 1950;39:349–354.

98. Song BL, Li HY, Peng DR: In vitro spermicidal activity of parabens against human spermatozoa. Contraception 1989;39:331–335.

99. Speth PA, Vree TB, Neilen NF, et al: Propylene glycol pharmacokinetics and effect after intravenous infusion in humans. Ther Drug Monit 1987;9:255–258.

100. Stajich GV, Lopez GP, Harry SW, et al: Iatrogenic exposure to mercury after hepatitis B vaccination in preterm infants. J Pediatr 2000;136:679–681.

101. Sturgill BC, Herold DA, Bruns DE: Renal tubular necrosis in burn patients treated with topical polyethylene glycol. Lab Invest 1982;46:81A.

102. Sweet AY: Fatality from intravenous nitrofurantoin. Pediatrics 1958;22:1204.

103. Tanaka M, Iwata Y, Kouzuki Y, et al: Effect of 2-hydroxypropyl-β-cyclodextrin on percutaneous absorption of methyl paraben. J Pharmacy Pharmacol 1995;47:897–900.

104. Tripathi BJ, Tripathi RC: Cytotoxic effects of benzalkonium chloride and chlorobutanol on human corneal epithelial cells in vitro. Lens Eye Toxicity Res 1989;6:395–403.

105. Unger AH, Sklaroff HJ: Fatalities following intravenous use of sodium diphenylhydantoin for cardiac arrhythmias. JAMA 1967;200:35–36.

106. United States Pharmacopeia 24/National Formulary 19, United States Pharmacopeial Convention, Inc., Rockville, MD, 2000.

107. Vernon J, Brummett R, Walsh T: The ototoxic potential of propylene glycol in guinea pigs. Arch Otolaryngol 1978;104:726–729.

108. Warner MA, Harper JV: Cardiac dysrhythmias associated with chemical peeling with phenol. Anesthesiology 1985;62:366–367.

109. Winder AF, Astbury NJ, Sheraidah GA, et al: Penetration of mercury from ophthalmologic preservatives into the human eye. Lancet 1980;2:237–239.

C. PSYCHOPHARMACOLOGIC MEDICATIONS

CHAPTER *57* CYCLIC ANTIDEPRESSANTS

Erica L. Liebelt / Paul D. Francis

A 2.5-year-old female was brought to the Emergency Department (ED) for evaluation of a seizure. The child was previously well and had no other medical problems. The young girl and her sibling ate dinner at a neighbor's house a couple of hours prior to this incident, and after returning home, the mother noticed she looked tired, and thus brought her to the living room to watch television. The mother then described that the girl had a generalized tonic-clonic seizure that lasted about 1 minute with drooling and eyes rolled back. The paramedics described the young girl as very lethargic and postictal, with a blood pressure of 90/50 mm Hg, a pulse of 160 beats/min, and respirations of 26 breaths/min. They attempted an intravenous line but failed and transported her to the hospital.

At the request of the paramedics and of the emergency department physician on medical control, the mother called the neighbor to determine whether there were any prescription medications or other pills that the girl could have accessed while in the house. The neighbor did reveal that her son's amitriptyline (which he took for attention deficit hyperactivity disorder) was on the table while they were eating dinner and she had noticed that the bottle had been spilled. According to the neighbor's count, one or two 75-mg amitriptyline tablets were missing.

In the ED 15 minutes later, the girl was still sleepy, but responded to the physician's questions and cried when the IV was placed. Vital signs were blood pressure, 90/50 mm Hg; pulse, 200 beats/min; respirations, 26 breaths/min; temperature, 37.6°C (99.7°F); and pulse oximeter, 97% oxygen saturation on room air. Physical examination demonstrated large pupils (6 mm) that were sluggishly reactive to light, slightly dry mucous membranes, no meningismus, tachycardia, and an altered mental status. Initial bedside glucose was 110 mg/dL. Arterial blood gas showed pH 7.28; Pco_2, 38 mm Hg; and Po_2, 94 mm Hg; HCO_3, 13 mEq/L. Blood was obtained for electrolytes, liver enzymes, complete blood count, and acetaminophen, salicylate, and amitriptyline levels. The cardiac monitor showed a regular wide-complex rhythm and a 12-lead electrocardiogram (ECG) was obtained, which confirmed a wide-complex tachycardia with a rate of about 200 beats/min and a variable QRS interval with a minimum duration of 220 msec (Fig. 57–1A). The girl then had another generalized tonic-clonic seizure, which lasted about 60 seconds. Blood pressure dropped to 60/30 mm Hg. Oxygen at 6 L/min was administered by face mask and an attempt was made to place an oral airway, but it was spit out by the patient. Lorazepam (0.1 mg/kg IV) was given, followed by an IV bolus of sodium bicarbonate (1 mEq/kg) over 3 minutes and by a 1-mg/kg bolus of lidocaine. A 20-mL/kg bolus of normal saline was administered through a second intravenous line and the blood pressure in-

creased to 88/47 mm Hg. The patient was intubated. Orogastric lavage was performed with a 24-French tube and activated charcoal was administered (1 g/kg).

Another 1 mEq/kg bolus of sodium bicarbonate was given because there was no change in the rhythm on the monitor. A second ECG was obtained 30 minutes after initial interventions, which showed a heart rate of 150 beats/min and narrowing of the QRS complex to 140 msec with a terminal R wave in lead aVR (R_{aVR}) of 6 mm (Fig. 57–1B). A continuous infusion of sodium bicarbonate and saline was administered at 60 mL/h by adding 100 mEq of hypertonic sodium bicarbonate (1 mEq/mL) to 5% dextrose/0.25% saline to give a cumulative sodium dose of 138 mEq/L. No further lidocaine was administered. Venous blood gas showed a pH of 7.43. Prior laboratory studies did not reveal any abnormalities except for a measured HCO_3 of 14 mEq/L. The patient was transferred to the pediatric intensive care unit of a tertiary care children's hospital for further management.

On arrival, the patient was intubated and sedated. She had a heart rate of 136 beats/min and blood pressure of 99/53 mm Hg. A fourth ECG obtained 10 hours after the initial ECG showed a heart rate of 120 beats/min, QRS interval of 80 msec, and a R_{aVR} of 4.5 mm (Fig. 57–1C) The patient was extubated within 6 hours and remained in the intensive care unit overnight for continuous ECG monitoring. The ECG abnormalities resolved and the last ECG showed a QRS duration of 80 msec and a R_{aVR} of 1 mm. The patient was awake, alert, and normotensive. A quantitative serum amitriptyline level obtained at the initial hospital returned at 1003 ng/mL. The patient was discharged home the next day after social service consultation and a total of 24 hours observation following extubation, the termination of sodium bicarbonate infusion, and the resolution of ECG abnormalities.

Cyclic antidepressants (CAs) comprise a group of pharmacologically related agents used in the treatment of depression as well as neuralgic pain, migraines, enuresis, and attention deficit hyperactivity disorder. Most CAs have at least three rings inherent in their chemical structure. They include the traditional tricyclic compounds imipramine, desipramine, amitriptyline, nortriptyline, doxepin, trimipramine, protriptyline, and clomipramine, as well as other cyclic compounds such as maprotiline and amoxapine (Table 57–1). These drugs share unique toxicologic characteristics that have led to an array of basic science and clinical research aimed primarily on innovative and optimal treatment modalities.

847

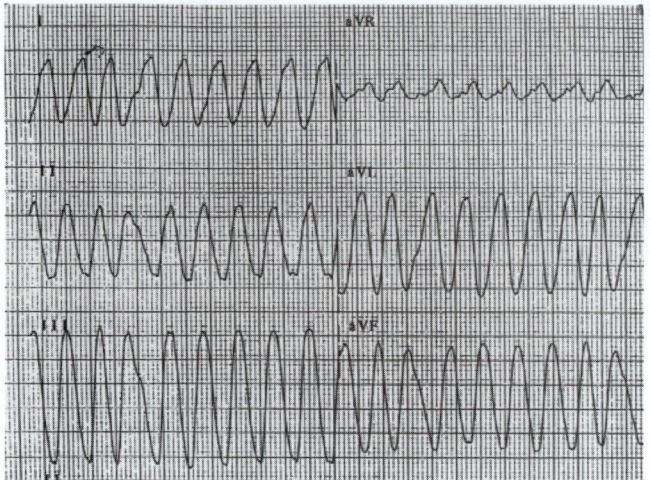

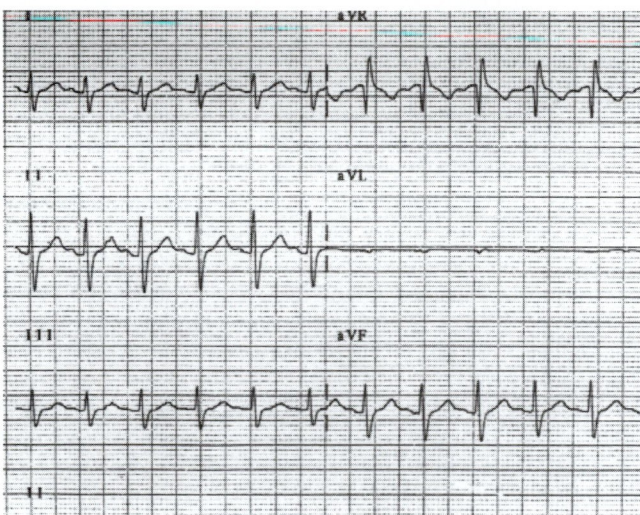

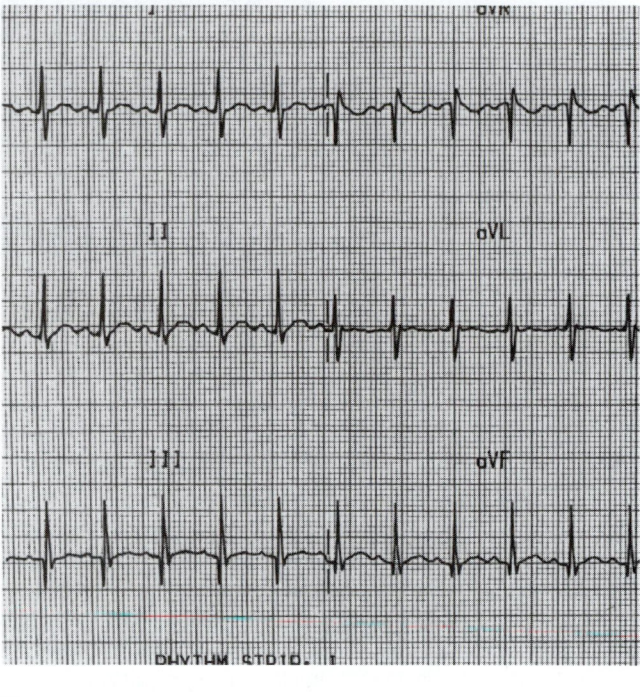

Figure 57–1. Case electrocardiograms. **A.** Initial ECG showing a wide-complex tachycardia with a variable QRS duration (minimum 220 msec). **B.** ECG 30 minutes after presentation shows narrowing of the QRS interval to a duration of 140 msec, and an amplitude of R_{aVR} of 6.0 mm. **C.** ECG 9 hours after presentation shows further narrowing of the QRS interval to 80 msec and decrease in the amplitude of R_{aVR} to 4.5 mm. *(Reproduced with permission from Liebelt EL: Targeted management strategies for cardiovascular toxicity from tricyclic antidepressant overdose: The pivotal role for alkalinization and sodium loading. Pediatr Emerg Care 1998;14:293–298.)*

HISTORY AND EPIDEMIOLOGY

Imipramine was the first tricyclic antidepressant (TCA) used for the treatment of depression in the late 1950s. However, the synthesis of iminodibenzyl, the "tricyclic" core of imipramine, and the description of its chemical characteristics date back to 1889.[7] Structurally related to the phenothiazines, imipramine originally was developed as a hypnotic agent for the sedation of agitated or psychotic patients and was serendipitously found to alleviate depression. From the 1960s until the late 1980s, the tricyclic antidepressants represented the major pharmacologic treatment for depression in the United States. However, by the early 1960s, the cardiovascular and central nervous system toxicity were also recognized as major complications of tricyclic antidepressant overdoses. The newer cyclic antidepressants were developed in the 1980s and 1990s to decrease some of the adverse effects seen with older TCAs, improve the therapeutic index, and hopefully reduce the incidence of serious toxicity. These included the tetracyclic

drug maprotiline and the dibenzoxapine drug amoxapine (Table 57–1).

The epidemiology of cyclic antidepressant poisoning has evolved significantly in the last 10 years as new indications for these drugs have emerged, aggressive prehospital care and excellent supportive medical care have developed, and the newer selective serotonin reuptake inhibitors (SSRIs) and other newer antidepressants have been introduced. The antidepressants are a leading cause of drug-related causes of self-poisoning in the world, primarily because of their ready availability to people with depression who by virtue of their depression are at high risk for overdose. In the United Kingdom between 1987 and 1992, the TCAs were associated with a significantly higher number of deaths (34) per million prescriptions, denoted as the Fatal Toxicity Index, than all of the other antidepressants taken together.[59,60] Also in the last 10 years, more medical indications for their use have emerged including chronic pain, obsessive-compulsive disorder, and in children, particularly, enuresis and attention deficit hyper-

TABLE 57–1. Cyclic Antidepressants—Classification by Chemical Structure

Tertiary Amines

Amitriptyline
Clomipramine
Doxepin
Imipramine
Trimipramine

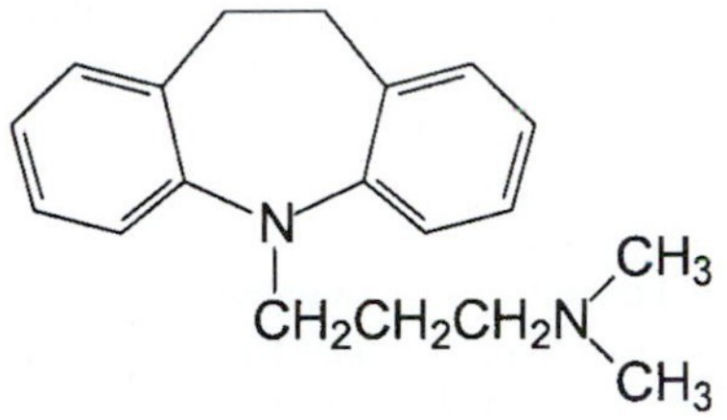

$CH_2CH_2CH_2N$ with CH_3 and CH_3

Imipramine

Secondary Amines

Desipramine
Nortriptyline
Protriptyline

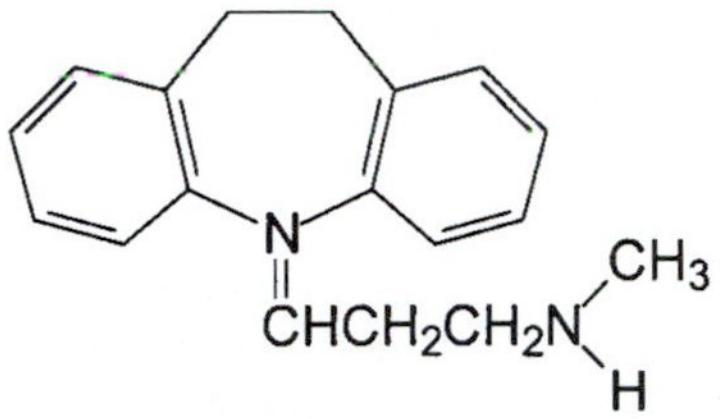

$CHCH_2CH_2N$ with CH_3 and H

Nortriptyline

Amoxapine

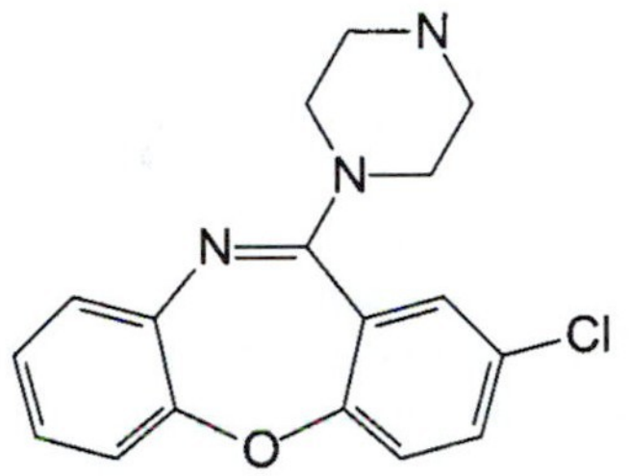

Cl

Maprotiline

$CH_2CH_2CH_2N$ with CH_3 and H

constant, although there has been a small decrease in the total number of CA exposures. What cannot be determined from these particular poison center data is whether prehospital deaths have declined and whether the total number of prescriptions for cyclic antidepressants has declined or remained constant, both factors that would contribute more meaning to the actual number of deaths. It was also recently demonstrated that there is a significant underreporting of deaths attributable to antidepressants through the AAPCC TESS data, making the significance of the actual numbers less clear.[64]

As the indications and uses for CAs, particularly TCAs, increase in children, there has been concern about whether the number of unintentional and intentional exposures has increased in this population. Children younger than 6 years of age have consistently accounted for about 13% of all CA exposures during the last 10 years. The number of younger children admitted for CA poisoning has also been increasing in the last 5 years.[39] Antidepressants (specifically TCAs) are the second most commonly prescribed psychotropic medication in preschool children, with a greater than 200% increase from 1991 to 1995.[171] Cyclic antidepressant ingestions will likely continue to have a greater fatality rate than the prototypical unintentional drug ingestion in younger children because only 1 or 2 pills can cause serious clinical toxicity in a small child. Furthermore, the numerous reports of sudden death in children on therapeutic doses of TCAs in the last 10 years contribute to the mortality associated with these drugs.

PHARMACOLOGY

In therapeutic doses the cyclic antidepressants exhibit numerous pharmacologic effects on the autonomic system, central nervous system, and cardiovascular system. However, they may be distinguished from each other by their relative potencies of each of these diverse biochemical effects, which are related to the modification of the basic cyclic chemical structure (Table 57–1). These pharmacologic differences appear to be unimportant at toxic doses as the clinical toxicity of most of the CAs is qualitatively and quantitatively similar with the exception of amoxapine and maprotiline, as noted below. The tricyclic antidepressants can be classified into tertiary and secondary amines based on the presence of a methyl group on the propylamine side chain (Table 57–1). The tertiary amines amitriptyline and imipramine are metabolized to the secondary amines nortriptyline and desipramine, respectively, which are themselves pharmacologically active and marketed as antidepressants.

The pharmacologic mechanisms of CAs include inhibition of neurotransmitter reuptake at central presynaptic terminals, central and peripheral anticholinergic effects, membrane depressant effects on the sodium channels of the distal conduction system, and inhibition of central sympathetic reflexes.[34] Cyclic antidepressants inhibit the reuptake of norepinephrine and/or serotonin and thus functionally increase the amount of these neurotransmitters at central nervous system (CNS) receptors. The tertiary amines, especially clomipramine, are more potent inhibitors of serotonin, whereas the secondary amines are more potent inhibitors of norepinephrine. These pharmacologic actions formed the basis of the monoamine hypothesis of depression in the 1960s. However, the mechanisms of action and antidepressant effects of these drugs appear to be much more complex than the simple inhibition of neurotransmitter reuptake.

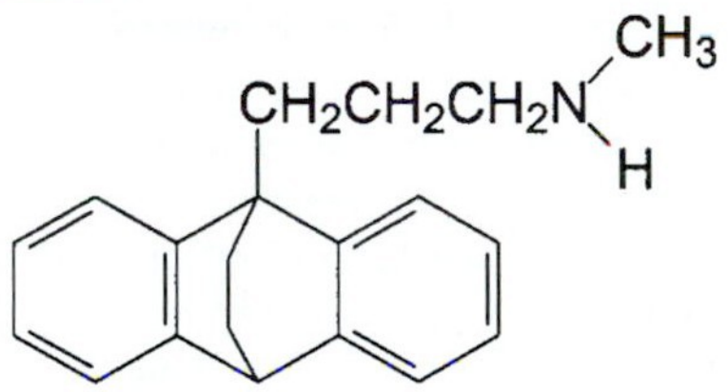

activity disorder, thus increasing their availability even more. In 1992, it was estimated that approximately 46 successful suicides would occur for every 1 million prescriptions written for tricyclic antidepressants in the United Kingdom.[59] Numerous epidemiologic studies, both in the United States and in Europe, demonstrate that the comparative risk of death is significantly greater with the tricyclic antidepressants as a group, as compared with the newer antidepressants, including the SSRIs.[60,69]

Based on data from the American Association of Poison Control Centers' (AAPCC) Toxic Exposure Surveillance System (TESS), cyclic antidepressants (primarily TCAs) were the leading cause of poisoning fatalities in the United States until 1993 when analgesics exceeded their position (page 1752 and Chap. 116). In the last 10 years, the number of deaths reported to poison centers that were caused by cyclic antidepressants has remained relatively

Extensive research in the last 10 years has led to the "receptor sensitivity hypothesis of antidepressant drug action," which postulates that alterations in the sensitivity of various receptors that occur only after chronic drug administration are directly related to their antidepressant effects. Chronic TCA administration appears to alter the number and/or function of central β-adrenergic and serotonin receptors.[122] In addition, TCAs modulate glucocorticoid receptor gene expression and cause alterations at the genomic level of other receptors.[9,82] All of these actions may play a role in their antidepressant effects.

All of the CAs are competitive antagonists of the muscarinic acetylcholine receptors although with different affinities. The acetylcholine blockade is responsible for the central and peripheral anticholinergic adverse effects, such as dry mouth, urinary retention, blurred vision, and sedation. The CAs also antagonize peripheral α_1-adrenergic receptors, which are responsible for orthostatic hypotension. With the exception of desipramine, they also have antihistaminic (H_1) properties accounting for their sedating properties. The membrane-stabilizing effect of CAs through sodium channel blockade is responsible for cardiac conduction abnormalities that occur even in therapeutic doses and is the primary mechanism of life-threatening cardiac toxicity.[50] Finally, animal research has demonstrated the interactions of CAs on the GABA-receptor chloride-ionophore complex in the brain. The effects of chronic TCA administration on chloride influx, chloride uptake, GABA transport, and specific GABA receptors may offer a novel mechanism of antidepressant drug action, as well as a mechanism of seizures seen in CA overdoses.[90,91,102,151]

Amoxapine is a dibenzoxapine cyclic antidepressant derived from the active antipsychotic loxapine. Although it has a three-ringed structure, this drug has little similarity to the other tricyclics. It is a potent norepinephrine reuptake inhibitor, has no effect on serotonin reuptake, and blocks dopamine receptors. Maprotiline is a tetracyclic antidepressant that predominantly blocks the reuptake of norepinephrine. Both of these CAs have a slightly different toxic profile than the traditional TCAs.

PHARMACOKINETICS AND TOXICOKINETICS

An understanding of selected pharmacokinetic properties of cyclic antidepressants is important when discussing their clinical toxicity and management strategies. These drugs are rapidly and almost completely absorbed from the gastrointestinal tract with peak concentrations 2–8 hours after administration of a therapeutic dose. However, in overdose, the decreased gastrointestinal motility caused by their anticholinergic effects and ionization in the acidic gastric juices alter these absorption kinetics, both factors causing further delay in absorption. Because of extensive first-pass metabolism by the liver, the oral bioavailability of CAs is low and variable, demonstrating the toxic potency of even small amounts of these drugs. However, metabolism may become saturated in overdose, increasing bioavailability. These properties contribute to the recommendations and rationale for gastrointestinal (GI) decontamination discussed later in the chapter.

Cyclic antidepressants are highly lipophilic and possess large and variable volumes of distribution (15–40 L/kg). These drugs are rapidly distributed to the heart, brain, liver, and kidney where the tissue:plasma ratio generally exceeds 10:1. In the canine my-

ocardium, CA levels exceed plasma levels by more than 200-fold.[67] Less than 2% of the ingested dose is present in blood several hours after overdose and serum TCA levels decline biexponentially.[114,135] The CAs are extensively bound to α_1-acid glycoprotein (AAG) in the serum, although there appears to be differential binding among the specific drugs.[2] Changes in the AAG concentration or pH can affect changes in binding and the percentage of free or unbound drug.[115,137] Specifically, a low blood pH (which often occurs in a severely poisoned patient) may increase the fraction of free/unbound drug, making it more available to exert its effects. Animal studies demonstrate that although the administration of AAG increases the concentration of total desipramine and protein-bound desipramine in the serum, the concentration of active free desipramine does not significantly decline.[115] Redistribution of CAs from tissues may account for this small change in the free fraction of the drug. All of these pharmacokinetic properties limit the value of antidepressant blood levels in assessing toxicity.

The CAs are metabolized in the liver by the cytochrome P450 (CYP) oxidative enzymes. The TCAs undergo demethylation, aromatic hydroxylation, and glucuronide conjugation of the hydroxy metabolites.[131] The tertiary amines imipramine and amitriptyline are demethylated to active metabolites desipramine and nortriptyline, respectively. The hydroxy metabolites of both tertiary and secondary amines are pharmacologically active and may contribute to toxicity after the first 12–24 hours. The glucuronide metabolites are inactive and this conjugation renders the lipophilic CAs more water soluble so they can subsequently be excreted by the kidney.

Genetically based differences in the activity of the CYP enzymes account for wide interindividual variability in metabolism and steady-state plasma concentrations.[131] Genetic polymorphisms of the CYP2D6 gene, which is responsible for the hydroxylation of imipramine and desipramine, are responsible for the slow metabolism in certain patients.[19,21,35] These "poor metabolizers" may recover more slowly from an overdose or demonstrate toxicity at therapeutic dosing.[16,149] This impaired metabolism is also postulated to cause death due to accumulation of parent drug and metabolites.[154] The metabolism of CAs may also be influenced by the concomitant ingestion of ethanol and other medications such as barbiturates, which may enhance their metabolism, or by drugs that inhibit the CYP2D6 isoenzyme (ie, SSRIs including fluoxetine, paroxetine, sertraline), which may increase the concentration of the CAs.[20,105,145] Patient variables such as age and ethnicity also affect CA metabolism. Increasing age reduces the renal clearance, accounting for much of the increased risk of toxicity in older patients.[131]

Elimination half-lives for therapeutic doses of CAs vary from 7 to 58 hours (54–92 hours for protriptyline), with even longer half-lives in the elderly.[122,135] The half-lives may be more prolonged in overdose as a result of saturable kinetics. A small fraction (15–30%) of CA elimination occurs through bile and gastric secretion.[47,92] The metabolites are then reabsorbed in the systemic circulation, resulting in enterohepatic and enterogastric circulation. There is little fecal excretion of these drugs. Finally, less than 5% of CAs are excreted by the kidney unchanged.[29,47]

The CAs have a low toxicity threshold, meaning a small increase over the therapeutic range may result in toxicity. Acute ingestions of 10–20 mg/kg of most CAs cause significant cardiovascular and central nervous system manifestations (therapeutic dose is 2–4 mg/kg/d). Thus, in adults, life-threatening overdose is usually associated with ingestions >1 g. However, in a 10-kg toddler, as few as two 50-mg imipramine tablets may cause significant toxicity (10 mg/kg).

PATHOPHYSIOLOGY

The CAs' effects on various neurotransmitters and the myocardial cells explain the pathophysiology of cardiac and central nervous system toxicity. Conduction delays, dysrhythmias, and hypotension characterize the cardiotoxicity caused by cyclic antidepressants. This toxicity results from drug effects on the myocardial action potential, direct effects on the vascular tone, and effects mediated by the autonomic nervous system.

The CAs block the rapid inward movement of sodium ions into the fast sodium channel, slowing phase 0 depolarization of the action potential in the distal His-Purkinje system, as well as the ventricular myocardium[50,163,166] (Figs. 57–2 and 21–6). Impaired depolarization within the conduction system slows the propagation of ventricular depolarization, which is manifested as prolongation of the QRS interval on the electrocardiogram. The right bundle branch has a relatively longer refractory period, and the subsequent intraventricular conduction delay and increased heart rate because of the anticholinergic effects disproportionately affect the right bundle.[108] This toxicity results in the rightward shift of the terminal QRS axis and right bundle-branch block that are seen in CA toxicity.

QT interval prolongation can occur in the setting of both therapeutic and toxic doses of CAs. This repolarization prolongation is a result of the CAs' effect on slowing repolarization and phase 4 (spontaneous) depolarization.[129] QT prolongation can predispose to the development of torsades de pointes. However, this dysrhythmia is probably more common in patients taking therapeutic doses of CAs than following overdose. Because torsades de pointes is more likely to occur in the setting of bradycardia, it is an unlikely finding in patients with acute CA toxicity.

Cyclic antidepressant–associated hypotension is multifactorial in its etiology. It is caused by direct myocardial depression secondary to the CA blockade of sodium entry into myocardial cells.[79] The inhibition of sodium entry into myocardial cells by the TCA blockade disrupts the subsequent coupling of calcium entry into the cells, thereby impairing myocardial contractility. Downregulation of adrenergic receptors with subsequent blunted physiologic responses to catecholamines is also suggested as another mechanism based on evidence of TCA-poisoned patients with actually normal to high serum catecholamine levels.[101] Peripheral vasodilation from TCAs' α-adrenergic blockade also contributes to the hypotension. The lack of efficacy of high doses of exogenous catecholamines suggests the mechanism of hypotension is not predominantly the depletion of norepinephrine.[101]

The most common dysrhythmia observed with CA toxicity is sinus tachycardia, which is primarily the result of peripheral cholinergic blockade. Norepinephrine reuptake inhibition also contributes to the tachycardia. Wide-complex tachycardia is the characteristic potentially life-threatening dysrhythmia observed in patients with severe CA toxicity and is probably multifactorial in etiology. By prolonging antegrade conduction, nonuniform conduction slowing may result, leading to reentry ventricular dysrhythmias.[163] Ventricular tachycardia may also occur in the setting of hypoxia and tissue ischemia, metabolic acidosis, and the use of β₁-adrenergic therapy. It is likely that most causes of wide-com-

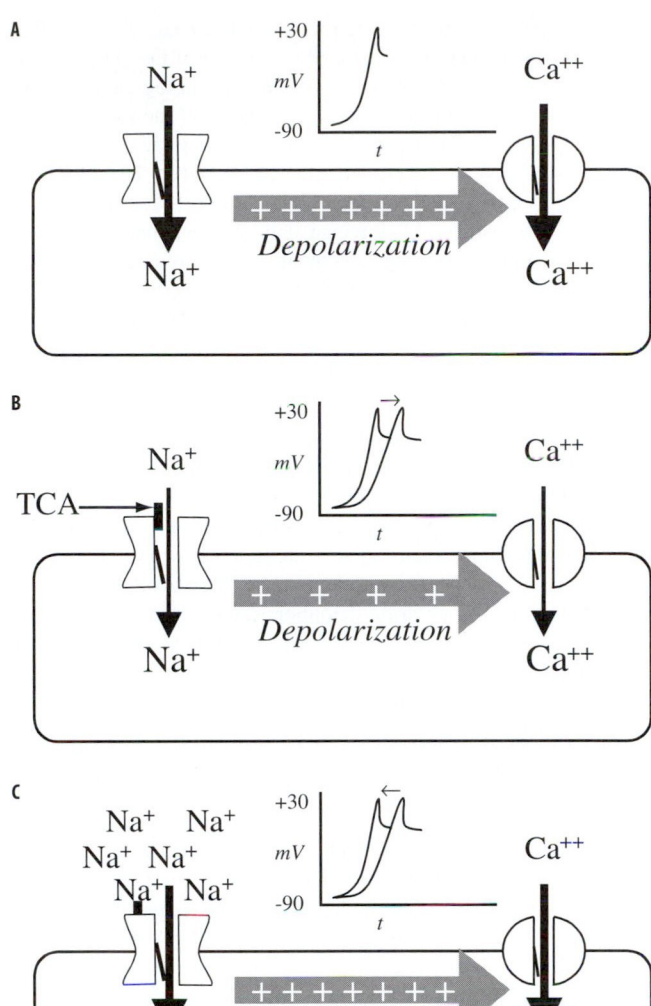

Figure 57–2. The effects of cyclic antidepressants (TCA) on the fast sodium channel. **A.** Sodium depolarizes the cell, which both propagates conduction allowing complete cardiac depolarization and opens voltage-dependent Ca^{2+} channels producing contraction. **B.** TCAs and other sodium channel blockers alter the conformation of the sodium channel, slowing the rate of rise of the action potential, which produces both negative dromotropic and inotropic effects. **C.** Raising the sodium ion gradient across the affected sodium channel speeds the rate of rise of the action potential, counteracting the drug-induced effects. See Figure 57–3 for the effects noted on the ECG.

plex tachycardia are actually sinus tachycardia with rate-dependent aberrancy. In such cases, the preceding P wave may not be apparent because of prolonged AV conduction, or widened QRS interval, or both. Electrophysiologic studies in a canine model demonstrate that QRS prolongation is rate dependent; that is, the faster the heart rate, the greater the conduction delay. In these studies, dogs could not accelerate their heart rate because they had a crushed sinus node and never developed "ventricular tachycardia."[3] Furthermore, induction of bradycardia through experimental pharmacologic agents prevented wide-complex tachycardia.[4] Earlier studies, however, demonstrated narrowing of the QRS interval with administration of propanolol.[134] This physiologic characteristic—use-dependent kinetics—is characteristic of the sodium channel blockade of Type IA antidysrhythmics (Chap. 52).

Attempts to find a causal relationship between TCA administration and myocardial disease through controlled trials have failed.[51,161] However, some recent data suggest that chronic tricyclic antidepressant drug treatment causes myocardial injury. Clinical studies using monoclonal antimyosin antibodies, a known marker for myocardial damage, demonstrate increased uptake of these antibodies in adults on long-term amitriptyline treatment.[94]

The agitation, delirium, and depressed sensorium characteristic of CNS toxicity are primarily caused by the central anticholinergic effects of the drug. The pathophysiology of CA-induced seizures has not been fully delineated and may be a result of a combination of increased levels of monoamines (particularly norepinephrine), antidopaminergic properties, anticholinergic properties, inhibition of neuronal sodium channels, and interactions with GABA receptors. Animal studies demonstrate that the interaction of CAs with the GABA-receptor chloride ionophore complex in the brain may be responsible for the convulsant effects of these drugs. Specifically, in drug-naïve rats, some CAs inhibited GABA-mediated chloride conductance, which was correlated with the frequency of seizures they induced.[90] A recent study in rats reported that amitriptyline actually augments chloride conductance in tissue.[91] This opposite action, may suggest yet another complex mechanism for seizures or may actually confer a protective anticonvulsant effect on patients who are chronically taking the drug prior to their overdose. The exact binding site of these drugs has not been elucidated, although some evidence suggests at least indirect activity at the picrotoxin binding site on the GABA chloride complex.[150]

CLINICAL MANIFESTATIONS OF TOXICITY

Cyclic antidepressant toxicity is characterized primarily by cardiovascular and central nervous system effects (Table 57–2). This toxic profile is qualitatively the same for all of the tricyclic antidepressants, but slightly different for some of the selected CAs, as noted below. The progression of clinical toxicity may be rapid and frequently unpredictable. It is common for a patient to present to the ED awake and alert and to then develop life-threatening cardiovascular and CNS toxicity within a couple of hours.

Acute Toxicity

Most clinical toxicity reported is derived from acute ingestions, especially in people who are chronically on the medication (acute on chronic ingestion). Clinical toxicity between these two cohorts of people does not appear to be different, although most studies do not distinguish between these two categories. It may be postulated that acute ingestions of smaller amounts of drug may result in toxicity more rapidly in people chronically taking these drugs because their organs may be more "vulnerable" to the drugs' effects.

Acute Cardiovascular Toxicity. Cardiovascular toxicity is responsible for the morbidity and mortality attributed to CAs. The characteristic features are conduction delays, dysrhythmias, and

TABLE 57–2. Clinical Manifestations of Toxicity Caused by Cyclic Antidepressants

Cardiovascular Toxicity

Conduction Delays	PR, QRS, QT interval prolongation
	T40-msec axis rightward rotation (120°–270°)
	Atrioventricular block
Dysrhythmias	Sinus tachycardia
	Supraventricular tachycardia
	Wide-complex tachycardia
	Sinus tachycardia with rate-dependent aberrancy
	Ventricular tachycardia
	Torsades de pointes
	Bradycardia
	Ventricular fibrillation
	Asystole
Hypotension	

Central Nervous System Toxicity

Altered mental status	Delirium
	Psychosis
	Lethargy
	Coma
Myoclonus	
Seizures	

Anticholinergic Toxicity

Altered mental status
Hyperthermia
Urinary retention
Paralytic ileus

hypotension. These toxic effects result from the drugs' effects on the myocardial cell's action potential, direct effects on the vascular tone, and effects mediated by the autonomic nervous system as described in detail below. Conduction delays include prolongation of the QRS interval and rightward shift of the terminal 40-msec QRS axis (T40-ms). PR, QRS, and QT interval prolongation can occur both in the setting of therapeutic and toxic doses of TCAs.[93] Second- and third-degree atrioventricular blocks are rare.

Sinus tachycardia (rate 120–160 beats/min in an adult) is the most common dysrhythmia associated with CA toxicity and usually does not cause hemodynamic compromise. Ventricular tachycardia is the most common lethal ventricular dysrhythmia although it may be difficult to distinguish this abnormal rhythm from supraventricular tachycardia with aberrant conduction or even markedly prolonged sinus tachycardia without visible P waves. Ventricular tachycardia occurs most often in patients with prolonged QRS interval and/or hypotension, and may be precipitated by seizures with accompanying acidosis.[88,156] Hypoxia, acidosis, hyperthermia, and β-adrenergic agonists may predispose the patient to ventricular tachycardia, which is associated with a high mortality. However, true fatal dysrhythmias are probably rare, as ventricular tachycardia and fibrillation occur in only about 4% of all cases.[53] Ventricular fibrillation, severe bradycardia and slow ventricular rhythms, and asystole are usually terminal dysrhythmias, although with prolonged administration of appropriate therapy they may be reversible. Prolonged cardiac massage may be necessary in cases of asystole due to CAs. Successful recovery has occurred in both children and adults receiving cardiopulmonary resuscitation despite periods of asystole exceeding 90 minutes.[110,147,158] Torsades de pointes is not common with acute TCA overdoses; it is more often found in people on therapeutic doses of CAs.

Refractory hypotension is probably the most common cause of death from CA overdose.[27,67,153] The etiology of CA-induced hypotension is multifactorial, as described previously. Hypoxia, acidosis, volume depletion, seizures, or the concomitant ingestion of other cardiodepressant or vasodilating drugs can exacerbate it.

Acute Central Nervous System Toxicity. Seizures and altered mental status are the primary manifestations of central nervous system toxicity. Delirium, disorientation, agitation, and/or psychotic behavior with hallucinations may be present. These alterations in consciousness are then usually followed by lethargy, rapidly progressing to obtundation and coma. The duration of coma is variable and does not necessarily correlate or occur concomitantly with electrocardiogram abnormalities. Coingestion of CNS depressants and/or concomitant hypotension may prolong the coma.

Cyclic antidepressant–induced seizures are usually generalized and brief and most often occur within 1 to 2 hours of presentation.[38,130] The incidence of seizures is estimated at 4% of patients presenting with overdose and 13% in fatal cases.[170] Uncontrolled seizures may result in metabolic acidosis, hyperthermia, rhabdomyolysis, and myoglobinuria with acute renal failure. Abrupt deterioration in hemodynamic status (hypotension, ventricular dysrhythmias) may develop during or within minutes after a seizure.[38,88,156] This rapid cardiovascular deterioration may be the result of a combination of seizure-induced acidosis and preexisting cardiovascular toxicity. The risk of seizures with CA overdoses may be increased in those patients on long-term therapy or who have other risk factors such as history of seizures, head trauma, or concomitant drug withdrawal.[146] Myoclonus and extrapyramidal symptoms may also occur in CA-poisoned patients.

Anticholinergic and Other Clinical Toxicity. Other anticholinergic toxicities include hyperthermia, urinary retention, paralytic ileus, dry flushed skin, and respiratory depression. Reported pulmonary complications include acute lung injury, aspiration pneumonitis, and the adult respiratory distress syndrome. Although pulmonary edema may not be correlated with hypotension, this clinical effect is most likely a result of coma, hypotension, pulmonary infection, and excessive fluid administration rather than the primary toxic effects of CAs.[141,142] Bowel ischemia, pseudo-obstruction, and pancreatitis are associated with CA overdose.[99,128,164]

Death directly caused by CA toxicity usually occurs in the first several hours after presentation for those patients who reach a healthcare facility. Late deaths (>1–2 days after presentation) are usually secondary to other factors such as aspiration pneumonitis, adult respiratory distress syndrome from refractory hypotension, and/or infection.[27]

Chronic Toxicity

Chronic CA toxicity does occur, and is usually manifested by exaggeration of adverse effects, such as sedation and sinus tachycardia, or defined by supratherapeutic drug concentrations in the blood in the absence of an acute overdose.[49] Unlike chronic theophylline and aspirin poisoning, this category of toxicity does not appear to cause the same acute life-threatening toxicity, although

there is little literature describing the clinical course of this cohort and it may even go unrecognized.

Several reports of sudden death in children taking therapeutic doses of TCAs have been published in the last 10 years.[121,126,127,160] The mechanism is unclear. QT prolongation with resultant torsades de pointes, advanced atrioventricular conduction delays, blood pressure fluctuations, and ventricular tachycardia are postulated mechanisms, although whether any of these effects contributed to the reported deaths is unknown. Prospective studies in children on therapeutic doses of TCAs by using 12-lead electrocardiograms, 24-hour ECG recordings, and Doppler echocardiography have failed to find any significant cardiac abnormalities as compared to children not on TCAs.[13,41] However, authors recommend that TCAs should not be initiated or continued on any child with a resting QT interval greater than 450 msec or bundle-branch block.[41]

Unique Toxicity from "Atypical" Cyclic Antidepressants

The CAs amoxapine and maprotiline have slightly different clinical toxic profiles.[165] Although the incidence of serious cardiovascular toxicity is lower with amoxapine overdoses, the incidence of seizures is significantly greater than for the traditional TCAs.[68,78,89] Moreover, seizures may be more frequent or status epilepticus may develop that is refractory to standard anticonvulsant therapy.[100] Similarly, the incidence of seizures, cardiac dysrhythmias, and duration of coma is greater with maprotiline toxicity as compared to the older TCAs.[33,77]

DIAGNOSTIC TESTING

Diagnostic testing for CA poisoning primarily relies on indirect bedside tests (ECG) and on other nonspecific laboratory analyses. Unlike acetaminophen evaluation, quantification of CA concentration provides little help for the acute management, but provides adjunctive information in supporting the diagnosis.

Electrocardiogram

The ECG is an easy and convenient bedside tool that can provide important diagnostic information in assessing patients, and in predicting clinical toxicity after a CA overdose. Cyclic antidepressant toxicity results in distinctive and diagnostic electrocardiographic changes that may allow early diagnosis and targeted therapy when the clinical history and physical examination may be unreliable. Furthermore, decisions about treatment and patient disposition must frequently be made in the emergency department without the benefit of other clinical parameters.

The maximal limb lead QRS interval duration is an easily measured ECG parameter that is a sensitive indicator of toxicity. One investigation reported that 33% of patients with a limb lead QRS interval of 100 msec or longer developed seizures and that 14% developed ventricular dysrhythmias.[17] There was a 50% incidence of ventricular dysrhythmias among patients with a QRS duration of 160 msec or longer. No ventricular dysrhythmias occurred in patients with a QRS duration of <160 msec. Subsequent studies have confirmed that a QRS duration >100 msec is associated with an increased incidence of serious toxicity including coma, need for intubation, hypotension, seizures, and dysrhythmias, making this ECG parameter a useful indicator of toxicity.[30,86]

A T40-ms axis between 120 and 270 degrees is also associated with TCA toxicity, and in one study, it was found to be a more sensitive indicator of general toxicity than the QRS interval alone.[30,108,168] A terminal QRS vector of 130–270 degrees discriminated between 11 patients with positive toxicology screens for TCAs and 14 patients with negative toxicology screens.[108] With further analyses, this report concluded that the positive and negative predictive values of this ECG parameter for TCA ingestions were 66% and 100%, respectively, in a population of 299 general overdose patients. A retrospective study reported that a TCA-poisoned patient was 8.6 times more likely to have a T40-ms axis of more than 120 degrees than was a non-TCA-poisoned patient.[168] Again, this parameter was a more sensitive indicator of TCA toxicity than the QRS interval. In both of these studies, patients with TCA ingestions/toxicity had altered mental status but not necessarily seizures and/or dysrhythmias specifically. However, the T40-ms axis is not easily measured in the absence of specialized computer-assisted analysis, limiting its practical utility. An abnormal rightward axis can be estimated by observing a negative deflection (terminal S wave) in lead I, and a positive deflection (terminal R wave) in lead aVR (Fig. 57–1B).

Easily quantifiable measurements in lead aVR on a routine ECG can also predict toxicity (Fig. 57–3). When prospectively studied, 79 patients with acute TCA overdoses demonstrated that the amplitude of the terminal R wave and R wave/S wave ratio in lead aVR (R_{aVR}, R/S_{aVR}) were significantly greater in those patients who developed seizures and ventricular dysrhythmias.[86] The sensitivity of $R_{aVR} \geq 3$ mm and $R/S_{aVR} \geq 0.7$ in predicting seizures and dysrhythmias was comparable to the sensitivity of a QRS $\geq$ 100 msec. In this study, an R_{aVR} of 3 mm or more was the only ECG variable that significantly predicted these complications.

Thus, specific ECG measurements such as the QRS interval duration and height of the R wave in lead aVR can be useful parameters in assessing and predicting CA toxicity, although neither is 100% sensitive in predicting cardiac and neurologic complications. Documenting the absence of these abnormalities on sequential ECGs, however, provides further evidence that cardiac toxicity is not developing. Serial ECGs should be obtained (at least three ECGs within the first 6 hours) to monitor for worsening of these parameters, which might signal the need for further interventions. Based on published data demonstrating ongoing changes of the QRS and T40-ms axis despite therapeutic interventions,[87] ECG parameters alone are not ideal and should be used in conjunction with the patient's clinical presentation, history, and course during the first several hours in decision making with regard to disposition and interventions.

Laboratory

Quantitative determination of CA plasma concentration has limited utility in the immediate evaluation and management of patients with acute overdoses. The CAs' pharmacologic properties—namely, large volumes of distributions, prolonged absorption phase, long distribution half-lives, pH-dependent protein binding, wide intrapatient variability of terminal elimination half-lives, and development of tolerance among people chronically on these medications—limit the value of plasma concentrations in predicting acute toxicity. Plasma concentrations usually do not correlate with acute clinical toxicity for these reasons. In one study, serum drug levels failed to predict the risk of seizures or ventricular dysrhythmias accurately.[17] Drug levels measured

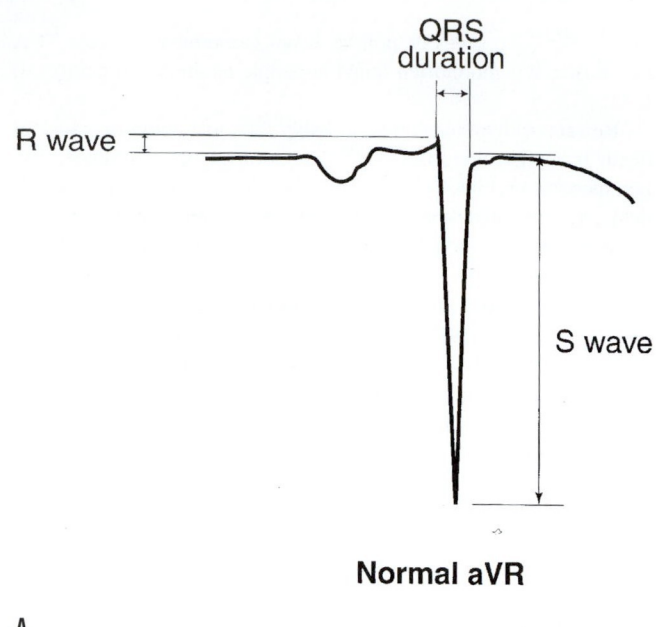

A

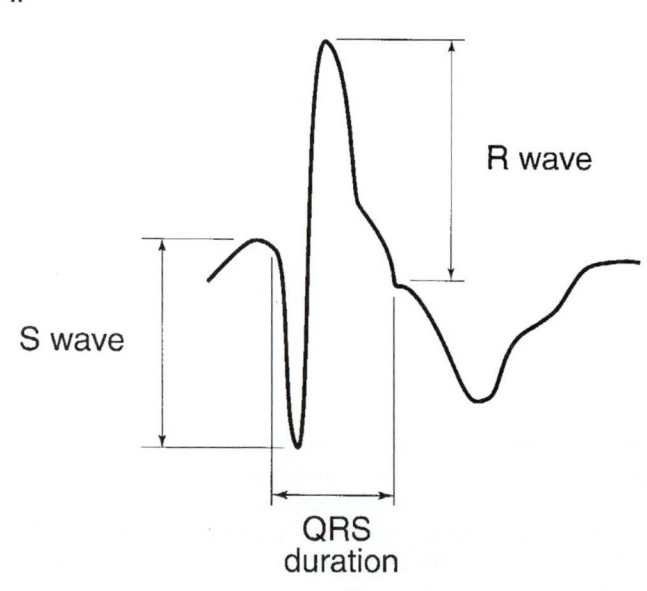

B

Figure 57–3. **A.** Normal QRS interval in lead aVR. **B.** Abnormal QRS interval in a patient with severe TCA poisoning. R_{aVR} is measured as the maximal height in millimeters of the terminal upward deflection in the QRS complex. The S wave is measured in millimeters as the depth of the initial downward deflection.

shortly after an overdose may be higher or lower than the final equilibrated level. Because of the high tissue:serum concentrations, the serum concentration does not accurately reflect the total body burden of the drug.

However, CA levels exceeding 1000 ng/mL are usually observed in patients with significant clinical toxicity (coma, seizures, and dysrhythmias), although life-threatening toxicity has also been observed in patients with levels less than 1000 ng/mL.[14,17,53,81,120,148] This serious toxicity at lower levels is probably a result of a number of factors, including the presence of coingestants, the circumstances of the ingestion (acute or acute on chronic), the timing of the level in relation to the ingestion, and the pharmacologic features as described above. Several studies demonstrate that both single and serial plasma levels are not predictive of clinical outcome or associated with clinical toxicity such as seizures and dysrhythmias and their resolution. Furthermore, quantitative levels are usually not readily obtainable in most hospital laboratories. Thus, evaluation and management should be guided by a combination of clinical signs and symptoms and the electrocardiogram.

Analyzing CA levels may be helpful in diagnosing chronic CA toxicity. Therapeutic CA concentrations (including active metabolites) are generally in the range of 50–300 ng/mL. Any level outside this range, when measured at the appropriate time in association with onset or increase in adverse effects (tachycardia, dizziness, prolonged QT on ECG), is an indication to decrease or stop the medication. Finally, quantitative levels may also be helpful in determining the cause of death in suspected overdose patients. Forensic studies have found lethal CA levels ranging from 1100 to 21,800 ng/mL. The measurement of liver drug concentrations or parent-to-metabolite drug ratios is preferable in the postmortem setting because CA levels may increase up to 5-fold[5,6] (Chap. 119).

Qualitative determination of the presence or absence of CAs may help to confirm a diagnosis in certain circumstances. It may also be helpful in making decisions regarding disposition and/or transfer in young children with unintentional ingestions who are asymptomatic. Cyclic antidepressants can be detected qualitatively in the urine by thin-layer chromatography or by high-performance liquid chromatography (HPLC). Bedside immunoassays are commercially available but have not been adequately studied.[136]

MANAGEMENT

Any person with a suspected or known ingestion of a CA requires immediate evaluation and treatment. Aggressive supportive care and hypertonic sodium bicarbonate are the mainstays of therapy (Table 57–3). The patient should be attached to a cardiac monitor and intravenous access should be secured. Early intubation is ad-

TABLE 57–3.   Treatment of Cyclic Antidepressant Toxicity

Toxic Effect	Treatment
Conduction Delays QRS > 100 msec $R_{aVR} \geq 3$ mm T40-ms axis > 130°	• $NaHCO_3$ —1 mEq/kg IV boluses to reverse the abnormality or to a target serum pH of no greater than 7.55 • Consider continuous $NaHCO_3$ infusion at 1.5 times maintenance IV fluid rate (150 mEq $NaHCO_3$ in 1 L of D_5W) • Controlled ventilation (if clinically indicated for hypoventilation)

Dysrhythmias
  Sinus tachycardia
  Wide-complex tachycardia/
    ventricular tachycardia
	• No treatment
	• $NaHCO_3$ —1 mEq/kg IV boluses to reverse the dysrhythmia or to a target serum pH of no greater than 7.55, and then consider continuous bicarbonate infusion
	• Controlled ventilation (if clinically indicated)
	• Correct hypoxia, acidosis, hypotension
	• Consider lidocaine—1 mg/kg slow IV bolus, followed by infusion of 20–50 μg/kg/min
	• Consider magnesium sulfate 25–50 mg/kg (maximum 2.0 g) IV over 20 minutes

Torsades de pointes	• Magnesium sulfate • Overdrive pacing
Hypotension	• Isotonic saline (0.9% NaCl) boluses (up to 30 mL/kg) • Trendelenburg position • Correct hypoxia, acidosis • $NaHCO_3$ —1 mEq/kg IV boluses to a target serum pH of 7.50–7.55, and then consider continuous bicarbonate infusion • Norepinephrine • Consider extracorporeal mechanical circulation (ECMO, cardiopulmonary bypass)
Seizures	• Benzodiazepines • Secure airway with intubation if necessary • Correct hypoxia, acidosis • Barbiturates if benzodiazepines fail • Continuous infusion of midazolam or propofol if barbiturates fail • Consider neuromuscular paralysis/general anesthesia if all other measures fail

Adapted with permission from Liebelt EL: Targeted management strategies for cardiovascular toxicity from tricyclic antidepressant overdose: The pivotal role for alkalinization and sodium loading. Pediatr Emerg Care 1998;14:293–298.

vised for patients with CNS depression and/or significant ECG changes (ie, wide-complex tachycardia) because of the potential for rapid clinical deterioration. A 12-lead electrocardiogram should be obtained on all patients. Laboratory tests including glucose and electrolytes should be sent on all patients with altered mental status, as well as an arterial blood gas to assess the degree of acidemia and to guide alkalinization therapy. Aggressive interventions for maintenance of blood pressure and peripheral perfusion must be performed early to avoid irreversible damage. The options for gastrointestinal decontamination should then be considered.

Gastrointestinal Decontamination

Ipecac-induced emesis is contraindicated, given the potential for precipitous neurologic and hemodynamic deterioration. Because of the potential lethality of large quantities of CAs, orogastric lavage should be considered in the symptomatic patient with an intentional overdose. Although the benefits of orogastric lavage for CA toxicity have not been substantiated by controlled trials, the potential benefits of removing significant quantities of a highly toxic drug must be weighed against the risks of the procedure.[18] Because the anticholinergic actions of some CAs may decrease gastric emptying, attempts at gastric lavage up to 12 hours after ingestion may yield unabsorbed drug. Patients with altered mental status or seizures should only undergo orogastric lavage after endotracheal intubation to protect the airway. The benefit of performing orogastric lavage in young children with unintentional ingestions of CAs may not be similar as in adults with intentional ingestions. These scenarios usually do not result in ingestion of large quantities of pills and the procedure may be associated with more risks and impracticalities (size of holes in pediatric tubes). Activated charcoal should be administered in all cases. An additional dose of charcoal several hours later is reasonable after a large ingestion or in a seriously poisoned patient where unabsorbed drug may still be in the GI tract, there may be desorption of CAs from activated charcoal, or if the patient may be a poor metabolizer. It is important to monitor for the development of a paralytic ileus to prevent abdominal complications from additional doses of activated charcoal.

Wide-Complex Dysrhythmias, Conduction Delays, and/or Hypotension

(Portions of this section are adapted with permission from Liebelt EL: Targeted management strategies for cardiovascular toxicity from tricyclic antidepressant overdose: The pivotal role for alkalinization and sodium loading. Pediatr Emerg Care 1998;14: 293–298.)

The mainstay therapy for treating wide-complex dysrhythmias, as well as for reversing conduction delays and hypotension, is the combination of serum alkalinization and sodium loading. This is probably best accomplished with hypertonic sodium bicarbonate (1 M solution, 1 mEq/mL, usually supplied as 8.4% solution giving 50 mEq per 50-mL ampule). In the late 1950s, alkalinization therapy with sodium lactate was proposed as a treatment for quinidine toxicity, which shares many of the CAs' cardiotoxic effects because of its similar mechanism of action.[11] French investigators recommended using sodium bicarbonate for treatment of tricyclic-induced dysrhythmias in the 1960s.[15,123] Uncontrolled clinical studies demonstrated that treatment with sodium lactate or sodium bicarbonate was effective in treating the cardiovascular effects associated with CA toxicity.[23] Subsequent controlled in vitro and in vivo studies in various animal models demonstrate that hypertonic $NaHCO_3$ is effective in reducing QRS prolongation, increasing blood pressure, and reversing or suppressing ventricular dysrhythmias caused by CA toxicity.[103,104,112,132–134] These studies also showed either equivalent or fewer beneficial effects of hyperventilation, sodium chloride, and other nonsodium buffer solutions as compared to $NaHCO_3$, suggesting multiple reasons for its effectiveness.

Several mechanisms are proposed for the beneficial effects of hypertonic sodium bicarbonate. First, elevating the blood pH through alkalinization increases the serum protein binding of CAs, thereby reducing the concentration of the unbound and pharmacologically active drug.[83] This mechanism probably contributes the least to the beneficial effects of sodium bicarbonate because only a very small fraction of the total CA dose is present in the serum, owing to its high lipid solubility and very large volume of distribution. Furthermore, animal studies examining the exogenous administration of binding proteins (AAG) to ameliorate TCA toxicity failed to demonstrate any significant differences in cardiotoxicity.[115] Second, increases in pH accelerate the recovery of sodium channels blocked by CAs by neutralizing the protonation of the drug-receptor complex, thereby facilitating the egress of the neutral form of the drug from the receptor site in the sodium channel.[133,134] Third, lowering of serum potassium levels in the presence of increased bicarbonate concentrations results in membrane hypopolarization, which, in turn, diminishes the blockade of sodium channels, which are voltage-dependent.[132]

Because underlying acidosis may exacerbate CA cardiotoxicity, an additional beneficial effect of $NaHCO_3$ lies in correction of acidosis. However, $NaHCO_3$ is also effective when the blood pH is normal, suggesting another predominant mechanism for its effects.[112,132] Increasing the extracellular concentration of sodium, or sodium loading, may overcome the blockade of the sodium channels through gradient effects (Fig. 57–2). This mechanism explains why in some animal studies $NaHCO_3$ was more effective in decreasing cardiotoxicity than were other sodium-free buffer solutions. Hypertonic sodium chloride loading reverses cardiotoxicity in several animal studies.[61,97,112] Hypertonic sodium chloride solution (15 mEq Na/kg) is highly efficacious in reversing QRS prolongation and hypotension, although an adequate direct comparison with $NaHCO_3$ is not available.[96] Unfortunately, no controlled human studies are attempting to dissect which mechanism of all those proposed is most important, although it is most likely a combination of all the mechanisms. Furthermore, no controlled studies demonstrate that sodium bicarbonate is effective; however, numerous reports and extensive clinical experience support its efficacy in treating serious CA cardiotoxicity.[22,23,62,63]

The optimal dosing and mode of administration of hypertonic $NaHCO_3$, as well as indications for initiating and terminating this treatment, are also unsupported by controlled clinical studies. Instead, this information is extrapolated from animal studies, clinical experience, and an understanding of the pathophysiologic mechanisms of CA toxicity. A bolus or rapid infusion over several minutes of $NaHCO_3$ (1 mEq/mL) at a dose of 1–2 mEq/kg should be administered initially.[23,96,112] Higher doses have been used successfully to treat patients, but experience is limited. Continuous ECG monitoring should be in place to follow the progression of the ECG abnormalities. Additional boluses may be administered until the QRS interval narrows, the amplitude of R_{aVR} decreases, the wide-complex tachycardia narrows, and the hypotension improves. Blood pH should be monitored after several bicarbonate boluses, aiming for a target pH of 7.50–7.55. Because there may be redistribution of the CA from the tissues into the blood over several hours for the reasons discussed previously, it may be reasonable to begin a continuous sodium bicarbonate infusion to maintain the pH in this range. Differences in outcomes between repetitive boluses alone and boluses with further bicarbonate infusions are not well studied. Although diluting $NaHCO_3$ in dextrose water or saline renders it less hypertonic, reducing the sodium gradient effect, the beneficial effects of pH elevation may still be warranted. The use of hypertonic saline solutions (3% NaCl) or combined $NaHCO_3$ and normal saline solutions (0.9%) for rapid infusion theoretically should be efficacious, although these modalities have not been adequately studied in humans.

Hyperventilation, although a more rapid and easily titratable method of serum alkalinization, is not as effective as a single modality in reversing cardiotoxicity.[72,96] Simultaneous hyperventilation and sodium bicarbonate administration may result in profound alkalemia and should be done only with extreme caution and careful monitoring of the pH.[169] Hyperventilation without bicarbonate administration may be indicated in patients with pulmonary edema or congestive heart failure where the administration of large quantities of sodium may be contraindicated.

Alkalinization and sodium loading with hypertonic $NaHCO_3$ along with controlled ventilation (if clinically indicated) should be administered in all overdose patients presenting with major cardiovascular toxicity. Indications include any conduction delays (QRS ≥100 msec, R_{aVR} ≥3 mm, and/or an unexplained or new right bundle-branch block), wide-complex tachycardia, and hypotension. Although the defined ECG parameters for conduction delays may be conservative indicators to start treatment, it is imperative to initiate treatment until CA toxicity can be excluded because of the risk for rapid and precipitous deterioration. The value of $NaHCO_3$ therapy for isolated sinus tachycardia, narrow-complex supraventricular tachycardia, and its prophylactic use without other signs of cardiotoxicity has not been studied. It is unclear whether the failure of the QRS complex to narrow with sodium bicarbonate treatment excludes CA toxicity. Treatment should not be empirically started because of the risks of hyperosmolarity.

Blood pH and resolution of ECG abnormalities have been suggested therapeutic endpoints for sodium bicarbonate therapy. Carefully monitoring and maintaining blood pH of 7.5–7.55 is a reasonable recommendation based on available evidence, avoiding profound alkalemia and its associated consequences. Some authors advocate for continuing alkalinization at least 12–24 hours after the ECG has normalized because of the drug's redistribution from the tissue. However, the time observed for resolution or normalization of conduction abnormalities is extremely variable, ranging from several hours to several days despite continuous bicarbonate infusion.[87] In some patients, clinical improvement occurred both before and during these ECG changes. Alkalinization is typically stopped or tapered when the patient has improved clinically and shown improvement of abnormal ECG findings. Additional therapeutic interventions for dysrhythmias and hypotension may be indicated if sodium bicarbonate and volume expansion with 0.9% NaCl are not effective.

Antidysrhythmic Therapy

Sodium bicarbonate therapy should be the first-line treatment for CA-induced ventricular dysrhythmias, although further therapeutic interventions may be necessary for those dysrhythmias refractory to this therapy.[104,134] By overcoming the sodium blockade, sodium bicarbonate can reverse the conduction slowing responsible for reentrant ventricular dysrhythmias. Lidocaine is the antidysrhythmic agent most commonly advocated for the treatment of CA-induced dysrhythmias, although there are no controlled clinical studies demonstrating its efficacy.[22,23,113] Because lidocaine has membrane-stabilizing properties similar to CAs, which may impair conductivity and decrease cardiac contractility, some investigators argue against its use in CA poisoning.[1] These theoretical concerns, however, are not well supported in the literature. The use of Class IA (quinidine, procainamide, disopyramide, and moricizine) and Class IC (flecainide, propafenone) antidysrhythmics is contraindicated because they have similar pharmacologic actions and thus may worsen the sodium channel inhibition caused by CAs and exacerbate cardiotoxicity. Class III antidysrhythmics (amiodarone, bretylium, and sotalol) prolong the QT interval and although unstudied, may be contraindicated as well.

Because of its antidysrhythmic properties, magnesium sulfate may be beneficial in the treatment of ventricular dysrhythmias. Animal studies of the effects of magnesium on CA-induced dysrhythmias have yielded conflicting results.[73,74] However, successful use of magnesium sulfate in the treatment of refractory ventricular fibrillation after TCA overdose has been reported.[76] The routine use of magnesium, however, needs further evaluation.

Based on electrophysiologic studies in animal models, the wide-complex tachycardia/ventricular tachycardia caused by CAs is rate-dependent.[3,133] Slowing the heart rate in the presence of CAs may allow more diastolic time for drug unbinding from sodium channels and might result in an improvement in ventricular conduction, which could then abolish the reentry mechanism for dysrhythmias. This mechanism was the rationale for the past use of physostigmine and propranolol. Thus, it is hypothesized that decreasing the sinus rate may itself be effective in abolishing ventricular dysrhythmias by eliminating rate-dependent conduction slowing. Propranolol terminated ventricular tachycardia in an animal model, but, unfortunately, also caused significant hypotension.[134] In one case series, patients developed severe hypotension or had a cardiac arrest shortly after receiving a β-adrenergic antagonist.[45] Other animal studies suggest that preventing or abolishing tachycardia by sinus node destruction, or by using bradycardic agents that impede sinus node automaticity without affecting myocardial repolarization or contractility, may successfully prevent CA-induced ventricular dysrhythmias.[3,4] The combined negative inotropic effects of β-adrenergic antagonists and CAs along with the significant cardiac and CNS effects reported with physostigmine use do not support their routine use in the management of CA-induced tachydysrhythmias at this time.

Phenytoin's use as an antidysrhythmic agent in CA toxicity has been extensively studied. Several animal and human studies advocate phenytoin's success in preventing or reversing some conduction abnormalities.[55,95] These studies show that phenytoin enhances atrioventricular and intraventricular conduction, as well as decreases ventricular automaticity. By increasing conduction velocity and membrane responsiveness, phenytoin could abolish reentrant dysrhythmias, making it a reasonable choice for CA-induced dysrhythmias. However, these studies are not well controlled for other confounding factors such as blood pH and sodium bicarbonate administration, they had very small numbers, and, in some, the cardiotoxicity was not severe. Other studies suggest phenytoin may have a proarrhythmogenic effect in the presence of

CAs, thus inducing or worsening ventricular dysrhythmias.[28] Based on available evidence, phenytoin is not recommended for wide-complex tachydysrhythmias associated with CAs.

Hypotension

Hypotension is the most common cause of death secondary to CA toxicity and is the most difficult complication to treat. Standard initial treatment for hypotension should include volume expansion with isotonic saline, placement of the patient in the Trendelenburg position, and alkalinization/sodium loading with hypertonic sodium bicarbonate (if conduction abnormalities are present also). Hypotension unresponsive to these therapeutic interventions necessitates the use of inotropic and/or vasopressor drug support and possibly extracorporeal cardiovascular support.

The choice of specific direct-acting or indirect-acting drug(s) to treat CA-associated hypotension is controversial because available data are limited and contradictory and because there is a theoretical concern that these drugs may precipitate potentially fatal dysrhythmias. Norepinephrine, epinephrine, dopamine, and dobutamine are proposed to be effective drugs for hypotension, but no controlled human studies are available. Furthermore, the pharmacologic properties of CAs complicate the choice of a specific agent. Specifically, CA blockade of neurotransmitter reuptake theoretically could result in a depletion of intracellular catecholamines. This blockade of norepinephrine and dopamine reuptake could then blunt the effect of dopamine, which is partially dependent on the release of endogenous norepinephrine for its inotropic activity.[25] Also, CAs blunt the dopamine-induced release of norepinephrine directly by preventing its neuronal uptake. These properties along with their α-adrenergic blockade and down-regulation of receptors suggest that a direct-acting vasopressor such as norepinephrine is more efficacious than an indirect-acting catecholamine such as dopamine. On the other hand, norepinephrine at high doses may be dysrhythmogenic and might exacerbate cardiovascular toxicity. Pure β-adrenergic agonists, such as isoproterenol and dobutamine, and even combination α- and β-adrenergic agonists such as dopamine, could theoretically result in unopposed β-adrenergic activity and may worsen the hypotension.

Animal data comparing various agents are conflicting and their direct applicability to clinical human poisoning is limited. In one study, norepinephrine (0.05–1.0 μg/kg/min) was more effective than dopamine (10–40 μg/kg/min) in an amitriptyline-induced hypotensive feline model; other investigators, however, found that dopamine was more effective in a similar model.[42,66] Another study showed that norepinephrine at doses of 0.25–1.0 μg/kg/min and high doses of dopamine at 15–30 μg/kg/min were equally effective in reversing amitriptyline-induced hemodynamic alterations in cardiac output, mean arterial pressure, and systemic vascular resistance.[162] A recent study reported that both norepinephrine and epinephrine increased the survival rate in TCA-poisoned rats.[75] In addition, epinephrine was superior to norepinephrine when used both with and without sodium bicarbonate, and the most effective treatment regimen in their study was epinephrine plus sodium bicarbonate—neither drug precipitated dysrhythmias. The authors propose that epinephrine is more efficacious because it augments myocardial perfusion more than norepinephrine and it improves the recovery of CA sodium channel blockade by hyperpolarization of the membrane potential through its stimulation of increased potassium intracellular trans-

port. These studies are limited because the effect of receptor down-regulation or catecholamine depletion cannot be assessed in the models of acute CA poisoning, which is different than many patients receiving chronic CA therapy prior to an acute ingestion. Furthermore, in all but one of these studies, animals were not treated with sodium bicarbonate, which is unlike clinical practice.

Limited clinical data have suggested that norepinephrine is more efficacious than dopamine.[157] In a retrospective study of 26 adult hypotensive patients, patients' response rates to norepinephrine (5–53 μg/min) were significantly better than response rates to dopamine (5–10 μg/kg/min).[159] Patients who failed to respond to dopamine at vasopressor doses (10–50 μg/kg/min) responded to norepinephrine (5–74 μg/min). However, the retrospective nature of this study and the subsequent lack of standard management therapies, indications for instituting vasoactive agents, and heterogeneity of the population limit its generalizability. In a case report of CA toxicity, glucagon is also reported to cause sustained increases in blood pressure.[139]

Based on the available data, pharmacologic effects, theoretical concerns, and experience, norepinephrine (0.1–0.2 μg/kg/min) is a sound choice for initial hypotension unresponsive to volume expansion and hypertonic sodium bicarbonate therapy. Central venous pressure and/or pulmonary artery catheterization may be necessary to guide the choice of additional vasopressor or inotropic agents, depending on the measured cardiac output and systemic vascular resistance, especially in the presence of other cardiodepressant drugs.

If pharmacologic measures fail to correct hypotension, extracorporeal life support measures should be considered. Extracorporeal membrane oxygenation (ECMO), extracorporeal circulation (ECC), and cardiopulmonary bypass are successful adjuncts for refractory hypotension and life support when maximum therapeutic interventions fail.[54,80,167] These modalities can provide critical perfusion to the heart and brain and maintain metabolic function while giving time for the body to metabolize and clear toxic concentrations of the drug by maintaining hepatorenal blood flow. Extracorporeal measures may then allow the impaired myocardium to recover. Further controlled studies are needed to evaluate these modalities and develop specific criteria for their use.

Central Nervous System Toxicity

Adequate airway protection with intubation should be initiated in any comatose patient or patient with a significantly depressed mental status because of acute CA toxicity. The use of flumazenil in the patient with a known or suspected CA ingestion is contraindicated. Several case reports of patients with CA overdoses have reported seizures following the administration of flumazenil.[56,84,98] Flumazenil antagonizes benzodiazepines at their receptor on the chloride ionophore of the GABA-receptor complex to reverse their pharmacologic effects. This action along with CAs' inhibition of GABA-mediated chloride influx may explain the increased risk of seizures in these people. Physostigmine is a short-acting cholinesterase inhibitor, that was used in the past to reverse the CNS toxicity of cyclic antidepressants.[26,106] However, physostigmine may increase the risk of cardiac toxicity and can cause bradycardia and asystole, as well as precipitate seizures in CA-poisoned patients, and thus is not recommended.[117]

Seizures caused by cyclic antidepressants are usually brief and may stop before treatment can be initiated. Recurrent seizures, prolonged seizures (>2 minutes), and status epilepticus need prompt treatment to prevent worsening acidosis, hypoxia, and the development of hyperthermia and rhabdomyolysis. Ensuring adequate ventilation and hydration may further minimize acidosis and prevent renal failure.[68] Benzodiazepines are effective as first-line therapy for seizures.[10] If this therapy fails, barbiturates should be administered. Failure to respond to barbiturates should lead to consideration of neuromuscular paralysis and general anesthesia with continuous EEG monitoring. Propofol controlled refractory seizures due to amoxapine toxicity.[100] Propofol also acts at the GABA-chloride ionophore complex.

The role of phenytoin as an anticonvulsant for CA-induced seizures is less clear. Some data demonstrate beneficial effects while other data question its efficacy. Phenytoin has been reported to reduce the incidence of amoxapine-induced seizures in dogs, but ineffective for imipramine-induced seizures in a rat study.[10,12] Furthermore, there are some animal studies demonstrating that phenytoin may potentiate ventricular dysrhythmias.[28] Based on this evidence, phenytoin is not recommended for seizures. The role of alkalinization and sodium loading in the treatment of CA-induced seizures has not been established, but is unlikely to be effective.

Elimination Enhancement

No specific treatment modalities have demonstrated efficacy in enhancing the elimination of CAs with subsequent improved clinical outcome. Some investigators propose multiple doses of activated charcoal to enhance CA elimination because of their small enterohepatic and enterogastric circulation.[92] Human volunteer studies and case series of patients with CA overdoses suggest that the half-life of CAs may be decreased by multiple-dose activated charcoal (MDAC).[32,70,109,155] MDAC reduced the apparent half-life of amitriptyline to 4–40 hours in overdose patients, as compared to previously published values of 30 to more than 60 hours in overdose.[155] Changes in the severity or duration of clinical toxicity, however, were not reported. Other investigators showed in human volunteers that MDAC reduced the half-life of therapeutic doses of amitriptyline about 20% as compared with no activated charcoal administration.[70] However, the methodologic flaws and equivocal findings of these studies along with the lack of any positive outcome data for this intervention from additional studies do not provide overwhelming evidence to support its use in this setting.[31,52] The pharmacokinetic properties of CAs discussed previously (large volumes of distribution, high plasma-protein binding) weighed against the small increases in clearance, and potential complications of MDAC, such as impaction, intestinal infarction, and perforation, do not warrant its routine use.[31] However, MDAC conceivably might shorten the duration of clinical toxicity in those patients who are "poor metabolizers." One additional dose of charcoal should be considered in patients with evidence of CNS and cardiovascular toxicity. Measures to enhance urinary CA excretion have a minimal effect on total clearance.[70]

Hemodialysis is ineffective in enhancing the elimination of CAs because of their large volumes of distribution, high lipid solubility, and extensive protein binding.[58] Hemoperfusion overcomes some of the limitations of hemodialysis, but should not be that effective because of the CAs' large volumes of distributions.[114] However, improvement in cardiotoxicity has been anecdotally reported during hemoperfusion in several uncontrolled case reports, although it may have been coincidental.[37] Currently, there is little substantial evidence to support the use of hemoperfusion in the management of CA overdose.

Investigational Therapies

Tricyclic antidepressant antibodies are showing great promise in providing additional emergent antidotal therapy. The development and investigation of antibodies to TCAs have been underway for more than 10 years.[65,71] An affinity-purified ovine polyclonal Fab fragment has sufficient affinity to remove TCAs (but not amoxapine or maprotiline) from serum and tissue receptors.[118,124,125,144] Because TCAs are lipophilic and have a large volume of distribution, toxic doses in humans are close to 100-fold larger as compared to digoxin, causing initial concern that immunotherapy for these drugs was perhaps not a rational modality of treatment. The amount of Fab fragments required for equimolar drug neutralization is enormous, which probably significantly impacts the cost, and possibly safety, of the drug. However, animal investigations clearly demonstrated that TCA immune Fab treatment was beneficial in reversing cardiovascular toxicity even when the dose was only about 10—30% of the equimolar dose of TCA.[24,36] Partial neutralization provided rapid improvement of QRS interval prolongation, hypotension, and heart rate in several independent animal models.

Initial clinical trials show favorable results with TCA-immune Fab treatment in improving both cardiovascular and central nervous system toxicity.[57] (Personal communication, Suzanne Ward PharmD, Protherics, Inc., Nashville, TN.) A Phase III clinical trial comparing TCA antibodies with standard treatment is currently being developed and is expected to be implemented in the future. This exciting new antidotal therapy will potentially impact on the mortality that is a result of TCA poisoning.

Experimental studies demonstrate that induction of ventricular tachydysrhythmias during tricyclic antidepressant toxicity is heart-rate-dependent.[3] A specific bradycardic agent, UL-FS 49, effectively impedes the marked sinus tachycardia and frequency-dependent ventricular conduction delay associated with amitriptyline toxicity in a canine model.[4] Pretreatment with this drug effectively prevented the onset of sustained ventricular tachydysrhythmias; thus, pretreated animals tolerated much higher serum concentrations of amitriptyline without adverse effect. In addition, unlike other β-adrenergic antagonists that have negative inotropic affects, UL-FS 40 did not appear to influence hemodynamics adversely, thereby potentially decreasing the risk of significant hypotension associated with its use. This investigational drug warrants further clinical studies in patients presenting with marked sinus tachycardia and conduction delays to determine its effectiveness in preventing wide-complex dysrhythmias and/or ventricular tachydysrhythmias.

Hospital Admission Criteria

All patients who present with a known or suspected CA ingestion should receive continuous cardiac monitoring and serial electrocardiograms for a minimum of 6 hours. Fears of delayed complications and inability to predict toxicity led clinicians in the past to adopt all-inclusive admission guidelines for the suspected CA ingestion. The once-standard practice of admitting all patients with CA ingestion for medical monitoring because of the risk of late complications or sudden death is not supported by the current literature. Most patients develop major clinical toxicity within several hours of presentation.[27] Several retrospective studies support a disposition algorithm which takes into account presenting clinical signs and symptoms.[8,27,44,158] If the patient is asymptomatic at presentation, undergoes gastrointestinal decontamination, has normal ECGs, or has sinus tachycardia (with normal QRS) which resolves, and remains asymptomatic in the healthcare facility for a minimum of 6 hours without any treatment interventions, the patient may be medically cleared for psychiatric evaluation (if appropriate) or discharged home, unless there are other medical issues.

A prospective study used the Antidepressant Overdose Risk Assessment (ADORA) criteria to identify patients who were at high risk for developing serious toxicity and thus proposed the following criteria for hospitalization.[43] In this study, the presence of a QRS interval >100 msec, cardiac dysrhythmias, altered mental status, seizures, respiratory depression, or hypotension on presentation to the ED (or within 6 hours of ingestion if the time was known) was 100% sensitive in identifying patients with significant toxicity and subsequent complications. Furthermore, none of the low-risk patients (defined as absence of all these criteria) developed any further toxicity or complications, supporting the decision for medical clearance and/or discharge. Table 57–4 presents proposed guidelines for hospitalization after a cyclic antidepressant ingestion, that are based on current epidemiologic and clinical evidence. These guidelines must be used in conjunction with knowledge of the patient's medical history and of the presence of coingestants that may present with similar signs and symptoms in making a decision for hospitalization or prolonged observation.

This guidelines and other studies also demonstrate that most serious or fatal CA ingestions will declare themselves within several hours after ingestion/presentation with these major signs of toxicity mandating admission. Criteria specifically for ICU admission (other than patients requiring ventilatory and/or blood pressure support) versus an inpatient bed with continuous cardiac monitoring are less clear and probably more institution dependent[152] (Chap. 104).

The disposition of patients with persistent isolated sinus tachycardia or prolonged QTc with no concomitant altered mental status or blood pressure changes is not clearly defined. Previous studies demonstrate that these two parameters alone are not predictive of subsequent clinical toxicity or complications.[43,44,53] In addition, the sinus tachycardia may persist for up to 1 week following ingestion.[107,140] However, another study of pure TCA-overdose patients reported that a heart rate >120 beats/min and a QTc interval >480 msec were associated with an increased likelihood of major toxicity.[30] These patients might be good candidates for observation units with continuous ECG monitoring and serial ECGs for 24 hours.

TABLE 57–4. Guidelines for Hospitalization after Cyclic Antidepressant Ingestion*

Altered mental status
Respiratory depression
Cardiac conduction defects
Cardiac dysrhythmias[†]
Seizures
Hypotension unresponsive to fluids

*Presence of any one of these signs at presentation or within 6 hours of the ingestion warrants admission.
[†]Presence of sinus tachycardia alone may warrant prolonged observation. See text for further explanation.

Qualitative toxicology testing demonstrating absence of CAs can provide additional support for discharging young children with questionable unintentional ingestions who remain asymptomatic earlier than 6 hours. Certainly for any patient, if there are any concerns about the accuracy of the ingestion history, psychosocial issues, or other coingestants with the potential for delayed toxicity, medical admission is warranted.

Inpatient Cardiac Monitoring

The duration of cardiac monitoring in any patient initially exhibiting signs of major clinical toxicity is dependent on many factors. Certainly the duration of CA cardiotoxicity and neurotoxicity may be prolonged as might be expected from the long serum half-life of CAs, in those patients who are slow hydroxylators, or in the presence of a coingestant that alters the metabolism of CAs or causes cardiac or neurologic toxicity. Recommendations from the older literature for 48–72 hours of ICU monitoring even in mild CA ingestions stem from isolated case reports of late-onset dysrhythmias, CNS effects, and sudden deaths.[46,48,116,138] However, review of these cases shows inadequate gastric decontamination, inadequate therapeutic interventions, and significant ongoing complications of overdose. Several retrospective studies demonstrate that late, unexpected complications in CA overdoses (such as seizures, dysrhythmias, and death) do not occur in patients who had few or no major signs of toxicity at presentation or a normal level of consciousness and normal ECG for 24 hours.[27,40,53,119,152] All fatalities due directly to CA toxicity occur in the first 12–24 hours.

Using normalization of ECG abnormalities as an endpoint for therapy and discharge is problematic and subject to discussion. Previous studies document the variable resolution and normalization of QRS prolongation and T40-ms axis rotation.[111,143] Small numbers of patients, inconsistent therapeutic interventions, and infrequent intervals at which serial ECGs were obtained flawed these studies. In a prospective observational study of 36 patients who had at least three ECGs in the first 8 hours, conduction abnormalities, specifically QRS interval prolongation and T40-ms axis rotation, varied widely in the time required for resolution, ranging from hours to days.[87] More importantly, these two parameters remained persistently abnormal despite standard therapeutic interventions, including GI decontamination and sodium bicarbonate therapy. Clinical improvement including mental status and hypotension occurred both before and during resolution of ECG abnormalities. Although this study was limited by the lack of premorbid baseline ECGs available for comparison, the data support the clinical impression that such patients are not at an increased risk for development of late complications.

Based on the available literature, it is reasonable to recommend that after the mental status and blood pressure have normalized, patients should be monitored an additional 24 hours off all therapy, including alkalinization, antidysrhythmics, and inotropics/vasopressors. If the patient shows improvement of ECG abnormalities with the above criteria, the patient may be discharged to a monitored bed on the ward with a low risk of further complications.

SUMMARY

Cyclic antidepressant poisoning continues to be a cause of serious morbidity and mortality worldwide. The distinctive characteristics of these drugs can cause significant central nervous system and cardiovascular toxicity, the latter being responsible for the mortality as a result of overdose of these drugs. Cardiovascular toxicity ranges from mild conduction abnormalities and sinus tachycardia to wide-complex tachycardia, hypotension, and asystole. Central nervous system toxicity may include delirium, lethargy, seizures, and coma. The ECG is a simple, readily available diagnostic test that can predict the development of significant toxicity, particularly seizures and/or dysrhythmias. Management strategies are based primarily on the pathophysiology of these drugs' toxicities—namely, sodium channel blockade in the myocardium. Alkalinization and sodium loading with sodium bicarbonate and isotonic saline are the principal modes of specific therapy for cardiovascular toxicity. Investigational immunotherapy with TCA antibodies has shown promising results in animal and initial clinical trials. Guidelines for observing or admitting patients to the hospital may be based on initial clinical presentation and/or development of clinical symptomatology and ECG changes.

REFERENCES

1. Ahmad S: Management of cardiac complications in tricyclic antidepressant poisoning [letter]. J R Soc Med 1980;73:79.
2. Amitai Y, Kennedy EJ, De Sandre P, Frischer H: Distribution of amitriptyline and nortriptyline in blood: Role of α_1-glycoprotein. Ther Drug Monit 1993;15:267–273.
3. Ansel GM, Coyne K, Arnold S, et al: Mechanisms of ventricular arrhythmia during amitriptyline toxicity. J Cardiovasc Pharmacol 1993;22:798–803.
4. Ansel GM, Meimer JP, Nelson SD: Prevention of tricyclic antidepressant-induced ventricular tachyarrhythmia by a specific bradycardic agent in a canine model. J Cardiovasc Pharmacol 1994; 24:256–260.
5. Apple FS: Postmortem tricyclic antidepressant concentrations: Assessing cause of death using parent drug to metabolite ratio. J Anal Toxicol 1989;13:197–198.
6. Apple FS, Bandt CM: Liver and blood postmortem tricyclic antidepressant concentrations. Am J Clin Pathol 1988;89:794–796.
7. Baldessarini RJ: Drugs and the treatment of psychiatric disorders. In: Gilman AG, Goodman IS, Rall TW, et al, eds: The Pharmacological Basis of Therapeutics, 4th ed. New York, Macmillan, 1985, pp. 387–445.
8. Banahan B, Schelkum P: Tricyclic antidepressant overdose: Conservative management in a community hospital with cost-saving implications. J Emerg Med 1990;8:451–454.
9. Barden N: Modulation of glucocorticoid receptor gene expression by antidepressant drugs. Pharmacopsychiatry 1996;29:12–22.
10. Beaubein AR, Carpenter DC, Mathieu LF, et al: Antagonism of imipramine poisoning by anticonvulsants in the rat. Toxicol Appl Pharmacol 1976;38:1–6.
11. Bellet S, Hamdan G, Somlyo A, et al: The reversal of cardiotoxic effects of quinidine by molar sodium lactate: An experimental study. Am J Med Sci 1959;237:165–176.
12. Bessen HA, Niemann JT, Haskell RJ, et al: Effect of respiratory alkalosis in tricyclic antidepressant overdose. West J Med 1983; 139;373–376.
13. Biederman J, Baldessarini RJ, Goldblatt A: A naturalistic study of 24-hour electrocardiographic recordings and echocardiographic findings in children and adolescents treated with desipramine. J Am Acad Child Adolesc Psychiatry 1993;32:805–813.
14. Biggs JT, Spiker DG, Petit JM, et al: Tricyclic antidepressant overdose—Incidence of symptoms. JAMA 1977;238:135–138.
15. Bismuth C, Bodin F, Pebay-Peroula F, et al: Intoxication par l'imipramine avec insuffisance cardiaque aigue. La Nouvelle Presse Medicale 1968;76:2277–2278.
16. Bluhm RE, Wilkinson GR, Shelton R, et al: Genetically determined drug-metabolizing activity and desipramine-associated cardiotoxicity: A case report. Clin Pharmacol Ther 1993;53:89–95.
17. Boehnert M, Lovejoy FH: Value of the QRS duration versus the serum drug level in predicting seizures and ventricular arrhythmias after an acute overdose of tricyclic antidepressants. N Engl J Med 1985;313:474–479.
18. Bosse GM, Barefoot JA, Pfeifer MP, et al: Comparison of three methods of gut decontamination in tricyclic antidepressant overdose. J Emerg Med 1995;13:203–209.
19. Brosen KD, Otton V, Gram LF: Imipramine demethylation and hydroxylation: Impact of the sparteine oxidation phenotype. Clin Pharmacol Ther 1986;40:543–549.
20. Brosen K, Skjelbo E: Fluoxetine and norfluoxetine are potent inhibitors of P450IID6—The source of the sparteine/debrisoquine oxidation polymorphism. Br J Clin Pharmacol 1991;31:136–137.
21. Brosen Z, Zeugin T, Myer UA: Role of P450IID6, the target of the sparteine/debrisoquin oxidation polymorphism, in the metabolism of imipramine. Clin Pharmacol Ther 1991;49:609–617.
22. Brown TCK: Sodium bicarbonate treatment for tricyclic antidepressant arrhythmias in children. Med J Aust 1976;2:380–382.
23. Brown TCK, Barker GA, Dunlop ME, et al: The use of sodium bicarbonate in the treatment of TCA-induced arrhythmias. Anaesth Intensive Care 1973;1:203–210.
24. Brunn GJ, Keyler DE, Pond SM, et al: Reversal of desipramine toxicity in rats using drug-specific antibody Fab fragment: Effect on hypotension and interaction with sodium bicarbonate. J Pharmacol Exp Ther 1992;260:1392–1399.
25. Buchman AL, Dauer J, Geiderman J: The use of vasoactive agents in the treatment of refractory hypotension seen in tricyclic antidepressant overdose. J Clin Psychopharmacol 1990;10:409–413.
26. Burks JS, Walker JE, Rumack BH, et al: Tricyclic antidepressant poisoning—Reversal of coma, choreoathetosis and myoclonus by physostigmine. JAMA 1974;230:1405–1407.
27. Callaham M, Kassel D: Epidemiology of fatal tricyclic antidepressant ingestion: Implications for management. Ann Emerg Med 1985; 14:1–9.
28. Callaham M, Schumaker H, Pentel P: Phenytoin prophylaxis of cardiotoxicity in experimental amitriptyline poisoning. J Pharmacol Exp Ther 1988;245:216–220.
29. Caraccio TR, Mofenson HC, Sturman K: Clinical toxicology of tricyclic antidepressants and cyclic antidepressants. N Y State J Pharm 1984;4:105–111.
30. Caravati EM, Bossart PJ: Demographic and electrocardiographic factors associated with severe tricyclic antidepressant toxicity. J Toxicol Clin Toxicol 1991;29:31–43.
31. Chyka P: Multiple-dose activated charcoal and enhancement of systemic drug clearance: Summaries of studies in animals and human volunteers. J Toxicol Clin Toxicol 1995;33:399–405.
32. Crome P, Dawling S, Braithwaite RA: Effect of activated charcoal on absorption of nortriptyline. Lancet 1977;1:1203–1205.
33. Crome P, Newman B: Poisoning with maprotiline and mianserin [letter]. Br Med J 1977;2:260.
34. Cusack B, Nelson A, Richelson E: Binding of antidepressants to human brain receptors: Focus on newer generation compounds. Psychopharmacology 1994;114:559–565.
35. Daly AK, Brockmoller J, Broly F, et al: Nomenclature for human CYP2D6 alleles. Pharmacogenetics 1996;6:193–201.
36. Dart RC, Sidki A, Sulllivan JB, et al: Ovine desipramine antibody fragments reverse desipramine cardiovascular toxicity in the rat. Ann Emerg Med 1996;27:309–315.
37. Diaz-Buxo JA, Farmer CD, Chandler JT: Hemoperfusion in the treatment of amitriptyline intoxication. Trans Am Soc Artif Intern Organs 1978;24:699–703.
38. Ellison DW, Pentel PR: Clinical features and consequences of seizures due to cyclic antidepressant overdose. Am J Emerg Med 1989;7:5–10.

39. Farrar HC, James LP: Characteristics of pediatric admissions for cyclic antidepressant poisoning. Am J Emerg Med 1999;17:495–496.

40. Fasoli R, Glauser F: Cardiac arrhythmias and ECG abnormalities in TCA overdose. J Toxicol Clin Toxicol 1981;18:155–163.

41. Fletcher SE, Case CL, Sallee FR, et al: Prospective study of the electrocardiographic effects of imipramine in children. J Pediatr 1993;122:652–654.

42. Follmer CH, Lum BK: Protective action of diazepam and of sympathomimetic amines against amitriptyline-induced toxicity. J Pharmacol Exp Ther 1982;222:424–429.

43. Foulke GE: Identifying toxicity risk early after antidepressant overdose. Am J Emerg Med 1995;13:123–126.

44. Foulke GE, Albertson TE, Walby WF: Tricyclic antidepressant overdose: Emergency department findings as predictors of clinical course. Am J Emerg Med 1986;4:496–500.

45. Freeman IW, Loughhead MG: Beta blockade in the treatment of tricyclic antidepressant overdosage. Med J Aust 1973;1:1233–1235.

46. Freeman JW, Mundy GR, Beattie RR, et al: Cardiac abnormalities in poisoning with tricyclic antidepressants. Br Med J 1969;2:610–613.

47. Gard H, Knapp D, Walle T, et al: Qualitative and quantitative studies on the disposition of amitriptyline and other tricyclic antidepressant drugs in man as it relates to the management of the overdosed patient. Clin Toxicol 1973;6:571–584.

48. Giles HM: Imipramine poisoning in childhood. Br Med J 1963;2:844–846.

49. Giller EL, Bialos DS, Docherty JP, et al: Chronic amitriptyline toxicity. Am J Psychiatry 1979;136:458–459.

50. Glassman AH: Cardiovascular effects of tricyclic antidepressants. Ann Rev Med 1984;35:503–511.

51. Glassman AH, Johnson LI, Giardina EGV, et al: The use of imipramine in depressed patients with congestive heart failure. JAMA 1983;250:1997–2001.

52. Goldberg MJ, Park GD, Spector R, et al: Lack of effect of oral activated charcoal on imipramine clearance. Clin Pharmacol Ther 1985;38:350–353.

53. Goldberg RJ, Capone RJ, Hunt JD: Cardiac complications following tricyclic antidepressant overdose—Issues for monitoring policy. JAMA 1985;254:1772–1775.

54. Goodwin DA, Lally KP, Null DM: Extracorporeal membrane oxygenation support for cardiac dysfunction from tricyclic antidepressant overdose. Crit Care Med 1993;21:625–627.

55. Hagerman GA, Hanashiro PK: Reversal of tricyclic-antidepressant-induced cardiac conduction abnormalities by phenytoin. Ann Emerg Med 1981;10:82–86.

56. Haverkos GP, DiSalvo RP, Imhoff TE: Fatal seizures after flumazenil administration in a patient with mixed overdose. Ann Pharmacother 1994;28:1347–1349.

57. Heard K, O'Malley GF, Dart RC: Treatment of amitriptyline poisoning with ovine antibody to tricyclic antidepressants. Lancet 1999;354:1614–1615.

58. Heath A, Wickstron I, Martensson E, et al: Treatment of antidepressant poisoning with resin hemoperfusion. Hum Toxicol 1982;1:361–371.

59. Henry JA, Alexander CA, Sener EK: Relative mortality from overdose of antidepressants. BMJ 1995;310:221–224.

60. Henry JA: Epidemiology and relative toxicity of antidepressant drugs in overdose. Drug Saf 1997;16:374–390.

61. Hoegholm A, Clementson P: Hypertonic sodium chloride in severe antidepressant overdosage. J Toxicol Clin Toxicol 1991;29:297–298.

62. Hoffman JR, McElroy CR: Bicarbonate therapy for dysrhythmias and hypotension in tricyclic antidepressant overdose. West J Med 1981;134:60–64.

63. Hoffman JR, Votey SR, Bayer M, et al: Effect of hypertonic sodium bicarbonate in the treatment of moderate-to-severe cyclic antidepressant overdose. Am J Emerg Med 1993;11:336–341.

64. Hoppe-Roberts JM, Lloyd LM, Chyka PA: Poisoning mortality in the United States: Comparison of national mortality statistics and poison control center reports. Ann Emerg Med 2000;35:440–448.

65. Hursting MJ, Opheim KE, Raisys VA, et al: Tricyclic antidepressant-specific Fab fragments alter the distribution and elimination of desipramine in the rabbit: A model for overdose treatment. J Toxicol Clin Toxicol 1989;27:53–66.

66. Jackson JE, Banner W: Tricyclic antidepressant overdose: Cardiovascular responses to catecholamines [abstract]. Vet Hum Toxicol 1981;23:361.

67. Jandhyala BS, Steenberg ML, Pered JM, et al: Effects of several tricyclic antidepressants on the hemodynamics and myocardial contractility of the anesthetized dogs. Eur J Pharmacol 1977;42:403–410.

68. Jennings AE, Levey AS, Harrington JT: Amoxapine associated with acute renal failure. Arch Intern Med 1983;143:1525–1527.

69. Kapur S, Mieczkowski T, Mann J: Antidepressant medications and the relative risk of suicide attempt and suicide. JAMA 1992;268:3441–3445.

70. Karkkainen S, Neuvonen PJ: Pharmacokinetics of amitriptyline influenced by oral charcoal and urine pH. Int J Clin Pharmacol Ther Toxicol 1986;24:326–332.

71. Keyler DE, Le Couteur DG, Pond SM, et al: Effects of specific antibody Fab fragments on desipramine pharmacokinetics in the rat in vivo and in the isolated, perfused liver. J Pharmacol Exp Ther 1995;272:1117–1123.

72. Kingston ME: Hyperventilation in tricyclic antidepressant poisoning. Crit Care Med 1979;7:550–551.

73. Kline JA, DeStefano AA, Schroeder JD, et al: Magnesium potentiates imipramine toxicity in the isolated rat heart. Ann Emerg Med 1994;24:224–232.

74. Knudsen K, Abrahamsson J: Effects of magnesium sulfate and lidocaine in the treatment of ventricular arrhythmias in experimental amitriptyline poisoning in the rat. Crit Care Med 1994;22:494–498.

75. Knudsen K, Abrahamsson J: Epinephrine and sodium bicarbonate independently and additively increase survival in experimental amitriptyline poisoning. Crit Care Med 1997;27:669–674.

76. Knudsen K, Abrahamsson J: Magnesium sulphate in the treatment of ventricular fibrillation in amitriptyline poisoning [letter]. Eur Heart J 1997;18:881–882.

77. Knudsen K, Heath A: Effects of self-poisoning with maprotiline. Br Med J 1984;288:601–603.

78. Kulig K, Rumack BH, Sullivan JB, et al: Amoxapine overdose: Coma and seizures without cardiotoxic effects. JAMA 1982;248:1092–1094.

79. Langou RA, Van Dyke C, Tahan SR, et al: Cardiovascular manifestations of tricyclic antidepressant overdose. Am Heart J 1980;100:458–464.

80. Larkin GL, Graeber GM, Hollingshed MJ: Experimental amitriptyline poisoning: Treatment of severe cardiovascular toxicity with cardiopulmonary bypass. Ann Emerg Med 1994;23:480–486.

81. Lavoie FW, Gansert GG, Weiss RE: Value of initial ECG findings and plasma drug levels in cyclic antidepressant overdose. Ann Emerg Med 1990;19:696–700.

82. Lesch KP, Manji HK: Signal-transducing G proteins and antidepressant drugs: Evidence for modulation of alpha subunit gene expression in rat brain. Biol Psychiatr 1992;32:549–579.

83. Levitt MA, Sullivan JB Jr, Owens SM, et al: Amitriptyline plasma protein building: Effect of plasma pH and relevance to clinical overdose. Am J Emerg Med 1986;4:121–125.

84. Lheureux P, Vranckx M, Leduc D, et al. Flumazenil in mixed benzodiazepine/tricyclic antidepressant overdose: A placebo-controlled study in the dog. Am J Emerg Med 1992;10:184–188.

85. Liebelt EL: Targeted management strategies for cardiovascular toxicity from tricyclic antidepressant overdose: The pivotal role for alkalinization and sodium loading. Pediatr Emerg Care 1998;14:293–298.

86. Liebelt EL, Francis PD, Woolf AD: ECG lead aVR versus QRS interval in predicting seizures and arrhythmias in acute tricyclic antidepressant toxicity. Ann Emerg Med 1995;26:195–201.

87. Liebelt EL, Ulrich A, Francis PD, et al: Serial electrocardiogram changes in acute tricyclic antidepressant overdoses. Crit Care Med 1997;25:1721–1726.

88. Lipper B, Bell A, Gaynor B: Recurrent hypotension immediately after seizures in nortriptyline overdose. Am J Emerg Med 1994;12:451–457.

89. Litovitz TL, Troutman WG: Amoxapine overdose: Seizures and fatalities. JAMA 1983;250:1069–1071.

90. Malatynska E, Knapp RJ, Ikeda M, et al: Antidepressants and seizure-interactions at the GABA-receptor chloride-ionophore complex. Life Sci 1988;43:303–307.

91. Malatynska E, Miller C, Schindler N, et al: Amitriptyline increases GABA-stimulated 36Cl-influx by recombinant (alpha 1 gamma) GABA A receptors. Brain Res 1999;851:277–280.

92. Manoguerra AS, Weaver LC: Poisoning with tricyclic antidepressant drugs. Clin Toxicol 1977;10:149–158.

93. Marshall JB, Forker AD: Cardiovascular effects of tricyclic antidepressant drugs: Therapeutic usage, overdose, and management of complications. Am Heart J 1982;103:401–414.

94. Martí V, Ballester M, Udina C, et al: Evaluation of myocardial cell damage by In-111-monoconcal antimyosin antibodies in patients under chronic tricyclic antidepressant drug treatment. Circulation 1995;91:1619–1623.

95. Mayron R, Ruiz E: Phenytoin: Does it reverse tricyclic antidepressant-induced cardiac conduction abnormalities? Ann Emerg Med 1986;15:876–880.

96. McCabe JL, Cobaugh DJ, Menegazzi JJ, et al: Experimental tricyclic antidepressant toxicity: A randomized, controlled comparison of hypertonic saline solution, sodium bicarbonate, and hyperventilation. Ann Emerg Med 1998;32:329–333.

97. McCabe JL, Menegazzi JJ, Cobaugh DJ, et al. Recovery from severe cyclic antidepressant overdose with hypertonic saline/dextran in a swine model. Acad Emerg Med 1994;1:111–115.

98. McDuffee AT, Tobias JD: Seizure after flumazenil administration in a pediatric patient. Pediatr Emerg Care 1995;11:186–187.

99. McMahon AJ: Amitriptyline overdose complicated by intestinal pseudo-obstruction and caecal perforation. Postgrad Med J 1989;65:948–949.

100. Merigian KS, Browning RG, Leeper KV: Successful treatment of amoxapine-induced refractory status epilepticus with propofol (Diprivan). Acad Emerg Med 1995;2:128–133.

101. Merigian KS, Hedges JR, Kaplan LA, et al: Plasma catecholamine levels in cyclic antidepressant overdose. J Toxicol Clin Toxicol 1991;29:177–190.

102. Nakashita M, Sasaki K, Sakai N, et al: Effects of tricyclic and tetracyclic antidepressants on the three subtypes of GABA transporter. Neurosci Res 1997;29:87–91.

103. Nattel S, Keable H, Sasyniuk BI: Experimental amitriptyline intoxication: Electrophysiologic manifestations and management. J Cardiovasc Pharmacol 1984;6:83–89.

104. Nattel S, Mittleman M: Treatment of ventricular tachyarrhythmias resulting from amitriptyline toxicity in dogs. J Pharmacol Exp Ther 1984;231:430–435.

105. Nemeroff CB, DeVane CL, Pollock BG: Newer antidepressants and the cytochrome P450 system. Am J Psychiatry 1996;153:311–320.

106. Newton RW: Physostigmine salicylate in the treatment of tricyclic antidepressant overdosage. JAMA 1975;231:941–943.

107. Nicotra MB, Rivera M, Pool JL, et al: TCA overdose: Clinical and pharmacologic observations. J Toxicol Clin Toxicol 1981;18:599–613.

108. Niemann JT, Bessen HA, Rothstein RJ, et al: Electrocardiographic criteria for tricyclic antidepressant cardiotoxicity. Am J Cardiol 1986;57:1154–1159.

109. Oppenheim RC, Stewart NF: Adsorption of tricyclic antidepressants by activated charcoal. I. Adsorption in low pH conditions. Aust J Pharm Sci 1975;4:79–84.

110. Orr DAK, Bramble MG: Tricyclic antidepressant poisoning and prolonged external cardiac massage during asystole. Br Med J 1981;283:1107–1108.

111. Pellinen TJ, Färkkilä M, Heikkilä J, et al: Electrocardiographic and clinical features of tricyclic antidepressant intoxication. Ann Clin Res 1987;19:12–17.

112. Pentel P, Benowitz N: Efficacy and mechanism of action of sodium bicarbonate in the treatment of desipramine toxicity in rats. J Pharmacol Exp Ther 1984;230:12–19.

113. Pentel PR, Benowitz NL: Tricyclic antidepressant poisoning—Management of arrhythmias. Med Toxicol 1986;1:101–121.

114. Pentel PR, Bullock ML, DeVane CL: Hemoperfusion for imipramine overdose: Elimination of active metabolites. J Toxicol Clin Toxicol 1982;10:239–248.

115. Pentel PR, Keyler DE: Effects of high dose alpha-1-acid glycoprotein on desipramine toxicity in rats. J Pharmacol Exp Ther 1988;246:1061–1066.

116. Pentel P, Olson KR, Becker CE, et al: Late complications of tricyclic antidepressant overdose. West J Med 1983;138:423–424.

117. Pentel P, Peterson CD: Asystole complicating physostigmine treatment of tricyclic antidepressant overdose. Ann Emerg Med 1980;9:588–590.

118. Pentel PR, Scarlett W, Ross CA, et al: Reduction of desipramine cardiotoxicity and prolongation of survival in rats with the use of polyclonal drug-specific antibody Fab fragments. Ann Emerg Med 1995;26:334–340.

119. Pentel P, Sioris L: Incidence of late arrhythmias following tricyclic antidepressant overdose. Clin Toxicol 1981;18:543–548.

120. Petit JM, Spiker DG, Ruwitch JF, et al: Tricyclic antidepressant plasma levels and adverse effects after overdose. Clin Pharmacol Ther 1977;21:47–51.

121. Popper CW, Ziminitzky B: Sudden death putatively related to desipramine treatment in youth: A fifth case and a review of speculative mechanisms. J Child Adolesc Psychopharmacol 1995;5:283–300.

122. Potter WZ, Manji HK, Rudorfer MW: Tricyclics and tetracyclics. In: Schatzberg AF, Nemeroff CB, eds: The American Psychiatric Press Textbook of Psychopharmacology, 2nd ed. Washington, DC, American Psychiatric Press, 1998, pp. 199–218.

123. Prudhommeaux JL, Lechat P, Auclair MC: Etude experimentale de l'influence des ions sodium sur la toxicite cardiaque de l'imipramine. Therapie (Paris) 1968;23:675–683.

124. Ragusi C, Boschi G, Risede P, et al: Influence of various combinations of specific antibody dose and affinity on tissue imipramine redistribution. Br J Pharmacol 1998;125:35–40.

125. Ragusi C, Scherrmann JM, Harrison K, et al: Redistribution of imipramine from regions of the brain under the influence of circulating specific antibodies. J Neurochem 1998;70:2099–2105.

126. Riddle MA, Geller B, Ryan N: Case study: Another sudden death in a child treated with desipramine. J Am Acad Child Adolesc Psychiatry 1993:32:792–797.

127. Riddle MA, Nelson JC, Kleinman CS, et al: Sudden death in children receiving Norpramin: A review of three reported cases and commentary. J Am Acad Child Adolesc Psychiatry 1991;30:104–108.

128. Roberge RJ, Martin TG, Hodgman M, Benitez JG: Acute chemical pancreatitis associated with a tricyclic antidepressant (clomipramine) overdose. J Toxicol Clin Toxicol 1994;32:425–429.

129. Rodriguez S, Tomargo J: Electrophysiological effects of imipramine on bovine ventricular muscle and Purkinje fibres. Br J Pharmacol 1980;70:15–23.

130. Rosenstein DL, Nelson JC, Jacobs SC: Seizures associated with antidepressants: A review. J Clin Psychiatry 1993;54:289–299.

131. Rudorfer MV, Potter WZ: Metabolism of tricyclic antidepressants. Cell Mol Neurobiol 1999;19:373–409.

132. Sasyniuk BI, Jhamandas V: Mechanism of reversal of toxic effects of amitriptyline on cardiac Purkinje fibers by sodium bicarbonate. J Pharmacol Exp Ther 1984;231:387–394.

133. Sasyniuk BI, Jhamandas V: Frequency-dependent effects of amitriptyline on V_{max} in canine Purkinje fibers and its alteration by alkalosis. Proc West Pharmacol Soc 1986;29:73–75.

134. Sasyniuk BI, Jhamandas V, Valois M: Experimental amitriptyline intoxication: Treatment of cardiac toxicity with sodium bicarbonate. Ann Emerg Med 1986;15:1052–1059.

135. Schulz P, Turner-Tamiysay K, Smith G, et al: Amitriptyline disposition in young and elderly normal men. Clin Pharmacol Ther 1983; 33:360–366.

136. Schwartz JG, Hurd IL, Carnahan JJ: Determination of tricyclic antidepressants for ED analysis. Am J Emerg Med 1994;12:513–516.

137. Seaberg DC, Weiss LD, Yeally DM, et al: Effects of alpha-1-acid glycoprotein on the cardiovascular toxicity of nortriptyline in a swine model. Vet Hum Toxicol 1991;33:226–230.

138. Sedal L, Korman M, Williams P, et al: Overdosage of tricyclic antidepressants. Med J Aust 1972;2:74–79.

139. Sener EK, Gabe S, Henry JA: Response to glucagon in imipramine overdose. J Toxicol Clin Toxicol 1995;33:51–53.

140. Serafimovski N, Thorball N, Asmussen I, et al: Tricyclic antidepressive poisoning with special references to cardiac complications. Acta Anaesthesiol Scand Suppl 1975;57:55–63.

141. Shannon M, Lovejoy FH: Pulmonary consequences of severe tricyclic antidepressant ingestion. J Toxicol Clin Toxicol 1987;25: 443–461.

142. Shannon MW, Merola J, Lovejoy FH Jr: Hypotension in severe tricyclic antidepressant overdose. Am J Emerg Med 1988;6:439–442.

143. Shannon MW: Duration of QRS disturbances after severe tricyclic antidepressant intoxication. J Toxicol Clin Toxicol 1992;30: 377–386.

144. Shelver WL, Keyler DE, Lin G, et al: Effects of recombinant drug-specific single-chain antibody Fv fragment on [3H]-desipramine distribution in rats. Biochem Pharmacol 1996;51:531–537.

145. Skjelbo E, Brosen K, Hallas J, Gram LF: The mephenytoin oxidation polymorphism is partially responsible for the *N*-demethylation of imipramine. Clin Pharmacol Ther 1991;49:18–23.

146. Skowron DM, Stimmel GL: Antidepressants and the risk of seizures. Pharmacotherapy 1992;12:18–22.

147. Southall DP, Kilpatrick SM: Imipramine poisoning: Survival of a child after prolonged cardiac massage. Br Med J 1974;4:508.

148. Spiker DG, Weiss AN, Chang SS, et al: Tricyclic antidepressant overdose: Clinical presentation and plasma levels. Clin Pharmacol Ther 1975;18:539–546.

149. Spina E, Henthorn TK, Eleborg L, et al: Desmethylimipramine overdose: Nonlinear kinetics in a slow hydroxylator. Ther Drug Monit 1985;7:239–241.

150. Squires RF, Saederup E: Antidepressants and metabolites that block GABA A receptors coupled to 35S-t-butylbicyclophosphorothionate binding sites in rat brain. Brain Res 1988;441:15–22.

151. Squires RF, Saederup E: Clozapine and several other antipsychotic/antidepressant drugs preferentially block the same "core" fraction of GABA (A) receptors. Neurochem Res 1998;23: 1283–1290.

152. Stern TA, O'Gara PT, Mulley AG: Complications after overdose with tricyclic antidepressants. Crit Care Med 1985;13:672–674.

153. Strom J, Sloth-Madsen P, Nygaard-Nielsen N: Acute self-poisoning with TCA in 295 consecutive patients treated in an ICU. Acta Anaesthesiol Scand 1984;28:666–670.

154. Swanson JR, Jones GR, Krasselt W, et al: Death of two subjects due to imipramine and desipramine metabolite accumulation during chronic therapy: A review of the literature and possible mechanisms. J Forensic Sci 1997;42:335–339.

155. Swartz CM, Sherman A: The treatment of tricyclic antidepressant overdose with repeated charcoal. J Clin Psychopharmacol 1984;4: 336–340.

156. Taboulet P, Michard F, Muszynski J, et al: Cardiovascular repercussions of seizures during cyclic antidepressant poisoning. J Toxicol Clin Toxicol 1995;33:205–211.

157. Teba L, Schiebel F, Dedhia HV, et al: Beneficial effect of norepinephrine in the treatment of circulatory shock caused by tricyclic antidepressant overdose. Am J Emerg Med 1988;6:566–568.

158. Tokarski GF, Young MJ: Criteria for admitting patients with tricyclic antidepressant overdose. J Emerg Med 1988;6:121–124.

159. Tran TP, Panacek EA, Rhee KJ, et al: Response to dopamine vs norepinephrine in tricyclic antidepressant-induced hypotension. Acad Emerg Med 1997;4:864–868.

160. Varley CK, McClellan J: Case study: Two additional sudden deaths with tricyclic antidepressants. Am Acad Child Adolesc Psychiatry 1997;36:390–394.

161. Veith RC, Raskid MA, Caldwell JH, et al. Cardiovascular effects of tricyclic antidepressants in depressed patients with chronic heart disease. N Engl J Med 1982;306:954–959.

162. Vernon DD, Banner W, Garrett JS, et al: Efficacy of dopamine and norepinephrine for treatment of hemodynamic compromise in amitriptyline intoxication. Crit Care Med 1991;19:544–549.

163. Vohra J, Burrows G, Hunt D, et al: The effect of toxic and therapeutic doses of tricyclic antidepressant drugs on intracardiac conduction. Eur J Cardiol 1975;3:219–227.

164. Wallace DE: Bowel ischemia in two patients following tricyclic antidepressant drugs [abstract]. Vet Hum Toxicol 1989;31:377.

165. Wedin GP, Oderda GM, Klein-Schwartz W: Relative toxicity of cyclic antidepressants. Ann Emerg Med 1986;15:797–804.

166. Weld FM, Bigger JT. Electrophysiological effects of imipramine on ovine cardiac Purkinje and ventricular muscle fibers. Circ Res 1980; 46:167–174.

167. Williams JM, Hollingshed MJ, Vasilakis A, et al: Extracorporeal circulation in the management of severe tricyclic antidepressant overdose. Am J Emerg Med 1994;12:456–458.

168. Wolfe TR, Caravati EM, Rollins DE, et al: Terminal 40-ms frontal plane QRS axis as a marker for tricyclic antidepressant overdose. Ann Emerg Med 1989;18:348–351.

169. Wrenn K, Smith BA, Slovis CM: Profound alkalemia during treatment of tricyclic antidepressant overdose: A potential hazard of combined hyperventilation and intravenous bicarbonate. Am J Emerg Med 1992;10:553–555.

170. Zaccara G, Muscas GC, Messori A: Clinical features, pathogenesis and management of drug-induced seizures. Drug Saf 1990;5: 109–151.

171. Zito JM, Safer DH, DosReis S, et al: Trends in the prescribing of psychotropic medications to preschoolers. JAMA 2000;283: 1025–1030.

SEROTONIN REUPTAKE INHIBITORS AND ATYPICAL ANTIDEPRESSANTS

Christine M. Stork

A 38-year-old female presented to the Emergency Department (ED) after a history of antidepressant overdose. She was drowsy, but initially responded to voice. The vital signs were blood pressure, 110/60 mm Hg; pulse, 110 beats/min; respiratory rate, 13 breaths/min; and temperature, 37°C (98.6°F). The physical examination was noncontributory with 4-mm reactive pupils, normal mucous membrane findings, and positive bowel sounds. The patient's ECG demonstrated a sinus tachycardia with a QRS duration of 90 msec.

The patient received 1 dose of oral activated charcoal. During observation, the patient experienced a brief 30-second generalized seizure. Repeat vital signs included blood pressure, 90 mm Hg by palpation; pulse, 120 beats/min; respiratory rate, 18 breaths/min; and temperature, 37.5°C (99.5°F). After an intravenous infusion of 2 L of 0.9% sodium chloride, her blood pressure returned to 120/60 mm Hg. The patient's electrocardiogram (ECG) remained unchanged. A 4-hour acetaminophen level was reported as negative, and the patient's mental status improved over the next 16 hours. A relative revealed that the patient had access to venlafaxine.

Many antidepressants inhibit the reuptake of serotonin as a means to achieve their therapeutic effect. The class of selective serotonin reuptake inhibitors (SSRIs) includes citalopram, fluoxetine, fluvoxamine, paroxetine, and sertraline (Fig. 58–1). Table 58–1 lists the pharmacology, therapeutic doses, and metabolism of the currently available SSRIs and other atypical antidepressants.

HISTORY AND EPIDEMIOLOGY

Initially marketed in the early 1980s, SSRIs are currently considered first-line therapy for the treatment of depressive disorders.[92] Since the finding that SSRIs are as effective as the tricyclic antidepressants for the treatment of major depression, they have become the largest prescribed class of medication for its treatment.[108,127] SSRIs are also used to treat obsessive/compulsive disorders, panic disorder, alcoholism, obesity, and various other medical and psychologic disorders.[36,95]

SSRIs differ from previously used antidepressants in that they have fewer adverse effects, particularly with respect to those characteristics that limit patient compliance, such as weight gain and anticholinergic effects[37] (Chap. 57). The relative safety of the SSRIs after overdose, when compared with traditional antidepressants, makes them desirable. This is particularly important prior to the onset of their therapeutic benefit, which can be delayed for up to 30 days. According to a study that summarized reports of SSRI toxicity using Medline 1985–1996, the American Association of Poison Control Centers (AAPCC) Toxic Exposure Surveillance System (TESS) data 1987–1996, and the U.S. Food and Drug Administration adverse event database through 1997, there were 57 SSRI-related deaths reported, only 6 of which could be attributed to the SSRI alone.[8] In those same years, there were more than 107,000 exposures to SSRIs reported to the AAPCC TESS (p. 1752 and Chap. 116).

PHARMACOLOGY

The modulation of serotonin neurotransmission has a definitive role in the treatment of depression.[113] However, the exact etiology of depression and the mechanism by which increased serotonergic neurotransmission attenuates symptoms remain unclear. Some postulated causes of depression include decreased overall serotonin neuronal storage, increased serotonin receptor sensitivity, and, finally, serotonin overactivity resulting in depressed dopamine neurotransmission.[113,132,144,146]

The SSRIs are distinct psychopharmaceutical agents capable of specifically inhibiting the reuptake of serotonin.[6] Their selectivity for serotonin reuptake may be structurally related to the p-trifluoromethyl substitution in some of these agents[147] (Fig. 58–1). By inhibiting serotonin reuptake, these drugs potentiate the activity of neuronally released serotonin and may subsequently alter the sensitivity of serotonin receptors. In addition, increased serotonergic activity, particularly at 5-HT$_{2A}$ receptors, may result in antidepressant activity through reduction of dopaminergic release.[146] Unlike tricyclic antidepressants and other atypical antidepressants, SSRIs have little direct interaction with cholinergic receptors, γ-amino butyric acid (GABA) receptors, sodium channels, or adrenergic reuptake (Table 58–2).

PHARMACOKINETICS AND TOXICOKINETICS

The SSRIs display diverse elimination patterns and have numerous active metabolites, which substantially increase both the duration of therapeutic effectiveness and the time during which drug interactions and adverse drug reactions can occur (Table 58–1).

Important pharmacokinetic and pharmacodynamic drug interactions are reported with therapeutic dosing. (Pharmacodynamic interactions are listed under "Serotonin Syndrome," later in this chapter.) The SSRIs and their active metabolites are both substrates for and potent inhibitors of cytochrome P450 (CYP) isoenzymes.[57,114] For example, fluoxetine, fluvoxamine, citalopram,

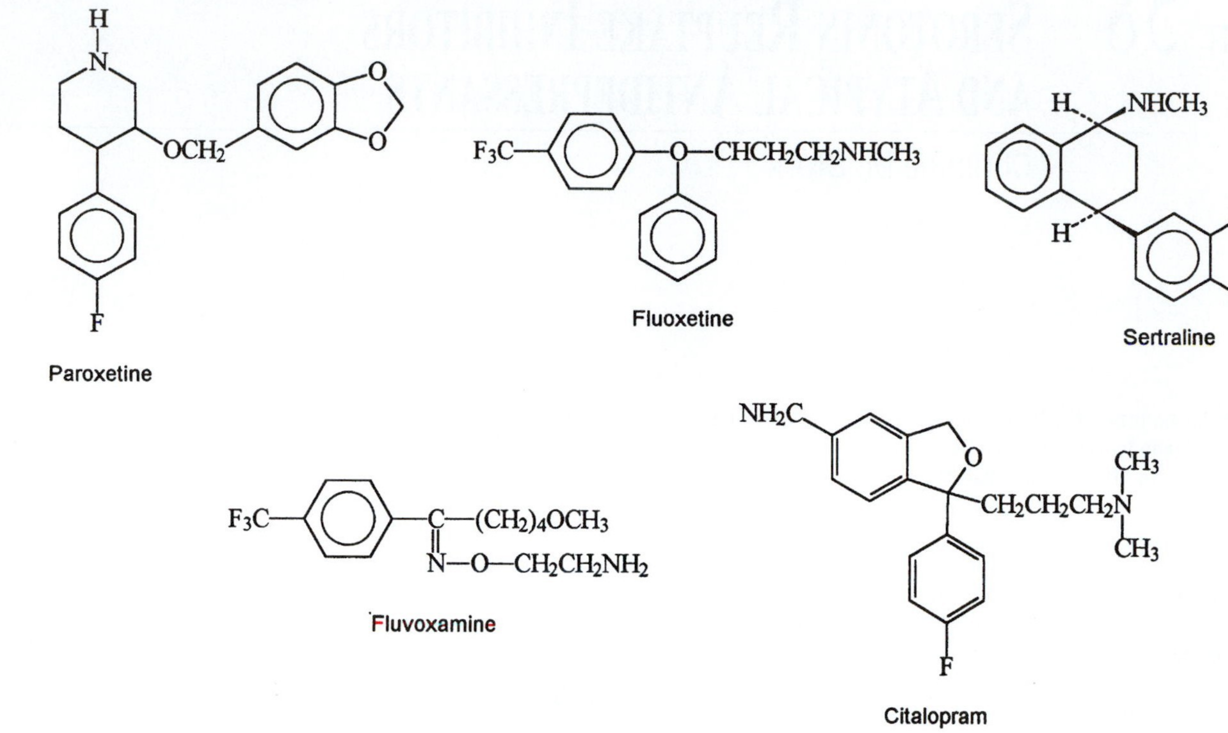

Figure 58–1. The structures of common selective serotonin reuptake inhibitors.

venlafaxine, mirtazapine, paroxetine, and sertraline are substrates for the CYP2D6 isoenzyme. Additionally, many of these also inhibit CYP2D6 (Table 58–1). The ability to inhibit CYP2D6 is greatest with paroxetine, followed by norfluoxetine, and finally fluoxetine.[27] The consequences of these interactions are manifest when the metabolism of drugs and toxins that rely on this isoenzyme for metabolic transformation is altered. This includes the aforementioned SSRIs that is substrates for this system. Chapter 11 discusses other cytochrome inhibitions.

OVERDOSE PATHOPHYSIOLOGY

The effects that occur following overdose are a direct extension of the pharmacologic activity of SSRIs in therapeutic doses. Excess serotonergic stimulation is prominent and nonselective.

CLINICAL MANIFESTATIONS

The acute manifestations of SSRI overdose include nausea, vomiting, dizziness, blurred vision, and, less commonly, central nervous system (CNS) depression and sinus tachycardia.[14,15] Hyponatremia, seizures, delayed seizures, and QRS complex prolongation are also reported, but are rare with most SSRIs, even after large overdoses[15,56,72] (Table 58–3).

Citalopram causes a widening of QT complexes and seizures in a dose-related manner. These effects typically occur in patients acutely exposed to more than 600 mg of citalopram, or in those with serum levels greater than 40 times the expected therapeutic levels.[58,104,105] In one case series, seizures were an early finding,

whereas the development of ECG abnormalities was delayed for as long as 24 hours following ingestion.[105] Although the mechanisms are unclear, experimental models suggest that the didesmethylcitalopram metabolite of citalopram prolongs the QT interval duration, whereas high levels of both the parent drug and this metabolite result in seizures and ventricular dysrhythmias.[13,21] In human case reports concurrent exposure to other drugs capable of producing these effects, such as tricyclic antidepressants, was not excluded by laboratory studies. Until further information is available, all patients exposed to citalopram should be carefully monitored for the development of ECG abnormalities and seizures.

MANAGEMENT

Treatment of patients with SSRI overdose is largely supportive. Dextrose and thiamine should be given to patients presenting with an alteration in mental status as indicated. Although cardiac manifestations after SSRI overdose are rare, a 12-lead ECG should be obtained to identify the effects of other, more life-threatening antidepressants to which the patient may have access (Chap. 57). Serum electrolytes and an acetaminophen level, and in females, a pregnancy test, may be useful for monitoring and treatment of patients with intentional overdose.

After the patient is stabilized, oral activated charcoal (1 g/kg) in a slurry may be useful to adsorb drug remaining in the gastrointestinal tract. Because of the potential for unexpected changes in mental status, syrup of ipecac should not be used in the management of these patients. Overdoses solely of SSRIs are rarely life-threatening; therefore, orogastric lavage is not generally indicated.

TABLE 58–1.   Drug Mechanism and Information for SSRIs and Atypical Antidepressants

Drug Mechanism and Example	Typical Daily Dose range (mg)	Vd (L/kg)	t½ (hr)	Metabolized Primarily by CYP	Major Active Metabolites	Major Metabolite t½	Drug (d) or Metabolite (m) Inhibits CYP (strong inhibitors are bold)
Selective Serotonin Reuptake Inhibitors (SSRIs)							
Citalopram (Celexa)	20–60	12–15	33–37	2C19, 3A4, 2D6	Monodesmethyl-citalopram, didesmethyl-citalopram	?	None
Fluoxetine (Prozac)	10–80	14–100	24–144	2C9, 2D6	Norfluoxetine	4–16 d	2D6 (d,m), 2C19 (d,m), **2D6 (d, m)**, 3A4 (m)
Fluvoxamine (Luvox)	100–300	25	15–23	1A2, 2D6	None	None	**1A2**, 2C9, **2C19**, 3A4
Paroxetine (Paxil)	10–50	8–28	2.9–44	2D6	None	None	**2D6**
Sertraline (Zoloft)	50–200	20	24	2C9, 2B6, 2C19, 2D6, 3A	Desmethylser-traline	62–104 h	2C19 (d,m)
Atypical Antidepressants							
Serotonin Reuptake Inhibitors (SRIs) with α-Adrenergic Antagonism:							
Trazodone (Desyrel)	50–600	0.47–1	3–9	2D6	Metachlorophenyl-piperazine	?	None
Nefazodone (Serzone)	300–600	0.22–0.87	3.5	3A4	Triazoledione, hydroxynefazo-done	2–33 h	**3A4 (d,m[hydroxy-nefazodone])**
SRI with Inhibition of Reuptake of Norepinephrine and Dopamine:							
Venlafaxine (Effexor)	75–375	6–7	3–4	2D6	O-desmethylvenla-faxine, depends on 3A4, and 2C19 for metabolism	10 h	None
SRI with α₂-Adrenergic Antagonism							
Mirtazapine (Remeron)	15–45	?	20–40	3A4	Desmethylmirta-zapine	?	None
SRI with Inhibition of Reuptake of Biogenic Amines or Dopamine							
Bupropion (Wellbutrin, Zyban)	150–450	20	9.6–20.9	2B6	Hydroxybupropion	24–37 h	None

Patients with small unintentional overdoses of SSRIs are not expected to develop significant signs and symptoms of poisoning. Those patients, frequently children, with well-defined small unintentional oral ingestions may be managed in the home with close observation.[94]

ADVERSE EFFECTS AFTER THERAPEUTIC DOSES

Adverse effects commonly attributed to therapeutic doses of SSRIs include gastrointestinal symptoms (anorexia, nausea, vomiting, diarrhea), sexual dysfunction in both males and females, headache, insomnia, jitteriness, dizziness, and fatigue.[149] Less common adverse effects include sedation, particularly following

citalopram and paroxetine as a result of their weak anticholinergic activity, and anxiety following fluoxetine treatment.[86]

Movement disorders, most commonly akathisia and dystonia, also occur after SSRI use.[1,44,46,87] These extrapyramidal side effects may be related to the complex interplay between serotonergic and dopaminergic activity. Predisposing factors for the development of movement disorders include preexisting neuromuscular disease and concomitant use of dopamine antagonists such as antipsychotics.[81]

The syndrome of inappropriate antidiuretic hormone (SIADH), in which severe hyponatremia may occur rapidly, is associated with SSRI use. In an animal model, the effect appears to be serotonin mediated with a dose-related increase in serum cortisol concentration, potentiation of oxitriptan-induced elevations in serum cortisol concentrations, and increased adrenocorticotropin

TABLE 58–2. Receptor Activity of SSRIs and Atypical Antidepressants

Drug	Mechanism	Serotonin Agonism	Dopamine Agonism	Peripheral α-Adrenergic Agonism
SSRIs				
Citalopram (Celexa)	SSRI, antimuscarinic	++++	0	0
Fluoxetine (Prozac)	SSRI	++++	0	0
Fluvoxamine (Luvox)	SSRI	++++	0	0
Paroxetine (Paxil)	SSRI, antimuscarinic	++++	0	0
Sertraline (Zoloft)	SSRI	++++	0	0
Atypical Antidepressants				
Bupropion (Wellbutrin, Zyban)	Inhibits reuptake of biogenic amines	+++	+++	+++
Duloxetine (investigational)	SRI, Norepinephrine reuptake inhibitor	++++	0	++
Mirtazapine (Remeron)	α₂-adrenergic antagonism, 5HT₂/5HT₃	++++	0	+++
Nefazodone (Serzone)	SRI, 5HT₂ receptor antagonism	++++	0	0
Reboxetine (Edronax, Vestra)	Selective Norepinephrine reuptake inhibitor	0	0	++++
Trazodone (Desyrel)	SRI, α-adrenergic antagonist	++++	0	+
Venlafaxine (Effexor)	SRI, norepinephrine and dopamine reuptake inhibitor	++++	0	++

SRRI: selective serotonin reuptake inhibitor; SRI: serotonin reuptake inhibitor; +: weak if any agonism; ++: weak agonism; +++: strong agonism; ++++: very strong agonism; 0: no effect.

(ACTH) and vasopressin concentrations.[40] A review of the literature identified females over age 70 who are concomitantly receiving diuretic therapy to be at greatest risk of SIADH.[77] The onset of symptoms can occur from 3 days to 4 months after the initiation of therapy, but most often occurs within the first 3 weeks of therapy.[148] Serotonin-mediated platelet dysfunction is also reported.[69]

Serotonin Syndrome

The SSRIs are associated with the development of the serotonin syndrome. This syndrome is also referred to as the serotonin behavioral or hyperactivity syndrome.[54] First described in animals, serotonin excess causes hyperactivity, forepaw-treading, head-weaving, hind-limb abduction, and an arched tail, in addition to tremor, rigidity, salivation, flushing, myoclonus, and seizures. In humans, the serotonin syndrome was first described in patients treated with monoamine oxidase inhibitors (MAOIs) who were given other drugs that enhance serotonergic activity.[25,101,131] It is characterized by an altered mental status, autonomic instability, and neuromuscular abnormalities resulting in hyperthermia.[88,97] However, ingestion of an MAOI is not required for this syndrome to develop, and its initiation is unpredictable (Table 58–4).

A prospective study of depressed inpatients given clomipramine demonstrated that 16 of 38 patients experienced symptoms consistent with the serotonin syndrome.[84] All except two cases spontaneously resolved within 1 week without discontinuation of therapy.

A study of 38 cases led to suggested diagnostic criteria for the serotonin syndrome. When other etiologies are excluded and an antipsychotic agent is not being concomitantly used, three of the following clinical findings should be present for a diagnosis of serotonin syndrome: altered mental status, agitation, myoclonus, hyperreflexia, diaphoresis, tremor, diarrhea, and incoordination.[137] These criteria, although not validated in human trials, can serve as a guide when evaluating potential cases of serotonin syndrome. Untreated patients may develop lactic acidosis, rhabdomyolysis, myoglobinuria, renal and hepatic dysfunction, disseminated intravascular coagulation, or adult respiratory distress syndrome.[89,137]

The pathophysiologic mechanism of the serotonin syndrome is not completely understood, but involves excessive selective stimulation of serotonin 5-HT₁A receptors. Serotonin 5-HT₂A agonism was initially thought to be involved as well. However, animal models found that specific stimulation of 5-HT₁A receptors resulted in signs and symptoms of serotonin syndrome even when 5-HT₂A receptors were inactivated.[30] The 5-HT₁D receptors, stimulated with antimigraine drugs such as sumatriptan, are not implicated in cases of serotonin syndrome. Cases of serotonin syndrome are associated with many agents that increase synaptic serotonin or enhance 5-HT₁A receptor stimulation.

TABLE 58–3. A Predictive Analysis of the Relative Potential for Seizures and QRS Prolongation of SSRIs and Atypical Antidepressants

Drug	Seizures	QRS Prolongation
Classic SSRIs		
Citalopram (Celexa)	+++	+++
Fluoxetine (Prozac)	+	+
Fluvoxamine (Luvox)	+	+
Paroxetine (Paxil)	+	+
Sertraline (Zoloft)	+	+
Others		
Bupropion (Wellbutrin, Zyban)	++++	+
Duloxetine (Investigational)	++++	Unknown
Mirtazapine (Remeron)	Unknown	++
Nefazodone (Serzone)	+	0
Reboxetine (Edronax, Vestra)	++++	Unknown
Trazodone (Desyrel)	+	0
Venlafaxine (Effexor)	++++	+++

0: does not cause; +: very rarely if ever causes; ++: rarely causes; +++: causes; ++++: very commonly causes.

TABLE 58–4. Potential Causes of Serotonin Syndrome

Drugs That Inhibit the Breakdown of Serotonin

Monamine oxidase inhibitors (nonselective)
  Phenelzine, moclobemide, clorgyline,
    isocarboxyzid [16,22,25,38,51,53,65,76,107,115,128,130,133,139,140]
  Ayahuasca preparations—psychoactive beverage for religious purposes
    in the Amazon and Orinoco River Basins (harmine and harmaline)[22]

Drugs That Block Reuptake of Serotonin

Dextromethorphan[115]
Meperidine[51]
SSRIs
Fluoxetine, citalopram, paroxetine, fluvoxamine,
  sertraline[4,9,11,16,26,34,38,45,49,53,55,61,71,85,93,102,107,111,119,128,129,136]
Clomipramine[79,107,117,133]
Nefazodone[18,71]
Pentazocine[61]
Trazodone[45,52,99,110,111]
Venlafaxine[29,65,80]
Cocaine[140]—weak reuptake inhibitor

Serotonin Precursors or Agonists

Buspirone[4,52]
Lithium[79,93,99]
L-Tryptophan[131,136]
Lysergic acid diethylamide (LSD)[126]
Valproic acid[18]

Drugs That Enhance Serotonin Release

MDMA (ecstasy)[76,130]
Mirtazapine[11]

The serotonin syndrome occurs most commonly following the use of combinations of serotonergic agents. This syndrome is also reported in patients following a single dose, high therapeutic doses, or overdoses of certain serotonergic agents in adults and children.[29,49,75,80,85,102,110,117]

Although selective MAO enzyme subtype A (MAO-A) inhibitor drug combinations at therapeutic doses are infrequently reported to cause serotonin syndrome, there are sporadic reports implicating selegiline or moclobemide when given in combination with SSRIs.[33,91]

The serotonin syndrome may also occur following the discontinuation of therapy of one serotonergic agent when an insufficient lag time occurs before initiating alternative therapy.[119,120] Some reasons for the development of the serotonin syndrome under these circumstances include residual pharmacologic effect, receptor down- or up-regulation, and the presence of active metabolites. For example, fluoxetine metabolism results in an active metabolite, norfluoxetine, with comparable pharmacologic effects and a half-life substantially longer than that of the parent drug. Residual effects of this metabolite may result in serotonin syndrome when another serotonergic agent, usually another antidepressant, is initiated prior to the complete elimination of norfluoxetine.[26]

Treatment for the serotonin syndrome begins with supportive care and a focus on decreasing muscle rigidity. Because this muscular rigidity is thought to be responsible for hyperthermia and death, rapid external cooling in conjunction with the aggressive use of benzodiazepines should limit the complications associated with prolonged hyperthermia. In severe cases, neuromuscular blockade should be considered to achieve rapid muscle relaxation.

The time course of the serotonin syndrome is variable and related to the time required to decrease drug levels of the offending agents. The serotonin syndrome resolves in most patients within 24 hours after removal of the offending drug, but can be prolonged when caused by drugs with long half-lives, protracted duration of effects, or active metabolites.

Several case reports suggest the successful use of the antihistamine, cyproheptadine (4 mg po) acting as a nonspecific antagonist at 5-HT$_{1A}$ and 5-HT$_2$ receptors.[55,82] The patients typically had mild to moderate symptoms of serotonin syndrome and were not hyperthermic. It is uncertain whether these patients would have responded to supportive care. However, pretreatment with nonspecific serotonin antagonists and serotonin 5-HT$_{1A}$-receptor antagonists prevents the development of the serotonin syndrome in animals.[48,67,135] Other drugs that are anecdotally reported to be successful in the treatment of symptoms caused by the serotonin syndrome include methysergide (2 mg twice daily), chlorpromazine, and propranolol.[50,52,59,121] Because all of these agents are of unproven utility, aggressive cooling and sedation with a benzodiazepine remain the basis of therapy.

Differential Diagnosis of the Serotonin Syndrome from the Neuroleptic Malignant Syndrome

There are many overlapping features between the serotonin syndrome and the neuroleptic malignant syndrome (NMS) (Chap. 59). Some authors call these "spectrum disorders" that can be caused by drugs with both antidopaminergic and/or proserotonergic effects.[90,150] Altered mental status, autonomic instability, and changes in neuromuscular tone that may result in hyperthermia characterize both syndromes. However, the implicated agents and pathophysiologic mechanisms are distinct. The development of NMS involves rapid blockade of dopaminergic neurons in the central nervous system, whereas the serotonin syndrome appears to result from acute overstimulation of serotonin receptors (5-HT$_{1A}$). 5-HT$_{2A}$ agonism results in an overall decrease in the release of neuronal dopamine, and some authors describe NMS with the use of serotonin-enhancing drugs. However, the levels of measured dopamine and serotonin metabolites in NMS patients support the hypothesis of central dopaminergic hypoactivity that is unrelated to increased serotonergic activity.[5,98]

In addition to the associated medications, the time courses of the two syndromes are substantially different. Signs and symptoms of the serotonin syndrome develop within minutes to hours after exposure to the offending agent, whereas NMS typically develops days to weeks after daily exposure to the drug in question.[53] Also, after symptoms develop and offending drugs are discontinued, the NMS can last for as long as a week, whereas the serotonin syndrome usually resolves within 24 hours. Patients with serotonin syndrome are also more likely to present with hyperreflexia and myoclonus, rather than with acute muscular "lead pipe" rigidity that occurs in those patients with NMS.[53,78]

ATYPICAL ANTIDEPRESSANTS

Atypical antidepressants are defined as not belonging to a set classification of antidepressants. As such, they are not selective serotonin reuptake inhibitors, tricyclic antidepressants, or monoamine oxidase inhibitors. In general, the atypical antidepressants are newer antidepressants that are developed in an attempt to decrease the undesirable side effects of traditional antidepressants.

Serotonin/Norepinephrine Reuptake Inhibitors

Venlafaxine

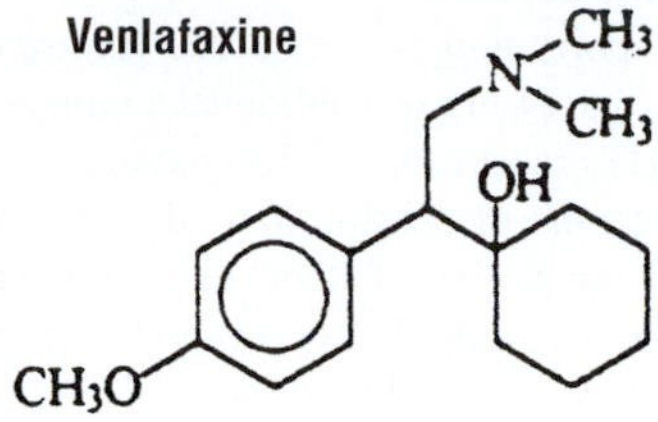

In addition to inhibiting the reuptake of serotonin, venlafaxine inhibits the reuptake of norepinephrine and dopamine. Venlafaxine produces a rapid down-regulation of central β-adrenergic receptors, which may result in a faster onset of antidepressant effect.[124] Patients acutely exposed to venlafaxine may present with nausea, vomiting, dizziness, tachycardia, central nervous system depression, hypotension, hyperthermia, hepatic enzyme elevations, and seizures.[68,145] QRS prolongation and ventricular tachycardia have resulted in death.[7,12,118,153] Although there are no clinical data on effectiveness, sodium bicarbonate may be theoretically helpful in attenuating these cardiotoxic effects. Similar investigational drugs are duloxetine and milnacipran,[19] which inhibit the reuptake of serotonin and norepinephrine. Overdose information is lacking, but clinical effects would be expected to be similar to venlafaxine overdose.

Norepinephrine Reuptake Inhibitors

Reboxetine

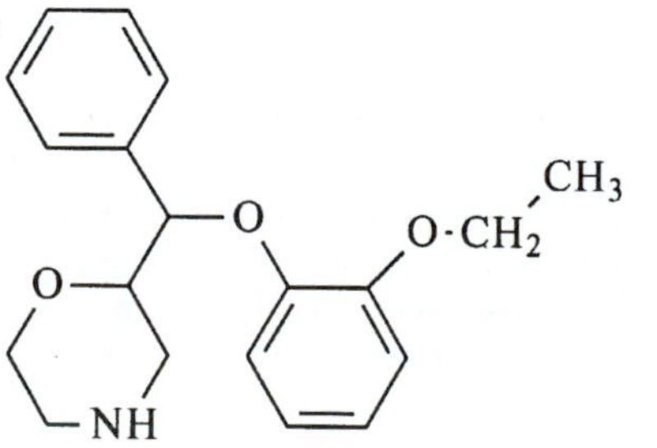

Reboxetine is a selective norepinephrine reuptake inhibitor.[143] Lack of experience precludes an analysis of overdose data. However, toxicity can be extrapolated from adverse effects reported in clinical trials and from experience with other drugs possessing similar pharmacologic characteristics. In particular, overdosed patients should be carefully monitored for tachycardia, hypotension, and the development of seizures.

Other Reuptake Inhibitors

Bupropion

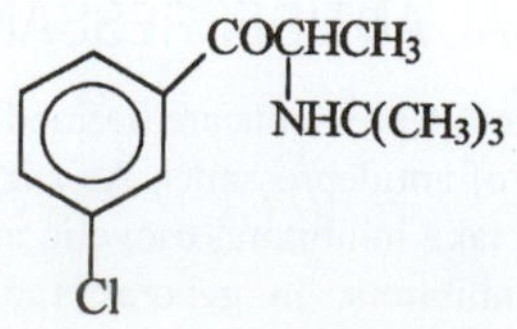

Bupropion is a unicyclic antidepressant. The exact pharmacologic mechanism of bupropion's action is unclear, but both the parent drug and an active metabolite may inhibit the reuptake of biogenic amines. Extended-release formulations of bupropion are frequently employed as adjuncts to enhance smoking cessation therapy.[70] At doses greater than 450–500 mg/d, there is a substantial risk of seizures.[31,73]

Acute large overdoses may result in seizure activity with and without QRS complex prolongation.[20,63,64,103,125,134,138] In some cases, these effects were delayed for up 10 hours, particularly after ingestion of sustained-release preparations.[62] Symptoms were reported to continue for up to 48 hours.

Several studies suggest that the seizures following either bupropion overdose or high therapeutic doses are caused by the metabolite hydroxybupropion.[39,106] Elevated hydroxybupropion levels were documented after seizures when bupropion levels were no longer detectable.[31,39,116]

Treatment, when required for seizures, should be supportive and include the judicious use of benzodiazepines, followed by barbiturates. If QRS prolongation occurs, the patient should be treated with sodium bicarbonate (Antidote in Depth: Sodium Bicarbonate). Other serious adverse effects reported after bupropion use include hepatic dysfunction, rhabdomyolysis, and isolated reports of dyskinesia, altered vestibular and sensory function, and serum sickness.[28,43,141,151]

Trazodone

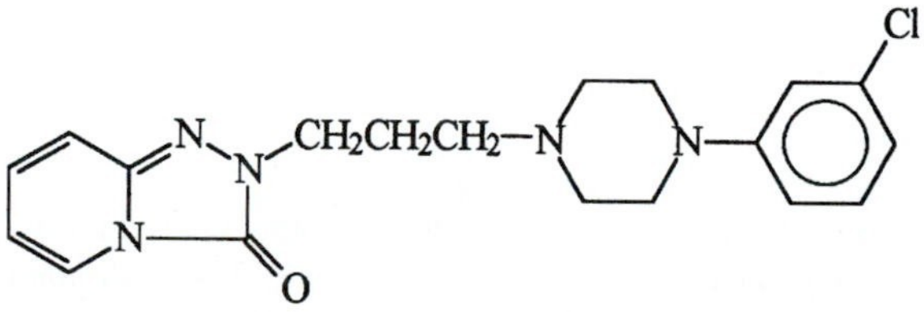

Trazodone is a serotonin agonist that acts through inhibition of serotonin reuptake. In addition, trazodone may have some peripheral α-adrenergic antagonist activity. Central nervous system depression and orthostatic hypotension are the most common complications after acute overdose of trazodone.[42] Trazodone is rarely reported to cause SIADH. This effect may be responsible for seizures, which are also rarely reported after acute overdose.[6,142] Priapism, reported with the therapeutic use of trazodone, may occasionally occur after overdose[23,42] (Chap. 30). Overdose management includes supportive care and fluids and vasopressors, if necessary.

Nefazodone

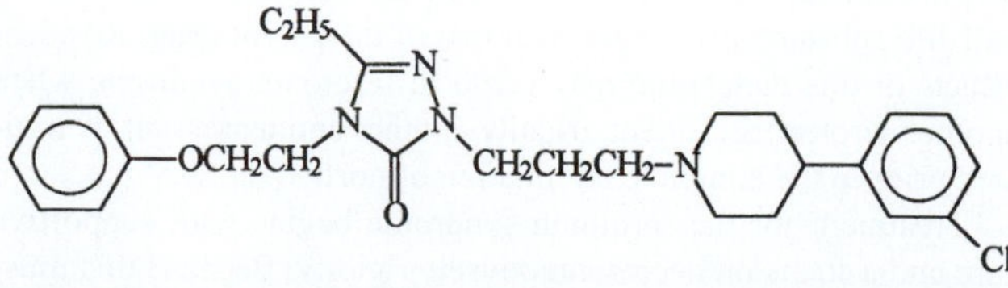

Nefazodone inhibits the reuptake of serotonin and is an antagonist of serotonin 5-HT$_2$ receptors.[3] Chronic therapeutic use of nefazodone over 14–24 weeks is reported to result rarely in centrilobular hepatic necrosis.[2] Experience with this drug in acute overdose is limited. Single cases of acute overdose show limited toxicity that includes CNS depression and hypotension, similar to trazodone.[24,41] Careful clinical monitoring is advised until more acute overdose information is available.

Mirtazapine

The mechanism of action of mirtazapine is unique in that it increases neuronal norepinephrine and serotonin through α_2-adrenergic antagonism.[32] Mirtazapine also blocks some subtypes of 5-HT receptors, including 5-HT$_2$ and 5-HT$_3$, which appear to have antidepressive effects.[100] The main effects that occur after acute overdoses of mirtazapine include the alteration of mental status and tachycardia.[17] Large overdoses or coingestants may be responsible for reports of respiratory depression and prolongation of the QT interval.[17,47,66,112] Because more overdose data are required before a precise constellation of symptoms can be attributed to this drug, careful clinical monitoring is advised. In therapeutic usage, mirtazapine caused a single case of reversible agranulocytosis.[96]

DRUG DISCONTINUATION SYNDROME

A drug discontinuation syndrome manifested by withdrawal manifestations is pharmacologically based. Like classic drug withdrawal, this syndrome also includes symptoms resulting from psychological withdrawal. Drug discontinuation syndromes are commonly reported after withdrawal of conventional antidepressants, including tricyclic antidepressants and monoamine oxidase inhibitors[83] (Chaps. 57 and 60). Selective serotonin reuptake inhibitors are reported to cause a discontinuation syndrome that typically begins within 5 days after drug discontinuation and that may last up to 3 weeks.[60] The most frequently reported symptoms include dizziness, lethargy, paresthesias, nausea, vivid dreams, irritability, and depressed mood.[122,152] The risk factors associated with the development of a discontinuation syndrome are not fully clarified, although it is more common with SSRIs with a shorter elimination half-life (paroxetine > fluvoxamine > sertraline > fluoxetine). In addition, those SSRIs with high-potency serotonin reuptake inhibition are more frequently implicated (paroxetine > sertraline > clomipramine > fluoxetine > venlafaxine > trazodone). Of the SSRIs, paroxetine most often results in discontinuation symptoms, which are estimated to occur at a rate of 300 cases per million prescriptions. Fluoxetine discontinuation syndrome occurred significantly less frequently at two cases per million prescriptions.[109] Fluoxetine's long elimination half-life and its active metabolite, norfluoxetine, probably decrease the incidence of discontinuation syndrome by providing a tapered effect after cessation.

The biochemical basis of the discontinuation syndrome is hypothesized to be a result of serotonin receptor down-regulation leading to alterations in serotonergic activity, including interactions with other neurotransmitters (γ-aminobutyric acid (GABA), norepinephrine, and dopamine); or biologic/cognitive sensitivity in individual patients.[123] Although postulated, antimuscarinic withdrawal seems an unlikely cause because in a human model, the antimuscarinic effects of desipramine failed to protect against paroxetine withdrawal.[35]

Treatment of patients exhibiting discontinuation symptoms should include supportive care and the reinitiation of the discontinued drug, if reinitiation of the drug is not contraindicated. The drug should then be tapered at a rate that allows for improved patient tolerance.

Many other antidepressants discussed in this chapter are also reported to result in discontinuation reactions. Symptoms appear similar to those reported after discontinuation of SSRIs and are treated in a similar manner[10,74] (Chap. 72).

SUMMARY

The toxicity of SSRIs or atypical antidepressants following acute overdose is usually not life-threatening, although a few agents produce seizures or cardiac toxicity. Treatment is generally supportive for all of these agents. There are, however, significant drug interactions and adverse drug reactions associated with serotonin reuptake inhibitors that may lead to acute life-threatening events. In addition, the management of these patients is frequently complicated because they are also likely to have concomitant access to more life-threatening antidepressants such as TCAs and MAOIs.

REFERENCES

1. Adler L, Angrist B: Paroxetine and akathisia. Biol Psychiatry 1995; 37:336–337.
2. Aranda-Michel J, Koehler A, Bejoaano PA, et al: Nefazodone-induced liver failure: Report of three cases. Ann Intern Med 1999; 130:285–288.
3. Augustin BG, Cold JA, Jann MW: Venlafaxine and nefazodone, two pharmacologically distinct antidepressants. Pharmacotherapy 1997; 17:511–530.
4. Baetz M, Malcolm D: Serotonin syndrome from fluvoxamine and buspirone. Can J Psychiatry 1995;40:428–429.
5. Bakheit AMO, Beehan PO, Prach AT, et al: A syndrome identical to the neuroleptic malignant syndrome induced by LSD and alcohol. Br J Addiction 1990;85:150–151.
6. Baldessarini RJ: Drugs and the treatment of psychiatric disorders. In: Hardman JG, Limbird LE, Molinoff PB, et al, eds: Goodman & Gilman's The Pharmacological Basis of Therapeutics, 9th ed. New York, McGraw-Hill, 1996, pp. 431–459.
7. Banham NDG: Fatal venlafaxine overdose. Med J Aust 1998;169: 445–448.
8. Barbey JT, Roose SP: SSRI safety in overdose. J Clin Psychiatry 1998:59(Suppl 15):42–48.
9. Bastani JB, Troester MM, Bastani AJ: Serotonin syndrome and fluvoxamine: A case study. Nebr Med J 1996;81:107–109.
10. Benazzi F: Mirtazapine withdrawal symptoms [letter]. Can J Psychiatry 1998;43:525.
11. Benazzi F: Serotonin syndrome with mirtazapine-fluoxetine combination [letter]. Int J Geriat Psychiatry 1998;13:493–496.
12. Blythe D, Hackett LP: Cardiovascular and neurological toxicity of venlafaxine. Hum Exp Toxicol 1999;18:309–313.
13. Boeck V, Fredricson OK, Svendsen O: Studies on acute toxicity and drug levels of citalopram in the dog. Acta Pharmacol Toxicol 1982; 50:169–174.

14. Borys DJ, Setzer SC, Ling LJ, et al: Acute fluoxetine overdose: Report of 234 cases. Am J Emerg Med 1992;10;115–120.

15. Braitberg G, Curry SC: Seizure after isolated fluoxetine overdose. Ann Emerg Med 1995;26:234–237.

16. Brannan SK, Talley BJ, Bowden CL: Sertraline and isocarboxazid cause of serotonin syndrome [letter]. J Clin Psychopharmacol 1994; 14:144–145.

17. Bremner JD, Wingard P, Walshe TA: Safety of mirtazapine in overdose. J Clin Psychiatry 1998;59:233–235.

18. Brazelton T, Blanc PD, Olson KR, Peak DA: Toxic effects of nefazodone [letter]. Ann Emerg Med 1997;20:550–551.

19. Briley M, Prost JF, Moret C: Preclinical pharmacology of milnacipran. Int Clin Psychopharmacol 1996;11(Suppl 4):9–14.

20. Bryant SG, Guernsey BG, Ingrim NB: Review of bupropion. Clin Pharm 1983;2:525–537.

21. Burgh Van Der M: Citalopram product monograph. Copenhagen, Denmark, H Lundbeck A/S, 1994, ISBN 87–88085–00–7.

22. Callaway JC, Grob CS: Ayahuasca preparations and serotonin reuptake inhibitors: A potential combination for severe adverse reactions. J Psychoactive Drugs 1998;30:367–369.

23. Carson CC III, Mino RD: Priapism associated with trazodone therapy. J Urol 1988;139:369–370.

24. Catalano G, Catalano MC, Tumarkin NBB: Nefazodone overdose: A case report. Clin Neuropharmacol 1999;22:63–65.

25. Cohen RM, Pickar D, Murphy DL: Myoclonus associated hypomania during MAO-inhibitor treatment. Am J Psychiatry 1980;137: 105–106.

26. Coplan JD, Gorman JM: Detectable levels of fluoxetine metabolites after discontinuation: An unexpected serotonin syndrome [letter]. Am J Psychiatry 1993;150:837.

27. Crewe HK, Lennard MS, Tucker GT, et al: The effect of selective serotonin reuptake inhibitors on cytochrome P4502D6 (CYP2D6) activity in human liver microsomes. Br J Clin Pharmacol 1992;34: 262–265.

28. Daniella D, Esquenazi J: Rhabdomyolysis associated with bupropion treatment [letter]. J Clin Psychopharmacol 1999;19:185–186.

29. Daniels RJ: Serotonin syndrome due to venlafaxine overdose. J Accid Emerg Med 1998;15:333–337.

30. Darmani NA, Zhao E: Production of serotonin syndrome by 8-OH DPAT in Cryptotis parva. Physiol Behavior 1998;65:327–331.

31. Davidson J: Seizures and bupropion: A review. J Clin Psychiatry 1989;50:256–261.

32. deBoer T: The pharmacologic profile of mirtazapine. J Clin Psychiatry 1996;57(Suppl 4):19–25.

33. Dingenmanse J, Wallnofer A, Gieschke R, et al: Pharmacokinetic and pharmacodynamic interactions between fluoxetine and moclobemide in the investigation of development of the "serotonin syndrome." Clin Pharmacol Ther 1998;63:403–413.

34. Dursun SM, Mathew VM, Reveley MA: Toxic serotonin syndrome after fluoxetine plus carbamazepine [letter]. Lancet 1993;342: 442–443.

35. Fava GA, Grandi S: Withdrawal syndromes after paroxetine and sertraline discontinuation [letter]. J Clin Psychopharmacol 1995;15: 374–375.

36. Ferguson JM, Feighrer JP: Fluoxetine-induced weight loss in overweight non-depressed humans. Int J Obesity 1987;11:163–170.

37. Finley PR: Selective serotonin reuptake inhibitors: Pharmacologic profiles and potential therapeutic distinctions. Ann Pharmacother 1994;28:1359–1369.

38. Fitzsimmons CR, Metha S: Serotonin syndrome caused by overdose with paroxetine and moclobemide. J Accid Emerg Med 1999;16: 293–295.

39. Friel PN, Logan BK, Fligner CL: Three fatal drug overdoses involving bupropion. J Anal Toxicol 1993;17:436–438.

40. Fuller R: Serotonergic stimulation of pituitary-adrenocortical function in rats. Neuroendocrinology 1985;32:118–120.

41. Gaffney PN, Schuckman HA, Beeson MS: Nefazodone overdose. Ann Pharmacother 1998;32:1249–1250.

42. Gamble DE, Peterson LG: Trazodone overdose: Four years of experience from voluntary reports. J Clin Psychiatry 1986;47:544–546.

43. Gardos G: Reversible dyskinesia during bupropion therapy. J Clin Psychiatry 1997;58:218.

44. George M, Trimble M: Dystonic reaction associated with fluvoxamine. J Clin Psychopharmacol 1993;13:220–221.

45. George TP, Godleski LS: Possible serotonin syndrome with trazodone addition to fluoxetine [letter]. Biol Psychiatry 1996;39: 384–385.

46. Gerber PE, Lynd LD: Selective serotonin reuptake inhibitor induced movement disorders. Ann Pharmacother 1998;32:692–698.

47. Gerritsen AW: Safety in overdose of mirtazapine: A case report [letter]. J Clin Psychiatry 1997;58:271.

48. Gerson SC, Baldessarini RJ: Motor effects of serotonin in the central nervous system. Life Sci 1980;27:1435–1451.

49. Gill M, LoVecchio F, Selden B: Serotonin syndrome in a child after a single dose of fluvoxamine. Ann Emerg Med 1999;33:457–459.

50. Gillman PK: The serotonin syndrome and its treatment. J Psychopharmacol 1999;12:100–109.

51. Gillman PK: Possible serotonin syndrome with moclobemide and pethidine [letter]. Med J Aust 1995;162:554.

52. Goldberg RJ, Huk M: Serotonin syndrome from trazodone and buspirone [letter]. Psychosomatics 1992;33:235–236.

53. Graber MA, Hoens TB, Perry PJ: Sertraline-phenelzine drug interaction: A serotonin syndrome reaction. Ann Pharmacother 1994;28: 732–735.

54. Grahame-Smith DC: Studies in vivo on the relationship between brain tryptophan, brain 5-HT synthesis and hyperactivity in rats treated with monoamine oxidase inhibitor and L-tryptophan. J Neurochem 1971;18:1053–1066.

55. Graudins A, Stearman A, Chan B: Treatment of the serotonin syndrome with cyproheptadine. J Emerg Med 1998;16:615–619.

56. Graudins A, Vossler C, Wang R: Fluoxetine-induced cardiotoxicity with response to bicarbonate therapy. Am J Emerg Med 1997;15: 501–503.

57. Greenblatt DJ, von Moltke LL, Harmatz JS, Shader RI: Human cytochromes and some newer antidepressants: Kinetics, metabolism, and drug interactions. J Clin Psychopharmacol 1999;19(Suppl 1): 23–35.

58. Grundemar L, Wohlfart B, Lagerstedt C, et al: Symptoms and signs of severe citalopram overdose [letter]. Lancet 1997;349:1602.

59. Guze BH, Baxter LR Jr: The serotonin syndrome: Case responsive to propranolol [letter]. J Clin Psychopharmacol 1986;6:119–120.

60. Haddad P: Newer antidepressants and the discontinuation syndrome. J Clin Psychiatry 1997;58(Suppl 70):17–22.

61. Hansen TE, Dieter K, Keepers GA: Interaction of fluoxetine and pentazocine. Am J Psychiatry 1990;147:949–950.

62. Harmon T, Jurta D, Krenzelok E: Delayed seizures from sustained-release bupropion overdose [abstract]. J Toxicol Clin Toxicol 1998;36:522.

63. Harris CR, Gualtieri J, Stark G: Fatal bupropion overdose. J Toxicol Clin Toxicol 1997;25:321–324.

64. Hebert S: Bupropion (Zyban, sustained-release tablets): Reported adverse reactions. Canadian Med Assoc J 1999;160:1050–1051.

65. Heisler MA, Guidry JR, Arnecke B: Serotonin syndrome induced by administration of venlafaxine and phenelzine [letter]. Ann Pharmacother 1996;30:84.

66. Hoes MJ, Zeijpveld JHB: First report of mirtazapine overdose [letter]. Int Clin Psychopharmacol 1996;11:147.

67. Hoes MJ, Zeijpveld JH: Mirtazapine as treatment for serotonin syndrome [letter]. Pharmacopsychiatry 1996;29:81.

68. Holliday SM, Benfield P: Venlafaxine: A review of its pharmacology and therapeutic potential in depression. Drugs 1995;49:280–294.

69. Humphries JE, Wheby MS, Vandenberg SR: Fluoxetine and the bleeding time. Arch Pathol Lab Med 1990;114:727–728.

70. Hurt RD, Sachs DPL, Glover ED, et al: A comparison of sustained-release bupropion and placebo for smoking cessation. N Engl J Med 1997;337:1195–1202.

71. John L, Perreault MM, Tao T, Blew PG: Serotonin syndrome associated with nefazodone and paroxetine. Ann Emerg Med 1997;29:287–289.

72. Johnsen CR. Hoejlyng N: Hyponatremia following acute overdose with paroxetine. Internat J Clin Pharmacol Ther 1998;36:333–335.

73. Johnson JA, Lineberry CG, Ascher JA, et al: A 102-center prospective study of seizure in association with bupropion. J Clin Psychiatry 1991;52:450–456.

74. Johnson H, Bouman WP, Lawton J: Withdrawal reaction associated with venlafaxine. BMJ 1998;317:787.

75. Kaminski CA, Robbins MS, Weibley RE: Sertraline intoxication in a child. Ann Emerg Med 1994;23:1371–1374.

76. Kaskey GB: Possible interaction between MAOI and "ecstasy." Am J Psychiatry 1992;149:411–412.

77. Kirchner V, Silver LE, Kelly CA: Selective serotonin reuptake inhibitors and hyponatremia: Review and proposed mechanisms in the elderly. J Psychopharmacol 1998;12:396–400.

78. Kline SS, Mauro LS, Scala-Barnett DM, Zick D: Serotonin syndrome versus neuroleptic malignant syndrome as a cause of death. Clin Pharmacol 1989;8:510–514.

79. Kojima H, Terao T, Yoshimura R: Serotonin syndrome during clomipramine and lithium treatment [letter]. Am J Psychiatry 1993;150:1897.

80. Kolecki P: Isolated venlafaxine-induced serotonin syndrome. J Emerg Med 1997;15:491–493.

81. Lane RM: SSRI-induced extrapyramidal side effects and akathisia: Implications for treatment. J Psychopharmacol 1998;12:192–214.

82. Lappin R, Auchincloss E: Treatment of serotonin syndrome with cyproheptadine. N Engl J Med 1994;331:1021–1022.

83. Lejoyeux M, Ades J: Antidepressant discontinuation: A review of the literature. J Clin Psychiatry 1997;58(Suppl 7):11–16.

84. Lejoyeux M, Roullion F, Ades J: Prospective evaluation of the serotonin syndrome in depressed inpatients treated with clomipramine. Acta Psychiatr Scand 1993;88:369–371.

85. Lenzi A, Raffaelli S, Marazziti D: Serotonin syndrome-like symptoms in patients with obsessive-compulsive disorder, following inappropriate increase in fluvoxamine dosage. Pharmacopsychiatry 1993;26:100–101.

86. Levinson ML, Lipsy RJ, Fuller DK: Adverse effects and drug interactions associated with fluoxetine therapy. Ann Pharmacother 1991;25:657–661.

87. Lewis CF, DeQuardo JR, Rajiv T: Dystonia associated with trazodone and sertraline. J Clin Psychopharmacol 1997;17:64–65.

88. Martin TG: Serotonin syndrome. Ann Emerg Med 1996;28:520–526.

89. Miller F, Friedman R, Tanenbaum J, Griffin A: Disseminated intravascular coagulation and acute myoglobinuric renal failure: A consequence of the serotonin syndrome [letter]. J Clin Psychopharmacol 1991;11:277–279.

90. Miyaoka H, Kamijima K: Encephalopathy during amitriptyline therapy: Are neuroleptic malignant syndrome and serotonin syndrome spectrum disorders? Int Clin Psychopharmacol 1995;10:265–267.

91. Montastruc JL, Charnontin B, Senard JM, et al: Pseudophaeochromocytoma in parkinsonian patients treated with fluoxetine plus selegiline [letter]. Lancet 1993;341:555.

92. Montgomery SA: Development of new treatments for depression. J Clin Psychiatry 1985;46:3–6.

93. Muly EC, McDonald W, Steffens D, Book S: Serotonin syndrome produced by a combination of fluoxetine and lithium [letter]. Am J Psychiatry 1993;150:1565.

94. Myers LB, Krenzelok EP: Paroxetine (Paxil) overdose: A pediatric focus. Vet Human Toxicol 1997;39:86–88.

95. Naranjo CA, Bremner KE: Clinical pharmacology of serotonin-altering medication for decreasing alcohol consumption. Alcohol Alcohol 1993;2:221–229.

96. Nelson JC: Safety and tolerability of the new antidepressants. J Clin Psychiatry 1997;58(Suppl 6):26–31.

97. Nierenberg DW, Semprebon M: The central nervous system serotonin syndrome. Clin Pharmacol Ther 1993;53:84–88.

98. Nisijima K, Ishiguro T: Cerebrospinal fluid levels of monoamine metabolites and gamma-aminobutyric acid in neuroleptic malignant syndrome. J Psychiatry 1995;29:233–244.

99. Nisijima K, Shimizu M, Abe T, Ishiguro T: A case of serotonin syndrome induced by concomitant treatment with low-dose trazodone and amitriptyline and lithium. Int Clin Psychopharmacol 1996;11:289–290.

100. Nutt D: Mirtazapine: Pharmacology in relation to adverse effects. Acta Psychiatr Scand 1997;96(Suppl 39):31–37.

101. Oates JA, Sjoerdsma A: Neurologic effects of tryptophan in patients receiving monamine oxidase inhibitor. Neurology 1960;10:1076–1078.

102. Pao M, Tipnis T: Serotonin syndrome after sertraline overdose in a 5-year-old girl. Arch Pediatr Adolesc Med 1997;151:1064–1067.

103. Paris PA, Saucier JR: ECG conduction delays associated with massive bupropion overdose. J Toxicol Clin Toxicol 1998;36:595–598.

104. Personne M, Persson H, Sjoberg G: Citalopram toxicity. Lancet 1997;350:518–519.

105. Personne M, Sjoberg G, Persson H: Citalopram overdose—Review of cases treated in Swedish hospitals. J Toxicol Clin Toxicol 1997;35:237–240.

106. Popli AP, Tanquary J, Lamparella V, Masand PS: Bupropion and anticonvulsant drug interactions. Ann Clin Psychiatry 1995;7:90–101.

107. Power BM, Pinder M, Hackett LP, Ilett KF: Fatal serotonin syndrome following a combined overdose of moclobemide, clomipramine and fluoxetine. Anaesth Intensive Care 1995;23:499–502.

108. Preskorn SH, Burke MJ: Somatic therapy for major depressive disorder: Selection of an antidepressant. J Clin Psychiatry 1992;53:5–18.

109. Price JS, Waller PC, Wood SM, et al: A comparison of the post-marketing safety of four selective serotonin re-uptake inhibitors, including the investigation of symptoms occurring on withdrawal. Br J Clin Pharmacol 1996;42:757–763.

110. Rao R: Serotonin syndrome associated with trazodone [letter]. Int J Geriatric Psychiatry 1997;12:129–132.

111. Reeves RR, Bullen JA: Serotonin syndrome produced by paroxetine and low-dose trazodone [letter]. Psychosomatics 1995;36:159–160.

112. Retz W, Maier S, Maris F, Rosler M: Non-fatal mirtazapine overdose. Int Clin Psychopharmacol 1998;12:277–279.

113. Richelson E: Biologic basis of depression and therapeutic relevance. J Clin Psychiatry 1991;52(Suppl 6):4–10.

114. Richelson E: Pharmacokinetic drug interactions of new antidepressants: A review of the effects on the metabolism of other drugs. Mayo Clin Proc 1997;72:835–847.

115. Rivers N, Horner B: Possible lethal interaction between Nardil and dextromethorphan [letter]. Can Med Assoc J 1970;103:85.

116. Rohrig TP, Ray NG: Tissue distribution of bupropion in a fatal overdose. J Anal Toxicol 1992;16:343–345.

117. Rosebush PI, Margetts P, Mazurek MF: Serotonin syndrome as a result of clomipramine monotherapy. J Clin Psychopharmacother 1999;19:285–287.

118. Rudolph RL, Derivan AT: The safety and tolerability of venlafaxine hydrochloride: Analysis of the clinical trials database. J Clin Psychopharmacol 1996;16(Suppl 2):54–61.

119. Ruiz R: Fluoxetine and the serotonin syndrome. Ann Emerg Med 1994;24:983–985.

120. Safferman AZ, Masiar SJ: Central nervous system toxicity after abrupt monoamine oxidase inhibitor switch: A case report. Ann Pharmacother 1992;26:337–338.

121. Sandyk R: L-Dopa-induced serotonin syndrome in a parkinsonian patient on bromocriptine [letter]. J Clin Psychopharmacol 1986;6:194–195.

122. Schatzberg AF, Haddad P, Kaplan EM, et al: Serotonin reuptake discontinuation syndrome: A hypothetical definition. J Clin Psychiatry 1997;58(Suppl 8):5–10.

123. Schatzberg AF, Haddad P, Kaplan EM, et al: Possible biological mechanisms of the serotonin reuptake inhibitor discontinuation syndrome. J Clin Psychiatry 1997;58(Suppl 7):23–27.

124. Schweizer E, Weise C, Clary C, et al: Placebo controlled trial of venlafaxine for the treatment of major depression. J Clin Psychopharmacol 1991;11:233–236.

125. Sigg T: Recurrent seizures from sustained-release bupropion [abstract]. J Toxicol Clin Toxicol 1998;37:634.

126. Silbergeld EK, Hurska RE: Lisuride and LSD: Dopaminergic and serotonergic interactions in the serotonin syndrome. Psychopharmacology 1979;65:233–257.

127. Simonsen LLP: Top 200 drugs: Rx prices still moderating as managed care grows. Pharm Times, April 1995:17–23.

128. Singer PP, Jones GR: An uncommon fatality due to moclobemide and paroxetine. J Analytical Toxicol 1997;21:518–520.

129. Skop BP, Finkelstein JA, Mareth TR, et al: The serotonin syndrome associated with paroxetine, an over-the-counter cold remedy, and vascular disease. Am J Emerg Med 1994;12:642–644.

130. Smilkstein MJ, Smolinske SC, Rumack BH: A case of MAO inhibitor/MDMA interaction: Agony after ecstasy. J Toxicol Clin Toxicol 1987;25:149–159.

131. Smith B, Prockop DJ: Central nervous system effects of ingestion of L-tryptophan by normal subjects. N Engl J Med 1962;267:1338–1341.

132. Snyder SH, Peroutka SJ: A possible role of serotonin receptors in antidepressant drug action. Pharmacopsychiatry 1982;15:131–134.

133. Spigset O, Mjorndal T, Lovheim O: Serotonin syndrome caused by a moclobemide-clomipramine interaction. BMJ 1993;306:248.

134. Spiller HA, Ramoska EA, Krenzelok EP: Bupropion overdose: A 3-year multi-center retrospective analysis. Am J Emerg Med 1994;12:43–45.

135. Sprouse JS, Aghajanian GK: (-)-Propranolol blocks the inhibition of serotonergic dorsal raphe cell firing by 5-HT1A selective agonists. Eur J Pharmacol 1986;128:295–298.

136. Steiner W, Fontaine R: Toxic reaction following the combined administration of fluoxetine and L-tryptophan: Five case reports. Biol Psychiatry 1986;21:1067–1071.

137. Sternbach H: The serotonin syndrome. Am J Psychiatry 1991;148:705–713.

138. Storrow AB: Bupropion overdose and seizure. Am J Emerg Med 1994;12:183–184.

139. Tackley RM, Tregaskis B: Fatality following a monamine oxidase inhibitor/tricyclic interaction. Anaesthesia 1987;42:760–763.

140. Tordoff SG, Stubbing JF, Linter SPK: Delayed excitatory reaction following interaction of cocaine and monoamine oxidase inhibitor (phenelzine). Br J Anaesth 1991;66:516–518.

141. Tripathi A, Greenberger PA: Bupropion hydrochloride induced serum sickness-like reaction. Ann Allergy Asthma Immunol 1999;83:165–166.

142. Vanpee D, Laloyaux P, Gillet JB: Seizure and hyponatremia after overdose of trazodone [Letter]. Am J Emerg Med 1999;17:430–431.

143. Versiani M, Mohammed A, Chouinard G: Double-blind, placebo-controlled study with reboxetine in inpatients with severe major depressive disorder. J Clin Psychopharmacol 2000;20:28–34.

144. Vetulani J, Stawarz RJ, Dingell JV, Sulser F: A possible common mechanism of action of antidepressant treatments: Reduction in the sensitivity of the noradrenergic cyclic AMP generating system in the rat limbic forebrain. Naunyn Schmiedebergs Arch Pharmacol 1976;293:109–114.

145. White CM, Hailey RA, Levin GM, Smith T: Seizure resulting from a venlafaxine overdose. Ann Pharmacother 1997;31:178–180.

146. Willner P: Dopamine and depression: A review of recent evidence. Brain Res Rev 1983;6:211–246.

147. Wong DT, Bymaster FP, Horng JS, Molloy BB: A new selective inhibitor for uptake of serotonin into synaptosomes of rat brain: 3-p-trifluoromethylphenoxy-N-methyl-3 phenylpropylamine. J Pharmacol Exp Ther 1975;193:804–811.

148. Woo MH, Smythe MA: Association of SIADH with selective serotonin reuptake inhibitors. Ann Pharmacother 1997;31:108–110.

149. Woodrum ST, Brown CS: Management of SSRI-induced sexual dysfunction. Ann Pharmacother 1998;32:1209–1215.

150. Yamada J, Sugimoto Y, Wakita H, Horisaka K: The involvement of serotonergic and dopaminergic systems in hypothermia induced in mice by intracerebroventricular injection of serotonin. Jpn J Pharmacol 1988;48:145–148.

151. Yolles JC, Armenta WA, Alao A: Serum sickness induced by bupropion. Ann Pharmacother 1999;33:931–933.

152. Zajecka J, Tracy KA, Mitchell S: Discontinuation symptoms after treatment with serotonin reuptake inhibitors: A literature review. J Clin Psychiatry 1997;58:291–297.

153. Zhalkovsky B, Walker D, Bourgeois JA: Seizure activity and enzyme elevations after venlafaxine overdose. J Clin Psychopharmacol 1997;17:490–491.

CHAPTER 59 ANTIPSYCHOTICS

Frank LoVecchio / Neal A. Lewin

A lethargic 40-year-old man was brought to the Emergency Department (ED) by paramedics. He was discovered slumped over a park bench with an empty pill container at his side. Bystanders at the scene stated that the patient had a history of chronic alcoholism, and had been hospitalized several times for "hallucinations." There was no other medical history available.

His vital signs were blood pressure, 90/50 mm Hg; pulse, 118 beats/min and regular; respirations, 10 breaths/min and regular; and rectal temperature, 95°F (35°C). The patient's skin revealed signs of compression where it was in contact with the park bench. There was no evidence of head trauma. Numerous carious teeth and gingivitis were noted. A gag reflex could not be elicited. His pupils were 4 mm, equal, and responsive to light. Oculocephalic reflexes were present. The optic discs were within normal limits. Coarse rales and rhonchi were heard over the right lower lung area. Heart sounds were normal with no audible murmurs. The patient's abdomen was distended with ascites and no palpable masses. Bowel sounds were diminished but present. Rectal examination was negative for occult blood. There was mild pitting edema in the extremities. Pulses were palpable and equal bilaterally. The patient was unresponsive to deep pain. Reflexes were normal and equal bilaterally. Plantar flexion was present bilaterally. There were no localizing neurologic findings.

As his airway and breathing were being assessed, bedside blood glucose was noted to be 130 mg/dL. Two successive 2-mg IV boluses of naloxone were administered with no subsequent response. Thiamine 100-mg was also given intravenously. The patient was successfully intubated with a cuffed 8.0-mm endotracheal tube and supplemental oxygen was administered. A 2-L intravenous infusion of 0.9% sodium chloride solution was administered rapidly and the blood pressure rose to 110/80 mm Hg. The initial room air arterial blood gas values were pH, 7.28; P_{CO_2}, 53 mm Hg; and P_{O_2}, 70 mm Hg. Blood samples were sent for electrolytes, glucose, serum calcium, acetaminophen, creatine phosphokinase (CPK), and complete blood count.

A nasogastric tube was inserted and 75 g of activated charcoal was instilled into the stomach. An electrocardiogram (ECG) revealed a sinus tachycardia with a prolonged QT interval and QRS duration of 110 msec. An abdominal radiograph suggested radiopaque material in the upper small bowel, and a chest radiograph demonstrated a right lower lobe infiltrate. The patient received broad-spectrum intravenous antibiotics following appropriate cultures. A bolus of 100 mEq of sodium bicarbonate (8.4%) was administered because of the slightly prolonged QRS interval. Shortly after its administration the QRS duration decreased to 90 msec. When the patient awoke 24 hours later in the intensive care unit (ICU), he admitted to ingesting a 1-month supply of mesoridazine pills. A CPK level peaked at 6500 U/L 20 hours after admission. Fifty hours after admission, he was transferred from the ICU to the psychiatric service for his depression.

HISTORY AND EPIDEMIOLOGY

Antipsychotic medication use has increased since their introduction in the 1950s.[9] More adverse reactions to psychotropic medications are to be anticipated with increased utilization, broader indications, and newer products. Newer products are a direct result of improved knowledge of pharmacologic mechanisms of these agents. These advances have stimulated research in identifying pathophysiologic changes of psychiatric diseases and the introduction of numerous "atypical" antipsychotics.

Mood and behavior modification in human beings was first attempted hundreds of years ago. One of the first formal reports occurred in 1845 when Moreau proposed a hashish model for mental illness research. Thirty years later, Freud presented his cocaine papers, followed shortly thereafter by Kraepelin, who founded the first laboratory of clinical pharmacology in Germany. In 1931, *Rauwolfia serpentina* was used in the treatment of insanity. Shortly thereafter, amphetamine-induced psychosis was used in an animal model to study psychosis. In 1943, Hofmann synthesized lysergic acid diethylamide (LSD).[42]

Treatment of psychosis with lithium salts was first reported in 1949, and chlorpromazine was synthesized the following year. The term *tranquilizer* was introduced shortly thereafter and was used to describe the psychic effects of reserpine. The years that followed led to the serendipitous recognition of monoamine oxidase inhibitor and antidepressant properties in antituberculous drugs such as iproniazid. Haloperidol was synthesized in 1958. In the next decades, research into the biologic basis of mental illness flourished.[42] This past decade saw the emergence of newer antipsychotics, which carry with them a hope of improved clinical effectiveness and decreased toxicity.

In addition to the treatment of the psychoses (schizophrenia and psychotic depression) antipsychotics are increasingly being used for nonpsychiatric conditions. Antipsychotics may be used for the chemical restraint of agitated patients, to control nausea and emesis, for relief of pain and/or nausea accompanying migraines, for the inhibition of hiccups, and for the management of various involuntary motor disorders such as Tourette syndrome or Huntington chorea.[48]

This chapter identifies the antipsychotic agents that are commonly used for the treatment of psychiatric illness and their adverse effects, as well as the manifestations of intentional and unintentional overdose.

PHARMACOLOGY

Classification of Antipsychotic Medications

In part because of their long and charged history, the terminology of the agents used in the management of psychosis is unfortunately complex. Antipsychotic agents encompass all drugs used in the resolution of psychosis and include both the neuroleptics and atypical antipsychotics. *Neuroleptics,* formerly called "major tranquilizers," are able to suppress spontaneous movements, but the term specifically contrasts the effects of agents such as chlorpromazine with those of the classic central nervous system depressants (ie, "minor tranquilizers"). These effects include the development of extrapyramidal movement disorders as well as the maintenance of spinal reflexes and antinociceptive-avoidance behaviors. It is currently appreciated that all neuroleptics have antipsychotic effects, but not all antipsychotics have neuroleptic effects. The term *antipsychotic* is a more general and hopeful term. We will attempt to exclusively use this term in this chapter, except where widespread use prohibits this clarification.

Prototypical antipsychotic agents include haloperidol and chlorpromazine. Sedation and antianxiety (sometimes difficult to notice in agitated patients) are common effects with antipsychotics. With the introduction of newer heterocyclic agents or atypical antipsychotics, such as clozapine and olanzapine, the use of the term neuroleptic is inappropriate for these medications because clozapine has well-defined antipsychotic effects with minimal extrapyramidal effects.[32,75]

Antipsychotics are divided into seven major classes: phenothiazines, thioxanthenes, butyrophenones, diphenylbutylpiperidines, dibenzodiazepines, dibenzoxazepines, and indoles (Table 59–1). The phenothiazines, commonly used in the treatment of various psychiatric disorders, have a basic three-ring structure (Fig. 59–1). Substitutions at position 2 and the nitrogen atom at position 10 in the middle ring yield compounds that can be divided into three major classes: the aliphatic (eg, chlorpromazine), piperidine (eg, thioridazine), and piperazine (eg, perphenazine) derivatives.[9] All three groups have similar central and peripheral dopaminergic-receptor blockade actions. The thioxanthenes are derivatives of the phenothiazines. A carbon atom replaces the nitrogen at position 10, with a double bond to the side chain. The thioxanthenes and the butyrophenones (such as haloperidol) are pharmacologically similar to the phenothiazines.

Atypical antipsychotics can be partitioned into various categories: (a) substantial selectivity for a dopamine receptor subtype, (b) significant selectivity for a nondopaminergic receptor, (c) atypical actions secondary to concomitant actions at two or more receptors, and (d) different functional effects when binding to the same receptor isoform in different cell types.[42,99a]

The phenothiazines have various inhibitory effects on a variety of receptors, including dopaminergic, cholinergic, α_1- and α_2-adrenergic, histaminic, and diverse serotonergic receptors.[9] Antipsychotic activity results from the dopamine-receptor-blocking activity in the limbic system and is probably mediated by serotonergic receptors. Excessive dopaminergic activity in the limbic system produces psychosis, such as schizophrenia, and addictive-drug-craving behavior.

The two basal ganglia sites identified as most important in dopaminergic effects are the substantia nigra, which is important in movement control, and the nucleus accumbens, which controls emotion and cognitive function.[10] Excessive dopaminergic activity in other areas, such as the striatum, may produce tics, acute choreoathetosis, or Tourette syndrome. Diminished dopaminergic activity in the basal ganglia produces various extrapyramidal disorders such as acute dystonias and parkinsonism.[81]

Further research will delineate which dopamine subtype receptors are responsible for manifestation and reversal of specific symptomatology. There are six distinct dopamine receptor subtypes: D_1,

TABLE 59–1.   Pharmacologic Classification of Typical and Atypical Antipsychotic Agents

Generic Name	Class	Sedation	D_2 Antagonism
Typical antipsychotics			
	Phenothiazine		
Chlorpromazine	Aliphatic	+++	+
Triflupromazine	Aliphatic	+	+++
Fluphenazine	Piperazine	+	+++
Perphenazine	Piperazine	++	++
Prochlorperazine	Piperazine	++	++
Trifluoperazine	Piperazine	+	+++
Thioridazine	Piperidine	+++	+
Mesoridazine	Piperidine	+	+
Thiothixene	Thioxanthene	++	+++
Haloperidol	Butyrophenone	+++	+++
Droperidol	Butyrophenone	++	++
Pimozide	Diphenylbutylpiperidine	+++	+++
Molindone	Dihydroindolone	++	++
Loxapine	Dibenzoxazepine	+	++
Atypical antipsychotics			
Clozapine	Dibenzodiazepine	++	+
Olanzapine	Thienobenzodiazepine	++	+
Quetiapine	Dibenzothiazepine	++	+
Risperidone	Benzisoxazole	++	+

+++, strong; ++, moderate; +, weak.

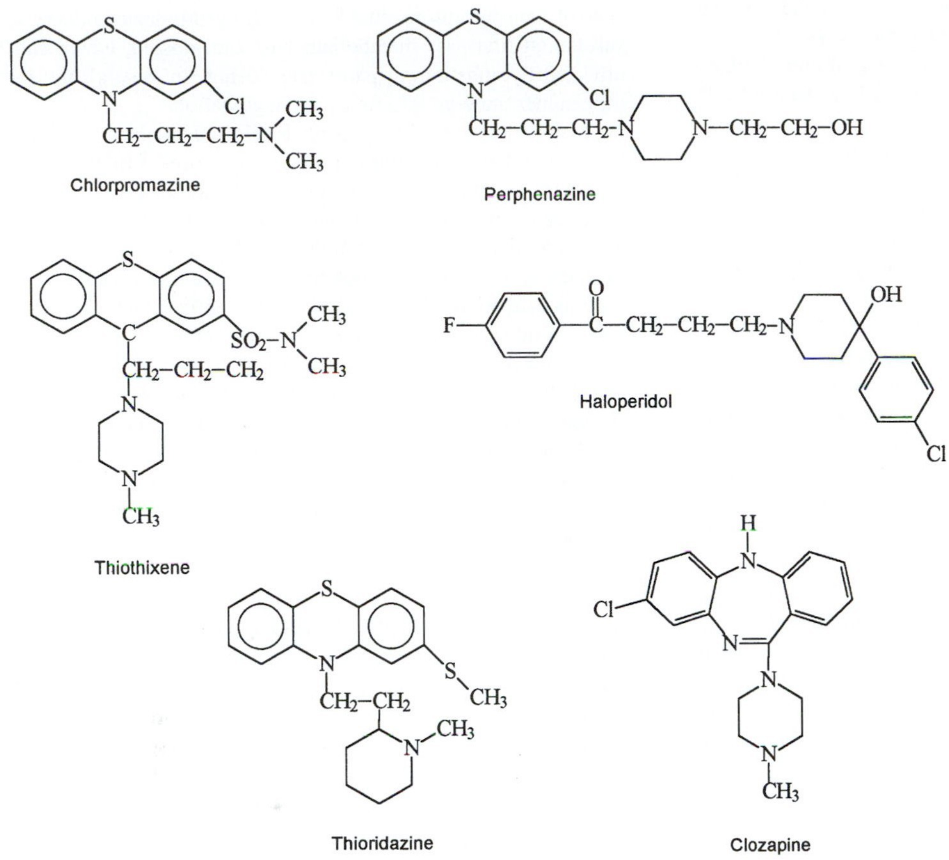

Figure 59–1. The structures of common antipsychotic drugs.

D_{2A}, D_{2B}, D_3, D_4, and D_5 (Table 59–2). Most clinically effective antipsychotic agents have a high affinity for D_2 and D_3 receptors. A strong correlation exists between clinical potencies of antipsychotic drugs and their ability to antagonize D_2 receptors.[96,97] Some antipsychotics, such as the thioxanthenes and phenothiazines, bind with high affinity to D_1, D_2, D_3, and D_4 receptors (Table 59–2). The heterocyclic substituted agents haloperidol and pimozide are high-

affinity antagonists for D_2 and D_3 dopamine receptors[72] and have variable affinity for D_4. The D_3 receptors are present in limbic areas of the CNS, and agents acting here would have fewer extrapyramidal effects than on dopamine receptors in the basal ganglia.[44] The effect of blocking D_1 or D_5 receptors remains unclear.[49]

Central glutamatergic effects show a net decrease following the administration of antipsychotics. The exact mechanism is unclear,

TABLE 59–2. **Effects of Antipsychotics on Postsynaptic Dopamine Receptors and Serotonin Receptors**

	D_1 and D_5	D_2	D_{2b}	D_3 and D_4	5-HT
Effect on cyclic AMP	Increases	Decreases	Increases phosphoinositide		
Agonists					
Dopamine	Full agonist (weak)	Full agonist (potent)	?	?	
Apomorphine	Partial agonist (weak)	Full agonist (potent)	?	?	
Antagonists					
Phenothiazines	Potent	Potent	?	?	
Thioxanthenes	Potent	Potent	?	?	
Butyrophenones	Weak	Potent	?		
Clozapine	Inactive	Weak	Weak	Potent	5-HT$_{2A}$
Olanzapine	Weak D_1	Moderate	?	?	5-HT$_{2A, C}$
Risperidone	Weak D_1	Moderate	?	?	5-HT$_{2A}$; weak 5-HT$_{1A, C, D}$
Quetiapine	Weak D_1	Moderate	?	?	Weak 5-HT$_{1A}$
Sertindole	Weak D_1	Moderate	?	?	5-HT$_{2A}$

with current theories suggesting that nigrostriatal dopamine neurons are antagonized by striatonigral GABA pathways.

An atypical antipsychotic agent with low risk of producing extrapyramidal reactions, such as clozapine, has a low affinity for D_2 receptors, but is also an active α-adrenergic antagonist. Clozapine and risperidone also have affinities for 5-HT$_2$ serotonin receptors. Clozapine has selectivity for D_4 dopamine receptors as well, but the significance of this subtype in the basal ganglia remains unknown. Although much of the information is unclear, the mechanism and receptor activities of some of the newer antipsychotics are discussed individually.

Olanzapine, a thienobenzodiazepine, has a potent affinity for D_1, D_2, D_4, 5-HT$_{2A}$, 5-HT$_{2C}$, 5-HT$_3$, α_1-adrenergic, histamine H$_1$, and muscarinic receptor subtypes. In comparison to other typical agents, olanzapine has less affinity for 5-HT$_1$ subtypes, GABA, β-adrenergic receptors, and benzodiazepine binding sites. Compared to clozapine, olanzapine has a high affinity for the dopamine D_4 receptor and less α_2-adrenoceptor activity. Olanzapine has a different binding profile from that seen with haloperidol, risperidone, and quetiapine.

Quetiapine is a dibenzothiazepine with affinity to 5-HT$_2$ and dopamine D_2 receptors. Quetiapine has affinity for H$_1$ and α_1- and α_2-adrenergic receptors, and mild affinity for dopamine D_1 receptors. In comparison to clozapine, quetiapine possesses less affinity for muscarinic cholinergic and benzodiazepine binding sites. Quetiapine and risperidone have stronger affinity for 5-HT$_2$ receptors than for D_2 receptors. Quetiapine has weak dopamine D_2 receptor affinity, akin to clozapine, whereas risperidone has higher dopamine D_2 receptor affinity, like haloperidol.

Risperidone is an benzisoxazole with greater affinity for the 5-HT$_2$ receptor in comparison to the D_2 receptor. Absolute affinity is high at both receptors. Risperidone is also a potent antagonist of α_1- and α_2-adrenergic and H$_1$ receptors. Risperidone has low to moderate affinity for 5-HT$_{1C}$, 5-HT$_{1D}$, and 5-HT$_{1A}$ receptors weak affinity for dopamine D_1 receptors. Risperidone has no affinity for cholinergic muscarinic or β_1- and β_2-adrenergic receptors.[42]

Sertindole is predominantly a 5-HT$_2$ antagonist with antagonist activity at α_1-adrenergic and dopamine D_2 and D_1 receptors. Sertindole has a low affinity for 5-HT$_{1A}$, α_2-adrenergic, β-adrenergic, H$_1$, and muscarinic receptors. Sertindole binds with high affinity to fewer receptors than either risperidone or clozapine. However, like risperidone and clozapine, sertindole binds with high affinity to D_2, 5-HT$_2$, and α_1-adrenergic receptors. Sertindole has no affinity for histamine receptors because risperidone and clozapine have high affinities. Clozapine also binds to muscarinic receptors with high affinity. Sertindole is more selective for the mesolimbic dopamine neurons than it is for the nigrostriatal dopaminergic neurons.[42]

PHARMACOKINETICS AND TOXICOKINETICS

The phenothiazines can be administered orally, intramuscularly, rectally, or intravenously. Gastrointestinal (GI) absorption is diminished because of drug binding in the intestinal wall.[49] Intramuscular absorption is variable, and some phenothiazines, such as chlorpromazine, may cause hypotension when administered intravenously or intramuscularly.[101] Chlorpromazine is mainly absorbed in the jejunum in a pH-dependent fashion; thus, concomitant therapy with H$_2$ antagonists results in decreased steady-state plasma chlorpromazine levels.[47] Chlorpromazine undergoes a substantial first-pass metabolism with oral dosing, which can be obviated by substituting parenteral dosing. In general, the butyrophenones undergo less first-pass degradation.

Peak chlorpromazine plasma levels are attained within 2–4 hours of oral administration of therapeutic doses.[20] In plasma, 99% of chlorpromazine is bound to albumin.[20] Biotransformation of this drug occurs in the liver by demethylation and hydroxylation.[20,22,73] There are more than 15 metabolites of this drug, half of which are excreted in the urine and stool. Several of the breakdown products, such as 7-hydroxychlorpromazine, have antipsychotic effects,[73,86] whereas others, such as chlorpromazine sulfoxide, are inactive.[59] The nonphenothiazine antipsychotics, such as the butyrophenones and the thioxanthenes, have no active metabolites. Half of the excretion of the phenothiazines occurs by conjugation of oxidized and hydroxylated metabolites with glucuronic acids and sulfates, after which the conjugated metabolites are excreted by the kidneys.[47,49] The remainder of phenothiazine excretion occurs via the enterohepatic system.

Metabolism of the phenothiazines by the liver microsomes may be enhanced by such cytochrome P450 enzyme inducers as barbiturates or rifampin.[21,37,50,70] Both concomitant lithium and antipsychotic therapy and cytochrome P450 enzyme drug interactions result in diverse neurotoxic manifestations.[11,24,37,79,95,106] Cardiac dysrhythmias are reported when lithium is discontinued following combined therapy with lithium and phenothiazines.[93,101]

Phenothiazine metabolites are lipophilic and have large volumes of distribution. Hence the breakdown products may be found in the urine up to 6 weeks after the last dose of the parent compound. There is little correlation between dose, serum level, and antipsychotic effect of phenothiazines.[21,77] Tolerance to the sedative and hypotensive effects occurs after several weeks of therapy. In general, optimum antipsychotic effects require approximately 1 month of therapy. Interestingly, chronic therapy with a constant dose results in lowered plasma levels. However, in spite of the lowered plasma levels of phenothiazines, tolerance to their antipsychotic effects typically does not occur for months.

PATHOPHYSIOLOGY AND CLINICAL MANIFESTATIONS

Toxicity of the antipsychotic agents can be broadly categorized into CNS and non-CNS effects (Table 59–3).[90] Toxic manifestations may occur with therapeutic doses, but are usually found in patients who have taken a consequential overdose or initiated therapy with a new drug but with totally different manifestations. The most common non-CNS complication is orthostatic hypotension, which commonly occurs during the initiation of therapy. The most likely cause of orthostatic hypotension is peripheral α-adrenergic blockade with contributing factors being direct vasodilation, central vasomotor reflex depression, and direct myocardial depression.[71]

The depressant action of phenothiazines on the heart is similar to that of the IA antidysrhythmic agents or tricyclic antidepressants. Through sodium and potassium channel blockade these drugs prolong the QRS and QTc intervals, respectively, and cause repolarization abnormalities (Chap. 52).[50,105] Supraventricular and ventricular tachydysrhythmias are also reported, but the majority of patients have sinus tachycardia and aberrant conductions simi-

TABLE 59–3. Toxic Effects of Antipsychotic Agents

Cardiovascular	Prolonged QT, QRS and PR intervals
	Nonspecific ST- and T-wave changes,
	Right-axis deviation (terminal 40 msec prolongation)
	Myocardial depression, orthostatic hypotension
Central nervous system	Akathisia
	Decreased sweating
	Decreased vasomotor reflexes
	Dystonia and related movement disorders
	Hyperthermia
	Potentially lower seizure threshold
	Impaired memory
	Parkinsonism or parkinson-like symptoms
	"Rabbit syndrome" (perioral tremor)
	Somnolence, coma
	Tardive dyskinesia
Endocrine	Amenorrhea and irregular menses
	Decreased ADH secretion
	Decreased gonadotrophins, ACTH, and growth hormone
	Increased prolactin secretion
Gastrointestinal	Dry buccal membranes
	Decreased gastrointestinal motility
Genitourinary	Ejaculation dysfunction
	Priapism
	Urinary retention
Ophthalmic	Miosis
	Mydriasis
	Blurred vision

lar to the tricyclic antidepressants (Chap. 57).[23,66,71] Of all the phenothiazines, thioridazine and mesoridazine are associated with the greatest cardiotoxicity because of their degree of sodium channel and potassium efflux blockade.[71] High-dose haloperidol and droperidol both orally and parenterally, is also associated with cardiac dysrhythmias including prolonged QTc-associated torsades de pointes.[14,33,46,52,66,80,108]

Respiratory effects are extremely rare. If they do occur, they are related to CNS depression.

The most commonly reported adverse effects of the antipsychotic medications involve the CNS and are generally reversible.[107] Sedation almost always accompanies the induction of antipsychotic therapy and tolerance to this effect develops within months. This effect led to the earlier classification of this group of agents as tranquilizers.

Clinical experience with overdose of the newer atypical agents is limited. Clozapine, with its profound anticholinergic effects, results in central nervous system depression and seizures,[94] but appears to be unlikely to cause cardiac conduction disturbances or agranulocytosis following acute ingestion. Clozapine has been associated with a case of nephritis.[30] Reports thus far with risperidone, olanzapine, and quetiapine suggest that patients should be monitored for obtundation, respiratory depression, and cardiac conduction abnormalities. A prospective poison center–based study with 31 presumed risperidone ingestions resulted in lethargy (23%) as the most common symptom with 1 death in a patient who also ingested imipramine.[1] Olanzapine has been associated with the neuroleptic malignant syndrome and lethargy.[35] Coma is reported after quetiapine ingestion.[45]

Movement Disorders

More troubling to the patient than sedation are the movement disorders. Three acute movement disorders occur within 1–60 days of initiating therapy: acute dystonia, parkinsonism, and akathisia (Table 59–4). An additional movement disorder, which occurs months to years after initiating therapy, is tardive dyskinesia[6,62–64] (Chap. 19).

Normal motor movement patterns depend on a delicate balance between dopamine and acetylcholine in the extrapyramidal system. Excessive stimulation of the cholinergic fibers that project from the basal ganglia to the thalamus results in hyperkinesis. The pathophysiology of acute dystonic reactions is not fully elucidated but at least a portion involves interference of neurotransmitters in the basal ganglia. Dopamine is an excitatory neurotransmitter, whereas GABA and acetylcholine, and to a lesser degree serotonin, act as inhibitors. Nigrostriatal dopamine neurons are antagonized by striatonigral GABA neurons and presynaptic serotonin receptors and inhibited by cholinergic striatal interneurons. Antipsychotics antagonize D_2 receptors, thus resulting in amplified acetylcholine release. Ironically, an acute dystonic reaction may be a result of enhanced dopamine discharge into supersensitive postsynaptic receptors. Acute administration of antipsychotics provokes increased dopamine synthesis and release from nigrostriatal neurons and postsynaptic receptor supersensitivity. These are compensatory attempts to surmount postsynaptic D_2 blockade. As drug concentrations decrease over hours to days, a state of dopamine surplus occurs and heightened muscular activity (dystonia) results.

Acute dystonic reactions typically occur within 48–72 hours of a single dose and are more common in males and children treated with butyrophenones and piperazines. The reactions may include oculogyric crisis (upward gaze paralysis); jaw, tongue, lip, and throat spasms; torticollis (neck twisting); retrocollis (back of neck spasm); opisthotonos (scoliosis); buccolingual (facial) grimacing; tortipelvis (abdominal wall spasm); and laryngeal dystonia, which is potentially life-threatening.[27,62,87] The anatomic localization for these effects varies according to individual susceptibility and cortical involvement. Significant hyperthermia may rarely be associated with dystonic reactions. Symptoms rapidly resolve with parenteral antihistamines, anticholinergics, or benzodiazepines. Recommended treatments in adults and children are diphenhydramine (Benadryl) IV or IM 1 mg/kg or benztropine mesylate (Cogentin) IV or IM 1–2 mg in adults and children older than 12 years of age. Intravenous administration has a more rapid onset. Diazepam 0.1 mg/kg IV may be used instead of anticholinergic agents when anticholinergics have failed or in agitated febrile patients who may have impaired thermoregulatory control.[6] Acute treatment should be followed with several days of oral benztropine mesylate (Cogentin) 1–2 mg twice daily, or diphenhydramine 1 mg/kg up to 50 mg four times daily.[68] If long-term therapy is needed, benztropine mesylate is the agent of choice. Rarely, patients may feign a movement disorder in order to receive their anticholinergic drug of choice.[25,83] The reason for the abuse of anticholinergics is unclear, but likely includes euphoria supported by the increased serotonin effects of Cogentin. Those over 40 year of age are more susceptible to the adverse effects of the antipsychotic agents, other than dystonic reactions, especially tardive dyskinesia (TD).[89] The prevalence of TD in patients older than 40 years of age is 3 times its prevalence in those patients who are younger than 40 years of age.

TABLE 59–4. Extrapyramidal Adverse Effects of Antipsychotic Agents

Effect and Time of Maximal Risk	Characteristics	Mechanism	Treatment
Dystonia (acute) (1–5 days)	Oculogyric crisis; torticollis; retrocollis; tortipelvis	Unknown; dopamine vs cholinergic imbalance; serotonin and GABA effects	Anticholinergics (diphenhydramine, benzotropine); benzodiazepines
Akathisia (5–60 days)	Restlessness; inability to sit	Unknown	Reduction in dose of antipsychotic agent; anticholinergics; benzodiazepines
Parkinsonism (5–30 days)	Bradykinesia; shuffling gait; resting tremor; rigidity; masked facies; perioral tremor ("rabbit" syndrome)	Antagonism of dopamine	Reduction in dose of antipsychotic agent; anticholinergics
Neuroleptic malignant syndrome (days to weeks)	Rigidity; autonomic dysfunction (unstable blood pressure); hyperthermia; altered mental status; catatonia; increased CPK	Antagonism of dopamine	Limit hyperthermia (rapid cooling); benzodiazepines; neuromuscular blockade; central dopamine agonists ? benefit (bromocriptine, amantadine)
Tardive dyskinesia (months to years)	Involuntary buccolinguomasticatory movements; choreoathetoid movements	Excess dopaminergic activity	Stop offending drug; addition of or increase in antipsychotic dose; cholinergic agents

Another toxic CNS effect of antipsychotic medications is akathisia, the subjective sensation of restlessness or muscle discomfort.[10] The severity and persistence of dyskinesia and akathisia increases with age.[10,89] Affected patients are usually elderly and may appear agitated, have restless legs, and are unable to sit still. Objective symptoms can persist. At times the patient may act violently. This symptom usually occurs early in treatment (5–60 days), especially with dosage increase. These symptoms are alleviated by reduction of the phenothiazine dose or by the addition of lorazepam, propranolol, or, to a lesser extent, antiparkinsonian drugs.[88]

Parkinsonism (bradykinesia) is another CNS effect of antipsychotic therapy.[29] In fact, it is the most common extrapyramidal effect, particularly in elderly women. Antipsychotic-induced parkinsonism occurs in 90% of susceptible patients within 72 days of initiating antipsychotic therapy and is characterized by a shuffling gait, resting tremor, rigidity, sialorrhea, pill rolling that is typically worse at rest, a masklike expression, fine-movement muscle weakness, postural instability, and bradykinesia. An atypical syndrome of perioral tremor (rabbit syndrome) may merely be a late parkinsonian variant.[56] The incidence of bradykinesia increases with age, but patients rarely develop symptoms if they have been maintained on the same dose for 3 months or more. When symptoms develop, they may be attenuated by reduction of dosage or by addition of antiparkinsonian agents.[4]

The most serious CNS toxic effect of antipsychotics is tardive dyskinesia, with a reported incidence ranging from 3% to 50%.[6] Its development appears to be much less frequent with use of the atypical antipsychotic agents. Also called *permanent dyskinesia*, tardive dyskinesia is characterized by involuntary, repetitive movements of the face, tongue, and lips (buccolinguomasticatory syndrome). Movements of the tongue typically appear first. Orofacial manifestations are more common in the elderly, whereas truncal movements are more common in young adults. The extremities and/or trunk may manifest choreoathetoid movements. Voluntary activity of the involved muscles may reduce the frequency of repetitive cycles and sleep typically abolishes all abnormal movements. Individuals on long-acting intramuscular depot therapy are more apt to develop the syndrome. Women who have been on butyrophenones or phenothiazine therapy for several years are more likely to develop the disorder perhaps secondary to higher doses if adjusted for weight. Tardive dyskinesia may first appear when drug dosage reductions are attempted after several years of therapy. Chronic dopamine receptor blockade results in receptor upregulation and increased dopamine secretion.[44,97] Reduction of phenothiazine dose may thus cause the movement disorder. Similarly, administration of L-dopa, the dopamine precursor, exacerbates the syndrome.[54]

The exact neuropathology of tardive dyskinesia is unknown. It is hypothesized that compensatory increases in dopamine neurotransmitter function may be involved. This hypothesis is supported by dissimilar therapeutic responses in patients with Parkinson disease from patients with tardive dyskinesia. In contrast to the similar responses of patients with choreoathetotic dyskinesias (ie, Huntington disease), other factors play a role as neuropathologic examination of patients with tardive dyskinesia does not reveal striatal damage. In addition, primate studies reveal that haloperidol, an agent commonly implicated in tardive dyskinesia, and its analogue (tetrahydropyridine) are metabolized to the potentially neurotoxic pyridinium metabolites haloperidol pyridinium (HPP$^+$) and reduced pyridinium (RHPP$^+$), respectively.[7,54] These metabolites are believed to cause nigrostriatal toxicity by inhibiting mitochondrial respiration and are similar to MPP$^+$ (1-methyl-4-phenylpyridium), a structurally related pyridinium neurotoxic metabolite of MPTP (Chap. 62). HPP$^+$ in rats is also a potent cytotoxin for dopaminergic and serotonergic neurons. Although the results are not confirmed in human beings, the authors suggest a potential link between HPP$^+$ and RHPP$^+$ neurotoxicity, which may result in tardive dyskinesias in haloperidol-treated patients.

Tardive dyskinesia may be permanent or show minimal improvement despite treatment. Preventive therapy in the form of "drug holidays" (periods of abstinence from drugs), which was thought to avert this complication, may not be as successful as previously reported.[68] Avoidance of high-dose, long-term daily therapy may also decrease its incidence.[56] Increase in dosage of antipsychotic medication may alleviate the symptoms. Haloperidol is commonly used for this purpose because of its potent blockade of dopamine receptors. In some patients, symptoms progressively disappear after stopping the antipsychotic agents, but psychotic symptoms may return. Piperazine phenothiazines or butyrophenones with little anticholinergic effect may be helpful in managing the psychosis, but not the tardive dyskinesia.[62–64]

Other medications have been used for the treatment of tardive dyskinesia with limited efficacy. Not only do anticholinergic medications not improve tardive dyskinesia, but they may, in fact, exacerbate the condition, as well as cause a psychosis. This would be the expected result if the postulated mechanism of dopaminergic overactivity with subsequent cholinergic underactivity were valid. Anticholinergics agents are commonly prescribed with antipsychotics to prevent parkinsonism, but some experts have expressed concern in that anticholinergics facilitate the development of tardive dyskinesia.[62–64] Another treatment approach is to decrease receptor stimulation by decreasing the amount of neurotransmitter available. Reserpine and meclofenoxate deplete catecholamine storage in synaptic vesicles by preventing reuptake of dopamine, thereby decreasing the amount of neurotransmitter available; however, long-term studies have not supported this therapy.[38,51,55,57,58]

Cholinergic stimulation using an anticholinesterase such as physostigmine may also help the ameliorate tardive dyskinesia.[105] The administration of choline, a precursor of acetylcholine, and lecithin, a dietary source of choline, has similarly exhibited short-term beneficial effects on the tardive dyskinesia.[4]

Neuroleptic Malignant Syndrome

Neuroleptic malignant syndrome (NMS) is characterized by hyperthermia, muscle rigidity, other extrapyramidal effects, autonomic dysfunction, and altered consciousness.[43,60,61,67,69] NMS is a rare sequela of antipsychotic treatment, with an estimated frequency of 0.02–2.4%.[57] Antipsychotics associated with NMS include phenothiazines, butyrophenones, thioxanthenes, loxapine, and olanzapine,[10] although all dopamine antagonists can potentially cause the syndrome. Of these, the medications with greater antidopaminergic activity seem to have a greater potential for causing NMS.[99]

This syndrome is an idiosyncratic, rare, and potentially fatal reaction, which usually occurs in the course of treatment with antipsychotic drugs. Typically, there is a history of a high initial dose with rapid escalation in dose.[39,98] A syndrome similar to NMS is described with the withdrawal of dopamine agonists in parkinsonian patients using lithium.[39,40,82,102] It has also been described with newer agents.[34] The mortality of this disorder was as high as 76% before 1976, but has since declined to about 20%, partly as a result of early recognition and rapid institution of appropriate therapy.[92] The current mortality is unknown.

The central dopamine blockade of NMS results in disequilibrium characterized by a constellation of clinical features including hyperthermia, muscle rigidity, autonomic instability, and alteration in mental status.[92] Unlike a febrile response to an underlying infection, where there is a hypothalamic-controlled elevation of the temperature set point, this is not the case in NMS-induced hyperthermia; therefore, the use of antipyretics is unwarranted.[60] The temperature rise can be mild or marked and is believed be caused by a combination of an altered dopamine response in the hypothalamus and amplified heat production from muscle hyperactiv-

ity.[26,94] The type of muscular activity accompanying or leading to NMS can vary and includes akinesia, choreoathetosis, tremors, myoclonus, dystonia, dyskinesia, dysphagia, dysarthria, opisthotonus, and "lead pipe" rigidity.[40] Alterations in mental status range from confusion and agitation to frank coma. There is no specific laboratory test for NMS, but abnormal findings, such as leukocytosis and creatine phosphokinase, and creatinine elevations are common.

The diagnosis of NMS is difficult to establish and is exclusionary. An essential point in the history is a recent change in antipsychotic dose or the addition of another dopamine antagonist. The differential diagnosis includes meningoencephalitis, tetanus, malignant hyperthermia, lethal catatonia, heatstroke, thyroid storm, serotonin syndrome, pheochromocytoma, strychnine poisoning, and toxicity from a variety of drugs, including anticholinergic poisoning. Perhaps the two syndromes most difficult to distinguish from NMS are serotonin syndrome and lethal catatonia, as all three feature fever and muscle rigidity. Malignant hyperthermia (Chap. 54) is associated with a history of anesthetic agent use, whereas lethal catatonia follows a period of manic hyperactivity and does not feature autonomic instability. If all of the manifestations of NMS are present, medical stabilization and rapid cooling takes precedence over the establishment of the diagnosis.

Treatment of NMS includes rapid external cooling with ice and intravenous benzodiazepines to decrease muscle rigidity, and discontinuation of antipsychotic agents.[94,103] In case reports, bromocriptine and amantadine are reported to be effective in treating NMS, presumably secondary to their central dopamine agonist effects.[5,41,78,81,85,104] However, significant clinical improvement typically does not occur for up to 3 days after initiation of these dopaminergic agents and therefore they are of limited use.[104] Dantrolene sodium, which inhibits the release of calcium from the sarcoplasmic reticulum, is reported as a treatment for NMS.[76,86] Dantrolene, a skeletal muscle relaxant is specifically indicated in the treatment of malignant hyperthermia. However, although its use is anecdotally reported in the treatment of NMS, it should not be considered as initial therapy. This is because NMS primarily involves the CNS, and there is no derangement of calcium transport in the skeletal muscle as in malignant hyperthermia.[67,104] Case reports suggest that the combination of pancuronium and sodium nitroprusside is effective in treating NMS.[16,91] The rationale for using a nondepolarizing agent such as pancuronium is that the muscle paralysis it causes would eliminate further muscle-induced heat generation. However, the use of nitroprusside to reverse any vasoconstriction is controversial and offers no clear advantage to supportive care. In addition, anticholinergic agents are ineffective in NMS and may contribute to increased morbidity and mortality.

The initial management of NMS should consist of good supportive care, aimed primarily at arresting muscle hyperactivity, and evaluation for other potentially life-threatening medical etiologies of hyperthermia. Intubation should be considered, and aggressive muscle relaxation should be pursued with intravenous benzodiazepines and a nondepolarizing agent as indicated. The offending pharmacologic agent should be discontinued. Based solely on the pathophysiology of the syndrome of central dopamine depletion, specific therapy with bromocriptine (2.5–5 mg PO tid), a dopamine agonist, is advocated for NMS. Most importantly, no agent should be considered a substitute for good supportive care. Aggressive supportive care has led to a reduction in mortality from NMS, as demonstrated by a prospective controlled clinical trial in which supportive therapy statistically reduced the duration of illness and incidence of complications compared to dantrolene or bromocriptine.[85]

The clinical course of NMS lasts usually about 10 days, and antipsychotic agents should not be restarted while symptoms of NMS persist. If antipsychotics are necessary, they should not be reintroduced until 1–2 weeks after symptoms resolve. The antipsychotic chosen should be from a different class than the one that precipitated NMS and should have minimal extrapyramidal effects. The atypical antipsychotic agents clozapine, risperidone, olanzapine, and quetiapine are recommended under these circumstances.[75]

DIAGNOSTIC TESTS

Plasma levels of antipsychotics do not correlate well with clinical signs and symptoms.[21,71,76,79] Historically, positive urine phenothiazine colorimetric testing, using the Forrest test, ferric chloride test, or Phenistix reagent strip test, can suggest the presence of phenothiazines.[36] An abdominal radiograph may help confirm a deliberate overdose, as some solid dosage forms of phenothiazines are radiopaque. However, radiographic findings are neither sensitive nor specific for the presence of phenothiazines. An electrocardiogram should be performed to look for cardiac abnormalities as discussed above.

MANAGEMENT

Patients with isolated acute antipsychotic ingestions generally have uncomplicated clinical courses. Deaths are rare and are most frequently associated with thioridazine and mesoridazine overdose,[8,18] or with overdoses of antipsychotics in combination with other drugs. In the management of patients with this overdose, sympathomimetic agents should be reserved for hypotensive patients refractory to intravenous fluids. Studies suggest that catecholamines modify impulse conduction, permitting reentry of delayed impulse within the conduction system and promoting dysrhythmias.[18,74]

Activated charcoal administered orally or via a nasogastric tube may be appropriate as a therapeutic intervention. Emesis, lavage, multiple-dose activated charcoal, cathartics, orogastric lavage, or gastric emptying is not ordinarily recommended for isolated antipsychotic overdoses for the risks of these agents or procedures outweigh the benefits. Because of the substantial protein binding and large volumes of distribution, hemoperfusion and hemodialysis are of no benefit in antipsychotic agent overdoses.[20]

Tachycardia is best managed with fluid resuscitation.[71] If a vasopressor is needed to manage refractory hypotension, a mixed α- and β-adrenergic receptor agonist such as dopamine should be avoided. Because the phenothiazines are potent α-adrenergic antagonists, β-adrenergic stimulation may enhance peripheral vasodilation, further exacerbating the blockade-induced vasodilation and hypotension. Direct-acting, as opposed to indirect-acting, α-adrenergic receptor agonists are preferred. The α-adrenergic receptor agonists phenylephrine, norepinephrine, and metaraminol are more appropriate drugs in this setting.[13] Hemodynamic monitoring will be required in hypotensive patients.

Dysrhythmias are most common with overdose of the piperidine class and are also seen with the butyrophenone agent haloperidol.[1–3,28] Electrocardiographic abnormalities should be treated, particularly if hemodynamic instability results.[15,21,31,53] These manifestations are similar to those of cyclic antidepressant-induced cardiac toxicity. For this reason, sodium bicarbonate may be an appropriate intervention to treat the Na$^+$ channel blockade–related cardiac toxicity from this drug (Antidotes in Depth: Sodium Bicarbonate). Supraventricular dysrhythmias can usually be managed supportively. Ventricular dysrhythmias should be treated with sodium bicarbonate and/or lidocaine. Class IA and IC antidysrhythmic agents are contraindicated because of their sodium channel–blocking effects. If torsades de pointes (polymorphic ventricular tachycardia) is present, magnesium, isoproterenol, or a pacemaker may be an effective treatment.

Treatment with physostigmine salicylate reverses central as well as peripheral anticholinergic abnormalities caused by phenothiazines (Antidotes in Depth: Physostigmine). However, because these clinical effects are rarely life-threatening and physostigmine may further impair cardiac conduction, its use is not typically recommended following antipsychotic drug overdose.[103]

SUMMARY

The use of antipsychotics has increased since their introduction in the 1950s. Adverse reactions are common, as are serious sequelae of intentional and unintentional overdoses. Physicians must be knowledgeable about the pharmacology of these agents and be aware of treatment modalities to be able to manage these potentially dangerous reactions.

ACKNOWLEDGMENTS

Eddy A. Bresnitz, MD, and Richard Y. Wang, MD, contributed to this chapter in a previous edition.

REFERENCES

1. Acri AA, Hentretig FM: Effects of risperidone in overdose. Am J Emerg Med 1998;16:498–501.
2. Aherwadkar SJ, Efendigil MC, Coulshed N: Chlorpromazine therapy and associated acute disturbances of cardiac rhythm. Br Heart J 1974;36:1251–1252.
3. Agelink MW, Majewski T, Wurthmann C, et al. Effects of newer atypical antipsychotics on autonomic neurocardiac function: A comparison between amisulpride, olanzapine, sertindole, and clozapine. J Clin Psychopharmacol. 2001;21:8–13
4. Akiyama K: Algorithms for antipsychotic-associated tardive movement disorders. Psychiatry Clin Neurosci 1999;53:S23–S29.
5. Amdurski S: A therapeutic trial of amantadine in haloperidol induced malignant antipsychotic syndrome [letter]. Curr Ther Res 1983;33:225.
6. American Psychiatric Association Task Force on Late Neurological Effects of Antipsychotic Drugs: Tardive dyskinesia. Am J Psychiatry 1980;137:1163–1172.
7. Avent KM, Etsuko U, Eyles DW, et al: Haloperidol and its tetrahydropyridine derivative (HPTP) are metabolized to potentially neurotoxic pyridinium species in the baboon. Life Sci 1996;59: 1473–1482.
8. Baker PB, Merigian KS, Roberts JR, et al: Hyperthermia, hypertension, hypertonia and coma in a massive thioridazine overdose. Am J Emerg Med 1988;6:346–349.
9. Andersson C, Chakos M, Mailman R, et al: Emerging roles for the novel antipsychotics medications in the treatment of schizophrenia. Psychiatr Clin North Am 1998;21:151–179.

10. Apple JE, Van Hauer G: Antipsychotic malignant syndrome associated with olanzapine therapy. Psychosomatics 1999;40:267–268.

11. Battaglia J, Thornton L, Young C: Loxapine-lorazepam-induced hypotension and stupor [letter]. J Clin Psychopharmacol 1989;9: 227–228.

12. Bausher J, Goldstein HS, Aronson MD, et al: Case report: "Pseudo-giant-p waves" and pericardial friction rub following chlorpromazine therapy. Am J Med Sci 1976;272:357–359.

13. Benowitz NL, Rosenberg J, Becker CE: Cardiopulmonary catastrophes in drug-overdosed patients. Med Clin North Am 1979;63: 127–140.

14. Bett JHN, Holt GW: Malignant ventricular tachyarrhythmia and Haldol. Br Med J 1983;287:1264.

15. Bigger JT: Cardiac electrophysiologic effects of moricizine hydrochloride. Am J Cardiol 1990;65:15D–20D.

16. Blue MG, Schneider SM, Noro S, et al: Successful treatment of NMS with sodium nitroprusside. Ann Intern Med 1986;104:56–57.

17. Caligiuri MR, Jeste DV, Lacro JP: Antipsychotic-Induced movement disorders in the elderly: Epidemiology and treatment recommendations [review]. Drugs Aging 2000;17:363–384.

18. Chouinard G, Ghadirian AM, Jones BD: Death attributed to ventricular arrhythmia induced by thioridazine in combination with a single Contact capsule. Can Med Assoc J 1978;119:729–730.

19. Conley RR, Metzer HY: Adverse events related to olanzapine [review]. J Clin Psychiatry 2000;61(Suppl 8):26–30.

20. Curry SH: Relation between binding to plasma protein, apparent volume of distribution, and rate constants of disposition and elimination for chlorpromazine in three species. J Pharm Pharmacol 1972;24: 818–819.

21. Curry SH, Davis JM, Janowsky DS, et al: Factors affecting chlorpromazine plasma levels in psychiatric patients. Arch Gen Psychiatry 1970;22:209–215.

22. Dahl SG, Strandjord RE: Pharmacokinetics of chlorpromazine after single and chronic dosage. Clin Pharmacol Ther 1976;21:437–438.

23. De Ponti F, Poluzzi E, Montanaro N, Ferguson J: QTc and psychotropic [letter]. Lancet 2000;356:75–76.

24. de la Gandara J, Dominguez RA: Lithium and loxapine: A potential interaction [letter]. J Clin Psychiatry 1988;49:126.

25. Demetropoulos S, Schauben JL: Acute dystonic reactions from "street Valium." J Emerg Med 1987;5:293–297.

26. Diamond BI, Borison RL: Basic and clinical studies of antipsychotic-induced supersensitivity psychosis and dyskinesia. Psychopharmacol Bull 1986;22:900–905.

27. Diamond SG, Markham CH, Baloh RW: Vestibular involvement in spasmodic torticollis: An old hypothesis with new data from otolith testing. Adv Otorhinolaryngol 1988;42:219–223.

28. Dorson PG, Crismon ML: Chlorpromazine accumulation and sudden death in a patient with renal insufficiency. Drug Intell Clin Pharm 1988;22:776–778.

29. Duvoisin R: History of parkinsonism. Pharmacol Ther 1987;32: 1–17.

30. Elias TJ, Bannister KM, Clarkson AR, et al: Clozapine-induced acute interstitial nephritis. Lancet 1999;354:1180–1181.

31. Ereshefsky L: Pharmacokinetics and drug interactions: Update for new antipsychotics [review]. J Clin Psychiatry 1996;57(Suppl 11): 12–25.

32. Ereshefsky L, Watanabe MD, Tran-Johnson TK: Clozapine: An atypical antipsychotic agent. Clin Pharm 1989; 8:691–709.

33. Fayer SA: Torsade de pointes ventricular tachyarrhythmia associated with haloperidol. J Clin Psychopharmacol 1986;6:375–376.

34. Filice GA, McDougall BC, Ercan-Fang N, et al: Antipsychotic malignant syndrome associated with olanzapine. Ann Pharmacother 1998;32:1158–1159.

35. Fogel J, Diaz JE: Olanzapine overdose [letter]. Ann Emerg Med 1998;32:275–276.

36. Forrest FM, Forrest IS, Mason AS: Review of rapid urine tests for phenothiazine and related drugs. Am J Psychiatry 1961;118: 300–307.

37. Forrest FM, Forrest IS, Serra MT: Modification of chlorpromazine metabolism by some other drugs frequently administered to psychiatric patients. Biol Psychiatry 1970;2:53–58.

38. Friedman JH: A case of progressive hemichorea responsive to high-dose reserpine. J Clin Psychiatry 1986;47:149–150.

39. Friedman JH, Feinberg SS, Feldman RG: A antipsychotic malignant-like syndrome due to levodopa therapy withdrawal. JAMA 1985; 254:2792–2795.

40. Fuller MA, Sajatovic M: Neurotoxicity resulting from a combination of lithium and loxapine. J Clin Psychiatry 1989;50:187–190.

41. Gangadhar BN, Desain G, Channabasarnana SM: Amantadine in the antipsychotic malignant syndrome. J Clin Psychiatry 1984;45: 526–529.

42. Baldessarini RJ: Drugs and the treatment of psychiatric disorders: Psychosis and anxiety. In: Hardman JG, Limbird LE, Molinoff PB, et al, eds: Goodman & Gilman's The Pharmacological Basis of Therapeutics, 9th ed. New York, McGraw Hill, 1996, pp. 399–430.

43. Guze BH, Baxter JR: Antipsychotic malignant syndrome. N Engl J Med 1985;313:163–166.

44. Hacksell U, Jackson DM, Mohell N: Does dopamine receptor subtype selectivity of antipsychotic agents provide useful leads for development of novel therapeutic agents? Pharmacol Toxicol 1995; 76:320–324.

45. Harmon TJ, Benitez JG, Krenzelok EP, et al: Loss of consciousness from acute quetiapine overdose. J Toxicol Clin Toxicol 1998;36: 599–602.

46. Henderson RA, Lane S, Henry JA: Life-threatening ventricular arrhythmia (torsade de pointes) after haloperidol overdose. Hum Exp Toxicol 1991;10:59–62.

47. Hicks R, Dysken MW, Davis JM, et al: The pharmacokinetics of psychotropic medication in the elderly: A review. J Clin Psychiatry 1981;42:374–385.

48. Hollister LE: Clinical Use of Psychotherapeutic Drugs. Springfield, IL, Charles C. Thomas, 1973.

49. Horacek J: Novel antipsychotics and extrapyramidal side effects. Theory and reality. Pharmacopsychiatry 2000;33(Suppl 1):34–42.

50. Howes CA, Pullar T, Sourindhrin I, et al: Reduced steady-state plasma concentrations of chlorpromazine and indomethacin in patients receiving cimetidine. Eur J Clin Pharmacol 1983;24:99–102.

51. Huang CC: Reserpine and alpha methyldopa in the treatment of tardive dyskinesia. Psychopharmacology 1981;33:359–362.

52. Hunt N, Stern TA: The association between intravenous haloperidol and torsade de pointes. Psychosomatics 1995;36:541–549.

53. Huston JF, Bell GE: The effect of thioridazine and chlorpromazine on the electrocardiogram. JAMA 1966;198:134–138.

54. Igarashi K, Matsubata K, Kasuya F, et al: Effect of a pyridinium metabolite derived from haloperidol on the activities of striatal tyrosine hydroxylase in freely moving rats. Neurosci Lett 1996;214: 183–186.

55. Izumi K, Tominaga H, Koja T, et al: Meclofenoxate therapy in tardive dyskinesia: A preliminary report. Biol Psychiatry 1986;21: 151–160.

56. Jeste DV, Wyatt RJ: Therapeutic strategies against tardive dyskinesia: Two decades of experience. Arch Gen Psychiatry 1982;39: 803–816.

57. Jeste DV, Wyatt RJ: In search of treatment for tardive dyskinesia: A review of the literature. Schizophr Bull 1979;5:251–293.

58. Jus K, Jus A, Gautier J, et al: Studies of the actions of certain pharmacological agents on tardive dyskinesia and on the rabbit syndrome. Int J Clin Pharmacol 1974;9:138–145.

59. Kaul PN, Whitfield LR, Clark ML: Chlorpromazine metabolism. VIII: Blood levels of chlorpromazine and its sulfoxide in schizophrenic patients. J Pharm Sci 1976;65:694–697.

60. Keck PE, Caroff SN, McElroy SL: Antipsychotic malignant syndrome and malignant hyperthermia: End of a controversy [review]? J Neuropsychiatry Clin Neurosci 1995;7:135–144.

61. Keck PE, Pope HG, Cohen BM, et al: Risk factors for antipsychotic malignant syndrome. Arch Gen Psychiatry 1989;46:914–918.

62. Klawans HL: Tardive dyskinesia: Review and update. Am J Psychiatry 1980;137:900–905.

63. Klawan HL, Tanner CM, Goetz CG: Epidemiology and pathophysiology of tardive dyskinesias [review]. Adv Neurol 1988;49:185–197.

64. Kobayashi RM: Drug therapy of tardive dyskinesia. N Engl J Med 1977;296:257–259.

65. Koek RJ, Pe EH: Acute laryngeal dystonic reactions to antipsychotics. Psychosomatics 1989;30:359–364.

66. Kriwisky M, Perry GY, Tarchitsky D, et al: Haloperidol-induced torsade de pointes. Chest 1990;98:482–484.

67. Lazarus A, Caroff SN, Mann SC: Beyond NMS: Management after the acute episode. Psychiatry Ann 1991;21:165–174.

68. Leckman JF, Peterson BS, Pauls DL, Cohen DG: Tic disorders. Psychiatr Clin North Am 1997;20(4):839–881.

69. Levenson JL: Antipsychotic malignant syndrome. Am J Psychiatry 1985;142:1137–1145.

70. Loga S, Curry SH, Lader M: Interactions of orphenadrine and phenobarbitone with chlorpromazine: Plasma concentrations and effects in man. Br J Clin Pharmacol 1975;2:197–208.

71. Lutz EG: Cardiotoxic effects of psychotropic drugs. J Med Soc NJ 1976;73:105–112.

72. Maclaren DC, Gambhir SS, Satamurthy N, et al: Repetitive, non-invasive imaging of the dopamine D2 receptor as a reporter gene in living animals. Gene Ther 1999;6:785–791.

73. Manian AA, Efran DH, Goldberg ME, et al: A comparative pharmacological study of a series of monohydroxylated and methoxylated chlorpromazine derivatives. Life Sci 1965;4:2425–2438.

74. Marrs-Simon P, Zell-Kanter M, Kendzierski DL, et al: Cardiotoxic manifestations of mesoridazine overdose. Ann Emerg Med 1988;17:1074–1078.

75. Matz R, Rich W, Oh D, et al: Clozapine: A potential antipsychotic agent without extrapyramidal manifestations. Curr Ther Res 1974;16:687–695.

76. May DC, Morris SW, Stewart RM, et al: Antipsychotic malignant syndrome: Response to dantrolene sodium. Ann Intern Med 1982;98:183–184.

77. May PRA, Van Putten T, Jenden DJ, et al: Chlorpromazine levels and the outcome of treatment in schizophrenic patients. Arch Gen Psychiatry 1981;38:202–207.

78. McCarron MM, Boettger ML, Peck JJ: A case of antipsychotic malignant syndrome successfully treated with amantadine. J Clin Psychiatry 1982;43:381–382.

79. McIntyre WT, Gershon S: Interpatient variations in antipsychotic therapy. J Clin Psychiatry 1985;46:3–16.

80. Mehta D, Mehta SH, Petit J, et al: Cardiac arrhythmia and Haldol. Am J Psychiatry 1979;136:1468–1469.

81. Moore NA: Behavioural pharmacology of the new generation of antipsychotic agents [review]. Br J Psychiatry Suppl 1999;38:5–11.

82. Mueller PS, Vester JW, Fermaglich J: Antipsychotic malignant syndrome-like state following a withdrawal of anti-parkinsonian drugs. J Nerv Ment Dis 1981;169:324–327.

83. Pullen GP, Best NR, Maguire J: Anticholinergic drug abuse: A common problem. Br Med J 1984;289:612–613.

84. Rivera-Calimlim L, Kerzner B, Karch FE: Effect of lithium on plasma chlorpromazine levels. Clin Pharmacol Ther 1978;23:451–455.

85. Rosebush PI, Stewart T, Mazurek MF: The treatment of antipsychotic malignant syndrome: Are dantrolene and bromocriptine useful adjuncts to supportive care? Br J Psychiatry 1991;159:709–712.

86. Rosenberg MR, Green M: Antipsychotic malignant syndrome. Arch Intern Med 1989;149:1927–1931.

87. Russell SA, Henner HM, Herson KJ, Stremski ES: Upper airway compromise in acute chlorpromazine ingestion. Am J Emerg Med 1996;14:467–468.

88. Sachdev P, Loneragan C: Intravenous benztropine and propranolol in tardive akathisia. Psychopharmacolgy 1993;1:119–122.

89. Saltz BL, Woemer MG, Kane JM, et al: Prospective study of tardive dyskinesia incidence in the elderly. JAMA 1991;266:2402–2406.

90. Saltz BL, Woemer MG, Robinson DG, et al: Side effects of antipsychotic drugs. Avoiding and minimizing their impact in elderly patients. Postgrad Med 2000;107:169–172, 175–178.

91. Sangal R, Dimitrijevic R: Antipsychotic malignant syndrome: Successful treatment with pancuronium. JAMA 1985;254:2795–2796.

92. Sekine Y, Rikihisa T, Ogata H, et al: Correlations between in vitro affinity of antipsychotics to various central neurotransmitter receptors and clinical incidence of their adverse drug reactions. Eur J Clin Pharmacol 1999;55:583–587.

93. Shalev A, Hermesh H, Munitz H: Mortality from antipsychotic malignant syndrome. J Clin Psychiatry 1989;50:18–25.

94. Shalev A, Munitz H: The antipsychotic malignant syndrome: Agent and host interaction. Acta Psychiatr Scand 1986;73:337–347.

95. Silvestri RC, Bromfield EB, Khoshbin S: Clozapine-induced seizures and EEG abnormalities in ambulatory psychiatric patients. Ann Pharmacother 1988;32:1147–1151.

96. Sletten I, Pichardo J, Korol B, et al: The effect of chlorpromazine on lithium excretion in psychiatric subjects. Curr Ther Res 1966;8:441–446.

97. Snyder SH: Receptors, neurotransmitters and drug responses. N Engl J Med 1979;300:465–472.

98. Snyder SH: Antischizophrenic drugs and the dopamine receptor. Drug Ther 1978;3:29–34.

99. Srinivassan AV, Murugappan M, Krishnamurthy SG, et al: Antipsychotic malignant syndrome. J Neurol Neurosurg Psychiatry 1990;53:514–516.

99a. Stahl SM: What makes an antipsychotic atypical? J Clin Psychiatry 1999;60:3–13.

100. Swett C, Cole JO, Hartz SC, et al: Hypotension due to chlorpromazine: Relation to cigarette smoking. Arch Gen Psychiatry 1977;34:661–663.

101. Toru M, Matsuda O, Maleiguchi K, et al: Antipsychotic malignant syndrome-like state following a withdrawal of antiparkinsonian drugs. J Nerv Ment Dis 1981;169:324–327.

102. Vassallo SU, Delaney KA: Pharmacologic effects on thermoregulation: Mechanisms of drug-related heatstroke. J Toxicol Clin Toxicol 1989;27:199–224.

103. Verhoeven WMA, Elderson A, Westernberg HC: Antipsychotic malignant syndrome: Successful treatment with bromocriptine. Biol Psychiatry 1985;20:680–684.

104. Ward A, Chaffman MO, Sorkin EM: Dantrolene: A review of its pharmacodynamic and pharmacokinetic properties and therapeutic use in malignant hyperthermia, the antipsychotic malignant syndrome and an update of its use in muscle spasticity. Drugs 1986;32:130–168.

105. Wech R, Chue P: Antipsychotic agents and QT changes [review]. J Psychiatry Neurosci. 2000;25:154–160.

106. Yassa R: A case of lithium chlorpromazine interaction. J Clin Psychiatry 1966;47:90–91.

107. Zaratzian VL: Psychotropic drugs: Neurotoxicity. Clin Toxicol 1980;17:231–270.

108. Zee-Cheng C, Mueller CE, Seifert CF, Gibbs HR: Haloperidol and torsade de pointes [letter]. Ann Intern Med 1985;102:418.

CHAPTER 60 MONOAMINE OXIDASE INHIBITORS

Lada Kokan

A 28-year-old woman ran into the Emergency Department (ED) clutching the back of her head, screaming that her head was going to explode. A brief history revealed that she was maintained on tranylcypromine for depression. Fifteen minutes before the onset of the headache she had been eating dinner in a restaurant and had eaten a salad with a yogurt dressing.

The initial evaluation revealed an alert, oriented, but agitated patient who was holding her head with both hands and had her eyes shut tightly. She was flushed and mildly diaphoretic. Her initial blood pressure was 200/110 mm Hg; her pulse was 90 beats/min and irregular; her respiratory rate was 28 breaths/min; and her temperature was 99°F (37.2°C). Cardiac auscultation suggested bigeminy. A neurologic evaluation revealed equal round and reactive pupils. She complained of photophobia. She was moving all four extremities equally and had no gross sensory deficits. The remainder of her physical evaluation was unremarkable. The cardiac monitor now demonstrated that the patient was in a normal sinus rhythm at a rate of 92 beats/min. Simultaneous with the placement of a peripheral intravenous (IV) line, the patient received 10 mg nifedipine sublingually.* She then vomited a large amount of undigested food. Repeat blood pressure was 190/100 mm Hg. The patient continued to complain of a severe throbbing occipital headache. Over 20 minutes the blood pressure stabilized at 130/80 mm Hg with some resolution of the headache.

On further questioning, the patient denied the ingestion of cheese or wine and denied the use of illicit drugs, specifically amphetamines or cocaine although she had used cocaine in the past. Because of the persistence of a mild headache and the risk of intracranial hemorrhage, a noncontrast head CT scan was obtained; it was normal. Although a lumbar puncture was considered, it was not performed as the patient's symptoms resolved completely with observation. Her mental status, vital signs, and neurologic examination remained normal subsequently and she was discharged home.

Her hypertensive MAOI interaction was likely caused by an unrecognized dietary indiscretion or undisclosed sympathetic drug use because the yogurt salad dressing is a food low in tyramine.

The monoamine oxidase inhibitors (MAOIs) were first used in the early 1950s to treat tuberculosis and hypertension. When their mood-elevating properties were recognized, they were then prescribed for the treatment of depression.[31] Despite their effectiveness, the use of MAOIs became limited by the potential food and

drug interactions, and in the 1970s, the MAOIs were largely replaced by tricyclic antidepressants.[3]

In the 1980s, there was a resurgence of MAOI use in the treatment of refractory depression, phobias, and anxiety disorders.[10,38] This trend corresponded to the reappearance of MAOI toxicity reports in the literature.[39,63] Subsequently, their use again declined following the appearance of the less toxic selective serotonin reuptake inhibitors (SSRIs) for treatment of depression. Recently, the emergence of a new generation of reversible and selective MAOIs again brings the MAOIs into focus. The new MAOIs are notably safer in overdose and have limited food and drug reactions.

EPIDEMIOLOGY

Few recent fatalities from MAOIs have been reported to the American Association of Poison Control Centers (p. 1752 and Chap. 116). MAOI use has declined as patients chosen for treatment are more carefully selected and greater care is taken to avoid interactions. The new generations of selective and reversible MAOIs are safer and are being prescribed more frequently than the older MAOIs. Extensive experience with the reversible MAOIs in Europe and Canada demonstrates that they have a wider therapeutic window and much less potential for food and drug interactions than the older nonselective MAOIs.

However, the irreversible MAOIs are still used and mortality has been reported from acute ingestions of as little as 170–680 mg of tranylcypromine and 375–1500 mg of phenelzine.[70] In contrast, ingestion of <2000 mg of moclobemide, one of the new reversible MAOIs, typically results in mild or no symptoms.[47]

PHARMACOLOGY

Although a chemically heterogeneous group of drugs, the MAOIs all have in common the ability to inhibit the enzyme monoamine oxidase. The nonselective MAOIs include the hydrazines, such as phenelzine (Nardil) and isocarboxazid (Marplan), as well as the amphetamine-derived tranylcypromine (Parnate). Newer MAOIs include the acetylenic agents pargyline, clorgyline, and selegiline (Deprenyl), as well as the benzamide derivative moclobemide (Manerex). Of these, isocarboxazid, phenelzine, tranylcypromine, and selegiline are currently available in the United States.

Monoamine oxidase (MAO) is a flavin-containing enzyme whose role is to deactivate biologically active monoamines. Monoamines, such as epinephrine, norepinephrine, dopamine, and

---

*Sublingual nifedipine is no longer routinely used.

serotonin, are molecules that contain a single amine group. Because monoamines are ubiquitous, MAO has an important role and is found in a wide variety of organs, particularly in the nerve terminals of the central nervous system (CNS) and in the mitochondrial membrane of hepatocytes and platelets.[25]

MAO degradation of monoamines helps regulate neurotransmitter stores at the nerve terminal (Fig. 60–1).[3] Therefore, MAO inhibition results in elevated synaptic neurotransmitter levels. This elevation is thought to be central to the antidepressant effects of MAOIs,[3] but this is difficult to prove. The antidepressant activity is approximately correlated with >85% inhibition of platelet MAO enzymatic activity and continues to rise linearly above this level of inhibition.[25,26,52]

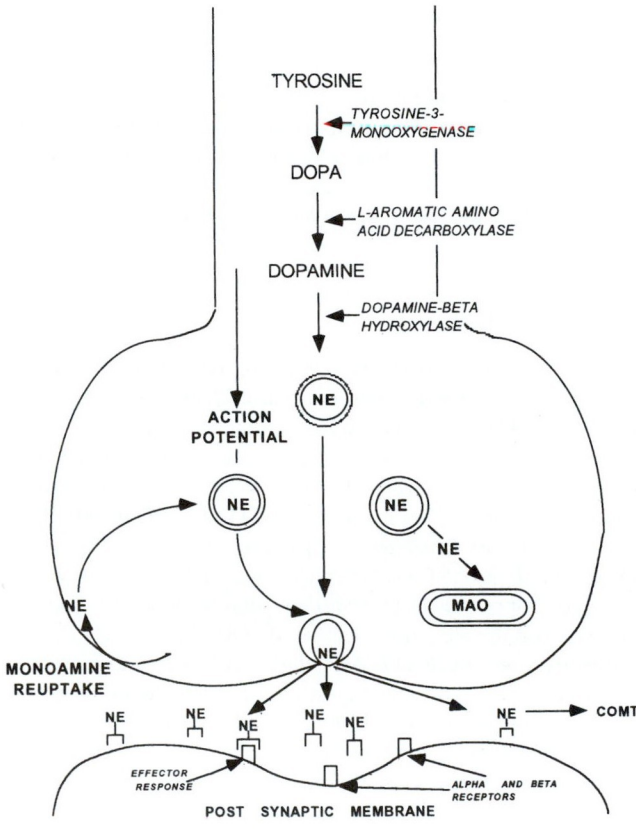

Figure 60–1. The sympathetic nerve terminal. Norepinephrine (NE) is synthesized in the sympathetic nerve cell and stored in vesicles. An action potential causes the vesicles to migrate to and fuse with the presynaptic membrane. NE diffuses across the synaptic cleft and binds with and activates postsynaptic α- and β-adrenergic receptors. NE is then taken back up into the neuron by the monoamine reuptake pump and repackaged into vesicles. NE that is taken up by the neuron but escapes repackaging is inactivated by mitochondrial monoamine oxidase (MAO). NE that diffuses away from the synaptic cleft is inactivated by catechol-O-methyl transferase (COMT). (Reprinted, with permission, from Lefkowitz RJ, Hoffman BB, Taylor P: Drugs acting at synaptic and neuroeffector junctional sites. In: Gilman AG, Rall TW, Nies AS, Taylor P, eds: Goodman and Gilman's The Pharmacologic Basis of Therapeutics, 8th ed. New York, Pergamon Press, 1990, pp. 84–121.)

There are two MAO enzyme subtypes, MAO-A and MAO-B. They are differentiated by their location in tissues, by the substrates that they preferentially degrade, and by their inhibitors[3] (Table 60–1).

MAO-A is found in the liver, in the gastrointestinal tract, and in monoaminergic neurons. Hepatic MAO-A is important in inactivating ingested monoamines such as tyramine, which can cause a significant systemic reaction if not inactivated by MAO-A in the gastrointestinal tract. The tyramine or "aged cheese" reaction is a food interaction that results when patients taking MAOIs ingest monoamines that cannot be metabolized by their inactivated MAO. The clinical manifestations of this reaction are discussed in more detail later in this chapter. Other substrates degraded primarily by MAO-A include epinephrine, norepinephrine, metanephrine, and serotonin, accounting for the negligible oral bioavailability of these monoamines. Circulating monoamines are also inactivated in the liver.

The MAO-B isoenzyme is found primarily in the brain and in platelets. Serotonergic neurons contain both MAO-A and MAO-B. Substrates degraded by MAO-B include dopamine, β-phenylethylamine, phenylethanolamine, and benzylamine.[3]

The active form of the enzyme MAO is a dimer consisting of two subunits. Each subunit is covalently bound with one flavin adenine dinucleotide (FAD), and has a molecular weight of approximately 60,000 daltons. Monoamine oxidase uses oxidative deamination to inactivate its substrates in two steps. First the monoamine is oxidized and FAD is reduced. Hydrolysis of the intermediate imine results in an aldehyde and $FADH_2$. In the second step $FADH_2$ is oxidized by O_2, forming H_2O_2 as a by-product.[18]

Substrates metabolized by both MAO subtypes include tyramine, dopamine, octopamine, and tryptamine.[73] Table 60–1 compares the various types of MAO inhibitors.

The nonselective MAOIs inhibit the MAO enzyme irreversibly. This means that new MAO must be synthesized before enzyme function can resume because of irreversible covalent binding to the enzyme, resulting in a prolonged pharmacologic half-life lasting several days to up to 2 weeks. Thus, until sufficient MAO is synthesized to metabolize monoamines normally, the patients taking irreversible MAOIs are at risk for significant morbidity and even mortality from drug-drug or drug-food interactions. Therefore, patients taking these drugs must be placed on a restrictive diet to avoid drug-food interactions and their use of prescription and nonprescription drugs must be closely monitored to avoid drug-drug interactions. For the same reason, severe morbidity and mortality are common after MAOI overdose.

Selegiline (Deprenyl, Eldepryl) is used for the treatment of Parkinson disease.[43] It is an irreversible inhibitor that selectively inhibits MAO-B at doses of less than 20 mg/d. Above this dose MAOI selectivity is lost, and findings in selegiline overdose may resemble those of the nonselective, irreversible MAOIs. An additional pharmacologic feature of selegiline is that it is metabolized to amphetamine and methamphetamine. This can result in hypomanic symptoms at therapeutic doses, as well as a hyperadrenergic state in overdose. Patients taking selegiline may also test positive for amphetamines on drug tests because of the metabolites.

The newer MAOIs, such as moclobemide, reversibly bind MAO in a competitive manner. Because the enzyme is bound reversibly and competitively by these drugs, some MAO is still available to metabolize ingested monoamines rapidly after moclobemide ingestion. This inhibition is competitive so that MAO

TABLE 60–1. Types of Monamine Oxidase

	MAO-A	MAO-B
Substrates	Serotonin	Benzylamine
	Epinephrine	Phenylethylamine
	Norepinephrine	Tyramine
	Metanephrine	β-Phenylethylamine
	Tryptamine	Tryptamine
	Dopamine	Dopamine
	Octopamine	Octopamine
Location	Gastrointestinal tract	Brain
	Liver	Platelets
	Exocrine pancreas	Pancreatic islets
	Monoaminergic neurons	Serotonergic neurons
	Serotonergic neurons	
Inhibitors: Irreversible	Clorgyline	Selegiline*†
	Tranylcypromine*	Pargyline*
	Phenelzine*	Tranylcypromine*
	Isocarboxazid*	Phenelzine*
		Isocarboxazid*
Reversible	Moclobemide	Lazabemide
	Brofaromine	
	Cimoxatone	
	Toloxatone	
	Harmaline	

*Currently available in the United States.
†Selective at doses up to 20 mg.

function can resume in hours in contrast to the older irreversible MAOIs, which require days, rather than hours, to replete deactivated MAO enzyme.

Consequently, these reversible inhibitors of MAOI-A (RIMAs) are much safer in overdose, require fewer food restrictions,[1,18,32,43,46] and have much less potential for drug interactions. Drug-drug interactions, although less common with RIMAs than with the older MAOIs, have been reported at therapeutic doses as well as in overdose.[47] These drugs include moclobemide (Manerex), brofaromine, cimoxatone, toloxatone, and befloxatone, and are not yet available in the United States.

Table 60–1 classifies the older irreversible MAOIs and the newer MAOIs, which inhibit the enzyme reversibly. It also classifies the selective and nonselective MAOIs. By classifying a given MAOI as reversible/irreversible and selective/nonselective to MAO-A or MAO-B, one can define much about the drug's pharmacology, toxicity, and interactions with food and drugs. These concepts are further discussed below.

Some less commonly encountered MAOIs include procarbazine (Matulane), which is a weak MAOI used as an antitumor agent for Hodgkin disease.[23] Clorgyline is an irreversible inhibitor of MAO-A.[73]

The enzymatic inhibitory action of MAOIs precedes their clinical effects by as long as 2 weeks,[3] an effect that is also seen with tricyclic antidepressants. The reason for this is not well characterized but may be related to down-regulation of CNS postsynaptic serotonin or its receptor. Several weeks after the initiation of MAO therapy, multiple changes in the CNS occur that affect neurotransmission. The number of β-adrenergic receptors decreases, and the activity of β-adrenergic, α_1- and α_2-adrenergic, and 5-HT$_1$

and 5-HT$_2$ receptors decreases.[45] Dopamine receptors are unaffected.[73] The initial increase in monoamine levels and the delayed receptor down-regulation may both contribute to the antidepressant activity of MAOIs via a mechanism of action that is not yet fully understood.

Other enzyme systems inhibited by MAOIs include diamine oxidase, pyridoxal phosphokinase, ceruloplasmin, dopa decarboxylase, L-glutamic acid decarboxylase, and other pyridoxine (B$_6$)-containing enzyme systems.[21] The clinical implications of the inhibition of these diverse enzyme systems other than MAO are poorly understood.

PHARMACOKINETICS AND TOXICOKINETICS

MAOIs are only available in oral form at present. They are well absorbed orally and peak levels are reached within 2–3 hours. MAOIs are hepatically metabolized primarily by acetylation and are excreted in the urine.[3] The therapeutic and toxic effects of MAOIs, however, lag behind their absorption and excretion characteristics, as discussed in the sections on pharmacology and clinical manifestations of overdose.

Recent studies with transdermal administration of selegiline show signs of clinical effectiveness in some patients within 1 week of administration.[13] Further clinical trials are ongoing with this method of administration that may challenge some of the currently proposed mechanisms of action and pharmacokinetics of MAOIs.[13]

Some MAOIs are structurally related to amphetamine and have amphetaminelike activity unrelated to the inhibition of MAO (Fig. 60–2).[35] In addition, selegiline is metabolized to amphetamine and methamphetamine.

MONOAMINE OXIDASE INHIBITOR OVERDOSE

The significant morbidity and mortality characteristic of overdose with the older irreversible MAOIs must be differentiated from that following overdose with the newer reversible MAOIs or RIMAs. The RIMAs have a much greater therapeutic window than the irreversible MAOIs, so that overdose with RIMAs characteristically results in a relatively benign course if no other drugs are ingested. Drug-drug interactions resulting in the serotonin syndrome greatly increase the danger from overdose with either type of MAOI.

Overdose from irreversible MAOIs is characterized by a spectrum of sympathetic hyperactivity that is followed by cardiovascular collapse in severe cases. These effects are attributed to the same elevation of monoaminergic neurotransmitter levels and amphetaminelike activity[35] that confers to MAOIs their antidepressant activity. Thus, presynaptic monoamines are released, stimulating postsynaptic adrenergic and serotonergic receptors and initiating a multiorgan sympathetic response. In addition, because of the lack of active MAO enzyme, the released monoamines are not adequately metabolized and the sympathetic response is greatly exaggerated.

In a limited or early phase of overdose with irreversible MAOIs, the patient typically appears irritable, anxious, flushed, diaphoretic, and tachycardic, and may complain of a headache. Characteristic symptoms of more severe overdose include hyperthermia, hypertonia, seizures, and marked hypertension. These severe cases may progress to cardiovascular collapse with hypotension and dysrhythmias, obtundation, and disseminated intravascular coagulopathy as the body's catecholamine stores are depleted and multiorgan failure occurs. Other symptoms may include tachypnea, nystagmus, mydriasis, hallucinations, trismus,

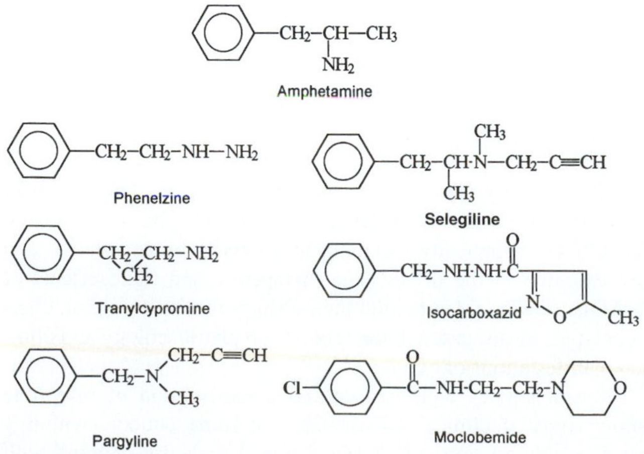

neuromuscular irritability, agitation, and delirium.[19,39] A predominance of sympathetic hyperactivity is expected to be associated with MAOIs that have amphetaminelike characteristics (see Fig. 60–2). Secondary problems resulting from CNS and hemodynamic hyperactivity may include rhabdomyolysis, renal failure, dehydration, intracranial hemorrhage, and ischemia (Chap. 18). There are many reports of delay in the onset of significant symptoms for as long as 12–32 hours after irreversible MAOI overdose.[4,39,42]

In contrast, the reversible inhibitors of MAO appear to be much less toxic in overdose. For example, moclobemide, a reversible inhibitor of MAO-A, has been ingested in doses of as much as 8000 mg, or 25 times the therapeutic dose, without causing significant toxicity. At doses as high as 8000 mg, fatigue, agitation, tachycardia, and hypertension were noted.[47] When interpreting the significance of these case reports, one must note that the patients who ingested the largest amount of moclobemide were lavaged early in their course; thus less drug may have been absorbed systemically, contributing to a more benign course. Whether the reversibility or some other pharmacologic property is responsible for this improved toxicity profile is unclear.

Therapy of patients with MAOI overdose should focus on emergency treatment of the airway followed by stabilization of the heart rate and blood pressure, and, subsequently, hyperthermia, seizures, and muscular rigidity.[19,39] Gastric decontamination should proceed after the patient is stabilized. This is especially important with overdose from irreversible MAOIs, which are characterized by a high potential for mortality and a delayed onset of clinical deterioration.

Because fluctuation of vital signs is characteristic of MAOI overdose, hemodynamic monitoring should be instituted even in patients who are initially stable. When supporting the patient's vital signs, preference should be given to titratable drugs with a rapid onset and termination of action because of the potential for rapid hemodynamic changes. Sodium nitroprusside and nitroglycerine are used to treat hypertension and can be rapidly stopped if hypotension develops. The short-acting α-adrenergic antagonist phentolamine given at 2–5 mg IV can also effectively control hypertension. However, β-adrenergic antagonists are not recommended for control of hypertension in this setting because of the potential for unopposed α-adrenergic effects, such as vasoconstriction, exacerbating the hypertension. Both α- and β-blocking antihypertensives are difficult to titrate and therefore increase the risk of iatrogenic hypotension in those patients with potentially unstable blood pressure. Although dopamine is the most familiar inotrope, it is not recommended in this situation because of its indirect effects on catecholamine release (see "Adverse Drug Events" below). Norepinephrine, a direct-acting agent, may be required in a hypotensive patient with an MAOI overdose who fails to respond to fluid therapy because the patient is likely to become catecholamine depleted.[47]

Hyperthermia must be aggressively treated (Chap. 18). The use of ice baths, cold water, and fans is the mainstay of treatment. Benzodiazepines help control muscular rigidity, seizures, and agitation that may be contributing to the hyperthermia and tachycardia. Phenobarbital and neuromuscular blocking agents may also be required for patients with ongoing seizures.[19,47] Vitamin B_6 should be given to replete potentially depleted stores in patients with refractory seizures, particularly if a hydrazine-derived MAOI such as phenelzine has been ingested. However, seizures are often con-

Figure 60–2. The structural similarities between amphetamine and the monoamine oxidase inhibitors.

trolled with first-line measures (Chap. 41 and Antidotes in Depth: Pyridoxine.).

Neuromuscular blockers are also essential for control of rigidity and hyperthermia if first-line treatment is unsuccessful. Dantrolene has been used in case reports to control neuromuscular rigidity and hyperthermia associated with MAOI overdose.[19,34] However, it should not be considered the standard of care, which remains the benzodiazepines and neuromuscular blocking agents.[19,34]

Atrial and ventricular dysrhythmias are a grave sign following MAOI overdose and are difficult to treat. Although standard Advanced Cardiac Life Support (ACLS) protocols should be followed, amiodarone use in this setting is unstudied. Theoretically, bretylium use could further deplete catecholamine stores, but this drug is not available.

After the initial components of patient stabilization have been completed, gastric decontamination should be performed.[19,39] Because of the potential for life-threatening toxicity in patients with MAOI overdose, even those with a delayed presentation should probably be given 1 g/kg activated charcoal and should also be lavaged with an orogastric lavage tube if there is potential for removing unabsorbed drug.

Finally, consideration should be given to the potential for mixed overdoses and concomitant medical problems. These should be diagnosed and treated in the usual manner.

Other treatment may be required for secondary problems associated with MAOI overdose. These include specific and symptomatic treatment of rhabdomyolysis, renal failure, diffuse intravascular coagulation (DIC), acute respiratory distress syndrome (ARDS), myocardial infarction, and intracranial hemorrhage.[39]

Asymptomatic patients with presumed MAOI overdose require 24 hours of monitoring and observation in the intensive care unit.

SEROTONIN SYNDROME

The serotonin syndrome is discussed in great detail in Chap. 58. The serotonin syndrome is also discussed below because of the importance of the MAOI-associated serotonin syndrome and because of its similarity to other MAOI drug interactions and overdoses.

Clinically, the serotonin syndrome is characterized by an altered mental status, hyperthermia, neuromuscular dysfunction (such as rigidity), and autonomic dysfunction (such as hypertension and/or hypotension and tachycardia).[60] Symptoms may also include shivering, disorientation, trismus, akathisia, coma, seizures, and later complications such as disseminated intravascular coagulation.[59,60]

Any patient taking an MAOI is at risk of developing the serotonin syndrome if the individual coingests an SSRI or another drug that raises CNS serotonin levels.[9,12,36,40] The reaction is not dose-dependent. Coingestion of a single dose of any prescription or nonprescription medicine that has the ability to elevate serotonin levels can result in symptoms. The half-life of the drugs involved determines the duration of risk for the development of the syndrome.

The serotonin syndrome is thought to result from overstimulation of CNS serotonin receptors, primarily 5-HT_{1A}. MAO degradation is normally an important pathway for degradation and control of CNS serotonin levels. Because other pathways are also involved, and because we neither measure total serotonin degradation nor CNS serotonin levels, the development of the serotonin syndrome is difficult to predict. However, the inhibition of enzymatic degradation by MAOIs may lead to increased serotonin levels, contributing to the serotonin syndrome, particularly when combined with drugs that are likely to raise serotonin levels via other pathways, such as inhibited serotonin reuptake by tricyclic antidepressants (see below).

Experimentally, the ability of various agents to cause hyperthermia in rabbits pretreated with an MAOI has been found to be in direct proportion to each agent's ability to block the reuptake of serotonin.[58] Both reversible and irreversible as well as selective and nonselective MAOIs are implicated.[49]

Nevertheless, in this respect as in overdose, moclobemide and the other reversible MAOIs appear to have a greater margin of safety and they appear to be safer than the older MAOIs to combine with SSRIs.[2] There are reports of the serotonin syndrome developing both with a combination of therapeutic agents and in overdose of moclobemide combined with SSRIs,[2,40,47,49,59] but these syndromes are mild with few fatalities reported.[47,59]

Although MAOIs and tricyclic antidepressants are sometimes used in combination for depressed patients,[74] this combination places patients at risk of developing the serotonin syndrome[50] as a consequence of the ability of tricyclics to inhibit serotonin reuptake. The degree of reuptake inhibition varies among the tricyclic antidepressants.

Other drugs that can inhibit serotonin reuptake, and that might result in the serotonin syndrome if combined with MAOIs, include meperidine (Demerol) and dextromethorphan, which is found in many nonprescription antitussives.[14] In contrast, morphine lacks the serotonin-potentiating effects in an animal model,[64] and in humans appears to be safe to use in combination with MAOIs.[58]

Treatment of the serotonin syndrome is similar in many respects to the treatment for MAOI overdose. Initial treatment focuses on control of the airway and vital signs. Attention should be focused on control of hyperthermia. An emphasis should be placed on hemodynamic monitoring and the use of titratable drugs that can be rapidly reversed when treating autonomic dysfunction such as hypertension.

After the patient is stabilized, gastric decontamination may be undertaken with activated charcoal. Gastric lavage probably has no role in patients who have developed signs and symptoms of the serotonin syndrome as by this time the drug is probably no longer in the stomach and has been distributed in the body.

Because of the long half-lives of the parent SSRI drug or active metabolite, a patient should discontinue SSRI therapy for at least 2 weeks, while the SSRI is "washed out" and levels fall, before initiating MAOI therapy so as to avoid an MAOI-SSRI interaction.[12] Fluoxetine has the longest half-life; in this case, the manufacturer recommends a 5-week washout period.[12] Similarly, at least 2 weeks is recommended before initiating SSRI therapy in a patient who had been taking the older MAOIs. A washout period is less important after therapy with the newer reversible MAOIs such as moclobemide.[68]

When switching from a tricyclic antidepressant to an MAOI, the standard recommendation is to wait 7–10 days between drugs. However, the prescribing practice of some psychiatrists is to switch from a tricyclic antidepressant (TCA) to an MAOI over a shorter period of time[33]; the community standard is in evolution.

TYRAMINE-RELATED MAOI-FOOD INTERACTIONS

Food interactions occur when pharmacologically active dietary monoamines such as tyramine, phenylethylamine, and histamine are ingested by patients taking MAOIs (Table 60–2).[56,66]

These monoamines are normally degraded by gastrointestinal and liver MAO-A before they enter the systemic circulation. However, with MAO inhibition, large quantities of monoamines may be absorbed in the systemic circulation. Protein-rich foods are particularly likely to contain decarboxylating bacteria that convert amino acids into pharmacologically active monoamines.[7,56] Tyramine acts in a manner similar to the indirect-acting sympathetic agents (Fig. 60–1). Stored norepinephrine is released into the nerve terminal, resulting in a hypertensive crisis.[16,27] Ingestion of as little as 6 mg of tyramine may result in a significant vasopressor effect in the MAO-inhibited patient.[30] This is 1–10% of the dose normally needed to achieve a vasopressor effect. Analysis of the tyramine content of food and beverages reveals that the amine composition of foods varies greatly even when the same type of cheese from different sources is analyzed.[16]

Less danger of a tyramine reaction occurs with the use of the reversible inhibitors of MAO (RIMAs), and patients taking these drugs can have an unrestricted diet.[28,68] Because of the reversible nature of MAO inhibition by these MAOIs, tyramine can compete effectively for MAO, more tyramine is degraded, and there is much less danger of a hypertensive reaction following ingestion of tyramine-rich foods.[28,57,65]

Symptoms of MAOI-food interactions reflect the hyperadrenergic state created by the nonmetabolized dietary monoamines. They include hypertension, tachycardia, and headache in early or minor reactions. Additional symptoms may include bradycardia, flushing, an altered mental status and seizures as well as secondary sequelae from uncontrolled hypertension, such as myocardial infarction and intracranial hemorrhage. However, these monoamines have a short half-life and the direct effects will have a rapid onset and abate within several hours.

Normotensive patients who experience severe hypertension after dietary interactions may be treated with the use of an α-adrenergic antagonist such as 2–5 mg IV of phentolamine.[27] Titratable drugs, such as nitroprusside, are an excellent choice to allow to enable controlled lowering of the blood pressure.

Treatment of individual symptoms in patients with MAOI-food interaction is similar to the symptomatic and supportive care described for MAOI overdose. However, these patients usually have early clinical manifestations rather than the delayed presentations characteristic of MAOI overdose. Therefore, patients with MAOI-food interactions may not require hospital admission if the interaction has been mild, resolution of symptoms has been complete, and the patient can be observed in the ED for 4–8 hours. Patients with an altered mental status, seizures, or suspected intracranial hemorrhage must be managed accordingly, have appropriate diagnostic studies, and be hospitalized for further studies and observation.

Table 60–3 compares the characteristics of MAOI overdose with symptoms following interactions of MAOIs with foods and indirect-acting sympathomimetic agents. It is notable that the syndromes overlap greatly. In fact, despite a few clinical differences, the most reliable way to tell them apart is by history.

ADVERSE DRUG EVENTS

There are several important adverse reactions that may occur during therapeutic use of MAOIs. Hepatotoxicity caused by hydrazine MAOIs is rare but serious, and has led to the discontinuation of the use of iproniazid.[6] Such hepatotoxicity results from cellular damage to the hepatic parenchyma and is rare with the MAOIs in current use. However, fatal hepatitis has also been reported after chronic therapeutic use of the reversible MAO-A inhibitor toloxatone. Peripheral neuropathy from vitamin B_6 depletion by the hydrazines can also occur. Orthostatic hypotension is common with pargyline.[6] The mechanism is thought to involve an alteration in synaptic amine stores in adrenergic neurons. Norepinephrine is replaced by the less potent dopamine, resulting in decreased adrenergic vasomotor tone. As an extension of their therapeutic effects, MAOIs may cause agitation and hypomanic behavior, insomnia, tremors and hyperhidrosis in therapeutic doses.[3] A variety of other effects, such as dry mouth, blurred vision, dizziness, difficulty with urination and ejaculation, and constipation, may also occur, particularly with phenelzine and tranylcypromine, especially when doses exceed 45 mg/d.[6]

Drug interactions with sympathomimetic agents are predictable and may occur when a patient taking an MAOI also takes one of the several types of drugs mentioned in Table 60–4.[4,40] Drug interactions may occur when the drug combinations are taken in therapeutic doses or in overdose. As with other MAOI-related interactions, they are more likely to occur in patients taking the older, nonspecific, irreversible inhibitors of MAO than with the RIMAs.[28,68] The serotonin syndrome has been discussed above. Other major types of drug interactions result from the indirect-acting sympathomimetic agents or from interactions caused by alteration of hepatic metabolism.

Indirect-acting sympathomimetic agents (Table 60–4) release norepinephrine stored in the peripheral sympathetic nerve terminal[27] (Fig. 60–1). Patients taking MAOIs have increased presynap-

TABLE 60–2. Dietary Considerations for Patients Taking MAOIs

High tyramine content
 Aged, mature cheeses (65–1500 mg/kg)
 Smoked, pickled, aged, putrefying meats or fish (0–470 mg/kg)
 Yeast and meat extracts (65–2250 mg/kg), including marmite
 Red wines (1.5–12 mg/kg)
 Broad beans

Moderate tyramine content
 Meat extracts (100–300 mg/kg)
 Pasteurized light and pale beers
 Ripe avocados

Low tyramine content
 Distilled alcohol
 Cottage cheese, cream cheese
 Sour cream
 Chocolate, caffeine-containing beverages
 Fruit
 Soy sauce
 Yogurt

Patients should avoid high tyramine content meals and eat small quantities of meals containing moderate amounts of tyramine. Patients may eat foods low in tyramine content.

TABLE 60–3. Characteristics of MAOI Reactions

	Serotonin Syndrome	Interaction Between Monoamine and Food or Drugs	MAOI Overdose
Onset of symptoms	Minutes to hours	Minutes to hours	Up to 24 hours
Signs and symptoms	Hypertension or hypotension Hyperthermia Muscle rigidity Disorientation Shivering Seizures	Severe hypertension Tachycardia or bradycardia Headache Flushing Seizures Intracranial hemorrhage	Hypertension or hypotension Diaphoresis Neuromuscular hyper- activity Opsoclonus Obtundation Seizures Intracranial hemorrhage Cardiovascular collapse
Symptom duration	Hours	Hours	Days

tic stores of norepinephrine because its degradation by MAO is inhibited. In a patient taking an MAOI, the norepinephrine release that is triggered by an indirect-acting sympathetic agent may result in a hyperadrenergic syndrome when a large amount of released norepinephrine stimulates postsynaptic α- and β-adrenergic and serotonergic receptors.

In contrast, direct-acting sympathetic agents such as epinephrine, norepinephrine, and isoproterenol are not potentiated by MAO inhibition and are relatively safely used in patients on MAOIs.[20,70] Rather than release a stored pool of norepinephrine, the direct-acting sympathetic agents bind directly with postsynaptic α- and β-adrenergic receptors and are not primarily degraded by MAO. Direct-acting and parenterally administered adrenergic agents are primarily cleared by cell reuptake and catechol-O-methyltransferase (COMT), a synaptic enzyme that is not inhibited by MAOIs.[37]

The hyperadrenergic syndrome that results from the interaction of an MAOI and an indirect-acting sympathetic drug may be difficult to distinguish from MAOI overdose or the serotonin syndrome. Fortunately, treatment is very similar and is based upon the same principles of supportive care of specific symptoms. Symp-

toms typically start within 4–8 hours of ingestion. Mild symptoms can include hypertension, tachycardia or reflex bradycardia, and headache. Severe reactions may occur with hyperthermia, an altered mental status, seizures, intracranial hemorrhage, and death.

Animal studies of MAOI-theophylline interactions implicate serotonin potentiation by theophylline via adenylate cyclase.[5,69] Human reports of interactions between MAOIs and theophylline are limited to reports with multiple coingestants that are known to interact with MAOIs.

Many cases of toxic reactions are reported in patients who were treated with MAOIs and given tryptophan for depression[51,67] or levodopa for Parkinson's disease.[55,65] The reaction appears to be similar to the tyramine-MAOI food interaction and includes hypertension, facial flushing, and a sensation of warmth. This reaction has been attributed to the administration of precursor amino acids in the setting of decreased degradation[24] (Table 60–3). Although there have been no reports of fatalities, these combinations should be avoided or used only with great caution. The use of selegiline, the specific inhibitor of MAO-B, with levodopa is considered safe in therapeutic doses.

Animal studies and human reports describe a potentiation of the hypoglycemic effects of insulin and sulfonylureas in the presence of MAO inhibition.[8] Tranylcypromine is a potent insulin secretagogue.[8] Persistent hypoglycemia with the use of selegiline is also reported.[55] Doses of hypoglycemic agents should be appropriately adjusted in patients on MAOIs because of the increased risk of hypoglycemic episodes. This hypoglycemic effect has not been observed with moclobemide.[28,68]

The MAOIs inhibit the mixed-function oxidase enzyme system of P450 that metabolizes and inactivates pentobarbital, amobarbital, and hexobarbital.[22] Doses of barbiturates should therefore be adjusted when MAOIs are used simultaneously. Similarly, the sedating effects of codeine may also be prolonged and potentiated in MAO-inhibited patients. Drugs in other classes that may necessitate dose adjustment because of prolonged and intensified effects in the setting of MAO inhibition include general anesthetics, sedatives, antihistamines, ethanol, and anticholinergic agents.[3]

When switching from one MAOI to another, a waiting period of 14 days is recommended to avoid hypertensive reactions that have been reported when switching from pargyline to tranyl-

TABLE 60–4. Sympathomimetic Agents

Indirect acting*	Direct acting
Amphetamine	Epinephrine
Hydroxyamphetamine	Norepinephrine
Benzphetamine	Isoetharine
Ritodrine	Ethylnorepinephrine
Methamphetamine	Isoproterenol
Phenylpropanolamine	Methoxamine
Fenfluramine	Phenylephrine
Propylhexedrine	Albuterol
Phentermine	
Tyramine	**Both direct and indirect acting***
	Dopamine
	Metaraminol
	Ephedrine
	Mephentermine

*High risk for adverse drug events with MAOIs.

cypromine. In some patients, more rapid switching or simultaneous administration may be safe.[72] However, it is impossible to predict who will have an adverse reaction and who will not.

Recently, attention has been drawn to the herbal medication St. John's wort, which is thought to be a weak MAO inhibitor and to increase CNS serotonin levels.[44,48,53] Although the mechanism of action requires further study, the concomitant use of St. John's wort with MAOIs should be avoided in order to avoid potentially harmful interactions.

In general, a patient on MAOIs should not use nonprescription medications without seeking the advice of a physician or pharmacist in order to avoid the potential for drug-drug interactions.

SUMMARY

MAOIs have been largely replaced by different classes of antidepressants with potentially less food and drug interactions. Fortunately, the newer, reversible MAOIs are emerging as safer drugs that will not necessitate dietary restrictions and that have less frequent drug-drug interactions. The newer indications for MAOI administration, such as anxiety and phobias, will lead to an increasing popularity of MAOIs and to their broader use. The complex pharmacology of MAOIs remains pertinent as treatment modalities in psychopharmacology evolve.

Acknowledgments

Diane Sauter contributed to this chapter in a previous edition. Thanks to Doson Chua B.Sc. (Pharm) for assistance with research.

REFERENCES

1. Amrein R, Allen SR, Guentert TW, et al: The pharmacology of reversible monoamine oxidase inhibitors. Br J Psych 1989;155(Suppl 6):66–71.
2. Amrein R, Guntert J, Dingemanse T, et al: Interactions of moclobemide with concomitantly administered medication: Evidence from pharmacological and clinical studies. Psychopharmacology 1992;106 (Suppl):S24–S31.
3. Baldessarini RJ: Depression and mania. In: Hardman JG, Limbird LE, Molinoff PB, Ruddon RW, Goodman AG, eds: Goodman and Gilman's The Pharmacological Basis of Therapeutics, 9th ed. New York, McGraw-Hill, 1996, pp. 431–460.
4. Baldridge ET, Miller LV, Haverbach JB, et al: Amine metabolism after an overdosage of a monoamine oxidase inhibitor. N Engl J Med 1962;267:421–426.
5. Berkowitz BA, Spector S, Pool W: The interaction of caffeine, theophylline and theobromine with monoamine oxidase inhibitors. Eur J Pharmacol 1971;16:315–321.
6. Bowman WC, Rand MJ: Psychotropic drugs. In: Textbook of Pharmacology, 8th ed. London, Blackwell Scientific Publications, 1980, pp. 15–19.
7. Bowman WC, Rand MJ: Psychotropic drugs. In: Textbook of Pharmacology, 8th ed. London, Blackwell Scientific Publications, 1980, pp. 43–50.
8. Bressler R, Vargas-Cordon M, Lebovitz HE: Tranylcypromine: A potent insulin secretagogue and hypoglycaemic agent. Diabetes 1968; 17:617–624.
9. Butler J, Leonard BE: Clinical and experimental studies on fluoxetine: Effects on serotonin uptake. Int Clin Psychopharmacol 1990;5:41–48.
10. Chaimowitz GA, Links PS, Padgett RW, et al: Treatment resistant depression: A survey of practice habits of Canadian psychiatrists. Can J Psychiatry 1991;36:353–356.
11. Christie JE, Crow TJ: Behavioral studies of the actions of cocaine, monoamine oxidase inhibitors and iminodibenzyl compounds on central dopamine neurons. Br J Pharmacol 1973;47:39–47.
12. Ciraulo DA, Shader RI: Fluoxetine drug-drug interactions: I. Antidepressants and antipsychotics. J Clin Psychopharmacol 1990;10:48–53.
13. Cromie WJ: Depression treated with skin patch. Harvard University Gazette, December 10, 1998.
14. Cuthbert MF, Greenberg MP, Morley SW: Cough and cold remedies: A potential danger to patients on monoamine oxidase inhibitors. Br Med J 1969;1:404–409.
15. Dally PJ: Fatal reaction with tranylcypromine and methylamphetamine. Lancet 1962;1:1235–1236.
16. Da Prada M, Zurchet G, Wuthrich I, et al: On tyramine, food, beverages and the reversible MAO inhibitor moclobemide. J Neurol Transm 1988;26(Suppl):31–56.
17. Dawson JK, Earnshaw SM, Graham CS: Dangerous monoamine oxidase inhibitor interactions are still occurring in the 1990s. J Accid Emerg Med 1995;12:49–51.
18. Dostert P: Can our knowledge of monoamine oxidase (MAO) help in the design of better MAO inhibitors? J Neural Transm 1994;41 (Suppl):269–279.
19. Erich JL, Shih RD, O'Connor RE: Ping-pong gaze in severe monoamine oxidase inhibitor toxicity. J Emerg Med;1995;13: 653–655.
20. Elis J, Laurence DR, Mattie H, et al: Modification by monoamine oxidase inhibitors of the effect of some sympathomimetics on blood pressure. Br Med J 1967;2:75–78.
21. Erspamer V: Recent research in the field of 5-hydroxytryptamine and related indole alkylamines. Prog Drug Res 1961;3:307–315.
22. Findlay JWA, Butz RF, Williams BB, et al: Effect of monoamine oxidase inhibitors on codeine disposition and pentobarbitone sleep-times in the rat. J Pharm Pharmacol 1981;33:34–47.
23. Foods interacting with MAO inhibitors. Abramowicz M (ed). Med Lett 1989;31:11–12.
24. Friend DG, Bell WR, Kline NS: The action of L-dihydroxyphenylalanine in patients receiving nialamide. Clin Pharmacol Ther 1965;6: 362–366.
25. Fritz RR, Malek-Ahmadi P, Rose RM, et al: Tranylcypromine lowers human platelet MAO-B activity but not concentration. Biol Psychiatry 1983;18:685–694.
26. Georgotas A, McCue RE, Friedman E, et al: Prediction of response to nortriptyline and phenelzine by platelet MAO activity: Am J Psychiatry 1987;144:339–340.
27. Hesselink JM: Safer use of MAOIs with nifedipine to counteract potential hypertensive crisis [letter]. Am J Psychiatry 1991;148:1616.
28. Hilton S, Ruch R: Moclobemide safety: Monitoring a newly developed product in the 1990s. J Clin Psychopharmacol 1995;14: 76S–83S.
29. Horler AR, Wynne NA: Hypertensive crisis due to pargyline and metaraminol. Br Med J 1965;2:460–461.
30. Horowitz D, Lovenberg W, Engelman K, et al: Monoamine oxidase inhibitors, tyramine and cheese. JAMA 1964;188:1108–1110.
31. Jacobsen E: The early history of psychotherapeutic drugs. Psychopharmacology 1986;89:138–144.
32. Jin YZ, Ramsay RR, Youngster SK, et al: A new class of powerful inhibitors of monoamine oxidase A. Biochem Biophysical Res Commun 1990;172:1338–1341.
33. Kahn D, Silver JM, Opler LA: The safety of switching rapidly from tricyclic antidepressants to monoamine oxidase inhibitors. J Clin Psychopharmacol 1989;9:198–202.
34. Kaplan RF, Feinglass NG, Webster WW et al: Phenelzine overdose treated with dantrolene sodium. JAMA 1986;255:5:642–644.
35. Keck PE JR, Buckovic A, Pope HG, et al: Acute cardiovascular response to monoamine oxidase inhibitors: A prospective assessment. J Clin Psychopharmacol 1989;9:203–206.
36. Keltner N: Serotonin syndrome: A case of fatal SSRI/MAOI interaction. Perspect Psychol Care 1994;30:26–31.

37. Kopin I, Axelrod J: The role of monoamine oxidase in the release and metabolism of norepinephrine. Ann N Y Acad Sci 1963;107:848–852.

38. Larsen JK: MAO inhibitors: Pharmacodynamic aspects and clinical implications. Acta Psychiatr Scand 1988;78(Suppl):74–80.

39. Linden CH, Rumack BH: Monoamine oxidase inhibitor overdose. Ann Emerg Med 1984;13:1137–1144.

40. Livingston MG, Livingston HM: Monoamine oxidase inhibitors. An update on drug interactions. Drug Saf 1996;14:219–227.

41. Low Beer GA, Tidmarsh D: Collapse after "Parstelin." Br Med J 1963;2:683–684.

42. Mallampalli R, Pentel PR, Anderson DC: Nonreactive pupils due to monamine oxidase inhibitor overdose. Crit Care Med 1987;15:536–537.

43. Mallinger AG, Smith E: Pharmacokinetics of monoamine oxidase inhibitors. Psychopharmacol Bull 1991;27:493–502.

44. Miller LG: Herbal medicinals: Selected clinical considerations focusing on known or potential drug-herbal interactions. Arch Intern Med 1998;158:2200–2211.

45. Mokler DJ, Stoudt KW, Rech RH: The 5-HT$_2$ antagonist pirenperone reverses disruption of FR-40 by hallucinogenic drugs. Pharmacol Biochem Behav 1985;22:677–682.

46. Moll E, Hetzl W: Moclobemide (Ro 11–1163) safety in depressed patients. Acta Psychiatr Scand 1990;360(Suppl):69–70.

47. Myrenfors PG, Eriksson T, Sandstedt CS, et al: Moclobemide overdose. J Intern Med 1993;233:113–115.

48. Neary JT, Bu Y: Hypericum L1 160 inhibits uptake of serotonin and norepinephrine in astrocytes. Brain Res 1999:916:358–363.

49. Neuvonen PJ, Pohojla-Sintonen S, Tacke U, et al: Five fatal cases of serotonin syndrome after moclobemide-citalopram or moclobemide-clomipramine overdoses [letter]. Lancet 1993;342:1419.

50. Penn RG, Rogers KJ: Comparison of the effects of morphine, pethidine and pentazocine in rabbits pretreated with a monoamine oxidase inhibitor. Br J Pharmacol 1971;42:485–492.

51. Pope HG, Jonas JM, Hudson JI, et al: Toxic reactions to the combination of monoamine oxidase inhibitors and tryptophan. Am J Psychiatry 1985;142:491–492.

52. Raft D, Davidson J, Wasik J, et al: Relationship between response to phenelzine and MAO inhibition in a clinical trial of phenelzine, amitriptyline and placebo. Neuropsychobiology 1981;7:122–126.

53. Roby CA, Anderson ED, Kantor E, et al: St. John's wort: Effect on CYP3A4 activity. Clin Pharmacol Ther 200;67:451–457.

54. Rowland MJ, Bransome ED Jr, Hendry LB: Hypoglycemia caused by selegiline, an antiparkinsonian drug: Can such side effects be predicted? J Clin Pharmacol 1994;34:80–85.

55. Sandyk R: L-Dopa-induced "serotonin syndrome" in a parkinsonian patient on bromocriptine. J Clin Psychopharmacol 1986;6:194–195.

56. Shulman KI, Walker SE, MacKenzie S, et al: Dietary restriction, tyramine and the use of monoamine oxidase inhibitors. J Clin Psychopharmacol 1989;9:397–402.

57. Silverstone T: New aspects in the treatment of depression. Int Clin Psychopharmacol 1992;6(Suppl 5):41–44.

58. Sinclair JG, Lo GF: The blockade of serotonin uptake and the meperidine monoamine oxidase inhibitor interaction. Proc West Pharmacol Soc 1977;20:373–374.

59. Singer PP, Graham RJ: An uncommon fatality due to moclobemide and paroxetine. J Anal Tox 1997;21:518–520.

60. Smilkstein MJ, Smolinske SC, Rumack BH: A case of MAO inhibitor/MDMA interaction. Agony after ecstasy. J Toxicol Clin Toxicol 1987;25:149–159.

61. Stack CG, Rogers P, Linter PK: Monoamine oxidase inhibitors and anaesthesia. Br J Anaesth 1988;60:222–227.

62. Stark DCC: Effects of giving vasopressors to patients on MAO inhibitors. Lancet 1962;2:1405–1406.

63. Sternbach H: The serotonin syndrome. Am J Psychiatry 1991;148:705–713.

64. Tanks CM, Lloyd AT: Hazards with monoamine oxidase inhibitors. Br Med J 1965;1:589.

65. Teychenne PF, Calne DB, Lewis PJ, et al: Interactions of levodopa with inhibitors of monoamine oxidase and L-aromatic acid decarboxylase. Clin Pharmacol Ther 1975;18:273–277.

66. Thakore J, Dinan TG, Kelleher M: Alcohol-free beer and the irreversible monoamine oxidase inhibitors. Int Clin Psychopharmacol 1992;7:59–60.

67. Thomas JM, Rubin EH: Case report of a toxic reaction from a combination of tryptophan and phenelzine. Am J Psychiatry 1984;141:281–283.

68. Tiller JWG, Johnson GFS, Franz CP, et al: Moclobemide for depression: An Australian psychiatric practice study. J Clin Psychopharmacol 1995;15:31S–34S.

69. Tobin AB, Osborne NN: Evidence for the presence of serotonin receptors negatively coupled to adenylate cyclase in the rabbit iris-ciliary body. J Neurochem 1989;53:686–691.

70. Tolefson GD: Monoamine oxidase inhibitors: A review. J Clin Psychol 1983;44:280–287.

71. Trinker FR, Flearn HJ, McCullock NW, et al: Experimental observations on the effects of adrenaline after treatment with antidepressant monoamine oxidase inhibitors (MAOI) drugs. Austr Dent J 1967;12:297–303.

72. True L, Alexander B, Carter B: Switching monoamine oxidase inhibitors. Drug Intell Clin Pharm 1985;19:825–827.

73. Wells DG, Bjorksten AR: Monoamine oxidase inhibitors revisited. Can J Anaesth 1989;36:64–74.

74. White K, Pistole T, Boyd JL: Combined monoamine oxidase inhibitor-tricyclic antidepressant treatment: A pilot study. Am J Psychiatry 1980;137:1422–1425.

CHAPTER 61 LITHIUM

Glendon C. Henry

Lithium
MW = 6.94 daltons
Lithium levels (serum):
  Therapeutic level for
    bipolar depression = 0.6–1.2 mEq/L (mmol/L)
Action level
    Acute toxicity = >4.0 mEq/L (mmol/L)
    Chronic toxicity = >1.5 mEq/L (mmol/L)
Values greater than or equal to the action level necessitate clinical intervention. Values less than this level may necessitate intervention based on the clinical condition of the patient.

A 36-year-old woman was rushed to the Emergency Department (ED) by her family because of a change in mental status. The patient was stuporous, but when aroused, she had slurred speech and complained of blurred vision. She was unable to provide any additional history at that time. According to the family and a clinic psychiatrist, the woman had manifested emotional problems for years and had been treated by numerous psychiatrists. The patient's purse contained bottles of phenothiazines, tricyclic antidepressants, lithium carbonate, and several analgesic combinations.

On examination, the patient was unkempt, diaphoretic, and poorly nourished. Her vital signs were blood pressure, 140/85 mm Hg; pulse, 110 beats/min; respirations, 18 breaths/min; temperature, 37.3°C (99.1°F); and oxygen saturation, 94% on room air. She had poor dentition and her mouth smelled of fresh vomitus. Horizontal nystagmus was present.

Her chest was normal to auscultation and percussion, heart rate was regular, and there were no murmurs, thrills, heaves, or gallops. Abdominal examination revealed hyperactive bowel sounds. Rectal examination revealed good sphincter tone, with no occult blood in the stool.

During the neurologic examination the patient became agitated with stimulation. She had a mild tremor and fasciculations in both upper extremities. There was no motor weakness, but the deep-tendon reflexes were hyperactive. Clonus of both lower extremities was noted and choreoathetoid movements were observed twice during the examination. All cranial nerves were normal, with the exception of the previously noted horizontal nystagmus. Low-flow oxygen was administered, and cardiac monitoring initiated. A large-bore intravenous catheter was inserted, and blood specimens were obtained for electrolytes, renal function, complete blood count (CBC), arterial blood gases (ABG), and serum lithium level. A bedside glucose determination was 120 mg/dL. The patient was administered 100 mg of thiamine HCl intravenously without response and an ampule of multivitamins was added to the first liter of 0.9% sodium chloride. The patient's clinical condition did not change.

The electrocardiogram (ECG) demonstrated a sinus tachycardia at 110 beats/min with normal P-R and QRS intervals, nonspecific ST segment and T-wave changes, and U waves. The chest radiograph was normal. A lumbar puncture was performed and all chemical and cytologic studies of the cerebrospinal fluid (CSF) were normal. Shortly thereafter, a serum lithium level of 3.6 mEq/L was reported by the laboratory. Other pertinent laboratory studies included a blood urea nitrogen (BUN) of 40 mg/dL and a creatinine of 1.9 mg/dL.

Following consultation with a nephrologist, hemodialysis was performed for 4 hours at a blood flow rate of 250 mL/min. During the procedure the patient became more alert and responsive. Her lithium level immediately postdialysis was reported as 0.6 mEq/L, but this rose to 2.1 mEq/L 4 hours later. A second hemodialysis treatment was performed the following day, and the patient's posttreatment and subsequent lithium levels remained below 0.1 mEq/L. She was now communicative and reported that her physician had started her on an angiotensin-converting enzyme (ACE) inhibitor 2 weeks earlier for mild hypertension. She denied acute ingestion or suicidal ideations and was discharged on a lower maintenance dose of lithium with close followup.

HISTORY

Lithium is the lightest metal known; it is a cation with an atomic number of 3 and a valence of +1. It is in the same column of the periodic table as sodium and potassium; thus, many of its actions are similar to those of sodium and potassium (Chap. 12). Although first prescribed as an antidepressant in 1970, lithium's use in medicine began much earlier.[1]

In the mid-19th century, because of the solubility of lithium urate, various lithium salts were used in the treatment of gouty arthritis and nephrolithiasis. At one time, it was a constituent in the soft drink Seven-Up. Later, lithium chloride was popularized as a table-salt substitute for the treatment of hypertensive patients.[1] However, in 1949, several deaths were attributed to lithium toxicity, leading the FDA to ban its use as a salt substitute. Ironically, this was about the time that a beneficial role for lithium in the treatment of mania was discovered. In 1970, lithium was recognized as the treatment of choice for patients with bipolar disorders.

In addition to its role in treating bipolar disorders, lithium carbonate is also prescribed in the prophylaxis and treatment of cluster headaches,[39] and as a "cell stimulator" in neutropenic patients.[44,52,54]

PHARMACOLOGY

Lithium's precise mechanism of action has not been fully elucidated. The actions of lithium are similar to those of sodium and potassium, with which it shares the same valence. The ionic radius of lithium is similar to that of magnesium; therefore, it may substitute for this ion as well.[47] Although lithium may alter some of the functions of magnesium and serve as a false ion for either sodium or potassium, its main effect may not be secondary to its substitution for any of these ions, but rather from its effect on phosphatidylinositol metabolism via a second messenger. After inositol is activated by a surface agonist,[9,19,53] it interacts with G proteins that then stimulate phospholipase C to cleave intracellular phosphatidylinositol to intracellular messengers 1,2-diacylglycerol (DAG) and inositol 1,4,5-triphosphate.[14,38] The latter is a direct stimulator for the release of intracellular calcium, while the former is an activator of protein kinase C. This is important because inositol does not cross the blood-brain barrier; thus, its concentration in the brain is maintained by regeneration and breakdown of phosphorylated components.[3,57] Lithium may inhibit the enzyme inositol monophosphatase, leading to an increase in inositol monophosphate and to a decrease in free inositol and the intermediate phosphatidylinositol 4,5-bisphosphate.[13,14,38] The final common pathway is a decrease in free brain inositol concentration, which is believed to result in both the desired and the adverse effects produced. Although this mechanism seems reasonable, lithium may also alter other pathways and its effects on protein kinase C and G proteins may be just as important as the depletion of inositol.[47] Norepinephrine activity may also be attenuated by lithium via a second messenger, cAMP.[7] Although its interactions with cAMP have been extensively evaluated, no definitive mechanism of action is yet elucidated. Its interactions with magnesium metabolism may play a vital role.[48] The numerous chemical interactions may explain various alterations in biologic functions brought about by lithium as well as its potential role in treating diverse disease processes.

Lithium may also effect neurotransmitters. It seems to increase the synthesis and turnover of serotonin,[46] while producing a down-regulation of the 5-HT$_{1A}$ receptors in the hippocampus[49] by diminishing serotonin binding to its receptors.[38] Although not as well established, lithium may also have an effect on the down-regulation of the α- and β-adrenergic receptors.[46] Similar net effects on dopaminergic receptors may occur because lithium may prevent up-regulation at the D$_2$ receptors.[2,75]

Lithium may cause other disorders such as nephrogenic diabetes insipidus[18,25] and hypothyroidism.[23] Diabetes insipidus may be the most problematic of all the complications induced by lithium because its development will invariably lead to further toxicity. Lithium may decrease cyclic adenosine monophosphate (cAMP) production in the renal collecting ducts by blocking the action of antidiuretic hormone (ADH)-sensitive adenylate cyclase, which produces a decrease in water reabsorption and polyuria. It

may also impair the expression or function of aquaporins, or water channels, in the renal tubules. The drug-induced diabetes insipidus creates a hyperosmolar state, which causes increased ADH secretion secondary to pituitary stimulation. This stimulation induces urinary prostaglandin secretion, which blocks ADH-sensitive cyclase, thereby decreasing water reabsorption.[18,25,28] Fortunately in the majority of the cases, the diabetes insipidus is reversible upon discontinuing lithium therapy.

Lithium is selectively concentrated in the thyroid gland, where long-term exposure produces hypothyroidism. The etiology of the hypothyroidism may be multifactorial and includes blocking of iodine uptake by the gland, reduced release of T3 and T4, or even decreased sensitivity of the gland to TSH.[58] In addition, lithium prevents the conversion of T4 to T3 and is associated with the formation of antithyroid antibodies. It is said that nearly one-third of all patients on chronic lithium therapy will have an increase in TSH, with one-third to one-half of those patients developing hypothyroidism.

TOXICOKINETICS

Immediate-release lithium is absorbed from the gastrointestinal tract within 1–2 hours, with peak levels achieved at 2–4 hours. Following ingestion of sustained-release preparations, initial absorption may be delayed for 6–12 hours with absorption completed after an additional 8 hours. In overdose, peak absorption may be delayed even longer. Lithium has a volume of distribution of 0.6–0.9 L/kg, which is slightly larger than total body water. Lithium is excreted via the kidney (95%), and its clearance is dependent on the glomerular filtration rate (GFR). Patients with a decreased GFR are at higher risk for toxicity.[63] Normally, 80% of the lithium handled by the kidney is reabsorbed, while 20% is excreted in the urine unchanged.[31,63,66,67] Lithium was believed to be solely reabsorbed in the proximal tubules following filtration,[51] but recent evidence suggests that some lithium is also reabsorbed in the loop of Henle, as well as in the distal tubules.[7,16,37] About 5% of lithium is secreted in sweat and saliva, and a small percentage is excreted in breast milk in the lactating female.[73]

After absorption, lithium undergoes a slow distribution as it traverses cell membranes in therapeutic and toxic doses.[34] Lithium enters the liver and kidney rapidly, while its passage into muscle, bone, and brain is much slower.[34] As lithium enters these outer compartments, its volume of distribution approaches 0.9 L/kg. The therapeutic elimination half-life for lithium is about 20–24 hours, but may be prolonged beyond that in patients who receive lithium therapy for extended periods of time or in those patients with reduced renal function.[30]

The CSF lithium levels range from 40% to 80% of that in the serum. Unfortunately, CSF levels do not correlate either with serum levels, therapeutic effect, or toxicity.[57,74]

CLINICAL MANIFESTATIONS

Signs and symptoms of chronic lithium toxicity are quite distinct from those resulting from single acute ingestions (Table 61–1). Similar to patients who ingest other metal salts, those patients with acute lithium overdose typically manifest early gastrointestinal symptoms such as nausea, vomiting, and diarrhea. Neurologic findings are delayed. Cardiovascular complaints, such as light-

TABLE 61–1. Toxicity of Lithium

	Acute	Chronic
Cardiovascular	Prolonged QT interval ST- and T-wave abnormalities	Myocarditis
Cutaneous	None	Dermatitis, ulcers, localized edema
Renal	Concentrating defects	Nephrogenic diabetes insipidus Interstitial nephritis Renal failure
Gastrointestinal	Nausea Vomiting	Minimal
Hematologic	Leukocytosis	Aplastic anemia
Neurologic		
Mild	Weakness, lightheadedness, fine tremor	Same
Moderate	Muscle twitching, tinnitus, drowsiness, hyperreflexia, slurred speech, apathy	Same
Severe	Confusion, clonus, coma, seizure, extrapyramidal symptoms (choreoathetoid movements)	Parkinson disease, psychosis, memory deficits, idiopathic intracranial hypertension
Endocrine	None	Hypothyroidism
Congenital	None	Hypothyroidism

headedness, dizziness, and orthostatic hypotension, are usually the result of excessive fluid loss rather than from a direct cardiotoxic effect. Electrocardiographic manifestations such as nonspecific T-wave changes may develop and are usually benign.[22] Although reported in the literature, malignant dysrhythmias and severe cardiac dysfunction are very rare.[68]

Neurologic abnormalities are the major manifestations of both acute and chronic lithium toxicity.[50,59,60] In the acute setting, the initial finding may be merely a fine tremor of the hands. As toxicity progresses, the patient will develop hyperreflexia followed by fasciculations, muscular irritability, choreoathetosis, clonus, agitation, and altered mental status. Confusion may be followed by lethargy, coma, and seizures. Dysarthria, nystagmus, and truncal ataxia may also occur.[21,50,55,70] The electroencephalogram (EEG) may show diffuse slowing.[59,61] Although the progression of these signs or symptoms may be orderly, the levels do not necessarily correlate with the toxic manifestations, which may be explained by the slow distribution time for lithium.[26,57,75]

Patients with chronic lithium toxicity rarely notice or manifest gastrointestinal symptoms and usually present with altered mental status. Toxicity typically results from either a dosing error, such as the continuation of high lithium doses following the control of a manic episode, or as a result of other predisposing factors, such as drug interactions, sodium restriction, or a decrease in renal lithium excretion. Numerous agents, such as the nonsteroidal anti-inflammatory agents, ACE inhibitors, serotonin reuptake inhibitors (SSRIs), and antipsychotic agents, may elevate lithium levels. Patients with a history of cardiovascular disease and anyone who uses a diuretic chronically are at increased risk for toxicity. Impaired elimination results from intrinsic renal dysfunction or diuretic therapy causing natruresis. Prerenal azotemia, or any condition that predisposes to a relative decrease in intravascular

volume or sodium, leads to a concomitant increased reabsorption of both sodium and lithium, as noted previously.

The toxicity of the patient chronically poisoned by lithium is almost exclusively neurologic and resembles the later stages of acute toxicity. An explanation for the difference in time between acute and chronic poisoning presentations is that with chronic use there is a high total body burden of lithium and therefore any additional increase in lithium intake results in immediate toxicity. By comparison, in the acute setting, there is a substantial delay in tissue distribution prior to the development of therapeutic or toxic effects.

Patients receiving chronic lithium therapy who also acutely ingest an excessive amount of lithium ("acute or chronic overdose") may be the most difficult to accurately diagnose and to properly manage because they may manifest signs and symptoms of both acute and chronic toxicity. Although neurologic signs may be present in this situation of a chronic overdose, acute gastrointestinal symptoms also occur, and toxicity may be more severe and prolonged (Table 61–1).

Patients who initially appear well may subsequently develop seizures and altered mental status.[50] Prolonged exposure of the central nervous system to excess lithium can cause permanent neurologic sequelae, even when enhanced extracorporeal clearance methods such as hemodialysis are used.[33,65] Long-term exposure to sustained toxic levels may result in memory deficits, neuromuscular weakness, change in personality, or tremors.[29,42,65,72] Hyperthermia is a grave marker of central nervous system (CNS) toxicity, necessitating immediate intervention. In addition, there are several reports linking lithium with the neuroleptic malignant syndrome (Chap. 18). Unfortunately, all of these cases describe patients who had ingested multiple agents, including at least one antipsychotic. There are no reports of NMS induced by lithium as the sole agent.[4,17] Lithium is frequently added after an antipsychotic is initiated and therefore it is difficult to determine what role lithium itself actually plays in this disorder.

DIAGNOSTIC TESTING

Laboratory studies should be sent for electrolytes, renal function, and a serum lithium level.[36,64] Not only will the renal function studies offer insight into the etiology of toxicity, but they will help predict the response to conservative therapy. A second and perhaps serial lithium levels are essential to assess both for ongoing absorption and for response to therapy. When polyuria or hypernatremia is present, simultaneous determinations of the serum and urine osmolarity may assist with the diagnosis of nephrogenic diabetes insipidus. Although not necessarily indicated, a leukocytosis is expected if a CBC is obtained. Similarly, thyroid function studies should be determined when clinical signs of hypothyroidism are suspected. The electrocardiograph should be performed while continuous monitoring is established. Continuous monitoring of the urine output may necessitate insertion of a Foley catheter in patients with significant toxicity.

MANAGEMENT

As in all toxicologic emergencies, it is important to define the nature of the patient's ingestion. It must be determined whether the ingestion is intentional or unintentional, whether one or more agents were ingested, and whether the agents are sustained- or regular-release products. With regard to lithium, it is essential to determine whether the ingestion is acute or chronic, or an acute ingestion following chronic treatment. These characteristics of the history may alter how the patient is treated and the eventual outcome. A risk assessment should be performed when the number of ingested pills is known. Each 300-mg lithium carbonate tablet contains approximately 8 mEq of lithium. Assuming a volume of distribution of nearly 1 L/kg and complete absorption for an 80-kg adult, each 300-mg tablet is expected to raise the serum lithium level approximately 0.1 mEq/L.

The patient's airway, breathing, and circulation must be assured; although lithium toxicity does not usually affect the airway or breathing, other coingestants may. Cardiovascular compromise and significant dysrhythmias are rarely associated with lithium poisoning, but can also occur in this setting as a result of excessive gastrointestinal and urinary fluid losses.

Gastrointestinal Decontamination

In a patient with an early presentation of an acute overdose, or of an acute overdose superimposed on a chronic overdose of lithium, orogastric lavage may remove pills remaining in the stomach if spontaneous emesis has not already occurred. However, immediate-release preparations are absorbed quickly and extended-release preparations may not pass through even the largest tube. Syrup of ipecac–induced emesis should be considered when the history and clinical presentation are consistent with very recent ingestion and a lack of coingestants. Because lithium is not significantly adsorbed to activated charcoal, its only utility is for the treatment of known or potential coingestants.[36,64] The use of a cathartic such as sorbitol has limited benefits and has the potential for complications because most consequential ingestions have spontaneous diarrhea.[55] Enhanced gastrointestinal clearance may be accomplished by initiating whole-bowel irrigation with a balanced polyethylene glycol-electrolyte solution (PEG-ELS). If the patient has ingested a sustained-release lithium preparation, such as Lithobid or Escalith CR, then whole-bowel irrigation is even more important.[62] When used, PEG-ELS should be administered at 2 L/h in the adult, or at 500 mL/h in a child. The endpoint of this therapy is a rectal effluent that has the same appearance as the instilled fluid (Antidotes in Depth: Whole-Bowel Irrigation).

Sodium polystyrene sulfonate (SPS) is a cation ionic exchange agent that is frequently used to treat severe hyperkalemia. Its ability to effectively bind potassium in exchange for sodium so that excessive potassium can be excreted in the stool has made SPS a very valuable agent. One reason that SPS is so effective for hyperkalemia is that the actual amount of potassium to be bound and excreted is small. Because of the similarities between lithium and potassium, a possible role for SPS in the treatment of lithium toxicity has been considered. Studies in dogs show that orally administered lithium is cleared more rapidly when SPS is administered.[45] Subsequent animal studies demonstrate the beneficial effects of SPS in reducing blood levels of intravenously administered lithium.[44] In fact, a human case report describes success in using SPS to treat lithium poisoning.[27]

There are substantial concerns with the use of SPS, however. In the rodent studies, extremely large doses (10 g/kg) of SPS were necessary to reduce significant amounts of lithium. Even the lower doses of SPS now under study are much larger than those usually

given to patients with renal failure. Another major concern is the effect of SPS on potassium. In mice, the hypokalemia induced can be significant; if extrapolated to humans, this electrolyte shift would contraindicate the use of SPS.[43] Thus far, studies in humans receiving single doses of SPS demonstrate conflicting effects in causing hypokalemia[11,69] and studies including multiple doses of SPS demonstrate the need for replacement potassium.[56] In summary, SPS in doses comparable to those effectively used to treat experimental lithium toxicity in animals will almost certainly induce hypokalemia in humans. Thus, the complications of hypokalemia, such as dysrhythmias, hypernatremia, and fluid overload, must be anticipated, as well as the substantial amount of SPS that will be needed to achieve success. These concerns make SPS less appealing.

Fluid and Electrolytes

During the evaluation of the patient it is prudent to begin hydration with 0.9% saline in order to promote good urine output to maximize the excretion of lithium.

In managing a patient with a lithium overdose, it is essential that the patient's fluid and electrolyte status be closely monitored and maintained. This approach may be obvious in the acutely poisoned patient who presents with nausea, vomiting, and diarrhea, but in the chronically overdosed patient, dehydration or an electrolyte disturbance may be the precipitating event for hospitalization. In all instances, collaboration and consultation with a nephrologist should be initiated early in the course of management if suspicion for toxicity is substantial.

In patients with normal renal function, osmotic and saline diuresis have limited roles and have not been shown to increase lithium clearance significantly.[37] When glomerular filtration is impaired, volume repletion with 0.9% sodium chloride solution followed by infusion at 1.5–2 times maintenance should be sufficient to maximize renal lithium clearance. Urinary alkalinization may have a limited beneficial effect on lithium excretion and clearance because sodium bicarbonate decreases lithium reabsorption in the proximal tubules. The use of sodium bicarbonate, however, is not recommended because of its potential to cause hypokalemia, alkalemia, and fluid overload, and because sodium bicarbonate does not significantly enhance elimination over that which can be accomplished by administering a balanced salt solution IV. Diuretics that act on the ascending limb of the loop of Henle or the distal tubule (eg, furosemide, ethacrynic acid, and the thiazides) have limited effects on lithium reabsorption, which maximally occurs in the proximal tubule.[51] Indeed, they may worsen lithium poisoning, particularly if the patient becomes salt- or water-depleted.

Three classes of agents shown to cause an initial increase in lithium excretion are osmotic agents (mannitol),[67] carbonic anhydrase inhibitors, and phosphodiesterase inhibitors (aminophylline). In each case, although the agent may initially produce a small increase in lithium excreted, these agents may result in dehydration resulting in sodium and lithium retention. Therefore, their use is not recommended for the treatment of lithium toxicity.

As noted, because chronic lithium therapy can induce diabetes insipidus, it can exacerbate its own toxicity. Amiloride has been shown to decrease the polyuria that is associated with lithium and therefore may help correct the fluid and electrolyte abnormalities as well as increase the excretion of lithium when nephrogenic diabetes insipidus is present. As with any potassium-sparing diuretic, dehydration must be prevented so as not to increase lithium reabsorption proximally, while simultaneously avoiding hyperkalemia. These are both rare events and patients are rarely given amiloride in the treatment of acute lithium toxicity.[10]

Extracorporeal Drug Removal

Peritoneal dialysis (PD), which had been used in the past, is no more efficacious than the endogenous lithium clearance by the kidneys;[15,77] thus, peritoneal dialysis is not indicated in the management of lithium overdoses in patients with functioning kidneys. The clearance of lithium by PD is between 10 and 15 mL/min, less than a normally functioning kidney.[76] Because of PD's potential to cause complications such as bowel perforation, peritonitis, or sepsis, PD's only benefit may be for a patient who has renal failure who is already receiving chronic PD and for the patient who has a working PD catheter in place. In this circumstance, PD could be started until more definitive therapy, such as hemodialysis, becomes available.

Definitive therapy for patients who manifest lithium toxicity and/or who cannot excrete lithium is extracorporeal removal by hemodialysis (HD). Because lithium is a small ion, has no protein binding, and has a relatively small volume of distribution, it is readily dialyzable.[15] Clearance of lithium by hemodialysis is solely dependent on blood flow, and ranges from 70 mL/min to 170 mL/min, which is far greater than that of the kidney.[20,24,35] Unfortunately, determining when to institute therapy is not always simple. Patients who are initially poisoned and have high lithium levels but no signs or symptoms may benefit the most from HD because lithium has not yet fully distributed to tissue compartments that are cleared less well than the plasma. Many of these patients will probably do well without HD, and the risks of the procedure must be considered before subjecting the patient to this invasive therapy. Conversely, after lithium has been distributed to the tissues, it is more difficult to remove by HD, and permanent sequelae may occur.[34]

Determining the need for HD should be based on a consideration of the probability that the patient may become toxic if elimination is not enhanced. Because lithium is not metabolized and is only renally excreted, all patients with potentially toxic lithium exposures and renal failure should undergo hemodialysis as soon as possible. These patients cannot clear lithium and may suffer long-term complications of toxicity. All patients with neurologic dysfunction, including altered mental status, should undergo hemodialysis.[61] Patients who are stable, but who may not be able to tolerate sodium repletion, such as those with congestive heart failure, pulmonary edema, or anasarca, should also be considered for early hemodialysis.

A patient who has only a mild tremor may not warrant HD, but must be monitored closely for further neurologic dysfunction. The most difficult decision regarding the initiation of HD relies on the interpretation of lithium levels. The definition of a "high" lithium level is arbitrary as well as dependent on the nature of the ingestion. After an acute ingestion, with no previous body burden of lithium, a level of ≥4.0 mEq/L should be considered an indication for HD regardless of the patient's clinical status.[34] At this level, as equilibration begins, some lithium will be excreted, and some will cross the cellular membrane, but it is unlikely that the patient will be able to excrete the lithium rapidly enough to prevent a significant amount from entering the central nervous system and causing

severe and potentially permanent neurologic toxicity.[6,33] However, a patient with an acute on chronic overdose or chronic overdose already has a body burden of lithium, and therefore may develop toxicity at a lower level than 4.0 mEq/L.[34] For these patients, a lithium level of ≥2.5 mEq/L and moderate to severe neurologic toxicity are reasonable indications for HD.[32]

A "rebound lithium level" is typically measured after hemodialysis because dialysis clears only the plasma; a significant amount of lithium is in the intracellular space and redistributes slowly into the plasma following treatment.[20,34] Lithium levels should therefore be drawn immediately after hemodialysis, and repeated 6 hours postdialysis. If either level is high, or if the patient continues to show signs of neurologic toxicity, a second course of hemodialysis may be needed. For this reason, the dialysis catheter should not be removed until a significant rebound effect can be excluded.

Recent studies indicate that continuous arteriovenous hemofiltration (CAVH) may serve as an alternate therapy to hemodialysis.[8,71] CAVH and continuous venovenous hemofiltration (CVVH) use essentially the same mechanism to remove toxins from the body, except that in CVVH, the patient has a pump connected to the circuit because of the lack of a gradient across the vessels. In CAVH, the difference in arterial and venous pressure serves as the pump that moves the blood around the circuit. Continuous arteriovenous hemofiltration works on the principle that as blood is constantly being filtered, any toxin that is present will be removed gradually from the body (Chap. 6). The benefits of CAVH over hemodialysis are that CAVH is a continuous process and although filtering takes place in a monitored setting, there is no need for specialized personnel, as there is for HD, and there may be fewer complications. In an effort to increase the efficiency in toxin removal, several studies now suggest continuous venous or arterial hemodiafiltration (CAVHDF) as the primary form of extracorporeal therapy. These forms of therapy are CAVH or CVVH with dialysis inserted into the circuit.[12,41] In a recent study,[41] seven patients with severe lithium toxicity were evaluated, four with acute and three with chronic overdoses. The acutely overdosed patients underwent CAVHDF, whereas the chronically overdosed were treated with CVVHDF. Clearances of 20–62 mL/min were achieved. Because the clearance is far less than that of HD, the total duration of the procedure must be longer to achieve similar total drug elimination. The authors found that CAVHDF and CVVHDF were both able to remove a significant amount of total body lithium burden and that all patients improved. In only one of their patients was there a rebound rise in the lithium level.[34,35] The authors concluded that either CAVHDF or CVVHDF may be excellent methods for removing lithium while preventing a rebound elevation of lithium following the procedure. A disadvantage of CAVHDF is the need to have the patient in a monitored setting for the entirety of the process. HD remains a better modality in terms of speed of toxin removal, and therefore may be better at preventing the gravest of complications, namely permanent neurologic deficits. Although more controlled studies must be performed, hemodiafiltration (HDF) may play an important role in treating patients with lithium toxicity, especially when HD is not available. In addition, HDF may be useful to attenuate the rebound effect in patients who have completed HD. Currently, CAVH and CVVH cannot be recommended as the sole extracorporeal therapeutic intervention for lithium removal if HD is available.

SUMMARY

Lithium plays an essential role in the psychopharmacologic armamentarium. Its use is extensive in diverse psychiatric and nonpsychiatric disorders. Lithium is available in various salt forms in controlled- and immediate-release preparations. Because of the profile of the patients using this drug, the diverse reasons for adverse drug effects, and the ease for developing toxicity (acute and/or chronic), the care for patients poisoned with lithium is complicated. Early recognition of poisoning and rapid use of hemodialysis are essential to decrease patient morbidity and mortality.

REFERENCES

1. Aita JF, Aita JA, Aita VA: 7-Up anti-acid lithiated lemon soda or early medicinal use of lithium. Nebr Med J 1990;75:277–279.
2. Alessi N, Naylor MW, Mohammad G, et al: Update on lithium carbonate therapy in children and adolescents. J Am Acad Child Psychiatry 1994;33:291–303.
3. Allison JH, Stewart MA: Reduced brain inositol in lithium treated rats. Nat New Biol 1971;233:267–268.
4. Amdisen A: Clinical features and management of lithium poisoning. Med Toxicol Adv Drug Exper 1988;3:18–32.
5. Anath J: Side effects in the neonate from psychotropic agents excreted through breast-feeding. Am J Psychiatry 1978;135:801–804.
6. Apte SN, Langston WJ: Permanent neurological deficits due to lithium toxicity. Ann Neurol 1983;13:452–455.
7. Atherton JC, Doyle A, Gee A, et al: Lithium clearance: Modification by the loop of Henle in man. J Physiol 1990;437:377–391.
8. Ayuso Gatell A, Leon Regidor MA, Mestre Saura J, et al: Acute lithium poisoning: Treatment with continuous arteriovenous hemofiltration. Rev Clin Exp 1989;185:195–197.
9. Baraban JM, Worley PF, Snyder SH: Second messenger and psychoactive drug action. Focus on the phosphoinositide system and lithium. Am J Psychiatry 1989;146:1251–1260.
10. Battle DC, Von Riote AB, Gaviaria M, et al: Amelioration of polyuria by amiloride in patient receiving long-term lithium therapy. N Engl J Med 1985;313:409–414.
11. Belanger DR, Tierne MG, Dickerson G: Effect of sodium polystyrene sulfonate on lithium availability. Ann Emerg Med 1992;21:1312–1315.
12. Bellomo R, Kearly Y, Parkin G: Treatment of life-threatening lithium toxicity with continuous arteriovenous hemodiafiltration. Crit Care Med 1991;19:836–837.
13. Berridge MJ, Downes CD, Hanley RR: Neurological and development action of lithium. A unifying hypothesis. Cell 1989;59:411–419.
14. Berridge MJ, Downes CP, Hanley RR: Lithium amplifies agonist-dependent phosphatidylinositol response in brain and salivary gland. Biochem J 1982;206:587–595.
15. Blye E, Lorch J, Cartell S: Extracorporeal therapy in the treatment of intoxication. Am J Kidney Dis 1984;3:321–338.
16. Boer WH, Koomans HA, Dorhout Mees EJ: Lithium clearances in healthy humans suggesting reabsorption beyond the proximal tubules. Kidney Int 1990;37:S39–S44.
17. Brust JC, Hammer JS, Challenor Y, et al: Acute generalized polyneuropathy accompanying lithium poisoning. Ann Neurol 1979;6:360–362.
18. Christensen EM, Kusano E, Yusufi ANK, et al: Pathogenesis of nephrogenic diabetes insipidus due to chronic administration of lithium in rats. J Clin Invest 1985;75:1969–1979.
19. Chuang DM: Neurotransmitter receptors and phosphoinositide turnover. Annu Rev Pharmacol Toxicol 1989;29:71–110.
20. Clendeninn NJ, Pond SM, Kaysen G, et al: Potential pitfalls in the evaluation of the usefulness of hemodialysis for the removal of lithium. Clin Toxicol 1982;19:341–352.
21. Demers R, Lukesh R, Prichard J: Convulsions during lithium therapy. Lancet 1970;2:315–316.
22. Demers RG, Heninger G: Electrocardiographic changes during lithium therapy. Dis Nerv Syst 1970;31:674–677.
23. Emerson GH, Dyson WL, Utiger RD: Serum thyrotropin and thyroxin concentrations in patients receiving lithium carbonate. J Clin Endocrinol Metab 1973;36:338–346.
24. Feneves AZ, Emmett M, White MG: Lithium toxicity associated with acute renal failure. South Med J 1984;77:1472–1474.
25. Forrest JN, Cohen AD, Torretti J, et al: On the mechanism of lithium induced diabetes insipidus in man and the rat. J Clin Invest 1974;53:1115–1123.
26. Frazer A, Mendel J, Secunda SK, et al: The prediction of brain lithium concentration from plasma or erythrocyte measure. J Psychiatr Res 1973;10:1–7.
27. Gehrke JC, Watling SM, Gehrke CW, et al: In-vivo binding of lithium using the cation exchange resin sodium polystyrene sulfonate. Am J Med 1996;14:37–38.
28. Gitten M: Lithium and the kidney. An updated review. Drug Saf 1999;3:231–243.
29. Goddard J, Bloom SR, Frackowiak RS, et al: Lithium intoxication. BMJ 1991;302:1267–1269.
30. Goodnick PJ, Fieve RR, Meltzer HC, et al: Lithium elimination half-life and duration of therapy. Clin Pharmacol Ther 1981;29:47–50.
31. Groth U, Prellwitz W, Jahnchen E: Estimation of pharmacokinetic parameter of lithium from saliva and urine. Clin Pharmacol Ther 1974;16:490–498.
32. Hansen HE, Amdisen A: Lithium intoxication. Q J Med 1978;14:123–144.
33. Hartitzch BV, Hoenich NA, Leigh RJ, et al: Permanent neurological sequelae despite hemodialysis. Br Med J 1972;4:757–759.
34. Jaeger A, Sauder P, Kopeferschmitt J, et al: When should dialysis be performed in lithium poisoning? A kinetic study in 14 cases of lithium poisoning. J Toxicol Clin Toxicol 1993;31:429–447.
35. Jaeger A, Sauder P, Kopeferschmitt J, et al: Toxicokinetics of lithium intoxication treated by hemodialysis. J Toxicol Clin Toxicol 1985;23:501–517.
36. Jones J, Mullen MJ, Dougherty J, et al: Repetitive doses of activated charcoal in the treatment of poisoning. Am J Emerg Med 1987;5:305–311.
37. Kirchner K: Lithium as a marker for proximal tubule delivery during low salt intake and diuretic infusion. Am J Physiol 1987;253:F188–F196.
38. Kofman O, Belmaker RH: Biochemical, behavior and clinical studies of the rate of inositol in lithium treatment and depression. Biol Psychiatry 1989;34:839–852.
39. Kudrow L: Lithium prophylaxis for cluster headache. Headache 1977;17:15–18.
40. Lapierre G, Stewart RB: Lithium carbonate and leukocytosis. Am J Hosp Pharm 1980;37:1525–1528.
41. LeBlanc M, Raymond M, Bonnardeaux A, et al: Lithium poisoning treated by high-performance continuous arteriovenous and venovenous hemodiafiltration. Am J Kidney Dis 1996;27:365–372.
42. Lewis DA: Unrecognized chronic lithium neurotoxic reactions. JAMA 1983;250:2029–2030.
43. Linakis JG, Hull KM, Lacouture PG, et al: Sodium polystyrene sulfonate treatment for lithium toxicity. Effects on serum potassium concentration. Acad Emerg Med 1996;3:333–337.
44. Linakis JG, Hull KM, Lee C, et al: Effects of delayed treatment with sodium polystyrene sulfate on serum lithium concentrations in mice. Acad Emerg Med 1995;2:681–685.
45. Linakis JG, Lacouture PG, Eisenberg MS, et al: Administration of activated charcoal or sodium polystyrene sulfonate (Kayexalate) as gas-

tric decontamination for lithium intoxication: An animal model. Pharmacol Toxicol 1989;65:387–389.

46. Manji HK, Hsaio JK, Risby ED, et al: The mechanism of action of lithium: Effects on serotonergic and noradrenergic systems in normal subjects. Arch Gen Psychiatry 1991;48:505–512.

47. Manji HK, Potter WZ, Lenox RH: Signal transduction pathways. Molecular targets for lithium's action. Arch Gen Psychiatry 1995; 52:531–543.

48. Mork A, Geiser A: Mode of action of lithium on the catalytic unit of adenylate cyclase from rat brain. Pharmacol Toxicol 1981;60: 241–248.

49. Odagaki Y, Koyama R, Matsubara S, et al: Effects of chronic lithium treatment on serotonin binding sites in rat brain. J Psychiatr Res 1990;24:271–277.

50. Okusa MD, Jovita L, Crystal T: Clinical manifestations and management of acute lithium intoxication. Am J Med 1994;97:383–389.

51. Petersen V, Hvidt S, Thomsen K, et al: Effect of prolonged thiazide treatment on renal lithium clearance. Br Med J 1974;3:143–145.

52. Prakash R: A review of the hematological side effects of lithium. Hosp Commun Psychiatry 1971:36:127–128.

53. Rana RS, Hokin LE: Role of phosphoinositides in transmembrane signaling. Physiol Rev 1990;70:115–164.

54. Richman CM, Makki MM, Weiser PA, et al: Effect of lithium carbonate on chemotherapy induced neutropenia and thrombocytopenia. Am J Hematol 1984;16:313–323.

55. Riegel JM, Becker CE: Use of cathartics in toxic ingestions. Ann Emerg Med 1981;10:254–258.

56. Roberge RJ, Martin TG, Schneider SM: Use of sodium polystyrene sulfonate in a lithium overdose. Ann Emerg Med 1993;22:1911–1915.

57. Sachs GS, Renshaw PF, Lafer B, et al: Variability of brain lithium levels during maintenance treatment: A magnetic resonance spectroscopy study. Biol Psychiatry 1995;38:422–428.

58. Salta R, Klein I: Effects of lithium on the endocrine system: A review. J Lab Clin Med 198;110:130–136.

59. Sansone MEG, Ziegler DK: Lithium toxicity: A review of neurologic complications. Clin Neuropharmacol 1985;8:242–248.

60. Saul RF, Hamburger HA, Selhorst JD: Pseudotumor cerebri secondary to lithium carbonate. JAMA 1985;253:2869–2870.

61. Schou M: Long-lasting neurological sequelae after lithium intoxication. Acta Psychiatr Scand 1984;70:594–602.

62. Smith SW, Ling LJ, Halstenson C: Whole-bowel irrigation as a treatment for acute lithium overdose. Ann Emerg Med 1991;20:536–539.

63. Sproule BA, Hardy BG, Schulman KI: Differential pharmacokinetics of lithium in elderly patients. Drugs Aging 2000;16:165–177.

64. Spyker DA: Activated charcoal reborn: Progress in poison management. Arch Intern Med 1985;145:43–44.

65. Strayhorn JM, Nash JL: Severe neurotoxicity despite "therapeutic" serum lithium levels. Dis Nerv Syst 1977;38:107–111.

66. Thomsen K, Bak M, Shirley DG: Chronic lithium treatment inhibits amiloride-sensitive sodium transport in the rat distal nephron. J Pharmacol Exp Ther 1999;289:443–447.

67. Thomsen K, Schou M: Renal lithium excretion in man. Am J Physiol 1968;215:823–827.

68. Tilkian AG, Schroeder JS, Kao JJ: Cardiovascular effects of lithium in man: A review of the literature. Am J Med 1976;61:665–670.

69. Tomaszewski C, Musso C, Pearson JR, et al: Lithium absorption prevented by sodium polystyrene sulfonate in volunteers. Ann Emerg Med 1992;21:1308–1311.

70. Vacaflor L, Lehmann HE, Ban TA: Side effects and teratogenicity of lithium carbonate treatment. J Clin Pharmacol J New Drugs 1970;10: 387–389.

71. Van Bommel EF, Kalmeijer MD, Possen HH: Treatment of high lithium toxicity with high-volume continuous venovenous hemofiltration. Am J Nephrol 2000;20:408–411.

72. Vestergaard L, Amdisen A, Schou M: Clinically significant side effects of lithium treatment. A survey of 237 patients in long term treatment. Acta Psychiatric Scand 1980:62:193–200.

73. Weinstein MR, Goldfield MD: Cardiovascular malformations with lithium use during pregnancy. Am J Psychiatry 1975;132:529–531.

74. White K, Cohen J, Nelson R, et al: Relationship between plasma, RBC and CSF lithium concentrations in human subjects. Int Pharmacopsychiatry 1979;14:185–189.

75. Whitworth P, Kendall DA: Effects of lithium on inositol phospholipid hydrolysis and inhibition of dopamine D1 receptors mediated cyclic AMP formation by carbachol in rat brain slices. J Neurochem 1989; 53:536–541.

76. Wilson JH, Donker AJ, van der Helm GK, et al: Peritoneal dialysis for lithium poisoning. Br Med J 1971;2:749–750.

77. Winchester JF: Evaluation of artificial organs: Extracorporeal removal of drugs. Artif Organs 1986;10:316–323.

Morphine

Emergency Medical Services (EMS) was called to provide assistance for a comatose 23-year-old man. EMS found the patient hypoventilating (2 breaths/min), cyanotic, and with prominent miosis. Earlier the same day the patient was evaluated in another hospital for a similar condition, and after supposedly having a dramatic response to naloxone, he was discharged.

In the current Emergency Department (ED), the patient was ventilated by bag-valve mask while preparations were made to perform endotracheal intubation. Naloxone, 0.4 mg, was administered intravenously and the patient became alert with a respiratory rate of 24. At that point the patient looked uncomfortable, he developed diaphoresis, and his pupils dilated. Physical examination revealed piloerection, hyperactive bowel sounds, and bilateral pulmonary rales with a normal cardiac examination. An electrocardiogram (ECG) demonstrated sinus tachycardia, and an arterial blood gas was reported as pH, 7.38; Pco_2, 28 mm Hg; and Po_2 (on 40% Venti-mask), 140 mm Hg. A portable chest radiograph showed diffuse patchy infiltrates.

The patient received continuous low-flow oxygen therapy for 24 hours in the intensive care unit (ICU), at all times maintaining his oxygen saturation in the normal range. Over the observation period his lungs cleared, and he was discharged after an additional day of observation with a referral back to his methadone maintenance treatment program.

HISTORY AND EPIDEMIOLOGY

The medicinal value of opium, the dried extract of the poppy plant (*Papaver somniferum*) is recorded around 1500 BC in the Ebers papyrus.[140] Raw opium is typically composed of at least 10% morphine, but extensive variability exists by growing region.[109] Although reformulated as laudanum (deodorized tincture of opium; 10 mg morphine/mL) by Paracelsus, as well as paregoric (camphorated tincture of opium; 0.4 mg/mL),[127] Dover's powder (pulvis Doveri), and Godfrey's cordial in later centuries,[140] their contents remained largely the same: phenanthrene poppy derivatives, such as morphine and codeine. Over the intervening centuries since the Ebers papyrus, opium and its components have

been exploited in two distinct manners: they have been used clinically to produce profound analgesia and nonmedicinally for their psychoactive effects.

To this day, opioids find their widest clinical application in the relief of acute or chronic suffering. Opioids are available in various formulations which allow administration by virtually any route: oral, parenteral (ie, SC/IV/IM), transdermal, transmucosal, epidural, intrathecal, rectal, and intranasal, as well as inhalational. Patients may also benefit from several of the nonanalgesic effects engendered by certain opioids. For example, codeine finds widespread use as an antitussive agent and diphenoxylate as an antidiarrheal drug. Unfortunately, the history of opium and its derivatives is marred by mankind's endless quest for drugs that produce pleasurable effects. Opium smoking was so problematic in China by the 1830s that the government attempted to prohibit its importation by the British East India Company. This act led to the Opium Wars with Britain. China eventually conceded and, in addition to allowing importation and sale of the drug, was forced to turn over Hong Kong to British rule. The euphoric and addictive potential of the opioids are immortalized in the works of several famous writers, such as Thomas de Quincey (*Confessions of an English Opium Eater*, 1821), Samuel Coleridge (*The Rime of the Ancient Mariner, 1798*), and Elizabeth Barrett Browning (*Aroura Leigh*, 1856).[11]

Because of mounting concerns of addiction and toxicity in the United States, the Harrison Narcotic Act was enacted in 1914, making the nonmedicinal use of opioids illegal. Since that time, the recreational and habitual use of heroin and other opioids remains at epidemic levels in the United States and worldwide despite massive attempts to curb their availability.

Morphine was isolated from opium by Armand Séquin in 1804,[140] and Charles Alder Wright synthesized heroin from it in 1874.[225] Ironically, heroin was developed and marketed in 1898 as an antitussive agent by Bayer, the German pharmaceutical company, which legitimized its medicinal role.[224] Subsequently, various agents with opioidlike effects have been marketed, each promoted for presumed advantages over morphine. In certain cases, such as fentanyl because of its pharmacokinetic profile, this assertion was realized, but generally, particularly with reference to abuse potential, the advantages have not been realized and fall short of expectations.

The terminology used in this chapter recognizes the broad range of agents commonly considered to be opiumlike. The term *opiate* specifically refers to the relevant alkaloids that are derived directly from the opium poppy: morphine and codeine, and, to some extent, thebaine and noscapine. *Opioids* are a much broader class of agents that are capable of producing opiumlike effects or of binding to opioid receptors (detailed below). Opioids include the naturally occurring peptides such as endorphin. A *semisynthetic opioid*, such as heroin or oxycodone, may by created by the modification of an opiate. Alternatively, *synthetic opioids* are newly synthesized chemical compounds that bear little overt structural similarity to the opiates yet are capable of producing opioid effects experimentally or clinically. Methadone and meperidine are examples of synthetic opioids. The term *narcotic* refers to a sleep-inducing agent and was initially used to connote the opioids. In its current use, however, law enforcement and the public use the term to indicate any illicit psychoactive substance. Consequently, the term opioid is used hereafter to encompass the opioids and the opiates.

PHARMACOLOGY

Opioid Receptor Subtypes

Despite nearly a century of studying opioids, the existence of specific opioid receptors was not proposed until the mid-20th century.[8] Beckett and Casy, synthetic chemists, noted a pronounced stereospecificity of existing opioids (only the *l*-isomer is active), and postulated the need for the drug to "fit" into a receptor. In 1963, after the study of the clinical interactions of nalorphine and morphine, the theory of receptor dualism was proposed,[144] which postulated the existence of two classes of opioid receptors. However, it was not until 1973 that such opioid binding sites were demonstrated experimentally.[183] Intensive experimental scrutiny using selective agonists and antagonists continues to permit refinement of receptor classification. The current, widely accepted schema postulates the coexistence of three major classes of opioid receptors, each with multiple subtypes, as well as several poorly defined minor classes.

Initially, it was unclear why such an elaborate system of receptors existed, because no endogenous ligand could be identified. However, evidence for the existence of just such endogenous ligands was uncovered in 1975 with the discovery of met- and leu-enkephalins,[99] and the subsequent identification of β-endorphin and dynorphin. As a group, these endogenous ligands for the opioid receptors are called endorphins (*endo*genous mor*phine*). Each is a 5-amino acid peptide, cleaved from a larger precursor peptide: proenkephalin, proopiomelanocortin, and prodynorphin, respectively.

All three major opioid receptors have been cloned and sequenced.[24] Each consists of seven transmembrane segments, along with an amino and a carboxy terminus. Significant sequence homology exists between the transmembrane regions of opioid receptors, and those of other members of the G-protein-binding receptor superfamily. However, the extracellular and intracellular segments differ from one another. These nonhomologous segments probably represent the ligand binding and signal transduction regions, respectively, which would be expected to differ

among the three classes of receptors. The individual receptors have distinct distribution patterns within the central nervous system and peripherally, and as described below, mediate unique, but not entirely understood, clinical effects. Until recently, researchers have used varying combinations of agonists and antagonists to pharmacologically distinguish the different receptor subtypes. However, molecular cloning technology, in which mutant mice lacking the genes for an individual opioid receptor ("knockout mice") are bred, promises new insights into this complex subject.

Because there are multiple opioid receptors and each elicits a different effect, determining which receptor an opioid agent binds to preferentially should allow prediction of a drug's clinical effects. However, the binding of a drug typically is not limited to one receptor type, and it is the relative affinity of a drug for differing receptors that accounts for its clinical effects (Table 62–1). Even the endogenous opioid peptides exhibit substantial crossover among the receptors.

Although the familiar pharmacologic nomenclature derived from the Greek alphabet is used throughout this textbook, the International Union of Pharmacology (IUPHAR) Committee on Receptor Nomenclature has recommended a nomenclature change to make opioid receptor names more consistent with those of other neurotransmitter systems.[51] In this new schema, the receptors are denoted by their endogenous ligand (opiates *p*eptides) with a subscript identifying their chronologic order of discovery. The δ receptor is therefore renamed as OP_1, κ is renamed as OP_2, and μ is renamed as OP_3. Interestingly, the IUPHAR has not incorporated subtype nomenclature into their scheme, but recommends using a subscripted letter for such distinctions (eg, OP_{3A} for μ_1).

TABLE 62–1. Clinical Effects Related to Opioid Receptors

Conventional Name	IUPHAR Name*	Important Clinical Effects of Receptor Agonists
μ_1	OP_{3a}	Supraspinal analgesia Peripheral analgesia Sedation Euphoria Prolactin release
μ_2	OP_{3b}	Spinal analgesia Respiratory depression Physical dependence Gastrointestinal dysmotility Pruritis Bradycardia Growth hormone release
κ_1	OP_{2a}	Spinal analgesia Miosis Diuresis
κ_2	OP_{2b}	Psychotomimesis Dysphoria
κ_3	OP_{2c}	Supraspinal analgesia
δ	OP_1	Spinal and supraspinal analgesia Modulation of μ-receptor function Inhibit release of dopamine

*International Union of Pharmacology, Committee on Receptor Nomenclature with recommended subtype additions.

Mu Receptor (μ or OP₃).   The early identification of the μ receptor as the *morphine binding site* gave this receptor its designation.[143] Although many exogenous agents produce supraspinal analgesia via μ receptors, an endogenous ligand has remained elusive. Although the likely candidate is β endorphin, the discovery of morphine and other morphinans in mammalian brain[55] raises the possibility of a role for these nonpeptide opioids. Although it is unclear whether the mammalian morphine is a dietary component[86] or is truly endogenous, a tentative biosynthetic pathway in the rat liver is described.[260] Additionally, and equally unexplainable, opioid peptides, such as morphicetin and casomorphin, may be found in cow's milk.[14]

Experimentally, there are two well-defined subtypes (μ₁ and μ₂), although there are currently no agents with sufficient selectivity to make this dichotomy clinically relevant. Experiments with knockout mice suggest that both subtypes derive from the same gene and that either posttranslational changes or local cellular effects subsequently differentiate them.[115] It is the μ₁ subtype that appears to be responsible for supraspinal (brain) analgesia, as well as for the pleasurable euphoria sometimes engendered by these agents. Although stimulation at the μ₂ subtype produces spinal-level analgesia, it also produces respiratory depression. All currently available μ agonists have some activity at the μ₂ receptor, and therefore produce some degree of respiratory compromise. It is not unexpected that μ receptors are localized to the regions of the brain involved in analgesia (periaqueductal gray, nucleus raphe magnus, medial thalamus[75]), euphoria and reward (mesolimbic system), and respiratory function (medulla).[157] Predictably, μ receptors are found in the medullary cough center, peripherally in the gastrointestinal tract, and on various sensory nerve endings including the articular surfaces (see the discussion of analgesia under "Clinical Manifestations" below).

Kappa Receptor (κ or OP₂).   Although it is now known that dynorphins are the endogenous ligands for κ receptors, these receptors were originally identified by their ability to bind ketocyclazocine; thus, the label κ.[143] Kappa receptors exist predominantly in the spinal cord of higher animals, although they are also found both in the antinociceptive regions of the brain[154] and in the substantia nigra.[262] Stimulation is responsible for spinal analgesia, miosis, and diuresis (via inhibition of antidiuretic hormone (ADH) release). Unlike μ, however, κ-receptor stimulation is not associated with significant respiratory depression or constipation. The κ receptor is currently subclassified into three subtypes. The κ₁ receptor subtype is responsible for spinal analgesia;[188] this analgesia is not reversed by μ selective antagonists,[154] supporting the role of κ receptors as independent mediators of analgesia. Although the function of the κ₂ receptor is largely unknown, stimulation of cerebral κ₂ receptors by agents such as pentazocine produces psychotomimesis in distinction to the euphoria evoked by μ agonists.[185] The κ₃ receptor is found throughout the brain and appears to participate in supraspinal analgesia. This receptor is primarily responsible for the action of nalorphine, an agonist-antagonist opioid.[181] Nalbuphine, another agonist-antagonist, exerts its analgesic effect via both κ₁ and κ₃ agonism, although both drugs are antagonists to morphine at the μ receptor.[187]

Delta Receptor (δ or OP₁).   Little is known about δ receptors, although the enkephalins are their endogenous ligands. Opioid peptides identified in the skin and brain of *Phyllomedusa* frogs,

termed dermorphin and deltorphin, respectively, are potent agonists at the δ receptor.[125] Delta receptors may be important in spinal and supraspinal analgesia, probably via a noncompetitive interaction with the μ receptor.[205,243] Delta receptors may also mediate dopamine release from the nigrostriatal pathway, where they modulate the motor activity associated with amphetamine.[104] Delta receptors do not modulate dopamine in the mesolimbic tracts and have little behavioral reinforcing role. Subpopulations, specifically δ₁ and δ₂, have been postulated based on in vitro studies, but are not presently confirmed in vivo.[243]

Nociceptin/Orphanin FQ Receptor (ORL₁ or OP₄).   The ORL₁ receptor was identified in 1994, based on sequence homology during screening for opioid receptor genes with DNA libraries.[19] It has a similar distribution pattern in the brain and uses similar transduction mechanisms as the other opioid receptor subtypes, and it binds many different opioid agonists and antagonists. However, its insensitivity to antagonism by naloxone, often considered the sine qua non of opioid character, delayed its acceptance as a valid opioid receptor subtype. Simultaneous identification of an endogenous ligand, called nociceptin by the French discoverers and orphanin FQ by the Swiss, allowed the designation OP₄.[19] A clinical role has yet to be defined, but anxiolytic and analgesic properties are described.[19]

Sigma Receptor (σ).   Although originally conceived as an opioid subtype,[143] the σ receptor is no longer considered to be opioid in character, and has not been given an IUPHAR OP designation. Investigation of this receptor revealed that it is insensitive to antagonism by naloxone, prefers ligands with a dextrorotatory stereochemistry, and has no endogenous ligand, all in contradistinction to the other opioid receptors. The effects of the σ receptor are nonetheless relevant to opioid pharmacology because certain opioids, such as dextromethorphan and pentazocine, are σ-receptor agonists. σ-Receptor stimulation is implicated in psychotomimesis and movement disorders, effects that are reported with both dextromethorphan and pentazocine independently.[161] Antipsychotic agents, such as haloperidol, are σ-receptor antagonists, which effect may account for at least part of their antipsychotic effects.[46,47]

Other Receptors (Epsilon (ε), Zeta (ζ)).   The current scheme of opioid receptors, although clinically useful, has some pharmacologic shortcomings. Two other opioid receptor subtypes, although largely uncharacterized in humans, may ultimately prove to be important. The ε receptor is postulated on the basis of in vivo binding assays and has no known clinical role.[167] The ζ receptor has been proposed, and may serve as an opioid growth factor receptor.[274]

Opioid Receptor Signal Transduction Mechanisms

Figure 62–1 illustrates opioid receptor signal transduction mechanisms. Continuing research into the mechanisms by which an opioid receptor induces an effect on the receptor-bearing cell has produced confusing, and often contradictory, results. Despite the initial theory that each receptor subtype was linked to a specific transduction mechanism, individual receptor subtypes may use one or more mechanisms, depending on several factors, including receptor localization (eg, presynaptic vs postsynaptic). As noted, all opioid receptor subtypes are members of a superfamily of membrane-bound receptors, which are coupled to GTP binding

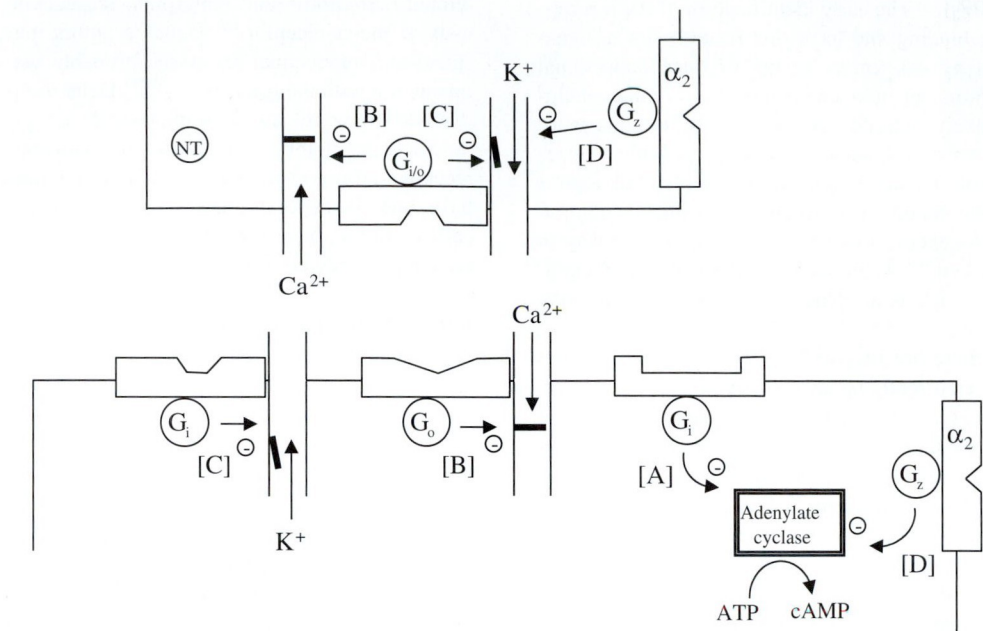

Figure 62–1. Opioid receptor signal transduction mechanisms. Upon binding of an opioid agonist to an opioid receptor, the respective G protein is activated. G proteins may (**A**) reduce the capacity of adenylate cyclase to produce cAMP; (**B**) close Ca^{2+} ion channels that reduce the signal to release neurotransmitters; (**C**) open K^+ channels and hyperpolarize the cell, which indirectly reduces cell activity. Each mechanism has been found coupled to each receptor subtype depending on location of the receptor (pre/postsynaptic) as well as of the neuron within the brain (see text). Note that α_2 receptors (**D**) mediate similar effects, using a different G protein (G_z). NT=neurotransmitter.

Adenylate cyclase/cAMP (A)

Inhibition of adenylate cyclase activity by G_i or G_o is the classic mechanism for postsynaptic signal transduction invoked by the inhibitory μ receptors.[245] However, this same mechanism has also been identified in cells bearing either δ or κ receptors.[27,269] Activation of cAMP production by adenylate cyclase, with subsequent activation of protein kinase A, occurs following exposure to very-low-dose opioid agonists and produces excitatory, antianalgesic effects.[37]

Calcium channels (B)

Presynaptic μ receptors inhibit norepinephrine release from the nerve terminals of cells of the rat cerebral cortex. Adenylate cyclase does not appear to be the modulator for these receptors because the inhibition of norepinephrine release is not enhanced by raising intracellular cAMP levels by various methods.[212] Opioid-induced blockade is, however, prevented by increased intracellular calcium levels that are induced either by calcium ionophores, which increase membrane permeability to calcium, or by raising the extracellular calcium concentration.[212] This implies a role for opioid-induced closure of N-type calcium channels, presumably via a G_o protein.[90] Reduced intraterminal concentrations of calcium prevent the neurotransmitter-laden vesicles from binding to the terminal membrane and releasing their contents. Nerve terminals containing dopamine appear to have an analogous relationship with inhibitory κ receptors, as do acetylcholine-bearing neurons with δ opioid receptors.[212]

Potassium channels (C)

Increased conductance through a potassium channel, generally mediated by G_i or G_o, results in membrane hyperpolarization with reduced neuronal excitability.[79,169] Alternatively, protein kinase A–mediated reduction in membrane potassium conductance enhances neuronal excitability.[37]

proteins, or G proteins.[157] The G protein is responsible for signaling the cell that the receptor has been activated and for the initiation of the desired cellular effects. The G proteins are generally of the pertussis-toxin-sensitive, inhibitory subtype known as G_i or G_o, although coupling to a cholera-toxin-sensitive, excitatory G_s subtype was recently described.[37] Regardless of subsequent effect, the G proteins consist of three conjoined subunits, α, β, and γ, from which the βγ subunit is liberated upon the binding of GTP to the α subunit. Upon dissociation from the βγ subunit, the α subunit modifies specific effector systems, such as phospholipase C or adenylate cyclase, or it may directly affect a channel or transport protein. The GTP is subsequently hydrolyzed by a GTPase intrinsic to the α subunit, which prompts its reassociation with the βγ subunit and termination of the receptor-mediated effect.[204]

CLINICAL MANIFESTATIONS

Table 62–2 outlines the clinical effects of opioids.

Therapeutic Effects

Analgesia. Although classical teaching attributes opioid analgesia solely to the brain, opioids actually appear to modulate cerebral cortical pain perception at supraspinal, spinal, and peripheral levels. The regional distribution of the opioid receptors confirms that μ receptors are responsible for most of the analgesic effects of morphine within the brain. They are found in highest concentration within areas of the brain classically associated with analgesia—the periaqueductal gray, nucleus raphe magnus, locus

TABLE 62–2. **Clinical Effects of Opioids**

Cardiovascular	Peripheral vasodilation
	Orthostatic hypotension
Dermatologic	Flushing (histamine)
	Pruritis
Endocrinologic	Reduced ADH release
	Reduced gonadotrophin release
Gastrointestinal	Reduced motility
	Reduced gastric acid secretion
	Increased biliary tract pressure
	Increased anal sphincter tone
Neurologic	Sedation, coma
	Seizures (meperidine, propoxyphene)
	Antitussive
Ophthalmic	Miosis
Pulmonary	Respiratory depression
	Bronchospasm (histamine)
	Pulmonary edema

ceruleus, and medial thalamus.[180] Microelectrode-induced electrical stimulation of these areas,[199] or iontophoretic application of agonists into these regions, results in profound analgesia.[12] Specifically, enhancement of inhibitory outflow from these supraspinal areas to the sensory nuclei of the spinal cord (dorsal roots) dampens nociceptive neurotransmission. Additionally, inactivation of the μ-opioid receptor gene in embryonic mouse cells results in offspring that are insensitive to morphine analgesia.[145] These mice maintain normal concentrations of other opioid receptor subtypes, which are able to bind ligands.

Interestingly, blockade of the N-methyl-D-aspartate (NMDA) receptor, a mediator of excitatory neurotransmission, enhances the analgesic effects of μ opioid agonists and may reduce the development of tolerance (see "Dextromethorphan" later in this chapter).[194] Even more intriguing is the finding that low-dose naloxone (0.25 μg/kg/h) actually improves the efficacy of morphine analgesia.[67] Administration of higher-dose, but still low-dose, naloxone (1 μg/kg/h) obliterated its opioid-sparing effect. Although undefined, the mechanism may relate to selective inhibition of G_s-coupled excitatory opioid receptors by extremely low concentrations of opioid receptor antagonist.[38]

Delta and κ receptors are responsible for mediation of analgesia as well, but they exert their analgesic effect predominantly in the spinal cord. Conceptually, these receptors modulate nociceptive impulses in transit to the thalamus via the spinothalamic tract to reduce the brain's perception of the pain. Agents with strong binding affinity for δ receptors in humans produce significantly more analgesia than morphine when both are individually administered intrathecally.[158] Indeed, the utility of spinal and epidural opioid analgesia is predicated on the direct administration of opioid near the κ and δ receptors in the spinal cord. Agonist-antagonist agents, with agonist affinity for the κ receptor and antagonist effects at the μ receptor, maintain analgesic efficacy.

Interestingly, communication between the immune system and the peripheral sensory nerves occurs in areas of tissue inflammation. In response to inflammatory mediators (eg, interleukin-1[210]), immune cells locally release opioid peptides, which bind and activate peripheral opioid receptors on sensory nerve terminals. Agonism at these receptors reduces afferent pain neurotransmission and may inhibit the release of other proinflammatory compounds such as substance P.[228] Of note, intra-articular morphine (1 mg)

administered to patients after arthroscopic knee surgery produces significant, long-lasting analgesia that can be prevented with intra-articular naloxone.[227] The clinical analgesic effect of 5 mg of intra-articular morphine is equivalent to 5 mg of morphine given intramuscularly.[29] Intra-articular analgesia is locally mediated by μ receptors.

Despite their well-defined analgesic properties and their recommendation by many clinical practice guidelines, opioids continue to be underprescribed for patients with acute and chronic pain. Reluctance often stems from the fear that patients may develop addiction or abuse. However, despite extensive investigation, this concern remains unfounded.[103,105] Furthermore, opioid analgesics are often better tolerated, safer, and less expensive than the alternatives.

Euphoria. The pleasurable effects of many of the drugs abused by humans appear to be mediated by the release of dopamine in the mesolimbic system.[9,52] This final common pathway is shared by all opioids that activate the μ/δ receptor complex in the ventral tegmental area, which, in turn, indirectly promotes the release of dopamine in the mesolimbic region.[163] Opioids may also have a direct reinforcing effect on their self-administration through μ receptors within the mesolimbic system.[89]

The sense of well-being and euphoria associated with strenuous exercise appears to be mediated by endogenous opioid peptides and μ receptors. This so-called "runners' high" is acutely reversible with naloxone,[44] and naloxone may also produce dysphoria in nonexercising, highly trained athletes. Even in normal individuals, high-dose naloxone (up to 4 mg/kg) may produce dysphoric symptoms.[32]

Exogenous opioids do not induce uniform psychological effects. Some, particularly the highly lipophilic agents such as heroin, result in euphoria and a sense of well-being, whereas morphine is largely devoid of such pleasurable effects.[221] Morphine, however, is analgesic, anxiolytic, and sedating. Because heroin has little affinity for opioid receptors and must be deacetylated to morphine for effect, it is likely that these seemingly incompatible properties relate to pharmacokinetic differences in blood-brain barrier penetration. Fentanyl produces effects that are noted to be subjectively similar to heroin by chronic users.[122] These pleasurable effects are suggested by the ascent of fentanyl abuse among anesthesiologists studied in the 1970s.[254] In distinction, certain opioids, such as pentazocine, produce dysphoria, an effect, as noted earlier, that relates to their affinity for κ or σ receptors.[185]

Antitussive. Codeine and dextromethorphan are two opioid agents with cough-suppressant activity. However, it is unlikely that cough suppression is mediated via the $μ_1$ opioid receptor because the ability of other opioids to suppress the medullary cough centers is not correlated with their analgesic effect. Various models suggest the possible involvement of the $μ_2$ or κ opioid receptor, the 5-HT_{1A} serotonin receptor, or perhaps the σ or NMDA receptors.[110]

Toxic Effects

When used correctly for medical purposes, opioids are remarkably safe and effective agents.[7,131] However, excessive dosing for any reason may result in serious toxicity. Most adverse or toxic effects are predictable based on the "opioid" pharmacodynamics (eg, respiratory depression), although several agents produce unexpected "nonopioid" or agent-specific responses. These drugs and effects are specifically addressed below. Determining that a patient is suffering from opioid toxicity is generally more important than identifying the specific agent involved. Notwithstanding some minor variations, patients poisoned by all available opioids predictably develop a constellation of signs known as the opioid toxidrome (Chap. 17); mental status depression, hypoventilation, miosis, and reduced bowel motility are the classical elements.

Respiratory Depression. Experimentally, using various opioid agonists and antagonists, μ_2 receptors are consistently implicated in the respiratory depressant effects of morphine.[132] Through these receptors, opioid agonists reduce ventilation by diminishing the sensitivity of the medullary chemoreceptors to hypercapnea.[257] In addition to the loss of hypercarbic stimulation, opioids also depress the ventilatory response to hypoxia.[257] The combined loss of hypercarbic and hypoxic drive leaves virtually no stimulus to breathe and apnea follows. Among the available opioid agonists, equianalgesic doses of all agents produce approximately the same degree of respiratory depression.[57,218] Patients chronically exposed to opioid agonists, such as those on methadone maintenance, experience chronic hypoventilation, although tolerance to the loss of hypercarbic drive may develop over several months.[141] However, such patients never develop complete tolerance to the loss of hypoxic stimulation.[209] Although some opioids, notably the agonist-antagonists, demonstrate a ceiling effect on respiratory depression, such sparing is generally at the expense of analgesic potency.[66] The different profiles of activity are likely a result of differential activities at the opioid receptor subtypes; that is, agonist-antagonists are predominantly κ-receptor agonists, and either partial agonists or antagonists at μ sites.

It is important to recognize that ventilatory depression may be secondary to either a reduction in respiratory rate or in tidal volume. Thus, although more accessible for clinical measurement, the respiratory rate is not an ideal index of ventilatory depression. In fact, in humans morphine-induced respiratory depression initially relates more closely with changes in tidal volume.[218] Escalating doses of opioids result in a reduction of respiratory rate as well.

Pulmonary Edema. Reports linking opioids with the development of pulmonary edema began to accumulate in the 1960s, although the first report was made by William Osler in 1880.[176] Virtually all opioids are implicated, and opioid-related pulmonary edema is reported in diverse clinical situations. Pulmonary edema may be an isolated finding or may occur in the setting of multisystem organ damage. Typically, the patient awakens from opioid coma, either spontaneously or following an opioid antagonist, and over the subsequent several minutes to hours develops hypoxemia and pulmonary rales. Occasionally, classic frothy, pink sputum is present in the patient's airway, or in the endotracheal tube of an intubated patient. Pulmonary edema was described in 71 out of 149 (48%) of 149 hospitalized heroin overdose patients in New York City,[56] and the outcome is generally dependent on comorbid conditions and delay to care.

No single mechanism can be consistently invoked in the genesis of opioid-associated pulmonary edema, and several prominent theories are each well supported by experimental data. Although several authors ascribe pulmonary edema to the administration of naloxone, the majority of affected patients had already suffered respiratory arrest and these patients were given naloxone to reestablish spontaneous breathing. In these patients it is likely that naloxone merely "uncovered" the clinical findings of acute lung injury that were not evident because of the inability to perform an adequate examination. Other evidentiary cases involve surgical patients given naloxone postoperatively who subsequently awoke with pulmonary edema. In addition to presumably receiving the naloxone for ventilatory compromise or hypoxia, these patients also received multiple intraoperative medications, further obscuring the etiology.[195,238] However, although naloxone is ordinarily safe when administered to nonopioid-tolerant individuals, the production of acute opioid withdrawal may be responsible for "naloxone-induced" pulmonary edema. In this situation, as in patients with "neurogenic" pulmonary edema, massive sympathetic discharge from the central nervous system occurs and produces pulmonary edema from the acute effects of catecholamines on the myocardium. Indeed, in an interesting series of experiments, precipitated opioid withdrawal in nontolerant dogs was associated with dramatic cardiovascular changes and abrupt elevation of serum catecholamine levels.[155,156] The effect was more dramatic in dogs with an elevated P_{CO_2} than in those with a normal or low P_{CO_2}, suggesting the need to adequately ventilate patients prior to reversal with naloxone.

However, even though abrupt precipitation of withdrawal by naloxone may contribute to the development of pulmonary edema, it cannot be the sole effect. Pulmonary edema was noted in 50–90% of the postmortem examinations performed on heroin overdose patients,[88,93] many of whom were declared dead before arrival to medical care and thus never received naloxone. In addition, neither naloxone nor any other opioid antagonist was available when Osler and others described their initial cases of pulmonary edema. Alternatively, the negative intrathoracic pressure generated by attempted inspiration against a closed glottis creates a large pressure gradient across the alveolar membrane and draws fluid into the alveolar space.[118] This mechanical effect, also known as the Müller maneuver, was invoked as the etiology of ventilator-associated pulmonary edema prior to the advent of demand ventilators and neuromuscular blockers. In the setting of opioid poisoning, glottic laxity may prevent adequate air entry during inspiration. This effect may be especially prominent at the time of naloxone administration, in which case breathing may be reinstituted before the return of adequate upper airway function.

Cardiovascular. Arteriolar and venous dilation secondary to opioid use may result in mild reduction in blood pressure.[255] This effect is clinically useful for the treatment of acute pulmonary edema. However, while patients do not typically develop significant supine hypotension, orthostatic changes in blood pressure and pulse routinely occur.[276] Bradycardia is unusual, although a reduction in heart rate is common as a result of the associated reduction in central nervous system stimulation. Opioid-induced hypotension appears to be mediated by histamine release,[63] although induction of histamine release does not appear to occur through interaction with an opioid receptor. It may be related to the nonspecific ability of certain compounds to activate mast cell G proteins,[6] which induce degranulation of histamine-containing vesicles. Many agents share this ability, which seems to be conferred by the presence of a positive charge on a hydrophobic molecule.[6] Accordingly, not all opioids are equivalent in their ability to release histamine.[6] After administration of one of four different opioids to 60 healthy patients, meperidine was noted to produce the most, and fentanyl the least, hypotension and elevation of plasma histamine levels.[65] The combination of H_1 and H_2 antagonists is effective in ameliorating the hemodynamic effects of opioids in humans.[186] Notwithstanding claims of efficacy, a beneficial role for naloxone may only occur with extremely high doses.

Prominent cardiovascular toxicity may occur with the use of propoxyphene, which causes wide-complex dysrhythmias and negative contractility through sodium channel antagonism similar to that of type IA antidysrhythmic agents (see "Propoxyphene" later in this chapter). Adulterants or coingestants may also produce significant cardiovascular toxicity. For example, quinine-adulterated heroin is associated with dysrhythmias;[137,217] cocaine, surreptitiously added to heroin, may cause significant myocardial ischemia or infarction.[97] Similarly, concern that naloxone administration may "unmask" cocaine toxicity in patients simultaneously using cocaine and heroin ("speedball") is probably warranted, although rarely reliably reported.[152]

Miosis. The mechanism by which opioids induce miosis remains controversial and support for each of several mechanisms may be found in the literature. Stimulation of parasympathetic pupilloconstrictor neurons in the Edinger-Westphal nucleus of the oculomotor nerve by morphine produces miosis. Additionally, morphine increases firing of pupilloconstrictor neurons to light,[126] which increases the sensitivity of the light reflex (central reinforcement of light reflex).[259] Although sectioning of the optic nerve may blunt morphine-induced miosis, the consensual reflex in the denervated eye is enhanced by morphine.[148] Because opioids classically mediate inhibitory neurotransmission, hyperpolarization of sympathetic nerves, or hyperpolarization of inhibitory neurons to the parasympathetic neurons (removal of inhibition), may ultimately be found to mediate the classic "pinpoint pupil" associated with opioid use.

Not all opioid-using patients present with miosis. Patients receiving meperidine[69] and propoxyphene regularly maintain normal pupillary size. Those using agents with predominantly κ-agonist effects (eg, pentazocine) may not develop miosis. Mydriasis may occur in severely poisoned patients secondary to hypoxic/anoxic brain insult. Additionally, concomitant drug use or the presence of adulterants may alter pupillary findings. For example, the combination of heroin and cocaine ("speedball") may produce virtually any size pupil, depending on the relative contribution by each drug. Similarly, patients ingesting Lomotil, or those patients using scopolamine-adulterated heroin,[182] routinely develop large, "anticholinergic" pupils.

Seizures. Seizures are a rare complication of the therapeutic use of most opioids. In patients with acute opioid overdose, they are most likely to be caused by hypoxia. However, experimental models in which morphine is microinjected into various brain regions of animals demonstrate a proconvulsant effect.[175] This effect is not inhibited by naloxone, suggesting that a mechanism other than opioid receptor binding is involved. In humans, morphine-induced seizures are only reported in neonates and may be related to incomplete formation of their blood-brain barrier.[119]

However, seizures should be anticipated in patients with meperidine, propoxyphene, or tramadol toxicity. These agents are discussed below. Naloxone antagonizes the convulsant effects of propoxyphene in mice, although it is not nearly as effective in preventing seizures from meperidine or its metabolite normeperidine.[70] Interestingly, naloxone potentiates the anticonvulsant effects of benzodiazepines and barbiturates, although in a single study it antagonized the effects of phenytoin.[101] The ability of fentanyl to induce seizures remains controversial. After several

reported cases of fentanyl-induced seizures,[198] electroencephalograms (EEGs) and electromyelograms (EMGs) were performed on 127 patients undergoing fentanyl anesthesia.[223] When assessed clinically and with EMG studies about one-third were considered to have seized. However, in no case did the corresponding EEG reveal epileptiform activity. It appears likely that the rigidity and myoclonus associated with fentanyl are readily misinterpreted as a seizure.

Movement Disorders. With rapid intravenous injection of certain high-potency opioids, especially fentanyl, patients may experience acute muscular rigidity. This rigidity primarily involves the trunk, and may impair chest wall movement and exacerbate hypoventilation. Although the mechanism is currently unclear, it may be related to blockade of dopamine receptors in the basal ganglia.[60] Indeed dopamine,[253] but not amantadine,[249] alleviates the rigidity. Additional experimental data suggest that the α_2-adrenergic receptor is also involved.[258] Chest wall rigidity is common in patients undergoing operative anesthesia and may necessitate administration of neuromuscular blocking agents to allow mechanical ventilation. Similar effects contribute to lethality during epidemics of fentanyl-adulterated heroin.[120] Opioid antagonists are generally therapeutic,[162] but may produce adverse hemodynamic effects, withdrawal phenomenon, or uncontrollable pain depending on the situation.

Interestingly, rapid escalation of methadone doses may produce choreoathetoid movements as a result of enhanced striatal dopamine release.[13] This may relate to the opposing effects on GABAergic interneurons produced by μ and κ receptors. Methadone, a μ agonist, inhibits the release of γ-aminobutyric acid (GABA), an inhibitory neurotransmitter, within the striatum and mesolimbic system, the ultimate effect of which is to enhance dopamine release. This possibility is intriguing given the developing concept that many forms of addiction result from the final common pathway of enhanced mesolimbic dopamine neurotransmission.[9]

Gastrointestinal Effects. Historically, the morphine analogue apomorphine was used as a rapidly acting emetic whose clinical utility was limited by its tendency to depress the patient's level of consciousness. Emesis induced by apomorphine is mediated through agonism at dopamine-2 receptor subtypes within the chemoreceptor trigger zone of the medulla. Many opioids, morphine in particular, produce significant nausea and vomiting when used therapeutically.[22] It is not clearly established whether these effects are inhibited by naloxone, but it is likely that they are not.

Although diphenoxylate and loperamide are widely used therapeutically to manage diarrhea, opioid-induced constipation is most frequently a bothersome side effect of both the therapeutic and recreational use of opioids. Mediated by μ_2 receptors within the smooth muscle of the intestinal wall, constipation is ameliorated by oral naloxone. Provided that the hepatic glucuronidative capacity is not exceeded (at doses of approximately 6 mg), enteral naloxone is poorly bioavailable and thus induces few, if any, opioid withdrawal symptoms.[149] A recently introduced quaternary ammonium agent, methylnaltrexone, is a bioavailable opioid that antagonizes the effects of opioids on the gastrointestinal tract, yet is unable to cross the blood-brain barrier.[272] Thus, the opioid withdrawal syndrome does not occur. This agent is not yet available in this country.

DIAGNOSTIC TESTING

Laboratory Considerations

Although it is always tempting to seek laboratory confirmation of an ingested substance in acutely poisoned patients, current laboratory methodology suffers from several important limitations and confounding variables. In general, the most apparent impediment to the use of laboratory testing in the acute care setting is the lack of timely reporting of results. Patients may suffer grave consequences if therapy is withheld pending test results. Opioid-poisoned patients, in particular, are amenable to rapid clinical diagnosis because of the uniqueness of the opioid toxidrome. Additionally, the availability of several distinct classes of agents capable of producing similar opioid effects limits the utility of laboratory tests, such as immunoassays, that rely on structural features to identify drugs. Furthermore, because there are remarkable differences in test availability, and because the accuracy and sensitivity of each test differ, interpretation of the test results may be difficult. Because opioids may be chemically detectable long after their clinical effects have resolved, assay results cannot be considered in isolation, and must be viewed in a clinical context. Several well-described problems with laboratory testing of opioids are described below and in Chapter 7.

Cross-Reactivity. Many opioids share remarkable structural similarities. Interestingly, structurally similar agents, such as methadone and propoxyphene, do not necessarily share the same clinical characteristics (Fig. 62–2). Because most assays depend on structural features to identify a drug, structurally similar agents may be detected in lieu of the desired drug. Whether a similar drug is noted by the assay depends on the sensitivity and specificity of the assay used, as well as the serum concentration of the agent. Some cross-reactivities are predictable, such as that of codeine with morphine on a variety of screening tests.[34] Other cross-reactivities are less predictable, as with the cross-reaction of dex-

tromethorphan and the phencyclidine (PCP) component of the fluorescence polarization immunoassay (Abbott TDx),[151,256] a widely used drug-of-abuse screening test (Chap. 7).

Congeners and Adulterants. Commercial opioid assays, which are specific for morphine, are unlikely to detect most of the semisynthetic and synthetic opioids. In some cases, epidemic fatalities involving fentanyl derivatives remained unexplained despite what appeared to be obvious opioid toxicity, until the ultrapotent fentanyl derivative, α-methylfentanyl, was specifically sought and identified by more sophisticated testing.[120] Oxycodone, hydrocodone, and other common morphine derivatives have variable detectability by different opioid screens.[223] Adulterants, such as scopolamine or quinine, are not detectable on an opioid screen.

Drug Metabolism. A fascinating dilemma may arise in patients who ingest moderate to large amounts of poppy seeds.[61,116] These seeds, which are widely used for culinary purposes, are derived from poppy plants similar to *P. somniferum*, and contain both morphine and codeine. Patients may develop dramatically elevated serum morphine and codeine concentrations,[61,214] and test positive for morphine. Because the presence of morphine on a drugs-of-abuse screen may suggest illicit heroin use, the implications are substantial. Federal workplace testing regulations thus require corroboration of a positive morphine assay with assessment of another heroin metabolite, 6-monoacetylmorphine, prior to reporting a positive result.[159] Humans cannot acetylate morphine and therefore cannot synthesize monoacetylmorphine, but readily deacetylate heroin, which is diacetylmorphine.

A similar problem may occur in patients taking therapeutic doses of codeine. Because codeine is demethylated to morphine, a morphine screen may be positive independently of the structural cross-reactivity described earlier. Thus, determination of the serum codeine or monoacetylmorphine level is necessary in these patients. Determination of the serum codeine is not foolproof,

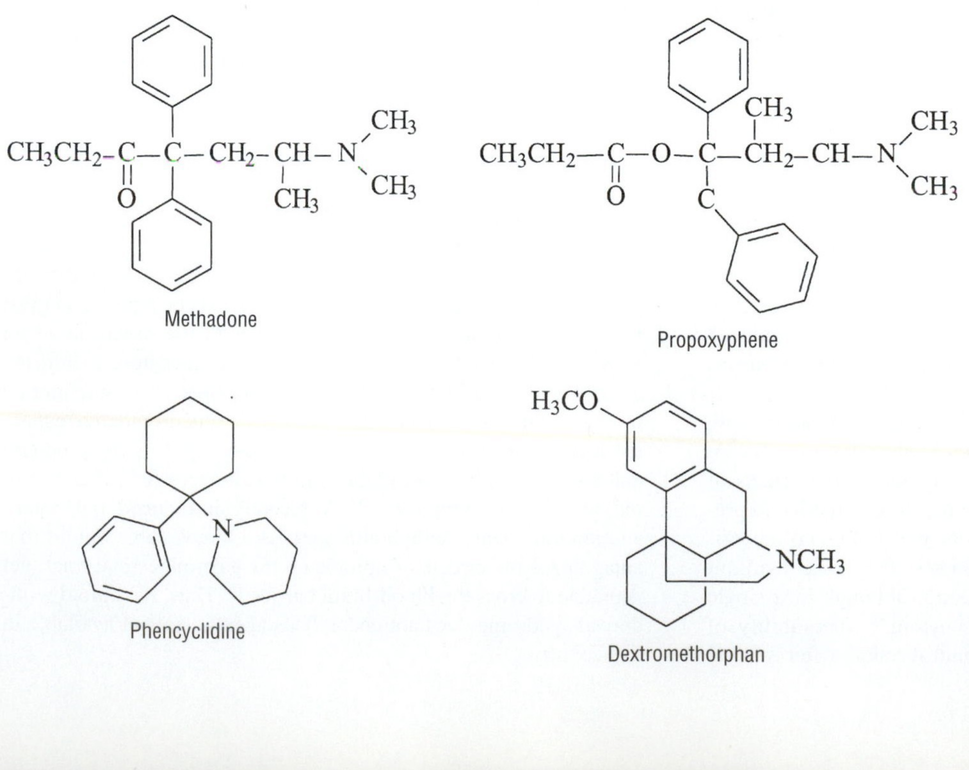

Methadone

Propoxyphene

Phencyclidine

Dextromethorphan

Figure 62–2. Structural similarity between methadone and propoxyphene and between phencyclidine and dextromethorphan.

however, because codeine is present in the opium preparation used to synthesize heroin.

MANAGEMENT

The consequential effects of acute opioid poisoning are central nervous system and respiratory depression. Although early support of ventilation and oxygenation is generally sufficient to prevent death, prolonged use of bag-valve mask ventilation and endotracheal intubation may be avoided by cautious administration of an opioid antagonist. Opioid antagonists, such as naloxone, competitively inhibit the binding of opioid agonists to the opioid receptors, allowing the patient to resume spontaneous respiration. Naloxone competes at all receptor subtypes, although not equally, and is effective at reversing almost all adverse effects mediated through opioid receptors. "Antidotes in Depth: Opioid Antagonists" has a complete discussion of naloxone and other opioid antagonists.

However, because most clinical findings associated with opioid poisoning are nonspecific, the diagnosis requires clinical acumen. Differentiating acute opioid poisoning from other etiologies with similar clinical presentations may be challenging. Patients manifesting the opioid toxidrome, those found in an appropriate environment, or those with characteristic physical clues such as fresh needle marks require little corroborating evidence. However, subtle presentations of opioid poisoning may be encountered and other entities superficially resembling opioid poisoning may occur. Hypoglycemia, hypoxia, and hypothermia are common, readily treatable clinical presentations that share features with opioid poisoning. Each may be rapidly diagnosed with routinely available, real-time testing. Other drugs responsible for similar clinical presentations include clonidine, PCP, phenothiazines, and sedative-hypnotic agents, primarily benzodiazepines. In such patients, however, clinical evidence is usually available to assist in diagnosis. For example, nystagmus is nearly always noted in PCP-intoxicated patients, hypotension or electrocardiographic abnormalities in phenothiazine-poisoned patients, and coma with virtually normal vital signs in those patients poisoned by benzodiazepines. Most difficult to differentiate on clinical grounds may be toxicity produced by the centrally acting antihypertensive agents such as clonidine (see "Clonidine" later in this chapter and Chap. 51). Additionally, a myriad of traumatic, metabolic, and infectious etiologies must always be considered and evaluated appropriately, and may occur simultaneously.

Antidote Administration

The goal of naloxone therapy is not necessarily complete arousal; rather, the goal is reinstitution of adequate spontaneous ventilation. Because precipitation of withdrawal is potentially detrimental and often unpredictable, the lowest practical naloxone dose should be administered initially with rapid escalation as warranted by the clinical situation. Most patients respond to 0.05 mg of naloxone administered intravenously, although, because the onset may be slower than with larger doses, the requirement for ventilatory assistance may be slightly prolonged. Administration in this fashion will effectively avert endotracheal intubation and allow timely identification of patients with nonopioid causes for their clinical condition, yet diminish the precipitation of acute opioid withdrawal. Subcutaneous administration may allow for smoother

arousal than the high-dose intravenous route,[250] but is unpredictable in onset and likely prolonged in offset. This can be a considerable disadvantage if the therapeutic goal is exceeded and the withdrawal syndrome develops.

In the absence of a confirmatory history or diagnostic clinical findings, the cautious empiric administration of naloxone may be both diagnostic and therapeutic. Naloxone, even at extremely high doses, has an excellent safety profile in patients with non-opioid-related indications, such as those with spinal cord injury[15] and acute ischemic stroke. Thus, administration in an empiric fashion to most non-opioid-poisoned patients is unlikely to be harmful. However, administration of naloxone to opioid-dependent patients may result in adverse effects; obviously, precipitation of an acute withdrawal syndrome should be anticipated. The obligatory agitation, hypertension, and tachycardia, while rarely life-threatening, may produce significant distress to both the patient and the clinical staff. Additionally, emesis, a common feature of acute opioid withdrawal, may be particularly hazardous in patients who do not rapidly regain consciousness after naloxone administration. For example, patients with concomitant ethanol or sedative-hypnotic exposure, or those with head trauma, are at substantial risk for the pulmonary aspiration of their vomitus if their airway is unprotected.

Identification of patients likely to respond to naloxone would conceivably reduce the unnecessary and potentially dangerous precipitation of withdrawal in opioid-dependent patients. Routine prehospital administration of naloxone to all patients with subjectively assessed altered mental status or respiratory depression was not beneficial in 92% of patients.[270] Alternatively, although not perfectly sensitive, a respiratory rate less than or equal to 12 breaths per minute in an unconscious patient presenting via EMS best predicted a response to naloxone.[94] Interestingly, in hospitalized patients, neither respiratory rate less than 8 per minute nor coma was able to predict a response to naloxone.[262] Whether the discrepancy between the latter two studies is a result of the demographics of the patient groups or whether patients with prehospital opioid overdose present differently than those patients with therapeutic misadventures is unclear. Regardless, relying on the respiratory rate to assess the need for ventilatory support or naloxone administration is not ideal because hypoventilation secondary to hypopnea may precede that caused by bradypnea.[201,218]

The decision to discharge a patient who awakens appropriately following naloxone administration is based on practical considerations. Patients presenting with profound hypoventilation or hypoxia are at risk for the development of acute lung injury or posthypoxic encephalopathy. Thus, it seems prudent to observe these patients for at least 24 hours in a medical setting. Those patients manifesting only moderate signs of poisoning who remain normal for at least several hours following parenteral naloxone are likely safe to discharge. However, the need for pyschosocial intervention in patients with uncontrolled drug use, or following a suicide attempt, may prevent discharge from an ED.

Patients with recurrent or profound poisoning by long-acting opioids, such as methadone, or patients with large gastrointestinal burdens (eg, "body packers" or sustained-release preparations) may require continuous infusion of naloxone to ensure continued adequate ventilation (Table 62–3). An hourly infusion rate of two-thirds of the initial reversal dose of naloxone is sufficient to prevent recurrence.[73] Titration of the dose may be necessary as the clinical situation indicates. Although repetitive bolus dosing of naloxone may be effective, it is labor intensive and subject to error.

TABLE 62–3.   How to Use a Naloxone Infusion

1. If a naloxone bolus is successful, administer two-thirds of the effective bolus dose per hour by IV infusion; frequently reassess the patient's respiratory status.
2. If respiratory depression is not reversed following the bolus dose:
   Intubate the patient, as clinically indicated, or
   Administer up to 10 mg of naloxone as an intravenous bolus. If the patient does not respond, do not initiate an infusion.
3. If the patient develops withdrawal following the bolus dose:
   Allow the effects of the bolus to abate.
   If respiratory depression recurs, administer one-half of the initial bolus dose, and begin an intravenous infusion at two-thirds of the initial bolus dose per hour. Frequently reassess the patient's respiratory status.
4. If the patient develops withdrawal signs or symptoms during the infusion:
   Stop the infusion until the withdrawal symptoms abate.
   Restart the infusion at one-half the initial rate; frequently reassess the patient's respiratory status.
   Exclude withdrawal from other substances.
5. If the patient develops respiratory depression during the infusion:
   Readminister one-half of the initial bolus and repeat until reversal occurs.
   Increase the infusion by one-half the initial rate; frequently reassess the patient's respiratory status.
   Exclude continued absorption, readministration of an opioid, or other etiologies for the respiratory depression.

Despite the availability of long-acting opioid antagonists, such as naltrexone and nalmefene,[111] that theoretically may permit single-dose reversal of methadone poisoning, the attendant risk of precipitating an unrelenting withdrawal syndrome hinders their use as agents for initial opioid reversal. However, these agents may have a clinical role in the maintenance of consciousness and ventilation in opioid-poisoned patients already awakened by naloxone. Expectedly, prolonged observation and perhaps antidote readministration may be required in order to match the pharmacokinetic parameters of the two agents. Otherwise well children who ingest short-acting opioids may be given a long-acting opioid antagonist initially, because they are not expected to develop a prolonged, potentially hazardous withdrawal. However, the same caveats remain regarding the need for extended observation periods if ingestion of methadone or other long-acting opioids is suspected.

Rapid and Ultrarapid Opioid Detoxification

Although not an emergent therapy of opioid poisoning or dependence, the concept of antagonist-precipitated opioid withdrawal has been promoted extensively as a "cure" for opioid (particularly heroin and oxycodone) addiction. Rather than slow, deliberate withdrawal, or detoxification, from opioids over several weeks, antagonist-precipitated withdrawal occurs over several hours or days.[192] The purported advantage of this technique is a reduced risk of relapse to opioid use because the duration of discomfort is reduced and a more rapid transition to naltrexone maintenance can be achieved. Mechanistic explanations include withdrawal-induced catecholamine depletion, rapid normalization of receptor regulation, and enhanced endogenous opioid release,[219] but each is based largely on circumstantial evidence.

Rapid opioid detoxification (ROD) techniques are usually offered by outpatient clinics and typically consist of naloxone- or naltrexone-precipitated opioid withdrawal tempered with varying amounts of clonidine, benzodiazepines, antiemetics, or other drugs. Ultrarapid opioid detoxification (UROD) uses a similar concept but involves the use of deep sedation or general anesthesia for greater patient control and comfort. Both techniques are costly; UROD under anesthesia commonly costs upward of $5000. Whether the reduced cost of short-term hospitalization for detoxification offsets this cost remains to be proven. Although most observational studies find excellent short-term results, relapse to drug use is very common following either technique. This may suggest a need for improved aftercare or may reflect a fundamental flaw in the mechanistic rationalization of the therapy.

The reported risks of these techniques are anecdotal and remain largely undefined but are of substantial conceptual concern. In one study, 10% of all patients who received UROD returned to the same hospital's ED for opioid withdrawal symptoms.[64] Transient pulmonary edema, renal insufficiency, and thyroid hormone suppression are reported following UROD, and many patients still manifest the opioid withdrawal 48 hours after the procedure.[81,184] Furthermore, the medical license of a physician performing UROD in New Jersey was suspended by state health authorities after their investigation into six deaths related to the procedure. In addition, selection bias, the lack of randomization, control groups, or blinding, and variations in treatment protocols and endpoints hinder the external applicability of much of the available research on antagonist-precipitated opioid withdrawal.[171]

OTHER OPIOIDS

Although the vast majority of opioid-poisoned patients will follow predictable clinical courses, certain opioids taken in overdose may produce atypical manifestations. Some of these effects can be anticipated, such as fentanyl-induced muscle rigidity, whereas others cannot. Therefore, careful clinical assessment and institution of empiric therapy is usually necessary to ensure proper management (Table 62–4).

Agonist-Antagonists

The opioid agonists in common clinical use tend to have specific binding affinity toward one class of opioid receptor, usually the μ class. The agonist-antagonist agents differ in that they interact with multiple receptor types at clinically relevant doses and may have different effects at each receptor. Thus, while most opioids typically produce either agonist or antagonist effects, these agents may have agonist effects at one receptor subtype and antagonistic effects at another receptor subtype. Pentazocine, for example, may elicit a withdrawal syndrome in a μ-opioid-tolerant individual because of antagonist or partial agonist effects at the μ receptor. This effect forms the basis of the claim offered by many methadone-dependent patients that they are "allergic to Talwin." However, this same drug can induce substantial analgesia in nontolerant patients through its agonist effects at κ_1 receptors. Although the clinical effects following overdose resemble the other opioid agents, they are significantly less likely to produce severe morbidity or mortality because of a ceiling effect on respiratory depression (see "Respiratory Depression" earlier in this chapter).

TABLE 62–4.   Classification, Potency, and Characteristics of Opioid Agents

Agent (Representative trade name)	Type[a]	Derivation	Analgesic dose (mg) (via route, equivalent to 10 mg morphine SC[b])	Comments[a,c]
Buprenorphine (Buprenex)	P/AA	Semisynthetic	0.4 IM	Opioid substitution therapy
Butorphanol (Stadol)	AA	Semisynthetic	2 IM	
Codeine	Ag	Natural	120 PO	Often combined with acetaminophen
Dextromethorphan (Robitussin DM)	NEC	Semisynthetic	Nonanalgesic (10–30 PO)	Antitussive; psychotomimetic via σ/NMDA receptor
Diphenoxylate (Lomotil)	Ag	Synthetic	Nonanalgesic (2.5 PO)	Antidiarrheal agent, combined with atropine; difenoxin is potent metabolite
Fentanyl (Sublimaze)	Ag	Synthetic	0.125 IM	Very-short-acting (<1 h)
Heroin (Diamorph)	Ag	Semisynthetic	5 SC	Diacetylmorphine, used therapeutically in some countries is not available in the United States
Hydrocodone (Hycodan, Vicodin)	Ag	Semisynthetic	10 PO	
Hydromorphone (Dilaudid)	Ag	Semisynthetic	1.3 SC	
LAAM (Orlaam)	Ag	Synthetic	(Flexible oral dosing[d])	L-α-Acetylmethadol or levomethadyl acetate; 3 times per week dosing for substitution therapy; long-acting, potent metabolites
Levorphanol (Levodromoran)	Ag	Semisynthetic	2 SC/IM	
Loperamide (Imodium)	Ag	Synthetic	Nonanalgesic (2 PO)	Antidiarrheal agent
Meperidine, Pethidine (Demerol)	Ag	Synthetic	75 SC/IM	Seizures caused by metabolite accumulation
Methadone (Dolophine)	Ag	Synthetic	10 IM	Very-long-acting (24 h)
Morphine	Ag	Natural	10 SC/IM	
Nalbuphine (Nubain)	AA	Semisynthetic	10 IM	
Nalmefene (Revex)	Ant	Semisynthetic	Nonanalgesic (0.1 IM)	Long-acting antagonist (4–6 h)
Nalorphine	AA	Semisynthetic	15 IM	Historically used as an opioid antagonist[a]
Naloxone (Narcan)	Ant	Semisynthetic	Nonanalgesic (0.1–0.4 IV/IM)	Short-acting antagonist (0.5 h)
Naltrexone (Trexan)	Ant	Semisynthetic	Nonanalgesic (50 PO)	Very-long-acting antagonist (24 h)
Oxycodone (Percocet, Oxycontin)	Ag	Semisynthetic	10 PO	Often combined with acetaminophen
Oxymorphone (Numorphan)	Ag	Semisynthetic	1 SC	
Paregoric (Parapectolin)	Ag	Natural	25 mL PO	Tincture of opium (0.4 mg/mL)
Pentazocine (Talwin)	AA	Semisynthetic	50 SC	Psychotomimetic via σ/NMDA receptor
Propoxyphene (Darvon)	Ag	Synthetic	65 PO	Seizures, dysrhythmias; combined with acetaminophen
Tramadol (Ultram)	Ag	Synthetic	50–100 PO	Seizures possible with therapeutic dosing

[a]Agonist antagonists, partial agonists, and antagonists may cause withdrawal in tolerant individuals.
[b]Typical dose (mg) for agents without analgesic effects is given in parentheses.
[c]Duration of therapeutic clinical effect ~3–6 hours unless noted; likely to be exaggerated in overdose.
[d]Although approximately equipotent with methadone, LAAM is not used as an analgesic.
Ag = full agonist (μ_1, μ_2, κ); AA = agonist-antagonist (κ agonist, μ antagonist); Ant = full antagonist (μ_1, μ_2, κ antagonist); P = partial agonist (μ_1, μ_2 agonist, κ antagonist); NEC = not easily classified.

Pentazocine.   Historically, patients abusing pentazocine (Talwin) administered it with tripelennamine, a blue capsule, accounting for the appellation "T's and Blues."[45] Although this mixture has largely fallen out of favor, pentazocine abuse still occurs[23] and newer combinations, such as pentazocine with methylphenidate, are reported.[21] At high doses, psychotomimetic effects may be noted, which are likely mediated by κ_2, or perhaps σ, receptors. Because pentazocine may be readily dissolved, intravenous injection was a preferred route for its abuse until the commercial formulation was altered in 1983 to include 0.5 mg naloxone (Talwin NX).[189] When ingested, the naloxone is eliminated by first-pass hepatic metabolism. However, if injected, naloxone prevents the pleasurable effects sought by users. Interestingly, potentiation of pentazocine analgesia by low-dose naloxone has been reported, and is likely a result of effects at either the κ^{129} or μ^{67} opioid receptor.

Heroin

Chemically, heroin is 3,6-diacetylmorphine, and its synthesis is performed relatively easily from morphine and acetic anhydride. Heroin has a lower affinity for the μ receptor than does morphine, but it is rapidly metabolized to 6-monoacetylmorphine, a more potent μ agonist than morphine. Users claim that heroin has an enhanced euphorigenic effect, often described as a "rush." This is likely related to the enhanced blood-brain barrier penetration occasioned by heroin's additional organic functional groups[174] and its subsequent metabolic activation within the central nervous system.

Heroin may be obtained in two distinct chemical forms: base or salt. The hydrochloride salt form is typically a white or beige powder and was the common form of heroin available prior to the 1980s.[106] Its high water solubility allows simple intravenous ad-

175. Olinger CP, Adams HP, Brott TG, et al: High-dose intravenous naloxone for the treatment of acute ischemic stroke. Stroke 1990; 21:721–725.

176. Osler W: Oedema of left lung—Morphia poisoning. Montreal Gen Hosp Rep 1880;1:291–293.

177. Oxman GL, Kowalski S, Drapela L, et al: Heroin overdose deaths— Multnomah County, Oregon, 1993–1999. MMWR Morb Mortal Wkly Rep 2000;49:633–636.

178. Parras F, Patier JL, Ezpeleta C: Lead-contaminated heroin as a source of inorganic-lead intoxication. N Engl J Med 1987;316:755.

179. Passaro DJ, Werner SB, McGee J, et al: Wound botulism associated with black tar heroin among injecting drug users. JAMA 1998; 279:859–863.

180. Pasternak GW: Multiple morphine and enkephalin receptors and the relief of pain. JAMA 1988;259:1362–1367.

181. Paul D, Pick CG, Tive LA, Pasternak GW: Pharmacological characterization of nalorphine, a kappa₃ analgesic. J Pharmacol Exp Ther 1991;257:1–7.

182. Perrone J, Hamilton R, Nelson L, et al: Scopolamine poisoning among heroin users. MMWR Morb Mortal Wkly Rep 1996;45: 457–460.

183. Pert CB, Snyder SH: Opiate receptor: Demonstration in nervous tissue. Science 1973;179:1011–1014.

184. Pfab R, Hirtl C, Zilker T: Opiate detoxification under anesthesia: No apparent benefit but suppression of thyroid hormones and risk of pulmonary and renal failure. J Toxicol Clin Toxicol 1999;37:43–50.

185. Pfeiffer A, Brantl V, Herz A, Emrich HM: Psychotomimesis mediated by κ opiate receptors. Science 1986;233:774–776.

186. Philbin DM, Moss J, Akins CW, et al: The use of H1 and H2 histamine antagonists with morphine anesthesia: A double-blind study. Anesthesiology 1981;55:292–296.

187. Pick CG, Paul, Pasternak GW: Nalbuphine, a mixed kappa₁ and kappa₃ analgesic in mice. J Pharmacol Exp Ther 1992;262: 1044–1050.

188. Piercey MF, Lahti RA, Schroeder LA, et al: U-50,488, a pure κ receptor agonist with spinal analgesic loci in the mouse. Life Sci 1982;31:1197–1200.

189. Poklis A: Decline in the abuse of pentazocine/tripelennamine (T's and Blues) associated with the addition of naloxone to pentazocine tablets. Drug Alcohol Depend 1984;14:135–140.

190. Poyhia R, Vainio A, Kalso E: A review of oxycodone's clinical pharmacokinetics and pharmacodynamics. J Pain Symptom Manage 1993;8:63–67.

191. Predergast ML, Grella C, Perry SM, Anglin MD: Levo-alpha-acetyl-methadol (LAAM): Clinical, research, and policy issues of a new pharmacotherapy for opioid addiction. J Psychoactive Drugs 1995; 27:239–247.

192. Presslich O, Loimer N: Opiate detoxification under general anesthesia by large doses of naloxone. J Toxicol Clin Toxicol 1989;27: 263–270.

193. Preston KL, Jasinski DR, Testa M: Abuse potential and pharmacological comparison of tramadol and morphine. Drug Alcohol Depend 1991;27:7–17.

194. Price DD, Mayer DJ, Mao J, Caruso FS: NMDA-receptor antagonists and opioid receptor interactions as related to analgesia and tolerance. J Pain Symptom Manage 2000;19(Suppl):S7–S11.

195. Prough DS, Roy R, Bumgarner J, Shannon G: Acute pulmonary edema in healthy teenagers following conservative doses of intravenous naloxone. Anesthesiology 1984;60:485–486.

196. Questel F, Dugarin J, Dally S: Thallium-contaminated heroin. Ann Intern Med 1996;124:616.

197. Raffa RB, Friderichs E, Reimann W, et al: Opioid and nonopioid components independently contribute to the mechanism of action of tramadol, an "atypical" opioid analgesic. J Pharmacol Exp Ther 1992;260:275–285.

198. Rao TLK, Mummaneni N, El-Etr AA: Convulsions: An unusual response to intravenous fentanyl administration. Anesth Analg 1982; 61:1020–1021.

199. Richardson DE, Akil H: Pain reduction by electrical brain stimulation in man. J Neurosurg 1977;47:178–183.

200. Riedel F, von Stockhausen HB: Severe cerebral depression after intoxication with tramadol in a 6-month-old infant. Eur J Clin Pharmacol 1984;26:631–632.

201. Rigg JRA, Rondi P: Changes in rib cage and diaphragm contribution to ventilation after morphine. Anesthesiology 1981;55:507–514.

202. Ripamonti C, Zecca E, Bruera E: An update on the clinical use of methadone for cancer pain. Pain 1997;70:109–115.

203. Risser D, Uhl A, Stichenwirth M, et al: Quality of heroin and heroin-related deaths from 1987 to 1995 in Vienna, Austria. Addiction 2000;95:375–382.

204. Ross EM: Pharmacodynamics: mechanisms of drug action and the relationship between drug concentration and effect. In: Hardman JGJ, Limbird LE, Molinoff PB, et al, eds: Goodman and Gilman's The Pharmacologic Basis of Therapeutics, 9th ed. New York, McGraw Hill, 1996, pp. 29–42.

205. Rothman RB, Holaday JW, Porreca F: Allosteric coupling among opioid receptors: Evidence for an opioid receptor complex. In: Herz A, Akil H, Simon EJ, eds: Opioids I, Handbook of Experimental Pharmacology, Vol 104/I. Berlin, Springer-Verlag, 1993, pp. 217–237.

206. Rubens R, Verhaegen H, Brugman J, Schuermans V: Difenoxin (R15403), the active metabolite of diphenoxylate (R1132). Arzneim-Forsch Drug Res 1972;22:526–529.

207. Rumack B, Temple A: Lomotil poisoning. Pediatrics 1974;53: 495–500.

208. Ruttenber AJ, Kalter HD, Santinga P: The role of ethanol abuse in the etiology of heroin-related death. J Forensic Sci 1990;35: 891–900.

209. Santiago TV, Pugliese AC, Edelman NH: Control of breathing during methadone addiction. Am J Med 1977;62:347–354.

210. Schafer M, Carter L, Stein C. Interleukin 1β and corticotropin-releasing factor inhibit pain by releasing opioids from immune cells in inflamed tissue. Proc Natl Acad Sci U S A 1994;91:4219–4223.

211. Schneider SM, Michelson EA, Boucek CD, Ilkhanipour K: Dextromethorphan poisoning reversed by naloxone. Am J Emerg Med 1991;9:237–238.

212. Schoffelmeer ANM, Van Vliet BJ, De Vries TJD, et al: Regulation of brain neurotransmitter release and of adenylate cyclase activity by opioid receptors. Biochem Soc Trans 1992;20:449–453.

213. Seaman SR, Brettle RP, Gore SM: Mortality from overdose among injecting drug users recently released from prison: Database linkage study. BMJ 1998;316:426–428.

214. Selavka CM: Poppy seed ingestion as a contributing factor to opiate-positive urinalysis results: The Pacific perspective. J Forensic Sci 1991;36:685–696.

215. Sempere AP, Posada I, Ramo C, Cabello A: Spongiform leucoencephalopathy after inhaling heroin. Lancet 1991;338:320.

216. Shaul WL, Wandell M, Robertson WO: Dextromethorphan toxicity: Reversal by naloxone. Pediatrics 1977;59:117–118.

217. Shesser R, Jotte R, Olshaker J: The contribution of impurities to the acute morbidity of illegal drugs of abuse. Am J Emerg Med 1991;9: 336–342.

218. Shook JE, Watkins WD, Camporesi EM: Differential roles of opioid receptors in respiration, respiratory disease, and opiate-induced respiratory depression. Am Rev Respir Dis 1990;142:895–909.

219. Simon DL: Rapid opioid detoxification using opioid antagonists. J Addictive Dis 1997;16:103–121.

220. Smith DA, Leake L, Loflin JR, Yealy DM: Is admission after intravenous heroin overdose necessary? Ann Emerg Med 1992;21: 1326–1330.

221. Smith GM, Beecher HK: Subjective effects of heroin and morphine in normal subjects. J Pharmacol Exp Ther 1962;136:47–52.

222. Smith M, Hughs R, Levine B, et al: Forensic drug testing for opiates. VI. Urine testing for hydromorphone, hydrocodone, oxymorphone, and oxycodone with commercial opiate immunoassays and gas chromatography-mass spectrometry. J Anal Toxicol 1995;19:18–26.

223. Smith NT, Benthuysen JL, Bickford RG: Seizures during opioid anesthetic induction—Are they opioid-induced rigidity? Anesthesiology 1989;71:852–862.

224. Sneader W: The discovery of heroin. Lancet 1998;352:1697–1699.

225. Sovner R, Wolfe J: Interaction between dextromethorphan and monoamine oxidase inhibitor therapy with isocarboxazid. N Eng J Med 1988;319:1671.

226. Spiller HA, Gorman SE, Villalobos D, et al: Prospective multicenter evaluation of tramadol exposure. J Toxicol Clin Toxicol 1997;35: 361–364.

227. Stein C, Comisel K, Haimerl E, et al: Analgesic effect of intraarticular morphine after arthroscopic knee surgery. N Engl J Med 1991; 325:1123–1126.

228. Stein C: The control of pain in peripheral tissues by opioids. N Engl J Med 1995;332:1685–1690.

229. Steinberg GK, Bell TE, Yenari MA: Dose escalation safety and tolerance study of the N-methyl-D-aspartate antagonist dextromethorphan in neurosurgery patients. J Neurosurg 1996;84:860–866.

230. Stork CM, Redd JT, Fine K, Hoffman RS: Propoxyphene-induced wide QRS complex dysrhythmia responsive to sodium bicarbonate—A case report. J Toxicol Clin Toxicol 1995;33:179–183.

231. Strain EC, Stitzer ML, Liebson IA, Bigelow GE: Dose-response effects of methadone in the treatment of opioid dependence. Ann Intern Med 1993;119:23–27.

232. Strain EC, Begelow GE, Leibson IA, et al: Moderate- vs. high-dose methadone in the treatment of opioid dependence. A randomized trial. JAMA 1999;281:1000–1005.

233. Strang J, Darke S, Hall W, et al: Heroin overdose: The case for take-home naloxone. BMJ 1996;312:1435–1436.

234. Strang J, Griffiths P, Gossop M: Heroin smoking by "chasing the dragon": Origins and history. Addiction 1997;92:673–683.

235. Strang J, Powis B, Best D, et al: Preventing opiate overdose fatalities with take-home naloxone: Pre-launch study of possible impact and acceptability. Addiction 1999;94:199–204.

236. Szekely JI, Sharpe LG, Jaffe JH: Induction of phencyclidine-like behavior in rats by dextrorphan but not dextromethorphan. Pharmacol Biochem Behav 1991;40:381–384.

237. Szeto HH, Inturrisi CE, Houde R, et al: Accumulation of normeperidine, an active metabolite of meperidine, in patients with renal failure or cancer. Ann Intern Med 1977;86:738–741.

238. Taff RH: Pulmonary edema following naloxone administration in a patient without heart disease. Anesthesiology 1983;59:576–577.

239. Tan TP, Algra PR, Valk J, Wolters EC: Toxic leukoencephalopathy after inhalation of poisoned heroin: MR findings. AJNR Am J Neuroradiol 1994;15:175–178.

240. Tennant FS, Rawson RA, Pumphrey E, et al: Clinical experiences with 959 opioid-dependent patients treated with levo-alpha-acetylmethadol (LAAM). J Subst Abuse Treat 1986;3:195–202.

241. Tighe TV, Walter FG: Delayed toxic acetaminophen level after initial four-hour nontoxic level. J Toxicol Clin Toxicol 1994;32: 431–434.

242. Tracqui A, Kintz P, Ludes B. Buprenorphine-related deaths among drug addicts in France: A report on 20 fatalities. J Anal Toxciol 1998;22:430–434.

243. Traynor JR, Elliot J. δ-Opioid receptor subtypes and cross-talk with μ receptors. Trends Pharmacol Sci 1993;14:84–86.

244. Turski WA, Czucawar SJ, Kleinrok Z, et al: Intra-amygdaloid morphine produces seizures and brain damage in rats. Life Sci 1983; 33:615–618.

245. Ueda H, Harada H, Nozaki M, et al: Reconstitution of rat brain μ opioid receptors with purified guanine nucleotide-binding regulatory proteins. Proc Natl Acad Sci U S A 1988;85:7013–1017.

246. Uhl GR, Javitch JA, Snyder SH: Normal MPTP binding in parkinsonian substantia nigra: Evidence for extraneuronal toxin conversion in human brain. Lancet 1985;i:956–957.

247. Ultram package insert. Ortho Pharmaceutical Corporation. Revised 3/12/96.

248. Utecht MJ, Facinelli Stone A, McCarron MM: Heroin body packers. J Emerg Med 1993;11:33–40.

249. Vacanti CA, Silbert BS, Vacanti FX: Fentanyl-induced muscle rigidity as affected by pretreatment with amantadine hydrochloride. J Clin Anesth 1992;4:282–284.

250. Wanger K, Brough L, Macmillan I, et al: Intravenous vs. subcutaneous naloxone for out-of-hospital management of presumed opioid overdose. Acad Emerg Med 1998;5:293–299.

251. Walsh SL, Johnson RE, Cone EJ, Bigelow GE: Intravenous and oral 1-alpha-acetylmethadol: Pharmacodynamics and pharmacokinetics in humans. J Pharmacol Exp Ther 1998;285:71–82.

252. Walsh SL, Preson KL, Bigelow GE, Stitzer ML: Acute administration of buprenorphine in humans: Partial agonist and blockade effects. J Pharmacol Exp Ther 1995;27:361–372.

253. Wand P, Kuschinsk K, Sontag KH: Morphine-induced muscular rigidity in rats. Eur J Pharmacol 1973;24:189–193.

254. Ward CF, Ward GC, Saidman LJ: Drug abuse in anesthesia training programs. JAMA 1983;250:922–925.

255. Ward JM, McGrath RL, Weil JV: Effects of morphine on the peripheral vascular response to sympathetic stimulation. Am J Cardiol 1972;29:659–666.

256. Warner A. Analyte of the month: Dextromethorphan. Am Assoc Clin Chem 1993;14:27–28.

257. Weil JV, McCullough BS, Kline JS, Sodal IE: Diminished ventilatory response to hypoxia and hypercapnia after morphine in normal man. N Engl J Med 1975;21:1103–1106.

258. Weinger MB, Chen DY, Lin T, et al: A role for CNS α-2-adrenergic receptors in opiate-induced muscle rigidity in the rat. Brain Res 1995;669:10–18.

259. Weinhold LL, Bigelow GE: Opioid miosis: Effects of lighting intensity and monocular and binocular exposure. Drug Alcohol Depend 1993;31:177–181.

260. Weitz CJ, Faull KF, Goldstein A: Synthesis of the skeleton of the morphine molecule by the mammalian liver. Nature 1987;330: 674–677.

261. Werling LL, Frattali A, Portoghese PS, et al: Kappa receptor regulation of dopamine release from striatum and cortex of rats and guinea pigs. J Pharmacol Exp Ther 1988;246:282–286.

262. Whipple JK, Quebbeman EJ, Lewis KS, et al: Difficulties in diagnosing narcotic overdoses in hospitalized patients. Ann Pharmacother 1994;28:446–450.

263. Whitcomb DC, Gilliam FR, Starmer CF, Grant AO: Marked QRS complex abnormalities and sodium channel blockade by propoxyphene reversed with lidocaine. J Clin Invest 1989;84:1629–1636.

264. Wiley JF, Wiley CC, Torrey SB, Henretig FM: Clonidine poisoning in young children. J Pediatr 1990;116:654–658.

265. Winek CL, Schweighardt FK, Fochtman FW, Collom WD: Quinine in urinalysis for heroin. JAMA 1971;217:1243–1244.

266. Wolfe TR, Caravati EM: Massive dextromethorphan ingestion and abuse. Am J Emerg Med 1995;13:174–176.

267. Wolters ECH, van Wijngaarden GK, Stam FC: Leucoencephalopathy after inhaling "heroin" pyrolysate. Lancet 1982;ii; 1233–1237.

268. Wu CH, Henry JA: Deaths on heroin addicts starting methadone maintenance. Lancet 1990;335:424.

269. Yasuda K, Raynor K, Kong H, et al: Cloning and functional comparison of kappa and delta opioid receptors from mouse brain. Proc Natl Acad Sci U S A 1993;90:6736–6740.

270. Yealy DM, Paris PM, Kaplan RM, et al: The safety of prehospital naloxone administration by paramedics. Ann Emerg Med 1990; 19:902–905.

271. Yen LM, Dao LM, Day NPJ, et al: Role of quinine in the high mortality of intramuscular injection tetanus. Lancet 1994;344: 786–787.

272. Yuan CS, Foss JF, O'Connor M, et al: Methylnaltrexone for reversal of constipation due to chronic methadone use: A randomized controlled trial. JAMA 2000;283:367–372.

273. Zador D, Sunjic S, Darke S: Heroin-related deaths in New South Wales, 1992: Toxicological findings and circumstances. Med J Aust 1996;164:204–207.

274. Zagon IS, Goodman SR, McLaughlin PJ: Demonstration and characterization of zeta (ζ), a growth-related opioid receptor, in a neuroblastoma cell line. Brain Res 1990;511:181–186.

275. Zawertailo LA, Kaplan HL, Busto UE, et al: Psychotropic effects of dextromethorphan are altered by the CYP2D6 polymorphism: A pilot study. J Clin Psychopharmacol 1998;18:332–337.

276. Zelis R, Mansour EJ, Capone RJ, Mason DT: The cardiovascular effects of morphine: The peripheral capacitance and resistance vessels in human subjects. J Clin Invest 1974;54:1247–1258.

277. Ziporyn T. A growing industry and menace: Makeshift laboratory's designer drugs. JAMA 1986;256:3061–3063.

ANTIDOTES IN DEPTH

Morphine

Naloxone

Naltrexone

Nalmefene

Opioid Antagonists
Mary Ann Howland

Naloxone, nalmefene, and naltrexone are pure competitive opioid antagonists at the mu (μ), kappa (κ), and delta (δ) receptors. Naloxone is used to reverse respiratory depression for patients manifesting opioid toxicity. The parenteral dose should be enough to maintain adequate airway reflexes and ventilation.[19] Dose titration, beginning with 0.05 mg and increasing as indicated to 0.4 mg, to 2 mg, and finally to 10 mg, will prevent abrupt opioid withdrawal and limit withdrawal-induced adverse effects such as vomiting and the potential for aspiration pneumonia. Naltrexone is used orally for patients following opioid detoxification to maintain opioid abstinence and also as an adjunct to achieve ethanol abstinence. Nalmefene is a parenteral agent whose duration of action falls between naloxone and naltrexone.

HISTORY

The effects of opium were recognized as early as the 3rd century BC.[55] By the 19th century, morphine (named for Morpheus, the god of dreams) was isolated from opium. In the 20th century, the presence of endogenous opioid peptides and families of opioid receptors including μ, δ, and κ were elucidated. The 20th century also witnessed an ever-evolving series of complications of opioid addiction and abuse. Awareness of these social problems resulting from opioid abuse and the ability to understand structure-activity relationships led to the synthesis of many new drugs in the hope of producing potent opioid agonists free of abuse potential. Although this has not been achieved, opioid antagonists and partial agonists were developed. *N*-allylnorcodeine was the first opioid antagonist synthesized, in 1915 by J. Pohl, and in the 1940s the pharmacology of *N*-allylnormorphine (nalorphine) was characterized.[35,63] In 1954, Lasagna and Beecher reported that nalorphine, a derivative of morphine, had both agonist and antagonist effects.[55] This eventually led to the development of levallorphan, naloxone, naltrexone, and nalmefene. Lewenstein and Fishman synthesized naloxone in 1960, and Matossian synthesized naltrexone in 1963.[7]

CHEMISTRY

Minor alterations can convert an agonist into an antagonist.[34] The substitution of the *N*-methyl group on morphine by a larger group led to nalorphine and also converted an agonist, levorphanol, to an antagonist, levallorphan.[55] Naloxone, naltrexone, and nalmefene are derivatives of oxymorphone.

PHARMACOLOGY

Naloxone, naltrexone, and nalmefene are pure competitive opioid antagonists at the μ (responsible for analgesia, miosis, euphoria, respiratory depression, and decreased GI motility), κ (responsible for weaker analgesia, miosis, respiratory depression, dysphoria, anxiety, nightmares, and hallucinations), and δ receptors. These antagonists are most potent at the μ receptor, often necessitating higher doses for effects at the κ and δ receptors. These agents bind to the opioid receptor in a competitive fashion, preventing the binding of agonists, partial agonists, or mixed agonist-antagonists without producing any action of their own. Naloxone, naltrexone, and nalmefene are similar in their potencies, but differ primarily in their pharmacokinetics, with both nalmefene and naltrexone having longer durations of action than naloxone. Naltrexone can be administered orally. Selective antagonists for μ, κ, and δ are available experimentally and are undergoing investigation.[38]

Both nalorphine and levallorphan are weak competitive antagonists at the μ receptor and agonists at the κ receptor. Nalorphine and levallorphan are no longer marketed because of undesirable κ agonist properties.

In the proper doses, pure opioid antagonists reverse all of the effects of endogenous and exogenous opioid agonists at the μ, κ, and δ receptors, except for those of buprenorphine, which has a very high affinity for and slow rate of dissociation from μ receptor.[53,55] Effects on other receptors and receptor subtypes are under investigation.[38] Effects reversed include CNS depression, respiratory depression, analgesia, miosis, inhibition of baroreceptor reflexes, some vasodilation, muscular rigidity, and laryngospasm (commonly seen with fentanyl use), and slowed gastrointestinal motility, all manifestations of opioid receptor effects.[23,55] Actions of opioid agonists that are not mediated by interaction with opioid receptors, such as direct mast-cell liberation of histamine or the sodium channel blocking effects of propoxyphene, are not reversed.[4] Opioid-induced seizures in animals tend to be antagonized by opioid antagonists with the exception of those caused by meperidine and tramadol.[8,29,55,62] A report of two newborns who developed seizures associated with a fentanyl and a morphine infusion demonstrated abrupt resolution following the administration of naloxone.[13] Both patients had electroencephalogram (EEG) monitoring during the seizures and the documented burst-suppression pattern was apparently terminated after naloxone administration.

It was recently discovered that opioids operate bimodally on opioid receptors.[11] At low concentrations, stimulation is excitatory and actually antianalgesic. This antianalgesic effect is modulated through a G_s protein and is usually less important clinically than the well-known inhibitory actions that result from coupling to a G_o protein at usual analgesic doses. Extremely low doses of opioid antagonists (ie, 0.25 μg/kg/h of naloxone) enhance the analgesic potency of the opioid and attenuate or prevent the development of tolerance and dependence.[11,28] Coadministration of these very low doses of antagonists or derivatives (ie, methylnaltrexone) with the opioid also limit opioid-induced adverse effects such as nausea, vomiting, constipation, and pruritus.[11,28,73] It is hypothesized that these beneficial effects result from modulating the opposing excitatory effects of opioids.

ADVERSE REACTIONS

Opioid antagonists prevent the actions of opioid agonists if administered as pretreatment, reverse the effects of endogenous and exogenous opioids, and unmask the manifestations of opioid withdrawal in opioid-dependent patients. Pure opioid antagonists produce very few effects in the non-opioid-dependent patient,

even when administered in high doses.[16,17,41,67] Adverse effects excluding withdrawal and resedation are rare. Patients tolerant to opioid agonists such as morphine exhibit opioid withdrawal reactions (yawning, lacrimation, diaphoresis, rhinorrhea, piloerection, mydriasis, vomiting, diarrhea, myalgias, mild elevations in heart rate and blood pressure, and insomnia) when exposed to opioid antagonists or agonist-antagonists such as pentazocine. Although ultrarapid heroin detoxification is associated with fatalities occurring in the postoperative period, opioid withdrawal ordinarily is not life-threatening. Opioid withdrawal is usually physically and psychologically disabling for the patient. In addition, if vomiting occurs because of withdrawal while the patient's airway is unprotected, aspiration pneumonia may complicate the patient's recovery. Resedation is a function of the relative duration of action of the opioid antagonist and the opioid agonist. Most opioid agonists have a duration of action longer than that of naloxone and shorter than that of naltrexone, whereas the relationship is variable with nalmefene. A long duration of action is advantageous when the antagonist is used to promote abstinence, but is unwanted when an inappropriately large dose is administered to an opioid-dependent patient.

Rare case reports describe acute lung injury (previously termed noncardiogenic pulmonary edema), hypertension, and cardiac dysrhythmias in association with naloxone administration.[3,12,25,45,54,57,59] However, acute lung injury clearly occurs following heroin overdose in the absence of naloxone. Because naloxone is administered to patients who have apparent opioid intoxication, it may be that naloxone is unmasking the acute lung injury previously induced by the opioid, but which is covert because of the patient's respiratory depression.[14]

Hypertension and cardiac dysrhythmias are most frequently reported following anesthesia and opioid reversal in patients with underlying cardiac or pulmonary disorders. The clinical complexities of the setting and case reports make it difficult to analyze and attribute these adverse effects solely to naloxone.[10] Unmasking an underlying clinical condition may also be a logical cause of cardiac dysrhythmias developing after naloxone-induced heroin reversal in a patient simultaneously abusing cocaine.[43] In view of the large number of naloxone doses administered, naloxone has a remarkably safe profile.

USE FOR OPIOID AND ETHANOL ABSTINENCE

Opioid dependence is managed by detoxification and prolonged opioid abstinence, or substitution with either methadone or naltrexone.[42] Any pure opioid antagonist could be substituted, but naltrexone is chosen because of its oral absorption and long duration of action as compared to that of naloxone or nalmefene.[36,41,56] One milligram of naloxone intravenously blocks 25 mg of intravenous heroin for an hour, whereas 50 mg of oral naltrexone blocks this dose of heroin for 24 hours; 100 mg has a blocking effect of 48 hours, and 150 mg is effective for 72 hours. Nalmefene blocks the actions of 2 μg/kg of intravenous fentanyl with a duration of action that is also dose dependent; 0.5 mg IV, 2 mg IV, and 50 mg orally last 4, 8, and 50 hours, respectively.[26,27] Before naltrexone can be administered, the patient must be detoxified from the opioid of dependence, and then naloxone is usually administered intravenously to confirm that the patient is no longer physically dependent. Should opioid withdrawal occur, it will be short-lived following naloxone, whereas it would be prolonged following naltrexone or nalmefene. Naltrexone does not produce tolerance, although prolonged treatment with naltrexone produces up-regulation of opioid receptors.[72]

Naltrexone is also used as adjunctive therapy in ethanol dependence based on the theory that the endogenous opioid system modulates the intake of ethanol.[51] Naltrexone reduces ethanol craving, the number of drinking days, and relapse rates.[51,69] Naltrexone induces moderate to severe nausea in 15% of these patients, possibly as a result of alterations in endogenous opioid tone induced by prolonged ethanol ingestion.[52]

MISCELLANEOUS USES

Endogenous opioids, including endorphins, dynorphins, and enkephalins, are involved in the regulation of many bodily functions, and opioid receptors are found not only in the central nervous system (CNS), but also throughout the body. Often these receptors and endogenous opioids work in concert with other neurotransmitter systems to modulate many effects.[20,22,65,67] For instance, during shock, the release of circulating endorphins produces an inhibition of central sympathetic tone by stimulating κ receptors within the locus ceruleus, resulting in vasodilation. Also, by stimulating the nucleus ambiguus, vagal tone is enhanced. However, the benefits from treatment of patients in septic shock with naloxone are variable.[15,61] Naloxone may have a temporizing effect through elevation of mean arterial pressure.[33]

Although promising in animal models of spinal cord injury, a human investigation of naloxone at doses about 100 times that used in the management of overdoses failed to demonstrate improvement in neurologic recovery.[9]

Opioid antagonists have been used in the management of overdoses with nonopioids such as ethanol,[5,18,48,58] clonidine,[71] captopril,[66] and valproic acid.[1,46] In none of these instances was improvement as dramatic or consistent as in the reversal of the toxic effects of an opioid.

PHARMACOKINETICS AND PHARMACODYNAMICS

Oral naloxone is poorly bioavailable because of extensive first-pass effect.[20] Naloxone is well absorbed by the intramuscular, subcutaneous, and endotracheal routes of administration. The onset of action after intravenous administration is extremely fast and occurs within 1–2 minutes. The distribution half-life of about 5 minutes is rapid because of its high lipid solubility, and the volume of distribution is 0.8–2.64 L/kg.[30,31,50] The elimination half-life is 60–90 minutes in adults, and approximately 2–3 times longer in neonates.[10,50] Naloxone is metabolized by the liver to several compounds, including a glucuronide.[10] The duration of action of naloxone is approximately 20–90 minutes[6,21] and depends on the dose of the agonist, the dose and route of administration of the naloxone, and the rate of elimination of the agonist and naloxone.

Naltrexone is rapidly absorbed, with peak plasma concentrations occurring at 1 hour and an oral bioavailability of 5–60%.[32,44,68,70] Distribution is rapid, with a volume of distribution of about 15 L/kg and low plasma-protein binding.[37,40] Naltrexone is metabolized in the liver to β-naltrexol (with 2–8% activity) and

2-hydroxy,3-methoxy-β-naltrexol.[67] Naltrexone has an enterohepatic cycle.[27,70] The plasma elimination half-life is 10 hours for naltrexone and 13 hours for β-naltrexol.[44,68,70] The terminal phase of elimination is 96 hours for naltrexone and 18 hours for β-naltrexol.[2]

Nalmefene is a derivative of naltrexone, with an oral bioavailability of 40%. After oral administration, peak plasma concentrations are usually reached within 1–2 hours.[16] Protein binding is approximately 45%.[16] Following oral administration, its half-life is 8–9 hours and demonstrates first-order kinetics up to 300-mg doses.[16] Although one study showed the half-life to be 108 ± 38 minutes after intravenous dosing, the study design may have been inadequate to determine the half-life.[30] Another study demonstrated a terminal half-life of 10.8 ± 5 hours after a 1-mg intravenous dose.[49] The apparent volume of distribution (V_d) is 3.9 L/kg for the central compartment and 8.6 L/kg at steady state. Nalmefene is metabolized in the liver to an inactive glucuronide conjugate that then probably undergoes enterohepatic recycling accounting for about 17% of the drug's reappearance in the feces. Less than 5% is excreted unchanged in the urine.

DOSING

The initial dose of antagonist is dependent on the dose of the agonist and the relative binding affinity of the agonist to the various opioid receptors in comparison to the antagonist. The presently available antagonists have a greater affinity for the μ receptor than for the κ or δ receptors. Therefore, the presence of an opioid with a greater affinity for the κ or δ receptor (eg, pentazocine, propoxyphene) requires a larger-than-ordinary dose of antagonist to cause reversal.[47] The dose of antagonist necessary for a child may equal the adult dose because antagonists are competitive and dependent on the size of the ingested dose of agonist. The duration of action of the antagonist depends on many drug and patient variables, such as the dose and clearance of both antagonist and agonist. Evaluation of the return of respiratory depression should be monitored continuously and resedation should be treated with either repeated rebolusing of the antagonist or, if necessary, with another bolus followed by a continuous infusion. What constitutes an observation period is dependent on many factors. Following the use of naloxone, observation for 4 hours should be adequate to determine whether respiratory depression will return. The experience with nalmefene is too limited to estimate an adequate observation time, although 24 hours seems prudent. An oral dose of 150 mg of naltrexone generally lasts 72 hours and this should be adequate for the majority of ingestions with the exception of those opioids, such as levo-α-acetylmethadol (LAAM), that have extremely long durations of action. Naltrexone should never be administered to a patient who is opioid dependent.[60] A challenge dose of naloxone to verify the lack of opioid dependency is strongly recommended before initiation of naltrexone.

A dose of naloxone of 0.4 mg IV will reverse the respiratory-depressant effects of most opioids and is an appropriate starting dose in the non-opioid-dependent patient. However, this dose in an opioid-dependent patient will usually produce withdrawal. Therefore, 0.05 mg is a practical starting dose in most patients, increasing to 0.4 mg, then to 2 mg, and finally to 10 mg. If there is no response to 10 mg, then an opioid is unlikely to be responsible for the respiratory depression. Return of respiratory depression requires repeated bolus doses or a continuous infusion.[39] Two-thirds of the bolus dose of naloxone that resulted in reversal, when given hourly, will usually maintain the desired effect.[58] This dose can be prepared for an adult by multiplying the effective bolus dose by 6.6, adding that quantity to 1000 mL, and administering the solution at a 100-mL/h IV infusion rate. Titration upward or downward is easily accomplished as necessary to maintain adequate ventilation and avoid withdrawal. A continuous infusion of naloxone is not a substitute for continued vigilance. An arbitrary length of time of 12–24 hours is often chosen for observation based on the presumed opioid, the route of administration, and the dosage form. The patient must be observed for about 2 hours after discontinuance of the naloxone to assure that respiratory depression will not recur. Body-packers are a unique subset of patients who must have special individualized management strategies (Chap. 62).

Naltrexone is administered orally in a variety of dosage schedules for the treatment of opioid dependence. Fifty milligrams daily, Monday through Friday, and 100 mg on Saturdays is a common dosing regimen. Alternatively, 100 mg every other day or 150 mg every third day can be administered.

The initial intravenous dose of nalmefene is 0.1 mg in a 70-kg person in whom opioid dependency is suspected. If withdrawal does not ensue, 0.5 mg can be given, followed by 1 mg in 2–5 minutes as necessary. If intravenous access is unavailable, the intramuscular or subcutaneous route may be used, but the onset of action is delayed by 5–15 minutes after a 1-mg dose. For the reversal of postoperative opioid depression, a starting dose of 0.25 µg/kg is used, followed by incremental doses of 0.25 µg/kg every 2–5 minutes to the desired effect or to a total of 1 µg/kg.

AVAILABILITY

Naloxone (Narcan) for intravenous, intramuscular, or subcutaneous administration is available in concentrations of 0.02 mg/mL, 0.4 mg/mL, and 1 mg/mL, with and without parabens, and in 1-mL and 2-mL ampules and in 10-mL multidose vials. Naloxone may be diluted in normal saline or 5% dextrose to facilitate continuous intravenous infusion. Any prepared solution should be used within 24 hours.

Nalmefene (Revex) is available in a blue-labeled 1-mL ampule containing 100 µg/mL and in a green-labeled 2-mL ampule containing 1 mg/mL.

Naltrexone is available as 50-mg pale yellow capsule-shaped tablets, scored and imprinted with DuPont on one side and the number 11 on the other side.

Acknowledgment

Richard S. Weisman, PharmD, contributed to this section in a previous edition.

REFERENCES

1. Alberto G, Erickson T, Popiel R, et al: Central nervous system manifestations of a valproic acid overdose responsive to naloxone. Ann Emerg Med 1989;18:889–891.
2. American Society of Health System Pharmacists Board of Directors, McEvoy G, ed: AMFS 1997 Drug Information—Nalmefene, Naloxone, Naltrexone. Bethesda, MD, American Society of Health System Pharmacists, 1997, pp. 1616–1619.
3. Andree RA: Sudden death following naloxone administration. Anesth Analg 1980;59:782–784.
4. Barke KE, Lindsay BH: Opiates, mast cells and histamine release. Life Sci 1993;18:1391–1399.
5. Barros S, Rodriguez G: Naloxone as an antagonist in alcohol intoxication [letter]. Anesthesiology 1981;54:174.
6. Berkowitz BA: The relationship of pharmacokinetics to pharmacologic activity: Morphine, methadone and naloxone. Clin Pharmacokinet 1976;1:219–230.
7. Blumberg H, Dayton HB: Naloxone, naltrexone, and related noroxymorphones. In: Costa E, Greengard P, Braude MC, et al, eds: Narcotic Antagonists: Advances in Biochemical Psychopharmacology, vol. 8. New York, Raven Press, 1973, pp. 33–44.
8. Bonfiglio MF: Naloxone in the treatment of meperidine induced seizures. Drug Intell Clin Pharm 1987;21:174–175.
9. Bracken MB, Shepard MJ, Collins WF, et al: A randomized, controlled trial of methylprednisolone or naloxone in the treatment of acute spinal cord injury. N Engl J Med 1990;322:1405–1411.
10. Chamberlain JM, Klein BL: A comprehensive review of naloxone for the emergency physician. Am J Emerg Med 1994;6:650–656.
11. Crain S, Shen K: Antagonists of excitatory opioid receptor functions enhance morphine's analgesic potency and attenuate opioid tolerance/dependence liability. Pain 2000;84:121–131.
12. Cuss FM, Colaco CB, Baron JH: Cardiac arrest after reversal of effects of opiates with naloxone. Br Med J 1984;288:363–364.
13. Da Silva O, Alexandrou D, Knoppert D, Yound GB: Seizure and electroencephalographic changes in the newborn period induced by opiates and corrected by naloxone infusion. J Perinatol 1999;19:120–123.
14. Dauberstein JL, Kaufman DM: A clinical study of an epidemic of heroin intoxication and heroin induced pulmonary edema. Am J Med 1971;51:704–714.
15. DeMaria A, Craven DE, Heffernan JJ, et al: Naloxone versus placebo in treatment of septic shock. Lancet 1985;1:1363–1365.
16. Dixon R, Gentile J, Hsu HB, et al: Nalmefene: Safety and kinetics after single and multiple oral doses of a new opioid antagonist. J Clin Pharmacol 1987;27:233–239.
17. Dixon R, Howes J, Gentile J, et al: Nalmefene: Intravenous safety and kinetics of a new opioid antagonist. Clin Pharmacol Ther 1986;39:49–52.
18. Dole VP, Fishman J, Goldfrank L, et al: Arousal of ethanol-intoxicated comatose patients with naloxone. Alcohol Clin Exp Res 1982;6:275–279.
19. Emergency Cardiovascular Care Guidelines. Part 8: Advanced challenges in resuscitation. Toxicology in ECC. Circulation 2000;102:1–223.
20. Evans CJ, Hammond DL, Frederickson RCA: The opioid peptides. In: Pasternak GW, ed: The Opiate Receptors. Clifton Park, NJ: Humana Press, 1988, pp. 23–71.
21. Evans JM, Hogg MJ, Lunn JN, Rosen M: Degree and duration of reversal by naloxone of effects of morphine in conscious subjects. Br Med J 1974;2:589–591.
22. Faden AI, Jacobs TP, Monsey E, et al: Endorphins in experimental spinal injury: Therapeutic effect of naloxone. Ann Neurol 1981;10:326–332.
23. Fahnenstich H, Steffan J, Kau N, Bartmenn P: Fentanyl-induced chest wall rigidity and laryngospasm in preterm and term infants. Crit Care Med 2000;28:836–839.
24. Fishman J, Roffwarg H, Hellman L: Disposition of naloxone-7,8,3H in normal and narcotic-dependent men. J Pharmacol Exp Ther 1973;183:575–580.
25. Flacke JW, Flacke WE, Williams GD: Acute pulmonary edema following naloxone reversal of high-dose morphine anesthesia. Anesthesiology 1977;47:376–378.
26. Gal TJ, DiFazio CA: Prolonged antagonism of opioid action with intravenous nalmefene in man. Anethesiology 1986;64:175–180.
27. Gal TJ, DiFazio CA, Dixon R: Prolonged blockade of opioid effect with oral nalmefene. Clin Pharmacol Ther 1986;40:537–542.

28. Gan T, Ginsberg B, Glass P, et al: Opioid-sparing effects of a low-dose infusion of naloxone in patient administered morphine sulfate. Anesthesiology 1997;87:1075–1081.

29. Gilbert PE, Martin WR: Antagonism of the convulsant effects of heroin, *d*-propoxyphene, meperidine, normeperidine and thebaine by naloxone in mice. J Pharmacol Exp Ther 1975;192:538–541.

30. Glass PS, Jhaveri RM, Smith LR: Comparison of potency and duration of action of nalmefene and naloxone. Anesth Analg 1994;78:536–541.

31. Goldfrank LR, Weisman RS, Errick JK, Lo MW: A dosing nomogram for continuous infusion intravenous naloxone. Ann Emerg Med 1986;15:566–570.

32. Gonzalez JP, Brogden RN: Naltrexone: A review of its pharmacodynamic and pharmacokinetic properties and therapeutic efficacy in the management of opioid dependence. Drugs 1988;35:192–213.

33. Hackshaw KV, Parker GA, Roberts JW: Naloxone in septic shock. Crit Care Med 1990;18:47–51.

34. Harris LS: Narcotic antagonists—Structure-activity relationships. In: Costa E, Greengard P, Braude MC, et al, eds: Narcotic Antagonists: Advances in Biochemical Psychopharmacology, vol. 8. New York, Raven Press, 1973, pp. 13–20.

35. Hart ER, McCawley EL: The pharmacology of *n*-allylnormorphine as compared with morphine. J Pharmacol Exp Ther 1944;82:339–348.

36. Kleber HD, Kosten TR, Gaspari J, Topazian M: Nontolerance to the opioid antagonism of naltrexone. Biol Psychiatry 1985;20:66–72.

37. Kogan MJ, Verebey K, Mule SJ: Estimation of the systemic availability and other pharmacokinetic parameters of naltrexone in man after acute and chronic oral administration. Res Commun Chem Pathol Pharmacol 1977;18:29–34.

38. Kramer TH, Shook JE, Kazmierski W, et al: Novel peptidic mu opioid antagonists: Pharmacologic characterization in vitro and in vivo. J Pharmacol Exp Ther 1989;249:544–551.

39. Lewis JM, Klein-Schwartz W, Benson BE, et al: Continuous naloxone infusion in pediatric narcotic overdose. Am J Dis Child 1984;138:944–946.

40. Ludden TM, Malspeis L, Baggot JD, et al: Tritiated naltrexone binding in plasma from several species and tissue distribution in mice. J Pharm Sci 1976;65:712–716.

41. Martin WR: Naloxone: Diagnosis and treatment; Drugs five years later. Ann Intern Med 1976;85:765–768.

42. Martin WR, Jasinski DR, Mansky PA: Naltrexone, an antagonist for the treatment of heroin dependence: Effects in man. Arch Gen Psychiatry 1973;28:784–790.

43. Merigian KS: Cocaine-induced ventricular arrhythmias and rapid atrial fibrillation temporally related to naloxone administration. Am J Emerg Med 1993;1:96–97.

44. Meyer MC, Straughn AB, Lo MW, et al: Bioequivalence, dose-proportionality and pharmacokinetics of naltrexone after oral administration. J Clin Psychiatry 1984;45:15–19.

45. Michaelis LL, Hickey PR, Clark TA, et al: Ventricular irritability associated with the use of naloxone hydrochloride. Ann Thorac Surg 1984;18:608–624.

46. Montero FJ: Naloxone in the reversal of coma induced by sodium valproate. Ann Emerg Med 1999;33:357–358.

47. Moore RA, Rumack BH: Naloxone: Underdosage after narcotic poisoning. Am J Dis Child 1980;134:156–158.

48. Moss LM: Naloxone reversal of nonnarcotic-induced apnea. JACEP 1973;2:46–48.

49. Nalmefene. Physician's Desk Reference. Montvale, NJ, Medical Economics, 1997, p. 1863.

50. Ngai SH, Berkowitz BA, Yang JC, et al: Pharmacokinetics of naloxone in rats and man: Basis for its potency and short duration of action. Anesthesiology 1976;44:398–401.

51. O'Malley SS, Jeffe AJ, Chang G, et al: Naltrexone and coping skills therapy for alcohol dependence. Arch Gen Psychiatry 1992;49:881–887.

52. O'Malley S, Krishinan-Sarin S, Farren C, O'Connor P: Naltrexone-induced nausea in patients treated for alcohol dependence: Clinical predictors and evidence for opioid mediated effects. J Clin Psychopharmacol 2000;20:69–76.

53. Pasternak GW: Pharmacological mechanisms of opioid analgesics. Clin Neuropharmacol 1993;16:1–18.

54. Prough DS, Roy R, Bumgarner J: Acute pulmonary edema in healthy teenagers following conservative doses of intravenous naloxone. Anesthesiology 1984;60:485–486.

55. Reisine T, Pasternak G: Opioid analgesics and antagonists. In: Hardman JG, Limbird LE, Molinoff PB, et al, eds: Goodman and Gilman's The Pharmacological Basis of Therapeutics, 9th ed. New York, McGraw-Hill, 1996, pp. 521–549.

56. Renault PF: Treatment of heroin dependent persons with antagonists: Current status. In: Willette RE, Barnett G, eds: Naltrexone: Research Monograph. Rockville, MD, National Institute on Drug Abuse, 1980;28:11–22.

57. Schwartz JA, Koenigsberg MD: Naloxone-induced pulmonary edema. Ann Emerg Med 1987;16:1294–1296.

58. Sorenson SC, Mattison K: Naloxone as an antagonist in severe alcohol intoxication [letter]. Lancet 1978;2:688–689.

59. Tanaka GY: Hypertensive reaction to naloxone. JAMA 1974;228:25–26.

60. Tornabene VW: Narcotic withdrawal syndrome caused by naltrexone. Ann Intern Med 1974;81:785–787.

61. Tuggle DW, Horton JW: Effects of naloxone on splanchnic perfusion in hemorrhagic shock. J Trauma 1989;29:1341–1345.

62. Umans JG, Inturrisi CE: Antinociceptive activity and toxicity of meperidine and normeperidine in mice. J Pharmacol Exp Ther 1982;223:203–223.

63. Unna K: Antagonistic effect of *n*-allyl-normorphine upon morphine. J Pharmacol Exp Ther 1943;79:27–31.

64. Van den Berg MH, Van-Giersbergen PL, Cox-Van-Put J, et al: Endogenous opioid peptides and blood pressure regulation during controlled stepwise hemorrhagic hypotension. Circ Shock 1991;35:102–108.

65. Van Giersbergen PL, Cox-Van-Put J, de-Jong W: Central and peripheral opiate receptors appear to be activated during controlled hemorrhagic hypotension. J Hypertens 1989;7(Suppl):2–27.

66. Varon J, Duncan SR: Naloxone reversal of hypotension due to captopril overdose. Ann Emerg Med 1991;20:1125–1127.

67. Verebey K, DePace A, Jukofsky D, et al: Quantitative determination of 2-hydroxy-3-methoxy-6β-naltrexol (HMN), naltrexone, and 6β-naltrexol in human plasma, red blood cells, saliva and urine by gas liquid chromatography. J Anal Toxicol 1980;4:33–37.

68. Verebey K, Volavka J, Mule SJ, Resnick RB: Naltrexone: Disposition, metabolism, and effects after acute and chronic dosing. Clin Pharmacol Ther 1976;20:315–328.

69. Volpicelli JR, Clay KL, Watson NT, O'Brien CP: Naltrexone in the treatment of alcoholism: Predicting response to naltrexone. J Clin Psychol 1995;56(Suppl 7):39–44.

70. Wall ME, Brine DR, Perez-Reyes M: Metabolism and disposition of naltrexone in man after oral and intravenous administration. Drug Metab Disposition 1981;9:369–375.

71. Wedin GP, Edwards LJ: Clonidine poisoning treated with naloxone. Am J Emerg Med 1989;7:343–344.

72. Yoburn BC, Markham CL, Pasternak GW, Inturrisi CE: Upregulation of opioid receptor subtypes correlates with potency changes of morphine and DADLE. Life Sci 1988;43:1319–1324.

73. Yuan C, Foss JF, O'Connor M, et al: Methylnaltrexone for reversal of constipation due to chronic methadone use. JAMA 2000;283:367–372.

CHAPTER 63 SEDATIVE-HYPNOTICS AGENTS

David C. Lee

Ambulance personnel brought a 23-year-old male into the Emergency Department (ED). He was found outside a bar lying on the street. He initially ambulated into the ambulance with help from the paramedics. He was lethargic and answered questions and followed commands intermittently. Initial vital signs included a heart rate of 55 beats/min, a blood pressure of 138/90 mm Hg, a respiratory rate of 12 breaths/min, an oral temperature of 36.8°C (98.3°F), and a room air pulse oximetry reading of 96%. His pupils were 2 mm and there were no signs of trauma. He had a good gag reflex and his exam was otherwise unremarkable. His bedside glucose test was normal. His electrocardiogram (ECG) revealed a sinus bradycardia at a rate of 53 beats/min. He was treated with 2 mg of intravenous naloxone and 100 mg of intravenous thiamine without response. He was placed on a stretcher in a hallway and was presumed to have alcohol intoxication. Thirty minutes later, he became cyanotic and he responded sluggishly to physical stimuli. His repeat vital signs were a heart rate of 50 beats/min, a blood pressure of 128/86 mm Hg, and a pulse oximetry reading of 88%. He was mechanically ventilated with a bag-valve mask. He became slightly more arousable. A decision was made to intubate him; however, the patient was very combative when attempts at intubation were made. When he was placed on 100% oxygen by mask, his pulse oximeter reading plummeted to 88% and he appeared apneic. Midazolam was given for sedation and intubation was performed successfully. Blood alcohol results returned with a level of 80 mg/dL. Urine toxicology screening for drugs-of-abuse was negative. Other routine laboratory screening was unremarkable.

Two hours later, he rapidly regained consciousness and self-extubated himself. He demanded to leave and appeared lucid and coherent. He admited to drinking a mixture of "Blue Nitro" (α-butyrolactone) and vodka. Although he had done this before, he stated he "may have taken an extra spoonful." He declined admission to a detoxification program and was released 6 hours later.

Sedative hypnotics refer to a loosely defined category of agents that are used to induce a calming effect and to limit excitability (sedative), or to induce drowsiness and sleep (hypnotic). *Anxiolytics* or *tranquilizers* are other medical terms that are used to describe these agents. Because many different types of drugs, botanicals, and foods are used for this effect, sedative-hypnotics actually encompass a wide range of agents. This chapter focuses on agents used solely for their sedative-hypnotic effects. Sedative-hypnotics can be divided into four major groups: barbiturates, ben-

zodiazepines, other pharmaceutical drugs, and nonpharmaceutical agents (Table 63–1).

HISTORY AND EPIDEMIOLOGY

Poisoning with sedative-hypnotic agents is one of the more common overdoses. According to data collected by the American Association of Poison Control Centers, sedative-hypnotics are consistently one of the top five agents associated with fatalities by overdose (p. 1752 and Chap. 116). With the ubiquitous worldwide use of sedative-hypnotics, this category of agents is probably involved in substantially more deaths than are reported. Several advocates of euthanasia favor suicide by sedative-hypnotic poisoning, specifically with barbiturates.[79]

Throughout history, sedative-hypnotic use and abuse have been commonplace. Mythology of ancient cultures is replete with stories of poisons or agents that cause sleep or a state of unconsciousness (Chap. 1). Overdoses of pharmaceutical sedative-hypnotics were reported soon after the commercial introduction of bromide in 1853. Other commercial agents that were subsequently developed include chloral hydrate, paraldehyde, sulfonyl, and urethane.

In 1903, the barbiturates were introduced and quickly replaced the older agents. This class of drugs dominated the market for sedative-hypnotics for the first half of the 20th century. Unfortunately, because barbiturates have a relatively small therapeutic index and substantial potential for abuse, they quickly became a major health problem. By the 1950s and 1960s, barbiturates were frequently implicated in self-poisonings and overdoses and were responsible for the majority of all drug-related suicides. As fatalities from barbiturates increased, attention shifted to curbing their abuse and finding safer alternatives.[26,147,157] These safer alternatives included methyprylon, glutethimide, ethchlorvynol, and methaqualone. Unfortunately, however, many of these agents also had significant undesirable effects. With the introduction of benzodiazepines in the early 1960s, barbiturates and the original alternatives were quickly supplanted.

Presently, benzodiazepines are the most commonly prescribed sedatives. First synthesized by Hoffman-LaRoche in 1955 and marketed in 1960, there are now more than 50 differing types of benzodiazepines marketed and thousands developed. In the 1980s, benzodiazepines captured more than 80% of the anxiolytic market and more than 50% of the hypnotic market.[80,162] As opposed to the barbiturates, the ingestion of a benzodiazepine alone accounts for relatively few deaths.[57] Most deaths blamed on benzodiazepines

TABLE 63–1.   Sedative-Hypnotics

Pharmaceutical
    Antihistamines
        Diphenhydramine
        Doxylamine
    Benzodiazepines*
    Barbiturates*
    Bromides•
    Chloral Hydrate*
    Cyclic antidepressants
        Amitriptyline
        Imipramine
        Maprotiline
    Ethchlorvynol (Placidyl)
    Glutethimide (Doriden)
    Meprobamate (Miltown)*
    Methyprylon (Noludar)•
    Methaqualone (Quaalude)*•
    Paraldehyde•
    Propofol*
    Sulfonal•
    Urethane•
    Zaleplon
    Zolpidem*
  Nonpharmaceutical
    Ethanol*
    Dietary supplements
        Botanicals
            Cypripedium calceolus (nerveroot)
            Primula veris (cowslip)
            Piscida piscipula (Jamaican dogwood)
            Humulus lupulus (hops)
            Passiflora incarnata (passion flower)
            Valeriana officinalis (valerian)*
        γ-Hydroxy butryrate (GHB)*•
            γ-Butyrolactone (GBL)*
            Furanone*
        Melatonin
        Tryptophan

*Documented interactions with the GABA system.
•Not marketed in the United States.

have occurred from mixed overdoses of benzodiazepines and other sedative-hypnotic agents.[71]

Although benzodiazepines represent most of the market for pharmaceutical sedatives by prescription, many nonprescription agents are used as hypnotics. There are also many "dietary supplements" and nonpharmaceutical agents that are promoted as sedative-hypnotics. With the exception of the antihistamines and γ-hydroxybutyrate (GHB) analogues, the majority of these are relatively nontoxic in the therapeutic or overdose settings.[7]

PHARMACOLOGY

All of the sedative-hypnotics can produce central nervous system (CNS) depression. Most clinically effective sedative-hypnotic agents produce their physiologic effects by enhancing the function of GABA system. This has been well described for benzodiazepines and barbiturates. With increasing understanding of this system, the mechanisms of action of many older agents have also been attributed to the GABA system (Table 63–1).

GABA$_A$ receptors are the primary mediators of inhibitory neurotransmission in the brain. The GABA$_A$ receptor is a pentameric structure composed of varying polypeptide subunits associated with a chloride channel on the postsynaptic membrane (see Fig. 10–9). These subunits are classified into three families: α, β, and γ. The most common GABA$_A$ receptor in the brain is composed of $\alpha_1\beta_2\gamma_2$ subunits.[38] Sedative-hypnotics alter the function of the chloride channel by increasing either its frequency or duration of opening. Indirect-acting agonists, such as the benzodiazepines, require the presence of GABA to affect the channel. Other agents, such as barbiturates and propofol, can directly open the channel at high doses without the presence of GABA.[136] This may explain the relatively high lethality seen with barbiturate overdoses as compared to benzodiazepine overdoses.

Toxicity of many of the sedative-hypnotics can be explained by their action on the various GABA receptor configurations. Differing sedative-hypnotics have unique affinities for certain GABA receptors with specific subunits. Variations in the five subunits of the GABA receptor confers the potency of its sedative, anxiolytic, hypnotic, amnestic, and muscle-relaxing properties.[119] Almost all sedative-hypnotics bind to GABA$_A$ receptors containing the α_1 subunit. Low doses of benzodiazepines are only affective at GABA$_A$ receptors with the γ_2 subunit.[38] Even within classes of sedative-hypnotics, there are varying affinities for differing subunits. This model helps explain why flunitrazepam has greater amnestic properties than diazepam, and why clonazepam has a greater anxiolytic property than both flunitrazepam and diazepam.[45]

There are also GABA$_B$ and GABA$_C$ receptors. GABA$_B$ receptors are coupled to a G protein and are located pre- and postsynaptically. Like GABA$_A$ receptors, GABA$_C$ receptors are also associated with a chloride channel; however, they are insensitive to barbiturates and benzodiazepines (Chap. 10). As such their function has not been clearly elucidated.[21,33,48]

Many sedative-hypnotics have activity at multiple differing receptor sites. Not only do sedative-hypnotics increase the effects of GABA-mediated inhibitory neurotransmission, many sedative-hypnotics decrease the affects of glutamate-mediated excitatory neurotransmission. Trichloroethanol, the active metabolite of chloral hydrate, decreases the effect of glutamate on *N*-methyl-D-aspartate (NMDA) receptors.[140] Barbiturates, etomidate, and propofol interact with NMDA and AMPA/kainate receptor function with barbiturates, markedly attenuating the excitatory effects of glutamate.[28,138,184] GHB also has affinity for inhibitory presynoptic GABA$_B$ receptors, which may explain the resultant muscular activity such as twitching. In addition there is evidence to suggest that there are also specific GHB receptor sites.[5,11,111]

Certain sedative-hypnotics will have specific sites that are concentrated in varying areas of the CNS. For example, benzodiazepines associated with GABA receptors tend to bind at specific areas in the CNS. There are two structurally different "central" benzodiazepine receptors found in the brain: type I (ω_1) and type II (ω_2). Type I receptors tend to be located throughout the brain and to contain the GABA$_A$ α_1 subunit.[45] Therefore, they are hypothesized to affect anxiety, sleep, and amnesia. Type II receptors tend to be concentrated in the hippocampus, striatum, and spinal cord, and are hypothesized to affect muscle relaxation and dependence. Zolpidem and zaleplon have greater affinity for type I receptors (specifically the α_1 subunit) and lower affinity for type II receptors than benzodiazepine hypnotics. For this reason, they are thought to have potent hypnotic affects and less addiction potential.[45,74,77]

Benzodiazepines also are active at certain types of benzodiazepine receptors that are not associated with the GABA receptor. These receptors differ structurally, pharmacologically, and physiologically from GABA-associated benzodiazepine receptors. Because the function and the structure of these receptors are not well defined, attempts to classify them are not satisfying. These sites have been labeled "peripheral" benzodiazepine receptors because of their predominant location on the outer membrane of the mitochondria, but they are also present in erythrocytes that lack mitochondria.[135,139] These receptors are prevalent throughout the body, with the greatest concentrations located in steroid-producing cells in the adrenal gland, the anterior pituitary gland, and the reproductive organs. The exact endogenous ligands or proteins that bind to these receptors are not clearly elucidated. Several types of endogenous benzodiazepinelike substances, endozepines, anthralin, porphyrins, and diazepam-binding inhibitors are proposed to bind to these receptors.[63]

Although the exact role of these receptors remains unclear, it is postulated that benzodiazepines may influence basic cellular functions such as mitochondrial respiratory control, cell growth, and cell differentiation. Peripheral benzodiazepine receptors also appear to affect several biologic systems that are designed to cope with stress, such as the hypothalamic-pituitary system, the sympathetic nervous system, the renin-angiotensin system, and the neuroendocrine-immune system.[63,183] These receptors may have a "neurosteroid" effect by modulating steroidogenesis. They are hypothesized to alleviate anxiety and stress without the presence of GABA by resulting in neurosteroid release in the adrenal glands.[41,114,132]

Peripheral benzodiazepine receptors may be of significance in modulating pathologic conditions such as hepatic encephalopathy, anxiety disorders, and abnormal immune function. Peripheral benzodiazepine receptors in the CNS are markedly decreased after neurotoxic insults caused by domoic acid, an excitatory amino acid, and the neurotoxins soman and 1-methyl-4-phenyl-1,2,3,6-tetrahydropyridine (MPTP).[77,91,92,97] These peripheral receptors are increased in the presence of encephalopathies caused by hepatic failure and thiamine deficiency.[27,99,103] Cardiac benzodiazepine receptor sites are linked to calcium channels (specifically, dihydropyridine sites) in animal tissues.[46,101,120–123] This mechanism may represent the theoretical support for the use of benzodiazepines in the treatment of the cardiac toxicity of agents such as chloroquine, cocaine, and sympathomimetics.[12,83,109,130]

PHARMACOKINETICS/TOXICOKINETICS

Most sedative-hypnotics are rapidly absorbed in the GI tract with the rate-limiting step being dissolution and dispersion of the drug. Barbiturates and benzodiazepines are primarily absorbed in the small intestine. Clinical effects are determined by the relative ability of these drugs to penetrate the blood-brain barrier. Agents that are highly lipophilic penetrate most rapidly. The ultrashort-acting barbiturates are clinically active in the most vascular parts of the brain (gray matter first) within 30 seconds of administration, resulting in sleep shortly thereafter.

After initial distribution, many of the sedative-hypnotics undergo a redistribution phase as they are dispersed to other body tissues, specifically fat. Drugs that are redistributed, such as the lipophilic (ultrashort-acting) barbiturates and some of the benzodiazepines (diazepam, midazolam), may have a brief clinical effect as the early peak concentrations in the brain rapidly decline. The clinical activity of many of these drugs is determined by their rapid distribution and redistribution (α phase) and not by their elimination (β phase) (Chap. 11; Table 63–2).

Many of the sedative-hypnotics are metabolized to pharmacologically active intermediates. This is particularly true for chloral hydrate and some of the benzodiazepines. The benzodiazepines can be hepatically demethylated, hydroxylated, or conjugated with glucuronide. Glucuronidation proceeds rapidly to the production of inactive metabolites. Benzodiazepines, such as diazepam, that undergo demethylation yield active intermediates that may possess more prolonged therapeutic half-lives than the parent compound. Because of the individual pharmacokinetics of sedative-hypnotics and the production of active metabolites, there is often no correlation between the therapeutic half-life and the biological half-life.

The majority of sedative-hypnotics, such as the highly lipid-soluble barbiturates and the benzodiazepines, are highly protein-bound. The kidney poorly filters the agents and elimination occurs principally by hepatic metabolism. Notable exceptions include chloral hydrate and meprobamate. Drugs with a low lipid-to-water partition coefficient, such as meprobamate and the longer-acting barbiturates, are poorly protein-bound and more subject to renal excretion, which can be influenced. Elimination can be increased with manipulation of urinary pH and hemodialysis (Chap. 6). Another mechanism is the use of multiple doses of activated charcoal (Antidotes in Depth: Activated Charcoal). Phenobarbital is a classic example of an agent whose elimination can be manipulated with these techniques. However, because of the high protein binding and high lipid solubility of most other agents, any attempts at acutely increasing the rate of elimination of the majority of sedative-hypnotics would be unsuccessful.

PHARMACODYNAMICS

Overdoses of multiple different types of sedative-hypnotics can be more lethal than an overdose of a single agent. These agents often act synergistically at the GABA site. For example, both barbiturates and benzodiazepines act on the GABA site, but barbiturates hold the ionophore open longer, while benzodiazepines increase the frequency of ionophore opening.[161] Varying sedative-hypnotics may increase the affinity of another agent at their respective binding sites. For example, pentobarbital increases the affinity of γ-hydroxybutyrate for its non-GABA binding site.[163] Propofol potentiates pentobarbital's effect on the chloride influx at the GABA receptor.[169] Propofol also increases the affinity and decreases the rate of dissociation of benzodiazepines to their site on the GABA receptor.[25,149] These actions cause an increased effect of each agent and clinically may lead to a deeper CNS and respiratory depression.

Another mechanism of increasing synergistic toxicity is the inhibition of elimination. The combination of ethanol and chloral hydrate, the infamous "Mickey Finn," has additive CNS depressant effects. Both drugs alter each other's metabolism. Chloral hydrate competes for alcohol dehydrogenase, thereby prolonging the half-life of ethanol. The metabolism of ethanol generates nicotinamide adenine dinucleotide (NADH), which is needed as a cofac-

TABLE 63–2.   Sedative-Hypnotic Agents

	Plasma Half-Life (hours)	Protein Binding (%)	Vd (L/kg)	Active Metabolites
Benzodiazepines				
Alprazolam	10–14	80	0.8	None
Chlordiazepoxide	5–15	96	0.3	Desmethylchlordiazepoxide, desmethyldiazepam, oxazepam
Clorazepate		97	0.9	Desmethyldiazepam, oxazepam
Clonazepam	18–50	85.4	3.2	None
Diazepam	20–70	98.7	1.0–1.5	Desmethyldiazepam, hydroxydiazepam, oxazepam
Estazolam	8–31	93		None
Flunitrazepam	16–35	80		7-Amino-flunitrazepam
Flurazepam	2.3	97.2	3.4	N-Hydroxymethyl-flurazepam, desalkylflurazepam
Lorazepam	9–19	90	0.8–1.3	None
Midazolam	3–8	95	1.0–1.5	1-Hydroxymethylmidazolam
Oxazepam	5–15		0.6	None
Temazepam	10–16	97	0.75–1.37	None
Triazolam	1.5–5.5	90	0.7–1.5	None
Barbiturates				
Ultrashort acting				
Methohexital	3–6	73	2.2	Unclear
Thiopental	8–10	72–86	1.5–3.5	None
Short acting				
Pentobarbital	15–48	60–70	0.5–1.0	None
Secobarbital	15–40	46–70		None
Intermediate acting				
Amobarbital	8–42			None
Aprobarbital	14–34	20		None
Butabarbital	35–50	26		None
Long acting				
Barbital	6–12	25		
Mephobarbital	10–70	40–60		Phenobarbital
Phenobarbital	48–144	20–45	0.5–0.6	None
Primidone	3.3–22.4	19	0.6–0.8	Phenobarbital, phenylethylmalonamide
Others				
Alcohols				
Chloral hydrate	4.0–9.5	35–40	0.6–1.6	Trichloroethanol
Ethchlorvynol	10–25	30–40	4	
Phenols				
Propofol	0.5–1 (initial)	98	2–10	
Imidazolecarboxylate				
Etomidate	1.25	76	2.5–4.5	
Piperidinediones				
Glutethimide	5–22	47–59	2.7	4-Hydroxy-glutethimide
Methyprylon	3–6	60	0.97	5–Methylpyrithyldione
Propanediols				
Meprobamate	6–16	20	0.75	None
Carisoprodol	8			Meprobamate
Quinazolines				
Methaqualone	19	80–90	5.8–6.0	4-Hydroxymethaqualone
Imidazopyridine				
Zolpidem	1.4–4.5	92	0.54	None
Pyrazolopyrimidine				
Zaleplon	1.0	60	1.4	None

tor for the metabolism of choral hydrate to trichloroethanol, an active metabolite. Finally, ethanol inhibits the conjugation of trichloroethanol, and trichloroethanol, in turn, inhibits the oxidation of ethanol (Fig. 63–1).[158,159]

Because of the greater variety of drugs, there are multiple drug-drug interactions that occur predominantly in the hospital setting that may also prolong the half-life of many sedative hypnotic agents. This may significantly increase their potency. For example, midazolam, which undergoes hepatic metabolism via CYP3A4, can have a dramatic increase in half-life in the presence of certain antifungal agents that have a similar metabolism.[134] The midazolam half-life undergoes a 400-fold rise when combined

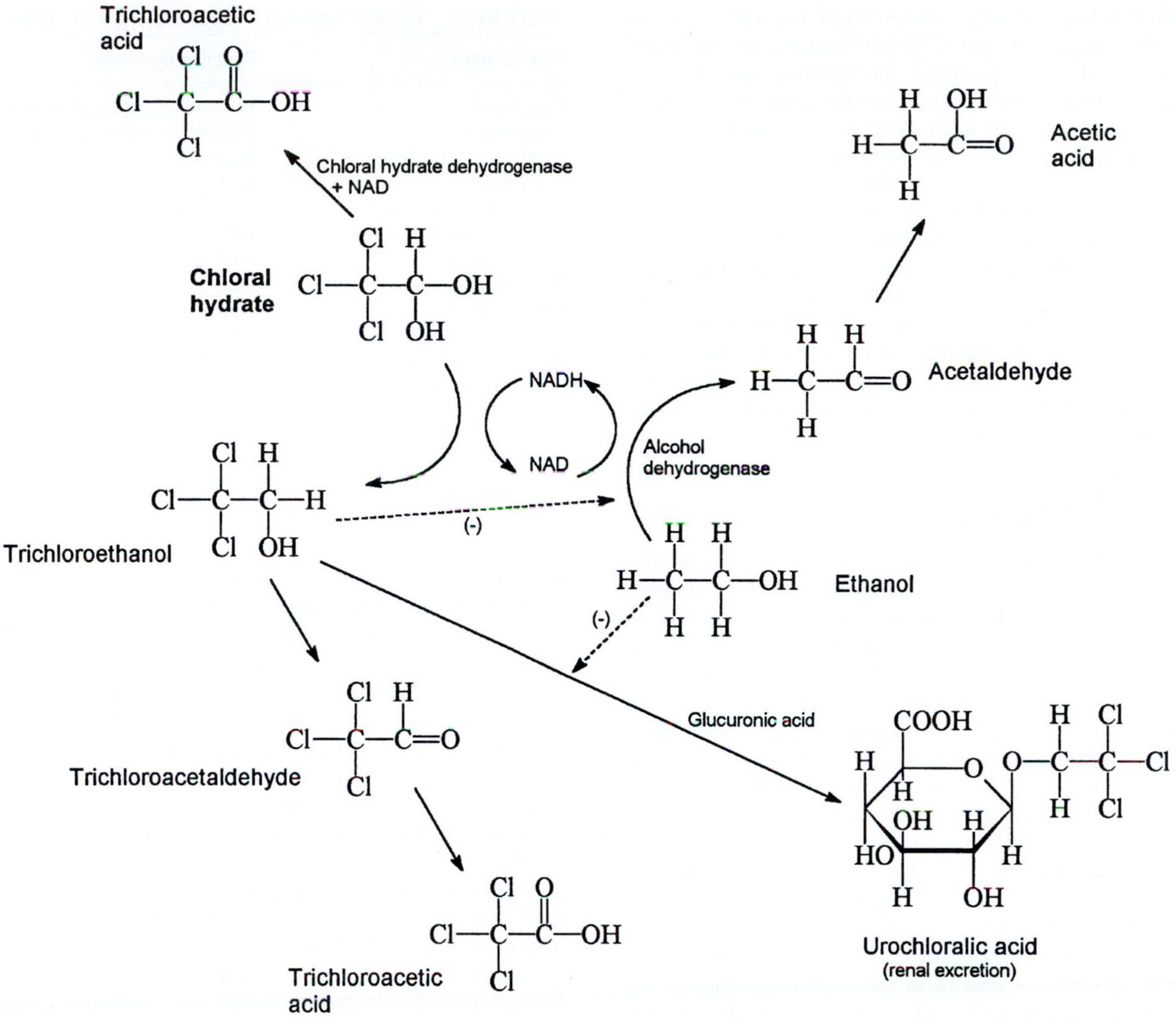

Figure 63–1. Metabolism of chloral hydrate and ethanol, demonstrating the interactions between chloral hydrate and ethanol metabolism. In particular, note the inhibitory (---) effects of ethanol on trichloroethanol metabolism and the converse. *(Adapted, with permission, from Sellers EM, Lang M, Koch-Weser J: Interaction of chloral hydrate and ethanol in man. I. Metabolism. Clin Pharmacol Ther 1972;13:40.)*

with itraconazole.[10] This finding is also related to the fact that intravenous administration of an agent bypasses the majority of enteric P450 cytochrome metabolism.

Tolerance

Ingestions of relatively large doses may not have the predicted effects in patients who chronically use sedative-hypnotics. These patients have often developed tolerance, the progressive diminution of effect of a particular drug with repeated administrations, often resulting in a need for greater doses to achieve the same effect. Tolerance can be secondary to pharmacodynamic and/or pharmacokinetic factors. However, in the majority of cases, tolerance to sedative-hypnotics is caused by pharmacodynamic changes.[162]

Pharmacodynamic tolerance occurs when there are adaptive neural and receptor changes ("plasticity") after repeated exposures. These changes include a decrease in number of receptors ("down-regulation"), reduction of firing of receptors ("receptor desensitization"), structural changes in receptors ("receptor shift"), and reduction of coupling of sedative-hypnotics and their respective GABA$_A$-related receptor site. In this setting, there is a decreased effect of a drug even though there are no significant changes in plasma or CNS drug levels. For example, benzodiazepine-dependent patients have decreased GABA$_A$ receptor density and sensitivity.[59,144] Pharmacodynamic tolerance to sedative-hypnotics can appear very quickly, even during short-term use. In one study, using an IV infusion of thiopental with a variable rate and a specific electroencephalogram (EEG) pattern, rapidly increasing thiopental levels were needed to produce a constant state of anesthesia.[13] The degree of acute tolerance can be directly proportional to the degree of CNS depression produced by the drug.[87] Thus, tolerance is dose related and can occur rapidly.

Pharmacokinetic tolerance occurs when metabolic changes cause a decreasing plasma and CNS level of a chronically administered drug. For example, chronic phenobarbital administration can result in pharmacokinetic tolerance. Repeated use of phenobarbital will induce hepatic microsomal enzyme function causing a decreasing half-life. Thus, increasing doses of phenobarbital may be required to achieve the same level.

Following termination of therapy, tolerance can be lost as the previously desensitized target receptors return to their original level of function. The rate at which this process occurs is governed by the biologic half-life of the particular sedative-hypnotic and any biologically active intermediates produced. Cross-tolerance readily exists among the sedative-hypnotics. Chronic use of benzodiazepines will not only decrease the activity of benzodiazepine binding sites on the GABA receptor, but it will also decrease the binding affinity of the barbiturate sites.[78]

Dependence and Withdrawal

Physical drug dependence refers to a condition in which a physiologic withdrawal state is induced when a drug is suddenly stopped. In animal models, dependence can be easily and rapidly achieved with the use of benzodiazepines.[94,95] Biologic theories of dependence are based on two main theories. The first involves actual decreases in endogenous production of a similar substance. Thus, when chronic sedative-hypnotic use occurs, the body reduces the amount of a similar endogenous substance. Although endogenous ligands are postulated for benzodiazepines, there has yet to be convincing confirmation of these agents. Presently, there is no proof that there is actual reduction of GABA or GABAergic agents during dependency. The second theory postulates that there are changes in the characteristic of the receptor. Similar to theories concerning tolerance, dependence is thought to mainly result from the "plasticity" of the receptor and the CNS. A molecular model of this theory describes a change in the protein subunits of the $GABA_A$ receptor, specifically replacing the α_1 and β_1 subunits with less active subunits, thereby decreasing the potency of sedative-hypnotics.[45]

When benzodiazepine use is diminished or discontinued, approximately one-third of chronic benzodiazepine users experience withdrawal, which can be life-threatening.[95] Similar to other withdrawal states, withdrawal from sedative-hypnotic agents is usually more severe and has a more rapid onset when the agent involved has a short half-life. Factors that contribute to the severity of withdrawal include shorter half-life of the agent, higher daily dosage, and underlying medical and psychologic illness (Chap. 72).

CLINICAL MANIFESTATIONS

Almost all patients with significant sedative-hypnotic overdoses will manifest slurred speech, ataxia, and incoordination similar to that which occurs with ethanol intoxication. Those with moderate to severe toxicity are stuporous or comatose, and the most severe cases may lose all neurologic responses. With increasing CNS depression, increasing respiratory depression occurs. Low minute and tidal volumes occur, causing signs of acute respiratory acidosis. Increasing hypoventilation and impending respiratory compromise contribute to cardiovascular depression. Cardiovascular

TABLE 63–3.   Clinical Findings of Sedative-Hypnotic Overdose

Clinical Signs	Sedative-Hypnotics
Hypothermia	Barbiturates, bromides, ethchlorvynol
Unique odors	Chloral hydrate, ethchlorvynol
Cardiac dysrhythmias	Meprobamate
Bradycardia	GHB
Tachydysrhythmias	Chloral hydrate
Muscular twitching	GHB, methaqualone, propofol
Acneiform rash	Bromides
Fluctuating coma	Glutethimide, meprobamate
GI bleeding	Chloral hydrate, methaqualone
Discolored urine	Propofol (green/pink)
Anticholinergic signs	Glutethimide

collapse can also be caused by direct depression of cardiac contractility, dilation of vascular smooth muscle, and medullary depression of cardiovascular regulation.

Although the physical examination can rarely be used to identify a particular sedative-hypnotic, it can give clues to the class of sedative-hypnotics (Table 63–3). Barbiturates cause fixed drug eruptions, which often are bullous eruptions over pressure-point areas. However, this phenomenon is not specific to barbiturates and is documented with other drugs, including carbon monoxide, methadone, imipramine, glutethimide, and benzodiazepines (nitrazepam, diazepam, oxazepam, and temazepam). Occasionally, the offending agent can be found in the aspirated fluid of these vesicles.

Benzodiazepine overdoses have unique characteristics in children. In a case series of benzodiazepine overdoses in children with a mean age of 36 months, the majority of patients presented with symptoms typical of a sedative-hypnotic overdose, such as lethargy and CNS depression. It was noteworthy that 17% solely manifested ataxia.[180]

The presentation of acute iatrogenic sedative-hypnotic toxicity in a hospital setting is identical to the nonhospital setting: CNS and respiratory depression. The main differences are related to the route of administration, the greater potency of agents used in the hospital setting, and their side effects.

There are other situations that differ between overdoses that occur in the hospital and in the community. In the critical care settings, large doses of sedative-hypnotics given chronically are associated with toxicities that are independent of the characteristics of the sedative-hypnotic. The toxicity maybe associated with the diluent of certain sedative-hypnotics, specifically propylene glycol. Multiple case reports document the development of hyperosmolar states, metabolic acidosis, and cardiovascular compromise in patients with prolonged use of lorazepam and etomidate.[96,104,148] Fatal reactions have also been attributed to the carrier base of intravenous propofol.[145]

An additional area of concern is the unrecognized development of dependence and the iatrogenic precipitation of withdrawal. In the critical care setting, potent, fast-acting, short-lived sedatives are commonly used. However, it is these same characteristics that increase the potential for dependence. Rapid weaning from these medications may precipitate withdrawal, often with a delayed presentation after extubation and cessation of sedation (Chap. 72).

DIAGNOSTIC TESTING

In the undifferentiated comatose patient without a clear history, when drug overdose is a primary concern, laboratory testing including electrolytes, renal profile (blood urea nitrogen (BUN) and creatinine), glucose, arterial blood gas analysis, and cerebrospinal fluid (CSF) analysis may be useful to exclude metabolic abnormalities. Diagnostic imaging studies such as a CT scan of the head to detect space-occupying lesions are often essential.

Routine laboratory screens for drugs of abuse are not helpful in the management of the undifferentiated comatose adult patient. These tests will vary in type, sensitivity, and specificity in differing institutions. Although almost all institutions will use immunoassay technology to screen drugs of abuse, different techniques in these clinical settings limit the ability to adequately identify many agents. Most will detect phenobarbital and certain benzodiazepines while many other sedative-hypnotics go undetected (Chap. 7).

Many benzodiazepines go undetected because they undergo significant metabolism that produces many differing active metabolites. The parent drug may not be found in urine specimens because of its presence in very low concentrations, while the patient may have significant symptoms due to the presence of multiple active metabolites. In addition, newer agents such as alprazolam and triazolam undergo minimal metabolism but are quite active at serum concentrations that may be too low to allow detection. Certain agents such as clonazepam and flunitrazepam that are 7-amino analogues may not be detected because most benzodiazepine screens only identify metabolites of 1,4-benzodiazepines such as oxazepam or desmethyldiazepam (Chap. 7).[50] On the other hand, screening may be useful in pediatric populations, especially if there is concern for child abuse.[13]

Specific laboratory levels may be helpful (ie, levels of ethanol or phenobarbital) to confirm or disprove overdoses of an agent, particularly if the etiology of the clinical condition is uncertain. However, specific levels of sedative-hypnotics other than phenobarbital are not routinely performed in most hospitals. Therefore, specific levels of sedative-hypnotics other than phenobarbital are rarely helpful in guiding management. Abdominal radiographs may be helpful if chloral hydrate is suspected because chloral hydrate is radiopaque (Chap. 8).

Although immediate identification of a particular sedative-hypnotic agent may be helpful in predicting the length of toxicity, it rarely affects the acute management of the patient. The exception may be for phenobarbital where urinary alkalization may alter management.

MANAGEMENT

With increasing doses, sedative-hypnotics typically produce drowsiness, CNS depression, unconsciousness, respiratory depression, cardiovascular collapse, and finally death. Treatments have been targeted to limit this progression. Historically, analeptics and other arousal agents (Antidotes in Depth: Antiquated Antidotes) were used with limited success. Similar to the majority of poisoned patients who present with unstable vital signs, the vast majority of patients with severe overdoses of sedative-hypnotics who present with unstable vital signs respond well to supportive care. Deaths secondary to sedative-hypnotic overdoses are a result of respiratory collapse and careful attention should be focused on monitoring and maintaining adequate airway and oxygenation.

As in the case of all critically ill patients, the airway should be controlled and adequate ventilation should be maintained. Supplemental oxygen, respiratory support, and prevention of aspiration are the cornerstones of treatment because mortality of sedative-hypnotic poisoning is secondary to respiratory failure. Hemodynamic instability is often a secondary or a delayed manifestation of sedative-hypnotic poisoning and typically follows respiratory collapse. Hypotensive patients should be resuscitated with volume expansion. Vasopressors should be used when patients do not respond to intravenous fluids or when there is evidence of pulmonary edema. There are significant concerns with regard to the development of lethal dysrhythmias from the use of β-adrenergic agonists in the setting of chloral hydrate overdose, because chloral hydrate is metabolized to the active halogenated hydrocarbon, trichloroethanol. In the setting of cardiac dysrhythmias, judicious use of β-adrenergic antagonists is proposed.[22,68,179]

Decontamination

All patients with significant ingestions should receive activated charcoal. The use of multiple-dose activated charcoal (MDAC) may not be effective in all poisonings. The use of MDAC has been extensively studied for phenobarbital; MDAC increases elimination of phenobarbital by 50–80%.[14,15,20,86,126,170] However, in the only controlled study, no difference could be demonstrated in outcome measures (time to extubation and length of hospitalization) in intubated patients with phenobarbital overdoses randomized to single-dose versus MDAC.[143] Although inconclusive, after ensuring an adequately protected airway, multiple doses of activated charcoal have potential benefits and limited adverse risks or costs (Antidotes in Depth: Activated Charcoal).

Although the efficacy of delayed orogastric lavage is controversial, orogastric lavage should be considered in patients who overdose with agents that may develop concretions, specifically, phenobarbital and meprobamate.[88,156]

There are no antidotes useful to counteract all sedative-hypnotic overdoses. Flumazenil, a competitive benzodiazepine antagonist, has been developed for benzodiazepines. However, the use of flumazenil has a poor risk/benefit ratio in patients who have an undifferentiated sedative-hypnotic overdose (Antidotes in Depth: Flumazenil).

There are very few situations when a patient with a sedative-hypnotic overdose will require extracorporeal methods of drug removal. The use of hemodialysis is exceptionally uncommon. Hemodialysis should be considered in patients with chloral hydrate overdoses who develop life-threatening cardiac manifestations and in patients with ingestions of extremely large quantities of phenobarbital and meprobamate who require prolonged intubation times.

Because the lethality of sedative-hypnotics is associated with the agent's ability to cause respiratory depression, asymptomatic patients can be downgraded to a lower level of care after a period of observation. Thus, patients who have been monitored in the intensive care unit (ICU) for a period of time (8–12 hours) without signs of respiratory depression can be transferred to a general medical floor. Long-acting agents, such as meprobamate and clonazepam, or agents that can have a significant enterohepatic circulation, such as glutethimide, will necessitate 24 hours of observation (Chap. 104).

SPECIFIC AGENTS
Barbiturates

In 1903, barbital became the first commercially available barbiturate. Many other barbiturates have been developed since then. These agents are all derivatives of barbituric acid (2,4,6-trioxo-hexa-hydropyrimidine), which by itself has no CNS depressant properties. Various side chains at the X, Y, and Z sites influence the individual barbiturate's lipophilicity, potency, and rate of elimination. Barbiturates with long side chains tend to have increased properties in all three areas. However, the observed clinical effects also depend on absorption, redistribution, and the presence or absence of active metabolites. For this reason, the durations of action of barbiturates (like those of benzodiazepines) do not correlate well with their biologic half-lives.

This family of agents can be divided into four categories based on their elimination half-lives (Table 63–2). In contrast to the long-acting barbiturates, the ultrashort-, short-, and intermediate-acting agents tend to be more lipid soluble and more protein bound; have a high pK_a, a more rapid onset, and a shorter duration of action; and are almost completely metabolized in the liver.

After ingestion, barbiturates are preferentially absorbed in the small intestine and are eliminated by hepatic and renal mechanisms. Typically, lipophilic barbiturates are protein bound and have less renal clearance. Renal excretion of unchanged drug can be significant for the long-acting barbiturates. Elimination of phenobarbital, a long-acting barbiturate with a relatively low pK_a (7.24), can be influenced with urinary alkalinization. Alkalinization of the urine with sodium bicarbonate to maintain a urinary pH of 7.5–8.0 can increase the amount of phenobarbital excreted 5–10-fold. This procedure is ineffective for the short-acting barbiturates, as they have higher pK_a values, are more protein bound, and are primarily metabolized by the liver with very little excretion by the kidneys (Chap. 6).

Barbiturates (especially the shorter-acting barbiturates) can accelerate their hepatic inactivation by enzyme autoinduction. Barbiturate use results in a marked increase in the enzyme content of the hepatic smooth endoplasmic reticulum and an increased rate of metabolism for a number of drugs and endogenous substances. Phenobarbital induces various hepatic cytochromes in the P450 system with the greatest effects on CYP3A.[90] A variety of drug interactions are reported following the use of barbiturates. As a result of enzyme induction, clinically significant interactions lead to increases in the metabolism of β-adrenergic antagonists, cortico-

steroids, doxycycline, estrogens, phenothiazines, quinidine, and theophylline. Agents such as valproic acid that compete for these hepatic cytochromes may also decrease phenobarbital metabolism.

Toxicity is manifested initially by slurred speech, ataxia, lethargy, nystagmus, headache, and confusion. As toxicity becomes more severe, the depth of coma increases, and severely poisoned patients may become anesthetized with total loss of neurologic function. Shock may occur as a result of medullary depression, peripheral vasodilation, or impairment of myocardial contractility. Hypothermia and cutaneous bullae are often present.[17,49] Early deaths caused by barbiturate ingestions are a result of respiratory arrest and cardiovascular collapse, while delayed deaths are a result of acute renal failure, pneumonia, pulmonary edema, cerebral edema, and multiorgan system failure.[4,70]

Benzodiazepines

Since the initial introduction of chlordiazepoxide in 1961 for anxiety, and of diazepam for seizure control in 1963,[50] benzodiazepines have become extremely popular. Benzodiazepines are used principally as anxiolytics and sedatives. Temazepam and triazolam are exceptions, and are used as hypnotics to produce sleep; clonazepam is the only benzodiazepine used as a chronic anticonvulsant agent and for the treatment of bipolar disorders. Benzodiazepines may rarely cause paradoxical psychological and CNS effects including nightmares, delirium, toxic psychosis, and transient global amnesia.[18,19,52,118,129] The incidence and intensity of CNS adverse events increases with age.[124]

The benzodiazepines are structurally organic bases with a benzene and a seven-member diazepine moiety. Similar to barbiturates, various side chains at R_1, R_2, R_2', R_3, R_4, and R_7 will influence potency, duration of action, metabolites, and rate of elimination. Benzodiazepines tend to be highly protein bound and lipophilic. They passively diffuse into the CNS, their main site of action. Because of their lipophilic nature, benzodiazepines are extensively metabolized via oxidation and conjugation in the liver prior to their renal elimination. Because they are mainly hepatically metabolized, the rate of elimination may not fluctuate in overdose.[6] Many of the benzodiazepines have active metabolites that are produced in various parts of the body. For example, metabolites of chlorazepate are formed in the gastrointestinal (GI) tract, while metabolites of diazepam are formed primarily in the liver.

A unique property of the benzodiazepine sedative-hypnotics is their relative safety even following substantial ingestion. The relatively safety of benzodiazepines is probably a result of their

GABA-receptor properties.[136] Unlike many other sedative-hypnotic agents, benzodiazepines do not open GABA channels independently at high tissue levels, and they do not result in "receptor desensitization," in which receptors limit their rate of activity in the constant presence of an agonist. Most obtunded patients become arousable within 12–36 hours following a benzodiazepine overdose because of the development of acute tolerance.[151] The duration of coma in elderly patients, however, may be prolonged. Benzodiazepines are not known to cause any specific systemic injury, and their long-term use has not been associated with specific organ toxicity. Deaths caused by benzodiazepine ingestions alone are extremely rare; deaths are usually secondary to combined overdoses.[71,160] Supportive care is the mainstay of treatment.

Tolerance to the sedative effects of the benzodiazepines occurs more rapidly than does tolerance to the antianxiety effects.[110,150] Abrupt withdrawal following long-term use of benzodiazepines may precipitate a benzodiazepine withdrawal syndrome, which can be characterized by changes in perception, paraesthesias, headaches, tremors, and weight loss. Withdrawal from benzodiazepines is common and almost a third of long-term users manifest withdrawal.[94] Alprazolam and lorazepam are associated with more severe withdrawal symptoms and more frequent recurrent symptoms as compared to chlordiazepoxide and diazepam.[94,95] Withdrawal can also occur when a chronic user of a particular benzodiazepine is switched to another benzodiazepine with a different receptor activity.[115]

In acute overdoses, drugs-of-abuse screens are of very limited value as they can have difficulty in identifying benzodiazepines, leading to false-positive and false-negative results.[43,50] Specific plasma concentrations of benzodiazepines also have no use in clinical management.[44]

Chloral Hydrate

Chloral hydrate (2,2,2,-trichloroethane-1,1-diol) belongs to the one of the oldest classes of pharmaceutical hypnotics, the chloral derivatives. This agent was introduced in 1832, and is still commonly used in the pediatric population.

Chloral hydrate is well absorbed, although irritating to the GI tract. It has a wide tissue distribution, rapid onset of action, and rapid hepatic metabolism. Trichloroethanol, the first active metabolite, is lipid soluble and is responsible for the majority of chloral hydrate's hypnotic effects. Chloral hydrate is metabolized by hepatic alcohol dehydrogenase (Fig. 63–1). Trichloroethanol has a plasma half-life of 4–12 hours and is metabolized to inactive trichloroacetic acid by alcohol and aldehyde dehydrogenases. It is then conjugated with glucuronide and excreted by the kidney as urochloralic acid. Less than 10% is excreted unchanged. This mechanism is inefficient in infants and neonates and the elimination half-lives of chloral hydrate and trichloroethanol are markedly increased in children younger than 2 years of age.

Chloral hydrate is currently used as a sedating agent for children prior to medical procedures in controlled situations.[1,112] Several comprehensive studies of clinical and pharmacologic characteristics of chloral hydrate use in neonates and infants suggest that even single-dose administration may result in prolonged chloral hydrate, trichloroethanol, and trichloroacetic acid half-lives.[117,146] This latter metabolite was still detectable at 6 days postadministration. These factors may be of concern in neonates and those infants exposed to repetitive doses.

Acute chloral hydrate poisoning causes other organ system toxicity atypical of the other sedative-hypnotics. Cardiac dysrhythmias appear to be the main cause of death.[68] The compound reduces myocardial contractility, and increases myocardial sensitivity to catecholamines.[23,29,167,179] Specifically, many halogenated hydrocarbons produce nonuniform changes in repolarization throughout the myocardium, predisposing to the development of reentrant circuits. A premature ventricular contraction, as occurs following release or injection of epinephrine, initiates this reentrant rhythm. Thus, persistent cardiac dysrhythmias (ventricular fibrillation, ventricular tachycardia, torsades de pointes) are common terminal events.[68] Standard antidysrhythmic agents are often ineffective. β-Adrenergic antagonists are currently considered the drug of choice for the treatment of most dysrhythmias secondary to chloral hydrate ingestions.[22,23,181] Chloral hydrate can also cause GI toxicity and overdoses can produce nausea, vomiting, hemorrhagic gastritis, and, rarely, gastric and intestinal necrosis, leading to perforation and esophagitis with stricture formation.[102,133,171]

Chloral hydrate is radiopaque and can be detected on radiographs. Few hospital-based laboratories have the capability to rapidly detect chloral hydrate or its metabolites.

Ethchlorvynol

Ethchlorvynol (1-chloro-3-ethyl-penten-4-yl-3-ol) was introduced in 1955 as a substitute for barbiturates. It is rapidly absorbed and lipid soluble. It is primarily hepatically metabolized and has a half-life of 25 hours. However, because of its high lipophilicity, it is readily stored in adipose tissue. Thus, its half-life can exceed 100 hours in overdoses. It is unclear whether its major metabolite, ethynyl 3,4-diol, is active. Stomach contents often reveal a pinkish (500-mg capsules) or greenish (750-mg capsules) tinged content. In addition, because of its volatility, it produces a characteristic pungent plastic or vinyl-like odor on the breath. As a result of its formulation, extraction of the compound and intravenous injection is an alternative route of abuse. Acute pulmonary edema often rapidly occurred following intravenous injection.[36]Symptoms and signs of ethchlorvynol overdoses can resemble barbiturate overdoses. These include prolonged coma, hypothermia, and bullous lesions. These lesions may be scattered and not confined to pressure points, and ethchlorvynol may be found in blister fluid.[58] Prolonged coma is a characteristic of ethchlorvynol poisoning.[165] Although hemodialysis increases the rate of removal of the drug from the plasma, complete plasma clearance during a 4–6-hour hemodialysis has little impact on total body clearance because of the significant lipid solubility and volume of distribution (4 L/kg). Hemoperfusion has been suggested as a better choice than hemodialysis, but either approach is rarely, if ever, indicated.[89]

Glutethimide

Glutethimide (3-ethyl-3-phenyl-2 l-2,6-piperidinedione) was introduced in 1954 as a substitute for barbiturates. It is poorly water-soluble and is slowly and erratically absorbed from the GI tract. Absorption may be significantly enhanced by coingestion of ethanol. Because of its lipophilic nature, it concentrates in fat-containing tissues. It is metabolized in the liver, and more than 14 metabolites have been identified, some of which are biologically active and may contribute to its toxicity.[38] High lipid solubility and delayed absorption may explain the cyclic variation in CNS depression that occurs in acute overdoses. In addition, the enterohepatic circulation of metabolites, especially of 4-hydroxyglutethimide (4-HG), which is more potent than the parent compound, may explain the fluctuating clinical course that occurs in severely intoxicated patients. Other active metabolites include 2-phenylglutarimide and γ-butyrolactone (an analogue of GHB). Profound, prolonged coma with a fluctuating mental status is the hallmark of glutethimide overdose. Unlike many of the other sedative-hypnotic agents, glutethimide can result in diverse anticholinergic symptoms such as dilated pupils.[69] It is also reported to produce thick and tenacious bronchial secretions with impairment of ventilation.[32] Toxic psychosis, seizures, cerebellar ataxia, and peripheral neuropathy are associated with the prolonged use of glutethimide.[32]

Methaqualone

Methaqualone (2-3-disubstituted quinazoline) was introduced in 1956 as another substitute for barbiturates. It has anticonvulsant, anesthetic, antihistaminic, and antispasmodic characteristics. Its effects as a tranquilizer and mood "elevator" have led to extensive abuse and led to its withdrawal from the market. The drug is

rapidly and completely absorbed from the GI tract within 2–3 hours. It is highly protein bound (70–90%), and almost exclusively metabolized in the liver to 4-hydroxymethaqualone, as well as to numerous other hydroxy metabolites.[24,81] Unlike many of the other sedative-hypnotics, hyperreflexia, clonus, and significant muscular hyperactivity can occur. Paresthesias and peripheral neuropathies can be a residual effect following overdose.[2,3]

Methyprylon

Methyprylon (3,3-diethyl-5-methyl-2,4-piperidinedione) was introduced in the 1950s and is used only as a hypnotic. It is rapidly absorbed from the gastrointestinal tract and is almost entirely hepatically metabolized by oxidation and dehydrogenation. Methyprylon is known to stimulate the hepatic microsomal enzyme system, as well as δ-aminolevulinic acid synthetase; therefore, it should be avoided in patients with intermittent porphyria. Because methyprylon is water soluble, hemodialysis has been used in severe cases, but this approach is rarely, if ever, indicated.[35,142]

Meprobamate/Carisoprodol

Meprobamate

Meprobamate (2-methyl-2-*n*-propyl-propane-1,3-diol-dicarbamate) was introduced in 1950 and is used for its muscle-relaxant characteristics. Carisoprodol, which was introduced in 1955, is metabolized to meprobamate. The propanediol carbamates, typified by meprobamate, have pharmacologic effects on the GABA$_A$ receptor similar to those of the barbiturates. They are both rapidly absorbed from the GI tract. The drug is metabolized in the liver to inactive hydroxylated and glucuronidated metabolites that are excreted almost exclusively by the kidney. Of all the nonbarbiturate tranquilizers, meprobamate is the most likely to produce euphoria.[84,85] Large masses or bezoars of pills have been noted in the stomach at autopsy.[156] Thus, in significant meprobamate ingestion, orogastric lavage with a large-bore tube and multiple-dose activated charcoal may be indicated. Whole-bowel irrigation may be helpful if multiple pills or small concretions are noted. Because patients can experience recurrent toxic manifestations as a result of concretion formation and delayed absorption, careful monitoring of the clinical course is essential even following initial improvement.

Bromides

Bromides were previously used as a "nerve tonic" and headache remedy. Although methylated bromides are still extensively used in the fumigation of soil and warehouses, and for fruits and vegetables, pharmaceutical bromides have largely disappeared from the US pharmaceutical market, and acute bromide intoxication is rare in the United States. Cases continue to occur in immigrants and travelers from other countries where bromides are still therapeutically employed. The drug is irritating to the GI tract and it is difficult to ingest and retain a sufficient amount to achieve a toxic level without vomiting. Bromide has a long plasma half-life (12 days) and toxicity typically occurs over a period of time as tissue levels increase. Bromide and chloride ions have a similar distribution pattern in the extracellular fluid. It is postulated that the preferential excretion of chloride results from the bromide ion moving across membranes slightly more rapidly than the chloride ion, with the result that it is more quickly reabsorbed in the renal tubules from the glomerular filtrate than is the chloride ion. Although osmolar equilibrium persists, CNS function is progressively impaired by a poorly understood mechanism, with resulting inappropriateness of behavior, headache, apathy, irritability, confusion, muscle weakness, anorexia, weight loss, thickened speech, psychotic behavior, tremulousness, ataxia, and eventually coma.[30,182] Delusions and hallucinations can occur. Bromide can also lead to hypertension, increased intracranial pressure, and papilledema. The chronic use of bromides can lead to dermatologic changes with the hallmark characteristic of a facial acneiform rash.[75,168] Toxicity with bromides during pregnancy may lead to fetal accumulation of bromide in the fetus.[141] A spurious hyperchloridemia may be found as a result of bromide's interference with the chloride assay (Chap. 24).

Zolpidem

Zolpidem (*N,N*,6-trimethyl-2-*p*-toyl-imidazopyridine-3-acetamide L-(+)-tartrate (2:1)) is an imidazopyridine hypnotic agent. Although zolpidem is structurally unrelated to the benzodiazepines, it binds preferentially to the type I benzodiazepine receptor subtype in the brain, specifically at the α_1 GABA$_A$ subunit.[45] Unlike benzodiazepines that prolong the first two stages of sleep and shorten stages 3 and 4 of rapid eye movement (REM) sleep, zolpidem has little effect on the stages of sleep. Because of its receptor selectivity, there appears to be a minimal effect at other sites on the GABA receptor that mediate anxiolytic, anticonvulsant, or muscle-relaxant effects.[98] It is suggested to have less abuse and addiction potential than benzodiazepines.[172] In overdoses, drowsiness and CNS depression are common, but coma and respiratory depression are exceptionally rare. Even at 40 times the therapeutic

dose, no biologic or electrocardiographic abnormalities have been reported.[62] Flumazenil has been used to reverse the effects of the drug,[105,178] although withdrawal has been documented with abrupt discontinuation.[176]

Deaths have occurred when zolpidem was taken in large amounts with other central nervous system depressants.[62]

Zaleplon

Zaleplon (N3,3 cyanopyrazolo-pyrmidinyl-phenyl-ethylacetamide) is a pyrazolopyrimidine hypnotic agent. In a manner similar to zolpidem, it binds to the α_1 subunit on the GABA$_A$ receptor and has many comparable clinical effects.[74] Although structurally different than benzodiazepines, benzodiazepine sedative properties are demonstrated in animals.[172] Animals given high doses chronically show dependence, and flumazenil can precipitate benzodiazepinelike withdrawal symptoms.[9] There have been no reports of the development of tolerance with zolpidem and zaleplon.[125]

SHORT-TERM ANESTHETIC/ SEDATIVE-HYPNOTICS

Propofol

Propofol (2,6-diisopropylphenol) is a rapidly acting intravenous sedative-hypnotic active at GABA$_A$ receptors. Propofol may also be active presynaptically, causing GABA release[131] and inhibiting dopamine release.[155] It is used for either the induction or maintenance of general anesthesia.

Propofol is highly lipid soluble and therefore crosses the blood-brain barrier rapidly. Onset of anesthesia usually occurs in less than 1 minute with duration of action lasting 3–8 minutes because of its rapid redistribution from the central nervous system.[50]

Propofol causes dose-related respiratory depression, and transient apnea may occur. The drug may also decrease systemic arterial pressure, and may cause myocardial depression. Although propofol typically does not cause dysrhythmias or myocardial ischemia, atropine-sensitive bradydysrhythmias have been noted, specifically sinus bradycardia and Mobitz type I atrioventricular block.[166,175] Prolonged infusions of propofol are associated with fatal fatty myocardial failure in children and young adults.[137] It is also associated with the development of profound lactic acidosis, especially in children.[72]

The unique nature of the carrier base, a milky soybean emulsion formulation, is associated with multiple adverse events. This carrier is a fertile medium for many organisms, such as enterococcal, pseudomonal, staphylococcal, streptococcal, and candidal strains. In 1990, the Centers for Disease Control (CDC) noted an infectious outbreak associated with *Staphylococcus aureus*-contaminated propofol. This carrier base is also associated with hypertriglyceridemia,[51,93,107] abnormalities in blood coagulability and platelet function,[8,40,76] and histamine-mediated anaphylactoid reactions.[47,100,116]

Etomidate

Etomidate is a nonbarbiturate hypnotic agent without analgesic properties that is primarily used as an induction agent. It is believed to be active at the GABA$_A$ receptor. The onset of action is less than 1 minute and its duration is less than 5 minutes. Etomidate has minimal effect on cardiac function, although rare cases of hypotension have been reported.[65–67,164] It has unique proconvulsant and anticonvulsant properties. Involuntary muscle movements are common during induction. This may be caused by etomidate interaction with glycine receptors at the level of the spinal cord.[39,127,128] Etomidate depresses adrenal production of cortisol and aldosterone even after a single dose.[152,173,174] This adverse effect is associated with an increase in mortality with long-term use.[177]

GHB (γ-Hydroxybutyrate)

GHB is a naturally occurring substance produced in mammalian brains. It has been described as a neurotransmitter and a neuromodulator with a four-carbon structure similar to GABA.[31] Medicinally, it has been used as an anesthetic, as a treatment for narcolepsy, and as a treatment for ethanol and opioid withdrawal.[16] GHB has gained popularity as a recreational drug of abuse and for its perception as a muscle-enhancing agent.

Although GHB has been available since the 1960s, its popularity dramatically increased in the 1980s with use by "bodybuilders"

in the belief that GHB use was associated with release of growth hormone. Its use rapidly spread to people seeking its mood-altering and sedative-hypnotic effects. The popularity of this drug also arose at the same time as the popularity of the Internet. Because this is a relatively simple structure that is easily produced, many recipes and sources for supplies developed on the Internet. Obtaining GHBlike compounds, as well as methods for producing these compounds, were readily available, which led to a new wave of drugs of abuse. This drug has been labeled as the "Internet Drug" and "Date Rape Drug."

In the early 1990s, the Food and Drug Administration (FDA) began to restrict the commercial availability of GHB. However, similar to designer amphetamine use of the 1970s and 1980s, chemical analogues to GHB were popularized. Drugs such as γ-butyrolactone (GBL), butanediol, and γ-valerolactone were promoted as alternatives. These were either analogues or precursors of GBH with similar effects and toxicities (Fig. 63–2). However, unlike the designer amphetamines, these analogues did not fall under the Controlled Substance Analogue Enforcement Act (the Designer Drug Law) that prohibits the commercial availability of analogues of illicit or "narcotic" agents.

After ingestion, GHB is rapidly absorbed and quickly crosses the blood-brain barrier. It is not protein bound and is rapidly metabolized and excreted through the lungs.[16] It has specific binding sites and selective brain distribution with the highest concentration in the basal ganglia. It indirectly interacts with GABA$_B$ and opioid receptors.[56,64,82,108] Because it is structurally similar to GABA, it is unclear whether GHB or its metabolites (see Fig. 63–2) possess the greatest activity.[53,73] Within the CNS, it causes increases in growth hormone and blunts central dopamine release. GHB may increase proenkephalin compounds.[153] Clinically, it modulates sleep by increasing slow-wave sleep and promoting REM sleep.[16,113] With larger doses, an anesthetic state occurs with deep

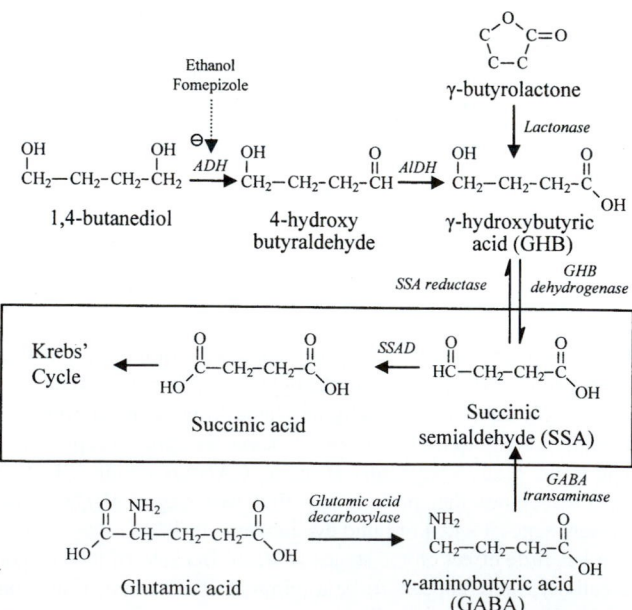

Figure 63–2. The metabolism of analogues and precursors of gamma-amino butyric acid. ADH, Alcohol dehydrogenase; AIDH, Aldehyde Dehydrogenase; SSAD, SSA dehydrogenase.

hypnosis, limited analgesia and amnesia, and no muscle relaxation. A characteristic random myoclonic motion of the extremities and face is often noted.

With its increasing popularity, reports of significant overdoses and death first appeared in the 1990s. Patients usually presented with profound CNS and respiratory depression. In a case series of 88 patients, more than a third of GHB abusers also developed an unexplained bradycardia.[34] However, unlike many other sedative-hypnotics, GHB overdoses were characterized by episodes of combativeness interspersed with episodes of obtundation.[106] Significant arousal and agitation occurred when intubation was attempted.[106] The majority of patients rapidly recover without sequelae with solely supportive care, usually within 6 hours.[34,106]

Although GHB indirectly interacts with opioid and GABA receptors, reversal agents such as naloxone and flumazenil are not consistently effective in arousing patients in the clinical setting,[106] nor animals in the laboratory setting.[42,154] The actual mechanisms whereby flumazenil and naloxone interact with GHB remain unclear. Flumazenil inhibits GHB-induced release of growth hormone and may reverse other effects of GHB, including the anxiolytic and neuromuscular effects.[154] Naloxone blunts the GHB-induced inhibition of central dopamine release.[54,55]

In controlled clinical trials of GBH for narcolepsy, withdrawal has not been documented. However, reports of withdrawal in patients who recreationally use GHB have been documented. Similar to withdrawal from GABAergic agents, anxiety, insomnia, disorientation, and auditory and visual hallucinations are reported.[60,61] However, unlike withdrawal from GABAergic agents, deaths have not been reported.[37]

SUMMARY

Sedative-hypnotics are among the leading causes of deaths caused by poisoning. Patients with sedative-hypnotic overdoses often present with the primary manifestation of CNS depression; however, death is typically a result of respiratory depression. Careful monitoring and supportive care are the cornerstones of treatment. Specific antidotes, such as flumazenil, and treatments, such as hemoperfusion, or hemodialysis, are rarely indicated.

ACKNOWLEDGMENT

Harold Osborn contributed to this chapter in a previous edition.

REFERENCES

1. American Academy of Pediatrics Committee on Drugs and Committee on Environmental Health: Use of chloral hydrate for sedation in children. Pediatrics 1993;92:471–473.
2. Anonymous. Does methaqualone cause neuropathy? Br Med J 1973; 3:307.
3. Abboud RT, Freedman MT, Rogers RM, et al: Methaqualone poisoning with muscular hyperactivity necessitating the use of curare. Chest 1974;65:204–205.
4. Afifi AA, Sacks ST, Liu VY, et al: Accumulative prognostic index for patients with barbiturate, glutethimide and meprobamate intoxication. N Engl J Med 1971;285:1497–1502.
5. Aizawa M, Ito Y, Fukuda H: Pharmacological profiles of generalized absence seizures in lethargic, stargazer and gamma-hydroxybutyrate-treated model mice. Neurosci Res 1997;29:17–25.
6. Allen MD, Greenblatt DJ, LaCasse Y, et al: Pharmacokinetic study of lorazepam overdosage. Am J Psychiatry 1980;137:1414–1415.
7. Allen MD, Greenblatt DJ, Noel BJ: Self-poisoning with over-the-counter hypnotics. Clin Toxicol 1979;15:151–158.
8. Aoki H, Mizobe T, Nozuch S, et al: In vivo and in vitro studies of the inhibitory effect of propofol on human platelet aggregation. Anesthesiology 1998;88:362–370.
9. Ator NA, Weerts EM, Kaminski BJ, et al: Zaleplon and triazolam physical dependence assessed across increasing doses under a once-daily dosing regimen in baboons Drug Alcohol Depend 2000;61: 69–84.
10. Backman JT, Kivisto KT, Olkkola KT, et al: The area under the plasma concentration-time curve for oral midazolam is 400-fold larger during treatment with itraconazole than with rifampicin. Eur J Clin Pharmacol 1998;54:53–58.
11. Banerjee PK, Snead OC 3rd: Presynaptic gamma-hydroxybutyric acid (GHB) and gamma-aminobutyric acid B (GABAB) receptor-mediated release of GABA and glutamate (GLU) in rat thalamic ventrobasal nucleus (VB): A possible mechanism for the generation of absence-like seizures induced by GHB. J Pharmacol Exp Ther 1995;273:1534–1543.
12. Baumann BM, Perrone J, Hornig SE, et al: Randomized, double-blind, placebo-controlled trial of diazepam, nitroglycerin, or both for treatment of patients with potential cocaine-associated acute coronary syndromes. Acad Emerg Med 2000;7:878–885.
13. Belson MG, Simon HK, Sullivan K, et al: The utility of toxicologic analysis in children with suspected ingestions. Pediatr Emerg Care 1999;15:383–387.
14. Berg MJ, Berlinger WG, Goldberg MJ, et al: Acceleration of the body clearance of phenobarbital by oral activated charcoal. N Engl J Med 1982;307:642–644.
15. Berg MJ, Rose JQ, Wurster DE, et al: Effect of charcoal and sorbitol-charcoal suspension on the elimination of intravenous phenobarbital. Ther Drug Monit 1987;9:41–47.
16. Beurdeley-Thomas A, Miccoli L, Oudard S, et al: The peripheral benzodiazepine receptors: A review. J Neurooncol 2000;46:45–56.
17. Beveridge GW: Bullous lesions in poisoning. Br Med J 1971;4: 116–117.
18. Bixler EO, Kales A, Brubaker BH, et al: Adverse reactions to benzodiazepine hypnotics: Spontaneous reporting system. Pharmacology 1987;35:286–300.
19. Boatwright DE: Triazolam, handwriting, and amnestic states: Two cases. J Forensic Sci 1987;32:1118–1124.
20. Boldy DA, Vale JA, Prescott LF: Treatment of phenobarbitone poisoning with repeated oral administration of activated charcoal. Q J Med 1986;61:997–1002.
21. Bormann J: The "ABC" of GABA receptors. Trends Pharmacol Sci 2000;21:16–19.
22. Bowyer K, Glasser, SP: Chloral hydrate overdose and cardiac arrhythmias. Chest 1980;77:232–235.
23. Brown AM, Cade JF: Cardiac arrhythmias after chloral hydrate overdose. Med J Aust 1980;1:28–29.
24. Brown SS, Goenechea S: Methaqualone: Metabolic, kinetic, and clinical pharmacologic observations. Clin Pharmacol Ther 1973;14: 314–324.
25. Bruner KR, Reynolds JN: Propofol modulation of [3H]flunitrazepam binding to GABAA receptors in guinea pig cerebral cortex. Brain Res 1998;806:122–125.
26. Buckley NA, Whyte IM, Dawson AH, et al: Correlations between prescriptions and drugs taken in self-poisoning. Implications for prescribers and drug regulation. Med J Aust 1995;162:194–197.
27. Butterworth RF: The astrocytic ("peripheral-type") benzodiazepine receptor: Role in the pathogenesis of portal-systemic encephalopathy. Neurochem Int 2000;36:411–416.
28. Cai Z, McCaslin PP: Acute, chronic and differential effects of several anesthetic barbiturates on glutamate receptor activation in neuronal culture. Brain Res 1993;611:181–186.

29. Capasso JM, Li PAnversa P: Myocardial mechanics predict hemodynamic performance during normal function and alcohol-induced dysfunction in rats. Am J Physiol 1991;261:H1880–H1888.

30. Carney MW: Five cases of bromism. Lancet 1971;2:523–524.

31. Cash CD: Gamma-hydroxybutyrate: An overview of the pros and cons for it being a neurotransmitter and/or a useful therapeutic agent. Neurosci Biobehav Rev 1994;18:291–304.

32. Chazan JA, Garella S: Glutethimide intoxication. A prospective study of 70 patients treated conservatively without hemodialysis. Arch Intern Med 1971;128:215–219.

33. Chebib M, Johnston GA: The "ABC" of GABA receptors: A brief review. Clin Exp Pharmacol Physiol 1999;26:937–940.

34. Chin RL, Sporer KA, Cullison B, et al: Clinical course of gamma-hydroxybutyrate overdose [see comments]. Ann Emerg Med 1998; 31:716–722.

35. Collins JM: Peritoneal dialysis for methyprylon intoxication [letter]. J Pediatr 1978;92:519–520.

36. Conces D, Kreipke D, Tarver R: Pulmonary edema induced by intravenous ethchlorvynol. Am J Emerg Med 1986;4:549–551.

37. Craig K, Gomez HF, McManus JL, et al: Severe gamma-hydroxybutyrate withdrawal: A case report and literature review. J Emerg Med 2000;18:65–70.

38. Curry SC, Hubbard JM, Gerkin R, et al: Lack of correlation between plasma 4-hydroxyglutethimide and severity of coma in acute glutethimide poisoning. A case report and brief review of the literature. Med Toxicol Adverse Drug Exp 1987;2:309–316.

39. Daniels S, Roberts RJ: Post-synaptic inhibitory mechanisms of anaesthesia—Glycine receptors. Toxicol Lett 1998;100–101:71–76.

40. De La Cruz JP, Paez MV, Carmona JA, et al: Antiplatelet effect of the anaesthetic drug propofol: Influence of red blood cells and leucocytes. Br J Pharmacol 1999;128:1538–1544.

41. Deutsch SI, Mastropaolo J, Hitri A: GABA-active steroids: Endogenous modulators of GABA-gated chloride ion conductance. Clin Neuropharmacol 1992;15:352–364.

42. Devoto P, Colombo G, Cappai F, et al: Naloxone antagonizes ethanol—But not gamma-hydroxybutyrate-induced sleep in mice. Eur J Pharmacol 1994;252:321–324.

43. Divanon F, Debruyne D, Moulin M, et al: Benzodiazepines: Toxic serum concentrations in positive enzyme immunoassay responses. J Anal Toxicol 1998;22:559–566.

44. Divoll M, Greenblatt DJ, Lacasse Y, et al: Benzodiazepine overdosage: Plasma concentrations and clinical outcome. Psychopharmacology 1981;73:381–383.

45. Doble A: New insights into the mechanism of action of hypnotics. J Psychopharmacol 1999;13:S11–S20.

46. Doble A, Benavides J, Ferris O, et al: Dihydropyridine and peripheral type benzodiazepine binding sites: Subcellular distribution and molecular size determination. Eur J Pharmacol 1985;119:153–167.

47. Ducart AR, Watremez C, Louagie YA, et al: Propofol-induced anaphylactoid reaction during anesthesia for cardiac surgery. J Cardiothorac Vasc Anesth 2000;14:200–201.

48. Duncan JS: Positron emission tomography receptor studies. Adv Neurol 1999;79:893–899.

49. Dunn C, Held JL, Spitz J, et al: Coma blisters: Report and review. Cutis 1990;45:423–426.

50. Dunn W: Various laboratory methods screen and confirm benzodiazepines. Emergency Medicine News, December 2000, pp. 21–24.

51. Eddleston JM, Shelly MP: The effect on serum lipid concentrations of a prolonged infusion of propofol—Hypertriglyceridaemia associated with propofol administration. Intensive Care Med 1991;17: 424–426.

52. Einarson TR, Yoder ES: Triazolam psychosis—A syndrome? Drug Intell Clin Pharm 1982;16:330.

53. Feigenbaum JJ, Howard SG: Gamma hydroxybutyrate is not a GABA agonist. Prog Neurobiol 1996;50:1–7.

54. Feigenbaum JJ, Howard SG: Naloxone reverses the inhibitory effect of gamma-hydroxybutyrate on central DA release in vivo in awake animals: A microdialysis study. Neurosci Lett 1997;224:71–74.

55. Feigenbaum JJ, Howard SG: Naloxone reverses the inhibitory effect of gamma-hydroxybutyrate on central DA release in vivo in awake animals: A microdialysis study. Neurosci Lett 1996;218:5–8.

56. Feigenbaum JJ, Simantov R: Lack of effect of gamma-hydroxybutyrate on mu, delta and kappa opioid receptor binding. Neurosci Lett 1996;212:5–8.

57. Finkle BS, McCloskey KL, Goodman LS: Diazepam and drug-associated deaths. A survey in the United States and Canada. JAMA 1979; 242:429–434.

58. Flemenbaum A, Gunby B: Ethchlorvynol (Placidyl) abuse and withdrawal (review of clinical picture and report of 2 cases). Dis Nerv Syst 1971;32:188–192.

59. Fujita M, Woods SW, Verhoeff NP, et al: Changes of benzodiazepine receptors during chronic benzodiazepine administration in humans. Eur J Pharmacol 1999;368:161–172.

60. Galloway GP, Frederick SL, Staggers F Jr: Physical dependence on sodium oxybate [letter]. Lancet 1994;343:357.

61. Galloway GP, Frederick SL, Staggers FE Jr, et al: Gamma-hydroxybutyrate: An emerging drug of abuse that causes physical dependence [see comments]. Addiction 1997;92:89–96.

62. Garnier R, Guerault E, Muzard D, et al: Acute zolpidem poisoning—Analysis of 344 cases. J Toxicol Clin Toxicol 1994;32:391–404.

63. Gavish M, Bachman I, Shoukrun R, et al: Enigma of the peripheral benzodiazepine receptor. Pharmacol Rev 1999;51:629–650.

64. Gerra G, Caccavari R, Fontanesi B, et al: Naloxone and metergoline effects on growth hormone response to gamma-hydroxybutyric acid. Int Clin Psychopharmacol 1995;10:245–250.

65. Gooding JM, Corssen G: Effect of etomidate on the cardiovascular system. Anesth Analg 1977;56:717–719.

66. Gooding JM, Corssen G: Etomidate: An ultrashort-acting nonbarbiturate agent for anesthesia induction. Anesth Analg 1976;55: 286–289.

67. Gooding JM, Weng JT, Smith RA, et al: Cardiovascular and pulmonary responses following etomidate induction of anesthesia in patients with demonstrated cardiac disease. Anesth Analg 1979;58: 40–41.

68. Graham SR, Day RO, Lee R, et al: Overdose with chloral hydrate: A pharmacological and therapeutic review [see comments]. Med J Aust 1988;149:686–688.

69. Greenblatt DJ, Allen MD, Harmatz JS, et al: Correlates of outcome following acute glutethimide overdosage. J Forensic Sci 1979;24: 76–86.

70. Greenblatt DJ, Allen MD, Harmatz JS, et al: Overdosage with pentobarbital and secobarbital: Assessment of factors related to outcome. J Clin Pharmacol 1979;19:758–768.

71. Greenblatt DJ, Allen MD, Noel BJ, et al: Acute overdosage with benzodiazepine derivatives. Clin Pharmacol Ther 1977;21:497–514.

72. Hatch DJ: Propofol-infusion syndrome in children [see comments]. Lancet 1999;353:1117–1118.

73. Hechler V, Ratomponirina C, Maitre M: γ-Hydroxybutyrate conversion into GABA induces displacement of GABAB binding that is blocked by valproate and ethosuximide. J Pharmacol Exp Ther 1997; 281:7537–7560.

74. Heydorn WE: Zaleplon—A review of a novel sedative hypnotic used in the treatment of insomnia. Expert Opin Investig Drugs 2000;9: 841–858.

75. Hezemans-Boer M, Toonstra J, Meulenbel J, et al: Skin lesions due to exposure to methyl bromide. Arch Dermatol 1988;124:917–921.

76. Hirakata H, Nakamura K, Yokubol B, et al: Propofol has both enhancing and suppressing effects on human platelet aggregation in vitro. Anesthesiology 1999;91:1361–1369.

77. Hoehns JD, Perry PJ: Zolpidem: A nonbenzodiazepine hypnotic for treatment of insomnia [published erratum appears in Clin Pharm 1993;12:881] [see comments]. Clin Pharm 1993;12:814–828.

78. Hu XJ, Ticku MK: Chronic benzodiazepine agonist treatment produces functional uncoupling of the gamma-aminobutyric acid-benzodiazepine receptor ionophore complex in cortical neurons. Mol Pharmacol 1994;45:618–625.

79. Humphrey D: Final Exit. Hemlock Society, Denver, CO, 1991.

80. Hutchinson MA, Smith PF, Darlington CL: The behavioural and neuronal effects of the chronic administration of benzodiazepine anxiolytic and hypnotic drugs. Prog Neurobiol 1996;49:73–97.

81. Ionescu-Pioggia M, Bird M, Orzack MH, et al: Methaqualone. Int Clin Psychopharmacol 1988;3:97–109.

82. Ito Y, Ishige K, Zaitsu E, et al: γ-Hydroxybutyric acid increases intracellular Ca^{2+} concentration and nuclear cyclic AMP-responsive element- and activator protein 1 DNA-binding activities through GABAB receptor in cultured cerebellar granule cells. J Neurochem 1995;65:75–83.

83. Jacob MK, White RE: Diazepam, gamma-aminobutyric acid, and progesterone open K(+) channels in myocytes from coronary arteries. Eur J Pharmacol 2000;403:209–219.

84. Jacobsen D, Frederichsen PS, Knutsen KM, et al: Clinical course in acute self-poisonings: A prospective study of 1125 consecutively hospitalised adults. Hum Toxicol 1984;3:107–116.

85. Jacobsen D, Frederichsen PS, Knutsen KM, et al: A prospective study of 1212 cases of acute poisoning: General epidemiology. Hum Toxicol 1984;3:93–106.

86. Jacobsen D, Wiik-Larsen E, Dahl T, et al: Pharmacokinetic evaluation of haemoperfusion in phenobarbital poisoning. Eur J Clin Pharmacol 1984;26:109–112.

87. Jaffe JH, Martin WR: Opioid analgesics and antagonists. In: Gilman AG, Goodman LS, Gilman A, eds: The Pharmacological Basis of Therapeutics. 6th edition. New York, Macmillan, 1980, pp. 513–514.

88. Johanson WG Jr: Massive phenobarbital ingestion with survival. JAMA 1967;202:1106–1107.

89. Kathpalia SC, Haslitt JH, Lim VS: Charcoal hemoperfusion for treatment of ethchlorvynol overdose. Artif Organs 1983;7:246–248.

90. Kemper B: Regulation of cytochrome P450 gene transcription by phenobarbital. Prog Nucleic Acid Res Mol Biol 1998;61:23–64.

91. Kuhlmann AC, Guilarte TR: The peripheral benzodiazepine receptor is a sensitive indicator of domoic acid neurotoxicity. Brain Res 1997;751:281–288.

92. Kuhlmann AC, Guilarte TR: Regional and temporal expression of the peripheral benzodiazepine receptor in MPTP neurotoxicity. Toxicol Sci 1999;48:107–116.

93. Kunst G, Bohrer H: Serum triglyceride levels and propofol infusion. Anaesthesia 1995;50:1101.

94. Lader M: Anxiolytic drugs: Dependence, addiction and abuse. Eur Neuropsychopharmacol 1994;4:85–91.

95. Lader M: Biological processes in benzodiazepine dependence. Addiction 1994;89:1413–1418.

96. Laine GA, Hossain SM, Solis RT, et al: Polyethylene glycol nephrotoxicity secondary to prolonged high-dose intravenous lorazepam. Ann Pharmacother 1995;29:1110–1114.

97. Lallement G, Delamanche IS, Pernot-Marino I, et al: Neuroprotective activity of glutamate receptor antagonists against soman-induced hippocampal damage: Quantification with an omega 3 site ligand. Brain Res 1993;618:227–237.

98. Langtry HD, Benfield P: Zolpidem. A review of its pharmacodynamic and pharmacokinetic properties and therapeutic potential. Drugs 1990;40:291–313.

99. Lavoie J, Layrargues GP, Butterworth RF: Increased densities of peripheral-type benzodiazepine receptors in brain autopsy samples from cirrhotic patients with hepatic encephalopathy. Hepatology 1990;11:874–878.

100. Laxenaire MC, Mata-Bermejo E, Moneret-Vautrin DA, et al: Life-threatening anaphylactoid reactions to propofol (Diprivan). Anesthesiology 1992;77:275–280.

101. Le Fur G, Mestre M, Carriot T, et al: Pharmacology of peripheral type benzodiazepine receptors in the heart. Prog Clin Biol Res 1985;192:175–186.

102. Lee DC, Vassalluzzo C: Acute gastric perforation in a chloral hydrate overdose [letter]. Am J Emerg Med 1998;16:545–546.

103. Leong DK, Le O, Oliva L, et al: Increased densities of binding sites for the "peripheral-type" benzodiazepine receptor ligand [3H]PK11195 in vulnerable regions of the rat brain in thiamine deficiency encephalopathy. J Cereb Blood Flow Metab 1994;14:100–105.

104. Levy ML, Aranda M, Zelman V, et al: Propylene glycol toxicity following continuous etomidate infusion for the control of refractory cerebral edema. Neurosurgery 1995;37:363–369; discussion 369–371.

105. Lheureux P, Debailleul G, De Witte O, et al: Zolpidem intoxication mimicking narcotic overdose: Response to flumazenil. Hum Exp Toxicol 1990;9:105–107.

106. Li J, Stokes SA, Woeckener A: A tale of novel intoxication: seven cases of gamma-hydroxybutyric acid overdose [see comments]. Ann Emerg Med 1998;31:723–728.

107. Lindholm M: Critically ill patients and fat emulsions. Minerva Anestesiol 1992;58:875–879.

108. Lingenhoehl K, Brom R, Heid J, et al: Gamma-hydroxybutyrate is a weak agonist at recombinant GABA(B) receptors. Neuropharmacology 1999;38:1667–673.

109. Lorente P, Lacampagne A, Pouzeratte Y, et al: γ-Aminobutyric acid type B receptors are expressed and functional in mammalian cardiomyocytes. Proc Natl Acad Sci U S A 2000;97:8664–8669.

110. Lucki I, Rickels K: The effect of anxiolytic drugs on memory in anxious subjects. Psychopharmacol Ser 1988;6:128–139.

111. Madden TE, Johnson SW: Gamma-hydroxybutyrate is a GABAB receptor agonist that increases a potassium conductance in rat ventral tegmental dopamine neurons. J Pharmacol Exp Ther 1998;287:261–265.

112. Malis DJ, Burton DM: Safe pediatric outpatient sedation: The chloral hydrate debate revisited. Otolaryngol Head Neck Surg 1997;116:535–537.

113. Mamelak M, Escriu JM, Stokan O: The effects of gamma-hydroxybutyrate on sleep. Biol Psychiatry 1977;12:273–288.

114. Marazziti D, Rotondo A, Martini C, et al: Changes in peripheral benzodiazepine receptors in patients with panic disorder and obsessive-compulsive disorder. Neuropsychobiology 1994;29:8–11.

115. Marks J: Techniques of benzodiazepine withdrawal in clinical practice. A consensus workshop report. Med Toxicol Adverse Drug Exp 1988;3:324–333.

116. Marone G, Stellato C, Mastronardi P, et al: Mechanisms of activation of human mast cells and basophils by general anesthetic drugs. Ann Fr Anesth Reanim 1993;12:116–125.

117. Marti-Bonmati L, Ronchera-Oms CL, Casillas C, et al: Randomised double-blind clinical trial of intermediate- versus high-dose chloral hydrate for neuroimaging of children. Neuroradiology 1995;37:687–691.

118. McKinnon NE: Triazolam intoxication [letter]. Can Med Assoc J 1982;126:893–894.

119. Mehta AK, Ticku MK: An update on GABAA receptors. Brain Res Brain Res Rev 1999;29:196–217.

120. Mestre M, Belin C, Uzan A, et al: Modulation of voltage-operated, but not receptor-operated, calcium channels in the rabbit aorta by PK 11195, an antagonist of peripheral-type benzodiazepine receptors. J Cardiovasc Pharmacol 1986;8:729–734.

121. Mestre M, Bouetard G, Uzan A, et al: PK 11195, an antagonist of peripheral benzodiazepine receptors, reduces ventricular arrhythmias during myocardial ischemia and reperfusion in the dog. Eur J Pharmacol 1985;112:257–260.

122. Mestre M, Carriot T, Belin C, et al: Electrophysiological and pharmacological evidence that peripheral type benzodiazepine receptors are coupled to calcium channels in the heart. Life Sci 1985;36:391–400.

123. Mestre M, Carriot T, Neliat G, et al: PK 11195, an antagonist of peripheral type benzodiazepine receptors, modulates Bay K8644 sensitive but not beta- or H2-receptor sensitive voltage operated calcium channels in the guinea pig heart. Life Sci 1986;39:329–339.

124. Meyer BR: Benzodiazepines in the elderly. Med Clin North Am 1982;66:1017–1035.

125. Mitler MM: Nonselective and selective benzodiazepine receptor agonists—Where are we today? Sleep 2000;23(Suppl 1):S39–S47.

126. Modi NB, Veng-Pedersen P, Wurster DE, et al: Phenobarbital removal characteristics of three brands of activated charcoals: A system analysis approach. Pharm Res 1994;11:318–323.

127. Modica PA, Tempelhoff R, White PF: Pro- and anticonvulsant effects of anesthetics (Part I). Anesth Analg 1990;70:303–315.

128. Modica PA, Tempelhoff R, White PF: Pro- and anticonvulsant effects of anesthetics (Part II). Anesth Analg 1990;70:433–444.

129. Morris HH, dEstes ML: Traveler's amnesia. Transient global amnesia secondary to triazolam. JAMA 1987;258:945–946.

130. Mullins ME: First-degree atrioventricular block in alprazolam overdose reversed by flumazenil. J Pharm Pharmacol 1999;51:367–370.

131. Murugaiah KD, IIcmmings HC Jr: Effects of intravenous general anesthetics on [3H]GABA release from rat cortical synaptosomes. Anesthesiology 1998;89:919–928.

132. Nudmamud S, Siripurkpong P, Chindaduangratana C, et al: Stress, anxiety and peripheral benzodiazepine receptor mRNA levels in human lymphocytes. Life Sci 2000;67:2221–2231.

133. Ogino K, Hobara T, Kobayashi H, et al: Gastric mucosal injury induced by chloral hydrate. Toxicol Lett 1990;52:129–133.

134. Olkkola KT, Backman JT, Neuvonen PJ: Midazolam should be avoided in patients receiving the systemic antimycotics ketoconazole or itraconazole. Clin Pharmacol Ther 1994;55:481–485.

135. Olson JM, Ciliax BJ, Mancini WR, et al: Presence of peripheral-type benzodiazepine binding sites on human erythrocyte membranes. Eur J Pharmacol 1988;152:47–53.

136. Orser BA, McAdam LC, Roder S, et al: General anaesthetics and their effects on GABA(A) receptor desensitization. Toxicol Lett 1998;100–101:217–224.

137. Parke TJ, Stevens JE, Rice AS, et al: Metabolic acidosis and fatal myocardial failure after propofol infusion in children: Five case reports [see comments]. BMJ 1992;305:613–616.

138. Patel PM, Goskowicz RL, Drummond JC, et al: Etomidate reduces ischemia-induced glutamate release in the hippocampus in rats subjected to incomplete forebrain ischemia. Anesth Analg 1995;80:933–939.

139. Pavese N, Giannaccini G, Betti L, et al: Peripheral-type benzodiazepine receptors in human blood cells of patients affected by migraine without aura. Neurochem Int 2000;37:363–368.

140. Peoples RW, Weight FF: Trichloroethanol potentiation of gamma-aminobutyric acid-activated chloride current in mouse hippocampal neurones. Br J Pharmacol 1994;113:555–563.

141. Pleasure JR, Blackburn MG: Neonatal bromide intoxication: Prenatal ingestion of a large quantity of bromides with transplacental accumulation in the fetus. Pediatrics 1975;55:503–506.

142. Polin RA, Henry D, Pippinger CE: Peritoneal dialysis for severe methyprylon intoxication. J Pediatr 1977;90:831–833.

143. Pond SM, Olson KR, Osterloh JD, et al: Randomized study of the treatment of phenobarbital overdose with repeated doses of activated charcoal. JAMA 1984;251:3104–3108.

144. Potokar J, Coupland N, Wilson S, et al: Assessment of GABA(A) benzodiazepine receptor (GBzR) sensitivity in patients on benzodiazepines. Psychopharmacology (Berl) 1999;146:180–184.

145. Reed MD, Blumer JL: Propofol bashing: The time to stop is now! Crit Care Med 1996;24:175–176.

146. Reimche LD, Sankaran K, Hindmarsh KW, et al: Chloral hydrate sedation in neonates and infants—Clinical and pharmacologic considerations. Dev Pharmacol Ther 1989;12:57–64.

147. Reynolds C: Alternatives to barbiturates. Oral Health 1966;56:253.

148. Reynolds HN, Teiken P, Regan ME, et al: Hyperlactatemia, increased osmolar gap, and renal dysfunction during continuous lorazepam infusion. Crit Care Med 2000;28:1631–1634.

149. Reynolds JN, Maitra R: Propofol and flurazepam act synergistically to potentiate GABAA receptor activation in human recombinant receptors. Eur J Pharmacol 1996;314:151–156.

150. Rickels K, Schweizer E, Csanalosi I, et al: Long-term treatment of anxiety and risk of withdrawal. Prospective comparison of clorazepate and buspirone. Arch Gen Psychiatry 1988;45:444–450.

151. Robins AH: The other side of the benzodiazepines. S Afr Cont Med Educ 1984;2:43–48.

152. Schenarts CL, Burton JH, Riker RR: Adrenocortical dysfunction following etomidate induction in emergency department patients. Acad Emerg Med 2001;8:1–7.

153. Schmidt-Mutter C, Gobaille S, Muller C, et al: Prodynorphin and proenkephalin mRNAs are increased in rat brain after acute and chronic administration of gamma-hydroxybutyrate. Neurosci Lett 1999;262:65–68.

154. Schmidt-Mutter C, Pain L, Sandner G, et al: The anxiolytic effect of gamma-hydroxybutyrate in the elevated plus maze is reversed by the benzodiazepine receptor antagonist, flumazenil. Eur J Pharmacol 1998;342:21–27.

155. Schulte D, Callado LF, Davidson C, et al: Propofol decreases stimulated dopamine release in the rat nucleus accumbens by a mechanism independent of dopamine D2, GABAA and NMDA receptors. Br J Anaesth 2000;84:250–253.

156. Schwartz HS: Acute meprobamate poisoning with gastrotomy and removal of a drug-containing mass. N Engl J Med 1976;295:1177–1178.

157. Scott DF: Alternatives to barbiturate hypnotics [letter]. Br Med J 1976;2:301.

158. Sellers EM, Carr G, Bernstein JG, et al: Interaction of chloral hydrate and ethanol in man. II. Hemodynamics and performance. Clin Pharmacol Ther 1972;13:50–58.

159. Sellers EM, Lang M, Koch-Weser J, et al: Interaction of chloral hydrate and ethanol in man. I. Metabolism. Clin Pharmacol Ther 1972;13:37–49.

160. Serfaty M, Masterton G: Fatal poisonings attributed to benzodiazepines in Britain during the 1980s [see comments]. Br J Psychiatry 1993;163:386–393.

161. Sivilotti L, Nistri A: GABA receptor mechanisms in the central nervous system. Prog Neurobiol 1991;36:35–92.

162. Smith PF, Darlington CL: The behavioural effects of long-term use of benzodiazepine sedative and hypnotic drugs: What can be learned from animal studies? N Z J Psychology 1994;23:48–63.

163. Snead OCD, Nichols AC, Liu CC: γ-Hydroxybutyric acid binding sites: Interaction with the GABA-benzodiazepine-picrotoxin receptor complex. Neurochem Res 1992;17:201–204.

164. Stowe DF, Bosnjak ZJ, Kampine JP: Comparison of etomidate, ketamine, midazolam, propofol, and thiopental on function and metabolism of isolated hearts. Anesth Analg 1992;74:547–558.

165. Teehan BP, Maher JF, Carey JJ, et al: Acute ethchlorvynol (Placidyl) intoxication. Ann Intern Med 1970;72:875–882.

166. Tramer MR, Moore RA, McQuay HJ: Propofol and bradycardia: Causation, frequency and severity. Br J Anaesth 1997;78:642–651.

167. Trulson ME, Ulissey MJ: Acute administration of chloral hydrate depletes cardiac enzymes in the rat. Acta Anat 1987;129:270–274.

168. Trump DL, Hochberg MC: Bromide intoxication. Johns Hopkins Med J 1976;138:119–123.

169. Uchida I, Li L,Yang, J: The role of the GABA(A) receptor alpha₁ subunit N-terminal extracellular domain in propofol potentiation of chloride current. Neuropharmacology 1997;36:1611–1621.

170. Veerman M, Espejo MG, Christopher MA, et al: Use of activated charcoal to reduce elevated serum phenobarbital concentration in a neonate. J Toxicol Clin Toxicol 1991;29:53–58.

171. Veller ID, Richardson JP, Doyle JC, et al: Gastric necrosis: A rare complication of chloral hydrate intoxication. Br J Surg 1972;59:317–319.

172. Wagner J, Wagner ML, Hening WA: Beyond benzodiazepines: Alternative pharmacologic agents for the treatment of insomnia. Ann Pharmacother 1998;32:680–691.

173. Wagner RL, White PF: Etomidate inhibits adrenocortical function in surgical patients. Anesthesiology 1984;61:647–651.

174. Wagner RL, White PF, Kan PB, et al: Inhibition of adrenal steroidogenesis by the anesthetic etomidate. N Engl J Med 1984;310: 1415–1421.

175. Warden JC, Pickford DR: Fatal cardiovascular collapse following propofol induction in high-risk patients and dilemmas in the selection of a short-acting induction agent [see comments]. Anaesth Intensive Care 1995;23:485–487.

176. Watsky E: Management of zolpidem withdrawal [letter]. J Clin Psychopharmacol 1996;16:459.

177. Watt I, Ledingham IM: Mortality amongst multiple trauma patients admitted to an intensive therapy unit. Anaesthesia 1984;39:973–981.

178. Wesensten NJ, Balkin TJ, Davis HQ, et al: Reversal of triazolam- and zolpidem-induced memory impairment by flumazenil. Psychopharmacology (Berl) 1995;121:242–249.

179. White JF, Carlson GP: Epinephrine-induced cardiac arrhythmias in rabbits exposed to trichloroethylene: Role of trichloroethylene metabolites. Toxicol Appl Pharmacol 1981;60:458–465.

180. Wiley CC, Wiley JF 2nd: Pediatric benzodiazepine ingestion resulting in hospitalization. J Toxicol Clin Toxicol 1998;36:227–231.

181. Zahedi A, Grant MH, Wong DT: Successful treatment of chloral hydrate cardiac toxicity with propranolol. Am J Emerg Med 1999;17: 490–491.

182. Zatuchni J, Hong K: Methyl bromide poisoning seen initially as psychosis. Arch Neurol 1981;38:529–530.

183. Zavala F: Benzodiazepines, anxiety, and immunity. Pharmacol Ther 1997;75:199–216.

184. Zhu H, Cottrell JE, Kass IS: The effect of thiopental and propofol on NMDA- and AMPA-mediated glutamate excitotoxicity. Anesthesiology 1997;87:944–951.

ANTIDOTES IN DEPTH

Flumazenil

Diazepam

Midazolam

Flumazenil
Mary Ann Howland

Flumazenil is a competitive benzodiazepine antagonist. It has no role in the unknown overdose because seizures and dysrhythmias may occur when the effects of a benzodiazepine are reversed in a mixed overdose. Flumazenil has the potential to induce benzodiazepine withdrawal symptoms, including seizures in patients who are benzodiazepine tolerant. Flumazenil does not reverse the respiratory depression induced by intravenous benzodiazepines, but does reverse the central nervous system (CNS) depression. Flumazenil is ideal for the few patients who are naïve to benzodiazepine and who overdose solely on a benzodiazepine. Because the duration of effect of flumazenil is shorter than that of most benzodiazepines, repeat doses may be necessary and vigilance is warranted. Flumazenil has no role in the management of ethanol intoxication and its role in the treatment of hepatic encephalopathy is under study. Recent case reports raise the possibility of a role for flumazenil for patients with paradoxical reactions to therapeutic doses of midazolam. Flumazenil is not expected to be effective in overdoses such as baclofen in which a benzodiazepine receptor is not involved.[9] However, it is effective for overdoses of zolpidem, an imidazopyridine derivative that interacts with ω_1 receptors, a subclass of central benzodiazepine receptors.[32,41]

HISTORY

Haefely and Hunkeler's initial work on synthesis of chlordiazepoxide led to an attempt to develop benzodiazepine derivatives that would act as antagonists.[23] This endeavor was initially unsuccessful, so they investigated the promising γ-aminobutyric acid (GABA) hypothesis of benzodiazepine mechanism of action. In 1977, the then-new technique of radioligand binding identified specific high-affinity benzodiazepine binding sites. Other investigators had simultaneously isolated a product produced by a *Streptomyces* species that had the basic 1,4-benzodiazepine structure; subsequently, synthetic compounds were derived from this mole-cule to act as potential tranquilizers. Hunkeler attempted to produce benzodiazepines with potent anxiolytic and anticonvulsant activity and diminished sedative and muscle-relaxing properties. Testing revealed that these derivatives had high in vitro binding affinities but lacked in vivo activity. An inability to enter the central nervous system was considered as an explanation for this discordance. During an experiment that attempted to demonstrate CNS penetration for these derivatives, it was noted that when diazepam was given to incapacitate the animals it surprisingly had a very weak effect. This lack of potency led to the discovery of a benzodiazepine antagonist. Further modifications led to the synthesis of RO-15–1788, flumazenil.

PHARMACOLOGY

Flumazenil is a water-soluble benzodiazepine analogue with a molecular weight of 303 daltons. It is a competitive antagonist with very weak agonist properties at the benzodiazepine receptor. The benzodiazepine receptor modulates the effect of GABA on the $GABA_A$ receptor by increasing the frequency of opening of the Cl channel, leading to hyperpolarization. Agonists such as diazepam stimulate the benzodiazepine receptor to produce anxiolytic, anticonvulsant, sedative, amnestic, and muscle-relaxant effects at low doses and hypnosis at high doses. Inverse agonists stimulate the benzodiazepine receptor and result in the opposite effects: anxiety, agitation, and seizures. Antagonists, such as flumazenil, competitively occupy the benzodiazepine receptor without causing any functional change and without allowing an agonist or inverse agonist access to the receptor. It has been suggested that the zero set point of intrinsic activity may be influenced by the activity of the GABA system or by chronic treatment with benzodiazepines.[18] Positron emission tomography (PET) investigations reveal that 1.5 mg of flumazenil leads to an initial receptor occupancy of 55%, whereas 15 mg causes almost total blockade of benzodiazepine receptor sites.[45]

The structures of flumazenil, diazepam, and midazolam are shown in the figure. Table 63–4 summarizes the physiochemical and pharmacokinetic properties of flumazenil.[28]

TABLE 63–4. Physicochemical and Pharmacologic Properties of Flumazenil

pK_a	Weak base
Partition coefficient at pH 7.4	14 (octanol/aqueous PO$_4$ buffer)
Volume of distribution	1.06 L/kg
Distribution half-life (t$_{1/2}\alpha$)	≤5 minutes
Metabolism	Hepatic: three inactive metabolites
	High clearance
Elimination	First order
Protein binding	54–64%
Half-life (t$_{1/2}\beta$)	53 minutes
Onset of action	1–2 minutes
Duration of action	Dependent on dose and elimination of benzodiazepine, time interval, dose of flumazenil, and hepatic function

Volunteer Studies

Volunteer studies demonstrate flumazenil's ability to reverse the effect of benzodiazepines.[13] Reversal is both immediate and dose dependent. Most individuals achieve complete reversal of benzodiazepine effect with a total IV dose of 1 mg.[1,8] A 3-mg IV dose produces similar effects that last approximately twice as long as the 1-mg dose.

Conscious Sedation

There are a number of studies evaluating patients undergoing conscious sedation for endoscopy or cardioversion who received diazepam or midazolam.[2,7,8,30,31] When a benzodiazepine is given to achieve conscious sedation during a procedure, flumazenil appears safe and effective in the reversal of sedation and the partial reversal of amnesia. Most patients respond to doses of 0.6–1 mg. Administering flumazenil slowly, at a rate of 0.1 mg/min, minimizes the disconcerting symptoms associated with rapid arousal, such as confusion, agitation, and emotional lability. Resedation occurs within 20–120 minutes, depending on the dose and pharmacokinetics of the benzodiazepine, as well as the dose of flumazenil. For this reason, patients must be carefully monitored, and subsequent doses of flumazenil given as needed. Because the amnestic effect of benzodiazepines is not consistently reversed, posttreatment instructions should be reinforced in writing and given to a responsible caretaker accompanying the patient.[12] Because of the risk of resedation, many endoscopists elect not to use flumazenil.

There are two case reports of patients undergoing endoscopy who developed seizures following benzodiazepine reversal.[48] One patient had a history of seizures and the other had no obvious etiology. Both recovered uneventfully.

Use for Paradoxical Reaction to Midazolam

Paradoxical reactions to benzodiazepines are uncommon.[20,37] The mechanism is unclear and has been attributed to a disinhibition reaction akin to ethanol intoxication or a perceived threat to oversedation with a protective response.[17] Management strategies include administering higher doses of the benzodiazepines, adding other agents such as opioids or droperidol, stopping the procedure, or using flumazenil.[27,43,49,50] Three patients undergoing endoscopy were premedicated with meperidine, droperidol, and midazolam in doses up to 10 mg.[17] Each patient exhibited paradoxical agitation and restlessness. Following flumazenil 0.5 mg IV the patients became calm and sedated, allowing successful completion of endoscopy. A satisfactory explanation has not been established.

Effects on Benzodiazepine-Induced Respiratory Depression

Flumazenil has not consistently reversed benzodiazepine-induced respiratory depression.[46] If respiratory depression is mediated through the benzodiazepine receptor, then flumazenil should be effective as a reversal agent, but this effect does not occur consistently.[10,21,35,39,46] Using oxygen saturation measurements and plethysmography to determine minute ventilation volumes, the effect of IV midazolam on respiratory depression was examined in patients undergoing endoscopy.[10] Flumazenil awakened patients rapidly but failed to affect minute ventilation and had little effect on oxygen saturation. When a benzodiazepine was used concomitantly with an opioid, the effects on ventilation were even more confusing.[54,56] Rebound respiratory depression and prolonged hypoxic episodes were documented. It is suggested that flumazenil may even have a slight respiratory depressant effect when combined with an opioid.[54] Clinical assessment of respiratory rate is inadequate to detect hypoxia. Benzodiazepine-induced apnea should be managed with fundamental procedures such as supplemental oxygen, airway stabilization, bag-valve mask ventilation, and endotracheal intubation, if indicated.

Use in the Overdose Setting

The use of flumazenil in the overdose setting has provoked substantial controversy. The first argument against its use is that benzodiazepines rarely cause morbidity and mortality. An analysis of 702 patients admitted to a medical intensive care unit (ICU) over a 14-year time period, who had taken benzodiazepines alone or in combination with ethanol or other drugs, resulted in 5 fatalities (0.7%) and 69 patients (9.8%) experienced complications.[26] By comparison, the fatality rate was 1.6% (55 of 3430) for patients with nonbenzodiazepine-related overdoses. In the pure benzodiazepine group, 2 patients died and 18 of 144 patients (12.5%) had complications, mostly aspiration pneumonitis and decubitus ulcers. Proponents of flumazenil therapy suggest that some of the 29 diagnostic procedures used in these patients would have been unnecessary, and possibly some of the complications that occurred could have been avoided. Opponents of flumazenil suggest that many of the cases of aspiration pneumonitis occurred prior to hospital admission and that these patients also often suffer from trauma and infectious disease, making most diagnostic procedures necessary in any event.

In an effort to develop indications for the safe and effective use of flumazenil, overdosed comatose patients were retrospectively assigned to either a low-risk or non-low-risk group.[22] Low-risk patients had CNS depression with normal vital signs, no other neurologic findings, no evidence of ingestion of a tricyclic antidepressant by history or electrocardiogram (ECG), no seizure history, and absence of an available history of chronic benzodiazepine ingestion. All other patients fell into the non-low-risk category. Of 35 consecutive comatose patients, 4 patients were assigned to the low-risk group. Flumazenil caused complete awakening in 3 patients, and partial awakening in the fourth patient, in the low-risk group with no adverse effects. In the non-low-risk group of 31 patients, flumazenil caused complete awakening in 4 patients, and partial awakening in 5 patients. Seizures occurred in 5 patients. Of the 5 patients with seizures, 1 had a history of seizures, all 5 were long-term benzodiazepine users, 4 had abnormal vital signs, and 3 had evidence of hyperreflexia or myoclonus. Therefore, although the use of flumazenil was safe and effective in the low-risk group, unfortunately very few patients met the criteria for inclusion in that risk group. The risk of seizures is substantial in the non-low-risk group.

In conclusion, the benefit of flumazenil appears to outweigh the risks in those patients for whom benzodiazepines are used therapeutically to perform a diagnostic or therapeutic procedure. When benzodiazepines are ingested alone in the overdose setting by non-benzodiazepine-dependent patients, as very rarely occurs in adults but might be expected in children, the risks associated with the use of flumazenil may be limited. Table 63–5 summarizes the indications for flumazenil in the overdose setting.

Adverse Effects and Safety Issues

Flumazenil has been studied in more than 3500 patients worldwide, including healthy volunteers and overdosed or consciously sedated patients. Its safety in healthy volunteers is well established, with no discernible objective or subjective effects.

The ability of flumazenil to precipitate acute benzodiazepine withdrawal seizures in a more controlled setting than the overdose setting was demonstrated by the reversal of long-term benzodiazepine sedation in the ICU. A study involving 1700 patients revealed that 14 patients developed adverse drug reactions with perhaps half related to abrupt arousal.[2] Two patients with a history of epilepsy developed tonic-clonic seizures and one patient developed myoclonic seizures.[2] A dose dependency toward inducing withdrawal reactions has been suggested. It may be that small doses of flumazenil (<1 mg) allow enough of the benzodiazepine receptor sites to be occupied with benzodiazepine so that abrupt withdrawal seizures are uncommon.

A study of 12 patients receiving midazolam sedation for 4 ± 3 days were administered 0.5 mg flumazenil as a rapid bolus. Norepinephrine and epinephrine plasma concentrations rose within 10 minutes, returned to baseline within 30 minutes, and correlated with an increase in heart rate, blood pressure, and myocardial oxygen consumption.[29]

Flumazenil causes a significant overshoot in cerebral blood flow and may cause a large increase in intracranial pressure in patients previously receiving midazolam for severe head injury.[60]

A review of 30 published case studies involving a total of 758 patients with drug overdoses was performed.[19] Three hundred eighty-seven patients were in double-blind study protocols and 371 patients were in open-label studies.[19] Fifty percent of cases were mixed overdoses. The doses of flumazenil utilized were from 0.2–5 mg. In all, there were 5 cases of seizures temporally related to flumazenil administration, all occurring after large bolus doses. Furthermore, in 3 of these 5 patients, tricyclic antidepressants were present in high concentrations in the blood. All of the seizures resolved without treatment or following administration of

a small dose of a benzodiazepine. In 2 patients given small doses of flumazenil, dysrhythmias developed, both presumed to be associated with the presence of an antidepressant. Of 497 patients enrolled in two clinical US studies sponsored by the manufacturer,[19] 6 patients developed seizures (5 had coingested tricyclic antidepressants) and 1 patient who had taken a tricyclic antidepressant and carbamazepine had a junctional tachycardia, which normalized after several minutes. Thus, in reviewing 1255 patients, 11 patients had seizures and 3 developed dysrhythmias, for an incidence of about 0.9%. The consensus of this group of authors was that (a) flumazenil is not a substitute for primary emergency care; (b) hypoxia and hypotension should be corrected before flumazenil is used; (c) small titrated doses of flumazenil should be used; (d) flumazenil should be avoided in patients with a history of seizures, evidence of seizures or jerking movements, or evidence of a cyclic antidepressant overdose; and (e) flumazenil should not be used by inexperienced clinicians.

An analysis of all seizures associated with flumazenil gathered from published cases or those reported to the manufacturer was published.[48] The total number of patients making up the denominator was approximately 3500. Forty-three patients seized and 6 patients died, but the author believed that none of the deaths were attributable to flumazenil.[48] Four patients developed status epilepticus; 2 of these were presumed to be caused by concomitant tricyclic antidepressant exposure, and the other 2 patients had received benzodiazepines to treat status epilepticus prior to flumazenil therapy. In 6 of 43 episodes of seizures, the relationship to flumazenil use was felt to be inadequately defined. The remaining 37 patients were stratified into five categories. In category 1, 7 patients were given flumazenil after they had received a benzodiazepine for treatment of a seizure disorder. Six of these 7 patients received more than 1 mg of flumazenil. In category 2, 20 patients received flumazenil for reversal of a benzodiazepine in a mixed-drug overdose. Many of these patients were shown to have coingested tricyclic antidepressants. Thirteen of these patients received more than 1 mg of flumazenil. Two of the patients in this group developed status epilepticus and died, possibly secondary to a severe tricyclic antidepressant overdose. Category 3 included 5 patients receiving benzodiazepines for suppression of non-drug-induced seizures. Two of these 5 patients received doses of flumazenil greater than 1 mg. Category 4 included 3 patients with acute benzodiazepine overdoses, in the presence of chronic benzodiazepine dependence. Category 5 included 2 patients receiving a benzodiazepine for conscious sedation. Therefore, the use of flumazenil may put the patient at risk for seizures by unmasking a toxic effect in mixed overdose, by removing the protective anticonvulsant effect in a patient with non-drug-induced seizures, or by precipitating acute benzodiazepine withdrawal.

The risks of flumazenil appear to greatly outweigh the potential benefits of reversal when benzodiazepines are used chronically or acutely to treat a seizure disorder. Flumazenil is best avoided in the overdose setting when there is evidence that a drug capable of causing seizures or dysrhythmias has been ingested. Any indication that theophylline, carbamazepine, chloral hydrate, chloroquine, and/or chlorinated hydrocarbons have been ingested is a contraindication to the use of flumazenil.[57] When there is a suggestion, based on history, clinical findings, or ECG findings (increased QRS, increased QT, or increased heart rate), that a cyclic antidepressant is involved, flumazenil should not be utilized.[25,34,40,57] In the event of flumazenil-induced seizures, a thera-

TABLE 63–5. Indications for Flumazenil in the Overdose Setting

Pure benzodiazepine overdose in a nontolerant individual who has:
- CNS depression
- Normal vital signs, including S_AO_2
- Normal ECG
- Otherwise normal neurologic examination

peutic dose of a benzodiazepine such as diazepam should be effective. Flumazenil is a competitive antagonist; higher doses of benzodiazepines will reverse higher doses of flumazenil. Table 63–6 summarizes the contraindications to the use of flumazenil.

Dosing

Slow IV titration (0.1 mg/min) to a total dose ≤1 mg seems most reasonable. Extravasation should be avoided because of the risk of local irritation. Resedation may occur at 20–120 minutes, and it may be necessary to readminister flumazenil. Although not FDA approved, a continuous intravenous infusion in saline or dextrose of 0.1–1.0 mg/h has been employed following the loading dose.[32,58,59]

Availability

Flumazenil is available as Romazicon in a concentration of 1 mg/mL.

FLUMAZENIL'S ROLE IN HEPATIC ENCEPHALOPATHY

Hepatic encephalopathy is considered to be a reversible metabolic encephalopathy characterized by a spectrum of CNS effects. Symptoms may progress from confusion and somnolence to coma. The current hypothesis implicates an increase in GABAergic tone in the development of encephalopathy.[5,47]

Animal studies of hepatic encephalopathy secondary to galactosamine or thioacetamide (hepatotoxins) demonstrate an increase in GABA effect, which is antagonized by flumazenil, bicuculline (a GABA-receptor antagonist), and isopropylbiclophosphate chloride (a calcium channel blocker).[6] Cerebrospinal fluid (CSF) from these animals contained a benzodiazepine receptor ligand with agonist activity. Rat studies involving hepatic encephalopathy resulting from acute liver ischemia showed only a slight response to flumazenil but significant improvement after administration of a partial inverse agonist.[6,55]

Human studies have also detected benzodiazepine-binding activity in the CSF, but not serum, of patients with hepatic encephalopathy. One group identified 4–19 peaks representing benzodiazepine-binding ligands from the frontal cortex of 11 patients who died of hepatic encephalopathy.[4] Two of the peaks were identified as diazepam and N-desmethyldiazepam. Six of the patients demonstrated brain concentrations of these substances that were 2–10 times higher than normal, and five patients had normal concentrations. There are several reports of patients with idiopathic recurring stupor who have measurable "endozepines" (endogenous benzodiazepine ligands) in serum and CSF.[44,52]

TABLE 63–6. Contraindications to the Use of Flumazenil

- Prior seizure history or current treatment of seizures
- History of ingestion of substance capable of provoking seizures or cardiac dysrhythmias
- Long-term use of benzodiazepines
- ECG evidence (terminal rightward 40 msec axis, QRS or QT prolongation) of cyclic antidepressants
- Abnormal vital signs; hypoxia

Flumazenil improves the clinical and electrophysiologic responses of patients with hepatic encephalopathy and idiopathic recurring stupor.[14,16,44,52] Some patients with encephalopathy have improved from stage IV to stage II encephalopathy after IV flumazenil. Maximal improvement after flumazenil lasts about 1–2 hours, and gradually dissipates within 6 hours. The response rate in case series averages approximately 65%. Not all patients respond, and the proposed explanations for this unresponsiveness include cerebral edema, hypoxia, other systemic diseases or complications, and irreversible CNS damage.

Animal and human data convincingly support the concept that increased GABAergic tone is responsible for hepatic encephalopathy. Evidence for endogenous benzodiazepine ligands that enhance GABA action has also been demonstrated. The source of these benzodiazepine receptor agonists is unclear, but diet and/or production by gut bacteria have been postulated.[5] Most authorities believe endogenous de novo synthesis to be unlikely. Flumazenil can lead to improvement in the clinical condition of a subgroup of patients with hepatic encephalopathy and may prove useful as an addition to conventional therapy.[3] Additional research is necessary to identify prospective responders, dosing considerations, and adverse effects.

FLUMAZENIL'S ROLE IN ETHANOL INTOXICATION

A number of animal studies indicate that many of the actions of ethanol are mediated through GABA neurotransmission.[51] Acute ethanol administration appears to enhance GABA transmission and inhibit N-methyl-D-aspartate (NMDA) excitation. Chronic ethanol administration leads to a down-regulation of the GABA system. Ethanol enhances $GABA_A$-induced chloride influx in a dose-dependent fashion without a direct effect on chloride. Flumazenil does not influence this action of GABA. Chronic ethanol use selectively increases the sensitivity to inverse benzodiazepine agonists, invoking a change in coupling or conformation of the receptor. These changes may explain the development of tolerance and the kindling and production of seizures that occur on withdrawal.

Two double-blind studies in patients with benzodiazepine or ethanol overdose evaluated the response to flumazenil. In one study involving 13 patients with suspected ethanol intoxication, 6 had no response to placebo when it was given first, while all 13 patients responded to 5 mg of flumazenil.[38] Improved consciousness occurred after 15 minutes and respiratory rates increased from 14 to 16 breaths/min. There was no effect on heart rate or blood pressure. This 5-mg dose of flumazenil was chosen because when 4 patients were studied with 1 mg of flumazenil, there was no improvement in mental status or vital signs.

Another comparable study demonstrated similar results.[33] One milligram of flumazenil administered to 9 ethanol-intoxicated patients produced the same effects as placebo. Subsequent administration of 2–5 mg of flumazenil in the open part of the study produced a clear improvement in the modified Glasgow coma scale in 5 of 11 patients. However, a closer inspection of phase 1 of this study reveals that an arousal reaction occurred in 7 of 9 patients after the flumazenil dose and in 5 of 9 patients following placebo administration. It is conceivable that the improvement in phase 2 was a continuation of this arousal reaction.

One case report indicates that ethanol-induced respiratory depression was reversed by flumazenil.[36] However, it is unclear whether the actual data support the authors' conclusions.

A randomized double-blind crossover study was conducted with eight male volunteers given IV ethanol to achieve a constant blood ethanol concentration of 160 mg/dL.[11] Once stabilized, the volunteers were given either placebo or 5 mg of flumazenil. A number of subjective and objective psychomotor tests were conducted, with no differences noted between volunteers given flumazenil and those volunteers given placebo. The probability of ethanol reversal at the suggested doses appears unlikely.

On the basis of this information it is unlikely that flumazenil has a significant effect on ethanol intoxication. Low doses of flumazenil (<1 mg) have had no effect, and doses of 5 mg are reported to produce favorable changes in sensorium, but these findings may be the result of confounding factors. Because we would never recommend 5 mg of flumazenil in the overdose setting because of the increased risk of adverse effects at this dose, flumazenil cannot be recommended to treat ethanol intoxication.

REFERENCES

1. Amrein R, Hetzel W, Hartmann D, Lorscheid T: Clinical pharmacology of flumazenil. Eur J Anaesth 1988;2:65–80.
2. Amrein R, Leishman B, Bentzinger C, Roncari G: Flumazenil in benzodiazepine antagonism: Actions and clinical use in intoxications and anaesthesiology. Med Toxicol 1987;2:411–429.
3. Barbaro G, Di Lorenzo G, Soldini M, et al: Flumazenil for hepatic encephalopathy grade III and IVa in patients with cirrhosis: An Italian multicenter double-blind, placebo-controlled, cross-over study. Hepatology 1998;28:374–378.
4. Basile AS, Hughes RD, Harrison PM, et al: Elevated brain concentrations of 1,4-benzodiazepines in fulminant hepatic failure. N Engl J Med 1991;325:473–478.
5. Benzodiazepine compounds and hepatic encephalopathy. N Engl J Med 1991;325:509–510.
6. Bosman DK, Van Den Buijs CACG, De Haan JC, et al: The effects of benzodiazepine-receptor antagonists and partial inverse agonists on acute hepatic encephalopathy in the rat. Gastroenterology 1991;101: 772–781.
7. Breheny FX: Reversal of midazolam sedation with flumazenil. Crit Care Med 1991;20:736–739.
8. Brogden RN, Goa KL: Flumazenil: A reappraisal of its pharmacological properties and therapeutic efficacy as a benzodiazepine antagonist. Drugs 1991;42:1061–1089.
9. Byrnes SMA, Watson GW, Hardy PAJ: Flumazenil: An unreliable antagonist in baclofen overdose. Anaesthesiology 1996;51:481–482.
10. Carter AS, Bell GD, Coady T, et al: Speed of reversal of midazolam-induced respiratory depression by flumazenil: A study in patients undergoing upper GI endoscopy. Acta Anaesth Scand 1990;34:59–64.
11. Clausen TG, Wolff J, Carl P, Theilgaard A: The effect of the benzodiazepine antagonist, flumazenil, on psychometric performance in acute ethanol intoxication in man. Eur J Clin Pharmacol 1990;38:233–236.
12. Discussion. Eur J Anaest 1988;2(Suppl):233–235.
13. Dunton AW, Schwam E, Pitman V, et al: Flumazenil: US clinical pharmacology studies. Eur J Anaesth 1988;2:81–95.
14. Ferenci P, Grimm G, Meryn S, Gangl A: Successful long-term treatment of portal-systemic encephalopathy by the benzodiazepine antagonist flumazenil. Gastroenterology 1989;96:240–243.
15. File SE, Pellow S: Intrinsic actions of the benzodiazepine receptor antagonist Ro 15–1788. Psychopharmacology 1986;88:1–11.
16. Flumazenil in the treatment of hepatic encephalopathy. Ann Pharmacother 1993;27:46–47.
17. Fulton SA, Mullen KD: Completion of upper endoscopic procedures despite paradoxical reaction to midazolam: A role for flumazenil? Arch J Gastroenterol 2000;95:809–811.
18. Gardner CR: Functional in vivo correlates of the benzodiazepine agonist-inverse agonist continuum. Prog Neurobiol 1988;31:425–476.
19. Geller E, Crome P, Schaller MD, et al: Risks and benefits of therapy with flumazenil (Anexate) in mixed drug intoxications. Eur Neurol 1991;31:241–250.
20. Greenblatt DJ, Shader RI: Benzodiazepines (first of two parts). N Engl J Med 1974;291:1011–1015.
21. Gross JB, Weller RS, Conard P: Flumazenil antagonism of midazolam-induced ventilatory depression. Anesthesiology 1991;75: 179–185.
22. Gueye PN, Hoffman JR, Taboulet P, et al: Empiric use of flumazenil in comatose patients: Limited applicability of criteria to define low risk. Ann Emerg Med 1996;27:730–735.
23. Haefely W, Hunkeler W: The story of flumazenil. Eur J Anaesth 1988;2:3–14.
24. Hart YM, Meinardi H, Sander JW, et al: The effect of intravenous flumazenil on interictal electroencephalographic epileptic activity: Results of a placebo-controlled study. J Neurol Neurosurg Pychiatry 1991;54:305–309.
25. Haverkos GP, DiSalvo RP, Imhoff TE: Fatal seizures after flumazenil administration in a patient with mixed overdose. Ann Pharmacother 1994;28:1347–1349.
26. Höjer J, Baehrendtz S: The effect of flumazenil (Ro 15–1788) in the management of self-induced benzodiazepine poisoning: A double-blind controlled study. Acta Med Scand 1988;224:357–365.
27. Honan VJ: Paradoxical reaction to midazolam and control with flumazenil. Gastrointest Endosc 1994;40:86–88.
28. Hunkeler W: Preclinical research findings with flumazenil (Ro 15–1788, Anexate): Chemistry. Eur J Anaesth 1988;2(Suppl):37–62.
29. Kamijo Y, Masuda T, Nishikawa T, et al: Cardiovascular response and stress reaction to flumazenil injection in patients under infusion with midazolam. Crit Care Med 2000;28:318–323.
30. Katz JA, Fragen RJ, Dunn KL: Flumazenil reversal of midazolam sedation of the elderly. Reg Anesth Pain Med 1991;16:247–252.
31. Kirkegaard L, Knudsen L, Jensen S, Kruse A: Benzodiazepine antagonist Ro 15–1788. Anaesthesia 1986;41:1184–1188.
32. L'heureux P: Continuous flumazenil for zolpidem toxicity—Commentary. J Toxicol Clin Toxicol 1998;36:745–746.
33. L'heureux P, Askenasi R: Efficacy of flumazenil in acute alcohol intoxication: Double-blind placebo controlled evaluation. Hum Exp Toxicol 1991;10:235–239.
34. L'heureux P, Vranckx M, Leduc D, Askenasi R: Flumazenil in mixed benzodiazepine/tricyclic antidepressant overdose: A placebo-controlled study in the dog. Am J Emerg Med 1992;10:184–188.
35. Lim AG: Death after flumazenil [letter]. BMJ 1989;299:858–859.
36. Linowiecki K, Paloucek F, Donnelly A, Leikin JB: Reversal of ethanol-induced respiratory depression by flumazenil. Vet Hum Toxicol 1992;34:417–419.
37. Litchfield NB: Complications of intravenous diazepam. Adverse psychological reactions. Anesth Prog 1980;27:175–183.
38. Martens F, Köppel C, Ibe K, et al: Clinical experience with the benzodiazepine antagonist flumazenil in suspected benzodiazepine or ethanol poisoning. J Toxicol Clin Toxicol 1990;28:341–356.
39. Mora CT, Torjman M, White PF: Effects of diazepam and flumazenil on sedation and hypoxic ventilatory response. Anesth Analg 1989; 68:473–478.
40. Mordel A, Winkler E, Almog S, et al: Seizures after flumazenil administration in a case of combined benzodiazepine and tricyclic antidepressant overdose. Crit Care Med 1992;20:1733–1734.
41. Patat A, Naef MM, Van Gessel E, et al: Flumazenil antagonizes the central effects of zolpidem, an imidazopyridine hypnotic. Clin Pharmacol Ther 1994;56:430–436.
42. Persson A, Pauli S, Halldin C, et al: Saturation analysis of specific [11]C Ro 15–1788 binding to the human neocortex using positron emission tomography. Hum Psychopharmacol 1989;4:21–31.

43. Rodrigo CR: Flumazenil reverses paradoxical reaction with midazolam. Anesth Prog 1991;38:65–68.

44. Rothstein JD, Guidotti A, Tinuper P, et al: Endogenous benzodiazepine receptor ligands in idiopathic recurring stupor. Lancet 1992; 340:1002–1004.

45. Savic I, Widen L, Stone-Eldaner S: Feasibility of reversing benzodiazepine tolerance with flumazenil. Lancet 1991;337:133–137.

46. Shalansky SJ, Naumann TL, Englander FA: Therapy update: Effect of flumazenil on benzodiazepine-induced respiratory depression. Clin Pharm 1993;12:483–487.

47. Skolnick P: The γ-aminobutyric acid A (GABA$_A$) receptor complex. In: Jones EA, moderator: The γ-aminobutyric acid A (GABA$_A$) receptor complex and hepatic encephalopathy: Some recent advances. Ann Intern Med 1989;100:532–546.

48. Spivey WH: Flumazenil and seizures: Analysis of 43 cases. Clin Ther 1992;14:292–305.

49. Thakker P, Gallagher TM: Flumazenil reverses paradoxical reaction to midazolam in a child. Anaesth Intensive Care 1996;24:505–507.

50. Thurston TA, Williams CG, Foshee SL: Reversal of a paradoxical reaction to midazolam with flumazenil. Anesth Analg 1996;83:192.

51. Ticku MK, Mhatre M, Mehta AK: Modulation of GABAergic transmission by ethanol. In: Biggio G, Costa E, eds: GABAergic Synaptic Transmission. New York, Raven, 1992, pp. 255–268.

52. Tinuper P, Montagna P, Cortelli P, et al: Idiopathic recurring stupor: A case with possible involvement of the gamma-aminobutyric acid (GABA)ergic system. Ann Neurol 1992;31:503–506.

53. Tobin JM, Lewis N: New psychotherapeutic agent chlordiazepoxide. JAMA 1960;174:1242–1249.

54. Tolksdorf W, Ney C, Ney R, Amberger M: The influence of flumazenil on respiration after midazolam and/or fentanyl [abstract]. Anesth Analg 1990;70:S409.

55. Van der Rijt CC, de Knegt RJ, Schalm SW, et al: Flumazenil does not improve hepatic encephalopathy associated with acute ischemic liver failure in the rabbit. Metab Brain Dis 1990;3:131–141.

56. Weinbroum A, Geller E: The respiratory effects of reversing midazolam sedation with flumazenil in the presence or absence of narcotics. Acta Anaesth Scand 1990;92:65–69.

57. Weinbroum A, Halpern P, Geller E: The use of flumazenil in the management of acute drug poisoning: A review. Intensive Care Med 1991;17:S32–S38.

58. Weinbroum MD, Rudick V, Sorkine P, et al: Use of flumazenil in the treatment of drug overdose: A double-blind and open clinical study in 110 patients. Crit Care Med 1996;24:199–206.

59. Winkler E, Shlomo A, Kriger D, et al: Use of flumazenil in the diagnosis and treatment of patients with coma of unknown etiology. Crit Care Med 1993;21:538–542.

60. Whitwan G, Amrein R: Pharmacology of flumazenil. Acta Anaesthesiol Scand 1995;39(Suppl 108):3–14.

D. ALCOHOLS AND DRUGS OF ABUSE

CHAPTER 64   ETHANOL

Luke Yip

A 44-year-old man was found unconscious in a homeless shelter. The report given to the paramedics was that the patient had a long history of alcoholism. He had been drinking heavily until 1–2 days previously when he was initially admitted to the shelter. Since then the patient had repeated bouts of vomiting and no significant oral intake. There was no further history available. The initial assessment by the paramedics was notable for a blood pressure of 100/72 mm Hg, a pulse of 120 beats/min, and a respiratory rate of 32 breaths/min. The patient was placed on high-flow oxygen, an intravenous (IV) line was established, blood samples were obtained for analysis, and a 0.9% NaCl fluid bolus was administered. The patient was given 2 mg of naloxone, 25 g of dextrose, and 100 mg of thiamine IV without clinical response. The patient was transported to the Emergency Department (ED).

On arrival at the ED, the patient had similar vital signs including a rectal temperature of 100.4°F (38°C), and an oxygen saturation by pulse oximetry of 100% on high-flow oxygen. His head was atraumatic. His sclera were anicteric. Pupils were 3 mm in size, equal, round, and reactive to light. Funduscopic examination was normal. His mucous membranes were dry and his gag reflex was intact. There was no definite odor to the patient's breath. There was no meningismus. Chest and abdominal examinations were normal except that the liver edge was palpable to three fingerbreadths below the costal margin. There was no splenomegaly and there was no testicular atrophy. Rectal tone was normal, stool was dark and negative for occult blood, and there was no bowel or bladder incontinence. The patient was stuporous. His corneal reflexes were intact. He had normal muscle tone, symmetric deep-tendon reflexes, plantar flexion was present, and there were no tremors, clonus, or fasciculations. There was a normal amount of axillary and pubic hair. There were no stigmata of chronic ethanol abuse such as palmar erythema, spider angiomata, and gynecomastia.

The blood glucose determined by a bedside rapid reagent test was 120 mg/dL (6.67 mmol/L). Electrocardiogram (ECG) showed sinus tachycardia without PR, QRS, or QTc, abnormalities. A portable chest radiograph showed haziness over both lung bases. A complete blood count (CBC) revealed leukocytes, 16,000/mm^3 without a left shift; hematocrit, 52%; platelets 150,000/mm^3. Blood chemistries were remarkable for sodium, 148 mEq/L; potassium, 2.9 mEq/L; chloride, 108 mEq/L; carbon dioxide, 9 mEq/L; glucose, 130 mg/dL; blood urea nitrogen (BUN), 50 mg/dL; creatinine, 1.6 mg/dL; aspartate aminotransferase (AST), 168 U/L; alanine aminotransferase (ALT), 80 U/L; and an elevated γ-glutamyl transpeptidase (GGTP) and alkaline phosphatase. The international normalized ratio (INR) and partial thromboplastin times were nor-

mal. The serum lipase was 90 U/L, serum ammonia was 70 μg/dL, and the serum lactate was 2.2 mEq/L. Blood ethanol level was undetectable. Urinalysis was remarkable for specific gravity of greater than 1.030, 1–2 ketones, and no crystals. Arterial blood gas analysis was remarkable for a pH of 7.08, a PCO$_2$ of 12 mm Hg, and a PO$_2$ of 110 mm Hg.

Intravenous fluid therapy with D$_5$WNS and supplemental potassium, folate, and multivitamins were initiated. Intravenous ceftriaxone 2 g and gentamicin 490 mg were administered for presumed aspiration pneumonitis. The patient was given an intravenous loading dose of ethanol followed by an ethanol infusion, while investigations were initiated into the etiologies of the patient's altered mental status and anion gap metabolic acidosis with severe acid-base derangement. A computed tomography (CT) scan of the patient's head was only remarkable for cerebral atrophy. Analysis of the cerebrospinal fluid from a lumbar puncture was unremarkable and specimens were sent for cultures. The investigation into the causes of an anion gap metabolic acidosis was unrewarding (Chaps. 24 and 66). The patient was admitted to the intensive care unit (ICU) where hemodialysis was performed because of persistent acid-base derangement in spite of supportive care. The patient recovered gradually. Alcoholic ketoacidosis was diagnosed by exclusion. The patient's blood was later confirmed to be negative for formate and glycolate.

Ethanol, or ethyl alcohol, is commonly referred to as *alcohol*. This term is somewhat misleading because there are numerous other alcohols whose varied toxicities are well described (see Antidotes in Depth: Thiamine Hydrochloride; Folic Acid and Leucovorin (Folinic Acid); Ethanol; Fomepizole; and Chap. 66). However, ethanol is probably the most commonly used and abused drug in the world. Its use is pervasive among all age groups and all socioeconomic groups, and represents a tremendous financial and social cost to society.

The ethanol content of alcoholic beverages is expressed by volume percent or by proof. Proof is a measure of the absolute ethanol content of distilled liquor, made at an index temperature by determining its specific gravity. In the United Kingdom, the Customs and Excise Act of 1952, declared proof spirits (100 proof) as those with weights of 12/13 the weight of an equal volume of distilled water at 11°C (51°F). Thus, proof spirits are 48.24% ethanol by weight or 57.06% by volume. Other spirits are designated over- or underproof, with the percentage of variance noted. In the United States, a proof spirit (100 proof) is one containing 50% ethanol by volume. The derivation of proof comes from the days when sailors in the British Navy suspected that the officers were diluting their rum (grog) ration and demanded "proof" that this was not the case. They achieved this by pouring a sample of grog on black granular gunpowder. If the gunpowder ignited by match or spark, the rum was up to standard, 100% proof that the liquor was 50% ethanol. This became shortened to 100 proof (Table 64–1). In addition to beverages, ethanol is present in hundreds of medicinal preparations as a diluent or solvent in concentrations ranging from 0.3% to 75%.[19,103,113] Mouthwashes may have up to 75% ethanol (150 proof) and colognes typically contain 40–60% ethanol (80–120 proof).[19,113] These products occasionally cause intoxication, especially in children.[22,35,66,84]

Veisalgia, "alcohol hangover," comes from the Norwegian *kveis*, "uneasiness following debauchery" and the Greek *algia*, "pain." The "hangover" syndrome has been attributed to congeners, substances that appear normally in alcoholic beverages in addition to ethanol and water.[18,23,24] The conventional listing of congeners includes fusel oil (a mixture containing amyl, butyl, propyl, and methyl alcohol), aldehydes, furfural, esters, low-molecular-weight organic acids, phenols, and other carbonyl compounds, tannins, solids, and a relatively large number of additional organic and inorganic compounds, usually in trace amounts.[18,24] Congeners contribute to the special characteristics of taste, flavor, aroma, and color of a beverage. The combinations and exact amounts of congeners vary with the type of beverage, ranging from 33 mg/L in vodka, to averages of 500 mg/L in some whiskies, and to as much as 29 g/L in specially aged whiskies or brandies.[18,23,24]

Consumption of illicitly produced ethanol ("moonshine") may result in lead or arsenic poisoning.[33,49] Incidental lead contamination is also reported in draught beers or wine contained in lead-capped bottles.[120,122] Of historic interest is that the addition of cobalt salts to beer to stabilize the "head" (foam) led to outbreaks of heart failure among heavy beer drinkers in Canada and Belgium in the 1960s. The "beer drinker's cardiomyopathy" was reported in heavy laborers who took most of their daily calories as beer and thus had associated protein malnutrition. These patients had a rapid deterioration in their clinical course after the onset of cardiomyopathy.[99,100] The clinical-pathologic pattern of this disease is distinct from the classic alcoholic cardiomyopathy.

EPIDEMIOLOGY

It is estimated that 5–10% of all drinkers of ethanol in the United States are ethanol dependent.[85,135] According to the National Longitudinal Alcohol Epidemiologic Survey (NLAES), the 1-year prevalence of combined ethanol abuse and dependence based on Diagnostic and Statistical Manual, 4th edition (DSM-IV) criteria was 7.41%, of 13,760,000 Americans.[56] The combined rate was almost 3 times higher among males than females and was also higher in persons under 45 years of age. The rates of ethanol abuse and dependence have been relatively stable since 1984. More than 200,000 Americans die annually of alcoholism, far more than die of all illicit drugs of abuse combined. Ethanol is the leading killer of persons aged 15–45 years. In this age group it is associated with 50% of traffic fatalities, 50% of deaths by fire, 67% of drownings, 67% of homicides, and 35% of suicides.[121] In 1998, there were 15,936 ethanol-related traffic fatalities in the United States that accounted for nearly 38% of total traffic fatalities.[107] Among 16–20-year-old male drivers, an increase of 20 mg/dL in blood ethanol concentration was estimated to be more than double the relative risk of fatal single-vehicle crash injury.[139] When the blood ethanol

---

TABLE 64–1.　Basic Information and Calculations for Ethanol

MW: 46 Daltons
Specific gravity: 0.7939 (~0.8) g/mL
Volume of distribution (Vd): (~0.6) L/kg

$$\text{Blood ethanol concentration (mg/dL)} = \frac{\text{dose (mg)}}{\text{Vd (L/kg)} \times \text{body weight (kg)} \times 10}$$

$$\text{mmol} = \frac{\text{mg}}{\text{MW}} = \frac{\text{mg}}{46}$$

$$\text{mmol/L} = \frac{\text{mg/dL}}{4.6}$$

For a 70-kg individual:

Dose of ethanol	Blood ethanol concentration
10 mL/kg of 10% (20 proof)	167 mg/dL (36.30 mmol/L)
3 mL/kg of 10% (20 proof)	50 mg/dL (10.87 mmol/L)
150 mL (5 "shots") of 40% (80 proof)	143 mg/dL (31.09 mmol/L)
30 mL (1 "shot") of 40% (80 proof)	27 mg/dL (5.87 mmol/L)

Level Consistent with Legal Intoxication = 10.87–21.74 mmol/L [50–100 mg/dL or 0.5–0.10 g/dL (%)]

Average reduction in blood ethanol level (elimination phase):
　　Nontolerant adult: 3.26–4.35 mmol/L/h (15–20 mg/dL/h, 100–125 mg/kg/h)
　　Tolerant adult: 6.52–8.70 mmol/L/h (30–40 mg/dL/h, 175 mg/kg/h)

concentration was 80–100 mg/dL (17.39–21.74 mmol/L), 100–150 mg/dL (21.74–32.61 mmol/L), and greater than 150 mg/dL (32.61 mmol/L), the relative risk was 52, 241, and 15,560, respectively. Twenty percent of the total national expenditure for hospital care is ethanol related, and the annual cost of health expenses and lost productivity is estimated to be $117 billion. Alcoholism is the leading cause of morbidity and mortality in the United States.[121]

For untreated alcoholics, life expectancy is decreased by 12–15 years as compared to the remainder of the population.[95] Mortality from the regular use of ethanol begins to increase when 3–5 drinks per day are consumed and rises sharply with the consumption of 7 or more drinks per day.[9] Although the daily consumption of 1 or 2 drinks per day may be "safe" for most people, it is unknown at the present time what is considered to be "safe" for pregnant women. The combination of a national tolerance of drinking and heavy advertising of ethanol makes it especially appealing to young people. In a country increasingly concerned with drug abuse, the excessive use of ethanol constitutes a serious and pervasive problem as well as a major health issue.

PHARMACOLOGY

Ethanol is a colorless, odorless liquid hydrocarbon. It is fully miscible in water and is both water soluble and lipid soluble. Ready diffusion across lipid membranes accounts for its pervasive effect on most organ systems.

Despite its long history of use and study, the mechanism of action for the intoxicating effect of ethanol remains the subject of debate.[74,112] Although most current research focuses on the interaction of ethanol with various proteins such as neurotransmitter-gated ion channels,[52,90,112] there is extensive evidence that ethanol interacts with a variety of neurotransmitters.[36,130,131] The major actions of ethanol involve enhancement of the effects of γ-aminobutyric acid (GABA) at $GABA_A$ receptors and blockade of the N-methyl-D-aspartate (NMDA) subtype of glutamate (excitatory amino acid (EAA)) receptor. NMDA receptors mediate neurotoxicity by increasing permeability to calcium currents and regulate neuronal long-term potentiation.[125] Animal studies indicate that the acute effects of ethanol are competitive inhibition of glycine's binding to the NMDA receptor and disruption of glutamatergic neurotransmission by inhibiting the response of the NMDA receptor. Persistent glycine antagonism and attenuation of glutamatergic neurotransmission by chronic ethanol exposure results in the compensatory up-regulation of NMDA receptors. Tolerance to ethanol results in enhanced EAA neurotransmission and NMDA receptor up-regulation,[69,129,130,131] which appears to involve selective increases in NMDA R2B subunit levels and other molecular changes in specific brain loci. Abrupt withdrawal of ethanol thus produces a hyperexcitable state that leads to the ethanol withdrawal syndrome and excitotoxic neuronal death.[131] In addition, chronic ethanol administration results in tolerance, dependence, and an ethanol withdrawal syndrome, mediated, in part, by desensitization and or down-regulation of $GABA_A$ receptors. GABA-mediated inhibition, which normally acts to limit excitation is diminished in effectiveness during ethanol withdrawal syndrome, and further intensifies this excitation. Augmentation of excitatory neurotransmission may lead to enhanced oxidative stress, which, in concert with reduced inhibitory neurotransmission, may con-

tribute to the ethanol withdrawal-associated neurotoxicity in humans.[69,130,131] In addition, NMDA receptors function to inhibit the release of dopamine in the nucleus accumbens and mesolimbic structures, which modulate the reinforcing action of addictive agents such as ethanol.[126] By inhibiting NMDA receptor activity, ethanol could increase dopamine release from the nucleus accumbens and ventral tegmental area and could thus create dependence (Chap. 10).

With chronic intake, the degree of tolerance that develops to ethanol is less than that occurring with opioids.[116] However, the withdrawal manifestations which occur with the abrupt cessation or relative diminution of ethanol intake are much more severe and potentially life-threatening as compared to that of opioid withdrawal (Chap. 72).

KINETICS AND METABOLISM

Ethanol is rapidly absorbed from the gastrointestinal (GI) tract, with about 20% being absorbed from the stomach and the remainder being absorbed from the small intestine.[1] Factors that enhance absorption include rapid gastric emptying, ethanol intake without food, the absence of congeners, dilution of ethanol (maximum absorption occurs at a concentration of 20%), and carbonation. Under optimal conditions for absorption, 80–90% of an ingested dose is fully absorbed within 60 minutes. Factors that delay ethanol absorption include high concentrations of ethanol (by causing pylorospasm), presence of food; coexistence of GI disease, coingestion of drugs; time taken to ingest the drink, and individual variation. When any of these latter factors is present, absorption may be delayed for 2–6 hours.

Alcohol dehydrogenase (ADH), specifically class IV ADH, located in the gastric mucosa, oxidizes a proportion of the ingested ethanol, thus reducing the amount available for absorption. This effect is more pronounced in men than in women, and in nonalcoholics than in alcoholics.[29,41] About 30% of Japanese are deficient in gastric ADH.[86]

In the liver, class I ADH (ADH2) metabolizes ethanol to acetaldehyde, which is converted to acetate by aldehyde dehydrogenase (ALDH). The mitochondrial form of aldehyde dehydrogenase (ALDH2) is the most important form for acetaldehyde metabolism. Approximately 40% of Asians, 80% of Native Americans, and as many as 29% of whites have an inactive ALDH2 enzyme because of a point mutation in the ALDH2 gene; consequently, they have a reduced capacity for acetaldehyde metabolism.[51,68] Approximately 90% of Asians also have a gain-of-function polymorphism of ADH2, called ADH2*2, which increases the rate at which acetaldehyde is produced. In affected individuals the accumulation of acetaldehyde with even modest ethanol consumption leads to a severe flushing reaction.[127,128,132] This is similar to that induced by disulfiram (Chap. 65).

For a typical 70-kg person, a "standard drink" containing 15 g of ethanol is defined as 1 oz (30 mL) of 100 proof liquor or about a 4-oz (120 mL) glass of wine (12% ethanol), or about a 10-oz bottle of beer (5% ethanol), raises blood ethanol level by 36 mg/dL (7.8 mmol/L). These figures represent the theoretical maximum serum ethanol concentration, based on instantaneous and complete ethanol absorption and no distribution or metabolism following a "standard drink" by a typical person.

Following complete distribution, ethanol is present in body tissues in a concentration proportional to that of the tissue water content. The concentration in the blood is maintained by back diffusion, which occurs whenever the level in the blood falls below that of the tissues. Ethanol freely passes through the placenta, exposing the fetus to ethanol levels comparable to those achieved by the mother.

Ethanol is primarily (>90%) eliminated by the liver via enzymatic oxidation, with 5–10% excreted unchanged by the kidneys, lungs, and sweat. Ethanol is unique among central nervous system (CNS) depressants in that it is principally metabolized by a cytosolic liver enzyme (ADH), whereas the other CNS depressants are metabolized by hepatic microsomal enzymes (P450). Ethanol is metabolized via at least three different pathways: the aforementioned ADH pathway located in the cytosol of the hepatocytes, the microsomal ethanol-oxidizing systems (MEOS; CYP2E1) located on the endoplasmic reticulum, and the peroxidase-catalase system associated with the hepatic peroxisomes[21,88] (Fig. 64–1).

The ADH system is the main pathway for ethanol metabolism in the body and is also the rate-limiting step. ADH is a zinc-containing enzyme that uses nicotinamide adenine dinucleotide (NAD$^+$) as a hydrogen acceptor to oxidize ethanol to acetaldehyde. In this process, hydrogen is transferred from ethanol to NAD$^+$, converting it to its reduced form, NADH. Similarly, hydrogen is transferred from acetaldehyde to NAD$^+$. Under normal conditions acetate is converted to acetylcoenzyme A (acetyl-CoA), which enters the Krebs cycle and is metabolized to carbon dioxide and water. The entry of acetyl-CoA into the Krebs cycle is indirectly dependent on adequate thiamine stores. Thiamine is an essential cofactor for enzymes that carry out decarboxylation reactions, such as pyruvate decarboxylase as well as for α-ketoglutarate dehydrogenase, and transketolase.[14,82] In addition, thiamine is required to maintain normal neuronal conduction.

The oxidation of ethanol generates an excess of reducing potential in the cytosol in the form of NADH with the ratio of NAD$^+$ to NADH being dramatically reduced. This ratio, also known as the redox potential, determines the ability of the cell to carry on various oxidative processes. The unfavorable change in redox potential because of ethanol metabolism contributes to the development of numerous metabolic abnormalities associated with alcoholism, such as alcoholic ketoacidosis, impaired gluconeogenesis, and alterations in fatty acid metabolism.

The MEOS system (CYP2E1) is responsible for very little ethanol metabolism in the novice or uninitiated drinker, but becomes more important as the ethanol concentration rises or as ethanol use becomes chronic (Fig. 64–1). CYP2E1 uses nicotinamide adenine dinucleotide phosphate (NADP$^+$) as a hydrogen acceptor to oxidize ethanol to acetaldehyde.[79] In this process, hydrogen is transferred from ethanol to NADP$^+$, converting it to its reduced form, NADPH. Similarly, acetaldehyde is further oxidized to acetate as hydrogen is transferred from acetaldehyde to NADP$^+$. The ability of ethanol to induce as well as to inhibit the MEOS system forms the basis for the well-established interactions between ethanol and a host of other drugs metabolized by this system.[28,40]

The capacity of the ADH enzyme system is saturated at relatively low blood ethanol levels. As the system is saturated, the metabolism moves from first-order to zero-order kinetics (Chap. 11). In adults, the average rate of ethanol metabolism is 100–125 mg/kg/h in occasional drinkers and up to 175 mg/kg/h in habitual drinkers.[12,50] As a result, the average-sized adult metabolizes 7–10 g/h and the blood ethanol level falls 15–20 mg/dL/h (3.26–4.35 mmol/L/h). Tolerant drinkers, by recruiting CYP2E1, may increase their clearance of ethanol to about 30 mg/dL/h (6.52 mmol/L/h).[12,50] Studies of ethanol-intoxicated patients indicate that although the average ethanol clearance rate is about 20 mg/dL/h (4.35 mmol/L/h), there is considerable individual variation (standard deviation of about 6 mg/dL/h (1.30 mmol/L/h).[12,50]

The excretion of ethanol by the lungs is first order and obeys Henry's law, in which the ratio between the concentration of ethanol in the alveolar air and the blood is constant. Although the alveolar air/blood constant is quite low (1:2100) and very little ethanol is excreted by this route, the fixed relationship forms the basis for the sampling of subjects' breath to reliably estimate their blood ethanol concentration.

CLINICAL PRESENTATION

The clinical features of acute ethanol intoxication are dependent on the degree of intoxication. Ethanol is a selective CNS depressant at low doses and a general depressant at high doses. It first depresses those areas of the brain that are involved with highly integrated functions. The cortex is released from integrated control, leading to animated behavior and the loss of restraint. The initial effect is paradoxical CNS stimulation caused by disinhibition.[25] In cases of mild intoxication, the signs of ethanol inebriation may be influenced by the individual's basic personality. The patient may be energized and loquacious, expansive, emotionally labile, and increasingly gregarious, or may appear to have lost self-control, exhibit antisocial behavior, and be ill tempered. As the degree of intoxication increases, there is successive inhibition and impairment of neuronal activity. The patient may become irritable, abusive, aggressive, violent, dysarthric, confused, disoriented, or lethargic. With severe intoxication, there is loss of protective reflexes, coma, and increasing risk of death from

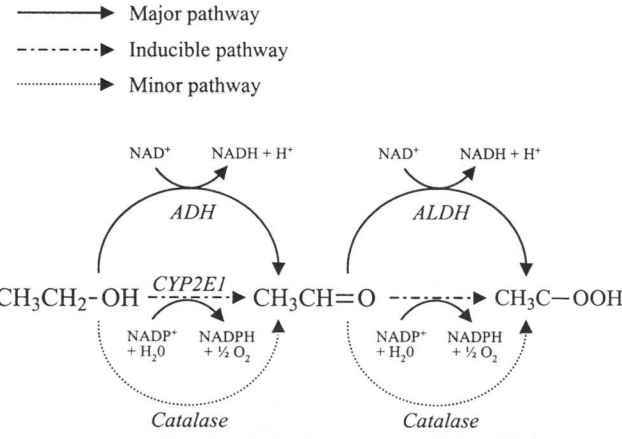

→ Major pathway

⇢ Inducible pathway

⋯⋯▸ Minor pathway

Figure 64–1. Ethanol oxidation. The major, minor and inducible pathways utilized for ethanol metabolism.

respiratory depression. An average non-alcoholic adult with a blood ethanol concentration of greater than 300 mg/dL (65.22 mmol/L) is usually comatose.[2]

The acute effects of ethanol ingestion also depend on the habituation of the drinker. This is mainly a consequence of the development of tolerance, which has a metabolic (pharmacokinetic) and a functional (pharmacodynamic) component.[125] Metabolic tolerance to ethanol is based on enhanced elimination by the ADH enzyme and the MEOS:CYP2E1 system. Functional tolerance (resistance to the effects of ethanol at the cellular level) is a more important determinant of habituation and may be mediated through alterations in glutamatergic, serotonergic, and adrenergic neurons.[73] Although individuals who are acutely intoxicated move through a progressive sequence of events, the association of a particular stage of intoxication with a specific blood ethanol level is not usually possible without knowing the pattern of ethanol use of the patient. In alcoholics, specific clinical manifestations of inebriation typically occur with significantly higher blood ethanol concentration than nontolerant individuals. Regardless, the absolute change above the baseline ethanol level may be important.

A patient may present with obvious signs and symptoms consistent with ethanol intoxication that include flushed facies, diaphoresis, tachycardia, hypotension, hypothermia, hypoventilation, mydriasis, nystagmus, vomiting, dysarthria, muscular incoordination, ataxia, altered consciousness, and coma. However, the presentation of an ethanol-intoxicated patient should also prompt the physician to carefully evaluate the patient for a variety of covert clinical and metabolic disorders. These coexisting disorders include hypoglycemia, head and neck injury, acid-base derangements, hypokalemia, hypomagnesemia, meningitis, sepsis, myopathy and neuropathy, bone marrow suppression, cardiomyopathy and dysrhythmias, gastrointestinal hemorrhages, pancreatitis, peptic ulcers, liver disease, and ingestion of ethylene glycol, methanol, or isopropanol. Diplopia, visual disturbances, and nystagmus may be evident, which may be a result of the toxic effects of ethanol or may represent Wernicke's encephalopathy. Hypothermia may be exacerbated by environmental exposure, by malnutrition and loss of carbohydrate or energy substrate, and by ethanol-induced vasodilation. Ethanol intoxication can impair cardiac output in patients with preexisting cardiac disease,[55] and cause or contribute to dysrhythmias such as atrial fibrillation and nonsustained ventricular tachycardia, as well as atrioventricular (AV) block, in binge drinkers.[32,57,58] Ethanol-induced angina is rarely described.[102] Hyperamylasemia may represent an underlying pancreatitis or salivary gland hyperplasia, which is also commonly associated with alcoholism and poor nutrition.[10] Ethanol-induced seizures are reported in adults, but are more frequent in children with ethanol-induced hypoglycemia.[67]

In the United States, according to National Highway Traffic Safety Administration (NHTSA) information, as of September 1999, 31 states legally defined driving under the influence of alcohol as a blood ethanol concentration above 100 mg/dL (21.74 mmol/L) whereas another 17 states and the District of Columbia used 80 mg/dL (17.39 mmol/L) as the legal limit.[107] Under these laws it is a crime to drive with a blood ethanol concentration at or above the proscribed level regardless of circumstances or behavior; Maryland and South Carolina do not have such a law but have set presumptive limits. In nontolerant individuals, blood ethanol concentrations as low as 20 mg/dL (4.35 mmol/L) have been demonstrated to impair driving-related skills.[108,140] Gross motor control and orientation may be significantly affected at concentra-

tions of 50 mg/dL (10.87 mmol/L).[21,104] Clinical ethanol intoxication is usually apparent at blood ethanol concentration of 50 mg/dL (10.87 mmol/L).

EVALUATION AND MANAGEMENT OF THE ETHANOL INTOXICATED PATIENT

Acute altered mental status in an alcoholic patient can be a consequence of a variety or combination of causes, including acute ethanol intoxication, hypoglycemia, therapeutic or illicit drug overdose, Wernicke-Korsakoff syndrome, head trauma, a postictal condition, infection, an intracranial hematoma (acute or chronic), hepatic encephalopathy, an electrolyte or acid-base disorder, or ethanol withdrawal. Acute ethanol intoxication occurs in habitual drinkers when they raise their ethanol level an equivalent amount above baseline (as described above). The intoxicated patient can present with a broad range of diagnostic possibilities. A meticulous and systematic approach to the evaluation and management of an inebriated patient helps the clinician avoid the potential pitfalls in such a situation.

Ethanol is rapidly absorbed from the gastrointestinal tract following oral ingestion. In situations in which recent ingestion (within 1 hour of presentation), delayed absorption, and concomitant ingestions are under consideration, gastric emptying may be a reasonable approach to the extremely intoxicated, comatose patient.[101] However, gastric emptying followed by the administration of activated charcoal is generally reserved for the unconscious patient with a history of a serious coingestion. Occasionally, the extremely intoxicated or comatose patient may have severe respiratory depression necessitating endotracheal intubation and ventilatory support.

The patient's fluid and electrolyte status should be assessed and abnormalities corrected. Multivitamins with folate (1–5 mg) and magnesium (2 g) should be added to the maintenance IV solution. Potassium and phosphate should be supplemented as indicated. Clinically significant abnormal coagulation profile may require administration of fresh-frozen plasma and vitamin K. The presence of fever should prompt a diligent search for, and treatment of, its etiology.

As with any patient presenting to the ED with an acute altered mental status, rapid but thorough investigation and treatment should be undertaken for reversible causes of acutely altered mental status such as hypoxia, hypoglycemia, or opioid effect. Supplemental oxygen should be administered as needed. Intravenous dextrose (0.5–1.0 g/kg), thiamine 100 mg, and naloxone 2 mg should be administered as clinically indicated. Abnormal vital signs should be noted, and the patient should be evaluated and treated accordingly. Patients who are combative and violent should be physically restrained and then chemically sedated with a benzodiazepine. Attempts by those who are clinically intoxicated to sign out against medical advice or who attempt to leave should also be prevented (Chap. 118). The presence or absence of an odor of ethanol on the breath is an unreliable means of ascertaining whether a person is intoxicated or whether ethanol has been consumed recently, even under optimum laboratory conditions.[106] A thorough physical examination should be performed to evaluate precipitating or coexisting medical or surgical illnesses.[43] While in the ED, the patient should be evaluated frequently. Laboratory and radiographic imaging studies should be obtained as clinically indicated.

A variety of techniques and agents have been advocated in the past either to reverse the intoxicating effects of ethanol or to enhance its elimination. Neither coffee nor caffeine itself counteracts the impaired psychomotor functions seen with acute intoxication.[109] Earlier anecdotal reports suggested a role for naloxone in reversing ethanol intoxication,[59,92] but the results could not be reliably reproduced.[110] The specific benzodiazepine antagonist flumazenil has no predictable effect on ethanol intoxication.[39] It is unlikely that a specific ethanol antagonist will be discovered because ethanol's mechanisms of action are complex and apparently are not mediated by a single receptor. Hemodialysis is an effective means of enhancing the systemic elimination of ethanol because of its small volume of distribution and low molecular weight. In severe ethanol poisoning resulting in respiratory failure or coma, hemodialysis may be an adjunct treatment to supportive care. However, this is rarely indicated or necessary.

Laboratory Testing

Blood tests that may be helpful include CBC, electrolytes, BUN, creatinine, ketones, acetone, lipase, liver enzymes, coagulation profile, ammonia, calcium, and magnesium. Total body magnesium may be depleted because of poor dietary intake, decreased GI absorption secondary to ethanol, and renal wasting as a consequence of the ethanol-related diuresis.[124] Patients with an anion gap metabolic acidosis should have urine ketones and a serum lactate level (Chaps. 24 and 66). Elevated serum or urinary ketones may be indicative of alcoholic ketoacidosis (AKA), starvation ketosis, or diabetic ketoacidosis. Because the laboratory nitroprusside reaction detects only ketones (acetone and acetoacetate) and not β-hydroxybutyrate, the assay for ketones in patients with AKA may be only mildly positive. High serum acetone levels may be indicative of isopropanol intoxication. A blood-ethanol level should be included in the initial laboratory studies.[66] If the blood-ethanol concentration is inconsistent with the patient's clinical condition, a prompt review of the patient's history is indicated, along with an exhaustive search for an underlying disorder, especially toxic-metabolic, trauma-related, neurologic, and infectious etiologies. Comatose patients with ethanol levels below 300 mg/dL (65.22 mmol/L) and patients with values in excess of 300 mg/dL (65.22 mmol/L) who fail to improve clinically during a limited period of close observation, should have a head CT scan, followed by a lumbar puncture if warranted. Because chronically ethanol-tolerant patients are prone to trauma and coagulopathies, both of which can cause intracerebral bleeding, the threshold for CT scanning these patients should be particularly low.

When blood methanol, ethylene glycol, and isopropanol levels are indicated but not readily available, a serum osmolality by freezing point depression may be helpful. A high osmol gap, the difference between the measured and the calculated serum osmolality, provides indirect evidence that osmotically active agents are present such as the toxic alcohols (Chap. 24). However, a "normal" osmol gap does not eliminate the toxic alcohols as being possible causes for an increased anion gap metabolic acidosis.[64] Ethanol itself will contribute to the measured serum osmolality and thus to the osmol gap. Ethanol's contribution to osmolality can be estimated by dividing the ethanol level in mg/dL by 4.6 (one-tenth the molecular weight of ethanol) and added to the calculated osmolarity.

There are numerous methodologies available to detect the presence of ethanol and quantitate its level. Blood-ethanol levels performed by immunoassay or gas chromatography are commonly used in hospitals. Although accurate, the results of these tests may be delayed several hours, and this delay may hamper decision-making and management in the emergency setting. Breath-alcohol analyzers, using microprocessors and infrared spectral analysis, are widely available and are routinely used by law-enforcement agencies as ethanol-screening devices. In the ED setting, they have been shown to accurately predict blood-ethanol levels.[134] Because, the unconscious or uncooperative patient may be unable to cooperate with the proper use of the breath-alcohol analyzer, attempts have been made to sample the breath of unconscious patients with breath-alcohol devices attached to mouth-cup and nasal tube adapters.[37,48] The normal blood/breath ethanol ratio also demonstrates individual and interindividual variations over time.[72] Other potential sources of error include recent use of ethanol-containing products, belching or vomiting of gastric ethanol contents, inadequate exhalation, obstructive pulmonary disease, and poor technique.[3,83] Furthermore, multidose inhalers (MDI) may contain a significant concentration of ethanol. Breath ethanol measurements with a mean ethanol level of 189 mg/dL (41.09 mmol/L) were recorded just after two puffs of Tornalate (bitolterol mesylate with 38% ethanol), Bronkometer (isoetharine mesylate with 30% ethanol), Primatene Mist (adrenaline with 34% ethanol), and salbutamol, while simultaneous blood-ethanol levels were undetectable.[8,53,89] Although MDIs may cause elevations of breath ethanol above the legal criteria for intoxication these effects are transient and may be prevented by a 10–15 minute interval between MDI use and breath-ethanol testing.[53,89]

Dipstick tests designed to detect ethanol in saliva are less reliable than breath tests and cannot be recommended at this time.[117] Determining fatty acid ethyl esters (FAEEs) may be a highly sensitive test for ethanol use.[30] Because FAEEs remain in the system for at least 24 hours, they may have a role as a marker of recent ethanol use, even after ethanol is completely metabolized. However, their availability is limited and their place in patient management is undefined.

Indications for Hospitalization

A patient with uncomplicated intoxication can be safely discharged from the ED after a period of careful observation. An individual should not be discharged while still clinically intoxicated. However, consideration may be given to a situation where the intoxicated patient is discharged to a protected environment under the supervision of a responsible adult. In this case the clinical assessment of the patient is more important than the blood ethanol level. Indications for hospital admission include persistently abnormal vital signs, persistently abnormal mental status with or without an obvious cause, a mixed overdose, concomitant serious trauma, consequential ethanol withdrawal, and an associated serious disease process such as pancreatitis or gastrointestinal hemorrhage.

Some alcoholics develop an organic brain syndrome that persists even when the person is sober. Many others are poor, lack social support, and lack the ability to comply with a treatment plan. Thus, the threshold for admission should be lower for chronic drinkers who are homeless, medically indigent, psychiatrically impaired, or otherwise disadvantaged. Alcoholics who are sober and who desire ethanol detoxification can be admitted for "drying out" and rehabilitation. Inpatient detoxification programs differ substantially from outpatient programs but their most consequential advantages may be that they enforce abstinence, provide more support and structure, and separate the patient from the social surroundings associated with drinking.[108] For patients who are not admitted, a referral may be offered to Alcoholics Anonymous or to another suitable ethanol rehabilitation program.

ETHANOL-INDUCED HYPOGLYCEMIA
Population at Risk and Associated Findings

Hypoglycemia associated with ethanol consumption usually occurs in malnourished chronic alcoholics and children (Chap. 40). It may also occur in binge drinkers and in occasional drinkers who stop eating. A 22% incidence of hypoglycemia was reported in one retrospective pediatric study of documented ethanol ingestion.[84] In a retrospective study of a pediatric and adolescent population, there was a 3.4% incidence of hypoglycemia (serum glucose concentration <67 mg/dL (3.72 mmol/L)) in patients with a mean blood-ethanol concentration of 138 mg/dL (30 mmol/L; interquartile range, 15–43 mmol/L).[35] Ethanol-intoxicated children younger than 5 years of age have an increased risk of developing hypoglycemia and it is the most common reported finding in this age group.[80,81]

Patients with ethanol-associated hypoglycemia usually present with an altered consciousness 2–10 hours following ethanol ingestion. Other physical findings may include hypothermia and tachypnea. Laboratory findings, in addition to hypoglycemia, usually include a positive blood ethanol level, ketonuria without glucosuria, and mild acidosis. Ethanol intoxication causes metabolic acidosis and respiratory depression in children. Mild respiratory or metabolic acidosis and mild hypokalemia are common findings.[80,81] Seizures are a particularly frequent occurrence in children with ethanol associated hypoglycemia.[22] In the newborn and young infants, hypoglycemia usually presents with irritability, feeding difficulties, lethargy, cyanosis, tachypnea, and/or hypothermia.[60,91] Management of ethanol-induced hypoglycemia is the same as any cause of hypoglycemia.

Mechanism of Ethanol-Associated Hypoglycemia

Hypoglycemia associated with ethanol consumption occurs when a low cellular redox state is established in the course of ethanol metabolism. This redox state favors the conversion of pyruvate to lactate, diverting pyruvate from gluconeogenesis (Fig. 64–2). Hypoglycemia typically occurs when there is a reduced caloric intake and only after the hepatic glycogen stores are depleted, as in an overnight fast. The mechanism by which hypoglycemia is associated with ethanol consumption in the well-nourished individual is less-well defined. Although the conditions that cause hypoglycemia in adults may also be present in infants and children, there is a more delicate balance that exists in the newborn and young child between glucose production and utilization.

ALCOHOLIC KETOACIDOSIS

The development of AKA requires a combination of physical and physiologic events to occur, each one of these conditions may be independent of one another. The normal response to starvation and depletion of hepatic glycogen stores is for amino acids to be converted to pyruvate. Pyruvate can serve as a substrate for gluconeogenesis, can be converted to acetyl-CoA and enter the Krebs cycle, or can undergo fatty acid synthesis. As described earlier, ethanol metabolism generates NADH, resulting in an excess of reducing potential. This low redox state favors the conversion of pyruvate

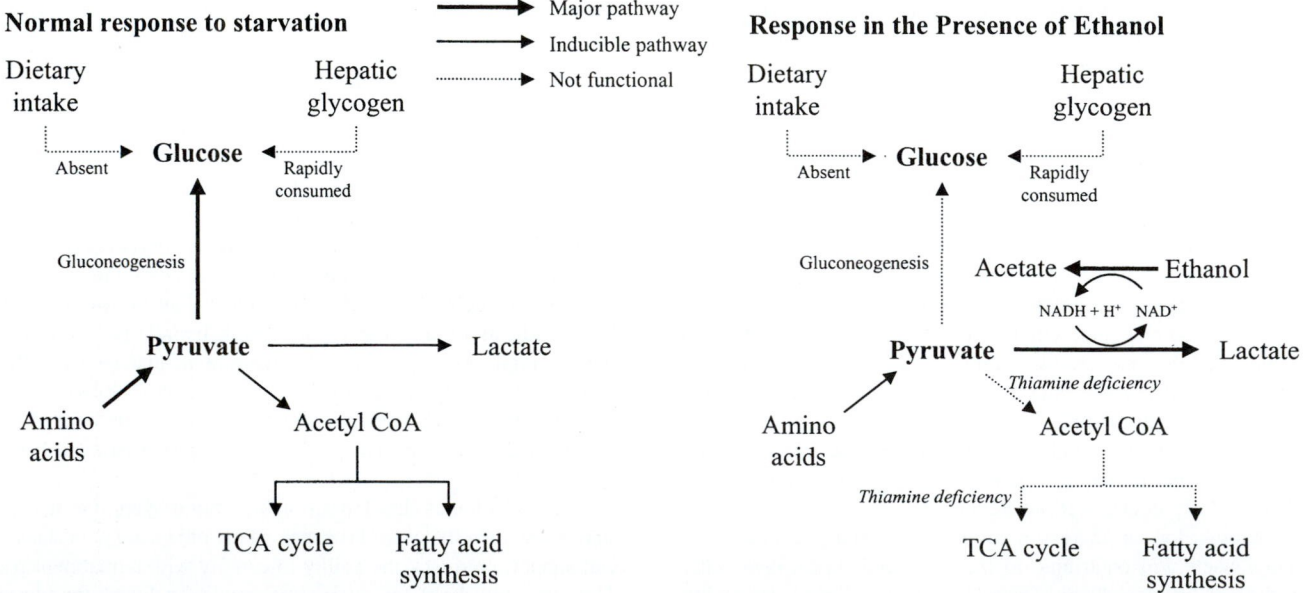

Figure 64–2. Central role of pyruvate in ethanol-induced hypoglycemia. TCA cycle = Tricarboxylic acid cycle. *(Modified, with permission, from Hoffman RS, Goldfrank LR: Ethanol-associated metabolic disorders in Endocrine metabolic disorders. Emerg Med Clin North Am 1989; 7:945.)*

to lactate, diverting pyruvate from being a substrate for gluconeogenesis. To compensate for the lack of normal metabolic substrates, the body mobilizes fat from adipose tissue and increases fatty acid metabolism as an alternative source of energy. This response is mediated by a decrease in insulin and an increased secretion of glucagon, catecholamines, growth hormone, and cortisol. Fatty acid metabolism results in the formation of acetyl-CoA and it combines with the excess acetate that is generated from ethanol metabolism to form acetoacetate[65] (Fig. 64–3). Most of the acetoacetate is reduced to β-hydroxybutyrate because of the excess reducing potential or low redox state of the cell. Volume depletion interferes with the renal elimination of acetoacetate and β-hydroxybutyrate, and contributes to the acidosis. Lactic acidosis caused by hypoperfusion or sepsis may coexist with the underlying ketoacidosis. Paradoxically, the arterial pH may be normal because of a compensatory respiratory alkalosis and a primary metabolic alkalosis resulting from vomiting (Chap. 24).

Clinical Features

A history of ethanol consumption combined with nausea, vomiting, electrolyte and acid-base abnormalities, anion gap metabolic acidosis, and altered mental status may represent AKA but is also consistent with a broad differential diagnosis, all of which should be considered and systematically excluded. The diagnosis of AKA is a diagnosis of exclusion.

Patients with AKA are typically chronic ethanol users, presenting after a few days of "binge" drinking. They become acutely starved because of cessation in oral intake as a result of nausea,

vomiting, abdominal pain from gastritis, hepatitis, pancreatitis, or a concurrent acute illness.[43,44,46] The patient may appear acutely ill with dehydration, tachypnea, tachycardia, and hypotension. The patient may be hypothermic or have a mildly elevated temperature. Sepsis, meningitis, pyelonephritis, or pneumonia may be present, and delirium tremens may develop.

The blood-ethanol level is usually low or undetectable because ethanol intake ceased substantially earlier in the clinical course. The hallmarks of AKA include a large anion gap metabolic acidosis with a serum lactate level unable to account for the gap. However, some patients have a normal blood pH or are alkalemic because of an associated metabolic alkalosis and respiratory alkalosis.[42] When patients with AKA were compared to patients with diabetic ketoacidosis (DKA), those with AKA tended to have a higher blood pH, lower serum potassium and chloride levels, and a higher serum bicarbonate level.[42,45] The anion gaps in patients with AKA and DKA are very similar, with β-hydroxybutyrate acting as the primary anion contributor and lactate having a less-consequential role.[45]

The nitroprusside test used to detect the presence of ketones in serum and urine may be only mildly positive in patients with AKA because the nitroprusside reaction only detects molecules containing a ketone moiety. These include acetone and acetoacetate but not β-hydroxybutyrate. Reliance on the nitroprusside test alone as a measure of ketoacidosis may lead to underestimation of the severity of the ketoacidosis. Specific assays for β-hydroxybutyrate may be performed, but are not readily available in most hospital laboratories. The blood glucose may be low or mildly elevated. Ethanol-induced hypoglycemia probably occurs first, causing increased levels of cortisol, growth hormone, glucagon, and epinephrine; correcting the hypoglycemia and mobilizing fatty acids, which are then converted to ketones.[26] Therefore, alcoholic hypoglycemia and alcoholic ketoacidosis may be sequential events of the same process depending on the point in this process at which the patient is evaluated.

The diagnostic criteria for AKA should include a recent history of ethanol intake with a relative or absolute decline in ethanol consumption for 24–72 hours before presentation, a history of vomiting, a blood glucose level less than 300 mg/dL (65.22 mmol/L), and a metabolic acidosis for which other causes have been excluded by clinical observations or laboratory studies.[123]

Management

Treatment should begin with adequate crystalloid fluid replacement, dextrose, and thiamine. Supplemental multivitamins, potassium, and magnesium should be instituted on an individual basis. The administration of dextrose will stimulate the release of insulin, decrease the release of glucagon, and reduce the oxidation of fatty acids. Exogenous glucose also facilitates the synthesis of adenosine triphosphate (ATP), which reverses the pyruvate-to-lactate and $NAD^+/NADH$ ratios. The provision of thiamine may facilitate pyruvate entry into the Krebs cycle, thus increasing ATP production. Volume replacement restores glomerular flow and improves excretion of organic acids. Administration of either exogenous administration of insulin or sodium bicarbonate in the management of AKA is usually unnecessary.[46]

During the recovery phase of AKA, β-hydroxybutyrate is converted to acetoacetate. As this process occurs, the nitroprusside test may become more positive because of higher levels of ace-

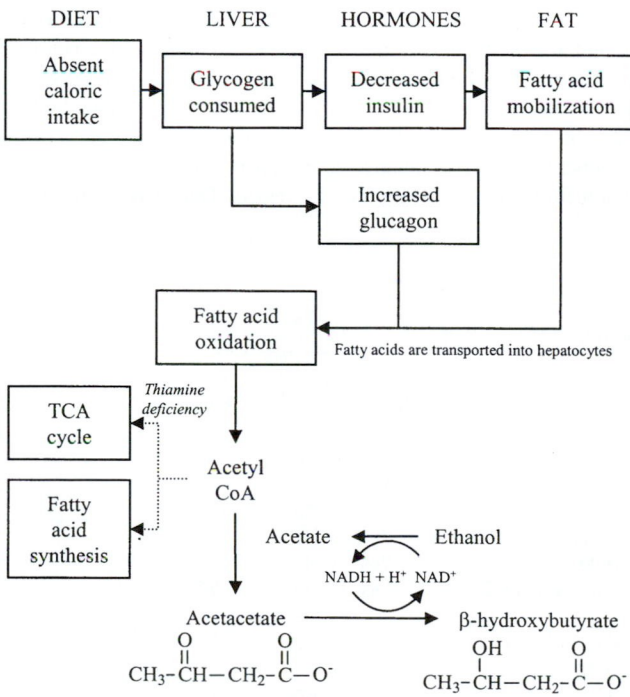

Figure 64–3. Mechanism of alcoholic ketoacidosis. *(Modified, with permission, from Hoffman RS, Goldfrank LR: Ethanol-associated metabolic disorders in endocrine metabolic disorders. Emerg Med Clin North Am 1989;7:952.)*

toacetate, resulting in a transient hyperketonemia that actually represents improvement of the metabolic status.

Mortality is rare from either ethanol-induced ketoacidosis or hypoglycemia. However, these patients may succumb to other precipitating or coexisting medical or surgical disorders,[43] such as occult trauma, pancreatitis, gastrointestinal hemorrhage, hepatorenal dysfunction, or infections.

ALCOHOLISM

Alcoholism has traditionally been defined as a chronic, progressive disease characterized by tolerance and physical dependence to ethanol and pathologic organ changes. Although alcoholism was historically considered to represent a defect in moral character, a more unified and enlightened view now considers it a multifactorial, genetically influenced disorder.[31,53] Alcoholism should be suspected in any patient who presents to the ED with unexplained trauma, seizures, or bizarre behavior. Suggestive physical findings associated with long-term alcoholism include flushed facies, parotid enlargement, gynecomastia, hepatomegaly, stigmata of cirrhosis, testicular atrophy, palmar erythema, Dupuytren's contractures, fluctuating mild hypertension, peripheral neuropathy, evidence of nutritional deficiencies, and repeated infections.

Concern for early detection and intervention with alcoholism led to attempts to create reliable diagnostic screening systems. The Brief Michigan Alcoholism Screening Test (MAST)[114] and the CAGE questions[97] represent two such devices (Tables 64–2 and 64–3). As can be seen from these screening devices, the presence of physical tolerance and/or dependence is not essential for a diagnosis of alcoholism. Instead, emphasis is placed on the social and behavioral concomitants of heavy drinking.[105] In the ED setting, questions concerning the patient's ability to function physically and psychologically are just as appropriate as quantifying the amount of ethanol consumed per day.

Alcoholism is commonly associated with affective disorders, especially depression,[96,119] and there is a higher rate of alcoholism among manic-depressives than in the general population.[138] Ethanol affects mood, judgment, and self-control, and creates a clinical condition conducive to self-injury and violence directed at others. Alcoholism is an important risk factor for suicide. Although many people drink in a misguided attempt to ameliorate their depression, all available evidence suggests that alcoholism adversely affects mood and cognitive ability. Research has pointed to an increased incidence of alcoholism in families,[20] and twin studies suggest that a tendency to drink is partly under genetic control.[7,61] Chromosomal linkage analysis has implicated chromosomes 4, 6, and 11 in the genetic predisposition to alcoholism.[11]

Although it is a serious disease with important health and economic consequences, alcoholism remains underdiagnosed and a treatment challenge in the United States. In one study, less than 10% of alcoholics referred for inpatient treatment were referred by physicians.[71] In general, healthcare providers tend to have an overly pessimistic view of the benefits of treating alcoholism. Particularly problematic is the apparent inability of most healthcare workers to effectively deal with the problem when it affects their colleagues. Success in the efforts to combat alcoholism requires increased public education and greater acceptance of alcoholism as a medical illness amenable to treatment.

Various strategies are employed to treat alcoholism. Treatment consists of psychosocial interventions, pharmacologic interventions, or both. A review of the evidence regarding the pharmacologic treatment of ethanol dependence was performed, focusing on 5 categories of drugs—the opioid antagonists naltrexone and nalmefene, acamprosate, disulfiram, various serotonergic agents, and lithium.[47] Naltrexone reduces the risk of relapse to heavy drinking and the frequency of drinking as compared with placebo, but does not substantially help maintain abstinence. Acamprosate reduces drinking frequency, although its effects on maintaining abstinence or reducing time to first drink are less clear. Controlled studies of disulfiram reveal a mixed outcome pattern. Some evidence suggests that drinking frequency is reduced, but there is minimal evidence to support improved continuous abstinence rates. There was limited data on serotonergic agents and the data is not encouraging. However, most studies were confounded by high rates of comorbid mood disorders. Lithium lacks efficacy in the treatment of primary ethanol dependence. The nonpharmacologic treatment for alcoholism is also successful. Data derived from sev-

---

TABLE 64–2. The Brief Michigan Alcoholism Screening Test

Question	Circle Correct Answer		Points
1. Do you feel you are a normal drinker?	Yes	No	N2
2. Do friends or relatives think you are a normal drinker?	Yes	No	N2
3. Have you ever attended a meeting of Alcoholics Anonymous?	Yes	No	Y5
4. Have you ever lost friends or girlfriends/boyfriends because of drinking?	Yes	No	Y2
5. Have you ever gotten into trouble at work because of drinking?	Yes	No	Y2
6. Have you ever neglected your obligations, your family, or your work for 2 or more days in a row because you were drinking?	Yes	No	Y2
7. Have you ever had delirium tremens (DTs) or severe shaking, or heard voices, or seen things that were not there after heavy drinking?	Yes	No	Y2
8. Have you ever gone to anyone for help about your drinking?	Yes	No	Y5
9. Have you ever been in a hospital because of drinking?	Yes	No	Y5
10. Have you ever been arrrested for drunk driving after drinking?	Yes	No	Y2

Score 6 = Probable diagnosis of alcoholism

Reprinted with permission, from Pokorny AO, Miller, BA, Kaplan HB: The Brief MAST. Am J Psychiatry 1972;129:342–345.

TABLE 64–3. **The CAGE Questions**

TABLE 64–3. **The CAGE Questions**

1. Have you ever felt you should **C**ut down on your drinking?
2. Have people **A**nnoyed you by criticizing your drinking?
3. Have you ever felt bad or **G**uilty about your drinking?
4. Have you ever had a drink first thing in the morning to steady your nerves or to get rid of a hangover (**E**ye-opener)?

Two or more affirmatives = probable diagnosis of alcoholism

Reprinted with permission, from West LJ, Maxwell DS, Noble EP, Soloman DH: Alcoholism. Ann Intern Med 1984;100:412–420.

eral studies and membership surveys indicate that recovery rates of 40–80% can be achieved in treatment programs based on the 12-step approach of Alcoholics Anonymous.[62,63,133]

COMMON ETHANOL-DRUG INTERACTIONS

Ethanol interacts with a variety of drugs[70] (Table 64–4). Although, the interaction between ethanol and disulfiram (Antabuse) can be life-threatening, this drug is occasionally used to prevent drinking recidivism (Chap. 65).

Acute intoxication with ethanol can transiently prolong the elimination of certain drugs (eg, phenytoin) because of competition for shared metabolic pathways such as the cytochrome P450 system. Alternatively, an increase in the MEOS system (CYP2E1)

TABLE 64–4. **Ethanol-Drug or Toxin Interactions**

Drugs	Adverse Effects
Acetaminophen	May increase hepatotoxicity*
Antihistamines	Enhanced CNS depression
Carbamates	Disulfiramlike effect
Cephalosporins	Disulfiramlike effect
Chloral hydrate	Enhanced CNS depression
Chloramphenicol	Disulfiramlike effect
Chlorpropamide	Disulfiramlike effect
Cimetidine	Increased alcohol level
Cocaine	Formation of cocaethylene
Coprinus mushrooms	Disulfiramlike effect
Disulfiram (Antabuse)	Nausea; vomiting; abdominal pain; flushing; diaphoresis; chest pain; headache; vertigo; palpitations
Griseofulvin	Disulfiramlike effect
Heroin	Enhanced CNS depression
Isoniazid	Increased incidence of hepatitis; increased isoniazid metabolism*
Methadone	Increased methadone metabolism*
Metronidazole	Disulfiramlike effect
Nitrofurantoin	Disulfiramlike effect
Phenytoin	Increased phenytoin metabolism
Ranitidine	Increased alcohol level
Sedative-hypnotics	Enhanced CNS depression
Thiuram derivatives	Disulfiramlike effect
Tolbutamide	Disulfiramlike effect; increased tolbutamide metabolism*
Warfarin	Increased warfarin metabolism*

*Effect possibly associated with chronic alcohol consumption.

with chronic drinking leads to accelerated metabolism and shortens the half-lives of drugs such as phenytoin, methadone, tolbutamide, isoniazid, and warfarin.[75]

Ethanol has additive sedative effects when ingested with antihistamines, cyclic antidepressants, phenothiazines, barbiturates, and other sedative-hypnotics such as glutethimide, opioids, and chloral hydrate ("Mickey Finn"). Ethanol can enhance the aspirin-induced increase in bleeding time.

Concomitant use of cocaine and ethanol leads to the formation of an active metabolite, cocaethylene, through transesterification of cocaine by the liver.[115] Cocaethylene has a longer half-life than cocaine itself (2 hours vs 48 minutes), which may explain some of the delayed cardiovascular effects attributed to cocaine use.[6,137] Both ethanol and cocaethylene inhibit the metabolism of cocaine, thereby prolonging the elimination of cocaine and enhancing its effects. (Chap. 67).[111]

Histamine$_2$ receptor antagonists such as cimetidine and ranitidine, but not famotidine, increase the bioavailability of imbibed ethanol.[5,13,16,38] This is a result of decreased first-pass metabolism caused by inhibition of the activity of alcohol dehydrogenase in the gastric mucosa.[27] In alcoholics and in those with higher ethanol levels, cimetidine may also delay ethanol clearance by inhibiting the MEOS system (CYP2E1). However, the increase in blood-ethanol level from such an interaction is of questionable clinical significance.[4,5,13,15]

Case reports and retrospective case series suggest chronic ethanol consumption may predispose a person to acetaminophen (APAP) hepatotoxicity[34,93,98,118,142] even when APAP has been used in accordance with the recommended dosage of not more than 4 g daily.[141] However, in a double-blind placebo control study in which confirmed alcoholics were given acetaminophen 4 g daily or placebo for 3 consecutive days, there were no clinical complications recognized and no differences between the two groups with regard to liver enzymes or to their coagulation profile.[78] Because ethanol induces cytochrome P450, the enzyme involved in the metabolism of acetaminophen to its hepatotoxic intermediate, NAPQI (*N*-acetyl-*p*-benzoquinoneimine), there is a theoretical basis for this concern. Recent fasting, common in alcoholics, was also associated with a predisposition to acetaminophen hepatotoxicity, probably due to depletion of glutathione[136] (Chap. 32). However, in a retrospective study, heavy drinkers did not develop more severe hepatotoxicity following APAP overdose than did nondrinkers.[94]

COMMON ETHANOL-RELATED DISEASES

Ethanol affects practically every organ system in the body (Table 64–5). In addition to the harmful effects of ethanol itself, there is evidence to suggest that its metabolite, acetaldehyde, is inherently toxic to biologic systems.[17,87] Acetaldehyde is associated with structural and functional alterations of mitochondria and hepatocytes,[76] interferes with phosphorylation, inactivates coenzyme A, and inhibits myocardial protein synthesis.[77] Acetaldehyde can be acutely toxic if its conversion to acetate is blocked because of congenital dysfunction of acetaldehyde dehydrogenase, or because of inhibition of the enzyme by disulfiram or other agents. Oxidation of ethanol results in the formation of excess NADH relative to NAD$^+$, and this altered redox potential has negative consequences for many cellular functions.

TABLE 64–5. Systemic Effects Associated with Ethanol Consumption

Cardiovascular	Diarrhea	Alcohol withdrawal
Cardiomyopathy	Hematemesis*	Central pontine myelinolysis
"Holiday heart"	Malabsorption	Cerebral atrophy (dementia)
(dysrhythmias)	Peptic ulcer	Cerebellar degeneration
"Wet" beriberi	Liver	CVA (SAH, infarction)
(thiamine deficiency)	Steatosis	"Dry" beriberi (Wernicke-
	Hepatitis	Korsakoff syndrome)
Endocrine and Metabolic	Cirrhosis	Wernicke's encephalopathy
Hypo-* or hyperglycemia	Pancreas	Korsakoff's psychosis
Hypophosphatemia	Pancreatitis (acute or chronic)	Intoxication*
Hypokalemia	Pancreatic pseudocyst	Marchiafava-Bignami disease
Hypomagnesemia		Myopathy
Hypothermia*	**Genitourinary**	Polyneuropathy
Hypertriglyceridemia	Hypogonadism	Pellegra
Hyperuricemia	Impotence	
Metabolic acidosis	Infertility	**Ophthalmic**
Malnutrition		Ophthalmoplegia ("dry" beriberi)
	Hematologic	Tobacco-alcohol amblyopia
Gastrointestinal	Coagulopathies	
Mouth	Folic acid, vitamin B$_{12}$, and iron,	**Psychiatric**
Cancer of the mouth,	deficiency anemias	Animated behavior*
pharynx, larynx	Hemolysis (Zieve's syndrome,	Loss of self-restraint*
Cheilosis	stomatocytosis, spur cell	Manic-depressive illness
Nutritional stomatitis	anemia)	Suicide and depression
Esophagus	Leukopenia	
Boerhaave's syndrome*	Thrombocytopenia	**Respiratory**
Cancer of the esophagus		Atelectasis
Diffuse-esophageal spasm*	**Neurologic**	Pneumonia*
Esophagitis*	Alcohol amnestic syndrome	Respiratory depression*
Mallory-Weiss tear*	Alcoholic hallucinosis	Respiratory acidosis*
Stomach and duodenum		
Gastritis*		
Chronic hypertrophic gastritis		

*Potential acute ethanol effects

SUMMARY

Acute ethanol intoxication and chronic alcoholism are among the most common and complex toxicologic and societal problems. These patients may present with a diversity of clinical problems that challenge the clinician to be meticulous and systematic in their evaluation and management of these patients.

REFERENCES

1. Abdulla A, Badawy B: The metabolism of alcohol. Clin Endocrinol Metab 1978;7:247–252.
2. Adinoff B, Gone GH, Linnoila M: Acute ethanol poisoning and the ethanol withdrawal syndrome. Med Toxicol Adverse Drug Exp 1988;3:172–196.
3. Alobaidi AA, Hill DW, Payne JP: Significance of variations in blood: Breath partition coefficient of alcohol. Br Med J 1976;2:1479–1481.
4. Amir I, Anwar N, Baraona E, et al: Ranitidine increases the bioavailability of imbibed alcohol by accelerating gastric emptying. Life Sci 1996;58:511–518.
5. Arora S, Baraona E, Lieber CS: Alcohol levels are increased in social drinkers receiving ranitidine. Am J Gastroenterol 2000;95:208–213.
6. Bailey DN, Bessler JB, Saucrey BA: Cocaine and cocaethylene-creatinine clearance ratios in humans. J Anal Toxicol 1997;21:41–43.
7. Ball DM, Murray RM: Genetics of alcohol misuse. BMJ 1994;50:18–35.
8. Barry PW, O'Callaghan C: New formulation metered dose inhaler increases breath-alcohol levels. Respir Med 1999;93:167–168.
9. Becker CE: Alcohol and drug use: Is there a safe amount? West J Med 1984;141:884–890.
10. Block RS, Weaver DW, Bowman DL: Acute alcohol intoxication: Significance of the amylase level. Ann Emerg Med 1983;12:294–296.
11. Blum K, Noble EP, Sheridan PJ: Allelic association of human receptor gene in alcoholism. JAMA 1990;263:2055–2060.
12. Brennan DF, Betzelos S, Reed R, Falk JL: Ethanol elimination rates in an ED population. Am J Emerg Med 1995;13:276–280.
13. Brown AS, James OF: Omeprazole, ranitidine, and cimetidine have no effect on peak blood ethanol concentrations, first-pass metabolism or area under the time-ethanol curve under "real-life" drinking conditions. Alimet Pharmacol Ther 1998;12:141–145.
14. Butterworth RF, Kril JJ, Harper CG: Thiamine-dependent enzyme changes in the brains of alcoholics: Relationship to the Wernicke-Korsakoff syndrome. Alcohol Clin Exp Res 1993;17:1084–1088.
15. Bye A, Lacey LF, Gupta S, et al: Effect of ranitidine hydrochloride (150 mg twice daily) on the pharmacokinetics of increasing doses of ethanol (0.15, 0.3, 0.6 g.kg^{-1}). Br J Clin Pharmacol 1996;41:129–133.

16. Caballeria J, Barbona E, Podamilens M, Lieber CS: Effects of cimetidine on gastric alcohol dehydrogenase activity and blood ethanol levels. Gastroenterology 1989;96:388–392.

17. Cederbaum AI, Lieber CS, Rubin E: Effects of chronic ethanol treatment on mitochondrial functions, I. Arch Biochem Biophys 1974;165:560–570.

18. Chapman LF: Experimental induction of hangover. Q J Stud Alcohol 1970;31:67–86.

19. Committee on Drugs, 1983–1984, American Academy of Pediatrics: Ethanol in liquid preparations intended for children. Pediatrics 1984;73:405–407.

20. Cotton NS: The familial incidence of alcoholism: A review. J Stud Alcohol 1979;40:89–93.

21. Crabb DW, Bosrom WF, Li TK: Ethanol metabolism. Pharmacol Ther 1987;34:59–73.

22. Cummins LH: Hypoglycemia and convulsions in children following alcohol ingestion. J Pediatr 1961;58:23–26.

23. Damrau F, Liddy E: Hangovers and whisky congeners: Comparison of whisky with vodka. J Natl Med Assoc 1960;52:262–264.

24. Damrau F, Goldberg AH: Adsorption of whisky congeners by activated charcoal. Southwest Med 1971;53:175–182.

25. David DJ, Spyker DA: The acute toxicity of ethanol: Dosage and kinetic nomograms. Vet Hum Toxicol 1979;21:272.

26. Devenyi P: Alcoholic hypoglycemia and alcoholic ketoacidosis: Sequential events of the same process? Can Med Assoc J 1982;127:513.

27. Di Padova C, Poine R, Frezza M, et al: Effects of ranitidine on blood alcohol levels after ethanol ingestion. JAMA 1992;267:83–86.

28. Djordjevic D, Nikolic J, Stefanovic V: Ethanol interactions with other cytochrome P450 substrates including drugs, xenobiotics, and carcinogens. Pathol Biol 1998;46:760–770.

29. Dohmen K, Baraona E, Ishibashi H, et al: Ethnic differences in gastric-alcohol dehydrogenase activity and ethanol first-pass metabolism. Alcohol Clin Exp Res 1996;20:1569–1576.

30. Doyle KM, Cluette-Brown JE, Dube DM, et al: Fatty acid ethyl esters in the blood as markers of ethanol intake. JAMA 1996;276:1152–1156.

31. Eckardt MJ, Harford IC, Kaelber CT: Health hazards associated with alcohol consumption. JAMA 1981;246:648–653.

32. Eilam O, Heyman SN: Wenckebach-type atrioventricular block in severe alcohol intoxication. Ann Emerg Med 1991;20:1170.

33. Ellis T, Lacy R: Illicit alcohol (moonshine) consumption in West Alabama revisited. South Med J 1998;91:858–860.

34. Embly DI, Fraser BN: Hepatotoxicity of paracetamol enhanced by ingestion of alcohol. S Afr Med J 1977;51:208–209.

35. Ernst AA, Jones K, Nick TG, et al: Ethanol ingestion and related hypoglycemia in a pediatric and adolescent emergency department population. Acad Emerg Med 1996;3:46–49.

36. Faingold CL, N'Gouemo P, Riaz A: Ethanol and neurotransmitter interactions—From molecular to integrative effects. Prog Neurobiol 1998;55:509–535.

37. Falkensson M, Jones W, Sorbo B: Bedside diagnosis of alcohol intoxication with a pocketsize breath-alcohol device: Sampling from unconscious subjects and specificity for ethanol. Clin Chem 1989;35:918–921.

38. Feely J, Wood AJ: Effects of cimetidine on the elimination and actions of ethanol. JAMA 1982;247:2819–2821.

39. Fluckiger A, Hartmann D, Leishman B, Zeigler WH: Lack of effect of the benzodiazepine antagonist flumazenil and the performance of healthy subjects during experimentally induced ethanol intoxication. Eur J Clin Pharmacol 1988;34:273–276.

40. Fraser AG: Pharmacokinetic interactions between alcohol and other drugs. Clin Pharmacokinet 1997;33:79–90.

41. Frezza M, DiRadova C, Pozzato G, et al: High blood alcohol levels in women: The role of decreased gastric alcohol dehydrogenase activity and first pass metabolism. N Engl J Med 1990;322:95–110.

42. Fulop M: Alcoholic ketoacidosis. Endocrinol Metab Clin North Am 1993;22:209–219.

43. Fulop M: Alcoholism, ketoacidosis, and lactic acidosis. Diabetes Metab Rev 1989;5:365–378.

44. Fulop M, Ben-Ezra J, Bock J: Alcoholic ketosis. Alcohol Clin Exp Res 1986;10:610–615.

45. Fulop M, Hoberman HD: Diabetic ketoacidosis and alcoholic ketosis. Ann Intern Med 1979;91:796–797.

46. Fulop M, Hoberman HD: Alcoholic ketosis. Diabetes 1975;24:785–790.

47. Garbutt JC, West SL, Carey TS, et al: Pharmacological treatment of alcohol dependence: A review of the evidence. JAMA 1999;281:1318–1325.

48. Gerberich SG, Gerberich BK, Fife D: Analysis of the relationship between blood alcohol and nasal breath alcohol concentrations. J Trauma 1989;29:338–343.

49. Gerhardt RE, Crecelius EA, Hudson JB: Moonshine-related arsenic poisoning. Arch Intern Med 1980;140:211–213.

50. Gershman H, Steper J: Rate of clearance of ethanol from the blood of intoxicated patients in the emergency department. J Emerg Med 1991;9:307–311.

51. Goedde HW, Harada S, Agarwal DP: Social differences in alcohol sensitivity. Hum Genet 1979;51:331–334.

52. Goldstein DB: The effect of drugs on membrane fluidity. Annu Rev Pharmacol Toxicol 1984;24:43–64.

53. Gomez HF, Moore L, McKinney P, et al: Elevation of breath ethanol measurements by metered-dose inhalers. Ann Emerg Med 1995;25:608–611.

54. Goodwin DW: Is Alcoholism Hereditary? New York, Oxford University Press, 1976, pp. 23–26.

55. Gould L: Hemodynamic effects of ethanol in patients with cardiac disease. Q J Stud Alcohol 1972;33:714–722.

56. Grant BF, Harford TC, Dawson DA, Chou P: Prevalence of DSM-IV alcohol abuse and dependence United States 1992. Alcohol Health Res World 1994;18:243–248.

57. Greenspon AJ: Provocation of ventricular tachycardia after consumption of alcohol. N Engl J Med 1979;301:1049–1156.

58. Greenspon AJ, Schaal SF: The "holiday heart": Electrophysiological studies of alcohol effects in alcoholics. Ann Intern Med 1983;98:135–140.

59. Guerin J, Friedberg G: Naloxone and ethanol intoxication. Ann Intern Med 1982;97:932–936.

60. Haymond MW: Hypoglycemia in infants and children. Endocrinol Metab Clin North Am 1989;18:211–252.

61. Hill SY, Goodwin DW, Cadoret R: Association and linkage between alcohol and eleven serological markers. J Stud Alcohol 1975;36:981–984.

62. Hoffman NG, Harrison PA, Belille CA: Alcoholics anonymous after treatment: Attendance and abstinence. Int J Addict 1983;18:311–313.

63. Hoffman NG, Miller NS: Treatment outcome for abstinence-based programs. Psych Ann 1992;22:402–407.

64. Hoffman RS, Smilkstein MJ, Howland MA, et al: Osmol gaps revisited: Normal values and limitations. J Toxicol Clin Toxicol. 1993;31:81–93.

65. Hoffman RS, Goldfrank LR: Ethanol-associated metabolic disorders. Emerg Med Clin North Am 1989;7:943–961.

66. Holt S, Stewart IC, Dixon JM: Alcohol and the emergency service patient. Br Med J 1980;281:638–640.

67. Hornfeldt CS: A report of acute ethanol poisoning in a child. J Toxicol Clin Toxicol 1992;30:115–121.

68. Hsu LC, Bendel RE, Yoshida A: Genomic structure of the human mitochondrial ALDH gene. Genomics 1988;2:57–65.

69. Hu X-J, Ticku MK: Chronic ethanol treatment upregulates the NMDA receptor function and binding in mammalian cortical neurons. Brain Res Mol Brain Res 1995;30:347–356.

70. Interactions of drugs with alcohol. Abramowicz M, (ed.). Med Lett Drugs Ther 1981;23:33–34.

71. Isselbacher KJ: Metabolic and hepatic effects of alcohol. N Engl J Med 1977;296:612–616.

72. Jones AW: Variability of the blood: Breath alcohol ratio in vivo. J Stud Alcohol 1978;39:1931–1939.

73. Kahanna JM, Kalant H, Le AD, et al: Role of serotonergic and adrenergic systems in alcohol tolerance. Prog Neuropsychopharmacol 1981;5:459–465.

74. Kalant H: Ethanol and the nervous system: Experimental neurophysiological aspects. Int J Neurol 1974;9:111–120.

75. Kater RM, Roggin G, Tobon F, et al: Increased rate of clearance of drugs from the circulation of alcoholics. Am J Med Sci 1969;258:35–39.

76. Kissin B, Degleiter H: The Biology of Alcoholism, Vol. 1. New York, Plenum, 1970, pp. 630–637.

77. Klatsky AL, Friedman GD, Sieglaub AB: Alcohol and mortality. Ann Intern Med 1981;95:139–144.

78. Kuffner E, Dart RC, Bogdan GM, et al: Effect of maximal daily doses of acetaminophen on the liver of alcoholic patients. Arch Intern Med 2001;161:2247–2252.

79. Kunitoh S, Imaoka S, Hiroi T, et al: Acetaldehyde as well as ethanol is metabolized by human CYP2E1. J Pharmacol Exp Ther 1997;280:527–532.

80. Lamminpaa A: Alcohol intoxication in childhood and adolescence. Alcohol Alcohol 1995;30:5–12.

81. Lamminpaa A, Vilska J: Acute alcohol intoxications in children treated in hospital. Acta Paediatr Scand 1990;79:847–854.

82. Lavoie J, Butterworth RF: Reduced activities of thiamine-dependent enzymes in brains of alcoholics in the absence of Wernicke's encephalopathy. Alcohol Clin Exp Res 1995;19:1073–1077.

83. Lester D: Breath tests for alcohol. N Engl J Med 1971;284:1269–1270.

84. Leung AK: Ethyl alcohol ingestion in children. Clin Pediatr 1986;25:617–619.

85. Lewis DC: Diagnosis and management of the alcoholic patient. RI Med J 1980;63:27–34.

86. Lieber CS: Alcohol and the liver: 1994 update. Gastroenterology 1994;106:1085–1105.

87. Lieber CS: Biochemical and molecular basis of alcohol-induced injury to the liver and other tissues. N Engl J Med 1988;319:1639–1644.

88. Lieber CS, DeCarli LM: Hepatotoxicity of ethanol. J Hepatol 1991;12:394–401.

89. Logan BK, Distefano S, Case GA: Evaluation of the effect of asthma inhalers and nasal decongestant sprays on a breath alcohol test. J Forensic Sci 1998;43:197–199.

90. Lovinger DM, White G, Weight FF: Ethanol inhibits NMDA-activated ion current in hippocampal neurons. Science 1989;243:1721–1724.

91. Lteif AN, Schwenk WF: Hypoglycemia in infants and children. Endocrinol Metab Clin North Am 1999;28:619–646.

92. Mackenzie AI: Naloxone in alcohol intoxication. Lancet 1979;1:733–736.

93. Maddrey WC: Hepatic effects of acetaminophen—Enhanced toxicity in alcoholics. J Clin Gastroenterol 1987;9:180–185.

94. Makin A, Williams R: Paracetamol hepatotoxicity and alcohol consumption in deliberate and accidental overdose. QJM 2000;93:341–349.

95. Malin H, Coakley J, Kaelber C: An Epidemiologic Perspective on Alcohol Use and Abuse in the U.S. Alcohol Consumption and Related Problems. Alcohol and Health Monograph no. 1, DHHS pub. no. ADM 82–1190. Washington, DC, U.S. Government Printing Office, 1982.

96. Mayfield D: Alcoholism and affective disorders: Experimental studies. In: Goodwin DW, Erickson CK, eds: Alcoholism and Affective Disorders. New York, SP Medical and Scientific, 1979, pp. 99–107.

97. Mayfield D, McLeod G, Hall P: More detailed interview screening. Am J Psychiatry 1974;131:1121–1126.

98. McClain CJ, Kromhout JP, Peterson FJ, Holtzman JL: Potentiation of acetaminophen hepatotoxicity. JAMA 1980;244:251–253.

99. McDermott PH, Delaney RL, Egon JD, et al: Myocarditis and cardiac failure in men. JAMA 1966;198:253–256.

100. Mercier G, Patry G: Quebec beer-drinkers' cardiomyopathy: Clinical signs and symptoms. Can Med Assoc J 1967;97:884–888.

101. Minocha A, Herold DA, Barth JT, Gideon DA: Activated charcoal in oral ethanol absorption: Lack of effect in humans. J Toxicol Clin Toxicol 1986;24:225–234.

102. Miwa K, Igawa A, Miyagi Y: Importance of magnesium deficiency in alcohol-induced variant angina. Am J Cardiol 1994;73:813–816.

103. Modell JG, Taylor JP, Lee JY: Breath alcohol value following mouthwash use. JAMA 1993;270:2955–2956.

104. Modell JG: Behavioral, neurologic, and physiologic effects of acute ethanol ingestion. In Fassler D, ed. The Alcoholic Patient: Emergency Medical Intervention. New York, Gardner Press, 1990, pp. 25–34.

105. Morse RM, Flarin DK: The definition of alcoholism. JAMA 1992;268:1012–1014.

106. Moskowitz H, Burns M, Ferguson S: Police officers' detection of breath odors from alcohol ingestion. Accid Anal Prev 1999;31:175–180.

107. National Highway Traffic Safety Administration. 1998 Traffic Fatalities Decline: Alcohol-Related Deaths Reach Record Low, Press Release No. 23–99, Washington, DC, Department of Transportation, 1999.

108. National Institute on Alcohol Abuse and Alcoholism. Alcohol and Health: Ninth Special Report to the US Congress, NIH Publication No. 97–4017, Rockville, MD, Department of Health and Human Services, 1997.

109. Nuotto E: Coffee and caffeine and alcohol effects on psychomotor function. Clin Pharmacol Ther 1982;31:68–72.

110. Nuotto E, Palva ES: Naloxone fails to counteract heavy alcohol intoxication. Lancet 1983;2:167–170.

111. Parker RB, Williams CL, Laizure SC, et al: Effects of ethanol and cocaethylene on cocaine pharmacokinetics in conscious dogs. Drug Metab Dispos 1996;24:850–853.

112. Peoples RW, Li C, Weight FF: Lipid vs. protein theories of alcohol action in the nervous system. Annu Rev Pharmacol Toxicol 1996;36:185–201.

113. Petroni NC, Cardoni AA: Alcohol content of liquid medicinals. Clin Toxicol 1979;14:407–432.

114. Pokorny AD, Miller BA, Kaplan HB: The brief MAST. Am J Psychiatry 1972;129:342–350.

115. Randall T: Cocaine, alcohol mix in body to form even longer lasting, more lethal drug. JAMA 1992;267:1043–1044.

116. Ritchie JM: The aliphatic alcohols. In: Gilman AG, Goodman LS, Rall TW, Murad F, eds: The Pharmacological Basis of Therapeutics, 7th ed. New York, Macmillan, 1985, pp. 372–387.

117. Rodenberg HD, Bennett JR, Watson WA: Clinical utility of a saliva alcohol dipstick estimate of serum ethanol concentrations in the emergency department. DICP Ann Pharmacother 1990;24:358–361.

118. Schiodt FV, Rochling FA, Casey DL, et al: Acetaminophen toxicity in an urban county hospital. N Engl J Med 1997;337:1112–1117.

119. Schuckit MA: Alcoholism and affective disorders: Diagnostic confusion. In: Goodwin DW, Erickson CK, eds: Alcoholism and Affective Disorders. New York, SP Medical and Scientific, 1979, pp. 9–19.

120. Sherlock JC, Pickford CJ, White GF: Lead in alcoholic beverages. Food Addit Contam 1986;3:347–354.

121. Sixth Special Report to Congress on Alcohol and Health. Department of Health and Human Services, National Institute on Alcohol Abuse and Alcoholism. DHHS pub. no. ADM 87–1519. Washington, DC, Department of Health and Human Services, 1987.

122. Smart GA, Pickford CJ, Sherlock JC: Lead in alcoholic beverages: A second survey. Food Addit Contam 1990;7:93–99.

123. Soffer A, Hamburger S: Alcoholic ketoacidosis: A review of 30 cases. J Am Med Wom Assoc 1982;37:106–110.

124. Sullivan JF, Wolpert PW, Williams R: Serum magnesium in chronic alcoholism. Ann N Y Acad Sci 1969;162:947–955.

125. Tabakoff B, Cornell N, Hoffman PL: Alcohol tolerance. Ann Emerg Med 1986;15:1005–1012.

126. Tabakoff B, Hoffman PL: Alcohol addiction: An enigma among us. Neuron 1996;16:909–912.

127. Takeshita T, Mao XQ, Morimoto K: The contribution of polymorphism in the alcohol dehydrogenase beta subunit to alcohol sensitivity in a Japanese population. Hum Genet 1996;97:409–413.

128. Takeshita T, Morimoto K, Mao X, et al: Characterization of the three genotypes of low Km aldehyde dehydrogenase in a Japanese population. Hum Genet 1994;94:217–223.

129. Thomas RJ: Excitatory amino acids in health and disease. J Am Geriatr Soc 1995;43:1279–1289.

130. Tsai GE, Ragan P, Chang R, et al: Increased glutamatergic neurotransmission and oxidative stress after alcohol withdrawal. Am J Psychiatry 1998;155:726–732.

131. Tsai GE, Coyle JT: The role of glutamatergic neurotransmission in the pathophysiology of alcoholism. Annu Rev Med 1998;49:173–184.

132. Tsutaya S, Shoji M, Sito Y, et al: Analysis of aldehyde dehydrogenase 2 gene polymorphism and ethanol patch test as a screening method for alcohol sensitivity. Tohoku J Exp Med 1999;187:305–310.

133. Walsh EC, Himpson RW, Merrigan DM: A randomized trial of treatment options for alcohol abusing workers. N Engl J Med 1991;325:775–782.

134. Wenzel J, McDermott FT: Accuracy of blood alcohol estimations obtained with a breath alcohol analyzer in a casualty department. Med J Aust 1985;142:627–628.

135. West LJ, Maxwell DS, Noble EP, Solomon DH: Alcoholism. Ann Intern Med 1984;100:405–406.

136. Whitcomb DC, Block GD: Association of acetaminophen hepatotoxicity with fasting and ethanol use. JAMA 1994;272:1845–1850.

137. Wilson LD, Hemming RJ, Suttheimer C, et al: Cocaethylene causes dose-dependent reductions in cardiac function in anesthetized dogs. J Cardiovasc Pharmacol 1995;26:965–973.

138. Winokur G, Clayton P: Family history studies: Sex differences and alcoholism in primary affective illness. Br J Psychiatry 1967;113:973–976.

139. Zador PL, Krawchuk SA, Voas RB: Alcohol-related relative risk of driver fatalities and driver involvement in fatal crashes in relation to driver age and gender: An update using 1996 data. J Stud Alcohol 2000;61:387–395.

140. Zador PL: Alcohol-related relative risk and fatal driver injuries in relation to driver age and sex. J Stud Alcohol 1991;52:302–310.

141. Zimmerman HJ, Maddrey WC: Acetaminophen (paracetamol) hepatotoxicity with regular intake of alcohol: analysis of instances of therapeutic misadventure. Hepatology 1995;22:767–773.

142. Zimmerman HJ: Effects of alcohol on other hepatotoxins. Alcoholism 1986;10:3–15.

ANTIDOTES IN DEPTH

Vitamin B₁
(thiamine hydrochloride)

Thiamine
Robert S. Hoffman

Thiamine (vitamin B_1) is a water-soluble vitamin that is essential in the creation and utilization of cellular energy. As a coenzyme in the pyruvate dehydrogenase complex, thiamine diphosphate, the active form of thiamine accelerates the conversion of pyruvate to acetyl-Coenzyme A (acetyl-CoA). This reaction is known to occur at thiamine's C2 atom, which is located between the nitrogen and sulfur atoms on the thiazolium ring.[21] In the presence of the protein-rich environment of the enzyme complex, this C2 atom is deprotonated to form a carbanion that rapidly attaches to the carbonyl group of pyruvate, thereby stabilizing it for decarboxylation.[21] In a series of subsequent reactions, the hydroxyethyl group that remains bound to thiamine diphosphate is transferred to lipoamide, where an acetyl group is later broken off and attached to CoA. This process links anaerobic glycolysis to the Krebs cycle, where subsequent aerobic metabolism produces 36 moles of adenosine triphosphate (ATP) from each mole of glucose (Fig. 64–4). When pyruvate cannot be converted to acetyl-CoA because of thiamine deficiency for example, only 2 moles of ATP can be generated, by anaerobic metabolism, from each mole of glucose. Thiamine is also required as a cofactor for a second enzyme in the Krebs cycle, α-ketoglutarate dehydrogenase, and for transketolase, an enzyme in the pentose phosphate pathway, in which nicotinamide adenine dinucleotide phosphate (NADPH) is formed for subsequent use in reductive biosynthesis. Thiamine also has an important role in the maintenance of normal neuronal conduction.[47,61]

Thiamine is available from natural sources, such as organ meats, yeast, eggs, and green leafy vegetables,[47] in a basic form composed of a substituted pyrimidine ring and a substituted thia-zole ring connected by a methylene bridge. This connection between the two rings is weak, and the molecule is unstable in an alkaline milieu and in a highly temperature environment. In addition, thiamine is highly water soluble, allowing it to leach out of foods that are washed or cooked in water for prolonged times. The synthesized thiamine hydrochloride salt, however, is usually quite stable. Thiamine requirements are determined by total caloric intake and energy demand, with a minimum daily requirement of 0.5 mg/1000 calories.[47]

Thiamine is well absorbed from the human gastrointestinal tract by a complex process.[25] At low concentrations, thiamine absorption occurs through a saturable mechanism, that is most effective in the duodenum, with absorption occurring to a lesser degree in the large bowel and stomach. As thiamine concentrations increase, however, the majority of absorption occurs through simple passive diffusion. Although more recently synthesized analogues such as thiamine propyl disulfide, benfotiamin, and fursultiamin have enhanced bioavailability, their use remains largely experimental.[13,54] Chronic liver disease, folate deficiency, steatorrhea, and other forms of malabsorption all significantly decrease thiamine's absorption. This malabsorption has even greater clinical relevance in the alcoholic population.[2,53] In experimental studies, when healthy volunteers were given small amounts of ethanol, a 50% reduction in gastrointestinal thiamine absorption resulted.[53]

Thiamine is eliminated from the body largely by renal clearance, which consists of a combination of glomerular filtration, flow-dependent tubular secretion, and saturable tubular reabsorption.[59] In an animal model furosemide, acetazolamide, chlorothiazide, amiloride, mannitol, and salt loading all significantly increased urinary elimination of thiamine.[29] This nonspecific flow-dependent elimination was confirmed in humans given small doses of furosemide.[41] Additionally, both furosemide and digoxin appear to inhibit thiamine uptake into myocardial cells.[64]

Mice develop signs of encephalopathy 10 days after being rendered thiamine deficient. Immunohistochemistry in these animals demonstrates a breakdown of the blood-brain barrier with resultant extravasation of albumin.[16] Similarly, rats also develop symptoms after 10 days of thiamine deficiency, and demonstrate deterioration of the blood-brain barrier with hemorrhage into the mammillary body and other areas of the brain in a pattern similar to findings described in humans with Wernicke's encephalopathy.[8,38] In other animal models of thiamine deficiency, neuronal tissues are also directly injured by oxidative stress and lipid peroxidation.[9] Finally, thiamine deficiency in rats produces 200–640% increases in levels of glutamate, an excitatory amino acid.[27] This excess of glutamate presumably results from blockade

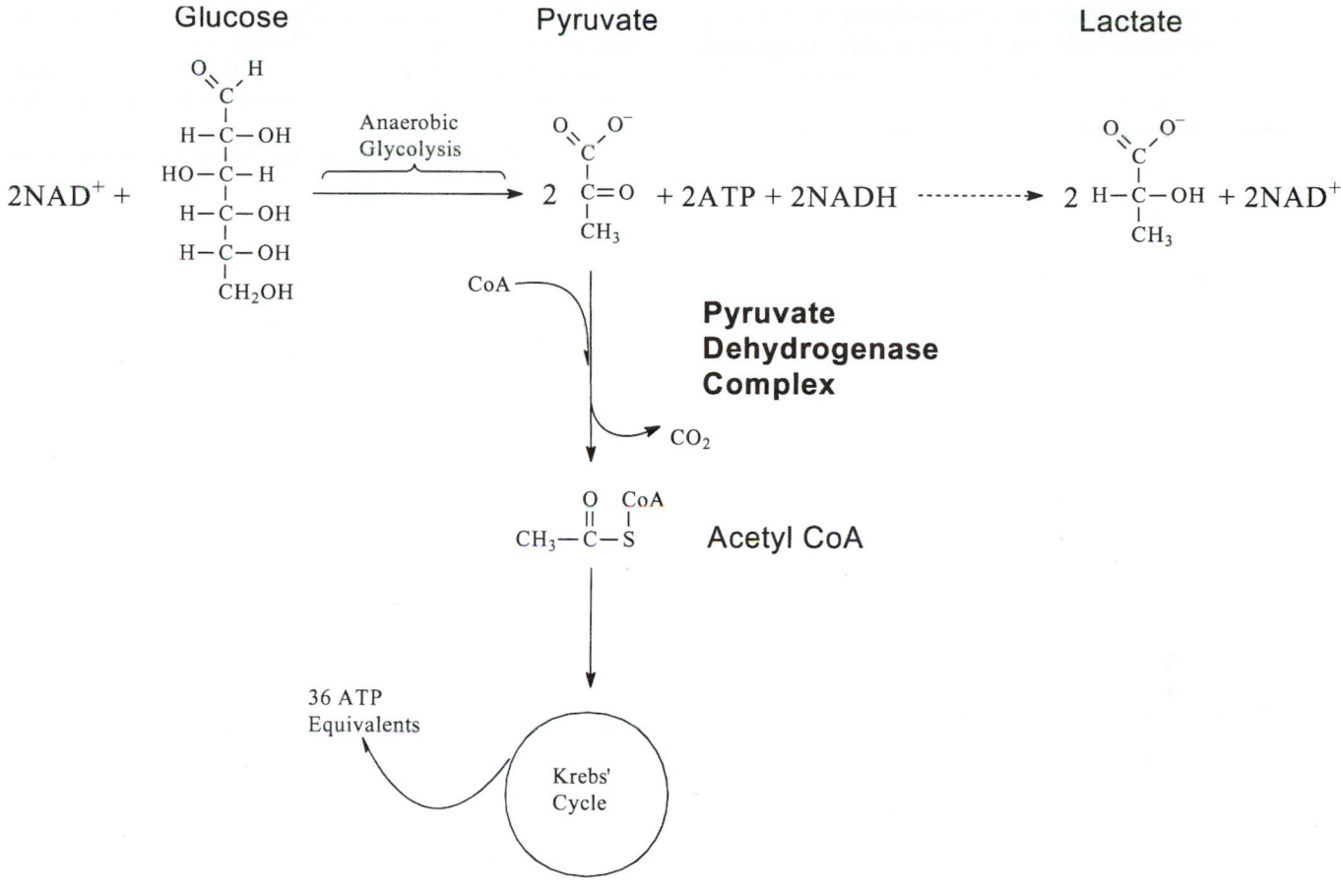

Figure 64–4. Thiamine links anaerobic glycolysis to the Krebs' cycle. Anaerobic glycolysis only yields 2 moles of adenosine triphosphate (ATP) as each mole of glucose is metabolized to 2 moles of pyruvate. To obtain the 36 additional ATP equivalents that can be derived as the Krebs' cycle converts pyruvate to CO_2 and H_2O, pyruvate must first be combined with Coenzyme A (CoA) to form acetyl-CoA and CO_2. This process requires the thiamine requiring enzyme system known as pyruvate dehydrogenase complex.

of α-ketoglutarate dehydrogenase, which shunts α-ketoglutarate, a natural precursor of glutamate away from the Krebs cycle. Rats subsequently develop increases in lactate in vulnerable regions of the brain marked by the induction of the protooncogene c-fos. Both the histochemical lesions and the gene induction can be blocked by the administration of the calcium channel blocker nicardipine.[32] This suggests a strong role for excitatory amino acid-induced alterations in calcium transport in the genesis of thiamine-deficient encephalopathy.

When thiamine is completely removed from the human diet, clinical manifestations of thiamine deficiency typically develop within 2–3 weeks, although tachycardia, the first sign of deficiency, may occur as early as 9 days after cessation of thiamine intake.[61] The clinical symptoms of thiamine deficiency present as two distinct patterns: "wet" beriberi or cardiovascular disease, and "dry" beriberi, the neurologic disease known as Wernicke-Korsakoff's syndrome. Although some patients display symptoms consistent with both disorders usually either the cardiovascular or the neurologic manifestations predominate. A genetic abnormality of transketolase activity, combined with low physical activity and low-carbohydrate diet, may predispose to neurologic symptoms,

whereas high-carbohydrate diets and increased physical activity lead to cardiovascular symptoms.[3,61]

Wet beriberi results from high-output cardiac failure that results from the peripheral vasodilation and the formation of arteriovenous fistulae secondary to thiamine deficiency. These patients complain of fatigue, decreased exercise tolerance, shortness of breath, and peripheral edema. The classic triad of oculomotor abnormalities, ataxia, and global confusion describes Wernicke's encephalopathy. Other manifestations include hypothermia and the absence of deep-tendon reflexes.[58] Additionally, patients develop a peripheral neuropathy with paresthesias, hypesthesias, and an associated myopathy, all related to axonal degeneration.[47] Laboratory studies may reflect a lactic acidosis brought on by excessive anaerobic glycolysis resulting from blocked entry of substrate into the Kreb's cycle.[20,26,42,58] Korsakoff's psychosis, an irreversible disorder of learning and processing of new information, characterized by a deficit in short-term memory and confabulation often occurs together with Wernicke's encephalopathy.[56] A 10–20% mortality rate is associated with Wernicke's encephalopathy, with survivors having an 80% risk of developing Korsakoff's psychosis.[40]

The exact cause of Wernicke's encephalopathy is unclear. In human autopsy studies, brain samples from alcoholic patients with Wernicke-Korsakoff's syndrome demonstrated decreased levels of pyruvate dehydrogenase, α-ketoglutarate dehydrogenase, and transketolase when compared to controls.[7] However, another controlled study demonstrated a similar decrease in enzyme activity of neuronal tissue of alcoholics who died from hepatic coma without ever manifesting signs of Wernicke's encephalopathy.[28] Thus, while thiamine deficiency is known to produce deficits in critical enzymes in humans, it is unclear whether these deficits are either necessary or sufficient to produce clinical disease.

In the United States, a healthy diet and mandatory thiamine supplementation of numerous food products protect most people from the manifestations of thiamine deficiency. This is, unfortunately, not true in other countries. A survey of the 17 major public hospitals in the Sydney, Australia area, identified more than 1000 cases of either acute Wernicke's encephalopathy or Korsakoff's psychosis between 1978 and 1993.[30] Similarly, a single Australian hospital identified 32 cases of Wernicke's encephalopathy during a 33-month period.[62] Mandatory supplementation of flour with thiamine in 1991 resulted in a dramatic reduction in hospitalized cases during 1992 and 1993,[30] as well as those subsequently identified by postmortem studies.[17]

The alcoholic patient, whose consumption of ethanol is his or her major source of calories, is the best described and most easily recognized patient at risk for thiamine deficiency.[40] Consequential thiamine deficiency is also described in inmates;[19] postoperative patients; in those patients with hyperemesis gravidarum or anorexia nervosa;[40,52] in those patients receiving parenteral nutrition;[10,20,24,26,42,57] in patients with acquired immunodeficiency syndrome (AIDS);[5,6,45] in patients with malignancies;[4,22,36,43,55] in the institutionalized elderly;[34,35] patients with congestive heart failure on furosemide therapy;[23,46] and in patients receiving hemodialysis;[11] among others. Thus, despite routine dietary supplementation, many people are still at risk because of dietary limitations, alcohol abuse, or underlying medical conditions.

Thiamine hydrochloride is included in the initial therapy for any patient with an altered mental status, potentially acting as both treatment and prevention of Wernicke's encephalopathy. Many patients with altered levels of consciousness have had or will have a poor nutritional status, or will be hospitalized without oral intake for a number of days because of gastrointestinal disorders or altered mental status. Although thiamine levels can be measured, either directly or functionally, by measuring their erythrocyte transketolase activity at baseline and in response to thiamine diphosphate,[18] these tests are unavailable for clinical use. Glucose loading increases thiamine requirements, which can exacerbate subtle thiamine deficiencies or even precipitate coma in the absence of parenteral thiamine supplementation.[40] Although it is commonly believed that acute glucose loading, in the form of a bolus of hypertonic dextrose, can precipitate Wernicke's encephalopathy over several hours in normal individuals, there is only evidence to support this effect in patients who already have grave manifestations of thiamine deficiency.[58] Previously healthy patients require prolonged dextrose administration in order to develop symptoms. Because the morbidity and mortality associated with Wernicke's encephalopathy are so severe, and treatment is both benign and inexpensive, thiamine hydrochloride should be included in the initial therapy for all patients who receive dextrose, for all patients with altered consciousness, and for every potential alcoholic or nutritionally deprived individual who presents to the emergency department or other clinical setting.

Adequate thiamine replacement consists of the immediate parenteral administration of 100 mg of thiamine hydrochloride, followed by the same dose on a daily basis. This can be given either intramuscularly or intravenously, but the oral route should be avoided because of its unpredictable absorption. In countries in which thiamine propyl disulfide (a lipid-soluble thiamine preparation) is available, the oral route may be considered equally efficacious for the replacement of serious thiamine deficiencies.[2,53,54] In some patients, symptoms such as ophthalmoplegia are reported to respond rapidly to as little as 2 mg of thiamine; however, the other neurologic and cardiovascular manifestations of thiamine deprivation may necessitate higher doses and may respond more slowly, if at all. Because of the safety of thiamine hydrochloride, and the urgency to correct the manifestations of thiamine deficiency, up to 1000 mg of thiamine hydrochloride can be used in the first 12 hours if a patient demonstrates persistent neurologic abnormalities.[33]

The practice of requiring the administration of parenteral thiamine prior to hypertonic dextrose in patients with altered consciousness is illogical.[14] Besides the fact that the first dose of dextrose is unlikely to cause thiamine deficiency, thiamine uptake into cells and activation of enzyme systems is slower than that of glucose uptake, which suggests that even pretreatment with thiamine offers little benefit over posttreatment.[51] Despite these limitations it is prudent to administer 100 mg of parenteral thiamine at the time of initial dextrose administration. The biochemical link between dextrose and thiamine is obvious, which demonstrates to the clinician the logic behind the administration of thiamine. Although thiamine is unlikely to offer immediate benefits for patients with altered consciousness, it will offer some long-term protection for these individuals and initiate therapy for an uncommon, serious, and easily overlooked disorder.

A supplementary indication for the administration of thiamine hydrochloride occurs in patients with ethylene glycol poisoning. As shown in Fig. 66–1 , a minor pathway for the elimination of glyoxylic acid involves its conversion to α-hydoxy-β-ketoadipate by α-ketoglutarate:glyoxylate carboligase, a thiamine and magnesium-requiring enzyme. There are no data to support an increase in α-hydoxy-β-ketoadipate formation following thiamine administration in ethylene glycol-poisoned animals or humans. However, animal models of primary hyperoxaluria show increases in urinary oxalate during thiamine deficiency, suggesting at least a potential importance of this pathway.[15,50] Because of the benignity of the therapy, it is prudent to administer standard doses of thiamine to patients with suspected or confirmed ethylene glycol poisoning. If magnesium supplementation is considered, caution is required because of the potential for renal compromise in ethylene glycol poisoned patients.

Very few complications are associated with the parenteral administration of thiamine. The older literature emphasized intramuscular administration because of numerous reports of anaphylactoid reactions associated with intravenous thiamine delivery.[12,39,44,49,60] It is generally believed that these reactions resulted from responses to the vehicle (chlorbutanol) or its contaminants rather than thiamine itself. Despite the availability of purer, aqueous preparations of thiamine, rare adverse reports still occur.[1,31,37,48] Although the intramuscular route is theoretically acceptable, many patients requiring thiamine may have diminished muscle mass or a coagulopathy, exacerbating the potential for pain and unpredictable absorption. The safety of thiamine use was evaluated in a large case series in which nearly 1000 patients received parenteral doses of up to 500 mg of thiamine without significant complications.[63] This study suggests that if anaphylaxis to thiamine exists, its occurrence is exceedingly rare, permitting the safe intravenous administration of thiamine to most patients.

REFERENCES

1. Assem ESK: Anaphylactic reaction to thiamine. Practitioner 1973; 211:565.

2. Baker H, Frank O: Absorption, utilization and clinical effectiveness of allithiamines compared to water-soluble thiamines. J Nutr Sci Vitaminol 1976;22(Suppl):63–68.

3. Blass JP, Gibson GE: Abnormality of a thiamine-requiring enzyme in patients with Wernicke-Korsakoff syndrome. N Engl J Med 1977; 297:1367–1370.

4. Burbato M, Rodriguez PJ: Thiamine deficiency in patients admitted to a palliative care unit. Palliat Med 1994;8:320–324.

5. Butterworth RF, Gaudreau C, Vincelette J, et al: Thiamine deficiency in AIDS [letter]. Lancet 1991;338:1086.

6. Butterworth RF, Gaudreau C, Vincelette J, et al: Thiamine deficiency and Wernicke's encephalopathy in AIDS. Metab Brain Dis 1991;6: 207–212.

7. Butterworth RF, Kril JJ, Harper CG: Thiamine-dependent enzyme changes in the brains of alcoholics: Relationship to the Wernicke-Korsakoff syndrome. Alcohol Clin Res 1993;17:1084–1088.

8. Calingasan NY, Baker H, Sheu KF, Gibson GE: Blood-brain barrier abnormalities in vulnerable brain regions during thiamine deficiency. Exp Neurol 1995;134:64–72.

9. Calingasan NY, Chun WJ, Park LC, et al: Oxidative stress is associated with region-specific neuronal death during thiamine deficiency. J Neuropathol Exp Neurol 1999;58:946–958.

10. Deaths associated with thiamine-deficient total parenteral nutrition. MMWR Morb Mortal Wkly Rep 1989;38:43–46.

11. Descombes E, Dessibourg CA, Fellay G: Acute encephalopathy due to thiamine deficiency (Wernicke's encephalopathy) in a chronic hemodialyzed patient: A case report. Clin Nephrol 1991;35: 171–175.

12. Eisenstadt WS: Hypersensitivity to thiamine hydrochloride. Minn Med 1942;85:861–863.

13. Greb A, Bitsch R: Comparative bioavailability of various thiamine derivatives after oral administration. Int J Clin Pharmacol Ther 1998;36: 216–221.

14. Hack JB, Hoffman RS: Thiamine before glucose to prevent Wernicke's encephalopathy: Examining the conventional wisdom [letter]. JAMA 1998;279:583–584.

15. Hannet B, Thomas DW, Chalmers AH, et al: Formation of oxalate in pyridoxine or thiamin deficient rats during intravenous xylitol infusions. J Nutr 1977;107:458–465.

16. Harata N, Iwasaki Y: Evidence for early blood-brain barrier breakdown in experimental thiamine deficiency in the mouse. Metab Brain Dis 1995;10:159–174.

17. Harper CG, Sheedy DL, Lara AI, et al: Prevalence of Wernicke-Korsakoff syndrome in Australia: Has thiamine fortification made a difference? Med J Aust 1998;168:542–545.

18. Herve C, Beyne P, Letteron P, Delacoux E: Comparison of erythrocyte transketolase activity with thiamine and thiamine phosphate ester levels in chronic alcoholic patients. Clin Chim Acta 1995;234: 91–100.

19. Jeyakumar D: Thiamine responsive ankle oedema in detention centre inmates. Med J Malaysia 1995;50:17–20.

20. Katamura K, Takahasi T, Tanaka H, et al: Two cases of thiamine deficiency-induced lactic acidosis during total parenteral nutrition. Tohoku J Exp Med 1993;171:129–133.

21. Kern D, Kern G, Neef H, et al: How thiamine diphosphate is activated in enzymes. Science 1997;275:67–70.

22. Kuba H, Inamura T, Ikezaki K, et al: Thiamine-deficient lactic acidosis with brain tumor treatment. Report of three cases. J Neurosurg 1998;89:1025–1028.

23. Kwok T, Falconer-Smith JF, Potter JF, Ives DR: Thiamine status of elderly patients with cardiac failure. Age Ageing 1992;21:67–71.

24. Lactic acidosis traced to thiamine deficiency related to nationwide shortage of multivitamins for total parenteral nutrition—United States, 1997. MMWR Morb Mort Wkly Rep 1997;46:523–528.

25. Laforenza U, Patrini C, Alvisi C, et al: Thiamine uptake in human intestinal biopsy specimens, including observations from a patient with acute thiamine deficiency. Am J Clin Nutr 1997;66:320–326.

26. Lange R, Erhard J, Eigler FW, Roll C: Lactic acidosis from thiamine deficiency during parenteral nutrition in a two-year-old boy. Eur J Pediatr Surg 1992;2:241–244.

27. Langlais PJ, Zhang SX: Extracellular glutamate is increased in thalamus during thiamine deficiency-induced lesions and is blocked by MK-801. J Neurochem 1993;61:2175–2182.

28. Lavoie J, Butterworth RF: Reduced activities of thiamine-dependent enzymes in the brains of alcoholics in the absence of Wernicke's encephalopathy. Alcohol Clin Exp Res 1995;19:1073–1077.

29. Lubetsky A, Winaver J, Seligmann H, et al: Urinary thiamine excretion in the rat: Effects of furosemide, other diuretics, and volume load. J Lab Clin Med 1999;134:232–237.

30. Ma JJ, Truswell AS: Wernicke-Korsakoff syndrome in Sydney hospitals: Before and after thiamine enrichment of flour. Med J Aust 1995; 163:531–534.

31. Morinville V, Jeannet-Peter N, Hauser C: Anaphylaxis to parenteral thiamine (vitamin B1). Schweiz Med Wochenschr 1998;128: 1743–1744.

32. Munujos P, Vendrell M, Ferrer I: Proto-oncogene c-fos induction in thiamine-deficient encephalopathy. Protective effects of nicardipine on pyrithiamine-induced lesions. J Neurol Sci 1993;118:175–180.

33. Nakada T, Knight RT: Alcohol and the central nervous system. Med Clin North Am 1984;68:121–131.

34. O'Keeffe ST, Tormey WP, Glasgow R, Lavan JN: Thiamine deficiency in hospitalized elderly patients. Gerontology 1994;40:18–24.

35. O'Rourke NP, Bunker VW, Thomas AJ, et al: Thiamine status of healthy and institutionalized elderly subjects: Analysis of dietary intake and biochemical study. Age Aging 1990;19:325–329.

36. Oriot D, Wood C, Gottesman R, Huault G: Severe lactic acidosis related to acute thiamine deficiency. J Parenteral Nutr 1991;12: 105–109.

37. Proebstle TM, Gall H, Jugert FK, et al: Specific IgE and IgG serum antibodies to thiamine associated anaphylactic reaction. J Allergy Clin Immunol 1995;95:1059–1060.

38. Rao VL, Butterworth RF: Thiamine phosphatases in human brain: Regional alterations in patients with alcoholic cirrhosis. Alcohol Clin Exp Res 1995;19:523–526.

39. Reingold IM, Webb FR: Sudden death following intravenous injection of thiamine hydrochloride. JAMA 1946;130:491–492.

40. Reuler JB, Girard DE, Cooney TG: Wernicke's encephalopathy. N Engl J Med 1985;312:1035–1037.

41. Rieck J, Halkin H, Almog S, et al: Urinary loss of thiamine is increased by low doses of furosemide in healthy volunteers. J Lab Clin Med 1999;134:238–243.

42. Romanski SA, McMahon MM: Metabolic acidosis and thiamine deficiency. Mayo Clin Proc 1999;74:259–263.

43. Rovelli A, Bonomi M, Murano A, et al: Severe lactic acidosis due to thiamine deficiency after bone marrow transplantation in a child with acute monocytic leukemia [letter]. Haematologica 1990;75: 579–581.

44. Schiff L: Collapse following parenteral administration of solution of thiamine hydrochloride. JAMA 1941;117:609.

45. Schramm C, Wanitschke R, Galle PR: Thiamine for the treatment of nucleoside analogue-induced severe lactic acidosis. Eur J Anaesthesiol 1999;16:733–735.

46. Seligmann H, Halkin H, Rauchfleisch S, et al: Thiamine deficiency in patients with congestive heart failure receiving long-term furosemide therapy: A pilot study. Am J Med 1991;91:151–155.

47. Skelton WP, Skelton N: Thiamine deficiency neuropathy: It's still common today. Postgrad Med 1989;85:301–306.

48. Stephen JM, Grant R, Yeh CS: Anaphylaxis from administration of intravenous thiamine. Am J Emerg Med 1992;10:61–63.

49. Stiles MH: Hypersensitivity to thiamine chloride with a note on sensitivity to pyridoxine hydrochloride. J Allergy 1941;12:507–509.

50. Takasaki E: The urinary excretion of oxalic acid in vitamin B1-deficient rats. Invest Urol 1969;7:150–153.

51. Tate JR, Nixon PF: Measurement of Michaelis constant for human erythrocyte transketolase and thiamine diphosphate. Anal Biochem 1987;160:78–87.

52. Tesfaye S, Achari V, Yang YC, et al: Pregnant, vomiting, and going blind. Lancet 1998;352:1594.

53. Thomson AD, Baker H, Leevy CM: Patterns of 35S-thiamine hydrochloride absorption in the malnourished alcoholic patient. J Lab Clin Med 1970;76:34–45.

54. Thomson AD, Frank O, Baker H, Leevy CM: Thiamine propyl disulfide: Absorption and utilization. Ann Intern Med 1971;74:529–534.

55. Van Zaanen HC, van der Lelie J: Thiamine deficiency in hematologic malignant tumors. Cancer 1992;69:1710–1713.

56. Victor M, Adams RD: The effect of alcohol on the nervous system. In: Meritt HH, Hare CC, eds: Metabolic and Toxic Diseases of the Nervous System. Baltimore, Williams & Wilkins, 1953, pp. 526–563.

57. Vortmeyer AO, Hagel C, Laas R: Haemorrhagic thiamine deficient encephalopathy following prolonged parenteral nutrition. J Neurol Neurosurg Psychiatry 1992;55:826–829.

58. Watson AJS, Walker JF, Tomkin GH, et al: Acute Wernicke's encephalopathy precipitated by glucose loading. Ir J Med Sci 1981;150:301–303.

59. Weber W, Nitz M, Looby M: Nonlinear kinetics of the thiamine cation in humans: Saturation of nonrenal clearance and tubular reabsorption. J Pharmacokinet Biopharm 1990;18:501–523.

60. Weigand CG: Reactions attributed to administration of thiamine chloride. Geriatrics 1950;5:274–279.

61. Wilson JD, Madison LL: Deficiency of thiamine (beriberi), pyridoxine, and riboflavin. In: Isselbacher KJ, Adams RD, Braunwald E, et al, eds: Harrison's Principles of Internal Medicine, 9th ed. New York, McGraw-Hill, 1980, pp. 425–429.

62. Wood B, Currie J: Presentation of acute Wernicke's encephalopathy and treatment with thiamine. Metab Brain Dis 1995;10:52–72.

63. Wrenn KD, Murphy F, Slovis CM: A toxicity study of parenteral thiamine hydrochloride. Ann Emerg Med 1989;18:867–870.

64. Zangen A, Botzer D, Zangen R, Shainberg A: Furosemide and digoxin inhibit thiamine uptake in cardiac cells. Eur J Pharmacol 1998;361:151–155.

Edwin K. Kuffner

$$C_2H_5 \quad \overset{S}{\underset{\|}{}} \quad \overset{S}{\underset{\|}{}} \quad C_2H_5$$
$$C_2H_5 \diagdown N-C-S-S-C-N \diagup C_2H_5$$
$$C_2H_5 \diagup \qquad\qquad\qquad \diagdown C_2H_5$$

Disulfiram

A 40-year-old female with a history of depression was found unresponsive by her husband. The husband stated that the patient had a strange garlic odor on her breath and she had complained of exhaustion and confusion for several days. The patient's medications included paroxetine, risperidone, and trazodone. The patient also had access to a supply of over-the-counter vitamins, herbal preparations, muscle liniments, and an unknown Mexican medication.

Emergency medical personnel transported the patient to the emergency department. A rapid reagent blood glucose was 130 mg/dL. Her mental status did not change following the intravenous administration of 2 mg of naloxone and 100 mg of thiamine. Her vital signs were: blood pressure, 178/100 mm Hg; pulse, 56 beats/min; respiratory rate, 18 breaths/min; rectal temperature, 94.8°F (34.9°C); room air pulse oximetry, 99% oxygen saturation.

The physical examination revealed the patient to be unresponsive with a Glasgow Coma Score (GCS) of 6. No evidence of trauma was noted. Pupils were 3 mm and sluggishly reactive to light. Cardiac, pulmonary, and abdominal examinations were unremarkable. Neurologic examination revealed flexion withdrawal to painful stimuli, areflexia, and occasional myoclonic jerks.

The etiology of this patient's CNS depression remained unclear. An intentional ingestion was suspected, but other life-threatening medical conditions were considered. The patient was intubated. Fifty grams of activated charcoal was administered via a nasogastric tube. The 12-lead electrocardiogram (ECG) revealed peaked T waves but did not reveal evidence of QRS widening or an R wave in AVR. The serum electrolytes were significant for a bicarbonate of 4 mEq/L, a potassium of 6.0 mEq/L and an anion gap of 26 mEq/L. The serum lactate was 16.9 mmol/L. Serum blood urea nitrogen (BUN), serum creatinine, and hepatic aminotransferases were normal. Serum acetaminophen, salicylate, and blood ethanol levels were undetectable. An arterial blood gas analysis on supplemental oxygen revealed a pH, 7.11, a P_{CO_2} of 6.7 mm Hg, and a P_{O_2} of 187 mm Hg. A complete blood count revealed a white blood cell count (WBC) of 15,600/mm^3 (89% neutrophils and 9% lymphocytes) with a normal hematocrit and platelet count. A computed tomography scan of the head, a chest radiograph, and a lumbar puncture were normal.

At this point, a diagnosis of either ethylene glycol or methanol toxicity was entertained. Blood was sent for ethylene glycol and methanol levels and the patient was treated with 50 mg of pyridoxine and 50 mg of folinic acid intravenously. Because fomepizole was unavailable, the patient was started on intravenous ethanol. A loading dose of 800 mg/kg of ethanol was followed by a continuous infusion to maintain the blood ethanol concentration between 100 and 120 mg/dL. Shortly after the loading dose of ethanol was administered, the patient developed generalized flushing, tachycardia with a pulse of 120 beats/min, and a systolic blood pressure of 70 mm Hg. The blood pressure did not respond to IV crystalloid, but did respond to norepinephrine. Hemodialysis was performed.

The ethylene glycol and methanol levels were eventually confirmed to be negative. The severe metabolic acidosis was corrected with hemodialysis. Within a few hours of discontinuing the ethanol infusion the patient's tachycardia and hypotension resolved.

Within 24 hours of presentation, the patient's mental status had returned to baseline. The patient admitted to ingesting the Mexican medication she had obtained over-the-counter in the United States from a Mexican pharmacist to help her with her alcoholism. The unknown medication was later identified as disulfiram confirming the clinical diagnosis.

A complete understanding of disulfiram toxicity is dependent upon understanding the distinction between the different forms of disulfiram toxicity that are associated with acute ingestions, chronic therapy, and disulfiram-ethanol reactions. The preceding case is unique in that it involves both toxicity from an acute overdose of disulfiram and toxicity from an iatrogenic disulfiram-ethanol reaction. This chapter emphasizes the distinctions between these three different forms of disulfiram toxicity.

HISTORY AND EPIDEMIOLOGY

Disulfiram, tetraethylthiuram disulfide, and related chemicals were used in the rubber industry as catalytic accelerators for the vulcanization (stabilization) of rubber by the addition of sulfur. In the early 1900s workers exposed to disulfiram developed adverse reactions when exposed to ethanol, which suggested at that time that disulfiram may be useful as an adjunct in the treatment of alcoholism.[117] In the 1940s, two Danish physicians, Hald and Jacobsen, who were ingesting disulfiram for its reputed antihelmintic properties became ill after consuming alcohol.[39] It was not until this time that disulfiram treatment for alcoholism gained popularity. Although the evidence to support the use of disulfiram therapy as part of a comprehensive alcohol treatment program is equivocal, even after standards of evidence-based medicine are applied, the use of disulfiram therapy is still common.[47]

It is difficult to obtain specific epidemiologic information about the three different forms of disulfiram toxicity when analyzing data from the American Association of Poison Control Centers (AAPCC). (See p. 1752 and Chapter 116).

In the past 15 years more than 8000 patients with exposures to disulfiram have been reported to the AAPCC. Fewer than 100 of these patients developed major adverse effects. Unlike many toxins reported to the AAPCC, the majority of the disulfiram exposures were in adults. There were only 8 deaths, all of whom were adults. Most of the deaths involved a disulfiram-ethanol reaction. In many of the deaths, coingestants, other than disulfiram and ethanol were involved.

The best studied and the most commonly reported life-threatening adverse effect of chronic disulfiram therapy is hepatotoxicity. The frequency of the spectrum of disulfiram-related hepatotoxicity is also difficult to determine. As many as 25% of all alcoholics treated with disulfiram develop subclinical elevations in their hepatic aminotransferase levels and the frequency of disulfiram-induced fatal hepatitis is 1 case in 25,000–30,000 patients treated per year.[35,89]

PHARMACOKINETICS AND TOXICOKINETICS

Therapeutic Ingestion of Disulfiram

Absorption. Disulfiram is highly lipid-soluble and very insoluble in water.[84] Following ingestion, disulfiram is either absorbed as the parent compound or converted to diethyldithiocarbamic acid (diethyldithiocarbamate) in the acid environment of the stomach. Diethyldithiocarbamic acid is also very unstable in this acid environment and rapidly undergoes absorption and spontaneous decomposition to carbon disulfide and diethylamine, or chelates copper, forming a bis(diethyldithiocarbamato) copper complex. The bis(diethyldithiocarbamato) copper complex is more stable than diethyldithiocarbamic acid and also can be absorbed as it passes through the upper gastrointestinal tract. In fact, most disulfiram is absorbed from the small intestine as this bis(diethyldithiocarbamato) copper complex. Approximately 70–90% of an ingested therapeutic dose of disulfiram is absorbed. The bioavailability of disulfiram varies with different preparations. In one study, the mean plasma disulfiram concentration in humans following a 250-mg dose was reported to be 0.38 ± 0.03 μg/mL.[28] Peak serum levels of disulfiram and its metabolites are achieved 8–10 hours following a 250-mg dose.[51]

Distribution. Approximately 96% of disulfiram itself and approximately 80% of disulfiram metabolites are protein bound.[51] Following absorption disulfiram and its metabolites are uniformly distributed throughout body tissues. A specific volume of distribution for disulfiram is not recognized.

Metabolism. Any absorbed disulfiram is rapidly converted to diethydithiocarbamic acid by erythrocyte glutathione reductase and endogenous thiols. It is difficult to detect the parent compound disulfiram in blood because of its rapid conversion to diethyldithiocarbamic acid. Diethyldithiocarbamic acid in the blood also chelates copper, forming a bis(diethyldithiocarbamato) copper complex. The bis(diethyldithiocarbamato) copper complex also undergoes conversion back to diethyldithiocarbamic acid. Diethyldithiocarbamic acid is metabolized by a number of different pathways including glucuronidation, methylation, nonenzymatic

degradation, and oxidation. Nonenzymatic degradation of diethyldithiocarbamic acid produces diethylamine and carbon disulfide. Carbon disulfide can be further oxidized to carbonyl sulfide, which can be further oxidized to carbon dioxide. Phase II methylation of diethyldithiocarbamic acid, which is mediated by an S-methyltransferase produces diethyldithiomethylcarbamic acid. Diethyldithiomethylcarbamic acid can be oxidized to diethylthiomethylcarbamic acid. Diethylthiomethylcarbamic acid is further oxidized to sulfoxide and sulfone metabolites and undergoes demethylation to form diethylthiocarbamic acid. Although diethyldithiocarbamic acid can be converted back to disulfiram and carbon disulfide and diethylamine can be converted back to diethyldithiocarbamic acid, these reactions are not clinically significant[26] (Fig. 65–1).

Elimination. Following a 250-mg dose, the half-lives of disulfiram, diethyldithiocarbamate and carbon disulfide are 7.3 ± 1.5 hours, 15.5 ± 4.5 hours, and 8.9 ± 1.4 hours, respectively.[84] Approximately 20% of disulfiram is excreted unchanged in the feces and another 20% or more is excreted by the lungs as carbon disulfide. The majority of disulfiram is excreted in the urine as the glucuronidated metabolite of diethyldithiocarbamic acid.[51] At 48 hours following a single 250-mg dose there is a negligible amount of disulfiram and metabolites detectable in the serum.[28]

Disulfiramlike Reaction

Disulfiram-ethanol reactions occur following exposure to disulfiram by either the oral or subcutaneous routes and to ethanol via either the oral, intravenous, dermal, or inhalation routes.[102] Patients taking disulfiram are at risk for disulfiram-ethanol reactions following exposure to ethanol contained in many products other than

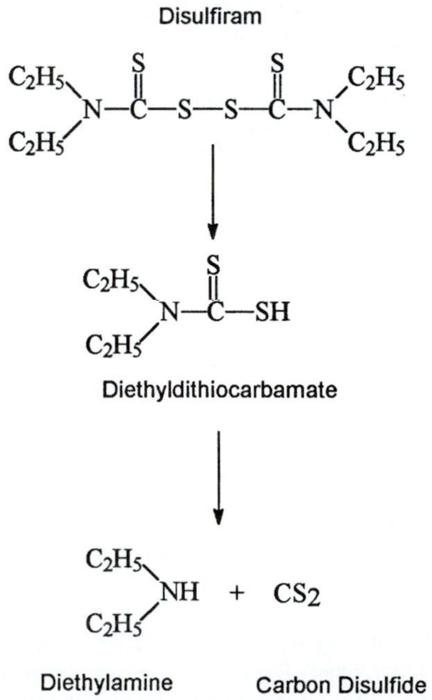

Figure 65–1. Disulfiram metabolism occurs in the liver and erythrocyte. The most consequential metabolites are diethyldithiocarbamate and carbon disulfide.

alcoholic beverages. Some common household products containing ethanol are listed in Table 65–1.

Most patients taking disulfiram who are exposed to ethanol develop symptoms of the disulfiram-ethanol reaction within 15 minutes. The symptoms usually peak within 30 minutes to 1 hour, and then gradually subside over the next few hours.

The duration of disulfiram's inhibition of aldehyde dehydrogenase is partially dependent upon the dose ingested and the route of administration. A 500-mg dose inhibits aldehyde dehydrogenase up to 3–4 days, a 1000-mg dose up to 5–6 days, and a 1500-mg dose up to 7–8 days.[39] Thus patients remain at risk for a disulfiram-ethanol reaction for up to 1 week following cessation of oral disulfiram therapy. There are also sustained-release and depot disulfiram preparations but none are readily available in the United States. Following a subcutaneous dose of 2 g of disulfiram, a patient reacted to oral ethanol at 21 days following the injection.[86] Although the severity of the disulfiram-ethanol reaction following subcutaneous disulfiram dosing is reported to be less than that following oral dosing, this has not been proved in a well controlled trial.

PHARMACOLOGY AND PATHOPHYSIOLOGY

Therapeutic doses of disulfiram used as part of a comprehensive alcohol treatment program usually range from 125–500 mg/d. Disulfiram's effectiveness in discouraging alcohol consumption is aversive in nature, as it is dependent on the patient's fear of developing a disulfiram ethanol reaction. Disulfiram does not have central nervous system effects that alter an alcoholic's drinking behavior.

Disulfiram-Ethanol Reaction

Understanding the metabolism of ethanol is critical to understanding the mechanism of action of disulfiram as it relates to the disulfiram-ethanol reaction (see Fig. 65–2). Disulfiram and its metabolites impair both cytosolic aldehyde dehydrogenase 1 (ALDH 1) and mitochondrial aldehyde dehydrogenase 2 (ALDH 2). Disulfiram's inhibition of ALDH 2 leads to a rise of acetaldehyde levels 5–10 times above baseline levels.[6] A few days of treatment with disulfiram can reduce baseline aldehyde dehydrogenase activity by 50%.[84] The degree of aldehyde dehydrogenase inhibition required to produce a severe disulfiram-ethanol reaction is well established. Although aldehyde dehydrogenase is present throughout the body, inhibition of hepatic mitochondrial aldehyde

TABLE 65–1.   Common Household Products that Contain Ethanol and May Cause a Disulfiram-Ethanol Reaction

Adhesives
Alcohols: denatured alcohol, rubbing alcohol
Detergents
Foods: liquor-containing desserts, fermented vinegar, some sauces
Nonprescription medications: analgesics, antacids, antidiarrheals, cough and cold preparations, topical anesthetics, vitamins
Personal hygiene products: after-shave lotions, colognes, deodorants, liquid soaps, mouthwashes, perfumes, skin liniments and lotions
Solvents

dehydrogenase is most important in the disulfiram-ethanol reaction.

The exact mechanism by which disulfiram and its metabolites inhibit ALDH 1 and ALDH 2 is still unclear. Disulfiram may inactivate aldehyde dehydrogenase by causing internal sulfur-sulfur bonds, or by competing for nicotinamide adenine dinucleotide.[113] Disulfiram's metabolites including, diethylthiomethylcarbamic acid and its sulfoxide and sulfone metabolites may also directly inhibit aldehyde dehydrogenase.[39,51,84] It is possible that different metabolites inactivate different isoenzymes of aldehyde dehydrogenase. Diethylthiocarbamic acid is believed to inactivate ALDH 2. Because aldehyde dehydrogenase inhibition is irreversible, new ALDH must be synthesized to metabolize acetaldehyde.[51]

Accumulation of acetaldehyde is responsible for many of the symptoms produced by the disulfiram-ethanol reaction. In fact, intravenous administration of acetaldehyde to humans produces similar symptoms as to those experienced by patients taking disulfiram who consume ethanol.[6] Acetaldehyde may increase the release of histamine, which may also be responsible for some of the effects of the disulfiram-ethanol reaction.

Disulfiram-Ethanollike Reactions

The term *disulfiramlike reaction* is commonly used to describe a presentation similar to the typical disulfiram-ethanol reaction when the patient has not been exposed to both disulfiram and ethanol. Most disulfiramlike reactions involve an exposure to ethanol.

Chemicals structurally similar to disulfiram (tetraethylthiuram disulphide) including carbon disulfide, tetramethylthiuram disulfide (thiram) and tetramethylthiuram monosulfide, were recognized in the early 1900s as causes of disulfiramlike reactions with ethanol.[40] Many of these chemicals were also used as catalytic accelerators for the vulcanization of rubber. Workers exposed to these chemicals who then consumed ethanol developed symptoms of the disulfiram-ethanol reaction.[117]

Thiram, the methyl analogue of disulfiram, is used as a fungicide, insecticide, larvicide, pesticide and seed disinfectant. Analogues of thiram used in agriculture include copper, mercuric and sodium diethyldithiocarbamate, zinc and ferric dimethyldithiocarbamate and zinc and disodium ethylenebis[dithiocarbamate]. Soaps and ointments containing thiram derivatives are also used for their scabicidal and bactericidal properties.[40] Exposure to thiram or its analogues in conjunction with ethanol precipitates disulfiramlike reactions.[94]

Calcium carbimide (citrated calcium carbimide) is another aldehyde dehydrogenase inhibitor also used in the management of alcoholic patients.[10] Although this agent may have fewer adverse effects than disulfiram, death can also occur from a calcium carbimide-ethanol reaction.[65,63]

Ingestion of ethanol following ingestion of various species of mushrooms can cause symptoms of a disulfiram-ethanol reaction. The classic mushroom species producing this reaction are the *Coprinus* mushrooms including *C. atramentarius, C. insignis, C. variegatus,* and *C. quadrifidus,* all of which contain the amino acid coprine.[95] The metabolite of coprine, 1-aminocyclopropanol, inhibits acetaldehyde dehydrogenase activity in a similar fashion to disulfiram. Other mushrooms that can produce a similar reaction with ethanol include *Boletus luridus, Clitocybe clavipes, Polyporus sulphureus, Pholiota squarosa, Morchella spp., Tricholoma aurantum,* and *Verpa bohemica*[20,103] (Chap. 76).

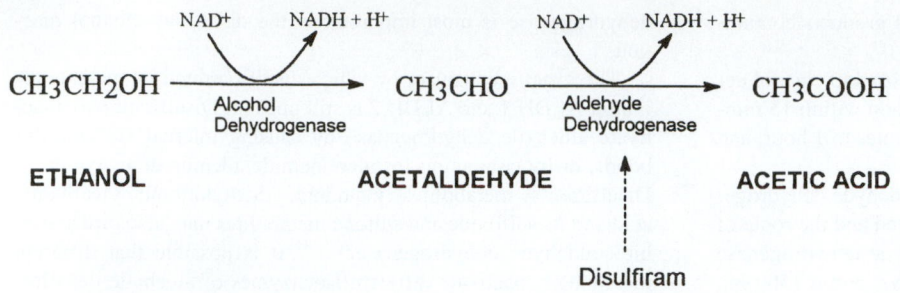

Figure 65–2. Disulfiram's site of action. The irreversible inactivation of aldehyde dehydrogenase results in an increased acetaldehyde level after ethanol is administered.

Some pharmaceutical preparations in combination with ethanol also produce symptoms of the disulfiram-ethanol reaction (see Table 65–2). Cephalosporins with this methylthiotetrazole (MTT) side chain, including cefotetan, cefoperazone, cefamandole, and cefmenoxine, are most commonly involved. Cephalosporins with the MTT side chain also cause hypoprothrombinemia and increased prothrombin times[58] (Chap. 46).

Alcohols other than ethanol and organic solvents including mineral spirits can also cause symptoms of a disulfiram-ethanol reaction.[101] Skin flushing without other more severe symptoms of the disulfiram-ethanol reaction occurs in workers who use the degreasing agent trichloroethylene and ingest ethanol. Skin flushing associated with trichloroethylene use has been termed "degreasers flush."[104] Interestingly, disulfiram inhibits the metabolism of trichloroethylene to trichloroethanol and trichloroacetic acid in

man.[8] Other organic solvents that cause a similar reaction with ethanol include dimethylformamide and carbon tetrachloride. This syndrome of skin flushing without other more severe symptoms of the disulfiram-ethanol reaction also occurs in patients with decreased baseline aldehyde dehydrogenase activity. Many Native Americans and Asians who have both increased alcohol dehydrogenase and decreased ALDH 2 activity caused by genetic polymorphism commonly experience skin flushing following exposure to ethanol. As many as 40–60% of some Asian populations experience this response, which may be prevented with H_2 antagonists but not H_1 antagonists. The former agents reduce the production of acetaldehyde by inhibiting alcohol dehydrogenase, an effect not possessed by the latter drugs. Some whites also have a similar reaction to ethanol.[33,46]

Other Enzymes Inhibited by Disulfiram

Disulfiram and its metabolites also inhibit other enzymes, especially those that contain sulfhydryl groups and metalloproteins.[79] Importantly, disulfiram inhibits norepinephrine synthesis in humans by inhibiting dopamine β-hydroxylase, an enzyme necessary for norepinephrine synthesis.[34,77] The mechanism for this inhibition may be the chelation of copper by diethyldithiocarbamate, which is necessary for dopamine β-hydroxylase activity.[96] Disulfiram also decreases urinary concentrations of vanillylmandelic acid in humans.[42] Decreased norepinephrine in conjunction with acetaldehyde, a vasodilator, may account for the hypotension associated with the disulfiram-ethanol reaction. Increased concentrations of dopamine as a consequence of dopamine β-hydroxylase inhibition may also explain the psychiatric effects following both acute disulfiram overdose and chronic disulfiram therapy. Although it has been theorized that some of the neurologic effects following both acute disulfiram overdose and chronic disulfiram therapy may be related to the metabolite carbon disulfide, this has not been confirmed in a well-controlled trial.[90]

Disulfiram and the Cytochrome P450 System

Disulfiram and its metabolites are known inhibitors of CYP2E1.[54] Single doses of disulfiram administered to healthy humans result in 50% inhibition of baseline CYP2E1 activity for at least 3 days, with some inhibition for greater than 1 week.[25,27] Although animal studies suggest that disulfiram alters acetaminophen metabolism, a human study found that disulfiram did not significantly alter the metabolism of a therapeutic dose of acetaminophen in either healthy patients or those with alcoholic liver disease.[87] Disulfiram may be an inducer of CYP2B1 and CYP2A1. Disulfiram does not appear to affect CYP2C9, CYP2C19, CYP2D6, or CYP3A4

TABLE 65–2. Agents Reported to Cause Disulfiramlike Reaction with Ethanol

Antimicrobial Agents
  Cephalosporins, especially those that contain a methylthiotetrazole (MTT) side chain, such as cefotetan, cefoperazone, cefamandole, and cefmenoxime.
  Metronidazole
  Moxalactam
  Trimethoprim-sulfamethoxazole
  Possible reactions with chloramphenicol, griseofulvin, quinacrine, procarbazine, phentolamine, nitrofurantoin
Sulfonylurea oral hypoglycemics
  Chlorpropamide
  Tolbutamide
Chemicals
  Calcium carbimide (citrated calcium carbimide)
  Carbon disulfide
  Carbon tetrachloride
  Chloral hydrate
  Dimethylformamide
  Nitrefazole
  Tetraethylthiuram disulfide (disulfiram)
  Tetramethylthiuram disulfide (thiram)
  Thiram analogs (fungicides)
    Copper, mercuric, and sodium diethyldithiocarbamate
    Zinc and ferric dimethyldithiocarbamate
    Zinc and disodium ethylenebis[dithiocarbamate]
  Trichlorethylene
Mushrooms
  Coprinus mushrooms including *C. atramentarius, C. insignis, C. variegatus,* and *C. quadrifidus, Boletus luridus, Clitocybe clavipes, Polyporus sulphureus, Pholiota squarosa, Morchella spp., Tricholoma aurantum,* and *Verpa bohemica*

activity.[51,54] Disulfiram inhibits the metabolism and/or decreases the clearance of phenytoin, theophylline and warfarin.[68,79,81,97] The effects of disulfiram on the cytochrome P450 system may be both dose and time dependent.

Disulfiram—Drug Interactions

Disulfiram decreases the clearance of amitriptyline, barbiturates, caffeine, chlordiazepoxide, diazepam, and imipramine. Combined therapy with omeprazole can cause catatonia.[37] Isoniazid and metronidazole may potentiate disulfiram's neuropsychiatric effects, producing confusion and psychosis.[98,116] Patients taking disulfiram therapeutically may develop hypotension following the administration of anesthetic agents.[24] Although animal studies suggest that disulfiram may increase the carcinogenicity of ethylene dibromide, this has not been proven in humans.[120]

CLINICAL MANIFESTATIONS

Acute Disulfiram Overdose

Acute overdose of disulfiram is uncommon and typically does not cause life-threatening toxicity. Most patients will develop symptoms within the first 12 hours following ingestion and resolution of symptoms within 24 hours of ingestion.[93]

Nausea, vomiting, and abdominal pain are common. A spectrum of central nervous system depression from drowsiness to coma may occur.[93] Metabolic acidosis is rare.[69] Dysarthria and movement disorders including myoclonus, ataxia, dystonia, and akinesia occur rarely. Movement disorders may be related to direct effects on the basal ganglia.[62,69] Sensorimotor neuropathy, subacute weakness, and psychosis are uncommon.[44,56,99,122] Hypotonia may be a prominent feature in children.[11] Persistent neurologic abnormalities lasting for weeks to months are rare, but are reported in both children and adults.[11,69,93]

Chronic Disulfiram Therapy

Most of the known adverse effects are derived from case reports. Despite the widespread international use of disulfiram, there are few well-controlled human trials evaluating chronic disulfiram toxicity. Toxicity from chronic disulfiram therapy correlates poorly with dose, and there is a wide variability in latency period between the time therapeutic dosing is initiated and symptoms develop. Side effects of chronic disulfiram therapy, unsurprisingly, occur most commonly in alcoholic patients.

Adverse effects most commonly involve the liver, the skin, or the central nervous system. Common effects include nausea, drowsiness, dizziness, headache, a metallic taste in the mouth, halitosis, and skin odor described as having a sulfur or garlic smell, decreased libido, impotence, and hypertension.[42,70,114]

Disulfiram therapy causes a spectrum of hepatotoxicity ranging from asymptomatic minor elevations of the aminotransferase levels to fulminant hepatic failure and death. The hepatotoxicity is clinically indistinguishable from alcoholic hepatitis. The mechanism of disulfiram induced hepatotoxicity is poorly understood and may be idiosyncratic. Injury may be caused by a hypersensitivity reaction, direct hepatotoxicity related to a metabolite or to an immunologic reaction.[31] Histologic patterns of toxicity are predominantly hepatocellular, specifically centrilobular in nature.[13]

The onset of hepatotoxicity usually varies from 2 weeks to 6 months after initiation of disulfiram therapy.[13] Although disulfiram-induced hepatotoxicity may be exacerbated by concurrent alcohol consumption, nonalcoholic patients taking disulfiram as a treatment for nickel dermatitis may also developed hepatotoxicity.[48,52,55]

Dermatoses associated with disulfiram therapy include exfoliative dermatitis, contact dermatitis, urticaria, pruritus, acne, and yellow palms.[7,71,100] Interestingly, thiram and its analogues, which are found in rubber, are also potent skin sensitizers.[103] Some patients with rubber sensitivity develop localized and generalized dermatitis following ingestion of disulfiram, whereas others can be treated with disulfiram without dermatologic complications.[80,116,118] Disulfiram can also cause flare-ups of nickel and cobalt dermatitis.[57,75] Disulfiram may exacerbate nickel dermatitis because diethyldithiocarbamate complexes with nickel and increases its absorption.[45]

Some reported neuropsychiatric side effects include headache; dizziness, confusion,[91] memory impairment,[70] ataxia, Parkinsonian symptoms,[64] seizures,[23] optic neuropathy,[1] coma,[70] peripheral neuropathypsychosis,[12,42,66] depression, catatonia,[30] and organic brain syndrome.[60,99] Confusion, memory impairment, peripheral neuropathy, and psychiatric diagnoses are common in alcoholic patients not taking disulfiram. Alcohol-induced and disulfiram-induced peripheral neuropathy are difficult to distinguish clinically. Disulfiram-induced peripheral neuropathy usually involves motor nerves more than sensory and autonomic nerves, is worse distally, and is usually bilateral. A small prospective study of alcoholics taking therapeutic doses of disulfiram did reveal abnormalities of peripheral nerve function.[82] Neurologic symptoms may be related to both dose and duration of therapy but these issues are not well studied.[27] Although case reports suggest an increased incidence of psychiatric complications, one prospective randomized study did not find an increased incidence of psychiatric complications in alcoholic patients taking disulfiram.[17]

Disulfiram therapy may result in increases in serum cholesterol.[72] Patients with occupational exposures to carbon disulfide have an increased risk of atherosclerosis and ischemic heart disease.[109] Although carbon disulfide is a metabolite of disulfiram, patients taking disulfiram do not have an increased risk of coronary artery disease. One case report suggests that disulfiram may cause thrombocytopenia.[111] Disulfiram is not believed to be teratogenic or carcinogenic.

Disulfiram-Ethanol Reaction

Signs and symptoms include facial and generalized body warmth and flushing, conjunctival injection, pruritus, urticaria, diaphoresis, lightheadedness, vertigo, headache, nausea, vomiting, and abdominal pain. Cardiac effects include palpitations, chest pain, and dyspnea. Tachycardia and hypotension are common. Orthostatic hypotension can cause syncope. ECG abnormalities consistent with myocardial ischemia are uncommon and usually occur in the setting of severe hypotension.[74] Rare complications include shock, hypertension, bronchospasm, and methemoglobinemia.[121] Esophageal rupture and intracranial hemorrhage secondary to vomiting may occur.[29,36,76,107,121] Deaths attributed to the disulfiram-ethanol reaction are very rare.[3,4,9,50,76] There is significant interindividual and intraindividual variation in the intensity and duration of a disulfiram-ethanol reaction.

DIAGNOSTIC TESTING

Disulfiram blood levels are not useful when managing most patients with suspected disulfiram toxicity following an acute overdose, chronic therapy, or a disulfiram-ethanol reaction. When interpreting a disulfiram blood level, it is important to note that only a small proportion of ingested disulfiram appears in the blood as the parent compound because of rapid metabolism. Metabolites of disulfiram including diethyldithiomethylcarbamic acid and diethylthiomethyl carbamic acid can also be measured in the plasma. Other markers of ingestion of disulfiram include carbon disulfide on the breath, and diethylamine in the urine. The activity of hepatic mitochondrial aldehyde dehydrogenase can be measured by liver biopsy, but this is impractical and dangerous. Leukocyte aldehyde dehydrogenase activity correlates most closely with hepatic mitochondrial aldehyde dehydrogenase activity. Decreased erythrocyte ALDH 1 activity and leukocyte ALDH 2 activity are markers of disulfiram exposure. Neither enzyme assay is commonly available.[84]

Chronic Disulfiram Toxicity

Monitoring serum aminotransferase levels, both before the initiation of therapy to establish a baseline and during the course of therapy, is recommended. Unfortunately, no well-controlled trial has specifically addressed the issue of the timing or frequency of routine serum aminotransferase monitoring. There is indirect evidence that the longer patients continue to take disulfiram in the face of elevated aminotransferase levels, the greater the risk of developing life-threatening hepatotoxicity.[31] If an alcoholic patient has increased aminotransferase levels from chronic alcohol use, it is appropriate to delay the administration of disulfiram until the aminotransferase levels have normalized. Aminotransferase levels should be measured if patients taking disulfiram develop clinical signs or symptoms of hepatitis. Common recommendations for asymptomatic patients include monitoring aminotransferase at 2 weeks following initiation of disulfiram therapy and at 3–6 months intervals thereafter. Some clinicians recommend monitoring aminotransferase levels more frequently.[119] Unfortunately, even conservative monitoring regimens may fail to detect patients who develop hepatitis during the testing intervals, so clinicians should educate patients about the signs and symptoms of hepatitis.

As a method of determining compliance with chronic disulfiram therapy, some have advocated using ethanol patch testing to produce cutaneous vasodilation. Studies demonstrate that patch testing is not a reliable measure of compliance with disulfiram therapy.[84] Measuring leukocyte aldehyde dehydrogenase activity or serum levels of disulfiram and/or its metabolites are better measures of compliance with disulfiram therapy.

Disulfiram-Ethanol Reaction

In most patients with suspected disulfiram-ethanol reactions it is important to confirm the presence of ethanol either with an exhaled ethanol concentration or a blood-ethanol level. Because only small amounts of ethanol can precipitate a disulfiram-ethanol reaction, some patients, especially those with small ingestions or dermal exposures, may not have clinically detectable ethanol levels at the time of evaluation. Elevated acetaldehyde concentrations in the blood will occur during a disulfiram-ethanol reaction, but acetaldehyde levels are not readily available, and therefore are not clinically useful when managing most patients.[41]

MANAGEMENT

Acute Disulfiram Overdose

Symptomatic and supportive care is the mainstay of treatment. There is no antidote for disulfiram toxicity. No studies specifically address gastrointestinal decontamination in the setting of an acute disulfiram overdose. Unless contraindicated, activated charcoal, 1 g/kg of body weight should be administered. It would be unusual for a patient with an isolated disulfiram ingestion to require either orogastric lavage or whole-bowel irrigation. Syrup of ipecac is not indicated, especially because some formulations contain ethanol, which could precipitate a disulfiram-ethanol reaction.

Chronic Disulfiram Therapy

If a patient on chronic disulfiram therapy develops toxicity related to disulfiram, the drug should be discontinued. In addition, patients should be instructed to have their serum aminotransferase levels measured if they develop any signs or symptoms of hepatitis, including anorexia, nausea, vomiting, abdominal pain, generalized weakness, malaise, fever, pruritus, scleral icterus, or jaundice.

If aminotransferase levels rise during therapy, the drug should be discontinued. Although rechallenge with disulfiram can, in some cases, confirm the role of disulfiram in causing hepatotoxicity, the benefit is not substantial enough to recommend this approach.[13] Because the evidence to support the use of disulfiram therapy as part of a comprehensive alcohol treatment program is equivocal using today's standards of evidence-based medicine, the risks of continuing disulfiram therapy usually outweigh the benefits. Following discontinuation of disulfiram therapy, hepatic aminotransferase levels usually return to baseline values. Rarely, patients may develop fulminant hepatic failure. Supportive care is the mainstay of treatment for disulfiram-induced hepatic failure. Liver transplantation has been successfully performed for disulfiram-induced hepatic failure.[89]

Disulfiram-Ethanol Reaction

Symptomatic and supportive care is the mainstay of treatment. It is unlikely that gastrointestinal decontamination aimed at removing ethanol will have any clinically significant effect on limiting the severity or duration of the disulfiram-ethanol reaction, because even small amounts of ethanol can cause toxicity in the presence of disulfiram. Additionally, because nausea and vomiting are common, patients often have spontaneous gastric emptying. Antiemetics may improve nausea and vomiting, and histamine (H_1) receptor antagonists, such as diphenhydramine, may improve cutaneous flushing.[106] Parenteral administration of medications is often necessary because of vomiting. Neither pharmacologic approach is well studied. Most patients with hypotension respond to Trendelenburg positioning and intravenous crystalloid administration. Symptomatic hypotension refractory to these measures rarely occurs. If hypotension is refractory to crystalloid administration a vasopressor should be administered. The initial vasopressor should be the one with which the clinician and the staff are most familiar administering. There is a theoretical benefit to administering a direct-acting vasopressor such as norepinephrine, because disulfiram inhibits dopamine β-hydroxylase, an enzyme necessary for norepinephrine synthesis. Because indirect-acting vasopressors, such as dopamine, require functioning dopamine β-hydroxylase to create a releasable pool of norepinephrine, they may be less effective in the setting of disulfiram toxicity. Patients with chest pain or cardiovascular instability should have an electrocardiogram performed.[74] Following resolution of symptoms most patients with a typical disulfiram-ethanol reaction who have normal vital signs can be safely discharged. More prolonged observation is essential for patients with persistent symptoms, ECG abnormalities, or any potentially life-threatening effect.

Fomepizole, an inhibitor of alcohol dehydrogenase prevents the metabolism of ethanol to acetaldehyde.[15] Theoretically, by preventing the production of acetaldehyde, fomepizole could limit the effects of the disulfiram-ethanol reaction. A patient on disulfiram experiencing a disulfiram-ethanol reaction was given fomepizole experimentally with an almost immediate decrease in the serum acetaldehyde level and a rapid clinical improvement.[67] Fomepizole normalized blood acetaldehyde levels and relieved the symptoms of the disulfiram-ethanol reaction in 4 volunteers given calcium carbimide and ethanol.[67] Fomepizole or hemodialysis should be considered for patients with life-threatening signs or symptoms of a disulfiram-ethanol reaction who are refractory to standard treatment. (see Antidotes Indepth: Fomepizole)

Use of Disulfiram as an Antidote

Case reports suggest that disulfiram may be useful for the treatment of nickel dermatitis.[21,22,52] However, small double-blind placebo-controlled study of patients with hand eczema and nickel allergy did not find a clinically significant difference between those treated with disulfiram and those treated with placebo.[52] Because some patients worsen with this therapy[57] and because patients treated for nickel dermatitis have developed disulfiram-induced hepatitis, this therapy is not generally indicated.[53]

Diethyldithiocarbamate, a disulfiram metabolite, is available as the chelator Dithiocarb. Although animal data and human case series suggest that diethyldithiocarbamate may be an effective chelator for the treatment of nickel carbonyl poisoning, no well-controlled human trial has evaluated this therapy. Because disulfiram increases nickel absorption in humans, it is prudent to only use diethyldithiocarbamate in the treatment of nickel carbonyl poisoning and not for the treatment of elemental or inorganic nickel poisoning.[16,108]

SUMMARY

Because disulfiram is still used in comprehensive alcohol treatment programs, it is critical to understand the distinction between the different forms of disulfiram toxicity, including toxicity from an acute overdose, chronic therapy, and from a disulfiram-ethanol reaction. Disulfiram toxicity following an acute overdose is unlikely to be life-threatening unless a massive amount is ingested, an event that usually occurrs in the setting of an intentional overdose by a suicidal adult. Although death is reported following disulfiram-ethanol reactions, most patients do not develop life-threatening toxicity. With the recent widespread availability of fomepizole, its role in treating life-threatening disulfiram-ethanol reactions requires further study. The most common adverse effects of disulfiram that most clinicians, including toxicologists, will en-

counter are secondary to chronic disulfiram therapy. These adverse effects on the liver and the central and peripheral nervous systems are often difficult to distinguish from the effects of chronic alcohol abuse. The effects, including life-threatening disulfiram-induced hepatotoxicity, are rare, and may be prevented by closely monitoring patients prescribed disulfiram and by discontinuing disulfiram therapy as soon as any evidence of toxicity develops.

REFERENCES

1. Acheson JF, Howard RS: Reversible optic neuropathy associated with disulfiram. Neuroopthalmology 1988;8:175–177.
2. Adams RM: Nickel. In: Adams RM, ed: Occupational Skin Disease. New York, Grune & Stratton, 1983, pp. 225–230.
3. Alha AR, Hjelt E, Tamminen V: Disulfiram-alcohol intoxication. Investigation of five fatal cases and the chemical determination of disulfiram and blood acetaldehyde. Acta Pharmacol Toxicol 1957; 13:277–288.
4. Amador E, Gazdar A: Sudden death during disulfiram-alcohol reaction. Q J Study Alcohol 1967;28:649–654.
5. Asmussen E, Hald J, Jørgenson G: Studies on the effect of tetraethylthiuram-disulfide (Antabuse) and alcohol on respiration and circulation in normal human subjects. Acta Pharmacol Toxicol 1948:4:297–304.
6. Asmussen E, Hald J, Larsen V: The pharmacological action of acetaldehyde on the human organism. Acta Pharmacol Toxicol 1948: 4:311–320.
7. Barefoot SW: Acneform eruption produced by the use of tetraethylthiuram disulfide [letter]. JAMA 1951;147:1653.
8. Bartonicek V, Teisinger J: Effect of tetraethylthiuram disulfide (disulfiram) on metabolism of trichloroethylene in man. Br Med J 1962;19:216–221.
9. Becker MC, Sugarman G: Death following "test drink" of alcohol in patients receiving Antabuse. JAMA 1952;149:568–571.
10. Bell RG: Clinical trial of calcium carbimide. Can Med Assoc J 1956; 74:797–798.
11. Benitz WE, Tatro DS: Disulfiram intoxication in a child. J Pediatr 1984;105:487–489.
12. Bennett AE, McKeever LG, Turk RE: Psychotic reaction during tetraethylthiuram disulfide (Antabuse) therapy. JAMA 1951;145: 483–484.
13. Berlin RG: Disulfiram hepatotoxicity: A consideration of its mechanism and clinical spectrum. Alcohol Alcohol 1989;24:241–246.
14. Billstein SA, Sudol TE: Disulfiram-like reactions rare with ceftriaxone [letter]. Geriatrics 1992;47:70.
15. Blomstrand R, Theorell H: Inhibitory effect on ethanol oxidation in man after administration of 4-methylpyrazole. Life Sci 1970;9: 631–640.
16. Bradberry SM, Vale JA: Therapeutic review: Do diethyldithiocarbamate and disulfiram have a role in acute nickel carbonyl poisoning? J Toxicol Clin Toxicol 1999;37:259–264.
17. Branchey L, Davis W, Lee KK, et al: Psychiatric complications of disulfiram treatment. Am J Psych 1987;144:1310–1312.
18. Brien JF, Loomis CW: Disposition and pharmacokinetics of disulfiram and calcium carbimide (calcium cyanamide). Drug Metab Rev 1983;14:113–126.
19. Brown KR, Guglielmo BJ, Pons VG, et al: Theophylline elixir, moxalactam, and a disulfiram reaction. Ann Intern Med 1982;97: 621–622.
20. Budmiger H, Kochler F: Hexenrohrling (Boletus luridus) Mit Alcohol: Ein Kaslitischer Beitrag. Schweiz Med Wsch 1982;112: 1179–1181.
21. Christensen OB: Disulfiram treatment of three patients with nickel dermatitis. Contact Dermatitis 1982;8:105–108.

22. Christensen OB, Kristensen M: Treatment with disulfiram in chronic nickel hand dermatitis. Contact Dermatitis 1982;8:59–63.

23. Daniel DG, Swallows A, Wolff F: Capgras delusion and seizures in association with therapeutic dosages of disulfiram. South Med J 1987;80:1577–1579.

24. Diaz JH, Hill GE: Hypotension with anesthesia in disulfiram-treated patients. Anesthesiology 1979;51:366–368.

25. Emery MG, Jubert C, Thymmel KE, et al: Duration of cytochrome P450 2E1 (CYP2E1) inhibition and estimation of functional CYP2E1 enzyme half-life after single-dose disulfiram administration in humans. J Pharmcol Exp Therp 1999;291:213–219.

26. Eneanya DI, Bianchine JR, Duran DO, et al: The actions and metabolic fate of disulfiram. Ann Rev Pharmacol Toxicol 1981;21:575–596.

27. Enghusen Poulsen H, Loft S, Andersen JR, et al: Disulfiram therapy-adverse drug reactions and interactions. Acta Psychiatr Scand Suppl 1992;369:59–66.

28. Faiman MD, Jensen JC, La Coursiere R: Elimination of disulfiram and metabolites in alcoholics after single and repeated doses. Clin Pharmacol Ther 1984; 36:520–526.

29. Fernandez D: Another esophageal rupture after alcohol and disulfiram [letter]. New Engl J Med 1972;286:610.

30. Fisher CM: "Catatonia" due to disulfiram toxicity. Arch Neurol 1989;46:798–804.

31. Forns X, Caballeria J, Bruguera M, et al: Disulfiram-induced hepatitis. Report of four cases and review of the literature. J Hepatol 1994;21:853–857.

32. Foster T, Raehl C, Wilson H: Disulfiram-like reactions associated with a parenteral cephalosporin. Am J Hosp Pharm 1980;37:858–859.

33. Goedde HW, Harada S, Agarwal DP: Racial differences in alcohol sensitivity: A new hypothesis. Hum Genet 1979;51:331–334.

34. Goldstein M, Anagnoste B, Lauber E, et al: Inhibition of dopamine-β-hydroxylase by disulfiram. Life Sci 1964;3:763–767.

35. Goyer PF, Major LF: Hepatotoxicity in disulfiram treated patients. J Stud Alcohol 1979;40:133–137.

36. Guarnaschelli JJ, Zapanta E, Pitts FW: Intracranial hemorrhage associated with the disulfiram-alcohol reaction. Bull Los Angeles Neurol Soc 1972;37:19–23.

37. Hajela R, Cunningham GM, Kapur BM, et al: Catatonic reaction to omeprazole and disulfiram in a patient with alcohol dependence. Can Med Assoc J 1990;143:1207–1208.

38. Hald J, Jacobsen E: A drug sensitizing the organism to ethyl alcohol. Lancet 1948;2:1001.

39. Hald J, Jacobsen E, Larsen V: The formation of acetaldehyde in the organism after ingestion of Antabuse (tetraethylthiuram disulfide) and alcohol. Acta Pharmacol Toxicol 1948;4:285–310.

40. Hald JE, Jacobsen E, Larsen V: The Antabuse effect of some compounds related to Antabuse and cyanamide. Acta Pharmacol Toxicol 1952;8:329–337.

41. Heath MJ, Pachar JV, Perez Martinez AL, et al: A exceptional case of lethal disulfiram-alcohol reaction. Forensic Sci Int 1992;56:45–50.

42. Heath RG, Nesselhof W, Bishop MP, et al: Behavioral and metabolic changes associated with administration of tetraethylthiuram disulfide (Antabuse). Dis Nerv Sys 1965;26:99–104.

43. Heelon MW, White M: Disulfiram-cotrimoxazole reaction. Pharmacotherapy 1998;18:869–870.

44. Hirschberg M, Ludolph A, Grotemeyer KH, et al: Development of a subacute tetraparesis after disulfiram intoxication. Case report. Eur Neurol 1987;26:222–228.

45. Hopfer SM, Linden JV, Rezuke WN, et al: Increased nickel concentrations in body fluids of patients with chronic alcoholism during disulfiram therapy. Res Commun Chem Pathol Pharmacol 1987;55:101–109.

46. Hsu LC, Bendel RE, Yoshida A: Genomic structure of the human mitochondrial ALDH gene. Genomics 1988;2:57–65.

47. Hughes JC, Cook CC: The efficacy of disulfiram: A review of outcome studies. Addiction 1997;92:381–395.

48. Iber FL, Lee K, Lacoursiere R, et al: Liver toxicity encountered in the Veterans Administration trial of disulfiram in alcoholics. Alcohol Clin Exp Res 1987;11:301–304.

49. Jensen JC, Faiman MD, Hurwitz A: Elimination characteristics of disulfiram in alcoholics after single and repeated doses. Clin Pharmacol Ther 1984; 36:500–506.

50. Jones RO: Death following ingestion of alcohol in Antabuse treated patient. Can Med Assoc J 1949;60:609–612.

51. Johansson B: A review of the pharmacokinetics and pharmacodynamics of disulfiram and its metabolites. Acta Psychiatr Scand Suppl 1992;369:15–26.

52. Kaaber K, Menne T, Veien N, et al: Treatment of nickel dermatitis with Antabuse: A double-blind study. Contact Dermatitis 1983;9:297–299.

53. Kaaber K, Menne T, Veien NK, et al: Some adverse effects of disulfiram in the treatment of nickel-allergic patients. Derm Beruf Umwelt 1987;35:209–211.

54. Kharasch ED, Hankins DC, Jubert C, et al: Lack of single-dose disulfiram effect on cytochrome P-450 2C9, 2C19, 2D6, and 3A4 activities: Evidence for specificity toward P-450 2E1. Drug Metab Dispos 1999;27:717–723.

55. Kirstensen ME: Toxic hepatitis induced by disulfiram in a non-alcoholic. Acta Med Scand 1981;209:335–336.

56. Kirubakaran V, Liskow B, Mayfield D, et al: Case report of acute disulfiram overdose. Am J Psychiatry 1983;140:1513–1514.

57. Klein LR, Fowler JF: Nickel dermatitis recall during disulfiram therapy for alcohol abuse. J Am Acad Derm 1992;26:645–646.

58. Kline SS, Mauro VF, Forney RB, et al: Cefotetan-induced disulfiram-type reactions and hypoprothrombinemia. Antimicrob Agents Chemother 1987;31:1328–1331.

59. Klink DD, Fritz RD, Franke GH: Disulfiram-like reaction to chlorpropamide. Wisconsin Med J 1969;68:134–136.

60. Knee ST, Razani J: Acute organic brain syndrome: a complication of disulfiram. Am J Psychiatry 1974;131:1281–1282.

61. Koff RS, Papadimas I, Honig EG: Alcohol in cough mixture, a hazard to disulfiram user. JAMA 1971;215:1988–1989.

62. Krauss JK, Mohadjer M, Wakhloo AK, et al: Dystonia and akinesia due to pallidoputamninal lesions after disulfiram intoxication. Mov Disord 1992;6:166–170.

63. Kupari M, Hillbom M, Lindros K, et al: Possible cardiovascular hazards of the alcohol-calcium carbimide interaction. J Toxicol Clin Toxicol 1982;19:79–86.

64. Laplane D, Attal N, Sauron B, et al: Lesions of the basal ganglia due to disulfiram neurotoxicity. J Neurol Neurosurg Psychiatry 1992;55:925–929.

65. Levy MS, Livingstone BL, Collins DM: A clinical comparison of disulfiram and calcium carbimide. Am J Psychiatry 1967;123:1018–1022.

66. Liddon SC, Satran R: Disulfiram (Antabuse) psychosis. Am J Psychiatry 1967;123:1284–1289.

67. Lindros KO, Stowell A, Pikkarainen P, et al: The disulfiram (Antabuse)-alcohol reaction in male alcoholics: Its efficient management by 4-methylpyrazole. Alcohol Clin Exp Res 1981;5:528–530.

68. Loi CM, Day JD, Jue SG et al: Dose-dependent inhibition of theophylline metabolism by disulfiram in recovering alcoholics. Clin Pharmacol Ther 1989;45:476–486.

69. Mahajan P, Lieh-Lai MW, Sarnaik A, et al: Basal ganglia infarction in a child with disulfiram poisoning. Pediatrics 1997;99:605–608.

70. Martensen-Larsen O: Five years experience with disulfiram in the treatment of alcoholics. Q J Stud Alcohol 1953;14:406–418.

71. Mathelier-Fusade P, Leynadier F: Occupational allergic contact reaction to disulfiram. Contact Dermatitis 1994;31:121–122.

72. Major LF, Goyer PF: Effects of disulfiram and pyridoxine on serum cholesterol. Ann Intern Med 1978;88:53–56.

73. McMahon F: Disulfiram-like reaction to a cephalosporin. JAMA 1980;243:2367.

74. McCabe ES, Wilson WW: Dangerous cardiac effects of tetraethylthiuram disulfide (Antabuse) therapy in alcoholism. Arch Intern Med 1954;94:259–263.

75. Meene T: Flare-up of cobalt dermatitis from Antabuse treatment. Contact Dermatitis 1985;12:53.

76. Motte S, Vincent JL, Gillet JB, et al: Refractory hyperdynamic shock associated with alcohol and disulfiram. Am J Emerg Med 1986; 4:323–325.

77. Musacchio JM, Goldstein M, Anagnoste B, et al: Inhibition of dopamine-β-hydroxylase by disulfiram in vivo. J Pharmacol Exp Ther 1966;152:56–61.

78. Neu HC, Prince AS: Interaction between moxalactam and alcohol [letter]. Lancet 1980;1:1422.

79. Olesen OV: Disulfiram (Antabuse) as inhibitor of phenytoin metabolism. Acta Pharmacol Toxicol 1966;24:317–322.

80. Olfson M: Disulfiram and allergy to rubber. Am J Psych 1988;145: 651–652.

81. O'Reilly RA: Interaction of sodium warfarin and disulfiram (Antabuse) in man. Ann Intern Med 1973;78:73–76.

82. Palliyath SK, Schwartz BD, Gant L: Peripheral nerve functions in chronic alcoholic patients on disulfiram: a six month follow-up. J Neurol Neurosurg Psychiatry 1990;53:227–230.

83. Pattison EM: Is there a formaldehyde-disulfiram reaction. J Stud Alcohol 1982;43:1257–1259.

84. Petersen EN: The pharmacology and toxicology of disulfiram an its metabolites. Acta Psychiatr Scand Suppl 1992;369:7–13.

85. Petroni NC, Cardoni AA: Alcohol content of liquid medicinals. Clin Toxicol 1979;14:407–432.

86. Phillips M: Persistent sensitivity to ethanol following a single dose of parenteral sustained-release disulfiram. Adv Alcohol Subst Abuse 1987;7:51–61.

87. Poulsen HE, Ranek L, Jorgensen L: The influence of disulfiram on acetaminophen metabolism in man. Xenobiotica 1991;21:243–249.

88. Product Information: Antabuse, disulfiram. Wyeth-Ayerst Laboratories, Philadelphia, PA, 1995.

89. Rabkin JM, Corless CL, Orloff SL, et al: Liver transplantation for disulfiram-induced hepatic failure. Am J Gastroenterol 1998;93: 830–831.

90. Rainey JM: Disulfiram toxicity and carbon disulfide poisoning. Am J Psychiatry 1977;134:371–378.

91. Rathod NH: Toxic effects of disulfiram therapy, with two case reports. Q J Study Alcohol 1958;19:418–427.

92. Refojo MF: Disulfiram-alcohol reaction caused by contact lens wetting solution. Contact Intraocul Lens Med J 1981;7:172.

93. Reichelderfer TE: Acute disulfiram poisoning in a child. Q J Study Alcohol 1969;30:724–728.

94. Reinl W: Alkoholüberempfindlichkeit nach Umgang mit dem Fungicid Tetramethylthiuramdisulfid (TMTD) [Sensitivity to alcohol from the fungicide tetramethylthiuram disulfide]. Arch Toxicol 1966;22: 12–15.

95. Reynolds WA, Lowe FH: Mushrooms and a toxic reaction to alcohol. N Engl J Med 1965;272:630–631.

96. Rogers WK, Benowitz NL, Wilson KM, et al: Effect of disulfiram on adrenergic function. Clin Pharmacol Ther 1979;25:469–477.

97. Rothstein E: Warfarin effect enhanced by disulfiram (Antabuse) [letter]. JAMA 1972;22:1052.

98. Rothstein E, Clancy DD: Toxicity of disulfiram combined with metronidazole. N Engl J Med 1969;280:1006–1007.

99. Ryan TV, Sciara AD, Barth JT: Chronic neuropsychological impairment resulting from disulfiram overdose. J Stud Alcohol 1993; 54:389–392.

100. Santonastaso M, Cecchetti E, Pace M et al: Yellow palms with disulfiram [letter]. Lancet 1997;350:1176.

101. Scott GE, Little FW: Disulfiram reaction to organic solvents other than ethanol. N Engl J Med 1985;312:790.

102. Shelly WB: Golf-course dermatitis due to thiram fungicide. JAMA 1964;188:115–117.

103. Spoerke DG, Rumack BH, eds: Handbook of Mushroom Poisoning—Diagnosis and Treatment. Boca Raton, FL, CRC Press, 1994.

104. Stewart RD, Hake CL, Peterson JE: "Degreasers flush," dermal response to trichloroethylene and ethanol. Arch Environ Health 1974; 29:1–5.

105. Stoll D, King LE Jr: Disulfiram-alcohol skin reaction to beer-containing shampoo. JAMA 1980;244:2045.

106. Stowell A, Johnson J, Ripel Å, et al: Diphenhydramine and the calcium carbimide-ethanol reaction: A placebo-controlled clinical trial. Clin Pharmacol Ther 1986;39:521–525.

107. Stransky G, Lambing MK, Simmons GT, et al: Methemoglobinemia in a fatal case of disulfiram-ethanol reaction [letter]. J Anal Toxicol 1997;21:178–179.

108. Sunderman FW: Use of sodium diethyldithiocarbamate in the treatment of nickel carbonyl poisoning. Ann Clin Lab Sci 1990;20: 12–21.

109. Sweetman PM, Taylor SWC, Elwood PC: Exposure to carbon disulphide and ischaemic heart disease in a viscose rayon factory. Br J Indust Med 1987;44:220–227.

110. Syed J, Moarefi G: An unusual presentation of a disulfiram-alcohol reaction [letter]. Del Med J 1995;67:183.

111. Thompson CC, Tacke RB, Woolley LH, et al: Purpuric oral and cutaneous lesions in a case of drug-induced thrombocytopenia. J Am Dent Assoc 1982;105:465–467.

112. Truitt EB, Puritz G, Morgan AM, et al: Disulfiram-like actions produced by hypoglycemic sulfonylurea compounds. Q J Stud Alcohol 1962;23:197–207.

113. Vallari RC, Pietruszko R: Human aldehyde dehydrogenase: Mechanism of inhibition of disulfiram. Science 1982;216:637–639.

114. Volicer L, Nelson KL: Development of reversible hypertension during disulfiram therapy. Arch Intern Med 1984;144:1294–1296.

115. Webb PK, Gibbs SC, Mathias CT, et al: Disulfiram hypersensitivity and rubber contact dermatitis [letter]. JAMA 1979;241:2061.

116. Whittington HG, Grey L: Possible interaction between disulfiram and isoniazid. Am J Psychiatry 1969;125:1725–1729.

117. Williams EE: Effects of alcohol on workers with carbon disulfide [letter]. JAMA 1937;109:1472–1473.

118. Wilson H: Side effects of disulfiram [letter]. Br Med J 1962;2:1610.

119. Wright C, Vafier JA, Lake CR: Disulfiram-induced fulminating hepatitis: Guidelines for liver-panel monitoring. J Clin Psychiary 1988; 49:430–434.

120. Yodaiken RE: Ethylene dibromide and disulfiram—A lethal combination [letter]. JAMA 1978;239:2783.

121. Zapata E, Orwin A: Severe hypertension and bronchospasm during disulfiram-ethanol test reaction. BMJ 1992;305:870.

122. Zorzon M, Mase G, Biasutti E, et al: Acute encephalopathy and polyneuropathy after disulfiram intoxication. Alcohol Alcohol 1995; 30:629–631.

CHAPTER 66 TOXIC ALCOHOLS

Adhi N. Sharma

Ethylene Glycol
MW	=	62 Daltons
Action serum level for Hemodialysis	=	>25 mg/dL with acidosis or renal insufficiency
	=	>4.03 mmol/L

Isopropanol
MW	=	60 Daltons

Methanol
MW	=	32 Daltons
Action serum level for Hemodialysis	=	>25 mg/dL
	=	>7.8 mmol/L

Values greater than or equal to the action level necessitate clinical intervention. Values less than this level may necessitate intervention based on the clinical condition of the patient.

A 35-year-old man was brought to the Emergency Department (ED) for bizarre behavior. According to his family, the patient stated that he wanted to kill himself. The patient was found holding a large fast-food beverage cup filled with a fluorescent green liquid. The patient, who was somnolent, said that he had been drinking this liquid for the last several hours. He appeared well nourished and well developed. Initial vital signs were blood pressure, 140/100 mm Hg; pulse, 80 beats/min; respiratory rate, 18 breaths/min; temperature 99.2°F (37.3°C).

His skin was dry, anicteric, and acyanotic. Examination of his head, ears, eyes, nose, and throat was unremarkable. Pupils were 5 mm and reactive, no nystagmus was noted, and funduscopy was normal. Chest, heart, and abdominal examinations were also noted to be normal.

An intravenous line was started with 0.9% NaCl solution and blood was drawn for glucose, electrolytes, blood urea nitrogen (BUN), creatinine, osmolality, ethanol, and acetaminophen levels. A urinary catheter was placed and a specimen was sent for analysis. An electrocardiogram (ECG) was performed and the patient was placed on a cardiac monitor.

Initial fingerstick glucose was 88 mg/dL and a urine specimen did not fluoresce under Wood's lamp examination. The patient was given 100 mg of thiamine HCl and 50 mg of pyridoxine intravenously. Activated charcoal was not administered. While awaiting results of the blood tests, the patient's clinical status remained stable.

Arterial blood gas determination on room air revealed pH, 7.01; P_{CO_2}, 15 mm Hg; and P_{O_2}, 95 mm Hg. His electrolytes were Na^+, 149 mEq/L; K^+, 6.0 mEq/L; Cl^-, 105 mEq/L; and HCO_3^-, 7 mEq/L. His other laboratory data were BUN, 9 mg/dL; Ca^{2+}, 9.2 mg/dL;

creatinine, 1.3 mg/dL; and glucose, 147 mg/dL. The calculated anion gap was 37 mEq/L (Chap. 24).

Serum osmolality was measured at 370 mOsm/kg and the calculated osmolarity was 300 mOsm/L (Chap. 24). Because the ethanol level was undetectable, the osmol gap was calculated to be 70 mOsm/L.

The patient was then loaded with 15-mg/kg of fomepizole and admitted to the medical intensive care unit (ICU). Within 5 hours of admission, he received his first hemodialysis treatment. The patient's initial serum ethylene glycol concentration was determined to be 222.6 mg/dL and his postdialysis level was 97.2 mg/dL. Therefore, he was dialyzed a second time, approximately 16 hours after admission. Appropriate psychiatric consultation was obtained and the patient had an uneventful recovery without evidence of sequelae on discharge from the hospital.

Alcohols are hydrocarbons that contain a hydroxyl (OH) group(s). Primary alcohols contain the hydroxyl group on a terminal carbon, as in the case of ethanol and methanol. In secondary alcohols, such as, isopropyl alcohol, the hydroxyl group is on a carbon bound to two other carbon atoms. A compound with two hydroxyl groups is commonly classified as a diol (butanediol), but may also be referred to as a glycol (ethylene glycol). All alcohols have potential toxicity, however, the term *toxic alcohols* commonly refers to ethylene glycol, methanol and isopropanol. Other less-common, but still consequential toxic alcohols include diethylene glycol, benzyl alcohol, and the glycol ethers, such as butoxyethanol (ethylene glycol butyl ether); and methoxyethanol (ethylene glycol methyl ether) (Chaps. 2 and 56).

Although used in a wide range of preparations, most alcohols are not intended for human consumption. The addition of ethylene glycol to water lowers the freezing point and raises the boiling point. Thus, more than a quarter of ethylene glycol produced is used in coolant mixtures, antifreeze for motor vehicles, and air-craft deicing solutions. Ethylene glycol is also used as a solvent in inks, pesticides, and adhesives. It is used in brake fluid and in heat exchangers and condensers. Ethylene glycol is used as a glycerin substitute in products such as cosmetics, paints, lacquers and detergents. Because most household exposures (particularly in children) to ethylene glycol result from the ingestion of automobile antifreeze, some companies have developed a propylene glycol product in an attempt to limit the potential toxicity.

Methanol is also used as antifreeze, specifically in window washer fluid (30%) or added to fuel as an anti-icing agent or octane booster ($\approx$100%). It is also used as an ethanol denaturant, an extraction agent and solvent, and as a fuel source, specifically for picnic stoves (4%) and soldering torches. Methanol is commonly used in varnish removers and paint, and as an industrial solvent. It is used in the manufacture of acetic acid, formaldehyde, methyl derivatives, and inorganic acids. Most household exposures result from the ingestion of windshield washing fluids and fuel deicing agents.

Isopropanol is produced from the hydration of propylene with sulfuric acid. It is a raw material used for the synthesis of acetone, glycerin, and other chemicals. Isopropanol is also used as a solvent for oils, gums, and resins and as a deicing agent for liquid fuels. Isopropanol is commonly used as rubbing alcohol in a 70% solution and as a solvent in hair-care products, skin lotion, and home aerosols. It is often ingested as an inexpensive and convenient substitute for ethanol.

Propylene glycol is commonly used as a diluent for parenteral preparations such as diazepam and phenytoin. It is also used as an environmentally safe alternative to ethylene glycol as automobile antifreeze or as a deicing agent, in food and cosmetic preparations, but it is more expensive to produce than ethylene glycol.

Diethylene glycol is used as a solvent and sprinkler antifreeze, and in paints and cosmetics. The ethylene glycol ethers, monomethyl [$CH_3OCH_2CH_2OH$] and monobutyl [$CH_3(CH_2)_3$ OCH_2CH_2OH] are two commonly used solvents called *cellu-solves*. They are found in paints, resins, and industrial coatings.

Alcohols have numerous applications and as such are contained in a myriad of household products. Ethanol is likely the world's commonest substance of abuse. Exposures to toxic alcohols may be intentional either as an ethanol substitute or for the purpose of self-harm. Unintentional exposures are often secondary to the ubiquitous nature of the products. Whatever the exposure, a thorough understanding of the pathophysiology and pharmacology is essential to providing appropriate therapy.

HISTORY AND EPIDEMIOLOGY

Although toxic alcohol ingestions usually involves a single patient, a number of mass exposures have occurred, often as a result of a failure of quality control. Diethylene glycol-contaminated glycerin has repeatedly been used in the preparation of medications in numerous developing countries including India, Bangladesh, Haiti, South Africa, and Nigeria.[27,45,72] These contaminated medications, usually acetaminophen elixirs, have led to the deaths of hundreds of children from renal failure in countries

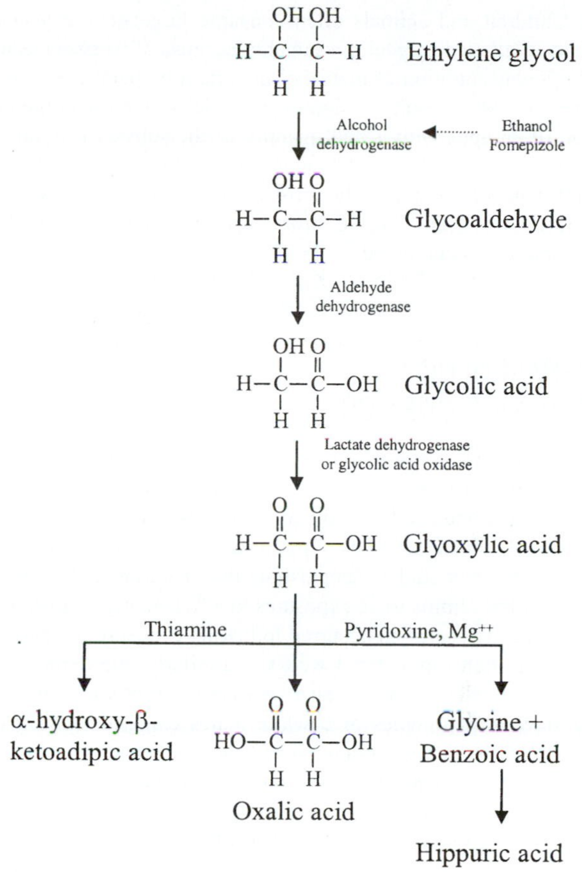

Figure 66–1. Major pathways of ethylene glycol metabolism.

where dialysis is not readily available. In the United States, a contaminated water supply containing 9% ethylene glycol led to an epidemic of poisoning in children who developed somnolence, ataxia, vomiting, hematuria, and crystalluria.[38] Death after hemodialysis has occurred because air conditioning cooling fluid, consisting of ethylene glycol, contaminated a hospital's water supply.[63] These types of exposures occur repeatedly and could be avoided with stricter quality control of pharmaceuticals and better engineering controls.

Because the glycol ethers have common commercial and industrial uses, occupational exposures account for the majority of toxicity. First introduced in the mid-1930s, the glycol ether methoxyethanol was used as a solvent in the garment industry in the production of stiffened or "fused" shirt collars. Shortly thereafter, reports were published describing encephalopathy and bone marrow suppression in workers exposed to methoxyethanol in the garment industry.[9] Since that time industrial use has grown exponentially, increasing the risk of toxicity to workers and necessitating specific safety protocols. Additionally, use of these solvents in household cleaning products (window cleaners) has resulted in a number of household exposures.[18]

Approximately 250 deaths attributable to toxic alcohol poisoning were reported to poison centers for the 10-year period from 1990–1999. Most of these deaths were related to methanol (134) and ethylene glycol (84) according to data from the American Association of Poison Control Centers (AAPCC) (see p. 1752, Chap.

116). Children and animals often consume larger-than-expected amounts of ethylene glycol, presumably because of its sweet taste. The high concentration of methanol in certain preparations (often in excess of 90%) results in significant toxicity, even with the ingestion of an apparently small quantity of the substance in question. Finally, the widespread availability and low cost of rubbing alcohol makes isopropanol the most frequently reported toxic alcohol exposure, accounting for more exposures than ethylene glycol and methanol combined.

PHARMACOLOGY AND TOXICOKINETICS

Exposure to toxic alcohols can occur via dermal, pulmonary, and gastrointestinal routes.[2,25,37,69] Most of the alcohols have a high vapor pressure and can be absorbed via inhalation, except for ethylene glycol, which has a low vapor pressure (0.6 mm Hg at 20°C (68°F)). Volunteer studies demonstrate that irritation of the upper respiratory tract limits toxic exposures to ethylene glycol mist and no evidence of absorption occurred following exposure of up to 27 parts per million (ppm) for 4 weeks.[73] Similarly, the dermal absorption of ethylene glycol is also very poor. An in vitro study of donor thigh skin samples of 3 white males exposed to 8 μg of ^{14}C-labeled ethylene glycol/cm^2 for 24 hours yielded an average flux of 0.009 μg/cm^2/h.[20] By contrast, dermal exposures to methanol, isopropanol and glycol ethers have led to toxicity.[2,42,69] All alcohols are absorbed rapidly from the gastrointestinal tract. The rate of absorption ranges from ethanol at 0.57 mg/cm^2/h to methanol at 8.4 mg/cm^2/h and the glycol ethers approximately 2.82 mg/cm^2/h.[21,41] Time to peak serum concentration ranges from 1 to 4 hours after ingestion of ethylene glycol and 30–60 minutes for methanol, the glycol ethers, and isopropanol.[3,56]

Alcohols share a common volume of distribution (see pharmacokinetics) with an approximate Vd of 0.6 L/kg (range 0.5–0.8 L/kg). Ethylene glycol, methanol, and isopropanol are all metabolized by oxidation via alcohol dehydrogenase (ADH) and aldehyde dehydrogenase (see Figs. 66–1, 66–2, and 66–3). Although ADH metabolizes all alcohols, enzyme-binding affinities vary. The affinity of ADH for ethanol is 4 times greater than its affinity for methanol and 8 times greater than its affinity for ethylene glycol. These variable affinities have significant therapeutic importance. Although peak methanol concentrations are achieved rapidly, metabolism may not be evident until 24 hours (range, 1–72 hours), delaying the development of acidosis and toxic symptoms.[6] In the liver, ADH metabolizes approximately 75–85% of methanol to formaldehyde, which is then oxidized by aldehyde dehydrogenase to formic acid. In the presence of folate, formic acid is converted to carbon dioxide and water.[52,53] This beneficial aspect of folate has been demonstrated both in mice and in nonhuman primates. Folate-deficient rats were more susceptible to methanol toxicity than were folate-rich rats.[66] Monkeys treated with folate after methanol ad-

ministration were relatively resistant to methanol toxicity, and when methanol toxicity was allowed to develop, it was reversed after folate treatment.[52,53] Because of its volatility, methanol can be eliminated unchanged by the lungs (10–20%) and about 3% is excreted unchanged via the kidneys. At low concentrations methanol metabolism follows zero-order kinetics at a rate of 8.5 mg/dL/h.[36] At much higher methanol concentrations first-order kinetics occur, possibly because of increased pulmonary elimination. In the presence of therapeutic levels of ethanol, the half-life ranges from 30 to 52 hours with a median of 43 hours.[55] In the presence of fomepizole, the mean half-life is 54 hours.[7]

Ethylene glycol is slowly metabolized over several hours (3–8) to glycoaldehyde.[57] Because it is a diol, it undergoes successive oxidations to yield glycolate, glyoxylate, and oxalate. As in the case of other aldehydes, glycoaldehyde is rapidly metabolized by aldehyde dehydrogenase to glycolate. The conversion of glycolate to glyoxylate is the rate-limiting step in this process.[50] Glyoxylate can follow alternate metabolic pathways; glycolic acid can be metabolized to hippurate in the presence of pyridoxine or to α-hydroxy-β-ketoadipic acid in the presence of magnesium and thiamine.[34,59] The majority of this elimination (80%) occurs in the liver. The remaining 20% is excreted unchanged by the kidneys. Virtually no ethylene glycol is eliminated via the lungs because of its chemical characteristics. The half-life of ethylene glycol and methanol have been described under various therapeutic conditions (see Table 66–1).[7,8]

Isopropanol is rapidly metabolized via alcohol dehydrogenase to acetone. However, as a result of its secondary alcohol characteristics, the initial oxidation forms a ketone and not an aldehyde, which permits no further oxidation or metabolism. Unlike the other alcohols, isopropanol follows first-order kinetics with regard to its elimination. This may be a consequence of the significant renal and pulmonary elimination of acetone. Approximately 80% of isopropanol is metabolized to acetone. The remainder is excreted unchanged in the urine with a small amount excreted through the lungs. The half-lives of isopropanol and acetone in adults are 2.9–16.2 hours and 7.6–26.2 hours, respectively.[17,56] The half-life of isopropanol can be doubled in the presence of ethanol, but there is no effect on acetone elimination. The kidneys excrete the majority of acetone, whereas the lungs excrete only a minority of acetone.

The metabolism of the glycol ethers varies substantially. ADH metabolizes monoalkyl ethers of ethylene glycol to their respective alkoxyacetic acids; for example, butoxyethanol is metabolized to butoxyacetic acid with butoxyacetaldehyde as an intermediate.[13,29] The metabolism of other glycol ethers and esters of ethylene glycol is not completely understood; some may undergo cleavage of the ether bond to produce ethylene glycol. This latter pathway is a speculative one based on reports of urinary oxalate crystals in 2 patients who ingested methoxyethanol and of a patient who ingested butoxyethanol.[51,58] None of these patients had detectable methanol levels, the other expected product of methoxyethanol cleavage. Most glycol ether exposures do not re-

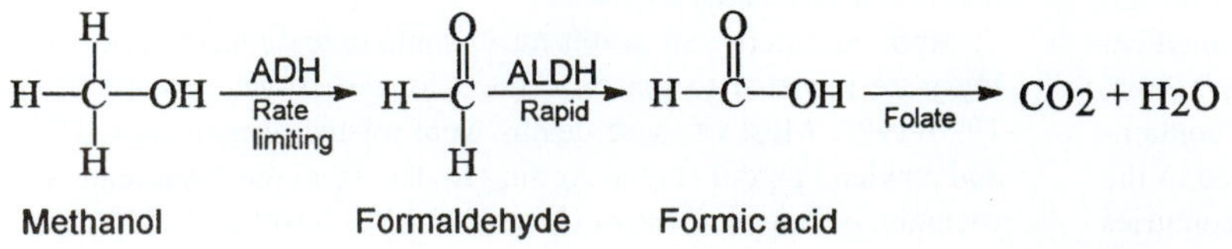

Figure 66–2. Methanol metabolism. Therapy is aimed at interfering with this conversion. Ethanol is a preferential substrate for alcohol dehydrogenase (ADH). 4-Methylpyrazole is a competitive inhibitor of the enzyme ADH. (ALDH = aldehyde dehydrogenase.)

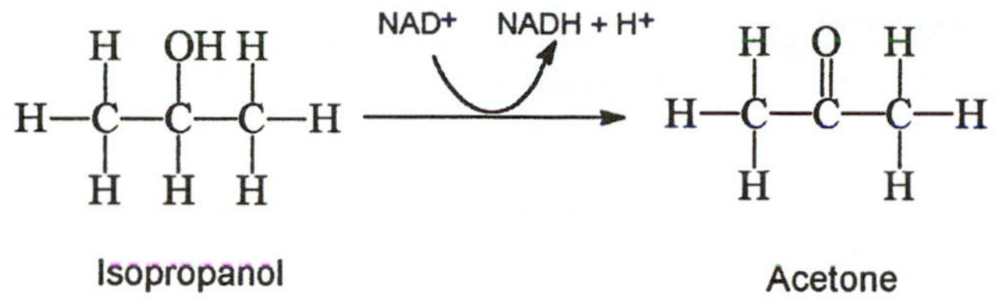

Figure 66–3. Isopropanol metabolism.

sult in the toxicity associated with ethylene glycol metabolism, suggesting that a different metabolic pathway exists (see examples of metabolism in Figure 66–4).

CLINICAL MANIFESTATIONS

Toxic alcohols have multiple effects. In general, the common symptoms are related to the parent alcohol and the specific effects are related to the resultant metabolites. Table 66–2 summarizes symptoms by systems and associated alcohols. It is important to remember that there may be an initial asymptomatic period following exposure. As a class, alcohols can cause inebriation, but the degree of inebriation present after consumption of a given amount of alcohol appears to be based on the number of carbon molecules present in its chemical structure.[71] Thus, methanol is less intoxicating than ethanol or ethylene glycol, which are less intoxicating than isopropanol. Inebriation can occur after ingestion of a toxic alcohol and may be the only presenting symptom. However, the absence of inebriation does not exclude significant toxic alcohol ingestion; thus, inebriation is an unreliable symptom. For example, a methanol level of 50 mg/dL may not result in inebriation, but it does have the potential for toxicity. However, a similar serum ethanol concentration may have obvious central nervous system (CNS) effects. All alcohols can cause CNS depression that may present as lethargy or coma and respiratory depression. The CNS depressant effect of isopropanol may be potentiated by its metabolism to acetone, a CNS depressant as well. Animal studies suggest that isopropanol is 2–3 times more potent than ethanol as a CNS depressant, while acetone's depressant effects are comparable to those of ethanol.[71] The ingestion of glycol ether has resulted in acute encephalopathy and may present as agitation, confusion, or coma. CNS depression occurred rapidly following the ingestion of butoxyethanol and ethanol, whereas a delay of 8–18 hours followed the ingestion of pure methoxyethanol.[9]

Alcohols are also vasodilators. As such, consumption can result in hypotension and reflex tachycardia. Occasionally, hypotension may be further exacerbated by bradycardia secondary to CNS depression.

TABLE 66–1. Apparent Plasma Half-lives (Hours) of Ethylene Glycol and Methanol Under Diverse Conditions

	Ethylene Glycol	Methanol
Alone	3–8.6*	zero order 8.5 mg/dL/h
With Ethanol	17–18	43
With Fomepizole	14–17*	54
With Ethanol and Dialysis	2.5–3.5	2.5–3.5

*With normal renal function

Additionally, the oxidation of an alcohol by ADH results in increased formation of nicotinamide adenine dinucleotide (NADH) resulting in a high NADH to NAD^+ ratio (Chap. 64). This low redox ratio favors the conversion of pyruvate to lactate, but rarely results in significant lactic acidosis. The decrease in pyruvate removes substrate form the Krebs' cycle, impairing energy production. This low redox effect combined with alcohol's inhibition of gluconeogenesis can cause hypoglycemia in susceptible individuals—small children and those with poor nutritional status such as alcoholics. The number of oxidative steps affects the NADH:NAD ratio and as such the effect is greater for ethylene glycol (4 oxidative steps) than for isopropanol (1 oxidative step).

An anion gap metabolic acidosis is another common feature of ethylene glycol and methanol toxicity. This acidosis is the result of the different organic acids formed from the metabolism of the parent compounds.[26] Although ethylene glycol is metabolized to glycolic, glyoxylic, and oxalic acid, glycolic acid is most responsible for the production of the acidosis.[50] Metabolic acidosis from methanol poisoning is caused by formic acid, but may be exacerbated by the increase in lactate production from formate's inhibition of the cytochrome oxidase chain. The alkoxyacetic acids formed from ADH metabolism of the monoalkyl ethers of ethylene glycol can also result in acidosis. For example, butoxyethanol metabolism results in butoxyacetic acid.[9]

Visual symptoms, if they develop, usually develop within 24 hours after methanol exposure.[46] The patient may complain of blurred or "snow field" vision. This is the result of formic acid-mediated retinal toxicity. In primate studies, formate produced retinal toxicity despite pH buffering, implicating the metabolite and not the associated acidosis in the development of the retinal effects.[48,49] If formate production persists, the toxin may result in permanent visual loss.[46,47] Ophthalmologic examination may reveal hyperemia of the optic disc and/or retinal edema.[5] Papilledema, ophthalmoplegia, and loss of pupillary light reflexes may be present. Rarely, these same symptoms may occur following exposure to ethylene glycol.

The oxalate formed form ethylene glycol metabolism can chelate calcium out of serum resulting in QT prolongation on the ECG and cardiac dysrhythmias secondary to hypocalcemia.[64] Furthermore, calcium oxalate precipitates in the renal tubules and can cause acute tubular necrosis within 12–48 hours after ingestion.[16] Multiple cranial nerve (CN) deficits may occur after ethylene glycol poisoning. In addition to pupillary deficits and ophthalmoplegia (CN II, III, and VI), facial paresthesias, facial weakness, hearing loss, dysarthria, and dysphagia (CN V, VII, VIII, IX, and X respectively), are reported.[68] These neurologic manifestations may resolve over a period of time from weeks to months. Postmortem analysis in 1 patient demonstrated dense crystals along the subarachnoid portion of CN VII and VIII.[1] Other authors suggest that an ethylene glycol-induced pyridoxine deficiency is responsible, but evidence is lacking.[68] The adult respiratory distress syndrome has been described in an ethylene glycol-poisoned patient, but this more likely represents a nonspecific complication of profound illness.[14]

As a result of its metabolic pathway, isopropanol does not manifest major toxicity unless extremely large doses are ingested. Patients with isopropanol ingestions manifest CNS depression, hemorrhagic gastritis, and tracheobronchitis.

Following exposure to monomethyl or monobutyl ethers of ethylene glycol the parent compound or its metabolite can result in acute tubular necrosis (without oxaluria), hepatitis, pancreatitis,

TABLE 66–2.   Signs and Symptoms of Toxic Alcohol Exposures

Organ System	Ethylene Glycol	Isopropanol	Methanol
Cardiovascular	Tachycardia	Tachycardia	Tachycardia
	Hypertension/hypotension	Hypotension	Hypotension
	Dysrhythmias	Myocardial depression	
	Myocarditis		
Central nervous	Ataxia	Areflexia	CNS depression
	Meningoencephalitis	Ataxia	Convulsions
	Convulsions	CNS depression	Dizziness
	CNS depression	Dizziness	Headache
	Inebriation	Headache	Hypothermia
	Myoclonus	Inebriation	Inebriation
		Muscle weakness	
		Hypothermia	
Gastrointestinal	Nausea, vomiting	Abdominal pain, cramping	Abdominal pain
		Gastritis	Anorexia
		Hematemesis	Gastritis
		Nausea, vomiting	Nausea, vomiting
			Pancreatitis
Ophthalmic	Ophthalmoplegia		"Snow fields"
	Nystagmus		Blurred vision
			Hyperemic optic discs
			Mydriasis
			Papilledema, blindness
Pulmonary	Hyperventilation, Tachypnea	Odor of acetone	Respiratory depression
	Pneumonitis	Respiratory depression	
	Respiratory depression	Hemorrhagic tracheobronchitis	
Renal	Crystalluria	Renal tubular acidosis	
	Renal insufficiency	Rhabdomyolysis	
Other		Hemolytic anemia	

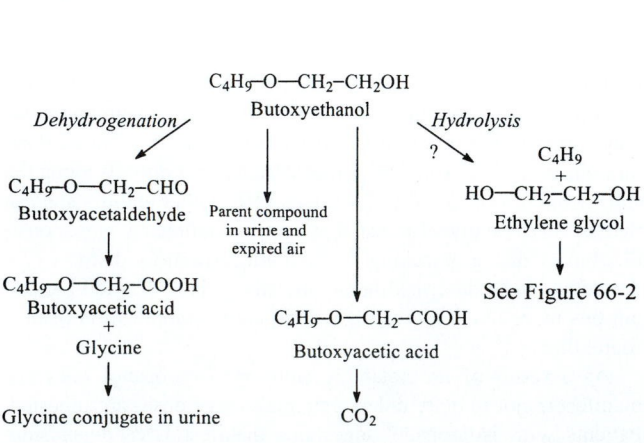

Figure 66–4.   The structure and metabolic fates of butoxyethanol (ethylene glycol butylether). In humans it appears that butoxyacetic acid is the primary pathway, but concern with regard to hydrolysis to ethylene glycol exists.

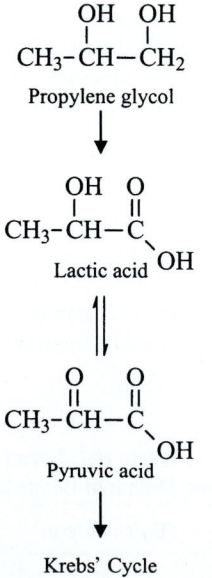

Figure 66–5.   Propylene glycol metabolism to lactic acid. Under normal conditions, lactate is converted to pyruvate which, following decarboxylation, enters the Krebs' cycle.

CNS depression, and metabolic acidosis. Bone marrow depression and toxic encephalopathy can result from the chronic inhalation of these ethers.[9,51,58] Butoxyacetic acid, the metabolite of butoxyethanol can result in hemolysis.[13]

Propylene Glycol and Benzyl Alcohol

$$H-C-OH$$

Benzyl alcohol

Propylene glycol is metabolized to lactic acid (Fig. 66–5). Profound lactic acidosis is reported following the infusion of large quantities of medications that employ propylene glycol as a diluent. Patients can develop hypotension, cardiac conduction abnormalities (QRS widening), dysrhythmias, and asystole when rapid IV infusions containing propylene glycol are administered. However, most propylene glycol ingestions result in a transient and clinically insignificant rise in serum lactate. Transdermal absorption of propylene glycol contained in silver sulfadiazine cream has resulted in hypoglycemia, seizures, and CNS depression in children with severe burns treated with this cream.[39]

Benzyl alcohol is interesting from a historical prospective. Most patients are exposed only to minimal amounts of benzyl alcohol, which is commonly used as a preservative for intravenous preparations.[43] However, use of these preparations in preterm neonates has resulted in lethal metabolic acidosis caused by the formation of hippuric acid and benzoic acid, the products of the hepatic oxidative metabolism of benzyl alcohol. Benzoic acid levels 12 times that of controls accounted for the demonstrated anion gap in neonates whose IVs had been flushed with bacteriostatic normal saline solution. These patients developed a symptom complex that included gasping reactions, hypotension, neurologic deterioration, hepatic and renal failure, and death.[28,44] For this reason benzyl alcohol is no longer used as an antimicrobial preservative in neonatal medicine (Chaps. 2 and 56).

DIAGNOSTIC TESTING

Several diagnostic tests are available to the clinician managing a patient with suspected toxic alcohol poisoning. The serum should be analyzed for BUN, creatinine, glucose, and electrolytes, including calcium. Ethylene glycol and methanol result in an anion gap metabolic acidosis, whereas isopropanol usually does not. Ethylene glycol can result in hypocalcemia or renal injury, and establishing baseline renal function in patients with any toxic alcohol ingestion is appropriate. Urine dipsticks can provide information as to the presence of ketones (suggesting isopropanol ingestion), while urine microscopy can determine the presence of crystals (Fig. 66–6). Calcium oxalate can form either monohydrate (spindlelike) or dihydrate crystals (envelope shaped). The dihydrate crystals are easily recognizable and diagnostic, whereas monohydrate spindles may be indistinguishable from hippurate crystals.[34] However, crystals are only present in approximately 50–65% of cases, therefore the absence of crystals is an unreliable finding.[8,34] In patients with normal renal function urine can be examined for the presence of fluorescence. Urinary fluorescence persists for only a few hours after ingestion of fluorescein containing radiator antifreeze. A volunteer study of 6 men who ingested fluorescein and then gave hourly urine samples, demonstrated that urinary fluorescence was short-lived, present 100% of the time at 2 hours, 60% of the time at 4 hours, and 20% of the time at 6 hours.[74] When present, it is best appreciated by examining urine on white gauze or filter paper with a black light (Wood's lamp).

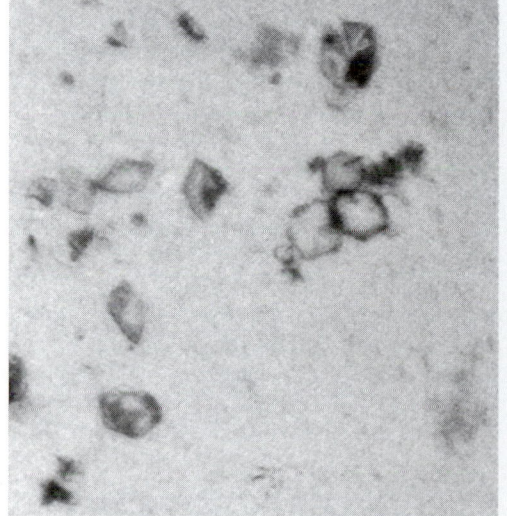

A

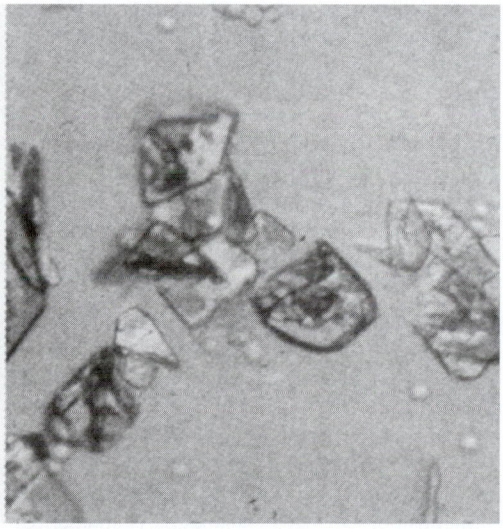

B

Figure 66–6. Calcium oxalate crystals (dehydrate forms) under low (**A**) and high (**B**) power, found in the urine of a patient following the ingestion of ethylene glycol.

Foley bags and urine tubes (glass or plastic) all possess inherent fluorescence and may result in false-positive results.

Osmol Gap

The ingestion of any toxic alcohol can raise the serum osmolality.[23,33] Since the calculated osmolarity consists of simply twice the serum sodium, in mEq, plus the molar sums of the glucose and BUN, it is not altered in the presence of additional osmotically active particles in the serum. However, these additional molecules raise the measured osmolality so that the gap between measured and calculated osmols increases. Laboratories should measure the osmolality by performing freezing-point depression studies as boiling-point elevation techniques volatilize many alcohols. The calculated serum osmolarity (Chap. 24) can then be subtracted from the measured osmolality resulting in the osmol gap. To avoid confusion any calculation of the serum osmolarity should also include ethanol, serum ethanol concentrations should be obtained on all patients with suspected toxic alcohol ingestion.[60] When the osmol gap is greater than 50 mOsm/L it should be considered nearly diagnostic of toxic alcohol ingestion. However, a normal or even negative osmol gap does not exclude the presence of toxic alcohols. This limitiation occurs because the range of normal osmol gaps within the population is large (perhaps −2 ± 6 mOsm/L) and it is the individual patient's change from baseline that is relevant. That is, if a patient has a baseline osmol gap of −2 mOsm/L and it is currently 8 mOsm/L (within the population norm), the patient actually has 10 mOsm/L of osmols left unaccounted. This may represent a methanol level of 32 mg/dL or an ethylene glycol level of 64 mg/dL, both of which are consequential.[70]

Additionally, a number of conditions create an increase in the osmol gap. One study found that both alcoholic ketoacidosis (AKA) and lactic acidosis raised the osmol gap by 10–11 mOsm/L. These authors found that an osmol gap greater than 25 mOsm/L was indicative of a toxic alcohol ingestion with a specificity of 88%.[62] Another study found that the osmol gap could be elevated in patients with chronic, but not acute renal failure.[65]

Acid-Base Status

Arterial blood gas analysis is a rapid way of determining serum pH, but this study's utility is limited by the presence of a normal serum bicarbonate during the first hours following toxic alcohol ingestion. This latter concept is of importance, as clinicians must recognize the temporal relationship between the anion and osmol gaps. Alcohols are effective osmols and raise the osmol gap. As the alcohols are metabolized to their acid products the body uses bicarbonate to buffer the serum pH. This results in a drop in serum bicarbonate and the development of an increased anion gap. As time passes and metabolism progresses, the osmol gap decreases while the anion gap increases. Abnormalities in the two gaps may or may not be present at the same time (see Fig. 66–7). Late in toxic alcohol ingestions the patient may have a large anion gap acidosis but a normal osmol gap. This explanation is another reason why both the osmol gap and anion gap are only useful when abnormal, but should never be used to exclude toxicity. Isopropanol causes a large osmol gap without an anion gap; this increased gap persists while metabolism to acetone occurs (a ketone, not an acid).

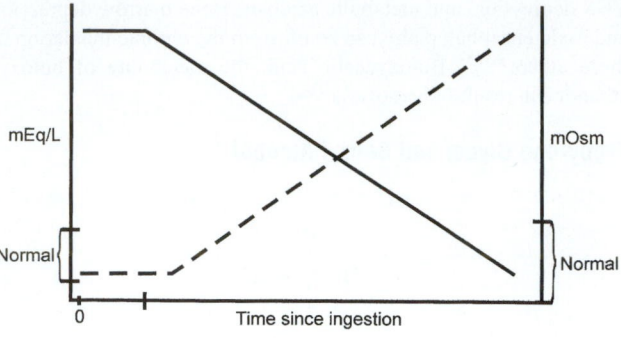

Figure 66–7. The relationship between the anion gap (−−−) and the osmol gap (−) over time.

QUANTITATIVE TESTING

When available, quantitative serum alcohol concentrations eliminate all of the guesswork from the management of a patient with a suspected toxic alcohol ingestion. Serum ethanol, methanol, and ethylene glycol concentrations; if rapidly available, can be used to determine the proper course of management, but may be less helpful if significant metabolism has already occurred. Substantially elevated serum ethanol concentrations can afford some protection to the patient and should always be determined.

Several techniques are available to obtain quantitative levels. The best method uses gas chromatography (GC) with flame ionization for the detection of toxic alcohols or their derivatives.[22] False-positive results can occur in the presence of propylene glycol (found in IV preparations such as phenytoin or diazepam), propionic acid, or 2,3 butanediol. For this reason, GC findings are often confirmed by mass spectrometry (MS). This technique also requires a dedicated GC column, which is a significant laboratory expense. Other techniques include variations on high-performance liquid chromatography and the GC method described.[67] The variation of the GC method has the advantage of limiting false-positive results, but this technique is not widely practiced (Chap. 7). An available enzymatic screening test utilizes glycerol dehydrogenase to catalyze the oxidation of ethylene glycol, producing NADH, which is then measured spectrophotometrically. While this enzymatic test has the advantage of being rapid and unaffected by methanol, ethanol, isopropanol, or the metabolites of ethylene glycol, it may cross-react with lactate, yielding false-positive results.[22] In addition, this screening test requires confirmation via GC-MS, limiting its usefulness.

Unfortunately, many hospital laboratories are not equipped to determine toxic alcohol levels rapidly and usually rely on reference laboratories for these assays. The delays involved in sending specimens to another site and awaiting results may prohibit timely management of these patients. Delayed testing is not of benefit in the initial management of toxic alcohol ingestion.

MANAGEMENT

The initial management should include airway stabilization, ventilation, establishing intravenous access, and attention to any vital sign aberrations. Decontamination can be attempted with nasogastric (NG) aspiration of a toxic liquid if the patient presents within several hours of ingestion. Activated charcoal (AC), syrup of ipecac, and orogastric lavage all have extremely limited roles in the management of toxic-alcohol-poisoned patients, but should be applied, as appropriate for any suspected or known coingestants. Although AC adsorbs alcohols to varying extents, the dose needed to approach a beneficial AC-to-drug ratio is usually in excess of tolerable amounts.[11,19] In addition to the risk of aspiration, orogastric lavage poses a risk of injury in patients who are most likely to ingest toxic alcohols, that is alcoholics who are at risk for esophageal injury. Moreover, NG aspiration may prove adequate to remove a liquid ingestion. Finally, syrup of ipecac offers little advantage over NG aspiration and carries with it the risk of esophageal injury.

Hypotensive patients should receive fluid resuscitation as guided by volume status and renal function prior to the institution of vasopressor therapy. When maintenance fluids are given, special attention should be paid to the addition of specific vitamins as adjuvant therapy. Thiamine and pyridoxine therapy should be administered to anyone suspected of ethylene glycol ingestion at doses of 100 mg and 50 mg IV every 6 hours, respectively (see Fig. 66–1 and Antidotes in Depth: Thiamine Hydrochloride and Pyridoxine). Thiamine will shift the metabolism of the intermediate glyoxylic acid to α-hydroxy-β-ketoadipic acid, reducing the production of oxalic acid.[34,59] Evidence suggests that pyridoxine, in the presence of magnesium, will promote the conversion of glyoxylic acid to glycine and benzoic acid, which can further be metabolized to hippuric acid. The net effect of these adjuvants is to decrease the total amount of oxalic acid formed. While theoretically beneficial, no human data exists that demonstrates benefit. In animal studies, folic acid enhances the metabolism of formic acid to CO_2 and water.[66] Thus, 50–75 mg of folate should be given IV every 4 hours for the first 24 hours of a suspected methanol ingestion or while elevated methanol levels are present.

In addition to vitamins, sodium bicarbonate should also be added to maintenance fluids or given as boluses, depending on the clinical situation. Sodium bicarbonate infusion can help correct a profound metabolic acidosis and should probably be used when the pH is less than 7.20 (see Antidotes in Depth: Sodium Bicarbonate). Because restoration of normal pH may require large volumes of bicarbonate, fluid and electrolyte balance should be monitored carefully. Additionally, alkalinization of serum is helpful in maintaining acids in the ionic form, which not only enhances the renal clearance of formate, but may also prevent formic acid from entering the CNS, particularly the optic nerves.[34]

The decision to inhibit the ADH-mediated metabolism of toxic alcohols should be made in any patient with a known (admitted or witnessed) ingestion; a high index of suspicion based on history, clinical manifestations of poisoning (ie, metabolic acidosis with normal serum lactate or elevated serum osmolality); or a serum concentration of a toxic alcohol (when possible) that exceeds treatment thresholds. The clinician must choose between ethanol and fomepizole as the ADH blocking agent to be administered (see Antidotes in Depth: Ethanol and Fomepizole).

Currently FDA approval for fomepizole exists for the treatment of ethylene glycol and methanol poisoning. As the availability and awareness of fomepizole has increased, its appropriate use has gained widespread acceptance as a first-line therapy for toxic alcohol ingestions.[3] Fomepizole has several benefits over an ethanol infusion. It is as effective as ethanol without the complications commonly associated with ethanol infusions.[35] That is, fomepizole does not cause hypotension, hypoglycemia, inebriation, pancreatitis, gastritis, or phlebitis. Fomepizole is administered every 12 hours, eliminating the need for monitoring a continuous ethanol infusion with its associated risks of supra- and subtherapeutic levels. Therefore, clinically stable patients treated with fomepizole will not necessitate intensive care, reducing this element of the cost of treatment. Although not specifically studied, fomepizole has been safely administered to children, including infants.[4,31] In this specific population the short term use is unlikely to be problematic. The dosing of fomepizole is simpler than that of ethanol in patients undergoing hemodialysis. The greatest limitation of fomepizole is its cost, which is substantially greater than ethanol, although when the total cost of treatment, including the therapeutic agent, ICU time, and hemodialysis, is considered, the difference in cost is less obvious. However, fomepizole is not a substitute for hemodialysis under many circumstances. Although fomepizole prevents the formation of toxic metabolites, it has no effect on those metabolites already formed and their resultant toxicity. In the META study (Methylpyrazole for Toxic Alcohols), 9 patients who had initially elevated serum creatinine levels had persistent renal compromise despite fomepizole therapy, although they had a decrease in urinary oxalate excretion following therapy.[8] Furthermore, the prolonged elimination of the parent compound following inhibition of its metabolism would require prolonged use of fomepizole, which is unstudied. Therefore, although it may be possible to treat patients with fomepizole alone, its use will be case dependent and the agent will not entirely replace hemodialysis.

Methanol or ethylene glycol concentrations greater than 25 mg/dL are considered traditional indications for hemodialysis.[15,30] Some authors suggest formate concentrations be used as an indication for hemodialysis of methanol poisoned patients.[36,54] However, in some situations, the clinical status of the patient is a better measure of when hemodialysis is indicated. Ideally, toxic alcohols should be dialyzed before they produce toxic manifestations. The early initiation of hemodialysis requires rapid determination of toxic alcohol concentration. Unfortunately, not all hospitals are capable of ascertaining toxic alcohol concentrations rapidly. Thus, the decision is often delayed until evidence of toxicity manifests.

When serum levels are not immediately available patients with established toxicity should be dialyzed.[32] These conditions exist for patients with significant metabolic acidosis in the absence of another cause of end-organ manifestations of toxicity (impaired vision or renal function), or when ADH inhibition is not possible, either because of the unavailability of an antidote or when patients cannot tolerate the antidote (ie, IV ethanol in the hypotensive patient). Current practice guidelines recommend considering hemodialysis for patients with the following: worsening vital signs despite intensive supportive care, significant persistent metabolic acidosis (pH <7.30), renal failure; and electrolyte disturbances unresponsive to therapy.[3] Patients with potential poisoning, as documented by history or ancillary testing should be dialyzed if either fomepizole is unavailable or obtaining a quantitative serum level is not possible. Hemodialysis can also be used as a necessary adjuvant to shorten the duration of therapy. When the metabolism of methanol is inhibited, methanol may have a long half-life (as long as 54 hours), necessitating treatment to continue for days to reach safe concentrations via endogenous elimination alone.[7,55]

Management of the other toxic alcohols varies somewhat. Isopropanol is less likely to be lethal, but does require identification and appropriate medical treatment, which usually involves supportive care and the exclusion of other pathologic conditions.[40]

Hemodialysis is rarely, if ever, required.[24,61] Management of the glycol ethers is not well established. The majority of case reports suggest that supportive care is sufficient. The half-life of butoxyacetic acid was decreased by hemodialysis in one case report, while in another report, no such effect was recognized.[9,10] Nonetheless, hemodialysis indications for the glycol ethers are generally similar to those for methanol and ethylene glycol.

Any patient requiring antidotal therapy should be hospitalized. Patients receiving ethanol infusions require extensive nursing supervision and laboratory analysis, often a level of care only achievable in an intensive care unit. Fomepizole therapy does not require monitoring of either an infusion or therapeutic levels. Therefore, clinically stable patients treated with fomepizole need not be admitted to intensive care units. However, any patient who is clinically unstable requires intensive care regardless of the antidote used.

Decisions with regard to the discharge of patients are much more difficult. Toxicity from methanol or ethylene glycol ingestion may not be manifest for hours because of delayed metabolism, which can be prolonged even further if the patient has consumed ethanol or another ADH inhibitor such as cimetidine.[12] These patients can appear intoxicated and may have normal routine laboratory values upon analysis, including an osmol gap, and specific levels of the alcohol are needed to make the diagnosis. It is easy to be lulled into a false sense of security if the assumption is made that the patient is "merely intoxicated." Seemingly insignificant exposures in children, such as a sip of a product that contains 100% methanol, may not lead to inebriation, but can result in significant toxicity if left untreated. For example, a 10-kg child need only ingest a teaspoon (5 mL) of gas line antifreeze (100% methanol) to potentially achieve a serum concentration of methanol of 83 mg/dL. Therefore, in the absence of serum concen-

trations of toxic alcohols, patients should be observed and undergo serial laboratory analysis, as described in the diagnostic testing section of this chapter, before disposition decisions can appropriately be made.

SUMMARY

Understanding several fundamental concepts of toxic alcohol poisoning will allow the physician to interpret clinical and laboratory data appropriately. Toxic alcohols behave as alcohols. The degree of inebriation for a given amount of alcohol increases with the number of carbons in the structure of the alcohol ingested.[71] Thus, patients often present inebriated in a manner that is indistinguishable from that associated with an ethanol ingestion. However, if a patient appears excessively inebriated for a given ethanol concentration, the diagnosis of toxic alcohol ingestion should be considered.

The toxicity of the toxic alcohols is dependent on their metabolites. These alcohols are metabolized via the same pathways as ethanol, with varying affinity for the enzymes involved. As such, toxicity will be delayed until a certain threshold of toxic metabolites has been formed. This makes early diagnosis without quantitative toxic alcohol levels difficult. The presence of ethanol can be protective in mixed ingestions, but may also obscure the diagnosis. Knowledge of the toxicity of these metabolites can allow the physician to predict the anticipated symptoms as well as which laboratory tests to order and enable proper interpretation of the results (Table 66–3).

Finally, the clinician needs a thorough understanding of both the osmol gap and the anion gap. An osmol gap greater than 50 mOsm/L should be considered secondary to a toxic alcohol until

TABLE 66–3.   Toxic Alcohols: Characteristics, Signs, and Symptoms of Toxicity

Substance	Formula	Half-life	Metabolites	High Anion Gap Acidosis	Ketosis	CNS Depression	Characteristic Findings	Commercial Sources
Benzyl alcohol	C_6H_6OH	?	Benzoic acid, hippuric acid	+	−	+	Neonatal "gasping syndrome"	Bacteriostatic preservatives
Ethanol[a]	CH_3CH_2OH	Zero-order kinetics 15–20 mg/dL/h	Acetaldehyde, acetic acid	+	+	+	Intoxication	Solvents, beverages, colognes
Ethylene glycol	CH_2OHCH_2OH	3–8.6h	Oxalic acid, glycolic acid	++	−	+	Renal failure, hypocalcemia, calcium oxalate crystals in urine	Antifreeze (95%), solvents, deicers, air-conditioning units
Glycol ether	$HOCH_2CH_2OR$	~3.1 h	Ethylene glycol and metabolites	+	−	+	Similar to ethylene glycol	Solvents, industrial coatings
Isopropanol	$CH_3CHOHCH_3$	2.5–3.5 h	Acetone	−	+	++	Ketosis without acidosis, hemorrhagic tracheobronchitis	Rubbing alcohol, solvents, lacquer
Methanol	CH_3OH	Zero-order kinetics 8.5mg/dL/h	Formaldehyde, formic acid	++	−	+	Blindness, pale edematous optic disc	Antifreeze, solvents, gasohol denaturant
Propylene glycol	$CH_2OHCHOHCH_3$	2–5 h	Lactic acid, pyruvic acid	+	−	+	Lactic acidosis	Solvents, deicers

+ = Presence and degree of symptoms; − = absence of symptoms.
[a]Only in the case of alcoholic ketoacidosis is there a high anion gap metabolic acidosis with ketonemia.

proven otherwise. However, a normal osmol gap does not exclude the diagnosis, or the need for extracorporeal toxin removal. A high anion gap does not develop until a certain degree of metabolism has occurred. Therefore, it is possible early after an ingestion to have an elevated osmol gap without an increased anion gap. Typically poisoning is discovered during an intermediate period when both gaps are abnormal.

Fomepizole and ethanol are competitive inhibitors of alcohol dehydrogenase and will inhibit the metabolism of methanol and ethylene glycol to their toxic metabolites. Hemodialysis removes methanol and ethylene glycol and their toxic metabolites.

A thorough understanding of these concepts can enable the clinician to manage toxic alcohol exposures appropriately. The presence of rapid quantitative toxic alcohol assays facilitates the management, but the use of the gaps discussed in this chapter is essential in the absence of such assays.

ACKNOWLEDGMENTS

Neal E. Flomenbaum, MD, Neal A. Lewin, MD, and Mary Ann Howland, PharmD, contributed to this chapter in previous editions.

REFERENCES

1. Anderson TJ, Shuaib A, Becker WJ: Neurologic sequelae of methanol poisoning. Can Med Assoc J 1987;136:1177–1179.

2. Aufderheide TP, White SM, Brady WJ, Stueven HA: Inhalational and percutaneous methanol toxicity in two fire fighters Ann Emerg Med 1993;22:1916–1918.

3. Barceloux DG, Krenzelok EP, Olson K Watson W: American Academy of Clinical Toxicology Practice Guidelines on the Treatment of Ethylene Glycol Poisoning. Ad Hoc Committee. J Toxicol Clin Toxicol 1999;37:537–560.

4. Baum CR, Langman CB, Oker EE, et al: Fomepizole treatment of ethylene glycol poisoning in an infant. Pediatrics 2000;106:1489–1491.

5. Baumbach GL: Methyl alcohol poisoning IV. Alterations of the morphological findings of the retina and optic nerve. Arch Ophthalmol 1977;95:1859–1865.

6. Bennett IL, Cary FH, Mitchell GL, Cooper MN: Acute methyl alcohol poisoning: A review based on experiences in an outbreak of 323 cases. Medicine 1953;32:431–463.

7. Brent J, McMartin K, Phillips S, Aaron C, Kulig K: Fomepizole for the treatment of methanol poisoning. N Engl J Med 2001;344:424–429.

8. Brent J, McMartin K, Phillips S, et al: Fomepizole for the treatment of ethylene glycol poisoning. N Engl J Med 1999;340:832–838.

9. Browning RG, Curry SC: Clinical toxicology of ethylene glycol monoalkyl ethers. Hum Exp Toxicol 1992;11:488–490.

10. Burkhart KK, Donovan JW: Hemodialysis following butoxyethanol ingestion. J Toxicol Clin Toxicol 1998;36:723–725.

11. Burkhart KK, Martinez MA: The adsorption of isopropanol and acetone by activated charcoal. J Toxicol Clin Toxicol 1992;30:371–375.

12. Caballeria J, Baraona E, Rodamilans M, Lieber CS: Effects of cimetidine on gastric alcohol dehydrogenase activity and blood ethanol levels. Gastroenterology 1989;96:388–392.

13. Carpenter CP, Pozzani UC, Weil CS, et al: The toxicity of butyl cellosolve solvent. AMA Arch Indust Health 1956;14:114–131.

14. Catchings TT, Beamer WC, Lundy L: Adult respiratory distress syndrome secondary to ethylene glycol ingestion. Ann Emerg Med 1985;14:594–596.

15. Cheng JT, Beysolow TD, Kaul B, et al: Clearance of ethylene glycol by kidneys and hemodialysis. J Toxicol Clin Toxicol 1987;25:95–108.

16. Clay KL, Murphy RC: On the metabolic acidosis of ethylene glycol intoxication. Toxicol Appl Pharmacol 1977;39:39–49.

17. Daniel DR, McAnalley BH, Garriott JC: Isopropyl alcohol metabolism after acute intoxication in humans. J Anal Toxicol 1981;5:110–112.

18. Dean BS, Krenzelok EP: Clinical evaluation of pediatric ethylene glycol monobutyl ether poisonings. J Toxicol Clin Toxicol 1992;30:557–563.

19. Decker WJ, Corby DCT, Hilburn RE, Lynch RE: Adsorption of solvents by activated charcoal, polymers and mineral sorbents. Vet Hum Toxicol 1981;235:44–46.

20. Driver J, Tardiff RG, Sedik L, et al: In vitro percutaneous absorption of [14C] ethylene glycol by man. J Exposure Anal Environ Epidemiol 1993;3:277–284.

21. Dugard PH, Walker M, Mawdssley SJ, Scott RC: Absorption of some glycol ethers through human skin in vitro. Environ Health Perspect 1984;57:193–197.

22. Eder AF, McGrath CM, Dowdy YG, et al: Ethylene glycol poisoning: Toxicokinetic and analytical factors affecting laboratory diagnosis. Clin Chem 1998;44:168–177.

23. Fligner CL, Jack R, Twiggs GA, Raisys VA: Hyperosmolality induced by propylene glycol: A complication of silver sulfadiazine therapy. JAMA 1985;253:1606–1609.

24. Freireich Aw, Cinque TJ, Xanthaky G, Landau D: Hemodialysis for isopropanol poisoning. N Engl J Med 1967;277:699–700.

25. Frenia ML, Schauben JL: Methanol inhalation toxicity. Ann Emerg Med 1993;22:1919–1923.

26. Gabow PA, Clay K, Sullivan JB, Lepoff R: Organic acids in ethylene glycol intoxication. Ann Intern Med 1986;105:16–20.

27. Geiling EMK, Cannon PR: Pathologic effects of elixir of sulfanilamide (diethylene glycol) poisoning. JAMA 1938;111:919–926.

28. Gershanik JJ, Boecler G, Ensley H, et al: The gasping syndrome and benzyl alcohol poisoning. N Engl J Med 1982;307:1384–1388.

29. Gershanik FP, Jenco M, Veulemans H, et al: Acute butylglycol intoxication: A case report. Hum Toxicol 1989;8:243–245.

30. Gonda A, Gault H, Churchill D, et al: Hemodialysis for methanol intoxication. Am J Med 1978;64:749–758.

31. Harry P, Jobard E, Briand M, et al: Ethylene glycol poisoning in a child treated with 4-methylpyrazole. Pediatrics 1998;102:E31.

32. Hylander B, Kjellstrand CM: Prognostic factors and treatment of severe ethylene glycol intoxication. Intensive Care Med 1996;22:546–552.

33. Jacobsen D, Bredesen JE, Eide I, Ostborg J: Anion and osmolal gaps in the diagnosis of methanol and ethylene glycol poisoning. Acta Med Scand 1982;212:17–20.

34. Jacobsen D, Hewlett TP, Webb R, et al: Ethylene glycol intoxication: Evaluation of kinetics and crystalluria. Am J Med 1988;84:145–152.

35. Jacobsen D, Sebastian CS, Blomstrand R, McMartin KE: 4-Methylpyrazole: A controlled study of safety in healthy human subjects after single, ascending doses. Alcohol Clin Exp Res 1988;12:516–522.

36. Jacobsen D, Webb R, Collins TD, McMartin KE: Methanol and formate kinetics in late diagnosed methanol intoxication. Med Toxicol 1988;3:418–423.

37. Kavet R, Nauss KM: The toxicity of inhaled methanol vapors. Crit Rev Toxicol 1990;21:21–50.

38. Kinde M, Johnson D, Holmes S, et al: Ethylene glycol intoxication due to contamination of water systems. MMWR Morb Mortal Wkly Rep 1987;36:611–614.

39. Kulick MI, Wong R, Okarma TB, et al: Prospective study of side effects associated with the use of silver sulfadiazine in severely burned patients. Ann Plast Surg 1985;14:407–419.

40. Lacouture PG, Wason S, Abrams A, Lovejoy FH Jr: Acute isopropyl alcohol intoxication: Diagnosis and management. Am J Med 1983;75:680–686.

41. Larese Filon F, Fiorito A, Adami G, et al: Skin absorption in vitro of glycol ethers. Int Arch Occup Environ Health 1999;72:480–484.

42. Lewin GA, Oppenheimer PR, Wingert WA: Coma from alcohol sponging. JACEP 1977;6:165–167.

43. Lopez-Herce J, Bonet C, Meana A, et al: Benzyl alcohol poisoning following diazepam intravenous infusion [letter]. Ann Pharmacother 1995;29:632.

44. Lovejoy FH: Fatal benzyl alcohol poisoning in neonatal intensive care units. Am J Dis Child 1982;136:974–975.

45. Malebranche R, Hecdivert C, Lassegue A, et al: Fatalities associated with ingestion of diethylene glycol-contaminated glycerin used to manufacture acetaminophen syrup—Haiti, November 1995–June 1996. MMWR Morb Mortal Wkly Rep 1996;45:649–650.

46. Martin-Amat G, McMartin KE, Hayrek SS, et al: Methanol poisoning: Ocular toxicity produced by formate. Toxicol Appl Pharmacol 1978; 45:201–208.

47. McCoy HG, Cipolle RJ, Ehlers SM, et al: Severe methanol poisoning. Am J Med 1979;67:804–807.

48. McMartin KE, Makar AB, Martin-Amat G, et al: Methanol poisoning I: The role of formic acid in the development of metabolic acidosis in the monkey and the reversal by 4-methylpyrazole. Biochem Med 1975;13:319–333.

49. McMartin KE, Martin-Amat G, Noker PE, Tephly TR: Lack of a role for formaldehyde in methanol poisoning in the monkey. Biochem Pharmacol 1979;28:645–649.

50. Moreau CL, Kerns II W, Tomaszewski CA, et al: Glycolate kinetics and hemodialysis clearance in ethylene glycol poisoning. META Study Group. J Toxicol Clin Toxicol 1998;36:659–666.

51. Nitter-Hauge S: Poisoning with ethylene glycol monomethyl ether. Acta Med Scand 1970;188:277–280.

52. Noker PE, Eells JT, Tephly TR: Methanol toxicity: Treatment with folic acid and 5-formyltetrahydrofolic acid. Alcohol Clin Exp Res 1980;4:378–383.

53. Noker PE, Tephly TR: The role of folates in methanol toxicity. Adv Exp Med Biol 1980;132:305–315.

54. Osterloh JD, Pond SM, Grady S, Becker CE: Serum formate concentrations in methanol intoxication as a criterion for hemodialysis. Ann Intern Med 1986;104:200–203.

55. Palatnick W, Redman LW, Sitar DS, Tenenbein M: Methanol half life during ethanol administration: Implications for management of methanol poisoning. Ann Emerg Med 1995;26:202–207.

56. Pappas AA, Ackerman BH, Olsen KM, Taylor EH: Isopropanol ingestion: A report of six episodes with isopropanol and acetone serum concentration time data. J Toxicol Clin Toxicol 1991;29:11–21.

57. Peterson C, Collins A, Mimes J, et al: Ethylene glycol poisoning: Pharmacokinetics during therapy with ethanol and hemodialysis. N Engl J Med 1981;304:21–23.

58. Rambourg-Schepens MO, Buffet M, Bertault R, et al: Severe ethylene glycol butyl ether poisoning. Kinetics and metabolic pattern. Hum Toxicol 1988;7:187–189.

59. Roberts JA, Seibold HR: Ethylene glycol toxicity in the monkey. Toxicol Appl Pharmacol 1969;15:624–631.

60. Robinson AG, Loeb JN: Ethanol ingestion: Commonest cause of elevated plasma osmolality? N Engl J Med 1971;284:1253–1255.

61. Rosansky SJ: Isopropyl alcohol poisoning treated with hemodialysis: Kinetics of isopropyl alcohol and acetone removal. J Toxicol Clin Toxicol 1982;19:265–271.

62. Schelling JR, Howard RL, Winter SD, Linas SL: Increased osmolal gap in alcoholic ketoacidosis and lactic acidosis. Ann Intern Med 1990;113:580–582.

63. Schultz S, Kinde M, Johnson D, et al: Ethylene glycol intoxication due to contamination of water systems. MMWR Morb Mortal Wkly Rep 1987;36:611–614.

64. Scully R, Galdabini J, McNealy B: Case records of the Massachusetts General Hospital. Weekly clinicopathological exercises. Case 38–1979. N Engl J Med 1979;301:650–657.

65. Sklar AH, Linus SL: The osmolal gap in renal failure. Ann Intern Med 1983;98:481–482.

66. Smith EN, Taylor RT: Acute toxicity of methanol in the folate-deficient acatalasemic mouse. Toxicology 1982;25:271–287.

67. Smith RA, Lang DG: Rapid determination of ethylene glycol and glycolic acid in biological fluids. Vet Hum Toxicol 2000;42:358–360.

68. Spillane L, Roberts JR, Meyer AE: Multiple cranial nerve deficits after ethylene glycol poisoning. Ann Emerg Med 1991;20:137–169.

69. Vicas IMO, Beck R: Fatal inhalational isopropyl alcohol poisoning in a neonate. J Toxicol Clin Toxicol 1993;31:473–481.

70. Walker JA, Schwartzbard A, Krauss EA, et al: The missing gap: A pitfall in the diagnosis of alcohol intoxication by osmometry. Arch Intern Med 1986;146:1843–1844.

71. Wallgren H: Relative intoxicating effects on rats of ethyl, propyl and butyl alcohols. Acta Pharmacol Toxicol 1960;16:217–222.

72. Wax PM: Elixirs, diluents and the passage of the 1938 Federal Food, Drug and Cosmetic Act. Ann Intern Med 1995;122:456–461.

73. Wills JH, Coluston F, Harris ES, et al: Inhalation of aerosolized ethylene glycol by man. Clin Toxicol 1974;7:463–476.

74. Winter ML, Ellis MD, Snodgrass WR: Urine fluorescence using a Wood's lamp to detect the antifreeze additive sodium fluorescein: A qualitative adjunctive test in suspected ethylene glycol ingestions. Ann Emerg Med 1990;19:663–667.

ANTIDOTES IN DEPTH

Folic Acid and Leucovorin (Folinic Acid)

Mary Ann Howland

Folic Acid

Folinic Acid

Leucovorin (folinic acid) is a primary antidote for a patient overdosed with methotrexate. Leucovorin is the biologically active, reduced form of folic acid, whose synthesis is prevented by methotrexate. Whereas only leucovorin is acceptable for a patient with methotrexate toxicity, either folic acid or leucovorin is acceptable in a patient poisoned with methanol. Folates enhance the elimination of formate following a methanol overdose.

PHARMACOLOGY

Folic acid (pteroylglutamic acid), an essential water-soluble vitamin, is a pteridine ring joined to PABA (*p*-aminobenzoic acid) and glutamic acid.[5] It is the most common pharmaceutical preparation of folate, although other congeners exist in foods. After absorption, folic acid is reduced by dihydrofolic acid reductase (DHFR)

to tetrahydrofolic acid, which accepts carbon groups at different positions on the molecule. Tetrahydrofolic acid therefore serves as the precursor for several biologically active forms of folic acid including 5-formyltetrahydrofolic acid (folinic acid, leucovorin, 5-FTHF, and 5-CHO-THF or citrovorum factor). These biologically active forms of folate are enzymatically interconvertible and function as cofactors, providing carbon groups necessary for many intracellular metabolic reactions, including the synthesis of thymidylate and purine nucleotides, which are DNA precursors. The minimum daily requirement of folate is normally 50 µg, but in pregnant women and nutritionally deprived acutely ill patients 100 to 200 µg may be required.[5]

ROLE IN METHANOL TOXICITY

Methanol toxicity in humans is currently believed to develop as a result of reduced formate metabolism when there is a relatively inadequate folate concentration. The rat model has not been useful in studying methanol toxicity because that species has a very well-developed folate metabolic system that rapidly oxidizes the toxic formic acid to nontoxic carbon dioxide at a rate 2–3 times faster than the rate demonstrated in monkeys. Primates and humans are not this fortunate. However, the administration of folic acid to monkeys speeds up formate metabolism.[16] Pretreatment with folic acid for 48 hours, or with leucovorin administered at 2 mg/kg IV at 0, 4, 8, 12, and 18 hours following methanol administration in monkeys, decreased formate levels and the accompanying metabolic acidosis, without affecting the rate of methanol elimination.[18] Leucovorin was still effective in hastening the elimination of formate when given 10 hours following methanol administration. Other studies demonstrate that rats and monkeys experimentally made folate-deficient develop methanol toxicity at lower methanol levels.[10]

Total folate, leucovorin, and 10-HCOH$_2$ folate dehydrogenase (which increases leucovorin levels) are all diminished in the livers of methanol-poisoned humans.[10] This finding further supports the hypothesis that methanol toxicity in humans develops as a result of reduced formate metabolism secondary to reduced folate levels.

In an analysis[7] of a single methanol-poisoned patient who was given folate and ethanol and hemodialyzed, the formate half-life was 1.1 hours.[19] In another methanol-poisoned patient treated without folate, the formate half-life was 2.8 hours.[7] This limited analysis by comparison may be inadequate to draw definitive conclusions, but appears to support the therapeutic role of folate.

ROLE IN METHOTREXATE TOXICITY

Methotrexate, an antimetabolite, is a structural analogue of folic acid, differing only in an amino group substituted for a hydroxyl group on the number 4 position of the pteridine ring (Chap. 47). Methotrexate binds to the active site of DHFR, rendering it incapable of reducing folic acid to its biologically active reduced forms, and incapable of regenerating the necessary active forms required for the synthesis of thymidylate, an essential precursor to DNA. Methotrexate's binding to DHFR is extremely tight at pH 6 with an inhibition constant of about 1 nmol/L. At physiologic pH the binding is more competitive, with an inhibition constant of about 1 μmol/L.[24] Leucovorin is a reduced, active form of folate that does not require DHFR for enzymatic interconversion to the form required for thymidylate formation. Folic acid would not be effective to counteract methotrexate toxicity because DHFR would be unavailable to convert folic acid to the necessary reduced and active forms.

LEUCOVORIN PHARMACOKINETICS

Leucovorin naturally formed in the body exists as the active (l) or (−) isomer, whereas the commercial preparation consists of equal amounts of the inactive (d) or (+) and active (l) or (−) isomers. The pharmacokinetics of the racemic mixture and its active metabolite were studied after IV infusion of 28 mg/m² over 5 minutes and 500 mg/m² per day (21 mg/m² per hour) as a constant infusion over 5.5 days in normal human volunteers.[28] The plasma half-life of the active (l) isomer was 35 minutes, considerably shorter than the 485 minutes of the inactive (d) isomer. During constant infusion the steady-state concentration for the active isomer was 2.33 μmol (1102 μg/L or 1.1 mg/L or 1.1 μg/mL), the half-life 35 minutes, and the volume of distribution 13.6 L. The inactive isomer achieved plasma concentrations 16-fold higher than the active form and was primarily cleared from the plasma by urinary excretion of unchanged drug. In contrast, the active isomer was metabolized to an active metabolite (L-5-CH3-THF) that achieved a plasma concentration of 4.85 μmol, a half-life of 412 minutes, and a volume of distribution of about 40 L; all of these values are greater than that of the parent compound. A more recent study detected no adverse effects of the inactive isomer on the intracellular uptake of the active isomer and concluded that giving the active isomer provided no pharmacokinetic advantage over the racemic mixture.[25]

The pharmacokinetics of orally administered leucovorin [(d,l)-5-formyltetrahydrofolate)] have been studied in healthy, fasted, male volunteers in single doses ranging from 20 mg to 100 mg, and 200 mg IV over 5 minutes as compared to 200 mg orally.[15] Bioavailability decreased from 100% for the 20-mg dose to 78% for the 40-mg dose, and ultimately to 31% for the 200-mg dose. A microbiologic assay was used to measure total tetrahydrofolates (reduced and active folates). The peak plasma concentrations for total reduced folates range from 318 ng/mL for 20 mg orally to 619 ng/mL for 100 mg orally. The 200-mg oral dose produced a peak plasma concentration of 859 ng/mL (1.82 μmol/L) as compared to 12,829 ng/mL (27.1 μmol/L) after the 200-mg IV dose. Normal plasma folate levels are in the range of 6–20 ng/mL or 13–43 nmol.

LEUCOVORIN DOSING FOR METHOTREXATE OVERDOSES

When a patient intentionally or unintentionally overdoses on methotrexate or is inadvertently administered methotrexate, a dose of leucovorin estimated to produce the same plasma concentration as the methotrexate dose should be given as soon as possible after the overdose, preferably within 1 hour. One mole of methotrexate weighs 455 daltons and 1 mole of leucovorin calcium weighs 511 daltons. In view of the safety of leucovorin and the toxicity of methotrexate, underdosing of leucovorin should be avoided. Plasma concentrations are often closely followed in patients on diverse oncologic methotrexate regimens. In the overdose setting, it is inappropriate to wait for a methotrexate plasma concentration before treatment with leucovorin is initiated. The toxic threshold for methotrexate is reported to be 2×10^{-8} mol/L (2×10^{-8} mol/L means 0.02×10^{-6} or 0.02 μmol/L or 20 nmol/L). Normal plasma folate levels are in the range of 13–43 nmol/L. One mole of methotrexate is 455 g/mol or 455 mg/mmol or 455 μg/μmol, or 455 ng/nmol. Therefore, 20 nmol equals 9100 ng (455 ng/nmol × 20 nmol) and 20 nmol/L equals 9100 ng/L or 9.1 ng/mL. In a patient not receiving methotrexate therapeutically, there is no need to permit any methotrexate to remain unantagonized by leucovorin. For example, if a child unintentionally ingests 100 2.5-mg methotrexate tablets for a total dose of 250 mg, only part of this dose is absorbed because methotrexate absorption is saturable. Methotrexate's bioavailability decreases from 100% with doses below 30 mg/m² to about 10–20% with doses above 80 mg/m². As a safety precaution, it should be assumed that a bioavailability of 50% would result in an absorbed dose of methotrexate of 125 mg. For this substantial exposure an intravenous dose of 125 mg of leucovorin could be given over 15–30 minutes. The dose should be repeated every 3–6 hours until the methotrexate level is less than 1×10^{-8} mol/L, and preferably close to zero. The methotrexate half-life may vary from 5 hours to 45 hours depending on the dose and the patient's renal function. For this reason leucovorin therapy should be continued for 12–24 doses (3 days) or longer. Patients with the potential of third-space storage in ascites or pleural effusion may also require leucovorin dosing for an extended period of time. Those patients with bone marrow toxicity require more prolonged dosing because plasma half-lives of methotrexate do not reflect persistent intracellular concentrations.

Unintentional overdose with intrathecal methotrexate is potentially quite consequential and is dose dependent. In these cases, intravenous leucovorin should be administered and intrathecal leucovorin should *not* be used.[9,12,23,30] Other modalities should also be utilized or considered, as should consultation with experienced hematologists/oncologists.[11] Intrathecal leucovorin was considered as a major factor in the death of a child given a slightly higher dose of intrathecal methotrexate than was prescribed.[9] Not all intrathecal overdoses require aggressive intervention, but consultation with experienced hematologists/oncologists is warranted.[11]

An intravenous leucovorin dose of 100 mg/m² every 6 hours should be effective in all but the most severe overdoses. A constant intravenous infusion of 21 mg/m²/h has been safely administered for 5 days. A transition to the oral administration of leucovorin depends on the plasma concentration of the methotrexate and whether adequate plasma concentrations of leucovorin can be achieved by that route. A 200-mg oral dose in an adult produces a peak plasma concentration of 1.82 μmol/L as compared to 27.1 μmol/L with a 200-mg IV dose. Administration of activated charcoal precludes the administration of oral leucovorin. In addition to leucovorin, other modalities to treat a methotrexate overdose should be performed (activated charcoal, urinary alkalinization), or considered (hemoperfusion, thymidine, carboxypeptidase G) under specific circumstances (Chap. 47).

AVAILABILITY

Folic acid is available parenterally in 10-mL multidose vials with 1.5% benzyl alcohol in concentrations of 5 or 10 mg/mL, from a variety of manufacturers. Once opened this vial must be kept refrigerated.

Leucovorin is available as a powder for injection in 50-, 100-, and 350-mg vials. Reconstitution with 5 mL to the 50-mg vial, or 10 mL to the 100-mg vial, with sterile water for injection results in a final concentration of 10-mg/mL. Adding 17 mL of sterile water for injection to the 350-mg vial results in a final concentration of 20 mg/mL. Because of the calcium content, the rate of intravenous administration should not be faster than 160 mg/min in adults. Leucovorin is also available orally in a variety of strengths including 5-, 10-, 15-, and 25-mg tablets.

ADVERSE EFFECTS AND SAFETY ISSUES

There are rare reports of reactions to parenteral injections of folic acid or leucovorin.[5] Seizures have rarely been associated with leucovorin administration.[17] The calcium content of leucovorin warrants a slow intravenous infusion at a rate not faster than 160 mg/min in adults. Leucovorin should not be administered intrathecally.

DOSING

The usual dose of leucovorin for methotrexate rescue ranges from 10 mg/m[2] IM or IV every 6 hours for 72 hours to 100 mg/m[2] every 3 hours in patients with renal compromise. If administration to neonates is necessary, a benzyl alcohol-free preparation must be used because of the toxicity of benzyl alcohol in neonates. For methotrexate overdoses, a dose of leucovorin equal to that of the ingested methotrexate dose should be administered as soon as possible intravenously over 15–30 minutes, but not faster than 160-mg/min in adults. This dose can be repeated every 3–6 hours for 1–3 days or longer depending on renal function, the presence of bone marrow toxicity, and the methotrexate serum concentrations.

Based on the convincing studies in monkeys and the benign nature of the therapy, folic acid or leucovorin should be administered parenterally at the first suspicion of methanol intoxication. Fifty to 70 mg of IV folate has been used every 4 hours for the first 24 hours to treat methanol-intoxicated patients without complications.[19] The precise dose is unknown, but 1–2 mg/kg every 4–6 hours is probably reasonable. It should be continued until the methanol and formate are eliminated. As the first dose is usually administered prior to hemodialysis, a second dose should be administered at the completion of hemodialysis, because hemodialysis probably removes this highly water-soluble vitamin. If leucovorin is not readily available, then folic acid should be given. Folic acid must never be substituted for folinic acid or leucovorin when a methotrexate-poisoned patient is being managed. Folic acid is inadequate treatment for methotrexate intoxication; leucovorin must be used.

REFERENCES

1. American College of Obstetricians and Gynecologists practice bulletin. Medical management of tubal pregnancy. Number 3, December 1998. Clinical management guidelines for obstetrician-gynecologists. Int J Gynaecol Obstet 1999;65:97–103.
2. Bleyer WA. New vistas for leucovorin in cancer chemotherapy [review]. Cancer 19898;63:995–1007.
3. Booser DJ, Walters RS, Holmes FA, Hortobagyi GN: Continuous-infusion high-dose leucovorin with 5-fluorouracil and cisplatin for relapsed metastatic breast cancer: A phase II study. Am J Clin Oncol 2000;23:40–41.
4. Gibbon BN, Manthey DE: Pediatric case of accidental oral overdose of methotrexate. Ann Emerg Med 1999;34:98–100.
5. Hillman RS: Vitamin B$_{12}$, folic acid and the treatment of megaloblastic anemias. In: Gilman AG, Goodman LS, Rall TW, Murad F, eds: Goodman and Gilman's The Pharmacological Basis of Therapeutics, 7th ed. New York, Macmillan, 1985, pp. 1323–1337.
6. Houben PF, Hommes OR, Knaven PJ: Anticonvulsant drugs and folic acid in young mentally retarded epileptic patients. A study of serum folate, fit frequency and IQ. Epilepsia 1971;12:235–247.
7. Jacobsen D, McMartin KE: Methanol and ethylene glycol poisonings: Mechanism of toxicity, clinical course, diagnosis and treatment. Med Toxicol 1986;1:309–334.
8. Janinis J, Papakostas P, Samelis G, et al: Second-line chemotherapy with weekly oxaliplatin and high-dose 5-fluorouracil with folinic acid in metastatic colorectal carcinoma: A Hellenic Cooperative Oncology Group (HeCOG) phase II feasibility study. Ann Oncol 2000;11:163–167.
9. Jardine LF, Ingram LC, Bleyer WA: Intrathecal leucovorin after intrathecal methotrexate overdose. J Pediatr Hematol Oncol 1996;18:302–304.
10. Johlin F, Fortman C, Nghiem D, et al: Studies on the role of folic acid and folate dependent enzymes in human methanol poisoning. Mol Pharmacol 1987;31:557–561.
11. Lampkin BC, Wells R: Intrathecal leucovorin after intrathecal methotrexate. J Pediatr Hematol Oncol 1996;18:249.
12. Lee ACW, Wong KW, Fong KW, So KT: Intrathecal methotrexate overdose. Acta Pediatr 1997;86:434–437.
13. Levitt M, Nixon PF, Pincus JH, et al: Transport characteristics of folates in cerebrospinal fluid; a study utilizing doubly labeled 5-methyltetrahydrofolate and 5-formyltetrahydrofolate. J Clin Invest 1971;50:1301–1308.
14. Lonardi F, Jirillo A, Bonciarelli G, et al: Toxicity of laevo-leucovorin and dose lowering [letter]. Eur J Cancer 1992;28A:1007–1008.
15. McGuire BW, Sia LL, Haynes JD, et al: Absorption kinetics of orally administered leucovorin calcium. NCI Monogr 1987;5:47–56.
16. McMartin KE, Martin-Amat G, Makar AB, et al: Methanol poisoning. V: Role of formate metabolism in the monkey. J Pharmacol Exp Ther 1977;201:564–572.
17. Metropol NJ, Creaven PJ, Petrelli N, et al: Seizures associated with leucovorin administration in cancer patients [letter]. J Natl Cancer Inst 1995;87:56–58.
18. Noker PE, Eells MS, Tephly TR: Methanol toxicity: Treatment with folic acid and 5-formyltetrahydrofolic acid. Alcohol Clin Exp Res 1980;4:378–383.
19. Osterloh J, Pond S, Grady S, et al: Serum formate concentrations in methanol intoxication as a criterion for hemodialysis. Ann Intern Med 1986;104:200–203.
20. Patel R, Newman EM, Villacorte DG, et al: Pharmacology and phase I trial of high-dose oral leucovorin plus 5-fluorouracil in children with refractory cancer: A report from the Children's Cancer Study Group. Cancer Res 1991;51:4871–4875.
21. Priest DG, Schmitz JC, Bunni MA, et al: Pharmacokinetics of leucovorin metabolites in human plasma as a function of dose administered orally and intravenously. J Natl Cancer Inst 1991;83:1806–1812.

22. Reynolds EH: Effects of folic acid on the mental state and fit-frequency of drug-treated epileptic patients. Lancet 1967;1:1086–1088.

23. Riva L, Conter V, Rizzari C, et al: Successful treatment of intrathecal methotrexate overdose with folinic acid rescue: A case report. Acta Paediatr 1999;88:780–782.

24. Salmon SE, Sartorelli AC: Cancer Chemotherapy. In: Katzung BG, ed: Basic and Clinical Pharmacology, 7th ed. Norwalk, CT, Appleton & Lange, 1998, pp. 889–891.

25. Schleyer E, Rudolph KL, Braess J, et al: Impact of the simultaneous administration of the (+)- and (−) − forms of formyl-tetrahydrofolic acid on plasma and intracellular pharmacokinetics of (−)-tetrahydrofolic acid. Cancer Chemother Pharmacol 2000;45:165–171.

26. Smith DB, Racusen LC: Folate metabolism and the anticonvulsant efficacy of phenobarbital. Arch Neurol 1973;28:18–22.

27. Stover P, Schirch V: The metabolic role of leucovorin. Trends Biochem Sci 1993;18:102–106.

28. Straw JA, Newman EM, Doroshow JH: Pharmacokinetics of leucovorin (dl-5 formyltetrahydrofolate) after intravenous injection and constant intravenous infusion. NCI Monogr 1987;5:41–45.

29. Tenenbein M: Recent advancements in pediatric toxicology. Pediatr Clin North Am 1999;46:1179–1788.

30. Trinkle R, Wu JK: Intrathecal leucovorin after intrathecal methotrexate overdose. J Pediatr Hematol Oncol 1997;19:267–268.

31. Weh HJ, Bittner S, Hoffknecht M, et al: Neurotoxicity following weekly therapy with folinic acid and high-dose 5-fluorouracil 24h infusion in patients with gastrointestinal malignancies [letter]. Eur J Cancer 1993;29A:1218–1219.

ANTIDOTES IN DEPTH

Ethanol

Mary Ann Howland

$$H-\underset{\underset{H}{|}}{\overset{\overset{H}{|}}{C}}-\underset{\underset{H}{|}}{\overset{\overset{H}{|}}{C}}-OH$$

Ethanol

Ethanol is a competitive antagonist of alcohol dehydrogenase. It is used to inhibit alcohol dehydrogenase, thus decreasing the metabolism of xenobiotics to toxic metabolites by alcohol dehydrogenase. Methanol and ethylene glycol are the two most common xenobiotics whose lethal synthesis is inhibited by ethanol. Other xenobiotics whose metabolism may be inhibited include short-chain polyethylene glycols such as di- and triethylene glycol.[41] Ethanol also affects the cytochrome P450 enzyme system, especially 2E1, for which it has biphasic properties as an inhibitor/inducer similar to fomepizole and isoniazid. Only the effect on alcohol dehydrogenase is used to therapeutic advantage, while the effect on the cytochrome P450 system often leads to unwanted drug interactions and pharmacokinetic tolerance after several days of ethanol administration.

AFFINITY FOR ALCOHOL DEHYDROGENASE

The dose of ethanol necessary to achieve competitive inhibition depends on the concentrations of the toxic alcohols and their affinity for the enzyme. A summary of in vitro experiments utilizing human liver demonstrate a K_m (affinity constant with the lower number indicating a stronger affinity) of 30 mM, 7 mM, 0.45 mM with ethylene glycol, methanol, and ethanol, and a K_i (inhibitory concentration) of 0.09 μmol with fomepizole.[22,33,34] This means that the affinity of ethanol for alcohol dehydrogenase is 67 times that for ethylene glycol and 15.5 times that for methanol. Studies in methanol-intoxicated monkeys revealed that when ethanol was administered at a molar ethanol-to-methanol (E/M) ratio of 1:4, the metabolism of methanol was reduced by 70%; at 1:1 E/M ratio, metabolism was reduced by >90%.[24] In these experiments, the dose of methanol was kept constant at about 1 g/kg (31 mmol/kg) while the dose of ethanol was varied. Although the methanol serum concentration was not measured, a calculation using the dose and a volume of distribution of 0.6 L/kg would predict a serum concentration of about 166 mg/dL. Methanol, even in molar ratios as high as 8:1, did not inhibit ethanol metabolism, and ethylene glycol did not inhibit methanol metabolism.[24] Even smaller amounts of ethanol are required to block the metabolism of ethyl-

ene glycol, as the affinity of ethylene glycol for alcohol dehydrogenase is less than that of methanol, and much less than that of ethanol.[16,22,33,34,36,39] Most authors[1,16,39] recommend a serum concentration of ethanol of 100 mg/dL, or at least a 1:4 molar ratio of ethanol to methanol or ethylene glycol, whichever is greater. One hundred mg/dL (≈22 mmol/L) protects against 88 mmol/L (286 mg/dL) of methanol and 88 mmol/L (546 mg/dL) of ethylene glycol. Inhibiting the metabolism of methanol and ethylene glycol impedes the formation of toxic metabolites and prevents the development of metabolic acidosis.[12,15,39] Renal, pulmonary, and extracorporeal routes of toxic alcohol removal then become the sole mechanisms for elimination.

CASE STUDIES

Case reports have attested to the efficacy of ethanol in preventing the sequelae of methanol and ethylene glycol poisoning when administered in a timely fashion after the ingestion and before the accumulation of the toxic metabolites.[4,6,18,31,43] Once blocked with ethanol, the half-life of ethylene glycol in two patients with normal kidney function was 17.5 hours, which was comparable to 17 hours in a case series of patients on fomepizole with normal kidney function.[4,31,37] Similarly, a methanol half-life of 46.5 hours was reported in a patient with methanol poisoning, which is quite similar to the 54 hours reported in a case series of patients treated with fomepizole.[2,18]

PHARMACOKINETICS AND DOSING

Ethanol can be given orally or IV (Tables 66–4 and 66–5). Concentrations of 20–30% (orally) and 5–10% IV are well tolerated. Intravenous administration has the advantage of complete absorption,[20] avoids gastrointestinal symptoms, and can be given to an unconscious or uncooperative patient. The disadvantages include the procurement of ethanol, the preparation of an intravenous solution, the hyperosmolarity of a 5% ethanol solution (about 950 mOsm/L), the possibility of osmotic dehydration and venous irritation. Ethanol can also be administered orally and is rapidly absorbed with peak concentrations achieved in about 1–1.5 hours.[5,11,40] The amount of ethanol absorbed after oral administration is dependent on a number of factors, but increases with fasting, nutritional status, accelerated gastric emptying, female gender, genetics, chronic alcoholism, lean body mass, increasing age, as well as in the presence of certain H_2 antagonists.[3,6,11,21,42,44] Sufficient concentrations are generally achieved when 0.8 g/kg of ethanol is given orally over 20 minutes.[3,5,6,11,21,40]

The objective, regardless of route, is rapidly to achieve and maintain a level of at least 100 mg/dL of ethanol, which proves adequate to achieve enzyme inhibition in most cases. Inhibition is best achieved by administering a loading dose of ethanol followed by a maintenance dose. The volume of distribution for ethanol is approximately 0.6 L/kg.[45] Therefore, the loading dose of ethanol is given by the following formula:

$$
\begin{aligned}
\text{Loading dose} &= C_p \times V_d \\
&= 1 \text{ g} / \text{L} \ (100 \text{ mg} / \text{dL}) \times 0.6 \text{ L} / \text{kg} \\
&= 0.6 \text{ g} / \text{kg} \\
C_p &= \text{plasma concentration which for this agent is} \\
&\quad \text{comparable to the serum concentration}
\end{aligned}
$$

For a 70-kg person, this would be 42 g (70 kg × 0.6 g/kg) of ethanol or 420 mL of 10% V/V ethanol. However, 0.8 g/kg or 8 mL/kg loading dose of a 10% ethanol solution is recommended in order to provide a margin of safety because of the variability in bioavailability and the ongoing metabolism that occurs during administration. The IV loading dose should be administered over 20–60 minutes as tolerated by the patient. The 10% ethanol concentration is preferable to the 5% concentration so as to limit the volume of fluid administered and is preferred to the more concentrated solutions thereby limiting local venous irritation and avoiding postinfusion phlebitis. Because of the free water content and significant hypertonicity of this solution, the patient should be closely observed for the development of hyponatremia. A second IV line using 0.9% sodium chloride solution may be necessary to avoid this complication which is not associated with oral administration.

To maintain an ethanol concentration of 100 mg/dL, enough ethanol has to be administered to replace that which is being eliminated (66–130 mg/kg/h). The average hourly dose for a 70-kg person is 4.6 g, but higher doses are required in chronic alcoholics (100–154 mg/kg/h) and in those undergoing hemodialysis (250–350 mg/kg/h; Chap. 6).[8,16,26,31]

Because ethanol elimination varies in each individual, frequent serum ethanol determinations should be made to ensure adequate dosing. Any increase in the anion gap or decrease in bicarbonate concentration implies that the ethanol dose is inadequate to achieve blockade of alcohol dehydrogenase.

Problems encountered with the administration of ethanol include further risk of central nervous system depression or ethanol related toxicities such as hepatitis and pancreatitis, hypoglycemia, dehydration, and fluctuating serum concentrations. Therefore, blood glucose and serum ethanol concentrations should be monitored and attention paid to adequate fluid management.

AVAILABILITY

A more practical problem often involves finding or preparing the ethanol to be given. Hospital pharmacies and emergency departments should stock ethanol for such a purpose. Commercial preparations of 5% ethanol in 5% dextrose are available for IV administration. Alternatively, sterile ethanol USP (absolute ethanol) can be added to 5% dextrose to make a solution of approximately 10% ethanol concentration. A 10% ethanol solution is preferred to limit the volume of fluid administered. Then 55 mL (not 50 mL) of absolute ethanol is added to 500 mL of 5% dextrose, to produce a total end volume of 555 mL (10% = 10 mL in 100 mL, in this case, 55 mL in 555 mL or 55/555). If oral administration is chosen, it is important to remember that 100-proof ethanol is 50% ethanol. Oral ethanol is preferable if this route is

TABLE 66–4. Intravenous Administration of 10% Ethanol

Loading Dose[c]	Volume (mL)[b] (given over 1 hour as tolerated)					
	10 kg	15 kg	30 kg	50 kg	70 kg	100 kg
Loading dose of 0.8 g/kg of 10% ethanol (infused over 1 hour as tolerated)	80	120	240	400	560	800

Maintenance Dose[a]	Infusion Rate[b] (mL/h for various weights)[d]					
	10 kg	15 kg	30 kg	50 kg	70 kg	100 kg
Normal Maintenance Range						
80 mg/kg/h	8	12	24	40	56	80
110 mg/kg/h	11	16	33	55	77	110
130 mg/kg/h	13	19	39	65	91	130
Approximate Maintenance Dose for Chronic Alcoholic						
150 mg/kg/h	15	22	45	75	105	150
Range Required During Hemodialysis						
250 mg/kg/h	25	38	75	125	175	250
300 mg/kg/h	30	45	90	150	210	300
350 mg/kg/h	35	53	105	175	245	350

[a]Infusion to be started immediately following the loading dose. Concentrations above 10% are not recommended for IV administration. The dose schedule is based on the premise that the patient initially has a zero ethanol level. The aim of therapy is to maintain a serum ethanol level of 100–150 mg/dL, but constant monitoring of the ethanol level is required because of wide variations in endogenous metabolic capacity. Ethanol will be removed by hemodialysis, and the infusion rate of ethanol must be increased during hemodialysis. Prolonged ethanol administration may lead to hypoglycemia.
[b]For a 5% concentration, multiply the amount by 2.
[c]A 10% V/V concentration yields approximately 100 mg/mL.
[d]Rounded to the nearest mL.
Reprinted, with permission, from Roberts JR, Hedges J, eds: Clinical Procedures in Emergency Medicine. Philadelphia, WB Saunders, 1985, pp.1073–1074.

TABLE 66–5. Oral Administration of 20% Ethanol

Loading Dose[b]	Volume (mL)					
	10 kg	15 kg	30 kg	50 kg	70 kg	100 kg
Loading dose of 0.8 g/kg of 20% ethanol, diluted in juice. May be administered orally or via nasogastric tube	40	60	120	200	280	400

Maintenance Dose[a]	mL/h for various weights[c,d]					
	10 kg	15 kg	30 kg	50 kg	70 kg	100 kg
Normal Maintenance Range						
80 mg/kg/h	4	6	12	20	28	40
110 mg/kg/h	6	8	17	27	39	55
130 mg/kg/h	7	10	20	33	46	66
Approximate Range for Chronic Alcoholic or Patient Receiving Continuous Oral Activated Charcoal						
150 mg/kg/h	8	11	22	38	53	75
Range Required During Hemodialysis						
250 mg/kg/h	13	19	38	63	88	125
300 mg/kg/h	15	23	46	75	105	150
350 mg/kg/h	18	26	53	88	123	175

[a]Concentrations above 30% (60 proof) are not recommended for oral administration. The dose schedule is based on the premise that the patient initially has a zero ethanol level. The aim of therapy is to maintain a serum ethanol level of 100–150 mg/dL, but constant monitoring of the ethanol level is required because of wide variations in endogenous metabolic capacity. Ethanol will be removed by hemodialysis, and the dose of ethanol must be increasing during hemodialysis. Prolonged ethanol administration may lead to hypoglycemia.
[b]A 20% V/V concentration yields approximately 200 mg/mL.
[c]Rounded to the nearest mL.
[d]For a 30% concentration, multiply the amount by 0.66.
Reprinted, with permission, from Roberts JR, Hedges J, eds: Clinical Procedures in Emergency Medicine. Philadelphia, WB Saunders, 1985, pp. 1073–1074.

acceptable. If there will be any delay in obtaining ethanol for intravenous use, oral therapy with ethanol should be initiated immediately.

COMPARISON TO FOMEPIZOLE

Although ethanol has been used as an antidote for years and has the advantages of easy access and low cost, fomepizole is a very potent inhibitor of alcohol dehydrogenase with many favorable attributes. Fomepizole does not produce central nervous system (CNS) depression. Fomepizole is easier to dose and does not require serum concentration monitoring. Adverse effects currently reported are limited and include nausea, dizziness, anxiety, headache, with fewer reports of rash, transient elevated aminotransferases, eosinophilia, and local reactions at the site of infusion when concentrated solutions are used (see Antidote in Depth: Fomepizole and Chap. 66).

SUMMARY

When administered appropriately, ethanol is an excellent first step in preventing further metabolism of methanol and ethylene glycol. This is particularly true when CNS depression is not an immediate concern. However, both fomepizole and ethanol do not affect the toxic metabolites that are already present in the body. Once alcohol dehydrogenase is blocked, the decision to use hemodialysis will depend on how much damage has been done to the eliminating organs, how well the body can eliminate the parent compound, and the amount of toxic metabolites already present in the body.

REFERENCES

1. Agner K, Hook O, Von Porat B: The treatment of methanol poisoning with ethanol. J Stud Alcohol 1949;9:515–522.
2. Brent J, McMartin K, Phillips SP, et al: Fomepizole for the treatment of methanol poisoning. N Engl J Med 2001;344:424–429.
3. Caballeria L: First-pass metabolism of ethanol: Its role as a determinant of blood alcohol levels after drinking. Hepatogastroenterology 1992;39:62–66.
4. Cheng JT, Beysolow TD, Kaul B, Weisman R, Feinfeld DA: Clearance of ethylene glycol by kidneys and hemodialysis. J Toxicol Clin Toxicol 1987;25:95–108.
5. Cobaugh DJ, Gibbs M, Shapiro DE, et al: A comparison of the bioavailabilities of oral and intravenous ethanol in healthy male volunteers. Acad Emerg Med 1999;6:984–988.
6. Cole-Harding S, Wilson JR: Ethanol metabolism in men and women. J Stud Alcohol 1987;48:380–387.
7. Davis DP, Bramwell KJ, Hamilton RS, Williams SR: Ethylene glycol poisoning: Case report of a record-high level and a review. J Emerg Med 1997;15:653–667.
8. Ekins BR, Rollins DE, Duffy DP, Gregory MC: Standardized treatment of severe methanol poisoning with ethanol and hemodialysis. West J Med 1985;142:337–340.
9. Faci A, Plaa GL, Sharkawi M: Chloral hydrate enhances ethanol-induced inhibition of methanol oxidation in mice. Toxicology 1998;131:1–7.

10. Fillmore MT, Vogel-Sprott M: Behavioral impairment under alcohol: Cognitive and pharmacokinetic factors. Alcohol Clin Exp Res 1998; 22:1476–1482.

11. Fraser AG, Hudson M, Sawyer AM, et al: Ranitidine, cimetidine, famotidine have no effect on post-prandial absorption of ethanol (0.8 g/kg) taken after an evening meal. Aliment Pharmacol Ther 1992;6: 693–700.

12. Grauer G, Thrall MA, Henre B, et al: Comparison of the effects of ethanol on 4-methylpyrazole on the pharmacokinetics and toxicity of ethylene glycol in the dog. Toxicol Lett 1987;35:307–314.

13. Hantson P, Wallemacq P, Brau M: Two cases of acute methanol poisoning partially treated by oral 4-methylpyrazole. Intensive Care Med 1999;25:528–531.

14. Hauser J, Szabo S: Extremely long protection by pyrazole derivatives against chemically induced gastric mucosal injury. J Pharmacol Exper Ther 1991;256:592–598.

15. Jacobsen D, Jansen H, Wiik-Larsen E, et al: Studies on methanol poisoning. Acta Med Scand 1982;212:5–10.

16. Jacobsen D, McMartin KE: Methanol and ethylene glycol poisonings: Mechanism of toxicity, clinical course, diagnosis and treatment. Med Toxicol 1986;1:309–334.

17. Jacobsen D, Sebastian CS, Barron SK, et al: Effects of 4-methylpyrazole, methanol/ethylene glycol antidote, in healthy humans. J Emerg Med 1990;8:455–461.

18. Jacobsen D, Webb R, Collins TD, McMartin KE: Methanol and formate kinetics in late diagnosed methanol intoxication. Med Toxicol 1988;3:418–423.

19. Jones AW, Jönsson KA, Kechagias S: Effect of high-fat, high-protein, and high-carbohydrate meals on the pharmacokinetics of a small dose of ethanol. Br J Clin Pharmacol 1997;44:521–526.

20. Julkunen RJ, Tannenbaum L, Baradna E, et al: First pass metabolism of ethanol: An important determinant of blood levels after alcohol consumption. Alcohol 1985;2:437–441.

21. Korman MG, Bolin TD: Alcohol and H₂-receptor antagonists. Med J Aust 1992;157:730–731.

22. Li TK, Theorell H: Human liver alcohol dehydrogenase: Inhibition by pyrazole and pyrazole analogs. Acta Chem Scand 1969;23:892–902.

23. Lieber CS: Gastric ethanol metabolism and gastritis: Interactions with other drugs, *Helicobacter pylori*, and antibiotic therapy (1957–1997)—A review. Alcohol Clin Exp Res 1997;21:1360–1366.

24. Makar AB, Tephly TR, Mannering GJ: Methanol metabolism in the monkey. Mol Pharmacol 1968;4:471–483.

25. Makar AB, Tephly TR: Inhibition of monkey liver alcohol dehydrogenase by 4-methylpyrazole. Biochem Med 1975;13:334–342.

26. McCoy HG, Cipolle RJ, Ehlers SM, et al: Severe methanol poisoning: Application of a pharmacokinetic model for ethanol therapy and hemodialysis. Am J Med 1979;67:804–807.

27. McKnight AJ, Langston EA, Marques PR, Tippetts AS: Estimating blood alcohol level from observable signs. Accid Anal Prev 1997;29: 247–255.

28. McMartin KE, Hedström K, Told B, et al: Studies on the metabolic interactions between 4-methylpyrazole and methanol using the monkey as an animal model. Archiv Biochem Biophys 1980;199:606–614.

29. McMartin KE, Makar AB, Palese MA, Tephly TR: Methanol Poisoning I. The role of formic acid in the development of metabolic acidosis in the monkey and the reversal by 4-methylpyrazole. Biochem Med 1975;13:319–333.

30. Papineau KL, Roehrs TA, Petrucelli N, et al: Electrophysiological assessment (the multiple sleep latency test) of the biphasic effects of ethanol in humans. Alcohol Clin Exp Res 1998;22:231–235.

31. Peterson C: Oral ethanol doses in patients with methanol poisoning. Am J Hosp Pharm 1981;38:1024–1027.

32. Peterson CD, Collins AJ, Himes JM, et al: Ethylene glycol poisoning: Pharmacokinetics during therapy with ethanol and hemodialysis. N Engl J Med 1981;304:21–23.

33. Pietruszko R: Human liver alcohol dehydrogenase inhibition of methanol activity by pyrazole, 4-methylpyrazole, 4-hydroxymethyl-pyrazole and 4-carboxypyrazole. Biochem Pharmacol 1975;24: 1603–1607.

34. Pietruszko R, Voigtlander K, Lester D: Alcohol dehydrogenase from human and horse liver—Substance specificity with diols. Biochem Pharmacol 1978;27:1296–1297.

35. Rainey PM: Relation between serum and whole-blood ethanol concentrations. Clin Chem 1993;39:2288–2292.

36. Roe O: Methanol poisoning: Its clinical course, pathogenesis and treatment. Acta Med Scand 1946;126(Suppl 182):1–253.

37. Sivilotti ML, Burns MJ, McMartin KE, Brent J: Toxicokinetics of ethylene glycol during fomepizole therapy: Implications for management. For the Methylpyrazole for Toxic Alcohols Study Group. Ann Emerg Med 2000;36:114–125.

38. Sullivan M, Chen C, Madden JF: Absence of metabolic acidosis in toxic methanol ingestion: A case report and review. Del Med J 1999; 71:421–426.

39. Tarr B, Winters L, Moore M, et al: Low-dose ethanol in the treatment of ethylene glycol poisoning. J Vet Pharm Ther 1985;8:254–262.

40. Tomaszewski C, Cline DM, Whitley TW, Grant T: Effect of acute ethanol ingestion on orthostatic vital signs. Ann Emerg Med 1995; 25:636–641.

41. Vassiliadis J, Graudins A, Dowsett RP: Triethylene glycol poisoning treated with intravenous ethanol infusion. J Toxicol Clin Toxicol 1999;37:773–776.

42. Vestal RE, McGuire EA, Tobin JD, et al: Aging and ethanol metabolism. Clin Pharmacol Ther 1975;21:343–353.

43. Wacker WE, Haynes H, Druyan R, et al: Treatment of ethylene glycol poisoning with ethyl alcohol. JAMA 1965;194:173–175.

44. Whitfield JB: ADH and ALDH genotypes in relation to alcohol metabolic rate and sensitivity. Alcohol Alcohol 1994;2:59–65.

45. Wilkinson P: Pharmacokinetics of ethanol: A review. Alcohol Clin Exp Res 1980;4:6–21.

46. Williams CS, Woodcock KR: Do ethanol and metronidazole interact to produce a disulfiram-like reaction? Ann Pharmacother 2000; 34: 255–257.

ANTIDOTES IN DEPTH

Fomepizole

Mary Ann Howland

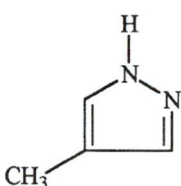

Fomepizole is a competitive inhibitor of alcohol dehydrogenase (ADH) that is useful in preventing the formation of toxic metabolites from ethylene glycol and methanol. It may also have a role in halting the disulfiram-ethanol reaction, and in limiting the toxicity from a variety of xenobiotics that rely on alcohol dehydrogenase for metabolism to toxic metabolites. In addition, as an inducer-inhibitor of certain cytochrome P450 isoenzymes it may lead to desirable or undesirable drug interactions.

HISTORY

In 1963, Theorell and associates described the inhibiting effect of pyrazole on the horse ADH-NAD$^+$ (nicotinamide adenine dinucleotide) enzyme-coenzyme system.[56] Pyrazole appeared to block ADH by complexation. Administration to rats and dogs previously poisoned with methanol and ethylene glycol improved survival.[58] However, pyrazole also inhibited other liver enzymes, including catalase and the microsomal ethanol-oxidizing system.[39] Additional adverse effects of pyrazole administration resulted in bone marrow, liver, and renal toxicity, and these effects were increased in the presence of ethanol and methanol.[48] These factors led to the search for less toxic compounds with comparable mechanisms of action.

In 1969, Li and Theorell found that pyrazole and 4-methylpyrazole (fomepizole) inhibited ADH found in human liver preparations.[38] Studies in rats and mice using fomepizole found the agent to be relatively nontoxic whether used alone or with ethanol.[6] Subsequent studies in monkeys and humans with methanol and ethylene glycol poisoning have demonstrated the inhibitory effect and relative safety of fomepizole.[10,11,48]

PHARMACOLOGY

Fomepizole has a molecular weight of 82 daltons and a pK_a of 2.91 at low concentrations and 3.0 at high concentrations. The freebase is chemically equivalent to the chloride and sulfate salts at physiologic pH.[14] The freebase is used in the United States, while the salts have been used in Europe.

Values for K_m have been estimated for the toxic alcohols along with the value for K_i with fomepizole. The smaller the K_m the

higher the affinity of the substrate for the enzyme and the lower the concentration of the substrate (ie, alcohol) that is needed to half saturate the enzyme. Studies in monkey liver and human liver demonstrate that fomepizole is a competitive inhibitor of alcohol dehydrogenase.[42,54] In monkey liver, fomepizole demonstrated very similar K_is for both ethanol and methanol at 7.5 and 9.1 µmol, respectively.[42] In this same model, the K_m was 3.2 for ethanol and 20.1 mmol for methanol, demonstrating a 6 times higher affinity of ethanol for alcohol dehydrogenase than methanol,[42] while the ratio was 15 times higher when human liver was used.[53] Studies in monkeys demonstrate that a concentration of fomepizole of about 9–10 µmol/L (74–82 µg/dL, 0.74–0.8 µg/mL) is needed to inhibit the metabolism of methanol to formate.[6,48] In human liver, the level needed to achieve inhibition is about 0.09–1 µmol.[38,53] The most recent trial that used intravenous fomepizole in the approved dosing regimen for patients poisoned with methanol, attempted to maintain a serum fomepizole concentration ≥0.8 µg/mL.

CYP2E1 isoenzyme oxidizes ethanol and a number of xenobiotics to toxic metabolites including acetaminophen, carbon tetrachloride, nitrosamines, and benzene. Fomepizole, like ethanol and isoniazid, has dual effects on this isozyme. Fomepizole induces this isoenzyme in rats in the liver and kidney but not in the lung through a posttranscriptional mechanism not involving increased mRNA. However, while fomepizole is present the isozyme is inhibited. After fomepizole is eliminated, the consequences of induction would be manifest.[8,60,61] In hepatocyte culture, fomepizole appears to stabilize and maintain the induced metabolic activity of the isoenzyme for about a week.[62]

PHARMACOKINETICS

Fomepizole has a volume of distribution of about 0.6–1 L/kg and is metabolized to 4-carboxypyrazole, an inactive metabolite that accounts for 80–85% of the administered dose. In a healthy human volunteer study, oral doses of fomepizole were rapidly absorbed and demonstrated saturation and nonlinear kinetics.[27] The K_m (concentration at which the maximum elimination rate is 50%) was estimated to be 75 µmol/L, as compared to 6 µmol/L in a dog model.[27,44] First-order kinetics were exhibited at concentrations below the K_m, while zero order elimination occured at concentrations 100–200% of the K_m.[27] The elimination of fomepizole at 10 mg/kg, 20 mg/kg, 50 mg/kg, and 100 mg/kg was 3.66, 5.05, 10.3, and 14.9 µmol/L/h, respectively.[27] Classical Michaelis-Menten kinetics predicts that the elimination rate is the same at the two higher doses, but this was not the case. The authors speculate that multiple metabolic pathways with different affinities exist and predominate at different fomepizole concentrations. After 20 mg/kg, the half-life of fomepizole calculated from the linear portion of the curve was 5.2 hours and occurred when serum concentrations were less than 100 µmol/L. Peak concentrations after oral administration were achieved within 2 hours and were 132, 326, 759, and 1425 µmol following 10, 20, 50, and 100 mg/kg doses, respectively. Every mg/kg oral dose of fomepizole raised the serum concentration 13–16 μmol.[27] The renal clearance was low (0.016 mL/min/kg), and only 3% of the administered dose was excreted unchanged in the urine.[27]

The pharmacokinetics of intravenous fomepizole were studied in 14 patients being treated for ethylene glycol toxicity.[45] A mean peak concentration of 342 μmol (200–400 μmol) was achieved following a loading dose of 15 mg/kg (183 μmol/kg). Supplemental doses of fomepizole of 10 mg/kg every 12 hours for 48 hours followed by 15 mg/kg every 12 hours until ethylene glycol levels were less than 20 mg/dL and every 4 hours during hemodialysis were administered.[45,55] The effect of simultaneous plasma ethanol concentrations was not analyzed. The lowest fomepizole plasma concentration of 105 μmol was present at 8 hours after the loading dose. The rate of elimination was determined to be zero order at 16 μmol/L/h as compared with a first-order elimination half-life of 3 hours during hemodialysis. Other authors have reported similar fomepizole clearances (12.99 μmol/L/h).[12] The plasma clearance of fomepizole during hemodialysis was 230 mL/min. Previous analysis using determinations of dialysis fluid revealed an extraction ratio of about 75% and a dialysance of 117 mL/min, which was very similar to a simultaneous ethylene glycol determination.[17] The Vd was 0.69 L/kg.[45] The dialysance of fomepizole was similar to urea in a pig model and suggests no significant protein binding of fomepizole.[28] The pharmacokinetic interactions between fomepizole and ethanol were studied in a double-blind crossover design in healthy human volunteers.[32] Fomepizole was given orally in doses of 10, 15, and 20 mg/kg 1 hour prior to oral ethanol at 0.5–0.7 g/kg as a 20% solution in orange juice. Fomepizole decreased the elimination rate of ethanol by about 40% from 12–16 mg/dL/h to about 7–9.5 mg/dL/h. When intravenous fomepizole was administered at 5 mg/kg over 30 minutes and ethanol in doses to achieve 50–150 mg/dL for 6 hours were administered orally beginning at the end of the fomepizole infusion, the elimination of fomepizole was decreased by about 50%.[32] This occurred without a change in the amount or fraction of unchanged fomepizole appearing in the urine. The authors suggested that the ethanol probably inhibited the metabolism of fomepizole to 4-carboxypyrazole by the cytochrome P450 system. A single low dose of fomepizole given to humans had a maximal effect on ethanol metabolism at 1.5–2 hours.[5] Therefore ethanol and fomepizole mutually inhibit the elimination of each other prolonging their respective plasma concentrations. Methanol also decreases the elimination of fomepizole by about 25% in the monkey.[48]

METHANOL

In Vitro and Animal Studies

Studies using human livers demonstrate the inhibitory effect of fomepizole on alcohol dehydrogenase.[53] Studies in monkeys, the animal species that most closely resembles humans in metabolizing methanol, also clearly demonstrates the inhibitory effect of fomepizole in preventing the accumulation of formate.[4,48,49]

Human Experience

The largest case series to date involved 11 patients given IV fomepizole in the approved US dosing regimen.[11] The formate levels in all patients administered fomepizole fell and the arterial pH increased.[11] Case reports demonstrate similar findings.[12,23,19]

Effect of Fomepizole on Methanol and Formate Concentrations

Methanol exhibits dose-dependent kinetics.[31] At low doses (0.08 g/kg), which achieve serum concentrations of about 10 mg/dL, methanol elimination is first order with a half-life of about 2.5–3 hours.[35,37] In concentrations of about 100–200 mg/dL, methanol exhibits zero-order kinetics and is eliminated at about 8.5–9 mg/dL/h in untreated humans[33] and 4.4–7 mg/dL/h in untreated monkeys.[16,51] At very high methanol doses in monkeys (3 g/kg), achieving serum concentrations of about 500 mg/dL, the elimination of methanol again exhibits apparent first-order kinetics. This alteration is likely caused by the greater contribution of other first-order pathways, such as pulmonary and urinary elimination, which may account for a greater fraction of the total body clearance under these circumstances.[33] Once fomepizole is administered in doses sufficient to achieve a minimum effective concentration to inhibit alcohol dehydrogenase the elimination of methanol becomes first order in humans and the half-life of methanol is about 54 hours.[11] When the metabolism of methanol to formate by alcohol dehydrogenase is blocked, formate is eliminated with a half-life dependent on dose and the uncertain effect of folate and bicarbonate therapies. In monkeys administered formate without the presence of methanol, the formate half-life is 30–50 minutes.[15] In monkeys given methanol followed by fomepizole, the formate levels decreased by more than 80% in 2 hours.[4]

ETHYLENE GLYCOL

In Vitro and Animal Studies

Monkeys given 3 g/kg of ethylene glycol intraperitoneally recovered without treatment, whereas those given 4 g/kg died without therapy and those given 4 g/kg with fomepizole all survived.[15]

Human Experience

The first 3 patients treated in France with oral fomepizole improved clinically and tolerated the therapy.[1] Subsequent case reports and case series utilizing fomepizole orally or IV with or without hemodialysis have also demonstrated its effectiveness in preventing glycolate accumulation.[2,7,10,22,24,34,50,55]

Effect of Fomepizole on Ethylene Glycol and Glycolate Concentrations in Humans

Kidney function is essential in the elimination of ethylene glycol. The half-life of ethylene glycol at low concentrations is about 8.6 hours.[55] Based on pooled human data, the half-life of ethylene glycol after alcohol dehydrogenase is blocked with fomepizole is about 14–17 hours in those patients with normal renal function, and about 49 hours in patients with impaired renal function.[1,24,55] Based on a limited number of determinations, the renal clearance of ethylene glycol averaged 31.5 mL/min during the first 2 days; the corresponding creatinine clearance was 112 mL/min and estimated total body clearance during fomepizole therapy was 57 mL/min.[2] These calculations suggest that the renal clearance of ethylene glycol accounted for only 55% of estimated total body clearance. Glycolate (MW 76 daltons) had a mean half-life of 10 ± 8 hours in patients treated with fomepizole before hemodialysis, and a mean half-life of less than 3 hours during hemodialysis,[50] although in this study, patient renal function is not defined nor is the amount of glycolate excreted unchanged by the kidneys described.

SAFETY AND ADVERSE EFFECTS

Because retinol dehydrogenase is an isozyme of ADH, and because it is responsible for converting retinol to retinal in the eye, it was essential to study whether fomepizole would inhibit this enzyme and subsequently produce retinal damage.[48] Studies in several species of monkeys and other animals demonstrate that fomepizole is relatively nontoxic, with no demonstrated signs of ocular toxicity.[4]

An oral placebo-controlled, double-blind, single-dose randomized sequential ascending-dose study was performed in healthy volunteers to determine fomepizole tolerance at 10–100 mg/kg.[31] There were no adverse effects in the 10 and 20 mg/kg groups, while at 50 mg/kg 3 of 4 subjects experienced slight to moderate nausea and dizziness within 2.5 hours of medication administration. All subjects reported comparable symptoms at 100 mg/kg. These symptoms lasted for 30 hours in 1 individual. There were no concomitant changes in any vital sign or laboratory parameter measured. Divided daily doses of fomepizole up to 20 mg/kg for 5 days have been administered without any demonstrable toxicity.[47] A transient elevation of aminotransferase levels was reported in 6 of 15 healthy volunteer subjects who received fomepizole.[30] The most common adverse effects reported by the manufacturer in a total of 76 patients and 63 volunteers were headache 12%, nausea 11%, and dizziness 7%. Other less commonly observed adverse effects include phlebitis, rash, fever, and eosinophilia. In the two largest cases series of fomepizole treatment for ethylene glycol toxicity and for methanol toxicity, there were no adverse events classified as definitely or probably related to fomepizole.[10,11] The LD_{50} of fomepizole in mice and rats is 3.8 mmol/kg after IV administration and 7.9 mmol/kg following oral administration.[41]

DISULFIRAM AND OTHER TOXINS

Fomepizole was successfully used to terminate the reactions (a) resulting from the use of an acetaldehyde inhibitor administered to volunteers pretreated with a small dose of ethanol and (b) occurring in a chronic alcoholic surreptitiously given disulfiram by his wife.[40] The intravenous administration of fomepizole prevented the accumulation of acetaldehyde by inhibiting its formation and allowing elimination to predominate thereby lessening the typical symptoms of facial flushing and tachycardia.[40] Pretreatment with oral fomepizole was successful in preventing the facial flushing and tachycardia typically associated with ethanol administration in ethanol sensitive Japanese subjects.[25,26] Limited animal studies and a few case reports suggest that fomepizole may be effective in limiting the toxicity secondary to diethylene glycol, triethylene glycol and 1,3-difluoro-2-propanol.[7,18,57]

COMPARISON TO ETHANOL

Ethanol has been used for years to inhibit the metabolism of methanol and ethylene glycol to their respective toxic metabolites. Although very inexpensive, ethanol has many disadvantages, including central nervous system depression that is at least additive

to that of the methanol or ethylene glycol; dosing difficulties as a result of its rapid and often unpredictable rate of metabolism; the development of tolerance; the lack of ready availability of an intravenous formulation; the necessity of closely monitoring serum concentrations; the hyperosmolarity of a 5% or 10% intravenous preparation;[63] and the potential for hypoglycemia or other ethanol-related adverse effects such as pancreatitis and hepatitis. Fomepizole has the advantage of being a very potent inhibitor of alcohol dehydrogenase without producing central nervous system (CNS) depression, having an easier dosing schedule without the need for serum concentration monitoring which allows every 12-hour dosing except during hemodialysis, when dosing should occur every 4 hours. Limited adverse effects include local reactions at the site of infusion when concentrations >25 mg/mL are employed, and nausea, dizziness, anxiety, headache, rash, transiently elevated aminotransferases, and eosinophilia.

DOSING

The loading dose is 15 mg/kg followed in 12 hours by 10 mg/kg every 12 hours for 4 doses, and then increased to 15 mg/kg every 12 hours for as long as necessary. The increase in the maintenance dose from 10 mg/kg to 15 mg/kg is recommended because fomepizole causes autoinduction, stimulating its own metabolism. Patients undergoing hemodialysis require additional doses of fomepizole to replace the amount removed during hemodialysis. The dose must be diluted in 100 mL of normal saline (NS) or D_5W prior to IV administration and then infused over 30 minutes to avoid local reactions.

AVAILABILITY

Fomepizole has received FDA approval and is now marketed as Antizol injection by Orphan Medical. Fomepizole is available in a tray pack containing 4 vials (1.5 mL vials of 1 g/mL) that can be diluted in 100 mL of D_5W or NS for adults to be administered intravenously over 30 minutes. Temperatures of <25°C (77°F) cause the fomepizole vials to solidify. Warming reliquifies the product.

SUMMARY

Fomepizole is a potent competitive inhibitor of alcohol dehydrogenase that is useful in inhibiting the metabolism of methanol and ethylene glycol and other substances that utilize alcohol dehydrogenase in the formation of toxic metabolites. Once alcohol dehydrogenase is blocked, the decision to use hemodialysis depends on how much damage has been done to the eliminating organs and how well the body can eliminate the parent compound as well as the already formed toxic metabolites. Fomepizole appears safe. Although fomepizole has been used successfully orally, only an intravenous dosing regimen is approved. Therefore, a formal oral bioavailability study and an approved oral regimen is appropriate for study.

REFERENCES

1. Baud F, Bismuth C, Garnier R, et al: 4-Methylpyrazole may be an alternative to ethanol therapy for ethylene glycol intoxication in man. J Toxicol Clin Toxicol 1986;24:463–483.

2. Baud F, Galliot M, Astier A, et al: Treatment of ethylene glycol poisoning with intravenous 4-methylpyrazole. N Engl J Med 1988;319: 97–110.

3. Blair AH, Vallee BL: Some catalytic properties of human liver alcohol dehydrogenase. Biochem 1966;5:2026–2034.

4. Blomstrand R, Ingelmansson S: Studies on the effect of 4-methylpyrazole on methanol poisoning using the monkey as an animal model: With particular reference to the ocular toxicity. Drug Alcohol Depend 1984;13:343–355.

5. Blomstrand R, Theorell H: Inhibitory effect on ethanol oxidation in man after administration of 4-methylpyrazole. Life Sci 1970;9: 631–640.

6. Blomstrand R, Wintzell H, Lof A, et al: Pyrazoles as inhibitors of alcohol oxidation and as important tools in alcohol research: An approach to therapy against methanol poisoning. Proc Natl Acad Sci U S A 1979;76:3499–3503.

7. Borron SW, Mégarbane B, Baud FJ: Fomepizole in treatment of uncomplicated ethylene glycol poisoning. Lancet 1999;354:831.

8. Brennan RJ, Mankes RF, Lefevre R, et al: 4-Methylpyrazole blocks acetaminophen hepatotoxicity in the rat. Ann Emerg Med 1994;23: 487–494.

9. Brent J, McMartin K, Phillips SP, et al: 4-Methylpyrazole (Fomepizole) therapy of methanol poisoning: Preliminary results of the meta trial. J Toxicol Clin Toxicol 1997;35:507.

10. Brent J, McMartin K, Phillips SP, et al: Fomepizole for the treatment of ethylene glycol poisoning. N Engl J Med 1999;340:832–838.

11. Brent J, McMartin K, Phillips SP, et al: Fomepizole for the treatment of methanol poisoning. N Engl J Med 2001;344:424–429.

12. Burns MJ, Graudins, Aaron CK, et al: Treatment of methanol poisoning with intravenous 4-methylpyrazole. Ann Emerg Med 1997;30: 829–832.

13. Cheng JT, Beysolow TD, Kaul B, et al: Clearance of ethylene glycol by kidneys and hemodialysis. J Toxicol Clin Toxicol 1987;25:95–108.

14. Chilukuri DM, Shah JC: pK_a of 4MP and chemical equivalence in formulations of free base and salts of 4MP. PDA J Pharm Sci Technol 1999;53:44–47.

15. Clay KL, Murphy RC, Watkins WD: Experimental methanol toxicity in the primate: Analysis of metabolic acidosis. Toxicol Appl Pharmacol 1975;13:319–333.

16. Eells JT, Makar AB, Noker PE, Tephly TR: Methanol poisoning and formate oxidation in nitrous oxide-treated rats. J Pharmacol Exp Ther 1981;217:57–61.

17. Faessel H, Houze P, Baud FJ, Scherrmann JM: 4-Methylpyrazole monitoring during haemodialysis of ethylene glycol intoxicated patients. Eur J Clin Pharmacol 1995;49:211–213.

18. Feldwick MS, Noakes PS, Prause U, et al: The biochemical toxicology of 1,3-difluoro-2-propanol, the major ingredient of the pesticide gliftor: The potential of 4-methylpyrazole as an antidote. J Biochem Mol Toxicol 1998;12:41–52.

19. Girault C, Tamion F, Moritz F, et al: Fomepizole (4-methylpyrazole) in fatal methanol poisoning with early CT scan cerebral lesions. J Toxicol Clin Toxicol 1999;35:777–780.

20. Goldfarb DS: Fomepizole for ethylene-glycol poisoning [letter]. Lancet 1999;354:1646.

21. Grauer GF, Thrall MAH, Henre BA, Hjelle JJ: Comparison of the effects of ethanol and 4-methylpyrazole on the pharmacokinetics and toxicity of ethylene glycol in the dog. Toxicol Lett 1987;35: 307–314.

22. Hantson PH, Hassoun A, Mahieu P: Ethylene glycol poisoning treated by intravenous 4-methylpyrazole. Intensive Care Med 1998;24: 736–739.

23. Hantson P, Wallemacq P, Brau M, et al: Two cases of acute methanol poisoning partially treated by oral 4-methylpyrazole. Intensive Care Med 1999;25:528–531.

24. Harry P, Turcant A, Bouachour G, et al: Efficacy of 4-methylpyrazole in ethylene glycol poisoning. Clinical and toxicokinetic aspects. Hum Exp Toxicol 1994;13:61–64.

25. Inoue K, Kera Y, Kiriyama T, Komura S: Suppression of acetaldehyde accumulation by 4-methylpyrazole in alcohol-hypersensitive Japanese. Jpn J Pharmacol 1985;38:43–48.

26. Inoue K, Fukunaga M, Kiriyama T, Komura S: Accumulation of acetaldehyde in alcohol-sensitive Japanese: Relation to ethanol and acetaldehyde oxidizing capacity. Alcoholism. Clin Exp Res 1984; 8:319–322.

27. Jacobsen D, Barron SK, Sebastian CS, et al: Nonlinear kinetics of 4-methylpyrazole in healthy human subjects. Eur J Clin Pharmacol 1989;37:599–604.

28. Jacobsen D, Østensen J, Bredesen L, et al: 4-Methylpyrazole (4-MP) is effectively removed by hemodialysis in the pig model. Vet Hum Toxicol 1992;34:362.

29. Jacobsen D, Øvrebo S, Østborg J, Sejersted OM: Glycolate causes the acidosis in ethylene glycol poisoning and is effectively removed by hemodialysis. Acta Med Scand 1984:216:409–416.

30. Jacobsen D, Sebastian CS, Barron SK, et al: Effects of 4-methylpyrazole, methanol/ethylene glycol antidote, in healthy humans. J Emerg Med 1990;8:455–461.

31. Jacobsen D, Sebastian CS, Blomstrand R, McMartin KE: 4-methylpyrazole: A controlled study of safety in healthy human subjects after single ascending doses. Alcohol Clin Exp Res 1988;12: 516–522.

32. Jacobsen D, Sebastian CS, Dies DF, et al: Kinetic interactions between 4-methylpyrazole and ethanol in healthy humans. Alcohol Clin Exp Res 1996;20:804–809.

33. Jacobsen D, Webb R, Collins TD, McMartin KE: Methanol and formate kinetics in late diagnosed methanol intoxication. Med Toxicol 1988;3:418–423.

34. Jobard E, Harry P, Turcant A, et al: 4-Methylpyrazole and hemodialysis in ethylene glycol poisoning. J Toxicol Clin Toxicol 1996;34: 373–377.

35. Jones AW: Elimination half-life of methanol during hangover. Pharmacol Toxicol 1987;60:217–220.

36. Knepshield JH, Shreiner GE, Lowenthal DT, et al: Dialysis of poisons and drugs: Annual review. Trans Am Soc Artif Intern Organs 1973; 19:590–633.

37. Leaf G, Zatman LJ: A study of the conditions under which methanol may exert a toxic hazard in industry. Brit J Indus Med 1952;9:19–31.

38. Li TK, Theorell H: Human liver alcohol dehydrogenase: Inhibition by pyrazole and pyrazole analogs. Acta Chem Scand 1969;23:892–902.

39. Lieber C, Rubin E, DeCarli L, et al: Effects of pyrazole on hepatic function and structure. Lab Invest 1970;22:615–621.

40. Lindros KO, Stowell A, Pikkarainen P, Salaspuro M: The disulfiram (Antabuse)-alcohol reaction in male alcoholics: Its efficient management by 4-methylpyrazole. Alcohol Clin Exper Res 1981;5:528–530.

41. Magnusson G, Nyberg J-A, Bodin N-O, Hansson E: Toxicity of pyrazole and 4-methylpyrazole in mice and rats. Experiencia 1972;28: 1198–1200.

42. Makar AB, Tephly TR: Inhibition of monkey liver alcohol dehydrogenase by 4-methylpyrazole. Biochem Med 1975;13:334–342.

43. Makar AB, Tephly TR, Mannering GJ: Methanol metabolism in the monkey. Mol Pharmacol 1968;4:471–483.

44. Mayersohn M, Owens, SM, Anaya AL, et al: 4-Methylpyrazole disposition in the dog: Evidence for saturable elimination. J Pharmaceutical Sci 1985;74:895–896.

45. McMartin KE, Brent J, Meta Study Group: Pharmacokinetics of fomepizole (4MP) in patients [abstract]. J Toxicol Clin Toxicol 1998; 36:450–451.

46. McMartin KE, Collins TD: Distribution of oral 4-methylpyrazole in the rat: Inhibition of elimination by ethanol. J Toxicol Clin Toxicol 1988;26:451–466.

47. McMartin KE, Heath A: The treatment of ethylene glycol poisoning with intravenous 4-methylpyrazole. N Engl J Med 1989;320:125.

48. McMartin KE, Hedstrom K-G, Tolf B, et al: Studies on the metabolic interactions between 4-methylpyrazole and methanol using the monkey as an animal model. Arch Biochem Biophys 1980;199:606–614.

49. McMartin KE, Makar AB, Martin A, et al: Methanol poisoning I. The role of formic acid in the development of metabolic acidosis in the monkey and the reversal by 4-methylpyrazole. Biochem Med 1975; 13:319–333.

50. Moreau CL, Kerns, W II, Tomaszewski CA, et al: Glycolate kinetics and hemodialysis clearance in ethylene glycol poisoning. J Toxicol Clin Toxicol 1998;36:659–666.

51. Noker PE, Eells JT, Tephly TR. Methanol toxicity: Treatment with folic acid and 5-formyl-tetrahydrofolic acid. Alcohol Clin Exp Res 1980;4:378–383.

52. Parry MF, Wallach R: Ethylene glycol poisoning. Am J Med 1974;57: 143–150.

53. Pietruszko R: Human liver alcohol dehydrogenase inhibition of methanol activity by pyrazole, 4-methylpyrazole, 4-hydroxymethyl-pyrazole and 4-carboxypyrazole. Biochem Pharmacol 1975;24: 1603–1607.

54. Pietruszko R, Voigtlander K, Lester D: Alcohol dehydrogenase from human and horse liver—Substrate specificity with diols. Biochem Pharmacol 1978;27:1296–1297.

55. Sivilotti M, Burns M, McMartin K, et al: Toxicokinetics of ethylene glycol during fomepizole therapy: Implications for management. Ann Emerg Med 2000;36:114–125.

56. Theorell H, Yonetani T, Sjoberg B: On the effects of some hetero-cyclic compounds on the enzymatic activity of liver alcohol dehydro-genase. Acta Chem Scand 1969;23:255–260.

57. Vassiliadis J, Graudins A, Dowsett RP: Triethylene glycol poisoning treated with intravenous ethanol infusion. J Toxicol Clin Toxicol 1999;37:773–776.

58. Van Stee E, Harris A, Horton M, et al: The treatment of ethylene gly-col toxicosis with pyrazole. J Pharmacol Exp Ther 1975;192:251–259.

59. Wacker WEC, Haynes H, Druyan R, et al: Treatment of ethylene gly-col poisoning with ethyl alcohol. JAMA 1965;194:1231–1233.

60. Wu D, Cederbaum AI: Induction of liver cytochrome P4502E1 by pyrazole and 4-methylpyrazole in neonatal rats. J Pharmacol Exp Ther 1993;263:1468–1473.

61. Wu D, Cederbaum AI: Characterization of pyrazole and 4-methyl-pyrazole induction of cytochrome P4502E1 in rat kidney. J Pharmacol Exp Ther 1994;270:407–413.

62. Wu DF, Clejan L, Potter B, et al: Rapid decrease of cytochrome P-45011E1 in primary hepatocyte culture and its maintenance by added 4-methylpyrazole. Hepatology 1990;12:1379–1389.

63. Zahlten RN: Cyclic AMP and corticosteroids [letter]. N Engl J Med 1974;290:743–744.

Judd E. Hollander / Robert S. Hoffman

A 22-year-old agitated male was brought to the hospital by ambulance after his family witnessed a "seizure." On arrival at the patient's apartment his family told paramedics that he had shaking movements of all of his extremities, his eyes rolled back, and he began to "foam at the mouth." The family did not know whether the patient had recently used any drugs because he had just returned from a trip to South America.

An intravenous line was started with 0.9% sodium chloride solution, and 100 mL of 50% dextrose in water ($D_{50}W$) and 100 mg of thiamine were given IV without any clinical response. High-flow oxygen was administered at 8 L/min. The patient was taken immediately to the hospital.

On arrival, the patient appeared to be a well-nourished, well-developed, markedly agitated man. His vital signs were: blood pressure, 215/130 mm Hg; pulse, 130 beats/min and regular; respiratory rate, 28 breaths/min; and rectal temperature, 103°F (39.4°C). His skin was diaphoretic and flushed. Examination of head, eyes, ears, nose, and throat revealed no head trauma. Blood was noted at the lateral aspect of the tongue. He had dilated (8-mm) pupils that reacted to light bilaterally. Extraocular movements were intact without nystagmus, and funduscopic examination was normal. Examination of the nose revealed an atrophic mucosa with a perforated nasal septum. A dry, white powder was noted on the patient's mustache. His neck was supple without thyromegaly and the trachea was midline. The chest was clear. The heart sounds revealed an S_4 gallop. Examination of his abdomen revealed high-pitched hyperactive bowel sounds, no organomegaly, and mild tenderness throughout without rebound. The patient subsequently vomited bilious material without blood or coffee grounds. On neurologic examination he was agitated, flailing all extremities with bilateral hyperactive reflexes and plantar flexion. Rectal examination was unremarkable and stool was negative for occult blood.

The electrocardiogram (ECG) revealed sinus tachycardia. The PR, QRS, and QTc intervals were within normal limits. Diffuse J-point and 0.5-mm ST-segment elevation was noted. Chest radiography was normal. A urine dipstick was positive for blood. The patient was treated with incremental doses of 5 mg of IV diazepam (total dose of 25 mg) until his vital signs approached normal. Repeat vital signs after 20 minutes of treatment were blood pressure, 140/80 mm Hg; pulse, 95 beats/min; respiratory rate, 20 breaths/min and regular; and rectal temperature, 101°F (38.3°C). Pupils were 4 mm, equal, and reactive, and the patient was less agitated. The patient stated that he had "snorted snow" and smoked a "joint" that his friends had given him.

Initial laboratory studies demonstrated: hematocrit, 45%; hemoglobin, 15 g/dL; white blood cell (WBC) count, 11,500/ mm^3 with a normal differential; and platelets, 200,000/mm^3. Arterial blood gas on room air revealed pH, 7.35; Pco$_2$, 28 mm Hg; and Po$_2$, 90 mm Hg. The serum electrolytes were sodium, 140 mEq/L; chloride, 105 mEq/L; bicarbonate, 13 mEq/L; potassium, 4.0 mEq/L; anion gap, 22 mEq/L; and calcium, 4.5 mg/dL. The blood urea nitrogen (BUN) and creatinine were normal, and blood glucose was 120 mg/dL. The creatine phosphokinase (CPK) was 1250 IU/L.

HISTORY AND EPIDEMIOLOGY

Cocaine is a natural alkaloid contained in the leaves of *Erythroxylon coca*, a shrub that grows abundantly in Mexico, South America, the West Indies, and Indonesia. In the 6th century, inhabitants of Peru chewed or sucked on the leaves for social and religious reasons. In the 1100s, the Incas used cocaine-filled saliva as local anesthesia for ritual trephinations.[68] Cocaine was identified as the active alkaloid in the coca leaf in 1857, and was first used as a local anesthetic in 1884.[91] In the early 20th century, cocaine was used briefly as an ingredient in Coca-Cola. Since 1975, cocaine use has increased, in part because of the increased production of the coca crops by international drug-trafficking cartels.

By 1990, more than 25 million Americans had tried cocaine at least once and 5 million Americans admitted to current cocaine use 1 or more times per month.[159] According to 1999 data, 3.7 million Americans had used cocaine in the previous year, and 1.5 million Americans used cocaine monthly.[188] The annual number of new users of any form of cocaine rose between 1994 and 1998 from 514,000 to 934,000, suggesting these numbers may continue to increase. Cocaine is the most frequent drug-related cause of emergency department visits in the United States.[187]

MEDICAL USES OF COCAINE

Cocaine is rarely used today as a topical anesthetic (in 4–10% solutions) for intranasal or bronchoscopic procedures. The older otolaryngologic literature implies that the maximal safe total dose of cocaine is 1–3 mg/kg body weight. More concentrated solutions (greater than 10%) are not advantageous clinically and have more adverse effects. Cocaine should be avoided in patients with hypermetabolic and febrile conditions, in patients receiving drugs that alter neurotransmitter metabolism (monoamine oxidase inhibitor (MAOI)), in those with hepatic impairment, and in patients with known plasma cholinesterase deficiency. It is the opinion of the authors that mucosal cocaine use is best limited to those extremely uncommon conditions when alternative agents are contraindicated.

A mixture of tetracaine, epinephrine, and cocaine (referred to as TAC) is still used by some clinicians as a topical anesthetic in children with scalp and facial lacerations. Pediatric deaths,[32] seizures,[33,34] respiratory distress,[218] and other significant systemic toxicities are reported.[44,65,191] As a result, we believe TAC should not be considered the anesthetic solution of choice in pediatric facial and scalp lacerations.[65]

PHARMACOLOGY

After extraction from the coca leaf, cocaine (benzoylmethylecgonine) is purified to the hydrochloride salt, a white crystal. Ecgonine is an aminoalcohol base that is closely related to tropine, the aminoalcohol in atropine. Cocaine is therefore best considered an ester-type local anesthetic of the tropane family.

The onset of action of cocaine depends on the dose and route of administration. Cocaine can be absorbed through the mucosa of the respiratory, gastrointestinal, and genitourinary tract, including less-common routes of absorption such as the urethra, bladder, and vagina. When insufflated, the onset of action is within 1–3 minutes, and its effects peak in 20–30 minutes. When used intravenously or smoked, the onset of action is within seconds and peak action occurs within 3–5 minutes.

Cocaine is a unique compound that produces many pharmacologic effects in humans. Through direct blockade of fast sodium channels, cocaine stabilizes the axonal membrane, producing a local anesthetic effect. Similar blockade of fast sodium channels on myocardial tissue imparts dose dependent type IA and IC antidysrhythmic properties to cocaine.[9,237] In addition, cocaine is the only local anesthetic that interferes with the uptake of neurotransmitters by the nerve terminals and simultaneously functions as a vasoconstrictor. These varied mechanisms interact to produce the wide clinical spectrum of cocaine toxicity.

Central nervous system (CNS) stimulation is probably the most prominent effect of cocaine. The CNS is stimulated in a rostral-to-caudal fashion. The cortex is stimulated first, which may result in restlessness, excitement, and increased motor activity. Later, stimulation of lower motor centers can result in tonic-clonic seizures. Cocaine's initial effect on the medullary response centers is an increase in respiratory rate with a subsequent depression resulting in respiratory failure. The vomiting center may also be initially stimulated, but emetic effects are usually self-limited.

The initial effect on the cardiovascular system is a transient bradycardia, secondary to stimulation of the vagal nuclei. The rapid onset and fleeting nature of this event reduces its relevancy outside of research settings. Tachycardia typically ensues, predominantly from increased central sympathetic stimulation. Cocaine's cardiostimulatory mechanism is to produce sensitization to epinephrine and norepinephrine, probably by preventing neuronal reuptake of these catecholamines, as well as by increasing the re-

lease of norepinephrine from adrenergic nerve terminals. The increased concentrations and persistence of catecholamines near the receptors of the effector organ lead to exaggerated sympathetic effects. Animal investigations reveal that the main vasopressor effects of cocaine are mediated by norepinephrine of sympathetic neural origin and that the main tachycardic effects of cocaine are mediated by direct release of epinephrine of adrenal medullary origin.[216]

Psychostimulant central nervous system effects secondary to cocaine are at least in part mediated through inhibition of dopamine reuptake in the nucleus accumbens.[73] Human subjects experience a subjective "high" when more than 47% of dopamine transporters are blocked.[225] Doses of cocaine that are able to produce typical psychostimulatory effects (0.3–0.6 mg/kg) block 60–77% of dopamine transporters.[225] Genetically engineered absence of the dopamine transporter totally prevents these psychostimulatory effects of cocaine in animals.[60] Cocaine also increases the concentrations of the excitatory amino acids, aspartate and glutamate, in the nucleus accumbens.[207] These excitatory amino acids further increase the extracellular concentrations of dopamine. Excitatory amino acid antagonists attenuate the effects of cocaine on extracellular dopamine[164] and block cocaine-induced convulsions and death.[183] Dopamine$_1$ (D$_1$) and dopamine$_2$ (D$_2$) receptor agonists have opposite effects on cocaine-seeking behavior. The D$_2$ agonists lead to cocaine-seeking behavior while D$_1$ agonists diminish craving for cocaine.[198]

In a human volunteer study, a selective dopaminergic antagonist blocked the development of euphoria, but not the cardiovascular effects, of cocaine.[184]

Cocaine is metabolized by liver esterases and plasma cholinesterase (pseudocholinesterase), and is also degraded nonenzymatically (Fig. 67–1).[210] Cocaine is rapidly hydrolyzed by esterases to its major metabolite, ecgonine methyl ester (EME), which accounts for 30–50% of the parent product. Nonenzymatic

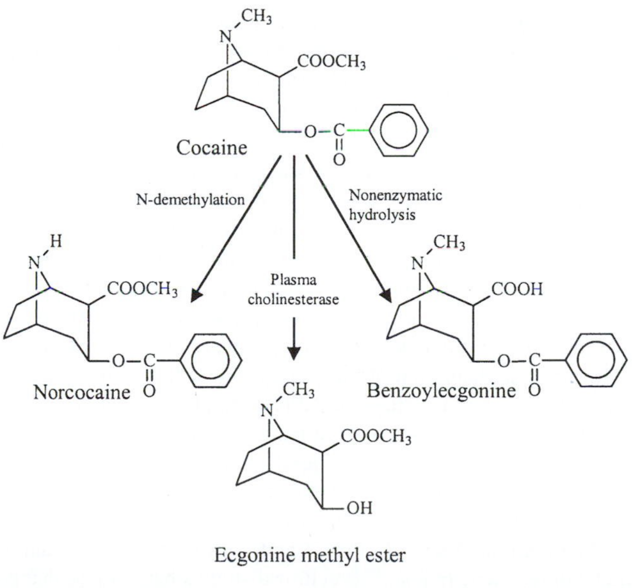

Figure 67–1. Metabolism of cocaine. The three principle metabolic pathways of cocaine are depicted.

hydrolysis results in the formation of the other major metabolite, benzoylecgonine, which accounts for approximately 40% of the parent product. Norcocaine and ecgonine are minor metabolites that constitute the remainder of cocaine's degradation products.

The activity of plasma cholinesterase determines the relative concentrations of the various metabolites, and quite possibly affects the degree of toxicity that develops. Serum from humans with plasma cholinesterase deficiency produce decreased concentrations of ecgonine methyl ester.[135] A similar effect is described in animals, and demonstrates a shift of the metabolite profile largely toward an increase in benzoylecgonine, with a smaller, but still substantial increase in norcocaine observed.[109] As a result, patients with plasma cholinesterase deficiency may have a greater potential for adverse reactions when compared to patients with normal metabolism.[41,80,163]

The biologic half-life of cocaine is 0.5–1.5 hours. A relatively minor amount is excreted unchanged in the urine.[107] Benzoylecgonine and EME are also excreted in the urine, with half-lives of 5–8 and 3.5–6 hours, respectively.[107] Because of its relative long elimination half-life, assays typically detect benzoylecgonine for 48–72 hours following cocaine use,[4] although in rare cases, benzoylecgonine has been detected in the urine up to 22 days following substantial cocaine use.[234]

Specific Effects of Cocaine Metabolites

The precise degree to which the parent compound and the major metabolites (Fig. 67–1) account for the observed clinical effects of cocaine remains unclear. Although older studies suggest that cocaine and norcocaine account for majority of the vascular effects of cocaine,[14] more recent studies demonstrate an active role for most metabolites. Cocaine, norcocaine, ecgonine, and benzoylecgonine all cause cerebrovascular vasoconstriction when suffused over the brain surface,[123] or when administered directly into the cerebral circulation,[193] although these studies have yielded conflicting results regarding the relative potencies of each of the various metabolites. Intravenous administration of cocaine and benzoylecgonine may also lead to cerebral vasoconstriction.[28] Most studies suggest that cocaine and norcocaine are the most potent vasoconstrictors, whereas benzoylecgonine and ecgonine have less of an effect. In some studies, however, EME produced mild vasodilatation of cerebral blood vessels,[137,193] and in a single model, was protective against cocaine lethality. With respect to proconvulsant effects, cocaine and norcocaine are most potent, but benzoylecgonine and EME administration may also lead to seizures in some models.[118,146] The sodium channel antagonist effects occur with the parent compound and with norcocaine, but do not result from the administration of benzoylecgonine or EME.[30]

The varying potencies of the major metabolites of cocaine explain why augmentation of the metabolism with the use of exogenous plasma cholinesterase may reduce the toxicity of cocaine by shunting degradation away from benzoylecgonine and norcocaine to less-toxic metabolites.[82] Rapid administration of butyrylcholinesterase to rats with severe cocaine toxicity ameliorated hypertension, QRS widening, seizures, and death.[135,140]

The combined use of ethanol and cocaine produces a unique metabolite, cocaethylene.[18] Preclinical studies have found that cocaethylene is equipotent to cocaine with regard to resultant behavioral effects, yet is more likely to result in lethality. Human studies demonstrate that relative to cocaine, cocaethylene produces milder subjective effects[168] and comparable hemodynamic effects. Co-

caethylene has a direct myocardial depressant effect[76] that is not mediated through coronary artery vasoconstriction.[172] Both cocaine and cocaethylene increase the permeability of human endothelial cells to low density lipoproteins.[119]

COCAINE PROCESSING AND USE

Cocaine exits as a hydrochloride salt or, in sulfated form, as a powder. When sold illicitly, it is adulterated with one or more of these compounds: mannitol, sucrose, lactose, caffeine, talc, amphetamine, heroin ("speedball"), phencyclidine (PCP), procaine, lidocaine, ergots, or strychnine.[199] When it is nasally insufflated various paraphernalia such as little spoons or straws are used.

"Free-basing" is the home conversion of the hydrochloride form of cocaine to the pure alkaloid cocaine. Unlike cocaine hydrochloride, free-base or crack can be smoked because it vaporizes rather than burns. Because it is lipophilic, it can readily cross the alveolar-capillary and blood-brain barriers. When smoked, it results in an intense euphoria comparable to that experienced with intravenous use. Cocaine base, cocaine paste, "pasta," and "bazooka" are also manufactured by an extraction process. The raw coca leaves are dried and then digested with sulfuric acid. Cocaine base is then extracted after precipitation with sodium bicarbonate. On assay, cocaine base contains between 40% and 85% cocaine sulfate. This similarity results in a great deal of confusion, both clinically and in the literature, where the terms cocaine, free-base, crack, and cocaine sulfate are often used synonymously. The distinction between pure free-base cocaine and cocaine sulfate occurs largely in the laboratory, as very few clinical differences can be definitively attributed to a particular form of the drug.

The availability of crack, a purified processed smokable form of cocaine, has increased access to cocaine. Crack acquired its name because of its rocklike appearance and the crackling sounds made when it is heated. It is available in small chips or rocks that are less expensive than the hydrochloride salt.

Cocaine free-base and crack are more stable to pyrolysis than is the hydrochloride salt, and therefore can be smoked either using a "coke pipe" or sprinkled on a cigarette or "joint." Crack and free-base cocaine are highly purified (85–90%). Crack is a greater risk to the user than is powdered cocaine because of its purity and high rate of absorption. Unlike nasal insufflation of cocaine hydrochloride—which exerts a vasoconstrictor effect on the nasal mucosa, thereby limiting its own absorption—crack smoking offers no such protection.

Crack users do not usually titrate or adjust their dosage, as do intranasal users.[203] Many free-base or crack users employ repetitive doses to achieve the rapid onset of euphoria (seconds) and to avoid the rapid dissipation and ensuing depression (5–7 minutes). They may continue this form of use for 12–24 hours before becoming exhausted and falling asleep. Intravenous injection and crack use both result in high drug concentrations and an associated euphoria leading to rapid drug dependence.

CLINICAL MANIFESTATIONS
Hyperthermia

By increasing psychomotor activity, cocaine augments heat production. There is also a decrease in heat dissipation resulting from cocaine-induced vasoconstriction (Chap. 18). Cocaine is postulated to have a direct stimulatory effect on thermoregulatory centers in the hypothalamic area, but this effect is not well substantiated. Finally, cocaine's stimulation of the calorigenic activity of the liver is believed to be an additional cause of hyperthermia.

Animal data demonstrate the clinical importance of cocaine-induced hyperthermia. One study compared the effects of hypertension and tachycardia, pH, acidosis, seizures, and hyperthermia on cocaine lethality. Only those agents that corrected hyperthermia improved survival.[22] In fact, reduced ambient temperature produced results that were equivalent to pharmacotherapy. In New York City, cocaine-related deaths increased when ambient temperatures were higher.[138]

Neurologic Effects

Cocaine is associated with an increased risk of stroke, which was documented in women to increase by 7-fold.[170] Cerebrovascular events—including subarachnoid hemorrhage,[131,196] intracerebral hemorrhage,[239] cerebral infarction,[62,129,130,197] transient ischemic attacks,[150] dystonic reactions,[21] toxic leukoencephalopathy,[139] migraine-type headache syndromes,[190] seizures,[27] cerebral vasculitis,[113,122] anterior spinal artery syndrome,[150] and varied psychiatric manifestations—are reported secondary to cocaine use. Most cocaine-toxic patients are anxious or agitated. This can be a transient effect of cocaine or it can reflect underlying organic or functional pathology.

Although some patients with neurologic catastrophes have had predisposing cerebrovascular disease[75,239] (for example, aneurysms or arteriovenous malformations), most have not. The pathophysiology of cerebrovascular infarction is probably similar to that of coronary arterial insufficiency[229] and includes hypercoagulability, impaired cerebrovascular autoregulation from increased cerebrovascular resistance,[129,130] vasoconstriction[112] and vasospasm,[62] embolism of particulate matter, and immunologically mediated arteritis or vasculitis.[20,122] In addition, the increased prevalence of anticardiolipin antibodies in cocaine users suggests that immunologic mechanisms may play a role in cocaine toxicity.[55]

Seizures may occur in the presence or absence of infarction or hemorrhage. Most seizures are single, generalized, induced by intravenous or crack cocaine, and are not associated with any lasting neurologic deficits. Multiple or focal seizures are usually associated with concomitant drug use or an underlying seizure disorder. A decreased level of consciousness and profound lethargy characterizes a "washed out" syndrome secondary to acute cocaine use. These patients are similar to patients with a prolonged postictal period except that they have a normal thought content. "Washed out" patients assume normal sleep postures and can occasionally be aroused to full orientation, in contrast to lethargic patients with subarachnoid hemorrhages or other intracranial catastrophes.

Cardiac Effects

Myocardial ischemia or infarction may occur secondary to cocaine insufflation, smoking, intravenous use, and even possibly during withdrawal.[5,35,59,88,90,92,98,128,147,156,222,242] The risk of myocardial infarction is increased 24-fold in the hour following cocaine use.[148] Myocardial infarctions typically occur in patients 19–60 years old without apparent massive exposures to cocaine or without concurrent seizures or agitation. Patients with cocaine-associated myocardial infarctions frequently have an atypical character to their

chest pain or pain that is delayed for hours to days after their most recent use of cocaine.[88,90,93,94,96] The ECGs of these patients may reveal abnormalities consisting of ST-segment elevation and T-wave inversions that often persist during hospitalization;[61,96,99] however, the electrocardiogram is less sensitive and less specific for myocardial infarction in patients who have recently used cocaine.[61,96,99] Cocaine induces vasoconstriction in both the left and right coronary arteries,[228] resulting in infarction within both distributions.[89,91,147] Q-wave and non-Q-wave infarctions occur with equal frequency.[5,89,91] Cocaine causes myocardial ischemia through a complex pathophysiology resulting from its acute and chronic effects.[86] Acutely, cocaine results in coronary artery vasoconstriction, tachycardia, systemic arterial hypertension, increased myocardial oxygen demand, platelet aggregation, and in situ thrombus formation.[88] Chronic cocaine users develop accelerated atherosclerosis and left ventricular hypertrophy, which can further exacerbate the oxygen supply-demand mismatch. There is no evidence to suggest that serum levels or route of administration alter the likelihood of developing ischemia.[91] Myocardial ischemia and infarction have occurred in patients without any underlying atherosclerotic disease or other evidence of preexisting heart disease.[29,102,105,147,166]

In patients with Prinzmetal's angina, ergonovine leads to a rise in systemic pressure, diffuse coronary artery narrowing, and focal vasospasm. In patients with cocaine-induced myocardial infarctions, however, administration of ergonovine uniformly fails to produce focal vasospasm.[102,105,166] One patient with a history of a cocaine-related ischemic event who had a negative ergonovine provocation test developed severe coronary vasospasm when provoked with intranasal cocaine.[104] Therefore, the absence of a response to this testing technique cannot exclude the possibility of cocaine-induced vasospasm.

With the use of ambulatory ECG (Holter) monitoring in patients admitted to an inpatient detoxification center, spontaneous episodes of ST-segment elevation occurred for up to 6 weeks after withdrawal of cocaine.[156] The researchers postulated that patients in cocaine withdrawal manifest a dopamine-depleted condition that results in intermittent coronary spasm. Myocardial infarction was documented in a 42-year-old man with normal coronary arteries, 3 days after his last use of cocaine.[35] Increased adrenergic-receptor sensitivity and catecholamine replenishment occurring during the cocaine withdrawal period were offered as an explanation. Further understanding of the pharmacologic characteristics of cocaine withdrawal may better explain these events.

Dysrhythmias.   Low-dose cocaine may result in bradycardias, whereas higher doses are associated with virtually all types of tachydysrhythmias. Sinus tachycardia; atrial fibrillation/flutter; other supraventricular tachycardias; ventricular premature contractions; accelerated idioventricular rhythms; ventricular tachycardia; torsades de pointes; and ventricular fibrillation may be the direct result of cocaine use. Laboratory studies demonstrate that high doses of cocaine result in infranodal and intraventricular conduction delays, and in lethal ventricular dysrhythmias secondary to prolonged QRS and QT intervals.[165,195] Clinical studies also have found a prolonged QT in patients with recent cocaine use.[99] These effects are similar to those observed with type IA and IC antidysrhythmic agents, and probably are mediated by the local anesthetic properties that result in sodium channel blockade. This may help to explain why increasing doses of cocaine appear to have a direct myocardial-depressant effect.[9,71,169,235] In addition to the local anesthetic effects, dysrhythmias may also occur as a result of cocaine-induced myocardial ischemia or infarction.[91,202]

Cardiomyopathy. Chronic cocaine use predisposes patients to the development of a dilated cardiomyopathy either from recurrent or diffuse ischemia with a subsequent "stunned" myocardium,[233] or from a direct effect on contractility independent of its ischemic effects.[108] Direct infusion of cocaine into human coronary arteries increases left ventricular end-diastolic pressures and end-systolic volume, as well as decreases left ventricular ejection fraction.[171] In some cases, the left ventricular systolic dysfunction may improve with cessation of cocaine use.[25] These results are comparable to the catecholamine-induced reversible cardiomyopathies associated with pheochromocytomas[103] and methamphetamine use.[101] Cocaine can also cause transplacental myocardial depression as evidenced by the fact that infants born to cocaine-using women had statistically lower cardiac outputs in the first day of life when compared with control infants.[226] The differences resolved by the second day of life.

Endocarditis and Endothelial Injury. An increased risk of upper extremity deep-vein thrombosis[132,133] and bacterial endocarditis[23] is associated with IV cocaine use. This risk of endocarditis seems to be increased over a similar population of IV heroin users and may result from the increased frequency of injections in cocaine users or from direct effects of cocaine on endovascular tissues and the immune system.[235]

Aortic Dissection. Several cases of cocaine-induced aortic dissection and rupture are reported.[178] Most, but not all patients had chronic cocaine use and were hypertensive. It is postulated that dissection and rupture result from the increased shear forces that are secondary to cocaine-induced hypertension, vasoconstriction, tachycardia. and possibly cocaine-induced vascular damage to media via effects on the vaso-vasorum.[178]

Pulmonary and Upper Airway Effects

Cocaine can result in a broad spectrum of acute pulmonary or upper airway complications.[69,218] These events range from asthma exacerbations, pneumothorax, pneumomediastinum,[127,201] acute lung injury,[31,78,114] diffuse alveolar hemorrhage,[153] recurrent pulmonary infiltrates with eosinophilia,[162] Goodpasture's syndrome,[56] and bronchiolitis obliterans with organizing pneumonia[167] to pulmonary vascular abnormalities[36,206,218] and upper airway burn and abscesses.[155] Cocaine may increase systemic vascular resistance with resultant left ventricular dysfunction and pulmonary edema.[47] Pulmonary artery hypertrophy, in the absence of foreign particle embolization, may also occur with chronic cocaine use.[154]

Chronic effects of cocaine on the lung appear to be related to the route of use, with crack smoking placing patients at highest risk.[2] Studies of pulmonary function in chronic cocaine users have not found significant long-term adverse effects on lung mechanics.[106,211,213,215] Heavy users of inhaled cocaine have normal spirometry; however, some studies have revealed a small decrease in the carbon monoxide-diffusing capacity (D_LCO), which is a physiologic marker of the integrity of the alveolar capillary membrane.[215] Chronic cocaine smokers might be at increased risk of lung cancer as early cellular abnormalities in the bronchial epithelium have been noted.[8] Acutely, smoked crack, but not intra-

venous cocaine, results in airway bronchoconstriction that may be mediated by foreign materials causing irritation or direct thermal injury.[214]

Skeletal Muscle Effects

Cocaine use can lead to severe rhabdomyolysis with massive elevations in creatine phosphokinase (CPK) levels, acute renal failure, profound hypotension, and hyperthermia.[6,16,77,144,145,163,185,186,205,236] Seizures, hyperthermia, hypotension, or prolonged unconsciousness are not necessary for the production of rhabdomyolysis.[241] Cocaine probably causes skeletal muscle ischemia through the same mechanisms by which it affects other vascular beds. Renal failure may result from both myoglobinuria and renal ischemia.[200]

Ophthalmic Effects

The visual system can be affected by cocaine both systemically and locally. Direct topical application of cocaine into the conjunctival sack denudes the corneal epithelium.[179] Particulate matter in smoke produces corneal abrasions and ulcerations ("crack eye").[142] Vascular effects, including central retinal artery occlusion and bilateral blindness from diffuse vasospasm, may also occur.[42,83]

Uteroplacental/Perinatal Effects

Maternal cocaine use decreases the likelihood of term deliveries and has an adverse effect on fetal growth and development.[1,24,26,43,136,161] An increased incidence of spontaneous abortions, abruptio placentae, fetal prematurity, and intrauterine growth retardation occurs. Experimental evidence in pregnant ewes demonstrated dose-dependent increases in maternal blood pressure with corresponding decreases in uterine blood flow.[152,240] Symptoms of neonatal cocaine withdrawal usually begin within 24–48 hours of birth. Withdrawal results in infants with jitteriness, irritability, poor eye contact, and vigorous sucking. In utero cocaine exposure also may result in infants with a small head circumference and low birth weight. Whether the decreased responsiveness and attentiveness observed in cocaine exposed neonates have long-term consequences is unknown.[49] At least one study suggests that prenatal cocaine exposure is not an additive risk for deficits in school-aged children with multiple other risk factors for slow development.[231] Both cocaine and cocaethylene bind to human milk and may be transmitted from nursing mothers to their infants.[7]

Gastrointestinal, Splenic, and Hepatic Vasculature

The intestinal vasculature is highly sensitive to catecholamines, because of the wide distribution of α-adrenergic receptors in the muscularis. Acute mucosal ischemia occurs following all common routes of cocaine use,[46,54,64,149,158] but is especially of concern following direct local toxicity in gastrointestinal drug smugglers (body packers).[158] Adverse consequences of cocaine occur in all age groups,[46,64,217] and with various clinical presentations, ranging from colitis to intestinal perforation.[51,126]

In various mouse models, cocaine is hepatotoxic, possibly through the formation of a species-specific reactive metabolite, norcocaine nitroxide,[63,110,116,117] or alternatively through the creation of a redox cycle that results in glutathione depletion.[115,116] Isolated hepatotoxicity in humans is uncommon. Hepatotoxicity usually manifests as elevations of aspartate aminotransferase (AST) and alanine aminotransferase (ALT) in the setting of hyperthermia or severe cardiovascular instability.

Psychological Effects

Tolerance and physical and psychological addiction to cocaine occur. Animal models, however, suggest that there also may be a "reverse tolerance" to the behavioral reactions of cocaine. It is theorized that the progressive effects of cocaine with use of smaller amounts may be related to "electrical kindling," a phenomenon in which "repetitive subthreshold electrical stimulation of the limbic system produces increasing effects on electrical activity and behavior, leading to seizures."[174]

The psychological or perceptual effects of cocaine can be disconcerting to the user. Some patients experience tactile hallucinations known as "cocaine bugs," or a crawling sensation under the skin with resultant self-excoriation, leading to irregular scratches and ulcers (Magnan's sign).

The stimulant abstinence syndrome follows a three-phase pattern of crash, withdrawal, and extinction, and typically occurs days after cocaine use, distinguishing it from the "washed out" syndrome that immediately follows acute cocaine toxicity. The crash is associated with intense depression, agitation, and anxiety. Withdrawal is marked by decreased energy, limited interest in the environment, and limited ability to experience pleasure. Extinction is the decrease in craving that occurs over time.[57]

DIAGNOSTIC TESTING

Most patients with mild cocaine toxicity do not require laboratory evaluation. The adrenergic effects of cocaine may be manifested on routine laboratory testing as leukocytosis, hyperglycemia, and hypokalemia. Patients with rhabdomyolysis, particularly if they are acidemic, may have hyperkalemia. The serum creatinine may be elevated in cases of rhabdomyolysis, renal failure, or renal infarction. Serial electrolyte determinations may be necessary in patients with rhabdomyolysis and/or renal insufficiency. The total CPK will be elevated in cases of rhabdomyolysis, and in almost half of patients with chest pain, most of whom will have myocardial infarction excluded by analysis with more specific cardiac markers.[96] Elevation of the myocardial fraction of CPK (CPK-MB) usually indicates a myocardial infarction (specificity is 75%), but false-positive elevations may occur.[97,143,222] Cardiac troponin I can confirm a myocardial infarction because it is more specific than CPK-MB (96%).[97,143] Chest radiography should be ordered if pneumonia, pulmonary infarction, pneumothorax, pneumomediastinum, or pneumopericardium are suspected.[48] Abdominal radi-

ography may detect cocaine packages (Chap. 8). Computerized tomography should be used to detect cerebrovascular events. Magnetic resonance imaging, angiography, or transesophageal echocardiography may be useful for the assessment of aortic dissection. Additional laboratory or diagnostic testing should be considered depending on the clinical condition. For example, lumbar puncture should be performed in patients with suspected subarachnoid hemorrhage and normal head CT scans; ventilation-perfusion scans or contrast spiral computerized tomography should be used in patients suspected of pulmonary infarction or embolus.

The initial electrocardiogram is less sensitive and less specific for identification of myocardial infarction in patients with cocaine-associated chest pain when compared to other patients with chest pain. Myocardial infarction can occur in both patients with normal and abnormal electrocardiograms. ST-segment elevation caused by early repolarization is common in young cocaine users without myocardial infarction.[61,96,99] ST-segment elevations that meet standard thrombolysis criteria are present in 11–43% of cocaine-associated chest pain patients who are not found to have infarctions.

Resting sestamibi scans can help risk stratify patients with cocaine associated chest pain syndromes.[120] In this group patients with normal resting images following injection during pain or patients with normal cardiac markers, normal or nonspecific electrocardiograms and an uneventful 9–12 hour period of observation can be safely released from the Emergency Department (ED) with followup arrangements.[86,120,121,232]

Nasal swabs and serum or urine analyses for cocaine can be performed. Laboratory tests available are gas chromatography (GC) and thin-layer chromatography (TLC) (benzoylecgonine in the serum or urine), as well as EMIT (enzyme-multiplied immunoassay techniques) and gas chromatography-mass spectrometry. Table 67–1 presents the relative sensitivity of the screening and definitive assays for cocaine and benzoylecgonine. Urine immunoassays for cocaine metabolites generally detect the major metabolite of cocaine, benzoylecgonine, at or above concentrations of 300 ng/mL. Usually, the presence of cocaine or its metabolites can be detected for 48–72 hours after use.[4] Rarely, using more sensitive methods (GC/MS), cocaine metabolites have been detected for up 3 weeks after the last use.[234] Because false-positive immunoassays are very unlikely, confirmation based upon GC/MS is largely performed only for legal reasons.

MANAGEMENT

Treatment of patients with cocaine toxicity requires an understanding of the underlying pathophysiology. The clinical approach to treatment requires an understanding of the acute and chronic ef-

TABLE 67–1.   Laboratory Assays for Cocaine and Benzoylecgonine (BE)

Laboratory Assay	Specimen	BE	Cocaine	Sensitivity
EMIT (enzyme-multiplied immunoassay technique)	Urine	X	—	200–300 ng/mL
RIA (radioimmunoassay)	Urine/blood	X	X	50–100 ng/mL
TLC (thin-layer chromatography)	Urine	X	—	1000 ng/mL
GC (gas chromatography)	Serum/urine	X	X	200–300 ng/mL
HPLC (high pressure liquid chromatography)	Serum/urine	X	X	200–300 ng/mL
GC-MS (gas chromatography-mass spectrometry)	Serum/urine	X	X	200–300 ng/mL

X = detectable.

fects of cocaine, both vascular and nonvascular effects, as well as the fact that cardiovascular and neurologic complications are inextricably linked (Fig. 67–2).

Nonvascular Manifestations

Because of the direct pharmacologic and toxicologic relationship between the neuropsychiatric and cardiovascular complications, successful management of the neuropsychiatric manifestations almost invariably has a salutary impact on resolution of the cardiovascular abnormalities, at least from an emergent or initial care perspective.

Agitation and Hyperthermia.   Animal studies uniformly demonstrate that the major causes of death from cocaine toxicity are psychomotor agitation and hyperthermia.[22,67] In these studies and in others, sedative-hypnotic agents are invariably successful for the treatment of cocaine toxicity and the prevention of lethality.[22,37,67] Figure 67–2 illustrates the predicted failure of therapeutic interventions directed solely at ameliorating the peripheral manifestations of cocaine toxicity. Thus, sedation with a benzodiazepine is chosen, because of demonstrable experimental efficacy[22,37,67] and substantial experience with their use in other clinical conditions associated with severe agitation and catecholamine excess, such as sedative-hypnotic or ethanol withdrawal. Interestingly, cocaine-associated chest pain syndromes respond as well to diazepam as they do to nitroglycerin.[10]

Agitation and seizures are managed in the standard manner, with a focus on rapid control of motor activity while protecting the patient's airway and achieving adequate ventilation and oxygenation. If possible, physical restraints should be avoided, but the initial transient use of restraints may be essential to secure intravenous access. If a restraining blanket is used, it should be constructed of a strong netting or mesh to avoid increasing the pa-

tient's temperature by preventing heat dissipation. Protecting the patient from hypoglycemia and hypoxia are critical; therefore, high-flow oxygen should be routinely administered and 0.5–1.0 g/kg of $D_{50}W$ and 100 mg of thiamine should be given as clinically indicated. If the patient manifests severe agitation, IV doses of a benzodiazepine should be used until sedation is achieved (Table 67–2). Most antipsychotic agents should be avoided, as they may confuse the clinical picture, impair heat dissipation, exacerbate an anticholinergic crisis, precipitate a dystonic reaction, or in some cases lower the seizure threshold and exacerbate cocaine-induced lethality.[22,39,67,238]

Diazepam, or another benzodiazepine such as lorazepam, should be used intravenously for initial management of seizures. Although no studies have compared barbiturates to phenytoin for control of cocaine-induced seizures, barbiturates are theoretically preferable because they also produce CNS sedation and are generally more effective for toxin-induced convulsions. If these agents are not rapidly effective, nondepolarizing neuromuscular blockade and general anesthesia may be indicated. Succinylcholine, a depolarizing neuromuscular-blocking agent, should be avoided because it may increase the risk of hyperkalemia in the setting of severe cocaine-induced rhabdomyolysis. In addition, the enzyme plasma cholinesterase is responsible for the metabolism of both succinylcholine and cocaine, so that, theoretically, if these two agents are used simultaneously, prolonged clinical effects of either or both agents might result.

Control of the patient's hyperthermia is best achieved by rapid cooling with an ice-water bath. Conduction and evaporation are rapidly efficacious. Control of the associated agitation, psychosis, or seizures is essential to maintain cooling while avoiding cerebral, hepatic, and skeletal muscle cellular destruction. There is no evidence that other pharmacologic agents (such as dantrolene) enhance the cooling process in patients with cocaine-related life-threatening hyperthermia.[53]

Dysrhythmias.   Atrial tachydysrhythmias that do not respond to sedative-hypnotic agents or control of the central sympathetic stimulus and cooling should respond to verapamil or diltiazem. The treatment of cocaine-induced ventricular dysrhythmias depends upon the time between cocaine use, dysrhythmia onset, and commencement of treatment. Ventricular dysrhythmias that develop rapidly following cocaine use should be presumed to occur from the local anesthetic effects of cocaine on the myocardium. Animal evidence overwhelmingly demonstrates the importance of these type I antidysrhythmic effects of cocaine.[9,11,66,237] In fact, in some animal models, cocaine-induced wide-complex dysrhythmias respond to the administration of sodium bicarbonate, in a manner similar to dysrhythmias associated with other type IA and type IC agents (Chaps. 52 and 57 and Antidote in Depth: Sodium Bicarbonate).[11,237] In addition, one animal model suggested that lidocaine exacerbated cocaine-induced seizures and dysrhythmias as a result of similar effects on sodium channels.[40] Although additive cardiac toxicities of lidocaine and cocaine might be anticipated because of lidocaine's IB antidysrhythmic effects, they have not been confirmed in other animal models.[66,74,237] Lidocaine has fast on-off sodium channel-binding kinetics, and might be expected to compete with cocaine (which has slow on-off kinetics) for binding to the sodium channel. Because lidocaine rarely affects QRS duration, QRS would be expected to shorten as lidocaine displaces cocaine from sodium channels. In humans with cocaine toxicity, wide-complex dysrhythmias are also reported.[105,230] Al-

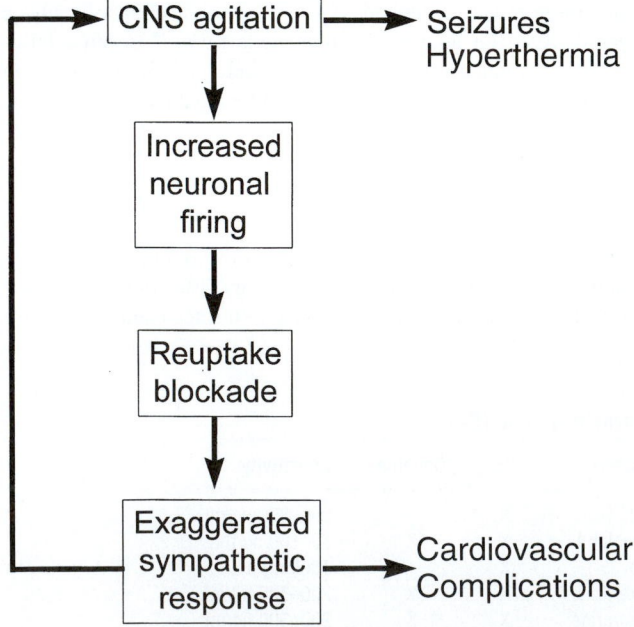

Figure 67–2.   Cocaine-induced CNS effects modulate peripheral events.

TABLE 67–2.   Treatment Summary for Specific Cocaine-Related Medical Conditions

Medical Condition	Treatments
Cardiovascular complications	
Dysrhythmias	
Sinus tachycardia	Observation
	Oxygen
	Diazepam 5–10 mg IV or lorazepam 1–2 mg IV titrated to effect
Supraventricular tachycardia	Oxygen
	Diazepam 5–10 mg IV or lorazepam 1–2 mg IV
	Diltiazem 20 mg IV or verapamil 5–10 mg IV
	Adenosine 6 mg or 12 mg IV
	Cardioversion if hemodynamically unstable
Ventricular dysrhythmias	Oxygen
	Sodium bicarbonate, 1–2 mEq/kg
	Lidocaine 1.5 mg/kg IV bolus followed by 2 mg/min infusion
	Defibrillation if hemodynamically unstable
	Diazepam 5–10 mg IV or lorazepam 1–2 mg IV
Acute coronary syndrome	Oxygen
	Diazepam 5–10 mg IV or lorazepam 1–2 mg IV
	Soluble aspirin 325 mg
	Nitroglycerin 1/150 mg sublingual × 3 every 5 minutes followed by an infusion titrated to a mean arterial pressure reduction of 10% or relief of chest pain.
	Morphine sulfate 2 mg IV q5min titrated to pain relief
	Phentolamine 1 mg IV; repeat in 5 minutes
	Verapamil 5–10 mg IV
	Heparin or low molecular weight heparin
	Percutaneous intervention (angioplasty and stent placement)
	Glycoprotein IIb/IIIa inhibitors
	Fibrinolytic therapy
Hypertension	Observation
	Diazepam 5–10 mg IV or lorazepam 1–2 mg IV titrated to effect
	Phentolamine 1 mg IV; repeat in 5 minutes
	Nitroglycerin or nitroprusside continuous infusion titrated to effect
Pulmonary edema	Furosemide 20–40 mg IV
	Morphine sulfate 2 mg IV q5min titrated to pain relief or respiratory status
	Nitroglycerin infusion titrated to blood pressure
	Consider phentolamine or nitroprusside
Hyperthermia	Sedation with benzodiazepines, monitor temperature
	Submersion in an ice bath
Neuropsychiatric symptoms	
Anxiety and agitation	Diazepam 5–10 mg IV or lorazepam 2–4 mg IV titrated to effect
Seizures	Diazepam 5–10 mg IV or lorazepam 2–4 mg IV titrated to effect
	Phenobarbital 25–50 mg/min up to 10–20 mg/kg
Intracranial hemorrhage	Neurosurgery consultation
Rhabdomyolysis	IV hydration to maintain urine output at 3 mL/kg/h
	Sodium bicarbonate titrated to an alkaline urine
	Hemodialysis, as necessary for renal failure
Cocaine washed-out syndrome	Supportive care
Body-packers	Activated charcoal
	Whole-bowel irrigation
	Admission to monitored setting even if asymptomatic
	Laparotomy or endoscopic retrieval for obstruction or cocaine-related symptoms

though bicarbonate therapy may be preferable, and has been used effectively,[230] lidocaine may also be beneficial, especially after benzodiazepines have been given to prevent the additive (cocaine and lidocaine) convulsant effects demonstrated in animals.[40,74] Although amiodarone is gaining popularity for routine management of ventricular dysrhythmias of other etiologies, it cannot be recommended for acute cocaine-induced tachydysrhythmias at this time because it is largely unstudied. In patients who present several hours after the last use of cocaine, the ventricular dysrhythmias may be generated by an ischemic myocardium, and standard management for ventricular dysrhythmias, including lidocaine[202] or possibly amiodarone, is indicated, and appears safe. Torsades de pointes is a rare complication of cocaine use.[194] It results from cocaine's ability to block potassium channels (Chaps. 9 and 21). Sodium bicarbonate therapy would not be indicated because the resultant hypokalemia would be expected to exacerbate this effect. Torsades de pointes resulting from cocaine toxicity should be managed with intravenous magnesium sulfate and overdrive pacing.

Rhabdomyolysis. Patients with significant elevation of CPK or myoglobinuria (rhabdomyolysis) require vigorous hydration to maintain a urine output of at least 3 mL/kg per hour; sodium bicarbonate to alkalinize the urine with careful monitoring of the serum potassium; and hemodialysis if renal failure occurs.

Vascular Manifestations

The vascular effects of cocaine occur through the acute stimulation of coronary artery vasoconstriction, in situ thrombus formation, platelet aggregation, decreased endogenous fibrinolysis, and increased myocardial oxygen demand secondary to hypertension and tachycardia. Chronic cocaine users may have more exaggerated oxygen supply-demand mismatch because of left ventricular hypertrophy and premature atherosclerosis. Other vascular beds may be involved based on identical mechanisms. Treatment of the vascular manifestations of cocaine toxicity should focus on the reversible causes of oxygen supply-demand mismatch: arterial vasoconstriction, platelet aggregation, thrombus formation, hypertension, and tachycardia. It is important to note that cocaine-induced vasoconstriction persists well beyond the time period of hypertension.[204]

Coronary Vasoconstriction. Studies in the cardiac catheterization laboratory have helped to elucidate the mechanisms of coronary artery vasoconstriction and have helped to evaluate several treatment options. In these studies, adults without prior cocaine use who were undergoing coronary catheterization for evaluation of underlying coronary artery disease were given 2 mg/kg of intranasal cocaine. Patients developed an increase in heart rate, blood pressure, and coronary vascular resistance. Coronary arterial diameter was diffusely narrowed by approximately 13%.[125] This effect of cocaine occurs in both the left and right coronary systems.[228] Following infusion of phentolamine (0.4 mg/min), an α-adrenergic antagonist, these parameters returned to baseline.[125] This suggests that cocaine-induced vasoconstriction is caused through an α-adrenergic mechanism and that phentolamine may be useful for treatment of cocaine-induced ischemia. At least one case report supports the use of phentolamine for patients with cocaine-induced myocardial ischemia.[90] The International Guidelines for Emergency Cardiovascular Care recommend α-adrenergic antagonists (phentolamine) for the treatment of cocaine-associated acute coronary syndrome.[219] Studies in the cardiac catheterization laboratory also demonstrate that nitroglycerin reverses cocaine-induced vasoconstriction.[17] In addition, a clinical case series found that nitroglycerin relieves cocaine-induced chest pain.[95] Chronic cocaine users, who may be more prone to atherosclerosis, might be at higher risk of ischemia because there is enhanced vasoconstriction at sites of significant coronary artery stenosis.[52] In addition, cigarette smoking enhances cocaine's vasoconstrictive effects.[88]

Coronary artery vasoconstriction was exacerbated by the administration of propranolol, a β-adrenergic antagonist, and resulted in anginal symptoms and ST-segment elevation in one of the study patients described previously.[124] Because propranolol inhibits the β_2-adrenergic receptors, an unopposed α-adrenergic receptor stimulation may occur, resulting in vasoconstriction and an increased blood pressure. This unopposed α-adrenergic effect was observed in some case series.[175–177] The increased afterload along with decreased left ventricular function might adversely effect systemic blood flow and tissue perfusion. These human observations

were confirmed in experimental animal models of cocaine toxicity, in which the use of β-adrenergic antagonists led to decreased coronary blood flow, increased seizure frequency, and high fatality rates.[22,67,208,209,227] The use of short acting β-adrenergic antagonists such as esmolol demonstrates similarly poor results,[173,189] with unopposed α-adrenergic effects resulting in significant increases in blood pressure for as many as 25% of patients. As a result of the compelling animal and human data, the use of β-adrenergic antagonists for the treatment of cocaine toxicity must be considered absolutely contraindicated.[72,87,88,219]

Labetalol does not appear to offer any advantages over pure β-adrenergic antagonists. Although some case reports fail to reproduce adverse outcomes,[45,58,111] labetalol has substantially more β-adrenergic antagonism than α-adrenergic antagonist effects.[212] Labetalol use results in unopposed α effects with severe hypertension in patients with pheochromocytomas,[15] increases the risk of seizure and death in animal models of cocaine toxicity,[208] and does not reverse cocaine-induced coronary artery vasoconstriction in humans.[13] The role, if any, for pure β and mixed α- and β-adrenergic antagonists in the treatment of cocaine toxicity has not been established. The choice of an antihypertensive agent that is rapid-acting, easily administered, and reliably controlled favors the use of vasodilating agents such as nitroprusside, nitroglycerin, or an α-adrenergic antagonist such as phentolamine.

Data regarding the efficacy of calcium channel blockers for the treatment of cocaine toxicity are contradictory. Some studies of cocaine-intoxicated animals that were pretreated with calcium channel blockers have yielded favorable results in a variety of end-points such as survival, seizures, and cardiac dysrrhythmias.[12,157,224] In contradistinction, other studies have found adverse effects in which these same outcomes were analyzed.[37] In experimental models of cocaine toxic animals that were not pretreated with calcium channel blockers, the subsequent administration of these agents has not been beneficial.[38,70,208] Using the human cardiac catheterization model of cocaine toxicity, verapamil does reverse cocaine-induced coronary artery vasoconstriction.[160] However, large-scale multicenter clinical trials of more than 5000 patients with myocardial ischemia unrelated to cocaine did not find beneficial effects of calcium channel blockers on important outcomes such as survival. As a result, the role of calcium channel blockers in patients with cocaine-induced vascular ischemia remains unclear.

Noncoronary Vasoconstriction. Cocaine-induced constriction of the cerebral,[20,112,130] ophthalmic,[83] pulmonary,[36,206] mesenteric,[54,158] and musculoskeletal[241] vascular beds is well-described in human case reports. Additionally, animal models describe cerebral vasoconstriction.[137] Although inadequately studied, all of these effects are presumed to occur by mechanisms similar to those described for cocaine-induced coronary vasoconstriction. As a result, the treatment strategies described should be initiated in patients with clinical signs and symptoms suggestive of vasoconstriction in noncoronary vascular beds.

Platelet and Thrombus Formation. Cocaine can directly injure the vascular endothelium, increase platelet aggregation through both direct and indirect pathways, and can impair normal fibrinolytic pathways by enhancing the effects of endogenous tissue plasminogen activator inhibitor.[151,180,181,192,221] As a result, the use of aspirin, heparin, and thrombolytic agents makes theoretical sense in the setting of vascular ischemia.[81,85,88,89] When considering the use of thrombolytic agents for acute myocardial infarction, the clinician must recognize that many young patients may have benign early repolarization and that only a small percentage of patients with cocaine-associated chest pain syndromes and J-point/ST-segment elevation are actually sustaining an acute infarction.[99] In addition, there are several case reports that document adverse outcomes following thrombolytic administration in patients with recent cocaine use.[19,100,134] The use of thrombolytic agents for vascular ischemia should be reserved for patients who are definitely having a myocardial infarction, who cannot have percutaneous interventions (angioplasty or stent placement), who fail to respond to vasodilator therapy, and who have low risk for cerebrovascular or other serious bleeding catastrophes.[81] The use of thrombolytic therapy for cocaine-induced cerebrovascular or mesenteric ischemia has not been studied. Limited experience with glycoprotein IIb/IIIa antagonists suggests that they may be useful in patients with cocaine-associated acute coronary syndromes.[50]

Hypertension and Tachycardia. These hemodynamic effects of cocaine rarely require specific treatment. Treatments aimed at the resolution of anxiety, agitation, hyperthermia, ischemia, and hypoxia will often lead to resolution of the abnormal hemodynamic parameters. When necessary, treatment aimed at the central effects of cocaine, such as benzodiazepines, will usually lead to reduction in blood pressure and heart rate. When hypertension fails to respond to sedation, it can be managed with sodium nitroprusside (0.5–10 μg/kg/min) titrated to achieve and maintain a normal blood pressure. Intravenous phentolamine at doses of 0.4 mg/min or nitroglycerin (starting at a dose of 10 μg/min) are effective vasodilators and may improve coronary perfusion.[17,125] Cocaine-toxic patients should be considered to have an acute elevation in blood pressure. Reduction of the blood pressure to a normal level should therefore occur, without concern of cerebral hypoperfusion, unless there is documentation or clinical evidence of long-standing hypertension.

The other cardiovascular end-organ manifestations of cocaine toxicity that may necessitate specific intervention are summarized in Table 67–2 which summarizes the general strategies for managing catecholamine excess, myocardial ischemia, and hypertension. These strategies allow for very case-specific approaches to complicated examples, such as aortic dissection, mesenteric ischemia, and abruptio placenta.

"BODY PACKERS" AND "BODY STUFFERS"

The act of swallowing containers, condoms, balloons, plastic bags, or packages filled with illegal drugs for the purpose of smuggling is called "body packing" and the individual who carries the pack-

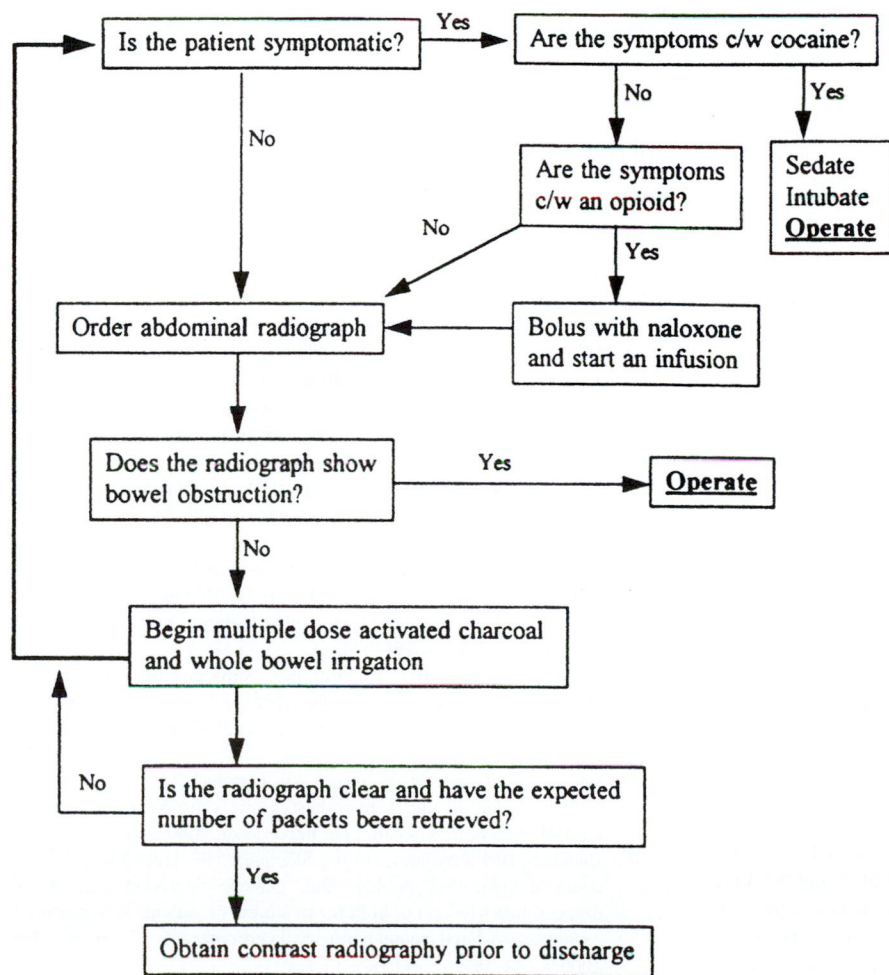

Figure 67–3. Algorithm for managing cocaine or heroin "body packers" (c/w = consistent with).

ages is called a "mule."[84,141] Body packers swallow large quantities of drugs. Patients being arrested who swallow illegal drugs to conceal the evidence are referred to as "body stuffers."[79,182] Unlike body packers, whose contraband is very carefully packaged to protect them and the drugs from gastrointestinal absorption, body stuffers do not take such precautions, and drug absorption is common, despite the fact that they ingest less drugs than body packers. Body stuffers also tend to ingest any and all the drugs they possess, potentially resulting in a polypharmaceutic overdose. Both body packers and body stuffers are unlikely to admit to their ingestion. Body packers may be discovered in airports having just arrived from a foreign country known to produce, export, or be a transit site for illegal drugs. Body stuffers are likely to be found near their homes.

Body stuffers may be seen before symptoms have developed. Activated charcoal should be given immediately; multiple-dose activated charcoal and a cathartic or whole-bowel irrigation may occasionally be indicated. In body packers, the drugs are usually located in the small and large bowel and are quite difficult to recover. Most body packers may be diagnosed by radiographic means, as the packages used to smuggle drugs are often radiopaque or have a distinct radiographic characteristic (Chap. 8).[141] Body stuffers are unlikely to be diagnosed by radiography.[79] The most success is seen with identification of crack vials or staples on the packaging materials. Most body packers will be asymptomatic unless leakage occurs. Symptomatic patients should be considered a medical emergency, and be evaluated for surgical removal of the packets. Both body packers and body stuffers should be treated with activated charcoal to limit cocaine absorption and whole-bowel irrigation may be considered to decrease gastrointestinal transit time.[84,223] They should be monitored in an intensive care unit setting until the cocaine bags have been eliminated, even if they are asymptomatic. Followup plain radiography and a barium swallow with small bowel follow-through offer definitive reassurance that all packages have been evacuated.[84] Figure 67–3 summarizes this treatment plan.

In approximately 3% of cases, surgical removal may be necessary for bowel obstruction or cocaine toxicity.[3] Obstruction at the ileocecal valve or splenic flexure may necessitate laparotomy with enterotomy. Although some physicians have operated on patients with gastric outlet obstruction, others have successfully retrieved a bag with endoscopic techniques.[84]

SUMMARY

The differential diagnosis of cocaine toxicity can be subdivided into three areas of consideration: the adrenergic toxidrome (Tables 17–1 and 67–3), specific complaints directly related to cocaine, and disease processes masked or confounded by cocaine.

Specific complaints directly related to cocaine may include such signs and symptoms as chest pain, abdominal pain, or shortness of breath. Although cocaine use can result in these symptoms, the differential diagnosis includes disease processes both related to and unrelated to cocaine. For example, chest pain may be caused by chest wall rhabdomyolysis, pneumothorax, or myocardial ischemia resulting from cocaine use, or it may be caused by pneumonia or pleurisy unrelated to cocaine. A history of recent cocaine use significantly increases the likelihood of serious etiologies for many otherwise common complaints. Although most cocaine-related adverse events occur within several hours of cocaine use,

TABLE 67–3. Differential Diagnosis of the Adrenergic Agent Toxidrome

Toxins
  Cocaine; phencyclidine; amphetamines; hallucinogens; caffeine; phenylpropanolamine; theophylline; ephedrine; pseudoephedrine; tyramine; MAO inhibitors
Metabolic disorders
  Pheochromocytoma; hypoglycemia; thyrotoxicosis
Neuropsychiatric disturbances
  Complex status epilepticus; schizophrenia; psychosis; mania
Drug withdrawal
  Ethanol; sedative-hypnotics

remote cocaine use (in the past several weeks) is also associated with vascular disasters in patients without other known predisposing factors.

Cocaine toxic patients may have concurrent ethanol ingestions, or mixed overdoses that mask some of the effects of cocaine. On the other hand, serious medical problems should not be falsely attributed to cocaine without excluding underlying medical pathology. For example, patients with an altered mental status may still need to undergo computerized tomography to exclude a subdural hematoma that may not have been caused directly by cocaine. Mental status changes caused by cocaine are short-lived. Waiting too long to determine whether the patient's mental status improves after cocaine is metabolized may have adverse consequences. Only a thoughtful and thorough evaluation of such patients will lead to the correct diagnosis.

REFERENCES

1. Acker D, Sachs BP, Tracey KJ: Abruptio placentae associated with cocaine use. Am J Obstet Gynecol 1983;146:220–221.
2. Albertson TE, Walby WF, Derlet RW: Stimulant-induced pulmonary toxicity. Chest 1995;108:1140–1149.
3. Aldrighetti L, Paganelli M, Giacomelli M, Villa G, Ferla G: Conservative management of cocaine-packet ingestion: Experience in Milan, the main Italian smuggling center of South American cocaine. Panminerva Med 1996;38:111–116.
4. Ambre J: The urinary excretion of cocaine and metabolites in humans: A kinetic analysis of published data. J Anal Toxicol 1985;9:241–245.
5. Amin M, Gabelman G, Karpel J, et al: Acute myocardial infarction and chest pain: Syndromes after cocaine use. Am J Cardiol 1990;66:1434–1437.
6. Anand V, Siami G, Stone WJ: Cocaine-associated rhabdomyolysis and acute renal failure. South Med J 1989;82:67–69.
7. Bailey DN: Cocaine and cocaethylene binding to human milk. Am J Clin Pathol 1998;110:491–494.
8. Barsky SH, Roth MD, Kleerup ED, Simmons M, Tashkin DP: Histopathologic and molecular alterations in bronchial epithelium in habitual smokers of marijuana, cocaine and/or tobacco. J Natl Cancer Inst 1998;90:1198–1205.
9. Bauman JL, Grawe JJ, Winecoff AP, Hariman RJ: Cocaine-related sudden cardiac death: A hypothesis correlating basic science and clinical observations. J Clin Pharmacol 1994;34:902–911.
10. Baumann BM, Perrone J, Hornig SE, Shofer FS, Hollander JE: Randomized controlled, double-blind, placebo-controlled trial of diazepam, nitroglycerin or both for treatment of patients with potential cocaine associated acute coronary syndromes. Acad Emerg Med 2000;7:878–885.

11. Beckman KJ, Parker RB, Hariman RJ, et al: Hemodynamic and electrophysiological actions of cocaine: Effects of sodium bicarbonate as an antidote in dogs. Circulation 1991;83:1799–1807.

12. Billman GE, Hoskins RS: Cocaine-induced ventricular fibrillation: Protection afforded by the calcium antagonist verapamil. FASEB J 1988;2:2990–2995.

13. Boehrer JD, Moliterno DJ, Willard JE, et al: Influence of labetalol of cocaine-induced coronary vasoconstriction in humans. Am J Med 1993;94:608–610.

14. Borne RF, Bedford JA, Buelke JL, et al: Biological effects of cocaine, derivatives I: Improved synthesis and pharmacologic evaluation of norcocaine. J Pharm Sci 1977;66:119–129.

15. Briggs RSJ, Birtwell AJ, Pohl JEF: Hypertensive response to labetalol in pheochromocytoma. Lancet 1978;1:1045–1046.

16. Brody SL, Wrenn KD, Wilber MM, Slovis CM: Predicting the severity of cocaine-associated rhabdomyolysis. Ann Emerg Med 1990;19:1137–1143.

17. Brogan WC, Lange RA, Kim AS, et al: Alleviation of cocaine-induced coronary vasoconstriction by nitroglycerin. J Am Coll Cardiol 1991;18:581–586.

18. Brookoff D, Rotondo MF, Shaw LM, et al: Cocaethylene levels in patients who test positive for cocaine. Ann Emerg Med 1996;27:316–320.

19. Bush HS: Cocaine associated myocardial infarction: A word of caution about thrombolytic therapy. Chest 1988;94:878.

20. Caplan LR, Hier DB, Banks G: Current concepts of cerebrovascular disease: Stroke and drug abuse. Stroke 1982;13:869–872.

21. Catalano G, Catalano MC, Rodriguez R: Dystonia associated with crack cocaine use. South Med J 1997;90:1050–1052.

22. Catravas JD, Waters IW: Acute cocaine intoxication in the conscious dog: Studies on the mechanism of lethality. J Pharmacol Exp Ther 1981;217:350–356.

23. Chambers HF, Morris DL, Tauber MG, Modin G: Cocaine use and the risk for endocarditis in intravenous drug users. Ann Intern Med 1987;106:833–836.

24. Chavez GF, Mulinare J, Cordero JF: Maternal cocaine use during early pregnancy as a risk factor for congenital urogenital anomalies. JAMA 1989;262:795–798.

25. Chokshi SK, Moore R, Pandian NG, et al: Reversible cardiomyopathy associated with cocaine intoxication. Ann Intern Med 1989;111:1039–1040.

26. Chouteau M, Namerow PB, Leppert P: The effect of cocaine abuse on birth weight and gestational age. Obstet Gynecol 1988;72:351–354.

27. Choy-Kwong M, Lipton RB: Seizures in hospitalized cocaine users. Neurology 1989;39:425–427.

28. Covert RF, Schreiber MD, Tebbett IR, Torgerson LJ: Hemodynamic and cerebral blood flow effects of cocaine, cocaethylene and benzoylecgonine in conscious and anesthetized fetal lambs. J Pharmacol Exp Ther 1994;270:118–126.

29. Cregler LL, Mark H: Relation of acute myocardial infarction to cocaine abuse. Am J Cardiol 1985;56:794.

30. Crumb WJ, Clarkson CW: Characterization of sodium channel blocking properties of the major metabolites of cocaine in single cardiac myocytes. J Pharmacol Exp Ther 1992;261:910–917.

31. Cucco RA, Yoo OH, Gregler L, et al: Non-fatal pulmonary edema after freebase cocaine smoking. Am Rev Resp Dis 1987;136:179–181.

32. Dailey RH: Fatality secondary to misuse of TAC solution. Ann Emerg Med 1988;17:159–160.

33. Daya MR, Burton BT, Schleiss MR, et al: Recurrent seizures following mucosal application of TAC. Ann Emerg Med 1988;17:646–648.

34. Dehner D, Hamilton GC: Seizures following topical applications of local anesthetics to burn patients. Ann Emerg Med 1984;13:456–458.

35. Del Aguila C, Rosman H: Myocardial infarction during cocaine withdrawal [letter]. Ann Intern Med 1990;112:712.

36. Delaney K, Hoffman RS: Pulmonary infarction associated with crack cocaine use in a previously healthy 23-year-old woman. Am J Med 1991;91:92–94.

37. Derlet RW, Albertson TE: Diazepam in the prevention of seizures and death in cocaine-intoxicated rats. Ann Emerg Med 1989;18:542–546.

38. Derlet RW, Albertson TE: Potentiation of cocaine toxicity with calcium channel blockers. Am J Emerg Med 1989;7:464–468.

39. Derlet RW, Albertson TE, Rice P: The effect of haloperidol in cocaine and amphetamine intoxication. J Emerg Med 1989;7:633–637.

40. Derlet RW, Albertson TE, Tharratt RS: Lidocaine potentiation of cocaine toxicity. Ann Emerg Med 1991;20:135–138.

41. Devenyi P: Cocaine complications and pseudocholinesterase [letter]. Ann Intern Med 1989;110:167–168.

42. Devenyi P, Schneiderman JF, Devenyi RG, Lawby L: Cocaine-induced central retinal artery occlusion. Can Med Assoc J 1988;138:129–130.

43. Doberczak TM, Shanzer S, Senie RT, et al: Neonatal neurologic and electroencephalographic effects of intrauterine cocaine exposure. J Pediatr 1988;113:354–358.

44. Dronen SC: Complications of TAC [letter]. Ann Emerg Med 1983;12:333.

45. Dusenberry SJ, Hicks MJ, Mariani PJ: Labetalol treatment of cocaine toxicity [letter]. Ann Emerg Med 1987;16:235.

46. Endress C, Kling GA: Cocaine-induced small-bowel perforation. Am J Roentgenol 1990;154:1346–1347.

47. Ettinger NA, Albin RJ: A review of the respiratory effects of smoking cocaine. Am J Med 1989;87:664–668.

48. Eurman DW, Potash HI, Eyler WR, et al: Chest pain and dyspnea related to "crack" cocaine smoking: Value of chest radiography. Radiology 1989;172:459–462.

49. Eyler FD, Behnke M, Conlon M, Woods NS, Wobie K: Birth outcome from a prospective, matched study of prenatal crack/cocaine use: II. Interactive and dose effects on neurobehavioral assessment. Pediatrics 1998;101:237–241.

50. Frangogiannis NG, Farmer JA, Lakkis NM: Tirofiban for cocaine induced coronary artery thrombosis. A novel therapeutic approach. Circulation 1999;100:1939.

51. Fishel R, Hamamoto G, Barbul A, et al: Cocaine colitis: Is this a new syndrome? Dis Colon Rectum 1985;28:264–266.

52. Flores ED, Lange RA, Cigarroa RG, et al: Effect of cocaine on coronary artery dimensions in atherosclerotic coronary artery: Enhanced vasoconstriction at sites of significant stenoses. J Am Coll Cardiol 1990;16:74–79.

53. Fox AW: More on rhabdomyolysis associated with cocaine intoxication [letter]. N Engl J Med 1989;321:1271.

54. Freudenberger RS, Cappell MS, Hutt DA: Intestinal infarction after intravenous cocaine administration. Ann Intern Med 1990;113:715–716.

55. Fritsma GA, Leikin JB, Maturen AJ, et al: Detection of anticardiolipin antibody in patients with cocaine abuse. J Emerg Med 1991;9:37–43.

56. Garcia-Rostan Y Perez GM, Bragado FG, Gil AMP: Pulmonary hemorrhage and antiglomerular basement membrane antibody-mediated glomerulonephritis after exposure to smoked cocaine (crack). A case report and review of the literature. Pathol Int 1997;47:692–697.

57. Gawin FH, Kleber HD: Abstinence symptomatology and psychiatric diagnosis in cocaine abusers. Arch Gen Psychiatry 1986;43:107–113.

58. Gay GR, Loper KA: The use of labetalol in the management of cocaine crisis. Ann Emerg Med 1988;17:282–283.

59. Gioia G, Manuel M, Russell J, et al: Myocardial perfusion pattern in patients with cocaine-induced chest pain. Am J Cardiol 1995;75:396–398.

60. Giros B, Jaber M, Jones S, et al: Hyperlocomotion and indifference to cocaine and amphetamine in mice lacking the dopamine transporter. Nature 1996;379:606–612.

61. Gitter MJ, Goldsmith ER, Dunbar DN, Sharkey SW: Cocaine and chest pain: Clinical features and outcome of patients hospitalized to rule out myocardial infarction. Ann Intern Med 1991;115:277–282.

62. Golbe LI, Merkin MD: Cerebral infarction in a user of freebase cocaine. Neurology 1986;36:1602–1604.

63. Gottfried MR, Kloss MW, Graham D, et al: Ultrastructure of experimental cocaine hepatotoxicity. Hepatology 1986;6:299–304.

64. Grafia A, Valverde JL, Borondo JC, et al: Vascular lesions in intestinal ischemia induced by cocaine-alcohol abuse: Report of a fatal case due to overdose. J Forensic Sci 1990;35:740–745.

65. Grant SA, Hoffman RS: Use of tetracaine, epinephrine and cocaine as a topical anesthetic in the emergency department. Ann Emerg Med 1992;21:987–997.

66. Grawe JJ, Hariman RJ, Winecoff AP, et al: Reversal of the electrocardiographic effects of cocaine by lidocaine, 2. Concentration-effect relationships. Pharmacotherapy 194;14:704–711.

67. Guinn MM, Bedford JA, Wilson MC: Antagonism of intravenous cocaine lethality in nonhuman primates. Clin Toxicol 1980;16:499–508.

68. Haddad LM: 1978: Cocaine in perspective. JACEP 1979;8:374–376.

69. Haim DY, Lippman ML, Goldberg SK, Walkenstein MD: The pulmonary complications of crack cocaine. A comprehensive review. Chest 1995;107:233–240.

70. Hale SL, Alker KJ, Rezkalla SH, et al: Nifedipine protects the heart from the acute deleterious effects of cocaine if administered before but not after cocaine. Circulation 1991;83:1437–1443.

71. Hale SL, Alker KJ, Rezkalla S, et al: Adverse effects of cocaine on cardiovascular dynamics, myocardial blood flow, and coronary artery diameter in an experimental model. Am Heart J 1989;118:927–933.

72. Haynes S, Stork CM, Hoffman RS, Goldfrank L: Beta-adrenergic blockade in cocaine toxicity [letter]. J Emerg Med 1995;13:537–538.

73. Heikkila RE, Orlansky H, Cohen G: Studies on the distinction between uptake inhibition and release of dopamine in rat brain tissue slices. Biochem Pharmacol 1975;24:847–852.

74. Heit J, Hoffman RS, Goldfrank LR: The effects of lidocaine pretreatment on cocaine neurotoxicity and lethality in mice. Acad Emerg Med 1994;1:438–442.

75. Henderson CE, Torbey M: Rupture of intracranial aneurysm associated with cocaine use during pregnancy. Am J Perinatol 1988;5:142–143.

76. Henning RJ, Wilson LD, Glauser JM: Cocaine plus ethanol is more cardiotoxic than cocaine or ethanol alone. Crit Care Med 1994;22:1896–1906.

77. Herzlich BC, Arsura EL, Pagala M, et al: Rhabdomyolysis related to cocaine abuse. Ann Intern Med 1988;109:335–336.

78. Hoffman CK, Goodman PC: Pulmonary edema in cocaine smokers. Radiology 1989;172:463–465.

79. Hoffman RS, Chiang WK, Weisman RS, et al: Prospective evaluation of "crack-vial" ingestions. Vet Hum Toxicol 1990;32:164–166.

80. Hoffman RS, Henry GL, Weisman RS, et al: Association between life-threatening cocaine toxicity and plasma cholinesterase activity. Ann Emerg Med 1991;21:247–253.

81. Hoffman RS, Hollander JE: Thrombolytic therapy in cocaine-induced myocardial infarction [editorial]. Am J Emerg Med 1996;14: 693–695.

82. Hoffman RS, Morasco R, Goldfrank LR: Administration of purified human plasma cholinesterase protects against cocaine toxicity in mice. J Toxicol Clin Toxicol 1996;34:259–266.

83. Hoffman RS, Reimer BI: "Crack" cocaine-induced bilateral amblyopia. Am J Emerg Med 1993;11:35–37.

84. Hoffman RS, Smilkstein MJ, Goldfrank LR: Whole-bowel irrigation and the cocaine "bodypacker": A new approach to a common problem. Am J Emerg Med 1990;8:523–527.

85. Hollander JE: Cocaine associated myocardial infarction [editorial]. J R Soc Med 1996;89:443–447.

86. Hollander JE: Cocaine associated myocardial ischemia [letter]. N Engl J Med 1996;334:536–537.

87. Hollander JE: Beta-adrenergic blockade in cocaine toxicity [letter]. J Emerg Med 1995:13:538–539.

88. Hollander JE: Management of cocaine-associated myocardial ischemia. N Engl J Med 1995;333:1267–1272.

89. Hollander JE, Burstein JL, Shih RD, et al: Cocaine associated myocardial infarction: Clinical safety of thrombolytic therapy. Chest 1995;107:1237–1241.

90. Hollander JE, Carter WC, Hoffman RS: Use of phentolamine for cocaine induced myocardial ischemia [letter]. N Engl J Med 1992; 327:361.

91. Hollander JE, Hoffman RS: Cocaine-induced myocardial infarction: An analysis and review of the literature. J Emerg Med 1992;10: 169–177.

92. Hollander JE, Hoffman RS, Burstein J, et al: Cocaine-associated myocardial infarction. Mortality and complications. Arch Intern Med 1995;155:1081–1086.

93. Hollander JE, Hoffman RS, Cocaine Associated Myocardial Infarction Study Group: Cocaine induced "micro-infarcts": A new clinical entity or false-positive CK-MB [abstract]? Vet Hum Toxicol 1994; 36:376.

94. Hollander JE, Hoffman RS, Gennis P, et al: Cocaine-associated chest pain: One-year follow-up. Acad Emerg Med 1995;2:179–184.

95. Hollander JE, Hoffman RS, Gennis P, et al: Nitroglycerin in the treatment of cocaine associated chest pain: Clinical safety and efficacy. J Toxicol Clin Toxicol 1994;32:243–256.

96. Hollander JE, Hoffman RS, Gennis P, et al: Prospective multicenter evaluation of cocaine associated chest pain. Acad Emerg Med 1994; 1:330–339.

97. Hollander JE, Levitt MA, Young GP, et al: The effect of cocaine on the specificity of cardiac markers. Am Heart J 1998;135(2):245–252.

98. Hollander JE, Lozano M Jr: Cocaine induced myocardial infarction secondary to a contaminant. Am J Emerg Med 1993;11:681–682.

99. Hollander JE, Lozano M Jr, Fairweather P, et al: "Abnormal" electrocardiograms in patients with cocaine-associated chest pain are due to "normal" variants. J Emerg Med 1994;12:199–205.

100. Hollander JE, Wilson LD, Leo PJ, Shih RD: Complications from the use of thrombolytic agents in patients with cocaine associated chest pain. J Emerg Med 1996;14:731–736.

101. Hong R, Matsuyama E, Nur K: Cardiomyopathy associated with the smoking of crystal methamphetamine. JAMA 1991;265:1152–1154.

102. Howard RE, Hueter DC, Davis GJ: Acute myocardial infarction following cocaine abuse in a young woman with normal coronary arteries. JAMA 1985;254:95–96.

103. Imperato-McGinley J, Gautier T, Ehlers HK, et al: Reversibility of catecholamine-induced dilated cardiomyopathy in a child with a pheochromocytoma. N Engl J Med 1987;316:793–796.

104. Isner JM, Chokshi SK: Cocaine and vasospasm. N Engl J Med 1989; 321:1604–1607.

105. Isner JM, Estes M, Thompson PD, et al: Acute cardiac events temporally related to cocaine abuse. N Engl J Med 1986;315:1438–1443.

106. Itkonen J, Schnoll S, Glassroth J: Pulmonary dysfunction in "freebase" cocaine users. Arch Intern Med 1984;144:2195–2197.

107. Jatlow PI: Drug of abuse profile: Cocaine. Clin Chem 1987;33: 66b–71b.

108. Johnson MN, Karas SP, Hursey TL, et al: Cocaine "binging" produces left ventricular dysfunction [abstract]. Circulation 1989;80(4 Suppl 2):15.

109. Kambam J, Mets B, Hickman RM, et al: The effects of inhibition of plasma cholinesterase and hepatic microsomal enzyme activity on cocaine, benzoylecgonine, ecgonine methyl ester, and norcocaine blood levels in pigs. J Lab Clin Med 1992;120:323–328.

110. Kanel GC, Cassidy W, Shuster L, et al: Cocaine induced liver injury: Comparison of morphologic features in man and experimental models. Hepatology 1990;11:646–651.

111. Karch SB: Managing cocaine crisis [letter]. Ann Emerg Med 1988; 18:228–229.

112. Kaufman MJ, Levin JM, Ross MH, et al: Cocaine induced cerebral vasoconstriction detected in humans with magnetic resonance imaging. JAMA 1998;279:376–380.

113. Kaye BR, Fainstat M: Cerebral vasculitis associated with cocaine abuse. JAMA 1987;258:2104–2106.

114. Kline JN, Hirasuna JD: Pulmonary edema after freebase cocaine smoking—Not due to an adulterant. Chest 1990;97:1009–1010.

115. Kloss MW, Cavagnaro J, Rosen GM, Rauckman EJ: Involvement of FAD-containing monooxygenase in cocaine-induced hepatotoxicity. Toxicol Appl Pharmacol 1982;64:88–93.

116. Kloss MW, Rosen GM, Rauckman EJ: Cocaine-mediated hepatotoxicity: A critical review. Biochem Pharmacol 1984;33:169–173.

117. Kloss MW, Rosen GM, Rauckman EJ: Evidence of enhanced in vivo lipid peroxidation after acute cocaine administration. Toxicol Lett 1983;15:65–70.

118. Konkol RJ, Erickson BA, Doerr JK, et al: Seizure induced by the cocaine metabolite benzoylecgonine in rats. Epilepsia 1992;33: 420–427.

119. Kolodgie FD, Wilson PS, Mergner WJ, Virmani R: Cocaine-induced increase in the permeability function of human vascular endothelial cell monolayers. Exp Mol Pathol 1999;66:109–122.

120. Kontos MC, Schmidt KL, Nicholson CS, et al: Myocardial perfusion imaging with technetium-99m sestamibi in patients with cocaine associated chest pain. Ann Emerg Med 1999;33:639–645.

121. Kushman SO, Storrow AB, Liu T, Gibler WB: Cocaine-associated chest pain in a chest pain center. Am J Cardiol 2000;85:394–396.

122. Krendel DA, Ditter SM, Frankel MR, Ross WK: Biopsy-proven cerebral vasculitis associated with cocaine abuse. Neurology 1990; 40:1092–1094.

123. Kurth CD, Monitto C, Albuquerque ML, et al: Cocaine and its metabolites constrict cerebral arterioles in newborn pigs. J Pharmacol Exp Ther 1993;265:587–591.

124. Lange RA, Cigarroa RG, Flores ED, et al: Potentiation of cocaine-induced coronary vasoconstriction by beta-adrenergic blockade. Ann Intern Med 1990;112:897–903.

125. Lange RA, Cigarroa RG, Yancy CW, et al: Cocaine-induced coronary-artery vasoconstriction. N Engl J Med 1989;321:1557–1561.

126. Lee HS, LaMaute HR, Pizzi WF, et al: Acute gastrointestinal perforations associated with use of crack. Ann Surg 1990;211:15–17.

127. Leitman BS, Greengart A, Wasser HJ: Pneumomediastinum and pneumopericardium after cocaine abuse. Am J Roentgenol 1988; 151:614.

128. Levine MAH, Nishakawa J: Acute myocardial infarction associated with cocaine withdrawal. Can Med Assoc J 1991;144:1139–1140.

129. Levine SR, Brust JCM, Futrell N, et al: Cerebrovascular complications of the use of the "crack" form of alkaloidal cocaine. N Engl J Med 1990;323:699–704.

130. Levine SR, Washington JM, Jefferson MF, et al: "Crack" cocaine-associated stroke. Neurology 1987;37:1849–1850.

131. Lichtenfeld PJ, Rubin DB, Feldman RS: Subarachnoid hemorrhage precipitated by cocaine snorting. Arch Neurol 1984;41:223–224.

132. Lisse JR, Davis CP, Thurmond-Anderle ME: Cocaine abuse and deep venous thrombosis [letter]. Ann Intern Med 1989;110:571–572.

133. Lisse JR, Davis CP, Thurmond-Anderle ME: Upper extremity deep venous thrombosis: Increased prevalence due to cocaine abuse. Am J Med 1989;87:457–458.

134. LoVecchio F, Nelson L: Intraventricular bleeding after the use of thrombolytics in a cocaine user. Am J Emerg Med 1996;14:663–664.

135. Lynch TJ, Mattes CE, Singh A, et al: Cocaine detoxification by human plasma butyrylcholinesterase. Toxicol Appl Pharmacol 1997; 145:363–371.

136. MacGregor SN, Keith LG, Chasnoff IJ, et al: Cocaine use during pregnancy: Adverse perinatal outcome. Am J Obstet Gynecol 1987; 157:686–690.

137. Madden J, Powers R: Effect of cocaine and cocaine metabolites on cerebral arteries in vitro. Life Sci 1990;47:1109–1114.

138. Marzuk PM, Tardiff K, Leon AC, et al: Ambient temperature and mortality from unintentional cocaine overdose. JAMA 1998;279: 1795–1800.

139. Maschke M, Fehlings T, Kastrup O, Wilhelm HW, Leonhardt G: Toxic leukoencephalopathy after intravenous consumption of heroin and cocaine with unexpected clinical recovery. J Neurol 1999;246: 850–851.

140. Mattes CE, Lynch TJ, Singh A, et al: Therapeutic use of butyrylcholinesterase for cocaine intoxication. Toxicol Appl Pharmacol 1997; 145:372–380.

141. McCarron MM, Wood JD: The cocaine body-packer syndrome. JAMA 1983;250:1417–1420.

142. McHenry JG, Zeiter JH, Madion MP, Cowden JW: Corneal epithelial defects after smoking crack cocaine. Am J Ophthalmol 1989; 108:732.

143. McLaurin MD, Apple FS, Henry TD, Sharkey SW: Cardiac troponin I and T concentrations in patients with cocaine-associated chest pain. Ann Clin Biochem 1996;33:183–186.

144. Menashe PI, Gottlieb JE: Hyperthermia, rhabdomyolysis, and myoglobinuric renal failure after recreational use of cocaine. South Med J 1988;81:379–381.

145. Merigian KS, Roberts JR: Cocaine intoxication: Hyperpyrexia, rhabdomyolysis and acute renal failure. J Toxicol Clin Toxicol 1987;25: 135–148.

146. Mets B, Virag L: Lethal toxicity from equimolar infusions of cocaine and cocaine metabolites in conscious and anesthetized rats. Anesth Analg 1995;81:1033–1038.

147. Minor RL, Scott BD, Brown DD, Winniford MD: Cocaine-induced myocardial infarction in patients with normal coronary arteries. Ann Intern Med 1991;115:797–806.

148. Mittleman MA, Mintzewr D, Maclure M, et al: Triggering of myocardial infarction by cocaine. Circulation 1999;99:2737–2741.

149. Mizrahi S, Loar D, Stamler B: Intestinal ischemia induced by cocaine abuse. Arch Surg 1988;123:394.

150. Mody CK, Miller BL, McIntyre HB, et al: Neurologic complications of cocaine abuse. Neurology 1988;38:1189–1193.

151. Moliterno DJ, Lange RA, Gerard RD, et al: Influence of intranasal cocaine on plasma constituents associated with endogenous thrombosis and thrombolysis. Am J Med 1994;96:492–496.

152. Moore TR, Sorg J, Miller L, et al: Hemodynamic effects of intravenous cocaine on the pregnant ewe and fetus. Am J Obstet Gynecol 1986;155:883–888.

153. Murray RJ, Albin RJ, Mergner W, et al: Diffuse alveolar hemorrhage temporally related to cocaine smoking. Chest 1988;93:427–429.

154. Murray RJ, Simialek J, Golle M, Albin RJ: Pulmonary artery medial hypertrophy in cocaine users without foreign particle microembolization. Chest 1989;96:1050–1053.

155. Nadel DM, Lyons KM: Shotgunning crack cocaine as a potential cause of retropharyngeal abscess. Ear Nose Throat J 1998;77:47–50.

156. Nademanee K, Gorelick DA, Josephson MA, et al: Myocardial ischemia during cocaine withdrawal. Ann Intern Med 1989;111: 876–880.

157. Nahas G, Trouve R, Demus JF, Von Sitron M: A calcium channel blocker as antidote to the cardiac effects of cocaine intoxication [letter]. N Engl J Med 1985; 313:519.

158. Nalbandian H, Sheth N, Dietrich R, Georgiou J: Intestinal ischemia caused by cocaine ingestion: Report of two cases. Surgery 1985;97: 374–376.

159. National Institute of Drug Abuse: National household survey on drug abuse. Population estimates, 1991. DHHS number (ADM) 92–1887. Rockville, MD, Department of Health and Human Services, 1992.

160. Negus BH, Willard JE, Hillis LD, et al: Alleviation of cocaine-induced coronary vasoconstriction with intravenous verapamil. Am J Cardiol 1994;73:510–513.

161. Ness RB, Grisso JA, Hirschinger N, et al: cocaine and tobacco use and the risk of spontaneous abortion. N Engl J Med 1999;340:333–339.

162. O'Donnell AE, Mappin G, Sepo TJ, et al: Interstitial pneumonitis associated with "crack" cocaine abuse. Chest 1991;100:1155–1157.

163. Om A, Ellahham S, Ornato JP, et al: Medical complications of cocaine: Possible relationship to low plasma cholinesterase enzyme. Am Heart J 1993;125:1114–1117.

164. Pap A, Bradberry CW: Excitatory amino acid antagonists attenuate the effects of cocaine on extracellular dopamine in the nucleus accumbens. J Pharmacol Exp Ther 1995;274:127–133.

165. Parker RB, Beckman KJ, Hariman RJI, et al: The electrophysiologic and arrhythmogenic effects of cocaine [abstract]. Pharmacotherapy 1989;9:176.

166. Pasternack PF, Colvin SB, Baumann FG: Cocaine-induced angina pectoris and acute myocardial infarction in patients younger than 40 years. Am J Cardiol 1985;55:847.

167. Patel RC, Dutta D, Schoenfeld SA: Free-base cocaine use associated with bronchiolitis obliterans organizing pneumonia. Ann Intern Med 1987;107:186–187.

168. Perez-Reyes M: Subjective and cardiovascular effects of cocaethylene in humans. Psychopharmacol 1993;113:144–147.

169. Perreault CL, Allen PD, Hague AN, et al: Differential mechanisms of cocaine-induced depression of contractile function in cardiac versus vascular smooth muscle [abstract]. Circulation 1989;80(4 Suppl 2):15.

170. Petitti DB, Sidney S, Quesenberry C, Bernstein A: Stroke and cocaine or amphetamine use. Epidemiology 1998;9:956–600.

171. Pitts WR, Vongpatannasin W, Cigoarroa JE, et al: Effects of intracoronary infusion of cocaine on left ventricular systolic and diastolic function in humans. Circulation 1998;97:1270–1273.

172. Pirwitz MJ, Willard JE, Landau C, et al: Influence of cocaine, ethanol, or their combination on epicardial coronary arterial dimensions in humans. Arch Intern Med 1995;155:1186–1191.

173. Pollan S, Tadjziechy M: Esmolol in the management of epinephrine and cocaine-induced cardiovascular toxicity. Anesth Analg 1989;69:663–664.

174. Post RM, Kopanda RT: Cocaine, kindling, and psychosis. Am J Psychiatry 1976;133:627–634.

175. Ramoska E, Sacchetti AD: Propranolol-induced hypertension in treatment of cocaine intoxication. Ann Emerg Med 1985;14:112–113.

176. Rappolt RT, Gay G, Inaba DS: Use of Inderal (propranolol-Ayerst) in 1-a (early stimulative) and 1-b (advanced stimulative) classification of cocaine and other sympathomimetic reactions. Clin Toxicol 1978;13:325–332.

177. Rappolt TR, Gay G, Inaba DS, Rappolt NR: Propranolol in cocaine toxicity [letter]. Lancet 1976;2:640–641.

178. Rashid J, Eisenberg MJ, Topol EJ: Cocaine induced aortic dissection. Am Heart J 1996;132:1301–1304.

179. Ravin JG, Ravin LC: Blindness due to illicit use of topical cocaine. Ann Ophthalmol 1979;11:863–864.

180. Rezkalla S, Mazza JJ, Kloner RA, et al: The effect of cocaine on human platelets. Am J Cardiol 1993;72:243–246.

181. Rinder HM, Ault KA, Jatlow PI, et al: Platelet alpha granule release in cocaine users. Circulation 1994;90:1162–1167.

182. Roberts J, Price D, Goldfrank L: The body stuffer syndrome: A clandestine form of drug overdose. Am J Emerg Med 1986;4:21–27.

183. Rockhold RW, Oden G, Ho IK, et al: Glutamate receptor antagonists block cocaine-induced convulsions and death. Brain Res Bull 1991;27:721–723.

184. Romach, MK, Glue P, Kampman K, et al: Attenuation of the euphoric effects of cocaine by the dopamine D1/D5 antagonist ecopipam (SCH 39166). Arch Gen Psychiatry 1999;56:1101–1106.

185. Roth D, Alarcon FJ, Fernandez JA, et al: Acute rhabdomyolysis associated with cocaine intoxication. N Engl J Med 1988;319:673–677.

186. Rubin RB, Neugarten J: Cocaine-induced rhabdomyolysis masquerading as myocardial ischemia. Am J Med 1989;86:551–553.

187. SAMHSA. Year End 1998 Emergency Department Data from the Drug Abuse Warning Network. Substance Abuse and Mental Health Services Administration, December 1999. Also available electronically at www.samhsa.gov or at www.health.org.

188. SAMHSA. 1999 National Household Survey on Drug Abuse Summary Findings. Available electronically at http://www.samhsa.gov/oas/oasftp.htm.

189. Sand IC, Brody SL, Wrenn KD, Slovis CM: Experience with esmolol for the treatment of cocaine-associated cardiovascular complications. Am J Emerg Med 1991;9:161–163.

190. Satel SL, Gawin FH: Migraine-like headache and cocaine use. JAMA 1989;261:2995–2996.

191. Schaffer DJ: Clinical comparison of TAC anesthetic solutions with and without cocaine. Ann Emerg Med 1975;14:1077–1080.

192. Schnetzer GW: Platelets and thrombogenesis—Current concepts. Am Heart J 1972;83:552–564.

193. Schreiber MD, Madden JA, Covert RF, Torgerson LJ: Effects of cocaine, benzoylecgonine and cocaine metabolites on cannulated pressurized fetal sheep cerebral arteries. J Appl Physiol 1994;77:834–839.

194. Schrem SS, Belsky P, Schwartzman D, Slater W: Cocaine-induced torsades de pointes in a patient with idiopathic long QT syndrome. Am Heart J 1990;120:980–984.

195. Schwartz AB, Janzen D, Jones RT, et al: Electrocardiographic and hemodynamic effects of intravenous cocaine in the awake and anesthetized dogs. J Electrocardiol 1989;22:159–166.

196. Schwartz KA, Cohen JA: Subarachnoid hemorrhage precipitated by cocaine snorting [letter]. Arch Neurol 1984;41:705.

197. Seaman ME: Acute cocaine abuse associated with cerebral infarction. Ann Emerg Med 1990;19:34–37.

198. Self DW, Barnhart WJ, Lehman DA, Nestler EJ: Opposite modulation of cocaine seeking behavior by D1- and D2-like dopamine receptor antagonists. Science 1996;271:1586–1589.

199. Shannon M: Clinical toxicity of cocaine adulterants. Ann Emerg Med 1988;17:1243–1247.

200. Sharff JA: Renal infarction associated with intravenous cocaine use. Ann Emerg Med 1984;13:1145–1147.

201. Shesser R, Davis D, Edelstein S: Pneumomediastinum and pneumothorax after inhaling alkaloidal cocaine. Ann Emerg Med 1981;10:213–215.

202. Shih RD, Hollander JE, Hoffman RS, et al: Clinical safety of lidocaine in cocaine associated myocardial infarction. Ann Emerg Med 1995;26:702–706.

203. Siegel RK: Cocaine smoking. J Psychoactive Drugs 1982;14:286–315.

204. Silverman DG, Kosten TR, Jatlow PI, et al: Decreased digital flow persists after the abatement of cocaine induced hemodynamic stimulation. Anesth Analg 1997;84:46–50.

205. Singhal P, Horowitz B, Quinnones MC, et al: Acute renal failure following cocaine abuse. Nephron 1989;52:76–78.

206. Smith GT, McClaughry PL, Purkey J, Thompson W: Crack cocaine mimicking pulmonary embolism on pulmonary ventilation perfusion scan. A case report. Clin Nucl Med 1995;20:65–68.

207. Smith JA, Mo Q, Guo H, et al: Cocaine increases extraneuronal levels of aspartate and glutamate in the nucleus accumbens. Brain Res Bull 1995;683:264–269.

208. Smith M, Garner D, Niemann JT: Pharmacologic interventions after an LD$_{50}$ cocaine insult in a chronically instrumented rat model: Are beta blockers contraindicated? Ann Emerg Med 1991;20:768–771.

209. Spivey WH, Schoffstall JM, Kirkpatrick R, et al: Comparison of labetalol, diazepam, and haloperidol for the treatment of cocaine toxicity in a swine model. Ann Emerg Med 1990;19:467–468.

210. Stewart DJ, Inaba T, Lucassen M, Kalow W: Cocaine metabolism: Cocaine and norcocaine hydrolysis by liver and serum esterases. Clin Pharmacol Ther 1979;25:464–468.

211. Suhl J, Gorelick DA: Pulmonary function in male freebase cocaine users [abstract]. Am Rev Resp Dis 1988;137:A488.

212. Sybertz EJ, Sabin CS, Pula KK, et al: Alpha and beta adrenoreceptor blocking properties of labetalol and its R,R-isomer, SCH 19927. J Pharmacol Exp Ther 1981;218:435–443.

213. Tashkin DP, Khalsa ME, Gorelick D, et al: Pulmonary status of habitual cocaine users. Am Rev Resp Dis 1992;145:92–100.

214. Tashkin DP, Kleerup EC, Koyal SN, et al: Acute effects of inhaled and IV cocaine on airway dynamics. Chest 1996;110:904–910.

215. Tashkin DP, Kleerup EC, Hoh CK, et al: Effects of "crack" cocaine on pulmonary alveolar permeability. Chest 1997;112:327–335.

216. Tella SR, Schindler CW, Goldberg SR: Cocaine: Cardiovascular effects in relation to inhibition of peripheral neuronal monoamine uptake and central stimulation of the sympathoadrenal system. J Pharmacol Exp Ther 1993;267:153–162.

217. Telsey AM, Merrit A, Dixon SD: Cocaine exposure in a term neonate. Clin Pediatr 1988;27:547–550.

218. Thadani PV: NIDA conference report on cardiopulmonary complications of crack cocaine use—Clinical manifestations and pathophysiology. Chest 1996;110:1072–1076.

219. The American Heart Association in Collaboration with the International Liaison Committee on Resuscitation (ILCOR). Guidelines for cardiopulmonary resuscitation and emergency cardiovascular care. Circulation 2000;102:I89.

220. Tipton GA, DeWitt GW, Eisenstein SJ: Topical TAC (tetracaine, adrenaline, cocaine) solution for local anesthesia in children: Prescribing inconsistency and acute toxicity. South Med J 1989;82:1344–1346.

221. Togna G, Tempesta E, Togna AR, et al: Platelet responsiveness and biosynthesis of thromboxane and prostacyclin in response to in vitro cocaine treatment. Haemostasis 1985;15:100–107.

222. Tokarski GF, Paganussi P, Urbanski R, et al: An evaluation of cocaine induced chest pain. Ann Emerg Med 1990;19:1088–1092.

223. Tomaszewski C, McKinney P, Phillips S, et al. Prevention of toxicity from oral cocaine by activated charcoal in mice. Ann Emerg Med 1993;22:1804–1806.

224. Trouve R, Nahas GG, Maillet M: Nitrendipine as an antagonist to the cardiac toxicity of cocaine. J Cardiovas Pharmacol 1987;9(Suppl 4):S49–S53.

225. Volkow ND, Wang GJ, Fischman MW, et al: Relationship between subjective effects of cocaine and dopamine transported occupancy. Nature 1997;386:827–830.

226. Van De Bor M, Walther FJ, Ebrahimi M: Decreased cardiac output in infants of mothers who abused cocaine. Pediatrics 1990;85:30–32.

227. Vargas R, Gillis RA, Ramwell PW: Propanolol promotes cocaine induced spasm of porcine coronary artery. J Pharmacol Exp Therap 1991;257:644–646.

228. Vongpatanasin W, Lange RA, Hillis LD: Comparison of cocaine-induced vasoconstriction of left and right coronary arterial systems. Am J Cardiol 1997;79:492–493.

229. Wallace EA, Wisniekski G, Zubal G, et al: Acute cocaine effects on absolute cerebral blood flow. Psychopharmacol 1996;128:17–20.

230. Wang R: pH-dependent cocaine cardiotoxicity [abstract]. J Toxicol Clin Toxicol 1996;34:561–562.

231. Wasserman GA, Kline JK, Bateman DA, et al: Prenatal cocaine exposure and school-age intelligence. Drug Alcohol Depend 1998;50:203–210.

232. Weber JE, Chudnofsky C, Bonzheim M, et al: Low risk of 30-day cardiovascular events following cardiac diagnostic unit observation for patients with cocaine-associated chest pain. Acad Emerg Med 2000;7:873–877.

233. Weiner RS, Lockhart JT, Schwartz RG: Dilated cardiomyopathy and cocaine abuse. Am J Med 1986;81:699–701.

234. Weiss RD: Protracted elimination of cocaine metabolites in long-term high-dose cocaine abuse. Am J Med 1988;85:879–880.

235. Weiss SH: Links between cocaine and retroviral infection. JAMA 1989;261:607–608.

236. Welch RD, Todd K, Krause GS: Incidence of cocaine associated rhabdomyolysis. Ann Emerg Med 1991;20:154–157.

237. Winecoff AP, Hariman RJ, Grawe JJ, et al: Reversal of the electrocardiographic effects of cocaine by lidocaine. Part 1. Comparison with sodium bicarbonate and quinidine. Pharmacotherapy 1994;14:698–703.

238. Witkin JM, Godberg SR, Katz JL: Lethal effects of cocaine are reduced by the dopamine-1 receptor antagonist SCH 23390 but not by haloperidol. Life Sci 1989;44:1285–1291.

239. Wojak JC, Flamm ES: Intracranial hemorrhage and cocaine use. Stroke 1987;18:712–715.

240. Woods JR, Plessinger MA, Clark KE: Effect of cocaine on uterine blood flow and fetal oxygenation. JAMA 1987;257:957–961.

241. Zamora-Quezada JC, Dinerman H, Stadecker MJ, Kelly JJ: Muscle and skin infarction after free-basing cocaine (crack). Ann Intern Med 1988;108:564–566.

242. Zimmerman JL, Dellinger RP, Majid PA: Cocaine associated chest pain. Ann Emerg Med 1991;20:611–615.

CHAPTER 68 AMPHETAMINES

William K. Chiang

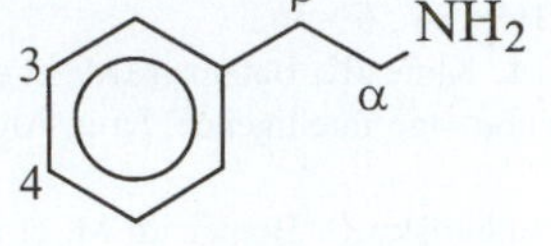

Phenylethylamine

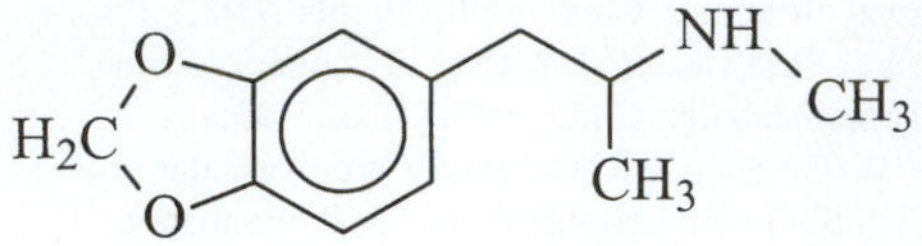

Methylenedioxymethamphetamine

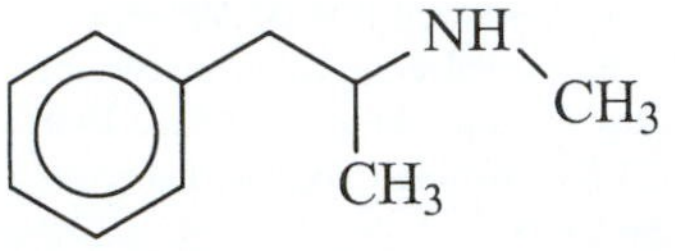

Methamphetamine

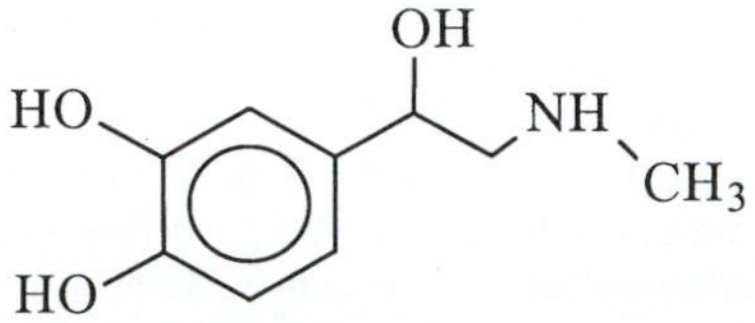

Epinephrine

A 25-year-old woman was brought to the Emergency Department (ED) by ambulance from a dance club. The paramedics reported that the patient became agitated in the club and had a generalized seizure. They also reported that the patient had used "Ecstasy" during the night. The woman was delirious, agitated, hallucinating, and paranoid. At times she was exceedingly hyperactive, jumping repeatedly on and off the stretcher. Frequently, she appeared to be involved with her hallucinations.

The physical examination revealed a blood pressure of 170/100 mm Hg; rectal temperature of 102.7°F (39.3°C); pulse of 120 beats/min and regular; respiratory rate of 18 breaths/min; and a pulse oximetry reading of 97% on room air. The patient appeared to be of normal habitus, acyanotic, and anicteric, but diaphoretic. Her head was normocephalic. Her pupils were dilated to 6 mm bilaterally, and they reacted slowly to light. The conjunctivae, extraocular movements, and the fundi were normal. Her neck was supple, exhibiting no thyromegaly. Examination of her heart was unremarkable, except for tachycardia. Her lungs were clear. The abdomen was soft, nontender, and without hepatomegaly; bowel sounds were normal. The extremities were normal, without any evidence of track marks, bruises, swelling, or rash. The patient moved all her extremities spontaneously and had normal symmetric deep-tendon reflexes with plantar flexion.

An immediate bedside glucose measurement demonstrated a serum glucose concentration of 95 mg/dL. She was treated with a total of 20 mg of diazepam IV for sedation and was placed on car-

diac monitoring. One and a half liters of normal saline were administered over 60 minutes for hydration. External cooling with ice packs around the axilla and groin was initiated. She became calm and less paranoid. Her rectal temperature decreased to 100°F (37.7°C) within 15 minutes.

On admission, her complete blood count was remarkable for an elevated white blood cell count of 15,000 cells/mm³. The serum electrolytes were remarkable for sodium of 109 mEq/L, potassium of 3.6 mEq/L, chloride of 81 mEq/L, bicarbonate of 20 mEq/L, blood urea nitrogen (BUN) 10 mg/dL, creatinine 1.1 mg/dL, and glucose of 105 mg/dL. The liver enzymes were normal. The urinalysis was negative for blood and protein, and the urine osmolality was 497 mOsm/kg. The chest radiograph was normal. The electrocardiogram (ECG) revealed a sinus tachycardia. A noncontrast head computed tomography (CT) scan performed was normal.

The presentation and physical findings in this case were entirely compatible with toxicity from a sympathomimetic agent, including 3,4-methylenedioxymethamphetamine (MDMA). However, hyponatremia is more consistent with MDMA usage or sympathomimetic agents with serotonergic effects (see "3,4-Methylenedioxymethamphetamine (MDMA)" later in this chapter). Therapy for this patient consisted of 3% saline, 50 mL/h for 6 hours with frequent serum sodium monitoring. The repeat serum sodium after 6 hours was 123 mEq/L. The patient's mental status improved and she had no further seizures. At this time, the patient was placed on free water restriction and her sodium slowly improved to 130 mEq/L by

1020

24 hours. The patient's mental status normalized. Her liver enzymes, renal function, and urinalysis remained normal. The patient was discharged from the hospital after 4 days without any sequelae.

Amphetamine is the trivial name and acronym for racemic β-phenylisopropylamine or *alpha-methylphenylethylamine* and belongs in the family of phenylethylamines. Numerous substitutions of the phenylethylamine structure are possible, resulting in different amphetaminelike compounds. Commonly, these compounds are referred to as amphetamines or amphetamine analogues, although phenylethylamines would be more precise. For the rest of this chapter, the term *amphetamines* refers to amphetamine analogues, and *amphetamine* specifically refers to β-phenylisopropylamine. Since the initial marketing of amphetamines, continued abuse and misuse have been substantial.[17,94,170] Amphetamines have been advocated by the medical communities for the treatment of depression, obesity, enuresis, postencephalitic parkinsonism, coma, and even alcoholism.[94,123] By 1970, the legal annual production of amphetamines was over 10 billion tablets, with the majority diverted for illicit usage.[94]

Currently, there are very limited medical indications for amphetamines, including narcolepsy, attention deficit hyperactivity disorder, and short-term weight reduction.[110] The prescriptive amphetamines include methylphenidate, pemoline, phentermine, phendimetrazine, amphetamine, dextroamphetamine, and methamphetamine. Because of structural differences, some amphetamines are marketed as nonamphetamine products in their package inserts. Despite the controlled status of amphetamines, there is a recent resurgence of amphetamine abuse, particularly with methamphetamine and MDMA.[43,92,191,193,249]

HISTORY AND EPIDEMIOLOGY

Edeleano first synthesized amphetamine (racemic β-phenylisopropylamine) in 1887. However, it was not rediscovered until the 1920s, when there was significant concern about the supply of ephedrine for asthma therapy. In the search for the synthesis for ephedrine, Alles from UCLA rediscovered dextroamphetamine and Ogata from Japan discovered methamphetamine (*d*-phenylisopropylmethylamine hydrochloride).[94] Amphetamine was marketed as Benzedrine inhaler, a nasal decongestant, by Smith, Kline, and French in 1932.[17] Amphetamine tablets were available in 1935 for the treatment of narcolepsy, and were advocated as anorexians in 1938. The stimulant and euphoric effects of amphetamines were widely recognized, resulting in diverse forms of abuse and misuse. Amphetamine abuse was reported as early as 1936.[123] Benzedrine inhalers, each containing 250 mg of amphetamine, were widely abused leading to a ban by the FDA in 1959. Propylhexedrine (Benzedrex) inhalers, a less potent amphetaminelike substance marketed in 1949 supplanted Benzedrine inhalers.[7] Propylhexedrine also resulted in significant misuse.[6]

Both amphetamine and methamphetamine were supplied as stimulants for soldiers and prisoners of war in World War II.[17,171] Widespread methamphetamine abuse in Japan persisted for more than a decade after the war. From 1950 to the 1970, there were sporadic periods of widespread amphetamine use and abuse in the United States. In the 1960s, various amphetamine derivatives such as methylenedioxyamphetamine (MDA) and *p*-methoxyamphetamine (PMA) were popularized as hallucinogens. Until 1971, only

a small proportion of the amphetamines produced by pharmaceutical companies was used for legitimate medical problems.[94,171] The Controlled Substance Act of 1970 placed amphetamines in Schedule II to regulate the diversion of pharmaceutical amphetamines for nonmedicinal uses.[48] Amphetamine abuse subsequently declined in the 1970s.[34,133,175]

In the 1980s, the so call "designer" amphetamines (see Table 68–1), mostly methylenedioxy-derivatives of amphetamine and methamphetamine came into vogue, as a mechanism of circumventing existing regulations. The most well known substances were MDMA and 3,4-methylenedioxyethamphetamine (MDEA), but more than 200 different derivatives have been described.[56,228] Before 1986, the Controlled Substances Act classified drugs as illegal only after they were synthesized and formally recognized by their structure, effects, or illegal usage. During this period any analogues (such as these "designer drugs") not yet formally classified could be sold legally. In 1986, the standard became prospective for any agent that was used as a stimulant, hallucinogen, or depressant, and for any agent designed as such.[25] In effect, this amendment eliminated the legal loophole that allowed the designer drug industry to flourish. Although the meaning of the term "designer drugs" has changed and is no longer legally relevant, many of these analogues are still widely illicitly available.[105,116,163]

From the late 1980s to the 1990s, a dramatic resurgence of methamphetamine abuse spread throughout much of the United States. A high purity preparation of methamphetamine hydrochloride was marketed in a large crystalline form termed "ice" by abusers.[9,38,59,170] In fact, methamphetamine surpassed cocaine and became the primary substance of abuse among those seeking care in the drug treatment programs of San Diego and San Francisco counties in the 1990s.[92,102] From 1991 to 1994, the number of methamphetamine-related deaths in the United States reported by medical examiners tripled from 151 to 433, with a disproportional distribution from the Los Angeles, San Diego, San Francisco, and Phoenix metropolitan areas. The number of methamphetamine-related emergency department visits also increased from 4900 in 1991 to 17,400 in 1994.[92] Although the initial source of methamphetamine was from Pacific Rim countries such as Korea and Taiwan, currently it is mostly produced in the United States, primarily in California and Oregon.[38,72] Methamphetamine is the most common illicit drug produced by clandestine laboratories in the United States at this time. Because of the ease and low cost of methamphetamine synthesis, the street value of methamphetamine is less than one-third that of cocaine.[72] Both the cost and the prolonged duration of effect may contribute to the increased popularity of methamphetamine. Methamphetamine continues to be a leading drug of abuse in the midwestern and western part of the United States.[92,135]

In the mid-1990s, MDMA became the amphetamines most widely used by college students and teenagers. MDMA is used by this population in large gatherings, known as "rave" or "techno" parties in England, Australia, and the United States.[198,199,249] Other MDMAlike analogues are often used or sold as MDMA in these gatherings.[10,249] While the trend of a particular amphetamine analogue waxes and wanes, use and abuse of amphetamines is likely to continue to be consequential.

Reports of methcathinone (a Khat-derived substance) use in the midwestern United States,[88,257] and a resurgence of 4-bromo-2,5-methoxyphenylethylamine (2CB) in dance clubs occurred in the 1990s.[70,82]

TABLE 68–1. Designer Amphetamines

Designer Drug	Clinical Manifestations	Structure
4-Bromo-2,5-dimethoxyamphetamine (DOB)	Marked psychoactive effect, potency > mescaline Sold as impregnated paper, like LSD Delayed onset of action, peak 3–4 h Fantasy, mood altering, for 10 h, resolution 12–24 h Agitation, sympathetic excess	
4-Bromo-2,5-methoxyphenyl-ethylamine (2CB, MFT)	Relaxation Sensory distortion Agitation Hallucinations Potency > mescaline	
Methcathinone (cat, Jeff, Khat, ephedrone)	Comparable to hallucinogenic and sympathetic effects of methamphetamine	
3,4-Methylenedioxyamphetamine (MDA, love drug)	Empathy, euphoria Agitation, delirium, hallucinations, death associated with sympathetic excess	
4-Methyl-2,5-dimethoxyamphetamine (DOM/STP) (serenity, tranquility, peace)	Narrow therapeutic index Euphoria, perceptual distortion Hallucinations, sympathetic stimulation	
3,4-Methylenedioxyethamphetamine (MDEA, Eve)	Comparable to MDMA Sympathetic excess	
3.4-Methylenedioxymethamphetamine (MDMA, Adam, ecstasy, XTC)	Psychotherapy "facilitator" Euphoria, empathy Nausea, anorexia Anxiety, insomnia Sympathetic excess	
Para-methoxyamphetamine (PMA)	Potent hallucinogen Marked stimulant effect	
2,4,5-Trimethoxyamphetamine	Similar to mescaline	

PHARMACOLOGY

The pharmacologic effects of amphetamines are complex but the primary mechanism of action is the release of catecholamines, particularly dopamine and norepinephrine, from the presynaptic terminals. Although there are conflicting mechanistic models of the amphetamines induction of catecholamine release, the variable results may be directly correlated with the different concentrations of amphetamines used in the studies. The best models to study the mechanism of action of amphetamines are based on dopaminergic neurons; similar mechanisms are invoked for norepinephrine and serotonin. Two storage pools exist for dopamine in the presynaptic terminals: the vesicular pool and the cytoplasmic pool. The vesicular storage of dopamine and other biogenic amines is maintained by the acidic environment inside the vesicles and the persistence of a stabilizing electrical gradient with respect to the cytoplasm. This environment is preserved by an ATP-dependent active proton transport system.[225] At low doses, amphetamines cause release of dopamine from the cytoplasmic pool by exchange diffusion at the dopamine uptake transporter site in the membrane. At moderate doses, amphetamines can also diffuse through the presynaptic terminal membrane and interact with the neurotransmitter transporter on the vesicular membrane to cause exchange release of dopamine into the cytoplasm. Dopamine is subsequently released into the synapse by reverse transport at the dopamine uptake site.[225,239] At high doses, an additional mechanism is invoked, as amphetamine diffuses through the cellular and vesicular membranes, alkalinizing the vesicles, permitting dopamine release from the vesicles and delivery into the synapse by reverse transport.[240,241]

Amphetamines may also block the reuptake of catecholamines similarly to other catecholamine-releasing agents by competitive inhibition.[95,110] However, the effects of this mechanism are considered to be minor. At higher doses, amphetamines can cause the release of serotonin (5-hydroxytryptamine, 5-HT) and affect central serotonin receptors. Certain amphetamines, such as MDMA and 4-bromo-2,5-dimethoxyamphetamine (DOB), have more significant serotonergic effects.[86,110] Amphetamines are structurally similar to nonhydrazine amine-derivative monoamine oxidase inhibitors such as phenelzine and tranylcypromine, and most also have weak monoamine oxidase inhibiting activities, but the significance of this inhibition is unknown.[195]

The most identifiable effects of amphetamines are those caused by catecholamine release and the resultant stimulation of peripheral α- and β-adrenergic receptors. The increased norepinephrine at the locus ceruleus mediates the anorectic and alerting effects, and some of the locomotor-stimulating effects as well.[95] The increase in central dopamine (particular at the neostriatum) mediates stereotypical behavior and some of the other locomotor activities.[47,86,95,126] The activity of dopamine in the neostriatum appears to be linked to glutamate release and inhibition of GABAergic efferent neurons.[86,125,126] Stimulation of the glutamatergic system contributes significantly to the stereotypical behavior, locomotor activities, and neurotoxicity of amphetamines.[18,23,125,126,236,237] The effects of serotonin and dopamine on the mesolimbic system alter perception and cause psychotic behavior.[86,109,172]

Because amphetamines directly interact with neurotransmitter transporters, minor modification of the molecule may significantly alter its pharmacologic profile.[114] The α-methyl group in amphetamines introduces chirality to the molecule. Except for MDMA and certain MDMA analogues, the *d*-enantiomers are much more potent (typically 4–10 times) than *l* forms of amphetamines. Substitution at different positions of the phenylethylamine molecule alters general clinical effects of amphetamines, as demonstrated by animal discrimination studies and human observations. Compounds with methyl substitution at the α carbon, such as amphetamine and methamphetamine, possess strong stimulant, cardiovascular, and anorectic properties.[83,181] Large group substitution at the α carbon reduces the stimulant and cardiovascular effects, but retains the anorectic properties (such as in phentermine).[12] Substitution at the para position of the phenyl ring enhances the hallucinogenic or serotonergic effects of amphetamines (such as in *p*-chloroamphetamine and MDMA).[12,83,181] Although some of these generalizations enable scientists to understand the effects of amphetamines, there are many exceptions, and such generalization may not apply when large doses of a particular molecule are employed.[67] In terms of the spectrum of activities, methamphetamine has the most potent cardiovascular effects, and DOB has the most potent hallucinogenic or serotonergic effects.[83,181]

Methamphetamine

Methamphetamine abuse in the United States is not new. From the 1950s to the 1970s, there were multiple epidemics of methamphetamine abuse.[17] Methamphetamine was and sometimes still is referred to as "crack," "speed," "yaba," and "go." The pharmacologic profile of methamphetamine is quite similar to amphetamine, although the effects on the central nervous system are more substantial.[38] "Ice," the most recent common name for methamphetamine, does not differ pharmacologically from other forms of methamphetamine. Methamphetamine is readily absorbed by the oral, parenteral, and inhalational routes. Because of a prolonged half-life of 19–34 hours, the duration of its acute effects can be greater than 24 hours.[38,59,60]

Since the 1990s, the activity and purity of methamphetamine available on the street is substantially higher than previous epidemics because of the method of synthesis.[146] Methamphetamine is now typically greater than 80–90% pure and almost exclusively in the dextroisomer form, which is most active on the central nervous system (CNS). The ephedrine method, using pharmaceutical grade L-ephedrine, produces a product with few contaminants that is stereochemically pure.[59,197] The production of the large crystal is possible by creating a supersaturated solution of methamphetamine hydrochloride.[59]

Methamphetamine can be easily synthesized with the proper chemicals and minimal equipment.[79] The primary ingredient of methamphetamine synthesis is ephedrine, which can be hydrogenated into methamphetamine. Phenyl-2-propanone (P2P), as an alternative ingredient, can be methylated into ephedrine and then into methamphetamine.[26] Because of the strict control of ephedrine and P2P, illicit chemists use phenylacetic acid to synthesize P2P.[26,51] Lead acetate, which is used as a substrate for the reaction, resulted in an epidemic of lead poisoning associated with methamphetamine abuse in Oregon.[3,36] Lead levels reported in drug users were as high as 513 μg/dL, and some samples of illicit manufactured methamphetamine had lead contents as high as 60% by weight.[36] Mercury contamination was also documented, although clinical mercury toxicity has not been reported.[26] The number of potential chemicals involved in the methamphetamine manufacturing process is significant, and without any legal monitoring, contamination of the product and the environment is inevitable.[4,26,113,139] In fact, 30% of the illicit methamphetamine manufacturing sites discovered in Oregon were discovered because of laboratory explosion. In California's San Bernadino County alone in 1995, 360 methamphetamine laboratories were identified and closed by drug enforcement agents.[72] Currently, sale of other potential amphetamine synthesis ingredients such as hydrochloric acid, hydrogen chloride gas, red phosphorous, and iodine are also monitored and restricted in the United States.

3,4-Methylenedioxymethamphetamine (MDMA)

MDMA was first synthesized in 1912, and was rediscovered in 1965 by Shulgin.[25] It is currently one of the most widely abused amphetamines by college students and teenagers.[43,191,249,253] It is commonly known as "ecstasy," "E," "Adam," "XTC," "M&M," and "MDM." Other structural relatives of MDMA, MDEA ("Eve") and MDA ("love drug"), are also used or distributed as MDMA in areas of MDMA use. These agents have similar clinical effects and acute and chronic toxicity. Recently, other MDMA-related substances are also found in "rave" scenes, 2CB, 2,4-dimethoxy-4-(n)-propylthiophenylethylamine (2C-T7), and N-methyl-1-(3,4-methylenedioxyphenyl)-2-butanamine (MBDB).[32,70,82,132] The term, "ecstasy" may also be used for all of these substances. Typically, MDMA is available in colorful and branded tablets, vary from 50 mg to 200 mg. MDMA and similar analogues are so-call entactogens (meaning touching within), capable of producing euphoria, inner peace, and a desire to socialize.[163,235] In addition, some psychologists used MDMA to enhance psychotherapy until the Controlled Substances Act of 1986.[182] People who use MDMA report that it enhances pleasure, heightens sexuality, and expands consciousness without the loss of control.[25,93,163] Negative effects reported with acute use included ataxia, restlessness, confusion, poor concentration, and memory problem.[235] MDMA has about one-tenth the CNS stimulant effect of amphetamine. Unlike amphetamine and methamphetamine, MDMA is a potent stimulus for the release of serotonin.[28,61,95,171] The concentration of MDMA required to stimulate the release of serotonin is 10 times less than that required for the release of dopamine or norepinephrine. In animal models, the stereotypic and the discriminatory effects of MDMA and its congeners can be distinguished from those of other amphetamines.[29,182]

The sympathetic effects of MDMA are mild in low doses. However, when a large amount of MDMA is taken, the clinical presentation is similar to that of other amphetamines and deaths can result from abuse.[66,104,105,177,253] Those patients at greatest risk developed dysrhythmias, hyperthermia, rhabdomyolysis, and disseminated intravascular coagulation.[66,105,230] Significant hyponatremia has been reported with MDMA use.[2,160,183] The increase in serotonin results in the excessive release of vasopressin (ADH).[103] Furthermore, large free-water intake combined with sodium loss from physical exertion (in dance clubs) may be crucial to the development of hyponatremia.

A major concern with MDMA usage is its long-term effects on the brain. In numerous animal models, acute administration of MDMA leads to serotonin transporter dysfunction, and repetitive administration of MDMA ultimately leads to permanent damage to serotonergic neurons.[161,164,166,173,184,203,205] Animal data suggest that MDMA induces hydroxyl free-radical generation and de-

creases antioxidants in serotonergic neurons.[207,227] When sufficient antioxidants are depleted, neuronal damage may occur. The evidence for these potential neurotoxic effects in humans is less clear. Indirect evidence of serotonergic effects in humans includes lower levels of 5-hydroxyindoleacetic acid (5-HIAA) in the cerebral spinal fluid (CSF) of MDMA users than in controls.[204] Case reports and studies of MDMA users demonstrate alteration in mood, sleep, anxiety, cognition, memory, and impulse control—all functions that are believed to be affected by serotonin.[5,162,165,167,171] Either single photon emission tomography (SPECT) or positron emission tomography (PET) demonstrates decreased serotonin transporter function in MDMA users.[185,201] Memory deficits appeared to persist even in abstinent MDMA users.[90,176] A major deficit in human studies is finding comparable control groups; it is possible that people with psychiatric problems are more likely to be MDMA users.[168] Another confounding variable is that MDMA users are more likely to use other drugs. Further studies are required to address the long-term neuropsychiatric effects of MDMA.

Propylhexedrine

Smith, Kline and French introduced propylhexedrine in 1949 as the primary active ingredient in Benzedrex nasal inhaler, to replace the widespread abuse of amphetamine in nasal inhalers.[7,77] Propylhexedrine is an alicyclic aliphatic sympathomimetic amine that is structurally similar to amphetamine, with a local vasoconstrictive effect and approximately 10% of the CNS stimulatory effect of amphetamine.[7] Propylhexedrine abuse became prevalent after the removal of amphetamine from nasal inhalers. The abusers disassembled the inhaler and ingested the cotton pledget vehicle of propylhexedrine itself, diluted it in beverages, or reconstituted the drug for intravenous injection. Numerous effects were reported with propylhexedrine abuse, including sudden death, myocardial infarction, cardiomyopathy, pulmonary hypertension, and acute psychosis.[6,7,49,63,77,147,156,157,251] Although propylhexedrine in nasal inhalers has largely been replaced by safer sympathomimetic agents (Chap. 35), the drug is still readily available and is abused as an inexpensive, legal "high."

Khat, Cathinone, and Methcathinone

Khat (also known as quat and gat), the fresh leaves and stems from the *Catha edulis* shrub, is one of the most commonly used drugs in eastern and central Africa, and in parts of the Arabian peninsula. Attention to khat was highlighted in the early 1990s by the media coverage of war in Somalia and Ethiopia. Khat is sold in small bundles of leaves in the local markets of these countries. The leaves and the tender stems are chewed or occasionally concocted into tea. Khat chewing has a significant role at social gatherings in these countries.[154] When the dried leaves and stems were studied, the primary active ingredient was thought to be cathine (norpseudoephedrine), present as 0.1–0.2% of the dried material. Cathine has about one-tenth the stimulant effects of D-amphetamine. Numerous other amphetaminelike compounds are also isolated, but occur in minute quantities.[122] When the fresh leaves are analyzed, however, cathinone (benzylketoamphetamine), a more potent psychoactive compound, was demonstrated to be the primary active agent.[84,98,122] As the leaves age, cathinone is degraded into cathine, which also explains why dried khat is neither popular nor widely distributed. Imported fresh khat must be consumed within a week before losing much of its potency. The primary effects of khat are increased alertness, insomnia, euphoria, anxiety, and hyperactivity. Significant adrenergic complications are much less frequent than those associated with amphetamine abuse.

Methcathinone, the methyl-derivative of cathinone, chemically synthesized from ephedrine, has been abused in the Soviet Union for many years. The potency of methcathinone is comparable to that of methamphetamine.[85,257] Methcathinone—also termed ephedrone, or sold under the street names of "cat" or "Jeff"—currently remains widely abused in Russia. Methcathinone abuse was first reported in Michigan in the early 1990s and is now reported in other states as well.[69]

Ephedrine or Ma-Huang Herbal Products

Ephedrine is commonly found in over-the-counter cold preparations. Ephedrine is also the active substance in the Chinese plant ma-huang, which has been used for centuries for the treatment of asthma. Although ephedrine is much less potent than amphetamine, when combined with other catecholamine-stimulating agents or when taken in large quantities, significant toxicity may occur.[24,30,192,221] In the United States, numerous ephedrine products, such as "go," "ultimate xphoria," "up your gas," and "herbal ecstasy," are marketed primarily to teenagers. Some of these products contain more than 500 mg of ephedrine, and this may be combined with pseudoephedrine, phenylpropanolamine, and caffeine; other products contain the plant extract ma-huang.[143,192,194] Many of these products are marketed as legal stimulants or safe herbal stimulants for a natural "high." Similarly, ma-huang is also widely marketed as a "safe" herbal weight-reducing product, especially when phenylpropanolamine was recently demonstrated to associate with brain hemorrhage in women.[130] Unfortunately, these products are linked to numerous deaths and adverse reactions.[98a,178,194,242a,254,259] Because these products are sold as food supplements, they are not regulated by the FDA. Only when the FDA can demonstrate a product's hazards, can the federal authority restrict these products (Chap. 77).

Sibutramine

Sibutramine (Meridia) is an amphetamine analogue (β-phenylethylamine analogue) with properties distinct from most amphetamines. Although originally investigated as an antidepressant, the FDA approved sibutramine in 1997 as a weight-reducing agent. Pharmacologically, sibutramine blocks the reuptake of serotonin, norepinephrine, and, to a lesser extent, dopamine, which are similar action those of many antidepressants.[155] Sibutramine has no direct affect or binding to α- or β-adrenergic, dopaminergic, and muscarinic receptors. Although sibutramine may increase the blood pressure of patients with hypertension, significant sympathomimetic effects are unexpected.[145] Sibutramine is extensively metabolized in the liver, especially by CYP3A4 into 2 active components.[145] Currently, overdose data are quite limited. Based on its

pharmacologic profile, altered mental status, seizures, and some serotonin symptoms may be expected with significant overdoses.

PHARMACOKINETICS AND TOXICOKINETICS

In general, amphetamines are relatively lipophilic and hence they can cross the blood-brain barrier readily. They have large volumes of distribution, varying from 3–5 L/kg for amphetamine and 3–4 L/kg for methamphetamine and phentermine, to 11–33 L/kg for methylphenidate. Pemoline is the exception as it has a small volume of distribution (0.2–0.6 L/kg).[11] Amphetamines differ from catecholamines in that they lack the catechol structure (hydroxyl groups at the 3 and 4 positions of the phenyl ring) and are resistant to metabolism by catechol-*O*-methyl transferase (COMT).[110] The α-methyl group in amphetamines makes them resistant to metabolism by monoamine oxidase. These characteristics permit better oral bioavailability and longer duration of effects.[181]

Amphetamine elimination may occur through multiple pathways, including diverse hepatic transformations and renal elimination. For MDMA and its analogues, *N*-dealkylation, hydroxylation, and demethylation are the dominant hepatic pathways.[39,40,159] Depending on the particular substance, active metabolites of secondary amphetamines and ephedrine derivatives may be formed.[11,39] *N*-Demethylation of methamphetamine and MDMA result in the formation of amphetamine and MDA, respectively.[39] Dealkylation and demethylation are mainly performed by cytochrome P450 isoenzymes, including CYP1A2, CYP2D6, and CYP3A4, but they are also performed by flavin monooxygenase (FMO).[159] Polymorphism of CYP2D6 in humans was discovered as a result of decreased *p*-hydroxylation of amphetamine in certain populations. Since its discovery, CYP2D6 polymorphism has been implicated in drug toxicity, substance use and abuse, and lack of drug efficacy in susceptible populations.[226] Increased amphetamine toxicity is a potential concern in patients with decreased CYP2D6 activity. Animal models with CYP2D6 deficiency are demonstrated to be more susceptible to MDMA toxicity; this has not been studied in human.[45] In general, because multiple enzymes and pathways (including renal) are involved in amphetamine elimination, it is less likely that CYP2D6 polymorphism or drug interaction with CYP3A4 alone will increase toxicity significantly. However, it is unclear if toxicity is enhanced when multiple mechanisms for altering drug metabolism and renal dysfunction are present simultaneously.

Renal elimination is substantial for amphetamine (30%), methamphetamine (40–50%), MDMA (65%), and phentermine (80%). Amphetamines are relatively strong bases with a typical pK_a range from 9–10, and renal elimination varies depending on the urine pH.[11] The half-life of amphetamines varies significantly: amphetamine, 8–30 hours; methamphetamine, 12–34 hours; MDMA, 5–10 hours; methylphenidate, 2.5–4 hours; and phentermine, 19–24 hours.[11,39] Repetitive administration, which occurs typically during binge use, may lead to drug accumulation and prolongation of the drug's half-life and duration of effect.[118]

CLINICAL MANIFESTATIONS

The clinical effects of amphetamines are largely related to the stimulation of central and peripheral adrenergic receptors. These clinical manifestations and complications are similar to those from cocaine use and may be indistinguishable except for the duration of effect of amphetamines, which tends to be longer (up to 24 hours).[59,74] Compared to cocaine, amphetamines are less likely to cause seizures, dysrhythmias, and myocardial ischemia. This may be related to the sodium channel blocking effects and to the thrombogenic effect of cocaine that do not result from amphetamine use.[87] Psychosis appears to be more likely with amphetamines than cocaine, which may be related to the more prominent dopaminergic effects of amphetamines.[8,86] Tachycardia and hypertension are the most common manifestations of cardiovascular toxicity. Most patients present to the emergency department, however, because of the CNS manifestations.[59,115,253] These patients are anxious, volatile, aggressive, and may have life-threatening agitation. Visual and tactile hallucinations, as well as psychoses, are common.[20,60,62,101,150,209,220] Other sympathetic findings include mydriasis, diaphoresis, and hyperthermia (Table 68–2).[60,66]

Death from amphetamine toxicity most commonly results from hyperthermia, dysrhythmias, and intracerebral hemorrhage.[35,55,73,121,128,149,189,210] Direct CNS effects may result in seizures. Tachycardia, hypertension, and vasospasm may lead to cerebral infarction,[89,138,213] intraparenchymal and subarachnoid hemorrhage,[52,100,112,127,238,258] myocardial ischemia or infarction,[76,190,246] aortic dissection,[52,65] pulmonary edema,[27,179,180] obstetrical complications, fetal death,[148] and ischemic colitis.[16,107,119] Dysrhythmias vary from premature ventricular complexes to ventricular tachycardia and ventricular fibrillation.[121,151] Agitation, increased muscular activity, and hyperthermia can result in metabolic acidosis, rhabdomyolysis,[50] acute tubular necrosis (acute renal failure), and coagulopathy.[66,81,120,129] Unless these systemic signs and symptoms are rapidly reversed, multiorgan failure and death ensue.

Amphetamine users seeking intense "highs" may go on "speed runs" for days to weeks. Because of the development of acute tolerance, they use increasing amounts of amphetamines during these periods, usually without much sustenance or sleep, attempting to achieve their desired euphoria.[17,48,140,232,242] Acute psychosis resembling paranoid schizophrenia may occur during these binges and has contributed to both amphetamine-related suicides and homicides.[68,136] Return to a normal sensorium occurs within a few days after discontinuation of the drug. Once an amphetamine user experiences psychosis, it is likely to be recurrent even after prolonged abstinence, which may be related to a kindling phenomenon.[17,74,186,242] Amphetamine-induced psychosis has contributed to the understanding of dopamine's function in schizophrenia. Typically after such binges, patients may sleep for prolonged periods, feeling hungry and depressed when awake. During this period of depression or withdrawal, the patient has continued craving for amphetamines.[101,137,143]

There are some direct neurologic effects of amphetamines. Compulsive repetitive behavior patterns are reported in humans and animals. Individuals may constantly pick at their skin, grind their teeth (bruxism), or perform repetitive tasks, such as constantly cleaning their house or car.[17] Choreoathetoid movements, although uncommon, are reported with acute and chronic amphetamine usage.[134,153,158,202,219,231] The etiology of the choreoathetoid movements may be related to increased dopaminergic activity at the striatal area.

Necrotizing vasculitis is associated with amphetamine abuse.[19,42] Angiography typically demonstrates beading and narrowing of the small and medium-sized arteries (see Fig. 8–23).[215,238] Progressive necrotizing arteritis[52] can involve multiple organ systems, including the central nervous, cardiovascular, gastrointestinal, and renal

systems. Complications include cerebral infarction and hemorrhage, coronary artery disease, pancreatitis, and renal failure.[42,99,152,215,218,238,258] The etiology of the arteritis remains unclear. Although various contaminants associated with parenteral drug use were postulated as potential etiologies, oral and IV amphetamine use in animal models is also associated with vasculitis, suggesting that this is a direct amphetamine effect.[216,217,243] Cardiomyopathy is also reported with acute and chronic amphetamine abuse.[19,111,188,234] Excessive catecholamine exposure in patients with pheochromocytomas and chronic cocaine use may be responsible for their associated cardiomyopathies; amphetamine-induced cardiomyopathy may be produced by similar mechanisms.[87,124,252]

Primary pulmonary hypertension, a rare and potentially fatal disease, is reported with chronic methamphetamine and propylhexedrine use.[6,63,141,222] However, substantial epidemiologic risk

---

TABLE 68–2. Amphetamine Toxicity

Acute toxicity

Cardiovascular System
Hypertension
Tachycardia
Dysrhythmias
Myocardial ischemia
Aortic dissection
Vasospasm

Central Nervous System
Hyperthermia
Agitation
Seizures
Intracerebral hemorrhage
Headache
Euphoria
Anorexia
Bruxism
Choreoathetoid movements
Hyperreflexia
Paranoid psychosis

Other Sympathetic Symptoms
Diaphoresis
Tachypnea
Mydriasis
Tremor
Nausea

Other Organ Systems
Rhabdomyolysis
Muscle rigidity
Acute lung injury
Ischemic colitis

Chronic toxicity

Vasculitis
Cardiomyopathy
Pulmonary hypertenion
Aortic and mitral regurgitation
Permanent damage to dopaminergic
  and serotonergic neurons

Laboratory abnormalities

Leukocytosis
Hyperglycemia
Hyponatremia
Elevated CPK
Elevated liver enzymes
Myoglobinuria

for primary pulmonary hypertension is demonstrated only with fenfluramine and aminorex (2-amino-5-phenyl-2-oxazoline).[22,96,229] Pulmonary hypertension was associated with the use of aminorex as an anorectic agent in Europe from 1965–1968.[97] In 1996, a case-controlled study substantiated the increased risk of pulmonary hypertension with the use of amphetamine appetite-suppressant drugs, particularly with fenfluramine.[1] The risk of pulmonary hypertension was increased 23-fold when the cumulative use of anorectic agents totaled more than 3 months.[1] Pulmonary hypertension may develop following exposure to anorectic agents that may be as brief as 3 weeks.[96] The exact cause of the pulmonary hypertension is unclear. Increased serotonin in the pulmonary vasculature is postulated to result in pulmonary vasoconstriction and endothelial proliferation.[108,179,212] Pulmonary hypertension is not currently reported with sibutramine. Pulmonary hypertension that develops following the use of anorectic drugs may be partially reversible after withdrawal of the agent, however, the median survival of patients studied during the European aminorex epidemic was 3.5 years from the time of diagnosis.[96] With current advances in therapy, improved survival is expected.[214]

Valvular heart disease is also associated with the use of the appetite-suppressants fenfluramine, dexfenfluramine, and phentermine, particularly if the duration of therapy is greater than 4 months.[46,78,117,131,250] The initial reports, in 1997, implicated significant aortic and mitral regurgitation with the use of these agents, and the prevalence was as high as 32%.[31] These reports resulted in the withdrawal of fenfluramine and dexfenfluramine. Subsequent studies demonstrated mostly mild aortic regurgitation and possible mitral regurgitation; the overall prevalence varies from study to study, ranging from 0.14% to 22.7%.[78,117,131,248] The highest risks appear to be in patients taking combination therapy with fenfluramine and phentermine, and those who utilized the agent for more prolonged periods (>4 months).[117] The dramatic differences in the overall prevalence rate in these studies may be related to differences in patient population, duration of therapy, and the timing of echocardiography (ie, during therapy or after the cessation of therapy). The echocardiographic findings usually improve following cessation of these agents.[106] The exact etiology of the valvular disease is unclear, but postulated to be related to the presence of increased serotonin levels. Similar valvular disorders are recognized in patients exposed to persistently increased serotonin levels with conditions such as malignant carcinoid syndrome.[211]

Although the chronic administration of MDMA and its analogues are better publicized and were discussed earlier, chronic administration of various amphetamines, including amphetamine and methamphetamine, to animals, depletes dopamine and serotonin in the neuronal synapses and produces irreversible destruction of those neurons.[15,80,205,206,208,224,255] The etiology of neuronal toxicity may be related to the generation of free oxygen radicals, resulting in the generation of toxic dopamine and serotonin metabolites and neuronal destruction.[80,142,223,255,256] Although not as well studied as MDMA, recent studies in former methamphetamine users demonstrated impaired memory and psychomotor functions, as well as corresponding dopamine transporter dysfunction and abnormal glucose metabolisms on PET scans.[244,245] The potential for permanent neurologic effects associated with chronic amphetamines use requires further study.

Finally, multiple medical complications can result from parenteral drug use and from the associated contaminants. Contami-

nation with infectious agents may result in HIV infection, hepatitis, and malaria. Bacterial and foreign body contamination may result in endocarditis, tetanus, wound botulism, osteomyelitis, and pulmonary and soft tissue abscesses[37] (Chaps. 8 and 109).

DIAGNOSTIC TESTING

Diagnosis by history is rarely reliable, and there is no readily available drug-specific serum analysis. The prevalence of amphetamine abuse in the local geographic region should heighten the suspicion of amphetamine toxicity. The physical and psychological assessment is nonspecific, and polydrug abuse is quite common. Qualitative urine immunoassay testing for amphetamines is available, but it is not valuable in the acute setting. Typically, the turnaround time for the test result is at least several hours, which is far too long to be clinically useful. Both false-positive and false-negative results are common. Many cold preparations contain structurally similar substances (pseudoephedrine, ephedrine, phenylpropanolamine, l-methamphetamine) that may cross-react with the available immunoassays.[44,64,75,196] In addition some immunoassays may not react with all amphetamines, resulting in false-negative results. MDMA frequently goes unrecognized on standardized testing.[16,44] Selegiline, a selective MAO-B inhibitor used for the treatment of parkinsonism, is metabolized to amphetamine and methamphetamine; patients taking selegiline will react positively with most amphetamine-testing techniques.[123] Even a true-positive result only means the patient has used an amphetamine analogue within the last several days. Management decisions must be determined by the clinical manifestations and impressions. Although newer, rapid, serum qualitative drug screens are available, false-positive and false-negative results remain common and may be misleading. The gold standard for drug testing, gas chromatography/mass spectrometry analysis, can misidentify isomeric substances such as l-methamphetamine, which is present in nasal inhalers, with d-methamphetamine if performed by inexperienced personnel.[233] In summary, the suspicion of amphetamine toxicity cannot be confirmed rapidly with a high level of reliability by the laboratory.

MANAGEMENT

Table 68–3 summarizes the therapeutic approach to a patient with amphetamine toxicity. The initial medical assessment of the agitated patient must include the vital signs and a rapid complete physical examination. An often-neglected vital sign is the rectal temperature. Hyperthermia, a frequent and rapidly fatal manifestation in patients with drug-induced delirium, requires immediate interventions to achieve cooling.[81,120,129] Some patients will require physical restraint to gain clinical control and prevent personal harm to themselves or others. Because agitation and resistance against physical restraint may lead to rhabdomyolysis and continued heat generation, intravenous chemical sedation should be instituted immediately. Blood specimens should be sent for glucose, BUN, and electrolyte assays. Hyponatremia should be considered for patient with altered sensorium and suspected MDMA usage (see Chap. 24). Intravenous (IV) glucose ($D_{50}W$, 0.5–1 g/kg) and thiamine 100 mg should be given as indicated. An ECG should be obtained to exclude ischemia, hyperkalemia, and drug toxicity (cyclic antidepressant), and cardiac monitoring should be initiated.

TABLE 68–3. Management of Patients with Amphetamine Toxicity

Agitation
Benzodiazepines (usually adequate for the cardiovascular manifestations)
Diazepam 10 mg (or equivalent) IV, repeat rapidly until the patient is calm (cumulative dose may be >100 mg of diazepam)

Seizures
Benzodiazepines
Barbiturates
Propofol

Hyperthermia
External cooling
Control agitation rapidly

Gastric decontamination and elimination
Activated charcoal for oral ingestions

Hypertension
Control agitation first
α-Adrenergic receptor antagonist (phentolamine)
Vasodilator (nitroprusside, nitroglycerin)

Delirium or hallucinations with abnormal vital signs
If agitated: benzodiazepines

Delirium or hallucinations with normal vital signs
Consider haloperidol or droperidol

A complete blood count, urinalysis, coagulation profile, chest radiograph, CT of the head, and lumbar puncture may be necessary, depending on the clinical presentation.

Because the clinician cannot accurately distinguish the diverse etiologies of drug-induced delirium, the choice of chemical sedation should be safe and effective regardless of the etiology. The most appropriate choice of sedation is a benzodiazepine because these agents have a high therapeutic index and good anticonvulsant activity. They are effective for the treatment of delirium induced by acute overdose of cocaine, amphetamines, and other agents, and the delirium associated with ethanol and sedative-hypnotic withdrawal.[57,60,87,187] The dose of benzodiazepine should be titrated rapidly intravenously until the patient is calm. In our clinical experience, cumulative benzodiazepine dosages required in the initial 30 minutes to achieve adequate sedation frequently exceeds 100 mg of diazepam or its equivalent. Antipsychotic agents, particularly potent dopamine antagonists such as haloperidol and droperidol, are frequently recommended by others for amphetamine-induced delirium. Antipsychotic agents may actually antagonize some of the effects of amphetamines via dopamine blockade.[57,58,71] In animal models, haloperidol may be superior to diazepam in preventing mortality from amphetamine toxicity.[33,54,57,58] In clinical experience, however, the benzodiazepines appear to be as efficacious as the antipsychotic agents in the management of amphetamine toxicity.[60] Antipsychotic agents may lower the seizure threshold, alter temperature regulation, may cause acute dystonia and cardiac dysrhythmias, and do not interact with the benzodiazepine–γ-aminobutyric acid (GABA)–chloride channel receptor complex. All of these effects may worsen the

clinical outcomes related to occult or concomitant cocaine toxicity and ethanol withdrawal.[87,91,187]

Rhabdomyolysis from amphetamine toxicity usually results from agitation and hyperthermia.[77,129] Sedation prevents further muscle contraction and heat production. External cooling should be instituted for significant hyperthermia. Adequate IV hydration and cardiovascular support should maintain urine output of 1–2 mL/kg/min. Although urinary acidification can significantly increase the elimination and decrease the half-lives of amphetamine or methamphetamine,[11,13,14,53] this pH manipulation does not decrease toxicity, and, in fact, may increase the risk of renal compromise and acute tubular necrosis from rhabdomyolysis. Acidification of the urine should not be considered because of the precipitation of ferrihemate in the renal tubules and increased risk of acute renal failure.[50] Patients with acute renal failure, acidemia, and hyperkalemia will likely require urgent hemodialysis.

Amphetamine body packers should be treated similarly to those who transport cocaine (Chap. 67). Any sympathomimetic symptoms suggesting leakage of the packets require surgical intervention.[247] Fluids, benzodiazepines, intubation, and external cooling may be necessary to stabilize these patients.

SUMMARY

Amphetamine usage is increasing dramatically throughout the United States. Similarly, ED visits, and morbidity and mortality related to amphetamines, parallel amphetamine usage. Many of these complications are similar to those of cocaine, such as agitation, hyperthermia, rhabdomyolysis, myocardial ischemia, and cerebral infarction. Physicians, more than ever, must understand the pathophysiology of amphetamines and be ready to diagnosis and treat its toxicity. The chronic effects of amphetamines as demonstrated in animal models pose serious concerns for humans, particularly as amphetamine usage becomes more prevalent; further studies are required to achieve prevention and management.

REFERENCES

1. Abenhaim L, Moride Y, Brenot F, et al: Appetite-suppressant drugs and the risk of primary pulmonary hypertension. N Engl J Med 1996;335:609–615.
2. Ajaelo I, Koenig K, Snoey E: Severe hyponatremia and inappropriate antidiuretic hormone secretion following ecstasy use. Acad Emerg Med 1998;5:839–840.
3. Allcott JV, Barnhart RA, Mooney LA: Acute lead poisoning in two users of illicit methamphetamine. JAMA 1987;258:510–511.
4. Allen A, Cantrell T: Synthetic reductions in clandestine amphetamine and methamphetamine labs. J Forensic Sci 1989;42:183–199.
5. Allen RP, McCann UD, Ricaurte GA: Persistent effects of (+)3,4-methylenedioxymethamphetamine (MDMA, "ecstasy") on human sleep. Sleep 1993;16:560–564.
6. Anderson RJ, Garza HR, Garriott JC, et al: Intravenous propylhexedrine abuse and sudden death. Am J Med 1979;67:15–20.
7. Anderson RJ, Reed WG, Hillis LD: History, epidemiology, and medical complications of nasal inhaler abuse. Clin Toxicol 1982;19:95–107.
8. Angrist B: Amphetamine psychosis: Clinical variation of the syndrome. In: Cho AK, Segal DS, eds: Amphetamines and Its analogs. Psychopharmacology, Toxicity, and Abuse. San Diego, CA, Academic Press, 1994, pp. 387–414.

9. Bailey DN, Shaw RF: Cocaine and methamphetamine-related deaths in San Diego County (1987): Homicides and accidental overdoses. J Forensic Sci 1989;34:407–422.

10. Baggott M, Heifets B, Jones RT, et al: Chemical analysis of ecstasy pills. JAMA 2000;284:2190.

11. Baselt RC, Cravey RH: Disposition of Toxic Drugs and Chemicals in Man, 3rd ed. Chicago, Year Book, 1989.

12. Battaglia G, DeSouza EB: Pharmacologic profile of amphetamine derivatives at various brain recognition sites: Selective effects on serotonergic systems. NIDA Res Monogr 1989;94:240–258.

13. Beckett AH, Rowland M: Urinary excretion kinetics of amphetamine in man. J Pharm Pharmacol 1965;17:628–639.

14. Beckett AH, Rowland M, Turner P: Influence of urinary pH on excretion of amphetamine. Lancet 1965;1:303.

15. Berger UV, Grzanna R, Molliver ME: Depletion of serotonin using p-chlorophenylalanine (PCPA) and reserpine protects against the neurotoxic effects of p-chloroamphetamine (PCA) in the brain. Exp Neurol 1989;103:111–115.

16. Beyer KL, Bicker JT, Butt JH: Ischemic colitis associated with dextroamphetamine use. J Clin Gastroenterol 1991;13:198–201.

17. Blum K: Central nervous system stimulants. In: Blum K, ed: Handbook of Arousable Drugs. New York, Gardner, 1984, pp. 305–347.

18. Borowski TB, Kirkby RD, Kokkinidis L: Amphetamine and antidepressant drug effects on GABA- and NMDA-related seizures. Brain Res Bull 1993;30:607–610.

19. Boswick DG: Amphetamine-induced cerebral vasculitis. Hum Pathol 1981;12:1031–1033.

20. Bowen JS, Davis GB, Kearney TE, Bardin J: Diffuse vascular spasm associated with 4-bromo-2,5-dimethoxyamphetamine ingestion. JAMA 1983;249:1477–1479.

21. Boyer EW, Quang L, Woolf, et al: Dextromethorphan and ecstasy pills. JAMA 2001;285:409–410.

22. Brenot F, Herve P, Petitpretz P, et al: Primary pulmonary hypertension and fenfluramine use. Br Heart J 1993;70:537–541.

23. Bristow LJ, Thorn L, Tricklebank MD, et al: Competitive NMDA receptor antagonists attenuate the behavioural and neurochemical effects of amphetamine in mice. Eur J Pharmacol 1994;264:353–359.

24. Bruno A, Nolte KB, Chapin J: Stroke associated with ephedrine use. Neurology 1993;43:1313–1316.

25. Buchanan JF, Brown CR: "Designer Drugs": A problem in clinical toxicology. Med Toxicol 1988;3:1–17.

26. Burton BT: Heavy metal and organic contaminants associated with illicit methamphetamine production. NIDA Res Monogr 1991;115:47–59.

27. Call TD, Hartneck J, Dickinson WA, et al: Acute cardiomyopathy secondary to intravenous amphetamine abuse. Ann Intern Med 1982;97:559–560.

28. Callaway CW, Johnson MP, Gold LH, et al: Amphetamine derivatives induce locomotor hyperactivity by acting as indirect serotonin agonists. Psychopharmacology 1991;104:293–301.

29. Callaway CW, Wing LL, Geyer MA: Serotonin release contributes to the locomotor stimulant effects of 3,4-methylenedioxymethamphetamine in rats. J Pharmacol Exp Ther 1990;254:456–464.

30. Capwell RR: Ephedrine-induced mania from an herbal diet supplement [letter]. Am J Psychiatry 1995;152:647.

31. Cardiac valvulopathy associated with exposure to fenfluramine or dexfenfluramine: US Department of Health and Human Services interim public health recommendations, November 1997. MMWR Morb Mortal Wkly Rep 1997;46:1061–1066.

32. Carter N, Rutty GN, Milroy CM, et al: Deaths associated with MBDB misuse. Int J Legal Med 2000;113:168–170.

33. Catravas JD, Waters IW, Davis WM, Hickenbottom JP: Haloperidol for acute amphetamine poisoning: A study in dogs. JAMA 1975;231:1340–1341.

34. Chambers CD: The epidemiology of stimulant abuse: a focus on the amphetamine-related substances. In: Smith DE, Wesson DR, Buxton ME, et al, eds: Amphetamine Use, Misuse, and Abuse. Boston, MA, GK Hall, 1979, pp. 92–103.

35. Chan P, Chen JH, Lee MH, et al: Fatal and nonfatal methamphetamine intoxication in the intensive care unit. J Toxicol Clin Toxicol 1994;32:147–155.

36. Chandler DB, Norton RL, Kauffman J, et al: Lead poisoning associated with intravenous methamphetamine use—Oregon, 1988. MMWR Morb Mortal Wkly Rep 1989;38:830–831.

37. Chiang WK, Goldfrank LG: Medical complications of drug abuse. Med J Aust 1990;152:83–88.

38. Cho AK: Ice: A new dosage form of an old drug. Science 1990;249:631–634.

39. Cho AK, Kumagai Y: Metabolism of amphetamine and other arylisopropylamines. In: Cho AK, Segal DS, eds: Amphetamines and Its Analogs. Psychopharmacology, Toxicity, and Abuse. San Diego, CA, Academic Press, 1994, pp. 43–77.

40. Cho AK, Wright J: Pathways of metabolism of amphetamine. Life Sci 1978;22:363–371.

41. Cimbura G: PMA deaths in Ontario. Can Med Assoc J 1974;110:1263–1267.

42. Citron BP, Halpern M, McCarron M, et al: Necrotizing angitis associated with drug abuse. N Engl J Med 1970;283:1003–1011.

43. Cloud J: It's all the rave. Time 2000;155:64–66.

44. Cody JT, Schwarzhoff R: Fluorescence polarization immunoassay of amphetamine, methamphetamine, and illicit amphetamine analogues. J Anal Toxicol 1993;17:23–33.

45. Colado MI, Williams JL, Green AR: The hyperthermic and neurotoxic effects of "Ecstasy" (MDMA) and 3,4-methylenedioxyamphetamine (MDA) in the Dark Agouti (DA) rat, a model of CYP2D6 poor metabolizer phenotype. Br J Pharmacol 1995;115:1281–1289.

46. Connolly HM, Crary JL, McGoon MD, et al: Valvular heart disease associated with fenfluramine-phentermine. N Engl J Med 1997;337:581–588.

47. Costall B, Naylor RJ: Extrapyramidal and mesolimbic involvement with the stereotypic activity of D- and L-amphetamine. Eur J Pharmacol 1974;15:121–129.

48. Council on Scientific Affairs: Clinical aspects of amphetamine abuse. JAMA 1978;240:2317–2319.

49. Croft CH, Firth BG, Hillis LD: Propylhexedrine-induced left ventricular dysfunction. Ann Intern Med 1982;97:560–561.

50. Curry SC, Chang D, Connor D: Drug- and toxin-induced rhabdomyolysis. Ann Emerg Med 1989;18:1068–1084.

51. Dal Carson TA, Angelos JA, Raney JK: A clandestine approach to the synthesis of phenyl-2-propanone from phenylpropenes. J Forensic Sci 1984;29:1187–1208.

52. Davis GG, Swalwell CI: Acute aortic dissections and ruptured berry aneurysms associated with methamphetamine abuse. J Forsensic Sci 1994;39:1481–1485.

53. Davis JM, Kopin IJ, Lemberger L, et al: Effects of urinary pH on amphetamine metabolism. Ann N Y Acad Sci 1971;179:493–501.

54. Davis MW, Logston DG, Hickenbottom JP: Antagonism of acute amphetamine intoxication by haloperidol and propranolol. Toxicol Appl Pharmacol 1974;29:397–403.

55. Delaney P, Estes M: Intracranial hemorrhage with amphetamine abuse. Neurology 1980;30:1125–1128.

56. Delliou D, Bromo DMA: New hallucinogenic drug [letter]. Med J Aust 1980;1:83.

57. Derlet RW, Albertson TE, Rice P: Antagonism of cocaine, amphetamine, and methamphetamine toxicity. Pharmacol Biochem Behavior 1990;36:745–749.

58. Derlet RW, Albertson TE, Rice P: Protection against d-amphetamine toxicity. Am J Emerg Med 1990;8:105–108.

59. Derlet RW, Heischober B: Methamphetamine. Stimulant of the 1990s? West J Med 1990;153:625–628.

60. Derlet RW, Rice P, Horowitz BZ, Lord RV: Amphetamine toxicity: Experience with 127 cases. J Emerg Med 1989;7:157–161.

61. De Souza EB, Battaglia G: Effects of MDMA and MDA on brain serotonin neurons: Evidence from neurochemical and autoradiographic studies. NIDA Res Monogr 1989;94:196–222.

62. Devan GS: Phentermine and psychosis. Br J Psychiatry 1990;156:442–443.

63. Di Maio VJM, Garriott JC: Intravenous abuse of propylhexedrine. J Forensic Sci 1977;22:152–158.

64. D'Nicoula J, Jones R, Levine B, et al: Evaluation of six commercial amphetamine and methamphetamine immunoassays for cross-reactivity to phenylpropanolamine and ephedrine in urine. J Anal Toxicol 1992;16:211–213.

65. Doflou J, Mark A: Aortic dissection after ingestion of "ecstasy" (MDMA). Am J Forensic Med Pathol 2000;21:261–263.

66. Dowling GP, McDonough ET, Bost RO: "Eve" and "ecstasy." A report of five deaths associated with the use of MDEA and MDMA. JAMA 1987;257:1615–1617.

67. Edison GR: Amphetamines: A dangerous illusion. Ann Intern Med 1971;74:605–610.

68. Ellinwood EH: Assault and homicide associated with amphetamine abuse. Am J Psychiatry 1971;127:1170–1175.

69. Emerson TS, Cisek JE: Methcathinone ("cat"): A Russian designer amphetamine infiltrates the rural Midwest. Ann Emerg Med 1993;22:1897–1903.

70. Erowid's psychoactive vaults. http://www.erowid.org/psychoactives/psychoactives.shtml.

71. Espelin DE, Done AK: Amphetamine poisoning. Effectiveness of chlorpromazine. N Engl J Med 1968;278:1361–1365.

72. Feinstein D: The Methamphetamine Control Act of 1996. http://www.senate.gov/member/ca/feinstein/general/meth.html.

73. Felgate HE, Felgate PD, James RA, et al: Recent paramethoxyamphetamine deaths. J Anal Toxicol 1998;22:169–172.

74. Fischman MW: Cocaine and the amphetamines. In: Meltzer HY, ed: Psychopharmacology: The Third Generation of Progress. New York, Raven, 1987, pp. 1543–1553.

75. Fitzgerald RL, Ramos JM Jr, Bogema SC, et al: Resolution of methamphetamine stereoisomers in urine drug testing: urinary excretion of R(−)-methamphetamine following use of nasal inhalers. J Anal Toxicol 1988;12:255–259.

76. Furst SR, Fallon SP, Reznik GN, et al: Myocardial infarction after inhalation of methamphetamine. N Engl J Med 1990;323:1147–1148.

77. Gal J: Amphetamines in nasal inhalers. Clin Toxicol 1982;19:577–578.

78. Gardin JM, Schumacher D, Constantine G, et al: Valvular abnormalities and cardiovascular status following exposure to dexfenfluramine or phentermine/fenfluramine. JAMA 2000;283:1703–1709.

79. Gary NE, Saidi M: Methamphetamine intoxication. A speedy new treatment. Am J Med 1978;64:537–540.

80. Gibb JW, Johnson M, Elayan I, et al: Neurotoxicity of amphetamines and their metabolites. NIDA Res Monogr 1997;173:128–145.

81. Ginsberg MD, Hertzman M, Schmidt-Nowara W: Amphetamine intoxication with coagulopathy, hyperthermia, and reversible renal failure. A syndrome resembling heatstroke. Ann Intern Med 1970;73:81–85.

82. Giroud C, Augsburger M, River L, et al: 2C-B: a new psychoactive phenylethylamine recently discovered in Ecstasy tablets sold on the Swiss black market. J Anal Toxicol 1998;22:345–354.

83. Glennon RA: Stimulus properties of hallucinogenic phenalkylamines and related designer drugs: Formulation of structure-activity relationship. NIDA Res Monogr 1989;94:43–67.

84. Glennon RA, Showwalter D: The effects of cathinone and several related derivatives on locomotor activity. Res Commun Subst Abuse 1981;2:186–191.

85. Glennon RA, Yousif M, Naiman N, et al: Methcathinone: A new and potent amphetamine-like agent. Pharmacol Biochem Behavior 1987;26:547–551.

86. Gold LHG, Geyer MA, Koob GF: Neurochemical mechanisms involved in behavioral effects of amphetamines and related designer drugs. NIDA Res Monogr 1989;94:101–126.

87. Goldfrank LR, Hoffman RS: The cardiovascular effects of cocaine. Ann Emerg Med 1991;20:165–175.

88. Goldstone MS: "Cat": Methcathinone—A new drug of abuse [letter]. JAMA 1993;269:2508.

89. Gospe SM Jr: Transient cortical blindness in an infant exposed to methamphetamine. Ann Emerg Med 1995;26:380–382.

90. Gouzoulis-Mayfrank E, Daumann J, Tuchtenhagen F, et al: Impaired cognitive performance in drug-free users of recreational ecstasy (MDMA). J Neurol Neurosurg Psych 2000;68:719–725.

91. Greenblatt DJ, Gross PL, Harris J, et al: Fatal hyperthermia following haloperidol therapy of sedative-hypnotic withdrawal. J Clin Psychiatry 1978;39:673–675.

92. Greenblatt JC, Gfroerer JC, Melnick D: Increasing morbidity and mortality associated with abuse of methamphetamine—United States, 1991–1994. MMWR Morb Mortal Wkly Rep 1995;44:882–886.

93. Greer G, Tolbert R: Subjective reports on the effects of MDMA in a clinical setting. J Psychoact Drugs 1986;18:319–327.

94. Grinspoon L, Bakalar JB: Amphetamines: Medical and health hazards. In: Smith DE, Wesson DR, Buxton ME, et al, eds: Amphetamine Use, Misuse, and Abuse. Boston, MA, GK Hall, 1979, pp. 18–34.

95. Groves PM, Ryan LJ, Diana M, et al: Neuronal actions of amphetamine in the rat brain. NIDA Res Monogr 1989;94:127–145.

96. Gurtner HP: Aminorex and pulmonary hypertension. Cor Vasa 1985;27:160–171.

97. Gurtner HP, Gertsch M, Salzmann C, et al: Haufen sich die primar vascularen Formen des chronischen Cor pulmonale? Schweiz Med Wochenschr 1968;98:1579–1589.

98. Halbach H: Medical aspects of the chewing of khat leaves. Bull WHO 1972;27:21–29.

98a. Haller CA, Benowitz NL: Adverse cardiovascular and central nervous system events associated with dietary supplements containing ephedra alkaloids. N Engl J Med 2000;343:1833–1838.

99. Hamer R, Phelphs D: Inadvertent intra-arterial injection of phentermine: A complication of drug abuse. Ann Emerg Med 1981;10:148–150.

100. Harrington H, Heller HA, Dawson D, et al: Intracerebral hemorrhage and oral amphetamine. Arch Neurol 1983;40:503–507.

101. Hart JB, Wallace J: The adverse effects of amphetamines. Clin Toxicol 1975;8:179–190.

102. Heischober B, Miller MA: Methamphetamine abuse in California. NIDA Res Monogr 1991;115:60–71.

103. Henry JA, Fallon JK, Kicman AT, et al: Low-dose MDMA ("ecstasy") induces vasopressin secretion. Lancet 1998;351:1784.

104. Henry JA, Hill IR: Fatal interaction between ritonavir and MDMA. Lancet 1998;325:1751–1752.

105. Henry JA, Jeffrey KJ, Dawling S: Toxicity and deaths from 3,4-methylenedioxymethamphetamine ("ecstasy"). Lancet 1992;340:384–387.

106. Hensrud DD, Connolly HM, Grogan M, et al: Echocardiographic improvement over time after cessation of use of fenfluramine and phentermine. Mayo Clin Proc 1999;74:1191–1197.

107. Herr RD, Caravati EM: Acute transient ischemic colitis after oral methamphetamine ingestion. Am J Emerg Med 1991;9:406–409.

108. Herve P, Launay J, Scrobohaci M, et al: Increased plasma serotonin in primary pulmonary hypertension. Am J Med 1995;99:249–254.

109. Hirata H, Ladenheim B, Rothman RB, et al: Methamphetamine-induced serotonin neurotoxicity is mediated by superoxide radicals. Brain Res 1995;677:345–347.

110. Hoffman BB, Lefkowitz RJ: Catecholamines, sympathomimetic drugs, and adrenergic receptor antagonists. In: Hardman JG, Limbird LE, Molinoff PB, et al, eds: Goodman and Gilman's The Pharmaco-

logical Basis of Therapeutics, 9th ed. New York, McGraw-Hill, 1996, pp. 199–227.

111. Hong R, Matsuyama E, Nur K: Cardiomyopathy associated with the smoking of crystal methamphetamine. JAMA 1991;265: 1152–1154.

112. Imanse J, Vanneste J: Intraventricular hemorrhage following amphetamine abuse. Neurology 1990;40:1318–1319.

113. Irvine GD, Chin L: The environmental impact and adverse health effects of the clandestine manufacture of methamphetamine. NIDA Res Monogr 1991;115:33–46.

114. Iversen L: Neurotransmitter transporters: Fruitful targets for CNS drug discovery. Mol Psychiatry 2000;5:357–362.

115. Jackson JG: Hazards of smokable methamphetamine [letter]. N Engl J Med 1989;321:907.

116. Jerrard DA: "Designer drugs"—A current perspective. J Emerg Med 1990;8:733–741.

117. Jick H, Vasilakis C, Weinrauch LA, et al: A population-based study of appetite-suppressant drugs and the risk of cardiac-valve regurgitation. N Engl J Med 1998;339:719–724.

118. Johnson LF, Anggaro E, Gunne LM: Blockade of intravenous amphetamine euphoria in man. Clin Pharmacol Ther 1971;12:889–896.

119. Johnson TD, Berenson MM: Methamphetamine-induced ischemic colitis. J Clin Gastroenterol 1991;13:687–689.

120. Jordan SC, Hampson F: Amphetamine poisoning associated with hyperpyrexia. Br J Med 1960;2:844.

121. Kalant H, Kalant OJ: Death in amphetamine users: Causes and rates. Can Med Assoc J 1975;112:299–304.

122. Kalix P: Pharmacological properties of the stimulant khat. Pharmacol Ther 1990;48:397–416.

123. Karch SB: Synthetic stimulants. In Karch SB: The pathology of drug abuse. Boca Raton, FL, CRC Press, 1993, pp. 165–218.

124. Karch SB, Billingham ME: The pathology and etiology of cocaine-induced heart disease. Arch Pathol Lab Med 1988;112:225–230.

125. Karler R, Calder LD, Thai LH, et al: The dopaminergic, glutamatergic, GABAergic bases for the action of amphetamine and cocaine. Brain Res 1995;671:100–104.

126. Karler R, Calder LD, Thai LH, et al: A dopaminergic-glutamatergic basis for the action of amphetamine and cocaine. Brain Res 1994; 658:8–14.

127. Kase CS, Foster TE, Reed JE, et al: Intracerebral hemorrhage and phenylpropanolamine use. Neurology 1987;37:399–404.

128. Katsumata S, Sato K, Kashiwade H, et al: Sudden death due presumably to internal use of methamphetamine. Forensic Sci Int 1993;62: 209–215.

129. Kendrick WC, Hull AR, Knochel JP: Rhabdomyolysis and shock after intravenous amphetamine administration. Ann Intern Med 1977;86:381–387.

130. Kernan WN, Viscoli CM, Brass LM, et al: Phenylpropanolamine and the risk of hemorrhagic stroke. N Engl J Med 2000;343:1826–1832.

131. Khan MA, Herzog CA, St. Peter JV, et al: The prevalence of cardiac valvular insufficiency assessed by transthoracic echocardiography in obese patients treated with appetite-suppressants drugs. N Engl J Med 1998;339:713–718.

132. Kintz P: Excretion of MBDB and BDB in urine, saliva, and sweat following single oral administration. J Anal Toxicol 1997;21: 570–575.

133. Klatt EC, Montgomery S, Nemiki T, et al: Misrepresentation of stimulant street drugs: A decade of experience in analysis program. J Toxicol Clin Toxicol 1986;24:441–450.

134. Klawans HL, Weiner WJ: The effects of D-amphetamine on choreiform movement disorder. Neurology 1974;6:312–318.

135. Koch crime institute: Methamphetamine trends in drug abuse, June 1998. http://www.kci.org/meth_info/june98_trends.htm.

136. Kojima T, Matsushima E, Iwama H, et al: Visual perception process in amphetamine psychosis and schizophrenia. Psychopharmacol Bull 1986;22:768–773.

137. Kokkinidis L, Zacharko RM, Anisman H: Amphetamine withdrawal: A behavioral evaluation. Life Sci 1968;38:1617–1623.

138. Kokkinos J, Levine SR: Possible association of ischemic stroke with phentermine. Stroke 1993;24:310–313.

139. Kram TC, Kram BS, Kruegel AV: The identification of impurities in illicit methamphetamine exhibits by gas chromatography/mass spectrometry and nuclear magnetic resonance spectroscopy. J Forensic Sci 1976;22:40–52.

140. Kramer JC, Fischman VS, Littlefield DC: Amphetamine abuse. Pattern and effects of high doses taken intravenously. JAMA 1967; 201:89–93.

141. Kringsholm B, Christoffersen P: Lung and heart pathology in fatal drug addiction. A consecutive autopsy study. Forensic Sci Int 1987; 34:39–51.

142. Kuhn DM, Geddes TJ: Molecular footprints of neurotoxic amphetamine action. Ann N Y Acad Sci 2000;914:92S–103S.

143. Lago JA, Kosten TR: Stimulant withdrawal. Addiction 1994;89: 1477–1481.

144. Lake C, Quirk R: Stimulants and look-alike drugs. Psychiatr Clin North Am 1984;7:689–701.

145. Lean MEJ: Sibutramine—a review of clinical efficacy. Int J Obesity 1997;21:S30–S36.

146. Lerner MA: The fire of ice. Newsweek, November 27, 1989, pp. 37–40.

147. Liggett SB: Propylhexedrine intoxication: Clinical presentation and pharmacology. South Med J 1982;76:250–251.

148. Little BB, Snell LM, Gilstrap LC: Methamphetamine abuse during pregnancy: Outcome and fetal effects. Obstet Gynecol 1988;72: 541–544.

149. Logan BK, Fligner CL, Haddix T: Cause and manner of death in fatalities involving methamphetamine. J Forensic Sci 1998;43: 28–34.

150. Lucas AR, Weiss M: Methylphenidate hallucinosis. JAMA 1971; 217:1079–1081.

151. Lucas BB, Gardner DL, Wolkowitz OM, et al: Methylphenidate-induced cardiac arrhythmias. N Engl J Med 1986;315:1485.

152. Lukes SA: Intracerebral hemorrhage from an arteriovenous malformation after amphetamine injection. Arch Neurol 1983;40:60–61.

153. Lundh H, Tunuing K: An extrapyramidal choreiform syndrome caused by amphetamine addiction. J Neurol Neurosurg Psych 1981; 44:728–730.

154. Luqman W, Danowski TS: The use of khat (Catha edulis) in Yemen social and medical observation. Ann Intern Med 1976;85: 246–249.

155. Luque CA, Rey JA: Sibutramine: A serotonin-norepinephrine reuptake-inhibitor for the treatment of obesity. Ann Pharmacother 1999; 33:968–978.

156. Mancusi-Ungaro HR, Decker WJ: Tissue injuries associated with parenteral propylhexedrine abuse. J Toxicol Clin Toxicol 1983–1984;21:359–372.

157. Marsden P, Sheldon J: Acute poisoning by propylhexedrine. Br Med J 1972;1:730.

158. Mattson RH, Calverley JR: Dextroamphetamine-sulfate–induced dyskinesis. JAMA 1968;204:108–110.

159. Maurer HH, Bickeboeller-Friedrich J, Kraemer T, et al: Toxicokinetics and analytical toxicology of amphetamine-derived designer drugs ("Ecstasy"). Toxicol Lett 2000;112–113:133–142.

160. Maxwell DL, Polkey MI, Henry JA: Hyponatremia and catatonic stupor after taking "ecstasy". BMJ 1993;307:1399.

161. McCann UD, Eligulashvilli V, Ricaurte GA: (+/−)3,4-Methylenedioxymethamphetamine ("'ecstasy'")-induced serotonin neurotoxicity: Clinical studies. Neuropsychology 2000;42:11–16.

162. McCann UD, Ricaurte GA: Lasting neuropsychiatric sequelae of methylenedioxymethamphetamine ("ecstasy") in recreational users. J Clin Psychopharmacology 1991;11:302–305.

163. McCann UD, Ricaurte GA: Use and abuse of ring-substituted amphetamines. In: Cho AK, Segal DS, eds: Amphetamines and Its

Analogs. Psychopharmacology, Toxicity, and Abuse. San Diego, CA, Academic Press, 1994, pp. 371–386.

164. McCann UD, Ridenour A, Shaham Y, et al: Serotonin neurotoxicity after 3,4-methylenedioxymethamphetamine (MDMA: "ectasy"): A controlled study in humans. Neuropsychopharmacology 1994;10:129–138.

165. McCann UD, Slate SO, Ricaurte GA: Adverse reactions with 3,4-methylenedioxymethamphetamine (MDMA; "ecstasy"). Drug Saf 1996;15:107–115.

166. McCann UD, Szabo Z, Scheffel U, et al: Positron emission tomographic evidence of toxic effect of MDMA ("ectasy") on brain serotonin neurons in human beings. Lancet 1998;352:1433–1437.

167. McGuire P: Long-term psychiatric and cognitive effects of MDMA use. Toxicol Lett 2000;112–113:153–156.

168. McGuire PK, Cope HM, Fahy T, et al: Diverse psychiatric morbidity associated with use of 3,4-methylenedioxymethamphetamine ("ectasy"). Br J Psychiatry 1994;165:391–394.

169. Miller MA: Trends and patterns of methamphetamine smoking in Hawaii. NIDA Res Monogr 1991;115:72–83.

170. Miller MA, Hughes AL: Epidemiology of amphetamine use in the United States. In: Cho AK, Segal DS, eds: Amphetamines and Its Analogs. Psychopharmacology, Toxicity, and Abuse. San Diego, CA, Academic Press, 1994, pp. 439–457.

171. Molliver ME: Serotonergic neuronal systems: What their anatomic organization tells us about function. J Clin Psychopharmacol 1987;7:3S–23S.

172. Molliver ME, Berger UV, Mamounas LA, et al: Neurotoxicity of MDMA and related compounds: Anatomic studies. Ann N Y Acad Sci 1990;600:640–661.

173. Morgan JP: Amphetamine and methamphetamine during the 1990s. Pediatr Rev 1992;13:330–333.

174. Morgan JP: The clinical pharmacology of amphetamine. In: Smith DE, Wesson DR, Buxton ME, et al, eds: Amphetamine Use, Misuse, and Abuse. Boston, MA, GK Hall, 1979, pp. 3–10.

175. Morgan JP, Kagan D: Street amphetamine quality and the controlled substances act of 1970. In: Smith DE, Wesson DR, Buxton ME, et al, eds: Amphetamine Use, Misuse, and Abuse. Boston, MA, GK Hall, 1979, pp. 73–91.

176. Morgan M: Memory deficits associated with recreational use of "ecstasy" (MDMA). Psychopharmacology 1999;141:30–36.

177. Mueller PD, Korey WS: Death by "ecstasy": The serotonin syndrome? Ann Emerg Med 1998;32:377–380.

178. Nadir A, Agrawal S, King PD, et al: Acute hepatitis associated with the use of a Chinese herbal product, ma-huang. Am J Gastroenterol 1996;91:1436–1438.

179. Naeije R, Wauthy P, Maggiorini M, et al: Effects of dexfenfluramine on hypoxic pulmonary vasoconstriction and emboli pulmonary hypertension in dogs. Am J Respir Crit Care Med 1995;151:692–697.

180. Nestor TA, Tamamoto WI, Kam TH: Acute pulmonary oedema caused by crystalline methamphetamine. Lancet 1989;2:1277–1278.

181. Nichols DE: Medicinal chemistry and structure-activity relationships. In: Cho AK, Segal DS, eds: Amphetamines and Its Analogs. Psychopharmacology, Toxicity, and Abuse. San Diego, CA, Academic Press, 1994, pp. 3–41.

182. Nichols DE, Oberlender R: Structure-activity relationships of MDMA-like substances. NIDA Res Monogr 1989;94:1–29 .

183. Nuvials X, Masclans JR, Peracaula R, et al: Hyponatremic coma after ecstasy ingestion. Intensive Care Med 1997;23:480.

184. Obradovic T, Imel KM, White SR: Repeat exposure to methylenedioxymethamphetamine (MDMA) alters nucleus accumbens neuronal responses to dopamine and serotonin. Brain Res 1998;785:1–9.

185. Obrocki J, Buchert R, Vaterlein O, et al: Ecstasy—Long-term effects on the human central nervous system revealed by positron emission tomography. Br J Psych 1999;175:186–188.

186. Ohmori T, Abekawa T, Muraki A, et al: Competitive and noncompetitive NMDA antagonists block sensitization to methamphetamine. Pharmacol Biochem Behav 1994;48:587–591.

187. Olmedo R, Hoffman RS: Withdrawal syndromes. Emerg Med Clin North Am 2000;18:273–288.

188. O'Neill ME, Arnolda LF, Coles DM, et al: Acute amphetamine cardiomyopathy in a drug addict. Clin Cardiol 1983;6:189–191.

189. Ong BH: Hazards to health. Dextroamphetamine poisoning. N Engl J Med 1962;266:1321–1322.

190. Packe GE, Garton MJ, Kennings K: Acute myocardial infarction caused by intravenous amphetamine abuse. Br Heart J 1990;64:23–24.

191. Pedersen W, Skrondal A: Ecstasy and new patterns of drug use: A normal population study. Addiction 1999;94:1695–1706.

192. Pentel P: Toxicity of over-the-counter stimulants. JAMA 1984;252:1898–1903.

193. Peroutka SJ: Incidence of recreational use of MDMA "ecstasy" on an underground campus. N Engl J Med 1987;317:1542–1543.

194. Perrotta DM, Coody G, Culmo C, et al: Adverse events associated with ephedrine-containing products—Texas, December 1993 to September 1995. MMWR Morb Mortal Wkly Rep 1996,45.689–693.

195. Pitts DK, Marwah J: Cocaine and central monoaminergic neurotransmission: A review of electrophysiological studies and comparison to amphetamine and antidepressants. Life Sci 1988;42:949–968.

196. Poklis A, Moore KA: Stereoselectivity of the TdxADx/FLx amphetamine/methamphetamine II amphetamine/methamphetamine immunoassay—Response of urine specimens following nasal inhaler use. Clin Toxicol 1995;33:35–41.

197. Puder KD, Kagan DV, Morgan JP: Illicit methamphetamine, analysis, synthesis, and availability. Am J Drug Alcohol Abuse 1988;14:463–473.

198. Randall T: Ecstasy-fueled "rave" parties become dances of death for English youths. JAMA 1992;268:1505–1506.

199. Randall T: "Rave" scene, ecstasy use, leap Atlantic. JAMA 1992;268:1506.

200. Rasmussen S, Cole R, Spiehler V: Methamphetamine prevalence in sheriff's crime lab samples. J Anal Toxicol 1989;12:263–267.

201. Reneman L, Booij J, Schmand B, et al: Memory disturbances in "ecstasy" users are correlated with an altered serotonin neurotransmission. Psychopharmacology 2000;148:322–324.

202. Rhee KJ, Albertson TE, Douglas JC: Choreoathetoid disorder associated with amphetamine-like drugs. Am J Emerg Med 1988;6:131–133.

203. Ricaurte GA, DeLanney LE, Irwin I, et al: Toxic effects of MDMA on central serotonergic neurons in the primate: Importance of route and frequency of drug administration. Brain Res 1988;446:165–168.

204. Ricaurte GA, Finnegan KF, Irwin I, et al: Aminergic metabolites in cerebrospinal fluid of humans previously exposed to MDMA: Preliminary observations. Ann N Y Acad Sci 1990;600:699–710.

205. Ricaurte GA, Finnegan KF, Nichols DE, et al: 3,4-Methylenedioxyethylamphetamine (MDE), a novel analogue of MDMA, produces long-lasting depletion of serotonin in the rat brain. Eur J Pharmacol 1987;137:265–268.

206. Ricaurte GA, Guillery RW, Seiden LS, et al: Dopamine nerve terminal degeneration produced by high doses of methylamphetamine in the rat brain. Brain Res 1982;235:93–103.

207. Ricaurte GA, McCann UD, Szabo Z, et al: Toxicodynamics and long-term toxicity of the recreational drug, 3,4-methylenedioxymethamphetamine (MDMA, "ecstasy"). Toxicol Lett 2000;112–113:143–146.

208. Ricaurte GA, Seiden LS, Schuster CR: Further evidence that amphetamines produce long-lasting dopamine neurochemical deficits by destroying dopamine nerve fibers. Brain Res 1984;303:359–364.

209. Richards KC, Borgstedt HH: Near fatal reaction to ingestion of the hallucinogenic drug MDA. JAMA 1971;218:1826–1827.

210. Riley I, Corson J, Haider I, et al: Fenfluramine overdosage. Lancet 1969;2:1162–1163.

211. Robiolio PA, Rigolin VH, Wilson JS, et al: Carcinoid heart disease: Correlation of high serotonin levels with valvular abnormalities de-

tected by cardiac catheterization and echocardiography. Circulation 1995;92:790–795.

212. Rothman RB, Ayestas MA, Dersch CM, et al: Aminorex, fenfluramine, and chlorphentermine are serotonin transporter substrates. Implications for primary pulmonary hypertension. Circulation 1999; 100:869–875.

213. Rothrock JF, Rubenstein R, Lyden PD: Ischemic stroke associated with methamphetamine inhalation. Neurology 1988;38:589–592.

214. Rubin LJ: Primary pulmonary hypertension. N Engl J Med 1997; 336:111–117.

215. Rumbaugh CL, Bergeron RT, Fang HCH, et al: Cerebral angiographic changes in drug abuse patient. Radiology 1971;101: 335–344.

216. Rumbaugh CL, Bergeron RT, Scanlan RL, et al: Cerebral vascular changes secondary to amphetamine abuse in the experimental animal. Radiology 1971;101:345–351.

217. Rumbaugh CL, Fang HCH, Higgins RE, et al: Cerebral microvascular injury in experimental drug abuse. Invest Radiol 1976;11: 282–294.

218. Salanova V, Taubner R: Intracerebral haemorrhage and vasculitis secondary to amphetamine use. Postgrad Med J 1984;60:429–430.

219. Sallee FR, Stiller RL, Perel JM, et al: Pemoline-induced abnormal involuntary movements. J Clin Psychopharmacol 1989;9:125–129.

220. Sato M: Psychotoxic manifestations in amphetamine abuse. Psychopharmacol Bull 1986;22:751–756.

221. Schaffer CB, Pauli MW: Psychotic reaction caused by proprietary oral diet agents. Am J Psychiatry 1980;137:1256–1257.

222. Schaiberger PH, Kennedy TC, Miller FC, et al: Pulmonary hypertension associated with long-term inhalation of "crank" methamphetamine. Chest 1993;104:614–616.

223. Seiden LS: Neurotoxicity of methamphetamine: Mechanisms of action and issues related to aging. NIDA Res Monogr 1991;115:24–32.

224. Seiden LS, Klever MS: Methamphetamine and related drugs: Toxicity and resulting behavioral changes in response to pharmacological probes. NIDA Res Monogr 1989;94:146–160.

225. Seiden LS, Sabol KE, Ricaurte GA: Amphetamine: Effects on catecholamine systems and behavior. Annu Rev Pharmacol Toxicol 1993;32:639–677.

226. Sellers EM, Otton SV, Tyndale RF: The potential role of the cytochrome P-450 2D6 pharmacogenetic polymorphism of drug abuse. NIDA Res Monogr 1997;173:9–26.

227. Shankaran M, Yamamoto BK, Gudelsky GA: Ascorbic acid prevents 3,4-methylenedioxymethamphetamine (MDMA)-induced hydroxyl radical formation and the behavioral and neurochemical consequences of the depletion of brain 5-HT. Synapse 2001;40:55–64.

228. Shulgin A, Shulgin A: PIHKAL: A chemical love Story. Berkeley, CA, Transform Press, 1991.

229. Simmonneau G, Fartoukh M, Sitbon O, et al: Primary pulmonary hypertension associated with the use of fenfluramine derivatives. Chest 1998;114:195S–199S.

230. Simpson DL, Rumack BH: Methylenedioxyamphetamine. Clinical description of overdose, death, and review of pharmacology. Arch Intern Med 1981;141:1507–1509.

231. Singh BK, Singh A, Chusid E: Chorea in long-term use of pemoline [letter]. Ann Neurology 1983;13:218.

232. Smith DE, Fisher CM: An analysis of 310 cases of acute high-dose methamphetamine toxicity in Haight Ashbury. Clin Toxicol 1970;3: 117–124.

233. Smith FP, Kidwell DA: Isomeric amphetamines—A problem for urinalysis? Forensic Sci Int 1991;50:153–165.

234. Smith HJ, Roche AHG, Herdson PB: Cardiomyopathy associated with amphetamine administration. Am Heart J 1976;91:792–797.

235. Solowij N, Hall W, Lee N: Recreational MDMA use in Sidney: A profile of "ectasy" users and their experiences with the drug. Br J Addict 1992;87:1161–1172.

236. Sonsalla PK: The role of N-methyl-D-aspartate receptors in dopaminergic neuropathology produced by the amphetamines. Drug Alcohol Depend 1995;37:101–105.

237. Sonsalla PK, Nicklas WJ, Heikkila RE: Role for excitatory amino acids in methamphetamine-induced nigrostriatal dopaminergic toxicity. Science 1989;243:398–400.

238. Stoessl AJ, Young GB, Feasby TE: Intracerebral haemorrhage and angiographic beading following ingestion of catecholaminergics. Stroke 1985;16:734–736.

239. Sudilovsky A: Disruption of behavior in cats by chronic amphetamine intoxication. Int J Neurol 1975;10:259–275.

240. Sulzer D, Chen TK, Lau YY, et al: Amphetamine redistributes dopamine from synaptic vesicles to the cytosol and promotes reverse transport. J Neurosci 1995;15:4105–4108.

241. Sulzer D, Pothos E, Sung HM, et al: Weak base model of amphetamine action. Ann N Y Acad Sci 1992;654:525–528.

242. Tadokoro S, Kuribara H: Reverse tolerance to the ambulation-increasing effect of methamphetamine in mice as an animal model of amphetamine-psychosis. Psychopharmacol Bull 1986;22:757–762.

242a. Traub SJ, Hoyek W, Hoffman RS: Dietary supplements containing ephedra alkaloids. N Engl J Med 2001;344:1095–1097.

243. Trugman JM: Cerebral arteritis and oral methylphenidate. Lancet 1988;1:584–585.

244. Volkow ND, Chang L, Wang G, et al: Association of dopamine transporter reduction with psychomotor impairment in methamphetamine abusers. Am J Psychiatry 2001;158:377–382.

245. Volkow ND, Chang L, Wang G, et al: Higher cortical and lower subcortical metabolism in detoxified methamphetamine abusers. Am J Psychiatry 2001;158:383–389.

246. Waksman J, Taylor RN Jr, Bodor GS, et al: Acute myocardial infarction associated with amphetamine use. Mayo Clin Proc 2001;76: 323–326.

247. Watson CJ, Thomson HJ, Johnston PS: Body-packing with amphetamines—An indication for surgery. J R Soc Med 1991;84: 311–312.

248. Wee CC, Phillips RS, Aurigemma G: Risk for valvular heart disease among users of fenfluramine and dexfenfluramine who underwent echocardiography before use of medication. Ann Intern Med 1998;129:870–874.

249. Weir E: Raves: A review of the culture, the drugs and the prevention of harm. CMAJ 2000;162:1829–1830.

250. Weissman NJ, Tighe JF Jr, Gottdiener JS, et al: An assessment of heart-valve abnormalities in obese patients taking dexfenfluramine, sustained-release dexfenfluramine, or placebo. N Engl J Med 1998; 339:725–732.

251. White L, DiMaio VJM: Intravenous propylhexedrine and sudden death [letter]. N Engl J Med 1977;297:1071.

252. Wiener RS, Lockhart JT, Schwartz RG: Dilated cardiomyopathy and cocaine abuse. Report of two cases. Am J Med 1986;81:699–701.

253. William H, Dratcu L, Taylor R, et al: "Saturday night fever": Ecstasy-related problems in a London accident and emergency department. J Accid Emerg Med 1998;15:322–326.

254. Wooten MR, Khangure MS, Murphy MJ: Intracerebral hemorrhage and vasculitis related to ephedrine use. Ann Neurol 1983;13: 337–340.

255. Wrona MZ, Yang Z, Zhang F, et al: Potential new insights into the molecular mechanism of methamphetamine-induced neurodegeneration. NIDA Res Monogr 1997;173:146–174.

256. Yamamoto BK, Zhu W: The effects of methamphetamine on the production of free radical and oxidative stress. J Pharmacol Exp Ther 1988;287:107–114.

257. Young R, Glennon RA: Cocaine-stimulus generalization to two new designer drugs: Methcathinone and 4-methylaminorex. Pharmacol Biochem Behavior 1993;45:229–231.

258. Yu YJ, Cooper DR, Wellenstein DE, et al: Cerebral angiitis and intracerebral hemorrhage associated with methamphetamine abuse. J Neurosurg 1983;58:109–111.

259. Zhinger KY, Dovensky W, Crossman A, et al: Ephedrone: 2-Methylamino-1-phenylpropan-1-one (Jeff). J Forensic Sci 1991;36: 915–920.

CHAPTER 69

PHENCYCLIDINE AND KETAMINE

Rueben Olmedo

Phencyclidine (PCP)   Ketamine

A 17-year-old male was brought to the Emergency Department (ED) by his school supervisor and two police officers. The boy was extremely agitated, with transient periods of blank staring and myoclonic movements of both arms. It took several members of the ED staff to keep him on a stretcher.

Initially, no history was obtainable from the patient, who responded to verbal stimuli with inappropriate physical gestures and a few nonsensical words. The school supervisor reported that the boy had become suddenly agitated and had created a disturbance in the lunchroom, throwing chairs about the room.

His vital signs were: blood pressure, 130/90 mm Hg; pulse, 110 beats/min; respiratory rate, 18 breaths/min; and temperature, 99.9°F (37.2°C). He was well developed and well nourished, anicteric, and acyanotic. The examination was normal except for a few pertinent findings. The skin was cool and diaphoretic. Conjunctivae were normal; extraocular movements were intact, but there was persistent vertical and horizontal nystagmus; pupils were equal at 4 mm and reactive to light; fundi were normal. The patient moved all extremities, had good strength and normal, symmetric deep-tendon reflexes; muscle tone seemed increased and there were periodic myoclonic jerks; plantar flexion was elicited; sensory examination could not be performed because of the patient's lack of response and agitation.

Blood was drawn for initial laboratory tests and an intravenous infusion of 5% dextrose in 0.45% sodium chloride solution was started at 200 mL/h. Fifty milliliters of 50% dextrose and 100 mg of thiamine were given IV. He was placed on 6 L of oxygen via nasal cannula. Fifty grams of activated charcoal with 50 g of sorbitol were administered by mouth.

The initial laboratory data, including complete blood count (CBC), electrolytes, arterial blood gas analysis, and urinalysis, were all normal. An electrocardiogram (ECG) revealed a sinus tachycardia at 110 beats/min and was otherwise normal.

By the time the physical examination and laboratory tests were completed, the patient had become calm and cooperative. He related that while at lunch, one of his friends had put mustard on his sandwich and that it tasted "terrific." He recalled finishing the sandwich and then slowly "freaking out," losing control of his mind and body.

The patient's clinical condition had significantly improved by the time his mother arrived in the ED. Within 3 hours after his arrival, he was cooperative and his neuropsychiatric examination was entirely normal. He was discharged home and arrangements were made for a followup examination with his pediatrician.

HISTORY AND EPIDEMIOLOGY

Phencyclidine (PCP) was discovered in 1926, but it was not until the 1950s, when Parke Davis, while searching for an ideal intravenous anesthetic that would rapidly achieve analgesia and anesthesia with minimal cardiovascular and respiratory depression, rediscovered PCP as a general anesthetic.[37] It was marketed under the name Sernyl because it rendered an apparent state of serenity when administered to laboratory monkeys. Its surgical use began in 1963, but was rapidly discontinued when a 10–30% incidence of postoperative psychoses and dysphoria was documented over the next 2-year period.[80] By 1967, the use of PCP was limited exclusively to veterinary medicine as a tranquilizer under the name Sernylan.

Simultaneously in the 1960s, PCP was evolving as a San Francisco street drug called "the PeaCe Pill."[63] The names subsequently applied to phencyclidine have been numerous and geographically diverse: on the West Coast it was "Angel Dust, PCP, crystal, crystal joints (CJs);" Chicago called it "THC" or "TAC;" and the East Coast opted for "the sheets" or "Hog" and "elephant tranquilizer."[107] The drug was initially unpopular with drug users because of its dysphoric effects and unpredictable oral absorption.[156] With time, though, its use spread in a similar geographic pattern to that of marijuana and LSD, from the coastal United States to the Midwest region.[63]

Phencyclidine abuse first became widespread during the 1970s.[26] The relatively easy and inexpensive synthesis coupled with the common masking of PCP as LSD, mescaline, psylocybin, cocaine, amphetamine, and/or "synthetic THC" (tetrahydrocannabinol), added to its allure and consumption.[107] By the late 1970s, PCP use had reached epidemic proportions.[7] The Drug Abuse Warning Network (DAWN) reported that the number of

PCP-related emergencies and deaths more than doubled in the 2 years from 1975 to 1977. In 1978, the National Institute of Drug Abuse (NIDA) reported that of young adults (18–25-years-old), 13.9% had used PCP.[50] The manufacture of phencyclidine was ultimately prohibited in 1978, when the drug was added to the Federal Controlled Substance Act of 1970. Classifying PCP as a Schedule II substance led to its decrease in availability and, therefore, use. The 1980s brought about a cocaine epidemic that eclipsed PCP; however, PCP has remained consistently available on the streets, primarily regionalized to large cities in the northeastern United States and Los Angeles,[96] where PCP use continues to rise and fall with various societal trends. Because many of PCP congeners made during the manufacturing process were being abused in place of PCP, the Controlled Substance Analogue Enforcement Act of 1986 made these derivatives illegal and established that the use of PCP's precursor, piperidine, necessitated mandatory reporting. With this new law in place, those possessing similar but not identical illegal substances could be prosecuted, leading to a further decline in the popularity of phencyclidine.

Laboratory investigation of phencyclidine derivatives led to the discovery of ketamine, a chloroketone analogue. Ketamine was introduced for general clinical practice in 1970 and marketed as Ketalar and Ketaject, and for veterinary use, as Ketavet. Ketamine has approximately one-tenth to one-twentieth the potency of PCP and a much shorter duration of action, it therefore provides greater control in clinical use. Thirty years of clinical experience have established that ketamine provides adequate surgical anesthesia, a rapid recovery, and less prominent emergence reactions than noted with PCP use.[54,77,139,169] Because of the simplicity and efficacy of its use, it is regularly employed in operating rooms, emergency departments, and throughout the developing world where little clinical monitoring is available during surgical and emergency procedures.[52,74,75,76,77,78,79,139,169]

Abuse of ketamine was first noted on the West Coast in 1971.[146] During the 1980s, there were reports of its abuse internationally, as well as among physicians.[3,65] The nonmedical use of dissociative anesthetics has continued to increase in the 1990s, in spite of the common complications associated with their use.[159] Presently ketamine, methylenedioxyamphetamine (MDA), and methylenedioxymethamphetamine (MDMA) are popular with today's youth. The same pharmacologic qualities that made ketamine more clinically popular than PCP are also responsible for its nonmedical popularity. Ketamine is regularly consumed at all-night "rave parties" and in nightclubs because of its reportedly "hallucinatory" and "out-of-body" effects, relatively inexpensive price, and short duration of effect (single snort lasting 15–20 minutes).[11,44,87,91,170]

The use of ketamine is not limited to the inner-city population. In the past 5 years, the media reports police arrests in affluent suburban communities for possession and sale of ketamine, as well as more in-depth and frequent reporting of the effects of its toxicity among users.[44,87,136,170] In contrast to PCP, ketamine is not manufactured illegally, but rather, obtained illicitly from medical, dental, and veterinary sources. Additionally, with the advent of the Internet, it is available nationwide; a sham "biotech" Internet company was seized by New York City police for selling so-called "date-rape drugs," including ketamine.[116] Adverse reactions do occur, although, there are few reports of fatalities secondary to ketamine during this period of increased use.[71,102,122] Because of its abuse potential, ketamine was also placed in Schedule III of the Controlled Substance Act in 1999.[138]

PHARMACOLOGY
General Chemistry

Phencyclidine's chemical name 1-(1-phenylcyclohexyl) piperidine provided the basis for its street acronym PCP. During its unlawful chemical synthesis, numerous analogues are made which have similar effects on the central nervous system (CNS) and which have been used as PCP substitutes. The "designer" arylcyclohexylamines are aliphatic or aromatic substituted amines, ketones, or halides, and appear similar to the parent compound. More than 60 psychoactive analogues are mentioned in the medical literature and the following salient points about the 5 most prevalent compounds are worth mentioning. TCP and PCC are piperidine derivatives. Piperidine, the synthetic precursor, was easily bought prior to 1986 for manufacturing PCP and its derivatives. TCP, a thiophene analog, (1-[1-(2-thienyl)cyclohexyl] piperidine), produces even more intense effects than PCP. An intermediate of PCP synthesis, PCC (1-piperidino-cyclohexanecarbonitrile) was a constituent of up to 20–22% of illicit drug preparations analyzed for phencyclidine; this is likely a result of a poor manufacturing process.[14,145] PCC degrades to piperidine, which may be recognized by its strong fishy odor. The presence of its carbonitrile group adds to its toxicity by generating cyanide on smoking.[12,14,152,153] The pyrrolidine derivative, PHP (phencyclohexylpyrrolidine), is comparable clinically to PCP and is not detected by the many drug screening methods available.[28,85] More potent than PCP, PCE (1-phenyl-cyclohexylethylamine) was commonly available on the street as a white powder indistinguishable from PCP.[145]

Ketamine and tiletamine, two legal congeners of PCP, are used clinically for sedation and anesthesia. In large quantities, both are also used in veterinary medicine for animal sedation. Ketamine is the only dissociative anesthetic product manufactured for use on humans for the purpose of anesthesia, conscious sedation, and the treatment of bronchospasm.

The molecular structure of ketamine, [2-(ortho-chlorophenyl)-2-methylaminocyclohexanone], contains a chiral center, producing a racemic mixture of two resolvable optical isomers or enantiomers, the D(+)-isomer and L(−)-isomer. Commercially available preparations of ketamine contain equal concentrations of the two enantiomers. These two molecules differ in their pharmacodynamic effects. In a randomized double-blind evaluation of these two enantiomers on patients undergoing surgery, the D(+)-isomer of ketamine was a more effective anesthetic, but manifested a higher incidence of psychotic emergence reactions than the L(−)-isomer. Other studies have also found differences in their effects on catecholamine reuptake.[139,169] The D(+)-isomer causes a greater increase in both blood pressure and pulse than the D(−)-isomer, as well as more bronchodilating effects.

Pharmacokinetics and Toxicokinetics

Phencyclidine is a white, stable solid that is readily soluble in both water and ethanol. It is a weak base with a pK_a between 8.6 and 9.4 and a high lipid to water partition coefficient. It is rapidly absorbed from the respiratory and the gastrointestinal tracts; as such, it is typically self-administered by oral ingestion, nasal insufflation, smoking, or intravenous and subcutaneous injection.

The effects of PCP are dependent on routes of delivery and dose. Its onset of action is most rapid from the intravenous and inhalational routes (2–5 minutes) and slowest (30–60 minutes) following gastrointestinal absorption.[42,43] Sedation is commonly produced by doses of 0.25 mg intravenously, whereas oral ingestion typically requires 1–5 mg to produce similar sedation. Signs and symptoms of abuse toxicity usually last 4–6 hours, and after large overdoses generally resolve within 24–48 hours, but may persist in a chronic user.[16,53,55,106,124,135] However, in the PCP-intoxicated patient, the relationships between dosage, clinical effects, and serum levels are not reliable or predictable.

There are several explanations for PCP's protracted CNS effects. It has a large volume of distribution of 6.2 L/kg.[42,174] Its high lipid solubility accounts for its entry and storage in the adipose and brain tissue. Also, upon reaching the acidic CSF, PCP becomes ionized. It is because of this ion-trapping that CSF levels are approximately 6–9 times higher than those of plasma.[118]

PCP undergoes first-order elimination over a wide range of doses. It has an apparent terminal half-life of 21 ± 3 hours under both controlled and overdose settings.[42,90] Prolonged signs or symptoms are demonstrated in those patients who "body-stuff" PCP in plastic bags.[90,176] Ninety percent of PCP is metabolized in the liver and 10% is excreted in the urine unchanged. Evidence indicates that PCP undergoes hepatic oxidative hydroxylation into 2 monohydroxylated and 1 dihydroxylated metabolites. All three of these compounds are conjugated to the more water-soluble glucuronide derivatives and are then excreted in the urine.

Urine pH is an important determinant of renal elimination of PCP. In acidic urine, the PCP molecule becomes ionized and reabsorption is blocked. Acidification of the urine thereby increases renal clearance of PCP from 1.98 ± 0.48 L/h to 2.4 ± 0.78 L/h.[42] Additional studies have found a much higher renal clearance (8.04 ± 1.56 L/h) if the urine pH was decreased to <5.0.[10] Although this may account for a substantial increase in the renal clearance, it only represents a 1.1% increase of the total drug clearance.

Similar to phencyclidine, ketamine is water soluble with a high lipid solubility that enables it to distribute to the CNS readily. It has a pK_a of 7.5 and a volume of distribution of 1.8 ± 0.7 L/kg. Ketamine has approximately one-tenth the potency of PCP,[77,92] and human trials demonstrate that its clinical effects, similar to PCP, are route and dose dependent.[46,49,54,154] Peak concentrations occur within 1 minute of IV administration and within 5 minutes of a 5-mg/kg IM injection.[169,177] Ketamine distributes immediately into the CNS with the duration of its hypnotic and anesthetic effects being principally a result of its redistribution from the brain to other tissues.[169] Recovery time averages 15 minutes for IV administration, but it is prolonged to between 30 and 120 minutes for intramuscular administration. Oral or rectal doses are not well absorbed and undergo substantial first-pass metabolism.[139,169] Symptoms after nasal administration last for 45–90 minutes, in contrast to oral administration of ketamine, where symptoms last 4–8 hours.

Ketamine is extensively metabolized in the liver by the cytochrome P450 isozymes. Its biotransformation is complex with numerous metabolites described.[2,139,169] The major pathway involves its N-demethylation to norketamine, a metabolite with one-third the anesthetic potency of ketamine. Norketamine is hydroxylated at different sites within the hexanone ring, producing varying second chiral centers. The majority of these diastereoisomers are glucuronidated to more water soluble derivatives that are then excreted in the urine.[77,139] As a minor metabolic pathway, ketamine also undergoes ring hydroxylation prior to N-demethylation. The elimination half-life, which reflects both metabolic and excretory phases, is 2.3 ± 0.5 hours and is prolonged when drugs requiring hepatic metabolism are coadministered.[104] Because of the enzymatic hepatic metabolism, tolerance, as well as enzyme induction following chronic administration, are reported.[77,139]

Available Forms

PCP is available on the street in a variety of forms, including powder, liquid, tablets, leaf mixtures, and rock crystal forms. Because its illegal manufacture is uncontrolled, the contents of PCP sold vary considerably, with powder often the purest form containing approximately 5 mg. Leaf mixtures are made by sprinkling approximately 1–10 mg of phencyclidine onto parsley, oregano, mint, tobacco, or marijuana. A typical PCP joint (known as "crystal joint," "KJ," or "supergrass"), is developed for smoking and contains about 1 mg per 150 mg of plant product.[7] Mentholated cigarettes dipped into liquid PCP are known as "supercools."

In the time period following PCP's inclusion in the Federal Controlled Substance Act of 1970, PCP was infrequently incorporated into marijuana cigarettes. Currently, there are reports of marijuana cigarettes again being adulterated with PCP. These are being sold on the street under varying names such as "Illy" in Connecticut, "Hydro" in New York City, "Dip" in New Jersey, "Wet" in Philadelphia, and "Fry" in Texas. The cigarettes are treated with "embalming fluid," allegedly to enhance the drug's euphoric effects. Embalming fluid, which contains formalin (formaldehyde in methanol), is used as a medium to ease a uniform distribution of PCP in these cigarettes.[86] It is difficult to discern whether this "enhanced" mixture is purchased intentionally or is placed in these cigarettes surreptitiously.

On the street and the Internet, ketamine is known as "vitamin K," "Special K," "Super K," "Ket," or simply "K." It is available in a liquid form that is dried into a pure white crystalline powder and typically self-administered by ingestion or insufflation in a fashion similar to PCP. It is rarely injected intravenously or intramuscularly in liquid form. Ketamine is primarily sold as tablets, capsules, or powder. These formulations are often adulterated with substances such as caffeine, MDMA, ephedrine, or methamphetamine. Exemplifying the commercial growth of ketamine, some of the tablets are even found to contain a "K" logo.[57] Common sedating doses are 75–300 mg orally (30–75 mg for insufflation). Higher doses, ranging between 300 and 450 mg orally (100–250 mg for insufflation), result in substantial CNS toxicity. These manifestations are similar to the clinical emergence reaction that patients experience when ketamine anesthesia is concluded.

PATHOPHYSIOLOGY

The arylcyclohexylamines, of which PCP and ketamine are prototypes, are a group of anesthetics that functionally and electrophysiologically "dissociate" the somatosensory cortex from higher centers.[46,168] This dissociation renders striking similarities to the symptoms of schizophrenia, which are not explained by the dopamine hypothesis. The precise mechanisms by which PCP and ketamine achieve these effects are complex and not fully understood; however, investigation of the nature of PCP-induced psychosis has led to a substantial identification of the various sites of PCP activity.

Most studies demonstrate that PCP and ketamine bind with high affinity to sites located in the cortex and limbic structures of the brain.[109] They block the *N*-methyl-D-aspartate (NMDA) receptors at serum concentrations encountered clinically.[165,178] Analogues of PCP (TCP, PCE, PHP, ketamine, and dizolcipine or MK-801) are also known to interact with the NMDA receptor in a dose-response manner that corresponds appropriately to their neurobehavioral effect.[27,142,171] The NMDA receptor is a Ca^{++}-mediated channel that is activated by the binding of the neurotransmitter glutamate, an excitatory amino acid. These dissociative agents bind to the NMDA receptor at a site independent of glutamate.[92,95,109,173] As such they antagonize glutamate's action on this channel noncompetitively and block Ca^{++} influx (see Fig. 10–14).

PCP and ketamine bind to the biogenic amine reuptake complex with one-tenth to one-fifth the affinity to which they bind to the NMDA receptor. This binding occurs at physiologic concentrations that normally take place after subanesthetic doses.[4,132] This weak inhibition of the norepinephrine and dopamine reuptake accounts for the respective sympathomimetic and psychomotor effects that occur clinically with dissociative agents. The initial studies on phencyclidine demonstrated that it consistently increased both the systolic and diastolic blood pressure (SBP and DBP) in a dose-dependent fashion.[37,55] (Doses of 0.06 mg/kg of PCP IV increased the SBP and DBP by 8 mm Hg, whereas 0.25 mg/kg produced a 26- and 19-mm increase in SBP and DBP, respectively.) PCP also increased the heart rate, but inconsistently.[80] Similarly ketamine produces mild increases in blood pressure, heart rate, and cardiac output via this same mechanism.[49,108,154,161,169] This effect is more pronounced by rapid intravenous infusion than intramuscular injection, and the D(+)-isomer has the greatest effect.[169]

In significant overdoses, PCP and ketamine also stimulate σ receptors at concentrations generally associated with coma, although with lower affinity.[155,172] Both D_2 and σ receptors demonstrate an inhibitory effect on the cholinergic receptor pathways.[172] At the higher concentrations typically associated with death, PCP and ketamine also bind to the nicotinic, opioid, and muscarinic cholinergic receptors.[164]

Data indicate that NMDA antagonists produce effects on behavior, sensation, and cognition that resemble aspects of endogenous psychoses, particularly schizophrenia.[93,129] These behavioral abnormalities were first observed in studies in the late 1950s when PCP, administered to healthy volunteers, generated a form of organic psychosis that mimicked schizophrenia. Also, when the drug was administered to schizophrenic patients it uniformly intensified their primary symptoms of profound disorganization, some of these symptoms lasting for weeks.[106] PCP-psychosis is so similar to schizophrenia that many psychiatrists cannot distinguish them without prior indication of drug abuse history.[151]

There is a connection between PCP psychosis and sensory processing. PCP and ketamine inhibit sensory perception in a dose-dependent manner. This processing in sensory information corresponds to their relative affinities to the NMDA receptor and not to the σ-receptor.[6,132] Clinically, it was encountered that the impairment of sensory input produced by PCP resembled that of patients who were deprived of sensory stimulation.[117] When external stimulation was reduced by environmental sensory deprivation, the psychotomimetic effects of PCP were diminished,[40] giving credence to the theory that it may not be anxiety that causes perceptual dysfunction in schizophrenia, but the converse.

Many of the NMDA antagonists, including PCP and ketamine, have a negative effect on cognition and memory. Both impair concentration, recall, learning, and retention of new information.[13,31,51,53,69,82–84,100,111,120,126] In a study of human cognition, it

was observed that learning and memory impairments in volunteers who were administered subanesthetic doses of ketamine (0.65 mg/kg), were independent of the subject's attention and related psychosis.[111] Accordingly, it is presumed that the NMDA receptor antagonists interfere with those functions that integrate interoceptive and exteroceptive input in which goal-directed action becomes possible similar to the organic psychosis in schizophrenia.

It was discovered that hypofunction of the NMDA receptor causes neuroanatomic and neurobehavioral toxicologic effects. Animals exposed to NMDA antagonists, such as PCP and dizocilpine, transiently demonstrated neuronal vacuolar degeneration in the retrosplenial cortex and the posterior cingulate areas of the brain.[127,128] Single high-doses or repeated exposure to NMDA receptor antagonists are associated with a higher incidence of cellular death.[45,59,60,127] This injury seems to be related to the induction of selective expression of individual heat shock proteins in this anatomic area.[144] The major function of cingulate cortical neurons is to mediate affective responses to pain,[166] and in patients with schizophrenia, structural abnormalities in the anterior cingulate cortex are described.[22] Additionally, transgenic mice with reduced NMDA receptor expression display behaviors similar to those of animal models of schizophrenia. These behavioral alterations are ameliorated by treatment with atypical antipsychotic drugs.[121]

Excitatory amino acids are also involved with mediating seizure activity in the brain. As NMDA inhibitors, the anticonvulsant properties of PCP and ketamine are theorized but the studies are inconclusive. Animals administered PCP or PCP analogues progress through dose-related clonic activity followed by tonic-clonic convulsions, as is typical of classic convulsant compounds.[132] Animal research also demonstrates wide interspecies variability of the electroencephalogram (EEG) effects of PCP.[55] In a murine seizure model, it was demonstrated that ketamine possessed selective anticonvulsant properties.[32] In humans, it is observed that although these dissociative agents induce excitatory activity in the thalamus and limbic areas, they do not affect cortical regions.[48,49,54,66] Excitation, muscle twitching, posturing,[119] and tonic clonic motor activity with or without EEG changes are reported with these subcortical EEG alterations.[35,47,66,119] In the clinical setting, many report ketamine to possess anticonvulsant properties at clinical doses that can be explained by an NMDA inhibitory effect.[35,47]

The NMDA receptor is also responsible for the development of the neuronal organization of the central nervous system.[88,89,147,148] It is linked to hypoxic/ischemic brain injury by mediating calcium influx, a final pathway in cell death. The uninhibited firing of NMDA afferent neurons secondary to brain injury causes their death as well as those of efferent neurons downstream. NMDA antagonists such as PCP are demonstrated to block hypoxic brain injury from stroke and trauma.[17,105] In a rat model of ischemic stroke, PCP had a protective effect on the brain, demonstrated by a decreased rate of seizure activity.[17] This effect is transient and has not been studied in human subjects.

Evidence from animal studies indicates that PCP produces modest tolerance in rats and squirrel monkeys. The development of tolerance is mostly secondary to PCP's pharmacologic effect, rather than to biodispositional changes. Dependence was also observed in monkeys who self-administered PCP (10 mg/kg/d to blood levels 100–300 ng/mL) over a month by the appearance of dramatic withdrawal signs when access was denied. Signs included vocalizations, bruxism, oculomotor hyperactivity, diarrhea, piloerection, difficulty remaining awake, tremors, and, in one case, convulsions.[15] These signs appeared within 8 hours of abstinence and were most severe at about 24 hours. When either PCP or ketamine (2.5 mg/kg/h) was readministered to the animals, PCP withdrawal symptoms were reversed, indicating cross-dependence from PCP to ketamine.[20,150]

Physiologic dependence in humans has not been studied formally. It is implied to occur by the observation that 68 chronic PCP users developed depression, anxiety, irritability, lack of energy, sleep disturbance, and disturbed thoughts after 1 day of abstinence from drug use.[137] It is additionally reported that neonates whose mothers used PCP developed jitteriness, vomiting, and hypertonicity that lasted for at least 2 weeks.[157] These symptoms may be represent PCP withdrawal or intrinsic teratogenic effects on neurologic development.[72,88] As there are few case reports of chronic ketamine use in the medical literature, it is unknown whether dependency occurs with ketamine as well. Although there are no controlled studies observing the physiologic symptoms of withdrawal in humans who chronically use PCP or ketamine, there is a definite psychological dependence on the sensations experienced during recreational use of the drugs.[146]

CLINICAL MANIFESTATIONS

The reported signs and symptoms of patients presenting to the emergency department with PCP toxicity are variable. The variations are a result of differences in dosage, the multiple routes of administration, concomitant drug use, and other associated medical conditions. In addition, individual differences in susceptibility to the drug's effects, the development of tolerance in chronic users, as well as contaminants in the drug manufacture may account for erratic clinical findings.

The majority of patients with PCP and ketamine toxicity who are brought to medical attention manifest diverse psychomotor abnormalities.[12,18,29,65,94,163] As dissociative anesthetics, these drugs produce a lack of response to external stimuli by functionally dissociating various elements of the brain. Consciousness, memory, perception, and motor activity appear dissociated from each other. This dissociation prevents the user from attaining cognition and properly assembling all this information to construct a reality. Clinically, the person may appear inebriated, either calm or agitated, and sometimes violent. In large overdoses, the drug's anesthetic effect causes patients to present in stuporous or comatose conditions. In recreational use, "dissociatives" are not taken for these effects, but rather for so-called "out of body" experiences. In addition, patients often have disordered thought processes, delirium (including disorientation to time, place, and person), amnesia, paranoia, and dysphoria.[64]

The manifestations of PCP and ketamine toxicity are better illustrated by results of their effects in controlled human studies. Volunteers who took these NMDA receptor antagonists in small doses (oral PCP doses of up to 7.5 mg/d, ketamine 0.1 mg/kg) exhibited inebriation, but higher doses (PCP above 10 mg/d; ketamine 0.5 mg/kg) generally caused a more severe impairment of mental function.[55,100] Neurologic, electroencephalographic, and pharmacologic testing demonstrates that intravenous doses of 0.1 mg/kg PCP[16,53,106,124,141] or 0.5 mg/kg of ketamine[100,132] causes diminution in all sensory modalities (pain, touch, proprioception, hearing, taste and visual acuity) in a dose-dependent fashion. Both drugs also cause feelings of apathy, depersonalization, hostility, isolation, and alterations in body image.[16,53,67,100,106,132] The deficits

in sensory modalities are evident prior to the development of the psychological effects of PCP, with pain perception disappearing first. This alteration in analgesic perception is the result of a blocking action on the thalamus and midbrain[124] (Fig. 69–1).

Abnormal stereognosis and proprioception occur in a dose-dependent manner. This disturbed perception results in body image distortions described as "numbness," "sheer nothingness," and "depersonalization." The decrease of proprioceptive sensation to gravity probably gives the sensation of "tripping" or "flying." Because all sensory modalities are affected, visual, auditory, and tactile illusions and delusions are common. Hallucinations are typically auditory rather than the visual type that is more common with LSD use. Ketamine's hallucinogenic effects on healthy human volunteers are linearly related at steady-state concentrations between 50 and 200 ng/mL.[24]

The reaction to the misperceived or disconnected reality may result in unintentional actions and violent behavior. The hallmark of PCP toxicity is the recurring delusion of superhuman strength and invulnerability resulting from both the anesthetic and dissociative properties of the drug. There are case reports of patients presenting with trauma either from jumping from high altitudes, fighting large crowds or the police, or self-mutilation. The true extent and incidence of violence, however, is probably less than previously suggested.[25]

Typically neurologic signs include nystagmus, ataxia, and altered gait. Initially, except for ataxia, motor movement is not impaired, until the patient becomes unconscious. On physical examination, use of dissociative agents typically produces relatively small pupils and (horizontal, vertical, and/or rotatory) nystagmus, and diplopia. In the largest case series reported to date, nystagmus and hypertension were noted in 57% of patients who had taken PCP.[114] Smaller and more limited studies have found an

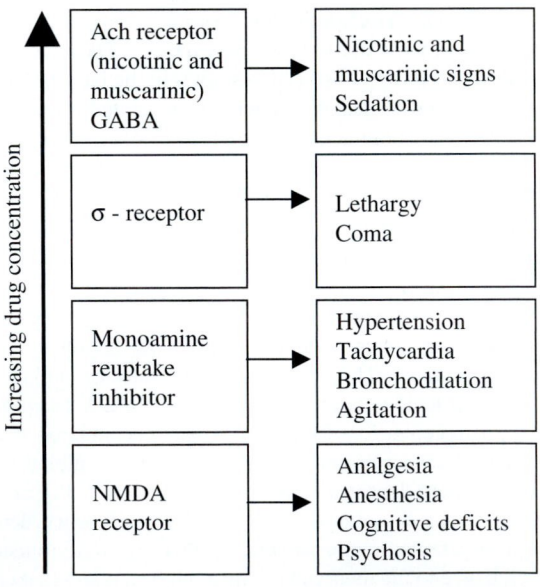

Figure 69–1. Clinical effects of phencyclidine and ketamine. Phencyclidine and ketamine bind to different receptors in the CNS with decreasing affinity that is an increasing concentration is necessary to cause the corresonding clinical effects. ACh = acetylcholine.

incidence of nystagmus of 89% or higher.[18] Other cerebellar manifestations were also encountered, most notably dizziness, ataxia, dysarthria, and nausea. A pooled data compilation of 35 reports demonstrated that emesis occurred 8.5% of the time.[77] In fact, internet chat groups devoted to substance abuse commonly direct users to "mix dissociatives with marijuana" for its antiemetic effect.

Larger doses of PCP produce loss of balance and confusion, the latter characterized by inability to repeat a set of objects, frequent loss of ideas, blocking, lack of concreteness, and disordered linguistic expression.[51,55,100,106,141] In general, dissociative anesthetics stimulate the central nervous system, but seizures rarely occur, except at high doses. The largest case series of PCP-intoxicated patients detected a 3.1% incidence of seizures.[114]

Although PCP- and ketamine-intoxicated patients also present with motor disturbances, it is not clear to what extent PCP and ketamine are actually responsible for these manifestations. The most common of the reported disturbances are dystonic reactions: opisthotonos, torticollis, tortipelvis, and risus sardonicus (facial grimacing). Myoclonic movements, tremor, hyperactivity, athetosis, stereotypies, and catelepsy are also associated with PCP and ketamine intoxication.[12,30,65,113] A slight increase in muscle tone is also observed, which is a result of its dopaminergic effect.[106] Laryngospasm has been reported after the use of ketamine anesthesia requiring intubation. The incidence of this complication is less than 0.017%,[77] which is 2% of the incidence following traditional general anesthesia.[130]

The acute psychosis, observed during the recovery phase of PCP anesthesia, limits its clinical use. This bizarre behavior, characterized by a confused state, vivid dreaming, and hallucinations, is termed an "emergence reaction." These reactions occur most frequently in middle-aged males with a reported incidence of 17–30%.[80,97] The most violent emergence reactions follow an intravenous dose of approximately 0.25 mg/kg (total 20 mg) of phencyclidine.[55] The mildest degrees of agitation produced by phencyclidine resemble the effects of ethanol intoxication. These same postanesthetic reactions also limit the clinical use of ketamine. The incidence of emergence reactions following ketamine administration may approximate 50% in adults and 10% in children.[77] Patients older than 10 years, females, and who normally dream frequently and/or have a prior personality disorder incur the greatest risk.[77] The incidence of the occurrence of emergence reactions appears to be exacerbated when the drugs are rapidly administered intravenously, and in those patients who are exposed to excessive stimuli during recovery. Although not proved in a controlled study, reducing external stimuli during the recovery phase may reduce emergence reactions.

Most PCP- and ketamine-intoxicated patients demonstrate mild sympathomimetic effects. Rarely, however, cardiovascular catastrophies are encountered.[58,115] These complications may result from direct vasospasm of blood vessels,[5,36] causing severe systemic hypertension[58] and cerebral hemorrhage.[23] Hypertension, abnormal behavior, and miosis in children strongly suggest PCP poisoning.[98]

The effect of PCP and ketamine on cardiac rhythm is controversial. Dysrhythmias are only observed in animals poisoned with very large doses of PCP. Ketamine is observed to both enhance and diminish epinephrine-induced dysrhythmias in animals.[21,56,81,99] The considerable experience in the use of ketamine anesthesia on humans undergoing surgery or cardiac catheterizations has not demonstrated prodysrhythmic effects.[62,125]

As these dissociative anesthetics were designed to retain normal ventilation, hypoventilation is uncommon. In clinical studies, PCP increased the minute ventilation, tidal volume, and respiratory rate of volunteers.[80] Clinically in PCP-intoxicated patients, irregular respiratory patterns occur with tachypnea much more common than bradypnea.[8,113] Hypoventilation, when present, is usually secondary to the use of particularly high doses of PCP. Pulmonary edema secondary to respiratory depression is also a rare occurrence. Large doses of PCP (20 mg/kg) administered to laboratory animals did produce respiratory depression.[37] Although respiratory depression in humans is an extremely rare event, it has been reported with fast or high dose infusions of ketamine.[73,169] In fact, because of its potent bronchodilating properties, ketamine has been used successfully to prevent intubation in patients with refractory asthma .[68,140,158,169]

Body temperature is rarely affected directly by PCP and ketamine. In one large series, only 2.6% of patients demonstrated hyperthermia (T >38.8°C/101.8°F).[114] In an experimental animal model, PCP failed to increase body temperature.[37,55] When hyperthermia does occur from severe psychomotor agitation, all the known complications including encephalopathy, rhabdomyolysis, myoglobinuria, electrolyte abnormalities and liver failure occur[8,19,39,133] (Chap. 18).

Both cholinergic and anticholinergic clinical manifestations occur in the PCP- or ketamine-intoxicated patient. Miosis, mydriasis, blurred vision, profuse diaphoresis, hypersalivation, bronchospasm, bronchorrhea, and urinary retention occur.[12,18,103,113,114] Clinically, ketamine stimulates salivary and tracheobronchial secretions; both of which are equally and effectively inhibited by atropine and glycopyrolate.[123] Furthermore, in a randomized double-blind trial, after infusion of 1.5 mg/kg of ketamine in healthy volunteers, physostigmine decreased nystagmus, blurred vision, and the time to recovery.[160]

Ironically, the very characteristics that were thought to make phencyclidine ideal for anesthesia—the preservation of muscle tone and cardiopulmonary function—magnify the difficulties in managing an individual who manifests dysphoria after an overdose. The course of delirium, stupor, and coma associated with PCP and ketamine is extremely variable, although the manifestations are much milder following ketamine use.

DIAGNOSTIC TESTING

Most hospital laboratories do not perform quantitative analysis of PCP, but many can do a qualitative test for the presence of the drug. The use of qualitative test for PCP is almost always more important than a quantitative determination, as the precise serum concentration does not correlate closely with the clinical effects. PCP may not be part of a routine toxicologic screening and it may therefore be necessary to request a specific analysis.

When a routine toxicologic screen is reported as negative this result should not lead to the erroneous conclusion that PCP exposure has been excluded. If it is necessary to confirm the suspicion that PCP is the offending agent, urine is most commonly utilized for analysis, although serum and possibly gastric contents can be employed. Rarely is it essential to make this determination.

PCP is qualitatively detected by an enzyme immunoassay at a sensitivity of 10 ng/mL. High-affinity antibodies were once studied as specific PCP antagonists to reverse PCP toxicity.[131,162] The detection of PCP is thus dependant on the concentration of PCP in the body fluid tested and the affinity of the antibody for the PCP molecule. As such, nonspecific antibody binding to a molecule similar in structure to PCP can produce analytic false-positive reactions. Metabolites of PCP, such as PCE, PHP, TCP, and its pyrrolidine derivative, TCPy, cross-react with the immunoassay at concentrations 30 times higher than those used to detect PCP. Because of its similar structure to PCP, dextromethorphan and its metabolite, dextrorphan, also cross-react with Syva EMIT (enzyme-multiplied immunoassay technique) and TDx PCP assays[167] (Chap. 7; Fig. 69–2).

Although nonspecific, laboratory findings resulting from PCP use may include leukocytosis, hypoglycemia, and elevation of muscle enzymes, myoglobin, BUN, and creatinine.[114] The EEG reveals diffuse slowing with theta and delta waves, which may return to normal before the patient improves clinically.

There is no commercially available immunoassay for ketamine. When necessary, ketamine is detected by gas chromatography and mass spectroscopy. There is anecdotal evidence that ketamine also cross-reacts with the urine PCP immunoassay because of their structural similarity.[143] Other authors, including the manufacturer who tests the reactivity of the commercially available PCP immunoassay with ketamine, do not confirm such results.[33,163]

MANAGEMENT

Agitation

Conservative management is indicated for PCP and ketamine intoxication and includes maintaining adequate respiration, circulation, and thermoregulation. The psychobehavioral symptoms observed during acute dissociative intoxication and during the emergence reaction are similar. To treat the symptoms of agitation and alteration of mental status of acutely intoxicated PCP patients, it is helpful to recognize that both pharmacologic[1,34,38,41,61,77,78,110,112] and behavioral[40,41,77,101] modalities have been employed to diminish agitation and emergence phenomena during conscious sedation with ketamine. To prevent self-injury, a common form of PCP-induced morbidity and mortality, the patient must be safely restrained, initially physically and then chemically. An intravenous line must be established and blood drawn for electrolytes, glucose, BUN, and creatinine determinations. The use of 0.5–1.0 g/kg (body weight) of dextrose and 100 mg of thiamine HCl intravenously should be considered following an immediate bedside determination of glucose.

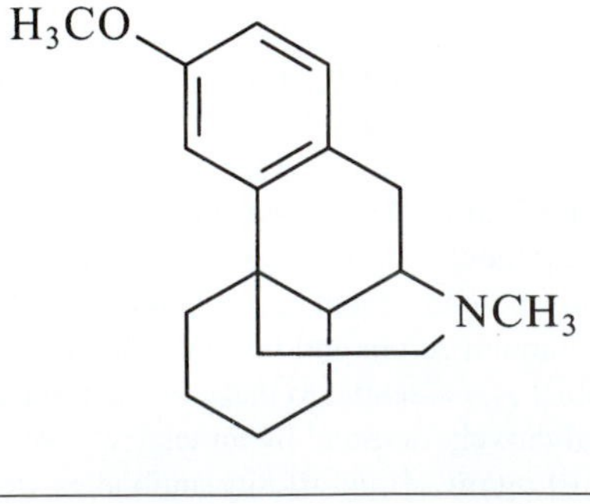

Figure 69–2. Dextromethorphan.

In the pharmacologic treatment of emergence reactions, antipsychotics and benzodiazepines are utilized, with benzodiazepines having the most success. A benzodiazepine such as diazepam, administered in titrated doses of up to 10 mg intravenously every 5–10 minutes until agitation is controlled, is usually safe and effective. Numerous studies demonstrate the benefits of benzodiazepines, although under certain conditions,[38,77] they may prolong recovery time. Midazolam may be more effective than diazepam under certain circumstances.[34,112] In contrast, phenothiazines may lower the seizure threshold, and both phenothiazines and butyrophenones may cause acute dystonic reactions. Phenothiazines may also cause significant hypotension, worsen hyperthermia, and exacerbate any anticholinergic effects from the drug.

Some behavioral modalities have also been implemented in the treatment. Early studies demonstrated that the psychotomimetic effects of PCP were diminished when external stimulation was reduced by environmental sensory deprivation.[40] The practice of placing patients in a quiet room with minimal sensory stimulation is recommended by many but has never been formally studied in a double-blind controlled trial. Conversely, it is observed in patients undergoing ketamine anesthesia that emergence reactions are less violent when patients are talked to or when music is played.[101,149]

Although it is always important to ask the patient the names, quantities, times, and route of all drugs taken, the information obtained from such a patient is notoriously unreliable. Even when the patient is trying to cooperate and give an accurate history, many street psychoactive agents are drug mixtures whose contents are unknown to the patient. Therefore pharmacologic management is complex and often sign or symptom dependent. Although some authors have attempted to define the appropriate therapy for specific PCP congeners,[70] we have not found such an approach to be beneficial.

Decontamination

Patients with a history of recent oral use of PCP are candidates for gastrointestinal decontamination, but they should be considered too unstable for the use of ipecac, as uncontrolled agitation or respiratory compromise may rapidly develop. Gastric lavage may be initiated with a nasogastric tube, but the patient may need to be sedated and the risk:benefit ratio considered. Activated charcoal, 1 g/kg, may be administered and repeated every 4 hours for several doses in the most symptomatic patients. Activated charcoal effectively adsorbs PCP and increases its nonrenal clearance; even without prior gastric evacuation this approach is usually adequate.[134] A single dose of a cathartic, such as sorbitol, may be given but its role is questionable.

Theoretically, toxic substances that are weak bases, such as PCP, can be eliminated more rapidly if the urine is acidified. Although urinary acidification with ammonium chloride was previously recommended,[9] we do not recommend this approach. The risks associated with acidifying the urine—simultaneously inducing a systemic acidosis, thereby potentially increasing urinary myoglobin precipitation—outweigh any perceived benefits (Chap. 6).

As opposed to the problems in applying ion-trapping to renal excretion, ion-trapping results in the active mobilization of PCP into gastric secretions. Phencyclidine is in a substantially ionized (and therefore nonlipid-soluble) form in the acid of the stomach and can be absorbed only when it reaches the more alkaline intestine. Gastric suction, therefore, can remove a significant amount of the drug and also interrupts the gastroenteric circulation (by which the drug is secreted into the acid environment of the stomach only to be reabsorbed again in the small intestine).[9] Continuous gastric suction, however, may also be dangerous and unnecessary. It should be reserved only for stuporous or comatose patients. Continuous suction may result in trauma to the patient as well as in fluid and electrolyte loss, which can further complicate management and possibly interfere with drug clearance by inhibiting the efficacy of activated charcoal. For these reasons the administration of multiple-dose activated charcoal rather than continuous nasogastric suction appears to be the safest and most effective way of removing ion-trapped drug from the stomach.

Most patients rapidly regain normal CNS function anywhere from 45 minutes to several hours after using the drug. However, those who have taken exceedingly high doses or who have an underlying psychiatric disorder may remain comatose or exhibit bizarre behavior for days or even weeks before returning to normal. Those who regain normal function rapidly should be monitored for several hours and then, after a psychiatric consultation, should receive drug counseling and any additional social support available. Patients whose recovery is delayed should be treated supportively and monitored carefully in an intensive care unit.

Many patients become depressed and anxious during the "post-high" period, and chronic users may manifest a variety of psychiatric disturbances.[175] These individuals typically present with repeated drug use, hospitalizations, and poor psychosocial functioning in the long-term.

The major toxicity of PCP appears to be behaviorally related: self-inflicted injuries, injuries resulting from exceptional physical exertion, and injuries sustained as a result of resisting the application of physical restraints are frequent. Patients appear to be unaware of their surroundings and are sometimes even oblivious to pain because of the agent's dissociative anesthetic effects. In addition to major trauma, rhabdomyolysis and resultant myoglobinuric renal failure account in large measure for the high morbidity and mortality associated with PCP intoxication. (Chapter 115 discusses indications and techniques of restraint application.)

If significant rhabdomyolysis[39,133] has occurred, myoglobinuria may be present. Early fluid therapy should be used to avoid deposition of pigment into the kidneys, leading to renal failure. Urinary alkalinization as part of the treatment regimen for rhabdomyolysis would potentially increase PCP reabsorption and deposition in fat stores, but this is only theoretical.

The clinical experience with recreational use of ketamine is limited, however, their manifestations appear to be similar yet milder and shorter-lived when compared to PCP. In a recent study of 20 patients who presented with acute ketamine intoxication, all were treated conservatively and successfully with intravenous hydration, and sedation with benzodiazepines.[163]

SUMMARY

As "dissociative" anesthetics became clinically available their abuse potential was also discovered. The popularity of PCP and ketamine results from their ability to produce an "out-of-body experience" with seemingly hallucinatory effects. The action of these agents is mediated by the NMDA receptor. Their toxicity, in great part neuropsychiatric in nature, is managed by supportive care. The popularity of ketamine may be related to its lesser toxicity and milder distortion of the personality.

Acknowledgment

Harold Osborn, MD, contributed to this chapter in a previous edition.

REFERENCES

1. Abajian JC, Page P, Morgan M: Effects of droperidol and nitrazepam on emergence reactions following ketamine anesthesia. Anesth Analg 1973;52:385–389.
2. Adams JD, Baillie TA, Trevor AJ, et al: Studies on the biotransformation of ketamine—Identification of metabolites produced in vitro from rat microsomal preparations. Biomed Mass Spec 1981;8:527–538.
3. Ahmed SN, Petchkovsky L: Abuse of ketamine. Br J Psychiatry 1980;137:303.
4. Akunne HC, Reid AA, Thurkuf A, et al: [3H]1-[2-(2-thienyl) cyclohexyl]piperidine-labeled two high-affinity binding sites associated with the biogenic amine reuptake complex. Synapse 1991;8:289–300.
5. Altura BT, Altura BM: Phencyclidine, lysergic acid diethylamide and mescaline: Cerebral artery spasm and hallucinogenic activity. Science 1981;212:1051–1052.
6. Anis NA, Berry SC, Burton NR, et al: The dissociative anaesthetics, ketamine and phencyclidine, selectively reduce excitation of central mammalian neurones by N-methyl-aspartate. Br J Pharm 1983;79:565–575.
7. Anonymous: Phencyclidine: The new American street drug. 1980;281:1511–1512.
8. Armen R, Kanel G, Reynolds T: Phencyclidine-induced malignant hyperthermia causing submassive liver necrosis. Am J Med 1984;77:167–172.
9. Aronow R, Done AK: Phencyclidine overdose: An emerging concept of management. JACEP 1978;7:56–59.
10. Aronow R, Miceli JN, Done AK: Clinical observations during phencyclidine intoxication and treatment based on ion-trapping. Res Monogr Ser 1978;21:218–228.
11. Awuonda M: Swedes alarmed at ketamine misuse. Lancet 1996;348:122.
12. Bailey DN: Clinical findings and concentrations in biological fluids after non-fatal intoxication. Am J Clin Pathol 1979;72:795–799.
13. Bakker CB, Amini FB: Observations on the psychotomimetic effects of Sernyl. Compr Psychiatry 1961;2:269–280.
14. Ballinger JR, Chow AYK, Downie RH, et al: GLC quantitation of 1-piperidinocyclohexanecarbonitrile (PCC) in illicit phencyclidine (PCP). J Anal Tox 1979;3:158–161.
15. Balster RL, Woolverton WL: Continuous access phencyclidine self-administration by rhesus monkeys leading to physical dependence. Psychopharmacology 1980;70:5–10.
16. Ban TA, Lohrenz JJ, Lehmann HE: Observations on the action of Sernyl—A new psychotropic drug. Can Psychiat Assoc J 1961;6:150–156.
17. Barone FC, Price WJ, Jakobsen S, et al: Pharmacological profile of a novel neuronal calcium channel blocker includes cerebral damage and neurological deficits in rat focal ischemia. Pharmacol Biochem Behav 1994;48:77–85.
18. Barton CH, Sterling ML, Vaziri ND: Phencyclidine intoxication: Clinical experience with 27 cases confirmed by urine assay. Ann Emerg Med 1981;10:243–246.
19. Barton CH, Sterling ML, Vaziri ND: Rhabdomyolysis and acute renal failure associated with phencyclidine intoxication. Arch Intern Med 1980;140:568–569.

20. Beardsley PM, Balster RL: Behavioral dependence upon phencyclidine and ketamine in the rat. J Pharmacol Exp Ther 1987;242: 203–211.

21. Bednarski RM, Sams RA, Majors LJ, et al: Reduction of the ventricular arrhythmogenic dose of epinephrine by ketamine administration in halothane-anesthetized cats. Am J Vet Res 1988;49:350–354.

22. Benes FM: Alterations in neural circuitry within layer II of anterior cingulate cortex in schizophrenia. J Psychiatr Res 1999;33:511–512.

23. Bessen HA: Intracranial hemorrhage associated with phencyclidine abuse. JAMA 1982;248:585–587.

24. Bowdle TA, Radant A, Cowley DS, et al: Psychedelic effects of ketamine in healthy volunteers: Relationship to steady-state plasma concentrations. Anesthesiology 1998;88:82–88.

25. Brecher M, Wang BW, Wong H, Morgan JP: Phencyclidine and violence: Clinical and legal issues. J Clin Psychopharmacol 1988;8: 397–401.

26. Brown JK, Malone III: Street drug analysis: Four years later. Clin Toxicol Bull 1974;4:139–160.

27. Browne RG: Discriminative stimulus properties of PCP mimetics. In: Cloudet D, ed: Phencyclidine: An update. NIDA Research Monograph 64. Rockville, MD, National Institute on Drug Abuse, 1986, pp. 134–147.

28. Budd RD: PHP, a new drug of abuse [letter]. N Engl J Med 1980;303:588.

29. Burns RS, Lerner SE, eds: Phencyclidine: A symposium. Clin Toxicol 1976;9:473–600.

30. Burrows FA, Seeman RG: Ketamine and myoclonic encephalopathy of infants (Kinsbourne syndrome). Anesth Analg 1982;61: 873–875.

31. Butelman ER: A novel NMDA antagonist, MK-801, impairs performance in a hippocampal-dependent spatial learning task. Pharmacol Biochem Behav 1989;34:13–16.

32. Buterbaugh GG, Michelson HB: Anticonvulsant properties of phencyclidine and ketamine. In: Cloudet D, ed: Phencyclidine: An update. NIDA Research Monograph 64. Rockville, MD, National Institute on Drug Abuse, 1986, pp. 67–79.

33. Caplan Y, Levine P: Abbott phencyclidine and barbiturates abused drug assays: Evaluation and comparison of Adx, FPIA, TDx, FPIA, EMIT and GC/MS methods. J Anal Toxicol 1989;289–292.

34. Cartwright PD, Pingel SM: Midazolam and diazepam in ketamine anesthesia. Anesthesia 1984;39:439–442.

35. Celesia GG, Chen RC, Bamforth BJ: Effects of ketamine in epilepsy. Neurology 1975;25:169–172.

36. Chen G, Ensor CR, Bohner B: An investigation on the sympathomimetic properties of phencyclidine by comparison with cocaine and desoxyephedrine. J Pharmacol Exp Ther 1965;149:71–78.

37. Chen G, Ensor CR, Russell D, et al: The pharmacology of 1-(1-phenylcyclohexyl) piperidine-HCl. J Pharmacol Exp Ther 1959;127: 241–250.

38. Chudnofsky CR, Weber JE, Stoyanoff PJ, et al: A combination of midazolam and ketamine for procedural sedation and analgesia in adult emergency department patients. Acad Emerg Med 2000;7: 228–235.

39. Cogen FC, Rigg G, Simmons JL, Domino EF: Phencyclidine-associated acute rhabdomyolysis. Ann Intern Med 1978;88:210–212.

40. Cohen BD, Luby ED, Rosenbaum G, et al: Combined Sernyl and sensory deprivation. Compr Psychiatry 1960;1:345–348.

41. Cohen S: Angel dust. JAMA 1977;238:515–516.

42. Cook CE, Brine DR, Jeffcoat AR, et al: Phencyclidine disposition after intravenous and oral doses. Clin Pharmacol Ther 1982;31: 625–634.

43. Cook CE, Brine DR, Quin GD, et al: Phencyclidine and phenylcyclohexene disposition after smoking phencyclidine. Clin Pharmacol Ther 1982;31:635–641.

44. Cooper M: "Special K: Rough catnip for clubgoers." The New York Times, 28 January 1996, sec. 13, p. 4.

45. Corso TD, Sesma MA, Tenkova TI, et al: Multifocal brain damage induced by phencyclidine is augmented by pilocarpine. Brain Res 1997;752:1–14.

46. Corssen G, Domino EF: Dissociative anesthesia: Further pharmacologic studies and first clinical experience with the phencyclidine derivative CI-581. Anesth Analg 1966;45:29–40.

47. Corssen G, Gutierez J, Reves J, et al: Ketamine in the anesthetic management of asthmatic patients. Anesth Analg 1972;51: 588–596.

48. Corssen G, Little SC, Tavakoli M: Ketamine and epilepsy. Anesth Analg 1974;53:319–333.

49. Corssen G, Miyasaka M, Domino EF: Changing concepts in pain control during surgery: Dissociative anesthesia with CI-581. A progress report. Anesth Analg 1968;47:746–759.

50. Crider R: Phencyclidine: Changing abuse patterns. In: Cloudet D, ed: Phencyclidine: An update. NIDA Research Monograph 64. Rockville, MD, National Institute on Drug Abuse, 1986:163–173.

51. Curran HV, Morgan C: Cognitive, dissociative and psychotogenic effects of ketamine in recreational users on the night of drug use and three days later. Addiction 2000;95:575–590.

52. Dachs RJ, Innes GM: Intravenous ketamine sedation of pediatric patients in the emergency department. Ann Emerg Med 1997;29: 146–150.

53. Davies BM, Beech HR: The effect of 1-arylcyclohexylamine (Sernyl) on twelve normal volunteers. J Mental Sci 1960;106: 912–924.

54. Domino EF, Chodoff P, Corssen G: Pharmacologic effects of CI-581, a new dissociative anesthetic in man. Clin Pharmacol Ther 1965;6:279–291.

55. Domino EF: Neurobiology of phencyclidine (Sernyl), a drug with an unusual spectrum of pharmacological activity. Int Rev Neurobiol 1964;6:303–347.

56. Dowdy EG, Kaya K: Studies of the mechanism of cardiovascular responses to CI-581. Anesthesiology 1968;29:931–943.

57. Drug Enforcement Association: Unusual tablet combination (ephedrine, caffeine, ketamine, and phencyclidine). Micrograms 2000; 33:311.

58. Eastman JW, Cohen SN: Hypertensive crisis and death associated with phencyclidine poisoning. JAMA 1975;231:1270–1271.

59. Ellison G, Switzer RC: Dissimilar patterns of degeneration in brain following four different addictive stimulants. Neuroreport 1993;5: 17–20.

60. Ellison G: Competitive and noncompetitive NMDA receptor antagonists induce similar limbic degeneration. Neuroreport 1994;5: 2688–2692.

61. Erbguth PH, Reiman B, Klein RL: The influence of chlorpromazine, diazepam, and droperidol on emergence from ketamine. Anesth Analg 1972;51:693–699.

62. Faithfull NS, Haider R: Ketamine for cardiac catheterization. Anaesthesia 1971;26:318–323.

63. Fauman B, Aldinger G, Fauman M, et al: Psychiatric sequelae of phencyclidine abuse. Clin Toxicol 1976;9:529–538.

64. Fauman B, Baker F, Coppleson LW: Psychosis-induced by phencyclidine. JACEP 1975;4:223–225.

65. Felser JM, Orban DJ: Dystonic reaction after ketamine abuse. Ann Emerg Med 1892;11:673–675.

66. Ferrer-Allado T, Brechner V, Dymond A, et al: Ketamine-induced electroconvulsive phenomena in the human limbic and thalamic regions. Anesthesiology 1973;38:333–344.

67. Fine J, Finestone SC: Sensory disturbances following ketamine anesthesia: Recurrent hallucinations. Anesth Analg 1973;52:428–430.

68. Fisher MM: Ketamine hydrochloride in severe bronchospasm. Anesthesia 1977;32:771–772.

69. Ghoneim MM, Hinrichs JM, Mewaldt SP, et al: Ketamine: Behavioral effects of subanaesthetics doses. J Clin Psychopharmacol 1985; 5:71–77.

70. Giannini AJ, Price WA, Loiselle RW, et al: Treatment of phenylcy-clohexylpyrrolidine (PHP) psychosis with haloperidol. J Toxicol Clin Toxicol 1985;23:185–189.

71. Gill JR, Stajic M: Ketamine in non-hospital and hospital deaths in New York City. J Forensic Sci 2000;45:655–658.

72. Golden NL, Sokol RJ, Rubin IL: Angel dust: Possible effects on the fetus. Pediatrics 1980;65:18–20.

73. Green SM, Clark R, Hostetler MA, et al: Inadvertent ketamine overdose in children: Clinical manifestations and outcome. Ann Emerg Med 1999;34:492–497.

74. Green SM, Clem KJ, Rothrock SG: Ketamine safety profile in the developing world: Survey of practitioners. Acad Emerg Med 1996; 3:598–604.

75. Green SM, Kuppermann N, Rothrock SG, et al: Predictors of adverse events with intramuscular ketamine sedation in children. Ann Emerg Med 2000;35:35–42.

76. Green SM, Rothrock SG, Lynch EL: Intramuscular ketamine for pediatric sedation in the emergency department: Safety profile in 1,022 cases. Ann Emerg Med 1998;31:688–697.

77. Green SM: Ketamine sedation for pediatric procedures: Part 2, Review and implications. Ann Emerg Med 1990,19:1033–1046.

78. Green SM: Ketamine sedation for pediatric therapy: Part 1, A prospective series. Ann Emerg Med 1990;19:1024–1032.

79. Green ST, Rothrock SG, Harris T, et al: Intravenous ketamine for pediatric sedation in the emergency department: Safety profile with 156 cases. Acad Emerg Med 1998;5:971–976.

80. Greifenstein FE, DeVault M, Yoshitake J, et al: A study of a 1-aryl cyclohexylamine for anesthesia. Anesth Analg 1958;37:283–294.

81. Hamilton IT, Bryson JS: The effect of ketamine on transmembrane potentials of Purkinje fibers of the pig heart. Br J Anaesth 1974; 46:636–642.

82. Harbourne GC, Watson FL, Healy DT, et al: The effects of subanesthetic doses of ketamine on memory, cognitive performance and subjective experience in healthy volunteers. J Psychophamacol 1996; 10:134–140.

83. Harris EW, Ganong AH, Cotman CW: Long-term potentiation in the hippocampus involves activation of *N*-methyl-D-aspartate receptors. Brain Res 1984;323:132–137.

84. Harris JA, Biersner RJ, Edwards D, et al: Attention, learning, and personality during ketamine emergence: A pilot study. Anesth Analg 1975;54:169–172.

85. Heveran JE: Radioimmunoassay for phencyclidine. J Forensic Sci 1980;25:79–87.

86. Holland JA, Nelson L, Ravikumar PR, et al: Embalming fluid-soaked marijuana. New high or new guise for PCP? J Psychoactive Drugs 1998;30:215–219.

87. Hubel JA. "Authorities cast a wary eye on raves." The New York Times. 29 June 1997, sec. 13LI, p. 15.

88. Ikonomidou C, Bosch F, Milsa M, et al: Blockade of NMDA receptors and apoptotic neurodegeneration in the developing brain. Science 1999;283:70–74.

89. Ishimaru MJ, Ikonomidou C, Jenkova TI, et al: Distinguishing excitotoxic from apoptotic neurodegeneration in the developing rat brain. J Comp Neurol 1999;408:461–476.

90. Jackson JE: Phencyclidine pharmacokinetics after a massive overdose. Ann Intern Med 1989;111:613–615.

91. Jansen KL: Non-medical use of ketamine. BMJ 1993;306;601–602.

92. Javitt DC, Zukin SR: Recent advances in the phencyclidine model of schizophrenia. Am J Psychiatry 1991;148:1301–1308.

93. Jentsch JD, Roth RH: The neuropsychopharmacology of phencyclidine: From NMDA receptor hypofunction to the dopamine hypothesis of schizophrenia. Neuropsychopharmacology 1999;20:201–225.

94. Johnson BD: Psychosis and ketamine. Brit Med J 1971;4:428.

95. Johnson KM, Snell LD, Sacaan AI, et al: Pharmacologic regulation of the NMDA receptor-ionophore complex. NIDA Res Monogr 1993;133:14–40.

96. Johnston LD, O'Malley PM, Bachman JG: National survey results on drug use from Monitoring the future survey, 1975–1993. NIH publication No. 93–3597. Bethesda, MD, NIDA, 1994.

97. Johnstone M, Evans V: Sernyl (C1–395) in clinical anaesthesia. Brit J Anaesth 1959;31:433–439.

98. Karp HN, Kaufman ND, Anand SK: Phencyclidine poisoning in young children. J Pediatr 1980;97:1006–1009.

99. Koehntop DE, Liao JC, Van Bergen FH: Effects of pharmacologic alterations of adrenergic mechanisms of cocaine, tropolone, aminophylline, and ketamine on epinephrine-induced arrhythmias during halothane-nitrous oxide anesthesia. Anesthesiology 1977;46: 83–93.

100. Krystal JH, Karper LP, Seibyl JP, et al: Subanesthetic effects of the noncompetitive NMDA antagonist, ketamine, in humans. Arch Gen Psychiatry 1994;51:199–214.

101. Kumar A, Bajaj A, Sarkar P, et al: The effect of music on ketamine-induced emergence phenomena. Anesthesia 1992;47:438–439.

102. Licata M, Pierini G, Popoli G: A fatal ketamine poisoning. J Forensic Sci 1994;39:1314–1320.

103. Liden CB, Lovejoy FH, Costello CE: Phencyclidine—Nine cases of poisoning. JAMA 1975;234:513–516.

104. Lo JN, Cumming JF: Interaction between sedative premedicants and ketamine in man and isolated perfused rat livers. Anethesiology 1975;43:307–312.

105. Lu Yf, Xing YZ, Pan BS, et al: Neuroprotective effects of phencyclidine in acute cerebral ischemia and reperfusion injury in rabbits. Chung Kuo Yao Li Hsueh Pao 1992;13:218–222.

106. Luby EG, Cohen BD, Rosenbaum G, et al: Study of a new schizophrenomimetic drug—Sernyl. AMA Arch Neurol 1959;129: 363–369.

107. Lundberg GD, Gupta RC, Montgomery SH: Phencyclidine: Patterns seen in street drug analysis. Clin Toxicol 1976;9:503–511.

108. Lundy PM, Lockwood PA, Thompson G, et al: Differential effects of ketamine isomers on neuronal and extraneuronal catecholamine uptake mechanisms. Anesthesiology 1986;64:359–363.

109. MacDonald JF, Barlett MC, Mody I, et al: The PCP site of the NMDA receptors complex. Adv Exp Med Biol 1990;268:27–33.

110. Magbagbeola JAO, Thomas NA: Effect of thiopentone on emergence reaction to ketamine anaesthesia. Can Anaesth Soc J 1974; 21:321–324.

111. Maholtra AK, Pinals DA, Weingartner H, et al: NMDA receptor function and human cognition: The effects of ketamine in healthy volunteers. Neuropsychopharmacology 1996;14:301–307.

112. Martinez-Aguirre E, Sansano C: Comparison of midazolam and diazepam as complement of ketamine-air anesthesia in children. Acta Anesthesiol Belg 1986;37:15–22.

113. McCarron M, Schulze BW, Thompson GA, et al: Acute phencyclidine intoxication: Clinical patterns, complications, and treatment. Ann Emerg Med 1981;10:290–297.

114. McCarron M, Schulze BW, Thompson GA, et al: Acute phencyclidine intoxication: Incidence of clinical findings in 1000 cases. Ann Emerg Med 1981;10:237–242.

115. McMahon B, Ambre J, Ellis J: Hypertension during recovery from phencyclidine intoxication. Clin Toxicol 1978;12:37–40.

116. Metro News Briefs; New York. "Police say web site was sham to sell drugs." The New York Times. 25 February 2000, sec. B, p. 6.

117. Meyer JS, Greifenstein F, Devault M: A new drug causing symptoms of sensory deprivation. Neurological, electroencephalographic and pharmacological effects of Sernyl. J Nerv Ment Dis 1959;129: 54–61.

118. Misra AL, Pontani RB, Bartolomeo J: Persistence of phencyclidine (PCP) and metabolites in brain and adipose tissue and implications for long-lasting behavioral effects. Res Commun Chem Path Pharmacol 1979;24:431–445.

119. Modica P, Tempelhoff R, White P: Pro and anticonvulsant effects of anesthetics (Part II). Anesth Analg 1990;70:433–444.

120. Moerschbaecher JM, Thompson DM: Differential effects of prototype opioid agonists on the acquisition of conditional discrimination in monkeys. J Pharmacol Exp Ther 1983;226:738–748.

121. Mohn AR, Gainetdinov RR, Caron MG, et al: Mice with reduced NMDA receptor expression display behaviors related to schizophrenia. Cell 1999;98:427–436.

122. Moore KA, Kilbane EM, Jones R, et al: Tissue distribution of ketamine in a drug fatality. J Forensic Sci 1997;2:1183–1185.

123. Morgensen F, Muller D, Valentin N: Glycopyrrolate during ketamine/diazepam anaesthesia: A double-blind comparison with atropine. Acta Anaesthesiol Scand 1986;30:332–336.

124. Morgenstern FS, Beech HR, Davies BM: An investigation of drug induced sensory disturbances. Psychopharmacologia 1962;3:193–200.

125. Morray JP, Lynn AM, Stamm SJ, et al: Hemodynamic effects of ketamine in children with congenital heart disease. Anesth Analg 1984;63:895–899.

126. Newcomer JW, Farber NB, Jevtovic-Todorovic V, et al: Ketamine-induced NMDA receptor hypofunction as a model of memory impairment and psychosis. Neuropsychopharmacology 1999;20:106–118.

127. Olney JW, Labruyere J, Price MT: Pathological changes induced in cerebrocortical neurons by phencyclidine and related drugs. Science 1989;244:1360–1362.

128. Olney JW, Labruyere J, Wang G, et al: NMDA receptor antagonist neurotoxicity: Mechanism and prevention. Science 1991;254:1515–1518.

129. Olney JW, Newcomer JW, Farber NB: NMDA receptor hypofunction model of schizophrenia. J Psych Res 1999;33:523–533.

130. Olsson GL, Hallen B: Laryngospasm during anesthesia. A computer-aided incidence study in 136,929 patients. Acta Anaesthesiol Scand 1984;28:567–575.

131. Owens SM, Mayersohn M: Phencyclidine-specific Fab fragments alter phencyclidine disposition in dogs. Drug Metab Dispos 1986;14:52–58.

132. Oye I, Paulsen O, Maurset A: Effects of ketamine on sensory perception: Evidence for a role of N-methyl-D-aspartate receptors. J Pharmacol Exp Ther 1992;260:1209–1213.

133. Patel R, Connor G: A review of thirty cases of rhabdomyolysis associated acute renal failure among phencyclidine users. J Toxicol Clin Toxicol 1985–1986;23:547–556.

134. Picchioni AC, Consroe PF: Activated charcoal: A phencyclidine antidote, or hog in dogs. N Engl J Med 1979;300:202.

135. Pradhan SN: Phencyclidine (PCP): Some human studies. Neurosci Biobehav Rev 1984;8:493–501.

136. Pristin T. "New Jersey Daily Briefing." The New York Times. 22 May 1996, sec. B, p. 1.

137. Rawson RA, Tennant FS, McCann MA: Characteristics of 68 chronic phencyclidine abusers who sought treatment. Drug Alcohol Depend 1981;8:223–227.

138. Rees DK, Wasem SE: The identification of ketamine hydrochloride. Microgram 2000;33:163–167.

139. Reich DL, Silvay G: Ketamine: An update on the first twenty-five years of clinical experience. Can J Anesth 1989;36:186–197.

140. Rock MJ, Reyes de la Rocha S, L'Hommedieu CS, et al: Use of ketamine in asthmatic children to treat respiratory failure refractory to conventional therapy. Crit Care Med 1986;14:514–516.

141. Rosenbaum G, Cohen BD, Luby ED, et al: Comparison of Sernyl with other drugs. AMA Arch General Psychiat 1959;1:651–657.

142. Shannon HE: Evaluation of phencyclidine analogues on the basis of discriminate stimulus properties in the rat. J Pharmacol Exp Ther 1981;216:543–551.

143. Shannon M: Letter to the Editors. Pediatr Emerg Care 1998;14:180.

144. Sharp FR, Jasper P, Hall J, et al: MK-801 and ketamine induce heat protein HSP72 in injured neurons in posterior cingulate and retrosplenial cortex. Ann Neurol 1991;30:801–809.

145. Shulgin AT, Maclean DE: Illicit synthesis of phencyclidine (PCP) and several of its analogs. Clin Toxicol 1976;9:553–560.

146. Siegel RK: Phencyclidine and ketamine intoxication: A study of four populations of recreational users. NIDA Res Monogr 21. In: Petersen RC, Stillman RC, eds: Phencyclidine (PCP) Abuse: An Appraisal. Rockville, MD, National Institute on Drug Abuse, 1978, pp. 119–147.

147. Singer W: Development and plasticity of cortical processing architecture. Science 1995;270:758–764.

148. Sircar R, Li CS: PCP/NMDA receptor-channel complex and brain development. Neurotoxicol Teratol 1994;16:369–373.

149. Sklar GS, Zukin SR, Reilly TA: Adverse reactions to ketamine anesthesia—Abolition by a psychological technique. Anesthesia 1981;36:183–187.

150. Slifer BL, Balster RL, Woolverton WL: Behavioral dependence produced by continuous phencyclidine infusion in rhesus monkeys. J Pharmacol Exp Ther 1984;230:399–406.

151. Snyder SH: Phencyclidine. Nature 1980;285:355–356.

152. Soine WH, Balster RL, Berglund KE, et al: Identification of a new phencyclidine analog, 1-(1-phenylcyclohexyl)-4-methylpiperidine, as a drug of abuse. J Anal Toxicol 1982;6:41–43.

153. Soine WH, Vincek WC, Agee DT: Phencyclidine contaminant generates cyanide. N Engl J Med 1979;301:438.

154. Stanley V, Hunt J, Willis KW, et al: Cardiovascular and respiratory function with CI-581. Anesth Analg 1968;47:760–768.

155. Steinpreis RE: The behavioral and neurochemical effects of phencyclidine in humans and animals: Some implications for modeling psychosis. Behav Brain Res 1996;74:45–55.

156. Stillman R, Petersen RC: The paradox of phencyclidine (PCP) abuse. Ann Intern Med 1979;90:428–429.

157. Strauss AA, Modanlou HD, Bosu SK: Neonatal manifestations of maternal phencyclidine (PCP) abuse. Pediatrics 1981;68:550–552.

158. Strube PJ, Hallam PL: Ketamine by continuous infusion in status asthmaticus. Anesthesia 1986;41:1017–1019.

159. Substance Abuse and Mental Health Services Administration. National Household Survey on Drug Abuse, 1996. USDHHS. http://www.samhsa.gov.

160. Toro-Matos A, Rendon-Platas AM, Avila Valdez E, et al: Physostigmine antagonizes ketamine. Anesth Analg 1980;59:764–767.

161. Tweed WA, Minuck M, Mymin D: Circulatory responses to ketamine anesthesia. Anesthesiology 1972;37:613–619.

162. Valentine JL, Mayersohn M, Wessinger WD, et al: Antiphencyclidine monoclonal Fab fragment reverse phencyclidine-induced behavioral effects and ataxia in rats. J Pharmacol Exp Ther 1996;278:709–716.

163. Viera L, Weiner A: Ketamine abusers presenting to the emergency department: A case series [abstract]. J Toxicol Clin Toxicol 2000;5:505.

164. Vincent JP, Cavey D, Kamenka JM, et al: Interaction of phencyclidine with muscarinic and opiate receptors in the central nervous system. Brain Res 1978;152:176–182.

165. Vincent JP, Kartalovski B, Geneste P, et al: Interaction of phencyclidine ("angel dust") with a specific receptor in rat brain membranes. Proc Natl Acad Sci U S A 1979;76:4678–4682.

166. Vogt BA: Cingulate cortex In: Peters A, Jones EG, eds: Cerebral Cortex. New York, Plenum, 1985, pp. 4:89–149.

167. Warner A: Dextromethorphan: Analyte of the month. In: American Association of Clinical Chemistry: In Service Training and Continuing Education. 1993;14:27–28.

168. Weingarten SM: Dissociation of limbic and neocortical EEG pattern in cats under ketamine anaesthesia. J Neurosurg 1972;37:429–433.

169. White PF, Way WL, Trevor AJ: Ketamine—Its pharmacology and therapeutic uses. Anesthesiology 1982;56:119–136.

170. Wilgoren J: "Police arrest 14 in drug raid at a nightclub in Manhattan." The New York Times, 18 April 1999, sec. 1, p. 41.

171. Willets J, Balster RL: Phencyclidine-like discriminate stimulus properties of MK-801 in rats. Eur J Pharmacol 1988;146:167–169.

172. Wolfe SA, De Souza EB: Sigma and phencyclidine receptors in the brain-endocrine-immune axis. NIDA Res Monogr 1993;133:95–123.

173. Wong EHF, Kemp JA: Sites for antagonism of *N*-methyl-D-aspartate receptor channel complex. Annu Rev Pharmacol Toxicol 1991;31: 401–425.

174. Woodworth JR, Owens SM, Mayersohn M: Phencyclidine (PCP) disposition kinetics in dogs as a function of dose and route of administration. J Pharmacol Exp Ther 1985;234:654–661.

175. Wright HH, Cole EA, Batey SR, Hanna K: Phencyclidine-induced psychosis: Eight-year follow-up of ten cases. South Med J 1988;81: 565–567.

176. Young JD, Crapo LM: Protracted phencyclidine coma from an intestinal deposit. Arch Intern Med 1992;152:859–860.

177. Zsigmond EK, Domino EF: Ketamine. Clinical pharmacology, pharmacokinetics and current clinical uses. Anesth Rev 1980;7:13–33.

178. Zukin SR, Zukin RS: Specific [3H]phencyclidine binding in rat central nervous system. Proc Natl Acad Sci U S A 1979;76:5372–5376.

CHAPTER 70

LYSERGIC ACID DIETHYLAMIDE AND OTHER HALLUCINOGENS

Jeffrey R. Tucker / Robert P. Ferm

Lysergic acid diethylamide

A 17-year-old male was brought to the Emergency Department (ED) by his friends because he was acting bizarrely on the way home from school. He told a friend that he had done "acid" after school and now could not stop staring at the bright lights. He kept telling his friends to join with him to enjoy the "peace of the lights."

Physical examination in the ED revealed an agitated male staring at the overhead lights. Vital signs were: blood pressure, 150/100 mm Hg; pulse, 112 beats/min; respiratory rate, 28 breaths/min; and oral temperature, 100.4°F (38°C). His skin was moist and pale. Examination of the eyes revealed slowly reactive 6-mm pupils without nystagmus. He had occasional faint, scattered end-expiratory wheezes. Cardiac auscultation was normal. The abdomen was soft and nontender, with hyperactive bowel sounds. There was no clubbing, cyanosis, or edema. The neurologic examination initially revealed an agitated, frightened, but oriented young male. He was frightened by the visual hallucinations and was "hearing purple and blue" from the overhead lights. The remainder of the neurologic examination was intact with the exception of a fine tremor. The patient admitted that he had taken LSD. He had previously used LSD at concerts with others, but this was the first time that he had used it alone. Although he knew where he was and that he was experiencing drug effects, he was frightened and extremely anxious of losing his mind. He was placed in a quiet location with minimal stimuli and an intravenous line was established. He received 10 mg diazepam by slow IV push. A rapid bedside blood glucose was 120 mg/dL. Pulse oximetry was 97%.

After approximately 8 hours observation, the patient was fully alert and oriented and was at his baseline functional status. His primary care provider was notified about this exposure, a referral was made for drug counseling, and he was discharged with family members.

Hallucinogens are a diverse group of drugs that alter and distort perception, thought, and mood without clouding the sensorium. To understand the effects of these drugs, an understanding of the concepts and definitions of altered perception, thought and mood is important. A hallucination is a false perception that has no basis in the external environment. The term is derived from the Latin "to wander in mind." An illusion is a mental impression that is derived from misinterpretation of an actual experience. The classic hallucinogens are also illusiogenic. Although many terms are used to describe the effects, the term "hallucinogens" often refers to the medical-legal context of these toxins, whereas psychedelic is used to describe the nonmedical and recreational use of these compounds. Other terms are used to describe the effects of these compounds, including entheogen (generating religious experience), oneirogen (producing dreams), psychotomimetic (producing psychosis), and phanerothyme (making feeling visible).[80]

EPIDEMIOLOGY

Hallucinogens have been used for thousands of years by different cultures, largely for religious experiences. Early hallucinogens were derived from fungi and plants. The ancient Indian holy book, *Rig-Veda,* written over 3500 years ago, describes a sacramental substance called Soma both as a god and as an intoxicating substance. The source of Soma is believed to be the juice of the mushroom *Amanita muscaria.*[65,71] The Aztecs used the psilocybin-containing teonanacatl (flesh of the gods), and ololiuqui (morning glory seeds) in their religious ceremonies. In AD 994, an epidemic of ergotism caused by the ingestion of contaminated rye and wheat product, which was produced by the fungus *Claviceps purpurea,* led to the deaths of 40,000 people in Europe. Ergotism has also been implicated as a cause of the behavior of the alleged witches of Salem, Massachusetts.[23]

Synthetic hallucinogen use is often said to have begun with the discovery and ingestion of LSD-25, commonly known as LSD. The synthesis of LSD was the result of extensive research at Sandoz laboratories with the ergot alkaloids from *Claviceps purpurea*. In 1938, while searching for a new analeptic agent, the Swiss chemist Albert Hofmann synthesized LSD-25. (The number 25 denotes that it was the 25th substance synthesized within the series.) LSD is the abbreviation of the German name Lysergsäurediäthylamide. LSD-25 was "tested" 5 years later when Hofmann unintentionally became exposed to the agent by the topical route and subsequently developed hallucinations.[41,77] In 1947, Sandoz began marketing LSD under the trademark Delysid. In the 1950s, psychiatrists used LSD as an adjunct for analytic psychotherapy and as an experimental model for schizophrenia.[83] It was thought that the administration of LSD could aid the patient in releasing repressed material. The Central Intelligence Agency experimented with the use of LSD as a tool for interrogating suspected communists and as a mind-control agent.[17,77]

In the 1960s, LSD became popular as a recreational drug with the concept of "fifth freedom": the right of all individuals to alter their consciousness as they saw fit. Timothy Leary popularized LSD as a way to "Tune in, Turn on, Drop out."[77] In 1966, because of concerns about the public health, a federal law banned LSD.[62] Initial reports of LSD-induced chromosomal breakage also appeared in the 1960s.[24,43,50] Further studies of pregnant women who had taken LSD did not show an increase risk of abortions or birth defects.[30,49]

Hallucinogen use diminished in the late 1970s and early 1980s, but over the last decade, there has been resurgence in hallucinogen use.[4] An annual survey of high school students showed a steady rise in use with a peak in 1996. In 1999, 14.2% of high school seniors claimed to have used LSD at least once in their life as compared to 9.9% in 1989.[44] LSD use is more prevalent in the suburbs than the in the inner city.[63,73] Hallucinogenic drugs were a regular experience at Grateful Dead Concerts for almost 30 years, are used at rave parties, and in the Acid House Movement.[28,61] In the late 1980s, the Acid House Movement appeared in Britain where LSD and methylenedioxymethamphetamine (MDMA) and "acid music" were used at all-night dance parties.[52]

Myths have been perpetuated regarding LSD toxicity. In an effort to reduce the use of LSD, it was reported that psychotic reactions occured in children after LSD blotter paper was stuck to their skin. In 1999, there was a rumor spread across the Internet that gang members were spreading a deadly mixture of LSD and strychnine on pay phone buttons. This combination was ironic because LSD and strychnine have long been associated with each other, as a result of unfounded concerns that strychnine was a by-product or contaminant in the production of LSD. Neither myth has credible evidence to support it.

LSD is classified as a Schedule I agent with high abuse potential, lack of established safety even under medical supervision, and no known use in medical treatment. However, after little research in the 1970s and 1980s, there was a revival of scientific interest in the 1990s. There are now several studies involving human subjects intended to clarify the mechanism of action and the basic physiologic and central nervous system effects of hallucinogens.[37,79] Although hallucinogens have been suggested as potential treatment

alternatives for patients with obsessive-compulsive disorder, controlled trials have not been conducted.[25]

CLASSIC HALLUCINOGENS

The major structural classes of hallucinogens are the lysergamides, indolealkyamines, phenylethylamines, and tetrahydrocannabinoids (Table 70–1). Lysergamides include LSD and lysergic acid hydroxyethylamide (olloliuqi) (Fig. 70–1). Psilocybin, N,N-dimethyltryptamine, and bufotenine are the major indolealkylamines (Fig. 70–2). The most significant phenylethylamines include mescaline and amphetamine derivatives such as MDMA (Chap. 68). Tetrahydrocannabinoids are discussed in Chap. 71.

Lysergamides

Lysergic acid diethylamide is the synthetic derivative of an ergot alkaloid. Although four LSD isomers exist, only the D(−) is active. Lysergic acid diethylamide is a water-soluble, colorless, tasteless, and odorless powder. Currently, most LSD is synthesized and typically sold as liquid-impregnated blotter paper, microdots, tiny tablets, "window pane" gelatin squares, liquid, powder, or tablets.[73] The minimum effective dose is 25 μg.[47] The Drug Enforcement Administration reports that the current street dose of LSD ranges from 20–80 μg which is lower than the 100–200 μg reported during the 1960s and early 1970s.[26]

TABLE 70–1. Agents Classified as Hallucinogens

Lysergamides
  D-Lysergic acid diethylamide (LSD)
  Lysergic acid hydroxyethylamide
    Ipomoea violacea
    Ololiuqui (South American morning glories)
  Ergine
    Argyreia (Wood rose)

Indolealkylamines/Tryptamine
  5-Methoxy-N,N-dimethyltryptamine
  Ibogaine
  N,N-Dimethyltryptamine
  Psilocin
  Psilocybin

Phenylethylamines
  Mescaline
  MDMA (3,4-methylenedioxymethamphetamine)
  DOB (4-bromo-2,5-dimethoxyamphetamine)
  PMA (paramethoxyamphetamine)

Tetrahydrocannabinoids (THC)
  Marijuana
  Hashish

Anticholinergics
  Belladonna alkaloids
    Jimsonweed (*Datura stramonium*)
    Mandrake (*Mandragora officinarum*)
    Henbane (*Hyoscyamus niger*)
    Deadly nightshade (*Atropa belladonna*)

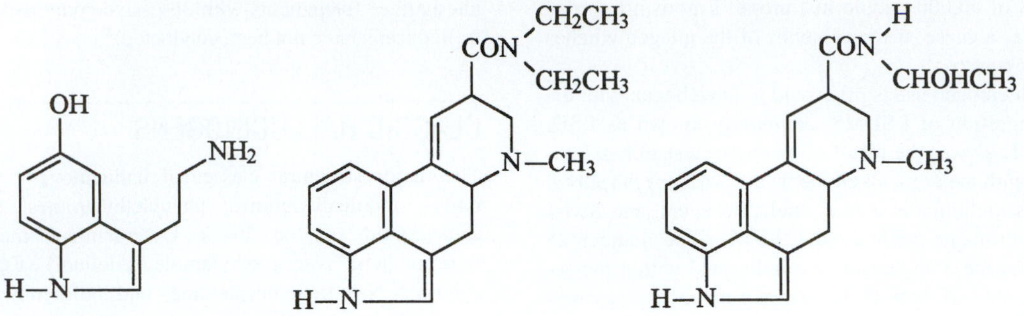

Serotonin LSD Ololiuqui Lysergic acid hydroxyethylamide

Figure 70–1. Hallucinogens of the lysergamide chemical class and their chemical similarity to serotonin.

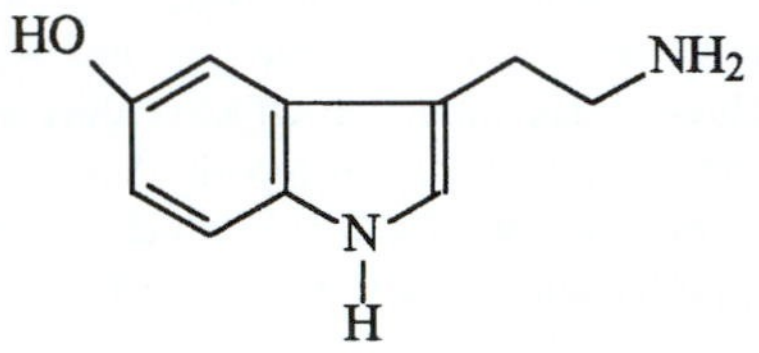

Serotonin

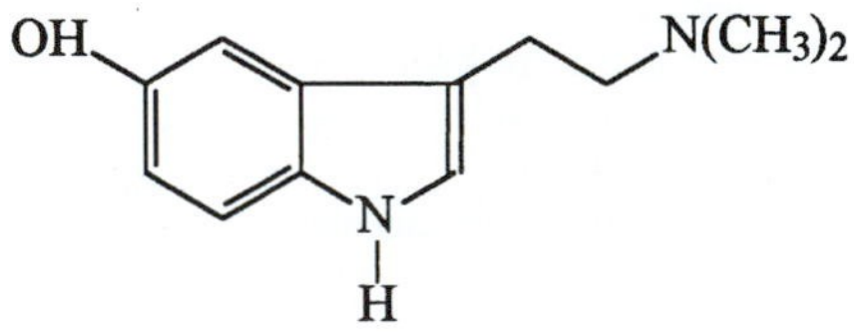

Bufotenine

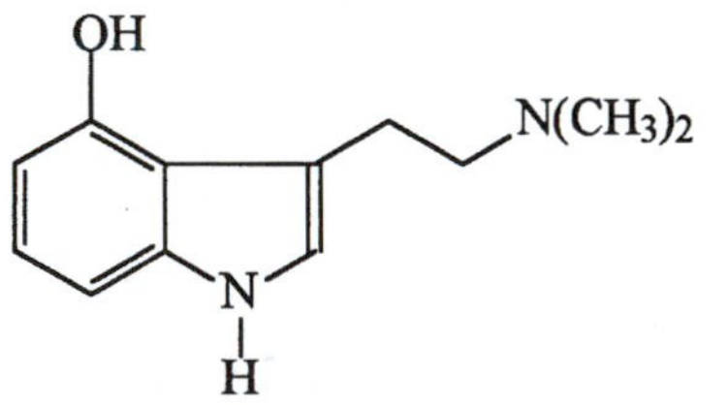

Psilocin

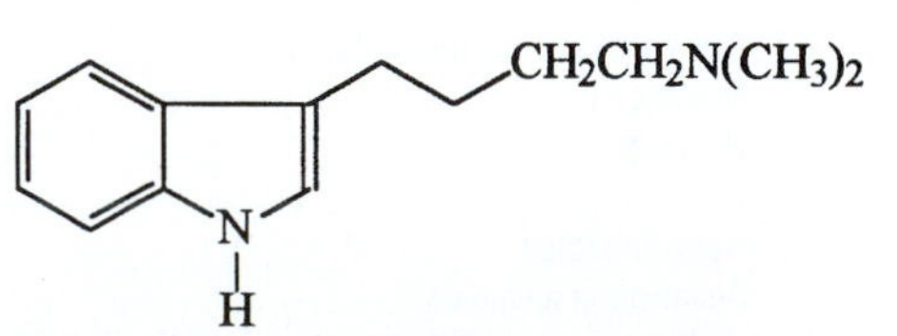

N,N-Dimethyltryptamine

Figure 70–2. Hallucinogens of the indolealkylamine chemical class and their chemical similarity to serotonin.

Lysergamides are also found naturally in several species of morning glory (*Rivea corymbosa*) or Hawaiian baby woodrose (*Ipomoea violacea*).[72] Morning glory seeds contain the toxin lysergic acid hydroxyethylamide, which has one-tenth the potency of LSD. Hallucinogenic effects require about 200–300 seeds. The seeds must be pulverized, because the intact seed coat prevents drug absorption.

Phenylethylamines

Peyote (*Lophophora williamsii*) is a small blue-green spineless cactus that grows in dry and rocky slopes throughout the southwestern United States and northern Mexico. Mescaline is the active hallucinogenic alkaloid found in the peyote cactus. Peyote buttons are the round fleshy tops of the cactus that have been sliced off and dried. The buttons are bitter tasting and nausea, vomiting, and diaphoresis often precedes the psychological effects. Six to 12 buttons (270–540 mg) are the common dose to produce hallucinogenic effects.[72] The legal use of peyote in the United States is restricted to the Native American Church where peyote buttons are used in religious ceremonies and as a medical treatment for physical and psychological ailments.[19,22]

MDMA

MDMA is an amphetamine analogue with stimulant and hallucinogenic properties. MDMA has one-tenth the central nervous system (CNS) stimulant effects of amphetamine, but unlike amphetamine and methamphetamine, it can cause release of serotonin. Proponents of MDMA believe it enhances pleasures, heightens sexuality and expands consciousness without loss of control.[74] It has a reputation as a safe drug. As its use has increased, there is an increasing recognition of significant toxicity: hyperthermia, dysrhythmias, hypertensive crisis, and disseminated intravascular coagulation (Chap. 68).

Indoles

Psilocybin is found in three major genera of mushrooms: *Psilocyba, Panaelous*, and *Conocybe* (Chap. 76).[71] Psilocybin-containing mushrooms are found in the southern United States, usually in cow pastures. The mushroom may be recognized by a greenish blue color that it assumes after bruising, but misidentification is common.[10] The active toxin, psilocybin, was first isolated in 1958 by Albert Hofmann. The effects are similar to LSD, but with a shorter duration of action of about 4 hours.

N,N-Dimethyltryptamine (DMT) is a potent short-acting hallucinogen. It is found naturally in the bark of the Yakee plant (*Virola calophylla*), which grows in the Amazon basin and is used by shamans as a hallucinogenic snuff to communicate with the spirits.[71] DMT is not absorbed from the gastrointestinal tract and is typically smoked, snorted, or injected. Because DMT is smoked or injected, it peaks in 5–20 minutes, with a duration of 30–60 minutes. This has earned it the name "businessman's trip." Current human hallucinogenic research involving DMT is being conducted to determine safety, specific receptor binding, and potential treatments.[80,81]

Bufotenine (5-hydroxydimethyltryptamine) is present in the secretions and skin of toads of the genus *Bufo*.[16] Although it is believed that bufotenine is a hallucinogen, there is controversy about its ability to cause altered perception.[51,66] Bufotenine does have peripheral effects on the heart rate and blood pressure, but does not cross the blood-brain barrier. In contrast, 5-methoxy-N,N-dimethyltryptamine (5-MeO-DMT) is a potent hallucinogen. The only species that produces 5-MeO-DMT is the *Bufo alvarius* (Colorado river toad).[66,85] Severe toxicity and death have occurred from the practice of toad licking in an attempt to experience the hallucinogen effects.[40,57,75]

Ibogaine is an indole alkaloid derived from the African shrub *Tabernanthe iboga*. It was initially used as a hallucinogen in religious ceremonies by indigenous people. In 1970, it was classified by the FDA as a Schedule I substance because of its illicit use.[35] The hallucinogenic effects have been divided into two phases. An acute phase of intense hallucinations develops 4–8 hours after ingestion, followed by a second stage lasting approximately 8–20 hours after ingestion.

Ibogaine's unique mechanism of action may allow a more complete understanding of the neurobiology of addiction. Ibogaine has a complex interaction with multiple receptors as opposed to simple replacement therapy, such as methadone.[6,42] Currently, Ibogaine is under investigation for the treatment of drug addiction involving opioids, ethanol, and nicotine, but significant side effects have limited its clinical benefit.[35,42] This has led to the development of safer and effective congeners such as 18-methoxycoronaridine to be tested as an antiaddictive medication.

PHARMACOKINETICS

Although the effects of the hallucinogens are similar, the onset of action, peak effect, and duration can be variable. The hallucinogens can be characterized by duration of action: ultrashort acting, short acting, intermediate acting, and long acting[80] (Table 70–2).

LSD has been the most studied hallucinogen and there is extensive information about its pharmacokinetics. Ingestion is the most common route of exposure. The gastrointestinal tract rapidly absorbs LSD. Other routes of administration include intranasal, parenteral, sublingual, smoking, and conjunctival instillation. Plasma protein binding is over 80% and volume of distribution is 0.28 L/kg. It is concentrated within the visual cortex and the limbic and reticular activating systems. It is metabolized in the liver via hydroxylation and glucuronidation, excreted predominately as a pharmacologically inactive compound, and has an elimination half-life of about 2.5 hours. Only small amounts are eliminated unchanged in the urine.

Tolerance to the psychological effects of LSD occurs within 2–3 days with daily dosing but rapidly dissipates if the drug is withheld for 2 or more days. Cross-tolerance among mescaline, psilocybin, and LSD has been reported in humans.[12] There is no evidence for physiologic tolerance, physiologic dependence, or a withdrawal syndrome with the classic hallucinogens. Cross-tolerance has not been documented between any members of that group and the amphetamines.[66] Limited tolerance is also demonstrated between psilocybin and cannabinoids such as marijuana.[18,64]

PHYSIOLOGY

Although the mechanism of action of the classic hallucinogens is incompletely understood, recent studies support a common site of action, on central serotonin receptors.[5,20,39,67] Serotonin, or 5-hydroxytryptamine (5-HT), is involved in the modulation of smooth muscle function in the gastrointestinal tract and cardiovascular system, in the regulation of platelet function, and as a neurotransmitter in the brain. Serotonin modulates many psychological and physiologic processes, including mood, personality, affect, appetite, motor function, sexual activity, temperature regulation, pain perception, sleep induction and ADH release.

The $5\text{-}HT_{2A}$ receptor is implicated in the modulation of hallucinations.[5,33,54,82,87] $5\text{-}HT_2$ receptors are located postsynaptically on certain subpopulations of neurons, predominately in the cerebral cortex. There is very good correlation between the affinity of both indolealkylamine and phenylethylamine hallucinogens for $5\text{-}HT_2$ receptors and hallucinogenic potency in humans.[34] Cortical involvement correlates with the substantial effect that hallucinogens cause on cognition, mood and perception, because this is the area of the brain that would mediate these effects. In the cerebral cortex, $5\text{-}HT_{2A}$ receptors are expressed in many areas with the highest density in the neocortex (layer Va) and the piriform cortex.[5] Also involved is the locus coeruleus, a subcortical area located bilaterally in the upper pons at the lateral border of the 4th ventricle that, projects throughout the entire neocortex and receives sensory

TABLE 70–2. **Pharmacokinetic Classification of Hallucinogens**

Classification	Toxin	Onset	Peak effect	Duration of effect
Ultrashort acting	DMT IV	1 min	5 min	30 min
Short acting	DMT IM	5–15 min	15–60 min	1–2 h
Intermediate acting	Psilocybin	15–30 min	1–3 h	6 h
Long acting	LSD; Mescaline	30–90 min	3–5 h	8–12 h
Ultralong acting	Ibogaine	2–4 h	4–8 h	18–24 h

input from all parts of the brain. This area is important in sympathetic nervous system regulation. Hallucinogens do not directly stimulate the locus coeruleus, but their actions are mediated through the 5-HT$_{2A}$ receptors. LSD is also an agonist at 5-HT$_{2C}$.[11,56,88]

Although the majority of investigation has focused on the role of serotonin for drug-induced hallucinations, other neurotransmitters are involved. Stimulation of 5-HT$_{2A}$ receptors enhances release of glutamate in the cortical layer V pyramidal cells.[5,9] Recent work indicates that LSD and other lysergamides stimulate both D$_1$ and D$_2$ dopamine receptors.[8,32,84] The psychological aspect of hallucinogens seems to represent a complex interaction between different neurotransmitters with the exact relationship of the serotonergic and dopaminergic systems still elusive.

CLINICAL EFFECTS

Physiologic changes accompany and often precede the perceptual changes. The physical effects may be caused by either direct drug effect or by a response to the disturbing or enjoyable subjective experience. Sympathetic effects mediated by the locus ceruleus include mydriasis, tachycardia, hypertension, tachypnea, hyperthermia, and diaphoresis. They occur shortly after ingestion and often precede the hallucinogenic effects. The sympathetic manifestations are mild in nature as compared to the effects of cocaine and amphetamines. Other clinical findings that are reported include piloerection, dizziness, hyperactivity, muscle weakness, ataxia, altered mental status, coma, and hippus, a spasmodic, rhythmical, pupillary dilation and constriction.[48] Nausea and vomiting often precede the psychedelic effects produced by psilocybin and mescaline. Potential life-threatening complications such as hyperthermia, coma, respiratory arrest, hypertension, tachcardia, and coagulopathy were described in a report of 8 patients with a massive LSD overdose.[45]

The psychological effects of LSD are dose related and affect changes in arousal, emotion, perception, thought process, and self-image. The response to the drug is related to the person's mindset, emotions, or expectations at the time and can be altered by the group or setting.[2] The person experiencing the effects of a hallucinogen is usually fully awake, alert, and oriented but confronted with diverse perceptual anomalies and varied sensations. The person may experience euphoria or dysphoria, can be emotionally labile, but generally realizes that he or she is under the influence of a drug. Perceptual distortions are common, typically involve loss of body image (people's faces and body parts appear distorted) and alteration in visual perceptions (objects undulate, their boundaries are lost and merge). There is acute attention to details with excessive attachment of meaning to ordinary objects and events. Usual thoughts seem novel and profound. Many people report an intensification of their sensory perceptions such as sound magnification and distortion; colors seem brighter with halolike lights around objects. Frequently, the person relates a sense of depersonalization and separation from the environment. The hallucinating person may perceive that he or she is observing an "out-of-body experience." Synesthesias, or sensory misperceptions, are frequent and include "hearing" color or "seeing" sounds. True hallucinations may occur and can be visual, auditory, tactile, or olfactory, although those of a visual nature are the most common.[86]

Acute adverse psychiatric effects of hallucinogens include panic reactions, true hallucinations, psychosis, and major depressive dysphoric reactions. Acute panic reactions, the most common adverse effect, present with frightening illusions, tremendous anxiety, apprehension, and a terrifying sense of loss of self-control. The acute depersonalization and perceptual alterations associated with hallucinogen use may be the stimulus for the decompensation.[46]

DIFFERENTIAL DIAGNOSIS

Hallucinosis is the abnormal organic mental condition of persistent hallucinations. The major causes of hallucinosis can be divided into structural, infectious, functional, and toxic-metabolic origins. The diagnosis of hallucinogen exposure often must be established on the basis of history and physical examination alone. Sympathomimetic effects such as mydriasis, tachycardia, hypertension, diaphoresis, and hyperactivity are generally less prominent in LSD ingestion than in phenylethylamine intoxication. The person who has ingested hallucinogens typically is oriented and will often give a history of drug use. This stands in stark contrast to patients with drug-induced delirium, in whom orientation is, by definition, altered.

Drugs such as amphetamine, cocaine, phencyclidine (PCP), and anticholinergics produce delirium or psychosis at doses capable of producing hallucinations. Patients with amphetamine toxicity typically present with elaborate and paranoid delusions as well as visual hallucinations. Psychiatric or "functional" causes of perceptual changes such schizophrenia typically present with auditory hallucinations. Patients with central anticholinergic toxicity usually present with disorientation, combative behavior, and incoherent mumbling, and may be unaware that the hallucinations are drug induced.[47] The presence of marked hyperthermia, uncontrollable behavior, or extreme agitation should suggest an alternative exposure such as cocaine, PCP, or amphetamines.

LABORATORY

The routine drug-of-abuse screens do not detect the classic hallucinogens such as LSD or DMT, but may detect MDMA or PCP. Although LSD exposure can be detected by radioimmunoassay, confirmation by high-performance liquid chromatography or gas chromatography is necessary. These tests are rarely used in the clinical setting, but are much more common for forsenic matters.[12,27]

TREATMENT

Most patients with hallucinogenic experiences are never brought to medical attention because they experience only the desired effect of the drug. In any patient who presents to the emergency department with disturbing hallucinations or psychosis, even if an ingestion of a hallucinogen is suspected, the basic approach for altered mental status should include consideration of the administration of dextrose, thiamine, and oxygen as indicated, and the vigorous search for other etiologies.

The patient with a dysphoric reaction can be placed in a quiet location with minimal stimuli. A nonjudgmental advocate should attempt to reduce the patient's anxiety, provide reality testing, and remind the individual that a drug was ingested and the effect will wear off in a couple of hours.[78] Significant agitation, dysphoria, or a "bad trip," combined with signs of autonomic instability, can usually be treated by the administration of a benzodiazepine.[1,73] Benzodiazepines remain the cornerstone of therapy, as the sedating effect will diminish both endogenous and exogenous sympathetic effects.[60] Phenothiazines have been used to treat acute psychotic reactions; however, there may be an increased incidence of hallucinogen persisting perception disorder, previously known as flashbacks, in those patients treated with phenothiazines.[3] Prolonged psychosis may require treatment with long-term antipsychotic therapy. Gastrointestinal decontamination with activated charcoal may be considered for asymptomatic patients with recent ingestions, but is probably not helpful after clinical symptoms appear, and attempts may lead to further agitation. Excessive physical restraint should be avoided because of concerns for hyperthermia and rhabdomyolysis.

Hallucinogens rarely produce life-threatening problems. Sedation with benzodiazepines is usually sufficient to treat autonomic instability and hyperthermia. In rare cases, hyperthermia may require more aggressive therapy with hydration, active external cooling, and muscle relaxants ranging from benzodiazepines to paralytic agents depending upon the severity of the individual's condition.[15] Morbidity and mortality typically result from the complications of hyperthermia including rhabdomyolysis and myoglobinuric renal failure, hepatic necrosis, and disseminated intravascular coagulopathy. For the most part, however, hydration, sedation, a supportive environment, and meticulous supportive care will prove adequate.[21]

Atypical antipsychotics such as clozapine and risperidone are antagonist at the 5-HT$_2$ receptors.[29] In animal model systems 5-HT$_2$ antagonists such as risperidone and ritanserin are effective in blocking the electrophysiologic and behavioral effects of hallucinogenic drugs. These agents may be a potential treatment for adverse reactions to hallucinogens, but require further before study they are used routinely.[58,59,68]

LONG-TERM EFFECTS

Long-term consequences of LSD use include prolonged psychotic reactions, severe depression, and exacerbation of preexisting psychiatric illness.[38,70] When LSD was initially popularized, some patients were noted to behave in a manner similar to schizophrenia and required admission to psychiatric facilities. In volunteer studies, panic reactions, hallucinogen persisting perception disorder, and extended psychoses were noted. When the drug was used for alleviation of anxiety and personality abnormalities, flashbacks and extended psychosis were reported.[31] It has been suggested that these individuals had preexisting compensated psychological disturbances.[5,53,76]

Hallucinogen persisting perception disorder (HPPD), previously known as flashbacks, is a chronic problem associated with LSD abuse and is characterized by transient recurrence of perceptual disturbances that were experienced in a previous hallucinogen experience.[7] These perceptions can be triggered during times of stress, illness, and exercise, and are often a virtual recurrence of the initial hallucinations. Common perceptual and visual disturbances in HPPD include geometric forms; false, fleeting perceptions in the peripheral fields; flashes of color; intensified color; and halos around objects.[53] hallucinogen persisting perception disorder may only last for several months, but some patients have re-

ported perceptual abnormalities up to 5 years. Reality testing is intact in patients with HPPD as opposed to patients with psychosis. The etiology of HPPD is unknown. Although, many drugs have been tried to treat patients with HPPD, most have not proven beneficial. Haloperidol and risperidone are associated with an exacerbation of panic and visual symptoms.[3] Clonidine may be an option. Patients who are on therapeutic doses of lithium are at risk for seizures or HPPD, whereas patients being treated with tricyclic antidepressants or a selective serotonin reuptake have an inconsistent altered response to the pyschotropic effects.[13,14,55] Although there are no reported case of serotonin syndrome reported with classic hallucinogens, there are cases associated with MDMA.

SUMMARY

Hallucinogens are a diverse group of drugs that alter and distort perception, thought, and mood without clouding the sensorium. Acute adverse psychiatric effects of hallucinogens include panic reactions, true hallucinations, psychosis, and major depressive dysphoric reactions. Hallucinogens rarely produce life-threatening problems. Long-term consequence of LSD use may include prolonged psychotic reactions, severe depression, exacerbation of preexisting psychiatric illness, and hallucinogen persisting perception disorder.

ACKNOWLEDGMENT

Cynthia K. Aaron, MD, contributed to this chapter in a previous edition.

REFERENCES

1. Abraham HD, Aldridge AM: Adverse consequences of lysergic acid diethylamide. Addiction 1993;88:1327–1334.
2. Abraham HD, Aldridge AM, Gogia P: The psychopharmacology of hallucinogens. Neuropsychopharmacology 1996;14:285–298.
3. Abraham, HD, Mamen A: LSD-like panic from risperidone in post-LSD visual disorder. J Clin Psychopharmacol 1996;16:238–241.
4. Adlaf EM, Ivis FJ: Recent findings from the Ontario student drug survey. CMAJ 1998;159:451–454.
5. Aghajanian GK, Marek GJ: Serotonin and hallucinogens. Neuropsychopharmacology 1999;21:16S–23S.
6. Alper KR, Lotsof HS, Frenken GM: Ibogaine in acute opioid withdrawal: An open label case series. Ann N Y Acad Sci 2000;909: 257–259.
7. American Psychiatric Association: Diagnostic and Statistical Manual of Mental Disorders, 4th ed. Washington, DC, American Psychiatric Association, 1994.
8. Antkiewicz-Michaluk L, Romanska I, Vetulani J: Ca^{2+} channel blockade prevents lysergic acid diethylamide-induced changes in dopamine and serotonin metabolism. Eur J Pharmacol 1997;332:9–14.
9. Arvanov VL, Liang X, Russo A, Wang RY: LSD and DOB: Interaction with 5-HT2A receptors to inhibit NMDA receptor-mediated transmission in the rat prefontal cortex. Eur J Neurosci 1999;11: 3064–3072.
10. Badham ER: Ethnobotany of psilocybin mushrooms, especially *Psilocybe cubensis*. J Ethnopharmacol 1984;10:249–254.
11. Backstrom JR, Chang MS, Niswender CM, et al: Agonist-directed signaling of serotonin 5-HT$_{2C}$ receptors: Difference between serotonin and lysergic acid diethylamide (LSD). Neuropsychopharmacology 1999;21:77S–81S.
12. Blaho K, Merigian K, Windberry S, et al: Clinical pharmacology of lysergic acid diethylamide: Case reports and review of the treatment of intoxication. Am J Ther 1997;4:211–221.

13. Bonson KR, Murphy DL: Alterations in responses to LSD in humans associated with chronic administration of tricyclic antidepressants, monoamine oxidase inhibitors or lithium. Neurosci Biobehav Rev 1996;73:229–233.

14. Bonson KR, Buckholtz JW, Murphy DL: Chronic administration of the serotonergic antidepressants attenuates the subjective effects of LSD in humans. Neuropsychopharmacology 1998;14:425–436.

15. Borowiak KS, Ciechanowski K, Waloszczyk P: Psilocybin mushroom intoxication with myocardial infarction. J Toxicol Clin Toxicol 1998; 36:47–49.

16. Brubacher JR, Lachmanen D, Ravikumar PR, Hoffman RS: Efficacy of digoxin-specific Fab fragments (Digibind) in the treatment of toad venom poisoning. Toxicon 1999;37:931–942.

17. Buchman J: Brainwashing, LSD, and CIA: Historical and ethical perspective. Int J Soc Psychiatry 1977;23:8–19.

18. Buckholtz NS, Zhou D, Freedman DX: Serotonin 2 agonist administration down-regulates rat brain serotonin 2 receptors. Life Sci 1988; 42:2439–2445.

19. Bullis RK: Swallowing the scroll: Legal implications of the recent Supreme Court peyote cases. J Psychoactive Drugs 1990;22:325–332.

20. Burris KD, Sanders-Bush E: Unsurmountable antagonism of brain 5-hydroxytryptamine-2 receptors by (+)-lysergic acid diethylamide and bromo-lysergic acid diethylamide. Mol Pharmacol 1992;42: 826–830.

21. Callaway CW, Clark RF: Hyperthermia in psychostimulant overdose. Ann Emerg Med 1994;24:68–76.

22. Calabrese JD: Spiritual healing and human development in the Native American Church: Toward a cultural psychiatry of peyote. Psychoanal Rev 1997;84:237–255.

23. Caporeal LR: Ergotism: The satan loosed in Salem? Science 1976; 192:21–26.

24. Cohen MM, Hirshhorn K, Frosch W: In vivo and in vitro chromosomal damage induced by LSD-25. N Engl J Med 1967;277:1043–1049.

25. Delgado PL, Moreno FA: Hallucinogens, serotonin and obsessive-compulsive disorder. J Psychoactive Drugs 1998;30:359–365.

26. Drug Enforcement Agency. Lysergic acid diethylamide (LSD). Department of Justice. [On-line] Available: www.usdoj.gov/dea/concern/lsd.htm (accessed 07/20/00).

27. Dupont RL, Verebey K: The role of the laboratory in the diagnosis of LSD and ecstasy psychosis. Psychiatr Ann 1994;24:142–144.

28. Erickson TB, Aks SE, Koenigsberg M, Bunney EB: Drug use patterns at major rock concerts events. Ann Emerg Med 1996;28:22–26.

29. Fink H, Morgenstern R, Oelssner W: Clozapine-A serotonin antagonist? Pharmacol Biochem Behav 1984;20:513–517.

30. Fody RP, Walker EM: Effects of drugs on the male and female reproductive systems. Ann Clin Lab Sci 1985;15:451–458.

31. Frankel FH: The concepts of flashbacks in historical perspective. Int J Clin Exp Hypn 1994;152:321–326.

32. Giacomelli S, Palmery M, Romanelli L, et al: Lysergic acid diethylamide (LSD) is partial agonist of D2 dopaminergic receptors and it potentiates dopamine-mediated prolactin secretion in lactrotrophs in vitro. Life Sci 1998;63:215–222.

33. Glennon RA: Do classical hallucinogens act as 5-HT$_2$ agonists or antagonists? Neuropsychopharmacology 1990;3:509–517.

34. Glennon RA, Titeler M, McKenney JD: Evidence for 5-HT$_2$ involvement in the mechanism of action of hallucinogenic agents. Life Sci 1984;35:2505–2511.

35. Glick SD, Maisonneuve IM: Mechanism of antiaddictive actions of ibogaine. Ann N Y Acad Sci 1998;844:214–226.

36. Glick SD, Maisonneuve IM: Development of novel medications for drug addiction: The legacy of an African shrub. Ann N Y Acad Sci 2000;909:88–103.

37. Gouzoulis-Mayfrank E, Hermle L, Thelen B, et al: History, rationale and potential of human experimental hallucinogenic drug research in psychiatry. Pharmacopsychiatry 1998;31:63S–68S.

38. Halpern JH, Pope HG: Do hallucinogens cause residual neuropsychological toxicity. Drug Alcohol Depend 1999;53:247–256.

39. Harrington MA, Zhong P, Garlow SJ, Ciarnello RD: Molecular biology of serotonin receptors. J Clin Psychiatry 1992;53(Suppl):8–27.

40. Hitt M, Ettinter DD: Toad toxicity. N Engl J Med 1986;314:517.

41. Hofmann A: History of the discovery of LSD. In: Pletscher A, Ladewig D, eds: 50 Years of LSD: Current Status and Perspective of Hallucinogens, New York, Parthenon, 1994, pp. 7–16.

42. House RV, Thomas PT, Bhargava HN: Comparison of the hallucinogenic indole alkaloids ibogaine and harmaline for potential immunomodulatory activity. Pharmacology 1995;51:56–65.

43. Jacobson CB, Berlin CM: Possible reproductive detriment in LSD users. JAMA 1972;222:1367–1373.

44. Johnston LD, O'Malley PM, Bachman: Drug trends in 1999 are mixed. University of Michigan and Information Services. Ann Arbor, MI. [On-line] Available: www.monitoringthefuture.org (accessed 02/15/00).

45. Klock JC, Boerner U, Becker CE: Coma, hyperthermia and bleeding associated with massive LSD overdose. West J Med 1973;120: 183–188.

46. Kulick AR, Ahmed I: Substance-induced organic mental disorders: A clinical and conceptual approach. Gen Hosp Psychiatry 1986;8: 168–172.

47. Kulig K: LSD. Emerg Med Clin North Am 1990;8:551–558.

48. Leikin JB, Krantz AJ, Zell-Kanter M, et al: Clinical features and management of intoxication due to hallucinogenic drugs. Med Toxicol Adverse Drug Exp 1989;4:324–350.

49. Li JH, Lin LF: Genetic toxicology of abused drugs: A brief review. Mutagenesis 1998;13:557–565.

50. Louria DB: Current concepts: Lysergic acid diethylamide. N Engl J Med 1968;278:435–438.

51. Lyttle T, Goldstein D, Gartz J: Bufo toads and bufotenine: Fact and fiction surrounding an alleged psychedelic. J Psychoactive Drugs 1996;28:267–290.

52. Lyttle T, Monagne M: Drugs, music and ideology: A social pharmacological interpretation of the acid house movement. Int J Addict 1992;27:1159–1177.

53. Madden JS: LSD and post-hallucinogen perceptual disorder. Addiction 1994;89:762–763.

54. Marek GJ, Aghajanian GK: Indoleamine and the phenethylamine hallucinogens: Mechanism of psychotomimetic action. Drug Alcohol Depend 1998;51:189–198.

55. Markek H, Lee A, Holmes RD, et al: Flashback syndrome exacerbated by selective serotonin reuptake inhibitor antidepressant in adolescents. J Pediatr 1994;125:817–819.

56. McClue SJ, Brazell C, Stahl SM: Hallucinogenic drugs are partial agonists of the human platelet shape change response: A physiological model of the 5-HT$_2$ receptors. Biol Psychiatry 1989;26:297–302.

57. McLeod WR, Sitaram BR: Bufotenine reconsidered. Acta Psychiatr Scand 1985;72:447–450.

58. Meert T, Clincke G: Evidence for a possible role of the 5-HT$_2$ antagonist ritanserin in drug abuse. Ann N Y Acad Sci 1992;654:483–486.

59. Meert TF, de Haes P, Janssen PAJ: Risperidone (R 64 766), a potent and complete LSD antagonist in drug discrimination by rats. Psychopharmacology 1989;97:206–212.

60. Miller PL, Gay GR, Ferris KC, Anderson S: Treatment of acute adverse psychedelic reactions: "I've tripped and I can't get down." J Psychoactive Drugs 1992;24:277–279.

61. Millman RB, Beeder AB: The new psychedelic culture: LSD, ectasy, "rave parties" and the Grateful Dead. Psychiatr Ann 1994;24: 145–147.

62. Neill JR: "More than medical significance": LSD and American Psychiatry 1953–1966. J Psychoactive Drugs 1979;19:39–45.

63. O'Malley PM, Johnston LD, Bachman JG: Adolescent substance use: Epidemiology and implications for public policy. Pediatr Clin North Am 1995;42:241–260.

64. Owens MJ, Knight DL, Ritchie JC, Nemeroff CB: The 5-hydroxytryptamine 2 agonist, (-1-(2,5-dimethoxy-4-bromophenyl)-2-aminopropane stimulates the hypothalamic-pituitary-adrenal (HPA) axis: II.

Biochemical and psychological evidence for the development of tolerance after chronic administration. J Pharmacol Exp Ther 1991;256: 795–800.

65. Riedlinger TJ: Wasson's alternative candidates for soma. J Psychoactive Drugs 1993;25:149–156.

66. Rivier L: Ethnopharmacology of LSD and related compounds. In: Pletscher A, Ladewig D, eds: 50 Years of LSD: Current Status and Perspective of Hallucinogens. New York, Parthenon 1994, pp. 43–55.

67. Roth BL, Willins DL, Kristiansen K, et al. 5-Hydroxytryptamine 2—Family receptors: Where structure meets function. Pharmacol Ther 1998;79:231–257.

68. Sadzot B, Baraban JM, Glennon RA, et al: Hallucinogenic drug interactions at human brain 5-HT$_2$ receptors: Implications for treating LSD-induced hallucinogenesis. Psychopharmacology 1989;98: 495–499.

69. Schechter M, Rosecrans J: Lysergic acid diethylamide (LSD) as a discriminative cue: Drugs with similar stimulus properties. Psychopharmacologia 1972;26:313–316.

70. Schneier FR, Siris SG: A review of psychoactive substance use and abuse in schizophrenia: Patterns of drug choice. J Nerv Ment Dis 1987;175:641–652.

71. Schultes RE: Hallucinogens of plant origin. Science 1969;163: 245–254.

72. Schultes RE, Hofmann A: Plants of the Gods. Rochester, VT: Healing Arts Press, 1992.

73. Schwartz RH: LSD. Its rise, fall and renewed popularity among high school students. Pediatr Clin North Am 1995;42:403–413.

74. Shannon M: Methylenedioxymethamphetamine (MDMA "Ecstacy"). Pediatr Emerg Care 2000;16:337–380.

75. Siegel DM, McDaniel SH: The frog prince: Tale and toxicology. Am J Orthopsychiatry 1991;61:558–562.

76. Smith DE, Seymour RB: LSD: History and toxicity. Psychiatr Ann 1994;24:145–147.

77. Stevens J: Storming Heaven. New York, Harper and Row, 1987.

78. Strassman RJ: Adverse reactions to psychedelic drugs: A review of the literature. J Nerv Ment Dis 1984;172:577–595.

79. Strassman RJ: Human hallucinogenic drug research: Regulatory, clinical, and scientific issues. NIDA Res Monogr 1994;146:92–123.

80. Strassman RJ: Hallucinogenic drugs in psychiatric research and treatment. J Nerv Ment Dis 1995;183:127–138.

81. Strassman RJ: Human psychopharmacology of N,N-dimethyltryptamine. Behav Brain Res 1996;73:121–124.

82. Titeler M, Lyon RA, Glennon RA: Radioligand binding evidence implicates the brain 5-HT$_2$ receptor as a site of action for LSD and phenylisopropylamine hallucinogens. Psychopharmacology 1988;94: 213–216.

83. Ulrich RF, Patten BM: The rise, decline and fall of LSD. Perspect Biol Med 1991;34:561–578.

84. Watts VJ, Lawler CP, Fox DR, et al: LSD and structural analogs: Pharmacological evaluation at D1 receptors. Psychopharmacology 1995;118:401–409.

85. Weil AT, Davis W: *Bufo alvarius*: A potent hallucinogen of animal origin. J Ethnopharmacol 1995;41:1–8.

86. Weller M, Wiedmann P: Visual hallucinations. Int Ophthalmol 1989; 13:193–199.

87. Wing LL, Tapson GS, Geyer MA: 5-HT$_2$ mediation of acute behavioral effects of hallucinogens in rats. Psychopharmacology 1990; 100:417–425.

88. Winter JC, Fiorella DJ, Timineri DM, et al: Serotonergic receptor subtypes and hallucinogen-induced stimulus control. Pharmacol Biochem Behav 1999;64:283–293.

CHAPTER 71   MARIJUANA

Edward J. Otten

Δ^9-tetrahydrocannabinol
(THC)

A 20-year-old male was brought to the Emergency Department (ED) by the police after they had stopped him for driving his automobile recklessly. The patient's car was weaving along the highway and had crossed the centerline several times. The police initially thought that the patient was intoxicated with alcohol, but breath analysis was negligible for ethanol. Because they felt that he might have some medical problem, he was taken to the emergency department.

Upon arrival the patient was drowsy but easily arousable to verbal stimuli. He stated that he had been to a party earlier that evening and thought that someone may have put something in his nonalcoholic drink. He insisted that he had not been drinking alcohol and did not use drugs in any form. He complained of a slight headache and inability to focus, but had no other complaints. His past medical history was negative. He had no known allergies and took no medications regularly.

The patient's vital signs were: blood pressure, 138/84 mm Hg; pulse, 112 beats/min; respiratory rate, 18 breaths/min; and temperature, 99.0°F (37.2°C). He was drowsy but arousable, oriented to person, place, time, and situation. Pupils were 5 mm, equal and reacted to light; conjunctivae were injected, and extraocular movements were normal without nystagmus. Lungs were clear to auscultation, and heart examination revealed a rapid, regular rhythm without murmur or rub. Neurologic examination was normal except for difficulty maintaining a normal erect posture. The patient's gait was normal as was his "finger-to-nose" examination. The patient remained difficult to arouse.

Oxygen saturation was 95% on room air and a fingerstick blood glucose was 120 mg/dL. A urine screen was positive for tetrahydrocannabinol. Upon further questioning the patient admitted to smoking several "joints" of marijuana prior to attempting to drive home. After 6 hours in the ED the patient was completely arousable and neurologic examination was completely normal. The patient was referred to outpatient drug counseling and discharged in the custody of his brother.

Marijuana is a common name for material obtained from the leaves and flowers of the Indian hemp plant, *Cannabis sativa*. Marijuana is one of many names for cannabis, which contains the psychoactive substance Δ^9-tetrahydrocannabinol (THC). THC is found in both the male and female plants. *Cannabis* has been cultivated for thousands of years for numerous purposes including medical, religious, and "recreational" use as well as for fiber. *Cannabis sativa* is the only species belonging to the genus *Cannabis*. Cultivated varieties of *Cannabis sativa* are used in the manufacture of fiber for rope and clothing, which have erroneously been thought to be separate species.

Cannabis sativa contains a number of active compounds known collectively as cannabinoids, including cannabidiol, cannabinol, cannabidiolic acid, cannibicyclol, and cannabigrol. In all, approximately 60 cannabinoids and 200 other chemical compounds have been identified in *Cannabis* plant material. Most of these constituents are found in small concentrations and have little or no psychoactive effects when compared to THC. These constituents do have chemical activity and may contribute to the acute and chronic medical problems resulting from marijuana use. Thus, THC is the primary constituent of marijuana, but not the only one; and THC is not pharmacologically equivalent to marijuana.

The percentage of the THC found in plants depends on ecotypic variables, including amount of light, moisture, soil type, trace elements, pH, and nutrients. Common misconceptions associated with potency of various types of marijuana that are based on origin, sex of the plant, and color are probably related to the phenotypic plasticity of the plants. The amount of active THC found in a sample deteriorates with time. Hashish and hashish oil are derivatives of the *Cannabis* plant that contain higher concentrations of THC; they are smoked either alone in pipes (hashish) or mixed with tobacco and smoked (hashish oil). Marijuana may also be ingested in food and is commonly used in conjunction with other drugs such as opium, alcohols, cocaine, heroin, phencyclidine, ketamine, and formaldehyde.[4,21,27]

EPIDEMIOLOGY

Nicotine, alcohol, caffeine, and marijuana are the most commonly used psychoactive substance in the world. In the United States, marijuana is the most frequently utilized illegal substance involving an estimated 20 million people.[45] Marijuana is thought by many to be a "gateway" drug, leading to use of other more dangerous substances such as heroin, cocaine, or amphetamines. Marijuana was shown to be a gateway drug in a study of 1265 New Zealand children over a 21-year period. In that study, those children using marijuana more than 50 times a year abused other drugs 140 times more often than did nonmarijuana users.[15] The United States Drug Enforcement Agency (DEA) has classified marijuana as a Schedule I substance.

Both the latest Centers for Disease Control and Prevention (CDC) statistics and National Institute on Drug Abuse (NIDA) data suggest a rise in the use of marijuana in the general population, particularly among teenagers. The NIDA survey on drug use showed an increase in the prevalence of reported marijuana usage in all groups of teenagers in 1994. Eighth grader use increased by 13%, 10th grader use increased by 25%, and 12th grader use increased by 31% as compared with 1993 estimates. From a historical peak of reported marijuana use in 1978, use decreased from 1979 to 1991. This trend was reversed in 1992, and the prevalence rate has increased annually since then. The Substance Abuse and Mental Health Services Administration (SAMHSA) National Household Survey on Drug Abuse, SAMHSA's Drug Abuse Warning Network (DAWN), and the National Institute of Justice Drug Use Forecasting (DUF) system data all suggest increases in marijuana use in 1998. National drug-related ED visits for marijuana increased 43%, from 152,433 in 1996 to 172,014 in 1998. The Youth Risk behavior Surveillance–National Alternative High School Youth Risk Behavior Survey, United States 1998 reported that 85% of students used marijuana once during their lifetime. Male students (88%) were more likely than female students (82%) to use marijuana and white students (89%) were more likely than African American students (77%) to use marijuana.[19] The Monitoring the Future Study for 1999 shows a trend of increasing marijuana use among high school students over a 20-year period. Not surprisingly, the higher the baseline use of marijuana in adolescents, the higher the probability of continued use.[18,24,25,28,41,45]

The number of motor vehicle or work-related injuries that are caused by marijuana use is unknown. Studies have implicated marijuana in motor vehicle fatalities, especially in the 15–30-year-old age group. After alcohol, marijuana was the most common drug found, being detected in 11–33% of the motor vehicle fatalities.[7,33,49] The federal government requires drug testing of the crew of any commercial carrier (planes, trains, buses) involved in major crashes.

PHARMACOLOGY AND PATHOPHYSIOLOGY

The onset of marijuana effects depend on the route of administration and the concentration of THC in the product used. Smoking marijuana usually leads to nearly immediate effects, whereas oral ingestion has a slow and unpredictable effect because of the instability of THC in the acidic environment of the stomach.[38] The smoking dynamics or manner in which the marijuana is smoked is the most important factor in determining the absorption of THC.[5,10] Depending on the initial concentration of THC, pyrolysis of THC, loss in sidestream smoke, and mucosal concentration, on average about half of the THC in the marijuana is delivered to the lungs. It takes about 15 seconds for the lungs to absorb the THC and to transport it to the brain.[40] A family of specific cannabinoid

receptors in the cerebral cortex may be responsible for the pharmacologic effects of marijuana.

The endocannabinoids, or naturally occurring ligands, 2-arachidonolyl-glycerol (Ara-G1) and anandamide, bind these same cannabinoid receptors.[3,8] These ligands produce effects similar to plant-derived THC with significant pharmacologic differences. Ara-G1 produces vasodilation and hypotension. Anandamide is 10-fold less potent and has a shorter duration of action.[36] Although the mechanisms for the synthesis and metabolism of anandamide are known, the physiologic role and the reason for the differences are unknown.[22,34,39] The CB1 receptors, found in the pain-processing areas of the brain and spinal cord, and the CB2 receptors located in the peripheral nerves, suggest a potential analgesic effect of THC. For these reasons it is suggested that the endogenous ligands may be important in pain modulation.

After smoking, the effects of marijuana peak in 10–30 minutes and may last for 1–4 hours, depending on the dose actually inhaled.[9] THC is lipophilic and therefore accumulated in lipid tissue; it is highly protein bound (97–99%), has a an apparent V_d of 10 L/kg, and it is enterohepatically recirculated. All of these characteristics result in slow elimination from the body. THC is oxidatively metabolized to the active compound 11-hydroxy-Δ^9-tetrahydrocannabinol, which is further oxidized to the inactive 11-nor-9-carboxy-Δ^9-THC.[10]

THC also has a dose-dependent effect in diminishing the cytolytic activity of large granular lymphocytes against K562 tumor cells, while decreasing the synthesis of tumor necrosis factor by macrophages. Both B- and T-cell activity are depressed by THC; however, cell-mediated immunity is more readily affected. Both CB1 and CB2 receptors have been identified in immune cells and modulate the effect of THC on the immune response. The CB2 receptor mediates the activation of mitogen-activated protein kinase, which may be the mechanism for the immunosuppressive effect.[30,39,46,54]

CLINICAL EFFECTS

Acute

The clinical effects of marijuana may be both physiologic and psychological, based partly on previous experience of the user.[9] The usual psychological effects are fairly predictable and include alterations in sensation, perception, cognition, and psychomotor functions.[29] Although users report enhanced perception and sensation, this enhancement is not observed experimentally. A sense of euphoria, relaxation, and various sensory alterations are generally the effects that are sought with marijuana use.[9] The true danger of acute marijuana toxicity results from the loss of motor skills and judgment. Airline pilots using a flight simulator were impaired for as long as 24 hours after a single dose of marijuana; the impairment was compounded by the pilot's age and the difficulty of the required flying tasks.[32] Perhaps as expected, the National Highway Traffic Safety Administration (NHTSA) study showed that a combination of marijuana and alcohol, even at low levels, impaired drivers more than either higher levels of marijuana or alcohol alone.[37] Marijuana affects performance of neuropsychiatric tests, especially digit recall and mathematical skills, and this appears to correlate with serum THC levels.[13,42]

An acute psychosis is associated with marijuana use; it is not clear whether preexisting psychopathology is responsible or whether this behavioral alteration is related to the dose of THC or the inexperience of the user. Studies of patients without prior psychopathology who developed acute psychotic reactions following marijuana use have shown that the reactions are usually transient.[35]

Although the psychological effects of marijuana may or may not be dose dependent, the physiologic effects are. Increase in heart rate is common, but blood pressure response is variable. Endocannabinoids cause vasodilation and hypotension in both humans and laboratory animals via the CB1 receptor. This effect may occur through inhibition of transmitter release or direct effects on smooth muscle cells.[22] Acutely, muscle tremors, and weakness, as well as bronchodilation occur. Conjunctival injection, increased appetite, decreased intraocular pressure, decreased testosterone levels, and urinary retention are all common sequelae of acute marijuana usage.[5,23,38] Pneumomediastinum and pneumothorax may occur following the alveolar overdistension and rupture from deep inhalation during marijuana smoking.[6] Dyspnea and chest pain may result, but are rarely life-threatening.

Chronic

Cannabinoids increase the activity of dopaminergic neurons in the mesolimbic pathway, which reinforces the abuse potential. Tolerance is associated with repeated use of marijuana. Similar to many other psychoactive drugs, tolerance can lead to both physiologic and psychological dependence, and a withdrawal syndrome. The withdrawal syndrome resulting from marijuana use can be reproduced experimentally and includes sleep disturbances, irritability, decreased appetite, nausea, and restlessness, all of which can be reversed by small doses of THC. Persistent consequential marijuana use produces residual neuropsychological effects that do not occur in light infrequent users.[1,20,42]

Smoking marijuana is implicated in chronic lung disease and carcinogenesis unrelated to tobacco smoking.[51] Marijuana smoking causes a 5-fold increase in blood carboxyhemoglobin level and a 3-fold increase in the amount of tar inhaled when compared with tobacco smoking.[53] Some studies indicate that because of the smoking dynamics associated with marijuana (ie, deep inhalations), a 4-fold greater respiratory burden of particulates occur compared to tobacco smoking, making marijuana inhalation potentially more dangerous to the lung than tobacco.[40] Marijuana seems to have a greater impact on central airway function, while the predominant effect of tobacco is on peripheral airways. Significantly worse values for specific airway conductance and airway resistance were found with marijuana smoking when compared with nonsmokers or tobacco smokers.[51] Bronchoalveolar lavage fluid from the lungs of marijuana smokers demonstrates an increase in macrophages and other inflammatory cells that is independent of, and additive to, that of tobacco.[44,51,53] Base fractions of marijuana are more mutagenic than tobacco, and high-dose base fractions were 7-fold more mutagenic than either tobacco or low-dose marijuana base fractions.[50]

Studies in pregnant female marijuana smokers demonstrate that there are a number of neonatal neurobehavioral disturbances that correlate with marijuana use during pregnancy; the effects seem to disappear during infancy and reappear later in early childhood.[2,12,16,43] Prenatal marijuana use by the mother significantly correlated with subsequent increased hyperactivity, impulsivity, increased delinquency, and inattention symptoms in the child.[17] Another study of subjects who started using marijuana before age 17 had smaller whole-brain and gray matter volumes and smaller stature.[52] THC interferes with testicular function by a number of mechanisms causing a decrease in sperm motility and numbers as well as an increase in abnormal morphology.[24]

MEDICAL USES

Marijuana may be used to treat symptoms, but not specific diseases. The Institute of Medicine evaluated a number of clinical studies of marijauna use.[26] As an antiemetic, although marijuana is useful in treating the nausea and vomiting associated with cancer chemotherapy, neither THC nor its analogues, nabilone and levonantradol, are as effective as standard antiemetics. Marijuana is useful in stimulating the appetite of HIV/AIDS patients and others, but was less effective than megestrol acetate. Some authors recommend the use of THC in the treatment of glaucoma, muscle spasticity, movement disorders, multiple sclerosis, and asthma, but there are no scientific studies supporting these recommendations. The dose of THC in marijuana that is smoked cannot be controlled, making scientific studies difficult to interpret as to efficacy and therapeutic drug levels. Currently, one prescription product, dronabinol (Marinol), contains synthetic THC. This drug has a standardized concentration of THC and therefore the amount that the patient receives can be controlled. Dronabinol is a Schedule II drug and can be prescribed for nausea and vomiting or anorexia. Animal studies show some promise for the use of THC as an analgesic, and clinical studies based on these findings are ongoing.[26]

In November 1996, California and Arizona passed propositions legalizing marijuana for medical purposes. The US Senate Judiciary Committee and the DEA have not supported these laws, and in 1997, the Arizona Senate passed a law nullifying a physician's right to prescribe Schedule I substances without federal approval. The DEA continues to prosecute in California, marijuana traffickers, and those arrested for criminal activities in the possession of marijuana under federal law.[4,31,47]

LABORATORY

All of the 20 metabolites of THC may cross-react with THC in the standard immunoassay used for the screening urine for marijuana. The screening test is designed to detect THC at either levels of 20, 50, or 100 ng/mL, depending on the purpose for which the test is performed. The gas chromatography-mass spectrometry (GC-MS) confirmation test for nor-9-carboxy-Δ^9-THC uses a cutoff level of 15 ng/mL.[23,48] The pattern of excretion is similar for most users of marijuana. The individual differences result from variable lengths of each phase of excretion, which depend on the individual pattern of usage. These variations result in screening and confirmation test results that may be positive for up to 70 or more days, depending on the cutoff levels used and the individual's lipid stores of THC. In general, THC can be detected for 1–3 days after a single acute use, and for 10 days to 4 weeks after daily use.[14] Passive exposure to marijuana smoke, depending on room air concentration, may give positive screening results for several days, even after a single exposure.[11] Rarely, false-positive results may occur after therapeutic use of naproxen, ibuprofen, and fenoprofen. False-negative results may occur from urine dilution, diuretic use, and the addition of table salt, or other contaminants to the urine. Concomitant testing of urine specific gravity, pH, temperature, and creatinine have eliminated most of these confounding variables.[23,48]

MANAGEMENT

The acute psychotic reaction involving paranoid delusions and hallucinations that may occur with marijuana usage can be managed effectively with benzodiazepines.[35] Patients presenting with dyspnea, chest pain, decreased breath sounds and or a low oxygen saturation may have a pneumothorax or pneumomediastinum and should be evaluated and managed accordingly. Patients with marijuana ingestions and overdoses of dronabinol should be treated with activated charcoal. Coingestants, such as PCP or cocaine, should be managed as indicated. There are no known cases of lethal marijuana intoxication.

SUMMARY

Patients with psychological manifestations can usually be treated supportively. Marijuana is a commonly used agent, often used with other toxins, but rarely associated with consequential overdoses. The role that marijuana plays in an individual's subsequent drug use remains highly debated, as does its role as a medicinal agent. Recent studies of marijuana's role in motor vehicle crashes and occupational injuries have initiated an increased focus on these substantial toxicologic complications.

REFERENCES

1. Ameri A: The effects of cannabinoids on the brain. Prog Neurobiol 1999;58:315–348.
2. Astley SJ, Little RE: Maternal marijuana use during lactation and infant development at one year. Neurotoxicol Teratol 1990;12:161–168.
3. Axelrod J, Felder CC: Cannabinoid receptors and their endogenous agonist anandamide. Neurochem Res 1998;23:575–581.
4. Beal JE, Olson R, Laubenstein L, et al: Dronabinol as a treatment for anorexia associated with weight loss in patients with AIDS. J Pain Symptom Manage 1995;10:89–97.
5. Benowitz NL, Jones RT: Cardiovascular and metabolic considerations in prolonged cannabinoid administration in man. J Clin Pharmacol 1981;21:214–223.
6. Brody SL, Anderson GV, Gutman JB: Pneumomediastinum as a complication of "crack" smoking. Am J Emerg Med 1988;6:241–243.
7. Brookoff D, Cook CS, Williams C, Mann CS: Testing reckless drivers for cocaine and marijuana. N Engl J Med 1994;331:518–522.
8. Calignano A, La Rana G, Giuffrida A, Piomelli D: Control of pain initiation by endogenous cannabinoids. Nature 1998;394:277–281.
9. Chait LD, Burke KA: Preference for high- versus low-potency marijuana. Pharmacol Biochem Behav 1994;49:643–647.
10. Chiang CN, Barnett G: Marijuana pharmacokinetics and pharmacodynamics. In: Redda KK, Walker CA, Barnett G, eds: Cocaine, Marijuana, Designer Drugs: Chemistry, Pharmacology, and Behavior. Boca Raton, FL, CRC Press, 1989, pp. 113–126.
11. Cone EJ, Johnson RE, Darwin WD, et al: Passive inhalation of marijuana smoke: Urinalysis and room air levels of delta-9-tetrahydrocannabinol. J Anal Toxicol 1987;11:89–96.
12. Day NL, Richardson GA, Goldschmidt L, et al: Effect of prenatal marijuana exposure on the cognitive development of offspring at age three. Neurotoxicol Teratol 1994;16:169–175.
13. Deadwyler SA, Heyse CJ, Michaelis RC, Hampson RE: The effects of delta-9-THC on mechanisms of learning and memory. In: Erinoff L,

ed: Neurobiology of Drug Abuse: Learning and Memory. NIDA research monograph 97. Washington, DC, USDHHS, 1990, pp. 79–93.
14. Ellis GM, Mann MA, Judson BA, et al: Excretion patterns of cannabinoid metabolites after last use in a group of chronic users. Clin Pharmacol Ther 1985;38:572–578.
15. Ferguson DM, Horwood LJ: Does cannabis use encourage other forms of illicit drug use? Addiction 2000;95:505–520.
16. Fried PA: Behavioral outcome in preschool and school-age children exposed prenatally to marijuana: A review and speculative interpretation. In: Wetherington CL, Smeriglio VL, Finnegan LP, eds: Behavioral Studies of Drug-Exposed Offspring: Methodological Issues in Human and Animal Research. NIDA research monograph 164. Washington, DC, USDHHS, 1996, pp. 242–260.
17. Goldschmidt L, Day NL, Richardson GA: Effects of prenatal marijuana exposure on child behavior problems at age 10. Neurotoxicol Teratol 2000;22:325–336.
18. Golub A, Johnson BD: The shifting importance of alcohol and marijuana as gateway substances among serious drug abusers. J Stud Alcohol 1994;55:607–614.
19. Grunbaum JA, Kann L, Kinchen SA, et al: Youth risk behavior Surveillance-National Alternative High School Youth Risk Behavior Survey, United States 1998. MMWR Morb Mortal Wkly Rep 1999; 48(SS-7):18–19.
20. Haney M, Ward AS, Comer SD, et al: Abstinence symptoms following smoked marijuana in humans. Psychopharmacology 1999;141: 395–404.
21. Hawks, RL: The constituents of Cannabis and the disposition and metabolism of cannabinoids. In: Hawks RL: The Analysis of Cannabinoids in Biological Fluids, NIDA research monograph 42. Washington, DC, USDHHS, 1982, pp. 125–317.
22. Hillard CJ: Endocannabinoids and vascular function. J Pharmacol Exp Ther 2000;294:27–32.
23. Huestis M: Pharmacology and toxicology of marijuana. Ther Drug Monit 1993;14:131–138.
24. Husain S: Marijuana abuse: Its pharmacology and effects on testicular function. In: Redda KK, Walker CA, Barnett G, eds: Cocaine, Marijuana, Designer Drugs: Chemistry, Pharmacology and Behavior. Boca Raton, FL, CRC Press, 1989, pp. 127–143.
25. Johnston LD, O'Malley PM, Bachman JG: National Survey Results on Drug Use from Monitoring the Future Study, 1975–1994. Washington, DC, USDHHS, 1996.
26. Joy JE, Watson SJ, Benson JA: The medical value of marijuana and related substances in marijuana and medicine: Assessing the science base. Washington DC, National Academy Press, 1999, pp. 137–192.
27. Joyce CRB, Curry SH: The Botany and Chemistry of Cannabis. London, J&A Churchill, 1970, pp. 1–60.
28. Kann L, Warren CW, Harris WA, et al: Youth risk behavior surveillance—United States, 1995. MMWR Morb Mortal Wkly Rep 1996; 45(SS4):1–83.
29. Kurzthaler I, Hummer M, Miller C, et al: Effects of cannabis on cognitive functions and driving ability. J Clin Psychiatry 1999;60: 395–399.
30. Kusher DI, Dawson LO, Taylor AC, Djeu, JY: Effect of the psychoactive metabolite of marijuana, delta-9-tetrahydrocannabinol (THC), on the synthesis of tumor necrosis factor by human large granular lymphocytes. Cell Immunol 1994;154:99–108.
31. Lane M, Vogel CL, Ferguson J, et al: Dronabinol and prochlorperazine in combination for the treatment of cancer chemotherapy-induced nausea and vomiting. J Pain Symptom Manage 1991;6: 352–359.
32. Leirer VO, Yesavage JA, Morrow DG: Marijuana, aging and task difficulty effects on pilot performance. Aviat Space Environ Med 1989;60:1145–1152.
33. Logan BK, Schwilke EW: Drug and alcohol use in fatally injured drivers in Washington State. J Forensic Sci 1996; 41:505–510.
34. Martin BR, Mechoulam R, Razdan RK: Discovery and characterization of endogenous cannabinoids. Life Sci 1999;65:573–595.

35. Mathers DC, Ghodse AH: Cannabis and psychotic illness. Br J Psychiatry 1992;161:648–653.

36. Matsuda LA, Lolait SJ, Brownstein MJ, Bonner TI: The THC receptor and its implications. In: Korenman SG, Barchas JD, eds: Biological Basis of Substance Abuse. Oxford, Oxford University Press, 1993, pp. 95–106.

37. National Highway Traffic Safety Administration: Marijuana and alcohol combined severely impede driving performance. Ann Emerg Med 2000;35:398–399.

38. Ohlsson A, Lingren JE, Wahlen A, et al: Plasma delta-9-tetrahydrocannabinol concentrations and clinical effects after oral and intravenous administration and smoking. Clin Pharmacol Ther 1980;28:409–416.

39. Parolaro D: Presence and functional regulation of cannabinoids receptors in immune cells. Life Sci 1999;65:637–644.

40. Perez-Reyes M: Marijuana smoking: Factors that influence the bioavailability of tetrahydrocannabinol. In: Chiang CN, Hawks RL, eds: Research Findings on Smoking of Abused Substances. NIDA research monograph 99. Washington, DC, USDHHS, 1990, pp. 42–62.

41. Perkonigg A, Lieb R, Hofler M, et al: Patterns of cannabis use, abuse and dependence over time: Incidence, progression and stability in a sample of 1228 adolescents. Addiction 1999;94:1663–1678.

42. Pope HG, Yurgelun-Todd D: The residual cognitive effects of heavy marijuana use in college students. JAMA 1996;275:521–527.

43. Richardson GA, Day NL, McGauhey PJ: The impact of prenatal marijuana and cocaine use on the infant and child. Clin Obstet Gynecol 1993;36:302–318.

44. Roth MD, Arora A, Barsky SH, et al: Airway inflammation in young marijuana and tobacco smokers. Am J Resp Crit Care Med 1998;157:928–937.

45. Rouse BA: Epidemiology of illicit and abused drugs in the general population, emergency department drug-related episodes, and arrestees. Clin Chem 1996;42:1330–1336.

46. Sarafian RA, Magallanes JA, ShauH, et al: Oxidative stress produced by marijuana smoke. An adverse effect produced by cannabinoids. Am J Respir Cell Mol Biol 1999;20:1286–1293.

47. Schwartz RH, Beveridge RA: Marijuana as an antiemetic drug: How useful is it today? Opinions from clinical oncologists. J Addict Dis 1994;13:53–65.

48. Schwartz RH, Hawks RL: Laboratory detection of marijuana use. JAMA 1985;254:788–792.

49. Soderstrom EA, Trifillis AL, Shankar BS, et al: Marijuana and alcohol use among 1023 trauma patients. Arch Surg 1988;123:733–737.

50. Sparacino CM, Hyldburg PA, Hughes TJ: Chemical and biological analysis of marijuana smoke condensate. In: Chiang CN, Hawks RL, eds: Research Findings on Smoking of Abused Substances. NIDA research monograph 99. Washington, DC, USDHHS, 1990, pp. 121–140.

51. Tashkin DP, Coulson AH, Clark VA, et al: Respiratory symptoms and lung function in habitual heavy smokers of marijuana alone, smokers of marijuana and tobacco, smokers of tobacco alone and nonsmokers. Am Rev Resp Dis 1987;135:209–216.

52 Wilson W, Mathew R, Turkington T, et al: Brain morphological changes and early marijuana use: A magnetic resonance and positron emission tomography study. J Addict Dis 2000;19:1–22.

53. Wu TC, Tashkin DP, Djahed B, Rose JE: Pulmonary hazards of smoking marijuana as compared with tobacco. N Engl J Med 1988;318:347–351.

54. Zheng ZM, Specter S, Friedman H: Inhibition by delta-9-tetrahydrocannabinol of tumor necrosis factor alpha production by mouse and human macrophages. Int J Immunopharmacol 1992;14:1145–1152.

CHAPTER 72 SUBSTANCE WITHDRAWAL

Richard J. Hamilton

Case 1. A 46-year-old male arrived in the Emergency Department (ED). He had been in police custody for 18 hours and requested evaluation by a physician because he had a seizure disorder and needed his daily dose of phenytoin. He stated that he was a frequent drinker but denied drug use. His seizures began 10 years ago, and he had been taking phenytoin ever since. He had been noncompliant with his phenytoin, possibly for 2 months. He denied any physical complaints and wanted to be seen and discharged.

His vital signs were: blood pressure, 130/80 mm Hg; respiratory rate, 12 breaths/min; pulse, 105 beats/min without orthostatic changes; and rectal temperature, 99.9°F (37.2°C). The man was well developed, poorly nourished, and appeared older than his stated age. He was garrulous and somewhat anxious. He was alert and oriented to time, place, and person. The pertinent positives on physical examination included a fine hand and tongue tremor, scattered spider hemangiomata, and hepatomegaly of 14 cm. The history and initial physical examination appeared consistent with the diagnosis of alcoholism and suspected alcohol withdrawal. Blood was drawn for a complete blood count, serum chemistries, liver function tests, and serum alcohol and phenytoin levels. The patient was to be observed while serum laboratory test results returned. A rapid reagent blood sugar was 70 mg/dL. One liter 0.9% sodium chloride was administered at 500 mL/h with multivitamins and 100 mg of thiamine. In addition, 25 mL of 50% dextrose solution was administered over 2 minutes.

One hour later, the patient began to shout at nursing staff that he was being held against his will and that he must leave. Repeat vital signs were blood pressure, 130/80 mm Hg; respiratory rate, 12 breaths/min; pulse, 130 beats/min; room air pulse oximetry, 98% saturation; and rectal temperature, 100.3°F (37.9°C). The patient was diaphoretic. The pupils were 5 mm, equal and briskly reactive. The tremor was now coarse. The patient demanded to be released and could not remember why he asked to be evaluated or who brought him to the hospital.

The patient's clinical condition was unchanged after 20 mg of diazepam was given as two 10-mg IV boluses 15 minutes apart. A portable chest radiograph was within normal limits. The electrocardiogram demonstrated a sinus tachycardia. A room air arterial blood gas analysis was reported as pH, 7.41; Pco_2, 37.4 mm Hg; Po_2, 73 mm Hg; Hco_3^-, 24 mEq; oxygen saturation, 95%. Diazepam was repeated as 10-mg IV boluses to a total of 100 mg, and the patient was placed in 4-point soft restraints after he began to remove his intravenous line and climb off the stretcher. His diaphoresis and tachycardia continued. He picked at the restraints, scratched his skin, and shouted nonsensical words occasionally.

Diazepam administered to a total dose of 220 mg did not improve the patient's agitation; the pulse was 110 beats/min; respiratory rate, 12 breaths/min; and temperature, 101.0°F (38.3°C). Toxicology consultation recommended phenobarbital intravenously. This was administered as 130-mg boluses over 3 minutes and repeated 4 times (520 mg total); the patient was sleeping, and the heart rate was 100 beats/min. The patient was electively intubated using thiopental and placed on a mechanical ventilator for airway protection. The patient remained sedate and required an additional 40 mg of diazepam over the next 24 hours. He developed a right lower lobe infiltrate on day 2 of his hospitalization and was treated with ampicillin/sulbactam. He recovered uneventfully and was extubated 48 hours later.

The central nervous system must balance excitation and inhibition to control physiologic function. The most intuitive way to balance this might be to increase excitatory nerve impulses for a physiologic action, and to increase inhibitory impulses whenever a physiologic action must be stopped. The central nervous system (CNS) uses a more efficient method: Excitatory neurons fire regularly, and inhibitory neurons inhibit the transmission of these impulses. Whenever action is required, the inhibitory neurons decrease their firing and permit the excitatory nerve impulses to travel to their end organs. Thus, all action in human neurophysiology is disinhibition.[101,185,204]

When administered chronically, many drugs and toxins affect the transmission of all classes of inhibitory neurons. Some act to increase the inhibitory effect with subsequent adaptive modulation (such as benzodiazepines and the $GABA_A$ receptor, opioids on the opioid receptor, or clonidine on the central α_2 receptor). Others act to block the inhibitory effect with subsequent adaptive modulation (caffeine on the adenosine receptor). Still others appear to increase the inhibitory effect with subsequent adaptive modulation of both inhibitory and excitatory neurons (ethanol and the $GABA_A$ and NMDA receptors respectively).[70,172] A withdrawal syndrome occurs when the drug or toxin is removed or reduced and the adaptive changes persist, producing dysfunction instead.

Thus, every withdrawal syndrome has two characteristics: (a) a preexisting physiologic adaptation to a drug or toxin, the continuous presence of which prevents withdrawal; and (b) decreasing concentrations of that substance. In contrast, simple tolerance to a drug is characterized as a physiologic adaptation that shifts the dose-response curve to the right. Patients with withdrawal syndromes have often developed tolerance, but tolerance does not require the continued presence of the drug to prevent withdrawal.

Finally, drugs and toxins that stimulate the excitatory neuronal pathways, such as cocaine, can produce a postintoxication syndrome that often results in lethargy, hypersomnolence, movement disorders, and irritability. Despite this syndrome meeting DSM-IV (Diagnostic and Statistical Manual of Mental Disorders 4th Edition) criteria for a withdrawal syndrome, it does not meet a toxicologic definition because the continuous use of this drug does not prevent withdrawal. This postintoxication syndrome, so called "crack crash" or "washed-out syndrome," is caused by prolonged use of the drug, and patients return to their premorbid function without intervention.[151,173,186,202] Withdrawal syndromes are best described and treated based on the class of receptors that are mostly affected. This concept organizes the approach to patient care as well.

HISTORY

Physicians have been faced with difficulties in treating ethanol withdrawal since Pliny the Elder in the 1st century BC. In his work *Naturalis Historia*, the alcoholic and alcohol withdrawal are described, ". . . drunkenness brings pallor and sagging cheeks, sore eyes, and trembling hands that spill a full cup, of which the immediate punishment is a haunted sleep and unrestful nights. . .".[147] An understanding of the relationship between alcohol and deterioration in health was obvious in that day. The appropriate treatment of ethanol withdrawal evolved over the course of the last century.

The era of modern medicine begins with Osler, and so it is fitting that we start with his remedies. His recommended treatment included confinement to bed, no restraints, withdrawal of alcohol, and judicious use of potassium bromide, chloral hydrate, hyoscine, and, possibly, opium.[140] He suggested that cold douches or baths be used to reduce fever and thereby produce sedation. He also emphasized the importance of feeding milk or broth. By using these methods, mortality was 14% according to several studies at the time.

In 1927, Cecil wrote that there were "no specific treatments," but that it was essential to produce sleep, stimulate the neurologic and circulatory systems, and feed the patient.[34] Paraldehyde, chloral hydrate, and hyoscyamine were considered acceptable hypnotics, but barbiturates were not recommended and morphine use was avoided. Strychnine and ergot were recommended for the treatment of tremor. Sheet restraints were suggested as humane replacements for "old-fashioned" canvas jackets. Sodium bicarbonate and cathartics were given hourly to patients with gastritis. Despite Cecil's innovations, mortality for uncomplicated cases approached that found in studies following Osler's recommendations. When severe alcohol withdrawal was associated with infections such as pneumonia, mortality was even higher; if associated with trauma, mortality reached 50%.

In 1929, the link between agitation, alcohol withdrawal, and hyperthermia was recognized.[23] Physical manifestations and complications of agitation were noted to be common to all markedly disturbed patients, regardless of the type of mental illness (alcohol or organic delirium, manic-depressive psychosis, schizophrenia, or dementia paralytica). Because of the severity of the agitation, febrile patients often received inadequate fluid replacement, resulting in dehydration. Further studies supported the benefits of

administration of carbohydrates, sodium chloride, and fluids were essential for a good outcome. By the mid-1930s at Boston City Hospital the fatality rate for all cases declined; an improvement largely attributed to improved nursing care.[130]

In the early 1950s, Victor and Adams, Mendelson and LaDou, and Isbell and coworkers correctly identified the etiology of delirium tremens (DTs) as alcohol withdrawal in a chronically (usually at least 2–3 weeks) dependent individual.[88,129,211] They determined that delirium tremens was not caused by alcohol intoxication, electrolyte or fluid disturbances, shock, infection, or trauma, as previously postulated, but only by withdrawal. All of these investigators noted the similarity of alcoholic DTs and barbiturate and paraldehyde withdrawal.

> Delirium tremens in its full-blown form is the most dramatic and gravest of all the alcoholic complications. It develops in a variety of settings. The patient, an excessive and steady drinker . . . may have been admitted for an unrelated illness, accident, operation, or infection . . . He may have suffered through several days of tremulousness, hallucinosis or seizures.
>
> The patient is restless and agitated, requiring restraints, . . . constantly pulling at his bed clothes, . . . swept over by a wave of apprehension and tremulousness, . . . conversation being garbled and unintelligible. Autonomic overactivity is manifested by dilated pupils, tachycardia, and an elevated temperature, attributable occasionally to no cause other than delirium. Drenching sweats may result in severe dehydration.[211]

The keen observations and classifications of the symptoms associated with withdrawal make worthwhile reading and can still contribute to the clinician's understanding of the natural history of this disorder. Much of the terminology used in these reports continues to this day and, unfortunately, adds to a confusing assortment of terms. The term "rum fit" appears to have originated as a description of the convulsions and/or behavior of sailors who were denied their daily rum rations. The term is used to describe a typical alcohol withdrawal seizure—brief, generalized, and occasionally recurrent. "Delirium tremens" was originally described as the "distinct clinical condition characterized by psychomotor, speech, and autonomic overactivity, disorientation, confusion, disordered sense perception, and frequently fatal outcome."[211]

In the late 1950s and early 1960s, clinicians examined the link between pharmacologic treatment choices and the impact on outcome. At the time, phenothiazines, paraldehyde and chloral hydrate were often employed in the treatment of DTs.[65] The phenothiazines were associated with slower control of fever and greater morbidity and mortality. A controlled study in 1964 demonstrated a 35% mortality rate with promazine and a 4.5% mortality rate with paraldehyde.[198] Causes of death were similar: fever, tachycardia, stupor, cyanosis, and cardiovascular collapse without defined pathology. These early studies established a clear improvement in outcome when sedative-hypnotics were compared to antipsychotics. Phenothiazines and butyrophenones are now generally considered inappropriate for any form of withdrawal, because they increase the incidence of hypotension, hyperthermia, seizures, and mortality.[20,71,75,76,140]

A comprehensive review of 39 fatal cases of DTs found dehydration in all cases in which volume status was noted.[197] The review included psychotic patients displaying mania or hyperactivity, and patients with DTs who also exhibited increased somatic activity (tremor, seizures) associated with dehydration. Approximately 50% of patients had temperatures greater than 40°C (104°F), including 9 of 12 patients with seizures; in 11 cases, hyperthermia was attributed solely to the delirium. Thus, regardless of etiology, hyperthermia, increased motor activity, and fluid depletion in the setting of DTs carried a grave prognosis. However, recognition and treatment of complications along with better fluid replacement and supportive care seemed to be the most important determinants of survival. Mortality at Philadelphia General Hospital decreased to 5.4% in the late 1950s (as compared to 18.5% in the early 1950s) using this approach.[196]

Finally, the benefits of benzodiazepines as the sedative-hypnotic of choice were first realized after controlled trial of diazepam and paraldehyde for severe DTs.[200] There was no mortality in diazepam-treated patients and sedation was achieved more rapidly. Adverse reactions and mortality, however, were significant with paraldehyde. The suggested diazepam regimen was 10 mg IV followed by 5 mg IV every 5 minutes until calm.

A quarter century later, our understanding of neurotransmitters and neurologic function makes a more precise understanding of this disorder possible. Alcohol withdrawal is a neurologic disorder with a continuum of progressively worsening symptoms caused by the effects of chronic ethanol on the central nervous system, and is often exacerbated by the clinical manifestations of alcoholism (nutritional depletion, impaired immunity, anemia, cirrhosis, head trauma).[108] The morbidity and mortality from this condition largely arise from inappropriate resuscitative efforts (failure to correct hypovolemia and lower temperature), inappropriate treatments (antipsychotics), and failure to identify concurrent illness (infection, CNS trauma). The 15% mortality observed by Victor and Adams largely occurred in the patients with concurrent illness. Half of all patients with delirium tremens and two-thirds of the patients with fatal delirium tremens had concurrent illness. This mortality was reduced to below 5% within a decade of their work when aggressive fluid resuscitation, cooling, and supportive care became the goal of therapy.[196,197] Finally, the development of the benzodiazepine class of sedative-hypnotics has lead to safe control of CNS manifestations without exacerbating concurrent illness or morbidity. Now, we only expect a fatal outcome if the underlying illness overcomes the patient.[176]

EPIDEMIOLOGY

Alcohol is the leading drug of abuse in the world. The National Institute for Alcohol Abuse and Alcoholism reports that roughly 5% of the US population has engaged in recent heavy drinking (5 or more drinks on 5 or more occasions within the past 30 days) and 15% of the population has engaged in recent binge drinking (5 or more drinks on at least 1 occasion within the past 30 days).[170]

Alcohol-withdrawal patients present to emergency departments for numerous reasons, but acute withdrawal is rarely the chief complaint. Many patients arrive at the hospital seeking care for the illness or circumstance that prevented them from drinking, such as an upper respiratory infection, trauma, or imprisonment.[69] Although we often consider alcoholism when we are confronted with patients with chronic diseases of the liver and pancreas, in fact, a greater percentage of patients admitted to the hospital with surgi-

cal diagnoses are likely to have a history of alcohol misuse and suffer from withdrawal.[132] In one Australian study of 2046 admitted patients of all types, 8% were at risk for alcohol withdrawal.[61] However, 16% of all postoperative patients and 31% of all trauma patients suffered some actual form of alcohol withdrawal during their admission. Half of all trauma patients are under the acute influence of alcohol at the time of the event. In general, alcohol-withdrawal patients are typically males in their third or fourth decade of life and patients who drink continuously, as opposed to "binge drinkers," are theoretically at highest risk for withdrawal.[149] However, characterizing alcohol withdrawal patients by age, sex, or otherwise will lead to a missed diagnosis more often than not. In fact, the severity of alcohol withdrawal does not diminish or increase with age, although patients over the age of 60 years are more likely to experience cognitive and functional impairments.[97] In addition, benzodiazepine requirements in the elderly relate to the severity of the withdrawal and do not diminish, and physicians should dose patients accordingly.

PATHOPHYSIOLOGY OF ALCOHOL AND OTHER GABAMINERGIC WITHDRAWAL SYNDROMES

Ethanol, benzodiazepines, and barbiturates enhance GABAminergic tone. This is the mechanism by which they produce sedation. γ-Aminobutyric acid $(GABA)_A$ receptors are postsynaptic receptors that, when activated, hyperpolarize the postsynaptic neuron by an inward chloride current without a G protein messenger.[101] These receptors have separate binding sites for GABA, barbiturates, benzodiazepines, and picrotoxin. Barbiturates and benzodiazepines bind to their receptor sites and enhance the affinity for GABA at its receptor site.[5] Chronic exposure to benzodiazepines appears to decrease $GABA_A$ receptor sensitivity.[110,195] Only high-dose barbiturates can open the GABA chloride channel without concomitant binding of a GABA molecule, and this has been specifically demonstrated with phenobarbital and pentobarbital.[64,82]

Many drugs (eg, ethanol, etomidate) have GABA-receptor activity without a clearly identified binding site. Ethanol, benzodiazepines, etomidate, and propofol are examples of drugs that merely enhance $GABA_A$ chloride channel activity and are classified as indirect GABA agonists. Traditional discussions suggest that acute exposure to ethanol affects membrane fluidity and cross-couples the 5 proteins that construct the GABA receptor, interact with a portion of the receptor, and enhance GABA release.[30,99,144,166,167] The result is an enhancement in GABA chloride channel activity, apparently without enhancing GABA binding to its recognition site on the receptor.[103] Recent research with chimeric reconstruction of GABA and NMDA channels demonstrates highly specific binding sites for ethanol. Ethanol binding to these sites enhances GABA and inhibits NMDA.[129a] The adaptation to chronic exposure to ethanol is a modified $GABA_A$ receptor function.[29,103,104,153,154,158,195] Chronic ethanol exposure first increases, and then ultimately decreases, messenger ribonucleic acid (mRNA) expression of certain $GABA_A$ subunit proteins.[29,95,103] These subunit proteins (α_1, α_3, α_6, γ_{2s}, γ_{2l}, and γ_3) are assembled in multiple combinations to form GABA receptor complexes with slightly different characteristics in different areas of the brain. Ultimately, withdrawal symptoms may represent the clinical manifestation of a change in GABA receptor complex characteristics, and thus cause diminished effectiveness, rather than a simple change in receptor numbers.[50] Genetic research using quantitative trait locus mapping and investigations examining $GABA_A$ receptor sensitivity suggest that a complex interaction between ethanol, production of $GABA_A$ subunits, and receptor modulation will ultimately explain many of the clinical characteristics of ethanol withdrawal.[31,93]

Although the exact mechanism is not completely known, what is clear is that during withdrawal, GABA synaptic activity is so diminished that inhibitory control of excitatory neurotransmitters and pathways such as glutamate, norepinephrine, and dopamine is lost.[60,164] This results in the clinical syndrome of withdrawal: CNS excitation (seizures, tremor, hallucinations) and autonomic stimulation (tachycardia, hypertension, hyperthermia, diaphoresis).[71,101]

Up-regulation in the excitatory neuronal pathways is also important in ethanol withdrawal, and the N-methyl-D-aspartate (NMDA) subtype of glutamate receptor (especially the MK-801 binding site) appears to be the major contributor.[84,206] Enhanced excitatory neurotransmission is a characteristic of ethanol withdrawal that appears to explain the "kindling" hypothesis, in which withdrawal events become progressively more severe.[12,17,22,27,210] The activity of an excitatory neuronal pathway increases the more it fires, a phenomenon known as long-term potentiation.[70] This may be a result of increased activity of mRNA and receptor protein expression.[46] Thus, as NMDA receptors increase in number and function, and $GABA_A$ receptor activity diminishes, withdrawal becomes more severe.[47,110,126,158] Knowledge of this phenomenon should prompt the clinician toward aggressive treatment of even minor withdrawal symptoms, in the hopes of attenuating the progression to subsequently more severe withdrawal episodes.[222]

CLINICAL CHARACTERISTICS OF ALCOHOL WITHDRAWAL

Alcohol withdrawal is a neurologic disorder with a continuum of progressively worsening symptoms caused by the effects of chronic ethanol on the central nervous system, and is often exacerbated by the clinical manifestations of alcoholism (nutritional depletion, impaired immunity, anemia, cirrhosis, head trauma).[108] In keeping with our model of withdrawal physiology, ethanol levels are falling or zero when clinical manifestations of withdrawal begin. For many patients, a brief alcohol withdrawal seizure (AWS) may be the first event. In others, a fine-motor tremor may develop (see Fig. 72–1). AWS, or rum fits, may occur without other signs of withdrawal and are characteristically brief tonic-clonic events with a short postictal period. They may recur, but status epilepticus is distinctly unusual in withdrawal (40% single seizures and 3% status epilepticus).[211]

A rapid recovery and normal mental status belie the seriousness of AWS. For one-third of all patients with alcohol withdrawal characterized by delirium (delirium tremens), the sentinel event is an isolated AWS. This seizure may occur despite the presence of an elevated serum ethanol level. In fact, an AWS that occurs despite an elevated ethanol level is a poor prognostic indicator because the relative protection of an elevated ethanol level will continue to be lost as the level drops.[210] They may even have a history of a seizure disorder and be taking anticonvulsant medica-

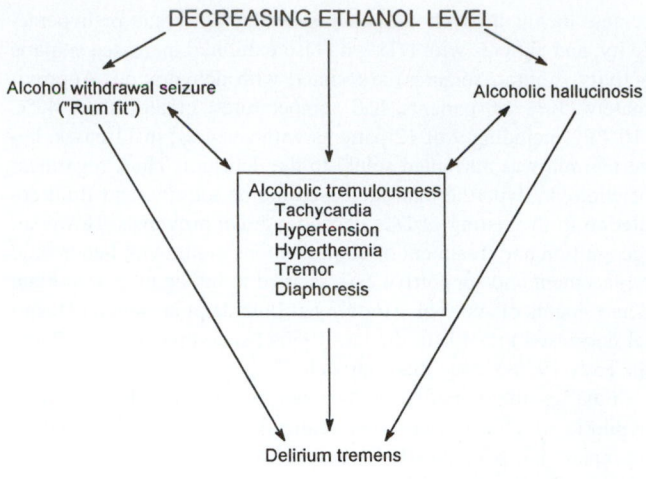

Figure 72–1. Representation of alcohol withdrawal. As ethanol levels fall, patients may develop alcohol withdrawal seizures ("rum fits"), alcoholic hallucinosis, or alcoholic tremulousness. Following this state, the patient can recover, develop another early manifestation of withdrawal, or progress to delirium tremens.

tions, largely because alcohol withdrawal seizures (AWS) cannot be differentiated from other acquired seizure disorders (eg, posttraumatic). An asymptomatic period after an alcoholic abstinence seizure may last for several hours, or the CNS excitation may progress without recovery.

Progressive CNS excitation characterizes the next phase of withdrawal. We suggest that patients with alcohol withdrawal be clinically classified into those with an intact and those with an altered consciousness. The advantage to this simple classification is that it avoids clinical descriptors that are only confusing, such as delirium, DTs, or florid DTs. Tachycardia, fever, and hypertension are identifiable markers for worsening withdrawal.

The central nervous system excitation begins as a fine intention tremor that can be detected in the outstretched hands or protruding tongue. This appears to be a variation of physiologic tremor except that patients with alcohol withdrawal have a tremor with a significantly higher amplitude as compared to the tremor normally associated with anxiety or emotional stress.

Formication, or the sensation of ants crawling on the skin, often promotes repeated itching and leads to excoriations. Disorders of thought, anxiety, agitation, and lability of mood also manifest to varying degrees. Hallucinations are largely visual and appear to occur especially in patients with inadequate thiamine stores.[85] When these CNS manifestations are present with normal vital signs, the patient may be anxious, display a fine tremor, and appear otherwise normal. Because these symptoms will invariably progress, all patients should be treated with sedation.

Patients with a history of alcoholism who develop CNS excitation and then manifest abnormal vital signs are experiencing clinical deterioration. Tachycardia, elevated temperature, hypertension, and diaphoresis mark the autonomic manifestations of this worsening withdrawal syndrome. If untreated or undertreated, the central nervous system excitation of these patients progresses to uncontrollable agitation, seizures, involuntary tremor, hyperthermia, rhabdomyolysis, and death.

MANAGEMENT FOR ALCOHOL AND OTHER GABAERGIC WITHDRAWAL SYNDROMES

There are four important principles in the management of the patient in withdrawal.

1. Restore inhibitory tone to the central nervous system by using long-acting benzodiazepines or barbiturates.
2. Identify and correct fluid, electrolyte, and nutritional deficiencies.
3. Evaluate the patient for concurrent illness including infection.
4. Allow the patient to rest peacefully without self-harm, decrease the need for restraints, and decrease the risk of rhabdomyolysis and hyperthermia while undergoing all necessary diagnostic studies.

The advantage of a neuropharmacologic approach to withdrawal is that it simplifies the treatment. Patients with alcohol withdrawal are disinhibited. They have amplified excitatory neuronal pathways and impaired inhibitory neuronal pathways that require the continuous presence of ethanol to approximate normal physiology. The goal of therapy is to rapidly restore the inhibitory tone—to reinhibit them.

Numerous studies support the "loading" and "symptom-triggered therapy" principles. In the "loading" approach, a benzodiazepine with active metabolites is administered in an escalating bolus fashion until the patient is brought to sedation. In the "symptom triggered" approach a fixed dose of benzodiazepine is repeated after interval reassessment until withdrawal symptoms are controlled.[121,168,214] Although the initial doses may be quite high in either approach, withdrawal is ultimately better managed with less total benzodiazepine, shorter duration of treatment, similar efficacy of treatment, and fewer adverse sequelae. This approach is in contradistinction to the fixed interval, fixed-dose technique, which administers benzodiazepine without consideration for the patients symptoms. This gives insufficient quantities of medication when withdrawal is severe and drug and active metabolites accumulates later as the withdrawal symptoms resolve. This causes lingering and excessive sedation. In addition, studies indicate that the hospital can realize a cost savings (50%) by using the loading dose regimen.[215] Properly sedated patients also improve staff perceptions of the safety of the environment because of a decrease in patient violence and agitation using the loading technique.[83]

Even with substantial benzodiazepine doses, respiratory compromise and the need for airway support are unlikely. Concerns about dosing benzodiazepines in patients with liver failure and the elderly are justified, but these patients also benefit from this approach, as the modest prolongation in half-life is not deleterious and patients do not have greater CNS depression but only a potentially more prolonged phase.[26,80,144,221]

The selection of a benzodiazepine is important to the success of this loading principle. Chlordiazepoxide and lorazepam have been used, but offer no unique benefits over diazepam.[92,137,159] In fact, it is precisely because large boluses of diazepam are metabolized to active metabolites (desmethyldiazepam) over the typical period of withdrawal (48–72 hours) that diazepam is the only benzodiazepine needed to treat this disorder.[3,223] A retrospective re-

view reported that the use of a single benzodiazepine rather than multiple benzodiazepines was a marker for treatment success in surgical patients experiencing alcohol withdrawal during surgical admission.[134] It is more important to rapidly sedate the patient with adequate doses of a single benzodiazepine, than to use multiple agents in hopes of finding an effective regimen.

When a loading dose is administered, and the patient is adequately sedated, minimal additional sedation is required. Diazepam and desmethyldiazepam have long half-lives, thus permitting the primary agent and the metabolite to be endogenously tapered and avoiding drug-induced cyclic variations.[2,3,150,176,177]

Ultimately, this approach has the added benefit of greatly simplifying management. The typical starting dose for a patient in alcohol withdrawal is 10 mg of diazepam given intravenously repeated every 5–15 minutes until the patient is sedated and the vital signs have improved. Twenty milligrams may be all that is needed for slightly more than one-third of the patients; 25% of all patients in ethanol withdrawal require 200 mg.[168] Patients who begin to experience withdrawal with an elevated ethanol level require the initial loading dose therapy and will likely require additional therapy as the ethanol level continues to decrease. An alcoholic can take as long as 6–8 hours to eliminate a serum ethanol level of 150 mg/dL (Chap. 64).

A portion of severe withdrawal patients can remain symptomatic despite doses of diazepam that approach 1 g.[109,136] In fact, doses can be so high (eg, gram quantities of diazepam) that the excipients such as propylene glycol may approach toxicity, although this has never been reported for a diazepam-loading regimen.[18,107,209] One report describes the use of 2335 mg of diazepam intravenously and 21,225 mg of oxazepam orally without control of agitation from alcohol withdrawal. There was no evidence of an abnormal pharmacokinetic profile.[220] When this level of benzodiazepine "resistance" is noted, it is more efficacious to add a barbiturate to attain a synergistic effect on the GABA$_A$ receptor chloride channel and bypass the ineffectual benzodiazepine receptor.[64,89]

There are several acceptable approaches to treating benzodiazepine-resistant withdrawal patients: intravenous phenobarbital or pentobarbital. Intravenous phenobarbital, a long-acting barbiturate, can be given as a bolus of 260 mg (phenobarbital is supplied in 130-mg ampules) over 5 minutes. Repeat dosing should be considered in 30 minutes. This is accomplished by giving a bolus of 130 mg of phenobarbital over 3 minutes. Studies and clinical experience with this drug show that most patients will require 8.5 mg/kg to achieve the endpoint of light sedation. Side effects of this drug regimen include hypotension (6%) that is easily reversed with fluid administration and respiratory depression that frequently requires ventilatory support. Phenobarbital levels are unnecessary, as the patient is loaded to a clinical effect and only treated as symptoms occur.[122,124]

Intravenous pentobarbital, a short-acting barbiturate, given as a 3–5-mg/kg bolus and 100-mg/h infusion should be an effective starting point and is a more aggressive and reliably effective technique for managing severe withdrawal. Symptoms dictate subsequent management and infusion rates. The initial pentobarbital bolus should be used as the induction agent for rapid sequence intubation and mechanical ventilation. Ultimately, very-high-dose anesthetic-type doses of barbiturates never fail to treat withdrawal because they directly open the GABA$_A$ chloride channel.[55,71] However, such therapy for prolonged periods (>24 hrs) alters the apparent pharmacokinetics of pentobarbited in such a way that it has a long duration of effect.

Propofol is an alternative agent for patients who do not respond to benzodiazepines. It has the advantage of easy titratability as well as a rapid offset of effect when the infusion is terminated. This latter effect uniquely allows periodic assessment of the patients' mental status. However, respiratory depression remains consequential and most patients require mechanical ventilation.[125] Although the mechanism of action is not completely understood, it appears to be both an GABA agonist and an NMDA receptor antagonist.

Seizures

Alcohol withdrawal seizures are brief, and recurrent, and rarely progress to status epilepticus. If seizure focality is evident, other CNS pathology is invariably present.[175] AWS are often first recognized in patients who are in their third and fourth decades. All other seizures should be considered to have a cause other than alcoholism itself.[211] All patients with first-time AWS should receive a thorough evaluation, including computed tomography (CT) scan of the brain, an electroencephalogram (EEG), and consideration for lumbar puncture. These studies have a high yield for identifying useful etiologic information such as evidence of CNS trauma and cortical atrophy, although intervention is uncommon.[53,98,105] Cortical atrophy is a common finding on a CT scan of the head in alcoholic patients, but temporal lobe volume deficits may correlate with AWS either as a cause or sequela.[193] It is unclear whether these AWS invariably progress to a permanent seizure disorder with chronic neurologic dysfunction or are merely a marker for the problems associated with severe alcoholism, such as recurrent head trauma, infections, and hypoxia, which cause CNS injury.[14] Phenytoin does not protect against AWS seizures and is, in fact, no better than placebo.[8,36,155] Alcoholics may be on phenytoin for primary epilepsy or a seizure disorder acquired from the manifestations of their disease (CNS infections, trauma, cortical atrophy).

Other Therapies

The use of antihypertensive agents, phenothiazines, antipsychotics, and sedative hypnotics other than benzodiazepines and barbiturates is without foundation. A number of studies that use vital signs as surrogate markers for severity of withdrawal support the use of clonidine and β-adrenergic antagonists.[16,86] However, these patients often experience more of the CNS manifestations of withdrawal, such as anxiety, agitation, and delirium.[3,213] The use of these drugs has largely arisen because of a lack of understanding of the pathophysiology of withdrawal. Although these drugs obviously will block the peripheral manifestations of alcohol withdrawal, they fail to treat the primary neurologic derangement responsible for these symptoms. For example, although the use of antipyretic agents are an important adjunct in treating patients with bacterial infection and fever, one would never consider reducing the dose of antibiotics if the fever resolved with acetaminophen. Vital sign abnormalities are the peripheral manifestations or markers for the severity of the neurologic derangement, and should be aggressively treated with drugs (benzodiazepines and barbiturates) that primarily affect the CNS. In addition, other therapies may actually exacerbate toxicity. Alcohol withdrawal treated with neuroleptics has a mortality rate of 6%.[11] These drugs lower the seizure threshold, impair heat regulation, and fail to correct the neurologic origin of this disorder.[9,14,20,75,76,207] Their use is only justified to treat underlying medical problems other than

withdrawal. Patients with CNS excitation with normal vital signs are candidates for oral benzodiazepines therapy, and can often be managed by an alcohol detoxification service.[19,79]

Alcohol withdrawal should not be fatal if the patient receives proper supportive care. Sedation (to produce calm, restful sleep), substrate repletion (dextrose, thiamine, folic acid), fluid and electrolyte balance, oxygen, and control of hyperthermia and agitation improve survival, although patients still die from complications such as trauma, CNS hemorrhage, pancreatitis, infection, liver disease, and electrolyte- or alcoholic cardiomyopathy-related dysrhythmias.[108,117] Aggressive evaluation for concurrent CNS infection and avoiding the pitfall of attributing fever solely to withdrawal symptoms prevents this morbidity. In general, the more severe the alcohol withdrawal, the more likely a concurrent illness.[58]

The effects of rapid cooling and hydration in combination with sedation have virtually eliminated mortality.[199] A similar approach to all agitated patients significantly reduces mortality and morbidity related to hyperthermia, rhabdomyolysis, and dehydration.[48,102] Hyperthermia in the agitated patient carries a particularly high risk. Unlike fevers of infectious etiologies, temperatures may exceed 106°F (41.1°C), with resultant tissue damage. Rapid cooling, titration of sedation with a benzodiazepine, and adequate hydration are essential early steps in the management of the agitated patient, regardless of the etiology.

A thorough evaluation of the alcohol withdrawal patient also includes fingerstick glucose, CBC, serum electrolytes, calcium and magnesium, chest radiograph, and urinalysis. The yield on these clinical investigations is extraordinarily high, and often reveals complications or phenomena associated with alcoholism that require treatment (occult infection, remote and/or recent head trauma, anemia, electrolyte abnormalities, and so forth).[59] Hypoglycemia is an important problem in alcohol withdrawal because of increased CNS glucose requirements and altered counterregulatory responses.[54] Thus, all patients with withdrawal require supplemental glucose and thiamine to assist in its transport and metabolism (Chap. 64).[216] Chest radiography often reveals evidence of chronic pulmonary infections, aspiration pneumonia, and cardiomyopathy. Magnesium supplementation continues to be a source of controversy in alcohol withdrawal. Though many reports suggest a beneficial effect and animal models point to a role in NMDA antagonism, prospective trials fail to find a benefit. Because deficiencies of this electrolyte can mimic ethanol withdrawal and alcoholics are often magnesium depleted, measuring magnesium levels and repleting a patient with a magnesium deficiency is important. There appears to be no defined role for its empiric use in this setting.[21,62,68,217]

CLINICAL CHARACTERISTICS AND TREATMENT OF BENZODIAZEPINE AND BARBITURATE WITHDRAWAL

The similarity between alcohol and barbiturate withdrawal was identified by Victor and Adams who noted the work of Isbell on chronic barbiturate intoxication and withdrawal.[87] Patients who are dependent on benzodiazepines, barbiturates, and other sedative-hypnotic drugs display withdrawal symptoms that are similar to alcohol withdrawal symptoms except that they may develop as late as 14 days after cessation of drug administration, depending on the pharmacokinetic profile of the abused drug. Diazepam, chlorazepate, and chlordiazepoxide are converted to active metabolites with half-lives of up to 200 hours. Phenobarbital's half-life is as long as 2–6 days. These patients may have symptoms such as anxiety or insomnia for many days before objective manifestations of withdrawal develop. Alprazolam is a short-acting benzodiazepine without active metabolites and can cause withdrawal symptoms within 24 hours of cessation of use.

Benzodiazepine withdrawal has most of the same characteristics as severe ethanol withdrawal, except the expected time course for resolution of withdrawal symptoms can last for 10 days. Patients develop the disinhibitory syndrome characterized by progressively worsening agitation, tachycardia, hypertension, fever, hyperthermia, and seizures.

No controlled studies have been done addressing the comparative efficacy of various treatment regimens. However, by considering this entity as another form of GABAminergic withdrawal, diazepam and barbiturates become the logical treatment regimen choices.

Some authors believe that phenobarbital is a useful first choice for patients with benzodiazepine withdrawal who still have normal vital signs, because patients perceive that the addicting drug has been eliminated. In addition, its long half-life allows an appropriate taper of drug levels without complicating management.[161] One approach is to start the patient on a phenobarbital dose that is considered a sedative-hypnotic equivalent (each 10 mg of diazepam is equated with 30 mg phenobarbital), and then each day the patient is administered 10% less of the total dose.

For benzodiazepine withdrawal with abnormal vital signs or seizures, diazepam loading in a fashion similar to ethanol withdrawal is an appropriate first choice. Phenobarbital loading can be used in this situation as well.[122]

Flumazenil is a short-acting benzodiazepine receptor antagonist that is capable of rapidly inducing a withdrawal syndrome in patients who are habituated to benzodiazepines, but not to alcohol (see Antidote in Depth: Flumazenil).[35] It is for this reason that flumazenil's use is discouraged in the overdose setting.[75,215,218] Flumazenil may have a role in reversing intoxications in pediatric patients, because the likelihood of chronic use is low. Flumazenil can produce seizures without the onset of consciousness, a particularly dangerous combination. The clinician should expect these seizures to require higher than normal doses of benzodiazepines because of the benzodiazepine receptor antagonism. This need for increased benzodiazepines can last from 1–2 hours, depending on the dose of flumazenil used. In refractory cases, intravenous pentobarbital intubation and mechanical ventilation may become necessary.

INHALANT WITHDRAWAL

Another poorly recognized but widespread source of drug abuse is inhalants. Solvents such as gasoline, ether, and toluene have well-established abuse potential, especially in adolescents. These chemicals are capable of producing deep anesthesia. Recent work has determined that anesthetics of this sort are active at the $GABA_A$ receptor and produce CNS inhibition. Elaboration of the mechanism specific for solvent of abuse awaits further study, although it is logical to assume they act in a similar fashion.[13]

Impoverished areas of the world suffer from higher rates of inhalant abuse and a case series from India highlights the sad facts

of this epidemic. These investigators describe 9 children with a mean age of 13.6 years, of low socioeconomic status, whose fathers abused alcohol. All subjects report a daily history of abuse of gasoline and a syndrome of irritability, psychomotor retardation, anhedonia, dry mouth, sleep disturbances, craving, and increase lacrimation with withdrawal of inhalant use. Further research is necessary to determine whether this is a true withdrawal syndrome or some other effect of inhalant abuse.[179]

$GABA_B$ WITHDRAWAL

Baclofen

$GABA_B$ receptors mediate presynaptic inhibition (by preventing Ca^{2+} influx) and postsynaptic inhibition (by increasing K^+ efflux). The postsynaptic receptors appear to have a similar inhibitory effect as the $GABA_A$ receptors. The presynaptic receptors provide feedback inhibition of GABA release. Unlike $GABA_A$ receptors, these are mediated through G protein messengers. Baclofen is the only clinically important $GABA_B$ agonist. The pre- and postsynaptic inhibitory properties of baclofen allow it, paradoxically, to cause seizures in both acute overdose and withdrawal. When the drug is withdrawn, a disinhibition similar to $GABA_A$ withdrawal occurs. This effect is probably a result of the reduction of the chronic inhibitory effect of baclofen on postsynaptic $GABA_B$ receptors. Although it is more typically sedating in overdose, baclofen also stimulates presynaptic $GABA_B$ autoreceptors to decrease release of $GABA_A$. The subsequent disinhibition leads to seizures, hypertension, and coma. Interestingly, many case reports of baclofen withdrawal describe hallucinations and psychosis as prominent symptoms. However, these may be no different than the withdrawal symptoms of $GABA_A$ agonists. That many patients experience double vision is difficult to explain.[160,182]

The development of this withdrawal syndrome typically occurs 24–48 hours after discontinuation of baclofen during an admission to the hospital for an unrelated medical problem. Case reports highlight the development of seizures, hallucinations, psychosis, dyskinesia, and visual disturbances. Intrathecal baclofen pumps have become an effective replacement for oral dosing, but withdrawal can occur following the use of this modality as well. Remember to consider withdrawal when patients are recovering from acute-on-chronic baclofen overdoses. Reinstatement of the prior baclofen-dosing schedule appears to resolve these symptoms within 24–48 hours. Benzodiazepines and $GABA_A$ agonists, not phenytoin, are the appropriate treatment for seizures induced by baclofen withdrawal.[143]

γ-HYDROXYBUTYRATE

γ-Hydroxybutyrate (GHB) is a compound found in mammalian brain, that has been investigated as an anesthetic and for treatment of narcolepsy, alcohol dependence, and opioid dependence. Along with its precursors, butanediol and γ-butyrolactone, they are abused for their euphoric, sedative, and purported anabolic effects. The mechanism of action of GHB is not fully known, but appears to have its effect, at least in part, on the GABA receptors. A withdrawal syndrome that resolves in 3–12 days has been reported that appears consistent with this mechanism—insomnia, anxiety, and tremor.[67] Occasionally, symptoms can be severe and require high doses of benzodiazepines.[42] Experience suggests that body builders commonly use GHB or its analogs several times daily, and hence are more likely to experience withdrawal than those who use them in a binge style for their euphoric effects.

Case 2. A 45-year-old male was brought to the ED by police officers. The patient was agitated, vomiting, diaphoretic, and complained that he was withdrawing from his methadone. He was incarcerated 24 hours earlier and had not received his methadone for 72 hours. His vital signs were blood pressure, 165/90 mm Hg; respiratory rate, 22 breath/min; pulse, 110 beats/min without orthostatic changes; and rectal temperature, 99.9°F (37.2°C). The man was well developed, well nourished, and appeared older than his stated age. He had mydriasis, profuse diaphoresis, hyperactive bowel sounds, piloerection, and diarrhea. He was given 10 mg of diazepam intravenously. Thirty minutes later he was noted to be sleeping, but was agitated when awakened. The remainder of his symptoms persisted. Methadone 10 mg was administered IM, and his vomiting, diarrhea, piloerection, and hyperactive bowel sound resolved.

PATHOPHYSIOLOGY OF OPIOID WITHDRAWAL

Opioids inhibit neurons and alleviate pain when they bind to an opioid receptor, activate G_s proteins, and stimulate K^+ efflux currents. The opioid receptors are also linked to the $G_{i/o}$ proteins. These act through adenyl cyclase and activate inward Na^+ current, thus enhancing the intrinsic excitability of a neuron (see Figure 72–2).[41]

Chronic exposure to opiates (only drugs directly derived from opium) and opioids (all drugs with opioid-receptor efficacy) results in a decreased efficacy of this receptor to open potassium channels by altering postreceptor, intracellular pathways. When chronic opioid use is present, the expression of adenyl cyclase increases through activation of the transcription factor cyclic adenosine monophosphate (cAMP) response element-binding protein (CREB). This results in an up-regulation of cAMP mediated responses such as the inward Na^+ channels responsible for intrinsic excitability. The net effect is that only higher levels of opioids result in analgesia and opioid effect. In the dependent patient, when opioid levels drop and this inward Na^+ flux is unchecked, the patient experiences withdrawal symptoms. These withdrawal symptoms are largely because of uninhibited activity at the locus ceruleus.[38,119,128,133]

Furthermore, opioid receptors and central α_2 receptors both exert a similar effect on the potassium channel in the locus ceruleus. Clonidine binds to the central α_2 receptor and stimulates potassium efflux as opioids do, and will create a partial sedative effect. This explains why clonidine has some efficacy in treating for opioid withdrawal. In addition, naloxone's antagonistic effect at the opioid receptor seems to reverse the effect clonidine has on this shared potassium efflux channel (Fig. 72–2).[72]

CLINICAL CHARACTERISTICS

Symptoms progress from drug craving, yawning, rhinorrhea, and piloerection to nausea, vomiting, diarrhea, diaphoresis, myalgias, arthralgias, anxiety, fear, and mild tachycardia. Chronicity relates to pharmacology of the opioid of abuse. Methadone withdrawal starts about 24 hours after the last dose and persists for 3–7 days. Heroin withdrawal begins approximately 6 hours after the last dose and is usually fully manifest at 24 hours. Withdrawal is physically and emotionally painful, but not life-threatening as long as adequate hydration and nutritional support are maintained and morbidity from emesis and dehydration can be minimized.

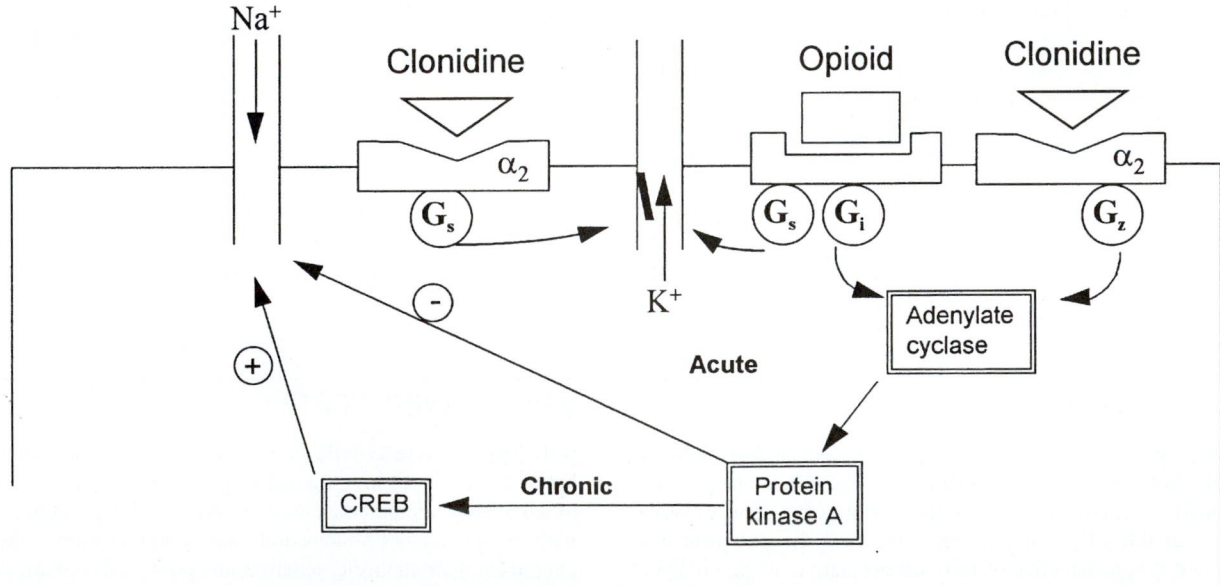

Figure 72–2. Immediate and long-term effects of opioids. The acute effects of both opioids and α_2-adrenergic agonists are to increase inhibition through enhanced potassium efflux and inhibited sodium influx. Chronic effects alter gene expression to enhance sodium influx and restore hemeostasis. CREB (cAMP response element-binding protein).

TABLE 72–1. Clinical Differentiation of Drug Withdrawal

	Opioids	Sedative-Hypnotics/Ethanol
Vital Signs		
Blood pressure	Hypertension, normal or orthostatic hypotension when volume depleted	Normal, hypertension, then orthostatic hypotension when volume depleted
Pulse	Tachycardia	Tachycardia
Respiratory rate	Tachypnea	Tachypnea
Temperature	Normal	Hyperthermia
Mental Status		
	Normal	Abnormal
	Anxiety	Restlessness
	Irritability	Irritability
		Psychosis, visual hallucinations more common than auditory
		Disorientation
Physical Signs and Symptoms		
	Yawning	Tremulousness
	Lacrimation	Muscle fasciculations
	Rhinorrhea	Diaphoresis
	Mydriasis	Seizures
	Tremor	
	Piloerection	
	Restlessness	
	Emesis, nausea	
	Diarrhea with increased bowel sounds	
	Seizures in neonates (only)	
	Muscle pain and spasm	

Table 72–1 compares opioid withdrawal with sedative-hypnotic or ethanol withdrawal.

TREATMENT

Treatment with methadone (10 mg IM or 20 mg po) is enough to blunt withdrawal symptoms without providing euphoria, although it may not eliminate drug craving. Maintenance programs often use higher daily doses to achieve this latter effect. Very high doses (greater than 100 mg of methadone per day) are used to flood opioid receptors so that intercurrent heroin abuse will not result in euphoria, thereby deterring drug-seeking behavior.[33,190,191]

Clonidine is an effective adjuvant in opioid withdrawal.[5,63,72] Doses start at 5–6 μg/kg/d and can get as high as 25 μg/kg/d. Clonidine is most useful in conjunction with methadone maintenance and a structured detoxification program. Clonidine can be considered as a therapeutic alternative in situations where hospital policy does not permit methadone administration. Clonidine, however, does not blunt craving for opioids.

Opioid withdrawal can be induced by the use of opioid receptor antagonists or mixed agonist-antagonists in opioid habituated patients. Often, this is the result of administering large doses of naloxone to opioid addicted patients who present with an opioid overdose. In patients suspected of chronic opioid use, use a low initial starting dose (0.05–0.2 mg of naloxone) and assist respiration as needed until a therapeutic effect is observed—usually within a few minutes. Readministration of the dose is based on clinical grounds. If withdrawal is induced, expect symptoms to resolve within 1 hour as the naloxone is eliminated and there is a reemergence of the primary opioid's effects. More severe withdrawal rarely may require administration of an opioid. This is generally only needed after inadvertent administration of a long-acting opioid antagonist such as naltrexone.

RAPID HEROIN DETOXIFICATION AND WITHDRAWAL

Naltrexone blocks the euphoric effects of opioid use and discourages recidivism by blunting drug craving.[73,96,114,115] Although the mechanism is not entirely clear, the speculation is that mere receptor occupancy by an antagonist is sufficient to blunt cravings. In theory, inducing opioid withdrawal under general anesthesia with high-dose opioid antagonists permits the transition from drug dependency to naltrexone maintenance without drug withdrawal symptoms.[111,112,113,157] However, studies demonstrate that withdrawal symptoms may be more intense and persist for up to 1 week after rapid detoxification.[174,184] Nonetheless, many patients are encouraged by the promise of a rapid transition to naltrexone maintenance from opioid dependence (Rapid Opioid Detoxification – ROD; Rapid Opioid Detoxification under Anesthesia – RODA; or Ultrarapid Opioid Detoxification – UROD). Many centers report success with this process, and tout it as a safe, comfortable, same day, outpatient treatment for heroin addiction.[6,25,74]

All studies suggest that the detoxification procedure is physiologically successful when opioid abstinence is measured by the response to antagonist challenge. However, recidivism ranges from 10% to 50% and outpatient psychosocial support is generally lacking.[116,171,189] In addition, these patients are sent home with potent medications, such as clonidine, baclofen, octreotide, ondansetron, benzodiazepines, and trazodone, to counter the continued withdrawal symptoms.

Instead of transitioning to oral naltrexone, an alternative approach is to compound the naltrexone into a pellet and implant it in the subcutaneous tissues.[74] This is not an FDA-approved route for the oral drug and there is no parenteral form available. However, emergency physicians and toxicologists may encounter patients who are in naltrexone-induced opioid withdrawal.

The literature contains a number of reports of ROD and UROD complications—death, prolonged respiratory depression, and an abstract of a case series of patients who experienced persistent withdrawal symptoms.[52,66,146,194] In addition, the use of naloxone may be associated with pulmonary edema, perhaps a result of the excessive release of catecholamines during unrecognized hypercarbia from hypoventilation.[10,37] To date, there is only 1 case report of complication of UROD with naltrexone pellet implant; in that case, the patient developed severe rhabdomyolysis.[188]

CLONIDINE WITHDRAWAL (α_2-ADRENERGIC RECEPTORS)

α_2-Adrenergic receptors are located in the central and peripheral nervous system. Clonidine is a central and peripheral α_2 agonist. Stimulation of peripheral postsynaptic α_2-adrenergic receptors results in vasoconstriction, bradycardia, and hypertension, and prevents acetylcholine release. This results in some anticholinergic symptoms, especially dry mouth. The peripheral effects manifest only in the initial period after a toxic dose. Stimulation of central presynaptic α_2-adrenergic receptors inhibits sympathomimetic output and results in bradycardia, and hypotension.[57]

Within 24 hours after the discontinuation of clonidine, norepinephrine levels rise as a result of enhanced efferent sympathetic activity.[165] Patients who use the clonidine patch may experience withdrawal later than 24 hours, if at all, because a reservoir of the drug in the skin generally allows levels to persist for days. Clonidine elimination half-life is 14 hours, and most patients who manifest withdrawal still have a low level of clonidine in the initial phase. Simultaneous use of β-adrenergic antagonists exacerbates withdrawal, as α-adrenergic receptor stimulation is unopposed by β-adrenergic antagonism.

The first symptoms occur 24 hours after discontinuation of clonidine and include headache, flushing, sweating, hallucinations, and anxiety.[26] Hypertensive encephalopathy and death have been reported in rare cases. Within 48 hours the patient's blood pressure rises to near or above pretreatment levels. There appears to be an association with high-dose therapy (greater than 1.2 mg/d) or concomitant β-adrenergic antagonism therapy and an increased likelihood and severity of withdrawal.[28,156] Treatment requires reinstatement of the drug by the oral route. Patients unable to swallow may be treated with sublingual clonidine. β-Adrenergic antagonists are absolutely contraindicated.

CAFFEINE (ADENOSINE$_1$ RECEPTORS)

The release of neurotransmitters is accompanied by passive release of adenosine as a by-product of adenosine triphosphate (ATP) breakdown. This adenosine acts on the presynaptic adenosine$_1$ autoreceptors to decrease further release of neurotransmitters, and on the postsynaptic adenosine$_1$ receptors to terminate neuronal transmission. Adenosine$_2$ receptors are found on the cerebral vasculature and peripheral vasculature and promote vasodilation[44] (Chap. 10).

Caffeine antagonizes the inhibitory effect of adenosine (Chap. 39). As a result, acute exposure results in increases in heart rate, ventilation, gastrointestinal motility, gastric acid secretion, and motor activity. Chronic exposure results in tolerance to the effects of large acute administration of the drug. This effect appears to be associated with caffeine's occupancy of adenosine$_1$ receptors. Chronic caffeine exposure regulates adenosine$_1$ receptors by a variety of theoretical mechanisms, such as increases in receptor number, increases in receptor affinity, or enhancing receptor coupling to the G protein. An animal study demonstrates that the adenosine receptor has a 3-fold increase in affinity for adenosine at the height of withdrawal symptoms. This model suggests that chronic caffeine administration results in increase in receptor affinity for adenosine, thus restoring a state of physiologic balance (normal motor inhibitory tone).

When caffeine is withdrawn, the enhanced receptor affinity results in a strong adenosine effect and clinical symptoms of withdrawal: headache (cerebral vasodilation), fatigue, and hypersomnia (motor inhibition).[183,190] Symptoms of anxiety, depression, headaches, sleepiness, and decreased alertness and activity peak at 24–48 hours and decrease over 1 week. Most patients correctly identify the source of their symptoms and medicate with the appropriate dose and preferred form of caffeine. Caffeine dependence and withdrawal have been demonstrated in patients who take as little as 129 mg/d of caffeine—the equivalent of an average 5 oz cup of coffee. Clinicians should consider this entity in the patient who is being evaluated for headache symptoms. Although 10% of caffeine users experience withdrawal symptoms, recent work suggests that 1% of men and 5% of women experience symptoms significant enough to interfere with daily acitivities.[49]

NICOTINE WITHDRAWAL

Nicotinic receptors are a type of acetylcholine receptors located in the autonomic ganglia, adrenal medulla, CNS, spinal cord, neuromuscular junction, and carotid and aortic bodies. Nicotinic receptors are fast-response cation channels that are not coupled to G proteins. This distinguishes them from muscarinic receptors, which are coupled to G proteins. They have both excitatory and inhibitory effects. Much remains unknown about these receptors and how they affect addiction and withdrawal (Chap. 73).[138,199]

Smoking cessation is the primary cause for nicotine withdrawal, although discontinuation of any tobacco product can lead to this syndrome. Cigarette craving is an important problem for hospitalized patients who are not permitted to smoke.

Nicotine withdrawal manifests largely as cigarette craving and subjective dysphoric symptoms. There are some symptoms of irritability, restlessness, and a decrease in heart rate and blood pressure. Cardiac symptoms resolve over 3–4 weeks, but cigarette craving may persist for months to years.

The nicotine transdermal system (patch) and nicotine polacrilex (gum) can be used to provide nicotine without the carcinogens in tobacco, and are now available over-the-counter. The patches utilize a stepwise reduction in subcutaneous delivery to gradually decrease the nicotine dose and appear to have greater compliance than the gum. Acute relief from withdrawal symptoms is most easily achieved with use of the gum, as rapid chewing releases an immediate dose of nicotine. However, the dose is approximately half of that which the average smoker receives in 1 cigarette, and the onset of action is 30 minutes instead of 10 minutes or less. These pharmacologic changes in delivery minimize the reinforcement and self-reward effects that are so prominent with the rapid nicotine delivery of cigarette smoking.

Bupropion has demonstrated efficacy for smoking cessation when administered at 300 mg/d and has a limited impact on anxiety and restlessness, but it does improve mood and concentration. Side effects include seizures at both therapeutic and toxic doses.[180]

SELECTIVE SEROTONIN REUPTAKE INHIBITOR WITHDRAWAL

Evidence has been building to support an SSRI withdrawal uptake inhibitor syndrome (Chap. 58). This syndrome complies with our definition of withdrawal syndromes in that symptoms begin when drug levels drop and reinstatement of the drug abates the syndrome. Most case reports point to venlafaxine as the most common drug involved in this syndrome. Headache, nausea, fatigue, dizziness, and dysphoria are commonly described symptoms. The condition appears to be uncomfortable but not life-threatening, and rapidly resolves with reinstatement of drug of the class and resolves when drug is discontinued after a more gradual taper.[4,43,98,118,142,225]

NEONATAL WITHDRAWAL SYNDROMES

Alcohol and GABA$_A$ Agonists

Maternal addiction to alcohol can result in a neonatal withdrawal syndrome that begins within 3 days after birth. It is characterized by varying degrees of tremor, nystagmus, clonus, opisthotonos, hypertonia, seizures, sleeplessness, crying, asymmetric or hyperactive reflexes, abnormal Moro reflex, excessive mouthing or rooting, diarrhea, vomiting, inability to feed, startle, sweating, and inability to thermoregulate. This syndrome is not directly correlated with the fetal alcohol syndrome. The syndromes are related to the use of alcohol at different times during pregnancy. Children of mothers addicted to benzodiazepines and barbiturates display the same symptoms.[39]

Neonatal alcohol withdrawal should be treated the same as adult alcohol withdrawal. The drug with the most clinical use for this condition in pediatrics is phenobarbital. The loading dose is 16 mg/kg over 24 hours to produce a 24-hour serum level of 20–30 mg/mL. This can be maintained with a dose of 2–8 mg/kg per 24 hours. Once withdrawal symptoms are controlled for 72 hours, the phenobarbital dose should be tapered at 10% per day. Elixirs of phenobarbital contain 14–25% ethyl alcohol; parenteral forms contain 67.8% propylene glycol, 10% ethyl alcohol, and 1.5% benzyl alcohol. Both of these preparations have potential risk to the neonate and should be considered possible explanations for metabolic abnormalities (Chaps. 56 and 105).[45,160]

Opioids

The neonatal opioid withdrawal syndrome shares characteristics of the adult opioid withdrawal syndrome: gastrointestinal distress (vomiting and diarrhea), irritability, yawning, sneezing, hypertonicity, hyperacusis, diaphoresis, lacrimation, and tremulousness. It typically occurs within 2 weeks of birth. In neonates, mottling, fever, myoclonic jerks, and seizures occur in addition to the usual adult opioid withdrawal symptoms. This latter symptom is only characteristic of opioid withdrawal in neonates and occurs in roughly 8% of children born to mothers on methadone maintenance and only 1% of those born to mothers who use heroin.[81,120] Paregoric appears to be more effective than diazepam in controlling and preventing these seizures while preserving the suck reflex. Paregoric is a combination of anhydrous morphine (0.4 mg/mL), camphor, alcohol 46%, and benzoic acid (4 mg/mL). Some clinicians prefer a 1:25 dilution of opium tincture because it contains only 0.7% alcohol and no camphor or benzoic acid. Dosage for either drug is 0.2 mL every 3 hours, increased by 0.05 mL at each dose until withdrawal symptoms are controlled, up to a maximum of 0.7 mL per dose. After the patient is stable, therapy is continued for 3–5 days and decreased gradually over a 2–4-week period. Withdrawal from maternal methadone can also be treated with tincture of opium, but special attention should be given to dose and interval, using small doses at short intervals to achieve rapid control of symptoms. Parenteral morphine should be reserved for short-term therapy of only severe withdrawal symptoms because it contains sodium bisulfite and phenol, which may cause anaphylactic reactions and hyperbilirubinemia, respectively, when administered chronically. Methadone has been used for neonatal withdrawal, but its use is discouraged because the long half-life (26 hours) makes dosing adjustments difficult.[9,91]

Caffeine

An infant with irritability, jitteriness, and vomiting may be suffering from caffeine withdrawal. One study detected caffeine in the serum of 6 of 8 infants with these symptoms. All mothers gave a history of heavy caffeine use and none were dependent on other drugs or alcohol. The children's symptoms persisted for several days and then resolved spontaneously.[127,128]

ACKNOWLEDGMENTS

Kathleen A. Delaney, MD, and Neal E. Flomenbaum, MD, contributed to this chapter in a previous edition.

REFERENCES

1. Aaronson LM, Hinman DJ, Okamoto M: Effects of diazepam on ethanol withdrawal. J Pharmacol Exp Ther 1982;221:319–325.
2. Adinoff B: Double-blind study of alprazolam, diazepam, clonidine, and placebo in the alcohol withdrawal syndrome: Preliminary findings. Alcohol Clin Exp Res 1994;18:873–878.
3. Adinoff B, Bone HGA, Linnoila M: Acute ethanol poisoning and the ethanol withdrawal syndrome. Med Toxicol 1988;3:172–196.
4. Agelink MW, Zitzelsberger A, Klieser E: Withdrawal syndrome after discontinuation of venlafaxine [letter]. Am J Psychiatry 1997;154:1473–1474.
5. Aghajanian GK: Tolerance of locus coeruleus neurons to morphine and suppression of withdrawal response to clonidine. Nature 1978;276:186–188.
6. Albanes AP, Gevirtz C, Oppenheim B, et al: Outcome and six-month follow-up of patients after Ultra Rapid Opiate Detoxification (UROD). J Addict Dis 2000;19:11–28.
7. Allan AM, Baier LD, Zhang X: Effects of lorazepam tolerance and withdrawal on GABA$_A$ receptor operated chloride channels in mice

selected for differences in ethanol withdrawal severity. Life Sci 1992;51:931–943.

8. Alldredge BK, Lowenstein DH, Simon RP: Placebo-controlled trial of intravenous diphenylhydantoin for short-term treatment of alcohol withdrawal seizures. Am J Med 1989;87:645–648.

9. American Academy of Pediatrics Committee on Drugs: Neonatal drug withdrawal. Pediatrics 1983:72;895–902.

10. Andree MA: Sudden death following naloxone administration. Anesth Analg 1980;59:782–784.

11. Athen D: Comparative investigation of chlormethiazole and neuroleptic agents in the treatment of alcoholic delirium. Acta Psychiatr Scand Suppl 1986;329:167–170.

12. Ballenger JC, Post RM: Kindling as a model for alcohol withdrawal syndromes. Br J Psychiatry 1978;133:1–14.

13. Balster RL: Neural basis of inhalant abuse. Drug Alcohol Depend 1998;51:207–214.

14. Bartolomei F, Suchet L, Barrie M, Gastaut JL: Alcoholic epilepsy: A unified and dynamic classification. Eur Neurol 1997;37:13–17.

15. Battaglia G, Napier TC: The effects of cocaine and the amphetamines on brain and behavior: a conference report. Drug Alcohol Depend 1998;52:41–48.

16. Baumgartner GR, Rowen RC: Clonidine vs chlordiazepoxide in the management of acute alcohol withdrawal syndrome. Arch Intern Med 1987;147:1223–1226.

17. Becker HC, Hale RL: Repeated episodes of ethanol withdrawal potentiate the severity of subsequent withdrawal seizures: An animal model of alcohol withdrawal "kindling." Alcohol Clin Exp Res 1993;17:94–98.

18. Bedichek E, Kirschbaum B: A case of propylene glycol toxic reaction associated with etomidate infusion. Arch Intern Med 1991; 151:2297–2298.

19. Beshai NN: Providing cost-efficient detoxification services to alcoholic patients. Public Health Rep 1990;105:475–481.

20. Blum K, Eubanks JD, Wallace JE, Hamilton H: Enhancement of alcohol withdrawal convulsions in mice by haloperidol. Clin Toxicol 1976;9:427–434.

21. Bluntzer ME, Blachley JD: Acid-base and electrolyte disturbances induced by alcohol. J Crit Illness 1986;1:19–26.

22. Booth BM, Blow FC: The kindling hypothesis: Further evidence from a US national study of alcoholic men. Alcohol Alcohol 1993; 28:593–598.

23. Bowman KM, Wortis H, Joliff E: Treatment of disturbed patients with sodium chloride orally and intravenously in hypertonic solutions. Arch Neurol Psychiatry 1939;41:702–710.

24. Boyd IW: Venlafaxine withdrawal reactions. Med J Aust 1998;169: 91–92.

25. Brewer C, Williams J, Carreno Rendueles E, Garcia JB: Unethical promotion of rapid opiate detoxification under anaesthesia (RODA) [letter]. Lancet 1998;351:218.

26. Brower KJ, Mudd S, Blow FC, et al: Severity and treatment of alcohol withdrawal in elderly versus younger patients. Alcohol Clin Exp Res 1994;18:196–201.

27. Brown ME, Anton RF, Malcom R, Ballenger JC: Alcohol detoxification and withdrawal seizures: Clinical support for a kindling hypothesis. Biol Psychiatry 1988;23:507–514.

28. Brown M, Salmon D, Rendell M: Clonidine hallucinations. Ann Intern Med 1980;93:456–457.

29. Buck KJ, Hahner L, Sikela J, Harris RA: Chronic ethanol treatment alters brain levels of gamma-aminobutyric acid A receptor subunit mRNAs: Relationship to genetic differences in ethanol withdrawal seizure severity. J Neurochem 1991;57:1452–1455.

30. Buck KJ, Harris RA: Benzodiazepine agonist and inverse agonist actions on GABA$_A$ receptor-operated chloride channels. II. Chronic effects of ethanol. J Pharmacol Exp Ther 1990;253:713–719.

31. Buck KJ, Hood HM: Genetic Association of a GABA(A) receptor gamma$_2$ subunit variant with severity of acute physiological dependence on alcohol. Mamm Genome 1998;9:975–978.

32. Cammarano WB, Pittet J, Weitz S, Schlobohm R, Marks JD: Acute withdrawal syndrome related to the administration of analgesic and sedative medications in adult intensive care unit patients. Crit Care Med 1998;26:676–684.

33. Caplehorn JR, Bell J, Kleinbaum DG, Gebski VJ: Methadone dose and heroin use during maintenance treatment. Addiction 1993; 88: 119–124.

34. Cecil RL: A Textbook of Medicine. Philadelphia, WB Saunders, 1927, pp 516–518.

35. Chan AW, Leong FW, Schanley DL, et al: Flumazenil (Ro155–788) does not affect ethanol tolerance and dependence. Pharmacol Biochem Behav 1991;39:659–663.

36. Chance JF: Emergency department treatment of alcohol withdrawal seizures with phenytoin. Ann Emerg Med 1991;20:520–522.

37. Chanmugam AS, Hengeller M, Ezenkwele U: Development of rhabdomyolysis after rapid opiate detoxification with subcutaneous naltrexone maintenance therapy. Acad Emerg Med 2000;7:303–305.

38. Christie MJ, Williams JT, North RA: Cellular mechanism of opioid tolerance: Studies in single brain neurons. Mol Pharmacol 1987;32: 633–638.

39. Coles CD, Smith IE, Fernhoff PM, et al: Neonatal ethanol withdrawal: Characteristics in clinically normal, nondysmorphic neonates. J Pediatr 1984:105;445–451.

40. Cucchia AT, Monnat M, Spagnoli J, et al: Ultra-rapid opiate detoxification using deep sedation with oral midazolam: short- and long-term results. Drug Alcohol Depend 1998;52:243–250.

41. Crain SM, Shen KF: Modulatory effects of Gs-coupled excitatory opioid receptor functions on opioid analgesia, tolerance, and dependence. Neurochem Res 1996;21:1347–1351.

42. Craig K, Gomes HF, McManus JL, Bania TC: Severe gamma-hydroxybutyrate withdrawal: A case report and literature review. J Emerg Med 2000;18:65–70.

43. Dallal A, Chouinard G: Withdrawal and rebound symptoms associated with abrupt discontinuation of venlafaxine. J Clin Psychopharmacol 1998;18:343–344

44. Daly JW, Fedholm BB. Caffeine—An atypical drug of dependence. Drug Alcohol Depend 1998;51:199–206.

45. D'Apolito KC, McRorie TI: Pharmacologic management of neonatal abstinence syndrome. J Perinat Neonat Nurs 1996;9:70–80.

46. Dave JR, Tabakoff B: Ethanol withdrawal seizures produce increased c-fos mRNA in mouse brain. Mol Pharmacol 1990;37: 367–371.

47. Davidson M, Shanley B, Wilce P: Increased NMDA-induced excitability during ethanol withdrawal: A behavioural and histological study. Brain Res 1995; 674:91–96.

48. Davies H, Chan NN, Dhiile WS, O'Shea D: Listeria meningoencephalitis masked by alcohol withdrawal. J R Soc Med 1999;92: 196–197.

49. Dews PB, Curtis GL, Hanford KJ, O'Brien CP: The frequency of caffeine withdrawal in a population based survey in a controlled, blinded pilot experiment. J Clin Pharmacol 1999;39:1221–1232.

50. Diamond I, Gordon AS: Cellular and molecular neuroscience of alcoholism. Physiol Rev 1977;77:1–20.

51. D'Onofrio G, Rathlev, NK, Ulrich AS, Fish SS, Freedland ES: Lorazepam for the prevention of recurrent seizures related to alcohol. N Engl J Med 1999;340:915–919.

52. Dyer C: Addict died after rapid opiate detoxification. BMJ 1998; 316:170.

53. Earnest MP, Yarnell PR: Seizure admissions to a city hospital: The role of alcohol. Epilepsia 1976;17:387–393.

54. Eckardt MJ, Campbell GA, Marietta CA, et al: Ethanol dependence and withdrawal selectively alter localized cerebral glucose utilization. Brain Res 1992;584:244–250.

55. Essig CF, Jones E, Lam RC: The effect of pentobarbital on alcohol withdrawal in dogs. Arch Neurol 1969;20:554–558.

56. Farfan Sedano A, Gomez Antunez M, Martinez Cilleros MC, Cuenca Carvajal C, Girones Pereze JM, Garcia Castano J: Alcohol

withdrawal syndrome: Clinical and analytical manifestations and treatment. An Med Interna 1997;14:604–606.

57. Farsang C, Kaposci J, Vajda L, et al: Reversal by naloxone of the antihypertensive action of clonidine: Involvement of the sympathetic nervous system. Circulation 1984;69:461–467.

58. Ferguson JA, Suelzer CJ, Eckert GJ, et al: Risk factors for delirium tremens development. J Gen Intern Med 1996;11:410–414.

59. Feussner KR: Computed tomography brain scanning in alcohol withdrawal seizures. Ann Intern Med 1981;94:519–524.

60. Fifkova E, Eason H, Bueltmann K, Lanman J: Changes in GABAergic and non-GABAergic synapses during chronic ethanol exposure and withdrawal in the dentate fascia of LS and SS mice. Alcohol Clin Exp Res 1994;18:989–997.

61. Foy A, Kay J: The incidence of alcohol-related problems and the risk of alcohol withdrawal in a general hospital population. Drug Alcohol Rev 1995;14:49–54.

62. Frankushen D: Significance of hypomagnesemia in alcoholic patients. Am J Med 1964;37:802–807.

63. Franz DN, Hare BD, McCloskey KL: Spinal sympathetic neurons: Possible site of opiate-withdrawal suppression by clonidine. Science 1982;215:1643–1645.

64. French-Mullen JMH, Barker JL, Rogawski MA: Calcium current block by pentobarbital, phenobarbital, and CHEB but not (+)pentobarbital in acutely isolated hippocampal CA1 neurons: Comparison with effects on GABA-activated Cl-current. J Neurosci 1993;13:3211–3221.

65. Friedhoff AJ, Zitrin A: A comparison of the effects of paraldehyde and chlorpromazine in delirium tremens. N Y State J Med 1959;59:1060–1063.

66. Fuasen GW, Nathan MS, Duyon S: Acute complications following ultra-rapid opiate detoxification. J Toxicol Clin Toxicol 1997:35;538–539.

67. Galloway GP, Frederick SL, Staggers FE Jr, et al: Gamma-hydroxybutyrate: An emerging drug of abuse that causes physical dependence. Addiction 1997;92:89–96.

68. Geiderman JM, Goodman SL, Cohen DB: Magnesium: The forgotten electrolyte. JACEP 1979;8:204–209.

69. Gentilello LM, Donovam DM, Dunn CW, Rivara FP: Alcohol interventions in trauma centers. JAMA 1992;267:2756–2759.

70. Glue P, Nutt D: Overexcitement and disinhibition. Dynamic neurotransmitter interactions in alcohol withdrawal. Br J Psychiatry 1990;157:491–499.

71. Golbert TM, Sanz CJ, Rose HD, et al: Comparative evaluation of treatments of alcohol withdrawal syndromes. JAMA 1967;201:99–102.

72. Gold MS, Redmond DE, Kleber HD: Clonidine blocks acute opiate withdrawal symptoms. Lancet 1978;2:599–602.

73. Gonzalez JP, Brogden RN: Naltrexone. A review of its pharmacodynamic and pharmacokinetic properties and therapeutic efficacy in the management of opioid dependence. Drugs 1988;35:192–213.

74. Gooberman L: Rapid opioid detoxification [letter]. JAMA 1998;279:1871.

75. Greenblatt DJ, Gross PL, Harris J, et al: Fatal hyperthermia following haloperidol therapy of sedative hypnotic withdrawal. J Clin Psychiatry 1978;39:673–675.

76. Greenland P, Southwick WH: Hyperthermia associated with chlorpromazine and full sheet restraint. Am J Psychiatry 1978;135:1234–1235.

77. Haverkos GP, DiSalvo RP, Imhoff TE: Fatal seizures after flumazenil administration in a patient with mixed overdose. Ann Pharmacother 1994;28:1347–1349.

78. Harris RA, Mihic SJ, Valenzuela CF: Alcohol and benzodiazepines: Recent mechanistic studies. Drug Alcohol Depend 1998;51:155–164.

79. Hayashida M, Alterman A, McLellan T, et al: Is inpatient medical alcohol detoxification justified? Results of a randomized, controlled study. NIDA Res Monogr 1988;81:19–25.

80. Heinala P, Piepponen T, Heikkinen H: Diazepam loading in alcohol withdrawal: Clinical pharmacokinetics. Int J Clin Pharmacol Ther Toxicol 1990;28:211–217.

81. Herzlinger RA, Kandall SR, Vaughan HG Jr: Neonatal seizures associated with narcotic withdrawal. J Pediatr 1977:91;638–641.

82. Hobbs RW, Rall TW, Verdoorn TA: Hypnotics and sedatives: Ethanol. In: Hardman JG, Limbird LE, Molinoff PB, Ruddon RW, eds: Goodman and Gilman's The Pharmacological Basis of Therapeutics, 9th ed. New York, Macmillan, 1996, pp. 374–377.

83. Hoey LL, Nahum A, Vance-Bryan K: A retrospective review and assessment of benzodiazepines in the treatment of alcohol withdrawal in hospitalized patients. Pharmacotherapy 1994;14:572–578.

84. Hoffman PL: Glutamate receptors in alcohol withdrawal-induced neurotoxicity. Metab Brain Dis 1995;10:73–79.

85. Holzbach E: Thiamine absorption in alcoholic delirium patients. J Stud Alcohol 1996;57:581–584.

86. Horwitz RI, Gottlieb LD, Kraus ML: The efficacy of atenolol in the outpatient management of the alcohol withdrawal syndrome. Results of a randomized clinical trial. Arch Intern Med 1989;149:1089–1093.

87. Isbell H, Altschul S, Kornetsky AB, et al: Chronic barbiturate intoxication: An experimental study. Arch Neurol Psychiatry 1950;64: 1–28.

88. Isbell H, Fraser HF, Wikler A, et al: An experimental study of the etiology of "rum fits" and delirium tremens. Q J Stud Alcohol 1955;16:1–33.

89. Ives TJ, Mooney AJ 3rd, Gwyther RE: Pharmacokinetic dosing of phenobarbital in the treatment of alcohol withdrawal syndrome. South Med J 1991;84:18–21.

90. Johnson H, Bouman WP, Lawton J: Withdrawal reaction associated with venlafaxine. BMJ 1998;317:787.

91. Jones HC: Shorter dosing interval of opiate solution shortens hospital stay for methadone babies. Fam Med 1999;31:327–330

92. Kaim SC, Klett CJ: Treatment of delirium tremens: A comparative evaluation of four drugs. Q J Stud Alcohol 1972;33:1065–1072.

93. Kang MH, Spigelman I, Olsen RW: Alteration in the sensitivity of GABA(A) receptors to allosteric modulatory drugs in rat hippocampus after chronic intermittent ethanol treatment. Alcohol Clin Exp Res 1998;9;2165–2173.

94. Kaplan GB, Greenblatt DJ, Kent MA, Cotreau-Bibbo MM: Caffeine treatment and withdrawal in mice: Relationships between dosage, concentrations, locomotor activity and A1 adenosine receptor binding. J Pharm Exp Ther 1993;266:1563–1571.

95. Keir WJ, Morrow AL: Differential expression of GABAA receptor subunit mRNAs in ethanol-naive withdrawal seizure resistant (WSR) vs. withdrawal seizure prone (WSP) mouse brain. Brain Res Mol Brain Res 1994;25:2000–2008.

96. Kirchmayer U, Davoli, Vester A: Naltrexone maintenance treatment for opioid dependence. Cochrane Database Syst Rev 2000: CD001333.

97. Kraemer KL, Mayo-Smith MF, Calkins DR: Impact of age on the severity, course, and complications of alcohol withdrawal. Arch Intern Med 1997;157:2234–2241.

98. Koranyi EK, Ravindran A, Seguin J: Alcohol withdrawal concealing symptoms of subdural hematoma—A caveat. Psychiatr J Univ Ott 1990;15:15–17.

99. Korpi ER: Role of GABAA receptors in the actions of alcohol and in alcoholism: Recent advances. Alcohol Alcohol 1994;29:115–129.

100. Kosobud AE, Crabbe JC: Sensitivity to N-methyl-D-aspartic acid-induced convulsions is genetically associated with resistance to ethanol withdrawal seizures. Brain Res 1993;610:176–179.

101. Krogsgaard-Larsen P, Scheel-Kruger J, Kofod H, eds: GABA-Neurotransmitters: Pharmacological, Biochemical, and Pharmacological Aspects. New York, Academic Press, 1979, pp. 102–103.

102. Kupari M, Koskinen P: Alcohol, cardiac arrhythmias and sudden death. Novartis Found Symp 1998;216:68–85.

103. Kuriyama K, Ueha T: Functional alterations in cerebral GABA$_A$ receptor complex associated with formation of alcohol dependence:

Analysis using GABA-dependent 36Cl⁻ influx into neuronal membrane vesicles. Alcohol Alcohol 1992;27:335–343.

104. Kuriyama K, Ueha T, Hirouchi M, et al: Functional alterations in GABAA receptor complex induced by ethanol. Alcohol Alcohol 1993:2(Suppl);321–325.

105. Lacy JR: Brain infarction and hemorrhage in young and middle-aged adults. West J Med 1984;141:329–335.

106. Legarda JJ, Gossop M. A 24-h inpatient detoxification treatment for heroin addicts: A preliminary investigation. Drug Alcohol Depend 1994;35:91–93.

107. Levy ML, Aranda M, Zelman V, Giannotta SL: Propylene glycol toxicity following continuous etomidate infusion for the control of refractory cerebral edema. Neurosurgery 1995;37:363–371.

108. Lieber CS: Medical disorders of alcoholism. N Engl J Med 1995; 333:1058–1065.

109. Lineaweaver WC, Anderson K, Hing DN: Massive doses of midazolam infusion for delirium tremens without respiratory depression. Crit Care Med 1988;16:294–297.

110. Little HJ: The benzodiazepines: Anxiolytic and withdrawal effects. Neuropeptides 1991;19(Suppl):11–14.

111. Loimer N, Lenz K, Schmid R, Presslich O: Technique for greatly shortening the transition from methadone to naltrexone maintenance of patients addicted to opiates. Am J Psychiatry 1991;148:933–935.

112. Loimer N, Linzmayer L, Schmid R, Grunberger J: Similar efficacy of abrupt and gradual opiate detoxification. Am J Drug Alcohol Abuse 1991;17:307–312.

113. Loimer N, Schmid R, Lenz K, Presslich O, Grunberger J: Acute blocking of naloxone-precipitated opiate withdrawal symptoms by methohexitone. Br J Psychiatry 1990;157:748–752.

114. Loimer N, Schmid W, Presslich O, Lenz K: Continuous naloxone administration suppresses opiate withdrawal symptoms in human opiate addicts during detoxification treatment. J Psychiatr Res 1989; 23:81–86.

115. Loimer N, Schmid R, Presslich O, Lenz K: Naloxone treatment for opiate withdrawal syndrome. Br J Psychiatry 1988;153:851–852.

116. Loimer N, Linzmayer L, Schmid R, Grunberger J: Similar efficacy of abrupt and gradual opiate detoxification. Am J Drug Alcohol Abuse 1991;17:307–312.

117. Lowenstein SR, Gabow PA, Cramer J, et al: The role of alcohol in new-onset atrial fibrillation. Arch Intern Med 1983;143:1882–1885.

118. Macbeth R, Rajagopalan M: Venlafaxine withdrawal syndrome [letter]. Aust N Z J Med 1998;28:218.

119. Maldonado R, Blendy JA, Tzavara E, et al: Reduction of morphine abstinence in mice with mutation in the gene encoding CREB. Science 1996;273:657–659.

120. Malpas TJ, Darlow BA, Lennox R, Horwood LJ: Maternal methadone dosage and neonatal withdrawal. Aust N Z J Obstet Gynaecol 1995;35:175–177.

121. Manikant S, Tripathi BM, Chavan BS: Loading dose diazepam therapy for alcohol withdrawal state. Indian J Med Res 1993;98: 170–173.

122. Martin PR, Bhushan CM, Kapur BM, et al: Intravenous phenobarbital therapy in barbiturate and other hypnosedative withdrawal reactions. Clin Pharmacol Ther 1979;26:256–264.

123. Matthes HWD, Maldonado R, Simonin F, et al: Loss of morphine-induced analgesia: Reward effect and withdrawal symptoms in mice lacking the m-opioid-receptor gene. Nature 1996;383:819–823.

124. Mayo-Smith MF: Pharmacologic management of alcohol withdrawal: A meta-analysis and evidence-based practice guideline. JAMA 1997;278:144–151.

125. McCowan C, Marik P: Refractory delirium tremens treated with propofol: A case series. Crit Care Med 2000:28;1781–1784.

126. McCown TJ, Breese GR: A potential contribution to ethanol withdrawal kindling: Reduced GABA function in the inferior collicular cortex. Alcohol Clin Exp Res 1993;17:1290–1294.

127. McGowan JD, Altman RE, Kanto WP Jr: Neonatal withdrawal symptoms after chronic maternal ingestion of caffeine. South Med J 1988;81;1092–1094.

128. McKim EM: Caffeine and its effects on pregnancy and the neonate. J Nurse Midwifery 1991;36:226–231.

129. Mendelson JH, LaDou J: Experimentally induced chronic intoxication and withdrawal in alcoholics: 2. Psychophysiological findings. Q J Stud Alcohol 1964;2(Suppl):14–39.

129a. Mihic SJ, Ye Q, Marilee JM, et al: Sites of alcohol and volatile anaesthetic action on GABA_A and glycine receptors. Nature 1997;389:385–389.

130. Milanov I, Toteva S, Georgiev D: Alcohol withdrawal tremor. Electromyogr Clin Neurophysiol 1996;36:15–20.

131. Moore M, Gray MG: Delirium tremens: A study of cases at the Boston City Hospital, 1915–1936. N Engl J Med 1939;220:953–956.

132. Moore RD, Bone LR, Geller G: Prevalence, detection, and treatment of alcoholism in hospitalized patients. JAMA 1989;261:403–407.

133. Nestler EJ: Under siege: The brain on opiates. Neuron 1996;16: 897–900.

134. Newman JP, Terris DJ, Moore M: Trends in the management of alcohol withdrawal syndrome. Laryngoscope 1995;105:1–7.

135. Nicol CF: Status epilepticus. JAMA 1975;234:419–420.

136. Nolop KB, Natow A: Unprecedented sedative requirements during delirium tremens. Crit Care Med 1985;13:246–249.

137. O'Brien JE, Meyer RE, Thoms DC: Double blind comparison of lorazepam and diazepam in the treatment of the acute alcohol abstinence syndrome. Curr Ther Res 1983;34:825–830.

138. Ochoa EL, Li L, McNamee MG: Desensitization of central cholinergic mechanisms and neuroadaptation to nicotine. Mol Neurobiol 1990;4:251–287.

139. O'Connor PG, Kosten TR: Rapid and ultrarapid opioid detoxification techniques. JAMA 1998;279:229–234.

140. Oldham AJ, Bott M: The management of excitement in a general psychiatric ward by high dosage of haloperidol. Acta Psychiatr Scand 1971;47:369–376.

141. Osler W: The Principles and Practice of Medicine, 8th ed. New York, Appleton, 1916, pp. 398–400.

142. Parker G, Blennerhassett J: Withdrawal reactions associated with venlafaxine. Aust N Z J Psychiatry 1998;32:291–294.

143. Peng CT, Ger J, Yang CC, Tsai WJ, Deng JF, Bullard MJ: Prolonged sever withdrawal symptoms after acute-on-chronic baclofen overdose. J Toxicol Clin Toxicol 1998;36:359–363.

144. Peppers MP: Benzodiazepines for alcohol withdrawal in the elderly and in patients with liver disease. Pharmacotherapy 1996;16:49–57.

145. Peris J, Coleman-Hardee N, Burry J, Pecins-Thompson M: Selective changes in GABAergic transmission in substantia nigra and superior colliculus caused by ethanol and ethanol withdrawal. Alcohol Clin Exp Res 1992;16:311–319.

146. Pfab R, Hirtl C, Zilken T: Opiate detoxification under anesthesia: No apparent benefit but suppression of thyroid hormones and risk of pulmonary and renal failure. J Toxicol Clin Toxicol 1999;37:43–50.

147. Picciotto M: Common aspects of the action of nicotine and other drugs of abuse. Drug Alcohol Depend 1998;51:165–172.

148. Plinius Secundus C: Naturalis historia. Book XIV, Chapter 22(28).

149. Pohorecky LA, Roberts P: Development of tolerance to and physical dependence on ethanol: Daily versus repeated cycles treatment with ethanol. Alcohol Clin Exp Res 1991;15:824–833.

150. Pond SM, Phillips M, Benowitz N, et al: Diazepam kinetics in acute alcohol withdrawal. Clin Pharmacol Ther 1979;25:832–836.

151. Prakash A, Das G: Cocaine and the nervous system. Int J Clin Pharmacol Ther Toxicol 1993;31:575–581.

152. Presslich O, Loimer N, Lenz K, Schmid R: Opiate detoxification under general anesthesia by large doses of naloxone. J Toxicol Clin Toxicol 1989;27:263–270.

153. Rassnick S, Krechman J, Koob GF: Chronic ethanol produces a decreased sensitivity to the response-disruptive effects of GABA receptor complex antagonists. Pharmacol Biochem Behav 1993;44: 943–950.

154. Rastogi SK, Thyagarajan R, Clothier J, Ticku MK: Effect of chronic treatment of ethanol on benzodiazepine and picrotoxin sites on the

154. GABA receptor complex in regions of the brain of the rat. Neuropharmacology 1986;25:1179–1184.

155. Rathlev N, D'Onofrio G, Fish S, et al: The lack of efficacy of phenytoin in the prevention of recurrent alcohol-related seizures. Ann Emerg Med 1994;23:513–518.

156. Reid JL, Dargie HJ, Davies DS, et al: Clonidine withdrawal in hypertension. Lancet 1977;1:1171–1174.

157. Resnick RB, Kestenbaum RS, Washton A, Poole D: Naloxone-precipitated withdrawal: A method for rapid induction onto naltrexone. Clin Pharmacol Therap 1977;21:409–413.

158. Ripley TL, Little HJ: Ethanol withdrawal hyperexcitability in vitro is selectively decreased by a competitive NMDA receptor antagonist. Brain Res 1995;699:1–11.

159. Ritson B, Chick J: Comparison of two benzodiazepines in the treatment of alcohol withdrawal: Effects on symptoms and cognitive recovery. Drug Alcohol Depend 1986;18:329–334.

160. Rivas DA, Chancellor MB, Hill K, Freedman MK: Neurological manifestations of baclofen withdrawal. J Urol 1993;150:1903–1905.

161. Robe LB, Gromisch DS, Iosub S: Symptoms of neonatal ethanol withdrawal. Curr Alcohol 1981;8:485–493.

162. Robinson GM, Sellers EM, Janacek E: Barbiturate and hypnosedative withdrawal by a multiple oral phenobarbital loading dose technique. Clin Pharmacol Ther 1981;30:71–76.

163. Rosen MI, Pearsall HR, Kosten TR: The effect of lamotrigine on naloxone-precipitated opiate withdrawal. Drug Alcohol Depend 1998;52:173–176.

164. Rossetti ZL, Carboni S, Brodie BB: Ethanol withdrawal is associated with increased extracellular glutamate in the rat striatum. Eur J Pharmacol 1995;283:177–183.

165. Rupp H, Maisch B, Brilla CG: Drug withdrawal and rebound hypertension: Differential action of the central antihypertensive drugs moxonidine and clonidine. Cardiovasc Drugs Ther 1996;10(Suppl 1):251–262.

166. Saito T, Hashimoto E: Membrane effects of ethanol in the brain. J Clin Exp Med 1990;154:869–873.

167. Saito T, Lee JM, Tabakoff B: Effects of chronic ethanol treatment on the beta-adrenergic receptor coupled adenylate cyclase system of mouse cerebral cortex. J Neurochem 1987;48:1817–1822.

168. Saitz R, Mayo-Smith MF, Roberts MS, et al: Individualized treatment for alcohol withdrawal. A randomized double-blind controlled trial. JAMA 1994;272:519–523.

169. Salloum IM, Cornelius JR, Daley DC, Thase ME: The utility of diazepam loading in the treatment of alcohol withdrawal among psychiatric inpatients. Psychopharmacol Bull 1995;31:305–310.

170. SAMHSA/OAS, National Household Survey on Drug Abuse: Main Findings 1997. DHHS Pub. No. (SMA)99–3295. Washington, DC, DHHS, 1999.

171. San L, Puig M, Bulbena A, Farre M: High risk of ultrashort noninvasive opiate detoxification. Am J Psychiatry 1995;152:956.

172. Sanna E, Serra M, Cossu A, et al: Chronic ethanol intoxication induces differential effects on GABAA and NMDA receptor function in the rat brain. Alcohol Clin Exp Res 1993;17:115–123.

173. Satel SL, Price LH, Palumbo JM, et al: Clinical phenomenology and neurobiology of cocaine abstinence: A prospective inpatient study. Am J Psychiatry 1991;148:495–498.

174. Scherbaum N, Klein S, Kaube H, Kienbaum P, Peters J, Gastpar M: Alternative strategies of opiate detoxification: Evaluation of the so-called ultra rapid detoxification. Pharmacopsychiatry 1998;31: 205–209.

175. Schwartz HS, Yarnell PR, VanderArk G: Focal motor seizures in patients with alcoholism. JACEP 1974;3:394.

176. Sellers EM: Clinical pharmacology and therapeutics of benzodiazepines. Can Med Assoc J 1978;118:1533–1538.

177. Sellers EM, Kalant H: Alcohol intoxication and withdrawal. N Engl J Med 1976;294:757–769.

178. Sellers EM, Naranjo CA, Harrison M, et al: Diazepam loading: Simplified treatment of alcohol withdrawal. Clin Pharmacol Ther 1983; 34:822–826.

179. Seoane A, Carrasco G, Cabre L, et al: Efficacy and safety of two new methods of rapid intravenous detoxification in heroin addicts previously treated without success. Br J Psychiatry 1997;171: 340–345.

180. Shar R, Vankar GK, Upadhaya HP: Phenomenology of gasoline intoxication and withdrawal symptoms among adolescents in India: A case series. Am J Addict 1999;8:254–257.

181. Shiffman S, Johnston JA, Khayrallah M, et al: The effect of bupropion on nicotine craving and withdrawal. Psychopharmacology 2000;148:33–40

182. Siegfried RN, Jacobson L, Chobal C: Development of an acute withdrawal syndrome following the cessation of intrathecal baclofen therapy in a patient with spasticity. Anesthesiology 1992;77: 1048–1050.

183. Silverman K, Evans SM, Strain EC, et al: Withdrawal syndrome after the double-blind cessation of caffeine consumption. N Engl J Med 1992;327:1109–1114.

184. Spangel R, Kirschke C, Tretter F, Holsboer F: Forced opiate withdrawal under anesthesia augments and prolongs the occurrence of withdrawal signs in rats. Drug Alcohol Depend 1998;52:251–256.

185. Spies CD, Nordmann A, Brummer G, et al: Intensive care unit stay is prolonged in chronic alcoholic men following tumor resection of the upper digestive tract. Acta Anaesthesiol Scand 1996;40:649–656.

186. Sporer KA, Lesser SH: Cocaine washed-out syndrome [letter]. Ann Emerg Med 1992;21:112.

187. Squires RF, ed: GABA and Benzodiazepine Receptors, Vol 1. Boca Raton, FL, CRC Press, 1991, pp. 2–10.

188. Stephenson J: Experts debate merits of 1-day opiate detoxification under anesthesia. JAMA 1997;277:363–364.

189. Stolerman IP, Shoaib M: The neurobiology of tobacco addiction. Trends Pharmacol Sci 1991;12:467–473.

190. Strain EC, Mumford GK, Silverman K, et al: Caffeine dependence syndrome. JAMA 1994;272:1043–1048.

191. Strain EC, Stitzer ML, Liebson IA, Bigelow GE: Dose-response effects of methadone in the treatment of opioid dependence. Ann Intern Med 1993;119:23–27.

192. Strain EC, Stitzer ML, Liebson IA, Bigelow GE: Methadone dose and treatment outcome. Drug Alcohol Depend 1993;33:105–117.

193. Sullivan EV, Marsh L, Mathalon DH, et al: Relationship between alcohol withdrawal seizures and temporal lobe white matter volume deficits. Alcohol Clin Exp Res 1996;20:348–354.

194. Taft RH: Pulmonary edema following naloxone administration in a patient without heart disease. Anesthesiology 1983;59:576–577.

195. Tamborska E, Marangos PJ: Brain benzodiazepine binding sites in ethanol dependent and withdrawal states. Life Sci 1986;38:465–472.

196. Tavel ME: A new look at an old syndrome: Delirium tremens. Arch Intern Med 1962;109:129–134.

197. Tavel ME, Davidson W, Batterton TD: A critical analysis of mortality associated with delirium tremens: Review of 39 fatalities in a 9-year period. Am J Med Sci 1961;242:58–69.

198. Thomas DW, Freedman DX: Treatment of alcohol withdrawal syndrome: Comparison of promazine and paraldehyde. JAMA 1964; 188:316–318.

199. Thompson WL: Management of alcohol withdrawal syndromes. Arch Intern Med 1978;138:278–283.

200. Thompson WL, Johnson AD, Maddrey WL, et al: Diazepam and paraldehyde for treatment of severe delirium tremens: A controlled trial. Ann Intern Med 1975;82:175–180.

201. Torrens M, Castillo C, San L, del Moral E, Gonzalez, ML, de la Torre R. Plasma methadone concentrations as an indicator of opioid withdrawal symptoms and heroin use in a methadone maintenance program. Drug Alcohol Depend 1998;52:193–200.

202. Trabulsy ME: Cocaine washed out syndrome in a patient with acute myocardial infarction. Am J Emerg Med 1995;13:538–539.

203. Treiman DM: The role of benzodiazepines in the management of status epilepticus. Neurology 1990;40(Suppl 2):32–42.

204. Tunniclif G, Raess BU: GABA Mechanism in Epilepsy. New York, Wiley, 1992, pp. 54–55.

205. Ulrichsen J, Bech B, Allerup P, et al: Diazepam prevents progression of kindled alcohol withdrawal behaviour. Psychopharmacology (Berl) 1995;121:451–460.

206. Ulrichsen J, Bech B, Ebert B, et al: Glutamate and benzodiazepine receptor autoradiography in rat brain after repetition of alcohol dependence. Psychopharmacology (Berl) 1996;126:31–41.

207. Uzbay IT, Akarsu ES, Kayaalp SO: Effects of bromocriptine and haloperidol on ethanol withdrawal syndrome in rats. Pharmacol Biochem Behav 1994;49:969–974.

208. Uzbay IT, Usanmaz SE, Tapanyigit EE, et al: Dopaminergic and serotonergic alterations in the rat brain during ethanol withdrawal: association with behavioral signs. Drug Alcohol Depend 1998;52: 39–47.

209. Van de Wiele B, Rubinstein E, Peacock W, Martin N: Propylene glycol toxicity caused by prolonged infusion of etomidate. J Neurosurg Anesthesiol 1995;7:259–262.

210. Veatch LM, Gonzalez LP: Repeated ethanol withdrawal produces site-dependent increases in EEG spiking. Alcohol Clin Exp Res 1996;20:262–267.

211. Victor M, Adams RD: The effect of alcohol on the nervous system. Res Publ Assoc Res Nerv Ment Dis 1953;32:526–573.

212. Vinson DC, Menezes M: Admission alcohol level: A predictor of the course of alcohol withdrawal. J Fam Pract 1991;33:161–167.

213. Wartenberg AA, Nirenberg TD, Liepman MR, et al: Detoxification of alcoholics: Improving care by symptom-triggered sedation. Alcohol Clin Exp Res 1990;14:71–75.

214. Wasilewski D, Matsumoto H, Kur E, et al: Assessment of diazepam loading-dose therapy of delirium tremens. Alcohol 1996;31: 273–278.

215. Watling SM, Fleming C, Casey P, Yanos J: Nursing-based protocol for treatment of alcohol withdrawal in the intensive care unit. Am J Crit Care 1995;4:66–70.

216. Weinbroum A, Rudick V, Sorkine P, et al: Use of flumazenil in the treatment of drug overdose: A double-blind and open clinical study in 110 patients. Crit Care Med 1996;24:199–206.

217. Williams HE: Alcoholic hypoglycemia and ketoacidosis. Med Clin North Am 1984;68:33–45.

218. Wilson A, Vulcano B: A double blind, placebo-controlled trial of magnesium sulfate in the ethanol withdrawal syndrome. Alcohol Clin Exp Res 1984;8:542–545.

219. Winkler E, Almog S, Kriger D, et al: Use of flumazenil in the diagnosis and treatment of patients with coma of unknown etiology. Crit Care Med 1993;21:538–542.

220. Wojnar M, Wasileski D, Matusmoto H, Cedro A. Differences in the course of alcohol withdrawal in women and men: A Polish sample. Alcohol Clin Exp Res 1997;21:1351–1355.

221. Woo E, Greenblatt DJ: Massive benzodiazepine requirements during acute alcohol withdrawal. Am J Psychiatry 1979;36:821–823.

222. Worner TM: Relative kindling effect of readmissions in alcoholics. Alcohol Alcohol 1996;31:375–380.

223. Wretlind M, Pilbrant A, Sundwall A, Vessman J: Disposition of three benzodiazepines after single oral administration in man. Acta Pharmacol Toxicol (Copenh) 1977;40:28–39.

224. Young GP, Rores C, Murohy C, Dailey RH: Intravenous phenobarbital for alcohol withdrawal and convulsions. Ann Emerg Med 1987; 16:847–850.

225. Zajecka J, Tracy KA, Mitchell S: Discontinuation symptoms after treatment with serotonin reuptake inhibitors: A literature review. J Clin Psychiatry 1997;58:291–297.

226. Zanis DA, Woody GE: One-year mortality rates following methadone treatment discharge. Drug Alcohol Depend 1998;52: 257–260.

CHAPTER 73

NICOTINE AND TOBACCO PREPARATIONS

Morton E. Salomon

Nicotine

MW	=	162 daltons
Toxic blood level	=	50 ng/mL
Toxic dose	=	1–2 mg (children)
	=	4–8 mg (adults)

Nicotine

At 8:15 AM an 11-month-old boy was found eating cigarette butts out of an ashtray. The parents cleaned his lips and mouth with cold water. Twenty minutes later the child vomited three times. The parents contacted their regional poison center, which advised them to bring the child immediately to an emergency department (ED). En route, via ambulance, the child vomited again. On presentation to the ED at 9:00 AM, the child was noted to be tremulous and diaphoretic with excessive salivation. He had a glassy-eyed look and did not interact with his parents. His vital signs were: blood pressure, 128/78 mm Hg; pulse, 150 beats/min; respiratory rate, 28 breaths/min; and temperature, 99.7°F (37.6°C). Pulse oximetry measured 96% saturation on room air.

Pupils were 3 mm and reactive to light. The skin was pale without rashes or bruises. The anterior fontanel was open (1 cm) and flat. The mouth was clear of particulate matter. Examination of the chest, heart, and abdomen was unremarkable. Pulses were strong. The neurologic examination was nonfocal.

At 9:10 AM, the child had a generalized seizure lasting less than 15 seconds. There was no incontinence, eye rolling, or focal features. The ED staff placed a 28-French orogastric tube into the stomach and lavaged with 100 mL aliquots of 0.9% sodium chloride. Lavaging produced a scant amount of brown particulate material along with other stomach contents. After the stomach contents were cleared, 10 g of activated charcoal were delivered through the orogastric tube, which was then replaced by a nasogastric tube.

Over the next 30 minutes, the child became increasingly lethargic. Neurologic examination demonstrated progressively more hypotonia, and his deep tendon reflexes became undetectable. His respiratory rate decreased to 18 breaths/min and he was breathing diaphragmatically with little intercostal muscle movement. The pulse had decreased to 84 beats/min and the blood pressure had decreased to 76/50 mm Hg. His skin was mottled and cool. The pulse oximeter registered 88–89%. An arterial blood gas analysis done prior to placing the child on oxygen showed pH, 7.44; P_{CO_2}, 46 mm Hg; and P_{O_2} 57 mm Hg. At 9:45 AM the child was intubated and placed on a ventilator. Copious clear secretions were noted from the mouth and endotracheal tube and the child was given 0.2 mg of atropine IV. The complete blood count (CBC), electrolytes, glucose, calcium, magnesium, and renal function tests done at the time of admission were within normal limits.

Four hours after presentation, the child was more alert and breathing more effectively and began fighting the ventilator. He was sedated with a continuous midazolam infusion, but was gradually weaned from the respirator and extubated 11 hours after the ingestion. He was discharged home 48 hours after ingestion in stable condition. Followup examination 15 days later revealed no apparent sequelae.

Fifty million Americans—25% of the adult population—smoke cigarettes despite antismoking public education campaigns, widespread knowledge of its health consequences, and decreasing social acceptance.[6,75] In the United States, 350,000 deaths annually are attributable to cigarette smoking, making it the single most important cause of preventable premature mortality.[54] It is now widely accepted that tobacco use is addictive and that nicotine is the component primarily responsible for dependency.[69]

Nicotine is a tertiary amine. It is a colorless, bitter-tasting, highly water-soluble, volatile liquid that is weakly alkaline (pK_a = 8.0–8.5).[6] The principal source of nicotine today is the tobacco plant, *Nicotiana tabacum*, from which nicotine was first isolated in 1826.[13] Nicotine also can be isolated from multiple plant species in the Solanaceae family. *Nicotiana tabacum* is not the only tobacco plant in this family. The first tobacco to be brought back from the New World to Europe was *Nicotiana rustica*, which contains a much higher concentration of nicotine (approximately 18%) and which is still used in "Turkish tobacco."[37] Nicotine is also found in small concentrations in plants outside the *Nicotiana* genus, and even in plants outside the Solanaceae family.

In addition, there are a number of alkaloids with chemical structures and physiologic activity similar to that of nicotine in tobacco plants and botanical species related to tobacco.[37] Nornicotine, anabasine, and anabatine are structurally similar alkaloids also found in tobacco. Anabasine is the principal alkaloid found in *Nicotiana glauca*.[62] Lobeline, derived from *Lobelia inflata*, or "Indian tobacco," is frequently used as a nicotine substitute.[31] Cystisine, found in mescal beans, is used for its mind-altering properties. Coniine, the lethal alkaloid in "poison hemlock," is also chemically related to nicotine.

HISTORY AND EPIDEMIOLOGY

The principal sources of nicotine exposure and poisoning are tobacco products: cigarettes, cigars, pipe tobacco, chewing tobacco, and snuff. Nicotine is also the essential component of smoking-cessation products such as nicotine gum, nicotine patches, and nicotine nasal and oral spray. Nicotine had a brief application as an animal tranquilizer and was used extensively as an agricultural insecticide in the 1920s and 1930s; formulations of this product are still used by "organic" gardeners.

Sources and Uses of Nicotine

Cigarettes. Cigarettes are the most widely used tobacco products in Western culture and the most likely culprit in nicotine poisoning. When a cigarette is burned, the smoker inhales both gaseous and particulate matter. Nicotine is found in the particulate phase of cigarette smoke, along with tar. The total nicotine content of a "regular" American cigarette varies between 13 and 20 mg. "Low nicotine" cigarettes contain half this amount, and many European cigarettes contain up to 30 mg of nicotine.[8,20,67] When a cigarette is smoked, more than half the nicotine escapes in the sidestream smoke and a large fraction remains in the butt and filter.[2] As a result, a typical cigarette delivers 0.5–2.0 mg of nicotine (average, 1.0 mg) to the smoker.[31] This amount depends on the total nicotine content of the cigarette as well as the individual's smoking technique. The nicotine content written on a cigarette package is determined by burning cigarettes on mechanical smoking machines in a standardized manner.[43] A smoker, on the other hand, extracts variable amounts of nicotine from a cigarette to maintain a steady blood nicotine level. Smokers vary the degree of nicotine extraction by altering the rate of puffing, the puff volume, the depth and duration of inhalation, and the size of the residual butt.[6,43] African Americans extract, on average, 30% more nicotine per cigarette smoked than whites.[55] When smokers switch from "regular" to "low-yield" cigarettes, they often maintain a similar nicotine intake by increasing the number of cigarettes they smoke and by puffing in a more vigorous manner[43] (see Table 73–1).

Not all cigarettes are made from pure tobacco. It is common, especially in Asia, to create cigarettes out of a mixture of tobacco and other products. "Kreteks" are cigarettes composed of 60% tobacco and 40% ground clove. In 1984, 66 billion of these cigarettes were sold worldwide. In the United States, they are especially popular with adolescents because of their pleasant odor and euphorigenic effect. Unfortunately, kreteks are more addicting than tobacco alone.[37] Moreover, eugenol, the major active ingredient in cloves, is believed to be the probable cause of the severe lower respiratory complications—acute lung injury and hemorrhage—that occurs in some users.[37]

Smokeless Tobacco. Smokeless tobacco, especially snuff, has regained popularity in the United States. Because smoking is not involved, the public generally believes that smokeless tobacco is more socially acceptable and less of a health risk.[23,37] In fact, in comparison to nonsmokers, there is as much as 48 times the risk of oropharyngeal cancers among long-time users of smokeless tobacco, in addition to other oral and nonoral health hazards.[12,13,37]

Smokeless tobacco comes in two varieties: chewing tobacco and snuff. Snuff is a finely cut tobacco powder packaged dry or moist. In Europe, especially England, small pinches of dry snuff are inhaled through the nostrils. In the United States, dry and wet snuff are usually "dipped." This involves placing a bite-size amount of tobacco (a "quid") between the mucous membranes and the gums. Chewing tobacco is generally packaged as "twists"—leaf tobacco twisted into ropelike portions—or "plugs"—shredded tobacco pressed into cakes. These forms are chewed or simply placed in the gingival recess. Generally, the nicotine from smokeless tobacco dissolves in the saliva and is absorbed through the mucous membranes of the mouth. However, approximately one-third of smokeless tobacco users swallow their saliva, absorbing additional nicotine in the intestinal tract.[12,13,66]

Snuff contains approximately 14 mg of nicotine per gram of tobacco. A typical quid contains 1.5–2.5 g of tobacco, which the user "dips" for 20–30 minutes. Ten percent of the available nicotine crosses the oral mucosa, producing a total nicotine dose of 2.0–3.5 mg/dip. Tobacco chewers use approximately 7 g of tobacco at a time. The nicotine content of a typical "chaw" is 7.8 mg/g of tobacco. Only 8% of this nicotine is absorbed through the oral mucosa, because the pH of chewing tobacco is only 6.5. Ultimately, the tobacco chewer gets approximately the same dose of nicotine or slightly more than the tobacco snuffer.[11] The smokeless tobacco user who takes 8–10 dips or chaws per day gets a nicotine dose equivalent to 30–40 cigarettes per day, and cotinine concentrations found in their urine are similar to those found in the urine of smokers.[5,11]

Less-Common Sources. Although poisoning from smokeless tobacco usually occurs by unintentional ingestion in children, 1 case report of nicotine poisoning occurred when a child licked the contents of a spittoon.[21] Another unusual source of nicotine poisoning is tobacco enemas. On occasion, tobacco has been soaked in water and the juice of this extract added to enemas for the treatment of pinworm. This practice has produced at least 1 reported case of severe nicotine poisoning.[20]

Green-leaf tobacco sickness (GTS) occurs when a tobacco harvester handles dew-laden tobacco leaves. The nicotine dissolves in the water and is absorbed through the worker's skin, if cutaneous precautions are not taken.[6,37] Transcutaneous nicotine poisoning is also reported in smugglers who hide tobacco leaves under their clothing.[37]

Nicotine salts such as nicotine sulfate were popular pesticides in the 1920s and 1930s. These compounds generally contain 40% nicotine; when they come in contact with moist skin, significant doses of nicotine are absorbed. Several cases of severe nicotine poisoning from insecticide skin exposure or ingestion, including deaths, have occurred.[9,37,52] Although industrial-scale manufacture of nicotine insecticides was discontinued by 1950, these products may still be available through catalogues and Web sites catering to the organic gardener.

TABLE 73–1. Sources of Nicotine

Source	Content (mg)	Delivered (mg)[a]
1 whole cigarette	13–30	0.5–2.0
1 low-yield cigarette	3–8	0.1–1.0
1 cigarette butt	5–7	—
1 cigar	15–40	0.2–1.0
1 g of snuff (wet)	12–16	2.0–3.5
1 g of chewing tobacco	6–8	2.0–4.0
1 piece of nicotine gum	2 or 4	1.0–2.0
1 nicotine patch	8.3–114	5.0–22/24 h
1 nicotine nasal spray	0.5	0.2–0.4

[a]Delivered through intended use of standard dose.

Gum. Nicotine is prepared in the form of gum to assist abstinent smokers with withdrawal symptoms. Nicotine resin gum (Nicorette) is packaged in two strengths, 2 mg and 4 mg per stick. It is designed to be chewed slowly and intermittently. When used correctly, blood concentrations of nicotine are less than those achieved through cigarette smoking, even when 4-mg gum is chewed. Because of alkaline buffers, approximately 53–72% of the nicotine in the gum is absorbed through the buccal mucosa. Additional amounts can be absorbed through swallowed saliva.[6] However, when the gum is chewed rapidly and vigorously, nicotine concentrations in the blood can rise rapidly, producing adverse effects, especially in children.[67] Severe nicotine poisoning in a 20-month-old child occurred from the use of nicotine gum.[65] Moreover, adverse effects are reported in adults who have used the gum while continuing to smoke.[48,67] If the gum is swallowed, it is less likely to be toxic because the nicotine is released and absorbed slowly during GI transit, producing low blood concentrations.[6]

Patches. There are currently four nicotine-releasing adhesive patches available to aid in the treatment of smoking cessation. These patches, designed for 16–24 hours of use, vary in size and nicotine release rates, and contain 8.3–114 mg of nicotine per patch. Only a portion of the total nicotine load of the patch is actually absorbed during the cutaneous application.

Nasal Spray and Inhaler. In 1996, a nicotine nasal spray (Nicotrol) was released in the United States as another treatment modality for withdrawal symptoms during smoking cessation. The metered-dose inhaler contains 100 mg of nicotine in a concentration of 10 mg/mL and is designed to deliver 200 equivalent puffs. Each puff contains 0.5 mg of nicotine of which slightly more than half will pass into the circulation through the nasal mucosa.[47] Absorption is diminished slightly by rhinitis and delayed by the use of α-adrenergic decongestants.[38] The recommended dose is 2 sprays (1 mg)—1 in each nostril—every 30–60 minutes. The user titrates the dosing frequency to withdrawal symptoms, using a maximum of 40 doses (80 puffs) per day and creating a steady-state serum nicotine level of 6–18 ng/mL.

A nicotine metered-dose oral inhaler for smoking cessation was recently released. The device is designed to mimic smoking by providing airway stimulation as well as nicotine replacement. Absorption of nicotine occurs primarily through the buccal and pharyngeal mucosa, but slow deep inhalation can redirect some nicotine into the pulmonary tree and achieve absorption there. An average steady-state serum nicotine level of 7 ng/mL was achieved in a 2-day trial of 15 subjects.[39]

PHARMACOLOGY AND PHARMACOKINETICS

Table 73–2 summarizes the pharmacologic characteristics of nicotine.

Absorption

The typical cigarette smoker will adjust his or her use of cigarettes and pattern of smoking to maintain an average nicotine concentration of 30 ng/mL.[6] Nicotine is readily absorbed from the buccal

TABLE 73–2. **Pharmacologic Characteristics of Nicotine**

Absorption	Lungs, oral mucosa, skin, intestinal tract, gastric acidity inhibits absorption
Volume of distribution	Approximately 1 L/kg
Protein binding	5–20%
Metabolism	80–90% metabolized in the liver, remainder in lung and kidney; principle metabolites are cotinine, nicotine-1'-*N*-oxide
Half-life	1–4 h, shorter in smokers (average, 2 h); half-life of cotinine is 19 h
Elimination	2–35% excreted unchanged in urine

mucosa, respiratory tract, intestinal tract, and skin. The usual site of absorption is the lungs. Inhaled nicotine from cigarette smoke reaches the brain in approximately 8 seconds, with central nervous system (CNS) levels of nicotine rising rapidly and then declining rapidly as the drug is redistributed to other tissues.[6,31] The cigarette smoker achieves a blood nicotine concentration of 5–30 ng/mL after a single cigarette.[6]

Nicotine from cigar and pipe tobacco as well as chewing tobacco, snuff, and nicotine resin chewing gum is generally absorbed through the buccal mucosa. Pipe and cigar tobacco are air-cured to achieve an alkaline pH of 8.50. Smokeless tobaccos and nicotine gum are buffered. The alkaline pH of all of these products enhances buccal absorption.[6] Smokeless tobacco users generally achieve nicotine concentrations comparable to those of cigarette smokers. Pipe and cigar smokers usually average lower nicotine concentrations, unless they inhale the smoke from these products.[6]

Ingested tobacco is poorly absorbed across the gastric mucosa because the acidic pH of the stomach keeps the nicotine ionized.[28,34] Nicotine absorption increases again in the alkaline milieu of the intestines.

Nicotine generally achieves a volume of distribution of 1 L/kg. It readily crosses the placenta and is also transmitted in small concentrations in breast milk.[6]

Metabolism/Elimination

Habitual tobacco users generally metabolize 80–90% of their nicotine intake, excreting 10–20% in urine unchanged. Metabolism takes place primarily in the P450 system of the liver, but also, to a lesser extent, in the kidney and lung.[9,31] The two major oxidative metabolites of nicotine are cotinine and nicotine–1-*N*-oxide. Both of these compounds are pharmacologically inactive and are excreted primarily by the kidney.[6,31]

The half-life of nicotine is 1–4 hours but generally averages 2 hours in chronic users.[6,31] Because nicotine metabolism in the liver is an inducible transformation, smokers metabolize the drug more rapidly than nonsmokers. The elimination half-life of cotinine is approximately 19 hours, making cotinine levels in the urine a better marker of recent tobacco use and total tobacco exposure.[6,31] Clearance of cotinine is slower in African Americans.[55]

Renal excretion of unchanged nicotine can vary from 2–35% of the total dose,[6] depending on urine flow and urine pH. Experimentally, acidification of the urine traps nicotine ions and enhances direct elimination.[6,20] Nonsmokers eliminate a larger proportion of nicotine unchanged in the urine because of their slower hepatic metabolism.[34]

Drug Interactions

A number of studies demonstrate that smokers have altered metabolism of many commonly used medications. Smokers metabolize the compounds listed in Table 73–3 more quickly than do nonsmokers.[31,34] Nicotine itself is metabolized more rapidly in smokers. The therapeutic effectiveness of opioids, benzodiazepines, nifedipine, and β-adrenergic antagonists is diminished in smokers.[31] Smokers with peptic ulcer disease are also more likely to fail treatment with H$_2$ antagonists and antacids.[6] The presumed mechanism for this change in drug metabolism is induction of microsomal enzyme systems. However, because there are 3000 components to tobacco smoke, it is difficult to know exactly which components affect metabolism. In all likelihood, nicotine is not responsible for the induction. For example, IV nicotine does not affect theophylline metabolism in humans.[6] It is more likely that polynuclear aromatic hydrocarbons (PAH), released by the combustion of tobacco, are responsible for the induction of P448 microsomal enzymes in the liver.[34] Drugs whose metabolism is affected by smoking are in part metabolized by this system. In contrast, drugs using the P450 system exclusively are not affected by chronic smoking.[34] This conclusion would be further supported by demonstrating the absence of drug interactions in users of smokeless tobacco, nicotine gum, and transdermal nicotine patches (TNP) users. Nicotine and ethanol are frequently used concomitantly. Animal studies demonstrate that pretreatment with ethanol exaggerates cardiovascular responses to IV nicotine. Heart rate and blood pressure increase in an additive way. Smokers are more apt to suffer from dysrhythmias and sudden death during alcohol use. It is likely that this is the result of increased oxygen demand triggered by additive cardiovascular stimulation.[7] Because ethanol does not influence the rate of nicotine metabolism, the etiology of this additive response is unclear.

PATHOPHYSIOLOGY

Nicotine binds stereospecifically to select acetylcholine receptors, generally referred to as nicotine receptors[6,31] (Chap. 10). There are nicotine receptors throughout the body, particularly in the autonomic ganglia, adrenal medulla, central nervous system, spinal cord, neuromuscular junctions, and chemoreceptors of the carotid and aortic bodies.[6,31] In the CNS, the highest density of nicotine receptors can be found in the limbic system, midbrain, and brainstem.[6] The physiologic effects on the CNS are similarly multiple, complex, and dose-dependent. At doses commonly encountered with tobacco use there is stimulation of the reticular activating system and an alerting pattern on electroencephalogram (EEG).[31,65] There is a facilitation of memory and attention, with a decrease in aggression and irritability.[31] Although nicotine might reduce skeletal muscular tone and decrease deep-tendon reflexes, its central and neuromuscular stimulatory effects can also produce

TABLE 73–3. Drugs with Enhanced Metabolism in Smokers

β Adrenergic antagonists (select agents)	Nicotine
Benzodiazepines	Opioids
Caffeine	Phenacetin
Cyclic antidepressants (select agents)	Theophylline
H$_2$ histamine antagonists	

tremor.[31,62] At very high doses, nicotine induces seizures. Studies in mice suggest that nicotine-induced seizures can be controlled by the neuroinhibitory agent 3-α-ol-20-one. It is therefore postulated that nicotine produces seizures at high doses by a CNS disinhibition mechanism at CNS nicotine receptor synapses.[40]

Gastrointestinal effects are probably mediated by nicotine stimulation of vagal centers in the medulla oblongata. Even at low doses, nicotine exposure produces nausea and vomiting in the inexperienced, nontolerant tobacco user. Nicotine also increases gastroesophageal reflux, probably by either lowering sphincter pressure or increasing acid secretion.[59] Diarrhea can be stimulated by larger doses of nicotine, which is probably mediated by both central and parasympathetic excitation.[20,31]

Nicotine exerts a number of endocrinologic effects either by acting directly on nicotine receptors in the endocrine gland or by stimulating neurohumoral pathways in the CNS. It enhances release of catecholamines. It also stimulates the production of vasopressin (antidiuretic hormone (ADH)), growth hormone, adrenocorticotropin (ACTH), cortisol, prolactin, serotonin, and β-endorphins. Nicotine also affects pancreatic exocrine functions. Rats pretreated with nicotine doses comparable to the exposure of moderate smokers exhibit increased amylase, trypsin, and chymotrypsin activity.[15] With repeated exposure, tolerance develops to many of these effects.[6]

Nicotine suppresses the appetite for food, especially sweet foods, while increasing basal energy expenditures. These effects explain why nicotine promotes weight loss. Smokers weigh, on average, 6–10 lbs less than nonsmokers. With repeated exposure, tolerance develops to many of these effects.[6,31] Habitual use of nicotine also decreases estrogen levels in female smokers, probably by promoting hydroxylation of estradiol. As a result, women who smoke are at increased risk for osteoporosis.

CLINICAL MANIFESTATIONS

More than 60% of reported nicotine exposures produce no toxicity and only 1% produced moderate to major toxicity. This low proportion of serious poisoning is not surprising, because 98% of exposures are unintentional and more than 90% occur in children younger than 6 years of age[8] (Chap. 116). Nonetheless, serious exposures do occur, even in young children, and seem to be dose related. In one report, approximately 45% of 51 childhood exposures to nicotine resulted in some degree of symptomatology. Only 8 (16%) of these 51 children required evaluation by a physician and only 4 children (8%) developed significant symptomatology (lethargy, unresponsiveness, limb jerking).[67] Similarly, another study reported that only 1 of 20 children who ingested nicotine became moderately ill and required 24 hours of hospitalization.[8] Most unintentional exposures in small children result from the ingestion of tobacco products. The tobacco itself usually induces spontaneous vomiting, which limits absorption of the toxin.

A child who ingests 1 or more cigarettes or 3 or more cigarette butts has a 90% chance of becoming symptomatic. Conversely, ingestion of smaller amounts will produce symptomatology only half the time.[75] In a retrospective review of 10 cigarette ingestions by children, the 4 children who became severely poisoned each ingested at least 2 whole cigarettes.[42] One-half piece or more of 2-mg nicotine chewing gum usually produces symptomatology in a child.[67]

Table 73–4 outlines the symptoms associated with acute nicotine exposure. Clinical signs of low concentrations of nicotine, such as those occurring routinely in smokers, include tremor and increased heart rate, respiratory rate, blood pressure, and alertness.

In marked contrast to these relatively mild effects associated with cigarette smoking, when nicotine is taken in "toxic" quantities, as in an insecticide exposure for example, the effects are more severe. The symptoms may follow a biphasic pattern in which there is initial stimulation followed quickly by inhibition.[62] Early symptoms of toxicity often include nausea, vomiting, diaphoresis, and increased salivation. Cardiovascular signs include tachycardia, hypertension, and pallor (secondary to vasoconstriction). Early neurologic manifestations include headache, dizziness, ataxia, and, in moderately severe cases, confusion as well as visual and auditory distortions.[8,62]

In the most severe exposures, these generally mild symptoms can be quickly overshadowed by signs of more extreme stimulation, such as seizures, muscle fasciculations, and atrial fibrillation.[8,62,65] Although seizures do occur, there are no reports of nicotine-induced status epilepticus in nonexperimental conditions. These symptoms are often succeeded by signs of multisystem depression, such as bradycardia and hypotension, and a curarelike neuromuscular blockade that leads to muscle paralysis, particularly respiratory paralysis.[52,62,65] Death is generally attributable to respiratory depression or paralysis (particularly of the intercostal muscles) complicated by increased bronchial secretions or to cardiovascular collapse.[9,52,62] Timely and adequate respiratory and cardiovascular support generally leads to full recovery without sequelae.[9,52]

Vomiting is the most common symptom of nicotine poisoning, occurring in more than 50% of symptomatic patients. However, it is not a reliable sign of toxicity.[67] Patients can present with lethargy and respiratory depression without prior vomiting or any other signs of CNS stimulation.[9] Moreover, nicotine chewing gum ingestions in children produce vomiting less frequently (20% incidence) than do those with cigarette ingestions.[67]

Following the ingestion of tobacco products, children usually manifest symptoms within 30–90 minutes. When children chew nicotine gum, symptoms are usually apparent within 15–30 minutes, a result of more rapid absorption through the buccal mucosa.[65,67] When death occurs, it usually occurs within 1 hour of exposure. With mild poisonings, symptoms generally last only 1–2 hours after exposure. With severe intoxication, however, full recovery might take 48–72 hours.[65]

As little as 1 mg of nicotine can produce symptoms in a small child. Four to 8 mg of nicotine might produce symptoms in an adult, especially a nonhabituated victim.[20] Forty to 60 mg of nico-

tine is generally accepted as the lethal dose in adults.[20,21,42] See Table 73–1 for the nicotine content of tobacco products and substitutes. In a prospective study of nicotine ingestions in children, the 3 most severely poisoned infants ingested a minimum of 1.4 mg/kg. The 25 asymptomatic children ingested a mean of 0.5 mg/kg, and all asymptomatic children ingested less than 1 mg/kg.[67] These numbers indicate a very narrow range between nontoxic and significantly toxic doses.

Green-leaf tobacco sickness generally produces a mild to moderate illness consisting of nausea, vomiting, headaches, dizziness, pallor, and diaphoresis.[6,37] However, in two recent outbreaks of green-leaf tobacco sickness in Kentucky, nearly 25% of the affected tobacco workers required hospitalization. A significant portion of these poisoned workers were under 18 years.[3,46]

One study exposed dogs transdermally and orally to three different commercially available nicotine patch systems. The topical administration provided 1–2 mg/kg over 24 hours, producing plasma concentrations as high as 43 ng/mL. Two of 12 topical applications elicited mild symptomatology (salivation and vomiting). Oral exposure up to 13 mg/kg produced maximal plasma concentrations of 73 ng/mL, with only mild symptoms (vomiting) in two of 12 oral challenges.[45]

Recently published reports from a 2-year postmarketing surveillance study by 34 poison centers describe toxicity from misuse or from unintentional exposure to TNPs. Transdermal application of 2–20 TNPs in 9 adults resulted in very serious toxicity. Eight patients were admitted to intensive care; 4 had refractory seizures; and 4 required assisted ventilation. However, 7 of the 9 patients ingested cointoxicants in suicide attempts, and the maximum nicotine level recorded was only 27 ng/mL.[78] Thirty-six exposures in children were less severe. Half the children had topical exposures, while half had bitten, chewed, or swallowed the patches. Nearly 40% developed symptoms, but only 27% required medical evaluation and only 5% were hospitalized for 24 hours or more.[77] It seems, therefore, that unintentional exposure to nicotine patches has not yet produced serious toxicity to date.

DIAGNOSTIC TESTING

Toxicologic assay for nicotine or its metabolites is of limited value in the management of a patient with an acute poisoning. The presence of nicotine or cotinine in the urine might reflect coincidental active or passive smoke exposure and therefore does not confirm nicotine as the cause of poisoning.[65] Serum nicotine levels must be determined shortly after exposure and are difficult to interpret. A serum nicotine level greater than 50 ng/mL generally predicts seri-

TABLE 73–4. Signs and Symptoms of Acute Nicotine Poisoning

	Gastrointestinal	Respiratory	Cardiovascular	Neurologic	
Early (15–60 min)	Abdominal pain Nausea Salivation Vomiting	Bronchorrhea Hyperpnea	Hypertension Tachycardia Pallor	Agitation/anxiety Ataxia/dizziness Blurred vision Confusion Distorted hearing	Headache Hyperactivity Muscle fasciculations Seizures Tremors
Delayed (0.5–4 h)	Diarrhea	Apnea Hypoventilation	Bradycardia Dysrhythmias Hypotension Shock	Coma Hyporeflexia Hypotonia	Lethargy Weakness Muscle paralysis

ous toxicity, but lower levels can also be significant in the nontolerant patient.[62]

MANAGEMENT

Unintentional ingestions of nicotine in small children almost invariably involve small amounts, with spontaneous vomiting providing adequate decontamination. Thus, many patients do not need medical evaluation. Individuals who ingest 1 or more whole cigarettes or 3 or more cigarette butts, who acquire their exposures from a more toxic source (a nicotine insecticide or a tobacco enema), who develop symptoms other than vomiting, or who are potentially suicidal, should be referred to an ED without delay. Patients with mild symptoms and no complicating circumstances can generally be observed for 4 hours in the ED and then released if symptoms have resolved.[62]

Initial Management

The patient with a significant recent oral exposure, who has not vomited prior to presentation, should be decontaminated by orogastric lavage. Emesis induced by syrup of ipecac should be avoided because nicotine poisoning may cause unexpected seizures or respiratory depression.[9,67] Activated charcoal effectively binds nicotine and should be used to reduce absorption in gastrointestinal (GI) exposures. Pharmacokinetic studies indicate that nicotine appears in the GI tract, even when administered IV.[67] Because this suggests that nicotine undergoes enteroenteric or enterohepatic circulation, multiple-dose activated charcoal should be administered in patients with serious exposures.

In cases of skin exposure to wet tobacco leaves, concentrated nicotine liquid, or nicotine pesticide powder, the patient's clothing should be promptly removed, bagged, and not returned to the patient and the skin thoroughly washed with soap and water. The medical staff must wear impervious gloves and gowns during these procedures to avoid secondary exposure.

Symptom-Directed Treatment

Because of the variety of stimulatory and depressant effects in the neuromuscular, sympathetic, parasympathetic, and central nervous systems, treatment of nicotine toxicity is a complex therapeutic problem. Treatment is based on a symptom analysis with primary emphasis on respiratory support. Seizures are usually treated with a benzodiazepine. Loading the patient with longer-acting anticonvulsants is generally unnecessary.[9,42,62] Cardiovascular compromise is treated with atropine for symptomatic bradycardia and fluids for hypotension.[62] If hypotension does not respond to fluids, a vasopressor such as dopamine or norepinephrine is recommended.[65] By reversing bradycardia with atropine, there is some risk of creating unopposed catecholamine effects. For this reason, some authors also suggest using concomitant phentolamine, an α-adrenergic antagonist, in the treatment of nicotine overdose.[20,62] Such combined therapy is unnecessary, however, as adrenergic stimulation is rarely life-threatening in nicotine poisoning, and adrenergic antagonism can exacerbate hypotension in the delayed phase. Respiratory compromise, caused by respiratory depression is generally treated with oxygen, intubation and positive pressure ventilation as indicated.

Enhancing Elimination

Although nicotine is a weak base ($pK_a = 8.0–8.5$) and excretion can theoretically be enhanced by acidification of the urine, this approach is not advisable.[9,62] The potential risks of acidification in a patient with seizures and possible rhabdomyolysis outweigh the theoretical benefits.[62] Furthermore, because the symptoms in nicotine poisoning are generally short-lived, acidification is unnecessary. Fluid diuresis may also enhance elimination and is safer but also is unnecessary due to the limited urinary elimination.[9]

Antidotes

There is no specific antidote for nicotine poisoning. Pempidine and mecamylamine demonstrate both competitive and noncompetitive antagonism to the central effects of nicotine,[44] and hexamethonium, a ganglionic blocking agent, prevents nicotine-induced seizures in animals.[62] None of these agents has been used, either experimentally or clinically, to treat overdoses in humans. Although their application is theoretically of interest, new approaches with these agents are not likely to be developed because severe nicotine poisoning is rare and nonspecific supportive measures are almost always adequate when initiated in a timely manner.

NICOTINE WITHDRAWAL AND TREATMENT

Tobacco use meets all of the World Health Organization (WHO) definitions of addiction. There is an overpowering compulsion to continue taking the drug. There is a tendency to develop tolerance to its effects and therefore keep increasing the dosage. Psychologic and physical dependency develops, and the absence of tobacco produces discomfort in the smoker. Finally, tobacco has detrimental consequences for both the individual user and society at large.[49]

Tobacco addiction occurs with forms of tobacco besides cigarettes, especially with smokeless tobacco. Of course, many smokeless tobacco users switch to this product to wean themselves from cigarettes.[49,56]

Individuals dependent on tobacco, like any other substance-dependent individuals, go through multiple cycles of quitting and relapsing. While spontaneous quitting without any special treatment program is the most common route to abstinence, the achievement rate by this method is only 1% of users per year.[6,35] Women cigarette smokers have a lower success rate than men.[53]

Smokers are much more likely than nonsmokers to have other substance dependencies.[35] Conversely, 80–95% of alcohol and drug abusers also smoke cigarettes. It has been suggested that nicotine use promotes the release of endogenous endorphins. Therefore, withdrawal from nicotine might have a strong biochemical resemblance to withdrawal from opioids.[16] In fact one study was able to precipitate withdrawal symptoms in nicotine-dependent rats with subcutaneous naloxone and then reverse the abstinence symptoms with morphine sulfate.[41] On the other hand, nicotine's neurochemical effects on the brain, and on other neurotransmitters such as dopamine, closely resemble that of other psychostimulants. (For an in-depth discussion of the physiology of withdrawal see Chap. 72.)

With so many substances involved in cigarette smoking, it is quite likely that tobacco dependency is a complex addiction, involving both psychological components, such as oral gratification, and physical dependency. It is now widely accepted that the primary addictive component of tobacco is nicotine,[50,56,75] but this is the subject of some controversy and is supported primarily by indirect evidence.

CLINICAL MANIFESTATIONS OF NICOTINE WITHDRAWAL

Manifestations of nicotine withdrawal can occur within 2–8 hours of the last cigarette. In fact, most moderate to heavy smokers experience some withdrawal symptoms as they wake up each morning. Withdrawal reaches maximum intensity at 24–48 hours, and then diminishes over a 2-week period of abstinence. After 1 month, symptoms are gone, except for the cravings for cigarettes and an increase in appetite.[6,63] Approximately 80% of smokers experience withdrawal symptoms when quitting, and withdrawal is nearly universal among smokers using 20 or more cigarettes per day.[6] Nicotine withdrawal is not confined to cigarette smokers alone. The same syndrome is reported in smokeless tobacco users and chronic users of nicotine chewing gum.[6,49]

Most of the symptoms associated with tobacco withdrawal are subjective, leading to an overall feeling of dysphoria. These manifestations, widely described in the literature, are summarized in Table 73–5.[14,27,31,36,49] The most dramatic and intense symptom of tobacco abstinence is a craving for cigarettes, which can continue for months to years.[6] Cravings for cigarettes are less intense and diminish more quickly in people who are totally abstinent, as compared to those who are only partially abstinent.[63]

One study evaluated 7 smokers in a battery of computerized performance tasks over a 24-hour period of abstinence. With increasing abstinence, the smoker's responses showed increased latencies and decreased accuracy.[68] Moreover, EEG studies evaluating smokers in withdrawal show a decrease in high-frequency activity and an increase in low-frequency activity, consistent with diminished arousal.[31]

TABLE 73–5.   Clinical Manifestations of Nicotine Withdrawal

Subjective	Objective
Anger/aggression/hostility	Decreased arousal pattern on EEG
Anxiety	Decreased blood pressure
Blurred vision	Decreased heart rate
Confusion	Diminished psychomotor performance
Constipation	Impaired short-term memory
Craving for cigarettes	Reduced plasma catecholamines
Drowsiness	Weight gain
Gastrointestinal upset	
Headache	
Hunger	
Impaired concentration	
Irritability/impatience	
Moodiness	
Restlessness	
Sleep disturbance	

The most common objective physical manifestation of nicotine abstinence is a decrease in heart rate by a mean of 9 beats/min within the first day of abstinence; it is a unique feature of nicotine withdrawal syndrome.[27] This decrease remains constant when measured over the next 5 weeks of abstinence, suggesting that heart rate reduction in tobacco abstinence reflects the absence of stimulation from nicotine, rather than withdrawal symptomatology.[76] Plasma levels of epinephrine and norepinephrine also decrease in abstinent smokers. This is probably another manifestation of the absence of nicotine effect and undoubtedly contributes to the reduction in mean heart rate.[17]

MANAGEMENT OF ACUTE NICOTINE WITHDRAWAL

In clinical practice, nicotine withdrawal syndrome is encountered when tobacco users attempt to quit in the interest of their long-term health or when acute illness forces abstinence. The discomfort is a primary obstacle to smoking cessation and contributes significantly, but not solely, to the low success rate of attempts to quit smoking. Therefore, any treatment approach that lessens nicotine withdrawal symptoms, without reinitiating the use of tobacco products, is more likely to aid the effort to quit, which in turn will have many long-term health benefits. An in-depth discussion of smoking cessation management falls outside the purview of a textbook on toxicologic "emergencies." However, a brief summary is included because of the current medical and public health significance of this subject.

Nicotine Replacement Therapy

One approach to the treatment of nicotine abstinence syndrome is to provide nicotine without tobacco. This therapy offers nicotine in a safer, more clinically controllable form that minimizes nicotine withdrawal symptoms. After the patient breaks the smoking habit, the nicotine replacement agent is gradually tapered.[60]

Nicotine gum is the oldest of the nicotine substitution therapies. It ameliorates many symptoms of nicotine withdrawal, especially feelings of irritability, aggression, and dysphoria. However, it seems less effective in eliminating cigarette craving and increased hunger.[10]

The effectiveness of nicotine chewing gum in promoting long-term smoking abstinence has been extensively studied.[32,71,72] A meta-analysis of all these studies, with special emphasis on double-blind, randomized, placebo-controlled trials with 1 or more years of followup study, indicates that nicotine chewing gum in conjunction with a formal program of behavioral therapy can produce 1-year abstinence rates of 29–49%.[1,6,74] On the other hand, when nicotine gum is used in general medical practice, without structured behavioral interventions, improvement in smoking abstinence is short-lived and smoking cessation rates at 6–12 months are similar to those of placebo-treated patients.[4,6,32]

Unfortunately, many smokers who use nicotine gum to quit develop dependency on the gum itself. As an adjuvant to smoking cessation nicotine gum should be used for a maximum of 3 months. However, several studies have reported continued use of the gum at 1-year followup (6–38% of users.).[6,25,26] Self-administration of the gum may reinforce some of the behavioral patterns that sustain smoking. It can be argued that the behavioral components of the addictive process must be decisively interrupted for successful treatment of the addiction.[56]

TNSs have supplanted chewing gum as the preferred nicotine replacement therapy. Because nicotine patches are easier to use (they require once-a-day application) compliance is better. The dose of nicotine delivered to the patient is more predictable, nicotine steady-state levels in the blood are higher, and the different-size patches make tapering easier to control. Finally, because no specific behavioral action is required of the patient, other than putting the patch on in the morning, a TNS does not require self-administration of nicotine by the user and therefore does not mimic oral smoking behavior.[56,60]

There are four patch systems currently available, each of which comes in several different doses of nicotine. Three of the patch systems are designed for 24-hour use, and the newest is made for 16-hour use to approximate more closely nicotine intake patterns of the smoker.[51] The patches generally deliver steady-state nicotine plasma concentrations of 10–15 ng/mL, which are maintained throughout the application of the patch.[24]

Several double-blind, placebo controlled studies have demonstrated that, at 6–12-month followup, TNS users achieve abstinence 2–4 times more frequently than placebo users.[14,19,22,74,75] And many studies have now demonstrated that this long-term efficacy is present even with little or no formal behavioral intervention accompanying the program.[1,14,74]

The most consistent adverse effect of the TNS is skin irritation at the site of the patch. In one trial, approximately 5% of patients withdrew from the study because they could not tolerate the cutaneous irritation.[1]

Both NNS and NOI reduce withdrawal symptoms and promote abstinence more effectively than placebo.[39,70,73] Both treatment modalities are based on the belief that airway stimulation will mimic smoking more closely and therefore be more effective in reducing cigarette cravings. Furthermore, the application of nicotine to mucous membranes provides a rapid transient rise in serum nicotine and thus reduces cigarette cravings more promptly than slower forms of nicotine delivery.[29] Although these characteristics are probably real, the replication of smoking's airway sensations might actually make long-term abstinence more difficult to achieve.

To date there have been no head-to-head comparisons of any of the NRTs. Both TNS and NNS seem to be more effective than nicotine gum in reducing cigarette craving and increased appetite.[29,60] A meta-analysis of 53 NRT trials, with data from more than 17,000 patients, concluded that all modalities were better than placebo in promoting abstinence at 6 or more months. The nicotine oral inhaler had the best abstinence odds ratio, but this is based on data from only 1 study, while nicotine gum had the lowest odds ratio.[64]

Clearly, nicotine replacement therapies are moderately effective in promoting smoking cessation, especially in the short run. To be successful, the patient must eventually face the inevitable—withdrawal from nicotine itself. Theoretically, if other treatment modalities effectively promote tobacco abstinence without the use of nicotine replacement they would have a substantial advantage.

Antidepressant Therapy

Antidepressant medications such as bupropion (Wellbutrin SR and Zyban) offer an encouraging alternative to nicotine replacement in smoking cessation. The idea of using antidepressants for smoking cessation grows out of the observations that nicotine has antidepressive effects; that anxiety and depression are frequent comorbid conditions in nicotine-addicted patients; that dysphoria is a common symptom of nicotine withdrawal; and that women have a more difficult time with nicotine abstinence.[30]

In a randomized double-blinded placebo-controlled comparison study of sustained-release bupropion, smoking abstinence at 52 weeks was 12% in the placebo group and 23% in the 300-mg per day bupropion group.[30] A subsequent trial, compared bupropion SR and nicotine patch, and both together, for smoking cessation efficacy in 893 subjects. The 1-year cessation rate was 16% in the patch group—roughly equivalent to placebo—but was 30% in the bupropion group and 35% in the bupropion-plus-patch group. The bupropion-plus-patch group also had the smallest weight gain.[33]

The sustained release bupropion dose currently recommended is 150 mg twice a day. Patients should be started on treatment at least 1 week prior to their smoking quit date and continued on treatment for 8 weeks. There is an increased seizure risk with bupropion, but generally not at the doses recommended for smoking cessation unless patients are otherwise seizure prone.[33]

SUMMARY

Nicotine, a tertiary amine from *Nicotiana tobacum* and other tobacco plants, is found commercially in a number smoking products and smoking-cessation treatment pharmaceuticals. It is commonly absorbed through the buccal mucosa or respiratory epithelium of the lungs, but can also be absorbed from the skin or intestine. Up to 90% of a nicotine "dose" is metabolized by an inducible P450 hepatic biotransformation, producing 2 inactive metabolites that are slowly excreted by the kidneys. It exerts its physiologic effects on selective acetylcholine receptors, primarily in neural tissue. While the vast majority of nicotine exposures are unintentional and occur in children producing mild or no toxicity, severe poisoning and even death can result, and there is a narrow range between non-toxic and significantly toxic doses. Clinical manifestations of consequential poisoning are complex but can be characterized as biphasic, with initial excitation followed quickly by inhibition. Management is symptom directed with special emphasis on seizure control and respiratory support.

In terms of smoking cessation management, it should be noted that, although several agents will reduce the severity of nicotine withdrawal, long-term smoking cessation is more difficult to achieve. In many approaches to smoking treatment, the overall mean 6–12-month success rate seems to be approximately 25%.[56] This is, of course, much better than the spontaneous abstinence rate of 1%, but as many as 70% of patients who achieve initial abstinence will be smoking again after 1 year.[16] Whatever approach one takes in treating tobacco abstinence, it seems the patient must start with a strong desire to quit, avoid unusually stressful situations, and have a social support network that encourages the effort to stop smoking. The most successful programs are multimodality treatments that combine counseling or other behavioral therapies with one or more pharmacologic interventions.

REFERENCES

1. Abelin T, Muller P, Buehler A, et al: Controlled trial of transdermal nicotine patch in tobacco withdrawal. Lancet 1989;1:7–10.

2. Armitage AK, Dollery CT, George CF, et al: Absorption and metabolism of nicotine from cigarettes. Br Med J 1975;4:313–316.

3. Ballard T, Ehler J, Freund E, et al: Green tobacco sickness: Occupational poisoning in tobacco workers. Arch Environ Health 1995;50: 384–389.

4. Benowitz NL: Nicotine replacement therapy during pregnancy. JAMA 1991;266:3174–3177.

5. Benowitz NL: Nicotine and smokeless tobacco. CA Cancer J Clin 1988;38:244–247.

6. Benowitz NL: Pharmacologic aspects of cigarette smoking and nicotine addiction. N Engl J Med 1988;319:1318–1330.

7. Benowitz NL, Jones RT, Jacob P: Additive cardiovascular effects of nicotine and ethanol. Clin Pharmacol Ther 1986;40:420–424.

8. Bonadio WA, Anderson Y: Tobacco ingestions in children. Clin Pediatr 1989;28:592–593.

9. Borys DJ, Seltzer SC, Ling LJ: CNS depression in an infant after the ingestion of tobacco: A case report. Vet Hum Toxicol 1988;30:20–22.

10. Cherek DR, Bennett RH, Grabowski J: Human aggressive responding during acute tobacco abstinence: Effects of nicotine and placebo gum. Psychopharmacology 1991;104:317–322.

11. Connolly GN, Orleans CT, Kogan M: Use of smokeless tobacco in major-league baseball. N Engl J Med 1988;318:1281–1284.

12. Consensus Conference: Health applications of smokeless tobacco use. JAMA 1986;255:1045–1048.

13. Council on Scientific Affairs: Health effects of smokeless tobacco. JAMA 1986;255:1038–1044.

14. Daughton DM, Heatley SA, Prendergast JJ, et al: Effect of transdermal nicotine delivery as an adjunct to low-intervention smoking cessation therapy. Arch Intern Med 1991; 151:749–752.

15. Dubick MA, Palmer R, Lau PP, et al: Altered exocrine pancreatic function in rats treated with nicotine. Toxicol Appl Pharmacol 1988; 96:132–139.

16. Edwards NB, Simmons RC, Rosenthal TL, et al: Doxepin in the treatment of nicotine withdrawal. Psychosomatics 1988;29:203–206.

17. Elgerot A: Psychological and physiological changes during tobacco-abstinence in habitual smokers. J Clin Psychol 1978;34:759–764.

18. Ernster VL, Grady DG, Greene JC, et al: Smokeless tobacco use and health effects among baseball players. JAMA 1990;264:218–224.

19. Fiore MC, Smith SS, Jorenby DE, Baker TB: Effectiveness of nicotine patch for smoking cessation. A meta-analysis. JAMA 1994;271: 1940–1947.

20. Garcia-Estrada H, Fischman C: An unusual case of nicotine poisoning. Clin Toxicol 1977;10:391–393.

21. Goepferd SJ: Smokeless tobacco: A potential hazard to infants and children. J Am Dent Assoc 1986;113:49–50.

22. Gourlay S: The pros and cons of transdermal nicotine therapy. Med J Aust 1994;160:152–159.

23. Gross JY, D'Alessandri R, Powell VL, Rodeheaver A: Smokeless tobacco: Health hazard on the rise. South Med J 1988;81:1089–1091.

24. Gupta SK, Okerholm RA, Coen P, et al: Single and multiple dose pharmacokinetics of Nicoderm. J Clin Pharmacol 1993;33:169–174.

25. Hajek P, Jackson P, Belcher M: Long-term use of nicotine chewing gum: Occurrence, determinants and effect on weight gain. JAMA 1988;260:1593–1596.

26. Hughes JR, Gust SW, Keenan R, et al: Long-term use of nicotine versus placebo gum. Arch Intern Med 1991;151:1993–1998.

27. Hughes JR, Higgins ST, Bickel WK: Nicotine withdrawal versus other drug withdrawal syndromes: Similarities and dissimilarities. Addiction 1994;89:1461–1470.

28. Hurt RD, Dale LC, Croghan GA, et al: Nicotine nasal spray for smoking cessation: Pattern of use, side effects, relief of withdrawal symptoms, and cotinine levels. Mayo Clin Proc 1998;73:118–125.

29. Hurt RD, Offord KP, Croghan IT, et al: Temporal effects of nicotine nasal spray and gum on nicotine withdrawal symptoms. Psychopharmacology 1998;140:98–104.

30. Hurt RD, Sachs D, Glover, ED, et al: A comparison of sustained-release bupropion and placebo for smoking cessation. N Engl J Med 1997;337:1195–1202.

31. Jaffe JH: Drug addiction and drug abuse. In: Gilman AG, Rall TW, Nies AS, Taylor P, eds: Goodman and Gilman's The Pharmacological Basis of Therapeutics, 8th ed. New York, Pergamon Press, 1990, pp. 545–549.

32. Jensen EJ, Schmidt E, Pedersen B, Dahl R: Effect of nicotine, silver acetate and ordinary gum in combination with group counseling on smoking cessation. Thorax 1990;45:831–834.

33. Jorenby DE, Leischow SJ, Nides MA, et al: A controlled trial of sustained-release bupropion, a nicotine patch, or both for smoking cessation. N Engl J Med 1999;340:685–691.

34. Jusko WJ: Influence of cigarette smoking on drug metabolism in man. Drug Metab Rev 1979;9:221–236.

35. Kazlowski LT, Wilkinson DA, Skinner W, et al: Comparing tobacco cigarette dependence with other drug dependencies. JAMA 1989; 261:898–901.

36. Kumar R, Cooke EC, Lader MH, Russell MAH: Is nicotine important in tobacco smoking? Clin Pharmacol Ther 1976;21:520–529.

37. Kunkel DB: The toxic emergency: Tobacco and friends. Emerg Med 1985;17:142–158.

38. Lunell E, Molander L, Andersson M: Relative bioavailability of nicotine from a nasal spray in infectious rhinitis and after use of a topical decongestant. Eur J Clin Pharmacol 1995;48:71–75.

39. Lunell E, Molander L, Leischow SJ, Fagerstrom KO: The effect of nicotine vapour inhalation on the relief of tobacco withdrawal symptoms. Eur J Clin Pharmacol 1995;48:235–240.

40. Luntz-Leybman V, Freund RK, Collins AC: 5-alpha-Pregnane-3 alpha-ol-20-one blocks nicotine-induced seizures and enhanced paired-pulse inhibition. Eur J Pharmacol 1990;185:239–242.

41. Malin DH, Lake JR, Carter VA, et al: Naloxone precipitates nicotine abstinence syndrome in the rat. Psychopharmacology 1993;112: 339–342.

42. Malizia E, Andreucci E, Alfani F, et al: Acute intoxication with nicotine alkaloids and cannabinoids in children from ingestion of cigarettes. Hum Toxicol 1983;2:315–316.

43. Marion DJ, Fortmann SP: Nicotine yield and measures of cigarette smoke exposure in a large population. Am J Public Health 1987;77: 546–549.

44. Martin TJ, Suchocki J, May EL, Martin BR: Pharmacological evaluation of the antagonism of nicotine's central effects by mecamylamine and pempidine. J Pharmacol Exp Ther 1990;251:45–51.

45. Matsushima D, Prevo ME, Gorsline J: Absorption and adverse effects following topical and oral administration of three transdermal nicotine products to dogs. J Pharm Sci 1995;84:365–369.

46. McKnight RH, Levine EJ, Rodgers GC: Detection of green tobacco sickness by a regional poison center. Vet Hum Toxicol 1994;36: 505–510.

47. McNeil Consumer Products Co: Manufacturer's Product Information. March 1996.

48. Mensch AR, Holden M: Nicotine overdose after a single piece of nicotine gum. Chest 1984;86:801–802.

49. Morse RM, Norvich RC, Graf JA: Tobacco chewing: An unusual case of drug dependence. Mayo Clin Proc 1977;52:358–360.

50. Mulligan SC, Masterson JG, Devane JG, Kelly JG: Clinical and pharmacokinetic properties of a transdermal nicotine patch. Clin Pharmacol Ther 1990;47:331–337.

51. Nicotine patches. Med Lett 1992;34:37–38.

52. Obsert BB, McIntyre RA: Acute nicotine poisoning. Pediatrics 1953; 11:338–340.

53. O'Hara P, Portser SA, Anderson BP: The influence of menstrual cycle changes on the tobacco withdrawal syndrome in women. Addict Behav 1989;14:595–600.

54. Ornish KA, Zisook S, McAdams LA: Effects of transdermal clonidine treatment on withdrawal systems associated with smoking cessation. Arch Intern Med 1988;148:2027–2031.

55. Perez-Stable EJ, Herrera B, Jacob P, et al: Nicotine metabolism and intake in black and white smokers. JAMA 1998;280:152–156.

56. Peters JA: Nicotine-replacement therapy in cessation of smoking. Mayo Clin Proc 1990;65:1619–1623.

57. Picciotto MR: Common aspects of the action of nicotine and other drugs of abuse. Drug Alcohol Depend 1998;51:165–172.

58. Pickworth WB, Fant RV, Butschky MF, Henningfield JE: Effects of transdermal nicotine delivery on measures of acute nicotine withdrawal. J Pharmacol Exp Ther 1996;279:450–456.

59. Rahal PS, Wright RA: Transdermal nicotine and gastroesophageal reflux. Am J Gastroenterol 1995;90:919–921.

60. Rose JE, Levin ED, Behm FM, et al: Transdermal nicotine facilitates smoking cessation. Clin Pharmacol Ther 1990;47:323–330.

61. Sach DP: Effectiveness of the 4-mg dose of nicotine polacrilex for the initial treatment of high-dependent smokers. Arch Intern Med 1995; 155:1973–1980.

62. Saxena K: Suicide plan by nicotine poisoning: A review of nicotine toxicity. Vet Hum Toxicol 1985;27:495–497.

63. Shiffman SM, Jarvik ME: Smoking withdrawal symptoms in two weeks of abstinence. Psychopharmacology 1976;50:35–39.

64. Silagy C, Mant D, Fowler G, Lodge M: The effectiveness of nicotine replacement therapies in smoking cessation. Online J Curr Clin Trials 1994; Doc# 113.

65. Singer J, Janz T: Apnea and seizures caused by nicotine ingestion. Pediatr Emerg Care 1990;6:135–137.

66. Smokeless Tobacco. Facts and Comparisons. Lawrence Review of Natural Products, June 1990.

67. Smolinske SC, Spoerke DG, Spiller SK, et al: Cigarette and nicotine chewing gum toxicity in children. Hum Toxicol 1988;7:27–31.

68. Sunder FR, Davis FC, Henninfield JE: The tobacco withdrawal syndrome: Performance decrements assessed on a computerized test battery. Drug Alcohol Depend 1989;23:259–266.

69. Surgeon General's Report: The health consequences of smoking. Nicotine addition: A report of the Surgeon General. Washington, DC, US Dept. of Health and Human Services, 1988.

70. Sutherland G, Stapleton JA, Russell MAH, et al: Randomized controlled trial of nasal nicotine spray in smoking cessation. Lancet 1992; 340:324–329.

71. Tonnesen P, Fryd V, Hansen M, et al: Effect of nicotine chewing gum in combination with group counseling on the cessation of smoking. N Engl J Med 1988;318:15–18.

72. Tonnesen P, Fryd V, Hansen M, et al: Two and four milligram nicotine chewing gum and group counseling in smoking cessation. Addict Behav 1988;13:17–27.

73. Tonnesen P, Norregaard J, Mikkelsen K, et al: A double-blind trial of a nicotine inhaler for smoking cessation. JAMA 1993;269: 1268–1271.

74. Tonnesen P, Norregaard J, Simonsen K, Sawe U: A double-blind trial of a 16-hour transdermal nicotine patch in smoking cessation. N Engl J Med 1991;325:311–315.

75. Transdermal Nicotine Study Group: Transdermal nicotine for smoking cessation. JAMA 1991;266:3133–3138.

76. West R, Schneider N: Drop in heart rate following smoking cessation may be permanent. Psychopharmacology 1988;94:566–568.

77. Woolf A, Burkhart K, Caraccio T, Litovitz T: Childhood poisoning involving transdermal nicotine patches. Pediatrics (electronic pages) 1997;99:724(e4).

78. Woolf A, Burkhart K, Caraccio T, Litovitz T: Self-poisoning among adults using multiple transdermal nicotine patches. J Toxicol Clin Toxicol 1996;34:691–698.

CHAPTER **74** **FOOD POISONING**

Michael G. Tunik / Lewis R. Goldfrank

Cases 1 and 2. A 30-year-old woman and her 32-year-old husband, on a scuba diving vacation in Puerto Rico, had a local dinner of rice, beans, a large red snapper, home-canned fruit preserves, and wine. That night, approximately 5 hours after dinner, abdominal discomfort and nausea, followed by vomiting and diarrhea, awakened them both. Although they were unsure of the order of events, a throbbing headache, rapid breathing, numbness of the arms, legs, and mouth ensued. Each patient described a feeling of bone and tooth pain with "deep aches in the joints." The woman stated that when she reached for a warm washcloth to rub on her "freezing skin," it seemed to her that the warm washcloth felt cold. This distressing symptom of temperature misinterpretation lasted for 2 days. The vomiting abated during the early morning hours, but the nausea and diarrhea continued for several days. Mild, crampy, abdominal pain persisted for approximately 4 days. The following morning, the couple spoke to some of the local inhabitants. Many of them described similar symptoms that would appear after they ate a large fish, such as sea bass, red snapper, grouper, or barracuda.

As so many people had the same symptoms, the couple did not seek medical help. On their return to the mainland 10 days later, there were no clinical or physical complaints, thus, they did not seek medical care.

The most common causes of foodborne disease are bacteria—*Salmonella spp., Shigella spp., Clostridium perfringens, Staphylococcus aureus, Campylobacter spp., Bacillus cereus, Escherichia coli,* group *A Streptococcus, Clostridium botulinum, Vibrio cholera*; viruses—hepatitis A, E, F, and G, Norwalk virus; parasites—*Entamoeba histolytica, Giardia lamblia, Trichinella spiralis*; fishborne toxins—scombrotoxin, ciguatoxin, paralytic shellfish; chemicals—heavy metals, monosodium glutamate; and plants—mushrooms[108] (Table 74–1).

FOODBORNE POISONING WITH NEUROLOGIC SYMPTOMS

The differential diagnosis of foodborne poisoning presenting with neurologic symptoms is vast (Tables 74–2 and 74–3). Many of these cases are ichthyosarcotoxic (involving toxins from the muscles, viscera, skin, gonads, and mucous surfaces of the fish); rarely, toxicity follows consumption of the fish blood or skeleton. Shellfish poisoning must also be considered. Most episodes of poisoning are not species specific, although particular forms of toxic-

ity from Tetraodontiformes (puffer fish), Gymnothoraces (moray eels), newts (*Taricha* and other species) have been recognized.

Deep-sea fish, eels, mussels, clams, and crabs are all implicated in diarrheal syndromes. In cases of ciguatera poisoning, the major symptoms are usually neurotoxic and the gastrointestinal (GI) symptoms are minor. Scombroid poisoning, which is exceptionally common, is not associated with neurologic manifestations, but facial flushing, headache, and dysphagia are its major signs and symptoms.

Knowing where the fish was caught is often helpful, but refrigerated transport of foods and rapid worldwide travel can complicate the assessment. Scombroid fish poisoning has occurred in the midwestern United States from frozen mahi mahi shipped there.[105] Travelers to Caribbean and Pacific islands, as well as individuals traveling within the United States, have suffered from ciguatera poisoning.[83] In geographically disparate regions of Canada,[116] individuals suffered from domoic acid intoxication caused by the ingestion of cultivated mussels from Prince Edward Island.

In the differential diagnosis of foodborne poisons presenting with neurologic symptoms, activities other than eating must always be considered. In particular, sport divers often perform their activities in high-risk areas (Florida, California, and Hawaii), and often during the high-risk periods (May through August), and in the process may sustain an unrecognized bite, sting (from a stingray tail), or laceration (from a deltoid or pectoral fin spine of a lion fish or stonefish) that can cause consequential marine toxicity (Chap. 103).

Ciguatera Poisoning

Ciguatera poisoning is one of the most commonly reported vertebrate fishborne poisonings, accounting for almost half of the reported cases in the United States.[108] It is endemic to warm-water, bottom-dwelling shore reef fish living around the globe between 35 degrees north and 35 degrees south latitude, including tropical areas such as the Indian Ocean, the South Pacific, and the Caribbean. Hawaii and Florida report 90% of all cases in the United States, most commonly during the spring and summer months, May through August.[57]

There are more than 500 fish species involved, with the barracuda, sea bass, parrot fish, red snapper, grouper, amber jack, kingfish, and sturgeon the most common sources. The common factor is the comparably large size of the fish involved.

Large fish (4–6 lb. or more) become vectors of ciguatera poisoning in accordance with complex feeding patterns inherent in aquatic life. Ciguatoxin can be found in blue-green algae, proto-

TABLE 74–1. Epidemiology[108] of Foodborne Poisoning Reported to the CDC (1993–1997)

Etiology	Cases	Outbreaks	Deaths
Salmonella	32,610	357	13
Escherichia coli[a]	3,260	84	8
Clostridium perfringens	2,772	57	0
Other parasitic	2,261	13	0
Other viral	2,104	24	0
Shigella	1,555	43	0
Staphylococcus aureus	1,413	42	1
Norwalk virus	1,233	9	0
Hepatitis A virus	729	23	0
Bacillus cereus	691	14	0
Other bacterial	609	6	1
Campylobacter	539	25	1
Scombrotoxin	297	69	0
Ciguatoxin	205	60	0
Streptococcus, group A	122	1	0
Listeria monocytogenes	100	3	2
Clostridium botulinum	56	13	1
Giardia lamblia	45	4	0
Vibrio parahaemolyticus	40	5	0
Other chemical	31	6	0
Yersinia enterocolitica	27	2	1
Mushroom poisoning	21	7	0
Brucella	19	1	0
Trichinella spiralis	19	2	0
Heavy metals	17	4	0
Streptococcus, other	6	1	0
Shellfish	3	1	0
Vibrio cholerae	2	1	0
Monosodium glutamate	2	1	0

[a]The fatality rate of E. coli 0157:H7 increased dramatically in the late 1990s.

zoa, and the free algae dinoflagellates. These plankton members of the phylum Protozoa are single-celled, motile, flagellated, pigmented organisms thriving through photosynthesis. Photosynthetic dinoflagellates such as *Gambierdiscus toxicus* and bacteria within the dinoflagellate are the origins of ciguatoxin.[36,64,91] These dinoflagellates are the main nutritional source for small herbivorous fish; as these small fish are the major food source for larger car-

TABLE 74–2. Differential Diagnosis of Possible Foodborne Poisoning Presenting with Neurologic Symptoms

Myasthenia gravis
Botulism
MSG (monosodium glutamate)
Poliomyelitis
Encephalitis
Tick paralysis
Carbon monoxide
Organic phosphorous compounds
Anticholinergic poisoning
Heavy metals
Diphtheria
Eaton-Lambert syndrome
Bacterial food poisoning
Plant ingestions (poison hemlock, Buckthorn)
Migraine
Bends type I, II, III (caisson disease)

nivorous fish, the ciguatoxin becomes increasingly concentrated in the flesh, adipose tissue, and viscera of larger and larger fish.[13]

Ciguatoxin is heat-stable, lipid-soluble, acid-stable, odorless, and tasteless. When purified, the toxin is a large (MW 1100 Da), complex ester that does not harm the fish but is stored in tissues.[90,121] The molecule binds to the sodium channel in diverse tissues and increases the sodium permeability of the channel.[12,122,149] Multiple ciguatoxins are identified in the same fish, perhaps explaining the variability of symptoms and differing severity.[91] People can be afflicted after eating fresh or properly frozen fish prepared by all common methods: boiling, baking, frying, stewing, or broiling.

The appearance, taste, and smell of the ciguatoxic fish are usually unremarkable. The majority of symptomatic episodes begin 2–6 hours after ingestion, 75% within 12 hours, and all but 4% within 24 hours.[13] Symptoms include acute onset of diaphoresis; abdominal pain with cramps, nausea, vomiting, a profuse watery diarrhea; and a constellation of dramatic neurologic symptoms.[166] Headaches are common. A sensation of loose, painful teeth may occur. Typically, dysesthesias and paresthesias predominate. Watery eyes, tingling, and numbness of the tongue, lips, throat, and perioral also occur. A strange metallic taste is frequently reported. A reversal of temperature discrimination is reported, but the pathophysiology remains to be elucidated.[27] Myalgias, most often in the lower extremities, arthralgias, ataxia, and weakness are commonly experienced.[13] Dysuria[50] and symptoms of dyspareunia and vaginal and pelvic discomfort may occur in women after sexual intercourse with men who are ciguatoxic.[82] Ciguatoxin may also be transmitted in breast milk,[22] and can cross the placenta.[114] Vertigo, seizures, and visual disturbances (eg, blurred vision, manifestations of scotomata, and transient blindness) are also described.

Bradycardia and orthostatic hypotension are also described.[45] The GI symptoms usually subside within 24–48 hours; however, cardiovascular and neurologic symptoms may persist for several days to weeks, depending on the amount of toxin ingested. Delayed symptoms may include protracted itching and hiccoughs. Although deaths are reported, none has yet been documented in the United States.[108] Mortality is a result of respiratory paralysis and seizures apparently managed without adequate life support.

Laboratory analysis using an ELISA (enzyme-linked immunosorbent assay) test for ciguatera toxin can be performed; alternatively, HPLC (high-pressure liquid chromatograph) is accurate. The original mouse bioassay was the standard, but was slow, involved the destruction of animals, and did not differentiate the variants in ciguatoxin structure. A rapid test is under development for field use, a dipstick immunobead assay, that will allow testing of fish without laboratory processing of the toxin-containing tissues.[12,62,113] A useful approach to diagnosis and management using laboratory testing is to exclude other diagnostic possibilities and determine the need for, or extent of, specific therapeutic interventions.

Initial treatment for victims of ciguatoxin poisoning include standard supportive care for a toxic ingestion.[84,166] In most patients, elimination of the toxin is accelerated if vomiting (40%) and diarrhea (70%) have occurred. Unless the patient develops symptoms and seeks medical care within 2 hours of the meal, syrup of ipecac is probably without benefit. There may be some benefit from the administration of activated charcoal and a cathartic. A cathartic (sorbitol, magnesium sulfate, or magnesium citrate) should be given only to patients who do not have diarrhea. In

TABLE 74–3. Common Foodborne Neurologic Diseases (Primary Presenting Symptoms)

	Onset/Duration*	Symptoms	Toxin Source/Toxin*/Mechanism•	Diagnosis/Therapy*
Ciguatera	2–30 h *Months to years	t,p n, v, d	Large reef fish: barracuda, snapper, parrot, sea bass, moray (dinoflagellate, source) *Ciguatoxin •Increased sodium channel permeability	Clinical, mouse bioassay, immunoassay *Supportive, mannitol
Tetrodotoxin	Minutes to hours *Days	p, r, ↓bp n, v, d	Puffer fish, *fugu,* blue-ringed octopus, newts, horseshoe crab *Tetrodotoxin •Blocks sodium channel	*Respiratory support
Neurotoxic shellfish poisoning	15 minutes to 18 hours *Days	b, t, n, v, d, p	Mussels, clams, scallops, oysters, *P. brevis:* "red tide" *Brevitoxin •↑ Sodium channel permeability	Clinical, mouse bioassay of food, HPLC
Paralytic shellfish poisoning	30 minutes *Days	r, p, n, v, d	Mussels, clams, scallops, oysters, *P. catanella, P. tamarensis* *Saxitoxin •Decreases sodium channel permeability	Clinical, mouse bioassay of food, HPLC *Respiratory support
Amnestic shellfish poisoning	15 minutes to 38 hours *Years	a n, v, d, p,r	Mussels, possibly other shellfish; *N. pungens;* *Domoic acid •Glutamate analog	Clinical, mouse bioassay of food, HPLC *Respiratory support
Botulism	12–73 h	r	Home canned foods, ? honey, corn syrups, *C. botulinum* *Botulinum toxin; •Binds to presynapse, blocks acetylcholine release	Immunoassay *Antitoxin, respiratory support

n = nausea; v = vomiting; d = diarrhea; p = paresthesias; r = respiratory depression; b = bronchospasm, t = temperature reversal sensation; a = amnesia, ↓bp = hypotension.

patients with significant GI fluid loss through vomiting and/or diarrhea, intravenous fluid and electrolyte repletion is essential. The orthostatic hypotension may respond to intravenous fluids, atropine, and sympathomimetic agents.

The use of IV mannitol may produce a marked decrease in neurologic and muscular dysfunctional symptoms associated with ciguatera. Gastrointestinal symptoms are less responsive to mannitol.[112,115] Mannitol should be used with caution, as it may cause hypotension. Vascular reexpansion and cardiovascular stability should be initial treatment priorities. A dose of 1 g/kg of mannitol over 30–45 minutes appears efficacious. Additional controlled clinical studies with mannitol are needed to define its mechanism(s) of action and therapeutic indications.

Admission to the hospital for cautious supportive care is essential when the diagnosis is uncertain, or when volume depletion, or any consequential manifestations are present. The differential diagnosis includes botulism, organic phosphorus compound poisoning, and other potentially life-threatening processes (Tables 74–2 and 74–3). The etiology of the symptoms must be rapidly identified to provide specific therapy, if available. Diaphoresis is a common clinical finding and an important factor in the differential diagnosis. Late in the course of ciguatera poisoning amitriptyline at 25 mg orally twice daily may alleviate symptoms.[23]

Ciguateralike Poisoning

Moray, conger, and anguillid eels carry a ciguatoxinlike neurotoxin in their viscera, muscles, and gonads that does not affect the eel itself. The toxin has a complex ester structure that may be structurally very similar to ciguatoxin, and which is thermostable.[107] These same eels also possess an ichthyohemotoxin that is resistant to drying but can be destroyed by heating to greater than 65°C (149°F). Individuals who eat these eels may

manifest neurotoxic symptomatology similar to that which occurs with ciguatoxin, or they may show signs of cholinergic toxicity, such as hypersalivation, nausea, vomiting, and diarrhea. Shortness of breath, mucosal erythema, and cutaneous eruptions may also occur. These findings may be present along with the neurotoxic symptoms.[58] Management is supportive. Mortality is related to the complications of neurotoxicity, such as seizures and respiratory paralysis.

Scombroid Poisoning

Scombroid poisoning was originally described with the Scombroidae fish (including the large dark meat marine tuna, albacore, bonito, mackerel, and skipjack). However, the most commonly ingested vectors identified by the Centers for Disease Control and Prevention are nonscombroid fish, such as mahi mahi and amber jack.[108] All of the implicated fish species live in temperate or tropical waters, particularly around California or Hawaii. The ingestion of bluefish in New Hampshire was the probable cause of scombroid poisoning in 5 people,[37] and mackerel the likely offender in 28 cases in a prison. The incidence of this disease is probably far greater than was originally perceived. This type of poisoning differs from other fishborne causes of illness in that it is entirely preventable if the fish is properly stored after it is removed from the water.

Scombroid poisoning results from eating cooked, smoked, canned, or raw fish. These fish all have a high concentration of histidine in their dark meat. *Morganella morganii, E. coli,* and *Klebsiella pneumoniae,* commonly found on the surface of the fish, contain a histidine decarboxylase enzyme that acts on a warm (not refrigerated), freshly killed fish to convert histidine to histamine, saurine, and other heat-stable substances. Saurine has been suggested as the causative toxin of scombroid poisoning. Chromatographic analysis demonstrates that histamine is found as histamine phosphate and saurine is merely histamine hydrochloride.[41,103] The term *saurine* originated from saury, a Japanese dried fish delicacy often associated with scombroid intoxication. The extent of spoilage usually correlates with histamine levels. Histamine levels in healthy fish are less than 0.1 mg/100 g of fish; left at room temperature this level rapidly increases, reaching toxic levels of 100 mg/100 g fish within 12 hours.

The appearance, taste, and smell of the fish is usually unremarkable.[8] Rarely, the skin has an abnormal "honeycombing" character, or a pungent, peppery taste that may be a clue to its toxicity (Chap. 28). Usually, within minutes to hours after eating the fish, the individual experiences numbness, tingling, or a burning sensation of the mouth, dysphagia, headache, and, of particular significance for scombroid poisoning, a peculiar flush characterized by an intense diffuse erythema of the face, neck, and upper torso.[73] Rarely, pruritus, urticaria, angioedema, or bronchospasm ensues. Nausea, vomiting, dizziness, palpitations, abdominal pain, diarrhea, and prostration may develop.[49,73,78,97]

The prognosis is good with appropriate supportive care and parenteral antihistamines such as diphenhydramine and any of the H_2-receptor antagonists such as ranitidine.[20] The toxic substance should be removed or absorbed from the gut. Inhaled β_2-adrenergic agonists and epinephrine may be necessary if bronchospasm is prominent. Patients usually show significant improvement within a few hours.

Elevated serum or urine histamine levels confirm the diagnosis. If any uncooked fish remains, the isolation of causative bacteria from the flesh is suggestive but not diagnostic. A capillary electrophoretic assay makes rapid histamine detection possible.[101] Levels of histamine greater than 50 mg/100 g of fish are considered hazardous by the FDA. Isoniazid may increase the severity of the reaction to scombroid fish by inhibiting enzymes that break down histamine.[66,161]

The patient may be reassured that he or she is not allergic to fish if other individuals experience a similar reaction to eating the same fish at the same time, or if any remaining fish can be preserved and tested for elevated levels of histamine. If this information is not available, an anaphylactic reaction to the fish must be considered. Table 74–4 lists the differential diagnosis of flushing, bronchospasm, and headache. Because many people often consume alcohol with fish, alcohol must be considered as an independent variable.

The differential diagnosis of the scombrotoxic flush apart from, a disulfiram like reaction, includes ingestion of niacin or nicotinic acid, carcinoid syndrome, Zollinger-Ellison syndrome, and pheochromocytoma. The history and clinical evolution usually establish the diagnosis quickly.

Shellfish Poisoning

Healthy mollusks living between 30 degrees north and 30 degrees south latitude ingest and filter large quantities of dinoflagellates. These dinoflagellates form the major source of available ocean food during the "non-R" months (May through August). During this time, these dinoflagellates are responsible for the "red tides" that may be seen from California to Alaska, from New England to St. Lawrence, and across the west coast of Europe.[95] The number of toxic dinoflagellates may be so overwhelming that birds and fish die, and humans who walk along the beach may suffer respiratory symptoms caused by aerosolized toxin.[96]

Ingestion of shellfish, including oysters, clams, mussels, and scallops, contaminated by dinoflagellates or algae may cause neurotoxic, paralytic, and amnestic symptoms. The dinoflagellates most frequently implicated are *Ptychodiscus brevis* (formerly *Gymnodinium breve*), the diatom causing neurotoxic shellfish poisoning; *Protogonyaulax catanella,* and *P. tamarensis*, which cause paralytic shellfish poisoning; and *Nitzschia pungens*, the diatom implicated in amnestic shellfish poisoning. Proliferation of *P. brevis* may cause a red tide, but shellfish poisoning may occur even in the absence of this extreme proliferation.

Paralytic shellfish poisoning (PSP) is caused by saxitoxin. Saxitoxin blocks the voltage-sensitive sodium channel in a manner identical to tetrodotoxin (see below). The shellfish implicated are usually clams, oysters, mussels, and scallops. An increased number of shellfish consumed is associated with more severe symptoms. Symptoms usually occur within 30 minutes of ingestion. Neurologic symptoms predominate and include paresthesias and

TABLE 74–4. Common Foodborne Disease Symptoms: Flushing, Bronchospasm, Headache (Primary Presenting Symptoms)

	Onset	Symptoms/Signs	Cause	Therapy
Anaphylaxis (anaphylactoid)	Minutes to hours	Urticaria, angioedema, bronchospasm, hypotension	Allergens—nuts, eggs, milk, fish, shellfish, peanuts, soy	Oxygen, epinephrine, Beta-$_2$ adrenergic agonist, Corticosteroids, volume expansion, H-$_1$ & H-$_2$ histamine blockers
MSG (mono sodium glutamate)	10–20 min	Flushing, ↓ BP, palpitations, facial pressure, headaches, bronchospasm Shivering (children)	Monosodium glutamate flavor enhancer, in Chinese and other fast food	Oxygen, β-$_2$ adrenergic agonists, volume expansion, avoidance
Metabisulfites	Minutes	Flushing, low BP, bronchospasm	Preservative used in: wines, salad (bars), fruit, juice, shrimp	See Anaphylaxis, Avoidance
Scombroid	Minutes to hours	Flushing, low BP, urticaria, headache, pruritis, GI symptoms	Large fish—poorly refrigerated; tuna, bonito, albacore, mackerel, mahi mahi (histidine)	See Anaphylaxis, Avoidance
Tyramine	Minutes to hours	Headache, hypertension (INH increases risk)	Wines, aged cheeses	Avoidance As for hypertension, migraines
Tartrazine	1–2 h	Urticaria, angioedema, bronchospasm	Yellow coloring Food additive	See Anaphylaxis, Avoidance

INH=isoniazid.

numbness of the mouth and extremities, a sensation of floating, headache, ataxia, vertigo, muscle weakness, paralysis, and cranial nerve dysfunction manifested by dysphagia, dysarthria, dysphonia, and transient blindness. Gastrointestinal symptoms are less common and include nausea, vomiting, abdominal pain, and diarrhea. Fatalities may occur due to respiratory failure, usually within the first 12 hours after symptom onset. Muscle weakness may persist for weeks.

Treatment is supportive, but with early intervention for respiratory failure. Orogastric lavage and cathartics have been used to remove unabsorbed toxin from the GI tract.[35,65,88,102,129] Antibodies against saxitoxin have reversed cardiorespiratory failure in animals,[15] but this therapy has yet to be used in humans. Assays for saxitoxin include a mouse bioassay, ELISA, and HPLC. HPLC has good interlaboratory accuracy,[163] but the differences in saxitoxin derivatives makes standardization of an analytic test difficult.[12,85]

Neurotoxic shellfish poisoning (NSP), is caused by brevetoxin. Brevetoxin, produced by *P. brevis*, is a lipid-soluble, heat-stable polyether toxin similar to ciguatoxin. It acts by stimulating sodium flux through the sodium channels of both nerve and muscle.[9,28] NSP is characterized by gastroenteritis with associated neurologic symptoms. Gastrointestinal symptoms include abdominal pain, nausea, vomiting, diarrhea, and rectal burning. Neurologic features include paresthesias, reversal of hot and cold temperature sensation, myalgias, vertigo, and ataxia. Other symptoms may include headache, malaise, tremor, dysphagia, bradycardia, decreased reflexes, and dilated pupils. Paralysis is not seen. The combination of bradycardia and mydriasis is unusual, but is also commonly seen with phenylpropanolamine toxicity. The incubation period is 3 hours (range, 15 minutes to 18 hours). The GI and neurologic symptoms appear simultaneously. Other manifestations of brevetoxin toxicity include respiratory irritation, cough, and bronchospasm, which occur when *P. brevis* is aerosolized by wave action during red tides. Duration of symptoms is on average 17 hours (range, 1–72 hours).[102]

Brevetoxins can be assayed using mouse bioassay or ELISA, and, more recently, by antibody radioimmunoassay (RIA) and reconstituted sodium channels.[118,158] Treatment is supportive and severe respiratory depression is very uncommon. Therapy includes removal of the patient from the environment and the administration of bronchodilators. NSP is not fatal.

Amnestic shellfish poisoning (ASP) is caused by domoic acid. The etiologic agent is domoic acid, a structural analogue of glutamic and kainic acids produced by the diatom *Nitzschia pungens*. The only documented outbreak occurred in Canada in 1987 and affected 107 individuals who had consumed mussels harvested from cultivated river estuaries on Prince Edward Island.[116] The possibility for other outbreaks exists, because the diatom *Pseudonitzschia australis* has been isolated in shellfish from other areas.[44] Pelican deaths caused by domoic acid-laden anchovies were reported in 1991. Canada instituted monitoring for domoic acid after this outbreak.[155] The death of 400 sea lions in California in 1998 was linked to domoic acid from the diatom *N. pungens f multiseries*.[135]

ASP is characterized by GI symptoms of nausea, vomiting, abdominal cramps, and diarrhea, and by neurologic symptoms of memory loss and, less frequently, coma, seizures, hemiparesis, ophthalmoplegia, purposeless chewing, and grimacing. Other symptoms include unstable blood pressure and cardiac dysrhythmias. The onset of symptoms after ingestion of mussels is 5 hours

(range, 15 minutes to 38 hours). The mortality rate is 2%, with death most frequently occurring in older patients, who suffer more severe neurologic symptoms. Ten percent of victims may suffer long-term antegrade memory deficits, as well as motor and sensory neuropathy. Postmortem examination has revealed neuronal damage in the hippocampus and amygdala.[154]

Tetrodon Poisoning

This type of fish poisoning involves only the order Tetraodontiformes. Although this order of fish is not restricted geographically, it is eaten most frequently in Japan, California, Africa, South America, and Australia.[58] Approximately 100 fresh- and saltwater species of this order fish exist, including a number of pufferlike fish such as the globe fish, balloon fish, blowfish, and toad fish.[104] Tetrodotoxin found in these fish is also isolated from the blue-ringed octopus[40] and the gastropod mullusc,[169] and has caused fatalities from ingestion of horseshoe crab eggs.[68] In Japan, a local variety of puffer fish, *fugu*, is considered a delicacy, but special licensing is required to prepare this exceedingly toxic fish. In 1989, the Food and Drug Administration legalized the importation of puffer fish, but prior to exportation from Japan, the fish must be laboratory tested and certified by two Japanese organizations to be tetrodotoxin-free. In addition, certain tetrodotoxin-containing newts (*Taricha,* notophthalmus, triturus, and cynops), in particular the *Taricha granulosa,* found in Oregon, California, and southern Alaska, can be fatal when ingested. Most newts and salamanders with bright colors and rough skins contain toxins.[24]

Tetrodotoxin is a heat-stable (except in alkaline milieu), water-soluble, nonprotein, aminoperhydroquanizole found mainly in the fish skin, liver, ovary, intestine, and, possibly, muscle.[58,132] The ovary has a high concentration of the toxin, and is most poisonous if eaten during the spawning season. Tetrodotoxin is detected by mouse bioassay. It is unstable when heated to 100°C (212°F) in acid, distinguishing it from saxitoxin. Tetrodotoxin may be detected using fluorescent spectrometry,[11] or detected in the urine of intoxicated patients using a combination of immunoaffinity chromatography with fluorometric high-performance liquid chromatography.[71] Neurotoxicity is produced by inhibition of sodium-potassium pump activity and blockade of neuromuscular transmission.[106]

Symptoms of tetrodon poisoning typically occur within minutes of ingestion. Headache, diaphoresis, dysesthesias, and paresthesias of the lips, tongue, mouth, face, fingers, and toes evolve rapidly. Buccal bullae and salivation may develop. Dysphagia, dysarthria, nausea, vomiting, and abdominal pain may ensue. Generalized malaise, loss of coordination, weakness, fasciculations, and an ascending paralysis (with risk of respiratory paralysis) occur in 4–24 hours. Other cranial nerves may be involved. In more severe toxicity, hypotension is present. In some studies, mortality has approached 50%.[141]

Therapy is supportive. Removal of the toxin and prevention of absorption are the essential measures. Supportive respiratory care emphasizing airway protection, including intubation, if necessary, is extremely important.

Less Common Poisonings: Echinoderms

The sea urchin usually causes toxicity by contact with its spinous processes, but this Caribbean delicacy is also toxic on ingestion. In preparing it as food, the venom-containing gonads should be removed, as they contain an acetylcholinelike substance that causes profuse salivation, abdominal pain, nausea, vomiting, and diarrhea. The starfish is also considered by some to be edible, although there are reports of an asteriotoxin with saponinlike activity that produces nausea and vomiting.

Other Types of Shellfish Poisoning

Oyster poisoning can be caused by a highly toxic venerupin extracted from dinoflagellates. Oyster poisoning has a high fatality rate and is localized to Japan. Callistin poisoning is caused by choline- or histaminelike substances, which generate an acute allergic reaction, and is localized to Japan. Adalone poisoning is caused by a photosensitizer that is extracted from Japanese seaweed. Red whelk poisoning is precipitated by a tetramine that produces curarelike symptoms and is reported in Japan.

PREVENTION OF MARINE FOODBORNE DISEASE

Careful evaluation of the symptoms and meticulous reporting to local and state health departments, as well as to the Centers for Disease Control and Prevention (CDC), will allow for more precise analysis of epidemics of poisoning from contaminated or poisonous food or fish. Many states and countries have developed rigorous health codes with regard to harvesting certain species of fish in certain areas at certain times. A review of foodborne intoxications reported to the CDC over a 5-year period may be representative of the number and severity of food poisoning in the United States (Table 74–1). Some examples of actions taken by state and foreign health agencies in controlling epidemics of fishborne food poisoning are:

- In 1972, the 3230-km Massachusetts coastline was noted to be unsafe for shellfish harvesting. A health emergency was declared because of a blooming of red tide. The state confiscated shellfish and prohibited the marketing, export, and serving of shellfish.[95]
- The Miami, Florida health code prohibits the sale of barracuda and warns against eating fillets from large and potentially toxic fish containing ciguatoxin.
- The Japanese closely regulate preparation and selling of the puffer fish ("fugu"), requiring special training and licensing of preparers.
- The Canadian government marks the location and time of harvesting of mussels, and mussels are tested for the presence of domoic acid.[44,116]

OTHER FORMS OF FISHBORNE POISONING

Filefish forms the toxin aluterin, which produces vomiting and diarrhea. Herring, sprat, sardines, and tarpon may contain clupeotoxin, which causes GI and neurologic symptoms. Ratfish, elephantfish, or chimeras may cause rapid central nervous system depression. Lampreys and hagfish may cause cyclostome poisoning with GI complications. Snek, mackerel, and castor-oil fish may cause gemblid poisoning, which is characterized by dramatic purgation. Mullet, goatfish, and rudderfish may cause hallucina-

tions. Sawara (mackerel) and ishingh (sea bass), two Japanese fish, and sandfish can cause hypervitaminosis A.

Case 3. A 4-year-old child presented to the Emergency Department with a history of diarrhea, vomiting, and intermittent abdominal pain for 1 week. The family became concerned when blood and mucus appeared in the stool after 4 days. At that time blood tests and stool cultures were obtained at another hospital. Antipyretics were prescribed for fever and instructions regarding hydration were given. No antibiotics or other therapy were offered, and the child's diarrhea and other symptoms began to resolve. The parents again became concerned when they noticed the child appeared pale, more irritable than usual, had a decreased urine output, and was uninterested in eating at a favorite fast food restaurant. The child was brought to the Emergency Department (ED) for evaluation after a brief generalized seizure. The child was otherwise healthy with no significant medical history, other medication use, or ingestions. The child was attending preschool.

Physical examination revealed an afebrile child with normal respirations, blood pressure 125/80 mm Hg, and heart rate 150 beats/min. The child appeared pale and irritable. The remainder of the physical examination was significant for a systolic flow murmur on cardiac auscultation, mild abdominal pain without rebound or guarding, and a liver edge palpable to 3 cm below the right costal margin. No meningeal signs were evident, and the neurologic examination was nonfocal. Laboratory studies were significant for a white blood count of 22,000/mm^3 and a hematocrit of 25%; platelet count of 80,000/mm^3. A peripheral blood smear revealed many schistocytes and helmet cells. Serum sodium was 128 mEq/L; potassium was 5.9 mEq/L; blood urea nitrogen (BUN) was 40 mg/dL; creatinine was 2.2 mg/dL; and alanine aminotransferase (ALT) was 180 U/L. Coagulation studies and cerebrospinal fluid (CSF) analysis were normal.

FOODBORNE POISONING ASSOCIATED WITH GASTROENTERITIS, ANEMIA, THROMBOCYTOPENIA, AND AZOTEMIA

This constellation of findings is typical for the hemolytic uremic syndrome (HUS), which is frequently caused by a bacterial gastroenteritis. The most common organism responsible is *E. coli* O157:H7. Other bacteria producing a Shigalike toxin can also cause the same findings. Other agents and toxins also implicated as causes of HUS include estrogen-containing oral contraceptives, mitomycin-C, cyclosporin-A, and radiation therapy.[117] Other nontoxicologic causes of this clinical picture include autoimmune disease, Kawasaki syndrome, eclampsia of pregnancy, and bacterial enteritis/sepsis leading to disseminated intravascular coagulopathy (DIC) and shock.

Laboratory findings typically include a microangiopathic hemolytic anemia, thrombocytopenia, and acute intrinsic renal failure. Other laboratory findings include hyperkalemia, metabolic acidosis, hyponatremia, and hypocalcemia. Liver aminotransferases may be elevated, and pancreatic involvement may produce hyperamylasemia, elevated pancreatic lipase, and hyperglycemia.

Most children with hemolytic uremic syndrome are younger than 6 years of age; many are younger than 2 years of age. HUS begins with a prodrome of diarrhea 90% of the time. The diarrhea lasts for 3–4 days and frequently becomes bloody. Abdominal pain because of colitis is also common. Other frequent findings include vomiting, altered mental status (irritability or lethargy), pallor, and low-grade fever. At the time of presentation, many children have oliguria or anuria. About 10% of children will present with a generalized seizure at the onset of HUS.[140] Postdiarrheal HUS is endemic in Argentina.[92] Frequent epidemics occur in North America, and many of these reports describe the association of enterohemorrhagic *E. coli* (EHEC) or *E. coli* O157:H7 with postdiarrheal HUS.[25,94,109,111,124,165] Postdiarrheal HUS is seen most frequently during the summer months, matching the peak incidence of positive stool cultures in cattle (the most common source of the organism).[59] Food products from cattle (ground beef, milk, yogurt, cheese) and water contaminated with fecal material are the common sources.[33,55,148] Contaminated water used in gardens and unpasteurized apple cider have also caused bloody diarrhea and HUS caused by EHEC.[17,30]

EHEC, including *E. coli* O157:H7, produces a toxin similar to the toxin produced by *Shigella dysenteriae* type I, referred to as Shigalike toxin (SLT) or verotoxin.[43,123] The proposed mechanism for SLT damage is intestinal absorption, bloodstream access to renal glomerular endothelium, intracellular adsorption via glycolipid receptors, ribosomal inactivation, and cell death.[111] In animal models, organ damage is more severe if endothelial cells have high concentrations of globotriaosylceramide receptors. This may explain the propensity for renal, gastrointestinal, and central nervous system involvement in children. Endothelial cell damage and other pathologic processes, including platelet and leukocyte activation, triggering of the coagulation cascade, as well as the production of cytokines, also occur.[70,162] More than one type of SLT exists; SLT-1, SLT-2 as well as variants on SLT-2 structure have been identified.[18]

Detection of *E. coli* O157:H7 through stool culture early in the course of disease is useful. The recovery decreases after the first week of illness.[117,151] *E. coli* O157:H7 almost always produces SLT; therefore, if stool cultures are negative, enzyme immunoassay (EIA) and polymerase chain reaction tests should be used to detect SLT in the stool.[26]

Treatment of HUS should focus on meticulous supportive care, with fluid and electrolyte balance being a priority. Peritoneal dialysis or hemodialysis should be instituted early for azotemia and for hyperkalemia, acidosis, or fluid overload. Red blood cells are transfused to maintain hemoglobin levels above 6 g/dL, and platelets to maintain hemostasis, especially before invasive procedures. Hypertension may be treated with short-acting calcium channel blockers (nifedipine 0.25–0.5 mg/kg/dose orally), and seizures with benzodiazepines. Many therapies have been used for HUS, including heparin, fibrinolytics, IV immunoglobulin, fresh-frozen plasma, vitamin E, and antiplatelet agents. None has been obviously beneficial and some have been deleterious.[137] Plasmapheresis has been used in nondiarrheal HUS and in recurrent HUS after renal transplants. In a controlled trial, antibiotics did not change the course or outcome of children with postdiarrheal HUS.[120] Anti-SLT-2 antibodies have protected mice from SLT-2 toxicity, but intravenous immunoglobulin with SLT-2 activity has not improved outcome in children with HUS. A phase 1 study of the feasibility of using synthetic SLT receptors attached to a chromosorb to prevent HUS is being performed.[7,157]

The mortality from HUS with good supportive care is approximately 5%; another 5% of victims suffer end-stage renal disease or cerebral ischemic events and chronic neurologic impairment. Prolonged anuria (more than 1 week) or oliguria (more than 2 weeks) or severe extrarenal disease may serve as markers for higher mortality and morbidity.[117]

Strategies to prevent the spread of *E. coli* O157:H7 and subsequent HUS include public education regarding thorough cooking of beef to achieve a well-done presentation, pasteurization of milk and apple cider, and thorough cleaning of vegetables. Public health measures include education of clinicians to consider *E. coli* O157:H7 in patients with bloody diarrhea, and routine capability of microbiology laboratories to culture *E. coli* O157:H7 and provide for EIA or PCR determination of SLT. Public health departments should provide active surveillance systems to identify early outbreaks of *E. coli* O157:H7 infection.

FOODBORNE POISONING ASSOCIATED WITH DIARRHEA AND AN ELEVATED TEMPERATURE

The initial differential diagnosis for acute diarrhea involves several etiologies: infectious (bacterial, viral, parasitic, and fungal), structural (including surgical), metabolic, functional, toxin-induced, and food-induced. The differential diagnosis is described in greater detail in Chap. 22.

An elevated temperature may be caused by invasive organisms, including *Salmonella spp.*, *Shigella spp.*, *Campylobacter spp.*, invasive *E. coli*, *Vibrio parahaemolyticus*, and *Yersinia spp.*, as well as some viruses. Episodes of acute gastroenteritis not associated with fever are usually caused by organisms producing toxins, including *S. aureus*, *B. cereus*, *C. perfringens*, enterotoxigenic *E. coli*, and viruses.[52, 99]

Fecal leukocytes are typically found in patients with shigellosis, salmonellosis, Campylobacter enteritis, typhoid fever, invasive *E. coli* colitis, *V. parahaemolyticus*, *Y. enterocolitica*, and ulcerative colitis. In all of these, except typhoid fever, the leukocytes are primarily polymorphonuclear, whereas in typhoid fever, they are mononuclear. No stool leukocytes are noted in cholera, viral diarrhea, noninvasive *E. coli* diarrhea, or nonspecific diarrhea.[61]

The timing of onset of diarrhea after exposure or the incubation period can be useful in differeniating its causes. Extremely short incubation periods of less than 6 hours are typical for Staphylococcus, *B. cereus* (type I), enterotoxigenic *E. coli*,[93,128,153] and preformed enterotoxins, as well as roundworm larvae ingestions. Intermediate incubation periods of 8–24 hours are found with *C. perfringens*, *B. cereus* (type II enterotoxin), enteroinvasive *E. coli*,[34,98] and salmonella. Longer incubation periods are seen in other bacterial causes of acute gastroenteritis (Table 74–5).

The three most likely etiologies are infectious, drug or chemical toxins, and foodborne. These three etiologies are not mutually exclusive. The differential diagnosis must be made among these groups when the time from exposure to onset of symptoms is brief, all of the nonbacterial infectious etiologies (viral, parasitic, fungal, and algal) except for upper GI invasion by roundworm larvae can be eliminated. The possibility of a bacterial etiology with enterotoxin production should be considered (Table 74–5).[42,52]

TABLE 74–5.   Common Foodborne Disease: Gastrointestinal (Primary Presenting Symptom)

Etiology	Onset	A	V	Di	Dy	F	Source	Pathogenesis	Therapy
Staphylococcus spp	2–6 h	+	+	+	−	−	Prepared foods: meats, pastries, salads	Heat-stable enterotoxin	Volume expansion
Bacillus cereus									
Type I	1–6 h	+	+	+	−	−	Fried rice	Heat-labile toxins	Volume expansion
Type II	12 h	+	−	+	−	−	Meats, vegetables	Heat-labile toxins	
Anasikiasis	1–12 h	+	+	−	−	−	Raw fish, sushi, Eustrongyloides, minnows, salmon, cod, herring, squid, tuna	Intestinal larvae	Endoscopy Laparotomy Removal
Clostridium perfringens	8–24 h	+	±	+	+	−	Poultry, heat-processed meats	Heat-labile enterotoxin	Volume expansion
Salmonella spp	8–24 h	±	±	+	±	+	Poultry, egg Pets (turtles, lizards, chicks)	Bacteria, endotoxin (Bacteremia)	Antibiotics
E. coli	24–72 h						Water, food	Enterotoxin, heat stable	Volume expansion
Enterotoxigenic		±	−	±	±	+	Enteric contact		Electrolytes
Invasive							Bacteria (invasive)		Antibiotics
Hemorrhagic							Shiga like toxin		Renal, hematologic support
Vibrio cholera	24–72 h	±	±	+	−	±	Water, food Enteric contact	Enterotoxin Heat labile	Electrolyte replacement
Shigella spp	24–72 h	+	±	+	+	±	Institutional food handler Household, preschool, enteric contact	Bacteria, Endotoxin	Antibiotics
Campylobacter jejuni	1–7 d	+	+	+	±	+	Milk, poultry Unchlorinated water Mimic appendicitis	Bacteria Heat-labile enterotoxin	Antibiotics
Yersinia spp	1–7 d	+	+	+	±	+	Pork, milk, pets: (arthritis pharyngitis); rash	Bacteria Enterotoxin	Antibiotics

A = abdominal pain; V = vomiting; Di = diarrhea; Dy = dysentery; F = fever.

EPIDEMIOLOGY

Epidemiologic analysis is of immediate importance, particularly when GI diseases strike more than one person in a group. The questions raised in Table 74–6 must be answered.[131] If available,

TABLE 74–6.   Epidemiologic Analysis of Gastrointestinal Disease

1. Is the occurrence of the disease in a large group significant enough to be consistent with foodborne disease (two or more cases)?
2. Is the symptomatology in affected individuals well defined and similar?
3. Is the onset, time, and duration of illness similar among affected group members (incubation)?
4. What are the possible modes of transmission (ie, contact, food, water)?
5. Is there a relationship between the time of exposure of the group and the mode of transmission?
6. Do attack rates differ for age, gender, or occupation?
7. Can it be determined which foods were served and to whom? Can the items which were not eaten by those who did not become ill be identified?
8. What is the food-specific attack rate?
9. How was the food procured? How was it stored?
10. Was cooking technique adequate?
11. Was personal hygiene acceptable?
12. Was there animal contamination?

an infectious disease consultant or infection control officer may be called for assistance. Alternatively, assistance from state and local health departments should be sought. Often only the Centers for Disease Control or state health department have the resources to investigate and confirm a presumptive diagnosis in an outbreak. Sophisticated techniques such as toxin detection, matching the organism in the food by phage type with a food handler, matching an organism by phage type with other persons, the isolation of 10 or more organisms per gram of implicated food,[34,42] or polymerase chain reaction (PCR) identification of bacterial or plasmid DNA are potentially useful, although generally not possible using the laboratory and personnel available in most hospitals.[51,63,146]

Structural, metabolic, and functional causes can often be eliminated. As in these diseases, neither a significant grouping of cases nor a limited clinical history is characteristic. Foodborne parasites such as *Trichinella spiralis* (trichinosis), *Toxoplasma gondii* (toxoplasmosis), and *G. lamblia* (giardiasis) must be considered although acute gastrointestinal symptoms are not usually prominent.

Staphylococcus Species

In cases of suspected food poisoning with a short incubation period, the physician should first assess the risk for staphylococcal causes. The usual foods associated with staphylococcal toxin production include milk products and other proteinaceous foods, cream-filled baked goods, potato and chicken salads, sausages, ham, tongue, and gravy. Piecrust can act as an insulator, maintaining the temperature of the cream filling and occasionally permitting toxin production even during refrigeration.[6] An assessment must routinely be made for the presence of lesions on the hand or nose of any food handlers involved. Unfortunately, "carriers" of enterotoxigenic staphylococci are difficult to recognize because they usually lack lesions and appear healthy.[63] A fixed association between a particular food and an illness would be most helpful epidemiologically, but clinically this rarely occurs. Factors such as environment, host resistance, nature of the agent, and dose make the results surprisingly variable.

Patients with staphylococcal food poisoning rarely have a significant temperature elevation, although in a review of 2992 documented cases, 16% had a subjective sense of fever.[63] Abdominal pain, nausea followed by vomiting, and diarrhea dominate the clinical findings. Diarrhea does not occur in the absence of nausea and vomiting. The mean incubation period is 4.4 hours with a mean duration of illness of 20 hours. Most enterotoxins are produced by *Staphyloccus aureas* coagulase-positive species. These enterotoxins initiate an inflammatory response in gastrointestinal mucosal cells and lead to cell destruction. These enterotoxins may have a dramatic effect on the emesis center in the brain and diverse other organ systems. Discrimination of unique *S. aureus* isolates from foodborne outbreaks can be made using restriction fragment length polymorphisms analysis by pulsed-field gel electrophoresis.[147]

Salmonella Species

Salmonella enteritidis infections are a great concern in the United States. Two particular outbreaks define very special problems. In the 1980s, there were recurrent outbreaks associated with grade A eggs or food containing such eggs. In the past, such outbreaks of salmonella enteritis were attributed to infection of the egg with salmonella (from the chicken's gastrointestinal tract) through cracks in the shell. More recently, outbreaks have involved non-cracked, nonsoiled eggs.[100] In these cases, presumably the salmonella has infected the eggs before the shell was formed. In either case, people who consume raw or undercooked eggs are most at risk for salmonella enteritis. Raw eggs may be found as ingredients of chocolate mousse, hollandaise sauce, eggnog, egg-creams, caesar salads, and homemade ice cream. Whole, partially cooked eggs may be eaten as sunny-side-up or poached eggs.[4,145] The second group of outbreaks was associated with raw milk,[119] which has become very popular in certain communities for unclear reasons. Inadequate microwave cooking also may cause small outbreaks.[38] Chronic diarrheal syndromes[110] of an ill-defined nature result. These outbreaks are of great concern because they frequently involve multiple-drug-resistant salmonella infections.[31] Campylobacteriosis, brucellosis, listeriosis, and tuberculosis also result from consuming raw milk. Drinking pasteurized milk may not be protective. An outbreak of salmonellosis resulting in more than 16,000 culture-proven cases was traced to one Illinois dairy. The probable cause of the outbreak was a transfer line connecting raw and pasteurized milk containment tanks.[127]

Additional concern has developed over the widespread use of antibiotics in animal feed. Meats, poultry, and manure-fertilized vegetables now frequently contain resistant bacterial strains that place virtually the entire population at risk.[31,127] Household pets known to harbor salmonella also places families at risk. Chicks, turtles, and iguanas carry salmonella and frequently transmit the organism to household contacts, including infants, who are at particular risk for invasive diseases.[2]

Campylobacter jejuni

Campylobacter jejuni, a curved gram-negative rod, is a major cause of bacterial enteritis. The organism is most commonly isolated in children younger than 5 years of age and in adults 20–40 years of age. Campylobacter enteritis outbreaks are more common in the summer months in temperate climates. Although most cases of Campylobacter enteritis are sporadic, outbreaks are associated with contaminated food and water.[152] The most frequent sources of Campylobacter in food are raw or undercooked poultry products[39] and unpasteurized milk.[168] Birds are a common reservoir, and small outbreaks are associated with contamination of milk by birds pecking milk-container tops.[142] Contaminated water supplies are also a frequent source of Campylobacter enteritis involving large numbers of individuals.[21] *C. jejuni* is heat-labile; cooking of food, pasteurization of milk, and chlorination of water prevent human transmission.

The incubation period for Campylobacter enteritis varies from 1 to 7 days (mean, 3 days). Typical symptoms include diarrhea, abdominal cramps, and fever. Other symptoms may include headache, vomiting, excessive gas, and malaise. The diarrhea may contain gross blood, and frequently leukocytes are present on microscopic examination.[39] Illness usually lasts 5–6 days (range, 1–8 days). Rarely, symptoms may last for several weeks. Severe presentations include lower GI hemorrhage, abdominal pain mimicking appendicitis, a typhoidlike syndrome, reactive arthritis, and meningitis. The organism may be detected by using polymerase chain reaction identification techniques.[48] Treatment is supportive consisting of volume resuscitation, and may include quinolone antibiotics in more severe cases.

Group A Streptococcus

Bacterial infections not usually associated with food or food handling may occasionally be transmitted by food or food handling. Streptococcal pharyngitis can be transmitted by food prepared by an individual with streptococcal pharyngitis.[32]

Clostridium botulinum

In the last 3 decades, a median of 4 cases of foodborne botulism, 3 cases of wound botulism, and 71 cases of infant botulism have been reported annually to the Centers for Disease Control.[139] Home-canned fruits and vegetables, as well as commercial fish products, are among the common foods causing botulism. The incubation period is usually 12–36 hours; typical symptoms include some initial GI symptoms, followed by malaise, fatigue, diplopia, dysphagia, and rapid development of small muscle incoordination.[86] In botulism, the toxin is irreversibly bound to the neuromuscular junction, where it impairs the presynaptic release of acetylcholine.[79] The diagnosis of botulism must be made immediately, and aggressive respiratory therapy must be initiated if the patient is to survive. Additional therapeutic measures include administering antitoxin (Chap. 75 and Antidote in Depth: Botulinum Antitoxin). The differential diagnosis of botulism includes myasthenia gravis, atypical Guillain-Barré syndrome, tick-induced paralysis, and certain chemical ingestions (see Tables 75–1 and 75–3).

Yersinia enterocolitica

Yersinia enterocolitica is a gram-negative coccobacillus that causes enteritis most frequently in children and young adults. Typical clinical features include fever, abdominal pain, and diarrhea, which usually contains mucus and blood.[10,150,164] Other associated symptoms include nausea, vomiting, anorexia, and weight loss. The incubation period may be 1 day to 1 week or more. Less-common features include prolonged enteritis, arthritis, pharyngeal and hepatic involvement, and rash. Yersinia is a common pathogen in many animals, including dogs and pigs. Sources of human infection include milk products, raw pork products, infected household pets, and person-to-person transmission.[19,56,87] Infections may be diagnosed based on cultures of food, stool, blood, and, less frequently, skin abscesses, pharyngeal cultures, or cultures from other organ tissues (mesenteric lymph nodes, liver). Yersinia may also be identified with polymerase chain reaction.[69] Therapy is usually supportive; however, patients with invasive disease (eg, bacteremia, bacterial arthritis) should be treated with intravenous antibiotics. Ciprofloxacin and third-generation cephalosporins are highly bacteriocidal against *Yersinia spp.*

Listeria monocytogenes

Listeriosis transmitted by food usually occurs in pregnant women, their fetuses, the elderly, and immunocompromised individuals (corticosteroid use, malignancy, diabetes, renal disease, HIV infection).[5,16,136,160] Typical food sources include unpasteurized milk, soft cheeses such as feta, and undercooked chicken. Individuals at risk should avoid the usual sources and should be evaluated for listeriosis if typical symptoms of fever, severe headache, muscle ache, and pharyngitis develop. Treatment with intravenous ampicillin or trimethoprim-sulfamethoxazole is indicated for systemic listerial infections.

Drug- and Toxin-Induced Diseases

Careful assessment of the possibility of a foodborne pesticide poisoning is essential. Aldicarb contamination has occurred in hydroponically grown vegetables, and watermelons contaminated with pesticides.[54] Eating malathion-contaminated chapatti and wheat flour has resulted in 60 intoxications and 1 death[29] (Chap. 89).

The possibility of unintentional acute heavy metal ingestion must also be considered. This type of poisoning most typically occurs when very acidic fruit punch is served in metal-lined containers. Antimony, zinc, copper, tin, or cadmium in a container may be dissolved by an acid food or juice medium. Insecticides, rodenticides, arsenic, lead, or fluoride preparations can be mistaken for a food ingredient. These poisonings usually have a rapid onset of signs and symptoms after the exposure.

Mushroom-Induced Disease

Some species produce major GI effects. *Amanita phalloides*, the most poisonous mushroom, usually causes GI symptoms as well as hepatotoxic effects with a delay to clinical manifestations. The rapid onset of symptoms may suggest some of the gastroenterotoxic mushrooms (Chap. 76).

Spicy Food

Certain religious or cultural customs, such as eating bitter herbs at a Passover seder[125] or wasabi[143] at a sushi bar, are associated with syncope. The precipitant in both instances is horseradish. Despite severe oropharyngeal or abdominal pain, no hematemesis, hematochezia, or fever is noted with horseradish. Gastric mucosal contact with pepperoni or jalapeño peppers (capsaicin) may produce a similar syndrome.[53]

Intestinal Parasitic Infections

The popularity of eating raw fish, usually from Japanese restaurants, has led to an increase in reported intestinal parasitic infections. The etiologic agents are typically roundworms (*Eustrongylidis anisakis*) or fish tapeworms (*Diphyllobothrium spp.*). Symptoms of anisakiasis, or eustrongylidiasis, that are localized to the stomach typically occur 1–12 hours after eating raw fish, whereas symptoms of lower intestinal involvement may be delayed for days or weeks. Typical gastric symptoms include nausea, vomiting, and severe crampy abdominal pain that may mimic a gastric ulcer; typical lower intestinal symptoms include abdominal cramping and, with perforation of the intestinal wall by the larvae, severe localized abdominal pain, rebound, and guarding, which may mimic an acute abdomen (appendicitis). Without an adequate dietary history (of eating raw fish), the diagnosis may be almost impossible to establish. Therapy would be directed toward the most likely diagnostic entity (gastric ulcer or appendicitis). Diagnosis is usually established on visual inspection of the larvae (on endoscopy, laparotomy, or pathologic examination), which are typically pink or red. Raw fish that may contain eustrongylides include minnows (*Fundulus spp.*) and other bait fish. *Anisakis simplex* and *Pseudotterranova decipiens* are Anisakidae that may be found in several types of frequently consumed raw fish, including mackerel, cod, herring, rockfish, and salmon, as well as yellowfin tuna and squid. Reliable methods of preventing ingestion of live anisakid larvae are freezing ($-4°F$ ($-20°C$) for 60 hours) or cooking ($140°F$ ($60°C$) for 5 minutes).[67,76,126,133,167]

Diphyllobothriasis (fish tapeworm disease) is caused by eating uncooked fish that harbor the parasite. Hosts include, but are not limited to, herring, salmon, pike, and whitefish. The symptoms are less acute than with intestinal roundworm ingestions, and usually begin 1–2 weeks after ingestion. Signs and symptoms include nausea, vomiting, abdominal cramping, flatulence, abdominal distension, diarrhea, and anemia (megaloblastic). Diagnosis is based on a history of ingesting raw fish and on identification of the tapeworm proglottids in stool.[159] Treatment with niclosamide, praziquantel, or paromomycin is usually effective.[1]

Monosodium Glutamate

The so-called "Chinese restaurant syndrome" is induced by ingestion of monosodium glutamate (L-sodium glutamate; MSG). Individuals present with burning, facial pressure, headache, flushing, chest pain, GI symptoms usually limited to nausea and vomiting, and, infrequently, life-threatening bronchospasm[3] and angioedema.[144] Intensity and duration of the symptoms are dose-related, with significant variation in individual responses to the amount ingested.[134,170] Monosodium glutamate causes "shudder attacks" or a seizurelike syndrome in young children. Absorption is more rapid following fasting, and the typical burning symptoms rapidly spread over the back, neck, shoulders, abdomen, and, occasionally, the thighs. Gastrointestinal symptoms are rarely prominent. Symptoms can usually be prevented by prior ingestion of food. When symptoms do occur, they usually last approximately 1 hour. The syndrome is not limited to patrons of Chinese restaurants. It is a reaction to MSG, which is used frequently in many restaurants. Monosodium glutamate is also marketed as an effective flavor enhancer.[14] Many sausages and canned soups contain heavy doses of MSG.

MSG (regarded as "safe" by the Food and Drug Administration) can also be the cause of other acute and bizarre neurologic symptoms. The pathophysiology has not been clarified, although studies implicate glutamate receptors.

Another foodborne toxin with gastrointestinal symptoms is also associated with Chinese restaurants and eating of reheated fried rice. *Bacillus cereus* type I is the causative organism, and bacterial overgrowth and toxin production causes consequential early onset nausea and vomiting. *Bacillus cereus* type II has a delayed onset of similar gastrointestinal symptoms, including diarrhea.[47]

Anaphylaxis and Anaphylactoid Presentations

Some foods and foodborne toxins may cause allergic or anaphylacticlike manifestations, that are also referred to as "restaurant syndromes"[138] (Table 74–4). The similarity of these syndromes complicates a patient's future approach to safe eating. Isolating the precipitant is essential so that the risk can be effectively assessed. Manufacturers of processed foods should provide an unambiguous listing of ingredients on package labels. Sensitive individuals (or their parents) must be rigorously attentive.[130,171] Confirmation may necessitate controlled double-blind oral challenge tests, and those with severe reactions should be protected by the immediate availability of epinephrine and antihistamine. Attempts to avoid allergic reactions to dairy products by avoiding dairy-containing foods may fail. Nondairy foods may still contain flavor enhancers of a dairy origin (partially hydrolyzed sodium caseinate and the like) and can cause morbidity and death in allergic individuals.[46] Individuals with known food allergies frequently fail to carry prescribed spring-injected epinephrine syringes, believing that the allergen is easily identifiable and avoidable.[72] Food additives to consider include antibiotics, aspartame, butylated hydroxyanisole (BHA), butylated hydroxytoluene (BHT), nitrates or nitrites, and parabens esters.[89] Regulation of these preservatives is limited, and agents such as sulfites are so ubiquitously used that it may be hard to predict which guacamole, cider, vinegar, fresh or dried fruits, wines or beers do or do not contain these sensitizing agents.

Vegetables and Plants

Plants, vegetables, and their diverse presentations are often involved in food poisonings.[60,74,75,80,81] Edible plants and plant products may be poorly cooked, prepared or contaminated. Extensive discussion is found in Chap. 78.

FOOD POISONING AND BIOTERRORISM

The threat of terrorist assaults has received increased attention recently and is discussed elsewhere in this text (Chap. 100). Food as a vehicle for intentional contamination with the intent of causing mass suffering or death has occurred in the United States.[77,156] In the first report,[77] 12 laboratory workers suffered gastrointestinal symptoms, primarily severe diarrhea, from consuming food served in the staff break room which had been purposefully contaminated

with *Shigella dysenteriae* type 2. Four were hospitalized, none had reported long-term sequelae. The Shigella strain is a rare one to cause endemic disease, and the identical strain, as identified by pulse-field gel electrophoresis, was found in 8 of the symptomatic workers, and in the pastries served in the break room, as well as and in the laboratory's stock culture of *Shigella dysenteriae*. This suggests purposeful poisoning of food eaten by laboratory personnel. The person responsible, and the motive, remain unknown.

The second cases series[156] describes a large community outbreak of food poisoning caused by *Salmonella typhimurium*. The outbreak occurred in the Dalles, Oregon area during the fall of 1984. A total of 751 people suffered salmonella gastroenteritis. The outbreak was caused by intentional contamination of restaurant salad bars and coffee creamer by members of a religious commune using a culture of *Salmonella typhimurium* purchased before the outbreak of food poisoning. A criminal investigation found a salmonella culture on the religious commune grounds that had *Salmonella typhimurium* identical to the salmonella strain found in food-poisoning victims, as identified by using antibiotic sensitivity, biochemical testing, and DNA restriction endonuclease digestion of plasmid DNA. It took more than a year for this purposeful salmonella outbreak to be linked to terrorist activity. Reasons for the delay in identifying the outbreak as a purposeful food poisoning include: (a) no apparent motive; (b) no claim of responsibility; (c) no pattern of unusual behavior in the restaurants; (d) no disgruntled restaurant employees identified; (e) epidemic exposure curves indicated multiple time points for contamination, suggesting a sustained source of contamination, not a single act; (f) no previous event of similar nature as a reference; (g) other possibilities seemed more likely (eg, repeated unintentional contamination by restaurant workers); and (h) fear that the publicity necessary to aid the investigation might generate copy cat criminal activity.

The delay in publication of the event (almost 10 years) was also due to fears of copycat activity. The activity of the Japanese cult Aum Shinrikyo and its use of biologic weapons appear to have provided the motivation to release this publication in the hopes that similar purposeful food poisoning patterns may be identified more quickly in the future.

The capacity for infecting large numbers of people with foodborne agents that are easy to obtain and disperse is clearly exemplified by the purposeful salmonella outbreak in Oregon, and the apparently unintentional salmonella outbreak which resulted in more than 16,000 culture-proven cases traced to contamination in 1 Illinois dairy where the probable cause of the outbreak was a transfer line connecting raw and pasteurized milk containment tanks.[127]

SUMMARY

The diversity of etiologies for food poisoning involves almost all aspects of toxicology. Our concerns represent the natural toxicity of a product such as a plant or animal, the contamination of these in the field or in the processing in a factory or in the home preparation or storage. These events may be intentional or unintentional, but they may alter our approaches to general nutrition and society. The current debates about the role of government in food preparation and protection range from bacteria such as *E. Coli* 0157:H7, to prions in Creutzfeldt-Jacob disease (bovine encephalopathy), to genetically altered materials such as corn. Future discussions of food poisonings and interpretations of the importance of these problems may dramatically alter our food sources and their preparation.

ACKNOWLEDGMENT

Robert H. Kirstein, MD contributed to this chapter in a previous edition.

REFERENCES

1. Abramowicz M, ed: Drugs for parasitic infections. Med Lett 1990; 32:29.
2. Ackman DM, Drabkin P, Birkhead G, Cieslak P: Reptile-associated salmonellosis in New York State. Pediatr Infect Dis J 1995;14: 955–959.
3. Allen DH, Baker GJ: Chinese restaurant asthma. N Engl J Med 1981;305:1154–1155.
4. Anonymous: Outbreaks of Salmonella serotype enteritidis infection associated with eating raw or undercooked shell eggs—United States,1996–1998. MMWR Morb Mortal Wkly Rep 2000;49:73–79.
5. Anonymous: Multistate outbreak of listeriosis—United States, 1998. MMWR Morb Mortal Wkly Rep 1998;7:1085–1086. .
6. Anunciacao LL, Linardi WR, do Carmo LS, Bergdoll MS: Production of staphylococcal enterotoxin A in cream-filled cake. Int J Food Microbiol 1995;26:259–263.
7. Armstrong GD, Rowe PC, Goodyer P, et al: A phase I study of chemically synthesized verotoxin (Shiga-like toxin) Pk-trisaccharide receptors attached to chromosorb for preventing hemolytic-uremic syndrome. J Infect Dis 1995;171:1042–1045.
8. Arnold SH, Brown WD: Histamine toxicity from fish products. Adv Food Res 1978;24:113–154.
9. Asai S, Krzanowski JJ, Lockey R, et al: The site of action of Ptychodiscus brevis toxin within the parasympathetic axonal sodium channel h gate in airway smooth muscle. J Allergy Clin Immunol 1984;73:824–828.
10. Attwood SE, Healy K, Caffarkey MT, et al: Yersinia infection and abdominal pain. Lancet 1987;1:529–533.
11. Baden DG, Fleming LE, Bean JA: Marine toxins. In: de Wolf FA, ed: Handbook of Clinical Neurology: Intoxication of the Nervous System. II. Clinical Toxins and Drugs. Amsterdam, Elsevier, 1994.
12. Baden DG, Melinek R, Sechet V, et al: Modified immunoassays for polyether toxins: Implications of biological matrixes, metabolic states, and epitope recognition. J AOAC Int 1995;78:499–508.
13. Bagnis R, Kubergki T, Laugier S: Clinical observations on 3,009 cases of ciguatera (fish poisoning) in the South Pacific. Am J Trop Med Hyg 1979;28:1067–1073.
14. Bellisle F: Effects of monosodium glutamate on human food palatability. Ann N Y Acad Sci 1998;855:438–441.
15. Benton BJ, Rivera VR, Hewetson JF, et al: Reversal of saxitoxin-induced cardiorespiratory failure by a burro-raised-STX antibody and oxygen therapy. Toxicol Appl Pharmacol 1994;124:39–51.
16. Berenguer J, Solera J, Diaz MD, et al: Listeriosis in patients infected with human immunodeficiency virus. Rev Infect Dis 1991;13: 115–119.
17. Besser RE, Lett SM, Weber JT, et al: An outbreak of diarrhea and hemolytic uremic syndrome from Escherichia coli O157:H7 in fresh-pressed apple cider. JAMA 1993;269:2217–2220.
18. Bitzan M, Ludwig K, Klemt M, et al: The role of Escherichia coli O157 infections in the classical (enteropathic) haemolytic uraemic syndrome: Results of a Central European, multicentre study. Epidemiol Infect 1993;110:183–196.
19. Black RE, Jackson RJ, Tsai T, et al: Epidemic Yersinia enterocolitica infection due to contaminated chocolate milk. N Engl J Med 1978;298:76–279.
20. Blalesly ML: Scombroid poisoning: Prompt resolution of symptoms with cimetidine. Ann Emerg Med 1983;12:104–106.
21. Blaser MJ, Keller LB: Campylobacter enteritis. N Engl J Med 1981; 305:1444–1452.
22. Blythe DG, Desilva DP: Mother's milk turns toxic following a fish feast. JAMA 1990;264:2074.
23. Bowman PB: Amitriptyline and ciguatera. Med J Aust 1984;140: 802.
24. Bradley SG, Klika LJ: A fatal poisoning from the Oregon rough-skinned newt (Taricha granulosa). JAMA 1981;246:247.
25. Brandt HR, Fouser LS, Watkins SL, et al: Escherichia coli O157:H7-associated hemolytic uremic syndrome after ingestion of contaminated hamburgers. J Pediatr 1994;125:519–526.
26. Brian MJ, Frosolono M, Murray BE, et al: Polymerase chain reaction for diagnosis of enterohemorrhagic Escherichia coli infection and hemolytic-uremic syndrome. J Clin Microb 1992;30:1801–1806.
27. Cameron J, Capra MF: The basis of the paradoxical disturbance of temperature perception in ciguatera poisoning. J Toxicol Clin Toxicol 1993;31:571–579.
28. Catterall WA, Trainer V, Baden DG: Molecular properties of the sodium channel: A receptor for multiple neurotoxins. Bull Soc Pathol Exot 1992;85:481–485. .
29. Chaudhry R, Lall SB, Baijayantimal M, et al: A foodborne outbreak of organophosphate poisoning. BMJ 1998;17:268–269.
30. Cieslak PR, Barrett TJ, Griffen PM, et al: Escherichia coli O157:H7 infection from a manured garden [letter]. Lancet 1993; 342:367.
31. Cody SH, Abbott SL, Marfin AA, Schulz B, et al: Two outbreaks of multidrug-resistant Salmonella serotype typhimurium DT104 infections linked to raw-milk cheese in northern California. JAMA 1999; 281:1805–1810.
32. Decker MD, Lavely GB, Hutcheson RH, Schaffner W: Food-borne streptococcal pharyngitis in a hospital pediatrics clinic. JAMA 1985; 253:679–681.
33. Deschenes G, Casenave C, Grimont F, et al: Clusters of haemolytic uremic syndrome due to unpasteurized cheese. Pediatr Nephrol 1996;10:203–205.
34. Dupont HL, Formal HB, Hornick RB, et al: Pathogenesis of Escherichia coli diarrhea. N Engl J Med 1971;285:1–289.
35. Eastaugh JE, Shepherd S: Infections and toxic syndromes from fish and shellfish consumption: A review. Arch Intern Med 1989;149: 1735–1740.
36. Endean R, Monks SA, Griffith JK, Llewellyn LE: Apparent relationships between toxins elaborated by the cyanobacterium Trichodesmium erythraeum and those present in the flesh of the narrow-barred Spanish mackerel Scomberomorus commersoni. Toxicon 1993;31:1155–1165.
37. Etkind P, Wilson ME, Gallagher K, et al: Bluefish associated scombroid poisoning. JAMA 1987;258:3409–3410.
38. Evans MR, Parry SM, Ribeiro CD: Salmonella outbreak from microwave cooked food. Epidemiol Infect 1995;115:227–230.
39. Finch MJ, Blake PA: Foodborne outbreaks of campylobacteriosis: The United States experience. Am J Epidemiol 1985;122: 262–267.
40. Flachsenberger WA: Respiratory failure and lethal hypotension due to blue-ringed octopus and tetrodotoxin envenomations observed and counteracted in animal models. J Toxicol Clin Toxicol 1987;24: 485–502.
41. Foo LY: Scombroid poisoning: Isolation and identification of saurine. J Sci Food Agric 1976;27:807–810.
42. Foster EM: Foodborne hazards of microbial origin. Fed Proc 1978; 37:2577–2581.
43. Fritsche TR, Tarr P: Shiga-like toxin-producing Escherichia coli in Seattle children: A prospective study. Gastroenterology 1993;105: 1724–1731.
44. Fritz L, Quillam MA, Walter JA, et al: An outbreak of domoic acid poisoning attributed to the pennate diatom Pseudonitzschia australis. J Phycol 1992;28:439–442.
45. Geller RJ, Benowitz NL: Orthostatic hypotension in ciguatera fish poisoning. Arch Intern Med 1992;152:2131–2133.

46. Gern JE, Yang E, Evrard HM, et al: Allergic reactions to milk-contaminated "nondairy" products. N Engl J Med 1991;324:976–979.

47. Giannella RA, Brasile A: Hospital food-borne outbreak of diarrhea caused by *Bacillus cereus*: Clinical, epidemiologic, and microbiologic studies. J Infect Dis 1979;139:366–370.

48. Giesendorf BA, Quint WG: Detection and identification of *Campylobacter spp.* using the polymerase chain reaction. Cell Mol Biol 1995;41:625–638.

49. Gilbert RJ, Hobbs G, Murray CK, et al: Scombrotoxic fish poisoning: Features of the first fifty incidents to be reported in Britain (1976–1979). Br Med J 1980;2:71–72.

50. Gillespie RJ, Lewis JH, Pearn ATC, et al: Ciguatera in Australia: Occurrence, clinical features, pathophysiology, and management. Med J Aust 1986;145:584–590.

51. Goossens H, Giesendorf BA, Vandamme P, et al: Investigation of an outbreak of *Campylobacter upsaliensis* in day care centers in Brussels: Analysis of relationships among isolates by phenotypic and genotypic typing methods. J Infect Dis 1995;172:1298–1305.

52. Grady GF, Keush GT: Pathogenesis of bacterial diarrheas. N Engl J Med 1971;285:831–841, 891–900.

53. Graham DY, Smith JL, Opekun AR: Spicy food and the stomach: Evaluation by endoscopy. JAMA 1988;260:3473–3475.

54. Green MA, Henmann MA, Wehr HM, et al: An outbreak of watermelon-borne pesticide toxicity. Am J Public Health 1987;77: 1431–1434.

55. Griffin PM, Tauxe RV: The epidemiology of infections caused by *Escherichia coli* O157:H7, other enterohemorrhagic *E. coli*, and the associated hemolytic uremic syndrome. Epidemiol Rev 1991;13: 60–98.

56. Gutman LT, Ottesen EA, Quan TJ, et al: An inter-familial outbreak of *Yersinia enterocolitica* enteritis. N Engl J Med 1973;288: 1372–1377.

57. Habekost RC, Fraser IM, Halstead BW: Observations on toxic marine algae. J Wash Acad Sci 1955;45:101–103.

58. Halstead BW: Poisonous and Venomous Animals of the World. Princeton, NJ, Darwin Press, 1978.

59. Hancock DD, Besser TE, Kinsel ML, et al: The prevalence of *Escherichia coli* O157.H7 in dairy and beef cattle in Washington State. Epidemiol Infect 1994;113:199–207.

60. Hardin JW, Arena JM: Human Poisoning from Native and Cultivated Plants. Chapel Hill, NC, Duke University Press, 1969, pp. 69–73.

61. Harris JC, Dupont HL, Hornic RB: Fecal leukocytes in diarrheal illness. Ann Intern Med 1972;76:697–703.

62. Hokama Y, Asahina AY, Shang ES, et al: Evaluation of the Hawaiian reef fishes with the solid phase immunobead assay. J Clin Lab Anal 1993;7:26–30.

63. Holmberg SD, Blake PA: Staphylococcal food poisoning in the United States: New facts and old misconceptions. JAMA 1984;251: 487–489.

64. Holmes MJ, Lewis RJ, Poli MA, et al: Strain-dependent production of ciguatera precursors (gambiertoxins) by *Gambierdiscus toxicus* (*Dinophyceae*) in culture. Toxicon 1991;29:761–765.

65. Hughs JM, Merson MH: Fish and shellfish poisoning. N Engl J Med 1976;295:1117–1120.

66. Hui JY, Taylor SL: Inhibition of in vivo histamine metabolism in rats by foodborne and pharmacologic inhibitors of diamine oxidase, histamine-*N*-methyl transferase, and monoamine oxidase. Toxicol Appl Pharmacol 1985;81:241–249.

67. Intestinal perforation caused by larval Eustrongyloides—Maryland. MMWR Morb Mortal Wkly Rep 1982;31:383–389.

68. Kanchanapongkul J, Krittayapoositpot P: An epidemic of tetrodotoxin poisoning following ingestion of the horseshoe crab *Carcinoscorpius rotundicauda*. Southeast Asian J Trop Med Public Health 1995;26:364–367.

69. Kapperud G, Vardund T, Skjerve E, et al: Detection of pathogenic *Yersinia enterocolitica* in foods and water by immunomagnetic separation, nested polymerase chain reactions, and colorimetric detection of amplified DNA. Appl Environ Microbiol 1993;59:2938–2944.

70. Karpman D, Andreasson A, Thysell H, et al: Cytokines in childhood hemolytic uremic syndrome and thrombotic thrombocytopenic purpura. Pediatr Nephrol 1995;9:694–699.

71. Kawatsu K, Shibata T, Hamano Y. Application of immunoaffinity chromatography for detection of tetrodotoxin from urine samples of poisoned patients. Toxicon 1999;37:325–333.

72. Kemp SF, Lockey RF, Wolf BL, Lieberman P: Anaphylaxis. A review of 266 cases. Arch Intern Med 1995;155:1749–1754.

73. Kim R: Flushing syndrome due to mahi mahi (scombroid fish) poisoning. Arch Dermatol 1979;115:963–964.

74. Kingsbury JM: Phytotoxicology: Major problems associated with poisonous plants. Clin Pharmacol Ther 1969;10:163–169.

75. Kingsbury JM: Poisonous Plants of the United States and Canada. Englewood Cliffs, NJ, Prentice-Hall, 1964.

76. Kliks MM: Human anisakiasis: An update [letter]. JAMA 1986; 255:2605.

77. Kolovacic SA, Kimura A, Simons SL, et al: An outbreak of Shigella dysenteriae type 2 among laboratory workers due to intentional food contamination. JAMA 1997;278:396–398.

78. Kow-Tong C, Malison MD: Outbreak of scombroid fish poisoning, Taiwan. Am J Public Health 1987;77:1335–1336.

79. Lamanna C, Carr CJ: The botulinal, tetanal and enterostaphylococcal toxins: A review. Clin Pharmacol Ther 1967;8:286–332.

80. Lampe KF: Rhododendrons, mountain laurel and mad honey. JAMA 1988;259:2009.

81. Lampe KF, McCann MA: AMA Handbook of Poisonous and Injurious Plants. Chicago, American Medical Association, 1985.

82. Lange WR, Lipkin KM, Yang GC: Can ciguatera be a sexually transmitted disease? J Toxicol Clin Toxicol 1989;27:193–197.

83. Lange WR, Snyder FR, Fudala PJ: Travel and ciguatera fish poisoning. Arch Intern Med 1992;152:2049–2053.

84. Lawrence DN, Enriquez MB, Lumish RM, Maceo A: Ciguatera fish poisoning in Miami. JAMA 1980;244:254–258.

85. Laycock MV, Thibault P, Ayer SW, Walter JA: Isolation and purification procedures for the preparation of paralytic shellfish poisoning toxin standards. Nat Toxins 1994;2:175–183.

86. Le Cour H, Ramos H, Almeida B, et al: Foodborne botulism: A review of 13 outbreaks. Arch Int Med 1988;148:578–580.

87. Lee LA, Gerber AR, Lonsway DR, et al: *Yersinia enterocolitica* 0:3 infections in infants and children associated with the household preparation of chitterlings. N Engl J Med 1990;322:984–987.

88. Levin R: Paralytic shellfish toxins: Their origin, characteristics and methods of detection: A review. J Food Biochem 1991;15:405–407.

89. Levine AS, Labuza TP, Morley JE: Food technology: A primer for physicians. N Engl J Med 1985;312:628–634.

90. Lewis RJ, Holmes MJ: Origin and transfer of toxins involved in ciguatera. Comp Biochem Physiol 1993;106:615–628.

91. Lewis RJ, Sellin M: Multiple ciguatoxins in the flesh of fish. Toxicon 1992;30:915–919.

92. Lopez EL, Contrini MM, Devoto S, et al: Incomplete hemolytic uremic syndrome in Argentinean children with bloody diarrhea. J Pediatr 1995;127:364–367.

93. Lumish RM, Ryder RW, Anderson DC, et al: Heat-labile enterotoxigenic *Escherichia coli*-induced diarrhea aboard a Miami-based cruise ship. Am J Public Health 1980;111:432–436.

94. Martin DL, MacDonald KL, White KE, et al: The epidemiology and clinical aspects of the hemolytic uremic syndrome in Minnesota. N Engl J Med 1990;323:1161–1167.

95. Massachusetts Department of Health: The red tide: A public health emergency. N Engl J Med 1973;288:1126–1127.

96. McCollum JPK, Pearson RCM, Ingham HR, et al: An epidemic of mussel poisoning in northeast England. Lancet 1968;2:767–770.

97. Merson MH, Baine WB, Gangarosa EJ, et al: Scombroid fish poisoning: Outbreak traced to commercially canned tuna fish. JAMA 1974;228:1268–1269.

98. Merson MH, Morris GK, Sack DA, et al: Travelers diarrhea in Mexico: A prospective study of physicians and family members attending a congress. N Engl J Med 1976;294:1299–1305.

99. Metcalf TG: Indication of viruses in shellfish-growing waters. Am J Public Health 1979;69:1093–1094.

100. Mishu B, Griffen PM, Tauxe RV, et al: Salmonella enteritidis gastroenteritis transmitted by intact chicken eggs. Ann Intern Med 1991; 115:190–194.

101. Mopper B, Sciacchitano CJ: Capillary zone electrophoretic determination of histamine in fish. J AOAC1994;77:881–884.

102. Morris PD, Campbell DS, Taylor TJ, et al: Clinical and epidemiological features of neurotoxic shellfish poisoning in North Carolina. Am J Public Health 1991;8:471–474.

103. Morrow JD, Margolis GR, Rowland J, et al: Evidence that histamine is the causative toxin of scombroid-fish poisoning. N Engl J Med 1991;324:716–720.

104. Mosher HS, Fuhrman FA, Buckwald HD, et al: Tarichatoxin-tetrodotoxin, a potent neurotoxin. Science 1964;144:1100–1110.

105. Murray LR, Edwards LC, Martin RJ, et al: Scombroid fish poisoning-Illinois, South Carolina. MMWR Morb Mortal Wkly Rep 1989; 38:140–141.

106. Narahashi T: Mechanism of action of tetrodotoxin and saxitoxin on excitable membranes. Fed Proc 1972;31:1117–1123.

107. Nukina M, Koyangi LM, Scheur PJ: Two interchangeable forms of ciguatoxin. Toxicon 1984;22:169–176.

108. Olsen SJ, Mackinnon LC, Goulding JS, et al: Surveillance for foodborne disease outbreaks-United States, 1993–1997. MMWR Morb Mortal Wkly Rep 2000;49:SS-1–SS51.

109. Orr P, Lorencz B, Brown R, et al: An outbreak of diarrhea due to verotoxin-producing Escherichia coli in the Canadian Northwest Territories. Scand J Infect Dis 1994;26:675–684.

110. Osterholm MT, MacDonald KL, White KE, et al: An outbreak of a newly recognized chronic diarrhea syndrome associated with raw milk consumption. JAMA 1986;256:484–490.

111. Ostroff SM, Kobayashi JM, Lewis JH: Infections with Escherichia coli O157:H7 in Washington state: The first year of statewide disease surveillance. JAMA 1989;262:355–359.

112. Palafox NA, Jain LG, Pinano AZ, et al: Successful treatment of ciguatera fish poisoning with mannitol. JAMA 1988;259:2740–2742.

113. Park DL: Evolution of methods for assessing ciguatera toxins in fish [review]. Rev Environ Contam Toxicol 1994;136:1–20.

114. Pearn J, Harvey P, De Ambrosis W, et al: Ciguatera and pregnancy. Med J Aust 1982;1:57–58.

115. Pearn JH, Lewis RJ, Ruff T, et al: Ciguatera and mannitol: Experience with a new treatment regimen. Med J Aust 1989;151:77–80.

116. Perl TM, Bedard L, Kosatsky T, et al: An outbreak of toxic encephalopathy caused by eating mussels contaminated with domoic acid. N Engl J Med 1990;322:1775–1780.

117. Pickering LK, Obrig TG, Stapleton FB: Hemolytic-uremic syndrome and enterohemorrhagic Escherichia coli. Pediatr Infect Dis J 1994;13:459–475.

118. Poli MA, Rein KS, Baden DG: Radioimmunoassay for PbTx-2-type brevetoxins: Epitope specificity of two anti-PbTx sera. JAOAC 1995;78:538–542.

119. Potter ME, Kaufman AF, Blake PA, Feldman RA: Unpasteurized milk: The hazards of a health fetish. JAMA 1984;252:2050–2054.

120. Proulx F, Turgeon JP, Delage G, et al: Randomized, controlled trial of antibiotic therapy for Escherichia coli O157:H7 enteritis. J Pediatr 1992;121:299–303.

121. Ragelis EP: Ciguatera seafood poisoning—Overview. In: Ragelis EP, ed: Seafood Toxins. ACS Symposium Series, 262. Washington, DC, American Chemical Society, 1984, pp. 25–36.

122. Rayner MD, Kosaki T, Felmeth EL: Ciguatoxin: More than an anticholinesterase. Science 1968;160:70–71.

123. Rowe PC, Orrbine E, Ogborn M, et al: Epidemic Escherichia coli O157:H7 gastroenteritis and hemolytic-uremic syndrome in a Canadian Inuit community: Intestinal illness in family members as a risk factor. J Pediatr 1994;124:21–26.

124. Rowe PC, Orrbine E, Wells GA, et al: Epidemiology of hemolytic uremic syndrome in Canadian children from 1987 to 1988. J Pediatr 1991;119:218–224.

125. Rubin HR, Wu AW: The bitter herbs of seder: More on horseradish horrors [letter]. JAMA 1988;259:1943.

126. Ruttenberg M: Safe sushi. N Engl J Med 1989;320:900–901.

127. Ryan CA, Nickels MK, Hargrett-Bean NT, et al: Massive outbreak of antimicrobial-resistant salmonellosis traced to pasteurized milk. JAMA 1987;258:3269–3274.

128. Sack DA, Kaminsky DC, Sack RB, et al: Enterotoxigenic Escherichia coli diarrhea of travelers: A prospective study of Peace Corps volunteers. Johns Hopkins Med J 1977;141:63–70.

129. Sakamoto Y, Lockey RF, Krzanowski JJ: Shellfish and fish poisoning related to the toxic dinoflagellates. South Med J 1987;80: 868–872.

130. Sampson HA, Mendelson L, Rosen J: Fatal and near fatal anaphylactic reactions to food in children and adolescents. N Engl J Med 1992;27:380–384.

131. Sartwell PE, ed: Maxcy-Rosenau Public Health and Preventive Medicine, 13th ed. Norwalk, CT, Appleton & Lange, 1992.

132. Schantz EJ, Johnson EA: Properties and use of botulinum and other microbial neurotoxins in medicine. Microbiol Rev 1989;56:80–99.

133. Schantz PM: The dangers of eating raw fish. N Engl J Med 1989;320:1143–1145.

134. Schaumburg HH, Byck R, Gerstl R, Mashman JH: Monosodium glutamate: Its pharmacology and role in the Chinese restaurant syndrome. Science 1969;163:826–828.

135. Scholin CA, Gulland F, Doucette GJ, et al: Mortality of sea lions along the central California coast linked to a toxic diatom bloom. Nature 2000;403:80–84.

136. Schuchat A, Deaver KA, Wenger JD, et al: Role of foods in sporadic listeriosis. I. Case control study of dietary risk factors. JAMA 1992;267:2041–2045.

137. Seigler RL: Management of hemolytic-uremic syndrome. J Pediatr 1988;112:1014–1020.

138. Settipane GA: The restaurant syndromes. Arch Intern Med 1986; 146:2129–2130.

139. Shapiro RL, Hatheway C, Swerdlow DL: Botulism in the United States: A clinical and epidemiologic review. Ann Int Med 1998; 129:221–228.

140. Siegler RL, Pravia AT, Christofferson RD, et al: A 20-year population-based study of postdiarrheal hemolytic uremic syndrome in Utah. Pediatrics 1994;94:35–40.

141. Sims JK, Ostman DC: Pufferfish poisoning: Emergency diagnosis and management of mild human tetrodotoxication. Ann Emerg Med 1986;15:1094–1098.

142. Southern JP, Smith RM, Palmer S: Bird attack on milk bottles: Possible mode of transmission of Campylobacter jejuni to man. Lancet 1990;336:1425–1427.

143. Spitzer DR: Horseradish horrors—Sushi syncope. JAMA 1988; 259:218–219.

144. Squire EN: Angioedema and monosodium glutamate. Lancet 1987; 1:988.

145. St. Louis ME, Morse D, Potter ME, et al: The emergence of grade A eggs as a major source of salmonella enteritis infections: New implications for the control of salmonellosis. JAMA 1988;259: 2103–2107.

146. Surveillance for epidemics. MMWR Morb Mortal Wkly Rep 1990; 38:694–696.

147. Suzuki Y, Saito M, Ishikawa N: Restriction fragment length polymorphisms analysis by pulsed-field gel electrophoresis for discrimination of Staphylococcus aureus isolates from foodborne outbreaks. Int J Food Microbiol 1999;46:271–274.

148. Swerdlow DL, Woodruff BA, Brady RC, et al: A waterborne outbreak in Missouri of Escherichia coli 0157:H7 associated with bloody diarrhea and death. Ann Intern Med 1992;117:812–819.

149. Swift AE, Swift TR: Ciguatera. J Toxicol Clin Toxicol 1993;31: 1–29.

150. Tacket CO, Ballard J, Harris N, et al: An outbreak of *Yersinia enterocolitica* infections caused by contaminated tofu (soybean curd). Am J Epidemiol 1985;121:705–710.

151. Tarr PI, Neill MA, Clausen CR, et al: *Escherichia coli* O157:H7 and the hemolytic uremic syndrome: Importance of early cultures in establishing the etiology. J Infect Dis 1990;162:553–556.

152. Tauxe RV, Hargrett-Bean N, Patton CM: Campylobacter isolates in the United States, 1982–1986. MMWR Morb Mortal Wkly Rep 1988;37:SS:1–13.

153. Taylor WR, Schell WL, Wells JG, et al: A foodborne outbreak of enterotoxigenic *Escherichia coli* diarrhea. N Engl J Med 1982;306: 1093–1095.

154. Teitelbaum JS, Zatorre RJ, Carpenter S, et al: Neurologic sequelae of domoic acid intoxication due to ingestion of contaminated mussels. N Engl J Med 1990;322:1781–1787.

155. Todd ECD: Domoic acid and amnesic shellfish poisoning—A review. J Food Prot 1993;56:69–83.

156. Torok TJ, Tauxe RV, Wise RP, et al: A large community outbreak of Salmonellosis caused by intentional contamination of restaurant salad bars. JAMA 1997;278:389–395.

157. Trachtman H, Christen E: Pathogenesis, treatment, and therapeutic trials in hemolytic uremic syndrome. Curr Opin Pediatr 1999;11: 162–168.

158. Trainer VL, Baden DG, Catterall WA: Detection of marine toxins using reconstituted sodium channels. J AOC Int 1995;78:570–573.

159. Turner JA, Sorvillo FJ, Murray RA, et al: Diphyllobothriasis associated with salmon. Morb Mortal Wkly Rep 1981;30: 331–338.

160. Update: Foodborne listeriosis United States, 1988–1990. Morb Mortal Wkly Rep 1992;41:251–252.

161. Uragoda CG, Kottegoda SR: Adverse reaction to isoniazid and ingestion of fish with a high histamine content. Tubercle 1977;58: 83–89.

162. van de Kar NC, van Hinsbergh VW, Brommer EJ, et al: The fibrinolytic system in the hemolytic uremic syndrome: In vivo and in vitro studies. Pediatr Res 1994;36:257–264.

163. van Egmond HP, van den Top HJ, Paulsch WE, et al: Paralytic shellfish poison reference materials: An intercomparison of methods for the determination of saxitoxin. Food Addit Contam 1994;11:39–56.

164. Vantrappen G, Geboes K, Ponette E: Yersinia enteritis. Med Clin North Am 1982;66:639–653.

165. Waters JR, Sharp JC, Dev VJ: Infection caused by *Escherichia coli* O157:H7 in Alberta, Canada and in Scotland: A five-year review, 1987–1991. Clin Infect Dis 1994;19:834–843.

166. Withers NW: Ciguatera fish poisoning. Annu Rev Med 1982;33: 97–111.

167. Wittner M, Turner JW, Jacquette G, et al: Eustrongylidiasis—A parasitic infection acquired by eating sushi. N Engl J Med 1989;320: 1124–1126.

168. Wood RC, MacDonald KL, Osterholm MT: Campylobacter enteritis outbreaks associated with drinking raw milk during youth activities. A 10-year review of outbreaks in the United States. JAMA 1992; 268:3228–3230.

169. Yang CC, Han KC, Lin TJ, et al: An outbreak of tetrodotoxin poisoning following gastropod mollusc consumption. Hum Exp Toxicol 1995;14:446–450.

170. Yang WH, Drouin MA, Herbert M, et al: The monosodium glutamate symptom complex: Assessment in a double-blind, placebo-controlled, randomized study. J Allergy Clin Immunol 1997;99: 757–762.

171. Yunginger JW, Sweeney KG, Sturner WQ, et al: Fatal food-induced anaphylaxis. JAMA 1988;260:1450–1452.

CHAPTER 75 BOTULISM

Lewis R. Goldfrank / Neal E. Flomenbaum

A 27-year-old woman was in excellent health until 3 days before admission, when her family gathered for dinner following the funeral of her mother-in-law. Shortly thereafter, the patient began experiencing dysphagia and dysarthria and seemed generally anxious. She saw her family physician, who prescribed diazepam. The day prior to her admission, the patient became dyspneic. She began to communicate by writing when talking became impossible. Writing soon became difficult as well, and the patient complained of having trouble walking and lifting her head. She would not eat and vomited food when she was force-fed. She then began to look straight ahead without moving her eyes.

The next day she was taken to the closest hospital, where the physicians in attendance noted the peculiarity of the symptoms, the fact that she was taking diazepam, and the temporal relationship to the funeral of her mother-in-law. The family physician was called from the emergency department and told of the new symptoms that had developed during the previous 2 days. Struck by the resemblance to the mother-in-law's symptoms prior to her death of a presumed myocardial infarction, he recommended an IM injection of saline as a placebo and discharge of the patient.

Shortly after the patient returned home, she became increasingly dyspneic and cyanotic, and then had a cardiopulmonary arrest. The husband initiated CPR until the paramedics arrived and took over.

Physical examination on admission revealed an apneic, intubated, comatose young woman with a blood pressure of 90/40 mm Hg, pulse of 80 beats/min, and rectal temperature of 97.0°F (36.1°C). Her left pupil was 4 mm in diameter, the right pupil was 3 mm, and both were sluggishly responsive to light.

The heart and lungs were unremarkable. The abdomen was soft, and bowel sounds were diminished. The stools were negative for occult blood. There was no response to painful stimuli or cold-water caloric testing. Her upper extremities were flaccid, with absent reflexes. The patient had increased extensor tone in her legs, 2+ patellar reflexes, ankle clonus, and generalized myoclonic jerks. Cerebrospinal fluid (CSF) examination was normal as was edrophonium (Tensilon) testing. An electromyogram (EMG) demonstrated increased muscle action potentials with rapid repetitive stimulation and posttetanic potentiation.

Botulism was diagnosed and the patient was given 2 vials of trivalent botulinal antitoxin and two 375-mg doses of guanidine over 6 hours. (The patient presented in 1974. Guanidine is rarely, if ever, used currently in the management of botulism. See discussion in the sixth edition of this work). However, her condition steadily deteriorated and she died 3 days after admission. Postmortem examination revealed cerebral edema and herniation. Examination of stomach contents revealed undigested mushrooms, from which *Clostridium botulinum* type B was isolated.

Because of the patient's presentation, the mother-in-law's hospitalization was reviewed: Twelve days before the daughter-in-law's first symptoms, the mother-in-law experienced nausea, vomiting, abdominal cramps, and distension, and she was treated with an antiemetic. Three days later, she complained of a dry throat, dysphagia, and chest pains. Two days after that, she had dyspnea as well. When an electrocardiogram (ECG) revealed inverted T waves in the precordial leads and occasional premature ventricular contractions, she was hospitalized to "rule out myocardial infarction."

The day after the mother-in-law's admission she was even more dyspneic and stuporous and was also noted to have dilated, sluggishly reactive pupils. She was then intubated and became more alert. However upon extubation the next day, she developed respiratory distress and required reintubation. A tracheostomy was then performed but she became febrile and died 2 days later.

Following the daughter-in-law's hospitalization and death, the body of the mother-in-law was exhumed, and an autopsy revealed bronchopneumonia, an enlarged heart, and mushroom fragments in the small intestines. The mushroom fragments yielded *C. botulinum* type B.

When the diagnosis of botulism was first considered, and before the mushrooms were implicated, all family members who had been at the funeral meal were admitted to the hospital for observation. At that time, a third member of the family reported having difficulty swallowing. This woman was the only other family member who had eaten mushrooms at the funeral meal. She was given 1 vial of trivalent botulinal antitoxin, and her symptoms resolved in 3 days. Her stool specimens later revealed *C. botulinum* type B. Twenty days after being given the antitoxin, the woman developed severe arthralgias and fever suggestive of serum sickness. Many of the other family members were understandably anxious and some complained of dry throat, headache, or tingling in their extremities, although none had eaten any of the mushrooms, and none had stools positive for *C. botulinum* type B. Most were discharged from the hospital within 24–48 hours.[39]

A carefully obtained history revealed that the mother-in-law canned her own peppers, eggplant, artichokes, and mushrooms without pressure-cooking. When these remaining canned foods were obtained from the house and examined, only the mushrooms were found to contain *C. botulinum* type B.

EPIDEMIOLOGY

Contrary to popular opinion, when botulism is diagnosed, multiple cases per occurrence do not necessarily follow. Between 1976 and 1988, hundreds of outbreaks occurred, involving more than 400 persons in total, but approximately 70% involved only 1 person, approximately 20% involved 2 persons, and only 10% involved more than 2 persons (mean number of 2.7 cases per outbreak).[103] It is of interest that when only sporadic patients were affected, they were more severely ill, with 85% requiring intubation as compared to only 42% requiring intubation in multiperson outbreaks. [103] There are approximately 1.25 cases of foodborne botulism per 10 million people annually in the United States.[52] Currently, the etiologies of botulism are 72% infant, 24% foodborne, 3% wound, and 1% adult type.[79]

Although only 4% of foodborne botulism is associated with food purchased in restaurants; these outbreaks usually affect large numbers of individuals and account for more than 40% of the total number of reported cases.[52] Commercial food processing accounts for only 2% of reported cases with vegetables (peppers, beans, mushrooms, tomatoes, and beets, with or without meat) thought to be the causative agents in about 70%, meat in 17%, and fish in 13% of cases.

Recently, concern was raised regarding minimally processed foods such as soft cheeses that lack sufficient quantities of intrinsic barriers to botulinum toxin production such as salt and acidifying agents.[73] These foods become high-risk agents when refrigeration standards are violated. The US Food and Drug Administration is reviewing recommendations for appropriate measures to take in processing such foods.[94,95] Common home-canning errors responsible for cases include failure to pressure-cook and allowing food to putrefy at room temperature.

In recent years, outbreaks of botulism have been associated with specialty foods consumed by different ethnic groups: chopped garlic in soy oil by Chinese in Vancouver, British Columbia;[62,86] fried lotus rhizome solid mustard in Japan;[64] uneviscerated salted fish—called *kapchunka*—eaten by Russian immigrants in New York City,[47,91] and the same food-called *faseikh*—eaten by Egyptians in Egypt.[100] Other outbreaks have involved fermented salmon eggs, seal, and whale skin consumed by Inuits and Native Americans in Alaska,[99] and heat-shrink-wrapped meat roll (Matambre) consumed in Argentina.[98]

It is important to be aware of new trends and unusual presentations or locations of botulism and to institute preventive education: although 90% of type E outbreaks have occurred in Alaska because of home-processed fish or meat from marine animals,[52] 1 incident occurred in New Jersey.[28] More recently, 3 cases of botulism involving members of the Native American church followed ingestion of a ceremonial tea made from the buttons of dried, alkaline-ground peyote cactus that had been prepared in a water-covered refrigerated jar. The resultant alkaline and anaerobic milieu presumably fostered the growth of toxin from naturally occurring spores.[35]

There is an ever increasing concern with regard to botulinum toxin as a biological weapon[4a]. The medical and public health issues associated with terrorism and botulinum toxin increase the relevance of this chapter in the twenty first century (see Chapter 100).

The case fatality ratio is about 12% for type A botulism and about 10% for types B and E.[49,61,90] Approximately 67% of patients with type A require intubation, as compared to 52% of patients with type B botulism and 39% of those with type E botulism.[103] Although the median incubation period for all patients is 1 day, it ranges from 0 to 7 days for type A, 0 to 5 days for type B, and 0 to 2 days for type E.[103] Physicians may need to respond more rapidly to a potential epidemic of type E, but they should be prepared for greater complication rates associated with type A.[103] When the type of toxin is unknown, the case fatality rate may remain as high as 50%, a figure comparable to general mortality rates in the past.[49,61,90] The improvement in case fatality rates for all types of botulism probably represents increasing awareness of the problem associated with earlier diagnosis and use of antitoxin, in conjunction with better and more easily accessible life-support techniques.

CHARACTERISTICS OF *CLOSTRIDIUM BOTULINUM*

Clostridium botulinum is a spore-forming, anaerobic, gram-positive bacillus. Although classified as a single species, it consists of three distinct genetic variants: *C. botulinum,* which produces toxin types A, B and E; *C. barati,* which produces toxin type F; and *C. butyricum,* which also produces toxin type E.[36,79] Rare instances of both adult and infant botulism are attributed to *C. barati* and *C. butyricum.*[58,65] Eight distinct toxins, designated types A through G, with C_α and C_β, have been identified to date. Although these toxins have slightly different mechanisms of action, the ultimate effects on vesicle release of acetylcholine and the resultant clinical syndromes are identical. All spores of this species are dormant and highly resistant to damage. They can withstand boiling at 100°C (212°F) for hours, although 30 minutes of moist heat at 120°C (248°F) usually destroys them. Germination of spores in food is promoted by a pH greater than 4.5, a sodium chloride content less than 3.5%, or a low nitrite level. Most viable organisms produce toxin in an anaerobic milieu with temperatures above 27°C (80.6°F), although some strains produce toxins even when conditions are not optimal. Type E botulinal organisms can produce toxin at temperatures as low as 5°C (41°F). To prevent spore germination, acidifying agents such as phosphoric or citric acid are employed in canning or bottling foods low in acid content, such as green beans, corn, beets, asparagus, chili peppers, mushrooms, spinach, figs, olives, and certain nonacidic tomatoes. As opposed to the spores, the toxin itself is heat-labile and can be destroyed by heating to 80°C (176°F) for 30 minutes or to 100°C (212°F) for 10 minutes. At high altitudes, the boiling point may be as low as 94.7°C (202.5°F), which may require a minimum of 30 minutes of boiling to destroy the toxin. Under high-altitude conditions, pressure cooking at 13–14 lb of pressure is often necessary to achieve appropriate temperatures to destroy the toxin.

Clostridium botulinum spores are ubiquitous and are present in soil, seawater, and air. Botulism outbreaks can occur anywhere in the world,[46,99] and in recent years, have been reported from such diverse areas as Iran, the former Soviet Union, Japan, France, Belgium, Portugal,[49] Scandinavia, and Canada. The general distribution of strains in the United States: type A strain is found west of the Mississippi,[12,54] type B is found east of the Mississippi particularly the Allegheny range,[8] and type E is found in the Pacific northwest.[83] Types A and B are typically found in poorly processed meats and vegetables and type E is commonly found in fish products. Type G has not been associated with naturally oc-curring disease.

Food contaminated with *C. botulinum* types A and B often do not look or smell normal and appear putrefied because of the action of proteolytic enzymes. In contrast, however, type E organisms are saccharolytic, not proteolytic, and therefore food contaminated with type E toxin may look and taste normal.

PATHOPHYSIOLOGY

Botulinum toxin is the most poisonous substance known. The LD_{50} for mice is 3 million molecules injected intraperitoneally. The oral human lethal dose is 1 µg (10^{-6} g) per kilogram. Because the toxin is often demonstrated only in the stool and is presumably biodegraded or inactivated in great part in the gastrointestinal tract, it is difficult to determine what percentage of the toxin is actually absorbed.[21] The toxin is a protein consisting of a single polypeptide chain, with a MW of 900,000 Da, which includes a nontoxic protein, and a 150,000 MW neurotoxic component. To become fully active, the 150,000 MW neurotoxin must undergo proteolytic cleavage to generate a heavy chain (MW 100,000) that is linked by a disulfide bond to a light chain (MW 50,000). It is the dichain form of the molecule that is responsible for both the toxicity and therapeutic benefits (see below).[36,81,82] The dichain form binds rapidly and irreversibly to the cell membrane and is uptaken by endocytosis. The heavy chain is responsible for cell membrane binding[67a]. Once inside the cell, the light chain acts as a zinc-dependent endoprotease to cleave polypeptides that are essential for exocytosis.[44,74] Different botulinum toxins share the mechanism of cell entry, but there appears to be a unique mechanism of preventing acetylcholine release for each individual botulinum toxin.[80] This reduction in presynaptic function impairs cholinergic transmission at all acetylcholine-dependent synapses in the peripheral nervous system (Fig. 75–1), but does not affect the central nervous system or axonal conduction.[82] Anticholinesterase (cholinergic) drugs, such as edrophonium (Tensilon), have no effect on the action of the toxin, but may affect

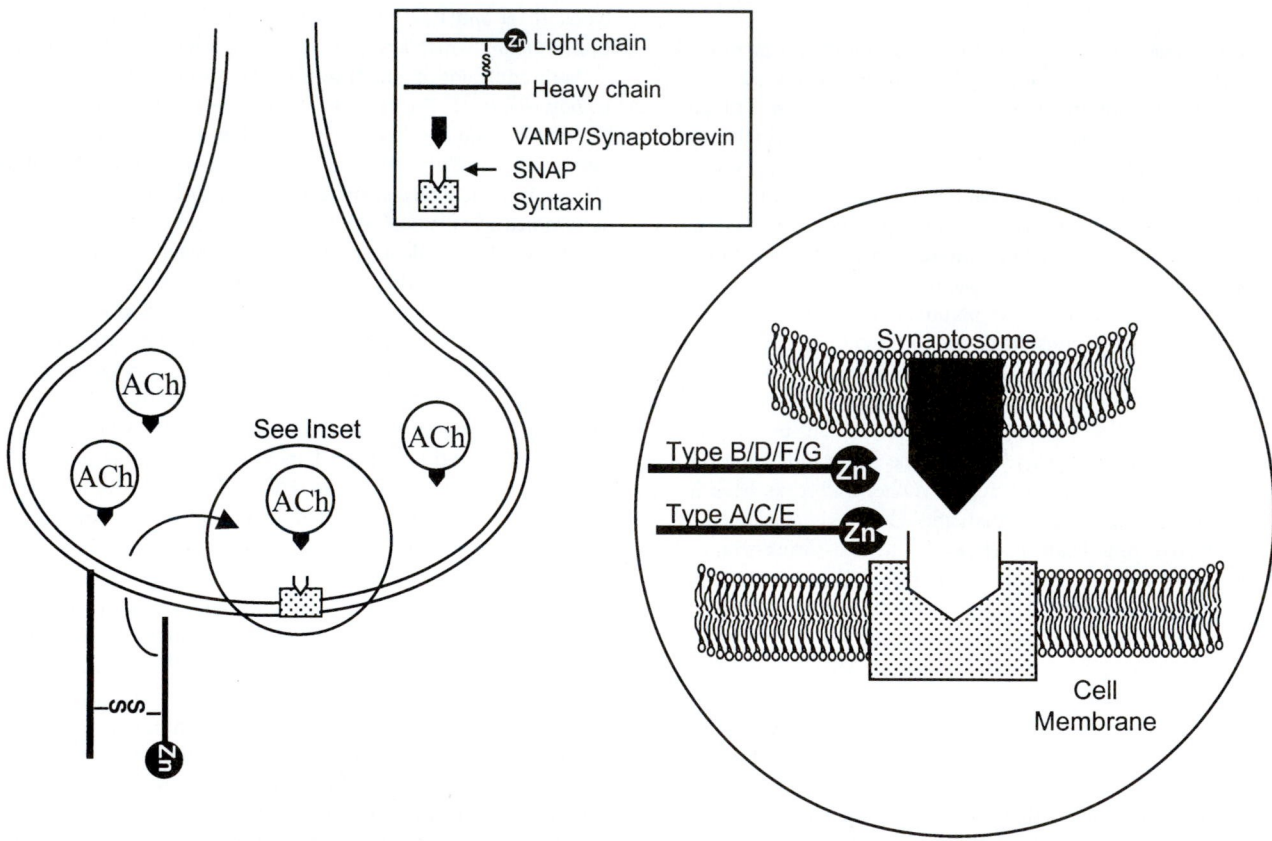

Figure 75–1. Botulinum toxin consists of two peptides linked by disulfide bonds. The heavy chain is responsible for specific binding to acetylcholine-containing neurons (the heavy chain of tetanus toxin is specific for glycine-containing neurons). Following binding to the cell surface, the entire complex undergoes endocytosis and subsequent translocation of the light chain into the nerve cell cytoplasm. The light chain, which is shared by tetanus toxin, contains a zinc-requiring endopeptidase, that cleaves proteins required by the docking/fusion complex critical to neuroexocytosis. Type B botulinum toxin and tetanus toxin target both VAMP/synaptobrevin, a docking protein located on the acetylcholine-containing synaptic vesicles (synaptosome). Type A and E botulism toxins proteolyse SNAP, a component of the presynaptic cell-membrane docking complex (associated with syntaxin). After destruction of these important components of the docking complex, neurotransmitter release cannot proceed, resulting in clinical findings consistent with acetylcholine (botulism) or glycine (tetanus) deficiency. The mechanism of action of tetanus toxin is identical to that of Type B botulinum toxin. VAMP vesicle-associated membrane protein; SNAP synaptosomal associated protein.

patients clinically if they still can release acetylcholine. The prolonged and variable period of recovery, that occurs after exposure to botulinum toxin, is directly related to the extent of the neuromuscular blockade and the neurogenic atrophy as well as the nerve ending and presynaptic membrane regeneration rates.[33,56]

SIGNS AND SYMPTOMS

Foodborne Botulism (Adult Type) (In Vitro)

Although botulism is the most dreaded of all food poisonings, the initial phase of the disease, which occurs during the first day following ingestion, is often so subtle as to go unnoticed. Unfortunately, botulism is often misdiagnosed on the first visit to a physician.[15,104] When gastrointestinal symptoms are striking, and food poisoning is suspected, the differential diagnosis should also include more acute poisonings, such as heavy metals, plants, mushrooms, and the common bacterial, viral, and parasitic agents discussed in Chap. 74.

Because the initial presentation of botulism is often subtle, and because physicians are so infrequently confronted with the disease (especially compared to the relatively more common diseases included in the differential diagnosis), there are often serious delays in initiating appropriate management (Table 75–1). This is particularly true of type E botulism, in which initial gastrointestinal signs may be much more prominent than neurologic signs.[5] The

first victim of an epidemic or an isolated victim is often misdiagnosed at a stage when the person could still be saved.[17,18] The definitive CDC criteria for the diagnosis of botulism are met when a patient presents with a neurologic disorder manifested by a descending paralysis and at least one of the following:

- electromyographic findings typical of botulism
- *C. botulinum* in stool or a wound
- botulinum toxin in serum, stool, or implicated food samples
- a compatible clinical illness in a person who is epidemiologically linked to a laboratory-confirmed case.[4a,52]

The early GI symptoms of botulism include nausea, vomiting, abdominal distension, and pain. There may or may not be a time lag (from 12 hours to several days, but typically not more than 24 hours) before one or more of the following symptoms appears, constipation, dry or sore mouth and throat, blurred vision and impaired accommodation, dysphonia (typically manifested by a nasal quality to the voice), dysarthria, diplopia, descending, bilaterally symmetric motor paralysis beginning with abducens (VI) or oculomotor (III) nerve palsy (frequently resulting in strabismus); dysphagia (at times predominant and severe); mydriasis (often fixed); respiratory insufficiency; and urinary retention (Table 75–2). Although many of these initial signs and symptoms are anticholinergic in nature, the mental status, sensory, and reflex examinations all usually remain normal. When medial rectus palsy, ptosis, and

TABLE 75–1. Botulism: Clues in the Various Phases of the Differential Diagnosis

Condition	Diagnostic Findings
Aminoglycoside poisoning	Postanesthetic paralysis, intraoperative exposure
Anticholinergic poisoning	Mydriasis, vasodilation, fever, tachycardia, ileus, dry mucosa, altered mental status
Buckthorn (*Karwinskia humboldtiana*)	Rapidly progressive ascending paralytic neuropathy with quadriplegia
Carbon monoxide	Headache, nausea, altered sensorium, tachypnea, elevated carboxyhemoglobin
Cerebrovascular accident (midbrain)	Asymmetric focal findings, abnormal CT
Diphtheria (polyneuritis)	Exudative pharyngitis, cranial polyneuropathy (late) cardiac manifestations, hypotension
Eaton-Lambert syndrome	Neoplasm, ophthalmoplegia (rare), no respiratory paralysis posttetanic facilitation on EMG, calcium channel blocking antibodies
Elapidae (coral snake) envenomation	Following envenomations: euphoria, lightheadedness, fasciculations, tremor, weakness, salivation, nausea, vomiting followed by bulbar palsy, paralysis including slurred speech, diplopia, ptosis, dysphagia, dyspnea, and respiratory compromise
Encephalitis	Fever, mental status abnormalities, seizures, elevated CSF protein, and pleocytosis
Food poisoning (bacterial)	Rapid onset of disease, absence of cranial nerve findings
Guillain-Barré syndrome (Miller-Fisher variant)	Acute inflammatory demyelinating polyneuropathy, absent deep-tendon reflexes, ataxia, elevated CSF protein without cells, denervation and prolonged nerve conduction velocity on EMG
Inflammatory myelopathies (acute myelitis, transverse myelitis)	Complete (transverse) or incomplete spinal syndrome: posterior column myelopathy with ascending paresthesias or ascending spinothalamic findings or Brown-Sequard syndrome. Typically follows viral illness, back pain, progressive paraparesis, asymmetric ascending paresthesias in legs. CSF: 5–50 lymphocytes/mm³
Magnesium toxicity	Oral or intravenous exposure to magnesium, respiratory compromise, diffuse flushing, weakness, hypermagnesemia
Multiple sclerosis	Weakness, visual blurring (optic neuritis), sensory disturbances, diplopia, ataxia. Lesions separated in space and time. Mononuclear cell pleocytosis in CSF. Evoked-reponse testing: slow or abnormal conduction in visual, auditory, somatosensory, or motor pathways; abnormal MRI with a paramagnetic dye (gadolinium)
Myasthenia gravis	Aggravation of fatigue with exercise, positive edrophonium (Tensilon) test, acetylcholine receptor antibodies
Organic phosphorous compounds	Salivation, lacrimation, urination, defecation, fasciculations, bronchorrhea
Paralytic shellfish poisoning	Incubation <1 h, dysesthesias, paresthesias, impaired mentation, respiratory paralysis
Poliomyelitis	Fever, GI symptoms, asymmetric neurologic findings, CSF pleocytosis, elevated CSF protein
Polymyositis	Insidious onset, proximal limb weakness, dysphagia, muscle tenderness, cramping, ↑ ESR, EMG: fibrillation and sharp waves
Tick (*Dermacentor spp*)-related paralysis	Ataxia, progressive large muscle weakness, ascending paralysis, absence of sensory loss, normal CSF analysis, presence of an embedded tick, and resolution upon removal

TABLE 75–2. Common Symptoms and Signs of Foodborne Botulism

General	Dizziness
	Fatigue
	Normal mental status
	Orthostatic hypotension
	Sore throat
Gastrointestinal	Abdominal distress
	Constipation (late)
	Diarrhea (early)
	Ileus
	Nausea
	Vomiting

Neurologic	**Symptoms**	**Signs**
	Blurred vision	Ataxia
	Difficulty urinating	Cranial nerve deficits
	Diplopia	Decreased gag reflex
	Dry mouth	Facial paresis
	Dysarthria	Lingual weakness
	Dysphagia	Ptosis
	Dyspnea	Extremity weakness
	Extremity weakness	Hyporeflexia
		Mydriasis (fixed)
		Nystagmus
		Ophthalmoplegia
		Paralysis, descending
		Urinary retention

TABLE 75–3. Differentiating Botulism From the Guillain-Barré Syndrome

	Botulism	Guillain-Barré Syndrome	Miller Fisher Variant of Guillain-Barré
Fever	Absent	May be present	May be present
Motor			
Pupils	Dilated or unreactive (50%)	Normal	Normal
Ophthalmoplegia	Present early	Present late	Present
Paralysis	Descending	Ascending	Descending
Deep-tendon reflexes	Present	Absent	Absent
Ataxia	Absent	Present	Present
Sensory			
Paresthesias	Absent	Present	Present
Laboratory			
CSF protein	Normal	Elevated	Elevated

sluggish pupillary reactivity occur, respiratory insufficiency usually follows. As weakness progresses, deep-tendon reflexes may diminish. The pulse is frequently normal or slow, and temperature in adults remains normal. The normal mental status and temperature in the presence of ophthalmoplegia that occurs with botulism but not anticholinergic poisoning should enable the clinician to rapidly institute appropriate management for this life-threatening biotoxin.[92] The most difficult and frequently encountered problem is differentiating between botulism and the Miller Fisher variant of the Guillain Barré syndrome (Table 75–3).

The index cases of botulism are usually the most seriously affected: such patients have generally been exposed to the greatest amount of toxin and therefore have the shortest incubation period. Conversely, a lack of symptoms in others is not necessarily reassuring that they were not exposed or will not ultimately develop serious sequelae.

Infant Botulism (In Vivo Infant Intestinal Colonization)

Infant botulism was first described in 1976 in California.[3,41,43,96] Several thousand hospital cases have now been confirmed across the world,[20,65] making this the most common form of botulism. Of these cases, 95% are reported in the United States, and 99% were from botulinum neurotoxin type A or B.[65] Affected children are always younger than 1 year of age (usually 1–3 months) and characteristically have normal gestations and births. The first signs of infant botulism are constipation, feeding difficulty, feeble crying, and a "floppy" baby with diffuse, decreased muscle tone, particularly apparent in the limbs and neck. Ophthalmoplegia, loss of facial grimacing, dysphagia, diminished gag reflex, poor anal

sphincter tone, and respiratory failure are also present, but fever and enteric symptoms do not occur. The differential diagnosis of infant botulism initially includes dehydration, failure to thrive, hypotonia of unknown etiology, sepsis, or a viral syndrome. Many of the syndromes cited in Table 75–1 are also relevant to the evaluation of sick children as are many rarer neurologic, myopathic, and congenital syndromes that occur in the first year of life.[43]

Only certain children are susceptible to infant botulism. Some infants may be immunologically unprepared for spore control, a deficiency that allows subsequent germination and toxin development. As opposed to the better-understood foodborne botulism variants, infant botulism may be the result of the ingestion of *C. botulinum* organisms with subsequent in vivo production of toxin followed by gut absorption. Also, an infant's gastrointestinal tract lacks bile acids and gastric acid, which, when present, may inhibit clostridial growth in the older child and adult. About 70% of cases of infant botulism occur in breast fed infants (only 45–50% of all infants are breast fed) possibly because bacterial growth associated with breast feeding may favor *Bifidobacterium* development whereas formula fed infants are rapidly colonized by *Coliforme spp.*, *Enterococcus spp.*, and *Bacteroides spp.*, all three of which may inhibit *C. botulinum*.[37,93] Conversely, the absence of these typical organisms in breast-fed infants may facilitate *C. botulinum* multiplication. Because the toxin in infant botulism is absorbed gradually as it is produced, the onset of clinical manifestations of botulism may be less abrupt than in severe cases of foodborne botulism, in which large amounts of preformed toxin are absorbed at one time.

Older studies suggested a correlation between the presence of both *C. botulinum* organisms and toxin and sudden infant death syndrome (SIDS).[84] However, in a prospective study of 248 infants with SIDS, not one child was found to have *C. Botulinum* on culture.[16] Both of these disorders have a common age distribution. However, the survival rate in infant botulism is approximately 98%,[77] which is quite different from that of "near SIDS."[4]

Although infant botulism is detected in approximately half of the states in the United States and all inhabited continents except Africa,[20] 50% of reported cases emanate from California, Utah,

Pennsylvania, and New Mexico.[102] In California, aggressive surveillance and educational efforts with regard to infant botulism have been practiced since 1976.

Cases of infant botulism must be managed in the hospital, preferably in a Pediatric Intensive Care Unit for at least the first week, when the risk of respiratory arrest is greatest. In a group of 57 affected infants aged 18 days to 7 months, 77% were intubated and 68% required mechanical ventilation. Loss of airway protection was the best indicator for aggressive management, whereas hypoxia and hypercarbia were unreliable indicators.[77]

Several children with infant botulism have had multiple respiratory arrests,[4] often associated with such procedures as lumbar punctures or while having a radiograph. Although nothing should ever take precedence over basic cardiopulmonary support, these functions often are unintentionally compromised during procedures.[43,50]

Wound Botulism (In Vivo)

Wound contamination was previously considered the least-common cause of botulism. The first case was not reported until 1943, and the total number of cases identified by the Centers for Disease Control and Prevention (CDC) currently approximates 100 cases, with most of the recent cases associated with the subcutaneous injection of heroin.[66] The "classic" presentation of wound botulism is that of a patient injured in an automobile crash who sustains a deep muscle laceration, crush injury, or compound fracture treated with open reduction. The wound is frequently quite dirty and usually associated with inadequate débridement, subsequent purulent drainage, and local tenderness, although in other cases, the wound may appear unremarkable. Four to 18 days later, cranial nerve palsies and the other neurologic findings typical of botulism (eg, dysphagia, dysphonia, dyspnea, and dysarthria) may appear.[59] Other classic signs of food-related botulism may be absent and there are no gastrointestinal manifestations.

In wound botulism, fever may be prominent and associated with the abscess, sinusitis, or other tissue infection presumed to harbor the clostridial organisms. Although in some cases the patients may need to be managed for wound-related problems, in other cases the wounds may appear healthy and uninfected. No particular vehicle, vector, or pathophysiology for wound botulism has been identified. Recognition of wound botulism as a potential complication of wound infections is essential for appropriate early and aggressive therapy.

In 1982 and 1983, 3 parenteral drug abusers presented to emergency departments in New York City with dysphagia, dysarthria, dry mouth, and progressive neurologic impairment. The symptoms were typical for botulism except that 1 patient lacked ocular symptoms and 2 had no cutaneous infections prior to the onset of cranial nerve dysfunction. In 1 case, a subcutaneous cystic lesion (the site of a previous attempted drug injection) yielded anaerobic gram-positive bacilli, that produced type B botulinum toxin. Remarkably, in all 3 cases, dysphagia was the most prominent symptom; in fact, 2 patients were initially admitted to otolaryngology services. The CDC evaluated 3 additional patients with botulism-like illnesses in whom no organism or toxin was found in serum, stool, or skin lesions.[53] The clinical courses and electromyographic patterns of all of these patients were compatible with botulism.

These 3 New York City cases were the first recognized to occur in parenteral drug users, but wound botulism has now become another substantial risk associated with septic parenteral drug use. More recently, cocaine[70,87] and heroin,[15] particularly subcutaneously injected "black tar heroin," have been associated with an increasing number of cases of wound botulism.[30,66] The marked increase in frequency associated with black tar heroin use appears to be related to its physical characteristics such as its viscosity, its potential to facilitate anaerobic growth, and its ability to devitalize tissue or inhibit wound resolution.[7,40,67]

Adult Infectious Botulism (In Vivo Adult Intestinal Colonization)

This fourth class of botulism established by the CDC includes any patient older than 1 year for whom it has been impossible to implicate a particular food source. Until the recent recognition of therapeutic botulism, adult infectious botulism was the rarest form of botulism with only 15 cases reported by 1997.[32,58] Some of the cases in this group may represent a variant form of infant botulism.[61] There is 1 well-documented case of an adult female with botulism resulting from the ingestion of a food source contaminated with *C. botulinum* type A organisms and no preformed toxin.[19] In this case, the combination of a long incubation period with toxin present in the serum and stool for 3 weeks after exposure and the absence of disease in the patient's spouse suggested in vivo intraluminal elaboration of toxin. This patient was a very unusual host in that she had peptic ulcer disease treated with truncal vagotomy, antrectomy, and a Billroth I anastomosis. She had also received perioperative antibiotics 5 weeks prior to the development of botulism. All of these factors may have compromised the gastric and bile acid barrier, gut flora, and motility, thus allowing spore germination, altered bacterial growth, and toxin development. Other cases of adult infectious botulism have occurred in patients with ileal bypass surgery and Crohn disease,[9] jejunoileal bypass for obesity,[23,27,57] gastroduodenostomy,[19,57] vagotomy and pyloroplasty,[58] and a necrotic volvulus.[52] The general risk factors favoring organism persistence and *C. botulinum* colonization include recent antibiotic therapy, gastric achlorhydria (surgically or pharmacologically induced) and previous intestinal surgery.

A single case report has demonstrated endogenous antibody production to botulinum toxin.[32] A 67-year-old male with long-standing Crohn disease who had previously undergone terminal ileum and right colonic resection presented with abdominal pain. Prior to admission the patient had experienced several episodes of poorly characterized diplopia. After admission systemic paralysis developed. Following the administration of two courses of equine trivalent botulinum antitoxin along with 81 days of antibiotic treatment, the patient had a prolonged recovery. In performing a mouse assay to determine the persistence of any previously administered antitoxin prior to administration of additional antitoxin, a particularly high level of antitoxin specific to type A toxin but not type B toxin was identified. An ELISA (enzyme-linked immunosorbent assay) test was next performed to distinguish equine from human antitoxin antibodies, and it demonstrated an endogenous human antitoxin response to the toxin. This response demonstrates a unique characteristic of adult infectious botulism, as other investigators have shown that antitoxin immunity does not generally develop in patients with foodborne botulism.

Therapeutic and Inadvertent Botulism (In Vitro)

The fifth and most recently recognized form of botulism is purely iatrogenic. Currently 10s to 100s of ngs botulinum toxin type A

(Botox or Oculinium) is injected under electromyographic control into extraocular muscles as a treatment for blepharospasm or as a supplement to corrective strabismus surgery.[42,81] This agent is also used to create the temporary weakness necessary to treat facial nerve disorders, achalasia, dystonia, torticollis, migraine headaches, voice and speech disorders (spasmodic dysphonia), and chronic anal fissures[14,55] The doses of botulinum toxin chosen are measured in functional units corresponding to the median lethal doses used for female Swiss Webster mice weighing 18–20 g. Doses range widely depending on the size of the muscle to be treated, the degree of weakness required and the commercial preparation of the toxin.[34] These injections irreversibly block the release of acetylcholine at the local neuromuscular junction. The affected muscles then weaken by atrophy over a 3-week period, but recover within 2–4 months as nerve transmission is restored through sprouting of new nerve endings and functional connections at motor endplates.[1,74] Repetitive doses may be indicated to prolong duration of action to several months.[34,42,51]

Because the toxin diffuses into local tissues, side effects typically occur locally,[72] but systemic manifestations are of concern if an inadvertent, excessive, or misdirected dose of toxin is administered. In addition, a number of studies demonstrate that even appropriately injected doses result in neuromuscular junction abnormalities throughout the body, infrequently producing autonomic dysfunction, but not muscle weakness.[29,48,63] Recently, however, two cases of iatrogenic botulism with muscle weakness and widespread EMG abnormalities resulted from intramuscular botulinum toxin injections in therapeutic doses.[6] Following repeated injections of therapeutic doses, patients develop neutralizing antibodies, which may subsequently limit the efficacy of the toxin.[13] Unfortunately, however, recurrent episodes of foodborne botulism occurring in one individual, suggest that clinically significant minute quantities of toxin exposure do not result in long-term immunity.[10,74]

DIAGNOSIS

Specific tests that are helpful in diagnosing botulism include the following:

Tensilon Test. Edrophonium (Tensilon) is a rapidly-acting anticholinesterase used to diagnose myasthenia gravis and occasionally used to differentiate myasthenia gravis from suspected botulism. An intravenous (IV) injection of 10 mg is prepared and then 1–2 mg are administered slowly, to avoid the nausea and vomiting commonly associated with larger doses. The remainder of the edrophonium is then given over the next 5 minutes. The strength of patients who have myasthenia gravis, but not botulism will dramatically improve within 30–60 seconds, and this improvement will last 3–5 minutes. This drug prevents the available acetylcholine from being metabolized, permitting continued reaction with the reduced number of postsynaptic acetylcholine receptors in myasthenia gravis. In rare cases, early in the course of botulism, there is a limited improvement in strength, which is far less dramatic than occurs in patients with myasthenia gravis.[22,70] Because the release of acetylcholine is impaired in botulism, the prevention of its metabolism is of limited importance.

Electromyography. The EMG pattern in all forms of botulism is characterized by brief, small, abundant motor unit action poten-

tials (BSAPs; or low-amplitude, short-duration potentials) (see Fig. 75–2 for a detailed explanation). Motor nerve conduction velocity remains normal, because axon conduction is not affected. Primary muscle diseases also produce normal conduction velocity and a BSAP pattern, but in botulism, serum levels of muscle enzymes and muscle biopsy are normal. Another typical EMG finding of botulism is an increment in small compound muscle action potential (CMAP) amplitude directly related to the release of acetylcholine following repetitive stimulation at 20–50 Hz.[44] Post-tetanic facilitation may be noted in cases of botulism as well as such other entities as the Eaton-Lambert paraneoplastic syndrome, aminoglycoside-associated paralysis, and hypermagnesemia. Although not pathognomonic, EMG findings interpreted in the light of the total clinical presentation can help to establish the diagnosis of botulism.[2,97]

Laboratory Testing. Samples of serum, stool, vomitus, gastric contents, and suspect foods should be subjected to anaerobic culture (*C. botulinum*) and toxin assay (botulinum toxins) (Table 75–4). If wound botulism is suspected, serum, stool, exudate, débrided tissue, and swab samples should be collected. For infant botulism, feces and serum samples should also be obtained. The specimens should be handled cautiously, refrigerated, and examined and tested as soon as possible after collection. The earlier that specimens are collected following the onset of illness, the more likely that toxin assay will be positive.[103] Later in the course of illness, stool culture is more likely to be positive. Serum samples should be taken prior to administration of antitoxin. Stool, serum and suspected food samples can be used for a mouse neutralization bioassay. The materials are injected into the mouse peritoneum and subsequent paralysis and death of the mouse are considered to be a positive test. Control animals receive portions of the specimen materials that have been boiled to destroy the toxin or previously incubated with antitoxin to achieve neutralization. Stool specimens are incubated anaerobically and then subcultured on an

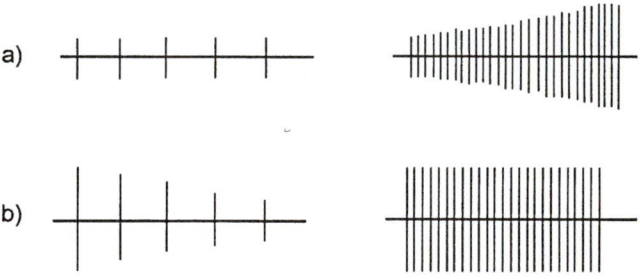

Figure 75–2. Electromyographic findings. Schematic representations of repetitive nerve stimulation at low (5/sec) and high (50/sec) frequencies. In botulism (a), repetitive stimulation produces a small-muscle action potential that facilitates (increases in amplitude) at higher frequencies. This effect results from increased acetylcholine release with high-frequency stimulation because of increased intracellular calcium concentration. In contrast, myasthenia gravis (b) is associated with a normal muscle action potential amplitude and a decremental response at low-frequency stimulation with a normal response at high-frequency stimulation. Myasthenia gravis, a disorder of the muscle endplate, produces this decremental response at low frequencies because the natural reduction in acetylcholine response with subsequent stimulation falls below threshold (see references 68 and 97).

TABLE 75–4. **Laboratory Assessment of Botulism**

Classification	Foodborne	Infant	Wound Infection	Adult Infectious
Toxin type	A, B, E, F, G in humans, C, D in animals	A, B, C, F	A, B	A?
Route	Ingestion	Ingestion	Wound, abscess (sinusitis)	Ingestion of bacteria and spores
Specimens	Stool: positive for bacteria/spores and toxin	Stool: positive for bacteria/spores and toxin for up to 8 wk after recovery	Wound site: Gram's stain, aerobic and anaerobic cultures	Stool: positive for bacteria/spores and toxin
Toxin in serum	Yes	Yes	Yes	Yes
Toxin, bacteria/ spores in food	Yes (all)	Bacteria/spores: yes Toxin: no	No	Bacteria/spores: yes Toxin: no
Family and friends	At risk if same foods were eaten	Unaffected	Unaffected (unless shared needle or similarly exposed)	Unaffected

egg yolk agar to search for lipase-producing gram-positive anaerobic rods.[53] Routine laboratory studies, including CSF analysis, are normal in botulism. Although polymerase chain reaction studies can be done to determine the presence of *Clostridum botulinum* in food, this test is not yet available for the study of human specimens.[24,89]

TREATMENT

Supportive Care

Respiratory compromise is the usual cause of death from botulism. To prevent or treat this complication, hospital admission of the patient and of all individuals suspected of exposure to a possible source is mandatory. Careful continuous monitoring of respiratory status by using parameters such as vital capacity, peak expiratory flow rate (PEFR), negative inspiratory force (NIF), pulse oximetry, and the presence or absence of a gag reflex is essential to determine the need for intubation or tracheostomy as the patient begins to manifest signs of bulbar paralysis.[76] The most reliable, readily obtainable test is the NIF, which can be used in most institutions to determine the need for intubation. In one study, approximately 80% of children with botulism required intubation for a reduced vital capacity and 25% of these children had frank respiratory compromise.[76] When suspicion of disease is high and the vital capacity is less than 30% of predicted, intubation should be strongly considered.[90]

Gastric Decontamination

An attempt should be made to remove the spores and toxin from the gut. Although most patients present after a substantial time delay, the etiologic agent may still be present hours or even days later. Activated charcoal should be a routine part of supportive care, as it adsorbs *C. botulinum* type A toxin in vitro.[31] Gastric lavage or emesis should be initiated only for an asymptomatic person who has very recently ingested a known contaminated food. If a cathartic is chosen, sorbitol is preferable to magnesium salts, which may potentially depress neuromuscular transmission and should therefore probably be avoided in this situation. Theoretically, whole-bowel irrigation also may have a role in decontamination, particularly if there is concern about initiating emesis, but

intervention other than activated charcoal has not been evaluated under these circumstances.

Wound Care

Thorough wound débridement is the most critical aspect of the management of wound botulism and should be performed promptly.[38,52] Antibiotic therapy alone is inadequate, as there are several case reports of disease despite antibiotic therapy. One of the 3 parenteral drug users (see the discussion under "Wound Botulism" earlier) also chronically used cocaine and had a purulent sinusitis, which may have been the source of the type A, *C. botulinum* toxin found in the serum, although nothing grew in cultures from sinus drainage or stool.

Botulinum Antitoxin

In humans the efficacy of the type specific antitoxin to type B strain toxin is unknown; whereas the type-specific antitoxins to A and E are probably beneficial.[46,90] Antitoxin can prevent paralysis but does not affect already paralyzed muscles. To be most effective, therefore, trivalent antitoxin to type A, B, or E must be employed immediately upon consideration of the disease in both symptomatic and asymptomatic individuals exposed to a presumptive source. However, the possible benefits of antitoxin must always be weighed against the high incidence of anaphylaxis and serum sickness from the equine antitoxin.

In a review of 132 cases of type A foodborne botulism, a lower fatality rate and a shorter course of illness were demonstrated for those patients who received trivalent (A, B, E) antitoxin, even after controlling for age and incubation period.[90] The earlier a patient received antitoxin, the shorter was the clinical course. In addition, no respiratory arrests occurred more than 5 hours after antitoxin was administered. In view of the high mortality rate associated with foodborne botulism and limited statistical data, the antitoxin should be given IV to all exposed patients. Botulinum antitoxins types A, B, AB (bivalent), E, ABE (trivalent), and F are available. The type-specific antitoxins are ineffective against any other antigen. Although specific foods tend to correlate relatively well with botulinum type, trivalent antitoxin (7500 U type A, 5500 U type B, and 8500 U type E) should be used until more specific type information is available. Each vial of trivalent antitoxin contains 10 mL (monovalent type E has 5000 IU/2 mL vial). The entire vial should be given as a 1:10 vol/vol dilution in 0.9% sodium chloride over several minutes. If epidemiologic investigation identifies the organism, subsequent type-specific antitoxin therapy may be instituted. Because antitoxin is an equine globulin preparation, hypersensitivity testing for horse serum is sometimes recommended, but there is no value to this testing. In any case, epinephrine should always be readily available to treat hypersensitivity reactions and anaphylaxis. The overall rate of adverse reactions including hypersensitivity and serum sickness[11] is 9–17%, with an incidence of anaphylaxis as high as 1.9%[5,61] (see Antidote in Depth: Botulinum Antitoxin).

Guanidine

In the past, guanidine was used to enhance acetylcholine release, although its merits had never been substantiated.[25,45,69] It is no longer recommended to treat botulism. (See previous editions of this text or p. 1183 in Goldfrank's *Toxicologic Emergencies,* 6th edition for a more extensive discussion.)

Penicillin

Penicillin G is one of many drugs with excellent in vitro efficacy against *C. botulinum* and is useful for wound botulism.[88] However, penicillin has no role in the management of botulism caused by preformed toxin, nor has it been shown to prevent gut spores from germinating. For these reasons penicillin is not considered useful in infant and adult infectious botulism nor is it considered adequate for wound botulism.

Treatment and Prevention of Infant Botulism

Whether there is any role for botulinum antitoxin or antibiotics in infant botulism is presently unclear. There are documented cases of children surviving without either antitoxin or parenteral antibiotics. Currently, antitoxin is not recommended, because circulating toxin is believed to be at very low levels and antitoxin has no effect on toxin-producing organisms in the gut.[43,50,75] Antitoxin therefore is not expected to halt syndrome progression. Moreover, in fully recovered children, both toxin and spores can be found for months in the stools, despite the use of oral or parenteral antibiotics and or antitoxin administration.

Measures employed to prevent infant botulism include limiting exposure to spores by thoroughly washing foods and objects that might be placed in a child's mouth. In addition, honey should not be given to infants. Epidemiologic studies indicate that ingestion of honey was associated with 34.7% of hospitalized cases of infant botulism worldwide. Moreover, of all nutritional items tested as possible epidemiologic sources, only honey was found to contain *C. botulinum* spores.[3] When *C. botulinum* spores were isolated from honey implicated in cases of infant botulism, the identical toxin serotype was isolated from the infant and, as noted previously, no preformed toxin was isolated. Testing of a human-derived botulism immune globulin (BIG) is under investigation and appears efficacious for the treatment of infant botulism[26,60] (see Antidote in Depth: Botulinum Antitoxin).

Prognosis

If the patient has had excellent respiratory support during the acute phase prior to hypoxia or aspiration pneumonitis and receives parenteral nutrition, residual neurologic disability may not occur. Although the initial course may be protracted, almost total functional recovery can follow within several months to a year. Common long-term sequelae are dysgeusia (Chap. 28), dry mouth, constipation, dyspepsia, arthralgia, exertional dyspnea, tachycardia, and easy fatigability.

The long-term status of 13 patients who survived a type B botulinum outbreak 2 years earlier was characterized by persistent dyspnea and fatigue, although surprisingly, pulmonary function tests had returned to normal in all patients.[101] Inspiratory muscle weakness persisted at two years in 4 of 13 patients. Maximal oxygen consumption and maximal workload during exercise were diminished in all patients and all had more rapid shallow breathing and a higher dyspnea score than controls. The reason for premature exercise termination may be multifactorial: Although persistent respiratory muscle weakness may be an explanation, most dyspnea and fatigue appeared to be related to reduced cardiovascular fitness, leg fatigue, and diminished nutrition. Nevertheless, because long-term prognosis can be so good, early recognition of the disease and supportive care are essential.

Pregnancy

There are now at least three reports of botulism occurring during pregnancy. One occurred during the second trimester,[71] and 2 cases occurred during the third trimester.[30,85] Although botulinum toxin or *C. botulinum* was isolated in the mother in 2 of the botulinum cases prior to antitoxin therapy, no detectable toxin was isolated from the neonate in either of the third-trimester cases. The large molecular weight of the neurotoxic component (150,000 Da) of the toxin makes passive diffusion unlikely[36] and, although theoretically possible, no active transport system has been identified.[85] In each of these three neonates, the abnormal neurologic findings noted at birth were most likely the result of complications of delivery, not botulinal disease in the infant. Appropriate care of the mother and preparation for maternal complications of delivery appears to assure the best potential outcome of a normal infant.

Epidemiologic and Therapeutic Assistance

Whenever botulism is suspected or proven, immediately contact the state health department or the Centers for Disease Control and Prevention Enteric Disease Branch, Bacterial Diseases Division, Bureau of Epidemiology, (404–639–2206 days or 404–639–2888 nights, weekends, or holidays). They can provide or facilitate diagnostic, consultative, and laboratory testing services, access to trivalent botulinum antitoxin, and assistance in epidemiologic investigations. Contact can be made by the local physician, hospital, or poison control center. All foods that may possibly be responsible for illness should be preserved for epidemiologic investigation. The merits of this surveillance and antitoxin release system were demonstrated in Argentina[98] where the CDC assisted in the establishment of comparable principles that are nation-specific, including local stocking of antitoxin, establishing mechanisms for distribution, emergency identification, response, and laboratory confirmation for suspect cases. Expansion of this system to other nations will enhance worldwide botulism surveillance for foodborne as well as potential terrorist dissemination of botulinum toxin.[78]

SUMMARY

Botulism remains one of the rarest poisonings, while its etiologies have become increasingly diverse. The incidence of wound botulism has dramatically increased, along with that of the adult infectious form of botulism. Previously unrecognized complications of therapeutic botulinum toxin now permit a better understanding of the effects of the toxin as well as a recognition of its potential complications. The international experience with botulism epidemics has allowed the CDC to enhance international epidemiologic surveillance and to prepare for the possible use of botulinum toxin as a biologic weapon. Further treatment strategies are being developed to include a F(ab′)₂ despeciated heptavalent immune globulin, human botulism immune globulin, a recombinant vaccine, and other creative advances (see Antidote in Depth: Botulinum Antitoxin).

Acknowledgment

Richard S. Weisman, PharmD, contributed to this chapter in a previous edition.

REFERENCES

1. Alderson K, Holds JB, Anderson RL: Botulinum induced alteration of nerve-muscle interactions in human orbicularis oculi following treatment for blepharospasm. Neurology 1991;41:1800–1805.
2. Argov MD, Mastaglia FL: Disorders of neuromuscular transmission caused by drugs. N Engl J Med 1979;301:409–413.
3. Arnon SS, Midura TF, Damus K, et al: Honey and other environmental risk factors for infant botulism. J Pediatr 1979;94:331–336.
4. Arnon SS, Midura TF, Damus K: Intestinal infection and toxin production by *Clostridium botulinum* as one cause of sudden infant death syndrome. Lancet 1978;1:1273–1277.
4a. Arnon SS, Schechter R, Inglesby TV, et al: Botulinum Toxin as a Biological Weapon: Medical and Public Health Management. JAMA 2001;285:1059–1070.
5. Badhey H, Cleri DJ, D'Amato RF, et al: Two fatal cases of type E adult foodborne botulism with early symptoms and terminal neurologic signs. J Clin Microbiol 1986;23:616–618.
6. Bakheit AMO, Ward CD, Mclellan DL: Generalised botulism-like syndrome after intramuscular injections of botulinum toxin type A: A report of two cases. J Neurol Neurosurg Psych 1997;62:198.
7. Bamberger J, Terplan M: Wound botulism associated with black tar heroin. JAMA 1998;280:1479–1480.
8. Barker WH, Weissman MD, Dowell VR, et al: Type B botulism outbreak caused by a commercial food product. JAMA 1977;237:456–459.
9. Bartlett JC: Infant botulism in adults. N Engl J Med 1986;315:254–255.
10. Beller M, Middaugh JP: Repeated type E botulism in an Alaskan Eskimo [letter]. N Engl J Med 1990;322:855.
11. Black RE, Gunn RA: Hypersensitivity reactions associated with botulinal antitoxin. Am J Med 1980;69:567–570.
12. Blake PA, Horwitz MD, Hopkins L, et al: Type A botulism from commercially canned beef stew. South Med J 1977;70:5–7.
13. Borodic GE, Pearce LB: New concepts in botulinum toxin therapy. Drug Saf 1994;11:145–152.
14. Brisinda G, Giorgio M, Bentivoglio AR, et al: A comparison of injections of botulinum toxin and topical nitroglycerin ointment for the treatment of chronic anal fissure. N Engl J Med 1999;341:65–69.
15. Burningham MD, Walter FG, Mechem C, et al: Wound botulism. Ann Emerg Med 1994;24:1184–1187.
16. Byard RW, Moore L, Bourne AJ, et al: *Clostridium botulinum* and sudden infant death syndrome: A 10-year prospective study. J Paediatr Child Health 1992;28:157–157.
17. Case records of the Massachusetts General Hospital, Case 48–1980. N Engl J Med 1980;303:1347–1355.
18. Cherington M: Botulism: Ten-year experience. Arch Neurol 1974;30:432–437.
19. Chia JK, Clark JB, Ryan CA, Pollack M: Botulism in an adult associated with foodborne intestinal infection with *Clostridium botulinum*. N Engl J Med 1986;315:239–241.
20. Cochran DP, Appleton RE: Infant botulism—Is it that rare? Dev Med Child Neurol 1995;37:274–278.
21. Dowell UR Jr, McCroskey LM, Hatheway CL, et al: Coproexamination for botulinal toxin and *Clostridium botulism*. JAMA 1977;238:1829–1832.
22. Edell TA, Sullivan CP Jr, Osborn KM, et al: Wound botulism associated with a positive Tensilon test. West J Med 1983;139:218–219.
23. English WJ II, Williams LP Jr, Bryant RE, Gillies MD: Case 48–1980: Botulism. N Engl J Med 1981;304:789–790.
24. Fach P, Gilbert M, Griffais R, et al: PCR and gene probe identification of botulinum neurotoxin A-, B-, E-, F-, and G-producing *Clostridium spp.* and evaluation in food samples. Appl Environ Microbiol 1995;61:1389–1392.
25. Faich GA, Graebner RW, Sato S: Failure of guanidine therapy in botulism A. N Engl J Med 1971;285:773–776.
26. Frankovich TL, Arnon SS: Clinical trial of botulism immune globulin for infant botulism. West J Med 1991;154:103.
27. Freedman M, Armstrong RM, Killian JM, Boland D: Botulism in a patient with jejunoileal bypass. Ann Neurol 1986;20:641–643.
28. French G, Pavlick A, Felsen A, et al: Outbreak of type E botulism associated with an uneviscerated, salt-cured fish product: New Jersey, 1992. MMWR Morb Mortal Wkly Rep 1992;41:521–522.
29. Girlanda P, Vita G, Nicolosi C, et al: Botulinum toxin therapy: Distant effects on neuromuscular transmission and autonomic nervous system. J Neurol Neurosurg Psychiatry 1992;55:844–845.
30. Gollober M, Beyer RA, Kwan S, et al: Wound botulism: California, 1995. MMWR Morb Mortal Wkly Rep 1995;44:889–892.
31. Gomez HF, Johnson R, Guven H, et al: Adsorption of botulinum toxin to activated charcoal with a mouse bioassay. Ann Emerg Med 1995;25:818–822.
32. Griffin PM, Hatheway CL, Rosenbaum RB, Sokolow R: Endogenous antibody production to botulinum toxin in an adult with intestinal colonization botulism and underlying Crohn's disease. J Infect Dis 1997;175:633–637.
33. Gutmann L, Pratt L: Pathophysiologic aspects of human botulism. Arch Neurol 1976;33:175–179.
34. Hallett M: One man's poison—Clinical applications of botulinum toxin. N Engl J Med 1999;341:118–120.
35. Hashimoto H, Clyde VJ, Parko KL: Botulism from Peyote. N Engl J Med 1998;339:203–204.
36. Hatheway Cl: Toxigenic clostridia. Clin Microbiol Rev 1990;3:66–98.
37. Hentges D: The intestinal flora and infant botulism. Rev Infect Dis 1979;1:668–673.
38. Hikes DC, Manoli A II: Wound botulism. J Trauma 1981;21:68–71.
39. Horwitz MA, Marr JS, Merson MH, et al: A continuing common-source outbreak of botulism in a family. Lancet 1975;2:861–863.
40. Horowitz B, Swensen E, Marquardt K: Wound botulism associated with black tar heroin [letter]. JAMA 1998;280:1479–1480.
41. Infant botulism: A newly recognized syndrome. Calif Morbid 1976;34(Suppl):1–2.
42. Jankovic J, Brin MF: Therapeutic use of botulinum toxin. N Engl J Med 1991;324:1186–1193.
43. Johnson RO, Clay SA, Arnon SS: Diagnosis and management of infant botulism. Am J Dis Child 1979;133:586–593.
44. Kao I, Drachman DB, Price DL: Botulinum toxin: Mechanism of presynaptic blockade. Science 1976;193:1256–1258.
45. Kaplan JE, Davis LE, Narayan V, et al: Botulism, type A, and treatment with guanidine. Ann Neurol 1979;6:69–71.
46. Koenig MG, Spickard A, Cardella MA, Rogers DE: Clinical and laboratory observations on type E botulism in man. Medicine 1964;43:517–545.

47. Kotev S, Leventhal A, Bashary A, et al: International outbreak of type E botulism associated with ungutted, salted white fish. MMWR Morb Mortal Wkly Rep 1987;36:812–813.

48. Lange DJ, Brin MF, Warner CL, et al: Distant effects of local injection of botulinum toxin. Muscle Nerve 1987;10:552–555.

49. LeCour H, Ramos H, Almeida B, Barbosa R: Food borne botulism: A review of 13 outbreaks. Arch Intern Med 1988;148:578–580.

50. Long SS: Botulism in infancy. Pediatr Infect Dis J 1984;3:266–271.

51. Ludlow CL: Treatment of speech and voice disorders with botulinum toxin. JAMA 1990;264:2671–2675.

52. MacDonald KL, Cohen ML, Blake PA: The changing epidemiology of adult botulism in the United States. Am J Epidemiol 1986;124:794–799.

53. MacDonald KL, Rutherford GW, Friedman SM, et al: Botulism and botulism-like illness in chronic drug users. Ann Intern Med 1985;102:616–618.

54. MacDonald KL, Spengler RF, Hatheway CL, et al: Type A botulism from sautéed onions: Clinical and epidemiologic observations. JAMA 1985;253:1275–1278.

55. Maria G, Cassetta E, Gui D, et al: A comparison of botulinum toxin and saline for the treatment of chronic anal fissure. N Engl J Med 1998;338:217–220.

56. Maselli RA, Ellis W, Mandler RN, Sheikh F, et al: Cluster of wound botulism in California: Clinical, electrophysiologic, and pathologic study. Muscle Nerve 1997;20:1284–1295.

57. McCroskey LM, Hatheway CL: Laboratory findings in four cases of adult botulism suggest colonization of the intestinal tract. J Clin Microbiol 1988;26:1052–1054.

58. McCroskey LM, Hatheway CL, Woodruff, et al: Type F botulism due to neurotoxigenic *Clostridium baratii* from an unknown source in an adult. J Clin Microbiol 1991;29:2618–2620.

59. Merson MH, Dowel VR: Epidemiologic, clinical and laboratory aspects of wound botulism. N Engl J Med 1973;289:1005–1010.

60. Metzger JF, Lewis GE Jr: Human derived immune globulin for the treatment of botulism. Rev Infect Dis 1979;1:689–692.

61. Morris JG Jr, Hatheway CL: Botulism in the United States, 1979. J Infect Dis 1980;142:302–305.

62. Morse DL, Pichard LK, Guzewich JT, et al: Garlic in oil associated botulism: Episode leads to product modification. Am J Public Health 1990;80:1372–1373.

63. Olney RK, Aminoff MJ, Gelb DJ, Lowenstein DH: Neuromuscular effects distant from the site of botulinum neurotoxin injection. Neurology 1988;38:1780–1783.

64. Otofugi T, Tokiwa H, Takahashi K: A food-poisoning incident caused by *Clostridium botulinum* toxin A in Japan. Epidemiol Infect 1987;99:167–172.

65. Paisley JW, Lauer BA, Arnon RS: A second case of infant botulism type F caused by *Clostridium baratii*. Pediatr Infect Dis J 1995;14:912–914.

66. Passaro DJ, Werner B, McGee J, et al: Wound botulism associated with black tar heroin among injecting drug users. JAMA 1998;279 859–863.

67. Passaro DJ, Werner B, Vugia DJ: Wound botulism associated with black tar heroin [letter]. JAMA 1998;280:1480.

67a. Pellizzari R, Rossetto O, Schiavo G, Montecucco C: Tetanus and Botulinum Neurotoxins: Mechanism of action and therapeutic uses. Phil Trans R Soc Lond B 1999;354:259–268.

68. Pickett JB III: AAEE case report #16: Botulism. Muscle Nerve 1988;11:1201–1205.

69. Puggiari M, Cherington M: Botulism and guanidine. JAMA 1978;240:2276–2277.

70. Rapoport S, Watkins PB: Descending paralysis resulting from occult wound botulism. Ann Neurol 1984;16:359–361.

71. Robin L, Herman D, Redett R: Botulism in a pregnant woman. N Engl J Med 1996;335:823–824.

72. Ross MH, Charness ME, Sudarsky L, Logigian EL: Treatment of occupational cramp with botulinum toxin: Diffusion of toxin to adjacent noninjected muscles. Muscle Nerve 1997;20:593–598.

73. Sacks HS: The botulism hazard. Ann Int Med 1997;126:918–919.

74. Schantz EJ, Johnson EA: Properties and use of botulinum toxin and other microbial neurotoxins in medicine. Microbiol Rev 1992;56:80–99.

75. Schmidt RD, Schmidt TW: Infant botulism: A case series and a review of the literature. J Emerg Med 1992;10:713–718.

76. Schmidt-Nowara WW, Samet JM, Rasario PA: Early and late pulmonary complications of botulism. Arch Intern Med 1983;143:451–456.

77. Schreiner MS, Field E, Ruddy R: Infant botulism: A review of 12 years experience at the Children's Hospital of Philadelphia. Pediatrics 1991;87:159–165.

78. Shapiro RL, Hatheway C, Becher J, Swerdlow DL: Botulism surveillance and Emergency Response. JAMA 1997;278:433–435.

79. Shapiro RL, Hatheway C, Swerdlow DL: Botulism in the United States: A clinical and epidemiologic review. Ann Intern Med 1998;129:221–228.

80. Sheridan RE: Gating and permeability of ION channels produced by *Botulinum* toxin types A and E in PC12 cell membranes. Toxicon 1998;36:703–717.

81. Simpson LL: Botulinum toxin: A deadly poison sheds its negative image. Ann Intern Med 1996;125:616–617.

82. Simpson LL: The origin, structure, and pharmacological activity of *Botulinum* toxin. Pharm Rev 1981;33:155–188.

83. Smith LDS: The occurrence of *Clostridium botulinum* and *Clostridium tetani* in the soil of the United States. Health Lab Sci 1978;15:74–80.

84. Sonnabend OAR, Sonnabend WFF, Krech V, et al: Continuous microbiological and pathological study of 70 sudden and unexpected infant deaths: Toxigenic intestinal *Clostridium botulinum* infection in 9 cases of sudden infant death. Lancet 1985;1:237–241.

85. St. Clair EH, DiLiberti JH, O'Brien ML: Observations of an infant born to a mother with botulism. J Pediatr 1975;87:658.

86. St. Louis ME, Peck SHS, Bowering D, et al: Botulism from chopped garlic, delayed recognition of a major outbreak. Ann Intern Med 1988;108:363–368.

87. Swedberg J, Wendel TH, Deiss F: Wound botulism. West J Med 1987;147:335–338.

88. Swenson JM, Thornsberry C, McCroskey LM, et al: Susceptibility of *Clostridium botulinum* to thirteen antimicrobial agents. Antimicrob Agents Chemother 1980;18:13–19.

89. Szabo EA, Pemberton JM, Gibson Am, Eyles MJ, Desmarchelier PM: Polymerase chain reaction for detection of *Clostridium botulinum* type A, B, and E in food, soil and infant faeces. J Appl Bacteriol 1994;76:39–45.

90. Tacket CO, Shandera WX, Mann JM, et al: Equine antitoxin use and other factors that predict outcome in type A foodborne botulism. Am J Med 1984;76:794–798.

91. Telzak EE, Bell EP, Kauter DA, et al: An international outbreak of type E botulism due to uneviscerated fish. J Infect Dis 1990;161:340–342.

92. Terranova W, Palumbo JN, Breman JG: Ocular findings in botulism type B. JAMA 1979;241:475–477.

93. Thompson JA, Glascow LA, Warpinski JR, et al: Infant botulism. Clinical spectrum and epidemiology. Pediatrics 1980;6:936–942.

94. Townes JM, Cieslak PR, Hatheway CL, et al: An outbreak of Type A botulism associated with a commercial cheese sauce. Ann Intern Med 1996;125:558–563.

95. Townes JM, Solomon HM, Griffin PM: The botulism hazard [letter]. Ann Intern Med 1997;126:919.

96. Turner HD, Brett EM, Gilbert RJ, et al: Infant botulism in England. Lancet 1978;1:1277–1278.

97. Valli G, Barbieri S, Scarlato G: Neurophysiological tests in human botulism. Electromyogr Clin Neurophysiol 1983;23:3–11.

98. Villar RG, Shapiro RL, Busto S, et al: Outbreak of type a botulism and development of a botulism surveillance and antitoxin release system in Argentina. JAMA 1999;281:1334–1338, 1340.

99. Wainwright RB, Heyward WL, Middaugh JP, et al: Foodborne botulism in Alaska, 1947–1985: Epidemiology and clinical findings. J Infect Dis 1988;157:1158–1162.

100. Weber JT, Hibbs RG, Darwish A, et al: A massive outbreak of type E botulism associated with traditional salted fish in Cairo. J Infect Dis 1993;167:451–454.

101. Wilcox P, Andofatto G, Fairbain MS, Pardy RL: Long-term follow-up of symptoms, pulmonary function, respiratory muscle strength and exercise performance after botulism. Am Rev Respir Dis 1989; 139:157–163.

102. Wilson R, Morris JG, Snyder JD, Feldman RA: Clinical characteristics of infant botulism in the United States: A study of the non-Californian cases. Pediatr Infect Dis 1982;1:148–150.

103. Woodruff BA, Griffin PM, McCroskey LM, Smart JF: Clinical and laboratory comparison of botulism form toxin types A, B, and E in the United States, 1975–1988. J Infect Dis 1992;166:1281–1286.

104. Wolfe L: Death by botulism: A medical mystery story. New York Magazine 1980;13:56–60.

ANTIDOTES IN DEPTH

Botulinum Antitoxin
Lewis R. Goldfrank

Trivalent (types A, B, and E) botulinum antitoxin is an equine globulin preparation that has been available in the United States since the late 1960s.[2] The production of antitoxin is complex, taking almost 2 years to immunize healthy horses against botulinum toxin, but excess product can be freeze-dried and preserved.[18] The resultant product is then defibrinated, digested, dialyzed, and purified as a 20% protein antitoxin.[3]

Botulinum antitoxin is distributed from the 9 regional centers of the Centers for Disease Control and Prevention (CDC) on a named patient basis after a probable diagnosis of botulism is established. Each 10-mL vial of the currently available trivalent botulinum antitoxin from Connaught Laboratories contains 7500 IU (2381 US units) of type A botulinum antitoxin, 5500 IU (1839 US units) of type B antitoxin, and 8500 IU (8500 US units) of type E antitoxin.[8] There is evidence substantiating the efficacy of types A and E antitoxin,[12,22] but the efficacy of type B antitoxin has not been established in clinical trials. The proportion and quantity of types A, B, and E antitoxin are assumed to be adequate to neutralize the quantities of circulating toxins suspected in cases of foodborne botulism.[3,8]

Currently there is only limited data available on the relationship of dose and route of administration, the amount of circulating antitoxin found in treated patients, the toxin-neutralizing capacity of this material, and the half-life of the antitoxin. Peak serum levels of antitoxin are 10–1000 times higher than the levels of antitoxin calculated to be necessary to achieve toxin neutralization. This excess was confirmed by the observation that there was a limited decrease of antitoxin when patients who had a quantified amount of circulating type A toxin prior to treatment were studied. In another patient, 90% of the activity of the equine antitoxin administered was detected when all the circulating toxin was neutralized.[9,14] The half-life for antitoxin persistence in a single patient was calculated at 6.5, 7.6, and 5.3 days for antitoxin types A, B, and E, respectively.[9] The prolonged half-life of the antitoxin and the exceedingly small quantities of toxin measured explain the limited decrease in antitoxin titres following toxin-antitoxin binding.

Like many other heterologous proteins, this horse serum-derived preparation results in substantial adverse effects.[13] Each patient treated during the initial decade that antitoxin was available (1967–1977) was studied to determine both hypersensitivity reaction rates and the efficacy of the antitoxin in preventing botulism. The overall rate of adverse reactions, including hypersensitivity and serum sickness, was 9–17%, with an incidence of anaphylaxis as high as 1.9%.[1,15] The issues of human sensitivity to equine proteins and conjunctival or intradermal testing of antitoxin preparations is discussed in detail in this text in Antidotes in Depth:

Antivenin (Crotalid and Elapid). However, after the need for botulinum antitoxin is established, hypersensitivity to equine proteins is not a contraindication to antitoxin administration, because botulism can be fatal. Anaphylaxis should be anticipated, and the clinician should be prepared to treat this complication immediately with epinephrine. The smaller quantities of botulinum antitoxin used for botulism present a far smaller risk for serum sickness[2] than do the larger amounts of antivenom used to treat snake envenomation. The risk of serum sickness from the refined serum proteins in botulinum antitoxin is approximately 4–10%.[2,8]

Patients who received antitoxin within the first 24 hours after exposure have a shorter clinical course of botulism without regression of symptoms, but a comparable mortality rate to those who received antitoxin later.[22] Reduced mortality can only be demonstrated in animal models.[16] Morbidity and mortality studies are difficult to perform for a disorder that is so rare and often recognized at a delayed stage, after the toxin is already tightly bound to the neuromuscular junction. Also, most of the reported case series involve patients who have received varying degrees of supportive care, further making evaluation or comparison unreliable.

Isolated human-derived type E botulinum antitoxin was used successfully to treat 100 Egyptians who presumably had ingested botulinum toxin-contaminated uneviscerated salted mullet fish.[7,25] Human-derived preparations of type E antitoxin were available as 5000 IU per 2-mL vials in Egypt as a consequence of the military preparedness for the 1991 Persian Gulf War. Prophylactic doses of the monovalent antitoxin were considered to be 1000–5000 IU administered IM, and were based on the estimated quantity of toxin ingested. The safety of this human-derived preparation allowed for repetitive dosing if clinical findings developed.[7] This small repetitive dosing regimen was based on the belief that effective treatment could be achieved when antitoxin doses that exceeded the level of toxin dose were administered before circulating toxin became tissue-bound.

In the presence of disease, 1 vial of the antitoxin is administered slowly IV over several minutes as a 1:10 vol/vol dilution in 0.9% sodium chloride. This dose may be complemented by an IM dose of a single vial given simultaneously. Subsequent doses may be given IV every 2–4 hours, depending on the progression of clinical findings.[3,8]

Numerous locally prepared botulinal antitoxins are available around the world. These agents lack international standardization. Future treatment for botulism may utilize additional types of immunotherapy.

Because of the lethality of botulinum toxin, the risk of adverse drug reaction for the antitoxin is considered acceptable for anyone with presumed illness, as well as for anyone potentially exposed to the toxin. Pregnancy is 0not a contraindication to antitoxin administration and antitoxin has been used successfully in this setting.[21]

A pentavalent toxoid (types A, B, C, D, and E) was developed at the US Army Medical Research Institute of Infectious Diseases at Fort Detrick, Maryland and has been studied for almost 40 years.[14] It remains investigational and its use is suggested only for laboratory personnel who do investigative work with *Clostridium botulinum.*

F(ab')$_2$ "despeciated" heptavalent (against toxin types A, B, C$_1$, D, E, F, and G) botulism immune globulin (dBIG) is also currently under investigation.[6] This equine immune globulin[5] is extensively purified to eliminate fibrinogen, plasminogen, and other proteins. Pepsin is used to remove the F$_c$ fragment of the immunoglobulin in order to reduce the potential for allergic manifestations should reexposure to horse protein occur.[10] When given prior to exposure, this F(ab')$_2$ immune globulin protected mice from inhaled toxin at doses 10 times that of the LD$_{50}$ and is fully protective when given after exposure, but prior to the onset of clinical signs.[11]

Ten of 45 patients given dBIG in the Egyptian type E botulism outbreak manifested adverse reactions; 9 were considered mild and 1 episode was classified as serum sickness.[10] In this botulism epidemic, the incidence of adverse effects of dBIG was compared to those of numerous other internationally available botulinal antitoxins. Although followup of individuals was limited, there was no evidence of any increased adverse effects associated with dBIG, and the agent appeared to be as safe as other commercially available antitoxins. Further investigations with regard to safety and efficacy are necessary.

Human derived botulism immune globulin (BIG) was developed for use in the treatment of infant botulism. This pentavalent (types A, B, C, D, and E) immune globulin is harvested by plasmapheresis from human donors who received multiple immunizations with pentavalent botulinal toxoid.[17,23] A longer biologic half-life with a prolonged effective level should be possible with BIG,[14] and the use of a human immune globulin obviously avoids the risk of hypersensitivity that is associated with foreign equine proteins. Both of these effects are substantial clinical advantages, particularly for the infant form of botulism, where toxin is slowly and continuously produced in the intestine and absorbed. Results of the orphan-drug infant botulism prevention clinical trial of the human BIG suggest many advantages over the current equine antitoxin therapy.[4]

BIG became available in California in 1991 for clinical trials.[4] Human BIG was used successfully in a 3-year-old child who developed altered gut microbial flora and botulism following bone marrow transplantation.[19]

Recombinant vaccines,[20] monoclonal antibodies, and drugs that act as metalloproteinase inhibitors thereby preventing toxin uptake, are all currently under investigation by the Department of Defense.[5]

SUMMARY

Consultation with a regional poison center, local health department, and the CDC (404-639-2206 days or 404-639-2888 nights, weekends, or holidays) or comparable agencies in other parts of the world provide improved access to rapid diagnostic tests for botulism and effective therapeutic modalities. This approach appears to be responsible for decreasing morbidity and for increasing survival after typical foodborne botulism.[18,24] Results of current research on infant botulism will demonstrate whether there is enough circulating toxin present in that variant to be amenable to antitoxin treatment. Antitoxin may be useful if a low level of absorbed toxin is present in these disorders as suggested.[14] After

these issues are clarified, it may be possible to provide adequate treatment for the infant form of botulism, which has become the most prevalent form of botulism.

REFERENCES

1. Badhey H, Cleri DJ, D'Amato RF, et al: Two fatal cases of type E adult foodborne botulism with early symptoms and terminal neurologic signs. J Clin Microbiol 1986;23:616–618.
2. Black RE, Gunn RA: Hypersensitivity reactions associated with botulinal antitoxin. Am J Med 1980;69:567–570.
3. Food and Drug Administration, Biological Products, Bacterial Vaccines and Toxoids: Implementation of efficacy review: Proposed rule. Fed Reg 1985;50:51002–51117.
4. Frankovich TL, Arnon SS: Clinical trial of botulism immune globulin for infant botulism. West J Med 1991;154:103.
5. Franz DR, Jahrling PB, Friedlander AM, et al: Clinical recognition and management of patients exposed to biological warfare agents. JAMA 1997;278:399–411.
6. Fries L, Sjogren M, McKee K, et al: Clearance kinetics and immunologic responses to "despeciated" equine botulinum antitoxin in human volunteers [abstract no 92]. In: Program and abstracts of the 31st Interscience Conference on antimicrobial agents and chemotherapy (Chicago). Washington, DC: American Society for Microbiology, 1991:114.
7. Goldsmith MF: Defensive biological warfare researchers prepare to counteract "natural enemies" in battle, at home. JAMA 1991;266:2522–2523.
8. Grabenstein JD: Immunoantidotes: II. One hundred years of antitoxins. Hosp Pharm 1992;27:637–646.
9. Hatheway CH, Snyder JD, Seals JE, et al: Antitoxin levels in botulism patients treated with trivalent equine botulism antitoxin to toxin types A, B, and E. J Infect Dis 1984;150:407–412.
10. Hibbs RG, Weber JT, Corwin A, et al: Experience with the use of an investigational F(ab')$_2$ heptavalent botulism immune globulin of equine origin during an outbreak of type E botulism in Egypt. Clin Infect Dis 1996;23:337–340.
11. Investigator's brochure. Botulinum F(ab')$_2$ antitoxin, heptavalent (equine derived). Document no. BB IND #3703. Ft. Detrick, Maryland: Office of the Surgeon General, Department of the Army, USAMRMC (MCMR-RCQ-HR).
12. Koenig MG, Spickard A, Cardella MA, Rogers DE: Clinical and laboratory observations on type E botulism in man. Medicine 1964;43:517–545.
13. Merson MH, Hughes JM, Dowell VR: Current trends in botulism in the United States. JAMA 1974;229:1305–1308.
14. Metzger JR, Lewis LE: Human-derived immune globulins for the treatment of botulism. Rev Infect Dis 1979;1:689–692.
15. Morris JG Jr, Hatheway CL: Botulism in the United States, 1979. J Infect Dis 1980;142:302–305.
16. Oberst FW, Crook JW, Cresthull P, House MJ: Evaluation of botulinum antitoxin, supportive therapy, and artificial respiration in monkeys with experimental botulism. Clin Pharmacol Ther 1968;9:209–214.
17. Pickett J, Berg B, Chaplin E, Brunstetter-Shafer MA: Syndrome of botulism in infancy: Clinical and electrophysiologic study. N Engl J Med 1976;295:770–772.
18. Shapiro RL, Hatheway C, Becher J, Swerdlow DL: Botulism surveillance and emergency response. JAMA 1997;278:433–435.
19. Shen WP, Felsing N, Lang D, et al: Development of infant botulism in a 3-year-old female with neuroblastoma following autologous bone narrow transplantation: Potential use of human botulism immune globulin. Bone Marrow Transplant 1994;13:345–347.
20. Smith LA: Development of recombinant vaccines for botulinum neurotoxin. Toxicon 1998;36:1539–1548.

21. St. Clair EH, DiLiberti JH, O'Brien ML: Observations of an infant born to a mother with botulism. J Pediatr 1975;87:658.

22. Tacket CO, Shandera WX, Mann JM, et al: Equine antitoxin use and other factors that predict outcome in type A foodborne botulism. Am J Med 1984;76:794–798.

23. Thilo EH, Townsend SF, Deacon J: Infant botulism at 1 week of age: Report of two cases. Pediatrics 1993;92:151–153.

24. Villar RG, Shapiro RL, Busto S, et al: Outbreak of type a botulism and development of a botulism surveillance and antitoxin release system in Argentina. JAMA 1999;281:1334–1338, 1340.

25. Weber JT, Hibbs RG, Darwish A, et al: A massive outbreak of type E botulism associated with traditional salted fish in Cairo. J Infect Dis 1993;167:451–454.

F. BOTANICALS

CHAPTER 76 MUSHROOMS

Lewis R. Goldfrank

A 58-year-old woman presented to the Emergency Department (ED) with severe, crampy, abdominal pain and profuse diarrhea. She had spent the summer morning picking wild mushrooms in a local park, as she had done for many years. She found numerous edible species and ate quite a few while picking them. Her symptoms began within 1 hour of returning from the park.

She explained that she was an expert in selecting edible mushrooms, that she picked at the same place every year, and that she never previously had trouble. Prior to coming to the United States she had foraged in the woods of Poland for years without difficulty. She insisted that the mushrooms could not be at fault as they were found growing on dead wood, and that slugs had mutilated several of the mushrooms.

The patient had diabetes mellitus, which was well controlled with chlorpropamide 500 mg daily, took no other medications, had no known allergies, and did not drink alcohol or smoke cigarettes. No other family members had been ill recently.

Physical examination revealed a pale, diaphoretic, dyspneic, and anxious woman who was persistently gagging. Her orthostatic vital signs were: blood pressure, 110/60 mm Hg and pulse, 120 beats/min supine; and 90/40 mm Hg and 145 beats/min upright. Her respiratory rate was 24 breaths/min and her temperature was 98.6°F (37°C).

The patient's head was atraumatic, her pupils were 4 mm, equal, and reactive; sclerae were anicteric; and her conjunctivae were pink. Her mucosa was moist with no excessive lacrimation or salivation, and her throat was unremarkable. There were no cutaneous abnormalities. Lungs were clear, heart sounds were normal, and abdominal examination revealed diffuse tenderness with hyperactive bowel sounds, but the liver and spleen were unremarkable. The extremities were normal.

When it was suggested that she stay in the hospital, the patient resisted vehemently. Her dizziness upon standing, however, convinced her to remain. Blood samples were drawn, an IV was started with 0.9% sodium chloride at 300 mL/h; a fingerstick glucose value of 180 mg/dL was obtained. The patient was admitted for observation and volume repletion.

As the patient prepared herself for admission, she gave her belongings and clothing to her daughter. At that point the staff noticed a large bag filled with mushrooms. The patient was so convinced of the quality of these mushrooms that she wanted to give them to her daughter to take home, but she was eventually persuaded to leave the mushrooms in the ED for further examination.

Her hematocrit was 42%, white blood cell count (WBC) was 8300/mm³ (72% polys, 20% lymphocytes, 4% monocytes, and 4% eosinophils), and prothrombin time was 13 seconds (control 12

seconds). Blood glucose was 220 mg/dL; blood urea nitrogen (BUN) was 21 mg/dL; sodium was 140 mEq/L; potassium was 3.7 mEq/L; chloride was 101 mEq/L; and bicarbonate was 30 mEq/L. The chest radiograph was normal and abdominal radiographs showed a nonspecific ileus pattern.

Despite the patient's certainty that the mushrooms were edible, her presentation persuaded the staff to have them investigated. Microscopic spore assessment methods to identify toxic mushrooms conducted by a mycologist confirmed that this patient had mistakenly picked the jack-o'-lantern (*Omphalotus illudens*), an orange, bioluminescent mushroom,[4] believing it to be the edible species of chanterelle (*Cantharellus cibarius*), a frequent error reported by others[26,74] (see Fig. 76–1).

EPIDEMIOLOGY

Unintentional exposures to mushrooms represent a small but relatively constant percentage of consultations requested from Poison Control Centers. (see citations for AAPCC data in Chap. 116) A summary of the 16 years of AAPCC data reveals that mushrooms represent <0.5% of the exposures to poisons. Combining data accumulated by the AAPCC and the Mushroom Poisoning Registry of the North American Mycological Association indicate that approximately 5 patient exposures to mushrooms per 100,000 population occur per year, with some variations a result of geographic and climatic conditions, as well as mycologic habitats.[72] Although the methods of analysis of patients with mushroom exposures have changed over the past 16 years, cumulative AAPCC Toxic Exposure Surveillance System (TESS) data consistently demonstrate the relative benignity of the vast majority of such ingestions. The inability of most healthcare providers to correctly identify the ingested mushroom, and the rarity of lethal ingestions, is also demonstrated by the accumulated data. In more than 95% of the cases, the exact species was unidentified,[72] and only about 10% of the toxin groups ingested were known; more than 50% of exposed individuals had no symptoms, 25% of the patients were treated in healthcare facilities annually, of whom 10–15% had minor manifestations of toxicity, less than 5% had moderate toxicity, and approximately 0.3% had major toxicity. During the 16-year period covered by TESS, only 17 of the patients were reported to die of their ingestions. Of all those mushrooms associated with a death, 12 were probably *Amanita* species, one was an hallucinogen, one was a *Boletus spp.*, and 3 were unidentified. All deaths occurred in adults. Of all the mushroom groups identified in poisonings, hallucinogens accounted for about 4.7%, gastrointestinal toxins ac-

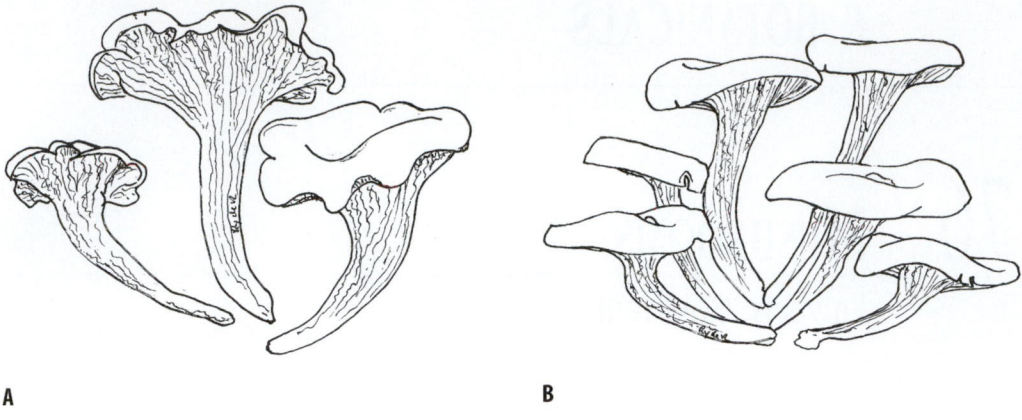

Figure 76-1. The Jack O'Lantern (*Omphalotus illudens*), an orange bioluminescent mushroom, (**A**) is often confused with its look-alike, the edible species of chanterelle (*Cantharellus cibarius*) (**B**).

counted for about 2.1%, miscellaneous nontoxins accounted for about 1.6%, and all the other groups represented less than 2% of the total. Because 90% of mushrooms involved in exposures are never identified, a strategy for making significant decisions with incomplete data is needed.

CLASSIFICATION AND MANAGEMENT

Because mushroom species vary widely in the toxins they contain and because identifying them with certainty is difficult, a clinical system of classification is more useful than a taxonomic system (Table 76–1). Ten groups of toxins are identifiable: cyclopeptides, gyromitrin, muscarine, coprine, ibotenic acid and muscimol, psilocybin, general gastrointestinal (GI) toxins, orellanine, and allenic norleucine and toxins inducing rhabdomyolysis.[28,38] In many cases, management and prognosis can be determined with a high degree of confidence from the history and initial symptoms.[28,38,39]

Group I: Cyclopeptide-Containing Mushrooms

α-Amanitin

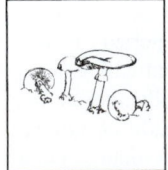

Most mushroom fatalities in North America are associated with the cyclopeptide-containing species.[5,84] These mushrooms include a number of *Amanita* species, including *A. verna, A. virosa,* and *A. phalloides,* as well as *Galerina autumnalis, G. marginata, G. venenata, Lepiota helveola, L. josserandi,* and *L.*

brunneoincarnata. Although not reflected in the AAPCC TESS data cited earlier, the mortality rate appears to be higher in children than in adults.[48]

Unfortunately, early differentiation of cyclopeptide poisonings from other types of mushroom poisoning is very difficult. Patients poisoned with cyclopeptides may present to an ED with a seemingly innocuous picture of nausea, vomiting, abdominal pain, and diarrhea, which is often attributed to other causes. Such patients may be sent home, only to return moribund on a subsequent day. The delayed onset of more serious symptoms is typical of cyclopeptide poisoning and is a critical consideration in assessing any potential poisoning.

Amanita phalloides contains 15–20 cyclopeptides of approximately 900 daltons, including the amatoxins (cyclic octapeptides), phallotoxins (cyclic heptapeptides), and virotoxins (cyclic heptapeptides). These 3 peptides appear to have the highest toxic potential.[17,36,80] Of these three chemically similar cyclopeptide molecules, phalloidin appears to be a rapid-acting toxin whereas amanitin tends to cause more delayed manifestations.[61] Phalloidin the principal phallotoxin, interrupts actin polymerization and impairs cell membrane function, but because of its limited absorption appears to have a limited toxicity, restricted mostly to gastrointestinal dysfunction. There is no evidence for virotoxin toxicity in human poisoning.

α-Amanitin is the principal amatoxin responsible for human toxicity following ingestion. Approximately 1.5–2.5 mg of amanitin can be obtained from 1 g of dry *Amanita phalloides,* and as much as 3.5 mg/g can be obtained from some *Lepiota spp.*[49,53,80] A 20-g mushroom therefore contains well in excess of the 0.1 mg/kg of amanitin considered lethal for humans.[16]

The amatoxins appear to be the most toxic of the cyclopeptides, leading to hepatic, renal, and central nervous system (CNS) damage. These polypeptides are heat stable, insoluble in water, and lose activity over a period of years after drying.[17] In vitro studies show that α-amanitin is cytotoxic on the basis of its interference with RNA polymerase II, preventing the transcription of DNA.[43,65] The LD$_{50}$ of β-amanitin in mice is 0.1–0.75 mg/kg and the LD$_{50}$ of β-amanitin in mice is 0.2–0.4 mg/kg,[16] suggesting comparable toxicity of both amanitins. The amanitins are poorly, but rapidly, absorbed from the GI tract,[32] and α-amanitin may be enterohepatically recirculated.[10] Target organs are those with the highest rate of cell turnover, including the gastrointestinal tract ep-

TABLE 76–1. **Mushroom Toxicity**

Genus/Species	Toxin	Time of onset of Symptoms	Primary Site of Toxicity	Symptoms	Mortality	Specific Therapy*

I.
Amanita phalloides,
  A. tennifolia, A. virosa
Galerina autumnalis
  G. marginata, G. veneata
Lepiota josserandii,
  L. helveola
	Cyclopeptides
	Amatoxins
	Phallotoxins
		5–24h	Hepatic	Phase I: GI toxicity-NVD
				
				Phase II: Quiescent,
				Phase III: gastroenteritis,
				  jaundice, ↑ AST, ↑ ALT
					10–30% lethal	Activated charcoal
						Hemoperfusion
						Penicillin G
						Silibinin

II. Gyromitra ambigua, G. esculenta, G. infula	Gyromitrin (metab- olite: mono- methylhydrazine)	5–10h	CNS	Seizures, abdominal pain, N/V, weakness, hepato- renal failure	Rare	Benzodiazepines, Pyridoxine, 70 mg/kg IV if indicated
III. Clitocybe dealbata, C. dilatata, C. illudens Most Inocybe spp.	Muscarine	0.5–2h	Autonomic nervous system	Muscarinic effects-saliva- tion, bradycardia, lacrimation, urination, defecation, diaphoresis.	Rare	Atropine: adults: 1–2 mg children: 0.02 mg/kg with a minimum of 0.1 mg
IV. Coprinus atramentarius	Coprine (metabo- lite: 1-aminocy- clopropanol)	0.5–2hr	Aldehyde dehydrogenase	Disulfiramlike effect with ethanol, tachycardia, N/V	Rare	—

V.
Amanita gemmata,
  A. muscaria,
  A. pantherina
	Ibotenic acid,
	muscimol
		0.5–2hr	CNS	GABAergic effects, rare
				delirium, hallucinations,
				dizziness, ataxia
					Rare	Benzodiazepines
						during excitatory
						phase

VI. Psilocybe caerulipes, P. cubensis Gymnopilus spectabilis Psathyrella foenisecii	Psilocybin, psilocin	0.5–1h	CNS	Ataxia, N/V, hyperkinesis, hallucinations	Rare	Benzodiazepines
VII. Clitocybe nebularis Chlorophyllum molyb- dites, C. esculentum, Lactarius sp. Paxillus involutus	Various GI irritants	0.5–3h	GI	Malaise, N/V/D,	Rare	—

VIII.
Cortinarius orellanus,
  C. speciosissimus,
  C. rainierensis
	Orelline, orellanine	>24h
		Days-weeks
			Renal	Phase I: N/V
				Phase II: Oliguria,
				  renal failure
					Rare	Hemodialysis for
						renal failure

IX. Amanita smithiana	Allenic norleucine	0.5–12h	Renal	Phase I: N/V Phase II: Oliguria, renal failure	None	Hemodialysis for renal failure
X. Tricholoma equestre	Unidentified myotoxin	24–72h	Muscle (peripheral and cardiac)	Fatigue, nausea, muscle weakness, myalgias (↑CPK), facial erythema, diaphoresis, myocarditis	25%	—

Adapted, with permission, from Lincoff G, Mitchel DH: Toxic and Hallucinogenic Mushroom Poisoning: A Handbook for Physicians and Mushroom Hunters. New York, Van Nostrand Reinhold, 1977, pp. 246–247.
*Supportive care-fluids, electrolyes, and antiemetics as indicated. N = nausea, V = vomiting D = diarrhea.

ithelium, hepatocytes, and kidneys. Pathologic manifestations include steatosis, central zonal necrosis, and centrilobular hemorrhage, with viable hepatocytes remaining at the rims of the larger triads. Lobular architecture remains intact.[5] Amatoxins show limited protein binding and are present in the plasma at low concentrations for 24–48 hours.[32] They are eliminated in the urine, gastroduodenal fluids, and feces for several days following ingestion, and can be detected by high-performance liquid chromatography,[32] thin-layer chromatography, and radioimmunoassay in gastroduodenal fluid, serum, urine, stool, and liver and kidney biopsies for several days following an ingestion.[10,16,17,35]

Some of the toxicokinetic analyses following unknown quantitative ingestions demonstrate 12–23 μg of amatoxin excretion in the urine, of which 60–80% occurred during the first 2 hours of collection. The extreme variability of the type and quantity of ingestant, the host, and the management make interpretations exceedingly difficult. Maximal urinary retrieval of 20 μg of amanitin was achieved in one series.[75] In another series, total maximal urinary α- and β-amanitin excreted were 3.19 mg and 5.21 mg, respectively. Two-thirds of the patients had a total excretion of greater than 1.5 mg amanitin toxins.[32]

Phase I of cyclopeptide poisoning resembles severe gastroenteritis, with profuse, watery diarrhea, not occurring until 5–24 hours after ingestion. Supportive fluid and electrolyte replacement leads to transient improvement during phase II, which occurs between 12 and 36 hours after ingestion.[53,84] However, despite such supportive care, phase III, manifested by hepatic,[5] renal,[5] and, rarely, pancreatic[20] toxicity and death, may ensue 2–6 days after ingestion. The initial hepatotoxicity begins within the second phase, but hepatic necrosis (Chap. 14) with elevated bilirubin, aspartate aminotransferase (AST), and alanine aminotransferase (ALT), hypoglycemia, jaundice, and coma are not manifest until 2–3 days after the ingestion.

Cyclopeptide poisoning alters the hormones that regulate glucose, calcium, and thyroid homeostasis resulting in widespread endocrine abnormalities.[33] Insulin and C-peptide concentrations may be elevated. Serum calcitonin concentrations may be elevated along with the presence of hypocalcemia. Thyroxine concentrations may be depressed and triiodothyronine concentrations undetectable, while thyroid-stimulating hormone concentrations may not be elevated. All of these findings were reported in a single study and therefore merit further investigation.[33]

In a series of 10 patients poisoned by diverse *Lepiota spp.*, 50% developed a mixed polyneuropathy. Most of the patients spontaneously recovered within 1 year, although a single patient progressively deteriorated.[55]

The search for treatments has been vigorously pursued in Europe because of the large number of victims each year and the current 20–30% mortality rate (previously 50–60%).[19] Thioctic (α-lipoic) acid was initially reported to be beneficial in treating the amatoxin-induced liver toxicity in several different animal models,[30] and a number of uncontrolled clinical trials in humans followed.[5] In 1963, thioctic acid, because of its potential effects as a coenzyme in the tricarboxylic acid cycle or as a free radical scavenger,[30] was credited for the survival of 39 of 40 patients poisoned by *Amanita phalloides*.[37] Hypoglycemia is a common feature of thioctic acid therapy for *Amanita* poisoning, although it is not clear whether it results from direct toxicity of the drug or is secondary to hepatic damage.

Thioctic acid was not effective in mouse[22] or dog models,[1,2] even with adequate glucose replacement.[21] Patients poisoned by *Amanita*

phalloides who received supportive care, fluid and electrolyte repletion, high-dose penicillin G, dexamethasone, and thioctic acid, have had survival rates between 70 and 90%.[19,31,46,47,84]

Several laboratory investigations in mice and rats suggest that 1 g/kg penicillin G (1 g = 1,600,000 units) may have a time- and dose-dependent protective effect.[24] These results are limited because the amatoxins were administered intraperitoneally, resulting in the demise of the untreated animals 12–24 hours later. Additional investigations demonstrated that 1 g/kg of penicillin G administered 5 hours after sublethal doses of α-amanitin decreased clinical and laboratory toxicity.[23] The mechanisms suggested include displacing α-amanitin from albumin, blocking its uptake from hepatocytes, binding circulating amatoxins, and preventing α-amanitin binding to RNA polymerase. None of these mechanisms is substantiated. Although the hepatoprotective effects of penicillin remain unclear, many authors recommend 1 million units of penicillin G/kg/d IV.[34,35,63] There is inadequate scientific or clinical data to recommend the use of penicillin.

Silibinin is one of three isomeric compounds (also silidianin and silicristin) initially thought to be the compound silymarin, which is extracted from the milk thistle *Silybum marianum*.[76,77] Silibinin may modify or occupy cell membrane receptor sites, thereby inhibiting hepatocellular penetration by α-amanitin. The use of silibinin in dogs at 50 mg/kg at 5 and 24 hours following exposure to α-amanitin suppressed chemical evidence of hepatotoxicity and lethality.[77] Silibinin is used at a dose of 5 mg/kg/d, but this agent is not FDA approved for use in the United States.[35] Although it is routinely available in health food stores, there is inadequate scientific or clinical evidence to support the use of this agent. Because of its hepatoprotective effects, *N*-acetylcysteine is also suggested as an antidote, but no evidence for any specific benefit has been demonstrated.

In animals cimetidine, a potent cytochrome P450 system inhibitor, may, by inhibiting metabolism, have a hepatoprotective effect against α-amanitin[59] but shows no protective affect against phalloidin toxicity.[61] Cimetidine is proposed as a therapeutic intervention,[60] but there is no available human data supporting its use.

Activated charcoal both adsorbs amanitin and improves survival in laboratory animals.[16] Emesis, lavage, and catharsis are not typically necessary, as the toxin usually induces emesis and catharsis. Activated charcoal is safe, logical, and a valuable part of any therapeutic strategy. Although the clinical presentation is often delayed, 1 g/kg body weight of activated charcoal orally every 2–4 hours (if the patient is not vomiting) or by continuous nasogastric infusion appears appropriate. Fluid and electrolyte repletion and treatment of hepatic compromise are essential. Sodium chloride (0.9%) solution, electrolytes, and $D_{50}W$ or $D_{10}W$ may be necessary because of substantial diarrheal volume loss and glycogen depletion.

Forced diuresis, hemodialysis, plasmapheresis, hemofiltration, and hemoperfusion[18] may be effective, but most studies offer no clinical evidence of benefit nor supportive pharmacokinetic data for any of these therapies.[35,52,53,75,79] Plasmapheresis does not remove more than 10 μg of amatoxin. Because of the absence of prospective controlled studies of exposure to amatoxins, in addition to the extreme variability of success with many regimens, multiple-dose activated charcoal and supportive care presently remain the standard therapy. Early recognition of definitive exposure to amanitin is an indication for hemoperfusion.

The criteria and timing for liver transplantation in this setting are far less established than for fulminant viral hepatitis where grade III or IV hepatic encephalopathy, marked hyperbilirubinemia, and azotemia are the well-established criteria for transplantation[51] (Chap. 14). Early identification of *Amanita*-induced liver toxicity is essential because of the rapid progression of hepatic failure and the difficulty inherent in obtaining a compatible liver. Successful transplantations were performed in individuals whose resected livers showed 0–30% hepatocyte viability. In these cases, the authors did not wait for progression past grade II encephalopathy, or for the development of azotemia or marked hyperbilirubinemia.[51] Criteria for patient selection is essential to avoid unnecessary risk while offering the potential for survival to appropriate candidates who have no functional liver. The grim prognosis[48,70] associated with hepatic coma secondary to *Amanita* poisoning has led several transplant groups to consider hepatic transplantation for encephalopathic patients with prolonged international normalized ratios (INRs), persistent hypoglycemia, metabolic acidosis, increased serum ammonia, increased AST, and hypofibrinogenemia.[27,34,51] There are now case reports of successful liver transplantation for fulminant hepatic failure from presumed *Amanita ocreata*,[34,83] *A. phalloides*,[32,51] *Lepiota helveola*,[45] and *L. brunneoincarnata* poisoning.[55]

Currently, the clinical use of an extracorporeal bioartificial liver (BAL) support system is being investigated. This BAL system consists of a high-flow plasma recirculation loop through a reservoir, an activated charcoal column, an oxygenator and a hepatocyte bioreactor consisting of cryoprecipitated viable porcine hepatocytes attached to collagen-coated dextran microcarriers in the extra fiber space of the bioreactor. The initial studies included patients with acetaminophen-induced fulminant hepatic failure who met criteria for liver transplantation and had a 90% predicted mortality without liver transplantation.[15] The 8 patients studied received standard medical measures including *N*-acetylcysteine, but they also underwent 6-hour daily BAL treatment. Of these patients, all manifested neurologic and metabolic improvement, while 5 recovered without transplantation and 3 received bridge therapy to liver transplantation. This study methodology is being continued at multiple clinical sites to evaluate the potential of extracorporeal hepatocyte perfusion as an intermediary stage in the management of toxin-induced hepatic failure.

Most studies suggest that no circulating amatoxins are present by the time it is evident that transplantation is indicated.[15] To enhance the likelihood of success several authors suggest that individuals who manifest symptoms suggestive of hepatotoxic *Amantia*, *Galerina*, or *Lepiota* species exposure should be told of the potential need for transplantation, and with their consent, rapidly transferred to a regional liver transplantation center should it be indicated.

Group II: Gyromitrin-containing Mushrooms

$$CH_3-CH=N-N \begin{cases} CH_3 \\ CHO \end{cases}$$

Gyromitrin

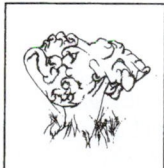

Members of the gyromitrin group include *G. esculenta*, *G. californica*, *G. brunnea*, and *G. infula*. *Gyromitra esculenta* is a good example of a mushroom with a "Jekyll and Hyde" personality, enjoying a reputation of being edible in the western United States but of being poi-

sonous in other areas. These mushrooms are found commonly in the spring under conifers, and are easily recognized by their brainlike appearance. Poisonings with these mushrooms are exceptionally uncommon in the United States, representing <1% of all recognized events, whereas these poisonings are considered more common in Europe. Certain cooking methods may eliminate the toxin, but inhalation of the fumes while cooking may cause poisoning. Because of the potential for toxicity, all members of this mushroom family should not be eaten. The most common error occurs in the spring, when an individual seeking the nongilled brainlike *Morchella esculenta* (morel) finds the similar *Gyromitra esculenta* (false morel) (see Fig. 76–2).

Gyromitra mushrooms contain gyromitrin (*N*-methyl-*N*-formyl hydrazone), which on hydrolysis splits into acetaldehyde and *N*-methyl-*N*-formyl hydrazine. This molecule, when subsequently hydrolyzed, yields monomethylhydrazine (CH_3NHNH_2). Gyromitrin is unstable and therefore unlikely to exist in its free form. The hydrazine moiety reacts with pyridoxine, resulting in inhibition of pyridoxal phosphate-related enzymatic reactions. This interference with pyridoxal phosphate disrupts the function of the inhibitory neurotransmitter, γ-aminobutyric acid (GABA).[38] The implications of this decrease in GABA, which is thought to contribute to intractable seizures associated with isoniazid or gyromitrin toxicity, is discussed in Antidotes in Depth: Pyridoxine.

The initial signs of toxicity for these mushrooms occur 5–10 hours after ingestion and include nausea, vomiting, diarrhea, and abdominal pain. The patients manifest headaches, weakness and diffuse muscle cramping. Most of these patients improve dramatically and return to normal function within several days. Rarely, patients develop delirium, stupor, convulsions, and coma. Infrequently, patients develop a hepatorenal syndrome and necessitate extensive in hospital care.

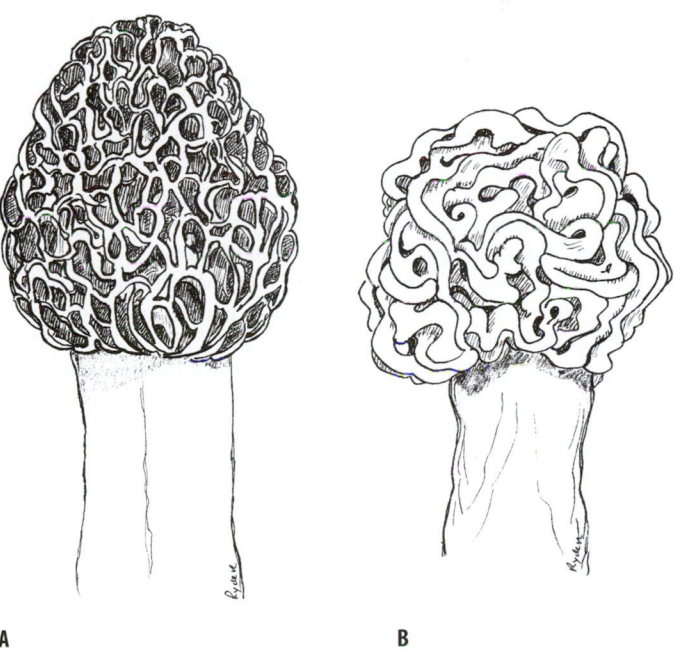

A   **B**

Figure 76–2. The edible morel (**A**) (*Morchella esculenta*) is confused with its look-alike the false morel (**B**) (*Gyromitra esculenta*).

Activated charcoal at 1 g/kg body weight should be given. Benzodiazepines such as diazepam are appropriate for the initial management of seizures. Under most circumstances supportive care is adequate treatment. Pyridoxine in doses of 70 mg/kg IV may be useful in limiting toxicity, particularly seizures (see Antidotes in Depth: Pyridoxine).

There are no rapid diagnostic strategies in the laboratory although thin-layer chromatography, gas-liquid chromatography, and mass spectrometry can be used for identification of the various hydrazine and hydrazone metabolites.

Group III: Muscarine-Containing Mushrooms

$$CH_3 - \overset{\overset{\textstyle O}{\|}}{C} - O - CH_2 - CH_2 - \overset{+}{N} \begin{matrix} CH_3 \\ - CH_3 \\ CH_3 \end{matrix}$$

Acetylcholine

Muscarine

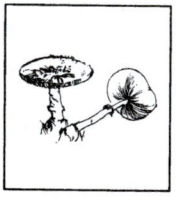

Mushrooms that contain muscarine include numerous members of the *Clitocybe* genus including *C. dealbata* (the sweater), *C. illudens* (*Omphalotus olearius*), and the *Inocybe* genus, including *I. Iacera* and *I. geophylla,* among others. Although *A. muscaria* and *A. pantherina* contain muscarine, the quantity is limited.

Muscarine and acetylcholine are similar structurally and have comparable clinical effects at the acetylcholine receptors. The peripheral manifestations typically include bradycardia, miosis, salivation, lacrimation, vomiting, diarrhea, bronchospasm, bronchorrhea, and micturition. Central muscarinic manifestations do not occur because muscarine, a quaternary ammonium compound, does not cross the blood-brain barrier (Chap. 10) and there are no nicotinic manifestations.

The effects of muscarine are often longer lasting than those of acetylcholine, because lacking an ester bond, the molecule is not susceptible to acetylcholinesterase hydrolysis. The clinical manifestations, which are typically mild, usually develop within 0.5–2 hours and last several additional hours. Significant toxicity is uncommon, limiting the need for more than supportive care. Rarely, atropine (1–2 mg given IV slowly for adults or 0.02 mg/kg with a minimum of 0.1 mg IV for children) can be titrated and repeated as frequently as indicated to reverse symptomatology.

There are no current, readily available, analytic techniques to identify muscarine although high-performance liquid chromatography would be appropriate for investigative purposes.

Group IV: Coprine-Containing Mushrooms

Coprine

1-aminocyclopropanol

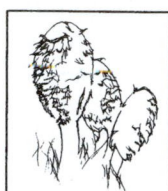

Coprinus mushrooms, particularly *C. atramentarius,* contain the toxin coprine. These mushrooms grow abundantly in temperate climates in grassy or woodland fields. They are known as "inky caps" because the gills autodigest into an inky liquid shortly after picking. The edible member of this group, *Coprinus comatus,* is nontoxic and probably its misidentification results in collector's errors. Coprine, an amino acid, or, more likely, its metabolite 1-aminocyclopropanol,[12,44,71] has a disulfiramlike effect. The inhibition of acetaldehyde dehydrogenase results in the buildup of acetaldehyde with its accompanying adverse effects. These effects occur if the patient ingests alcohol concomitantly or for as long as 48–72 hours after the mushroom ingestion. Within 0.5–2 hours of ingestion, an acute disulfiram effect is noted, with tachycardia, flushing, nausea, and vomiting. Interestingly, alcohol ingested simultaneously does not result in clinical manifestations since the inhibition of aldehyde dehydrogenase is slightly delayed while coprine metabolism occurs. Treatment is symptomatic with fluid repletion and antiemetics such as metoclopramide, although the clinical manifestations are usually mild and resolve within several hours. This group of mushrooms rarely causes fatalities (Chap. 65 for further discussion of disulfiram).

Group V: Ibotenic Acid- and Muscimol-Containing Mushrooms

GABA

Ibotenic acid

Muscimol

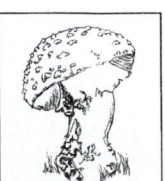

Most of the mushrooms in this class are primarily in the *Amanita* genus, which includes *Amanita muscaria, A. pantherina,* and *A. gemmata.* They exist singly and are scattered throughout the US woodlands. The brilliant red or tan cap (pileus) is easily recognized in the fields during summer and fall, as well as a mushroom commonly depicted in children's books.

Small quantities of the isoxazole derivative ibotenic acid and muscimol, its decarboxylated metabolite are found in these mushrooms which have been used throughout history in ancient religious customs. Ibotenic acid is structurally similar to the stimulatory neurotransmitter glutamic acid. The stereochemistry of muscimol is very similar to that of the neurotransmitter GABA and may act as a GABA agonist, with typical GABA manifestations.

Most patients who develop symptoms have intentionally ingested large quantities of these mushrooms while seeking an hallucinatory experience. Within 0.5–2 hours of ingestion, these compounds produce the GABAergic manifestations of somnolence, dizziness, hallucinations, dysphoria, and delirium in adults, whereas the excitatory glutamatergic manifestations of myoclonic movements, seizures, and other neurologic findings predominate in children.[6] There are no clinical anticholinergic manifestations.

Treatment is invariably supportive. Most symptoms respond solely to supportive care, although benzodiazepines such as diazepam are appropriate for any of the excitatory central nervous system manifestations.

Group VI: Psilocybin-Containing Mushrooms

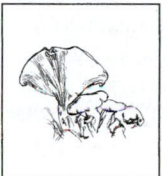

Psilocybin

Psilocin

Serotonin

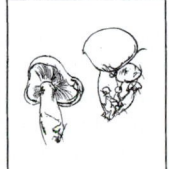

Psilocybin-containing mushrooms include *Psilocybe caerulescens, Psilocybe cubensis, Conocybe cyanopus, Panaeolus foenisecii, Gymnopilus spectabilis,* and *Psathyrella foenisecii.* Domestic cultivation of these so-called "magic mushrooms" is an infamous part of the drug culture. One popular drug culture magazine regularly advertises mail-order kits containing *Psilocybe cubensis* spores to grow at home. These mushrooms have been used for native North and South American religious experiences for thousands of years. They grow abundantly in warm, moist areas of the United States.

Toxicity from this group is very common because of the popularity of hallucinogens.[7] Psilocybin is rapidly and completely hydrolyzed to psilocin in vivo. Serotonin, psilocin, and psilocybin are very similar structurally and presumably act at a similar 5-HT$_2$ receptor site. The effects of psilocybin as a serotonin agonist and antagonist are discussed in Chaps. 10 and 70.

The psilocybin and psilocin indoles, like those of lysergic acid diethylamide (LSD), rapidly (within 1 hour of ingestion) produce CNS effects, including ataxia, hyperkinesis, and hallucinations.[29] Rare cases of renal failure,[25,54] seizures, and cardiopulmonary arrest[7] are associated with psilocybin containing species. Such associations should always be questioned however when reported in a substance using population potentially simultaneously exposed to other toxins.

In most instances, patients who take several mushrooms orally manifest tachycardia, anxiety, dysphoria, tremor, and dysesthesias, and may have mydriasis. One patient who used an extract of *Psilocybe* mushrooms intravenously experienced chills, weakness, dyspnea, headache, severe myalgias, vomiting associated with hyperthermia, hypoxemia, and mild methemoglobinemia.[14]

Treatment for the hallucinations is usually supportive, although benzodiazepines such as diazepam may be necessary when reassurance proves inadequate.

Group VII: Gastrointestinal Toxin-Containing Mushrooms

By far the largest group of mushrooms is a diverse group that contains a variety of ill-defined GI toxins. Many of the hundreds of mushrooms in this group fall into the "little brown mushroom" category. Some *Boletes, Lactarius spp., Omphalotus olearius, Rhodophyllus spp., Tricholoma spp., Chlorophyllum molybdites,* and *C. esculentum* are mistaken for edible or hallucinogenic species. The toxins associated with this group have not been identified, and some suggest that malabsorption of proteins and sugars such as trehalose, or allergy, may be responsible for symptoms. Gastrointestinal toxicity occurs 0.5–3 hours after ingestion when epigastric distress, malaise, nausea, vomiting, and diarrhea are evident. Treatment is supportive with regard to fluid resuscitation, vomiting, and diarrhea. The clinical course is brief and the prognosis excellent.

Rarely, clinical presentations can be life-threatening, with hypovolemic shock necessitating fluids and vasopressors.[66] Resolution of symptoms usually occurs within 6–24 hours. The clinical courses associated with specific mushroom ingestions are variable.[6]

Others have described a *Paxillus* syndrome, which may be associated with one of its constituents, involutin.[35] A small number of patients with ingestions of *Paxillus involutus,* and possibly *Clitocybe claviceps* and *Boletus luridus,* develop an immune-mediated hemolytic anemia, hemoglobinuria, oliguria, and renal failure. IgG antibodies to a *Paxillus* extract were detected by a hemagglutination test in these patients.[81,82] Death is rare.

Group VIII: Orelline- and Orellanine-Containing Mushrooms

Orellanine

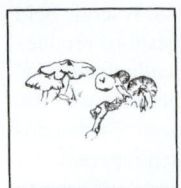

Cortinarius mushrooms, such as *Cortinarius speciosissimus* and *C. orellanus,* are commonly found throughout Europe. The *C. orellanus* toxins, orelline and orellanine, are bipyridyl agents that are also present in the North American species *C. rainierensis.*[11,62] The toxic compound orellanine is a hydroxylated and amine oxidized bipyridine compound activated by its metabolism through the P450 system. Toxicologically, these molecules are similar to paraquat and diquat. Other nephrotoxins, such as cortinarines, are also isolated from certain *Cortinarius* species.[69] These agents result in tubular damage, as well as in interstitial nephritis and fibrosis.

The initial symptoms occur 24–36 hours after ingestion and include headache, chills, anorexia, nausea, and gastritis. Several days to weeks after the initial symptoms, oliguric renal failure may develop and hepatotoxicity is rarely reported.[8] Nephrotoxicity is characterized by interstitial nephritis with tubular damage and early fibrosis of injured tubules with relative glomerular sparing.[11,62] Hemoperfusion, hemodialysis, and renal transplantation are employed in treatment.[8] There is no evidence to suggest that secondary detoxification by plasmapheresis or hemoperfusion is of any benefit.[35,56] The data are inadequate to define management or prognosis precisely, as most patients improve rapidly, while some (4 of 26 in one series) demonstrate months of chronic renal failure.[8] There are no laboratory or clinical parameters to assist in predicting the individual reactions to the toxins.

Thin-layer chromatography on renal biopsy material can detect orellanine long after clinical exposure.[56,57] Orellanine is rapidly concentrated in the urine in a soluble form, and is detected in the plasma at the time of clinical symptoms by some investigators,[56] but not by other investigators.[57]

Group IX: Allenic Norleucine-Containing Mushrooms

$$CH_2{=}C{=}CH{-}CH_2{-}CH{-}COOH$$
$$|$$
$$NH_2$$

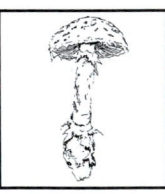

This relatively new diagnostic group is currently associated solely with the ingestion of *Amanita smithiana.* The 13 cases of *A. Smithiana* poisoning reported have all occurred in the Pacific Northwest.[40,73,78] Because the mature specimen often lacks any evidence of a partial or universal veil, these mushrooms are not recognized as *Amanita* species. It appears that all of the poisoned individuals were seeking the edible pine mushroom matsutake (*Tricholoma magnivalere*), a highly desirable look-alike (see Fig. 76–3). The *A. smithiana* and *A. abrupta* possess two aminoacid toxins: allenic norleucine (amino-hexadienoic acid) and possibly L-2-amino-4-pentynoic acid.[13,50,85] In vitro, renal epithelial tissue cultured with allenic norleucine developed morphologic changes similar to those seen following *A. smithiana* ingestion.[50] The in vitro model also demonstrated a more rapid onset of renal cellular toxicity with allenic norleucine (12 hours) compared to that of orellanine (24 hours).[50] In mice the extract of *Amanita abrupta* was also hepatotoxic which suggests that other agents in addition to the two described amino acids were present.[85]

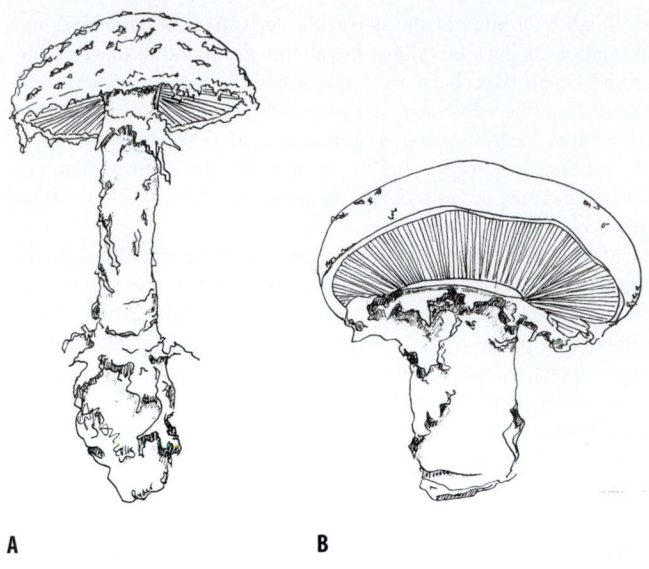

A   **B**

Figure 76–3. The edible pine mushroom, the matsutake (**B**) (*Tricholoma magnivalare*), is a highly desirable mushroom that is often confused with the nephrotoxic look-alike *Amanita smithiana* (**A**).

The initial symptoms were noted from 30 minutes to 12 hours following ingestion of raw or cooked specimens. Gastrointestinal manifestations, including anorexia, nausea, vomiting, abdominal distress, and diarrhea, occurred frequently, accompanied by malaise, sweating, and dizziness. In some cases, vomiting and diarrhea persisted. The patients were oliguric or anuric upon presentation. Acute renal failure manifests 4–6 days following ingestion with marked elevation of BUN and creatinine. ALT and lactate dehydrogenase levels were frequently elevated, whereas amylase, AST, alkaline phosphatase, and bilirubin were only infrequently abnormal.

Risk of toxicity was greatest in older patients and in those patients with underlying renal insufficiency. Although several patients did not require hemodialysis, those who did were dialyzed 2–3 times per week for approximately 1 month. None of the patients in the 3 series died. The clinical course for this poisoning has led us to suggest an alteration in the initial approach to patients in the American northwest who have early onset (0.5–3 hours) of gastrointestinal distress following mushroom ingestion. Until now, all patients who had early onset of nausea, vomiting, diarrhea, and abdominal cramps were presumed to be poisoned by a member of the groups containing either the gastrointestinal toxins or muscarine. However, a better understanding of *A. smithiana* led us to abandon the use of an algorithm we and others frequently employed in the past (see *Goldfrank's Toxicologic Emergencies,* 6th ed., Fig. 75–1).

There is no known antidote for these nephrotoxins. Activated charcoal, although of no proven benefit, should be used in standard doses when a patient in the American northwest presents with early gastrointestinal manifestations. The clinician will be forced to consider the circumstances of ingestion to assess the probability of an *Amanita smithiana* (group IX) instead of the ingestion of mushrooms containing a gastrointestinal toxin.

In view of the substantial morbidity associated with *A. smithiana* ingestions, historic, clinical and or temporal evidence of this ingestion should lead to charcoal hemoperfusion or hemodialysis when the patient presents in the early phase of exposure. There is no evidence with regard to activated charcoal's potential to adsorb allenic norleucine. When a patient presents with renal compromise, the history of early as opposed to delayed gastrointestinal manifestations may allow the clinician to differentiate *Amanita smithiana* from a *Cortinarius spp.* exposure.

Group X: Rhabdomyolysis Associated Mushrooms

Twelve patients who ingested *Tricholoma equestre (T. flavorvirens)* mushrooms for three consecutive days developed potentially lethal rhabdomyolysis.[5a] All patients developed fatigue, muscle weakness and myalgias 24–72 hours following the last mushroom meal. The individuals also developed facial erythema, nausea without vomiting and profuse sweating. The mean maximal creatine phosphokinase (CPK) was 226,067 U/L in women and 34,786 U/L in men. Electromyography revealed muscle injury, with myotoxic activity. The biopsied showed myofibrillar injury and edema consistent with an acute myopathy.

In the three patients who died dyspnea, muscle weakness, pulmonary congestion, acute myocarditis, dysrhythmias, cardiac failure and death ensued. Autopsy demonstrated myocardial lesions identical to those found in the peripheral muscles. The authors reproduced the muscle toxicity using *Tricholoma equestre* extracts in a mouse model, but the etiology of the toxicity is not as yet defined. Triterpenoids, sterols, indoles and acetylenic compounds extracted from these mushrooms were previously assumed to be without toxicity.

MANAGEMENT

Because the ingestion of certain mushrooms may lead to toxicity with substantial mortality, patients with suspected mushroom ingestions require rigorous management. A serious effort at precise identification of the genus and species involved will make assessment, management, and followup easier and more logical. Initially, the basic regimen of emesis, adsorption, and catharsis should be followed unless the unknown mushroom toxins produce sufficient emesis to obviate the need for gastric evacuation. If nausea and vomiting persist, an antiemetic may be used to ensure that the patient can be given activated charcoal, 1 g/kg. Appropriate life-support measures should be instituted as necessary: Fluid, electrolyte, and glucose repletion are essential because of the wide variability in quantity and type of toxin present in mushrooms according to both geography and local conditions as well as individual susceptibility. The routine use of specific antidotes should be avoided, as they are usually unnecessary and may result in an unanticipated adverse reaction.

DISPOSITION

It is important to remember that many patients with mushroom ingestions present with signs and symptoms suggestive of mixed poisonings. Whereas some ingestions produce "purer" symptom complexes than others, some ingestions, such as those of *A. muscaria*, produce muscarinic, GI, and CNS effects, and still other ingestions, such as of *Cortinarius* species, have acute gastroin-

testinal and delayed renal manifestations. Treatment or partial treatment may further complicate the assessment. In addition, it is essential to remember that any acute gastrointestinal disorder may actually represent mushroom toxicity. In the spring and fall in areas with moderate weather and humidity, it is particularly important to consider exposure to intentional or unrecognized mushroom toxins, although in the absence of a precise history a logical approach to management is impossible.

Because the clinical course of mushroom poisoning can be deceptive, all patients who manifest early symptoms (<3 hours) and remain symptomatic despite supportive care (Tables 76–1 and 76–2) should be admitted to the hospital. In this group of patients, *Amanita smithiana* should be of particular concern. Those patients whose delayed initial presentation (>5 hours) is suggestive of amatoxin exposure should be hospitalized, as should any patient postingestion who cannot be followed safely or reliably as an outpatient. Tables 76–1 and 76–2 show the characteristic times of appearance and evolution of symptoms caused by mushroom toxins and groups. Confusion may result from atypical clinical manifestations or, commonly, the ingestion of several different mushrooms species, some of which may produce early symptoms and others delayed toxicity. Patients with certain types of ingestions may appear to improve initially with only supportive care. This latency period, which is characteristic of *Amanita spp.*, may not be appreciated when several species are eaten simultaneously. However, because hepatotoxicity leading to death may not appear until 3–6 days after ingestion (amatoxins) and because nephrotoxicity may not appear for 3–21 days (orellanine and allenic norleucine), all patients with symptoms require subsequent followup.

Unfortunately, we are still very dependent on visualizing and analyzing the gross, microscopic, or chemical characteristics of the mushroom ingested. When the mushroom or parts are unavailable, the diagnosis must be based on the clinical presentation. There are no rapidly available studies in emergency departments or clinical chemistry laboratories to assist our management. The development of a rapid clinical test for amatoxins,[35] gyromitrin, orellanine, and allenic norleucine would be useful and might permit early use of hemoperfusion and greater vigilance with regard to the use of hemodialysis. We have not yet achieved the ability to use thin-layer chromatography, high-performance liquid chromatography, gas chromatography, or gas chromatography-mass spectrometry for clinically relevant circumstances.

TABLE 76–2. Mushroom Toxicity: A Correlation Between Symptomatology and Time of Onset of Symptoms

	Early <3hr	Middle 5–24hr	Late >24hr
Gastrointestinal	muscarine gastrointestinal toxins allenic norleucine	amatoxin allenic norleucine gyromitrin	orelline & orellanine
Hepatic			amatoxin gyromitrin
Neuropsychiatric	ibotenic acid & muscimol psilocybin	gyromitrin	
Renal			orelline & orellanine allenic norleucine

LYCOPERDONOSIS

Lycoperdonosis is not related to either the toxic or hallucinogenic characteristics of a mushroom. This syndrome occurs following the acute inhalation of spores as a folk medical therapy for epistaxis,[67] or by adolescents for various experimental reasons.[68] Puffball mushrooms (*Lycoperdon perlatum, L. pyriforme,* or *L. gemmatum*) which are edible in the fall, can, upon decay or drying, release large numbers of spores by compression or agitation. Massive inhalation, insufflation, and chewing of spores can, within hours, lead to the development of nasopharyngitis, nausea, vomiting, and pneumonitis. Over a period of several days, cough, shortness of breath, myalgias, fatigue, and fever develop. Several patients required intubation because of pulmonary compromise associated with the diffuse reticulonodular infiltrates. Lung biopsy demonstrated an inflammatory process with the presence of *Lycoperdon* spores.[67] Patients treated with prednisone and antifungal agents such as amphotericin B recovered within several weeks without sequelae.

IDENTIFICATION

General

Although mushroom identification is a difficult science, this section may be helpful to the clinician dealing with a suspected case of mushroom toxicity. However, it is generally best to rely on symptomatology, not mushroom appearances, to confirm a diagnosis. As a general rule, positive identification of the mushroom should be left to the mycologist or qualified toxicologist.

The most important anatomic features of both edible and poisonous mushrooms are their pileus, stipe, lamellae or gills, and volva.

- Pileus—the broad, caplike structure from which hang the gills (lamellae), tubes, or teeth.
- Stipe—the long stalk or stem that supports the cap; the stipe is not present in some species.
- Lamellae—the platelike or gill-like structures on the undersurface of the pileus that radiate out like the spokes of a wheel. The spores are found on the lamellae. Some mushrooms have pores or toothlike structures on their pilei, which contain the spores. The mode of attachment of the lamellae to the stipe is noteworthy in making an identification (Fig. 76–4).
- Volva—the partial remnant of the veil found around the base of the stipe in some species.
- Veil—a membrane that may completely or partially cover the lamellae, depending on the stage of development. The "universal" veil covers the underside, the spore-bearing surface of the pileus.
- Annulus—the ringlike structure that may surround the stipe at some point below the junction with the cap which is a remnant of the partial veil.
- Spores—microscopic reproductive structures, resistant to extremes in temperature and dryness, produced in the millions on the spore-bearing surface (see lamellae, above). Of all the characteristics of a mushroom, spores are the least variable, although many mushrooms have similar-appearing spores. A spore print is helpful in establishing an identification (Fig. 76–5). A spore print viewed microscopically is comparable to

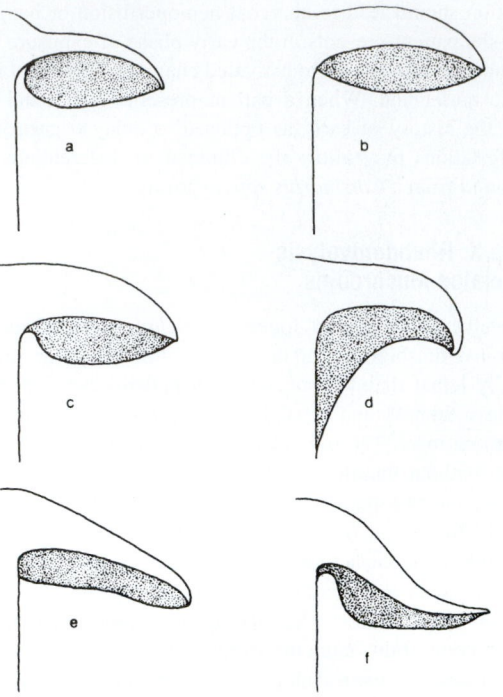

Figure 76–4. Gill attachment. The way the gill approaches and joins the stem is often specific for certain genera and most species. Any gills will be of one of the following types (or a combination fo two types, such as sinuate-decurrent): (**a**) free: (**b**) adnexed (just reaching the stem); (**c**) sinuate (with sudden notch or upward curve by the stem; emarginate); (**d**) decurrent (running down the stem to a greater or lesser extent); (**e**) adnate (joined to the stem by the full depth of the gill, but not running down the stem); (**f**) sinuate, with a decurrent "tooth" running down the stem. *(Reprinted, with permission, from Kibby G: Mushrooms and Toadstools: A Field Guide. Oxford, Oxford University Press, 1979, p. 16).*

a bacterial Gram's stain. Colors of spores range from white to black, and include shades of pink, salmon, buff, brown, and purple. Spore color is, in general, constant for a species.

The Unknown Mushroom

1. The most important determinant is whether the ingested mushroom could be one of the deadly varieties, especially *Amanita.* Outside of the Pacific Northwest, the onset of GI symptoms within 3 hours of ingestion is not the result of an *amatoxin* poisoning. In the Pacific Northwest, it may represent an *A. Smithiana* (allenic norleucine) poisoning (see Tables 76–1 and 76–2).
2. Attempt to obtain either the mushrooms collected or a detailed description of their features. Arrange for transport of the mushroom in a dry paper bag (not plastic); ensure that the mushroom is neither moistened nor refrigerated, either of which will alter its structure. Also remember that gastric contents may contain spores that can be crucial for analysis.
3. If the mushroom cap is available, make a spore print by placing the pileus spore-bearing surface side down on a piece of paper for at least 4–6 hours in a windless area. The spores that collect on the paper can then be analyzed for color. White spore prints can be more easily visualized on white paper by

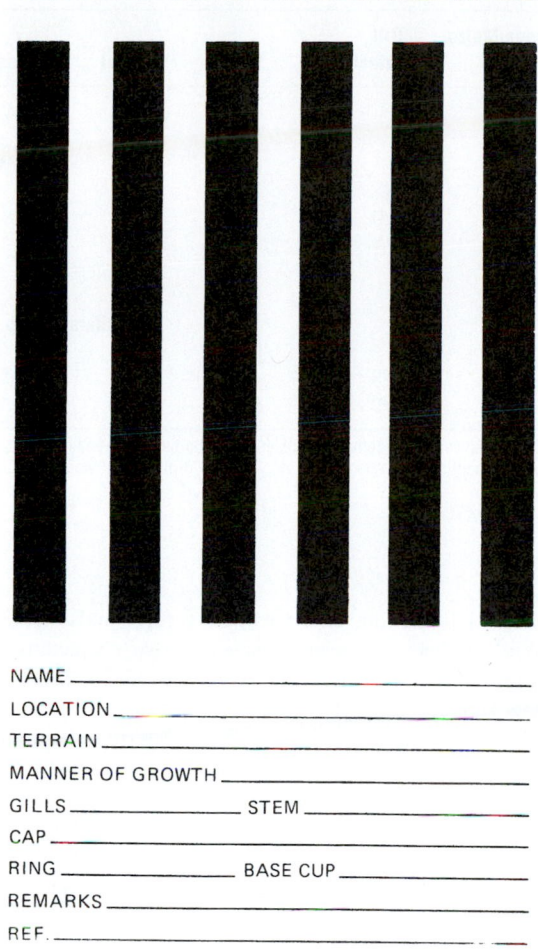

NO._____ DATE _____

NAME _____

LOCATION _____

TERRAIN _____

MANNER OF GROWTH _____

GILLS _____ STEM _____

CAP _____

RING _____ BASE CUP _____

REMARKS _____

REF. _____

Figure 76–5. Spore print format. To make the print, cut off the stem (stipe) from the cap (pileus) as close to the cap underside as possible. Lay the cap, underside down, on the pattern. Cover with a bowl or can overnight. In the absence of air currents, the spores will drift down onto the paper rather than blowing away. After several hours usually a sufficient pileup of loose spores will be quite visible. The print may be "fixed" onto the paper with artist's fixative or hair spray. It is wise to enter any data on the print sheet before cutting off the stipe. *(The spore print format was invented by D. A. Wolfthal; it was first reported briefly in* The Mycophile, *published by the North American Mycological Association, and then completely presented in* The Journal of Wild Mushrooming. *Published with inventor's permission.)*

tilting the paper and looking at it from an angle. (For details of a slightly more refined technique, see Fig. 76–5.)

4. Concomitant with step 3, contact a mycologist and use the best resources available for identification. A botanical garden usually has expert mycologists on staff, or a local mycology club can locate a mycologist for you. Alternatively the North American Mycological Association can furnish this information. Also a regional poison control center can almost always provide this expertise or locate an expert for you.

5. In the event that none of the resources in step 4 is accessible, Melzer's reagent can be useful in differentiating look-alike species, and in defining the presence of an amatoxin. A positive reaction is the development of a dark blue color, when

touched with Melzer's reagent.[42] Melzer's reagent is a solution of 20 mL of water, 1.5 g of potassium iodide, 0.5 g of iodine, and 20 g of chloral hydrate. Staining a sample of the spores with 1 drop of reagent and then viewing it under a microscope helps to determine whether the mushroom is a deadly *Amanita*, with bluish black "amyloid" reacting round spores (Table 76–3).

6. An additional test used by some is the Meixner reaction. The application of several drops of 10–12N hydrochloric acid to an amatoxin-containing spore sample also gives a blue reaction.[39] The reliability of this test remains in doubt, and most mycologists prefer to use Melzer's reagent.

POISONING PRINCIPLES: MYTHS AND SCIENCE

Differentiating myths from science is a difficult task in any field of medicine. This effort is even more complex when discussing mushrooms. The following principles are of great value in developing a logical approach to a potential ingestion.

1. Wild mushrooms should never be eaten unless an experienced mycologist can absolutely identify the mushroom. Even experts have trouble identifying some mushrooms, yet some foragers boldly imply that distinguishing edible from toxic mushrooms is "as easy as telling brussels sprouts from broccoli." Remember the saying, "There are old mushroom hunters, and bold mushroom hunters; but there are no old, bold mushroom hunters."

2. The toxicology of any species may vary depending on geographic location.

3. If poisoning is suspected, attempt to find examples of the mushrooms eaten and identify them. Every ED should have a readily available resource on mushrooms such as one of the major mycology field guides.[3,9,41,42,58,64] In any case, identification is still best made with the aid of the poison center's consultant mycologist.

4. Mushrooms are often implicated as the cause of an illness when, in fact, infections or other diseases are responsible. Other etiologies include the mode of preparation (the sauce or wine) or the cooking utensil.

5. There are no absolute generic approaches for evaluating the potential toxicity of a mushroom. Myths suggesting the safety or lack of it by the staining of silver, the presence of insects or slugs, peeling off the mushroom cap, or the area of growth are unreliable or false. Neither odor nor taste is a good predictor of toxicity. Pure white mushrooms, little brown mushrooms, large brown mushrooms, and red- or pink-pored boletes (a mushroom without lamellae) should be considered potentially toxic.

6. Cooking may inactivate some toxins but not others. In general, no wild mushroom should be eaten raw or in large quantities. Examples of toxicity associated with lack of cooking include *Armillariella mellea* (honey mushroom), which is usually well tolerated cooked but not raw, and *Verpa bohemica* (a morel-like mushroom), which is edible but a cause of illness if eaten in excess.

7. Associated phenomena may be responsible for or contribute to toxicity. Could insecticides have been sprayed on the

TABLE 76–3. Physical Characteristics of Common Toxic Mushrooms

Name	Color of Pileus	Spore Print Color	Spore Shape/Melzer Reaction	Gill Attachment	Veils	Habitat	Season
Amanita muscaria	Red to red orange to yellow orange	White	E/–	F	U±;P±	G	A/W
Amanita phalloides	Yellow green to green blue	White	R/amyloid	F	U;P±	G	A
Amanita smithiana	White	White	E/amyloid	F	U;P±	G/W	A/W
Amanita virosa	White	White	R/amyloid	F	U;P±	G	A
Clitocybe	White	White/Yellow	E/–	A/D	—	G	P
Coprinus	Gray brown	Black	E/–	F/A	U±;P±	G/W/D	P
Cortinarius orellanus	Orange brown	Rust	Oval-r/-	A	U±;P	G (conifers)	P
Galerina	Brown	Brown	Er/–	A	P±	G/W	
Gyromitra	Brown Rust	Brown	E/–			G (conifers)	Sp
Inocybe	Variable: white to gray brown	Brown	E/–	A	P±	G	A
Paxillus involutus	Brown	Clay brown	E/–	D/S	—	G/W	S/A
Psilocybe	Brown	Purple brown	E/–	A/D	P±	G/W/D	A

E = ellipsoid, R = round, r = roughened, F = free, A = attached, D = decurrent, S = stipeless and shelflike, P = partial veil or veil remnants present, P± = partial veil or veil remnants present in some species, U = universal veil or veil remnants present, U± = universal veil or veil remnants present in some species, – = no veils, G = ground, W = wood, D = dung, A = autumn, Sp = spring, W = winter, S = summer, P = perennial.
Adapted, with permission, from Lincoll GH: The Audubon Society Field Guide to North American Mushrooms, New York, 1981.

mushrooms? Is it an alcohol-related response? Besides the well-known disulfiram reaction involving *C. atramentarius*, other good edibles, including the black morel (*Morchella angusticeps*) and the sulfur polypore (*Laetiporus sulfureus*), can cause adverse reactions if consumed with alcohol. The etiology of these adverse reactions is not understood.

8. "Edible" mushrooms, allowed to deteriorate, become toxic. Therefore, only young, recently matured specimens should be eaten when adequate mycological support is available.

9. The finding that only some people who ate a mushroom species manifested characteristic toxicity should not exclude the diagnosis of mushroom poisoning. The degree of toxicity may be dose-related or genetically determined, or a person may have a pathologic predisposition to toxicity.

10. Mushroom allergy can manifest as anaphylaxis.

11. Most poisonous mushrooms resemble edible mushrooms at some phase of their growth. For this reason even careful ex-

amination of the ring, cap, consistency, form, and color may not reliably identify the edible species. Also, characteristic features of specific toxic mushrooms may not be present under certain conditions. Although the deadly *A. phalloides* and *A. virosa* usually have remnant patches of tissue from the universal veil that envelops the mushroom in its "button" stage, rain may wash these remnants away. Similarly, a subterranean basal cup may not be noticed if the mushroom is cut at the ground level by a novice forager (Fig. 76–6).

12. Even the new in vogue "wild mushrooms" in the fanciest markets may not be entirely safe.

ACKNOWLEDGMENTS

Alan G. Kulberg, MD, Kenneth E. Lampe, PhD (deceased), and Eddy A. Bresnitz, MD, contributed to this chapter in a previous edition. Pamela Ryder, Nurse Practitioner, contributed the mushroom illustrations.

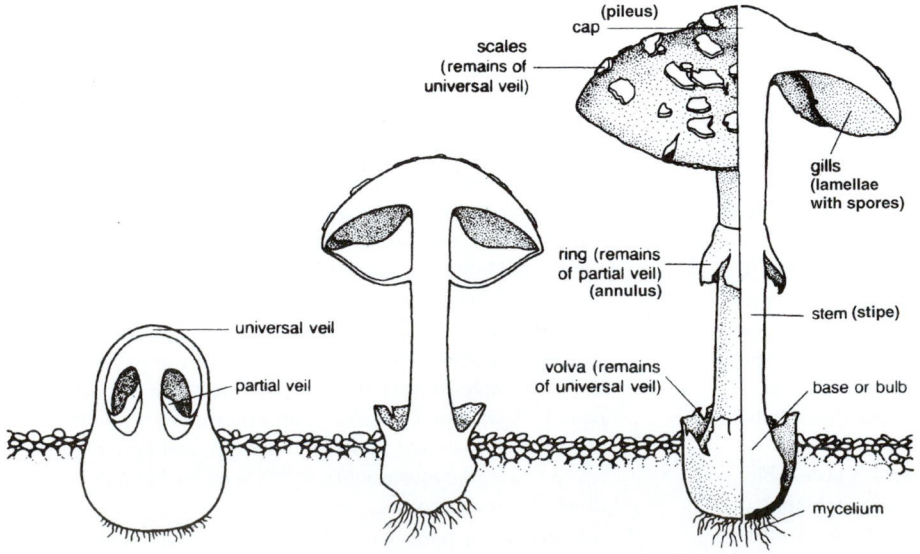

Figure 76–6. In the more highly specialized and evolved mushrooms, various protective tissues cover the fruit body and its constituent parts during its development. In the toadstool shown, an *Amanita* species, two veils of tissue are involved—one an outer enclosing bag, the universal veil, which ruptures as the fruit body expands to leave a volva at the base and fragments on the cap, the other an inner partial veil covering the developing gills, which is pulled away as the cap opens to leave a ring on the stem. (*Reprinted, with permission, from Kibby G: Mushrooms and Toadstools, A Field Guide. Oxford, Oxford University Press, 1979, p. 14.*)

REFERENCES

1. Alleva FR: Thioctic acid and mushroom poisoning [letter]. Science 1975;187:216.

2. Alleva FR, Balazs T, Sager AO, et al: Failure of thioctic acid to cure mushroom-poisoned mice and dogs, Abstract 155. Presented at 14th Annual Meeting of the Society of Toxicology, Williamsburg, VA, 1975.

3. Ammirati JF, Traquair JA, Horgen PA: Poisonous Mushrooms of the Northern United States and Canada. Minneapolis, University of Minnesota Press, 1985.

4. Ayer WA, Browne LM: Terpenoid metabolites of mushrooms and basidiomycetes. Tetrahedron 1981;37:2199–2248.

5. Becker CE, Tong TG, Boerner U: Diagnosis and treatment of *Amanita phalloides*-type mushroom poisoning: Use of thioctic acid. West J Med 1976;125:100–109.

5a. Bedry R, Baudrimont I, Deffieux G, et al: Wild mushroom intoxication as a cause of rhabdomyolysis. N Engl J Med 2001;345:798–802.

6. Benjamin DR: Mushroom poisoning in infants and children: The *Amanita pantherina/muscaria* group. J Toxicol Clin Toxicol 1992;30:13–22.

7. Borowiak KS, Ciechanowski K, Waloszczyk P: Psilocybin mushroom (*Psilocybe semilanceata*) intoxication with myocardial infarction. J Toxicol Clin Toxicol 1998;36:47–49.

8. Bouget J, Bousser J, Pats B, et al: Acute renal failure following collective intoxication by *Cortinarius orellanus*. Intensive Care Med 1990;16:506–510.

9. Bresinsky A, Besl H: A Colour Atlas of Poisonous Fungi. Wurzburg, Germany, Wolfe, 1990.

10. Busi C, Fiume L, Costantino D, et al: *Amanita* toxins in gastroduodenal fluid of patients poisoned by the mushroom *Amanita phalloides* [letter]. N Engl J Med 1979;300:800.

11. Carder CA, Wojciechlowski NJ, Skoutakis VA: Management of mushroom poisoning. Clin Toxicol Consult 1983;5:103–118.

12. Carlson A, Henning P, Lindberg P, et al: On the disulfiram-like effect of coprine, the pharmacologically active principle of *Coprinus atramentarius*. Acta Pharmacol Toxicol 1978;42:292–297.

13. Chilton WS, Tsou G, Kirk L, Benedict RG: A naturally-occurring allenic amino acid. Tetrahedron Lett 1968;60:6283–6284.

14. Curry SC, Rose MC: Intravenous mushroom poisoning. Ann Emerg Med 1985;14:900–902.

15. Detry O, Arkadopoulos N, Ting P, et al: Clinical use of a bioartificial liver in the treatment of acetaminophen-induced fulminant hepatic failure. Am Surg 1999;65:934–938.

16. Faulstich H: New aspects of *Amanita* poisoning. Klin Wochenschr 1979;57:1143–1152.

17. Faulstich H: Structure of poisonous components of *Amanita phalloides*. Curr Probl Clin Biochem 1977;7:2–10.

18. Feinfeld DA, Mofenson HC, Caraccio T, Kee M: Poisoning by amatoxin-containing mushrooms in suburban New York—Report of four cases. J Toxicol Clin Toxicol 1994;32:715–721.

19. Floersheim GL: Treatment of human amatoxin mushroom poisoning: Myths and advances in therapy. Med Toxicol 1987;2:1–9.

20. Floersheim GL: Treatment of mushroom poisoning. JAMA 1984;252:3130–3132.

21. Floersheim GL: Antagonistic effects against single lethal doses of *Amanita phalloides*. Naunyn Schmiedebergs Arch Pharmacol 1976;293:171–174.

22. Floersheim GL: Rifampicin and cysteamine protect against the mushroom toxin phalloidin. Experientia 1974;30:1310–1311.

23. Floersheim GL, Eberhard M, Tschumi P, Buchert F: Effects of penicillin on liver enzymes and blood clotting factors in dogs given a boiled preparation of *Amanita phalloides*. Toxicol Appl Pharmacol 1978;46:455–462.

24. Floersheim GL, Schneeberger J, Bucher K: Curative potencies of penicillin in experimental *Amanita phalloides* poisoning. Agents Actions 1971;2:138–141.

25. Franz M, Regele H, Kirchmair M, et al: Magic mushrooms: Hope for a "cheap high" resulting in end-stage renal failure. Nephrol Dial Transplant 1996;11:2324–2327.

26. French AL, Garrettson LK: Poisoning with the North American jack-o'-lantern mushroom: *Omphalotus illudens*. J Toxicol Clin Toxicol 1988;26:81–88.

27. Galler GW, Weisenberg E, Brasitus TA: Mushroom poisoning: The role of orthotopic liver transplantation. J Clin Gastroenterol 1992;15:229–232.

28. Hanrahan JP, Gordon MA: Mushroom poisoning: Case reports and a review of therapy. JAMA 1984;251:1057–1061.

29. Hatfield GM, Brady LR: Toxins of higher fungi. Lloydia 1975;38:36–55.

30. International Symposium on Thioctic Acid, Naples, 1955: Thioctic acid, physics, chemistry, and biology. Chem Abstr 1957;51:8153–8155.

31. Jacobs J, Von Behren J, Kreutzer R: Serious mushroom poisonings in California requiring hospital admission 1990–1994. West J Med 1996;165:283–288.

32. Jaeger A, Jehl F, Flesch F, et al: Kinetics of amatoxins in human poisoning: Therapeutic implications. J Toxicol Clin Toxicol 1993;31:63–80.

33. Kelner MJ, Alexander NM: Endocrine hormone abnormalities in *Amanita* poisoning. J Toxicol Clin Toxicol 1987;25:21–37.

34. Klein AS, Hart J, Brems JJ, et al: *Amanita* poisoning: Treatment and the role of liver transplantation. Am J Med 1989;86:187–193.

35. Koppel C: Clinical symptomatology and management of mushroom poisoning. Toxicon 1993;31:1513–1540.

36. Kostansek EC, Lipscomb WN, Yocum RR, et al: The crystal structure of the mushroom toxin β-amanitin. J Am Chem Soc 1977;99:1273–1274.

37. Kubicka J: Neue Moglichkeiten in der behandlung von vergiftung mit dem grunen Knollenblatterpilz—*Amanita phalloides*. Mykol Mitteil 1963;7:92–94.

38. Lampe KF: Toxic fungi. Annu Rev Pharmacol Toxicol 1979;19:85–104.

39. Lampe KF, McCann MA: Differential diagnosis of poisoning by North American mushrooms with particular emphasis on *Amanita phalloides*-like intoxication. Ann Emerg Med 1987;16:956–962.

40. Leathem AM, Purssell RA, Chan VR, Kroeger PD: Renal failure caused by mushroom poisoning. J Toxicol Clin Toxicol 1997;35:67–75.

41. Lincoff GH: The Audubon Society Field Guide to North American Mushrooms. New York, Knopf, 1981.

42. Lincoff G, Mitchel DH: Toxic and Hallucinogenic Mushroom Poisoning: A Handbook for Physicians and Mushroom Hunters. New York, Van Nostrand Reinhold, 1977.

43. Lindell TJ, Weinberg F, Morris PW, et al: Specific Inhibition of nuclear RNA polymerase II by alpha-amanitin. Science 1970;170:447–449.

44. Marchner H, Tottmar O: A comparative study on the effects of disulfiram, cyanamide, and 1-aminocyclopropanol on the acetaldehyde metabolism in rats. Acta Pharmacol Toxicol 1978;43:219–232.

45. Meunier BC, Camus CM, Houssin DP, et al: Liver transplantation after severe poisoning due to amatoxin containing *Lepiota*—report of three cases. J Toxicol Clin Toxicol 1995;33:165–171.

46. Moroni F, Fantozzi R, Masini E, Mannaioni PF: A trend in the therapy of *Amanita phalloides* poisoning. Arch Toxicol 1976;36:111–115.

47. Olson KR, Pond SM, Seward J, et al: *Amanita phalloides*-type mushroom poisoning. West J Med 1982;137:282–289.

48. Paaso B, Harrison DC: A new look at an old problem: Mushroom poisoning—Clinical presentations and new therapeutic approaches. Am J Med 1975;58:505–508.

49. Paydas S, Kocak R, Erturk F, et al: Poisoning due to amatoxin containing *Lepiota* species. Br J Clin Pract 1990;44:450–453.

50. Pelizzri V, Feifel E, Rohrmoser MM, Gstraunthaler G, Moser M: Partial purification and characterization of a toxic component of *Amanita smithiana*. Mycologia 1994;86:555–560.

51. Pinson CW, Daya MR, Benner KG, et al: Liver transplantation for severe *Amanita phalloides* mushroom poisoning. Am J Surg 1990;159:493–499.

52. Piqueras J, Duran-Suarez JR, Massuet L, Hernandez-Sanchez JM: Mushroom poisoning: Therapeutic apheresis or forced diuresis. Transfusion 1987;27:116–117.

53. Pond SM, Olson KR, Woo OF, et al: Amatoxin poisoning in northern California, 1982–1983. West J Med 1986;145:204–209.

54. Raff E, Halloran PF, Kjellstrand CM: Renal failure after eating "magic" mushrooms. Can Med Assoc J 1992;147:1339–1341.

55. Ramirez P, Parrilla P, Sanchez-Bueno F, et al: Fulminant hepatic failure after *Lepiota* mushroom poisoning. J Hepatol 1993;19.51–54.

56. Rapior S, Delpech N, Andary C, Huchard G: Intoxication by *Cortinarius orellanus*: Detection and assay of orellanine in biological fluids and renal biopsies. Mycopathologia 1989;108:155–161.

57. Rohrmoser M, Kirchmair M, Feifet E, et al: Orellanine poisonings: Rapid detection of the fungal toxin in renal biopsy material. J Toxicol Clin Toxicol 1997;35:63–66.

58. Rumack BH, Salzman E, eds: Mushroom Poisoning: Diagnosis and Treatment. Boca Raton, FL, CRC Press, 1978.

59. Schneider SM, Borochovitz D, Krenzelok EP: Cimetidine protection against alpha-amanitin hepatotoxicity in mice: A potential model for the treatment of *Amanita phalloides* poisoning. Ann Emerg Med 1987;16:1136–1140.

60. Schneider SM, Cochran KW, Knenzelok EP: Mushroom poisoning: Recognition and emergency management. Emerg Med Rep 1991;12:81–88.

61. Schneider SM, Vanscoy G, Michelson EA: Failure of cimetidine to affect phalloidin toxicity. Vet Hum Toxicol 1991;33:17–18.

62. Schumacher T, Hoiland K: Mushroom poisoning caused by species of the genus *Cortinarius* fries. Arch Toxicol 1983;53:87–106.

63. Serné EH, Toorians AW, Geitema JA, Bronsveld W, Haagsma EB: *Amanita phalloides*, a potentially lethal mushroom: Its clinical presentation and therapeutic options. Neth J Med 1996;49:19–23.

64. Smith AH: The Mushroom Hunter's Field Guide. Ann Arbor, University of Michigan Press, 1969. (Essential for anyone who wants to be sure out in the field; good descriptions and color photographs of common poisonous and edible species.)

65. Sperti S, Montanaro L, Fiume L, Mattioli A: Dissociation constants of the complexes between RNA polymerase II and amanitins. Experientia 1973;29:33–34.

66. Stenklyft PH, Augenstein WL: Chlorophyllum molybdites: Severe mushroom poisoning in a child. J Toxicol Clin Toxicol 1990;28:159–168.

67. Strand RD, Neuhauser EBD, Sornberger CF: Lycoperdonosis. N Engl J Med 1967;277:89–90.

68. Taft TA, Cardillo RC, Letzer D, et al: Respiratory illness associated with inhalation of mushroom spores. Wisconsin, 1994. MMWR Morb Mortal Wkly Rep 1994;43:525–526.

69. Tebbett IR, Caddy B: Mushroom toxins of the genus *Cortinarius*. Experientia 1984;40:441–446.

70. Teutsch C, Brennan RW: *Amanita* poisoning with recovery from coma: A case report. Ann Neurol 1978;3:177–179.

71. Tottmar O, Lindberg P: Effect on rat liver acetaldehyde dehydrogenases *in vitro* and *in vivo* by coprine, the disulfiram-like constituent of *Coprinus atramentarius*. Acta Pharmacol Toxicol 1977;40:476–481.

72. Trestrail JH III: Mushroom poisoning in the United States: An analysis of 1989 United States Poison Center Data. J Toxicol Clin Toxicol 1991;29:459–465.

73. Tulloss RE, Lindgren JE: *Amanita smithiana*—Taxonomy, distribution, and poisonings. Mycotaxon 1992;45:373–387.

74. Vander Hoek TL, Erickson T, Hryhorczuk D, et al: Jack-o'-lantern mushroom poisoning. Ann Emerg Med 1991;20:559–561.

75. Vesconi S, Langer M, Iapichino G, et al: Therapy of cytotoxic mushroom intoxication. Crit Care Med 1985;13:402–406.

76. Vogel G: The anti-*Amanita* effect of silymarin. In: Faulstich H, Kommerell B, Wieland T, eds: Amanita Toxins and Poisoning: International Amanita Symposium, Heidelberg. Baden-Baden, Gerhard Witzstrock, 1980, pp. 180–189.

77. Vogel G, Tuchweber B, Trost W, Mengs U: Protection by silibinin against *Amanita phalloides* intoxication in beagles. Toxicol Appl Pharmacol 1984;73:355–362.

78. Warden CR, Benjamin DR. Acute renal failure associated with suspected *Amanita smithiana* mushroom ingestions: A case series. Acad Emerg Med 1998;5:808–812.

79. Wauters JP, Rossel C, Farquet JJ: *Amanita phalloides* poisoning treated by early charcoal hemoperfusion. Br Med J 1978;2:1465.

80. Wieland TH, Faulstich H: Amatoxins, phallotoxins, phallolysin, and antamanide: The biologically active components of poisonous *Amanita* mushrooms. CRC Crit Rev Biochem 1978;5:185–260.

81. Winkelmann M, Borchard F, Stangel W, Grabensee B: Todlich verlaufene immunhamolytische anamie nach genuß des kahlen kremplings (*Paxillus involutus*). Dtsch Med Wschr 1982;107:1190–1194.

82. Winkelmann M, Stangel W, Schedel I, Grabensee B: Severe hemolysis caused by antibodies against the mushroom *Paxillus involutus* and its therapy by plasma exchange. Klin Wochenschr 1986;64:935–938.

83. Woodle ES, Moody RR, Cox KL, et al: Orthotopic liver transplantation in a patient with *Amanita* poisoning. JAMA 1985;253:69–70.

84. Yamada EG, Mohle-Boetani J, Olson KR, Werner SB: Mushroom poisoning due to amatoxin. Northern California, winter 1996–1997. West J Med 1998;169:380–384.

85. Yamaura Y, Fukuhara M, Takabatake E, Ito N, Hashimoto T: Hepatotoxic action of a poisonous mushroom, *Amanita abrupta,* in mice and its toxic component. Toxicol 1986;38:161–173.

Oliver L. Hung / Neal A. Lewin / Mary Ann Howland

A 21-year-old female, 5–6 weeks pregnant by dates, presented to the Emergency Department (ED) complaining of 2 days of abdominal pain and bilious vomiting. She reported that she purchased several abortifacients from an herbalist, including "slippery elm" powder to be brewed as a tea, "blue cohosh" tincture for ingestion, and "parsley" and "slippery elm" douches. For 4 days, she ingested approximately 15 cups/d of slippery elm tea and 10–20 doses/d of blue cohosh. She had also used the parsley and slippery elm douches the day before presentation. The patient denied any history of medical illness, allergies, or medications. She denied cigarette smoking.

On examination, the patient was flushed and diaphoretic. Vital signs were: temperature (rectal), 39°C (102.2°F); blood pressure 149/62 mm Hg; pulse 148 beats/min; and respiratory rate 24 breaths/min. Her heart sounds were normal and her lungs were clear to auscultation. She was noted to have fasciculations of her abdominal muscles. The gynecologic examination was unremarkable. Neurologic examination revealed diffuse muscular weakness. Her pupils were equal, reactive, and normal size. Laboratory tests including serum electrolytes and complete blood count were normal. The electrocardiogram (ECG) revealed a sinus tachycardia without conduction abnormalities; urinalysis revealed large ketones. The patient was admitted to the hospital for intravenous hydration. An ultrasound revealed an intrauterine gestation. With appropriate advice with regard to her desire for termination of her pregnancy and social services followup, she was discharged home without complications the following day.

The patient's clinical presentation is consistent with poisoning by a nicotinelike agent. The recent use of herbal preparations in a previously healthy women suggest that the poisoning may be related to a toxic constituent of one or several of these preparations. Although the popularity of herbal preparations may in part be related to the belief that they are safe, one of the herbal products used by this patient is known to have toxic side effects. Blue cohosh (*Caulophyllum thalictroides*) is also known as squaw root and papoose root. It is a traditional native American herb found in the woods of eastern North America. Historically, blue cohosh was used by the American Indians to facilitate childbirth. It continues to be used today as a uterine stimulant, antispasmodic, antirheumatic, emmenagogue, and an abortifacient.[13] The oxytocic activity of the plant is believed to be caused by the glycosides caulosaponin and caulophyllosaponin, derivatives of the saponin hederagenin. The plant also contains the nicotinelike alkaloid methylcytisine, which has one-fortieth the potency of nicotine.[13] Many other herbal preparations are popularly used as abortifa-

cients, including aloe; bitter melon; black cohosh; cantharidin; compound Q; ergots; feverfew; juniper; mugwort; nutmeg; pennyroyal oil; quinine; rue; sage; and white cohosh.

DEFINITION

The botanical definition of the term *herb* is specific for certain leafy plants without woody stems. However, herbal preparations often include nonherb plant materials, even animal and mineral products. The definition of herbal preparation is unclear. Broadly, it includes any "natural" or "traditional" remedy, but these terms are poorly defined. Although these products are often called medications, this may be inaccurate and misleading. Many herbal preparations are used for their nonspecific "adaptogenic" properties (help the body return to a normal state by resisting stress) and lack any medicinal or disease-specific effects. Because many herbal users and herbalists do not consider herbal preparations as medications, the use of the term *herbal medicine* by the clinician may convey a different, and perhaps unintended, meaning. For these reasons, it may be inappropriate and unhelpful to refer to these products as medications.

Herbal preparations are a subset of alternative medical therapies. These are defined as interventions neither widely taught in medical schools nor generally available in US hospitals.[58] Alternative medical therapies are divided into several major domains: alternative medical systems (eg, Ayurveda, homeopathy), mind-body interventions (eg, prayer, hypnosis), biologic-based therapies (eg, herbal preparations, diet therapies), manipulative and body-based methods (eg, chiropractic, massage), and energy therapies (eg, therapeutic touch).[106] When these therapies are used in conjunction with conventional medical therapies, alternative medical therapies are also known as complementary medical therapies.

For regulatory purposes, herbal preparations are recognized by the Food and Drug Administration (FDA) as a type of dietary supplement, which reflects their classification as nutrients with nondrug status.[46] However, not all dietary supplements are herbal preparations. Many nonherbals, such as vitamins, minerals, nutritional supplements, and food additives, are also dietary supplements.

The study of herbal preparations is complicated by a lack of standardized nomenclature. The diversity of common and botanical names may increase confusion. A single plant preparation may have many common names in addition to a botanical name. For example, *Datura stramonium* is also known as Jimson Weed, Angel's trumpet, datura, stramonium, apple of Peru, Jamestown weed, thornapple, and tolguacha. Likewise, a common name for a plant such as gordolobo may refer to several botanical plants such as *Verbascum thapsus* and *Gnaphalium macounii*.[77] Thus, an accurate classification of herbal preparations is very difficult, which limits effective study.

HISTORICAL BACKGROUND

Since ancient times, and perhaps since prehistoric times, people of all cultures have used herbal preparations to treat disease and to promote health.[41] A 60,000-year-old Iraqi burial site contained 8 different medicinal plants, suggesting very early historical usage.[137] The earliest surviving written account of medicinal plants is the Egyptian Ebers papyrus ca. 1500 BC, which lists dozens of medicinal plants and uses. In India, the *Vedas*, epic poems written in about 1500 BC, contain references to herbal preparations of the time. In China, the *Divine Husbandman's Classic,* written in the 1st century AD, lists 252 herbal preparations. In ancient Europe, herbal medicines were also the mainstay of healing. In the 1st century, the Greek physician Dioscorides wrote one of the first European herbal books, *De Materia Medica*, which listed 600 herbals and was translated into many languages. Shamans and folk healers from America, Africa, and Asia continue to include herbals for spiritual and medicinal purposes based on oral traditions passed from generation to generation.

During the Scientific Revolution, European scientists began to isolate purified extracts of plant products for use as medicinal agents. In 1806 and 1832, morphine and codeine were isolated from the sap of the poppy plant, *Papaver somniferum*.[125] In the mid-18th century, Edward Stone described the success of the bark of the willow tree in the cure of "agues" (fever) in a letter to the president of the Royal Society of Medicine.[78] Later, in 1829, salicin, the active ingredient of the willow bark, was identified and its derivative sodium salicylate was marketed in 1875 as a treatment for rheumatic fever and as an antipyretic. The enormous success of this drug led to the synthesis of acetylsalicylic acid in 1899. The original brand name, aspirin (*acetyl spiric* acid), is said to have been derived from *Spirea*, the plant genus from which salicylic acid was once prepared. Prescriptions from plant-derived medicines accounted for 25% of prescriptions dispensed in the United States between 1959 and 1980.[2] At least 60% of over-the-counter medicines still contain one or more natural products as ingredients.[50]

Today, herbal preparations continue to be the dominant form of healing in the developing world because of the high cost of "Western" medical treatment and the scarcity of "Western"-trained medical personnel.[49,86,90,101] The World Health Organization estimates that 4 billion people, 80% of the world population, use herbal preparations for some aspect of primary healthcare.[2] In the developed world, there appears to be a resurgence of herbal preparation usage.[57] In 1991, a US survey determined that 2.5% of respondents had used herbal preparations in the prior year.[57] The same survey, repeated in 1997, determined that reported herbal usage in the previous year increased to 12.1%.[58]

Factors attributed to this resurgence include lower cost and ease of purchase when compared to prescription medications, consumer empowerment, dissatisfaction with conventional therapies, and the perception that herbals are better and safer. Herbal preparations and other dietary supplements are no longer sold exclusively in health food stores, but are now available for sale in mainstream outlets such as grocery stores, drug stores, complementary practitioners offices, mail order companies, the Internet, and even gasoline stations. Sales of herbal preparations in the United States, in 1999, were estimated at approximately $4 billion and are growing at an annual rate of 18% a year.[16] US herbal sales are expected to peak at $6–8 billion per year by 2003.[71] For the first time, large pharmaceutical companies have entered the herbal/botanical market. In 1998, Bayer Consumer Care, Warner-Lambert, and Whitehall-Robbins (American Home Products) each launched a line of herbal products. Other companies, including SmithKline Beecham and McNeil, reportedly have test-marketed herbal products and are expected to enter this market in the future.[5]

Although the FDA does not classify these preparations as medications, they are often used to prevent or treat medical illness. Despite reports of toxicity associated with their usage, no systematic evaluation of herbal efficacy or safety is required.

Because patients often do not consider herbal preparations as medications, they may not provide a history of usage unless directly questioned. In one recent study, 21.7% of respondents in an urban ED survey reported the use of herbal preparations. For 15.6% of these users, the herbal preparation was being used specifically to treat aspects of the patient's presenting chief complaint. Thirty-seven percent of herbal users reported that their physicians were unaware of their herbal preparation usage.[75]

Herbal preparation use appears to vary greatly, depending on the community surveyed. Rural areas of Mississippi and southwestern West Virginia reported that 71% and 73% of respondents respectively, used herbal remedies in the past year.[33,45] Among Chinese Americans in New York City and Hispanic Americans in West Texas, herbal preparation use was also reported to be very high, 43% and 50%, respectively.[97,118] Herbal preparations use also appears to be higher among populations with chronic illness such as AIDS, rheumatoid arthritis, and cancer.[81,82,100,148] In the United States, increased herbal preparation usage is associated with multiple factors including concurrent illness and diverse socioeconomic and cultural influences.

Although poorly studied, there is growing evidence that herbal preparations may be beneficial in the treatment of certain medical conditions. For example, *Ginkgo biloba* may delay the mental deterioration resulting from Alzheimer's disease.[89] Saw palmetto may be as effective as finasteride in the treatment of benign prostatic hyperplasia.[152] Glucosamine and chondroitin may be useful in the treatment of osteoarthritis.[99] St. John's wort may be effective in treating mild and moderate depression.[94] Finally, Chinese herbal medicines may be effective in the treatment of irritable bowel syndrome.[11] However, these represent preliminary studies. Additional scientific evidence is required to prove their effectiveness by current scientific standards.

In 1998, Congress established the National Center for Complementary and Alternative Medicine (NCCAM) at the National Institutes of Health to stimulate, develop, and support research in complementary and alternative medicines.[98] NCCAM is currently investigating the use of St. John's wort for the treatment of depression, *Ginkgo biloba* for delaying the progression of dementia, glucosamine and chondroitin for osteoarthritis, and shark cartilage for lung cancer. NCCAM is planning additional trials, including milk thistle for the treatment of hepatic disease, valerian root for insomnia, feverfew for the treatment of migraine headaches, and echinacea for the treatment/prevention of upper respiratory infections.[98]

REGULATION OF HERBAL PREPARATIONS

There is very little federal regulation of the herbal industry. In 1994, Congress passed the Dietary Supplement and Health Education Act (DSHEA), which reduced the Food and Drug Administration's (FDA) oversight of products categorized as dietary supplements.[62] Dietary supplements include vitamins, minerals, herbals, amino acids, and any product that had been sold as a "supplement" before October 15, 1994. As a result, the FDA has very little authority regulating herbal products.[46]

Ingredients that were used in dietary supplements in the United States prior to October 15, 1994, were automatically "grandfathered" by DHSEA as safe products. After this date, any new ingredient intended for use in dietary supplements require notification and approval by the FDA at least 75 days in advance of marketing. The FDA must review within this time period whether the proposed ingredient is reasonably expected to be safe under the intended conditions for use. Because most ingredients contained in dietary supplements were in use prior to 1994, the vast majority of dietary supplements are not subject to premarket safety evaluations. In 1993, the FDA established a monitoring system to identify unanticipated or unintended safety problems with marketed dietary supplements through the use of its Special Nutritionals Adverse Event Monitoring System (SNAEMS). From January 1993 until October 1998, 2621 adverse events involving over 3100 products, including 101 deaths, were reported.[144]

If the FDA determines that a manufactured dietary supplement is unsafe, the agency can warn the public, suggest changes to make the supplement safer, urge the manufacturer to recall the product, recall the product, or ban the product. To ban a dietary supplement from the marketplace, the FDA must prove that the product is unsafe. Since the passage of DSHEA in 1994, the FDA has not succeeded in banning any dietary supplements, although it has tried on several occasions without success (eg, ephedrine, Cholestin).

Because the FDA considers dietary supplements food products, quality control issues and production methods concerning dietary supplements are governed by the Current Good Manufacturing Practices regulations for foods.[145] However, these regulations only ensure that dietary supplements are produced under sanitary conditions and do not guarantee the purity or efficacy of the product.

Herbal products can be marketed without any proof of testing for efficacy or safety. Although packaging claims to cure or prevent a specific disease are not permitted unless approved, claims detailing how a product affects the "body's structure or function" are permissible. Substantiation of these claims is required, but their methodology and requirements have not been defined. In reality, no proof is necessary unless the manufacturer is challenged by regulators.[145]

In March 1999, the FDA implemented new dietary supplement labeling rules. All dietary supplement labels must provide a statement of identity (eg, ginseng); net quantity of contents (eg, 60 capsules); structure-function claims with disclaimers that the product has not been evaluated by the FDA; directions for use (eg, "Take 1 capsule daily"); supplements fact panel (list of serving size, amount, and active ingredients); other ingredients list; and name and place of business of manufacturer, packer, or distributor.

In February 2000, the FDA advised dietary supplement manufacturers not to make claims related to pregnancy on their products.

BACKGROUND OF HERBAL TOXICOLOGY

There is a growing awareness of the widespread use of herbal preparations in the United States. Frequently, it is only after the patient demonstrates toxicity that the physician seeks information about the use of these products. Some well-publicized examples of toxicity from herbal preparation usage include 6 cases of anticholinergic poisoning in New York City in 1994, from contaminated Paraguay tea;[22,74] 3 cases of life-threatening bradycardia in Colorado in 1993, following consumption of *Jin Bu Huan* tablets;[27] and 4 cases of agranulocytosis with 1 death following consumption of *Chui Fong Tou Ku Wan* in San Francisco in 1975.[128] Although few studies have examined this issue, most herbal preparations used in developed countries appear to be safe. In Hong Kong, in 1990, Chinese herbal medicines and proprietary medicines accounted for only 0.2% of all acute medical admissions despite their use by 40–60% of the population. Western medications were responsible for 4.4% of acute medical admissions.[36,37] From 1983 to 1989, the National Poisons Unit, London, received 1070 inquiries following exposures to herbal extracts, of which 270 (25.2%) cases were symptomatic. They were able to demonstrate a probable association between exposure and effect in only 32 of the 270 cases.[119] In the United States, a multicenter poison control center study in 1998 collected 2253 calls involving dietary supplements including herbals—493 patient exposures were determined to be caused by dietary supplement and were associated with 5 deaths, 13 seizures, 8 cases of coma, and 9 cases of hepatotoxicity.[115] The overall severity outcome among dietary supplement cases was greater when compared to outcomes of other poison center-reported exposures.[115] However in developing countries, the toxicity from herbal preparation usage may be much higher. It was reported in South Africa that traditional medicines account for 15.8% of acute poisonings, and were responsible for 51.7% of all deaths from acute poisonings.[79]

PHARMACOLOGIC PRINCIPLES

The pharmacologic activity of herbal preparations (plant containing) can be classified by 5 active constituent classes: volatile oils, resins, alkaloids, glycosides, and fixed oils.[138]

- **Volatile oils** are odorous plant ingredients. They are also called ethereal or essential oils, because they evaporate at room temperatures. Most are mucous membrane irritants with some central nervous system activity. Examples of herbs containing volatile oils include pennyroyal oil *(Mentha pulegium)*, catnip *(Nepata cataria)*, chamomile *(Chamomilla recutita)*, and garlic *(Allium sativum)*.
- **Resins** are complex chemical mixtures of acrid resins, resin alcohols, resinol, tannols, esters, and resenes. These substances are often strong gastrointestinal irritants. Examples of resin-containing herbs include dandelion *(Taraxacum officinale)*,

elder (*Sambucus spp.*), and black cohosh root (*Cimicifuga racemosa*).

■ **Alkaloids** are a heterogeneous group of alkaline, organic, and nitrogenous compounds. The alkaloid compound is usually found throughout the plant. They are often the most pharmacologically active and most toxic compounds. Their pharmacologic actions may be central nervous system (CNS) depression or stimulation. However, the pyrrolizidine alkaloids, present in thread-leafed groundsel (*Senecio longilobus*) and comfrey (*Symphytum officinale*), cause hepatic venoocclusive disease. Other examples of alkaloid-containing herbs include Aconitum (*Aconitum napellus*), Goldenseal (*Hydrastis canadensis*), and Jimson Weed (*Datura stramonium*).

■ **Glycosides** are esters that contain a sugar component (glycol) and a nonsugar (aglycone), which yields one or more sugars during hydrolysis. These include the anthroquinones, saponins, cyanophores, and lactone glycosides. The anthroquinones (senna (*Cassia acultifolia*) and aloe (*Aloe vera*)) are irritating cathartics. Saponins (licorice (*Glycyrrhiza lepidata*) and ginseng (*Panax ginseng* and *quinquefolium*)) are mucous membrane irritants, cause hemolysis, and have steroid activity. Cyanophores found in apricot, cherry, and peach pits release cyanide. Lactone glycosides (tonka beans (*Dipteryx odorata*)) have anticoagulant activities.

■ **Fixed oils** are esters of long-chain fatty acids and alcohols. Herbs containing fixed oils are generally used as emollients, demulcents, and bases for other agents. Generally, these are the least active and dangerous of all herbal preparations. Examples include olive (*Olea europaea*), and peanut (*Arachis hypogaea*) oil.

FACTORS CONTRIBUTING TO HERBAL TOXICITY

The toxicity of a plant may vary widely and depends on certain conditions.[77] The time of year or developmental stage at which the plant is collected may affect its toxicity. For example, the pyrrolizidine alkaloid content of *Senecio* leaves varies widely from month to month and year to year.[77] In some cases, only selective parts of a plant used to prepare an herbal preparation may be responsible for its toxicity. For example, the pyrrolizidine content of comfrey-pepsin capsules varies from 270 mg/kg to 2900 mg/kg, depending on whether the leaves or roots were used in the preparation.[76] The area in which the plant is collected may affect its toxicity. *Senecio longilobus* from Gardner Canyon, Arizona, may contain up to 18% pyrrolizidine alkaloids by dry weight, the highest level recorded for any *Senecio* plant species (normal concentration is 0.5%). Finally, conditions of storage and length of storage may affect its toxicity. The toxicity of *Crotalaria* decreases with storage because of the breakdown of pyrrolizidines.

Few poisonings are likely to result from the inherent toxicity of the herbal (see Table 77–1). Most poisonings are likely to result from the misuse, misidentification, misrepresentation, or contamination of the product. Heavy-metal poisonings from lead, cadmium, mercury, copper, zinc, and arsenic are associated with herbal preparation usage.[37,48,52,55,117,119,124] High levels of these elements may be the result of contamination during the manufacturing process of some herbal or patent medications. In some cases, such as cinnabar (mercuric sulfide) and calomel (mercurous chloride), these ingredients are intentionally included for purported

medicinal benefit.[80] Patent medications may also contain pharmaceutical medications, such as acetaminophen, aspirin, antihistamines, or corticosteroids.[38,52] Many of these medicines are unlisted on the packaging and may not even by approved for use in the United States. For example, 4 cases of agranulocytosis followed consumption of *Chui Fong Tou Ku Wan*, a preparation containing aminopyrine (which is not approved for over-the-counter sales in the United States) and phenylbutazone, but not listed on the packaging.[128] Both aminopyrine and phenylbutazone are associated with agranulocytosis.

CLASSIFICATION OF TOXICITY

Herbal preparations are associated with a wide variety of toxicologic manifestations (Table 77–2). In addition, many individual herbal preparations are associated with multiple types of toxicologic effects. To better understand these effects, it may be useful to organize herbal toxicity into several general categories.[51]

Indirect Health Risks

Herbal usage may result in toxicity by altering previous conventional medication therapy. A patient may discontinue or become less compliant with previous therapy with untoward consequences. Alternatively, the addition of an herbal preparation may affect the pharmacologic effect (eg, bioavailability or clearance) of concurrent conventional therapy with resulting increase risk of toxicity. For example, coadministration of St. John's wort with the protease inhibitor indinavir may result in decreased plasma indinavir concentrations and potentially decreased antiretroviral activity.[122]

Direct Health Risks

Direct health risks include pharmacologically predictable and dose-dependent toxic reactions, idiosyncratic toxic reactions, long-term toxic effects, and delayed toxic effects. For example, ingestion of aconite tea, containing aconite, in the appropriate dosage, predictably results in tachydysrhythmias and hypotension in all patients. Idiosyncratic toxic reactions cannot be predicted on the basis of principal pharmacologic properties. For example, ingestion of chamomile tea results in anaphylaxis in a small subset of patients. Long-term toxic effects result only after chronic usage. For example, long-term use of herbal anthranoid laxatives results in muscular weakness from hypokalemia. Delayed toxic effects include carcinogenicity and teratogenicity. For example, sassafras root contains safrole that is a hepatocarcinogen in laboratory animals.

TOP SELLING HERBAL SUPPLEMENTS

The top selling herbal supplements in the United States for 1998, are listed below in order of sales.

■ Ginkgo (*Ginkgo biloba*) ($138 million)—This herbal contains ginkgo flavone glycoside ginkgolides that are reputed to have antioxidant properties, to inhibit platelet aggregation, and to increase circulation. It is a popular remedy for Alzheimer disease and for peripheral vascular disease. In appropriate doses,

TABLE 77–1. Laboratory Analysis and Treatment Guidelines for Specific Herbal Preparations and Their Critical Contaminants

Herbal Preparation	Suggested Laboratory Analysis	Antidote
Cardiac Toxins		
Ch'an Su	Serum digoxin, potassium	Digoxin Fab
Foxglove	Serum digoxin, potassium	Digoxin Fab
Oleander	Serum digoxin, potassium	Digoxin Fab
Squill	Serum digoxin, potassium	Digoxin Fab
Central Nervous System Toxins		
Henbane	None	Physostigmine
Jimsonweed (Datura)	None	Physostigmine
Mandrake	None	Physostigmine
Gastrointestinal Toxins		
Aloe	Serum electrolytes	Potassium repletion
Buckthorn	Serum electrolytes	Potassium repletion
Cascara	Serum electrolytes	Potassium repletion
Fo-Ti	Serum electrolytes	Potassium repletion
Senna	Serum electrolytes	Potassium repletion
Heavy Metals	Ag, As, Au, Cd, Cr, Cu, Hg, Pb, Th, or Zn	Metal chelator
	Abdominal radiograph	
Hematologic Toxins		
Dong Quai	INR	Vitamin K_1
Tonka bean	INR	Vitamin K_1
Woodruff	INR	Vitamin K_1
Hepatotoxins		
Pennyroyal oil	AST/ALT	*N*-Acetylcysteine
Pyrrolizidine Alkaloids	AST/ALT	None available
Salicylates		
Medicated oils, etc.	Serum salicylate	Sodium bicarbonate, multiple-dose activated charcoal, hemodialysis
Cellular Toxins		
Apricot pits (cyanide)	Lactate	Cyanide antidote kit
Autumn crocus (colchicine)	WBC, BUN	? Glutamic acid
Elder (cyanide)	Lactate	Cyanide antidote kit
Periwinkle (vincristine)	WBC, BUN	? Glutamic acid
Podophyllum (podophylline)	WBC, BUN	? Glutamic acid
Miscellaneous		
Licorice	Serum potassium	Potassium repletion
Quinine	None	Sodium bicarbonate, magnesium

ginkgo appears to be safe. Ginkgo may increase the risk of bleeding for individuals who are also taking antiplatelet agents or anticoagulants.[65,102,112]

- St. John's wort (*Hypericum perforatum*) ($121 million)— St. John's wort is a popular herbal remedy for the treatment of depression and as topical remedy for cuts, bruises, and wounds. It is also used as an herbal AIDS treatment. The active ingredient, hypericin, is a weak monoamine oxidase inhibitor that also possesses antiretroviral activity in vitro and hyperforin modulates serotonin. Acute toxicity appears limited to photosensitization reactions. St. John's wort induces CYP 3A4 and may interact with medications metabolized by this enzyme (eg, indinavir, oral contraceptives, cycloserine).[89] St. John's wort may also interact with selective serotonin reuptake inhibitors.[122]

- Ginseng (*Panax ginseng*) ($98 million)—This herb is popular for its adaptogenic properties. It also used to enhance memory and physical performance, to increase energy, and to decrease stress. The active ingredients are triterpene saponins called

ginsenosides. Long-term use is associated with the development of ginseng abuse syndrome.[67]

- Garlic (*Allium sativum*) ($84 million)—Garlic is a popular remedy to reduce blood pressure and cholesterol. It is also used as a treatment for infections and cancer. The active ingredient is allicin which is an antibacterial and an antioxidant. Garlic also contains ajoene, which is an antiplatelet agent. Garlic may increase the risk of bleeding for individuals who are also taking antiplatelet agents or anticoagulants.[66]

- Echinacea (*Echinacea purpurea, augustifolia*) ($33 million)— Echinacea is a reputed immunostimulant and is a popular herbal remedy for cold and flu symptoms. In appropriate doses, echinacea appears to be safe.[70]

- Saw palmetto (*Serenoa repens*) ($27 million)—Saw palmetto is a popular remedy for benign prostatic hypertrophy. Saw palmetto appears to inhibit 5-α-reductase. In appropriate doses, saw palmetto appears to be safe.[102,112]

- Grape seed extract (*Vitis vinifera*) ($11 million)—Grape seed extracts contain the antioxidant compounds procyanidins. It is

TABLE 77–2. Selected Herbal Preparations, Popular Use, and Potential Toxicities

Herbal Preparation	Scientific Name	Other Common Names	Traditional and Popular Usage	Toxic or Active Ingredient(s)	Adverse Effects
Aconite	Aconitum napellus, kusnezoffi, carmichael	Monkshood, wolfbane caowu, chuanwu, bushi	Topical analgesic, neuralgia, asthma, and heart disease	Aconite alkaloids (C19 diterpenoid esters)	Gastrointestinal distress, cardiac dysrhythmias
Agrimony	Agrimonia eupatoria	Cocklebur, stickwort, liverwort	Catarrh, gall bladder disease, astringent		Photodermatitis
Alfalfa	Medicago sativa		Arthritis, diabetes	L-Canavanine	High doses: lupus, pancytopenia
Aloe	Aloe vera and other spp.	Cape, Zanzibar, Socotrine, Curacao, Carrisyn	Heals wounds, emollient, laxative, abortifacient	Anthraquinones, barbaloin, isobarbaloin	Gastrointestinal distress, dermatitis
Apricot pits	Prunus armeniaca	Laetrlle	(Laetrile) cancer remedy	Amygdalin	Cyanide poisoning
Aristolochia	Aristolochia clematis	Birthwort, heartwort, fangchi	Uterine stimulant	Aristolochic acid	Nephrotoxin
Artemisa	Artemisa vulgaris, dracunculus, lactiflora	Mugwort, felon herb, moxa, guizhou	Depression, dyspepsia, menstrual disorder, abortifacient		Gastrointestinal distress
Atractylis	Atractylis gummifera		Chewing gum, antipyretic, diuretic, gastrointestinal remedy	Potassium atractylate and gummiferin: mitochondrial toxin	Hepatitis, altered mental status, seizures, vomiting, hypoglycemia
Autumn crocus	Colchicum autumnale	Crocus, fall crocus, meadow saffron, mysteria, vellorita	Gout, rheumatism, prostate, hepatic disease, cancer, gonorrhea	Colchicine	Gastrointestinal distress, renal disease, agranulocytosis
Bee pollen, royal jelly	Derived from Apis mellifera	—	Increase stamina, athletic ability, longevity		Allergic reactions, anaphylaxis
Bee venom	Derived from Apis mellifera	—	Immunomodulator		Allergic reactions, anaphylaxis
Betel nut	Areca catechu	Areca nut, pinlang, pinang	Stimulant	Arecoline	Acute: bronchospasm Chronic: associated with leukoplakia and squamous cell carcinoma
Bitter melon	Momordica charantia	MAP-30 (protein extract)	Abortifacient, diabetes, gastrointestinal disorder, diabetes, cancer, and HIV therapy	—	None
Black cohosh	Cimicifuga racemosa	Black snakeroot, squawroot, bugbane, baneberry	Abortifacient, menstrual irregularity, astringent, dyspepsia		Dizziness, nausea, vomiting, headache
Blue cohosh	Caulophyllum thalictroides	Squaw root, papoose root	Abortifacient, menstrual disorders, antispasmodic	Methylcytisine (1/40 potency of nicotine)	Nicotinic toxicity
Borage	Borago officinalis	—	Diuretic, antidepressant, antiinflammatory	Pyrrolizidine alkaloids, amabiline	Hepatotoxicity
Boron		Boron	Topical astringent, wound remedy	Boron	Dermatitis, gastrointestinal distress, renal and hepatic toxicity, seizures, coma, death
Boneset	Eupatorium perfoliatum	Thoroughwort, vegetable antimony, feverwort	Antipyretic	Pyrrolizidine alkaloids identified	Hepatotoxicity dermatitis, milk sickness
Broom	Cytisus scoparius	Bannal, broom, broom top	Cathartic, diuretic, induces labor, drug of abuse	L-Sparteine	Nicotinelike poisoning
Buchu	Barosma betulina	Bookoo, buku, diosma, bucku, bucco	Diuretic, stimulant, carminative, urine infections, insect repellent	—	None
Buckthorn	Rhamnus frangula		Laxative	Anthraquinones	Diarrhea, weakness

TABLE 77–2. Selected Herbal Preparations, Popular Use, and Potential Toxicities

Herbal Preparation	Scientific Name	Other Common Names	Traditional and Popular Usage	Toxic or Active Indredient(s)	Adverse Effects
Burdock root	*Arctium lappa, Arctium minus*	Great burdock, gobo, lappa, beggar's button, hareburr, niu bang zi	Diuretic, cholerectic, induces sweating, skin disorders and burn remedy	Atropine (possible contaminant)	Anticholinergic toxicity
Calendula	*Calendula officinalis*	Marigold, garden marigold, pot marigold, gold bloom, holligold	Wounds, dysmenorrhea, fever, pesticide	—	None
Cantharidin	*Cantharidin* beetle	Spanish fly, blister beetles	Aphrodisiac, abortifacient, blood purifier	Terpenoid: cantharidin	Gastrointestinal distress, urinary tract and skin irritant, renal toxicity
Caraway	*Umbellifarae carvi*		Antispasmodic, carminative		
Cascara	*Cascara sagrada*		Laxative	Anthraquinones	Diarrhea, weakness
Cat's claw	*Uncaria tomentosa Uncaria guianensis*	Uña de gato	AIDS, cancer, arthritis, ulcers, menstrual cramps, wounds, contraceptive	—	None
Catnip	*Nepeta cataria*	Cataria, catnep, catmint	Indigestion, colic, sedative, headaches, emmenagogue	Nepetalactone	Sedative
Chamomile	*Chamomilla recutita Chamomilla nobile*	In Mexico, manzanilla	Digestive disorders, skin disorders, cramps	Allergens	Contact dermatitis, allergic reaction, anaphylaxis
Carp bile (raw)	*Ctenopharyngodon idellus, Cyprinus carpio*	Grass carp Common carp	Improve visual acuity and health	? cyprinol, C27 bile alcohol	Hepatitis, renal failure
Ch'an Su	*Bufo bufo gargarizans Bufo bufo melanosticus*	Stone, lovestone, black stone, rock hard, chu an wu, kyushin	Topical anesthetic, aphrodisiac, cardiac medication	Bufodienolides, bufotenin	Cardiac dysrhythmias, hallucinations
Chaparral	*Larrea tridentata*	Creosote bush, greasewood, hediondilla	Bronchitis, analgesic, retard aging, cancer treatment	Nondihydroguaiaretic acid (NDGA)	Hepatotoxicity
Chestnut	*Aesculus spp.*	Horse chestnut, California buckeye, Ohio buckeye, buckeye	Arthritis, rheumatism, varicose veins, hemorrhoids.	Esculin, nicotine, quercitin, quercitrin, rutin, saponin, shikimic acid	Fasciculations, weakness, incoordination, gastrointestinal distress, paralysis, stupor
Clove	*Syzgium aromaticum*	Caryophyllum	Expectorant, antiemetic, counterirritant, antiseptic, carminative	Eugenol (4-allyl-2-methoxyphenol)	Pulmonary toxicity (cigarettes)
Coltsfoots	*Tussilago farfara*	Coughwort, horse-hoof, kuandong hua	Dry cough, throat irritation, asthma, bronchitis	Pyrrolizidine alkaloid, senkirkine	Allergy, potential hepatotoxicity, hepatic tumors (rats)
Comfrey	*Symphytum officinale* and other species *S. x uplandicum*	Knitbone, bruisewort, blackwort, slippery root, Russian comfrey	Ulcers, hemorrhoids, bronchitis, heal burns, sprains, swelling, bruises	Pyrrolizidine alkaloids: symphytine, echimidine, lasiocarpine	Hepatic venoocclusive disease, hepatocellular adenomas (rats)
Compound Q	*Trichosanthes kirilowii*	Gualougen, GLQ-223, Chinese cucumber root	Fevers, swelling, expectorant, abortifacient, diabetes, AIDS	Trichosanthin	Pulmonary and cerebral edema, cerebral bleed, seizures, fevers
Chuenlin	*Coptis chinensus, japonicum*	Huanglien, Ma Huang	Infant tonic	Berberine: displace bilirubin from protein	Neonatal hyperbilirubinemia
Damiana	*Tumera diffusa var aphrodisiaca*		Stimulant, purgative, aphrodisiac, antidepressant		Genitourinary irritation
Dandelion	*Taraxacum officinale*		Diuretic, detoxifying remedy, bitter	—	None
Dong Quai	*Angelica polymorpha*	Tang kuei, dang gui	Blood purifier, menstrual disorders, improve circulation	Coumarin, psoralens, safrole in essential oil	Anticoagulant effects, photodermatitis, carcinogenic (oil)
Echinacea	*Echinacea angustifolia Echinacea purpurea*	American cone flower, purple cone flower, snakeroot	Infections, immunostimulant	—	None

TABLE 77–2. Selected Herbal Preparations, Popular Use, and Potential Toxicities

Herbal Preparation	Scientific Name	Other Common Names	Traditional and Popular Usage	Toxic or Active Ingredient(s)	Adverse Effects
Elder	*Sambucus spp.*	Elderberry, sweet elder, sambucus	Diuretic, laxative, astringent, cancer	Cyanogenic glycoside sambunigrin in leaves	Vomiting, abdominal cramps, weakness if ingesting uncooked leaves
Ephedra	*Ephedra spp.*	Ma-Huang, Mormon tea, yellow horse, desert tea, squaw tea	Stimulant, bronchial disorder therapy, diet aid	Ephedrine, pseudo-ephedrine	Headache, insomnia, dizziness, palpitations, seizures, cerebro-vascular accidents, myocardial infarction, death
Evening Primrose	*Oenothera biennis*	Oil of evening primrose	Premenstrual syndrome, rheumatoid arthritis, diabetes, eczema	—	None
Fennel	*Foeniculum vulgare*	Common, sweet, or bitter fennel	Gastroenteritis, expectorant, emmenagogue, stimulate lactation	Volatile oils: transanethole, fenchone estrogens: dianethole and photoanethole	Ingestion of volatile oils: vomiting, seizures, pulmonary edema, dermatitis, estrogen effects
Feverfew	*Tanacetum parthenium*	Featherfew, altamisa, bachelor's button, featherfoil, febrifuge plant, midsummer daisy, nosebleed, wild quinine	Migraine headache, menstrual pain, asthma, dermatitis, arthritis, antipyretic, abortifacient		Oral ulcerations, "postfeverfew syndrome": rebound of migraine symptoms, anxiety, and insomnia following cessation of use
Fo-Ti	*Polygonum multiflorum*	Climbing knotwood, ho shou-wu	Scrofula, cancer, constipation therapy, promote longevity	Anthraquinones: chrysophaol and emodin	Cathartic effects
Foxglove	*Digitalis purpurea* *Digitalis lanata* *Digitalis lutea* other *Digitalis spp.*	Purple foxglove, throatwort, fairy finger, fairy cap, lady's thimble, scotch mercury, witch's bells, dead man's bells	Asthma therapy, sedative and diuretic/cardiotonic. In India, used to treat wounds and burns	Digitalis glycosides (eg, digitoxin, gitoxin, digoxin, digitalin, gitaloxin)	Blurred vision, gastrointestinal distress, dizziness, muscle weakness, tremors, cardiac dysrhythmias
Garlic	*Allium sativum*	Allium, stinking rose, rustic treacle, nectar of the gods, da suan	Therapy for infections and coronary artery disease, antihypertensive agent	Active: allicin, allin Toxic: ajoene	Contact dermatitis, gastroenteritis, antiplatelet effects
Gentian	*Gentiana lutea* *Gentiana spp.*	Bitter root, gall weed longdancao	Bitter, digestive stimulant, emmenagogue	—	None
Germander	*Teucrium chamaedrys*	Wall germander	Relief of fever, abdominal disorders, wounds, diuretic, choleretic		Hepatitis, cirrhosis
Ginkgo	*Ginkgo biloba*	Maidenhair tree, kew tree, tebonin, tanakan, rokan, kaveri	Dementia, asthma, chillblains, digestive aid		Extracts: gastrointestinal distress, headache, skin reaction, whole plants: allergic reactions, potential risk for bleeding
Ginseng	*Panax ginseng, quinquefolium, pseudoginseng*	Ren shen	Respiratory illnesses, gastrointestinal disorders, impotence, fatigue, stress, adaptogenic, external demulcent		Ginseng abuse syndrome
Glucomannan	*Amorphophallus konjac*	Konjac, konjac mannan	Weight reducing agent: "grapefruit diet"	Polysaccharides to increase viscosity and decrease gastric emptying	Esophageal and lower gastrointestinal obstruction
Glucosamine	2-amino-2-deoxyglucose	Chitosamine	Wound-healing polymer, antiarthritic	—	None
Goat's rue	*Galega officinalis*	French lilac, French honeysuckle	Antidiabetic	Galegine, paragalegine	Hypoglycemia

TABLE 77–2. **Selected Herbal Preparations, Popular Use, and Potential Toxicities (continued)**

Herbal Preparation	Scientific Name	Other Common Names	Traditional and Popular Usage	Toxic or Active Ingredient(s)	Adverse Effects
Goldenseal	Hydrastis canadensis	Orange root, yellow root, turmeric root	Astringent, gastrointestinal disorder and menstrual bleeding therapy		Gastrointestinal distress, paralysis, and respiratory failure in large ingestions
Gordolobo yerba	Senecio longiloba, aureus, vulgaris, spartoides	Groundsel liferoot	Gargle and cough medicine emmenagogue	Pyrrolizidine alkaloids	Hepatic veno-occlusive disease
Gotu Kola	Centella asiatica	Hydrocotyle, Indian pennywort, talepetrako	Wound healing, tonic		Contact dermatitis
Grape seed	Vitis vinifera		Antioxidant: anti-aging, peripheral vascular disease		None
Hawthorn	Crataegus oxyacantha	English hawthorn, haw, maybush, whitethorn	Blood pressure and dysrhythmia therapy, antispasmodic, sedative	Dehydrocatechins	Hypotension and sedation
Heliotrope	Crotalaria specatabulis, Heliotropium europeaum	Rattlebox, groundsel, viper's bugloss, bush tea		Pyrrolizidine alkaloids	Hepatic venoocclusive disease
Henbane	Hyoscyamus niger	Fetid nightshade, poison tobacco, insane root, stinky nightshade	Sedative, painkiller, antispasmodic, asthma remedy	Hyoscyamine, hyoscine	Anticholinergic toxicity
Holly	Ilex aquifolium Ilex opaca Ilex vomitoria	Holly, English holly, Oregon holly, and American holly	Tea: emetic, CNS stimulant, coronary artery disease therapy	Saponins	Gastrointestinal distress
Hydrangea	Hydrangea paniculata	Seven bark, wild hydrangea	Diuretic, stimulant, carminative, cystitis, renal calculi, and asthma therapy	Hydrangin	Dizziness, chest pain, gastrointestinal distress
Iboga	Tabernanthe iboga	Ibogaine	Aphrodisiac, stimulant, hallucinogen, addiction treatment	Indole alkaloid: ibogaine	Hallucinations, cholinergic hyperactivity
Impila	Callipesis laureola		Zulu traditional remedy	Potassium atractylate-like compound	Vomiting, hypoglycemia, centrilobular hepatic necrosis
Jalap	Ipomoea purga	—	Cathartic	Convolvulin	Profuse watery diarrhea
Jimson weed	Datura stramonium	Datura, stramonium, apple of Peru, Jamestown weed, thornapple, tolguacha	Asthma remedy	Atropine, scopolamine, hyoscyamine	Anticholinergic toxicity
Juniper	Juniperus communis	Oil of sabinol	Tonic, diuretic, urinary antiseptic, emmena-gogue, abortifacient	Oil: terpenen-4-ol	Renal irritation
Kava kava	Piper methysticum	Awa, kava-kava, kew, tonga	Relaxation beverage, uterine relaxation, headaches, colds, wounds, aphrodisiac	Kava lactones Flavokwain A and B	Mild euphoria, sedation, muscle weakness, skin discoloration
KH-3	Procaine hydrochloride	Gerovital-H3, GH-3, Gero-vita	Cerebral atherosclerosis, dementia, arthritis, hair loss, hypertension	Procaine	Procaine toxicity
Khat	Catha edulis	Qut, kat, chaat, Kus es Salahin, Tchaad, Gat	CNS stimulant, depression, fatigue, obesity, and ulcers remedy	Cathine and cathinine	Euphoria, dysphoria, stimulation, sedation, psychological dependence
Kola nut	Cola acuminata	Botu cola, cola nut	Digestive aid, tonic, aphrodisiac, headache remedy, diuretic	Caffeine	None
Kombucha	Mixture of bacteria and yeast	Kombucha tea, kom-bucha mushroom, Manchurian tea	Memory loss, premenstrual syndrome, cancer therapy		Possible metabolic acidosis and hepatitis
Levant berry	Anamirta cocculus	Fish killer, fishberry, hockle elderberry, Indian berry, louse-berry, poisonberry	Vermifuge, symptomatic relief for malaria	Picrotoxin	Stimulant, gastro-intestinal distress

(continued)

TABLE 77–2. Selected Herbal Preparations, Popular Use, and Potential Toxicities (continued)

Herbal Preparation	Scientific Name	Other Common Names	Traditional and Popular Usage	Toxic or Active Ingredient(s)	Adverse Effects
Licorice	*Glycyrrhiza glabra*	Spanish licorice, Russian licorice, gancao	Gastric irritation	Glycoside glycyrrhizin	Flaccid weakness, hypokalemia, lethargy
Lobelia	*Lobelia inflata*	Indian tobacco	Antispasmodic, respiratory stimulant, relaxant	Pyridine-derived alkaloids (lobeline)	Nicotine toxicity
Mace	*Myristica fragrans*	Mace, muscade, seed cover of nutmeg	Diarrhea, mouth sores, insomnia, rheumatism	Myristicin (methoxysafrole)	Hallucinations
Mandrake	*Mandragora officinarum*		Hallucinogen	Scopolamine, hyoscyamine	Anticholinergic toxicity
Mate	*Ilex paraguayensis*	Paraguay tea	Stimulant (caffeine)	Caffeine	None
Milk thistle	*Carduus marianus* *Silybum marianum*	Mary thistle	Liver disease, antidepressant, HIV therapy	Silymarin, silybinin	None
Mistletoe	*Viscum album,* *Phoradendron leucarpum*	Iscador	Antispasmodic, calmative, cancer and HIV therapy	Viscotoxins, pharotoxins	Gastrointestinal distress, bradycardia, delirium
Morning glory	*Ipomoea purpurea*	Heavenly blue, blue star, flying saucers	Drug of abuse	LSD	LSD toxicity
Myrrh	*Commiphora molmol*	Mulmul, ogo, heerabol	Astringent, antiseptic, emmenagogue, antispasmodic, cancer	—	None
Nutmeg	*Myristica fragrans*	Mace, rou dou kou	Hallucinogen, abortifacient, aphrodisiac, gastrointestinal disorders, emmenagogue	Myristicin	Hallucinogen, gastrointestinal distress
Oleander	*Nerium oleander*	Adelfa, laurier rose, rosa laurel, rose bay, rose francesca	Cardiac illness, asthma, corns, cancer, and epilepsy	Oleanrin, neriin, gentiobiosyloeandrin, odoroside A	Gastrointestinal distress, diarrhea, dysrhythmias
Ostrich fern	*Matteuccia struthipteris*	—	Laxative	—	Gastrointestinal distress if eaten undercooked
Parsley	*Petroselinum crispum*	Rock parsley, garden parsley	Diuretic, uterine stimulant, abortifacient	Myristicin, apiol, furocoumarin, psoralen	Uterine stimulant Photosensitization
Passion flower	*Passiflora incarnata*	Passiflora, maypop	Insomnia, analgesic	Vitexin	None
Pau d'Arco	*Tabebuia spp.*	Ipe roxo, lapacho, taheebo tea	Tonic, blood builder, cancer remedy, AIDS therapy	Naphthoquinone derivative: lapachol	Gastrointestinal distress, anemia, bleeding
Pennyroyal oil	*Hedeoma pulegioides,* *Mentha pulegium*	American pennyroyal, squawmint, mosquito plant	Abortifacient, regulate menstruation, digestive tonic	Pulegone, menthofuran	Hepatotoxicity
Periwinkle	*Catharanthus roseus*	Red periwinkle, Madagascar or Cape periwinkle, old maid, church-flower, ramgoat rose, "myrtle," magdalena	Ornamental; used to treat ocular inflammation, diabetes and hemorrhage, insect stings, cancers	Vincristine, vinblastine	Vincristine/vinblastine toxicity
Podophyllum	*Podophyllum peltatum* *Podophyllum hexandrum* *Podophyllum emodi*	Mandrake, mayapple, American podophyllum, Indian podophyllum, guijiu	Cathartic, purgative	Podophyllin	Podophyllin toxicity
Pokeweed	*Phytolacca americana* *Phytolacca decandra*	American nightshade, cancer jalap, inkberry, poke, scoke	Chronic rheumatisms, arthritis, emetic, purgative	Saponins: phytolaccigenin, jaligonic acid, phytolaccagenic acid, pokeweed mitogen	Gastroenteritis, blurry vision, weakness, respiratory distress, seizures, leukocytosis
Quinine	*Cinchona succirubra* *Cinchona calisya* *Cinchona ledgeriana*	Red bark, Peruvian bark, Jesuit's bark, China bark, cinchona bark, quinaquina, fever tree	Malaria, fever, indigestion, cancer, hemorrhoids, varicose veins, abortifacient	Quinine	Cinchonism
Red Bush Tea	*Aspalathus linearis*	Rooibos tea	Common tea substitute	—	None

TABLE 77–2. Selected Herbal Preparations, Popular Use, and Potential Toxicities (continued)

Herbal Preparation	Scientific Name	Other Common Names	Traditional and Popular Usage	Toxic or Active Ingredient(s)	Adverse Effects
Rehmennia	*Rehmannia glutinosa*	Sheng di huang, Chinese foxglove root	Longevity herb, lowers blood pressure, kidney and liver tonic	—	None
Rue	*Ruta graveolens*	Herb of grace, herb grass	Emmenagogue, antispasmodic, abortifacient	Furocoumarins, bergapten and xanthoxanthin	Photosensitization
Sage	*Salvia officinalis*	Garden sage, true sage, scarlet sage, meadow sage	Antiseptic, astringent, hormonal stimulant, carminative, abortifacient	Thujone	None
Saint John's Wort	*Hypericum perforatum*	Klamath weed, John's wort, goatweed, sho-ren-gyo	Anxiety, depression, gastritis, insomnia, promote healing, AIDS	—	Occasional photosensitization drug interaction: CYP 3A4
Sassafras	*Sassafras albidum*	—	Stimulant, antispasmodic, purifier	Safrole	Hepatotoxicity, carcinogen (?)
Saw Palmetto	*Serenoa repens*	Sabal, American dwarf palm tree, cabbage palm	Genitourinary disorders, increase sperm production, sexual vigor	—	Diarrhea
Schisandra	*Schisandra chinensis*	Wu zei zi	Tonic, aphrodisiac, liver treatment, sedative	—	None
Scullcap	Scutellaria laterifolia	Skullcap, helmetflower, hood wort	Reputed tranquilizer, tonic, antispasmodic	—	None
Senna	*Cassia acutifolia* *Cassia angustifolia*	Alexandrian senna	Stimulant, laxative, diet tea	Anthraquinone glycosides (sennosides)	Diarrhea, CNS effects
Shark cartilage	eg, *Squalus acanthias*, *Sphyrna lewini*	—	Cancer cure-inhibit tumor angiogenesis	—	None
Siberian ginseng	*Acanthopanax senticos*	Devil's shrub, eleuthra, eleutherococ	Adaptogens. blood pressure therapy, immune system stimulant	—	None
Slippery Elm	*Ulmus rubra* *Ulmus fulva*	Elm, elm bark, red elm	Acne, boils, indigestion, abortifacient	Oleoresin	Contact dermatitis
Soapwort	*Saponaria officinalis*	Bruisewort, bouncing bet, dog cloves, fuller's herb, latherwort	Acne, psoriasis, eczema, boils, used to make natural soaps	Saponins	(IV) highly toxic (PO) none
SOD	Superoxide dismutase	Orgotein, ormetein, palosein	Improve health, lengthen lifespan, chronic bladder disease, paraquat poisoning	—	None
Squill	*Urginea maritima*, *Urginea indica*	Sea onion	Diuretic, emetic, cardiotonic, expectorant	Cardiac glycoside: scillaren A	Emesis
Tonka bean	*Dipteryx odorata* *Dipteryx oppositifolia*	Tonquin bean, cumaru	Food and cosmetics	Coumarin	Anticoagulant effect
T'u-san-chi	*Gynura segetum*	—	Herbal tea	Pyrrolizidine alkaloids	Hepatic venoocclusive disease
Tung seed	*Aleurities moluccana*	Tung, candlenut, candleberry, barnish tree, balucanat, otaheite	Wood preservative (oil), purgative (oil), asthma treatment (seed)		Gastrointestinal distress, hyporeflexia, death, latex dermatitis
Valerian	*Valeriana officinalis* and other *spp.*	Radix valerianae, Indian valerian, red valerian	Anxiety, insomnia, antispasmodic	Valerenic acid, bornyl acetate	CNS depression
White cohosh	*Actaea alba* *Actaea rubra*	Baneberry, snakeberry, doll's eyes, coralberry	Emmenagogue	Toxic glycosides	Headache, gastrointestinal distress, delirium, circulatory failure
Wild lettuce	*Lactuca virosa*	Lettuce opium, prickley lettuce	Sedative, cough suppressant, narcotic substitute	—	None
Woodruff	*Galium odoratum*	Sweet woodruff	Wound healing, tonic, varicose vein treatment, antispasmodic	Coumarin	None

(continued)

TABLE 77–2. Selected Herbal Preparations, Popular Use, and Potential Toxicities (continued)

Herbal Preparation	Scientific Name	Other Common Names	Traditional and Popular Usage	Toxic or Active Ingredient(s)	Adverse Effects
Wormwood	*Artemisia absinthium*	Absinthem	Sedative, analgesic, antihelminthic	Thujone	Psychosis, hallucinations, seizures
Yarrow	*Achillea millefolium*	Bloodwort, carpenter's grass, dog daisy, nosebleed	Heal wounds, cold and flu remedy, digestive disorder treatment, diuretic		Contact dermatitis
Yew	*Taxus baccata* and other *spp.*	Yew	Antispasmodic, cancer remedy	Taxine (Na-K channel blocker)	Dizziness, dry mouth, bradycardia, cardiac arrest
Yohimbe	*Pausinystalia yohimbe*	Yohimbi, yohimbehe	Body building, aphrodisiac, hallucinogen	Alkaloid yohimbine from bark	Hypotension, abdominal pain, weakness, paralysis

a popular antiaging and arthritis remedy. In appropriate doses, grape seed extracts appear to be safe.

■ Kava kava (*Piper methysticum*) ($8 million)—Kava kava is a popular sleeping aid, stress reliever, and muscle relaxant. Kavalactones are the active ingredients. In appropriate doses, kava kava appears to be safe. Kava kava may potentiate sedation in patients taking sedative-hypnotics.[102]

■ Evening primrose (*Oenthoera biennis*) ($8 million)—Evening primrose contain cis-γ-linoleic acid (GLA), a prostaglandin E_1 precursor. This herbal is a popular remedy for premenstrual syndrome, diabetes, eczema, and rheumatoid arthritis. In appropriate doses, evening primrose appears to be safe. This herbal may lower the seizure threshold in epilepsy.[102]

■ Goldenseal (*Hydrastis canadensis)* ($8 million)—Goldenseal is a popular remedy for colds and flu symptoms and dyspepsia. It is also a popular topical remedy for canker sores, sore gums, and sore throat. In appropriate doses, goldenseal appears to be safe.[68]

■ Cranberry (*Vaccinium macrocarpon*) ($8 million)—Cranberry is a popular remedy for the treatment of urinary tract infections. In appropriate doses, cranberry appears to be safe.[8]

■ Valerian (*Valeriana officinalis*) ($8 million)—Valerian is a popular remedy for anxiety and is also used as a sleeping aid. In appropriate doses, valerian appears to be safe. Valerian may potentiate sedation in patients taking sedative-hypnotics.[112]

TOXICITY OF SPECIFIC HERBAL PREPARATIONS

Cardiovascular Toxins

Aconite. Aconites (Caowu and Chuanwu) are the dried rootstocks of the *Aconitum* plant.[140] In China, aconite is usually derived from *A. carmichaeli* (chuanwu) or *A. kuznezoffii* (caowu). In Europe and the United States, aconite is derived from *A. napellus*, commonly known as monkshood or wolfsbane. The tubers are the most toxic part of the plant, and when ingested, both cardiac and neurologic symptoms occur. Aconite poisoning is far more common in Asia, especially China.[40] In Hong Kong, it is responsible for the majority of serious poisonings from Chinese herbal preparations.[38,40]

Aconite toxicity is caused by C19 diterpenoid-ester alkaloids, including aconitine, mesaconitine, and hypoaconitine.[19] Mechanis-

tically, aconitine increases sodium influx through the sodium channel, increasing inotropy, while delaying the final repolarization phase of the action potential and promoting premature excitation.[73] Sinus bradycardia and ventricular dysrhythmias can occur.[39] Symptoms can occur from 5 minutes to 4 hours after ingestion. Paresthesias of the oral mucosa and entire body may be followed by nausea, vomiting, diarrhea, and hypersalivation, and then by progressive skeletal muscle weakness. Fatalities may occur with doses as low as 5 mL of aconite tincture, 2 mg of pure aconite, or 1 g of dried plant. Atropine may be of value in treating bradycardia or hypersalivation.[140] Although there is no antidote available, anecdotal reports suggest the use of amiodarone, flecainide, bretylium, and procainamide for tachydysrhythmias.[140] Pharmacologic principles would support the use of these sodium channel blockers. One case of aconite-induced refractory tachydysrhythmias was successfully managed with a ventricular assist device.[61]

Ch'an Su. Ch'an Su is a traditional herbal remedy derived from the secretions of the parotid and sebaceous glands of a toad, *Bufo bufo gargarizans* or *Bufo melanosticus*. This remedy is traditionally used as a treatment for congestive heart failure.[84] Ch'an Su contains two groups of toxic compounds: digoxinlike cardioactive steroids consisting of bufadienolides, and a hallucinogenic compound, bufotenin. Clinical findings following ingestion are similar to digoxin poisoning, including gastrointestinal symptoms and dysrhythmias. It is also marketed as an aphrodisiac for its purported topical anesthetic effects and is sold under names such as "Stone," "Love Stone," "Black Stone," and "Rock Hard." Between 1993 and 1996 in New York City, several fatalities were associated with the ingestion of Ch'an Su marketed as a topical aphrodisiac.[24] Severe toxic reactions or death are also reported after mouthing toads, "toad licking," and eating an entire toad, toad soup, or toad eggs.[17] Assays for serum digoxin unpredictably cross-react with bufadienolides, but may qualitatively assist in making a presumptive diagnosis (see Table 77–1). Similarly, digoxin-specific Fab (Digibind) was successfully used to treat Ch'an Su poisoning and should be empirically administered for any suspected case of Ch'an Su cardiotoxicity.[17]

Central Nervous System Toxins

Absinthe. Wormwood (*Artemisia absinthium*) extract is the main ingredient in absinthe, a toxic liquor that is outlawed in the

United States since 1912. This volatile oil is a mixture of α- and β-thujone (see Table 77–3).[154] Both tetrahydrocannabinol, the active ingredient in marijuana, and thujone have an affinity for a common CNS receptor binding site and for similar oxidative metabolic pathways.[154]

Chronic absinthe use caused absinthism, which was characterized by psychosis, hallucinations, intellectual deterioration, and seizures. The most famous victim of absinthism may have been Vincent Van Gogh, who is thought to have suffered from this disorder in the later part of his life. He is suggested to have had pica, eating paint and drinking turpentine and camphor for its terpene content when he craved absinthe.[6] A thujone-free wormwood extract is now used in flavoring vermouth. A case of wormwood-induced seizures, rhabdomyolysis, and acute renal failure was recently described involving a patient who purchased and consumed approximately 10 mL of essential oil of wormwood from the Internet, assuming it was absinthe liquor.[150] Treatment remains supportive.

Anticholinergic Agents: Henbane, Jimson weed, Mandrake.

Many plants contain the belladonna alkaloids: atropine (*dl*-hyoscyamine), hyoscyamine, and scopolamine (*l*-hyoscine). They may be used therapeutically as an asthma remedy or as a natural hallucinogen. Occasionally, these plants are mistakenly included in herbal teas.[34] Examples of plants with anticholinergic properties include: henbane, Jimson weed, and mandrake. Signs and symptoms of anticholinergic poisoning include mydriasis, diminished bowel sounds, urinary retention, dry mouth, flushed skin, tachycardia, and agitation. Mildly poisoned patients usually require only supportive care and central nervous system sedation with intravenous benzodiazepines. Intravenous physostigmine reverses anticholinergic poisoning; however, its use should be limited for

TABLE 77–3.   Psychoactive Substances Used in Herbal Preparations

Labeled Ingredient	Scientific Name	Usage	Active Ingredients	Effects
Broom	*Cytisus spp.*	Smoked for relaxation	Sparteine	Sedative-hypnotic
California poppy	*Eschscholtzia californica*	Smoked as marijuana substitute	Alkaloids and glucosides	Euphoriant
Catnip	*Nepeta cataria*	Smoke or tea as marijuana substitute	Nepetalactone	Euphoriant
Ch'an Su	*Bufo bufo gargarizans* *Bufo bufo melanosticus*	Smoke or licked for hallucinations	Bufotenin	Hallucinogen
Cinnamon	*Cinnamomum camphora*	Smoked with marijuana	?	Stimulant
Cloves	*Syzgium aromaticum*	Smoked in cigarette/"kreteks"	Eugenol	Euphoriant
Damiana	*Turnera diffusa*	Smoke as marijuana substitute	?	Stimulant/hallucinogen
Goldenseal	*Hydrastis canadensis*	Ingested to mask detection of opioid, marijuana, or cocaine in urine drug screen	—	No evidence
Hops	*Humulus lupulus*	Smoke or tea as sedative and marijuana substitute	Humulone, lupulone → methylbutenol	Sedative (mild)
Hydrangea	*Hydrangea paniculata*	Smoke as marijuana substitute	Hydrangin, saponin	Stimulant
Ibogaine	*Tabernanthe iboga*	Stimulant, hallucinogen	Ibogaine	Hallucinogen
Juniper	*Juniper macropoda*	Smoke as hallucinogen	?	Hallucinogen
Kava kava	*Piper methysticum*	Smoke or tea as marijuana subtsitute	Kava lactones	Hallucinogen
Kola nut	*Cola spp.*	Smoke, tea, or capsules as stimulant	Caffeine, theobromine, kolanin	Stimulant
Lobelia	*Lobelia inflata*	Smoke or tea as marijuana substitute	Lobeline	Euphoriant
Mandrake	*Mandragora officinarum*	Tea as hallucinogen	Atropine, scopolamine	Hallucinogen
Mate	*Ilex parguayensis*	Tea as stimulant	Caffeine	Stimulant
Mormon Tea	*Ephedra nevadensis*	Tea as stimulant	Ephedrine	Stimulant
Morning glory	*Ipomoea violacea*	Seeds have hallucinogens	D-lysergic acid amide (ergine)	Hallucinogen
Nutmeg	*Myristica fragrans*	Tea as hallucinogen	Myristicin	Hallucinogen
Passion flower	*Passiflora incarnata*	Smoke, tea, or capsules as marijuana substitute	Harmala alkaloids	Stimulant (mild)
Periwinkle	*Catharanthus roseus*	Smoke or tea as euphoriant	Indole alkaloids	Hallucinogen
Prickly poppy	*Argemone mexicana*	Smoke as euphoriant	Protopine, bergerine, isoquinolones	Analgesic
Snakeroot	*Rauwolfia serpentina*	Smoke or tea as tobacco substitute	Reserpine	Tranquilizer
Thorn apple	*Datura stramonium*	Smoke or tea as tobacco substitute or hallucinogen	Atropine, scopolamine	Hallucinogen
Tobacco	*Nicotiana spp.*	Smoke as tobacco	Nicotine	Stimulant
Valerian	*Valeriana officinalis*	Tea or capsules	Chatinine, velerine alkaloids	Tranquilizer
Wild lettuce	*Lactuca sativa*	Smoke as opium substitute	Unknown	Analgesic (mild)
Wormwood	*Artemisia absinthium*	Smoke or tea as relaxant	Thujone	Analgesic
Yohimbe	*Pausinystalia yohimbe*	Smoke or tea as stimulant	Yohimbine	Hallucinogen (mild)

Adapted from Siegel RK: Herbal intoxication. JAMA 1976;236:473–476.

selected moderate to severe cases because inappropriate use may cause seizures and dysrhythmias.

Ephedra. Members of the genus *Ephedra* are generally erect evergreen plants resembling small shrubs. Common names include sea grape, ma-huang, yellow horse, desert tea, squaw tea, and Mormon tea. Ephedra species have a long history of use as stimulants and for the management of bronchospasm. They contain the alkaloids, ephedrine and, in some species, pseudoephedrine.[143] In large doses, ephedrine causes nervousness, headache, insomnia, dizziness, palpitations, skin flushing, tingling, vomiting, anxiety, restlessness, mania, and psychosis. Cases of seizures, stroke, myocardial infarction, and death have been described following the ingestion of pills known as "herbal ecstacy." These pills contained ephedra and were sold as safe and natural stimulants.[21] The treatment is similar to that for other CNS stimulants (see Chap. 68).

Khat. A common form of drug abuse in East Africa involves chewing the leaves and stems of the khat plant (*Catha edulis*) and swallowing the juice.[56,95] Khat is used by herbalists to treat depression, fatigue, obesity, and gastric ulcers. The two active compounds in khat are cathine (norpseudoephedrine) and cathinone (α-aminopropiophenone), the more active stimulant. More than 30 other minor compounds are also found in khat. Red khat contains more cathinone than white khat, and is a more potent stimulant. This herb produces euphoria, dysphoria, stimulation, and sedation. The two major components have a direct action on neuromuscular junctions and also interact with dopaminergic pathways. It is suggested that these amphetaminelike compounds have a stimulatory effect with potencies between that of caffeine and amphetamine. True psychotic reactions are rare and physical dependency is not reported, but psychological dependence is common in chronic abusers. Chronic abuse is implicated in causing hypertension in young adults, which is reversible with cessation of khat. Stomatitis, constipation, esophagitis, and gastritis result from ingestion of khat tannins found in the plant. Norpseudoephedrine is found in the urine and breast milk of women who use khat. Severe adverse effects of khat use include myocardial infarction, cerebral hemorrhage, and pulmonary edema. Cirrhosis, decreased libido, anorexia, and impotence are also reported. Oral carcinomas are described in khat chewers in Saudi Arabia.

Nicotinic Agents: Betel Nut, Blue Cohosh, Broom, Chestnut, Lobelia, Tobacco. Betel (*Areca catechu*) is chewed by an estimated 200 million people worldwide for its euphoric effect. The active ingredient is arecoline, a direct-acting nicotinic agonist. The betel leaf also contains a phenolic volatile oil and an alkaloid capable of producing sympathomimetic reactions. Arecoline is a bronchoconstrictor, although it is weaker than methacholine, and may cause exacerbation of bronchospasm in asthmatic patients chewing betel nut.[142] Treatment for betel nut toxicity is supportive. Long-term use of betel nut is associated with leukoplakia and squamous cell carcinoma of the oral mucosa.[109]

Many other herbal preparations have nicotinic-effects. Examples of plants and their nicotinic ingredient include blue cohosh, methylcytisine; broom, *l*-sparteine; chestnut, esculin; lobelia, lobeline; and tobacco, nicotine.

Nutmeg and Mace. Nutmeg and mace are products of the evergreen tree *Myristica fragrans*, indigenous to the Spice Islands and cultivated in the Caribbean. The fruits of *M. fragrans* resemble apricots or peaches. When ripe, the husk splits open and a single glossy brown nut (nutmeg) is revealed, enclosed by a scarlet netlike aril, which, when dried, is called mace.

Nutmeg has been used by herbalists to treat dyspepsia, musculoskeletal and arthritic disorders, psychiatric conditions, and narcosis, and as an emmenagogue and abortifacient. Nutmeg ingestions have been reported among prisoners, college students, and adolescents attempting to achieve euphoria, although intoxications have occurred with the unintentional misuse of the herbal preparation.[116,151] The essential oil is thought to be the active component, containing alkylbenzene derivatives and terpenes. The nutmeg contains 5–15% of this volatile oil, depending on the geographic region. Myristicin, one of the components of the oil, was initially considered the active compound; it has weak monoamine oxidase inhibitor properties that are responsible for some of the cardiovascular symptoms.[1,111,134] However, myristicin alone does not account for the total effects of nutmeg. It may be metabolized in vivo to the psychotomimetic amphetaminelike compound 3-methoxy-4,5-methylenedioxyamphetamine (MMDA), and elemicin, another ingredient in the oil, is converted to 3,4,5-trimethoxyamphetamine (TMA).[111,134] Eugenol, isoeugenol, borneol, safrole, and linalol are also active components.

Symptoms of nutmeg poisoning, including nausea, vomiting, and CNS effects, occur within several hours of ingesting 5–15 g of nutmeg. Within 24 hours, after an acute delirium and subsequent deep sleep, the patient usually recovers uneventfully. With exceedingly large doses, symptoms may persist for days. Hypothermia may be a consequence of ingesting large amounts of nutmeg.[134]

Gastrointestinal Toxins

Goldenseal. Goldenseal (*Hydrastis canadensis*) was originally used by the Cherokees and other Native Americans as a dye and an internal remedy.[68] Today, it is used as an astringent, a remedy for mucous membranes or gastrointestinal tract disorders, and as a treatment for menorrhagia. Goldenseal is reputed to mask the presence of illicit drugs on urine drug screens. This myth originated in the murder-mystery *Stringtown on the Pike* (1900), which was written by an internationally known plant pharmacist, Uri Lloyd. In this novel, one of the major characters is accused of murder by poisoning with strychnine, but is posthumously exonerated with evidence that hydrastine (the active alkaloid in goldenseal) and morphine cross-react to produce a false-positive color assay for strychnine.[63] Multiple studies indicate that goldenseal does not affect the results of urinary drug screens.[43,106,114] Appropriate usage of this herbal is thought to be safe, but large ingestions can cause vomiting, diarrhea, convulsions, paralysis, and respiratory failure. In those cases, the patient should receive supportive care.

Pokeweed. Pokeweed (*Phytolacca americana* or *Phytolacca decandra*) is also known as inkberry, Virginia poke, scoke, pigeon berry, garget, and American cancer. It is often mistaken for horseradish, parsnips, or Jerusalem artichoke. Gastrointestinal effects are very common after ingestion; in severe cases, there may also be neurologic symptoms, such as decreased vision, respiratory depression, seizures, and weakness, and cardiac dysrhythmias. The root is the most toxic part of the plant, although the leaves, stems, and berries also possess enterotoxins, including triterpenes, saponins, and glycoproteins.[92] Pokeweed can cause mitotic and morphologic changes in lymphocytes and plasma cells by a non-specific mitogenic effect. Diagnosis can be aided by observing for a marked lymphocytosis in affected patients. Symptoms typically begin within several minutes of exposure and last 24–48 hours. Treatment remains supportive.

Hepatotoxins

Pennyroyal. Pennyroyal oil is a volatile oil extract from the leaves of *Mentha pulegium* and *Hedeoma pulegioides* plants. Herbalists use pennyroyal oil as an abortifacient and to regulate menstruation. The abortive effect is thought to be caused by irritation and contraction of the uterus.[139] Pennyroyal is usually ingested as a strong tea prepared from the leaves or as the oil itself. It is cited as the causative agent in several well-documented cases of hepatic failure following ingestion of as little as 15 mL of the oil.[4] The postulated mechanism is direct hepatotoxicity following glutathione depletion from the cyclohexanone pulegone, and its cytochrome P450-dependent toxic metabolites that include menthofuran. Pulegone and menthofuran also cause neurotoxicity, renal toxicity, and bronchiolar epithelial cell destruction. Other effects of pennyroyal ingestion include a minty odor on the breath, GI bleeding, seizures, hematuria, and vaginal bleeding. On autopsy, vacuolization of the white matter of the midbrain is reported in both a fatal human exposure and in animal models.[8,113] Because pulegone depletes hepatic glutathione stores, *N*-acetylcysteine treatment may be beneficial. Hepatotoxicity was reportedly prevented by early administration of *N*-acetylcysteine after a pennyroyal ingestion.[4,18] *N*-Acetylcysteine treatment similar to the dosing regimen used in acetaminophen overdose should be considered as first-line therapy for patients with pennyroyal-associated hepatotoxicity.

Pyrrolizidine Alkaloids. Pyrrolizidine alkaloids are hepatotoxins found in many plants. *Heliotropium*, *Senecio*, *Crotolaria*, and *Symphytum* are the most common sources of pyrrolizidine alkaloids.[121,126] Conversion to the toxic, active metabolites probably occurs in vivo and most likely involves metabolism in the liver to pyrroles, which serve as biologic alkylating agents.[76] The pyrroles cause hepatic sinusoidal hypertrophy and venous occlusion resulting in hepatic venoocclusive disease, hepatomegaly, and cirrhosis, and possibly hepatic carcinoma. Chronic low doses may cause pulmonary toxicity resulting in pulmonary artery hypertension and right ventricular hypertrophy. Consumption of "bush" tea, prepared from the leaves of the *Crotolaria* plant from the surrounding scrubland, is considered an endemic problem in Jamaica. Epidemics have also occurred in Afghanistan and India, where ingestion of contaminated cereals containing *Heliotropium* and *Crotolaria* seeds resulted in reports of 1632 and 60 cases of venoocclusive disease, respectively.[104,141] In Western countries, ingestion of herbal products containing *Senecio* and comfrey have led to several cases of hepatic venoocclusive disease.[121] Treatment of hepatic venoocclusive disease is supportive, but may require liver transplantation in severe cases. Examples of other plants and products containing pyrrolizidine alkaloids include borage (*Borago officinalis*), coltsfoot (*Tussilago farfara*), and T'u-san-chi'i (*Gynura segetum*).[76,85,127]

Other Hepatotoxins

Several herbal preparations are also associated with hepatotoxicity. These include chaparral (*Larrea tridentata*),[23,69] german-der (*Teucrium chamaedrys*),[89] impilia (*Callilepsis laureola*),[87] Atractylis (*Atractylis gummifera*), and sassafras (*Sassafras albidum*).[132]

Metals

Poisonings by metals, including arsenic, cadmium, lead, and mercury, may occur following consumption of various types of herbal preparations.[28,48,127] Treatment consists of cessation of the herbal product and use of an appropriate chelating agent when indicated.

Hai Ge Fen (clamshell powder) was contaminated with copper, chromium, arsenic, or lead in several case reports.[72,96] Pay-Loo-Ah, a red and orange powder used by the Hmong people as a fever and rash remedy, was contaminated with lead in one case report.[25] Ghasard, Bola Goli, Kandu, Moha Yogran Guggulu, traditional Indian remedies for abdominal pain, are associated with lead poisoning.[28,131] One fatality from lead poisoning from Ghasard, Bola Goli, and Kandu is reported from the United States.[28] Ayurvedic remedies often intentionally contain metals such as gold, silver, copper, zinc, iron, lead, tin, and mercury.[124]

Azarcon (lead tetroxide) and Greta (lead oxide) are used by an estimated 7.2–12.1% of Mexican-Hispanic families for treatment of *empacho*. In Spanish, *empacho* means "blocked intestine" but it refers to any type of chronic digestive problem, including diverse symptoms such as constipation, diarrhea, nausea, vomiting, anorexia, apathy, and lethargy.[30,33] Azarcon and Greta are fine powders with total lead contents varying from 70% to greater than 90%.[14,31]

Surma and Kohl, eye makeup used in India, Middle East, and Africa, contain over 50% lead.[3,7,124,135] Lead poisoning and fatalities have been reported. Herbal balls, hand-rolled mixtures of herbs and honey produced in China, are often associated with arsenic and mercury contamination.[60] Examples include An Gong Niu Huang Wan, Da Huo Luo Wan, and Niu Huang Chiang Ya Wan.

Colloidal silver products, which are suspensions of finely-divided metallic silver, are promoted by health food stores as antimicrobials, immune system stimulants, and antiinflammatory agents. Silver toxicity, or argyria may occur with chronic usage and is associated with a bluish skin discoloration,[64] neurologic deficits, silver deposition in visceral organs, and renal damage.[64]

Renal Toxins

Aristolochia. Aristolochia (*Aristolochia fangchi*), also known as birthwort, heartwort, and fangji, produces progressive interstitial renal fibrosis. An epidemic occurred in Belgium when this herbal was substituted for another Chinese herbal, *Stephania tetranda*, in the formulation of a weight loss regimen.[146,147] Of 70 identified cases of renal fibrosis, 30 patients developed chronic renal failure. Aristolochia contains aristolochic acid, which is a known nephrotoxin and carcinogen. The fibrosing process typically becomes clinically apparent 12–24 months after the initial injury. Patients with aristolochia-induced nephropathy also have an increased risk for developing urothelial cancer.[108]

Miscellaneous

Garlic. Garlic (*Allium sativum*) has been used as a food and a medicine since ancient times.[66] The intact cells of garlic contain the odorless, sulfur-containing amino acid derivative (+)-S-allyl-L-cysteine sulfoxide, also known as alliin. When crushed, alliin is converted to allicin (diallyl thiosulfinate), which has antibacterial activity and gives the herb its characteristic odor and flavor. Garlic is used as a traditional remedy for a host of infections and as a treatment for hypertension, colic, and cancer. Side effects of garlic extracts include contact dermatitis, gastroenteritis, nausea, and vomiting. Patients who are already taking anticoagulant medications should consume garlic with caution because of its antiplatelet metabolite ajoene.[66] Treatment remains supportive.

Ginseng. Ginseng is the common name for deciduous, perennial plants of the genus *Panax*. *Panax ginseng* is native to Korea, China, Japan, and Russia. *Panax quinquefolium* is the common ginseng species in North America, and grows abundantly throughout the central and eastern regions of Canada and the United States. Ginseng preparations have been used in China for the treatment of respiratory illnesses, gastrointestinal disorders, impotence, fatigue, and stress ("adaptogenic effect"). It is regarded as a tonic and panacea (hence the name Panax—"all healing"). Its only recognized use in America is as an external demulcent.[64,87,98] However, an estimated 6 million people regularly ingest ginseng in herbal teas or apply it as a cosmetic. Ginseng provides a good example of the complexity of the biochemistry and pharmacologic effects of herbs. The active components of ginseng are called ginsenosides and include panaxin, panax acid, panaquilin, panacen, sapogenin, and ginsenin. Its general metabolic effects include a decrease in serum glucose levels and serum cholesterol levels; increases in erythropoiesis, hemoglobin production, and iron absorption from the gut; increases in blood pressure and heart rate, and GI motility and CNS stimulation. Because of the lack of oversight in the health food industry, many ginseng products may not contain significant quantities of ginsenosides. In one study of 54 ginseng products, 60% of those analyzed contained pharmacologically insignificant amounts of ginseng and 25% contained no ginsenosides at all.[93] Long-term use of ginseng is associated with

Ginseng Abuse Syndrome (GAS), consisting of hypertension, nervousness, sleeplessness, and morning diarrhea.[133]

Chamomile Tea. Chamomile tea is a popular herbal drink made from chamomile flower heads. Anaphylactic reactions can occur in patients allergic to ragweed, asters, chrysanthemums, or other members of the *Compositae* family.[10,21] Such reactions are rare, but can be life-threatening. The patient need not have severe allergies or be highly atopic to experience a cross-reaction.

Rattlesnake Capsules. Rattlesnake capsules are a common Mexican folk remedy used to treat cancer, arthritis, and skin disorders. These capsules contain dried, pulverized rattlesnake powder and are sold under various names—vibora de cascabel, polvo de vibora, and carne de vibora—without prescriptions. Infection with *Salmonella arizonae* is described following ingestion.[12,44,110,129,149]

Chinese Patent Medications

Chinese patent medicines, a component of traditional Chinese medicine, comprise multiple products including plant, animal parts, and minerals, which are formulated into tablets, capsules, syrups, powders, ointments, and plasters for easy use. These products appear to be very susceptible to adulteration or contamination. Poorly regulated Chinese pharmaceutical companies produce most of the Chinese patent medicines (see Table 77–4). They are often sold by nonherbalists in convenience stores in packages that are not labeled in English. In 1998, the California Department of Health Services investigated 260 Asian patent medications for adulterants and determined that 32% contained undeclared pharmaceutics or heavy metals.[83]

Jin Bu Huan is a traditional Chinese preparation used as a sedative and analgesic.[153] The active ingredient, an isoquinoline alkaloid levo-tetrahydropalmatine (L-THP), is responsible for the

TABLE 77–4.   **The 20 Most Popular Asian Patent Medicines That Contain Toxic Ingredients**

Product Name	Manufacturer	Toxic Ingredients
Ansenpenaw Tablets	Chung Lien Drug Works (Hankow, China)	Mercuric chloride
Bezoar Sedative Pills	Lanzhou Fo Ci Pharmaceutical Factory (Lanzhou, China)	Mercuric chloride 2% or 10%
Compound Kangweiling	Wo Zhou Pharmaceutical Factory (Zhe Jiang, China)	Centipede (scolopendra) 10%
Dahuo Luodan	Beijing Tun Jen Tang (Beijing, China)	Centipede (scolopendra)
Danshen Tabletco	Shanghai Chinese Medicine Works (Shanghai, China)	Borneol
Fructus Persica Compound Pills	Lanzhou Fo Ci Pharmaceutical Factory (Lanzhou, China)	Cannabis indica seed
Fuchingsung-N Cream	Tianjin Pharmaceutical Corp. (Tianjin, China)	Fluocinolone acetanide
Kwei Ling Chi	Changchun Chinese Medicines and Drugs Manufactory (Chang Chun, China)	Mercuric chloride
Kyushin Heart Tonic	Kyushin Seikyaku Co., Ltd. (Tokyo, Japan)	Toad venom, borneol
Laryngitis Pills	China Dzechuan Provincial Pharmaceutical Factory (Chengtu Branch, China)	Borax 30%, toad-cake 10%
Leung Pui Kee Cough Pills	Leung Pui Kee Medical Factory (Hong Kong)	Dover's powder (opium powder)
Lu-Shen-Wan	Shanghai Chinese Medicine Works (Shanghai, China)	Toad secretion
Nasalin	Kwangchow Pharmaceutical Industry Co. (Kwangchow, China)	Centipede 5%
Nui Huang Chieh Tu Pien	Tung Jen Tang (Beijing, China)	Borneo camphor
Nui Huang Xiao Yan Wan Bezoar Antiphlogistic Pills	Soochow Chinese Medicine Works (Kiangsu, China)	Realgar 19.23%
Pak Yuen Tong Hou Tsao Powder	Kwan Tung Pak Yuen Tong Main Factory (Hong Kong)	Scorpion 10%
Po Ying Tan Baby Protector	Po Che Tong Poon Mo Um (Hong Kong)	Camphor 20%
Superior Tabellae Berberini HCl	Min-Kang Drug Manufactory (I-Chang, China)	Berberini HCl
Watson's Flower Pagodo Cakes	A.S. Watson & Co., Ltd. (Hong Kong)	Piperazine phosphate
Xiao Huo Luo Dan	Lanzhou Fo Ci Pharmaceutical Factory (Lanzhou, China)	Aconite 42%

From Appendix E. Alternative Medicine: Expanding Medical Horizons. A report to the National Institutes of Health on alternative medical systems and practices in the United States. Presented under the auspices of the workshop on alternative medicine. Chantilly, Virginia. Sept. 14–16, 1992.

morphinelike properties of Jin Bu Huan. In two case reports, 3 pediatric patients developed life-threatening bradycardia and 7 adult patients developed hepatitis while using Jin Bu Huan.[26,27] Hepatotoxicity may be related to L-THP, which is structurally similar to the hepatotoxic pyrrolizidine alkaloids.[153] Although the package insert for Jin Bu Huan in these cases indicate that *Polygala chinensis* was the plant source for L-THP, *Polygala chinensis* does not contain L-THP. Plants from the genera *Stephania* and *Corydalis* are also known as Jin Bu Huan and contain appreciable amounts of L-THP. It is probable that this product was simply mislabeled by the manufacturer.

Nan Lien Chiu Fong Toukuwan (now withdrawn from the market) was found to variably contain aminopyrine, phenacetin, phenylbutazone, indomethacin, mefenamic acid, diazepam, hydrochlorothiazide, dexamethasone, mercuric sulfide, lead, and cadmium, depending on the manufacturer.[38] Several cases of agranulocytosis were reported following ingestion of this preparation.[128] Dr. Tong Shap Yee's asthma pills were found to contain theophylline.[38] Leng Pui Kee cough pills were found to contain bromhexine.[38]

Tung Shueh, also known as black ball, contains diazepam and mefenamic acid and is associated with acute interstitial nephritis.[53] Gan Mao Tong Pian, an herbal cold remedy, contains phenylbutazone and caused aplastic anemia in one child.[107] Chui Feng Su Ho Wan, which contains *Glycyrrhiza glabra*, was associated with hypokalemia-induced torsade de pointes in an elderly woman.[38]

Several Chinese patent medicines contain the mercurials cinnabar (mercuric sulfide) and calomel (mercurous chloride). Tse Koo Choy and Qing Fen, which contain calomel, are associated with several cases of mercury poisoning.[80]

Many Chinese medicated oils contain oil of wintergreen, which is composed of methylsalicylate. Although these oils are intended for external use, it is a common practice to ingest a few drops undiluted or in a hot drink as a general tonic or specific remedy. Examples of medicated oils include White Flower Medicine Oil (40% oil of wintergreen, 30% menthol, 6% camphor), Red Flower Oil (67% oil of wintergreen, 22% turpentine oil), and Kwan Loong Medicated Oil (menthol 25%, methyl salicylate 15%, camphor 10%).[38]

Herbal Preparations and AIDS Therapies

Many patients infected with human immunodeficiency virus (HIV) have turned to alternative treatments in the hope of finding less-toxic therapy than the conventional modalities currently available. In a study of 114 HIV-positive patients in a university-based AIDS clinic, 22% used one or more herbal products in a 3-month period.[81] Twenty-four percent of these patients were unable to state which herbs they were taking. Adverse effects included dermatitis, nausea, vomiting, diarrhea, thrombocytopenia, coagulopathies, altered mental status, hepatotoxicity, and electrolyte imbalances. Twenty percent of patients stated their physicians were unaware of their use of herbs.

Two herbals currently used for AIDS therapy are St. John's wort (*Hypericum perforatum*) and Chinese cucumber (*Trichosanthes kirilowii*).[42,130] St. John's wort is a perennial, that is native to Europe but which is also found in the United States and Canada. Herbalists have used the plant since the Middle Ages. Recently, it was used to treat anxiety and depression, as a diuretic, and for gastritis. It contains tannin, hypericin, hyperforin, a red dianthrone pigment, rutin, flavinoids, and hyperoside. Studies are currently

being conducted with hypericin as an immunomodulator in patients with AIDS. Acute toxicity appears to be limited to photosensitization reactions. St. John's wort appears to be an inducer of CYP 3A4 pathway which may produce significant drug interactions with other medications metabolized by CYP 3A4. In addition to decreasing indinavir plasma concentrations, St. John's wort also appears to decrease cyclosporine levels in transplant patients and to cause breakthrough bleeding for woman taking oral contraceptives.[59] Consequently, use of St. John's wort should be avoided in those patients taking medications metabolized by the CYP 3A4 pathway (see Table 77–5).

Chinese cucumber, or Compound Q, is employed in Chinese medicine to reduce fevers, swelling, and coughing, to control diabetes, and as an abortifacient.[42] Trichosanthin appears to be synonymous with Compound Q. It has also been called Gualougen and GLQ-223. According to some herbalists, this compound blocks HIV replication in infected T4 cells and destroys HIV-infected macrophages. Extracts of Chinese cucumber are extremely toxic with reports of pulmonary and cerebral edema, cerebral hemorrhage, and myocardial damage resulting from parenteral administration.[42] Seizures and fever occurred in patients with AIDS who had used Chinese cucumber parenterally.[42]

Other herbal preparations, including *lactobacillus acidophilus*; adrenal cortex, aloe vera, *Astragalus*, blue-green algae, *Allium sativum*, Artemisia, astragalus, bitter melon, Bioperine, cat's claw, Chlorella, chromium picolinate, coenzyme Q10, curcumin, dandelion root, DHEA (dehydroepiandrosterone), Echinacea, elderberry, evening primrose oil, flaxseed oil, garlic, germanium, *Ginkgo biloba*, ginseng, glutamine, glutathione, glycyrrhizin, grapeseed, saw palmetto, Siberian ginseng, and silymarin have been used for the treatment of HIV infection.[15,47,54,100]

TREATMENT

A specific treatment strategy should emphasize identification of the specific herbal preparation(s) used by the patient, concurrent medication(s), and medical illness(es). Because herbal preparation toxicity varies greatly depending on the preparation used, careful examination may be aided by knowledge of the herbal preparation. In most cases, supportive care and discontinuation of the herbal preparation(s) is sufficient. Some herbal toxicities may require specific laboratory analysis and therapy (Table 77–1).

All adverse events associated with herbal preparations should be reported to the local poison control center or to FDA Medwatch by phone at 1–800-FDA-1088 or online at https://www.accessdata.fda.gov/scripts/medwatch/.

SUMMARY

The popularity of herbal preparations is expected to increase for the foreseeable future. Although most herbal users will suffer no ill effects, both herbal users and clinicians should be aware that these preparations are pharmacologically active with the potential for toxicity. They may interact with prescription medications to increase the toxicity of the medication or to decrease its therapeutic effect. Patients with specific medical conditions may have increased risk of toxicity when using herbal preparations.

Herbal users should be aware that these preparations are poorly studied. Scientific proof of efficacy is lacking for many prepara-

TABLE 77–5. Herbal Drug Interactions

Herbal	Drug	Effect
Bitter melon (*Momordica charantia*)	Sulfonylureas	Hypoglycemia
Coenzyme Q	Warfarin	Decreased INR
Danshen (*Salvia miltiorrhiza*)	Warfarin	Increased INR
Devil's Claw	Warfarin	Purpura
Dong Quai	Warfarin	Increased INR
Ephedra	Decongestants, stimulants	Sympathomimetic toxicity
	MAO inhibitors	Potential serotonin syndrome
Evening Primrose Oil	Anticonvulsants	Lower seizure threshold
Feverfew	Aspirin, antiplatelet agents, warfarin	Increased risk of bleeding
Garlic	Aspirin, antiplatelet agents, anticoagulants	Increased risk of bleeding
Ginkgo biloba	Aspirin, antiplatelet agents, anticoagulants	Increased risk of bleeding
Gossypol	Diuretics	Hypokalemia
	Digoxin, quinidine	Potentiates drug toxicity
Hops	Sedative-hypnotic	Potentiates sedation
Kava Kava	Alcohol, sedative-hypnotics	Potentiates sedation
Kelp	Thyroxine	Hyperthyroidism
Kola nut	Caffeine, theophylline	CNS stimulation
Licorice	Diuretics	Hypokalemia
	Digoxin, quinidine	Potentiates drug toxicity
	Corticosteroids	Potentiates effect
Papaya	Warfarin	Increased INR
Psyllium	Lithium	Decreased serum lithium concentration
	Digoxin	Decreased serum digoxin concentration
Shankapulshpi	Phenytoin	Decreases phenytoin level
St. John's wort	P450 (oral contraceptives cyclosporine, indinavir); digoxin	Decreased effectiveness
	MAO inhibitor, SSRI	Potential serotonin syndrome
Tonka beans	Warfarin	Increased INR
Valerian	Alcohol, sedative-hypnotics	Potentiates sedation
Woodruff	Warfarin	Increased INR
Wormwood	Anticonvulsants	Lowers seizure threshold
Yohimbine	MAO inhibitor, SSRI	Possible serotonin syndrome
	Antihypertensives, caffeine decongestants	Hypertension or hypotension

Adapted from Fugh-Berman A: Herb-drug interactions. Lancet 2000; 355: 134–138; and Miller LG: Selected clinical considerations focusing on known or potential drug-herb interactions. Arch Intern Med 1998;158:2200–2211.

tions. In the United States, no standards exist for their manufacture. Many herbal products do not contain the purported amount of the active ingredient. Some herbal products do not contain the correct active ingredient. Many herbal products are adulterated with prescription medications or contain contaminants such as heavy metals.

Many herbal stores are staffed by untrained personnel who may dispense incorrect medical advice and unfounded claims concerning their products.[120] Trained herbalists (eg, Chinese herbal-ists) may dispense traditional remedies with potential for serious toxicity as the result of improper identification of the correct herbal or improper preparation of the herbal product by the herbalist or herbal user.[38] Most herbal users and many herbalists may be unaware of their product's potential for toxicity.

Clinicians should be familiar with herbal preparations and their potential for drug interactions and adverse effects. Every patient history should include questions assessing the concurrent or recent past use of herbal preparations.

REFERENCES

1. Abernethy MK, Becker L: Acute nutmeg intoxications. Am J Emerg Med 1992;10:429–430.
2. Akerele O: Summary of WHO guidelines for the assessment of herbal medicines. HerbalGram 1993;28:13–20.
3. Ali A, Smales O, Aslam M: Surma and lead poisoning. Br Med J 1978;2:915–916.
4. Anderson IB, Mullen WH, Meeker JE, et al: Pennyroyal toxicity: Measurement of toxic metabolite levels in two cases and review of the literature. Ann Intern Med 1996;124:726–734.
5. Annual Industry Overview 1998. Nutrition Business Journal 1998; 3(9):5–6.
6. Arnold WN: Vincent van Gogh and the thujone connection. JAMA 1988;260:3042–3044.
7. Aslam M, Healy MA, Daris SS, et al: Surma and blood lead in children. Lancet 1980;1:568–569.
8. Avorn J, Monane M, Gurwitz JH, et al: Reduction of bacteriuria and pyuria after ingestion of cranberry juice. JAMA 1994;271:751–754.
9. Bakerink JA, Gospe SM, Dimand RJ, et al: Multiple organ failure after ingestion of pennyroyal oil from herbal tea in two patients. Pediatrics 1996;98:944–947.
10. Benner M, Lee H: Anaphylactic reaction of chamomile tea. J Allergy Clin Immunol 1973;52:307–308.
11. Bensoussan A, Talley NJ, Hing M, et al: Treatment of irritable bowel syndrome with Chinese herbal medicine: A randomized controlled trial. JAMA 1998;280:1585–1589
12. Bhatt BD, Zuckerman MJ, Foland JA, et al: Rattlesnake meat ingestion—A common Hispanic folk remedy. West J Med 1988; 149:605.
13. Blue cohosh. Review of Natural Products. Levittown, PA, Pharmaceutical Information Associates, May 1985.
14. Bose A, Vashishta K, O'Loughlin BJ: Azarcon por emphacho—Another cause of lead toxicity. Pediatrics 1983;72:106–110.
15. Braun JF, Powderly WG, Steinberg CL, et al: A guide to underground AIDS therapies. Patient Care 1993;27:53–70.
16. Breevoort P: The booming US botanical market: A new overview. HerbalGram 1998;44:33–56.
17. Brubacher JR, Ravikumar PR, Bania T, et al: Treatment of toad venom poisoning with digoxin-specific Fab fragments. Chest 1996; 110:1282–1288.
18. Buechel DW, Haverlah, VC, Gardner ME: Pennyroyal oil ingestion: report of a case. J Am Osteopath Assoc 1983;82:793–794.
19. But PP, Tai YT, Young K: Three fatal cases of herbal aconite poisoning. Vet Hum Toxicol 1994;34:212–215.
20. Casterline C: Allergy to chamomile teas. JAMA 1980;244:330–331.
21. CDC: Adverse events associated with ephedrine-containing products—Texas. Morb Mortal Wkly Rep 1996;45:689–693.
22. CDC: Anticholinergic poisoning associated with an herbal tea—New York City. Morb Mortal Wkly Rep 1995;44:193–195.
23. CDC: Chaparral-induced toxic hepatitis—California and Texas. Morb Mortal Wkly Rep 1992;41:812–814.
24. CDC: Deaths associated with a purported aphrodisiac—New York City. Morb Mortal Wkly Rep 1995;44:853–861.

25. CDC: Folk remedy-associated lead poisoning in Hmong children. MMWR Morb Mortal Wkly Rep 1983;32:555–556. also JAMA 1983;250;3149–3150.

26. CDC: Jin Bu Huan Toxicity in adults—Los Angeles. MMWR Morb Mortal Wkly Rep 1993;42:920–922.

27. CDC: Jin Bu Huan Toxicity in children—Colorado. MMWR Morb Mortal Wkly Rep 1993;42:633–636.

28. CDC: Lead poisoning associated death from Asian Indian folk remedies—Florida. Morb Mortal Wkly Rep 1984;33:638–645.

29. CDC: Lead poisoning associated with traditional ethnic remedies—California, 1991–1992. Morb Mortal Wkly Rep 1993;42: 521–524

30. CDC: Lead poisoning from lead tetroxide used as a folk remedy—Colorado. MMWR Morb Mortal Wkly Rep 1982;30:647–648.

31. CDC: Lead poisoning from Mexican folk remedies-California. MMWR Morb Mortal Wkly Rep 1983;32:554. also JAMA 1983; 250:3149.

32. CDC: Self-treatment with herbal and other plant-derived remedies—Rural Mississippi, 1993. Morb Mortal Wkly Rep 1995; 44: 204–207.

33. CDC: Use of lead tetroxide as a folk remedy for gastrointestinal illness. MMWR Morb Mortal Wkly Rep 1981;30:546–547.

34. Chan JCN, Chan TYK, Chan KL, et al: Anticholinergic poisoning from Chinese herbal medicines [letter]. Aust N Z J Med 1994; 24:317.

35. Chan TYK: Aconitine poisoning: A global perspective. Vet Hum Toxicol 1994;36:326–328.

36. Chan TYK, Chan AYW, Critchley JAJH: Hospital admissions due to adverse reactions to Chinese herbal medicines. J Trop Med Hyg 1992;95:296–298.

37. Chan TYK, Chan JCN, Tomlinson B, et al: Chinese herbal medicines revisited: A Hong Kong perspective. Lancet 1993;342–1532–1534.

38. Chan TYK, Critchley JAJH: Usage and adverse effects of Chinese herbal medicines. Hum Exp Toxicol 1996;15:5–12.

39. Chan TYK, Tomlinson B, Chan WWM, et al: A case of acute aconitine poisoning caused by chuanwu and caowu. J Trop Med Hyg 1993;96:62–63.

40. Chan TYK, Tse LKK, Chan JCN, et al: Aconitine poisoning due to Chinese herbal medcines: A review. Vet Hum Toxicol 1994;36: 452–455.

41. Chevalier A: The Encyclopedia of Medicinal Plants. New York, DK Publishing, 1996.

42. Chinese cucumber. Review of Natural Products. Levittown, PA, Pharmaceutical Information Associates, April 1990.

43. Combie J, Nugent TE, Tobin T: Inability of goldenseal to interfere with the detection of morphine in urine. Equine Veterinary Science, Jan/Feb 1982, pp. 16–21.

44. Cone LA, Boughton WH, Cone LA, et al: Rattlesnake capsule-induced Salmonella arizonae bacteremia. West J Med 1990;153; 315–316.

45. Cook C, Baisden D: Ancillary use of folk medicine by patients in primary care clinics in southwestern West Virginia. South Med J 1986;79:1098–1101.

46. Cowley G: "Herbal Warning." Newsweek, May 6, 1996, pp. 60–65.

47. Critical path AIDS project. AIDS alternative treatment. http://www. critpath.org/alt.htm.

48. D'Arcy PF: Adverse reactions and interactions with herbal medicines. Adverse Drug React Toxicol Rev 1991;10:189–208.

49. Danesi MA, Adetunji JB: Use of alternative medicine by patients with epilepsy: A survey of 265 epileptic patients in a developing country. Epilepsia 1994;35:344–351.

50. Der Marderosian A: Promising practices in the use of medicinal plants in the United States. In: Tomlinson TR, Akerele O, eds: Medicinal Plants, Their Role in Health and Biodiversity. Philadelphia, PA, University of Pennsylvania Press, 1998, pp. 177–190.

51. DeSmet PA: Health risks of herbal remedies. Drug Saf 1995;13: 81–93.

52. DeSmet PA: Toxicological Outlook on the Quality Assurance of Herbal Remedies. Adverse Effects Herb Drugs 1992;1:1–72.

53. Diamond JR, Pallone PL: Acute interstitial nephritis following use of Tung Shueh pills. Am J Kidney Dis 1994;24:219–221.

54. Direct AIDS Alternative Information Resources: Buyer's Club Product Catalog, February 2000.

55. Dolan G. Blumsohn A: Lead poisoning due to Asian ethnic treatment for impotence. J R Soc Med 1991;84:630–631.

56. Duke JA: CRC Handbook of Medicinal Herbs. Boca Raton, FL, CRC Press, 1985.

57. Eisenberg DM, Kessler RC, Foster C, et al: Unconventional medicine in the United States. N Engl J Med 1993;328:246–252.

58. Eisenberg DM, Davis RB, Ettner SL: Trends in alternative medicine use in the United States, 1990–1997: Results of a follow-up national survey. JAMA 1998;280:1569–1575.

59. Ernst E: Second thoughts about safety of St. John's wort. Lancet 1999;354:2014–2016.

60. Espinoza EO, Mann MJ, Bleasdell B: Arsenic and mercury in traditional Chinese herbal balls [letter]. N Engl J Med 1995;333: 803–804.

61. Fitzpatrick AJ, Crawford M, Allan RM, et al: Aconite poisoning managed with a ventricular assist device. Anaesth Intensive Care 1994;22:714–717.

62. Food and Drug Administration: Federal Register. Part II 21 CFR Part 101. Food labeling; Final rule and proposed rules. December 28, 1995.

63. Foster S: Goldenseal: Masking of drug tests. HerbalGram 1989;21: 7–8.

64. Fung MC, Weinbraub M, Bowen DL: Colloidal silver proteins marketed as health supplements [letter]. JAMA 1995;274:1196–1197.

65. Fugh-Berman: Herb-drug interactions. Lancet 2000;355:134–138.

66. Garlic. Review of Natural Products. Levittown, PA, Pharmaceutical Information Associates, Apr. 1994.

67. Ginseng. Review of Natural Products. Levittown, PA, Pharmaceutical Information Associates, Sept. 1990.

68. Goldenseal. Review of Natural Products. Levittown, PA, Pharmaceutical Information Associates, May 1994.

69. Gordon DW, Rosenthal G, Hart, J, et al: Chaparral ingestion. JAMA 1995;273:489–490.

70. Grimm W. Muller HH: A randomized controlled trial of the effect of fluid extract of *Echinacea purpurea* on the incidence and severity of colds and respiratory infections. Am J Med 1999;106:138–143.

71. HerbWorld News Online. US herbal market nearing saturation. September 29, 1999. http://www.herbs.org/current/herbsaturation.html.

72. Hill GJ: Lead poisoning due to Hai Ge Fen. JAMA 1995;273:24–25.

73. Honerjager P and Meissner A: The positive inotropic effect of aconitine. Arch Pharmacol 1983;322:49–58.

74. Hsu CK, Leo P, Shastry D, et al: Anticholinergic poisoning associated with herbal tea. Arch Intern Med 1995;155:2245–2248.

75. Hung OL, Shih RD, Chiang WK, et al: Herbal preparation usage among urban emergency department patients. Acad Emerg Med 1997;4:209–213.

76. Huxtable RJ: Herbal teas and toxins: novel aspects of pyrrolizidine poisoning in the United States. Perspect Biol Med 1980;24:1–14.

77. Huxtable RJ: The harmful potential of herbal and other plant products. Drug Saf 1990;5(Suppl 1):126–136.

78. Insel PA: Analgesic-antipyretic and antiinflammatory agents and drugs employed in the treatment of gout. In: Hardman JG, Limbird LE, eds: Goodman and Gilman's The Pharmacological Basis of Therapeutics, 9th ed. New York, McGraw-Hill, 1996;617

79. Joubert PH: Poisoning admissions in black South Africans. J Toxicol Clin Toxicol 1990]28:85–94.

80. Kang-Yum E, Oransky SH: Chinese patent medicine as a potential source of mercury poisoning. Vet Hum Toxicol 1992;34:235–238.

81. Kassler WJ, Blanc P, Greenblatt R: The use of medicinal herbs by human immunodeficiency virus-infected patients. Arch Intern Med 1991;151:2281–2288.

82. Kestin M, Miller L, Littlejohn G, et al: The use of medicinal herbs by human immunodeficiency virus-infected patients. Arch Intern Med 1991;151:2281–2288.

83. Ko RJ: Adulterants in Asian patent medicines. N Engl J Med 1998;339:847.

84. Ko RJ, Greenwald MS, Loscutoff SM, et al: Lethal ingestion of Chinese herbal tea containing Ch'an Su. West J Med 1996;164:71–75.

85. Kumana CR, Ng M, Lin HJ, et al: Herbal tea induced hepatic veno-occlusive disease: Quantification of toxic alkaloid in adults Gut 1985;26: 101–104.

86. Lam CL, Catarivas MG, Munro C, et al: Self-medication among Hong Kong Chinese. Soc Sci Med 1994;39:1641–1647.

87. Larrey D, Pageaux GP: Hepatotoxicity of herbal remedies and mushrooms. Semin Liver Dis 1995;15:183–188.

88. Larrey D, Vial T, Pauwels A, et al: Hepatitis after germander (*Teucrium chamaedrys*) administration: Another instance of herbal medicine hepatotoxicity. Ann Intern Med 1992;117:129–132.

89. LeBars PL, Katz MM, Berman N, et al: A placebo-controlled, double-blind, randomized trial for an extract of *Ginkgo biloba* for dementia. JAMA 1997;278:1327–1332.

90. LeGrand A, Sri-Ngernyuang L, Streefland PH: Enhancing appropriate drug use: The contribution of herbal medicine promotion. Soc Sci Med 1993;36:1023–1035.

91. Lewis W: Ginseng revisited. N Engl J Med 1980;243:31.

92. Lewis WH, Smith P: Poke root herbal tea poisoning. JAMA 1979;242:2759–2760.

93. Liberti LE and DerMarderosian A: Evaluation of commercial ginseng products. J Pharm Sci 1978;67:1487–1489.

94. Linde K, Ramirez G, Mulrow CD, et al: St. John's wort for depression—An overview and meta-analysis of randomised clinical trials. BMJ 1996;313:253–258.

95. Louman W, Danouske MD: The use of khat (Catha edulis) in Yemen social and medical observations. Ann Intern Med 1976;85:246–249.

96. Markowitz SB, Nunez CM, Klitzman S, et al: Lead poisoning due to Hai Ge Fen. The porphyric content of individual erythrocytes. JAMA 1994;271:932–934.

97. Marsh WW, Hentges K: Mexican folk remedies and conventional medical care. Am Fam Physician 1988;37:257–262.

98. Marwick C: New center director state complementary agenda. JAMA 2000;293:990–991.

99. McAlindon TE, LaValley MP, Gulin JP, et al: Glucosamine and chondroitin for treatment of osteoarthritis: A systematic quality assessment and meta-analysis. JAMA 2000;283:1469–1475.

100. McKnight I, Scott M: HIV and complementary medicine. Med J Aust 1996;165:143–145.

101. Michie CA: The use of herbal remedies in Jamaica. Ann Trop Paediatr 1992;12:31–36.

102. Miller LG: Herbal medicinals: Selected clinical considerations focusing on known or potential drug-herb interactions. Arch Intern Med 2000;158:2200–2211.

103. Minor JR: Ginseng: Fact or fiction. Hosp Form 1979;186–192.

104. Mohabbat O, Younos MS, Merzad AA, et al: An outbreak of hepatic veno-occlusive disease in northwestern Afghanistan. Lancet 1976;2:269–271.

105. National Center for Complementary and Alternative Medicine: Major domains of complementary and alternative medicine. June 1, 2000. http://nccam.nih.gov/nccam/fcp/classify/.

106. Nebelkopf E: Herbal therapy in the treatment of drug use. Int J Addict 1987;22:695–717.

107. Nelson L, Shih R, Hoffman R: Aplastic anemia-induced by an adulterated herbal preparation. J Toxicol Clin Toxicol 1995;33:467–470.

108. Nortier JL, Martinez MCM, Schmeiser HH, et al: Urothelial carcinoma associated with the use of a Chinese herb (Aristolochia fangchi). N Engl J Med 2000;342:1686–1692.

109. Norton SA: Betel: consumption and consequences. J Am Acad Dermatol 1998;38:81–88.

110. Noskin GA, Clarke JT: Salmonella arizonae bacteremia as the presenting manifestation of human immunodeficiency virus infection following rattlesnake meat ingestion. Rev Infect Dis 1990;12:514–517.

111. Nutmeg. The Review of Natural Products. Levittown, PA, Pharmaceutical Information Associates, September 1987.

112. O'Hara MA, Kiefer D, Farrell K, et al: A review of 12 commonly used medicinal herbs. Arch Fam Med 1998;7:523–536.

113. Olsen P, Thorup I: Neurotoxicity in rats dosed with peppermint oil and pulegone. Arch Toxicol (Suppl) 1984;7:408–409.

114. Ostrenga UJ, Perry D: Goldenseal. PharmChem Newsletter 4 (January 1975).

115. Palmer ME, Haller C, McKinney P, et al: Adverse events from botanical and other dietary supplements. Acad Emerg Med 2000;7:499.

116. Panayotopoulos DJ, Chisholm DD: Hallucinogenic effect of nutmeg. Br Med J 1970;698:754.

117. Parsons JS: Contaminated herbal tea as a potential source of chronic arsenic poisoning. NCMJ 1981;42:38–39.

118. Pearl WS, Leo P, Tseng WO: Use of Chinese therapies among Chinese patients seeking emergency department care. Ann Emerg Med 1995;26:735–738.

119. Perharic L, Shaw D, Colbridge M, et al: Toxicological problems resulting from exposure to traditional remedies and food supplements. Drug Saf 1994;11:285–294.

120. Phillips LG, Nichols MH, King WD: Herbs and HIV: The health food industry's answer. South Med J 1995;88:911–913.

121. Pillans PI: Toxicity of herbal products. N Z Med J 1995;108:469–471.

122. Piscitelli SC, Burstein AH, Chaitt D, et al: Indinavir concentrations and St. John's wort. Lancet 2000;355:547–548.

123. Pontifex AH, Gary AK: Lead poisoning from an Asian Indian folk remedy. Can Med Assoc J 1985;133:1227–1228.

124. Prpic-Majic D, Pizent A, Jurasovic J, et al: Lead poisoning associated with the use of Ayurvedic meta-mineral tonics. J Toxicol Clin Toxicol 1996;34:417–423.

125. Reisine T, Pasternak G: Opioid analgesics and antagonists. In: Hardman JG, Limbird E, eds: Goodman and Gilmans' The Pharmacological Basis of Therapeutics, 9th ed. New York, McGraw-Hill, 1996; 521–555.

126. Ridker PM, Ohk'uma S, McDermott WV, et al: Hepatic veno-occlusive disease associated with the consumption of pyrrolizidine-containing dietary supplements. Gastroenterology 1985;88:1050–1054.

127. Ridker PM: Toxic effects of herbal teas. Arch Environ Health 1987;42:133–136.

128. Ries CA, Sahud MA: Agranulocytosis caused by Chinese herbal medicines. JAMA 1975;231:352–355.

129. Riley KB, Antoniskis D, Maris R, et al: Rattlesnake capsule-associated Salmonella arizonae infections. Arch Intern Med 1988;148:1207–1210.

130. Saint John's Wort. Review of Natural Products. Levittown, PA, Pharmaceutical Information Associates, Jan 1995.

131. Saryan LA: Surreptitious lead exposure from an Asian Indian medication. J Anal Toxicol 1991;15:336–338.

132. Segelman AB, Segelman FP, Karliner J, et al: Sassafras and herb tea: Potential health hazards. JAMA 1976;236:477.

133. Siegel RK: Ginseng abuse syndrome. JAMA 1979;241:1614–1615.

134. Siegel RK: Herbal intoxication: Psychoactive effects from herbal cigarettes, tea, and capsules. JAMA 1976;236:473–476.

135. Snodgrass G, Ziderman D, Gulati V, et al: Cosmetic plumbism. Br Med J 1973;27:230.

136. Snow LG: Folk medical beliefs and their implications for care of patients: A review based on studies among black patients. Ann Intern Med 1974;81:82–96.

137. Solecki RS: Shanidar IV, a Neanderthal flower burial of northern Iraq. Science 1975;190:880.

138. Spoerke DG: Herbal medication: Use and misuse. Hosp Form 1980; 941–951.

139. Sullivan JB, Rumack BH, Thomas H, et al: Pennyroyal oil poisoning and hepatotoxicity. JAMA 1979;242:2873–2874.

140. Tai YT, But PP-H, Young K, et al: Cardiotoxicity after accidental herb-induced aconite poisoning. Lancet 1992;340:1254–1256.

141. Tandon BN, Handon HD, Tandon RK, et al: An epidemic of veno-occlusive disease of liver in central India. Lancet 1976;2:271–272.

142. Taylor RFH, Al-Jarad N, John LME, et al: Betel nut chewing and asthma. Lancet 1992;330:1134–1136.

143. The Ephedras. Review of Natural Products. Levittown, PA, Pharmaceutical Information Associates, Nov 1995.

144. US Food and Drug Administration: The Special Nutritionals Adverse Event Monitoring System. October 20,1998. http://vm.cfsan.fda.gov/~dms/aemsfull.html.

145. US Food and Drug Administration: FDA Guide to Dietary Supplements. January 1999. http://vm.cfsan.fda.gov/~dms/fdsupp.html.

146. Vanhaelen M, Vanhaelen-Fastre R, But P, et al: Identification of aristolochic acid in Chinese herbs [letter]. Lancet 1994;343:174.

147. Vanherweghem JL, Depierreux M, Tielemans C, et al: Rapidly progressive interstitial renal fibrosis in young woman: Association with slimming regimen including Chinese herbs. Lancet 1993;341: 387–391.

148. Verhoef MJ, Sutherland LR, Brkich L: Use of alternative medicine by patients attending a gastroenterology clinic. CMAJ 1990;142: 121–125.

149. Waterman SH, Juarez G, Carr SJ, et al: *Salmonella arizonae* infections in Latinos associated with rattlesnake folk medicine. Am J Public Health 1990;80:286–289.

150. Weisbord SD, Soule JB, Kimmel PL: Brief report: Poison online—Acute renal failure caused by oil of wormwood purchased through the Internet. N Engl J Med 1997;337:825–827.

151. Weiss G: Hallucinogenic and narcotic-like effects of powdered myristica (nutmeg). Psychiatr Q 1960;34:346–356.

152. Wilt TJ, Ishani A, Stark G: Saw palmetto extracts for treatment of benign prostatic hyperplasia. JAMA 1998;280:1604–1609.

153. Woolf GM, Petrovic JM, Rojter SE: Acute hepatitis associated with the Chinese herbal product Jin Bu Huan. Ann Intern Med 1994; 121:729–735.

154. Wormwood. Review of Natural Products. Levittown, PA, Pharmaceutical Information Associates, Apr 1991.

155. Chevalier A: The Encyclopedia of Medicinal Plants. New York, DK Publishing, 1996.

156. Foster S, Tyler VE: Tyler's Honest Herbal: A Sensible Guide to the Use of Herbs and Related Remedies, 4th ed. New York, Haworth Press, 1999.

157. The Review of Natural Products monograph system (ISSN 0734–4961). Levittown, PA, Pharmaceutical Information Associates.

158. Lewis WH, Elvin-Lewis MP: Medical Botany: Plant Affecting Man's Health. New York, Wiley, 1977.

159. Robbers, JE, Speedie MK, and Tyler VE: Pharmacognosy and Pharmacobiotechnology. Philadelphia, Williams and Wilkins, 1996.

160. Robbers JE, Tyler VE: Tyler's Herbs of Choice: The Therapeutic Use of Phytomedicinals, 2nd ed. New York, Haworth Press, 1999.

CHAPTER 78 PLANTS

Mary Palmer / Joseph M. Betz

Quick Index: Plants That May Be Life-Threatening in Single Ingestion and the Organ System Affected

Common Name (Scientific Name)	Organ System Affected				Page
	Cardiac	Neurologic	GI/Hepatic**	Other	
Ackee (*Blighia sapida*)		Seizures, encephalopathy	Vomiting	Hypoglycemia, acidemia	1166
Aconitum, monkshood, and larkspur (*Aconitum* or *Delphinium spp.*)	Bradycardia, dysrhythmias	Paresthesias, mental status change	Nausea, vomiting		1169
Autumn crocus (*Colchicum autumnale*)			Gastroenteritis	Antimitotic, multi-system failure	1171
Apricot seed kernels (*Prunus armeniaca*) and pits from seeds of other members of *Prunus* genus such as plum, pear, cherry, almond, and peach, as well as apple (*Malus spp.*)	Tachycardia	Coma	Nausea, vomiting	Multisystem failure, lactic acidemia	1162
Azalea, mountain laurel, and rhododendron* (*Azalea, Kalmia,* and *Rhododendron spp.*)	Bradycardia, dysrhythmias	Paresthesias, mental status change	Nausea, vomiting	Concentrated in honey	1171
Buckthorn, coyatillo, and tullidora (*Karwinskia humboldtiana*)		Ascending motor neuropathy like Guillan-Barré		Respiratory failure	1167
Blue green algae or Cyanobacteria		Paresthesias, paralysis possible	Hepatic failure	Cholinergic signs, neuropathy	1166
Castor beans (*Ricinus communis*), (*Jatropha curcas*); rosary pea (*Abrus precatorius*), Chinese cucumber (*Trichosanthes spp.*), and other lectins			Gastroenteritis	Multisystem failure associated with volume loss	1165
Climbing or bittersweet nightshade* (*Solanum dulcamara*)	Tachycardia	Hallucinations, agitation	Diminished GI motility		1159
False hellebore, others (*Veratrum viride, spp.*); *Zigadenus* and *Amianthium spp.*	Bradycardia, dysrhythmias		Nausea, vomiting		1170
Foxglove (*Digitalis spp.*); strophanthus (*Strophanthus spp.*), squills (*Urginea spp.*) and other cardiac glycosides	Bradycardia, dysrhythmias		Nausea, vomiting	Hyperkalemia	1162
Jimsonweed, (*Datura stramonium*); belladonna (*Atropa belladonna*), European or true mandrake (*Mandragora officinarium*), henbane, and hyoscyamus (*Hyoscyamus niger*)	Tachycardia	Hallucinations, agitation	Diminished GI motility	Anticholinergic toxicity	1158
May apple (*Podophyllum peltatum*)		Encephalopathy	Nausea, vomiting	Antimitotic, multisystem failure	1171
Oleander* and yellow oleander (*Nerium* and *Thevetia spp.*) and other cardiac glycosides	Bradycardia, dysrhythmias		Nausea, vomiting		1162
Poison hemlock (*Conium maculatum*)	Bradycardia, tachycardia (biphasic dose response)	Ascending paralysis	Nausea, vomiting	Nicotinic toxicity, rhabdomyolysis, renal failure	1159
Pokeweed, American pokeweed* (*Phytolacca americana*)			Severe gastroenteritis		1162
Yew* (*Taxus spp.*)	Bradycardia, dysrhythmias		Nausea, vomiting		1170
Water hemlock (*Cicuta maculata*)		Seizures	Nausea, vomiting, diarrhea	Cholinergic toxicity, rhabdomyolysis, renal failure	1168

*Denotes plants both commonly reported (Table 78–2) and potentially life-threatening.
**Any plant ingestion may produce nonspecific gastrointestinal distress.

A 25-year-old male was found unconscious with a sustained ventricular tachycardia. He was found with a printout from a Web page describing the use of *Aconitum spp.* (monkshood) from horticultural sources as a means of committing suicide. His vital signs were blood pressure, 60/palpable mm Hg; pulse, 120–170 beats/min; respiratory rate, 22 breaths/min; temperature 99° F (37.3° C); and 100% oxygen saturation on pulse oximetry breathing 28% oxygen. His dysrhythmia was responsive to sodium bicarbonate and 100 mg lidocaine IV bolus followed by a 2-mg/min infusion. His cocaine, amphetamine, salicylate, and acetaminophen screens were negative. Upon awakening, he would not describe what he had done. Although both urine and serum specimens were obtained, local public health and medical examiner laboratories, as well as three commercial natural product laboratories, were unable to analyze these specimens for aconitine, the active ingredient probably responsible for his symptoms.

HISTORY AND CURRENT TASK OF PLANT TOXICOLOGY

Some plants produce powerful toxins, most of which are discussed below. Aconitine, from monkshood, exemplifies the rich history of plant toxicology because it was believed by the Greeks to be the first poison—"lycotonum"—created by the goddess Hecate from foam of the river Cerebrus.[18] Plant toxicology did not become an organized discipline in the United States until 1894, when the US Department of Agriculture responded to concern over significant livestock losses from plant poisonings.[428] Since that time, poison control centers in the United States, Europe, and elsewhere have emerged as primary managers and reporters of plant poisonings in humans.

The difficult task at this point in the history of human plant toxicology is delineation of hazard versus risk for plant exposures. Hazard is defined as the set of circumstances in which the user comes to harm, while risk is the probability that harm will result from a hazard (examples, Chap. 120).[475] Increasingly, evaluations of risk are being based on poison center data and usually cite the numerous calls without consequence as a part of the risk equation (Chap. 116).[234–239,294,430] While these "evidence-based" studies may to some extent free us from wasteful overreaction and overspending on negligible risks, it is important to remember that poison center data are dominated by pediatric cases and other unsubstantiated cases (Chap. 116)[170]. These cases often represent small or nonexistent exposures, and their inclusion in the database may mask real risks by diluting "true" hazardous exposures with trivial or nonexistent exposures. Risk is also affected by likelihood of encountering a hazardous plant. For instance, if a highly hazardous plant is encountered rarely, the risk may be assessed as low as a less hazardous plant encountered and reported more frequently. Equally troublesome, risks from a particular plant may be overstated by misidentification of the plant or by poor documentation and followup. Chemically, plants are exceedingly complex, and factors such as seasonal variability, geography, plant part, local environmental stresses, and methods of processing can affect the potential for harm. All of these factors must be weighed when considering human/plant interactions to decide whether any given plant exposure warrants alarm or reassurance.

CLASSIFICATION OF PLANT TOXINS AND THE APPROACH TO THE POISONED PATIENT

The science of pharmacognosy traditionally defines active constituents according to the class of organic molecules to which they belong. The toxicology of plants is defined by such an approach herein (Table 78–1) because it offers understanding of plant toxicology by chemical constituents and their attendant mechanisms (when understood), which may or may not be taxonomically faithful.

Such classification varies depending on the pharmacognosist, and the "science" is understandably vague because differentiation of chemical class is not simple. For instance, cardiac glycosides are actually "steroidal glycosides" and could be equally well classified with steroids as with glycosides, while kava lactones such as kawain, yangonin, and methysticin are mono- or diunsaturated α-pyrones, as well as members of the enormous group of plant phenols. The approach employed in this chapter borrows primarily from two groups of authors.[109,344]

From the standpoint of plant evolution, various toxins are presumably selected because the plants that contain them are relatively protected from predation. Some toxins are narrowly distributed within taxa, while others jump taxonomic lines between species, genera, families, and orders. For instance, belladonna alkaloids are restricted to the Solanaceae family. On the other hand, pyrrolizidine alkaloids are found in a number of families and phylogenetic groups,[254] suggesting either that these groups underwent convergent evolution, or that the morphologic basis of taxonomy awaits integration with chemotaxonomy and the techniques of molecular biology.

From the point of view of the toxicologist, the taxonomic context of the toxin is important because rapid identification of the plant can be helpful to management and disposition decisions, especially in symptomatic patients. Communication with an expert botanist or poison center is highly recommended. In general, building a crude knowledge of the families can help exclude the few severely life-threatening plants. For instance, if the flower does not have a flat top that looks like a carrot or dill flower, it is probably not in the Umbelliferae family and unlikely to be a hemlock; if the flower does not look like a shooting star like those belonging to potato or tomato plants, it is unlikely to be in the Solanaceae family and unlikely to produce anticholinergic toxicity.

In addition, by simply comparing the plant in question with pictures or descriptions from a field guide of flora, it is possible to exclude its identity as one of the life-threatening or concerning plants listed in the quick index. Photographs of poisonous plants are available on the World Wide Web and in books.[132] Faxing a photocopy or transmitting a digital image of the suspect plant to an expert is a more specific tool that can help in a timely manner.[274] Several computer database systems have been developed to help with plant identification;[73,425,427] if an herbarium is easily accessible, the plant can be compared to voucher specimens of plants known to produce toxicity.[458,460] Furthermore, if a plant identification is made but the toxicity of the plant cannot be readily established by consultation with standard reference works, the PLANTOX database (http://vm.cfsan.fda.gov/~djw/readme.html) managed by the Food and Drug Administration contains more

TABLE 78–1. Active Ingredients Classified Using a Pharmacognosy Approach with Examples and Selected Symptoms

Alkaloid	Plant Sources	Common Name	Family	Symptoms/Notes
Aconitine and related compounds	*Aconitum napelius* and other *Aconitum spp.*	Monkshood and others	Ranunculaceae (buttercup)	Sodium channel opener, cardiac and neurologic toxicity
Anagyrine	*Lupinus latifolius* and other *Lupinus spp.*	Lupin	Fabaceae	Nicotinic effects; teratogenic
Arecoline	*Areca catechu*	Betel	Aracaceae	Buccal carcinoma; cholinergic effects
Belladonna alkaloids: atropine, hyoscyamine, scopolamine	*Atropa belladonna, Mandragora officinarium, Datura stramonium, Hyoscyamus niger*	Belladonna; European or true mandrake, stramonium, locoweed, Jimson weed; henbane, hyoscyamus	Solanceae	Anticholinergic effects
Berberine	*Hydrastis canadensis, Mahonia spp., Derberis spp., Coptis spp.,* and others	Goldenseal, Oregon grape, barberry, goldthread, others	Ranunculaceae	High-dose cardiac depression and uterine stimulation in animals
Caffeine	*Coffee arabica, Camellia sinensis, Cola nitida,* and other *Cola spp; Paullinia cupana; Ilex paraguariensis*	Coffee, tea, kola nut, guarana, maté, yerba maté or Paraguay tea	Rubiaceae, Theaceae, Sterculiaceae, Sapindaceae, Aquifoliaceae	CNS stimulation
Cathinone	*Catha edulis*	Khat	Celastaceae	CNS stimulant
Cocaine	*Erythroxylon coca*	Coca	Erythroxylaceae	CNS stimulation
Colchicine	*Colchicum autumnale, Gloriosa superba,* others	Autumn crocus, meadow saffron, others	Liliaceae	Antimitotic with multiorgan system toxicity
Coniine	*Conium maculatum*	Poison hemlock	Umbelliferae (Apiaceae)	Nicotinic effects
Cytisine	*Laburnum anagyroides* (syn. *Cytisus laburnum*)	Golden chain, laburnum	Fabaceae	Nicotinic effects
Emetine/cephaline	*Cephaelis ipecacuanha, C. acuminata*	Ipecac	Rubiaceae	Emesis and cardiotoxicity
Ephedrine and related compounds	*Ephedra spp.,* especially *sinensis, Sida cordafolia*	Ephedra, ma huang	Ephedraceae/Gnetaceae= gymnosperm	CNS stimulant
Ergotamine and related compounds	*Claviceps purpurea, C. paspali*	Ergot	Claviciptaceae	Vasospastic, oxytocic; fungus infesting certain pasture grasses (livestock) and rye (*Secale cereale*)
Hydrastine	*Hydrastis canadensis*	Goldenseal	Ranunculaceae	Strychninelike movement disorders in high dose
Lobeline	*Lobelia inflata*	Indian tobacco	Campanulaceae	Nicotinic effects
Lysergic acid	*Ipomoea tricolor* and other *Ipomoea spp., Argyreia spp.*	Morning glory	Convolvulaceae	Hallucinogenic
Lycorine, homolycorine	*Narcissus spp.* and other Amaryllidaceae	Narcissus	Liliaceae (Amarilladaceae)	Mechanical trauma with calcium oxalate raphides that introduce cytotoxic lycorine
Mescaline	*Lophophora williamsii*	Peyote or mescal buttons	Cactaceae	Hallucinogenic
Methylaconitine and related compounds	*Delphinium spp.*	Larkspur and others	Ranunculaceae (buttercup)	Sodium channel opener, cardiac and neurologic toxicity
n-Methylcytisine and related compounds	*Caulophyllum thalictroides*	Blue cohosh	Berberidaceae	Nicotinic effects
Morphine/other opium derivatives	*Papaver somniferum*	Poppy with opium derivatives	Papaveraceae	CNS sedative
Nicotine	*Nicotiana tabacum* and other *Nicotiana spp.*	Tobacco	Solanceae	Nicotinic effects
Physostigmine	*Physostigma venenosum*	Calabar bean, ordeal bean	Fabaceae	Cholinergic effects (cholinesterase inhibitor)
Pilocarpine	*Pilocarpus jaborandi, P. pinnatifolius*	Jaborandi	Rutaceae	Muscarinic agonist
Pyrrolizidine alkaloids like symphytine, lycopsamine, senecionine and ridelliine	*Symphytum spp., Borago officinalis, Heliotropium spp.; Senecio spp., Tussilago farfara, Crotalaria spp.*	Comfrey, borage, ragwort; groundsel, coltsfoot; rattlebox	Boraginaceae, Compositae, Fabaceae	Hepatotoxicity

(continued)

TABLE 78–1. **Active Ingredients Classified Using a Pharmacognosy Approach with Examples and Selected Symptoms (continued)**

Alkaloid	Plant Sources	Common Name	Family	Symptoms/Notes
Quinine	*Cinchona* spp., *Remijia pedunculata*	Cinchona, Cuprea bark	Rubiaceae	Cinchonism; cardiac dysrhythmias
Reserpine	*Rauwolfia serpentina*	Rauwolfia, snakeroot	Apocynaceae	CNS and cardiac depression
Sanguinarine	*Sanguinaria canadensis, Argemone mexicana*	Sanguinaria, bloodroot, Mexican pricklepoppy	Papaveraceae	Multiple systems including carditis
Solanine, chaconine	*Solanum americanum, S. nigrum, S. dulcamara, S. carolinense, S. tuberosum, Lycopersicon esculentum*	Nightshade, black nightshade, deadly nightshade, horse nettle, potato, bittersweet, tomato, woody nightshade	Solanaceae	Hemolytic, cytotoxic
Sparteine	*Cytisus scoparius*	Broom, Scotch broom	Fabaceae	Nicotinic effects; oxytocic
Strychnine and brucine	*Strychnos nux-vomica, S. ignatii*	Nux vomica, Ignatia, St. Ignatius bean, vomit button	Loganiaceae	Movement disorders; tetany; convulsions
Swainsonine	*Astragulus* spp., *Swainsonia* spp., *Oxytropis* spp., *Hedysarium alpinum*	Locoweed, *Hedysarium alpinum*=wild potato	Fabaceae	Lysosomal storage disorder
Synephrine	*Citrus aurantium*	Bitter orange	Rutaceae	CNS stimulant
Taxine	*Taxus baccata, Taxus brevifolia*, other *Taxus* spp.	English yew, Pacific yew, yew	Taxaceae	Sodium channel blocker; cardiac and neurologic toxicity
Theobromine	*Theobroma cacao*	Cocoa	Sterculiaceae	CNS stimulant
Theophylline	*Camellia sinensis*	Tea, green tea	Theaceae	CNS stimulant
Tubocurarine	*Chondrodendron* spp., *Curarea* spp., *Strychnos* spp.	Tubocurare, curare	Menispermaceae, Loganaceae	"Curare"=crude extract containing quaternary compounds and alkaloids; paralytic
Veratridine	*Veratrum viride, V. album, V. californicum*	False, green, European, and California hellebore	Liliaceae	Sodium channel opening
Vincristine	*Catharanthus roseus* (formerly *Vinca rosea*)	Vinca, Madagascar periwinkle	Apocynaceae	Antimitotic effects; binds tubules
Yohimbine	*Pausinystalia yohimbe, Corynanthe yohimbe*	Yohimbe	Rubiaceae	α_2-Adrenergic receptor stimulation, cholinergic (bronchospastic) effects
Glycosides ***Cardiac glycosides (CGs)***				
Asclepin and related cardenolides	*Cryptostegia grandifolia; Ascliepias* spp.; *Caloltropis* spp.	Pink allamanda, rubber vine, milk weed, crown flower	Asclepidaceae	Cardiac dysrhythmias
Adonitoxin	*Adonis vernalis*	Pheasant's eyes	Ranunculaceae	See above
Cheiranthosides, strophadogenin, others	*Cheiranthus* spp., *Erysimum* spp.	Wall flower	Brassicaceae	See above
Convallatoxin	*Convallaria majalis*	Lily of the valley	Liliaceae	Cardiac glycosides; nausea, vomiting, cardiac conduction disturbances and increased automaticity
Cymarin	*Apocynum cannabinum, Strophanthus kombe, Adonis vernalis*	Black Indian hemp, dogbane, Canadian hemp, Apocynum; see above	Apocynaceae, Ranunculaceae	See above
Digitoxin	*Digitalis purpurea, D. lanata*	Purple foxglove, Grecian foxglove	Scrophularaceae	See above
Digoxin, lanatosides A-E	*Digitalis lanata*	Grecian foxglove	Scrophularaceae	See above
Euomonoside and related glycosidesHellebrin	*Euonymus europaeus*	Spindle tree	Celastraceae	See above
	Helleborus niger	Black hellebore	Ranunculaceae	See above
Oleandrin	*Nerium oleander*	Oleander	Apocynaceae	See above
Scillaren A, B	*Urginea maritima, U. indica*	Red, white, or Mediterranean squill, Indian squill	Liliaceae	See above
Strophanthin	*Strophanthus kombe* and spp., *Convallaria majalis, Adonis vernalis*	Strophanthus, see above	Apocynaceae, Liliaceae, Ranunculaceae	See above

(continued)

TABLE 78–1.   Active Ingredients Classified Using a Pharmacognosy Approach with Examples and Selected Symptoms (continued)

Alkaloid	Plant Sources	Common Name	Family	Symptoms/Notes
Thevetin	*Thevetia peruviana*	Yellow oleander	Apocynaceae	See above
Cyanogenic glycosides				
Amygdalin, emulsin	*Prunus armeniaca, Prunus spp.; Malus spp.*	Apricot seed pits, wild cherry, peach, plum, pear, almond, apple and other seed kernels	Rosaceae	Cyanide toxicity
Anthracyanins	*Sambucus spp.*	Elderberry		
Linamarin	*Manihot esculenta*	Cassava, manihot, tapioca	Euphorbiaceae	Spastic paresis and vision disturbances with chronic use
Glucosinolates (isothiocyanate glycosides)				
Sinigrin	*Brassica nigra*	Black mustard	Brassicaceae	Mustard dermal irritant
Progoitrin	*Brassica olearacea* var. *capitata*	Cabbage	Brassicaceae	Glycosidic precursor to goitrin, antithyroid compound
Anthraquinone glycosides				
Barbaloin, iso-barbaloin, aloinosides	*Aloe barbadensis, A. vera* others	Aloe	Liliaceae (Amaryllidaceae)	Cathartic and aloe gel
Cascarosides, *O*-glycosides, emodin	*Cascara sagrada, Rhamnus purshiana, R. cathartica*	Cascara, sacred bark, chittem bark, common buckthorn	Rhamnaceae	Cathartic
Frangulins	*Rhamnus frangula*	Frangula bark, alder, buckthorn	Rhamnaceae	Cathartic
Rhein anthrones	*Rheum officinale, Rheum spp.*	Rhubarb	Polygonaceae	Cathartic (root)
Sennosides	*Cassia senna, C. angustifolia*	Senna	Fabaceae	Cathartic
Saponin glycosides				
Steroidal saponins: aglycones are smilagenin, sarsaspogenin	*Agave lecheguilla*	Agave	Amaryllidaceae	Contact dermatitis
Steroidal saponins (aglycones: diosgenin, yamogenin, and others	*Tribulus terrestris*	Tribulus terrestris	Fabaceae	Hematogenous photosensitivity in animals
Glycyrrhizin	*Glycyrrhiza glabra*	Licorice	Fabaceae	Pseuodhyperaldosteronism
Other types of glycosides				
Atractyloside, gummiferine	*Atractylis gummifera*	Thistle	Compositae	Hepatotoxicity
Ranunculin, protoanemonin	*Ranunculus spp., Pulsatilla spp.*	Pilewort and other buttercups, Pulsatilla	Ranunculaceae	Contact dermatitis
Salicin	*Salix spp., Populus spp.*	Willow and poplar species	Salicaceae	Cinchonism
Terpenoids including resins and oleoresins				
Ginkgolides A-C, M	*Ginkgo biloba*	Ginkgo	Ginkgoaceae	Inhibit platelet-activating factor and thiamine
Gossypol	*Gossypium spp.*	Cotton, cotton seed oil	Malvaceae	Classified also as polyphenol; inhibits spermatogenesis
Grayanotoxins	*Rhododendron spp., Azalea spp. Kalmia spp.*	Rhododendron, azaleas, Mountain laurel	Ericaceae	Sodium-channel effects
Hyperforin	*Hypericum perforatum*	St. John's Wort	Hypericaceae (Clusiaceae)	Inhibits cytochrome P450
Kawain, methysticin yangonin and other kava lactones	*Piper methysticum*	Kava kava	Piperaceae	CNS depression
Lantadene A and B, phylloerythrin	*Lantana camara*	Lantana camara	Verbenaceae	Photosensitivity; fatalities
Myristicin, elemicin	*Myristica fragrans*	Nutmeg, mace	Myristicaceae	Hallucinogenic
Phorbal esters	*Euphorbia pulcherrima, E. spp.*	Poinsettia	Euphorbiaceae	Irritant, contact dermatitis

(continued)

TABLE 78–1.   Active Ingredients Classified Using a Pharmacognosy Approach with Examples and Selected Symptoms (continued)

Alkaloid	Plant Sources	Common Name	Family	Symptoms/Notes
Ptaquiloside	*Pteridum spp.*	Bracken fern	Polypodiaceae	Norsesquiterpene glycoside, thiaminase inhibition, alkylating agent/bladder and GI carcinogen
Pulegone	*Mentha pulegium, Hedeoma pulegioides*	Pennyroyal	Lamiaceae	Abortifacient; hepatoxic, renal failure; spongiform encephalopathy
Sesquiterpene lactones	*Chrysanthemum spp., Taraxacum officinale,* others	Chrysanthemum, dandelion, other Compositaceae	Compositae	Allergic contact dermatitis
Tetrahydrocannibinol	*Cannibis sativa*	Cannibis, marijuana, Indian hemp, hashish, pot	Moraceae	CNS euphoriant; substance of abuse
Thujone	*Artemisia absinthium, Tanacetum vulgare, Chrysanthemum vulgare*	Absinthe, tansy	Compositae	CNS seizures, hallucinations; acute and chronic absinthism
Urushiol oleoresin	*Toxicodendron radicans, T. toxicarium, T. diversilobum, T. vernix, Ginkgo biloba, Anacardium occidentale,* many others	Poison ivy, oak and sumac; ginkgo; cashew, and many others	Anacardaceae; Ginkgoaceae; others	Allergic contact dermatitis

Phenols or phenylpropanoids including lignans, flavonoids, tannins

Asarin	*Acorus calamus*	Sweet flag, rat root, flag root, calamus	Araliaceae	β-Asarone; gastrointestinal distress
Bergamottin, naringenin or naringen	*Citrus paradisi*	Grapefruit	Rutaceae	Inhibits cytochrome P450
Capsaicin	*Capsicum frutescens, C. annuum*	Capsicum, cayenne pepper	Solanaceae	Dermal irritant
Coumarin	*Dipteryx odorata, D. oppositifolia, Meliotus spp., Trifolium pratense, Anthoxanthum odoratum; Gallium triflorum*	Tonka beans, sweet clover, red clover, sweet vernal, grass, sweet-scented bedstraw	Lamiaceae, Poaceae, Rubiaceae, others	Anticoagulation by inhibition of vitamin K activation (at vitamin K 2-3 reductase)
Esculoside (6-β-ᴅ-glucopyranosyloxy-7-hydroxycoumarin)	*Aesculus hippocastanum*	Horse chestnut	Hippocastanaceae	Anticoagulation
Podophyllotoxin	*Podophyllum peltatum, P. emodi*	Mayapple, wild mandrake	Berberidaceae	Lignan; antimitotic with purgative, neuropathy and multiorgan system failure
Primin	*Primula obconica*	Primrose	Primulaceae	Allergin
Psoralens	Multiple	Multiple	Umbelliferae, Rutaceae, Solanaceae, others	Photosensitivity
Tannic acid	*Quercus spp.*	Oak	Fagaceae	Oak toxicosis in livestock
Toxin T-454, others	*Karwinskia humboldtiana*	Buckthorn, wild cherry, tullidora, coyatillo, capulincillo, others	Rhamnaceae	Polyneuropathy

Lipids and fixed oils

Croton oil	*Croton tiglium* and *spp.*	Croton	Eurphorbiaceae	Contains tropane alkaloids and diterpenes; carcinogenic, cathartic

Proteins, lectins, peptides, amino acids

Abrin	*Abrus precatorius*	Prayer beans, rosary pea, Indian bean, crab's eye, jequirty pea	Euphorbiaceae	Toxalbumin, inhibits protein synthesis; purgative
β-N-Oxalylamino-L-alanine (BOAA); β-aminopropionitrile (BAPN)	*Lathyrus sativus*	Grass pea, chick pea	Fabaceae	Lathyrism with spastic paresis or bone degeneration
Cystatin	*Wisteria floribunda*	Wisteria	Fabaceae	Lectin that binds N-acetylgalctosamine; gastrointestinal toxicity
Hypoglycin	*Blighia sapida*	Ackee fruit	Sapindaceae	Hypoglycemia, hepatotoxicity, encephalopathy, seizures

(continued)

TABLE 78–1. Active Ingredients Classified Using a Pharmacognosy Approach with Examples and Selected Symptoms (continued)

Alkaloid	Plant Sources	Common Name	Family	Symptoms/Notes
Microcystin	*Microcystis* and *Anabaena spp.*	Blue-green algae	Planktonic cyanobacteria	Hepatotoxicity; photo-sensitivity
Phoratoxin, ligatoxin	*Phoradendron spp.*	American mistletoe	Loranthaceae or Viscaceae	Gastrointestinal toxicity; antimitotic
Phytolaccotoxin	*Phytolacca americana*	Poke Weed, Indian poke, poke, inkberry, scoke, pigeonberry, garget, American cancer	Phytolaccaceae	Lectin with single chain that inactivates rRNA and protein systhesis; gastrointestinal toxicity
Ricin, curcin	*Ricinus communis, Jatropha curcas*	Castor or rosary seeds, purging nuts, physic nut, tick seeds	Euphorbiaceae	Toxalbumin, lectins inhibit protein synthesis; purgative
Trichosanthine	*Trichosanthes kirilowii, T. anguina*	Chinese cucumber, snake gourd	Cucurbitaceae	Polypeptide inhibits protein synthesis like ricin; abortifacient
Unnamed lectin	*Robinia pseudacacia*	Black locust	Fabaceae	Lectin with 2 chains that binds N-acetyl-D-galactosamine; gastrointestinal toxicity
Viscumin	*Viscum album*	European mistletoe	Loranthaceae or Viscaceae	Lignan; polypeptides; gastrointestinal toxicity; antimitotic
Alcohols				
Cicutoxin	*Cicuta maculata*	Water hemlock	Umbelliferae	Highly potent and usually fatal: seizures, vomiting, diarrhea, salivation
Carboxylic acids				
Oxalates	*Rheum* and *Rumex spp., Spinacia oleracea,* others	Rhubarb and dock species, spinach	Polygonaceae, Chenopodiaceae	Nephrolithiasis,
Oxalate raphides	*Philodendron, spp., Dieffenbacia spp., Brassaia spp., Schefflera* spp., *Caladium spp., Epipremnum aureum, Spathiphyllum spp.*	Philodendron, dieffenbachia, umbrella tree, caladium, devil's Ivy, pathos, peace lily	Araceae	Mechanical plant dermatitis; chemical and allergic irritants
Carbohydrates				
Musilage	*Ulmus rubra, Althaea officinalis*	Slippery elm	Ulmaceae, Malvaceae	Inert; vehicle for abortifacients
Psyllium	*Plantago spp.* seed husks	Plantago	Plantaginaceae	Bulking laxative, contamination with *Digitalis lanata*
Other				
Aristolochic acid	*Aristolochia reticulata, A. spp.*	Texan or Red River snake root	Aristolochiaceae	Renal failure and carcinoma; related to alkaloids as derivative of isothebaine
Mixture: Alkaloids, polyphenols, saponins, steroids, triterpenoids	*Ilex spp.* berries	Holly	Aquifoliaceae	Gastrointestinal distress
Sauropus toxins	*Sauropus androgenous*	Sauropus	Euphorbiaceae	Bronchiolitis obliterans torsades de pointes
Saxitoxin like agent	*Anabaena* and *Aphanixzomenon*	Blue green algae	Planktonic cyanobacteria	Guanidium compound; sodium channel blockade
Tremitone	*Eupatorium rugosum, Haplopappus, Heterophyllus*	Snake root, rayless goldenrod	Asteraceae (Compositae)	Milk sickness

than 18,000 bibliographic references to plant poisonings.[73,426,428] Finally, plant material or patient tissue samples can be analyzed by chemical methods,[138] but accessibility to natural product laboratories may be limited[314] or may carry a high cost of both money and time.

Emphasis is placed on flowering plants (angiosperms) and on exposures directly or indirectly related to foraging, dietary, or occupational contact with plants. Where appropriate, it includes some gymnosperms or algae and, rarely, medicinal contact (a medicinal use is discussed in Chap. 77). Because our understanding of plant toxicity is a poor relative to that of pharmaceutical agents, animal research is included to provide a more comprehensive foundation for comparison to human experiences. As with any animal research, the relevance to humans will be borne out with time and provides a background that heightens our understanding of potential toxicity in humans that may otherwise go unrecognized without such precedent. In addition, the complexity of plant chemistry and secondary metabolites should be remembered while relating the simplified chemical schemes with patient pathology (Table 78–1) because plants do contain more than one chemical or chemicals from more than one class. The most common exposures reported to poison centers in the United States over the last 10 years should provide the most frequently requested applications for the pharmacologic approach in clinical practice

(Table 78–2). Finally, because there is sometimes overlap in prominent pharmacologic activities among structurally dissimilar toxins, some toxins are categorized by some chemical and clinical features such as sodium/calcium channel effects or antimitotic and dermal effects, rather than by their pharmacognosy classification. In addition, drug interactions provide another grouping of effects that cross lines among active ingredients.

ACTIVE CONSTITUENTS IN PLANTS, TAXONOMIC ASSOCIATIONS, AND SELECTED SYMPTOMS

Alkaloids: Toxidromes and Other Manifestations

The term *alkaloid* was originally used to designate natural substances that reacted like bases or alkalis. There is no simple and precise definition of the term, although it has come to refer to nitrogen-containing basic substances of natural origin and limited distribution. The nitrogen atom is generally part of a heterocyclic system and most alkaloids possess significant pharmacologic activity. These compounds represent the largest and most chemically diverse group of toxic constituents responsible for plant-induced

TABLE 78–2. Plants Associated with Exposures Commonly Reported to Poison Control Centers 1989–1998 and the Organ System Primarily Affected (see Chap 116)

Common Name (Scientific Name)	Cardiac	Neurologic	GI/Hepatic**	Other
African violet (*Saintpaulia spp.*)				Nontoxic
Azalea, mountain laurel, or rhododendron* (*Azalea, Kalmia,* or *Rhododendron spp.*)	Dysrhythmias	Paresthesias, mental status change	Nausea, vomiting	Concentrated in honey
Cactus (*Cactus spp.*)				Mechanical dermatitis
Caladium (*Caladium spp.*)			Mucosal irritation	Dermal: oxalate raphides
Christmas cactus (*Schlumbergera bridgesii*)				Nontoxic
Chrysanthemum (*Chrysanthemum spp.*)				Allergic dermatitis
Climbing or bittersweet nightshade* (*Solanum dulcamara*)	Tachycardia	Hallucinations, agitation		Anticholinergic toxicity
Dumbcane (*Dieffenbachia spp.*)			Gastric mucosal irritation	Dermal: oxalate raphides
English ivy (*Hedera helix*)				Dermal
Eucalyptus (*Eucalyptus globus* or *spp.*)				Dermal
Holly (*Ilex spp.*)			Gastroenteritis	
Jade plant (*Crassula spp.*)				Nontoxic
Pathos, devil's ivy (*Epipremnum aureum*)			Gastric mucosal irritation	Dermal: oxalate raphides
Peace lily (*Spathiphyllum spp.*)			Gastric mucosal irritation	Dermal: oxalate raphides
Pepper (*Capsicum annum*)			Gastric mucosal irritation	Dermal and ocular: phenlypropanoids
Philodendron (*Philodendron spp.*)			Gastroc mucosal irritation	Dermal: oxalate raphides
Poinsettia (*Euphorbia pulcherrima*)			Nausea, vomiting	Dermal: phorbal esters
Poison ivy (*Toxicodendron radicans*)				Dermal: urushiol resins
Spider plant (*Chlorophytum comosum*)				Nontoxic
Umbrella tree (*Brassaia spp., Schefflera spp.*)			Gastric mucosal irritation	Dermal: oxalate raphides
Weeping fig tree (*Ficus benjamina*)				Nontoxic

*Denotes plants both commonly reported and potentially life-threatening.
**Any plant ingestion may produce nonspecific gastrointestinal distress.

deaths. They figure prominently in human history, ranging from epidemics of poisoning caused by ergot-infested rye bread in the Middle Ages to addictions to cocaine, heroin, and nicotine in contemporary time. Most of these compounds are insoluble in water, form salts (typically crystalline) in reaction with acid, and are readily isolated from their plant source. They usually have a bitter taste. Alkaloids are widely distributed within members of the Liliaceae and Amaryllidaceae, but may also be found in the Solanceae, Apocynaceae, Papaveraceae, Ranunculaceae, Rubiaceae, and Berberidaceae. Numerous examples of toxic constituents of these families are given in the discussion below, which begins with a description of every major toxidrome that involves alkaloids. A number of life-threatening alkaloids are discussed in the section on sodium and calcium channel effects under "Effects Shared by Diverse Ingredients" later in this chapter.

Belladona Alkaloids: Atropine, Scopolamine, Hyoscyamine, Mandragorine, and Others

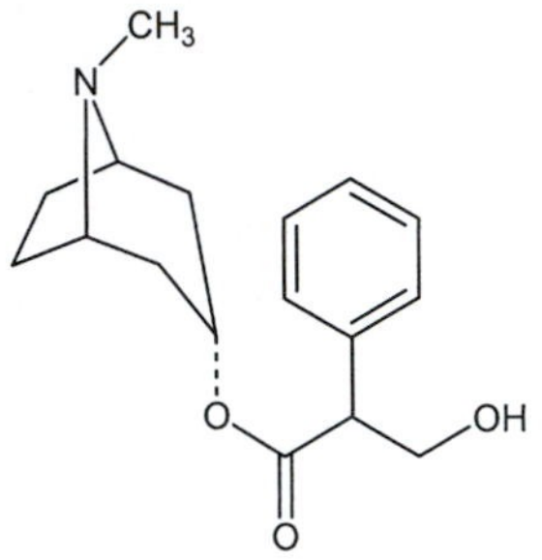

Atropine

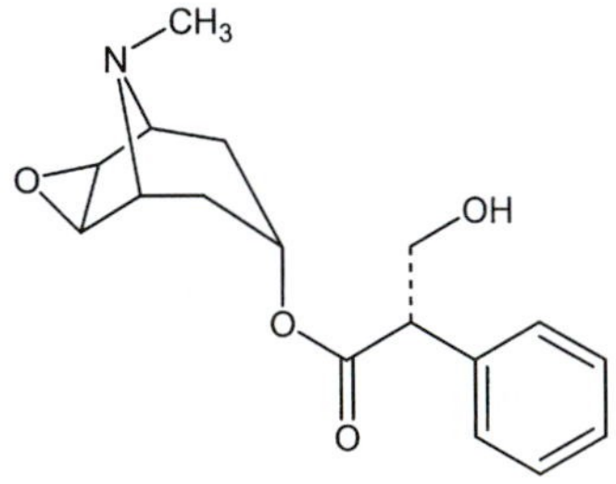

Scopolamine

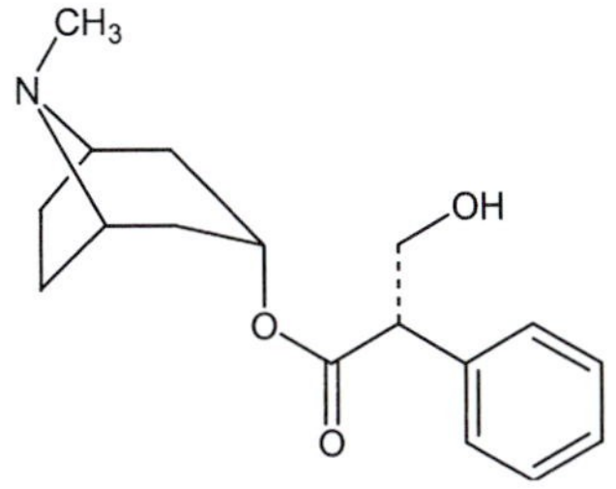

Hyoscyamine

The belladonna alkaloids are solanaceous alkaloids (from the family Solanaceae; Table 78–1). These alkaloids have potent antimuscarinic effects and produce some, if not all, of the classic signs of this toxidrome following ingestion: tachycardia, hypertension, hyperthermia, dry skin and mucous membranes, skin flushing, diminished bowel sounds, urinary retention, agitation, disorientation, and hallucinations (Chap. 17). Atropos was the fate who could cut the threads of life and who lent his name to "atropine." The anticholinergic plant henbane wreathed the heads of dwellers of Hades, while belladonna poisoned Mark Antony's troops in the Parthenium Wars in 38 AD. The toxic fruits of *Datura sanguinea*,

imbibed by Peruvian indians, produced violent convulsions, which the indians believed let them "speak to the mighty gods confidentially."[293] Since the 1970s, the quest for recreational "highs" has surpassed unintentional ingestions as the main source of toxicity. Hallucinatory effects are sought in seeds and teas, especially in late summer, the time that jimsonweed (*Datura stramonium*) seeds become available.[50,51,72,128,157,163,224,322,371,378,399,403] One hundred of these seeds contain up to 6 mg of atropine, but other plant parts contain varying degrees of alkaloids as well.

Although various species and plants within species bear differing concentrations of a range of compounds, the clinical effects are the same,[335,410,412] Onset of symptoms typically occurs 1–4 hours postingestion, or more rapidly if the plants are smoked or consumed as an infusion. The duration of effect is in part dose-dependent and may last from a few hours to 2 weeks.[157] The time course of anticholinergic poisoning can be shortened by the use of physostigmine, which may require repetitive dosing necessitating observation and hospitalization. Physostigmine may be life-saving in the face of hyperthermia, seizures, and severe agitation (Antidotes in Depth: Physostigmine). Anticholinergic toxicity may be produced without detectable atropine, scopolamine, or hyoscyamine levels and is better left as a clinical and not a laboratory diagnosis.[54,371,378]

Other Solanaceous Alkaloids: Solanine, Nicotine, Lobeline, Sparteine, *N*-Methylcytisine, Cytisine, and Coniine

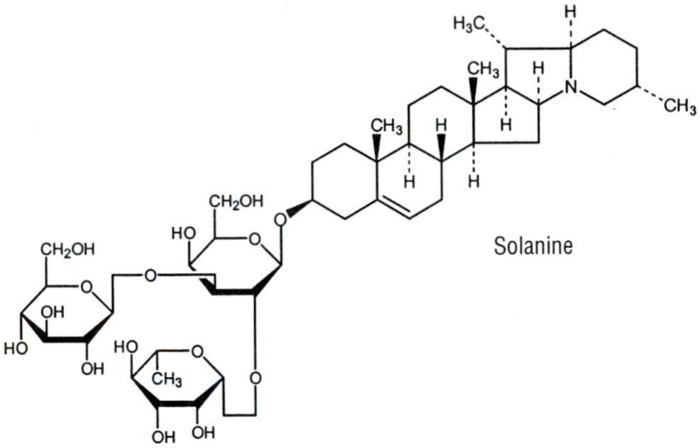

Solanine

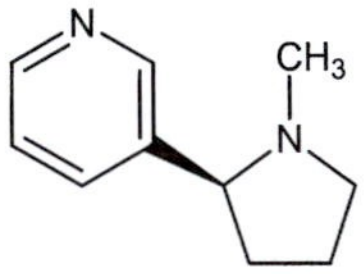

Nicotine

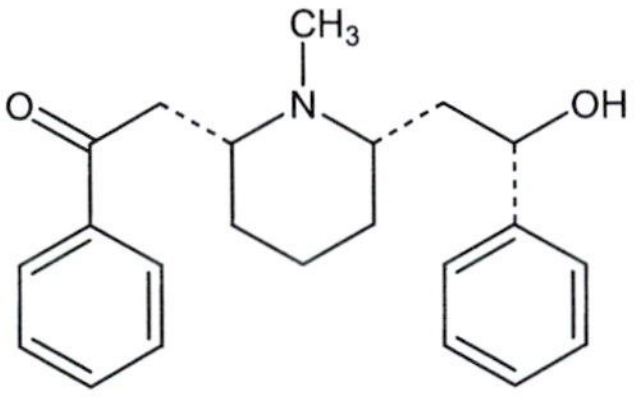

Lobeline

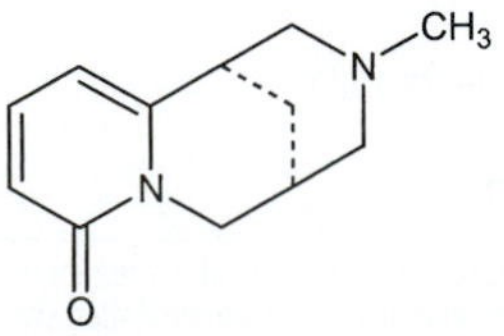

N-Methylcytisine

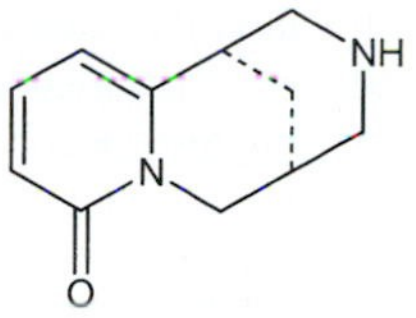

Cytisine

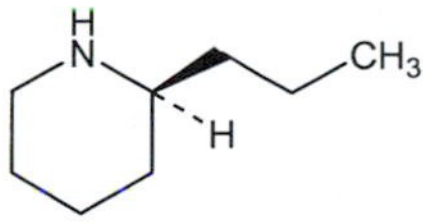

Coniine

Solanine inhibits cholinesterase in vitro, although cholinergic symptoms are not noted clinically. Nonetheless, solanine-induced central nervous system (CNS) toxicity includes hallucinations, delirium, and coma.[54,275] On the other hand, symptomatic patients more typically develop nausea, vomiting, diarrhea, and abdominal pain that begins 2–24 hours after ingestion, which, in addition to the CNS toxicity, may persist for several days.[81,318] Although present in most of the 1700 species in the genus *Solanum*, solanine toxicity in humans is uncommonly encountered. Green potatoes and green potato tops are most commonly associated with symptoms, which is not surprising because that is where the alkaloids are most concentrated. Most of the reports of deaths are from the older literature,[5,173] and consumption of 2–5 g/kg body weight per day is not predicted to cause acute toxicity.[324]

Nicotine toxicity (other than from inhaled sources) occurs via ingestion of leaves of *Nicotiana tabacum*, cigarette remains, and transdermally among farm workers harvesting tobacco (green tobacco sickness).[142,146,332] Patients develop antecedent nausea and vomiting.[269] Overstimulation of the nicotinic receptors by high doses of nicotine produces a toxidrome that progresses from gastrointestinal symptoms to diaphoresis, mydriasis, fasciculations, tachycardia, hypertension, hyperthermia, and seizures, respiratory depression, and death (Chap. 73). Wearing of protective clothing by tobacco farm workers best prevents green tobacco sickness.

This toxidrome is also produced by alkaloids other than nicotine. Modern accounts of nicotinic toxicity from lobeline (found in all parts of *Lobelia inflata*) cannot be located, but its overenthusiastic use by medical botanist Samuel Thomson in the 18th century resulted in morbidity and mortality of his patients.[46]

Sparteine from broom (*Cytisus scoparius*)[413,444] and *N*-methylcytisine from blue cohosh (*Caulophyllum thalictroides*)[337] provide additional examples of nicotinelike alkaloids that may also be teratogenic.[213] Laburnum (*Cytisus laburnum*) contains cytisine that when ingested (even as little as 0.5 mg/kg, or a few peas) is reportedly responsible for mass poisonings and fatalities in children and adults who eat them.[136,291,311,341] Unfortunately, such reports have resulted in thousands of unnecessary hospital admissions for patients without morbidity and mortality after ingestion of this plant, demonstrating the difficulty in separating hazard from risk and in obtaining accurate dose-response information in the setting of plant and human variability.[29,126]

The most famous description of the end stages of nicotinic toxicity dates from about 2400 years ago by an observer of Socrates' fatal ingestion of a decoction of poison hemlock (*Conium maculatum*)[401]:

. . . the person who had administered the poison went up to him and examined for some little time his feet and legs, and then squeezing his foot strongly asked whether he felt him.

Socrates replied that he did not and said to us when the effect of the poison reached his heart, Socrates would depart.

According to the book of Exodus, quail feeding on seeds (presumably from poison hemlock) became toxic and passed the toxicity on to the Israelites who ate the fowl.[25] Birds do not experience coniine toxicity but provide a vector for poisoning. Even in the 20th century, people have succumbed to hemlock poisoning following their avian repasts; this is especially well documented in Italy, where the toxic alkaloid coniine was subsequently detected in the bird meat, as well as in the blood, urine, and tissue of some of the victims.[342,363] Age of the plant, usually found at water's edge or in disturbed areas, correlates with a high concentration of coniine, while the toxin γ-coniceine occurs in greater amounts in new growth, distributing the plant's toxicity over the length of the growing season.[76,95,139] Fatal poisonings are reported on multiple continents, including North America and Australia.[95,130,138] In the case series described above, the 17 poisoned Italian patients had elevated liver aminotransferases and myoglobin levels, and 5 of the 17 patients had acute tubular necrosis.[342] These cases demonstrate that death can develop 1–16 days following ingestion, despite gastric emptying, forced diuresis, peritoneal or hemodialysis, and respiratory support.[343]

Cholinergic Alkaloids: Arecoline, Physostigmine, and Pilocarpine

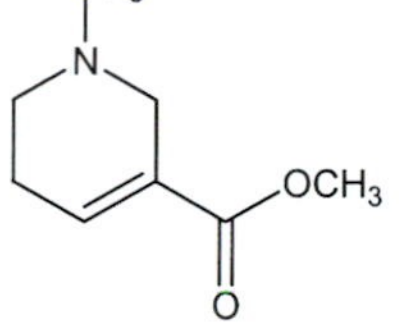

Arecoline

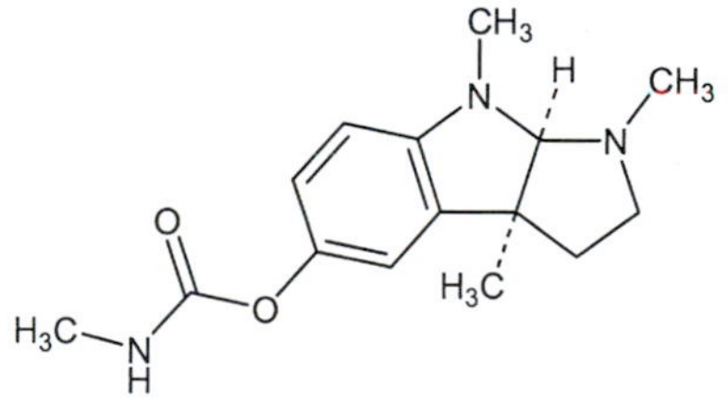

Physostigmine

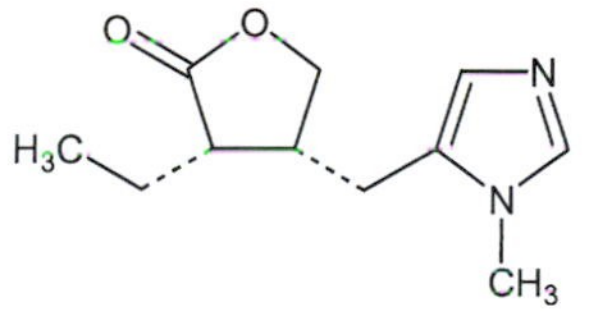

Pilocarpine

Betel chewing has been a habitual practice in the East since ancient times. The "quid" is a masticatory consisting of betel nut (*Areca catechu*) and other ingredients. Effects of acute exposure to arecoline, the major alkaloid, include sweating, salivation, hyperthermia, possible exacerbation of asthma, and exacerbation of extrapyramidal signs in patients treated with anticholinergic medications. Prolonged use is also associated with dental decay and buccal cancer.[66,86,93,109,366] Physostigmine is an alkaloid derived from the Calabar bean (*Physostigma venenosum*), in which it is present in concentrations of 0.15%. It was used historically as an "ordeal poison" in West Africa.[109] The miotic effects of this compound have been used to reverse mydriatic agents, and its cholinesterase-inhibiting properties make it a valuable antidote in anticholinergic poisoning (Antidotes in Depth: Physostigmine). Pilocarpine is derived from *Pilocarpus jaborundi* from South America and possesses stimulatory effects on muscarinic receptors that oppose those of atropine. It is of value in treatment of glaucoma.[109] Reversal of toxicity can be achieved by atropine

Psychotropic Alkaloids: Lysergic Acid and Mescaline

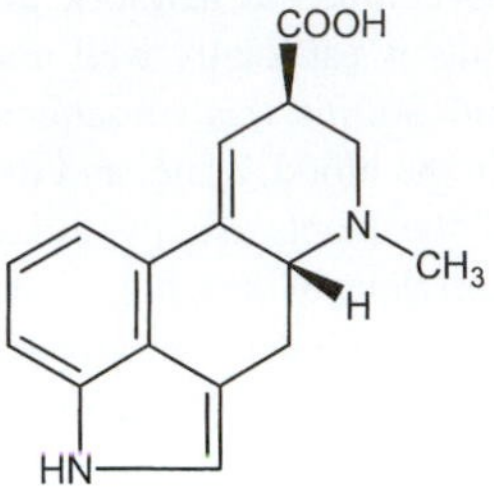

Lysergic acid

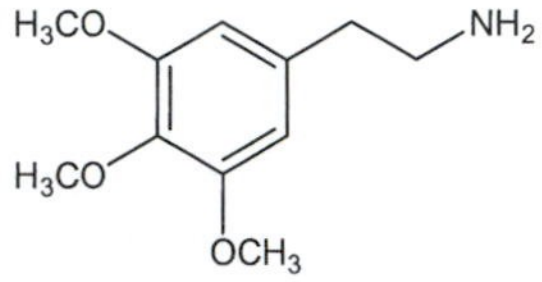

Mescaline

Hallucinations from the direct serotonin effects of lysergic acid derivatives and from the amphetaminelike serotonin effects of the mescaline alkaloids are reported following ingestion of morning glory seeds (*Ipomea spp.*) and peyote cactus (*Lophophora williamsonii*), respectively (Chap. 70). Ingestion of at least 150 morning glory seeds produces troubling nausea and vomiting that limit any potential pleasures of the "psychedelic" experience.[69,123,196,437]

Alkaloidal CNS Stimulants and Depressants: Ephedrine, Synephrine, and Cathinone

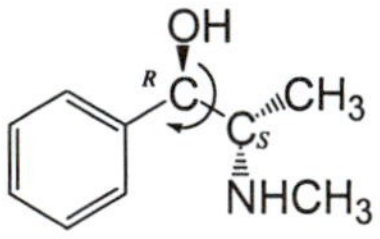

Ephedrine

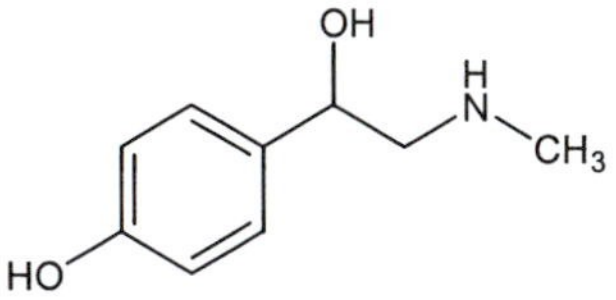

Synephrine

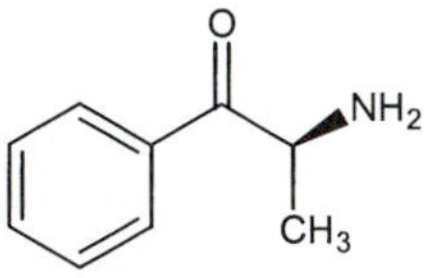

Cathinone

One medicinal plant worth noting is the traditional Chinese medicinal plant ma huang. A number of alkaloid-containing Asian species, belonging to the genus *Ephedra*, have a 5000-year history of use as asthma medications. Prehistoric use is suggested by the discovery of this plant in a Neanderthal gravesite.[255] Modern usage of these plants falls outside of the traditional indications for asthma to include intended use to increase energy, enhance athletic performance, and aid weight loss. The alkaloid-producing species

contain (−)-ephedrine and 5 structurally related compounds: (+)-pseudoephedrine, (−)-norephedrine, (−)-N-methylephedrine, (+)-norpseudoephedrine, and (+)-N-methylpseudoephedrine. In recent years, a disturbing number of reports involving morbidity and mortality have called into question the safety profile of the herb. Adverse events in both the popular[36,161,162] and, increasingly, the medical literature include cerebral vascular accidents, hepatotoxicity, myocardial infarction, myocarditis, renal calculi, and death.[169,198,206,296,329,388,400,415,446]

Ephedrine is also identified in certain varieties of *Sida cordifolia,* and synephrine, another compound structurally related to ephedrine, occurs in *Citrus aurantium*. In addition to commercial formulations, deaths are reported following ingestion of *C. aurantium* rinds by children.[271] Another plant ingested for its CNS stimulant activity is khat (*Catha edulis*). The plant contains cathinone (α-aminopropiophenone) as well as cathine ((+)-norpseudoephedrine).

Pyrrolizidine Alkaloids

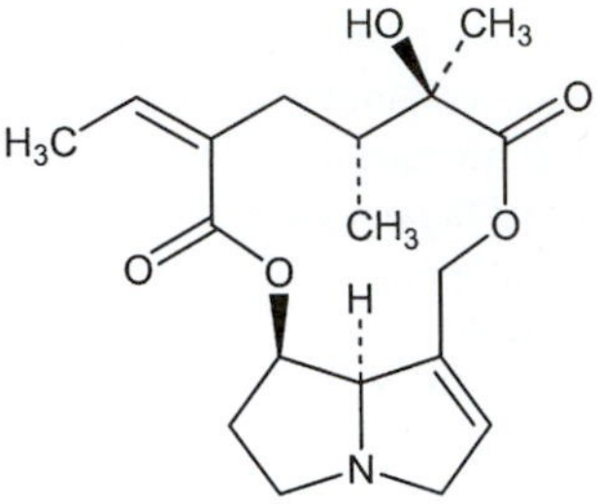

Senecionine

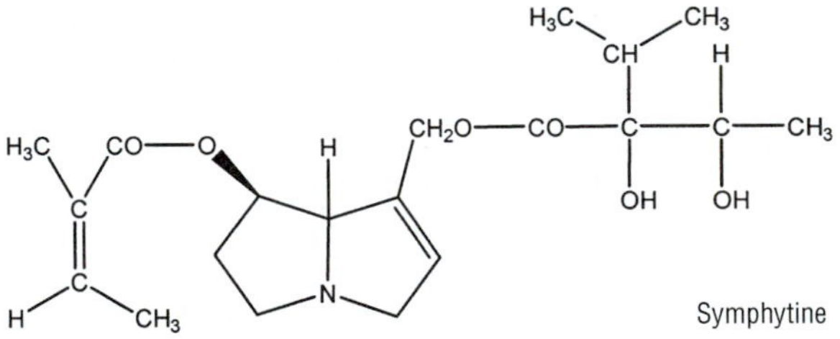

Symphytine

Pyrrolizidine alkaloids are widely distributed both botanically and geographically, and about half of the approximately 350 different alkaloids that have been characterized to date are toxic. Pyrrolizidine alkaloids are found in 6000 plants and in 13 plant families, but are most heavily represented within the Boraginaceae, Compositae, and Fabaceae. Within these families, the genera *Heliotropium, Senecio,* and *Crotalaria,* respectively, are particularly notable for their content of toxic pyrrolizidine alkaloids.[387] These hepatotoxic alkaloids all contain a 1-hydroxymethyl pyrrolizidine system unsaturated in the 1,2-position, and at least one esterified hydroxyl group.[438] The hepatic cytochrome P450 system converts these compounds to highly reactive pyrroles in vivo. Chronic exposures to these toxic pyrroles cause hepatic venoocclusive disease by stimulating proliferation of the intima of hepatic vasculature. Most poisonings occur as a result of contamination of food grain with seeds of pyrrolizidine alkaloid–containing plants or by use of pyrrolizidine alkaloid–rich plants for medicinal purposes. Acute poisoning is probably caused by hepatic necrosis associated with an overwhelming oxidant effect.[71,159] It is estimated that 20% of patients with acute pyrrolizidine alkaloid poisoning die, 50% recover completely, and the rest develop a subacute or chronic variation of hepatic venooc-clusive disease.[14] Pyrrolizidine alkaloids are teratogenic and are transmitted through breast milk.[349] Other types of plant-associated hepatic disorders are discussed in "Effects Shared by Diverse Ingredients" later in this chapter, and it is reasonable to give a course of *N*-acetylcysteine for such cases (Antidotes in Depth: *N*-Acetyl-cysteine).

Isoquinoline Alkaloids: Sanguinarine, Berberine, and Hydrastine

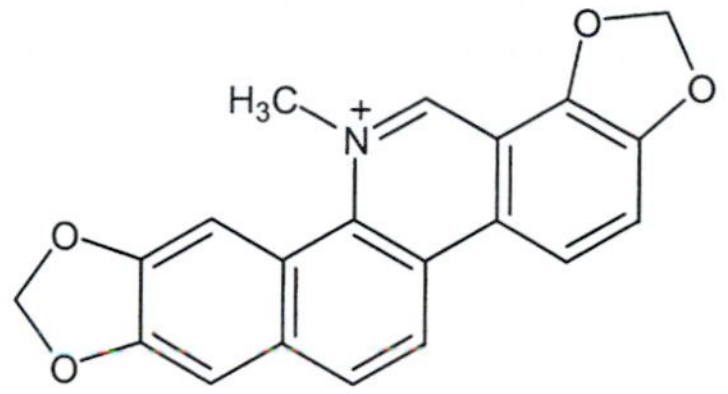

Sanguinarine

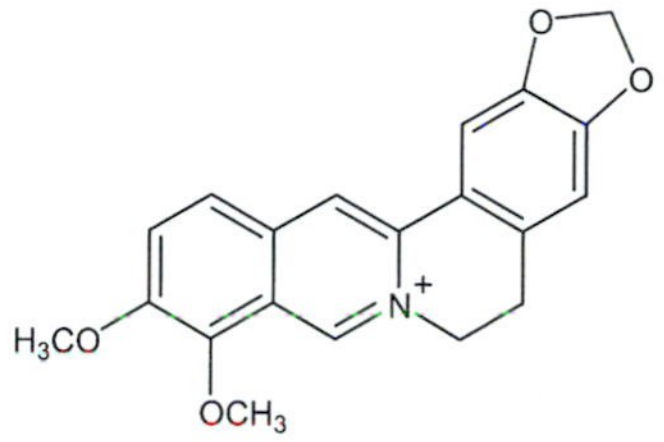

Berberine

Sanguinarine was recently detected in 26 family members who consumed a mustard oil contaminated with seeds of *Argemone mexicana*.[374] All patients suffered gastrointestinal distress followed by lower extremity edema, skin darkening, erythema, sarcoidlike skin depositions, perianal itching, anemia, and hepatomegaly. Ascites developed in 12%, while carditis and congestive heart failure were experienced in about a third of the affected individuals.[374] Medicinally, sanguinarine is used for dental hygiene.[176] In North America, sanguinarine is found in blood root (*Sanguinaria canadensis*), which, like *Argemone,* is in the Ranuculaceae family.

Berberine is closely related to sanguinarine and reportedly also has cardiac depressant effects. It is said to depress respiration and to stimulate smooth muscles in vasculature and the uterus.[271] A number of medicinal plants contain berberine, including gold-enseal (*Hydrastis canadensis*), Oregon grape (*Mahonia spp.*), and barberry (*Berberis spp.*). In addition, strychninelike movement disorders are described following the ingestion of hydrastine,[242] which is found in a 4% concentration in goldenseal.

Other Alkaloids: Emetine/Cephaline, Strychnine/Curare, and Swainsonine

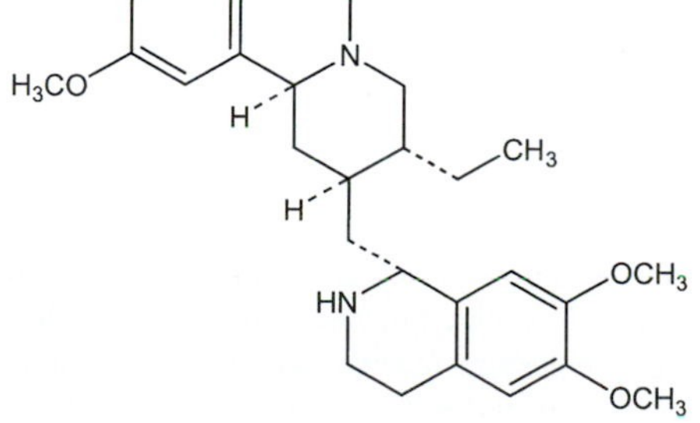

Emetine

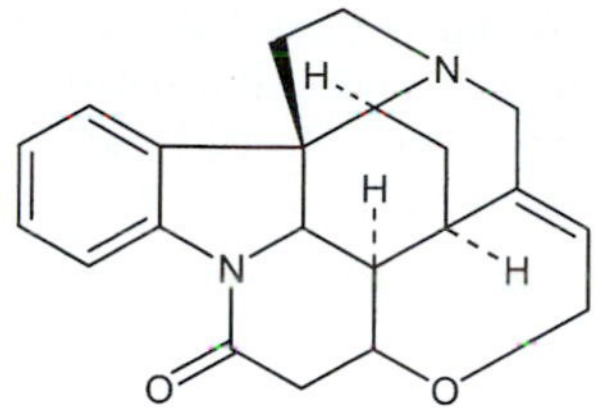

Strychnine

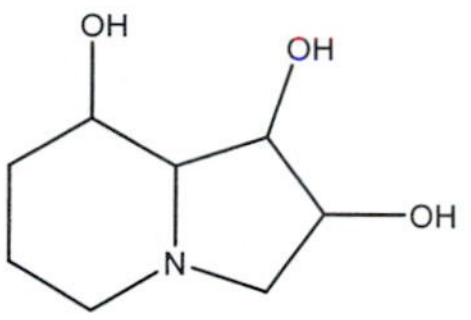

Swainsonine

Emetine and cephaline are derived from *Cephaelis ipecacuanha*, a tropical plant native to the forests of Bolivia and Brazil. They are the principal active constituents in syrup of ipecac, and as emetine's name suggests, it produces emesis. Chronic use, typically by patients with eating disorders or Munchausen by proxy,[13,114] can lead to cardiomyopathy, smooth-muscle dysfunction, myopathies, electrolyte and acid-base disturbances related to excessive vomiting, and death.[364] Classic cardiac pathology demonstrates Z-band streaming in the myocardium and fine cytoplasmic inclusion bodies detectable on ultrastructural microscopy, while other muscle pathology includes vacuolar degeneration with myofibrillolysis and fine cytoplasmic body formation.[166,241,402] The clinical course may be reversible if ipecac is withdrawn prior to extensive tissue damage.[190] Liquid chromatographic analysis of urine for emetine can confirm the diagnosis when history is unrevealing.[240] Emetine poisoning in patients ingesting plant material is not reported, but the potential exists.

Strychnine and curare, although both derived from plants of the *Strychnos* genus, possess very different clinical effects. The alkaloid strychnine is derived from the seeds of *Strychnos nux-vomica* and results in peripheral neuromuscular effects by postsynaptic glycine antagonism. Curare is the name given to the unstandardized extract of the bark of certain members of the genera *Strychnos* and *Chondodendron*. The physiologically active principal of curare is (+)-tubocurarine chloride, a competitive antagonist of acetylcholine at nicotinic receptors in the neuromuscular junction. The pharmacology and potential applications of curare are great, as it is the molecule from which most nondepolarizing agents are derived. Records of plant poisoning are restricted to its traditional use as arrow and fish poisons.[24,254,330]

After subsisting on seeds containing swainsonine for nearly 4 months, a naturalist forager manifested profound muscular weakness and died in the wilderness.[232] The compound is also believed to be responsible for birth defects in livestock and at least partly responsible for the defeat of George Armstrong Custer at Little Big Horn because the horses of troops sent to reinforce him appeared to suffer from locoism.[187] Swainsonine inhibits the glycosylation of glycoproteins by α-mannosidase II of the Golgi apparatus, which results in a lysosomal storage disease. The compound is isolated from *Swainsonia canescens*, *Astragalus lentiginosus* (spotted locoweed), other species of *Swainsonia* and *Astragalus,* several species belonging to the genera *Oxytropis* and *Ipomoea,* and several fungi.[70] Most reports of swainsonine poisoning are in grazing livestock, which manifest a syndrome called *locoism*, a chronic neurologic disease marked by staggering gait, incoordination, difficulty eating and drinking, an abnormal behavior, and a rough coat. Swainsonine was used with some success in clinical trials for the treatment of advanced neoplasms,[155] but adverse effects among treated patients included hepatic and pancreatic dysfunction, shortness of breath, lethargy, and nausea.

Glycosides

Glycosides are defined as organic compounds that yield a sugar or sugar derivative (the glycone) and a nonsugar moiety (the aglycone) upon hydrolysis. The chemical structure or the biologic activity of the aglycone is often the basis of subclassification of the glycosides. Examples include cardioactive steroids (cardiac glycosides) and cyanogenic, anthraquinone, and saponin glycosides.

Cardiac Glycosides: Digoxin, Digitoxin, Oleandrin, and Others

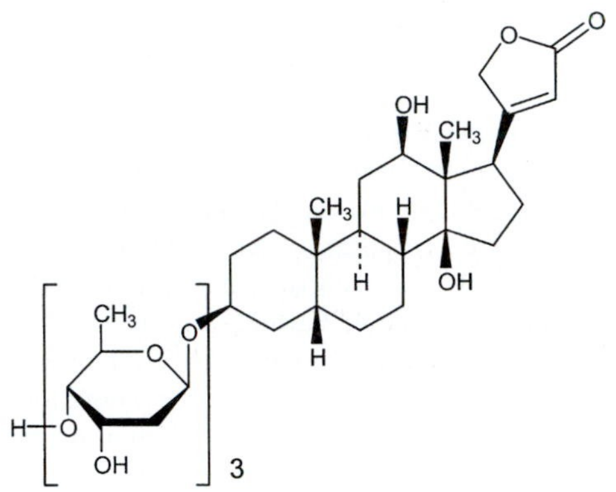

Digoxin

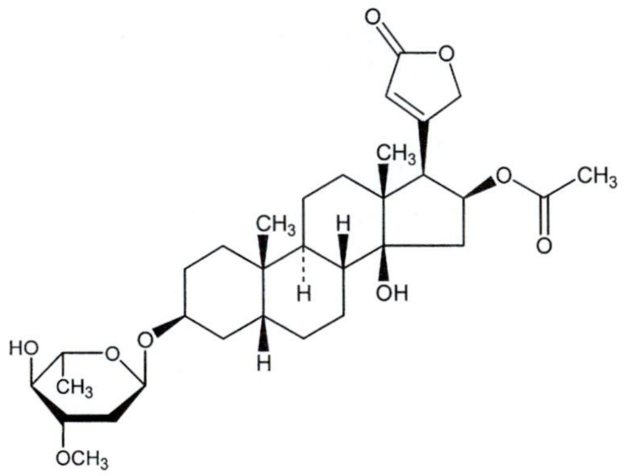

Oleandrin

Poisoning by virtually all cardiac glycosides is clinically indistinguishable from poisoning by digoxin (Chap. 48), which is itself derived from *Digitalis lanata*.[344] However, compared to pharmaceutical digoxin toxicity, toxicity resulting from cardiac glycoside plant ingestions may be associated with markedly different pharmacokinetics. For example, digitoxin found in *Digitalis* species has a plasma half-life as long as 192 hours (average, 168 hours).

The clinical and pharmacologic properties are true across taxonomic boundaries.[359] Reports of poisoning by *Digitalis spp.*,[184,334,340,376] squill (*Urginea spp.*),[127,406] lily of the valley (*Convallaria spp.*),[102,236,244] oleander (*Nerium spp.*),[8,97,165,236,249,365,373,411] and yellow oleander (*Thevetia spp.*)[27,100,101,359,360] are remarkably similar. The potency of these effects depends on the plant and dose. For instance, lily of the valley is rarely associated with morbidity or mortality,[102,252,244] whereas the ingestion of only 2 seeds of yellow oleander by adults can produce severe symptoms, and expected outcome is grave if more than 4 seeds are consumed.[359] Poisonings by oleander and yellow oleander occur predominantly

in the Mediterranean and in the Near and Far East. However, these plants are attractive ornamental plants and are popular in the United States and Europe, and poisoning in some of these regions is common.[82]

Patients experience nausea, vomiting within several hours, followed by hyperkalemia, conduction delays, and increased automaticity (bradycardia and tachydysrhythmias) caused by inhibition of the membrane Na^+-K^+ ATPase. Interestingly, the cardiac effects are indistinguishable from plants with sodium or calcium channel effects (see below). Empiric treatment with digoxin-specific antibody and activated charcoal should not be delayed in the face of uncertain plant identity. In addition, various cardiac glycosides respond differently to the therapeutic use of digoxin-specific antibody. Use of very large doses of digoxin-specific antibody (up to 37 vials reported in one case[340]) may increase the opportunity for therapeutic cross-reactivity between antibody and the nondigoxin cardiac glycosides.[32,82,354,373] Likewise, these may respond variably to diagnostic digoxin assays in clinical use. In particular, use of monoclonal instead of polyclonal antibody digoxin detection assays may miss the presence of nondigoxin molecules altogether, and give a false conclusion that cardiac glycosides are not present.

Cyanogenic Glycosides: Amygdalin, Linamarin, (*S*)-Sambunigrin

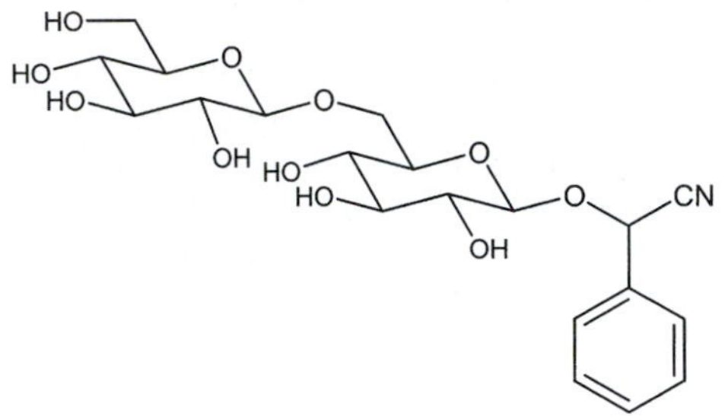

Amygdalin

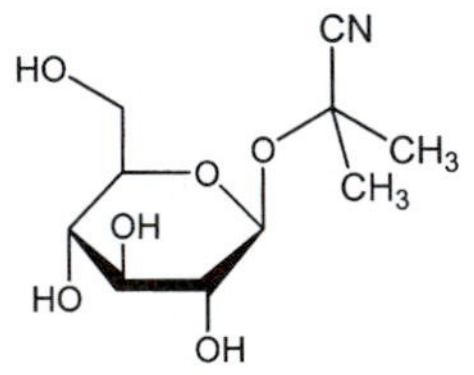

Linamarin

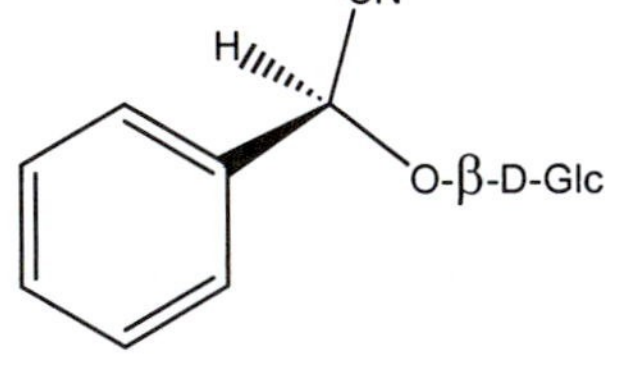

(*S*)-Sambunigrin

Cyanogenic glycosides are compounds that yield a hydrogen cyanide on complete hydrolysis. These glycosides are represented in a broad range of taxa and in about 2500 plant species.[419] The amount of glycoside in the plant varies with the species, stage of plant development, and plant part. The species that are most important to humans are cassava (*Manihot esculenta*), which contains linamarin, and *Prunus* species, which contain amygdalin. There are rare reports of cyanide poisoning associated with European elderberry seed ingestion (*Sambucus nigra*; sambunigrin), and these are more severe when these ingestions include leaves as well as berries.[40,52] While plants in the genera *Pyracantha*, *Passiflora*, *Hydrangea*, and many others are readily available cyanogenic plants in North America, these either contain stable cyanogenic glycosides that are not consumed in quantities sufficient to induce poisoning, or poisonings are underreported.[153]

Reports of acute and chronic cyanide toxicity (including deaths) associated with consumption of inadequately prepared cassava (*M. esculenta*) are worldwide (Chap. 98).[2,351] Chronic manifestations include visual disturbances (amblyopia), upper motor neuron disease with spastic paraparesis, and hypothyroidism. These findings are associated with protein-deficient states and use of tobacco and alcohol. The ataxic neuropathy resembles that produced by lathyrism (see "Lectins" later in this chapter). A unifying hypothesis about the etiology of these two similar diseases from seemingly very different sources is that thiocyanate accumulation may lead to degeneration of the AMPA (α-amino-3-hydroxy-5-methyl-isoxazole-4-propionic acid)-containing neurons that are first stimulated and then destroyed in neurolathyrism.[381,384]

Acute human cyanide toxicity from plant sources in the United States is predominantly caused by seeds of members of the Rosacea family, such as apricot (*Prunus armeniaca*), bitter almond (*Prunus amygdalus*), peach (*Prunus persica*), pear (*Pyrus communis*), apple (*Malus sylvestris*), and plum (*Prunus domestica*).[44] The fleshy fruit is nontoxic, but the leaves, bark and seed kernels contain amygdalin, which is metabolized to cyanide by the enzyme emulsin.

Amygdalin was the active ingredient of Laetrile, an apricot pit extract, promoted for its supposed selective toxicity to tumor cells, that was popular in the 1970s. Its sale was restricted in the United States because it lacked efficacy and safety.[290] However, patients continued to travel to other countries for Laetrile therapy, also marketed as "vitamin B-17," and it is now available again through alternative medicine providers.[439] Ingestions of *Prunus* seeds continues today, and they are available from health food sources, as well as from the fruits themselves. Poisonings continue to occur because of a lack of understanding of the toxic nature of the seeds, belief in amygdalin as a health-promoting substance, or attempts at suicide.[167,321,352,372,392,409] Poisoning is caused by cyanide, and is characterized by metabolic acidosis, lactic acidosis, headache, dizziness, vertigo, stupor, coma, seizures, and hyperthermia. Survivors may suffer parkinsonism as a consequence of effects on the basal ganglia.[321] Treatment of acute poisoning involves use of the cyanide antidote kit (Antidotes in Depth: Cyanide Antidotes) and activated charcoal.

Saponin Glycosides: Glycyrrhizin

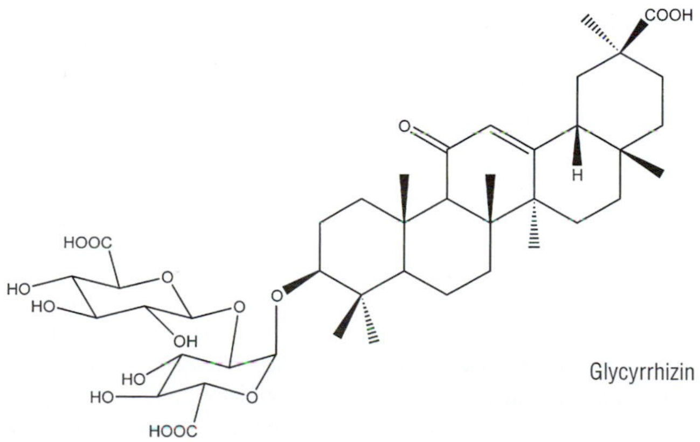

Glycyrrhizin

Saponin refers to a steroid-type structure as seen in the structure of glycyrrhizin, which is derived from *Glycyrrhiza glabra* (licorice) and other *Glycyrrhiza* species. This glycoside inhibits 11-β-hydroxysteroid dehydrogenase, an enzyme that converts cortisol to cortisone. When large amounts of licorice root are chronically consumed, the resultant high levels of cortisol activate mineralocorticoid receptors in the kidney with the same binding affinity as aldosterone and produce pseudohyperaldosteronism.[111] Chronic use eventually leads to hypokalemia with muscle weakness, sodium and water retention, hypertension, or dysrhythmias.[78,107,111,302] Care involves evaluation of fluid and electrolytes, support for cardiac disturbances, particularly potassium replacement, and abstinence from further ingestion of root materials.

Holly berries (from over 300 *Ilex spp.*) are a common and attractive ingestant among children, especially during winter holidays.[418] They contain a mixture of alkaloids, polyphenols, saponins, steroids, and triterpenes.[435] Saponins appear to be responsible for the gastrointestinal (GI) symptoms such as nausea, vomiting, diarrhea, and abdominal cramping that result from ingestion of the berries. Experimental data in animals describe hemolysis and cardiotonic effects similar to those of digoxin.[15,429] CNS depression was reported in a case in which a child consumed a "handful" of berries; however, this child was also treated with syrup of ipecac.[346] One recent study stated that no untoward effects are to be expected for ingestions of less than six berries,[430] while others suggest a minimal toxic dose of two berries.[132] Treatment is supportive and symptoms may be expected to be restricted to GI effects.

Anthraquinone Glycosides: Sennoside and Others

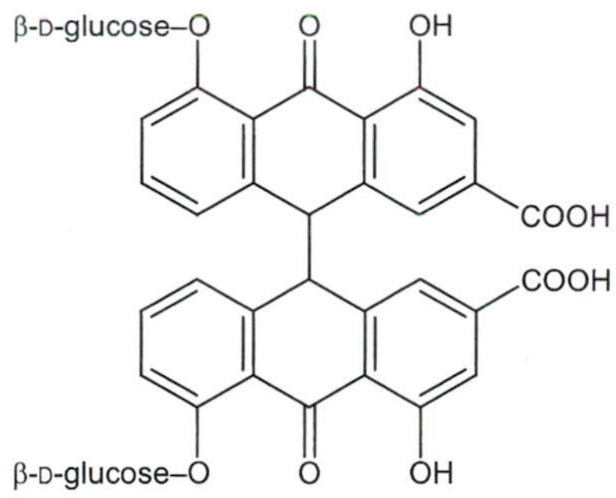

Sennoside A

Anthraquinone laxatives are both regulated as nonprescription pharmaceutical ingredients and as dietary supplements. These glycosides, for example sennoside, are metabolized in the bowel to produce derivatives that stimulate colonic motility, probably by inhibiting Na^+/K^+ ATPase in the intestine. They also promote accumulation of water and electrolytes in the gut lumen, producing fluid and electrolyte shifts that can be life-threatening.[113]

Other Glycosides: Salicin and Atractyloside

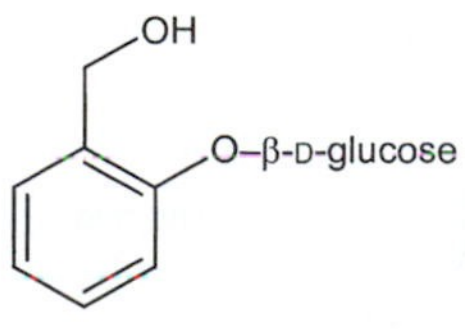

Salicin

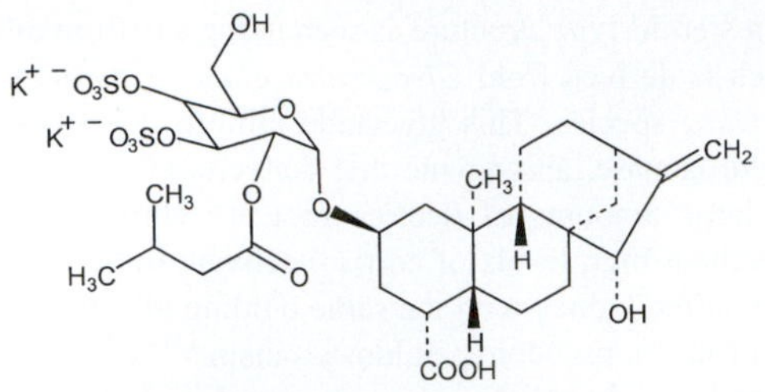

Atractyloside

Gossypol

Salicin is an inactive glycoside that must be hydrolyzed to produce salicylic acid (Chap. 33). The glycosidic bond is relatively resistant to stomach acid, and the hydrolysis must be accomplished by gut flora. There are distinct differences in the ability of the flora of individual humans to produce the necessary enzymes, thus resulting in variable therapeutic effects. However, enough hydrolysis occurs in all individuals to be concerned with regard to hypersensitivity. When hydrolyzed, salicin (MW 286) is stoichiometrically converted to salicylic acid (MW 138).

Atractylis gummifera was a favorite agent of homicide during the reign of the Borgias. Atractyloside, the active ingredient, decreases levels of cytochrome P450.[178] These compounds inhibit oxidative phosphorylation in the liver by inhibiting transport of adenosine 5′-diphosphate (ADP) into hepatic mitochondria (Chap. 14). Death as a result of liver failure was reported in four children, and severe illness was reported in two others, following ingestion of an unknown quantity of the plant.[252] Hepatorenal disease also results from ingestion.[304] Treatment should include *N*-acetylcysteine (Antidotes in Depth: *N*-Acetylcysteine).

The effects of the glycosides sinigrin (from *Brassica nigra* seed and *Alliaria officinalis* (horseradish) root) and naringen (a polyphenolic glycoside from the grapefruit *Citrus paradisi*)) are discussed in the sections "Plant Dermatitides" and "Plant-Drug Interactions," respectively, later in this chapter).

Terpenoids and Resins: Ginkgolides, Ptaquiloside/Thiaminase, Kava Lactones, Methysticin Thujone, and Gossypol

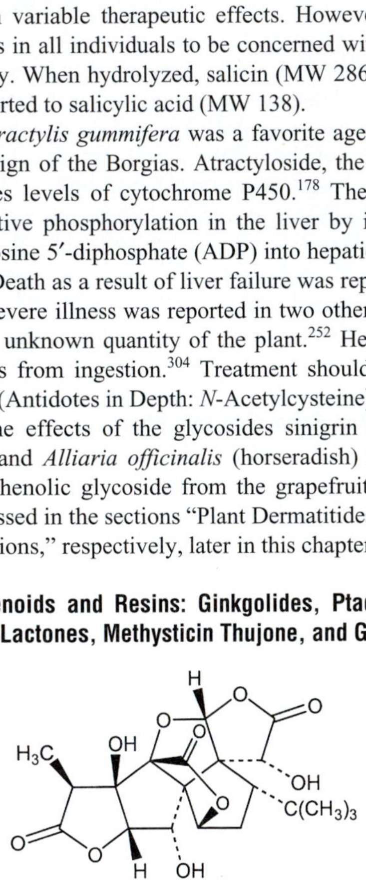

Ginkgolide B

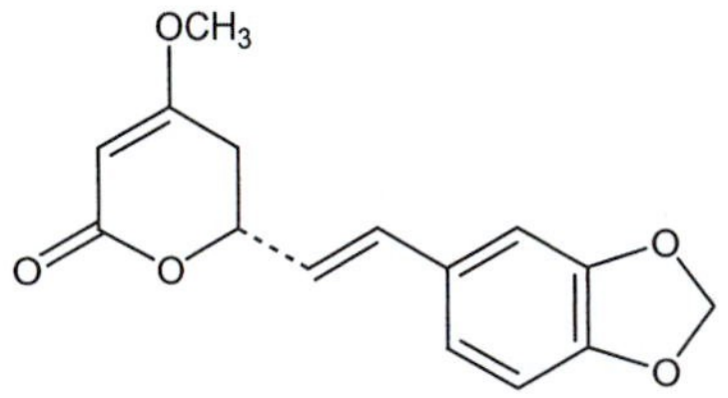

Methysticin

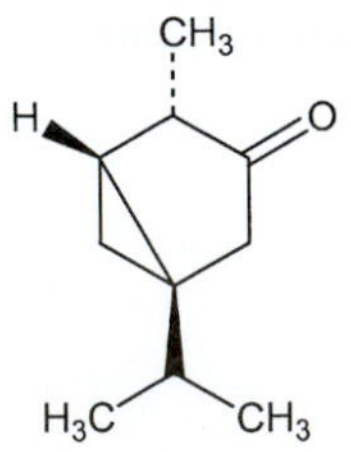

Thujone

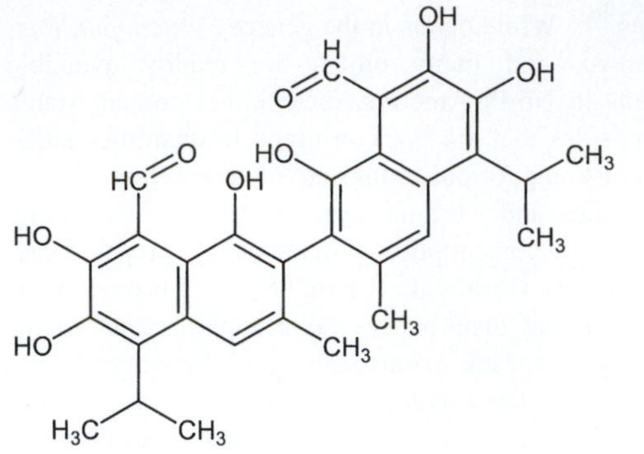

Terpenes are organic compounds formed by the assembly of a number of 5-carbon units (isoprene, C_5H_8). Monoterpenes are composed of two such units ($C_{10}H_{16}$) and are common elements of essential oils. Sesquiterpenes are composed of three ($C_{15}H_{24}$) isoprene units; diterpenes are composed of four ($C_{20}H_{32}$) isoprene units; triterpenes are composed of six ($C_{30}H_{48}$) isoprene units; and tetraterpenoid carotenoids are composed of eight ($C_{40}H_{60}$) isoprene units. Terpenes represent the largest group of secondary metabolites, with about 20,000 having been identified to date. The metabolites contain a number of functional groups, including alcohols, phenols, ketones, and esters, and they play a prominent role in plant defense. Examples include hyperforin, grayanotoxins, phorbol esters, and urushiol resins, which are discussed with plant-drug interactions, the sodium channel effectors, and plant dermatitides later in this chapter.

A risk of bleeding and thiaminase effects in humans are demonstrated following ingestion of certain parts of *Ginkgo biloba*. Ginkgolides are associated with antiplatelet aggregation effects, probably through antiplatelet-activating-factor (anti-PAF) effects. Three reports of spontaneous bleeding associated with ingestion of *Ginkgo* leaf products as an herbal medicine are perhaps explained by this property.[348,350,416] Although not a terpenoid, another component found only in the seed—4′-methoxypyridoxine—was associated with seizures in a child who ingested the seeds. A mechanism similar to isoniazid-induced seizures is plausible.[423] This case suggests the role of pyridoxine as a possible treatment should cases develop in the future (Chap. 43 and Antidotes in Depth: Pyridoxine). The dermal effects of *Ginkgo* are discussed later in the section "Plant Dermatitides."

Animal ingestions of terpenes in bracken ferns (*Pteridium aquilinum*) result in hemorrhage associated with profound thrombocytopenia related to ptaquilosides and cerebral disease related to the thiaminases.[110,377] Although no acute human poisonings have been reported, the increases in worldwide range and density suggest substantial risk if humans are susceptible. Chronic toxicity through transmission in cow's milk is suggested by an increased prevalence of gastric and esophageal cancer in areas in which the fern is endemic and consumed by cows whose milk is not diluted in large enough volumes with the milk from unexposed cows. Pulmonary adenomas are associated with spore inhalation in animals.[440]

Nervous system effects are also produced by a series of terpene lactones found in kava kava (*Piper methysticum*) and by thujone-containing plants (Table 78–1) such as *Artemisia absinthium*. Kava kava has enjoyed a long ceremonial history among islanders of the South Pacific, and observers visiting Oceania have recorded its acute and chronic effects (both pleasant and unpleasant) over the centuries. Importation of kava kava to Australia in 1983 was a measure to assist Aborigines with alcohol-abuse problems; however, the kava kava itself became abused and its subsequent ban has resulted in growth of a black market.[12,49] Proposed mechanisms to explain the effects of kava lactones include effects at GABA$_A$ and GABA$_B$ receptors,[84,204] or local anesthetic effects.[149,315] Acute symptoms following ingestion include peripheral numbness, weakness, and sedation, while chronic use leads to kava dermopathy and weight loss.[35,180]

Thujone is one of many terpenes associated with seizures.[34] It is found in the wormwood plant (*Artemisia absinthium*) and its derivative absinthe, and in some strains of tansy (*Tanacetum vulgare*). Absinthism is characterized by seizures and hallucinations, permanent cognitive impairment, and personality changes. Acute and chronic absinthism led to a worldwide ban of the alcoholic beverage absinthe, which contained thujone, in the early 1900s. The essential oil of wormwood is composed almost exclusively of thujone. Wormwood oil is currently available over the Internet and is responsible for at least two reports of adverse reactions in people seeking its hallucinatory or euphoriant effects[21,434]; α and β isomers of thujone are believed to act much like camphor to produce CNS depression and seizures. The use of the structural similarity of thujone to one of the terpenoids of marijuana, tetrahydrocannabinol (THC) to explain the psychoactive effects is controversial,[88,282] (see Chap. 71).

(+/−)-Gossypol is a multifunctional sesquiterpene that is derived from cottonseed oil. It is used experimentally as a reversible male contraceptive. The mechanism for its spermicidal effects[75] is unclear, but has been attributed to inhibition of plasminogen activation and plasmin activity in acrosomal tissue.[394] These effects are not currently reported to produce systemic bleeding. Gossypol also inhibits 11-β-hydroxysteroid dehydrogenase, as does glycyrrhizin, but typically results in only isolated hypokalemia.[75]

Proteins and Peptides

Lectins

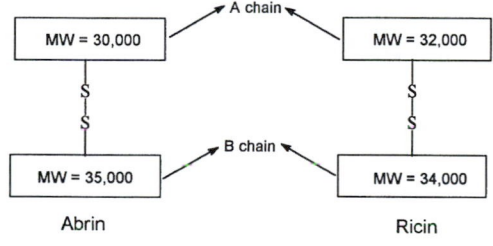

Abrin Ricin

Lectins are glycoproteins that are classified according to binding affinity for specific carbohydrate ligands—in particular, galactosamines—and by the number of protein chains linked by disulfide bonds. A number of lectins produce severe gastritis and are associated with hemagglutination and mitogenic properties. Other lectins are neurotoxins. Many have been explored for antiviral, antibacterial, immune stimulatory, contraceptive, abortifacient, and anticancer potential. Toxalbumins such as ricin and abrin are lectins that are potent cytotoxins.

Ricin. The potency of this toxin was hypothesized in the 1978 assassination of Georgi Markov, an exiled Bulgarian broadcaster.

While waiting for a London bus, Markov was jabbed in the back of the thigh with an umbrella. Over the next 3 days, he developed a severe gastroenteritis and high fevers, which eventually led to his death. On autopsy, a 1.5-mm-diameter metallic sphere with a volume of 0.28 mm^3 was recovered from the wound. Toxin was released through two tiny holes in the sphere and ricin was considered to be one of the only agents potent enough to produce the gastrointestinal symptoms. The coroner was able to recreate the scenario by injecting a similar dose of ricin into a pig that died in a similar fashion within 26 hours.[231] Ricin is potent enough to be considered a possible biologic warfare agent (Chap. 100).

Ricin, extracted from the castor bean (*Ricinus communis*), exerts its cytotoxicity by two separate mechanisms. The compound is a large molecule that consists of two polypeptide chains bound by disulfide bonds, and must enter the cell to exert its toxic effect. The B chain binds to the terminal galactose of cell surface glycolipids and glycoproteins. The bound toxin then undergoes endocytosis and is transported via endosomes to the Golgi apparatus and the endoplasmic reticulum.[357] There the A chain is translocated to the cytosol where it stops protein synthesis by inhibiting the 60 S ribosome. In addition to the gastrointestinal manifestations of vomiting, diarrhea, and dehydration, ricin can cause cardiac, hematologic, hepatic, and renal toxicity. All contribute to death in humans[9,55,207,226,231,313,338,431] and animals.[3] Despite the obvious toxicity of this compound, death can probably be prevented by early and aggressive fluid and electrolyte replacement. Allergic reactions to some of these lectin-bearing plants have been noted, in particular to *R. communis*.[300] Occupational exposures to castor oil present a particular hazard,[86,407] and the plant's pollen may also be a pneumoallergen.[140]

But just how lethal are ingestions of the ornamental seeds? The highest concentration of toxin is in the hard, brown-mottled seeds. These are both tempting and available, even to children in the United States, because they are attractive enough to be used to make jewelry, and their parent plants are showy enough to have been exported for horticultural purposes outside of their native India (including to the United States).[183,218] While mastication of one seed in a child is enough to produce death,[226] this outcome (or even serious toxicity) is uncommon, even if the seeds are chewed, probably because GI absorption of the toxin is poor.[9,220,221,231,338] Activated charcoal should be administered promptly.

Other Ricinlike Lectins. *Abrus precatorius* (jequirity pea, rosary pea),[17,83,179] *Jatropha spp.*,[253] *Trichosanthes spp.* (eg, *kirilowii* or Chinese cucumber),[38,63,205,230] *Robinia pseudoacacia* (black locust),[74,247,279,303] *Phoradendron spp.* (American mistletoe) and *Viscum spp.* (European mistletoe),[99,105,389] and *Wisteria spp.* (wisteria)[188,347] all produce at least one double-chain lectin that binds to galactose-containing structures in the gut or inhibits protein synthesis in a manner similar to that of ricin. Pokeweed mitogen (PWM) of *Phytolacca americana* (pokeweed) is a single-chain protein that inhibits ribosomal RNA by removing purine groups.[195,336] Given their mechanisms, it is not surprising that the above-mentioned lectins are all capable of producing gastrointestinal symptoms, and they otherwise have toxic profiles with variable degrees of overlap in pattern and severity with ricin in humans and animals. Seizures and hallucinations are reportedly associated with *Abrus*, mistletoe, and *Trichosanthes* species. Additional focus is given below to the clinical presentation of poisoning from pokeweed and mistletoe because these represent relatively common North American exposures.

Pokeweed. The most commonly ingested toxic plant lectins in the United States are probably from pokeweed, but like ricin, these ingestions rarely cause death. Phytolaccatoxin and pokeweed mitogen are found in all plant parts, but the highest concentrations are found in the plant root. The mature deep purple berries are less toxic.[246] Pokeweed leaves are consumed following boiling without toxic effect if water is changed between the first and second boiling. When this detoxification technique is not followed—such as in preparation of poke salad or pokeroot tea—violent gastrointestinal effects can ensue 0.5–6 hours after ingestion. Nausea, vomiting, abdominal cramping, diarrhea, hemorrhagic gastritis, and death may occur. In addition, bradycardia and hypotension, perhaps induced by an increase in vagal tone, may be associated with nausea and vomiting.[171,345] More often than not, toxicity is limited to the GI tract. The mitogen produces a lymphocytosis 2–4 days after ingestion that may take up to 10 days to clear, but this is without clinical consequence.

Mistletoe. Mistletoe berries, both American and European, can produce severe gastroenteritis, especially when delivered as teas or extracts, or particularly as parenteral antineoplastic medicinal agents in Europe. As festive holiday plants they become seasonally available for children. Ingestion of more than three to five berries or one to five leaves of the American species may cause toxicity.[234,382] Despite single reports of seizure, ataxia, hepatotoxicity, and death,[168,179,382] most authors performing such retrospective examinations[168,179,250,382] conclude that mistletoe ingestions are not a very consequential risk.

Hypoglycin and Ackee Fruit

Hypoglycin A

Hypoglycin A (β-methylene cyclopropyl-L-α-aminopropionic acid) and hypoglycin B (dipeptide of hypoglycin A and glutamic acid) are found in the unripe fruit (ackee) and seeds of *Blighia sapida* (Euphorbiaceae). The tree is native to Africa but was imported to Jamaica in 1778 by botanist Thomas Clarke. The scientific name of the plant derives from Captain William Bligh, the British explorer.[31] The tree is also naturalized in Central America, southern California, and Florida. Epidemics of illness (Jamaican vomiting sickness) associated with consumption of the unripe fruit (raw and cooked) occur in Africa, but are more common in Jamaica, where it is the national dish.[53,277,396] The most toxic part is the yellow oily aril of the fruit, which contains three large shiny black seeds.[61] Cases in the United States are usually associated with canned fruit.[60,276] Hypoglycin A is metabolized to methylene cyclopropyl acetic acid (MCPA), which competitively inhibits the carnitine-acyl CoA transferase system.[1,30,31] This prevents importation of long-chain fatty acids into the mitochondria, preventing their β-oxidation to precursors of gluconeogenesis. β-Oxidation and gluconeogenesis are further arrested by inhibition of various enzymes,[30,106] such as inhibition of glutaryl CoA dehydrogenase, which blocks the malate shunt (Chap. 13). In addition, increased levels of glutaric acid may inhibit the glutamic acid decarboxylase that produces GABA from glutamic acid. This not only depletes GABA, but also increases levels of excitatory glutamate to produce seizures.[1,211] Insulin levels remain unaffected by hypoglycin

and metabolites.[285] Carboxylic and other organic acid substrates build up in the urine and serum as a result of these metabolic perturbations. Detection of these acids can help corroborate the diagnosis.[150,395]

Jamaican vomiting sickness is characterized by epigastric discomfort and the onset of vomiting starting 2–6 hours after ingestion. Convulsions, coma, and death can ensue, with death occurring approximately 12 hours following consumption. Laboratory findings are notable for profound hypoglycemia with reports of glucose levels close to zero mg/dL, hepatic enzyme and bilirubin abnormalities, and aciduria and acidemia without ketonemia. Cholestatic hepatitis can also occur, and has been reported in chronic use.[250] Autopsy reveals fatty degeneration of liver and other organs with depletion of glycogen stores.[187] Untreated, patient mortality reaches 80%, with 85% of the fatal cases suffering seizures. Anaphylaxis can also occur with exposure to the fruit.[251] Treatment with glucose and fluid replacement is essential. Benzodiazepines can control seizures, perhaps directly if the seizures are related to depletion of GABA. L-Carnitine therapy may exert a theoretical therapeutic role similar to that noted with valproic acid toxicity,[26,106,256] whereas glycine therapy shows some beneficial effects in rats (Chap. 41).[370]

Lathyrins. β-*N*-Oxalylamino-L-alanine (BOAA) and β-aminopropionitrile (BAPN) are peptides from the grass pea (*Lathyrus sativus*) that produce neurolathyrism (seeds) and osteolathyrism (leaves), respectively, in individuals with a dietary dependence on this plant. Neurolathyrism is clinically indistinguishable from spastic paresis associated with consumption of improperly prepared cassava ("Cyanogenic Glycosides: Amygdalin, Linamarin, and (*S*)-Sambunigrin" earlier in this chapter), and thiol oxidation with depletion of nicotinamide adenine dinucleotide (NADH) dehydrogenase at the level of neuronal mitochondria (such as excitatory AMPA receptors) may be the common etiology.[277,312,381,412] Epidemics occur in Bangladesh, Ethiopia, Israel, and India.[144,145,200,258,286] BOAA exposure results in a degeneration of corresponding corticospinal pathways that becomes irreversible if consumption of undetoxified grass peas is not stopped early. BOAA stimulates the α-amino-3-hydroxy-5-methyl-isoxazole-4-propionic acid (AMPA) class of glutamate receptors to provide constant neuronal stimulation, eventual degeneration, and hence, spasticity. BAPN affects bone matrix and leads to bone pain and skeletal deformities that develop in adulthood.[89,174] These diseases occur in areas where the plants are endemic, the food is consumed for 2 months or more, and when diets are otherwise poor in protein and possibly in zinc.[243]

Microcystins. Several Cyanobacteria (blue-green algae) belonging to various species of the genera *Microcystis*, *Anabaena*, *Nodularia*, *Nostoc*, and *Oscillatoria* elaborate a series of peptide toxins called microcystins and nodularins (*Nodularia spumigena*). These compounds produce hepatotoxicity by causing deterioration of the microfilament function in hepatocytes, leading to cell shrinkage and bleeding into the hepatic sinusoids.[45] There is also evidence that these peptides are carcinogenic to humans.[45,93] While most cases of untoward effects from blue-green algae occur in animals, the potential for harm was demonstrated by the use of contaminated water in a dialysis unit in Brazil.[202] Unfiltered water was identified as the risk factor for liver disease in 100 patients who attended the dialysis center (Chap. 6). Fifty of these patients died from acute liver failure following early signs of nausea, vomiting, and visual disturbances. Microcystins were detected in the water of the reservoir and of the dialysis center, as well in serum and liver tissue of the patients. No patients were affected at another dialysis center that used water from the same source but after chlorination and filtration. The concern for poisoning is heightened because certain species of Cyanobacteria are harvested and consumed as health foods.[43,148,209] The chief concern is unintentional inclusion of toxigenic species with the harvested material. In addition to the sodium channel and acetylcholine esterase effects discussed below, ingestion of the genus *Microcystis* is also associated with photosensitization.[124]

Phenols and Phenylpropanoids

Quercetin

Coumarin

These represent one of the largest groups of secondary metabolites. As suggested by their name, the latter compounds contain a phenyl ring attached to a propane side chain, devoid of nitrogen. For instance, one class, the *flavonoids,* have a side chain derived from phenylalanine and another aromatic side chain that is a condensation product of three molecules of malonyl CoA. Flavonoids such as quercetin are among the most widely distributed compounds among plants, with more than 2000 identified either as free compounds or bound as glycosides.

Coumarins and their isomers are lactone phenylpropanoids derived from cinnamic acids produced via the shikimic acid pathway. Some coumarins are warfarinlike in their activity (Chap. 42) and are capable of producing a bleeding diathesis when plants are consumed in large enough quantities.[192,245]

Lignans are formed when phenylpropanoid side chains react to form bisphenylpropanoid derivatives. *Lignins* are high-molecular-weight polymers of phenylpropanoids that bind to cellulose and provide strength to the cell walls of plant stems and bark. *Tannins* are polymers that bind to proteins, and are classified into two groups: hydrolysable or condensed.[109,344] Condensed tannins such as karwinol are termed *proanthocyanidins.*

Capsaicin

Capsaicin

Derived from *Capsicum annuum* or other species of chile or cayenne peppers, capsaicin is a simple phenylpropanoid that causes release of the neuropeptide substance P from sensory C-type nerve fibers. The immediate response to capsaicin is the initial period of intense local irritation and is the rationale for pepper

spray or mace. Eventual depletion of substance P prevents local transmission of pain impulses from these receptors to the spinal cord, blocking perception of pain by the brain. Factors affecting the degree of pain experienced include length of exposure, individual sensitivity, and size of the area of skin involvement.[421,433]

Painful exposures to capsaicin-containing peppers are among the most common plant-related exposures presented to poison centers. They cause burning or stinging pain to the skin, and if ingested in large amounts by adults or small amounts by children, can produce nausea, vomiting, abdominal pain, and burning diarrhea.[92,421,432,433] Eye exposures produce intense tearing, pain, conjunctivitis, and blepharospasm.[405]

Skin irrigation, dermal aloe gel, analgesics, or oral antacids are therapeutic agents that may be helpful as appropriate, but patients can be reassured that the effects are transitory and produce no long-term damage. Irritated eyes can be treated with irrigation and local analgesia, but generally resolve without sequelae within 24 hours.[158,203]

***Karwinskia* Toxins.** Buckthorn, coyotillo, tullidora, wild cherry, or capulincillo are among the many common names for *Karwinskia humboldtiana,* whose toxins are identified by their molecular weights (T-514, T-496, T-516, T-544). Toxicity has been known for more than 200 years. In 1920, an epidemic of deaths was reported after 20% of 106 Mexican soldiers died following ingestion of foraged *Karwinskia* fruits.[215,266] The fruits are attractive to children, and epidemic poisonings have been reported in Central America[11] and are possible wherever the shrub is found (in semidesert areas throughout the southwestern United States and Caribbean, as well as Mexico and Central America). Recently, poisonings from this plant in Mexico have increased from a total of 72 cases reported between 1990 and 1994 to 40 cases a year currently reported in northern Mexico.[266,299] Uncoupling of oxidative phosphorylation or dysfunction of peroxisome assembly and integrity is described for Schwann cells.[418,436] Each toxin exhibits similar cytotoxic effects at the cellular level, but with trophism for different organs in animal models.[266]

Within a few days of ingestion, a symmetric motor neuropathy ascends from the lower extremities to produce a bulbar paralysis that may lead to death. Deep-tendon reflexes are abolished in affected areas, but cranial nerve findings are absent. Distinction of this demyelinating motor neuropathy from Guillain-Barré, poliomyelitis, toxic solvent, and other polyneuropathies is best assisted by detection of T-514 in the blood of the affected patients.[28,215,266] The other recognized toxins are not detected in blood. Occasionally, axonal damage is observed, but demyelination is the predominant finding on biopsy. Nerve-conduction studies always demonstrate loss or abolishment of function in fast-conducting axons. Cerebrospinal fluid demonstrates normal protein, glucose, and cytology. Treatment is supportive, with mechanical ventilation as needed, and recovery typically slow.

Other Phenylpropanoids: Bergamottin/Naringenin, Hyperforin, Asarin, NDGA, and Esculoside

α-Asarone

Nordihydroguaiaretic acid (NDGA)

Esculoside

Other phenylpropanoids include bergamottin and naringenin derived from grapefruit, which are inhibitors of CYP3A4 in gut and liver.[135] Grapefruit juice consumption can increase circulating drug levels, including terfenadine, carbamazepine, felodipine, and some of the other drugs metabolized by that enzyme system. These effects are maximally achieved by a single glass of grapefruit juice.[260] On the other hand, hyperforin, another phenylpropanol, diminished levels of the anti-HIV drug indinavir in a clinical trial on healthy volunteers and of cyclosporin in organ transplant patients. Induction of CYP3A4 has been proposed as the mechanism by which this reduction occurs, although several alternative hypotheses have been suggested.[325,353]

Asarin is found in the sweet flag plant tuber (*Acorus calamus*). Putative euphoric and hallucinogenic effects that motivate ingestion are in contrast to confirmed reports of unpleasant gastrointestinal effects.[417] Hepatotoxicity is associated with ingestions of chaparral (*Larrea tridentata*), which contains nordihydroguaiaretic acid (NDGA),[367,369] and such cases of hepatotoxicity warrant use of *N*-acetylcysteine (Antidotes in Depth: *N*-Acetylcysteine). Podophyllin and psoralens are discussed in the sections "Antimitotic Alkaloids and Resins" and "Plant Dermatitides and Ocular and Local Mucous Membrane Effects" later in this chapter, respectively.

A triterpene saponin, esculoside (also called esculin or aesculin) is believed to be the toxic component in horse chestnut (*Aesculus hippocastanum*). Horse chestnut extracts are used medicinally in venous insufficiency, and its therapeutic use at high doses (>340 µg/kg) is associated with renal failure.[182] A lupuslike syndrome manifested by recurrent fever, myalgias, arthralgias, pleuritis, pericarditis, myocarditis and the presence of antimitochondrial antibodies is reported.[160] Leaves, twigs, or horse chestnuts ingested by children or infused as teas result in a syndrome that resembles nicotine intoxication, including vomiting, diarrhea, muscle twitching, weakness, lack of coordination, dilated pupils, paralysis, and stupor.[297] The mechanism of this toxicity is not defined, but ingestion of chestnut weighing approximately 1% of a child's weight is suggested to be poisonous to a child.[175] Horse chestnut pollen may produce hypersensitivity.[328]

Carboxylic Acids: Oxalic Acid and Oxalate Raphides

Oxalic acid

Oxalic acid is the strongest of the carboxylic acids found in living organisms, and it forms poorly soluble chelates with calcium and other divalent cations. Higher plants vary in their ability to accu-

mulate these products of metabolism. Oxalates are mainly found in certain plant families such as the Araceae, Chenopodiaceae, Polygonaceae, Amaranthaceae, and several of the grass families. Human dietary sources include rhubarb, spinach, strawberries, chocolate, tea, and nuts.[267] The human consumption of soluble oxalate-rich foods correlates with kidney stone formation;[185] however, nephrolithiasis, chronic renal failure, and hypocalcemia are better demonstrated in animals than in people.

The insoluble calcium oxalate raphides that are present in certain plants, usually in the Araceae family, are found in conjunction with a protein toxin that increases the painful irritation to skin or mucous membranes. This special manifestation is covered in more detail under "Plant Dermatitides and Ocular and Local Mucous Membrane Effects" later in this chapter.

Alcohols: Cicutoxin

Cicutoxin

Cicutoxin, a diacetylenic diol, is found in the water hemlock, *Cicuta maculata,* and other *Cicuta spp.* Ingestion of any part of this plant constitutes the most common form of lethal plant ingestion in the United States. In a series of 83 ingestions from 1900–1975, the case fatality rate was 30%, and it dominated plant-related fatalities among the most recent 10-year reviews of the Toxic Exposure Surveillance System (TESS) and Centers for Disease Control (CDC) plant-poisoning records (p. 1752 and Chap. 116).[133,239,284] In contrast to most plant exposures in humans (which tend to be pediatric), these ingestions usually involve adults who incorrectly identify the plant as wild parsnip, turnip, parsley, or ginseng. All plant parts are poisonous at all times, but the tuber is especially toxic, and more so during the winter and early spring.[152,284] Absorption of cicutoxin is rapid and occurs through the skin as well as through the gut.[219] Ingestion of as little as a 2-cm section of the sweet-tasting root of *Cicuta* can produce fatal status epilepticus; a child's use of a stem as a toy whistle caused the child's death. The cause of seizures is not clear but may be from central cholinergic overstimulation, sodium channel effects, or blockade of potassium-dependent channels.[42,48,306,391]

Symptoms of mild or early poisonings consist of gastrointestinal symptoms (nausea, vomiting, epigastric discomfort) and begin as early as 15 minutes after ingestion. Emesis may diminish the toxic load in the gut. Diaphoresis, flushing, dizziness, excessive salivation, bradycardia, hypotension, bronchial secretions with respiratory distress, and cyanosis occur, and rapidly progress to violent seizures that are the probable cause of death. Complications include rhabdomyolysis with renal failure and severe acidemia.[42] Immediate gastric evacuation should be performed by whatever means are available and benzodiazepines should be administered for seizures. In addition, treatments with hemodialysis, anticholinergic therapy, and sodium thiopentone infusion are recommended in separate case reports as potential life-saving measures.[228,306,342,385] Analytical methods are available.[138,379]

Miscellaneous and Unidentified Toxic Ingredients

Fixed Oils

Ricinoleic acid

Fixed oil toxicity is generally not caused by the oils themselves, although there are exceptions. For example, the glycerides of ricinoleic and isoricinoleic acids from castor oil are hydrolyzed in the gut to the purgative ricinoleic acid. The oils usually act as carriers of lipophilic active toxins. For instance, the hypersensitivities associated with the use of castor oil were discussed earlier, and croton oil is a carrier of the skin irritant and tumor-promoting diphorbol esters of the plant *Croton tiglium*.[87]

Sauropus androgynus. In 1994, it became fashionable among Taiwanese to ingest cooked and uncooked *Sauropus androgynus* or "weight-loss vegetables." While indeed an effective dieting agent, its consumption led to over 200 cases of bronchiolitis obliterans. Despite its long history of use in Malaysian cooking, it was used in much smaller quantities. The toxin responsible for producing pulmonary manifestations associated with consumption of *Sauropus androgynus* (Euphorbiaceae) has never been identified. The effects were dose-related—usually about 100 g/d—and manifested themselves by the seventh month after approximately 10 weeks of use.[194] The epidemic was associated with at least four deaths, and, in addition to pulmonary disease, included three cases of torsades de pointes.[62,259,443] This last complication is consistent with the plant's high concentration of papaverine, a toxin that produces dysrhythmias in animals.[441] Steroid and bronchodilator therapy consistently failed to improve symptoms, and lung transplantation remains the only effective treatment for advanced cases.[259]

Tremetone

Tremetone

Milk sickness is the name given to a particular toxidrome caused by transmission of toxins from white snakeroot (*Eupatorium rugosum*) to humans via the milk of grazing animals.[19,20,368] Mary Todd Lincoln experienced it and her symptoms fit the description:

> A patient with milk sickness usually became extremely weak, nauseated, thirsty, and constipated, sometimes with a burning sensation in the stomach. The breath was foul, like turpentine or acetone, a symptom that sometimes occurred even before more obvious signs of illness. Skillful doctors claimed they could smell this distinctive odor as they entered a sickroom. Fever was low or absent, separating milk sickness from malaria, typhoid, and other febrile diseases. Death could come in as little as two days or as late as ten days, or the patient might recover, then relapse and die after exertion. Many, but not all, survivors remained weakened for months or years.[45]

Tremetol, a mixture of novel alcohols concentrated in the leaves, stems, and, possibly, flowers of the plant, was thought for many years to be the toxic entity. Attention has subsequently shifted to the arylene ketone tremetone. The toxicity of tremetone was not established until recently, when it was demonstrated that this nontoxic compound is transformed into a toxic entity by hepatic microsomal enzymes.[20] The structure of the unstable toxin that arises from tremetone has not yet been elucidated, but toxicity is cumulative.

It is one of several natural plant toxicants transmitted in milk, including pyrrolizidine alkaloids, ptaquiloside, and nitrates, that result in methemoglobinemia.[210,316,375] Whether poisoning is caused by ingestion of the plant or toxic milk, white snakeroot produces trembling, sweating, depression, stiff gait, heart failure, cholestatic jaundice, and death in the affected animal. Onset of symptoms occurs in 1 day to 3 weeks, and death is almost certain once symptoms develop.[273,368] This delay in onset of symptoms after ingestion of the plant by the animal causes human consumption of the contaminated milk and fatalities prior to the recognition of the lactating animal's illness.

EFFECTS SHARED BY DIVERSE INGREDIENTS

Plant-Drug Interactions

Hawthorn (*Craetagus spp.*) used medicinally for cardiac disorders may produce an additive effect when taken concomitantly with digoxin, producing bradycardia.[191,271] Excessive intake of broccoli provides enough vitamin K to interfere with coumarin.[80] Hyperforin has been tentatively identified as the compound responsible for the interaction between St. John's wort and indinavir,[350] and cytochrome P450 effects of bergamottin and naringenin from grapefruit were discussed earlier. Identification of active ingredients that cause an increase or decrease in drug effect is rare, although a number of plants have been suggested to cause plant-drug interactions.[80,87,134,177,283,380]

Effectors at Sodium Channels: Alkaloids, Terpenoids, and Guanidinium Compounds

Disturbances of sodium and calcium homeostasis may result in similar clinical presentations. Ironically, this occurs whether the channels become more (aconitine, veratridine) or less (taxine, saxitoxin) permeable to sodium, calcium, or both (grayanotoxin, *Aconitum* alkaloids other than aconitine).

Aconitine

Aconitine

Aconitine from *Aconitum spp.* or *Delphinium spp.* has the most persistent toxicity and lowest therapeutic index among the many active alkaloid ingredients of the toxin called aconite. Some of these related alkaloids are controlled medicinal substances in the People's Republic of China and Taiwan.[91] Aconite is used for its psychoactive effects[112] and for homicide.[445] Properly processed aconite is supposedly less cardiotoxic than unprocessed material, as processing results in the production of the less toxic dehydroaconitine. Because aconite is an increasingly popular Asian herbal medicine and plant exposures occur in non-Asian cultures, suspicion of this ingredient should be raised in potentially poisoned patients who manifest cardiac toxicity, paresthesias, and seizures.[56–59,112,311,404]

The mechanism of action depends on the individual alkaloid. Some compounds block and others activate sodium channels.[6,362] Aconitine itself binds to the voltage-dependent sodium channel at binding site 2 of the α subunit, prolongs sodium current influx, slows repolarization, and permanently activates cardiac muscle and voltage-dependent nervous tissue receptors. It also has calcium channel–opening effects. About 1 teaspoon of the root (2–5 mg) may cause death by paralysis of the respiratory center or cardiac muscle. The alkaloid is used for treatment of dysrhythmias and of pain by producing inexcitable sensory neurons. Central release of acetylcholine may be responsible for bradycardia,[216] but the role of acetylcholine is unclear because aconitine toxicity is successfully treated with both atropine and physostigmine (the latter only reported in animals).[323]

The aconitine alkaloids are rapidly absorbed from the GI tract, and cardiovascular and central nervous system symptoms are usually obvious prior to arrival in the emergency department. Cardiac, central nervous, and gastrointestinal system manifestations are dose dependent and typically progress from bradycardia and hypotension to tachydysrhythmias and cardiac arrest; from paresthesias to CNS depression, respiratory muscle depression, paralysis, and seizures; and from nausea, vomiting, and diarrhea to abdominal cramping, respectively.[56–59,112,229,281,302,311,445] The cardiac toxicity resembles that caused by cardiac glycosides, with atrioventricular conduction blockade and increased ventricular automaticity resulting in a variety of rapid ventricular rates, from multifocal premature ventricular contractions to ventricular fibrillation and torsades de pointes. A history of paresthesias may be useful in differentiating aconitine toxicity from that caused by a cardiac glycoside, but empiric use of digoxin-specific antibodies should not be delayed if there is any doubt. These antibodies, however, are ineffectual against aconitine. Orogastric lavage, activated charcoal, and preparation for cardiac pacing, bypass, or balloon pump assist are warranted given the potential for rapid cardiovascular deterioration.[122,308] Bradycardia is usually responsive to atropine. Use of sodium bicarbonate has theoretical disadvantages given the sodium load in the presence of sodium-channel opening. No controlled clinical trials guide treatment, but there are reports of success with amiodarone.[442] Analytical methods are available, and alkaloids are detectable in serum for the first day postingestion, and in urine for up to 6 days after ingestion.[138,288,307]

Taxine

Taxine A

Taxine is another alkaloid mixture of sodium channel effectors. It is derived from the yew (*Taxus baccata*), an ornamental evergreen shrub with attractive red berries. The yew's toxicity has been known since antiquity—Julius Caesar reported its use for suicide by the king of Eburones.[138] Although a large quantity of leaves is needed to produce poisoning, suicidal death from leaves was described in *Lancet* in 1836,[138] as well as more recently.[294,375,386] Paclitaxel (taxol) is an alkaloid component of the relatively rare Pacific yew (*Taxus brevifolia*) that is used as an antitumor chemotherapeutic agent because of its ability to promote the assembly of microtubules and to inhibit the tubulin disassembly process in mitotic cells.

Taxine's mechanism of action is postulated to be inhibition of both sodium and calcium currents.[317,398] Whereas the fleshy red-orange aril of the fruit is devoid of alkaloid, the alkaloid is contained in the relatively large hard seed within the fruit. Toxicity can occur if whole berries with the seeds are ingested. The low rate of toxicity[235,430] in reported cases is probably related to the presumed small unintentional ingestions by children attracted to the appealing berries. Poisoning from ingestion of other parts of these plants has not been reported in humans, although the veterinary literature is rich with reports of animals poisoned by the plant. Toxicity progresses within an hour after ingestion from nausea, abdominal pain, bradycardia, and cardiac conduction delays to wide-complex ventricular dysrhythmias, paresthesias, ataxia, and mental status changes.[115,305,365] Four prisoners who drank an extract of yew experienced profound hypokalemia and two died from cardiac arrest.[115,365] The ingestion of yew has also been associated with anaphylaxis.[33] Management following poisoning should follow that suggested for aconitine if the findings are suggestive of the toxicity noted with a sodium channel–opening agent. An animal model indicates that bradycardia is responsive to atropine.[332] Analytical methods for the taxines are published and are thus available as diagnostic tools.[138,222]

Veratridine

Veratridine

Use of veratrum alkaloids (from *Veratrum viride*) is also historically grounded in North American plant lore. Its therapeutic use by the apothecary who attended George Washington predates its use by allopathic physicians in the 1950s for its antihypertensive effects. Its use as a test of endurance among American Indian braves and its withdrawal from modern pharmacopoeias were the result of its toxicity.[41,233] In Europe, confusion of veratridine-containing plants with gentian (*Gentiana lutea*) used for teas and wines is a common foraging error because of their similar appearance.[119,141,333] This may account for the high incidence of poisonings by this genus in Europe.[193,201] Inhalational exposures to veratrum alkaloids in commercial European sneezing powders has caused toxicity, particularly in children, and has led to the withdrawal of sneezing powders from the market.[41,125,237] In the United

States, foraging errors result from confusion in appearance of the roots with those of leeks (*Allium porrum*), another member of the lily family.[331]

Veratridine derivatives were used therapeutically or investigationally in the United States as pesticides and for treatment of eclampsia, hypertension, congestive heart failure, and myasthenia gravis.[109,131] Overdoses were more commonly reported when these derivatives were used as pesticides and antihypertensive medications.[41]

Veratridine and related steroidal alkaloids, such as protoveratrine, veratramine, and jervine (from the rhizome of *Veratrum album* and other *Veratrum spp.*), also prolong sodium current and calcium current, and are thus associated with increased levels of excitatory amines.[94,116,278,309,339,414] These effects are not as prolonged as those of aconitine. Although severe toxicity is reported, deaths are rare. Cardiac depression, and not stimulation, is often attributed to the mechanism of veratridine and related alkaloids, but the clinical manifestations among sodium channel effectors are indistinguishable, whether acting by blocking or enhancing ion flow. For instance, some cases of veratridine toxicity suggest either ectopy or increased automaticity similar to that produced by aconitine.[141,264,331] The compound is rapidly absorbed with resultant gastrointestinal distress and vomiting occurring within 30 minutes of ingestion. Bradycardia and hypotension follow, and treatment with atropine and vasopressors is usually successful.[77,199,264]

Zygacine. Toxic effects of veratridine alkaloids, notably vomiting, hypotension, and bradycardia, are also produced by other alkaloid-containing members of the lily family, such as *Zigadenus spp.* (death camus) and probably *Amianthium muscitoxicum* (fly poison). Fatalities among Native Americans in the western United States caused by *Zigadenus* were recorded after interviews conducted in the 19th century.[424] Its toxic principle compound ingredient is a steroidal alkaloid called zygacine.[263] Symptoms begin 1–2 hours after ingestion.[181,383] Based on animal data, it is believed that four to five bulbs—such as a meal of supposed onions—could produce death in a child, although other plant parts are highly toxic and symptoms have been produced with as little as half a bulb.[411,457] Atropine is effective for treatment of bradycardia.

Grayanotoxins

Grayanotoxin

Grayanotoxins (formerly termed andromedotoxins) are a series of 18 toxic diterpenoids present in leaves of the various species of *Rhododendron*, *Kalmia*, and *Leucothoe* (Ericaceae). They exert their toxic effects via sodium channels, which they open or close, depending on the toxin.[298] Grayanotoxin I increases membrane permeability to sodium and affected calcium channels in a manner similar to that of veratridine (and batrachotoxin; Chap. 101).[96,137,217] This toxicity is most clearly seen in poisoning by the honey of plants in the family Ericaceae (Table 78–1), such as *Rhododendron* and *Azalea*, which demonstrate higher concentrations than plant parts.[223] Accounts of poisoning by honey date

back to at least 401 BC, when Xenophon's troops were incapacitated after eating honey made from nectar of *Rhododendron luteum*. These reports are echoed by modern accounts of toxic honey in the same region.[23,143,332,393,422,444] Bradycardia, hypotension, gastrointestinal manifestations, mental status changes ("mad honey"), and seizures are described in patients suffering grayanotoxin toxicity.[156,246]

Antimitotic Alkaloids and Resins

Colchicine

Podophyllotoxin

Consumption of colchicine from plant sources such as autumn crocus (*Colchicum autumnale*) produces a spectrum of symptoms, including nausea, vomiting, watery diarrhea, hypotension, bradycardia, electrocardiogram (ECG) abnormalities, diaphoresis, alopecia, bone marrow depression, renal failure, hepatic necrosis, hemorrhagic pulmonary edema (acute lung injury), convulsions, and death.[4,154,225,280] Colchicine-induced deaths from ingestion of *Gloriosa superba* are the commonest of plant-associated fatalities in Sri Lanka.[118] Confusion of the bulbs or leaves of this plant with those of wild onions or garlic has occurred as a foraging error, while unintentional pediatric consumption, or ingestion with suicidal intent, accounts for the other cases involving morbidity or mortality. The mechanism of toxicity is disruption of microtubule formation in mitotic cells.[22]

Vincristine and vinblastine are two other indole alkaloids that are used as antineoplastics and isolated from the Madagascar periwinkle (*Catharanthus roseus*). No reports of poisoning by these alkaloids following ingestion of the plant could be found, but adverse effects produced by the drugs during chemotherapy are reported (Chap. 47).

Poisoning by podophyllum resin disrupts tubulin formulation to produce multisystem organ failure. Podophyllum resin is the dry, alcoholic extract of the rhizomes and roots of mayapple (*Podophyllum peltatum*). The dry resin consists of up to 20% podophyllotoxin, α- and β-peltatin, desoxypodophyllotoxin, and dehydropodophyllotoxin. These compounds are originally present in the plant as β-D-glucosides. Podophyllum resin containing podophyllin is available by prescription for topical treatment of venereal warts, and its medicinal derivatives, such as etoposide, are used for a range of neoplastic diseases. It is used as a popular traditional Chinese medicine, which may produce toxicity even in "therapeutic" doses.[209] Poisonings are caused by misidentification and adulteration, possibly because the list of common names by which it is known includes mayapple as well as mandrake, wild mandrake, and American and European mandrake.[37,129] Catharsis is prominent after ingestion, but onset of symptoms may be delayed (10 hours in a fatal ingestion[47]). Acute severe sensorimotor neuropathy and bone marrow suppression following transient leukocytosis can occur even after one-time acute exposures, and may be directly related to the inhibition of microtubule assembly. Lethargy, confusion, encephalopathy, autonomic instability, sensory ataxia, and death are described following large exposures.[301] Podophyllum resin is teratogenic by both the oral and dermal routes of exposure, and should never be used in pregnant women. Glutamic acid has been used to prevent vincristine-induced peripheral neuropathy and it would be a reasonable therapy following podophyllin ingestion.[197] Hemoperfusion is reportedly unsuccessful in treatment of podophyllin intoxication.[47]

Plant Dermatitides, and Ocular and Local Mucous Membrane Effects

A large number of plants result in undesirable dermal effects (Chap. 29), and these are the commonest plant-associated reports to US poison centers and occupational health centers. Dermatitides may be categorized[108,287,358,361,390] as those that produce (a) mechanical injury from, for instance, thorns or oxalates (calcium oxalate raphides); (b) irritant dermatitis, such as those caused by contact with phorbol esters, some glycosides, or the phenylpropanoid capsaicin (discussed earlier); (c) allergic dermatitis; and (d) photosensitivity reactions, such as those from phenylpropanoid linear coumarins called psoralens.

There is much overlap between these categories (some plants are capable of producing all types) and clinicians may have difficulty distinguishing between them and skin disorders,[22,268,270] or between them and pseudophytodermatitides caused by arthropods, pesticides, or wax (used in fruit and vegetable packaging).[390] Agents that cause adverse skin reactions would also cause eye and local gastric mucosal irritation.

Mechanical Dermal Injury. Dermatitis from mechanical injury is often combined with primary or allergic contact dermatitis. Stinging nettles (*Urtica dioica* and other species) have a specialized apparatus in the form of an elongated silicious cell (glandular trichome) that acts like a hypodermic syringe to deliver irritant chemicals into the skin. Contact with these stinging hairs shears off the tip of the hair, producing micromechanical injury and releasing irritant contents: acetylcholine, histamine, and 5-OH-tryptamine.[310] A proteinase, mucanain, is released from the barbed trichomes of *Mucuna* species (cowhage),[108] and workers who handpick pineapples are subject to fissuring and loss of fingerprints after bromelain is introduced following dermal abrasion by raphides.[227]

Exposures to commonly available household plants such as dumbcane (*Dieffenbachia spp.*), *Philodendron spp.*,[294] and *Narcissus* bulbs can lead to mechanical injury and painful microtrauma produced by bundles of tiny needlelike calcium oxalate crystals called raphides. Packages of hundreds of raphides called idioblasts contain proteolytic enzymes. *Dieffenbachia* (more than 30 species) exposures are commonly reported household or malicious plant exposures.[10,326] These exposures are rarely serious.[320] When the leaves are chewed, immediate pain and swelling occur. Severe oral exposures can be excruciating and progress to profuse salivation, dysphagia, and loss of speech. Soothing liquids, ice, par-

enteral opioids, corticosteroids, and airway protection may be indicated, but antihistamines contribute little relief. The edema and pain typically take 4–8 days to begin to subside.[246] Ocular exposure to the sap may produce a chemical conjunctivitis, corneal abrasions, and, rarely, permanent corneal opacifications. Exposures to *Caladium spp.* can also be serious for similar reasons. Other exposures to common oxalate raphide-containing household plants in the same family (*Philodendron, Brassaia, Epipremnum aureum, Spathiphyllum,* and *Scheflera spp.*) are not as painful, presumably because the crystals are packaged differently and do not simultaneously deliver proteolytic enzymes. Ingestion is generally associated with the immediate onset of symptoms: mucosal irritation, local swelling, and GI irritation.[227,292] One exception is a report of the death of an 11-month-old following complications arising from esophageal lesions induced by philodendron.[272]

Irritant Dermatitis

Protoanemonin

Sinigrin

Low-molecular-weight substances such as phorbal esters (Euphorbiaceae) and glycoside hydrolysis products (hydrolysis of ranunculin gives rise to protoanemonin and then to anemonin in Ranunculaceae; hydrolysis of sinigrin from various Brassicaceae yields allyl isothiocyanate) may penetrate through the skin directly without preliminary mechanical injury to produce primary contact dermatitis. Although one death as a result of prolonged contact with sinigrin in mustard plaster is reported,[287] exposures to primary irritants in Brassicaceae and Ranuculaceae are usually mild or only of concern in livestock.[39,212,214,263,295,355]

Larger compounds may enter cells via micropunctures. Variations in susceptibility are multifactorial, depending on plant factors, climate, skin anatomy, duration, size, and intensity of exposure. Dermatitis can also occur without contact, and a number of substances are identified as causative agents for airborne contact dermatitis (ABCD). Exposure to these substances leads to swelling of exposed sites, mostly the upper eyelids, neck, exposed extremities, including antecubital fossae, and other skin folds[65,358] (Chap. 29).

On the other hand, the phorbol esters found in spurges (Euphorbiaceae) present a wider range of problems. These plants produce an irritating milky sap that is capable of producing erythema, desquamation, and bullae. The saps of some species are more irritating than others.[104] For instance, the manchineel tree (*Hippomane mancinella*), found in the Caribbean and Florida, was once planted on graves to deter grave robbers, and juice from the tree has been used to brand animals and to blind people.[287] In addition to dermal and ocular injury, ingestion of some spurges can induce severe gastrointestinal injury. Poinsettia (*Euphorbia pulcherrima*), crown-of-thorns (*E. splendens*), candelabra cactus (*E. lacteal*), and pencil tree (*E. tirucalli*) are spurges found in the home as holiday or other ornamentation that rarely produce serious injury, despite reputations to the contrary. The poinsettia plant, for instance, gained a reputation of significant toxicity based on a single, inadequately documented case report from Hawaii in 1919, involving the death of a 2-year-old child. In a subsequent case, an 8-month-old child developed oral mucosal burns after chewing poinsettia.[103] Contact dermatitis, and even GI complaints such as nausea, vomiting, and abdominal pain,[79] are rare findings among the many reported exposures to poinsettia.[238]

Allergic Dermatitis

Urushiols

Allergic contact dermatitis results from type IV hypersensitivity response to plant exposures and, unlike dermatitis caused by primary irritants, requires repeat exposures to the agent before symptoms manifest themselves. The most infamous of these substances are the urushiol oleoresins derived from catechols that are found in *Ginkgo biloba* (Ginkgoaceae), and members of the Proteaceae (eg, *Macadamia integrifolia*) and the Anacardaceae.[108] The latter family is notable because it includes poison ivy (*Toxicodendron radicans*), poison oak (*T. toxicarium, T. diversilobum*), and poison sumac (*T. vernix*),[68,120,121,265,397] as well as mango (*Mangifera indica*), pistachio (*Pistacia vera*), cashew (*Anacardium occidentale*), Indian marking nut "Bhilawanol" (*Semecarpus anacardium*),[151] and others. Upon first exposure, the urushiol resins penetrate the skin and react with proteins to form antigens to which the body forms antibodies. When these antigens are formed following reexposure, a classic allergic reaction ensues, with release of inflammatory mediators and physiologic sequelae, such as urticaria, itching, swelling, and pain. In extreme cases, these reactions can progress to type I hypersensitivity, as demonstrated by a 6% rate of anaphylaxis to mango among 580 patients who had previously had mango-induced contact dermatitis.[7] Cross-reactivity between allergens is possible, and particular vigilance is required in sensitive individuals.[117,172,262] Prevention by removal of exposed objects that act as fomites for the oils and the use of protective ointments is appropriate.[265,420] Therapy includes washing with soap and water and corticosteroid creams, and for those frequently exposed, desensitization (see Chap. 29).[120,289]

Allergic contact dermatitis/urticaria is the most common of the plant-induced occupational injuries. For instance, in the United States, 1 in 3 of 462 floral shops surveyed reported that at least one employee had developed contact dermatitis, while 1% of all patch-tested patients over a 15-year period in Amsterdam showed an allergic response to plants.[358] Reactions are reported following exposure to *Narcissus* and Peruvian lily (*Alstroemeria spp.*). The dry, painfully fissured hyperkeratosis of fingertips ("tulip fingers") observed in horticultural workers chronically handling tulips are a result of exposure to the glycoside tuliposide A.[189] Upon hydrolysis, this compound yields α-methylene-butyrolactone, the true allergen. *Alstroemeria* species, a common ornamental, also contains tuliposide A, and can thus be expected to cause cross-reactive allergic contact dermatitis in people sensitive to tulips. Primin (2-methoxy-6-*n*-pentyl-*p*-benzoquinone) from members of the Primulaceae[22,64,257] was responsible for the most

frequently reported allergic plant dermatitis in northern Europe until workers refused to stock primroses.

The "wood cutters dermatitis" of loggers occurs with the development of sensitivity to compounds in liverwort (*Frullania spp.*) that is cross-reactive to ursinic acid in lichens and mosses found on the wood.[358] In addition, sensitivity to Compositae involves more than 600 sesquiterpene lactones (particularly those with an α-methylene attached to the lactone) in at least 200 of the 25,000 species in the family, and is as ubiquitous as the distribution of species. *Chrysanthemum* allergy is a common occupational hazard in Europe,[164,390] and sensitivity to *Parthenium hysterophorus* in India takes a toll on weedpullers.[408] Cross-reactivity with common weeds such as ragweed (*Ambrosia spp.*) or dandelion (*Taraxaacum spp.*) initiate the risk. A myriad of other types of plants are involved in producing occupational dermatitides.[139,207,208,319,356]

Photosensitivity Dermatitis

Psoralen

A photosensitivity response is produced when compounds such as psoralen (a linear furocoumarin) interacts with sunlight. These photosensitizing agents are activated by ultraviolet A (320–400 nm) to produce singlet oxygen and DNA adducts. In addition to severe sunburnlike symptoms, hyperpigmentation lasting for several months may result from exposure to these compounds. The mechanism by which this reaction is produced is unknown, but it is postulated that depletion of glutathione may indirectly stimulate melanogenesis by disinhibition of the normally suppressant tyrosinase.[90,358]

Primary photosensitization is produced by furanocoumarins that act either by direct contact (absorption through the skin) or by blood-borne transfer to dermal capillary beds following their ingestion.[67] More than 200 of these compounds have been identified in at least 15 plant families, including Compositae, Fabaceae, Rosaceae, Rutaceae (citrus fruits), Solanaceae, and Umbelliferae. Humans using St. John's wort may be susceptible to this syndrome.[98,147,225,248] Although there is a report of a 45-year-old woman who died from complications of severe burns received in a tanning salon following exposure to psoralen,[90] most other human reactions are sequelae to handling of crop plants or retail produce belonging to the Umbelliferae (anise, caraway, carrot, celery, chervil, dill, fennel, parsley, and parsnip), Rutaceae (grapefruit, lemon, lime, bergamot, and orange), Solanaceae (potato), or Moraceae (figs) family.[261,358] Photodermatitis in humans is an epidermal reaction characterized by bullous or vesicular lesions, pigmentation, and erythema. These begin hours after exposure, usually peaking at 12–36 hours and persisting for many days. Healing with characteristic hyperpigmentation is almost pathognomonic.

Hepatogenous photosensitivity is produced when a substance that is normally harmlessly ingested, absorbed, and hepatically excreted gains access to the peripheral circulation through failure of a liver excretion or detoxification mechanism. An example is the photosensitivity that occurs when phylloerythrin, a product of chlorophyll digestion normally eliminated in the bile, accumulates in the blood as a result of liver dysfunction. The cyanobacterium *Microcystis aeruginosa,* as well as the plants *Lantana camara,*

Tribulus terrestris, and *Agave lecheuilla*, are reported to cause this type of photosensitization in animals.[124]

SUMMARY

Plant toxins, as well as therapeutic ingredients, can be organized using a pharmacognosy approach. Examples are provided in which the toxin has therapeutic use (colchicine, taxine, physostigmine, pilocarpine, and others). Some toxins act directly or are metabolized to toxic principals (tremetone), whereas others are toxic through secondary contact in animal meat or milk (coniine, tremetone, nitrates, pyrollizidine alkaloids). This analysis should not lead to the false conclusion that all toxic plants, all toxins in plants, or all toxic mechanisms are known (see the section "Miscellaneous and Unidentified Toxic Ingredients" earlier in this chapter). Some reassurance can be achieved by excluding the exposure to most life-threatening plants and plant toxins or ascertaining whether a common exposure is toxic. This determination can be aided by basic taxonomy while awaiting expert input. Management should balance the relative risks of using invasive gastric emptying and use of activated charcoal if the plant induces sedation or vomiting, or is nontoxic. Potentially fatal ingestions from sodium channel effectors, cicutoxin, or high-dose belladonna alkaloids may require cardiac support devices, dialysis, or physostigmine, respectively, as well as gastric emptying, and similar to ingestion with all life-threatening plant toxins, may warrant use of activated charcoal and other supportive measures. Seizures can be controlled with benzodiazepines as long as it is remembered that some plants have the potential to reduce pyridoxine (Ginkgo seeds) or thiamine (gingolides; ptaquiloside, although its effects are not known in humans), which suggests empiric emergency replacement should seizures be associated with direct ingestion or milk intake. Hepatotoxicity should be treated empirically with *N*-acetylcysteine. Other toxin-specific measures are noted throughout this chapter, but most require supportive management, the intensity of which is dictated by the patient's condition and plant identification. Laboratory diagnostic assays are published for many plant toxins, but in most cases, are impractical to perform.

REFERENCES

1. Addae JT, Melvill GN: A re-examination of the mechanism of ackee induced vomiting sickness. West Ind Med J 1988;37:6–8.
2. Akintonwa A, Tunwashe OL: Fatal cyanide poisoning from cassava-based meal. Hum Exp Toxicol 1992;11:47–49.
3. Albretsen JC, Gwaltney-Brant SM, Khan SA: Evaluation of castor bean toxicosis in dogs: 98 cases. J Am Anim Hosp Assoc 2000;36:229–233.
4. Aleem HM: *Gloriosa superba* poisoning. J Assoc Physicians India 1992;40:541–542.
5. Alexander RF, Forbes GB, Hawkins ES: A fatal case of solanine poisoning. Br Med J 1948;2:518.
6. Ameri A: The effects of Aconitum alkaloids on the central nervous system. Prog Neurobiol 1998;56:211–235.
7. Andre F: Role of new allergens and of allergens consumption in the increased incidence of food sensitizations in France. Toxicology 1994;93:77–83.
8. Ansford AJ, Morris HP: Fatal oleander poisoning. Med J Aust 1981;1:360–362.
9. Aplin PJ, Eliseo T: Ingestion of castor oil plant seeds. Med J Aust 1997;167:260–261.
10. Arditti J, Rodriguez E: *Dieffenbachia*: Uses, abuses, and toxic constituents: A review. J Ethnopharmacol 1982;5:293–302.
11. Ascherio A, Bermudez CS, Garcia D: Outbreak of buckthorn paralysis in Nicaragua. J Trop Pediatr 1992;38:87–89.
12. Australian Broadcasting Corporation: December 30, 1998, http://abc.net.au/ra/newsarchive/1998/dec/rael-30dec1999–74.htm.
13. Bader AA, Kerzner B: Ipecac toxicity in "Munchausen syndrome by proxy." Ther Drug Monit 1999;21:259–260.
14. Bah M, Bye R, Pereda RM: Hepatotoxic pyrrolizidine alkaloids in the Mexican medicinal plant *Pachera candidissima* (*Asteraceae: Senecioneae*). J Ethnopharmacol 1994;43:19–30.
15. Balansard J, Flandrin P: Heterosides of the leaves of the holly tree (*Ilex aquifolium*). Chem Abstr 1951;45:7307.
16. Barker BE, Farnes P, LaMarche PH: Peripheral blood plasmacytosis following systemic exposure to *Phytolacca Americana* (pokeweed). Pediatrics 1966;38:490–493.
17. Barri ME, el Dirdiri NI, Abu Damir H, et al: Toxicity of *Abrus precatorius* in Nubian goats. Vet Hum Tox 1990;32:541–545.
18. Baumann, H: The Greek World in Myth, Art and Literature. Portland, OR, Timber Press, 1993.
19. Beier RC, Norman JO: The toxic factor in white snakeroot: Identity, analysis and prevention. Vet Hum Toxicol 1990;32:81–88.
20. Beier RC, Norman JO, Reagor JC, et al: Isolation of the major component in white snakeroot that is toxic after microsomal activation: Possible explanation of sporadic toxicity of white snakeroot plants and extracts. J Nat Toxins 1993;1:286–293.
21. Berlin R, Smilkstein M: Wormwood Oil@Toxic.ing [abstract]. J Tox Clin Tox 1996;34:583.
22. Bhushan M, Beck MH: Allergic contact dermatitis from primula presenting as vitiligo. Contact Dermatitis 1999;41:292–293.
23. Biberoglu S, Biberoglu K, Biberoglu B: Mad honey [letter]. JAMA 1988;269:1943.
24. Bisset NG: War and hunting poisons of the New World. Part 1. Notes on the early history of curare. J Ethnopharmacol 1992;36:1–26.
25. Blythe WB: Hemlock poisoning, acute renal failure, and the Bible. Ren Fail 1993;15:653.
26. Borum PR: Carnitine. Annu Rev Nutr 1983;3:233–259.
27. Bose TK, Basu RK, Biswas B, et al: Cardiovascular effects of yellow oleander ingestion. J Indian Med Assoc 1999;97:407–410.
28. Bovanova L, Brandsteterova E, Caniova A, et al: High-performance liquid chromatographic determination of peroxisomicine A1 (T-514) in genus *Karwinskia*. J Chromatogr B Biomed Sci Appl 1999;732:405–410.
29. Bramley A, Goulding R: Laburnum "poisoning." Br Med J 1981;283:1220–1221.
30. Bressler R, Corredor C, Brendel K: Hypoglycin and hypoglycin-like compounds. Pharmacol Rev 1969;21:105–127.
31. Bressler R: The unripe ackee—Forbidden fruit. N Engl J Med 1976;295:500–501.
32. Brubacher JR, Padinjarekuttu RR, Bania T, et al: Treatment of toad venom poisoning with digoxin-specific Fab fragments. Chest 1996;10:1282–1288.
33. Burke MJ, Siegel D, Davidow B. Anaphylaxis: Consequence of yew (Taxus) needle ingestion. N Y State J Med 1979;79:1576–1578.
34. Burkhard PR, Burkhardt K, Haenggeli CA, Landis T: Plant-induced seizures: Reappearance of an old problem. J Neurol 1999;246:667–670.
35. Burnham, TH, ed: *Piper methysticum* Frost. The Review of Natural Products. St. Louis, MO, Facts and Comparisons, 1996.
36. Burros M, Jay S: Concern is growing over an herb that promises a legal high. New York Times, April 10, 1996, B1.
37. But PP: Herbal poisoning caused by adulterants or erroneous substitutes. J Trop Med Hyg 1994;97:371–374.
38. Byers VS, Levin AS, Waites LA, et al: A phase I/II study of trichosanthin treatment of HIV disease. AIDS 1990;4:1189–1196.

39. Calnan CD: Contact urticaria from cabbage (*Brassica*). Contact Dermatitis 1981;7:279.

40. Cao G, Prior RL: Anthocyanins are detected in human plasma after oral administration of an elderberry extract. Clin Chem 1999;45:574–576.

41. Carlier P, Efthymiou ML, Garnier R, et al: Poisoning with *Veratrum*-containing sneezing powders. Hum Toxicol 1983;2(2):321–325.

42. Carlton BE, Tufts E, Girard DE: Water hemlock poisoning complicated by rhabdomyolysis and renal failure. Clin Toxicol 1979;14:87–92.

43. Carmichael WW: The toxins of Cyanobacteria. Sci Am 1994:78–86.

44. Carter JH, Goldman P: Bacteria-mediated cyanide poisoning by apricot kernels in children from Gaza. Pediatrics 1981;68:5–7.

45. Duffy DC: Land of milk and poison. Nat Hist 1990;July:4–8.

46. Norton S: Toxic effects of plants. In: Klaassen CD, ed: Casarett & Doull's Toxicology, The Basic Science of Poisons, 5th ed. New York, McGraw-Hill, 1996:841–853.

47. Cassidy DE, Drewry J, Fanning JP: Podophyllum toxicity: A report of a fatal case and a review of the literature. J Toxicol Clin Toxicol 1982;19:35–44.

48. Catterall WA: Neurotoxins that act on voltage-sensitive sodium channels in excitable membranes. Annu Rev Pharmacol Toxicol 1980;20:15–43.

49. Cawte J: Parameters of kava used as a challenge to alcohol. Aust N Z J Psychiatry 1986;20:70–76.

50. Centers for Disease Control: Anticholinergic poisoning associated with an herbal tea—New York City, 1994. MMWR Morb Mortal Wkly Rep 1995;44:193–195.

51. Centers for Disease Control: Jimson weed poisoning—Texas, New York, and California, 1994. Morb Mortal Wkly Rep 1995;44:41–44.

52. Centers for Disease Control: Leads from MMWR. Poisoning from elderberry juice. JAMA 1984;251:2075.

53. Centers for Disease Control: Toxic hypoglycemic syndrome—Jamaica, 1989–1991. Morb Mortal Wkly Rep 1992;41:53–55.

54. Fugr U: Drug interactions with grapefruit juice. Extent, probable mechanism and clinical relevance. Drug Saf 1998;18:251–272.

55. Challoner KR, McCarron MM: Castor bean intoxication. Ann Emerg Med 1990;19:1177–1183.

56. Chan TY, Tomlinson B, Critchley JA, Cockram CS: Herb-induced aconite poisoning presenting as tetraplegia. Vet Hum Toxicol 1994;36:133–134.

57. Chan TY: Aconitine poisoning: A global perspective. Vet Hum Toxicol 1994;36:326–328.

58. Chan TYK, Tomlinson B, Critchley JAJH: Aconitine poisoning following the ingestion of Chinese herbal medicines: A report of eight cases. Aust N Z J Med 1993;23:268–271.

59. Chan TYK, Tomlinson B, Tse LKK, et al: Aconitine poisoning due to Chinese herbal medicines: A review. Vet Human Toxicol 1994;36:452–455.

60. Chase GW Jr, Landen WO Jr, Gelbaum LT, Soliman AG: Ion-exchange chromatographic determination of hypoglycin A in canned ackee fruit. J Assoc Off Anal Chem 1989;72:374–377.

61. Chase GW Jr, Landen WO Jr, Soliman AG: Hypoglycin A content in the aril, seeds, husks of ackee fruit at various stages of ripeness. J Assoc Off Anal Chem 1990;73:318–319.

62. Chen IC, Chang KC, Hsieh YK, Wu D: Torsade de pointes due to consumption of *Sauropus androgynus* as a weight-reducing vegetable. Am J Cardiol 1996;78:1186–1187.

63. Chow LP, Chou MH, Ho CY, et al: Purification, characterization and molecular cloning of trichoanguin, a novel type I ribosome-inactivating protein from the seeds of *Trichosanthes anguina*. Biochem J 1999;338:211–219.

64. Christensen LP, Larsen E: Direct emission of the allergen primin from intact *Primula obconica* plants. Contact Dermatitis 2000;42:149–153.

65. Christensen LP: Direct release of the allergen tulipalin A from Alstroemeria cut flowers: A possible source of airborne contact dermatitis? Contact Dermatitis 1999;41:320–324.

66. Chu NS: Betel chewing increases the skin temperature: Effects of atropine and propranolol. Neurosci Lett 1995;194:130–132.

67. Clare NT: Photosensitization in Diseases of Domestic Animals, Review Series #3 of the Commonwealth Bureau of Animal Health, Commonwealth Agricultural Bureaux, Farnham Royal, Bucks, England, 1952, p. 11.

68. Cohen LM, Cohen JL: Erythema multiforme associated with contact dermatitis to poison ivy: Three cases and a review of the literature. Cutis 1998;62:139–142.

69. Cohen S: Suicide following morning glory seed ingestion Am J Psychiatry 1964;120:1024–1025.

70. Colegate SM, Dorling PR: Bioactive indolizidine alkaloids. In: D'Mello JPF, ed: Handbook of Plant and Fungal Toxicants. Boca Raton, FL, CRC Press, 1997.

71. Cook BA, Sinnhuber JR, Thomas PJ, et al: Hepatic failure secondary to indicine N-oxide toxicity. A Pediatric Oncology Group study. Cancer 1983;52:61–63.

72. Coremans P, Lambrecht G, Shepens P, et al: Anticholinergic intoxication with commercially available thorn apple tea. J Toxicol Clin Toxicol 1994;32:589–592.

73. Cornell J, Weathers P, Pokras M: Poisonous plant identification: A comparison of databases designed for veterinary use. Vet Hum Toxicol 1995;37:482–485.

74. Costa Bou X, Soler I Ros JM, Seculi Palacios JL: Poisoning by *Robinia pseudoacacia*. An Esp Pediatr 1990;32:68–69.

75. Coutinho EM, Athayde C, Atta G, et al: Gossypol blood levels and inhibition of spermatogenesis in men taking gossypol as a contraceptive. A multicenter, international, dose-finding study. Contraception 2000;61:61–67.

76. Cromwell BT: The separation, micro-estimating and distribution of the alkaloids of hemlock (*Conium maculatum* L.). Biochem J 1956;64:259–266.

77. Crummett D, Bronstein D, Weaver Z 3d: Accidental *Veratrum viride* poisoning in three "ramp" foragers. N C Med J 1985;46:469–471.

78. Cumming AM, Boddy K, Brown JJ, et al: Severe hypokalaemia with paralysis induced by small doses of liquorice. Postgrad Med J 1980;56:526–529.

79. D'Archy WG: Severe contact dermatitis from poinsettia. Arch Dermatol 1974;109:909–910.

80. D'Arcy PF: Adverse reactions and interactions with herbal medicines. Part 2—Drug interactions. Adverse Drug React Toxicol Rev 1993;12:147–62.

81. Dalvi RR, Bowie WC: Toxicology of solanine: An overview. Vet Hum Toxicol 1983;25:13–15.

82. Dasgupta A, Hart AP: Rapid detection of oleander poisoning using fluorescence polarization immunoassay for digitoxin. Effect of treatment with digoxin-specific Fab antibody fragment (bovine). Am J Clin Pathol 1997;108:411–416.

83. Davies HH: *Abrus precatorius* (rosary pea): The most common lethal plant poison. J Fla Med Assoc 1978;65:188–191.

84. Davies LP, Drew CA, Duffield PH, et al: Kava pyrones and resin: Studies on GABA$_A$, GABA$_B$, and benzodiazepine binding sites in rodent brain. Pharmacol Toxicol 1992;71:120–126.

85. Davison AG, Britton MG, Forrester JA, et al: Asthma in merchant seamen and laboratory workers caused by allergy to castor beans: Analysis of allergens. Clin Allergy 1983;13:553–561.

86. Deahl M: Betel nut-induced extrapyramidal syndrome: An unusual drug interaction. Mov Disord 1989;4:330–332.

87. De Smet PAGM: Health risks of herbal remedies. Drug Saf 1995;13:81–93.

88. Del Castillo J, Anderson M, Rubottom GM: Marijuana, absinthe and the central nervous system. Nature 1975;253:365–366.

89. Di Cesare PE, Nimni ME, Yazdi M, Cheung DT: Effects of lathyritic drugs and lathyritic demineralized bone matrix on induced and sustained osteogenesis. J Orthop Res 1994;12:395–402.

90. Diawara MM, Trumble JT: Linear furanocoumarins. In: D'Mello JPF, ed. Handbook of Plant and Fungal Toxicants. Boca Raton, FL, CRC Press, 1997.

91. Dickens, P, Tai YT, But PP, et al: Fatal accidental aconitine poisoning following ingestion of Chinese herbal medicine: A report of two cases. Forensic Sci Int 1994;67:55–58.

92. Diehl AK, Bauer RL: Jalaproctitis. N Engl J Med 1978;299:1137–1138.

93. Ding W-X, Shen H-M, Zhur H-G, Lee B-L, Ong C-N: Genotoxicity of microcystic Cyanobacteria extract of a water source in China. Mutat Res 1999;442:69–77.

94. Dobrev D, Milde AS, Andreas K, Ravens U: The effects of verapamil and diltiazem on N-, P- and Q-type calcium channels mediating dopamine release in rat striatum. Br J Pharmacol 1999,127: 576–582.

95. Drummer OH, Roberts AN, Bedford PJ: Three deaths from hemlock poisoning. Med J Aust 1995;162:592–593.

96. Duch DS, Hernandez A, Levinson SR, Urban BW: Grayanotoxin-I-modified eel eletroplax sodium channels. Correlation with batrachotoxin and veratridine modifications. J Gen Physiol 1992:100:623–645.

97. Durakovic Z, Durakovic A, Durakovic S: Oleander poisoning treated by resin haemoperfusion. J Indian Med Assoc 1996;94:149–150.

98. Duran N, Song P-S: Hypericin and its photodynamic action. Photochem Photobiol 1986;43:677–680.

99. Eck J, Langer M, Mockel B, et al: Cloning of the mistletoe lectin gene and characterization of the recombinant A-chain. Eur J Biochem 1999;264:775–784.

100. Eddleston M, Ariaratnam CA, Sjostrom L, et al: Acute yellow oleander (*Thevetia peruviana*) poisoning: Cardiac arrhythmias, electrolyte disturbances, and serum cardiac glycoside concentrations on presentation to hospital. Heart 2000;83:301–306.

101. Eddleston M, Rajapakse S, Rajakanthan, et al: Anti-digoxin Fab fragments in cardiotoxicity induced by ingestion of yellow oleander: A randomized controlled trial. Lancet 2000;355:967–972.

102. Edgerton PH: Symptoms of digitalis-like toxicity in a family after accidental ingestion of lily of the valley plant. J Emerg Nurs 1989;15:220–223.

103. Edwards N: Local toxicity from a poinsettia plant: A case report. J Pediatr 1983;102:404–405.

104. Eke T, Al-Husainy S, Raynor MK: The spectrum of ocular inflammation caused by Euphorbia plant sap. Arch Ophthalmol 2000;118:13–16.

105. Endo Y, Oka T, Turugi K, Franz H: The mechanism of action of the cytotoxic lectin from *Phoradendron californicum*: The RNA N-glycosidase activity of the protein. FEBS Lett 1989;248:115–118.

106. Entman M, Bressler R: The mechanism of action of hypoglycin on long-chain fatty acid oxidation. Mol Pharmacol 1967;3:333–340.

107. Epstein MT, Espiner EA, Donald RA, Hughes H: Liquorice toxicity and the renin-angiotensin-aldosterone axis in man. Br Med J 1977;1:209–210.

108. Evans FJ, Schmidt RJ: Plants and plant products that induce contact dermatitis. Planta Med 1980;4:289–316.

109. Evans WC, ed: Trease and Evans' Pharmacognosy, 14th ed. London, WB Saunders, 1998.

110. Evans WC, Evans IA, Humphreys DJ, et al: Induction of thiamine deficiency in sheep, with lesions similar to those of cerebrocortical necrosis. J Comp Pathol 1975;85:253–267.

111. Farese RV, Biglieri EG, Shackleton CHL, et al: Licorice-induced hyperminerlocorticoidism. N Engl J Med 1991;325:1223–1227.

112. Fatovich DM: Aconite: A lethal Chinese herb. Ann Emerg Med 1992;21:309–311.

113. Food and Drug Administration Center for Food Safety and Applied Nutrition: Minutes of the special working group on stimulant laxative substances in foods of the FDA Food Advisory Committee. http://vm.cfsan.fda.gov/~dms/ds-lax1.html, 1995.

114. Feldman KW, Christopher DM, Opheim KB: Munchausen syndrome/bulimia by proxy: Ipecac as a toxin in child abuse. Child Abuse Negl 1989;13:257–261.

115. Feldman R, Chrobak J, Liberek Z, Szafewski J: 4 cases of poisoning with the extract of yew (*Taxus baccata*) needles. Pol Arch Med Wewn 1988;79:26–29.

116. Ferger B, Boonen G, Haberlein H, Kuschinsky K: In vivo microdialysis study of (+/−)-kavain on veratridine-induced glutamate release. Eur J Pharmacol 1998;347:211–214.

117. Fernandez C, Fiandor A, Marinez-Garate A, Martinez Quesada J: Allergy to pistachio: Cross-reactivity between pistachio nut and other anacradiaceae. Clin Exp Allergy 1995;25:1254–1259.

118. Fernando R, Fernando DN: Poisoning with plants and mushrooms in Sri Lanka: A retrospective hospital-based study. Vet Hum Toxicol 1990;32:579–581.

119. Festa M, Andreetto B, Ballaris MA, Panio A, Piervittori R: A case of Veratrum poisoning. Minerva Anestesiol 1996;62:195–196.

120. Fisher AA: Poison ivy/oak dermatitis. Part I: Prevention-soap and water, topical barriers, hyposensitization. Cutis 1996;57:384–385.

121. Fisher AA: Poison ivy/oak dermatitis. Part II: Specific features. Cutis 1996;58:22–24.

122. Fitzpatrick AJ, Crawford M, Allan RM, Wolfenden H: Aconite poisoning managed with a ventricular assist device. Anaesth Intensive Care 1994;22:714–717.

123. Flach C: A case of morning glory (*Ipomoea*) seed psychosis. Nord Psykiatr Tidsskr 1967;21:313–321.

124. Flaoyen A, Froslie A: Photosensitization disorders. In: D'Mello JPF, ed. Handbook of Plant and Fungal Toxicants. Boca Raton, FL, CRC Press, 1997.

125. Fogh A, Kulling P, Wickstrom E: Veratrum alkaloids in sneezing powder—A potential danger. J Toxicol Clin Toxicol 1983;20:175–179.

126. Forrester RM: Have you eaten laburnum? Lancet 1979;1:1073.

127. Foukaridis GN, Osuch E, Mathibe L, Tsipa P: The ethnopharmacology and toxicology of *Urginea sanguinea* in the Pretoria area. J Ethnopharmacol 1995;49:77–79.

128. Francis PD, Clarke CF: Angel trumpet lily poisoning in five adolescents: Clinical findings and management. J Paediatr Child Health 1999;35:93–95.

129. Frasca T, Brett AS, Yoo SD: Mandrake toxicity. A case of mistaken identity. Arch Intern Med 1997;157:2007–2009.

130. Fraser NC: Accidental poisoning deaths in British children 1958–1977. Br Med J 1980;280:1595–1598.

131. Freis ED: "New" treatment for congestive heart failure. Am Heart J 1979;97:127–128.

132. Frohne D, Pfander HJ: A Colour Atlas of Poisonous Plants. A Handbook for Pharmacists, Doctors, Toxicologists, and Biologists. London, Wolf Publishing Company, 1983.

133. Fugh-Berman A: St. John's wort and major depression. JAMA 2001;286:43–45.

134. Fugh-Berman A: Herb-drug interactions. Lancet 2000;355:134–138.

135. Fugr U: Drug interactions with grapefruit juice. Extent, probable mechanism and clinical relevance. Drug Saf 1998;18:251–272.

136. Furet Y, Ernouf D, Brechot JF, et al: Collective poisoning by flowers of laburnum. Presse Med 1986;15:1103–1104.

137. Furue T, Yakehiro M, Seyama I: Differential effects of lipid-soluble toxins on sodium channels and L-type calcium channels in frog ventricular cells. Hiroshima J Med Sci 1997;46:43–50.

138. Gaillard Y, Pepin G: Poisoning by plant material: Review of human cases and analytical determination of main toxins by high-performance liquid chromatography-(tandem) mass spectrometry. J Chromatogr B Biomed Sci Appl 1999;733:181–229.

139. Garcia M, Fernandez E, Navarro JA, et al: Allergic contact dermatitis from *Hedera helix* L. Contact Dermatitis 1995;33:133–134.

140. Garcia-Gonzalez JJ, Bartolome-Zavala B, Del Mar Trigo-Perez M, et al: Pollinosis to *Ricinus communis* (castor bean): An aerobiological, clinical and immunochemical study. Clin Exp Allergy 1999;29:1265–1275.

141. Garnier R, Carlier P, Hoffelt J, Savidan A: Acute dietary poisoning by white hellebore (*Veratrum album* L.). Clinical and analytical data. Apropos of 5 cases. Ann Med Interne 1985;136:125–128.

142. Gehlbach SH, William WA, Perry LD, et al: Green tobacco sickness: An illness of tobacco harvesters. JAMA 1974;229:1880–1883.

143. Geroulanos S, Attinger B, Cakmakci M: Honey-induced poisoning. Schweiz Rundsch Med Prax 1992;81:535–540.

144. Getahun H, Haimanot RT: Psychosocial assessment of lathyrism patients in rural Esti district of South Gondar, northern Ethiopia. Ethiop Med J 1998;36:9–18.

145. Getahun H, Mekonnen A, Teklehaimanot R, Lambein F: Epidemic of neurolathyrism in Ethiopia. Lancet 1999;354:306–307.

146. Ghosh SK, Gokani VN, Doctor PB, et al: Intervention studies against "green symptoms" among Indian tobacco harvesters. Arch Environ Health 1991;46:316–317.

147. Giese AC: Hypericism. In: Smith KC, ed., Photochem Photobiol Rev, Vol. 5. New York, Plenum Press, 1980, pp. 229–255.

148. Gilroy DJ, Kauffman KW, Hall RA, Huang X, Chu FS: Assessing potential health risks from microcystin toxins in blue-green algae dietary supplements. Environ Health Perspect 2000;108:435–439.

149. Gleeitz J, Beile A, Peters T: (+)-Kawain inhibits veratridine-activated voltage-dependent Na+-channels in synaptosomes prepared from rat cerebral cortex. Neuropharmacology 1995;34(9):1133–1138.

150. Golden KD, Kean EA, Terry SI: Jamaican vomiting sickness: A study of two adult cases. Clin Chim Acta 1984;142:293–298.

151. Goldsmith NR: Dermatitis from *Semecarpus anacardium* (Bhilawanol or the marking nut). JAMA 1957;123:27–28.

152. Gomperzt LM: Poisoning with water hemlock (*Cicuta maculata*). A report of 17 cases. JAMA 1926;87:1277–1278.

153. Goonasekera CD, Vasanthathilake VW, Ratnatunga N, Seneviratne CA: Is Nai Habarala (*Alocasia cucullata*) a poisonous plant? Toxicon 1993;31:813–816.

154. Gooneratne BW: Massive generalized alopecia after poisoning by *Gloriosa superba*. Br Med J 1966;5494:1023–1024.

155. Goss PE, Baptiste J, Fernandes B, et al: A phase I study of swainsonine in patients with advanced malignancies. Cancer Res 1994;54:1450–1457.

156. Gossinger H, Hruby K, Haubenstock A: Cardiac arrhythmias in a patient with grayanotoxin-honey poisoning. Vet Hum Toxicol 1983;25:328–329.

157. Gowdy JM: Stramonium intoxication: A review of symptomatology in 212 cases. JAMA 1972;221:585–587.

158. Grant WM: Toxicology of the Eye, 3rd ed. Springfield, IL, Charles C. Thomas, 1986.

159. Griffin DS, Segall HJ: Genotoxicity and cytotoxicity of selected pyrrolizidine alkaloids, a possible alkenyl metabolite of the alkaloids, and related alkenyls. Toxicol Appl Pharmacol 1986;86:227–234.

160. Grob PJ, Muller-Schoop JW, Hacki MA, Joller-Jemelka HI: Drug-induced pseudolupus. Lancet 1975;2:144–148.

161. Gugliotta G: Health concerns grow over herbal aids. Washington Post, March 19, 2000, A1.

162. Gugliotta G: Woman using herbal aid has stroke. Washington Post, April 20, 2000, A2.

163. Guharoy SR, Barajas M: Atropine intoxication from the ingestion and smoking of Jimson weed (*Datura stromonium*). Vet Hum Toxicol 1991;33:588–589.

164. Guin JD, Beaman JH: Clinics in Dermatology, Vol 4: Plant Dermatitis. Philadelphia, JB Lippincott, 1986.

165. Gupta A, Joshi P, Jortani SA, et al: A case of nondigitalis cardiac glycoside (oleander) toxicity. Ther Drug Monit 1997;19:711–714.

166. Halbig L, Gutmann L,Goebel HH, Brick JF, Schochet S: Ultrastructural pathology in emetine-induced myopathy. Acta Neuropathol 1988;75:577–582.

167. Hall AH, Linder CHJ, Kulig KW, et al: Cyanide poisoning from laetrile ingestion: Role of nitrite therapy. Pediatrics 1986;78: 269–272.

168. Hall AH, Spoerke DG, Rumack BH: Assessing mistletoe toxicity. Ann Emerg Med 1986;105:1320–1323.

169. Haller CA, Benowitz NL: Adverse cardiovascular and central nervous system events associated with dietary supplements containing ephedra alkaloids. N Engl J Med 2000;343:1833–1838.

170. Hamilton RJ, Goldfrank LR: Poison center data and the Pollyanna phenomenon. J Toxicol Clin Toxicol 1997;35:21–23

171. Hamilton RJ, Shih RD, Hoffman RS: Mobitz type I heart block after pokeweed ingestion. Vet Hum Toxicol 1995;37:66–67.

172. Hamilton TK, Zug KA: Systemic contact dermatitis to raw cashew nuts in a pesto sauce. Am J Contact Dermat 1998;9:51–54.

173. Hansen AA: Two fatal cases of potato poisoning. Science 1925;61: 348–349.

174. Haque A, Hossain M, Lambein F, Bell EA: Evidence of osteolathyrism among patients suffering from neurolathyrism in Bangladesh. J Nat Toxins 1997;5:43–46.

175. Hardin JW, Arena JM: Human Poisoning from Native and Cultivated Plants. Kingsport, TN, Duke University Press, 1974.

176. Harkrader RJ, Reinhart PC, Rogers JA, et al: The history, chemistry and pharmacokinetics of Sanguinaria extract. J Can Dent Assoc 1990;56:7–12.

177. Heck AM, DeWitt BA, Lukes AL: Potential interactions between alternative therapies and warfarin. Am J Health Syst Pharm 2000;57: 1221–1227.

178. Hedili A, Warnet JM, Thevenin M, et al: Biochemical investigation of *Atractylis gummifera* L hepatotoxicity in the rat. Biological monitoring of exposures and the response at the subcellular level to toxic substances. Arch Toxicol 1989;13:312–315.

179. Hegde R, Podder SK: A- and B-subunit variant distribution in the holoprotein variants of protein toxin abrin: Variants of abrins I and II have constant toxic A subunits and variant B subunits. Arch Biochem Biophys 1997;344:75–84.

180. Heiligenstein E, Guenther G: Over-the-counter psychotropics: A review of melatonin, St. John's wort, valerian, and kava-kava. J Am Coll Health 1998;46:271–276.

181. Heilpern KL: Zigadenus poisoning. Ann Emerg Med 1995;25: 259–262.

182. Hellberg K, Ruschewski W, de Vivie R: Drug induced acute renal failure after heart surgery. Scanning Microsc 1975;23:396–399.

183. Henry GW, Schwenk GR, Bohnert GA: Umbrellas and mole beans: A warning about acute ricin poisoning. J Indiana State Med Assoc 1981;74:572–573.

184. Hess T, Stucki P, Barandum S, et al: Treatment of a case of lanatoside C intoxication with digoxin-specific F(ab)2 antibody fragments. Am Heart J 1979;98:767–771.

185. Hesse A, Siener R, Heynck H, Jahnen A: The influence of dietary factors on the risk of urinary stone formation. Scanning Microsc 1993;7:1119–1127.

186. Hill KR, Bras G, Clearkin KP: Acute toxic hypoglycemia occurring in the vomiting sickness of Jamaica. Morbid anatomical aspects. West Indian Med J 1955;33:323–328.

187. Hintz HF, Thompson LJ: Custer, selenium and swainsonine. Vet Hum Toxicol 2000;42:242–243.

188. Hirashiki I, Ogata F, Yoshida N, et al: Purification and complex formation analysis of a cysteine proteinase inhibitor (cystatin) from seeds of *Wisteria floribunda*. J Biochem 1990;108:604–608.

189. Hjorth N, Wilkinson DS: Contact dermatitis. IV. Tulip fingers, hyacinth itch and lily rash. Br J Dermatol 1968; 80:696–698.

190. Ho PC, Dweik R, Cohen MC. Rapidly reversible cardiomyopathy associated with chronic ipecac ingestion. Clin Cardiol 1998;2: 780–783.

191. Hobbs C, Foster S: Hawthorn: A literature review. HerbalGram 1990;22:19–33.

192. Hogan III RP: Hemorrhagic diathesis caused by drinking an herbal tea. JAMA 1983;49:2679–2680.

193. Hruby K, Lenz K, Kerausler J: *Veratrum album* poisoning (Austrian Poison Information Centre). Wien Klin Wochenschr 1981;93: 517–519.

194. Hsiue TR, Guo YL, Chen KW, et al: Dose-response relationship and irreversible obstructive ventilatory defect in patients with consumption of *Sauropus androgynus*. Chest 1998;113:71–76.

195. Hudak KA, Wank P, Tumer NE: A novel mechanism for inhibition of translation by pokeweed antiviral protein: Depurination of the capped RNA template. RNA 2000;6:369–380.

196. Ingram AL Jr: Morning glory seed reaction. JAMA 1964;190: 1133–1134.

197. Jackson DV, Rosenbaum DL, Carlisle LJ, et al: Glutamic acid modification of vincristine toxicity. Cancer Biochem Biophys 1984,7. 245–252.

198. Jacobs KM, Hirsch KA: Psychiatric complications of ma-huang. Psychosomatics 2000;41:58–62.

199. Jaffe AM, Gephardt D, Courtemanche L: Poisoning due to ingestion of *Veratrum viride* (false hellebore). J Emerg Med 1990;8:161–167.

200. Jahan K, Ahmad K: Studies on neurolathyrism. Environ Res 1993; 60:259–266.

201. Jaspersen-Schib R, Theus L, Guirguis-Oeschger M, et al: Serious plant poisonings in Switzerland 1966–1994. Case analysis from the Swiss Toxicology Information Center. Schweiz Med Wochenschr 1996;126:1085–1098.

202. Jochimsen EM, Carmichael WW, An JS, et al: Liver failure and death after exposure to microcystins at a hemodialysis center in Brazil. N Engl J Med 1998;338:873–878.

203. Jones LA, Tandberg D, Troutmann WG: Household treatment for "chile burns" of the hands. J Toxicol Clin Toxicol 1987;25:483–491.

204. Jussogie A, Scmiz A, Heimke C: Kava pyrone extract enriched from *Piper methysticum* as modulator of the GABA binding site in different regions of the rat brain. Psychopharmacology 1994;116: 469–474.

205. Kahn JO, Kaplan LD, Gambertoglio JG, et al: The safety and pharmacokinetics of GLQ223 in subjects with AIDS and AIDS-related complex: A phase I study. AIDS 1990;4:1197–1204.

206. Kalix P: The pharmacology of psychoactive alkaloids from Ephedra and Catha. J Ethnopharmcol 1991;32:201–208.

207. Kanerva L, Alanko K, Pelttari M, Estlander T: Occupational allergic contact dermatitis from Compositae in agricultural work. Contact Dermatitis 2000;42:238–239.

208. Kanerva L, Makinen-Kiljunen S, Kiistala R, Granlund H: Occupational allergy caused by spather flower (*Spathiphyllum wallisii*). Allergy 1995;50:174–178.

209. Kao WF, Hung DZ, Tsai WJ, Lin KP, Deng JF: Podophyllotoxin intoxication: Toxic effect of Bajiaolian in herbal therapeutics. Hum Exp Toxicol 1992;11:480–487.

210. Kaplan M, Vreman HJ, Hammerman C, et al: Favism by proxy in nursing glucose-6-phosphate dehydrogenase-deficient neonates. J Perinatol 1998;18:477–479.

211. Kean EA: Commentary on a review on the mechanism of ackee-induced vomiting sickness. West Indian Med J 1988;37:139–141.

212. Kelch WJ, Kerr LA, Adair HS, Boyd GD: Suspected buttercup (*Ranunculus bulbosus*) toxicosis with secondary photosensitization in a Charolais heifer. Vet Hum Toxicol 1992;34:238–239.

213. Kennelly EJ, Flynn TJ, Mazzola EP, et al: Detecting potential teratogenic alkaloids from blue cohosh rhizomes using an in vitro rat embryo culture. J Nat Prod 1999;62:1385–1389.

214. Kern JR, Cardellina JH 2d: Native American medicinal plants. Anemonin from the horse stimulant *Clematis hirsutissima*. J Ethnopharmacol 1983;8:121–123.

215. Kim HL, Stipanovic RD: Isolation of karwinol A from coyotillo (*Karwinskia humboldtiana*) fruits. In: Garland T, Barr AC, eds:

Toxic Plants and Other Natural Toxicants. New York, CAB International, 1998.

216. Kimura I, Takada M, Hojima H: Aconitine induces bradycardia through a transmission pathway including the anterior hypothalamus in conscious mice. Biol Pharm Bull 1997;20:856–860.

217. Kimura T, Kinoshita E, Yamaoka K, et al: On-site of action of grayanotoxin in domain 4 segment 6 of rat skeletal muscle sodium channel. FEBS Lett 2000;465:18–22.

218. Kinamore PA: Abrus and ricinus ingestion: Management of three cases. Clin Toxicol 1980;17:401–405.

219. King LA, Lewis MJ, Parry D, Twitchett PJ, Kilner EA: Identification of oenanthotoxin and related compounds in hemlock water dropwort poisoning. Hum Toxicol 1985;4:355–364.

220. Kingsbury JM: Phytotoxicology I: Major problems associated with poisonous plants. Clin Pharmacol Ther 1969;10:163–169.

221. Kingsbury JM: Poisonous Plants in the United States and Canada. Englewood Cliffs, NJ, Prentice-Hall, 1964.

222. Kite GC, Lawrence TJ, Dauncey EA: Detecting Taxus poisoning in horses using liquid chromatography/mass spectrometry. Vet Hum Toxicol 2000;42:151–154.

223. Klein-Schwartz W, Litovitz T: Azalea toxicity: An over-rated problem? J Toxicol Clin Toxicol 1985;23:91–101.

224. Klein-Schwartz, Oderda GM: Jimson weed intoxication in adolescents and young adults. Am J Dis Child 1984;138:737–739.

225. Klintschar M, Beham-Schmidt C, Radner H, et al: Colchicine poisoning by accidental ingestion of meadow saffron (*Colchicum autumnale*): Pathological and medicolegal aspects. Forensic Sci Int 1999;106:191–200.

226. Knight B: Ricin: A potent homicidal poison. Br Med J 1979;1: 350–351.

227. Knight TE: Philodendron-induced dermatitis: Report of cases and review of the literature. Cutis 1991;48:375–378.

228. Knutsen OH, Pazkowski P: New aspects in the treatment of water hemlock poisoning. J Toxicol Clin Toxicol 1984;22:157–166.

229. Kolev ST, Leman P, Kite GC, et al: Toxicity following accidental ingestion of Aconitum containing Chinese remedy. Hum Exp Toxicol 1996;15:839–842.

230. Kondo T, Mizukami H, Takeda T, Ogihara Y: Amino acid sequences and ribosome-inactivating activities of karasurin-B and karasurin-C. Biol Pharm Bull 1996;19:1485–1489.

231. Kopferschmitt J, Flesch F, Lungnier A, et al: Acute voluntary intoxication by ricin. Hum Toxicol 1983;2:239–242.

232. Krakauer J: Into the Wild. New York, Doubleday, 1996.

233. Kreig MB: Green Medicine. Chicago, Rand-McNally, 1975.

234. Krenzelok EP, Jacobsen TD, Aronis J: American mistletoe exposures. Am J Emerg Med 1997;15:516–520.

235. Krenzelok EP, Jacobsen TD, Aronis J: Is the yew really poisonous to you? J Toxicol Clin Toxicol 1998;36:219–223.

236. Krenzelok EP, Jacobsen TD, Aronis JM: Lily of the valley (*Convallaria majalis*) exposures: Are the outcomes consistent with the reputation [abstract]? J Toxicol Clin Toxicol 1996; 34:601.

237. Krenzelok EP, Jacobsen TD, Aronis JM: Hemlock ingestions: The most deadly plant exposures [abstract]. J Toxicol Clin Toxicol 1996; 34:601–602.

238. Krenzelok EP, Jacobsen TD, Aronis JM: Poinsettia exposures have good outcomes—Just as we thought. Am J Emerg Med 1996;14: 671–674.

239. Krenzelok EP, Jacobsen TD: Plant exposures—A national profile of the most common plant genera. Vet Hum Toxicol 1997;39: 248–249.

240. Lachman MF, Romeo R, McComb RB: Emetine identified in urine by HPLC, with fluorescence and ultraviolet/diode array detection, in a patient with cardiomyopathy. Clin Chem 1989;35:499–502.

241. Lacomis D: Case of the month. June 1996—Anorexia nervosa. Brain Pathol 1996;6:535–536.

242. Laidlaw PP: The action of some isoquinoline derivatives. Biochem J 1910;5:243–265.

243. Lambein F, Haque R, Khan JK, et al: From soil to brain: Zinc deficiency increases the neurotoxicity of *Lathyrus sativus* and may affect the susceptibility for the motorneuronal disease neurolathyrism. Toxicon 1994;32:461–466.

244. Lamminpaa A, Kinos M: Plant poisonings in children. Hum Exp Toxicol 1996;15:245–249.

245. Lamnaouer D: Anticoagulant activity of coumarins from *Ferula communis* L. Therapie 1999;54:747–751.

246. Lampe KF: Rhododendrons, mountain laurel, and mad honey. JAMA 1988;259:2009.

247. Landolt G, Feige K, Schoberl M: Poisoning of horses by the back of the false acasia. Schweiz Arch Tierheilkd 1997;139:363–366.

248. Lane-Brown MM: Photosensitivity associated with herbal preparations of St. John's wort. Med J Aust 2000;172:302.

249. Langford SD, Boor PJ: Oleander toxicity: An examination of human and animal toxic exposures. Toxicology 1996;109:1–13.

250. Larson J, Vender R, Camuto P: Cholestatic jaundice due to ackee fruit poisoning. Am J Gastroenterol 1994;89:1577–1578.

251. Lebo DB, Ditto AM, Boxer MB, et al: Anaphylaxis to ackee fruit. J Allergy Clin Immunol 1996;98:997–998.

252. Lemaigre G, Tebbi Z, Galinsky R, et al: Hepatite fulminante par intoxication due au chardon a glu (*Atractylis gummifera* L.). Nouvelle Presse Med 1975;4:2865–2868.

253. Levin Y, Sherer Y, Bibi H, et al: Rare *Jatropha multifida* intoxication in two children. J Emerg Med 2000;19:173–175.

254. Lewis WH, Elvin-Lewis MPF: Medical Botany: Plants Affecting Man's Health. New York, John Wiley & Sons, 1977.

255. Lietava J: Medicinal plants in a Middle Paleolithic grave: Shanidar IV? J Ethnopharmacology 1992;35:263–266.

256. Lieu YK, Hsu BY, Price WA, et al: Carnitine effects on coenzyme A profiles in rat liver with hypoglycin inhibition of multiple dehydrogenases. Am J Physiol 1997;272:E359–E366.

257. Lleonart Bellfill R, Casas Ramisa R, Nevot Faolco S: Primula dermatitis. Allergol Immunopathol (Madr) 1999;27:29–31.

258. Ludolph AC, Spencer PS: Toxic models of upper motor neuron disease. J Neurol Sci 1996;139:53–59.

259. Luh SP, Lee YC, Chang YL, et al: Lung transplantation for patients with end-stage *Sauropus androgynus*-induced bronchiolitis obliterans (SABO) syndrome. Clin Transplant 1999;13:496–503.

260. Lundahl JU, Regardh CG, Edgar B, Johnsson G: The interaction effect of grapefruit juice is maximal after the first glass. Eur J Clin Pharmacol 1998;54:75–81.

261. Lutchman L, Inyang V, Hodgkinson D: Phytophotodermatitis associated with parsnip picking. J Accid Emerg Med 1999;16:453–454.

262. Maillard H, Machet L, Meurisse Y, et al: Cross-allergy to latex and spinach. Acta Derm Venereol 2000;80:51.

263. Makeiff D, Majak W, McDiarmid RE, Reaney B, Benn MH: Determination of zygacine in *Zygadenus venenosus* (Death camas) by image analysis on thin-layer chromatography. J Agric Food Chem 1997;45:1209–1211.

264. Marinov A, Koev P, Mirchev N: Electrocardiographic studies of patients with acute hellebore (*Veratrum album*) poisoning. Vutr Boles 1987;26:36–39.

265. Marks JG Jr, Fowler JF Jr, Sheretz EF, Rietschel RL: Prevention of poison ivy and poison oak allergic contact dermatitis by quaternium-18 bentonite. J Am Acad Dermatol 1995;33:212–216.

266. Martinez HR, Bermudez MV, Rangel-Guerra RA, de Leon Flores L: Clinical diagnosis in *Karwinskia humboldtiana* polyneuropathy. J Neurol Sci 1998;154:49–54.

267. Massey LK, Sutton RAL: Modification of dietary oxalate and calcium reduces urinary oxalate in hyperoxaluric patients with kidney stones. J Am Diet Assoc 1993;93:1305–1307.

268. Massmanian A: Contact dermatitis due to *Euphorbia pulcherrima Willd*, simulating a phototoxic reaction. Contact Dermatitis 1998;38:113–114.

269. McGee D, Brabson T, McCarthy J, Picciotti M: Four-year review of cigarette ingestions in children. Pediatr Emerg Care 1995;11:13–16.

270. McGovern TW, LaWarre SR, Brunette C: Is it, or isn't it? Poison ivy look-a-likes. Am J Contact Dermat 2000;11:104–110.

271. McGuffin M, Hobbs C, Upton R Goldberg A, eds: American Herbal Products Association's Botanical Safety Handbook. Boca Raton, FL, CRC Press, 1997.

272. McIntire MS, Guest JR, Porterfield JF: Philodendron—An infant death. J Toxicol Clin Toxicol 1990;28:177–183.

273. McKeever GE: Milk sickness: A disease of the Middle West. Mich Med 1973;72:775–780.

274. McKinney PE, Gomez HF, Phillips S, Brent J: The fax machine: A new method of plant identification [letter]. J Toxicol Clin Toxicol 1993;31:663–665.

275. McMillan M, Thompson JC: An outbreak of suspected solanine poisoning in schoolboys: Examination of solanine poisoning. Q J Med 1979;48:227–243.

276. McTague JA, Forney R Jr: Jamaican vomiting sickness in Toledo, Ohio. Ann Emerg Med 1994;23:1116–1118.

277. Meda HA, Diallo B, Buchet JP, et al: Epidemic of fatal encephalopathy in preschool children in Burkina and consumption of unripe ackee (Blighia sapida) fruit. Lancet 1999;353:536–540.

278. Meder W, Fink K, Zentner J, Gothert M: Calcium channels involved in K+- and veratridine-induced increase of cytosolic calcium concentration in human cerebral cortical synaptosomes. J Pharmacol Exp Ther 1999;290:1126–1131.

279. Mejia MJ, Morales MM, Llopis A, Martinez I: School children poisoning by ornamental trees. Aten Primaria 1991;8:88, 90–91.

280. Mendis S: Colchicine cardiotoxicity following ingestion of *Gloriosa superba* tubers. Postgrad Med J 1989;65:752–755.

281. Merchant HD, Choksi ND, Ramamoorthy K, et al: Aconite poisoning and cardiac arrhythmias. Report of 3 cases. Indian J Med Sci 1963;17:857.

282. Meschler JP, Howlett AC: Thujone exhibits low affinity for cannabinoid receptors but fails to evoke cannabimimetic responses. Pharmacol Biochem Behav 1999;62:473–480.

283. Miller LG: Herbal medicinals: Selected clinical considerations focusing on known or potential drug-herb interactions. Arch Intern Med 1998;158:2200–2211.

284. Miller MM: Water hemlock poisoning. JAMA 1933;101:852–853.

285. Mills J, Melville GN, Bennett C, et al: Effect of hypoglycin A on insulin release. Biochem Pharmacol 1987;36:495–497.

286. Misra UK, Sharma VP, Singh VP: Clinical aspects of neurolathyrism in Unnao, India. Paraplegia 1993;31:249–254.

287. Mitchell J, Rook A: Botanical Dermatology: Plants and Plant Products Injurious to the Skin. Vancouver, BC, Canada, Greenglass Ltd, 1979.

288. Mizugaki M, Ito K, Ohyama Y, et al: Quantitative analysis of Aconitum alkaloids in the urine and serum of a male attempting suicide by oral intake of aconite extract. J Anal Toxicol 1998;22:336–340.

289. Moe JF: How much steroid for poison ivy? Postgrad Med 1999;106:21–24.

290. Moertel CG, Fleming TR, Rubin J, et al: A clinical trial of amygdalin (Laetrile) in the treatment of human cancer. N Engl J Med 1982;306:201–206.

291. Morkovsky O, Kucera J: Mass poisoning of children in a nursery school by the seeds of *Laburnum anagyroides*. Cesk Pediatr 1980;35:284–285.

292. Mrvos R, Dean BS, Krenzelok EP: Philodendron/dieffenbachia ingestions: Are they a problem? J Toxicol Clin Toxicol 1991;29:485–491.

293. Muller JL: Love potions and the ointment of witches: Historical aspects of the nightshade alkaloids. J Toxicol Clin Toxicol 1998;36:617–627.

294. Musshoff F, Jacob B, Fowinkel C, Daldrup T: Suicidal yew leaves ingestion—Phloroglucindimethylether (3,5-dimethylphenyl) as a marker for poisoning from *Taxus baccata*. Int J Legal Med 1993;106:45–50.

295. Nachman RJ, Olsen JD: Ranunculin: A toxic constituent of the poisonous range plant bur buttercup (*Ceratocephalus testiculatus*). J Agric Food Chem 1983;31:1358–1360.

296. Nadir A, Agrawal S, King PD, Marshall JB: Acute hepatitis associated with the use of a Chinese herbal product, ma-huang. Am J Gastroenterol 1996;91:1436–1438.

297. Nagy M: Human poisoning from horse chestnuts. JAMA 1973;226:213.

298. Narahashi T: Modulators acting on sodium and calcium channels: Patch-clamp analysis. Adv Neurol 1986;44:211–224.

299. Nava ME, Castellanos JL, Casteneda ME: Geographical factors in the epidemiology of intoxication with *Karwinskia* (tullidora) in Mexico. Cad Saude Publica 2000;16:255–260.

300. Navarro-Rouimi R, Charpin D: Anaphylactic reaction to castor bean seeds. Allergy 1999;54:1117.

301. Ng THK, Chan YW, Yu YL, et al: Encephalopathy and neuropathy following ingestion of a Chinese herbal broth containing podophyllin. J Neurol Sci 1991;101:107–113.

302. Nielsen I, Pedersen RS: Life-threatening hypokalaemia caused by liquorice ingestion. Lancet 1984;1:1305.

303. Nishiguchi M, Yoshida K, Sumizono T, Tazaki K: Studies by site-directed mutagenesis of the carbohydrate-binding properties of a bark lectin from *Robinia pseudoacacia*. FEBS Lett 1997;403:294–298.

304. Nogue S, Sanz P, Botey A et al: Insuffance renale aigue due a une inoxication par le chardon a glu (*Atractylis gummifera* L.) [letter]. Presse Med 1992;21:130.

305. Nora M, Elsner G, Purdy C, Zipes DP: Wide QRS rhythm due to taxine toxicity. J Cardiovasc Electrophysiol 1993;4:59–61.

306. North DS, Nelson RB; Anticholinergic agents in cicutoxin poisoning. West J Med 1985;143:250.

307. Ohta H, Seto Y, Tsunoda N: Determination of Aconitum alkaloids in blood and urine samples. I. High-performance liquid chromatographic separation, solid-phase extraction and mass spectrometric confirmation. J Chromatogr B Biomed Sci Appl 1997;691:351–356.

308. Ohuchi S, Izumoto H, Kamata J, Kawase T, et al: A case of aconitine poisoning saved with cardiopulmonary bypass. Kyobu Geka 2000;53:541–544.

309. Okuyama K, Kiuchi S, Okamoto M, et al: T-477, a novel Ca 2+ and Na+ channel blocker, prevents veratridine-induced neuronal injury. Eur J Pharmacol 2000;398:209–216.

310. Oliver F, Amon EU, Breathnach A, et al: Contact urticaria due to the common stinging nettle (*Urtica dioica*)—Histological, ultrastructural and pharmacological studies. Clin Exp Dermatol 1991;16:1–7.

311. Ortuno AF, Salaverria GI, Vazquez RS, Blesa Malpica AL: Fatal poisoning caused by aconitine alkaloid. Rev Clin Esp 1999;199:861.

312. Pai KS, Ravidranath V: L-BOAA induces selective inhibition of brain mitochondrial enzyme, NADH-dehydrogenase. Brain Res 1993;621:215–221.

313. Palatnick W, Tenebein M: Hepatotoxicity from castor bean ingestion in a child. J Toxicol Clin Toxicol 2000;38:67–69.

314. Palmer M, O'Donnell R, Ye M. Kava's methysticin: Protection from strychnine and veratridine [abstract]. J Toxicol Clin Toxicol 1999;35:609.

315. Palmer M, Rao RB: Problems evaluating contamination of dietary supplements [letter]. N Engl J Med 1999;340:568.

316. Panter KE, James LF: Natural plant toxicants in milk: A review. J Anim Sci 1990;68:892–904.

317. Panter KE, Molyneux RJ, Smart RA, et al: English yew poisoning in 43 cattle. J Am Vet Assoc 1993;202:1476–1477.

318. Patil BC, Sharma RP: Evaluation of solanine toxicity. Food Cosmet Toxicol 1972;10:395–398.

319. Paulsen E, Skov PS, Andersen KE: Immediate skin and mucosal symptoms from pot plants and vegetable in gardeners and greenhouse workers. Contact Dermatitis 1998;39:166–170.

320. Pedaci L, Kernzelok EP, Jacobsen TD, Aronis J: Dieffenbachia species exposures: An evidence-based assessment of symptom presentation. Vet Hum Toxicol 1999;41:335–358.

321. Pentore R, Venneri A, Nichelli P: Accidental choke-cherry poisoning: Early symptoms and neurological sequela of an unusual case of cyanide intoxication. Ital J Neurol Sci 1996;17:233–235.

322. Pereira CA, Nishioka S de D: Poisoning by the use of Datura leaves in a homemade toothpaste. J Toxicol Clin Toxicol 1994;32:329–331.

323. Pfister JA, Panter KE, Manners GD, Cheney CD: Reversal of tall larkspur (*Delphinium barbeyi*) poisoning in cattle with physostigmine. Vet Hum Toxicol 1994;36:511–514.

324. Phillips BJ, Hughes JA, Phillips JC, et al: A study of the toxic hazard that might be associated with the consumption of green potato tops. Food Chem Toxicol 1996;34:439–448.

325. Piscitelli SC, Burstein AH, Chaitt D, et al: Indinavir concentrations and St. John's wort. Lancet 2000;355:547–548.

326. Pohl RW: Poisoning by Dieffenbachia. JAMA 1961;177:812–813.

327. Polunin I: Pineapple dermatosis Br J Dermatol 1951;63:441–455.

328. Popp W, Horak F, Jager S, et al: Horse chestnut (*Aesculus hippocastanum*) pollen: A frequent cause of allergic sensitization in urban children. Allergy 1992;47:380–383.

329. Powell T, Hsu FF, Turk J, Hruska K: Ma-huang strikes again: Ephedrine nephrolithiasis. Am J Kidney Dis 1998;32:153–159.

330. Prance G: The poisons and narcotics of the Amazonian Indians. J R Coll Physicians Lond 1999;33:368–376.

331. Prince LA, Stork CM: Prolonged cardiotoxicity from poison lily. Vet Hum Toxicol 2000;42:282–285.

332. Quandt SA, Arcury TA, Preisser JS, Norton D, Austin C: Migrant farmworkers and green tobacco sickness: New issues for an understudied disease. Am J Ind Med 2000;37:307–315.

333. Quatrehomme G, Bertrand F, Chauvet C, Ollier A: Intoxication from *Veratrum album*. Hum Exp Toxicol 1993;12:111–115.

334. Radford DJ, Gillies AD, Hinds JA, Duff P: Naturally occurring cardiac glycosides. Med J Aust 1986;144:540–544.

335. Raffauf RF: A Handbook of Alkaloids and Alkaloid-Containing Plants. New York, Wiley-Interscience, 1970.

336. Rajamohan F, Venkatachlam TK, Irvin JD, Uckun FM: Pokeweed antiviral protein isoforms PAP-I, PAP-II, and PAP-III depurinate RNA of human immunodeficiency virus (HIV)-1. Biochem Biophys Res Commun 1999;260:453–458.

337. Rao RB, Hoffman RS, Desiderio R, et al: Nicotinic toxicity from tincture of blue cohosh (*Caulophyllum thalictroides*) used as abortifacient [abstract]. J Toxicol Clin Toxicol 1998;36:455.

338. Rauber A, Heard J: Castor bean toxicity re-examined. Vet Hum Toxicol 1985;27:498–502.

339. Ravens U, Himmel HM: Drugs preventing Na+ and Ca2+ overload. Pharmacol Res 1999;39:167–174.

340. Rich SA, Libera JM, Locke RJ: Treatment of foxglove extract poisoning with digoxin-specific Fab fragments. Ann Emerg Med 1993;22:1904–1907.

341. Richards HG, Stephens A: A fatal case of laburnum seed poisoning. Med Sci Law 1970;10:260–266.

342. Rizzi D, Basile L, DiMaggio A, et al: Clinical spectrum of accidental hemlock poisoning: Neurotoxic manifestations, rhabdomyolysis and acute tubular necrosis. Nephrol Dial Transplant 1991;6:939–943.

343. Rizzi D, Basile L, DiMaggio A, et al: Rhabdomyolysis and acute tubular necrosis in coniine (hemlock) poisoning. Lancet 1989;2:1461–1462.

344. Robbers JE, Speedie MK, Tyler VE, eds: Pharmacognosy and Pharmacobiotechnology. Baltimore, MD, Williams & Wilkins, 1996.

345. Roberge R, Brader E, Martin ML, et al: The root of evil pokeweed intoxication. Ann Emerg Med 1986;15:470–473.

346. Rodrigues TD, Johnson PN, Jeffrey LP: Holly berry ingestion: Case report. Vet Hum Toxicol 1984;26:157–158.

347. Rondeau ES: Wisteria toxicity. J Toxicol Clin Toxicol 1993;31:107–112.

348. Rosenblatt M, Mindel J. Spontaneous hyphema associated with ingestion of *Ginkgo biloba* extract. N Engl J Med 1997;336:1108.

349. Roulet M, Laurini R, Rivier L, Calame A: Hepatic veno-occlusive disease in newborn infant of a woman drinking herbal tea. J Pediatr 1988;112:433–436.

350. Rowin J, Lewis SL. Spontaneous bilateral subdural hematomas associated with chronic *Ginkgo biloba* ingestion. Neurology 1996;46:1775–1776.

351. Ruangkanchanasetr S, Wananukul V, Suwanjutha S: Cyanide poisoning, 2 case reports and treatment review. J Med Assoc Thai 1999;82:S162–S167.

352. Rubino MJ, Davidoff F: Cyanide poisoning from apricot seeds. JAMA 1979;241:359.

353. Ruschitzka F, Meier PJ, Turnina M, et al: Acute heart transplant rejection due to Saint John's wort. Lancet 2000;355:548–549.

354. Safadi R, Levy I, Amitai Y, et al: Beneficial effect of digoxin-specific Fab antibody fragments in oleander intoxication. Arch Intern Med 1995;155:2121–2125.

355. Sanchez-Guerrero IM, Escudero AI: Occupational contact dermatitis to broccoli. Allergy 1998;53:621–622.

356. Sanchez-Perez J, Garcia-Diez A: Occupational allergic contact dermatitis from eugenol, oil of cinnamon and oil of cloves in a physiotherapist. Contact Dermatitis 1999;41:346–347.

357. Sandvig K, van Deurs B: Endocytosis and intracellular transport of ricin: Recent discoveries. FEBS Lett 1999;452:67–70.

358. Santucci B, Picardo M: Occupational contact dermatitis to plants. Clin Dermatol 1992;10:157–165.

359. Saraswat DK, Garg PK, Saraswat M: Rare poisoning with *cerebra thevetia* (yellow olcander). Review of 13 cases of suicidal attempt. J Assoc Physicians India 1992;40:628–629.

360. Saravanapavananthan N, Ganeshamoorthy J: Yellow oleander poisoning—A study of 170 cases. Forensic Sci Int 1988;36:247–250.

361. Sasseville D: Phytodermatitis. J Cutan Med Surg 1999;3:263–279.

362. Sauviat MP: Effect of neurotoxins on the electrical activity and contraction of the heart muscle. C R Seances Soc Biol Fil 1997;191:451–471.

363. Scatizzi A, Di Maggio A, Rizzi D, et al: Acute renal failure due to tubular necrosis caused by wildfowl-mediated hemlock poisoning. Ren Fail 1993;15:93–96.

364. Schiff RJ, Wurzel CL, Brunson SC, et al: Death due to chronic syrup of ipecac use in a patient with bulimia. Pediatrics 1986;78:412–416.

365. Schulte T: Lethal intoxication with leaves of the yew tree. Arch Toxicol 1975;34:153–158.

366. Sen S, Talukder G, Sharma A: Betel cytotoxicity. J Ethnopharmacol 1989;26:217–247.

367. Shad JA, Chinn CG, Brann OS: Acute hepatitis after ingestion of herbs. South Med J 1999;92:1095–1097.

368. Sharma OP, Dawra RK, Kurade NP, Sharma PD: A review of the toxicosis and biological properties of the genus Eupatorium. J Nat Toxins 1998;6:1–14.

369. Heikh NM, Philen RM, Love LA: Chaparral-associated hepatotoxicity. Arch Intern Med 1997;157:913–919.

370. Sherratt HAS, Al-Bassam SS: Glycine in ackee poisoning [letter]. Lancet 1976;2:1243.

371. Shervette RE 3d, Schydlower M, Lampe RM, et al: Jimson "loco" weed abuse in adolescents. Pediatrics 1979;63:520–523.

372. Shragg TA, Albertson TE, Fisher CJ Jr: Cyanide poisoning after bitter almond ingestion. West J Med 1982;136:65–69.

373. Shumaik GM, Wu AW, Ping AC, et al: Oleander poisoning: Treatment with digoxin-specific FAB antibody. Ann Emerg Med 1988;17:732–735.

374. Singh R, Faridi MM, Singh K, Siddiqui R, Bhatt N, Karna S: Epidemic dropsy in the eastern region of Nepal. J Trop Pediatr 1999;45:8–13.

375. Sinn LE, Porterfield JF: Fatal taxine poisoning from yew leaf ingestion. J Forensic Sci 1991;36:599–601.

376. Slifman NR, Obermeyer WR, Aloi BK, et al: Contamination of botanical dietary supplements by *Digitalis lanata*. N Engl J Med 1998;339:806–811.

377. Smith BL: The toxicity of bracken fern (genus Pteridium) to animals and its relevance to man. In: D'Mello JPF, ed: Handbook of Plant and Fungal Toxicants. Boca Raton, FL, CRC Press, 1997.

378. Smith EA, Mellan CE, Pickell JA, Oehme FW: Scopolamine poisoning from homemade "moon flower" wine. J Anal Toxicol 1991;15:216–219.

379. Smith RA, Lewis D: Cicuta toxicosis in cattle: Case history and simplified analytical method. Vet Hum Toxicol 1987;29:240–241.

380. Smolinske SC: Dietary supplement-drug interactions. J Am Med Womens Assoc 1999;54:191–192, 195.

381. Spencer PS: Food toxins, AMPA receptors and motor neuron diseases. Drug Metab Rev 1999;31:561–587.

382. Spiller HA, Willias DB, Gorman SE, Sanftleban J: Retrospective study of mistletoe ingestion. J Toxicol Clin Toxicol 1996;34:405–408.

383. Spoerke DG, Spoerke SE: Three cases of Zigadcnus (death camus) poisoning. Vet Hum Toxicol 1979;21:346–347.

384. Sriram K, Shankar SK, Boyd MR, Ravindranath V: Thiol oxidation and loss of mitochondrial complex I precede excitatory amino acid-mediated neurodegeneration. J Neruosci 1998;18:10287–10296.

385. Starreveld E, Hope E: Cicutoxin poisoning (water hemlock). Neurology 1975;25:730–734.

386. Stebbing J, Simmons HL, Hepple J: Deliberate self-harm using yew leaves (*Taxus baccata*). Br J Clin Pract 1995;49:101.

387. Stegelmeier BL, Edgar JA, Colegate SM, et al: Pyrrolizidine alkaloid plants, metabolism and toxicity. J Nat Toxins 1999;8:95–116.

388. Stickel F, Egerer G, Seitz HK: Hepatotoxicity of botanicals. Public Health Nutr 2000;3:113–124.

389. Stirpe F: Mistletoe toxicity. Lancet 1983;1:295.

390. Stoner JG, Rasmussen JE: Plant dermatitis. J Am Acad Dermatol 1983;9:1–15.

391. Strauss U, Wittstock U, Schubert R, et al: Cicutoxin from *Cicuta virosa*—A new and potent potassium channel blocker in T lymphocytes. Biochem Biophys Res Commun 1996;219:332–336.

392. Suchard JR, Wallace KL, Gerkin RD: Acute cyanide toxicity caused by apricot kernel ingestion. Ann Emerg Med 1998;32:742–744.

393. Sutlupinar N, Mat A, Satganoglu Y: Poisoning by toxic honey in Turkey. Arch Toxicol 1993;67:148–150.

394. Taitzoglou IA, Tsantarliotou M, Kouretas D, Kokolis NA: Gossypol-induced inhibition of plasminogen activator activity in human and ovine acrosomal extract. Andrologia 1999;31:355–359.

395. Tanaka K, Isselbacker KJ, Shih V: Isovaleric and alpha methylbutyric acidemias induced by hypoglycin A: Mechanism of Jamaican vomiting sickness. Science 1972;175:69–71.

396. Tanaka K, Kean EA, Johnson B: Jamaican vomiting sickness. N Engl J Med 1976;295:461–467.

397. Tanner TL: Rhus (*Toxocodendron*) dermatitis. Prim Care 2000;27:493–502.

398. Tekol Y, Kameyama M: Electrophysiology of the mechanisms of action of the yew toxin, taxine, on the heart. Arzneimittelforschung 1987;37:428–431.

399. Thabet H, Brahmi N, Amamou M, et al: Datura stramonium poisonings in humans. Vet Hum Toxicol 1999;41:320–321.

400. Theoharides TC: Sudden death of a healthy college student related to ephedrine toxicity from a ma huang-containing drink. J Clin Psychopharmacol 1997;17:437–439.

401. Thompson CJS: Poisons and Poisoners. New York, Macmillan, 1931.

402. Thyagarajan D, Day BJ, Wodak J, et al: Emetine myopathy in a patient with an eating disorder. Med J Aust 1993;159:757–760.

403. Iongson J, Salen P: Mass ingestion of Jimson Weed by eleven teenagers. Del Med J 1998;70:471–476.

404. Tomassoni AJ, Snook CP, McConvill BJ, Siegel EG: Recreational use of delphinium—An ancient poison revisited [abstract]. J Toxicol Clin Toxicol 1996;121:598.

405. Tomlinack RL, Spyker DA: Capsicum and capsaicin—A review: Case report of the use of hot peppers in child abuse. J Toxicol Clin Toxicol 1987;25:591–601.

406. Tongcok Y, Kozan O, Cavdar C, Guven H, Fowler J: *Urginea maritime* (squill) toxicity. J Toxicol Clin Toxicol 1995;33:83–86.

407. Topping MND, Henderson RTS, Luczynska CM, et al: Castor bean allergy among workers in the felt industry. Allergy 1982;37:603–608.

408. Towers GHN, Mitchell JC: The current status of the weed *Parthenium hysterophorus* as cause of allergic contact dermatitis. Contact Dermatitis 1983;9:465–469.

409. Townsend WA, Boni B: Cyanide poisoning from ingestion of apricot kernels. MMWR Morb Mortal Wkly Rep 1975;24:428.

410. Trabattoni G, Visintini D, Terzano GM, et al: Accidental poisoning with deadly nightshade berries: A case report. Hum Toxicol 1984;3:513–516.

411. Tracqui A, Kintz P, Branche F, Ludes B: Confirmation of oleander poisoning by HPLC/MS. Int J Legal Med 1998;111:32–34.

412. Tugrul L: Abuse of henbane by children in Turkey. Bull Narc 1985;37:75–78.

413. Tyler VE: The Honest Herbal—A Sensible Guide to the Use of Herbs and Related Remedies, 3rd ed. New York, Pharmaceutical Products Press, 1993.

414. Ulbricht W: Effects of veratridine on sodium currents and fluxes. Rev Physiol Biochem Pharmacol 1998;133:1–54.

415. Vahedi K, Domigo V, Amarenco P, Bousser MG: Ischaemic stroke in a sportsman who consumed ma huang extract and creatine monohydrate for body building. J Neurol Nuerosurg Psychiatry 2000;68:112–113.

416. Vale S: Subarachnoid haemorrhage associated with *Ginkgo biloba*. Lancet 1998;352:36.

417. Vargas CP, Wolf LR, Gamm SR, Koontz K: Getting to the root (*Acorus calamus*) of the problem. J Toxicol Clin Toxicol 1998;36:259–260.

418. Vargas-Zapata R, Torres-Gonzalez V, Sepulveda-Saavedra J, et al: Peroxicomicine A1 (plant toxin-514) affects normal peroxisome assembly in the yeast *Hansenula polymorpha*. Toxicon 1999;37:385–398.

419. Vetter J: Plant cyanogenic glycosides. Toxicon 2000;38:11–36.

420. Vidmar DA, Iwane MK: Assessment of the ability of the topical skin protectant (TSP) to protect against contact dermatitis to urushiol (Rhus) antigen. Am J Contact Dermat 1999;10:190–197.

421. Vogl TP: Treatment of Hunan hand [letter]. N Engl J Med 1982;306:178.

422. Von Malottki K, Wiechmann HW: Acute life-threatening bradycardia: Food poisoning by Turkish wild honey. Dtsch Med Wochenschr 1996;121:936–938.

423. Wada K, Ishigaki S, Ueda K, Sakata M, Haga M: An antivitamin B6, 4'-methoxypyridoxine, from seed of *Ginkgo biloba* L. Chem Pharm Bull 1985;33:3555–3557.

424. Wagstaff DJ, Case AA: Human poisonings by Zigadenus. J Toxicol Clin Toxicol 1987;25:361–367.

425. Wagstaff DJ, Lellinger DB, Wiersema JH: Retrospective searching for poisonous plant vouchers. Vet Hum Toxicol 1999;41:158–161.

426. Wagstaff DJ, Raisbeck M, Wagstaff AT: Poisonous plant information system (PPIS). Vet Hum Toxicol 1989;31:237–238.

427. Wagstaff DJ, Wiersema JH, Lellinger DB: Poisonous plant vouchers. Vet Hum Toxicol 1999;41:162–164.

428. Wagstaff DJ: Genesis to genesis: A historic perspective of plant toxicology. In: Garland T, Barr AC, eds: Toxic Plants and Other Natural Toxicants. New York, CAB International, 1998.

429. Waud RA: A digitalis-like action of extracts made from holly. J Pharmacol Exp Ther 1932;45:279.

430. Wax PM, Cobaugh DJ, Lawrence RA: Should home ipecac-induced emesis be routinely recommended in the management of toxic berry ingestions? Vet Hum Toxicol 1999;41:394–397.

431. Wedin GP, Neal JS, Everson GW, et al: Castor bean poisoning. Am J Emerg Med 1986;4:259–261.

432. Weidner J: Possible harmful effects from a capsaicin base aerosol dog repellent. Vet Hum Toxicol 1980;22:18–19.

433. Weinberg RB: Hunan hand [letter]. N Engl J Med 1981;305:1020.

434. Weisbord SD, Soule JB, Kimmel PL: Poison online—Acute renal failure caused by oil of wormwood purchased through the Internet. N Engl J Med 1997;337:825–827.

435. West LG, McLaughlin JL, Eisenbeiss GK: Saponins and triterpenes from *Ilex opaca*. Phytochemistry 1977;16:1846–1847.

436. Wheeler MH, Camp BJ: Inhibitory and uncoupling actions of extracts from *Karwinskia humboltiana* on respiration and oxidative phosphorylation. Life Sci 1971;10:41–51.

437. Whelan FJ, Bennett FW, Moeller WS: Morning glory seed intoxication: A case report. J Iowa Med Society 1968;58:946–948.

438. WHO International Programme on Chemical Safety: Pyrrolizidine Alkaloids. Geneva, World Health Organization, 1988, p. 61

439. Wilson B: The rise and fall of laetrile. Nutr Forum 1988;5:33–40.

440. Wilson D, Donaldson LJ, Sepai O: Should we be frightened of bracken? A review of the evidence. J Epidemiol Community Health 1998;52:812–817.

441. Wilson RF, White CW: Serious ventricular dysrhythmias after intracoronary papaverine. Am J Cardiol 1988;62:1301–1302.

442. Winslow E: Hemodynamic and arrhythmogenic effects of aconitine applied to the left atria of anesthetized cats. Effects of amiodarone and atropine. J Cardiovasc Pharmacol 1981;3:87–100.

443. Wu C-L, Hsu W-H, Chiang C-D, et al: Lung injury related to consuming *Sauropus androgynus* vegetable. J Toxicol Clin Toxicol 1997;35:241–248.

444. Yavuz H, Ozel A, Akkus I, Erkul I: Honey poisoning in Turkey. Lancet 1991;337:789–790.

445. Yoshioka N, Gonmori K, Tagashira A, et al: A case of aconitine poisoning with analysis of aconitine alkaloids by GC/SIM. Forensic Sci Int 1996;81:117–123.

446. Zaacks SM, Klein L, Tan CD, et al: Hypersensitivity myocarditis associated with ephedra use. J Toxicol Clin Toxicol 1999;37:485–489.

G. HEAVY METALS

CHAPTER **79** ## ARSENIC

Marsha Ford

Arsenic (inorganic)
MW	=	74.9 daltons
Normal range (whole blood)	=	<5 µg/L
	=	<0.665 µmol/day
Normal range (24 h urine)	=	<50 µg/day
	=	<6.65 µmol/day
Action level (24 h urine)	=	>100 µg/day
	=	>13.3 µmol/day

Values greater than or equal to the action level necessitate clinical intervention. Values less than this level may necessitate intervention based on the clinical condition of the patient.

A 55-year-old Asian female was hospitalized for diarrhea, nausea, vomiting, and weakness of unknown etiology. The patient had diabetes and had been in her usual state of health until 5 weeks earlier when, after eating noodle paste, she and her husband developed persistent nausea, vomiting, and diarrhea. Both were admitted with dehydration and hypokalemia and treated for 1 week. On discharge, the patient's weakness necessitated the use of a cane for walking. Approximately 3 weeks later, the patient's husband complained of weakness, then vomited and had a syncopal episode. He was resuscitated with intravenous (IV) fluids and admitted to the hospital. The following day he suddenly became hypotensive, had a cardiopulmonary arrest, and died. Four days later, the wife again developed nausea, vomiting, diarrhea, and weakness. She also noted numbness in her hands and feet, described as "pins and needles." She distinguished this from the numbness in her toes previously ascribed to diabetic neuropathy. The patient had also been bedridden for the past 10 days because of weakness and inability to walk. There were no further neurologic complaints.

Her past medical history revealed adult onset diabetes for 3 years, hypertension, and an episode of an unknown heart dysrhythmia. Her medications included NPH insulin, digoxin, ranitidine, multivitamins, and thiamine. There was no history of alcohol abuse. Review of systems was pertinent for a 20-lb weight loss over the past month and diffuse tissue swelling. Physical examination revealed a weak Asian female lying in bed. Vital signs were blood pressure, 120/75 mm Hg; pulse, 90 beats/min; respirations, 20 breaths/min; and temperature, 100.4°F (38°C). Examination of the head, ears, eyes, nose, and throat demonstrated periorbital edema and bilateral carotid bruits. Lungs were clear to auscultation, and the cardiac examination revealed normal rate with a 2/6 systolic ejection murmur radiating to the aortic region. Abdominal examina-

tion revealed mild distension with bowel sounds present, with no tenderness or organomegaly. Pulses were 1+ in all the extremities. Neurologic exam revealed orientation to person, place, and time; cranial nerves II–XII intact; motor examination with muscle strength 4–5/5 except for quadriceps and iliopsas strength of 3/5 bilaterally; and deep tendon reflexes 1+ biceps with absent brachioradialis, knee, and ankle reflexes. Plantar reflexes were normal. Sensory examination revealed absent position sense, decreased vibration and pinprick in the lower extremities, and decreased vibration, position sense, and pinprick in the upper extremities.

During the next 3 days the patient's muscle strength diminished in a caudal-to-rostral pattern, and she was transferred to the intensive care unit (ICU) with a diagnosis of Guillain-Barré syndrome. Review of the records from the first hospitalization revealed a prolonged QTc interval on routine electrocardiogram (ECG) and a finding of mild hypotension requiring 6 days of intravenous crystalloid infusions, an unusual requirement for the presumed diagnosis of gastroenteritis. In the ICU, laboratory examination revealed a hemoglobin (Hb) of 8.1 g/dL, with a mean corpuscular volume (MCV) of 93.3 µm^3, and a white blood count (WBC) of 2400 cells/mm^3. Other laboratory tests were within normal limits, including serum iron, cortisol, vitamin B$_{12}$, folate, and thyroid function tests. Westergren sedimentation rate was normal at 19 mm/h. Her ECG demonstrated a normal sinus rhythm, QRS axis of +60 degrees, and a QTc of 0.61 seconds. Lumbar puncture measured a normal opening pressure of 135 mm H$_2$O and the cerebrospinal fluid (CSF) contained 5 WBC/mm^3, 0 red blood cells (RBC)/mm^3, protein 0.42 g/L, and glucose 98 mg/dL. Radiopaque material was noted on a plain abdominal radiograph. The toxicologic consultant ordered a stat spot urine for arsenic, which measured 16,422 µg/L. The patient underwent chelation therapy until the urinary arsenic was less than 50 µg /L.

During recovery the patient experienced extreme pain with even light touch to the extremities. Ten months later the patient had gradually recovered from her peripheral neuropathy to the point that she could feed herself.

Arsenic is a metalloid that exists in multiple forms: elemental, gaseous (arsine), organic, and inorganic (As(III) [trivalent, or arsenite] and As(V) [pentavalent, or arsenate]). Sources of and facts about arsenic are listed in Tables 79–1 and 79–2. This chapter discusses the properties and toxicity of inorganic arsenic, the most prevalent toxic form. Arsenic metal is considered nonpoisonous because of its insolubility in water or bodily fluids,[146] and the toxicity of exogenous organic forms is low. The gaseous form, which is highly toxic, is discussed in Chap. 25.

HISTORY/EPIDEMIOLOGY

Arsenicals in the form of arsphenamine for syphilis and Fowler solution for asthma once featured prominently in a physician's therapeutic armamentarium, and today arsenic continues to fill a therapeutic need in the form of melarsoprol for trypanosomiasis and rarely arsenic trioxide for acute promyelocytic leukemia (discussed below). Arsenic poisoning can be unintentional, iatrogenic, suicidal, homicidal, occupational, or environmental.[66,81,82,105,120] Mass poisonings have occurred. Nearly 400 residents of Hong

TABLE 79–1.   Sources of Arsenic Exposure

Inorganic
  Occupational/manufacturing
    Animal feed (additive)
    Brass/bronze
    Ceramics/glass
    Computer chips
    Dyes/paints
    Electron microscopy
    Fireworks (Chinese)
    Fossil fuel combustion—coal
    Herbicides
    Insecticides/pesticides
    Metallurgy
    Mining
    Rodenticides
    Semiconductors (gallium arsenide)
    Smelting—copper, lead, zinc, sulfide minerals
    Soldering
    Wood preservatives
  Medicines/contaminated drugs
    Chemotherapy (acute promyelocytic leukemia)
    Depilatory
    Herbals/alternative medicines
    Homeopathic remedies
    Kelp
    "Moonshine" ethanol
    Opium
  Other
    Contaminated well water
Organic
  Melarsoprol (trypanocidal)
  Parasitic therapy (veterinary)
  Seafood (arsenobetaine)

TABLE 79–2.   Established Standards for Occupational Arsenic Exposure

	Arsenic
MW	74.9 daltons
MCL	10 ppb
Occupational	
ACGIH	
TLV-TWA	0.01 mg/m³
(elemental, inorganic compounds, arsenous acid, arsenic acid)	
TLV-STEL	Not established
OSHA	
PEL-TWA	
• Organic compounds	0.5 mg/m³
• Inorganic compounds	0.01 mg/m³
PEL-STEL	Not established
NIOSH	
REL-TWA	Not established
REL-STEL (inorganic compounds)	0.02 mg/m³ (15-minute ceiling)

ACGIH = American Conference of Governmental Industrial Hygienists; OSHA = Occupational Safety and Health Administration; NIOSH = National Institute for Occupational Safety and Health; MW = molecular weight; MCL = maximum contaminant level of drinking water, US Environmental Protection Agency; TLV = threshold limit values; TWA = time weighted average; STEL = short-term exposure limit; PEL = permissible exposure limits; REL = recommended exposure limits.

Kong fell ill after eating contaminated bread from the Esing Bakery in 1857; two bakery foremen are thought to have tampered with the recipe![64] In England, the Staffordshire Beer Epidemic saw 6000 beer drinkers fall ill and 70 die from beer brewed with sugar made with arsenic contaminated sulfuric acid.[143] In 1998, nearly 70 people were poisoned by eating maliciously contaminated curry at a festival in Wakayama, Japan.

Contaminated soil, water, and food are the primary sources of arsenic for the general population. Pentavalent arsenic is the most common inorganic form in the environment.[35] The primary form of arsenic in seafood is an organic arsenical, arsenobetaine, although arsenosugars can be found in crustaceans and seaweed[97]; less than 1% is inorganic arsenic.[41] However, inorganic arsenic is found in larger amounts in other foodstuffs, such as rice and produce.[147]

In the past 2 decades, consumption of contaminated water has emerged as the primary cause of large-scale outbreaks of chronic arsenic toxicity. Arsenic leaches from various minerals and ores as well as from industrial waste.[66] In Bangladesh, millions of people have been poisoned by drinking water from tubewells contaminated with arsenic leached from ground minerals.[153] Ironically, the wells were dug to obtain safer groundwater. Hydroarsenicism has also been reported in Chile, Taiwan, Thailand, India, Mexico, and Argentina. In the United States, the Environmental Protection Agency recommended, and President Clinton signed, a regulation to decrease the maximum contaminant level (MCL) of arsenic in drinking water from 50 parts per billion (ppb) (0.050 mg/L) to 10 ppb (0.010 mg/L).[43] This recommendation was made after applying statistical models to data compiled in a study of the risk of bladder and lung cancer in a Taiwanese population.[24,43] Extrapolating these data and models to the United States population, the currently acceptable level of 50 ppb appears to be associated with an increased risk of lung and bladder cancer. This level of 10 ppb is also in line with the World Health Organization provisional guide limit. After further review, the Environmental Protection Agency ultimately adopted the MCL of 10 ppb in October 2001.

PHARMACOLOGY

Arsenic has limited therapeutic uses in humans. Melarsoprol (Mel B; Arsobal), the arsenoxide derivative of an organic arsenical, is used to treat the meningoencephalitic stage of West African (Gambian) and East African (Rhodesian) trypanosomiasis. The drug concentrates in trypanosomes via a purine transporter. Its target is trypanothione, the primary reducing agent in trypanosomes. Melarsoprol binds to trypanothione to produce *Mel T*, a competitive inhibitor of trypanothione reductase that is responsible for maintaining adequate levels of trypanothione. The resulting decrease in trypanothione leads to a loss of reducing capacity with subsequent lysis of the parasite.[163]

More recently, arsenic trioxide (As_2O_3) (Trisenox) has emerged as a treatment for relapsed acute promyelocytic leukemia (APL)[154] and is being investigated for treatment of other malignancies.[21] Daily intravenous doses of 10–15 mg, or 0.15 mg/kg, are administered initially, with subsequent daily intravenous courses consisting of 0.15 mg/kg administered for 25 days per course. It induces nonterminal APL cell differentiation,[187] proteolytic degradation of the *PML-RAR-α* fusion gene that results from the chromosomal translocation characteristic of APL,[150] and apoptosis in leukemic cells by inducing procaspases 2 and 3 and the activation of caspases 1 and 3.[154]

PHARMACOKINETICS/TOXICOKINETICS

Inorganic arsenic is tasteless and odorless and is well absorbed by the gastrointestinal, respiratory, intravenous, and mucosal routes. Gastrointestinal (GI) absorption is facilitated by increased solubility and smaller particle size, and occurs predominantly in the small intestine, followed by the colon.[119] Poorly soluble compounds such as arsenic trioxide (As_2O_3) are less well absorbed[169] than soluble compounds such as trivalent and pentavalent compounds that, in aqueous solution, have a GI absorptive capacity greater than 90%.[123] However, when placed in an aqueous solution, As_2O_3 is more toxic than an identical dose of undissolved As_2O_3 eaten in food.[169] A rodent experiment demonstrated approximately 70% GI absorption of dimethylarsinic acid (cacodylic acid).[157] Systemic absorption via the respiratory tract depends on the particulate size, as well as the arsenic compound and its solubility. Large, nonrespirable particles are cleared from the airways by ciliary action and swallowed, allowing GI absorption to occur. Respirable particles lodging in the lungs can be absorbed over days to weeks or remain unabsorbed for years.[18,177] Penetration of arsenic through intact skin does not pose a risk for acute toxicity, but may represent a risk following chronic application. Arsenic acid (H_3AsO_4) applied to intact skin in rhesus monkeys resulted in absorption of a mean of 2.0–6.4% of the applied dose.[178] Skin irritation and damage may increase systemic absorption.[52,140]

Studies in humans receiving intravenous radioarsenic isotope (As^{74}) show that arsenic is cleared from the blood in three phases:

Phase 1 (2–3 hours)—Arsenic is rapidly cleared with a half-life of 1–2 hours; more than 90% may be cleared during this phase.

Phase 2 (3 hours to 7 days)—A more gradual decline occurs, with an estimated half-life of 30 hours; by 10 hours postinfusion the arsenic is concentrated in RBCs by a 3:1 ratio as compared to plasma.

Phase 3 (10 or more days)—Clearance continues slowly with an estimated half-life of 300 hours.[112]

The rapid clearance in Phases 1 and 2 explains why blood testing for arsenic is unreliable, except in the early phase of an acute poisoning.

Initial distribution is predominantly to liver, kidney, muscle, and skin. The skin is rich in sulfhydryl groups; its elimination half-life of arsenic was estimated to be 1 month in a rabbit study.[39] Distribution to brain occurs quickly; in the As^{74} study, 0.30% percent of the administered dose was found in brain biopsy samples in the first hour postinfusion. This peak declined to 0.16% by day 7.[112] Ultimately, arsenic distributes to all tissues. Arsenic crosses the placenta and accumulates in the fetus[14,104] but is not appreciably excreted in breast milk.[31]

Metabolism by adding methyl groups occurs primarily in the liver but also in the kidneys, testes, and lungs (Fig. 79–1). If the arsenic is pentavalent, approximately 50–70% will first be reduced to trivalent arsenic.[159,170] This bioactivation step requires the oxidation of glutathione[36] and can begin less than 15 minutes following exposure.[170] S-Adenosylmethionine (SAM) is the primary methyl donor, although cyanocobalamin (vitamin B_{12}), 5′-deoxyadenosyl-cobalamin (coenzyme B_{12}), and methylcobalamin (methyl B_{12}) can donate.[19,108] Dietary and vitamin deficiencies as well as high doses of inorganic arsenic may diminish the ability to methylate arsenic,[107,168,172] although the theory that large concentrations of arsenic can overwhelm the methylation process is debated.[75] In the case of pentavalent arsenic, decreased methylation might result in increased production of the trivalent arsenic.[170] Addition of a methyl group produces monomethylarsonic acid (MMA), and a sec-

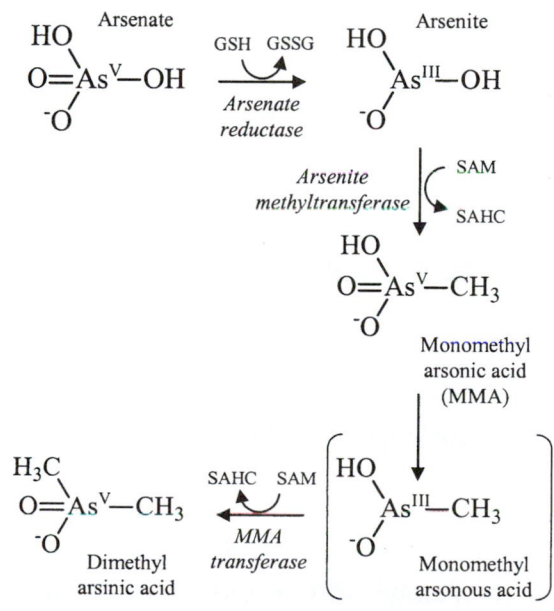

Figure 79–1. Metabolism of arsenate [As(V)] and arsenite [As(III)]. GSH, glutathione; SAM, S-adenosylmethionine; SAHC, S-adenosylhomocysteine; MMA, monomethylarsonic acid; DMA, dimethylarsinic acid.

ond methyl group forms dimethylarsinic acid (DMA). These steps are catalyzed by methyltransferases that apparently occur in the same protein, but which have different optimal substrates and pH.[185] Trivalent intermediates of MMA and DMA occur, but their potential to produce toxicity is unknown.[170] Methylation decreases the toxicity of arsenic and increases its elimination. For humans, the estimated LD_{50} of arsenic trioxide is 1.43 mg/kg; that of MMA is 50 mg/kg, and that of DMA is 500 mg/kg.

Urinary elimination of unchanged arsenic and its methylated metabolites occurs via glomerular filtration, tubular secretion, and active reabsorption.[165,173] Human studies demonstrate renal arsenic elimination of 46–68.9% in the first 4–5 days postingestion.[20,84,127,169] Approximately 30% is eliminated with a half-life of greater than 1 week, while the remainder is slowly excreted with a half-life of greater than 1 month.[20,111] Human fecal elimination is minimal, with reported amounts ranging from 0.21–6.1%.[112,161]

Arsenobetaine is also well absorbed and is excreted unchanged in the urine.[170] Elimination occurs more rapidly than with inorganic arsenic. In human volunteers, 25% is excreted in the first 2–4 hours, 50% by 20 hours, and 70–83.7% after 166 hours. A two-compartment exponential model shows nearly 50% of the arsenobetaine eliminated with a first component half-life of 6.9–11.0 hours, while the second component half-life is 75.7 hours.[84]

PATHOPHYSIOLOGY

The mechanisms of inorganic arsenic toxicity differ for the trivalent and pentavalent forms. The primary biochemical lesion of As(III) is inhibition of the pyruvate dehydrogenase (PDH) complex (Fig. 79–2). Normally, dihydrolipoamide is recycled to lipoamide, a necessary cofactor in the conversion of pyruvate to acetyl coenzyme A (acetyl CoA). As(III) binds the sulfhydryl groups of dihydrolipoamide, blocking lipoamide regeneration.[133,135] Acetyl

CoA is a central molecule in metabolism, and the resulting decrease leads to several deleterious effects:

- Decreased citric acid cycle activity and, thus, decreased adenosine triphosphate (ATP) production.
- Decreased gluconeogenesis that can worsen hypoglycemia—pyruvate carboxylase catalyzes the conversion of pyruvate to oxaloacetate (initial step in gluconeogenesis) and this reaction requires the carboxylation of biotin, a CO_2 carrier attached to pyruvate carboxylase; biotin cannot be carboxylated unless acetyl CoA is attached to the enzyme.[134,135,160]

In the citric acid cycle, oxidation of α-ketoglutarate to succinyl coenzyme A uses an α-ketoglutarate dehydrogenase complex that contains the same cofactors as the PDH complex, including lipoamide. Arsenic also blocks the dihydrolipoamide-lipoamide recycling in this complex, thus interfering with citric acid cycle activity at a second point. Succinyl CoA is necessary for production of porphyrins and amino acids,[284] and deficiency may contribute to anemia and wasting seen with chronic arsenic poisoning. Arsenic inhibition of thiolase, the catalyst for the final step in fatty acid oxidation, also impairs ATP production. Diminished fatty acid oxidation results in decreased acetyl CoA and in the loss of nicotinamide adenine dinucleotide (NADH) and flavin adenine dinucleotide (reduced form) ($FADH_2$), electron carriers reduced during fatty acid breakdown whose subsequent oxidation yields ATP.[138] Trivalent arsenic also inhibits glutathione synthetase, glucose 6-phosphate dehydrogenase (required to produce NADPH), and glutathione reductase.[5,149] These inhibitions result in decreased levels of reduced glutathione, which is required to facilitate arsenic metabolism, protect RBCs from oxidative damage, maintain hemoglobin in the ferrous state, and scavenge hydrogen peroxide and other organic peroxides.[158]

Animal experiments with phenylarsine oxide, a trivalent arsenical, demonstrate inhibition of insulin-induced glucose trans-

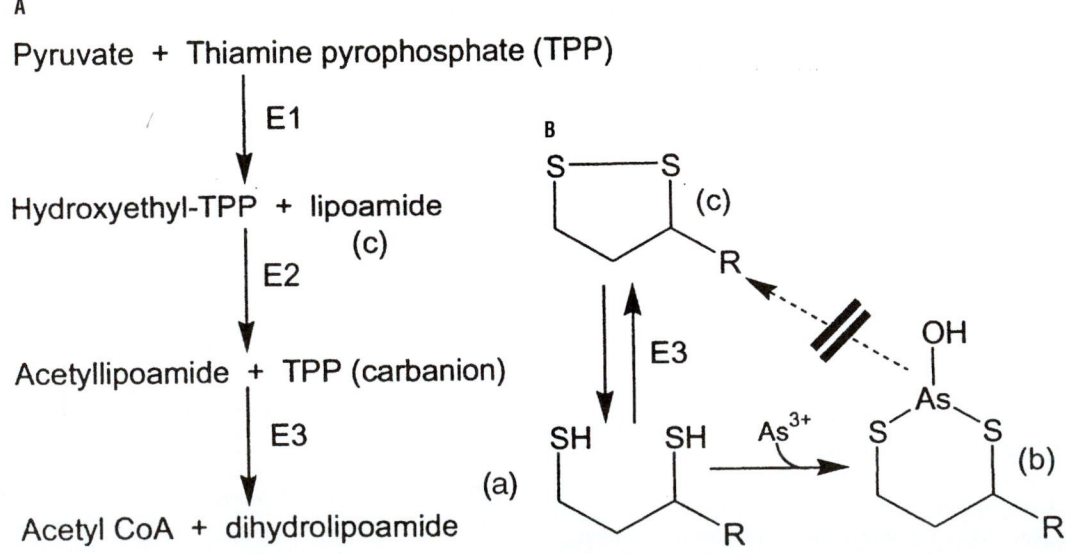

Figure 79–2. Effect of trivalent arsenicals (As^{3+}) on pyruvate dehydrogenase complex (PDH). **A.** The normal PDH complex. **B.** Effects of As^{3+} on dihydrolipoamide regeneration. (a) = dihydrolipoamide, (b) = arsenic binding preventing the regeneration of lipoamide, (c) = lipoamide, E1 = pyruvate dehydrogenase, E2 = dihydrolipoamide acetyltransferase, E3 = dihydrolipoamide dehydrogenase.

port (involving vicinal sulfhydryl groups) and β-cell damage in pancreatic islets (attributed to inhibition of the α-ketoglutarate dehydrogenase complex).[15,50,68] These findings support a link between exposure to arsenic and the development of diabetes mellitus.[94,128] The impaired glucose transport and inhibited gluconeogenesis can lead to glycogen depletion and hypoglycemia;[135] several animal experiments indicate improved central nervous system (CNS) glucose content[134] and an increase in survival time with glucose treatment.[136,137]

Toxicity from pentavalent [As(V)] arsenic may occur by several mechanisms. Toxicity may occur from its transformation to trivalent arsenic [As(III)].[79,171] It also resembles phosphate chemically and structurally,[158] may share a common transport system for cellular uptake with phosphate,[79] and can uncouple oxidative phosphorylation by substituting for inorganic phosphate (P_i) in the glycolysis reaction catalyzed by glyceraldehyde 3-phosphate dehydrogenase (Fig. 79–3).[158] The resulting unstable product, 1-arseno-3-phosphoglycerate, spontaneously hydrolyzes to 3-phosphoglycerate, so glycolysis continues. But the ATP normally produced during conversion of 1,3-bisphosphoglycerate to 3-phosphoglycerate is lost. Uncoupling may also occur if adenosine diphosphate (ADP) forms ADP-arsenate instead of ATP in the presence of As(V). The ADP-arsenate rapidly hydrolyzes, thus uncoupling oxidative phosphorylation.[63]

Effects on RBCs include decreased membrane fluidity and ATP depletion.[179,188] Chronic arsenic exposure is associated with vascular disease; in vitro studies demonstrate inhibition of endothelial cell proliferation and glycoprotein synthesis and lipid peroxidation.[25,103] Proposed mechanisms by which arsenic can induce cancer include DMA-induced DNA damage, gene amplification, replacing phosphate in DNA during replication, and increased cell proliferation.[23,182,183] Experimental evidence and human studies support a number of etiologic or contributing factors for skin keratosis and cancer: (a) chronic stimulation of ker-

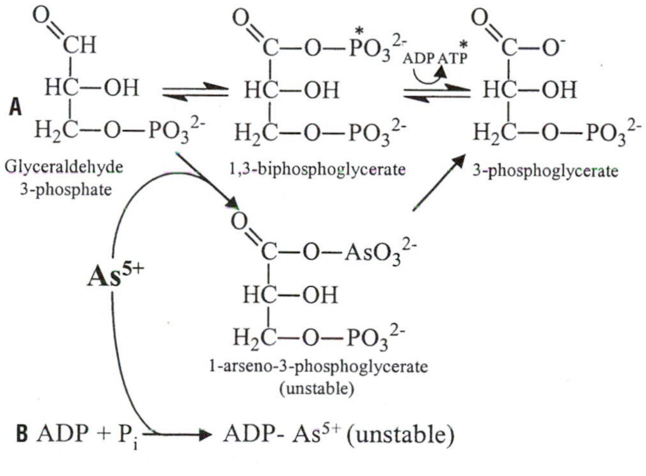

Figure 79–3. Pathophysiologic effects of pentavalent arsenic [As(V), As^{5+}]. **A.** As^{5+} substitutes for inorganic phosphate (*) in glycolysis, bypassing the formation of 1,3-bisphosphoglycerate (1,3-BPG) and thus losing the ATP formation that occurs when 1,3-BPG is metabolized to 3-phosphoglycerate. **B.** Uncoupling of oxidative phosphorylation (see Fig. 13–1). Energy loss also occurs if As^{5+} substitutes for P_i and blocks the formation of ATP + AMP from two ADPs. ATP—adenosine triphosphate; ADP—adenosine diphosphate; AMP—adenosine monophosphate.

atinocyte-derived growth factors such as transforming growth factor-α (TGF-α),[54,55] impaired methylation,[27,77] mutation in the p53 tumor suppressor gene,[76] inhibition of poly(ADP-ribose) polymerase, vital for DNA repair,[114] or interference with mitotic spindle and microtubular function.[129,181] Pigmentary changes also occur, and hyperpigmentation is thought to be a consequence of increased melanin.[181]

CLINICAL MANIFESTATIONS

Inorganic Arsenicals

Toxic manifestations vary depending on the amount and form of arsenic ingested, as well as the chronicity of ingestion. Other influencing factors include individual variations in methylation and excretion. Larger doses of a potent compound such as arsenic trioxide will rapidly produce manifestations of acute toxicity, while chronic ingestion of substantially lower amounts of pentavalent arsenic in groundwater will slowly result in different clinical manifestations. Subacute toxicity can develop in a patient who survives an acute exposure, and some of the same features may occur in patients who are slowly poisoned environmentally. The physician must be aware of these differences in order to avoid misdiagnosis.

Acute Toxicity. Gastrointestinal signs and symptoms of nausea, vomiting, abdominal pain, and diarrhea are the earliest manifestations of acute poisoning by the oral route. They occur 10 minutes to several hours following ingestion; the diarrhea has been compared to that seen with cholera and may resemble "rice water."[26,70,81,87,142] Severe multisystem illness can ensue in the severest cases. Cardiovascular signs ranging from sinus tachycardia and orthostatic hypotension to shock can develop. Reported cases have mimicked myocardial infarction or systemic inflammatory response syndrome (SIRS), with intravascular volume depletion, capillary leak, myocardial dysfunction, and diminished systemic vascular resistance.[13,22,59,85,148] Acute encephalopathy can develop and progress over several days, with delirium, coma, and seizures attributed to cerebral edema and microhemorrhages.[34,47,148] Seizures or syncope may be secondary to dysrhythmias, and the underlying cardiac rhythm should be assessed. In three cases, seizures secondary to torsades de pointes associated with a prolonged QTc developed 4 days to 5 weeks after acute arsenic ingestion.[13,58,156] Pulmonary edema, acute respiratory distress syndrome (ARDS) and respiratory failure, hepatitis, hemolytic anemia, acute renal failure, rhabdomyolysis, other ventricular dysrhythmias, and death can occur.[14,44,45,57,62,101,113,145] Three individuals died after suddenly developing bradycardia followed by asystole.[14,85,105] Fever may develop, misleading the practitioner to diagnose sepsis.[40,85] Hepatitis can occur and may be caused by altered intrahepatic heme metabolism resulting in increased synthesis of bilirubin or by altered protein transport between hepatocytes.[3,100] Acute renal failure may be secondary to ischemia caused by hypotension, tubular deposition of myoglobin or hemoglobin, renal cortical necrosis, and direct renal tubular toxicity.[17,53,85,145,166] Glutathione depletion may be contributory.[73] Unusual complications include phrenic nerve paralysis, unilateral facial nerve palsy, pancreatitis, pericarditis, and pleuritis.[10,186] Fetal demise has been reported, with toxic levels of arsenic found in the fetal organs.[14,104]

Acutely poisoned patients with less severe illness may experience persistent gastroenteritis and mild hypotension, necessitating hospitalization and intravenous fluids for days.[96] These manifestations are atypical for most viral and bacterial enteric illnesses, and should alert the physician to consider arsenic toxicity, especially if there is a pattern of repetitive gastrointestinal illnesses. A metallic taste or oropharyngeal irritation can occur; the latter can mimic pharyngitis.[14,70] The garlicky breath odor attributed to inorganic arsenicals has also been reported with exposure to arsine gas. Gastrointestinal ulcerative lesions and hemorrhage may be seen.[47,59] Toxic erythroderma and exfoliative dermatitis result from a hypersensitivity reaction to arsenic.[162]

Reported adverse effects of arsenic trioxide therapy for leukemia include fluid retention, nausea and vomiting, prolonged QTc and torsades de pointes, rash, hyperpigmentation and keratosis, pleural and pericardial effusions, hepatitis, renal failure, muscular atrophy, peripheral neuropathy, pseudotumor cerebri, and chronic neuromuscular degeneration.[51,78,80,167]

Subacute Toxicity. In the days and weeks following an acute exposure, prolonged or additional signs and symptoms in the nervous, gastrointestinal, hematologic, dermatologic, pulmonary, and cardiovascular systems can occur. Encephalopathic symptoms of headache, confusion, decreased memory, personality change, irritability, hallucinations, delirium, and seizures may develop or persist.[40,49] Sixth cranial nerve palsy and bilateral sensorineural hearing loss have been reported.[1,30,58] Peripheral neuropathy typically develops 1–3 weeks after acute poisoning, although in one series, nine patients developed maximal neuropathy within 24 hours of exposure.[30,70,83,96] Sensory symptoms develop first, and diminished to absent vibratory sense may be found on physical examination.[118] Progressive symptoms and signs include numbness, tingling, and formication, with physical findings of diminished to absent pain, touch, temperature, and deep-tendon reflexes in a stocking glove distribution. Superficial touch of the extremities may elicit severe or deep-aching pains, a finding also seen with thallium poisoning. Motor weakness may then develop. The worst cases manifest an ascending flaccid paralysis mimicking Guillain-Barré syndrome, as occurred with our patient.[30,38,70,83,96,126] Respiratory problems can include dry cough, rales, hemoptysis, chest pain, and patchy interstitial infiltrates.[70,125] These may be misinterpreted as viral or bronchitic disease. Leukopenia, and less commonly anemia and thrombocytopenia, occur from days to 3 weeks after an acute exposure, but will resolve as bone marrow function returns.[92,100,105]

Dermatologic lesions can include patchy alopecia, oral herpetiform lesions, a diffuse pruritic macular rash, and a brawny nonpruritic desquamation.[40,70,120,124] Diaphoresis and edema of the face and extremities can develop.[1,70,120] Mees lines (transverse striate leuconychia) are 1–2 mm wide, horizontal white nail bands that represent disturbed nail matrix keratinization. They occur uncommonly in arsenic poisoning—one series of 74 patients with acute and chronic toxicity found Mees lines in only 5% of patients—and are not pathognomonic, having also been reported with thallium poisoning, chemotherapy, Hodgkin disease, helminthic infections, renal failure, and systemic lupus erythematosus.[1,181] A minimum of 30–40 days after exposure is required for the lines to extend visibly beyond the nail lunulae. Contact dermatitis has been reported from topical exposure in an occupational setting.[11] Other possible toxic manifestations include nephropathy,

fatigue, anorexia with weight loss, torsades de pointes, and persistence of gastrointestinal symptoms.[9,109]

Chronic Toxicity. Chronic low-level exposure typically occurs from occupational or environmental sources. Multiple dermatologic lesions have been reported in populations suffering from hydroarsenicism.[66,121,128,181] Alterations in pigmentation occur first, with hyperpigmentation being the most common. Hypopigmentation with a "raindrop" pattern can also occur. Hyperkeratoses typically develop on the palms and soles, but can be diffuse. Squamous and basal cell carcinomas and Bowen disease occur; Bowen disease usually proliferates in multiple sites, especially on the trunk, and is noted for developing on sun-protected areas. Latency periods for developing keratoses, Bowen disease, and squamous cell carcinoma were 28, 39, and 41 years, respectively, in 17 patients chronically exposed to environmental or medicinal arsenic.[180] Gastrointestinal symptoms of nausea, vomiting, and diarrhea are less likely but can occur.[16,65] Hepatomegaly was present in 190 of 248 patients with hydroarsenicism; liver biopsy in 69 cases revealed noncirrhotic portal fibrosis in 91.3%.[144] Portal hypertension and hypersplenism have occurred.[65,116] Hepatic angiosarcomas have been linked to arsenic exposure.[86,95,131,139] Population studies in areas of Bangladesh and Taiwan where the water is contaminated with arsenic show an increased prevalence of diabetes mellitus.[94,128] Restrictive lung disease was reported in 9 of 17 patients, and a restrictive plus obstructive pattern was seen in another 7 cases.[66] Aplastic anemia and agranulocytosis have been documented in patients exposed to arsenic.[40] A dose-response relationship between arsenic exposure and vascular disease has been reported in several populations. After adjusting for age, sex, hypertension, diabetes mellitus, cigarette smoking, and alcohol consumption, a significant relationship was observed with cerebrovascular disease in a region of Taiwan.[29] Blackfoot disease, an obliterative arterial disease of the lower extremities occurring in Taiwan, is linked with chronic arsenic exposure.[25,164] Raynaud phenomenon and vasospasm were reported to be increased in smelter workers exposed to arsenic as compared to a control group.[93] Encephalopathy and peripheral neuropathy are the neurologic manifestations most commonly reported.[12,69,188] Electromyographic studies of 33 patients with chronic ingestion of arsenic-contaminated water revealed 10 patients with findings consistent with sensory neuropathy. The minimum time for exposure was 2 years; interestingly, three patients consumed water whose arsenic concentration slightly exceeded the former US permissible contaminant level of 50 ppb.[72] Arsenic has been classified as a definite carcinogen by the International Agency for Research on Cancer (IARC, Group 1) and the National Toxicology Program (NTP). Cancers known to develop include lung (adenocarcinomas and oat cell carcinomas) and skin. Bladder carcinoma is strongly associated.[28,98,152] Finally, a critical literature review of animal and human studies found that exposure to environmental arsenic was unlikely to cause reproductive or developmental toxicity.[37]

Melarsoprol. Many of the toxic effects seen with inorganic arsenic can occur with the therapeutic use of melarsoprol, including fever, encephalopathy, and acute cerebral edema with seizures and coma. Whether these effects are caused by drug toxicity or by an immune reaction elicited by trypanosomal antigens is unknown.[122,163] Other adverse effects include vomiting, abdominal pain, peripheral neuropathy including Guillain-Barré syndrome, hypersensitivity reactions, hypertension, myocardial damage, and albuminuria.[56] Hemolysis can occur in patients with glucose-6-phosphate dehydrogenase (G6PD) deficiency, and erythema nodosum in patients with leprosy.[163] In a study of the utility of melarsoprol to treat refractory or advanced leukemia, reported adverse effects included fatigue, vomiting, diarrhea, vertigo, fever, seizures, headache, back pain, and injection site pain.[155]

DIAGNOSTIC TESTING

The utility of laboratory diagnostic studies depends on whether the exposure is acute, subacute, chronic, or remote with residual clinical effects. Failure to understand the time course of arsenic metabolism, clearance, and effect on laboratory parameters can mislead the physician in assessing a case of possible arsenic toxicity. Abdominal radiographs may demonstrate gastrointestinal radiopaque material soon after an ingestion[2,26,59,60,71]; however, an acute ingestion with negative abdominal radiographs is reported.[33] The incidence of visualizing radiopaque material after an ingestion is unknown, and the absence of this finding should not eliminate arsenic as a diagnostic consideration.

Diagnosis ultimately depends on finding an elevated urinary arsenic level. In an emergency, a spot urine may be sent prior to beginning chelation therapy. An elevated arsenic level verifies the diagnosis, whereas a low level does not exclude arsenic toxicity.[175] In nine acute, symptomatic patients, initial spot urine arsenic levels ranged from 192,000 to 198,450 µg/L.[87] Because urinary excretion of arsenic is intermittent, definitive diagnosis hinges upon finding a concentration equal to or greater than 50 µg/L, 100 µg/g creatinine, or 100 µg total arsenic in a 24-hour urine collection (see below for a discussion of elevated urinary arsenic caused by arsenicals in food). All urine specimens should be collected in metal-free containers. If testing is performed by an outside reference laboratory, specimens from acutely ill patients should be sent via express transportation with a request for a rapid analysis.

Laboratory evaluation of chronic toxicity, including laboratory parameters that become abnormal within days to weeks following an acute exposure, should focus on complete blood count (CBC), renal and liver function tests, and urinalysis (UA), as well as on 24-hour urinary arsenic determinations. CBC findings can include a normocytic, normochromic, or megaloblastic anemia; an initial leukocytosis followed by leukopenia, with neutrophils depressed more than lymphocytes, and a relative eosinophilia; thrombocytopenia; and a rapidly declining hemoglobin indicative of hemolytic anemia or a gastrointestinal hemorrhage.[9,92,176] Basophilic stippling of RBCs may be seen;[92] this can occur in other toxic and clinical disorders. Karyorrhexis, a rupture of the RBC cell nucleus with chromatin disintegration into granules that are extruded from the cell, and dyserythropoiesis are reported in both lead- and arsenic-toxic patients. Both findings are a result of inhibition of DNA synthesis and damage to the nuclear envelope.[42] The karyorrhexis can occur within 4 days and resolve by 2 weeks after poisoning and may be an early indication of arsenic toxicity.[92] Elevated serum creatinine, aminotransferases, and bilirubin and depressed haptoglobin levels may develop. Urinalysis may reveal proteinuria, hematuria, and pyuria.[9] Cerebral spinal fluid examination in patients with CNS findings can be normal or exhibit mild protein elevation to 0.265 g/L.[70] Urinary arsenic excretion in subacute and chronic cases varies inversely with the postexposure time period, but low-level excretion may continue for months after exposure.[32,70] In a study of 41 cases of arsenic-induced peripheral neuropathy, most patients with a neuropathy of 4–8 weeks duration had total 24-hour urinary arsenic measurements of 100–400 µg.[70] In cases of suspected arsenic toxicity in which the urinary arsenic measurements fall below accepted toxic levels, analysis of hair and nails may permit a diagnosis. Arsenic can be detected in the proximal portions of hair within 30 hours of ingestion.[184] Hair grows at a rate of 0.4 mm per day, while nail grows at a rate of 0.1 mm per day. Total replacement of a fingernail requires 3–4 months of growth, whereas toenails require 6–9 months of growth.[67] These facts, plus the frequency of hair cutting, should be considered when estimating the utility of measuring arsenic levels in these tissues. Reference laboratory normal values should be used to determine the presence of elevated arsenic levels. In cases of remote toxicity, hair and nail arsenic measurements may or may not be elevated, depending on the time elapsed since exposure. Sequential hair analysis to assess the time(s) of exposure to arsenic can be performed on pulled hairs whose roots demonstrate the anagen (growing) phase.

When interpreting slightly elevated urinary arsenic levels, laboratory findings must be correlated with the clinical findings because the nontoxic organoarsenicals in seafood transiently elevate urinary arsenic excretion up to 1700 µg/L.[8] When seafood arsenic is a consideration or when findings do not correlate with those of the laboratory, speciation of arsenic can be requested from a reference laboratory. This test is accomplished either by using liquid chromatography separation followed by graphite furnace atomic absorption analysis[117] or by ion chromatography with inductively coupled plasma mass spectrometry.[141] These techniques separate the organoarsenicals arsenobetaine, arsenocholine, MMA, and DMA from As (III) and As (V). Alternatively, the patient can be retested after a 1-week abstinence from seafood. If the history suggests an episode of poisoning several months earlier, hair and nails can be anlayzed.

Electrophysiologic testing in patients with neuropathy shows slowed sensory conduction; motor conduction can also be diminished, with findings compatible with axonal degeneration. Sural nerve biopsy in nine patients with peripheral neuropathy revealed axonal degeneration and decreased myelinated fibers.[118]

MANAGEMENT
General

Acute arsenic toxicity is life-threatening and mandates aggressive treatment. Advanced life-support monitoring and therapies should be initiated when necessary, with a few caveats. Careful attention to fluid balance is important, because cerebral and pulmonary edema may be present. Agents that prolong the QTc, such as the class IA, IC, and III antidysrhythmic agents, should be avoided. Potassium, magnesium, and calcium levels should be maintained within normal range to avoid exacerbating a prolonged QTc. Glucose levels and glycogen stores should be maintained parenterally with dextrose and hyperalimentation solutions or with enteral feedings, given the experimental evidence suggesting carbohydrate depletion in arsenic poisoning, with a beneficial effect of glucose.[102,136,137,160] Arsenic poorly adsorbs to activated charcoal, cholestyramine, or bentonite.[132] In view of the potential benefit of activated charcoal adsorption, this agent should be given for arsenic ingestions until further precise data describing adsorptive characteristics are available. If radiopaque material is seen in the gastrointestinal tract, whole-bowel irrigation can be administered until the radiopaque material is no longer seen on a repeat abdominal radiograph. Continuing nasogastric suction may be important in removing arsenic resecreted in the gastric or biliary secretions. In three patients, arsenite was still detectable in the gastric aspirate 5–7 days following an ingestion.[107] There is no clinical experience with the use of *N*-acetylcysteine to increase glutathione levels, although an animal experiment suggested a protective effect.[130]

In cases of chronic toxicity the patient should be removed from the arsenic source and gastric decontamination performed if there is evidence of arsenic in the gastrointestinal tract. Arsenic can be readily removed from skin with soap, water, and vigorous scrubbing.[178] For all cases, if homicidal intent is suspected, patients should be advised against accepting food or drink from anyone. Hospital visitors should be closely monitored and outside nutritional products should be forbidden.[81]

When to Begin Chelation Therapy

When to begin chelation therapy depends on the clinical condition of the patient, as well as on the laboratory results for arsenic in urine, hair, or nails. A severely ill patient with known or suspected acute poisoning should be chelated immediately, before laboratory confirmation is received. In a series of 33 patients with coma, seizures, or both, 24 patients were treated with BAL (British Anti-Lewisite) within 6 hours (mean = 1 hour) and 75% survived, while the survival rate was 45% in 9 patients treated late (range, 9–72 hours; mean = 30 hours).[40] Cases of subacute and chronic toxicity can await rapid laboratory confirmation prior to beginning chelation, unless the clinical condition deteriorates.

Specific

Chelators. Dimercaprol (British Anti-Lewisite, or BAL) and meso-2,3-dimercaptosuccinic acid (Succimer) are the two chelators available in the United States. A third drug, sodium 2,3-dimercapto-1-propane sulfonate (DMPS), is currently commercially unavailable in the United States, but is distributed by Heyl, a German pharmaceutical company, as Dimaval. All contain vicinal dithiol moieties that bind arsenic to form stable 1,2,5-arsadithiolones (Fig. 79–4), and all are most effective when

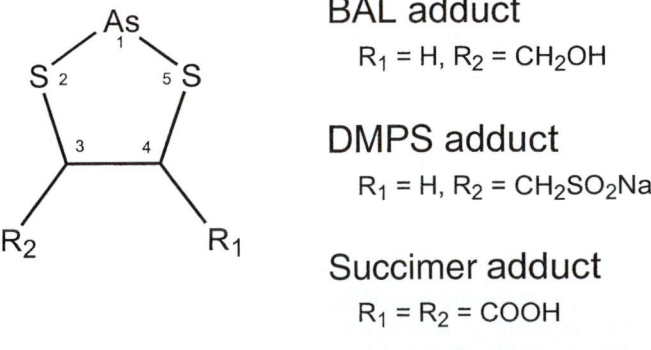

BAL adduct
$R_1 = H$, $R_2 = CH_2OH$

DMPS adduct
$R_1 = H$, $R_2 = CH_2SO_2Na$

Succimer adduct
$R_1 = R_2 = COOH$

Figure 79–4.   1,2,5-arsadithiolane adducts with BAL, DMPS, and succimer.[115]

TABLE 79–3.   Adverse Effects of Chelating Agents Used for Arsenic Poisoning

Chelating Agent Dosage	Adverse Effects
BAL 3–5 mg/kg every 4–6 hours	Hypertension Febrile reaction, diaphoresis Nausea, vomiting, salivation Lacrimation, rhinorrhea Headache
Endpoint: 24-hour urinary arsenic <50 μg/L or until another agent is substituted	Painful injection, injection site sterile abscess Hemolysis in G-6-PD-deficient patients BAL-iron complex very toxic Chelation of essential metals (prolonged course)
Succimer 10 mg/kg per dose every 8 hours for 5 days, then 10 mg/kg per dose every 12 hours	Nausea, vomiting, diarrhea Abdominal gas, pain Transient elevations in hepatic aminotransferases, and alkaline phosphatase
Endpoint: 24-hour urinary arsenic <50 μg/L	Rash, pruritus Sore throat, rhinorrhea Drowsiness, paresthesias Thrombocytosis, eosinophilia
DMPS 5 mg/kg per dose IM, administered as a 5% solution Day 1: q 6–8h (3–4 doses) Day 2: q 8–12 h (2–3 doses) Day 3 and thereafter: q 12–24 h (1–2 doses daily)	Allergic reactions Increased copper and zinc excretion Nausea Pruritus Vertigo Weakness
Endpoint: 24-hour urinary arsenic <50μg/L	

administered in doses equimolar to the arsenic burden.[115] Table 79–3 lists the dosing regimens and adverse effects.

In the United States, BAL remains the initial chelating drug for acute arsenical toxicity, and perhaps for poisoning with lipophilic organoarsenicals such as oxophenarsine as well.[115] It is the only intracellular/extracellular chelator available in the United States, and it can be administered parenterally to patients whose gastrointestinal motility may be decreased. Its therapeutic:toxic ratio is narrow, with adverse effects likely to occur in patients receiving doses of ≥4 mg/kg. It is administered intramuscularly in peanut oil; the injections are painful and can lead to sterile skin abscesses. In a cellular study of glucose uptake impaired by a lipophilic arsenical, BAL was superior to succimer and DMPS in restoring cellular equilibrium.[115] An older human case series found increased survival with early use of BAL and improvement in encephalopathy within 24 hours of initiating therapy.[40] However, other acute cases treated promptly with BAL developed peripheral neuropathy.[96] In a study of subacute cases with peripheral neuropathy, BAL accelerated recovery, but did not affect the overall recovery rate.[30] Despite BAL therapy being started 8 hours postingestion, a man who consumed 2.15 g of arsenic developed severe toxicity and neurologic deficits.[46] Most concerning are the animal experiments indicating that BAL shifts arsenic into the brain and testes, two organs that have blood-organ barriers susceptible to this lipophilic drug.[6,74,91,115] It is clear that BAL has limitations, and that there is need for a safer, more effective parenteral chelator with both intracellular and extracellular efficacy.

Succimer is an oral hydrophilic analogue of BAL and is the chelator of choice for subacute and chronic toxicity. It has proven effective in animal studies and in reported human cases.[6,48,88,90,99,106,151] In mice exposed to sodium arsenite, it was more effective than DMPS or BAL in protecting from lethality, and it was more potent than BAL in restoring activity in the pyruvate dehydrogenase complex.[6] It is equal or superior to BAL in speeding arsenic elimination.[115] Liver function tests and essential metal levels should be monitored in patients requiring prolonged therapy.[48,61]

DMPS is also a water-soluble analogue of BAL. It can be administered by the oral, intravenous, or intramuscular routes. It is eliminated from the body more slowly than succimer and has the advantage of intracellular as well as extracellular distribution.[4] Two brothers ingested nearly pure arsenic trioxide (1 and 4 g each) and were treated with intravenous and oral DMPS. The brother who ingested 4 g developed hypotension, renal failure, respiratory insufficiency, and asystolic cardiac arrest. DMPS was started 32 hours postingestion, and the patient survived with normal renal function and no neurologic dysfunction. His sibling had a milder course; DMPS was started 48 hours postingestion, and there were no neurologic sequelae on followup.[113] DMPS significantly increased biliary excretion of arsenic in a guinea pig model, but did not increase fecal excretion, most likely because of enterohepatic recirculation of the DMPS-As complex.[132]

D-Penicillamine has not demonstrated efficacy in chelating or reversing the biochemical lesions of arsenic[7,89] and should not be used. Its previous advantage of oral administration has been rendered moot by the availability of succimer.

Hemodialysis. Hemodialysis removes negligible amounts of arsenic, with or without concomitant BAL therapy, and is not indicated in patients with normal renal function. In patients with renal failure, hemodialysis clearance rates range from 76 to 87.5 mL/min, with or without concomitant BAL therapy.[110,174] In two acutely toxic patients with renal failure, total arsenic removed during a 4-hour dialysis measured 4.68 mg in patient 1 and 3.36 mg in patient 2. Concomitant 24-hour urinary arsenic excretions were 3.12 mg and 2.03 mg, respectively. When renal function returned, however, the 24-hour urinary excretion of arsenic far exceeded that recovered by dialysis, with totals of 18.99 mg (patient 1) and 75 mg (patient 2) reported.[174] There is no published experience with hemodialysis removal of a water-soluble complex, such as DMPS-As.

SUMMARY

Arsenicals produce multisystem toxicity by various pathophysiologic mechanisms. A thorough understanding of inorganic arsenic metabolism and excretion, as well as of the diverse clinical manifestations of acute, subacute, and chronic toxicity, is necessary to avoid misdiagnosis. Chelation therapy with BAL in the United States, or with DMPS where available, should be started immediately in the symptomatic patient. Treatment can await laboratory results for patients with no acute symptoms or with subacute or chronic toxicity, unless clinical deterioration intervenes.

REFERENCES

1. Abernathy CO, Ohanian EV: Non-carcinogenic effects of inorganic arsenic. Environ Geochem Health 1992;14:35–41.
2. Adelson L, George RA, Mandel A: Acute arsenic intoxication shown by roentgenograms. Arch Intern Med 1961;107:401–404.
3. Albores A, Cebrian ME, Bach PH, Connelly JC, Hinton RH, Bridges JW: Sodium arsenite induced alterations in bilirubin excretion and heme metabolism. J Biochem Toxicol 1989;4:73–78.
4. Aposhian HV: Mobilization of mercury and arsenic in humans by sodium 2,3-dimercapto-1-propane sulfonate (DMPS). Environ Health Perspect 1998;106(Suppl 4):1017–1025.
5. Aposhian HV, Aposhian MM: Newer developments in arsenic toxicity. J Am Coll Toxicol 1989;8:1297–1305.
6. Aposhian HV, Carter DE, Hoover TD, Hsu CA, Maiorino RM, Stine E: Succimer, DMPS, and DMPA as arsenic antidotes. Fundam Appl Toxicol 1984;4:S58–S70.
7. Aposhian HV, Tadlock CH, Moon TE: Protection of mice against lethal effects of sodium arsenite—A quantitative comparison of a number of chelating agents. Toxicol Appl Pharmacol 1981;61:385–392.
8. Arbouine MW, Wilson HK: The effect of seafood consumption on the assessment of occupational exposure to arsenic by urinary arsenic speciation measurements. J Trace Elem 1992;6:153–160.
9. Armstrong CW, Stroube RB, Rubio T, et al: Outbreak of fatal arsenic poisoning caused by contaminated drinking water. Arch Environ Health 1984;39:276–279.
10. Bansal SK, Haldar N, Dhand UK, Chopra JS: Phrenic neuropathy in arsenic poisoning. Chest 1991;100:878–880.
11. Barbaud A, Mougeolle JM, Schmutz JL: Contact hypersensitivity to arsenic in a crystal factory worker. Contact Dermatitis 1995;33:272–273.
12. Beckett WS, Moore JL, Keogh JP, Bleecker ML: Acute encephalopathy due to occupational exposure to arsenic. Br J Industrial Med 1986;43:66–67.
13. Beckman KJ, Bauman JL, Pimental PA, et al: Arsenic-induced torsade de pointes. Crit Care Med 1991;19:290–291.
14. Bolliger CT, van Zijl P, Louw JA: Multiple organ failure with the adult respiratory distress syndrome in homicidal arsenic poisoning. Respiration 1992;59:57–61.
15. Boquist L, Boquist S, Ericsson I: Structural beta-cell changes and transient hyperglycemia in mice treated with compounds inducing inhibited citric acid cycle enzyme activity. Diabetes 1988;37:89–98.
16. Borgono JM, Vincent P, Venturino H, Infante A: Arsenic in the drinking water of the city of Antofagasta: Epidemiological and clinical study before and after the installation of a treatment plant. Environ Health Perspect 1977;19:103–105.
17. Bouletreau P, Ducluzeau R, Bui-Xuan B, et al: Acute renal complications of acute intoxications. Acta Pharmacol Toxicol 1977;41(Suppl):49–63.
18. Brune D, Nordberg G, Wester PO: Distribution of 23 elements in the kidney, liver and lungs of workers from a smeltery and refinery in north Sweden exposed to a number of elements and of a control group. Sci Total Environ 1980;16:13–35.
19. Buchet JP, Lauwerys R. Study of inorganic arsenic methylation by rat liver in vitro: Relevance for the interpretation of observations in man. Arch Toxicol 1985;57:125–129.
20. Buchet JP, Lauwerys R, Roels H: Comparison of the urinary excretion of arsenic metabolites after a single oral dose of sodium arsenite, monomethylarsonate or dimethylarsinate in man. Int Arch Occup Environ Health 1981;48:71–79.
21. Calleja EM, Gabrilove JL, Warrell RP Jr: Arsenic trioxide inhibits cell survival in a variety of cancer cell types [abstract]. Proc Am Soc Clin Oncol 1988;17:218a.

22. Campbell JP, Alvarez JA: Acute arsenic intoxication. Am Fam Physician 1989;40:93–97.

23. Chan PC, Huff J: Arsenic carcinogenesis in animals and in humans: Mechanistic, experimental, and epidemiological evidence. Environ Carcino Ecotox Revs 1997;C15:83–122.

24. Chen C-J, Chuang Y-C, Lin T-M, Wu HY: Malignant neoplasms among residents of a blackfoot disease-endemic area in Taiwan: High-arsenic artesian well water and cancers. Cancer Res 1985; 45:5895–5899.

25. Chen GS, Asai T, Suzuki Y, et al: A possible pathogenesis for black-foot disease: Effects of trivalent arsenic (As_2O_3) on cultured human umbilical vein endothelial cells. J Dermatol 1990;17:599–608.

26. Chernoff AI, Hartroft WS: Acute gastroenteritis. Am J Med 1956; 21:282–291.

27. Chiou HY, Hsueh YM, Hsieh LL, et al: Arsenic methylation capacity, body retention, and null genotypes of glutathione S-transferase M1 and T1 among current arsenic-exposed residents in Taiwan. Mutat Res 1997;386:197–207.

28. Chiou HY, Hsueh YM, Liaw KF, et al: Incidence of internal cancers and ingested inorganic arsenic: A seven-year follow-up study in Taiwan. Cancer Res 1995;55:1296–1300.

29. Chiou HY, Huang WI, Su CL, et al: Dose-response relationship between prevalence of cerebrovascular disease and ingested inorganic arsenic. Stroke 1997;28:1717–1723.

30. Chuttani PN, Chawla LS, Sharma TD: Arsenical neuropathy. Neurol 1967;17:269–274.

31. Concha G, Vogler G, Nermell B, Vahter M: Low-level arsenic excretion in breast milk of native Andean women exposed to high levels of arsenic in the drinking water. Int Arch Occup Environ Health 1998;71:42–46.

32. Copeman PR, Bodenstein JC: An investigation of cases of arsenical poisoning. J Forensic Med 1955;2:196–216.

33. Cullen NM, Wolf LR, St Clair D: Pediatric arsenic ingestion. Am J Emerg Med 1995;13:432–435.

34. Danan M, Dally S, Conso F: Arsenic-induced encephalopathy. Neurology 1984;34:1524.

35. Del Razo LM, Arellano MA, Cebrian ME: The oxidation states of arsenic in well-water from a chronic arsenicism area of northern Mexico. Environ Pollut 1990;64:143–153.

36. Delnomdedieu M, Basti MM, Otvos JD, Thomas DJ: Reduction and binding of arsenate and dimethylarsinate by glutathione: A magnetic resonance study. Chem Biol Interact 1994;90:139–155.

37. Desesso JM, Jacobson CF, Scialli AR, et al: An assessment of the developmental toxicity of inorganic arsenic. Reprod Toxicol 1998; 12:385–433.

38. Donofrio PD, Wilbourn AJ, Albers JW, et al: Acute arsenic intoxication presenting as Guillain-Barré-like syndrome. Muscle Nerve 1987;10:114–120.

39. Du Pont O, Ariel I, Warren SL: The distribution of radioactive arsenic in the normal and tumor-bearing (Brown-Pearce) rabbit. Am J Syph Gonorrhea Vener Dis 1941;26:96–118.

40. Eagle H, Magnuson HJ: The systemic treatment of 227 cases of arsenic poisoning (encephalitis, dermatitis, blood dyscrasias, jaundice, fever) with 2,3-dimercaptopropanol (BAL). J Clin Invest 1946; 25:420–441.

41. Edmonds JS, Shibata Y, Francesconi KA, et al: Arsenic transformations in short marine food chains studied by HPLC-ICP MS. Appl Organomet Chem 1997;11:281–287.

42. Eichner ER: Erythroid karyorrhexis in the peripheral blood smear in severe arsenic poisoning: A comparison with lead poisoning. Am J Clin Pathol 1984;81:533–537.

43. Environmental Protection Agency: National primary drinking water regulations; arsenic and clarifications to compliance and new source contaminants monitoring. Proposed rules. 40 CFR Parts 141 and 142. Fed Reg 2000 (Oct. 20);65(204):63027–63035.

44. Fanton L, Duperret S, Guillaumee F, et al: Fatal rhabdomyolysis in arsenic trioxide poisoning. Hum Exp Toxicol 1999;18:640–641.

45. Fernandez-Sola J, Nogue S, Grau JM, Casademont J, Munne P: Acute arsenical myopathy: Morphological description. J Toxicol Clin Toxicol 1991;29:131–136.

46. Fesmire FM, Schauben JL, Roberge RJ: Survival following massive arsenic ingestion. Am J Emerg Med 1988;6:602–606.

47. Fincher R-ME, Koerker RM: Long-term survival in acute arsenic encephalopathy: Follow-up using newer measures of electrophysiologic parameters. Am J Med 1987;82:549–552.

48. Fournier L, Thomas G, Garnier R, et al: 2,3-Dimercaptosuccinic-acid treatment of heavy metal poisoning in humans. Med Toxicol 1988;3:499–504.

49. Freeman JW, Couch JR: Prolonged encephalopathy with arsenic poisoning. Neurology 1978;28:853–855.

50. Frost SC, Lane MD: Evidence for the involvement of vicinal sulfhydryl groups in insulin-activated hexose transport by 3T3-L1 adipocytes. J Biol Chem 1985;260:2646–2652.

51. Galm O, Fabry U, Osieka R: Pseudotumor cerebri after treatment of relapsed acute promyelocytic leukemia with arsenic trioxide[letter]. Leukemia 2000;14:343–344.

52. Garb LG, Hine CH: Arsenical neuropathy: Residual effects following acute industrial exposure. J Occup Med 1977;19:567–568.

53. Gerhardt RE, Hudson JB, Rao RN, Sobel RE: Chronic renal insufficiency from cortical necrosis induced by arsenic poisoning. Arch Intern Med 1978;138:1267–1269.

54. Germolec DR, Spalding J, Yu HS, et al: Arsenic enhancement of skin neoplasia by chronic stimulation of growth factors. Am J Pathol 1998;153:1775–1785.

55. Germolec DR, Yoshida T, Gaido K, et al: Arsenic induces overexpression of growth factors in human keratinocytes. Toxicol Appl Pharmacol 1996;141:308–318.

56. Gherardi RK, Chariot P, Vanderstigel M, et al: Organic arsenic-induced Guillain-Barré-like syndrome due to melarsoprol: A clinical, electrophysiological, and pathological study. Muscle Nerve 1990; 13:637–645.

57. Giberson A, Vaziri D, Mirahamadi K, Rosen SM: Hemodialysis of acute arsenic intoxication with transient renal failure. Arch Intern Med 1976;136:1303–1304.

58. Goldsmith S, From AHL: Arsenic-induced atypical ventricular tachycardia. N Engl J Med 1980;303:1096–1098.

59. Gousios AG, Adelson L: Electrocardiographic and radiographic findings in acute arsenic poisoning. Am J Med 1959;27:659–663.

60. Gray JR, Khalil A, Prior JC: Acute arsenic toxicity—An opaque poison. Can Assoc Radiol J 1989;40:226–227.

61. Graziano JH, Cuccia D, Friedheim E: The pharmacology of 2,3-dimercaptosuccinic acid and its potential use in arsenic poisoning. J Pharmacol Exp Ther 1978;207:1051–1055.

62. Greenberg C, Davies S, McGowan T, et al: Acute respiratory failure following severe arsenic poisoning. Chest 1979;76:596–598.

63. Gresser MJ: ADP-arsenate: Formation by submitochondrial particles under phosphorylating conditions. J Biol Chem 1981;256: 5981–5983.

64. Griffin JP: The Easing Baker, Hong Kong. Adverse Drug React Toxicol Rev 1997;16:79–81.

65. Guha Mazumder DN, Chakraborty AK, Ghose A, et al: Chronic arsenic toxicity from drinking tubewell water in rural West Bengal. Bull WHO 1988;66:499–506.

66. Guha Mazumder DN, Das GJ, Santra A, et al: Chronic arsenic toxicity in west Bengal—The worst calamity in the world. J Indian Med Assoc 1998;96:4–7, 18.

67. Habiv TP: Nail Disease in Clinical Dermatology: A Color Guide to Diagnosis and Therapy, 3rd ed. St. Louis, Mosby, 1996.

68. Henriksen EJ, Holloszy JO: Effects of phenylarsine oxide on stimulation of glucose transport in rat skeletal muscle. Am J Physiol 1990; 258(4 Pt 1):C648–C653.

69. Hessl SM, Berman E: Severe peripheral neuropathy after exposure to monosodium methyl arsonate. J Toxicol Clin Toxicol 1982;19: 281–287.

70. Heyman A, Pfeiffer JB, Willett RW: Peripheral neuropathy caused by arsenical intoxication: A study of 41 cases with observations on the effects of BAL (2,3-dimercaptopropanol). N Engl J Med 1956; 254:401–409.

71. Hilfer RJ, Mandel A: Acute arsenic intoxication diagnosed by roentgenograms. N Engl J Med 1962;266:663–664.

72. Hindmarsh JT, McLetchie OR, Heffernan LPM, et al: Electromyographic abnormalities in chronic environmental arsenicalism. J Anal Toxicol 1977;1:270–276.

73. Hirata M, Tanaka A, Hisanaga A, Ishinishi N: Effects of glutathione depletion on the acute nephrotoxic potential of arsenite and on arsenic metabolism in hamsters. Toxicol Appl Pharmacol 1990;106: 469–481.

74. Hoover TD, Aposhian HV: BAL increases the arsenic-74 content of rabbit brain. Toxicol Appl Pharmacol 1983;70:160–162.

75. Hopenhayn-Rich C, Smith AH, Goeden HM: Human studies do not support the methylation threshold hypothesis for the toxicity of inorganic arsenic. Environ Res 1993;60(2):161–177.

76. Hsu CH, Yang SA, Wang JY, et al: Mutational spectrum of p53 gene in arsenic-related skin cancers from the blackfoot disease endemic area of Taiwan. Br J Cancer 1999;80:1080–1086.

77. Hsueh YM, Chiou HY, Huang YL, et al: Serum beta-carotene level, arsenic methylation capability, and incidence of skin cancer. Cancer Epidemiol Biomarkers Prev 1997;6:589–596.

78. Huan SY, Yang CH, Chen YC: Arsenic trioxide therapy for relapsed acute promyelocytic leukemia: A useful salvage therapy. Leuk Lymphoma 2000;38:283–293.

79. Huang R-N, Lee T-C: Cellular uptake of trivalent arsenite and pentavalent arsenate in KB cells cultured in phosphate-free medium. Toxicol Appl Pharmacol 1996;136:243–249.

80. Huang SY, Chang CS, Tang JL, et al: Acute and chronic arsenic poisoning associated with treatment of acute promyelocytic leukaemia. Br J Haematol 1998;103:1092–1095.

81. Hunt E, Hader SL, Files D, Corey GR: Arsenic poisoning seen at Duke Hospital, 1965–1998. N C Med J 1999;60:70–74.

82. Hutton JT, Christians BL, Dippel RL: Arsenic poisoning. N Engl J Med 1982;307:1080.

83. Jenkins RB: Inorganic arsenic and the nervous system. Brain 1966; 89:479–498.

84. Johnson LR, Farmer JG: Use of human metabolic studies and urinary arsenic speciation in assessing arsenic exposure. Bull Environ Contam Toxicol 1991;46:53–61.

85. Jolliffe DM, Budd AJ, Gwilt DJ: Massive acute arsenic poisoning. Anaesthesia 1991;46:288–290.

86. Kasper ML, Schoenfield L, Strom RL, Theologides A: Hepatic angiosarcoma and bronchioloalveolar carcinoma induced by Fowler's solution. JAMA 1984;252:3407–3408.

87. Kersjes MP, Maurer JR, Trestrail JH: An analysis of arsenic exposures referred to the Blodgett regional poison center. Vet Hum Toxicol 1987;29:75–78.

88. Kosnett MJ, Becker CE: Dimercaptosuccinic acid as a treatment for arsenic poisoning [abstract]. Vet Hum Toxicol 1987;29:462.

89. Kreppel H, Reichl FX, Forth W, Fichtl B: Lack of effectiveness of D-penicillamine in experimental arsenic poisoning. Vet Hum Toxicol 1989;31:1–5.

90. Kreppel H, Reichl FX, Kleine A, et al: Antidotal efficacy of newly synthesized dimercaptosuccinic acid (SUCCIMER) monoesters in experimental arsenic poisoning in mice. Fundam Appl Toxicol 1995;26: 239–245.

91. Kreppel H, Reichl FX, Szinicz L, et al: Efficacy of various dithiol compounds in acute As₂O₃ poisoning in mice. Arch Toxicol 1990; 64:387–392.

92. Kyle RA, Pease GL: Hematologic aspects of arsenic intoxication. N Engl J Med 1965;273:18–23.

93. Lagerkvist BE, Linderholm H, Nordberg GF: Arsenic and Raynaud's phenomenon. Vasospastic tendency and excretion of arsenic in smelter workers before and after the summer vacation. Int Arch Occup Environ Health 1988;60:361–364.

94. Lai MS, Hsueh YM, Chen CJ, et al: Ingested inorganic arsenic and prevalence of diabetes mellitus. Am J Epidemiol 1994;139:484–492.

95. Lander JJ, Stanley RJ, Sumner HW, et al: Angiosarcoma of the liver associated with Fowler's solution (potassium arsenite). Gastroenterology 1975;68:1582–1586.

96. Le Quesne PM, McLeod J. Peripheral neuropathy following a single exposure to arsenic: Clinical course in four patients with electrophysiological and histological studies. J Neurol Sci 1977;32: 437–451.

97. Le XC, Cullen WR, Reimer KJ: Human urinary arsenic excretion after one-time ingestion of seaweed, crab, and shrimp. Clin Chem 1994;40:617–624.

98. Lee-Feldstein A. Cumulative exposure to arsenic and its relationship to respiratory cancer among copper smelter employees. J Occup Med 1986;28(4):296–302.

99. Lenz K, Hruby K, Druml W, et al: 2,3-Dimercaptosuccinic acid in human arsenic poisoning. Arch Toxicol 1981;47:241–243.

100. Lerman BB, Ali N, Green D: Megaloblastic, dyserythropoietic anemia following arsenic ingestion. Ann Clin Lab Sci 1980;10:515–517.

101. Levin-Scherz JK, Patrick JD, Weber FH, Garabedian C Jr: Acute arsenic ingestion. Ann Emerg Med 1987;16:702–704.

102. Liebl B, Muckter H, Doklea E, et al: Influence of glucose on the toxicity of oxophenylarsine in MDCK cells. Arch Toxicol 1995;69: 421–424.

103. Lin TH, Huang YL, Tseng WC: Arsenic and lipid peroxidation in patients with blackfoot disease. Bull Environ Contam Toxicol 1995; 54(4):488–493.

104. Lugo G, Cassady G, Palmisano P: Acute maternal arsenic intoxication with neonatal death. Am J Dis Child 1969;117:328–330.

105. Mackell MA, Gantner GE, Poklis A, Graham M: An unsuspected arsenic poisoning murder disclosed by forensic autopsy. Am J Forensic Med Pathol 1985;6:358–361.

106. Maehashi H, Murata Y: Arsenic excretion after treatment of arsenic poisoning with SUCCIMER or DMPS in mice. Jpn J Pharmacol 1986; 40:188–190.

107. Mahieu P, Buchet JP, Roels HA, Lauwerys R: The metabolism of arsenic in humans acutely intoxicated by As₂O₃: Its significance for the duration of BAL therapy. Clin Toxicol 1981;18:1067–1075.

108. Marafante E, Vahter M: The effect of methyltransferase inhibition on the metabolism of [74As]arsenite in mice and rabbits. Chem Biol Interact 1984;50:49–57.

109. Massey EW, Wold D, Heyman A: Arsenic: Homicidal intoxication. South Med J 1984;77:848–851.

110. Mathieu D, Mathieu-Nolf M, Germain-Alonso M, et al: Massive arsenic poisoning—Effect of hemodialysis and dimercaprol on arsenic kinetics. Intensive Care Med 1992;18:47–50.

111. McKinney JD: Metabolism and disposition of inorganic arsenic in laboratory animals and humans. Environ Geochem Health 1992; 14:43–48.

112. Mealey J, Brownell GL, Sweet WH: Radioarsenic in plasma, urine, normal tissues, and intracranial neoplasms. Arch Neurol Psychiatr 1959;8:310–320.

113. Moore DF, O'Callaghan CA, Berlyne G, et al: Acute arsenic poisoning: Absence of polyneuropathy after treatment with 2,3-dimercaptopropanesulphonate (DMPS). J Neurol Neurosurg Psychiatry 1994; 57:1133–1135.

114. Moore MM, Harrington-Brock K, Doerr CL: Relative genotoxic potency of arsenic and its methylated metabolites. Mutat Res 1997; 386:279–290.

115. Muckter H, Liebl B, Reichl FX, et al: Are we ready to replace dimercaprol (BAL) as an arsenic antidote? Hum Exp Toxicol 1997; 16:460–465.

116. Nevens F, Fevery J, Van Steenbergen W, et al: Arsenic and non-cirrhotic portal hypertension: A report of eight cases. J Hepatol 1990; 11:80–85.

117. Nixon DE, Moyer TP: Arsenic analysis II. Rapid separation and quantification of inorganic arsenic plus metabolites and arsenobetaine from urine. Clin Chem 1992;38:2479–2483.

118. Oh SJ: Electrophysiological profile in arsenic neuropathy. J Neurol Neurosurg Psychiatry 1991;54:1103–1105.

119. Otani K: Studies on the absorption and distribution of arsenic (English summary). Sappori Igaku Zasshi 1957;11:285–294.

120. Park MJ, Currier M: Arsenic exposures in Mississippi: A review of cases. South Med J 1991;84:461–464.

121. Pazirandeh A, Brati AH, Marageh MG: Determination of arsenic in hair using neutron activation. Appl Radiat Isot 1998;49:753–759.

122. Pepin J, Milord F: African trypanosomiasis and drug-induced encephalopathy: Risk factors and pathogenesis. Trans R Soc Trop Med Hyg 1991;85:222–224.

123. Pershagen G, Vahter M: Arsenic: A Toxicological and Epidemiological Appraisal. Stockholm, Department of Environmental Hygiene of the Karolinska Institute and the National (Swedish) Environment Protection, 1979.

124. Peters HA, Croft WA, Woolson EA, et al: Hematological, dermal and neuropsychological disease from burning and power sawing chromium-copper-arsenic (CCA)-treated wood. Acta Pharmacol Toxicol (Copenh) 1986;59 Suppl 7:39–43.

125. Peters HA, Croft WA, Woolson EA, et al: Seasonal arsenic exposure from burning chromium-copper-arsenate treated wood. JAMA 1984;251:2393–2396.

126. Poklis A, Saady JJ: Arsenic poisoning: Acute or chronic? Suicide or murder? Am J Forensic Med Pathol 1990;11:226–232.

127. Pomroy C, Charbonneau SM, McCullough RS, Tam GK: Human retention studies with ^{74}As. Toxicol Appl Pharmacol 1980;53: 550–556.

128. Rahman M, Tondel M, Ahmad SA, Axelson O: Diabetes mellitus associated with arsenic exposure in Bangladesh. Am J Epidemiol 1998;148:198–203.

129. Ramirez P, Eastmond DA, Laclette JP, Ostrosky-Wegman P: Disruption of microtubule assembly and spindle formation as a mechanism for the induction of aneuploid cells by sodium arsenite and vanadium pentoxide. Mutat Res 1997;386:291–298.

130. Ramos O, Carrizales L, Yanez L, et al: Arsenic increased lipid peroxidation in rat tissues by a mechanism independent of glutathione levels. Environ Health Perspect 1995;103(Suppl 1):85–88.

131. Regelson W, Kim U, Ospina J, Holland JF: Hemangioendothelial sarcoma of liver from chronic arsenic intoxication by Fowler's solution. Cancer 1968;21:514–522.

132. Reichl F-X, Hunder G, Liebl B, et al: Effect of DMPS and various adsorbents on the arsenic excretion in guinea pigs after injection with As_2O_3. Arch Toxicol 1995;69:712–717.

133. Reichl F-X, Kreppel H, Forth W: Pyruvate and lactate metabolism in livers of guinea pigs perfused with chelation agents after repeated treatment with As_2O_3. Arch Toxicol 1991;65:235–238.

134. Reichl F-X, Kreppel H, Szinicz L, et al: Effect of glucose treatment on carbohydrate content in various organs in mice after acute As_2O_3 poisoning. Vet Hum Toxicol 1991;33:230–235.

135. Reichl F-X, Szinicz L, Kreppel H, Forth W: Effects of arsenic on carbohydrate metabolism after single or repeated injection in guinea pigs. Arch Toxicol 1988;62:473–475.

136. Reichl F-X, Kreppel H, Szinicz L, et al: Reduction of arsenic trioxide toxicity in mice by repeated treatment with glucose. Arch Toxicol Suppl 1991;14:225–227.

137. Reichl FX, Szinicz L, Kreppel H, et al: Effect of glucose in mice after acute experimental poisoning with arsenic trioxide (As_2O_3). Arch Toxicol 1990;64:336–338.

138. Rein K-A, Borrebaek B, Bremer J: Arsenite inhibits β-oxidation in isolated rat liver mitochondria. Biochim Biophys Acta 1979;574: 487–494.

139. Roat JW, Wald A, Mendelow H, Pataki KI: Hepatic angiosarcoma associated with short-term arsenic ingestion. Am J Med 1982;73: 933–936.

140. Robinson TJ: Arsenical polyneuropathy due to caustic arsenical paste. Br Med J 1975;3:139.

141. New LC-ICP-MS Techniques. Glen Ellyn, IL, Tower Conference Management Company, 1989.

142. Roses OE, Garcia Fernandez JC, Villaamil EC, et al: Mass poisoning by sodium arsenite. J Toxicol Clin Toxicol 1991;29:209–213.

143. Royal Commissioners: The final report of the Royal Commission on arsenical poisoning. Lancet 1903;2:1674–1676.

144. Santra A, Das GJ, De BK, et al: Hepatic manifestations in chronic arsenic toxicity. Indian J Gastroenterol 1999;18:152–155.

145. Sanz P, Corbella J, Nogue S, et al: Rhabdomyolysis in fatal arsenic trioxide poisoning. JAMA 1989;262:3271.

146. Savory J, Sedor FA: Arsenic poisoning. In: Brown SS, ed: Clinical Chemistry and Chemical Toxicology of Metals. New York, Elsevier/North Holland, 1977, pp. 271–286.

147. Schoof RA, Yost LJ, Eickhoff J, et al: A market basket survey of inorganic arsenic in food. Food Chem Toxicol 1999;37(8):839–846.

148. Schoolmeester WL, White DR: Arsenic poisoning. South Med J 1980;73:198–208.

149. Shaebar FZ, Yannai S: In vitro effects of cadmium and arsenite on glutathione peroxidase, aspartate and alanine aminotransferase, cholinesterase and glucose-6-phosphate dehydrogenase activities in blood. Vet Hum Toxicol 1989;31:528–531.

150. Shao W, Fanelli M, Ferrara FF, et al: Arsenic trioxide as an inducer of apoptosis and loss of PML/RAR alpha protein in acute promyelocytic leukemia cells. J Natl Cancer Inst 1998;90:124–133.

151. Shum S, Whitehead J, Vaughn L, Hale T: Chelation of organoarsenate with dimercaptosuccinic acid. Vet Hum Toxicol 1995;37: 239–242.

152. Smith AH, Goycolea M, Haque R, Biggs ML: Marked increase in bladder and lung cancer mortality in a region of northern Chile due to arsenic in drinking water. Am J Epidemiol 1998;147:660–669.

153. Smith AH, Lingas EO, Rahman M: Contamination of drinking water by arsenic in Bangladesh: A public health emergency. Bull WHO 2000;78:1093–1103.

154. Soignet SL, Maslak P, Wang ZG, et al: Complete remission after treatment of acute promyelocytic leukemia with arsenic trioxide. N Engl J Med 1998;339:1341–1348.

155. Soignet SL, Tong WP, Hirschfeld S, Warrell RP Jr: Clinical study of an organic arsenical, melarsoprol, in patients with advanced leukemia. Cancer Chemother Pharmacol 1999;44:417–421.

156. St. Petery J, Gross C, Victorica BE: Ventricular fibrillation caused by arsenic poisoning. Am J Dis Child 1970;120:367–371.

157. Stevens JT, Hall LL, Farmer JD, et al: Disposition of ^{14}C and/or ^{74}As-cacodylic acid in rats after intravenous, intratracheal, or peroral administration. Environ Health Perspect 1977;19:151–157.

158. Stryer L: Biochemistry, 4th ed. New York, WH Freeman, 1995.

159. Styblo M, Yamauchi H, Thomas DJ: Comparative in vitro methylation of trivalent and pentavalent arsenicals. Toxicol Appl Pharmacol 1995;135:172–178.

160. Szinicz L, Forth W: Effect of As_2O_3 on gluconeogenesis. Arch Toxicol 1988;61:444–449.

161. Tam GK, Charbonneau SM, Bryce F, et al: Metabolism of inorganic arsenic (74As) in humans following oral ingestion. Toxicol Appl Pharmacol 1979;50:319–322.

162. Tay CH, Seah CS: Arsenic poisoning from anti-asthmatic herbal preparations. Med J Aust 1975;2:424–428.

163. Tracy JW, Webster LT Jr: Drugs used in the chemotherapy of protozoal infections (continued). In: Hardman JG, Limbird LE, eds: Goodman & Gilman's The Pharmacologic Basis of Therapeutics, 9th edition. New York, McGraw-Hill, 1996, pp. 987–1008.

164. Tseng CH, Chong CK, Chen CJ, Tai TY: Dose-response relationship between peripheral vascular disease and ingested inorganic arsenic among residents in blackfoot disease endemic villages in Taiwan. Atherosclerosis 1996;120:125–133.

165. Tsukamoto H, Parker HR, Gribble DH: Metabolism and renal handling of sodium arsenate in dogs. Am J Vet Res 1983;44:2331–2335.

166. Tsukamoto H, Parker HR, Gribble DH, et al: Nephrotoxicity of sodium arsenate in dogs. Am J Vet Res 1983;44:2324–2330.

167. Unnikrishnan D, Dutcher JP, Varshneya N, et al: Torsade de pointes in 3 patients with leukemia treated with arsenic trioxide. Blood 2001;97:1514–1516.

168. Vahter M: Biotransformation of trivalent and pentavalent inorganic arsenic in mice and rats. Environ Res 1981;25:286–293.

169. Vahter M: Metabolism of arsenic. In: Fowler BA, ed: Biological and Environmental Effects of Arsenic. New York, Elsevier, 1983, pp. 171–198.

170. Vahter M: Methylation of inorganic arsenic in different mammalian species and population groups. Sci Prog 1999;82(Pt 1):69–88.

171. Vahter M, Marafante E: Intracellular interaction and metabolic fate of arsenite and arsenate in mice and rabbits. Chem Biol Interact 1983;47:29–44.

172. Vahter M, Marafante E: Effects of low dietary intake of methionine, choline or proteins on the biotransformation of arsenite in the rabbit. Toxicol Lett 1987;37:41–46.

173. Vahter M, Norin H: Metabolism of [74]As-labeled trivalent and pentavalent inorganic arsenic in mice. Environ Res 1980;21:446–457.

174. Vaziri ND, Upham T, Barton CH: Hemodialysis clearance of arsenic. Clin Toxicol 1980;17:451–456.

175. Wagner SL, Weswig P: Arsenic in blood and urine of forest workers. Arch Environ Health 1974;28:77–79.

176. Weinberg SL: The electrocardiogram in acute arsenic poisoning. Am Heart J 1960;60:971–975.

177. Wester PO, Brune D, Nordberg G: Arsenic and selenium in lung, liver, and kidney tissue from dead smelter workers. Br J Industrial Med 1981;38:179–184.

178. Wester RC, Maibach HI, Sedik L, et al: In vivo and in vitro percutaneous absorption and skin decontamination of arsenic from water and soil. Fundam Appl Toxicol 1993;20:336–340.

179. Winski SL, Carter DE: Arsenate toxicity in human erythrocytes: Characterization of morphologic changes and determination of the mechanism of damage. J Toxicol Environ Health A 1998;53:345–355.

180. Wong SS, Tan KC, Goh CL: Cutaneous manifestations of chronic arsenicism: Review of seventeen cases. J Am Acad Dermatol 1998;38(2 Pt 1):179–185.

181. Woollons A, Russell-Jones R: Chronic endemic hydroarsenicism. Br J Dermatol 1998;139:1092–1096.

182. Yamanaka K, Hasegawa A, Sawamura R, Okada S: Dimethylated arsenics induce DNA strand breaks in lung via the production of active oxygen in mice. Biochem Biophys Res Comm 1989;165:43–50.

183. Yamanaka K, Hasegawa A, Sawamura R, Okada S: Cellular response to oxidative damage in lung induced by the administration of dimethylarsinic acid, a major metabolite of inorganic arsenics, in mice. Toxicol Appl Pharmacol 1991;108:205–213.

184. Young EG, Smith RP: Arsenic content of hair and bone in acute and chronic arsenical poisoning: Review of 2 cases examined posthumously from medico-legal aspect. Br Med J 1942;1:251–253.

185. Zakharyan R, Wu Y, Bogdan GM, Aposhian HV: Enzymatic methylation of arsenic compounds: Assay, partial purification, and properties of arsenite methyltransferase and monomethylarsonic acid methyltransferase of rabbit liver. Chem Res Toxicol 1995;8:1029–1038.

186. Zaloga GP, Deal J, Spurling T, et al: Case report: Unusual manifestations of arsenic intoxication. Am J Med Sci 1985;289:210–214.

187. Zhang T, Westervelt P, Hess JL: Pathologic, cytogenetic and molecular assessment of acute promyelocytic leukemia patients treated with arsenic trioxide (As_2O_3). Mod Pathol 2000;13:954–961.

188. Zhang TL, Gao YX, Lu JF, Wang K: Arsenite, arsenate and vanadate affect human erythrocyte membrane. J Inorg Biochem 2000;79(1–4):195–203.

ANTIDOTES IN DEPTH

Dimercaprol (BAL)
Mary Ann Howland

$$
\begin{array}{c}
\text{H} \\
| \\
\text{H--C--OH} \\
| \\
\text{H--C--SH} \\
| \\
\text{H--C--SH} \\
| \\
\text{H}
\end{array}
$$

2,3-Dimercaptopropanol (BAL)

Dimercaprol (British Anti-Lewisite; BAL; 2,3-dimercaptopropanol) is an effective metal chelator used clinically in the treatment of inorganic mercury (not methyl mercury) and arsenic (not arsine) toxicity, and in conjunction with edetate calcium disodium (CaNa$_2$EDTA) for lead encephalopathy and severe lead toxicity. The dose and duration of BAL therapy depend on the metal being chelated and the severity of toxicity.[19,26]

OVERVIEW OF PRINCIPLES OF CHELATION

According to the theory of chelating metals, soft metals such as Hg^{2+}, Au$^+$, Cu$^+$, and Ag$^+$ form the most stable complexes with sulfur donors[1,5,28] (see Chap. 12 for further details). Soft metals are therefore referred to as sulfur seekers and have large atomic radii with a large number of electrons in the outer shell. The chelator or ligand, in this case a sulfur-containing compound such as BAL, forms a coordinate bond with the metal by donating a pair of free electrons. Hard metals such as Na$^+$, K$^+$, Mg^{2+}, Ca^{2+}, and Al^{3+} are referred to as oxygen seekers and form the best complexes with hard ligands containing a COO$^-$ group such as CaNa$_2$EDTA. Borderline metals, such as Pb^{2+}, Cd^{2+}, Cu^{2+}, As^{3+}, and Zn^{2+}, prefer nitrogen-donating ligands but will also react with hard or soft ligands. Antidotes for metal poisoning often contain more than one type of donating group, making them effective for more than one type of metal. BAL has two adjacent sulfur groups, thus the term *dithiol*; the presence of these two sulfur groups permits the formation of a ring structure with the metal, thereby enhancing chelator stability.[1,5,28]

The most useful chelators have a relatively low order of toxicity, form stable complexes with the chelated metals, have tissue distribution characteristics similar to the metal to be chelated, and effect a favorable outcome.[1,5,28] Desirable aspects of the metal-chelator complex are elimination from the body without breakdown, lack of redistribution to the brain or other critical organs, and a low order of toxicity. Unfortunately, there is no currently available chelator with all of these attributes. Also, there are no published double-blind, randomized, placebo-controlled trials evaluating outcome issues with the use of metal chelators such as

dimercaprol, CaNa$_2$EDTA, or succimer with lead, arsenic, or mercury poisoning in humans. The majority of evidence accumulated to date for efficacy comes from animal studies, several case series compared to historical controls, and several case reports. Redistribution characteristics of metal chelator complexes are being rigorously investigated in animal models, because redistribution to vital tissues such as the brain is of great concern. Although BAL has been in use since the late 1940s,[20] much of our practice relies on opinion and historical precedence and many questions with regard to pharmacokinetics and toxicokinetics remain to be addressed.

HISTORY

Investigation into the use of sulfur donors as antidotes was precipitated by the World War II threat of chemical warfare with lewisite (dichloro-(2-chlorovinyl)-arsine) and mustard gas (dichloro-diethyl-sulfide), vesicant gases that resulted in tissue damage when combined with protein sulfhydryl (SH) groups[31] (Chap. 100). These investigations led to the discovery of the dithiol 2,3-dimercaptopropanol, called British Anti-Lewisite. BAL combined with lewisite forms a stable 5-membered ring.

CHEMISTRY

The molecular weight of BAL is 124.2 daltons and it has a specific gravity of 1.21.[32] BAL is an oily liquid with only 6% weight/volume water solubility, 5% weight/volume peanut oil solubility, and a disagreeable odor. Aqueous solutions are easily oxidized and therefore unstable. Peanut oil stabilizes BAL, while the addition of benzyl benzoate in the ratio of 1 part BAL to 2 parts of benzyl benzoate renders the BAL miscible with peanut oil in all proportions.[32]

ARSENIC
Animal Studies

The assumption that lewisite would be sprayed over the land and its population, causing skin lesions, led researchers to believe that the limited water solubility and high lipid solubility of BAL would be valuable for potential cutaneous application.[36] In a rodent model, topical BAL was very effective at low concentrations in preventing lewisite-induced toxicity and in reversing toxicity when administered within 1 hour of skin exposure.[29,31] In rabbits, topical BAL proved effective in preventing ocular destruction if applied within 20 minutes of exposure.[19] Urinary arsenic concentrations were significantly increased after the application of topical BAL.[31]

The effectiveness against lewisite and other arsenicals of both parenteral single-dose and multiple-dose BAL was studied in rabbits. When begun within 2 hours of lewisite exposure, BAL injections of 4 mg/kg given every 4 hours led to a 50% survival of exposed rabbits. This dose regimen was demonstrated to be one-seventh of the maximum tolerated dose of BAL.[13]

The most recent studies in a variety of animal models demonstrate that although dimercaprol has a beneficial effect in increasing the LD_{50} of sodium arsenite, the therapeutic index is low and arsenic redistribution to the brain occurs.[2,4,3,16,33] In these animal models, succimer and the investigational agent dimercaptopropane sulfonate (DMPS) also beneficially increase the LD_{50}, but with a better therapeutic index and with no redistribution to the brain. Chapter 79 discusses the significant controversy with regard to in vitro and in vivo studies on the facilitation of arsenic entry into the cells.

Human Studies

Experiments in human volunteers given minute amounts of arsenic demonstrated the ability of BAL to increase urinary arsenic concentration by about 40%, with maximum excretion occurring within 2–4 hours after BAL administration.[38] Dimercaprol was subsequently used in the treatment of arsenical dermatitis resulting from syphilis therapy with organic arsenicals. When applied to affected skin, topical BAL produced erythema, pruritus, and dysesthesias, but had no adverse effects on unaffected skin. Abscesses occasionally resulted, whether or not the BAL was given IM through affected or unaffected skin. Intramuscular BAL produced both subjective and objective improvement, limited the duration of the arsenical dermatitis, and was accompanied by elevated urinary arsenic levels.[9,23,24]

In a study of 227 patients with inorganic arsenic poisoning, maximal efficacy and minimal toxicity were achieved when BAL was administered intramuscularly at 3 mg/kg every 4 hours for 48 hours and then twice daily for 7–10 days. This regimen resulted in complete recovery in 6 of 7 patients with severe arsenic-induced encephalopathy and demonstrated the importance of administering BAL as soon as possible after the exposure. Of 33 patients with severe arsenic-induced encephalopathy, 18 of 24 treated within 6 hours survived, versus only 4 of 9 treated after a lapse of 72 or more hours.[12] Furthermore, the effectiveness of BAL was also demonstrated in three patients who were treated successfully with appropriate doses of BAL after mistakenly receiving 10–20 times the therapeutic dose of Mapharsen (oxophenarsine hydrochloride). A fourth patient, treated with inadequate doses of BAL, died.[12] This study also supported the effectiveness of BAL in treating arsenic-induced agranulocytosis, encephalopathy, dermatitis, massive overdose of Mapharsen, and probably arsenical fever.[12]

When dimercaprol first became more widely available, 42 children who were treated following arsenic ingestions were compared to a historical group of 111 other children who had ingested arsenic.[39] The percentage of children exhibiting symptoms on presentation were similar between groups (46%), but there were fewer deaths (0 vs 3), a shorter average hospital stay (1.6 vs 4.2 days), and fewer individuals with persistent symptoms at 12 hours (0% vs 29.3%) in the treated patients.

Ocular damage caused by lewisite is partly a result of the liberation of hydrochloric acid, which results in an acid injury causing localized superficial opacity of the cornea and deep penetration of lewisite into the cornea and aqueous humor with resultant rapid necrosis. A 5% BAL ointment or solution applied within 2 minutes of exposure prevented the development of a significant reaction; application at 30 minutes lessened the reaction, but did not prevent permanent damage.[17]

MERCURY

Because mercury also reacts with sulfhydryl groups, animal studies were performed to assess the affinity and ability of thiols to competitively chelate inorganic mercury and prevent toxicity. As in the case of arsenic exposure, the dithiols BAL and BAL glucoside were more effective than the monothiol 1-thiosorbitol in preventing mercury-induced death and uremia.[15] The clinical efficacy of BAL in treating inorganic mercury poisoning was substantiated in patients who ingested mercury bichloride.[22,21] Thirty-eight patients ingesting more than 1 g of mercuric chloride who were treated with dimercaprol within 4 hours of exposure were compared to historical controls.[21] There were no deaths in the 38 patients treated with BAL as compared to 27 deaths in the 86 untreated patients. Death was a result of hemorrhagic gastritis and renal failure.[21] BAL is particularly useful for patients who have ingested a mercuric salt, as their associated gastrointestinal toxicity limits the potential of an orally administered antidote such as succimer.

Animal models demonstrate that when BAL is administered to chelate mercury following poisoning from elemental mercury vapor or exposure to short-chain organic mercury compounds, brain levels of mercury may increase.[6,8] However, in a rat model, the initiation of BAL therapy within 1 day of exposure to short-chain organic mercury compounds prevented neurologic toxicity.[40] When treatment was delayed for 12 days, no effect on established neurotoxicity could be demonstrated. We do not recommend BAL therapy when patients are exposed to short-chain organic mercury compounds because it may increase brain concentrations of methyl mercury.[5,19]

LEAD

BAL is used in combination with $CaNa_2EDTA$ to treat patients with severe lead poisoning; otherwise, succimer has become the lead chelator of choice. When lead encephalopathy is present, it is very important to administer the dimercaprol first, followed by the $CaNa_2EDTA$ 4 hours later, together with the second dose of BAL. This regimen is used to prevent the $CaNa_2EDTA$ from facilitating the redistribution of lead into the brain.[10,11] Providing two different chelators also reduces the blood lead level significantly faster than $CaNa_2EDTA$ alone, and maintains a better molar ratio of chelator to lead.[10] Once the mobilization of lead has begun, it is important to provide uninterrupted therapy to prevent redistribution of lead to the brain.[10] Because cerebral edema is often a critical complication of lead encephalopathy, meticulous attention must be made to restrict fluids and lower elevated intracranial pressure.

ADVERSE EFFECTS AND SAFETY ISSUES

The LD_{50} of BAL by SC administration is 110 mg/kg (0.88 mmol/kg) in rats[19] and 183 mg/kg (1.48 mmol/kg) IP (intraperitoneal) in mice.[4] The toxicity of BAL in humans is dose-dependent and affected by urinary pH. An acidic urine allows dissociation of the BAL-metal chelate. For patients who received 2.5 mg/kg every 4–6 hours for 4 doses, less than 1% of 700 intramuscular injections resulted in minor reactions such as pain at the injection site.[12] When doses of 4 mg/kg and 5 mg/kg were given, the incidence of adverse effects rose to 14% and 65%, respectively.[12] At these higher doses the following symptoms were reported in decreasing order of frequency: nausea; vomiting; headache; burning sensation of lips, mouth, throat, and eyes; lacrimation; rhinorrhea; salivation; muscle aches; burning and tingling of extremities; tooth pain; diaphoresis; chest pain; anxiety; and agitation.[23] These effects were maximal within 10–30 minutes of exposure, and usually subsided within 30–50 minutes.[12] Elevations in systolic and diastolic blood pressure and tachycardia commonly occur and are correlated with increasing doses.[19,26] Thirty percent of children given BAL may develop a fever that can persist throughout the therapeutic period.[19] A transient reduction in the percentage of polymorphonuclear leukocytes may also occur.[19] Doses above 5 mg/kg should not be administered. Doses above 25 mg/kg can be expected to produce a hypertensive encephalopathy with convulsions and coma.[39]

BAL is not very effective in the presence of arsenic-induced liver damage.[24] Moreover, in rats, preexistent liver hepatotoxicity was exacerbated when BAL was used for treatment of arsenic poisoning. Therefore, unless the hepatotoxicity is considered arsenic-induced, hepatic dysfunction is a contraindication to BAL use.[31] Dimercaprol should not be used for patients poisoned by methyl mercury because animal studies demonstrate a redistribution of mercury to the brain.[5,19]

Since dissociation of the BAL-metal chelate will occur in an acid urine, the urine of patients receiving BAL should be alkalinized to prevent renal liberation of the metal.[19] Dimercaprol should be used with caution for patients with glucose-6-phosphate dehydrogenase (G6PD) deficiency, as it may cause hemolysis.[18] In these cases, a risk-to-benefit analysis must be made because G6PD-deficiency syndromes are variably expressed in young cells. In addition, chelators are relatively nonspecific and may bind metals other than those desired, thus causing deficiency of an essential metal. For example, BAL given to mice increased copper elimination to 3 times normal.[7] Dimercaprol is formulated in peanut oil; therefore, the patient should be evaluated for peanut allergy. There is limited evidence to suggest that iron supplements should not be given to patients who are receiving BAL because the BAL-iron complex appears to cause severe vomiting and decreases metal chelation.[10,11,14]

Unintentional intravenous infusion of a methylprogesterone product in peanut oil resulted in a syndrome comparable to that associated with fat embolization. Lipoid pneumonia, pleural effusions, and hypoxia ensued, with resolution over a 2-week period.[34] A similar syndrome would be expected from the intravenous use of dimercaprol.

PHARMACOKINETICS

There are no recent pharmacokinetic studies with BAL. The limited amount of information available dates back to the late 1940s. Blood concentrations of BAL peak about 30 minutes after IM administration and distribution occurs quickly.[32,35] After IM administration to rabbits, blood levels drop quickly after 2 hours. Urinary excretion of BAL metabolites, perhaps partially as glucuronic acid conjugates, accounted for nearly 45% of the dose within 6 hours and for 81% within 24 hours.[32,34] Very little is excreted unchanged in the urine.[32] BAL is concentrated in the kid-

ney, liver, and small intestine.[30] BAL can also be found in the feces, pleading for an enterohepatic circulation. Hemodialysis may be useful in removing the BAL-metal chelate in cases of renal failure.[19,25,37]

DOSING

The dose of BAL for lead encephalopathy is 75 mg/m^2 IM every 4 hours for 5 days.[10,11] As noted earlier, the first dose of dimercaprol should precede the first dose of CaNa$_2$EDTA by 4 hours. Thereafter, intravenous CaNa$_2$EDTA in a dose of 1500 mg/m^2/d as a continuous infusion, or divided into 2–4 doses, should be administered. These daily doses are equimolar.

The dose of BAL for severe inorganic arsenic poisoning has not been established. One regimen uses 3 mg/kg IM every 4 hours for 48 hours and then twice daily for 7–10 days.[12] Another regimen uses 3–5 mg/kg IM every 4–6 hours on the first day and then tapers the dose and frequency depending on the patient's symptomatology. A third regimen reduces the number of injections by day 2, terminating therapy within 5–7 days.[39]

The dose of dimercaprol for patients exposed to inorganic mercury salts is 5 mg/kg IM initially, followed by 2.5 mg/kg every 8–12 hours for 1 day, followed by 2.5 mg/kg every 12–24 hours until the patient appears clinically improved, up to a total of 10 days.

Commercially available BAL is a yellow, viscous liquid with a sulfur odor. It is available in 3-mL ampules containing 100 mg/mL of BAL, 200 mg/mL of benzyl benzoate, and 700 mg/mL of peanut oil. This agent should only be administered by deep IM injection.

REFERENCES

1. Aaseth J: Recent advances in the therapy of metal poisonings with chelating agents. Hum Toxicol 1983;2:257–272.
2. Aposhian HV, Tadlock CH, Moon TE: Protection of mice against the lethal effects of sodium arsenite—A quantitative comparison of a number of chelating agents. Toxicol Appl Pharmacol 1981;61: 385–392.
3. Aposhian HV, Mershon MM, Brinkley FB, et al: Anti-Lewisite activity and stability of meso-dimercaptosuccinic acid and 2,3-dimercapto-1-propanesulfonic acid. Life Sci 1982;31:2149–2156.
4. Aposhian HV, Carter DE, Hoover TD, et al: DMSA, DMPS, and DMPA as arsenic antidotes. Fundam Appl Toxicol 1984;4:S58–S70.
5. Aposhian HV, Maiorino RM, Gonzalez-Ramirez D, et al: Mobilization of heavy metals by newer, therapeutically useful chelating agents. Toxicology 1995;97:23–38.
6. Berlin M, Ullberg S: Increased uptake of mercury in mouse brain caused by 2,3-dimercaptopropanol. Nature 1963;197:84–85.
7. Cantilena LR, Klaassen CD: The effect of chelating agents on the excretion of endogenous metals. Toxicol Appl Pharmacol 1982;63: 344–350.
8. Canty AJ, Kishimoto R: British anti-lewisite and organ-mercury poisoning. Nature 1972;253:123–125.
9. Carleton AB, Peters RA, Stocken LA, et al: Clinical uses of 2,3-dimercaptopropanol (BAL): VI. The treatment of complications of arseno-therapy with BAL. J Clin Invest 1946;25:497–527.
10. Chisolm JJ Jr: The use of chelating agents in the treatment of acute and chronic lead intoxication in childhood. J Pediatr 1968;73:1–38.
11. Committee on Drugs: Treatment guidelines for lead exposure in children. Pediatrics 1995;96:155–160.

12. Eagle H, Magnuson HJ: The systemic treatment of 227 cases of arsenic poisoning (encephalitis, dermatitis, blood dyscrasias, jaundice, fever) with 2,3-dimercaptopropanol (BAL). Am J Syph Gonor Ven Dis 1946;30:420–441.

13. Eagle H, Magnuson HJ, Fleischman R: Clinical uses of 2,3-dimercaptopropanol (BAL): I. The systemic treatment of experimental arsenic poisoning (Mapharsen, lewisite, phenyl arsenoxide) with BAL. J Clin Invest 1946;25:451–466.

14. Edge WD, Somers GF: The effect of dimercaprol (BAL) in acute iron poisoning. Q J Pharm Pharmacol 1948;21:364–369.

15. Gilman A, Allen RP, Philips FS, et al: Clinical uses of 2,3-dimercaptopropanol (BAL): X. The treatment of acute systemic mercury poisoning in experimental animals with BAL, thiosorbitol and BAL glucoside. J Clin Invest 1946;25:549–556.

16. Hoover TD, Aposhian HV: BAL Increases the arsenic-74 content of rabbit brain. Toxicol Appl Pharmacol 1983;70:160–162.

17. Hughes WF: Clinical uses of 2,3-dimercaptopropanol (BAL): IX. The treatment of lewisite burns of the eye with BAL. J Clin Invest 1946; 25:541–548.

18. Janakiraman N, Seeler RA, Royal JE, et al: Hemodialysis during BAL chelation therapy for high blood lead levels in two G6PD-deficient children. Clin Pediatr 1978;17:485–487.

19. Klaassen CD: Heavy metals and heavy metal antagonists. In: Hardman JG, Limbird LE, eds: The Pharmacological Basis of Therapeutics, 10th ed. New York, Macmillan, 2001, pp. 1851–1875.

20. Kosnett MJ: Unanswered questions in metal chelation. J Toxicol Clin Toxicol 1992;30:529–547.

21. Longcope WT, Luetscher JA: The use of BAL (British Anti-Lewsite) in the treatment of the injurious effects of arsenic, mercury and other metallic poisons. Ann Intern Med 1949;31:545–554.

22. Longcope WT, Luetscher JA, Calkins F, et al: Clinical uses of 2,3-dimercaptopropanol (BAL): XI. The treatment of acute mercury poisoning by BAL. J Clin Invest 1946;25:557–567.

23. Longcope WT, Luetscher JA, Wintrobe MM, et al: Clinical uses of 2,3-dimercaptopropanol (BAL): VII. The treatment of arsenical dermatitis with preparations of BAL. J Clin Invest 1946;25:528–533.

24. Luetscher JA, Eagle H, Longcope WT: Clinical uses of 2,3-dimercaptopropanol (BAL): VIII. The effect of BAL on the excretion of arsenic in arsenical intoxication. J Clin Invest 1946;25:534–540.

25. Maher JF, Schreiner GE: The dialysis of mercury and mercury-BAL complex. Clin Res 1959;7:298.

26. Mahieu P, Buchet JP, Roels HA, et al: The metabolism of arsenic in humans acutely intoxicated by As_2O_3: Its significance for the duration of BAL therapy. J Toxicol Clin Toxicol 1981;18:1067–1075.

27. Oehme FW: British anti-lewisite (BAL): The classic heavy metal antidote. Clin Toxicol 1972;5:215–222.

28. Pearson RG: Hard and soft acids and bases; NSAB. Part II. Underlying theories. J Chem Educ 1968;45:643–648.

29. Peters RA: Biochemistry of some toxic agents. J Clin Invest 1955;34: 1–20.

30. Peters RA, Spray GH, Stocken LA, et al: The use of British anti-lewisite containing radioactive sulfur for metabolism investigations. Biochem J 1947;41:370–373.

31. Peters RA, Stocken LA, Thompson RM: British anti-lewisite (BAL). Nature 1945;156:616–618.

32. Randall RV, Seeler AO: BAL. N Engl J Med 1948;239:1004–1009, 1040–1048.

33. Schafer B, Kreppel H, Reichl FX, et al: Effect of oral treatment with BAL, DMPS or DMSA arsenic in organs of mice injected with arsenic trioxide. Arch Toxicol 1991;14(Suppl):228–230.

34. Seifert SA, Dart RC, Kaplan EH: Accidental, intravenous infusion of a peanut oil-based medication. J Toxicol Clin Toxicol 1998;36: 733–736.

35. Spray GM, Stocken LA, Thompson RMS: Further investigations on the metabolism of 2,3-dimercaptopropanol. Biochem J 1947;41: 363–366.

36. Stocken LA, Thompson RM: Reactions of British-lewisite with arsenic and other metals in living systems. Physiol Rev 1949;29: 168–194.

37. Vaziri ND, Upham T, Barton CM: Hemodialysis clearance of arsenic. Clin Toxicol 1980;17:451–456.

38. Wexler J, Eagle M, Tatum MJ, et al: Clinical uses of 2,3-dimercaptopropanol (BAL): II. The effect of BAL on the excretion of arsenic in normal subjects after minimal exposure to arsenical smoke. J Clin Invest 1946;25:467–473.

39. Woody NC, Kometani JT: BAL in the treatment of arsenic ingestion of children. Pediatrics 1948;1:372–378.

40. Zimmer LJ, Carter DE: The effect of 2,3-dimercaptopropanol and D-penicillamine on methyl mercury-induced neurological signs and weight loss. Life Sci 1978;23:1025–1034.

CHAPTER 80 LEAD

Fred M. Henretig

Lead

MW	=	207 daltons
Normal range (whole blood)	=	<10 μg/dL
	=	<0.48 μmol/L
Action level (children)	=	10 μg/dL
	=	>0.48–0.62 μmol/L

Values greater than or equal to the action level necessitate clinical intervention. Values less than this level may necessitate intervention based on the clinical condition of the patient.

A 3-year-old boy was rushed to the Emergency Department (ED) by the rescue squad after having had a 20-minute seizure at home. He initially appeared postictal, with flaccid muscle tone and minimal response to painful stimulation. His blood pressure was 130/80 mm Hg with a heart rate 110 beats/min; respirations were shallow, at a rate of 10 breaths/min; and temperature was 98.6°F (37°C). Pulse oximetry was 85% on room air. The child improved with suctioning, placement of a nasopharyngeal airway, and 40% oxygen was administered by facemask. Intravenous lines were placed, blood for laboratory studies drawn, and intravenous fluid administered. The electrocardiogram (ECG) monitor revealed a normal sinus rhythm. An effort was made to elicit more history of the child's illness and to perform a more systematic examination, but within a few minutes the child began to convulse. Diazepam 0.2 mg/kg IV was infused, with prompt cessation of seizure activity. However, respiratory effort also diminished, and the child underwent endotracheal intubation. A rapid bedside test for glucose estimated the blood glucose at 194 mg/dL. Arterial blood gas determination after intubation revealed normal ventilation and oxygenation, with a minimal metabolic acidosis. Five minutes later, another generalized seizure occurred, but it resolved immediately with a second dose of 0.2 mg/kg of diazepam.

Further history revealed that this child had been in his usual state of health until 3 days prior to admission, when he developed symptoms of an upper respiratory infection. Two days later he developed tactile fever, vomited once, and appeared less active. On the day of admission, he seemed drowsy, vomited several times, and in the evening developed twitching and abnormal eye movements, prompting a call to the rescue squad.

His past medical history was notable for developmental delay, primarily in the speech and personal/social spheres. He spoke only single words, was not toilet trained, and was unable to dress himself. The mother denied any history of head trauma or recent ingestion, but did comment that 3 weeks previously she had had to remove paint chips from the child's mouth.

Physical examination revealed an intubated child with blood pressure of 84/50 mm Hg, heart rate of 120 beats/min, a manually ventilated respiratory rate of 25 breaths/min, and temperature of 100.9°F (38.3°C). There were no signs of external trauma. Cardiac, pulmonary, and abdominal examinations were normal. The neuro-logic examination revealed an obtunded child with intermittent withdrawal to pain. At times, tonic extensor posturing was noted. Pupils were 3 mm and sluggishly reactive, with normal fundi. Deep tendon reflexes were 3+ to 4+ on the left leg and 2+ to 3+ on the right leg. There was bilateral sustained ankle clonus. Plantar extension was present on the left and the response was equivocal on the right.

The patient went immediately to CT scan, which revealed diffuse cerebral edema and loss of gray-white matter differentiation (Fig. 80–1). Recurrent seizure activity necessitated phenobarbital loading first and then midazolam infusion. The child was also treated with modest hyperventilation and dexamethasone for presumed increased intracranial pressure, and empirically with ceftriaxone and acyclovir for possible central nervous system (CNS) infection. A lumbar puncture was performed, revealing opening pressure of 46 cm H$_2$O (N = 10–28 cm H$_2$O) clear, colorless fluid, and closing pressure of 15 cm H$_2$O. The cell count was 3 white blood cells (WBC)/mm^3 and 0 red blood cells (RBC)/mm^3, with cerebrospinal fluid (CSF) protein of 96 mg/dL and glucose of 108 mg/dL. One dose of mannitol was given after the lumbar puncture confirmed elevated intracranial pressure. The results of other admission laboratory tests included a white blood count, 11,300/mm^3; hemoglobin, 6.6 g/dL; mean corpuscular volume (MCV), 50 μm^3; platelet count, 473,000/ mm^3; peripheral blood smear positive for RBC basophilic stippling; sodium 139 mEq/L; potassium, 4.3 mEq/L; chloride, 105 mEq/L; bicarbonate, 22 mEq/L; blood urea nitrogen (BUN), 15 mg/dL; creatinine, 0.3 mg/dL; glucose, 170 mg/dL; calcium, 9.4 mg/dL; magnesium, 1.8 mg/dL; phosphorus, 3.5 mg/dL; ammonia, 44 μmol/L; alanine aminotransferase (ALT), 83 U/L; and aspartate aminotransferase (AST), 118 U/L. Urinalysis revealed 4+ glucose, 5–10 WBCs, 0–5 RBCs, and 1+ protein. Radiographic studies were negative for radiopaque foreign bodies of the abdomen, but positive for dense metaphyseal bands at the wrist (Fig. 80–2). Blood lead level was 220 μg/dL, and erythrocyte protoporphyrin was 649 μg/dL.

Despite anticonvulsant therapy with phenytoin, phenobarbital, and midazolam infusion, a continuous reading electroencephalogram demonstrated periodic epileptiform activity. Pentobarbital was added to the therapeutic regimen, resulting in intermittent burst suppression of up to 40-second duration. The child underwent chelation therapy with dimercaprol (British Anti-Lewisite, BAL) and

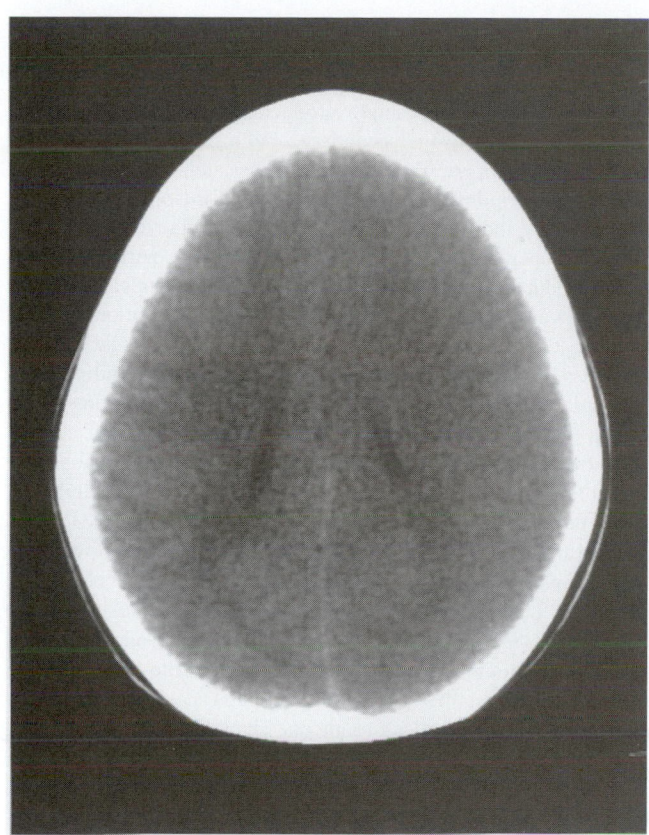

Figure 80–1. Computerized tomography scan of the brain reveals diffuse cerebral edema and loss of gray-white matter differentiation. *(Courtesy of Department of Radiology, St. Christopher's Hospital for Children, Philadelphia, PA.)*

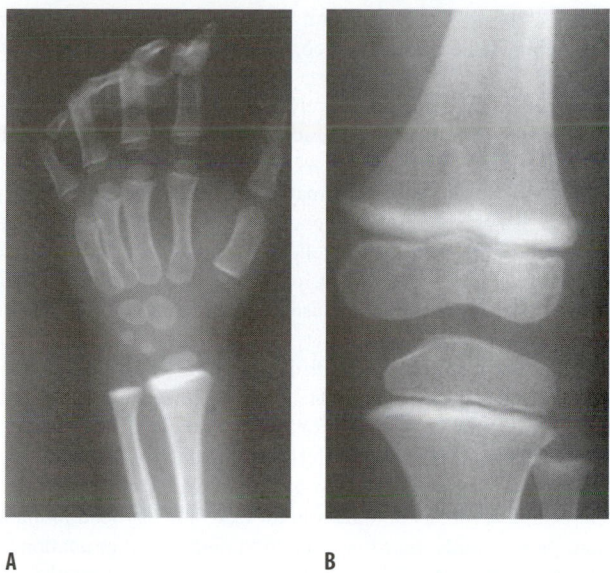

Figure 80–2. **A.** Radiograph of the wrist reveals increased bands of calcification: "lead lines." *(Courtesy of Department of Radiology, St. Christopher's Hospital for Children, Philadelphia, PA.)* **B.** Similar radiographic findings in another patient at the knee. *(Courtesy of Richard Markowitz, MD, Department of Radiology, Children's Hospital of Philadelphia, Philadelphia, PA.)*

edetate calcium disodium (CaNa$_2$EDTA). The BAL was dosed at 75 mg/m^2/dose IM every 4 hours for 5 days. The CaNa$_2$EDTA was begun with the second dose of BAL, as a continuous infusion of 1500 mg/m^2/d diluted in normal saline to a concentration of 0.5%, and continued also for 5 days. After a 2-day interval, the child received a second 5-day course of chelation, resulting in a blood lead level of 33 μg/dL.

Despite chelation, the patient required high-dose pentobarbital for 6 days and continuous midazolam infusion for 14 days in order to suppress seizure activity. He was hospitalized for 23 days prior to transfer to a chronic care rehabilitative facility. His neurologic examination prior to transfer was notable for choreoathetoid movements and generalized hypotonia, inability to localize visual or auditory stimuli, and nonpurposeful movements of the extremities. An MRI on day 22 revealed cerebral and cerebellar cortical atrophy with multiple areas of infarction involving the frontal and parietal lobes (Fig. 80–3).

PHYSICAL PROPERTIES

Lead is a silvery-gray, soft, metal with an atomic weight of 207.21 and an atomic number of 82. It has a low melting point, 327.4°C (621.3°F), and boils at 1620°C (2948°F) at atmospheric pressure. It is widely distributed geologically, and occurs principally as two

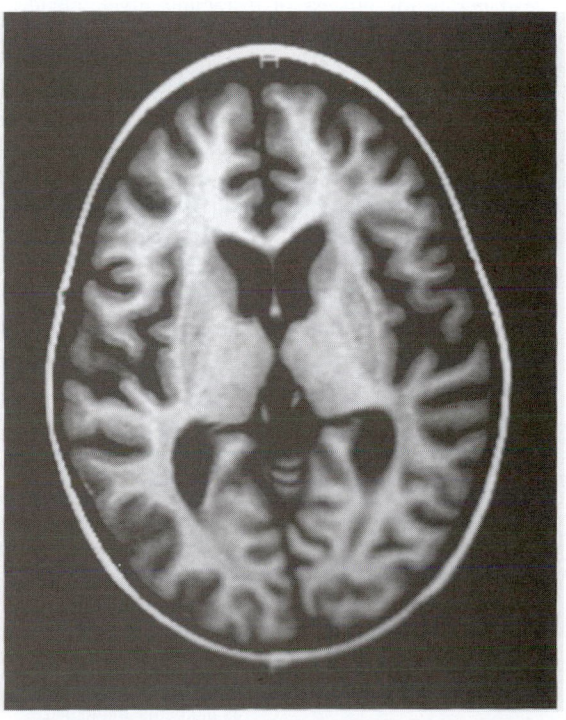

Figure 80–3. Magnetic resonance image of the brain reveals cortical atrophy and multiple areas of cerebral infarction. *(Courtesy of Eric Faerber, MD, Department of Radiology, St. Christopher's Hospital for Children, Philadelphia, PA.)*

isotopes, [206]Pb and [208]Pb. Natural lead ore deposits are found in Canada, the United States, Mexico, and Peru, as well as in Europe, Asia, and Australia. The most abundant lead ore is galena (PbS).[293] Metallic lead is relatively insoluble in water and dilute acids, but will dissolve in nitric, acetic, and hot, concentrated sulfuric acids. In compounds, lead assumes valence states of +2 and +4. Inorganic lead compounds may be brightly colored and vary widely in water solubility; several are used extensively as pigments such as lead chromate (yellow) and lead oxide (red). Lead also forms organic compounds, of which two, tetramethyl and tetraethyl lead, had commercial use as gasoline additives.[148] These are essentially insoluble in water, but readily soluble in organic solvents.[249] Lead complexes with ligands containing sulfur, oxygen, or nitrogen as electron donors. It thus forms stable complexes with several ligands common to biologic molecules, including $-OH$, $-H_2PO_3$, $-SH$, and $-NH_2$. Complexes with sulfhydryl ($-SH$) groups are thought to be of most toxicologic importance. There is no known physiologic role for lead, and any lead found in human body fluids represents environmental contamination.[214] Table 80–1 summarizes several of the major lead compounds.

HISTORY

Lead's low melting point and malleability made it one of the first metals smelted and used by human society.[16,301] Lead-based ocher paints were recovered from the Neanderthal-era Mousterian burial mounds dating to approximately 40,000 BC. Lead artifacts were unearthed in a Neolithic site in Turkey dating to 6200 BC. Ancient Egyptians and Hebrews used lead, and the Phoenicians established lead mines in Spain circa 2000 BC. The Greeks and Romans produced lead during the process of extracting silver intended for coinage. Roman society found many uses for lead, including pipes, cooking utensils, and ceramic glazes, and a common practice was to use sapa, a grape syrup simmered down in lead vessels, as a sweetener and preservative.[206,300] Postindustrial lead use increased dramatically, and today, lead is the most widely used nonferrous metal, with global production on the order of 9 million tons annually. The US annual production of lead averages 1.1 million tons, of which about 0.5 million tons are newly mined and 0.6 million tons are recycled from scrap metal.[148,311] Lead is used widely in industry for its waterproofing and electrical- and radiation-shielding properties. Both metallic lead (as grids) and lead

oxide (in paste) are used in electric storage batteries, and these account for almost two-thirds of annual US use. Because batteries last only 27 months on average, and about 80% of battery lead is resmelted as scrap, this single product accounts for the largest source of raw lead to the secondary smelting and refining industry.[249] Lead alloys are used to shield power and telephone cables, in the printing industry to produce type, and in solders. Solder is used in many industries, including tin can production, plumbing and repair operations, and the automobile industry, particularly radiator production and repair. Sheet lead lines chemical reaction containers and is used in medical and industrial radiation shields. Metallic lead is also used for ammunition manufacturing, bronze and brass production, and for annealing, galvanizing, and plating. Inorganic lead compounds have historically been considered among the highest-quality paint pigments for their bright colors, durability, and weather resistance, and are still used today for nonresidential outdoor paints. Lead compounds are used as stabilizers in the production of polyvinylchloride plastics, in glazes for ceramic ware, and in the manufacture of glass intended for crystal, optical, and electronic applications, such as color television picture tubes. Lead azide and styphnate are used in explosives.[148,249] Use of both lead-based paint for house paint and leaded gasoline has been essentially eliminated by regulation in the United States since the 1980s, but persistence of lead paint in older houses still constitutes an enormous environmental challenge.[6,193]

The problem of human poisoning from lead, known as plumbism, dates back to antiquity. Dioscorides, a Greek physician in the 2nd century BC, observed that lead makes the mind "give way."[167] Pliny cautioned the Romans of the danger of inhaled fumes from lead smelting.[196] Modern authors have suggested that extensive use of sapa in Roman aristocratic society contributed to the downfall of Roman dominance.[206] Lead poisoning was also recognized in Colonial times. Benjamin Franklin observed, in 1763, the "dry gripes" (abdominal colic) and "dangles" (wrist drop) that afflicted tinkers, painters, and typesetters, as well as the "gripes" caused by rum distillation in leaden condensing coils.[180] Lead salts, particularly lead acetate (sugar of lead), were used medicinally in the early 19th century for control of bleeding and diarrhea; recent examination of hair samples from Andrew Jackson identified elevated lead levels, compatible with his described chronic affliction of "bilious colic," a syndrome including constipation and severe, cramping abdominal pain. Jackson was frequently treated with lead acetate by his physicians, and in addition harbored two retained bullets—one in his left lung and one in his left shoulder.[82] With the 19th-century Industrial Revolution, lead poisoning became a common occupational disease. Charles Dickens's account of lead mill workers in his 1863 *The Uncommercial Traveler* is haunting. Dickens visits a home near the mill, sees a woman bent over in a corner, and inquires of his guide as to her condition:

And tis the lead, sur.
  The what?
  The lead, sur. Sure, tis the lead-mills, where the woman gets took on at eighteen-pence a day, sur . . . and her constitooshun is lead-poisoned, bad as can be, sur; and her brain is coming out her ear and it hurts her dreadful. . . .[85,196]

The reproductive effects of lead poisoning were also noted by the turn of the 20th century. A 1911 article described the high rate

TABLE 80–1. Representative Lead Compounds

Compound	Molecular Formula	Major Use/Comment
Lead arsenate	$Pb_3(AsO_4)_2$	Insecticide
Lead azide	$Pb(N_3)_2$	Cartridge primers, primer cord
Lead carbonate	$2PbCO_3Pb(OH)_2$	Paint pigment (basic white lead)
Lead chromate	$PbCrO_4$	Paint pigment (chrome yellow)
Lead oxide	Pb_3O_4	Paint pigment (red lead) commonly used as primer for rust protection on metal. Other oxides used as pigments and in glazes.
Lead silicate	$PbSiO_3$	Glazes for china, porcelain, tiles
Lead sulfide	PbS	Most abundant lead ore (galena); responsible for gingival lead line
Tetraethyl lead	$Pb(C_2H_5)_4$	Antiknock additive to gasoline

Adapted and compiled, with permission, from references 148, 249.

of stillbirths, infertility, and abortions among women in the pottery industry, or who were married to pottery workers.[207]

The modern history of childhood plumbism can be traced to the recognition of lead-paint poisoning in Brisbane, Australia, in 1897.[289] By 1914, a law banning the use of leaded house paint was passed in Australia. Lead poisoning was reported in US children in 1917,[28] but it took another 54 years for a similar law to be effected in the United States.[196] A classic article by Byers and Lord, in 1943, established that children who recovered from clinical plumbism were frequently left with neurologic sequelae and intellectual impairment.[38] Symptomatic childhood lead poisoning was a frequent occurrence in US pediatric medical centers throughout the 1950s and 1960s, a period during which much research established effective chelation therapy protocols with BAL and CaNa$_2$EDTA.[62,65,66] In the 1970s and 1980s, the research thrust in childhood lead poisoning centered on the recognition and quantification of more subtle neurocognitive impairment due to subclinical lead poisoning.[163,196,197] Over this time period, the US Centers for Disease Control and Prevention (CDC) have steadily revised downward the definitions of blood lead level (BLL) in children representing undue absorption and lead poisoning. The CDC definition of lead poisoning was 60 μg/dL in the early 1960s, while currently 10 μg/dL represents undue absorption (elevated BLL), and BLL >15 μg/dL suggests the need for medical case management.[52]

EPIDEMIOLOGY

Although substantial progress was made in its prevention as a consequence of hazard reduction and early screening, specific diagnostic tests, and treatment, lead poisoning remains a pervasive environmental and toxicologic problem today. Lead poisoning affects persons of all ages, but tends to cluster into several distinct at-risk populations. The scope and clinical significance of the problem are most severe in young children, aged 1–6 years, whose primary source of exposure is deteriorated lead paint in their home. The US Department of Health and Human Services has declared such childhood lead poisoning "the most important environmental health problem for young children."[6] The second, large, affected group is adults, exposed at their place of work, whose occupation involves lead smelting or reclamation, construction or demolition, or the manufacture or repair of lead-containing materials.[36,83,249] General environmental exposures from contaminated air, water, and food are uncommon in advanced societies today, but may still affect an entire community under special circumstances. Exotic sources are also reported sporadically, including exposures to contaminated folk medications, cosmetics, ingested lead foreign bodies, retained bullets, artists' or other hobby materials, firing ranges, illicit distilled alcoholic beverages, and substances of abuse.[240]

POPULATION SURVEYS

Several recent national and regional surveys have evaluated current US population-based trends in BLLs and sociodemographic correlates. The Third National Health and Nutrition Examination Survey (NHANES III) examined more than 13,000 US citizens of ages 1 to beyond 70 years, in a nationally representative cross-

sectional survey.[36] The survey, done between 1988 and 1991, determined mean BLLs and their sociodemographic correlates. The mean BLL for this sample of the US population was 2.8 μg/dL, with the highest mean BLLs observed in 1–2-year-olds (4.1 μg/dL). Among adults, elderly persons had higher mean BLLs than did younger adults, with a mean of 4.0 μg/dL in the 50–69-year-olds and >70-year-olds. In general, BLLs were higher for males, blacks, central-city residents, persons of low income and educational attainment, and residents of the Northeast region of the United States. The estimated prevalence of BLLs >10 μg/dL for children aged 1–5 years was 8.9%, or approximately 1.7 million children; however, this prevalence rose to 36.7% for non-Hispanic black children residing in central cities of >1 million population. When these findings are compared to the previous NHANES II survey carried out in 1976–1980,[141] a 78% decline in BLLs overall is observed.[225]

Such a dramatic improvement might be interpreted as evidence that the general problem of environmental lead pollution is largely conquered in the United States. The current overall mean BLL in the United States is comparable to that measured in children living in the relatively pristine environment of the Himalayas.[221,223] Further, several studies of urban and suburban private fee-for-service or health maintenance organization pediatric practices confirm the relative infrequency (<5%) of finding middle- to upper-income children with elevated BLLs.[27,202,283] Nevertheless, for young minority children and the poor who reside in our nation's deteriorating central cities, the battle is far from won.[49,109] In 1997, the CDC reported that there were still nearly 900,000 children younger than 6 years of age with elevated BLLs.[45] With further analysis, the CDC reported in 2000 that children enrolled in Medicaid had a prevalence of elevated BLLs 3 times greater than those not in Medicaid.[43] In Philadelphia in 1999, 27% of all screened young children had elevated BLLs, and 4.5% had BLLs ≥20 μg/dL.[219] More than 40% of children attending an inner-city West Philadelphia clinic were recently found to have elevated BLLs.[40]

The CDC estimates that 95% of adults with BLLs above 25 μg/dL are exposed primarily through occupational exposure.[50] Nevertheless, NHANES III demonstrated similar demographic correlates for adults as for children, and thus urbanization and poverty are likely important factors for adult lead poisoning as well.[36] The Adult Blood Lead Epidemiology and Surveillance program of the CDC reported a nearly 20% prevalence of BLLs ≥25 μg/dL in tested adults.[44]

SOURCES

Numerous sources of lead exposure exist. Environmental exposures affect the entire population, particularly young children, and include leaded paint, soil and dust contaminated by lead paint, leaded gasoline automobile exhaust, industrial waste, airborne lead from automobile exhaust and industrial emissions, water contaminated via lead pipes and lead solder, and food contaminated via lead-soldered cans (Table 80–2). Adults with occupational or recreational exposure to lead constitute another large group of persons at risk. For convenience, these categories of lead exposure are discussed separately, though there is considerable overlap. For example, workers who fail to change lead dust–covered work clothes or shoes may bring this lead hazard home to affect their children.[15,240]

TABLE 80–2. Environmental Lead Sources

Source	Comment
Leaded paint	Especially pre-1978 homes
Dust	House dust from deteriorated lead paint
Soil	From yards contaminated by deteriorated lead paint, lead industry emissions, roadways with high leaded gasoline usage
Water	Leached from leaded plumbing (pipes, solder), cooking utensils, water coolers
Air	Leaded gasoline (pre-1976 US, still prevalent worldwide), industrial emissions
Food	Lead solder in cans (pre-1991 US, still prevalent in imported canned foods); "natural" calcium supplements; "moonshine" whiskey; lead-foil covered wines; contaminated flour, paprika
Exotic	Folk remedies, cosmetics; ingested lead foreign bodies, retained lead bullets; illicit substance abuse (heroin, methamphetamine, leaded gasoline "huffing"); burning batteries, leaded paper, or wood for fuel; use of lead-glazed ceramics; hand–mouth contact with pool cue chalk, glazes, leaded ink; vinyl miniblinds

Environmental Sources

Paint. Lead pigments (typically lead carbonate) account for 50% by weight of many white house paints in the pre-World War II era. Thus, a thumbnail-sized chip of this paint might contain up to 200 mg of lead (vs a typical dietary intake of <2 μg/day for a young child).[32,69] Since 1978, paint intended for interior or exterior residential surfaces, toys, or furniture may contain no more than 0.06% lead.[6] However, an estimated 3 million tons of lead remain in 57 million existing US homes built prior to 1980 and painted with lead-based paint.[292] Most dangerous are the 3.8 million homes with deteriorated paint in which 2 million young children reside.[6,193] This aging housing stock has created an enormous environmental hazard of lead exposure to these children, and to adult homeowners, house painters, and construction workers who become involved in sanding, scraping, and restoration of painted surfaces in these homes. Further, lead-based paint is still allowed for industrial, military, marine, and some outdoor uses such as structural components of bridges and highways; occasionally, some of this paint is inadvertently used in homes.[52] Attempts to abate lead-painted outdoor structures can pollute entire communities.[156]

Paint-derived lead exposure to children has historically been blamed on pica, the common pediatric behavior of eating nonfood items, and attributed to ingestion of macroscopic paint chips. Unproven inferences were made suggesting such children were victims of inadequate parenting.[196] A more recent understanding is that, while pica may play a role for some children, most lead paint exposure in childhood relates to the crumbling, peeling, flaking, or chalking of aging paint.[52,64] These fine paint particles are incorporated into household dust and yard soil, where ordinary childhood hand-mouth activity results in ingestion.[56,250] Seasonal variations in house dust lead content occur, with higher levels in the summer months. This correlates well with predictable increases in BLLs in preschool children. This may reflect, in part, increased exposure to leaded street dust and soil while playing outdoors, and/or increased contamination of windowsills and floors by outdoor dust gaining entrance through open windows.[313]

Lead paint is typically found in these older homes on kitchen and bathroom walls, and particularly on any painted wood surfaces, including window frames and sills.[65,97] Dilapidated homes in the inner city are not the only source of lead-paint hazard. Pre-1960 dwellings in any area, particularly if paint is visibly deteriorated or the home is undergoing renovation, are likely to be hazardous.[47,64,257] Adults, as well as children, may develop lead poisoning when homeowners renovate Victorian-era homes[77] in rural[173] or regentrifying urban neighborhoods (the latter has been dubbed "yuppie plumbism").[7,251]

Soil. Closely related to the exposure from lead-based paint is that of soil contaminated by residue of deteriorated exterior house paint and leaded gasoline emissions. In addition, some communities are further contaminated by proximity to lead smelters or lead-using industries.[1] Children's BLLs rise 3–7 μg/dL for every 1000 parts per million (ppm) rise in their environmental soil or dust concentrations.[1,33]

Water. Ground and surface water generally have low lead levels. Lead contaminates drinking water via lead-based plumbing, connectors, lead-soldered joints, and/or lead-containing brass faucets. Water that is low in mineral content (soft), acidic, and hot is more likely to leach lead; the time of standing in contact with lead piping or solder is also correlated with higher lead content.[1] Many homes in the United States built prior to 1920 have lead pipes, and many newer homes have lead-containing solder or brass fixtures. An estimated 16% of household water supplies have lead in excess of 20 μg/L (the current standard is 15 μg/L).[91] Older watercoolers in schools and public buildings also may contain lead solder, with resulting high water lead levels. Their intermittent use, with water standing for some time (eg, over a weekend), may exacerbate this phenomenon.[52] Elevated lead levels in infancy are associated with the use of hot tap water that has been further boiled down to prepare infant formula,[266] as has water boiled in an imported Iranian kettle.[103]

Air. The regulated removal of lead from gasoline in the United States between 1976 and 1990, and EPA standards for industrial emissions, has resulted in dramatic decreases in overall air lead content, with concomitant decreases in mean US BLLs, as noted earlier.[225,249] Remaining sources of airborne lead in the United States include point sources such as mines and smelters and the allowed use of leaded gasoline in agricultural vehicles.[240] Unfortunately, many third-world and Eastern European countries are not yet able to institute leaded-gasoline and industrial-emission controls.[52,269]

Food. Lead in food is the result of several factors, including atmospheric lead falling onto leafy vegetables, soil lead being taken up by plants, and lead solder in food cans leaching into contents. Declines in leaded gasoline use have indirectly decreased food lead exposure, and further dramatic reduction in food exposure can be attributed to the regulation of lead-soldered cans.[32,52,193,263] Lead-soldered food or soft-drink cans have not been manufactured in the United States since November 1991, but some foreign cans still have lead-soldered seams.[193]

Food supplements and beverages may be contaminated with lead. Table 80–2 summarizes such exposures.

Other Environmental Sources

A number of additional, somewhat "exotic," sources of lead exposure resulting in occasional cases of lead poisoning have been described; several examples are noted in Table 80–2.[52,142,193] One such source is ethnic folk remedies or cosmetics that are common to immigrant populations in the United States.[48] Hispanic Americans have used metal-containing remedies for an illness often referred to as "empacho" (colic or gastroenteritis symptoms). Two such remedies are azarcon, which is an orange, 86–95% lead tetroxide powder, and greta, which may also contain mercury.[34] Other names for azarcon and greta include alarcon, coral, rueda, liga, and Maria Luisa.[240] Lead-containing ethnic folk remedies used by Asian communities include paylooah, which can contain arsenic and is used for rash and fever, and chuifong tokuwan, ghasard, bali goli, and kandu.[48,240] A lead-contaminated Chinese herbal tea is hai ge fen.[178] Similarly, Middle Eastern and Indo-Pakistani remedies and eye cosmetics that contain lead are maha yogran guggulu, surma, kohl, alkohl, saoott, satrinj, bint dahab, cebagin, and "Indian plants."[20,248,312] Of note, many families are initially hesitant to report these remedies when their child's history is taken, or fail to consider them as "medicine" at all. It may enhance reporting to specifically ask about them by their common name.[48]

Another significant group of unusual exposures relates to ingestion or mouthing of metallic lead objects or gunshot wounds with retained lead ammunition.[142] Several cases have been reported of pediatric lead toxicity caused by lead curtain weight, bullet, or fishing weight ingestions, or by repetitive mouthing of imported leaded necklaces (Fig. 80–4).[127,130,142,169] Ingested single, large, foreign bodies do not generally cause toxicity unless they are retained in the intestinal tract for 2 weeks or more.[89] However, a recent report highlighted the danger of acute lead toxicity resulting from the ingestion of multiple small diameter lead pellets from a strap-on ankle weight.[182] Lead poisoning from retained lead bullets, shrapnel, or shot after gunshot wounds is an uncommon complication of gunshot wounds.[126,281] Most cases result from lead

ammunition particles being bathed by acidic synovial, serosal, or, possibly, cerobrospinal fluids.[87,183,258,281] The surface area of lead fragments exposed to body fluids also appears to influence the rapidity of developing elevated blood levels.[87,258] One small study suggests that ED patients with x-ray evidence of retained lead shrapnel have an increased risk of elevated BLLs as compared to controls.[98]

Numerous additional exposures are reported as lead hazards, including exotic parenteral,[2,213] oral,[52,68,102,184,229,297] and inhalational[88,146,209] exposures (Table 80–2). New environmental sources continue to arise and create notoriety; one of the more recent new sources was the discovery of the lead hazard secondary to vinyl miniblind exposure in the late 1990s.[203]

Occupational and Recreational Sources

It is estimated that more than 1 million workers in the United States, employed in more than 100 occupations, are exposed to lead.[240] The most important route of absorption in occupational settings is inhalation of lead dust and fumes. In addition, workers may eat, drink, or smoke in lead-dust–contaminated areas, resulting in some ingestion as well. However, presence of lead in the workplace, per se, does not imply a significant risk of poisoning. The risk is correlated with several factors that contribute to the occurrence of respirable lead fumes or dust particles (<5 μm in diameter) in the worksite atmosphere.[249] There are three general categories of such factors. The first relates to the degree of hazard inherent in the work process itself, including high temperatures (eg, >1000°C/1832°F); significant aerosol, dust, or fume production; and less mechanized technology. Second, the adequacy of dust elimination, such as local and general ventilation, is critical. The third category is that of worksite and personal hygiene, including proper use of protective clothes and equipment, and thorough housekeeping. In general, small shops employing few workers are more hazardous than large factories with hundreds or thousands of employees. The small, sometimes "backyard" operations are less likely to adhere to industry safety regulations, are

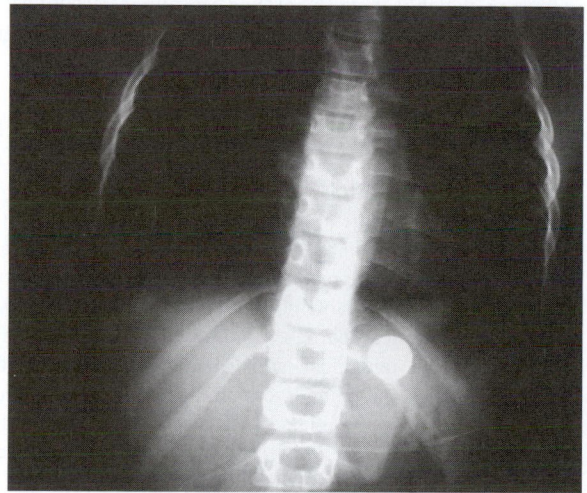
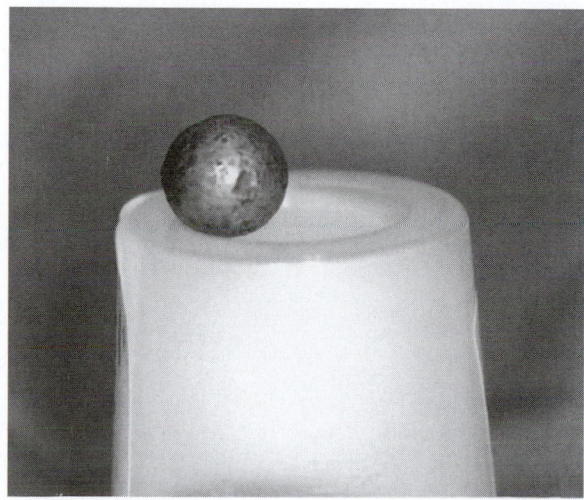

A

B

Figure 80–4. **A.** Radiograph of the abdomen reveals ingested metallic foreign body. **B.** The ingested foreign body was a Civil War era musketball from the collection of the patient's father. *(Courtesy of Evaline Alessandrini, MD, Division of Emergency Medicine, Children's Hospital of Philadelphia, Philadelphia, PA.)*

less automated, and have less environmental control, and the relatively few workers are less educated about potential risks and protective equipment usage.[83,162,194] Despite the risk factors that may be specific to each worksite, there are some types of lead-related work that are more hazardous than others, based on actual surveys of BLLs and reported incidence of clinical poisoning (Table 80–3).[171,240,249]

The highest risk group of occupational exposures include any that involve welding, cutting, or burning of metallic lead or lead-coated materials.[99,110,124,136,172,179] In moderate-risk occupations, exposure potential is significant, but typical job circumstances result in relatively low incidence of clinical poisoning and/or prevalence of elevated biologic markers of excessive body lead burden.[100,249] Several occupations occasion lead exposure beyond normal background levels, but with minimal health risk.[148,249] Finally, hobbies and recreational pursuits using lead-containing materials under circumstances similar to occupational exposures are a source of potential risk.[52,157,265]

TABLE 80–3. Occupational and Recreational Lead Sources

High-Risk Occupations
  Shipbreaking
  Metal welders, cutters (includes bridge and highway reconstruction workers)
  Lead smelters, refiners
  Storage battery manufacturers, repairers, recyclers
  Painters, construction workers (sanding, scraping, spraying of lead paint; demolition of lead-painted sites)
  Polyvinyl chloride plastic manufacturers
  Crystal glass makers
  Automobile radiator repairers
  Firing range instructors, bullet salvagers
Moderate-Risk Occupations
  Lead miners
  Welders
  Solderers
  Plumbers
  Wire and cable workers
  Type founders
  Ship repairers
  Automobile factory workers and mechanics
  Glass blowers
  Pottery glazers
  Enamelers
  Varnish makers
  Shot makers
Low-Risk Occupations
  Traffic police officers, taxi drivers, garage workers, turnpike tollbooth operators, gas station attendants (exposed to leaded gasoline exhaust fumes)
  Rubber product manufacturers
  Electronics manufacturers
  Jewelers
  Pipefitters
  Printers
Recreational and Hobby Sources
  Crafters of ceramics
  Repair of automobiles, boats
  Home remodeling, refinishing
  Furniture refinishing, restoring
  Stained glass making
  Painting (fine artists' pigments)
  Target shooting, recasting lead for bullets

TOXICOLOGY

Pharmacokinetics

Absorption. Lead is absorbed primarily through inhalation and ingestion. In adults with occupational exposures, inhalation is the predominant form of absorption, whereas for children, gastrointestinal absorption is the predominant form of absorption.

Inhaled particles <0.5–1 μm in size are most likely to reach the alveoli, where they are almost completely absorbed.[97,98] Larger particles deposit in airways, are cleared by mucociliary activity, and are eventually swallowed and may be absorbed. The overall absorption of inhaled lead averages 30–40%. Of note, both minute ventilation and the concentration of lead in air determine airborne lead exposure, and thus a worker engaged in vigorous physical activity will absorb considerably more lead than a person in the same atmosphere at rest. Likewise, children, with relatively greater volume of inhaled air per unit of body size because of higher metabolic rates, are proportionally at greater risk in a given degree of atmospheric lead pollution. It is estimated that children have a 2.7-fold higher lung deposition rate of lead than do adults.[1]

Gastrointestinal (GI) absorption is less efficient than pulmonary absorption. Adults absorb an estimated 10–15% of ingested lead in food, and children have a higher GI absorption rate, averaging 40–50%.[1,116] However, it should be noted that fasting and diets deficient in iron, calcium, and zinc enhance GI absorption of lead, factors that are frequent among groups of young children.[116,165] A study of adults under fasting conditions found a lead absorption rate from beverage consumption of almost 60%.[134] The role of essential trace elements in decreasing lead absorption is assumed to be a consequence of competitive absorption processes; an iron-binding protein, mobilferrin, initially identified in rat duodenum, is also found in human duodenal mucosa and competitively binds lead.[70]

Cutaneous absorption of inorganic lead is low; one study found an average absorption of 0.06% through intact skin.[190] Alkyl leads may have appreciable cutaneous absorption that is capable of causing toxicity.[249]

Transplacental lead transfer is critical in fetal and neonatal lead exposure, which is under increasing scrutiny in recent years. Lead readily crosses the placental barrier throughout gestation, and lead uptake is cumulative until birth.[230]

Distribution. Absorbed lead enters the bloodstream where at least 99% is bound to erythrocytes.[115] From blood, lead is distributed into both a relatively labile soft tissue pool and into a more stable bone compartment. The classic three-compartment model may be somewhat of an oversimplification. Currently, at least two bone compartments are recognized, a more labile pool in trabecular bone, and a more stable pool in cortical bone. In adults, about 95% of the body lead burden is stored in bone, versus only 70% for children. The remainder is distributed to the major soft tissue lead storage sites, including liver, kidney, bone marrow, and brain. Most of the toxicity associated with lead is a result of soft tissue uptake, so that the relative decrease in bone storage is another comparative disadvantage for lead-poisoned children.

Lead uptake into soft tissues occurs in a complex fashion that depends on numerous factors, including blood lead levels, external exposure factors, and specific tissue kinetics.[1] In general, tissue lead content in populations without very excessive exposure averages 200–500 parts per billion (ppb); rises above this with excessive exposure rapidly produce overt toxicity. For example, brain lead content in humans with overt encephalopathy is on the order of 1–2 ppm or less (eg, only twice the above-noted range). BLLs of only 100–150 ppb (10–15 μg/dL) are now recognized as associated with subtle toxic effects in critical target organs.

Lead in the central nervous system (CNS) is of particular toxicologic importance, and studies have addressed specific storage sites. Lead preferentially concentrates in gray matter and certain nuclei.[115] Fetal brain uptake is relatively higher than with postnatal exposure in animal models.[239] The highest brain concentrations are found in hippocampus, cerebellum, cerebral cortex, and medulla.

Unlike soft tissue storage, bone lead accumulates throughout life. Bone storage begins in utero, and occurs across all ranges of exposure, so that there is no threshold for bone lead uptake.[1] Total body accumulation of lead may range from 200 mg to over 500 mg in workers with heavy occupational exposure.[115] Bone lead is thought to be relatively metabolically inert, but recent evidence suggests that it can be mobilized from the more labile compartment and contributes as much as 50% of the blood lead content. This may be of particular importance during pregnancy and lactation, in elder persons with osteoporosis,[271] and in children with immobilization because of fracture or neurologic disease.[177] Lead also accumulates in teeth, particularly the dentine of children's teeth, a phenomenon that has been used to quantify cumulative lead exposure in young children.[197,199]

Excretion.   Absorbed lead that is not retained is excreted primarily in urine (about 65%) and bile (about 35%).[1] A miniscule amount is lost via sweat, hair, and nails. Children excrete less of their daily uptake than adults, with an average retention of 33% versus 1–4%, respectively.[314] Biologic half-lives for lead are estimated as follows:[1,169,231] blood (adults, short-term experiments), 25 days; blood (children, natural exposure), 10 months; soft tissues (adults, short-term exposure), 40 days; bone (labile, trabecular pool), 90 days; and bone (cortical, stable pool), 10–20 years.

Alkyl lead compounds have unique pharmacokinetics that are less-well characterized.[31] Tetraethyl lead is lipid soluble, easily absorbed through intact skin, and distributed widely to lipophilic tissues including the brain. Tetraethyl lead is metabolized to triethyl lead, which is believed to be the major toxic compound. Alkyl leads may slowly release lead as the inorganic form, with subsequent kinetics as noted above.

PATHOPHYSIOLOGY

General Effects

Lead, similar to many heavy metals, is a complex toxin exerting numerous pathophysiologic effects in many organ systems.[115] At the biomolecular level, lead functions in three general ways. First, its affinity for biologic electron-donor ligands, especially sulfhydryl groups, allows it to bind and impact numerous enzymatic, receptor, and structural proteins. Second, lead is chemically similar to calcium and interferes with numerous metabolic pathways, particularly in mitochondria and in second messenger systems regulating cellular energy metabolism. Lead may function as an inhibitor or agonist of calcium-dependent processes. For example, lead inhibits neuronal voltage-sensitive calcium channels[13] and membrane-bound Na^+-K^+-ATPase,[274] but activates calcium-de-

pendent protein kinase C.[174] Third, lead exhibits mutagenic and mitogenic effects in mammalian cells in vitro and is carcinogenic in rats and mice.[189] Evidence for human carcinogenicity is lacking, however.[93] Genetic polymorphism may impact on individual susceptibility to lead. Recent evidence suggests that this occurs for at least two genes, those coding for δ-aminolevulinic acid dehydratase and the vitamin D receptor.[210]

CNS Neurotoxicity

Overt acute neurotoxicity classically manifests as an acute encephalopathy. The pathogenesis of this syndrome involves failure of the blood-brain barrier.[113] When lead accumulates in brain microvasculature above a critical level, capillary function is disrupted by alteration of cellular calcium metabolism, resulting in separation of the tight intercellular junctions that normally seal endothelial cells. Animal models also demonstrate that the immature endothelium lining capillaries of the developing brain allow greater egress of lead into astrocytes and neurons.[112,286]

Proteinaceous fluid extravasates, and because brain tissue is without lymphatic drainage, brain edema occurs rapidly. The cerebellum and cerebral occipital lobes are effected predominantly, but the process is widespread, resulting in increased intracranial pressure, coma, seizures, and permanent neuronal loss.

More subtle neurotoxic effects, such as those that underlie cognitive impairment without overt symptomatology, are less well understood but probably include altered neurotransmitter function in both children and adults and subtle morphologic changes, particularly in the developing brain in utero and in early childhood.[111,116] Neuronal cell bodies of the cerebral cortex and basal ganglia begin to form during the first trimester of gestation and migrate to their adult location by the end of the second trimester.[111,270] At birth, synaptic connections are sparse, however. Over the first 2 years of life, the multiple connections and neural networks characteristic of the mature brain rapidly develop and are actually twice as dense at age 2 years as in adulthood. The next several years of life, through late childhood, allow considerable postnatal reorganization and progressive "pruning" of synapses.[140] Synapse persistence is likely determined by individual synapse activity, which, in turn, is determined by environmental factors involving motor and sensory stimulation, as well as nutritive and toxic influences.[19] These events are all taking place at precisely the time that the brain lead content is peaking in lead-exposed young children.

Lead impacts on cell differentiation and several biochemical pathways that may interfere with this postnatal reorganization of brain microanatomy. In rodent models, lead decreases oligodendrite density, myelin deposition, and cortical synaptogenesis.[218] Lead induces glial cells to undergo precocious differentiation, potentially altering the migration path of neurons.[71] Lead blocks voltage-sensitive calcium channels, and thus may reduce stimulated synaptic conduction.[13] At the same time, lead either facilitates calcium entry or functions as a calcium agonist within nerve terminals, resulting in enhanced background release of neurotransmitters.[186] Thus, stimulated neurotransmitter release is decreased while spontaneous neurotransmitter release is facilitated, resulting in a decreased "signal-to-noise" ratio in the developing brain.[111] Synaptic pruning may become disorganized, leaving a cortex with approximately normal synaptic density but suboptimal architecture. Such changes are likely to be long lasting, if not permanent.

An additional consideration is the impact of lead on protein kinases. These important intracellular enzymes involved as second messengers influence neurotransmitter function in several ways, including regulation of release, ion flux, and gene activation involved in memory function.[135] Low levels of lead directly stimulate brain protein kinases.[174] This effect could also alter synapse development and pruning. Lead-induced changes in brain capillary endothelial cells that are less severe than occur in patients with encephalopathy may also allow altered fluid dynamics and cellular milieu in astrocytes and neurons. Thus, lead may exert both direct effects on neurons and indirect effects via the brain's support system that result in abnormal synaptic anatomy and function.[111]

Lead exerts neurotoxicologic effects that may be relevant to cortical function in both developing and mature nervous systems. Lead impairs several neurotransmitter systems, including the classic acetylcholine-, dopamine-, norepinephrine-, γ-aminobutyrate (GABA)-, glutamate-, and N-methyl-D-aspartate–dependent systems.[72,115] Lead also interferes with normal neural cell adhesion molecule sialylation, and thus impairs cell-cell adhesion and learning in adult animal models.[232]

Low-level lead exposure is also toxic to the auditory and visual neural systems, as well as to neuromotor performance and fine-motor coordination. Elevated BLLs are associated with hearing deficits in children.[256] Recent studies reveal a higher threshold for auditory nerve action potentials, and segmental demyelination and axonal degeneration of the cochlear nerve in lead-exposed animals. Similar deficits of retinal function are observed in rats with lead levels <20 μg/dL.[211] Studies of 6-year-old children with modest lead burdens (mean BLL at age 2 years of 17 μg/dL, range 6–49 μg/dL) found an association of higher lead levels with poorer performance in bilateral coordination, visual-motor control, upper-limb speed and dexterity, and overall fine-motor coordination.[86]

Peripheral Neuropathy

Peripheral neuropathy is a classic effect of occupational lead poisoning. It is caused by Schwann cell destruction, followed by segmental demyelination and axonal degeneration.[115] Sensory nerves are less affected than motor nerves. Using a sensitive test such as nerve conduction velocity, peripheral nerve dysfunction can be demonstrated at BLLs as low as 40 μg/dL.[262] Peripheral neuropathy is rare in children, but occasionally occurs in those with sickle hemoglobinopathy.[95]

Hematologic

Lead is a potent inhibitor of several enzymes in the heme biosynthetic pathway, as well as of other enzymes of hematologic importance. Lead poisoning results in anemia, which is believed a result of both decreased erythrocyte survival and decreased hemoglobin synthesis. Some authors further postulate a defect in erythropoietin function secondary to associated renal damage.[125,238]

Shortened erythrocyte life span is believed due to increased membrane fragility. Inhibition of Na$^+$-K$^+$-ATPase and pyrimidine-5′-nucleotidase may impair erythrocyte membrane stability by altering energy metabolism. The inhibition of pyrimidine-5′-nucleotidase is also thought to underlie the appearance of basophilic stippling in erythrocytes, representing clumping of degraded RNA, which is normally eliminated by this enzyme.[212]

Several steps in the heme synthesis pathway are impaired (Fig. 80–5).The most sensitive effect of lead is inhibition of the mitochondrial enzyme δ-aminolevulinic acid dehydratase (ALA-D). This decrease in ALA-D activity is observed at BLLs in the mini-

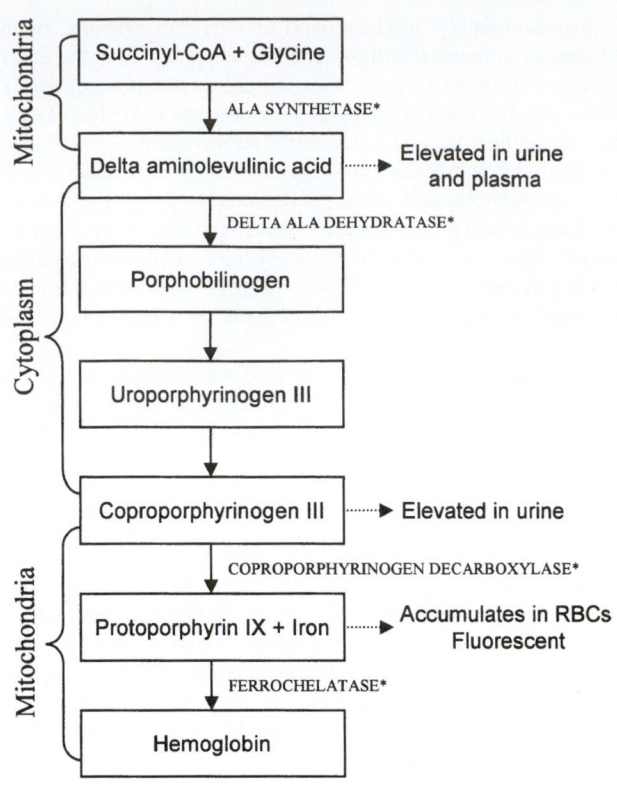

Figure 80–5.   The heme synthesis pathway. The enzymatic steps inhibited by lead are marked with an asterisk (*).

mally elevated range, >10 μg/dL, and results in accumulation of δ-aminolevulinic acid (δ-ALA) in blood and urine. Genetic polymorphism of the ALA-D gene (alleles D^1 and D^2) may contribute to individual sensitivity to lead-induced heme synthetic failure, with the D^2 allele increasing sensitivity to lead.[12] Lead also depresses function of coproporphyrinogen oxidase and ferrochelatase. The former effect results in elevated urinary coproporphyrin III, a phenomenon that, in the past, was used in a bedside test for acute plumbism. The ferrochelatase inhibition results in decreased heme formation and increased erythrocyte protoporphyrin concentration. The latter is complexed with zinc in vivo, at the site normally occupied by iron. Erythrocytes with increased zinc protoporphyrin fluoresce intensely, and the quantification of this effect serves as the basis of a commonly used screening test and marker of lead's hematologic toxicity.[222] Erythrocyte protoporphyrin is also increased in iron-deficiency anemia, caused by a lack of available iron for incorporation into heme, and the rare condition erythropoietic protoporphyria. Iron deficiency is a common concomitant of lead exposure, as noted above, and probably contributes significantly to much of the hypochromic, microcytic anemia actually observed in childhood plumbism.[67]

The reduced heme body pool may also impact other organ systems, but for convenience in the context of understanding lead's impairment of heme synthesis, it is commented on here. It is suggested that impaired heme synthesis might impair several heme-dependent metabolic systems, including decreased cytochrome function with resultant impaired energy metabolism in the CNS, reduced 1,25-(OH)$_2$-vitamin D synthesis with consequent alterations in calcium metabolism, and reduced activity of liver enzymes resulting in altered xenobiotic detoxification and endogenous agonist metabolism.[1,117] Elevations of δ-ALA per se may be neurotoxic at higher levels, impacting GABA receptors.[35]

Renal

Nephropathy is one of the oldest described toxic effects of lead. It is typically a hazard for the heavily exposed adult worker,[115] and is inconsistently reported in adult survivors of severe childhood plumbism.[90] Lead is a renal carcinogen in rodent models, but its status in humans is uncertain.[93,115]

Functional changes associated with acute lead nephropathy include decreased energy-dependent transport, resulting in a Fanconilike syndrome of aminoaciduria, glycosuria, and phosphaturia. These changes are believed related to disturbed mitochondrial respiration and phosphorylation, and are reversible with discontinuation of exposure and/or treatment.[121] An additional microscopic finding is characteristic nuclear inclusion bodies in renal tubular cells, composed of lead-protein complex. These may be present in shed renal cells in the urinary sediment of heavily exposed workers. When affected persons are chelated, these inclusion bodies disappear coincident with increased urinary lead excretion. It is thought that these inclusion bodies account for the major fraction of renal intracellular lead and provide a significant pathway for lead excretion.[119] As lead nephropathy becomes more chronic, inclusion bodies become less common, and renal tubules begin to atrophy with the progressive appearance of interstitial fibrosis. These morphologic changes are typically associated with mild azotemia and decreased creatinine clearance. This progression from acute, reversible nephropathy to chronic, irreversible fibrosis noted in rodent models has not been clearly demonstrated in humans.[118]

There does not appear to be a specific biologic marker for lead nephropathy. Chronic pathologic changes are usually observed in workers with BLLs >60 μg/dL. Some studies found a correlation between markers of renal dysfunction such as urinary N-acetyl-β-D-glucosaminadase, and blood and urinary β2-microglobulin with elevated BLLs, but these findings are not consistent.[106] One study found markers of altered renal eicosanoid synthesis (decreased urinary 6-keto-prostaglandin F1 and increased thromboxane) in exposed workers with normal renal function,[42] while another study found urinary α1-microglobulin to correlate with chronic lead exposure,[58] suggesting potential future value for such tests.

The association of plumbism with gout ("saturnine gout") was noted more than 100 years ago by a pioneer in occupational medicine, the English physician Garrod.[105] Lead decreases renal uric acid excretion, with resulting elevated blood urate levels and urate crystal deposition in joints. Renal function is virtually always impaired. Patients with saturnine gout and renal disease have higher lead excretions after chelation than do patients with gout who are free of renal dysfunction (Table 80–4).[16,18]

Increased blood pressure is probably the most prevalent adverse health effect observed from lead exposure in adults. Several epidemiologic studies document significant associations between hypertension and body lead burdens.[94,226] The association is particularly strong for adult men aged 40–59 years, with an approximate 1.5–3.0-mm Hg rise in systolic pressure for every doubling of BLL beginning at 7 μg/dL.[290] A recent finding from the Harvard longitudinal Nurses' Health Study also found a significant association between patellar lead and risk of hypertension in middle-

TABLE 80–4.   Relation of Lead Burden, Renal Insufficiency, Gout, and Hypertension

	N	Age (y)	SCr (mg/dL)	BPb (μg/dL)	EDTA Provocation (μg lead/3 day)
Gout, no RI	22	53	1.3	24	470
Gout and RI	22	57	3.0[a]	26	806[b]
HTN, no RI	21	55	1.2	18	340
HTN and RI	27	57	3.2[a]	19	860[a]
RI of known etiology (controls)	22	54	3.4	15	440

[a] $p < 0.001$ compared to HTN, no RI and controls.
[b] $p < 0.005$ compared to gout, no RI and controls.
SCr = serum creatinine; BPb = blood lead; RI = renal insufficiency; HTN = hypertension. Values given are group means.
Adapted, with permission, from Batuman V: Lead nephropathy, gout and hypertension. Am J Med Sci 1993;305:241–247.

aged women.[129] Hypertension does not appear to be consistently associated with elevated lead levels in children.[260] As noted above for gout, lead excretion after chelation challenge is higher in patients with decreased renal function and hypertension than in patients with hypertension alone, or renal failure of known, but not lead-related, etiology (Table 80–4).[16] The primary mechanism of lead-related hypertension is believed to be altered calcium-activated changes in contractility of vascular smooth muscle cells, secondary to decreased Na+-K+-ATPase activity and stimulation of the Na+-Ca2+ exchange pump. Lead may also affect vessels by altering neuroendocrine input or sensitivity to such stimuli. Elevated plasma renin activity is found in persons after periods of modest exposure, although levels may drop to normal or lower in chronic severe exposure.[298] Lead increases Na+-lithium countertransport in vitro (a phenomenon believed linked to renal Na+-hydrogen exchange) in erythrocytes from healthy normotensive persons.[17] Similar findings are also observed in patients with essential hypertension, suggesting that there may be some common pathophysiologic mechanisms, as well as that some proportion of "essential" hypertension may actually represent occult lead nephropathy.[16]

Reproductive System

Impairment of both male and female reproductive function is long associated with overt plumbism. Historically, infertility and stillbirths were common among heavily exposed women lead workers. Gametotoxic effects in animals of both sexes and chromosomal abnormalities in workers with BLLs above 60 μg/dL are reported.[115,280] More recent studies found reduced sperm counts, impaired sperm motility, and abnormal morphology in battery workers with BLLs >40 μg/dL,[11] and increased incidence of menstrual irregularity and spontaneous abortion in lead-exposed female workers in China.[141] Prematurity is more common in children of pregnancies associated with elevated maternal lead levels.[193] Testicular endocrine hypofunction occurs in smelter workers with BLLs in the 60-μg/dL range.[237]

Congenital anomalies are reported after maternal lead exposure. An infant with the VACTERL association (vertebral anomalies, anal atresia, cardiac defect, tracheoesophageal fistula, renal and limb anomalies) was born to a mother with high first-trimester lead levels.[158] At least two young infants are reported, who presented at ages 2 days[107] and 2 months,[261] respectively, with convulsions and very high BLLs believed to be a consequence of intrauterine exposure. In addition, the 2-month-old infant manifested an unusual finding of "metallic brownish" fingernail discoloration, and was found to have an extremely elevated nail lead content of 4157 $\mu g/g$.

Endocrine

Reduced thyroid and adrenopituitary function are reported in adult lead workers.[245,246] Children with elevated lead levels have depressed secretion of human growth hormone and insulinlike growth factor.[139]

Skeletal System

In addition to the skeletal system's importance as the largest repository of lead body burden, recent studies suggest that bone metabolism is adversely affected by lead as well. Hormonal response is altered by reduced 1,25-dihydroxyvitamin D_3 levels and by inhibition of osteocalcin. Both new bone formation and coupling of normal osteoblast and osteoclast function may thus be impaired.[39,115] Bands of increased metaphyseal density on radiographs of long bones in young children with heavy lead exposure demonstrate increased calcium deposition in the zones of provisional calcification (Fig. 80–2). Impaired bone growth and shortened stature are associated with childhood lead poisoning.[255] Impaired calcium or cyclic AMP messenger systems may underlie these cellular effects.[115]

Gastrointestinal

Gastrointestinal symptoms typically appear with higher levels of blood lead and include abdominal pain, anorexia, vomiting, and the constipation of "lead colic." These symptoms may be partly explained by spasmodic contraction of intestinal wall smooth muscle, analogous to that believed to occur in vascular walls.[249] Hepatitis and pancreatitis are reported in association with an acute intravenous exposure to lead,[205] and in cases of acute ingestion of lead compounds.[204] A metallic taste is described in patients with lead poisoning.[128] A purple-blue gingival "lead line," or Burton line, representing precipitation of lead sulfide, is also observed occasionally in adults with lead exposure and poor gingival hygiene.[3]

Cardiac

Rarely, myocarditis and cardiac dysfunction are reported in both adult[153] and pediatric[196,272] patients with clinical plumbism. Animal models demonstrate increased sensitivity to norepinephrine-induced dysrhythmias and decreased myocardial contractility, protein phosphorylation, and high-energy phosphate generation.[151] Electrocardiographic abnormalities include atrial dysrhythmias, tachycardia, and inverted T waves.[272] A study comparing bone lead content and ECG findings in men (average age 68 years; range, 48–93) found significant associations between bone lead and longer QT and QRS intervals, an increased risk of intraventricular blocks in those younger than 65 years of age, and an increased risk of atrioventricular block in those older than 65 years of age.[57] Recent descriptions of cardiac toxicity are scarce, although one adult worker with a BLL of 213 $\mu g/dL$ developed frequent multifocal premature ventricular contractions in addition to colic and anemia.[234] It seems plausible that lead-induced impair-

ment of intracellular calcium metabolism is likely to impact cardiac electrophysiology.

CLINICAL PRESENTATION

Inorganic Lead

The numerous observed lead-induced pathophysiologic effects accurately predict that the clinical manifestations of lead poisoning are diverse. These manifestations of lead toxicity are often characterized as falling into distinct syndromes of acute and chronic symptomatology. In most cases, these distinctions really describe a continuum of severity, with more severely exposed persons manifesting the classic "acute" lead toxicity syndrome. Rarely, patients with massive acute inhalational exposure, intentional overdose of soluble lead compounds, or intravenous administration of lead-contaminated substances of abuse present with clinical findings that are somewhat unique, but overlap considerably with the more severe cases of chronic lead exposure. By far, the most important contexts of lead toxicity in the United States today are related to chronic environmental exposure in children and chronic occupational exposure in adult workers. These are sufficiently distinct in epidemiology, clinical manifestations, and current recommended management approaches that they are described separately (Tables 80–5 and 80–6). Severe symptomatic poisoning is rare today among persons of all ages, although it is still reported. There were 139 deaths attributed to lead poisoning in the United States between 1979 and 1988, with the majority occurring among adults, in whom the primary reported exposure was illegal moonshine whiskey.[278] However, the largest public health concern currently is the detection and management of persons with asymptomatic but potentially toxic elevated lead levels.

It should be first reemphasized that the occurrence of overt clinical symptoms in lead-exposed persons is in most cases the

TABLE 80–5. Clinical Manifestations of Lead Poisoning in Children

Clinical Severity	Typical Blood Lead Levels ($\mu g/dL$)
Severe	>70–100
CNS: Encephalopathy (coma, altered sensorium, seizures, bizarre behavior, ataxia, apathy, incoordination, loss of developmental skills; papilledema, cranial nerve palsy, signs of increased ICP)	
GI: Persistent vomiting	
Heme: Pallor (anemia)	
Mild/Moderate (preencephalopathic)	
CNS: Hyperirritable behavior, intermittent lethargy, decreased interest in play, "difficult" child	>50–70
GI: Intermittent vomiting, abdominal pain, anorexia	
Asymptomatic	
CNS: Impaired cognition, behavior	>10
PNS: Impaired fine-motor coordination	
Misc: Impaired hearing, growth	

CNS = central nervous system; ICP = intracranial pressure; PNS = peripheral nervous system; GI = gastrointestinal; Heme = hematologic; Misc = miscellaneous.

TABLE 80–6. Clinical Manifestations of Lead Poisoning in Adults

Clinical Severity	Typical Blood Lead Levels (μg/dL)
Severe	>100–150
CNS: Encephalopathy (coma, seizures, obtundation, delirium, focal motor disturbances, headaches, papilledema, optic neuritis, signs of increased ICP)	
PNS: Foot drop, wrist drop	
GI: Abdominal colic	
Heme: Pallor (anemia)	
Renal: Nephropathy	
Moderate	>80
CNS: Headache, memory loss, decreased libido, insomnia	
GI: Metallic taste, abdominal pain, anorexia, constipation	
Renal: Nephropathy with chronic exposure	
Misc: Mild anemia, myalgias, muscle weakness, arthralgias	
Mild	>40
CNS: Tiredness, somnolence, moodiness, lessened interest in leisure activities	
Misc: Impaired psychometrics, reproduction; hypertension	

CNS = central nervous system; ICP = intracranial pressure; PNS = peripheral nervous system; GI = gastrointestinal; Heme = hematologic; Misc = miscellaneous.

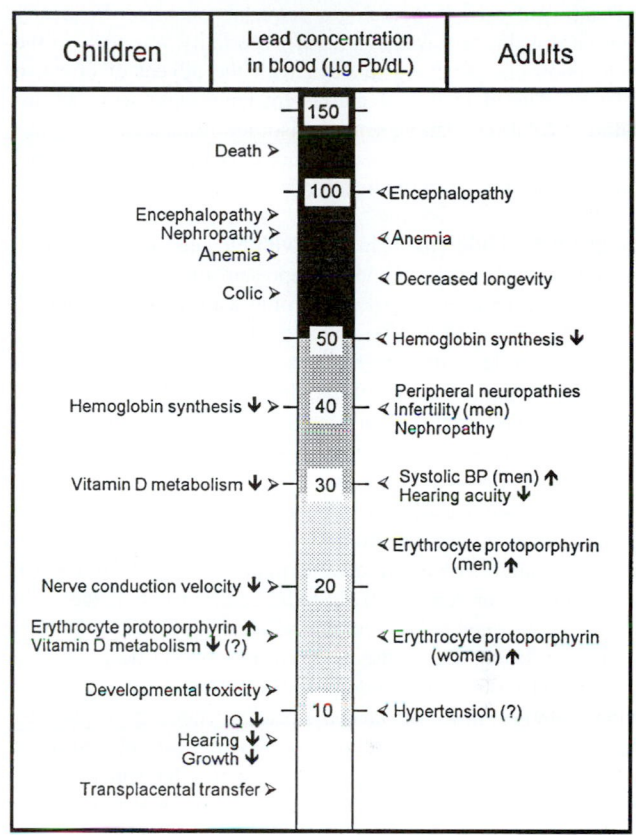

Figure 80–6. The biochemical and clinical effects of lead in children and adults. (*Modified from Royce SE, Needleman HL: Case Studies in Environmental Medicine. Lead Toxicity. Atlanta, Agency for Toxic Substances and Disease Registry, 1992.*)

culmination of a long history of lead exposure. As total dose increases, these symptoms are almost always preceded first by measurable biochemical and physiologic impairment, followed, in turn, by subtle prodromal clinical effects that may only become apparent in hindsight (Fig. 80–6). In general, it is considered that children are more susceptible than adults to toxicity for a given dose (eg, measured blood lead level); however, the data for this regard primarily concern effects on the CNS, reflecting the aforementioned issues of blood-brain barrier immaturity and early childhood neurodevelopment.

Symptomatic Children. Acute lead encephalopathy is the most severe presentation of pediatric plumbism. Encephalopathy is characterized by pernicious vomiting and apathy, bizarre behavior, loss of recently acquired developmental skills, ataxia, incoordination, seizures, altered sensorium, or coma. Physical examination may reveal papilledema, oculomotor or facial nerve palsy, diminished deep-tendon reflexes, or other evidence of increased intracranial pressure.[51,307] There may be pallor if there is coexisting anemia in patients with more chronic exposure. Encephalopathy usually occurs in children aged 15–30 months, is associated with BLLs >100 μg/dL although it is reported with BLLs as low as 70 μg/dL,[224] and tends to occur more commonly in summer months.[65] The reason for this seasonal prevalence is poorly understood, although it may reflect the increase in lead dust exposure that typically occurs during warm summer months.[313] Milder but ominous symptoms that may portend incipient encephalopathy include sporadic vomiting, hyperirritable or aggressive behavior, periods of lethargy interspersed with lucid intervals, and decreased

interest in play activities. Many patients seek medical advice for vomiting and lethargy during the 2–7 days prior to onset of frank encephalopathy.[65] Additional symptoms include anorexia, constipation, and intermittent abdominal pain.[62,224] Physical examination of such children is usually without specific abnormalities.

Subencephalopathic symptomatic plumbism usually occurs in children 1–5 years old and is associated with BLLs >70 μg/dL, but may occur with levels as low as 50 μg/dL. Unfortunately, common complaints in well children of this age ("terrible two's," with functional constipation and who don't eat as much as parents expect) often overlap with the milder range of reported symptoms of lead poisoning. It is not infrequent that parents whose child was diagnosed by routine blood screening recognize milder symptoms only in hindsight, after chelation treatment ("it seemed as if the child was going through a phase").[104] This is especially true currently, when symptomatic plumbism is rarely reported.[51,52] Other uncommon clinical presentations are described,[62] including isolated seizures without encephalopathy (indistinguishable from idiopathic epilepsy), chronic hyperactive behavior disorder, isolated developmental delay, progressive loss of cortical function simulating degenerative cerebral disease, peripheral neuropathy (reported particularly in children with sickle-cell hemoglobinopathy),[95] and a syndrome of colicky abdominal pain, vomiting, constipation, and myalgias of trunk and proximal girdle muscles.

Death and serious neurologic sequelae occurred frequently when encephalopathy was common.[63] Mortality was 65% in the prechelation era, dropping to <5% with the advent of effective chelation. The incidence of permanent neurologic sequelae, including mental retardation, seizure disorder, blindness, and hemiparesis, is 25–30% in patients who develop encephalopathic symptoms prior to onset of chelation.[62]

Asymptomatic Children. Children with elevated body lead burdens but without overt symptoms represent the largest group of persons believed to be at risk of chronic lead toxicity. Almost 1 million children aged 1–5 years have BLLs >10 μg/dL, the currently accepted level of concern.[45] As noted previously in the discussion of pathophysiologic effects, the subclinical toxicity of lead in this population centers around subtle effects on growth, hearing, and neurocognitive development. This last effect, in particular, is the subject of intense research interest and scrutiny.[81]

Numerous studies attempt to elucidate and quantify cognitive and behavioral deficits in children with BLLs below those typically associated with symptomatic plumbism (<50–70 μg/dL). Cross-sectional or retrospective studies carried out in the early 1970s demonstrated subtle but statistically significant deficits in cognitive performance, in the range of a 1–5-point decrement on standardized IQ tests, in children with elevated BLLs.[80,217] Many of these studies, however, lacked sufficient numbers of patients, adequate markers of lead burden, or sufficiently careful controls to be fully convincing. The first large, well-controlled study that addressed the majority of methodologic criticisms was reported by Needleman et al in 1979.[197] These authors compared the neurocognitive performance of 58 children in whom the dentine of shed primary teeth showed a high lead content (top 10th percentile) versus that of 100 control children with the lowest 10th percentile lead content. The subjects were Boston first- and second-grade schoolchildren, and none had been identified as having had lead poisoning. The high- and low-lead-content groups were carefully controlled for confounding variables, including medical history; parental education, social class, and IQ; and parental attitudes toward education and school. There was a 4-point deficit in IQ in the high-lead group (102.1 vs 106.6). In addition, more than 2000 children with known dentine levels were blindly evaluated by teachers in ratings of several classroom behaviors. The occurrence of nonadaptive behaviors, such as distractibility and impulsiveness, was associated in dose-related fashion to dentine lead content. Of note, prior BLLs were determined from medical record review for some of the study participants and averaged 23.8 μg/dL for 23 of 50 in the low-lead cohort and 35.5 μg/dL for 58 of 100 in the high-lead cohort. Both the strength and dose-response effect of these associations were impressive, particularly because the study population was a large random sample of ostensibly normal school children. Despite these strengths, criticisms of the Boston study are noted.[96] These include lack of concordance on multiple dentine lead analyses, high subject exclusion rate, focus on one measure of cognitive performance, the IQ test, rather than including tests of academic achievement, and failure to correct for confounders in the analysis of classroom behavior by teachers. However, a number of similar cross-sectional studies using a variety of controls for potential confounders and either blood lead or tooth lead as markers of body burden have found similar associations.[52,116,242,309]

The Boston researchers provided an 11-year followup on these schoolchildren.[200] Persistent high-lead effects included failure to graduate high school, higher frequency of learning disability, and lower class rank. Australian researchers note similar findings in children aged 11–13 years, despite substantial declines in BLLs after age 2.[287] Recently, antisocial or delinquent behavior, in addition to IQ per se, was correlated with body lead burden measured by K x-ray fluorescence spectroscopy of the tibia in schoolchildren.[85] Similar behavioral correlates are noted when utilizing lifetime average BLL as the exposure marker.[37]

Additional studies have attempted to extend the potential lower threshold for both body lead burden and critical age by using a longitudinal design and enrolling children at birth, or even prenatally. Bellinger et al[21] reported on 249 Boston children from birth to 2 years of age and found a 4.8-point IQ deficit between high- and low-lead-exposure groups. However, they subsequently reported that by age 5 years, the association between prenatal lead exposure and cognitive index diminished greatly, except in children with higher concurrent lead exposure.[22] The persistence of cognitive deficit was related primarily to higher postnatal lead exposure and less favorable markers of socioeconomic status. Similar studies and results were found in Cincinnati and Cleveland in the United States and Sydney and Port Pirie in Australia (the latter is a smelter town with rural surroundings).[14,116,227] An effort to rigorously evaluate all three types of modern (since 1979), carefully done studies of the low-lead and intelligence association (cross-sectional studies with blood or tooth lead, and prospective studies) and combine their results with a statistical meta-analysis technique has been reported.[227] The overall finding was that, while the majority of individual studies failed to achieve statistical significance, taken together, there was a significant inverse association between lead exposure and IQ, on the order of 1–2 IQ points for a doubling of body lead burden (BLL increase from 10–20 μg/dL or tooth lead from 5–10 μg/g). Figure 80–7 presents an overview of several representative lead-intelligence relationship studies.

It should be noted that several issues relating to the ability of observational epidemiologic studies to infer causality need to be considered in interpreting these findings. On the one hand, they share several features of classic epidemiologic criteria for such inference: temporal relationship, strong statistical association, dose-

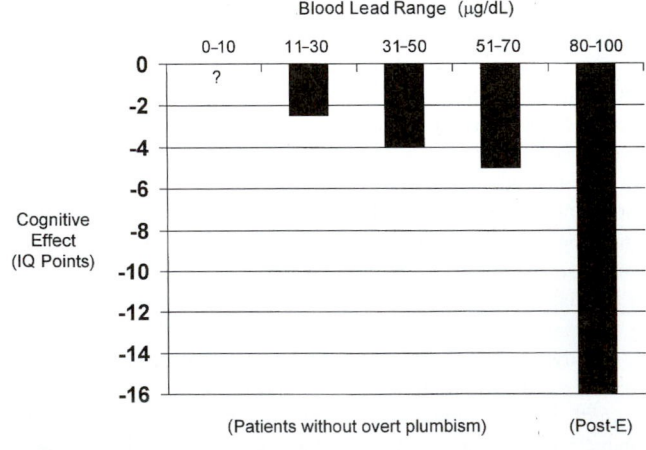

Figure 80–7. The relationship between blood lead and neurocognitive impairment. IQ = full-scale intelligence quotient scores; Post-E = postencephalopathic children. *(Adapted from reference 116. Composite data from references 80, 81, 197, 227, 242, 309.)*

response gradient, control for confounding variables, relatively consistent findings across studies, and biologic plausibility (including support from animal studies). On the other hand, it is difficult to control for all confounders, especially those that relate to individual parent-child and other minienvironmental factors. In this regard, the possibility of reverse causality should also be considered. It is possible that children with lower IQ manifest behaviors that would enhance lead absorption. This has been evaluated statistically, using data derived from many of the aforementioned studies, and reveals that every 10-point decrement in IQ is associated with a 1.5–3.0% increase in BLL, a relatively small but obviously important effect, were it to occur.[227] While many questions remain for future research, the cumulative weight of these studies certainly adds to the conviction that occult lead poisoning is a potential cause of cognitive deficit. These results are those of populations, not individuals, and the magnitude of change may seem small for the majority of exposed children. However, mean population changes on the order of 4 IQ points result in a marked decrease in the number of children who score in the superior range (IQ >125), and an approximate 4-fold increase in those with a severe deficit (IQ <80).[116,196] This obviously represents an enormous societal loss. Additional subtle clinical findings in asymptomatic children with elevated lead burdens is alluded to in the discussion of pathophysiologic effects. These findings do not usually present as recognized concerns in individual patients, but to review, have included measurable deficits in growth,[255] hearing,[256] and fine-motor coordination.[86]

Adults. Adults with occupational lead exposure may manifest numerous signs and symptoms representing disorders of several organ systems. True acute poisoning occurs rarely, after very high respiratory,[148] large oral,[204] or intravenous exposures.[1,205] Such patients may present with colic, hepatitis, pancreatitis, hemolytic anemia, and encephalopathy over days or weeks. Most adult plumbism is related to chronic respiratory exposure, although some authors have used the term *acute poisoning* to include patients with such exposure whose symptoms are severe and of relatively recent onset (within 6 weeks of presentation) and whose exposure is relatively brief (average 1 year or less).[76]

Acute encephalopathy is rarely reported in adults since the 1920s.[76] The majority of modern cases are not associated with occupational exposures, but rather with ingestion of illicit "moonshine" whiskey. Of fatal adult cases in the United States between 1979 and 1988, moonshine was the lead source in 22 of 25 patients for which the lead source was identified.[278] Encephalopathy in adults is manifested by seizures (75% of cases), obtundation, confusion, focal motor disturbances, papilledema, headaches, and optic neuritis.[305] Encephalopathy is characterized by diffuse pathologic changes and cerebral edema and is usually associated with very high BLLs (typically >150 µg/dL). Other manifestations of symptomatic lead poisoning in adults involve CNS, peripheral nerve, hematologic, renal, gastrointestinal, rheumatologic, and endocrine/reproductive findings.[148,240,249] Subencephalopathic CNS findings include changes in mood and cognition. Subtle neurocognitive abnormalities demonstrable by neuropsychiatric testing are being found in adults as well as children with modest elevations in blood lead. Such studies have documented abnormal psychometrics and nerve conduction in workers recently exposed to lead as BLLs rose to above 30 µg/dL.[168] Early symptoms, at BLLs of 40–80 µg/dL, include increased tiredness at the end of the day, disinterest in leisure-time pursuits, falling asleep easily, moodiness,

and irritability. As for children, these early symptoms may be so subtle as to be recognized only in hindsight after the patient is away from the exposure. Subclinical effects on reproductive function and blood pressure may be apparent in this range of exposure, as detailed earlier. As exposure increases (BLL >80 µg/dL, or air levels of 0.3–0.5 mg/m³), new symptoms develop, including headache, memory loss, decreased libido, and insomnia. Gastrointestinal effects may appear, including metallic taste, abdominal pain, decreased appetite, weight loss, and constipation. Musculoskeletal and rheumatologic complaints at this stage include muscle pain, muscle weakness (especially upper extremity, dominant side), joint tenderness, numbness of the legs, occasional paresthesias, tremor, and hyperreflexia. Many patients at this stage have mild anemia. Patients with prolonged exposure at this level are at risk for chronic nephropathy. As exposure increases further (BLLs >100 µg/dL), attacks of colic may appear, anemia is virtually always present, and the patient is at significant risk for peripheral nerve palsy or encephalopathy.

Physical examination findings will vary with degree of severity. Mild and moderate symptoms usually occur in patients with normal examination findings.[83] In encephalopathic patients, typical changes of stupor, coma, posturing, and papilledema are noted. Milder abnormal neurologic findings include dominant wrist or hand weakness, paresthesia, or tremor. Grayish stippling of the retina circumferential to the optic disk is described by one author,[277] but disputed by others.[215] A bluish-purple gingival lead line (Burton line), representing lead sulfide precipitation, is described rarely in adult patients with poor oral hygiene. Abdominal guarding and tenderness are occasionally observed. Patients with gout may have typical joint findings of acute arthritis. Severely anemic patients may exhibit pallor. Careful neuropsychologic testing may reveal abnormalities of memory span, rapid motor tapping, visual motor coordination, and grip strength.[76] Table 80–6 summarizes the spectrum of symptoms and signs associated with adult lead poisoning.[240]

Organic Lead

Clinical symptoms of tetraethyl lead (TEL) toxicity are usually nonspecific initially, and include insomnia and emotional instability.[31,249] Nausea, vomiting, and anorexia may occur. The patient may exhibit tremor and increased deep-tendon reflexes. In more severe cases, these symptoms progress to an encephalopathy with delusions, hallucinations, and hyperactivity, which may resolve or deteriorate to coma and, occasionally, death. Severe cases may also develop hepatic and renal injury. Of note, in contrast to inorganic lead poisoning, patients with significant TEL toxicity do not consistently manifest hematologic abnormalities or elevations of heme synthesis pathway biomarkers. In addition, there is not a close correlation of neurotoxicity severity with measured BLL.[132]

ASSESSMENT
Clinical Diagnosis in Symptomatic Patients

The physician must consider the diagnosis of lead poisoning in order to recognize this uncommon condition. For all patients in whom plumbism is considered, based on clinical manifestations, the medical evaluation should first include a comprehensive past medical history, including that of foreign body ingestions or gunshot wounds with retained bullets. Further inquiry should elicit occupational and recreational history of all home occupants, family use of ethnic folk medicines, use of imported, glazed ceramics, age and condition of residence and/or any recent renovation activity, source and use of drinking water, and proximity of residence to lead-using industry. Children may be at further risk if they are 1–5 years of age and have persistent vomiting, lethargy, irritability, clumsiness, or loss of recently acquired developmental skills; afebrile seizures; a strong history of pica, including acute unintentional ingestions,[131] or aural, nasal, or esophageal foreign bodies;[308] residence in a pre-1960s-built home, especially with deteriorated paint, or one that has undergone recent remodeling; a family history of lead poisoning; iron deficiency anemia; or evidence of child abuse or neglect.[101,259]

The differential diagnosis of plumbism is broad. Adult patients may be misdiagnosed as having carpal tunnel syndrome, Guillain-Barré syndrome, sickle-cell crisis, acute appendicitis, renal colic, and infectious encephalitis. Children are often initially considered to have viral gastroenteritis, or even to have insidious symptoms passed off as a difficult developmental phase.

The patient who presents to the ED with acute encephalopathy that may represent lead poisoning presents the physician with a dilemma: severe lead toxicity requires urgent diagnosis, but confirmatory blood lead assays are usually not available on an immediate basis.[137] For adults, a history of occupational exposure is often available from past medical records or family members, and lead encephalopathy can be strongly considered with positive supportive laboratory findings (usually available on urgent basis) such as anemia, basophilic stippling, elevated erythrocyte protoporphyrin (especially >250 μg/dL), and abnormal urinalysis. In this context, it would probably be appropriate to institute presumptive chelation therapy while awaiting lead levels. In children, a similar indication for presumptive treatment would be suggested by a constellation of clinical features and ancillary studies: age 1–5 years, a prodromal illness of several days' to weeks' duration (suggestive of milder lead-related symptoms), occurrence in summer, history of pica and source of lead exposure, the laboratory features noted above, which are equally helpful in young children, radiologic findings of dense metaphyseal "lead lines" at wrists or knees (Fig. 80–2), and/or evidence of recent pica for lead paint particles on abdominal radiographs (Fig. 80–8). In both adults and children, the decision to institute empiric chelation treatment should not deter additional emergent diagnostic efforts to exclude or to confirm other important entities while blood lead levels are pending. An important consideration in this context may be the suspicion of an acute, potentially treatable CNS infection (eg, bacterial meningitis or herpetic encephalitis). Lumbar puncture may be dangerous in patients with lead encephalopathy because of the risk of cerebral herniation. If immediate lumbar puncture is thought to be highly desirable, a computed tomography scan would allow determination of severe cerebral edema, midline shift, or other evidence of especially high risk for herniation. If performed, the minimal amount of fluid necessary for diagnosis (<1 mL) should be removed through a small-gauge needle. Alternatively, empiric treatment for infectious processes can be initiated while the lead level is pending, and delayed lumbar puncture can be performed if blood lead level is normal.

Laboratory Considerations

Laboratory testing is used to augment the evaluation of both lead exposure and lead toxicity. Traditionally, the direct measurement of lead in blood was costly and posed technical obstacles; thus, a reliance developed on using biomarkers derived from lead-induced abnormalities of the heme synthesis pathway and on using

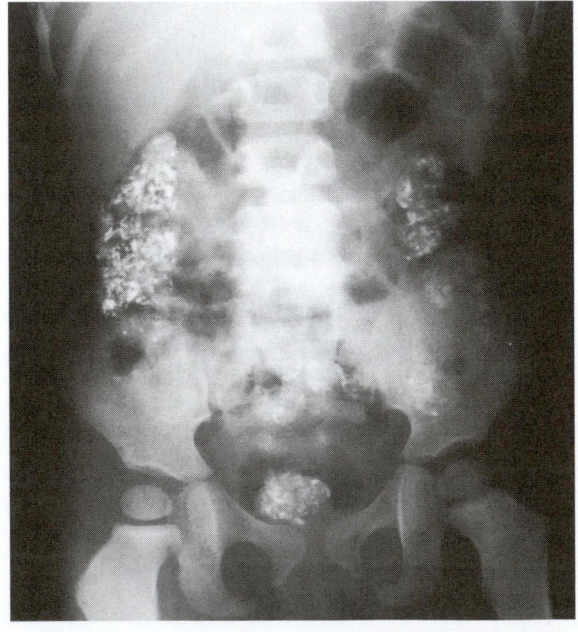
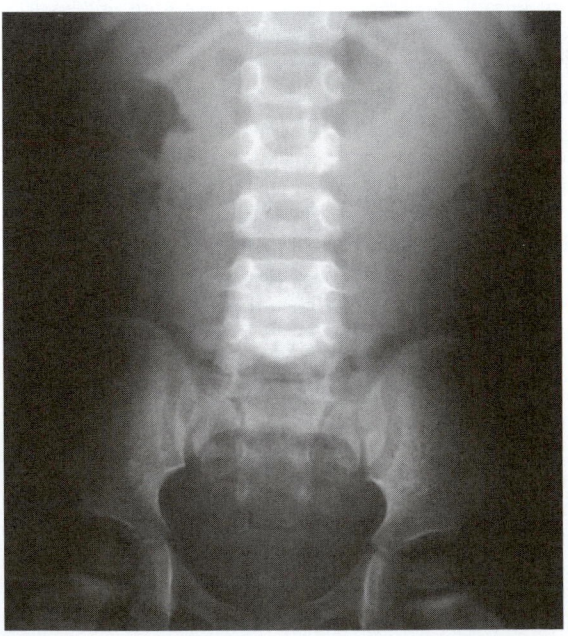

A

B

Figure 80–8. **A.** Abdominal radiograph of a child who had massive paint chip ingestion. **B.** Followup radiograph after whole-bowel irrigation. *(Courtesy of Department of Radiology, St. Christopher's Hospital for Children, Philadelphia, PA.)*

enhanced urine lead excretion after chelating agent administration. These indirect assays have waned in utility as levels of concern for lead exposure have decreased concomitantly with technical advances in direct blood lead measurement.[122] Several of the indirect biomarkers are reviewed briefly here; for a more in-depth discussion the interested reader is referred to several comprehensive reviews.[122,220]

Routine Laboratory Tests. As detailed in the sections on hematologic and renal pathophysiolgic effects, lead may cause several changes in routine complete blood count, urinalysis, or renal function tests. These are usually observed only in moderate to severe degrees of exposure. The patient may manifest normochromic or hypochromic microcytic anemia and red blood cell stippling. The urinalysis may be positive for protein and glucose. Renal function tests may reveal elevated blood urea nitrogen and creatinine in patients with chronic lead nephropathy.

Radiographic evaluation may be helpful occasionally. The growing long bones, particularly at wrists and knees, in children about 9 months to 5 years of age may reveal characteristic "lead lines" of increased calcification in the zone of provisional calcification (Fig. 80–2). These dense metaphyseal bands take 4–8 weeks of heavy exposure to develop. They are more likely to be significant if the smaller ulna and fibula are involved as well as the larger radius and tibia.[29] Lead lines may also be present in flat bones such as ribs, clavicles, and the iliac crest.[312] Abdominal radiographs may reveal radiopacities representing lead paint chips or particles and, rarely, lead-containing folk medicines or foreign bodies (Figs. 80–4 and 80–8).[34] These findings are usually present for 24–36 hours postingestion.[220] One survey found that 26% of children with lead levels >55 µg/dL had abdominal radiopacities.[181]

Biomarkers of Lead Exposure and Toxicity. The effect of lead on the heme synthesis pathway (Fig. 80–5) and the ease of sampling blood and urine have led to several tests based on enzyme inhibition or accumulation of substrates. The erythrocyte δ-aminolevulinic acid dehydratase activity is a sensitive marker of lead exposure and shows 50% inhibition at lead levels of only 15 µg/dL. However, the enzyme must be assayed within 24 hours of blood sampling and is so sensitive it cannot distinguish between moderate and severe exposure.[122,201] The measurement of accumulated ALA in urine may serve as a useful tool for tracking lead exposure in occupational settings, but today is considered relatively insensitive because it does not rise appreciably until blood lead is >40 µg/dL. The relatively low-cost test of urine ALA continues its value in areas of the world with extensive lead contamination but limited financial resources.[122,257]

Erythrocytes accumulate protoporphyrin in the presence of iron deficiency or inhibition of heme synthetase by lead. The red cell has an average life span of 120 days, so that erythrocyte protoporphyrin (EP) levels reach a steady state over 3 months and reflect relatively long-term lead exposure.[220] A simple fluorometric technique for assaying red cell EP was developed in the early 1970s,[222] and for 2 decades this test became the method of choice for lead surveillance. It could utilize a fingerstick drop of blood, was not influenced by surface lead-dust contamination, and also screened for iron deficiency, another prevalent condition of young children. Of note, the terms EP, free erythrocyte protoporphyrin (FEP), and zinc protoporphyrin (ZPP) have often been used interchangeably in the past. This reflects a confusion based on older extraction techniques of measuring red cell protoporhyrins.[220] In lead-poisoned or iron-deficient red cells, most of the increased EP is bound to zinc. Most current tests measure total red cell EP and obviate the need for extraction and for distinguishing FEP from ZPP. The EP first increases at lead levels of about 17 µg/dL, and thus is also insensitive to lead levels in the 10–25-µg/dL range.[122] As such, it is no longer recommended as a surveillance test for childhood lead poisoning. The EP may still be useful for tracking response to therapy and distinguishing acute from chronic lead exposure and as an adjunct to the emergency diagnosis of symptomatic plumbism.

Chelatable Lead. The baseline excretion of lead in urine is not generally considered a sensitive biomarker of lead exposure. However, lead excretion after a single dose of the chelator CaNa$_2$EDTA is correlated with blood lead and several heme pathway markers.[61,122] A lead "challenge," "mobilization," or "provocative" test was developed to evaluate the size of the mobilizable pool of body lead burden, with the hope of pinpointing which asymptomatic patients with modestly elevated blood lead levels would most benefit from a full course of chelation therapy.[244] Standardized doses of CaNa$_2$EDTA were administered and 24-hour[244] or 8-hour[176] urine collections tested for lead excretion, with various formulas proposed for a "positive" test. Several assumptions about the validity of this test are not obvious.[122] It is not clear whether positive responders will continue to excrete more lead than poor responders. Conversely, it is not clear that negative tests would imply lack of any value for subsequent chelation. One large series of lead mobilization tests found that the test was positive in only 28% of children with blood lead levels of 40–49 µg/dL, and 66% of children with lead levels of 50–69 µg/dL.[303] Most authorities would currently recommend chelation for all patients in the latter group, and many of those in the former.[52] It is also possible that single doses of CaNa$_2$EDTA may translocate lead from less vulnerable sites, such as bone, to more vulnerable sites, such as the brain; this is demonstrated in rats.[61,74] Finally, the test is cumbersome, difficult technically in children who are not toilet trained, and requires parenteral drug administration, and thus is not risk free. This test is no longer recommended by the American Academy of Pediatrics,[5] and seems to be falling out of favor in occupational medicine practice as well.[83,122,249]

Blood Lead. For many years the use of blood lead as a biomarker for lead exposure was avoided by researchers and clinicians.[122] As noted earlier, blood lead has complex kinetics, reflecting the redistribution of lead from other compartments, primarily bone, to blood. Blood sampling required relatively large volumes (5–7 mL) and was costly and technically difficult. However, recently several factors favor the use of whole blood as the primary biomarker for both research and clinical practice. The evolution of atomic absorption spectrophotometry (AAS) allows reliable, sensitive determinations of blood lead as low as 1 µg/dL. The equipment is widely available and some techniques (eg, graphite furnace AAS) require only 0.25 mL blood; newer modifications also allow application to capillary blood samples.[249] All the alternative biomarkers discussed above have some inherent limitations, particularly lack of sensitivity at the lower body lead burdens currently of concern. Lastly, virtually all of the recent research associating low-level lead exposure with adverse clinical outcomes, especially neurocognitive deficits in children or renal function in adults, have utilized blood lead as the primary bio-marker.[122]

Whole venous blood for lead testing may be collected, after careful skin preparation, through standard stainless-steel needles into special lead-free (tan top) or trace element–free (dark blue top) evacuated tubes (eg, Vacutainers from Becton Dickinson Co). If these are not readily available, standard heparinized tubes (green top) may be used, but elevated values should probably be verified.[249] The blood should be mixed thoroughly as soon as possible to ensure anticoagulation. Pediatric blood-lead testing is often hampered by the requirement for venipuncture and relatively large blood volumes. An alternative is the use of capillary sampling by fingerstick puncture. This technique is safe and quick and can be applied to mass screening. Its principal drawback is the potential for contamination by lead-soiled fingertips, and thus an excessive rate of false-positive testing. At least in a controlled research protocol, capillary test results were highly correlated with matched venous samples, with mean capillary-venous differences of less than 1 μg/dL.[252] It is imperative that fingers be swabbed thoroughly with alcohol prior to puncture. Fingerstick blood may be collected in capillary tubes or as a dried blood spot on filter paper.[279] Venous confirmation of elevated capillary lead levels is still considered mandatory prior to chelation or other significant interventions. The capillary test is considered too inaccurate, because of frequent false-positives, to be of value in the context of adult occupational exposure.[249]

Other Lead Assays

Lead can also be quantified in urine, teeth, and hair. Urine assays are considered insensitive, and hair is unreliable because of surface contamination.[220] Shed primary teeth are used in research studies as biomarkers of cumulative childhood lead exposure,[197] but are obviously impractical in clinical patient management.

Research Methodologies. X-ray fluorescence (XRF) technology estimates tooth[30] and bone[138] lead, and thus indirectly is a cumulative measure of body lead exposure in epidemiologic studies. Protocols have not yet achieved the standardization that would be required for a clinically useful test. The tests are relatively costly and require the patient to remain still for up to 30 minutes, involve low-dose radiation exposure, and are not widely available.[122] The XRF technique may have promise in research studies of issues concerning past chronic heavy lead exposure and a variety of current health outcomes.[302]

SCREENING

Children

As evidence accumulated in the 1970s and 1980s that low-level lead exposure was a significant pediatric public health issue, it simultaneously became apparent that the only way to detect elevated lead burdens early in childhood would be to screen widely.[53] In October 1991, the CDC recommended that every child in the United States be screened at age 1 year, and, preferably, at age 2 years as well, by whole-blood lead determination. A blood lead of >10 μg/dL was defined as the intervention level.[52] However, over the next few years, numerous studies appeared that found a very low prevalence of elevated lead levels in selected communities.[27,202,283] Several of these found that a few simple questions re-

garding housing age and condition were predictive for the few children who did have elevated lead levels.[27,133,202] Concern grew that overemphasis and misappropriation of resources on universal screening would further compromise higher-priority efforts for targeted screening of the most at-risk populations.[133,253] A 1994 national survey found that only 29% of children living in homes built prior to 1960, and only 30% of children in families earning less than $20,000 per year, had been screened.[26] At the same time, remarkable cases of extremely elevated blood lead levels (>100 μg/dL) detected on routine screening continued to be reported, especially in minority, inner-city children.[79] In response to these developments, the CDC proposed new recommendations in 1997 and 2000,[43,46] which were recently endorsed by the American Academy of Pediatrics,[4] and are outlined in Table 80–7. This approach emphasizes targeted screening and followup for most children from low-prevalence communities. A recent study examined cost-effectiveness of this recommended approach, and found that only universal screening would detect all BLLs >10 μg/dL and was cost-effective in high prevalence areas. Targeted screening of venous blood was more cost-effective but less sensitive in low- or medium-prevalence communities. In both contexts, venous blood

---

TABLE 80–7. Pediatric Screening and Followup Guidelines

Screening

Screen
1. All high-risk children at 1 and 2 y (3–6 y if not previously screened)
2. Selected low-risk children (any affirmative answer to risk questions) (high-risk community = 12% of young children with elevated BPb, 27% of homes built before 1950; all children enrolled in Medicaid)

Personal Risk Questionnaire
1. Does your child live in or regularly visit a home built before 1950?
2. Does your child live in or regularly visit a home built before 1978 undergoing remodeling or renovation (or has been within 6 mo)?
3. Specific exposure questions:
   Personal, family history of lead poisoning
   Occupational, industrial, hobby exposures
   Proximity to major roadway
   Hot tap water for consumption
   Cultural exposures (folk remedies, cosmetics, ceramic food containers, trips, residence outside US, international adoptees)
   Migrant farm workers, receipt of poverty assistance
   History of pica for paint chips, dirt
   History of iron deficiency

Followup

BPb (μg/dL)	Recommended Action
< 9	Retest in 1 y
10–14	Retest in 3 mo; education
15–19	Retest in 2 mo; education; if 15–19 twice, refer for case management
20–44	Clinical evaluation; education; environmental investigation
45–69	Clinical evaluation and case management within 48 h; education; environmental investigation; chelation therapy
≥70	Hospitalize child; immediate chelation therapy; education; environmental investigation

BPb = venous blood lead.
Educational interventions as per Table 80–9.
Chelation therapy as per Tables 80–10.
Reprinted, with permission, from Centers for Disease Control and Prevention: Screening Young Children for Lead Poisoning: Guidance for State and Local Public Health officials. US Dept of Health and Human Services, Public Health Service, Federal Register, Feb 21, 1997.

testing would be more cost-effective than capillary testing.[147] The optimal approach to screening in low- to medium-prevalence communities is still unknown, and this issue remains controversial.[195] However, there is a broad consensus that universal screening is still required in low-income children, and it is recommended by the CDC for all children enrolled in Medicaid, at ages 12 and 24 months (or 36–72 months if not previously tested).[43]

Adults

The Occupational Safety and Health Administration (OSHA) developed a lead standard for US workers in 1978 that was formulated to reduce workplace exposure to lead, to decrease symptomatic lead poisoning, and to provide quality medical care to workers with elevated blood lead levels.[296] This regulation requires employers to ensure workplace standards for environmental control and employee education, to regularly monitor environmental contamination and employee lead status, and to provide free medical surveillance and necessary treatment, while continuing the salary of any worker removed from the worksite because of lead exposure. The OSHA permissible exposure level for lead in worksite air is 50 μg/m^3 averaged over an 8-hour day. Employees at risk for the action level of 30 μg/m^3 for >30 days per year must be screened periodically, as outlined in Table 80–8.[295] It is illegal to provide medicinal dietary interventions or prophylactic chelation prior to routine screening. It should be noted that the law's intent is not simply to remove lead-poisoned workers from the worksite, only to replace them with newer employees whose lead burdens are less extensive, but rather to recognize an opportunity to improve workplace hygiene.[249] Where the lead standard is being invoked, such as the lead smelting and battery manufacturing industries, clinical lead poisoning and average blood lead levels have decreased impressively.[295] In 1993, the lead standard was extended to the construction industry,[294] but it is not yet applied to agricultural workers.

TREATMENT

There are several caveats about the treatment of lead poisoning. First, the most important aspect of treatment is removal from exposure to lead. Unfortunately, effective implementation of this therapy is often beyond the control of the clinician, but rather depends on a complex interplay of public health, social, and political actions. Currently, the ability to control exposure is generally more applicable to adults with occupational exposures than to children exposed to residential hazards. Second, in children for whom some residual lead exposure continues, optimization of nutritional status is vital in order to minimize absorption. Finally, pharmacologic therapy with chelation agents, while a mainstay of therapy for symptomatic patients, is an inexact science, with numerous unanswered questions despite almost 50 years of clinical use.[5,9,154] The rationale for chelation therapy of lead-poisoned patients is that chelating drugs complex with lead, forming a chelate that is excreted in urine, feces, or both. Chelation therapy does increase lead excretion, reduce blood levels, and reverse hematologic markers of toxicity during therapy. Reports from the 1950s found symptomatic improvement of adults chelated for lead colic.[299] The institution of effective combination chelation treatment of childhood lead encephalopathy in the 1960s certainly contributed to the dramatic decline in mortality and morbidity of that devastating degree of plumbism.[62] However, the same era saw major advances in pediatric critical care in general, and medical management of increased intracranial pressure in particular.[154] The situation of chelation therapy for asymptomatic patients with mildly to moderately increased body burdens of lead is even less clear. Questions asked today include: (a) Do chelating drugs materially decrease body burdens of lead in the context of chronic exposure, or merely enhance excretion briefly, only to be subsequently offset by slowed "natural" excretion?[175] (b) To what degree does increased excretion of a toxic metal reverse established toxicity?[120,154] (c) Does the process of chelation result in dangerous redistribution of metal from less vulnerable (eg, bone) to more vulnerable target organs (eg, brain)?[61,154] (d) Are there potential adverse health effects related to aggressive chelation therapy (which, for example, might contribute to excretion or redistribution of physiologically important trace metals and thus impact on normal growth and development)? [276,288,316]

Long-term reduction of target tissue lead content or reversal of toxicity is not demonstrated in human trials.[175,192] For example, two recent studies examined the impact of CaNa$_2$EDTA therapy on neurotoxic effects of low to moderate lead exposure. A study in rats failed to find improvement in a lever-pressing-for-food model,[73] and a study in children found modest improvement in cognitive index after treatment, but failed to demonstrate any additional benefit of CaNa$_2$EDTA per se over dietary supplementation and home abatement.[241] Furthermore, a recent study of succimer therapy in lead-exposed adult rhesus monkeys found that chelation did not lower brain lead content, while cessation of exposure did.[75]

Decreasing Exposure

All patients with significantly elevated lead levels warrant specific environmental interventions. In adults, this usually involves changes in their worksite, and the discussion above on screening.[83,249] Remedial actions might include improvements in ventilation, modification of personal hygiene habits, and optimal use of respiratory apparatus. It is vital to prohibit smoking, eating, and drinking in a lead-exposed work area. Work clothes should be changed after each shift and should not be lockered together with street clothes.

Table 80–9 summarizes several specific educational guidelines that may be offered to parents of lead-exposed children.[6,52,64,254] While home lead-paint abatement, or relocation, is mandatory, renovations must be done by trained and experienced workers,

TABLE 80–8. **OSHA Adult Lead Standard Screening and Followup Summary**

BPb (μg/dL)	Recommended Action
>60 on a single test; or average >50 of last 3 samples, or all samples over prior 6 mo (requires confirmation within 2 wk)	Immediate removal from worksite; BPb every month
>40–60	Repeat BPb in 2 mo
<40	Repeat BPb in 6 mo; BPb at which a worker who has been medically removed from the worksite may return (requires confirmation BPb within 2 wk)

BPb = blood lead (μg/dL).
Compiled, with permission, from references 83 and 296.

TABLE 80–9. Reducing Lead Exposure

Adults
Implement OSHA lead standard
Improve ventilation
Use respiratory apparatus
Wear protective clothing; change from workclothes before leaving worksite
Modify personal hygiene habits
Prohibit eating, drinking, smoking in worksite

Children
Notify local health department
Home lead paint abatement (professional contractors if possible; use plastic sheeting, low dust-generating paint removal; replacement of lead-painted windows, floor treatment; final cleanup with high-efficiency particle air vacuum, wet-mopping)
Avoid most hazardous areas of home, yard
Dust control: wet-mopping, sponging with high-phosphate detergent; frequent hand, toy, pacifier washing
Soil lead exposure reduction by planting grass, shrubs around house
Use only cold, flushed tap water for consumption
Optimize nutrition: avoid fasting; iron, calcium sufficient diet; iron and/or calcium supplementation as necessary
Avoid food storage in open cans
Avoid imported ceramic containers for food, beverage use
Evaluate parental occupations, hobbies

with the family out of the home, and with appropriate cleanup instituted prior to the family's return. In many communities, assistance with home inspection and abatement is available through public health agencies.[92,291] In addition, simple, inexpensive home dust-reduction techniques correlate with decreased blood lead levels.[55,149] Recent research into the efficacy of such environmental interventions in the homes of young children shows relatively mixed results, with a few general themes emerging:[41,155,235] lead hazard control interventions do have a modest impact on reducing children's BLLs, generally in the range of a 6–25% decline from baseline—the effect is more pronounced with higher baseline BLLs, and the interventions must be performed carefully (preferably by trained staff). Simple efforts to decrease soil lead exposure may also help, such as planting grass or large shrubs in affected areas (usually close to the house).[52] Formal soil removal and replacement is very costly (average $9600 per home) and minimally effective (average decline in blood lead of 1 μg/dL).[304] Nutritional evaluation and counseling to optimize diet will minimize lead absorption. Evidence suggests that dietary iron may inhibit lead absorption, but might also diminish excretion of an existing body lead burden. Thus, all lead-exposed children should be tested for concomitant iron deficiency and treated with pharmacologic iron preparations as necessary, although iron therapy for iron-replete patients without ongoing lead exposure is not recommended.[310] Even in the absence of overt iron deficiency, or after successful treatment, a diet rich in iron, calcium, and frequent nutritious snacks is optimal[247] (Table 80–9). Recently, a nutritional role for ascorbic acid in the prevention of lead toxicity has been postulated. For example, an inverse relationship between blood ascorbate levels and BLLs was found in the NHANES III data.[273]

Chelation Therapy

The indications for and specifics of chelation therapy are determined by patient age, blood-lead level, and clinical symptomatol-

ogy (Table 80–10). Three chelation agents are currently recommended as drugs of choice for the treatment of lead poisoning: BAL and CaNa$_2$EDTA are used parenterally for more severe cases, and succimer (dimercaptosuccinic acid) is available for oral therapy.[78] Pharmacologic profiles of these three agents are detailed in the corresponding Antidotes in Depth discussions on dimercaprol (BAL), edetate calcium disodium, and succimer. Table 80–3 presents capsule summaries in relation to therapeutic adverse effects and monitoring issues.

A fourth drug, D-penicillamine, has been used orally for patients with mild to moderate excess lead burdens, and its use is described here briefly. Since 1991, the role of D-penicillamine in lead poisoning treatment has been largely replaced by succimer. Chelation using D-penicillamine shares the advantage of oral administration with succimer. Typical dosing regimens begin with one dose of 10 mg/kg/d, increased as tolerated in a week to 20 mg/kg/d (in two doses) and then a week or more later to 30 mg/kg/d (in two or three doses).[159] Unfortunately, D-penicillamine has a toxicity profile that includes serious, life-threatening hematologic disorders and reversible, but serious, dermatologic and renal effects, although these are reported primarily in adults on high-dose treatment. In children, adverse effects may occur in up to 33% of patients, but are milder, with gastrointestinal upset, reversible leukopenia or thrombocytopenia, rash, and proteinuria/hematuria dominating.[159,267] A recent report suggests that a lower dosage regimen (15 mg/kg/d) maintains efficacy with a lower incidence of adverse effects.[268] Nevertheless, courses of therapy average 10 weeks in duration, and it seems unlikely that patients unable to successfully complete succimer therapy will do better with D-penicillamine. It is our practice to use inpatient CaNa$_2$EDTA chelation with the rare child who fails succimer treatment; the American Academy of Pediatrics recommends D-penicillamine use only when unacceptable adverse reactions to both succimer and CaNa$_2$EDTA occur, and yet it remains important to continue chelation.[5]

Chelation is not a panacea for lead poisoning. It is a relatively inefficient process, with a typical course of therapy decreasing body content of heavy metal by 1–2%.[154,192] Furthermore, there is little evidence that chelating agents have significant access to critical sites in target organs, particularly in the brain.[75] Assumptions that reducing blood lead level will improve subtle neurocognitive dysfunction or other subclinical organ toxicity are appealing theoretically, but unproven.[288]

Pediatric Therapy. Lead encephalopathy is an acute life-threatening emergency and should be treated under the guidance of a multidisciplinary team in the intensive care unit of a hospital experienced in the management of critically ill children. Encephalopathy requires treatment by combination parenteral chelation therapy with maximum-dose BAL and CaNa$_2$EDTA and meticulous supportive care.[5,52,62,66] Such combination therapy has a dramatic effect on decreasing BLL, with typical declines, in percent change compared to baseline, of 50% or more within 15 hours, and 75–80% by 48–72 hours. It is far superior to monotherapy with CaNa$_2$EDTA in this regard.[62] The development of combined chelation therapy for childhood lead encephalopathy, reported by Chisolm[62] and Coffin[66] in the mid-1960s, had an equally dramatic impact on reducing mortality, and must be hailed as one of the outstanding milestones in clinical pediatrics of our time.

Chelation is instituted with intramuscular (IM) BAL 75 mg/m^2/d (or 25 mg/kg/d) in six divided doses.[5,52] The second dose

TABLE 80–10.   Chelation Therapy Guidelines[a]

Condition, BPb (μg/dL)	Dose	Regimen/Comments
Adults		
Encephalopathy	BAL 450 mg/m²/d[a]	75 mg/m² IM every 4 h for 5 d
	CaNa₂EDTA 1500 mg/m²/d[a]	Continuous infusion, or 2–4 divided IV doses, for 5 d (start 4 h after BAL)
Symptoms suggestive of	BAL 300–450 mg/m²/d[a]	50–75 mg/m² every 4 h for 3–5 d
encephalopathy or > 100	CaNa₂EDTA 1000–1500 mg/m²/d[a]	Continuous infusion, or 2–4 divided IV doses, for 5 d (start 4 h after BAL)
		Base dose, duration on BPb, severity of symptoms (see text)
Mild symptoms or 70–100	Succimer 700–1050 mg/m²/d	350 mg/m² tid for 5 d, then bid for 14 d
Asymptomatic and < 70	Usually not indicated	Remove from exposure
Children		
Encephalopathy	BAL 450 mg/m²/d[a]	75 mg/m² IM every 4 h for 5 d
	CaNa₂EDTA 1500 mg/m²/d[a]	Continuous infusion, or 2–4 divided IV doses, for 5 d (start 4 h after BAL)
Symptomatic, or > 70	BAL 300–450 mg/m²/d[a]	50–75 mg/m² every 4 h for 3–5 d
	CaNa₂EDTA 1000–1500 mg/m²/d[a]	Continuous infusion, or 2–4 divided IV doses, for 5 d (start 4 h after BAL)
		Base dose, duration on BPb, severity of symptoms (see text)
Asymptomatic: 45–69	Succimer 700–1050 mg/m²/d	350 mg/m² tid for 5 d, then bid for 14 d
	or CaNa₂EDTA, 1000 mg/m²/d[a]	Continuous infusion, or 2–4 divided IV, for 5 d (see text)
	(or rarely, D-penicillamine)	
20–44	Routine chelation not indicated	Await current studies (eg, NIEHS TLC)
	(see text)	If succimer used, same regimen as per above group
< 20	Chelation not indicated	See Table 80–9
	Attempt exposure reduction	

[a]Doses expressed mg/kg: BAL 450 mg/m² (24 mg/kg); 300 mg/m² (18 mg/kg). CaNa₂EDTA 1000 mg/m² (25–50 mg/kg); 1500 mg/m² (50–75 mg/kg) adult maximum 2–3 g/d). Succimer 350 mg/m² (10 mg/kg).
Subsequent treatment regimens based on postchelation BPb and clinical symptoms (see text). BPb = blood lead (μg/dL); EP = erythrocyte photoporphyrin; IM = intramuscular; IV = intravenous; NIEHS TLC = National Institute of Environmental Health Sciences supported multicenter study: Treatment of lead-exposed children.
Compiled, with permission, from references 5, 52, 148, 192, 224, and 228.

of BAL is given 4 hours later, followed immediately by intravenous (IV) CaNa₂EDTA, in maximum concentration of 0.5% solution, at 1500 mg/m²/d (or 50 mg/kg/d)[5] as a continuous infusion over several hours or in divided-dose infusions.[5,52,224] The delay in initiating CaNa₂EDTA infusion is based on past observations of clinical deterioration in encephalopathic patients treated with this agent alone.[5,62] Therapy is typically continued with both agents for 5 days, although in milder cases with prompt resolution of encephalopathy and decrease of BLL to <50 μg/dL, BAL may be discontinued after 3 days, with continuation of CaNa₂EDTA alone for 2 more days.

The presence of radiopaque material in the gastrointestinal tract on radiography has raised concern that parenteral chelation might enhance absorption of residual gut lead. This issue is not settled fully,[61,143] but most experts advocate initiation of chelation without delay in seriously symptomatic patients. It seems reasonable to simultaneously attempt bowel decontamination,[5] as with a whole-bowel irrigation solution (Fig. 80–8). A recent case report described the successful use of chelation therapy begun with parenteral BAL and CaNa₂EDTA and then enteral succimer (initiated after 3 days of whole-bowel irrigation) for a child with lead encephalopathy and an extraordinarily high BLL of 550 μg/dL.[114] Generally, oral fluids, feedings, and medications are withheld for at least the first several days. Careful provision of adequate intravenous fluids optimizes renal function while avoiding overhydration and the risk of exacerbating cerebral edema. Appropriate fluid therapy is approximated by basal fluid requirements (1 mL/kcal/d; kcal = 100/kg for first 10 kg, plus 50/kg for next 10 kg, plus 20/kg thereafter) and replacement of ongoing losses. Such a regimen should result in the desired urine output of 0.5 mL/kcal/d (or 350–500 mL/m²/d).[62,137] The occurrence of inappropriate secretion

of antidiuretic hormone syndrome (SIADH) may be associated with lead encephalopathy,[62,254,282] so that urine volume, specific gravity, and serum electrolytes should be closely monitored, especially as fluids are gradually liberalized with clinical improvement. Were SIADH to occur, with significant hyponatremia, strict fluid restriction is usually indicated (Chap. 24). In the context of lead encephalopathy, this approach would need to be tempered by the requirement for maintaining good urine output to optimize chelation efficacy. Mannitol administration has been reported helpful in a few selected cases.[62]

Seizure control is usually accomplished with benzodiazepines (pediatric dosing: diazepam 0.1–0.3 mg/kg, or lorazepam 0.05–0.1 mg/kg). Rarely, continuous infusions of midazolam or high-dose pentobarbital therapy may be necessary.[307] Ongoing anticonvulsant therapy is typically continued with phenytoin or phenobarbital.

Recent advances in management of cerebral edema and increased intracranial pressure are not critically evaluated in the currently rare context of lead encephalopathy. Lumbar puncture should be avoided if lead encephalopathy is highly suspected, and acute infectious processes are not. It seems reasonable that noninvasive measures such as modest hyperventilation, low-dose mannitol or glycerol hyperosmotic therapy, and steroids might have a salutary effect at minimal risk of increased iatrogenic morbidity.[5,62,66,307] Whether more aggressive measures such as intracranial pressure monitoring, induced hypothermia, or pentobarbital coma would decrease mortality or morbidity further is unknown.

Children with milder symptoms, or who are asymptomatic, with BLL >70 μg/dL, should be chelated with a regimen similar to that recommended for encephalopathy. It is likely that this group of patients will require only 2–3 days of BAL, in addition to 5 days of CaNa$_2$EDTA. The asymptomatic patients in this group might also be adequately treated with DMSA (succimer) and CaNa$_2$EDTA, or even DMSA alone, but these regimens have not been studied to date in such children. Intensive care monitoring may be prudent for such patients as well, at least during the initiation of chelation therapy.[192,224]

Chelation therapy is widely recommended for asymptomatic children with BLLs between 45 and 70 µg/dL.[5,9,52,192] Children without overt symptoms may be treated with succimer, which has documented efficacy in lowering BLLs and short-term safety since its FDA approval in 1991.[24,60,124,160,192] Succimer is initiated at 30 mg/kg/d (or 1050 mg/m^2/d) orally in three divided doses; this is continued for 5 days, then decreased to 20 mg/kg/d (or 700 mg/m^2/d) in two divided doses for 14 additional days.[5,123] The original data establishing this empiric dosing regimen were based on surface area rather than body weight.[123] For younger children, the alternative dosing by body weight results in suboptimal dosing.[236] Although the ability to chelate children orally with succimer makes it tempting to prescribe this medication routinely for outpatient therapy, and some animal evidence suggests succimer does not enhance enteral lead absorption,[145] clinical reports suggest that children must be protected from continued lead exposure during succimer chelation.[59,60] Home abatement and reinspection should be accomplished before initiation of ambulatory succimer therapy; if this is not feasible, then hospitalization is still warranted. Alternative regimens (for rare patients with succimer intolerance or allergy, or parental noncompliance) would include inpatient parenteral chelation with CaNa$_2$EDTA at 25 mg/kg/d for 5 days,[5] or an outpatient oral course of D-penicillamine. Combination chelation therapy with either BAL and CaNa$_2$EDTA or succimer and CaNa2EDTA for patients with lead levels in this range produced comparable reductions in BLLs with both regimens.[25] Neither regimen was compared to monotherapy with succimer alone, but the mean decline in postrebound BLLs for the combined succimer and CaNa$_2$EDTa group was significantly better than is typically achieved with succimer alone (−38.5% vs −20% to −30%).[24,25]

After initial chelation therapy, decisions to retreat are based on clinical symptoms and followup BLLs. Patients with encephalopathy or any severe symptoms, or initial BLL >100 µg/dL, will often require repeated courses of treatment. It is suggested that at least 2 days elapse before restarting chelation. The precise regimen and dosing of chelating agents are determined by ongoing symptomatology and the repeat BLLs (Table 80–10). A third course of chelation should rarely be necessary sooner than 5–7 days after the second course ends.[224] For patients with milder degrees of plumbism (eg, asymptomatic, initial BLL <70 µg/dL), it is reasonable to allow 10–14 days of reequilibration before restarting treatment.[5]

The management of children with BLLs of 20–44 µg/dL is controversial.[23,108,159,170,191,288] Current CDC[46] and American Academy of Pediatrics[5] recommendations include aggressive environmental and nutritional interventions with close monitoring of blood lead levels, but not routine chelation therapy, for asymptomatic children with this degree of elevated body lead burden. To assess potential additional benefit of chelation therapy for these children, the National Institute of Environmental Health Sciences is currently sponsoring a multicenter, randomized, placebo-controlled study of succimer therapy in children aged 12–32 months with BLLs of 20–44 µg/dL, the Treatment of Lead-exposed Children (TLC) trial.[288] Both study groups of patients enrolled in TLC

received nutritional supplementation and home lead hazard-reduction interventions. Preliminary results from this trial were recently published and suggest modest efficacy in reducing BLL while confirming short-term safety of succimer use. The mean area-under-the-curve BLL of the succimer-treated group was 4.5 µg/dL lower than the placebo group during the 6-month period, and 2.7 µg/dL lower during the 12-month period following start of therapy. However, no benefit was noted in treated patients at 3 years postenrollment on measures of cognition, neuropsychiatric function, or behavior.[315] Furthermore, small but statistically significant decrements in growth velocity were noted in the treatment group, which might reflect trace mineral depletion.[316] The study has been extended, and outcomes will be measured for 7 years postenrollment to ascertain any subtle changes in neurocognitive function that might emerge. Until the final results of this and similar studies are available, the optimal approach to chelation for these children is unknown, but there is no evidence to recommend it at this time. Potential indications for chelation treatment in this group were proposed and included BLLs at the higher end of the range (eg, 35–44 µg/dL), BLLs that remain the same or rise over several months after rigorous environmental controls are instituted, younger children (eg, <2 years old), evidence of biochemical toxicity (elevated EP, after iron supplementation if necessary), or any hint of subtle symptoms.[192] These indications may now require reevaluation in light of the preliminary TLC findings.

BLLs of 10–19 µg/dL are defined by CDC as representing excessive exposure to lead, but do not require chelation therapy. Close monitoring (for the 10–14-µg/dL range) and careful environmental investigation and interventions as necessary (particularly for the 15–19 µg/dL range) are appropriate and sufficient (Table 80–7).[5,52] The educational approaches outlined earlier (Table 80–9) should be included in the case management of all children with even modestly elevated lead levels.

Adult Therapy. The first principle in the treatment of adults with lead poisoning is that chelation therapy may not substitute for adherence to OSHA lead standards at the worksite and should never be given prophylactically.[83,148] In addition to the guidelines for decreasing lead exposure noted earlier, chelation therapy is indicated in adults with significant symptoms (encephalopathy, abdominal colic, severe arthralgias or myalgias) and evidence of target organ damage (neuropathy or nephropathy) and possibly in asymptomatic workers with markedly elevated BLLs and/or evidence of biochemical toxicity or increased chelatable lead.[228,233,249,264] Table 80–10 outlines chelation therapy regimens for adults. Recent reports support the use of succimer in adult patients with mild to moderate plumbism after environmental and occupational remedies were insituted.[161,228] Treatment of patients with tetraethyl lead toxicity is largely supportive, with sedation as necessary. If blood lead levels are significantly elevated, chelation as described above may be considered, but it has not been found clinically efficacious.[249,284]

An area of particular concern in the management of adult plumbism involves decisions regarding therapy during pregnancy. As noted previously, lead freely passes the placental barrier and accumulates in the fetus throughout gestation.[230] Chelation therapy during early pregnancy poses theoretical problems of teratogenicity, particularly that caused by enhanced fetal excretion of potentially vital trace elements (see also the relevant Antidotes in Depth sections). Symptomatic pregnant women with elevated BLLs certainly warrant chelation therapy. There are few published reports, however, from which to draw guidance as to the optimum approach. Three cases are described[8,216,285] in which CaNa$_2$EDTA (actually, "CaEDTA" in one case[216]) was administered in late (8th to 9th month) pregnancy without overt harm to the fetus, and a normal-appearing infant was born in each case. In two of these cases, it is reported that maternal BLLs declined from about 80 µg/dL to 26 µg/dL, while the newborn's BLL was 60 µg/dL and 79 µg/dL, respectively, suggesting poor efficacy for fetal chelation. However, it should be noted that the newborn's hemoglobin level was generally much higher than the mother's, and thus some of the maternal-neonatal difference in lead levels may simply reflect this difference in hemoglobin level and hence total blood lead content. More recently, two cases of prenatal chelation have been reported in abstract format, one also using CaNa$_2$EDTA and one using succimer.[187,188,208] Again, both newborns appeared normal and had higher BLLs at birth than did the mother. In general, there currently seems little support for routine chelation therapy in pregnant women who wouldn't otherwise warrant treatment based on their own symptoms or degree of elevated BLL. Postnatally, infant BLLs may decline over time without chelation, but this occurs very slowly.[243] In two of the neonates exposed to prenatal maternal chelation described above, who were then monitored for 2 weeks postpartum, the BLL remained stable or rose until chelation therapy was instituted.[216,285] In two additional cases of neonates whose mothers were not treated prepartum, BLLs also remained stable or rose for 17 days to 3 weeks.[107,275] Thus, postpartum chelation therapy may be warranted for neonates, depending on BLLs, as per the guidelines described above for older children.

SUMMARY

Lead is a ubiquitous element in the earth's crust that has long been used by humans for a variety of purposes. Metallic lead finds many uses for its waterproofing and electrical and radiation shielding properties. Lead compounds are used as paint pigments and find many applications in the manufacture of plastics, ceramics, glass, and explosives.

Lead poisoning, or plumbism, has an equally long history, dating back to antiquity. Today, lead poisoning is primarily an important environmental health problem for young children exposed to deteriorated lead paint, and as an occupational exposure for adult workers, although numerous other exotic exposures are continually reported.

Lead has toxic effects on multiple organs, involving especially the hematologic and neurologic systems in patients of all ages, and renal injury with hypertension in adults. This can result in a broad spectrum of clinical effects, ranging from vague constitutional symptoms without overt physical signs to an acute encephalopathy with potentially fatal cerebral edema and increased intracranial pressure. Several techniques have been used to estimate increases in body lead burden, but currently the measurement of whole-blood lead level (BLL) is favored.

The mainstays of treatment are removal from exposure and chelation therapy for those patients with symptoms or significantly elevated body lead burdens. Defining a group of asymptomatic patients that will benefit from chelation therapy has been difficult and controversial. Parenteral chelation with CaNa$_2$EDTA and BAL has been proven efficacious in lowering BLLs and reducing mortality and morbidity from severe lead poisoning. Recently, succimer, an oral chelator, has also had considerable clinical experience demonstrating efficacy in reducing BLLs in asymptomatic children.

REFERENCES

1. Agency for Toxic Substances and Disease Registry: The nature and extent of lead poisoning in children in the United States: A report to Congress. Atlanta, ATSDR, 1988.
2. Allcott JV III, Barnhart RA, Mooney LA: Acute lead poisoning in two users of illicit methamphetamine. JAMA 1987;258:510–511.
3. Aly MH, Kim HC, Renner SW, et al: Hemolytic anemia associated with lead poisoning from shotgun pellets and the response to succimer treatment. Am J Hematol 1993;44:280–283.
4. American Academy of Pediatrics, Committee on Environmental Health: Screening for elevated blood lead levels. Pediatrics 1998; 101:1072–1078.
5. American Academy of Pediatrics, Committee on Drugs: Treatment guidelines for lead exposure in children. Pediatrics 1995;96: 155–160.
6. American Academy of Pediatrics, Committee on Environmental Health: Lead poisoning: From screening to primary prevention. Pediatrics 1993;92:176–183.
7. Amitai Y, Graef JW, Brown MJ, et al: Hazards of "deleading" homes of children with lead poisoning. Am J Dis Child 1987;141: 758–760.
8. Angle CR, McIntire MS. Lead poisoning during pregnancy. Am J Dis Child 1964;108:436–439.
9. Angle CR: Childhood lead poisoning and its treatment. Annu Rev Pharmacol Toxicol 1993;32:409–434.
10. Appel BR, Kahlon JK, Ferguson J, et al: Potential lead exposures from crystal decanters. Am J Public Health 1992;82:1671–1673.
11. Assennato G, Paci C, Molinini R, et al: Sperm count suppression without endocrine dysfunction in lead-exposed men. Annu Rev Pharmacol Toxicol 1986;41:387–390.
12. Astrin KH, Bishop DF, Wetmur JG, et al: Delta-aminolevulinic acid dehydratase isoenzymes and lead toxicity. Ann N Y Acad Sci 1987; 514:23–29.
13. Audesirk G: Electrophysiology of lead intoxication: Effects on voltage-sensitive ion channels. Neurotoxicology 1993;14:137–147.
14. Baghurst P, McMichaelm A, Wigg N, et al: Environmental exposure to lead and children's intelligence at the age of 7 years. N Engl J Med 1992;327:1279–1284.
15. Baker EL Jr, Folland DS, Taylor TA, et al: Lead poisoning in children of lead workers: Home contamination with industrial dust. N Engl J Med 1977;296:260–261.
16. Batuman V: Lead nephropathy, gout and hypertension Am J Med Sci 1993;305:241–247.
17. Batuman V, Dreisbach A, Chun E, Naumoff M: Lead increases red cell sodium-lithium countertransport. Am J Kidney Dis 1989;14: 200–203.
18. Batuman V, Maesaka JK, Haddad B, et al: The role of lead in gout nephropathy. N Engl J Med 1981;304:520–523.
19. Bear MF, Cooper LN, Ebner E: A physiologic basis for a theory of synapse modification. Science 1987;237:42–48.
20. Beigel Y, Ostfeld I, Schoenfield N: A leading question. N Engl J Med 1998;339:827–830.
21. Bellinger D, Leviton A, Waternaux C, et al: Longitudinal analyses of prenatal and postnatal lead exposure and early cognitive development. N Engl J Med 1987;316:1037–1043.
22. Bellinger D, Sloman J, Leviton A, et al: Low-level lead exposure and children's cognitive function in the pre-school years. Pediatrics 1991;87:219–227.
23. Berlin CM, Banner W: Treatment of lead-exposed children [letter]. Pediatrics 1996;98:163.
24. Besunder JB, Anderson RL, Supeer DM: Short-term efficacy of oral dimercaptosuccinic acid in children with low to moderate lead intoxication. Pediatrics 1995;96:683–687.

25. Besunder JB, Sunder DM, Anderson RL: Comparison of dimercaptosuccinic acid and calcium disodium ethylenediaminetetraacetic acid versus dimercaptopropanol and ethylenediaminetetraacetic acid in children with lead poisoning. J Pediatr 1997;130:966–971.

26. Binder S, Matte TD, Kresnow M, et al: Lead testing of children and homes: Results of a national telephone survey. Public Health Rep 1996;111:342–346.

27. Binns HJ, LeBailly SA, Poncher J, et al: Is there lead in the suburbs? Risk assessment in Chicago suburban pediatric practices. Pediatrics 1994;93:164–171.

28. Blackfan KD: Lead poisoning in children with special reference to lead as a cause of convulsions. Am J Med Sci 1917;153:877–887.

29. Blickman JG, Wilkinson RF, Graef JW: The radiologic "lead band" revisited. Am J Radiol 1986;146:245–247.

30. Bloch P, Garavaglia G, Mitchell G, et al: Measurement of lead content of children's teeth in situ by x-ray fluorescence. Phys Med Biol 1976;20:56–63.

31. Bolanowska W, Piotrowski J, Garczynski H: Triethyl lead in the biologic material in cases of acute tetraethyl lead poisoning. Arch Toxicol 1967;22:278–282.

32. Bolger PM, Carrington CD, Capar SG, Adams MA: Reductions in dietary lead exposure in the United States. Chem Speciation Bioavailability 1991;3:3–36.

33. Bornschein RL, Succop PA, Krafft KM, et al: Exterior surface dust lead, interior house dust lead and childhood exposure in an urban environment. In: Hemphill D, ed: Trace Substances in Environmental Health. Columbia, MO, University of Missouri, 1986, pp. 322–332.

34. Bose A, Vashistha K, O'Loughlin BJ: Azarcon por empacho—Another cause of lead toxicity. Pediatrics 1983;72:106–108.

35. Brennan MJW, Cantrill RC: Delta-aminolevulinic acid is a potent agonist for GABA receptors. Nature 1979;280:514–515.

36. Brody DJ, Pirkle JL, Kramer RA, et al: Blood lead levels in the US population. Phase 1 of the Third National Health and Nutrition Examination Survey (NHANES III, 1988 to 1991). JAMA 1994;272:277–283.

37. Burns JM, Baghurst PA, Sawyer MG, et al: Lifetime low-level lead exposure to environmental lead and children's emotional and behavioral development at ages 11–13 years. The Port Pirie Cohort Study. Am J Epidemiol 1999;149:740–749.

38. Byers RK, Lord EE: Late effects of lead poisoning on mental development. Am J Dis Child 1943;66:471–483.

39. Caffey J. Lead poisoning associated with rickets: Report of a case with absence of lead lines in the skeleton. Am J Dis Child 1937;55:798–806.

40. Campbell C, Tobin R, Webb D, et al: Prevalence of lead screening and elevated lead levels in Philadelphia children [abstract]. Presented at the 127th Annual Meeting, American Public Health Association, Chicago, IL, Nov 7–11, 1999.

41. Campbell C, Osterhoudt KC: Prevention of childhood lead poisoning. Curr Opin Pediatr 2000;12:428–437.

42. Cardenas A, Roels H, Bernard AM, et al: Markers of early renal changes induced by industrial pollutants. II. Application to workers exposed to lead. Br J Ind Med 1993;50:28–36.

43. Centers for Disease Control and Prevention: Recommendations for blood lead screening of young children enrolled in Medicaid: Targeting a group at high risk. MMWR Morb Mort Wkly Rep 2000;49:1–13.

44. Centers for Disease Control and Prevention: Adult blood lead epidemiology and surveillance—United States, second and third quarters, 1998, and annual 1994–1997. MMWR Morb Mort Wkly Rep 1999;48:213–223.

45. Centers for Disease Control and Prevention: Blood lead levels—United States, 1991–1994. MMWR Morb Mort Wkly Rep 1997;46:141–146.

46. Centers for Disease Control and Prevention: Screening young children for lead poisoning: Guidance for state and local public health officials. US Dept of Health and Human Services, Public Health Service, Federal Register, Feb 21, 1997.

47. Centers for Disease Control and Prevention: Children with elevated blood lead levels attributed to home renovation and remodeling activities—New York, 1993–1994. MMWR Morb Mort Wkly Rep 1996;45:1120–1123.

48. Centers for Disease Control and Prevention: Lead poisoning associated with use of traditional ethnic remedies—California, 1991–1992. MMWR Morb Mort Wkly Rep 1993;42:521–524.

49. Centers for Disease Control and Prevention: Blood lead levels among children in high-risk areas—California, 1987–1990. MMWR Morb Mort Wkly Rep 1992;41:291–294.

50. Centers for Disease Control and Prevention: Elevated blood lead levels in adults—United States, second quarter, 1992. MMWR Morb Mort Wkly Rep 1992;41:715–716.

51. Centers for Disease Control and Prevention: Fatal pediatric poisoning from leaded paint—Wisconsin, 1990. MMWR Morb Mort Wkly Rep 1991;40:193–195.

52. Centers for Disease Control and Prevention: Prevention of lead poisoning in young children: A statement by the Centers for Disease Control. Atlanta, US Dept of Health and Human Services, Public Health Service, 1991.

53. Centers for Disease Control and Prevention: Strategic plan for elimination of childhood lead poisoning. US Dept of Health and Human Services, Public Health Service, 1991.

54. Centers for Disease Control and Prevention: Elevated blood lead levels associated with illicitly distilled alcohol—Alabama, 1990–1991. MMWR Morb Mort Wkly Rep 1992;41:294.

55. Charney E, Kessler B, Farfel M, Jackson D: Childhood lead poisoning: A controlled trial of the effect of dust-control measures on blood lead levels. N Engl J Med 1983;309:1089–1093.

56. Charney E, Sayre J, Coulter M: Increased lead absorption in innercity children: Where does it come from. Pediatrics 1980;65:226–231.

57. Cheng Y, Schwartz J, Vokonas PS, et al: Electrocardiographic conduction disturbances in association with low-level lead exposure (the Normative Aging Study). Am J Cardiol 1998;82:594–599.

58. Chia KS, Jeyaratnam J, Lee J, et al: Lead-induced nephropathy: Relationship between various biologic exposure indices and early markers of nephrotoxicity. Am J Ind Med 1995;27:883–895.

59. Chisolm JJ Jr: BAL, EDTA, DMSA, and DMPS in the treatment of lead poisoning in children. J Toxicol Clin Toxicol 1992;30:493–504.

60. Chisolm JJ Jr: Safety and efficacy of meso-2,3-dimercaptosuccinic acid (DMSA) in children with elevated blood lead concentrations. J Toxicol Clin Toxicol 2000;38:365–375.

61. Chisolm JJ Jr: Mobilization of lead by calcium disodium edetate: A reappraisal. Am J Dis Child 1987;141:1256–1257.

62. Chisolm JJ Jr: The use of chelating agents in the treatment of acute and chronic lead intoxication in childhood. J Pediatr 1968;73:1–38.

63. Chisolm JJ Jr, Barltrop D: Recognition and management of children with increased lead absorption. Arch Dis Child 1979;54:249–362.

64. Chisolm JJ Jr, Farfel MR: Environmental control and deleading. Pediatr Ann 1994;23:627–633.

65. Chisolm JJ Jr, Harrison HE: The treatment of acute lead encephalopathy in children. Pediatrics 1957;19:2–20.

66. Coffin R, Phillips JL, Staples WI, Spector S: Treatment of lead encephalopathy in children. J Pediatr 1966;69:198–206.

67. Cohen AR, Trotzky MS, Pincus D: Reassessment of the microcytic anemia of lead poisoning. Pediatrics 1981;67:904–906.

68. Cohen N, Modai D, Golik A, et al: An esoteric occupational hazard for lead poisoning. J Toxicol Clin Toxicol 1986;24:59–67.

69. Colorado Department of Health: Colorado Disease Bulletin, Vol XV, Issue 9, May 1, 1987.

70. Conrad ME, Umbrier JN, Moore EG, Rodning CR: Newly identified iron-binding protein in human duodenal mucosa. Blood 1992;79:244–247.

71. Cookman GR, Hemmens SE, Keane GJ, et al: Chronic low-level lead exposure precociously induces rat glial development in vitro and in vivo. Neurosci Lett 1988;86:33–37.

72. Corey-Slechta DA: Relationships between lead-induced learning impairments and changes in dopaminergic, cholinergic, and glutamatergic neurotransmitter system functions. Annu Rev Pharmacol Toxicol 1995;35:391–415.

73. Corey-Slechta DA, Weiss B: Efficacy of the chelating agent CaEDTA in reversing lead-induced changes in behavior. Neurotoxicology 1989;10:685–698.

74. Corey-Slechta DA, Weiss B, Cox C: Mobilization and redistribution of lead over the course of CaEDTA chelation therapy. J Pharmacol Exp Ther 1987;243:804–813.

75. Cremin JJ, Luck M, Laughlin N, Smith DR: Efficacy of succimer chelation for reducing brain lead in a primate model of human lead exposure. Toxicol Appl Pharmacol 1999;161:283–293.

76. Cullen MR, Robins JM, Eskenazi B: Adult inorganic lead intoxication: Presentation of 31 new cases and a review of the literature. Medicine (Baltimore) 1983;62:221–247.

77. Curran JP, Nunez JR: Lead poisoning during home renovation. N Y State J Med 1989;89:679–680.

78. Dart RC, Hurlbut KM, Maiorino RM, et al: Pharmacokinetics of meso-2,3-dimercaptosuccinic acid in patients with lead poisoning and in healthy adults. J Pediatr 1994;125:309–316.

79. Davoli CT, Serwint JR, Chisolm JJ Jr: Asymptomatic children with venous lead levels >100 µg/dL. Pediatrics 1996;98:965–968.

80. De la Burde B, Choate MS: Early asymptomatic lead exposure and development at school age. J Pediatr 1975;87:637–642.

81. De la Burde B, Choate MS: Does asymptomatic lead exposure in children have latent sequelae? J Pediatr 1972;81:1088–1096.

82. Deppisch LM, Centeno JA, Gemmel DJ, Torres NL: Andrew Jackson's exposure to mercury and lead: Poisoned president? JAMA 1999;282:569–571.

83. DeRoos FJ: Smelters and metal reclaimers. In: Greenberg MI, Hamilton R, Phillips S, eds: Occupational, Industrial and Environmental Toxicology. St. Louis, Mosby-Year Book, 1997, pp. 291–301.

84. Dey PM, Burger J, Gochfeld M, Reuhl KR. Developmental lead exposure disturbs expression of synaptic neural cell adhesion molecules in herring gull brains. Toxicology 2000;146:137–147.

85. Dickens C: The Uncommercial Traveler: A Collection of Short Stories. London, T. Nelson & Sons, 1861.

86. Dietrich KN, Berger OG, Succop PA: Lead exposure and the motor developmental status of urban six-year old children in the Cincinnati prospective study. Pediatrics 1993;91:301–307.

87. Dillman RO, Crumb CK, Lidsky MJ: Lead poisoning from a gunshot wound. Am J Med 1979;66:509–514.

88. Dolcourt JL, Finch C, Coleman GD, et al: Hazard of lead exposure in the home from recycled automobile storage batteries. Pediatrics 1981;68:225–229.

89. Durback LF, Wedin GP, Seidler DE: Management of lead foreign body ingestion. J Toxicol Clin Toxicol 1989;27:173–182.

90. Emmerson BT: Chronic lead nephropathy. Kidney Int 1973;4:1–5.

91. Environmental Protection Agency: Maximum contaminant level goals and national primary drinking water regulations for lead and copper. Fed Reg 1991;56:26469–26470.

92. Environmental Protection Agency: Strategy for reducing lead exposures: Report to Congress. Washington, DC, EPA, 1991.

93. Environmental Protection Agency: Evaluation of Potential Carcinogenicity of Lead and Lead Compounds. EPA/600/8–89/0454A. Office of Health and Environmental Assessment. Washington, DC, US Environmental Protection Agency, 1989.

94. Environmental Protection Agency: Supplement to the 1986 Air Quality Criteria for Lead. Addendum EPA/600/8–89/049A. Office of Health and Environmental Assessment. Washington, DC, US Environmental Protection Agency, 1989;1:A1–A67.

95. Erenberg G, Rinsler SS, Fish BG: Lead neuropathy and sickle cell disease. Pediatrics 1974;54:438–441.

96. Ernhardt CB, Landa B, Schell NB: Lead levels and intelligence [letter]. Pediatrics 1981;68:903–905.

97. Farfel MR, Chisolm JJ Jr: Health and environmental outcomes of traditional and modified practices for abatement of residential lead-based paint. Am J Pub Health 1990;80:1240–1245.

98. Farrell SE, Vandevander P, Schoffstall JM, Lee DC: Blood lead levels in emergency department patients with retained lead bullets and shrapnel. Acad Emerg Med 1999;6:208–212.

99. Fishbein A: Lead poisoning: I. Some clinical and toxicological observations on the effects of occupational lead exposure among firearms instructors. Isr J Med Sci 1992;28:560–572.

100. Fishbein A, Thornton J, Blumberg WE, et al: Health status of cable splicers with low-level exposure to lead: Results of a clinical survey. Am J Public Health 1980;70:697–700.

101. Flaherty EG: Risk of lead poisoning in abused and neglected children. Clin Pediatr 1995;34:128–132.

102. Franco G, Cottica D, Minoia C: Chewing electric wire coatings: An unusual source of lead poisoning. Am J Ind Med 1994;25:291–296.

103. Frankel M, Rogers P, Pursell R, et al: Severe lead intoxication in an infant from an imported kettle [abstract]. Vet Hum Toxicol 1992; 34:355.

104. Friedman JA, Weinberger HL: Six children with lead poisoning. Am J Dis Child 1990;144:1039–1044.

105. Garrod AB: A Treatise on Gout and Rheumatic Gout (Rheumatoid Arthritis), 3rd ed. London, Longmans, Green & Co., 1876.

106. Gennart JP, Bernard A, Lauwerys R: Assessment of thyroid, testis, kidney, and autonomic nervous system function in lead-exposed workers. Int Arch Occup Health 1992;64:49–58.

107. Ghafour SY, Khuffash FA, Ibrahim HS, Reavey PC: Congenital lead intoxication with seizures due to prenatal exposure. Clin Pediatr 1984;23:282–283.

108. Glotzer DE: Management of childhood lead poisoning: Strategies for chelation. Pediatr Ann 1994;23:606–615.

109. Goldman LR, Carra J: Childhood lead poisoning in 1994. JAMA 1994;272:315–316.

110. Goldman RH, Baker El, Hannan M, et al: Lead poisoning in automobile radiator mechanics. N Engl J Med 1987;317:214–218.

111. Goldstein GW: Neurologic concepts of lead poisoning in children. Pediatr Ann 1992;21:384–388.

112. Goldstein GW: Lead poisoning and brain cell function. Environ Health Perspect 1990;89:91–94.

113. Goldstein GW: Brain capillaries: A target for inorganic lead poisoning. Neurotoxicology 1984;5:167–175.

114. Gordon RA, Roberts G, Amin Z, et al: Aggressive approach in the treatment of acute lead encephalopathy with an extraordinarily high concentration of lead. Arch Pediatr Adolesc Med 1998;152: 1100–1104.

115. Goyer RA: Toxic effects of metals. In: Klaassen CD, ed: Casarett and Doull's Toxicolgy: The Basic Science of Poisons, 5th ed. New York, McGraw-Hill, 1996, pp. 691–709.

116. Goyer RA: Lead toxicity: Current concerns. Environ Health Perspect 1993;100:177–187.

117. Goyer RA: Lead toxicity: From overt to subclinical to subtle health effects. Environ Health Perspect 1990;86:177–181.

118. Goyer RA: Lead and the kidney. Curr Topics Pathol 1971;55: 147–176.

119. Goyer RA: Lead toxicity: A problem in environmental pathology. Am J Pathol 1971;64:167–182.

120. Goyer RA, Cherian MG, Jones MM, Reigart JR: Role of chelating agents for prevention, intervention and treatment of exposures to toxic metals. Environ Health Perspect 1995;103:1048–1052.

121. Goyer RA, Rhyne B: Pathologic effects of lead. Int Rev Exp Pathol 1973;12:1–77.

122. Graziano JH: Validity of lead-exposure markers in diagnosis and surveillance. Clin Chem 1994;40:1387–1390.

123. Graziano JH, LoIacono NJ, Meyer P: Dose-response study of oral 2,3-dimercaptosuccinic acid in children with elevated blood lead concentrations. J Pediatr 1988;113:751–757.

124. Graziano JH, Lolacono LJ, Moulton T, et al: Controlled study of meso-2,3-dimercaptosuccinic acid for the management of childhood lead intoxication. J Pediatr 1992;120:133–139.

125. Graziano JH, Slavkovic V, Factor-Litvak P, et al: Depressed serum erythropoietin in pregnant women with elevated blood lead. Arch Environ Health 1991;46:347–350.

126. Greenough FB: A case of probable lead poisoning, resulting fatally from a bullet lodged in the knee joint twelve years previously. Boston Med Surg J 1874;91:472.

127. Greensher J, Mofenson HC, Balakrishnan C, et al: Lead poisoning from ingestion of lead shot. Pediatrics 1974;54:641–643.

128. Grimsley EW, Adams-Mount L: Occupational lead intoxication: Report of four cases. South Med J 1994;87:689–691.

129. Grondona C: Lead revisited: A case study on lead exposed painters. AAOHN J 1993;41:33–38.

130. Hagelmeyer CD, Moorehead JC, Horenblas L, Bayer MJ: Fatal lead encephalopathy following foreign body ingestion: Case report. J Emerg Med 1988;6:397–400.

131. Hammer LD, Ludwig S, Henretig F: Increased lead absorption in children with accidental ingestions. Am J Emerg Med 1985;3: 301–304.

132. Hansen KS, Sharp FR: Gasoline sniffing, lead poisoning and myoclonus. JAMA 1978;240:1375–1376.

133. Harvey B: Should blood lead screening recommendations be revised? Pediatrics 1994;93:201–204.

134. Heard MJ, Chamberlain AC: Effect of minerals and food on uptake of lead from the gastrointestinal tract in humans. Hum Toxicol 1982; 1:411–415.

135. Hemings HC, Nairn AC, McGuinness TL, et al: Role of protein phosphorylation in neuronal signal transduction. FASEB J 1989;3: 1581–1592.

136. Henretig F, Osterhoudt K, Greenberg M, et al: Acute lead encephalopathy in a bullet salvager[abstract]. J Toxicol Clin Toxicol 1997;35:525.

137. Henretig FM, Shannon MW: Toxicologic emergencies. In: Fleisher GR, Ludwig S, eds: Textbook of Pediatric Emergency Medicine, 3rd ed. Baltimore, Williams & Wilkins, 1993, pp. 779–781.

138. Hu H, Milder FL, Burger DE: The use of K x-ray fluorescence for measuring lead burden in epidemiological studies: High and low lead burdens and measurement uncertainty. Environ Health Perspect 1991;94:107–110.

139. Huseman CA, Varma MM, Angle CR: Neuroendocrine effects of toxic and low blood lead levels in children. Pediatrics 1992;90: 186–189.

140. Huttenlocher PR, de Courten C: The development of synapses in striate cortex of man. Hum Neurobiol 1987;6:1–9.

141. Jiang X, Liang Y, Wang Y: Studies of lead exposure on reproductive system: A review of work in China. Biomed Environ Sci 1992;5: 266–275.

142. Jones TF, Moore WL, Craig AS, et al: Hidden threats: Lead poisoning from unusual sources. Pediatrics 1999;104:1223–1225.

143. Jugo S, Malikovic T, Kostial K: Influence of chelating agents on the gastrointestinal absorption of lead. Toxicol Appl Pharmacol 1975; 34:259–263.

144. Kakosy T, Hudak A, Naray M: Lead intoxication epidemic caused by ingestion of contaminated ground paprika. J Toxicol Clin Toxicol 1996;34:507–511.

145. Kapoor SC, Wielopolski L, Graziano JH, LoIacono NJ: Influence of 2,3-dimercaptosuccinic acid on gastrointestinal lead absorption and whole body lead retention. Toxicol Appl Pharmacol 1989;97: 525–529.

146. Kaufman A, Wiese W: Gasoline sniffing leading to increased lead absorption in children. Clin Pediatr 1978;17:475–477.

147. Kemper AR, Bordley WC, Downs SM. Cost-effectiveness analysis of lead poisoning screening strategies following the 1997 guidelines of the Centers for Disease Control and Prevention. Arch Pediatr Adolesc Med 1998;152:1202–1208.

148. Keogh JP: Lead. In: Sullivan JB Jr, Krieger GR, eds: Hazardous Materials Toxicology: Clinical Principles of Environmental Health. Baltimore, Williams & Wilkins, 1992, pp. 834–844.

149. Kimbrough RD, LeVois M, Webb DR: Management of children with slightly elevated lead levels. Pediatrics 1994;93:188–191.

150. Kocak R, Anarat A, Altinas G, et al: Lead poisoning from contaminated flour in a family of 11 members. Hum Toxicol 1989;8: 385–386.

151. Kopp SJ, Glonek T, Erlander M, et al: The influence of chronic low-level cadmium and/or lead feeding on myocardial contractility related to phosphorylation of cardiac myofibrillar proteins. Toxicol Appl Pharmacol 1980;54:48–56.

152. Korrick SA, Hunter DJ, Rotnitzky A, Speizer FE: Lead and hypertension in a sample of middle-aged women. Am J Public Health 1999;89:330–335.

153. Kosmider S, Petelenz T: Electrocardiographic changes in elderly patients with chronic lead poisoning. Pol Arch Med Wewn 1962;32: 437–442.

154. Kosnett MJ: Unanswered questions in metal chelation. J Toxicol Clin Toxicol 1992;30:529–547.

155. Lanphear BP, Howard C, Eberly S, et al: Primary prevention of childhood lead exposure: A randomized trial of dust control. Pediatrics 1999;103:772–777.

156. Landrigan PJ, Baker EL Jr, Himmelstein JS, et al: Exposure to lead from the Mystic River bridge: The dilemma of deleading. N Engl J Med 1982;306:673–676.

157. Lecos CW: Pretty poison: Lead and ceramic ware. FDA Consumer July/August 1987:6–9.

158. Levine F, Muenke M: VACTERL association with high prenatal lead exposure: Similarities to animal models of lead teratogenicity. Pediatrics 1991;87:390–392.

159. Liebelt EL, Shannon MW: Oral chelators for childhood lead poisoning. Pediatr Ann 1994;23:616–626.

160. Liebelt EL, Shannon M, Graef JW: Efficacy of oral meso-2,3 dimercaptosuccinic acid therapy for low-level childhood plumbism. J Pediatr 1994;1214:313–317.

161. Lifshitz M, Hashkanazi R, Phillip M: The effect of 2,3-dimercaptosuccinic acid in the treatment of lead poisoning in adults. Ann Med 1997;29:83–85.

162. Lilis R, Fischbein A, Eisinger J, et al: Prevalence of lead disease among secondary lead smelter workers and biologic indicators of lead exposure. Environ Res 1977;14:255–285.

163. Lin-Fu JS: Undue absorption of lead among children—A new look at an old problem. N Engl J Med 1972;286:702–710.

164. Lyons JD, Filston HC: Lead intoxication from a pellet entrapped in the appendix of a child: Treatment considerations. J Pediatr Surg 1994;29:1618–1620.

165. Mahaffey KR: Nutrition and lead: Strategies for public health. Environ Health Perspect 1995;103:191–196.

166. Mahaffey KR, Annest JL, Roberts J, Murphy RS: National estimates of blood lead levels: United States 1976–1980. N Engl J Med 1982; 307:573–579.

167. Major RH: A History of Medicine. Springfield, IL: Charles C Thomas, 1954.

168. Mantere P, Hanninen H, Hernberg S, Luukkonen R: A prospective follow-up study on psychological effects in workers exposed to low levels of lead. Scand J Work Environ Health 1984;10:43–50.

169. Marcus AH: Multicompartment kinetic modules for lead: Linear kinetics and variable absorption in humans without excessive lead exposures. Environ Res 1985;36:459–472.

170. Marcus SM: Treatment of lead-exposed children [letter]. Pediatrics 1996;98:161–162.

171. Marcus SM: Lead poisoning from industrial exposure. Occup Med 1978;1:1–4.

172. Marino PE, Franzblau A, Lilis R, et al: Acute lead poisoning in construction workers: The failure of current protective standards. Arch Environ Health 1989;44:140–145.

173. Marino PE, Landrigan PJ, Graef J, et al: A case report of lead paint poisoning during renovation of a Victorian farmhouse. Am J Public Health 1990;80:1183–1185.

174. Markovac J, Goldstein GW: Picomolar concentrations of lead stimulate brain protein kinase C. Nature 1988;334:71–73.

175. Markowitz ME, Bijur PE, Ruff H, Rosen JF: Effects of calcium disodium versenate (CaNa$_2$EDTA) chelation in moderate childhood lead poisoning. Pediatrics 1993;92:265–271.

176. Markowitz ME, Rosen JF: Assessment of lead stores in children: Validation of an 8-hour CaNa$_2$EDTA provocation test. J Pediatr 1984;104:337–341.

177. Markowitz ME, Weinberger HL: Immobilization-related lead toxicity in previously lead-poisoned children. Pediatrics 1990;86: 455–457.

178. Markowitz SB, Nunez CM, Klitzman S, et al: Lead poisoning due to hai ge fen: The porphyrin content of individual erythrocytes. JAMA 1994;271:932–934.

179. McCallum RI, Sanderson JT, Richards AE: The lead hazard in ship-breaking: The prevalence of anemia in burners. Ann Occup Hyg 1968;11:101–113.

180. McCord CP: Lead and lead poisoning in early America. Benjamin Franklin and lead poisoning. Industr Med Surg 1953;22:394–399.

181. McElvaine MD, DeUngria EG, Matte TD, et al: Prevalence of radiographic evidence of paint chip ingestion among children with moderate to severe lead poisoning, St. Louis, Misssouri, 1989 through 1990. Pediatrics 1992;89:740–742.

182. McKinney PE: Acute elevation of blood lead levels within hours of ingestion of large quantities of lead shot. J Toxicol Clin Toxicol 2000;38:435–440.

183. Meggs WJ, Gerr F, Aly M, et al: The treatment of lead poisoning from gunshot wounds with succimer (DMSA). J Toxicol Clin Toxicol 1994;32:377–385.

184. Miller MB, Curry S, Kunkel D, et al: Pool cue chalk: A source of environmental lead. Pediatrics 1996;97:916–917.

185. Miller SA: Lead in calcium supplements. JAMA 1987;257:1810.

186. Minnema DJ, Michelson IA, Cooper GP: Calcium efflux and neurotransmitter release from rat hippocampal synaptosomes exposed to lead. Toxicol Appl Pharmacol 1988;92:351–357.

187. Mirkin D, Sudakin D, Parker S, et al: Plumbism in pregnancy treated with DMSA [abstract]. J Toxicol Clin Toxicol 2000;38:547.

188. Mirkin D, Sudakin D, Parker S, et al: Lead chelation in the neonate [abstract]. J Toxicol Clin Toxicol 2000;38:548.

189. Moore MR, Meredith P: The carcinogenicity of lead. Arch Toxicol 1979;42:87–94.

190. Moore MR, Meredith PA, Watson WS, et al: The percutaneous absorption of lead-203 in humans from cosmetic preparations containing lead acetate, as assessed by whole-body counting and other techniques. Food Cosmet Toxicol 1980;18:399–405.

191. Mortensen ME: Succimer chelation: What is known? J Pediatr 1994;125:233–234.

192. Mortensen ME, Walson PD: Chelation therapy for childhood lead poisoning—The changing scene in the 1990s. Clin Pediatr 1993;32:284–291.

193. Mushak P, Davis JM, Crocewtti AF, Grant LD: Pre-natal and post-natal effects of low-level lead exposure: Integrated summary of a report to the US Congress on childhood lead poisoning. Environ Res 1989;50:11–36.

194. National Institute for Occupational Safety and Health: Recommendations for control of occupational safety and health hazards—Foundries. Washington, DC, US Government Printing Office, Sept 1985.

195. Needleman HL: Childhood lead poisoning: The promise and abandonment of primary prevention. Am J Public Health 1998;88:1871–1877.

196. Needleman HL: The persistent threat of lead: Medical and sociological issues. Curr Probl Pediatr 1988;18:702–744.

197. Needleman HL, Gunnoe C, Leviton A, et al: Deficits in psychological and classroom performance of children with elevated dentine lead levels. N Engl J Med 1979;300:689–695.

198. Needleman HL, Riess JA, Tobin MJ, et al: Bone lead levels and delinquent behavior. JAMA 1996;275:363–369.

199. Needleman HL, Shapiro IM: Dentine lead levels in asymptomatic Philadelphia school children: Subclinical exposure in high and low risk groups. Environ Health Perspect 1974;7:27–31.

200. Needleman HL, Schell A, Bellinger D, et al: The long-term effects of exposure to low doses of lead in childhood: An 11-year follow-up report. N Engl J Med 1990;322:83–88.

201. Nieburg PI, Weiner LS, Oski BF, Oski FA: Red blood cell-aminolevulinic acid dehydratase activity. Am J Dis Child 1974;127:348–350.

202. Nordin JD, Rolnick SJ, Griffen JM: Prevalence of excess lead absorption and associated risk factors in children enrolled in a midwestern health maintenance organization. Pediatrics 1994;93:172–177.

203. Norman EH, Hertz-Piccioto I, Salmen DA, Ward TH: Childhood lead poisoning and vinyl miniblind exposure. Arch Pediatr Adolesc Med 1997;151:1033–1037.

204. Nortier JWR, Sangster B, Van Kestern RG: Acute lead poisoning with hemolysis and liver toxicity after ingestion of red lead. Vet Hum Toxicol 1980;22:145–147.

205. Norton RL, Weinstein L, Rafalski T, et al: Acute intravenous lead poisoning in a drug abuser: Associated complications of hepatitis, pancreatitis, hemolysis and renal failure [abstract]. Vet Hum Toxicol 1989;31:340.

206. Nriagu JO: Saturnine gout among Roman aristocrats. N Engl J Med 1983;308:660–663.

207. Oliver P: A lecture on lead poisoning and the race. Br Med J 1911;1:1096–1098.

208. Olmedo RE, Rella JG, Hoffman RS, Nelson L: Lead poisoning in late pregnancy due to maternal pica [abstract]. J Toxicol Clin Toxicol 1999;37:626.

209. Oski FA, Perkins KC: Elevated blood lead in a six-month old breast-fed infant: The role of newsprint logs. Pediatrics 1976;57:426–427.

210. Onalaja AO, Claudio L: Genetic susceptibility to lead poisoning. Environ Health Perspect 2000;108(Suppl 1):23–28.

211. Otto DA, Fox DA: Auditory and visual dysfunction following lead exposure. Neurotoxicology 1993;14:191–207.

212. Paglia DE, Valentine WN, Dahlgner JG: Effects of low level lead exposure on pyrimidine-5′-nucleotidase and other erythrocyte enzymes. J Clin Invest 1976;56:1164–1169.

213. Parras F, Patier JL, Ezpeleta C: Lead-contaminated heroin as a source of inorganic lead intoxication [letter]. N Engl J Med 1987;316:755.

214. Patterson CC: Contaminated and natural lead environments of man. Arch Environ Health 1965;11:344–348.

215. Pearce WG: More on retinal stippling [letter]. N Engl J Med 1964;270:533–534.

216. Pearl M, Boxt LM: Radiographic findings in congenital lead poisoning. Radiology 1980;136:83–84.

217. Perino J, Ernhardt CB: The relation of subclinical lead levels to cognitive and sensorimotor impairment in black preschoolers. J Learn Disabil 1974;7:616–620.

218. Petit TL, LeBoutillier JC: Effects of lead exposure during development on neocortical dendritic and synaptic structure. Exp Neurol 1979;64:482–492.

219. Philadelphia Department of Public Health, Childhood Lead Poisoning Prevention Program: Venous lead levels. Quarterly report, April 1, 1999 to June 30, 1999.

220. Philip AT, Gerson B: Lead poisoning—Part II: Effects and assay. Clin Lab Med 1994;14:651–670.

221. Piomelli S: Childhood lead poisoning in the 90s. Pediatrics 1994;93:508–510.

222. Piomelli S: A micromethod for free erythrocyte protoporphyrins: FEP test. J Lab Clin Med 1973;81:932–940.

223. Piomelli S, Corash L, Corash MB, et al: Blood lead concentrations in a remote Himalayan population. Science 1980;210:1135–1137.

224. Piomelli S, Rosen JF, Chisolm JJ Jr, Graef JW: Management of childhood lead poisoning. J Pediatr 1984;105:523–532.

225. Pirkle JL, Brody DJ, Gunter EW, et al: The decline in blood lead levels in the United States. The National Health and Nutrition Examination Surveys (NHANES). JAMA 1994;272:284–291.

226. Pirkle JL, Schwartz J, Landis JR, Harlan WR: The relationship between blood lead levels and blood pressure and its cardiovascular risk implications. Am J Epidemiol 1985;121:246–258.

227. Pocock SJ, Smith M, Baghurst P: Environmental lead and children's intelligence: A systematic review of the epidemiological evidence. Br Med J 1994;309:1189–1197.

228. Porru S, Alessio L: The use of chelating agents in occupational lead poisoning. Occup Med 1996;46:41–48.

229. Raasch FO, Rosenberg JH, Abraham JL: Lead poisoning from hair spray ingestion. Am J Forensic Med Pathol 1983;4:159–164.

230. Rabinowitz MB, Needleman HL: Temporal trends in the lead concentrations of umbilical cord blood. Science 1982;216:1429–1431.

231. Rabinowitz MB, Wetherill GW, Kopple JD: Kinetic analysis of lead metabolism in healthy humans. J Clin Invest 1976;58:260–270.

232. Regan CM: Neural cell adhesion molecules, neuronal development and lead toxicity. Neurotoxicology 1993;14:69–74.

233. Rempel D: The lead-exposed worker. JAMA 1989;262:532–534.

234. Restek-Samarzija N, Samarzija M, Momcilovic B: Ventricular arrhythmia in acute lead poisoning: A case report [abstract]. Presented at the EAPCCT XVI International Congress, Vienna, Austria, April, 1994.

235. Rhoads GG, Ettinger AS, Weisel CP, et al: The effect of dust lead control on blood lead in toddlers: A randomized trial. Pediatrics 1999;103:551–555.

236. Rhoads GG, Rogan WJ: Treatment of lead-exposed children [letter]. Pediatrics 1996;98:162–163.

237. Rodamilans M, Martinez-Osaba MJ, To-Figueras J, et al: Lead toxicity on endocrine testicular function in an occupationally exposed population. Hum Toxicol 1988;7:125–128.

238. Romeo R, Aprea C, Boccalon P, et al: Serum erythropoietin and blood lead concentrations. Int Arch Occup Environ Health 1996;69:73–75.

239. Rossouw J, Offermeier J, von Rooyen JM: Apparent central neurotransmitter receptor changes induced by low-level lead exposure during different developmental phases in the rat. Toxicol Appl Pharmacol 1987;91:132–139.

240. Royce SE, Needleman HL: Case Studies in Environmental Medicine. Lead Toxicity. Atlanta, Agency for Toxic Substances and Disease Registry, 1992.

241. Ruff H, Bijur PE, Markowitz M, et al: Declining blood lead levels and cognitive changes in moderately lead-poisoned children. JAMA 1993;269:1641–1646.

242. Rummo JH, Routh DK, Rummo NJ, Brown JF: Behavioral and neurological effects of symptomatic and asymptomatic lead exposure in children. Arch Environ Health 1979;34:120–124.

243. Ryu JE, Ziegler EE, Fomon SJ: Maternal lead exposure and blood lead concentration in infancy. J Pediatr 1978;93:476–478.

244. Saenger P, Rosen JF, Markowitz M: Diagnostic significance of edetate disodium calcium testing in children with increased lead absorption. Am J Dis Child 1983;136:312–315.

245. Sandstead HH, Orth DN, Abe K, et al: Lead intoxication: Effect on pituitary and adrenal function in man. Clin Res 1970;18:76.

246. Sandstead HH, Stant EG, Brill AB, et al: Lead intoxication and the thyroid. Arch Intern Med 1969;123:632–635.

247. Sargent JD: The role of nutrition in the prevention of lead poisoning in children. Pediatr Ann 1994;23:636–642.

248. Saryan LA: Surreptitious lead exposure from an Asian Indian medication. J Anal Toxicol 1991;15:336–338.

249. Saryan LA, Zenz C: Lead and its compounds. In: Zenz C, Dickerson OB, Horvath EP Jr, eds: Occupational Medicine, 3rd ed. St. Louis, Mosby, 1994, pp. 506–541.

250. Sayre JW, Charney E, Vostal J, Pless IB: House and hand dust as a potential source of childhood lead exposure. Am J Dis Child 1974;127:167–170.

251. Schaeffer SJ, Campbell JR: The new CDC and AAP lead poisoning recommendations: Consensus versus controversy. Pediatr Ann 1994;23:592–599.

252. Schlenker TL, Fritz CJ, Mark D, et al: Screening for pediatric lead poisoning: Comparability of simultaneously drawn capillary and venous blood samples. JAMA 1994;271:1346–1348.

253. Schoen EJ: Childhood lead poisoning: Definitions and priorities. Pediatrics 1993;91:504–505.

254. Schultz B, Pawel D, Murphy A: A retrospective examination of in-home educational visits to reduce childhood lead levels. Environ Res 1999;80:364–368.

255. Schwartz J, Angle C, Pitcher H: Relationship between childhood blood lead levels and stature. Pediatrics 1986;77:281–288.

256. Schwartz J, Otto D: Blood lead, hearing thresholds, and neurobehavioral development in children and youth. Arch Environ Health 1987;42:153–164.

257. Selander S, Cramer K: Interrelationships between lead in blood, lead in urine and ALA in urine during lead work. Br J Ind Med 1970;27:28–39.

258. Selbst SM, Henretig F, Fee MA, et al: Lead poisoning in a child with a gunshot wound. Pediatrics 1986;77:413–416.

259. Selbst SM, Henretig FM, Pierce J: Lead encephalopathy in a child with sickle cell disease. Clin Pediatr 1985;24:280–285.

260. Selbst SM, Sokas RK, Henretig FM, et al: The effect of blood lead on blood pressure in children. J Environ Pathol Toxicol Oncol 1993;12:213–218.

261. Sensirivatana R, Supachadhiwong O, Phancharoen S, Mitrakul C: Neonatal lead poisoning: An unusual clinical manifestation. Clin Pediatr 1983;22:582–584.

262. Seppalainen AM, Hernberg S: Subclinical lead neuropathy. Am J Ind Med 1989;1:413–420.

263. Settle DM, Patterson CC: Lead in albacore: Guide to lead pollution in Americans. Science 1980;207:1167–1176.

264. Seward JP: Occupational lead exposure and management. West J Med 1996;165:222–224.

265. Shannon M: Lead poisoning in adolescents who are competitive marksmen. N Engl J Med 1999;341:852.

266. Shannon MW, Graef JW: Lead intoxication in infancy. Pediatrics 1992;89:87–90.

267. Shannon MW, Graef J, Lovejoy FH Jr: Efficacy and toxicity of D-penicillamine in low-level lead poisoning. J Pediatr 1988;112:799–804.

268. Shannon MW, Townsend MK: Adverse effects of reduced-dose D-penicillamine in children with mild-to-moderate lead poisoning. Ann Pharmacother 2000;34:15–18.

269. Shen X, Rosen JF, Guo D, Wu S: Childhood lead poisoning in China. Sci Total Environ 1996;181:101–109.

270. Sidman RL, Rakie P: Neuronal migration, with special reference to developing human brain. Brain Res 1973;62:1–35.

271. Silbergeld EK, Scwartz J, Mahaffey K: Lead and osteoporosis: Mobilization of lead from bone in post-menopausal women. Environ Res 1988;47:79–94.

272. Silver W, Rodriguez-Torres R: Electrocardiographic studies in children with lead poisoning. Pediatrics 1968;41:1124–1127.

273. Simon JA, Hudes ES: Relationship of ascorbic acid to blood lead levels. JAMA 1999;281:2289–2293.

274. Simons TJB: Cellular interactions between lead and calcium. Br Med Bull 1986;42:431–434.

275. Singh N, Donovan CM, Hanshaw JB: Neonatal lead intoxication in a prenatally exposed infant. J Pediatr 1978;93:1019–1021.

276. Smith DR, Calacsan C, Woolard D, et al: Succimer and the urinary excretion of essential elements in a primate model of childhood lead exposure. Toxicol Sci 2000;54:473–480.

277. Sonkin N: Stippling of the retina—A new physical sign in the early diagnosis of lead poisoning. N Engl J Med 1963;269:779–780.

278. Staes C, Matte T, Staeling N, et al: Lead poisoning deaths in the United States, 1979–1988 [letter]. JAMA 1995;273:847–848.

279. Stanton NV, Jones R: Evaluation of filter paper blood lead methods: Results of a pilot proficiency testing program. Clin Chem 1999; 45:2229–2235.

280. Stowe HD, Goyer RA: The reproductive ability and progeny of F_1 lead-toxic rats. Fertil Steril 1971;22:755–760.

281. Stromberg BV: Symptomatic lead toxicity secondary to retained shotgun pellets: Case report. J Trauma 1990;30:356–357.

282. Suarez CR, Black LE 3d, Hurley RM: Elevated lead levels in a patient with sickle cell disease and inappropriate secretion of antidiuretic hormone. Pediatr Emerg Care 1992;8:88–90.

283. Taubman B, Wiley C, Henretig F: Prevalence of elevated blood lead levels in a suburban middle class private practice. Arch Pediatr Adol Med 1994;148:757–760.

284. Tenenbein M: Leaded gasoline abuse: The role of tetraethyl lead. Hum Exp Toxicol 1997;16:217–222.

285. Tinapu AE, Amin JS, Casalino MB, Yuceoglu AM: Congenital lead intoxication. J Pediatr 1979;94:765–767.

286. Toews AD, Kolber A, Hayward J, et al: Experimental lead encephalopathy in the suckling rat: Concentration of lead in cellular fractions enriched in brain capillaries. Brain Res 1978;147:131–138.

287. Tong S, Baghurst PA, Sawyer MG, et al: Declining blood lead levels and changes in cognitive function during childhood: The Port Piric Cohort Study. JAMA 1998;280:1915–1919.

288. Treatment of Lead-Exposed Children (TLC) Trial Group: Safety and efficacy of succimer in toddlers with blood lead levels of 20–44 µg/dL. Pediatr Res 2000;48:593–599.

289. Turner AJ: Lead poisoning among Queensland children. Aust Med Gazette 1897;16:475–479.

290. Tyroler HA: Epidemiology of hypertension as a public health problem: An overview as background for evaluation of blood lead-blood pressure relationship [symposium]. Environ Health Perspect 1988; 78:3–8.

291. US Department of Housing and Urban Development: A comprehensive and workable plan for the abatement of lead-based paint in privately owned housing. Report to Congress. Washington, DC, Housing and Urban Development, 1990.

292. US Department of Housing and Urban Development: Lead-based paint: Interim guidelines for hazard identification and abatement in public and Indian housing. Fed Reg 1990;55:14556–14614.

293. US Department of the Interior: Minerals Yearbook for 1990, Vol 1. Washington, DC, Government Printing Office, 1991.

294. US Department of Labor, Occupational Safety and Health Administration: Lead exposure in construction—Interim final rule. 29 CFR part 1926.62. Fed Reg 5/4/93.

295. US Department of Labor, Occupational Safety and Health Administration: Lead standard, 20 CFR 1910.1025 (revised July 1, 1990). Washington, DC, US Government Printing Office, 1990.

296. US Department of Labor, Occupational Safety and Health Administration: Occupational health and safety standard: Occupational exposure to lead (29 CFR 1910.1025). Fed Reg 1978;42:52952–53014.

297. Vance MV, Curry SC, Bradley JM, et al: Acute lead poisoning in nursing home and psychiatric patients from the ingestion of lead-based ceramic glazes. Arch Intern Med 1990;150:2085–2092.

298. Vander AJ: Chronic effects of lead on renin-angiotensin system. Environ Health Perspect 1988;78:77–83.

299. Wade JF, Burnum JF: Treatment of acute and chronic lead poisoning with disodium calcium versenate. Ann Intern Med 1955;42:251–259.

300. Waldron HA: Lead poisoning in the ancient world. Med Hist 1973;17:391–399.

301. Wedeen RP: Poison in the Pot: The Legacy of Lead. Carbondale, IL, Southern Illinois University Press, 1984.

302. Wedeen RP, Ty A, Udasin I, et al: Clinical application of in vivo tibial K-XRF for monitoring lead stores. Arch Environ Health 1995; 50:355–361.

303. Weinberger HL, Post EM, Schneider T, et al: An analysis of 248 initial mobilization tests performed on an ambulatory basis. Am J Dis Child 1987;141:1266–1270.

304. Weitzman M, Aschengrau A, Bellinger D, et al: Lead-contaminated soil abatement and urban children's blood lead levels. JAMA 1993; 269:1647–1654.

305. Whitfield CL, Ch'ien LT, Whitehead JD: Lead encephalopathy in adults. Am J Med 1972;52:289–297.

306. Wiley JF II, Bell LM, Rosenblum LS, et al: Lead poisoning: Low rates of screening and high prevalence among children seen in inner-city emergency departments. J Pediatr 1995;126:392–395.

307. Wiley J, Henretig F, Foster R: Status epilepticus and severe neurologic impairment from lead encephalopathy, November, 1994 [abstract]. J Toxicol Clin Toxicol 1995;33:529–530.

308. Wiley JF II, Henretig FM, Selbst SM: Blood lead levels in children with foreign bodies. Pediatrics 1992;89:593–596.

309. Winneke G, Brockhaus A, Ewers U, et al: Results from the European multicenter study on lead neurotoxicity in children: Implications for risk assessment. Neurotoxicol Teratol 1990;12:553–559.

310. Wright RO, Shannon MW, Wright RJ, Hu H: Association between iron deficiency and low-level lead poisoning in an urban primary care clinic. Am J Public Health 1999;89:1049–1053.

311. Woodbury WD: Lead. In: Minerals Yearbook, 1987. Washington, DC, Bureau of Mines, US Department of Commerce, 1987, pp. 541–567.

312. Woolf DA, Riach ICF, Deerwesh A, et al: Lead lines in young infants with acute lead encephalopathy: A reliable diagnostic test. J Trop Pediatr 1990;36:90–93.

313. Yiin LM, Rhoads GG, Lioy PJ: Seasonal influences on childhood lead exposure. Environ Health Perspec 2000;108:177–182.

314. Ziegler EE, Edwards BB, Jensen RL, et al: Absorption and retention of lead by infants. Pediatr Res 1978;12:29–34.

315. Rogan W, Dietrich K, Ware J, Dockery D, et al, for the Treatment of Lead-Exposed Children (TLC) Trial Group: The effect of chelation therapy with succimer on neuropsychological development in children exposed to lead. N Engl J Med 2001;344:1421–1426.

ANTIDOTES IN DEPTH

SUCCIMER

Mary Ann Howland

Succimer
(2,3-dimercaptosuccinic acid)

DMPS
(2,3-dimercapto-1-propanesulfonic acid)

Succimer (meso-2,3-dimercaptosuccinic acid, succimer) is an orally active metal chelator that is FDA approved for the treatment of lead poisoning in children with blood lead levels above 45 μg/dL. Succimer is also being used to treat lead-poisoned adults, children with blood lead levels less than 45 μg/dL, and patients poisoned with arsenic and organic and inorganic mercury. Succimer has many advantages over dimercaprol and edetate calcium disodium (CaNa$_2$EDTA), the two other agents used for similar clinical problems. These advantages include oral administration, limited effects on trace metals such as zinc, enhanced patient tolerance, limited toxicity, the ability to coadminister iron, if needed, and the lack of a contraindication in glucose-6-phosphate dehydrogenase (G6PD)-deficient individuals.[24] Additionally, in contrast to CaNa$_2$EDTA, succimer does not redistribute lead to the brain of poisoned animals.[9,26] The role of succimer alone and in conjunction with other chelators to treat lead encephalopathy continues to be defined.

HISTORY

Succimer was initially synthesized in 1949 in England.[66] In 1954, antimony-a,a′-dimercapto-potassium succinate (TWSb) was developed to treat schistosomiasis.[38] TWSb is antimony bound to the potassium salt of succimer in a 2:3 ratio, forming a water-soluble drug with 50 times less toxicity than the previously used antimony compound, tartar emetic. Several years later, a group from Shanghai demonstrated the ability of the sodium salt of succimer to increase the LD$_{50}$ of tartar emetic 16-fold in mice.[97] An early review of the Chinese experience with IV succimer in the treatment of occupational lead and mercury poisoning suggested efficacy similar to IV CaNa$_2$EDTA in increasing urinary lead and to IM DMPS (racemic-2,3-dimercapto-1-propanesulfonic acid, unithiol) for mercury with little observed toxicity.[95] This experience, subsequent widespread use in Asia[70,73,83,95,96,99] and Europe,[16,30,36,39,58,91] and the realization that succimer could be used orally[3,45] led the way for US-based animal experiments, human trials, and FDA approval in 1991 for the treatment of lead-poisoned children.

CHEMISTRY

Succimer is a white crystalline powder with a molecular weight of 182 daltons and a characteristic sulfur odor and taste. Succimer is the meso form of 2,3-dimercaptosuccinic acid; the racemic form is being investigated.[33] Because it contains four ionizable hydrogen ions, succimer has four different pK$_a$s—2.31, 3.69, 9.68, and 11.14—with the dissociation of the two lower values representing the carboxyl groups and the two higher values the sulfur groups.[4] Lead and cadmium bind to the adjoining sulfur and oxygen atoms, while arsenic and mercury bind to the two sulfur moieties forming pH-dependent water-soluble complexes[79] (see Fig. 80–9). Succimer is highly protein-bound to albumin through a disulfide bond. Subhuman primate studies of IV and oral[20] C-succimer indicate that following an IV dose, radiolabel is eliminated almost exclusively via the kidney, with only trace amounts (<1%) excreted via feces or expired air.[66] Following the administration of a single oral dose of 10 mg/kg, succimer is rapidly and extensively metabolized.[61] Approximately 20% of the administered dose is recovered in the urine, presumably reflecting the quantity of drug absorbed from the gut. Eighty-nine percent of the total drug eliminated in the urine is altered and in the form of disulfides of L-cysteine. The majority of the altered succimer is in the form of a mixed disulfide with two L-cysteine residues per succimer molecule and a small amount containing one L-cysteine residue per succimer molecule. The remaining 11% is excreted as unaltered free succimer.[61] Maximal excretion of succimer occurs in urine specimens collected between 2 and 4 hours after administration. Surprisingly, the blood only contains albumin-bound succimer and no evidence of the altered disulfide moieties.

LEAD

In addition to precise analysis of metal elimination kinetics, measures of clinical outcome are essential for an understanding of the utility of this agent. The treatment of lead-exposed children (TLC) trial is a step in that direction.[93] The TLC trial is a randomized, multicenter, double-blind, placebo-controlled, ongoing study to examine the effects of succimer on cognitive development, behavior, stature, and blood pressure in children 1–3 years old with blood lead levels between 20 and 44 μg/dL.

In the meantime, several groups, including the environmental toxicology group from the University of California, are studying the efficacy of succimer in reducing blood, brain, and tissue lead by using rat and nonhuman primate models of childhood and adult lead poisoning.[84,85,87] Monkeys most closely resemble humans in their lead-associated toxicity but their use is costly.[72] The rat model is economical but of limited use because of the species differences with regard to lead and succimer metabolism and efficacy. In addition, a 21-day succimer-chelation treatment period in the rat model extrapolates to a much longer time frame in humans. The primate experiments are exciting, but one substantial criticism is the lack of comparison groups with regard to dimercaprol and CaNa$_2$EDTA treatment. It is notable that the animal evidence sug-

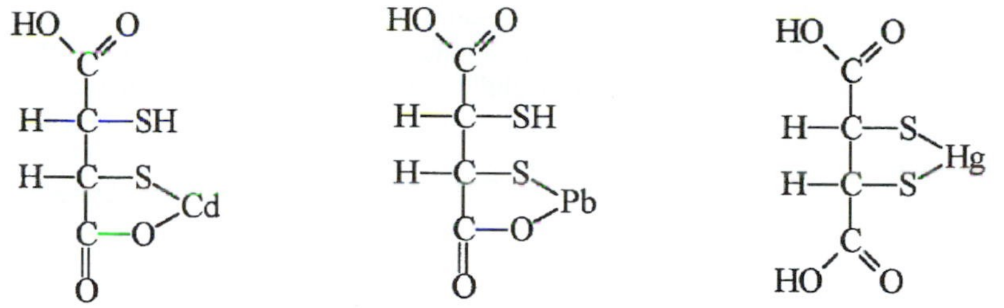

Figure 80–9. The chelation of cadmium, lead, and mercury with succimer (DMSA).

gests that isolated blood lead levels do not accurately reflect brain levels. If this finding is also true in humans, the importance and ability to interpret blood lead levels will be significantly altered. It is hoped that future animal studies will assess the rebound phenomenon and compare followup brain and blood lead levels several weeks and months following cessation of lead exposure with and without succimer chelation therapy.

The validity of using blood lead levels as a marker of brain lead was studied in adult rhesus monkeys that were administered lead orally for 5 weeks to achieve a target blood lead level of 35–40 µg/dL.[28] Five days after lead exposure ceased, succimer chelation in the currently approved dosage regimen was initiated. Two IV doses of radioactive lead tracer were administered prior to succimer chelation to study the kinetics of recent as compared to chronic lead uptake and distribution. Four areas of the brain, as well as blood and bone, were assayed for lead. Merely stopping further lead exposure significantly reduced both blood and brain lead levels, 63% and 34%, respectively, as compared with pretreatment levels, and was not statistically different than halting exposure followed by succimer treatment. However, when an integrated area-under-the-curve (AUC) blood analysis over the 19-day succimer treatment course was used instead of a single blood lead level, the differences between succimer and control were statistically significant. It is unclear how clinically significant these differences are. Succimer showed the biggest drop in blood lead levels over the first 5 days, while a similar endpoint was gradually achieved in the control. Both the lead from recent exposure (radioactive tracer lead) and chronic exposure declined to the same extent independent of treatment with succimer. A better correlation existed between brain prefrontal cortex lead levels and an integrated blood lead analysis than with a single blood lead measurement. This study clearly demonstrates the importance and efficacy of eliminating all exposure to lead.

Similarly, a study in neonatal rats demonstrates that going from 7 to 21 days of succimer chelation decreased brain lead levels without a corresponding decrease in blood lead levels.[84] The authors propose that a slow rate of egress of brain lead to the blood is responsible for the demonstrable benefit of prolonging therapy from 7 to 21 days. In this study, succimer decreased blood lead by about 50% when compared to the vehicle as control and this difference persisted for the 21 days of treatment. Succimer decreased brain lead 38% at 7 days and 68% at 21 days. Previous animal studies have demonstrated succimer's ability to enhance urinary lead elimination [37,45,87] and to reduce blood,[14,26,34,35,50,76,85,87,88,90] brain,[14,26,76,89,90] liver,[87] and kidney lead levels[14,26,35,50,76,90] while reducing[14,50,76,90] or showing no effect on bone lead levels.[26,87] One study suggested preferential effects of succimer in male mice.[88] These studies differ in the amounts and duration of lead administration prior to chelation as well as in route, dose, and duration of chelation. It is noteworthy that several months following a course

of succimer chelation, tissue lead levels were similar to pretreatment values, indicating that the short-term effects were not persistent.[26] Given the limited absolute amount of lead that is actually eliminated by chelation in comparison to the total body burden, particularly bone, these transient effects are not surprising.

Under a variety of experimental conditions in animals, succimer prevents the deleterious effect of lead on heme synthesis,[14,45,76] blood pressure,[54] and behavior.[88]

Published studies of succimer in children and adults with chronic lead poisoning demonstrate consistent findings.[17,24,46,47,48,59,71] During the first 5 days of succimer chelation (1050 mg/m^2/d in children, or 30 mg/kg/d in adults in three divided doses) blood lead drops precipitously by about 60–70%. This blood lead level remains unchanged during the next 14–23 days of continued therapy, with two-thirds of the initial daily dose divided twice a day. Increases in urinary lead excretion coincide with the drop in blood lead level with maximal excretion occurring on day 1.[24,47] Calculations indicate that urinary lead excretion exceeds estimated blood content. This suggests that some lead is being removed from soft tissues as a concentration gradient is established from tissue to blood to urine.[24,48] Typically, 2 weeks after the completion of succimer, blood lead rebounds to values 20–40% lower than pretreatment values. In the one randomized, double-blind, placebo-controlled trial of succimer in children with pretreatment blood lead levels of 30–45 µg/dL, followup at 1 month and at 6 months showed no difference between succimer and control.[71] Succimer restores red cell δ-aminolevulinic acid dehydratase (ALA-D) activity, decreases erythrocyte protoporphyrin, and decreases urinary excretion of δ-aminolevulinic acid and coproporphyrin.[17,24,47,48,71]

There is a large body of evidence reporting the usage and safety of succimer in adults with chronic lead poisoning.[11,16,36,39,43,92,94] The published foreign experience with oral succimer for metal poisoning includes nearly 100 adult cases and contributes considerably to the supporting evidence. At least 74 additional individuals have been successfully treated parenterally (IM or IV) with the sodium salt of succimer.[11,16,36,39]

LEAD ENCEPHALOPATHY

The experience with succimer in severely lead-poisoned subjects, including those with encephalopathy, is very limited.[36,39,47] Three children with a mean blood lead level >70 µg/dL treated with 5 days of succimer achieved comparable declines in blood lead to two similar children treated previously with BAL for 3 days combined with 5 days of CaNa$_2$EDTA.[47] In three adult patients with encephalopathy, significant improvement was reported following succimer chelation.[36] In a 3-year-old with a massive lead exposure superimposed on chronic lead poisoning and a blood lead of 550 µg/dL, BAL and CaNa$_2$EDTA were administered for 5 days, whole-bowel irrigation (WBI) was performed on the first 3 days, and succimer was started following WBI on day 3 and continued for 19 days. The blood lead level dropped from 550 μg/dL to 70 μg/dL on day 5, but rebounded to 99 μg/dL 2 days after BAL and CaNa$_2$EDTA were stopped, although succimer therapy had continued.[42]

ARSENIC

Succimer has been used in China and the Soviet Union since 1965 for arsenic toxicity.[3,11] Animal studies with sodium arsenite and lewisite demonstrate succimer's ability to produce an improved LD$_{50}$ with a good therapeutic index, lack of redistribution of arsenic to the brain as compared to BAL or control, and reduced kidney and liver arsenic concentrations.[3,11,57,80] A few case reports attest to the ability of succimer to enhance the urinary excretion of arsenic.[27,81] A randomized placebo-controlled trial of succimer in treating 21 patients with chronic arsenic poisoning in India, demonstrated improved clinical results and enhanced urinary excretion in both groups, but no statistical differences could be demonstrated.[65] In a comparison between BAL, succimer, and DMPS as arsenic antidotes, the higher therapeutic indexes of succimer and DMPS favor them over BAL in chronic arsenic poisoning.[69] The authors speculated that the lipophilic nature of BAL might make it preferable for acute toxicity, especially that involving lipophilic organoarsenicals. This point needs further investigation.

MERCURY

Succimer also enhances the elimination of mercury and has been used to treat patients poisoned with inorganic, elemental, and methyl mercury. Succimer improves survival, decreases renal damage, and enhances elimination of mercury following inorganic mercury[4,20,50,53,62,78,98] and methyl mercury exposure in animals.[1,2,7,63] However, one study in mice subjected to intraperitoneal mercuric chloride demonstrated an enhanced deposition of mercury in motor neurons following chelation with succimer or DMPS.[32] Of 53 construction workers who were exposed to mercury vapor, 11 received succimer and N-acetyl-d,l-penicillamine in a crossover study.[19] Mercury elimination was increased during the period of succimer administration when compared to the period of N-acetyl-d,l-penicillamine administration. Because the chelators were administered for only 2 weeks late in the clinical course, therapeutic benefit could not be evaluated. When succimer was given to victims of an extensive Iraqi methyl mercury exposure, blood methyl mercury half-life decreased from 63 days to 10 days.[3]

ADVERSE EFFECTS AND SAFETY ISSUES

Succimer is generally well tolerated with few serious adverse events reported.[24,25] Common adverse effects are gastrointestinal including nausea, vomiting, flatus, diarrhea, and a metallic taste in 10–20% of patients. Mild elevations in aspartate aminotransferase (AST) and alanine aminotransferase (ALT) are reported.[23,25,48,59,74] A single patient with severe hyperthermia and

hypotension reportedly related to succimer administration has been described.[74] Rarely, chills, fever, urticaria, rash, reversible neutropenia, and eosinophilia are reported.[17,24,25,43] Apparently unrelated adverse events during the latest open-labeled prospective study in children included an elevation in bone-derived alkaline phosphatase, eosinophils, and elevated serum aminotransferases.[24]

The Chinese, however, have reported a high incidence of more serious adverse effects (including dizziness and weakness) in response to IV or IM succimer.[96,99] This discrepancy is undoubtedly related to succimer's relatively low (approximately 20%)[66] oral bioavailability as a result of first-pass metabolism. Therefore, parenteral administration delivers a substantially greater dose.

Incidental chelation of essential elements is always a concern with chelating agents. A number of studies with succimer demonstrate either no rise in urinary zinc, copper, iron, or calcium,[24,39,46] or a small rise in zinc, copper, or calcium.[36,39,47,48] Urinary excretion of essential elements was the focus of a recent study in a primate model of childhood lead exposure.[85] Infant rhesus monkeys were exposed to lead for the first year of life to achieve blood lead levels of 40–50 μg/dL. Succimer was administered in the standard dosage regimen and complete urine collections over the first 5 days were analyzed for calcium, cobalt, copper, iron, magnesium, manganese, nickel, and zinc. Only when the data were analyzed collectively for all eight elements for all 5 days was there a statistically significant increased urinary elimination. This raises the possibility that children with nutritional deficiencies or repeated succimer chelation may be at risk for enhanced elimination of some essential elements.[24,85,87] An obvious limitation concerning the safety of succimer is that there is still relatively limited clinical experience with the drug, particularly with regard to long-term administration.

One concern with administering succimer orally is that outpatient management might permit unintentional continued lead exposure and the possibility for succimer-facilitated lead absorption. Studies with D-penicillamine, dimercaprol,[51] and IV CaNa$_2$EDTA do demonstrate enhanced lead absorption and elevated blood lead levels. Animal studies suggest that succimer does not promote lead retention in the face of continued exposure unless lead exposure is overwhelming.[45,52,76] A radiolabeled lead tracer administered to adult volunteers suggested that succimer increased the net absorption of lead from the gastrointestinal tract and may have distributed it to other tissues, as well as having enhanced urinary elimination.[86] Absorption is bimodal and consistent with an initial phase followed by a delayed increase attributable to an enterohepatic effect. It may be that succimer-enhanced urinary lead elimination often exceeds enhanced lead absorption. One recent study reported two children with environmental exposure and dramatic rises in blood lead while receiving succimer.[24] In the event of unintentional exposure to a new lead source, decontamination of the gastrointestinal tract should complement oral succimer.[67]

While iron supplementation cannot be given concomitantly with BAL because the BAL-iron complex may be a potent emetic, iron has been given concomitantly to patients receiving oral succimer without any adverse effects.[49] The prevalence of both iron deficiency and elevated blood lead levels is highest among poor, inner-city children.[60] Because heme is a constituent of all cells, including those of the brain, it appears clinically prudent to provide iron supplementation during chelation therapy, when the heme pathway is freed of the inhibitory effects of lead. It is recommended to separate the timing of administration of the iron from the succimer.[24]

Most blood lead is measured by graphite furnace atomic absorption spectrophotometry, in which case succimer does not interfere with the measurement. However, in the event that blood lead levels were to be measured by anodic stripping voltametry, succimer would affect the results by chelating the mercury in the electrode.[24]

There is a single case report of a 3-year-old patient who reportedly ingested 185 mg/kg of succimer. He remained asymptomatic.[82] There was a dose-dependent effect of succimer on early and late fetal resorption and fetal body weight and length when succimer was administered to pregnant mice during organogenesis. No observed teratogenic effects were noted when 410 mg/kg, or approximately 5% of the acute LD_{50}, of succimer was administered subcutaneously.[31] Doses of succimer of 30–60 mg/kg/d by gavage were administered from day 6 to day 21 of gestation to lead-poisoned rats.[22] These doses of succimer decreased embryonic and fetal blood lead levels and normalized offspring body weight at 13 weeks. And although succimer was able to reverse some lead-induced immunotoxic effects, succimer itself caused problems with the immune system that persisted into adulthood.[22] A leading authority strongly recommends against the use of succimer in pregnancy.[24]

PHARMACOKINETICS

The pharmacokinetics of a single oral dose of succimer were determined in three children and three adults with lead poisoning, and in five healthy adult volunteers.[29] Children received 350 mg/m² of succimer, and adults received 10 mg/kg of succimer. The peak level and the time to peak blood concentration of total succimer (parent and altered oxidized metabolites) were similar for all three groups. The half-life of total succimer was 1.5 times longer in the children than in either adult group. The renal clearance of total succimer was greater in healthy adults than in lead-poisoned patients. Distribution of succimer (parent and/or oxidized metabolites) into erythrocytes appeared greater in poisoned patients than in the healthy adults.[29]

The metabolism of succimer was studied in lead-poisoned children, and then in normal adults.[13] The results indicate that succimer undergoes an enterohepatic circulation facilitated by gastrointestinal (GI) microflora. Similar to the previous pharmacokinetic study, moderate lead exposure impaired the renal elimination of succimer.

COMBINED CHELATION THERAPY

It has been proposed that succimer be combined with $CaNa_2EDTA$ to take advantage of the ability of succimer to remove lead from soft tissues, including the brain, while capitalizing on the ability of $CaNa_2EDTA$ to mobilize lead from bone.[26] A number of rodent models have examined this combination and found the combination to be superior in enhancing the elimination of lead, reducing tissue levels of lead, and in restoring some lead-induced biochemical abnormalities.[34,35,89] Although the addition of succimer to $CaNa_2EDTA$ prevented the redistribution of lead to the brain caused by $CaNa_2EDTA$ alone, the combination also increased urinary excretion of zinc, calcium, and iron.[89,90] A retrospective review comparing dimercaprol plus CaEDTA to succimer plus $CaNa_2EDTA$ in children with blood lead levels >45 μg/mL

demonstrated a similar reduction in blood lead levels at the end of treatment and at 14 and 33 days following the termination of treatment.[18] Blood lead level reductions were approximately 75%, 40%, and 37% at the end of therapy, and at 14 and 33 days posttreatment, respectively. The succimer plus $CaNa_2EDTA$ combination was better tolerated.[18]

DMPS

DMPS (racemic-2,3-dimercapto-1-propanesulfonic acid, Na salt) is an investigational metal chelator which, like succimer, is a water-soluble analogue of BAL.[3,7,21] A dose of 15 mg/kg of DMPS is equimolar to 12 mg/kg of succimer. DMPS has been used in the Soviet Union since the late 1950s and is marketed in both oral and parenteral forms in Germany as Dimaval. DMPS seems promising in mercury and arsenic poisoning.[3,7,9,12,21,41] DMPS is associated with an increase in the urinary excretion of copper and the development of Stevens-Johnson syndrome.[23] Like succimer, DMPS does not appear to redistribute mercury or lead to the brain. More research needs to be done to determine whether DMPS is more advantageous than succimer given its lower LD_{50} in rodents (5.22 mmol/kg vs 16.5 mmol/kg for succimer).

DOSING

Succimer (Chemet) is available as 100-mg bead-filled capsules. In patients who cannot swallow the capsule whole, the capsule can be separated immediately prior to use and sprinkled into a small amount of juice or on apple sauce, ice cream, or soft food, or put on a spoon and followed by a fruit drink. The dosage is 350 mg/m² in children 3 times a day for 5 days followed by 350 mg/m² twice a day for 14 days. In adults, the dosage is 10 mg/kg in the same regimen as above. Using 10 mg/kg in children rather than dosing based upon body surface area, as was done during the premarketing trials, may result in patient underdosing.[68]

UNANSWERED QUESTIONS

In spite of the epidemic of lead poisoning, there is a paucity of rigorous data defining the role of succimer. There are many unanswered questions regarding clinical efficacy, pharmacokinetics, and dosage regimens.[56,68] These questions include: How exactly does succimer bind lead in the blood? Is it succimer, its active disulfide cysteine metabolites, or both that bind lead? What happens to the cysteine conjugates? How do the kidneys handle the lead chelate? What exactly is reabsorbed in the enterohepatic circulation, succimer, the cysteine metabolites, or the lead chelated form? Should a longer succimer-dosing regimen be used? And, the most important question of all, does succimer chelation improve clinical outcome?

REFERENCES

1. Aaseth J: Treatment of mercury and lead poisonings with dimercaptosuccinic acid and sodium dimercaptopropanesulfonate. Analyst 1996; 120:853–854.
2. Aaseth J, Friedheim EA: Treatment of methyl mercury poisoning in mice with 2,3-dimercaptosuccinic acid and other complexing thiols. Acta Pharmacol Toxicol 1978;42:248–252.

3. Aposhian HV, Carter DE, Hoover TD, et al: succimer, DMPS and DMPA as arsenic antidotes. Fundam Applied Tox 1984;4:S58–S70.

4. Aposhian HV: succimer and DMPS—Water-soluble antidotes for heavy metal poisoning. Annu Rev Pharmacol Toxicol 1983;23: 193–215.

5. Aposhian HV, Aposhian MM: Meso-2,3-dimercaptosuccinic acid: Chemical, pharmacological and toxicological properties of an orally effective metal chelating agent. Annu Rev Pharmacol Toxicol 1990; 30:279–306.

6. Aposhian HV, Maiorino RM, Dart RC, et al: Urinary excretion of meso-2,3 dimercaptosuccinic acid in human subjects. Clin Pharmacol Ther 1989;45:520–526.

7. Aposhian HV, Maiorino RM, Gonzalez-Ramirez D, et al: Mobiliza-tion of heavy metals by newer, therapeutically useful chelating agents. Toxicology 1995;97:23–38.

8. Aposhian HV, Maiorino RM, Rivera M, et al: Human studies with the chelating agents, DMPS and succimer. J Toxicol Clin Toxicol 1992;30: 505–528.

9. Aposhian M, Maiorano R, Xu Z, Aposhian HV: Sodium 2,3-dimer-capto-1-propanesulfonate (DMPS) treatment does not redistribute lead or mercury to the brain of rats. Toxicol 1996;109:49–55.

10. Aposhian HV, Mershon MM, Brinkley, Hsu CA: Anti-lewisite activ-ity and stability of meso-dimercaptosuccinic acid and 2,3-dimercapto-1-propanesulfonic acid. Life Sci 1982;31:2149–2156.

11. Aposhian HV, Taklock CH, Moon TE: Protection of mice against the lethal effects of sodium arsenite: A quantitative comparison of a num-ber of chelating agents. Toxicol Appl Pharmacol 1981;61:385–392.

12. Aposhian HV, Zheng B, Aposhian M, et al: DMPS-Arsenic challenge test. Toxicol Appl Pharmacol 2000;165:74–83.

13. Asiedu P, Moulton T, Blum CB, et al: Metabolism of meso-2,3-dimer-captosuccinic acid in lead-poisoned children and normal adults. Envi-ron Health Perspect 1995;103:734–739.

14. Bankowska J, Hine C: Retention of lead in the rat. Arch Environ Con-tam Toxicol 1985;14:621–629.

15. Bhattacharya A, Smelser D, Berger O, et al: The effect of succimer therapy in lead intoxication using postural balance as a measure: A case study in a nine-year-old child. Neurotoxicology 1998;19: 57–64.

16. Bentur Y, Brook JG, Behar R, Taitelman U: Meso-2,3-dimercaptosuc-cinic acid in the diagnosis and treatment of lead poisoning. J Toxicol Clin Toxicol 1987;25:39–51.

17. Besunder JB, Anderson RL, Super DM: Short-term efficacy of oral dimercaptosuccinic acid in children with low to moderate lead intoxi-cation. Pediatrics 1995;96:683–687.

18. Besunder JB, Super DM, Anderson R: Comparison of dimercaptosuc-cinic acid and calcium disodium ethylenediaminetetraacetic acid versus dimercaptopropanol and ethylenediaminetetraacetic acid in children with lead poisoning. J Pediatr 1997;130:966–971.

19. Bluhm RE, Bobbitt RG, Welch LW, et al: Elemental mercury vapour toxicity, treatment, and prognosis after acute, intensive exposure in chloralkali plant workers. I: History, neuropsychological findings and chelator effects. Hum Exp Toxicol 1992;11:201–210.

20. Buchet JP, Lauwerys RR: Influence of 2,3 dimercaptopropane-1-sul-fonate and dimercaptosuccinic acid on the mobilization of mercury from tissues of rats pretreated with mercuric chloride, phenylmercury acetate or mercury vapors. Toxicology 1989;54:323–333.

21. Campbell JR, Clarkson TW, Omar MD: The therapeutic use of 2,3-dimercaptopropane-1-sulfonate in two cases of inorganic mercury poisoning. JAMA 1986;256:3127–3130.

22. Chen S, Golemboski KA, Sanders FS, et al: Persistent effect of in utero meso-2,3-dimercaptosuccinic acid (succimer) on immune func-tion and lead-induced immunotoxicity. Toxicology 1999;132:67–69.

23. Chisolm JJ: BAL, EDTA, succimer and DMPS in the treatment of lead poisoning in children. J Toxicol Clin Toxicol 1992;30:493–504.

24. Chisolm JJ: Safety and efficacy of meso-2,3-dimercaptosuccinic acid (succimer) in children with elevated blood lead concentrations. J Toxicol Clin Toxicol 2000;38:365–375.

25. Committee on Drugs: Treatment guidelines for lead exposure in chil-dren. Pediatrics 1995;96:155–160.

26. Cory-Slechta DA: Mobilization of lead over the course of succimer chelation therapy and long-term efficacy. J Pharmacol Exp Ther 1988; 246:84–91.

27. Cullen NA, Wolf LR, St. Clair D: Pediatric arsenic ingestion. Am J Emerg Med 1995;13:432–435.

28. Cremin JD, Luck ML, Laughlin NK, Smith DR: Efficacy of succimer chelation for reducing brain lead in a primate model of human expo-sure. Toxicol Appl Pharmacol 1999;161:283–293.

29. Dart RC, Hurlbut KM, Maiorino RM, et al: Pharmacokinetics of meso-2,3-dimercaptosuccinic acid in patients with lead poisoning and in healthy adults. J Pediatr 1994;125:309–316.

30. Devars DuMayne JF, Prevost C, Gaudin B, et al: Lead poisoning treated with 2,3-dimercaptosuccinic acid. Presse Med 1984;13:2209.

31. Domingo JL, Paternain JL, Llobet JM, Corbella J: Developmental toxicity of subcutaneously administered meso-2,3-dimercaptosuccinic acid in mice. Fundam Appl Toxicol 1986;11:715–722.

32. Ewan KB, Pamphlett R: Increased inorganic mercury in spinal motor neurons following chelating agents. Neurotoxicology 1996;17: 343–349.

33. Fang X, Fernando Q: Synthesis, structure, and properties of *rac*-2,3-dimercaptosuccinic acid, a potentially useful chelating agent for toxic metals. Chem Res Toxicol 1994;7:148–156.

34. Flora SJS, Bhattacharya R, Vijayaraghavan R: Combined therapeutic potential of meso-2,3-dimercaptosuccinic acid and calcium disodium versenate on the mobilization and distribution of lead in experimental lead intoxication in rats. Fundam Appl Toxicol 1995;25:233–240.

35. Flora GJS, Seth PK, Prakash AO, Mathur R: Therapeutic efficacy of combined meso-2,3-dimercaptosuccinic acid and calcium disodium edetate treatment during acute lead intoxication in rats. Hum Exp Toxicol 1995;14:410–413.

36. Fournier L, Thomas G, Garnier R, et al: 2,3-Dimercaptosuccinic acid treatment of heavy metal poisoning in humans. Med Toxicol 1988; 3:499–504.

37. Friedheim E, Crovi C, Wakker CH: Meso-dimercaptosuccinic acid, a chelating agent for the treatment of mercury and lead poisoning. J Pharm Pharmacol 1976;28:711–712.

38. Friedheim E, DaSilva JR: Treatment of schistosomiasis mansonii with antimony a,a'-dimercapto-potassium succinnate (TWSb). Am J Trop Med Hyg 1954;3:714–727.

39. Friedheim E, Graziano JH, Popovac D, et al: Treatment of lead poi-soning by 2,3-dimercaptosuccinic acid. Lancet 1978;2:1234–1235.

40. Glotzer DE: The current role of 2,3-dimercaptosuccinic acid (suc-cimer) in the management of childhood lead poisoning. Drug Saf 1993;9: 85–92.

41. Gonzalez-Ramirez D, Zuniga-Charles M, Narro-Juarez A, et al: DMPS (2,3-dimercaptopropane-1-sulfonate, Dimaval) decreases the body burden of mercury in humans exposed to mercurous chloride. J Pharm Exp Ther 1998;287:8–12.

42. Gordon R, Roberts G, Amin Z, et al: Aggressive approach in the treat-ment of acute lead encephalopathy with an extraordinarily high con-centration of lead. Arch Pediatr Adolesc Med 1998;152:1100–1104.

43. Grandjean P, Jacobsen IA, Jorgensen PJ: Chronic lead poisoning treated with dimercaptosuccinic acid. Pharmacol Toxicol 1991;68: 266–269.

44. Graziano JH: Role of 2,3-dimercaptosuccinic acid in the treatment of heavy metal poisoning. Med Toxicol 1986;1:155–162.

45. Graziano JH, Leong JK, Friedheim E: 2,3-Dimercaptosuccinic acid: A new agent for the treatment of lead poisoning. J Pharm Exp Ther 1978;206:696–700.

46. Graziano JH, LoIacono N, Meyer P: A dose-response study of oral 2,3-dimercaptosuccinic acid (succimer) in children with elevated blood lead concentrations. J Pediatr 1988;113:751–757.

47. Graziano JH, LoIacono NJ, Moulton T, et al: Controlled study of meso-2,3-dimercaptosuccinic acid for the management of childhood lead intoxication. J Pediatr 1992;120:133–139.

48. Graziano JH, Siris E, LoIacono N, et al: 2,3-Dimercaptosuccinic acid as an antidote for lead intoxication. Clin Pharmacol Ther 1985;37: 431–438.

49. Haust HL, Inwood M, Spence JD, et al: Intramuscular administration of iron during long-term chelation therapy with 3,2-dimercaptosuccinic acid in a man with severe lead poisoning. Clin Biochem 1989; 22:189–196.

50. Jones M, Basinger M, Gale G, Atkins L, Smith A, Stone A: Effect of chelate treatment on kidney, bone, and brain levels of lead-intoxicated mice. Toxicology 1994;89:91–100.

51. Jugo S, Maljkovic T, Kostial K: Influence of chelating agents on the gastrointestinal absorption of lead. Toxicol Appl Pharmacol 1975; 34:259–263.

52. Kapoor SC, Wielopolski L, Graziano JH, LoIacono NJ: Influence of 2,3-dimercaptosuccinic acid on gastrointestinal lead absorption and whole body lead retention. Toxicol Appl Pharmacol 1989;97: 525–529.

53. Keith RL, Setiarahardjo I, Fernando Q, et al: Utilization of renal slices to evaluate the efficacy of chelating agents for removing mercury from the kidney. Toxicology 1997;116:67–75.

54. Khalil-Manesh F, Gonick HC, Weiler EW, et al: Effect of chelation treatment with dimercaptosuccinic acid (succimer) on lead-related blood pressure changes. Environ Res 1994;65:86–99.

55. Klaassen CD: Heavy metals and heavy-metal antagonists. In: Gilman AG, Goodman LS, Rall TW, Murad F, eds: Goodman and Gilman's The Pharmacological Basis of Therapeutics, 7th ed. New York, Macmillan, 1985, pp. 1605–1627.

56. Kosnett MJ: Unanswered questions in metal chelation. J Toxicol Clin Toxicol 1992;304:529–547.

57. Kreppel H, Paepcke U, Thiermann H, et al: Therapeutic efficacy of new dimercaptosuccinic acid (succimer) analogues in acute arsenic trioxide poisoning in mice. Arch Toxicol 1993;67:580–585.

58. Lenz K, Hruby K, Druml W, et al: 2,3-Dimercaptosuccinic acid in human arsenic poisoning. Arch Toxicol 1981;47:241–243.

59. Liebelt E, Shannon M: Oral chelators for childhood lead poisoning. Pediatr Ann 1994;23:616–626.

60. Mahaffey KR: Factors modifying susceptibility to lead. In: Mahaffey KR, ed: Dietary and Environmental Lead: Human Health Effects. New York, Elsevier, 1985, pp. 373–419.

61. Maiorino RM, Bruce DC, Aposhian HV: Determination and metabolism of dithiol chelating agents: VI. Isolation and identification of the mixed disulfides of meso-2,3-dimercaptosuccinic acid with L-cysteine in human urine. Toxicol Appl Pharmacol 1989;97:338–349.

62. Magos L: The effects of dimercaptosuccinic acid on the excretion and distribution of mercury in rats and mice treated with mercuric chloride and methylmercury chloride. Br J Pharmacol 1976;56:479–484.

63. Magos L, Peristianis GC, Snowden RT: Postexposure preventive treatment of methylmercury intoxication in rats with dimercaptosuccinic acid. Toxicol Appl Pharmacol 1978;45:463–475.

64. Mann KV, Travers JD: Succimer, an oral lead chelator. Clin Pharm 1991;10:914–922.

65. Mazumder DN, Das Gupta J, Santra A, et al: Chronic arsenic toxicity in west Bengal—the worst calamity in the world. J Indian Med Assoc 1998;96:4–7, 18.

66. McGown EL, Tillotson JA, Knudsen JJ, Dumlao CR: Biological behavior and metabolic fate of the BAL analogues succimer and DMPS. Proc West Pharmacol Soc 1984;27:169–176.

67. McKinney PE: Acute elevation of blood lead levels within hours of ingestion of large quantities of lead shot. J Toxicol Clin Toxicol 2000;38:435–440.

68. Mortensen ME: Succimer chelation: What is known? J Pediatr 1994; 125:233–234.

69. Muckter H, Leibl B, Reichl FX: Are we ready to replace dimercaprol (BAL) as an arsenic antidote? Hum Exp Toxicol 1997;16: 460–465.

70. Ni W, Feng Y, Yu J, et al: A study of oral succimer in the treatment of lead poisoning. Personal communication, 1989.

71. O'Connor ME, Rich D: Children with moderately elevated lead levels: Is chelation with succimer helpful? Clin Pediatr (Phila) 1999;38: 325–331.

72. O'Flaherty EJ, Inskip MJ, Yagiminas AP, Franklin CA: Plasma and blood lead concentrations, lead absorption and lead excretion in subhuman primates. Toxicol Appl Pharmacol 1996;138:121–130.

73. Okonishnokova IE, Rosenberg EE: Succimer as a means of chemoprophylaxis against occupational poisonings of workers handling mercury. Gig Tr Prof Zabol 1971;15:29–32.

74. Okose P, Jennis T, Honcharuk L: Untoward effects of oral dimercaptosuccinic acid in the treatment of lead poisoning [abstract]. Vet Hum Toxicol 1991;33:376.

75. Pappas JB, Ahlquist T, Winn P, et al: The effect of oral succimer on ongoing exposure to lead [abstract]. Vet Hum Toxicol 1992;34:361.

76. Pappas JB, Ahlquist JT, Allen EM, Banner W: Oral dimercaptosuccinic acid and ongoing exposure to lead: Effects on heme synthesis and lead distribution in a rat model. Toxicol Appl Pharmacol 1995; 133:121–129.

77. Piomelli S, Rosen JF, Chisolm JJ Jr, Graef JW: Management of childhood lead poisoning. J Pediatr 1984;105:523–532.

78. Planas-Bohne F: The influence of chelating agents on the distribution and biotransformation of methylmercuric chloride in rats. J Pharmacol Exp Ther 1981;217:500–504.

79. Rivera M, Zheng W, Aposhian HV, Fernando Q: Determination and metabolism of dithiol-containing agents VIII. Metal complexes of meso-dimercaptosuccinic acid. Toxicol Appl Pharmacol 1989;100: 96–106.

80. Schafer B, Kreppel H, Reichl FX, et al: Effect of oral treatment with BAL, DMPS or succimer in organs of mice injected with arsenic trioxide. Arch Toxicol 1991;14(Suppl):228–230.

81. Shum S, Whitehead J, Vaughn L: Chelation of organoarsenate with dimercaptosuccinic acid. Vet Hum Toxicol 1995;37:239–242.

82. Sigg T, Burda A, Leikin JB, et al: A report of pediatric succimer overdose. Vet Hum Toxicol 1998;40:90–91.

83. Singh PK, Jones MM, Xu Z, et al: Mobilization of lead by esters of meso-2,3-dimercaptosuccinic acid. J Toxicol Environ Health 1989;27: 423–434.

84. Smith D, Bayer L, Strupp B: Efficacy of succimer chelation for reducing brain Pb levels in a rodent model. Environ Res 1998;78:168–176.

85. Smith DR, Calacsan C, Woodlard D, et al: Succimer and the urinary excretion of essential elements in a primate model of childhood lead exposure. Toxicol Sci 2000;54:473–480.

86. Smith DR, Ilustre RP, Osterloh JD: Methodological considerations for the accurate determination of lead in human plasma and serum. Am J Ind Med 1998;33:430–438.

87. Smith DR, Woolard D, Luck ML, et al: Succimer and the reduction of tissue lead in juvenile monkeys. Toxicol Appl Pharmacol 2000;166:230–240.

88. Stewart PW, Blaine C, Cohen M, et al: Acute and longer term effects of meso-2,3 dimercaptosuccinic acid (succimer) on the behavior of lead-exposed and control mice. Physiol Behav 1996:59:849–855.

89. Tandon SK, Singh S, Jain V: Efficacy of combined chelation in lead intoxication. Chem Res Toxicol 1994;7:585–589.

90. Tandon SK, Singh S, Prasad S, Mathur N: Mobilization of lead by calcium versenate and dimercaptosuccinate in the rat. Clin Exper Pharmacol 1998;25:686–692.

91. Thomas G, Fournier L, Garnier R, Dally S: Nail dystrophy and dimercaptosuccinic acid. J Toxicol Clin Exp 1987;7:285–287.

92. Thomas PS, Ashton C: An oral treatment for lead toxicity. Postgrad Med J 1991;67:63–65.

93. Treatment of Lead Exposed Children Trial Group: The treatment of lead-exposed children (TLC) trial: Design and recruitment for a study of the effect of oral chelation on growth and development in toddlers. Ped Perinatal Epidem 1998;12:313–333.

94. Tuntunji MF, al-Mahasneh QM: Disappearance of heme metabolites following chelation therapy with meso 2,3-dimercaptosuccinic acid (succimer). J Toxicol Clin Toxicol 1994;32:267–276.

95. Wang SC, Ting KS, Wu CC: Chelating therapy with NaDMS in occupational lead and mercury intoxication. Chin Med J (Engl) 1965; 84:437–439.

96. Xue H, Ni W, Xie Y, Cao T: Comparison of lead excretion of patients after injection of five chelating agents. Chung Kuo Yao Li Hsuch Pao 1982;3:41–44.

97. Yu-I L, Chiao-Chen C, Yea-Lin T, Kuang-Sheng T: Studies on antibilharzial drugs VI: The antidotal effects of sodium dimercaptosuccinate and BAL-glucoside against tartar emetic. Acta Physiol Sinica 1957;21:24–32.

98. Zalups RK: Influence of 2,3-dimercaptopropoane-1-sulfonate (DMPS) and meso-2,3-dimercaptosuccinic acid (succimer) on the renal disposition of mercury in normal and uninephrectomized rats exposed to inorganic mercury. J Pharmacol Exp Ther 1993;267:791–799.

99. Zhang J: Clinical observations in ethyl mercury chloride poisoning. Am J Ind Med 1984;5:251–258.

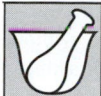

ANTIDOTES IN DEPTH

Edetate Calcium Disodium (CaNa₂EDTA)

Mary Ann Howland

NaOOC—CH₂   CH₂—COONa
        CH₂CH₂
    N   N
H₂C   Ca   CH₂
    CH₂   CH₂
    COO   OOC

Edetate calcium disodium (ethylenediamine tetraacetic acid, CaNa₂EDTA) is a chelating agent used for the management of lead poisoning. It has largely been supplanted by succimer for mild to moderate lead toxicity. Although it retains a role for the management of serious lead poisoning and lead encephalopathy in conjunction with dimercaprol, even this role is being challenged by succimer.

CHEMISTRY

Edetate calcium disodium belongs to the family of polyaminocarboxylic acids. It has a molecular weight of 374 daltons. It is capable of chelating many heavy metals, but is used primarily in the management of lead poisoning. The term *chelate* has its origin in the Greek word *chele*, which means "claw," implying an ability to tightly grasp the metal.[38] Implicit in chelation is the formation of a ring-structured complex. When CaNa₂EDTA chelates lead, the calcium is displaced and the lead takes its place, forming a stable-ring compound.[23]

PHARMACOKINETICS

Calcium disodium EDTA is an ionic, water-soluble compound. The volume of distribution is small because of its polar nature and approximates that of the extracellular fluid compartment in normal individuals.[19,23] The volume of distribution is even smaller in patients with renal dysfunction (0.05–0.23 L/kg).[29] CaNa₂EDTA appears to penetrate cells, such as erythrocytes, poorly.[2,19] Less than 5% of CaNa₂EDTA gains access to the spinal fluid.[19,23] Oral administration is of limited value because of an oral bioavailability of less than 5%. Renal elimination approximates the glomerular filtration rate,[28] which correlates with creatinine clearance,[29] and results in the excretion of 50% of CaNa₂EDTA in the urine in 1 hour and more than 95% in 24 hours.[19,23] Dosage adjustments are necessary if CaNa₂EDTA is used in patients with renal dysfunction.[28,29] The half-life is about 20–60 minutes.[3,19,23] When

CaNa₂EDTA combines with lead extracted from soft tissues and body fluids, it forms a stable, soluble, nonionized compound that is subsequently excreted in the urine. Following CaNa₂EDTA administration, urinary lead excretion is increased 20–50-fold.

LEAD

Humans

CaNa₂EDTA is capable of reducing blood lead levels during therapy, enhancing renal excretion of lead, and reversing the effects of lead on hemoglobin synthesis.[11] Blood lead levels rebound considerably days to weeks following the cessation of CaNa₂EDTA, as is the case after termination of other chelators.[1,2,20] Although CaNa₂EDTA has been used clinically since the 1970s, no rigorous clinical studies have ever been performed to evaluate whether CaNa₂EDTA is capable of reversing the neurobehavioral effects of lead. Chelators including CaNa₂EDTA are incapable of dramatically decreasing the body burden of lead, because only several milligrams of lead are eliminated during chelation.[8,9,31] A study of children with blood lead levels of 25–50 μg/dL who were given 5 days of CaNa₂EDTA revealed very little difference in blood lead, bone lead, or erythrocyte protoporphyrin levels when compared to pretreatment values.[25] Another study in children demonstrated no additional benefits of CaNa₂EDTA on cognitive performance beyond that which was achieved by limiting further lead exposure and correcting an iron deficiency anemia.[30] A followup study in children with initial blood lead levels about 30 μg/dL by the same authors suggested an improvement in perceptual motor performance over a 6-month period beyond that which was achieved by the treatment of the iron deficiency anemia.[33] However, CaNa₂EDTA failed to reverse lead-induced learning deficits in the rat model.[13]

Animals

Animal studies demonstrate a decrease in tissue lead stores including brain levels when measurements are performed at the end of CaNa₂EDTA therapy.[21] However a rat study that examined the effect of CaNa₂EDTA on brain lead levels following a single dose demonstrated a significant increase in brain lead levels,[14] suggesting that CaNa₂EDTA may initially mobilize lead and facilitate redistribution to the brain. Further doses are then able to enhance lead elimination, reduce blood lead levels and subsequently reduce brain lead levels. This phenomenon may explain why some case reports demonstrate a deterioration in lead encephalopathy when CaNa₂EDTA is used without concomitant dimercaprol therapy.

CaNa₂EDTA MOBILIZATION TEST

The CaNa₂EDTA mobilization test for diagnostic purposes was recently scrutinized[7] and considered obsolete by some authorities.[11] Criticisms include difficulties with administration, unreliability as a predictor of total body lead burden, expense, and the risk of worsening toxicity through redistribution of lead to either the kidney or brain.[11,12] Advocates suggest that the CaNa$_2$EDTA lead mobilization test is cost saving if it can be used to identify the one-third of moderately lead-poisoned children (25–45 µg/dL) who are most able to excrete lead at an enhanced rate.[24] The advocates of the test suggest that the use of outpatient 6–8-hour protocols minimizes administration difficulties,[26] and that the potential risk of redistribution of lead to the brain has only been demonstrated in rats,[12] and is purely theoretical in humans.[26] There are no data to support a detrimental central nervous system (CNS) effect of the CaNa$_2$EDTA challenge test in moderately poisoned children.

ROLE IN THE TREATMENT OF ATHEROSCLEROSIS

The treatment of atherosclerosis with disodium EDTA cannot be recommended. Although proponents cite the theoretical benefit of chelating calcium from atherosclerotic plaques, there is no scientific evidence to support this approach.

ADVERSE EFFECTS AND SAFETY ISSUES

The principal toxicity of CaNa$_2$EDTA is related to the metal chelate. In mice, the LD$_{50}$ values of various CaNa$_2$EDTA metal chelates when administered intraperitoneally (IP) are CaNa$_2$EDTA, 14.3 mmol/kg; lead EDTA, 3.1 mmol/kg; and mercury EDTA, 0.01 mmol/kg.

When CaNa$_2$EDTA is given to patients with lead poisoning, the sites of major renal toxicity are the proximal tubule and, to a lesser extent, the distal tubule and glomeruli.[23] This toxicity may be caused by the release of lead in the kidneys during excretion.[23] Of 210 children who received dimercaprol and CaNa$_2$EDTA, 3% developed acute oliguric renal failure, which resolved over time without hemodialysis, and 21% had biochemical evidence of nephrotoxicity.[24] Other studies failed to demonstrate any cases of renal failure in more than 1000 patient courses of therapy when CaNa$_2$EDTA was given in divided daily doses of 1000 mg/m^2 IV over 1 hour, every 6 hours.[26] Lead toxicity also causes renal damage independent of chelation. It is therefore important to monitor renal function closely during CaNa$_2$EDTA administration and to adjust the dose and schedule appropriately.[28,29] Nephrotoxicity may be minimized by limiting the total daily dose of CaNa$_2$EDTA to 1 g in children or 2 g in adults, although doses may need to be higher to treat lead encephalopathy. Widely spaced, small doses, while maintaining good hydration seem to increase efficacy and decrease toxicity.[28] Other adverse effects of CaNa$_2$EDTA include malaise, fatigue, thirst, chills, fever, myalgias, dermatitis, headache, anorexia, urinary frequency and urgency, sneezing, nasal congestion, lacrimation, glycosuria, anemia, transient hypotension, increased prothrombin times, and inverted T waves.[23] Mild increases in alanine aminotransferase (ALT) and aspartate aminotransferase (AST) (usually reversible) and decreases in alkaline phosphatase are frequently reported. Extravasation may result in the development of painful calcinosis at the injection site.[34] Depletion of endogenous metals, particularly zinc, iron, and manganese,

may result from chronic therapy.[5,37] A decrease in serum dopamine β-hydroxylase, a copper-dependent enzyme, without any demonstrable decrease in serum copper occurred after a single injection of calcium disodium edetate in three adult lead welders.[15] The clinical relevance of this is unknown.[15] The administration of disodium EDTA can lead to life-threatening hypocalcemia.[2] Because CaNa$_2$EDTA has replaced sodium EDTA as the EDTA preparation of choice, hypocalcemia has disappeared as a clinical concern.

An animal study suggests that gastrointestinal lead absorption may be enhanced by the intraperitoneal or oral administration of CaNa$_2$EDTA.[20] Obviously, removal of lead from the child's environment should remain the first strategy in the management of lead toxicity. In the event of unintentional exposure to a new lead source, decontamination of the gastrointestinal tract should complement chelation.[27]

The safety of CaNa$_2$EDTA has not been established in pregnancy, and a risk-to-benefit analysis must be made if its use is considered. In a model of lead poisoning in pregnant rats, fetal resorption decreased and the number of live fetuses increased when CaNa$_2$EDTA was used, although the placental levels of lead were increased.[17] Zinc levels were not affected. Another study, however, found that when CaNa$_2$EDTA was given to pregnant rats not poisoned with lead, increases in submucous clefts, cleft palate, adactyly/syndactyly, curly tail, and abnormal ribs and vertebrae occurred.[4] These teratogenic effects occurred with doses of CaNa$_2$EDTA comparable to human doses and without causing noticeable changes in the mother except for weight gain. Use of zinc calcium EDTA and zinc EDTA preparations in pregnant rats caused no teratogenic effects at low dose but resulted in the development of submucous cleft palates in 30% of the offspring receiving the higher dose of zinc calcium EDTA.[4] This suggests that the incorporation of zinc into EDTA may be protective in pregnant rats.

DOSING AND ADMINISTRATION

The dose of CaNa$_2$EDTA is determined by the patient's body surface area or weight (up to a maximum dose) and the severity of the poisoning and renal function (Chap. 80 and Table 80–10).[11,25,30] For patients with lead encephalopathy, the dose of CaNa$_2$EDTA is 1500 mg/m^2/d to be given by continuous IV infusion starting 4 hours after the first dose of dimercaprol and after an adequate urine flow is established.[10] Combined dimercaprol-CaNa$_2$EDTA therapy is given for 5 days, followed by a rest period of at least 2–4 days, which permits lead redistribution. There is limited evidence to suggest that folic acid, pyridoxine, and thiamine increase the antidotal properties of CaNa$_2$EDTA.[35] Before a blood lead concentration is measured, the CaNa$_2$EDTA infusion should be interrupted for 1 hour to avoid a falsely elevated value.

For symptomatic children without lead encephalopathy, the dose of CaNa$_2$EDTA is 1000 mg/m^2/d in addition to dimercaprol at 50 mg/m^2 every 4 hours. However, because of the FDA approval and the demonstrated ability of succimer to reduce brain lead levels in animals, this agent is increasingly replacing the role of CaNa$_2$EDTA in this lead-poisoned pediatric population.[9]

Because of the pain associated with IM administration, most clinicians recommend that CaNa$_2$EDTA be administered at concentrations ≤0.5% by continuous IV infusion over 24 hours in 5% dextrose or 0.9% NaCl. Concentrations ≥0.5% may lead to thrombophlebitis and should be avoided. CaNa$_2$EDTA is not compatible with other solutions. Careful attention to total fluid requirements in children and patients who have or who are at risk for lead encephalopathy is paramount.[23,30] Rapid intravenous infusions may worsen lead encephalopathy associated with cerebral edema and increased intracranial pressure. Starting BAL 4 hours prior to CaNa$_2$ EDTA appears to be more effective than starting CaNa$_2$EDTA prior to and simultaneously with BAL in children with acute lead encephalopathy.[6] As noted, CaNa$_2$EDTA alone, without BAL, may promote redistribution of lead from soft tissue to brain.[11,12,14] Treating with two chelators also reduces the blood lead level significantly faster than does CaNa$_2$EDTA alone, while maintaining a better molar ratio of chelator to lead.[6]

If CaNa$_2$EDTA is to be administered IM to avoid the use of an IV and fluid overload, then procaine sufficient to produce a final concentration of 0.5% is added to the CaNa$_2$EDTA at 1 mL of a 1% procaine solution for each mL of chelator.[23] The procaine minimizes pain at the injection site.

COMBINATION THERAPY WITH SUCCIMER OR DMPS

The possible benefit of combining CaNa$_2$EDTA with succimer or 2,3-dimercapto-1-propane-sulfonic acid (DMPS) is under investigation in animals.[16,18,36] The combination of CaNa$_2$EDTA with succimer appears more potent than either individual agent in promoting urine and fecal lead excretion, and decreasing blood and liver lead levels, but this approach may increase nephrotoxicity and zinc depletion.

AVAILABILITY

Calcium disodium EDTA is available as Calcium Disodium Versenate in 5-mL ampules containing 200 mg of CaNa$_2$EDTA per milliliter (1 g per ampule).[23] Disodium edetate (sodium EDTA) should not be considered an alternative to CaNa$_2$EDTA because of the risk of life-threatening hypocalcemia by using sodium EDTA.

SUMMARY

CaNa$_2$EDTA reduces blood lead levels, enhances urinary lead excretion, and reverses lead-induced hematologic effects. Studies evaluating long-term effects in reversing lead-induced neurotoxicity have not been performed. CaNa$_2$EDTA remains the standard of care for patients with lead encephalopathy when used in conjunction with dimercaprol. CaNa$_2$EDTA as a diagnostic aid in determining which patients are appropriate candidates for chelation is no longer recommended.[11,14] Recommended doses and dosage schedules should not be exceeded and should be reduced when the creatinine clearance is reduced. Patients should be well hydrated to achieve an adequate urine flow prior to and during CaNa$_2$EDTA therapy.

REFERENCES

1. Angle CR: Childhood lead poisoning and its treatment. Ann Rev Pharmacol Toxicol 1993;32:409–434.

2. Aposhian HV, Maiorinao RM, Gonzalez-Ramirez D, et al: Mobilization of heavy metals by newer, therapeutically useful chelating agents. Toxicology 1995;97:23–38.

3. Bowazzi P, Lanzoni J, Marcussi F: Pharmacokinetic studies of EDTA in rats. Eur J Drug Metab Pharmacokinet 1981;6:21–26.

4. Brownie CF, Brownie C, Noden D, et al: Teratogenic effect of Ca EDTA in rats and the protective effect of zinc. Toxicol Appl Pharmacol 1986;82:426–443.

5. Cantilena LR, Klaassen CD: The effect of chelating agents on the excretion of endogenous metals. Toxicol Appl Pharmacol 1982;63:344–350.

6. Chisolm JJ Jr: The use of chelating agents in the treatment of acute and chronic lead intoxication in childhood. J Pediatr 1968;73:1–38.

7. Chisolm JJ Jr: Mobilization of lead by calcium disodium edetate. Am J Dis Child 1987;141:1256–1257.

8. Chisolm JJ Jr: BAL, EDTA, DMSA and DMPS in the treatment of lead poisoning in children. J Toxicol Clin Toxicol 1992;30:493–504.

9. Chisolm JJ Jr: Safety and efficacy of meso-2,3-dimercaptosuccinic acid (DMSA) in children and elevated blood lead concentrations. J Toxicol Clin Toxicol 2000;38:365–375.

10. Coffin R, Phillips LJ, Staples WL, et al: Treatment of lead encephalopathy in children. J Pediatr 1966;69:198–206.

11. Committee on Drugs: Treatment guidelines for lead exposure in children. Pediatrics 1995;96:155–160.

12. Cory-Slechta D, Weiss B, Cox C: Mobilization and redistribution of lead over the course of calcium disodium ethylenediamine tetraacetate chelation. J Pharmacol Exp Ther 1994;13:253–256.

13. Cory-Slechta DA, Weiss B: Efficacy of the chelating agent CaEDTA in reversing lead-induced changes in behavior. J Toxicol Neuro Toxicol 1989;10:685–698.

14. Cory-Slechta DA, Weiss B, Cox C: Mobilization and redistribution of lead over the course of calcium disodium ethylenediamine tetraacetate chelation therapy. J Pharmacol Exp Ther 1987;243:804–813.

15. Deparis P, Caroldi S: In vivo inhibition of serum dopamine B hydroxylase by CaNa$_2$EDTA injection. Hum Exp Ther 1994;13:253–256.

16. Flora GJS, Seth PK, Prakas A, et al: Therapeutic efficiency of combined meso-2,3-dimercaptosuccinic acid and calcium disodium edetate treatment during acute lead intoxication in rats. Hum Exp Toxicol 1995;14:410–413.

17. Flora SJ, Tandon SK: Influence of calcium disodium edetate on the toxic effects of lead administration in pregnant rats. Indian J Physiol Pharmacol 1987;31:267–272.

18. Flora SJS, Bhattacharga R, Vijayaraghauan R: Combined therapeutic potential of meso-2,3-dimercaptosuccinic acid and calcium disodium edetate on the mobilization and distribution of lead in experimental lead intoxication in rats. Fundam Appl Toxicol 1995;25:233–240.

19. Foreman H, Trujillo T: The metabolism of ^{14}C labeled ethylenediaminetetra-acetic acid in human beings. J Lab Clin Med 1954;43:566–571.

20. Graziano JH, Leong JK, Friedheim E: 2,3-Dimercaptosuccinic acid: A new agent for the treatment of lead poisoning. J Pharmacol Exp Ther 1978;206:696–700.

21. Jones MM, Basinger MA, Gale GR, et al: Effect of chelate treatments on kidney, bone and brain lead levels of lead-intoxicated mice. Toxicology 1994;89:91–100.

22. Jugo S, Maljkovic T, Kostial D: Influence of chelating agents on the gastrointestinal absorption of lead. Toxicol Appl Pharmacol 1975;34:259–263.

23. Klaassen CD: Heavy metals and heavy metal antagonists. In: Gilman AG, Goodman LS, Rall TW, Murad F, eds: Goodman and Gilman's The Pharmacological Basis of Therapeutics, 9th ed. New York, McGraw-Hill, 1996, pp. 1664–1665.

24. Kumark, N: Reversible nephrotoxic reactions to a combined 2,3 dimercapto-1-propanol and calcium disodium ethylene diaminetetraacetic acid regimen in asymptomatic children with elevated blood lead levels. Pediatrics 1982;70:259–262.

25. Markowitz M, Bijur P, Ruff M, et al: Effects of calcium disodium versenate (CaNa$_2$-EDTA) chelation in moderate childhood lead poisoning. Pediatrics 1993;92:265–271.

26. Markowitz M, Rosen J, Piomelli S, Weinberger H: Personal communication, 1995.

27. McKinney PE: Acute elevation of blood lead levels within hours of ingestion of large quantities of lead shot. J Toxicol Clin Toxicol 2000; 38:435–440.

28. Morgan JW: Chelation therapy in lead nephropathy. South Med J 1975;68:1001–1006.

29. Osterloh J, Becker CE: Pharmacokinetics of CaNa$_2$-EDTA and chelation of lead in renal failure. Clin Pharmacol Ther 1986;40:686–693.

30. Piomelli S, Rosen JF, Chisolm JJ Jr, Graef JW: Management of childhood lead poisoning. J Pediatr 1984;105:523–532.

31. Rosen JF, Markowitz ME: Trends in the management of childhood lead poisonings. Neurotoxicology 1993;14:211–217.

32. Ruff HA, Bijur PE, Markowitz M, et al: Declining blood levels and cognitive changes in moderately lead-poisoned children. JAMA 1993;269:1641–1646.

33. Ruff H, Markowitz M, Bijur P, Rosen J: Relationships among blood lead levels, iron deficiency, and cognitive development in two-year-old children. Environ Health Perspect 1996;104:180–185.

34. Schumacher HR, Osterman AL, Choi SJ, et al: Calcinosis at the site of leakage from extravasation of calcium disodium edetate intravenous chelator therapy in a child with lead poisoning. Clin Orthop 1987;219: 221–225.

35. Tandon SK, Flora ST, Singh S: Chelation in metal intoxication: Influence of various components of vitamin B complex on the therapeutic efficacy of Ca EDTA in lead intoxication. Pharmacol Toxicol 1987; 60:62–65.

36. Tandon SK, Singh S, Jain VK: Efficiency at combined chelation in lead intoxication. Chem Res Toxicol 1994;7:585–589.

37. Thomas DJ, Chisolm J: Lead, zinc, copper decorporation during Ca EDTA treatment of lead poisoned children. J Pharmacol Exp Ther 1986;229:829–835.

38. Williams DR, Halstead BW: Chelating agents in medicine. J Toxicol Clin Toxicol 1982–1983;19:1081–1115.

CHAPTER 81 MERCURY

Young-Jin Sue

Mercury

MW	=	200.59 daltons
Normal levels		
Blood	=	<10 µg/L (<50 nmol/L)
Urine	=	<20 µg/L (<100 µnmol/L)
Action levels		
Blood	=	>35 µg/L (>175 nmol/L)
Urine	=	>150 µg/L (>750 nmol/L)

Values greater than or equal to the action level necessitate clinical intervention. Values less than this level may necessitate intervention based on the clinical condition of the patient.

A 16-year-old male presented to the Emergency Department approximately 40 minutes after having intentionally ingested "several teaspoons" of mercuric oxide (HgO) from his chemistry set. On arrival, he was alert and oriented but diaphoretic and vomiting. He complained of midepigastric pain and a metallic taste in his mouth. Initial vital signs were blood pressure, 130/80 mm Hg; pulse, 110 beats/min; respiratory rate, 18 breaths/min; and rectal temperature, 99.7°F (37.6°C). Physical examination revealed an anxious, somewhat pale young man who was repeatedly vomiting blood-tinged, nonbilious material. He had no respiratory distress or drooling. Other than a grayish discoloration of the buccal mucosa, examination of the oropharynx was unremarkable. The lungs were clear. The cardiac examination was normal except for a sinus tachycardia. The abdominal examination revealed a nondistended, soft abdomen, moderately tender to deep palpation in the epigastric region; no masses or organomegaly were appreciated. Rectal examination revealed no trace of blood. Examination of the skin was unremarkable. The neurologic examination was normal except for mild tremulousness.

A cardiac monitor was attached to the patient, and he was given 1 L of 0.9% sodium chloride solution (IV) over the subsequent 15 minutes. Results of a complete blood count (CBC), electrolytes, blood urea nitrogen (BUN), creatinine, glucose, prothrombin time (PT), partial thromboplastin time (PTT), and liver enzymes were within normal limits. Blood was obtained for whole-blood mercury levels, and the bladder was catheterized to collect urine for 24-hour urine mercury quantification. Initial spot urinalysis revealed 2⁺ proteinuria.

Because mercuric oxide may be caustic, endoscopic examination of the upper gastrointestinal (GI) tract was recommended. However, based on this patient's clinical presentation, the treating physician decided that he was at low risk for penetrating mucosal injury and did not request endoscopy. Gastric lavage via nasogastric tube with milk followed by 0.9% sodium chloride solution was performed, and after lavage, 1 g/kg of activated charcoal was instilled.

The electrocardiogram (ECG) was normal except for sinus tachycardia. Upright chest and abdominal radiographs revealed the presence of a radiopaque substance scattered throughout the GI tract but no extraluminal air. Figures 81–1A and B are abdominal radiographs of a patient with a similar exposure. Whole-bowel irrigation with polyethylene glycol electrolyte lavage solution was begun. The rectal effluent contained flecks of blood. A subsequent abdominal radiograph after whole-bowel irrigation revealed no radiopaque densities.

HISTORY AND EPIDEMIOLOGY

The toxicologic manifestations of mercury have become known as a result of thousands of years of medicinal applications, industrial use, and environmental disasters.[49,70] Mercury occurs naturally in small amounts as the elemental silver-colored liquid (quicksilver); as inorganic salts, eg, mercuric sulfide (cinnabar), mercurous chloride (calomel), mercuric chloride (corrosive sublimate), and mercuric oxide; and in organic compounds, (methylmercury). In recent centuries, mercury preparations were widely used to treat both syphilis and constipation. The musician Paganini was among the famous persons whose gingivitis, dental decay, ptyalism, and erethism from mercury therapy are described.[56] In the 1800s, the United States witnessed an epidemic of "hatters' shakes" or "Danbury shakes" and "mercurial salivation" in hat industry workers.[79] Danbury, CT, was a US center of felt hat manufacturing in which mercury nitrate was used to mat animal furs to make felt ("carrotting").[70,79]

In the early 1900s, acrodynia, or "pink disease," was described in children who received calomel for ascariasis or teething discomfort.[15] One of the most devastating epidemics of mercury poisoning occurred as the result of a decade of contamination of Minamata Bay by a nearby vinyl chloride plant during the 1940s. Methylmercury accumulated in the Japanese bay's marine life and resulted in the poisoning of the local fishing community. Although officially only 121 victims were counted initially, thousands more are believed to have been affected by what has subsequently been named Minamata disease.[59,72] The largest outbreak of methylmercury poisoning to date occurred in Iraq in late 1971. Approximately 95,000 tons of seed grain intended for planting and treated with methylmercury as a fungicide were baked into bread for di-

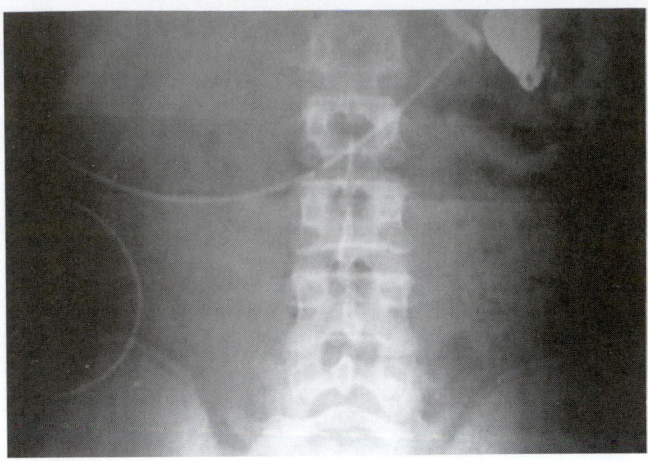

A

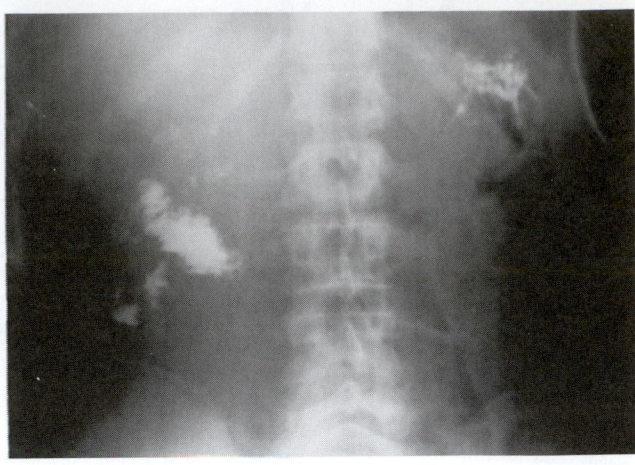

B

Figure 81–1. A chemist ingested mercuric oxide in a suicide attempt. **A.** Initial plain abdominal radiograph reveals the radiopaque liquid in the stomach. **B.** A second radiograph shows progrssion of the toxin through the bowel. The patient was followed radiographically as the substance was eventually expelled into the feces.

rect consumption, resulting in widespread neurologic symptoms, 6530 hospital admissions, and more than 400 deaths.[5,18,62] In 1997, a scientist succumbed to delayed, progressive neurologic deterioration following dermal exposure to a minute quantity of dimethylmercury.[54] Contemporary controversies involving mercury include the potential for toxicity from mercury-containing dental amalgams and mercury-based preservatives (thimerosal) in childhood immunizations. Tables 81–1 and 81–2 show the potential occupational and nonoccupational risks for mercury exposure.

FORMS OF MERCURY AND KINETICS

The three important classes of mercury compounds differ with respect to toxicodynamics and toxicokinetics (Table 81–3). Each of the three classes of mercurials produces distinct clinical patterns of poisoning stemming in part from unique and kinetic features

(Table 81–4). Within each class, the specific poisoning manifestations are determined by route of exposure (eg, inhalational, oral, dermal, or parenteral), rate of exposure, distribution and biotransformation of mercury within the body, and relative accumulation or elimination of mercury by the target organ systems.

Absorption

Elemental Mercury. Elemental mercury (Hg^0) gains access to the circulation primarily via inhalation of vapor, although slow absorption following aspiration, subcutaneous deposition, and direct intravenous embolization is reported.[42,53,76,82] Although elemental mercury is moderately volatile at room temperature, volatilization increases significantly when it is heated. Vaporization may also be hastened by aerosolization. Both occur when elemental mercury is vacuumed.[28,64] When inhaled by human volunteers, 75–80% of a stable and radioactive mercury vapor mixture is retained.[33,46] Because elemental mercury is negligibly absorbed from normally

TABLE 81–1. Potential Occupational Exposures to Mercury

Elemental	Salts	Organic
Amalgam	Disinfectants	Bactericide makers
Barometers	Dye makers	Drug makers
Bronzers	Explosives	Embalmers
Ceramic workers	Fireworks makers	Farmers
Chlorine workers	Fur processors	Fungicides
Dentists	Laboratory workers	Histology technicians
Electroplaters	Tannery workers	Pesticides
Jewelers	Taxidermists	Seed handlers
Mercury refiners	Vinyl chloride makers	Wood preservatives
Paint makers		
Paper pulp workers		
Photographers		
Thermometers		

TABLE 81–2. Nonoccupational Exposures to Mercury

Medicinal	Food	Other
Antiseptics	Fish	Button batteries
Calomel teething powders	Grains and seed, treated	Chemistry sets
Dental amalgam	Livestock, fed treated grain	Home amalgam extraction
Diuretics		Lightbulbs
Laxatives		Self-injection
Sphygmomanometers		Preservatives
Stool fixatives		"Magico-religious" use
Thermometers		
Weighted nasogastric tubes		

TABLE 81–3. Classes of Mercury Compounds

	Formula	Example
Elemental mercury	Hg^0	Quicksilver
Inorganic mercury salts	Hg^+	Mercurous ion
	HgCl	Calomel
	Hg^{2+}	Mercuric ion
	$HgCl_2$	Mercuric chloride
Organic mercury compounds	Short-chain, alkyl-mercury compounds	Methylmercury Ethylmercury
	Long-chain, aryl-mercury compounds	Methoxyethylmercury Phenylmercury

functioning gut, it is usually considered nontoxic when ingested. Abnormal gastrointestinal (GI) motility prolongs mucosal exposure to elemental mercury and increases subsequent ionization to more readily absorbed forms. Similarly, anatomic GI abnormalities such as fistulae or perforation may be associated with extravasation of mercury into the peritoneal space where elemental mercury is oxidized to more readily absorbed inorganic forms.

Inorganic Mercury Salts. The principal route of absorption for inorganic mercury salts is the GI tract. Inorganic mercury salts are absorbed after dissociation of ingested soluble divalent mercuric salts such as mercuric chloride ($HgCl_2$). Approximately 10% of such compounds is absorbed from the gut.[46] Absorption of a relatively insoluble monovalent mercurous compound, such as calomel (HgCl), is thought to depend on its oxidation to the divalent form.[55] Mercuric oxide, a poorly water-soluble compound commonly found in disc batteries, was well-absorbed from ligated gastrointestinal segments of rats, possibly following conversion to chlorides in gastric acid.[24] Inorganic mercury salts are also absorbed across skin and mucous membranes, as evidenced by urinary excretion of mercury following the dermal application of mercurial ointments and powders containing HgCl.[78] The degree

of dermal absorption varies by concentration of mercury, skin integrity, and the lipid solubility of the vehicle. With substantial dermal exposures to inorganic mercury salts, skin absorption may be difficult to distinguish from concomitant absorption via other routes, such as ingestion.

Organic Mercury Compounds. As with inorganic mercury salts, organic mercury compounds are primarily absorbed from the GI tract. Methylmercury, considered the prototype of the short-chain alkyl compounds, is about 90% absorbed from the gut.[46] Aryl and long-chain alkyl compounds have been reported to have greater than 50% gastrointestinal absorption.[55] Although both dermal and inhalational absorption of organic mercury compounds have been reported, precise quantitation and exclusion of concomitant absorption by ingestion are difficult to determine.[20,23,80,81]

Distribution and Biotransformation

After it is absorbed, mercury distributes widely to all tissues, predominantly the kidneys, liver, spleen, and central nervous system (CNS). The initial distributive pattern into nervous tissue of elemental and organic mercury differs from that of the inorganic salts because of their greater lipid solubility.

Elemental Mercury. Although peak levels of elemental mercury are delayed in the CNS as compared to other organs (2–3 days vs 1 day),[11] significant accumulation in the CNS may occur following an acute, intense exposure to elemental mercury vapor. Conversion of elemental mercury to the charged mercuric cation within the CNS favors retention and local accumulation of the metal there. As Hg^0 does not covalently bind to other compounds, its toxicity depends on its oxidation initially to the mercurous ion (Hg^+) and then to the mercuric ion (Hg^{2+}) by the enzyme catalase (Table 81–5).[46] Because this oxidation-reduction reaction favors the mercuric cation at steady state, the distribution and late manifestations of metallic mercury toxicity eventually resemble those of inorganic mercury salt poisoning. Conversely, and to a lesser extent, inorganic mercuric ions are reduced to the elemental state, although the site and mechanism of this reaction are not well understood.[11,55]

Inorganic Mercury Salts. The greatest concentration of mercuric ions is found in the kidneys, particularly within the renal tubules. Very little mercury is found as free mercuric ions. At least in animal studies, administration of mercury induces the renal synthesis of metallothionein, a compound that binds to and detoxifies mercuric ions.[10] In blood, mercuric ions are found within the red blood cells and are bound to plasma proteins in approximately equal proportions. Blood concentrations are greatest immediately following inorganic mercury exposure, with rapid waning as distribution to other tissues occurs. Although penetration of the blood-brain barrier is poor because of low lipid solubility, slow elimination and prolonged exposure contribute to consequential CNS accumulation of mercuric ions. Within the CNS, mercuric ions are concentrated in the cerebral and cerebellar cortices. Although inorganic

TABLE 81–4. Differential Characteristics of Mercury Exposure

	Elemental	Inorganic (Salt)	Organic (Alkyl)
Primary route of exposure	Inhalation	Oral	Oral
Primary tissue distribution	CNS, kidney	Kidney	CNS, kidney, liver
Clearance	Renal, GI	Renal, GI	Methyl:GI Aryl: renal, GI
Clinical effects CNS	Tremor	Tremor, erethism	Paresthesias, ataxia, tremor, tunnel vision, dysarthria
Pulmonary	+++	—	—
Gastrointestinal	+	+++(caustic)	+
Renal	+	+++(ATN)	+
Acrodynia	+	++	—
Therapy	BAL, DMSA	BAL, DMSA	DMSA (early)

TABLE 81–5. Oxidation States of Mercury

$2Hg^0$ [elemental]	←catalase→	$(Hg^+)_2$ (unstable) [mercurous]	↔	$2Hg^{2+}$ [mercuric]

mercurials undergo organification in marine life (see the earlier description of the Minamata Bay disaster), the importance of this conversion in humans is unknown.[20] Animal studies demonstrate that the placenta functions as an effective barrier to mercuric ions.[55]

Organic Mercury Compounds.   Once absorbed, aryl and long-chain alkyl mercury compounds differ from the short-chain organic mercury compounds (ie, methylmercury) in an important way. The former possess a labile carbon-mercury bond, which is cleaved shortly following absorption, releasing the inorganic mercuric ion. Thus, the distribution pattern and toxicologic manifestations produced by the aryl and long-chain alkyl compounds beyond the immediate postabsorptive phase are comparable to those of the inorganic mercury salts, but the organification has facilitated absorption and reduced the caustic effects. In contrast, short-chain alkyl mercury compounds possess relatively stable carbon-mercury bonds and are very slowly converted to the mercuric cation.[80] Because it is lipophilic, methylmercury readily penetrates the blood-brain barrier and is easily transferred across the placenta. An important consequence of the combination of both of these properties is the devastating neurologic degeneration seen in prenatally exposed infants with Minamata disease.

After methylmercury is absorbed in brain tissue, its fate is uncertain. Animal evidence supports the conversion of methylmercury to inorganic mercury in brain tissue.[44] Primates fed oral methylmercury daily for periods exceeding 1 year and then killed within a few days of termination of exposure demonstrated an average brain inorganic mercury fraction of only 19%. When the postexposure period was extended to between 150 and 650 days, the inorganic mercury fraction was increased to 88%. Similarly, greater quantities of inorganic mercury relative to total mercury were found in brains of long-term survivors of methylmercury poisoning.[21] In one patient who survived 22 years following methylmercury ingestion, autopsy results revealed that the brain mercury was nearly completely in the inorganic form.

Methylmercury concentrates in red blood cells (RBCs) to a much greater degree than do mercuric ions, with an RBC to plasma ratio of about 10:1.[55] Despite its apparent affinity for nervous tissue and red blood cells, the kidneys and liver are the sites of greatest methylmercury concentration. Because of its extensive sulfhydryl bonds, the deposition of methylmercury in hair at concentrations approximately 250 times that found in whole blood has encouraged attempts to quantify degree of exposure to methylmercury by hair analysis.[29,39,71]

Elimination

Elemental Mercury/Inorganic Mercury Salts.   Mercuric ions are excreted through the kidney by both glomerular filtration and tubular secretion, and in the GI tract by transfer across gut mesenteric vessels into feces. Small amounts are reduced to elemental mercury vapor and volatilized from skin and lungs. The total-body half-life of elemental mercury and inorganic mercury salts is estimated at approximately 30–60 days.[17,46]

Organic Mercury Compounds.   In contrast to elemental mercury and inorganic mercury salts, the elimination of short-chain alkyl mercury compounds is predominantly fecal. Enterohepatic recirculation contributes to its somewhat longer half-life of about 70

days. Less than 10% of methylmercury is excreted in urine and feces as the mercuric cation.[80]

PATHOPHYSIOLOGY

Mercury's pervasive disruption of normal cell physiology is believed to arise from its avid covalent binding to sulfur, replacing the hydrogen ion in the body's ubiquitous sulfhydryl groups. Mercury also reacts with phosphoryl, carboxyl, and amide groups, resulting in widespread dysfunction of enzymes, transport mechanisms, membranes, and structural proteins. Mercury deposits in all tissues. Not surprisingly, the clinical manifestations of mercury toxicity involve multiple organ systems with variable features and intensity.

Necrosis of the gastrointestinal mucosa and proximal renal tubules, which occurs shortly after mercury salt poisoning, is thought to result from direct oxidative effect of mercuric ions. An immune mechanism is attributed to the membranous glomerulonephritis and acrodynia associated with the use of mercurial ointments.[13,31]

Neurologic manifestations of methylmercury poisoning correlated with pathologic findings in the brains of both adults and children believed to have been prenatally exposed.[48,72] Grossly, atrophy of the brain was more severe in children when methylmercury was either prenatally or postnatally acquired, when compared with the brains of most adult cases. In the adult brain, neuronal necrosis and glial proliferation were most prominent in the calcarine cortex of the cerebrum and in the cerebellar cortex. In fetal Minamata disease, similar lesions were present but in a more diffuse and severe form. Atrophy of the cerebellar hemispheres, postcentral gyri, and calcarine area of the brain on magnetic resonance images in organic mercury-poisoned patients correlated with clinical findings of ataxia, sensory neuropathy, and visual field constriction, respectively.[41]

CLINICAL SYNDROMES

Elemental Mercury

Symptoms of acute elemental mercury inhalation occur within hours of exposure and consist of cough, chills, fever, and shortness of breath. Gastrointestinal complaints include nausea, vomiting, and diarrhea, accompanied by a metallic taste, dysphagia, salivation, weakness, headaches, and visual disturbances. Chest radiography during the acute phase may reveal interstitial pneumonitis and both patchy atelectasis and emphysema. Symptoms may resolve or progress to pulmonary edema, respiratory failure, and death. Survivors of severe pulmonary manifestations may develop interstitial fibrosis and residual restrictive pulmonary disease. The acute respiratory symptoms may occur concomitantly with or lead to the development of subacute inorganic mercury poisoning manifested by tremor, renal dysfunction, and gingivostomatitis. Thrombocytopenia may also occur during the acute phase.[28,64]

While acute exposure to elemental mercury vapor occurs most commonly in the occupational setting, poisonings caused by mishandling of the metal in the home are reported.[36,52,68,73] Numerous attempts at home metallurgy with metallic mercury have resulted in fatalities. In such a home environment, ambient air concentrations of mercury were found to be as high as 900 μg/m³, ultimately necessitating demolition of the home after futile attempts at decontamination.[50] The lethal dose of inhaled elemental mercury has not been determined. As with other inhaled toxins, younger individuals may possess greater sensitivity to the pulmonary toxicity of mercury vapor. A 7-month-old infant and the family's young kitten were the first to succumb to fumes generated during attempts to heat metallic mercury on the kitchen stove.[52] Although respiratory toxicity from elemental mercury usually results from inhalation of vapor, massive endobronchial hemorrhage followed by death has occurred following direct aspiration of metallic mercury into the tracheobronchial tree.[84]

Gradual volatilization of elemental mercury has resulted in chronic toxicity, both in the occupational setting and in the home, from improper handling, such as vacuuming spilled mercury.[51,64,73] In a typical case of poisoning following domestic exposure to elemental mercury, two siblings presented with ataxia several weeks after approximately 20 mL of elemental mercury was spilled in their home. Evaluation revealed distal paresthesias, mild weakness, and absent deep-tendon reflexes.[73] One child had persistent weakness, visual field defects, and emotional lability despite chelation.

The clinical importance of volatilized metallic mercury from dental amalgams for both the dentist and patient has been a point of contention for years. The preponderance of evidence currently refutes the idea that mercury poisoning results from dental amalgams. Several comprehensive reviews of the subject conclude that (a) occupational exposure to mercury from dental amalgam is acceptably low provided that recommended preventive measures (eg, adequate ventilation) are adhered to; (b) the quantity of mercury vaporized from dental amalgam by mechanical forces such as chewing is clinically insignificant; and (c) in very rare cases, hypersensitivity to mercury amalgam may necessitate removal of the amalgam.[22,25,26,27,43,67]

Unusual cases of chronic toxicity have resulted from intentional subcutaneous or intravenous injection of elemental mercury (Figs. 8–6 and 81–2).[35,53] Aside from management specific to mercury toxicity, local wound care and excision of deposits of mercury were additional therapeutic challenges presented by these cases. Radiographs are useful in guiding the removal of the radiopaque deposits.

Inorganic Mercury Salts

Acute ingestion of mercuric salts produces a characteristic spectrum from severe irritant to caustic gastroenteritis. Immediately, a grayish discoloration of mucous membranes and metallic taste may accompany local oropharyngeal pain, nausea, vomiting, and diarrhea in addition to abdominal pain, hematemesis, and hematochezia. The lethal dose of mercuric chloride has been estimated at 30–50 mg/kg.[11] The hallmarks of severe acute mercuric salt ingestion are hemorrhagic gastroenteritis, massive fluid loss resulting in shock, and acute tubular necrosis. A 27-year-old man presented with hematemesis 24 hours after reportedly ingesting 6 g of mercuric chloride in a suicide attempt. Shortly after admission, he developed hypotension and oliguric renal failure, and then underwent gastrectomy for total gastric necrosis. He remained on hemodialysis until he died of sepsis 3 months later.[63]

Oropharyngeal injury, nausea, hematemesis, hematochezia, and abdominal pain were prominent symptoms in a series of 54 patients who presented after ingesting up to 4 g of mercuric chlo-

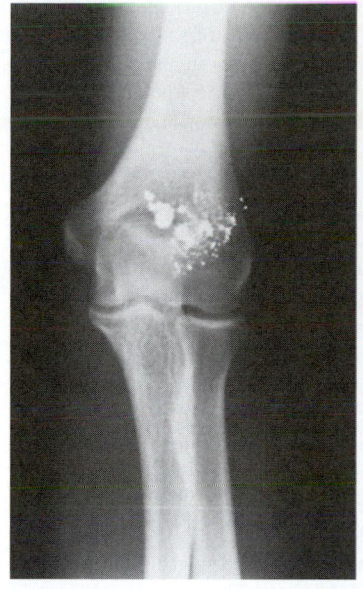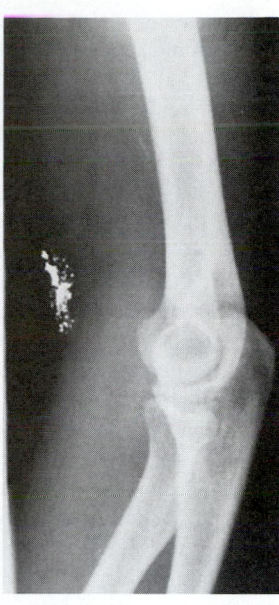

A   **B**

Figure 81–2.   A-P (**A**) and lateral (**B**) view of the elbow after an unsuccessful suicidal gesture involving an attempted intravenous injection of mercury in the antecubital fossa. Note extensive mercury deposition, which was partially removed by surgical intervention. (Courtesy of Diane Sauter, MD.)

ride.[74] In this group, a fatal outcome was associated with the early development of oliguria (within 3 days). The development of anuria appeared to be related to the dose of mercuric chloride ingested. The histopathologic finding of proximal tubular necrosis following mercuric salt poisoning is thought to result from both direct toxicity to renal tubules by mercuric ions and from renal hypoperfusion caused by shock, suggesting that aggressive fluid therapy may be useful.[31]

Acute ingestion of mercuric salts is usually intentional, but unintentional ingestion occurs sporadically in children as well as adults.[37] A 2-year-old girl developed melena 2 days after swallowing a mercuric oxide–containing disc battery.[47] Abdominal radiograph revealed two battery halves surrounded by radiopaque material in the stomach and proximal gut. During surgical removal of the battery fragments, areas of ulceration and bleeding were found in the gastric mucosa. Although ingestion of button batteries containing mercuric oxide is associated with a greater incidence of fragmentation than with other batteries, clinical systemic mercury toxicity by this route has not been reported.[45]

Mercuric chloride–containing stool preservatives are also a potential source of unintentional inorganic mercury poisoning. Two young children presented with bloody gastroenteritis and proteinuria after ingesting 10–20 mL of a polyvinyl alcohol preservative that contained 4.5% mercuric chloride.[65] One child had a relatively benign course and was discharged following 5 days of oral chelation. The other required dialysis for renal failure but subsequently recovered without apparent sequelae. Ethnic medicines are yet another source of unintentional inorganic mercury poisoning.[38] Because they are not subject to FDA regulation and available without prescription, these substances are often inadequately labeled and of variable composition (Chap. 77).

Subacute or chronic mercury poisoning occurs after (a) inhalation, aspiration, or injection of elemental mercury; (b) ingestion or application of inorganic mercury salts; or (c) ingestion of aryl or long-chain alkyl mercury compounds. Slow in vivo oxidation of elemental mercury and dissociation of the carbon-mercury bond of aryl or long-chain alkyl mercury compounds result in the production of the inorganic mercurous and mercuric ions.

The predominant manifestations of subacute or chronic mercury toxicity include gastrointestinal symptoms, neurologic abnormalities, and renal dysfunction. Gastrointestinal symptoms consist of a metallic taste and burning sensation in the mouth, loose teeth and gingivostomatitis, hypersalivation, and nausea.[78] The neurologic manifestations of chronic inorganic mercurialism are described by tremor and the overlapping syndromes of neurasthenia and erethism. Neurasthenia is a symptom complex that includes fatigue, depression, headaches, hypersensitivity to stimuli, psychosomatic complaints, weakness, and loss of concentrating ability. Erethism, derived from the Greek word *red*, describes the easy blushing and intense shyness of the sufferer. In addition, the symptoms include anxiety, emotional lability, irritability, insomnia, anorexia, weight loss, and delirium. The mercurial tremor is well described in numerous case reports as a central intention tremor that is abolished during sleep. In the most severe forms of mercury-associated tremor, choreoathetosis and spasmodic ballismus may be present. Other neurologic manifestations of inorganic mercurialism include a mixed sensorimotor neuropathy, ataxia, concentric constriction of visual fields ("tunnel vision"), and anosmia.

Chronic poisoning with mercuric ions is associated with renal dysfunction, which ranges from asymptomatic, reversible proteinuria to nephrotic syndrome with edema and hypoproteinemia. Renal histology of patients with mercury-associated nephrotic syndrome is suggestive of an immune glomerulonephritis.[13] Postmortem examination of the kidneys from two women who died following chronic abuse of mercurous chloride–containing laxatives revealed severe proximal tubular atrophy and mercury deposition within the cortical interstitium and renal macrophages.[77]

An idiosyncratic hypersensitivity to mercury ions is thought to be responsible for acrodynia or "pink disease," which is an erythematous, edematous, and hyperkeratotic induration of the palms, soles, and face, and a pink papular rash seen largely in a subset of children exposed to mercurous powders. The rash is described as morbilliform, urticarial, vesicular, and hemorrhagic. This symptom complex also includes excessive sweating, tachycardia, irritability, anorexia, photophobia, insomnia, tremors, paresthesias, decreased deep-tendon reflexes, and weakness. The acral rash may progress to desquamation and ulceration. The prognosis is favorable after withdrawal from mercury exposure. Acrodynia was vividly described 50 years ago in 41 children, many of whom were treated with mercurous chloride calomel-containing powders or ointments.[78] The authors observed that the development of acrodynia following exposure to mercury was more common in younger children, did not seem to correlate with dose, and was not necessarily related to urine concentrations of mercury.

Childhood acrodynia has become uncommon since the abandonment of mercurial teething powders and diaper rinses. Occasional case reports are still noted, however. An 8-year-old child developed acrodynia with a scarlatiniform rash, irritability, and myalgias after playing with elemental mercury for several days.[3] Particularly striking were the presence of an unremittingly pruritic, vesicular eruption of the hands and feet, profuse diaphoresis which necessitated four or five changes of clothes each day, and

the child's maintenance of a rigid fetal position. A 23-month-old child developed acrodynia following exposure to mercury from shattered fluorescent light bulbs,[75] and a 4-year-old boy developed acrodynia and increased urinary mercury excretion 10 days after the interior of his home was painted with phenylmercuric acetate–containing paint. The paint used was subsequently found to contain approximately 3 times the concentration of mercury recommended by the Environmental Protection Agency (EPA). In 1990, the EPA banned mercury-containing compounds from interior paints.[2] However, mercury-containing paints manufactured prior to that ruling or marketed for outdoor use can still be sold.

Thimerosal is an example of an aryl or long-chain alkyl mercury compound that results in chronic inorganic mercury toxicity. It is a compound that is widely used as a preservative in the pharmaceutical industry (Chap. 56). Although initial kinetics suggest a stable ethyl-mercury bond, the later elimination phase more closely resembles that of the inorganic mercury compounds. Thimerosal is approximately 50% mercury by weight. Although it is generally considered safe, toxicity and death can occur following both intentional overdose and excessive therapeutic application of Merthiolate (0.1% thimerosal or 600 μg/mL mercury). An 18-month-old child with chronic otitis media and bilateral tympanostomy tubes developed neurologic symptoms after receiving a total of 1.2 L of Merthiolate as an ear irrigant over a period of 4 weeks. A substantial amount was believed to have been swallowed after draining through the tympanostomy tubes.[61] Examination of the child revealed irritability, ataxia, tremors, and opisthotonic posturing. Despite chelation with *N*-acetyl penicillamine (NAP), the child died 3 months after hospitalization. A 44-year-old man developed gastritis, renal failure, delirium, and polyneuropathy following intentional ingestion of 5 g of thimerosal.[58] He survived with supportive care and the use of oral chelating agents, dimercaptopropane sulfonate (DMPS) and dimercaptosuccinic acid (DMSA).

Recent concern that the cumulative dose of thimerosal in childhood immunizations may exceed federally recommended maximum mercury doses (Environmental Protection Agency, 0.1 μg/kg/d; Agency for Toxic Substances and Disease Registry, 0.3 μg/kg/d; Food and Drug Administration, 0.4 μg/kg/d) led to a call by the American Academy of Pediatrics to reduce or eliminate thimerosal from vaccines. Currently, vaccinations contain 25 μg or less of mercury per 0.5 mL of vaccine.[4] Many immunizations contain no thimerosal. Although sensitization following use in vaccinations has been reported in atopic children,[57] clinical mercury toxicity is not reported in appropriately immunized children. A rise in blood mercury levels following a single dose of hepatitis B vaccine was demonstrated in preterm infants.[69] This rise, while greater than that seen in a control group of term infants, has uncertain clinical significance. Until an alternate preservative is developed for use in childhood vaccines, the use of thimerosal is required for vaccines distributed in multidose vials, an economic necessity in developing countries. At the present time, there is clearly more evidence for risk to child health from the diseases targeted for prevention by the vaccines than from thimerosal. For infants born to hepatitis B surface antigen–negative mothers, the Academy recommends that initiation of the vaccine series should be deferred until the infant is 2–6 months of age.

Organic Mercury Compounds

In contrast to the inorganic mercurials, methylmercury produces an almost purely neurologic disease that is usually permanent except in the mildest of cases. Although the predominant syndrome associated with methylmercury is that of a delayed neurotoxicity, acutely, gastrointestinal symptoms, tremor, respiratory distress, and dermatitis may occur.[20,80] Characteristically, clinical manifestations follow the initial poisoning by a latent period of weeks to months. Consequently, the lethal dose is difficult to determine for methylmercury. The Agency for Toxic Substances and Disease Registry minimal risk level with respect to developmental effects is set at 0.04 µg/kg for acute oral exposure.[11] The lipophilic property and slower elimination of methylmercury may contribute to its profound neurologic effects.[23]

Infants exposed prenatally to methylmercury were the most severely affected individuals in the Minamata Bay environmental catastrophe. Often born to mothers with little or no manifestation of methylmercury intoxication themselves, exposed infants exhibited decreased birth weight and muscle tone, profound developmental delay, seizure disorders, deafness, blindness, and severe spasticity. The development of neurologic symptoms in infants exclusively breast-fed by women exposed to methylmercury after delivery and the detection of mercury in the milk of lactating women are very strong evidence for the risk of mercury poisoning via breast milk.[23,40]

Several weeks after ingesting the methylmercury-contaminated grain in Iraq, cases of paresthesias involving the lips, nose, and distal extremities began to appear. Symptomatic patients also noted headaches, fatigue, and tremor. More serious cases progressed to ataxia, dysarthria, visual field constriction, and blindness. Other neurologic deficits included hyperreflexia, hearing disturbances, movement disorders, salivation, and dementia. The most severely affected patients lay in a mute rigid posture punctuated only by spontaneous crying, primitive reflexive movements, or feeding efforts.[62]

While the outlook for methylmercury neurotoxicity is generally considered dismal, observations over the subsequent 2 years in 49 Iraqi children poisoned during the 1971 outbreak revealed complete resolution or at least partial improvement in all but the most severely affected.[5] Of 40 symptomatic children, 33 mildly to severely affected children showed partial to complete resolution of symptoms. The 7 children classified as "very severely poisoned" remained physically and mentally incapacitated.

While neurologic disease is by far the dominant manifestation of methylmercury poisoning, dermatitis, electrocardiographic abnormalities (ST segment changes), and renal tubular dysfunction are also associated with this poisoning.[23,34]

Dimethylmercury is another short-chain organic mercury compound. Its extreme toxicity was tragically demonstrated by the delayed fatal neurotoxicity that developed in a chemist who inadvertently spilled dimethylmercury on her gloved hands. Over a period of several days, she developed progressive difficulty with speech, vision, and gait. Despite chelation and exchange transfusion, she died within several months of the exposure.[54] Neuropathologic examination of her brain revealed lesions in the cerebellum, temporal lobe, and visual cortex.[66]

INITIAL MANAGEMENT

After initial assessment and stabilization, the early toxicologic management of mercury poisoning includes termination of exposure by removal from vapors; washing exposed skin; gastrointestinal decontamination; supportive measures such as hydration and humidified oxygen; baseline diagnostic studies such as serum laboratories, radiographs, and electrocardiogram; consideration of cointoxicants; and meticulous monitoring.

Inhalation of mercury vapors or aspiration of metallic mercury may result in life-threatening respiratory failure, and in this situation, stabilization of cardiorespiratory function is the initial priority. Postural drainage and endotracheal suction may be effective in removing aspirated metallic mercury. Parenteral deposition of subcutaneous or intramuscular mercury may be amenable to surgical excision if well localized (Fig. 81–2).

Ingestion of inorganic mercuric salts may lead to cardiovascular collapse caused by severe gastroenteritis and third-space fluid loss. Gastrointestinal decontamination of ingested inorganic salts of mercury is particularly problematic because of the salts' caustic nature and risk for perforating injury. Endoscopic examination of the upper gastrointestinal tract is suggested by some prior to attempts at gastric emptying and lavage. However, one series of mercuric chloride poisonings reported recovery without long-term gastrointestinal sequelae in patients who did not succumb to renal failure.[74] Therefore, unless there is high suspicion for penetrating gastrointestinal mucosal injury, removal of mercury from absorptive surfaces should take priority over endoscopic evaluation.

Lavage with protein-containing solutions such as milk or egg whites has been advocated in the belief that mercury may be bound to the administered sulfhydryl-containing proteins and thereby be more readily removed by subsequent lavage.[8] Until this is rigorously studied, it is probably not harmful and may be of benefit. Metals are among the substances that are often stated to be poorly adsorbed to activated charcoal. Nevertheless, the serious nature of late sequelae following mercury absorption, the typically small quantities of mercury ingested, and evidence that inorganic mercuric compounds have substantial adsorption to activated charcoal (800 mg mercuric chloride to 1 g activated charcoal in one in vitro study[6]) justify administration of the adsorbent. Whole-bowel irrigation with polyethylene glycol solution may be useful in removing residual mercury, and therefore should be used and followed by obtaining serial radiographs.

Included in the initial management of mercury poisoning is consideration for environmental decontamination. Elemental mercury spilled onto solid surfaces should be adsorbed to sand and the resulting mixture then be swept into tightly sealed containers. Ideally, a mercury decontamination kit should be used. The kit consists of calcium polysulfide, which contains excess sulfur to convert mercury to water-insoluble mercuric sulfide (cinnabar). Absorbent surfaces, such as carpets, should be removed. Spilled mercury compounds should not be vacuumed because vacuuming could volatilize the substances.[16] Guidance for decontamination of major spills and disposal of materials can be provided by local and federal hazardous materials agencies.

LABORATORY

The dual findings of unexplained neuropsychiatric and renal abnormalities in an individual should alert the examiner to the possibility of mercurialism, as should an at-risk occupation or access by the patient to a mercurial product (Tables 81–1 and 81–2).

Occupational or environmental exposure and a consistent clinical scenario may be suggestive of mercury poisoning, but demonstration of mercury in blood, urine, or tissues is necessary for confirmation of exposure. Of the many methods available to measure mercury, cold atomic absorption spectrometry is rapid, sensitive, and accurate, but cannot distinguish the various forms of mercury. Thin-layer and gas chromatographic techniques can be used to distinguish organic from inorganic mercury.[20] Blood should be collected into a trace-element collection tube obtained from the laboratory performing the assay. Urine should be collected for 24 hours into an acid-washed container obtained from the laboratory. Attempts to measure or otherwise handle the specimen should be avoided to prevent contamination.

There is considerable overlap among concentrations of mercury found in the normal population, asymptomatic exposed individuals, and patients with clinical evidence of poisoning. There is no definitive correlation between either blood or urine mercury levels and mercury toxicity.[11,29] However, mercury is virtually undetectable in the nonpoisoned individual, and levels less than 10 μg/L and 20 μg/L for whole blood and urine, respectively, are generally considered normal. Following long-term exposure to mercury vapor, levels as low as 35 μg/L for blood and 150 μg/L for urine may be associated with nonspecific symptoms of mercury poisoning.[30]

Urine mercury levels may correlate roughly with exposure severity and neuropsychiatric symptoms associated with inorganic mercury poisoning,[11,60] but the relationship to total body burden is probably poor. Urine mercury values have their greatest utility in confirming exposure and monitoring the efficacy of chelation therapy. Whole-blood mercury levels may acutely reflect inorganic mercury load, but become less reliable as redistribution to tissues takes place.

Because of the very minimal urinary excretion of organic mercury, urine mercury levels are not useful in evaluating methylmercury poisoning. Because of the relative concentration of methylmercury in red blood cells, total body methylmercury burden may be best reflected by blood levels.[20] Blood levels may well correlate with acute toxicity of methylmercury. However, as methylmercury distributes to and accumulates in brain, the severity of clinical manifestations probably more closely reflects the degree of the irreversible neuronal destruction that has taken place rather than the current body burden of mercury. Correlation of increasing blood mercury levels with prevalence of paresthesias was suggested in a population of Iraqis studied early in the course of methylmercury poisoning.[19] However, in another group of patients, blood levels did not correlate with severity of methylmercury poisoning.[62] This apparent discrepancy may have resulted from the finding that paresthesias are among the earliest reported symptoms of methylmercury poisoning.

Because mercury accumulates in hair, hair analysis may be a tool for measuring mercury burden. The reliability of this method is questionable because metal incorporation reflects past exposure, and hair avidly binds mercury from the environment. Nevertheless, some authors support its use.[39] One analysis comparing organic mercury concentrations in the distal scalp hairs to other organs of cadavers demonstrated significant correlation, with correlation coefficients ranging from 0.59 to 0.82 for the cerebrum and from 0.65 to 0.76 for the kidney.[71] The hair was prepared by washing in a nonionic detergent followed by acid digestion. In addition to mercury assays, neuropsychiatric testing, nerve conduction studies, and urine assays for N-acetyl β-D-glucosaminidase and β₂-microglobulin are advocated for early detection of subclinical inorganic and organic mercury toxicity.[26,34,60]

TREATMENT

After initial stabilization and decontamination early institution of chelating agents may minimize or prevent widespread effects of mercury resulting from its affinity for essential cellular sulfhydryl groups. A high degree of protein binding and distribution to the brain are responsible for the lack of efficacy of other measures such as peritoneal dialysis and hemodialysis to increase mercury clearance.[63] Hemodialysis may nevertheless be ultimately necessary because of the acute renal failure that often follows mercuric chloride poisoning.

Chelating agents themselves have thiol groups that are believed to compete with endogenous sulfhydryl groups for the binding of mercury. They thereby prevent inactivation of sulfhydryl-containing enzymes and other essential proteins (Antidotes in Depth: Dimercaprol and Antidotes in Depth: Succimer for further discussion). A history of significant mercury exposure and the presence of typical symptoms of mercury poisoning are sufficient indications for the institution of chelation therapy. Elevated blood and urine mercury concentrations can help support the decision to begin chelation therapy in unclear cases and may also be used to guide duration of therapy.

For clinically significant acute inorganic mercury poisoning, dimercaprol (BAL) may be administered for 10 days in decreasing dosages, eg, 5 mg/kg IM once, 2.5 mg/kg IM every 8–12 hours for 1 day, and then 2.5 mg/kg IM every 12–24 hours thereafter until clinical improvement occurs. This dosing regimen of BAL, derived from the use of BAL in lead poisoning, may be adjusted according to clinical response and the occurrence of adverse reactions. Some animal evidence suggests that BAL may increase mercury mobilization into the brain. However, in that instance, phenylmercury and BAL were administered simultaneously. It is unclear whether the increased brain mercury represented altered distribution as a result of a phenylmercury-BAL complex or a BAL-driven redistribution of inorganic mercury.[14]

When a patient is able to take oral medications, BAL therapy may be augmented with 2,3-dimercaptosuccinic acid (DMSA) at 10 mg/kg orally 3 times a day for 5 days. Adverse effects such as headache, nausea, vomiting, abdominal pain, and diaphoresis may result from the primary ingestion as well as from the chelation therapy, especially when BAL is used. For patients who are not acutely ill or who have been chronically poisoned, initiation of therapy with oral DMSA is recommended, as the adverse effects and pain of administration of BAL are probably not warranted.

D-Penicillamine (DPCN) is an orally administered monothiol with adverse effects that include gastrointestinal distress, rashes, leukopenia, thrombocytopenia, and proteinuria (Chap. 82C). Although uncommon when therapeutic doses are used, these adverse effects may seriously limit the utility of the drug. The use of DPCN has largely been supplanted by DMSA. Because the DPCN-mercury chelation compound is excreted exclusively into urine, other agents should be used in the presence of renal failure. N-Acetyl-d,l-penicillamine (NAP), an investigational analogue of DPCN, has been used with variable success for mercury poisoning.[9,32] NAP is thought to be a more effective chelator of mercury than DPCN, perhaps because of its greater stability.[7] The penicillamines should be administered only after complete gastrointestinal decontamination, as the absorption of mercury may theoretically be enhanced following chelation by penicillamine.

The neurotoxicity of methylmercury and other organic mercury compounds is relatively resistant to treatment, and the optimum mode of therapy is not clear. In rats treated with BAL or DPCN following injection with methylmercury, both agents were effective at reducing tissue mercury and preventing neurologic toxicity if administered within the first day of a methylmercury injection.[83] However, neither agent reversed neurologic toxicity when administered 12 days after injection of methylmercury despite a decrease of tissue mercury in rats treated with DPCN. DMPS or 2,3-dimercapto-1-propanesulphonate, an investigational water-soluble analogue of BAL, led to a striking reduction of blood half-life of mercury, ie, 10 days versus 60 days, when compared with DPCN, NAP, and a thiolated resin (half-lives of 24 days, 23 days, and 19 days, respectively) during the outbreak of methylmercury poisoning in Iraq in 1971.[19] Clinical improvement was not observed in any treatment group, but it is reasonable to postulate that reducing the total body burden of methylmercury may prevent or limit progression of disease. When studied in mice poisoned with methylmercury,[1] DMSA was superior to NAP, DMPS, and a thiolated resin in decreasing brain mercury and increasing urinary excretion. Brain mercury was decreased to 35% of control, and total body burden fell to 19%. A nonabsorbed polythiol resin may reduce the elimination half-life of methylmercury, presumably by interrupting its enterohepatic reabsorption.[19,23]

Oral N-acetylcysteine enhanced urinary excretion and decreased tissue concentrations of methylmercury in mice.[12] A similar effect was not demonstrated for inorganic mercury. The mice were treated for only 48 hours following intraperitoneal injection with methylmercury. The generalizability of these findings to more long-standing human poisonings is unclear.

As the neurologic impairment associated with methylmercury is both profound and essentially irreversible, early recognition of poisoning and prevention of neurotoxicity are essential to a successful outcome. Although further investigation is necessary, DMSA may prove to be the treatment of choice for methylmercury poisoning because of its apparently low toxicity and reported efficacy in animal trials.

SUMMARY

Mercury poisoning is a complex toxicologic problem associated with a large variety of clinical presentations. An ever-present awareness of the problem, coupled with the knowledge of its differing clinical forms, may serve to guide recognition and treatment. Although some chelating agents do show promise in the treatment of mercury poisoning, neurologic sequelae, particularly those resulting from organic mercury exposures, remain largely irreversible. Promotion of public education regarding the dangers of mercury may aid in the prevention of mercury poisoning.

REFERENCES

1. Aaseth J, Friedheim EAH: Treatment of methyl mercury poisoning in mice with 2,3-dimercaptosuccinic acid and other complexing thiols. Acta Pharmacol Toxicol 1978;42:248–252.
2. Agocs MM, Etzel RA, Parrish G, et al: Mercury exposure from interior latex paint. N Engl J Med 1990;323:1096–1100.
3. Alexander JF, Rosario R: A case of mercury poisoning: Acrodynia in a child of 8. Can Med Assoc J 1971;104:929–930.
4. American Academy of Pediatrics, Committee on Infectious Diseases and Committee on Environmental Health: Thimerosal in vaccines—An interim report to clinicians. Pediatrics 1999;104(3 Pt 1):570–574.
5. Amin-Zaki L, Majeed MA, Clarkson TW, Greenwood MR: Methylmercury poisoning in Iraqi children: Clinical observations over two years. Br Med J 1978;1:613–616.
6. Andersen AH: Experimental studies on the pharmacology of activated charcoal; III. Adsorption from gastrointestinal contents. Acta Pharmacol 1948;4:275–284.
7. Aposhian HV, Aposhian MM: N-acetyl-d,l-penicillamine, a new oral protective agent against the lethal effects of mercuric chloride. J Pharmacol 1959;126:131–135.
8. Arena JM: Treatment of mercury poisoning. Mod Treat 1971;8:619–625.
9. Aronow R, Fleischmann LE: Mercury poisoning in children. Clin Pediatr 1976;15;936–945.
10. Asano S, Eto K, Kurisaki E, et al: Acute inorganic mercury vapor inhalation poisoning. Pathol Int 2000;50:169–174.
11. ATSDR: Toxicologic profile for mercury. Atlanta, GA, USDHHS, 1992. Draft.
12. Ballatori B, Lieberman MW, Wang W: N-Acetylcysteine as an antidote in methylmercury poisoning. Environ Health Perspect 1998;106(5):267–271.
13. Becker CG, Becker EL, Maher JF, Schreiner GE: Nephrotic syndrome after contact with mercury. Arch Intern Med 1962;110:178–186.
14. Berlin M, Rylander R: Increased brain uptake of mercury induced by 2,3-dimercaptopropanol (BAL) in mice exposed to phenylmercuric acetate. J Pharmacol Exp Ther 1964;146:236–240.
15. Black J: The puzzle of pink disease. J R Soc Med 1999;92:478–481.
16. Campbell D, Gonzales M, Sullivan JB: Mercury. In: Sullivan JB, Krieger GR, eds: Hazardous Material Toxicology. Baltimore, Williams & Wilkins, 1992, pp. 824–833.
17. Clarkson TE: Mercury. J Am Coll Toxicol 1989;8(7):1291–1296.
18. Clarkson TW, Amin-Zaki L, Al-Tikriti SK: An outbreak of methylmercury poisoning due to consumption of contaminated grain. Fed Proc 1976;35:2395–2399.
19. Clarkson TW, Magos L, Greenwood MR, et al: Tests of efficacy of antidotes for removal of methylmercury in human poisoning during the Iraq outbreak. J Pharmacol Exp Ther 1981;218:74–83.
20. Dales LG: The neurotoxicity of alkyl mercury compounds. Am J Med 1972;53:219–232.
21. Davis LE, Kornfeld M, Mooney HS, et al: Methylmercury poisoning: Long-term clinical, radiological, toxicological, and pathological studies of an affected family. Ann Neurol 1994;35:680–688.
22. Eley BM, Cox SW: Mercury from dental amalgam fillings in patients. Br Dent J 1987;163:221–225.
23. Elhassani SB: The many faces of methylmercury poisoning. J Toxicol Clin Toxicol 1982–1983;19:875–906.
24. Endo T, Nakaya S, Kimura R, Murata T: Gastrointestinal absorption of inorganic mercuric compounds in vivo and in situ. Toxicol Appl Pharmacol 1984;74:223–229.
25. Englund GS, Dahlquist R, Lindelof B, et al: DMSA administration to patients with alleged mercury poisoning from dental amalgams—A placebo-controlled study. J Dent Res 1994;73:620–628.
26. Eti S, Weisman RS, Hoffman RS, Reidenberg MM: Slight renal effect of mercury amalgam fillings. Pharmacol Toxicol 1995;76:47–49.
27. Fung YK, Molvar MP: Toxicity of mercury from dental environment and from amalgam restorations. J Toxicol Clin Toxicol 1992;30:49–61.
28. Fuortes LJ, Weismann DN, Graeff ML, et al: Immune thrombocytopenia and elemental mercury poisoning. J Toxicol Clin Toxicol 1995;33:449–455.
29. Gosselin RE, Smith RP, Hodge HC: Mercury. In: Gosselin RE, Smith RP, Hodge HC, eds: Clinical Toxicology of Commercial Products, 5th ed. Baltimore, Williams & Wilkins, 1984, pp. 262–275.

30. Goyer RA: Toxic effects of metals. In: Amdur MO, Doull J, Klaassen CD, eds: Casarett and Doull's Toxicology: The Basic Science of Poisons, 4th ed. New York, Pergamon Press, 1991, pp. 623–680.

31. Hewitt WR, Goldstein RS, Hook JB: Toxic responses of the kidney. In: Amdur MO, Doull J, Klaassen CD, eds: Casarett and Doull's Toxicology: The Basic Science of Poisons, 4th ed. New York, Pergamon Press, 1991, pp. 354–382.

32. Hryhorczuk DO, Meyers L, Chen G: Treatment of mercury intoxication in a dentist with N-acetyl-d,l-penicillamine. Clin Toxicol 1982; 19:401–408.

33. Hursh JB, Clarkson TW, Cherian MG, et al: Clearance of mercury (Hg-197, Hg-203) vapor inhaled by human subjects. Arch Environ Health 1976;31:302–309.

34. Iesato K, Wakashin M, Wakashin Y, Tojo S: Renal tubular dysfunction in Minamata disease: Detection of renal tubular antigen and beta-2-microglobulin in the urine. Ann Intern Med 1977;86:731–737.

35. Johnson HRM, Koumides O: Unusual case of mercury poisoning. Br Med J 1967;1:340–341.

36. Jung RC, Aaronson J: Death following inhalation of mercury vapor at home. West J Med 1980;132:539–543.

37. Kahn A, Denis R, Blum D: Accidental ingestion of mercuric sulphate in a 4-year-old child. Clin Pediatr 1977;16:956–958.

38. Kang-Yum E, Oransky SH: Chinese patent medicine as a potential source of mercury poisoning. Vet Hum Toxicol 1992;34:235–238.

39. Katz SA, Katz RB: Use of hair analysis for evaluating mercury intoxication of the human body: A review. J Appl Toxicol 1992;12:79–84.

40. Koos BJ, Longo LD: Mercury toxicity in the pregnant woman, fetus, and newborn infant: A review. Am J Obstet Gynecol 1976;126: 390–409.

41. Korogi Y, Takahashi M, Shinzato J, Okajima T: MR findings in seven patients with organic mercury poisoning (Minamata disease). Am J Neuroradiol 1994;15:1575–1578.

42. Krohn IT, Solof A, Mobini J, Wagner DK: Subcutaneous injection of metallic mercury. JAMA 1980;243:548–549.

43. Langan DC, Fan PL, Hoos AA: The use of mercury in dentistry: Critical review of the recent literature. J Am Dent Assoc 1987;115: 867–879.

44. Lind B, Friberg L, Nylander M: Preliminary studies on methylmercury biotransformation and clearance in the brain of primates: II. Demethylation of mercury in brain. J Trace Elem Exp Med 1988; 1:49–56.

45. Litovitz T, Schmitz BF: Ingestion of cylindrical and button batteries: An analysis of 2382 cases. Pediatrics 1992;89:747–757.

46. Magos L: Mercury. In: Seiler HG, Sigel H, eds: Handbook on Toxicity of Inorganic Compounds. New York, Marcel Dekker, 1988, pp. 419–436.

47. Mant TGK, Lewis JL, Mattoo TK, et al: Mercury poisoning after disc-battery ingestion. Hum Toxicol 1987;6:179–181.

48. Matsumoto H, Koya G, Takeuchi T: Fetal Minamata disease: A neuropathological study of two cases of intrauterine intoxication by a methyl mercury compound. J Neuropathol Exp 1964;24:563–574.

49. Maurissen JPJ: History of mercury and mercurialism. N Y State J Med 1981;81:1902–1909.

50. Acute, chronic poisoning, residential exposures to elemental mercury –Michigan, 1989–1990. Morb Mortal Wkly Rep 1991;40: 393–395.

51. Mortensen ME, Powell S, Sferra TJ: Elemental mercury poisoning in a household. Morb Mortal Wkly Rep 1990;39:424–425.

52. Moutinho ME, Tompkins AL, Rowland TW, et al: Acute mercury vapor poisoning. Am J Dis Child 1981;135:42–44.

53. Murray KM, Hedgepeth JC: Intravenous self-administration of elemental mercury: Efficacy of dimercaprol therapy. Drug Intell Clin Pharm 1988;22:972–975.

54. Nierenberg DW, Nordgren RE, Chang MB, et al: Delayed cerebellar disease and death after accidental exposure to dimethylmercury. N Engl J Med 1998;338:1672–1676.

55. Nordberg GF, Skerfving S: Metabolism. In: Friberg L, Vostal J, eds: Mercury in the Environment: An Epidemiological and Toxicological Appraisal. Cleveland, CRC Press, 1972, pp. 29–90.

56. O'Shea JG: Was Paganini poisoned with mercury? J R Soc Med 1988;81:594–597.

57. Patrizi A, Rizzoli L, Vincenzi C, Trevisi P, Tosti A: Sensitization to thimerosal in atopic children. Contact Dermatitis 1999;40:94–97.

58. Pfab R, Muckter H, Roider G, Zilker T: Clinical course of severe poisoning with thimerosal. Clin Toxicol 1996;34(4):453–460.

59. Powell PP: Minamata disease: A story of mercury's malevolence. South Med J 1991;84:1352–1358.

60. Rosenman KD, Valciukas JA, Glickman L, et al: Sensitive indicators of inorganic mercury toxicity. Arch Environ Health 1986;41:208–215.

61. Royhans J, Walson PD, Wood GA, MacDonald WA: Mercury toxicity following Merthiolate ear irrigations. J Pediatr 1984;104:311–313.

62. Rustam H, Hamdi T: Methyl mercury poisoning in Iraq. Brain 1974; 97:499–510.

63. Sauder PH, Livardjani F, Jaeger A, et al: Acute mercury chloride intoxication: Effects of hemodialysis and plasma exchange on mercury kinetic. J Toxicol Clin Toxicol 1988;26:189–197.

64. Schwartz JG, Snider TE, Montiel MM: Toxicity of a family from vacuumed mercury. Am J Emerg Med 1992;10:258–261.

65. Seidel J: Acute mercury poisoning after polyvinyl alcohol preservative ingestion. Pediatrics 1980;66:132–134.

66. Siegler RW, Nierenberg DW, Hickey WF. Fatal poisoning from liquid dimethylmercury: A neuropathologic study. Hum Pathol 1999;30: 720–723.

67. Snapp KR, Boyer DB, Peterson LC, Svare CW: The contribution of dental amalgam to mercury in blood. J Dent Res 1989;68:780–785.

68. Snodgrass W, Sullivan JB, Rumack BH, Hashimoto C: Mercury poisoning from home gold ore processing. JAMA 1981;246:1929–1931.

69. Stajich GV, Lopez GP, Harry SW, Sexson WR: Iatrogenic exposure to mercury after hepatitis B vaccination in preterm infants. J Pediatr 2000;136:679–681.

70. Sunderman FW: Perils of mercury. Ann Clin Lab Sci 1988;18: 89–101.

71. Suzuki T, Hongo T, Yoshinaga J, et al: The hair-organ relationship in mercury concentration in contemporary Japanese. Arch Environ Health 1993;48:221–229.

72. Takeuchi T: Pathology of Minamata disease. Acta Pathol Jpn 1982; 32:73–99.

73. Taueg C, Sanfilippo DJ, Rowens B, et al: Acute and chronic poisoning from residential exposures to elemental mercury—Michigan, 1989–1990. J Toxicol Clin Toxicol 1992;30:63–67.

74. Troen P, Kaufman SA, Katz KH: Mercuric bichloride poisoning. N Engl J Med 1951;244:459–463.

75. Tunnessen WW, McMahon KJ, Baser M: Acrodynia: Exposure to mercury from fluorescent light bulbs. Pediatrics 1987;79:786–789.

76. Wallach L: Aspiration of elemental mercury—Evidence of absorption without toxicity. N Engl J Med 1972;287:178–179.

77. Wands JR, Weiss SH, Yardley JH, Maddrey WC: Chronic inorganic mercury poisoning due to laxative abuse. Am J Med 1974;57:92–101.

78. Warkany J, Hubbard DM: Adverse mercurial reactions in the form of acrodynia and related conditions. Am J Dis Child 1951;81:335–373.

79. Wedeen RP: Were the hatters of New Jersey "mad"? Am J Ind Med 1989;16:225–233.

80. Winship KA: Organic mercury compounds and their toxicity. Adv Drug React Ac Pois Rev 1986;3:141–180.

81. Yeh TF, Pildes RS, Firor HV: Mercury poisoning from mercurochrome treatment of an infected omphalocele. Clin Toxicol 1978; 13:463–467.

82. Yotsuyanagi T, Yokoi K, Sawada Y: Facial injury by mercury from a broken thermometer. J Trauma 1996;40:847–849.

83. Zimmer LJ, Carter DE: The effect of 2,3-dimercaptopropanol and D-penicillamine on methyl mercury induced neurological signs and weight loss. Life Sci 1978;23:1025–1034.

84. Zimmerman JE: Fatality following metallic mercury aspiration during removal of a long intestinal tube. JAMA 1969;208:2158–2160.

CHAPTER 82 METALS

Robert S. Hoffman

The immediately preceding chapters of this text provide in-depth discussions of the toxicities of arsenic, lead, and mercury, as does the chapter on thallium that follows. These metals were selected for placement in individual chapters because of their historical relevance, their well-recognized clinical toxicity, and the volume of toxicologic data available for review. Virtually all other metal salts and some elemental forms (Chap. 12) have the potential for acute or chronic toxicity. For many, the available data involve limited animal experiments and rare human case reports, and discussion would not be useful in a text focusing on toxicologic emergencies.

This chapter contains three subsections that highlight cadmium, copper, and bismuth. Much like the metals discussed in previous chapters, these three toxins were selected because of their clinical relevance to acute toxicity in humans. For discussions of other metals, the reader is referred to a series of monographs by Donald Barceloux,[1–8] as well as Chap. 81 in the 6th edition of this text.

As the following three sections are reviewed, the reader should concentrate on similarities that exist between the toxicologic effects of these and other metal salts. Multiple organ system involvement, including gastrointestinal, neurologic, and renal effects, characterize typical toxicity. Although these common manifestations underlie the principles of acute metal toxicity, unique effects such as the pulmonary manifestations of cadmium, the hematologic and hepatic effects of copper, and the characteristic neurologic effects of bismuth are distinctive.

REFERENCES

1. Barceloux DG: Chromium. J Toxicol Clin Toxicol 1999;37:173–194.
2. Barceloux DG: Cobalt. J Toxicol Clin Toxicol 1999;37:201–206.
3. Barceloux DG: Manganese. J Toxicol Clin Toxicol 1999;37:293–307.
4. Barceloux DG: Molybdenum. J Toxicol Clin Toxicol 1999; 37: 231–237.
5. Barceloux DG: Nickel. J Toxicol Clin Toxicol 1999;37:239–258.
6. Barceloux DG: Selenium. J Toxicol Clin Toxicol 1999;37:145–172.
7. Barceloux DG: Vanadium. J Toxicol Clin Toxicol 1999;37:265–278.
8. Barceloux DG: Zinc. J Toxicol Clin Toxicol 1999;37:279–292.

CHAPTER 82A BISMUTH

Rama B. Rao

Bismuth
MW = 208.9 daltons
Normal Levels
  Blood = 2–11 µg/L (9–52 nmol/L)
  Urine = <4 µg/L (<20 nmol/L)
Action Level
  Blood = 100 µg/L (478 nmol/L)
Values greater than or equal to the action level necessitate clinical intervention. Values below this level may necessitate intervention based on the clinical condition of the patient.

Bismuth is commonly utilized for treatment of peptic ulcer disease, traveler's diarrhea, nausea, and vomiting, as well as for treatment of the flatus and odor associated with ileostomies and colostomies.[13] It is an active ingredient in both prescribed and over-the-counter oral preparations, as well as in bismuth-impregnated surgical packing paste.[8,51]

In the gastrointestinal tract, bismuth binds to sulfhydryl groups and decreases fecal odor through formation of bismuth sulfide.[44] Sulfhydryl binding is also the proposed mechanism of bismuth's antimicrobial effect, causing lysis of *Helicobacter pylori*, the causative bacteria in peptic ulcer formation. Bismuth may also inhibit bacterial enzyme function, as well as prevent adhesion of *H. pylori* to the gastric mucosa.[50]

This chapter reviews the history and manifestations of bismuth-related complications, and the toxicity and therapy of acute and chronic overdose of currently available bismuth-containing compounds.

HISTORY AND EPIDEMIOLOGY

Nearly 300 years ago, bismuth was recognized as medicinally valuable. It was included in topical salves and oral preparations for various gastrointestinal ailments. Renal toxicity was described as early as 1802. In the early 20th century, cases of renal failure were reported in pediatric patients administered intramuscular bismuth for the treatment of gingivostomatitis.[6,24,43] Administration of bismuth thioglycollate and its related water-soluble compounds, triglycollamate and trithioglycollamate, was responsible for the renal failure.[7,11,28,49] Affected children would typically present with abdominal pain, oliguria or anuria, malaise, and vomiting. Renal failure occurred sometimes after just one or two medication doses. Alterations in consciousness usually abated with treatment or resolution of the uremia. As the use of intramuscular injections was mostly abandoned, this form of bismuth-induced renal failure became uncommon.

Historically, syphilis was also treated with intramuscular bismuth. A rash known as "erythema of the 9th day" occasionally occurred. This consisted of a diffuse macular rash of the trunk and extremities that resolved without intervention.[15]

Hepatic failure, in patients administered "Analbis" antipyretic rectal suppositories, was described histopathologically as yellow atrophy with vacuolization.[2,21] An investigation of the suppositories suggested that diallylacetic acid, and not bismuth, was the hepatotoxic molecule. This agent is no longer marketed.

More recently, epidemics of bismuth-induced encephalopathy, particularly among patients with ileostomies or colostomies, were reported in France, Britain, and Australia. As a result, some countries banned or restricted bismuth preparations to prescription only. Bismuth subsalicylate is still widely available in the United States as a nonprescription agent, and encephalopathy is still periodically reported.[14] Other reported episodes of bismuth-induced encephalopathy include systemic absorption from bismuth-impregnated surgical packing paste and transdermal absorption from chronic application of a bismuth-containing skin cream.

TOXICOKINETICS

Bismuth is present in nature in both the trivalent and pentavalent forms. The trivalent form of bismuth is employed for all medicinal uses, as the bismuthyl (BiO) moiety. Most of orally administered bismuth remains in the gastrointestinal (GI) tract, being excreted in the feces. Only about between 0.16 and 0.28 % is systemically absorbed. The peak absorption ranges between 15–60 minutes with high intra- and interindividual variation.[22,24] The plasma-to-blood ratio of bismuth is 1.55.[3]

The distribution and elimination of orally administered bismuth follows a complex, multicompartmental model. The volume of distribution in humans is unknown.

Once in the circulation, bismuth binds to α_2-macroglobulin, IgM, β-lipoprotein, and haptoglobin. It rapidly penetrates liver, kidney, lungs, and bone. Bismuth can cross the placenta and enter the amniotic fluid and fetal circulation. It also readily crosses the blood-brain barrier. In animal models, bismuth is identified in the fenestrated membranes of synaptosomes,[35,38] localizing in the thalamus and cerebellum. This is similar to human reports, which also describe diffuse cortical uptake in toxic exposures.[24] Ninety percent of systemic bismuth is eliminated through the kidneys, where it induces its own metal-binding protein.

Some authors propose three different half-lives to describe the pharmacokinetics of orally administered bismuth. The first, a distribution half-life, is approximately 1–4 hours. The second, the plasma half-life, lasts 5–11 days. The third is the half-life of urinary excretion lasting between 21 and 72 days[3] with bismuth detected as late as 5 months after the last oral dose.[22]

PATHOPHYSIOLOGY

Like other metals, bismuth toxicity involves multiple organ systems. The effect of different bismuth salts can be categorized into four groups based upon the solubility and gastrointestinal absorption of the agent[40] (Table 82–1).

The mechanism of bismuth-induced encephalopathy is thought to be related to neuronal sulfhydryl binding. The gray-matter concentration of bismuth is nearly twice that of white matter in patients who die of bismuth encephalopathy.[24] In an encephalopathic patient dying from concomitant sepsis, the autopsy revealed loss of cerebellar Purkinje cells not expected from sepsis alone.[25] The factors predisposing some individuals to bismuth encephalopathy from group II agents, however, are not well defined. Age, gender, and duration of therapeutic use do not predict the likelihood of developing encephalopathy.

CLINICAL MANIFESTATIONS

Acute

Acutely, massive overdoses of bismuth may result in abdominal pain and oliguria or anuria. Acute renal failure can occur from acute massive overdose of bismuth salts and is not limited to the water-soluble compounds (group III). In reported cases, overdoses of colloidal bismuth subsalicylate or tripotassium dicitratobismuthate (TDC) caused acute tubular necrosis.[1,17,19,43,46] Histopathologically, bismuth causes degeneration of the proximal tubule, similar to other heavy metals. While these substances are potentially neurotoxic, signs of encephalopathy are generally absent. In one case, a patient with bismuth-induced renal failure was described as having diminished deep-tendon reflexes, muscle weakness, and myoclonus, without an alteration in consciousness.[17]

Chronic

The most common toxicologic finding associated with repeated therapeutic doses of oral bismuth compounds is a diffuse, progressive encephalopathy. Affected patients exhibit neurobehavioral changes, such as apathy and irritability. With continued exposure, these patients may develop difficulty concentrating, diminished short-term memory, and occasionally, visual hallucinations.[26,27] A movement disorder characterized by muscle twitching, myoclonus, ataxia, and tremors may ensue. Weakness and, rarely, seizures may advance to immobility.[29,30] Ultimately these patients can lapse into coma and die with continued bismuth administration.

Rarely, patients recovering from severe encephalopathy may complain of scapular, humeral, or vertebral pain because of fractures caused by severe neuromuscular manifestions.[12]

Like several other heavy metals, bismuth can cause a generalized pigmentation of skin. Deposition of bismuth sulfide into the mucosa causes a blue-black discoloration of gums.[52] This can occur in the absence of toxic effects. Formation of the same compound in the gastrointestinal tract causes blackening of the stool.

Liver failure is rarely reported, except in patients with multisystem organ failure from fatal neurotoxicity.

DIAGNOSIS

The clinician must have an index of suspicion based on the acute or chronic nature of the exposure. Patients with acute massive overdoses should be observed and evaluated for possible renal failure. Serum chemistries in these patients may demonstrate uremia. A patient with a urinalysis positive for red and white blood cells and elevated protein may suggest signs of renal injury earlier than the serum studies. Formation of nuclear inclusion bodies can be identified on renal biopsy or on postmortem examination of the kidney.[11,37]

The diagnosis of bismuth-induced encephalopathy is based on a history of exposure coupled with diffuse neuropsychiatric and motor findings.[27] Other causes of encephalopathy should be entertained and excluded (Table 82–2). An abdominal radiograph will likely demonstrate radiopacities of bismuth in the intestines. Stool will be black, but will test negative for occult blood.

The presence of bismuth in the blood is confirmatory, but absolute concentrations are poorly correlated with the risk and severity of disease. In a review of 310 patients with encephalopathy in France, 288 patients (93%) had a blood concentration >100 ng/mL, with the majority of these blood concentrations between 100 ng/mL and 1000 ng/mL.[26] Twenty-two patients suffered encephalopathy at blood concentrations below 100 ng/mL.[26] In another report, two patients with encephalopathy had blood concentrations of 900 ng/mL and 2500 ng/mL, both of whom recovered when the concentration fell below 500 ng/mL.[5] Just as blood concentrations do not reflect severity of illness, tissue concentrations may also poorly correlate to severity of illness. An example

TABLE 82–1. Bismuth Salts Grouped by Absorption Characteristics [41]

Group	Examples	Chemistry	Toxicity
I	Bismuth subnitrate Bismuth subcarbonate	Insoluble in water	Minimal
II	Bismuth subgallate	Lipid soluble Organic	Potentially neurotoxic
III	Bismuth triglycollamate	Water soluble Organic	Potentially nephrotoxic
IV	Bictropeptide	Hydrolyzable Water soluble Organic	Minimal

TABLE 82–2. Differential Diagnosis of Bismuth Encephalopathy

Creutzfeld-Jacob disease
Ethanol withdrawal
Lithium toxicity
Neurodegenerative leukoencephalopathies
Nonketotic hyperosmolar coma
Postanoxic and posthypoglycemic encephalopathies
Progressive multifocal ataxia
Viral encephalopathies

was noted in a patient who recovered from a severe encephalopathy. On discharge, he had low blood bismuth concentrations and died 3 months later of unrelated trauma. At autopsy he was found to have an elevated central nervous system (CNS) bismuth burden.[9]

The electroencephalographic (EEG) findings of encephalopathic patients generally demonstrate nonspecific slow wave changes.[14,17] In one study, the EEG findings were described in association with blood concentrations. At less than 50 ng/mL, the EEG was normal or demonstrated diffuse slowing. In patients with blood concentrations of less than 1500 ng/mL, the findings of sharp wave abnormalities were noted. At higher concentrations (>2000 ng/mL), neurologic events, such as myoclonic jerks, did not have corresponding EEG changes. The authors proposed that an elevated body burden might have an inhibitory effect on the cerebral cortex.[9]

Imaging studies, such as computed tomography, demonstrate a diffuse cortical hyperdensity of gray matter in encephalopathic patients with blood concentrations >2000 ng/mL. These findings resolve with recovery. Magnetic resonance imaging was normal in another encephalopathic patient.[14]

TREATMENT

Typically, supportive care, including hemodialysis for renal failure, results in a complete recovery. Some authors suggest GI decontamination with activated charcoal and polyethylene glycol solution.[43] While the evidence for this is lacking, it is a reasonable first gesture. Chelation therapy with British Anti-Lewisite (BAL) is beneficial in experimental models,[41a] reportedly beneficial in humans,[29a] and often recommended, but clear evidence of efficacy is lacking. BAL undergoes biliary elimination, a major advantage over other chelators in patients, such as these, who are expected to develop renal insufficiency. Some authors recommend the addition of dimercaptopropane sulfonate (DMPS), citing that BAL with hemodialysis did not affect clearance, whereas the addition of DMPS to hemodialysis was effective.[43] It is uncertain whether the clinical course of the patient was improved. In human volunteers using colloidal bismuth subcitrate, dimercaptosuccinic acid (DMSA) and DMPS, both at a dose of 30 mg/kg, increased urinary elimination of bismuth by 50-fold.[41b] However, as resolution of renal toxicity is generally observed with supportive care only, the use of chelating agents or hemodialysis in acute overdose without neurotoxicity is probably not indicated.

Typically, withdrawal of the source of bismuth results in reversal of symptoms, even in patients with severe encephalopathy. Recovery may take days to weeks, but is usually complete.

In an animal model, D-penicillamine was most efficacious in enhancing elimination of bismuth. In a human volunteer model that used therapeutic doses of tripotassium-dicitrato-bismuthate, however, a single dose of D-penicillamine did not enhance urinary excretion.[31] It is uncertain how these agents affect the course of encephalopathic patients.

Prevention is the most valuable tool in avoiding neurotoxicity. Patients and their families should be taught to recognize the more subtle changes produced by bismuth-induced neurotoxicity as laboratory testing is limited. While blood concentrations of bismuth are not routinely performed, a bismuth concentration above 100 ng/mL or symptoms at lower levels warrant withdrawal of bismuth therapy.

Bismuth Drug Interactions and Reactions

Ranitidine, which is frequently prescribed with bismuth compound for dyspepsia or ulcer disease, does not affect the pharmacokinetics of bismuth absorption.[22] In the United States, where bismuth subsalicylate is the most common oral bismuth-containing compound, up to 90% of the salicylate is absorbed and detectable by salicylate screening.[34] Salicylate toxicity has been reported and salicylate concentrations should be performed in both acute and chronic exposures.

Methemoglobinemia from subnitrate salt of bismuth is also described, but uncommon.[20]

SUMMARY

Presently, the most likely manifestations of bismuth toxicity are either neurologic or renal, depending upon the type of compound and whether therapeutic or acute massive overdose occurred. The factors predisposing some individuals to neurotoxicity from therapeutic use of oral bismuth compounds are poorly understood. Thus, patients using therapeutic bismuth with new movement disorders or alterations in mental status should be assessed for possible bismuth-induced encephalopathy.

REFERENCES

1. Akpolat I, Kahraman H, Akpolat T, et al: Acute renal failure due to overdose of colloidal bismuth. Nephrol Dial Transplant 1996;11:1890–1898.
2. Barnett RN: Reactions to a bismuth compound. Toxic manifestations following the use of the bismuth salt of heptadienecarboxylic acid in suppositories. JAMA 1947;135:28–30.
3. Benet LZ: Safety and pharmacokinetics: Colloidal bismuth subcitrate. Scand J Gastroenterol 1991;25(Suppl 185):29–35.
4. Bennet JE, Wakefield JC, Lacey LF: Modeling trough plasma bismuth concentrations. J Pharmacokinet Biopharm 1997;25:79–106.
5. Bes A, Caussanel JP, Geraud G, et al: Encephalopathie toxique par les sels de bismuth. Rev Med Toulouse 1976;12:810–813.
6. Bierer DW: Bismuth subsalicylate: History chemistry, and safety. Rev Infect Dis 1990;12:S3–S8.
7. Boyette DP, Ahiskie NC: Bismuth nephrosis with anuria in an infant. J Pediatr 1946;28:493–497.
8. Bridgeman AM, Smith AC: Iatrogenic bismuth poisoning: Case report. Aust Dental J 1994;39:279–281.
9. Buge A, Supino-Viterbo V, Rancurel G, Pontes C: Epileptic phenomena in bismuth toxic encephalopathy. J Neurol Neurosurg Psychiatr 1981;44:62–67.
10. Burns R, Thomas DW, Barron VJ. Reversible encephalopathy possibly associated with bismuth subgallate ingestion. Br Med J 1974;1:220–223.
11. Czerwinski AW, Ginn HE: Bismuth nephrotoxicity. Am J Med 1964;37:969–975.
12. Emile J, De Bray JM, Bernat M, et al: Osteoarticular complications in bismuth encephalopathy. Clin Toxicol 1981;18:1285–1290.
13. Goldenberg MM, Honkomp LJ, Davis CS: Antinauseant and antiemetic properties of bismuth subsalicylate in dogs and humans. J Pharmacol Sci 1976;65:1398–1400.
14. Gordon MF, Abrams RI, Rubin DB, et al: Bismuth subsalicylate toxicity as a cause of prolonged encephalopathy with myoclonus. Mov Disord 1995;10:220–222.
15. Gryboski JD, Gotoff SP: Bismuth nephrotoxicity. N Engl J Med 1961;265:1289–1291.

16. Hasking GJ, Duggan JM: Encephalopathy from bismuth subsalicylate. Med J Aust 1982;2:167.

17. Hudson M, Mowat NAG: Reversible toxicity in poisoning with colloidal bismuth subcitrate. BMJ 1989;299:159.

18. Hundal O, Bergseth M, Gharehnia B, et al: Absorption of bismuth from two bismuth compounds before and after healing of peptic ulcers. Hepatogastroenterology 1999;46:2882–2886.

19. Huwez F, Pall A, Lyons D, Stewart MJ: Acute renal failure after overdose of colloidal bismuth subcitrate. Lancet 1992;340:1298.

20. Jacobsen JB, Huttel MS: Methemoglobin after excessive intake of a subnitrate containing antacid. Ugeskr Laeger 1982;144:2340–2350.

21. Karelitz S, Freedman AD: Hepatitis and nephrosis due to soluble bismuth. Pediatrics 1951;8:772–776.

22. Koch KM, Kerr BM, Gooding AE, Davis IM. Pharmacokinetics of bismuth and ranitidine following multiple doses of ranitidine bismuth citrate. Br J Clin Pharmacol 1996;42:207–211.

23. Kruger G, Thomas DJ, Weinhardt F, Hoyer S: Disturbed oxidative metabolism in organic brain syndrome caused by bismuth in skin creams. Lancet 1976;1:485–487.

24. Lambert JR: Pharmacology of bismuth-containing compounds. Rev Infect Dis 1991;13:S691–S695.

25. Liessens JL, Monstrey J, Vanden Eeckhout E, Djudzman R, Martin JJ: Bismuth encephalopathy. Act Neurol Belg 1978;78:301–309.

26. Martin-Bouyer G, Foulon G, Guerbois H, Barin C: Epidemiological study of encephalopathies following bismuth administration per os. Characteristics of intoxicated subjects: Comparison with a control group. Clin Toxicol 1981;18:1277–1283.

27. Martin-Bouyer G, Weller M: Neuropsychiatric symptoms following bismuth intoxication. Postgrad Med J 1988;64:308–310.

28. McClendon SJ: Toxic effects with anuria from a single injection of a bismuth preparation. Am J Dis Child 1941;61:339–341.

29. Mendelowitz PC, Hoffman RS, Weber S: Bismuth absorption and myoclonic encephalopathy during bismuth subsalicylate therapy. Ann Intern Med 1990;112:140–141.

29a. Molina JA, Calandre L, Bermego F: Myoclonic encephalopathy due to bismuth salts: Treatment with dimercaprol and analysis of CSF transmitters. Acta Neurol Scand 1989;79:200–203.

30. Monseu G, Struelens M, Roland M: Bismuth encephalopathy. Acta Neurol Belg 1976;76:301–308.

31. Nwokolo CU, Pounder RE: D-Penicillamine does not increase urinary bismuth excretion in patients treated with tripotassium dicitrato bismuthate. Br J Clin Pharmacol 1990;30:648–650.

32. O'Brien D: Anuria due to bismuth thioglycollate. Am J Dis Child 1959;97:384–386.

33. Pamphlett R, Stoltenberg M, Rungby J, Danscher G: Uptake of bismuth in motor neurons of mice after single oral doses of bismuth compounds. Neurotoxicol Teratol 2000;22:559–563.

34. Pickering LK, Feldman S, Ericsson CD, Cleary TG: Absorption of salicylate and bismuth from a bismuth subsalicylate containing compound (Pepto-Bismol). J Pediatr 1981;99:654–656.

35. Pollet S, Albouz S, Le Saux F, et al: Bismuth intoxication: Bismuth level in pig brain lipids and in subcellular fractions. Toxicol Eur Res 1979;2:123–125.

36. Randall RE, Osheroff RJ, Bakerman S, Setter JG: Bismuth nephrotoxicity. Ann Intern Med 1972;77:481–482.

37. Rodilla V, Miles AT, Jenner W, Hawksworth GM: Exposure of human cultured proximal tubule cells to cadmium, mercury, zinc, and bismuth: Toxicity and metallothionein induction. Chem Biol Interact 1998;115:71–83.

38. Ross JF, Broadwell RD, Poston MR, Lawhorn GT: Highest brain bismuth levels and neuropathology are adjacent to fenestrated blood vessels in mouse brain after intraperitoneal dosing of bismuth subnitrate. Toxicol Appl Pharmacol 1994;124:191–200.

39. Sainsbury SJ: Fatal salicylate toxicity from bismuth subsalicylate. West J Med 1991;155:637–639.

40. Serfontein WJ, Mekel R: Bismuth toxicity in man II. Review of bismuth blood and urine levels in patients after administration of therapeutic bismuth formulations in relation to the problem of bismuth toxicity in man. Res Commun Chemical Pathol Pharmacol 1979;26:391–411.

41. Serfontein WJ, Mekel R, Bank S, et al: Bismuth toxicity in man I: Bismuth blood and urine levels in patients after administration of a bismuth protein complex (bictropeptide). Res Commun Chem Pathol Pharmacol 1979;26:383–389.

41a. Slikkerveer A, Jong HB, Helmich RB, de Wolff FA: Development of a therapeutic procedure for bismuth intoxication with chelating agents. J Lab Clin Med 1992;119:529–537.

41b. Slikkerveer A, Noach LA, Tytgat GN, et al: Comparison of enhanced elimination of bismuth in humans after treatment with meso-2,3 dimercaptosuccinic acid and D,L-2,3-dimercaptopropane-1-sulfonic acid. Analyst 1998;123:91–92.

42. Stevens PE, Bierer DW: Bismuth subsalicylate: History chemistry, and safety. Rev Infect Dis 1990;12:S3–S8.

43. Stevens PE, Moore DF, House IM, et al: Significant elimination of bismuth by haemodialysis with a new heavy metal chelating agent. Nephrol Dial Transplant 1995;10:696–698.

44. Suarez FL, Furne JK, Springfield J, Levitt MD: Bismuth subsalicylate markedly decreases hydrogen sulfide release in the human colon. Gastroenterology 1998;114:923–929.

45. Szymanska JA, Zelazowski AJ, Kawiorski S: Some aspects of bismuth metabolism. Clin Toxicol 1981;18:1291–1298.

46. Taylor EG, Klenerman P: Acute renal failure after bismuth subcitrate overdose. Lancet 1990;335:670–671.

47. Thompson HE, Steadman LT, Pommeranke WT: The transfer of bismuth into fetal circulation after maternal administration of sobisimol. Am J Syp 1941;25:725–730.

48. Tremaine WJ, Sandborn WJ, Wolff BG, et al: Bismuth carbomer foam enemas for chronic pouchitis: A randomized, double-blind, placebo-controlled trial. Aliment Pharmacol Ther 1997;11: 1041–1046.

49. Urizar R, Vernier RL: Bismuth nephropathy. JAMA 1966;198: 207–209.

50. Walsh JH, Peterson WL: Drug therapy: The treatment of *Helicobacter pylori* infection in the management of peptic ulcer disease. N Engl J Med 1995;333:984–991.

51. Wilson APR: The dangers of BIPP. Lancet 1994;334:1313–1314.

52. Zala L, Hunziker T, Braathen LR: Pigmentation following long-term bismuth therapy for pneumatosis cystoides intestinalis. Dermatology 1993;187:288–289.

CHAPTER 82B CADMIUM

Stephen J. Traub / Robert S. Hoffman

Cadmium

MW	=	112.4 daltons
Normal Levels		
Blood	=	<5 µg/L (0.004 µmol/L)
Urine	=	<3 µg/g creatinine (0.0026 µmol/g creatinine)
Action Levels		
Blood	=	>15 µg/L (0.133 µmol/L)
Urine	=	>15 µg/g creatinine (0.133 µmol/g creatinine)

Values greater than or equal to the action levels necessitate clinical intervention. Values below this level may necessitate intervention based on the clinical condition of the patient.

A 53-year-old male who performed metalwork as a hobby became ill approximately 6 hours after welding in his shop. He developed a violent cough, and sought care from a local physician. The physician, who elicited the history of metalwork, diagnosed the patient with metal fume fever, reassured him that his symptoms would pass, and discharged him home.

The next morning the patient's condition worsened, and he presented to a local emergency department complaining of severe shortness of breath. Vital signs were pulse, 117 beats/min; blood pressure, 105/64 mm Hg; respiratory rate, 22 breaths/min and labored; and temperature, 101.3°F (38.5°C). Lung examination revealed diffuse rales. Pulse oxygenation was 87% on room air. The patient was placed on supplemental oxygen, and his oxygen saturation improved to 94%. Arterial blood gas analysis and cooximetry confirmed the patient's hypoxia and excluded methemoglobinemia and carboxyhemoglobinemia. A chest radiograph showed diffuse interstitial alveolar filling. Further history revealed that the patient had been welding with a cadmium-containing solder without appropriate respiratory precautions. A working diagnosis of cadmium pneumonitis was established.

The patient's respiratory status slowly declined over the course of the next 24 hours, necessitating endotracheal intubation. He was treated with intravenous steroids (dexamethasone 10 mg IV every 6 hours) and broad-spectrum antibiotics (ceftriaxone, 1 g IV every 12 hours), but continued to deteriorate despite aggressive and appropriate supportive care. He expired on hospital day 4.

Cadmium, atomic number 48, is a transitional metal in group IIB of the periodic table. In its pure atomic form, it is a bluish solid at room temperature. It is readily oxidized to a divalent ion, Cd^{++}. Naturally occurring cadmium commonly exists as cadmium sulfide (CdS), a trace contaminate of zinc-containing ores.[38]

Cadmium sulfide, cadmium oxide, and other cadmium-containing compounds are refined to produce elemental cadmium, which is then used for industrial purposes. When combined with other metals, cadmium forms alloys of relatively low melting points, which accounts for its extensive historical use as a component of solders and brazing rods. Today, the majority of cadmium is used in the production of nickel-cadmium batteries. Other current and historical uses of cadmium include its role as a reagent in electroplating, as a pigment, as part of the phosphorescent system in black and white televisions, and as a neutron absorber in nuclear reactors. Cadmium salts have also been used as veterinary antihelminthics.[13] Much like lead, there is no known biologic role for cadmium.

HISTORY AND EPIDEMIOLOGY

As cadmium processing increased in the last century, so, too, did cadmium toxicity. Cadmium exposure with resultant toxicity usually occurs in one of three settings: environmental, occupational, or hobby work.

Environmental Exposure

Environmental exposure to cadmium generally occurs through the consumption of foods grown in cadmium-contaminated areas. Because cadmium is fairly common as an impurity in ores (particularly those containing zinc), areas that mine or refine ores are at highest risk for contamination. Although many countries (such as Sweden[46] and Belgium[12]) have reported on environmental cadmium exposure, the most remarkable historical example of environmental cadmium pollution occurred in Japan.

In the 1950s, a mine near the Jinzu river basin in the Toyama prefecture was discharging large amounts of cadmium into the environment, contaminating the rice that was a staple of the local food supply. An epidemic of painful osteomalacia followed, affecting hundreds of people, mostly postmenopausal multiparous women.[62] The afflicted were prone to develop pathologic fractures, and were reported to call out "itai-itai" (literally, "ouch-ouch") as they walked, because of the severity of their pain.[29] These symptoms were ultimately linked to the cadmium.

Environmental exposure also occurs in smokers, who have higher blood cadmium levels than do nonsmokers.[84] Although this elevation is probably a result of soil contamination in the areas where the tobacco is grown, tobacco smoking is not established as an independent risk factor for cadmium toxicity.

Occupational Exposure

Welders, solderers, and other metalworkers (eg, jewelry workers) who use cadmium-containing alloys are at risk of developing acute cadmium toxicity through the inhalation of cadmium oxide fumes. Other workers (such as in battery factories) who do not work with metals per se may develop significant chronic cadmium toxicity through exposure to cadmium-containing dust. A better understanding of the health effects of cadmium has led to improvements in working conditions and significantly decreased workplace cadmium exposure.

Hobby Exposure

Hobbyists who are exposed to cadmium are generally exposed to cadmium oxide through metalwork with cadmium solders, similar to the exposures of occupational metalworkers. Significant cadmium toxicity in this population invariably results from metalworking in a closed space with inadequate ventilation and/or improper respiratory precautions.

TOXICOKINETICS

The bioavailability of elemental cadmium (cadmium metal) is unknown. Cadmium salts are poorly (5–20%) bioavailable via the gastrointestinal (GI) route, but cadmium fumes (cadmium oxide) are readily bioavailable (up to 90%) via the pulmonary route.[93] Because the only data on cadmium toxicokinetics come from work with cadmium salts, "cadmium" in this discussion should be construed as referring to inorganic cadmium salts unless otherwise noted.

After exposure, cadmium is taken up into the bloodstream, where it is bound to α_2-macroglobulin and albumin.[95] It is then quickly and preferentially redistributed to the liver and kidney. Although other organs such as the pancreas, spleen, heart, lung, and testes can accumulate part of an acute cadmium load, they do so much less avidly.[26]

After it is incorporated in the liver and kidney, cadmium is complexed with metallothionein, an endogenous thiol-rich protein that is produced in both organs. Metallothionein binds and sequesters cadmium. Slowly, over time, hepatic stores of the cadmium-metallothionein complex (Cd-MT) are released. Circulating Cd-MT is then filtered by the glomerulus, and a significant amount is reabsorbed by, and concentrated in, the proximal tubule cells.[79,80] Cadmium is renally concentrated by this mechanism, which is one of the reasons that the kidney is the principal target organ in cadmium toxicity.

There is no evidence that cadmium ions are oxidized, reduced, methylated, or otherwise biotransformed. The volume of distribution (Vd) of cadmium is unknown, but is presumably quite large as a consequence of significant hepatic sequestration. Cadmium distribution and elimination are complex, and an eight-compartment kinetic model is proposed.[52] The slow release of cadmium from metallothionein-complexed hepatic stores accounts for its very long half-life of 10 or more years.

PATHOPHYSIOLOGY
Cellular Pathophysiology

Cadmium is very quickly and efficiently complexed to metallothionein in vivo, which raises the question of whether free cadmium or the cadmium-metallothionein complex is the ultimate toxicant. It appears, however, that unbound cadmium mediates cellular damage[26,36,58,61,80]; metallothionein is unquestionably protective[23,58] and functions as a natural chelating agent with a strong affinity for cadmium.[19,53] Although metallothionein may play a role in proximal tubular concentration of cadmium, renal damage is reduced by metallothionein, as metallothionein-deficient mice demonstrate more toxicity after cadmium exposure than controls.[58]

The exact mechanism by which cadmium interferes with cellular function is poorly understood. Cadmium exerts at least some of its toxic effect via the binding of sulfhydryl groups and the subsequent denaturing of proteins and/or inactivation of enzymes. The mitochondrion is one of the organelles most effected by this process,[1] which may result in a greater susceptibility to oxidative stress in cadmium-poisoned cells. Cadmium may also interfere with E-cadherin, an important protein in some cell-cell junctions[68]; this interference may play a role in the development of acute lung injury. The demonstrated interference of cadmium with calcium transport mechanisms[89,90] might lead to intracellular hypercalcemia and, ultimately, to cell death.

Specific Organ System Pathophysiology

Kidney. The pathophysiology of cadmium-related renal disease has been thoroughly studied and is well understood. Animals exposed to cadmium develop evidence of biochemical dysfunction and morphologic abnormalities of the kidney within 10 weeks when exposed to subcutaneous cadmium,[26] and within 8 hours when given intraperitoneal cadmium.[79] In humans, the renal damage caused by cadmium usually develops over years.

Proteinuria is by far the most common renal abnormality caused by cadmium. Proteinuria usually begins with proximal tubular dysfunction, which manifests as urinary loss of low-molecular-weight proteins such as β_2-microglobulin and retinol binding protein. This low-molecular-weight proteinuria is usually more significant than, and generally precedes glomerular dysfunction, which manifests as urinary loss of higher-molecular-weight proteins such as albumin and transferrin. Some cadmium-exposed workers, however, have predominantly glomerular proteinuria.[7] There appears to be a dose-response relationship between total body cadmium burden and urinary dysfunction,[12,45,46,64,88] although some authors refute such a relationship, especially at low doses.[41] As noted earlier, proteinuria develops because of injury to the proximal convoluted tubule, which concentrates cadmium by reabsorbing the cadmium-metallothionein complex.[79,80]

Cadmium also appears to produce hypercalcuria,[75] possibly via damage to the proximal tubule.

Bone. Cadmium causes osteomalacia, probably through abnormalities of calcium and phosphate homeostasis. In one autopsy study, the severity of osteomalacia in a cadmium-exposed population correlated with a decline in the serum [calcium] × [phosphate] product.[83] These electrolyte imbalances are, in turn, probably a result of renal proximal tubular dysfunction.

Lung. The pathophysiology of acute cadmium pneumonitis is not well established. Human autopsy studies[33,67,76,96] generally show degeneration of, and/or loss of, bronchial and bronchiolar epithelial cells; most patients also had proteinaceous pulmonary edema. The mechanism by which these findings develop is not clear.

Gastrointestinal Tract. Based on case reports,[9,97] cadmium salts appear to be caustic substances with the potential to induce significant GI symptoms (nausea, vomiting, and abdominal pain) and result in GI hemorrhage, necrosis, and perforation. In this respect, cadmium salts appear to be similar to mercuric chloride (HgCl$_2$).

CLINICAL MANIFESTATIONS

Acute Poisoning

Oral/Cadmium Salts. Although most acute cadmium exposures are pulmonary, acute oral exposures also occur. In one case,[9] a 17-year-old female ingested approximately 150 g of cadmium chloride and presented to the emergency department with hypotension and edema of the face, pharynx, and neck. Her condition quickly deteriorated, and she suffered a respiratory arrest. She was intubated, underwent orogastric lavage, chelation with an unspecified agent, and charcoal hemoperfusion. Multisystem organ failure ensued, and she died within 30 hours of presentation. At autopsy, the most significant finding was hemorrhagic necrosis of the upper GI tract, consistent with a caustic ingestion. Although her blood cadmium level was more than 2000 times normal, it is not clear whether her demise was related to the cellular effects of cadmium or to the caustic nature of the ingestion.

In a second case,[97] a 23-year-old male ingested approximately 5 g of cadmium iodide in a suicide attempt and presented with acute hemorrhagic gastroenteritis. His condition deteriorated, and despite treatment with ethylenediamine-tetraacetic acid (EDTA) and supportive measures, he died on hospital day 7. Autopsy did not reveal a specific cause of death.

Pulmonary/Cadmium Fumes. Cadmium pneumonitis results from acute inhalation of cadmium oxide fumes during metalwork. The acute phase of cadmium pneumonitis may mimic metal fume fever (Chap. 95), but the two entities are distinctly different. Whereas metal fume fever is benign and self-limited, acute cadmium pneumonitis can progress to hypoxia, respiratory insufficiency, and death.

Case reports of patients who develop acute cadmium pneumonitis[4,5,33,67,76,86,96,98] are striking in their similar presentations. Patients were generally in good health until they began soldering or brazing with cadmium alloy in a closed space or without appropriate respiratory precautions. Within 6–12 hours, they developed constitutional symptoms, such as fever and chills, as well as a cough and respiratory distress, for which they sought care.

On initial presentation to a healthcare provider, these patients may not appear ill; they may have a normal physical examination, oxygenation status, and chest radiograph. This apparent normalcy may lead to some confusion about the severity of the patient's illness, and misdiagnosis (with metal-fume fever or some other non-specific pulmonary ailment) is common. As the pneumonitis progresses to acute lung injury (ALI; Chap. 95), rales and rhonchi develop, oxygenation becomes impaired, and the chest radiograph develops a pattern consistent with pulmonary edema. Death despite aggressive supportive care is reported, and usually occurs within 3–5 days.[33,67,76,96]

Patients who survive an episode of acute cadmium pneumonitis are described as developing various chronic pulmonary ailments, including restrictive lung disease,[4,5] diffusion abnormalities,[4] and pulmonary fibrosis.[86] Patients may recover without apparent sequelae.[98] Given the small number of patients, lack of controls, and lack of uniformity of care, the findings of long-term sequelae in case reports of patients with a history of acute cadmium pneumonitis should be considered associations at best.

Chronic Poisoning

Chronic cadmium poisoning generally occurs through occupational exposure, although instances of mass environmental exposure, such as occurred in Japan,[29,62] are reported. Unfortunately, studies of chronic cadmium poisoning in humans are retrospective, and thus imperfectly controlled. In addition, especially in the industrial setting, cadmium exposure may serve simply as a marker for other exposures, such as toxic vapors, other heavy metals, or solvents, which may contribute to or cause the pathologic condition in question. Nonetheless, a great deal of data about the chronic toxicity of cadmium is available.

Nephrotoxicity. The most common finding in chronic cadmium poisoning is proteinuria. This proteinuria is generally felt to be irreversible even after removal from exposure,[40,50,71] although some small studies suggest a potential for clinical improvement.[87] The question of whether renal dysfunction progresses after removal from exposure, however, is less clear. One large study of an environmentally exposed population found no progression of proteinuria or decrease in glomerular filtration rate (GFR) over time,[40] whereas a study of a different environmentally exposed population showed slowly progressive renal dysfunction over a 10-year period.[43] In an occupationally exposed cohort, followup studies showed a progressive decrease in GFR over time.[70,71] It is important to note that the route and duration of exposure, as well as blood and urine cadmium concentrations, differ markedly within these studies, limiting the importance and breadth of applicability of any analysis.

Occupational cadmium exposure is also associated with nephrolithiasis,[44,74] quite likely because of hypercalcuria.[75]

Pulmonary Toxicity. Large studies of cadmium-exposed workers failed to demonstrate consistent results regarding chronic occupational cadmium exposure and chronic lung disease. In one study of 57 workers occupationally exposed to enough cadmium to produce renal dysfunction, there was no evidence of pulmonary dysfunction, even in those individuals with the greatest cadmium exposure.[28] Conversely, other studies demonstrate both restrictive[17] and obstructive[22,73] changes on pulmonary function tests. Interestingly, a followup study of the group with restrictive lung disease showed improvements after cadmium exposure was reduced.[16] The discrepancy in these results may be partly a result of markedly different degrees of exposure among the various groups.

Cadmium may be associated with pulmonary neoplasia; the carcinogenicity of cadmium is discussed separately (below).

Musculoskeletal Toxicity. Osteomalacia, one of the most prominent features of the itai-itai epidemic, is a condition in which inadequate mineralization of mature bone predisposes these bones to pathologic fractures. Interestingly, osteomalacia is generally not a prominent feature of most populations occupationally exposed to cadmium, although it is mentioned in case reports.[10,50] The bias toward men in occupational cadmium studies (whereas the original itai-itai epidemic consisted largely of women), as well as differences in cumulative dosing, may account for some of this discrepancy.

Hepatotoxicity. Although the liver stores as much cadmium as any other organ, hepatotoxicity is not a prominent feature of human cadmium exposure.[42] The liver can certainly be a target organ, however, and hepatotoxicity is easily inducible in animals.[1,26,27,69]

Neurologic Toxicity. Evidence suggests that cadmium may be a neurotoxin. Cadmium exposure has been linked to olfactory disturbances,[72,82] impaired higher cortical function,[91] Parkinson syndrome,[65,91] and sensory peripheral neuropathy.[91,92]

Other Organ Systems. Cadmium induces hypertension in rats,[57] but human studies have not shown a convincing link.[32,66] Although there is evidence that cadmium may cause immunosuppression affecting both humoral and cell-mediated immunity in animals,[25] a single human study showed no overt immunopathology in an occupationally exposed cohort.[49] The testes are clearly a target organ in animal exposures,[56] but the testes are not considered a major target organ in humans.

Cancer. Cadmium is capable of inducing tumors in multiple tissues in animals. These effects seem to be exacerbated by zinc deficiency.[93] In humans, the only well-established site of carcinogenicity is the lung, and even those studies demonstrating an increased rate of lung cancer have methodologic flaws, such as coexposure to arsenic, a known pulmonary carcinogen.[11,51] The preponderance of evidence, however, indicates that cadmium is a human carcinogen, and it is designated as such by the International Agency for Research on Cancer and the US National Toxicology Program.

DIAGNOSTIC TESTING

Other than to confirm exposure, cadmium levels have limited utility in the management of the acutely exposed patient. Diagnosis and treatment are based on the patient's history, physical examination, and symptoms. Ancillary tests, such as arterial blood gas analysis and chest radiograph in a patient exposed to cadmium oxide fumes, are more useful than cadmium levels.

In the patient chronically exposed to cadmium, both cadmium levels and ancillary testing may prove helpful. Workers at high risk for cadmium toxicity should undergo regular urinalysis for proteinuria, and the development of proteinuria should prompt a reassignment to a low-exposure or no-exposure area. In the asymptomatic patient, the acceptable level for cadmium-exposed workers without proteinuria is 15 μg Cd/g urinary creatinine, although renal dysfunction has occurred at levels as low as 5 μg Cd/g urinary creatinine.[21,45] Urinary cadmium levels, which reflect the slow, steady-state turnover and release of metallothionein-bound cadmium from the liver, are a better reflection of total body cadmium burden than blood levels. It is for this reason that urine cadmium levels are used for occupational monitoring.

MANAGEMENT

Acute Exposure

Oral/Cadmium Salts. After airway, breathing, and circulation have been assessed, attention can be given to gastrointestinal decontamination. Although oral exposures are rare, they can prove fatal.[9,97] In light of this, even in the absence of any evidence, gastric lavage seems appropriate. A small nasogastric tube should suffice, as inorganic cadmium salts are powders, not pills. There are no data regarding the use of activated charcoal in acute oral cadmium toxicity; however, activated charcoal is a relatively benign intervention and is clearly indicated in the treatment of ingestion of some metals, such as thallium and mercury (Chap. 82). In light of this, activated charcoal should be given in the absence of any contraindications (such as known perforation or pending endoscopy).

Given the lack of experience with acute oral cadmium poisoning, all patients should be admitted to the hospital for supportive care, monitoring of renal and hepatic function, and consideration of evaluation of the gastrointestinal tract for evidence of caustic damage. Suggestions for the evaluation of a patient with a potential caustic injury are found elsewhere in this text (Chap. 87).

Although it seems logical to chelate any patient with an acute life-threatening ingestion of a metal compound, the benefit of chelation in acute cadmium exposure is unproven. Multiple chelating agents have been tried, all in animal models, and frequently with conflicting results.

The ideal chelating agent for treatment of oral cadmium toxicity would be well tolerated, would decrease gastrointestinal absorption of cadmium, would decrease the concentration of cadmium in organs such as the kidney and liver, and would not lead to increased cadmium levels in other critical organs such as the brain. Of the chelating agents studied for cadmium toxicity thus far, 2,3-dimercaptosuccinic acid (DMSA, succimer) comes closest to fulfilling these criteria. In models of acute oral cadmium toxicity, DMSA decreases the gastrointestinal absorption of cadmium[3,6] and improves survival[6,48] without increasing cadmium burdens in target organs.[2,6] In a patient thought to have ingested potentially lethal amounts of cadmium (5 g is the lowest reported human toxic dose), treatment with DMSA would be reasonable given the low toxicity and apparent efficacy of this agent. It must be stressed, however, that the data supporting the use of DMSA are promising but not definitive, and are only derived from animal models. Furthermore, the Food and Drug Administration has not approved DMSA for this indication. It would be reasonable to use doses of DMSA that are well tolerated (10 mg/kg/dose three times a day), although dosing in human exposures is completely unstudied.

Other chelating agents that may have some benefit in treating cadmium toxicity, but for which further investigation is warranted, include diethylenetriaminepentaacetic acid (DTPA)[6,14] and 2,3-dimercaptopropane sulfonate (DMPS),[14,48] both of which reduce tissue burdens and increase survival.

Many other chelating agents have been studied for treatment of acute cadmium toxicity and were found to be ineffective or detrimental. 2,3-Dimercaptopropanol (British Anti-Lewisite, BAL) increases whole-body cadmium excretion,[47] but may increase renal tissue levels.[14,47] BAL probably reduces acute toxicity modestly, but at the expense of potentiating chronic toxicity.[20] Penicillamine does not appear to increase cadmium excretion or reduce tissue levels and may increase renal cadmium levels,[14] as well as speed the development of nephrotoxicity.[59] Cyclic tetramines (such as CYCLAM and TACPD, which have shown promise in nickel chelation) are theoretically beneficial in cadmium toxicity,[37] but have yielded discouraging results thus far.[81] Detergent formula chelating agents such as sodium tripolyphosphate (STPP) and nitrilotriacetic acid (NTA) appear to enhance both tissue uptake and lethality of cadmium as compared to controls.[30,31] Data regarding calcium disodium EDTA are conflicting; although both mortality[39] and renal concentrations[14] were reduced in some models, there is also evidence that EDTA may potentiate toxicity.[60] Dithiocarbamates decrease renal and hepatic concentrations,[77,94] although some members of this class promote the uptake of cadmium into the CNS.[3,34]

The ability to draw conclusions about the above chelating agents in acute toxicity is difficult, for a number of reasons. Although some agents, such as EDTA and some dithiocarbamates, show promise, these agents may potentially prove harmful by redistributing cadmium to target organs. Furthermore, multiple models of acute cadmium exposure (oral, subcutaneous, intraperitoneal, and intravenous), multiple routes of administration of the chelating agent (oral, intraperitoneal, and intravenous), and multiple animal models (mouse, rat, and toad) are employed by various authors. Comparisons between studies are thus difficult, if not impossible. In addition, there is no evidence that the animal models being used are of any significance with regard to human toxicokinetics or toxicodynamics.

Perhaps most significantly, most of the studies in question administer chelating agents within 30 minutes of exposure, which is an unrealistic time frame for the management of most human cadmium poisonings. The issue of rapidity of initiation of treatment is crucial, because cadmium is so rapidly cleared from the blood and redistributed to target organs that small delays may render chelating agents ineffective. One important study established that a variety of chelating agents (including EDTA, DTPA, and a dithiocarbamate) were effective in promoting cadmium excretion and reducing critical organ levels of cadmium when given immediately after cadmium exposure. However, in the second part of this study, when administration of these agents was delayed by only 2 hours, excretion fell by 90%, and concentrations of cadmium in target organs were indistinguishable from the control group.[15]

In summary, DMSA appears to have the most benefit in preventing morbidity and mortality in animal models of acute cadmium toxicity. DTPA and DMPS have also been shown to be effective, but the data are less convincing than for DMSA. Studies examining other agents, such as BAL, penicillamine, cyclic tetramines (CYCLAM and TACPD), detergent formula chelating agents (STPP and NTA), EDTA, and some dithiocarbamates, have found that these agents either have a mixed safety profile or are outright deleterious.

Pulmonary/Cadmium Fumes. The patient who is ill after exposure to cadmium fumes (generally cadmium oxide) will invariably present with respiratory complaints and, usually, with constitutional symptoms as well. The patient should be removed from the exposure; the airway should then be assessed and appropriate oxygenation assured, although hypoxia may not be a problem acutely. Steroids are frequently used, but there are no studies to prove their efficacy. Because cadmium inhalation injuries are neither benign nor self-limited, all patients with acute inhalational exposures to cadmium should be admitted to the hospital for observation and supportive care until respiratory symptoms have resolved. All such patients should have long-term followup arranged with a pulmonologist to assess the possibility of chronic lung injury, even in instances of single exposures.

Chelation should never be entertained as an option for patients acutely exposed to cadmium fumes. Although large studies are lacking, these patients do not appear to be at risk for extrapulmonary injury.[4,5,86,98]

Chronic Exposure

Patients chronically exposed to cadmium frequently come to attention during routine screening, as cadmium is a known industrial toxin and most patients who work with cadmium are under close medical surveillance. Usually, patients have developed proteinuria or less commonly, chronic pulmonary complaints.

The management of such patients is challenging. Reduction (and preferably elimination) of cadmium exposure is the first intervention. However, as mentioned earlier, chronic cadmium-induced renal and pulmonary changes may have a largely irreversible component.

Chelation of patients with chronic cadmium toxicity is not currently recommended for a number of reasons. First, there is no evidence that chelation of chronically poisoned animals improves long-term outcomes, although some agents may lessen short-term organ dysfunction.[55] Second, the majority of cadmium in a chronically exposed patient is bound to intracellular metallothionein, which greatly reduces its toxicity. Any attempt to remove cadmium from these deposits risks redistributing cadmium to other organs, possibly exacerbating toxicity; for instance, BAL may potentiate nephrotoxicity.[24] Finally, many typical chelating agents (such as DMSA and DTPA[35]) do not remove significant amounts of cadmium, possibly because they cannot cross cell membranes to access the intracellular cadmium or because these agents do not have a high enough affinity for cadmium to dislodge it from metallothionein.

Of all chelating agents tested thus far in animal models of chronic cadmium toxicity, the dithiocarbamates have shown the most success in reducing total body cadmium burdens in chronically poisoned animals. Unfortunately, the most effective agents, which are highly lipophilic, also tend to cause redistribution of cadmium to the brain; their lipophilicity allows them to cross cell membranes into hepatocytes, but also promotes their uptake into the lipid-rich central nervous system.[35] Numerous dithiocarbamates have been synthesized and studied with regard to cadmium decorporation, however, and several species effectively reduce whole-body, renal, and hepatic cadmium levels without an increase in CNS cadmium.[55,78] At this time, there are no FDA-approved dithiocarbamate preparations.

Further research into the subject of chelation for chronic cadmium poisoning is ongoing, and may in the future suggest an agent which is not only safe, but reduces the risk of exacerbating end-organ toxicity. However, there is insufficient evidence at this time to justify the use of any chelating agent in the treatment of chronic cadmium toxicity.

SUMMARY

Cadmium is a potent toxin with different effects based on the time course and route of exposure. In the acute oral exposure, gastrointestinal injury may predominate; in acute inhalation, a severe chemical pneumonitis may ensue. In chronic environmental or occupational exposure, nephrotoxicity (usually manifest by proteinuria) is the most significant finding, although other organ systems, such as the lungs, can be affected. Treatment for all patients with suspected cadmium poisoning, acute or chronic, consists of removal from the source, decontamination if possible, and supportive care. In the rare instance of acute cadmium salt ingestion, treatment with DMSA may be warranted; there is insufficient evidence to recommend chelation in the chronically cadmium poisoned patient at this time.

REFERENCES

1. Al-Nasser IA: Cadmium hepatotoxicity and alterations of the mitochondrial function. J Toxicol Clin Toxicol 2000;38:407–413.

2. Andersen O, Nielsen JB: Oral cadmium chloride intoxication in mice: Effects of penicillamine, dimercaptosuccinic acid and related compounds. Pharmacol Toxicol 1988;63:386–389.

3. Anderson O, Nielsen JB, Svendsen P: Oral cadmium chloride intoxication in mice: Diethyldithiocarbamate enhances rather than alleviates acute toxicity. Toxicology 1988;52:331–342.

4. Anthony JS, Zamel N, Aberman A: Abnormalities in pulmonary function after brief exposure to toxic metal fumes. Can Med Assoc J 1978;119:586–588.

5. Barnhart S, Rosenstock L: Cadmium chemical pneumonitis. Chest 1984;86:791.

6. Basinger MA, Jones MM, Hoscher MA, et al: Antagonists for acute oral cadmium chloride intoxication. J Toxicol Environ Health 1988;23:77–89.

7. Bernard A, Roels H, Hubermont G, et al: Characterization of the proteinuria of cadmium-exposed workers. Int Arch Occup Environ Health 1976;38:19–30.

8. Bernard A, Roels H, Thielemans N, et al: Assessment of the causality of the cadmium-protein relationships in the urine of the general population with reference to the Cadmibel study. IARC Sci Publ 1992;118:341–346.

9. Buckler HM, Smith WD, Rees WD: Self-poisoning with oral cadmium chloride. Br Med J 1986;292:1559–1560.

10. Blainey JD, Adams RG, Brewer DB, et al: Cadmium-induced osteomalacia. Br J Ind Med 1980;37:278–284.

11. Bofetta P: Methodological aspects of the epidemiological association between cadmium and cancer in humans. IARC Sci Publ 1992;118:425–434.

12. Buchet JP, Lauwerys R, Roels H, et al: Renal effects of cadmium body burden of the general population. Lancet 1990;336:699–702.

13. Budavari S, O'Neil MJ, Smith A, et al, eds: The Merck Index. Whithouse Station, NJ, Merck & Company, 1996, p. 1665.

14. Cantilena LR, Klaassen CD: Comparison of the effectiveness of several chelators after single administration on the toxicity, excretion, and distribution of cadmium. Toxicol Appl Pharmacol 1981;58:452–460.

15. Cantilena LR, Klaassen CD: Decreased effectiveness of chelation therapy with time after acute cadmium poisoning. Toxicol Appl Pharmacol 1982;63:173–180.

16. Chan OY, Poh SC, Lee HS, et al: Respiratory function in cadmium battery workers—A follow-up study. Ann Acad Med Singapore 1988;17:283–287.

17. Chan OY, Poh SC, Tan KT, Kwok SF: Respiratory function in cadmium battery workers. Singapore Med J 1986;27:108–119.

18. Cherian MG: Chelation of cadmium with BAL and DTPA in rats. Nature 1980;287:871–872.

19. Cherian MG, Goyer RA, Delaquerriere-Richardson L: Cadmium-metallothionein-induced nephropathy. Toxicol Appl Pharmacol 1976;38:399–408.

20. Cherian, MG, Rodgers K: Chelation of cadmium from metallothionein in vivo and its excretion in rats repeatedly injected with cadmium chloride. J Pharmacol Exp Ther 1982;222:699–703.

21. Chia KS, Tan AL, Chia SE, et al: Renal tubular function of cadmium exposed workers. Ann Acad Med Singapore 1992;21:756–759.

22. Cortona G, Apostoli P, Toffoletto F, et al: Occupational exposure to cadmium and lung function. IARC Sci Publ 1992;118:205–210.

23. Coyle P, Niezing G, Shelton TL, et al: Tolerance to cadmium toxicity by metallothionein and zinc: In vivo and in vitro studies with MT-null mice. Toxicology 2000;150:53–67.

24. Dalhamn T, Friberg L: Dimercaprol (2,3-dimercaptopropanol) in chronic cadmium poisoning. Acta Pharmacol Toxicol 1955;11: 68–71.

25. Dan G, Lall SB, Rao DN: Humoral and cell-mediated immune response to cadmium in mice. Drug Chem Toxicol 2000;23:349–360.

26. Dudley RE, Gammal LM, Klaassen CD: Cadmium-induced hepatic and renal injury in chronically exposed rats: Likely role of hepatic cadmium-metallothionein in nephrotoxicity. Toxicol Appl Pharmacol 1985;77:414–426.

27. Dudley RE, Svoboda DJ, Klaassen CD: Acute exposure to cadmium causes severe liver injury in rats. Toxicol Appl Pharmacol 1982;65:302–313.

28. Edling C, Elinder CG, Randma E: Lung function in workers using cadmium containing solder. Br J Ind Med 1986;43:657–662.

29. Emmerson BT: "Ouch-ouch" disease: The osteomalacia of cadmium nephropathy. Ann Intern Med 1970;73:854.

30. Engstrom B: Influence of chelating agents on toxicity and distribution of cadmium among proteins of mouse liver and kidney following oral or subcutaneous exposure. Acta Pharmacol Toxicol 1981;48:108–117.

31. Engstrom B, Nordberg GF: Effects of detergent formula chelating agents on the metabolism and toxicity of cadmium in mice. Acta Pharmacol Toxicol 1978;43:387–397.

32. Engvall J, Perk J: Prevalence of hypertension among cadmium-exposed workers. Arch Environ Health 1985;40:185–190.

33. Fuortes L, Leo A, Ellerbeck PG, Friell LA: Acute respiratory fatality associated with exposure to sheet metal and cadmium fumes. J Toxicol Clin Toxicol 1991;29:279–283.

34. Gale GR, Atkins LM, Walker EM, et al: Comparative effects of diethyldithiocarbamate, dimercaptosuccinate, and diethylenetri-aminepentaacetate on organ distribution and excretion of cadmium. Ann Clin Lab Sci 1983;13:33–44.

35. Gale GR, Atkins LM, Walker EM, et al: Mechanism of diethyldithiocarbamate, dihydroxyethyldithiocarbamate, and dicarboxymethyldithiocarbamate action on distribution and excretion of cadmium. Ann Clin Lab Sci 1983;13:474–481.

36. Goyer RA, et al: Non-metallothionein-bound cadmium in the pathogenesis of cadmium nephrotoxicity in the rat. Toxicol Appl Pharmacol 1989;101:232–244.

37. Gulumian M, Casimiro E, Linder PW, et al: Evaluation of a new chelating agent for cadmium: A preliminary report. Hum Exp Toxicol 1993;12:247–251.

38. Hammond, CR: Cadmium. In: Lide DR, ed: CRC Handbook of Chemistry and Physics, 80th ed. Boca Raton, FL, CRC Press, 1989, pp. 4–8.

39. Hilmy AM, El-Domaity N, Daabees AY: Toxicity of cadmium administration to the toad and the treatment of its poisoning with EDTA. Comp Biochem Physiol C 1986;85:249–252.

40. Hotz P, Buchet JP, Bernard A, et al: Renal effects of low-level environmental cadmium exposure: 5-year follow-up of a subcohort from the Cadmibel study. Lancet 1999;354:1508–1513.

41. Ikeda M, Moon CS, Zhang ZW, et al: Urinary alpha1-microglobulin, beta2-microglobulin, and retinol-binding protein levels in general populations in Japan with references to cadmium in urine, blood, and 24-hour food duplicates. Environ Res 1995;70:35–46.

42. Ikeda M, Watanabe T, Zhang Z-W, et al: The integrity of the liver among people environmentally exposed to cadmium at various levels. Int Arch Occup Environ Health 1997;69:379–385.

43. Iwata K, Saito H, Moriyama M, Nakano A: Renal tubular function after reduction of environmental cadmium exposure: A ten-year follow-up. Arch Environ Health 1993;48:157–163.

44. Jarup L, Elinder CG: Incidence of renal stones among cadmium exposed battery workers. Br J Ind Med 1993;50:598–602.

45. Jarup L, Elinder CG: Dose-response relations between urinary cadmium and tubular proteinuria in cadmium-exposed workers. Am J Ind Med 1994;26:759–769.

46. Jarup L, Hellstrom L, Alfven T, et al: Low level exposure to cadmium and early kidney damage: The OSCAR study. Occup Environ Med 2000;57:668–672.

47. Jones MM, Cherian MG, Singh PK, et al: A comparative study on the influence of vicinal dithiols and a dithiocarbamate on the biliary excretion of cadmium in rat. Toxicol Appl Pharmacol 1991;110:241–250.

48. Jones MM, Weater AD, Weller WL: The relative effectiveness of some chelating agents as antidotes in acute cadmium poisoning. Res Commun Chem Pathol Pharmacol 1978;22:581–588.

49. Karakaya A, Yucesoy B, Sardas OS: An immunological study on workers occupationally exposed to cadmium. Hum Exp Toxicol 1994;13:73–75.

50. Kazantis G: Renal tubular dysfunction and abnormalities of calcium metabolism in cadmium workers. Environ Health Perspect 1979;28:155–159.

51. Kazantis G, Blanks RG, Sullivan KR: Is cadmium a human carcinogen? IARC Sci Publ 1992;118:435–446.

52. Kjellstrom T, Nordberg GF: A kinetic model of cadmium metabolism in the human being. Environ Res 1978;16:248–269.

53. Klaassen CD, Liu J, Choudhuri S: Metallothionein: An intracellular protein to protect against cadmium toxicity. Annu Rev Pharmacol Toxicol 1999;39:267–294.

54. Kojima S, Kaminaka K, Kiyozumi M, et al: Comparative effects of three chelating agents on distribution and excretion of cadmium in rats. Toxicol Appl Pharmacol 1986;83:516–524.

55. Kojima S, Ono H, Kiyozumi M, et al: Effect of N-benzyl-D-glucamine dithiocarbamate on the renal toxicity produced by subacute exposure to cadmium in rats. Toxicol Applied Pharmacol 1989;98:39–48.

56. Kojima S, Sugimura Y, Hirukawa H, et al: Effects of dithiocarbamates on testicular toxicity in rats caused by acute exposure to cadmium. Toxicol Appl Pharmacol 1992;116:24–29.

57. Lall SB, Das N, Rama R, et al: Cadmium-induced nephrotoxicity in rats. Indian J Exp Biol 1997;35(2):151–154.

58. Liu J, Liu Y, Habeebu SS, Klaassen CD: Susceptibility of MT null mice to chronic CdCl$_2$-induced nephrotoxicity indicates that renal injury is not mediated by the CdMT complex. Toxicol Sci 1998;46:197–203.

59. Lyle WH, Green JN, Gore V, et al: Enhancement of cadmium nephrotoxicity by penicillamine in the rat. Postgrad Med J 1968;Suppl:18–21.

60. McGivern J, Mason J: The effect of chelation on the fate of intravenously administered cadmium in rats. J Comp Pathol 1979;89:1–9.

61. Min K-S, Onosaka S, Tanaka K: Renal accumulation of cadmium and nephropathy following long-term administration of cadmium-metallothionein. Toxicol Appl Pharmacol 1996;141:102–109.

62. Murata I, Hirono T, Saeki Y, et al: Cadmium enteropathy, renal osteomalacia ("itai itai" disease in Japan). Bull Soc Int Chir 1970;29:34–42.

63. Nishio H, Hayashi C, Lee MJ, et al: Itai-itai disease is not associated with polymorphisms of the estrogen receptor alpha gene. Arch Toxicol 1999;73:496–498.

64. Nogawa K, Kido T, Shaikh ZA: Dose-response relationship for renal dysfunction in a population environmentally exposed to cadmium. IARC Sci Publ 1992;118:311–318.

65. Okuda B, Iwamoto Y, Tachibana H, Sugita M: Parkinsonism after acute cadmium poisoning. Clin Neurol Neurosurg 1997;99:263–265.

66. Ostergaard K: Cadmium and hypertension. Lancet 1977;8013:677–678.

67. Patwardhan JR, Finckh ES: Fatal cadmium-fume pneumonitis. Med J Aust 1976;1(25):962–966.

68. Prozialec WC: Evidence that e-cadherin may be a target for cadmium toxicity in epithelial cells. Toxicol Appl Pharmacol 2000;164:231–249.

69. Rikans LE, Yamano T: Mechanisms of cadmium-mediated acute hepatotoxicity. J Biochem Mol Toxicol 2000;14:110–117.

70. Roels H, Djubgang J, Buchet JT, et al: Evolution of cadmium-induced renal dysfunction in workers removed from exposure. Scand J Work Environ Health 1982;8:191–200.

71. Roels HA, Lauwerys RR, Buchet JP, et al: Health significance of cadmium-induced renal dysfunction: A five-year follow-up. Br J Ind Med 1989;46:755–764.

72. Rose CS, Heywood PG, Costanzo RM: Olfactory impairment after chronic occupational cadmium exposure. J Occup Med 1992;34:600–605.

73. Sakurai H, Omae K, Toyama T, et al: Cross-sectional study of pulmonary function in cadmium alloy workers. Scand J Work Environ Health 1982;8S1:122–130.

74. Scott R, Cunningham C, McLelland A, et al: The importance of cadmium as a factor in calcified upper urinary tract stone disease—A prospective 7-year study. Br J Urol 1982;54:584–589.

75. Scott R, Patterson PJ, Burns R, et al: Hypercalciuria related to cadmium exposure. Urology 1978;11:462–465.

76. Seidal K, Jorgensen N, Elinder CG, et al: Fatal cadmium-induced pneumonitis. Scand J Work Environ Health 1993;19:429–431.

77. Shimada H, Funakoshi T, Kiyozumi M, et al: Comparison of the effectiveness of dithiocarbamates on the excretion and distribution of cadmium in mice. Res Commun Chem Pathol Pharmacol 1991;73:249–252.

78. Singh PK, Jones SG, Gale GR, et al: Selective removal of cadmium from aged hepatic and renal deposits: N-substituted talooctamine dithiocarbamates as cadmium mobilizing agent. Chem Biol Interact 1990;74:79–91.

79. Squibb KS, Pritchard JB, Fowler BA: Cadmium-metallothionein nephropathy: Relationships between ultrastructural/biochemical alterations and intracellular cadmium binding. J Pharmacol Exp Ther 1984;229:311–321.

80. Squibb KS, Ridlington JW, Carmichael NG, Fowler BA: Early cellular effects of circulating cadmium-thionein on kidney proximal tubules. Environ Health Perspect 1979;28:287–296.

81. Srivasta RC, Gupta S, Ahmad N, et al: Comparative evaluation of chelating agents on the mobilization of cadmium: A mechanistic approach. J Toxicology Environ Health 1996;47:173–182.

82. Surunda AJ: Measuring olfactory dysfunction from cadmium in an occupational and environmental medicine office practice. J Occup Environ Med 2000;42:337.

83. Takebayashi S, Jimi S, Segawaa M, Kiyoshi Y: Cadmium induces osteomalacia mediated by proximal tubular atrophy and disturbances of phosphate reabsorption. A study of 11 autopsies. Pathol Res Pract 2000;196:653–663.

84. Telisman S, Jurasovic J, Pizent A, et al: Cadmium in the blood and seminal fluid of nonoccupationally exposed adult male subjects with regard to smoking habits. Int Arch Occup Environ Health 1997;70:243–248.

85. Thun MJ, et al: Nephropathy in cadmium workers: Assessment of risk from airborne occupational exposure to cadmium. Br J Ind Med 1989;46:689–697.

86. Townshend RH: Acute cadmium pneumonitis: A 17-year follow up. Br J Ind Med 1982;39:411–412.

87. Tsychya K: Proteinuria of cadmium workers. J Occup Med 1976;18:463–466.

88. van Sittert NJ, Ribbens PH, Huisman B, Lugtengurg D: A nine-year follow-up study of renal effects in workers exposed to cadmium in a zinc ore refinery. Br J Ind Med 1993;50:603–612.

89. Verbost PM, Filk G, Pang PKT, et al: Cadmium inhibition of the erythrocyte Ca2+ pump. J Biol Chem 1989;264:5613–5615.

90. Verbost PM, Senden MHMN, van Os CH: Nanomolar concentrations of Cd2+ inhibit Ca2+ transport systems in plasma membranes and intracellular Ca2+ stores in intestinal epithelium. Biochem Biophys Acta 1987;902:247–252.

91. Viaene, MK, Masschelein R, Leenders J, et al: Neurobehavioural effects of occupational exposure to cadmium: A cross-sectional epidemiological study. Occup Environ Med 2000;57:19–27.

92. Viaene, MK, Roels HA, Leenders J, et al: Cadmium: A possible etiological factor in peripheral polyneuropathy. Neurotoxicology 1999; 20:7–16.

93. Waalkes MP: Cadmium carcinogenesis in review. J Inorg Biochem 2000;79:241–244.

94. Wang, C, Fany Y, Peng S, et al: Synthesis of novel chelating agents and their effect on cadmium decorporation. Chem Res Toxicol 1999; 12:331–334.

95. Watkins SR, Hodge RM, Cowman DC, Wickham PP: Cadmium-binding serum protein. Biochem Biophys Res Commun 1977;74: 1403–1410.

96. Winston RM: Cadmium fume poisoning. Br Med J 1971;758:401.

97. Wisniewska-Knypl JM, Jablonska J, Myslak Z: Binding of cadmium on metallothionein in man: An analysis of a fatal poisoning by cadmium iodide. Arch Toxicol 1971;28:46–55.

98. Yates DH, Goldman KP: Acute cadmium poisoning in a foreman plant welder. Br J Ind Med 1990;47:429–431.

Lewis S. Nelson

Copper

MW	=	63.5 daltons
Normal Levels		
Blood, total	=	70–140 µg/dL (11–22µmol/L)
Serum, total	=	120–145 µg/dL (18.9–22.8 µmol/L)
Serum free	=	4–7 µg/dL (0.63–1.1 µmol/L)
Urine	=	30–50 µg/L (0.47–0.79 µmol/L)
Ceruloplasmin	=	25–50 µg/dL
Action Levels		
Blood	=	100 µg/dL (15.7 µmol/L)

Values greater than or equal to the action level necessitate clinical intervention. Values less than this level may necessitate intervention based on the clinical condition of the patient.

A 16-year-old boy presented to the hospital 3 days after reportedly ingesting 1 tablespoon of K77 Root Killer in an attempt to gain needed attention from his aunt. The patient denied suicidality and stated that he did not know that the granules, which were in his home to halt the growth of tree roots into the home's septic system, were toxic. Immediately after ingesting the product, he was given milk by his aunt. According to the patient this prompted four episodes of blue-colored emesis, containing crystals of the ingested substance. Although he had abdominal pain for the next 72 hours, the patient did not seek medical care because he assumed these symptoms would be transient. There was no suggestion that this was indeed a suicide attempt.

Ultimately, the patient presented to the hospital because he developed dark brown discoloration of his urine, yellowing of his eyes, and worsening abdominal pain. He denied throat discomfort, hematemesis, or melena. His presenting vital signs were blood pressure, 102/52 mmHg; pulse, 86 beats/min; respirations, 18 breaths/min; and he was afebrile. His physical examination was significant for the presence of scleral and sublingual icterus, although dermal jaundice was not appreciated. His oropharynx was normal and his chest was clear. On abdominal examination there was moderate tenderness over the left upper quadrant and left costovertebral angle. There was no involuntary guarding or rebound. Stool obtained by rectal examination was guaiac negative. The patient's neurologic examination was normal.

A chest radiograph was normal. His initial laboratory assessment was remarkable for a hematocrit of 20%, and normal chemistries (anion gap, 5) and renal function (blood urea nitrogen (BUN), 15 mg/dL; creatinine, 0.8 mg/dL). Hepatic profiling revealed an aspartate aminotransferase (AST) of 54 IU/L, alkaline phosphatase of 77 IU/L, and a total bilirubin of 5.2 mg/dL with an indirect bilirubin of 0.2 mg/dL.

The patient was started on D-penicillamine, 500 mg every 6 hours orally, and was hydrated aggressively with intravenous 0.9% sodium chloride. His clinical status improved over the next 72 hours and no blood transfusion was required.

Copper is among the more frequently reported metals with which patients are poisoned. It routinely ranks third, behind lead and arsenic, in nonmedicinal metal exposures (such as iron or lithium) reported to US Poison Control Centers (Chap. 116). Still, acute symptomatic poisoning remains relatively rare in this country. In India, copper sulfate ingestion is a leading cause of suicide.[23,67] In that country, copper sulfate poisoning is reportedly responsible for nearly a third of all poisonings requiring hemodialysis, and is the most common nephrotoxic indication for dialysis.[6,21] The dramatic clinical presentations and potential for poor outcome without appropriate treatment highlight the toxicologic significance of copper.

Copper, in its various forms, is still used intensively in our society. As the metal, it is extensively used in both wiring and plumbing. Its use in coinage, at least in the United States, fell dramatically with its replacement by zinc in the penny. Copper salts, alternatively, are widely used in fungicides, algicides, and plant growth regulators (Table 82–3). They are also important as catalysts, particularly in the petroleum industry. Throughout this chapter, unless otherwise noted, discussion of toxicologically important aspects of copper refers to inorganic, or ionic, copper.

HISTORY AND EPIDEMIOLOGY

Copper is available naturally, either as native copper or as one of its sulfide or oxide ores. Important ores include malachite ($CuCO_3 (OH)_2$), chalcocite (Cu_2S), cuprite (Cu_2O), and chalcopyrite ($CuFeS_2$ or $Cu_2S\ Fe_2S_3$). Chalcopyrite, a yellow sulfide ore, is the source of 80% of the world's copper production. The smelting of copper ores began about 7000 years ago; copper metal gradually assumed its current level of importance at the start of the Bronze Age around 3000 BC. Smelting, or the separation of the ore components, begins with roasting to dry the ore concentrate, which is then further purified by electrolysis to a 99.5% level of purity. The sulfide ores have a naturally high arsenic content that is released

TABLE 82–3.   Important Copper Products

Chemical Name	Chemical Structure	Common Name	Notes
Chalcopyrite	$CuFeS_2$	Copper iron sulfide	Copper ore; source of 80% of world's copper
Chromated cupric arsenate	1% copper oxide 47% chromium oxide 34% arsenic pent-oxide	CCA	Wood preservative [34]
Copper triethanolamine complex	$Cu((HOCH_2CH_2)_3N)_2$	Chelated copper	Algicide
Cupric acetoarsenite	$Cu(C_2H_3O_2)_2.3Cu(AsO_2)_2$	Paris or Vienna green	Insecticide, wood preservative, pigment*
Cupric arsenite	$CuHAsO_3$	Swedish or Scheele green	Wood preservative insecticide*
Cupric hydroxide	$Cu(OH)_2$		Fungicide
Cupric chloride	$CuCl_2$		Catalyst in petrochemical industry
Cupric chloride, basic	$CuCl_2 + CuO$	Basic copper chloride; copper oxychloride	Fungicide
Copper octanoate		Copper soap	Fungicide in paint, rot-proof rope, and roofing
Cupric oxide	CuO	Black copper oxide; tenorite	Glass pigment, flux, polishing agent
Cupric sulfate	$CuSO_4$	Roman vitriol, blue vitriol, bluestone, hydrocyanite	Fungicide, plant growth regulator, whitewash, home-grown crystals
Cupric sulfate, basic	$CuSO_4 + CuO$	Bordeaux solution	Fungicide
Cuprous cyanide	$CuCN$	Cupricin	Electroplating solutions
Cuprous oxide	Cu_2O	Red copper oxide, cuprite	Antifouling paint

*No longer used in United States.

during the extraction process, posing a risk for those who perform copper smelting.

Although, as noted, acute copper poisoning is uncommon in the United States, copper's historical role as a pharmacotherapeutic agent remains noteworthy. Copper sulfate was used in burn wound débridement until cases of systemic poisoning were reported.[35] Interestingly, in one report, each wound débridement procedure was associated with a fall in the child's hematocrit by 8–10%. In the 1960s, copper sulfate (250-mg dose, containing 100 mg copper ion) was ironically a recommended emetic agent, typically for use in children, following potentially toxic exposures.[40] It was recognized for its rapid onset and effectiveness, and it compared favorably with syrup of ipecac. However, this was rapidly identified to be a highly dangerous practice and its use was discontinued.[36,72] Copper salts are still administered in religious rituals as a green-colored "spiritual water," containing 100–150 g/L of copper sulfate as an emetic to expel one's sins.[7,71]

Acute or chronic copper poisoning occurs when copper ions are leached from copper pipes or copper containers. This occurs most frequently when carbon dioxide gas, used for postmix soft drink carbonation, backflows into the tubing transporting water to the soda dispensers, creating an acidic solution of carbonic acid.[83] Similarly, storage of acidic potable substances, such as orange or lemon juice, in copper vessels may cause copper poisoning.[84] A particularly dangerous situation occurs when acidic water is inadvertently used for hemodialysis.[26,48] In this circumstance, the leached copper avoids the normal gastrointestinal barrier and is delivered directly to the patient's circulation. In one reported series, the copper level in the dialysis water was 650 µg/L, causing several poisonings and the death of a patient with a whole-blood copper level of 2095 µg/L.[26] Similarly, stagnant water or hot water,[63] even if not highly acidic, may accumulate copper ions and cause poisoning.[8,27]

Metallic copper is ideal for electrical wiring because it is highly malleable, can be drawn into fine wire, and has an electrical conductivity only exceeded by silver. Similarly, its excellent heat conductivity accounts for its widespread use in cookware. Although the metal is reactive with air, it forms a resistant layer of insoluble copper carbonate on its surface. It is this water- and air-resistant compound that accounts for the green coloration of ornamental roofing and statues. Because copper is a soft metal it must be strengthened prior to use in structural applications or as a coinage metal. This is most commonly done by the creation of copper alloys. Brass is an alloy of copper compounded with as much as 35% zinc. Similarly, bronze contains copper combined with up to 14% zinc. Gunmetal is an alloy that contains 88% copper, 10% tin, and 2% zinc. Sterling silver and white gold also contain copper.

CHEMICAL PRINCIPLES

Metallic copper (Cu^0) has an oxidation state of zero and, although not in itself poisonous, it may release copper ions in acidic environments. The copper intrauterine device (IUD) for contraception derives its efficacy from the effects of the local release of copper ions.[12] Similarly, metallic copper bracelets, worn by patients with rheumatoid arthritis, purportedly derive their far-reaching anti-inflammatory effect through dermal copper ion absorption and distribution to affected tissues.[80] Ingestion of large amounts of metallic copper, for example as coins, may rarely produce acute copper poisoning.[86] Poisoning in this situation is caused by release of large amounts of copper ion from copper alloy by the acidic gastric content. Also, finely divided metallic copper dust or bronze powder used in industry and for gilding, although not systemically bioavailable, may produce life-threatening bronchopulmonary irritation, presumably as a consequence of the local release of ions.[33]

As noted, most patients who are suffering from acute copper poisoning are exposed to ionic copper. In copper (II) sulfate, also known as cupric sulfate, the copper atom is in the +2 oxidation state. Copper sulfate is used as a fungicide and algicide and to eradicate tree roots that invade septic or sewage systems. Copper sulfate is the most readily available form and that which is involved in the majority of nonindustrial copper salt exposures. Copper sulfate was a favorite ingredient in many home chemistry sets because of its brilliant blue color when dissolved in water. Although serious poisoning, particularly in children,[81] led regulatory agencies in the United States to restrict its use, it still accounts for most chemistry set–related exposures in other countries.[53] Home-grown copper sulfate crystals kits are occasionally responsible for fatal poisonings.[30]

Cuprous salts, containing copper in the +1 oxidation state, are unstable in water and readily oxidize to the cupric form. Regardless of oxidation state, there are numerous copper salts used in industry and agriculture (Table 82–3), many of which are not poisonous. Because those salts that are water soluble are more likely to be toxic, it is important to determine the nature of the implicated copper product in poisoned patients. Analogously, when examining the medical literature, it is critical to discern which form of copper is involved in the experiment or case report before understanding and application of the results can occur.

PHARMACOLOGY/PHYSIOLOGY

Copper is one of eight essential metals that our body stores in milligram amounts (100–150 mg). Daily requirements of copper are approximately 50 µg/kg in infants and 30 µg/kg in adults. The daily requirement is satisfied by nuts, fish, and green vegetables such as legumes, although our largest source is generally from drinking water. Although most natural water contains a small quantity (4–10 µg/L), most copper is tightly bound to organic matter and therefore not orally bioavailable. Copper pipes typically add about 1 mg of copper to the daily intake of an adult. The Environmental Protection Agency guidelines permit up to 1.3 mg/L of copper in drinking water, although in some areas concentrations may intermittently be as high as 60 mg/L. Copper in water may be tasted at concentrations of 1–5 mg/L and a blue-green discoloration is imparted when the levels are greater than 5 mg/L. Acute gastrointestinal symptoms occur when water contains more than 25 mg/L, although levels as low as 3 mg/L are often considered "toxic" by regulatory agencies. Copper deficiency is exceedingly rare even in the poorest communities and is most frequently a result of excessive zinc intake or to a genetic aberration such as Menkes disease.

Copper is absorbed by an active process involving a Cu-ATPase in the small intestinal mucosal cell membrane, also known as the Menkes ATPase (see below). Although the gastrointestinal absorption varies with the copper intake and is as low as 12% in patients with high copper intake, in the presence of damaged mucosa, such as following acute overdose, the fractional absorption is likely to be significantly higher. Once absorbed, copper is rapidly bound to albumin and amino acids, such as histidine, for transport to the liver and other tissues. Its half-life in the plasma is approximately 15 minutes. Copper uptake by the hepatic cells occurs via a specific uptake pump after being released locally in the reduced state from its carrier (albumin or ceruloplasmin). This process, which is facilitated by the reducing agent ascorbic acid, provides a potential window, however brief, for detoxification of the ion by chelating agents.

In the hepatocyte complex, trafficking systems exist involving ceruloplasmin, metallothionein, and other metallochaperones within the cytoplasm to prevent copper toxicity and to aid delivery to the appropriate enzymes.[18] A distinct Cu-ATPase, located on certain subcellular organelles such as the trans-Golgi network or pericanalicular lysosomes, assists in the appropriate localization and elimination, respectively, of the metal.[18] By this mechanism, copper is either incorporated into enzymes or released, as a metallothionein-copper complex, directly into the biliary system for fecal elimination.

Some copper is released from the liver bound primarily to ceruloplasmin, an α_2-sialoglycoprotein with a molecular weight of 132,000 daltons. Ceruloplasmin-bound copper accounts for approximately 90–95% of serum copper. Ceruloplasmin is a multifunctional protein that binds six atoms of copper per molecule, and copper bound to this carrier has a plasma half-life of approximately 24 hours. Ceruloplasmin is also involved in the mobilization of iron from its storage sites and it serves an analogous role as a ferrioxidase during the ferrous-ferric conversion. Copper (I) is oxidized directly by ceruloplasmin, thereby avoiding the generation of reactive oxygen species. About 5–10% of serum copper is bound to albumin under normal conditions, but following acute poisoning, the majority of the excess copper binds to albumin. The albumin-copper complex represents the "free" or toxicologically active copper. The amount of unbound copper in the blood under normal circumstances is well below 1%. The volume of distribution of copper is 2.0 L/kg and the half-life of erythrocyte copper is 26 days.

There are several important copper-containing enzymes in humans (Table 82–4). The common link among these enzymes is their participation in redox reactions in which a molecule, typically oxygen, donates or shares its electrons with another com-

TABLE 82–4. Important Copper-Containing Enzymes and Their Functions

Enzyme	Function
Alcohol dehydrogenase	Metabolism of alcohols
Catalase	Detoxifies peroxide
Ceruloplasmin	Copper transport, ferrioxidase
Cytochrome c oxidase	Electron transport chain
Dopamine β-hydroxylase	Converts dopamine to norepinephrine
Factor V	Coagulation cascade
Lysyl oxidase	Cross-links collagen and elastin
Monoamine oxidase	Deamination of primary amines
Superoxide dismutase	Detoxifies free radicals
Tyrosinase	Melanin production

pound. In this respect, the physiology, chemistry, and toxicology of copper are most similar to those of iron. In fact, "blue-blooded" animals, such as octopi and spiders, use copper in hemocyanin, a blue pigment, in a manner analogous to how "red-blooded" animals use iron in hemoglobin. When all of the various roles of copper are compiled, it is understandable why a genetic defect in intestinal copper absorption, or Menkes "kinky hair" syndrome, is characterized by mental retardation, thermoregulatory dysfunction, hypopigmentation, connective tissue abnormalities, and pili torti (kinky hair).

The elimination of copper occurs predominantly through biliary excretion following complexation with ceruloplasmin. Biliary excretion approximates gastrointestinal absorption, and averages 1000 μg/24h (35–305 μg/L).[5] Renal elimination under normal conditions is trivial, accounting for approximately 5–25 μg/24h (2.7–30 μg/L).[5]

TOXICOLOGY/PATHOPHYSIOLOGY

Redox Chemistry

In acute overdose, a high fraction of the serum copper remains bound to low-affinity proteins, such as albumin, and thus is biologically active. Because, as a transition metal, copper is capable of assuming one of several different oxidation, or valence, states, it is an active participant in reduction-oxidation, or redox, reactions. In particular, participation in the Fenton reaction and Haber-Weiss cycle explains the toxicologic effects of copper as a generator of oxidative stress and inhibitor of several key metabolic enzymes (Chap. 12). In particular, the mitochondrial electron transport chain and lipid membranes serve as ready sources of electrons for copper reduction, establishing a chain of events that ultimately leads to mitochondrial or membrane dysfunction, respectively.[55]

Erythrocytes

Copper (II) ion inhibits sulfhydryl groups on enzymes in important antioxidant systems, including glucose-6-phosphate dehydrogenase and glutathione reductase.[76] While support for these effects is only indirect, intraerythrocytic levels of reduced glutathione fall following copper exposure. This effect is presumably part of the protective role that glutathione, a nucleophile or reducing agent, normally has on oxidants, in this case, either cupric ions[50] or the reactive oxygen species they generate.[49,77] Thus, in the setting of copper poisoning, in which excessive quantities of oxidants are produced, the depletion of glutathione presumably allows peroxidative membrane damage.

In the presence of sulfhydryl-rich cell membranes, such as those on erythrocytes, cupric ions are reduced to cuprous ions, which are capable of generating superoxide radicals in the presence of oxygen.[44] This one electron reduction of oxygen regenerates the cupric ion, allowing redox cycling and continuous generation of reactive oxygen species (Fig. 82–1). The importance of hemoglobin-derived reactive oxygen species is demonstrated by the lack of hemolysis in the presence of anaerobic conditions or in an environment saturated with carbon monoxide.[10] The in vitro hemolytic activity of copper sulfate is reduced by albumin and several sulfhydryl-containing compounds, including D-penicillamine and succimer.[1] Interestingly, dimercaptopropane sulfonate (DMPS), another sulfhydryl-containing compound that is often

$$2\ Cu^{2+} \xrightarrow{\substack{GSH \quad GSSG \\ or \\ DMPS \quad Ox\text{-}DMPS}} 2\ Cu^+ + 2\ H^+$$

$$Cu^+ + H_2O_2 \longrightarrow Cu^{2+} + OH^- + OH^\bullet$$
Fenton reaction

$$Cu^+ + O_2^{\bullet-} + H_2O_2 \longrightarrow O_2 + OH^- + OH^\bullet$$
Haber-Weiss reaction

Figure 82–1. Copper, in the cupric or Cu^{2+} state, is reduced by sulfhydryl-containing compounds, such as glutathione (GSH) or dimercaptopropane sulfonate (DMPS), to its cuprous form (Cu^+); in the process, disulfide links are formed. Oxidized glutathione (GSSG) is subsequently enzymatically reduced by glutathione reductase to regenerate GSH. Superoxide anions (O_2^-), formed when molecular oxygen (O_2) acquires an additional electron, are continually generated by mitochondria. Both the Fenton and the Haber-Weiss reactions use the cuprous form of copper as a catalyst to convert the superoxide radical into the more biologically consequential hydroxyl radical ($OH^\bullet$).[14,73]

used as a chelator, worsens copper-induced hemolysis. This paradoxical effect is variably ascribed to concomitant inhibition of superoxide dismutase, an important antioxidant enzyme, or to its ability to efficiently reduce either membrane dithiols to thiols or cupric to cuprous ion, in either case increasing the generation of superoxide.[2]

Hemolysis frequently occurs within the first 24 hours in patients with acute copper poisoning.[68] This time of onset differs markedly from hemolysis that follows most other oxidant stressors and is likely a consequence of the differing nature of the erythrocyte insult. That is, the hemolysis following most oxidant exposures is caused by precipitation of hemoglobin as Heinz bodies and subsequent erythrocyte destruction by the reticuloendothelial system. This may occur in the setting of acute copper poisoning, particularly following less substantial exposure. More consequently, and accounting for the early hemolysis, copper also directly oxidizes the erythrocyte membrane, thereby initiating red cell lysis independently of the reticuloendothelial system. Oxidant-induced disulfide cross-links in the erythrocyte membrane reduce its stability and flexibility, thereby predisposing to early cell rupture.[4,62]

Liver

Although most of the accumulated copper in hepatocytes is rapidly complexed with metallothionein or otherwise used, failure to completely sequester copper ions allows their participation in redox reactions. Hepatic cells are protected from copper toxicity in vitro by prior induction of metallothionein with zinc or cadmium or by the infusion of metallothionein. These hepatic protective effects support the toxicologic significance of free intracellular copper ions. These findings also explain the therapeutic use of zinc acetate in patients suffering from Wilson disease,[16] because copper itself is not a good inducer of metallothionein in humans.

Copper ions also generate hydroxyl radicals, which are potent inducers of lipid peroxidation, as well as other reactive oxygen species. Lipid peroxidation is confirmed in hepatocytes by the measurement of increased production of lipid-conjugated dienes and other products.[69] The peroxidative effects on biologic membranes are worse in animals deficient in vitamin E and are prevented by vitamin E replacement, presumably because of its role as a membrane-localized free radical scavenger.[39,69] These effects are most pronounced in mitochondria, perhaps because of the reduction of cupric to cuprous ion in these organelles.[29,70] Copper ions also accumulate in the cellular nuclei, where localized production of hydroxyl radicals may form DNA adducts and cause apoptosis.[61] Histologically, liver damage follows a centrilobular pattern of necrosis.

The sequelae of copper's potent hepatotoxic effects are not isolated to the liver. After liver necrosis occurs, typically at liver concentrations greater than 50 mg/g dry weight, massive release of copper into the blood occurs, which may be of sufficient magnitude to cause hemolysis. This sequence of events is common during the crises of Wilson disease, and may allow for an understanding of a delayed secondary episode of hemolysis that occurs in some copper-poisoned patients.

Kidney

The kidneys bioaccumulate copper. Although primarily bound to metallothionein, when available, copper is otherwise free to participate in oxidant-generating reactions in a manner analogous to iron. Thus, reactive oxygen species are probably responsible for the nephrotoxic effects of copper. Pathologic analysis of the kidneys of oliguric or anuric patients typically reveals tubular necrosis, and some demonstrate hemoglobin casts. These findings suggest that renal failure may result indirectly from the hemoglobinuria induced by the massive release of free extracellular hemoglobin. The urinary hemoglobin, like myoglobin, may undergo conversion to ferriheme or its release of iron, either of which results in oxidative stress on the renal tubular epithelial cell.[87] Additionally, free intravascular hemoglobin, through the local scavenging of nitric oxide within the renal arterioles, may cause renal vasoconstriction.[79]

Central Nervous System

Although charged entities such as copper ions do not readily cross the blood-brain barrier, elevated cerebrospinal fluid copper concentrations are characteristic of chronic copper overload conditions such as Wilson disease.[74] This accumulation is accomplished through carrier-mediated transport of albumin-bound, not ceruloplasmin-bound, copper into the central nervous system.

CLINICAL MANIFESTATIONS
Acute Copper Salt Poisoning

Gastrointestinal irritation is the most common initial manifestation of copper salt poisoning. This syndrome includes the rapid onset of emesis and abdominal pain, possibly followed by gastroduodenal ulceration, hemorrhage, or perforation.[23,46] Blue coloration of the vomitus may occur following the ingestion of certain copper salts, particularly copper sulfate.[30,65,81] Blue vomitus is not, however, pathognomonic for copper poisoning, and also occurs in patients who ingest boric acid, methylene blue, or food dyes. Other common symptoms include retrosternal chest pain and a metallic taste. The lethal dose of copper sulfate is suggested to be 0.15–0.3 g/kg, but this is unverified. Intravenous injection of copper sulfate reportedly produces a clinical syndrome identical to that following ingestion.[58]

Given its location and function within the gastrointestinal tract, the liver receives the initial and most substantial exposure to any ingested copper product. Hepatotoxicity is therefore a frequent, although rarely an isolated,[37] manifestation of acute copper sulfate poisoning, typically occurring in the patients with more severe poisoning. Jaundice, while among the common clinical and biochemical findings following overdose, may be hepatocellular or hemolytic.[9]

Hemolysis is more common than hepatotoxicity, and is present in most patients with liver damage.[51,68] As noted, copper-induced hemolysis occurs earlier and may be more severe than hemolysis induced by conventional toxins (see "Pathophysiology" earlier in this chapter). Additionally, copper-induced oxidation of the heme iron within the erythrocyte produces methemoglobinemia.[54] In most reported cases, the discovery of significant methemoglobinemia occurs early in the patient's clinical course and is rapidly followed by hemolysis.[20] Because the methemoglobin is released within the plasma, methylene blue should not be expected to reduce the ferric iron because this reaction requires an intact erythrocyte. Because free methemoglobin is filterable, methemoglobinuria may occur, although it cannot be differentiated from other heme forms in the urine without specialized testing. In addition, many reports document an abnormal glucose-6-phosphate dehydrogenase (G-6-PD) activity, suggesting causation for methemoglobinemia or hemolysis. However, interpretation of this test result is difficult because high levels of copper interfere with the measurement of G-6-PD.

Renal and pulmonary toxicity occur occasionally and represent extraerythrocytic manifestations of the oxidative effects of the copper ions. In spite of massive intravascular hemolysis,[22] hemoglobinuric renal failure is uncommon in patients who receive adequate volume replacement therapy.

Hypotension and cardiovascular collapse occur in patients with the most severe poisoning and are likely multifactorial in origin. Undoubtedly, intravascular volume depletion from vomiting and diarrhea is involved. However, the poor patient outcome despite appropriate volume loading suggests that direct effects of copper on vascular and cardiac cells are present. Sepsis due to transmucosal invasion may also be partially responsible.[24]

Depressed mental status, ranging from lethargy to coma, or seizures following acute poisoning are likely epiphenomena related to damage to other organ systems. These findings are particularly common in patients with hepatic failure, and are comparable to those of hepatic encephalopathy from other causes. In patients with chronic poisoning, such as Wilson disease, neurologic manifestations are prominent (see below) and typically involve movement disorders.

Although not strictly a form of copper poisoning, inhalation of copper oxide fumes, generated during welding or other industrial processes, may produce metal fume fever, a syndrome historically called "brass chills" or "foundry workers' ague." Patients with this syndrome present with cough, chills, chest pain, or fever that are most likely immunologic and not toxicologic in origin (Chap. 95). However, copper oxide formation, unlike zinc oxide, only occurs at extremely high temperatures, accounting for the relative infrequency of the copper-induced metal fume fever.

Chronic Copper Poisoning

Although hepatolenticular degeneration, known as Wilson disease, is a condition of chronic copper overload, there are qualitative similarities to acute copper poisoning. Wilson disease is an inherited, autosomal-recessive disorder of copper metabolism affecting approximately 1/40,000 persons. The gene implicated in this disease (ATP7B) codes for a hepatocyte membrane-bound copper-binding protein that is required for the maturation of ceruloplasmin and the biliary excretion of copper. The resultant increase in hepatic copper concentrations produces continuing oxidative stress on the hepatocyte and cellular necrosis with the inevitable development of cirrhosis. Patients undergo periodic fluctuations in the extent of their copper-induced hepatitis, and episodes of severe hepatitis are frequently associated with hemolysis as stored copper is released from dying hepatocytes. The adverse effects of copper on the lenticular nucleus in the basal ganglia causes movement disorders such as ataxia, tremor, parkinsonism, dysphagia, and dystonia.[56] None of the other forms of copper poisoning are associated with substantial or direct neurotoxicity. Psychiatric manifestations, such as behavioral changes or mood disorders, may also occur.[16] Accumulation of copper within the cornea accounts for the characteristic green-brown Kayser-Fleischer rings. Although patients' serum copper levels are decreased, they typically have a reduced ceruloplasmin concentration caused by the failure of copper incorporation into ceruloplasmin and release from the liver and an elevated urinary copper concentration.[16] Treatment involves lifelong therapy with D-penicillamine, trientine (triethylene tetramine), or molybdenum salts; if patients are D-penicillamine sensitive they can receive either trientine or molybdenum salts. Zinc acetate, FDA approved as a maintenance therapy, induces the formation of intestinal metallothionein and thereby blocks copper absorption by effecting intestinal mucosal cell sequestration.

Chronic exogenous copper poisoning is uncommon in adults, but is reported following the use of copper-containing dietary supplements.[57] However, chronic exposure is common in children in some parts of the world. This condition, commonly called childhood cirrhosis in India or idiopathic copper toxicosis elsewhere, generally occurs in the setting of excessive dietary intake of copper because of copper-contaminated water or from brass vessels used to store milk. In these children, there may be a genetic predisposition to copper accumulation as signs of chronic liver disease develop by several months of age and progress rapidly.[64,66] Both serum copper and ceruloplasmin levels are markedly elevated, which differentiates this disease from Wilson disease. The incidence of the disease has fallen dramatically, probably as a consequence of improved nutrition and replacement of copper utensils and storage containers with those made of steel.

"Vineyard sprayers lung," first described in 1969, refers to the occupational pulmonary disease that occurred among Portuguese vineyard workers applying Bordeaux solution, a 1–2% copper sulfate solution neutralized with hydrated lime ($Ca(OH)_2$).[59] The patients developed interstitial pulmonary fibrosis, which included histiocytic granulomas containing copper. Many of these workers also developed lung adenocarcinoma, hepatic angiosarcoma, and micronodular cirrhosis, raising the possibility of a carcinogenic effect of chronic copper exposure. There is also a suggestion of an increased incidence of pulmonary adenocarcinoma among smelters, who are, however, exposed to many other toxins, including arsenic, a known carcinogen.[47] Copper is not on the list of suspected carcinogens compiled by the International Agency of Research on Cancer (IARC).

Ocular effects of copper salts, primarily following occupational exposure, include irritation of the corneal, conjunctival, or adnexal structures. Chronic ocular exposure to particulate elemental copper or one of its alloys may result in chalcosis lentis, from the Greek word *chalkos*, or copper. This chronic exposure manifests as a green-brown discoloration of the lens or cornea similar to Kayser-Fleischer rings.

DIAGNOSTIC TESTING

Real-time testing for copper is impractical and almost all management decisions must be based on clinical criteria. Copper levels are often obtained for confirmatory or investigative purposes. Although never adequately studied, whole-blood copper levels may better correlate with clinical findings than serum copper concentrations.[23] The rapid movement of copper from serum into the erythrocyte presumably explains this finding. However, while there is a statistical relationship between the whole-blood copper levels and the severity of poisoning, there is little correlation between clinical findings at any given copper concentration regardless of what biologic tissue is measured.[23,77] Similarly, other than at extremely high or low values, there is no defined value at which the prognosis may be established with certainty. Reported serum copper concentrations in patients with hemolysis range from 96 to 747 µg/dL, and those following severe poisoning include values of 6600 µg/dL[30] and 8267 µg/dL.[20] Serum copper levels in 11 patients with copper-induced acute renal failure ranged from 115 to 390 µg/dL.[21] The normal urinary copper value is approximately 25 µg/24h, and is reportedly as high as 628 µg/24h in patients with copper poisoning.[28]

Occasionally, serum copper levels reveal a secondary rise, likely because of release during hepatocellular necrosis. This secondary rise typically occurs only in patients with life-threatening poisoning, and clinical evaluation is far more practical than serial copper levels.[68]

Elevated copper levels are also noted in patients with inflammatory conditions, biliary cirrhosis, and pregnancy. These conditions are associated with an elevated ceruloplasmin, and the fraction of bound copper in the serum remains normal. Although the hepatic copper content of patients with Wilson disease is elevated, their serum copper levels are generally below normal unless hepatic necrosis is occurring.

Although serum ceruloplasmin levels rise in patients with acute copper poisoning,[78] presumably reflecting increased hepatic synthesis, the ceruloplasmin cannot be used to define the patients' prognosis. Metallothionein levels may also rise rapidly,[46] but the implications of this finding are not defined.

Routine laboratory testing following acute copper salt poisoning should include an assessment for both hemolysis and hepatotoxicity. Differentiation of these etiologies as a cause for jaundice is made by standard methodology, such as comparison of the bilirubin fractions. That is, indirect bilirubin is proportionally elevated in patients with hemolysis, whereas the direct fraction rises in patients with hepatocellular necrosis. An assessment of the patients' electrolyte and hydration status is warranted. The international normalized ratio (INR) may be prolonged in the absence of liver injury or diffuse intravascular coagulation (DIC), and may be a result of a direct effect of free copper ions on the coagulation cascade.[54]

The utility of radiographs to identify copper solutions is unstudied. However, even though copper metal embedded in the skin is clearly visible, topically applied copper salts are not visualized.[13] The diagnostic implications of these findings following copper salt ingestion are undefined. Thus, obtaining an abdominal radiograph, while probably of low clinical yield, may be justified if it occasionally alters management.

MANAGEMENT

Optimal and aggressive supportive care is the cornerstone to the effective management of patients with acute copper poisoning. Attention to antiemetic therapy, fluid and electrolyte correction, and normalization of vital signs is the critical first step before consideration of chelation therapy. Gastrointestinal decontamination is of limited concern because the onset of emesis is generally within minutes of ingestion. A dose of oral activated charcoal, while of unproved benefit, is unlikely to be harmful and may have potential adsorptive capacity for copper. Advanced therapy for patients with renal failure may include hemodialysis, and liver transplantation may be needed for patients with life-threatening hepatic failure.

Chelation Therapy

Chelation therapy should be initiated when hepatic or hematologic complications are present or the patient is severely poisoned. Studies on the efficacy of chelation therapy following acute copper salt poisoning are limited. Even when administered early and appropriately, organ damage and death still occur. Application of the data from the existing literature is complex because of the lack of controlled therapeutic studies of human copper poisoning. Although experimental animal models and uncontrolled human data exist, the results are frequently contradictory. Three agents are clinically available, and most dosing and efficacy data derive either from their use in the treatment of patients with Wilson disease or from their effects on copper elimination during chelation of other metals.

Most patients with copper poisoning are initially treated with intramuscular BAL.[75,81] Although BAL may be less effective than D-penicillamine its use is probably appropriate in patients in whom vomiting or gastrointestinal injury prevents oral D-penicillamine administration. Furthermore, because the BAL-copper complex primarily undergoes biliary elimination, it is useful in patients with renal failure. When tolerated, D-penicillamine therapy should be started simultaneously or shortly after the initiation of therapy with BAL.

Calcium disodium ethylenediamine tetraacetate (CaNa$_2$-EDTA) reduces the oxidative damage induced by copper ions in experimental models.[85] However, when used for the chelation of other metals, it does not greatly enhance the elimination of copper.[76] In addition, even with short-term use CaNa$_2$-EDTA inactivates dopamine β-hydroxylase in humans, presumably by chelating its copper moiety.[25] However, because the in vivo activity of this enzyme is restored upon the addition of exogenous copper, the detrimental effect on the formation of neuronal

norepinephrine during the treatment of acute poisoning is debatable.

D-Penicillamine (D-β-β-dimethylcysteine, Cuprimine), a structurally distinct metabolite of penicillin, is an orally bioavailable monothiol chelating agent. It is used in the treatment of lead, mercury, and copper toxicity, as well as in the management of rheumatoid arthritis and scleroderma. D-Penicillamine is effective in preventing copper-induced hemolysis in patients with Wilson disease and in reducing hepatotoxicity in those with Indian childhood cirrhosis.[11] Its protective mechanism is primarily mediated through chelation of unbound copper ions, rendering them unable to participate in redox reactions.[42] The D-penicillamine-copper complex undergoes rapid renal clearance in patients with competent kidneys. The use of D-penicillamine is not formally studied in patients with acute copper salt poisoning, but case studies suggest that copper elimination is enhanced.[35] The recommended dose is 1–2 g/d in adults and 20–30 mg/kg in children, in both cases given orally in four divided doses.[11]

Although D-penicillamine appears effective, it is associated with several significant complications. For example, D-penicillamine is associated with a worsening of neurologic findings in nearly 50% of patients treated for Wilson disease.[15] Subacute toxicities of D-penicillamine include aplastic anemia, agranulocytosis, and renal and pulmonary disease. Long-term use of D-penicillamine is also associated with various cutaneous lesions and immune system dysfunction. However, in the brief treatment necessary for acutely poisoned patients, the major risk is the potential for hypersensitivity reactions that occur in 25% of patients who are penicillin allergic. This hypersensitivity reaction is likely related to contamination of the pharmaceutical preparation with penicillin rather than immunologic cross-reactivity. The use of D-penicillamine during pregnancy is associated with congenital abnormalities, although all of the data are derived from women with Wilson disease who had long-term therapy.

Succimer, or dimercaptosuccinic acid, is sometimes described as being an ineffective copper chelator, although it is able to triple the baseline copper elimination in a murine model.[19] Given its ease of use, relative safety, and benefit in experimental models, succimer may be used in lieu of D-penicillamine in patients with mild or moderate poisoning. Under these circumstances, the use of standard lead poisoning dosing regimens is warranted.

Dimercaptopropane sulfonate (DMPS), an experimental chelating agent that is gaining popularity for the treatment of lead poisoning, prevents acute tubular necrosis in copper-poisoned mice.[52] DMPS proved to be the most effective of a panel of chelators in a murine model of copper sulfate poisoning.[38] However, DMPS, unlike D-penicillamine, forms intramolecular disulfide bridges, each of which liberates an electron. This property, which accounts for its potency as a reducing agent, also probably explains its propensity to worsen copper-induced hemolysis in vitro.[1,3] Because an adequate analysis of risk versus benefit is unavailable, DMPS should probably not be used to chelate copper-poisoned patients.

Trientine, an orally bioavailable agent, is the second-line agent for patients with Wilson disease. As with zinc therapy, which is also of proven efficacy in Wilson disease, these agents have no known role in acute copper poisoning. Although unstudied in such patients, the need for several weeks of zinc therapy prior to realizing full efficacy makes its acute therapeutic use questionable. Although large oral doses of zinc salts may limit the absorption of copper ion, the concomitant gastrointestinal corrosive effects of zinc ion make this therapy impractical.[32]

Extracorporeal Elimination

Limited data exist regarding the extent to which copper ion is eliminated by various extracorporeal means. Exchange transfusion, a conceptually beneficial method of copper removal from the body, is of undefined, but probably limited, benefit in acute copper sulfate poisoning.[24] Hemodialysis membranes undoubtedly allow copper ion to cross based upon the recognized association of hemodialysis actually resulting in copper poisoning.[26] Although copper should be similarly cleared by hemodialysis, its relatively large volume of distribution makes this unlikely. Furthermore, copper ions are highly protein bound, and the dialyzable concentration (ie, albumin bound) is less than 1 pmol/L, suggesting that hemodialysis would have little clinical utility. This fact is supported by case reports in which serum or dialysate concentrations of copper are assessed.[58] Furthermore, given the propensity of hemodialysis to lyse erythrocytes, which may release stored copper and worsen toxicity, hemodialysis is not recommended.[31]

Peritoneal dialysis is not useful in patients with fulminant Wilson disease.[45] Peritoneal dialysis removed less than 0.7 mg in a copper sulfate-poisoned child whose copper concentration was 207 µg/dL.[31] However, in the same patient, the addition of albumin to the dwell removed 9 mg of copper at a time when the child's serum copper concentration was lower.[24]

Recently, continuous hemofiltration (CVVH) using albumin dialysis or plasma exchange enhanced the elimination of copper in patients with fulminant Wilson disease.[41,43] Copper removal averaged 17 mg and 7 mg per treatment, respectively, but it is unclear whether this removal would be beneficial following an ingestion of a substantial gram quantity of copper sulfate.

Management of the hepatic toxicity requires little more than standard supportive care. The potential benefit of *N*-acetylcysteine is unstudied, although it is used in many forms of fulminant hepatic failure. Liver transplantation should be considered, but specific criteria for transfer to a specialized liver unit or for transplant, other than those that are applicable for Wilson disease[60] or other more common, noncopper etiologies, are undefined.

There are no controlled data on the treatment of acute copper poisoning in pregnancy. The available data on pregnant women with Wilson disease document that D-penicillamine is teratogenic and that zinc may be the preferred agent.[17]

SUMMARY

Acute copper poisoning is rare in the United States, but it is associated with dramatic toxicologic effects, primarily hemolysis and hepatitis. Copper's toxicologic effects are primarily mediated by oxidative stress on the erythrocyte and hepatocyte, and this similarity to iron salt poisoning adds a framework for the conceptual understanding of the disease. The infrequency of acute copper poisoning severely limits our ability to perform controlled studies on its management. Fortunately, exhaustive research into diseases of copper metabolism, particularly Wilson disease, which has periodic exacerbations similar to acute copper poisoning, provides insight into managing patients with acute copper salt poisoning.

REFERENCES

1. Aaseth J, Skaug V, Alexander J: Haemolytic activity of copper as influenced by chelating agents, albumine and chromium. Acta Pharmacol Toxicol 1984;54:304–310.
2. Aaseth J, Ribarov S, Bochev P: The interaction of copper (Cu2+) with the erythrocyte membrane and 2,3-dimercaptopropanesulphonate in vitro: A source of activated oxygen species. Pharmacol Toxicol 1987; 61:250–253.
3. Aaseth J, Benov L, Ribarov S: Mercaptodextran—A new copper chelator and scavenger of oxygen radicals. Acta Pharmacol Sinica 1990;11:363–367.
4. Adams KF, Johnson G, Hornowski E, et al: The effect of copper on erythrocyte deformability. A possible mechanism of hemolysis in acute copper intoxication. Biochem Biophys Acta 1979;550:279–287.
5. Adelstein SJ, Vallee BL: Copper metabolism in man. N Engl J Med 1961;265:892–897.
6. Agarwal SK, Tiwari SC, Dash SC: Spectrum of poisoning requiring haemodialysis in a tertiary care hospital in India. Int J Artif Organs 1993;16:20–22.
7. Akintonwa A, Mabadeje AFB, Odutola TA: Fatal poisoning by copper sulfate ingested from "Spiritual Water." Vet Hum Toxicol 1989; 31:453–454.
8. Arens P: Factors to be considered concerning the corrosion of copper tubes. Eur J Med Res 1999;28:243–245.
9. Ashraf I: Hepatic derangements (biochemical) in acute copper sulphate poisoning. J Indian Med Assoc 1970;55:341–342.
10. Barnes G, Frieden E: Oxygen requirement for cupric ion-induced hemolysis. Biochem Biophys Res Commun 1983;115:680–684.
11. Bavdekar AR, Bhave SA, Pradhan AM, et al: Long-term survival in Indian childhood cirrhosis treated with D-penicillamine. Arch Dis Child 1996;74:32–35.
12. Beltran-Garcia MJ, Espinosa A, Herrera N, et al: Formation of copper oxychloride and reactive oxygen species as causes of uterine injury during copper oxidation of Cu-IUD. Contraception 2000;61:99–103.
13. Bentur Y, Koren G, McGuigan M, Speilberg SP: An unusual exposure to copper: Clinical and pharmacokinetic evaluation. J Toxicol Clin Toxicol 1988;26:371–380.
14. Bergendi L, Benes L, Durackova Z, et al: Chemistry, physiology and pathology of free radicals. Life Sci 1999;65:1865–1874.
15. Brewer GJ, Terry CA, Aisen AM, Hill GM: Worsening of neurologic syndrome in patients with Wilson's disease with initial penicillamine therapy. Arch Neurol 1987;44:490–493.
16. Brewer GJ: Recognition, diagnosis and management of Wilson's disease. Proc Soc Exp Biol Med 2000;223:39–46.
17. Brewer GJ, Johnson VD, Dick RD, et al: Treatment of Wilson's disease with zinc. XVII: Treatment during pregnancy. Hepatology 2000; 31:364–370.
18. Camakaris J, Voskoboinik I, Mercer JF: Molecular mechanisms of copper homeostasis. Biochem Biophys Res Commun 1999;261: 225–232.
19. Cantilena LR, Klaassen CD: The effect of chelating agents on the excretion of endogenous metals. Toxicol Appl Pharmacol 1982;63: 344–350.
20. Chugh KS, Singhal PC, Sharma BK: Methemoglobinemia in acute copper sulfate poisoning. Ann Intern Med 1975;82:226–227.
21. Chugh KS, Sharma BK, Singhal PC, et al: Acute renal failure following copper sulphate intoxication. Postgrad Med J 1977;53:18–23.
22. Chugh KS, Singhal PC, Sharma BK, et al: Acute renal failure due to intravascular hemolysis in the North Indian patients. Am J Med Sci 1977;274:139–146.
23. Chuttani HK, Gupta PS, Gulati S, et al: Acute copper sulfate poisoning. Am J Med 1965;39:849–854.
24. Cole DEC, Lirenman DS: Role of albumin-enriched peritoneal dialysate in acute copper poisoning. J Pediatr 1978;92:955–957.

25. De Paris P, Caroldi S: In vivo inhibition of serum dopamine-beta-hydroxylase by CaNa₂ EDTA injection. Hum Exp Toxicol 1994;13:253–256.

26. Eastwood JB, Phillips ME, Minty P, et al: Heparin inactivation, acidosis and copper poisoning due to presumed acid contamination of water in a hemodialysis unit. Clin Nephrol 1983;20:197–201.

27. Eife R, Weiss M, Muller-Hocker M, et al: Chronic poisoning by copper in tap water: II. Copper intoxications with predominantly systemic symptoms. Eur J Med Res 1999;28:224–228.

28. Fairbanks VF: Copper sulfate-induced hemolytic anemia. Arch Intern Med 1967;120:428–432.

29. Gu M, Cooper JM, Butler P, et al: Oxidative-phosphorylation defects in liver of patients with Wilson's disease. Lancet 2000;356:469–474.

30. Gulliver JM: A fatal copper sulfate poisoning. J Anal Toxicol 1991;15:341–342.

31. Hamlyn AN, Gollan JL, Douglas AP, et al: Fulminant Wilson's disease with haemolysis and renal failure: Copper studies and assessment of dialysis regimens. Br Med J 1977;2:660–663.

32. Hantson P, Lievens M, Mahieu P: Accidental ingestion of a zinc and copper sulfate preparation. J Toxicol Clin Toxicol 1996;34:725–730.

33. Harris GBC, Haggarty RJ: Toxic hazards: Bronze-powder inhalation. N Engl J Med 1957;256:40–41.

34. Hay E, Derazon H, Eisenberg Y, et al: Suicide by ingestion of a CCA wood preservative. J Emerg Med 2000;19:159–163.

35. Holtzman NA, Elliot DA, Heller RH: Copper intoxication: Report of a case with observations on ceruloplasmin. N Engl J Med 1966;275:347–352.

36. Holtzman NA, Haslam RHA: Elevation of serum copper following copper sulfate as an emetic. Pediatrics 1968;42:189–193.

37. Jantsch W, Kulig K, Rumack BH: Massive copper sulfate ingestion resulting in hepatotoxicity. J Toxicol Clin Toxicol 1984;85: 585–588.

38. Jones MM, Basinger MA, Tarka MP: The relative effectiveness of some chelating agents in acute copper intoxication in the mouse. Res Commun Chem Pathol Pharmacol 1980;27:571–577.

39. Kadiiska MB, Hanna PM, Jordan SJ, Mason RP: Electron spin resonance evidence for free radical generation in copper treated vitamin E and selenium-deficient rats: In vivo spin-trapping investigation. Mol Pharmacol 1993;44:222–227.

40. Karlsson B, Noren L: Ipecacuanha and copper sulphate as emetics in intoxications in children. Acta Paediatrica Scand 1965;54:331–335.

41. Kiss JE, Berman D, Van Thiel D: Effective removal of copper by plasma exchange in fulminant Wilson's disease. Transfusion 1998;38:327–331.

42. Klein D, Lichtmannegger J, Heinzmann U, et al: Dissolution of copper-rich granules in hepatic lysosomes by D-penicillamine prevents the development of fulminant hepatitis in Long-Evans cinnamon rats. J Hepatol 2000;32:193–201.

43. Kreymann B, Seige M, Schweigart U: Albumin dialysis: Effective removal of copper in a patient with fulminant Wilson disease and successful bridging to liver transplantation. J Hepatol 1999;31:1080–1085.

44. Kumar SK, Rowse C, Hochstein P: Copper-induced generation of superoxide in human red cell membrane. Biochem Biophys Res Commun 1978;83:587–592.

45. Kuno T, Hitomi T, Zaitu M, et al: Severely decompensated abdominal Wilson disease treated with peritoneal dialysis: A case report. Acta Paediatr Jpn 1998;40:85–87.

46. Kurisaki E, Kuroda Y, Sato M: Copper-binding protein in acute copper poisoning. Forensic Sci Int 1988;38:3–11.

47. Lubin JH, Pottern LM, Stone BJ, et al: Respiratory cancer in a cohort of copper smelter workers: Results from more than 50 years of follow-up. Am J Epidemiol 2000;151:554–565.

48. Manzler AD, Schreiner AW: Copper-induced acute hemolytic anemia. A new complication of hemodialysis. Ann Intern Med 1970;73:409–412.

49. Metz EN, Sagone AL: The effect of copper on the erythrocyte hexose monophosphate shunt pathway. J Lab Clin Med 1972;80:405–413.

50. Milne L, Nicotera P, Orrenius S, et al: Effects of glutathione and chelating agents on copper-mediated DNA oxidation: Pro-oxidant and antioxidant properties of glutathione. Arch Biochem Biophys 1993;304:102–109.

51. Mital VP, Wahal PK, Bansal OP: Study of erythrocytic glutathione in acute copper sulphate poisoning. Indian J Pathol Bacteriol 1966;9:155–162.

52. Mitchell WM, Basinger MA, Jones MM: Antagonism of acute copper (II)-induced renal lesions by sodium 2,3-dimercaptopropanesulfonate. Johns Hopkins Med J 1982;151:283–285.

53. Mucklow ES: Chemistry set poisoning. Int J Clin Pract 1997;51:321–323.

54. Nagaraj MV, Rao PV, Susarala S: Copper sulphate poisoning, hemolysis and methemoglobinemia. J Assoc Physcians India 1985;33:308–309.

55. Nakatani T, Spolter L, Kobayashi K: Redox state in liver mitochondria in acute copper sulfate poisoning. Life Sci 1994;54:967–974.

56. Oder W, Prayer L, Grimm G, et al: Wilson's disease: Evidence of subgroups derived from clinical findings and brain lesions. Neurology 1993;43:120–124.

57. O'Donohue J, Reid M, Varghese A, et al: A case of adult chronic copper self-intoxication resulting in cirrhosis. Eur J Med Res 1999;28:252.

58. Oldenquist G, Salem M: Parenteral copper sulfate poisoning causing acute renal failure. Nephrol Dial Transplant 1999;14:441–443.

59. Pimentel JC, Marques F: "Vineyard sprayer's lung": A new occupational disease. Thorax 1969;24:678–688.

60. Robles R, Parrilla P, Sicilia J, et al: Indications and results of liver transplants in Wilson's disease. Transplant Proc 1999;31:2453–2454.

61. Sagripanti JL, Goering PL, Lamanna A: Interaction of copper with DNA and antagonism by other metals. Toxicol Appl Pharmacol 1991;110:477–485.

62. Salhany JM, Swanson JC, Cordes KA, et al: Evidence suggesting direct oxidation of human erythrocyte membrane sulfhydryls by copper. Biochem Biophys Res Commun 1978;82:1294–1298.

63. Salmon MA, Wright T: Chronic copper poisoning presenting as pink disease. Arch Dis Child 1971;46:108–110.

64. Scheinberg IH, Sternlieb I: Is non-Indian childhood cirrhosis caused by excess dietary copper? Lancet 1994;344:1002–1004.

65. Schwartz E, Schmidt E: Refractory shock secondary to copper sulfate ingestion. Ann Emerg Med 1986;15:952–954.

66. Sethi S, Grover S, Khodaskar MB: Role of copper in Indian childhood cirrhosis. Ann Trop Paediatr 1993;13:3–5.

67. Singh S, Sharma BK, Wahi PL, et al: Spectrum of acute poisoning in adults (10-year experience). J Assoc Physicians India 1984;32:561–563.

68. Singh MM, Singh G: Biochemical changes in blood in cases of acute copper sulphate poisoning. J Indian Med Assoc 1968;50:549–555.

69. Sokol RJ, Devereaux M, Mierau GW, et al: Oxidant injury to hepatic mitochondrial lipids in rats with dietary copper overload. Gastroenterology 1990;90:1061–1071.

70. Sokol RJ, Devereaux M, O'Brien K, et al: Abnormal hepatic mitochondrial respiration and cytochrome c oxidase activity in rats with long-term copper overload. Gastroenterology 1993;105:178–187.

71. Sontz E, Schwieger J: The "Green Water" syndrome: Copper-induced hemolysis and subsequent acute renal failure as a consequence of a religious ritual. Am J Med 1995;98:311–315.

72. Stein RS, Jenkins D, Korns ME: Death after use of cupric sulfate as emetic. JAMA 1976;235:801.

73. Stohs SJ, Bagchi D: Oxidative mechanisms in the toxicity of metal ions. Free Radic Biol Med 1995;18:321–336.

74. Stuerenburg HJ: CSF copper concentrations, blood-brain barrier function, and coeruloplasmin synthesis during the treatment of Wilson's disease. J Neural Transm 2000;107:321–329.

75. Takeda T, Yukioka T, Shimazaki S: Cupric sulfate intoxication with rhabdomyolysis, treated with chelating agents and blood purification. Intern Med 2000;39:253–255.

76. Thomas DJ, Chisolm J: Lead, zinc and copper decorporation during calcium disodium ethylenediamine tetraacetate treatment of lead-poisoned children. J Pharmacol Exp Ther 1986;239:829–835.

77. Wahal PK, Mehrotra MP, Patney NL, et al: A study of haemolytic jaundice in acute copper sulphate poisoning. J Assoc Physicians India 1976;24:103–108.

78. Wahal PK, Mehrotra MP, Kishore B, et al: A study of serum ceruloplasmin levels in acute copper sulphate poisoning. J Assoc Physicians India 1978;26:983–987.

79. Wakabayashi Y, Kikawada R: Effect of L-arginine on myoglobin-induced acute renal failure in the rabbit. Am J Physiol 1996;270:F784–F789.

80. Walker WR, Keats DM: An investigation of the therapeutic value of the "copper bracelet"—Dermal assimilation of copper in arthritic/rheumatoid conditions. Agents Actions 1976;6:454–459.

81. Walsh FM, Crosson FJ, Bayley M, et al: Acute copper intoxication: Pathophysiology and therapy with a case report. Am J Dis Child 1977;131:149–151.

82. Walshe JM: Penicillamine: A new oral therapy for Wilson's disease. Am J Med 1956;21:487–495.

83. Witherell LE: Outbreak of acute copper poisoning due to soft drink dispenser [letter]. Am J Public Health 1980;70:1115.

84. Wyllie J: Copper poisoning at a cocktail party. Am J Public Health 1957;47:617.

85. Yamamoto H, Hirose K, Hayasaki Y, et al: Mechanism of enhanced lipid peroxidation in the liver of Long-Evans cinnamon (LEC) rats. Arch Toxicol 1999;73:457–464.

86. Yelin G, Taff ML, Sadowski GE: Copper toxicity following massive ingestion of coins. Am J Forensic Med Pathol 1987;8:78–85.

87. Zager RA, Burkhart KM, Conrad DS, et al: Iron, heme oxygenase, and glutathione: Effects on myohemoglobinuric proximal tubular injury. Kidney Int 1995;48:1624–1634.

Maria Mercurio / Robert S. Hoffman

Thallium

MW	=	204.39 daltons	
Normal Levels			
Blood	=	<2µg/L	(<9.78 nmol/L)
Urine	=	<5µg/L	(<24.5 nmol/L)
Action Levels			
Blood	=	>100 µg/L	(>0.490 µmol/L)
Urine	=	>200 µg/L	(>0.980 µmol/L)

Values greater than or equal to the action level necessitate clinical intervention. Values below this level may necessitate intervention based on the clinical condition of the patient.

A 21-year-old female college student developed mild, but persistent abdominal pain with intermittent severe colicky pain. Three days after the initial painful episode, her hair began to fall out. She became constipated, and noted a delay in the onset of her menses. Within 5 days of her initial symptoms, she was completely bald. On day 18, she was hospitalized, where routine physical examination only revealed horizontal white (Mees) lines on her fingernails. Her routine blood chemistries and several special studies for autoimmune disease were all normal. Her overall condition responded to nutritional support, her symptoms gradually resolved, her hair regrew, and she was discharged almost 2 months after the onset of symptoms, but without a clear diagnosis.

The patient returned to school. One month later, she felt pain in both her hands and feet, and developed difficulty speaking, dizziness, blurred vision, and vertigo. She was taken to the hospital once again. On admission, her blood pressure was 140/110 mm Hg; other vital signs were normal. Examination of her extremities showed good muscular strength in her legs but poor muscle coordination, and hyperesthesias in a stocking-and-glove distribution. Her deep-tendon reflexes were hypoactive in both legs, but normal in her upper extremities. Cranial nerve examination revealed horizontal and vertical nystagmus, and palsies of the abducens (VI) and facial (VII) cranial nerves. Routine chemistries and a lumbar puncture were normal.

Four days later, still without a diagnosis, her symptoms of vertigo and tremulousness worsened. Her doctors noted that she was showing signs of oculogyric crisis, and her mental status deteriorated. Her alopecia returned. A magnetic resonance image (MRI) of her brain was interpreted as normal, and an electroencephalogram (EEG) was felt to be nondiagnostic. Her condition progressed very rapidly with the development of bulbar palsy, involuntary chewing movements of her mouth, and spastic clonus of both upper limbs. Her level of consciousness changed from mild agitation to lethargy. Tonic movements of both upper extremities and episodic oculogyric crisis were noted.

Five days after her hospitalization, she became comatose. Investigative studies for arsenic, antinuclear antibody, antidouble-stranded DNA antibody, rheumatoid factor, HIV, and Lyme disease were negative. Routine urinalysis was normal. She was treated with several broad-spectrum antibiotics, antiviral agents, hormones, and intravenous injections of γ-globulin, none of which had any appreciable effect on her signs and symptoms.

Because her spontaneous respiratory efforts became progressively weaker and irregular, a tracheostomy was performed and she was placed on a ventilator. At that point, the diagnosis of acute disseminated encephalomyelitis was considered. Plasmapheresis was initiated and seven exchanges, for a total of 10 L, were completed over the following 3 weeks. No change in her condition was noted.

Ultimately, the diagnosis of thallium toxicity was considered. Blood, urine, and cerebrospinal fluid (CSF) thallium levels were reported as 275, 532, and 31 µg/L, respectively. Nail and hair levels were 22,824 and 532 µg/kg, respectively. The patient was started on a regimen of intravenous potassium (100 mEq/d), oral Prussian blue (250 mg/kg/d divided q4h in 50 mL of 15% mannitol), and daily hemodialysis. Her symptoms slowly improved. About 2 months after hospitalization she began to intermittently regain consciousness.

One year after the initial event, her orientation and memory improved and her IQ was estimated at 128, with good mathematical and verbal abilities. The patient was able to sit in a wheelchair for a prolonged period of time and could move herself 20–30 meters. She still could not move her legs. Her vision remained poor, but periodically she was able to see clearly.

HISTORY AND EPIDEMIOLOGY

Thallium, a metal with atomic number 81, is located between mercury and lead on the periodic table. Thallium is a commonly found constituent of granite, shale, volcanic rock, and pyrites (which are used to make sulfuric acid), and is also recovered as flue dust from iron, lead, cadmium, and copper smelters. Thallium is a soft pliable metal-like lead that melts at 300°C (572°F), boils at 1482°C (2699.6°F), and is essentially nontoxic. However, thallium forms univalent thallous and trivalent thallic salts, which are highly toxic. It has been used in alloys as an anticorrosive, in optical lenses to increase the refractive index, in artists' paints, in lamps to improve tungsten filaments, in imitation jewelry, as a catalyst, and in fireworks.

In the early 1900s, thallium salts were used medicinally to treat syphilis, gonorrhea, tuberculosis, and ringworm of the scalp, and as a depilatory.[4,56] Although the usual oral dose given for epilation in the treatment of ringworm of the scalp was 7–8 mg/kg, fatal doses ranged from 6 to 40 mg/kg.[10,47] Many cases of severe thallium poisoning (thallotoxicosis) resulted from the treatment of ringworm, with one author summarizing nearly 700 cases and 46 deaths.[58]

Because thallium sulfate is odorless and tasteless, it was also successfully used as a rodenticide. Commercially available as Thalgrain, Echol's Roach Powder, Mo-Go, Martin's Rat Stop liquid, and Senco Corn Mix, thallium sulfate was very efficient at killing rats, prairie dogs, and other unwanted rodents. In response to numerous case reports of unintentional poisonings,[59,68] its use as a household rodenticide was restricted in the United States in 1965. Ultimately, even the commercial use of thallium salts as a rodenticide was banned in the United States in 1975, because of continued reports of human toxicity.

Unfortunately, life-threatening unintentional poisoning continues in other countries where thallium salts are still commonly used as rodenticides.[66,85] Additional cases of thallium poisoning are reported in this and other countries as a result of its use as a homicidal agent,[15,51,55,61] and through contamination of herbal products[72] and illicit drugs such as heroin[65] and cocaine.[33] Although occupational exposures to consequential amounts of thallium salts are uncommon, toxicity is well described in this setting as well.[28] Presently, trace amounts of thallium salts are used as a radioactive contrast agent to image tumors and to visualize cardiac function.[56]

The following discussion of thallium toxicity actuality refers to toxicity resulting from exposure to inorganic thallium salts, because this source represents virtually the entire literature on thallium poisoning.

TOXICOKINETICS

Exposures usually occur via one of three routes: *inhalation* of dust, *ingestion,* and *absorption* through intact skin. Thallium is rapidly absorbed following all routes of exposure, distributed throughout most of the body following three-compartment toxicokinetics[67] (Chap. 11), and eliminated slowly via the kidneys and gastrointestinal tract. The volume of distribution for thallium is very large, and is estimated to be about 3.6 L/kg.[14] Although thallium is found in all organs, it is distributed unevenly, with higher concentrations found in the large and small intestine, liver, kidney, heart, brain, and muscles.[4,43]

The toxicokinetics of thallium can be described in the following three-phase model. In the first phase, which occurs rapidly in the 4 hours following exposure, thallium is distributed to a central compartment and to well-perfused peripheral organs such as the kidney, liver, and muscle. In the second phase, which can last between 4 and 48 hours, thallium is distributed into the central nervous system.[67] Whereas traditional sources suggest that this distribution phase is generally completed within 24 hours of ingestion,[67] a recent human case suggests slower distribution into the CNS as evidenced by increasing CSF levels days following exposure when blood levels were declining.[75] The third, or elimination, phase starts about 24 hours after ingestion. The primary mecha-

nism of thallium elimination is secretion into the intestine, but enteral reabsorption of the thallium that was initially present in the bile subsequently reduces the fecal elimination.[13,55] The duration of the elimination phase depends on the route of exposure, dose, and treatment. Unlike many other metals such as lead, thallium does not have a major anatomic reservoir. As such, reported elimination half-lives are as short as 1.7 days in humans with thallium poisoning.[31]

Thallium is excreted primarily via the feces (51.4%) and the urine (26.4%).[46] It is glomerularly filtered, and approximately 50% is reabsorbed in the tubules. Furthermore, thallium is secreted into the tubular lumen in a manner similar to potassium.[2]

PATHOPHYSIOLOGY

The mechanism of toxicity of thallium is not well established. In the body, thallium behaves biologically like potassium because of their similar ionic radii (0.147 nm for thallium and 0.133 nm for potassium). Because cell membranes cannot differentiate between thallium and potassium ions, thallous ions accumulate in areas with high potassium concentrations such as central and peripheral nervous, hepatic, and muscular tissues.[53,85] This accumulation is the fundamental principle that governs the use of radioactive thallium in cardiac imaging studies. Thallium replaces potassium in the activation of potassium-dependent enzymes.[53] In low concentrations, thallium stimulates these enzyme systems, but in high concentrations, it inhibits them.[54] Thallium also inhibits several potassium-dependent systems. Pyruvate kinase, a magnesium-dependent glycolytic enzyme that requires potassium to achieve maximum activity, has 50 times greater affinity for thallous ions than potassium ions.[38] Succinate dehydrogenase, an essential enzyme in the Krebs cycle, is inhibited by small doses of thallium in rats.[26] Sodium-potassium ATPase, which is responsible for active transport of monovalent ions across cell membranes, can use thallous ions at extremely low concentrations because of an affinity that is 10-fold greater than that of potassium ions,[6,21] but is inhibited by thallium at higher concentrations.[34] Thallium also impairs depolarization of muscle fibers.[56] Mitochondrial energy is decreased as a result of the inhibition of pyruvate kinase and succinate dehydrogenase, resulting in a decrease of adenosine triphosphate (ATP) generation via oxidative phosphorylation. Enzymatic destruction results in swelling and vacuolization of the mitochondria after exposure to thallium.[76] At low levels, thallium can activate other potassium-dependent enzymes such as phosphatase, homoserine dehydrogenase, vitamin B_{12}–dependent diol dehydrogenase, L-threonine dehydrogenase, and adenosine monophosphate (AMP) deaminase.[56]

Thallous ions have been used to isolate riboflavin from milk in the form of a reversible precipitate. Thallous ions may also form insoluble complexes and cause intracellular sequestration of riboflavin in vivo.[8] Riboflavin is the vitamin precursor of the flavin coenzyme FAD (flavin adenine dinucleotide). Because of a decrease in riboflavin, metabolic reactions dependent upon flavoproteins will decrease, causing disruption of the electron transport chain and a subsequent further decrease or impairment in the generation of cellular energy.[8] This decrease in cellular energy may lead to a decrease in mitotic activity and cessation of hair follicle formation resulting in the clinical sign of alopecia. Subsequent hair loss is the result of combined arrested formation and local destruction of hairshaft cells in the hair bulb.[8,68] Unfortunately, riboflavin supplementation was ineffective in one animal model of thallium poisoning.[3] Data also demonstrate that the dermatologic, neurologic, and cardiovascular effects of thallium toxicity mirror the side effects of thiamine deficiency (beri beri), highlighting the inhibitory effect of thallium on glycolytic enzymes.[8,56] It is unclear whether thiamine administration has any beneficial effect in patients with thallium poisoning.

Thallium, like many other metals, has a high affinity for sulfhydryl groups. Sulfhydryl groups, present in enzymes and other proteins, form complexes with thallium. Keratin, a structural protein, consists of many cysteine residues that cross-link and form disulfide bonds. These disulfide bonds add strength to keratin. Thallium interferes with the formation of disulfide bonds, which may lead to the development of alopecia and defects in nail growth resulting in Mees lines.[23,56,61,71] Additionally, the complexation of sulfhydryl groups with thallium results in a decrease in glutathione production (secondarily to a decrease in cysteine). This results in the accumulation of lipid peroxides in the brain, specifically the cerebellum, which appear as dark, pigmented, lipofuscinlike areas.[25] The complexity and presumable multifactorial nature of thallium poisoning are again highlighted by the inability of N-acetylcysteine–induced augmentation of glutathione stores to protect against toxicity in an animal model.[3]

Thallium also adversely affects protein synthesis in animals by damaging ribosomes, particularly the 60S subunit.[32] Although ribosomes are primarily dependent on potassium and magnesium, thallium will be used if present. In an experimental model, low concentrations of thallium are protective against hypokalemia-induced ribosomal inactivation. As thallium concentrations increase, the protective effects diminish, resulting in progressive destabilization and destruction of the ribosomes. Ribosomal destruction can also be produced with exposure to potassium concentrations of 4.5–20 times higher than the thallium concentrations necessary to achieve the same effect.[32]

Pathologic studies of the central nervous system in patients with thallium poisoning reveal localized areas of edema found in the cerebral hemispheres and brainstem. Chromatolytic changes are prominent in neurons of the motor cortex, third-nerve nuclei, substantia nigra, and pyramidal cells of the globus pallidus. In chronic exposures, there are signs of edema of the pial and arachnoidal membranes, and changes in the ganglion cells of the ventral and dorsal horns of the spinal cord, consisting of chromatolysis, swelling, and fatty degeneration.[4,68]

The peripheral nervous system, which is usually clinically affected before the central nervous system, exhibits axonopathy in a classic dying back or wallerian degeneration pattern.[4,17] Fragmentation and degeneration of associated myelin sheaths are accompanied by activation of Schwann cells.[4,8,9] Because thallium affects the longer peripheral fibers—first sensory, then motor, and finally the shorter fibers—toxic effects occur initially in the lower extremities.

CLINICAL MANIFESTATIONS

Many of the effects of thallium poisoning are somewhat nonspecific and occur over a variable time course.[44] When combined, however, a clear toxidrome can be defined (Table 83–1). Alopecia and the painful ascending peripheral neuropathy are the most characteristic findings.[19,55] Because of the delayed development of alopecia, the diagnosis of thallotoxicosis is often overlooked. In fact, with acute exposures, a dose-dependent latent period of hours to days may precede initial symptoms.[44,56] When death occurs, it is usually the result of coma, respiratory paralysis, and cardiac arrest.

Unlike most other metal salt poisonings, in cases of thallium toxicity, gastrointestinal symptoms are usually modest or may even be absent.[10] The most common symptom is abdominal pain, which is sometimes accompanied by vomiting and either diarrhea or constipation.[15,44,41,54,71,86] Constipation may be a result of decreased intestinal motility and peristalsis caused by direct involvement of the vagus nerve.[10,56] Rarely, severe symptoms, such as hematemesis, bloody diarrhea, or ulceration of the mucosal lining, can occur.

Pleuritic chest pain was described in one small series of poisoned patients.[51] Another patient was reported to have developed "chest tightness" shortly after drinking thallium-poisoned tea.[55] No etiology for this finding has been proposed.

Tachycardia and hypertension frequently occur in patients with thallotoxicosis and usually develop during the first or second week following an acute ingestion. A poor prognosis may be associated with a persistent and pronounced tachycardia. No exact mechanism has been determined for these cardiovascular effects of thallium toxicity. Some authors theorize that they result from autonomic neuropathic dysfunction directly related to vagus nerve involvement, but others have noted early electrocardiographic changes, such as T-wave flattening or inversion and nonspecific ST-segment abnormalities, which might suggest direct myocardial damage.[5,9,54,56] Another theory suggests that a stimulating effect of thallium on ATPase in the chromaffin cells can lead to increased output of catecholamines, resulting in sinus tachycardia.[2,55]

Neurologic effects usually appear 2–5 days postexposure. Patients may present with severely painful, rapidly progressive ascending peripheral neuropathies.[4,5,17,51] Pain and paresthesias are present in lower extremities (especially the soles of the feet), and although numbness is present in fingers and toes, there is also decreased sensation to pinprick, touch, temperature, vibration, and proprioception.[5,72] The weight of the bedsheets on the lower extremities may be sufficient to cause excruciating pain.[51] Motor weakness is always distal in distribution, with the lower limbs more affected than the upper limbs.[9,56]

Symptoms of confusion, delirium, psychosis, hallucinations, seizures, headache, insomnia, anxiety, tremor, ataxia, and choreoathetosis are common. Onset is variable, and most likely dependent on dose. Ataxia can develop within 48 hours after ingestion. Insomnia occurs in almost every patient and may progress to total reversal of sleep rhythm. Coma may occur, especially with larger exposures.[9,44,56,71] All cranial nerves—with the possible exception of I, V, and VIII—can be affected by thallium. Third cranial nerve involvement, as evidenced by ptosis, is common, and may be present asymmetrically.[9] Nystagmus, another common finding, demonstrates fourth and sixth cranial nerve involvement.[9] Neuropsychologic findings may indicate focal injury, and have been reported to persist for months after exposure.[49]

Thallium is toxic to both the retinal fibers and the neural retina.[73] In cases of a large single ingestion of thallium, approximately 25% of patients may develop severe lesions of the optic nerve.[56,71] Optic neuropathies can lead to optic atrophy and a permanent decrease in visual acuity. In early stages, the optic disk shows signs of neuritis, which is red and poorly defined, and later develops pallor from resultant optic nerve atrophy. In patients exposed to multiple small doses, nearly 100% suffer optic injury.[54] Visual complaints may be delayed in comparison to other neuro-

TABLE 83–1. Clinical Manifestations of Acute Thallium Poisoning

Organ System	Onset of Effects			Residual Effects
	Immediate (<6 hours)	Intermediate (Rarely in the first few days; within 2 weeks)	Late (>2 weeks)	
Gastrointestinal				
Nausea	†			
Vomiting	†			
Diarrhea	†			
Constipation	†	†		
Cardiovascular				
Nonspecific ECG changes	†	†		
Hypertension		†		
Tachycardia		†		
Respiratory				
Pleuritic chest pain	†	†		
Respiratory depression		†	†	
Renal				
Albuminuria		†		
Renal insufficiency		†		‡
Dermatologic				
Dry skin		†		
Alopecia		†		‡
Mees lines			†	‡
Neurologic				
Painful ascending sensory neuropathy		†	†	‡
Motor neuropathy		†	†	‡
Cranial nerve abnormalities		†		
Altered mental status		†		‡
Seizures		†	†	
Optic neuritis				‡
Memory and cognitive deficits				‡

† = typical onset of symptoms.
The time course outlined above may be accelerated with extremely large doses.
When "†" appears in two adjacent columns, the time course is highly variable and may be dose-dependent.
With small ingestions, many effects listed above may not be evident.
‡ = effects that may persist long after exposure, and possibly permanently.

logic findings,[73] and can include decreased acuity and central scotomata. Other ophthalmic effects that have been described are noninflammatory keratitis, cataracts, and the color vision defect of tritanomaly (blue color defect).[79,80]

Renal function may remain normal in mild cases of thallium poisoning, even though the kidney bioaccumulates thallium more than any other organ. Changes in renal function in patients with severe thallotoxicosis include oliguria, diminished creatinine clearance, elevated blood urea nitrogen, and albuminuria.[2,51,54,56] These findings correlate with morphologic studies in thallium-poisoned rats, demonstrating abnormalities in the renal medulla, mainly in the thick ascending limb of the loop of Henle, that occur by the second day after exposure and resolve by the tenth day.[2]

Alopecia is the most common and classic manifestation of thallium toxicity.[55,82] Typically occurring as the presenting symptom in patients with chronic exposures, following an acute exposure, epilation begins in approximately 10 days and total hair loss usually occurs within a month.[19,55] Facial and axillary hair, especially the inner one-third of the eyebrows, may be spared, but in some cases, full beards, as well as all scalp hair, are lost.[68] Microscopic studies show thallium deposition as dark brown or black pigmentation located in the roots of hair samples. These deposits can be found within 3–5 days of initial exposure.[7,54] In patients with chronic exposures, several bands may be noted on the hair shaft, demonstrating multiple exposures. Initial hair regrowth is very fine and unpigmented, but usually returns to normal following mild exposure.[54] In patients with severe exposures, alopecia may be permanent. Dermatologic effects that have been observed include acne, palmar erythema, and dry scaly skin that results from damage to the sebaceous glands.[82] Mees lines appear within 2–4 weeks after exposure.[55,61,71]

Other less common findings include hepatic injury[33] and hypochloremic metabolic acidosis.[71] Anemia and thrombocytopenia are occasionally reported.[45,71]

Special Concerns: Teratogenic Effects

In animal models, thallium is teratogenic.[22,24] One study evaluated 297 children born in an area in which thallium levels were higher than normal because of industrial contamination.[16] Urine thallium levels in the exposed children were as high as 76.5 µg/L. Although these children had a slightly higher than expected incidence of congenital abnormalities, no causal relationship could be established with regard to thallium exposure.[16]

There are few human reports of acute thallium poisoning during pregnancy. A comprehensive literature review demonstrated 25 cases, which included acute and chronic exposures that occurred during all trimesters.[30] Thallium crosses the placenta, albeit slowly, and is able to cause characteristic fetal toxicity,[18,60] which manifests initially as decreased fetal movement, possibly as a consequence of fetal paralysis. The classic adult signs and symptoms of thallium poisoning have been described in the neonate following delivery and the fetus following abortion.[18,54,60,66] However, outcome of the pregnancy may be normal despite significant maternal toxicity.[18,35] The only consistent finding is a trend toward prematurity and low birth weight, especially in those children exposed during the first trimester.[30] At least one author recommends continuing the pregnancy as long as the mother is clinically improving.[18] It is reasonable to conclude that a fetus exposed during organogenesis has the potential for permanent injury. Those exposed later in the pregnancy may recover without deficit if their exposures are limited and the mother recovers. If the exposure occurs closer to term, the child may be born with overt toxicity such as alopecia, dermatitis, nail growth disturbances, and permanent central nervous system lesions.[54] Because thallium is eliminated in breast milk, nursing children have an additional risk of exposure.[30]

These few case reports and animal studies provide confusing and sometimes contradictory results. It seems that fetal outcome is determined both by the stage of pregnancy and the extent of maternal toxicity. However, because there are insufficient data to predict the outcome of pregnancy complicated by maternal thallium poisoning, all patients should receive individualized care.

ASSESSMENT

Most patients with acute and consequential thallium toxicity present to the Emergency Department soon after exposure with the alterations in gastrointestinal, cardiovascular, and neurologic function described previously. Establishing the correct diagnosis at this early stage is essential to assure a satisfactory outcome. Unfortunately, many patients with either smaller acute exposures or chronic thallium poisoning first present for healthcare days to weeks after their initial exposure, and diagnosis is often delayed. In these instances, obtaining valuable aspects of the exposure history may be difficult. Gastrointestinal symptoms may not have occurred, or may have been dismissed because of their mild and transient nature. Those patients with small acute or chronic exposures usually present for healthcare because of alopecia or the acute onset of neuropathy.

The differential diagnosis of the neuropathy includes disorders such as poisoning by arsenic, colchicine, and vinca alkaloids; botulism; thiamine deficiency; and Guillain-Barré syndrome. Both the sensory neuropathy and the preservation of reflexes help differentiate thallium-induced neuropathy from Guillain-Barré syndrome and most other causes of acute neuropathy.[9] When gastrointestinal symptoms are present along with neuropathy and other end-organ effects, poisoning with metal salts such as arsenic and mercury should be considered (Chaps. 79 and 81). The differential diagnosis of abrupt and complete alopecia is more restricted and includes arsenic, selenium, colchicine, and vinca alkaloid poisoning (Chap. 29). When Mees lines are present, they indicate past exposure to metals, mitotic inhibitors, or antimetabolites, and as such are nonspecific for thallium (Chaps. 29, 79, and 81).

Diagnostic Testing

Radiographs of tampered food products[51] and the abdomen[23] can document the presence of a heavy metal such as thallium, which is radiopaque. Although abdominal radiography may be useful shortly after a suspected exposure, the sensitivity and specificity of this test is unknown. Similarly, the yield from other routine studies, such as the complete blood count, electrolytes, urine analysis, and ECG, is limited in that these other studies are often normal, or demonstrate nonspecific findings at best.

Microscopic inspection of the hair reveals a diagnostic pattern of black pigmentation of the hair roots of the scalp in approximately of 95% of poisoned patients.[7,55,71,82] However, to the untrained observer this test is likely to be inconclusive.

The definitive clinical diagnosis of thallium poisoning can only be established by demonstrating elevated thallium levels. Thallium can be recovered in the hair, nails, feces, saliva, blood, and urine, and standard assays and normal values for most of these sources can be found.[56] Urine spot tests notoriously give false-negative results, require the use of dangerous materials that are not routinely available (20% nitric acid), and should therefore be avoided.[71] The standard toxicologic method is to obtain a 24-hour urine sample for thallium to be assayed by atomic absorption spectroscopy.[11,87] Normal urine values are below 5 µg/L. Some authors suggest a potassium mobilization test to enhance urinary elimination (similar to the ethylenediaminetetraacetic acid (EDTA) mobilization test) to assist in the diagnosis of thallium exposure.[7,33,71] We advise against this practice because of its lack of proven utility and its potential to exacerbate neurologic toxicity (see the discussion of potassium in the next section of this chapter).

MANAGEMENT

The treatment goals for a patient with thallium poisoning are identical to those of all poisoned patients: initial stabilization, prevention of absorption, and enhanced elimination. Following the initial assessment and stabilization of the patient's airway, breathing, and circulatory status, gastrointestinal decontamination should be instituted in patients with known thallium ingestions because of the significant morbidity and mortality associated with a significant exposure.

Decontamination

Patients who present for healthcare shortly after ingestion should be considered candidates for ipecac-induced emesis or for orogastric lavage (Chap. 5). If the patient presents more than a few hours after ingestion, or has had considerable spontaneous emesis, these techniques should be avoided. Thallium salts are substantially adsorbed to activated charcoal in vitro.[41,29] Additionally, because thallium undergoes enterohepatic recirculation, activated charcoal may be useful both to prevent absorption following a recent ingestion and to enhance elimination of thallium in patients who present in the postabsorptive phase.[81] In fact, a rat model of thallium poisoning demonstrated that multiple-dose activated charcoal (given as 0.5 g/kg twice daily for 5 days) increased the fecal elimination of thallium by 82% and produced a substantial improvement in survival.[46] Other data demonstrate that activated charcoal alone is superior to either forced diuresis or potassium chloride therapy.[42] In patients with severe thallium toxicity constipation is common, such that the addition of mannitol[48] or another cathartic to the first dose of activated charcoal seems logical. While no studies address the utility of whole-bowel irrigation with polyethylene glycol electrolyte lavage solution, this technique may prove useful, especially when radiopaque material is demonstrated in the gastrointestinal tract by an abdominal radiograph.

Potassium

The similarities between the cellular handling of potassium and thallium ions led to the natural investigation of a role for potassium in the treatment of thallium poisoning. In humans, potassium administration is associated with an increase in urinary thallium elimination.[10,20,62] The magnitude of this increase is reported to be on the order of 2–3-fold.[62] This is supported by animal models that demonstrate some benefit in terms of either enhanced thallium elimination or survival.[21,42,46] It is believed that potassium administration blocks tubular reabsorption of thallium and mobilizes thallium from tissue stores, thereby raising thallium levels available for glomerular filtration.[57,71] However, it is this second mechanism that is of concern. Many authors report either the development of acute neurologic toxicity or the severe exacerbation of neurologic symptoms during potassium administration.[5,20,51,62,70,83] Others cite data demonstrating that potassium's augmentation of thallium elimination in humans is quite limited.[39] Additionally, some animal models demonstrate that potassium loading enhances lethality[50] and permits thallium redistribution into the CNS.[26] For these reasons, the routine use of potassium should be considered potentially dangerous. Some authors recommend forced diuresis, especially in conjunction with potassium chloride.[13,81] However, no convincing experimental evidence can support the use of forced diuresis with or without potassium at this time.

Once again, the similarities between thallium and potassium might suggest a role for administration of sodium polystyrene sulfonate (SPS) as a sodium-thallium exchange resin. Although in vitro binding between thallium and SPS is excellent, it is unlikely to be clinically useful because of preferential binding between potassium and SPS.[29]

Chelation

Thallium toxicity does not respond to traditional chelation therapy. Studies demonstrate that the use of EDTA and diethylenetriamine pentaacetic acid are without benefit.[56,71] Dimercaprol (British Anti-Lewisite, BAL) and D-penicillamine also fail to enhance thallium excretion in experimental models.[56,71] In one model in which D-penicillamine was able to enhance thallium elimination, it did so at the cost of substantial thallium redistribution into vital organs.[69] Similarly, sulfur-containing compounds such as cysteine or N-acetyl cysteine (NAC) have not been demonstrated to be beneficial.[46,52] Another chelator, diphenylthiocarbazone (dithizone), forms a minimally toxic complex with thallium, resulting in a 33% increase in fecal elimination of thallium in rats.[74] Unfortunately, dithizone is goitrogenic and diabetogenic in animal studies.[46,56,81] Dithiocarb (sodium diethyldithiocarbamate), an intermediate metabolite of tetraethylthiuram disulfide (disulfiram, or Antabuse) (Chap. 65), also increases the urinary excretion of thallium.[74,78] Prior to thallium elimination, however, the formation of a lipophilic thallium-diethyldithiocarbamate complex can result in the redistribution of thallium into the central nervous system.[36,78] After decomposition of the chelate complex, thallium may remain

in the central nervous system, potentially exacerbating neurologic symptoms.[36,78] Because of the significant adverse effects of dithizone and the redistribution of thallium following dithiocarb use, neither agent is recommended in the treatment of patients with thallium toxicity.

Prussian Blue

Prussian blue is a crystal lattice of potassium ferric hexacyanoferrate ($KFe(Fe(CN)_6)$) and can be used as a chelator for thallium toxicity.[40] In vitro thallium is more effectively adsorbed to Prussian blue than to activated charcoal.[29,37,40] When given orally, Prussian blue acts as an ion exchanger for univalent cations, with its affinity increasing as the ionic radius of the cation increases. As such, Prussian blue interferes with the enterohepatic circulation by exchanging potassium ions, from its lattice, for thallium ions in the gastrointestinal tract. This results in the formation of a concentration gradient causing an increased movement of thallium into the gut.

Oral Prussian blue reduces the half-life of elimination of thallium in rats by 50%.[67] Other animal studies overwhelmingly support both the safety and the superiority of Prussian blue as an antidote over all other agents in thallium poisoning.[27,36,40,50,52,69] Humans with thallium poisoning are routinely given Prussian blue, which appears to result in clinical benefits, enhanced fecal elimination, and falling thallium concentrations.[11,12,14,51,64,76,83,84,86] One series of 11 thallium-poisoned patients demonstrated both the safety of Prussian blue and its ability to substantially increase fecal thallium elimination.[77] Unfortunately, because there are no controlled trials in humans that compare Prussian blue to other agents, and many of the patients reported above received multiple therapies, the true utility of Prussian blue is unknown.

Reports suggest that Prussian blue is not absorbed from the gastrointestinal system,[32,77] but our clinical experience demonstrates that prolonged therapy results in blue discoloration of the sweat and tears. Currently, Prussian blue is neither commercially available as a pharmaceutical agent, nor approved for use in the United States by the Food and Drug Administration. It is available from chemical supply companies, in various forms with varying degrees of efficacy.[40,77] The colloidal, or soluble, form seems to be more efficacious than the insoluble form.[77] The dose of Prussian blue is 250 mg/kg/d orally via a nasogastric tube in 2–4 divided doses per day.[77] If patients are constipated, the Prussian blue may have greater utility if dissolved in 50 mL of 15% mannitol.[81] Although any cathartic may be appropriate, most authors have used mannitol, possibly because of concerns regarding repeated magnesium use in patients with neurologic findings and sorbitol in patients with poor gastrointestinal mobility.

Extracorporeal Drug Removal

Extracorporeal drug removal may have a limited beneficial role in patients with thallium toxicity, especially if begun shortly after the initial exposure while serum concentrations remain high prior to effective tissue distribution. A frequently quoted review attests to the benefits of hemodialysis.[54] The actual data, however, show that hemodialysis at various stages of poisoning is no better than forced diuresis.[12,63] Reported thallium removal rates by hemodialysis are trivial: 143 mg of thallium were removed by 120 hours,[64] 222.8 mg were removed by 121 hours,[12] and 128 mg were removed by 54 hours of hemodialysis.[12] These values can be placed in perspective knowing that the minimum lethal adult dose of thallium is estimated to be on the order of 1 g,[56] and that many reported cases involve ingestions 10 times greater than the minimum lethal dose. Data from a more recent hemodialysis experience suggest that by using high blood flow rates (300 mL/min), clearances as high as 90–150 mL/min could be obtained.[48] Although clearances seem encouraging, this must be kept in the perspective of thallium's large volume of distribution. With lower blood flow rates, charcoal hemoperfusion may be 2–3 times more efficient than hemodialysis, providing clearance rates as high as 139 mL/min.[12] Furthermore, combined hemoperfusion and hemodialysis were used in several cases[1,12,14] and were reported to remove as much as 93 mg of thallium within 3 hours of therapy.[1] While extracorporeal therapy alone is probably insufficient for patients with significant poisoning, and unnecessary in those with small exposures, it may have some utility in combination with other therapies, especially in patients with renal insufficiency or those with early massive and presumed lethal exposures. As is the case with other toxins, the use of peritoneal dialysis is probably ineffective in removing thallium.[39] Table 83–2 summarizes the suggested therapy for thallium-poisoned patients.

SUMMARY

The elimination of thallium salts from common use as depilatories and rodenticides substantially reduced the incidence of both intentional and unintentional thallium toxicity in the United States. Despite this fact, cases of significant poisoning still occur in countries in which thallium-containing rodenticides remain in use, and in this country as well, from attempted homicide and by intentional contamination of foods and illicit drugs. Early recognition of the thallium toxidrome and prompt initiation of safe and appropriate therapy will substantially improve the patient's prognosis. When recognition and subsequent treatment are delayed, morbidity and mortality can be consequential.[61]

TABLE 83–2. Treatment for Thallium Poisoning

Early (patients who present in the first hours postexposure)
- Stabilize airway, breathing, and circulation if necessary
- Consider ipecac-induced emesis or orogastric lavage if the patient has not vomited
- Consider whole-bowel irrigation with polyethylene glycol electrolyte lavage solution for patients with large ingestions or the presence of radiopaque material on abdominal radiograph
- Begin multiple-dose activated charcoal therapy; add a cathartic to the first dose if the patient does not have diarrhea
- Give Prussian blue 250 mg/kg/d in 2 or 4 divided doses, dissolved in water, or 50 mL of 15% mannitol if the patient does not have diarrhea
- Consider simultaneous charcoal hemoperfusion and hemodialysis, especially if the patient has renal insufficiency

Late (patients who present more than 24 hours postexposure or with chronic toxicity)
- Stabilize airway, breathing, and circulation if necessary
- Begin multiple-dose activated charcoal therapy; add a cathartic to the first dose if the patient does not have diarrhea
- Give Prussian blue 250 mg/kg/d in 2 or 4 divided doses, dissolved in water, or 50 mL of 15% mannitol if the patient does not have diarrhea

REFERENCES

1. Aoyama H, Yoshida M, Yamamura Y: Acute poisoning by intentional ingestion of thallous malonate. Hum Toxicol 1986;5:389–392.
2. Appenroth D, Gambaryan S, Winnefeld K, et al: Functional and morphological aspects of thallium-induced nephrotoxicity in rats. Toxicology 1995;96:203–215.
3. Appenroth D, Winnefeld K: Is thallium-induced nephrotoxicity in rats connected with riboflavin and/or GSH?—Reconsideration of hypotheses on the mechanism of thallium toxicity. J Appl Toxicol 1999;19:61–66.
4. Bank WJ, Pleasure DE, Suzuki K, et al: Thallium poisoning. Arch Neurol 1972;26:456–464.
5. Bank WJ: Thallium. In: Spencer PS, Schaumburg HH, eds: Experimental and Clinical Neurotoxicology. Baltimore, Williams & Wilkins, 1980, pp. 570–577.
6. Britten JS, Blank M: Thallium activation of the (Na+-K+)-activated ATPase of rabbit kidney. Biochim Biophys Acta 1968;159:160–166.
7. Burnett JW: Thallium poisoning. Cutis 1990;46:112–113.
8. Cavanagh JB, Fuller NH, Johnson HRM, Rudge P: The effects of thallium salts with particular reference to the nervous system changes. Q J Med 1974;43:293–319.
9. Cavanagh JB: What have we learned from Graham Frederick Young? Reflections on the mechanism of thallium neurotoxicity. Neuropath Appl Neurobiol 1991;17:3–9.
10. Chamberlain PH, Stavinoha WB, Davis H, et al: Thallium poisoning. Pediatrics 1958;12:1170–1182.
11. Chandler HA, Archbold GPR, Gibson JM, et al: Excretion of a toxic dose of thallium. Clin Chem 1990;36:1506–1509.
12. De Backer W, Zachee P, Verpooten GA, et al: Thallium intoxication treated with combined hemoperfusion-hemodialysis. Clin Toxicol 1982;19:259–264.
13. De Groot G, van Heijst ANP, van Kesteren RG, Maes RAA: An evaluation of the efficacy of charcoal hemoperfusion in the treatment of three cases of acute thallium poisoning. Arch Toxicol 1985;57:61–66.
14. De Groot G, van Heijst ANP: Toxicokinetic aspects of thallium poisoning: Methods of treatment by toxin elimination. Sci Total Environ 1988;71:411–418.
15. Desenclos JC, Wilder MH, Coppenger GW, et al: Thallium poisoning: An outbreak in Florida, 1988. South Med J 1992; 85:1203–1206.
16. Dolgner R, Brockhaus A, Ewers U, et al: Repeated surveillance of exposure to thallium in a population living in the vicinity of a cement plant emitting dust-containing thallium. Int Arch Occup Environ Health 1983;52:79–94.
17. Dumitru D, Kalantri A: Electrophysiologic investigation of thallium poisoning. Muscle Nerve 1990;13:433–437.
18. English JC: A case of thallium poisoning complicating pregnancy. Med J Aust 1954;1:780–782.
19. Feldman J, Levisohn DR: Acute alopecia: Clue to thallium toxicity. Pediatr Dermatol 1993;10:29–31.
20. Gastel B: Clinical conferences at Johns Hopkins Hospital. Thallium poisoning. Johns Hopkins Med J 1978;142:27–31.
21. Gehring PJ, Hammond T: Prussian blue: The interrelationship between thallium and potassium in animals. Pharmacol Exp Ther 1967; 155:187–201.
22. Gibson JE, Becker BA: Placental transfer, embryotoxicity, and teratogenicity of thallium sulfate in normal and potassium-deficient rats. Toxicol Appl Pharmacol 1970;16:120–132.
23. Grunfeld O, Hinostroza G: Thallium poisoning. Arch Intern Med 1964;114:132–138.
24. Hall BK: Critical periods during development as assessed by thallium-induced inhibition of growth of embryonic chick tibiae in vitro. Teratology 1985;31:353–361.
25. Hasan M, Ali SF: Effects of thallium, nickel, and cobalt administration on the lipid peroxidation in different regions of the rat brain. Toxicol Appl Pharmacol 1981;57:8–13.

26. Hasan M, Chandra S, Dua PR, et al: Biochemical and electrophysiological effects of thallium poisoning on the rat corpus striatum. Toxicol Appl Pharmacol 1977;41:353–359.

27. Heydlauf H: Ferric-cyanoferrate (II): An effective antidote in thallium poisoning. Eur J Pharmacol 1969;6:340–344.

28. Hirata M, Taoda K, Ono-Ogasawara M, et al: A probable case of chronic occupational thallium poisoning in a glass factory. Ind Health 1998;36:300–303.

29. Hoffman RS, Stringer JA, Feinberg RS, Goldfrank LR: Comparative efficacy of thallium adsorption by activated charcoal, Prussian blue, and sodium polystyrene sulfonate. J Toxicol Clin Toxicol 1999;37: 833–837.

30. Hoffman RS: Thallium poisoning during pregnancy: A case report and comprehensive literature review. J Toxicol Clin Toxicol 2000;38: 765–773.

31. Hologgitas J, Ullucci P, Driscoll J: Thallium elimination kinetics in acute thallotoxicosis. J Anal Toxicol 1980;4:68–73.

32. Hultin T, Naslund PH: Effects of thallium (I) on the structure and functions of mammalian ribosomes. Chem Biol Interact 1974:8: 315–328.

33. Insley BM, Grufferman S, Ayliffe HE: Thallium poisoning in cocaine users. Am J Emerg Med 1986;4:545–548.

34. Inturrisi CE: Thallium-induced dephosphorylation of a phosphorylated intermediate of the (sodium+thallium-activated) ATPase. Biochim Biophys Acta 1969;78:630–633.

35. Johnson W: A case of thallium poisoning during pregnancy. Med J Aust 1960;47:540–542.

36. Kamerbeek HH, Rauws AG, ten Ham M, van Heijst ANP: Dangerous redistribution of thallium by treatment with sodium diethyldithiocarbamate. Acta Med Scand 1971;189:149–154.

37. Kamerbeek HH, Rauws AG, ten Ham M, van Heijst ANP: Prussian blue therapy in thallotoxicosis. Acta Med Scand 1971;189:321–324.

38. Kaye JF: Thallium activation of pyruvate kinase. Arch Biochem Biophys 1971;143:232–239.

39. Koshy PM, Lovejoy FK: Thallium injection with survival: Ineffectiveness of peritoneal dialysis and potassium chloride diuresis. Clin Toxicol 1981;18:521–525.

40. Krazov J, Rios C, Altagracia M, et al: Relationship between physicochemical properties of Prussian blue and its efficacy as antidote against thallium poisoning. J Appl Toxicol 1993;13:213–216.

41. Lehmann PA, Favare L: Parameters for the absorption of thallium ions by activated charcoal and Prussian blue. J Toxicol Clin Toxicol 1984;22:331–339.

42. Leloux MS, Lich NP, Claude JR: Experimental studies on thallium toxicity in rats. J Toxicol Clin Exp 1990;10:147–156.

43. Leung KM, Ooi VE: Studies on thallium toxicity, its tissue distribution and histopathological effects in rats. Chemosphere 2000;41: 155–159.

44. Lovejoy FH: Thallium. Clin Toxicol Rev 1982;4:1–2.

45. Luckit J, Mir N, Hargreaves M, et al: Thrombocytopenia associated with thallium poisoning. Hum Exp Toxicol 1990;9:47–48.

46. Lund A: The effect of various substances on the excretion and the toxicity of thallium in the rat. Acta Pharmacol Toxicol 1956;12:260–268.

47. Lynche GR, Lond MB, Scovell JMS: The toxicology of thallium. Lancet 1930;12:1340–1344.

48. Malbrain MLNG, Lambrecht GLY, Zandijk E, et al: Treatment of severe thallium intoxication. J Toxicol Clin Toxicol 1997;35:97–100.

49. McMillan TM, Jacobson RR, Gross M: Neuropsychology of thallium poisoning. J Neurol Neurosurg Psychiatry 1997;63:247–250.

50. Meggs WJ, Goldfrank LR, Hoffman RS: Effects of potassium in a murine model of thallium poisoning [abstract]. J Toxicol Clin Toxicol 1995;33:559.

51. Meggs WJ, Hoffman RS, Shih RD, et al: Thallium poisoning from maliciously contaminated food. J Toxicol Clin Toxicol 1994;32: 723–730.

52. Meggs WJ, Morasco RC, Shih RD, et al: Effects of Prussian blue and N-acetylcysteine on thallium toxicity in mice. J Toxicol Clin Toxicol 1997;35:163–166.

53. Melnick RL, Monti LG, Motzkin SM: Uncoupling of mitochondrial oxidative phosphorylation by thallium. Biochem Biophys Res Comm 1976;69:68–73.

54. Moeschlin S: Thallium poisoning. Clin Toxicol 1980;17:133–146.

55. Moore D, House I: Thallium poisoning: Diagnosis may be elusive but alopecia is the clue. Br Med J 1993;306:1527–1529.

56. Mulkey JP, Oehme FW: A review of thallium toxicity. Vet Hum Toxicol 1993;35:445–453.

57. Mullins LJ, Moore RD: The movement of thallium ions in muscle. J Gen Physiol 1960;43:759–773.

58. Munch JC, Ginsburg HM, Nixon CE: The 1932 thallotoxicosis outbreak in California. JAMA 1933;100:1315–1319.

59. Munch JC: Human thallotoxicosis. JAMA 1934;102:1929–1933.

60. Neal JB, Appelbaum E, Gaul LE, Masselink RJ: An unusual occurrence of thallium poisoning. N Y State J Med 1935;35:657–659.

61. Pai V: Acute thallium poisoning: Prussian blue therapy in 9 cases. West Indian Med J 1987;36:256–258.

62. Papp JP, Gay PC, Dodson VN, Pollard HM: Potassium chloride treatment in thallotoxicosis. Ann Intern Med 1969;71:119–123.

63. Paulson G, Vergara G, Young J, Bird M: Thallium intoxication treated with dithizone and hemodialysis. Arch Intern Med 1972;129: 100–103.

64. Pedersen RS, Olesen AS, Freund LG, et al: Thallium intoxication treated with long-term hemodialysis, forced diuresis and Prussian blue. Acta Med Scand 1978;204:429–432.

65. Questel F, Dugarin J, Dally S: Thallium-contaminated heroin [letter]. Ann Intern Med 1996;124:616.

66. Rangel-Guerra R, Martinez HR: Thallium poisoning: Experience with 50 patients. Gac Med Mex 1990;126:487–494.

67. Rauws AG: Thallium pharmacokinetics and its modification by Prussian blue. Arch Pharmacol 1974;284:295–306.

68. Reed D, Crawley J, Faro SN, et al: Thallotoxicosis: Acute manifestations and sequelae. JAMA 1963;183:516–522.

69. Rios C, Monroy-Noyola A: D-Penicillamine and Prussian blue as antidotes against thallium intoxication in rats. Toxicology 1992;74:69–76.

70. Roby DS, Fein AM, Bennett RH, et al: Cardiopulmonary effects of acute thallium poisoning. Chest 1984;84:236–240.

71. Saddique A, Perterson CD: Thallium poisoning: A review. Vet Hum Toxicol 1983;25:16–22.

72. Schaumberg HH, Berger A: Alopecia and sensory polyneuropathy from thallium in a Chinese herbal medication [letter]. JAMA 1992; 268:2430–2431.

73. Schmidt D: A case of localized retinal damage in thallium poisoning. Int Ophthalmol 1997;21:143–147.

74. Schwetz BA, O'Neil PV, Voelker FA, Jacobs DW: Effects of diphenylthiocarbazone and diethyldithiocarbamate on the excretion of thallium by rats. Toxicol Appl Pharmacol 1967;10:79–88.

75. Sharma AN, Nelson LS, Hoffman RS: Evaluation of CSF thallium levels. J Toxicol Clin Toxicol 2001;39:237–238.

76. Spencer PS, Peterson ER, Madrid RA, et al: Effects of thallium salts on neuronal mitochondria in organotypic cord ganglia-muscle combination cultures. J Cell Biol 1973;58:79–85.

77. Stevens W, van Peteghem C, Heyndrickx A, Barbier F: Eleven cases of thallium intoxication treated with Prussian blue. Int J Clin Pharmacol 1974;10:1–22.

78. Sunderman FW: Diethyldithiocarbamate therapy of thallotoxicosis. Am J Med Sci 1967;2:107–118.

79. Tabandeh H, Crowston JG, Thompson GM: Ophthalmologic features of thallium poisoning. Am J Ophthalmol 1994;117:243–245.

80. Tabandeh H, Thompson GM: Visual function in thallium toxicity [letter]. BMJ 1993;307:324.

81. Thompson DF: Management of thallium poisoning. Clin Toxicol 1981;18:979–990.

82. Tromme I, Van Neste D, Dobbelaere F, et al: Skin signs in the diagnosis of thallium poisoning. Br J Dermatol 1998;138:321–325.

83. Van Der Merwe CF: The treatment of thallium poisoning: A report of 2 cases. S Afr Med J 1972;46:960–961.

84. Vergauwe PL, Knockaert DC, Van Tittelboom TJ: Near fatal subacute thallium poisoning necessitating prolonged mechanical ventilation. Am J Emerg Med 1990;8:548–550.

85. Villanueva E, Hernandez-Cueto C, Lachica E, et al: Poisoning by thallium: A study of five cases. Drug Saf 1990;5:384–389.

86. Wainwright AP, Kox WJ, House IM, et al: Clinical features and therapy of acute thallium poisoning. Q J Med 1988;69:939–944.

87. Wakid NW, Cortas NK: Chemical and atomic absorption methods for thallium in urine compared [letter]. Clin Chem 1984;30:587–588.

H. HOUSEHOLD TOXINS

CHAPTER **84** ANTISEPTICS, DISINFECTANTS, AND STERILANTS

Paul M. Wax

A 60-year-old woman was brought to the Emergency Department (ED) from home 3 hours after drinking an unknown liquid. Apparently, the woman had ingested a few ounces of a liquid from an old liquor bottle that was stored in the garage. The patient had a past medical history that was significant for ethanol abuse. She was not taking any known medications.

In the ED, the patient was unresponsive to voice but responded to deep pain. According to a family member, the patient had gone to the garage, looking for a bottle of rum. She was later discovered lying next to the bottle, having vomited several times. The bottle was also brought into the ED. Her vital signs were: blood pressure, 80/40 mm Hg; pulse, 130 beats/min and regular; respiratory rate, 14 breaths/min; and temperature, 98.6°F (37°C). The patient was disheveled but otherwise well appearing. An unusual, somewhat sweetish odor was noted on her breath. Examination of the head, eyes, ears, nose, and throat was otherwise unremarkable. The neck was supple. The chest was clear to auscultation bilaterally and cardiac examination revealed a rapid heart rate. Abdominal examination was soft and nontender, with normoactive bowel sounds. Rectal examination was negative for occult blood. Extremity examination was normal. Neurologically, the patient was comatose and had normal muscle tone and symmetric reflexes. Her initial electrocardiogram (ECG) showed sinus tachycardia with normal conduction and no evidence of ischemia.

In the ED, the patient continued to vomit. She underwent endotracheal intubation for airway protection. The patient was treated with aggressive fluid resuscitation, including 3 L 0.9% NaCl, during the first 2 hours. Her blood pressure gradually improved, but she did exhibit episodes of atrial fibrillation and was given two intravenous doses of 0.25-mg digoxin. The patient was admitted to the intensive care unit (ICU). Pertinent initial laboratory studies revealed serum sodium, 134 mEq/L; potassium, 3.8 mEq/L; chloride, 98 mEq/L; bicarbonate, 18 mEq/L; blood urea nitrogen (BUN), 15 mg/dL; creatinine, 1.1 mg/dL; and glucose, 90 mg/dL. The arterial blood gas on room air showed pH 7.28; Pco_2, 50 mm Hg; and Po_2, 70 mm Hg. Urine toxicology screen was negative for drugs of abuse. Serum ethanol level was 30 mg/dL. The old liquor bottle that the patient had drunk from was noted to have a disinfectantlike odor that resembled formaldehyde. Given this formaldehydelike odor, the remaining liquid from the bottle was sent to the medical examiners office for a formaldehyde level.

In the ICU, the patient remained comatose for the first 48 hours. Esophagogastroscopy revealed gastric inflammation, but no ulcerations or deep burns. There were no further dysrhythmias. The patient began to awaken during the third day of hospitalization and

was extubated and fully awake within 96 hours of the ingestion. The patient now admitted that she had run out of liquor in her house and had gone out to the garage, looking for other sources of ethanol. She believed that she had been drinking from an old rum bottle. A month after discharge, the medical examiner's report of the analysis of the liquid from the old bottle revealed the presence of phenol. No formaldehyde, ethanol, or other chemicals were detected.

Antiseptics, disinfectants, and sterilants are a diverse group of antimicrobial agents used to prevent infection (Table 84–1). Although these terms are sometimes used interchangeably (and some of these agents are used for both antisepsis and disinfection), the distinguishing characteristics between the groups are important to emphasize. An antiseptic is a chemical agent that is applied to living tissue to kill or inhibit microorganisms. Iodophors, chlorhexidine, and the alcohols (ethanol and isopropanol) are commonly used antiseptics. A disinfectant is a chemical or physical agent that is applied to inanimate objects to kill microorganisms. Chlorine bleach (sodium hypochlorite), phenolic compounds, and formaldehyde are examples of currently used disinfectants. A sterilant is a chemical or physical agent that is applied to inanimate objects to kill all living organisms, including spores. Ethylene oxide and glutaraldehyde are examples of sterilants. Neither antiseptics nor disinfectants have complete sporicidal activity. Not surprisingly, many of these chemicals that are used to kill microbiologic organisms also demonstrate considerable human toxicity.[20,64]

Although sulfur, vinegar (acetic acid), and mercurial compounds were used as antiseptics as long as 2000 years ago, it was not until the 19th century that the use of antiseptics became commonplace. Some of the epochal figures in medicine were the first to extol the importance of antiseptics. Semmelweis implemented the practice of hand washing with chloride of lime as a means of preventing the dreaded puerperal fever. Lister experimented extensively with phenol as an antiseptic. Koch used mercury bichloride. Other agents introduced as antiseptics during the 19th century include tincture of iodine (used extensively during the Civil War), hydrogen peroxide, isopropanol, and ethanol.[64]

The use of these agents evolved during the 20th century as their toxicity and the principles of microbiology became better understood. Two of the more toxic antiseptics—iodine and phenol—were gradually replaced by the less toxic iodophors and substituted phenols. Mercury bichloride was superseded by the organic mercurials (eg, merbromin, thimerosal), which also proved

TABLE 84–1.   Antiseptics, Disinfectants, Sterilants, and Related Compounds

Chemical	Commercial Product	Use	Toxic Effects	Therapeutics and Evaluation
Acids				
Boric acid	Borax	Antiseptic	Blue-green emesis and diarrhea	GI decontamination
	Sodium perborate	Mouthwash	Boiled lobster appearance	Hemodialysis (rare)
	Dobell's solution	Eyewash		
		Roach Killer	CNS; renal	
Alcohols				
(Chaps. 64,66)				
Ethanol	Rubbing alcohol	Antiseptic	CNS depression	Supportive
	(70% ethanol)	Disinfectant	Respiratory depression	
Isopropyl alcohol	Rubbing alcohol	Antiseptic	CNS depression	Hemodialysis (rare)
	(70% Isopropanol)	Disinfectant	Respiratory depression	
			Ketonemia, ketonuria	
			GI irritation/bleeding	
			Hemorrhagic tracheobronchitls	
Aldehydes				
Formaldehyde	Formalin	Disinfectant	Caustic gastroenteritis	Gastric lavage
	(37% formaldehyde,	Fixative	CNS depression	Hemodialysis
	12–15% methanol)	Urea insulation		Sodium bicarbonate
Glutaraldehyde	Cidex (2% glutaraldehyde)	Sterilant	Mucosal and dermal irritant	
Chlorhexidine	Hibiclens	Antiseptic	GI irritation	
Chlorinated Compounds				
Chlorine		Disinfectant	Irritant	
Chlorophors	Chlorine bleach	Disinfectant	Mild GI irritation	Endoscopy (rare)
(Sodium Hypochlorite)	(5% NaOCl)			
	Dakin's solution			
	(1 part 5% NaOCl,			
	10 parts H$_2$O)			
Ethylene Oxide		Sterilant	Irritant	
		Plasticizer	CNS depression	
			Peripheral neuropathy	
			Carcinogen ?	
Organic Mercurials	Merbromin 2%	Antiseptic	CNS	(Chap. 81)
(Chaps. 56, 81)	(Mercurchrome)	(obsolete)	Renal	
	Thimerosal (Merthiolate)			
Iodinated Compounds				
Iodine	Tincture of Iodine	Antiseptic	Caustic gastroenteritis	Milk, starch
	(2% I$_2$, 24% NaI,			Sodium thiosulfate
	50% ethanol)			Endoscopy
	Lugol's solution (5% I$_2$)			
Iodophors	Providone-iodine	Antiseptic	Limited	Same as iodine if symptomatic
	(Betadine) (0.001% I$_2$)			
Iodide	SSKI (100% KI)	Expectorant	Iodism	Steroids for significant salivary
				gland enlargement
Oxidants				
Chlorates	Sodium chlorate	Antiseptic	Hemolytic anemia	Methylene blue?
	Potassium chlorate		Methemoglobinemia	Exchange transfusion
		Matches	Renal failure	Hemodialysis
		Herbicide		
Hydrogen peroxide	H$_2$O$_2$ 3%—household	Disinfectant	Oxygen emboli	Lavage
	H$_2$O$_2$ 30%—industrial		GI caustic	Radiographic evaluation
				Endoscopy
Potassium permanganate		Antiseptic	Oxidizing agent, caustic	Decontamination
			Manganese elevation	Endoscopy as needed
Phenols				
Nonsubstituted	Phenol (carbolic acid)	Disinfectant	Caustic gastroenteritis	Decontamination:
			Dermal burns	Polyethylene glycol or water
			Cutaneous absorption	Endoscopy as needed
			CNS effects	
Subsituted	Hexachlorophene	Disinfectant	CNS disturbances	
Quaternary Ammonium				
Compounds				
Benzalkonium chloride	Zephiran	Disinfectant	GI caustic at high concentrations	Endoscopy if significant GI symptoms

toxic. More recently, newer compounds, such as quaternary ammonium compounds, ethylene oxide, and glutaraldehyde, were introduced.

PHENOL

Phenol, also known as carbolic acid, is one of the oldest antiseptic agents. Although at one time it was the standard antiseptic to which other antiseptics were compared and was used as a preoperative antiseptic and in wound dressings, phenol's toxicity limited its usefulness. It is rarely used as an antiseptic today and has been replaced by the many phenolic derivatives. Currently, phenol is used as a disinfectant, chemical intermediary, and nail cauterizer. The last application uses a highly concentrated 89% solution. Phenol is also a component (0.1–4.5%) of various lotions, ointments, gels, gargles, lozenges, and throat sprays.[64] Campho-Phenique and Chloraseptic contain 4.7% and 1.4% phenol, respectively. Although many cases of phenol poisoning were reported in the past, acute oral overdoses of phenol-containing solutions are relatively uncommon today.[58]

Phenol acts as a general protoplasmic poison. Toxicity is a result of its ability to cause cell wall disruption, protein denaturation, and coagulation necrosis. Intentional ingestion of concentrated phenol, ingestion of phenol-containing water, occupational exposure to aerosolized phenol, dermal contact, and parenteral administration may all result in symptomatic phenol poisoning. Phenol demonstrates excellent skin penetrance.[16] Severe dermal burns from phenol with resultant phenol absorption have resulted in systemic toxicity, and even death within minutes to hours.[16,99] Parenteral administration of phenol has also resulted in death.[102] The lethal dose may be as little as 1 g.[77]

Clinical manifestations can be divided into local and systemic symptoms. Systemic symptoms from gastrointestinal (GI) or dermal absorption of phenol are usually more dangerous than the local effects and can result in significant morbidity and mortality. Manifestations of systemic toxicity include central nervous system (CNS) and cardiac symptoms. CNS effects include central stimulation, seizures, lethargy, and coma.[60] In a study of patients who had ingested Creolin (26% phenol), CNS symptoms predominated.[158] Nine of 52 patients evaluated at the hospital developed lethargy, and 2 patients developed coma. Seizures were not reported. Cardiac symptoms from phenol include tachycardia, bradycardia, and hypotension.[60] Excessive dermal absorption of phenol during chemical peeling procedures was associated with dysrhythmias.[179]

Other systemic symptoms that may develop include pulmonary disturbances, hypothermia, metabolic acidosis, methemoglobinemia, and rabbit syndrome.[14,77,86] "Phenol marasmus" was a term used in the 19th century to describe patients (usually physicians) who developed a typical characteristic syndrome after chronic exposure to aerosolized phenol. These symptoms included anorexia, weight loss, vertigo, headache, and salivation. A brown, or even black, discoloration of the urine was usually noted.[111] Dark urine (bilirubin-negative) was also a prominent feature in a more recent case of occupational exposure to vaporized phenol.[111]

Local toxicity to the GI tract from the ingestion of phenol may result in nausea, vomiting, bloody diarrhea, and severe abdominal pain. Serious GI burns are uncommon, and strictures are rare.[73,147] White patches in the oral cavity may be detected. In the Creolin study cited above, only 1 of 17 patients who underwent endoscopy

had a significant esophageal burn.[158] Ingestions of phenol-contaminated water are associated with the development of nausea, vomiting, diarrhea, burning sensation in the mouth, mouth sores, and dark urine.[8,84] Dermal exposures to phenol usually result in a light brown staining of the skin.

Markedly elevated blood and urine levels of phenol may be detected after ingestion, or dermal absorption, of phenol and phenol-containing compounds (eg, Campho-Phenique).[16,77,93]

A variety of solutions have been suggested for dermal and gastric decontamination of phenol. Olive oil was recommended in the past as an irrigant fluid because it was thought to dissolve phenol and prevent absorption.[55] Animal studies, however, show that systemic phenol absorption is actually increased when olive oil is used as a decontaminant.[35] A study employing a rat model showed that cutaneous decontamination with a low-molecular-weight polyethylene glycol solution decreased mortality, systemic effects, and dermal burns.[22] Although this study suggested that polyethylene glycol was superior to water as a decontamination agent, a subsequent study using a swine model could not demonstrate a difference between these two agents.[135] Given the lack of definitive efficacy data, either low-molecular-weight polyethylene glycol (eg, PEG 300 or 400), if it is readily available in the ED, or water is currently recommended for dermal irrigation and careful gastric decontamination. Appropriate endoscopic evaluation, as needed to determine the extent of GI injury, and good supportive care are also recommended.

SUBSTITUTED PHENOLS AND OTHER RELATED COMPOUNDS

Hexachlorophene

Substituted phenols are also used as antiseptic and disinfectant agents. Hexachlorophene (pHisoHex), a trichlorinated bis-phenol, is one of the best known substituted phenols. Hexachlorophene is considered generally less tissue-toxic than phenol. This agent was formerly used extensively as a detergent in hospitals. During the 1970s, an association was observed between repetitive whole-body washing of premature infants with 3% hexachlorophene and the development of vacuolar encephalopathy and cerebral edema.[109] There were multiple reports of significant neurologic toxicity and death in children who became toxic after ingesting hexachlorophene.[71] Fatalities also occurred after patients absorbed substantial amounts of hexachlorophene during the treatment of burn injuries.[30] Since these reports, the use of hexachlorophene has declined significantly.

pHisoDerm, another antiseptic agent with a similar sounding name to pHisoHex, contains sodium octylphenoxyethoxyethyl ether sulfonate and lanolin. These chemicals act as soaps and detergents. No reports of significant toxicity from pHisoDerm can be found in the literature. Irritative effects (nausea, vomiting, diarrhea) would be the main problems to anticipate with oral exposure.

In a study of poisoning admissions to Hong Kong hospitals, the ingestion of Dettol liquid, a household disinfectant that contains 4.8% chloroxylenol, 9% pine oil, and 12% isopropanol, accounted for 10% of admissions.[28] Aspiration (perhaps, in part, because of the pine oil) occurred in 8% of these patients, resulting in upper airway obstruction, pneumonia, and acute respiratory distress syndrome. More common symptoms included nausea, vomiting, sore mouth, sore throat, drowsiness, abdominal pain, and fever. Dermal contact with Dettol may result in full-thickness chemical burns.[41]

Cresol, a mixture of three isomers of methylphenol, has better germicidal activity than phenol and is a commonly used disinfectant. Exposure to concentrated cresol may result in significant local tissue injury, hemolysis, renal injury, hepatic injury, and CNS and respiratory depression.[41,65,186] Phenol levels, as well as cresol levels, serve as markers of exposure.[186]

FORMALDEHYDE

Formaldehyde is a water-soluble, highly reactive gas at room temperature. Formalin consists of an aqueous solution of formaldehyde, usually containing about 37% formaldehyde and 12–15% methanol. Formaldehyde is quite irritating to the upper airways, and its odor is readily detectable at low concentrations. Lethality in adults begins to occur following ingestion of 1–2 ounces of formalin.[46]

Although formaldehyde was once widely used as a disinfectant and fumigant, its role as a disinfectant is now largely confined to the disinfection of hemodialysis machines. Nonetheless, formaldehyde has many other applications. Healthcare workers are probably most familiar with the use of formaldehyde as a tissue fixative and embalming agent. Formaldehyde is also used in the textile industry and in the production of resins and plastics. Formaldehyde is a major component of urea formaldehyde foam, used extensively for insulation.[25]

Formaldehyde is a protoplasmic poison and potent caustic. The acute ingestion of formaldehyde (as formalin) may result in both local and systemic symptoms. It causes coagulation necrosis, protein precipitation, and tissue fixation. Ingestions of formalin may result in significant gastric injury, including hemorrhage, diffuse necrosis, perforation, and stricture.[4,11,143] The most extensive damage appears in the stomach, with only occasional involvement of the small intestine and colon.[89] Chemical fixation of the stomach may occur.[165] Esophageal involvement is not very prominent, and, if present, is usually limited to its distal segment.[89]

The most striking systemic manifestation of formaldehyde poisoning is acidosis, resulting from the conversion of formaldehyde to formic acid. This reaction occurs rapidly. On initial presentation, the patient may already have a profound acidemia, accompanied by a large anion gap. Although the methanol component of the formalin solution is readily absorbed and has resulted in methanol levels of 40 mg/dL,[23,46] the rapid metabolism of formaldehyde to formic acid appears to be responsible for much of the acidosis (Chap. 66). The development of extensive tissue necrosis leading to lactate production may also be a factor. Blindness due to the accumulation of formate, a retinal toxin, is not reported. This is likely due to the lethality of the dose of formaldehyde necessary to cause retinal toxicity.

Patients presenting after acute formaldehyde ingestions complain of the rapid onset of severe abdominal pain, which may be accompanied by vomiting and diarrhea. Altered mental status and coma usually follow rapidly. Examination may demonstrate epigastric tenderness, hematemesis, cyanosis, hypotension, and tachypnea. Hypotension may be profound. Decreased myocardial contractility, as well as hypovolemic shock, contributes to the cardiovascular instability.[72,167] Early endoscopic findings include ulceration, necrosis, perforation, and hemorrhage of the stomach, with little esophageal involvement. Acute intravascular hemolysis is described in hemodialysis patients whose dialysis equipment contained residual formaldehyde after undergoing routine cleaning.[126,136]

Occupational and environmental exposure to formaldehyde receives considerable attention. In particular, there is concern over the potential off-gassing of formaldehyde from the widely used urea formaldehyde building insulation, such as particle boards.[124] Headache, nausea, skin rash, sore throat, nasal congestion, and eye irritation are associated with the use of these polymers.[38] Formaldehyde, at concentrations as low as 1 ppm, may cause significant irritation to mucous membranes of the upper respiratory tract and conjunctivae.[75,104] Formaldehyde is also a potential sensitizer for immune-mediated reversible bronchospasm.[69] The exact immunologic mechanism is not yet elucidated, although it is likely that formaldehyde acts as a hapten. In addition, formaldehyde is thought to be a dermal sensitizer.[156] Although both animal and human data suggest that formaldehyde exposure is associated with an increased incidence of nasopharyngeal carcinoma,[3,142] its role in the pathogenesis of cancer in humans is unproven.[1,128]

Acute chemical pneumonitis occurs after significant inhalational exposure.[134] Hepatotoxicity is also related to formaldehyde exposure.[13] Membranous nephropathy is also associated with occupational or environmental formaldehyde exposure.[21] Significant neurobehavioral impairment and seizures are also associated with long-term occupational exposure to formaldehyde (although phenol exposure may have contributed to the problems).[87]

The initial management of a patient with a significant formaldehyde exposure should include immediate dilution with water. Although such an approach may be useful in reducing the caustic effect, strong evidence for a beneficial result is lacking. Careful gastric aspiration with a small-bore nasogastric tube may limit systemic absorption. The role of activated charcoal is not studied and it probably should not be used if endoscopy is considered likely. Significant acidemia should be treated with sodium bicarbonate and folinic acid. Immediate hemodialysis may remove the accumulating formic acid, as well as the parent molecules: formaldehyde and methanol.[46] An ethanol infusion or 4-methylpyrazole may block the metabolism of methanol, but neither of these agents will block the conversion of formaldehyde to formic acid (Chap. 66). Early endoscopy is recommended for all patients with significant GI symptoms to assess the degree of burn injury. Surgical intervention may be required for those with severe burns. Emergent gastrectomy, as well as late surgical intervention to relieve formaldehyde-induced gastric outlet obstruction, has sometimes been required.[66,91]

IODINE AND IODOPHORS

Iodine usually refers to molecular iodine, also known as I_2, free iodine, or elemental iodine. This chemical is the active ingredient of iodine-based antiseptics. The poor solubility of I_2 in water is increased by adding iodide (I^-). Alternatively, the use of ethanol as the solvent (eg, tincture of iodine) allows substantially more concentrated forms of I_2 to be available. Iodophors are substances in which molecular iodine is compounded to a high-molecular-weight carrier or to a solubilizing agent. Povidone-iodine (Betadine), a commonly used iodophor, consists of iodine linked to polyvinylpyrrolidone (povidone). Problems associated with the use of iodine include unpleasant odor, skin irritation, allergic reactions, clothes staining, and poor stability. Iodophors, which limit the release of molecular iodine and are generally less toxic, are the standard iodine-based antiseptic preparations. Iodophor preparations are formulated as solutions, ointments, foams, surgical scrubs, wound-packing gauze, and vaginal preparations. The most common preparation is a 10% povidone-iodine solution that contains 1% "available" iodine (referring to all oxidizing iodine species), but only 0.001% free iodine (referring only to molecular iodine).[20,64]

Iodine is one of the oldest topical antiseptics. It is also used to disinfect medical equipment and drinking water. Iodine is an effective antiseptic against bacteria, viruses, protozoa, and fungi, and is used both prophylactically and therapeutically.[43] Iodine is cytotoxic and an oxidant. It is thought to work by binding amino and heterocyclic nitrogen groups, oxidizing sulfhydryl groups, and saturating double bonds. Iodine also iodinates tyrosine groups.[64]

Iodine ingestions are much less common than in the past as a result of the change in antiseptic use from iodine to iodophor antiseptics.[45] During the early part of the 20th century, however, iodine ingestions were quite routine. A study at Boston City Hospital from 1915 to 1936 revealed that iodine ingestions (usually tincture of iodine) were the most common cause of poisoning, accounting for 27% of all patients admitted for suicide attempts.[115] Molecular iodine may cause severe caustic injury of the gastrointestinal (GI) tract, similar to what occurs following exposure to a strong alkali or acid (Chap. 87). A 1937 study reported 18 cases of oral iodine ingestions, usually involving tincture of iodine, that resulted in death.[48] The amount ingested was recorded in 9 of these cases, and ranged from 30 to 250 mL (0.6–5.0 g of iodine). Symptoms consisted of vomiting, diarrhea, abdominal pain, GI bleeding, delirium, anuria, and vasomotor collapse. Death usually occurred within the first 48 hours after ingestion and resulted from gastrointestinal injury, hypovolemia, and circulatory collapse. Gastrointestinal strictures can also occur after the ingestion of tincture of iodine.[182]

There may be significant systemic absorption of iodine from topical iodine or iodophor preparations.[129] Markedly elevated iodine levels do occur in patients who receive topical iodophor treatments to areas of dermal breakdown, such as burn injuries.[96] Significant absorption occurs when iodophors are applied to the vagina, perianal fistulas, umbilical cords, and the skin of low-birth-weight neonates.[177] A fatality following intraoperative irrigation of a hip wound with povidone-iodine is reported.[39] The serum iodine level, reported at necropsy, in this case, was 1000 times normal (normal, 5–8 μg/dL).

Until recently, reports of adverse consequences from iodophor ingestions could not be found in the literature. In a recent single case report, however, a 9-week-old infant died within 3 hours of receiving povidone-iodine by mouth.[92] In this unusual case, the child was administered 15 mL of povidone-iodine mixed with 135 mL of polyethylene glycol by nasogastric tube over a 3-hour period for the treatment of infantile colic. Postmortem examination showed an ulcerated and necrotic intestinal tract. A blood iodine level of 14,600 μg/dL was recorded. Significant toxicity from intentional ingestions of iodophors in adults is not documented.

Acid-base disturbances are among the most significant abnormalities associated with iodine and iodophors. Metabolic acidosis occurred in several burn patients after receiving multiple applications of povidone-iodine ointment.[96,131] These patients had elevated serum iodide concentrations and normal lactate levels. The exact etiology of the acidosis remains unclear. Postulated mechanisms for the acidosis have included the povidone-iodine itself (pH 2.43), bicarbonate consumption from the conversions of I_2 to NaI, or decreased renal elimination of H^+ as a consequence of iodine toxicity.[131] Metabolic acidosis associated with a high lactate level after iodine ingestion likely reflects tissue destruction.[43]

Electrolyte abnormalities may also occur following the absorption of iodine. A patient with decubitus ulcers who received prolonged wound care with povidone-iodine–soaked gauze developed metabolic acidosis, renal failure, hypernatremia, and hyperchloremia.[43] The hyperchloremia was thought to be caused by a spurious elevation of measured chloride ions as a consequence of iodine's interference with the chloride assay. This interference occurs on the Technicon STAT/ION autoanalyzer, but does not occur when the silver halide precipitation assay is used.[43] Spurious hyperchloremia from iodine (or iodide) may result in the calculation of a low or negative anion gap (Chap. 24).[26,49]

Other problems associated with topical absorption of iodine-containing preparations include hypothyroidism (particularly in neonates),[26,155] hyperthyroidism, elevated liver enzymes, neutropenia, and hypoxemia.[43] Because of the lack of consistency between iodine levels and symptomatology, and because many of these patients had significant secondary medical problems that may have accounted for their symptoms, the exact relationship between iodine absorption and the development of a specific clinical syndrome remains speculative. However, a recent clinical controlled trial that compared preterm infants exposed to either topical iodinated antiseptic agents or to chlorhexidine-containing antiseptics showed that the infants exposed to topical iodine–containing antiseptics were more likely to have higher thyrotropin levels and elevated urine iodine levels than was the chlorhexidine group.[101] Contact dermatitis can result from repetitive applications of iodophors.[108] A fatal case of exfoliative dermatitis from repeated local applications of tincture of iodine has also been described.[148]

The patient who ingests an iodine preparation requires expeditious evaluation, stabilization, and decontamination. Careful nasogastric aspiration and lavage may be performed to limit the caustic effect of the iodine if signs of perforation are absent. Irrigation with a starch solution will convert iodine to the much less toxic iodide, and, in the process, turn the gastric effluent dark blue-purple. This change in color may serve as a useful guide in determining when lavage can be terminated. If starch is not available, milk may be a useful alternative. Instillation of 100 mL of a solution of 1–3% sodium thiosulfate may also convert any remaining iodine to iodide. Activated charcoal binds iodine and may be useful.[42] Whether any one of these suggested agents offers a distinct advantage over the others is not studied. Minimal GI absorption of iodine occurs because of its conversion to iodide in the GI tract.[33] Early endoscopy may help assess the extent of the gastrointestinal injury. Judicious use of corticosteroids for circumferential second-degree burn injuries may be helpful in preventing stricture formation (Chap. 87).

Most patients with iodophor ingestion require only supportive management. The use of starch or sodium thiosulfate may be considered in symptomatic patients. Endoscopy is recommended in patients with persistent symptoms.

IODIDES

Iodide, as noted, refers to the reduced form of iodine, I^-. Iodide is most commonly found in the salts, potassium iodide and sodium iodide. Potassium iodide is used as an expectorant and in the treatment of hyperthyroidism and radiation exposure. Saturated solution of potassium iodide (SSKI), containing 1 g/mL, is an example of a potassium iodide preparation. Sodium iodide is found as a dietary supplement in iodized table salt. Although iodides by themselves are not used as antiseptics, they are discussed in this section because iodine-containing antiseptic compounds may consist of a mixture of molecular iodine and an iodide salt. Lugol's iodine solution, for instance, consists of 5% iodine and 10% potassium iodide. Tincture of iodine consists of 2% iodine, 2.4% sodium iodide, 47% alcohol, and water. Iodine is much more toxic than iodide because of its propensity to cause significant local tissue injury. Because iodide is not caustic, treatment of iodine ingestions includes conversion of iodine to the less toxic iodide.

The organic iodides are another group of iodine-containing compounds. Radiologic contrast agents such as diatrizoate meglumine (Hypaque; 282 mg I_2/mL) are examples of commonly used organic iodides. Other iodine-containing compounds include the antidysrhythmic amiodarone (75 mg in a 200 mg tablet) and the antifungal Vioform (clioquinol; 12 mg in 1 gm of cream). Isotopes of iodine are another group of agents that contain iodine. The most commonly used isotope, I^{131}, is employed in the diagnosis of thyroid disorders and treatment of hyperthyroidism.

Iodism, first described in 1902, refers to a variety of reactions to iodides. The term has been used to describe both dose-dependent reactions and hypersensitivity reactions ("iodine idiosyncrasy").[24,78] The duration of exposure is most often chronic, but iodism may occur following acute exposures.

The most noticeable manifestations of chronic dose-dependent iodide toxicity include skin eruptions (ioderma), salivary gland swelling, and goiter. Acute parotitis may be the most recognizable finding; hence, this syndrome is referred to as "iodide mumps."[24,62] Salivary swelling is thought to be caused by ductal inflammation and blockage. Significant salivary gland enlargement may result in dysphagia and possible airway obstruction.[18] Other manifestations of iodism include metallic taste, gingivitis, sialorrhea, bronchorrhea, coryza, nausea, and vomiting.[18,78] Drug-induced fever is also attributed to iodide administration.[171] Pure iodide ingestions do not produce GI injuries.

Hypersensitivity reactions from the ingestion of small therapeutic doses of iodides may also occur. Manifestations of these idiosyncratic reactions include eosinophilia, lymphadenopathy, arthralgias, submucosal hemorrhages, arthritis, diverse cutaneous manifestations, hematuria, proteinuria, fever, and rapid onset of acute painful salivary gland swelling (sialoadenitis).[24,62,180] A periarteritis nodosa type of reaction from iodide exposure is also described.[138]

Ioderma refers to the protean group of dermal lesions usually associated with chronic exposure to iodides. These skin eruptions are quite varied, ranging from pustular/bullous eruptions to generalized erythema and urticaria.[148] Although ioderma is usually related to iodide exposure, it is also reported to occur as a systemic manifestation of povidone-iodine exposure from wound irrigation.[19]

Subacute and chronic exposure to excess iodides are also implicated in a variety of thyroid disorders, including goiter,[184] thyrotoxicosis (Jod-Basedow phenomenon),[50] and myxedema.[116]

Acute exposure to iodide in patients with normal thyroid glands generally results in blockade of thyroid hormone production (Wolff-Chaikoff effect). This is the basis for the administration of SSKI following exposure to radioactive fallout. Acute overdose of iodide medications is rare and typically of limited clinical consequence. In one case, a patient inadvertently ingested 15 g of potassium iodide and developed myocardial irritability and face, neck, and mouth swelling within 12 hours of ingestion.[172] Subsequent recovery was uneventful.

Reactions to intravenous iodinated radiologic contrast agents are well known.[36] Anaphylactoid reactions are idiosyncratic in nature and not dose dependent. Salivary gland swelling is also described as a sequela to intravenous urography using these agents.[168] The use of iodides, such as radiologic contrast media in early pregnancy, is potentially teratogenic and may lead to cretinism.

Management of acute iodide ingestions is basically supportive. Activated charcoal may be considered in patients with large ingestions. Because absorbed iodide competes with chloride in the proximal tubule, sodium chloride diuresis may enhance the elimination of iodide. As a result of the conversion of iodine to iodide, patients treated for iodine ingestions may be at risk for subsequent iodide toxicity. Systemic corticosteroids have been used with success in the management of iodide-induced sialoadenitis[180] and ioderma.[5]

CHLORHEXIDINE

Chlorhexidine

Chlorhexidine is another commonly used antiseptic agent that is especially useful as a dental antiseptic. This cationic biguanide compound has been in use since the early 1950s. It is found in a variety of skin cleansers, usually as a 4% emulsion (eg, Hibiclens), and may also be found in mouthwash. Chlorhexidine is reported to have low toxicity.

Few cases of deliberate oral ingestion of chlorhexidine can be found in the literature. Symptoms are usually mild and gastrointestinal irritation is the most likely effect after oral ingestion.[27] Chlorhexidine has poor enteral absorption. In one case, ingestion of 150 mL of a 20% chlorhexidine gluconate solution resulted in oral cavity edema and significant irritant injury of the esophagus.[110] In the same case, liver function tests rose to 30 times normal on the fifth day after ingestion. Liver biopsy showed lobular necrosis and fatty degeneration. Subsequently, the liver function tests normalized. In another case, the ingestion of 30 mL of a 4% solution by an 89-year-old woman did not result in any GI injury.[47]

Intravenous administration of chlorhexidine is associated with hemolysis, although this may be caused by the hypotonicity of the injected solution.[29] Inhalation of vaporized chlorhexidine is reported to cause methemoglobinemia due to the conversion of chlorhexidine to *p*-chloraniline.[175] The rectal administration of 4% chlorhexidine resulted in one patient in acute ulcerative colitis.[63]

Topical absorption of chlorhexidine is negligible. Contact dermatitis is reported in up to 8% of patients who received repetitive topical applications of chlorhexidine.[64] More ominously, anaphylactic reactions, including shock, are associated with dermal application.[7,123] Eye exposure may result in corneal damage.[169]

Treatment guidelines for chlorhexidine exposure are similar to those for other potentially caustic agents. Patients with significant symptoms may require endoscopy, but the need for such extensive evaluation is quite uncommon.

THE ALCOHOLS

Isopropanol and ethanol are commonly used as skin antiseptics. Sold as rubbing alcohol, the standard concentration for these solutions is usually 70%. Their antiseptic action is thought to be a result of their ability to coagulate proteins. Isopropanol is slightly more germicidal than ethanol.[64] These agents have limited efficacy against viruses or spores. Isopropanol tends to be more irritating than ethanol and may cause more pronounced central nervous system depression.[178] The greater toxicity of isopropanol has caused some emergency departments to switch rubbing alcohol formulations from isopropanol to ethanol (Chaps. 64 and 66).

CHLORINE AND CHLOROPHORS

Chlorine, one of the first antiseptics, is still used in the treatment of the community water supply and in swimming pools. Chlorine is a potent pulmonary irritant and may cause severe bronchospasm and pulmonary edema. Chapter 95 further discusses chlorine.

Sodium hypochlorite, found in chlorine bleach (eg, Clorox) and Dakin solution, remains a commonly used disinfectant. First used in the late 1700s to bleach clothes, its utility arises from its oxidizing capability, measured as "available chlorine," and its ability to release hypochlorous acid slowly. It is used to clean blood spills and to sterilize certain medical instruments. Toxicity from hypochlorite is mainly a result of its irritant effects. The ingestion of large amounts of household liquid bleach (5% sodium hypochlorite) on rare occasions can result in esophageal burns with subsequent stricture formation.[51] In a cat model of bleach ingestion, a high incidence of mucosal injury and stricture formation was noted.[181] However, the vast majority of household bleach ingestions in humans do not cause significant GI injuries.[94,132] Accordingly, aggressive evaluation with endoscopy is usually not warranted when assessing most patients with household liquid bleach ingestions. The ingestion of a more concentrated "industrial strength" bleach preparation increases the likelihood of local tissue injury and should be managed accordingly (Chap. 87).

Although direct inhalation of sodium hypochlorite vapors is usually not problematic, the erroneous mixing of sodium hypochlorite bleach with ammonia or acids can lead to the production of toxic vapors resulting in significant pulmonary symptomatology. Mixing sodium hypochlorite (NaOCl) with ammonium hydroxide (NH$_3$OH) produces chloramine; mixing sodium hypochlorite with acid-containing toilet bowl cleaners (eg, hydrochloric acid, phosphoric acid) produces chlorine. When chloramine comes in contact with the moist mucous membranes of the pulmonary tree, hypochlorous acid (HOCl) and oxygen free radicals are produced. Hypochlorous acid subsequently decomposes to hydrochloric acid and oxygen. Chlorine contact with moist airway tissues also produces hypochlorous acid, hydrochloric acid, and oxygen (Chap. 95).

QUATERNARY AMMONIUM COMPOUNDS

Quaternary ammonium compounds are a type of cationic surfactant (surface-active agent) used as disinfectants, detergents, and sanitizers. Chemically, the quaternary ammonium compounds are synthetic derivatives of ammonium chloride. They are structurally similar to other quaternary ammonium derivatives, such as the cholinesterase inhibitors (eg, neostigmine) and the neuromuscular blockers (eg, succinylcholine). Other cationic surfactants include the pyridinium compounds and the quinolinium compounds. Benzalkonium chloride (Zephiran) was one of the most commonly employed quaternary ammonium compounds in the past, but with the development of many newer quaternary ammonium compounds over the years, its use has substantially decreased. However, nebulized solutions used for the treatment of asthma, including albuterol and ipratropium bromide, may contain small amounts of benzalkonium chloride. Newer quaternary ammonium compounds are currently used as hospital disinfectants, including Coverage 256, which contains 6% alkyl dimethyl ammonium chloride and 5% octyldecyldimethyl ammonium chloride, and Render, which contains 5% alkyl dimethyl benzyl ammonium chloride.

Quaternary ammonium compounds generally have a low order of toxicity as compared to phenol or formaldehyde. Of the infrequent complications that are described, most result from ingestions of benzalkonium chloride. Complications of these ingestions include burns to the mouth and esophagus, CNS depression, elevated liver enzymes, metabolic acidosis, and hypotension.[2,174,183] Muscle paralysis is also occasionally described as a complication of these ingestions and is presumably a result of cholinesterase inhibition at the neuromuscular junction.[58] Chronic inhalational exposure is associated with occupational asthma.[17] Topical use of the quaternary ammonium compounds can cause contact dermatitis.[151] Few data are available on the toxicity of the newer quaternary ammonium compound ingestions.

Ingestions of other cationic surface-active agents, such as the pyridinium agent cetrimonium bromide (Cetrimide), are associated with caustic burns to the mouth, lips, and tongue.[117] Peritoneal irrigation with cetrimonium bromide can produce metabolic abnormalities, hypotension, and methemoglobinemia.[9,114]

Treatment recommendations following the ingestion of the quaternary ammonium compounds and other cationic surface-active agents are similar to those for other potentially caustic ingestions. Emergency department evaluation should be considered for all patients who ingest more than a taste of a dilute (less than 1%) solution. Therapy is mainly supportive. Endoscopy may be warranted if symptoms suggest the possibility of a burn injury.

POTASSIUM PERMANGANATE

Potassium permanganate (KMnO$_4$) is a violet water-soluble compound that is usually sold as crystals or tablets. Historically, it was used as an abortifacient, urethral irrigant, lavage fluid for alkaloid poisoning, and snakebite remedy. Currently, potassium permanganate is most often used a dermal antiseptic, particularly for patients with eczema.

Potassium permanganate is a strong oxidizing agent and poisoning may result in local and systemic toxicity.[157] Upon contact with mucous membranes, potassium permanganate reacts with water to form manganese dioxide, potassium hydroxide, and molecular oxygen. Local tissue injury is the result of contact with the nascent oxygen, as well as the caustic effect of potassium hydroxide. A brown-black staining of the tissues occurs from the manganese dioxide.

Following ingestion, initial symptoms include nausea and vomiting. Laryngeal edema and ulceration of the mouth, esophagus, and, to a lesser extent, the stomach may result from the caustic effects. Fatal gastrointestinal perforation and hemorrhage may occur.[113,125] Esophageal strictures and pyloric stenosis may be late complications.

Although potassium permanganate is not well absorbed from the GI tract, systemic absorption may occur, resulting in life-threatening toxicity. Systemic effects include hepatotoxicity, renal damage, methemoglobinemia, hemolysis, hemorrhagic pancreatitis, acute respiratory distress syndrome, disseminated intravascular coagulation, and cardiovascular collapse.[107,113,125] Elevation in blood or serum manganese concentration may also occur, confirming systemic absorption (normal levels: blood manganese 3.9–15.0 µg/L, serum manganese 0.9–2.9 µg/L).

Chronic ingestion of potassium permanganate may result in classic manganese poisoning (manganism). A 66-year-old man who mistakenly ingested 10 g of potassium permanganate over a 4-week period (because of medication mislabeling) developed impaired concentration and autonomic and visual symptoms. He also developed abdominal pain, gastric ulceration, and alopecia. Serum manganese was elevated. Nine months later, the patient's neurologic examination displayed extrapyramidal signs consistent with parkinsonism (Chap. 19).[76]

Since the consequential effects of KMnO₄ ingestion are due to its liberation of strong alkalis, the initial treatment of such a patient should include assessment for evidence of airway compromise. For similar reasons, syrup of ipecac–induced emesis is not recommended. Dilution with milk or water may be useful. The use of neutralizing agents, such as egg whites or sodium hypochlorite, is reported but unproved.[157] The efficacy of activated charcoal is unknown.

Patients with symptoms consistent with caustic injury should undergo early endoscopy. Corticosteroid agents along with antibiotics may be warranted in some cases, especially if laryngeal edema is present. Liver enzymes, BUN, creatinine, amylase, serum manganese, and methemoglobin levels should be performed when systemic toxicity is suspected. Methemoglobinemia should be treated with methylene blue. Dermal irrigation with dilute oxalic acid may be successful in removing cutaneous staining.[157]

HYDROGEN PEROXIDE

Hydrogen peroxide, an oxidizing agent with weak antiseptic properties, has been used for many years as an antiseptic and a disinfectant. This agent is generally available in two strengths: dilute hydrogen peroxide, with a concentration of 3–9% by weight (usually 3%), sold for home use; and concentrated hydrogen peroxide, with a concentration greater than 10%, used primarily for industrial purposes. Commercial-strength hydrogen peroxide is most commonly found as a 27.5–70% solution. Home uses for dilute hydrogen peroxide include ear cerumen removal, mouth gargle, vaginal douche, enema, and hair bleaching. Dilute hydrogen peroxide is also sometimes used as a veterinary emetic. Commercial

uses of the more concentrated solutions include bleaching and cleansing textiles and wool, and producing foam rubber and rocket fuel. In the last few years, 35% hydrogen peroxide became available to the general public in health food stores and is sold as "hyperoxygenation therapy." This potentially dangerous therapy is touted as a treatment for a variety of conditions, including AIDS and cancer.[79]

Hydrogen peroxide has two main mechanisms of toxicity: local tissue injury and gas formation. The extent of local tissue injury is determined by the strength of the hydrogen peroxide. Dilute hydrogen peroxide is an irritant and concentrated hydrogen peroxide is a caustic. Gas formation results when hydrogen peroxide interacts with tissue catalase, liberating molecular oxygen and water. While 1 mL of 3% hydrogen peroxide liberates 10 mL of oxygen at standard temperature and pressure, 1 mL of the more concentrated 35% hydrogen peroxide liberates more than 100 mL of oxygen. Gas formation can result in life-threatening embolization. Gas embolization may be due to dissection of gas under pressure into the tissues or may result from liberation of gas in the tissue or blood following absorption. The use of hydrogen peroxide in closed spaces, such as operative wounds, or its use under pressure during wound irrigation, increases the likelihood of embolization.

Symptoms consistent with sudden oxygen embolization include rapid deterioration in mental status, cyanosis, acute respiratory failure, seizures, and ischemic ECG changes.[52] A 2-year-old boy died after ingesting 4–6 oz (120–180 mL) of 35% hydrogen peroxide.[31] Antemortem chest radiograph showed gas in the right ventricle, mediastinum, and portal venous system. Portal vein gas is also a prominent feature in other cases.[106] Arterialization of gas oxygen embolization may result in cerebral infarction.[150] Bilateral hemispheric infarctions detected by MRI imaging may occur after ingestion of concentrated hydrogen peroxide.[80]

The combination of local tissue injury and gas formation from the ingestion of concentrated hydrogen peroxide may cause GI disturbances, such as vomiting, hematemesis, abdominal pain, and abdominal bloating.[79,106] Endoscopy may show significant gastric mucosal erosions; esophageal injury is usually minimal. Airway compromise manifested by stridor, drooling, apneic episodes, and radiographic evidence of subepiglottic narrowing may occur.[44] Death from intravenous injection of 35% hydrogen peroxide is also reported.[98]

Clinical sequelae from the ingestion of dilute hydrogen peroxide are usually much more benign.[44,70] Nausea and vomiting are the most common symptoms.[44] A whitish discoloration may be noted in the oral cavity. Gastrointestinal injury is usually limited to superficial mucosal irritation, but multiple gastric and duodenal ulcers, accompanied by hematemesis, are reported.[70] Portal venous gas embolization may occur as a result of the ingestion of 3% hydrogen peroxide.[32,137]

The use of 3% hydrogen peroxide for wound irrigation may result in significant complications. Extensive subcutaneous emphysema occurred after a dog bite to a human's face was irrigated under pressure with 60 mL of 3% hydrogen peroxide.[154] Systemic oxygen embolism, causing hypotension, ischemic ECG changes, and coma, resulted from the intraoperative irrigation of an infected herniorrhaphy wound.[12] Gas embolism, resulting in intestinal gangrene, was reported to occur following colonic lavage with 1% hydrogen peroxide during surgical treatment of meconium ileus.[149] Multiple cases of acute colitis are reported as a complication of administering 3% hydrogen peroxide enemas.[112] The use of 3%

hydrogen peroxide as a mouth rinse is associated with the development of oral ulcerations.[139] Ocular exposures may result in conjunctival injection, burning pain, and blurry vision.[44]

A careful examination should be performed to detect any evidence of gas formation. A chest radiograph may reveal gas in the cardiac chambers, mediastinum, or pleural space. An abdominal radiograph may show gas in the GI tract or portal system and define the extent of bowel distension. MRI and computed tomography (CT) scan may be useful to detect brain lesions secondary to gas embolism.[6,80] Endoscopic evaluation may be necessary in patients who ingest concentrated hydrogen peroxide to determine the extent of burn injury.

The treatment of patients with hydrogen peroxide ingestions depends to a large degree on whether the patient has ingested a dilute or concentrated solution. Those with ingestions of concentrated solutions require expeditious evaluation. Dilution with milk or water, although unstudied, is unlikely to be helpful. Careful nasogastric aspiration of hydrogen peroxide may be helpful if the patient presents immediately after ingestion. Syrup of ipecac–induced emesis is contraindicated and activated charcoal offers no antidotal benefit. Patients with abdominal distension from gas formation should be treated with nasogastric suctioning. Those with clinical or radiographic evidence of gas in the heart should be placed in the Trendelenburg position to prevent gas from blocking the right ventricular outflow tract. Careful aspiration of intracardiac air through a central venous line may be attempted in patients in extremis.[31] Although randomized controlled trials are not available, case reports suggest that hyperbaric therapy may be useful in cases of life-threatening gas embolization after hydrogen peroxide ingestion.[106,118] Asymptomatic patients who unintentionally ingest small amounts of 3% hydrogen peroxide can be safely watched at home.

BORIC ACID

Boric acid is an odorless, transparent crystal although it is most commonly available as a finely ground white powder. It is also commonly found as a 2.5–5% aqueous solution. Boric acid (H_3PO_3), prepared from borax (sodium borate; $Na_2B_4O_7 \cdot 10\,H_2O$), was first used as an antiseptic agent by Lister in the late 19th century. Although used extensively over the years for antisepsis and irrigation, boric acid is only weakly bacteriostatic. As a result of its germicidal limitations and its inherent toxicity, boric acid is obsolete in modern antiseptic therapy. Nonetheless, it continues to be used as an antimicrobial to treat such conditions as vulvovaginal candidiasis.[176] Boric acid is also employed in the treatment of cockroach infestation and as a soap, contact lens solution, toothpaste, and food preservative.

Boric acid is readily absorbed through the GI tract, wounds, abraded skin, and serous cavities. Absorption does not occur through intact skin. Boric acid is predominantly eliminated unchanged by the kidney. Small amounts are also excreted into sweat, saliva, and feces.[53] Boric acid is concentrated in the brain and liver.

The exact mechanism of action of boric acid's toxicity remains unclear. Although it is an inorganic acid, it does not behave as a caustic agent. Local effects are limited to tissue irritation.

Over the years, boric acid has developed a reputation as an exceptionally potent toxin. This reputation was derived in great part from a series of reports involving neonatal exposures to boric acid resulting in high morbidity and mortality. Life-threatening toxicity resulted from the repetitive topical application of boric acid for the treatment of diaper rash or the use of infant formulas unintentionally contaminated with boric acid.[53,185] Fatality rates greater than 50% were reported in some series.[185] Although infants appear to be the most sensitive to the toxic effects of boric acid, many cases of significant adult toxicity are also reported. These cases date predominantly from the time when boric acid was widely used as an irrigant. Routes of exposure to boric acid, resulting in fatalities, include wound irrigation, pleural irrigation, rectal washing, bladder irrigation, and vaginal packing.[130,173]

Classic boric acid poisoning, as described in these reports, usually involved multiple exposures over a period of days. Gastrointestinal, dermal, CNS, and renal manifestations predominate. The initial symptoms—nausea, vomiting, diarrhea, and occasionally crampy abdominal pain—may be confused with an acute gastroenteritis. At times, the emesis and diarrhea are greenish blue.[185] Following the onset of GI symptoms, the majority of patients develop a characteristic intense generalized erythroderma.[185] This rash, described as producing a "boiled lobster" appearance, may appear indistinguishable from toxic epidermal necrolysis or staphylococcal scalded skin syndrome in the neonate.[144] The rash may be especially noticeable on the palms, soles, and buttocks.[53] Typically, extensive desquamation takes place within 1–2 days. At times, prominent mucous membrane involvement of the oral cavity and conjunctivae is also apparent.[185] At about the time of the development of the erythroderma, patients, particularly young infants, may develop prominent signs of CNS irritability, resembling meningeal irritation. Seizures, delirium, and coma can occur.[53] Renal injury is common, a result of the renal elimination of this compound and prerenal azotemia from GI losses.[53] Other complications of boric acid poisoning include hepatic injury, hyperthermia, and cardiovascular collapse. The abandonment of boric acid as an irrigant and particularly its removal from the nursery setting have led to a marked decrease in the incidence of significant boric acid poisoning.

Two retrospective studies on boric acid ingestions suggest that a single acute ingestion of boric acid is generally quite benign.[100,103] In these studies, 79–88% of patients remained asymptomatic. Symptoms, when present, primarily consist of GI irritative symptoms, such as nausea and vomiting. None of the 1184 patients in these two studies manifested the generalized erythroderma so commonly described in previous reports. Central nervous system manifestations of acute overdose were infrequent and limited to occasional lethargy and headache. Renal toxicity did not occur following single acute ingestions.

Several reports suggest, however, that significant toxicity from massive acute ingestion of boric acid can occur. Fatality resulted from a single ingestion of two cups (280 g) of boric acid crystals by a 45-year-old man.[140] Symptoms on presentation (two days after ingestion) included nausea, vomiting, green diarrhea, lethargy, hypotension, renal failure, and a prominent "boiled lobster" rash on his trunk and extremities. In another case, the ingestion of 30 g of boric acid by a 77-year-old man resulted in similar symptoms and death 63 hours postingestion, despite hemodialysis.[81]

Long-term chronic exposure to boric acid results in alopecia in adults and seizures in children.[56,127,166] A 32-year-old woman who chronically ingested mouthwash containing boric acid over a

7-month period developed progressive hair loss.[166] The chronic application of a borax and honey mixture to pacifiers resulted in the development of recurrent seizures in nine infants, which resolved after the mixture was withheld.[56,127]

The diagnoses of boric acid poisoning can be confirmed with the measurement of blood or serum boric acid levels (nl = 1.4 nmol/mL), but this test is not routinely available. Treatment of boric acid toxicity is mainly supportive. Activated charcoal is not recommended because of its relatively poor adsorptive capacity for boric acid.[42] In cases of massive oral overdose or renal failure, hemodialysis, or perhaps exchange transfusion in infants, may be helpful in shortening the half-life of boric acid.[103,170,185]

MERCURIALS

Both inorganic mercurials, such as mercury bichloride, and organic mercurials, such as merbromin (Mercurochrome) or thimerosal (Merthiolate), were used in the past as topical antiseptic agents. Thimerosal contains 49% mercury. Their relatively weak bacteriostatic properties, along with the many problems associated with mercury toxicity, significantly limit their usefulness (Chap. 81). Repeated application of topical mercurials may result in significant absorption and systemic toxicity.[119,141,] The use of high-dose hepatitis B immunoglobulin (HBIG) may cause mercury toxicity because of the use of thimerosal as a preservative in the HBIG preparation.[105] In one case, a 44-year-old male patient received 250 mL of HBIG (containing about 30 mg thimerosal) over 9 days following liver transplantation.[150] He developed speech difficulties, tremor, and chorea. His blood mercury level was 104 µg/L (normal <10µg/L). Increased mercury levels in both preterm and term infants, following immunizations with thimerosal-containing hepatitis B vaccine, have also generated much concern and led to the call to reduce or eliminate the mercury content of vaccines (Chaps. 56 and 81).[61,159]

CHLORATES

Sodium chlorate is a strong oxidizing agent. At one time, the chlorate salts, sodium chlorate and potassium chlorate, were used as medicinal agents to treat inflammatory and ulcerative lesions of the oral cavity and could be found in various mouthwash, toothpaste, and gargle preparations.[160] Although their use as local antiseptics is obsolete, chlorates are used as herbicides and in the manufacture of matches, explosives, and dyestuffs.[82] More recent cases of chlorate poisoning resulted from the ingestion of the sodium chlorate–containing weed killers, or dispensing errors that confused sodium chlorate with sodium sulfate or sodium chloride.[82,88] Sodium chlorate in the form of white crystals has also been mistaken for table sugar.[67] A case of significant toxicity from the inhalation of atomized chlorates is also reported.[82]

Sodium chlorate is rapidly absorbed from the GI tract and eliminated predominantly unchanged from the kidneys.[83] Its systemic effects are chiefly hematologic and renal. Chlorate's major mechanism of toxicity is its ability to oxidize hemoglobin and increase red blood cell membrane rigidity.[152] Consequently, significant methemoglobinemia and hemolytic anemia may result. Chlorates may also be directly toxic to the proximal renal tubule.[97] The hemolytic anemia and the resultant hemoglobinuria may secondarily cause disseminated intravascular coagulation and potentiate renal toxicity. The worsening renal function is especially problematic because of its adverse effect on chlorate elimination. The methemoglobinemia may be severe and cause significant hypoxic stress. Earlier reports suggested that methemoglobinemia was predominantly extracellular, occurring only after the development of significant hemolysis,[57] but subsequent reports suggest that methemoglobinemia may occur prior to hemolytic anemia.[121,163] Chlorates may also act locally as a GI irritant, and cause mild CNS depression after absorption.[58]

Clinical signs and symptoms of chlorate poisoning usually begin 1–4 hours after ingestion.[90] The earliest symptoms are GI, including nausea, vomiting, diarrhea, and crampy abdominal pain. Subsequently, the patient may exhibit cyanosis from the methemoglobinemia and black-brown urine from the hemoglobinuria. Anuria may ensue. Laboratory studies may show methemoglobinemia, anemia, Heinz bodies, ghost cells, fragmented spherocytes, decreased platelet count, and abnormal coagulation. Hyperkalemia may be particularly problematic if the patient ingests potassium chlorate preparations.[40]

Treatment of a patient with a significant chlorate ingestion should include gastric lavage and the use of activated charcoal.[67] It has been suggested that administration of sodium thiosulfate may inactivate the chlorate ion by reducing it to the chloride ion,[67] but an in vitro study did not confirm this hypothesis.[164] Although methylene blue may be used in the treatment of symptomatic methemoglobinemia in an attempt to reduce methemoglobin to hemoglobin, its efficacy in the treatment of chlorate-induced methemoglobinemia may be limited, as compared to its efficacy in the treatment of other oxidant-induced methemoglobinemias.[121,163] This may be a consequence of the inactivation by chlorates of glucose-6-phosphate dehydrogenase, an enzyme that is required for methylene blue's reduction of methemoglobin.[153] Exchange transfusion, peritoneal dialysis, and hemodialysis have all been advocated in the treatment of patients with severe chlorate poisoning.[121,163] Because the chlorate ion is easily dialyzable, hemodialysis (or peritoneal dialysis if hemodialysis is unavailable) is capable of removing this toxin, as well as treating any concomitant renal failure that may have developed.[82,90,97]

ETHYLENE OXIDE

Ethylene oxide

Ethylene oxide is a gas that is commonly used to sterilize heat-sensitive material in healthcare facilities. Unlike antiseptics and disinfectants, which generally do not exhibit full sporicidal activity, sterilants, such as ethylene oxide, inactivate all organisms. Ethylene oxide is also used in the synthesis of many chemicals, including ethylene glycol, surfactants, rocket propellants, and petroleum demulsifiers, and has been used as a pesticide fumigant. Chemically, ethylene oxide has a cyclic ester structure, known as an epoxide. It acts as an alkylating agent, reacting with most cellular components, including DNA and RNA.

Medical attention regarding ethylene oxide toxicity has centered on its mutagenic and possible carcinogenic effects.[95] Approximately 270,000 workers (including 96,000 hospital workers) in the United States are at risk for occupational exposure to ethylene oxide.[162] Retrospective studies suggest a possible excess incidence of leukemia and gastric cancer in ethylene oxide–exposed workers.[74,162] These studies are inconclusive, and the carcinogenicity of ethylene oxide remains subject to debate. It is also suggested that an increased incidence of spontaneous abortions may be associated with occupational exposure to ethylene oxide (Chap. 110).[68]

The acute toxicity of ethylene oxide is mainly a result of its irritant effects. Conjunctival, upper respiratory tract, GI, and dermal irritation may occur. Dermal burns from acute exposure to ethylene oxide are described. Acute exposure to a broken ethylene oxide ampule by a 43-year-old recovery room nurse resulted in nausea, lightheadedness, malaise, syncope, and recurrent seizures.[146] There were no long-term complications. In another case of acute exposure, coma was followed by an irreversible parkinsonism.[10]

Chronic exposure to ethylene oxide may cause motor and sensory neuropathies.[59,122]

Treatment for patients with ethylene oxide exposure is supportive.

GLUTARALDEHYDE

Glutaraldehyde

Glutaraldehyde is a liquid solution used in the cold sterilization of nonautoclavable endoscopic, surgical, and dental equipment. It is also employed as a tissue fixative, embalming fluid, preservative, and tanning agent, in radiographic solutions, and in the treatment of warts.[54] Glutaraldehyde is a dialdehyde with two active carbonyl groups. It kills all microorganisms, including viruses and spores. It is prepared as a 2% alkaline solution in 70% isopropanol (Cidex). Approximately 35,000 workers are occupationally exposed to glutaraldehyde (Chap. 110).[133]

Data on human toxicity from glutaraldehyde are limited. Clinical signs and symptoms are thought to be comparable to those of formaldehyde exposure. However, animal studies show that glutaraldehyde administered enterally or topically is less toxic than an equal amount of formaldehyde.[145]

No reported cases of deliberate or unintentional ingestion of glutaraldehyde are available. Glutaraldehyde is a mucosal irritant. Coryza, epistaxis, headache, asthma, chest tightness, palpitations, tachycardia, and nausea are all associated with glutaraldehyde vapor exposure.[15,34,120] Contact dermatitis and ocular inflammation may also occur.[37,54,85]

Preliminary animal evidence suggests that glutaraldehyde, like formaldehyde, may be a potent nasal carcinogen.[161] Additional research is needed in this controversial area. Treatment recommendations are similar to those for patients with formaldehyde exposure.

SUMMARY

A chemically diverse group of antiseptic, disinfectant, and sterilant agents have been reviewed. Many of the more toxic agents—such as iodine, phenol, and chlorates—are no longer commonly used as cleansing agents but have not disappeared and may still be available in some settings. Formaldehyde exposures, while also uncommon, can also cause significant problems. Frequently employed antiseptics, such as chlorhexidine, pHisoDerm, and many of the currently used quaternary ammonium compounds, have a relatively low degree of toxicity. Ingestions of the iodophors do not usually cause significant toxicity, but absorption through other routes may still produce significant adverse effects. Ingestions of hydrogen peroxide, particularly the more concentrated formulations, may be more problematic.

REFERENCES

1. Acheson ED, Gardner MJ, Pannett B, et al: Formaldehyde in the British chemical industry: An occupational cohort study. Lancet 1984;1:611–616.
2. Adelson L, Sunshine I: Fatal poisoning due to a cationic detergent of the quaternary ammonium compound type. Am J Clin Pathol 1952;22:656–661.
3. Albert RE, Sellakumar AR, Laskin S, et al: Gaseous formaldehyde and hydrogen chloride induction of nasal cancer in the rat. J Natl Cancer Inst 1982;68:597–603.
4. Allen RE, Thoshinsky MJ, Stallone RJ, Hunt TK: Corrosive injuries of the stomach. Arch Surg 1970;100:409–413.
5. Aquilina JT: Fungating ioderma treated with hydrocortisone. JAMA 1955;158:727–728.
6. Ashdown BC, Stricof DD, May M, Sherman SJ, Carmody RF: Hydrogen peroxide poisoning causing brain infarction: Neuroimaging findings. AJR Am J Roentgenol 1998;170:1653–1655.
7. Autegarden JE, Pecquet C, Huet S, Bayrou O, Leynadier F: Anaphylactic shock after application of chlorhexidine to unbroken skin. Contact Dermatitis 1999;40:215.
8. Baker EL, Landrigan PJ, Bertozzi PE, et al: Phenol poisoning due to contaminated drinking water. Arch Environ Health 1978;33:89–94.
9. Baraka A, Yamut F, Wakid N: Cetrimide-induced methaemoglobinemia after surgical excision of hydatid cyst. Lancet 1980;2:88–89.
10. Barbosa ER, Comerlatti LR, Haddad MS, Scaff M: Parkinsonism secondary to ethylene oxide exposure. Arq Neuropsiquiatr 1992;50:531–533.
11. Bartone NF, Grieco V, Herr BS: Corrosive gastritis due to ingestion of formaldehyde. JAMA 1968;203:50–51.
12. Bassan MM, Dudai M, Shalev O: Near-fatal systemic oxygen embolism due to wound irrigation with hydrogen peroxide. Postgrad Med J 1982;58:448–450.
13. Beall JR, Ulsamer AG: Formaldehyde and hepatotoxicity: A review. J Toxicol Environ Health 1984;13:1–21.
14. Bennett IL, James DF, Golden A: Severe acidosis due to phenol poisoning: Report of two cases. Ann Intern Med 1950;32:324–327.
15. Benson WG: Exposure to glutaraldehyde. J Soc Occup Med 1984;34:63–64.
16. Bentur Y, Shoshani O, Tabak A, et al: Prolonged elimination half-life of phenol after dermal exposure. J Toxicol Clin Toxicol 1998;36:707–711.
17. Bernstein JA, Stauder T, Bernstein DI, Bernstein IL: A combined respiratory and cutaneous hypersensitivity syndrome induced by work exposure to quaternary amines. J Allergy Clin Immunol 1994;94:257–259.

18. Bianco RP, Smith PJ, Keen RR, Jordan JE: Iodide intoxication: Report of a case. Oral Surg 1974;32:876–880.

19. Bishop ME, Garcia RL: Ioderma from wound irrigation with povidone-iodine. JAMA 1978;240:249–250.

20. Block SS: Definition of terms. In: Block SS, ed: Disinfection, Sterilization, and Preservation, 4th ed. Philadelphia, Lea & Febiger, 1991, pp. 18–25.

21. Breysse P, Couser WG, Alpers CE, et al: Membranous nephropathy and formaldehyde exposure. Ann Intern Med 1994;120:396–397.

22. Brown VK, Box VL, Simpson BJ: Decontamination procedures for skin exposed to phenolic substances. Arch Environ Health 1975; 30:1–6.

23. Burkhart KK, Kulig KW: Formate levels following a formalin ingestion. Vet Hum Toxicol 1990;32:135–137.

24. Carter JE: Iodide "mumps." N Engl J Med 1961;264:987–988.

25. Casteel SW, Vernon RJ, Bailey EM: Formaldehyde: Toxicology and hazards. Vet Hum Toxicol 1987;29:31–33.

26. Chabrolle JP, Rossier A: Goiter and hypothyroidism in the newborn after cutaneous absorption of iodine. Arch Dis Child 1978; 53:495–498.

27. Chan TY: Poisoning due to Savlon (cetrimide) liquid. Hum Exp Toxicol 1994;13:681–682.

28. Chan TYK, Lau MSW, Critchley JA: Serious complications associated with Dettol poisoning. Q J Med 1993;86:735–738.

29. Cheung J, O'Leary JJ: Allergic reaction to chlorhexidine in an anaesthetized patient. Anaesth Intensive Care 1985;13:429–439.

30. Chilcote R, Curley A, Loughlin HH, et al: Hexachlorophene storage in burn patients associated with encephalopathy. Pediatrics 1977; 59:457–459.

31. Christensen DW, Faught WE, Black RE, et al: Fatal oxygen embolization after hydrogen peroxide ingestion. Crit Care Med 1992; 20:543–544.

32. Cina SJ, Downs JC, Conradi SE: Hydrogen peroxide: A source of lethal oxygen embolism. Am J Forensic Med Pathol 1994;15:44–50.

33. Cohn BN: Absorption of compound solution of iodine from the gastrointestinal tract. Arch Intern Med 1932;49:950–956.

34. Connaughton P: Occupational exposure to glutaraldehyde associated with tachycardia and palpitations [letter]. Med J Aust 1993;159:567.

35. Conning DM, Hayes MJ: The dermal toxicity of phenol: An investigation of the most effective first-aid measures. Br J Ind Med 1970; 27:155–159.

36. Crocker D, Vandam LD: Untoward reactions to radiodiagnostic contrast media. Clin Pharmacol Ther 1963;4:654–662.

37. Dailey JR, Parnes RE, Aminlari A: Glutaraldehyde keratopathy. Am J Opthalmol 1993;115:256–258.

38. Dally KA, Hanrahan LP, Woodbury MA, Kanarek MS: Formaldehyde exposure in nonoccupational environments. Arch Environ Health 1981;36:277–284.

39. D'Auria J, Lipson S, Garfield JM: Fatal iodine toxicity following surgical débridement of a hip wound: Case report. J Trauma 1990; 30:353–355.

40. Davies P: Potassium-chlorate poisoning with oliguria. Lancet 1956; 1:612–613.

41. DeBono R, Laitung G: Phenolic household disinfectants—further precautions required. Burns 1997;23:182–185.

42. Decker WJ, Combs HF, Corby DG: Adsorption of drugs and poison by activated charcoal. Toxicol Appl Pharmacol 1968;13:454–460.

43. Dela Cruz F, Brown DH, Leikin JB, et al: Iodine absorption after topical administration. West J Med 1987;146:43–45.

44. Dickson KF, Caravati EM: Hydrogen peroxide exposure—325 exposures reported to a regional poison control center. J Toxicol Clin Toxicol 1994;32:705–714.

45. Dyck RF, Bear RA, Goldstein MB, Halperin ML: Iodine/iodide toxic reaction: Case report with emphasis on the nature of the metabolic acidosis. Can Med Assoc J 1979;120:704–706.

46. Eells JT, McMartin KE, Black K, et al: Formaldehyde poisoning: Rapid metabolism to formic acid. JAMA 1981;246:1237–1238.

47. Emerson D, Pierce C: A case of a single ingestion of 4% Hibiclens. Vet Hum Toxicol 1988;30:583.

48. Finkelstein R, Jacobi M: Fatal iodine poisoning: A clinicopathologic and experimental study. Ann Intern Med 1937;10:1283–1296.

49. Fischman RA, Fairclough GF, Cheigh JS: Iodide and negative anion gap. N Engl J Med 1978;298:1035–1036.

50. Fradkin JE, Wolff J: Iodide-induced thyrotoxicosis. Medicine (Baltimore) 1983;62:1–20.

51. French RJ, Tabb HG, Rutledge LJ: Esophageal stenosis produced by ingestion of bleach: Report of two cases. South Med J 1970;63: 1140–1144.

52. Giberson TP, Kern JD, Pettigrew DW, et al: Near-fatal hydrogen peroxide ingestion. Ann Emerg Med 1989;18:778–779.

53. Goldbloom RB, Goldbloom A: Boric acid poisoning: A report of four cases and a review of 109 cases from the world literature. J Pediatr 1953;43:631–643.

54. Goncalo S, Brandao M, Pecegueiro M, et al: Occupational contact dermatitis to glutaraldehyde. Contact Dermatitis 1984;10:183–184.

55. Goodman L, Geiger AJ: Therapy in carbolic acid poisoning: With special reference to the use of oil antidotes. Am J Med Sci 1935;190: 206–219.

56. Gordon AS, Prichard JS, Freedman MH: Seizure disorders and anemia associated with chronic borax intoxication. Can Med Assoc J 1973;108:719–724.

57. Gordon S, Brown JA: Potassium chlorate poisoning: Report of a case. Lancet 1947;2:503–504.

58. Gosselin RE, Smith RP, Hodge HC: Clinical Toxicology of Commercial Products, 5th ed. Baltimore, Williams & Wilkins, 1984.

59. Gross JA, Haas ML, Swift TR: Ethylene oxide neurotoxicity: Report of four cases and review of the literature. Neurology 1979;29: 978–983.

60. Haddad LM, Dimond KA, Schweistris JE: Phenol poisoning. JACEP 1979;8:267–269.

61. Halsey NA: Limiting infant exposure to thimerosal in vaccines and other sources of mercury. JAMA 1999;282:1763–1766.

62. Harden RM: Submandibular adenitis due to iodide administration. Br Med J 1968;1:160–161.

63. Hardin RD, Tedesco FJ: Colitis after Hibiclens enema. J Clin Gastroenterol 1986;8:572–575.

64. Harvey SC: Antiseptics and disinfectants; fungicides; ectoparasiticides. In: Gilman AG, Rall TW, Nies AS, Taylor P, eds: Goodman and Gilman's The Pharmacological Basis of Therapeutics, 7th ed. New York, Pergamon Press, 1985, pp. 959–979.

65. Hashimoto T, Iida H, Dohi S: Marked increases of aminotransferase levels after cresol ingestion. Am J Emerg Med 1998;16:667–668.

66. Hawley CK, Harsch HH: Gastric outlet obstruction as a late complication of formaldehyde ingestion: A case report. Am J Gastroenterol 1999;94:2289–2291.

67. Helliwell M, Nunn J: Mortality in sodium chlorate poisoning. Br Med J 1979;1:1119.

68. Hemminki K, Mutanen P, Saloniemi I, et al: Spontaneous abortions in hospital staff engaged in sterilizing instruments with chemical agents. Br Med J 1982;285:1461–1463.

69. Hendrick DJ, Land DJ: Occupational formalin asthma. Br J Ind Med 1977;34:11–18.

70. Henry MC, Wheeler J, Mofenson HC, et al: Hydrogen peroxide 3% exposures. J Toxicol Clin Toxicol 1996;34:323–327.

71. Herskowitz J, Rosman NP: Acute hexachlorophene poisoning by mouth in a neonate. J Pediatr 1979;94:495–496.

72. Hilbert G, Gruson D, Bedry R, Cardinaud JP: Circulatory shock in the course of fatal poisoning by ingestion of formalin. Intensive Care Med 1997;23:708.

73. Hodge GE, Scharfe EE: Stricture of the esophagus. Can Med Assoc J 1937;37:541–547.

74. Hogstedt C, Aringer L, Gustavsson A: Epidemiologic support for ethylene oxide as a cancer-causing agent. JAMA 1986;255: 1575–1578.

75. Holness DL, Nethercott JR: Health status of funeral service workers exposed to formaldehyde. Arch Environ Health 1989;44:222–228.

76. Holzgraefe M, Poser W, Kijewski H, Beuche W: Chronic enteral poisoning cause by potassium permanganate. J Toxicol Clin Toxicol 1986;24:235–244.

77. Horch R, Spilker G, Stork GB: Phenol burns and intoxications. Burns 1994;20:45–50.

78. Horn B, Kabins SA: Iodide fever. Am J Med Sci 1972;64:467–471.

79. Humberston CL, Dean BS, Krenzelok EP: Ingestions of 35% hydrogen peroxide. J Toxicol Clin Toxicol 1990;28:95–100.

80. Ijichi T, Itoh T, Sakai K, et al: Multiple brain gas embolism after ingestion of concentrated hydrogen peroxide. Neurology 1997;48:277–279.

81. Ishii Y, Fujizuka N, Takahashi T, et al: A fatal case of acute boric acid poisoning. J Toxicol Clin Toxicol 1993;31:345–352.

82. Jackson RC, Elder WJ, McDonnell H: Sodium-chlorate poisoning complicated by acute renal failure. Lancet 1961;2:1381–1383.

83. Jansen H, Zeldenrust J: Homicidal chronic sodium chlorate poisoning. Forensic Sci 1972;1:103–105.

84. Jarvis SN, Straube RC, Williams AL, Bartlett CL: Illness associated with contamination of drinking water supplies with phenol. Br Med J 1985;290:1800–1802.

85. Jordan WP, Dahl MV, Albert HL: Contact dermatitis from glutaraldehyde. Arch Dermatol 1972;105:94–95.

86. Kamijo Y, Soma K, Fukuda M, et al: Rabbit syndrome following phenol ingestion. J Toxicol Clin Toxicol 1999;37:509–511.

87. Kilburn KH: Neurobehavioral impairment and seizures from formaldehyde. Arch Environ Health 1994;49:37–44.

88. Klendshoj NC, Burke WJ, Anthone R, Anthone S: Chlorate poisoning. JAMA 1962;180:1133–1134.

89. Kline BS: Formaldehyde poisoning. Arch Intern Med 1925;36:220–228.

90. Knight RK, Trounce JR, Cameron JS: Suicidal chlorate poisoning treated with peritoneal dialysis. Br Med J 1967;3:601–602.

91. Koppel C, Baudisch H, Schneider V, Ibe K: Suicidal ingestion of formalin with fatal complications. Intensive Care Med 1990;16: 212–214.

92. Kurt TL, Morgan ML, Hnilica V, et al: Fatal iatrogenic iodine toxicity in a 9-week old infant. J Toxicol Clin Toxicol 1996;34:231–234.

93. Lahoud CA, March JA, Proctor DD: Campho-Phenique ingestion: An intentional overdose. South Med J 1997;90:647–648.

94. Landau G, Saunders WH: The effect of chlorine bleach on the esophagus. Arch Otolaryngol 1964;80:174–176.

95. Landrigan PJ, Meinhardt TJ, Gordon J, et al: Ethylene oxide: An overview of toxicologic and epidemiologic research. Am J Ind Med 1984;6:103–115.

96. Lavelle KJ, Doedens DJ, Kleit SA, Forney RB: Iodine absorption in burn patients treated topically with povidone-iodine. Clin Pharmacol Ther 1975;17:355–362.

97. Lee DB, Brown DL, Baker LR, et al: Haematological complications of chlorate poisoning. Br Med J 1970;2:31–32.

98. Leiken J, Sing K, Woods K: Fatality from intravenous use of hydrogen peroxide for home "superoxygenation therapy" [abstract]. Vet Hum Toxicol 1993;35;342.

99. Lewin JF, Cleary WT: An accidental death caused by the absorption of phenol through skin: A case report. Forensic Sci Int 1982;19:177–179.

100. Linden CH, Hall AH, Kulig KW, Rumack BH: Acute ingestions of boric acid. J Toxicol Clin Toxicol 1986;24:269–279.

101. Linder N, Davidovitch N, Reichman B: Topical iodine-containing antiseptics and subclinical hypothyroidism in preterm infants. J Pediatr 1997;131:434–439.

102. Litovitz TL, Holm KC, Bailey KM, et al: 1991 Annual report of the American Association of Poison Control Centers national data collection system. Am J Emerg Med 1992;10:452–505.

103. Litovitz TL, Klein-Schwartz W, Oderda GM, Schmitz BF: Clinical manifestations of toxicity in a series of 784 boric acid ingestions. Am J Emerg Med 1988;6:209–213.

104. Loomis TA: Formaldehyde toxicity. Arch Pathol Lab Med 1979;103:321–324.

105. Lowell JA, Burgess S, Shenoy S, et al: Mercury poisoning associated with hepatitis-B immunoglobulin [letter]. Lancet 1996; 347:480.

106. Luu TA, Kelley MT, Strauch JA, Avradopoulos K: Portal vein gas embolism from hydrogen peroxide ingestion. Ann Emerg Med 1992; 21:1391–1393.

107. Mahomedy MC, Mahomedy YH, Canham PA, et al: Methemoglobinemia following treatment dispensed by witch doctors: Two cases of potassium permanganate poisoning. Anesthesia 1975;30:190–193.

108. Marks JG: Allergic contact dermatitis to povidone-iodine. J Am Acad Dermatol 1982;6:473–475.

109. Martinez AJ, Boehm V, Hadfield MG: Acute hexachlorophene encephalopathy: Cliniconeuropathological correlation. Acta Neuropathol 1974;28:93–103.

110. Massano G, Ciocatto E, Rosabianca C, et al: Striking aminotransferase rise after chlorhexidine self-poisoning [letter]. Lancet 1982; 1:289.

111. Merliss RR: Phenol marasmus. J Occup Med 1972;14:55–56.

112. Meyer CT, Brand M, DeLuca VA, Spiro HM: Hydrogen peroxide colitis: A report of three patients. J Clin Gastroenterol 1981;3:31–35.

113. Middleton SI, Jacyna M, McClaren D, et al: Hemorrhagic pancreatitis—A cause of death in severe potassium permanganate poisoning. Postgrad Med J 1990;66:657–658.

114. Momblano P, Pradere B, Jarrige N, et al: Metabolic acidosis induced by cetrimonium bromide. Lancet 1984;2:1045.

115. Moore M: The ingestion of iodine as a method of attempted suicide. N Engl J Med 1938;219:383–388.

116. Morgans ME, Trotter WR: Two cases of myxedema attributed to iodide administration. Lancet 1953;2:1335–1337.

117. Mucklow ES: Accidental feeding of a dilute antiseptic solution (chlorhexidine 0.05% with cetrimide 1%) to five babies. Hum Toxicol 1988;7:567–569.

118. Mullins ME, Beltran JT: Acute cerebral gas embolism from hydrogen peroxide ingestion successfully treated with hyperbaric oxygen. J Toxicol Clin Toxicol 1998;36:253–256.

119. Mullins ME, Horowitz BZ: Iatrogenic neonatal mercury poisoning from Mercurochrome treatment of a large omphalocele. Clin Pediatr 1999;38:111–112.

120. Norback D: Skin and respiratory symptoms from exposure to alkaline glutaraldehyde in medical services. Scand J Work Environ Health 1988;14:366–371.

121. O'Grady J, Jarecsni E: Sodium chlorate poisoning. Br J Clin Pract 1971;25:38–39.

122. Ohnishi A, Murai Y: Polyneuropathy due to ethylene oxide, propylene oxide, and butylene oxide. Environ Res 1993;60:242–247.

123. Okano M, Nomura M, Hata S, et al: Anaphylactic symptoms due to chlorhexidine gluconate. Arch Dermatol 1989;125:50–52.

124. Olsen JH, Dossing M: Formaldehyde induced symptoms in day care centers. Am Ind Hyg Assoc J 1982;43:366–370.

125. Ong KL, Tan TH, Cheung WL: Potassium permanganate poisoning—A rare cause of fatal self-poisoning. J Accid Emerg Med 1997; 14:43–45.

126. Orringer EP, Mattern WD: Formaldehyde-induced hemolysis during chronic hemodialysis. N Engl J Med 1976;294:1416–1420.

127. O'Sullivan K, Taylor M: Chronic boric acid poisoning in infants. Arch Dis Child 1983;58:737–749.

128. Partanen T, Kauppinen T, Nurminen M, et al: Formaldehyde exposure and respiratory and related cancer. Scand J Work Environ Health 1985;11:409–415.

129. Pennington JA: A review of iodine toxicity reports. J Am Diet Assoc 1990;90:1571–1581.

130. Pfeiffer CC, Hallman LF, Gersh I: Boric acid ointment: A study of possible intoxication in the treatment of burns. JAMA 1945;128:266–273.

131. Pietsch J, Meakins JL: Complications of povidone-iodine absorption in topically treated burn patients. Lancet 1976;1:280–282.

132. Pike DG, Peabody JW, Davis EW, Lyons WS: A reevaluation of the dangers of Clorox ingestion. J Pediatr 1963;63:303–305.

133. Pinnas JL, Meinke GC: Other aldehydes. In: Sullivan JB, Krieger GR, eds: Hazardous Materials Toxicology. Baltimore, Williams & Wilkins, 1992, pp. 981–986.

134. Porter JA: Acute respiratory distress following formalin inhalation. Lancet 1975;2:603–604.

135. Pullin TG, Pinkerton MN, Johnston RV, Kilian DJ: Decontamination of the skin of swine following phenol exposure: A comparison of the relative efficacy of water versus polyethylene glycol/industrial methylated spirits. Toxicol Appl Pharmacol 1978;43:199–206.

136. Pun KK, Yeung CK, Chan TK: Acute intravascular hemolysis due to accidental formalin intoxication during hemodialysis. Clin Nephrol 1984;21:188–190.

137. Rackoff WR, Merton DF: Gas embolization after ingestion of hydrogen peroxide. Pediatrics 1990;85:593–594.

138. Rasmussen H: Iodide hypersensitivity in the etiology of periarteritis nodosa. J Allergy 1955;26:394–407.

139. Rees TD, Orth CF: Oral ulcerations with use of hydrogen peroxide. J Peridontol 1986;57:689–692.

140. Restuccio A, Mortensen ME, Kelley MT: Fatal ingestion of boric acid in an adult. Am J Emerg Med 1992;10:545–547.

141. Rohyans J, Walson PD, Wood GA, MacDonald WA: Mercury toxicity following Merthiolate ear irrigations. J Pediatr 1984;104:311–313.

142. Roush GC, Walrath J, Stayner LT, et al: Nasopharyngeal cancer, sinonasal cancer, and occupations related to formaldehyde: A case-control study. J Natl Cancer Inst 1987;79:1221–1224.

143. Roy M, Calonje MA, Mouton R: Corrosive gastritis after formaldehyde ingestion. N Engl J Med 1962;266:1248–1250.

144. Rubenstein AD, Musher DM: Epidemic boric acid poisoning simulating staphylococcal toxic epidermal necrolysis of the newborn infant: Ritter's disease. J Pediatr 1970;77:884–887.

145. Rumack B: Glutaraldehyde: POISINDEX, 1998.

146. Salinas E, Sasich L, Hall DH, et al: Acute ethylene oxide intoxication. Drug Intell Clin Pharm 1981;15:384–386.

147. Schulenburg CA: Corrosive stricture of the stomach without involvement of esophagus. Lancet 1941;2:367–368.

148. Seymour WB: Poisoning from cutaneous application of iodine. Arch Intern Med 1937;59:952–966.

149. Shaw A, Cooperman A, Fusco J: Gas embolism produced by hydrogen peroxide. N Engl J Med 1967;277:238–241.

150. Sherman SI, Boyer LV, Sibley WA: Cerebral infarction immediately after ingestion of hydrogen peroxide solution. Stroke 1994;25:1065–1067.

151. Shmunes E, Levy EJ: Quaternary ammonium compound contact dermatitis from a deodorant. Arch Dermatol 1972;105:91–93.

152. Singelmann E, Steffen C: Increased erythrocyte rigidity in chlorate poisoning. J Clin Pathol 1983;36:719.

153. Singelmann E, Wetzel E, Adler G, Steffen C: Erythrocyte membrane alterations as the basis of chlorate toxicity. Toxicology 1984;30:135–147.

154. Sleigh JW, Linter SP: Hazards of hydrogen peroxide. Br Med J 1985;291:1706.

155. Smerdely P, Boyages SC, Wu D, et al: Topical iodine-containing antiseptics and neonatal hypothyroidism in very-low-birthweight infants. Lancet 1989;2:661–664.

156. Sneddon IB: Dermatitis in an intermittent haemodialysis unit. Br Med J 1968;1:183–184.

157. Southwood T, Lamb CM, Freeman J: Ingestion of potassium permanganate crystal by a three-year-old boy. Med J Aust 1987;146:639–640.

158. Spiller HA, Quadrani-Kushner DA, Cleveland P: A five-year evaluation of acute exposure to phenol disinfectant. J Toxicol Clin Toxicol 1993;31:307–313.

159. Stajich GV, Lopez GP, Harry SW, Sexson WR: Iatrogenic exposure to mercury after hepatitis B vaccination in preterm infants. J Pediatr 2000;136:679–681.

160. Stavrou A, Butcher R, Sakula A: Accidental self-poisoning by sodium chlorate weed-killer. Practitioner 1978;221:397–399.

161. St. Clair MD, Gross EA, Morgan KT: Pathology and cell proliferation induced by intra-nasal instillation of aldehydes in the rat: Comparison of glutarealdehyde and formaldehyde. Toxicol Pathol 1990;18: 353–361.

162. Steenland K, Stayner L, Greife A, et al: Mortality among workers exposed to ethylene oxide. N Engl J Med 1991;324:1402–1407.

163. Steffen C, Seitz R: Severe chlorate poisoning: Report of a case. Arch Toxicol 1981;48:281–288.

164. Steffen C, Wetzel E: Pathophysiological aspects of chlorate poisoning. Hum Toxicol 1985;4:541–542.

165. Steigmann F, Dolehide RA: Corrosive (acid) gastritis. N Engl J Med 1956;254:981–986.

166. Stein KM, Odom RB, Justice GR, Martin GC: Toxic alopecia from ingestion of boric acid. Arch Dermatol 1973;108:95–97.

167. Strubelt O, Brasch H, Pentz R, Younes M: Experimental studies on the acute cardiovascular toxicity of formalin and its antidotal treatment. J Toxicol Clin Toxicol 1990;28:221–223.

168. Sussman RM, Miller J: Iodide "mumps" after intravenous urography. N Engl J Med 1956;255:433–434.

169. Tabor E, Bostwich DC, Evans CC: Corneal damage due to eye contact with chlorhexidine gluconate. JAMA 1989;261:557–558.

170. Teshima D, Morishita K, Ueda Y, et al: Clinical management of boric acid ingestion: Pharmacokinetic assessment of efficacy of hemodialysis for treatment of acute boric acid poisoning. J Pharmacobiodyn 1992;15:287–294.

171. Thurm RH, Finkel HE: Drug fever due to potassium iodide. N Y State J Med 1965;65:2263–2265.

172. Tresch DD, Sweet DL, Keelan MH, Lange RL: Acute iodide intoxication with cardiac irritability. Arch Intern Med 1974;134:760–762.

173. Valdes-Dapena MA, Arey J: Boric acid poisoning: Three fatal cases with pancreatic inclusions and a review of the literature. J Pediatr 1962;61:531–546.

174. Van Berkel M, de Wolff FA: Survival after acute benzalkonium chloride poisoning. Hum Toxicol 1988;7:191–193.

175. Van der Vorst MM, Tamminga P, Wijburg FA, Schutgens RB: Severe methaemoglobinaemia due to para-chloraniline intoxication in premature neonates [letter]. Eur J Pediatr 1990;150:73.

176. Van Slyke KK, Michel VP, Rein MF: Treatment of vulvovaginal candidiasis with boric acid powder. Am J Obstet Gynecol 1981;141:145–148.

177. Vorherr H, Vorherr UF, Mehta P, et al: Vaginal absorption of povidone-iodine. JAMA 1988;244:2628–2629.

178. Wallgren H: Relative intoxicating effects of ethyl, propyl and butyl alcohol. Acta Pharmacol Toxicol 1960;16:217–220.

179. Warner MA, Harper JV: Cardiac dysrhythmias associated with chemical peeling with phenol. Anesthesiology 1985;62:366–367.

180. Waugh WH: Use of cortisone by mouth in prevention and therapy of severe iodism. Arch Intern Med 1954;93:299–303.

181. Weeks RS, Ravitch MM: Esophageal injury by liquid chlorine bleach: Experimental study. J Pediatr 1969;74:911–916.

182. Wilensky AO, Kaufman PA: Pyloric stenosis following the ingestion of tincture of iodine. Am J Surg 1939;43:779–782.

183. Wilson JT, Burr IM: Benzalkonium chloride poisoning in infant twins. Am J Dis Child 1975;129:1208–1209.

184. Wolff J: Iodide goiter and the pharmacologic effects of excess iodide. Am J Med 1969;47:101–124.

185. Wong LC, Heimbach MD, Truscott DR, Duncan BD: Boric acid poisoning: Report of 11 cases. Can Med Assoc J 1964;90:1018–1023.

186. Wu M, Tsai W, Yang C, Deng J: Concentrated cresol intoxication. Vet Human Toxicol 1998;40:341–343

Naphthalene   Paradichlorobenzene   Camphor

A normally healthy 2-year-old female had a few days of fever, non-productive cough, clear rhinorrhea, and nonbloody diarrhea. The mother had rubbed a fragrant yellow oil that she had purchased from a local herbalist for relief of respiratory congestion on the patient's chest 3–4 times per day for 2 days. A baby-sitter unfamiliar with the intended route of administration mistakenly administered 1 teaspoon of the oil to the child by mouth. Within 15 minutes the child vomited and within 30 minutes she had a generalized tonic-clonic seizure that resolved spontaneously. The baby-sitter called emergency medical personnel and the child was transported to the Emergency Department (ED) without incident.

Upon arrival she was irritable, moaning, and smelled "like a mothball." Her vital signs were blood pressure, 88/42 mm Hg; pulse, 132 beats/min; respiratory rate, 27 breaths/min; rectal temperature, 99.1°F (37.3°C); and pulse oximetry of 100% on oxygen. A rapid reagent blood sugar was 88 mg/dL. There was no evidence of trauma. Her pupils were 5 mm and reactive. There was no nystagmus. Cardiac, pulmonary, and abdominal examinations were unremarkable. Neurologic examination revealed normal motor strength without tremor, dysmetria, or ataxia. The child remained irritable.

Shortly after arrival, the child had a second generalized tonic-clonic seizure that lasted less than 1 minute. She was treated with 5 mg (0.5 mg/kg) of intravenous diazepam.

The complete blood count and serum electrolytes were normal. The baby-sitter brought the bottle of oil to the emergency department. The label read "Camphorated Oil" and "Harmful if swallowed." The label did not contain the concentration.

The child was admitted to the hospital for further observation. No more seizure activity was noted and within a few hours postingestion she returned to her baseline mental status.

Many different products have historically been used as moth repellents. In the United States, paradichlorobenzene has largely replaced both camphor and naphthalene as the most common component of mothballs and moth flakes because it is less toxic. Because paradichlorobenzene is widely available and because life-threatening camphor and naphthalene toxicity still occur, these agents still deserve discussion.

CAMPHOR

History and Epidemiology

Camphor was first produced by distilling bark from the camphor tree, *Cinnamomum camphora*. Today, most camphor is synthesized from the hydrocarbon pinene, a derivative of turpentine oil. Camphor has been used as an aphrodisiac, contraceptive, abortifacient, suppressor of lactation, analeptic, cardiac stimulant, antiseptic, cold remedy, muscle liniment, and drug of abuse.[32,38,45,52,69]

Camphorated oil and camphorated spirits contain varying concentrations of camphor. Historically, most camphorated oil was 20% weight (of solute) per weight (of solvent) (w/w) camphor with cottonseed oil and most camphorated spirits contained 10% w/w camphor with isopropyl alcohol. Toxicity and death following ingestion of camphorated oil, which was commonly confused with castor oil and cod liver oil, prompted the FDA to ban the nonprescription sale of camphorated oil in the United States in 1983.[4,25,45,72,89] Today, based on the 1983 FDA ruling, nonprescription camphor products may not contain greater than an 11% concentration of camphor. Camphorated oil is still used as an herbal remedy and muscle liniment, and products containing greater than 11% camphor can still be purchased legally outside of the United States.[86]

Common camphor-containing products include cold sore ointments (usually <1% camphor), muscle liniments, rubefacients (usually 4–7% camphor), and camphor spirits (usually 10% camphor). Paregoric, camphorated tincture of opium, contains a combination of anhydrous morphine (0.4 mg/mL), alcohol (46%), and benzoic acid (4 mg/mL) but only a small amount of camphor.[50] Occupational exposures to camphor occur during the manufacture of plastic, celluloid, lacquer, varnish, explosives, embalming fluids, and numerous pharmaceuticals and cosmetics.[39]

Although products containing lower concentrations of camphor are safer, life-threatening toxicity and death still result, usually from misuse or intentional overdose. Most cases of acute camphor poisoning follow unintentional ingestion of camphor-containing liquids mistaken for other medications.[4,45,61,71,87] According to data obtained by the American Association of Poison Control Centers (AAPCC), over the past 15 years there have been only four deaths attributed to camphor, all in adults, two of which occurred in the setting of an intentional suicidal overdose. Chapter 116 has complete references and discussion of the AAPCC data.

Pharmacology and Pathophysiology

Camphor (2-bormanone, 2-camphonone) is a cyclic ketone of the terpene group. Camphor's pharmacologic activity is not well studied and its mechanism of action remains unclear. More importantly, the therapeutic benefit of camphor has not been proven in a well-controlled clinical trial. It is unlikely that camphor has true therapeutic benefit as an expectorant or an anti-infective agent. Camphor may provide some local analgesic and antipruritic effects, but much safer drugs are available for these indications.

Pharmacokinetics and Toxicokinetics

There are limited data on camphor's pharmacokinetics and toxicokinetics. Camphor toxicity is reported following ingestion, dermal application, inhalation, intranasal instillation, intraperitoneal administration, and transplacental transfer.[16,67,73,75,77,83,84,91] Ingestion of solid camphor also causes toxicity.[21] Liquid camphor preparations are rapidly absorbed from the gastrointestinal tract. Camphor can be detected in the blood within 15–20 minutes postingestion.[67,73] Camphor is highly lipid soluble and is predominantly metabolized in the liver where it undergoes hydroxylation followed by conjugation with glucuronic acid. Inactive metabolites, including campherol, borneol, hydroxy-camphor, and camphoglycuronic acid, are excreted by the kidneys.[74]

As with most toxins, the toxic dose of camphor reported in the medical literature is highly variable.[34,45,82] The majority of reported cases of toxicity in both adults and children have resulted from ingestion of 20% camphorated oil, which is no longer widely available in the United States. As little as 1 teaspoon (1 g) of 20% camphorated oil has been reported to cause death in an infant.[82]

Clinical Manifestations

Exposure to camphor can often be detected by its characteristic aromatic odor (Chap. 28). Ingestion of camphor typically produces oropharyngeal irritation, nausea, vomiting, and abdominal pain. Generalized tonic-clonic seizures may be the first sign of camphor toxicity, usually occurring within minutes to 1–2 hours postingestion.[6,9] Most seizures are brief and self-limited, although some patients may have a more protracted course.[6,54,83] Central nervous system (CNS) depression is common, but rarely compromises respiratory function.[16,53,67] Other neurologic effects include headache, lightheadedness, transient visual changes, confusion, myoclonus, and hyperreflexia.[19,51,73,77] Psychiatric effects include agitation, anxiety, and hallucinations.[34,51,53] Subcutaneous injections of camphor produce variable cardiovascular effects.[38] Dermal effects include flushing and petechial hemorrhages.[16,38,84]

Case reports suggest that acute ingestion of camphor can cause transient elevations of the liver enzymes.[4,47,71,73,77] Chronic administration of camphor to a child caused altered mental status and elevated hepatic aminotransferase levels suggestive of Reye syndrome.[47] Although camphor toxicity does not produce morphologic changes of the liver characteristic of Reye syndrome, camphor toxicity should be considered in the differential diagnosis of acute hepatic encephalopathy. Albuminuria may also occur.[82]

Camphor crosses the placenta. Both fetal demise and delivery of healthy neonates are reported in mothers experiencing camphor toxicity within 24 hours of term delivery.[10,73,91]

Inhalation and dermal exposure to camphor usually produces only mucous membrane irritation and dermal irritation, respectively.[33]

Death occurs secondary to respiratory failure or seizures.[8,16,21,67] Pathologic changes following ingestion include cerebral edema, neuronal degeneration, fatty changes, centrolobular congestion of the liver, and hemorrhagic lesions in the skin, gastrointestinal tract, and kidneys.[47,82,91]

Diagnostic Testing

When managing most patients with camphor toxicity, no specific diagnostic testing is indicated. Camphor and hydroxylated metabolites can be identified in blood.[52] Camphor and camphoglycuronic acid can be identified in urine.[38,74] However, these camphor levels are not useful when managing most patients with camphor toxicity because they are not rapidly available and do not correlate well with clinical toxicity.

Management

After an acute ingestion, patients who should be evaluated in a healthcare facility include those who have signs or symptoms consistent with camphor toxicity, patients who have recently ingested more than 1 g of camphor (1 teaspoon of 20% camphorated oil), suicidal patients, and any patient with a large occupational exposure.

Gastric decontamination is not well studied in patients who ingest camphor. Nasogastric suctioning and lavage seem preferable to orogastric lavage following recent ingestion of most liquid preparations of camphor. Because liquid camphor preparations are so rapidly absorbed, the benefit of gastrointestinal decontamination is expected to diminish as the time following ingestion increases. Syrup of ipecac should not be administered because camphor-induced seizures can occur prior to the onset of ipecac-induced emesis, raising the risk of pulmonary aspiration when vomiting does subsequently occur. Administration of activated charcoal, 1 g/kg, is likely to be safe although its efficacy is not studied.

There is no antidote for camphor toxicity. Most patients survive with supportive care. Case reports suggest that most patients who will develop life-threatening camphor toxicity will develop symptoms within a few hours postexposure.

Specific management of seizures in the setting of camphor toxicity is not well studied. Patients with camphor-induced seizures should be treated with benzodiazepines and/or barbiturates. No human study has investigated or compared the efficacy of either benzodiazepines or barbiturates in preventing or controlling camphor-induced seizures. Because most healthcare providers are familiar with the use of benzodiazepines for the treatment of seizures, benzodiazepines are the first-line treatment for most causes of toxin-induced seizures, including camphor. Toxin-induced seizures rarely respond to administration of phenytoin. Repeat doses of benzodiazepines may be needed to control seizures. If benzodiazepines fail to control seizures, a barbiturate, such as phenobarbital, should be administered.

In case reports, hemodialysis with a lipid dialysate and either hemoperfusion using an Amberlite resin or charcoal hemoperfusion successfully removed camphor.[4,30,53,54,60] Neither isolated lipid hemodialysis nor lipid dialysis in combination with hemoperfusion is recommended or widely available, or demonstrated to improve outcome in a well-controlled clinical trial.

NAPHTHALENE

History and Epidemiology

Naphthalene is a bicyclic aromatic hydrocarbon that is pure white and has a noxious odor. Naphthalene toxicity has resulted from its historical use as an antihelminthic and an antiseptic.[81] Toilet-bowl and diaper-pail deodorizers containing naphthalene have also caused toxicity.[15,95] Occupational exposures to naphthalene may occur during the manufacture of dyes, synthetic resins, celluloid, solvents, and fuels. Naphthalene is the single most abundant component of coal tar and exposures occur during coal-tar processing.

Most unintentional exposures to naphthalene-containing mothballs occur in children and do not cause life-threatening toxicity. There are no published statistics estimating the incidence of either hemolysis or methemoglobinemia following exposure to naphthalene. Patients with known glucose-6-phosphate dehydrogenase deficiency are at increased risk for hemolysis. Populations with an increased incidence of glucose-6-phosphate dehydrogenase deficiency include Africans, African-Americans, and patients of Mediterranean and Asian descent.[13] Patients at increased risk of methemoglobinemia include newborn infants who have fetal hemoglobin, which is more susceptible to the formation of methemoglobin, and decreased nicotinamide adenine dinucleotide (NADH) methemoglobin reductase activity, which impairs the reduction of methemoglobin to hemoglobin.[48]

Pharmacology/Pharmacokinetics and Toxicokinetics

Naphthalene toxicity is reported following ingestion, dermal application, and inhalation.[17,22,24,76,90] Naphthalene's absorption is not well studied. Highly lipid-soluble compounds may increase naphthalene's oral and dermal absorption.[68] There is a theoretical risk of increasing naphthalene absorption following the ingestion of milk and/or fatty foods. Naphthalene is slowly metabolized in the liver to α- and β-naphthol and to α- and β-naphtholoquinone.[59,72] The oxidant stress responsible for naphthalene-induced hemolysis and methemoglobinemia is caused by the hepatic metabolites of naphthalene and not by the parent compound.[72] α-Naphthol is the metabolite that is predominantly responsible for naphthalene's hematologic toxicity.[59,94] Similar to most toxins, the toxic dose of naphthalene reported in the medical literature is highly variable. As little as one naphthalene mothball has resulted in toxicity in an infant.[29,95]

Pathophysiology

To understand naphthalene-induced hemolysis and methemoglobinemia, it is important to understand how oxidant stress affects erythrocytes and the normal mechanisms erythrocytes use to prevent and reverse the effects of oxidant stress.

Normal hemoglobin consists of four polypeptide (globin) chains: two α and two β chains. Each globin chain protects a central heme group composed of four porphobilinogen molecules and an iron atom in the reduced ferrous state (Fe^{+2}). Erythrocytes produce energy by either anaerobic metabolism (Embden-Meyerhoff pathway/glycolysis), which generates NADH, or by aerobic metabolism (hexose monophosphate shunt), which generates NADPH. Erythrocyte energy production is limited by lack of both the tricarboxylic acid (Krebs) cycle and the cytochrome electron transport chain (Chap. 25).

Oxidant stress can cause methemoglobinemia and/or hemolysis. When oxidant stress causes any one of the iron atoms from any of hemoglobin's four globin chains to be oxidized from the ferrous state (Fe^{+2}) to the ferric state (Fe^{+3}) state, methemoglobin is formed (Chap. 94). A simple change in the oxidation renders methemoglobin incapable of carrying oxygen. When oxidant stress causes hemoglobin denaturation, the heme groups and the globin chains dissociate and precipitate in the erythrocyte, forming Heinz bodies. An erythrocyte with denatured hemoglobin is more susceptible to hemolysis and to removal by the reticuloendothelial system.

Erythrocytes prevent toxicity from oxidant stress by a number different enzymatic and nonenzymatic mechanisms. Ascorbic acid, glutathione, and proteins with sulfhydryl groups combine directly with toxins with oxidizing potential before they react with hemoglobin. In addition, catalase limits the toxicity of hydrogen peroxide by converting it to water and oxygen. The most important protective mechanism, though, involves the generation of reduced nicotine adenine dinucleotide phosphate (NADPH), which is used to maintain a supply of reduced glutathione, the major intracellular reducing agent. Reduced glutathione, in the presence of glutathione peroxidase, combines with toxins with oxidizing potential before they combine with hemoglobin. The hexose monophosphate shunt is used to produce NADPH. NADPH is formed when glucose-6-phosphate dehydrogenase converts glucose-6-phosphate to 6-phosphogluconate. Patients with varying degrees of glucose-6-phosphate dehydrogenase deficiency do not generate as much NADPH and therefore have decreased levels of reduced intracellular glutathione (Fig. 94–5). Theoretically, patients with glucose-6-phosphate dehydrogenase deficiency are at increased risk of both hemolysis and methemoglobinemia following oxidant stress. In practice, patients with glucose-6-phosphate deficiency are at much greater risk of toxin-induced hemolysis than toxin-induced methemoglobinemia.[20]

Patients with decreased glutathione stores, including newborns, are at increased risk of naphthalene-induced hemolysis.[94] Patients with decreased glucose-6-phosphate dehydrogenase (G6PD) activity are also more susceptible to naphthalene-induced hemolysis because they have decreased glutathione stores.[88] There are many different variants of glucose-6-phosphate deficiency. The gene that codes for G6PD is X-linked; therefore, males may be affected more than females.[49]

Red blood cells have two different methemoglobin reductase enzyme systems that reduce methemoglobin back to normal hemoglobin. The NADH-methemoglobin reductase system and the NADPH-methemoglobin reductase system are normally responsible for reducing about 95% and 5% of methemoglobin back to hemoglobin, respectively. The NADPH-methemoglobin reductase system is important during the treatment of methemoglobinemia with methylene blue (Chap. 94 and Antidotes in Depth: Methylene Blue).

Clinical Manifestations

Acute and chronic exposures to naphthalene result in similar toxicity.[15,94] Ingestion and inhalational exposures to naphthalene commonly cause headache, nausea, vomiting, diarrhea, abdominal pain, fever, and altered mental status.[15,35,57,65] Dermal exposure has caused dermatitis.[24] Cataracts have also been reported.[27]

Oral, inhalation, and dermal naphthalene exposures can produce oxidant stress that causes two distinct hematologic disorders.

Hemolysis and methemoglobinemia occur independently or simultaneously in both children and adults with normal and deficient glucose-6-phosphate dehydrogenase activity.[29,35,44,58,59,90,95]

When hemolysis or methemoglobinemia occurs, they usually become clinically evident within 1–2 days postexposure due to the time delay necessary for metabolism. Patients with ongoing exposure to naphthalene following ingestion or dermal exposure may have persistent methemoglobinemia and/or hemolysis over a few days postexposure. Anemia secondary to hemolysis often does not reach its nadir until 3–5 days postexposure.

Signs and symptoms of hemolysis and methemoglobinemia are nonspecific and include tachycardia, tachypnea, shortness of breath, generalized weakness, decreased exercise tolerance, and altered mental status. Methemoglobinemia may produce cyanosis, whereas hemolysis may produce pallor and jaundice (Chap. 94). Renal failure as a complication of naphthalene-induced hemolysis and hemoglobinuria is reported.[14] A case report associated the development of aplastic anemia with chronic exposure to both naphthalene and paradichlorobenzene.[37]

Naphthalene pica during pregnancy causes maternal and fetal toxicity. Naphthalene or its metabolites cross the placenta.[5] Children born to mothers who were experiencing naphthalene toxicity at the time of delivery have developed hemolytic anemia believed to be related to the maternal naphthalene exposure.[94]

Diagnostic Testing

When managing most patients with naphthalene toxicity, no specific diagnostic testing is indicated. Both naphthalene and its metabolites can be identified in blood and urine. Identification of 1-naphthol and 2-naphthol in the urine can confirm exposure to naphthalene.[66] Qualitative or quantitative testing for naphthalene or its metabolites is rarely indicated when managing a case of an acute overdose.

Naphthalene-induced hemolysis is similar in presentation to hemolysis from other toxins that cause oxidative stress. A decreased hemoglobin concentration and a decreased hematocrit are the hallmarks of hemolysis. Hyperbilirubinemia from hemolysis is characterized by an elevation of the indirect bilirubin (unconjugated bilirubin). The direct bilirubin (conjugated bilirubin) is relatively normal unless the patient has hepatic or biliary dysfunction, which would not be expected with naphthalene. Serum haptoglobin is usually low because the haptoglobin-hemoglobin complex is cleared by the kidneys. Both the direct and indirect Coombs test are negative in naphthalene-induced hemolytic anemia. Lactate dehydrogenase is usually elevated. Gross or microscopic hemoglobinuria is confirmed by a urine dipstick that reacts strongly positive for hemoglobin with a paucity of red blood cells on microscopic examination. This should be differentiated from myoglobinemia by measuring the serum creatine phosphokinase, which will be elevated in patients with rhabdomyolysis and myoglobinuria.

Examination of a peripheral blood smear can reveal evidence of hemolysis before a patient develops clinical or laboratory evidence of anemia.[35] The peripheral smear may reveal red blood cell (RBC) fragmentation, anisocytosis, microspherocytosis, reticulocytosis, nucleated RBCs, basophilic stippling, and Heinz body formation (Chap. 25). Peripheral smear abnormalities and anemia may occur within the first 24 hours following ingestion.[15,35,78,94,95]

Testing for glucose-6-phosphate dehydrogenase activity is not recommended during an acute episode of hemolysis following naphthalene exposure. Newly formed erythrocytes have higher glucose-6-phosphate dehydrogenase activity than do older red blood cells. If glucose-6-phosphate dehydrogenase activity is measured during an episode of hemolysis when many of the older red blood cells that are more susceptible to hemolysis have already been hemolyzed, the glucose-6-phosphate dehydrogenase activity may be falsely elevated. It is best to delay testing for glucose-6-phosphate dehydrogenase activity for a few months following an episode of hemolysis.[40] Family members of patients with life-threatening glucose-6-phosphate dehydrogenase deficiency should also be tested.

Naphthalene-induced methemoglobinemia is similar in presentation to methemoglobinemia from other toxins that cause oxidative stress. The percentage of methemoglobin can only be determined using a cooximeter (Chap. 94).

Management

Most patients with an unintentional exposure to one or part of one naphthalene-containing mothball do not require healthcare evaluation. Patients who should be evaluated in a healthcare facility following an acute ingestion include those who recently ingested more than one naphthalene-containing mothball, anyone with signs or symptoms of hemolysis and/or methemoglobinemia, patients with known or suspected G6PD deficiency, all intentional ingestions, and patients with large inhalational exposures, especially those occurring in an occupational setting.

Gastrointestinal decontamination is not well studied in patients who ingest naphthalene. Most patients with unintentional exposures do not require gastrointestinal decontamination. Syrup of ipecac may be useful following ingestion of multiple naphthalene-containing mothballs in children, provided it can be administered within 30 minutes to 1 hour postingestion. Administration of activated charcoal, 1 g/kg, although not of proven efficacy, is also reasonable for patients with large ingestions since it is considered safe. Repeat doses of activated charcoal 0.5 g/kg and/or whole-bowel irrigation with polyethylene glycol is indicated for patients with evidence of hemolysis and/or methemoglobinemia who are suspected to have ongoing absorption of naphthalene within the gastrointestinal tract as these therapies may reduce absorption of the naphthalene.

Patients with signs or symptoms of hemolysis and/or methemoglobinemia should undergo diagnostic testing. Patients who present asymptomatic and within the first 24 hours following exposure do not have any clinical or laboratory evidence of hemolysis or methemoglobinemia are still at risk for delayed toxicity. If based upon the history it is determined that an asymptomatic patient is at risk for toxicity, diagnostic testing within the first 24 hours following exposure may detect the onset of methemoglobinemia and/or hemolysis before the patient becomes symptomatic. Most asymptomatic patients who are at low risk for toxicity can usually be managed on an outpatient basis if reevaluation within 24 hours can be arranged. Patients who are discharged should be instructed to return if they develop signs or symptoms of hemolysis or methemoglobinemia. Patients with laboratory evidence of hemolysis and/or methemoglobinemia and patients who cannot reliably be managed on an outpatient basis should be admitted.

Patients with life-threatening hemolysis and anemia should be treated with packed red blood cell transfusions. However, most patients with functioning bone marrow who are able to compensate for the hemolysis by increasing reticulocytosis will not require a transfusion. Patients with significant methemoglobinemia should receive methylene blue, 1–2 mg/kg (0.1–0.2 mL/kg of a 1% solution) intravenously. Repeat doses may be necessary (Antidotes in Depth: Methylene Blue).

PARADICHLOROBENZENE

History and Epidemiology

Today, paradichlorobenzene is the most common component of moth repellents. Paradichlorobenzene is also a common component of deodorizers and disinfectants and is also used widely in the chemical industry. As such, exposure to paradichlorobenzene in the United States is extremely common. A 1995 study suggested that 98% of the US population had 2,5-dichlorophenol, a metabolite of paradichlorobenzene, detectable in the urine.[41]

Most unintentional exposures to paradichlorobenzene-containing mothballs occur in children and do not cause toxicity.

Pharmacology/Pharmacokinetics and Toxicokinetics/Pathophysiology

Paradichlorobenzene is pure white and has a noxious odor. The mechanism for paradichlorobenzene's effects, its pharmacology, and its toxicokinetics have not been extensively studied. Paradichlorobenzene toxicity results from ingestion and inhalation.[43,62]

Clinical Manifestations

Inhalation of paradichlorobenzene may cause nausea and vomiting, headache, and mucous membrane irritation.[18,43]

Only a single case report links acute ingestion of paradichlorobenzene with hemolysis, but upon close examination there are weaknesses to this claim. The supposed causation is very tenuous. A 3-year-old child developed jaundice, methemoglobinemia, and hemolysis after exposure to "demothing crystals." The patient had 2,5-dichlorophenol and 2,5-dichloroquinol detected in the urine, and on this basis it was concluded that the moth repellent was paradichlorobenzene. The demothing agent itself was not confirmed to be paradichlorobenzene. This information places the reported hemolytic properties of paradichlorobenzene in question.[36]

Case reports associate chronic exposure to paradichlorobenzene with weight loss, ataxia, pulmonary granulomatosis, dyspnea, hepatotoxicity, anemia, and fixed drug eruptions.[12,18,26,62,63,85,92] A large, well-controlled study of chronic paradichlorobenzene exposures in humans has not been performed.

Diagnostic Testing

Both paradichlorobenzene and its metabolite, 2,5-dichlorophenol, can be identified in blood and urine following exposure. Identification of 2,5-dichlorophenol can confirm exposure to paradichlorobenzene.[41] However, because such a large proportion of the US population has detectable urinary metabolites of paradichlorobenzene from everyday exposures, detecting paradichlorobenzene in the urine should not necessarily be used to confirm an exposure following an ingestion of a mothball. Quantifying the amount of paradichlorobenzene in the urine of workers may be useful for monitoring occupational exposures.[28] Qualitative or quantitative testing for paradichlorobenzene or its metabolites is not indicated when managing a patient with an acute overdose.

Management

Referral to a Healthcare Facility.
Most unintentional exposures to paradichlorobenzene do not cause life-threatening toxicity. Most asymptomatic patients with unintentional exposures can be managed as outpatients. Patients who should be evaluated in a healthcare facility include those with any life-threatening signs or symptoms, suicidal patients, and any patient with a large exposure, especially those occurring in an occupational setting.

Gastrointestinal Decontamination.
Gastrointestinal decontamination is not well studied in patients who ingest paradichlorobenzene. Most patients with unintentional exposures do not require gastrointestinal decontamination. Administration of activated charcoal, 1 g/kg, although not studied, is reasonable for patients with large, intentional ingestions given its well-documented safety.

MOTHBALL RECOGNITION

Healthcare providers occasionally must determine whether a mothball is made of naphthalene, paradichlorobenzene, or camphor. When the container from which a mothball was taken is unavailable, as is often the case, mothballs made of naphthalene, paradichlorobenzene, and camphor are difficult to distinguish based upon either appearance, odor, texture, or size. Although most new paradichlorobenzene mothballs are slightly larger than most new naphthalene mothballs, all mothballs decompose when exposed to air, making size an unreliable differentiating characteristic. Blood and urine tests that identify camphor, naphthalene, paradichlorobenzene, and their metabolites are time-consuming, costly, and not readily available to most clinicians. Identifying a mothball as paradichlorobenzene can often lead to outpatient management, saving both money and undue worry. The following tests may allow rapid identification of the component of an unknown mothball. When performing these tests it is most helpful to have camphor, naphthalene, and paradichlorobenzene controls available for comparison (Table 85–1).

Most mothballs are white, crystalline, and have a noxious odor.[93] Camphor mothballs are more oily than both naphthalene and paradichlorobenzene mothballs. If controls are available, mothballs can often be differentiated based upon their odor and texture.[2] Even if a mothball can be identified by its physical characteristics, it is recommended that a confirmatory analytic test still be performed.

The easiest way to differentiate camphor mothballs from either naphthalene or paradichlorobenzene mothballs is to place the mothball in water. Mothballs made of naphthalene or paradichlorobenzene sink, whereas mothballs made of camphor float. Naphthalene mothballs can then be differentiated from paradichlorobenzene mothballs by placing the mothball in water that is saturated with table salt (sodium chloride). Naphthalene and camphor mothballs float, whereas paradichlorobenzene mothballs sink.[55]

Both naphthalene and paradichlorobenzene mothballs are radiopaque. Although paradichlorobenzene mothballs are more radiopaque than naphthalene mothballs, this difference is not clinically reliable enough to differentiate between them (Fig. 85–1).

Paradichlorobenzene and naphthalene have different melting points, 53.5°C (128.3°F) and 80.2°C (176.4°F), respectively. A

TABLE 85–1. Mothballs: Laboratory Differentiation

	Naphthalene	Paradichlorobenzene	Camphor
Weight	3.6 g/mothball	5.0 g/mothball	Available in cake form
Appearance	Clear, white, dry crystalline balls	Clear white, wet, oily crystalline balls	Wet, oily crystalline
Specific gravity[29]	1.094–1.100	1.429–1.437	0.999
Radiography[93]	Faintly opaque	Densely opaque	—
Flotation in water[55]	Sinks	Sinks	Floats
Flotation in saturated solution table salt[55]	Floats	Sinks	Floats
Chloroform + aluminum chloride test[2]	Immediate blue color	No reaction	Not tested
Bunsen burner test: touch crystals to copper wire[2]	Initial flame yellow-orange	Initial yellow-orange, then bright green	Not tested
Differentiation by melting point by placing in 60°C water bath[70]	Solid until 80°C (176°F)	Early liquefaction in 3 min at >60°C (127.4°F)	Solid until 178°C (352.4°F)
Solubility in turpentine	Poor (64–75%) Incomplete at 60 min	Excellent (98%) Complete at 60 min	Not tested
Solubility in water	None	None	None
Differential solubility in alcohols[93] (methanol, ethanol, isopropanol)	None	None	None
Odor (have reference mothballs available)	Pungent aromatic	Pungent aromatic	Pungent aromatic

small amount of an unknown mothball should be placed in a covered test tube in a 60°C (140°F) water bath. A mothball made of paradichlorobenzene readily melts at 60°C (140°F).[70] When chloroform is added to naphthalene, an intense blue color is produced. No color change is seen with paradichlorobenzene and chloroform. It is inadvisable to use or store chloroform in acute care environments where improper handling or misuse can result in toxicity.

When paradichlorobenzene and naphthalene are placed on a hot copper wire and placed in a flame they both initially produce a yellow-orange flame. The paradichlorobenzene then produces a bright green flame, whereas the naphthalene does not. Another distinguishing feature is solubility in turpentine. Paradichlorobenzene solubilizes faster in turpentine than naphthalene.[93]

SUMMARY

Historically the most common components of moth repellents have been camphor, naphthalene, and paradichlorobenzene. In the United States, paradichlorobenzene has largely replaced both camphor and naphthalene as the most common component of mothballs and moth flakes because it is less toxic. If an unknown moth repellent can be identified as paradichlorobenzene, limited toxicity would be expected following an acute exposure. It is important for clinicians to understand how to use simple tests to identify the component of an unknown mothball. Because life-threatening camphor and naphthalene toxicity are still reported, it is important for clinicians to understand how to manage patients exposed to these toxins.

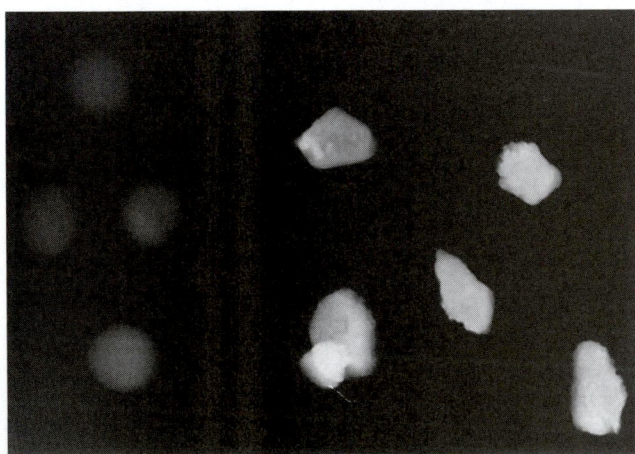

Figure 85–1. Radiograph of mothballs. Paradichlorobenzene (on the right) is densely radiopaque, whereas naphthalene (on the left) is faintly radiopaque.

REFERENCES

1. Abelson SM, Henderson AT: Mothball poisoning. US Armed Forces Med J 1951;11:491–493.
2. Ambre J, Ruo TI, Smith-Coggins R: Mothball composition: Three simple tests for distinguishing paradichlorobenzene from naphthalene. Ann Emerg Med 1986;15:724–726.
3. Anonymous: Ortho, meta and para-dichlorobenzene. Rev Environ Contam Toxicol 1988;106:51–68.
4. Antman E, Jacob G, Volpe B, et al: Camphor overdosage. Therapeutic considerations. N Y Med J 1978;78:896–897.
5. Anziulewicz JA, Dick HJ, Chiarvili EE: Transplacental naphthalene poisoning. Am J Obstet Gynecol 1959;78:519–521.
6. Aronow R, Spigiel RW: Implications of camphor poisoning. Drug Intell Clin Pharm 1976;10:631–634.
7. Azouz WM, Parke DV, Williams RT: Studies in detoxification. The metabolism of halogenobenzenes. Ortho- and paradichlorobenzenes. Biochem J 1955;59:410.
8. Barker F: A case of poisoning by camphorated oil [letter]. Br Med J 1910;1:921.
9. Benz RW: Camphorated oil poisoning with no mortality. Report of twenty cases. JAMA 1919;72:1217–1218.

10. Blackmon WP, Curry HB: Camphor poisoning: Report of a case occurring during pregnancy. J Florida Med Assoc 1957;43:999–1000.

11. Blair J: Camphorated oil poisoning. Ohio St Med J 1929;25:808–809.

12. Campbell DM, Davidson RJ: Toxic haemolytic anemia in pregnancy due to a pica for paradichlorobenzene. J Obstet Gynaecol Br Commonw 1970;77:657–659.

13. Childs B, Zinkman WH, Browne EA, et al: A genetic study of a defect in glutathione metabolism of the erythrocyte. Bull Johns Hopkins Hosp 1958;102:21.

14. Chugh KS, Singhal PC, Sharma BK, et al: Acute renal failure due to intravascular hemolysis in the North Indian patients. Am J Med Sci 1977;274:139–144.

15. Chusid E, Fried CT: Acute hemolytic anemia due to naphthalene ingestion. Am J Dis Child 1955;89:612–614.

16. Clark TL: Fatal case of camphor poisoning [letter]. Brit Med J 1924; 1:467.

17. Cock TC: Acute hemolytic anemia in the neonatal period [letter]. AMA J Dis Children 1957;94:77.

18. Cotter LH: Paradichlorobenzene poisoning from insecticides. N Y State J Med 1953;53:1690–1699.

19. Craig JO: Poisoning by the volatile oils in childhood [letter]. Arch Dis Child 1953;28:475.

20. Curry S: Methemoglobinemia. Ann Emerg Med 1982;11:214–221.

21. Davies R: A fatal case of camphor poisoning [letter]. Br Med J 1887;1:726.

22. Dawson JP, Thayer WW, Desforges JF: Acute hemolytic anemia in the newborn infant due to naphthalene poisoning: A report of two cases with investigations into the mechanism of the disease. Blood 1958;13:1113–1125.

23. Emery DP, Corban JG: Camphor toxicity. J Paediatr Child Health 1999;35:105–106.

24. Fanburg SJ: Exfoliative dermatitis due to naphthalene. Arch Derm Syph 1940;42:53–58.

25. Food and Drug Administration: Proposed rules: External analgesic drug products for over-the-counter human use; tentative final monograph. Fed Reg 1983;48:5852–5869.

26. Frank SB, Cohen HJ: Fixed drug eruption due to paradichlorobenzene. N Y State J Med 1961;61:4079.

27. Ghetti G, Mariani L: Eye changes due to naphthalene. Med Lav 1956; 47:524–530.

28. Ghittori S, Imbriani M, Pezzagno G, et al: Urinary elimination of *p*-dichlorobenzene (*p*-DCB) and weighted exposure concentration. G Ital Med Lav 1985;7:59–63.

29. Gidron E, Leurer J: Naphthalene poisoning. Lancet 1956;1:228–233.

30. Ginn HE, Anderson KE, Mercier RK, et al: Camphor intoxication treated by lipid dialysis. JAMA 1968;203:230–231.

31. Gouin S, Patel H: Unusual cause of seizure. Pediatr Emerg Care 1996; 12:298–300.

32. Greene RR, Ivy AC: The effect of camphor oil on lactation. JAMA 1938;110:641–642.

33. Gronka PA, Bobkoskie RL, Tomchick GJ, et al: Camphor exposure in a packaging plant. Am Ind Hyg Assoc J 1969;30:276–279.

34. Haft HH: Camphor liniment poisoning [letter]. JAMA 1925;84:1571.

35. Haggerty RJ: Toxic hazards: Naphthalene poisoning. N Engl J Med 1956;255:919–920.

36. Hallowell M: Acute haemolytic anaemia following the ingestion of para-dichlorobenzene. Arch Dis Child 1959;34:74–75.

37. Harden RA, Baetjer MA: Aplastic anemia following exposure to paradichlorobenzene and naphthalene. J Occup Med 1978;20:820–822.

38. Heard JD, Brooks RC: A clinical and experimental investigation of the therapeutic value of camphor. Am J Med Sci 1913;145:238–253.

39. Herrmann AP Jr: Camphorated oil: Health, history and hazard. Am Pharm 1978;18:15.

40. Herz F, Kaplan E, Scheye ES: Diagnosis of erythrocyte glucose-6-phosphate dehydrogenase deficiency in the Negro male despite hemolytic crisis. Blood 1970;35:90–93.

41. Hill RH, Ashley DL, Head SL, et al: *p*-Dichlorobenzene exposure among 1,000 adults in the United States. Arch Environ Health 1995; 50:277–280.

42. Hockwald RS, Arnold J, Clayman CB, et al: Status of primaquine. 4. Toxicity of primaquine in Negroes. JAMA 1952;149:1568.

43. Hollingsworth RL, Rowe VK, Oyen F, et al: Toxicity of para-dichlorobenzene: Determinations on experimental animals and human subjects. Arch Indust Health 1956;14:138–147.

44. Jacobziner H, Raybin HW: Accidental chemical poisonings. Naphthalene poisoning. N Y State J Med 1964;1762–1766.

45. Jacobziner H, Raybin HW: Camphor poisoning. Arch Pediatr 1962; 79:28.

46. Jacobziner H: Accidental chemical poisonings. N Y J Med 1963: 3575–3577.

47. Jimenez JF, Brown AL, Arnold WC, et al: Chronic camphor ingestion mimicking Reye's syndrome. Gastroenterology 1983;84:394–398.

48. Johnson CJ, Bonrud PA, Dosch TL, et al: Fatal outcome of methemoglobinemia in an infant. JAMA 1987;257:2796–2797.

49. Kattamis CA: Glucose-6-phosphate dehydrogenase deficiency in female heterozygotes and the X-inactivation hypothesis. Acta Pediatr Scand 1967;172(Suppl):103–109.

50. Kauffman RE, Banner W, Berlin CM, et al: Camphor revisited: Focus on toxicity. Committee on Drugs. American Academy of Pediatrics. Pediatrics 1994;94:127–128.

51. Klingensmith WR: Poisoning by camphor. JAMA 1934;102: 2182–2183.

52. Köppel C, Tenczer J, Schirop T, et al: Camphor poisoning, abuse of camphor as a stimulant. Arch Toxicol 1982;51:101–106.

53. Köppel C, Martens F, Schirop T, Ibe K: Hemoperfusion in acute camphor poisoning. Intensive Care Med 1988;14:431–433.

54. Kopelman R, Miller S, Kelly R, et al: Camphor intoxication treated by resin hemoperfusion. JAMA 1979;241:727–728.

55. Koyama K, Yamashita M, Ogura Y, et al: A simple test for mothball component differentiation using water and a saturated solution of table salt: Its utilization for poison information service. Vet Hum Tox 1991;33:425–427.

56. Lahoud CA, March JA, Proctor DD: Campho-Phenique ingestion: An intentional overdose. South Med J 1997;90:647–648.

57. Linick M: Illness associated with exposure to naphthalene in mothballs. MMWR Morb Mortal Wkly Rep 1983;32:34–35.

58. MacGregor RR: Naphthalene poisoning from ingestion of mothballs. Can Med Assoc J 1954;70:313–314.

59. Mackell JW, Rieders F, Brieger H, et al: Acute hemolytic anemia due to the ingestion of naphthalene mothballs. Pediatrics 1951;7:722–728.

60. Mascie-Taylor BH, Widop B, Davison AM: Camphor intoxication treated by charcoal hemoperfusion. Postgrad Med J 1981;57:725–726.

61. Miller DGM: The toxicity of camphor (camphorated oil) [letter]. JAMA 1914;63:579.

62. Miyai I, Hirono N, Fujita M, et al: Reversible ataxia following chronic exposure to paradichlorobenzene. J Neurol Neurosurg Psychiatry 1988;51:453–454.

63. Nalbandian RM, Pearce JF: Allergic purpura induced by exposure to *p*-dichlorobenzene. Confirmation by indirect basophil degranulation test. JAMA 1965;194(7):238–239.

64. Nash FL: Naphthalene poisoning. Br Med J 1903;1:251–259.

65. Ostlere R, Amos R, Wass JAH: Haemolytic anaemia associated with ingestion of naphthalene-containing anointing oil. Clin Toxicol 1988; 64:444–446.

66. Owa JA, Izedonmwen OE, Ogundaini AO, et al: Quantitative analysis of 1-naphthol in urine of neonates exposed to mothballs: The value in infants with unexplained anaemia. Afr J Med Med Sci 1993;22: 71–76.

67. Phelan WJ: Camphor poisoning: Over-the-counter dangers. Pediatrics 1976;57:428–431.

68. Picchioni AL: Mothball poisoning in children. Am J Hosp Pharm 1950;17:303–304.

69. Rabl W, Katzgraber F, Steinlechner M: Camphor ingestion for abortion. Forensic Sci Int 1997;89:137–140.

70. Reeves RR, Pendarvis RO: Mothball melting points. Ann Emerg Med 1986;15:1377.

71. Reid FM: Accidental camphor ingestion. JACEP 1979;8:339–340.

72. Rieders F, Brieger H: Hemolytic action of naphthalene and its oxidation products. Pediatrics 1951;7:725–727.

73. Riggs J, Hamilton R, Homel S, et al: Camphorate oil intoxication in pregnancy: Report of a case. Obstet Gynecol 1965;25:255–258.

74. Robertson JS, Mussain M: Metabolism of camphors and related compounds. J Biochem 1969;113:57–64.

75. Rübsamen W: Tödliche Kamfervergiftung nach Anwendung von offizinellem Kampferöl zur postoperativen Peritonitisprophylaxe. Zentralbl F Gynäk 1912;36:1009–1015.

76. Schafer WB: Acute hemolytic anemia related to naphthalene. Report of a case in a newborn infant. Pediatrics 1951;7:172–174.

77. Seife M, Leon JL: Camphor poisoning following ingestion of nose drops. JAMA 1954;155:1059–1060.

78. Shannon K, Buchanan GR: Severe hemolytic anemia in black children with G-6 PD deficiency. Pediatrics 1982;70:364–369.

79. Siegel E, Wason S: Camphor toxicity. Pediatr Clin North Am 1986; 33:375–379.

80. Siegel E, Wason S: Mothball toxicity. Pediatr Clin North Am 1986; 33:369–374.

81. Smillie WG: Betanaphthol poisoning in the treatment of hookworm disease. JAMA 1920;74:1503–1506.

82. Smith AG, Margolis G: Camphor poisoning, anatomical and pharmacologic study; report of a fatal case; experimental investigation of protective action of barbiturate. Am J Pathol 1954;30:857–868.

83. Skoglund RR, Ware L, Schkanberger JE: Prolonged seizures due to contact and inhalation exposure to camphor. Clin Pediatr 1977;16: 901–902.

84. Summers GD: Case of camphor poisoning. Br Med J 1947;2: 1009–1010.

85. Sumers J: Hepatitis with concomitant esophageal varices following exposure to mothball vapors. N Y State J Med 1952;52:1048–1049.

86. Theis JG, Koren G: Camphorated oil: Still endangering the lives of Canadian children. CMAJ 1995;152:1821–1824.

87. Tidcombe FS: Severe symptoms following the administration of a small teaspoonful of camphorated oil [letter]. Lancet 1897;2:660.

88. Todisco V, Lamour J, Finberg L: Hemolysis from exposure to naphthalene mothballs [letter]. N Engl J Med 1991;325:1660.

89. Trestrail JH, Spartz ME: Camphorated and castor oil confusion and its toxic results. Clin Toxicol 1977;11:151–158.

90. Valaes T, Doxiadis SA, Fessas P: Acute hemolysis due to naphthalene inhalation. J Pediatr 1963;63:904–915.

91. Weiss J, Catalano P: Camphorated oil intoxication during pregnancy. Pediatrics 1973;52:713–716.

92. Weller RW, Crellin AJ: Pulmonary granulomatosis following extensive use of paradichlorobenzene. AMA Arch Intern Med 1953;91: 408–413.

93. Winkler JV, Kulig K, Rumack BH: Mothball differentiation: Naphthalene from paradichlorobenzene. Ann Emerg Med 1985;14:30–32.

94. Zinkham WJ, Childs B: A defect of glutathione metabolism in erythrocytes from patients with a naphthalene-induced hemolytic anemia. Pediatrics 1958;22:461–471.

95. Zuelzer WW, Apt L: Acute hemolytic anemia due to naphthalene poisoning: Clinical and experimental study. JAMA 1949;141:185–190.

CHAPTER 86 HYDROCARBONS

David D. Gummin / Daniel O. Hryhorczuk

A 26-year-old Hispanic male presented to the Emergency Department (ED) with 3 weeks of increasing bilateral lower extremity weakness. His family expressed concern that he was now beginning to fall several times daily. He also complained that his hands had become "clumsy" over the past week, and he noted an inability to grasp objects. He denied any recent head or neck trauma, recent acute illness, or immunizations. Past medical and surgical histories were negative; he took no medications and had no allergies. He admitted to occasional alcohol and intermittent tobacco use, but denied the use of illicit drugs. He was unemployed for several years. On examination, he appeared disheveled and cachectic. Vital signs were: blood pressure, 132/89 mm Hg; heart rate, 102 beats/min; respirations, 20 breaths/min; and temperature, 37.1°C (98.8°F). He had bitemporal wasting and horizontal nystagmus. The heart, lung, abdominal, and extremity examinations were remarkable only for diffuse atrophy, most notably in the thenar and hypothenar eminences. Right upper extremity strength was 5/5. Motor strength in the left upper extremity flexors was 5/5, while strength in the left wrist extensors was 4/5, as was the strength in the left-hand intrinsic muscles. Strength in the hamstrings was 4/5, and in the ankles it was 0/5 bilaterally for both dorsiflexion and plantar flexion. Bilateral foot drop was noted. Sensation to pinprick, proprioception, and vibration, and the deep-tendon reflexes were preserved. Plantar flexion was present bilaterally. He was too ataxic to ambulate. The complete blood count, electrolytes, electrocardiogram, and chest radiograph were unremarkable. A computed tomography (CT) scan of the brain showed diffuse cerebral and cerebellar atrophy.

At that point, a resident noted paint stains on the patient's clothing, and queried the patient about his hobbies. With time and persistence, the patient admitted to 12 years of chronic recreational solvent abuse. Further questioning revealed that the patient had a 35-year-old brother who had died from complications of paint sniffing 1 year previously. Nerve conduction studies were consistent with a length-dependent polyneuropathy, predominantly motor. The patient admitted that he had run out of money to buy paint 3 months earlier, and had switched to sniffing unleaded gasoline. He remained nonambulatory during his hospitalization, and was transferred to a short-term rehabilitation facility, after which he was lost to followup.

Organic chemistry was born during the industrial revolution and evolved rapidly with advances in coal-tar chemistry. The discovery of aniline dye led to the large-scale distillation of coal tar to obtain crude naphtha, which was the source of useful aromatic hydrocarbons such as benzene. Other coal-tar distillation products included light oil, creosote oil, anthracene oil, road tar, and pitch.

Eventually, petroleum distillation replaced coal tar as the major source of fossil fuels, naphtha, aromatic solvents, and other organic compounds. In addition to their uses as fuels, the large family of petroleum distillate compounds has a myriad of other uses in industry, including uses as solvents, lubricating oils, and chemical feedstocks and intermediates. They also have common household applications such as paint thinners, furniture polish, lamp oils, and lubricants (Table 86–1).

While hydrocarbons (HCs) represent a diverse group of chemicals, their commonality rests primarily in their use. Most of the products in everyday use, such as gasoline, kerosene, or fuel oils, are variable mixtures of hydrocarbons obtained as distillation fractions. This complicates the assessment of their toxicity. As a result, in discussing hydrocarbon toxicology, generalities are often used to discuss the behavior of these complex mixtures. This chapter highlights the toxicology of individual hydrocarbons when they are commercially present as the individual compounds or when they present unique toxicologic issues.

DEFINITIONS

A *hydrocarbon* is an organic compound made up primarily of carbon and hydrogen atoms, typically ranging from 1 to 60 carbon atoms. This definition includes products derived from plants (pine oil, vegetable oil), animal fats (cod liver oil), natural gas, petroleum, and coal tar. There are two basic types of hydrocarbon molecules: *aliphatic* (straight or branched chains) and *cyclic* (closed ring), each with its own subclasses. The aliphatics include the *paraffins* (*alkanes*, with a generic formula C_nH_{2n+2}), the *olefins* (*alkenes* have one double bond and *alkadienes* have two double bonds), the *acetylenes* (generic formula C_nH_{2n-2} with a triple bond), and the *acyclic terpenes* (polymers of isoprene, C_5H_8). Some aliphatic compounds have branches in which the subchain also contains carbon atoms—both chains are essentially straight.

Solvents are a heterogenous class of chemical compounds used to dissolve and to provide a vehicle for delivery of other chemical substances. Probably the most common industrial solvent is water. The common solvents most familiar to toxicology are the *organic solvents* (containing one or more carbon atoms), and most of these are hydrocarbons. Most are liquids under the conditions in which they are used. Specifically named solvents (Stoddard solvent, white naphtha, ligroin) represent mixtures of hydrocarbon compounds, emanating from a common distillation fraction.

Saturated hydrocarbons contain carbon atoms only in their most reduced state, with each carbon bound to either hydrogen or to another carbon. No double or triple bonds are present. Con-

TABLE 86–1. Household Products Containing Hydrocarbons

Adhesives (glues)	Mothballs
Baby oil	Motor oils
Car waxes	Naphtha
Cod liver oil	Paint removers
Contact cement	Paint thinners
Furniture polishes	Paraffin
Furniture refinishers	Paste waxes
Gasoline	Petroleum jelly
Home heating fuel	Pine oils
Kerosene	Plastic cement
Kitchen waxes	Solvents
Lacquers	Stain removers
Laxatives	Sterno fuel
Lighter fluids	Stoddard solvent
Liquid solder	Turpentine
Liquid steel	Typewriter correction fluids
Mineral oil	Varnish removers
Mineral seal oil	Wax
Mineral spirits	

versely, *unsaturated* compounds are those with hydrogens removed, and higher-order (double or triple) bonds present.

The cyclic hydrocarbons include the *alicyclics* (three or more carbon atoms in a ring structure, with properties similar to those of aliphatics), *aromatics,* and *cyclic terpenes.* The alicyclics are further divided into the *cycloparaffins* (*naphthenes*) such as cyclohexane and the *cycloolefins* (two or more double bonds) such as cyclopentadiene.

The aromatic hydrocarbons are divided into the *benzene* group (one ring), the *naphthalene* group (two rings), and the *anthracene* group (three rings). *Polycyclic aromatic hydrocarbons* (polynuclear aromatic hydrocarbons) have multifused benzene rings. Aromatic organic compounds may also be *heterocyclic* (eg, where oxygen or nitrogen substitutes for carbon in the ring). Structurally, these molecules are flat, with reactive electron clouds above and below the ring.

The *cyclic terpenes* are the principal components of a variety of plant-derived essential oils, often providing color, odor, and flavor. *Limonene* in lemon oil, *menthol* in mint oil, *pinene* in turpentine, and *camphor* are all terpenes.[160]

The physical properties of hydrocarbons vary by the number of carbon atoms and molecular structure (Table 86–2). Unsubstituted aliphatic hydrocarbons containing up to 4 carbons are gaseous at room temperature, those with 5–19 carbon molecules are liquid, and those with longer-chain molecules tend to be tars or solids. Branching of chains tends to destabilize intermolecular forces, so that less energy is required to separate the molecules. The result is that, for a given molecular size, highly branched molecules have lower boiling points and tend to be more volatile.[157]

As discussed previously, most commercial hydrocarbon products are variable mixtures of individual hydrocarbon compounds. An illustrative example of a *mixture* is gasoline. Gasoline is a mixture of alkanes, alkenes, naphthenes, and aromatic hydrocarbons, predominantly 5–10 carbon molecules in size.[237] Natural gasoline is separated from crude oil in a common distillation fraction. However, most commercially available gasolines are actually blends of up to eight component fractions from refinery processors. More than 1500 individual compounds may be present in commercial grades, but most analytical methods are only able to isolate 150–180 compounds from gasoline. Notably, *n*-hexane is present at up to 6%, and benzene is present at 1–6%, depending upon the grade and the place of origin of the product. In addition, a number of additives may go into the final formulation: alkyl leads, ethylene dichloride, and ethylene dibromide in leaded gasoline, and oxygenates such as methyl t-butyl ether (MTBE), as well as methanol and ethanol.

Organic halides contain one or more halogen atoms (fluorine, chlorine, bromine, iodine), which are usually substituted for hydrogen atoms in the parent structure. Examples include chloroform, trichloroethylene (TCE), and the freons.

Oxygenated hydrocarbons demonstrate toxicity specific to the oxidation state of the carbon, as well as to the atoms adjacent to it (the "R" groups). The *alcohols* are widely used as solvents in in-

TABLE 86–2. Physical Properties of Common Hydrocarbon Compounds

Compound	Carbon Atoms/Formula	Common Uses	Boiling Point (°C)	Viscosity (SSU)*
Aliphatics				
Gasoline	4–10	Motor vehicle fuel	30–210	30
Naphtha	8–12	Charcoal lighter fluid	100–200	29
Kerosene	5–15	Heating fuel	200–300	35
Turpentine	$C_{10}H_{16}$	Paint thinner	155	33
Mineral spirits	9–12	Paint and varnish thinner	110–200	30–35
Mineral seal oil	13–17	Furniture polish	300–500	30–35
Heavy fuel oil	20–45	Heating oil	325–540	>450
Aromatics				
Benzene	C_6H_6	Solvent, reagent, gasoline additive	80	31
Toluene	C_7H_8	Solvent, spray paint solvent	111	28
Xylene	C_8H_{10}	Solvent, paint thinner, reagent	144(o), 139(m), 138(p)	28
Halogenated				
Methylene chloride	CH_2Cl_2	Solvent, paint stripper, propellant	40	27
Carbon tetrachloride	CCl_4	Solvent, propellant, refrigerant	77	30
Trichloroethylene	$HClC=CCl_2$	Degreaser, spot remover	87	27
Tetrachloroethylene	$Cl_2C=CCl_2$	Dry cleaning solvent, chemical intermediate	121	28

*Direct values for kinematic viscosity in Saybolt seconds universal (SSU) were not available for the following compounds: naphtha, xylene, methylene chloride, carbon tetrachloride, trichloroethylene, perchloroethylene, and toluene. SSU was calculated by converting from available measurements in centipoise viscosity and/or centistokes viscosity using the following conversions: the value in centistokes is estimated by dividing centipoise by density at 20°C; SSU is approximated from centistokes using $y = 3.2533x + 26.08$ ($R^2 = 0.9998$). Centipoise viscosity for naphtha was estimated from the value for butylbenzene. Centipoise viscosity for xylene is the average of *o-*, *m-*, and *p*-xylene.

dustry and in household products. Their toxicities are discussed in Chaps. 64 and 66. *Ethers* contain an oxygen bound on either side by a carbon atom. Acute toxicity tends to mirror that of the corresponding alcohols. *Aldehydes* and *ketones* contain a single carbon-oxygen double bond (C=O)—the former at the terminal carbon, the latter somewhere in the middle. Organic *acids, esters, amides,* and *acyl halides* represent more oxidized states of carbon; human toxicity is agent specific.

Phenols consist of benzene rings with an attached hydroxyl (alcohol) group. The parent compound, phenol, has only one hydroxyl group attached to benzene. The toxicity of phenol can be dramatically altered by addition of other functional groups to the benzene ring (Chap. 84). Cresols, catechols, and salicylate are examples of substituted phenols.

A variety of organic amines, amides, nitroso, and nitro compounds, as well as phosphates, sulfites, and sulfates, are used commercially and in industry. The addition of these functional groups to hydrocarbons dramatically alters the toxicity of the compound.

Figure 86–1 and Chap. 12 present the chemical structures of some of the more commonly encountered hydrocarbons.

BACKGROUND AND EPIDEMIOLOGY

The process of obtaining hydrocarbons from coal involves distillation of bituminous (soft) coal to remove *coal gas*, which can then be separated into a variety of natural gases. A large amount of distillant residue from the heating process remains as *coal tar*, which can be separated into kerosene and a variety of other hydrocarbon mixtures. The principal commercial source of hydrocarbons today involves distillation of crude oil. Petroleum is heated to fixed temperatures in a large-scale distillation procedure, allowing separation of hydrocarbons into distillation fractions by vapor (boiling) point. Because of the relationship between boiling point and molecular weight, this process roughly divides substances into like-sized mixtures. The most volatile fractions come off early, as gas, and are used primarily for heating. The least volatile fractions (larger than about 10 carbons) are used chiefly for fuel and/or lubricants, paraffins, petroleum jelly, and asphalt. The remaining volatile hydrocarbon fractions (C_5 to C_{10}) form the fractions most commonly used as solvents.

Longer alkanes are often submitted to an industrial process known as *cracking* in which they are superheated in a chamber, with catalytic pyrolysis, into shorter-chain alkanes and alkenes. Refineries then typically employ processes such as *catalytic isomerization*, to increase the amount of branching in the hydrocarbon chain (which increases the "octane" of the fuel), and *catalytic reforming*, which converts alkanes and cycloalkanes into aromatic compounds.[157]

Occupations at risk for solvent exposure include petrochemical workers, plastics and rubber workers, printers, laboratory workers, painters, and hazardous waste workers. But exposures are ubiquitous in many occupations, and even in everyday life. In fact, the Occupational Safety and Health Administration estimates nearly 238,000 American workers are exposed annually to significant concentrations of benzene alone.[106] Hydrocarbons are so common in our society that exposures and illnesses are typically hidden in databases according to the product implicated, and not merely as "hydrocarbon" or "solvent" exposure. This makes the epidemiology of hydrocarbon exposure and hydrocarbon-related illness particularly difficult to analyze. Because a common property of organic solvents is their volatility, inhalational exposure and even dermal exposure and absorption may occur.[94] Most exposure does not involve ingestion—it may range from pumping your own gasoline to painting one's home or applying or removing fingernail polish. Tables 86–1 and 86–2 list frequently encountered hydrocarbon-containing compounds.

In the years 1995–1999, an average of 65,804 annual human exposures to hydrocarbon compounds were reported to American poison centers that contribute to the Toxic Exposures Surveillance System (TESS) database of the American Association of Poison Control Centers (AAPCC). These exposures resulted in an average of 13 deaths per year over the same period, and accounted for 3% of the total human exposures reported to AAPCC. The incidence of both exposures and deaths has not changed dramatically in this database since the first AAPCC report in 1983. Reliably, 40–50% of exposures are unintentional exposures in children younger than 6 years of age. The overwhelming majority of exposures in this age group are categorized as unintentional (page xx and Chap. 116). However, even within the TESS database, many thousands of hydrocarbon exposures are not listed as such, but are ascribed to "chemicals, pesticides, personal care products, cleaning substances, paints, automotive products," and the like. Certainly these numbers dramatically underestimate North American exposures.

Of greater concern is the trend toward increased intentional abuse of volatile solvents by young people. Data from the Monitoring the Future (MTF) study for the National Institute on Drug Abuse (NIDA) indicate that children in 8th to 12th grades have steadily increased their volatile inhalant use since the 1970s. Although this trend has leveled since 1995, as many as 10.3% of 8th graders and 5.6% of 12th graders have tried inhalants. Five percent of 8th graders say they have abused inhalants in the past

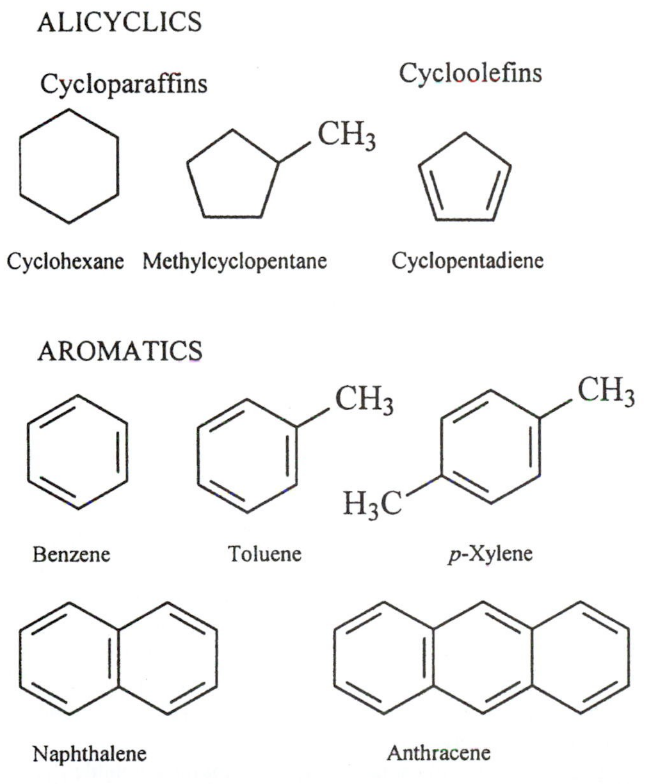

ALICYCLICS

Cycloparaffins   **Cycloolefins**

Cyclohexane   Methylcyclopentane   Cyclopentadiene

AROMATICS

Benzene   Toluene   *p*-Xylene

Naphthalene   Anthracene

Figure 86–1. Basic hydrocarbon structures.

month. This survey almost certainly underestimates true use patterns, as high school dropouts are not surveyed.[116] Similarly, the 1999 National Household Survey on Drug Abuse (NHSDA) estimates that 17 million Americans (7.8%) have abused inhalants at least once. The highest incidence of use is among 12–17-year-olds; but even among adults age 18–25 years, the rate of first use more than doubled between 1990 and 1998 (from 4.6 to 11.2 per 1000 potential new users). Overall, there was an increase of nearly a million new inhalant users in 1998, an increase of 154% over 1990.[212]

Medical examiner data reported to the Drug Abuse Warning Network (DAWN) from 1993–1998 implicate inhalants, solvents, and aerosols in an average of 135 drug-related deaths per year. These constitute 1.4–1.5% of the annual drug-related deaths reported into this system. While DAWN is biased in receiving the bulk of its reports from the large metropolitan areas, the problem permeates nonurban areas as well.[113,202] As is the case in other datasets, children demonstrate particular risk: Although decedents age 6–17 years accounted for only 0.8% of drug mentions, this age group had 6% of mentions of inhalants/solvents/aerosols.[225] The only Western nation that routinely tracks deaths from inhalant abuse (Great Britain) documents two deaths per week.[175]

In summary, three populations appear to be at risk for hydrocarbon-related illness: children with unintentional exposures, often ingestions; workers with occupational exposures, often dermal and inhalational; and adolescents/young adults who intentionally abuse solvents through inhalation.

PHARMACOLOGY

Hydrocarbon use has a colorful history in medicine. Essential oils (or volatile oils) are typically fragrant hydrocarbon plant extracts. Examples are menthol, eucalyptus oil, clove oil, sassafras oil, and pennyroyal oil, among others. These oils have been used from antiquity for a variety of medicinal reasons, and are enjoying a resurgence with recent popularity of herbal supplements (Chap. 77). Mineral oil, castor oil, and glycerin are commonly used as laxatives. Hydrocarbon-based ointments, petroleum jelly, and camphor are used topically on skin and mucous membranes. Phenol and substituted phenols are common medical disinfectants (Chap. 84). Diethyl ether and halogenated hydrocarbon compounds such as chloroform were among the first general anesthetics; they were used more than 150 years ago.[143,190] Cyclopropane and TCE have been widely used as general anesthetics.[143]

The toxicity of inhaled hydrocarbon solvent vapors relates primarily to their ability to alter consciousness. In fact, acute central nervous system (CNS) toxicity of solvent vapors in the settings of occupational overexposure or inhalational abuse can be predicted with analogy to the pharmacology of inhaled general anesthetics.[198] The concentration of a volatile anesthetic that will produce loss of nociception in 50% of patients is defined as the minimum alveolar concentration (MAC) required to induce anesthesia. Inhaled solvent vapor similarly produces unconsciousness when the agent's partial pressure in the lung reaches its ED_{50}. Essentially all patients are anesthetized when the partial pressure is increased 30% above the MAC (MAC × 1.3). The dose-response curves suggest that essentially no individual is rendered unconscious by an inhaled dose 30% below the MAC. However, acute impairment of

cognitive and motor function may occur at much lower exposures.[24]

Lipid-soluble solvents, such as aromatic, aliphatic, or chlorinated hydrocarbons, are more likely to cause both acute and chronic CNS effects than are water-soluble hydrocarbons such as alcohols, ketones, and esters.[138] The property of an inhaled anesthetic that correlates most closely with its ability to extinguish nociception is its lipid solubility.[95] The Meyer-Overton hypothesis, proposed more than 100 years ago, implies that an anesthetic agent dissolves into some crucial lipid compartment of the CNS, causing inhibition of neuronal transmission.[143] Unfortunately, this hypothesis really correlates agent characteristics with efficacy more than it elucidates a mechanism of action. This relationship may simply reflect delivery of the agent to its effector site(s), and may have little bearing on the therapeutic or toxic mechanism within the CNS. On the other hand, the lack of specific structural similarities or functional groups between various hydrocarbons, all of which induce similar clinical CNS effects, implies a non-receptor-mediated mechanism of action. Nonspecific inhibition of neuronal transmission through membrane or membrane protein conformational changes may occur.[187,195]

At least some hydrocarbons may have specific cellular sites of action within the CNS.[17] Volatile anesthetics, for example, can affect ligand-gated ion channels. They interact with acetylcholine receptors to increase neurotransmitter binding[75] and to potentiate nicotinic blockade.[30] They stimulate γ-amino butyrate (GABA$_A$) activity,[135,154] as do toluene and trichloroethane (TCE),[22] and they inhibit GABA catabolism.[48] Some agents stimulate glutamate release.[103] Toluene, on the other hand, inhibits neurotransmission at glutamate N-methyl-D-aspartate receptors. Toluene and TCE enhance glycine receptor function. Prolonged exposure to toluene can perturb dopaminergic transmission.[22] General anesthetic effects are modulated by adenosine[192] and by central α$_2$-adrenergic agonism.[191] This line of mechanistic research suggests that the Meyer-Overton hypothesis may be too simplistic to explain the differences in pharmacologic profiles observed with this wide class of specific chemicals.

TOXICOKINETICS

Human toxicokinetic data are lacking for most hydrocarbons, and much of our understanding of the kinetics of this large family of chemicals comes from animal studies. Hydrocarbons are variably absorbed through ingestion, inhalation, or dermal routes of exposure, depending on their structure and chemical properties. Partition coefficients, in particular, are useful predictors of the rate and extent of the absorption and distribution of hydrocarbons into tissues. A partition coefficient for a given chemical is the ratio of concentrations achieved between two different media at equilibrium. The blood:air and tissue:air or tissue:blood coefficients directly relate to the pulmonary uptake and distribution of hydrocarbons. The tissue:blood partition coefficient is commonly determined by dividing the tissue:air coefficient by the blood:air coefficient.[81,172] Table 86–3 presents partition coefficients for commonly encountered hydrocarbons. Where human data are limited, rat data are presented in the table. However, human and rat data correlate closely.[172]

Inhalation is a major route of exposure for most volatile hydrocarbons. The dose through the respiratory route is determined by

TABLE 86–3. **Kinetic Parameters of Selected Hydrocarbons**

Agent	Partition Coefficients		$t_{1/2}$		Elimination	Relevant Metabolites
	Blood/Air	Fat/Air	α	β		
Aliphatics						
n-Hexane	2.29*	159*	11 min	99 min	10–20% exhaled; liver metabolism by P450	2–Hexanol, 2, 5-hexa-nedione, γ-valerolactone
Paraffin/tar	Not absorbed or metabolized					
Aromatics						
Benzene	8.19	499*	8 h	90 h	12% exhaled; liver metabolism to phenol	Phenol, catechol, hydroquinone, and conjugates
Toluene	18.0*	1021*	4–5 h	15–72 h	Extensive liver extraction and metabolism	80% metab. to benzyl alchol; 70% renally excreted as hippuric acid
o-Xylene	34.9	1877*	30–60 min	20–30 h	Liver P450 oxidation	Toluic acid, methyl hippuric acid
Halogenated						
Methylene chloride	8.94	120*	Apparent $t_{1/2}$ of COHb 13 h	40 min	92% exhaled unchanged. Low doses metabolized; high doses exhaled. Two liver metabolic pathways	(a) P4502E1 to CO and CO_2 (b) Glutathione transferase to CO_2, formaldehyde, formic acid
Carbon tetrachloride	2.73	359*	84–91 min*	91–496 min*	Liver P450, some lung exhalation (dose-dependent)	Trichloromethyl radical, trichloromethyl peroxy radical, phosgene
TCE	8.11	554*	3 h	30 h	Liver P450—epoxide intermediate; trichloroethanol is glucuronidated and excreted	Chloral hydrate, trichloroethanol, trichloroacetate
1, 1, 1- Trichloroethane	2.53	263*	44 min	53 h	91% exhaled; liver P450	Trichloroacetate, trichloroethanol
Tetrachloroethylene	10.3	1638*	160 min	33 h	80% exhaled; liver P450	Trichloroacetate, trichloroethanol

*Noted: Fat/blood partition coefficient is obtained by dividing the fat/air coefficient by the blood/air coefficient. As determined in rat models. All coefficients are determined at 37°C (98.6°F).

the air concentration, duration of exposure, minute ventilation, and the blood:air partition coefficient. Most hydrocarbons cross the alveolus through passive diffusion. The driving force for passive diffusion across the alveolus is the difference in vapor concentration between the alveolus and the blood. Hydrocarbons that are highly soluble in blood and tissues are readily absorbed through inhalation, and blood concentrations rise rapidly following inhalation exposure. Although aromatic hydrocarbons are generally well absorbed through inhalation, for aliphatic hydrocarbons, absorption through inhalation varies by molecular weight; aliphatic hydrocarbons with between 5 and 16 carbons are readily absorbed, whereas those with more than 16 carbons are not as readily absorbed.[3]

Absorption of aliphatic hydrocarbons through ingestion is inversely related to molecular weight, ranging from complete absorption at lower molecular weights to about 60% for C_{14} hydrocarbons, 5% for C_{28} hydrocarbons, and essentially no absorption for aliphatic hydrocarbons with >32 carbons.[3] Oral absorption of aromatic hydrocarbons with between 5 and 9 carbons ranges from 80% to 97%. Oral absorption data for aromatic hydrocarbons with greater than 9 carbons are limited. While some hydrocarbons can be absorbed from the gastrointestinal tract in amounts sufficient to produce systemic toxicity, it is imperative to weigh the oral toxicity (oral LD_{50}) of the hydrocarbon against the aspiration hazard (intratracheal LD_{50}) when considering gastric decontamination.

While the skin is a common area of contact with solvents, for most hydrocarbons the dose received from dermal exposure is a small fraction of the dose received through other routes, such as inhalation. The skin is composed of both hydrophilic (proteinaceous portion of cells) and lipophilic (cell membranes) regions. While many hydrocarbons can remove lipids from the stratum corneum, permeability is not simply a result of lipid removal; permeability is also increased with hydration of the skin. When compounds have near equality in the water/lipid partition coefficient, their rate of skin absorption is increased. Solvents that contain both hydrophobic and hydrophilic moieties (eg, glycol ethers, dimethylformamide, dimethylsulfoxide) are particularly well absorbed.[138] Other factors, in addition to the partition coefficient and permeability constant, that determine penetration across the skin include the thickness of the skin layer, the difference in concentration of the solvent on both sides of the epithelium, the diffusion constant, and skin integrity (ie, normal vs cut or abraded).

The dose received via skin absorption also depends on the surface area of the skin exposed and the duration of contact. Although highly volatile compounds may have a short duration of skin contact because of evaporation, skin absorption can also occur from contact with hydrocarbon vapor. In studies with human volunteers exposed to varying concentrations of hydrocarbon vapors, the dermal dose accounted for only 0.1–2% of the inhalation dose. With massive exposure (eg, immersion), dermal absorption may contribute significantly to toxicity.[94] Significant absorption with resultant toxicity has been described with carbon tetrachloride,[115] tetrachloroethylene,[94] and phenol.[134]

After they are absorbed into the central compartment, hydrocarbons are distributed to target and storage organs based on their tissue:blood partition coefficients and on the rate of perfusion of the tissue with blood. During the onset of systemic exposure, hydrocarbons accumulate in tissues, such as fat, that have coefficients between tissue and blood that are greater than 1 (eg, for toluene, the fat:blood partition coefficient is 60). Table 86–3 presents the distribution half-lives of selected hydrocarbons.

Hydrocarbons can be eliminated from the body unchanged, eg, through expired air, or can be metabolized to more polar compounds, which are then excreted through urine or bile. Table 86–3 presents the blood elimination half-lives (for first-order elimination processes) and metabolites of selected hydrocarbons. Some hydrocarbons are metabolized to toxic metabolites (eg, methylene chloride, carbon tetrachloride, n-hexane, methyl-n-butyl ketone). The specific toxicities of these metabolites are discussed under "Special Cases," later in this chapter.

PATHOPHYSIOLOGY

Pulmonary

For years, the medical literature held the stage for debate over the pathogenesis of lung injury after hydrocarbon exposure. Early investigators debated whether pulmonary toxicity was caused by gastrointestinal absorption of hydrocarbons with subsequent pulmonary toxicity, or caused by direct aspiration into pulmonary parenchyma.[28,60,66,82,105,133,177,180,233] The rat and baboon models made it clear that hydrocarbons are absorbed in the gastrointestinal tract and can be recovered from lung and many other tissues.[15,140] Based upon the amounts absorbed in these animal studies, however, the volume of ingested hydrocarbon needed to cause pulmonary toxicity is enormous. A number of other animal models (dogs, monkeys, and baboons) employing gastric instillation of hydrocarbon demonstrated lack of pulmonary toxicity when aspiration did not occur.[63,105,242,248] It is currently held that aspiration is the main route of injury from ingested hydrocarbons.

The mechanism of pulmonary injury, however, is not completely understood. Intratracheal instillation of small amounts (0.2 mL/kg) of kerosene causes physiologic abnormalities in lung mechanics (decreased compliance and total lung capacity) and pathologic changes such as interstitial inflammation, polymorphonuclear exudates, intra-alveolar edema and hemorrhage, hyperemia, bronchial and bronchiolar necrosis, and vascular thrombosis.[82,83,92,100,184,185] These changes most likely reflect both direct toxicity to pulmonary tissue and disruption of the lipid surfactant layer.[86,193,240]

Several factors are associated with pulmonary toxicity after hydrocarbon ingestion. These include specific physical properties of the hydrocarbon ingested (Table 86–2) and historical information involving the volume ingested and the occurrence of vomiting. The properties of *viscosity*, *surface tension*, and *volatility* of a particular hydrocarbon are the main determinants of its aspiration potential (Table 86–2).[84,105]

Viscosity is the measurement of a fluid's resistance to flow. *Kinematic viscosity* is the absolute viscosity divided by the fluid's density, usually expressed in stokes or in centistokes (mm^2/sec).

One method of quantifying viscosity is by the agent's rate of flow through a calibrated orifice. This is measured in Saybolt seconds universal (SSU). At a given temperature, viscosity values can be converted from SI units of kinematic viscosity (eg, the stoke or the centistoke) to SSU. Substances with low viscosities (SSU <60: turpentine, gasoline, naphtha) are associated with a higher tendency for aspiration in animal models. The US Consumer Products Safety Commission (CPSC) is currently considering proposing the labeling of hydrocarbon products as an aspiration hazard if the viscosity is <100 SSU; the European Union defines aspiration risk as <45 SSU.

Surface tension is a cohesive force generated by attraction— van der Waals forces—between molecules.[170] This influences adherence of a liquid compound along a surface ("its inability to creep"), and is measured using a modified Wilhelmy balance.[105] In theory, the lower the surface tension, the higher the aspiration risk.[84,105]

Volatility is the tendency for a liquid to become a gas. Hydrocarbons with high volatility tend to vaporize, displace oxygen, and lead to transient hypoxia.

It is not clear which of the physical properties of the hydrocarbon is most important in predicting toxicity. Several studies have examined the risk of pulmonary toxicity relative to the amount of hydrocarbon ingested, with or without vomiting. Some authors have found an association between the volume ingested and risk for pulmonary toxicity, whereas other authors have not.[21,26,55] Similar discrepancies hold for presence of vomiting.[21,26,39,164,166] Moreover, the validity of these studies has been questioned because of retrospective methodology and poor response rates regarding the volume ingested. Only one prospective study addressed these issues: the Co-Operative Kerosene Poisoning Study (COKP). Forty-six hospitals participated in this series of 760 cases. Of these, 54% had clear estimates of the amount ingested. Twenty-nine percent of patients reportedly ingested more than 30 mL of hydrocarbon, 35% ingested 10–30 mL, and 35% ingested less than 10 mL. No association was found between amount of hydrocarbon ingested and the age of the patient. In patients who ingested more than 30 mL, there was a 52% chance of developing pulmonary complications.[173] Those patients who ingested this amount of hydrocarbon were found to have a higher chance of developing central nervous system complications than did those who ingested less than 30 mL. Regarding spontaneous vomiting, the cooperative study was able to provide data on only 273 of the 760 patients. There was a 54% incidence of pulmonary toxicity when vomiting occurred, and a 39% incidence of pulmonary toxicity when there was no history of vomiting.[173] Although these features may be useful for predicting the possibility of hydrocarbon-induced pulmonary toxicity, none of these parameters are 100% predictive. Serious poisoning is less likely with agents that have higher viscosity and higher surface tension, such as mineral oil. However, severe hydrocarbon pneumonitis has been associated with "low-risk" hydrocarbons as well.[183] Furthermore, patients have been severely injured with low-volume (<5 mL) ingestions, as well as by ingestions without a history of coughing, gagging, or vomiting.[10]

Intravenous (IV) and subcutaneous injections of hydrocarbons are reported.[224,226] Severe hydrocarbon pneumonitis may occur following intravenous exposure. Animal experiments show that intravascular hydrocarbons injure the first capillary bed encountered.[28] Intravenous injection expectedly causes pulmonary toxicity, and portal vein injection leads to direct hepatic injury.[28,60,105,180,244,248] The clinical course after IV hydrocarbon injection mirrors that of aspiration injury.

Cardiac

Exposure to hydrocarbons may cause cardiotoxicity. Halogenated hydrocarbons and benzene are most frequently implicated, although toluene and gasoline may also induce dysrhythmias.[19] Atrial fibrillation, ventricular fibrillation, and sudden cardiac death are reported.[90,163,178] Myocardial depression occurs by an unclear mechanism.[11] A canine model demonstrated ventricular premature beats and/or ventricular fibrillation after inhalation of trichloroethane followed by intravenous injection of epinephrine.[179] Dysrhythmia-induced sudden death, termed the "sudden sniffing death syndrome," is well-described after inhalation of chlorinated hydrocarbons, but also for aromatic compounds.[126] Classically, sudden death occurs after an episode of sudden exertion.[20,78,178] The mechanism of dysrhythmia induction appears to be sensitization of the myocardium to endogenous catecholamines.[20,78,126,178,179] Tachydysrhythmias, cardiomegaly, and myocardial infarction are uncommonly reported after exposure by ingestion.[111,204] A retrospective followup cohort of exposed methylene chloride workers did not find evidence of excess long-term cardiac disease.[168]

Central Nervous System

The specific mechanism of CNS depression from hydrocarbon intoxication is unclear. It is enticing to propose that specific channel inactivation or stimulation of inhibitory channels is responsible (see "Pharmacology" section earlier in this chapter). To date, however, no unifying theory or evidentiary support for specific receptor binding explains the acute CNS impairment seen with either volatile anesthetic or other hydrocarbon inhalation. In cases of hydrocarbon aspiration, hypoxia from pulmonary damage may contribute to the CNS depression.[140,245]

The CNS toxicity of chronic toluene abuse is well described, and illustrates the ability of some hydrocarbons to produce pathologic changes in the CNS. Prolonged, moderate-to-heavy exposure to hydrocarbons, as seen in volatile solvent abuse, can lead to irreversible CNS damage. The primary pathologic process is white matter degeneration, or *leukoencephalopathy*. Autopsy studies of the brains of chronic toluene abusers show profound atrophy and mottling of the white matter. Microscopic examination shows a consistent pattern of myelin and oligodendrocyte loss with relative preservation of axons.[125] Animal studies of toluene poisoning also reveal biochemical changes, including diminished norepinephrine and dopamine concentrations, and alterations in various neurotransmitter levels.[186]

Peripheral Nervous System

Peripheral neuropathy is well described following occupational exposure to *n*-hexane or methyl-*n*-butyl ketone (MnBK).[27] Methyl ethyl ketone (MEK) may exacerbate this neurotoxicity, probably by interfering with metabolic pathways of *n*-hexane and MnBK but MEK is not itself neurotoxic.[8,182] This toxic axonopathy appears to be caused by a common metabolic intermediate—2,5-hexanedione. The mechanism by which this intermediate causes peripheral neuropathy may relate to decreased phosphorylation of neurofilament proteins, with disruption of the axonal cytoskeleton (see "Special Cases" later in this chapter). Other organic solvents, such as carbon disulfide, acrylamide, and ethylene oxide, may cause a similar peripheral axonopathy.[89]

Cranial and peripheral neuropathies have been reported after acute and chronic exposure to TCE.[37,117,132,213] Pathologically, TCE appears to induce myelinopathy, rather than the axonopathy that occurs with hexane or MnBK.[71,89]

Hepatic

Chlorinated hydrocarbons (Table 86–2) are particularly hepatotoxic. In most cases, this occurs via Phase I activation to a reactive intermediate (Chap. 14). In the case of carbon tetrachloride, this intermediate is the trichloromethyl radical. This toxic metabolite forms covalent bonds with hepatic macromolecules, and may initiate lipid peroxidation.[29] Hepatic injury, manifested as aminotransferase elevation and hepatomegaly, is usually reversible, except in massive overexposures (see "Special Cases" later in this chapter). Hepatotoxicity in animals has been ranked for common hydrocarbons as follows: carbon tetrachloride >> benzene, trichloroethylene > pentane.[241]

Dermal

Most hydrocarbon solvents cause nonspecific irritation of the skin and mucous membranes. Repeated, prolonged contact can dry and crack the skin. Contact dermatitis and blistering may progress to partial and even full-thickness burns.[96] Severity is proportional to duration of exposure. The mechanism of dermal injury appears to be defatting of the lipid layer of the stratum corneum. As many as 9% of workers may develop eczematous lesions from dermal contact.[249] Limonene and turpentine contain sensitizers that rarely can result in contact allergy (Chap. 29).

Immunologic

Hydrocarbons disturb the integrity of membrane lipid bilayers, causing swelling and increased permeability to protons and other ions. This alters the structural and functional integrity of the membrane. Changes in the lipid composition of the membrane occur, and membrane lipopolysaccharides and proteins are disturbed.[195] Resultant toxicity may directly destroy capillary endothelium.[28] Additionally, there appears to be derangement of basement membranes, which is postulated to underlie both alveolar and glomerular toxicity of hydrocarbons.[206] Immune mechanisms may account for basement membrane dysfunction in chronic exposures. In fact, inhalation of hydrocarbons is linked to Goodpasture syndrome (immune dysfunction causing both pulmonary damage and glomerulonephritis).[25]

CLINICAL MANIFESTATIONS
Pulmonary

Most patients who develop pulmonary toxicity after hydrocarbon ingestion have an episode of coughing, gagging, and choking. This occurs shortly after ingestion, usually within 30 minutes, and is presumptive evidence of aspiration.[141] Absence of tachypnea on initial evaluation has an 80% negative predictive value for aspiration pneumonitis.[234] More severely affected patients may rapidly develop progressive pulmonary toxicity over the subsequent hours to days. Pulmonary toxicity manifests as rales, rhonchi, bronchospasm, tachypnea, hypoxemia, hemoptysis, pulmonary edema (hemorrhagic or nonhemorrhagic), or signs of respiratory distress.[220] Cyanosis develops in approximately 2–3% of patients.[147] This may be a consequence of simple asphyxiant effects from volatilized hydrocarbons, ventilation-perfusion mismatch, or, rarely, a result of methemoglobinemia (aniline, nitrobenzene, nitrite-containing hydrocarbons). Clinical findings often worsen over several days, but typically resolve within 5–7 days. Death is rare (<2%), and is typically caused by severe progressive respiratory insult marked by hypoxia, ventilation-perfusion mismatch, and barotrauma.[20,69,102,146,199,232,252]

Radiographic evidence of pneumonitis develops in 40–88% of admitted patients.[18,21,26,66,133,166,177] Findings can develop as early as 15 minutes or as late as 24 hours after exposure (Fig. 86–2).[55,79,100,118,173,228] Ninety percent of patients who develop radiographic abnormalities develop evidence of pneumonitis by 4 hours postingestion.[55] The majority of patients who have respiratory signs and symptoms beyond the initial history of gagging, choking, and coughing develop radiographic pneumonitis.[10] Clinical signs of pneumonia (rales, rhonchi, and so on) are evident in 40–50% of patients.[66] A small percentage (<5%) will be completely asymptomatic after a period of observation but have radiographic findings.[10] Chest radiographs performed immediately on initial presentation are not useful in predicting pneumonia in either symptomatic or asymptomatic patients.[234]

Specific radiologic findings include perihilar densities, bronchovascular markings, bibasilar infiltrates, and pneumonic consolidation.[18,85] Right-sided involvement occurs in 75% of cases, and bilateral involvement in approximately 50% of cases. Upper lobe involvement is uncommon.[18,33,101] Pleural effusions develop in 3% of cases,[144] with one-third appearing within 24 hours. Pneumothorax, pneumomediastinum, and pneumatoceles are uncommonly reported.[16,23,41,64,130,189,243] Initial radiographs after ingestion may reveal two liquid densities in the stomach, known as the "double-bubble" sign.[56] This represents an air-fluid and a hydrocarbon-water interface, as the hydrocarbon is not miscible with gastric fluids (primarily water) and may have a specific gravity less than water.

Radiographic changes often progress over several days, typically reaching a maximum at 5–7 days with resolution over several weeks. Radiographic resolution does not correlate with clinical improvement, usually lagging behind by several days to weeks.[82] Long-term followup in patients with hydrocarbon pneumonitis is limited.[33,79,93,177,216,224] Frequent respiratory tract infections are described in individuals after hydrocarbon pneumonitis, but these studies are poorly controlled.[79,178,220] Bronchiectasis and pulmonary fibrosis are reported, but appear to be uncommon.[89,145,177] In one study, 82% of patients seen 8–14 years after hydrocarbon-induced pneumonitis had asymptomatic minor pulmonary function abnormalities.[93] The abnormalities were consistent with small-airway obstruction and loss of elastic recoil. The authors hypothesized that this group may be predisposed to chronic obstructive pulmonary disease.

Cardiac

The most worrisome cardiotoxicity associated with hydrocarbon exposure is that of myocardial sensitization and dysrhythmias.[19,179] This phenomenon is well described for halogenated hydrocarbons, and less so for aromatic compounds. Sudden death can occur after exposure to high concentrations of volatile inhalants or inhaled anesthetics, apparently resulting from tachydysrhythmias (see "Pathophysiology" section earlier in this chapter).

Central Nervous System

Transient CNS excitation may occur initially after acute hydrocarbon inhalation or ingestion.[126] More commonly, CNS depression or general anesthesia occurs; it may be profound.[66] Coma and seizures are reported in 1–3% of cases.[133,166,177,251] Chronic occupational exposure or volatile substance abuse may lead to a chronic neurobehavioral syndrome—painter's syndrome—most completely described after chronic toluene overexposure. The clinical features include ataxia, spasticity, dysarthria, and dementia, consistent with a leukoencephalopathic syndrome.[73] The severity and reversibility of this syndrome depend on the intensity and duration of toluene abuse.[186] Infrequent exposure may produce no clinical neurologic signs, whereas heavy (eg, daily) use can lead to significant neurologic impairment after as little as 1 year, but more commonly after 2–4 years of use. The specific cognitive and neuropsychologic findings in toluene-induced dementia have been termed a "white matter dementia."[73]

Initial findings include behavioral changes, impaired sense of smell, impaired concentration, and mild unsteadiness of hand movements and gait. Further exposure leads to slurred speech, head tremor, poor vision, deafness, stiff-legged and staggering gait, and dementia. Physical findings can include nystagmus, ataxic tremor, spasticity with hyperreflexia and abnormal Babinski reflexes, deafness, impaired vision, and a broad-based, staggering gait. An abnormal brainstem auditory-evoked response (BAER) appears to be a sensitive indicator of toluene-induced CNS damage. Electroencephalograms can show mild, diffuse slowing. Computed tomography in severe cases shows mild to moderate cerebellar and cortical atrophy. MRI findings are consistent with white matter disease. Chronic toluene use is addictive and can produce withdrawal. Most cases show significant clinical improvement after 6 months of abstinence, although with moderate to severe abuse, improvement may not be complete.[186]

In the occupational setting, exposures are rarely as high as those seen with volatile substance abuse. Given the significantly lower exposures, the findings among workers overexposed to solvents (ie, exposed above permissible exposure limits) are often subclinical, and detected primarily through neurobehavioral testing. In rare cases, however, a worker may be acutely overexposed to solvent concentrations that can produce central nervous system depression. Repeated symptomatic overexposures over long periods of time have the potential to lead to a chronic encephalopathy as evident from the experience with solvent abusers.

Peripheral Nervous System

Peripheral neuropathy may occur after exposure to *n*-hexane or MnBK, and possibly to toluene.[27,99,121,211] The axonopathy typically begins in the distal extremities and progresses proximally (a classic "dying-back" neuropathy), and should be considered in the assessment and differential diagnosis of the patient with Guillian-Barré syndrome.[196] The longest axons appear to be affected initially, so that the patient manifests a "length-dependent polyneuropathy." With discontinuation of exposure many of the effects reverse over weeks to months.[101,121,174,250] However, the phenomenon of "coasting" may occur, in which neuropathy progresses for a time (weeks to months) after discontinuation of the toxic insult.[196] A reversible peripheral neuropathy occurring in 40% of

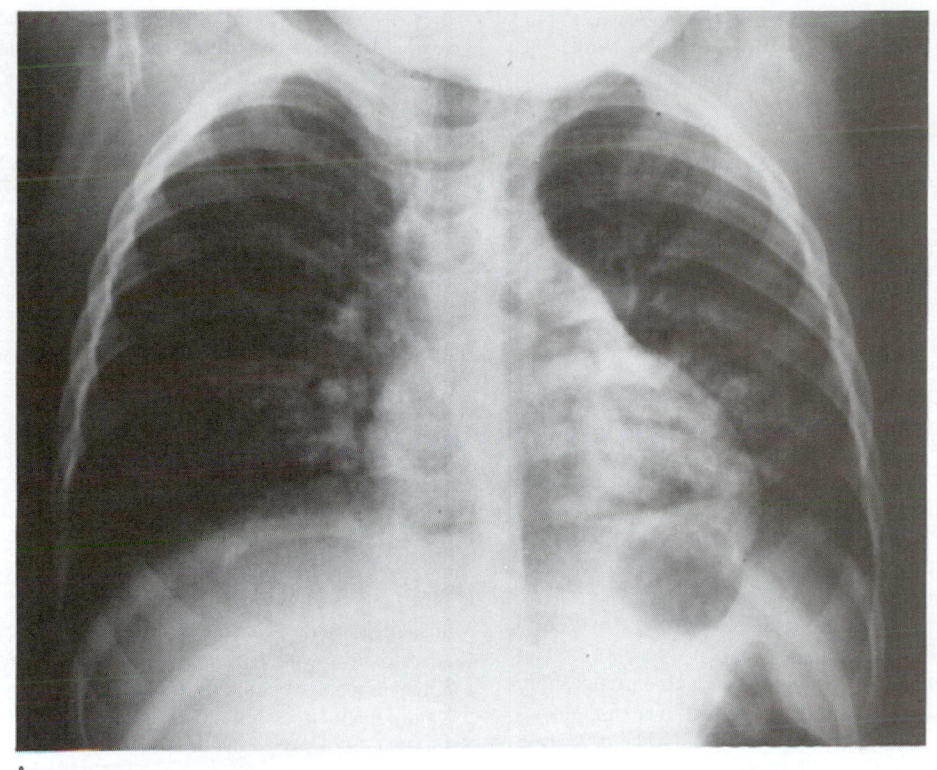

A

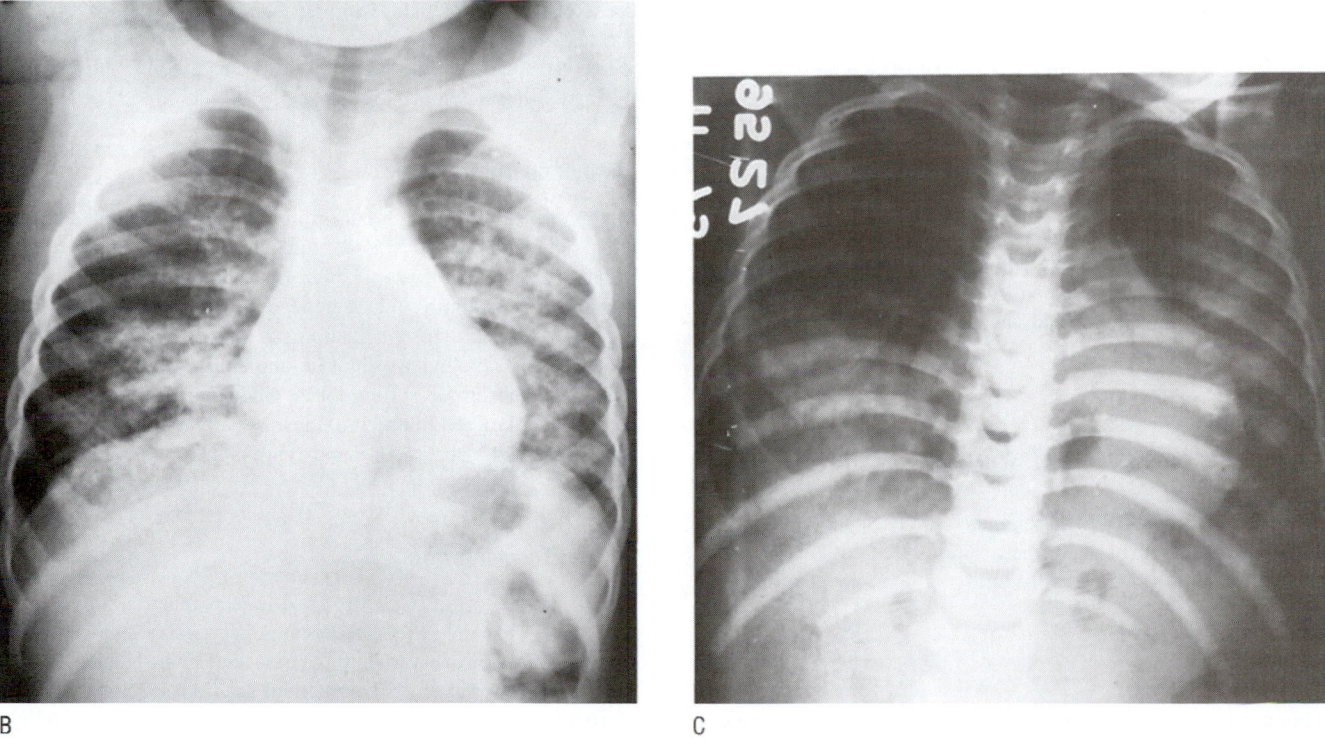

B

C

Figure 86–2. Three sequential radiographs of a young girl with severe hydrocarbon aspiration pneumonitis. **A.** Initial: Patchy densities appear in basilar areas of both lung fields with increased interstitial markings and peribronchial thickening. **B.** Day 2: More extensive diffuse alveolar infiltrates are apparent. **C.** Day 6: Dense consolidation and atelectasis are evident in the right lower lobe. *(Courtesy of Nancy Genieser, MD, Professor of Radiology, New York University.)*

chronic toluene abusers is manifested by severe motor weakness, without sensory deficits or areflexia.[211] It is unclear whether the toluene in these early series may have been contaminated by *n*-hexane or by MnBK.[8,197]

Trichloroethylene is associated with trigeminal neuralgia.[37,46,70,132] Trigeminal nerve damage was documented by evoked potentials following 15 minutes of TCE inhalation.[132] Some evidence suggests that decomposition products or impurities in TCE may be responsible for cranial neuropathy.[46,70]

Gastrointestinal

Hydrocarbons are irritants to the gastrointestinal mucous membranes. Nausea and vomiting are common after ingestion. As discussed earlier, vomiting may be associated with increased risk of pulmonary toxicity.[26,164,166,183] Hematemesis can occur, and was reported in 5% of cases in one study.[164] Gastrointestinal ulcerations have been found in animal studies.[15,122]

Hepatic

Hepatic injury may occur after exposure to halogenated hydrocarbons, particularly carbon tetrachloride. Carbon tetrachloride can produce fatal centrilobular necrosis by inhalational, oral ingestion, or dermal exposure.[149] Vinyl chloride is a known liver carcinogen. Trichloroethylene, tetrachloroethylene, and 1,1,1-trichloroethane are considered less hepatotoxic.[149,218] Hepatotoxicity may uncommonly follow ingestion of petroleum distillates.[114] Aminotransferase elevation typically resolves with cessation of exposure, except in extreme poisoning.

Renal

Halogenated hydrocarbons are also nephrotoxic. Examples include chloroform, carbon tetrachloride, ethylene dichloride, tetrachloroethane, and 1,1,1-trichloroethane. Acute renal failure and distal renal tubular acidosis occur in some painters and volatile substance abusers especially those who use toluene.[120,214] Toluene may precipitate a renal tubular acidosis (see "Special Cases" later in this chapter). Human studies of nephrotoxicity are confounded by other exposures, and the findings in animal studies are conflicting.[2]

Hematologic

Hemolysis has been sporadically reported to occur after hydrocarbon ingestion.[1,7,209] One retrospective study of 12 patients showed hemolysis in 3 patients and disseminated intravascular coagulation in another patient.[7] Although one of these three patients required transfusion, hemolysis is usually mild and does not require RBC transfusion.

Dermatologic

Hydrocarbons are irritating to skin. Acute, prolonged exposure can cause dermatitis, as well as full-thickness burns.[96] Chronic exposure to kerosene or diesel fuel can cause oil folliculitis.[57,224] A specific skin lesion called *chloracne* is associated with exposure to chlorinated aromatic hydrocarbons with highly specific stereochemistry (eg, dioxins, polychlorinated biphenyls). "Degreaser's flush," is a disulfiramlike reaction associated with concomitant ethanol and trichloroethylene exposure.

Soft-tissue injection of hydrocarbon is locally toxic, leading to necrosis. Secondary cellulitis, abscess formation, and fasciitis can occur. Infectious complications are treated by meticulous wound care, with surgical débridement as necessary. A particularly destructive injury involves high-pressure injection gun injury. These injuries typically involve the extremities, with high-pressure injection of grease or paint into the fascial planes and tendon sheaths. Emergent surgical débridement is necessary in most of these cases.[72,159]

SPECIAL CASES

n-Hexane

Hexane is a six-carbon simple aliphatic hydrocarbon. The straight-chain isomer, normal hexane or *n*-hexane, is rarely used commercially because of its toxicity. However, it is a contaminant of many hydrocarbon mixtures, including commercial-grade gasoline. It is also used as the solvent in rubber cement preparations, which may contain up to 90% *n*-hexane. Human exposure occurs primarily by inhalation. Both *n*-hexane and MnBK are well-known peripheral neurotoxins, which cause a classic "dying-back" peripheral polyneuropathy, beginning in a "stocking-glove" distribution.[27,47] Neurotoxicity does not appear to be directly caused by the parent compounds; rather, it results from a common metabolic intermediate—2,5-hexanedione. Toxicity appears related to the ability of this intermediate to form a ringed pyrrole structure, which causes decreased phosphorylation of neurofilament proteins, disrupting the axonal cytoskeleton.[88] Similar five-, six-, and seven-carbon species do not induce similar neurotoxicity, except those which are direct precursor intermediates in the metabolic pathway producing 2,5-hexanedione (Fig. 19–2).[88,215]

Methylene Chloride

Methylene chloride is perhaps most commonly encountered in paint removers, but it is also found in cleaning and degreasing agents, and in aerosol propellants. Like other halogenated hydrocarbons, it can rapidly induce general anesthesia by inhalation or ingestion. Myocardial sensitization can occur. Unlike other hydrocarbon agents, methylene chloride and similar halomethanes (eg, methylene dibromide, bromoform, chloroform) are metabolized by liver P450 mixed function oxidase to carbon monoxide. Significant, delayed, and prolonged carboxyhemoglobinemia may occur[4,62,176,205,208] (Table 86–3).

Carbon Tetrachloride

Carbon tetrachloride (CCl_4) is used as an industrial solvent and reagent. Its use in the United States has declined dramatically since recognition of its toxicity caused the Environmental Protection Agency to restrict its commercial use.[3] Absorption occurs by all routes. It is an irritant to skin and mucous membranes, and is a potent gastric irritant when ingested. As with other halogenated hydrocarbons, aspiration can result in pneumonitis, and systemic absorption may result in ventricular dysrhythmias.[65]

More unique to CCl_4 exposures are hepatotoxicity and nephrotoxicity. Both occur more commonly with repetitive exposure (eg, occupational exposures).[49,217] Carbon tetrachloride is likely the most hepatotoxic of the known hydrocarbons. Hepatotoxicity may even occur following dermal exposure.[115] Toxicity is believed to follow Phase I activation of the parent compound, with free radical formation and subsequent lipid peroxidation and production of protein adducts.[29] Localization of specific Phase I hepatic enzymes in the centrilobular area of the liver results in regionalized (Zone 3) centrilobular injury after CCl_4 exposure (Chap. 14). Hepatotoxicity is typically manifested as reversible aminotransferase elevation with or without hepatomegaly. Cirrhosis is reported in both animal models and in humans with prolonged overexposures. Nephrotoxicity is less well studied, but may result from a similar mechanism.[34] The proximal convoluted tubule and the loop of Henle appear to be specifically targeted.[74] Carbon tetrachloride is a suspected human carcinogen.[3]

Benzene

Benzene is hematotoxic, and is associated with hemolysis, aplastic anemia, and acute myelogenous leukemia.[5,127,148,171] Aplastic anemia may be delayed.[87] Other aromatic hydrocarbons have been reported to cause similar hematologic effects in animals. These effects are most likely caused by benzene contamination of the other compounds. An excess risk has not been demonstrated in groups with long-term exposure to toluene, xylene, or other aromatic hydrocarbons.[14,59,181,229,239] Other hematologic malignancies may be linked to benzene as well, including chronic myelocytic leukemia, myelodysplastic syndromes, and lymphoma.[219] Chromosomal changes are believed to provide a marker for carcinogenicity.[223] Because of the carcinogenic risk, most benzene-based solvents have been unilaterally removed from the US market, and the Occupational Safety and Health Administration (OSHA) has limited the permissible worker exposure level to 1 part per million.[106]

Toluene

Toluene has essentially replaced benzene as the primary solvent in many commercial products such as oil paints and stains. As such, it is readily available and heavily abused as an inhalant. The CNS sequelae of chronic solvent inhalation are most frequently related to chronic toluene exposure (see above).

Chronic toluene abuse can cause transient distal renal tubular acidosis (RTA). Although the mechanism of this RTA is incompletely understood, a significant contributor to the metabolic acidosis is the formation of hippuric acid[43,119] (Table 86–3). Continued sodium loss in the urine may transform the initial nongap metabolic acidosis into a positive anion gap metabolic acidosis.[43] Renal potassium loss may be severe, and can result in symptomatic hypokalemia.[119] In one series, distal RTA was seen in 44% of hospitalized paint sniffers.[230] Clinical findings are a hyperchloremic metabolic acidosis, hypokalemia, and aciduria. There is typically an associated transient renal azotemia, as well as proteinuria and an active urine sediment.[211,230] Rarely, proximal RTA or the Fanconi syndrome may occur.[158,230] The metabolic acidosis is believed to be multifactorial, involving RTA, accumulation of toluene metabolites, and tissue hypoxia.

Pine Oil and Terpenes

Pine oil is an active ingredient in many household cleaning products. It is a mixture of unsaturated hydrocarbons comprised of terpenes, camphenes, and pinenes. The major components are terpenes, which are found in plants and flowers. Wood distillates are products derived from pine trees and include pine oil and turpentine. Patients who ingest pine oil often emit a strong pine odor. Wood distillates are readily absorbed, and ingestion may cause CNS and pulmonary toxicity.

Toxicity after gastrointestinal absorption appears to be limited.[31,53,68,109,124,200,201] Aspiration pneumonitis remains the primary clinical concern. Acute toxicity is similar to that of petroleum distillate ingestion, and management is similar. Rare reported complications of wood distillate ingestion include turpentine-associated thrombocytopenic purpura, acute renal failure, and hemorrhagic cystitis.[128,231]

Tar and Asphalt Injuries

Tar and asphalt injuries are common occupational hazards among construction workers. These hot hydrocarbon mixtures can cause severe cutaneous burns. The material quickly hardens and is very difficult to remove. Immediate cooling with cold water is important to limit further thermal injury. Complete removal is essential to ensure proper burn management and to limit infectious complications. Attempts to mechanically remove hardened tar or asphalt often cause further damage. Dissolving the material with mineral oil, petroleum jelly, or antibacterial ointments (Neosporin, Polysporin) has met with variable success. Surface-acting agents combined with an ointment (De-Solv-it, Tween-80, Polysorbate 80) are more effective.[61,210,222]

Asphalt workers are additionally at risk for toxic gas exposure. Roofing asphalt is typically cooled in large ventilated tanks into which the asphalt releases a number of toxic gases. Without proper dispersion of these gases, high concentrations of hydrogen sulfide, carbon monoxide, propane, methane, and volatilized hydrocarbons may accumulate with potential for overexposure.[104]

Volatile Inhalant Abuse

Aromatic and short-chained hydrocarbons readily volatilize at room temperature. Inhalation of the hydrocarbon vapors is rapidly intoxicating, and products containing these hydrocarbons are inexpensive and readily and legally obtainable. They are commonly abused by adolescents and young adults.[202,212] The hydrocarbon is typically poured into a container for *sniffing*, into a rag or sock for *huffing*, or into a plastic/paper bag for *bagging*. The concentration of inhaled hydrocarbon increases from sniffing to huffing to bagging. Consequently, abusers often begin with sniffing lower concentrations and progress to huffing and bagging with higher levels of exposure.[136] Volatilized hydrocarbons are readily absorbed in the alveoli and rapidly distribute to the CNS. One or two huffs will begin to intoxicate the user in several seconds, and the effects persist for several minutes. Chronic users can maintain a prolonged high with periodic inhalations every few hours. Some chronic abusers maintain the high throughout their waking hours over years of abuse.

Many types of inhalants are abused (Table 86–4). However, the most commonly abused inhalants are toluene from paints and adhesives, gasoline, butane from cigarette lighter fluids, butyl and isobutyl nitrite, and halogenated hydrocarbons from typewriter correction fluids, propellants, and dry-cleaning fluids.[50,51,77,136,167,202]

The most concerning emergent toxicities from volatile inhalant abuse are cardiac and neurologic.[44,45] Central nervous system effects include stupor, lethargy, excitation, agitation, hallucinations (auditory and visual), seizures, ataxia, headache, dizziness, nys-

TABLE 86–4. Composition of Abused Hydrocarbon Solvents

Inhalant	Chemical Constituents
Acrylic paint	Toluene
Aerosol propellant	Fluorocarbons (chlorodifluoromethane, dichlorodifluoromethane), trichlorofluoromethane, nitrous oxide
Anesthetics	Enflurane, halothane, isoflurane, nitrous oxide
Dyes	Acetone, methylene chloride
Fire extinguishing agent	Bromochlorodifluoromethane (BCF)
Gas (bottled), torches	Propane, butane, acetylene
Gasoline	Hydrocarbons
Glues/adhesives	Toluene, benzene, xylene, acetone, naphtha, *n*-hexane, trichlorethylene, ethyl acetate, tetrachloroethylene, trichloroethane, carbon tetrachloride, methylethyl ketone
Lighter fluid	Butane
Nail polish remover	Acetone, amyl acetate, isopropanol
Paint stripper	Methylene chloride
Paints/varnishes/lacquers	Trichloroethylene, toluene, mineral spirits
Polystyrene cements	Acetone, toluene, trichloroethylene, *n*-hexane
Refrigerants	Flourochloromethanes
Rubber cement	Benzene, *n*-hexane, trichloroethylene
Shoe polish	Chlorinated hydrocarbons, toluene
Solvent (laboratory)	Carbon tetrachloride, chloroform, diethyl ether, *n*-hexane, methyl isobutyl ketone
Spot remover	Trichloroethane, trichloroethylene, carbon tetrachloride
Typewriter correction fluid	Trichloroethane, trichloroethylene, perchloroethylene

Modified, with permission, from Meredith TJ, Ruprah M, Liddle A, Flanagan RJ: Diagnosis and treatment of acute poisoning with volatile substances. Human Toxicol 1989: 8:277–286; and Wyse DG: Deliberate inhalation of volatile hydrocarbons: A review. Can Med Assoc J 1973;108:71–74.

tagmus, and respiratory depression.[202] Cardiac effects are the most acutely hazardous. High concentrations of hydrocarbons sensitize the myocardium to catecholamines, producing dysrhythmias and sudden death.[20,78,178,179] Less common acute effects include methemoglobinemia from amyl and isobutyl nitrites,[44,51,54] carbon monoxide toxicity from methylene chloride,[62,176,205,208] hepatitis from chlorinated hydrocarbons, and muscle weakness, metabolic acidosis, rhabdomyolysis, renal tubular acidosis, and hypokalemia from toluene.[52,67,76,131,150,211,214] Lead poisoning associated with gasoline abuse was associated with the prior use of tetraethyl lead.[80] The incidence of lead toxicity from gasoline has decreased substantially with the reduction of lead content in gasoline (Chap. 80).

DIAGNOSTIC TESTING

Laboratory and ancillary testing for hydrocarbon toxicity should be guided by available information regarding the specific agent, the route of exposure, and the best attempt at quantifying the exposure. Inhalation or ingestion of hydrocarbons associated with pulmonary aspiration is most likely to result in pulmonary toxicity. The use of pulse oximetry and arterial blood gas testing is clinically indicated. Timing and interpretation of radiographic studies is addressed above under "Clinical Manifestations." Early radiography may be prognostically indicated in patients who are severely symptomatic; however, radiographs performed immediately after hydrocarbon ingestion demonstrate a low predictive value for the occurrence of aspiration pneumonitis. In the asymptomatic patient, early radiography is not cost-effective. Patients observed for 6 hours after an ingestion who demonstrate no abnormal pulmonary findings, who have adequate oxygenation, who are not tachypneic, and who have a normal chest film after the observa-

tion period have a good prognosis with very low risk of subsequent deterioration.[10,234]

Specific diagnostic testing for hydrocarbon poisoning can include (a) bioassays for the specific hydrocarbon or its metabolites in blood, breath, or urine or (b) assessment of toxicity or function of the hydrocarbon's target organ. Bioassays for a hydrocarbon are seldom necessary for diagnosis or management of hydrocarbon poisoning in the emergency setting. Exceptions may include testing to assist in differential diagnosis (eg, testing for carbon tetrachloride in a comatose patient with unexplained hepatorenal syndrome or a carboxyhemoglobin determination in a paint stripper with chest pain), testing for worker compensation purposes (eg, testing for urinary trichloroethanol and trichloroacetic acid in a worker exposed to trichloroethylene with unexplained bouts of dizziness), or for forensic purposes (eg, sudden death in a huffer).

When deciding whether to obtain a bioassay for a hydrocarbon, the clinician should determine: (a) What is the most informative biologic sample (blood, urine, breath) and how should it be collected, handled, and stored? (b) What are the kinetics of the hydrocarbon and the timing of exposure, and how should the results be interpreted in light of these kinetics? and (c) What ranges of concentrations are associated with toxicity? Only a few, specialized clinical laboratories perform most hydrocarbon bioassays. The analytic laboratory toxicologist can often assist the clinician in determining the appropriate choice and timing of a bioassay. Table 86–3 provides useful information on the elimination kinetics of selected hydrocarbons and on their common metabolites.

The choice of specific diagnostic laboratory tests to assess organ system toxicity or function depends on the type, dose, and route of exposure and on the assessment of the patient's clinical condition. Depending on the above, useful tests may include pulse oximetry, arterial blood gases, chest radiograph, electrocardiogram, electrolytes, and/or CPK. Acute poisoning with benzene has been reported to produce an altered electroencephalogram (EEG) pattern (paroxysmal slow waves).[169] If a hydrocarbon has specific target organ toxicities (eg, benzene/bone marrow, carbon tetrachloride/liver, or *n*-hexane/peripheral nervous system), evaluation and monitoring of target organ system function is indicated.

Chronic overexposures to hydrocarbons, as occur with volatile substance abuse, can result in persistent damage to the central nervous system. In addition to the clinical and mental status exam, this damage can be detected using neuroimaging methods such as magnetic resonance imaging (MRI) or positron emission tomography (PET). Major MRI findings in patients with chronic toluene abuse include atrophy, white matter T2 hyperintensity, and T2 hypointensity involving the basal ganglia and thalamus.[40] Neurobehavioral testing detects subtle central nervous system effects following chronic occupational overexposures.

MANAGEMENT

Hydrocarbons are a diverse family of compounds with a wide spectrum of toxicities. Moreover, many exposures deal with mixtures of hydrocarbons rather than with individual agents. As such, identification of the specific type, route, and amount of hydrocarbon exposure is essential to effective management.

Decontamination is one of the cardinal principles of emergency toxicology, with priority that is second only to stabilization of the cardiopulmonary status. Safe decontamination can avoid further absorption of toxicant(s), and avoids secondary casualties in those attempting to provide care (Chap. 93). Protection of rescuers with appropriate personal protective equipment and rescue protocols is paramount, especially in situations in which the victim has lost consciousness. The principle of removing the patient from the exposure (eg, vapor or gaseous hydrocarbon) or the exposure from the patient (eg, hydrocarbon liquid on skin or clothing), while protecting the rescuer, necessitates that personal protective equipment be considered at each level of the healthcare delivery system.

While systemic toxicity is unlikely from cutaneous absorption of hydrocarbons, absorption can occur after external exposure.[207] Further absorption or inhalation of hydrocarbons from grossly contaminated clothing can worsen systemic toxicity. Proper disposal of contaminated clothing and other articles is indicated. This poses a strong argument for competent field decontamination of victims, particularly in mass casualty situations. Decontamination of the skin should have high priority in massive hydrocarbon exposures, particularly those involving highly toxic hydrocarbons such as those referred to in the mnemonic CHAMP (Table 86–5). Water may be ineffective to decontaminate most hydrocarbons, but early decontamination with soap and water may be adequate. All exposed clothing should be removed, and exposed skin areas should be irrigated with copious amounts of water and then washed with soap. The caregiver should remain aware that most hydrocarbons are highly flammable, posing a fire risk to hospital staff (Chap. 93).

Despite decades of vigorous debate, the role of gastric decontamination after hydrocarbon ingestion remains controversial.[19,60,152,153,165,246,248] Early arguments focused on the controversy over whether gastrointestinal absorption and subsequent lung secretion was the mechanism by which hydrocarbon-induced pulmonary toxicity occurred. Many clinical studies have addressed the efficacy of gastric lavage versus ipecac-induced emesis to pre-

vent pulmonary toxicity.[10,21,39,55,161,162,164,166,173] Results of these studies are equivocal, but the studies were predominantly retrospective and nonrandomized. It is likely that patients manifesting greater toxicity underwent gastric emptying more frequently, and that this biased early studies against a demonstrable benefit from gastric emptying. Moreover, spontaneous vomiting was frequently included in the gastric emptying group.[55] This may have further biased these studies, as vomiting appears to increase risk of pneumonitis.[55,173]

Two studies prospectively randomized patients who underwent gastric lavage. Neither study had uniform indications for lavage. One of these, the COKP trial, was only able to randomize patients at 7 of 46 hospitals. In the subset of randomized lavage patients, 44% had pulmonary complications, versus 47% who were not lavaged. The other study reported pulmonary complications in 47% of the lavaged group, versus 61% of controls. Available studies do not offer a definitive answer to the debate over gastric emptying after hydrocarbon ingestion, although many authors offer an opinion.[12,13,82,137,152,153,235,238]

When there are no contraindications, gastric emptying may be potentially useful in several circumstances: (a) when the hydrocarbon has inherent severe toxicity, (b) when the hydrocarbon is used to solubilize a potent toxicant or is coingested with a more potent toxicant, or (c) when a large volume of hydrocarbon is ingested (>30 mL) (Table 86–5). Patients who have no symptoms at home or on initial medical evaluation generally do not need gastric emptying. Two studies suggest that these patients do not develop subsequent toxicity.[10,139] For patients who do require gastric emptying, it is unclear whether gastric lavage or induced emesis is the superior method.[161,162,173] If emesis is chosen, the patient must be awake, alert, and able to protect his or her airway. Toxic coingestants that may suddenly affect mental status or airway protection represent a contraindication for use of this procedure. If gastric lavage is performed, a small nasogastric tube (18-French, not a large-bore tube) should be employed. If there is no gag reflex in a patient with an altered level of consciousness, an endotracheal tube (preferably cuffed) should be placed prior to lavage (Chap. 5). In summary, gastric emptying is probably indicated after massive (eg, intentional, suicidal) ingestions, or after ingestion of severely toxic hydrocarbons, such as those denoted in the mnemonic CHAMP (Table 86–5).

Activated charcoal has limited ability to decrease gastrointestinal absorption of hydrocarbons.[128,155] As discussed earlier, gastrointestinal absorption plays a small role in hydrocarbon toxicity. Furthermore, activated charcoal administration may distend the stomach and predispose patients to vomiting and aspiration.[236] Its

---

TABLE 86–5. Gastric Emptying For Hydrocarbon Ingestion

Contraindications
- Occurrence of spontaneous vomiting
- Asymptomatic intially and at initial medical evaluation

Indications
- Large volume of hydrocarbon ingested: (>30 mL)
- Intentional ingestions
- A hydrocarbon with inherent systemic toxicity (CHAMP)
  - C: camphor
  - H: halogenated hydrocarbons
  - A: aromatic hydrocarbons
  - M: hydrocarbons compounds containing metals
  - P: pesticides in a hydrocarbon vehicle

use may be justified in patients with mixed overdoses, but its role in isolated hydrocarbon ingestions appears limited.

Giving olive oil or mineral oil with hydrocarbon ingestion was suggested in the past.[21,79,251] These hydrocarbon oils have very high viscosities and low aspiration potential. Theoretically, adding these oils to ingested hydrocarbon raises the viscosity of the resultant combination, thereby decreasing aspiration risk. Animal models do not show any benefit,[155] and these additives can sometimes cause hydrocarbon pneumonitis and lipoid pneumonia themselves.[58] The addition of these agents may distend the stomach and increase the risk of vomiting and aspiration. Currently, there is no role for olive or mineral oil administration in hydrocarbon ingestions.

The use of cathartics for hydrocarbon ingestions has not been well studied in the laboratory or in clinical trials. Because hydrocarbon absorption plays little role in toxicity, their theoretical use is not justified. A single study showed that baboons administered metoclopramide had less hydrocarbon in their stomach 2 hours after gastric instillation as compared to controls. The authors suggest that the promotility effect coupled with the antiemetic effect may decrease aspiration risk when administered in this setting.[244] Further study is needed to delineate the role of this agent in acute hydrocarbon ingestions.

Antibiotics are frequently administered in the setting of hydrocarbon pneumonitis to treat possible bacterial superinfection.[55,105,107,164,173,194,228] In experimental models, superinfection occurs as rapidly as 7 hours after aspiration.[105] Using radiolabeled *Staphylococcus aureus*, by 4 hours after insult, hydrocarbon-injured lungs were shown to have a decreased ability to clear bacteria.[36]

Animal models, including guinea pigs, dogs, and baboons, demonstrate no efficacy of prophylactic antibiotics.[32,203,244] One of these studies showed that administered antibiotic altered bacterial lung flora to predominantly gram-negative organisms, as compared to gram-positive lung cultures in the controls.[32] These studies led to decreased use of prophylactic antibiotics, so that clinical evidence of infection dictated therapy for most clinicians.[66] This approach, however, is not without limitations. Abnormal lung auscultation, fever, leukocytosis, and abnormal radiographic findings are the initial manifestations of both bacterial pneumonia and hydrocarbon pneumonitis. Abnormal temperatures are reported to occur in 50–90% of patients with hydrocarbon toxicity.[21,39,55,82,133,164,166] An elevated temperature is often initially noted, with the temperature reaching maximum at 8–12 hours and then declining over several days.[55,166] Leukocytosis is frequently reported, being present in as many as 50–60% of patients who aspirate hydrocarbons.[133,164,166,177]

Antibiotic administration may be justified in severely poisoned patients. Ideally, sputum cultures should direct antibiotic use. These, however, are often delayed and are not useful in critically ill patients. Some authorities recommend prophylactic antibiotics in all cases. Others recommend close observation of temperature and blood leukocyte count, as delayed elevation (24 hours after presentation) of temperature and/or leukocytes may signal bacterial superinfection. No human studies are available to support either approach and this issue remains controversial.

Corticosteroids, like antibiotics, have been prophylactically administered in the setting of hydrocarbon pulmonary toxicity.[42,89,108,112,145,151,173,227] The rationale for their use is prevention and limitation of the inflammatory response in the lungs after hydrocarbon injury. Animal models do not show any benefit of corticosteroid administration.[6,32,203,247] In fact, one study showed that

corticosteroids increase risk for bacterial superinfection with or without concomitant antibiotics.[131] Furthermore, two controlled human trials failed to show a benefit from corticosteroid administration.[97,142] It is clear that corticosteroid use does not improve the acute course of hydrocarbon pulmonary toxicity, but some authors purport improved outcome with delayed corticosteroid therapy in similar types of devastating acute lung injury (eg, 5–10 days after onset of acute respiratory distress syndrome).[123] None of the experimental or human studies, however, address long-term effects such as pulmonary fibrosis, chronic obstructive pulmonary disease, or bronchiectasis. The incidence of long-term effects is poorly studied, but they appear to be relatively uncommon. Coupled with the possible increased risk of bacterial superinfection, corticosteroid administration in this setting is not recommended.

Patients with severe hydrocarbon toxicity pose unique problems for management. Respiratory distress requiring mechanical ventilation in this setting may be associated with a large ventilation-perfusion mismatch. The use of positive end-expiratory pressure (PEEP) is often beneficial.[183,252] However, very high levels of PEEP may be required with subsequent increased risk of barotrauma.[183,252] High-frequency jet ventilation, using very high respiratory rates (220–260) with small tidal volumes, is useful for decreasing the need for PEEP.[38,183,252] Patients who continue to have severe ventilation-perfusion mismatch despite PEEP and then high-frequency jet ventilation have benefitted from extracorporeal membrane oxygenation.[98,110,252] Extracorporeal membrane oxygenation appears to be a useful option in severe pulmonary toxicity after other treatments have failed.

As discussed, the toxic mechanism for hydrocarbon-induced pulmonary damage may in part be caused by detrimental effects on surfactant.[86] Several commercial surfactant preparations are available and are useful for other disease conditions associated with inadequate surfactant function. One animal model did not show benefit, whereas another showed increased survival and improved pulmonary function after exogenous surfactant.[193,240] No studies are currently available to assess the clinical effectiveness in human toxicity, and further study is warranted.

Cyanosis is uncommon after hydrocarbon toxicity. Although this is most often a result of severe hypoxia, methemoglobinemia associated with hydrocarbon exposure is reported.[54,129] The potential for methemoglobinemia should be investigated in patients who remain cyanotic following normalization of arterial oxygenation.

Hypotension in severe hydrocarbon toxicity raises additional concerns. The etiology of hypotension in this setting is often compromise of cardiac output because of high levels of PEEP. Hydrocarbons do not have significant direct cardiovascular effects, and decreasing the PEEP may improve hemodynamics. The use of catecholamines (dopamine, epinephrine, isoproterenol, norepinephrine, and the like) should be avoided if possible, as hydrocarbons can sensitize myocardium and predispose to dysrhythmias.[20,78,178,179]

Management of dysrhythmias associated with hydrocarbon toxicity should include consideration of electrolyte and acid-base abnormalities (eg, hypokalemia and acidosis from toluene), hypoxemia, hypotension, and hypothermia. Ventricular fibrillation poses a specific concern, as common resuscitation algorithms recommend epinephrine administration to treat this rhythm. If it is ascertained that the dysrhythmia emanates from myocardial sensitization by a hydrocarbon solvent, catecholamines should be avoided. In this setting, lidocaine has been used successfully, as has β blockade.[156]

The use of hyperbaric oxygen (HBO) was studied in a rat model of severe kerosene-induced pneumonitis.[188] HBO at 4 atmospheres absolute (ATA) showed some benefit in 24-hour survival rates. No followup studies have been performed. Hydrocarbon poisonings associated with carbon tetrachloride, however, may include a role for HBO[35,221] (Antidotes in Depth: Hyperbaric Oxygen).

In the past, hospital admission was routinely recommended for patients who had ingested hydrocarbons because of concern over possible delayed symptom onset and progression of toxicity.[39,55,91] Several reports documented patients with relatively asymptomatic presentations who rapidly decompensated with respiratory compromise.[10,91,139] However, progression of symptoms after hydrocarbon ingestion is rare.[10,139] In a retrospective study of 950 patients, only 14 (1.5%) had progression of pulmonary toxicity.[10] Of these, half had persistence of symptoms for less than 24 hours. Eight hundred patients, who were asymptomatic on initial evaluation with normal chest radiographs remained asymptomatic after 6–8 hours of observation and had a normal repeat radiograph. No patients in this group had progressive symptoms, and all were discharged without clinical deterioration. Seventy-one of the 950 patients had initial respiratory symptoms but were asymptomatic at initial medical evaluation. Of the 71 patients, 36 had radiographic evidence of pneumonitis. Among these 36 patients, 2 (6%) developed progression of pulmonary symptoms during their 6-hour observation period. Of the 35 who had a normal radiograph, 2 (6%) developed pulmonary symptoms and radiographic pneumonitis during the 6-hour observation period. The four patients who were hospitalized for progression of symptoms became asymptomatic over the next 24 hours and had no complications.

A separate poison center–based study evaluated 120 asymptomatic patients for an 18-hour telephone followup period.[139] Sixty-two patients had initial pulmonary symptoms that quickly resolved. One of these 62 patients (1.6%) developed progressive pulmonary toxicity. This patient was hospitalized and had resolution of symptoms within 24 hours without complications.

It is clear that the vast majority of patients exposed to a hydrocarbon will not need to be hospitalized[10,139] (Chap. 116 has further references from TESS). A number of investigators suggest protocols for determining which patients can be safely discharged.[10,13,122,137,139] None of these protocols have been prospectively validated. However, rational guidelines for hospitalization can be recommended. Those patients who have clinical evidence of toxicity, and most individuals with intentional ingestion should be hospitalized. Patients who do not have any initial symptoms, have normal chest radiographs at 6 hours after ingestion, and who do not develop symptoms during the 6-hour observation period can be safely discharged. Care should be individualized for patients who are asymptomatic but who have radiographic evidence of hydrocarbon pneumonitis, and for patients who have initial respiratory symptoms but quickly become asymptomatic during medical evaluation. Reliable patients may be considered for possible discharge with next-day followup.

SUMMARY

Hydrocarbons are a diverse group of chemical agents and can cause toxicity by inhalation, ingestion, or dermal absorption. Most hydrocarbons occur as mixtures of several chemical species. Ubiquitous use of hydrocarbons in our society means that exposures are extremely common. Populations at particular risk for toxicity include children who ingest hydrocarbon compounds, workers who are occupationally exposed by inhalation or dermal absorption, and youths who intentionally inhale volatile hydrocarbons.

Toxicity is largely determined by the route of exposure and is agent specific. Acute systemic toxicity is unlikely to occur in the absence of CNS effects such as excitation or sedation. Most hydrocarbons are capable of producing profound CNS depression, even general anesthesia. Aspiration pneumonitis is the primary concern after hydrocarbon ingestion.

Specific agents may demonstrate specific organ toxicity: the halogenated hydrocarbons are cardiotoxic, hepatotoxic, and nephrotoxic. Most are also acutely toxic to the CNS and some are also peripheral neurotoxicants. Diagnosis is predominantly clinical. Diagnostic studies are rarely specific, and agent-specific studies are seldom helpful in the acute setting. Skin decontamination is important in massive dermal exposures. Gut decontamination, as well as the use of prophylactic antibiotics or corticosteroids, remains controversial. Management is largely supportive, and no specific antidotes are available.

ACKNOWLEDGMENT

Richard D. Shih contributed to this chapter in a previous edition.

REFERENCES

1. Adler R, Robinson RG, Binkin NJ: Intravascular hemolysis: An unusual complication of hydrocarbon ingestion. J Pediatr 1976;89:679–680.
2. Agency for Toxic Substances and Disease Registry (ATSDR): Toxicological Profile for Toluene. Washington, DC, US Public Health Service, 1994.
3. Agency for Toxic Substances and Disease Registry (ATSDR): Toxicological Profile for Total Petroleum Hydrocarbons. Washington, DC, US Public Health Service, 1998.
4. Ahmed AE, Kubic VL, Stevens JL, et al: Halogenated methanes: Metabolism and toxicity. Fed Proc 1980;39:3150–3155.
5. Aksoy M, Erdem S, Dincol G, et al: Aplastic anemia due to chemicals and drugs: A study of 108 patients. Sex Transm Dis 1984;11(4 Suppl):347–350.
6. Albert WC: The efficacy of steroid therapy in the treatment of experimental kerosene pneumonitis. Am Rev Respir Dis 1968;98:888–889.
7. Algren JT, Rodgers GC: Intravascular hemolysis associated with hydrocarbon poisoning. Pediatr Emerg Care 1992;8:34–35.
8. Altenkirch H, Stoltenburg G, Wagner HM: Experimental studies on hydrocarbon neuropathies induced by methyl-ethyl-ketone (MEK). J Neurol 1978;219:159–170.
9. American Conference of Government Industrial Hygienists (ACGIH): 1998 TLVs and BEIs: Threshold Limit Values for Chemical Substances and Physical Agents and Biological Exposure Indices. Cincinnati, OH, ACGIH, 1998.
10. Anas N, Namasonthi V, Ginsburg CM: Criteria for hospitalizing children who have ingested products containing hydrocarbon. JAMA 1981;246:840–843.
11. Anene O, Castello FV: Myocardial dysfunction after hydrocarbon ingestion. Crit Care Med 1994;22:528–530.
12. Arena J: Hydrocarbon poisoning—Current management. Pediatr Ann 1987;16:879–883.
13. Arena J: Petroleum distillate ingestion [letter]. Pediatr Ann 1978;7:513.
14. Ashford NA: New scientific evidence and public health imperatives. N Engl J Med 1987;316:1084–1085.

15. Ashkenazi AE, Berman SE: Experimental kerosene poisoning in rats: Use of C^{14} labeled hendecane as indicator of absorption. Pediatrics 1961;26:642–649.

16. Baldachin BJ, Melmed RN: Clinical and therapeutic aspects of kerosene poisoning: A series of 200 cases. Br Med J 1964;2:28–30.

17. Balster RL: Neural basis of inhalant abuse. Drug Alcohol Depend 1998;51:207–214.

18. Barbour O: Kerosene poisoning. JAMA 1926;87:488.

19. Bass M: Death from sniffing gasoline [letter]. N Engl J Med 1978; 299:203.

20. Bass M: Sudden sniffing death. JAMA 1970;212:2075–2079.

21. Beamon RF, Siegel CJ, Landers G, et al: Hydrocarbon ingestion in children: A six-year retrospective study. JACEP 1976;5:771–775.

22. Beckstead MJ, Weiner JL, Eger EI, et al: Glycine and gamma-aminobutyric acid$_A$ receptor function is enhanced by inhaled drugs of abuse. Mol Pharmacol 2000;57:1199–1205.

23. Bergeson PS: Pneumatoceles following hydrocarbon ingestion. Am J Dis Child 1975;129:49–54.

24. Bleecker ML, Bolla KI, Agnew J, et al: Dose-related subclinical neurobehavioral effects of chronic exposure to low levels of organic solvents. Am J Ind Med 1991;19:715–728.

25. Bombassei GJ, Kaplan AA: The association between hydrocarbon exposure and anti-glomerular basement membrane antibody-mediated disease (Goodpasture's syndrome). Am J Ind Med 1992;21: 141–153.

26. Bonte FJ, Reynolds J: Hydrocarbon pneumonitis. Radiology 1958;71:391–397.

27. Bos PM, de Mik G, Bragt PC: Critical review of the toxicity of methyl n-butyl ketone: Risk from occupational exposure. Am J Ind Med 1991;20:175–194.

28. Bratton L, Haddon JE: Ingestion of charcoal lighter fluid. J Pediatr 1975;87:633–636.

29. Brent JA, Rumack BH: Role of free radicals in toxic hepatic injury: II. Are free radicals the cause of toxin-induced liver injury? J Toxicol Clin Toxicol 1993;31:173–196.

30. Brett RS, Dilger JP, Yland KF: Isoflurane causes "flickering" of the acetylcholine receptor channel: Observations using the patch clamp. Anesthesiology 1988;69:161–170.

31. Brook MP, McCarron MM, Mueller JA: Pine oil cleaner ingestion. Ann Emerg Med 1989;18:391–395.

32. Brown J III, Burke B, Dajani AS, et al: Experimental kerosene pneumonia: Evaluation of some therapeutic regimens. J Pediatr 1974;84: 396–401.

33. Brunner S, Rovsing H, Wulf H: Roentgenographic change in the lungs of children with kerosene poisoning. Am Rev Respir Dis 1964;89:250–254.

34. Budavari S, ed: The Merck Index, 11th ed. Rahway, NJ, Merck & Co, Inc., 1989.

35. Burkhart KK, Hall AH, Gerace R, et al: Hyperbaric oxygen treatment for carbon tetrachloride poisoning. Drug Saf 1991;6:332–338.

36. Burley S, Huber G: The effect of toxic agents commonly ingested by children on antibacterial defenses in the lung. Proc Soc Pediatr Res 1971;16:83.

37. Buxton PH, Hayward M: Polyneuritis cranialis associated with industrial trichloroethylene poisoning. J Neurol Neurosurg Psychiatry 1967;30:511–518.

38. Bysani GK, Rucoba RJ, Noah ZL: Treatment of hydrocarbon pneumonitis. High frequency jet ventilation as an alternative to extracorporeal membrane oxygenation. Chest 1994;106:300–303.

39. Cachia EA, Fenech FF: Kerosene poisoning in children. Arch Dis Child 1964;39:502.

40. Caldemeyer KS, Armstrong SW, George KK, et al: The spectrum of neuroimaging abnormalities in solvent abuse and their clinical correlation. J Neuroimaging 1996;6:167–173.

41. Campbell JB: Pneumatocele formation following hydrocarbon ingestion. Am Rev Respir Dis 1970;101:414–418.

42. Carithers HA: Accident prevention in childhood—The kerosene hazard. JAMA 1955;159:109–111.

43. Carlisle EJ, Donnelly SM, Vasuvattakul S, et al: Glue-sniffing and distal renal tubular acidosis: Sticking to the facts. J Am Soc Nephrol 1991;1:1019–1027.

44. Carpenter C: Animal and human response to vapors of Stoddard solvent. Toxicol Appl Pharmacol 1975;32:282–297.

45. Carpenter CP, Geary DL, Myers RC, et al: Petroleum hydrocarbon toxicity studies: XIII. Animal and human response to vapors of toluene concentrate. Toxicol Appl Pharmacol 1976;36: 473–490.

46. Cavanagh JB, Buxton PH: Trichloroethylene cranial neuropathy: Is it really a toxic neuropathy or does it activate latent herpes virus? J Neurol Neurosurg Psychiatr 1989;52:297–303.

47. Chang YC: Neurotoxic effects of n-hexane on the human central nervous system: Evoked potential abnormalities in n-hexane polyneuropathy. J Neurol Neurosurg Psychiatry 1987;50:269–274.

48. Cheng SC, Brunner EA: Effects of anesthetic agents on synaptosomal GABA disposal. Anesthesiology 1981;55:34–40.

49. Clayton GD, Clayton FE, eds: Patty's Industrial Hygiene and Toxicology, Volume 2B: Toxicology, 3rd ed. New York, John Wiley & Sons, 1981.

50. Cohen S: Glue sniffing. JAMA 1975;231:653–654.

51. Cohen S: The volatile nitrites. JAMA 1979;241:2077–2078.

52. Cohr KH, Stolkholm J: Toluene: A toxicologic review. Scand J Work Environ Health 1979;5:71–90.

53. Cubells JM, Martinez RA, Youssef W: Poisoning by spirits of turpentine or turpentine oil: Review of its treatment. Ann Esp Pediatr 1952;83:446–453.

54. Curry S: Methemoglobinemia. Ann Emerg Med 1982;11:214–221.

55. Daeschner CW, Blattner RJ, Collins VP: Hydrocarbon pneumonitis. Pediatr Clin North Am 1957;4:243–253.

56. Daffner RH, Jimenez JP: The double gastric fluid level in kerosene poisoning. Pediatr Radiol 1973;106:383–384.

57. Das M, Misra MP: Acne and folliculitis due to diesel oil. Contact Dermatitis 1988;18:120–121.

58. De la Rocha SR, Cunningham JC, Fox E: Lipoid pneumonia secondary to baby oil aspiration: A case report and review of the literature. Pediatr Emerg Care 1985;1:74–80.

59. Decoufle P, Blattner WA, Blair A: Mortality among chemical workers exposed to benzene and other agents. Environ Res 1983;30: 16–25.

60. Deichmann WB, Kitzmiller KV, Witherup S, et al: Kerosene intoxication. Ann Intern Med 1944;21:803–823.

61. Demling RH, Buerstatte WR, Perea A: Management of hot tar burns. J Trauma 1980;20:242.

62. Di Vincenzo GD, Kaplan CJ: Uptake, metabolism and elimination of methylene chloride vapors by humans. Toxicol Appl Pharmacol 1981;59:130–140.

63. Dice WH, Ward G, Kelley J, et al: Pulmonary toxicity following gastrointestinal ingestion of kerosene. Ann Emerg Med 1982;11: 138–142.

64. Dragsted PJ: Pseudocysts of the lungs in kerosene poisoning. Dis Chest 1965;48:87–90.

65. Dreisbach RH, Robertson WO, eds: Diagnosis and evaluation of poisoning. In: Handbook of Poisoning, 12th ed. Norwalk, CT, Appleton & Lange, 1987.

66. Eade NR, Taussig LM, Marks MI: Hydrocarbon pneumonitis. Pediatrics 1974;54:351–357.

67. Echeverria D, Fine L, Langolf G, et al: Acute neurobehavioral effects of toluene. Br J Industr Med 1989;46:483–495.

68. Erickson T, Popiel R, Hryhorczuk DO, et al: Pine oil cleaners in prison. Ann Emerg Med 1990;19:445–448.

69. Farabaugh JC: Kerosene poisoning. Minn Med 1936;19:780–781.

70. Feldman RG, Chirico-Post J, Proctor SP: Blink reflex latency after exposure to trichloroethylene in well water. Arch Environ Health 1988;43:143–148.

71. Feldman RG, White RF, Currie JN, Travers PH, Lessell S: Long-term follow-up after single toxic exposure to trichloroethylene. Am J Ind Med 1985;8:119–126.

72. Fialkov JA, Freiberg A: High pressure injection injuries: An overview. J Emerg Med 1991;9:367–371.

73. Filley CM, Franklin GM, Heaton RK, Rosenberg NL: White matter dementia: Clinical disorders and implications. Neuropsychiatry Neuropsychol Behav Neurol 1988;1:239–254.

74. Finkel AJ, ed: Hamilton and Hardy's Industrial Toxicology, 4th ed. Boston, John Wright, 1983.

75. Firestone LL, Sauter JF, Braswell LM, Miller KW: Actions of general anesthetics on acetylcholine receptor-rich membranes from *Torpedo californica*. Anesthesiology 1986;64:694–702.

76. Fischman C, Oster VR: Toxic effects of toluene. JAMA 1979;241:1713–1715.

77. Flanagan RJ, Ruprah M, Meredith TJ, Ramset JR: An introduction to the clinical toxicology of volatile substances. Drug Saf 1990;5:359–383.

78. Flowers NC, Horan LG: Nonanoxic aerosol arrhythmias. JAMA 1972;219:23–27.

79. Foley JC, Dreyer NB, Soule AB, et al: Kerosene poisoning in young children. Radiology 1954;62:817–829.

80. Fortenberry JD: Gasoline sniffing. Am J Med 1985;79:740–744.

81. Gargas ML, Burgess RJ, Voisard DE, et al: Partition coefficients of low-molecular-weight volatile chemicals in various liquids and tissues. Toxicol Appl Pharmacol 1989;98:87–99.

82. Geehr E: Management of hydrocarbon ingestions. Top Emerg Med 1979;1:97–110.

83. Gerarde HW: Toxicological studies on hydrocarbons: V. Kerosene. Toxicol Appl Pharmacol 1959;1:462–469.

84. Gerarde HW: Toxicological studies on hydrocarbons: IX. The aspiration hazard and toxicity of hydrocarbons and hydrocarbon mixtures. Arch Environ Health 1963;6:329–341.

85. Gershon-Cohen J, Bringhurst LS, Byrne RN: Roentgenography of kerosene poisoning. Am J Roentgenol 1953;69:557.

86. Giammona ST: Effects of furniture polish on pulmonary surfactant. Am J Dis Child 1967;113:658–663.

87. Gosselin RE, Smith RP, Hodge HC, eds: Clinical Toxicology of Commercial Products, 5th ed. Baltimore, Williams & Wilkins, 1984.

88. Graham DG: Neurotoxicants and the cytoskeleton. Curr Opin Neurol 1999;12:733–737.

89. Graham JR: Pneumonitis following aspiration of crude oil and its treatment by steroid hormones. Trans Am Clin Climatol Assoc 1955–56;67:104–112.

90. Greenberg MD, Robinson T, Birrer R: Atrial fibrillation after intravenous administration of gasoline. Am Heart J 1993;125:1438–1439.

91. Griffin JW, Daeschner CV, Collins VP, et al: Hydrocarbon pneumonitis following furniture polish ingestion. J Pediatr 1954;13:13–26.

92. Gross P: Kerosene pneumonitis: An experimental study with small doses. Am Rev Resp Dis 1963;88:656–663.

93. Gurwitz D, Katten M, Levison H, et al: Pulmonary function abnormalities in symptomatic children after hydrocarbon pneumonitis. Pediatrics 1978;62:789–794.

94. Hake CL, Stewart RD: Human exposure to tetrachloroethylene: Inhalation and skin contact. Environ Health Perspect 1977;21:231–238.

95. Halsey, MJ: Physical chemistry applied to anaesthetic action. Br J Anaesth 1974;46:172–180.

96. Hansbrough JF, Saputa-Sirvent R, Dominic W, et al: Hydrocarbon contact injuries. J. Trauma. 1985;25:250–252.

97. Hardman G, Tolson R, Hadhdassarian O: Prednisone in the management of kerosene pneumonia. Indian Practitioner 1960;13:615–620.

98. Hart LM, Cobaugh DJ, Dean BS, et al: Successful use of extracorporeal membrane oxygenation (ECMO) in the treatment of refractory respiratory failure secondary to hydrocarbon aspiration [abstract]. Vet Hum Toxicol 1991;33:361.

99. Hawkes CH, Cavanagh JB, Fox AJ: Motoneuron disease: A disorder secondary to solvent exposure? Lancet 1989;2:73–76.

100. Heacock CH: Pneumonia in children following the ingestion of petroleum products. Radiology 1949;53:793.

101. Herskowitz A, Ishii N, Schaumburg H: *n*-Hexane neuropathy: A syndrome occurring as a result of industrial exposure. N Engl J Med 1971;285:82–85.

102. Higgins JM: Rapidly fatal result in a child from ingestion of kerosene. Penn Med J 1932;36:526–527.

103. Hirose T, Inoue M, Uchida M, Inagaki C: Enflurane-induced release of an excitatory amino acid, glutamate, from mouse brain synaptosomes. Anesthesiology 1992;77:109–113.

104. Hoidal CR, Hall AH, Robinson ND, et al: Hydrogen sulfide poisoning from toxic inhalations of roofing asphalt fumes. Ann Emerg Med 1986;15:826–830.

105. Ikeda K: Oil aspiration pneumonia (lipoid pneumonia): Clinical, pathologic and experimental consideration. Am J Dis Child 1935;49:985–1006.

106. International Programme on Chemical Safety: Benzene: Environmental Health Criteria, Publication 150. Geneva, World Health Organization, 1993, pp. 28–43.

107. Jacobziner H: Accidental chemical poisonings, kerosene, and other petroleum distillate poisonings. N Y State J Med 1963;63:3428.

108. Jacobziner H, Raybin HW: Mixture of tranquilizers, lighter fluid, paint thinner, and iodine poisonings. N Y State J Med 1962;62:862.

109. Jacobziner H, Raybin HW: Turpentine poisoning. Arch Pediatr 1961;78:357–364.

110. Jaeger RW, Scalzo AS, Thompson MW: ECMO in hydrocarbon aspiration [abstract]. Vet Hum Toxicol 1987;29:485.

111. James FW, Kaplan S, Bensing G: Cardiac complications following hydrocarbon ingestion. Am J Dis Child 1971;121:431–433.

112. Jamison KE, Wallace ER: Kerosene pneumonitis treated with adrenal steroids. Calif Med 1964;100:43.

113. Janofsky M: Fatal crash reveals inhalants as danger to youth. The New York Times, March 2, 1999, p. A12.

114. Janssen S, van der Geest S, Meijer S, et al: Impairment of organ function after oral ingestion of refined petrol. Intensive Care Med 1988;14:238–240.

115. Javier Perez A, Courel M, Sobrado J, Gonzalez L: Acute renal failure after topical application of carbon tetrachloride. Lancet 1987;1(8531):515–516.

116. Johnston LD, O'Malley PM, Bachman JG: The Monitoring the Future National Results on Adolescent Drug Use: Overview of Key Findings, 1999. NIH Publication 00–4690. Bethesda, MD, National Institute on Drug Abuse, 2000.

117. Joron GE, Cameron DG, Halpenny GW: Massive necrosis of the liver due to trichloroethylene. Canad Med Assoc J 1955;73:890–891.

118. Karlson KH: Hydrocarbon poisoning in children. South Med J 1982;75:839–840.

119. Kao KC, Tsai YH, Lin MC, et al: Hypokalemic muscular paralysis causing acute respiratory failure due to rhabdomyolysis with renal tubular acidosis in a chronic glue sniffer. J Toxicol Clin Toxicol 2000;38:679–681.

120. Kaysen GA: Renal toxicology. In: La Dou J, ed: Occupational Medicine. Norwalk, CT, Appleton & Lange, 1994, pp. 259–260.

121. King PJ, Morris JG, Pollard JD: Glue sniffing neuropathy. Aust N Z J Med 1985;15:293–299.

122. Klein BL, Simon JE: Hydrocarbon poisonings. Pediatr Clin North Am 1986;33:411–419.

123. Kollef MH, Schuster DP: The acute respiratory distress syndrome. N Engl J Med 1995;332:27–37.

124. Koppel C, Tenczer J, Tonnesmann U, et al: Acute poisoning with pine oil—Metabolism of monoterpenes. Arch Toxicol 1981;49:73–78.

125. Kornfeld M, Moser AB, Moser HW: Solvent vapor abuse leukoencephalopathy. Comparison to adrenoleukodystrophy. J Neuropathol Exp Neurol 1994;53:389–398.

126. Kulig K, Rumack B: Hydrocarbon ingestion. Curr Top Emerg Med 1981;3:1–5.

127. Kwong YL, Chan TK: Toxic occupational exposures and paroxysmal nocturnal haemoglobinuria. Lancet 1993;341:443.

128. Laass W: Therapy of acute oral poisonings by organic solvents: Treatment by activated charcoal in combination with laxatives. Arch Toxicol 1980;4(Suppl):406–409.

129. Lareng L: Acute toxic methemoglobinemia from accidental ingestion of nitrobenzene. Eur J Toxicol 1974;7:12–16.

130. Lavenstein AF: Ingestion of kerosene complicated by pneumonia, pneumothorax, pneumopericardium, and subcutaneous emphysema. J Pediatr 1945;26:395–400.

131. Lazar RB, Ho SU, Melen O, et al: Multifocal central nervous system damage caused by toluene abuse. Neurology 1983;33:1337–1340.

132. Leandri M, Schizzi R, Scielzo C, et al: Electrophysiological evidence of trigeminal root damage after trichloroethylene exposure. Muscle Nerve 1995;18:467–468.

133. Lesser LI, Weens HS, McKey JD: Pulmonary manifestations following ingestion of kerosene. J Pediatr 1943;23:352–364.

134. Liao JT, Oehme FW: Literature reviews of phenolic compounds: I. Phenol. Vet Hum Toxicol 1980;22:160–164.

135. Lin L-H, Whiting P, Harris RA: Molecular determinates of general anesthetic action: Role of GABA$_A$ receptor structure. J Neurochem 1993;60:1548–1553.

136. Linden CH: Volatile substances of abuse. Emerg Med Clin North Am 1990;8:559–578.

137. Litovitz TL: Hydrocarbon ingestions. Ear Nose Throat J 1983;62:142–147.

138. Lundberg I, Hogstedt C, Liden C, Nise G: Organic solvents and related compounds. In: Rosenstock L, Cullen MR, eds: Clinical Occupational and Environmental Medicine. Philadelphia, WB Saunders, 1994, pp. 766–784.

139. Machado B, Cross K, Snodgrass WR: Accidental hydrocarbon ingestion cases telephoned to a regional poison center. Ann Emerg Med 1988;17:804–807.

140. Mann MD, Pirie DJ, Wolfsdorf J: Kerosene absorption in primates. J Pediatr 1977;91:495–498.

141. Marandian MH, Youssefian H, Saboury M, et al: Intoxication accidentelle par ingestion de petrole chex l'enfant: Etude clinique, radiologique, biologique et anatomopathologique, a propos de 3462 cas. Ann Pediatr (Paris) 1981;28:601–609.

142. Marks MI, Chicoine L, Legere G, et al: Adrenocorticosteroid treatment of hydrocarbon pneumonia in children—A cooperative study. J Pediatr 1972;81:366–369.

143. Marshall BE, Longnecker DE: General anesthetics. In: Goodman LS, Limbird LE, Milinoff PB, et al, eds: Goodman & Gilman's The Pharmacological Basis of Therapeutics, 9th ed. New York, McGraw-Hill, 1996, pp. 307–330.

144. Matsumoto T, Koga M, Sata T, et al: The changes of gasoline compounds in blood in a case of gasoline intoxication. J Toxicol Clin Toxicol 1992;30:653–662.

145. Mayock RL, Zinsser HF: Kerosene pneumonitis treated with adrenal steroids. Ann Intern Med 1961;54:559.

146. McLean CC: Kerosene poisoning [letter]. JAMA 1933;101:1987.

147. McNally WD: Kerosene poisoning in children. J Pediatr 1956;48:296–299.

148. Mehlman MA: Benzene health effects: Unanswered questions still not addressed. Am J Ind Med 1991;20:707–711.

149. Meredith TJ, Ruprah M, Liddle A, et al: Diagnosis and treatment of acute poisoning with volatile substances. Hum Toxicol 1989;8:277–286.

150. Meulenbelt J, De Groot G, Savelkoul TJF: Two cases of toluene intoxication. Br J Ind Med 1990;47:417–420.

151. Mintz AA: Furniture polish intoxication. South Med J 1966;59:1010–1014.

152. Mofenson HC: The new correct answer to an old question on kerosene ingestion [letter]. Pediatrics 1977;59:788.

153. Mofenson HC, Greensher J: Controversies in the prevention and treatment of poisonings. Pediatr Ann 1977;6:717–725.

154. Moody EJ, Suzdak PD, Paul SM, Skolnick P: Modulation of the benzodiazepine/gamma-aminobutyric acid receptor chloride channel complex by inhalation anesthetics. J Neurochem 1988;51:1386–1393.

155. Morgan DP: Effectiveness of activated charcoal, mineral oil, and castor oil in limiting gastrointestinal absorption of a chlorinated hydrocarbon pesticide. Clin Toxicol 1977;11:61–70.

156. Moritz F, de La Chapelle A, Bauer F, et al: Esmolol in the treatment of severe arrhythmia after acute trichloroethylene poisoning [letter]. Intensive Care Med 2000;26:256.

157. Morrison RT, Boyd RN: Organic Chemistry, 6th ed. Englewood Cliffs, NJ, Prentice Hall, 1992, pp. 92–118.

158. Moss AH, Gabow PA, Kaehny WD, et al: Fanconi's syndrome and distal renal tubular acidosis after glue sniffing. Ann Intern Med 1980;92:69–70.

159. Mrvos R, Dean BS, Krenzelok EP: High pressure injection injuries: A serious occupational hazard. J Toxicol Clin Toxicol 1987;25:297–304.

160. Nelson DL, Cox MM, eds: Lehninger Principles of Biochemistry, 3rd ed. New York, Worth Publishing, 2000.

161. Ng RC: Using syrup of ipecac for ingestion of petroleum distillates. Pediatr Ann 1977;6:708–710.

162. Ng RC, Darwish H, Stewart DA: Emergency treatment of petroleum distillate and turpentine ingestion. Can Med Assoc J 1974;3:537–538.

163. Nierenberg DW, Horowitz MB, Harris KM, et al: Mineral spirits inhalation associated with hemolysis, pulmonary edema, and ventricular fibrillation. Arch Intern Med 1991;151:1437–1440.

164. Nouri L, Al-Rahim K: Kerosene poisoning in children. Postgrad Med J 1970;46:71–75.

165. Nunn JA, Martin FM: Gasoline and kerosene poisoning in children. JAMA 1934;103:472–475.

166. Olstad RB, Lord RM Jr: Kerosene intoxication. Am J Dis Child 1952;83:446–453.

167. Osterloh J: Butyl nitrite abuse and overdose [abstract]. Vet Hum Toxicol 1984;26:416.

168. Ott MG, Skory LK, Holder BB, et al: Health evaluation of employees occupationally exposed to methylene chloride. Scand J Work Environ Health 1983;9(Suppl 1):1–38.

169. Ottelio C, Giagheddu M, Marrosu F: Altered EEG pattern in aromatic hydrocarbon intoxication: A case report. Acta Neurol 1993;15:357–362.

170. Padday JF: Theory of surface tension. In: Matijevic E, ed: Surface and Colloid Science, Vol. 1. New York, Wiley-Interscience, 1969.

171. Paustenbach DJ, Bass RD, Price P: Benzene toxicity and risk assessment, 1972–1992: Implications for future regulation. Environ Health Perspect 1993;101(Suppl 6):177–200.

172. Pierce CH, Dills RL, Silvey GW, et al: Partition coefficients between human blood or adipose tissue and air for aromatic solvents. Scand J Work Environ Health 1996;22:112–118.

173. Press E: Cooperative kerosene poisoning study: Evaluation of gastric lavage and other factors in the treatment of accidental ingestion of petroleum distillate products. Pediatrics 1962;29:648–674.

174. Prockop L: Neurotoxic volatile substances. Neurology 1979;29:862–865.

175. Ramsey J, Anderson HR, Bloor K, Flanagan RJ: An introduction to the practice, prevalence and chemical toxicology of volatile substance abuse. Hum Toxicol 1989;8:261–269.

176. Ratney RS, Wegman DH, Elkins HB: In vivo conversion of methylene chloride to carbon monoxide. Arch Environ Health 1974;28:223–236.

177. Reed ES, Leikin S, Kerman HD: Kerosene intoxication. Am J Dis Child 1950;79:623–632.

178. Reinhardt CF, Aza A, Maxfield ME, et al: Cardiac arrhythmias and aerosol sniffing. Arch Environ Health 1971;22:265–279.

179. Reinhardt CF, Mullin LS, Maxfield ME: Epinephrine-induced cardiac arrhythmia potential of some common industrial solvents. J Occup Med 1973;15:953–955.

180. Richardson JA, Pratt-Thomas HR: Toxic effects of varying doses of kerosene administered by different routes. Am J Med Sci 1951;221:531–536.

181. Rinsky RA, Smith AB, Hornung R, et al: Benzene and leukemia: An epidemiologic risk assessment. N Engl J Med 1987;316:1044–1050.

182. Saida K, Mendell JR, Weiss HS: Peripheral nerve changes induced by methyl n-butyl ketone and potentiation by methyl ethyl ketone. J Neuropathol Exp Neurol 1976;35:207–225.

183. Scalzo AJ, Weber TR, Jaeger RW, et al: Extracorporeal membrane oxygenation for hydrocarbon aspiration. Am J Dis Child 1990;144:867–871.

184. Scharf SM, Heimer D, Goldstein J: Pathologic and physiologic effects of aspiration of hydrocarbons in the rat. Am Rev Respir Dis 1981;124:625–629.

185. Scharf SM, Prinsloo I: Pulmonary mechanics in dogs given different doses of kerosene intratracheally. Am Rev Respir Dis 1982;126:695–700.

186. Schaumburg HH: Toluene. In: Spencer PS, Schaumburg HH, eds: Experimental and Clinical Neurotoxicology, 2nd ed. New York, Oxford University Press, 2000, pp. 1183–1189.

187. Schoenborn BP: Binding of cyclopropane to sperm whale myoglobin. Nature 1967;214:1120–1122.

188. Schwartz SI, Breslau RC, Kutner F, et al: Effects of drugs and hyperbaric oxygen environment on experimental kerosene pneumonitis. Dis Chest 1965;47:353–359.

189. Scott EP: Pneumonia, pneumothorax and emphysema following ingestion of kerosene. J Pediatr 1944;25:31–34.

190. Secher O: Physical and chemical data on anaesthetics. Acta Anaesthesiol Scand Suppl 1971;42:1–95.

191. Segal IS, Jarvis DJ, Duncan SR, et al: Clinical efficacy of oral-transdermal clonidine combinations during the perioperative period. Anesthesiology 1991;74:220–225.

192. Seitz PA, Riet M, Rush W, Merrell J: Adenosine decreases the minimum alveolar concentration of halothane in dogs. Anesthesiology 1990;73:990–994.

193. Shih RD, Mercurio M, Morasco R, et al: Artificial surfactant administration in an animal model of severe hydrocarbon-induced pulmonary toxicity [abstract]. J Toxicol Clin Toxicol 1996;34:139.

194. Shirkey HC: Treatment of petroleum distillate ingestion. Mod Treatment 1967;4:580–592.

195. Sikkema J, de Bont JA, Poolman B: Mechanisms of membrane toxicity of hydrocarbons. Microbiol Rev 1995;59:201–222.

196. Smith AG, Albers JW: n-Hexane neuropathy due to rubber cement sniffing. Muscle Nerve 1997;20:1445–1450.

197. Snyder R, ed: Toluene. In: Ethel Browning's Toxicity and Metabolism of Industrial Solvents, Volume I: Hydrocarbons, 2nd ed. New York, Elsevier Science Publishing, 1987.

198. Snyder R, Andrews LS: Toxic effects of solvents and vapors. In: Klaassen CD, ed: Casarett and Doull's Toxicology: The Basic Science of Poisons, 5th ed. New York, McGraw-Hill, 1996, pp. 737–771.

199. Soule AB, Foley JC: Poisoning from petroleum distillates. The hazards of kerosene and furniture polish. J Maine Med Assoc 1957;48:103–110.

200. Sperling F: In vivo and in vitro toxicology of turpentine. Clin Toxicol 1969;2:21–35.

201. Sperling F, Marcus W, Collins C, et al: Acute effects of turpentine vapor on rats and mice. Toxicol Appl Pharmacol 1967;10:8–20.

202. Spiller HA, Krenzelak EP: Epidemiology of inhalant abuse reported to two regional poison centers. J Toxicol Clin Toxicol 1997;35:167–173.

203. Steele RW, Conklin RH, Mark HM: Corticosteroids and antibiotics for the treatment of fulminant hydrocarbon aspiration. JAMA 1972;219:1434–1437.

204. Steiner MM: Syndromes of kerosene poisoning in children. Am J Dis Child 1947;74:32–44.

205. Stevens JL, Ratnayake JH, Anders MW: Metabolism of dihalomethanes to carbon monoxide: Studies in isolated rat hepatocytes. Toxicol Appl Pharmacol 1980;55:484–489.

206. Stevenson A, Yaqoob M, Mason H, et al: Biochemical markers of basement membrane disturbances and occupational exposure to hydrocarbons and mixed solvents. Q J Med 1995;88:23–28.

207. Stewart RD, Dodd HC: Absorption of carbon tetrachloride, trichloroethylene, tetrachloroethylene, methylene chloride and 1,1,1-trichloroethane through human skin. Am Ind Hyg Assoc J 1964;25:439–446.

208. Stewart RD, Fisher TN, Hosko MJ, et al: Experimental human exposure to methylene chloride. Arch Environ Health 1972;25:342–348.

209. Stockman JA: More on hydrocarbon-induced hemolysis [letter]. J Pediatr 1977;90:848.

210. Strata RJ, Saffle JR, Kravitz M, et al: Management of tar and asphalt injuries. Am J Surg 1983;146:766–769.

211. Streicher HZ, Gabow PA, Moss AH, et al: Syndromes of toluene sniffing in adults. Ann Intern Med 1981;94:758–762.

212. Substance Abuse and Mental Health Services Administration (SAMHSA): National Household Survey on Drug Abuse: Main Findings 1999. Rockville, MD, DHHS, August, 2000. Available electronically at www.samhsa.gov.

213. Szlatenyi CS, Wang RY: Encephalopathy and cranial nerve palsies caused by intentional trichloroethylene inhalation. Am J Emerg Med 1996;14:464–466.

214. Taher SM, Anderson RJ, McCartney R, et al: Renal tubular acidosis associated with toluene sniffing. N Engl J Med 1974;290:765–768.

215. Takeuchi Y, Ono Y, Hisanaga N, et al: A comparative study on the neurotoxicity of n-pentane, n-hexane, and n-heptane in the rat. Br J Ind Med 1980;37:241–247.

216. Taussig LM, Castro E, Landau LI, et al: Pulmonary function 8–10 years after hydrocarbon pneumonitis. Clin Pediatr 1977;16:57–59.

217. Tomenson JA, Baron CE, O'Sullivan JJ, et al: Hepatic function in workers occupationally exposed to carbon tetrachloride. Occup Environ Med 1995;52:508–514.

218. Torkelson TR: Halogenated aliphatic hydrocarbons. In: Clayton GD, Clayton FE, eds: Patty's Industrial Hygiene and Toxicology, 4th ed. New York, John Wiley & Sons, 1994.

219. Travis LB, Li CY, Zhang ZN, et al: Hematopoietic malignancies and related disorders among benzene-exposed workers in China. Leuk Lymphoma 1994;14:91–102.

220. Truemper E, Reyes de la Rocha SR, Atkinson SD: Clinical characteristics, pathophysiology, and management of hydrocarbon ingestion: Case report and review of the literature. Pediatr Emerg Care 1987;3:187–193.

221. Truss CD, Killenberg PG: Treatment of carbon tetrachloride poisoning with hyperbaric oxygen. Gastroenterology 1982;82:767–769.

222. Tsou TJ, Hutson HR, Bear M, et al: De-solv-it for hot paving asphalt burn: Case report. Acad Emerg Med 1996;3:88–89.

223. Turkel B, Egeli U: Analysis of chromosomal aberrations in shoe workers exposed long-term to benzene. Occup Environ Med 1994;51:50–53.

224. Upreti RK, Das M, Shanker R: Dermal exposure to kerosene. Vet Hum Toxicol 1989;31:16–20.

225. US Department of Health and Human Services (DHHS): Drug Abuse Warning Network (DAWN) Annual Medical Examiner Data, 1996. Series D-4, Publication (SMA) 98–3228, Rockville, MD, July, 1998. Available electronically at www.samhsa.gov.

226. Vaziri ND, Smith PJ, Wilson A: Toxicity with intravenous injection of naphtha in man. Clin Toxicol 1980;16:335–343.

227. Verhulst HL, Page LA: Adrenocortical steroids in the treatment of kerosene pneumonia. New Drugs 1961;1:147–153.

228. Victoria MS, Nangia BS: Hydrocarbon poisoning: A review. Pediatr Emerg Care 1987;3:184–186.

229. Vigliano EC, Saita G: Benzene and leukemia. N Eng J Med 1964; 271:872–876.

230. Voights A, Kaufman CE: Acidosis and other metabolic abnormalities associated with paint sniffing. South Med J 1983;76:443–452.

231. Wahlberg P, Nyman D: Turpentine and thrombocytopenic purpura. Lancet 1969;2:215–216.

232. Waldowski D, Meyer RJ: Hydrocarbon poisoning: A continuing childhood hazard. Virg Med Monthly 1967;94:409–411.

233. Waring JI: Pneumonia in kerosene poisoning. Am J Med Sci 1933; 185:325–330.

234. Wason S, Katona B: A review of symptoms, signs and laboratory findings predictive of hydrocarbon toxicity [abstract]. Vet Hum Toxicol 1987;29:492.

235. Wasserman GS: Hydrocarbon poisoning. Crit Care Q 1982;4:33–41.

236. Watson WA, Weinman SA, ACE Study Group: Activated charcoal (AC) dosing and the prevalence and predictors of emesis [abstract]. J Toxicol Clin Toxicol 1995;33:489–490.

237. Weaver NK. Gasoline. In: Sullivan JB, Krieger GR, eds: Hazardous Materials Toxicology: Clinical Principles of Environmental Health. Philadelphia, Williams & Wilkins, 1992, pp. 807–817.

238. White LE, Driggers DA, Wardinsky TD: Poisoning in childhood and adolescence: A study of 111 cases admitted to a military hospital. J Fam Pract 1980;11:27–31.

239. White MC, Infante PF, Chu KC: A quantitative estimate of leukemia mortality associated with occupational exposure to benzene. Risk Anal 1982;2:195–204.

240. Widmer LR, Goodwin SR, Berman LS, et al: Artificial surfactant for therapy in hydrocarbon-induced lung injury in sheep. Crit Care Med 1996;24:1524–1529.

241. Wirtschafter ZT, Cronyn MW: Relative hepatotoxicity. Arch Environ Health 1964;9:1980–1985.

242. Wolfe BM, Brodeur AE, Shields JB: The role of gastrointestinal absorption of kerosene in producing pneumonitis in dogs. J Pediatr 1970;76:867–873.

243. Wolfe RR: Pneumatoceles complicating hydrocarbon pneumonitis. J Pediatr 1967;71:711–714.

244. Wolfsdorf J: Experimental kerosene pneumonitis in primates: Relevance to the therapeutic management of childhood poisoning. Clin Exp Pharmacol Physiol 1976;3:539–544.

245. Wolfsdorf J: Kerosene intoxication: An experimental approach to the etiology of the CNS manifestations in primates. J Pediatr 1976;88: 1037–1040.

246. Wolfsdorf J: Massive ingestion of kerosene: A study of gastric clearance in primates. Clin Exp Pharm Physiol 1975;2:405–409.

247. Wolfsdorf J, Kundig H: Dexamethasone in the management of kerosene pneumonia. Pediatrics 1974;53:86–90.

248. Wolfsdorf J, Kundig H: Kerosene poisoning in primates. S Afr Med J 1972;46:619–621.

249. Yakes B, Kelsey KT, Seitz T, et al: Occupational skin disease in newspaper pressroom workers. J Occup Med 1991;33:711–717.

250. Yamamura Y: n-Hexane polyneuropathy. Folia Psychiatr Neurol Jap 1969;23:45–57.

251. Zieserl E: Hydrocarbon ingestion and poisoning. Compr Ther 1979; 5:35–42.

252. Zucker AR, Berger S, Wood LDH: Management of kerosene-induced pulmonary injury. Crit Care Med 1986;14:303–304.

CHAPTER 87 CAUSTICS AND BATTERIES

Rama B. Rao / Robert S. Hoffman

A 34-year-old male ingested a cup of liquid drain opener (sodium hydroxide) in an attempted suicide. He vomited once and presented to the Emergency Department (ED) 30 minutes later complaining of chest and abdominal pain. His vital signs were blood pressure, 130/80 mm Hg; heart rate, 100 beats/min; respiratory rate 22 breaths/min; and temperature, 99°F (37.2°C). His oropharynx was only mildly erythematous. There was no stridor, and his lungs were clear. His heart was regular in rhythm without murmurs or gallops. Bowel sounds were present, and the abdomen was soft with mild left-upper-quadrant tenderness. His stool was negative for occult blood. The patient's extremities were warm and well perfused, and his neurologic examination was unremarkable.

Two large-bore intravenous lines were started with 0.9% sodium chloride at 250 mL/h. Blood was sent for serum electrolytes, CBC, platelet count, coagulation profile, type and cross-match, and arterial blood gas analyses. A fiber-optic inspection of the nasopharynx revealed a patent airway with no edema of the larynx. Chest and abdominal radiographs were unremarkable. Over the next few hours his vital signs remained unchanged, as did the rest of his physical examination. The arterial blood gas analyses was pH, 7.30; P_{CO_2}, 30 mm Hg; and P_{O_2}, 88 mm Hg. Upper gastrointestinal endoscopy performed 4 hours after the ingestion revealed a second-degree noncircumferential burn of the midesophagus and third-degree circumferential burn of the distal esophagus with significant necrosis precluding safe passage of the endoscope into the stomach. Repeat vital signs at that time were blood pressure, 90/60 mm Hg; heart rate, 120 beats/min; respiratory rate, 26 breaths/min; and temperature, 100°F (37.8°C). His examination became significant for inspiratory rales in the left lower lung field, and a repeat chest radiograph revealed a small effusion at the left lung base. His abdomen remained soft with the same degree of tenderness as he had on presentation.

The patient was taken to the operating room for exploratory surgery. A bronchoscopy, done simultaneously, was unremarkable. Laparotomy revealed dark discoloration and necrosis of the serosal surface of the gastric antrum, necessitating resection. Further evaluation of the esophagus by thoracotomy revealed a perforation of the distal esophagus above the lower esophageal sphincter. The patient underwent esophagogastrectomy with placement of bilateral chest tubes for drainage, and placement of a jejunostomy tube for subsequent feeding. Postoperatively, the patient developed pneumonia and responded well to antibiotic therapy. He had intensive medical and psychiatric care in the hospital. After several weeks in the hospital, he was discharged with postoperative and psychiatric followup care organized.

Caustic agents cause histologic and clinical damage on contact with tissue surfaces. There are many caustic agents available in home products (Table 87–1). These may come in solid and liquid forms with different viscosities and concentrations of solution.

As early as 1927, the United States mandated warning labels on lye- and acid-containing products. The subsequent development of poison prevention education, safety packaging, and lowering of available household concentrations of caustics led to a dramatic decrease in the incidence of unintentional caustic injuries in children. One study noted that although children comprised 39% of admissions for caustic ingestions, adults comprised 81% of patients requiring treatment.[69] Unfortunately, children in developing nations may not benefit from these interventions, as such safety considerations are not globally used.

In adults, sources of caustic exposures can be industrial or household products that result in occupational exposure or are used in suicide attempts. Less commonly, poorly labeled containers may be mistaken for a beverage. Lye is also used criminally to splash a victim's face and cause skin deformities and blindness.

Unfortunately, the severity of a caustic injury may not be immediately evident in patients who present shortly after an exposure. Predicting which patients will require immediate interventions to prevent morbidity and mortality requires multiple clinical and laboratory parameters. This chapter reviews the pathophysiology and approach to patients with potentially serious caustic exposures.

PATHOPHYSIOLOGY

A caustic agent is a substance that causes both functional and histologic damage on contact with body surfaces. Although there are many ways to categorize caustic agents, they are most typically classified as acids or alkalis. An acid is a proton donor and causes significant injury, generally at a pH below 3. An alkaline agent is a proton acceptor causing significant caustic injury, generally at a pH above 11. The injury is incurred as neutralization of the substance takes place at the expense of the tissues, which also releases thermal energy and induces burns. The extent of injury is determined by duration of contact; ability of the substance to penetrate tissues; volume, pH, and concentration of the agent; and a property known as titratable acid or alkaline reserve (TAR). TAR quantifies the amount of neutralizing substance needed to bring the pH of a caustic to that of physiologic tissues. The larger the

TABLE 87–1. Sources of Common Caustic Chemicals

Chemical Agent	Commercial Applications
Acetic acid	Permanent wave neutralizers, photographic stop bath
Acids (tungstic, picric, tannic)	Industrial use
Ammonia (ammonium hydroxide)	Toilet bowl cleaners, metal cleaners and polishes, hair dyes and tints, antirust products, jewelry cleaners, floor strippers, glass cleaners, wax removers
Benzalkonium chloride	Detergents
Boric acid	Roach powders, water softeners, germicide
Cantharides (Spanish fly)	Aphrodisiac (in animals), hair tonic, illicit abortifacient
Formaldehyde, formic acid	Deodorizing tablets, plastic menders, fumigant, embalming agent
Hydrochloric acid (muriatic acid)	Metal and toilet bowl cleaners
Hydrofluoric acid	Antirust products, glass etching, microchip etching
Iodine	Antiseptics
Mercuric chloride (HgCl$_2$)	Preservative
Methylethyl ketone peroxide	Industrial synthetic agent
Oxalic acid	Disinfectants, household bleach, metal cleaning liquids, antirust products, furniture polish
Phenol (creosol, creosote)	Antiseptics, preservatives
Phosphoric acid	Toilet bowl cleaners
Phosphorous	Matches, rodenticides, fireworks, insecticides
Potassium permanganate	Illicit abortifacient, antiseptic solution
Selenious acid	Gun bluing
Sodium hydroxide	Detergents, Clinitest tablets, paint removers, drain cleaners and openers, oven cleaners
Sodium borates, carbonates, phosphates, and silicates	Detergents, electric dishwasher preparations, water softeners
Sodium hypochlorite	Bleaches, cleansers
Sulfuric acid	Automobile batteries, drain cleaners
Zinc chloride	Soldering flux

titratable alkaline reserve, the more caustic or damaging the agent.[7,26,53,66,72] Some agents with a pH between 3 and 11 can cause severe burns because of the molecular properties of the substance and its TAR. Both zinc chloride and phenol are examples of caustics with a near physiologic pH. These factors, along with the presence or absence of food in the stomach, may play a role in the severity of injury sustained by caustic exposure.[149]

A grading system based on endoscopic visualization describes esophageal burns in a classification similar to that applied to dermal burns. Grade I burns are generally accepted as hyperemia or edema of the mucosa without evidence of ulcer formation.[38,86,207] Grade II burns include submucosal lesions, ulcerations, and exudates. Some studies have further divided grade II lesions into grade IIa, noncircumferential lesions, and grade IIb, near-circumferential injuries.[33] Grade III burns are defined as deep ulcers and necrosis into the periesophageal tissues.[56,60,68,86] A small amount of necrosis is defined by one author as grade IIIa, with extensive necrosis as IIIb.[207]

Alkalis

Alkaline agents saponify tissues, causing deep and progressive damage while penetrating mucosal surfaces.[7,66] The injury is histologically described as liquefactive necrosis. Animal studies demonstrate that within seconds of contact there is the erythema and edema of the mucosa and a subsequent inflammatory reaction extending to the submucosa and muscular layers of the esophagus. Ulcers may form. On microscopic inspection, there is evidence of transmural thrombosis. Cell death occurs early in this necrotic phase.[7,88,101,184]

Experimental animal models, human case reports, postmortem studies, and histologic inspection of surgical specimens reveal a consistent pattern of injury and repair.[1,54,61,117,133,158] As wound healing progresses, neovascularization and fibroblast proliferation take place, laying down new collagen and replacing the damaged esophageal layers with granulation tissue. Ulcers may persist for up to 8 weeks as remodeling occurs. The esophagus subsequently undergoes shortening.[197] If the initial injury penetrates deeply enough, there is progressive narrowing of the esophageal lumen. The dense scar formation presents clinically as a stricture.[41,66] Strictures can evolve over a period of weeks to months, leading to dysphagia and significant nutritional deficits.[153,161,197] Grade I burns carry no risk of stricture formation.[38,86,207] Grade II circumferential burns lead to stricture formation in about 75% of cases. Grade III burns invariably progress to stricture formation and are also at a high risk of perforation.[4,69,133,195] Significant complications can occur at various stages of wound recovery. Most importantly, these include airway compromise, perforations of the gastrointestinal tract with the development of mediastinitis or peritonitis, and other overwhelming infections from bacteria residing in the oropharynx. Other complications reported include motility abnormalities of the pharynx and esophagus,[42] formation of aorto- and tracheoesophageal fistulas, delayed massive hemorrhage from erosion into a great vessel, and pulmonary thrombosis.[18,69,86,140,147,166,168] Long-term survivors of moderate and severe injury of the esophagus have a risk of esophageal carcinoma that is 1000 times higher than the general population and appear to present with a 40-year latency.[6]

Acids

Acid-induced lesions differ histologically from those following alkali ingestions. A cat model of the effects of sulfuric acid on the esophagus revealed a coagulative necrosis of the mucosa with whitish discoloration of the tissues and underlying smooth muscle spasm.[7] On gross inspection an inflammatory response ensues,[119] and edema, mucosal sloughing, motility dysfunction, and esophageal shortening are demonstrated in other animal models.[172,175] The subsequent burns are not unlike those occurring with alkali ingestion. Acid ingestions frequently give rise to gastric damage with pooling of the agent in the antrum probably secondary to pylorospasm.[32,39,44,45,63, 78,89,99,119,139,179,180,200,207] In most series, both the gastric and esophageal mucosa are equally affected.[45,78,208] On occasion, the esophagus may be spared damage while severe injury is noted in the stomach.[39,63,69,181] This tends to be a rarer finding than concomitant injury to both stomach and esophagus, and is probably related to the rapid transit time of liquid acids through the upper gastrointestinal tract. Skip lesions from acid ingestions may be a function of viscosity and contact time.[69]

In addition, acids tend to disproportionally damage extraintestinal organs such as the spleen, liver, biliary tract, and pancreas because of the absorption characteristics of these agents.[29,74,193,197] A patient who survives the acute injury may subsequently develop stricture formation, gastric atony, decreased acid secretion, pseudodiverticuli, and gastric outlet obstruction.[28,59,89,144,179,208] As with alkali injuries, grade II and grade III circumferential burns are at risk for stricture formation.

The subsequent risk of carcinoma after acid ingestions is not adequately studied, but three patients developed squamous cell cancer of the stomach (a rare form of stomach cancer) years after their initial injuries.[48]

Clinical Presentation and Predictors of Injury

A patient's skin, eyes, gastrointestinal tract, and respiratory tract can all be sites of caustic injury. By far, the most life-threatening and long-term morbidity of caustic exposure results from oral ingestion. In general, patients who have ingested alkaline or acid agents have similar initial presentations.

Patients usually experience severe pain on contact. Depending upon the amount of agent swallowed and its formulation (solid vs liquid), the patient may complain of oropharyngeal, throat, chest, or abdominal pain. Spontaneous vomiting may occur, followed by rapid airway compromise if significant burns of the oropharynx or aspiration of caustic has occurred. Accordingly, patients may be tachypneic or hyperpneic due to airway injury, or as a compensatory response to the lactic acidosis generated from necrotic tissue.

As grade II and grade III burns can progress to more severe complications, several studies have attempted to identify patients with these potential injuries. A prospective study of alkali ingestions by both adults and children found that stridor was 100% specific for significant esophageal injury, but was unfortunately based on only three patients with this sign. No other single sign or symptom was predictive of the presence of an esophageal injury.[60]

The presence or absence of oropharyngeal burns identified on examination has repeatedly been found to be a poor predictor of distal esophagogastric injury.[2,27,38,56,60,151,192] In one study there was a 37.5% incidence of esophageal lesions in the absence of oropharyngeal lesions, and 22.2% of these were second- and third-degree burns.[151]

A retrospective study of 378 children admitted for a caustic injury found that signs or symptoms could not be used to predict significant esophageal injury.[56] In a prospective study of 79 children evaluated for vomiting, drooling, or stridor, a combination of two or more of these signs was found to be a predictor of significant esophageal injury as visualized on endoscopy.[38]

The abdominal examination is likewise an unreliable indicator of the severity of injury. The presence of abdominal pain suggests tissue injury of variable grades, but the absence of pain or findings on abdominal examination does not preclude life-threatening gastrointestinal damage.[51,78,153,166,204] Peritoneal signs and mental status changes are more ominous findings, usually indicating severe injury.

Patients surviving the first few hours may develop precipitous hemodynamic instability secondary to vascular or viscous perforations, or septic shock.

Those patients surviving a few weeks after a grade II or III injury may subsequently present with dysphagia and vomiting from stricture formation or motility disorders.

DIAGNOSTIC TESTING

Laboratory

All patients with presumed caustic exposure necessitate blood for type and crossmatch, baseline, hemoglobin, and electrolytes, and a urinalysis. An elevated INR and partial thromboplastin times are associated with severe caustic injury.[204]

A prospective study of serum pH as a predictor of significant injury in patients with alkali ingestions has yet to be undertaken, but it may be a useful indicator of the extent of injury, as significant tissue necrosis would be expected to generate a lactic acidosis.[166] In some cases of acid injury, a systemic acidemia may be noted due to systemic absorption of nonionized acid from the stomach mucosa. Hydrochloric acid ingestions may initially result in a nonanion gap metabolic acidosis, as both the hydrogen and chloride ions dissociate in the serum and are both accounted for in the measurement of the anion gap. Other acids, such as sulfuric acid, may also be absorbed and precipitate an elevated anion gap metabolic acidosis as the anion, sulfate (SO_4^{-2}), for example, in this case, is not directly measured in the calculation of the anion gap.

Obtaining gastric fluid to test pH was performed in one study. A gastric pH greater than 7.30 correlated retrospectively with severe alkaline injury. The prospective utility of this information is limited, as obtaining gastric secretions without direct visualization may be dangerous.

Radiology

Both chest and abdominal radiographs can provide information in the initial stages of management only if radiographic findings are present (Fig. 87–1). Pneumomediastinum, pleural effusion, and pneumoperitoneum are indicators of viscus perforation. An upright lateral chest radiograph may be more sensitive than a pos-

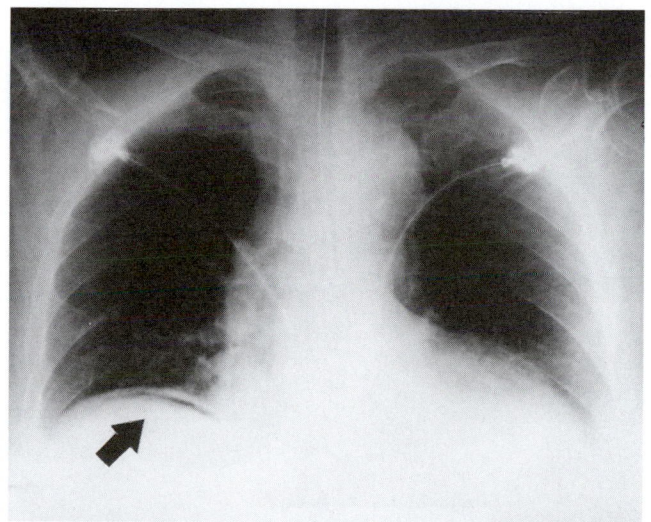

Figure 87–1. Chest radiograph demonstrating free air under the right hemidiaphragm. This patient ingested concentrated hydrochloric acid and had a perforated viscus. The patient required emergent laparotomy for repair. (*Courtesy of the New York City Poison Center Toxicology Fellowship.*)

teroanterior film in detecting free peritoneal air.[203] In general, however, these studies have a low sensitivity, and an absence of radiographic findings does not preclude presence of perforations of the upper gastrointestinal tract.[204] Even contrast studies can fail to detect perforations,[78] but dye extravasation outside of the gastrointestinal tract is diagnostic when present.[208] In patients with grade III injuries in which the presence of perforation is uncertain or where circumferential burns of the esophagus 0preclude visualization of the remainder of the upper GI tract, water-soluble contrast is recommended as it is less irritating to tissues in cases of perforation.[54]

Esophageal dilation, displacement of the pleural reflection, and widening of the pleuroesophageal line are suggestive of significant necrosis and impending perforation.[117] In general, the results should be interpreted within the context of the patient's clinical status, as the information can be unreliable.[18,35,65,78,117] There may be a role for computed tomography (CT), although the use of CT has yet to be formally investigated in acute caustic ingestions (Fig. 87–2).

The most valuable use of radiographic procedures is to noninvasively follow the patient after initial evaluation and stabilization have occurred. In a group of patients followed with serial contrast studies, radiographic findings included blurred esophageal margins or "scalloped and straightened margins," linear collections of contrast materials corresponding to intramural dissection and ulcers, retained contrast secondary to esophageal dysmotility, dilatation of the esophagus, and displacement of the pleural reflection.[117] Esophageal narrowing develops later (Fig. 87–3).[117] This information can be utilized in management of patients, and one author recommends routine use of contrast radiography to follow patients postoperatively.[185]

Other radiographic studies recently reported in the management of patients with caustic ingestion include esophageal ultrasound to determine the depth of injury,[138] and chest contrast tomography of strictures to determine width as a potential indicator for response to dilation.[99]

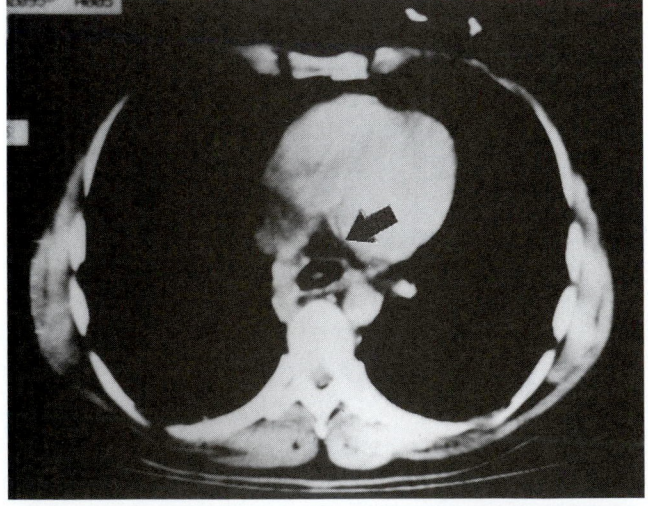

Figure 87–2. Computed tomograph of a patient who ingested an acid. This transverse view through the chest demonstrates mediastinal air (arrow) from a perforated esophagus that was not evident on plain radiographs. *(Courtesy of the New York City Poison Center Toxicology Fellowship.)*

MANAGEMENT
Initial Stabilization

The primary goal of initial management is airway assessment and stabilization followed by obtaining a thorough history of the exposure. For both adults and children, simple inspection of the oropharynx, vital signs, and mental status and assessment for stridor or respiratory distress are critical to preparing for the treatment of airway compromise. Large-bore intravenous access in adults is crucial, and blood work should be sent for type and crossmatch, hematocrit, coagulation parameters, and electrolytes, as these patients may require emergent surgical intervention.

Direct visual inspection of the vocal cords with a fiberoptic nasopharyngoscope will provide additional information regarding the need for intubation. Any signs of airway edema or depressed mentation should prompt airway protection, as edema may rapidly evolve over a period of minutes to hours making subsequent attempts at intubation or bag-valve mask ventilation difficult. Patients who clearly have a need for intubation are best served by direct visualization of the airway, as perforation of edematous tissues of the pharynx and larynx is a grave complication. Fiberoptic intubation or orotracheal intubation with a laryngoscope may be attempted. Paralytic agents for induction are best avoided, if possible, as airway edema and bleeding may distort the ability to successfully intubate or ventilate via bag-valve mask. Patients with significant ingestions may require emergent surgical airway intervention. These decisions are dependent upon the status of the patient, the ability to endotracheally or nasotracheally intubate via fiberoptic scope, and the comfort of the physician in performing the technique of a surgical airway. If airway involvement is significant enough to warrant intubation, electively or otherwise, it is best to mobilize a team of the most skilled physicians early in the event of unforeseen complications in attempting to gain control of the airway. Nonsurgical airway placement is recommended whenever possible, as it is less likely to interfere with the surgical field if esophageal repair is required.[204] Subsequent assessment of heart rate and blood pressure will provide some information regarding the severity of the ingestion, and should be followed serially.

Decontamination, Dilution, and Neutralization

The ability to decontaminate patients with alkaline ingestions is limited. Gastric emptying via blind passage of an orogastric or nasogastric tube carries the risk of perforation of damaged tissues and thus should be avoided in all unknown or definitively identified alkaline agents. In patients with large intentional ingestions of acid who present within 30 minutes, consideration can be given to cautious placement of a narrow nasogastric tube suction to remove remaining acid in the gut.[149] This technique has never been studied in this group of patients, and although there is a risk of perforation, the outcome for these patients is often grave and options for treatment limited. Therefore, early removal of some portion of the ingested acid may have potential benefit.

Activated charcoal is contraindicated, as it will interfere with tissue evaluation by endoscopy and preclude a subsequent management plan. Additionally, most caustics are not adsorbed to activated charcoal. Syrup of ipecac is also contraindicated, as it may cause reintroduction of the caustic agent to the upper gastrointestinal tract and airway.

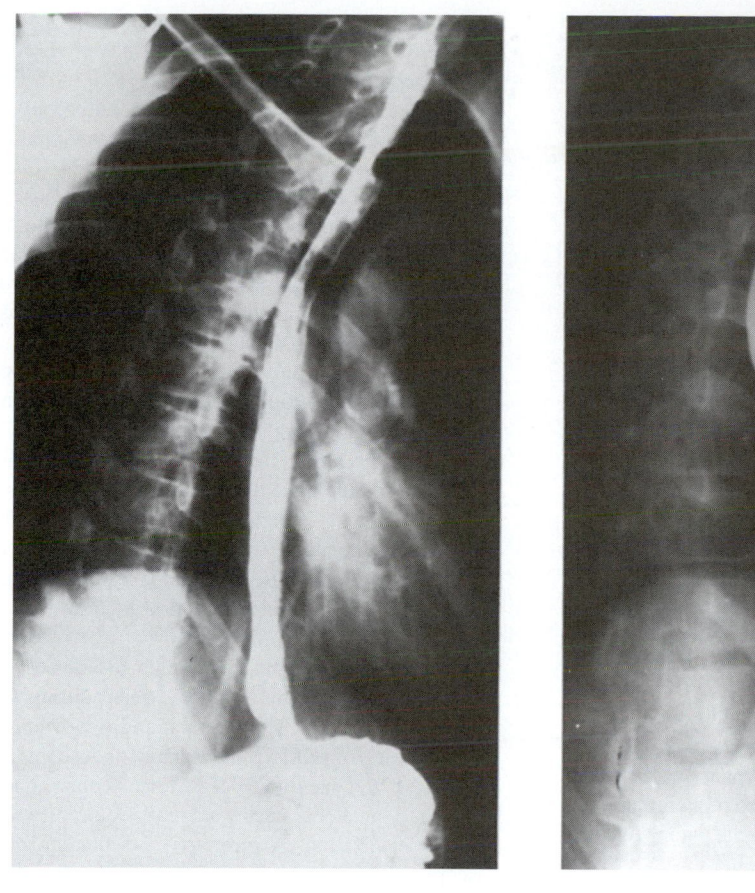

A   B

Figure 87–3. **A.** Barium swallow several days after ingestion of liquid lye shows the esophagus to be atonic. There is poor coating of the esophagus, suggesting edema and intramural penetration. Note that the initial evaluation immediately following a caustic ingestion to assess the extent of injury is esophagoscopy, rather than a contrast esophagram. **B.** Four months later, a repeat barium esophagram shows a severe stricture below the middle third of the esophagus. The barium barely passes the stricture and the remainder of the esophagus is pencil thin. (*Courtesy of Emil J. Balthazar, MD, Professor of Radiology, New York University.*)

The use of dilutional therapy has been examined in both in vitro and in vivo models in an attempt to attenuate caustic injury. Early in vitro models demonstrated a dramatic increase in temperature when either water or milk was added to crystal Drano or Clinitest tablets.[163] Another in vitro model of dilution found smaller changes in temperature and pH despite large volumes of diluent. It was suggested that dilution would have limited utility.[118] An in vivo canine model of alkaline injury demonstrated that water dilution did not cause an increase in either temperature or intraluminal pressures.[77] Alternatively, an ex vivo study of harvested rat esophagi examined the histopathologic effects of saline dilution after an alkali injury and found that damage occurred to tissue within seconds to minutes and was attended by an increase in temperature. The utility of dilution appeared to decrease as time from exposure lengthened, with minimal efficacy noted in as little as 30 minutes.[74,75]

The extrapolation of these variable results to humans with caustic exposures is limited, and suggests that histologic damage can only be attenuated by milk or water when administered within the first seconds to minutes following the ingestion.[7,74–77,101,184] For solid substances, such as crystal lye or Clinitest tablets, there may be some value for dilution later than for liquid caustics, as tissue

contact time is increased with solid agents and their concentration is usually 100% over a small surface area. Milk may be the best agent with regard to its ability to attenuate the heat generated.[181] Caution should be used in advising patients or family members about the use of dilutional agents. A child who refuses to swallow or take oral liquids should not be forced to do so. There is concern about the airway, extent of damage, potential for nausea, abdominal distension, and vomiting that may worsen the injury.[163]

The use of milk or water should be limited to patients within the first few minutes after exposure who have no airway compromise or vomiting, who are alert and not complaining of significant abdominal pain or nausea, and who are old enough and able to speak.

Attempts at neutralizing caustics should be avoided. This technique has the potential to worsen tissue damage by forming gas and generating an exothermic reaction. In vitro and ex vivo models demonstrate that neutralization of caustics generates heat, requires a large volume to attain a physiologic pH, and may have limited utility in preventing histologic damage after the first few minutes postexposure.[73,118,163] In an in vivo canine model, orange juice was used to neutralize sodium hydroxide–induced gastric injury and demonstrated no change in temperature or intraluminal pressure.[77] There are no other data demonstrating that clinical outcome is improved. Accordingly, neutralization is not recommended at this time.

Surgical Management

After airway assessment, a complete physical examination should be performed, and the patient should be placed on continuous hemodynamic monitoring. Hypotension is a grave finding and often indicates perforation or significant blood loss. Intravenous fluids and assessment for operative intervention should be considered. Surgical intervention can include laparotomy for inspection and resection or repair of perforations, or possibly laparoscopy for tissue visualization, although laparoscopy may not allow inspection of the posterior aspect of the stomach. Gastrostomy or enterostomy can also be performed to provide a nutritional conduit.

The decision to perform emergent surgery for patients with caustic ingestions is most obvious in those who have evidence of perforation either on endoscopic examination or radiographic studies,[204] severe abdominal rigidity, or persistent hypotension. Many patients, however, will not have such evidence, and yet may be in grave danger of perforation, necrosis, sepsis, or delayed hemorrhage during recovery, all of which may be avoided if surgery is performed early in the management.[143]

Identifying such surgical candidates in a timely fashion is challenging. Some studies demonstrate increased morbidity and mortality for patients who have delayed surgical repair.[51,78,81,157,166] In some cases, these patients did not have evidence of significant tissue damage earlier in their clinical course, and the parameters utilized for surgical intervention were variable.[78,166,204] Some surgeons advocate laparotomy for all patients with second- and third-degree burns of the esophagus identified on endoscopy.[51,132] This aggressive approach allows for direct inspection of serosal surfaces and an opportunity for repair.[51,132]

Several retrospective and prospective series of surgical patients with caustic ingestions found that patients with large ingestions of caustics (greater than 150 mL), shock, agitation, acidemia, or coagulation disorders tend to have severe findings on surgical exploration. The abdominal examination was frequently unreliable in predicting the need for surgery.[166,204,208] Patients with severe acid injuries may lack abdominal pain, abdominal tenderness on examination, and radiographic findings.[45,78,208] Large-volume ingestions, ranging between 40 and 200 mL, and a delay in surgical repair are associated with increased mortality.[45,78,204]

One author used a stepwise approach of bronchoscopy, endoscopy, and abdominal sonography to provide additional information regarding extent of injury prior to surgery. Hemoglobinuria, respiratory distress, ascites, pleural fluid, and a serum pH below 7.2 were used as indications for surgery.[204]

It is clear that no single criterion can determine which patients without obvious perforation require surgery. Serial clinical evaluation of the mental status, vital signs, acid-base status, radiographs, coagulation studies, history of a massive or intentional ingestion, and type of caustic agent may collectively aid in the decision to operate. A timely decision for those patients who need surgery appears to improve outcome following acid ingestions,[31] and it is likely that the same holds true for those with alkaline ingestions.

Endoscopy

The majority of adult patients with caustic ingestions have injury without immediate life-threatening manifestations. Their assessment subsequently requires direct inspection of the esophagus by endoscopy.

Endoscopy is a standard diagnostic tool in the management of caustic ingestions. The candidates for endoscopy include all patients with stridor (after the airway is stabilized), children with both vomiting and drooling (and potentially just one of these symptoms), and adults with intentional ingestions. Any adult with an unintentional ingestion who manifests symptomatology potentially related to the exposure should probably undergo endoscopy as well, because this group has not been adequately studied.

Children with unintentional caustic ingestions who remain completely asymptomatic and tolerate liquids after a few hours of observation can probably be discharged from the hospital. Further evaluation by endoscopy should be considered in pediatric patients with a single symptom (pain, vomiting, drooling) and definitively provided if more than one symptom is present.[38]

Patients should have the procedure performed within 12 hours and preferably no later than 24 hours postingestion. Numerous case series demonstrate that the procedure is safe during this period; it offers a rapid means of obtaining diagnostic and treatment information, and shortens the period of time that patients forego nutritional support.[33,41,44,51,65,68,94,109,132,166,167,195,198,207] There is a period of wound softening beginning on the second or third day postinjury and lasting for roughly 2 weeks during which time there is an increased risk of perforation if endoscopy is performed.

The choice of rigid versus flexible endoscopy is dependent on the comfort and experience of the endoscopist. The flexible endoscope has a smaller diameter but may require gentle insufflation of air for visualization. A prospective evaluation of fiberoptic endoscopy recommends the following guidelines for a safe approach: (a) direct visualization of the esophagus prior to advancing the instrument, (b) minimal insufflation of air, (c) passage into the stomach unless there was a severe esophageal burn (particularly circumferential burns), and (d) no retroversion or retroflexion of the instrument within the esophagus.[207] Adherence to this regimen should minimize the risk of iatrogenic perforation of the upper gastrointestinal tract.

Most cases of perforation clearly linked to endoscopy have occurred when the endoscope was advanced through a severely eroded esophagus.[195] The advantage of visualization of the gastric mucosa is demonstrated by several case reports of patients with minimal esophageal damage, yet severe necrosis and ulceration of the stomach, sometimes necessitating surgical resection.[132,181,192,207] Some authors advocate the presence of a surgeon during endoscopy to assist in the assessment for potential surgical intervention.[166]

Endoscopy even in hemodynamically stable patients may be of limited utility. Significant circumferential burns to the esophagus may preclude the visualization of distal portions of the upper GI tract, which may contain more severe lesions. In addition the injury may evolve, and although most endoscopies performed early give an adequate idea of the grading, continued tissue damage may occur. Perforations, in fact, often occur during the remodeling phase between days 7 and 14.[184] Endoscopy is also an operator-dependent procedure in which distinguishing between a grade II and grade III injury can be difficult. The endoscopist is only able to appreciate the mucosal surface, and not the serosal side, limiting the utility of the results. This is especially evident in stomach ulcerations, which may appear black and necrotic from a true burn through the layers of the stomach, or from the effect of stomach acid on the blood exposed from a shallower lesion. Only direct serosal inspection allows for the distinction, and in questionable circumstances, surgical inspection provides the definitive evaluation.

After Endoscopy

The extent of tissue injury dictates the subsequent management and disposition of patients. Patients with isolated grade I injuries of the esophagus do not develop strictures and are not at increased risk of carcinoma. Their diet can be resumed as tolerated. They can potentially be discharged from the hospital after this diagnosis is established with endoscopy, they are able to eat and drink,[14,192] and their psychiatric status is defined as stable. No additional therapies are required.

If the endoscopy reveals grade IIa lesions of the esophagus and sparing of the stomach, a soft diet can be resumed as tolerated, or a nasogastric tube can be passed to provide interim enteral support. Patients with higher grades of injury must be followed for the complications of perforation, infection, and stricture. The metabolic demands of these burn patients increase significantly,[176] and oral intake may be poorly tolerated or contraindicated if there is a risk of perforation. For these patients feeding via gastrostomy, jejunostomy, or total parenteral nutrition can be instituted as indicated.

Patients with grade IIb lesions often develop strictures, and interventions such as corticosteroids, with antibiotics or stents for lesional bypass, can be entertained. Corticosteroid therapy for treatment of caustic injury was first investigated in animals in the 1950s. The theory was to arrest the process of inflammatory repair and potentially prevent stricture formation. Unfortunately, most animals given steroids died of overwhelming sepsis. However, when combined with antibiotic therapy, the death rate diminished.[161]

Adequate human data demonstrating the efficacy of corticosteroids with or without antibiotics have yet to be generated. There are multitudes of case series that use different criteria for the institution of corticosteroid and antibiotic therapy. Most of these are retrospective and do not differentiate the outcome of second- and third-degree lesions.[4,35,79,133,135,166,195]

Third-degree burns as described in different studies have variable definitions, and there is some evidence that they may progress to stricture regardless of therapy.[4,69,133,195] Third-degree burns also have a high degree of complication, including fistula formation, infection, and perforation. Corticosteroids may mask infection and make the friable, necrotic tissue more prone to perforation. A meta-analysis of the efficacy of corticosteroid therapy in 361 patients with caustic injury found that patients with second- and third-degree burns, strictures formed in 24% of the corticosteroid-treated group and 52% of the untreated group. The authors concluded that prospective trials are necessary to better define the role of corticosteroids in caustic injury.[79]

The only prospective, randomized study of corticosteroid efficacy for caustic injury of the esophagus spanned an 18-year period during which a total of only 60 children could be randomized to corticosteroid therapy plus antibiotics or no corticosteroid therapy. In this study, third-degree burns were distinguished from second-degree burns by their circumferential pattern. The incidence of stricture was not different between the treated and untreated groups, and it appeared that the circumferential burns were more likely to develop strictures than were the ulcerative noncircumferential lesions.[4] Although the study failed to have the power to detect a meaningful difference between the treatment and nontreatment groups, no other study has prospectively enrolled sufficient patients to answer the question of corticosteroid efficacy. The most suitable group to receive corticosteroids (with antibiotics) is probably that group of patients with grade IIb injuries. When corticosteroids are employed, the appropriate dose is 2 mg/kg/d of prednisolone or its equivalent in children, and methylprednisolone 40 mg every 8 hours in adults. The course of therapy is 14–21 days followed by a corticosteroid taper. Concomitant antibiotic therapy is indicated after corticosteroids are begun. The antibiotic chosen should treat oral flora, including anaerobic bacteria. Intravenous penicillin, ampicillin, or clindamycin are appropriate for infectious prophylaxis.[66,161]

No major outcome studies have investigated the use of antibiotics alone as prophylactic treatment for stricture or burns, although some case series include antibiotics in the therapeutic regimen. Fever and infection may indicate a potential or impending perforation and may be masked by the prophylactic use of antibiotics alone. It is probably best to reserve antibiotics for an identified source of infection unless corticosteroids are being employed as therapy.

In general, patients with grade III injuries progress to stricture formation that is not altered by corticosteroids. Severely injured tissue (grade IIIb) is at a high risk of complications, including perforations and infections, which may be masked or worsened by corticosteroid therapy. This group needs close attention to several clinical parameters to aid in deciding on the need for surgery. Endoscopy can be used to follow the progress of patients provided they remain stable and other imaging procedures such as contrast radiography or computed tomography are used during the period of wound softening. Patients with stricture formation require long-term endoscopic followup for the presence of neoplastic changes of the esophagus that may occur with a delay of several decades.[6]

STRICTURES

Stricture formation is a debilitating complication of both acid and alkaline ingestions that can evolve over a period of weeks or months (Fig. 87–3). A variety of management strategies have been used in an attempt to prevent strictures or to minimize the sequelae of esophageal obstruction. The placement of intraluminal stents and nasogastric tubes may have some potential benefit.[134,198] Both animal models[155] and human case series[71,134,154] report the use of silicone rubber tubing to maintain the patency of the esophageal lumen. The stent is placed by direct visualization and attached to a feeding tube secured in the nasopharynx. The internal diameter is 3/8 inch in adults, and 1/4 inch in children, allowing the patient to receive feedings through the stent without interference in esophageal repair. The device is left in place for 3 weeks,[154,155] and these patients are given corticosteroids as well as antibiotics. Outcomes are variable in the prevention of strictures. In animal models, the use of a stent for 3 weeks appears to be superior in maintaining patency to corticosteroids with antibiotics alone.[155] The potential disadvantage is the concomitant mechanical trauma of the stent or tube at the site, and the potential for increased reflux, which may inhibit repair.[175] A cat model of stented sodium hydroxide burns also reported deaths from aspiration and mediastinitis.[155] Large series of human exposures managed with stents and corticosteroids are lacking.

The more common approach is endoscopic dilation, which is usually done over a wire with a device designed for esophageal dilation. There are a variety of types of dilators, and generally, multiple dilations are required. The safest time for dilation is after confirmation of stricture formation and after acute repair of the esophagus has taken place so that the risk of perforation is decreased. This is usually no earlier than 4 weeks postingestion. Contrast CT can be used to determine maximal esophageal wall thickness as a predictor of response to dilation.[99] In one study, patients with a maximal esophageal wall thickness of 9 mm or greater required more than seven sessions to achieve adequate dilation. This was significantly higher than in patients with a smaller maximal wall thickness.[99] Measurement of maximal wall thickness may be useful in determining the long-term followup, the type of nutritional support, and the potential need for surgical repair as an alternative to dilations. It may also provide an indication for those who should undergo dilations under fluoroscopy to limit the risk of perforation.

The risk of perforation from dilation is well reported in several series.[69,86,99,152,195] Following perforation, patients may complain of dyspnea or chest pain and may have subcutaneous emphysema or pneumomediastinum. A CT scan or contrast radiograph may identify the perforation and provide information for emergent surgical repair if the diagnosis is unclear.[99,152]

The natural repair of tissue causes collagen production, which increases scar formation and can ultimately result in stricture formation. Lathyrogens such as β-amino proprionitrile (BAPN), penicillamine, and other agents, such as *N*-acetylcysteine (NAC) and colchicine, interfere with collagen synthesis and/or breakdown. These agents have been examined as treatment for the prevention of strictures in various animal models. Colchicine, which increases collagen synthesis as well as collagenase activity, did not prevent stricture formation in rabbits with sodium hydroxide–induced esophageal burns.[186] Both penicillamine and NAC were of some benefit in preventing strictures in rats and rabbits.[57,108,186] BAPN was examined in a dog model in conjunction with dilation, and there was some suggestion that it was useful.[113] More recently, rats treated with epidermal growth factor and interferon-γ had decreased collagen production and stenosis following sodium hydroxide burns.[13]

All of these modalities are still experimental for the treatment of caustic burns, and their routine use cannot be advocated in human exposures at this time.

UNIQUE CAUSTIC INGESTIONS

Clinitest Tablets

Clinitest tablets are used to test for glucosuria by directly adding the tablet to the urine. The reagent contains copper sulfate, sodium carbonate, sodium hydroxide, and citric acid. In the presence of glucose and moisture, cupric sulfate is converted to cupric oxide, inducing a detectable color change in the urine and releasing carbon dioxide and heat.[24,98,145] Unfortunately, this tablet formulation can be easily misinterpreted as an oral medication and can be ingested unintentionally or in an attempted suicide with the potential for severe alkaline caustic injury. As the tablet takes minutes to dissolve, the tissue destruction incurred is generally well localized, especially if minimal fluid is ingested and the tablet is lodged in the upper gastrointestinal tract. The range of reported toxicity is

highly variable. One patient who swallowed at least 47 tablets over several days secondary to misunderstanding the use of the pills had relatively benign findings and outcome,[114] yet unintentional ingestion of just one pill has also resulted in death from an aortoesophageal fistula induced by the burn.[143] Single-tablet ingestions in children frequently result in stricture formation, perhaps because they are often consumed without fluids.[24,58,147] Gastroduodenal ulcers are also reported.[36,194]

Patients can present with vomiting, chest and abdominal pain, and, rarely, oral lesions, which are unreliable indicators of the severity of exposure.[114,145] A case of fatal laryngeal edema was reported.[114] Management of these injuries is similar to those caused by other caustic alkaline agents. The airway should be quickly assessed. Dilutional therapy should be considered in an attempt to decrease the local concentration of the caustic components. An in vitro study noted that the heat released on contact with water is increased when less water is present, or when the number of tablets in solution is increased. Orange juice appeared to minimize the pH elevation of the resulting solution most efficaciously.[98] An extrapolation of these results warrants at least cold tap-water dilution, and, if possible, cold orange juice, but only if the patient is alert and can tolerate fluids. Subsequent management includes endoscopic evaluation of the upper gastrointestinal tract. Fortunately, Clinitest use has decreased dramatically as safer glucose testing of capillary blood has become more widely available.

Ammonia (Ammonium Hydroxide)

Ammonia products are weak bases that can cause significant esophageal burns depending on the concentration and volume ingested.[14,69,166,181,184] Household ammonium hydroxide ranges in concentration from 3% to 10%. Management of these patients should proceed similarly to other alkaline ingestions. Strictures have evolved in patients who ingested 28% ammonia solutions.[142] For exposures to gases resulting from ammonium hydroxide combined with bleach see Chapter 95.

Sodium Hypochlorite (Bleach)

Sodium hypochlorite is the major component in most industrial and household bleach preparations. Large case series and reports have found that grade II and grade III injuries occur only in patients with large-volume ingestions of concentrated bleach products.[44] A series of 393 household bleach ingestions reported no stricture formation,[100] and a canine model found that although regurgitation was a common effect of bleach, no esophageal lesions were noted, and perforation only occurred with prolonged contact.[100] Most patients do well with supportive care.[14,33,69,180] Patients who complain of pain, or who have either high-concentration or high-volume ingestions, should have endoscopic evaluation of the esophagus, as there are little data regarding these severe exposures.

Phenols

Phenols have historically been used as antiseptic agents and are currently present in household cleaning agents and disinfectants in 2–5% solutions.[80] Phenolic compounds are strongly acidic agents that can induce severe dermal and mucosal injury. The acidity attributed to phenols is not from the ability to donate protons, but rather the ability to accept an electron pair to form a covalent bond. The aromatic ring in phenol confers a property known as resonance stabilization, which allows the electron pair to reside at different sites on the molecule (Chap. 12). As such the potential energy in the compound can cause caustic injury, including liquefactive necrosis. Phenols are insoluble in water, and irrigation with water can potentially increase tissue penetration. If water is the only irrigant immediately available for dermal burns, it can be employed, preferably with soap, and then followed by low-molecular-weight polyethylene glycol (PEG) solution or isopropyl alcohol when available.[80,137,177] Oral ingestion of phenol has caused significant esophageal burns.[10,14,177] Concentrated phenol ingestion has resulted in coma and severe acidosis, most likely from tissue destruction.[10] One retrospective study found that patients presented with cough, vomiting, a change in urine color to dark green, stridor, and, in three cases, coma of rapid onset.[177] Endoscopy and supportive care are recommended.

Detergents

Household detergents contain silicates, carbonates, and phosphates, and have the potential to induce caustic burns and strictures even when ingested unintentionally.[34,181] Airway compromise can occur,[34,49,115] but the majority of unintentional exposures result in minor toxicity.[93] These agents are frequently present in laundry powders and automatic dishwashing detergents.

Cationic detergents include quinilinium compounds, pyridinium compounds, and quaternary ammonium agents. These are frequently found in products for industrial use, as well as household fabric softeners. A concentration of greater than 7.5% of the agent can cause severe burns.[110] These agents bind well to activated charcoal;[110] however, because no large series have been evaluated with this therapy, all patients with symptoms or signs of caustic injury, intentional ingestions, or exposures to concentrations greater than 7.5% should be evaluated endoscopically and activated charcoal should be avoided.[110]

Zinc Chloride and Mercuric Chloride

Zinc chloride ($ZnCl_2$) and mercuric chloride ($HgCl_2$) are corrosive agents with severe systemic toxicity.[30,128,129,150] Ingestion of these substances causes life-threatening illness from cationic metal exposure. The local corrosive effects, though of great concern, are less consequential than the manifestations of systemic absorption. For this reason, aggressive decontamination with gentle nasogastric tube aspiration and placement of activated charcoal serve as primary gestures in the initial management of patients with these ingestions, as there are some in vitro data to suggest adequate charcoal binding of Hg^{2+}.[3] Some of these patients will also require chelation therapy. The local effects of these agents can be managed supportively and directly assessed after systemic absorption has been prevented or treated.

Ophthalmic Exposures

Ophthalmic exposures to caustic agents frequently occur from splash injuries, and, more recently, from the alkaline byproducts of sodium azide release in automobile air bag deployment.[196] The mainstay of therapy for these patients is immediate irrigation of the eye for a minimum of 15 minutes with normal saline, lactated Ringer solution, or tap water, if it is the only agent available. Acid exposures can be severe, but the tissue damage is usually self-limited after irrigation is complete, as the coagulative necrosis tends to prevent further penetration into deeper layers of the eye. Alka-

line injuries are of considerable concern as the liquefactive necrosis and saponification of the tissue allow for deep penetration of the substance. Several liters of irrigation fluid are recommended for these patients. The normal pH of ophthalmic secretions is close to 7.40. This can be tested colorimetrically by using a urine dipstick, which can test a range of pH from 5 to 9 using a color chart.[130] Litmus paper can be used in the same fashion. Another option is Nitrazine paper, which changes color from yellow to dark blue at a pH above 6.5,[55] and may be especially useful in acid exposures. These different test strips can be applied to the ocular secretions to test the baseline pH, and followed with intermittent evaluations after 15 minutes to determine the adequacy of irrigation. If these agents are not readily available, irrigation should not be delayed, as the depth of penetration of the caustic agent can determine outcome. Anterior chamber irrigation may be required and is performed emergently by an ophthalmologist. A thorough eye examination should be completed and followup should be arranged (Chap. 27).

Button Batteries

Button batteries present a unique problem of both foreign body ingestion and potential caustic injury. Button or disk batteries are found in small devices such as hearing aids, watches, and handheld calculators and computer games. These batteries range in size from 6.8 to 23 mm, and they are easily ingested by children.[107] Each contains a metal salt and a variety of caustic alkaline substances, such as sodium and potassium hydroxide, that can induce significant burns and subsequent strictures if the contents leak.[96,174]

Older, in vitro models of button batteries placed in a liquid with a pH of 5.5 led to an increase in pH to 11.5 with a brownish discoloration when leakage occurred from the seal or crimp of the two sides of the battery.[159,193] Animal models of button batteries placed on esophageal surfaces result in serosal edema, tissue discoloration, and burns with severity associated with duration of contact.[120,159,193]

A review of 2382 cases of button battery ingestions revealed that the majority of batteries pass uneventfully in the stool, with 86% completing the transit through the gastrointestinal tract within 4 days.[107] Two patients in the series developed strictures and 10% of the batteries had dissolution of the crimp or seal. Unfortunately, fatal cases of transesophageal fistula and perforation of the aortic arch were reported in two patients with a significant delay in diagnosis.[15,169] For this reason, a thorough evaluation and followup of patients with button battery ingestion are mandatory.

Initial management includes airway assessment and stabilization followed by anteroposterior and lateral chest radiographs that visualize the neck, chest, and abdomen, in that order, particularly in children.[170] Patients with batteries in the airway or lower respiratory tract are usually symptomatic and require emergent removal via bronchoscopy. Intact batteries located past the pylorus in patients who are asymptomatic can be followed at home with serial stool examinations checking for battery passage, as 99% will be eliminated within 7 days.[106] Patients should return to the healthcare setting for abdominal pain, vomiting, fever, or failure of the battery to pass within 7 days. The use of hand-held metal detectors is not investigated in these patients.

For children younger than 6 years of age in whom the battery is located in the stomach, battery size should be assessed on the radiograph, as batteries greater than 15 mm are less likely to pass the pylorus spontaneously.[170] These patients should be reassessed in 48 hours by physical examination and repeat radiograph to check for movement of the battery past the pylorus. Endoscopic retrieval of the battery should be considered when the battery has failed to pass the pylorus.[164,170] The role of polyethylene glycol solution for whole-bowel irrigation has not been adequately investigated, although its use can be considered in patients with batteries in the stomach or with poor mobility in the intestines.[182]

If the battery is visualized in the esophagus, it requires immediate endoscopic removal by forceps or magnet.[201] There are no studies of the use of glucagon or other agents to lower the esophageal sphincter pressure and allow movement of the battery into the stomach. Glucagon should be used with caution, as it can induce vomiting and nausea, and patients are at risk of battery aspiration. Other means of battery removal have been attempted, such as syrup of ipecac or Foley balloon passage to retrieve the battery, but these procedures have met with little success and incur the risk of foreign body aspiration. Endoscopy allows for both battery removal and tissue inspection (Fig. 87–4).[163,201]

Leakage of mercury was reported in patients with a concomitant elevation in urine mercury excretion.[9,95] Although metal poisoning is a potential concern, especially when the battery is split on the radiograph, there have been no reported cases of symptomatic metal poisoning from these exposures.

In addition to leakage of battery contents, pressure necrosis and an electrical gradient across the moist tissue from the battery surfaces may contribute to damage, but this appears to be less significant than the alkaline exposure of battery contents.

Tissue damage can occur at other sites of battery placement including the nares and ear canal. These exposures have resulted in severe otorhinologic burns and perforations.[83] These, too, should be removed when identified.

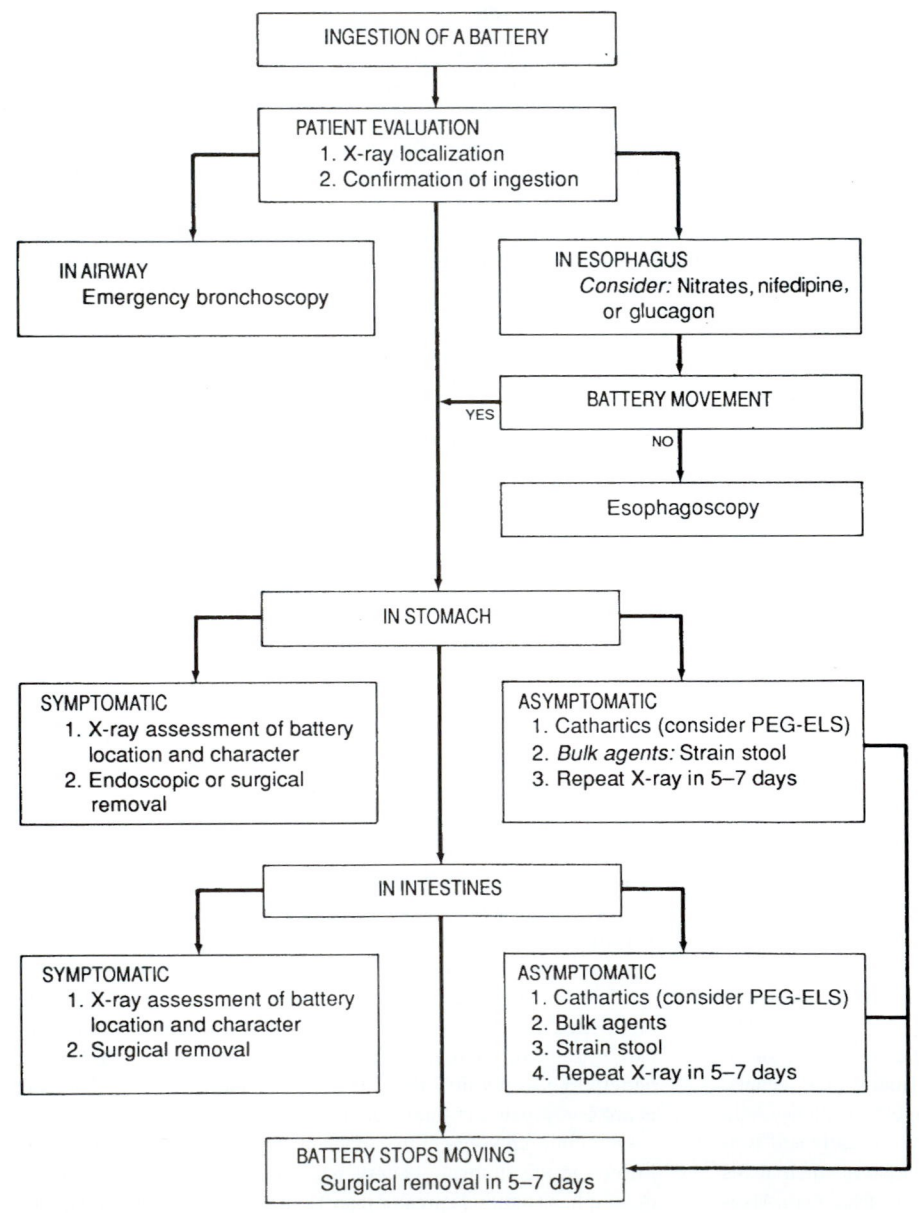

Figure 87–4. Algorithm for the management and assessment of patients with button battery ingestions.

SPECIAL CONSIDERATIONS

Hydrofluoric Acid

Hydrofluoric acid (HF) is used for glass etching, brick cleaning, etching chips in the semiconductor industry, electroplating, leather tanning, rust removal, and the cleaning of porcelain.[43,85]

HF has unique properties that can cause life-threatening complications following seemingly trivial exposure. The less common anhydrous form is greater than 70% hydrofluoric acid and used almost exclusively for industrial purposes. More common, in both industry and household products, is the aqueous form of HF, which generally ranges in concentrations from 3% to 40%.

Pathophysiology.   Hydrofluoric acid is formed as the product of gaseous sulfuric acid and calcium fluoride, which is subsequently cooled to a liquid.[111] The pK_a of aqueous HF is 3.5×10^{-4}, behaving in part as a weak acid. As such, it is roughly 1000 times less dissociated than equimolar hydrochloric acid. A permeability coefficient of 1.4×10^{-4} cm/sec allows it to penetrate deeply into tissues prior to dissociating into hydrogen ions and highly electronegative fluoride ions.[64] These fluoride ions avidly bind to intracellular stores of calcium and magnesium, ultimately leading to cellular dysfunction and cell death.[16,104,123]

There are several theories regarding the fate of the calcium and fluoride ions in the tissues. Formation of insoluble calcium fluoride is proposed as the etiology for both the precipitous fall in serum calcium and the severe pain associated with tissue toxicity. There is also some in vitro evidence that fluorapatite $[3(Ca_3(PO_4)_2 Ca(F_2)]$ is formed in the presence of phosphate and hydroxyapatite and may be a more likely pathway for deposition of the fluoride ion.[16]

Exposures to hydrofluoric acid occur via dermal, ocular, inhalation, and oral routes with one reported case of toxicity from an HF enema.[25] Fatal dermal exposures are reported from burns of 2.5% body surface area with exposure to concentrated (anhydrous) HF.[183] Because of the ability of HF to penetrate tissues, systemic toxicity can occur via any route, and this poses a greater threat than local injury to the patient if not rapidly decontaminated and treated.[17,22,62,165,171,187,188] The natural histories of these fatal exposures share the similar features of hypocalcemia hypomagnesemia, and, in most cases, hyperkalemia as preterminal events.[8,19,62,97,111,116,125,126,183] In some circumstances, the hypocalcemia is so severe that the coagulation cascade is disrupted and patients are noted to be coagulopathic on postmortem examination.[116,127,131]

Patients who die invariably do so from sudden-onset myocardial conduction failure and ventricular fibrillation. The evidence regarding the mechanism of myocardial irritability is variable. Some postmortem cases reveal significant myocardial injury.[127] These findings are inconsistently encountered in humans, but dog studies in which animals die of cardiac arrest have not demonstrated any histologic abnormalities of the myocardium.[40,122] Most theories regarding myocardial irritability relate to the hypocalcemia causing an efflux of potassium ions into the extracellular space.[40,104,127] The subsequent hyperkalemia may alter the automaticity and resting potential of the heart, making it more prone to fatal dysrhythmias.[126] Dogs treated with quinidine, a potassium efflux blocker, seem to be protected from fatal doses of intravenous sodium fluoride.[40] However, the mechanism of toxicity may be much more complicated.[205] A child with systemic fluoride toxic-

ity, who was appropriately repleted with calcium, and who had reportedly "normal electrolytes," still experienced ventricular fibrillation and was successfully resuscitated.[17,205] Perhaps this is because serum potassium, calcium, and magnesium levels only partly represent levels near the tissues.[16,17,40,125,126]

Assessing Severity of Exposures.   Determining which exposures are life-threatening can be achieved by following certain historical and clinical features of an exposure. All oral ingestions and inhalational exposures should be considered potentially fatal, as well as burns of the face and neck regardless of HF concentration. Inhalational exposure should be assumed for all skin burns with a body surface area greater than 5%, soaked clothing, HF concentration greater than 50%, and head and neck burns.[84] Inhaled hydrogen fluoride is a particular risk with greater concentrations. Patients presenting with altered mental status are critically ill and necessitate rapid therapy.

Concentrations of greater than 20% HF have a great potential for toxicity irrespective of the extent of surface area exposed. As a general rule, patients who experience severe pain within minutes of contact are most likely exposed to a very high concentration of HF and can deteriorate rapidly. An otherwise well-appearing patient may have a precipitous demise without any clinical manifestations of hypocalcemia. In some reported cases, this may be because these findings were not sought, and in other cases, the signs did not exist, despite a very low serum calcium. In other reports carpal spasm and Chvostek sign were present.[62,165] Electrocardiographic findings of both hypocalcemia (prolonged QT) and hyperkalemia (peaked T wave), in both human case reports and in dog studies, may be more reliable indicators of toxicity.[8,22,62,131,144,183]

Not all exposures to HF are fatal; in fact, the vast majority of exposures are to the surfaces of fingertips with low concentrations of the agent. Most household rust removal products have concentrations ranging between 6 and 12%, and the time to evolution of pain at the site of contact may be delayed as long as 24 hours.[191] These presentations are much less likely to result in life-threatening systemic toxicity. The extent of tissue injury in dermal exposures is determined by the volume, concentration, and contact time with the tissues.

Clinical Presentation.   Patients with inhalational exposures can present in a variety of ways depending upon the HF concentration. Thirteen oil refinery workers exposed to low-concentration hydrofluoric acid mist experienced minor upper respiratory tract irritation.[102] Alternatively, in a mass exposure to HF in a community in Texas, throat burning and shortness of breath were among the common chief complaints.[202] Some patients showed evidence of altered pulmonary function tests and hypoxemia on arterial blood gas analysis. Sixteen percent of patients had hypocalcemia from the gaseous exposure. Stridor, wheezing, and rhonchi, as well as erythema and ulcers of the upper respiratory tract, were described on the physical examinations of these patients. Eye pain was another complaint noted with these patients, and it can occur simultaneously with gaseous HF exposure.[102,121,136,160,202]

Intentional ingestion of concentrated hydrofluoric acid (or NaF, which results in the formation of HF when mixed with stomach acid) causes significant gastritis while often sparing the remainder of the GI tract. Patients may present with vomiting and abdominal pain. Systemic absorption is rapid and usually fatal. A patient with an ingestion of a low concentration of HF suffered multiple episodes of ventricular fibrillation was successfully resuscitated and discharged to home.[178] Accordingly, patients surviving to reach the hospital may present with a depressed mental status and are at risk for dysrhythmias and airway compromise.[19,105,116,178]

Following dermal exposure, it is usually recognized that the higher the concentration of HF, the more rapid the onset of excruciating pain at the site of contact.[50,111,183] For household products, there is often a delay of several hours before patients develop pain.[50,173,190,191] The initial site may appear benign despite the complaints of the patient. Over time the tissue may become hyperemic, with subsequent blanching with whitish discoloration and coagulative necrosis of the tissue as calcium is precipitated.[141] Ulcerations may form at a rate dependent on the concentration and duration of contact.[43,87,112]

Initial Stabilization.   For all types of exposures, the mainstay of management is to prevent or limit systemic absorption, assess for systemic toxicity, and rapidly correct any electrolyte imbalances. To prevent absorption from dermal, oral, or inhalational routes, a solution of calcium or magnesium salt is delivered to the affected area to prevent HF penetration and to provide an alternative source of cations for the damaging electronegative fluoride ions. Intravenous access should be obtained. An ECG should be examined for signs of hypocalcemia and hyperkalemia. The patient should be placed on continuous cardiac monitoring, and have a rapid assessment of serum electrolyte concentrations.

If there is a clinical suspicion of severe toxicity by the parameters described, then the immediate administration of calcium and magnesium is recommended. Intravenous preparations of calcium are available in two forms: calcium gluconate and calcium chloride. Ten percent calcium gluconate contains 0.45 mEq/mL and comes in 10-mL vials of 1 g/vial. It can safely be administered in a peripheral line at 1 g over 5 minutes, or by rapid intravenous push if the patient suddenly deteriorates. Ten percent calcium chloride contains 1.36 mEq/mL of solution. It is also available in 10-mL vials of 1 g each. It is considerably more irritating to the tissues and may be more appropriately administered through a central venous access site (Antidotes in Depth: Calcium). Patients can require several grams of calcium to treat HF toxicity.[62,178] Intravenous magnesium can be administered to adults as 20 mL of a 20% solution (4 g) over 20 minutes. An approach that uses intravenous calcium, magnesium, and calcium or magnesium gels locally to limit absorption may protect against life-threatening hypocalcemia. Ionized calcium should be monitored serially along with magnesium and potassium.[62] Serial screening with both the electrocardiogram and physical examination can help to guide the extent and nature of therapy. Additional information may be obtained from an arterial blood-gas analysis. As systemic toxicity progresses, there is potential for development of metabolic acidosis.[16] An animal model of hydrogen fluoride toxicity found that maintaining a normal acid-base balance was protective against HF toxicity;[156] Thus it may be beneficial to correct any significant acidemia with hydration and intravenous sodium bicarbonate. This treatment may simultaneously protect against life-threatening hyperkalemia.

Rapid airway assessment and protection should occur early in patients with potential inhalation injury, respiratory distress, or burns significant enough to cause a change of mental status. Patients with symptomatic inhalational injuries can be treated with nebulized calcium gluconate. A report of patients exposed to a low concentration of HF and treated with 4 mL of a 2.5% nebulized solution demonstrated no adverse effects to treatment, with some subjective reports of decreased irritation.[102]

In patients with intentional ingestion of hydrofluoric acid, gastric emptying via nasogastric tube is indicated, because these exposures are almost universally fatal.[8,19,116,131] Because aqueous hydrofluoric acid is a weak acid, the risk of perforation by passage of a nasogastric tube is significantly lower than the risk of death from systemic absorption.[8,116] In the acidic environment of the stomach more of the weak acid solution remains unionized, penetrating the gastric mucosa and causing rapid systemic poisoning. An oral calcium- or magnesium-containing solution should be delivered to the stomach as soon as gastric emptying is complete. Magnesium citrate (standard cathartic dose), magnesium sulfate, or any of the calcium solutions can be administered orally to prevent absorption. There have been no controlled trials of this therapy in animals or humans, but there may be a potential benefit in limiting absorption of HF. These patients should be assessed for systemic HF poisoning.

A Foley catheter should be placed to follow urine output, as most of the fluoride ions are eliminated renally.[12,82,92,165] If renal function is compromised, then hemodialysis should be considered in the patient with severe HF poisoning. There is one reported case of successful clearance of fluoride ions via hemodialysis.[12] The clearance rate, however, was not significantly different than that of normally functioning kidneys and therefore is not recommended in cases in which renal function is preserved. The use of quinidine, although protective in dogs,[127] has not been studied or used in humans, and at this time is inappropriate treatment for severe HF poisoning.

For patients dying from overwhelming dermal exposure, both the intravenous calcium and magnesium treatment described and the local decontamination should occur simultaneously. This can be achieved by the topical application of a calcium-containing gel, or by intradermal injection of calcium, which is described later. There is a case report of a woman dying from severe HF toxicity with multiple manifestations of systemic toxicity who was treated surgically by amputation of the affected limb, and who subsequently survived. Although not routinely recommended, this may be an alternative measure for patients who are not responding adequately to all other therapeutic modalities.[21,91]

Ocular exposures from liquid splashes or hydrogen fluoride gas result in pain, corneal opacification, sloughing of the cornea, revascularization, and, sometimes, keratoconjunctivitis sicca (dry eye) as a long-term complication.[11,124,162] Patients with ocular exposures should receive vigorous irrigation of 1 L of normal saline, lactated Ringer solution, or water to the affected eye.[124] Although there are limited data, repetitive irrigation is described as causing a worsened outcome.[120] A complete ophthalmic examination should be performed after the patient is deemed stable, and an ophthalmic consultation should be obtained. One case report demonstrated a good outcome of ocular HF exposure with the use of 1% calcium gluconate eyedrops.[11] This has yet to be adequately studied and is not indicated at this time. There is no role for gel therapy or intraocular injection in these patients, because most calcium and magnesium preparations are potentially toxic to ocular tissues and may actually worsen outcome.[124]

The most important therapy for skin exposures is rapid removal of clothing and irrigation of the affected area with copious amounts of water or saline, whichever is more readily available.[5,92,103,112] For high-concentration HF or a >5% body surface area burn, electrocardiographic monitoring and large-bore intravenous access should be established, and laboratory studies sent for calcium, magnesium, serum electrolytes, type, cross-match, and coagulation profiles. Topical calcium gel should be applied to the affected area. This is prepared by mixing 3.5 g of calcium gluconate powder in 5 ounces of sterile water-soluble lubricant, or 25 mL of 10% calcium gluconate in 75 mL of sterile water-soluble lubricant.[5,23,84] If calcium gluconate is unavailable, calcium chloride or calcium carbonate can be used in a similar formulation.[29] If none of these are available, a sterile magnesium solution (3.48 g of magnesium gluconate in 5 ounces of lubricating jelly) has also demonstrated some efficacy in the treatment of HF burns.[23] Topical therapy for both severe and non-life-threatening exposures may scavenge the fluoride ions prior to dermal penetration. An animal study examining the efficacy and mechanism of topical calcium gel therapy found the fluoride ion concentration of the gel significantly higher than in the non-calcium-containing gel controls. Although a limited study, these animals also had a decrease in urinary fluoride ion concentration as compared to controls, suggesting less overall absorption of the HF into the tissues.[92] Quaternary ammonium compounds, such as topical benzalkonium chloride, have also been advocated in the treatment of HF burns and can be used when available[112]; however, calcium-containing gels appear to be more efficacious. Intradermal injection of calcium and magnesium salts and intravenous infusions of magnesium may also be therapeutic.

Hand exposures are by far the most common presentation of hydrofluoric acid exposure. Several therapy options have been studied and described in animal models for treatment of topical HF burns. Unfortunately, many study designs use histologic or subjective wound inspection as outcome parameters,[23,146] some with unblinded inspection.[20,47,91,92] These animal models do not address the parameters of pain reduction, cosmesis, and functionality that are important clinically. There are four types of therapies that have had variable success in human exposures. These include the application of calcium via topical, intradermal, intravenous, and intra-arterial routes.

After irrigation, a gel solution of calcium carbonate or gluconate can be mixed directly into a sterile surgical glove and then placed onto the patient's hand for 30 minutes. Two case series report limited success with this therapy.[5,29] Some patients describe prompt and dramatic relief of pain within minutes. Magnesium hydroxide and magnesium gluconate gel used in rabbit models also show some histologic evidence of efficacy,[23] but their use has not been reported in humans.

Alternatively or simultaneously, analgesics can be administered orally or intravenously as needed, but preferably not to the point of sedation, because local pain response will guide therapy. Digital blocks with subcutaneous lidocaine or bupivacaine can be used for patients presenting 12–24 hours after the injury from a low concentration of HF and no systemic signs of toxicity.[46]

All patients with digital exposures should be observed over 4–6 hours, as the pain is likely to recur and reapplication of the gel or alternative therapy may be necessary. In addition, wound margins may become apparent and require débridement, and even if successful pain control is achieved, the patient will require specialized followup or wound care.

If topical gel therapy fails within the first few minutes of application, consideration should be given to intradermal therapy with calcium gluconate, because the benefit in pain control often occurs immediately. This treatment may have limited utility, however, in small spaces, such as fingertips. Histologic studies in animal models demonstrate that 10% calcium chloride solution can be damaging to the tissues and should be avoided.[46,67] The preferable method is to approach the wound from a distal point of injury and inject intradermally no more than 0.5 mL/cm^2 of 5% calcium gluconate. One author recommends a palmar fasciotomy whenever this method of treatment is used.[5] This seems extreme, and is not currently recommended unless a compartment syndrome is present, as the potential for iatrogenic injury is increased. The limits of intradermal injection include potential to increase soft-tissue damage without adequate relief, infection, and inadequate space to safely inject without causing a compartment syndrome. This is especially problematic under the nail. Some authors have recommended removal of the nail. This has some advantages in accessing the affected area; however, it is a painful procedure that is often cosmetically undesirable and the outcome is not always significantly improved.

If the wound is large or in a section of the fingerpad or an area that is not amenable to intradermal injections, then consideration should be given to the use of intra-arterial calcium gluconate. This procedure delivers calcium directly to the affected tissue from a proximal artery. Placement should be ipsilateral and proximal to the affected area, usually in the radial or brachial artery. The method of obtaining access is somewhat debated. Because of the potential to sclerose and damage the endothelial lining of the artery, and because extravasation can have potentially devastating consequences, the placement of an intra-arterial infusion line was originally recommended with confirmation of an arteriogram or placement under direct visualization of the vessel. This is still recommended in cases in which cannulation of the artery is expected to be difficult because of prior surgery or deformity. If the arterial line is carefully placed in a single attempt, and a good confirmatory arterial tracing is obtained, the infusate can be started. The recommended drip consists of 10 mL of 10% calcium gluconate in either 40 mL of D$_5$W or normal saline to run over 4 hours.[5,90,148,173,190,191] This gives a 2% calcium gluconate solution for arterial infusion. An animal model examined the effect of undiluted 10% calcium gluconate intra-aortically in rats. Although the model did not include HF, there was significant tissue injury in the vessel wall as compared to 2% calcium gluconate.[46] Calcium chloride has also been used successfully, although the potential for vessel injury may increase and complications of calcium chloride extravasation can lead to significant tissue necrosis itself.[189,206] The overall complications of intra-arterial calcium infusion in several case series were relatively benign, including radial artery spasm, hematoma, and inflammation at the puncture site, and, in some cases, a fall in serum magnesium.[173,190]

After the drip is initiated, patients typically experience significant pain relief. Patients requiring an arterial line for treatment should be admitted to the hospital, as the majority will require more than one treatment, and some patients may require as many as five separate infusions of calcium gluconate. In addition, wounds may require débridement,[5] and one author suggests that after the drip, tissue can be salvaged that initially would not have been considered viable.[191] There have been no reported cases of clinically significant hypercalcemia with this therapy, although serum calcium levels were not recorded in every series.

Other reported therapies have included an intravenous Bier block technique that uses 25 mL of 2.5% calcium gluconate. The effects lasted 5 hours and there were no adverse events.[70] This technique is not reported as being used in a substantial number of patients, and has yet to be studied as an alternative therapy.

A rabbit model of empiric intravenous magnesium therapy for the management of dermal HF burns suggested an efficacy for wound healing when compared to untreated controls.[37] Another animal model suggested a potential benefit to wound healing with empiric therapy as well.[199] Both of these models are limited, and this therapy has never been well examined in humans. An approach of both local and systemic therapy with calcium and magnesium may be required to provide adequate relief for patients with HF hand injuries.

SUMMARY

Assessing the severity of injuries in patients with caustic exposures can be clinically challenging. For all ingestions, primary consideration should be given to airway assessment and stabilization. The clinician must then consider multiple bedside, laboratory and radiographic factors to decide how best to inspect the tissues of the gastrointestinal tract. Ideally, the gastroenterologists and surgeons are involved in the care of the patient early, so that any surgical intervention deemed necessary can be performed promptly. Other types of exposures to the skin and eyes require rapid decontamination with simple irrigants such as normal saline solution.

Household and industrial exposures to caustic agents constitute a potentially life-threatening global health concern. Public health efforts to decrease access to high concentrations of caustic agents should be encouraged, especially in developing nations.

REFERENCES

1. Aceto T, Terplan K, Fiore RR, Munschauer RW: Chemical burns of the esophagus in children and glucocorticoid therapy. J Med 1970;1: 101–109.
2. Alford BR, Harris HH: Chemical burns of the mouth, pharynx and esophagus. Ann Otol Rhinol Laryngol 1959;68:122–128.
3. Andersen AH: Experimental studies on the pharmacology of activated charcoal. III. Adsorption from gastro-intestinal contents. Acta Pharmacol 1948;4:275–284.
4. Anderson KD, Rouse TM, Randolph JG: A controlled trial of corticosteroids in children with corrosive injury of the esophagus. N Engl J Med 1990;323:637–640.
5. Anderson WJ, Anderson JR: Hydrofluoric acid burns of the hand: Mechanism of injury and treatment. J Hand Surg 1988;13:52–57.
6. Appelqvist P, Salmo M: Lye corrosion carcinoma of the esophagus: A review of 63 cases. Cancer 1980;45:2655–2658.
7. Ashcraft KW, Padula RT: The effect of dilute corrosives on the esophagus. Pediatrics 1974;53:226–232.
8. Baltazar RF, Mower MM, Reider R, et al: Acute fluoride poisoning leading to fatal hyperkalemia. Chest 1980;78:660–663.
9. Bass DH, Millar AJW: Mercury absorption following button battery ingestion. J Pediatr Surg 1992;27:1541–1542.
10. Bennet IL, James DF, Golden A: Severe acidosis due to phenol poisoning: Report of two cases. Ann Intern Med 1950;32:324–327.
11. Bentur Y, Tannenbaum S, Yaffe Y, Halpert M: The role of calcium gluconate in the treatment of hydrofluoric acid eye burn. Ann Emerg Med 1993;22:1488–1490.
12. Berman L, Taves D, Mitra S, Newmark K: Inorganic fluoride poisoning: Treatment by hemodialysis. N Engl J Med 1973;289:922.
13. Berthet B, Di Costanzo J, Arnaud C, et al: Influence of epidermal growth factor and interferon gamma on healing of oesophageal corrosive burns in the rat. Br J Surg 1994;81:395–398.
14. Bikhazi HB, Thompson ER, Shumrick DA: Caustic ingestions—Current status: A report of 105 cases. Arch Otolaryngol 1969;89: 112–115.
15. Blatnik BS, Toohill RJ, Leman RH: Fatal complications from alkaline foreign body in the esophagus. Ann Otol Rhinol Laryngol 1977; 86:611–615.
16. Boink ABTJ, Wemer J, Meulenbelt J, et al: The mechanism of fluoride-induced hypocalcemia. Hum Exp Toxicol 1994;13:149–155.
17. Bordelon BM, Saffle JR, Morris SE: Systemic fluoride toxicity in a child with hydrofluoric acid burns: Case report. J Trauma 1993;34: 437–439.
18. Borja AR, Ransdell HT, Thomas TV, Johnson W: Lye injuries of the esophagus: Analysis of ninety cases of lye ingestion. J Thorac Cardiovasc Surg 1969;57:533–538.
19. Bost RO, Springfield A: Fatal hydrofluoric acid ingestion: A suicide case report. J Anal Toxicol 1995;19:535–536.
20. Bracken WM, Cuppage F, McLaury RL, et al: Comparative effectiveness of topical treatments for hydrofluoric acid burns. J Occup Med 1985;27:733–739.
21. Buckingham FM: Surgery: A radical approach to severe hydrofluoric acid burns—A case report. J Occup Med 1988;30:873–874.
22. Burke WJ, Hoegg UR, Philips RE: Systemic fluoride poisoning resulting from a fluoride skin burn. J Occup Med 1973;15:39–41.
23. Burkhart KK, Brent J, Kirk MA, et al: Comparison of topical magnesium and calcium treatment for dermal hydrofluoric acid burns. Ann Emerg Med 1994;24:9–13.
24. Burrington JD: Clinitest burns of the esophagus. Ann Thorac Surg 1975;20:400–404.
25. Cappell MS, Simon T: Fulminant acute colitis following a self-administered enema. Am J Gastroenterol 1993;88:122–126.
26. Cardona JC, Daly JF: Current management of corrosive esophagitis: An evaluation of results in 239 cases. Ann Otol Rhinol Laryngol 1971;80:521–526.
27. Cello JP, Fogel RP, Boland CR: Liquid caustic ingestion—Spectrum of injury. Arch Intern Med 1980;140:501–504.
28. Chaudhary A, Puri AS, Dhar P, et al: Elective surgery for corrosive-induced gastric injury. World J Surg 1996;20:703–706.
29. Chick LR, Borah G: Calcium carbonate gel therapy for hydrofluoric acid burns of the hand. Plastic Reconstr Surg 1990;86:935–939.
30. Chobanian SJ: Accidental ingestion of liquid zinc chloride: Local and systemic effects. Ann Emerg Med 1981;10:91–93.
31. Chodak GW, Passaro E: Acid ingestion—Need for gastric resection. JAMA 1978;238:225–226.
32. Chong SC, Beahrs OH, Payne WS: Management of corrosive gastritis due to ingested acid. Mayo Clin Proc 1974;49:861–865.
33. Christensen BT: Prediction of complications following unintentional caustic ingestion in children. Is endoscopy always necessary? Acta Paediatr 1995;84:1177–1182.
34. Clausen JO, Nielsen TLF, Fogh A: Admission to Danish hospitals after suspected ingestion of corrosives. Dan Med Bull 1994;41: 234–237.
35. Cleveland WW, Thorton N, Chesney JG, Lawson RB: The effect of prednisone in the prevention of esophageal stricture following the ingestion of lye. South Med J 1958;51:861–864.
36. Colbert PM, Sanders PD, Frankl H: Isolated antral ulceration from ingestion of a single Clinitest tablet. Gastrointest Endosc 1977;24: 82–83.
37. Cox RD, Osgood KA: Evaluation of intravenous magnesium sulfate for the treatment of hydrofluoric acid burns. J Toxicol Clin Toxicol 1994;32:123–136.
38. Crain EF, Gershel JC, Mezey AP: Caustic ingestions—Symptoms as predictors of esophageal injury. Am J Dis Child 1984; 138:863–865.
39. Cullen ML, Klein MD: Spontaneous resolution of acid gastric injury. J Pediatr Surg 1987;22:550–551.
40. Cummings CC, McIvor ME: Flouride-induced hyperkalemia—The role of calcium-dependent potassium channels. Am J Emerg Med 1986;6:1–3.

41. Daly JF, Cardona JC: Acute corrosive esophagitis. Arch Otolaryngol 1961;74:41–46.

42. Dantas RO, Mamede RCM: Esophageal motility in patients with esophageal caustic injury. Am J Gastroenterol 1996;91:1157–1161.

43. Dibbell DG, Iverson RE, Jones W, et al: Hydrofluoric acid burns of the hand. J Bone Joint Surg 1970;52:931–936.

44. Di Costanzo J, Noirclerc M, Jouglard J, et al: New therapeutic approach to corrosive burns of the upper gastrointestinal tract. Gut 1980; 21:370–375.

45. Dilawari JB, Singh S, Rao PN, Anand BS: Corrosive acid ingestion in man—A clinical and endoscopic study. Gut 1984;25:183–187.

46. Dowbak G, Rose K, Rohrich RJ: A biochemical and histological rationale for the treatment of hydrofluoric acid burns with calcium gluconate. J Burn Care Rehabil 1994;15:323–327.

47. Dunn BJ, MacKinnon MA, Knowlden NF, et al: Hydrofluoric acid dermal burns—An assessment of treatment efficacy using an experimental pig model. J Occup Med 1992;34:902–909.

48. Eaton H, Tennekoon GE: Squamous carcinoma of the stomach following corrosive acid burns. Br J Surg 1972;59:382–387.

49. Einhorn A, Horton L, Alticri M, et al: Serious respiratory consequences of detergent ingestions in children. Pediatrics 1989;84: 472–474.

50. El Saadi MS, Hall AH, Hall PK, et al: Hydrofluoric acid dermal exposure. Vet Hum Toxicol 1989;31:243–247.

51. Estrera A, Taylor W, Mills LJ: Corrosive burns of the esophagus and stomach: A recommendation for an aggressive surgical approach. Ann Thorac Surg 1986;41:276–283.

52. Forsen JW, Muntz HR: Hair relaxer ingestion: A new trend. Ann Otol Rhinol Laryngol 1993;102:781–784.

53. Friedman EM, Lovejoy FH Jr: The emergency management of caustic ingestions. Emerg Med Clin North Am 1984;2:77–86.

54. Gago O, Ritter FN, Martel W, et al: Aggressive surgical treatment for caustic injury of the esophagus and stomach. Ann Thorac Surg 1972;13:243–250.

55. Garite TJ, Spellacy WN: Premature rupture of membranes. In: Scott JR, DiSaia PJ, Hammond CB, Spellacy WN, eds: Danforth's Obstetrics and Gynecology, 7th ed. Philadelphia, Lippincott, 1994, p. 30.

56. Gaudreault P, Parent M, McGuigan MA, et al: Predictability of esophageal injury from signs and symptoms: A study of caustic ingestion in 378 children. Pediatrics 1983;71:767–770.

57. Gehanno P, Geudon C: Inhibition of experimental esophageal lye strictures by penicillamine. Arch Otolaryngol 1981;107:145–147.

58. Genieser NB, Becker MH: "Clinitest strictures" of the esophagus. Clin Pediatr 1969;8:17A–19A.

59. Gillis DA, Higgins G, Kennedy R: Gastric damage from ingested acid in children. J Pediatr Surg 1985;20:494–496.

60. Gorman RL, Khin-Maung-Gyi MT, Klein-Schwartz W, et al: Initial symptoms as predictors of esophageal injury in alkaline corrosive ingestions. Am J Emerg Med 1992;10:189–194.

61. Gossot D, Safarti E, Celerier M: Early blunt esophagectomy in severe caustic burns of the upper digestive tract: Report of 29 cases. J Thorac Cardiovasc Surg 1987;94:188–191.

62. Greco RJ, Hartford CE, Haith LR, Patton ML: Hydrofluoric acid induced hypocalcemia. J Trauma 1988;28:1593–1596.

63. Gupta S: A technique of repairing acid burns of the stomach. Ann R Coll Surg Engl 1988;70:74–75.

64. Gutknecht J, Walter A: Hydrofluoric and nitric acid transport through lipid bilayer membranes. Biochim Biophys Acta 1981;644:153–156.

65. Haller JA, Andrews HG, White JJ, et al: Pathophysiology and management of acute corrosive burns of the esophagus: Results of treatment in 285 children. J Pediatr Surg 1971;6:578–583.

66. Haller JA, Bachman K: The comparative effect of current therapy on experimental caustic burns of the esophagus. Pediatrics 1964;34: 236–245.

67. Harris JC, Rumack BH, Bregman DJ: Comparative efficacy of injectable calcium and magnesium salts in the therapy of hydrofluoric acid burns. Clin Toxicol 1981;18:1027–1032.

68. Hawkins DB: Dilatation of esophageal strictures: Comparative morbidity of anterograde and retrograde methods. Ann Otol Rhinol Laryngol 1988;97:460–465.

69. Hawkins DB, Demeter MJ, Barnett TE: Caustic ingestion: Controversies in management: A review of 214 cases. Laryngoscope 1980;90: 98–109.

70. Henry JA, Hla KK: Intravenous regional calcium gluconate perfusion for hydrofluoric acid burns. J Toxicol Clin Toxicol 1992;30:203–207.

71. Hill JL, Norberg HP, Smith MD, et al: Clinical technique and success of the esophageal stent to prevent corrosive strictures. J Pediatr Surg 1976;11:443–450.

72. Hoffman RS, Howland MA, Kamerow HN, Goldfrank LR: Comparison of titratable acid/alkaline reserves and pH in potentially caustic household products. J Toxicol Clin Toxicol 1989;27: 241–261.

73. Homan CS, Maitra SR, Lane BP, et al: Effective treatment for acute alkali injury to the esophagus using weak-acid neutralization therapy: An ex-vivo study. Acad Emerg Med 1995;2:952–958.

74. Homan CS, Maitra SR, Lane BP, et al: Histopathologic evaluation of the therapeutic efficacy of water and milk dilution for esophageal acid injury. Acad Emerg Med 1995;2:587–591.

75. Homan CS, Maitra SR, Lane BP, et al: Therapeutic effects of water and milk for acute alkali injury of the esophagus. Ann Emerg Med 1994;24:14–19.

76. Homan CS, Maitra SR, Lane BP, Geller ER: Effective treatment of acute alkali injury of the rat esophagus with early saline dilution therapy. Ann Emerg Med 1993;22:178–182.

77. Homan CS, Singer AJ, Henry MC, Thode HC: Thermal effects of neutralization therapy and water dilution for acute alkali exposure in canines. Acad Emerg Med 1997;4:27–32.

78. Horvath OP, Olah T, Zentai G: Emergency esophagogastrectomy for the treatment of hydrochloric acid injury. Ann Thorac Surg 1991;52: 98–101.

79. Howell JM, Dalsey WC, Hartsell FW, Butzin CA: Steroids for the treatment of corrosive esophageal injury: A statistical analysis of past studies. Am J Emerg Med 1992;10:421–425.

80. Hunter DM, Timerding BL, Leonard RB, et al: Effects of isopropyl alcohol, ethanol, and polyethylene glycol/industrial methylated spirits in the treatment of acute phenol burns. Ann Emerg Med 1992;21: 1303–1307.

81. Hwang TL, Shen-Chen SM, Chen MF: Nonthoracotomy esophagectomy for corrosive esophagitis with gastric perforation. Surg Gynecol Obstet 1987;164:537–540.

82. Juncos LI, Donadio JV: Renal failure and fluorosis. JAMA 1972;222:783–785.

83. Kavanaugh K, Litovitz T: Miniature battery foreign bodies in auditory and nasal cavities. JAMA 1986;255:1470–1472.

84. Kirkpatrick JR, Burd DAR: An algorithmic approach to the treatment of hydrofluoric acid burns. Burns 1995;21:495–499.

85. Kirkpatrick JR, Enion DS, Burd DAR: Hydrofluoric acid burns: A review. Burns 1995;21:483–493.

86. Kirsch MM, Peterson A, Brown JW, et al: Treatment of caustic injuries of the esophagus: A ten-year experience. Ann Surg 1978;188: 675–678.

87. Klauder JV, Shelanski L, Gabriel K: Industrial uses of compounds of fluorine and oxalic acid. Arch Environ Health 1955;12:412–419.

88. Knox WG, Scott JR, Zintel HA, et al: Bougienage and steroids used singly or in combination in experimental corrosive esophagitis. Ann Surg 1967;166:930–940.

89. Kocchar R, Mehta S, Nagi B, Goenka MK: Corrosive acid-induced esophageal intramural pseudodiverticulosis—A study of 14 patients. J Clin Gastroenterol 1991;13:371–375.

90. Kohnlein HE, Achinger R: A new method of treatment of the hydrofluoric acid burns of the extremities. Chir Plast 1982;6:297–305.

91. Kohnlein HE, Merkle P, Springorum HW: Hydrogen fluoride burns: Experiments and treatment. Surg Forum 1973;24:50.

92. Kono K, Yoshida Y, Watanabe M, et al: An experimental study on the treatment of hydrofluoric acid burns. Arch Environ Contam Toxicol 1992;22:414–418.

93. Kost KM, Shapiro RS: Button battery ingestion—A case report and review of the literature. J Otolaryngol 1987;16:252–254.

94. Krenzelok EP: Liquid automatic dishwashing detergents: A profile of toxicity. Ann Emerg Med 1989;18:60–63.

95. Kuhn JR, Tunell WP: The role of cineesophagoscopy in caustic esophageal injury. Am J Surg 1983;146:804–806.

96. Kulig K, Rumack C, Rumack B, Duffy J: Disk battery ingestion—Elevated urine mercury levels and enema removal of battery fragments. JAMA 1983;249:2502–2504.

97. Kwok MC, Svancarek WP, Creer M: Fatality due to hydrofluoric acid exposure. J Toxicol Clin Toxicol 1987;25:333–339.

98. Lacouture PG, Gaudreault P, Lovejoy FH: Clinitest tablet ingestion: An in vitro investigation concerned with initial emergency management. Ann Emerg Med 1986;15:143–146.

99. Lahoti D, Broor SL, Basu P, et al: Corrosive esophageal strictures: Predictors of response to endoscopic dilatation. Gastrointest Endosc 1995;41:196–200.

100. Landau GD, Saunders WH: The effect of chlorine bleach on the esophagus. Arch Otolaryngol 1964;80:174–176.

101. Leape LL, Ashcraft KW, Scarpelli DG, Holder TM: Hazard to health—Liquid lye. N Engl J Med 1971;284:578–581.

102. Lee DC, Wiley JF, Snyder JW: Treatment of inhalational exposure to hydrofluoric acid with nebulized calcium gluconate [letter]. J Occup Med 1993;35:470.

103. Leonard LG, Scheulen JJ, Munster AM: Chemical burns: Effect of prompt first aid. J Trauma 1982;22:420–423.

104. Lepke S, Paasow H: Effects of fluoride on potassium and sodium permeability of the erythrocyte membrane. J Gen Physiol 1968;51:365S–372S.

105. Lidbeck WL, Hill IB, Beeman JA: Acute sodium fluoride poisoning. JAMA 1943;121:826–827.

106. Litovitz T, Butterfield AB, Holloway RR, Marion LI: Battery ingestion: Assessment of therapeutic modalities and battery discharge state. J Pediatr 1984;105:868–873.

107. Litovitz T, Schmitz BF: Ingestion of cylindrical and button batteries: An analysis of 2382 cases. Pediatrics 1992;89:747–757.

108. Liu A, Richardson M, Robertson WO: Effects of N-acetylcysteine on caustic burns. Vet Hum Toxicol 1985;28:316.

109. Lowe JE, Graham DY, Boisaubin EV, Lanza FL: Corrosive injury to the stomach: The natural history and role of fiberoptic endoscopy. Am J Surg 1979;137:803–806.

110. Mack RB: Decant the wine, prune back your long-term hopes. N C Med J 1987;48:593–595.

111. MacKinnon MA: Hydrofluoric acid burns. Dermatol Clin 1988;6:67–74.

112. MacKinnon MA: Treatment of hydrofluoric acid burns [letter]. J Occup Med 1986;28:804.

113. Madden JW, Davis WM, Butler C, Peacock EE: Experimental esophageal lye burns II: Correcting established strictures with beta-aminoproprionitrile and bougienage. Ann Surg 1973;178:277–284.

114. Mallory A, Schaefer JW: Clinitest ingestion. Br Med J 1977;2:105–107.

115. Mandarikan BA: Ingestion of dishwasher detergent by children. Br J Clin Pract 1990;44:35–36.

116. Manoguerra AS, Neuman TS: Fatal poisoning from acute hydrofluoric acid ingestion. Am J Emerg Med 1986;4:362–363.

117. Martel W: Radiologic features of esophagogastritis secondary to extremely caustic agents. Diagn Radiol 1972;103:31–36.

118. Maull KI, Osmand AP, Maull CD: Liquid caustic ingestions: An in vitro study of the effects of buffer, neutralization, and dilution. Ann Emerg Med 1985;14:1160–1162.

119. Maull KI, Scher LA, Greenfield LJ: Surgical implications of acid ingestion. Surg Gynecol Obstet 1979;148:895–898.

120. Maves MD, Carrithers JS, Brick HG: Esophageal burns secondary to disc battery ingestion. Ann Otol Rhinol Laryngol 1984;93:364–369.

121. Mayer L, Guelich J: Hydrogen fluoride (HF) inhalation and burns. Arch Environ Health 1963;7:445–447.

122. Mayer TG, Gross PL: Fatal systemic fluorosis due to hydrofluoric acid burns. Ann Emerg Med 1985;14:149–153.

123. McClure FJ: A review of fluorine and its physiologic effects. Physiol Rev 1933;13:277–300.

124. McCulley JP, Whiting DW, Petitt MG, Lauber SE: Hydrofluoric acid burns of the eye. J Occup Med 1983;25:447–450.

125. McIvor ME: Delayed fatal hyperkalemia in a patient with acute fluoride intoxication. Ann Emerg Med 1987;16:1165–1167.

126. McIvor M, Baltazar RF, Beltran J, et al: Hyperkalemia and cardiac arrest from fluoride exposure during hemodialysis. Am J Cardiol 1983; 51:901–902.

127. McIvor ME, Cummings CE, Mower MM, et al: Sudden cardiac death from acute fluoride intoxication: The role of potassium. Ann Emerg Med 1987;16:777–781.

128. McKinney PE: Zinc chloride ingestion in a child—Exocrine pancreatic insufficiency. Ann Emerg Med 1995;25:562.

129. McKinney PE, Brent J, Kulig K: Acute zinc chloride ingestion in a child—Local and systemic effects. Ann Emerg Med 1994;23:1383–1387.

130. McNeely MDD: Urinalysis. In: Sonnenwirth AC, Jarrett L, eds: Gradwohl's Clinical Laboratory Methods and Diagnosis. St. Louis, Mosby, 1980, p. 483.

131. Menchel SM, Dunn WA: Hydrofluoric acid poisoning. Am J Forensic Med Pathol 1984;5:245–248.

132. Meredith W, Kon ND, Thompson JN: Management of injuries from liquid lye ingestion. J Trauma 1988;28:1173–1180.

133. Middelkamp JN, Ferguson TB, Roper CL, Hoffman FD: The management and problems of caustic burns in children. J Thorac Cardiovasc Surg 1969;57:341–347.

134. Mills LJ, Estrera AS, Platt MR: Avoidance of esophageal stricture following severe caustic burns by the use of an intraluminal stent. Ann Thorac Surg 1979;28:63–65.

135. Mitani M, Hirata K, Fukuda M, Kaneko M: Endoscopic ultrasonography in corrosive injury of the upper gastrointestinal tract by hydrochloric acid. J Clin Ultrasound 1996;24:40–42.

136. Moazam F, Talbert JL, Miller D, Mollitt DL: Caustic ingestion and its sequelae in children. South Med J 1987;80:187–190.

137. Morris JB, Smith FA: Regional deposition and absorption of inhaled hydrogen fluoride in the rat. Toxicol Appl Pharmacol 1982;62:81–89.

138. Mozingo DW, Smith AA, McManus WF, et al: Chemical burns. J Trauma 1988;28:642–647.

139. Muhletaler CA, Gerlock AJ, de Soto L, Halter SA: Acid corrosive esophagitis: Radiographic findings. Am J Radiol 1980;134:1137–1140.

140. Mutaf O, Avanoglu A, Ozok G: Management of tracheoesophageal fistula as a complication of esophageal dilatations in caustic esophageal burns. J Pediatr Surg 1995;30:823–826.

141. Noonan T, Carter EJ, Edelman PA, Zawacki BE: Epidermal lipids and the natural history of hydrofluoric acid (HF) injury. Burns 1994;20:202–206.

142. Norton RA: Esophageal and antral strictures due to ingestion of household ammonia—Report of two cases. N Engl J Med 1960;262:10–12.

143. Ochi K, Ohashi T, Sato S, et al: Surgical treatment for caustic ingestion injury of the pharynx, larynx, and esophagus. Acta Otolaryngol 1996;522(Suppl):116–119.

144. O'Connor HJ, Dixon MF, Grant AC, et al: Fatal accidental ingestion of Clinitest in an adult. J R Soc Med 1984;77:963–965.

145. O'Neil K: A fatal hydrogen fluoride exposure. J Emerg Nurs 1994;20:451–453.

146. Paley A, Seifter J: Treatment of experimental hydrofluoric acid corrosion. Proc Soc Exp Biol Med 1941;46:190–192.

147. Payten RJ: Clinitest tablet stricture of the esophagus. Br Med J 1972;4:728–729.

148. Pegg SP, Siu S, Gillett G: Intra-arterial infusions in the treatment of hydrofluoric acid burns. Burns 1985;11:440–443.

149. Penner GE: Acid ingestion—Toxicology and treatment. Ann Emerg Med 1980;9:374–379.

150. Potter JL: Acute zinc chloride ingestion in a young child. Ann Emerg Med 1981;10:267–269.

151. Previtera C, Guisti F, Guglielmi M: Predictive value of visible lesions (cheeks, lips, oropharynx) in suspected caustic ingestion: May endoscopy reasonably be omitted in completely negative pediatric patients? Pediatr Emerg Care 1990;6:176–178.

152. Ragheb MI, Ramadan AA, Khalia MA: Management of corrosive esophagitis. Surgery 1976;79:494–498.

153. Ray JF III, Myers WO, Lawton BR, et al: The natural history of liquid lye ingestion—Rationale for an aggressive surgical approach. Arch Surg 1974;109:436–439.

154. Reyes HM, Hill JL: Modification of the experimental stent technique for esophageal burns. J Surg Res 1976;20:65–70.

155. Reyes HM, Lin CY, Schlunk FF, Repogle RL: Experimental treatment of corrosive esophageal burns. J Pediatr Surg 1974;9:317–327.

156. Reynolds KE, Whitford GM, Pashley DH: Acute fluoride toxicity: The influence of acid-base status. Toxicol Appl Pharmacol 1978;45:415–427.

157. Ribet ME: Esophagogastrectomy for acid injury. Ann Thorac Surg 1992;53:738–742.

158. Ritter FN, Newman MH, Newman DE: A clinical and experimental study of corrosive burns of the stomach. Ann Otol Rhinol Laryngol 1968;77:830–842.

159. Rivera EA, Maves MD: Effects of neutralizing agents on esophageal burns caused by disk batteries. Ann Otol Rhinol Laryngol 1987;96:362–366.

160. Rose L: Further evaluation of hydrofluoric acid burns to the eye [letter]. J Occup Med 1984;26:483.

161. Rosenberg N, Kunderman PJ, Vroman L, Moolten SE: Prevention of experimental esophageal stricture by cortisone II. Arch Surg 1953;66:593–598.

162. Rubinfeld RS, Silbert DI, Arentsen JJ, Laibson PR: Ocular hydrofluoric acid burns. Am J Ophthalmol 1992;114:420–423.

163. Rumack BH, Burrington JD: Caustic ingestions: A rational look at diluents. Clin Toxicol 1977;11:27–34.

164. Rumack CM, Rumack BH: Battery ingestions. Pediatrics 1992;89:771–772.

165. Sadove R, Hainsworth D, Van Meter W: Total body immersion in hydrofluoric acid. South Med J 1990;83:698–700.

166. Safarti E, Gossot D, Assens P, Celerier M: Management of caustic ingestion in adults. Br J Surg 1987;74:146–148.

167. Schild JA: Caustic ingestion in adult patients. Laryngoscope 1985;95:1199–1201.

168. Scott JC, Jones B, Eisele DW, Ravich WJ: Caustic ingestion injuries of the upper aerodigestive tract. Laryngoscope 1992;102:1–8.

169. Shabino CL, Feinberg AN: Esophageal perforation secondary to alkaline battery ingestion. JACEP 1979;8:360–362.

170. Sheikh A: Button battery ingestions in children. Pediatr Emerg Care 1993;224–229.

171. Sheridan RL, Ryan CM, Quinby WC Jr, et al: Emergency management of major hydrofluoric acid exposures. Burns 1995;21:62–64.

172. Shirazi S, Schulze-Delrieu K, Custer-Hagen T, et al: Motility changes in opossum esophagus from experimental esophagitis. Dig Dis Sci 1989;34:1668–1676.

173. Siegel DC, Heard J: Intra-arterial calcium infusion for hydrofluoric acid burns. Aviat Space Environ Med 1992;63:206–211.

174. Sigalet D, Lees G: Tracheoesophageal injury secondary to disc battery ingestion. J Pediatr Surg 1988;23:996–998.

175. Sinar DR, Fletcher JR, Cordova CC, et al: Acute acid-induced esophagitis impairs esophageal peristalsis in baboons. Gastroenterology 1981;80:1286.

176. Souba WW: Nutritional support. N Engl J Med 1997;336:41–48.

177. Spiller HA, Quadrani-Kushner DA, Cleveland P: A five-year evaluation of acute exposures to phenol disinfectant (26%). J Toxicol Clin Toxicol 1993;31:307–313.

178. Stremski ES, Grande GA, Ling LJ: Survival following hydrofluoric acid ingestion. Ann Emerg Med 1992;21:1396–1399.

179. Subbarao KSVK, Kakar AK, Chandrasekhar V, et al: Cicatricial gastric stenosis caused by corrosive ingestion. Aust N Z J Surg 1988;58:143–146.

180. Sugawa C, Lucas CE: Caustic injury of the upper gastrointestinal tract in adults: A clinical and endoscopic study. Surgery 1989;106:802–807.

181. Sugawa C, Mullins RJ, Lucas CE, Leibold WC: The value of early endoscopy following caustic ingestion. Surg Gynecol Obstet 1981;153:553–556.

182. Tenenbein M: Whole-bowel irrigation for toxic ingestions. J Toxicol Clin Toxicol 1985;23:177–184.

183. Tepperman PB: Fatality due to acute systemic fluoride poisoning following a hydrofluoric acid skin burn. J Occup Med 1980;22:691–692.

184. Tewfik TL, Schloss MD: Ingestion of lye and other corrosive agents—A study of 86 infant and child cases. J Otolaryngol 1980;9:72–77.

185. Thompson JN: Corrosive esophageal injuries I: A study of nine cases of concurrent accidental caustic ingestions. Laryngoscope 1987;97:1060–1066.

186. Thompson JN: Corrosive esophageal injuries II: An investigation of treatment methods and histochemical analysis of esophageal strictures in a new animal model. Laryngoscope 1987;97:1191–1202.

187. Trevino MA, Hermann GH, Sprout WL: Treatment of severe hydrofluoric acid exposures. J Occup Med 1983;25:861–863.

188. Upfal M, Doyle C: Medical management of hydrofluoric acid exposure. J Occup Med 1990;32:727–731.

189. Upton J, Mulliken JB, Murray JE: Major intravenous extravasation injuries. Am J Surg 1979;137:497–506.

190. Vance MV, Curry SC, Kunkel DB, et al: Digital hydrofluoric acid burns: Treatment with intraarterial calcium infusion. Ann Emerg Med 1986;15:890–896.

191. Velvart J: Arterial perfusion for hydrofluoric acid burns. Hum Toxicol 1983;2:233–238.

192. Viscomi GJ, Beekhuis GJ, Whitten CF: An evaluation of early esophagoscopy and corticosteroid therapy in the management of corrosive injury of the esophagus. J Pediatr 1961;59:356–360.

193. Votteler TP, Nash JC, Rutledge JC: The hazard of ingested alkaline disc batteries in children. JAMA 1983;249:2504–2506.

194. Warren JB, Grifin DJ, Olson RC: Urine sugar reagent tablet ingestion causing gastric and duodenal ulceration. Arch Intern Med 1984;144:161–162.

195. Webb WR, Koutras P, Ecker RR, Sugg WL: An evaluation of steroids and antibiotics in caustic burns of the esophagus. Ann Thorac Surg 1970;9:95–101.

196. White JE, McClafferty K, Orfon RB, et al: Ocular alkali burn associated with automobile air bag activation. Can Med Assoc J 1995;153:933–934.

197. Wiesskopf A: Effects of cortisone on experimental lye burn of the esophagus. Ann Otol Rhinol Laryngol 1952;61:681–691.

198. Wijburg FA, Beukers MM, Heymans HS, et al: Nasogastric intubation as sole treatment of caustic esophageal lesions. Ann Otol Rhinol Laryngol 1985;94:337–341.

199. Williams JM, Hammad A, Cottington EC, Harchelroad FC: Intravenous magnesium in the treatment of hydrofluoric acid burns in rats. Ann Emerg Med 1994;23:464–469.

200. Wilson DAB, Wormald PJ: Battery acid—An agent of attempted suicide in black South Africans. S Afr Med J 1994;84:529–531.

201. Wilson JA, Phillips EM: Endoscopic retrieval of a miniature battery [letter]. Gut 1985;26:215.

202. Wing JS, Sanderson LM, Brender JD, et al: Acute health effects in a community after a release of hydrofluoric acid. Arch Environ Health 1991;46:155–159.

203. Woodring JH, Heiser MJ: Detection of pneumoperitoneum on chest radiographs: Comparison of upright lateral and posteroanterior projections. Am J Radiol 1995;165:45–47.

204. Wu MH, Lai WW: Surgical management of extensive corrosive injuries of the alimentary tract. Surg Gynecol Obstet 1993;177:12–16.

205. Yolken R, Konecny P, McCarthy P: Acute fluoride poisoning. Pediatrics 1976;58:90–93.

206. Yosowitz P, Ekland DA, Shah RC, Parsons RW: Peripheral intravenous infiltration necrosis. Ann Surg 1975;182:553–556.

207. Zargar SA, Kochhar R, Mehta S, Mehta SK: The role of fiberoptic endoscopy in the management of corrosive ingestion and modified endoscopic classification of burns. Gastrointest Endosc 1991;37: 165–169.

208. Zargar SA, Kochhar R, Nagi B, et al: Ingestion of corrosive acids: Spectrum of injury to upper gastrointestinal tract and natural history. Gastroenterology 1989;97:702–707.

ANTIDOTES IN DEPTH

Calcium

1 mg/dL = 0.25 mmol/L = 0.5 mEq/L

Normal Range
Total
    8.4–10.2 mg/dL
    2.10–2.55 mmol/L
    4.20–5.10 mEq/L
Ionized
    4.48–4.92 mg/dL
    1.12–1.23 mmol/L
    2.24–2.46 mEq/L

Calcium

Mary Ann Howland

In the clinical practice of medical toxicology, there is good evidence to support the administration of calcium to overcome the effects of calcium channel blockers (CCBs), to correct the hypocalcemia induced by ethylene glycol and the fluoride from hydrofluoric acid exposures, to complex with fluoride to limit tissue destruction, to treat iatrogenic magnesium poisoning, and to counteract the cardiac effects of hyperkalemia (except when associated with cardiac glycoside toxicity). The use of calcium in the management of β-adrenergic antagonist overdoses is being investigated, and the role of calcium to counteract muscle spasms resulting from black widow spider envenomations is being questioned.

PHYSIOLOGY

Calcium is essential in maintaining the normal function of the heart, vascular smooth muscle, skeletal system, and nervous system. It is vital to many enzymatic reactions, intimately involved in neurohormonal transmission, and critical for the maintenance of cellular integrity.[22,37] The endocrine system keeps the serum calcium concentration within the physiologic range. Approximately half of the total serum calcium is ionized and active, and the rest is bound primarily to albumin. Excess calcium raises the threshold for nerve and muscle excitation, resulting in muscle weakness, lethargy, and coma.[22] Insufficient calcium facilitates stimulation of nerves and muscles, resulting in tetany and seizures.[22]

CALCIUM CHANNEL BLOCKERS

Calcium channel blocker overdoses result in hypotension, myocardial depression, bradycardia, sinus arrest, arteriovenous (AV) block, shock, pulmonary edema, altered mental status, nausea, vomiting, constipation, metabolic acidosis with hyperglycemia, and, rarely, seizures.[42] Calcium may enter a cell in numerous ways; of these the voltage-dependent L-types channels in cardiac and smooth muscles are inhibited by calcium channel antagonists with varying degrees of selectivity depending on the agent.[2,53] Calcium channel blockers do not alter receptor-operated channels, the release of calcium from intracellular stores, or serum calcium concentrations.[57] In patients who overdose with CCBs, the serum calcium concentration therefore remains normal.

Intravenous administration of small doses of calcium to dogs poisoned with verapamil or diltiazem improves cardiac output secondary to an increase in inotropy.[2,21] Heart rate and cardiac conduction are affected minimally, if at all, unless greater amounts of calcium are given.[19,21,49] Case reports and reviews of the literature suggest similar findings in humans.[1,9,18,24,33,45,46,55]

Calcium should be administered to symptomatic patients with CCB overdoses and often produces a beneficial response. Unfortunately, the sickest patients usually respond inadequately, and other measures are required. Calcium administered to a patient with digoxin toxicity could prove quite harmful. In the event of concurrent overdose with both digoxin and a calcium channel blocker, early use of digoxin-specific antibody fragments should make the subsequent use of calcium less dangerous.

The amount of calcium needed to treat overdoses with CCBs is unknown. In animal experiments, there appears to be a dose-related improvement.[9,21] The customary approach is to administer an initial intravenous dose of 1 g of calcium chloride or 3 g of calcium gluconate, both about 4 mg/kg in a 70-kg adult, and to repeat this dose every 10–20 minutes for 3–4 additional doses, as needed.[42] Therapy in children is based on the current recommended pediatric dose of calcium for hypocalcemia, which is 5–7 mg/kg of elemental calcium infused slowly at a rate ≤100 mg/min and repeated once in 10 minutes. Calcium chloride 10% contains 27.2 mg/mL of elemental calcium, and calcium gluconate 10% contains 9 mg/mL of elemental calcium. Therefore, a starting dose in children should be about 0.6 mL/kg of calcium gluconate 10%. To avoid hypercalcemia, serum calcium concentration should be monitored when more than 2 doses are administered. However, calcium administration may not be as consequential as feared. One author successfully used 6 g of calcium gluconate intravenously over 20 minutes, followed by 6 g over the second hour and then 2 g/h for a total of 30 g of calcium gluconate without adverse effects in a CCB overdose.[9] Another author administered 18 g of calcium gluconate over 3 hours to a patient who overdosed on sustained-release verapamil. The serum calcium rose to 3.04 mmol/L without obvious toxicity and the patient survived.[32]

ETHYLENE GLYCOL

Ethylene glycol poisoning results in the generation of toxic metabolites that frequently produce central nervous system, cardiovascular, renal, and metabolic abnormalities. The generation of oxalic acid, which complexes with calcium and subsequently precipitates in the kidneys, brain, and elsewhere, is believed to account for the hypocalcemia that occurs with this poisoning.[1,25,41,53,56] After exposure to ethylene glycol, serum calcium should always be monitored. Signs of hypocalcemia include widening of the QT interval of the electrocardiogram (ECG), the presence of Chvostek and Trousseau signs, and tetany. Intravenous calcium should be administered in the customary doses (see above) to patients with these findings, accompanied by frequent monitoring of serum calcium.

HYDROFLUORIC ACID

Any body contact with hydrofluoric acid can result in severe burns and death, depending on the concentration of hydrofluoric acid and duration of exposure. The pathophysiologic derangements result from (a) release of free hydrogen ions; (b) complexation of fluoride with calcium and magnesium to form insoluble salts, which cause cellular necrosis; (c) liberation of potassium ions; and (d) cellular dehydration.[5,6,10,17,34,36,38,58] Following hydrofluoric acid exposure, the gluconate salt of calcium is used topically and subcutaneously to manage minor to moderate cutaneous burns, intravenously to treat systemic hypocalcemia and intra-arterially to manage significant burns.[1,5,7,10–12,15,17,20,34,36,38,43,48,50,52,58–60,62] The chloride salt is acceptable for topical therapy. Experimental studies demonstrate that when concentrated hydrofluoric acid burns are immediately flushed with water and then covered with 2.5% calcium gluconate gel or topical dimethyl sulfoxide (DMSO)/10% calcium gluconate plus subcutaneous 10% calcium gluconate, there is a significant reduction in burn size.[7,58] Unfortunately, neither DMSO nor a commercial calcium gluconate gel is readily available. A topical calcium gel can be prepared from calcium carbonate tablets or calcium gluconate powder or solution, and a water-soluble jelly such as K-Y Jelly (mix 3.5 g calcium gluconate powder or 25 mL of calcium gluconate 10% solution or 10 g of calcium carbonate tablets with 5 ounces of K-Y Jelly). Calcium chloride should not be injected subcutaneously or allowed to extravasate as it may lead to tissue necrosis.

Deaths from hypocalcemia secondary to skin, gastrointestinal, and inhalational hydrofluoric acid toxicity are documented in the literature.[11,20] In severe hydrofluoric acid exposures, aggressive administration of intravenous or intra-arterial calcium may be required, along with frequent serum calcium determinations in addition to other therapies as indicated, such as antidysrhythmic therapy (Chap. 87). To facilitate the availability of maximum amounts of calcium, simultaneous administration of oral and nebulized 2.5% calcium gluconate should also be given if there are no contraindications. To prepare nebulized calcium gluconate, mix 1.5 mL of 10% calcium gluconate solution with 4.5 mL of sterile water or saline to make a 2.5% solution. One patient who was massively exposed to hydrofluoric acid required a total of 267 mEq of calcium over 24 hours.[20] An ingestion of 30 mL of 70% hydrofluoric acid theoretically generates 660 mEq of fluoride. For moderate to severe burns (generally from hydrofluoric acid concentrations greater than 10%) of the fingers and hands, an intra-arterial calcium infusion may be more effective than local (or IV) therapy, although it is more invasive[43,52,59,60] and more hazardous.[52] One group successfully used 10 mL of 10% calcium gluconate solution mixed in 40–50 mL of 5% dextrose infused intra-arterially over 4 hours followed by subsequent 40-mL infusions after 4 hours when pain persisted.[59] Serum calcium and serum magnesium concentrations should be carefully monitored in all severely poisoned patients.[52,59]

HYPERMAGNESEMIA

Hypermagnesemia causes both direct and indirect depression of skeletal muscle, resulting in neuromuscular blockade, loss of reflexes, and profound muscular paralysis.[22] Excess magnesium also causes widening of the PR interval and QRS complex on the ECG and slows the sinoatrial (S-A) node, ultimately resulting in cardiac arrest. Intravenous calcium serves as a physiologic antagonist to the effects of magnesium.

HYPERKALEMIA

Hyperkalemia causes significant myocardial depression. On ECG, the height of the T wave increases, and the PR interval and QRS complex widen; impulse generation and conduction are depressed, and cardiac arrest occurs.[22] Calcium may make the membrane threshold potential less negative so that a greater stimulus is required to depolarize the cell. This amounts to a stabilization effect, which may antagonize the hyperexcitability caused by modest hyperkalemia. When hyperkalemia is severe, voltage-gated sodium channels are inactivated and cannot be depolarized, regardless of the strength of the impulse. Calcium may transform the voltage sensor of the sodium channel from inactive to closed, thus allowing the sodium channel to be opened with depolarization.[23] However, if hyperkalemia is secondary to the toxic effects of digoxin on the Na^+-K^+-ATPase pump, then intravenous calcium would potentially exacerbate an already excessive intracellular calcium concentration and is therefore contraindicated.

BETA-ADRENERGIC ANTAGONISTS

In vitro studies suggest that the negative inotropic action of propranolol and analogues is related to interference with both the forward and reverse transport of calcium in the sarcoplasmic reticulum and to inhibition of microsomal and mitochondrial calcium uptake.[16,30,36] In a canine model of propranolol poisoning, the administration of a bolus of calcium chloride followed by a continuous infusion improved mean arterial pressure, maximal left ventricular pressure change over time, and peripheral vascular resistance, but had no effect on bradycardia or QRS prolongation.[31] Several case reports attest to the beneficial effects of calcium in β-adrenergic antagonist overdose.[8,26,44,51] As long as no contraindications exist, a trial of intravenous calcium seems reasonable.

BLACK WIDOW SPIDER ENVENOMATION

Envenomation by a black widow spider (*Latrodectus spp.*) leads to local and systemic symptoms. Severe abdominal or back pain that begins within several hours of envenomation is the most common finding among symptomatic exposures.[13] How the venom exerts its effects is unclear, but the release of synaptic transmitters, including norepinephrine and acetylcholine, is believed to be involved.[47] Intravenous calcium, along with analgesics, benzodiazepines, and muscle relaxants, is used to successfully relieve the pain and muscle spasms.[13,27] Rarely, antivenom may be indicated. Animal studies suggest that the venom induces changes in the permeability of calcium that may be overcome by increasing the extracellular concentration of calcium.[28,40] One prospective study noted improvement in 6 of 13 patients treated with calcium gluconate.[27] However, a large retrospective study of 163 patients casts doubt on the effectiveness of calcium.[13] Very few patients in the study had received adequate pain relief from calcium, and all but one patient had also required opioids.[13] More research is necessary to clarify the role of calcium, if any, in the management of black widow spider envenomation.

SAFETY ISSUES AND CALCIUM PREPARATIONS

Severe hypercalcemia is defined by a serum calcium concentration greater than 3.5 mmol/L in a patient with a normal albumin concentration. The adverse effects of hypercalcemia (independent of the rate of administration) include nausea, vomiting, constipation, hypertension if intravascular volume is maintained, shortened QT interval on ECG, polyuria, polydipsia, cognitive difficulties, hyporeflexia, coma, and enhanced sensitivity to digitalis.[3] Significant hypercalcemia may lead to myocardial depression. The symptoms exhibited depend on the patient's age, rate of increase in the serum calcium, and duration of the hypercalcemia.[3]

A variety of calcium salts are available for parenteral administration. The two most commonly used are calcium chloride and calcium gluconate (Table 87–2). Calcium chloride is an acidifying salt and is extremely irritating to tissue. It should never be given intramuscularly, subcutaneously, or perivascularly.[22,37] Calcium gluconate is less irritating, but care should also be taken to avoid extravasation. The best reason for choosing calcium gluconate in almost all clinical situations is that the tissue risk is far less. Equal doses of calcium chloride and calcium gluconate produce similar serum ionized calcium measurements, with peaks occurring within 30 seconds and accompanied by similar measured hemodynamic values.[35] These measurements support the idea that simple dissociation of calcium from gluconate is responsible for releasing calcium, rather than hepatic metabolism. Earlier evidence suggesting that infusions of intravenous calcium chloride produce slightly larger increases in ionic calcium than do infusions of calcium gluconate has been challenged.[35,61] Intravenous calcium must be administered slowly, at a rate not exceeding 0.7–1.8 mEq/min or one 10-mL vial of calcium chloride over 10 minute in adults. In cases of extreme life-threatening hypocalcemia or for a patient in extremis, faster rates may be required. More rapid administration may lead to vasodilation, hypotension, bradycardia, dysrhythmias, syncope, and cardiac arrest.[4,14,29,37,54]

SUMMARY

In summary, intravenous calcium is an effective remedy for the hypocalcemia induced by ethylene glycol and hydrofluoric acid. It serves as a physiologic antagonist to the cardiac and/or neurologic effects of hypermagnesemia and hyperkalemia (except when associated with cardiac glycosides) and counteracts the effects of calcium channel antagonist overdoses. It may have some benefit in the treatment of β-adrenergic receptor antagonist overdoses. The efficacy of calcium in the management of patients with black widow spider envenomation has yet to be clarified. Great care must be taken to avoid extravasation. Calcium chloride, in particular, can be quite toxic to tissue. Equal doses of calcium gluconate and calcium chloride deliver equal amounts of ionic or active calcium. Electrocardiographic monitoring and frequent serum calcium determinations are required to prevent iatrogenic toxicity. Although most clinical experience involves intravenous use, advances in intra-arterial topical and inhalational calcium therapy offer unique potential advantages in certain circumstances.

TABLE 87–2.   The Two Most Commonly Used Calcium Salts

	Calcium Chloride	Calcium Gluconate
10% solution	10 mL = 1 g of calcium chloride = 1.36 mEq/mL elemental calcium = 27.2 mg/mL elemental calcium	10 mL = 1 g of calcium gluconate = 0.45 mEq/mL elemental calcium = 9 mg/mL elemental calcium

Adult dose	10 mL of 10 % solution
	Repeat dose q10–20 min for
	   3–4 doses as needed
	Infuse ≤0.7–1.8 mEq/min or
	10 mL of 10% CaCl$_2$ over 10 min
	Monitor serum calcium
		30 mL of 10% solution over 10 min
		Repeat dose q10–20 min for
		   3–4 doses as needed
		Infuse ≤0.7–1.8 mEq/min
		or 30 mL of 10% Ca gluconate over 10 min
		Monitor serum calcium

Pediatric dose*	5–7 mg/kg elemental calcium
	0.2–0.25 mL/kg of 10% solution
	Infuse slowly over several min;
	   repeat dose in 10 min if needed
	Monitor serum calcium
		5–7 mg/kg elemental calcium
		0.6–0.8 mL/kg of 10% solution
		Infuse slowly over several min; repeat dose
		   in 10 min if needed
		Monitor serum calcium

*Not to exceed adult dose.

REFERENCES

1. Anderson WJ, Anderson JR: Hydrofluoric acid burns of the hand: Mechanism of injury and treatment. Am J Hand Surg 1988;13:52–57.
2. Bean BP: Classes of calcium channels in vertebrate cells. Annu Rev Physiol 1989;51:367–384.
3. Belezekian JP: Management of acute hypercalcemia. N Engl J Med 1992;326:1196–1215.
4. Berliner K: The effect of calcium injections on the human heart. Am J Med Sci 1936;191:117–121.
5. Bertolini JC: Hydrofluoric acid: A review of toxicity. J Emerg Med 1992;10:163–168.
6. Boink ABTJ, Wemer J, Meulenbelt J, et al: The mechanism of fluoride-induced hypocalcemia. Hum Exp Toxicol 1994;13:149–155.
7. Bracken WM, Cuppage F, McLaury RL, et al: Comparative effectiveness of topical treatments for hydrofluoric acid burns. J Occup Med 1985;27:733–739.
8. Briacombe JR, Scully M, Swainston R: Propranolol overdose. A dramatic response to calcium chloride. Med J Aust 1991;155:267–268.
9. Buckley N, Dawson AH, Howarth D, Whyte IM: Slow-release verapamil poisoning. Med J Aust 1993;158:202–204.
10. Caravati EM: Acute hydrofluoric acid exposure. Am J Emerg Med 1988;6:143–150.
11. Chan KM, Svancarek WP, Creer M: Fatality due to acute hydrofluoric acid exposure. J Toxicol Clin Toxicol 1987;25:333–339.
12. Chick LR, Borah G: Calcium carbonate gel therapy of hydrofluoric acid burns of the hand. Plast Reconstr Surg 1990;86:935–940.
13. Clark RF, Wathern-Kestner S, Vance M, Gerkin R: Clinical presentation and treatment of black widow spider envenomation: A review of 163 cases. Ann Emerg Med 1992;21:782–787.
14. Clarke NE: The action of calcium on the human electrocardiogram. Am Heart J 1941;22:367–373.
15. Conway EE, Sockolow R: Hydrofluoric acid burn in a child. Pediatr Emerg Care 1991;7:345–347.
16. Dhalla NS, Lee SL: Comparison of the actions of acebutolol, practolol, and propranolol on calcium transport by heart microsomes and mitochondria. Br J Pharmacol 1976;57:215–221.
17. Edinburg M, Swift R: Hydrofluoric acid burns of the hands: A case report and suggested management. Aust N Z J Surg 1989;59:88–91.
18. Erickson F, Ling L, Grande G, et al: Diltiazem overdose? Case report and review. J Emerg Med 1991;9:357–366.
19. Gay R, Algeo S, Lee R, et al: Treatment of verapamil toxicity in intact dogs. J Clin Invest 1986;77:1805–1811.
20. Greco RJ, Hartford CE, Haith LR, Patton ML: Hydrofluoric acid-induced hypocalcemia. J Trauma 1988;28:1593–1596.
21. Hariman RJ, Mangiardi LM, McAllister RG, et al: Reversal of the cardiovascular effects of verapamil by calcium and sodium: Differences between electrophysiologic and hemodynamic responses. Circulation 1979;59:797–804.
22. Hayes RC: Agents affecting calcification: Calcium, parathyroid hormone, calcitonin, vitamin D, and other compounds. In: Gilman AG, Rall T, Nies A, Taylor P, eds: Goodman and Gilman's The Pharmacologic Basis of Therapeutics, 8th ed. New York, Pergamon, 1990, pp. 1496–1501.
23. Hille B: Ionic Channels of Excitable Membranes. Sunderland MA, Sinauer Associates, 1984.
24. Hofer CA, Smith JK, Tenholder MF: Verapamil intoxication: A literature review of overdoses and discussion of therapeutic options. Am J Med 1993;95:431–438.
25. Introna F Jr, Smialek JE: Antifreeze (ethylene glycol) intoxications in Baltimore: Report of six cases. Acta Morphol Hung 1989;37:245–263.
26. Jones JL: Metoprolol overdose. Ann Emerg Med 1982;11:114–115.
27. Key GF: A comparison of calcium gluconate and methocarbamol (Robaxin) in the treatment of latrodectism (black widow spider envenomations). Am J Trop Med Hyg 1981;30:273–277.

28. Kobernick M: Black widow spider bites. Am Fam Physician 1984; 29:241–245.
29. Kuhn M: Severe bradyarrhythmias following calcium pretreatment. Am Heart J 1991;121:1812–1813.
30. Langemeijer J, de Wildt D, de Groot G, Sangster B: Calcium interferes with the cardiodepressive effects of beta-blocker overdose in isolated rat hearts. J Toxicol Clin Toxicol 1986;24:111–133.
31. Love J, Hanfling D, Howell J: Hemodynamic effects of calcium chloride in a canine model of acute propranolol intoxication. Ann Emerg Med 1996;28:1–6.
32. Luscher TF, Noll G, Sturmer T, Muser B, et al: Calcium gluconate in severe verapamil intoxication [letter]. N Engl J Med 1994;330: 718–719.
33. MacDonald D, Alguire P: Case reports: Fatal overdose with sustained release verapamil. Am J Med Sci 1992;303:115–117.
34. MacKinnon MA: Hydrofluoric acid burns. Dermatol Clin 1988;6: 67–74.
35. Martin T, Kang Y, Robertson K, et al: Ionization and hemodynamic effects of calcium chloride and calcium gluconate in the absence of hepatic function. Anesthesiolgy 1990;73:62–65.
36. McCulley JP: Ocular hydrofluoric acid burns: Animal model, mechanism of injury and therapy. Am Ophthalmol Soc 1990;88:649–683.
37. McEvoy G, ed: AHFS Drug Information, 1997. Baltimore, American Society of Hospital Pharmacists, 1997.
38. Mistry DG, Wainwright DJ: Hydrofluoric acid burns. Am Fam Physician 1992;45:1748–1754.
39. Noack E, Kurzmack M, Verjovski-Almeida Sand Inesi G: The effect of propranolol and its analogs on Ca− transport by sarcoplasmic reticulum vesicles. J Pharmacol Exp Ther 1978;206:281–288.
40. Pardel JF: Influence of calcium on 3H-noradrenaline release by Lactrodectus venom gland extract on arterial tissue of the rat. Toxicon 1979;17:455–465.
41. Parry MF, Wallach R: Ethylene glycol poisoning. Am J Med 1974;57: 143–150.
42. Pearigen PD, Benowitz NS: Poisoning due to calcium antagonists: Experience with verapamil, diltiazem and nifedipine. Drug Saf 1991; 6:408–430.
43. Pegg SP, Siu S, Gillet G: Intra-arterial infusions in the treatment of hydrofluoric acid burns. Burns 1985;11:440–443.
44. Pertoldi F, D'Orlando L, Mercanto W: Electromechanical dissociation 48 hours after atenolol overdose. Usefulness of calcium chloride. Ann Emerg Med 1998;31:777–781.
45. Proano L, Chiang WK, Wang RY: Calcium channel blocker overdose. Am J Emerg Med 1995;13:444–450.
46. Ramoska EA, Spiller HA, Winter M, Borys D: A one-year evaluation of calcium channel blocker overdoses: Toxicity and treatment. Ann Emerg Med 1993;22:196–200.
47. Rauber A: Black widow spider bites. J Toxicol Clin Toxicol 1983–1984;21:473–485.
48. Roberts JR, Merigian KS: Acute hydrofluoric acid exposure. Am J Emerg Med 1989;7:125–126.
49. Sabatier J, Pouyet T, Shelvey G, Cavero I: Antagonistic effects of epinephrine, glucagon and methylatropine but not calcium chloride against atrio-ventricular conduction disturbances produced by high doses of diltiazem in conscious dogs. Fundam Clin Pharmacol 1991;5: 93–106.
50. Sadove R, Hainsworth D, Van Meter W: Total body immersion in hydrofluoric acid. South Med J 1990;83:698–700.
51. Sangster B, de Wildt D, van Dijk A: A case of acebutolol intoxication. J Toxicol Clin Toxicol 1983;20:69–77.
52. Siegel DC, Heard JM: Intra-arterial calcium infusion for hydrofluoric acid burns. Aviat Space Environ Med 1992;63:206–211.
53. Simpson E: Some aspects of calcium metabolism in a fatal case of ethylene glycol poisoning. Ann Clin Biochem 1985;22:90–93.
54. Smallwood RA: Some effects of the intravenous administration of calcium in man. Aust Acad Med 1967;16:126–131.

55. Spiller HA, Meyers A, Ziemba T, Riley M: Delayed onset of cardiac arrhythmias from sustained release verapamil. Ann Emerg Med 1991; 20:201–203.

56. Tarr BD, Winters LJ, Moore MP, et al: Low dose ethanol in the treatment of ethylene glycol poisoning. J Vet Pharmacol Ther 1985;8: 254–262.

57. Triggle DJ: Calcium-channel antagonists: Mechanisms of action, vascular selectivities, and clinical relevance. Cleve Clin J Med 1992;59: 617–626.

58. Upfal M, Doyle C: Medical management of hydrofluoric acid exposure. J Occup Med 1990;32:726–731.

59. Vance MV, Curry SC, Kunkel DB, et al: Digital hydrofluoric acid burns: Treatment with intraarterial calcium infusion. Ann Emerg Med 1986;15:890–896.

60. Velvart J: Arterial perfusion for hydrofluoric acid burns. Hum Toxicol 1983;2:233–238.

61. White RD, Goldsmith RS, Rodriquez R, et al: Plasma ionic calcium levels following injection of chloride, gluconate, and gluceptate salts of calcium. J Thorac Cardiovasc Surg 1976;71:609–613.

62. Zachary LS, Reus W, Gottlieb J, et al: Treatment of experimental hydrofluoric acid burns. J Burn Care 1986;7:35–39.

I. PESTICIDES

CHAPTER 88 INSECTICIDES: ORGANIC PHOSPHORUS COMPOUNDS AND CARBAMATES

Richard F. Clark

A 40-year-old suicidal male was brought by relatives into the Emergency Department (ED) after drinking two sips of 50% malathion about 3 hours earlier. The patient was awake but confused and extremely diaphoretic. He had the odor of hydrocarbons, although there was no evidence that the liquid had spilled onto his clothes. His initial vital signs in the ED were: blood pressure, 210/120 mm Hg; pulse, 100 beats/min; respiratory rate, 22 breaths/min; temperature, 98.6°F (37°C); and oxygen saturation, 95% on room air. Physical examination demonstrated midsized pupils, coarse crackles in all lung fields, and copious vomiting and diarrhea. The patient was drooling between episodes of vomiting.

The patient was completely undressed and his clothing placed in bags for hazardous materials. His skin was thoroughly washed with soap and water. Oxygen was administered by facemask, an intravenous line was inserted, and normal saline was infused.

Even with supplemental oxygen applied, the victim's oxygenation began to fall several minutes after arrival in the ED. His heart rate also rapidly increased to 120 beats/min, and an electrocardiogram (ECG) demonstrated a prolonged QTc duration (560 msec). A portable chest radiograph showed bilateral pulmonary edema with normal heart size. The Poison Control Center (PCC) was contacted immediately and recommended administration of atropine and pralidoxime. After administration of atropine 3 mg and pralidoxime 1 g intravenously, his breath sounds improved. But, despite therapy, his oxygenation continued to fall to 87%, and he began coughing up pink-tinged, frothy sputum and continued having large amounts of vomiting and diarrhea. A pralidoxime infusion at 200 mg/h was initiated, with recommendations to increase the rate to 300–500 mg/h if rapid improvement was not noted. The PCC advised giving additional 2-mg atropine doses every 5–15 minutes as needed to control his secretions.

Although the quantity of emesis, diarrhea, and bronchorrhea improved after a total of 20 mg of atropine, the clinicians elected to intubate the patient for airway protection. He was sedated with midazolam and paralyzed with vecuronium. His oxygen saturation following intubation was 98% on 100% FIO₂ at an intermittent mechanical ventilation (IMV) rate of 16, and his vital signs were blood pressure, 175/90 mm Hg; and pulse, 125 beats/min. A nasogastric tube was inserted and lavage of stomach contents performed followed by administration of 75 g of activated charcoal. He was transferred to the intensive care unit (ICU).

In the ICU, the pralidoxime infusion was increased to 500 mg/h, and atropine was administered intermittently throughout the first 24 hours of admission for a total dose of 30 mg. Hematologic studies were normal except for a white blood cell count (WBC) of 19,000/mm³. His other laboratory studies were remarkable for a glucose of 195 mg/dL, potassium of 3.2 mEq/L, and serum bicarbonate of 20 mEq/L. The chest radiograph dramatically improved over the first 24 hours, and by the second day was only remarkable for a right-upper-lobe infiltrate. The patient was kept sedated with midazolam and intubated for another 24 hours to better monitor pulmonary status. His ECG gradually improved by the second day, with a heart rate of 105, and normalization of his QTc interval.

On hospital day 2, because oxygenation was normal on room air, his sedation was terminated and he was extubated. His nausea and vomiting had largely improved, and no further frothy sputum was observed. Diaphoresis and diarrhea had resolved, but he continued to smell of solvents. Cholinesterase measurements sent initially showed virtually no detectable red blood cell (RBC) or butyrylcholinesterase (plasma) activity. All other laboratory results had normalized by the second day. He was transferred to a stepdown unit for observation, and did not require any further atropine that day. The pralidoxime infusion was maintained at 500 mg/h, and penicillin was begun for presumed aspiration pneumonia. With continued hydrocarbon odor present, it was advised to continue to wash the victim's skin and hair at least on a daily basis.

On hospital day 3, the patient reported feeling much better. His pralidoxime infusion was stopped and he was evaluated by the psychiatric service. That afternoon, he reported two episodes of diarrhea and some nausea, and was again administered atropine 2 mg IV and restarted on pralidoxime with resolution of symptoms once again.

He required no further atropine during his hospitalization. Pralidoxime infusion was stopped successfully on hospital day 5, and he was discharged to a psychiatric facility on hospital day 7.

EPIDEMIOLOGY

Organic phosphorus compounds and carbamates are the two groups of cholinesterase-inhibiting pesticides that produce human toxicity. Poisoning from these agents results in a rise in the concentration of acetylcholine (ACh) at muscarinic and nicotinic cholinergic receptors, which, in turn, leads to the syndrome of cholinergic excess. Although the term *organophosphate* has traditionally been used in clinical practice and in the literature to refer to all phosphorus-containing pesticides that inhibit cholinesterase, not all of these chemicals contain ester side chains off the phosphorus molecule. Some of these chemicals, such as parathion, contain thioesters, whereas others are vinyl esters. The more correct term, and the one that is used in this chapter, is *organic phosphorus compound*.

During the past 5-year period of 1995–2000, the American Association of Poison Control Centers recorded more than 75,000 exposures to organic phosphorus compounds and more than 25,000 exposures to carbamates, with 44 fatalities, ranking these agents as the most lethal insecticides in use in the United States, and among the most lethal poisonings (Chap. 116). In Taiwan, where insecticides are often more accessible than medications in rural areas, fatality rates with exposures to these compounds are as high as 23%.[134] The World Health Organization estimates that at least 1 million unintentional poisonings and 2 million suicide attempts occur annually from these agents.[13] However, these figures may neglect numerous unreported and possibly unrecognized illnesses resulting from environmental exposure to these chemicals.

Patients may present following unintentional or suicidal ingestion of anticholinesterase insecticides or after working in areas recently treated with these compounds.[55] Children and adults can develop toxicity while playing in or inhabiting a residence recently sprayed or fogged with organic phosphorus agents by a pesticide applicator.[158] Direct dermal contact with these insecticides may be rapidly poisonous. Outbreaks of mass poisoning have occurred from contamination of crops or food.[13,28,36,105,129,130] Organic phosphorus agents have also been used for homicide.[105,106]

HISTORY

The first potent synthetic organic phosphorus anticholinesterase was tetraethyl pyrophosphate (TEPP), which was synthesized by Clermont in 1854. Clermont's report described the taste of the compound, which is remarkable, because a few drops should be rapidly fatal.[57] In 1932, Lange and Krueger published an account of choking and blurred vision following inhalation of dimethyl and diethyl phosphorofluoridates.[65] This report inspired Schrader to begin investigating these agents, initially as pesticides, and later for use in warfare (Chap. 100). During this research, Schrader's group synthesized hundreds of compounds, including the popular pesticide parathion and the chemical warfare agents sarin, soman, and tabun. Allied scientists were also motivated during the same period by the work of Lange and Krueger, and independently discovered other extremely toxic compounds such as diisopropyl phosphofluoridate (DFP).[144] Since that time, it is estimated that more than 50,000 organic phosphorus compounds have been synthesized and screened for pesticidal activity, with dozens being produced commercially.[12]

The history of carbamates was first recognized by Westerners in the 19th century when the Calabar bean (*Physostigma venenosum Balfour*) was used in tribal cultural practice in West Africa.[143] These beans were imported to Great Britain in 1840, where, by 1864, Jobst and Hesse isolated an active alkaloid component that they named "physostigmine."[143] Physostigmine was first medicinally used to treat glaucoma in 1877.[58,66] In the 1930s, the synthesis of aliphatic esters of carbamic acid led to the development and introduction of carbamate pesticides, marketed initially as fungicides.[145] The Union Carbide Corporation developed and first mar-

keted carbaryl in 1953, which was the agent prepared at Bhopal, India (Chap. 1).[90]

PHARMACOLOGY

Organic Phosphorus Compounds

Figure 88–1 shows the basic formula for cholinesterase-inhibiting organic phosphorus compounds. The "X" or "leaving group" determines many of the characteristics of the compound and provides a means of classifying organic phosphorus agents into four main groups (Table 88–1). Group 1 substances contain a quaternary nitrogen at the X position, and are collectively termed phosphorylcholines. In addition to being powerful cholinesterase inhibitors, these chemicals can also directly stimulate cholinergic receptors. Phosphorylcholines are among the most potent anticholinesterases, originally developed as war gases.[43] Group 2 compounds are called fluorophosphates because they possess a fluorine molecule as the leaving group. Like group 1 agents, these compounds are volatile and highly toxic, making them well-suited for chemical warfare. The leaving group of group 3 compounds is a cyanide molecule or a halogen other than fluorine. The most well-known agents in this group are cyanophosphates such as tabun. The fourth group is the broadest and comprises various subgroups based on the configuration of the R_1 and R_2 groups, with the majority falling into the category of either a dimethoxy or diethoxy compound. Most of the insecticides in use today fall into this last class.[43]

"Direct"-acting organic phosphorus agents can inhibit acetylcholinesterase (AChE) without being structurally altered by the body. Many of the more popular pesticides, such as parathion and malathion, are "indirect" inhibitors requiring partial metabolism (to paraoxon and malaoxon, respectively) within the body to become active. Most of the indirect inhibitors undergo oxygenation in the intestinal mucosa and liver following absorption to form the more active "oxone" metabolites.[74] The active form is able to combine with cholinesterase. The covalent bond is completed as the leaving group of the organic phosphorus compound is split off by AChE, resulting in a stable but reversible bond between the remaining substituted phosphate of the organic phosphorus agent and AChE, effectively inactivating the enzyme (Fig. 88–2). Although the splitting of the choline-enzyme bond in normal ACh metabolism is completed within microseconds, the severing of the organic phosphorus compound–enzyme bond can require as much as 1000 hours.[43,137] In organic phosphorus compound poisoning,

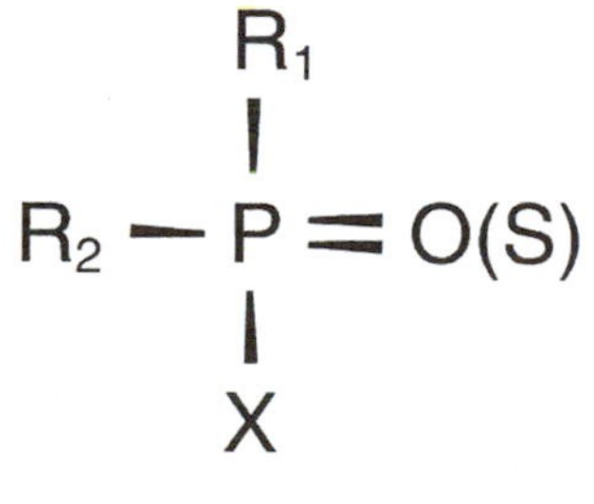

$$R_2 - \underset{\underset{X}{|}}{\overset{\overset{R_1}{|}}{P}} = O(S)$$

Figure 88–1. General structure of organic phosphorus insecticides. X represents the leaving group. R_1 and R_2 may be aromatic or aliphatic groups that can be identical.

TABLE 88–1. The Classification of Organic Phosphorus Agents by Groups.[43] Leaving Groups and Examples of Each Group Are Included.

Group 1–phosphorylcholines
Leaving group: substituted quarternary nitrogen
    Echothiophate iodide

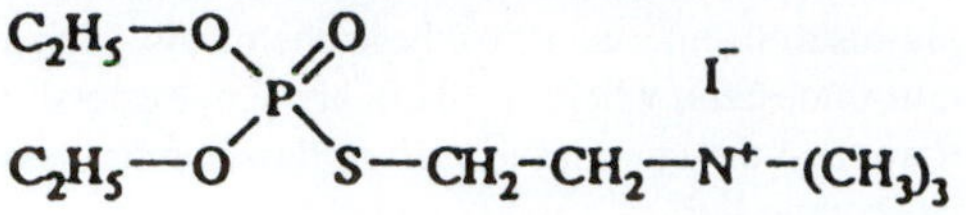

Group 2–fluorophosphates
Leaving group: fluoride
    Dimefox, sarin, mipafox

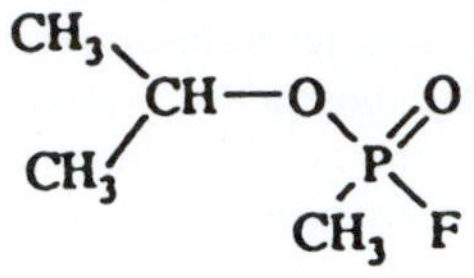

Group 3–cyanophosphates, other halophosphates
Leaving group: CN, SCN, OCN, halogen other than fluoride
    Tabun

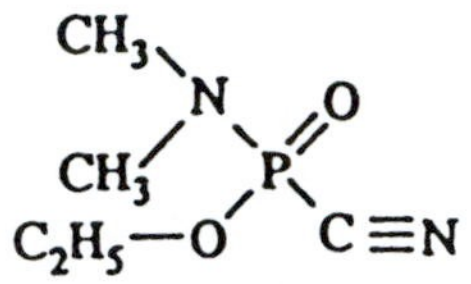

Group 4–multiple constituents
Leaving group:
  Dimethoxy
    Azinphos-menthyl, bromophos, chlorothion,
    crotoxyphos, dicapthon, dichlorvos, dicrotophos,
    dimethoate, fenthion, malathion, mevinphos,
    parathion-methyl, phosphamidon, temephos,
    trichlorfon

  Diethoxy
    Carbophenothion, chlorfenvinphos, chlorpyriphos,
    coumaphos, demeton, diazinon, dioxathion,
    disulfoton, ethion, methosfolan, parathion,
    phorate, phosfolan, TEPP

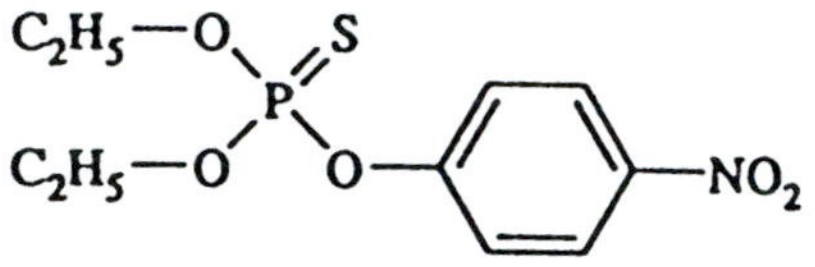

  Other dialkoxy
    Isopropyl paraoxon, isopropyl parathion

  Diamino
    Schradan

  Chlorinated and other substituted dialkoxy
    Haloxon

  Trithioalkyl
    Merphos

  Triphenyl and substituted triphenyl
    Triorthocresyl phosphate (TOCP)

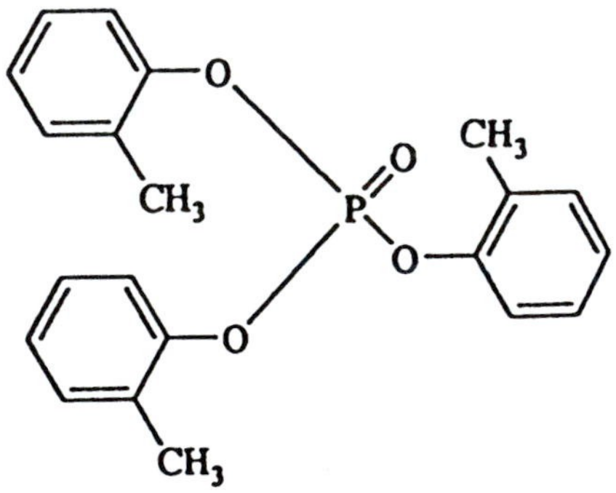

  Mixed substituent
    Crufomate, cyanofenphos

Echothiophate iodide

Sarin

Tabun

Parathion

Triorthocresyl phosphate (TOCP)

the complex becomes irreversibly bound during the next 24–72 hours when one of the R groups leaves the phosphate molecule. This step is termed "aging."[127] De novo synthesis of AChE is required to replenish its supply once aging has occurred.[120,143,152]

Carbamates

Carbamate insecticides are *N*-methyl carbamates derived from carbamic acid (Fig. 88–3). Medicinal carbamate compounds include physostigmine, pyridostigmine, and neostigmine. Medications such as meprobamate and various urethanes are carbamate derivatives, but do not cause cholinesterase inhibition.[143] Thiocarbamate fungicides and herbicides (eg, Maneb, Zineb, Nabam, Mancozeb) also do not inhibit AChE and do not produce cholinergic poisoning.

When exposed to carbamate compounds, AChE undergoes carbamylation in a manner similar to phosphorylation by organic phosphorus agents, allowing ACh to accumulate in synapses.[153]

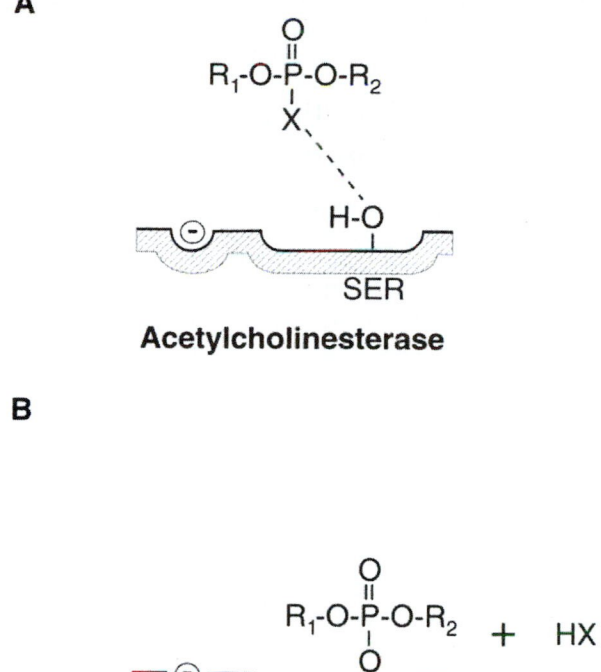

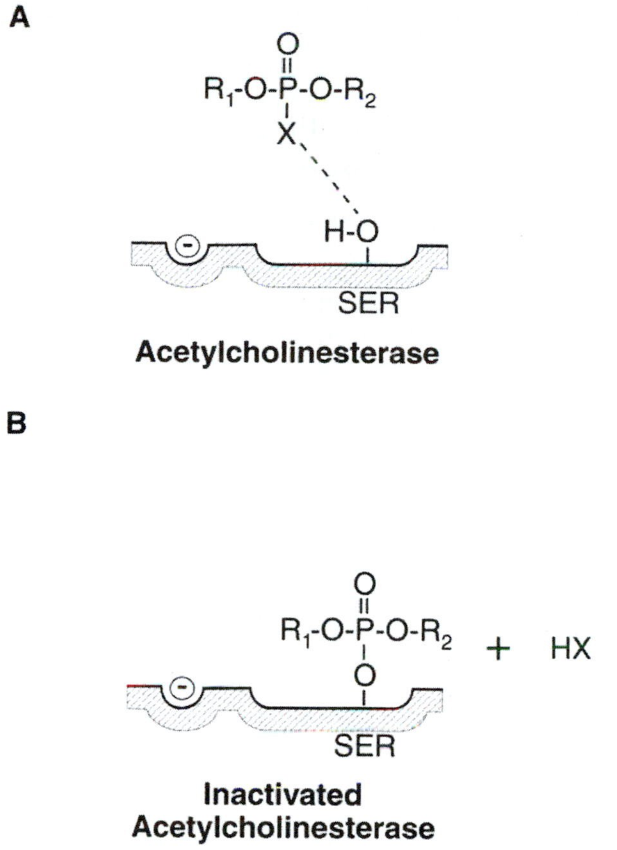

Figure 88–2. Mechanism of inhibition of acetylcholinesterase by an organic phosphorous compound. The HX is the leaving group. A serine residue at the active site of the enzyme gives up a hydrogen atom to combine with the leaving group, while the active site undergoes phosphorylation and inhibition. This initial inhibition is reversible with pralidoxime. However, as the inhibited phosphorylated enzyme "ages," one of the R groups is lost. The aged phosphorylated enzyme is unable to be rejuvenated by pralidoxime.

However, because aging cannot occur, the carbamate-AChE bond hydrolyzes spontaneously, resulting in reactivation of the enzyme. As such, the duration of toxic symptoms in carbamate poisoning is generally less than 24 hours.

PHARMACOKINETICS
Organic Phosphorus Compounds

Organic phosphorus agents are extremely well absorbed from the lungs, gastrointestinal tract, skin, mucous membranes, and con-

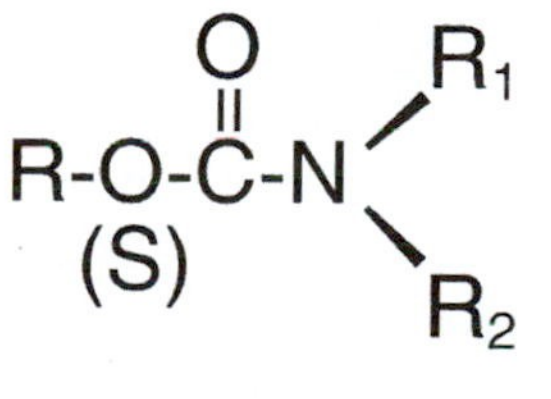

Figure 88–3. General structure of carbamate insecticides.

junctiva following inhalation, ingestion, or topical contact.[43,69,87] Intravenous and subcutaneous injections[99,118,155] and percutaneous exposure may cause severe toxicity.[15,69,116] The presence of broken skin and dermatitis and higher environmental temperatures enhances cutaneous absorption.[43]

Cholinesterase-inhibitor poisonings can be chronic or acute, although the differentiation has little clinical relevance. The difficulty in removing these compounds from the skin and clothing may explain some chronic poisonings.[15] Inadequate skin and respiratory protection during pesticide application may be responsible for many of these cases.

Most organic phosphorus agents are lipophilic.[143] Radiolabeled parathion injected into mice distributes most rapidly into the cervical brown fat and salivary glands, with high levels also measured in the liver, kidneys, and ordinary adipose tissue.[39] Adipose tissue gradually accumulates the highest levels. Cholinergic crisis may recur in patients when fat stores of unmetabolized organic phosphorus agents are mobilized.[42,43] The more lipophilic compounds such as fenthion and chlorfenthion are particularly susceptible to this phenomenon.[149]

Peak levels of organic phosphorus agents are measured 6 hours after oral ingestion in man.[112] Although serum half-lives of these compounds range from minutes to hours,[65] prolonged absorption or redistribution from fat stores may allow for measurement of circulating insecticide concentrations for up to 48 days.[18,44,65,124]

Organic phosphorus agents are thought to be metabolized by various mixed function oxidases in the liver and intestinal mucosa, but the exact pathways are not yet well understood.[43,74,139] The phosphorylating ability of these substances is lost when any of the side chains are hydrolyzed. Certain indirect-acting agents are activated to a more toxic compound by this initial metabolism. Particularly, lipophilic organic phosphorus compounds may be protected from metabolism by fat storage, markedly prolonging their elimination half-life.[18,43,94] Inactive metabolites of these agents are excreted in the urine.[43]

Carbamates

Carbamate insecticides are well absorbed across skin and mucous membranes, as well as by inhalation and ingestion. Peak serum levels of some compounds are measured 30–40 minutes following ingestion.[10] Most carbamates undergo hydrolysis, hydroxylation, and conjugation in the liver and intestinal wall, with 90% excreted in the urine within 3 days.[113] There are two main pharmacokinetic characteristics that distinguish carbamates from organic phosphorus compounds. First, carbamate insecticides do not easily cross into the central nervous system (CNS).[43] CNS effects of carbamates are thus limited, although CNS dysfunction may still occur in massive poisonings or may result from hypoxia secondary to pulmonary toxicity and paralysis. Second, the carbamate-cholinesterase bond does not "age" as in organic phosphorus compound poisoning; thus it is reversible, with spontaneous hydrolysis occurring within several hours.

PATHOPHYSIOLOGY

Acetylcholine is a neurotransmitter found at both parasympathetic and sympathetic ganglia, skeletal neuromuscular junctions, terminal junctions of all postganglionic parasympathetic nerves, postganglionic sympathetic fibers to most sweat glands, and at some nerve endings within the central nervous system (Fig. 88–4).[43] As the axon terminal is depolarized, vesicles containing ACh rupture, releasing ACh into the synapse or neuromuscular junction. Acetylcholine then binds postsynaptic receptors leading to activation (G proteins for muscarinic receptors and ligand-linked ion channels for the nicotinic receptors). Activation alters the flow of K^+, Na^+, and Ca^{2+} ionic currents, and alters membrane potential of the postsynaptic membrane, resulting in propagation of the action potential.[9]

Acetylcholinesterase is an enzyme that hydrolyzes ACh into two inert fragments: acetic acid and choline. Under normal circumstances, virtually all ACh released by the axon is hydrolyzed almost immediately, with choline being reuptaken into the presynaptic terminal and used to resynthesize ACh.[43,114,143] Organic phosphorus agents and carbamates are powerful inhibitors of carboxylic ester hydrolases within the body, including chymotrypsin, AChE, plasma or butyrylcholinesterase (pseudocholinesterase), plasma and hepatic carboxylesterases (aliesterases), paraoxonases (A-esterases), and other nonspecific proteases. Acetylcholinesterase is found in human nervous tissue and skeletal muscle, and on erythrocyte (RBC) cell membranes. RBC cholinesterase activity levels correlate with functioning nervous system AChE. Butyrylcholinesterase is a hepatic-derived protein that is found in human plasma, liver, heart, pancreas, and brain. Although the function of this enzyme is not well understood, its activity can be easily measured and has important clinical implications in anesthesia (Chap. 54).

CLINICAL MANIFESTATIONS
Organic Phosphorus Compounds

Clinical findings in organic phosphorus pesticide poisoning are typical of those caused by excessive stimulation of muscarinic and nicotinic cholinergic receptors by ACh in the central and autonomic nervous systems, as well as at skeletal neuromuscular junctions (Fig. 88–4). Although the classically described patient with organic phosphorus insecticide poisoning is unresponsive with pinpoint pupils, muscle fasciculations, diaphoresis, emesis, diarrhea, salivation, lacrimation, urinary incontinence, and an odor of garlic, most presentations are not so typical. The onset of symptoms varies according to the agent, the route, and the degree of exposure. Patients suffering massive ingestions have become symptomatic as quickly as 5 minutes following ingestion, and deaths have occurred within 15 minutes of ingestion.[43,82] Most victims of acute poisonings become symptomatic within 8 hours of exposure, and nearly all are symptomatic within 24 hours.[105] The longest delays may occur with agents requiring metabolic activation, such as malathion, or very lipid-soluble agents such as fenthion. Symptoms may last for variable lengths of time, again based

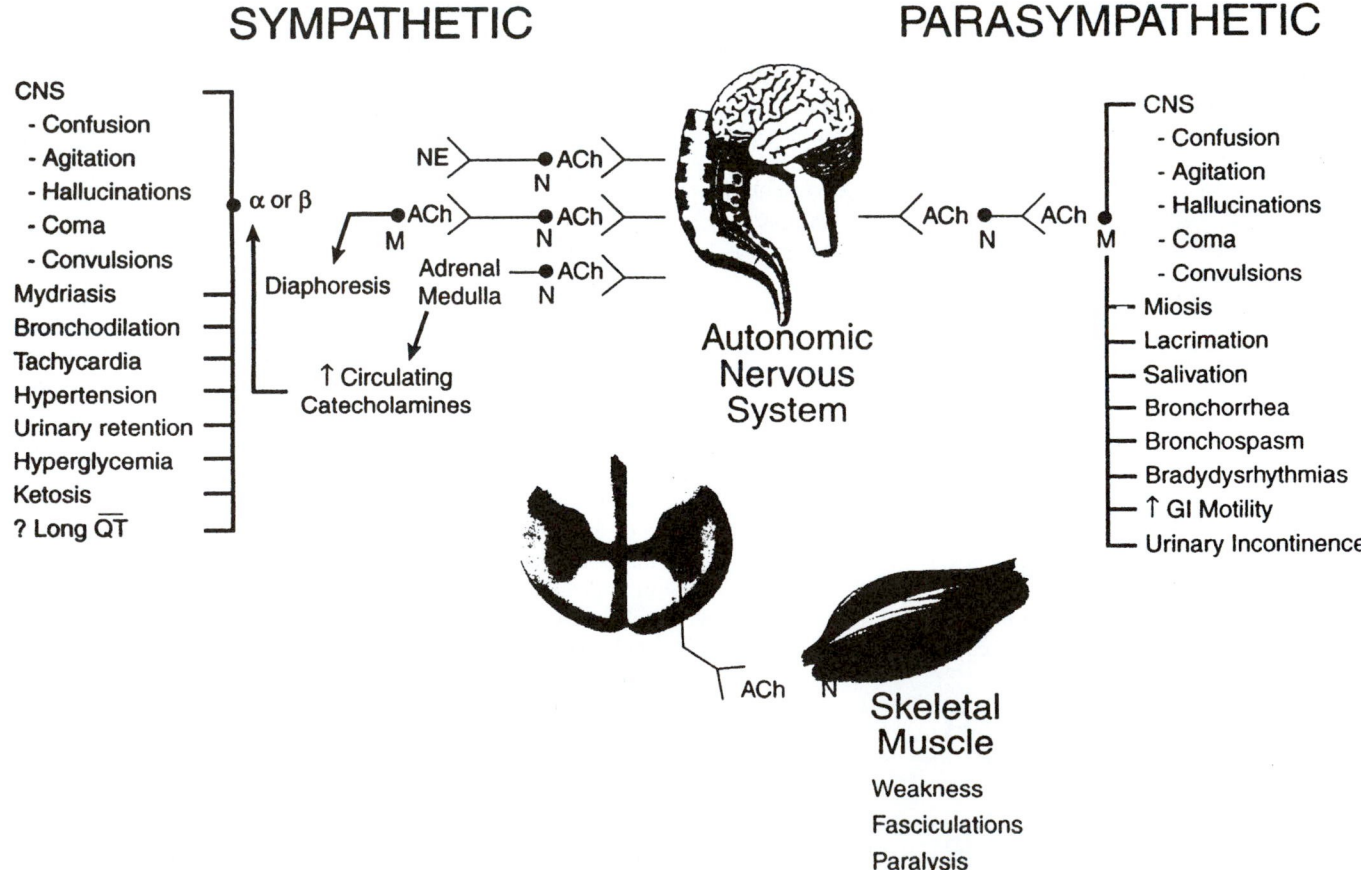

Figure 88–4. Pathophysiology of cholinergic syndrome as it affects the autonomic and somatic nervous systems.

on the agent and the circumstances of the exposure. For example, the more lipophilic compounds, such as dichlofenthion, can cause cholinergic effects for several days following oral ingestion.[18]

A variety of CNS findings are reported after organic phosphorus compound exposure. Many patients present awake and alert, complaining of anxiety, restlessness, insomnia, headache, dizziness, blurred vision, depression, tremors, or other nonspecific symptoms.[105] The victims' level of consciousness may deteriorate rapidly to confusion, lethargy, and coma, and they may display inappropriate behavior or convulsions.[105]

The effects of excessive ACh on the autonomic nervous system may be variable because cholinergic receptors are found in both the sympathetic and parasympathetic nervous systems (Fig. 88–4). Excessive muscarinic activity can be characterized by various mnemonics, including "SLUD" (salivation, lacrimation, urination, defecation) and "DUMBBELS" (defecation, urination, miosis, bronchospasm or bronchorrhea, emesis, lacrimation, salivation). Of these, miosis may be the most consistently encountered sign. Bronchorrhea can be so profuse that it mimics pulmonary edema.[105]

Although muscarinic findings are emphasized in these mnemonics, muscarinic signs usually do not overwhelmingly or initially predominate, except in very severe poisonings. In many cases, excessive autonomic activity from stimulation of nicotinic adrenal receptors (resulting in catecholamine release) and postganglionic sympathetic fibers offsets parasympathetic findings.[143] Mydriasis is reported in as many as 13% of cases, presumably from nicotinic stimulation of sympathetic receptors.[36] Bronchodilation and urinary retention can occur as a result of sympathetic activity on smooth muscle.[143] Excessive adrenergic influences on metabolism result in glycogenolysis with hyperglycemia and ketosis that is occasionally mistaken for diabetic ketoacidosis.[33,93] Hypoglycemia can also be seen, although the mechanism is unclear.[60] Increased sympathetic activity usually precipitates demargination, resulting in leukocytosis.[105] Hyperamylasemia is occasionally reported in cases of severe organic phosphorus pesticide poisoning, and although pancreatitis may result from spasm of the sphincter of Oddi,[31,89] this finding is most often the result of salivary gland stimulation and not the result of pancreatic dysfunction.[79] Elevations in hepatic enzymes can also occur following organic phosphorus pesticide exposures.[43,86,117]

The cardiovascular manifestations of organic phosphorus compound toxicity also reflect mixed effects on the autonomic nervous system.[85] Increased sympathetic tone is usually initially present, and most patients manifest a sinus tachycardia,[85,105] and sometimes hypertension. As toxicity becomes more severe, bradycardia with a prolonged PR interval and atrioventricular blocks of various degrees occur because of excessive parasympathetic tone, and possibly because of reduced coronary blood flow.[26,73,85,105,107] Unequal sympathetic stimulation of myocardial cells is likely responsible for the occasional prolonged QT interval.[85,102,126] This prolongation in QT interval can be associated with polymorphous ventricular tachycardia (torsades de pointes).[8,70,85,147]

Liquid preparations of organic phosphorus compounds are usually dissolved in a hydrocarbon. Pulmonary aspiration following ingestion is common in severe poisoning, and hydrocarbon pneumonitis may complicate the clinical course.

Acetylcholine stimulation of nicotinic receptors also governs skeletal muscle activity. Excessive cholinergic stimulation at these sites behaves like a depolarizing neuromuscular blocking agent (similar to succinylcholine) and initially results in fasciculations

or weakness. This effect is considered by some to be the most reliable signs of organic phosphorus pesticide toxicity.[106] As the severity of poisoning progresses, paralysis ensues. Paralysis of the respiratory muscles in combination with bronchorrhea, bronchoconstriction, and CNS depression lead to hypoxemia and respiratory arrest, the most common cause of death in poisoning with organic phosphorus chemicals.[105,142] Rarely, patients may present only with paralysis from nicotinic effects without other signs and symptoms suggestive of organic phosphorus agent toxicity.[38,46] Respiratory depression is in part centrally mediated.[105] Extrapyramidal effects such as rigidity and choreoathetosis occur uncommonly after severe anticholinesterase poisoning but can persist for several days after cholinergic features have resolved.[63]

Carbamates

Poisoning from carbamate insecticides appears identical to that of organic phosphorus compounds except for the two main factors listed above regarding the lack of CNS penetration and rapid hydrolyzation of the carbamate-AChE bond. However, CNS abnormalities may occur in victims of severe carbamate poisonings, some of which may result from hypoxia caused by respiratory insufficiency or severe bronchorrhea.

DIAGNOSTIC TESTING
Organic Phosphorus Compounds

When confronted with a patient in cholinergic crisis who presents with a history of acute excessive exposure to an anticholinesterase insecticide, the diagnosis is at times straightforward. However, when the history is unreliable or does not suggest cholinesterase inhibitor poisoning, the physician must turn to other means to confirm the diagnosis of organic phosphorus or carbamate insecticide poisoning.

The most reliable and appropriate laboratory test for confirming cholinesterase inhibition by insecticides measures specific insecticides and active metabolites in biologic tissues. Unfortunately, such tests or results are rarely obtainable within a few minutes or hours, and normal ranges or toxic levels are not established for most agents. If available, another useful test is the measurement of AChE activity in neuronal tissue, but this requires CNS or neuronal tissue biopsies and, even then, is not very useful unless the baseline activity is known. Thus, the diagnostic study of necessity for verifying anticholinesterase poisoning is the measurement of cholinesterase activity in readily accessible tissue, such as the plasma and erythrocytes.[43,105]

Butyrylcholinesterase is able to metabolize various exogenous compounds, including succinylcholine and cocaine. Erythrocytes contain a form of "true AChE," similar to the enzyme found in neuronal tissue, that is specific for ACh.[14] It should be remembered that inhibition of the red blood cell and butyrylcholinesterase serves as a marker for anticholinesterase poisoning, and inhibition of these enzymes does not directly contribute to signs and symptoms of insecticide poisoning.

After a significant exposure to an organic phosphorus or carbamate insecticide, butyrylcholinesterase activity usually falls first, followed rapidly by a decrease in red blood cell cholinesterase activity. The sequence may be highly variable, but by the time patients present with acute symptoms, both cholinesterase activities have usually fallen well below baseline values, and often have fallen below detectable limits.[105]

Butyrylcholinesterase activity usually recovers before that of the red blood cell, often returning to normal within a few days if there is no repeat exposure to the inciting agent.[16] However, butyrylcholinesterase activity is less specific for exposure to these insecticides than is red cell cholinesterase activity.[43] Low butyrylcholinesterase activity is frequently found in patients with a number of disorders, including hereditary deficiency of the enzyme, malnutrition, hepatic parenchymal disease, chronic debilitating illnesses, and iron deficiency anemia.[43] Drugs such as cocaine, succinylcholine, morphine, and codeine may cause butyrylcholinesterase activity to fluctuate, presumably by their effect on acetylcholine release from nerve terminals, but the mechanism is still unclear.[110] High butyrylcholinesterase activity occurs in some individuals with nephrotic syndrome because an inverse correlation exists between enzyme activity and the concentration of serum albumin.[43] Additionally, day-to-day variation in enzyme activity in healthy individuals may be as high as 20%.[43]

Red blood cell cholinesterase activity is thought to more accurately reflect nervous tissue AChE activity than butyrylcholinesterase because of the presence of true AChE in red blood cells. Some authors suggest that clinical organic phosphorus pesticide poisoning occurs when red blood cell cholinesterase activity falls 50% below baseline values.[98,105] While these statements are generally true, there are several potential pitfalls in interpreting cholinesterase laboratory values. First, it is AChE inhibition in nervous tissue that causes toxicity, and red blood cell and butyrylcholinesterase activity may not always reflect neuronal enzyme activity. Organic phosphorus insecticides vary in their ability to inhibit butyrylcholinesterase or red blood cell cholinesterase. This variation may lead to some patients presenting highly symptomatic after minimal reductions in red blood cell cholinesterase, while others can be asymptomatic after losing 50% activity.[16,55,97] The wide normal range of red blood cell and butyrylcholinesterase activity also allows for patients with high normal values to suffer significant falls in cholinesterase activity, yet still register "normal" levels of cholinesterase activity on laboratory assay.[16,55,97]

Red blood cell cholinesterase regenerates more slowly than AChE found in neurons.[105] To completely replenish the supply, red blood cells in circulation must be replaced, or pralidoxime administered. It is estimated that an average of 66 days may be necessary for red blood cell cholinesterase to stop declining following severe inhibition[16] (assuming no treatment with pralidoxime), and activity may take up to 120 days to return to normal. The patient may have completely recovered neuronal activity of AChE and resolved all cholinergic symptoms, yet still have low red blood cell cholinesterase laboratory values. For this reason, in subacute poisoning with organic phosphorus agents, it is difficult to accurately predict the time of onset or length of exposure from red blood cell cholinesterase activity alone. In fact, the ability of red blood cell cholinesterase activity to serve as a historical marker for excessive exposure to organic phosphorus insecticides provides the basis for monitoring red blood cell cholinesterase activity in pesticide workers.[17,27,77]

Depressed red blood cell cholinesterase activity can be noted for reasons other than insecticide poisoning, such as in antimalarial therapy and pernicious anemia. Genetic and circadian variations are also common, with daily fluctuations within the same individual as high as 10%.[156] In addition, levels are normally slightly lower in children younger than 4 months of age, probably

increasing as hepatic function matures.[68] Oral contraceptives raise red blood cell cholinesterase activity.

The most important aspect to consider when interpreting cholinesterase activity as reported by a laboratory is how it compares with baseline values in the individual (Table 88–2). Because baseline values are usually unavailable in most cases of acute and chronic cholinesterase inhibitor poisoning, laboratories report out a "reference range" of activity. This range is based on the central 95% of values of cholinesterase activity for the general population. Our laboratory uses standard reference range intervals of 18–29 U/g Hgb for red blood cell cholinesterase, and 5200–12,800 U/L for butyrylcholinesterase, but these ranges may vary significantly with different assays.

Blood samples for cholinesterase activity should be obtained in the appropriate blood tubes. Gray-top or other tubes containing fluoride will permanently inactivate the enzyme, yielding falsely low activity levels, and should not be used. Specimens for red blood cell cholinesterase are usually drawn into tubes containing a chelating anticoagulant such as ethylenediaminetetraacetic acid (EDTA) to prevent clot formation. Butyrylcholinesterase does not require an anticoagulant and can be drawn into a tube without chelators or anticoagulants. Because laboratory color coding systems for blood tubes vary, laboratory personnel should be contacted to determine the appropriate venipuncture container. If either test will not be immediately performed, tubes should be spun and frozen.

Carbamates

Carbamates inhibit neuronal and red blood cell AChE, as well as butyrylcholinesterase. The relative ease with which spontaneous decarbamylation of cholinesterase takes place may result in the measurement of relatively normal red cell cholinesterase activity despite severe cholinergic symptoms if the assay is not performed

TABLE 88–2. Interpreting Cholinesterase Values

	Red Blood Cell Cholinesterase	Butyrylcholinesterase
Advantage	Better reflection of synaptic inhibition	Easier to assay, declines faster
Site	RBC (reflects CNS gray matter, motor end plate)	CNS white matter, plasma, liver, pancreas, heart
Regeneration (untreated)	1%/day	25–30% in first 7–10 days
Normalization (untreated)	35–49 days	28–42 days
Use	Unsuspected prior exposure with elevated plasma cholinesterase	Acute exposure
False depression	Pernicious anemia, hemoglobinopathies, antimalarial treatment, oxalate blood tubes	Liver dysfunction (cirrhosis), malnutrition, hypersensitivity reactions, drugs (succinylcholine, codeine, morphine), pregnancy, genetic deficiency

within several hours of sampling.[34] Just as in organic phosphorus pesticide poisoning, the wide "normal" range of cholinesterase values may make interpretation of cholinesterase activity difficult at times without knowing the patient's baseline values. Unlike organic phosphorus agents, carbamates generally do not produce persistent depressed red blood cell and butyrylcholinesterase activities.

Atropine Challenge

An atropine sulfate challenge may be helpful in diagnosing cholinergic poisoning in a patient who presents with findings suggestive of this disorder, but in whom no history is available to suggest excessive exposure to an organic phosphorus or carbamate insecticide. A test dose of 1–5 mg of atropine in adolescents or adults, or 0.05 mg/kg in children up to an adult dose, should produce classic antimuscarinic findings such as mydriasis, tachycardia, and dry mucous membranes. The persistence of cholinergic signs and symptoms after an atropine challenge strongly suggests the presence of organic phosphorus compound or carbamate poisoning.[72,105] However, some patients suffering from mild to moderate anticholinesterase poisoning may respond to these doses of atropine. Therefore, the reversal of cholinergic findings does not exclude poisoning by one of these agents.

Electromyogram (EMG) Studies

Although measuring cholinesterase levels is most often used to estimate tissue and neuronal AChE activity, studies support the use of repetitive nerve stimulation testing as an accurate method of quantifying AChE inhibition at the neuromuscular junction.[5,6,19] Spontaneous repetitive potentials or fasciculations following single-nerve stimulation resulting from persistent ACh at nerve terminals can be a sensitive indicator of AChE inhibition at the motor endplate, and may be useful in the early diagnosis of anticholinesterase poisoning.[6] This type of evaluation may also be of benefit in early detection of rebound cholinergic crisis caused by continued insecticide absorption or redistribution from adipose, or onset of an intermediate syndrome (see below).[5,19]

Differential Diagnosis

The differential diagnosis for cholinergic poisoning is divided into three main categories (Table 88–3). The first group comprises other noninsecticidal anticholinesterase agents. In addition to organic phosphorus and carbamate insecticides, this includes the medicinal anticholinesterases neostigmine, pyridostigmine, physostigmine, and echothiophate iodide. The most common population to suffer cholinergic poisoning syndrome from medicinal anticholinesterases is patients with myasthenia gravis who are administered excessive pyridostigmine. This group of medicinals and toxins should all produce low butyrylcholinesterase or red blood cell AChE activity. Some of these agents, like neostigmine, will not cross the blood-brain barrier and would only cause peripheral symptoms in overdose. Newer agents used to treat Alzheimer disease, such as tacrine, are also organic phosphorous compounds, but symptomatic overdose of these agents has not yet been reported.

The next category of compounds producing a cholinergic poisoning syndrome contains agents with cholinomimetic activity. These compounds directly stimulate muscarinic or nicotinic cholinergic receptors, but do not inhibit AChE. In this case, bu-

TABLE 88–3.   Categories of Cholinergic Poisoning

Anticholinesterase agents
  Organic phosphorus insecticides
  Organic phosphorus ophthlamic preparations
  Carbamate insecticides
  Carbamate medicinal preparations

Cholinomimetics
  Pilocarpine
  Carbachol
  Aceclidine
  Methacholine
  Bethanechol
  Muscarine-containing mushrooms

Nicotine alkaloids
  Coniine
  Lobeline
  Nicotine

tyrylcholinesterase and red blood cell cholinesterase activity should be normal. Cholinomimetic medicinal agents include preparations of carbachol, aceclidine, methacholine, pilocarpine, and bethanechol. Muscarine-containing mushrooms can be cholinomimetic, and some patients ingesting them can present with salivation, diaphoresis, and vomiting (Chap. 76). Finally, poisonings from nicotine alkaloids (eg, nicotine, lobeline, and coniine) cause CNS, autonomic, and skeletal muscle symptoms similar to those occurring in organic phosphorus and carbamate toxicity (Chap. 73).

MANAGEMENT

Organic Phosphorus Compounds

The earliest cause of death from organic phosphorus or carbamate poisoning is from respiratory failure and hypoxemia as a consequence of coma and convulsions, nicotinic effects on skeletal muscles, such as weakness and paralysis, and excessive muscarinic effects on the cardiovascular and pulmonary system causing bronchospasm, bronchorrhea, aspiration, bradydysrhythmias, and hypotension. Initial treatment is directed at ensuring an adequate airway and ventilation, and at reversing excessive muscarinic effects. Convulsions not secondary to hypoxemia are treated with standard anticonvulsants (benzodiazepines, barbiturates).

Maintenance of the patient's airway is best assured by early endotracheal intubation and positive pressure ventilation in comatose victims, in those patients with significant weakness, or in those patients unable to handle copious secretions that may accompany the poisoning. Only a nondepolarizing neuromuscular blocking agent should be used to induce pharmacologic paralysis. The metabolism of the depolarizing agent succinylcholine will be extended in the presence of low butyrylcholinesterase activity, resulting in paralysis that can be prolonged up to 24 hours or more.[128]

The second priority in management is to control excessive muscarinic activity. Atropine sulfate competitively antagonizes ACh at muscarinic receptors to reverse excessive secretions, miosis, bronchospasm, vomiting, diarrhea, diaphoresis, and urinary incontinence.[65,105] Intravenous doses should begin at 1–5 mg in adolescents and adults, and at 0.05 mg/kg in children up to adult doses, and should be repeated every 2–3 minutes until atropinization occurs.[43,105,158] Atropinization is present when the patient exhibits dry skin and mucous membranes, decreased or absent bowel sounds, tachycardia, reduced secretions, no bronchospasm (in absence of other causes such as aspiration), and, usually, mydriasis. An improvement in pulmonary secretions should be the target in atropine therapy and can be guided by following lung sounds and oxygenation. Tachycardia is not a contraindication to atropine therapy. Although the pupils are often helpful in gauging the need for atropine, the miosis encountered in severe ingestions and by direct ocular exposure to organic phosphorus agents may respond only to topical ophthalmic atropine.[123] Isolated pulmonary manifestations may respond to administration of nebulized atropine or ipratropium, and this treatment can accompany parenteral administration of these agents.

Large doses of atropine may be needed to reverse the bronchospasm, bronchorrhea, bradycardia, and heart block associated with severe organic phosphorus pesticide toxicity.[43,50,87,106] Some patients with mild symptoms need only 1 or 2 mg of atropine for reversal of cholinergic toxicity, but the moderately poisoned adolescent or adult commonly requires doses as large as 40 mg.[32,63] Severe poisonings may necessitate even higher doses. In severely ill adults, 5-mg boluses of atropine repeated every 2–3 minutes for stabilization may be used. Adults have received over 1000 mg of atropine in 24 hours (with pralidoxime) without producing antimuscarinic effects,[32,148] and total doses as large as 11,000 mg during the course of treatment have been reported.[59] Children have been managed with continuous infusions of atropine starting at 0.025 mg/kg/h,[7,78] and continuous infusions have been used for as long as 32 days in severely poisoned patients.[44] Adult infusions of atropine can begin at 0.5–1 mg/h and should be titrated as needed.

Atropine is not effective for reversing excessive nicotinic effects. Therefore, the patient who improves after receiving atropine must still be closely monitored in an intensive care setting for impending respiratory failure.

When antimuscarinic CNS toxicity becomes evident, yet peripheral cholinergic findings necessitate the administration of more atropine (eg, bradycardia, bronchorrhea, vomiting), glycopyrrolate bromide can be substituted for atropine because its quaternary ammonium structure limits CNS penetration. The intravenous dose of glycopyrrolate is 1–2 mg, repeated as needed in adolescents and adults, or 0.025 mg/kg in children up to adult doses. Although scopolamine has also been used in place of atropine, it may cause more pronounced CNS effects. A urinary catheter should be inserted in all atropinized patients to prevent urinary retention.

Pralidoxime

Although phosphorylated AChE undergoes hydrolytic regeneration at a very slow rate, this process can be markedly enhanced by using an oxime such as pralidoxime chloride (2-PAM) (Fig. 88–5).[151] In addition to rejuvenating AChE, pralidoxime may also reverse organic phosphorus compound toxicity by directly inactivating free organic phosphorus molecules and by exhibiting an apparent antimuscarinic effect on nervous tissue.[43,71] Regeneration of AChE lowers ACh concentrations to normal levels, reversing both muscarinic and nicotinic effects. An immediate rise in red blood cell cholinesterase activity, presumably paralleling a rise in neuronal AChE activity, is often noted after the administration of pralidoxime. Unfortunately, pralidoxime is unable to rejuvenate

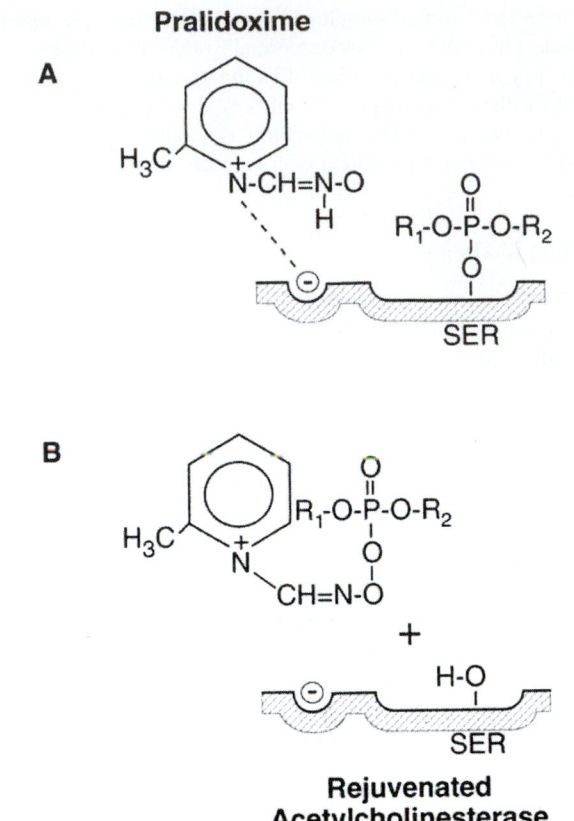

Figure 88–5. Mechanism of rejuvenation of acetylcholinesterase by pralidoxime. The positively charged aromatic nitrogen of pralidoxime is "attracted" to the anionic site of acetylcholinesterase, allowing the reactive oxime portion of the molecule to position itself over the phosphorylated active site of the enzyme. Pralidoxime then becomes phosphorylated, rejuvenating acetylcholinesterase.

active enzyme from the organic phosphorus compound–AChE complex that has undergone aging.[32,54] Therefore, pralidoxime therapy is most effective if started early in the course of toxicity.[30,127]

It is presumed that most phosphorylated AChE will be aged within 24–48 hours of exposure.[43,143] The actual rate of aging, however, varies significantly among organic phosphorus agents. In addition, circulating organic phosphorus pesticide concentrations have been measured for as long as 48 days after exposure,[18,44] either because of prolonged absorption from the GI tract or, more likely, because of redistribution from fat stores.[7,32,43,44,105] Therefore, some AChE may still be undergoing new inhibition for days or weeks after ingestion in symptomatic patients, and such inhibition may be reversible by pralidoxime.[149] Case reports support this by noting dramatic effects in reversing paralysis, weakness, and cholinergic symptoms after late administration of pralidoxime.[19–21,23,94,105,109]

The initial dose of pralidoxime in adolescents and adults is 1–2 g intravenously over 10–15 minutes (30–50 mg/kg IV over 10–15 minutes in children up to adult doses).[65] Minimal plasma concentrations of 4 μg/mL are estimated to be necessary for maintenance of enzyme reactivation.[140] Bolus dosing of pralidoxime every 4–8 hours is ineffective in maintaining these levels,[92] and a constant infusion appears to be more appropriate. Present recommendations in adults are to begin the infusion at 250–500 mg/h, titrating to symptoms.[65] Alternative dosing by weight in other studies suggests 4–5 mg/kg as a loading dose over 15–30 minutes, followed by a continuous infusion of 2–4 mg/kg/h to maintain serum concentrations.[92,150] Pharmacokinetics of pralidoxime in children are extremely variable and different from adults.[125] Reports suggest that loading doses in children should be 25–50 mg/kg of pralidoxime intravenously over 15–30 minutes (not to exceed adult doses, unless clinically indicated), followed by a continuous infusion of 10–20 mg/kg/h. This regimen is efficacious in treating symptoms associated with organic phosphorus pesticide poisoning and does not result in pralidoxime-associated toxicity.[37,125]

Side effects of pralidoxime are usually minimal at normal doses.[47,108] Severely poisoned patients have received 0.5 g/h for weeks without adverse effects.[44,105] Rapid infusion can cause mild cholinergic effects because of transient blockade of AChE[105] and has resulted in neuromuscular blockade and central respiratory depression.[65,143]

Some effects of pralidoxime are not well understood. Unlike atropine, the quaternary ammonium compound structure of pralidoxime should prevent it from crossing the blood-brain barrier.[105] But case reports of organic phosphorus compound toxicity describe pralidoxime-induced reversal of convulsions and improvements in mental status and electroencephalograms not attributable to improved ventilation or perfusion.[35,41,52,53,67,83,84,110]

Pralidoxime is not equally effective in reversing cholinergic symptoms in all types of organic phosphorus compound poisonings.[65,105] It is particularly efficacious in reversing toxicity from parathion, diazinon, methyl parathion, EPN, TEPP, dimethoate, and dichlorvos.[43] Dimethoxy compounds, such as malathion and methyl demeton, can be more resistant to reversal.[43]

Diazepam may improve survival in victims of severe organic phosphorus pesticide poisoning. Animal studies demonstrate that administering diazepam with oximes in the treatment of organic phosphorus nerve gases (sarin, soman, tabun, VX) can increase survival and decrease the incidence of seizures and neuropathy.[71,72,76,84,103,122] Diazepam can also decrease cerebral morphologic damage resulting from organic phosphorus compound–related convulsions.[91,136]

Decontamination

Rapid cutaneous absorption of organic phosphorus pesticides and carbamates necessitates removal of all clothing. Medical personnel should avoid self-contamination by wearing neoprene or nitrile gloves. Double-gloving with standard vinyl gloves may be protective for short intervals. Skin should be triple-washed with water, soap, and water, and rinsed again with water. Although alcohol-based soaps are sometimes recommended to dissolve hydrocarbons,[40] these products can be difficult to find, and expeditious skin cleansing should be the primary goal. Cutaneous absorption can also occur as a result of contact with vomitus and diarrhea if the initial exposure was through ingestion. Oily insecticides may be difficult to remove from thick or long hair, even with repeated shampooing, and shaving scalp hair may be necessary.

In acute ingestions, if emesis has not occurred, evacuation of stomach contents is recommended. Because the onset of coma, seizures, and paralysis can be rapid, lavage is the only option if gastric emptying is desired, and induced emesis should be avoided. Although there are data suggesting that activated char-

coal may adsorb some organic phosphorus insecticides, there are no studies evaluating whether repeat administration of activated charcoal changes the outcome or clinical course of patients with organic phosphorus pesticide poisoning. Thus, it is recommended that patients with anticholinesterase poisoning receive a single dose of 1 g/kg activated charcoal because ileus may develop during atropine therapy.

Disposition

Even after atropinization, patients with anticholinesterase poisoning should be continuously observed for evidence of deteriorating neurologic function and the potential for paralysis. It is common for patients to develop confusion and agitation following large doses of atropine as a consequence of the central antimuscarinic effects.

Red blood cell and butyrylcholinesterase activities should be measured intermittently after the institution of pralidoxime therapy.[64,76,135,149,154] Butyrylcholinesterase may not normalize with pralidoxime therapy because this enzyme does not contain an anionic site to attract the compound. Red blood cell cholinesterase activity may be markedly depressed long after neuronal AChE levels have returned to normal. Therefore, it is not unusual to send a patient home with subnormal cholinesterase activity as long as the individual remains asymptomatic. A significant fall in cholinesterase activity may reflect redistribution of insecticide from fat stores or prolonged absorption and may be accompanied by the redevelopment of cholinergic symptoms 3 or 4 days after initial resolution of symptoms.[32,43,94] Further deterioration of cholinesterase activity should be treated by reinstituting a pralidoxime infusion, even though the patient may still be asymptomatic. After another 24 hours of pralidoxime, assuming the patient is still asymptomatic, pralidoxime can be halted again, and red blood cell and butyrylcholinesterase activities monitored. When available, electromyographic studies detecting signs of motor endplate dysfunction and early AChE inhibition may be a more sensitive method for identifying recurrent cholinergic toxicity.[6]

When a patient becomes asymptomatic and has not needed pralidoxime and atropine for 1–2 days, and the cholinesterase activity is documented to be stable (independent of AChE activity), the patient may be discharged. It is important that the patient not wear clothing home that was worn when the poisoning occurred.

Carbamates

The treatment of patients with carbamate poisoning is identical to that of organic phosphorus compound poisoning with two exceptions. First, it has been suggested to avoid pralidoxime in monomethylcarbamate exposure because animal data imply that pralidoxime may increase AChE inactivation in carbaryl poisoning.[43,75,81] However, other studies and subsequent anecdotal experience have found that pralidoxime is useful in treating intoxications with the less common dimethylcarbamates such as isolan,[43] and may not adversely impact monomethylcarbamate poisoning in humans. Comparative human data investigating the use of pralidoxime in carbamate poisonings are lacking. Fortunately, because of the rapid hydrolysis of the carbamate-AChE complex, symptoms, including weakness and paralysis, usually resolve within 24–48 hours without pralidoxime therapy. Administering pralidoxime to a poisoned patient in a cholinergic crisis is appropriate if it is unknown whether the patient is suffering from organic phosphorus or carbamate pesticide poisoning. If the poisoning is from a carbamate pesticide, pralidoxime therapy may not be necessary, but should not prove detrimental.

Second, significant inhibition of red blood cell and butyrylcholinesterase by carbamates generally does not last for more than 1–2 days, assuming absorption is complete. Patients usually have normal red blood cell and butyrylcholinesterase values by the time of discharge. There are no reported cases of recurrent or delayed poisonings following carbamate insecticide intoxication. Therefore, repeating cholinesterase tests after patients are asymptomatic is usually unnecessary.

Chronic Toxicity

Illness may also result from chronic exposure to excessive amounts of organic phosphorus insecticides. Chronic organic phosphorus compound poisoning is most common in workers regularly coming in contact with these substances, but it may also occur in individuals who have repeated exposures to excessive amounts of organic phosphorus insecticides in their living environments. Cholinergic ophthalmic preparations can lead to toxicity in this manner.[88] Although tolerance to all systemic effects (including death in rats) of these compounds may be observed with long-term exposures,[43] persons undergoing such contact may become symptomatic after variable lengths of time. Symptoms can range from vague neurologic complaints, such as weakness and blurred vision, to miosis, nausea, vomiting, diarrhea, diaphoresis, and other cholinergic effects.[88,96,119] Red blood cell cholinesterase activity is the most sensitive measure of chronic poisoning.[43,56]

Delayed Syndromes

Intermediate Syndrome. Delayed muscle weakness without fasciculations or cholinergic features can be noted in patients 24–96 hours after acute organic phosphorus compound poisoning.[51,65,111,115,121,131] This phenomenon was first described in 1987, and is termed the "intermediate syndrome" (IMS).[131] The majority of reported cases of IMS presented initially with cholinergic signs and symptoms that improved with atropine and oxime therapy over the first day or two after the exposure. Relapse with peripheral neurologic impairment caused by IMS is usually recorded around 48 hours after presentation. IMS is seen most often in patients poisoned with parathion, methylparathion, diazinon, malathion, fenthion, monocrotophos, dimethoate, and methamidophos.[51,131] A redistribution of the lipophilic pesticide from adipose tissue is suggested as an etiology,[19,21–25,42,80,133] but there are no data suggesting that the syndrome is caused by anticholinesterase activity. There is growing speculation that IMS may result from inadequate oxime therapy,[19–21] although recent case reports question this theory.[138]

The most frequently encountered clinical findings of IMS include weakness, cranial nerve palsies, and areflexia. Fasciculations are seen in some cases. Level of consciousness is rarely affected. The muscle weakness in these patients can progress to respiratory distress and paralysis.[51,115,121,131] The most commonly affected muscles are the facial, extraocular, palatal, respiratory, and those of the proximal limbs.[51,121,131]

Clinical examination remains the most reliable means of predicting the occurrence of IMS.[21] Electromyograms will often show tetanic fade in these patients, and suggest both pre- and postsynaptic involvement.[65] However, repetitive nerve stimulation may not always accurately predict the occurrence or severity of IMS.[21]

The treatment of IMS is largely supportive with airway protection and ventilatory assistance. There are no substantial data demonstrating that pralidoxime or atropine is effective in the treatment of this disorder, although patients may be on these medications for control of cholinergic symptoms. The weakness and paralysis commonly resolve in 5–18 days.[51,65,131]

Encephalopathy and Peripheral Neuropathies. Peripheral neuropathies can occur after chronic organic phosphorus pesticide exposures and several days or weeks after acute exposures. This disorder appears to result from inhibition of an enzyme within nervous tissue named neurotoxic esterase or neuropathy target esterase (NTE).[61,65,111] Symptoms appear to be initiated by the phosphorylation of this enzyme, or perhaps of some related compound, followed by aging of the complex.[157] Such neuropathies may even result from exposure to organic phosphorus compounds that do not inhibit red blood cell cholinesterase or produce clinical cholinergic toxicity.[11] Some of the more commonly implicated chemicals include triaryl phosphates, such as triorthocresyl phosphate (TOCP), and dialkyl phosphates, such as merphos, mipafox, and chlorpyrifos.[62,105] Pathologic findings in anticholinesterase neuropathy demonstrate effects primarily on large distal neurons, with axonal degeneration preceding demyelination.[104]

Contaminated foods and beverages can be responsible for epidemics of organic phosphorus compound–induced delayed polyneuropathies and encephalopathy. In the 1930s, thousands of individuals in the United States became weak or paralyzed after drinking rum containing triorthocresyl phosphate, an outbreak nicknamed "Jamaican ginger paralysis."[3,95,100,101] Contaminated cooking and mineral oils were connected with outbreaks of delayed polyneuropathies in Vietnam and Sri Lanka.[28,129,130] Vague distal muscle weakness and pain are often the presenting symptoms, but weakness may progress to paralysis.[38,49] The onset and clinical course of these symptoms do not seem to be altered by the administration of atropine or pralidoxime.[38,105,146] Pyramidal tract signs may appear weeks to months after exposure.[65,146] Electromyograms and nerve conduction studies may be helpful in diagnosing this disorder and differentiating it from similar presentations such as Guillain-Barré syndrome.[1,133] Recovery in these patients is variable over months to years, with residual deficits common.[4,101,132]

Delayed neuropathies are not usually associated with carbamate insecticides. One reason for this difference is presumed to be that aging of the complex is a requirement for neuron degeneration. Ironically, studies suggest that subgroups of carbamates may actually bind NTE and exert a protective effect against more toxic organic phosphorus compounds.[2] However, several cases of possible delayed neuropathy associated with carbamates have been reported.[29,145,157] These cases involve ingestions of carbaryl, m-tolyl methylcarbamate, and carbofuran, include both sensory and motor tracts, and tend to resolve over 3–9 months. EMG findings in these subjects are variable.

Behavioral Toxicity

Behavioral changes may also occur after acute and chronic exposure to organic phosphorus compounds.[65] Symptoms include confusion, psychosis, anxiety, drowsiness, depression, fatigue, and irritability.[43,94,128,141] Changes may be noted on the electroencephalogram of these patients and can last for weeks.[43,48,56] Single photon emission computed tomography (SPECT) scanning revealed morphologic changes in the basal ganglia of one child following anticholinesterase poisoning.[7] Even though no specific treatment is effective, most psychological abnormalities resolve within a year.[45] Behavioral toxicity following carbamate exposure is extremely rare.

SUMMARY

Anticholinesterase compounds are increasingly popular as pesticides. As the use of these agents expands, instances of both acute and chronic exposure are likely to become more common. The clinical presentation of toxicity from these compounds relates to their ability to stimulate the parasympathetic, and, to a lesser extent, the sympathetic branches of the autonomic nervous system. The early clinical findings in anticholinesterase poisoning may be mixed, with signs and symptoms that can include weakness, fasciculations, tachycardia, hypertension, vomiting, diaphoresis, diarrhea, salivation, small (or less often large) pupils, and either micturition or urinary retention. As acetylcholine concentrations continue to rise, the clinical course usually changes to mainly reflect muscarinic, skeletal muscle, and CNS abnormalities, with bradycardia, heart block, hypotension, bronchorrhea, bronchospasm, salivation, diaphoresis, lacrimation, vomiting, diarrhea, urinary incontinence, miosis, fasciculations and paralysis, hyperglycemia, and ketosis. Secretions may become copious from every orifice and hinder resuscitation efforts. With supportive care, some patients with anticholinesterase poisoning improve rapidly with signs and symptoms resolving within 2 or 3 days. In other cases, redistribution and absorption of these chemicals may continue for days, leading to prolonged or recurrent cholinergic symptoms and lengthy hospitalizations. Although measuring cholinesterase activity can be helpful when the diagnosis of anticholinesterase poisoning is not clear, most laboratories are unable to rapidly produce results of these tests. Expeditious recognition of cholinergic syndrome and appropriate therapy with atropine to control muscarinic activity and an oxime to regenerate acetylcholinesterase (in the case of organic phosphorus pesticides) can be coupled with supportive care to improve clinical outcome.

REFERENCES

1. Abou-Donia MB, Lapadula DM: Mechanisms of organophosphorus ester-induced delayed neurotoxicity: Type I and type II. Annu Rev Pharmacol Toxicol 1990;30:405–440.
2. Ahmed MM, Glees P: Neurotoxicity of tricresylphosphate (TCP) in slow loris (nycticebus coucang). Acta Neuropathol (Berl) 1971;19:94–98.
3. Aring CD: The systemic nervous affinity of triorthocresyl phosphate (Jamaica ginger palsy). Brain 1942;65:34–47.
4. Barrett DS, Oehme FW: A review of organophosphorus ester-induced delayed neurotoxicity. Vet Hum Toxicol 1985;27:22–37.
5. Benson BJ, Tolo D, McIntire M: Is the intermediate syndrome in organophosphate poisoning the result of insufficient oxime therapy? J Toxicol Clin Toxicol 1992;30:347–349.
6. Besser R, Gutmann L, Dillmann U, et al: End-plate dysfunction in acute organophosphate intoxication. Neurology 1989;39:561–567.
7. Borowitz SM: Prolonged organophosphate toxicity in a twenty-six-month-old child. J Pediatr 1988;112:302–304.
8. Brill DM, Maisel AS, Prabhu R: Polymorphic ventricular tachycardia and other complex arrhythmias in organophosphate insecticide poisoning. J Electrocardiol 1984;17:97–102.
9. Brown JH, Taylor J: Muscarinic receptor agonists and antagonists. In: Hardman JG, Limbird LE, Molinoff PB, et al, eds: Goodman & Gilman's The Pharmacological Basis of Therapeutics, 9th ed. New York, McGraw-Hill, 1996, pp. 141–160.
10. Casper HH, Pekas JC: Absorption and excretion of radiolabeled 1-naphthyl-N-methylcarbamate (carbaryl) by the rat. N Y Acad Sci 1971;24:160–166.
11. Cavanagh JB, Davies DR, Holland P, Lancaster M: Comparison of the functional effects of dyflos, tri-o-cresyl phosphate and tri-p-ethylphenyl phosphate in chickens. Brit J Pharmacol 1961;17:21–27.
12. Chadwick JA, Oosterbaan RA: Actions on insects and other invertebrates. In: Koelle GB, ed: Cholinesterases and Anticholinesterase Agents. Handbook Experimental Pharmak, Vol. 15. Berlin, Springer-Verlag, 1963, pp. 299–373.
13. Chaudhry R, Lall SB, Baijayantimal M, Dhawan B: A foodborne outbreak of organophosphate poisoning. BMJ 1998;17:268–269.
14. Clay C, Stewart GO: Two unusual presentations of organophosphate poisoning. Anaesth Intensive Care 1982;10:279–280.
15. Clifford NJ, Nies AS: Organophosphate poisoning from wearing a laundered uniform previously contaminated with parathion. JAMA 1989;262:3035–3036.
16. Coye MJ, Barnett PG, Midtling JE, et al: Clinical confirmation of organophosphate poisoning by serial cholinesterase analyses. Arch Intern Med 1987;147:438–442.
17. Coye MJ, Barnett PG, Midtling JE, et al: Clinical confirmation of organophosphate poisoning of agricultural workers. Am J Ind Med 1986;10:399–409.
18. Davies JE, Barquet A, Freed VH, et al: Human pesticide poisonings by a fat-soluble organophosphate insecticide. Arch Environ Health 1975;30:608–613.
19. DeBleecker JL: The intermediate syndrome in organophosphate poisoning: An overview of experimental and clinical observation. J Toxicol Clin Toxicol 1995;33:683–686.
20. DeBleecker JL: Intermediate syndrome: Prolonged cholinesterase inhibition. J Toxicol Clin Toxicol 1993;31:197–199.
21. DeBleecker J, Van Den Neucker K, Colardyn F: Intermediate syndrome in organophosphorus poisoning: A prospective study. Crit Care Med 1993;21:1706–1711.
22. DeBleeker JL: Multiple system organ failure: Link to intermediate syndrome indirect. J Toxicol Clin Toxicol 1996;34:249–250.
23. DeBleecker J, Van Den Neucker K, Willems J: The intermediate syndrome in organophosphate poisoning: Presentation of a case and review of the literature. J Toxicol Clin Toxicol 1992;30:321–329.
24. DeBleecker J, Vogelaers D, Ceuterick C, et al: Intermediate syndrome due to prolonged parathion poisoning. Acta Neurol Scand 1992;86:421–424.
25. DeBleecker J, Willems J, Van Den Neucker K, et al: Prolonged toxicity with intermediate syndrome after combined parathion and methyl parathion poisoning. J Toxicol Clin Toxicol 1992;30:333–345.
26. Dekker M: Organophosphate insecticide poisoning. Clin Toxicol 1979;15:189–191.
27. Dellinger JA: Monitoring the chronic effects of anticholinesterase pesticides in aerial applicators. Vet Hum Toxicol 1985;27:427–430.
28. Dennis DT: Jake Walk in Vietnam. Ann Intern Med 1977;86:665–666.
29. Dickoff DJ, Gerber O, Turovsky Z: Delayed neurotoxicity after ingestion of carbamate pesticide. Neurology 1987;37:1229–1231.
30. DiKart WL, Kiestra SH, Sangster B: The use of atropine and oximes in organophosphate intoxication: A modified approach. J Toxicol Clin Toxicol 1988;26:199–208.
31. Dressel TD, Goodale RL, Arneson MA, Borner JW: Pancreatitis as a complication of anticholinesterase insecticide intoxication. Ann Surg 1979;189:199–204.
32. Du Toit PW, Muller FO, Van Tonder WM, Ungerer MJ: Experience with intensive care management of organophosphate insecticide poisoning. S Afr Med J 1981;60:227–229.

33. Durrant W: Massive glycosurea and ketonuria in organophosphorous poisoning. Centr Afr J Med 1978;24:253.

34. Ecobichon DJ, Joy RM: Pesticides and Neurological Diseases. Boca Raton, FL, CRC Press, 1982.

35. Erdmann WD, Sakai F, Scheler F: Erfarungen bei der spezifischen Behandlung einer E605-Vergiftungen mit Atropine und dem Esteraseaktivator PAM. Dtsch Med Wochenschr 1958;83:1359.

36. Etzel RA, Forthal DN, Hill RH, Demby A: Fatal parathion poisoning in Sierra Leone. Bull WHO 1987;65:645–649.

37. Farrar HC, Wells TG, Kearns GL: Use of continuous infusion of pralidoxime for treatment of organophosphate poisoning in children. J Pediatr 1990;116:658–661.

38. Fisher JR: Guillain-Barré syndrome following organophosphate poisoning. JAMA 1977;238:1950–1951.

39. Fredricksson T, Bigelow JK: Tissue distribution of P32-labeled parathion. Arch Environ Health 1961;2:663–667.

40. Fredricksson T: Percutaneous absorption of parathion and paraoxon, IV: decontamination of human skin from parathion. Arch Environ Health 1961;3:185–188.

41. Funckes AJ: Treatment of severe parathion poisoning with pyridine aldoxime methiodide (2-PAM). Arch Environ Health 1960;1: 404–406.

42. Gadoth N, Fisher A: Late onset of neuromuscular block in organophosphorus poisoning. Ann Intern Med 1978;88:654–655.

43. Gallo MA, Lawryk NJ: Organic phosphorus pesticides. In: Hayes WJ, Laws ER, eds: Handbook of Pesticide Toxicology. San Diego, Academic Press, 1991, pp. 917–1090.

44. Gerkin R, Curry S: Persistently elevated plasma insecticide levels in severe methylparathion poisoning [abstract]. Vet Hum Toxicol 1987; 29:483–484.

45. Gershon S, Shaw FH: Psychiatric sequelae of chronic exposure to organophosphate insecticides. Lancet 1961;1:1371–1374.

46. Goldman H, Teitel M: Malathion poisoning in a 34-month-old child following accidental ingestion. J Pediatr 1958;52:76–78.

47. Grob D, Johns RJ: Use of oximes in the treatment of intoxication by anticholinesterase compounds in normal subjects. Am J Med 1958; 24:497–511.

48. Grob D, Harvey AM, Langworthy OR, Lilienthal JL: The administration of diisopropyl fluorophosphate (DFP) to man. Effect on the central nervous system with special reference to the electrical activity of the brain. Bull Johns Hopkins Hosp 1947;81:257.

49. Gross D: Clinical aspects: Diagnosis and symptomatology. In: Albertini AV, Gross D, Zinn WM, eds: Triaryl-Phosphate Poisoning in Morocco 1959. Stuttgart, George Thieme, 1968, pp. 53–81.

50. Hayes MM, Van Der Westhuizen NG, Gelfan M: Organophosphate poisoning in Rhodesia. S Afr Med J 1978;54:230–234.

51. He F, Xu H, Qin F, Xu L, et al: Intermediate myasthenia syndrome following acute organophosphate poisoning—An analysis of 21 cases. Hum Exp Toxicol 1998;17:40–45.

52. Hiraki K, Namba T, Yamada M, et al: Progress in the management of parathion poisoning: Introduction of cholinesterase reactivator, PAM. Nippon Iji Shimpo 1956;1702:10–14.

53. Hiraki K, Namba Y, Taniguchi Y, Okazaki S: Effect of 2-pyridine aldoxime methiodide (PAM) against parathion (Folidol) poisoning: Analysis of 39 cases. Naika Ryoiki 1958;6:84–97.

54. Hobbiger F: Protection against the lethal effects of organophosphates by pyridine-2-aldoxime methiodide. Br J Pharmacol 1957;12: 438–446.

55. Hodgson M, Parkinson D: Diagnosis of organophosphate poisoning [letter]. N Engl J Med 1985;313:329.

56. Holmes JH: Organophosphorus insecticides in Colorado. Arch Environ Health 1964;9:445–453.

57. Holmstedt B: Structure-activity relationship of the organophosphorus anticholinesterase agents. In: Koelle GB, ed: Handbuch der Experimentellen Pharmakologie. Berlin, Springer-Verlag, 1963, pp. 428–485.

58. Holmstedt B: The ordeal bean of Old Calabar: the pageant of *Physostigmata venenosum* in medicine. In: Swain T, ed: Plants in the Development of Modern Medicine. Cambridge, Harvard University Press, 1972, pp. 303–360.

59. Hopmann G, Wanke H: Maximum dose atropine treatment in severe organophosphate poisoning. Dtsch Med Wochenschr 1974;99: 2106–2108.

60. Hruban Z, Schulman S, Warner NE, et al: Hypoglycemia resulting from insecticide poisoning. JAMA 1963;184:590–593.

61. Johnson MK: The delayed neurotoxic effect of some organophosphorus compounds: Identification of the phosphorylation site as an esterase. Biochem J 1969;114:711–717.

62. Johnson MK: Organophosphates and delayed neuropathy—Is NTE alive and well? Toxicol Appl Pharmacol 1990;102:385–399.

63. Joubert J, Joubert PH: Chorea and psychiatric changes in organophosphate poisoning. S Afr Med J 1988;74:32–34.

64. Kaliste-Korhonen E, Ryhanen R, Ylitalo P, Hanninen O: Cold exposure decreases the effectiveness of atropine-oxime treatment in organophosphate intoxication in rats and mice. Gen Phamacol 1989: 20:805–809.

65. Karalliedde L, Senanayake N: Organophosphorus insecticide poisoning. Br J Anaesth 1989;63:736–750.

66. Karczmar AG: History of the research of anticholinesterase agents. In: Karczmar AG, ed: Anticholinesterase Agents, Vol. 1. International Encyclopedia of Pharmacology and Therapeutics, Sect. 13. Oxford, Pergamon Press, Ltd, 1970, pp. 1–44.

67. Karlog O, Nimb M, Paulson E: Parathion (Bladan) forgiftning, behandlet med 2-PAM (pyridyl-2-aldoxime-N-metyljodid). Ugeskr Laeg 1958;120:177.

68. Karlsen RL, Sterri S, Lyngaas S, Fonnum F: Reference values for erythrocyte acetylcholinesterase and plasma cholinesterase activities in children, implications for organophosphate intoxication. Scand J Clin Lab Invest 1981;41:301–302.

69. Kipling RM, Cruickshank AN: Organophosphate insecticide poisoning. Anaesthesia 1985;40:281–284.

70. Kiss Z, Fazekas T: Organophosphates and torsade de pointes ventricular tachycardia. J R Soc Med 1983;76:984–985.

71. Koplovitz I, Mento R, Matthews C, et al: Dose-response effects of atropine and HI-6 treatment of organophosphorus poisoning in guinea pigs. Drug Chem Toxicol 1995;18:119–136.

72. Koplovitz I, Gresham VC, Dochterman LW, et al: Evaluation of the toxicity, pathology, and treatment of cyclohexylmethylphosphonofluoridate (CMPF) poisoning in rhesus monkeys (GF). Arch Toxicol 1992;66:622–628.

73. Krop S, Kunkel AM: Observations on pharmacology of the anticholinesterases sarin and tabun. Proc Soc Exp Biol Med 1954;86: 530–533.

74. Kubistova J: Parathion metabolism in female rat. Arch Int Pharmacodyn Ther 1959;118:308–315.

75. Kurtz PH: Pralidoxime in the treatment of carbamate intoxication. Am J Emerg Med 1990;8:68–70.

76. Kusic R, Jovanovic D, Randjelovic S, et al: HI-6 in man: Efficacy of the oxime in poisoning by organophosphorus insecticides. Hum Exp Toxicol 1991;10:113–118.

77. Larsen K, Hanel HK: Effect of organophosphorus compounds on S-cholinesterase in workers removing poisonous depots. Scand J Work Environ Health 1982;8:222–226.

78. LeBlanc FN, Benson BE, Gilg AD: A severe organophosphate poisoning requiring the use of an atropine drip. J Toxicol Clin Toxicol 1986;24:69–76.

79. Lee WC, Yang CC, Deng JF, et al: The clinical significance of hyperamylasemia in organophosphate poisoning. J Toxicol Clin Toxicol 1998;36:673–681.

80. Leon SFE, Pradilla AG, Gamboa N, et al: Multiple system organ failure, intermediate syndrome, congenital myasthenic syndrome, and anticholinesterase treatment: The linkage is puzzling. J Toxicol Clin Toxicol 1996;34:245–246.

81. Lieske CN, Clark JH, Maxwell DM, et al: Studies of the amplification of carbaryl toxicity by various oximes. Toxicol Lett 1992;62: 127–137.

82. Lokan H, Ross J: Rapid death by mevinphos poisoning while under observation. Forensic Sci Int 1981;23:179–182.

83. Lotti M, Becker CE: Treatment of acute organophosphate poisoning: evidence of a direct effect on central nervous system by 2-PAM (pyridine-2-aldoxime methyl chloride). J Toxicol Clin Toxicol 1982;19:121–127.

84. Lotti M: Treatment of acute organophosphate poisoning. Med J Aust 1991;154:51–55.

85. Ludomirsky A, Klein HO, Sarelli P, et al: Q-T prolongation and polymorphous ("torsade de pointes") ventricular arrhythmias associated with organophosphorus insecticide poisoning. Am J Cardiol 1982;49:1654–1658.

86. Lutterotti A: Leberschadigung bei Vergiftung mit Insektiziden aus der Reine der Cholinesterase-Blocker. Med Welt 1961;46:2430–2433.

87. Mackey CL: Anticholinesterase insecticide poisoning. Heart Lung 1982;11:479–484.

88. Manoguerra A, Whitney C, Clark RF, Anderson B, Turchen S: Cholinergic toxicity resulting from ocular instillation of echothiophate iodide eyedrops. J Toxicol Clin Toxicol 1995;33:463–465.

89. Marsh WA, Vukov GA, Conradi EC: Acute pancreatitis after cutaneous exposure to an organophosphate insecticide. Am J Gastroenterol 1988;83:1158–1160.

90. Matzumura F: Toxicology of Insecticides. New York, Plenum Press, 1975.

91. McDonough JH, Jaax NK, Crowley RA, et al: Atropine and/or diazepam therapy protects against soman-induced neural and cardiac pathology. Fundam Appl Toxicol 1989;13:256–276.

92. Medicis JJ, Stork CM, Howland MA, et al: Pharmacokinetics following a loading plus a continuous infusion of pralidoxime compared with the traditional short infusion regimen in human volunteers. J Toxicol Clin Toxicol 1996;34:289–295.

93. Meller D, Fraser I, Kryger M: Hyperglycemia in anticholinergic poisoning. Can Med Assoc J 1981;124:745–748.

94. Merrill DG, Mihm FG: Prolonged toxicity of organophosphate poisoning. Crit Care Med 1982;10:550–551.

95. Merritt HH, Moore M: Peripheral neuritis associated with ginger extract ingestion. N Engl J Med 1980;203:4–12.

96. Metcalf RL, Swift TR, Sikes RK: Neurological findings among workers exposed to fenthion in a veterinary hospital: Georgia. MMWR Morb Mortal Wkly Rep 1985;34:402–403.

97. Midtling JE, Barnett PG, Coye MJ, et al: Clinical management of field worker organophosphate poisoning. West J Med 1985;142:514–518.

98. Milby TH: Prevention and management of organophosphate poisoning. JAMA 1971;216:2131–2133.

99. Moody SB, Terp DK: Dystonic reaction possibly induced by cholinesterase inhibitor insecticides. Drug Intell Clin Pharm 1988;22:311–312.

100. Morgan DP: Recognition and Management of Pesticide Poisonings, 3rd ed. Washington, DC, US Environmental Protection Agency, 1982.

101. Morgan JP, Penovich P: Jamaica ginger paralysis: Forty-seven-year follow-up. Arch Neurol 1978;35:530–532.

102. Moss AJ, McDonald J: Unilateral cervicothoracic sympathetic ganglionectomy for the treatment of long QT interval syndrome. N Engl J Med 1971;285:903–904.

103. Murphy MR, Blick DW, Dunn MA, et al: Diazepam as a treatment for nerve agent poisoning in primates. Aviat Space Environ Med 1993;64:110–115.

104. Mutch E, Blain PG, Williams FM: Interindividual variations in enzymes controlling organophosphate toxicity in man. Human Exp Toxicol 1992;11:109–116.

105. Namba T, Nolte CT, Jackrel J, Grob D: Poisoning due to organophosphate insecticides. Am J Med 1971;50:475–491.

106. Namba T: Diagnosis and treatment of organophosphate poisoning. Medical Times 1972;100:100–126.

107. Namba T, Greenfield M, Grob D: Malathion poisoning: A fatal case with cardiac manifestations. Arch Environ Health 1970;21:533–541.

108. Namba T, Okazaki S, Taniguchi Y, et al: Toxicity of PAM (pyridine-2-aldoxime methiodide). Naika Ryoiki 1958;6:437–439.

109. Namba T, Hiraki K: PAM (pyride-2-aldoxime methiodide) therapy for alkylphosphate poisoning. JAMA 1958;166:1834–1839.

110. Nelson TC, Burritt MF: Pesticide poisoning, succinylcholine induced apnea and pseudocholinesterase. Mayo Clin Proc 1986;61:750–755.

111. Nisse P, Forceville X, Cezard C, et al: Intermediate syndrome with delayed distal polyneuropathy from ethyl parathion poisoning. Vet Hum Toxicol 1998;40:349–352.

112. Nolan RJ, Rick DL, Freshour NL, Saunders JH: Chlorpyrifos: Pharmacokinetics in human volunteers. Toxicol Appl Pharmacol 1984;73:8–15.

113. Nye DE, Dorough HW: Fate of insecticides administered endotracheally to rats. Bull Environ Contam Toxicol 1976;15:291–296.

114. O'Brien RD: Phosphorylation and carbamylation of cholinesterase. Ann N Y Acad Sci 1969;169:204–214.

115. Parker PE, Brown FW: Organophosphate intoxication: Hidden hazards. South Med J 1989;82:1408–1410.

116. Peiris JB, Fernando R, De Abrew K: Respiratory failure from severe organophosphate toxicity due to absorption through the skin. Forensic Sci Int 1988;36:251–253.

117. Prellwitz W, Schuster HP, Schylla G, et al: Differential diagnosis of organ involvement in exogenous intoxications with the aid of clinical and clinical-chemical examinations. Klin Wochenschr 1970;48:51–53.

118. Rao AVR: An unusual case of diazinon poisoning. Indian J Med Sci 1965;19:768–770.

119. Rosenberg J, Quenon SG: Organophosphate toxicity associated with flea-dip products: California. MMWR Morb Mortal Wkly Rep 1988;37:329–336.

120. Rotenberg M, Shefi M, Dany S, et al: Differentiation between organophosphate and carbamate poisoning. Clin Chim Acta 1995;234:11–21.

121. Routier RJ, Lipman J, Brown K: Difficulty in weaning from respiratory support in a patient with the intermediate syndrome of organophosphate poisoning. Crit Care Med 1989;17:1075–1076.

122. Rump S, Raszewski W, Gidynska T, Galecka E: Effects of CGS 9896 in acute experimental intoxication with fluostigmine (DFP). Arch Toxicol 1990;64:412–413.

123. Sachs A, Cameron GR, Cruikshank JD, et al: Medical Manual of Chemical Warfare. New York, Chemical Publishing, 1956.

124. Sakamoto T, Sawada Y, Nishide K, et al: Delayed neurotoxicity produced by an organophosphorous compound (Sumithion). Arch Toxicol 1984;56:136–138.

125. Schexnayder S, James LP, Kearns GL, Farrar HC: The pharmacokinetics of continuous infusion pralidoxime in children with organophosphate poisoning. J Toxicol Clin Toxicol 1998;36:549–555.

126. Schwartz PJ: Cardiac sympathetic innervation and the sudden infant death syndrome: A possible pathogenic link. Am J Med 1976;60:167–172.

127. Segall Y, Waysbort D, Barak D, et al: Direct observation and elucidation of the structures of aged and nonaged phosphorylated cholinesterases by 31P NMR spectroscopy. Biochemistry 1993;32:13441–13450.

128. Selden BS, Curry SC: Prolonged succinylcholine-induced paralysis in organophosphate insecticide poisoning. Ann Emerg Med 1987;16:215–217.

129. Senanayake N, Jeyaratnam J: Toxic polyneuropathy due to ginger oil contaminated with tri-cresyl phosphate affecting adolescent girls in Sri Lanka. Lancet 1981;1:88–89.

130. Senanayake N: Tri-cresyl phosphate neuropathy in Sri Lanka: A clinical and neurophysiological study with a three-year follow up. J Neurol Neurosurg Psychiatry 1981;44:775–780.

131. Senanayake N, Karalliedde L: Neurotoxic effects of organophosphate insecticides: An intermediate syndrome. N Engl J Med 1987; 316:761–763.

132. Senanayake N: Tri-cresyl phosphate neuropathy in Sri Lanka: A clinical and neurophysiological study with a three-year follow up. J Neurol Neurosurg Psychiatry 1981;44:775–780.

133. Senanayake N, Sanmuganathan PS: Extrapyramidal manifestations complicating an organophosphorus poisoning. Hum Exp Toxicol 1995;14:600–604.

134. Sheu JJ, Wang JD, Wu YK: Determinants of lethality from suicidal pesticide poisoning in metropolitan Hsin Chu. Vet Hum Toxicol 1998;40:332–336.

135. Shih TM: Comparison of several oximes on reactivation of soman-inhibited blood, brain, and tissue cholinesterase activity in rats. Arch Toxicol 1993;67:637–646.

136. Sidell FR, Borak J: Chemical warfare agents: II. Nerve agents. Ann Emerg Med 1992;21:865–871.

137. Smith PW: Bulletin: Medical problems in aerial applications. Washington, DC, Office of Aviation Medicine, Federal Aviation Administration, 1982.

138. Sudakin DL, Mullins ME, Horowitz BZ, Abshier V, Letzig L: Intermediate syndrome after malathion ingestion despite continuous infusion of pralidoxime. J Toxicol Clin Toxicol 2000;38:47–50.

139. Sultatos LG, Shao M, Murphy SD: The role of hepatic biotransformation in mediating the acute toxicity of the phosphorothioate insecticide chlorpyrifos. Toxicol Appl Pharmacol 1984;73:60–68.

140. Sundwall A: Minimum concentrations of N-methylpyridinium-2-aldoxime methane sulphonate (P2S) which reverse neuromuscular block. Biochem Pharmacol 1961;8:413–417.

141. Tabershaw IR, Cooper C: Sequelae of acute organic phosphate poisoning. J Occup Med 1966;8:5–20.

142. Takahashi H, Kojima T, Ikeda T, et al: Differences in the mode of lethality produced through intravenous and oral administration of organophosphorus insecticides in rats. Fundam Appl Toxicol 1991; 16:459–468.

143. Taylor P: Anticholinesterase agents. In: Hardman JG, Limbird LE, Molinoff PB, et al, eds: Goodman & Gilman's The Pharmacological Basis of Therapeutics, 9th ed. New York, Macmillan, 1996, pp. 161–176.

144. Tisdale WH, Flenver AL: Derivatives of dithiocarbamic acid as pesticides. Ind Eng Chem 1942;34:501–506.

145. Umehara F, Izumo S, Arimura K, Osame M: Polyneuropathy induced by m-tolyl methyl carbamate intoxication. J Neurol 1991;238: 47–48.

146. Vasilescu C, Alexianu M, Dan A: Delayed neuropathy after organophosphorus insecticide (Dipterex) poisoning: A clinical, electrophysiological and nerve biopsy study. J Neurol Neurosurg Psychiatry 1984;47:543–548.

147. Wang MH, Tseng CD, Bair SY: Q-T interval prolongation and pleomorphic ventricular tachycardia ("torsade de pointes") in organophosphate poisoning: Report of a case. Hum Exp Toxicol 1998; 17:587–590.

148. Warriner RA, Nies AS, Hayes WJ: Severe organophosphate poisoning complicated by alcohol and turpentine ingestion. Arch Environ Health 1977;32:203–205.

149. Willems JL, De Bisschop HC, Verstraete AG, et al: Cholinesterase reactivation in organophosphorus poisoned patients depends on the plasma concentrations of the oxime pralidoxime methylsulphate and of the organophosphate. Arch Toxicol 1993;67:79–84.

150. Willems JL, Langenberg JP, Verstaete AG, et al: Plasma concentrations of pralidoxime methylsulphate in organophosphorus poisoned patients. Arch Toxicol 1992;66:260–266.

151. Wilson IB: Molecular complementarity and antidotes for alkylphosphate poisoning. Fed Proc 1959;18:752–758.

152. Wilson IB, Hatch MA, Ginsburg S: Carbamylation of acetylcholinesterase. J Biol Chem 1960;235:2312–2315.

153. Winteringham FW, Fowler KS: Substrate and dilutional effects on the inhibition of acetylcholinesterase by carbamates. Biochem J 1966;101:127–134.

154. Woodard CL, Calamaio CA, Kaminskis A, et al: Erythrocyte and plasma cholinesterase activity in male and female rhesus monkeys before and after exposure to sarin. Fundam Appl Toxicol 1994;23: 342–347.

155. Wulfsohn NL, Smith JC, Foldes FF: Acute phospholine intoxication after intracutaneous injection. Clin Pharmacol Ther 1966;7:44–47.

156. Yager J, McLean H, Hudes M, Spear RC: Components of variability in blood cholinesterase assay results. J Occup Med 1976;18: 242–244.

157. Yang PY, Tsao TCY, Lin JL, Lyu RK, Chiang PC: Carbofuran-induced delayed neuropathy. J Toxicol Clin Toxicol 2000;38:43–46.

158. Zwiener RJ, Ginsburg CM: Organophosphate and carbamate poisoning in infants and children. Pediatrics 1988;81:121–126.

ANTIDOTES IN DEPTH

Pralidoxime

Mary Ann Howland

Pralidoxime

Obidoxime
(Toxigonin)

Asoxime (HI-b)

Pralidoxime (2-hydroxyiminomethyl-1-methyl pyridinium chloride; 2-PAM) is the only currently available cholinesterase-reactivating agent in the United States.[24] It is employed with atropine in the management of patients poisoned with organic phosphorus pesticides and, at times, in the management of patients poisoned with carbamate pesticides. Administration should be initiated as soon as possible after pesticide exposure, but pralidoxime may remain effective for days, and should be administered to all symptomatic patients independent of delay. Continuous infusion is preferable to intermittent administration for patients with serious toxicity and a prolonged therapeutic course may be required.

CHEMISTRY

Pralidoxime is a quaternary ammonium oxime with a molecular weight of 173 daltons. The chloride salt exhibits excellent water solubility and physiologic compatibility.

REACTIVATION OF CHOLINESTERASES FOLLOWING ORGANIC PHOSPHORUS COMPOUND POISONING

Organic phosphorus pesticides are powerful inhibitors of carboxylic esterase enzymes, including acetylcholinesterase (true cholinesterase, found in red blood cells, nervous tissue, and skele-

tal muscle) and pseudocholinesterase or butyrlcholinesterase (found in plasma, liver, heart, pancreas, and brain).[36] The organic phosphorus compound binds firmly to the serine-containing esteratic site on the enzyme, inactivating it by phosphorylation.[22,36,51] This reaction results in the accumulation of acetylcholine at muscarinic, nicotinic, and central nervous system (CNS) synapses, leading to the manifestations of organic phosphorus poisoning. After the organic phosphorus pesticide binds to cholinesterase, the enzyme is inactivated and can undergo one of three processes: endogenous hydrolysis of the phosphorylated enzyme; reactivation by a strong nucleophile, such as 2-PAM; and biochemical changes that render the phosphorylated molecule inactive ("aged").

Endogenous hydrolysis of organic phosphorus compounds can be extremely slow and, for the most part, is considered insignificant. The positively charged quaternary nitrogen of pralidoxime is attracted to the negatively charged anionic site on the phosphorylated enzyme, bringing it in close proximity to the phosphorous moiety. Pralidoxime exerts a nucleophilic attack on the phosphate moiety, successfully competing for it and releasing it from the acetylcholinesterase enzyme.[35] This action liberates the enzyme and permits enzymatic function.

EFFICACY RELATED TO TIME OF ADMINISTRATION AFTER POISONING

Early in vitro evidence suggested that to be successful, cholinesterase reactivators must be administered within 24–48 hours of exposure to the organic phosphorus compounds; otherwise the acetylcholinesterases would be irreversibly inactivated. It is no longer believed that there is a true time limitation on reactivator function. The 48-hour limit was derived from in vitro experiments using a small number of tightly bound compounds and reactivators such as nicotinehydroxamic acid methiodide (NHA), monoisonitrosoacetone (MINA), and oximes (obidoxime and pralidoxime methiodide). These studies used data from plasma pseudocholinesterase enzyme activity, which is now recognized to be relatively unaffected by oxime nucleophilic attack. The early data were accepted without adequate consideration of numerous factors such as relevance to human systems, the use of newer and less tightly bound compounds, temperature and pH variation, blood flow, fat solubility, and species specificity. Fat-soluble organic phosphorus compounds redistribute from fat stores over time, acting similarly to sustained-release products. They have not aged and they continue to reinhibit acetylcholinesterase for days. An in vitro experiment assessed the effect of aging on the ability of pralidoxime to regenerate rat erythrocyte and brain cholinesterases using three different organic phosphorus compounds.[55] The rate of reactivation of erythrocyte and brain cholinesterases by pralidoxime was significantly decreased over time for fenitrothion and methylparathion, with no reactivation occurring at 48 hours. In contrast, a very high reactivation rate for ethylparathion was still apparent at 48 hours. This demonstrates that the structure of the organic phosphorus compound plays a significant role in the rate of aging and reactivation with pralidoxime. Fenitrothion and methylparathion are both O'O dimethylorganic phosphorus compounds, whereas ethylparathion is an O'O diethylorganic phosphorus compound.[55] Other studies also suggest that 2-PAM and obidoxime are effective long after the previously suggested 48-hour window of therapy.[2,4,7,10,11,13,18,19,31,33]

CARBAMATES

Acetylcholinesterase inactivated by carbamates spontaneously reactivates with plasma elimination half-lives of 1–2 hours, with clinical recovery in several hours, and rarely in more than 24 hours.[25] Although pralidoxime is rarely indicated for carbamate poisoning, it was previously suggested that pralidoxime was contraindicated following exposure to a carbamate. This approach was based solely on data derived from the study of a single carbamate—carbaryl (Sevin)—and inappropriately generalized to all carbamates. In vitro experiments demonstrated that pralidoxime had no effect on the reactivation of erythrocyte acetylcholinesterase carbamylated by aldicarb, methoxyl, and carbaryl.[27] Pralidoxime decreased the rate of carbamylation by 16 insecticidal carbamates and only modestly increased the rates for 3, 1 of which was carbaryl.[12] Animal studies demonstrated the beneficial effects of pralidoxime and obidoxime in doubling the lethal dose for a number of carbamate insecticides.[37,48] However, with carbaryl (Sevin), obidoxime and pralidoxime mesylate worsened intoxication, possibly because the carbamate-oxime complex may be a more potent cholinesterase inhibitor than carbaryl alone.[17,37,44,48] Even in the presence of carbaryl, atropine and the oxime resulted in survival data comparable to that of atropine alone.[17] This evidence suggests that although pralidoxime is not usually a necessary adjunct to atropine in a pure carbamate overdose, it may occasionally improve morbidity and mortality.[8] Pralidoxime should always be used in conjunction with atropine and should not be the sole therapy. Pralidoxime should not be withheld in a seriously poisoned patient because of the possibility that the agent may be a carbamate.

PHARMACOLOGY

Pralidoxime's action is most striking at nicotinic sites, often improving muscle strength within 10–40 minutes after administration.[36,51] Pralidoxime is effective at muscarinic sites and may demonstrate synergism with atropine at these sites.[14] The primary effect of atropine is to block the muscarinic and CNS symptoms of organic phosphorus compound poisoning. Because pralidoxime and atropine work synergistically, 2-PAM should rarely be used alone.[14] Some organic phosphorus compounds respond much better to 2-PAM than do other compounds; it depends on the affinity of pralidoxime for the particular type of phosphorylated enzyme and its reactivating ability.[59]

The CNS effects of 2-PAM, a quaternary nitrogen compound,[36] are controversial, as the molecule is not expected to cross the blood-brain barrier.[30,36] Animal studies offer conflicting results, possibly because of the use of brain homogenate models rather than cortical slices.[32] Rat studies using radiolabeled pralidoxime demonstrated a lack of any radioactivity in the CNS after IV administration.[54] Following exposure to IV fenitrothion, intravenous administration of pralidoxime in rats failed to improve survival or to reactivate brain cholinesterase, whereas intramedullary prali-

doxime partially restored brain cholinesterase and eliminated fatalities.[54] Clinical observations have certainly suggested a CNS action, with a return of consciousness in some cases.[35,36,40,57] A 3-year-old child who was comatose from parathion intoxication was given 500 mg of 2-PAM IV over 15 minutes with continuous electroencephalographic (EEG) monitoring. Within 2 minutes there was a dramatic response on the EEG, followed by normalization of consciousness.[28]

Early work with cats led to a proposal that 4 μg/mL was a desired therapeutic concentration for pralidoxime.[50] Recent in vitro work with human erythrocytes and a mouse hemidiaphragm model suggests that much higher serum concentrations are actually needed.[59] Twenty percent reactivation was achieved with serum concentrations of 10 μg/mL, and 70% reactivation was achieved with concentrations of 17 μg/mL using paraoxon as the inhibitor.[59]

The understanding of the pathophysiology of the intermediate syndrome is inadequate to determine whether pralidoxime can prevent the development of the syndrome.[49] Certain organic phosphorus pesticides may lead to the development of delayed onset neurotoxicity that cannot be prevented by pralidoxime treatment.

OTHER REVERSAL AGENTS

To improve the central effect of pralidoxime, the dihydropyridine derivative of pralidoxime (2-PAM) was synthesized.[5] This derivative, known as pro-2-PAM, acts as a "prodrug," or drug carrier, which allows passage through membranes such as the blood-brain barrier. Once across the membranes, in vivo oxidation converts pro-2-PAM to the active species, demonstrating a 13-fold higher level of 2-PAM in the brain than PAM administered under similar conditions. Further experiments supported the significantly increased central effects of pro-2-PAM.[43] The use of sugar oximes (the molecular combination of glucose with 2-PAM derivatives) to promote CNS penetration appears promising.[41] Obidoxime (Toxogenin) is an oxime used outside the United States that contains two active sites per molecule and is considered by some to be more effective than 2-PAM.[14,59] An in vitro study utilizing human erythrocyte acetylcholinesterase supported the superiority of obidoxime to pralidoxime in reactivating acetylcholinesterase inhibited by the dimethylphosphoryl and diethylphosphoryl organic phosphorus compounds paraoxon, mevinphos, and malaoxon. Obidoxime is approximately 4 times more active in reactivating acetylcholinesterase than is pralidoxime.[59] The H series of oximes (named after Hagedorn) were developed to act against the chemical warfare nerve agents. These agents have superior effectiveness against certain chemical warfare agents (ie, sarin, VX) but they are less efficacious in organic phosphorus insecticide poisoning, and their toxicity profile is inadequately defined.[9,23,26,29,42,59] In addition to reactivating acetylcholinesterases, these agents have direct central and peripheral anticholinergic effects.[42]

DURATION OF TREATMENT

The signs and symptoms of organic phosphorus compound poisoning are usually manifest within 12–24 hours.[36] Delayed manifestations occur with the fat-soluble organic phosphorus compounds, such as fenthion or chlorfenthion, and other compounds requiring metabolic conversion to active agents, such as parathion, which undergoes hepatic conversion to paraoxon. The route of exposure may also influence the onset of systemic symptoms; for example, there may be a delay following dermal contact, which does not occur following ingestion or inhalation. When symptoms are delayed or prolonged, or when treatment is delayed, prolonged therapy with 2-PAM may be indicated.[1,7,33] In one case of poisoning with the fat-soluble organic phosphorus compound fenthion, there was a 5-day delay before cholinergic symptoms appeared, and some symptoms persisted for 30 days.[33] Pralidoxime and atropine were administered continuously in varying doses for most of that period.

PHARMACOKINETICS AND PHARMACODYNAMICS

Pralidoxime pharmacokinetics are characterized by a two-compartment model. Pharmacokinetics vary depending on whether calculations are determined in healthy volunteers or poisoned patients. In volunteers, the steady-state volume of distribution is about 0.8 L/kg and the half-life is 75 minutes.[20,47] Pralidoxime is renally excreted, and within 12 hours, 80% of the dose has been recovered unchanged in the urine.[47] Thiamine administered intravenously at 100 mg/h for 2.5 hours prolonged the half-life, increased the volume of distribution and peak plasma concentrations, and decreased the plasma, intercompartmental, and renal clearances when pralidoxime (5 mg/kg) was given intravenously.[21] Thiamine and pralidoxime are both strong bases, and thiamine might decrease renal clearance through competition for renal secretion.[21] The benefit of using thiamine in poisoned patients to prolong the plasma half-life of pralidoxime has never been tested.

A dose of 10 mg/kg of 2-PAM IM or IV to volunteers results in peak plasma concentrations of 6 µg/mL (reached 5–15 minutes after IM injection) and a plasma half-life of approximately 75 minutes.[47] Animal data suggest that a plasma level greater than 4 µg/mL is effective against nicotinic symptoms, but recent studies suggest that even higher levels may be necessary.[6,50,59] Following a standard IV 30-minute infusion dose of 1 g of 2-PAM in a 70-kg man, the plasma level was less than 4 µg/mL at 1.5 hours. In a simulated model, a continuous infusion of 500 mg/h of 2-PAM leads to a level greater than 4 µg/mL after 15 minutes, which can be maintained throughout the infusion.[52] In a human volunteer study, an intravenous loading dose of 4 mg/kg over 15 minutes followed by 3.2 mg/kg/h for a total of 4 hours maintained pralidoxime serum concentrations greater than 4 µg/mL for 257 minutes. The same total dose, 16 mg/kg, administered over 30 minutes only maintained those concentrations for 118 minutes.[31]

In poisoned patients, and in those patients receiving continuous infusions of pralidoxime as opposed to intermittent infusions, the volume of distribution and the half-life are increased. A volume of distribution of 2.77 L/kg, an elimination half-life of 3.44 hours, and a clearance of 0.57 L/kg/h have been reported in poisoned adults administered a mean loading dose of 4.4 mg/kg followed by an infusion of 2.14 mg/kg/h.[57] In poisoned children and adolescents, the volume of distribution varied with severity of poisoning from 8.8 L/kg in the severely poisoned patients compared with 2.8 L/kg in those moderately poisoned.[45] After a mean loading dose of 29 mg/kg followed by a continuous infusion of about 14 mg/kg/h, a steady-state serum concentration of 22 µg/mL, a half-life of 3.6 hours, and a clearance of 0.88 L/kg/h were calculated.[45]

Oral administration of salts of 2-PAM (not used clinically because of anticholinesterase poisoning–induced vomiting) demonstrated peak concentrations at 2–3 hours, a biologic half-life of 1.7 hours, and an average urine recovery of 27% of unchanged 2-PAM.[25]

ADVERSE EFFECTS

Adverse effects of therapeutic doses of 2-PAM in humans are minimal and may not be evident unless plasma levels are exceptionally high at >400 µg/mL.[15,16,34–36,40,52] Transient dizziness, blurred vision, and elevations in diastolic blood pressure may be related to the rate of administration.[20,21,31] Rapid IV administration has produced sudden cardiac and respiratory arrest.[38,46,58]

DOSING AND ADMINISTRATION

The optimal dosage regimen for pralidoxime is unknown. Traditionally the recommended initial adult dose is 1–2 g in 100 mL of 0.9% sodium chloride solution given intravenously over 15–30 minutes.[39] Rapid administration (bolus or >200 mg/min in adults) can lead to respiratory and cardiac arrest. The pediatric dose is 20–40 mg/kg as a loading dose given intravenously over 30 minutes. These initial doses can be repeated in 1 hour if muscle weakness and fasciculations are not relieved. Thereafter, additional doses may be needed every 3–8 hours as long as signs of poisoning recur.[39]

Alternatively, a loading dose followed by a continuous maintenance infusion has been reported to be safe and effective in a limited number of adults and children.[45,53,56,57] Serious intoxication may require continuous infusion of 500 mg/h in adults and 10–20 mg/kg/h in children. One author suggests a loading dose of 25–50 mg/kg in children, depending on the severity of the poisoning, to be followed by a continuous infusion of 10–20 mg/kg/h.[45] Continuous infusion may be more effective than multiple single injections.[34,36] In the case of pulmonary edema, the dose can be given as a 5% solution (concentrations above 35% w/v produce muscle necrosis in animals).[47] Long-term dosing may be necessary, depending on the patient's clinical condition.

AVAILABILITY

Pralidoxime chloride (Protopam) is supplied in 20-mL vials containing 1 g of powder, ready for reconstitution with sterile water for injection.[24]

SUMMARY

Pralidoxime is an effective reactivator of acetylcholinesterase in many organic phosphorus compound poisonings. It primarily reverses neuromuscular manifestations, but has some CNS effects. New oximes may improve CNS penetration and efficacy. Pralidoxime and atropine are synergistic and should be used together in the management of organic phosphorus poisonings. If a patient requires multiple doses of atropine for muscarinic symptoms, then the use of 2-PAM is indicated. In symptomatic patients, acetylcholinesterase is partially inactivated and will remain so until new enzyme is synthesized or inactivated enzyme is reactivated. The resolution of all signs or symptoms with atropine alone indicates only that inactivation is less than 50% and that endogenous hydrolysis of phosphorylated enzyme is sufficient to eliminate symptoms. This clinical response does not mean, however, that the enzyme systems are fully active; patients may still benefit from enzyme regeneration with the safe and effective antidote pralidoxime.

Finally, because newer fat-soluble organic phosphorus pesticides are currently available, it may be necessary to administer atropine and 2-PAM for more prolonged periods of time than previously suggested.[50]

ACKNOWLEDGMENT

Cynthia K. Aaron contributed to this discussion in a previous edition.

REFERENCES

1. Aaron CK, Smilkstein M: Intermediate syndrome or inadequate therapy [abstract]. Vet Human Toxicol 1988;30:370.
2. Amos WC Jr, Hall A: Malathion poisoning treated with Protopam. Ann Intern Med 1965;62:1013–1016.
3. Blaber LC, Creasey NH: The mode of recovery of cholinesterase activity in vivo after organophosphorus poisoning: I. Erythrocyte cholinesterase. Biochem J 1960;77:591–596.
4. Blaber LC, Creasey NH: The mode of recovery of cholinesterase activity in vivo after organophosphorus poisoning: II. Brain cholinesterase. Biochem J 1960;77:597–604.
5. Bodor N, Shek E, Higuchi T: Delivery of a quaternary pyridinium salt across the blood-brain barrier by its dihydropyridine derivative. Science 1975;190:155–156.
6. Bokowjic D, Jovanovic D, Jokanovic M, et al: Protective effects of oximes HI-6 and PAM 2 applied by osmotic minipumps in quinalphos poisoned rats. Arch Int Pharmacodyn Ther 1987;288:309–318.
7. Borowitz SM: Prolonged organophosphate toxicity in a twenty-six-month-old child. J Pediatr 1988;112:303–304.
8. Burgess JL, Bernstein JN, Hurlbut K: Aldicarb poisoning—A case report with prolonged cholinesterase inhibition and improvement after pralidoxime therapy. Arch Intern Med 1994;154:221–224.
9. Clement JG, Bailey DG, Madill HD, et al: The acetylcholinesterase oxime reactivator HI-6 in man: Pharmacokinetics and tolerability in combination with atropine. Biopharm Drug Dispos 1995;16:415–425.
10. Davies DR, Green AL: The kinetics of reactivation, by oximes, of cholinesterase inhibited by organophosphorus compounds. Biochemistry 1956;63:529–535.
11. Davison AN: Return of cholinesterase activity in the rat after inhibition by organophosphorus compounds: I. Diethyl p-nitrophenyl phosphate (E600, Paraoxon). Biochem J 1953;54:583–590.
12. Dawson RM: Oximes in treatment of carbamate poisoning [letter]. Vet Rec 1994;134:687.
13. Durham WF, Hayes WJ Jr: Organic phosphorus poisoning and its therapy. Arch Environ Health 1962;5:21–47.
14. Finkelstein Y, Taitelman U, Biegon A: CNS involvement in acute organophosphate poisoning: Specific pattern of toxicity, clinical correlates and antidotal treatment. Ital J Neurol Sci 1988;9:437–446.
15. Grob D, Jones RJ: Use of oximes in the treatment of intoxication by anticholinesterase compounds in normal subjects. Am J Med 1958; 24:497–511.
16. Hagerstrom-Portnoy G, Jones R, Adams AJ, Jampolsky A: Effects of atropine and 2-PAM chloride on vision and performance in humans. Aviat Space Environ Med 1987;10:47–53.
17. Harris LW, Talbot BG, Lennox WJ, et al: The relationship between oxime-induced reactivation of carbamylated acetylcholinesterase and antidotal efficacy against carbamate intoxication. Toxicol Appl Pharmacol 1989;98:128–133.
18. Hobbinger F: Chemical reactivation of phosphorylated human and bovine true cholinesterase. Br J Pharmacol 1956;11:295–303.
19. Hobbinger F: Effect of nicotinehydroxamic acid methiodide on human plasma cholinesterase inhibited by organophosphates containing dialkylphosphate groups. Br J Pharmacol 1955;10:356–362.
20. Jager BV, Staff GN: Toxicity of diacetyl monoxime and of pyridine-2-aldoxime methiodide in man. Bull Johns Hopkins Hosp 1958;102:203–211.
21. Josselson J, Sidell FR: Effect of intravenous thiamine on pralidoxime kinetics. Clin Pharmacol Ther 1978;24:95–100.
22. Karczmar A: Invited review: Anticholinesterases: Dramatic aspects of their use and misuse. Neurochem Int 1998;32:401–411.
23. Kassa J, Cabal J: A comparison of the efficacy of a new asymmetric bispyridinium oxime BI-6 with currently available oximes and H oximes against soman in in vitro and in vivo methods. Toxicology 1999;132:111–118.
24. Kastrup E, ed: Facts and Comparisons. Philadelphia, JB Lippincott, 1983.
25. Kondritzer A, Zvirblis P, Goodman A, Paplanus S: Blood plasma levels and elimination of salts of 2-PAM in man after oral administration. J Pharm Sci 1968;57:1142–1145.
26. Kusic R, Jovanovic D, Randjelovic A, et al: HI-6 in man: Efficacy of the oxime in poisoning by organophosphorus insecticides. Hum Exp Toxicol 1991;10:113–118.
27. Lifshitz M, Rotenberg M, Sofer S, et al: Carbamate poisoning and oxime treatment in children: A clinical and laboratory study. Pediatrics 1994;93:652–655.
28. Lotti M, Becker C: Treatment of acute organophosphate-poisoning: Evidence of a direct effect on central nervous system by 2-PAM (pyridine-2-aldoxime methyl chloride). J Toxicol Clin Toxicol 1982;19:121–127.
29. Lundy PM, Hansen AS, Hand BT, Boulet CA: Comparison of several oximes against poisoning by soman, tabun and GF. Toxicology 1992; 72:99–105.
30. Matin M, Siddiqui R: Modification of the level of acetylcholinesterase activity by two oximes in certain brain regions and peripheral tissues of paraoxon treated rats. Pharmacol Res Commun 1982;4:241–246.
31. Medicis JJ, Stork CM, Howland MA, et al: Pharmacokinetics following a loading plus a continuous infusion of pralidoxime compared with the traditional short infusion regimen in human volunteers. J Toxicol Clin Toxicol 1996;34:289–295.
32. Milosevic MP, Andjelkovic D: Reactivation of paraoxon-inactivated cholinesterase in the rat cerebral cortex by pralidoxime chloride. Nature 1966;210:206.
33. Merrill D, Mihm F: Prolonged toxicity of organophosphate poisoning. Crit Care Med 1982;10:550–551.
34. Namba T: Diagnosis and treatment of organophosphate insecticide poisoning. Med Times 1972;100:100–126.
35. Namba T, Hiraki K: PAM (pyridine-2-aldoxime methiodide) therapy for alkyl-phosphate poisoning. JAMA 1958;166:1834–1839.
36. Namba T, Nolte C, Jackrel J, Grob D: Poisoning due to organophosphate insecticides: Acute and chronic manifestations. Am J Med 1971;50:475–492.
37. Natoff IL, Reiff B: Effect of oximes on the acute toxicology of acetylcholinesterase carbamates. Toxicol Appl Pharmacol 1973;25:569–575.
38. Pickering EN: Organic phosphate insecticide poisoning. Can J Med Technol 1966;28:174–179.
39. Protopam chloride. Package Insert (revised 1996). Ayerst Labs. Physician's Desk Reference, 55th ed. Montvale, NJ, Medical Economics, 2001, pp. 3442–3443.
40. Quimby G: Further therapeutic experience with pralidoximes in organic phosphorus poisoning. JAMA 1963;187:202–206.

41. Rachaman E, Ashani Y, Leader H, et al: Sugaroximes, new potential antidotes against organophosphorus poisoning. Arzneimittelforschung 1979;29:875–876.

42. Rousseaux CG, Du AK: Pharmacology of HI-6, an H-series oxime. Can J Physiol Pharmacol 1989;67:1183–1189.

43. Rump S, Faff J, Borkowska G, et al: Central therapeutic effects of di-hydro-derivative of pralidoxime (pro-2-PAM) in organophosphate in-toxication. Arch Int Pharmacodyn Ther 1978;232:321–331.

44. Sanderson DM: Treatment of poisoning by anticholinesterase insecti-cides in the rat. J Pharm Pharmacol 1961;13:435–442.

45. Schexnayder S, James L, Kearns G, Farrar H: The pharmacokinetics of continuous infusion pralidoxime in children with organophosphate poisoning. J Toxicol Clin Toxicol 1998;36:549–555.

46. Scott RJ: Repeated asystole following PAM in organophosphate self-poisoning. Anesth Intensive Care 1986;4:458–460.

47. Sedell FR, Groff WA: Intramuscular and intravenous administration of small doses of 2-pyridinium aldoxime methylchloride to man. J Pharm Sci 1971;60:1224–1228.

48. Sterri S, Rognerud B, Fiskum S, Lyngaas S: Effect of toxogenin and P2S on the toxicity of carbamates and organophosphorus compounds. Acta Pharmacol Toxicol 1979;45:9–15.

49. Sudakin D, Mullins M, Horowitz Z, et al: Intermediate syndrome after malathion ingestion despite continuous infusion of pralidoxime. J Toxicol Clin Toxicol 2000;38:47–50.

50. Sundwall A: Minimum concentrations of n-methyl pyridinium-2-aldoxime methane sulphonate (PS2) which reverse neuromuscular block. Biochem Pharmacol 1961;8:413–417.

51. Taylor P: Anticholinesterase agents. In: Hardman JG, Limbind LE, Molinoff PB, Ruddoev RW, eds: Goodman and Gilman's The Phar-macological Basis of Therapeutics, 9th ed. New York, Macmillan, 1996, pp. 100–119.

52. Thompson DF, Thompson GD, Greenwood RB, Trammel HL: Thera-peutic dosing of pralidoxime chloride. Drug Intell Clin Pharm 1987; 21:1590–1593.

53. Tush G, Anstead M: Pralidoxime continuous infusion ion the treat-ment of organophosphate poisoning. Ann Pharmacother 1997;31: 441–444.

54. Uehara S, Hiromori T, Isobe N, et al: Studies on the therapeutic effect of 2-pyridine aldoxime methiodide (2-PAM) in mammals following organophosphorous compound (op)-poisoning (report III): Distribu-tion and antidotal effect of 2-PAM in rats. J Toxicol 1993;18: 265–275.

55. Uehara S, Hiromori T, Suzuki T, et al: Studies on the therapeutic ef-fect of 2-pyridine aldoxime methiodide (2-PAM) in mammals follow-ing organophosphorous compound (op)-poisoning (report II): Aging of op-inhibited mammalian cholinesterase. J Toxicol 1993;18: 179–183.

56. Willems JL, BeBisschop HC, Verstraete AG, et al: Cholinesterase re-activation in organophosphorus poisoned patients depends on the plasma concentrations of the oxime pralidoxime methylsulfate and of the organophosphate. Arch Toxicol 1993;97:79–84.

57. Willems JL, Langenberg JP, Verstraete AC, et al: Plasma concentra-tions of pralidoxime methyl sulfate in organophosphorus poisoned pa-tients. Arch Toxicol 1992;66:260–266.

58. Wislicki L: Differences in the effect of oximes on striated muscle and respiratory centre. Arch Int Pharmacodyn Ther 1960;120:1–19.

59. Worek F, Backer M, Thiermann H, et al: Reappraisal of indications and limitations of oxime therapy in organophosphate poisoning. Hum Exp Toxicol 1997;16:466–472.

CHAPTER 89

INSECTICIDES: ORGANOCHLORINES, PYRETHRINS, AND DEET

Michael G. Holland

A 2-year-old boy (weight, 15 kg) was brought to the Emergency Department (ED) after vomiting and having a witnessed seizure at home. The only history available was that the child had a cold and a "skin condition." By pursuing the connection between seizures and a skin condition, the poison information specialist obtained further history that implicated lindane. The child's grandmother was unable to read the instructions on the bottle, and had given him 1 teaspoon (5 mL, or 50 mg) of 1% lindane orally 3 times a day, rather than applying topically. The child probably received a total of 6 doses (300 mg over 2 days, or 20 mg/kg), the last dose being approximately 3 hours prior to admission.

On examination, the child was alert, asymptomatic, with normal vital signs. He was given 1 g/kg (15 g) of activated charcoal aqueous slurry to adsorb any lindane remaining in the gastrointestinal tract. The child was observed in an intensive care setting for 12 hours. He remained asymptomatic, had no recurrence of seizures, and was discharged home in good condition.

ORGANOCHLORINES

Organochlorine pesticides are complex, cyclic chlorinated hydrocarbons having molecular weights generally in the range of 300–550 Da. They are solids at room temperature (ie, nonvolatile). Most organochlorines have a negative temperature coefficient, making them more insecticidal at lower temperatures, and less toxic to warm-blooded organisms.[102] Most act as central nervous system (CNS) stimulants.

In contrast, chlorinated hydrocarbon solvents and fumigants are low molecular weight, alkyl compounds that are volatile liquids or gases, and that generally have CNS depressant effects (Chap. 86).[19]

The organochlorine pesticides are grouped into four categories based on their chemical structures and similar toxicities: (a) hexachlorocyclohexane (lindane, the γ isomer; with the commonly used misnomer γ-benzene hexachloride), the primary organochlorine pesticide still in common clinical and agricultural use in the United States. Isomerism is important, because the β and Δ isomers are CNS depressants and have no insecticidal properties.[1,16,67] (b) Dichlorodiphenyltrichloroethane (DDT) and related analogues; (c) cyclodienes (the related isomers aldrin, dieldrin, and endrin; as well as heptachlor, endosulfan), and related compounds (toxaphene, dienochlor); and (d) mirex and chlordecone (Table 89–1; Fig. 89–1). These compounds differ substantially, both between and within groups, with respect to toxic doses, skin absorption, fat storage, metabolism, and elimination.[18] The signs and symptoms of toxicity in humans, however, are remarkably similar within each group.

Historical Perspectives

Until the 1940s, commonly available pesticides included highly toxic arsenicals, mercurials, lead, sulfur, and nicotine.[81] When Nobel Prize-winning chemist Paul Müller demonstrated the insecticidal properties of DDT in the early 1940s, a whole new class of pesticides was introduced.[25] The organochlorine insecticides were inexpensive to produce, nonvolatile, environmentally stable, and had relatively low acute toxicity when compared to previous insecticides (see Table 89–1). Widespread use of these compounds occurred from the 1940s until the mid-1970s. They were highly effective and revolutionized modern agriculture, allowing unprecedented output from each acre of arable land. Because of their stability, organochlorines were used extensively in structural protection and soil treatments. Medical and public health applications of DDT and its analogues were also found in the control of typhus and eradication of malaria.[18] By 1953, DDT alone was credited for saving an estimated 50 million lives, and with averting 1 billion cases of human disease.[26] It has been suggested that because of this unprecedented impact on human health, DDT is the single most important factor in the population explosion that occurred between 1950 and 1970.[26]

However, the properties that made these chemicals such effective insecticides also made them environmental hazards: they are slowly metabolized, lipid soluble, chemically stable, and environmentally persistent. In her 1962 book *Silent Spring*, Rachel Carson, a biologist with the US Fish and Wildlife Service, demonstrated that organochlorines are bioconcentrated and biomagnified up the food chain.[10] The organochlorine residues in predatory birds, most notably grebes, peregrine falcons, bald eagles, and pelicans, caused eggshell thinning and decreased reproductive success.[32] These facts, and the finding of DDT residues in humans, led to the severe restriction or total ban of many organochlorines in North America and Europe.[18] However, because they are still highly effective and very inexpensive, the organochlorines are widely used in developing countries, and will be for the foreseeable future.

Toxicokinetics of the Organochlorine Insecticides

Absorption. All of the organochlorine pesticides are well absorbed orally and by inhalation; transdermal absorption is variable, depending on the particular compound. Absorption by any route may be affected by the vehicle, as well as the physical state (solid or liquid) of the pesticide. None of the organochlorines are water-soluble, and are usually either dissolved in organic solvents or manufactured as powders for dusting.

TABLE 89–1. Classification of Organochlorine Pesticides

Classes	CAS[1] Registry #	Brand Name(s)	Current U.S. EPA Registration	Acute Oral Toxicity	Dermal Absorption	Lipid Storage	Specific Characteristics
Hexachloro-cyclohexanes	Lindane (γ isomer) 58-89-9	Kwell	Topical scabicide; seed treatment: RED[2] 2001	Moderate	High	Low	Topical scabicide: seizures, CNS excitation; musty odor
DDT and analogues	DDT-Dichlorodi-phenyltrichlor-oethane 50-29-3	Neocid, Ixodex, Anofex, others	Canceled 1972	Low to moderate	Low	Highest	Tremors, CNS excitation; odorless
	Methoxychlor 72-43-5	Marlate	Suspended 1/14/2000	Low	Low	Moder-ate	Less toxic DDT substitute
	Dicofol 115-32-2	Kelthane	Residential use banned 1998; cotton, citrus, apple	Low	Low	Low	
	Chlorbenzilate 510-15-6	Benzilan, Benzo-Chlor	Citrus miticide	Low	Low	Low	Much less environmental persistence than DDT
Cyclodienes and related compounds, toxaphene	Aldrin 309-00-2	Aldrex, Octalene, Toxadrin	Canceled 1974	High	High	High	Rapidly metabolized to dieldrin; mild "chemical" odor
	Dieldrin 60-57-1	Dieldrite, Octalox, Quintox	Canceled 1974	High	High	High	Stereoisomer of endrin; early and late seizures; odorless
	Endrin 72-20-8	Hexadrin	Canceled 1974	Highest	High	None	Most toxic organochlorine; rapid onset seizures; status epilepticus
	Chlordane 57-74-9	Octachlor, Toxichlor, others	Canceled 1988	Moderate	High	High	Early and late seizures occur
	Endosulfan 115-29-7	Thiodan, Cyclodan, others	RED 2000	High	High	Low	Strong sulfur odor
	Heptachlor 76-44-8	Drinox	Restricted: fire ant control; soil treat-ment	Moderate	High	High	Toxic metabolite heptachlor epoxide; odor of camphor
	Isobenzan 297-78-9	Telodrin	Never registered in US	High	Moderate	High	Also inhibits Mg^{++}-ATPase; mild "chemical" odor
	Dienochlor 2227-17-0	Pentac	Canceled	NA	Low	Low	Toxic metabolite binds to GSH
	Toxaphene (Polychlori-nated Cam-phene) 800-35-2	Alltox, Chemphene, Toxakil, others	Canceled 1982	Moderate-high	Low	Low	Seizures; terpene odor, often mixed with parathion
Chlordecone and Mirex	Chlordecone 143-50-0	Kepone	Canceled 1977	Moderate	High	High	"Kepone shakes"; seizures not seen; structurally similar to mirex
	Mirex 2385-85-5	Dechlorane	Canceled 1976	Low	High	High	(?) Converted to chlorde-cone; toxicity identical

1. Cas: Chemical Abstracts Service # provided here to facilitate Toxline, Medline database searches
2. RED: Registration Eligibility Decision

Dichlorodiphenyltrichloroethane (DDT) and its analogues methoxychlor, dicofol, and chlorbenzylate are very poorly absorbed transdermally, unless the pesticide is dissolved in a suitable hydrocarbon solvent.[72] DDT has limited volatility, so that air concentrations are usually low, and toxicity by the respiratory route is unlikely.

All of the cyclodienes have significant transdermal absorption rates. In fact, cutaneous absorption of dieldrin is so high that toxicity by the dermal route is approximately 50% that of the oral route.[18] Oral absorption of the cyclodienes is high, and significant poisonings have occurred when foodstuffs were contaminated with these pesticides;[4] in addition, consuming pesticide residues

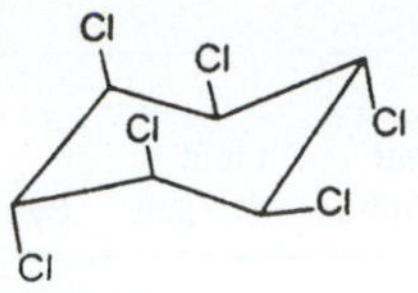

Lindane (γ hexachlorocyclohexane)

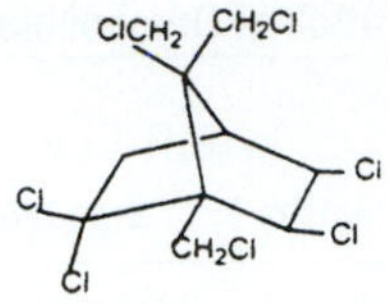

Toxaphene

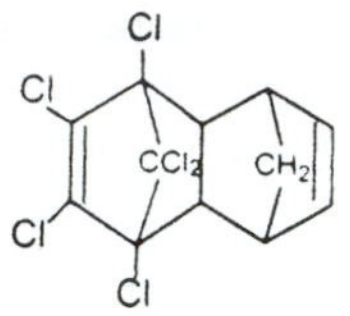

Aldrin (metabolized to dieldrin)

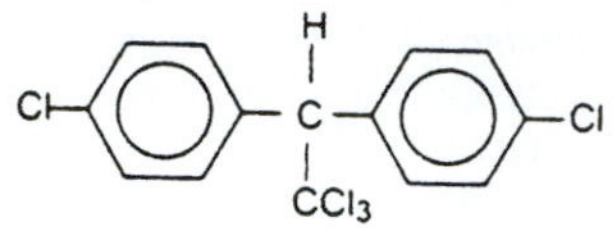

DDT

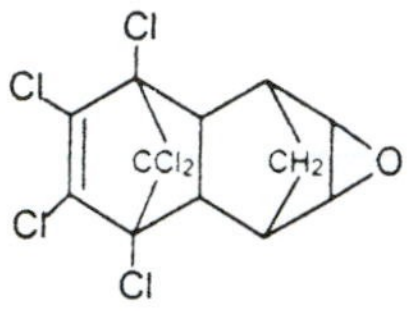

Dieldrin (metabolite of aldrin)

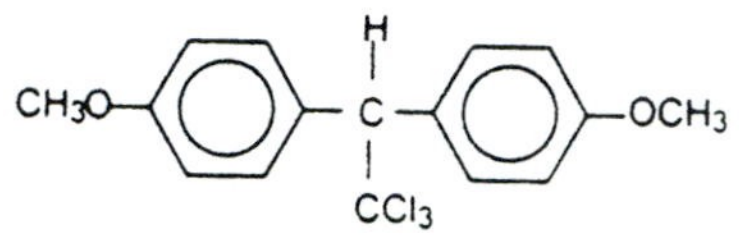

Methoxychlor

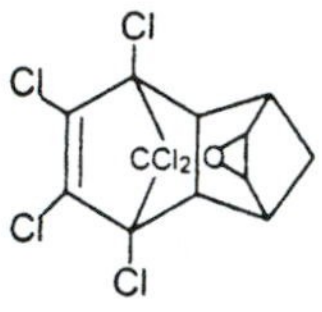

Endrin (stereoisomer of dieldrin)

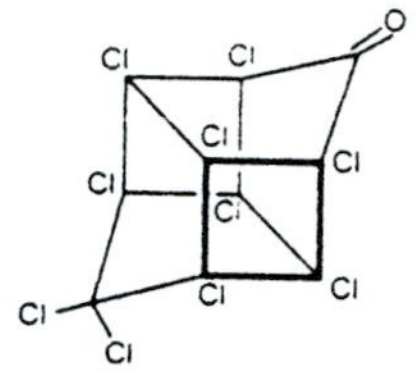

Chlordecone

Figure 89–1. Structures of various organochlorine Pesticides.

on feed sources has killed livestock and wild animals.[86] Toxaphene is poorly absorbed through the skin in both acute and chronic exposures.[80]

Lindane is well absorbed after skin application, and has a documented forearm skin absorption rate in adults of 9.3% of a topically applied dose over 24 hours.[28] Anatomic sites vary in their absorptive capacities: axillary rates are 3.6 times greater, while scrotal absorption is 42 times greater than that of forearm rates.[9,31,43,87] Animal studies and case reports suggest that the young, the malnourished, and those who receive repeated topical doses may have increased accumulation and increased risk for seizures.[68] Hot baths, the vehicle for the lindane, and a disturbed cutaneous integrity all enhance dermal penetration.[88] Additionally, occlusive clothing or bandages substantially increases absorption, as does application to abraded or irritated skin,[87] or to skin affected by dermatoses. The state of hydration of the skin also affects the amounts absorbed, so that bathing just prior to application can enhance absorption and increase the likelihood of toxicity.[56,87] Lindane is a stable compound, and volatilizes easily when heated. It was used extensively in the past in home vaporizers, and toxicity was common via inhalation, as well as when these tablets were unintentionally ingested by children.[18] Review of data when lindane was ingested therapeutically as an anthelmintic demonstrates that 40 mg/d for 3–14 days often produced no symptoms.[18] An epidemic of lindane poisoning related to the unintentional substitution of lindane powder for sugar in coffee demonstrated a delay of 20 minutes to 3 hours before the onset of nausea, vomiting, dizziness, facial pallor, severe cyanosis of the face and extremities, collapse, convulsions, and hyperthermia. Affected patients ingested an average of 86 mg/kg of lindane in a single dose.[18]

Mirex and chlordecone are efficiently absorbed via skin, by inhalation, and orally.[27]

Distribution. All organochlorines are lipophilic, a property that allows penetration to their sites of action in the nerves of both target and nontarget species.[13] The fat-to-serum ratios at equilibrium are high, in the range of 660:1 for chlordane;[35] 220:1 for lindane;[81] and 150:1 for dieldrin.[19] Central nervous system redistribution of the organochlorines to the blood and then to fat may account for the apparent rapid CNS recovery in spite of the persistent substantial total body burden. In the rat model, there is a relationship between the concentration of DDT or dieldrin in the brain and the clinical signs produced after a single dose of the insecticide.[18,22]

Serum lindane levels peak at 6 hours, and have a half-life of 18 hours after topical application.[29]

Metabolism. The high lipid solubility and very slow metabolic disposition of DDT, DDE (metabolite of DDT), dieldrin, heptachlor, chlordane, mirex, and chlordecone causes significant adipose tissue storage and increasing body burdens in chronically exposed populations.[27,72] Organochlorines that are rapidly metabolized and eliminated, such as endrin (an isomer of dieldrin), endosulfan, lindane, methoxychlor, dienochlor, chlorbenzilate, dicofol, and toxaphene tend to have less persistence in body tissues, despite being highly lipid soluble.[72]

Most organochlorines are metabolized by the hepatic microsomal enzyme systems. They are dechlorinated, oxidized, and then conjugated. However, metabolism may result in the production of a more toxic metabolite, such as heptachlor to heptachlor epoxide, chlordane to oxychlordane, and aldrin to dieldrin.

Animal studies show that most organochlorine pesticides are capable of inducing the hepatic microsomal enzyme systems.[17,81,104] Enzyme induction has led to changes in biodegradation of the pesticide in rodents,[93] and in certain animal models the acute toxicity of organic phosphorus compounds and carbamates may be reduced by the administration of organochlorines. This protective effect is presumably induced by the hepatic microsomal metabolism of the organic phosphorus compound because administering piperonyl butoxide, an inhibitor of the liver microsomal enzyme system, can block it.[18,104] However, induction of hepatic enzymes has not been described in man, except in rare cases of massive exposure that had concomitant neurologic findings.[27,35]

Elimination. The elimination half-life of lindane is 21 hours in adults. Because of its rapid metabolism, it does not seem to bioaccumulate in tissues.[57] The half-lives of fat-stored compounds such as DDT and chlordecone are measured in months or years. The primary route of excretion of the organochlorines is in the bile, but most also have detectable urinary metabolites. However, as with other compounds excreted in bile, most of the organochlorines have significant enterohepatic recirculation. There are also significant enterohepatic and enteroenteric recirculations of mirex and chlordecone.[8,15,27] All of these lipophilic toxins are excreted in maternal milk.[73]

Mechanisms of Toxicity

The same neurotoxic properties that make the organochlorines lethal to the target insects make them potentially toxic to higher animals. The organochlorines exert their effects in various areas of the nervous system, most importantly in the CNS.[26] Electrophysiologic studies demonstrate that the organochlorine insecticides affect the neuronal membrane by either interfering with repolarization, by prolonging depolarization, or by impairing the maintenance of the polarized state of the neuron. The end result is hyperexcitability of the nervous system and repetitive neuronal discharges.

DDT primarily affects the axon, by causing the voltage-dependent Na^+ channels to remain open after depolarization, allowing repetitive action potentials to travel down the axon.[60,89] Low-level stimuli cause exaggerated responses, seen clinically as prominent tremors and abnormal startle reflexes in test animals.[41,98] Evidence of this mechanism of action is the amelioration of DDT-induced tremor by pretreatment with phenytoin, a sodium channel blocker, which reduces the ability of voltage-dependent Na^+ channels to recover from inactivation.[42,97]

The cyclodienes and lindane are γ-aminobutyric acid (GABA) antagonists. They inhibit the $GABA_A$-dependent chloride channels at the GABA-receptor-chloride ionophore complex in the CNS by interacting at the picrotoxinin binding site.[1,5,16,30,34,37,61,67] In fact, the degree of binding at this site correlates well with the amount of Cl^- influx inhibited and the relative neurotoxicity of each insecticide[6,34] (see graphic of $GABA_A$ receptor [Figs. 10–9, 10–10, and 89–2]). Indeed, development of cyclodiene resistance seems to be related to alterations of the $GABA_A$ receptor in these affected insects.[7,59] This also explains the efficacy of GABA agonists, such as benzodiazepines and phenobarbital, in treating the seizures and neurotoxicity of the cyclodienes[38] and lindane.[105] Similarly, toxaphene seems to exert its principal toxicity by inhibiting the $GABA_A$ receptor-chloride ionophore complex.[80]

The mechanisms of action of mirex and chlordecone are not as well understood. They appear to inhibit the Na^+,K^+-ATPase, as well as the Ca^{+2}-ATPase "pumps." However, lindane, DDT, and the cyclodienes also inhibit these enzymes yet have very different symptoms of toxicity. Phenytoin and serotonin agonists exacerbate the prominent tremor seen with chlordecone intoxication, but conversely attenuate the tremors in DDT poisoning.[27] Mirex and chlordecone are poor inhibitors of the GABA-dependent chloride

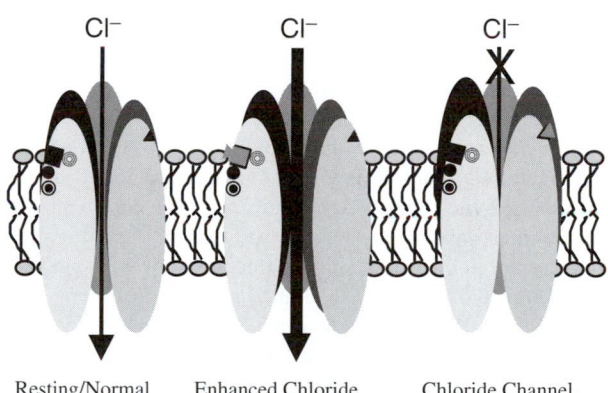

$GABA_A$ chloride channel complex

Resting/Normal   Enhanced Chloride Channel Opening   Chloride Channel Closed

◎ Benzodiazepine binding site
● Barbiturate binding site
◉ Volatile anesthetics binding site
◀ Picrotoxin binding site
■ GABA binding site
◀ Picrotoxin, also lindane, cyclodienes
▣ GABA

Figure 89–2. Chloride channel. Under resting conditions, a tonic influx of chloride maintains the nerve cell in a polarized state. Binding of GABA or an indirect acting GABA agonist (benzodiazepine, barbiturate, volatile anesthetic) opens the chloride channel. The subsequent chloride influx hyperpolarizes the cell membrane, making the neuron less likely to propagate an action potential in response to a stimulus. GABA antagonists, such as picrotoxin, close the chloride channel reducing chloride influx. The resulting decreased membrane polarity causes the neuron to become hyperexcitable to even to those stimuli that are normally subthreshold in nature. For a further discussion of the chloride channel see Chap. 10.

channel, suggesting that their mechanism of action is not at this site.[6] Seizures have not been described with mirex or chlordecone.

Organochlorines cause sensitization of the myocardium to endogenous catecholamines and predispose test animals to dysrhythmias, presumably in a fashion similar to the chlorinated hydrocarbon solvents (Chap. 86).[72]

Drug Interactions

There are theoretical consequences of liver enzyme induction, such as enhanced metabolism of therapeutic drugs and/or reduced efficacy. Dysfunctional uterine bleeding was attributed to enhanced oral contraceptive metabolism induced by chlordane, but this was in a single patient with weeks of excessive exposure to chlordane.[35] A large group of workers poisoned by chlordecone over many months had some increased hepatic microsomal activity, but no evidence of drug interactions or adverse clinical effects.[27] Thus, induction of the hepatic microsomal enzyme system by organochlorines probably occurs only with extended, heavy exposure.[72] There are no definitive reports of enhanced metabolism of therapeutic drugs or adverse reactions because of microsomal enzyme induction in man.

Laboratory Testing

Blood levels document exposure, but may have no other clinical value, and are not readily available. Most humans studied have measurable levels of DDT in adipose tissue. In a study of a community with a very large exposure to DDT, serum DDT levels continued to increase with age. These increasing levels were not associated with any apparent adverse health effects, but were associated with increasing levels of the liver enzyme GGT.[50] In a group of factory workers with a prolonged exposure to chlordecone, clinical signs and symptoms of toxicity seemed to correlate with blood levels.[15] Again serum lindane levels document exposure, and most laboratories report toxic ranges. Lindane-exposed workers with chronic neurologic symptoms showed a blood lindane level of 0.02 mg/L.[3,39] A limited series of acute oral ingestions suggests that a serum level of 0.12 mg/L correlates with sedation, and that 0.20 mg/L is associated with seizures and coma.[3] However, after cutaneous application, lindane levels in the CNS–the site of its major toxic effect–are 3–12 times higher than serum levels.[24,87]

Clinical Manifestations

Acute Exposure. In sufficient doses, organochlorine pesticides lower the seizure threshold and produce CNS stimulation, with resultant seizures, respiratory failure, and death.[4,11,14,25,37,38,46,47,74,76] In the case of DDT, tremor may be the only initial manifestation. Nausea, vomiting, hyperesthesia of the mouth and face, paresthesias of face, tongue, and extremities, headache, dizziness, myoclonus, leg weakness, agitation, and confusion may subsequently occur. Seizures only occur after high doses.[25,38,47] However, with lindane, the cyclodienes, and toxaphene, there often are no prodromal signs or symptoms, and more often than not, the first manifestation of toxicity is a generalized seizure.[4,11,25,26,38,47,74,91] If seizures develop, they often occur within 1–2 hours of ingestion when the stomach is empty, but may be delayed as much as 5–6 hours when the ingestion follows a substantial meal.[38]

Seizures related to dermal application of 1% lindane for treatment of ectoparasitic diseases may occur following a single inappropriate application,[52,68,95] or, more commonly, after repetitive prolonged exposures.[48,70] The time from application to seizure onset can vary from hours to days. The seizures are often self-limited, but may recur and result in status epilepticus.

The cyclodienes are notable for their propensity to cause seizures for several days following an acute exposure. If the seizures are brief and hypoxia has not occurred, recovery is usually complete. Electroencephalographic (EEG) abnormalities have been recorded before, during, and sometimes following seizures.[47] Fever secondary to central mechanisms, increased muscle activity, and/or aspiration pneumonitis is common.[26]

The ingestion of combinations of agents may result in significantly increased toxicity because of synergy. This has been demonstrated for DDT and lindane.[39] Single, acute, oral doses of 10 mg/kg or more of DDT are usually necessary to produce symptoms.[38]

Risks of Toxicity from Therapeutic Use of Lindane. Patients are at risk for developing central nervous system toxicity caused by 1% lindane from improper topical therapeutic use such as exceeding recommended application times or amounts, repeated applications, application following hot baths, and use of occlusive dressings or clothing after application. Toxicity also occurs after unintentional oral ingestion, as the illustrative case in this chapter demonstrates. Rarely, toxicity occurs after proper therapeutic use.[3,20,29,48,52,63,68,70,88,94,95]

An evaluation of published English-language case reports and those submitted to the Food and Drug Administration divided toxicity into those associated with concentrations of lindane greater than or less than 1%.[48] Only 6 of 26 cases could be considered probably related to 1% lindane; 4 of these 6 cases were secondary to ingestion or inappropriate skin application.

Young children appear at greatest risk, possibly because of greater skin permeability, increased ratio of body surface area to mass, immature liver enzymes, and oral absorption from licking the skin. Impaired hepatic metabolism may be contributory.[39] The elderly may also be at risk. Three of 19 elderly patients treated topically with 1% lindane developed a single seizure of 5–10 minutes duration within 4–5 days of application.[95] Although it was not recommended, all of the patients received a hot bath prior to lindane application, and they may have been given up to twice the recommended dose. This combined with atrophic skin, a generalized dermatitis in one patient, and perhaps an age-related increased sensitivity, may have predisposed these patients to seizures.

Patients with preexisting conditions making them more prone to seizures may be at risk of developing toxicity from therapeutic use. This includes chlorpromazine treatment, CNS disease, skin absorption changes, bathing just prior to and dressing immediately after application.[87]

Chronic Exposure. Chlordecone, unlike the other organochlorines, produces an insidious picture of chronic toxicity related to its extremely long persistence in the body. Because of poor industrial hygiene practices in a makeshift chlordecone factory in Hopewell, VA, 133 workers were heavily exposed for 17 months in 1974–1975. They developed toxicity, which became known as the "Hopewell epidemic," and consisted of a constellation of symptoms, most notably a prominent tremor of the hands, but also a fine tremor of the head and trembling of the entire body, known as the "Kepone Shakes." Other symptoms included weakness, opsoclonus (rapid, irregular, dysrrhythmic ocular movements), ataxia, mental status changes, rash, weight loss, and elevated liver enzymes.[27] Pseudotumor cerebri, oligospermia, and decreased sperm motility were also found in these factory workers.[15] Severely affected workers even exhibited an exaggerated startle response, remarkably similar to that seen in animal studies.[27] The exposures were so intense that some workers went home covered with chlordecone, and several workers' wives developed neurologic symptoms, presumably from exposures while laundering their husbands' work clothes.

Organochlorines and Breast Cancer.

DDT and other organochlorine insecticides were shown to have estrogenic effects in several assays.[21,90] These environmental estrogenic compounds adversely affect birds because differentiation of the avian reproductive system is estrogen dependent.[32] Breast cancer incidence rates in the United States have steadily climbed 1% per year since the 1940s, coinciding with the worldwide use of DDT. Because lifetime exposure to excess estrogen is a known risk factor for human breast cancer, women who have higher levels of estrogenic organochlorines may be at risk for developing breast cancer.[78,79,107]

Several small case-control studies of women with breast cancer showed that women with the disease had higher average body burdens of DDT, DDE, and polychlorinated biphenyls (PCBs) than their age-matched controls. These studies implicated the organochlorines as a cause of human breast cancer. However, more recently, larger studies have shown no increased risk of breast cancer due to exposure to organochlorines, and that currently accepted hereditary and lifestyle risk factors were present in the patients with cancer.[44,49,77,78] In addition, other natural dietary estrogens such as flavenoids, ligans, sterols, and fungal metabolites are present in the human diet, and the organochlorine contribution is probably minimal by comparison.[33]

Some reports suggest an association between long-term exposure to organochlorine pesticides and aplastic anemia.[71,75] Chlordane and heptachlor exposures are weakly associated with leukemias and drug-induced thrombocytopenic purpura.[38] The organochlorines can induce liver tumors in mice, but have not been shown to do so in rats or hamsters.[39] There is no convincing evidence that any of these agents are carcinogenic in humans. Workers heavily exposed to DDT and dieldrin do not have an increased incidence of neoplasms.[39] Epidemiologic evidence suggests that the incidence of deaths from liver cancer has steadily decreased since 1930, which includes the more than 50 years since the introduction of the organochlorines.[38] There is some evidence that DDT can be a facilitator of carcinogenesis induced by other agents, such as aflatoxin, and that chlordane may have the same facilitative character with regard to diethylnitrosamine.[38] A recent comprehensive review found no evidence of human cancer risk from exposure to aldrin or dieldrin.[92]

Diagnostic Clues

The history of exposure to an organochlorine pesticide is the most critical piece of information, because exposure is otherwise rare. By law, the package label of these products must list the ingredients, the concentrations, and the vehicle. The EPA-registered use of the insecticide may be helpful in determining which agent is involved (Table 89–2). The presence of an unusual odor in the mouth, in the vomitus, or on the skin may be helpful. Toxaphene,

TABLE 89–2. Common Household Pesticides

Pest	Usual Recommendation
Ants	Baygon, bendiocarb, chlorpyrifos, diazinon, permethrin, resmethrin, silica gel-pyrethrum, baits containing boric acid
Bedbugs	Permethrin
Cockroaches	Baygon, bendiocarb, chlorpyrifos, diazinon, permethrin, resmethrin, silica gel pyrethrum, tetramethrin, boric acid
Fleas	Baygon, bendiocarb, chlorpyrifos, d-limonene, permethrin, pyrethrins, silica gel pyrethrum, resmethrin, tetramethrin
Flies (house)	Allethrin, pyrethrum, resmethrin, tetramethrin
Mosquitoes	Allethrin, pyrethrum, pyrethrins, resmethrin, tetramethrin
Silverfish	Baygon, bendiocarb, boric acid, chlorpyrifos, diazinon, silca gel pyrethrum
Spiders	Baygon, bendiocarb, chlorpyrifos, diazinon, permethrin, pyrethrins, resmethrin, tetramethrin
Termites	Effective pesticides restricted in use for application by certified applicators
Ticks	Baygon, chlorpyrifos, diazinon, malathion, tetramethrin

Reproduced, with permission, from Guide to Safe Pest Management Around the Home. New York State College of Agriculture and Life Sciences of Cornell University, 1997/1998, Misc Bull 74 Media Services at Cornell University.

a chlorinated pinene, has a mild turpentinelike odor, and endosulfan has a unique "rotten egg" sulfur odor (see Table 89–1). An abdominal radiograph may reveal the presence of a radiopaque chlorinated pesticide, because radiopacity may correlate with the number of chlorine atoms per molecule (Chap. 8).[23] A large number of other toxins lead to seizures as the first manifestation of toxicity, and must be considered in the differential of an unknown exposure (Chaps. 10 and 19).

Laboratory Tests

Gas chromatography can detect organochlorine pesticides in serum, adipose tissue, and urine.[19,44] If confirmation is necessary for legal purposes, it may be necessary to measure concentrations of organochlorines. If the patient's history and toxidrome are obvious, then laboratory evaluation is unnecessary, as this determination will not alter the course of management, and these blood tests are not available on an emergent basis. At present, there are no data correlating health effects and tissue concentrations. Routine surveillance of serum levels in the occupationally exposed is not currently performed.[19]

Management

Organochlorine poisoning may result in hypoxia secondary to seizures, aspiration of vomitus, or respiratory failure. Hyperthermia as a consequence of seizures or from a central mechanism may occur. As with any patient who presents with an altered mental status, dextrose and thiamine should be administered. Skin decontamination is essential, especially in the case of topical lindane. Clothing should be removed and placed in a plastic bag and the skin washed with soap and water. Healthcare providers should be protected with rubber gloves and aprons. Because these pesticides are almost invariably liquids, a nasogastric tube can be used to suction and lavage gastric contents. This is most appropriate if the ingestion occurred within several hours. Activated charcoal can be used after or instead of gastric lavage, when lavage is not indicated.[38,56] The ability of activated charcoal to bind various organochlorines has never been adequately studied. A murine model of lindane toxicity following intragastric administration showed a trend, but not a statistically significant benefit, of activated charcoal.[45] The use of cholestyramine, a nonabsorbable bile acid-binding anion exchange resin, in the same murine model did show a statistically significant benefit by raising both the convulsive dose and the lethal dose.[45] The doses of activated charcoal or cholestyramine were 2.25 g/kg, or about 12–28 times the lethal and convulsive doses of lindane, respectively. Oil-based cathartics should never be used, as they may facilitate absorption.

Seizures should be controlled with a benzodiazepine followed by phenobarbital if further intervention is indicated. Phenytoin is probably less effective in these cases, particularly with the GABA antagonists lindane, toxaphene, and the cyclodienes.[52,80,97] If these measures are inadequate, more aggressive measures should be instituted rapidly, such as a pentobarbital infusion and, if necessary, neuromuscular blockade to control the peripheral manifestations of seizures, thereby preventing metabolic acidosis and rhabdomyolysis. Hyperthermia should be managed aggressively with external cooling.

Cholestyramine should be administered to all patients symptomatic from chlordecone, and possibly other organochlorines. Chlordecone undergoes both enterohepatic and enteroenteric recirculation, which can be interrupted by cholestyramine at a dosage of 16 g/d.[15] Cholestyramine increased the fecal elimination of chlordecone 3–18-fold in industrial workers exposed during the Hopewell epidemic.[15] The extent of toxicity appears to be related to the tissue levels of chlordecone and improves following cholestyramine therapy.

PYRETHRINS AND PYRETHROIDS

The pyrethrins are the active extracts from the flower *Chrysanthemum cinerariaefolium*. These insecticides are important historically, having been used in China since the 1st century AD,[18] and developed for commercial application by the 1800s. They are produced by organic solvent extraction from ground Chrysanthemum flowers. The resulting concentrates have greater than 90% purity. Pyrethrum, the first pyrethrin identified, consists of 6 esters derived from chrysanthemic acid and pyrethric acid. These insecticides are highly effective contact poisons, and their lipophilic nature allows them to readily penetrate insect chitin (exoskeleton), and paralyze their nervous systems through Na^+ channel blockade.[13,59,72,89] When applied properly, they have essentially no systemic mammalian toxicity because of their rapid hydrolysis. Pyrethrins break down rapidly in light and in water, and therefore have no environmental persistence or bioaccumulation. This fact makes them expensive to use, as they must be constantly reapplied.

The pyrethroids are the synthetic derivatives of the natural pyrethrins (see Table 89–3 and Fig. 89–3). They were developed in an effort to produce more environmentally stable products. The development of the pyrethroids can be divided into "generations," based on efficacy and dates of introduction.[102] The first generation began in 1949, with the development of allethrin. The second generation began in 1965, with the introduction of tetramethrin. The major advance of the second generation was pyrethroids with potencies many times that of the pyrethrins. The third generation, introduced in the 1970s and including fenvalerate and permethrin, were the first pyrethroids with practical agricultural use. They

TABLE 89–3. Synthetic Pyrethroids

Class	Generic Name, CAS #	Brand Names
Type I*	Allethrin 584-79-2	Pynamin
	Bioallethrin 584-79-2	D-trans
	Dimethrin 70-38-2	Dimetrin
	Phenothrin 26002-80-2	Fenothrin, Forte, Sumithrin
	Resmethrin 10453-86-8	Benzofluroline, Chrysron, Crossfire, Premgard, Pynosect, Pyretherm, Synthrin,
	Bioresmethrin 28434-01-7	
	Tetramethrin 7696-12-0	Neo-Pynamin
	Permethrin 52645-53-1	Ambush, Biomist, Dragnet, Ectiban, Elimite, Ipitox, Ketokill, Nix, Outflank, Perigen, Permasect, Persect, Pertox, Pounce, Pramex, etc
	Bifenthrin 82657-04-3	Capture, Talstar
	Prallethrin 23031-36-9	SF, Etoc
	Imiprothrin 72963-72-5	Multicide, Pralle, Raid Ant & Roach
Type II	Fenvalerate 51630-58-1	Belmark, Evercide, Extrin, Fenkill, Sanmarton, Sumicidin, Sumifly, Sumipower, Sumitox, Tribute
	Acrinathrin 103833-18-7	Rufast
	Cyfluthrin 68359-37-5	Baythroid, Bulldock, Cyfoxylate, Eulan SP, Solfac, Tempo 2
	Cyhalothrin 91465-08-6	Demand, Karate, Ninja 10WP, Scimitar, Warrior
	Cypermethrin 52315-07-8	Ammo, Barricade, CCN52, Cymbush, Cymperator, Cynoff, Cypercopal; Cyperkill, Cyrux, Demon, Flectron, KafilSuper, Ripcord, Siperin, others
	Deltamethrin 52918-63-5	Butoflin, Butox, Crackdown, Decis, DeltaDust, DeltaGard, Deltex, K-Othrine, Striker, Suspend
	Esfenvalerate 66230-04-4	Asana, Asana-XL, Sumi-alpha,
	Fenpropathrin 39515-41-8	Danitol, Herald, Meothrin, Rody
	Flucythrinate 70124-77-5	AASTAR, Cybolt, Fluent, Payoff
	Fluvalinate 102851-06-9	Evict, Fireban, Force, Mavrik, Raze, Yardex
	Tefluthrin 19538-32-2	Demand, Force, Karate, Scimitar
	Tralomethrin 66841-25-6	Dethmor, SAGA, Scout, Scout X-tra, Tralex

*These agents are listed in their approximate order of introduction and potency.

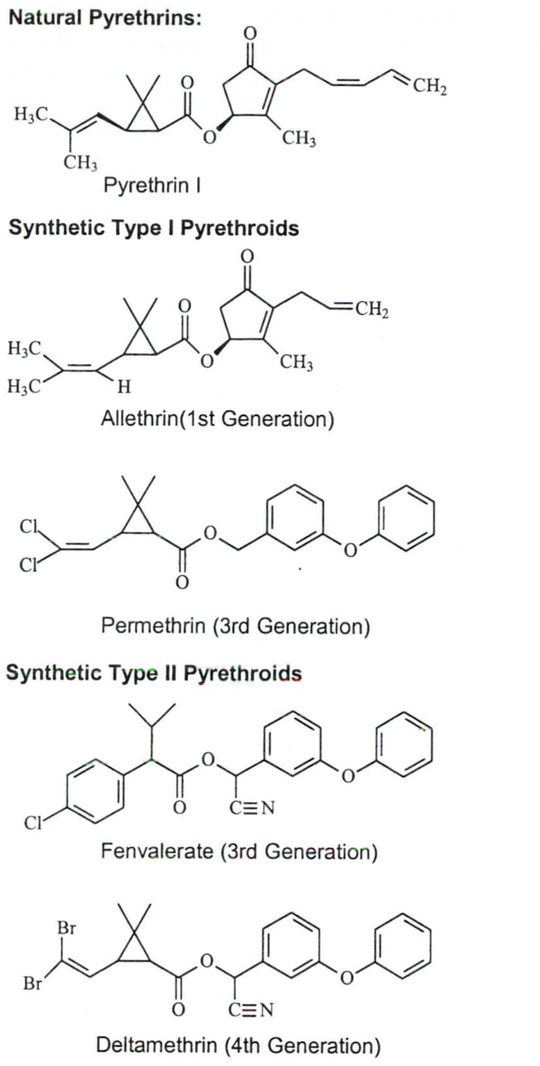

Natural Pyrethrins:

Pyrethrin I

Synthetic Type I Pyrethroids

Allethrin(1st Generation)

Permethrin (3rd Generation)

Synthetic Type II Pyrethroids

Fenvalerate (3rd Generation)

Deltamethrin (4th Generation)

Figure 89–3. Representative structures of Pyrethrin and Pyrethroids.

were more potent, as well as more environmentally stable, with efficacious crop residues lasting 4–7 days. The current fourth generation includes mostly type II pyrethroids, which have even greater insecticidal activity, as well as environmental stability for nearly 10 days after application.[55,102]

There are more than 1000 pyrethroids, of which 6–10 are in widespread use today.[18,26,66] Pyrethrins and pyrethroids are found in more than 2000 commercially available products. These insecticides have a rapid paralytic effect ("knock down") on insects. Most mammalian species are relatively resistant, because the pyrethrins can be rapidly detoxified by ester cleavage and oxidation.[66] Toxicity of the pyrethrins and pyrethroids is enhanced in insects by combination with synergists such as piperonyl butoxide or *N*-octyl bicycloheptene dicarboximide, which inhibit microsomal enzymes and further impairs the capacity of the insect to metabolize the pyrethrins.

The pyrethroids can be divided into two types based on their structures and their clinical manifestations in overdose. Type I

pyrethroids (permethrin, allethrin, tetramethrin, fenothrin) lack a cyano group, whereas the type II agents (cypermethrin, deltamethrin, fenpropathrin, fluvalinate, fenvalerate) have a cyano group at the ester linkage, and are generally more potent and toxic than the type I pyrethroids (see Fig. 89–3).[26,55,72]

Permethrin (Elimite, Nix), a type I pyrethroid, is used medicinally for topical treatment of ectoparasitic conditions in humans, as well as impregnated in clothing for its insect repellant properties. There have been no seizures or other serious toxicities with permethrin. Because of its excellent safety profile, permethrin may well replace lindane (Kwell) as the drug of choice for these conditions.

During the summer of 2000, the identification of West Nile virus in dead birds throughout New York State led to pesticide spraying for mosquito control in various counties. Fourteen human West Nile virus cases were diagnosed in the New York City area. The primary pesticides used for mosquito control efforts were pyrethroids, which included sumithrin (Anvil) and resmethrin (Scourge). Preliminary review of surveillance data did not reveal any indications of fatalities or widespread acute health effects from these pesticide applications. More detailed review of the data is ongoing (personal communication, Matthew P. Mauer, DO, MPH; NYS Department of Health, Bureau of Occupational Health; January 19, 2001).

Toxicokinetics

The oral toxicity of pyrethrins in mammals is extremely low, because they are so readily hydrolyzed into inactive compounds, and therefore have an extremely high LD_{50} in humans. Their dermal toxicity is even lower, owing to their slow penetration and rapid metabolism.[26,66]

The pyrethroids are more stable than the natural pyrethrins, and systemic absorption by the oral route resulting in toxicity has occurred.[40] Absorption probably also occurs through the oral mucosa, as noted by a large study of Chinese insecticide sprayers who frequently used their mouths to clear clogged spray nozzles.[12] Most exposures are from dermal absorption, the rate of which may vary depending on the solvent vehicle. Direct absorption of pyrethroids through the skin to the peripheral sensory nerves probably accounts for the facial paresthesias that occur in these cases, as symptoms were prominent in areas of direct contact.[12,53] The pyrethroids are also absorbed via inhalation; however, in this same large study of sprayers, inhalation was not found to be a clinically significant route of exposure by breathing zone assays.[12]

The pyrethroids and pyrethrins are lipophilic and as such are rapidly distributed to the site of toxicity, the central nervous system.[26] Because they are rapidly metabolized, there is no storage or bioaccumulation, and this limits chronic toxicity.[25] There is no evidence of enterohepatic recirculation.

The microsomal monooxygenase system efficiently detoxifies the pyrethroids in animals and man. Piperonyl butoxide, a monooxygenase inhibitor, acts as a synergist to enhance the potency of pyrethroids 10–300-fold to target insects. It is often added to ensure lethality, as the initial "knock down" effect of a pyrethroid alone is not always lethal to the insect.[25]

Parent compounds, as well as metabolites of the pyrethroids, are found in the urine.[72] Deltamethrin disappeared from the urine of exposed workers within 12 hours, and fenvalerate disappeared within 24 hours.[12]

Pathophysiology

Like DDT, pyrethrins and pyrethroids prolong the inactivation of the voltage-dependent sodium channel by binding to it in the open state, causing a prolonged depolarization[30,59,60] (Chap. 10). Type I pyrethroids induce repetitive discharges more readily than type II, but type II agents cause the Na^+ channel to remain open longer, and allow a greater degree of depolarization.[89,101] Type II agents are thus more potent, and lead to significant after-potentials, which can produce repetitive depolarizations and eventual nerve conduction block. Some studies show some interference of the type II agents with the GABA-mediated inhibitory chloride channels, but only in high concentrations.[13,59] It is now generally accepted that suppression of the GABA chloride channels has no significant role in pyrethroid toxicity.[59] Type I pyrethroids have a negative temperature coefficient, similar to DDT, and are more selectively toxic to nonwarm-blooded target species. Type II agents have a positive temperature coefficient, which makes them more insecticidal at higher ambient temperatures.[102] However, this property partly explains the greater mammalian toxicity of type II agents as compared to type I.[59]

Clinical Manifestations

Pyrethrum has an LD_{50} of well over 1 g/kg in man, extrapolated from animal data. Most cases of toxicity associated with the pyrethrins are the result of allergic reactions.[66,103] At highest risk are patients who are sensitive to ragweed pollen, 50% of whom may cross-react with chrysanthemums (ragweed and chrysanthemum are in the same botanical genus). These allergic reactions actually may result from other natural components present in the extracts.[72] The synthetic pyrethroids generally do not induce allergic reactions.[66]

In animals, type I pyrethroid poisoning most closely resembles that of DDT, with extensive tremors, twitching, increased metabolic rate, and hyperthermia. Excluding the rare possibility of skin irritation or allergy, the type I agents are unlikely to cause systemic toxicity in humans. The type II agents are generally more potent, and cause profuse salivation, ataxia, coarse tremor, choreoathetosis, and seizures in animals. In humans, type II agents cause paresthesias (secondary to sodium channel effects in sensory nerves), salivation, nausea, vomiting, dizziness, fasciculations, altered mental status, coma, seizures, and pulmonary edema.[40,53] A review of more than 500 cases of acute pyrethroid poisoning from China highlights some similar manifestations between a massive acute type II pyrethroid overdose and an organic phosphorus compound overdose.[40] However, serious atropine toxicity and death has resulted when poisoning from a type II pyrethroid was mistaken for an organic phosphorus compound, and treatment was directed at these seemingly cholinergic signs.[40] Although the type II agents contain a cyanide moiety, cyanide poisoning does not occur and cyanide antidotal therapy is not indicated.

Treatment

Initial treatment should be directed toward skin decontamination, as most poisonings occur from exposures by this route. Patients with large oral ingestions of a type II pyrethroid should be treated with a single standard dose of activated charcoal. Contact dermatitis and acute systemic allergic reactions should be treated in the usual manner, utilizing corticosteroids, β-adrenergic agonists, and epinephrine as clinically indicated.

Treatment of systemic toxicity is entirely supportive and symptomatic, because no specific antidote exists. Benzodiazepines should be used for tremor and seizures. Topical vitamin E oil (dl-α-tocopheryl) is especially effective in preventing and treating the cutaneous paresthesias seen in these exposures.[18,66]

DEET

The topical insect repellant, N,N-diethyl-3-methylbenzamide (DEET, former nomenclature N,N-diethyl-m-toluamide), was patented by the US Army in 1946, and marketed in the United States since 1956. Currently, it is used worldwide by more than 200 million persons annually. The EPA estimates that 38% of the US population uses DEET each year.

It can be purchased without prescription in concentrations ranging from 5% to 100%, and in multiple formulations of solutions, creams, lotions, gels, and aerosol sprays. DEET seems to repel insects by interfering with the chemoreceptors that attract the insects to their hosts.[30]

Toxicokinetics

DEET is extensively absorbed via the gastrointestinal tract.[69] Skin absorption is significant, depending on the vehicle and the concentration. It does not bind to stratum corneum, and only 0.08% or less of a dose remains in the skin 8 hours after application.[69] DEET is lipophilic, and skin absorption usually occurs within 2 hours, although it is eliminated from plasma within 4 hours. The volume of distribution is large, in the range of 2.7–6.21 L/kg in animal studies. DEET is extensively metabolized by oxidation and hydroxylation by the hepatic microsomal enzymes. DEET is excreted in the urine within 12 hours, mainly as metabolites, with 15% or less appearing as the parent compound.[30,69]

Pathophysiology

The exact mechanism of DEET toxicity is unknown. A recent review of adverse reactions to DEET showed 26 cases had major morbidity including N, encephalopathy, ataxia, convulsions, respiratory failure, hypotension, anaphylaxis or death, particularly after ingestion or dermal exposure to large amounts.[30,62,64,96,99] These primarily neurologic adverse reactions occurred mainly in children, and most involved prolonged use and excessive dosing beyond what is currently recommended. One fatal case involved a child who was known to be heterozygous for ornithine carbamoyl transferase (OCT) deficiency, and death was due to a Reyelike syndrome with hyperammonemia. This child had experienced prior episodes of hyperammonemia unrelated to DEET use, and DEET does not appear to affect OCT activity in humans.[65] There is currently no evidence that enzyme polymorphism affects DEET metabolism or influences individual susceptibility to toxicity.

Although single, large, acute oral doses (1–3 g/kg) in rats produced seizures and CNS damage,[100] smaller acute doses (500 mg/kg and less) and chronic multigenerational dosing in another rat study produced no obvious toxicity.[82] Teratogenicity studies in rats and rabbits fail to demonstrate toxicity except at the highest doses,[83,106] and DEET was not found to be carcinogenic.[84] In view of the millions of applications, the number of reports of toxicity appears exceedingly small, and suggests a remarkably wide margin of safety.[30,36,69,65]

Clinical Manifestations

Most calls to poison control centers regarding DEET exposures involve minor or no symptoms, and symptomatic exposures occur primarily when DEET is sprayed in the eyes or inhaled.[99] Except for suicidal ingestions, most serious reactions consist of seizures in children overexposed via the dermal route; in fact, some of these cannot be definitely attributed to DEET.[36,65] Most symptoms resolve without treatment and the majority of the cases of serious toxicity recover fully with supportive care.

Treatment

DEET poisonings are treated with supportive care aimed at the primarily neurologic symptoms. In cases of dermal exposures skin decontamination should be a priority to prevent further absorption. Oral ingestions should receive a single dose of activated charcoal if clinically indicated.

Avoiding the overuse of DEET seems prudent. The American Academy of Pediatrics recommends DEET concentrations of 10% or less for use on children,[85] and most commercial formulations marketed for use on children are approximately 5–7%. One application lasts 4–6 hours or more, so frequent reapplication is unnecessary. Soaking the skin is not more effective and may contribute to toxicity. DEET should be applied only to exposed skin. One should avoid abraded skin, or skin with rashes. Care should be taken to avoid exposure to eyes and sensitive skin areas. Avoid use on children's hands, so that the child does not wipe on eyes, mouth, genitalia, and so on. Adults should apply DEET to their own hands and then wipe onto the child's face, rather than spraying onto a child's face. Because mosquitoes are most active for a few hours preceding and following dusk, DEET should be promptly washed off the child's skin when protection is no longer needed (ie, after going indoors). Avoid using combination products such as sunscreen mixed with DEET, when the repellant component is not needed. Other options for protection include mechanical means, such as mosquito netting.

INSECTICIDES, DEET, AND THE GULF WAR SYNDROME

During operations Desert Shield/Desert Storm, nearly 700,000 Americans served in the Persian Gulf. Some returning troops began reporting a variety of symptoms and illnesses they attributed initially to exposure to burning oil well fires in Kuwait. Approximately 10% of these veterans, or 67,000, have registered with the Persian Gulf Registry Health Examination Program. This program was initiated to study whether veterans were experiencing adverse health effects related to exposures encountered in the Persian Gulf War. The most common symptoms are largely nonspecific and multiorgan and include fatigue, rashes, headache, muscle aches, memory problems, dyspnea, insomnia, and gastrointestinal (GI) symptoms. Multiple studies and expert panels have been unable to identify a causative agent responsible for this "Persian Gulf syndrome."

Some investigators have suggested that combinations of DEET, permethrin, and pyridostigmine have additive neurotoxic effects and could be a cause of the symptoms.[51] Although there is laboratory evidence of synergy of these agents in causing neurotoxicity in test animals,[2,54] it is difficult to apply this to human experience in the Gulf War. The exposures in the veterans were primarily dermal, except for the pyridostigmine tablets, whereas the experimental animals were either gavaged or injected with the insecticides. In addition, the pyridostigmine was only taken for 2 weeks or less during cooler weather when biting insects were dormant, so concomitant use with permethrin and DEET would have been low. It appears unlikely that these compounds were used together at toxic dosages for any sustained time period. Given the diversity and multisystem nature of symptoms experienced by these veterans, it is unlikely that use of these chemicals is responsible for the illnesses. Further study is ongoing.[58]

LEGAL STANDARDS FOR AN INSECTICIDE LABEL

The Federal Insecticide, Fungicide and Rodenticide Act of 1962 (Table 88–4) established criteria for a "signal word" on an insecticide label, which implies the degree of toxicity based on an oral LD_{50}. Also, the label on the original container of these products is usually instructive and should always be brought to the medical facility. The label provides the following information:

- Brand name
- Intended product use
- Active and inert ingredients and their percent composition
- Directions for use
- Pests to be controlled; crops, animals, or sites to be treated
- Dosage, time interval, and method of application
- Warnings to protect users, consumers of treated foods, beneficial plants, animals, and endangered species
- "Keep out of reach of children"
- Antidotes and first-aid instructions
- Net content
- Name and address of manufacturer
- EPA registration number and signal word based on the LD_{50}

Consumers asking for help in choosing the most effective and safest pesticides should be told to contact their county agricultural or cooperative extension agents. It is important to choose an effective pesticide as well as a product formulated for use in the requisite area (indoors vs outdoors), because concentrations and residues vary. Instructions must always be read carefully and followed, as failure to do so may lead to toxicity (Table 89–4).

SUMMARY

The ideal insecticide is one that has low acute toxicity to humans and nontarget species (pyrethroids, DDT), is inexpensive to apply and produce (organic phosphorus compounds, DDT), but would have no environmental persistence or bioaccumulation (organic phosphorus compounds, pyrethroids). With mass production techniques, some of the newer pyrethroids may come closer to this

TABLE 89–4. Criteria Established by the Federal Insecticide, Fungicide, and Rodenticide Act of 1962

Signal Word	Toxicity	Oral LD$_{50}$ mg/kg
Danger Poison Skull and crossbones figure Call physician immediately Keep out of reach of children	High	0–50
Warning No antidote Keep out of reach of children	Moderate	50–500
Caution No antidote Keep out of reach of children	Low	500–5000
No Signal Word Keep out of reach of children	Relatively safe	> 5000

ideal than those most commonly used today. Until that goal is achieved, the neurotoxic organochlorines will continue to be used. In January 2000, the Associated Press reported that 21 people in Iran were poisoned, and 3 died, when DDT powder was inadvertently used in food preparation instead of flour. Although banned in North America and Europe, organochlorine pesticides are still widely used in other parts of the world, and will have important implications for toxicologists for some time to come.

REFERENCES

1. Abalis IM, Eldefrawi ME, Eldefrawi AT: Effects of insecticides on GABA-induced chloride influx into rat brain microsacs. J Toxicol Environ Health 1986;18:13–23.
2. Abou-Donia M, Wilmarth K, Jensen K, et al: Neurotoxicity resulting from coexposure to pyridostigmine bromide, DEET, and permethrin: Implications of Gulf War chemical exposures. J Toxicol Environ Health 1996;48:35–56.
3. Aks SE, Krantz A, Hryhorczuk DO, et al: Acute accidental lindane ingestion in toddlers. Ann Emerg Med 1995;26:647–651.
4. Anonymous: Acute convulsions with endrin poisoning: Pakistan. Morb Mortal Wkly Rep 1986;33:687–688, 693.
5. Bloomquist JR: Intrinsic lethality of chloride-channel-directed insecticides and convulsants in mammals. Toxic Lett 1992;60:289–298.
6. Bloomquist JR, Adams PM, Soderlund DM: Inhibition of gamma-aminobutyric acid-stimulated chloride flux in mouse brain vesicles by polychlorocycloalkane and pyrethroid insecticides. Neurotoxicology 1986;7:11–20.
7. Bloomquist JR, French-Constant RH, Roush RT: Excitation of central neurons by dieldrin and picrotoxinin in susceptible and resistant *Drosophila melanogaster*. Pesticide Sci 1991;32:463–470.
8. Boylan JJ, Cohn WJ, Egle JL, et al: Excretion of chlordecone by the gastrointestinal tract: Evidence for a nonbiliary mechanism. Clin Pharmacol Ther 1979;25:579–585.
9. Brisson, P: Percutaneous absorption. Can Med Assoc J 1974;110:1182–1185.
10. Carson R: Silent Spring. Boston, Houghton Mifflin Company, 1962.
11. Carvalho WA, Matos GB, Cruz SLB, Rodrigues DS: Human aldrin poisoning. Braz J Med Biol Res 1991;24:883–887.
12. Chen S, Zhang Z, He F, et al: An epidemiological study on occupational acute pyrethroid poisoning in cotton farmers. Br J Ind Med 1991;48:77–81.
13. Coats JR: Mechanisms of toxic action and structure-activity relationships for organochlorine and synthetic pyrethroid insecticides. Environ Health Perspect 1990;87:255–262.
14. Coble Y, Hildebrandt P, Davis J, et al: Acute endrin poisoning. JAMA 1967; 202:153–157.
15. Cohn WJ, Boylan JJ, Blanke RV, et al: Treatment of chlordecone (kepone) toxicity with cholestyramine. N Engl J Med 1978;298:243–248.
16. Cole LM, Casida JE: Polychlorocycloalkane insecticide-induced convulsions in mice in relation to disruption of the GABA-regulated chloride ionophore. Life Sci 1986;39:1855–1862.
17. Conney AH, Welch RM, Kuntzman R, Burns JJ: Effects of pesticides on drug and steroid metabolism. Clin Pharmacol Ther 1966;8:1–10.
18. Costa, LG: Basic Toxicology of pesticides. In: Keifer MC, ed: Occupational Medicine: State of the Art Reviews. Human Health Effects of Pesticides. Philadelphia, Hanley and Belfus, 1997, pp. 251–268.
19. Coye MJ, Lowe JA, Maddy KJ: Biological monitoring of agricultural workers exposed to pesticides: II. Monitoring of intact pesticides and their metabolites. J Occup Med 1986;28:628–636.
20. Crosby AD, D'Andrea GH, Geller RJ: Human effects of veterinary biological products. Vet Hum Toxicol 1986;28:569–571.
21. Cummings AM: Methoxychlor as a model for environmental estrogens. Crit Rev Toxicol 1997;27:367–379.
22. Dale WE, Gaines TB, Hayes WJ: Poisoning by DDT: Relationship between clinical signs and concentrations in rat brain. Science 1963;142:1474–1476.
23. Dally S, Garnier R, Bismuth C: Diagnosis of chlorinated hydrocarbon poisoning by x-ray examination. Br J Ind Med 1987;44:424–425.
24. Davies JE, Dedhia HV, Morgade C, Barquet A, Maibach HI: Lindane poisonings. Arch Dermatol 1983;119:142–144.
25. Ecobichon DJ: Toxic effects of pesticides. In: Klaassen CD, ed: Casarett and Doull's Toxicology: The Basic Science of Poisons, 5th ed. New York, Macmillan, 1996, pp. 643–669.
26. Ecobichon DJ, Joy RM: Pesticides and Neurological Diseases, 2nd ed. Boca Raton, FL, CRC Press, 1994.
27. Faroon O, Kueberuwa S, Smith L, DeRosa C: ATSDR evaluation of health effects of chemicals II. Mirex and chlordecone: Health effects, toxicokinetics, human exposure, and environmental fate. Toxicol Ind Health 1995;11:1–188.
28. Feldmann RJ, Maibach HI: Percutaneous penetration of some pesticides and herbicides in man. Toxicol Appl Pharmacol 1974;28:126–132.
29. Fischer TF: Lindane toxicity in a 24-year-old woman. Ann Emerg Med 1994;24:972–974.
30. Fradin MS: Mosquitoes and mosquito repellents: A clinician's guide. Ann Intern Med 1998;128:931–940.
31. Franz TJ: Kinetics of cutaneous drug penetration. Int J Dermatol 1983;22:499–505.
32. Fry MD: Reproductive effects in birds exposed to pesticides and industrial chemicals. Environ Health Perspect 1995;103:165–171.
33. Gaido K, Dohme L, Wang F, et al: Comparative estrogenic activity of wine extracts and organochlorine pesticide residues in food. Environ Health Perspect 1998;106:1347–1351.
34. Gant D, Eldefrawi ME, Eldefrawi AT: Cyclodiene insecticides inhibit GABA$_A$ receptor-regulated chloride transport. Toxicol Appl Pharmacol 1987;88:313–321.
35. Garrettson LK, Guzelian PS, Blanke RV: Subacute chlordane poisoning. J Toxicol Clin Toxicol 1984–85;22:565–571.
36. Goodyer L, Behrens R: Short report: The safety and toxicity of insect repellents. Am. J Trop Med Hyg 1998;59:323–324.
37. Grutsch JF, Khasuwinah A: Signs and mechanisms of chlordane intoxication. Biomed Environ Sci 1991;4:317–326.
38. Hayes WJ: Chlorinated hydrocarbon insecticides. In: Hayes WJ, Lawes ER, eds: Pesticides Studied in Man. San Diego, Academic Press, 1991, pp. 731–868.

39. Hayes WJ, Lawes ER, eds: Handbook of Pesticide Toxicology. San Diego, Academic Press, 1991.

40. He F, Wang S, Liu L, et al: Clinical manifestations and diagnosis of acute pyrethroid poisoning. Arch Toxicol 1989;63:54–58.

41. Herr DW, Gallus JA, Tilson HA: Pharmacological modification of tremor and enhanced acoustic startle by chlordecone and *p,p'*-DDT. Psychopharmacology 1987;91:320–325.

42. Hong JS, Herr DW, Hudson PM, Tilson HA: Neurochemical effects of DDT in rat brain in vivo. Arch Toxicol 1986;9:14–26.

43. Idson B: Vehicle effects in percutaneous absorption. Drug Metab Rev 1983;14:207–222.

44. Hunter DJ, Hankinson SE, Laden F, et al: Plasma organochlorine levels and the risk of breast cancer. N Engl J Med 1997;337:1253–1258.

45. Kassner JT, Maher TJ, Hull KM, Woolf, AD: Cholestyramine as an adsorbent in acute lindane poisoning: A murine model. Ann Emerg Med 1993;22:1392–1397.

46. Kintz P, Baron L, Tracqui A, et al: A high endrin concentrate in a fatal case. Forensic Sci Int 1992;54:177–180.

47. Klaassen CD: Nonmetallic environmental toxicants. In: Hardman JG, Limbird LE, Molinoff PB, and Ruddon RW, eds. Goodman and Gilman's The Pharmacologic Basis of Therapeutics, 9th ed. New York, McGraw-Hill, 1996, pp. 1684–1699.

48. Kramer MS: Operational criteria for adverse drug reactions in evaluating suspected toxicity of a popular scabicide. Clin Pharmacol Ther 1980;27:149–155.

49. Krieger N, Wolff MS Hiatt RA, et al: Breast cancer and serum organochlorines: A prospective study among white, black, and Asian women. J Natl Cancer Inst 1994;86:589–599.

50. Kriess K, Zack MM, Kimbrough RD, et al: Cross-sectional study of a community with exceptional exposure to DDT. JAMA 1981;245:1926–1930.

51. Kurt TL: Epidemiological association in US veterans between Gulf War illness and exposures to anticholinesterases. Toxicol Lett 1998;102–103, 523–526.

52. Lee B, Groth P: Scabies transcutaneous poisoning during treatment. Pediatrics 1977;59:643.

53. Le Quesne PM, Maxwell IC, Butterworth STG: Transient facial sensory symptoms following exposure to synthetic pyrethroids: A clinical and electrophysiological assessment. Neurotoxicology 1980;2:1–11.

54. McCain WC, Lee R, Johnson MS et al: Acute oral toxicity study of pyridostigmine bromide, permethrin, and DEET in the laboratory rat. J Toxicol Environ Health 1997;50:113–124.

55. Mestres R, Mestres G: Deltamethrin: Uses and environmental safety. Rev Environ Contam Toxicol 1992;124:1–18.

56. Morgan DP, Dotson TB, Lin LI: Effectiveness of activated charcoal, mineral oil, and castor oil in limiting gastrointestinal absorption of a chlorinated hydrocarbon pesticide. Clin Toxicol 1977;11:61–70.

57. Mortensen ML: Management of acute childhood poisonings caused by selected insecticides and herbicides. Pediatr Clin North Am 1986;33:421–445.

58. Murphy FM, ed: A Guide to Gulf War Veterans' Health: 1998 Continuing Medical Education Program. St. Louis, MO, Department of Veterans Affairs, 1998.

59. Narahashi T: Nerve membrane Na+ channels as targets of insecticides. Trends Pharmacol Sci 1992;13:236–241.

60. Narahashi T, Frey JM, Ginsburg KS, Roy ML: Sodium and GABA-activated channels as the targets of pyrethroids and cyclodienes. Toxicol Lett 1992;64/65:429–436.

61. Obata T, Yamamura HI, Malatynska E et al: Modulation of GABA-stimulated chloride influx by bicycloorthocarboxylates, bicyclophosphorus esters, polychlorocycloalkanes and other cage convulsants. J Pharmacol Exp Ther 1988;244:802–806.

62. Oransky S, Roseman B, Fish D, et al: Seizures temporally associated with use of DEET insect repellent—New York and Connecticut. Morb Mortal Wkly Rep 1989;38:678–680.

63. Ortiz Martinez A, Martinez-Conde E: The neurotoxic effects of lindane at acute and subchronic dosages. Ecotoxicol Environ Saf 1995;30:101–105.

64. Osimitz TG, Grothaus RH: The present safety assessment of DEET. J Am Mosq Control Assoc 1995;11:274–278.

65. Osimitz TG, Murphy JV: Neurological effects associated with use of the insect repellent *N,N*-diethyl-*m*-toluamide (DEET). Clin Toxicol 1997;35:435–441.

66. Paton DL, Walker JS: Pyrethrin poisoning from commercial strength flea and tick spray. Am J Emerg Med 1988;6:232–235.

67. Pomes A, Rodriquez-Farre E, Sunol C: Disruption of GABA-dependent chloride flux by cyclodienes and hexachlorocyclohexanes in primary cultures of cortical neurons. J Pharmacol Exp Ther 1994;271:1616–1623.

68. Pramanik A, Hansen R: Transcutaneous gamma benzene hexachloride absorption and toxicity in infants and children. Arch Dermatol 1979;115:1224–1225.

69. Qiu H, Jun HW, McCall JW: Pharmacokinetics, formulation, and safety of insect repellent *N,N*-diethyl-3-methylbenzamide (DEET): A review. J Am Mosq Control Assoc 1998;14:12–27.

70. Rasmussen J: The problem of lindane. J Am Acad Dermatol 1981;3:507–516.

71. Rauch A, Kowalsky S, Lesar T, et al: Lindane (Kwell)-induced aplastic anemia. Arch Intern Med 1990;150:2393–2395.

72. Reigart JR, Roberts JR, eds: Recognition and Management of Pesticide Poisonings, 5th ed. Washington, DC, Environmental Protection Agency, 1999.

73. Rogan WJ: Pollutants in breast milk. Arch Pediatr Adolesc Med 1996;150:981–990.

74. Rowley DL, Rab MA, Hardjutunojo W, et al: Convulsions caused by endrin poisoning in Pakistan. Pediatrics 1987;79:928–934.

75. Rugman FP, Cosstick R: Aplastic anemia associated with organochlorine pesticide: Case reports and review of evidence. J Clin Pathol 1990;43:98–101.

76. Runhaar EA, Sangster B, Greve PA, Voortman M: A case of fatal endrin poisoning. Hum Toxicol 1985;4:241–247.

77. Safe SH: Environmental and dietary estrogens and human health: Is there a problem? Environ Health Perspect 1995;103:346–351.

78. Safe SH: Xenoestrogens and breast cancer. N Engl J Med 1997;337:1303–1304.

79. Safe SH: Is there an association between exposure to environmental estrogens and breast cancer? Environ Health Perspect 1997;105:675–678.

80. Saleh MA: Toxaphene: Chemistry, biochemistry, toxicity and environmental fate. Rev Environ Contam Toxicol 1991;118:2–85.

81. Schenker MB, Louie S, Mehler LN, Albertson TE: Pesticides. In: Rom WN, ed: Environmental and Occupational Medicine, 3rd ed. Philadelphia, Lippincott-Raven, 1998, pp. 1157–1172.

82. Schoenig GP, Hartnagel RE, Schardein JL, Vorhees CV: Neurotoxicity evaluation of *N,N*-diethyl-*m*-toluamide in rats. Fundam Appl Toxicol 1993;22:355–365.

83. Schoenig GP, Neeper-Bradley TL, Fisher LC, Hartnagel RE: Teratologic evaluations of *N,N*-diethyl-*m*-toluamide (DEET) in rats and rabbits. Fundam Appl Toxicol 1994;23:63–69.

84. Schoenig GP, Osimitz TG, Gabriel KL, Hartnagel R, Gill MW, Goldenthal EI: Evaluation of the chronic toxicity and oncogenicity of *N,N*-Diethyl-*m*-Toluamide (DEET). Toxicol Sci 1999;47:99–109.

85. Shelov SP, ed. Caring for Your Baby and Young Child: Birth to Age 5. New York, Bantam Books, 1994.

86. Smith RA, Lewis D: A potpourri of pesticide poisonings in Alberta in 1987. Vet Hum Toxicol 1988;30:118–120.

87. Solomon BA, Haut SR, Carr EM, Shalita AR: Neurotoxic reaction to lindane in an HIV-seropositive patient. J Fam Pract 1995;40:291–295.

88. Solomon L, Fahrner L, West D: Gamma benzene hexachloride toxicity. Arch Dermatol 1977;113:353–357.

89. Song J, Nagata K, Tatebayashi H, Narahashi T: Interactions of tetramethrin, fenvalerate and ddt at the sodium channel in rat dorsal root ganglion neurons. Brain Res 1996;708:29–37.

90. Soto AM, Chung KL, Sonnenschein C: The pesticides endosulfan, toxaphene, and dieldrin have estrogenic effects on human estrogen-sensitive cells. Environ Health Perspect 1994;102:380–383.

91. Starr M, Clifford N: Acute lindane intoxication. Arch Environ Health 1972;25:374–375.

92. Stevenson DE, Walborg EF Jr, North DW, et al: Reassessment of human cancer risk of aldrin/dieldrin [monograph]. Toxicol Lett 1999;109:123–186.

93. Street JC, Chadwick RW: Ascorbic acid requirements and metabolism in relation to organochlorine pesticides. Ann N Y Acad Sci 1975;258:132–143.

94. Telch J, Jarvis DA: Acute intoxication with lindane (gamma benzene hexachloride). Can Med Assoc J 1982;126:662–663.

95. Tennebein M: Seizures after lindane therapy. J Am Geriatr Soc 1991;39:394–395.

96. Tenenbein M: Severe toxic reactions and death following the ingestion of diethyltoluamide-containing insect repellents. JAMA 1987;258:1509–1511.

97. Tilson HA, Hong JS, Mactutus CF: Effects of 5,5 diphenylhydantoin (phenytoin) on neurobehavioral toxicity of organochlorine pesticides and permethrin. J Pharmacol Exp Ther 1985;233:285–289.

98. Tilson MA, Shaw S, McLamb RL: The effects of lindane, DDT and chlordecone on avoidance responding and seizure activity. Toxicol Appl Pharmacol 1987; 88:57–65.

99. Veltri JC, Osimitz TG, Bradford DC, Page BC: Retrospective analysis of calls to poison control centers resulting from exposure to the insect repellent N,N-diethyl-m-toluamide (DEET) from 1985–1989. J Toxicol Clin Toxicol 1994;32:1–16.

100. Verschoyle RD, Brown AW, Nolan C, et al: A comparison of the acute toxicity, neuropathology, and electrophysiology of N,N-diethyl-m-toluamide and N,N-dimethyl-1,2-diphenylacetamide in rats. Fundam Appl Toxicol 1992;18:79–88.

101. Vijverberg HPM, van den Bercken J: Neurotoxicological effects and the mode of action of pyrethroid insecticides. Crit Rev Toxicol 1990;21:105–126.

102. Ware GW: An Introduction to Insecticides, 3rd ed. http://www.ipmworld. umn.edu/chapters/ware.htm last modified 12/23/99; accessed 11/2001.

103. Wax PM, Hoffman RS, Goldfrank LR: Fatality associated with inhalation of a pyrethrin insecticide. J Toxicol Clin Toxicol 1994;32: 457–460.

104. Williams CH, Casterline JL: Effects on toxicity and on enzyme activity of the interactions between aldrin, chlordane, piperonyl butoxide and banol in rats. Proc Soc Exp Biol Med 1970;135:46–49.

105. Woolley DE: Differential effects of benzodiazepines, including diazepam, clonazepam, Ro 5–4864 and devazepide, on lindane-induced toxicity. Proc West Pharmacol Soc 1994;37:131–134.

106. Wright DM, Hardin BD, Goad PW, Chrislip DW: Reproductive and developmental toxicity of N,N-diethyl-m-toluamide in rats. Fundam Appl Toxicol 1992;19:33–42.

107. Wolf MS, Toniolo PG, Lee EW, et al: Blood levels of organochlorine residues and the risk of breast cancer. J Nat Cancer Inst 1993; 85:648–652.

Neal E. Flomenbaum

A 52-year-old HIV positive man with a CD4 count of 600/mm^3 and no previous history of opportunistic infections presented to the Emergency Department (ED) with a complaint of gross hematuria. He reported ingesting 8 boxes of rodenticide 6 days prior to presentation, in an attempted suicide. He was taking fluoxetine and clonazepam for depression, and his other medications included methylphenidate and testosterone injections.

On physical examination, he was well developed, well appearing, and in no apparent distress. Vital signs were: blood pressure 170/70 mm Hg, pulse 76 beats/min, respiratory rate 18 breaths/min, and temperature 36.1°C (97°F). Examination of the head, eyes, ears, nose, and throat revealed only mild bleeding from the gingival mucosa. His chest, heart, abdomen, back, and genitalia were unremarkable. Rectal examination and testing for occult blood were negative. The skin and extremities were normal with no evidence of petechiae or ecchymoses.

Initial laboratory studies showed a white blood cell (WBC) count of 11.3×10^3/mm^3, hemoglobin of 15.6 g/dL, and hematocrit of 44.9%; platelets were normal. The initial prothrombin time (PT) was 79.2 seconds (international normalized ratio (INR) of 38.2), and activated partial thromboplastin time (PTT) was 101.3 seconds. Specific factor analysis demonstrated factor II 12%, factor V 17%, factor VIII less than 1%, and factor IX 6%. Urinalysis revealed greater than 100 red blood cells (RBCs)/high-power field.

The patient was immediately treated with 2 units of fresh-frozen plasma, and 150 mg of oral vitamin K$_1$ initially and every 6 hours. Serial coagulation profiles and factor II and factor VII levels were monitored. After approximately 40 hours of oral vitamin K$_1$ therapy, factor levels were considered adequate for normal coagulation. Oral vitamin K$_1$ was continued for 5 more days and after appropriate psychiatric evaluation and care, the patient was discharged home.

The patient continued taking an oral maintenance dose of 150 mg of vitamin K$_1$ every 6 hours as an outpatient and was monitored with periodic PT/PTT levels; all values remained within normal range and the dose of vitamin K$_1$ was tapered over the following 40 days. Vitamin K$_1$ was eventually discontinued completely after day 46 without a clinically significant change in either the PT or specific factor levels.[12]

(This case was adapted with permission from Bruno GR, Howland MA, McMeeking A, Hoffman RS: Long-acting anticoagulant overdose: Brodifacoum kinetics and optimal vitamin K dosing. Ann Emerg Med 2000; 36:262–267.)

EPIDEMIOLOGY

The above case is an example of the most frequently encountered serious rodenticide exposure in the United States today. Each year, the American Association of Poison Control Centers (AAPCC)/Toxic Exposure Surveillance System (TESS) reports between 13,000 and 16,000 exposures to long-acting anticoagulants—the 4 hydroxycoumarins, brodifacoum, and difenacoum, and the indandione derivatives chlorphacinone. Although the vast majority of such exposures are asymptomatic ingestions by children, approximately 250–300 ingestions yearly result in various degrees of coagulopathy.

Unlike the case presented above, rodenticide exposures are most commonly associated with young children. Between 1995 and 1999, 17,000–20,000 rodenticide exposures were reported annually to AAPCC/TESS, over 85% of which involved children younger than 6 years of age (see Chapter 116 and p. 1752). Remarkably, despite the very large number of exposures, no more than 6 deaths are reported annually. The rodenticide categories identified and tracked by AAPCC/TESS are: α-naphthyl thiourea (ANTU); anticoagulant standard and long-acting, barium carbonate; cyanide, monofluoroacetate, strychnine, Vacor, "other", and "unknown." Long-acting anticoagulants and strychnine account for all of the deaths caused by *known* rodenticides, whereas the "other and unknown" categories combined account for about 14% of exposures and almost 40% of the deaths per year. Unfortunately, exposures to cholecalciferol and bromethalin, the two newest rodenticides marketed for general use in the United States, are not tracked by TESS and therefore, it is not possible to determine at present any trends in usage or related toxicity. Also not explicit in the database are exposures to compounds not specifically used as rodenticides. An example of this is *Tres Pasitos,* an illegally imported agent used by certain ethnic groups in the New York City region. The active ingredient is the carbamate cholinesterase-inhibitor aldicarb, which in used legally in some parts of the US as an insecticide. However it is not registered for use as a rodenticide and is sold covertly for such use in local shops. Poisoning by this highly potent agent may produce fulminant cholinergic poisoning, a syndrome that is not expected following exposure to conventional rodenticides.[58a]

In addition to children, suicidal persons, potential homicide victims, pest control operators, and intoxicated, psychiatric, and impaired-elderly persons are at risk of intentional or unintentional rodenticide exposures. The large number of unintentional ingestions of rodenticides placed in food containers or dishes illustrates the danger of marketing toxic substances in such dishes or transferring a toxic substance to another container.

THE DEFINITION AND CLASSIFICATION OF RODENTICIDES

A rodenticide is any product commercially marketed to kill rodents, mice, squirrels, gophers, and other small animals. The "perfect rodenticide," one that effectively kills rodents but is not toxic to humans or nonrodent pets, has yet to be discovered or synthesized. Instead, a wide variety of less-than-perfect rodenticides are commercially available differing from one another in chemical composition, mechanism for killing rodents, and toxicity to humans.[34,47,48,58,65] In addition to the commonly available warfarin and cholecalciferol rodenticides, and to the more toxic, but rarely used types discussed below, new, purportedly "effective and harmless" products are occasionally introduced, only to be subsequently withdrawn when the true human toxicities become known. Some of these products may remain in basements, on hardware store shelves, or in use by professional pest control operators long after they are officially withdrawn from sale. The most important information necessary to deal effectively with rodenticide exposures therefore, are the full name or type of rodenticide involved, and the quantity, nature (acute or repetitive ingestions, inhalation, skin contact, and so on) and time of exposure.

Rodenticides are a disparate group of organic and inorganic compounds and substances bearing little or no relationship to one another apart from their usage—currently or historically—as rodenticides. Rodenticides have been classified in several ways: (a) inorganic and organic compounds; (b) animal selectivity; (c) nature and onset of symptoms; and (d) LD_{50} in rats.

Inorganic and Organic Compounds

Inorganic compounds include the salts of arsenic, thallium (sulfate), phosphorus, barium (carbonate), and zinc (phosphide); whereas *organic compounds* include sodium fluoroacetate, ANTU, warfarin, red squill, strychnine, norbormide, and Vacor (or PNU).[5]

Animal Selectivity

The cardiac glycoside and potent emetic, red squill, was promoted as a rodenticide because, unlike humans, rats do not vomit and therefore would be expected to experience the cardiotoxic effects of red squill whereas humans and other animals presumably would vomit the poison *prior* to experiencing any cardiotoxic effects. Norbormide, an irreversible smooth-muscle constrictor, causes widespread ischemic necrosis and death in rats but does not appear to affect other animals or humans, because it acts on a specific smooth muscle-norbormide receptor found only in rats. ANTU a *relatively* selective rodenticide is a derivative of phenylthiourea, without the bitter taste characteristic of the thiourea. ANTU causes pulmonary edema in rats that have not developed tolerance to it. ANTU, however, is only *relatively* selective: although the rats are more sensitive to it than other animals, large doses (>4 g/kg) can also be lethal to primates.

All of the rodenticides classified as inorganic, as well as organic rodenticides such as strychnine and sodium fluoroacetate, are nonselective and of extreme concern when ingested by humans and domestic animals. For the most part, use of this entire group of rodenticides is restricted to commercial pest control operators and government agencies.

Nature and Onset of Symptoms

Although a rodenticide classification system based purely on the nature and onset of symptoms seems very appealing, such a system may be unreliable, may create a false sense of security, and may result in inappropriate management and/or inadequate followup. Many different rodenticides cause neurologic and/or gastrointestinal signs and symptoms, whereas characteristic or pathognomonic signs such as "risus sardonicus" from strychnine, or alopecia from thallium, may not be recognized, do not always occur consistently (especially after ingesting small amounts), or, as in the case of thallium-induced alopecia, will not occur until days after an acute ingestion. Classifying rodenticides by the *time of onset of symptoms* may similarly lump together within a late-onset group some of the least toxic (regular warfarin type, cholecalciferol) and most toxic, (long-acting warfarin type, thallium) rodenticides.

LD_{50} in Rats

Probably the most clinically useful way of classifying rodenticides at present is by toxicity based on LD_{50} data in rats. With a few noteworthy exceptions, the relative degree of toxicity per kilogram and the characteristic adverse effects generally hold among different mammals, allowing the healthcare provider the opportunity to consider a combination of historical and characteristic physical evidence to diagnose or exclude various rodenticides and to decide on an optimal management plan. The limitations of this classification system, however, must be understood in order to use it appropriately: (a) in rare cases, the LD_{50} may vary unpredictably among species (eg, Vacor); and (b) repeated ingestions of less toxic rodenticides (eg, short-acting anticoagulants, cholecalciferol) may, in fact, make them highly toxic (Table 90–1).

HIGHLY TOXIC RODENTICIDES (SIGNAL WORD: "DANGER")

According to the Federal Insecticide, Fungicide, and Rodenticide Act (FIFRA), highly toxic rodenticides are those substances with a single-dose LD_{50} of less than 50 mg/kg body weight. The label "Danger" is the strongest warning by the Consumer Product Safety Commission for a potential toxic hazard. Lower hazard levels are denoted by "Warning" and "Caution" (Table 90–1 and Table 91–1). How well do current FIFRA testing guidelines protect infants and children who may be more sensitive than adults to the effects of many rodenticides? Based on the experience with lead testing in setting human exposure levels, FIFRA levels may be below current regulatory action levels even without the additional protection provided by the more recently enacted Food Quality Protection Act (FQPA).[69] The highly toxic "Danger" group includes thallium, sodium monofluoroacetate (SMFA, compound 1080), fluoroacetamide (compound 1081), strychnine, zinc phosphide, elemental phosphorus, arsenic, barium carbonate, and Vacor.

Thallium

Thallium sulfate is an odorless, tasteless compound absorbed easily by inhalation, through unbroken skin, and via the gastrointestinal tract.[34] It may also cause death secondarily, that is, when a thallium-poisoned animal is eaten.[9] Although the use of thallium as a commercial rodenticide ended in 1965, it is still used by industry and is an ingredient in some homeopathic remedies; currently, the most common setting for cases of thallium poisoning are attempted suicides or homicides.[21,22,35,40,49,57,59,64] Thallium has a volume of distribution estimated to range between 3.6 L/kg in humans to 20 L/kg in rats, is excreted by both the kidneys and liver, and has a human elimination half-life of 2–15 days.[49,58] Gas-

TABLE 90–1. **Management of Specific Rodenticide Ingestions**

Toxin Name	Physical Characteristics	Toxic Mechanism	Estimated Fatal Dose	Diagnostic Presenting Signs and Symptoms	Onset	Antidote and/or Treatment*
Highly Toxic Signal word: DANGER[a] (LD$_{50}$ < 50 mg/kg)						
Thallium (see ch 83)	White, crystalline, odorless, tasteless	Combines with mitochondrial sulfhydryl groups, interfering with oxidative phosphorylation	14 mg/kg	Anorexia, abdominal pain, diarrhea, painful neuropathy, delirium, coma, seizures, alopecia (late), Mees line	GI symptoms acutely, other symptoms 12–14 h delay	Activated charcoal, ferric ferrocyanide, (Berlin or Prussian blue)
Sodium monofluoroacetate (SMFA, compound 1080);	White, crystalline, odorless, tasteless, water soluble	Fluoroacetate to fluorocitrate; interferes with Krebs cycle	3–7 mg/kg	Seizures, coma, tachycardia, PVCs, VT, VF, ST-T wave changes	2–20 h	Experimental regimens: see text
Sodium fluoroacetamide (compound 1081)	Same as SMFA	Same as SMFA; fluoride toxicity	13–14 mg/kg	Same as SMFA	Same as SMFA	Same as SMFA
Strychnine	Bitter taste	Competitive glycine antagonism at the postsynaptic spinal cord motor neuron	Children: 15 mg Adults: 1–2 mg/kg	Restlessness, anxiety, twitching, hyperextension alternating with relaxation, intense pain, trismus or facial grimacing ("risus sardonicus"), inability to swallow, opisthotonos	10–20 min	Quiet room, IV, benzodiazepines, neuromuscular blockade
Zinc phosphide	Heavy, gray crystalline line powder, water insoluble, "rotten fish" or "phosphorus" odor; normally used as 1% concentration	Releases phosphine on contact with water or acid or in GI tract	40 mg/kg in rats	"Rotten fish" breath odor, black vomitus, GI and cardiovascular toxicity, pulmonary edema, agitation, coma, seizures, hepatic/renal toxicity	Within hours; inhalation may have delayed onset	Dilution with water, milk, or NaHCO$_3$
Elemental phosphorus (yellow or white phosphorus)	Yellow, waxy paste, fat soluble, water insoluble	Local irritation and burns on contact followed by GI, liver, and renal damage, and interferes with clotting	1 mg/kg (more toxic if dissolved in alcohol, fats, oils)	Skin and GI burns, "smoking" luminescent vomitus and stools with garlic odor, jaundice, dyshythmias, coma, delirium, seizures, cardiac arrest	1–2 h	Supportive care
Arsenic trioxide (see ch 79)	White, crystalline powder	Combines with sulfhydryl groups and interferes with a variety of enzymatic reactions	1–4 mg/kg	Dysphagia, nausea and vomiting, bloody diarrhea cardiovascular collapse, garlic odor, altered mental status, late sensory/motor neuropathy	Symptoms: 1 h Death: 1–24 h	Succimer, dimercaprol until urine arsenic level: <50 μg/24 h. Hemodialysis to remove chelation compound if renal failure.
Barium (soluble forms: carbonate, chloride, hydroxide)	Yellow, white, slightly lustrous lump	Hypokalemia neuromuscular blockade.	20–30 mg/kg	Headache, paresthesias, peripheral weakness, paralysis, nausea, vomiting, diarrhea, abdominal pain, ECG abnormalities, dysrhythmias, cardiac and pulmonary failure	1–8 h	Orogastric lavage with Na$_2$SO$_4$, potassium replacement
PNU (N-3-pyridylmethyl-N'-p-nitrophenyl urea, Vacor)	Yellow, resembling cornmeal or yellow-green powder in bait; odor: peanuts	Interferes with nicotinamide metabolism in pancreas (destroying pancreatic beta cells), central and peripheral nervous system, and heart	5 mg/kg	Nausea and vomiting abdominal pain, severe orthostatic hypotension, hyperglycemia with or without ketoacidosis, GI perforations, pneumonia, neuropathy	4–48 h	Nicotinamide (Niacinamide) 500 mg IV or IM followed by 200 mg IV or IM every 2 h to a total of 3 g/24 h. 100 mg PO 3 times/d for 2 weeks. Manage diabetic ketoacidosis with insulin

(continued)

TABLE 90–1. **Management of Specific Rodenticide Ingestions (continued)**

Toxin Name	Physical Characteristics	Toxic Mechanism	Estimated Fatal Dose	Diagnostic Presenting Signs and Symptoms	Onset	Antidote and/or Treatment*
Moderately Toxic Signal Word: WARNING[a] (LD$_{50}$, 50–500 mg/kg)						
Alpha-naph-thylthiourea (ANTU)	Odorless, slightly bitter, fine, blue-gray powder, water-insoluble	Acute lung injury	>4 g/kg	Dyspnea, rales, clear pulmonary froth, cyanosis, hypothermia	?	Supportive care
Cholecalciferol (vitamin D$_3$)	0.075% pellets, 364 pellets/oz; (1 pellet = 2308 U vitamin D)	Hypercalcemia	?	Headache, lethargy, weakness, fatigue, renal injury and failure, "metastatic" calcifications, due to hypercalcemia	Hours to days	Fluids; if severe: furosemide, prednisone, calcitonin, biphosphates
Low Toxicity Signal Word: CAUTION[a] (LD$_{50}$, 500–5000 mg/kg)						
Red squill	Bitter taste	Cardiac glycoside; poisoning	?	Mycocardial irritability, blurred vision, hyperkalemia	30 min–6 h	Digoxin-specific Fab, atropine; see Chap. 48
Norbormide (dicarboxi-mide)	Yellow cormeal bait, peanut butter, 1% concentration	Vasoconstriction and ischemia in rats only via specific norbormide receptor in rat smooth muscle	?	Transient hypothermia and hypotension with doses up to 300 mg	?	Supportive care
Bromethalin	7.5% concentrate, green pellets, with Bitrex (denatonium benzoate)	Uncouples oxidative phosphorylation; interrupts nerve impulse conduction	?	Muscle tremors, myoclonic jerks, flexion of major muscles, coma?, ataxia, focal motor seizures	Immediate	Supportive care
Anticogulants: Short Acting						
Warfarin	Yellow cornmeal, rolled oats (0.025%)	Anticoagulation via interference with clotting factors II, VII, IX, X; death from hemorrhage	> 5–20 mg/d for > 5 d	Bleeding with elevated INR	12–48 h	Vitamins K$_1$, fresh frozen plasma (FFP) as indicated
Prolin	Warfarin (0.025%) plus sulfaquinoxalin (0.025%)	Anticoagulant antibiotic combination eliminates intestinal vitamin K producing organisms				
Anticoagulants: Long Acting						
Hydroxycoumarins						
4-Hydroxy-coumarin (Brodifa-coum, Difena-coum)	0.005% grain-based bait	Anticoagulant	?	Bleeding with elevated INR	Delayed several days	Vitamin K$_1$, fresh frozen plasma (FFP) as indicated
Warfacide (Couma-furyl)	0.5% for dilution to 0.025% white powder, tasteless, odorless					
Indandiones						
Pindone (Pival)	Moldy, acrid odor, fluffy yellow powder, concentrations 0.005–2.5%	Anticoagulant	?	Chronic ingestion possibly produces cardiac and neurologic symptoms as well as bleeding with elevated INR	Delayed several days`	Vitamin K$_1$, fresh frozen plasma (FFP) as indicated
Pivalyn	0.5%					
Diphacinone	0.005–2.0%					
Chloropha-cinone	0.005–2.5%					
Valone	0.005–2.5%					

[a]The LD$_{50}$ values used in this table are derived from data on acute oral ingestions of the commercial product by rats. In some cases the commercial product contains a very small percentage of active ingredient. The signal words that appear on labels of registered products may differ from the signal word assigned to the acute oral LD$_{50}$ test because the label may also reflect another study (acute dermal or inhalational LD$_{50}$) requiring a more severe signal word. See Chapters 89–4 and 91–1 for the Consumer Product Safety Commission definitions and use of signal words as indicators of potential hazard of toxicity. Peacock D, Biologist, Registrations Division Office of Pesticide Programs, EPA, Washington, DC.

*Gastrointestinal decontamination should be provided as appropriate (Chap. 5); only unique or controversial aspects are discussed in this table.

trointestinal signs appear 0.5–2 days following ingestion or exposure and include nausea, vomiting, hematemesis, bloody diarrhea, abdominal pain, and, later, ileus. Neurologic sequelae typically occur 2–5 days after exposure and include headache, lethargy, muscle weakness, painful paresthesias in the extremities, tremors, ptosis, ataxia, myoclonus, seizures, delirium, and coma. Nonfatal exposures have resulted in long-term neurologic impairment such as painful neuropathies, paresis, optic nerve atrophy, ataxia, choreiform movements, and dementia. Another characteristic long-term effect is alopecia (Chap. 83).

Sodium Monofluoroacetate (SMFA, Compound 1080)

The development and commercial use of sodium monofluoroacetate (SMFA, compound 1080), another highly toxic rodenticide (LD_{50} 2 mg/kg), was the result of efforts in this country during the 1940s to find an effective rodenticide not subjected to the shortages caused by World War II.[34] Since its introduction in 1946, the use of SMFA in the United States has been limited to commercial exterminators.

Originally marketed as a liquid mixed with a dye to be placed in shallow paper cups in areas inaccessible to humans, by 1949 at least 12 deaths were recorded. The deaths included 5 small children who had chewed on the poison cups, 3 juveniles who encountered the poison in a soft drink bottle, and 4 adult suicides. An additional 4 deaths in children were probably caused by SMFA.[34]

SMFA is derived from *Palicourea spp.* (South America), *Acacia spp.* (Australia), *Dichapetalum cymosum* (Africa), and a few other plants, it is a white, odorless, water-soluble salt, with an appearance similar to that of flour or baking soda. SMFA is reported to be tasteless as a powder but tasting weakly like vinegar in dilute solution.[34]

Unlike thallium, SMFA cannot be absorbed through unbroken skin. However, it is toxic when ingested, inhaled in dusts, or absorbed through open wounds. The toxicity of SMFA is related primarily to its interference with the Krebs cycle rather than because of its fluoride content.[34,66,73] All ω-monofluoro amino acids with an odd number of carbon atoms and ω-monofluoro alkanoic acids with an even number of carbon atoms are toxic.[34] The toxic effects of SMFA occur 1 to several hours after exposure and result from the conversion of the nontoxic fluoroacetate ions to fluorocitric acid which, in turn, blocks the tricarboxylic acid cycle essential to energy production in mammalian cells (Figure 13–2).[66] The term "lethal synthesis" was first coined to describe these in vivo effects of fluoroacetic acid.[34,66]

Toxic effects of SMFA, primarily involving the CNS and the heart, include nausea and apprehension followed by cardiac dysrhythmias, seizures, and coma, with death resulting from ventricular tachycardia and ventricular fibrillation or respiratory failure secondary to pulmonary edema or bronchopneumonia.[16,32,73] Animals dying of SMFA poisoning rapidly develop a characteristic extensor rigor mortis and are subsequently found with extremities in hyperextension.

Investigators from Taiwan retrospectively analyzed 38 consecutive cases of SMFA poisoning, including 7 deaths, that occurred

between 1988 and 1993. Of the 38 patients, 74% had nausea or vomiting—the most common finding; 65% had hypokalemia; and 42% had hypocalcemia. The most common ECG pattern was a nonspecific, ST-T and T-wave abnormality. Hypotension, elevated serum creatinine, and acidemia were the most accurate prognostic indicators of subsequent death.[18] The hypotension or shock after SMFA poisoning may be a result of diminished systemic vascular resistance and increased cardiac output.[19]

There is no known antidote for SMFA. Orogastric lavage followed by the use of activated charcoal and a sorbitol cathartic are recommended, although adsorption by activated charcoal is probably not significant. Glycerol monoacetate as a substrate in the blocked Krebs cycle has been used experimentally in monkeys at doses of 0.1–0.5 mL/kg body weight IV, or 0.55 g/kg IM every half hour for several hours.[17] In an attempt to inhibit the conversion of fluoroacetate to fluorocitrate, 500 mL of 10% acetamide in 5% dextrose over 30 minutes every 4 hours, or a 10% solution of ethyl alcohol, have been used experimentally with limited success.[16,17] An ethanol-loading regimen is described in Antidotes in Depth: Ethanol. A combination of calcium gluconate (to correct hypocalcemia) and sodium succinate (to supplement the blocked trichloroacetic acid cycle) has reduced mortality from sodium fluoroacetate in mice, but only when the calcium gluconate and sodium succinate were administered simultaneously.[62]

Fluoroacetamide

Fluoroacetamide (compound 1081) is a fluoroacetate derivative similar to sodium monofluoroacetate but with a slightly higher LD_{50} (13–14 mg/kg)[34] and a somewhat slower onset of symptoms. In 2 cases of fluoroacetamide poisoning, both the life-threatening dysrhythmias and the prolonged QT intervals that preceded them responded to calcium chloride therapy, suggesting that fluoride content plays a role in fluoroacetamide toxicity.[87] An acute inhalation toxicity experiment exposing rats to *aerosolized* 2-fluoroacetamide resulted in desquamation and necrosis of the respiratory epithelium, marked hypertrophy of hepatocytes, and renal damage.[85] Because of the extreme toxicities of both fluoroacetamide and sodium monofluoroacetate, they are rarely used, even by licensed pest control operators.

Strychnine

Strychnine is a naturally occurring alkaloid from the seeds of the tree *Strychnos nux vomica,* which is a small poisonous tree with ovate leaves and yellowish-white tubular flowers indigenous to India, Indochina, northern Australia and Hawaii. The yellow-orange hard shelled fruit is 1.5 inches in diameter and contains greyish seeds 0.5 inches in diameter, which in turn contain 1.1 to 1.4% strychnine.[41a,65a] Strychnine, a highly toxic substance that had been used as a rodenticide since the 16th century, is generally encountered as an odorless, colorless crystal or bitter white powder that can be absorbed through the gastrointestinal tract or nasal mucosa.[12] Strychnine is a CNS stimulant that causes muscle twitching, extensor spasm, opisthotonos, trismus or a characteristic facial grimacing known as "risus sardonicus", painful "seizures" during which the patient is conscious, and medullary paralysis resulting in death.[60,61,86,89]

Ironically, considering its extreme danger to humans, strychnine is not even an effective rodenticide because rats appear to quickly learn to avoid the bitter taste it imparts to the bait. For both of these reasons, strychnine is virtually never used today as a rodenticide. However, it may still be encountered as a component of homeopathic tonics and cathartic pills,[63] and as recently as 1979, had been proposed as a treatment for nonketotic hyperglycinemia in infants.[37] A traditional Cambodian remedy for gastrointestinal disorders known as "slang nut" or "poisonous nut", which is the fruit of the Strychos nux vomica, has been implicated in one recent case of strychnine poisoning[41a] and a different Cambodian herbal preparation was implicated in another.[46a] Crimidene, another rodenticide that is a synthetic chlorinated pyrimidine compound related to strychnine, produces similar CNS signs and symptoms.[74]

The adult lethal dose of strychnine is reportedly between 50 and 100 mg, or 1–2 mg/kg of body weight,[63,65a,74] and signs and symptoms of strychnine poisoning often begin within 15–20 minutes of ingestion. There is very little protein binding, the half-life is 10–16 hours, and detoxification and elimination are primarily by hepatic metabolism.[37,62a,74,80] Although initial studies involving small doses of strychnine suggested that up to 20% was excreted unchanged in the urine,[58,93] more recent pharmacokinetic studies indicate that less than 1% is excreted in the urine after larger ingestions.[37,62a,80] Only three published studies of strychnine exposures include multiple blood levels: In one (nonfatal) case study, 19 determinations were made including a peak level of 1.6 mg/L about 4 hours postingestion. In this instance, a $t_{1/2}$ of 10 hours was calculated by first-order kinetics.[28] Results from a fatal case with 4 determinations and a peak level of 3.8 mg/L suggested both a large volume of distribution (13 L/kg) for strychnine and nonlinear, Michaelis-Menten elimination.[37] More recently, another fatal case with 18 strychnine determinations between 20 minutes to 52 hours post ingestion indicated a $t_{1/2}$ of 10–16 hours by first order kinetics similar to the findings in the nonfatal case.[62a]

Strychnine causes competitive antagonism of the inhibitory neurotransmitter glycine at the postsynaptic spinal cord motor neuron.[37,44] Victims of strychnine poisoning may remain awake with relaxed muscles between episodes of opisthotonos and muscle contractions that are triggered by minimal sensory stimuli.[37]

Complications of strychnine-induced muscle spasm include hypoxia, hyperthermia, cardiac arrest, rhabdomyolysis, acute renal failure, and hyperthermia.[37] Postmortem findings in the case with the 3.8 mg/L peak level included extensive necrosis of the cerebral cortex and brainstem, and bilateral lower lobe bronchopneumonia.[37]

The differential diagnosis of confusion accompanied by episodic muscle rigidity includes phencyclidine toxicity, the neuroleptic malignant syndrome, viral encephalitis, epilepsy, tetanus[46a] and isoniazid toxicity. Tetanus, in particular, has much

in common with strychnine poisoning such as the facial muscle grimacing known as "risus sardonicus", sudden painful tonic muscle contractions and decorticate posturing during which time the patient remains conscious. However, strychnine poisoning typically results in more prominent alterations in mental status.[46a]

Early useful interventions advocated for strychnine poisoning include activated charcoal[3,4] and orogastric lavage with aggressive airway management.[37] However, once symptoms appear, any manipulation or excitement may precipitate opisthotonos or tonic-clonic "seizures," and for this reason, a quiet environment and benzodiazepines have been advocated.[34]

The extensor spasm, opisthotonos, and seizures associated with strychnine poisoning may be controlled initially by a benzodiazepine such as diazepam (0.1–0.5 mg/kg, IV slowly)—which acts as an indirect GABA agonist—followed by a barbiturate such as pentobarbital (another GABA agonist). If these measures prove ineffective, immediate induction of general anesthesia and/or neuromuscular blockade with a nondepolarizing neuromuscular blocking agent should be considered.[37,86] The latter is recommended because strychnine seizures are thought to originate at the level of the spinal cord and not at the cerebral cortex.[37] Intubation and mechanical ventilation will permit safer gastric evacuation by orogastric lavage, and maintenance of adequate urine output with fluid and diuretic therapy may reduce the risk of acute renal failure from rhabdomyolysis.[37]

Acidification of the urine theoretically may enhance excretion of strychnine after ingestion of minimal amounts, but after significant exposures, renal excretion appears to be insignificant, and any benefit of acidification will almost certainly be outweighed by the risk of exacerbating the profound lactic acidosis and myoglobinuria secondary to rhabdomyolysis that have been documented in these cases.[13] Chapter 69 discusses urinary acidification and rhabdomyolysis.

Orogastric lavage (or even worse, emesis) in the unintubated victim of strychnine poisoning may be extremely dangerous because of the potential for generalized muscle contractions. Therefore, activated charcoal alone, administered by a nasogastric tube, may be the safest and most effective initial measure.

Zinc and Aluminum Phosphide

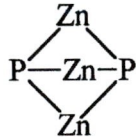

Both zinc and aluminum phosphide are still used as rodenticides in developing nations because they are both cheap and effective. Zinc phosphide's dark gray color, "rotten fish odor," and bad taste reportedly make it unattractive to animals other than rats. Typically mixed with tartar emetic, zinc phosphide is highly toxic because it releases phosphine and zinc on contact with water and acid. Phosphine inhibits cytochrome oxidase and the electron transport system,[20] and causes widespread cellular toxicity, injury and necrosis to the gastrointestinal tract, liver and kidneys.[27] Patients poisoned by zinc phosphide manifest, in 4 days to 2 weeks, nausea and vomiting, excitement, chills, chest tightness, cough, hypotension, dyspnea, pulmonary edema, circulatory collapse, cardiac dysrhythmias, convulsions and coma, renal damage, anuria, tetany (hypocalcemia), leukopenia, and death.[2,20] Inhalation of zinc phosphide dust may induce pulmonary edema. Long-term occupational exposure results in a constellation of neuropsychiatric, cardiac, pulmonary, renal, and hepatic findings.[2] Treatment advocated for zinc phosphide poisoning includes dilution with sodium bicarbonate, milk, or water, orogastric lavage, and administration of activated charcoal, a cathartic, and possibly a proton pump inhibitor type of antacid (such as omeprazole).

Yellow Phosphorus

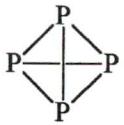

Elemental
phosphorus

Yellow (or "white") phosphorus, the form of elemental phosphorus still used as a rodenticide in some parts of the world, is highly poisonous—a human ingestion of 50 mg or 1 mg/kg may be fatal.[23,77,84] The other commonly available form of elemental phosphorus, red phosphorus, is the only form of phosphorus still used in matches today and, in contrast to yellow phosphorus, is relatively harmless. When used as a rodenticide, yellow phosphorus is usually mixed with molasses or peanut butter and spread on bread as bait for rodents or roaches. For obvious reasons, rodenticides deployed in this manner may be unintentionally ingested by children or compromised adults.

Contact with yellow phosphorus causes second- and third-degree skin burns within minutes to hours. Yellow phosphorus is most immediately toxic to the gastrointestinal tract and liver and ingestions are usually followed by a peculiar type of vomiting, described as "smoking," luminescent, and with a garlicky odor. Resultant stools may also be luminescent and "smoking."[84]

Delirium, coma, and death from cardiovascular collapse may ensue.[68,88] Yellow phosphorus has a direct toxic effect on the myocardium and peripheral vessels. Experimentally, acute phosphorus poisoning depresses rat myocardial protein synthesis.[88]

Patients who survive the acute effects of yellow phosphorus poisoning may then have a relatively symptom-free period lasting for a few weeks, only to experience a third stage of systemic toxicity involving the gastrointestinal tract, liver, heart, kidney, and central nervous system.

Treatment for yellow phosphorus poisoning in the past has included orogastric lavage with potassium permanganate 0.1% solution, or 3% hydrogen peroxide diluted to a 2% solution to oxidize the phosphorus to harmless phosphates, followed by the use of activated charcoal and possibly a cathartic. These approaches have not been adequately investigated. Neither corticosteroids, which had been previously recommended, nor exchange transfusions appear to be useful; in one group of 49 suicidal patients from Colombia, corticosteroids did not prevent coma or death from hepatic injury.[50] In another group of 15 patients with hepatic encephalopathy, 3 of 5 patients treated with exchange transfusions survived, as compared to 3 of 10 untreated patients.[50]

Red phosphorus is nonvolatile, insoluble, not absorbed through the gastrointestinal tract, and, therefore, relatively harmless when ingested.[84]

Arsenic

Another highly toxic element still in rare use as a rodenticide is arsenic. Arsenic trioxide is a white, crystalline powder that causes dysphagia, muscle cramps, convulsions, vomiting, and bloody diarrhea following ingestion. Death from arsenic poisoning is a result of cardiovascular collapse. Immediate treatment recommendations for arsenic poisoning include orogastric lavage followed by activated charcoal and a cathartic. Succimer (Dimercaptosuccinic acid, DMSA)[43,81] or dimercaprol may be used to chelate this heavy metal after it is absorbed. Between 1956 and 1974, arsenicals were identified as the single most common cause of unintentional rodenticide-related deaths. However, because of its extreme toxicity, pest control operators have avoided using arsenic for many years (Chap. 79).

Barium Carbonate

Barium carbonate is a highly toxic soluble salt previously used as a rodenticide. Another toxic soluble barium salt, barium sulfide is currently used as a male depilatory.[82] Insoluble forms of barium, such as the barium sulfate commonly used in radiographic procedures, are harmless. But, soluble forms of barium—such as the acetate, carbonate, chloride, hydroxide, nitrate, and sulfide forms—cause profound weakness and gastrointestinal, neurologic, cardiovascular, pulmonary, and possibly renal dysfunction.[67,94]

Most of the toxic effects of barium result from its direct stimulation of all types of muscle, including cardiac muscle, and from its ability to cause a profound reduction in serum potassium together with an increase in intracellular potassium.[76,82,94] Death results from hypokalemia, cardiac dysrhythmias, congestive heart failure, and pulmonary toxicity.

A similar mechanism has been proposed for the hypokalemic paralysis that results from barium poisoning, chronic potassium deficiency, and thyrotoxicosis:[45] the large, active and passive influx of extracellular potassium into the muscle turns off the Na^+-K^+-ATPase pump causing depolarization and paralysis. However, in 1 case report involving barium carbonate, the degree of weakness correlated with the plasma barium concentrations and not the potassium concentrations.[67] The author suggests that barium itself is responsible for membrane depolarization by causing release of acetylcholine[83] and by competitively reducing the permeability of all membranes to potassium,[45] with the resultant intensity of neuromuscular blockade correlating directly with the plasma barium concentrations.

One case of renal toxicity and acute renal failure following ingestion of a teaspoonful of barium chloride may have resulted from treatment with intravenous $MgSO_4$, saline, and furosemide (in addition to the previously recommended oral $MgSO_4$).[94] The intravenous combination of medications may have caused barium sulfate to precipitate out into the renal tubules.

Treatment for the ingestion of soluble forms of barium includes emesis, if it can be accomplished rapidly outside of the hospital, or orogastric lavage with 5–10 g of sodium sulfate added to the lavage solution in the hope of converting the barium carbonate to barium sulfate.[5,65] Instilling $MgSO_4$ 30 g, through a nasogastric tube in 1 instance appears to have been effective in precipitating the barium as the insoluble sulfate.[55] The most important aspect of management is rapid, aggressive potassium replacement intravenously as indicated by frequent serum potassium monitoring,[34,65,94] together with vigilance for subsequent hyperkalemia resulting from rhabdomyolysis and extracellular return during recovery.[82]

Vacor (N–3-pyridylmethyl-N′-p-nitrophenyl urea, PNU)

The quest for a safe, highly effective single-dose rodenticide occasionally leads to the introduction of extremely toxic substances with tragic consequences to humans who are exposed to them. One of the most unfortunate examples is N–3-pyridylmethyl-N′-p-nitrophenyl urea (Vacor, PNU), which was introduced in 1975 with labeling indicating that it was safe for human consumption. Shortly after its introduction, 7 South Koreans died after eating Vacor-contaminated rice. In the United States, more than 100 poisonings and at least 12 deaths caused by Vacor occurred between 1975 and 1980, with deaths resulting from the ingestion of as little as a single (30-g) package. The manufacturer withdrew Vacor from sale in June 1979, with a request to return all unsold Vacor, but no public recall was ever issued. Information in this section regarding the management of Vacor poisoning may also be applicable to pentamidine, alloxan, and streptozotocin exposures, all of which destroy pancreatic β cells.

Although more than 20 years have elapsed since Vacor was withdrawn from the market, AAPCC/TESS continues to report between 1 and 7 Vacor exposures annually with adverse outcomes rated from none to moderate, but no major adverse effects or deaths. These continuing reports of Vacor exposures without the serious sequelae seen in the 1970s suggest either an overreporting of unconfirmed exposures or a large reservoir of Vacor packets in the environment. The last confirmed exposure to Vacor reported in the medical literature occurred in 1986, when a patient ingested the contents of a package that had been sold and placed many years earlier; at the time of the exposure, the recommended antidote, niacinamide was no longer available.[38]

Vacor is a structural analogue of alloxan and streptozotocin and, as noted above, all three destroy pancreatic β cells.[42] Pentamidine toxicity also results in islet cell necrosis without an accompanying lymphocytic infiltrate.[33] Vacor, alloxan, and streptozotocin all interfere with niacinamide metabolism in pancreatic β cells, liver, and brain cells.[36,41,46] In vitro studies demonstrate that these toxins are incorporated into various intracellular nucleotides, which are then unable to act as hydrogen carriers in oxidoreductase systems, thereby inhibiting the activities of certain enzyme systems. When these nucleotides are substituted for niacinamide in the synthesis of nicotinamide adenine dinucleotide (NADH) or nicotinamide adenine dinucleotide phosphate (NADPH), major abnormalities of the pentose phosphate pathway result, causing defects in intermediary metabolism and RNA production.[36]

Recently, investigators who incubated mitochondria and submitochondrial particles from beef, rat heart, and rat liver with various concentrations of Vacor demonstrated that it specifically inhibits the NADH-ubiquinone reductase activity of respiratory complex I in mammalian mitochondria, in turn correlating quantitatively with the inhibition of insulin release from insulinoma cells and pancreatic islets. This inhibition was entirely consistent with the dose effects of Vacor that had been reported in human poisonings.[29]

In other rat experiments, electron microscopy of the thickened glomerular basement membranes that developed within 7 days of Vacor ingestion revealed increased collagen, laminin, fibronectin, neutral polysaccharides, and chondroitin sulfate proteoglycan.[79] Electrophysiologic studies on a peripheral motor nerve-skeletal system of Vacor-treated rats showed decreased amplitude of muscle action potential with corresponding structural studies demonstrating degenerative changes in the axon terminal at the neuromuscular junction.[1]

Humans who ingested Vacor developed, within hours, an insulin-deficient hyperglycemia or diabetic ketoacidosis, accompanied by severe postural hypotension and sensorimotor peripheral and autonomic neuropathies.[41,46,54,70,72] Reported deaths were caused by ketoacidosis, gastrointestinal perforation, cardiac dysrhythmias, and pneumonia.

Patients who survived Vacor ingestions after manifesting symptoms, almost invariably required insulin therapy to manage their newly acquired diabetes. The major long-term management problem however, was the neuropathy, especially the resultant postural hypotension which is both severe and extremely resistant to therapy.

Based on the in vitro studies noted and on an in vivo rat study, a treatment plan for acute Vacor (and presumably, alloxan and streptozotocin) ingestions was formulated, calling for 500 mg of niacinamide (nicotinamide) IM or IV, immediately followed by 100–200 mg IM or IV every 4 hours for up to 48 hours, increased to every 2 hours if signs of toxicity develop. Under this treatment plan, the maximum total dose of niacinamide is 3 g/d for an adult. For small children, approximately one-half of the adult dose was recommended. When the patient was able to take oral medications, 100 mg of niacinamide was recommended 3–5 times daily for 2 weeks. Fludrocortisone was frequently necessary for persistent postural hypotension.

In the past, investigators cautioned against substituting niacin (nicotinic acid) for niacinamide (nicotinamide), out of concern that (a) the vasodilatory effects of nicotinic acid would exacerbate the hypotensive effects of Vacor;[46] (b) niacin is less effective than niacinamide; and (c) niacin causes and exacerbates glucose intolerance.[56] However, when intravenous niacinamide became unavailable in this country, substituting niacin as the only available alternative was advocated. Niacinamide in capsule form may still be found at various nutritional supplement outlets.

In addition to giving niacinamide (nicotinamide), emesis, or orogastric lavage, activated charcoal and cathartic administration were recommended. Ketoacidosis should be managed with insulin, and silent, nonpainful, gastrointestinal perforation should be anticipated and rigorously searched for.

The reasons that Vacor continues to be of more than historical interest over two decades after its withdrawal include the insights it provides into the limitations of product testing techniques and of postmarketing surveillance: Because of widely varying LD$_{50}$s, perhaps resulting from a common gene not shared by other animals, rats and humans appear to be the most susceptible to Vacor toxicity.[34] Vacor is also providing new insights into possible environmental etiologies of diseases—in this case, diabetes mellitus—just as MPTP (see Chap 62) has demonstrated a link between environmental toxins and parkinsonism.

Vacor poisoning may be a biochemical paradigm for the metabolic induction of insulin-dependent diabetes mellitus, as well as some of its associated vascular and neurologic problems: Vacor-induced diabetes mellitus closely mimics the "naturally occurring" disease. Of 18 patients who had developed diabetes mellitus after Vacor ingestions, 44% also developed retinopathy, 28% developed proteinuria, and all developed (muscle) capillary membrane thickening similar to that seen in insulin-dependent diabetes after a mean duration of 6.2 years postingestion.[31]

MODERATELY TOXIC RODENTICIDES (SIGNAL WORD: "WARNING")

Moderately toxic rodenticides, those with an LD_{50} of 50–500 mg/kg body weight, include the "selective" rodenticide ANTU and cholecalciferol (vitamin D_3), one of the newest and increasingly popular rodenticides.

α-Naphthyl-Thiourea

ANTU kills rats by causing pulmonary edema and pleural effusion, probably because of damage to the lung capillaries resulting in increased permeability.[10,75] Young rats and rats exposed initially to small, nonlethal doses are relatively resistant to the lethal effects of ANTU, possibly by developing pulmonary cell hyperplasia in response to the small doses.[8] The heart appears to be unaffected by ANTU.[10,75] There are no well-documented cases or series of human ANTU ingestions from which human toxicity can be accurately determined. In several older series of combined ANTU + chloralose ingestions, it appears that the respiratory symptoms were more severe from the combination than from chloralose alone, suggesting pulmonary effects of ANTU in humans. Of the 14 patients poisoned by the combination, 11 required intubation because of tracheobronchial hypersecretion.[30,34] Recommended treatment for ANTU ingestions is orogastric lavage followed by administration of activated charcoal.[58]

Cholecalciferol

Cholecalciferol (vitamin D_3) was first registered and marketed in the United States in late 1984. It is now widely used by professional pest control operators as Quintox, and by the general public as Rampage. Cholecalciferol mobilizes calcium from the bones of rodents and rabbits and in toxic doses produces hypercalcemia, osteomalacia, and metastatic calcification of the cardiovascular system, kidneys, stomach, and lungs; death typically occurs in 2–5 days.[51–53] All animals are susceptible to the effects of cholecalciferol, but because of their size, rats and mice succumb to much lower doses than do larger animals such as cats and dogs.[51–53] Cholecalciferol appears to be an effective rodenticide either when a large amount is consumed in one meal or when smaller amounts are consumed over a 2–3-day period.[53,71] Because death is not immediate and the cholecalciferol does not impart unusual characteristics to the bait, the bait shyness seen with zinc phosphide, ANTU, strychnine, and other rodenticides does not occur with cholecalciferol.[51–53] The closely related calciferol (vitamin D_2 or ergocalciferol) has been used as a rodenticide in Europe and Canada since 1978, with no genetic resistance reported to date.[51–53]

Although rats manifest the signs of severe acute hypercalcemia, including lethargy and ultimately death from myocardial infarction in 2–5 days,[71] no serious human toxicity or death from the rodenticide form of cholecalciferol has been reported to date. All of the advice for managing human ingestions is based on experience with treating therapeutic forms of vitamin D poisoning and hypercalcemia. One case of cholecalciferol poisoning in an industrial setting may be particularly relevant because, as in the case of a child who might repeatedly ingest small amounts of rodenticide, the exposure described was two small doses over a 32-day period and resulted in prolonged hypercalcemia.[39]

Immediate intervention after a large acute ingestion should include gastric emptying by emesis or orogastric lavage followed by gastric decontamination with activated charcoal and possibly sorbitol. Repetitive dosing of activated charcoal has been recommended, but data are insufficient to confirm its usefulness.

Treatment for moderate to severe degrees of hypercalcemia (greater than 11.5 mg/dL) include IV fluid therapy with 0.9% sodium chloride solution if the patient is hypovolemic and can tolerate a fluid load. Potassium and magnesium levels should be monitored and maintained. Furosemide should be administered. Prednisone (0.5–1.0 mg/kg daily) appears to be particularly effective for hypercalcemia secondary to vitamin D poisoning. Calcitonin (salmon calcitonin, Calcimar) 4–8 IU/kg SC or IM every 6–12 hours may reduce serum calcium levels by 1–3 mg/dL over a few hours by inhibiting osteoclastic bone resorption while promoting calciuria. Bisphosphonates (such as pamidronate) can be used concomitantly with calcitonin to produce a prolonged effect.

A normal serum calcium level obtained 48 hours after an acute ingestion almost certainly excludes any significant toxicity.

LOW-TOXICITY RODENTICIDES (SIGNAL WORD: "CAUTION")

The remaining rodenticides, with one exception, are of low toxicity (LD_{50}, 500–5000 mg/kg). This category includes red squill (*Urginea maritima*) and norbormide, along with the "warfarin-type" anticoagulant rodenticides, which are still the most commonly used rodenticides today.

Red Squill

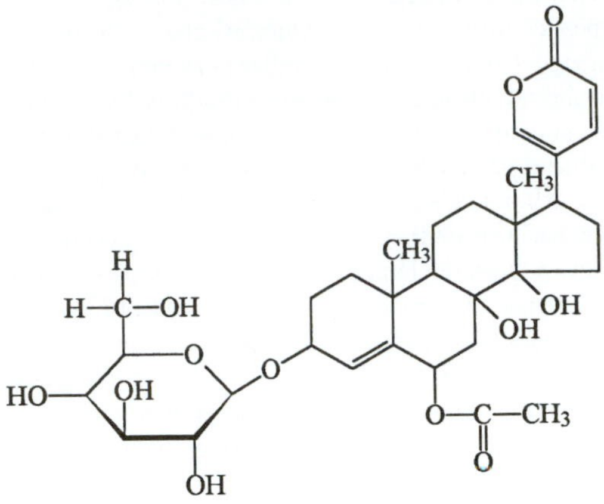

Red squill is a naturally occurring rodenticide found in the sea onion plant *Urginea maritima* of the *Liliaceae* family. It contains scillaren A and B, which are cardiac glycosides. The effects of red squill on humans are chiefly gastrointestinal: abdominal pain, nausea, and vomiting. Red squill is considered to be so potent an emetic in humans, that the expected cardiotoxicity (ie, ventricular irritability, premature ventricular contractions, ventricular fibrillation, and so on) is rarely, if ever, seen as a result of ingesting the commercial rodenticide. However, a 1995 case report of a human who ingested two bulbs of the plant, documents the subsequent nausea, vomiting, seizures, hyperkalemia, atrioventricular block, ventricular dysrhythmias, and death that would be expected after a massive cardiac glycoside poisoning.[90]

Evaluation should include cardiac monitoring, electrolyte (particularly potassium) analysis, and a digoxin assay with which these cardiac glycosides may cross-react. There are no specific data indicating the degree of cross-reactivity demonstrated by red squill, but this concept and the consequent utility of obtaining a "digoxin" level is discussed for many other plant and animal cardiac glycosides in Chap. 48.

When present, the cardiotoxicity of red squill is probably best treated with digoxin-specific antibody fragments [see Antidotes in Depth: Digoxin-Specific Antibody Fragments (Fab)].[78]

Norbormide

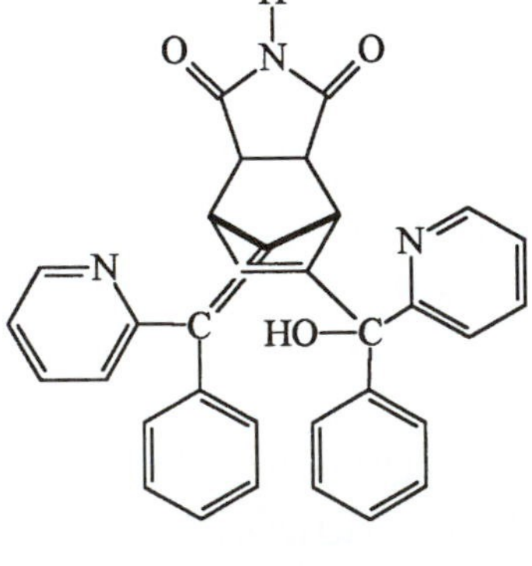

Norbormide

Norbormide, the irreversible smooth-muscle constrictor, appears to be specific for rats and has no known human toxicity. Rats die as a result of intense generalized vasoconstriction, resulting in tissue anoxia.[58] In vitro norbormide promotes calcium entry into smooth-muscle cells, inducing a myogenic contraction selective for the small vessels in rats, whereas in the arteries of other mammals (and in the rat aorta), norbormide behaves like a calcium channel entry blocker.[11] Although emesis and catharsis may be considered if they can be easily performed, it is probably quite sufficient to achieve gastric decontamination with activated charcoal and possibly a cathartic, especially when dealing with an uncooperative patient.

Anticoagulants

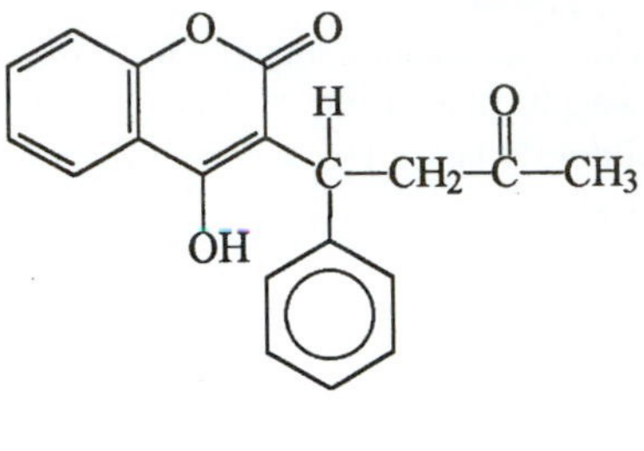

Warfarin

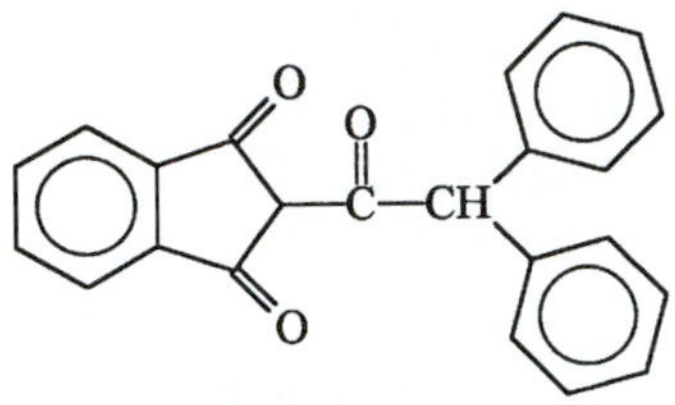

Diphacinone

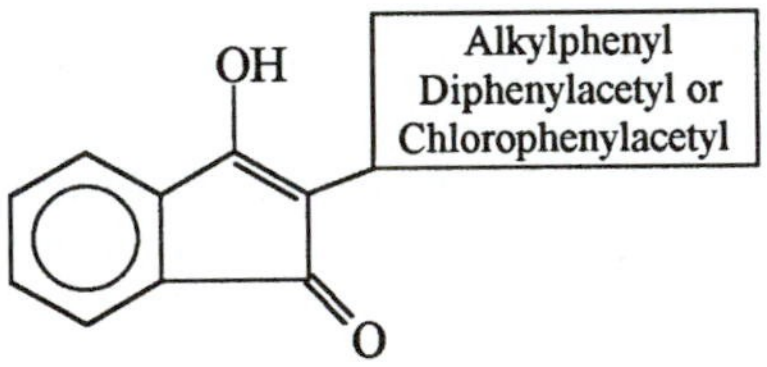

4-Hydroxycoumarins

The anticoagulant, or warfarin-type rodenticides are far and away the most commonly implicated in rodenticide related calls to poison centers (see Chapter 116 and p. 1752). Prior to the 1980s, both human and rodent toxicity from the anticoagulant rodenticides depended on repeated exposure to relatively small doses. Although there was virtually no toxicity to humans after a single exposure from this type of rodenticide, the inability to ensure repetitive ingestions by rats made warfarin-type anticoagulants less effective as rodenticides. In addition, a selection process led to the prevalence of resistant rats ("super rats") in some areas. For both of these reasons, more toxic rodenticides continued to be used and introduced.

In the 1980s, newer types of anticoagulant rodenticides were marketed that are both lethal to rats and toxic to humans after a single acute ingestion. Use of these potent long-acting anticoagulant rodenticides continues to increase. A single ingestion of a "superwarfarin" rodenticide such as difenacoum or brodifacoum, may result in marked anticoagulation effects for up to 7 weeks. The case presented at the beginning of this chapter demonstrates the severity and duration of brodifacoum toxicity.[12] Chapter 42 has a detailed discussion on the classification, mechanism of action, diagnosis, and treatment of warfarin and long-acting anticoagulants.

Appropriate management of patients exposed to anticoagulant rodenticides begins with an appreciation of the time required before clinical effects become apparent. Because acute single-dose ingestions of currently available anticoagulant rodenticides typically do not result in immediate toxic effects, initially there are no clinical findings. The history then becomes essential in attempting to exclude or diagnose an exposure; if the details of the history are in doubt, baseline complete blood count (CBC) and PT determinations are important. Additionally, when an acute exposure to a long-acting anticoagulant is under consideration, a factor analysis for factors II and VII may be very useful, if available. An abnormal PT or INR and/or diminished levels of factors II and VII will serve to identify either the chronic ingester of a short-acting anticoagulant or a patient who presents several hours or days after exposure to a long-acting coumarin.[7] In either case, an abnormal PT or INR and/or decreased factor levels should prompt a careful search for bleeding complications. For patients with active blood loss, fresh-frozen plasma (FFP) is the initial treatment of choice, followed by Vitamin K_1 for long-term control of the PT or INR.

Bromethalin

Bromethalin is the newest rodenticide and is considered to be of low toxicity in its commercial product (LD_{50} of >500 mg/kg in rats.) Bromethalin was registered with the EPA in 1982, became available in 1986, and is currently available commercially in the United States as green pellets mixed with cornmeal (which gives it a fresh corn odor) and Bitrex. Of all the currently used rodenticides, less is known about bromethalin, marketed as Assault or Vengeance, than about any of the other rodenticides. From the time bromethalin became available, concern was expressed about its potential toxicity.[51] However, the first possible bromethalin-induced case of human toxicity was not reported until 1996,[14] perhaps because as late as 1997 bromethalin had been registered in only 6 states; in 2 of these states, California and New York, bromethalin first became available in 1996.

Bromethalin is considered to be a highly effective, single-feeding rodenticide with a mode of action reportedly involving the uncoupling of oxidative phosphorylation in the mitochondria, resulting in decreased ATP production, increased fluid accumulation, and consequent increased pressure on nerve axons interrupting nerve impulse conduction.[52]

The pathologic changes resulting from a 1.5 mg/kg oral dose of bromethalin administered to cats, included spongy changes, hypertrophied fibrous astrocytes, and hypertrophied oligodendrocytes in the white matter of the cerebrum, cerebellum, brainstem, spinal cord, and optic nerve.[24,26] Prior to sacrifice of the animal, the clinical manifestations of bromethalin poisonings included ataxia, focal motor seizures, decerebrate posture, decreased proprioception, and depressed level of consciousness. Dogs given oral doses of 6.25 mg/kg of bromethalin developed hyperexcitability, tremors, seizures, depression, and death within 15–63 hours of exposure.[25] Death in animals is also usually preceded by paralysis and loss of tactile sensation.[91,92]

In 1996, the first case of possible bromethalin-induced human toxicity was reported. A 28-year-old male was found unconscious with open packages of two different rat poisons—Velsicol (diphacinone 0.005%) and Vengeance (bromethalin 0.01%), carisoprodol, and alcohol. Tactile stimulation produced muscle tremors and severe myoclonic jerks with flexion of major muscle groups. The patient was intubated, attached to a respirator and lavaged; he was given phenytoin, mannitol, dexamethasone, and diazepam. Blood and urine analyses were positive for his prescribed fluoxetine in therapeutic levels and negative for carisoprodol and ethanol. EEG demonstrated only bihemispheric slowing with a normal head computed tomography (CT) scan. After 24 hours, the patient responded to noxious stimuli and was free of tremors and myoclonus. He was discharged 2 days later.[14]

Because there is no known antidote for bromethalin, it is hoped that the symptomatic and supportive care provided to the patient described above will prove to be sufficient to achieve a good outcome after other significant human exposures. In rats, administration of a commercially available extract of *Gingko biloba* immediately after 1.0 mg/kg ingestion of bromethalin resulted in a statistically significant decrease in the severity of adverse neurologic effects.[24]

MANAGING THE PATIENT EXPOSED TO AN UNKNOWN RODENTICIDE

For the patient exposed to an unknown rodenticide, the approach is more complicated than for a patient who ingests a known common commercial rodenticide such as warfarin or cholecalciferol. First, as always, adequate breathing and circulation must be assured and the patient briefly examined. If the patient is initially stable, the next priority is to make every effort to fully identify the type and quantity of rodenticide ingested.

If the rodenticide and its package material are not brought with the patient, someone should be sent to bring them back to the ED. Identifying a harmless rodenticide ingestion early on is more cost effective and less traumatic to the patient than treating for an unknown ingestion. If the rodenticide container is labeled, and the information is telephoned back to the ED, care should be taken to obtain the *full* name, not just the brand name. For example, until 1986, there was a line of rodenticides all carrying the "Pied Piper" name on a variety of very different products: Pied Piper for Rats and Mice contained ANTU and warfarin; whereas Pied Piper Kwik-Kill Mouse Seed contained strychnine; and Pied Piper Rodenticide contained red squill. Many manufacturers still use similar names for dissimilar poisons.

While awaiting full identification of the rodenticide, a careful physical examination should be performed, searching for toxic signs that indicate specific rodenticides:

- Gastrointestinal symptomatology, paresthesias, and the late onset of hair loss are characteristic of *thallium*.
- Irritability or "apprehension" followed by seizures, coma, and death from respiratory failure or ventricular tachycardia and fibrillation are produced by *SMFA* and *fluoroacetamide*.
- Central nervous system stimulation, opisthotonos, prolonged recurrent motor seizures or convulsions, and medullary paralysis followed by death suggest *strychnine* poisoning.
- Hypotension, vomitus with a rotten or "fishy" odor, cardiopulmonary collapse, coma, renal damage, and leukopenia suggest *zinc phosphide* poisoning.
- Oral and skin burns, luminescent "smoking" vomitus, and stools with a garlic odor, and gastrointestinal and biliary damage characterize *yellow phosphorus* poisoning.

■ Dysphagia, muscle cramps, seizures, hematemesis, and bloody diarrhea followed by cardiovascular collapse suggest *arsenic*.

■ The combination of striking hyperglycemia with or without ketoacidosis, and severe postural hypotension, autonomic and peripheral neuropathies, ileus, and esophageal or GI perforation characterize *PNU or Vacor* poisoning.

■ Muscle tremors, myoclonic jerks with flexion of major muscle groups, and unresponsiveness may be the human manifestations of *bromethalin* poisoning.

■ Dyspnea, rales, pulmonary edema, pleural effusions, and hypothermia are seen with massive ingestions of *ANTU*.

■ Nausea, vomiting, diarrhea, and abdominal pain will probably be the only effects of ingesting *red squill*, but when those effects are combined with signs of ventricular irritability (premature ventricular contractions and ventricular fibrillation), then this potent emetic and cardiac glycoside is certainly identified.

■ Signs or symptoms of a bleeding disorder and abnormal PT or INR, or low levels of coagulation factors, point to either a large acute ingestion of a *superwarfarin rodenticide*, such as brodifacoum, or repeated (chronic) ingestion of a *regular warfarin-type* rodenticide.

■ Finally, evidence of hypercalcemia following (massive or chronic) rodenticide ingestion suggests a new and popular product, *cholecalciferol (vitamin D₃)*.

If a toxic syndrome is identified, aggressive management, including the use of specific antidotes, may be necessary (see Table 90–1). Immediately following an ingestion and prior to the development of signs and symptoms of toxicity, there is no rodenticide currently in use for which lavage followed by activated charcoal, and possibly a cathartic, is *contraindicated*, although they may be unnecessary for the older warfarin-type rodenticides and most unintentional exposures. After the patient is symptomatic, however, orogastric lavage, activated charcoal, and catharsis must be individualized according to the specific toxin and the patient's clinical condition.

If every effort to identify the rodenticide fails, the following diagnostic evaluation may be indicated: A CBC or hemoglobin (Hgb)/hematocrit (Hct) determination and INR (prothrombin time) will help diagnose and manage repetitive ingestions of the older warfarin-type rodenticide, chronic ingestions of the newer *superwarfarin anticoagulant* rodenticides, and a large single ingestion of a superwarfarin a few days after ingestion. Repetitive ingestions of the otherwise harmless older warfarins is an important consideration for children who have pica, as well as for institutionalized, emotionally disturbed adults who may nibble grainlike rodenticides repeatedly. Serum glucose, potassium, and bicarbonate determinations will identify hyperglycemia and ketoacidosis caused by *Vacor*, and an elevated serum calcium concentration suggests *cholecalciferol (vitamin D₃)* ingestion. Liver enzymes, blood urea nitrogen (BUN), and creatinine are useful baseline determinations for rodenticides that cause renal or hepatic damage (eg, *zinc phosphide, yellow phosphorus, cholecalciferol*). A serum sample and 50 mL of urine should be obtained and sent to the toxicology laboratory with the request to hold it for possible heavy metals screening, especially if the patient is vomiting. Finally, if indicated by history or symptomatology, additional specimens may be collected for specific rodenticide determinations (eg, *thallium, strychnine*); chest and abdominal radiographs may be useful because of the radiopaque nature of some of the uncommonly used rodenticides (Chap. 8).

If there is any doubt about either the nature of the rodenticide or the reliability of the patient (or parents) after the diagnostic evaluation, the patient may be admitted or held in the ED for observation. No matter what type of rodenticide was ingested, a determination should be made as to whether the ingestion was unintentional, a suicide gesture or attempt, or a manifestation of abuse or neglect.[7] A psychiatric assessment is, of course, indicated for any possible suicide attempt.

If the patient is a child or infant, the emergency physician should review the principles of poison prevention with the parents (Chap. 4) and should consider the possibility that the incident represents child abuse or neglect. The emotional state of the parents must be taken into consideration when the physician is contemplating sending the child home for continued observation in the absence of history, physical, or laboratory evidence suggesting a serious exposure.

In summary, the key to managing the patient who ingested a rodenticide is to identify the rodenticide, the quantity ingested, its potential toxicity, and any available specific antidote. Toxic ingestions should be excluded or treated immediately; conversely, patients with the most common acute anticoagulant or cholecalciferol exposures should not be overtreated.

ACKNOWLEDGMENTS

Mary Ann Howland, PharmD, and Richard S. Weisman, PharmD, contributed to this chapter in a previous edition.

REFERENCES

1. Ahn JS, Lee TH, Lee MC: Ultrastructure of neuromuscular junction in Vacor-induced diabetic rats. Korean J Intern Med 1998;13:47–50.
2. Amr MM, Abbas EZ, El-Samra M, et al: Neuropsychiatric syndromes and occupational exposure to zinc phosphide in Egypt. Environ Res 1997;73:200–206.
3. Anderson AH: Experimental studies on the pharmacology of activated charcoal: III. Absorption from gastrointestinal contents. Acta Pharmacol 1948;4:275–284.
4. Anderson AH: Experimental studies on the pharmacology of activated charcoal: I. Absorption power of charcoal in aqueous solutions. Acta Pharmacol 1946;2:69–78.
5. Arena JM, Drew RH: Rodenticides, fungicides, herbicides, fumigants and repellents. In: Arena JM, Drew RH, eds: Poisoning: Toxicology, Symptoms, Treatment, 5th ed. Springfield, IL, Charles C Thomas, 1986, pp. 222–251.
6. Arneson D, Chi'en LT, Chance P, Wilroy RS: Strychnine therapy in nonketotic hyperglycinemia. Pediatrics 1979;63:369–373.
7. Babcock J, Hartman K, Pedersen A, et al: Rodenticide-induced coagulopathy in a young child. A case of Münchausen syndrome by proxy. Am J Pediatr Hematol Oncol 1993;15:126–130.
8. Barton CC, Bucci TJ, Lomax LG, et al: Stimulated pulmonary cell hyperplasia underlies resistance to alpha-naphthylthiourea. Toxicology 2000;143:167–181.
9. Ben-Assa B: Indirect thallium poisoning in a Bedouin Family. Harefuah 1962;62:378–380.
10. Bohm GM: Changes in lung arterioles in pulmonary oedema induced in rats by alpha-naphthyl-thiourea. J Pathol 1973;110:343–345.
11. Bova S, Travis L, Debetto P, et al: Vasorelaxant properties of norbormide, a selective vasoconstrictor agent for the rat microvasculature. Br J Pharmacol 1996;117:1041–1046.

12. Bruno CR, Howland MA, McMeeking A, Hoffman RS: Long-acting anticoagulant overdose: Brodifacoum kinetics and optimal vitamin K dosing. Ann Emerg Med 2000;36:262–267.

13. Boyd RE, Brennan PT, Deng JF, et al: Strychnine poisoning: Recovery from profound lactic acidosis, hyperthermia, and rhabdomyolysis. Am J Med 1983;74:507–512.

14. Buller G, Heard J, Gorman S: Possible bromethalin-induced toxicity in a human [abstract]. A case report. J Toxicol Clin Toxicol 1996; 34:572.

15. Chefurka W, Kashi KP, Bond EJ: The effect of phosphine on electron transport in mitochondria. Pestic Biochem Physiol 1976;6:65–82.

16. Chenoweth MB: Monofluoroacetic acid and related compounds. Pharm Rev 1949;1:383–424.

17. Chenoweth MB, Kandel A, Johnson LB, Bennett DR: Factors influencing fluoroacetate poisoning: Practice treatment with glycerol monoacetate. J Pharmacol Exp Ther 1951;102:31–49.

18. Chi CH, Chen KW, Chan SH, et al: Clinical presentation and prognostic factors in sodium monofluoroacetate intoxication. J Toxicol Clin Toxicol 1996;34:707–712.

19. Chi CH, Lin TK, Chen KW: Hemodynamic abnormalities in sodium monofluoroacetate intoxication. Hum Exp Toxicol 1999;18: 351–353.

20. Chugh SN, Aggarwal HK, Mahajan SK: Zinc phosphide intoxication symptoms: Analysis of 20 cases. Int J Clin Pharmacol Ther 1998;36: 406–407.

21. DeBacker W, Zachee P, Verpooten GA, Majelyne W: Thallium intoxication treated with combined hemoperfusion-hemodialysis. J Toxicol Clin Toxicol 1982;19:259–264.

22. Desenclos JC, Wilder MH, Coppenger GW, et al: Thallium poisoning: An outbreak in Florida, 1988. South Med J 1992;85:1203–1206.

23. Diaz-Rivera RS, Collazo PJ, Pons ER, et al: Acute phosphorus poisoning in man: A study of 56 cases. Medicine 1950;29:269–298.

24. Dorman DC, Cote LM, Buck WB: Effects of an extract of Gingko biloba on bromethalin-induced cerebral lipid peroxidation and edema in rats. Am J Vet Res 1992;53:138–142.

25. Dorman DC, Simon J, Harlin KA, Buck WB: Diagnosis of bromethalin toxicosis in the dog. J Vet Diagn Invest 1990;2:123–128.

26. Dorman DC, Zachary JF, Buck WB: Neuropathologic findings of bromethalin toxicosis in the cat. Vet Pathol 1992; 29:138–144.

27. Ecobichon DJ: Toxic effects of pesticides. In: Klaassen CD, ed. Casarett and Doulls' Toxicology: The Basic Science of Poisons, 5th ed. New York, McGraw-Hill, 1996, pp. 681.

28. Edmunds M, Sheehan TMT, Van't Hoff W: Strychnine poisoning: Clinical and toxicological observations on a non-fatal case. J Toxicol Clin Toxicol 1986;24:245–255.

29. Esposti MD, Myers MA: Inhibition of mitochondrial complex I may account for IDDM-induced by intoxication with the rodenticide Vacor. Diabetes 1996;45:1531–1534.

30. Favarel-Garrigues JC, Boget JC: Intoxications aigues par les raticides a' base de chloralose et d'ANTU. Concours Med 1968; 90:2289– 2298.

31. Feingold KR, Lee TH, Chung MY, Sipehstein MD: Muscle capillary basement membrane width in patients with Vacor-induced diabetes mellitus. J Clin Invest 1986;78:102–107.

32. Gajdusek DC, Luther G: Fluoroacetate poisoning: A review and report of a case. Am J Dis Child 1950;79:310–320.

33. Hauser L, Sheehan P, Simpkins H: Pancreatic pathology in pentamidine-induced diabetes in acquired immunodeficiency syndrome patients. Hum Pathol 1991;22:926–929.

34. Hayes WJ: Pesticides Studied in Man. Baltimore, Williams & Wilkins, 1982.

35. Heath A, Ahlmen J, Branegard B, et al: Thallium poisoning: Toxin elimination and therapy in three cases. J Toxicol Clin Toxicol 1983; 20:451–463.

36. Herken H: Antimetabolic action of 6-amino-nicotinamide on the pentose phosphate pathway in the brain. In: Aldridge N, ed: Mechanism of Toxicity. London, St. Martin's, 1970, p. 189.

37. Heiser JM, Daya MR, Magnussen AR, Norton RL: Massive strychnine intoxication: Serial blood levels in a fatal case. J Toxicol Clin Toxicol 1992;30:269–283.

38. Howland MA, Weisman R, Sauter D, Goldfrank L: Nonavailability of poison antidotes. N Engl J Med 1986;314:927–928.

39. Jibani M, Hodges NH: Prolonged hypercalcemia after industrial exposure to vitamin D₃. Br Med J 1985;290:748–749.

40. Kamerbeek HH, Rauws AG, Ham MT, et al: Dangerous redistribution of thallium by treatment with sodium diethyldithiocarbamate. Acta Med Scand 1971;189:149–154.

41. Karam JH, LeWitt PA, Young CH, et al: Insulinopenic diabetes after rodenticide (Vacor) ingestion: A unique model of acquired diabetes in man. Diabetes 1980;29:971–978.

41a. Katz J, Prescott K, Woolf AD: Strychnine poisoning from a Cambodian traditional remedy. Am J Emerg Med 1996;14:475–477.

42. Kenney RM, Michaels IAL, Flomenbaum NE, Yu GSM: Poisoning with N-3-pyridylmethyl-N'-p-nitrophenyl urea (Vacor). Arch Pathol Lab Med 1981;105:367–370.

43. Kosnett MJ, Becker CE: Dimercaptosuccinic acid: Utility in acute and chronic arsenic poisoning [abstract]. Vet Hum Toxicol 1988; 30:369.

44. Kuno M, Weakly JN: Quantal components of the inhibitory synaptic potential in spinal mononeurones of the cat. J Physiol (Lond) 1972; 224:287–303.

45. Layzer RB: Periodic paralysis and the sodium-potassium pump. Ann Neurol 1982;11:547–552.

46. LeWitt PA: The neurotoxicity of the rat poison Vacor: A clinical study of 12 cases. N Engl J Med 1980;302:73–77.

46a. Libenson MH, Yang JM: Weekly clinicopathological exercises: Case 12–2001: A 16-year-old boy with an altered mental status and muscle rigidity. N Eng J Med 2001;344:1232–1239.

47. Lisella FS, Long KR, Scott HG: Toxicology of rodenticides and their relation to human health. J Environ Health 1970;33:231–237.

48. Lisella FS, Long KR, Scott HG: Toxicology of rodenticides and their relation to human health. J Environ Health 1970;33:361–365.

49. Lovejoy FH: Thallium. Clin Toxicol Rev 1982;5:1–2.

50. Marin GA, Mantoya CA, Sierra JL, Senior JR: Evaluation of corticosteroid and exchange transfusion treatment of acute yellow phosphorous intoxication. N Engl J Med 1961;284:125–128.

51. Marsh R: Personal communication, June 29, 1993.

52. Marsh RE: Currrent (1987) and future rodenticides for commensal rodent control. Bull Soc Vector Ecol 1988;13:102–107.

53. Marsh R, Tunberg A: Characteristics of cholecalciferol: Rodent control—Other options. Pest Control Technol 1986;14:43–45.

54. Miller LV, Stokes JD, Silpipat C: Diabetes mellitus and autonomic dysfunction after Vacor rodenticide ingestion. Diabetes Care 1978;1: 73–76.

55. Mills K, Kunkel D: Prevention of severe barium carbonate toxicity with oral magnesium sulfate [abstract]. Vet Hum Toxicol 1993; 35:342.

56. Molner GD, Berge KG, Rosenveas JW, et al: The effect of nicotinic acid in diabetes mellitus. Metabolism 1974;13:181–189.

57. Moore D, House I, Dixon A, et al: Grand rounds, Guy's Hospital—Thallium poisoning. Br Med J 1993;306:1527–1529.

58. Morgan DP: Recognition and Management of Pesticide Poisonings, 4th ed. Washington, DC, United States Environmental Protection Agency, 1989.

58a. Nelson LS, Perrone J, DeRoos F, et al. Aldicarb poisoning by an illicit rodenticide imported into the United States: Tres Pasitos. J Toxicol Clin Toxicol 2001;39:447–452.

59. Nogué S, Mas A, Parés A, et al: Acute thallium poisoning: An evaluation of different forms of treatment. J Toxicol 1982;19:1015–1021.

60. Oberpaur B, Donoso A, Claveria C, et al: Strychnine poisoning: An uncommon intoxication in children. Pediatr Emerg Care 1999;15: 264–265.

61. O'Callaghan WA, Joyce N, Counihan HE, et al: Unusual strychnine poisoning and its treatment: Report of 8 cases. Br Med J 1982; 285:478.

62. Omara F, Sisodia CS: Evaluation of potential antidotes for sodium fluoroacetate in mice. Vet Hum Toxicol 1990;32:427–431.

62a. Palatnick W, Meatherall R, Sitar D, Tenenbein M: Toxicokinetics of acute strychnine poisoning. J Toxicol Clin Toxicol 1997;35:617–620.

63. PDR for Herbal Medicines, 2nd ed. Montvale, NJ, Medical Economics, 2000.

64. Pedersen RS, Olesen AS, Freund LG, et al: Thallium intoxication treated with long-term hemodialysis, forced diuresis and Prussian blue. Acta Med Scand 1978;204:429–432.

65. Pelfrene AF: Synthetic rodenticides. In: Hayes WJ, Laws ER, eds: Handbook of Pesticide Toxicology. San Diego, Academic Press, 1991, pp. 1271–1316.

65a. Perper JA: Fatal strychnine poisoning–a case report and review of the literature. J Forensic Sci 1985;30:1248–1255.

66. Peters RA: Lethal synthesis. Proc Roy Soc Lond 1952;13:139–143.

67. Phelan DM, Hagley SR, Guerin MD: Is hypokalaemia the cause of paralysis in barium poisoning? Br Med J 1984;289:882.

68. Pietras RJ, Stavrakos C, Gunnar RM, Tobin JR: Phosphorus poisoning stimulating acute myocardial infarction. Arch Intern Med 1968; 122:430–434.

69. Plunkett LM: Do current FIFRA testing guidelines protect infants and children? Lead as a case study. Federal Insecticide, Fungicide, and Rodenticide Act. Regul Toxicol Pharmacol 1999;29:80–87.

70. Pont A, Rubino JM, Bishop D, Peal R: Diabetes mellitus and neuropathy following Vacor ingestion in man. Arch Intern Med 1979;139: 185–187.

71. Product Information Sheet. Quintox. Madison, WI, Bell Laboratories, 1985.

72. Prosser PR, Karm JH: Diabetes mellitus following rodenticide ingestion in man. JAMA 1978;239:1148–1150.

73. Reigart JR, Brueggeman JL, Keil JE: Sodium fluoroacetate poisoning. Am J Dis Child 1975;129:1224–1226.

74. Reigart JR, Roberts JR: Recognition and Management of Pesticide Poisonings, 5th ed. Washington, DC, United States Environmental Protection Agency, 1999.

75. Richter CP: The development and use of alpha-naphthyl-thiourea (ANTU) as a rat poison. JAMA 1945;129:927–931.

76. Roza O, Berman LB: The pathophysiology of barium, hypokalemia and cardiovascular effects. J Pharmacol Exp Ther 1971;177:433–439.

77. Rubitsky HJ, Myerson RM: Acute phosphorus poisoning. Arch Intern Med 1949;83:164–178.

78. Sabouraud AE, Ortizberea M, Cano N, et al: Specific anti-digoxin Fab fragments: An available antidote for proscillaridin and scilliroside poisoning. Hum Exp Toxicol 1990;9:191–193.

79. Seon YD, Lee TH, Lee MC: Changes of glomerular basement membrane components in Vacor-induced diabetic nephropathy. Korean J Intern Med 1999;14:77–84.

80. Sgaragli GP, Mannaioni PF: Pharmacokinetic observations on a case of massive strychnine poisoning. Clin Toxicol 1973;6:533–540.

81. Shum S, Whitshead J, Vaughan L, et al: Chelation of organoarsonate with dimercapton succinic acid. Vet Hum Toxicol 1995;37:239–242.

82. Sigue G, Gamble L, Pelitere M, et al: From profound hypokalemia to life-threatening hyperkalemia. A case of barium sulfide poisoning. Arch Intern Med 2000;160:548–551.

83. Silinsky EM: On the role of barium in supporting the asynchronous release of acetylcholine quanta by motor nerve impulses. J Physiol 1978;274:157–171.

84. Simon FA, Pickering LK: Acute yellow phosphorus poisoning. JAMA 1976;235:1343–1366.

85. Singh M, Vijayaraghavan R, Pant SC, et al: Acute inhalation toxicity study of 2-fluoroacetamide in rats. Biomed Environ Sci 2000;13: 90–96.

86. Smith BA: Strychnine poisoning. J Emerg Med 1990;8:321–325.

87. Taitelman U, Roy A, Hoffer E: Fluoroacetamide poisoning in man: The role of ionized calcium. Arch Toxicol Suppl 1983;6:228–231.

88. Talley RC, Linhart JW, Trevino AJ, Moore L: Acute elemental phosphorous poisoning in man: Cardiovascular toxicity. Am Heart J 1972; 84:139–140.

89. Teitelbaum DT, Ott JE: Acute strychnine intoxication. Clin Toxicol 1970;2:267–273.

90. Tuncok Y, Kozan O, Caudar C, et al: Urginea maritima (squill) toxicity. J Toxicol Clin Toxicol 1995;33:83–86.

91. Van Lier RBL, Ottosen D: Studies on the mechanism of toxicity of bromethalin, a new rodenticide. Theoret Toxicol 1981;1:114.

92. Velsicol Chemical Corp: Vengeance Rodenticide Technical Manual. St. Louis City, Michigan 1986, p. 19.

93. Weiss S, Hatcher RA: Studies on strychnine. J Pharm Exper Therap 1922;14:419–482.

94. Wetherill SF, Guarino MJ, Cox RW: Acute renal failure associated with barium chloride poisoning. Ann Intern Med 1981;95:187–188.

Rebecca L. Tominack / Susan M. Pond

H3C—N+⟨pyridyl⟩—⟨pyridyl⟩—N+—CH3

Paraquat

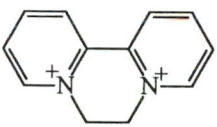

Diquat

A 22-year-old 60-kg male was brought to the Emergency Department (ED) at 2 AM, about 1 hour after deliberately swallowing about 200 mL of an unknown herbicide. He was drinking heavily and had not eaten for about 12 hours. He vomited several times soon after the ingestion and was found by relatives, who brought him to the hospital. In the ED, he was cooperative but restless and agitated. He complained of burning in the mouth, throat, and stomach and shortness of breath. He kept repeating "I want to die." His pulse was 105 beats/min, blood pressure 170/70 mm Hg, respiratory rate 24 breaths/min, and temperature, 97.3°F (36.3°C). Physical examination was normal except for superficial buccal ulcerations, pharyngeal erythema, and epigastric and abdominal tenderness.

An intravenous line was inserted. Gastrointestinal decontamination was initiated with 100 g of activated charcoal mixed into a slurry with 100 mL of 70% sorbitol by mouth. The patient vomited most of the dose and became increasingly agitated and uncooperative. To proceed further with therapy, the patient was paralyzed, intubated, and ventilated with room air. Another dose of charcoal/sorbitol was administered via a nasogastric tube. He was transferred to the Intensive Care Unit (ICU).

The admission chest radiograph was normal, and the electrocardiogram (ECG) showed sinus tachycardia. The complete blood count revealed a moderate leukocytosis, serum electrolytes were normal except for a potassium level of 3.4 mEq/L, liver enzymes were abnormal with a slight increase in alanine aminotransferase and an increased lactate dehydrogenase. An arterial blood gas on room air showed pH 7.43, P_{CO_2} 29 mm Hg, P_{O_2} 98 mm Hg, and bicarbonate 21.5 mEq/L.

At 10 AM an upper gastrointestinal (GI) endoscopy was performed. The pharynx was edematous and inflamed. There were erythema and superficial ulcerations, some oozing blood, in the esophagus and stomach. The treatment plan was aggressive supportive care. By 5 PM, his blood pressure had fallen precipitously to 80/50 mm Hg but responded to a bolus of intravenous 0.9% NaCl and vasopressors. However, arterial oxygenation deteriorated at this time, requiring increasing inspired oxygen tensions to maintain an acceptable P_{O_2} level above 60 mm Hg. Crackles were heard at the lung bases, and acute lung injury was diagnosed. Positive end-expiratory pressure was added to the ventilator settings. His blood

pressure fell again to 70/30 mm Hg and urine output declined to less than 5 mL/h. A Swan-Ganz catheter was inserted to manage his fluid status, which revealed a low cardiac output despite a normal intravascular volume. The peripheral vascular resistance also decreased over the ensuing hours. The patient died at 9 PM from cardiogenic shock, 19 hours after admission.

INTRODUCTION

Definitions and Regulations

Herbicides are chemical agents intended to kill unwanted vegetation or regulate some aspect of the growth cycle of plants. In the United States, the Environmental Protection Agency (EPA) regulates all pesticide products, including herbicides, which are sold or distributed in commerce under the Federal Insecticide, Fungicide and Rodenticide Act (FIFRA). Table 91–1 demonstrates the EPA toxicity classification. Registration is based on scientific studies that demonstrate that these agents can be used without posing unreasonable risks to people or the environment. Aspects of regulation cover all facets of pesticide development and use, including approval to use on a crop-by-crop basis, usage rates, labeling, protective measures for workers, and whether actual application is restricted to those who are specially certified by training in proper handling techniques ("restricted-use pesticides"). In addition, the EPA establishes tolerances (maximum levels) of pesticide residues in raw agricultural commodities and in food or feed products under the Federal Food, Drug, and Cosmetic Act. Under the Food Quality Protection Act of 1996, when establishing tolerances the EPA must consider the higher vulnerability of children to pesticide residues, aggregate exposures of the public to residues from all sources, and sum the effects of agents with a common mechanism of toxicity. Other Federal Agencies (Food and Drug Administration, US Department of Agriculture) and individual states cooperate with the EPA in various aspects of regulation of pesticides. Most of the developed world operates equally stringent pesticide approval and registration systems. Because of this intense, ongoing regulatory oversight, pesticide chemicals are among the best-studied chemicals in modern society.

TABLE 91–1. EPA Toxicity Classifications

Category and Signal Word	Oral LD$_{50}$ (mg/kg)	Dermal LD$_{50}$ (mg/kg)	Inhalation LC$_{50}$ (mg/L)	Eye Irritation	Skin Irritation
I Danger Poison	0–50	0–200	0–0.05	Corrosive: corneal opacity not reversible within 21 days	Corrosive
II Warning	50–500	200–2000	0.05–0.5	Corneal opacity reversible within 8–21 days; irritation persisting for 7 days	Severe irritation at 72 hours
III Caution	500–5000	2000–20,000	0.5–5.0	Corneal opacity; irritation reversible within 7 days	Moderate irritation at 72 hours
IV None	>5000	>20,000	>5.0	Irritation cleared within 24 hours	Mild or slight irritation at 72 hours

History, Chemistry, and Epidemiology

Before the increase in knowledge of organic chemistry in the late 1800s, farmers had few options for weed control. Often there was no attempt to control weeds at all; crop seeds were scattered in a field, nature took its course, and separation of mature weeds from crop was done at the harvest. Smothering weeds before planting by turning the soil with a plough was a standard agricultural practice that only recently is being replaced with an alternative "no-till" practice. In the early 1700s farmers began sowing seed in rows to facilitate mechanical weed removal after the crop emerged. However, pulling weeds by hand or chopping them with a hoe are prohibitively labor-intensive solutions, particularly for field crops. The first serious attempts to find chemical agents for weed control originated in the success of Bordeaux mixture (copper sulfate and lime) and Paris Green (copper acetoarsenite) in controlling fungal diseases affecting the French vineyards. Heavy metal salts such as iron sulfate, copper nitrate, and arsenates and various inorganic chemicals such as borates and chlorates were investigated and found marginally acceptable, primarily to control broadleaf weeds among cereal grain crops on small, intensively cultivated farms. Thus, before the second World War, only a limited number of chemicals were available as herbicides, and these were of relatively low potency, relatively high toxicity to nontarget species, and undesirably persistent in the environment.

In the 1940s the first herbicidal chemical based specifically on plant physiology was discovered, 2,4-dichlorophenoxyacetic acid (2,4-D). This agent interferes with growth-regulating compounds called auxins produced by the plant. It was a great success because of its efficiency against broadleaf weeds in crops, low cost, higher potency, lower toxicity, and lack of persistent residues. Since this success in the 1940s there has been a steady introduction of active herbicide ingredients into the marketplace. At present, there are approximately 180 chemical agents registered for use as herbicides in the United States, 55 introduced in the 1990s alone.

Typical classification schemes organize herbicides by mechanism of action on the plant and subcategorize by general chemical structure. Agents within the same chemical group usually share qualitatively similar toxicologic profiles.

Most contemporary herbicides are organic chemicals, and some of a herbicide's behavior in plants, animals, and the environment can be predicted from its organic chemistry. Aliphatic chain structures with polar, nonhalogen substitutions (N, O, P, S) tend to be readily degraded in the environment by microbiota. Aromatic structures, particularly if halogenated, tend to be more difficult to degrade and might persist in the environment. Although some degree of herbicide persistence may be desirable for crops with a long growing season, persistence from one growing season to another or any bioaccumulation is generally undesirable.

Many herbicide structures include an organic acid or other polar groups that can participate in salt formations. The parent acids are often not sufficiently water soluble for water-based application. Organic salts, often amine, ammonium, sodium, or potassium ionize in water and are more often encountered commercially. Salts are also relatively nonvolatile, which prevents loss to the atmosphere and adds an increased margin of safety against inhalation exposure by the applicator.

The worldwide use of herbicide active ingredients is estimated to have been 2.25 billion pounds in 1997. Thus, herbicides account for approximately 40% of the worldwide total pesticide use of 5.68 billion pounds. The United States market accounted for 25% of world herbicide use (568 million pounds). The largest sector of US use is agriculture, accounting for 83% of total herbicide poundage applied. The highest-use agricultural herbicides in pounds for 1997 were atrazine, 78 million pounds; metolachlor, 66 million; glyphosate, 36 million; acetochlor, 33 million; and 2,4-D, 31 million pounds. In the home and garden market, much smaller by poundage but significant for potential human exposures, the top-use herbicides were 2,4-D, 8 million pounds; glyphosate, 6 million; dicamba, 4 million; mecoprop, 4 million; and trifluralin, 2 million pounds.[2]

FORMULATIONS AND ADJUVANTS

Herbicide formulations generally require multiple ingredients to allow mixing, dilution, application, and stability of the herbicidal chemical. Formulation ingredients are generally not individually disclosed on the label, material safety data sheet (MSDS), or other product information. In the United States, they are lumped under the FIFRA designation "inert ingredients" or "other ingredients." Although often significantly less toxic than active ingredients, they can be present in quantities that pose some risk of adverse health effect. Surfactants, organic solvents, and preservatives should be considered in any exposure, whether a large volume intentional ingestion of product concentrate or a topical exposure to products diluted with water for use. In addition, tank mix additives are adjuvant ingredients sold separately for addition to a commercial herbicide formulation by the applicator at the time of dilution and use. Particularly in occupational exposures, it is important to inquire about tank mix additives in order to assess the entire spectrum of potential toxic or irritant action.

A variety of formulation types are marketed, including emulsifiable or water-soluble solution concentrates, suspension or microencapsulated concentrates, gels, wettable powders, water-dispersible granules, dusts, pellets, and other novel formulations. Most are concentrated liquids or solids that produce solutions, suspensions, or emulsions of the active ingredient when diluted with water for spray. These concentrates carry high proportions of active ingredients (25–65%) and adjuvants compared to the concentrations in the intended use dilution. The toxic and irritant properties of the water dilution are usually more benign than those of the original concentrate. Prediluted products ("ready to use") are purchased at the proper use concentration and invariably contain some type of preservative to prevent mold or bacterial growth. Thus, they may carry some risk of allergic contact dermatitis.

Wettable powders and water-dispersible granules form water based suspensions for spray application. Dusts and granules are broadcast by application directly out of the bag by hand or by mechanized distribution. They characteristically contain relatively low concentrations of the active ingredient (2–25%) because they are not further diluted before use. However, they are dusty, which increases exposure risk to the worker.

Solvents

Aqueous solution concentrates and gels use water as the primary solvent and occasionally alcohols or glycols as cosolvents. Lipid-soluble active ingredients to be delivered in liquid formulations such as emulsifiable concentrates generally require an organic solvent system comprised of a primary solvent and one or more cosolvents. Organic solvents may impart flammability risk as well as their own vapor and ingestion toxicity risk to a formulation. Common solvent classes include vegetable oils, various aromatic and aliphatic hydrocarbons, esters, alcohols, ketones, methyl esters of C_{8-18} fatty acids, and solvents with low vapor pressure such as - cyclohexanone, isophorone, alkyl pyrrolidones, and alkyl biphenyls.

Surfactants and Emulsifiers

Herbicides intended for land-based plants (not natural waterways) usually contain surface-active agents or require surfactant tank mix additives. The health professional must assume the presence of significant surfactant in any herbicide concentrate until proven otherwise. Surface-active agents are critical to the formation and stability of the diluted spray and to enhance the biologic activity of the herbicide by aiding the spread of the spray droplets onto the leaf surface to maximize the area of contact. Because tropical vegetation is often protected by a very thick waxy cuticle, the surfactant content of herbicides used in tropical areas may be markedly increased compared to those used in temperate climates.

Nonionic surfactants are the most commonly used class, followed by anionic agents; cationic surfactants are hardly used at all. Many nonionic surfactants can be easily recognized by their ethoxylated structure. Anionic surfactants can be easily recognized by a sulfate, sulfonate, or phosphate moiety as well as a cation for salt formation. Surfactants can be irritating on skin and eye exposure and cause irritant contact dermatitis with prolonged or repeated exposures. Ethoxylated nonionic surfactants rapidly oxidize on storage and with exposure to air or to hydroperoxides,

peroxides, and a variety of aldehydes, including formaldehyde, to levels that are capable of inducing or inciting allergic contact dermatitis.[46] Surfactants are considered to contribute significantly to the overall clinical picture of large volume ingestions of an herbicide concentrate as occurs in suicidal gestures. Systemic surfactant effects include pharyngeal, esophageal, and gastrointestinal irritation and ulceration, hypotension, hypoxemia, and acute lung injury.

Preservatives and Others

Preservatives to deter mold, fungal, and bacterial growth in the formulation include isothiazolones, parabens, propionic acid, sodium sulfite, sorbic acid, and carbamates, some of which are contact sensitizers. The manufacturer may reduce the concentration of a sensitizing preservative below the guinea pig sensitization threshold. However, because many of the agents are in widespread use across a number of product classes, it is possible for the patient to be sensitized from another source and then react to the low levels in any particular herbicide product.

Other adjuvants provide a variety of functions on an as-needed basis in a particular formulation. Such functional additions include structured polymers, dispersants, binders, wetting agents, disintegrants, fillers and carriers, acid scavengers, hydrotropes, milling aids, densifiers, crystal promoters, effervescents, bittering agents, dyes and dye stabilizers, pH adjusters and buffers, seed preservatives, nitrogen fertilizers, and antifreeze agents.

REGULATORY STATUS OF FORMULATION ADJUVANTS IN THE UNITED STATES

Over a decade ago the EPA initiated a graduated Inerts Regulatory Strategy. This is a major effort aimed to reduce the potential for adverse effects to public health and the environment from pesticides containing potentially toxic inert ingredients. It requires data showing the safety of the material in the amounts and patterns of expected use. Inert ingredients present in pesticide formulations under registration at the time were placed in one of four lists: List 1, Inerts of Toxicologic Concern; List 2, Potentially Toxic Inerts with High Priority for Testing; List 3, Inerts of Unknown Toxicity; and List 4, Minimal-Risk Inerts. Once a material is on List 4, it can be used without additional regulatory burden. Data on the materials on Lists 1, 2, and 3 are being systematically reviewed to either reclassify the material to List 4 or to cancel its use as an inert in pesticides. Once an ingredient is canceled from List 1 or 2, it will likely never be approved for use in the future. New additions to List 4 desired by a manufacturer will eventually require submission and review of a data package. The long-term goal is to have only List 4 inerts in registered pesticides.

List 1 inerts (Toxicologic Concern) were so designated for known carcinogenicity, reproductive or developmental toxicity, neurologic or other chronic effects, ecologic effects, or bioaccumulation. Most were voluntarily withdrawn by manufacturers, and those desired for continued use must have data provided that support the safety of their use.

List 2 inerts (Potentially Toxic, High Priority for Testing) have similar structures to chemicals on List 1. Supporting safety data will be also required to move these items to List 4b.

List 3 inerts (Unknown Toxicity) were so designated because of lack of data to classify them on other lists. Their ultimate disposition is reclassification or, of course, attrition or withdrawal.

List 4 inerts (Minimal Risk) were subdivided into List 4a, GRAS (generally recognized as safe), such as cookie crumbs and corn cobs, and 4b, sufficient data to substantiate that current patterns of use in pesticide products will not adversely affect public health and the environment. List 4b contains chemicals such as isopropyl alcohol, petrolatum, and the majority of surfactants used.

Current categorized lists of the inerts by Chemical Abstracts Service (CAS) number as well as changes over time in the lists can be accessed on the EPA's web page (*www.epa.gov/opprd001/inrts/lists.html*).

HERBICIDE FORMULATION INFORMATION RESOURCES

In the United States, the label will usually identify only the active ingredient, often by its full chemical name rather than a common name. The MSDS usually repeats the ingredient information found on the label. However, any material on the SARA 313 Hazardous Materials List must be identified in the MSDS if it is present at >1% in the formulation or at >0.1% for a carcinogen. Check the hazard identification section of the MSDS for this.

A call to the manufacturer is unlikely to yield a full accounting of the formulation. The persons attempting to answer the inquiry may not themselves have access to the Confidential Statement of Formulation (CSF) that represents the recipe and variations approved by the EPA. A state law in Iowa requires that the manufacturer, within 15 minutes of the call, reveal to a health professional or poison center the exact composition of the pesticide formulation in the event of a human exposure. If the exposure occurs in an occupational setting, the OSHA Hazard Communication Standard, CFR 1910. 1200 (i), requires the manufacturer to reveal the exact identify of all chemicals in the product that may pose a health hazard for the purposes of emergency patient assessment and care. This includes any material claimed to be a trade secret, and it must be revealed *immediately* on request. However, the manufacturer may require the health care professional to keep the trade secrets as secret and may make that request in writing after the urgent situation has passed. For nonemergency inquiries regarding an occupational exposure to a material with trade secret chemicals, the request may have to be made in writing, following the guidelines issued in the standard.

Some global hazard information may be gleaned from the so-called "signal word" (Danger, Caution, Warning) plus other hazard statements on a pesticide label. The EPA requires a signal word appropriate to the classification of the most severe toxic effect found in animal testing of skin irritancy, eye irritancy, or lethality (oral LD_{50}, dermal LD_{50}, or inhalation LC_{50}). Keep in mind that the categories refer only to the concentrated product before dilution. A herbicide product that is Category I for eyes will not be corrosive once it is diluted for spray use.

When assessing any exposure to a pesticide, a series of standard questions often yields useful information in assessing the hazard and risk to the particular patient as well as in forming the treatment options (see Table 91–2).

In dermal or eye exposure, the primary concern will be local irritation. Allergic contact is possible if the formula contains a sen-

TABLE 91–2 Questions that Should Be Asked About Exposure to a Pesticide Product

Name of product and manufacturer
Type of formulation if known (such as emulsifiable concentrate, wettable powder)
Concentration of active ingredient
Presence and concentration of significant inerts, especially surfactants, solvents, preservatives
Dilution to which patient was exposed (may differ significantly from the product in the bottle)
Amount ingested or other quantification of dermal or inhalation exposures
Name and amount of any additives used at the time of mixing, if diluted
Route(s) of exposure
Circumstances of exposure, especially unintentional or suicidal
Time since exposure
Timing and extent of vomiting after ingestion
Age and prior medical conditions of the patient
Any first-aid measures taken by the patient before medical contact

sitizing active or adjuvant ingredient or an ethoxylated surfactant that has formed sensitizing aldehydes and other oxidation products. The results of the guinea pig sensitization test are not necessarily to be relied on in evaluating such a possibility. Because most herbicide active ingredients are water soluble, their penetration through the skin is usually minimal.

In potential spray exposure, the droplet size generated by the equipment is a primary consideration in evaluating extent of airborne exposure. Spray equipment and nozzles used in agriculture are intended to deliver relatively large droplets, which fall quickly to minimize spray drift onto nontargeted plants. Generally more than 95% of droplets generated are larger than 100 μm and are not considered respirable particles, capable of being retained by the lung.[32] Most particles over 10 μm are filtered out by impacting in the nasopharynx and large airways. However, during heavy, prolonged, or overhead spraying, sufficient numbers of large mist droplets can enter the nose and mouth and may result in symptoms such as bad taste and irritated nose and throat. These symptoms are usually self-limiting. Use of an inexpensive, easily obtainable dust/mist respirator will reduce this problem.

Ingestion of most herbicides that have been diluted with water for use is unlikely to cause severe toxicity, even in relatively large quantity. Ingestion of concentrated formulations that carry high loads of active ingredient, solvent, surfactant, and other adjuvants may result in significant toxicity that may be life-threatening. Target organ damage inherent to the active ingredient as well as systemic surfactant effects must be anticipated.

PARAQUAT

Paraquat is the classic example of a herbicide that is safe when used as directed but is capable of dramatic toxicity when misused. Because of its low cost, rapid action, and favorable environmental characteristics, it remains a widely used herbicide throughout the world. The combination of ready availability and high toxicity results in continued appearance of severe and fatal poisonings, many from suicidal intent. Once the free radical–initiated pulmonary fibrosis is under way, even heroic medical interventions fail to salvage the patient. Poor worker protection practices are also problematic in subacute and chronic toxicity.

Characteristics

Paraquat (1,1'-dimethyl-4,4'-bipyridylium dichloride, CAS 1910–42–5) was synthesized in 1882. As methyl viologen it has been used as a color indicator for oxidation-reduction reactions since 1932. This indicator use is based on its reduction to a blue radical by alkaline sodium dithionite,[14] which is also the basis for a colorimetric urine screen for paraquat exposure. Paraquat's herbicidal action was serendipitously recognized when a field observation in the 1950s recorded that a quaternary salt used as a surfactant for a test herbicide was itself herbicidal.[13] Synthesis of more active compounds led to the rediscovery of both paraquat and diquat and their introduction to the market in the early 1960s.[13] Paraquat is a nonselective contact herbicide, desiccant (harvest aid), defoliant, and plant growth regulator primarily used on field crops, fruit and nut crops, and nonagricultural areas such as airports, commercial buildings, and storage yards.

Paraquat rapidly damages and kills plants through contact action by intercepting electrons moving through photosystem I, the photosynthesis pathway in plants that generates reducing equivalents. In the presence of light, it generates reactive oxygen radicals including hydrogen peroxide that disrupt cell membrane integrity. It is rapidly inactivated by adsorption to soil. Because only the contacted leaves are affected, regrowth can occur from the roots of perennials.

Paraquat dichloride is marketed most commonly as an aqueous solution concentrate containing 200 g paraquat dichloride/L (20% w/v), sometimes in combination with diquat or other herbicides. In the United States, paraquat is registered as a Restricted Use Pesticide available in concentrations from 23 to 43.5% dichloride salt. Spray dilutions are typically in the range of 1 to 5 g/L (0.1 to 0.5% w/v). The aqueous concentrates also contain appropriate adjuvant agents as described above and sometimes deterrent adjuvants to prevent unintentional ingestion or reduce the amount swallowed and absorbed. If no blue dye is added, the concentrate is dark brown like cola, for which it can be mistaken, especially if decanted into a soft drink bottle.

Epidemiology

Most cases of paraquat poisoning result from the deliberate ingestion of one of the liquid formulations containing 20 to 40% paraquat.[73] Thousands of deaths have been reported since paraquat was first marketed in 1962, mostly in adults with intentional ingestions. Unintentional ingestions can occur, particularly when the product has been handled or stored incorrectly.[30,73] Death has also been reported from homicidal use, massive dermal exposure, intravenous administration, and prolonged occupational spraying.[20,30,48,73,100]

Suicidal ingestion of paraquat has been a disproportionate problem in some countries including the United Kingdom, Western Samoa, Fiji, Sri Lanka, Malaysia, and Japan.[73] Measures taken by the manufacturer and by regulatory agencies have curbed the incidence of unintentional ingestions and reduced the mortality rate.[107] These have included thickened or gel formulations with reduced paraquat concentration, capping the maximum concentration allowed in commerce and for spray application, restrictions on open sale and availability, improved product labeling, education programs about correct use, marker blue dyes, pyridine stenchant additives to make the product smell bad and taste worse, and emetics. Comparing the 4-year periods immediately before and

after the 1988 institution of the color change from brown to blue and addition of a stenchant and emetic to paraquat formulations in the United States, there was a nearly 50% decline in the proportion of all pesticide exposures represented by paraquat ingestion. This indicates that such measures indeed have an impact on unintentional exposures. However, they are unlikely to influence those truly intent on suicide.

Toxicokinetics

Absorption. Splash or diluted spray mist exposure to skin, eyes, and upper airways leads to minimal systemic absorption despite the risk of local tissue damage. Repeated or continuous dermal contact, especially to a concentrated solution, may lead to some absorption into the bloodstream if the integrity of the stratum corneum is impaired.[4,67,100]

Following ingestion, systemic absorption of paraquat begins rapidly but is incomplete (<30% of the dose). Absorption occurs predominantly from the small intestine and is facilitated by active transport of the herbicide across the mucosal cells.[37] If the GI mucosa is compromised, the percentage absorbed is likely to be higher because of additional absorption by passive diffusion. Peak plasma concentrations of paraquat generally occur within 2 hours after ingestion.[87]

Paraquat's volume of distribution is about 1 to 2 L/kg.[39] It distributes rapidly to most tissues, with highest concentrations in the kidneys and the lungs.[87] Higher renal levels reflect the role of the kidney in the elimination of paraquat. The high concentrations in the lung result from time- and energy-dependent uptake of paraquat by type I and II alveolar epithelial cells via the polyamine uptake pathway. The uptake results from the structural similarity between paraquat and endogenous diamines and polyamines such as putrescine and spermidine.[87] These are taken up actively into the lung by a membrane transport system that has specificity for molecules with two positively charged quaternary nitrogen atoms separated by a distance of approximately 0.6 to 0.7 nm (Fig. 91–1).[27]

Elimination. More than 90% of the absorbed dose of paraquat is eliminated by the kidneys as the parent compound within the first 12 to 24 hours after the ingestion.[10] Even in patients who have ingested a toxic dose, renal function and paraquat clearance remain unaffected for several hours. When renal function is normal, the renal clearance of paraquat is higher than that of creatinine because of net tubular secretion of the molecule. As renal function deteriorates, clearance of paraquat falls concurrently, and the half-life becomes prolonged, from about 12 hours to more than 24.[39] Redistribution from lung and muscle into the bloodstream is slow, with a half-life of about 24 hours,[87] and accounts for the detection of low concentrations of paraquat in the urine for several days after the ingestion.[10]

Toxicodynamic Mechanism

Ingestion of formulated paraquat produces tissue damage in the mouth and upper GI tract. Damage to organs such as kidney, heart, liver, pancreas, and muscle is assumed to be related to redox cycling and oxygen toxicity, but this has not been proven. The mechanism of toxicity has been determined most clearly in the lung when it is exposed to lower concentrations consistent with an ingested dose of 20 to 40 mg cation/kg (equivalent to 27 to 54

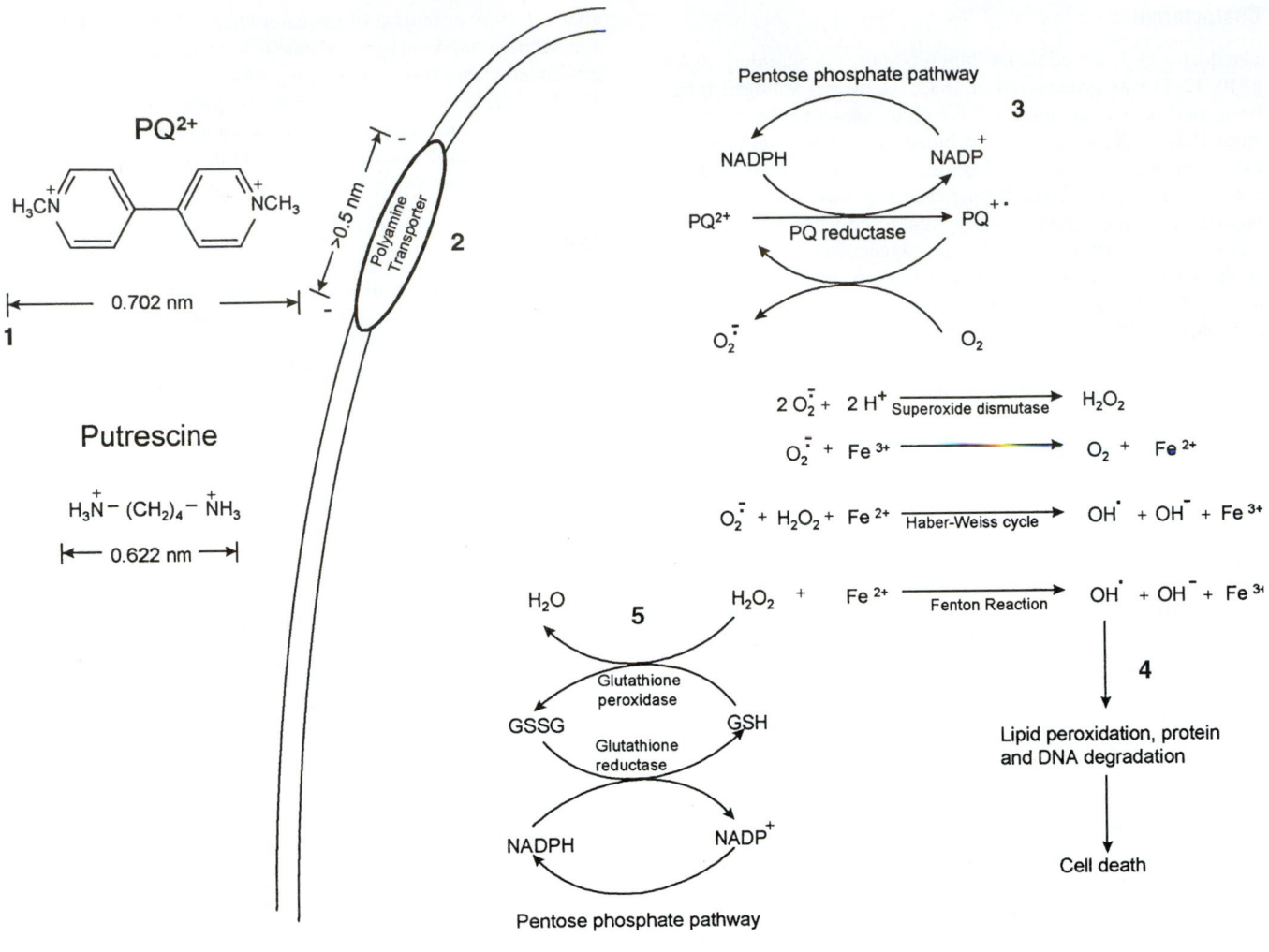

Figure 91–1. Mechanisms of toxicity of paraquat in the type II alveolar epithelial cell. **1.** Structure of paraquat and putrescine, showing the distance between the two nitrogen atoms of each. **2.** Putative receptor responsible for the active uptake of paraquat by the alveolar epithelial cells. **3.** Redox cycling of paraquat and oxygen. **4.** Formation of the OH radical. **5.** Detoxification of hydrogen peroxide (H_2O_2). *(Reprinted, with permission, from Smith LL: Mechanism of paraquat toxicity in lung and its relevance to treatment. Hum Toxicol 1987;6:31–36.)*

mg/kg of the dichloride salt found in 10–20 mL of the 20% concentrate).

Once actively transported inside the pneumocyte, paraquat is reduced by an NADPH-dependent reaction to the monocation radical (PQ$^+$; Fig. 91–1).[87] This radical spontaneously reacts with molecular oxygen to form a superoxide radical ($O_2\bullet$) as well as regenerating the original paraquat dication, which now can undergo this reduction–oxidation cycle again. The nearly inexhaustible supply of electrons and oxygen in the lung sustain this redox cycling. It is further augmented over time by an increasing supply of paraquat molecules to participate in this process as they are accumulated from the blood against a concentration gradient and sequestered in the lung. The recycling participation of paraquat in activating molecular oxygen explains why oxygen enhances the toxicity of paraquat and paraquat enhances the toxicity of oxygen.[47,87]

Many superoxide radicals initially formed in the reaction of oxygen with PQ$^+$ can transfer their free electrons, forming other free radicals and resulting in chain reactions that are very damaging to cellular structures. For example, two superoxide radicals can be catalyzed by superoxide dismutase to hydrogen peroxide (H_2O_2), which in turn can be detoxified by catalases or peroxidases to nontoxic water molecules. On the other hand, in the presence of iron both the initial superoxide and hydrogen peroxide can also be catalyzed to yield the potent hydroxyl radical (OH$\bullet$), which is thought to be the ultimate toxic free radical species derived from paraquat. The OH$\bullet$ generates further free radicals by interacting with biomolecules such as proteins or membrane fatty acids. For example, OH$\bullet$ can take a hydrogen atom from polyunsaturated fatty acids, forming a lipid radical and subsequently lipid peroxides or hydroperoxide. These in turn pass on the free electron to other lipids, and a chain reaction of lipid damage occurs (see Chapters 12 and 13). This process, known as lipid peroxidation, leads to degradation of cell membranes. The reactive oxygen species formed by the initial interaction with PQ$^+$ interact with molecular sites on DNA, proteins, and cell membranes, disrupt cellular functions, and cause cell death. Cascading free radical production explains why the cellular injury from paraquat and other free radical generators far exceeds that produced by the initial reaction products.

NADPH is consumed during the initial reduction of paraquat to PQ^+ and by the glutathione peroxidase and reductase enzyme systems as they detoxify the superoxide radicals and their products.[87] In response, the pentose phosphate and fatty acid synthesis pathways are activated to regenerate NADPH. Restoration of NADPH cellular reducing equivalents promotes the continuous redox reaction involving paraquat and oxygen and thus the continuous generation of more toxic oxygen species.

Antioxidant systems, such as the enzymes superoxide dismutase, catalase, and glutathione peroxidase and vitamins C and E, cannot respond in the same way, and so their capacity to extinguish the runaway free radical chain reaction is limited.[87] This imbalance explains why the dose–response curve for paraquat toxicity is very steep. Once a threshold dose is attained that begins to overwhelm the antioxidant defense system and damage cells, it requires very little increase in dose to attain the maximum toxic effect in a test population.

Clinical Manifestations

The clinical features of paraquat poisoning are summarized in Table 91–3.[7,8,79,88,89,100] Ocular exposure causes gradually developing irritation that reaches a maximum about 12 to 24 hours after exposure as a result of stripping of the superficial epithelium of the cornea and conjunctiva. The severity of the injury is directly proportional to the concentration of the formulation. Dermatitis and nail damage can follow dermal contact with paraquat, particularly if it is not washed off quickly.[79] The nails can become deformed by white bands, ridging, disruption of the nail bed, and impaired growth. Spray mist droplets impacting on the upper respiratory tract mucosa can produce inflammation, epistaxis, cough, and chest pain.

The severity of paraquat ingestion poisoning can be divided into three categories.[100] Patients classified as having mild poisoning may be asymptomatic or develop only GI tract effects such as oral mucosal ulceration and diarrhea. They recover without sequelae. Mild poisoning usually results from an ingestion of 10 mL or less of 20% paraquat dichloride concentrate in a 70-kg person. This is equivalent to 20 mg paraquat cation/kg or 28.6 mg paraquat dichloride salt/kg.

Patients who ingest between 20 and 40 mg paraquat cation/kg (10 to 20 mL of the 20% concentrate in a 70-kg person) usually die 5 days to several weeks after the ingestion. The most characteristic features of toxicity in these patients are the early development of upper GI tract corrosion and acute renal tubular necrosis and the delayed but progressive development of pulmonary fibrosis, which is the cause of death. The characteristic proliferative lesion, pulmonary fibrosis, may not become evident until a week or more after the ingestion, even though destructive phase of cellular damage from free radicals begins immediately.[87] The destructive phase is characterized by loss of type I and II alveolar cells, loss of surfactant, infiltration by inflammatory cells, and hemorrhage. Patients can develop hemorrhagic pulmonary edema. The subsequent proliferative phase is characterized by loss of alveolar integrity, proliferation of fibroblasts, and deposition of collagen in the interstitium and alveolar spaces. The fibrosis, which is in part cytokine mediated,[3] is not specific for paraquat-induced injury but is seen in response to acute alveolitis induced by many pulmonary toxins.

Patients who ingest more than 40 mg paraquat cation/kg (>20 mL of 20% concentrate in a 70-kg person) usually die within 1 to 5 days after ingestion from multiorgan failure, shock, or tissue destruction in the GI tract. Death from esophageal perforation and mediastinitis can occur within 2 to 3 days of the ingestion.

If a history of paraquat ingestion is unsuspected, the diagnosis can be missed. Such patients have been treated for spurious illness such as diphtheria, as was the case in three patients who presented with prominent membranes on the tongue and pharynx.[88]

Diagnostic Testing

Urine and plasma should be sent to the laboratory promptly for qualitative and, if available, quantitative determination of paraquat concentrations. If possible, specimens should be shipped in plastic containers because paraquat binds to glass. Treatment of the patient should continue until the results are available.

Rapid, qualitative analysis in urine is performed by reducing paraquat to its blue monocation radical with sodium dithionite under alkaline conditions and comparing the result with appropriate positive and negative controls.[11,14] A fresh alkaline sodium dithionite solution is made by adding 100 mg of sodium dithionite (nonoxidized) to 5 mL of 5 M NaOH. An aliquot sample (250 μL) of this solution is added to 1 mL urine. If paraquat is present in a

---

TABLE 91–3. Clinical Features of Paraquat Poisoning By Organ System

Cardiovascular
Hypovolemia, shock, dysrhythmias

Central nervous
Coma, convulsions, cerebral edema

Dermatologic
Corrosion of skin, nails, cornea, conjunctiva, and nasal mucosa

Endocrine
Adrenal insufficiency caused by adrenal necrosis as part of multiple organ failure

Gastrointestinal
Oropharyngeal ulceration and corrosion; nausea, vomiting, hematemesis, diarrhea, dysphagia, perforation of esophagus, pancreatitis, centrilobular hepatic necrosis, cholestasis

Genitourinary
Oliguria or nonoliguric renal failure caused by acute tubular necrosis; proximal tubular dysfunction

Hematopoietic
Polymorphonuclear leukocytosis early, anemia late

Respiratory
Cough, aphonia, prominent pharyngeal membranes (pseudodiphtheria), mediastinitis, pneumothorax, hemoptysis, pulmonary edema, and hemorrhage, pulmonary fibrosis

concentration of 2 μg/mL or greater, a concentration-dependent blue to black color is evident. Diquat is reduced similarly to form a yellow-green color.

Plasma or urine paraquat concentrations can be measured quantitatively by a variety of techniques, the most common being radioimmunoassay, gas chromatography, spectroscopy, and high-performance liquid chromatography.[11,26,84] It is usually relatively easy to identify a laboratory that can perform the spot test but more difficult to find one to do the quantitative measurements. Many manufacturers support a 24-hour emergency service that should provide this information for each country. The telephone number for the service can be found either on the product label or via a poison center or other emergency facility. In many countries and areas, quantitative assays are not available in a timely manner to assist with management of the patient. In this case, the management must be guided by the clinical and other laboratory findings.

Clinical chemistry abnormalities reflect the development of acute renal tubular necrosis and necrosis of the liver, lung, pancreas, and muscle.[87] Monitoring plasma creatine kinase is useful in diagnosing the delayed onset of type 1 skeletal muscle fiber damage.[91] If paraquat concentrations in blood exceed about 10 mg/L, measured values of creatinine and LDH may be elevated artificially because of interference with the colorimetric methods used to measure them.[24] Hematologic abnormalities, if any, are usually nonspecific and related to bleeding, infection, or stress. Methemoglobinemia with hemolysis has been reported[65] but was thought to be caused by the monolinuron in the formulation, not the paraquat.[75]

Tissue destruction injury to the esophagus and mediastinum can be associated with pneumomediastinum and pneumothorax.[20] The changes in the lung parenchyma are obvious on the chest radiograph, first as cystic and linear opacities and later as consolidation, particularly in the perihilar regions.[42] A chest radiograph, taken on the ninth day after the ingestion of paraquat in a patient who died 3 days later, is shown in Fig. 91–2. It shows diffuse consolidation most marked in the perihilar regions.

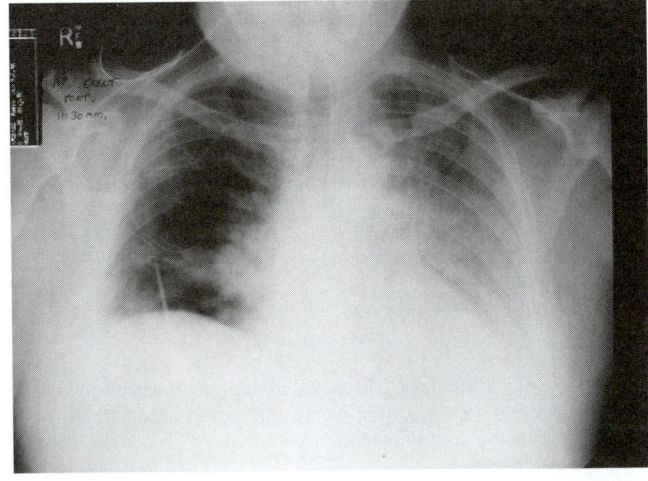

Figure 91–2. Chest radiograph taken 9 days after the ingestion of 70 mL of 20% paraquat, demonstrating diffuse alveolar consolidation, most marked in the perihilar regions.

Management

Early treatment is a very important determinant of survival in paraquat-poisoned patients. Therefore, any patient who has been exposed to paraquat should be treated as a medical emergency, even if there are no symptoms or signs of toxicity at the time of presentation. This is particularly true when the patient has been exposed to one of the concentrated liquid formulations or there has been an ingestion either alone or as a component of a splash exposure with dermal or ocular contact. An accurate history should be taken as for any agrichemical ingestion.

If there has been dermal exposure, either primarily or secondarily from contact with contaminated vomitus, the clothing should be removed immediately and the skin washed gently but thoroughly with soap and water. Harsh scrubbing should not be conducted because the resultant skin abrasion could actually increase the transdermal absorption of paraquat. If the eyes have been splashed, ocular irrigation with copious amounts of water should continue for 15 minutes. These patients should be seen by an ophthalmologist for further management.

Gastric Emptying. If paraquat was ingested only minutes earlier, measures to remove it or prevent its absorption from the gastrointestinal tract should be instituted immediately. Spontaneous vomiting is a near certainty in significant ingestions of paraquat concentrate because of its irritant effects and the emetic added to many formulations. If it has not yet occurred, consideration should be given to inducing vomiting, assuming there are no contraindications. Alternatively, a slurry of activated charcoal, Fuller's earth, bentonite, or garden clay can be considered in the field as a first aid measure, especially if there will be a substantial delay in reaching a medical facility. In most developed countries, resorting to nonpharmaceutical clay will not need to be seriously considered. Even if the patient has already vomited, further gastrointestinal decontamination should be considered. Once the patient has presented for medical care, induced emesis with syrup of ipecac should not be employed because of the time delay involved between its administration and subsequent emesis. This time is better spent by administering an oral adsorbent as quickly as possible.[64]

Adsorbents. Oral adsorbent options include 1 to 2 g/kg of activated charcoal, 1 to 2 g/kg of Fuller's earth in a 15% (w/L) aqueous suspension, or 1 to 2 g/kg bentonite in a 7% (w/v) aqueous slurry. All three adsorbents bind and retain paraquat effectively, but activated charcoal is used most frequently because of its ready availability. In some countries, the manufacturer provides hospitals or local company representatives with kits containing Fuller's earth and a cathartic. The adsorbent may be given with a cathartic such as a magnesium salt or 70% sorbitol (2 mL/kg). If the patient vomits the first dose of the adsorbent, another should be given, through a nasogastric tube if necessary. Rapid control of repeated vomiting with antiemetics and promotility agents is essential when the patient cannot retain the adsorbent.

Lavage. Naso- or orogastric lavage may be relatively ineffective in reducing absorption. Spontaneous vomiting may have already emptied the stomach, leaving little for lavage to affect. Paraquat, in liquid formulation, empties into the small bowel relatively rapidly and may be substantially out of reach by the time lavage can be performed. During the time spent in lavage, paraquat absorption is proceeding rapidly from the bowel. In cats, absorption of paraquat was reduced more by an oral adsorbent than by lavage.[19] In addition, substantial mucosal damage in the esophagus and stomach caused by paraquat formulation places these structures at risk for perforation by the large-bore lavage tube.

Extracorporeal Removal. Methods to maintain or increase the rate of elimination of paraquat from the body should be considered. Forced diuresis and peritoneal dialysis are not effective.[10] Hemodialysis can equal or exceed renal clearance of paraquat, particularly when renal function is impaired, but has not reduced mortality.[34] Therefore, hemodialysis should be performed for the usual indications in patients with acute renal failure and considered only when hemoperfusion is not available.[22]

Hemoperfusion, across a cartridge containing activated charcoal, enhances elimination of paraquat from the blood. When hemoperfusion was performed once in dogs 2 to 12 hours after an LD_{50} or LD_{100} dose of paraquat, mortality was reduced significantly.[33,105] On the other hand, there is no clinical evidence that hemoperfusion is efficacious in humans.[34] Many factors may account for this. Most patents ingest many multiples of a potentially fatal dose; even if hemoperfusion removes an amount equivalent to several fatal doses, many fatal doses still remain in the body. Many patients present hours after ingestion; during this time the paraquat is actively removed from the blood and sequestered in the lung, where it is inaccessible to hemoperfusion. When renal function is normal, hemoperfusion contributes very little additional clearance, so it has proportionately less effect on survival. Likewise, most of the absorbed dose is eliminated by the kidneys during the first 12 hours after the ingestion; hemoperfusion after this time has little proportional effect on total clearance. Last, the slow redistribution phase from the muscles and lung to plasma limits the removal rate of paraquat.[71] Because of these factors, we recommend that charcoal hemoperfusion be begun and continued for 6 to 8 hours only if it can be initiated *within 4 hours* of ingestion. Based on current clinical and experimental evidence, there is no indication for repeated hemoperfusion.

Although continuous arteriovenous hemofiltration can reduce the marked rebound in plasma paraquat concentrations that occurs after hemoperfusion as a result of redistribution of paraquat from the tissues,[70] no clinical benefit of this procedure has been demonstrated.

Fluids and Oxygen. Fluids and electrolytes should be administered IV in sufficient volume to replace GI tract losses and maintain high normal urine output and normal hemodynamics.

Supportive and palliative care are most important components of the management of paraquat-poisoned patients. Attention should be paid to analgesia for the pain associated with the mucosal ulceration. Patients should be monitored frequently for the development and progression of renal and respiratory failure. Supplemental oxygen is a two-edged sword in that it accelerates paraquat-induced oxygen radical toxicity as it temporarily relieves the distress of hypoxia. Generally, supplemental oxygen is withheld until the arterial oxygen tension falls below 50 mm Hg and/or the patient expresses respiratory distress. Its potential contribution to the pathologic process and the ultimate decline of the patient should be acknowledged.

Investigational Management Strategies

None of the proposed "antidotes" for paraquat toxicity have demonstrable clinical efficacy.[5,7] Failed treatments examined experimentally, and in some cases clinically, include those that could prevent the accumulation of paraquat by the lung (various polyamines, *d*-propranolol), increase efflux of paraquat from the lung (cyclophosphamide, *d*-propranolol), reduce or prevent the consequences of the redox cycling (reduction of F_IO_2, vitamin E, superoxide dismutase, ascorbic acid, deferoxamine, selenium, niacin, or N-acetylcysteine), or reduce the extent of pulmonary fibrosis (corticosteroids, immunosuppressive agents, fibrinolytic agents, colchicine, and radiotherapy).

Some groups administer vitamin C (4000 mg/d) and vitamin E (250 mg/d) routinely;[95] these have very few contraindications or side effects, even if efficacy is unproved. Few controlled trials of these approaches have been performed. In one study, when 33 patients given high doses of cyclophosphamide and dexamethasone were compared prospectively with 14 patients given standard therapy (gastrointestinal decontamination and fluids) there was no significant difference in the mortality in the two groups (63 and 61%, respectively).[68] In another study, 16 patients comparable to 17 conventionally treated control patients in age, gender, urine dithionite results, and time since ingestion were given pulse therapy with cyclophosphamide and methylprednisolone. The pulsed-therapy group had a 25% mortality compared to the group treated conventionally (71%).[57]

Despite having theoretical benefit or demonstrated effectiveness in animal models,[25,77] reduction of inspired oxygen concentration in paraquat-poisoned patients has not been demonstrated to be effective clinically. Low-dose inhaled nitric oxide reduces the intrapulmonary shunt in a paraquat-poisoned patient, and anecdotal survival cases exist in which the multifaceted treatment included nitric oxide inhalation. These findings are preliminary and do not justify use of nitric oxide; it may actually add to the toxicity by reacting with the superoxide anion forming the peroxynitrite anion and the hydroxyl radical.[6,23,61]

Paraquat-specific IgG antibodies and their paraquat Fab reduce the in vitro uptake and toxicity of paraquat in type II pneumocytes.[18] However, in vivo use of intact antibodies or Fab fragments is complicated by their reduction of the renal clearance of paraquat because of the protein–paraquat complex formation and the protein load of antibody required to reduce or prevent toxicity. Assuming that a 70-kg patient ingested 30 mg paraquat ion/kg, the absorbed dose to be "neutralized" (5% absorption) would be 105 mg. Thus, a stoichiometric dose of paraquat Fab would be 28 g. If less than a stoichiometric dose can shift the patient's position on the dose toxicity curve to the left, sufficiently far to prevent death, the dose would be less. It would be even less for a recombinant, single-chain antibody (sFv), which is half the molecular weight of Fab. The volume of a 14-g (0.2 g/kg) dose of a sFv corresponds to 200 mL of plasma. In addition, compared to intact IgG and Fab, the volume of distribution (V_d) and renal clearance of sFvs are larger.[21] These kinetic properties would be advantageous for treatment of paraquat poisoning because of its large V_d and high renal clearance. It may be possible to deliver lower doses of anti-PQ sFv by inhalation, more or less topically to the target cells. Unfortunately, such therapy with sFvs has not been developed clinically to date because of the prohibitive costs of manufacturing sufficient amounts of such recombinant products even to test in animals.

Any efficacy of such antibody therapy, however, will be limited by the practical issues such as the length of time before the patient presents to a medical facility. The "window of opportunity" for any effective treatment of paraquat poisoning is very short, only a few hours at most.

Lung Transplantation

Lung transplantation has been performed in a few patients, but only one has survived.[44,63,80,102] In that case, a single lung was transplanted 44 days after paraquat ingestion; recovery was complicated by subsequent removal of the other poisoned native lung, and severe myopathy prevented weaning from mechanical ventilation.[102] Therefore, single or bilateral lung transplantation can be considered if a patient survives for 3 weeks or longer with end-stage respiratory failure and otherwise meets criteria for transplantation. In this context of prolonged medically supported survival, other serious, long-term effects of paraquat are revealed. For example, patients given lung transplants who survived for several months after paraquat exposure have developed progressive toxic myopathy, which proved fatal in one case.[80,102]

Prognosis

Not all patients who ingest paraquat die, but the mortality in some series of patients has been as high as 75%.[7,83,100] Typically a patient who survives does not develop pulmonary injury and has no residual effects. There have been a few survivors reported with residual pulmonary fibrosis, and some have progressively improved over time.[9,40]

The outcome is dose-dependent. Patients who ingest paraquat intentionally usually take a higher dose than those who ingest it unintentionally and therefore have a worse prognosis. Similarly, the incidence of death is higher the more concentrated the formulation ingested.

Plasma concentrations of paraquat measured within 28 hours after the ingestion are useful in estimating the prognosis according to the nomogram presented in Fig. 91–3.[36,74] This nomogram was derived empirically from clinical data and not by statistical means. Thus, it is not infallible. Patients with higher concentrations than those expected from the nomogram to be associated with survival have survived; conversely, some with lower concentrations have died.[74] When experience with the nomogram in 166 cases was reviewed, it correctly predicted the outcome in 93% of cases who died and in 64% who survived.[74] Therefore, reports in the literature of unexpected survival in individual patients as determined on the nomogram should be attributed only with caution to one or another innovative treatment because of the imperfections of the predictive line. The extension of this nomogram beyond 28 hours[83,84] has similar predictive efficacy. It appears that whenever the initial plasma concentration of paraquat exceeds 3 mg/L, mortality is 100%.[34] The mode of death is cardiogenic shock within 24 hours of the ingestion in those whose paraquat levels exceed 10 μg/mL.[74]

Additionally, concentrations of paraquat in urine obtained within the first 24 hours of ingestion can be used to estimate prognosis.[83,84] Of 53 patients studied, 15 who had urinary concentrations of paraquat below 1 μg/mL within the first 24 hours survived. Urinary concentrations in those who died within 24 hours ranged from approximately 10 to 10,000 μg/mL; concentrations in those who died later from pulmonary fibrosis were between 1 and 1000 μg/mL.

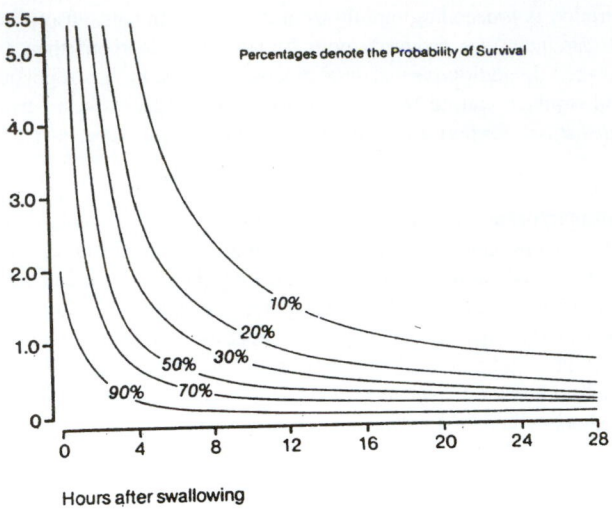

Figure 91–3. Nomogram showing the relationship among the plasma concentrations of paraquat on the *ordinate* (μg/mL), time after ingestion on the *abscissa*, and the probability of survival. *(Reprinted, with permission, from Hart RB, Nevitt A, Whitehead A: A new statistical approach to the prognostic significance of plasma paraquat concentrations [Letter]. Lancet 1984;2:1222–1223.)*

Several compilations of indices using physiologic and clinical data[76,84,90] have been proposed and have predictive efficacy comparable to the nomogram of plasma paraquat level against time. The rate of increase in plasma creatinine over a 5-hour period has also been proposed as a predictor of outcome but has not yet been subsequently validated.[76] One group prospectively studied routine lung scintigraphy changes in 13 paraquat-poisoned patients using [97]Tc-labeled diethylenetriamine pentaacetate aerosol inhalation compared to volunteer controls. The four patients showing normal alveolar permeability survived, and the nine with abnormal alveolar permeability died.[45]

Several factors can moderate the amount of paraquat absorbed and thus the plasma and urinary concentrations. When paraquat is swallowed on a full stomach, its absorption is reduced because of delayed gastric emptying and the adsorption of the herbicide by the food.[8] The presence of ulceration in the upper gastrointestinal tract is a poor prognostic sign because it may reflect the concentration and the dose of paraquat in the formulation. In one series of patients who had upper GI endoscopy between 3 hours and 3 days after the ingestion, 9 of 14 patients with gastric and esophageal ulcerations died.[8] Conversely, all six who had no gastric ulcerations survived.

The development of renal failure heralds a poor prognosis. Of 20 patients in one series who developed renal failure, 19 died.[8]

DIQUAT

Diquat (1,1′-ethylene-2,2′-dipyridylium dibromide)[12] is used agriculturally for the same purposes as paraquat as well as for the control of aquatic weeds; it is combined with paraquat in several formulations. The LD[50] of the two compounds in animals is of the same order of magnitude.[89] In terms of caustic effects, kinetics, and mechanisms of toxicity, diquat is similar to paraquat[89] with one important exception. Diquat lacks the structural features necessary for active transport by the polyamine uptake pathway into the lungs. Therefore, the extent of pulmonary injury and fibrosis in patients who take toxic doses of diquat is much less than that after paraquat. In comparison to paraquat, there have been relatively few cases of diquat poisoning. In a review of 11 cases the lethal adult human dose of diquat was 6 to 12 g.[8] Effects from massive ingestion include severe gastrointestinal damage, airway compromise, respiratory failure, renal failure, seizures, and hemodynamic collapse. Most died despite treatment such as forced diuresis, hemoperfusion, and the administration of antioxidants.[35,60,72,85,101,106] In one fatal case, the serum diquat level 4 hours after ingestion of 60 g of diquat cation was 64 μg/mL. The patient exhibited progressive anuria, coma, and seizures and died 26 hours after ingestion from cardiovascular collapse. Extracorporeal removal techniques yielded 1.09 g of diquat. Postmortem analysis revealed marked renal tubular damage.[45] Another patient ingested 200 mL of diquat dibromide diluted to 1.84% and remained asymtomatic until 8 hours afterward. He subsequently developed esophagitis, epiglottitis, and acute renal failure, from which he slowly recovered.[98] Intravaginal instillation of 20 mL of concentrated diquat formulation resulted in local corrosion, renal failure, diffuse slowing on EEG, and a 3-month spastic tetraparesis, from which she eventually recovered.[78]

Treatment of diquat-exposed patients proceeds along the same lines as for those exposed to paraquat regarding gastric decontamination, adsorbents, hemodialysis and perfusion, and supportive care. Diquat may introduce an artifact in the laboratory assay for serum creatinine.[85]

GLYPHOSATE

| Glutamic acid | Glufosinate | Glyphosate |

History and Epidemiology

Glyphosate (*N*-phosphonomethyl glycine) was originally synthesized by a French chemist and logged into a chemical bank. In the late 1960s an American company acquired and screened this bank of compounds and discovered glyphosate's remarkable herbicidal activity. After nearly 30 years of commercial availability, glyphosate is one of the most widely used and studied herbicides in the world. Growth in use has averaged approximately 20% per year. Use continues to increase largely because of its suitability for "no-till" soil preparation before planting of crops. This conservation measure preserves topsoil; over half of the world's 650 million arable acres will use no-till planting by 2002. Glyphosate is also one of the nonselective herbicides for which genetically engineered resistant crops have been developed, and this may eventually become the largest driver to further increase in use.

Glyphosate is registered for use in over 100 countries. The original glyphosate formulation concentrate (Roundup Herbicide,

Monsanto) contained the isopropylamine salt of glyphosate (41% w/v), a polyethoxylated tallow amine surfactant (15.4% w/v), and water. Over 100 different brand names comprised of many formulations have been sold worldwide by this company. In addition, other companies may now market the glyphosate molecule, and it is estimated to appear in thousands of other herbicide products. Some products contain the original isopropylamine salt, but some contain the monoammonium, sodium sesqui-, or other salts of glyphosate. Some products are dry formulations; some contain different surfactant systems, or greater or lesser amounts of total surfactant, or no surfactant at all. Glyphosate may also be sold in combination with other herbicides including various chlorphenoxy compounds, simazine, linuron, and picloram or with a fertilizer to boost plant growth, thereby enhancing lethality.

A related chemical is glyphosine [*N*,*N*-bis(phosphonomethyl) glycine], which is a plant growth regulator. It is a dimer of glyphosate.

Agronomic Mechanism and Toxicity

Glyphosate is applied after the plant has emerged from the soil ("postemergent") and is nonselective in its action, killing any green plant. It inhibits the enzyme 5-enolpyruval shikimic acid 3-phosphate (EPSP) synthetase, which is important in the biosynthesis of aromatic amino acids. The lethal effects in the plant can be reversed by supplying L-phenylalanine and L-tyrosine. There is no equivalent enzyme in animal systems; thus, this is the mechanism of its selective toxicity. In addition, it has a minor activity as a nonspecific metal chelator, an effect that does not appear important clinically.

Glyphosate's environmental profile is considered quite favorable. It displays a relative lack of volatility, lack of residual soil activity, lack of soil migration, rapid environmental biotic degradation to basic elements ($t_{1/2}$ in soil = 60 days), and no bioaccumulation. Its mammalian safety profile is also quite favorable. It is noncarcinogenic (US EPA category E), nonmutagenic, and devoid of developmental toxicity. There is no serious chronic toxicity in 2-year animal feeding studies, and its acute oral toxicity is relatively low (rat oral LD_{50} = 5600 mg/kg).

The formulated glyphosate is practically devoid of systemic toxicity from dermal exposure. The moderate skin irritation of the original Roundup formulation is caused by the polyethoxylated tallow amine surfactant, which is corrosive to skin in animal tests when applied without dilution. As the surfactant content is progressively reduced in the concentrated formulation or by dilution, the potential for irritation declines.

Toxicokinetics

Absorption. Glyphosate kinetics and metabolic fate have been extensively characterized in animals, and human clinical data appear to follow the same general patterns. Rats orally dosed with ^{14}C-labeled glyphosate acid in water absorbed 20 to 30% and excreted the remainder in the feces. A 10-fold higher dose resulted in 30-fold higher blood concentrations, suggesting an enhanced absorption ratio at higher doses. Pretreatment of rats with surfactant and glyphosate in drinking water did not increase the subsequent absorption of the labeled glyphosate.[16]

Dermal absorption has been determined experimentally in an in vitro human skin model using ^{14}C-labeled glyphosate in formulated herbicide. After 16 hours, not more than 2.3% of the applied dose was recovered in the plasma receptor fluid. In vivo dermal absorption studies in rhesus monkeys confirmed poor absorption; total urinary recovery of labeled glyphosate was only 0.4% of applied dose in 24 hours and 2% in 7 days. Water or soap and water washing removed the applied glyphosate; 50% was still recoverable by washing at 24 hours.[104] Several worker-biomonitoring studies verify poor dermal absorption by failing to find detectable levels of glyphosate in the urine.[43,55]

Elimination. Glyphosate is not metabolized in mammalian systems; a minor metabolite, aminomethyl phosphonic acid, may be detected in amounts <0.5% of glyphosate and is theorized to originate from colonic bacterial metabolism. It is rapidly excreted unchanged in the urine. Experience in human poisoning suggests an elimination half-life from the blood of 2 to 3 hours, assuming renal function is normal. Half-life becomes prolonged as renal function progressively deteriorates. Following IV dosing of labeled glyphosate in rats, 90% was recovered in urine in 6 hours, and essentially all within 24 hours.[16] IV dosing of glyphosate in dogs resulted in a V_d of 0.28 L/kg, an average elimination half-life of 82 minutes, and a renal clearance of 2.5 ± 0.5 ml/min/kg.[81] The absorption, distribution, and disposition of the polyethoxylated tallow amine surfactant are not known. It comprises a related assortment of large molecules that are unlikely to be absorbed intact from the normal gut.

Clinical Manifestations

Several large published series have characterized the range of clinical effects produced by ingestion of the classic Roundup formulation in Pacific area countries.[56,66,82,94,99] These are irritation, edema, and erosions of the oropharynx and GI tract; nausea, vomiting, diarrhea, and midchest and abdominal pain; leukocytosis, metabolic acidosis, elevated salivary amylase, tachypnea, hypoxia, acute lung injury, and volume-responsive hypotension followed by cardiovascular hypotension unresponsive to fluids and pressor amines. Secondary organ dysfunction may occur in the CNS, liver, and kidneys. Some cases are complicated with aspiration pneumonitis. Fatality rates in the large published series range from 7.5 to 16%. Those who ingest large volumes of concentrate (>200 mL) and those developing acute lung injury or cardiogenic shock are at more risk of a fatal outcome. In a series of 50 patients evaluated with upper endoscopy, esophageal injury was noted in 68%, gastric injury in 72%, and duodenal injury in 16%. Severity of esophageal injury (Zagar grade 2 or 3) was correlated with length of hospital stay and complication rate.[17] In a series of 53 patients evaluated by laryngoscopy, 36 (68%) showed significant laryngeal injury, which was correlated with longer length of hospital stay and risk of aspiration pneumonitis.[41]

Oral and gastrointestinal irritation (burning of mouth and throat, vomiting, abdominal pain) develop rapidly after ingestion. Hypotension may develop within hours of very large ingestions. Some patients may appear to be relatively stable for the first 8 to 12 hours and then develop hypotension and respiratory distress.

It is difficult to correlate ingested amount with severity of clinical effect because of the unmeasured loss through vomiting. However, in general, severity follows a dose-related trend. In one large series, there were 11 fatalities among 41 cases (27%) who ingested an estimated 150 mL or more of concentrated formulation (41% isopropylamine glyphosate, 15% ethoxylated tallow amine surfactant) but none among 51 who ingested <150 mL.[99] In another large series, an average ingestion of 17 ± 16 mL (range

5–50 mL) produced no symptoms; 58 ± 52 mL (5–150 mL), mild symptoms; 128 ± 114 mL (20–500 mL), moderate symptoms; and 184 ± 70 mL (85–200 mL), severe symptoms or death.[82] Risk of death appears to be higher in older patients.[17, 41]

Once diluted for use, the various glyphosate formulations offer little risk of adverse effects except temporary, minor eye, membrane, or skin irritation. The potential for adverse systemic effect is essentially nil. Some dry formulations may contain sodium sulfite, which could cause bronchospasm in sulfite-sensitive patients. Allergic contact dermatitis is possible if a sensitizing preservative such as 3-iodo-2- propanyl butyl carbamate or a benzisothiazalone is contained in the particular formulation. The latter preservatives are also phototoxic. Additionally, recent experimental evidence has shown that the ethoxylated surfactants undergo decomposition with time to release a variety of aldehydes including formaldehyde. This is known to be a potent contact sensitizer and may account for many skin rashes previously judged to be unrelated to glyphosate herbicide formulations.[8]

Mechanism of Toxicity of Formulated Glyphosate

The surfactant is suspected to be the primary culprit of this toxic syndrome, but the relative contribution of the surfactant and the glyphosate to the toxic syndrome remains controversial. Many of the clinical features identified in glyphosate-surfactant poisonings occur regularly with reported cases of large-volume ingestion of herbicide concentrates irrespective of the active ingredient. This is observational evidence that a systemic surfactant syndrome accompanies many serious herbicide ingestion poisonings and is a primary determinant of the toxic symptoms in the early phase of acute poisoning. Although it is described as nonionic, its tertiary nitrogen is largely protonated at physiologic pH, and it clinically produces effects more traditionally associated with a cationic surfactant. Clinical descriptions of ingestion of benzalkonium chloride, a quaternary ammonium cationic surfactant, share striking similarities with those of the tallow amine-containing original Roundup formulation. These include superficial necrosis of mucous membranes, severe GI tract irritation with erosions, glottic edema, pulmonary edema, profound hypotension, oliguria, renal failure, and cardiovascular collapse.[28]

An in vivo intravenous study in dogs confirmed the surfactant's role in causing hypotension through myocardial depression at exposure levels comparable to human poisonings.[92] It compared the cardiovascular physiologic effects of infusions of equivalent doses of isopropylamine glyphosate alone, polyethoxylated tallow amine surfactant alone, or the two combined as in the formulated herbicide. The endpoint of infusion was a 50% fall in mean arterial pressure. Both the surfactant alone and the combination reduced mean arterial pressure, heart rate, cardiac output, and left ventricular stroke work index and elevated peripheral vascular resistance, whereas the glyphosate infused alone did not. These findings suggest that the hypotension produced was primarily related to myocardial depression and was caused by surfactant.

It is theoretically possible that isopropylamine itself may exhibit cardiac or other actions. It represents 30% by weight of the isopropylamine salt of glyphosate, is used as an emulsifying agent and wax remover, and has a rat oral LD_{50} of 820 mg/kg.

Issues of relative contribution of various formulation ingredients to the clinical effects have not been fully investigated; current understanding remains limited. Soon after the first large suicidal ingestion series were published, the amount of surfactant in the original Roundup formulation sold in the United States was significantly reduced; thus, the published literature probably overstated the toxic potential to humans who might have ingested this revised formula. The myriad of different glyphosate formulations currently sold as options to the original formulation share this tenuous connection to the literature. Publications based on a particular archaic glyphosate formulation may become largely irrelevant to contemporary clinical information needs on glyphosate because the marketed formulations continue to change and diversify. However, as clinical descriptions of agrichemical *surfactant* poisonings, the literature will have enduring applicability.

Laboratory

In some fatal cases serum glyphosate levels have been reported to exceed 3000 mg/L, although many are significantly lower.[92] However, serum levels are not useful clinically in assessing the severity of exposure or poisoning. Furthermore, glyphosate analysis is not readily available. Patient status can be assessed by serum determinations of oxygenation status, renal and hepatic function, electrolytes, and acid–base balance. Leukocytosis and increased serum amylase may be noted. The chest x-ray may be normal or show evidence of acute lung injury or aspiration. The electrocardiogram shows no abnormalities specific to the ingestion but may document possible abnormalities in patients with severe cardiorespiratory compromise.

Treatment

Gastric Decontamination. Ingestion of less than two mouthfuls of concentrated herbicide in an adult are unlikely to cause serious illness, and ingestions of nearly any amount of dilute (<2% glyphosate) solution are inconsequential other than risk of bad taste, nausea, and perhaps vomiting. In significant ingestions of herbicide concentrate, spontaneous vomiting usually occurs rapidly and obviates the need for gastric lavage. The potential risk to the patient who may have suffered severe mucosal damage to the esophagus and stomach as well as the timing of the procedure relative to ingestion must be considered before lavage is attempted.

Activated charcoal has been shown indirectly to adsorb the fatal toxin in formulated herbicide. Pretreatment of rats with activated charcoal before administration of an LD$_{100}$ oral dose of the original Roundup formulation or an equivalent dose of surfactant prevents mortality. Likewise, in vitro mixing of either with activated charcoal and administration of the supernatant is not lethal. This suggests that the primary toxic principal is adsorbed by activated charcoal and is probably the surfactant.[81] The binding characteristics of glyphosate and activated charcoal are unknown.

Extracorporeal Removal. Hemodialysis and resin hemoperfusion are effective in removing glyphosate from blood. Activated charcoal hemoperfusion of cow blood in an in vitro system failed to remove glyphosate.[81] It is not expected that hemodialysis would remove surfactant because of its large molecular size. Because of the rapid elimination of glyphosate by normal kidneys and its uncertain role in the toxic syndrome, there is no proven benefit to accelerating glyphosate removal by hemodialysis. This should be reserved for renal indications. Although, theoretically, resin hemoperfusion may remove surfactant, this has not been proven experimentally or in patients, largely because the surfactant composition

does not permit analysis. Neither has improved clinical outcome been demonstrated for hemoperfusion. This technique cannot be recommended without some evidence of efficacy.

Supportive Care. There are no specific therapies or antidotal measures for glyphosate-surfactant poisoning. It does not inhibit acetylcholinesterase and is not an organic phosphorus agent but a phosphonate. Atropine and oxime reactivators are not indicated and should be avoided. Fluids and electrolytes should be administered IV in sufficient volume to replace GI tract losses and maintain high normal urine output and normal hemodynamics. However, in severe poisoning, hypotension from cardiovascular compromise may supervene; fluid overload may precipitate or worsen hypoxemia and respiratory distress. In such cases, hemodynamic monitoring may be necessary to optimize management.

Hypoxemia occurs frequently even in the absence of abnormal chest x-ray and should be monitored and corrected, with patients endotracheally intubated and mechanically ventilated if necessary.

Prognosis

Fatalities generally occur in the first 2 days after ingestion. Development of respiratory distress requiring intubation, renal failure requiring dialysis, and shock are poor prognostic signs.[56] Recovery in survivors is complete.

GLUFOSINATE AND BIALAPHOS
Description and Toxic Mechanism

The soil fungus *Streptomyces hydroscopicus* produces the tripeptide phosphinothricin-alanine-alanine, which is metabolized in plants and animals to phosphinothricin. This unique amino acid, also known as glufosinate (2-amino-4-hydroxymethylphosphinyl butanoic acid), is an analogue of glutamic acid. It exerts a nonselective herbicidal action by inhibiting glutamine synthetase, an enzyme important in amino acid metabolism, nitrogen transformation, and detoxification of ammonia. The accumulation of ammonium is phytotoxic. Bialaphos (phosphinothricin-alanyl-alanine) is the original tripeptide parent molecule and has limited commercialization as a herbicide. It is metabolized in plants to glufosinate. Its active moiety, glufosinate, is synthesized and used in many world areas for control of weeds and weedy grasses, especially among permanent crops as in plantations, forests, orchards, and vineyards, and to desiccate certain crops to facilitate harvest.

Glufosinate is marketed as the ammonium salt (CAS 5127–47–2) in various products including Basta®, Ignite®, Challenge®, Finale®, and Hayabusa®. Basta's surfactant has been characterized as anionic, sodium polyoxyethylene alkyl ether sulfate. Bialaphos is marketed in Japan as Herbiace.

Because of its structural similarity to glutamate, glufosinate was investigated in laboratory animals for activity on various enzyme systems utilizing glutamate. Glufosinate inhibits mammalian glutamine synthetase in various tissues but causes accumulation of ammonia and glutamate only when administered at near-lethal levels. The mammalian system, unlike plants, apparently can compensate for inhibition of glutamine synthetase by other metabolic pathways.[29] Glufosinate also inhibits glutamate decarboxylase, leading to a decrease in GABA.

Toxicokinetics

Glufosinate and bialaphos are absorbed orally, at least to some extent. Onset of serious CNS symptoms is delayed several hours after a large volume ingestion of herbicide concentrate. Glufosinate is excreted renally unchanged. The serum glufosinate concentration was measured every 3–6 hours in a 65-year-old male who ingested an estimated 60 grams as 300 ml of a 20%w/v concentrate. Total urinary excretion was measured every 24 hours. The distribution half life ($T_{1/2}$ alpha) was 1.84 hours and the elimination half life ($T_{1/2}$ beta) was 9.6 hours. The apparent volume of distribution was estimated to be 1.4 liters/kg. Renal clearance was calculated as 78 ml/min, and represented nearly all of whole body clearance.[38]

Pathophysiology

Glufosinate and bialaphos are centrally neurotoxic in man. The exact mechanism of central perturbation is unclear but both seizures and profound CNS depression can occur concurrently. Clinical improvement lags behind the physical elimination of the compound, implying prolonged effect at the target site(s).

The circulatory failure noted in patients with severe acute oral poisoning is most likely due to systemic surfactant syndrome. This was experimentally demonstrated in an in vivo and in vitro animal model by induction of the characteristic vasodilatation and cardiac depression effects caused by either the surfactant alone or the formulated herbicide containing the surfactant but not by glufosinate alone.[51]

Clinical Manifestations

Early symptoms of the systemic surfactant syndrome may appear very soon after ingestion of concentrate and include oral irritation, nausea and vomiting. Death from cardiovascular failure has occurred in at least two patients who ingested at least 300 mL of the surfactant-formulated herbicide.[52] Onset of CNS symptoms may be delayed for 4 to 8 hours after large ingestion; in one patient it occurred 34 hours after ingestion.[52] CNS symptoms may continue to progress for 24–48 hours. Typical CNS symptoms include drowsiness, ataxia, disordered eye movement, disorientation, tremor, stupor, deep coma, and central apnea and respiratory arrest.[38, 50,52,96] Convulsions are a late manifestation of poisoning and appear in only approximately 50% of those seriously poisoned.[53] Case reports note seizure onset 7.5 to 29 hours after ingestion.[50,93,96] They are always preceded by loss of consciousness and in fact may begin after the patient is beginning to awaken from deep coma.[96] Seizures are repetitive and can be prolonged; status epilepticus is possible. They may occur for several days, although their duration and frequency will diminish.[96]

Secondary organ damage may manifest as a result of seizure activity including fever, acute muscle damage, and post–status epilepticus myopathy.

In the recovery period, loss of short-term memory (both retrograde and anterograde amnesia) may occur.[103] This effect is also a feature of amnestic shellfish poisoning, which involves domoic acid, another excitatory amino acid neurotransmitter. Recovery from glufosinate poisoning is prolonged; extubation may be delayed for a week or more. Normalization of higher functions may require weeks. Some patients have required discharge into a rehabilitation facility.

Well-documented central diabetes insipidus developed approximately 14 hours after admission in one reported case of glufosinate poisoning. The peak urine output was >300 mL/h, serum sodium 167 mEq/L, plasma osmolality 332 mOsm/kg, urine osmolality 200 mOsm/kg, and plasma antidiuretic hormone abnormally low. The patient responded to intranasal desmopressin given 40 hours after admission, with normalization of affected physiologic parameters within 48 hours.[93]

Ingestions of the related chemical bialaphos are less frequent because of its limited commercial availability. In one well-documented case of ingestion of 100 mL of 32%w/v bialaphos plus ethanol, the patient exhibited early vomiting, respiratory distress, and metabolic acidosis. Ten hours after ingestion he developed nystagmus, which lasted for 19 days. Respiratory arrest occurred 36 hours after ingestion. Seizure episodes lasting 80 seconds, followed by 40 hours of complete apnea, developed 44 hours after ingestion. The patient recovered and was discharged without apparent sequalae.[62]

Laboratory

There is no readily available laboratory test to document ingestion of glufosinate or bialaphos or determine serum levels. HPLC has been used in research settings to measure glufosinate in plasma, urine, and CSF. Serum should be monitored for elevations of amylase and hepatic transaminases, and creatine phosphokinase monitored in patients with multiple seizures. Clinicians should be aware of the potential for diabetes insipidus and suspect it if the urine output, serum sodium, and serum osmolarity become abnormally high without attendant concentration of urine. There are no clinical data on serum ammonia levels.

Management

In one series, five patients who reportedly ingested 0.3 to 1.8 mL/kg (~20–100 mL) of 18.5% glufosinate ammonium formulation remained asymptomatic, but six who ingested 1.7 to 9.1 mL/kg (100–500 mL) developed CNS dysfunction 8 to 34 hours later. The acute neurotoxic dose of glufosinate was thereby estimated to be approximately 300 mg/kg. Ingestion in adults of more than one or two mouthfuls of concentrate should be evaluated in a health care facility because CNS dysfunction onset may occur 24 hours or more later.

Gastric Decontamination. Orogastric or nasogastric lavage and activated charcoal may be indicated in any particular patient according to accepted guidelines for use of gastric decontamination in oral poisoning (see Chapter 31). Spontaneous vomiting is a feature of significant ingestions of formulated herbicide because of the surfactant content; it may be unnecessary to attempt gastric lavage. Particular attention must be exercised in protecting the airway because of the obtundation and coma that may develop many hours after ingestion. Gastric lavage plus extracorporeal removal failed to prevent progression of CNS effects to coma and seizures in two patients who presented 30 minutes and 3.5 hours after ingestion.[96]

Extracorporeal Removal. Hemodialysis has been shown to be superior to charcoal hemoperfusion in eliminating glufosinate from blood in vitro.[97] However, several clinical authorities perform both procedures in tandem in a herbicide-poisoned patient.[86,93,96] In theory, any circulating surfactant would more likely be removed by hemoperfusion, and any water-soluble herbicide is more likely to be removed by dialysis. Neither proof of the theory nor an improved clinical outcome has been demonstrated for this practice. Early hemodialysis/hemoperfusion with documented significant reductions in plasma glufosinate levels failed to avert the progression of CNS pathology or hasten recovery. In one case the serum glufosinate level was reduced from 3.11 μg/mL to 0.91μg/mL. In the other case it was reduced from 1.56 μg/mL to 0.68 μg/ml. Midpoint in this dialysis, the concentration was 0.75 μg/mL at the inlet and 0.10 μg/mL at the outlet.[96] Several authors have noted that onset and resolution of clinical symptoms lag behind serum glufosinate levels.[38,96] Thus, serum levels appear to underestimate the degree of toxic effect at the tissue target level.

Supportive Care

Central respiratory failure and arrest may develop suddenly and require emergent intubation and ventilation. Prophylactic intubation is indicated for any glufosinate- or bialaphos-poisoned patient who becomes stuporous. In addition, hypotension, airway edema, or acute lung injury may develop in patients with large-volume herbicide ingestion as a result of systemic surfactant syndrome. Patients should be carefully monitored for adequate organ perfusion, respiratory effort, and oxygenation.

Seizures respond to intravenous benzodiazepines. The single published case of diabetes insipidus responded to intranasal desmopressin.[93]

Prognosis

There were six fatalities among 34 glufosinate poisonings reported by the Japanese Poison Center.[97] Recovery may be prolonged, but other than anterograde memory loss, appears to be complete. More clinical experience is required to better understand this poisoning.

ATRAZINE AND OTHER CHLOROTRIAZINES

Atrazine
6-chloro N² ethyl N⁴ isopropyl-1,3,5-triazine-2,4-diamine

The chloro-S-triazine herbicides, including atrazine, simazine, cyanzine, and others, comprise the most extensively used herbicide class in the United States. Despite this magnitude of use, there are few reports of acute human toxicity related to any of these agents in the published medical literature.[58,69]

Atrazine is classified in the United States as a Restricted Use Pesticide because of its potential to contaminate groundwater; it may be purchased and applied only by certified applicators. Its primary uses are to control broadleaf and grassy weeds in crops such as corn, sugar cane, and conifers and for nonselective weed control in noncrop rights of way and industrial land. Application is

either preemergence or early postemergence when weeds are young and growing. Formulations include wettable powders, water-dispersible granules, dry flowables, and flowable liquids; some concentrations contain as much as 80 to 90% atrazine. Additionally, it is present in many multiple-ingredient products. Liquid formulations are likely to contain a hydrocarbon solvent.

Toxicokinetics

In vitro experimentation with human skin preparations showed that up to 16.4% of dermally applied atrazine is eventually absorbed beyond the skin surface. In the first 20 hours, less than 5% of the applied dose was fully absorbed and recovered in the receptor fluid. The largest recovered fraction (12% of dose) was within the dermal layers analyzed.[1] Six atrazine manufacturing workers evaluated by urinary biomonitoring showed that only 1 to 2% of the external dose encountered per workshift was excreted in the urine, primarily as metabolites.[15]

Atrazine is well absorbed after ingestion, 80% following single-dose administration to rats. The average plasma protein binding of atrazine in rats was 26% (range 18–37%) and was independent of total plasma concentration within the studied ranged of 30 to 400 μg/L.[59]

Atrazine is extensively metabolized by hepatic isoenzyme P450 1A2 to a variety of metabolites,[54] which are then renally excreted. Only 2% is excreted unchanged, and 80% as the dealkyl; 10% as the deisopropyl, and 8% as the deethyl metabolites. The half-life of elimination of metabolites in urine was approximately 8 hours.[15] Cutaneous metabolism of atrazine by dermal cytochrome P450 occurs during dermal absorption to several metabolites; deisopropyl atrazine represents 50% of the total metabolized fraction.[1]

Clinical Manifestations

A single case report is published of intentional atrazine ingestion of 500 mL of a concentrate containing 100 g atrazine, 25 g amitrole, and 25 g ethylene glycol plus an uncharacterized amount of surfactant.[69] The 38-year-old male patient was admitted 7 hours after ingestion with coma, shock, metabolic acidosis and gastrointestinal bleeding. Initially the shock was hyperdynamic with increased cardiac output and and low systemic vascular resistance. Later in the brief course, left ventricular failure supervened, and renal failure, hepatic necrosis, and disseminated intravascular coagulation developed. The patient died on the third day despite aggressive treatment including hemodialysis and ethanol. It is unlikely that the estimated 22 mL of ethylene glycol in the formulation contributed substantially to the clinical course. The systemic surfactant syndrome symptoms are evident (GI bleeding, peripheral followed by cardiogenic shock, and renal failure). Effects possibly attributable to atrazine and amitrole include hepatic and renal damage and disseminated intravascular coagulopathy.

Acute poisoning in ruminant animals produced weakness, ataxia, fever, respiratory distress, severe diarrhea, and death; dogs also exhibited renal and hepatic injury.[49] The rat oral LD$_{50}$ of atrazine is 1780 mg/kg.

Atrazine is capable of inducing cell-mediated sensitivity after prolonged or repeated contact with the skin. It is mildly to moderately irritant to skin, eyes, and mucous membranes.

Atrazine is associated with mammary tumors (fibroadenomas and adenocarcinomas) in some animal studies, acting by an epigenetic, hormonally mediated mechanism. It does not itself have direct estrogenic effects but acts through neuroendocrine pathways in the hypothalamus. Because of this limited evidence for carcinogenicity in experimental animals and inadequate evidence of carcinogenicity in humans, IARC rates atrazine as Category 3—unclassifiable as to carcinogenicity in humans. The US EPA classifies atrazine as a Group C possible human carcinogen.

Management

The toxic dose of atrazine or other triazine herbicides in their various formulations is unknown, but is apparently relatively high. Orogastric or nasogastric lavage and activated charcoal may be indicated in any particular patient according to accepted guidelines for use of gastric decontamination in oral poisoning (Chapter 31). Because liquid formulations are likely to be emulsifiable concentrates containing both surfactant and a hydrocarbon solvent, precautions must be taken to avoid both aspiration and esophageal trauma.

Hemodialysis removed only 120 mg of atrazine in 4 hours in a man who had ingested a total of 100 g. The initial atrazine plasma concentration was only 2 μg/mL, and the mean clearance over 4 hours was estimated at 250 mL/hour.[69] Hepatic metabolites, which represent the majority of renally excreted atrazine molecules, were not assayed in this case. Unless renal impairment intervenes, it is unlikely that hemodialysis will materially affect the clinical course. There are no data on hemoperfusion.

Experience with acute toxicity is too limited to permit adequate characterization of effects or treatment. There are no antidotes or specific treatment measures. Hypotension, airway edema, or acute lung injury may develop in patients with large-volume herbicide ingestion as a result of systemic surfactant syndrome. Patients should be carefully monitored for adequate organ perfusion, respiratory effort, and oxygenation.

Analysis of atrazine in biologic specimens is not routinely available.

SUMMARY

The diverse worldwide agricultural role of herbicides has led to their increasing risks and availability as suicidal or unintentional agents of great potential concern.

The exposure of various populations to paraquat and diquat has led to unique toxicologic emergencies. Glyphosate, glufosinate, and atrazine are additional examples of high-risk herbicides. The formulations emphasizing their exceptionally diverse characteristics and the novel components are discussed. The evaluation of the scientific understanding of the supposedly inert components of these formulations are emphasized. The increasing interest in the toxic potential of these agents is timely, particularly as society attempts to assess the risks and benefits of these agents.

REFERENCES

1. Ademola J, Sedik L, Wester R, Maibach H: In vitro percutaneous absorption and metabolism in man of 2-chloro-4-ethylamino-6-isopropylamino-s-triazine (atrazine). Arch Toxicol 1993;67:85–91.
2. Aspelin A, Grube A: Pesticides Industry Sales and Usage 1996 and 1997 Market Estimate. Nov 1999; US EPA 733-R-99-001.
3. Barabás K, Serényi P, Selypes A: Inhibition of lung damage caused by paraquat with lymphokines or cytokines. Exp Pathol 1990;38:189–195.
4. Bataller R, Bragulat E, Nogue S, et al: Prolonged cholestasis after acute paraquat poisoning through skin absorption. Am J Gastroenterol 2000;95:1340–1343.
5. Bateman DN: Pharmacological treatments of paraquat poisoning. Hum Toxicol 1987;6:57–62.
6. Berisha HI, Pakbaz H, Absood A, Said SI: Nitric oxide as a mediator of oxidant lung injury due to paraquat. Proc Natl Acad Sci USA 1994;91:7445–7449.
7. Bismuth C, Garnier R, Baud FJ, et al: Paraquat poisoning. An overview of the current status. Drug Saf 1990;5:243–251.
8. Bismuth C, Garnier R, Dally S, et al: Prognosis and treatment of paraquat poisoning: A review of 28 cases. J Toxicol Clin Toxicol 1982;19:461–474.
9. Bismuth C, Hall AHG, Baud FJ, Borron S: Pulmonary dysfunction in survivors of acute paraquat poisoning. Vet Hum Toxicol 1996;38:220–222.
10. Bismuth C, Scherrmann JM, Garnier R, et al: Elimination of paraquat. Hum Toxicol 1987;6:63–67.
11. Braithwaite RA: Emergency analysis of paraquat in biological fluids. Hum Toxicol 1987;6:83–86.
12. Brian RC, Homer RF, Stubbs J, Jones RL: A new herbicide: 1,1′-ethylene-2,2′-dipyridylium dibromide. Nature 1958;191:446–447.
13. Calderbank A, Brian RC, Allen HP, et al: Bipyridylium herbicides. In: Peacock FC, ed: Jealott's Hill. Fifty Years of Agricultural Research 1928-1978. Birmingham, Kynock Press, 1978:67–86.
14. Calderbank A, Farrington JA: The chemistry of paraquat and its radical. In: Bismuth C, Hall AH, eds: Paraquat Poisoning. Mechanisms, Prevention, Treatment. New York, Marcel Dekker, 1995:89–106.
15. Catanacci G, Franco B, Maurizio B, et al: Biological monitoring of human exposure to atrazine. Toxicol Lett 1993;69:217–222.
16. Chan P, Mahler J: NTP Technical report on toxicity studies of glyphosate administered in dosed feed to F344/N rats and B6C3F1 mice. National Toxicology Program Toxicity Report Series No. 16. NIH 92-3135T, 1992.
17. Chang CY, Peng YC, Hung DZ, et al: Clinical impact of upper gastrointestinal tract injuries in glyphosate-surfactant oral intoxication. Hum Exp Toxicol 1999;18:475–478.
18. Chen N, Bowles MR, Pond SM: Prevention of paraquat toxicity in suspensions of alveolar type II cells by paraquat-specific antibodies. Hum Exp Toxicol 1994;13:551–557.
19. Clark DG: Inhibition of the absorption of paraquat from the gastrointestinal tract by adsorbents. Br J Indust Med 1971;28:186–188.
20. Daisley H, Simmons V: Homicide by paraquat poisoning. Med Sci Law 1999;39:266–269.
21. Devlin CM, Bowles MR, Gordon RB, Pond SM: Production of a paraquat-specific murine single chain Fv fragment. J Biochem 1995;118:480–487.
22. Drault JN, Baelen E, Mehdaoui H, et al: Massive paraquat poisoning. Favorable course after treatment with N-acetylcysteine and early hemodialysis. (in French). Ann Fr Anesth Reanim 1999;18:534–537.
23. Eisenman A, Armali Z, Raikhlin-Eisenkarft B, et al: Nitric oxide inhalation for paraquat-induced lung injury. J Toxicol Clin Toxicol 1998;36:575–584.
24. Fairshter RD, Miyada DS, Ulich TR, Tipper P: The effects of paraquat dichloride on clinical chemistry measurements. J Anal Toxicol 1986;10:162–164.
25. Fogt F, Zilker T: Total exclusion from external respiration protects lungs from development of fibrosis after paraquat intoxication. Hum Toxicol 1989;8:465–474.
26. Fuke C, Ameno K, Ameno S, et al: A rapid, simultaneous determination of paraquat and diquat in serum and urine using second-derivative spectroscopy. J Anal Toxicol 1992;16:214–216.
27. Gordonsmith RH, Brooke-Taylor S, Smith LL, Cohen GM: Structural requirements of compounds to inhibit pulmonary diamine accumulation. Biochem Pharmacol 1983;32:3701–3709.

28. Gosselin R, Smith R, Hodge H, eds: Benzalkonium Chloride in Clinical Toxicology of Commercial Products, 5th ed. Baltimore, Williams & Wilkins, 1984 III-63–66.

29. Hack R, Ebert E, Ehling G, Leist K: Glufosinate ammonium—some aspects of its mode of action in mammals. Food Chem Toxicol 1994; 32:461–470.

30. Hall AH, Becker CE: Occupational health and safety considerations in paraquat handling. In: Bismuth C, Hall AH, eds: Paraquat Poisoning. Mechanisms, Prevention, Treatment. New York, Marcel Dekker, 1995:249–266.

31. Hall AW: Paraquat and diquat exposures reported to US poison centers, 1983-1992. In: Bismuth C, Hall AH, eds: Paraquat Poisoning. Mechanisms, Prevention, Treatment. New York, Marcel Dekker, 1995:33–64.

32. Hall FR, Fox RD: The reduction of pesticide drift. In: Foy CL, Pritchard DW, eds: Pesticide Formulation and Adjuvant Technology. Boca Raton, CRC Press, 1996:209–239.

33. Hampson ECGM, Effeney DJ, Pond SM: Efficacy of single or repeated hemoperfusion in a canine model of paraquat poisoning. J Pharmacol Exp Ther 1990;254:732–740.

34. Hampson ECGM, Pond SM: Failure of hemoperfusion and hemodialysis to prevent paraquat poisoning. A retrospective review of 42 patients. Med Toxicol 1988;3:64–71.

35. Hanston P, Wallemacq P, Mahieu P: A fatal case of diquat poisoning: toxicokinetic data and autopsy findings. J Toxicol Clin Toxicol 2000;38:149–152.

36. Hart TB, Nevitt A, Whitehead A: A new statistical approach to the prognostic significance of plasma paraquat concentrations. Lancet 1984;2:1222–1223.

37. Heylings JR: Gastrointestinal absorption of paraquat in the isolated mucosa of the rat. Toxicol Appl Pharmacol 1991;107:482–493.

38. Hirose Y, Kobayashi M, Koyama K, et al: A toxicokinetic analysis in a patient with acute glufosinate poisoning. Hum Exp Toxicol 1999;18:305–308.

39. Houzé P, Baud FJ, Mouy R, et al: Toxicokinetics of paraquat in humans. Hum Exp Toxicol 1990;9:5–12.

40. Hudson M, Patel SB, Ewen SWB, et al: Paraquat induced pulmonary fibrosis in three survivors. Thorax 1991;46:201–204.

41. Hung DZ, Deng JF, Wu TC: Laryngeal survey in glyphosate intoxication: a pathophysiological investigation. Hum Exp Toxicol 1997;16:596–599.

42. Im J-G, Lee KS, Han MC, et al: Paraquat poisoning: Findings of chest radiography and CT in 42 patients. Am J Radiol 1991;157: 697–701.

43. Jauhiainen A, Rasanen K, Sarantila R, et al: Occupational exposure of forest workers to glyphosate during brush saw work. Am Ind Hyg Assoc J 1991;52:61–64.

44. Kalmholz S, Veith FJ, Mollenkopf F, et al: Single lung transplantation in paraquat intoxication. NY State J Med 1984;84:81–85.

45. Kao CH, Hsieh JF, Ho YJ, et al: Acute paraquat intoxication: using nuclear pulmonary studies to predict patient outcome. Chest 1999; 116(3):709–714.

46. Karlberg A-T, Bergh M, Shao LP, Nilsson J: Common surfactants form contact allergens at normal handling and storage. Am J Indust Med Suppl 1999;1:134–135.

47. Keeling PL, Pratt IS, Aldridge WN, Smith LL: The enhancement of paraquat toxicity in rats by 85% oxygen: Lethality and cell-specific lung damage. Br J Exp Pathol 1981;62:643–654.

48. Kishimoto T, Fujioka H, Yamadori I, et al: Lethal paraquat poisoning caused by spraying in a vinyl greenhouse causing pulmonary fibrosis with hepatorenal dysfunction (in Japanese). Nihon Kokyuki Gakkai Zasshi 1998;36:347–352.

49. Kobel W, Sumner DD, Campbell JB, et al: Protective effect of activated charcoal in cattle poisoned with atrazine. Vet Hum Toxicol 1985;27:185–188.

50. Koyama K, Andou Y, Saruki K, Matsuo H: Delayed and severe toxicities of an herbicide containing glufosinate and surfactant. Vet Hum Toxicol 1994;36:17–18.

51. Koyama K, Koyama K, Goto K: Cardiovascular effects of an herbicide containing glufosinate and a surfactant: in vitro and in vivo analyses in rats. Toxicol Appl Pharmacol 1997:145:409–414.

52. Koyama K, Matuso H, Saruki K, Andou Y: The acute oral toxic dose of an herbicide containing glufosinate. Abstract. J Toxicol Clin Toxicol 1995;33:519.

53. Koyama K: Glufosinate and a surfactant: Which component produces effects on the central nervous system in acute oral Basta poisoning? Vet Hum Toxicol 1999;41:341.

54. Lang D, Rettie A, Boecker R: Identification of enzymes invloved in the metabolism of atrazine, terbuthylazine, ametryne, and terbutryne in human liver microsomes. Chem Res Toxicol 1997;10:1037–1044.

55. Lavy T, Cowell J, Steinmetz J, Massey J: Conifer seedling nursery worker exposure to glyphosate. Arch Environ Contam Toxicol 1992; 22:6–13.

56. Lee HL, Chen KW, Chi CH, et al: Clinical presentations and prognostic factors of a glyphosate-surfactant herbicide intoxication: A review of 131 cases. Acad Emerg Med 2000;8:906–910.

57. Lin JL, Wei MC, Liu YC: Pulse therapy with cyclophosphamide and methylprednisolone in patients with moderate to severe paraquat poisoning: a preliminary report. Thorax 1996;51:661–663.

58. Loosli R: Epidemiology of atrazine. Rev Environ Contam Toxicol 1995;143:47–57.

59. Lu C, Anderson LC, Morgan MS, Fenske R: Salivary concentrations of atrazine reflect atrazine plasma levels in rats. J Toxicol Environ Health 1998;53:283–292.

60. Mahieu P, Bonduelle Y, Bernard A, et al: Acute diquat intoxication. Interest of its repeated determination in urine and the evaluation of renal proximal tubule integrity. J Toxicol Clin Toxicol 1984;22: 363–369.

61. Maruyama K, Takeuchi M, Chikusa H, Muneyuki M: Reduction of intrapulmonary shunt by low-dose inhaled nitric oxide in a patient with late-stage respiratory distress associated with paraquat poisoning. Intensive Care Med 1995;21:778–779.

62. Matsukwa, Hachisuka H, Sawada S, et al: Bialaphos poisoning with apnea and metabolic acidosis. J Toxicol Clin Toxicol 1991:29: 141–146.

63. Matthew H, Logan A, Woodruff MFA, Heard B: Paraquat poisoning. Lung transplantation. Br Med J 1968;3:759–763.

64. Meredith TJ, Vale JA: Treatment of paraquat poisoning in man: methods to prevent absorption. Hum Toxicol 1987;6:49–55.

65. Ng LL, Naik RB, Polak A: Paraquat ingestion with methemoglobinemia treated with methylene blue. Br Med J 1982;284:1445-1446.

66. Ong HC, Tsai WJ, Deng JF: An analysis if the clinical findings observed in the cases of glyphosate ingestion poisonings. Abstract presented, International Congress of the European Association of Poison Control Centers, Milano, Italy, Sept. 1990.

67. Papiris SA, Maniati MA, Kyriakidis V, Constantopoulos SH: Pulmonary damage due to paraquat poisoning through skin absorption. Respiration 1995;2:101–103.

68. Perriëns JH, Benimadho S, Kiauw IL, Wisse J, et al: High-dose cyclophosphamide and dexamethasone in paraquat poisoning: A prospective study. Hum Exp Toxicol 1992;11:129–134.

69. Pommery J, Mathieu M, Mathieu D, Lhermitte M: Atrazine in plasma and tissue following atrazine-animotriazole-ethylene glycol-formaldehyde poisoning. J Toxicol Clin Toxicol 1993:31:323–331.

70. Pond SM, Johnston SC, Schoof DD, et al: Repeated hemoperfusion and continuous arteriovenous hemofiltration in a paraquat poisoned patient. J Toxicol Clin Toxicol 1987;25:305–316.

71. Pond SM, Rivory LP, Hampson ECGM, Roberts MS: Kinetics of toxic doses of paraquat and the effects of hemoperfusion in the dog. J Toxicol Clin Toxicol 1993;31:229–246.

72. Powell D, Pond SM, Allen TB, Portale AA: Hemoperfusion in a child who ingested diquat and died from pontine infarction and hemorrhage. J Toxicol Clin Toxicol 1983;20:405–420.

73. Pronczuk de Garbino J: Epidemiology of paraquat poisoning. In: Bismuth C, Hall AH, eds: Paraquat Poisoning. Mechanisms, Prevention, Treatment. New York, Marcel Dekker, 1995:37–52.

74. Proudfoot A: Predictive value of early plasma paraquat concentrations. In: Bismuth C, Hall AH, eds: Paraquat Poisoning. Mechanisms, Prevention, Treatment. New York, Marcel Dekker, 1995: 275–284.

75. Proudfoot AT: Methemoglobinemia due to monolinuron—not paraquat. Br Med J 1982;285:812.

76. Ragoucy-Sengler C, Pileire B. A biological index to predict patient outcome in paraquat poisoning. Hum Exp Toxicol 1996;15:265–268.

77. Rhodes ML, Zavala DC, Brown D: Hypoxic protection in paraquat poisoning. Lab Invest 1976;5:496–500.

78. Rudez J, Sepcic K, Sepcic J: Vaginally applied diquat intoxication. J Toxicol Clin Toxicol 1999;37:877–879.

79. Samman PD, Johnston ENM: Nail damage associated with handling of paraquat and diquat. Br Med J 1969;1:818–819.

80. Saunders NR, Alpert HM, Cooper JD: Sequential bilateral lung transplantation for paraquat poisoning. A case report. J Thorac Cardiovasc Surg 1985;89:734–742.

81. Sawada K, Yamanouchi T, Yamashita M: A comparative study between direct hemoperfusion and hemodialysis for removing glyphosate. Jpn J Toxicol 1989;2:393–396.

82. Sawada Y, Nagai Y: Roundup poisoning: its clinical observations and possible involvement of surfactant. J Clin Exp Med (Jpn) 1987; 143:25–27.

83. Scherrmann JM, House P, Bismuth C, Bourdon R: Prognostic value of plasma and urine paraquat concentration. Hum Toxicol 1987;6:91–93.

84. Scherrmann JM: Analytical procedures and predictive value of late plasma and urine concentrations. In: Bismuth C, Hall AH, eds: Paraquat Poisoning. Mechanisms, Prevention, Treatment. New York, Marcel Dekker, 1995:285–298.

85. Schmidt DM, Neale J, Olson KR: Clinical course of a fatal ingestion of diquat. J Toxicol Clin Toxicol 1999;37:881–884.

86. Shinohara M, Tsuchida A, Abe Y, et al: Hemodialysis and hemoperfusion in successful treatment of a poisoning with an herbicide containing glufosinate ammonium and a surfactant. Clin Nephrol 1997;48:61.

87. Smith LL: The toxicity of paraquat. Adv Drug React Pois Rev 1988;1:1–17.

88. Stephens DS, Walker DH, Schaffner W, et al: Pseudodiphtheria: Prominent pharyngeal membrane associated with fatal paraquat ingestion. Ann Intern Med 1981;94:202–204.

89. Stevens JT, Sumner DD: Herbicides. In: Hayes WJ, Laws ER, eds: Handbook of Pesticide Toxicology, Vol. 3. Classes of Pesticides. Boston, Academic Press, 1991:1356–1408.

90. Suzuki K, Takasu N, Arita S, et al: A new method for predicting the outcome and survival period in paraquat poisoning. Hum Toxicol 1989;8:33–38.

91. Tabata N, Morita M, Mimasaka S, et al: Paraquat mypoathy: report on two suicide cases. Forensic Sci Int 1999;100: 117–126.

92. Tai T, Yamahita M, Wakimore H: Hemodynamic effects of Roundup, glyphosate and surfactant in dogs. Jpn J Toxicol 1990;3:63–68.

93. Takahashi H, Toya T, Matsumiya N, Koyama K: A case of transient diabetes insipidus associated with poisoning by an herbicide containing glufosinate. J Toxicol Clin Toxicol 2000;38: 153–156.

94. Talbot A, Shiaw MH, Huang JS, et al: Acute poisoning with a glyphosate-surfactant herbicide (Roundup): a review of 93 cases. Hum Exp Toxicol 1991:10:1–8.

95. Talbot AR, Barnes MR, Ting RS: Early radiotherapy in the treatment of paraquat poisoning. Br J Radiol 1988;61:405–408.

96. Tanaka J, Yamashita M, Matsuo H, Yamamoto T: Two cases of glufosinate poisoning with late onset convulsions. Vet Hum Toxicol 1998;40:219–222.

97. Tanaka J, Yamashita M, Yamamoto T: A comparative study of direct hemoperfusion and hemodialysis for the removal of glufosinate ammonium. J Toxicol Clin Toxicol 1995;33:691–694.

98. Tanen DA, Curry SC, Laney RF: Renal failure and corrosive airway and gastrointestinal injury after ingestion of diluted diquat solution. Ann Emerg Med 1999;34:542–545.

99. Tominack R, Yang GY, Tsai WJ, Chung HM, Deng JF: Taiwan national poison center survey of glyphosate-surfactant herbicide ingestions. J Toxicol Clin Toxicol 1991;29:91–109.

100. Vale JA, Meredith TJ, Buckley BM: Paraquat poisoning: clinical features and immediate general management. Hum Toxicol 1987;6:41–47.

101. Vanholder R, Colardyn F, DeRueck J, et al: Diquat intoxication. Report of two cases and review of the literature. Am J Med 1981;76:1267–1271.

102. Walder B, Brundler MA, Spiliopoulos A, Romand JA: Successful single-lung transplantation after paraquat intoxication. Transplantation 1997;64:789–791.

103. Watananbe T, Sano T: Neurological effects of glufosinate poisoning with a brief review. Hum Exp Toxicol 1998;17:35–39.

104. Wester RC, Melendres J, Sarason R, et al: Glyphosate skin binding, absorption, residual tissue distribution, and skin decontamination. Fundam Appl Toxicol 1991;16:725–732.

105. Widdop BM, Medd RK, Braithwaite RA: Charcoal hemoperfusion in the treatment of paraquat poisoning. Proc Eur Soc Toxicol 1976;18:156–159.

106. Williams PF, Jarvie DR, Whitehead AP: Diquat intoxication: treatment by charcoal hemoperfusion and description of a new method of diquat measurement in plasma. J Toxicol Clin Toxicol 1986;24: 11–20.

107. Yoshioka T, Sugimoto T, Kinoshita N, et al: Effects of concentration reduction and partial replacement of paraquat by diquat on human toxicity: a clinical survey. Hum Exp Toxicol 1992;11:241–245.

CHAPTER **92**

INDUSTRIAL POISONING
Information and Control

Peter H. Wald

Three workers engaged in the production of mercuric acetate were admitted to hospital within 22 calendar days of each other, 30, 48, and 5 days, respectively, after their last working day. The workers served the same reactor in which elemental mercury was oxidized by peroxide to mercuric oxide, and mercuric acetate was formed by the reaction of mercuric oxide with acetic acid. They all presented with neurologic findings including ataxia, dysarthria, tremor, deteriorating vision, and cerebellar signs. The first two had rapidly progressive downhill courses to coma that ended in death. The diagnosis of mercury vapor intoxication of the first two patients was established 21 and 16 days after their admission, when the third patient was admitted and hospitals were informed about their exposure. Blood mercury levels were on the order of 2000 µg/L with low urine mercury levels. All patients were chelated with penicillamine without any noticeable effect.

Organic mercury was probably formed as an unintended byproduct of this reaction. Similar to the reaction that occurred in Minamata, an acetate fragment reacted with mercury in the presence of an oxidizer to form organic mercury. In this reaction, methyl mercury acetate could have been formed, which is 5.4 times more volatile than mercury vapor. The incorrect diagnosis of mercury vapor exposure in these cases was established despite the facts that (1) the observed signs of a rapid irreversible downhill course, ataxia, dysarthria, and constriction of visual fields are rarely present in mercury vapor poisoning and are characteristic of organic mercury poisoning; (2) the degree of deterioration after removal from exposure further implicated organic mercury, not mercury vapor; (3) blood mercury concentrations were in the range associated with severe poisoning in the Iraq methyl mercury epidemic; (4) there was little response to treatment with penicillamine, the opposite of what would be expected with mercury vapor; and (5) the blood-to-urinary mercury concentration ratios were high, whereas this ratio is usually below 0.5 in mercury vapor toxicity or in workers exposed to mercury vapor.

The other important facet of these cases is the public health implications of this sentinel health event. There were three employees in this workplace who were affected by this exposure. Were there any others?

These cases illustrate three important problems associated with the diagnosis and treatment of occupational or environmentally caused diseases: (1) the ability to establish the diagnosis correctly, (2) the ability to treat the condition correctly, and (3) the ability to act correctly on any public health issues related to the exposure. The following discussion allows the clinician to assemble an adequate database to achieve the appropriate diagnosis and treatment.

TAKING AN OCCUPATIONAL HISTORY

Because time spent at work is a large percentage of many people's day, the occupational health history should be a routine part of any medical history and physical examination. This is especially true of patients presenting to a physician with potential chemical exposures at work or unusual symptoms. The history should include several brief survey questions. Positive responses then lead to a more detailed occupational and environmental history, which is composed of three elements: present work, past work, and nonoccupational exposures.

The Brief Occupational Survey

There are three questions that should be incorporated into the occupational survey:

- Exactly what kind of work do you do?
- Are you exposed to any physical (radiation, noise, extremes of temperature or pressure), chemical (liquids, fumes, vapors, dusts, or mists), or biologic hazards at work? (Table 92–1)
- Are your symptoms related in any way to starting or being off work? For example, do they occur when you arrive at work at the beginning of the day or week, or when you work at a specific location, or during a specific process at work?

Present Work

Collected data on a person's present job reveals what his or her present exposures may be, which can help formulate the differen-

TABLE 92–1.   Hazard Classes, Hazard Types, and Several Common Examples Found in the Workplace

Hazard Class	Hazard Type	Examples
Physical hazards	Man–machine interfaces	Repetitive motion Lifting Vibration Mechanical trauma, electric shock
	Physical environment	Temperature Pressure Long/rotating shifts
	Energy	Ionizing radiation: x-ray, ultraviolet Non-ionizing radiation: infrared, microwave, magnetic fields Lasers Noise
Chemical hazards	Solvents	Aliphatics, aromatics, alcohols, ketones, ethers, aldehydes, acetates, peroxides, halogenated compounds
	Metals	Lead, mercury, cadmium
	Gases	Combustion products, irritants, simple and chemical asphyxiants
	Dusts	Organic (wood) and inorganic (asbestos/silica)
	Pesticides	Organochlorine, organicphosphorous, carbamate
	Epoxy resins and polymer systems	Toluene diisocyanate, phthalates
Biologic hazards	Bacteria	*Bacillus anthracis, Legionella pneumophila, Borrelia burgdorferi*
	Viruses	Hepatitis, human immunodeficiency virus, hantavirus
	Mycobacteria	*Mycobacterium tuberculosis*
	Rickettsia and *Chlamydia*	*Chlamydia psittaci, Coxiella brunetti*
	Fungi	*Histoplasma capsulatum, Coccidioides immitis*
	Parasites	*Echinococcus* spp, *Plasmodium* spp
	Envenomations	Arthropod, marine, snake
	Allergens	Enzymes, animals, dusts, insects, latex, plant pollen dusts

TABLE 92–2.   Components of an Occupational Health History

Current work history
  Specifics of the job
    Employer's name
    Type of industry
    Duration of employment
    Employment location, hours, and shift changes
    Description of work process
    Unusual activities of the job that are occasional (maintenance)
    Adjacent work processes
  Hazardous exposures (Table 92–1)
  Possible health effects
    Suspicious health problems
    Temporality of symptoms
    Specific distribution of symptoms (rash, paresthesias)
    Affected coworkers
    Presence or absence of known risk factors (smoking, alcohol)
  Workplace sampling and monitoring
    Individual and/or area air monitoring
    Surface sampling
    Biologic monitoring
    Medical surveillance records
  Exposure controls
    Administrative controls
    Process engineering controls
      Enclosure
      Shielding
      Ventilation
      Electrical and mechanically controlled interlocks
    Personal protective equipment
      Respirators
      Protective clothing
      Earplugs, glasses, gloves, face shields, head and foot protection
Past work history
  Review current work history for all past employment
Nonoccupational exposures
  Secondary employment
  Hobbies
  Outdoor activities
  Residential exposures
  Community contamination
  Habits

tial diagnosis for the employee's complaints. These data can be systematically collected by focusing on four areas: specifics of the job, hazardous exposures, health effects, and control measures (Table 92–2).

Specifics of the Job

It is not sufficient simply to inquire what the patient does for a living. Like healthcare professionals, workers in other industries have their own jargon. When asked for a job title, a patient may respond with one that has meaning only in his or her trade. Even if the job title is recognizable, it may not provide any useful information and, in fact, may be misleading. A secretary working in a small plastics manufacturing plant may have occupational exposures quite different from the secretary who works for a law firm.

The important specific information requested should include name of employer, type of industry, duration and location of employment, hours and shift changes, process description including unusual occasional activities, and adjacent processes. The employer may be able to provide information about materials used at the plant. Always obtain the patient's permission before calling the employer. A patient may be fired or otherwise discriminated against (despite legal protections) for suggesting that health problems are work-related.

It is important to learn what actually happens in the patient's immediate work environment because nearby work processes may contribute other exposures. If possible, the patient should be asked for a diagram of the work area. The patient should also be questioned about job process changes. A previously safe job may have been changed to a potentially dangerous one without a change in the patient's job title.

The patient should describe exactly what he or she does on any given day and for how long. Unusual and nonroutine tasks, such as those performed during overtime, maintenance, or in an emergency, should also be described. The primary job may not involve chemicals, but the patient may nevertheless perform tasks that entail unprotected exposure to a toxic chemical.

Hazardous Exposures

The names and/or types of all chemicals or substances to which the patient may be exposed are important in determining potential adverse effects and any relationship to the patient's complaints. It is important to elicit any recent changes in suppliers of these products, as even a slight change in the formulation of a chemical may cause adverse effects in an individual who had no problems working with that compound previously. This information may be obtained from the material safety data sheet (MSDS), an important but not always reliable source of information about the chemical. In addition to adverse health effects, it contains information on chemical reactivity, safety precautions, and other data. As an initial step, it should be requested and reviewed; however, information provided on health effects should be crosschecked with other resources. Four major concerns result from relying solely on MSDS sheets: (1) some are excellent, but others are incomplete and inadequate; (2) components of a product that are regarded as "trade secrets" do not have to be revealed; (3) components that have important health effects (such as solvent or solid carriers of the "active ingredients") may often be grouped together under "inert ingredients" without being specifically named; and (4) process intermediates or unintended by-products of a manufacturing process may not be identified. However, if a chemical is believed to be related to a health effect, manufactures are required to release all information to a physician including trade secrets and inert components.

Exposures to physical and biologic agents can be elicited during the review of the job processes. Most patients know what they are, or have been, exposed to, even if they do not know the exact name of the substance or its medical effects.

Health Effects

Significant occupational exposures usually cause medical effects, although some do so only after a substantial latency period. Key areas of interest include suspicious health problems, temporality of symptoms, and affected coworkers. These data, combined with workplace monitoring and sampling data, can help in determining whether the patient is suffering a work-related illness (Table 92–3). Patients may suspect that their illness or complaint is work-related, especially when symptoms occur at the workplace and improve or disappear over the weekend or during a vacation. Specific distribution of findings such as a rash in a bilateral glove pattern is also supportive of an occupational etiology. Coworkers with similar complaints (not necessarily of the same severity) should raise suspicion that a workplace exposure is responsible for a particular symptom complex. Finally, diseases such as lung cancer or hepatitis, occurring in the absence of known risk factors such as smoking and alcohol, are also important.

Workplace Sampling, Monitoring, and Control

Control of workplace hazards begins with an industrial hygiene monitoring program. Employers are required to give results of both area and individual sampling to employees. A medical surveillance program that includes periodic spirometry and respiratory questionnaires usually indicates that the patient works with a potential respiratory toxin. A medical surveillance program that includes biologic monitoring for a specific substance may also provide an immediate clue to what may be causing the patient's complaints. Finally, if the patient knows exactly what he or she is working with, the physician can usually determine quickly whether any of the substances are compatible with the patient's complaints. Many companies do not perform routine industrial hygiene monitoring or medical surveillance. Individuals who became sick or ill at work are often sent to the local hospital's emergency department. In situations such as this, emergency departments must be prepared to develop the type of occupational history outlined above or be able to consult or refer immediately to appropriate individuals or clinics.

Portions of Table 92–2 and the following section on evaluation and control of workplace hazards detail the types of controls that are usually used in workplaces. It is important to determine whether the workplace employs any control measures, engineering controls, work practice protocols, administrative controls, and personal protective equipment. The existence of control measures usually indicates that the employer recognizes and has attempted to deal with a hazardous exposure.

PAST WORK

It is important not to limit the occupational history to the patient's current workplace and job. Many occupational diseases have long latency periods between exposure to a toxic agent(s) and initial development of clinical symptoms. In addition, patients may have been exposed to substances at work that make them more sensitive to other environmental agents. Thus, for example, someone who developed asthma secondary to a previous workplace exposure may suffer asthma attacks on exposure to simple irritants in the current workplace. When taking an in-depth occupational history, explore issues relevant to the current work history for each previous job.

NONOCCUPATIONAL EXPOSURES

Workers may be exposed to toxic substances in the course of pursuing secondary employment, hobbies, or outdoor activities in contaminated or industrial areas. Residential exposures, such as those from gas and wood stoves, chemically treated furniture and

TABLE 92–3. Evidence Supporting Work-Relatedness of Occupational Disease

Known or documented exposure to a causative agent
Symptoms consistent with suspected workplace exposure
Suggested or diagnostic physical signs
Similar problems in coworkers or workers in related occupations
Temporal relationship of complaints related to work
Confirmatory environmental or biologic monitoring data
Scientific biologic plausibility
Absence of a nonoccupational etiology
Resistance to maximum medical treatment because employee continues to be exposed at work

fabrics, and pest control, may also be relevant. It is important to ask patients about these potential exposures before focusing entirely on exposures in their primary place of employment. This obviously includes relevant issues from the social history such as tobacco, alcohol, and drug use.

EVALUATION AND CONTROL OF WORKPLACE HAZARDS

Initial Workplace Evaluation

The Occupational Safety and Health Act places legal responsibility for providing a safe and healthy workplace on the employer. The rationale for this is that the employer is in the best position to make any modifications necessary to prevent additional work-related illness and injury. The physician may wish to initiate a dialogue with a patient's employer to promote preventive action but should do so only with the patient's informed consent. The initial treating physician may also refer to an occupational medicine specialist, who is specifically trained to manage work-related exposures and diseases and initiate prevention programs.

Because the initial contact may influence subsequent events, it is important to identify the appropriate person, such as someone in the company medical department, the patient's supervisor, the plant's safety officer, or the shop manager. If management is willing to examine the hazardous conditions, a plant walk-through inspection can provide unique insight and information usually unavailable in an office setting. A walk-through makes it easier to understand the work environment, identify safety and health hazards, assess control measures, and recognize opportunities for prevention and also facilitates a good working relationship with key personnel in management and labor. The physician with a number of patients who work in the plant or who provides health services to the workers through the company or labor union may wish to be involved in the walk-through. Assistance with plant inspections can be obtained from occupational health specialists, such as occupational physicians or industrial hygienists.

Industrial Hygiene Sampling and Monitoring

Equipment exists to measure airborne concentrations of toxic chemicals, noise levels, radiation levels, temperature, and humidity. Employees can be fitted with pumps and other devices to measure individual exposure levels at the breathing zone, where, depending on what controls are used, concentrations may vary from those in the general work area. These results can then be compared with OSHA and other available standards to help determine the extent of the hazard and to formulate a control plan. OSHA requires that employers monitor the levels of only a few specific hazards, including asbestos, formaldehyde, lead, vinyl chloride, noise, and ethylene oxide; ongoing sampling of the remaining estimated 60,000 chemicals in use in the workplace is not required. Where industrial hygiene sampling has been performed, OSHA's medical access standard gives any exposed worker or his or her representative the right to review and copy all sampling data.

Control of Workplace Hazards

Workplace hazard control has traditionally relied on a hierarchy of methods to protect workers from exposure. The preferred solution is complete elimination of the hazard by *substitution*. Where this is not possible, controls that shield workers or reduce their exposure are the next preferred method. Finally, personal protective equipment, which requires a positive action from the worker, is the least favored method.

Engineering Controls

Health and safety professionals prefer, and OSHA regulations require, where feasible, the use of engineering controls to reduce worker exposure to hazardous substances or agents. Engineering controls are preferred because they intercept hazards at their source or in the workplace atmosphere before they reach the worker.

Engineering controls include redesign or modification of process or equipment to reduce hazardous emissions, isolation of a process through enclosure, automation of an operation, and installation of exhaust systems that remove hazardous dusts, fumes, and vapors. Local exhaust systems, such as hoods, are preferable to general dilution ventilation because the former removes contaminants closer to their source and at relatively high rates.

Engineering controls have several advantages over control measures focused on the worker. Properly installed and maintained engineering controls are reliable and consistent, and their effectiveness does not depend on human supervision or interaction. They can limit exposure through several routes, such as inhalation and skin absorption, simultaneously. In addition, engineering controls do not place a burden on the worker or interfere with worker comfort or safety.

Work Practices

Work practices are procedures that the worker can follow to limit exposure to hazardous agents. Examples are the use of high-powered vacuum cleaners instead of compressed air cleaning and pouring techniques that direct hazardous material away from the worker. Although not as effective as engineering controls, work practice can be a useful component of an overall hazard control program.

Administrative Controls

Administrative controls reduce the duration of exposure for any individual worker or reduce the total number of workers exposed to a hazard. Examples are rotation of workers into and out of hazardous areas so that no one worker is exposed full time and scheduling procedures likely to generate high levels of exposure, such as cleaning or maintenance activities, during nights or weekends. Administrative controls sometimes have the side effect of exposing more workers to a hazard, albeit at lower doses that, it is hoped, do not cause health effects.

Personal Protective Equipment

Personal protective equipment, such as respirators, earplugs, gloves, and hard hats, is the least effective but most commonly used control method. Employers may often favor personal protective equipment over the institution of more costly engineering and administrative controls.

Respirators and other forms of personal protective equipment are often hot, uncomfortable, and awkward to wear and may make it difficult for workers to breathe, speak, or hear, depending on the equipment involved. Consequently, workers often remove or refuse to wear the protection. Respirators put extra stress on the heart and the lungs. Both respirators and earplugs limit conversation and therefore present a safety hazard in themselves.

Because personal protective equipment does not stop a hazard from getting into the environment, if it fails, the worker is entirely vulnerable to exposure. In addition, generally only one route of exposure is protected. For example, the commonly used half-mask respirator still leaves the skin and eyes exposed.

Choosing the right piece of personal protective equipment can be difficult and may depend on the nature and extent of the hazard. For example, each type of respirator is rated for the amount of protection it provides; as would be expected, the cost of a respirator increases with its protection factor. Use of the wrong type of respirator can leave the worker insufficiently protected.

Half-mask respirator cartridges are available in various colors, coded to the contaminant filtered out of the breathing environment. If the wrong cartridge is used, the worker is effectively unprotected from the hazardous contaminant. To be effective, a respirator must be meticulously fit to the individual worker. Failure to achieve a proper seal negates the respirator's usefulness. High cheekbones, dentures, scars, perspiration, talking, head movements, and facial hair can prevent a proper seal. This is often ignored or overlooked by an employer who adopts a "one-size-fits-all" policy.

Even if each employee is provided the proper respirator, the respiratory protection program may not be effective. OSHA requires that employers institute a program of proper fit testing, cleaning, maintenance, and storage of respirators, which can be at least as costly as the institution of engineering controls.

In some instances, the use of personal protective equipment may be unavoidable. An employer may need to control a hazardous exposure through a combination of measures, such as engineering controls and personal protective equipment. Ideally, the employer is using personal protective equipment as a control of last resort and in strict compliance with OSHA standards.

Worker Education and Training

Regardless of the control measures employed, workers and supervisors need to be educated in the recognition and control of workplace hazards and the prevention of work-related illness and injury. The OSHA Hazard Communication Standard requires that employers train workers in ways to detect the presence or release of hazardous chemicals, their physical and health hazards, methods of protection against the hazards, and proper emergency procedures, as well as how to read the labeling system and how to read and use an MSDS.

With the passage of federal, state, and local right-to-know laws, many consulting companies now offer hazard communication training. These programs are of uneven quality. Those that focus on acute hazards, ignore chronic effects, and emphasize personal protective equipment over other control measures may not be effective in training workers to recognize and control chemical hazards.

Medical Monitoring

Together with worker education and industrial hygiene, a medical program can form the foundation of an effective occupational disease prevention regimen. Medical monitoring, however, is fraught with technical and ethical pitfalls. Medical monitoring encompasses both medical screening and medical surveillance.

Medical screening refers to the cross-sectional testing of a population of workers for evidence of excessive exposure or early stages of disease that may or may not be related to work and that may or may not influence the ability to tolerate or perform work.

Preemployment and preplacement physical examinations are another type of medical screening, often favored by employers. The new Americans with Disabilities Act (ADA) regulates the timing, scope, content, and use of these examinations and the information gathered. Comprehensive resources for information on the ADA are available at *http://www.adata.org*. The ADA prohibits "pre-employment" medical examinations and inquiries. After a job offer has been made, "preplacement" examinations and inquiries can be conducted to determine whether an applicant can perform a job safely and effectively. The physician evaluates past medical history, current symptoms, and physical laboratory findings to determine whether an individual currently has the physical or mental abilities necessary to perform the essential functions of the job and whether the individual can do so without posing a "direct threat" to the health or safety of self or others. This threat must be more than theoretic and cannot be based on some future time; the threat must be concrete and relatively immediate.

There are few tests and few conditions that are good predictors of either ability to perform a task or increased susceptibility to a particular exposure. Many workers and their advocates view preplacement examinations as a way for employers to choose the "fittest" worker and to avoid their legally mandated obligation to provide a safe and healthy workplace for all workers. This is not true for most employers. Physicians asked by an employer to perform preplacement examinations should be sure that each component of the examination relates to the actual job the individual is being hired to perform and the actual risks he or she will encounter on the job. Both the law and sound occupational medical practice dictate that the employer's attention and efforts be directed toward redesign of the job and its hazards so that it is safe and healthy for all workers to perform.

Medical surveillance refers to the ongoing evaluation, by means of periodic examinations, of high-risk individuals or potentially exposed workers to detect early pathophysiologic changes indicative of significant exposure. OSHA requires little in the way of medical surveillance, although several OSHA standards require employers to institute medical surveillance programs, for example, for workers exposed to asbestos, arsenic, vinyl chloride, lead, and ethylene oxide. Depending on the potential exposure, medical surveillance can include a history and physical examination, chest radiograph, pulmonary function test, blood and urine tests, and other laboratory evaluations.

A medical surveillance program can also include biologic monitoring, the purpose of which is not to identify the occurrence of disease but to measure the uptake or presence of a particular substance or its metabolites in body fluids or organs. Ideally, this occurs before any pathophysiologic damage is done. Consequently, biologic monitoring is potentially a primary preventive measure. For example, several volatile organic compounds, such as benzene and toluene, if inhaled or absorbed through the skin, produce metabolites that can be measured in urine.

Biologic monitoring can have some advantages over air monitoring because it measures the *actual* absorption of a substance by the body as opposed to ambient levels in the workplace. The amount of a chemical absorbed may not be closely correlated to ambient levels in the workplace for several reasons, including differences in individual work habits, use and effectiveness of personal protective equipment, dermal absorption of chemicals unrelated to their concentration in the air, and nonoccupational exposures.

Biologic monitoring, however, has several very significant limitations. For most chemicals, there are no standards of "normal" or "safe" levels against which results can be compared. Obtaining specimens may be difficult, expensive, and invasive (eg, fat biopsies to detect dioxin). The timing of specimen collection is critical, as different chemicals have different biologic half-lives. The storage and handling of specimens and interpretation of results are also vulnerable to error. Nevertheless, if carefully designed and implemented, biologic monitoring can be a useful complement to a comprehensive industrial hygiene program.

With the exception of biologic monitoring, medical monitoring programs identify disease processes already under way and are, therefore, at best a form of secondary prevention. Employers use results to remove workers instead of remediating the hazard abuse medical and biologic monitoring programs. To be an effective preventive measure, these programs must be coordinated with environmental monitoring programs that identify the nature, source, and extent of workplace hazards; implementation of engineering controls and other measures that control hazards as close as possible to the source; and worker education programs that, at a minimum, inform workers of exposures, their effects, and proper control measures.

Both medical monitoring programs and preplacement examinations raise issues of doctor–patient confidentiality. Employee medical records should be available only to the corporate medical or first-aid department, and not to the personnel office and general management. Unless required by statute, employers should never be told the results of history, physical, or diagnostic examinations unless the patient gives his or her written consent. The examining physician need only inform the employer that an individual is or is not capable of performing a particular job with or without specified restrictions; the physician should not disclose diagnostic information about medical conditions.

INFORMATION RESOURCES

Healthcare professionals require information on industrial toxins in a number of situations, ranging from caring for an acutely ill patient in an ED, when information must be obtained quickly, to caring for a patient with chronic symptoms that may reflect an occupational disease. The American College of Occupational and Environmental Medicine publishes a *Suggested Reading List* (http://www.acoem.org) that provides reference sources for information on toxicology, acute and chronic health effects, diagnosis, and treatment; assists in screening and surveillance; and provides information on groups at risk, product uses, and sources of further information. However, the use of these resources depends on the proper identification of the substance in question; if the substance, its generic name, and ingredients are not known, the research process becomes more difficult.

The practitioner should take a logical approach to seeking information about industrial toxins. First, the substance must be identified by its generic name. This can be done by reviewing the MSDS or contacting poison control centers, the employer, manufacturer, unions, or government agencies. MSDSs are also available for searching online. MSDS Online (www.msdsonline.com) is a good starting point, but typing "MSDS" into any online search engine will yield a number of sites offering data sheets.

Poison Control Centers

Regional poison control centers (PCCs) can provide assistance even when the exact chemical name is unknown because information on toxic substances and their management may be cross-referenced by trade name and manufacturer. Moreover, PCC personnel can usually suggest additional resources. Most PCCs have computerized listings of poisons that are updated regularly. The best-known system is Poisindex (Micromedex, Englewood, CO). Subscribers to this system receive quarterly updates of an alphabetically organized listing of approximately 500,000 industrial and nonindustrial chemicals and compounds. The system includes trade names, the components, and their concentrations, when available, of each compound listed. These are then crossreferenced to management protocols. The name of the manufacturer is also listed.

Employers and Manufacturers

Many state and federal laws require manufacturers to generate, retain, and disclose information that may help physicians care for persons with work-related health problems. Scientific information, exposure data, information on health effects, and collected medical data are included in the types of information that must be retained.

The Chemical Transportation Emergency Center (CHEMTREC; 1–800–424–9300; www.chemtrec.org), sponsored by the Chemical Manufacturers Association, has as its primary responsibility to provide information to healthcare practitioners responding to hazardous spills. However, it will also provide information on commercial products found in a patient's workplace. Employers are required to furnish this information to employees in the form of MSDSs.

Worker's Compensation Insurance Carriers

Smaller companies often lack internal health and safety staffs. Worker's compensation or company risk insurance carriers may have valuable information about exposures and controls in the workplace. As a service to their clients, carriers will often do walk-throughs and hazards evaluations for clients that lack these resources and suggest appropriate engineering controls. Healthcare professionals can contact the carrier directly to see what additional information is available.

Regulatory Agencies

The Occupational Safety and Health Act requires chemical manufacturers to create a MSDS for each chemical they produce, and employers who use chemicals must retain the MSDSs in the workplace. Required information includes chemical and common names; physical, safety, and health-hazard data; exposure limits; precautions for safe handling and use; generally applicable control measures; and emergency and first-aid procedures. The OHSA Hazardous Communication Standard requires individual employers to provide employees with information on the chemical and physical agents used in their workplaces. With the patient's permission, a call to the plant manager, foreperson, or safety officer may be all that is necessary to determine the name of the substance in question. Employers may also be able to provide information on exposure levels in the patient's work environment. In addition, company medical departments (where they exist) may have results of medical testing done on the patient.

There is an important point to reiterate about MSDSs: healthcare providers should not rely on these sheets as the sole source of information. The MSDSs are created by the chemical manufacturers as they generate scientific and health data in the course of seeking approval from the Environmental Protection Agency (EPA) to manufacture chemical substances and mixtures and will not be a complete product evaluation. In addition, Section 8(c) of the Toxic Substances Control Act (TSCA) requires chemical manufacturers to report records of significant adverse reactions to human health or the environment. When contacting chemical manufacturers, physicians should ask to speak with a toxicologist, chemist, or someone in the products information department.

Unions

Labor unions, where they exist, can also be excellent sources of information on toxic exposures. At the local level, union officers, health and safety committee members, and shop stewards may be able to provide material safety data sheets, exposure data, medical and epidemiologic information, and reports of incidents or cases of interest in a particular plant. The health and safety department of the American Federation of Labor and Congress of Industrial Organizations (AFL-CIO, *www.aflcio.org*) in Washington, DC, can provide information on occupational health and safety activities as well as advice on which member unions may be of specific help. At the international level, unions often have well-trained health and safety professionals, who may provide or suggest sources of helpful information. In addition, some cities have a coalition of occupational safety and health groups that may provide information about other known exposed or affected workers.

Government Agencies

There are a myriad of agencies that have some regulatory authority over manufacturing and services industries. These agencies, and their important regulatory authority are listed in Table 92–4.

The Occupational Safety and Health Administration of the US Department of Labor (*www.osha.gov*) is responsible for setting and enforcing workplace health and safety standards. It is empowered to investigate occupational health and safety complaints and can inspect work sites and levy fines for violations of its standards. In approximately half of the 50 states, the OSHA program is implemented by a state agency. Individual workers, their representatives (unions), or their physicians can file a complaint with the state or federal OSHA program and request an inspection. OSHA regulations protect workers from discrimination and punishment by their employer, who may be angered by their filing a complaint.

Some state OSHA agencies have separate enforcement and consultation arms. This means that companies can request assistance from the occupational health specialists in the consultation branch without fear of reprisal from the enforcement branch. Healthcare workers should be familiar with the functions of their state agency and workers' rights under the law.

The National Institute for Occupational Safety and Health (NIOSH) of the US Department of Health and Human Services is part of the Centers for Disease Control (*www.cdc.gov/niosh*). It is not a regulatory agency. NIOSH is responsible for researching the causes of occupational disease and injury and methods for their prevention and control; evaluating workplace conditions; recom-

mending exposure limits to OSHA for standard setting; and training occupational health and safety professionals. It is empowered to conduct on-site evaluations of health hazards in response to requests from employee representatives or employers. After conducting these evaluations, NIOSH investigators immediately contact OSHA, the employees, and the employer if they find that the workers are in imminent danger.

As part of the process of recommending exposure standards to OSHA, NIOSH develops comprehensive documents that critically evaluate all available scientific data on particular chemicals. These "criteria documents" review the chemical's properties, production methods, uses, and workers at risk as well as studies of exposure effects in humans and animals. Methods of screening, surveillance, and control are presented. The agency periodically issues technical reports and special occupational hazard reviews of specific occupations. In conjunction with OSHA, NIOSH develops and disseminates health hazard alerts to inform employers, employees, and healthcare professionals of serious health effects of particular chemicals.

The EPA (*www.epa.gov*) is charged with protecting the nation's land, air, and water. The agency administers a number of laws designed to preserve the public health and environment, one of which is the Toxic Substances Control Act (TSCA). This act authorizes the EPA to collect information on chemical risks from manufacturers and processors and to review information on new chemicals and new uses of chemicals before they are manufactured. Unless designated a trade secret, this information is subject to disclosure and is, therefore, available. The TSCA assistance office may be most useful when resource materials and government documents contain no information about the chemicals or processes in question.

The National Toxicology Program (NTP) (*http://ntp-server.niehs.nih.gov*) is a federal program established in 1978 to develop scientific information on exposure to toxic chemicals.

The Agency for Toxic Substances and Disease Registry (ATSDR) (*www.atsdr.cdc.gov*) is part of the Public Health Service created by Congress to implement the health-related sections of laws that protect the public from hazardous wastes and environmental spills of hazardous substances. In 1986, the Superfund Amendments and Reauthorization Act (SARA) made amendments to the initial enabling legislation of 1980 and broadened ATSDR's responsibilities in the areas of health assessment, toxicologic databases, information dissemination, and medical education. One of its offices, the Office of Health Assessment, provides emergency response for toxic and environmental disasters, consults in public health emergencies, assesses hazardous waste sites, provides technical assistance to agencies and organizations, and estimates health risks to humans from exposure to hazardous substances. The program areas in which ATSDR operates include health assessments, toxicologic profiles, emergency response, and exposure and disease registries.

On-Line Databases

Printed material is often adequate to determine the adverse health effects of chemical exposures, but some resources may be unavailable to physicians, and textbook publication usually lags 2 years or more behind new information. As a result, up-to-date findings and reports may be missed if the practitioner relies solely on printed material. The National Library of Medicine (*www.nlm.nih.gov*) now sponsors Internet searching of both Medline and a

TABLE 92–4. Government Agencies and Their Important Regulatory Authority of the Workplace—a Timeline

Regulation	Agency	Authority
Occupational Safety and Health Act (OSHA, 1970)	Department of Labor	Congress passed the Occupational and Safety Health Act and created the Occupational Safety and Health Administration to ensure worker and workplace safety. Their goal was to make sure employers provide their workers a place of employment free from recognized hazards to safety and health, such as exposure to toxic chemicals, excessive noise levels, mechanical dangers, heat or cold stress, or unsanitary conditions. In order to establish standards for workplace health and safety, the Act also created the National Institute for Occupational Safety and Health (NIOSH) as the research institution for the Occupational Safety and Health Administration. Part 1910.1200 of the Act established the Hazardous Communication Standard (HazCom). The purpose of this section is to ensure that the hazards of all chemicals produced or imported are evaluated and that information concerning their hazards is transmitted to employers and employees. This transmittal of information is to be accomplished by means of comprehensive hazard communication programs, which are to include container labeling and other forms of warning, material safety data sheets, and employee training.
Resource Conservation and Recovery Act (RCRA, 1976)	Environmental Protection Agency (EPA)	RCRA (pronounced "rick-rah") gave the EPA the authority to control hazardous waste from "cradle to grave." This includes the generation, transportation, treatment, storage, and disposal of hazardous waste. RCRA also set forth a framework for the management of nonhazardous wastes. The 1986 amendments to RCRA enabled the EPA to address environmental problems that could result from underground tanks storing petroleum and other hazardous substances. RCRA focuses only on active and future facilities and does not address abandoned or historic sites (see CERCLA). HSWA (pronounced "hiss-wa"), the Federal Hazardous and Solid Waste Amendments, are the 1984 amendments to RCRA that required phasing out land disposal of hazardous waste. Some of the other mandates of this strict law include increased enforcement authority for the EPA, more stringent hazardous waste management standards, and a comprehensive underground storage tank program.
Toxic Substances Control Act (TSCA, 1976)	EPA	TSCA was enacted by Congress to give the EPA the ability to track the 75,000 industrial chemicals currently produced or imported into the United States. The EPA repeatedly screens these chemicals and can require reporting or testing of those that may pose an environmental or human-health hazard. EPA can ban the manufacture and import of those chemicals that pose an unreasonable risk. Reporting requirements include: (1) premanufacturing notification for new chemicals, (2) allegation of significant adverse reactions, (3) reporting of health and safety studies, and (4) notification of suspicion of substantial risk to health.
Comprehensive Environmental Response, Compensation, and Liability Act (CERCLA, 1980)	EPA	The Comprehensive Environmental Response, Compensation, and Liability Act (CERCLA), commonly known as the Superfund, was enacted by Congress on December 11, 1980. This law created a tax on the chemical and petroleum industries and provided broad federal authority to respond directly to releases or threatened releases of hazardous substances that may endanger public health or the environment. Over 5 years, $1.6 billion was collected, and the tax went to a trust fund for cleaning up abandoned or uncontrolled hazardous waste sites. CERCLA: (1) established prohibitions and requirements concerning closed and abandoned hazardous waste sites, (2) provided for liability of persons responsible for releases of hazardous waste at these sites, and (3) established a trust fund to provide for cleanup when no responsible party could be identified. The law authorizes two kinds of response actions: (1) short-term removals, where actions may be taken to address releases or threatened releases requiring prompt response, and (2) long-term remedial response actions that permanently and significantly reduce the dangers associated with releases or threats of releases of hazardous substances that are serious but not immediately life threatening. These actions can be conducted only at sites listed on the EPA's National Priorities List (NPL).
Superfund Amendments and Reauthorization Act (SARA, 1986)	EPA	SARA reflected the EPA's experience in administering the complex Superfund program during its first 6 years and made several important changes and additions to the program. SARA: (1) stressed the importance of permanent remedies and innovative treatment technologies in cleaning up hazardous waste sites, (2) required Superfund actions to consider the standards and requirements found in other state and federal environmental laws and regulations, (3) provided new enforcement authorities and settlement tools, (4) increased state involvement in every phase of Superfund, (5) increased the focus on human health problems posed by hazardous waste sites, (6) encouraged greater citizen participation in making decisions on how sites should be cleaned up, and (7) increased the size of the trust fund to $8.5 billion. SARA also required the EPA to revise the Hazard Ranking System (HRS) to ensure that it accurately assessed the relative degree of risk to human health and the environment posed by uncontrolled hazardous waste sites that may be placed on the National Priorities List (NPL). Emergency Planning and Community Right-to-Know Act (EPCRA), also known as Title III of *SARA,* was enacted by Congress as the national legislation on community safety. This law was designated to help local communities protect public health, safety, and the environment from chemical hazards. The law requires manufacturers to report the amount of toxic substances released each year (Toxic Release Inventory, TRI) To implement EPCRA, Congress required each state to appoint a State Emergency Response Commission (SERC). The SERCs were required to divide their states into Emergency Planning Districts and to name a Local Emergency Planning Committee (LEPC) for each district.
Americans with Disabilities Act (ADA, 1990)	Department of Labor	ADA was enacted by Congress to establish clear and comprehensive prohibition of discrimination on the basis of disability. The act specifically covers discrimination in the areas of: (1) employment, (2) public services, (3) public accomodations and services operated by private entities, and (4) telecommunications.

number of databases in the Toxicology Data Network (TOXNET) that are very useful for finding information about industrial chemicals. Additional databases are also available for searching on the OSHA, NIOSH, EPA, and ATSDR websites.

OBLIGATIONS OF THE HEALTHCARE PROVIDER TO THE INDIVIDUAL PATIENT, COWORKERS, EMPLOYER, GOVERNMENT, AND COMMUNITY

Occupational diseases and injuries are, in principle, preventable. Physicians who diagnose a work-related disease or injury have an opportunity, and even an ethical obligation, to participate in the identification and control of workplace hazards and the prevention of further occupational illness and injury. Physicians can choose from a range of possible followup measures, the goals of which are to prevent recurrence or worsening of the disease or injury in the patient and to prevent the development of disease or injury in other potentially exposed workers. Some of these activities may necessitate contact with occupational medicine physicians, toxicologists, industrial hygienists, lawyers, journalists, government officials, management personnel, and union officials.

Obligations to the Patient

Inform the Patient That the Illness May Be Work-Related. When it is determined that the workplace is a factor in the etiology or aggravation of the patient's illness, this fact and its implications should be discussed with the patient. It should never be assumed that the patient is fully aware of the health risks associated with any workplace exposure. He or she should be provided information regarding the nature of workplace hazards, their health risks, and preventive measures as well as recommendations regarding continued exposure.

Suggest How the Patient Can Reduce the Exposure. In some cases the patient can take steps to reduce exposure. Adjustments in work habits that may be helpful may include using a respirator or other personal protective equipment provided by the employer, using workplace shower and change rooms to avoid carrying toxic chemicals from the workplace to the home, and avoiding ingestion of workplace toxins by careful handwashing before eating or smoking and by taking lunch, coffee, and smoking breaks away from the work station. Obviously, these recommendations assume that the employer provides the appropriate equipment and facilities, which is not always the case. The most effective hazard-control measures require significant commitment by and cooperation from the employer.

Suggest that the Patient Remove Himself or Herself from the Exposure. The employer may be willing to transfer the patient to a location away from the offending hazard. This may result in a reduction in pay, seniority, or other benefits, which may be compensable under Workers' Compensation. The employment provisions of the ADA require employers to make "reasonable accommodations" for both work- and non-work-related disabilities. Nevertheless, the employer may not be able to accommodate the patient. The patient should be counseled carefully, and other options should be explored.

Advise the Patient to Notify the Employer. Patients who are suffering from a work-related illness may be entitled to Workers' Compensation benefits, Social Security disability, or other government-sponsored benefit programs. In addition, they may have a valid claim against the manufacturer of a chemical, a defective product, or another third party. The degree of disability necessary to bring a successful claim varies.

Once a patient is informed that he or she has a work-related illness, strict time limits are set in motion, and failure to meet them can preclude the patient from successfully filing a claim or receiving needed benefits. The patient should be advised to provide written notice immediately to his or her employer of a work-related illness (supported by a physician's letter) and to seek advice about statutes of limitations and other requirements. This information is generally available from the State Workers' Compensation Board and is usually required to be provided to the employee by the employer. If there is a union at the workplace, it may be able to advise and assist the patient.

Obligations to Coworkers

A patient with a work-related illness should be advised to inform coworkers about his or her condition. If the patient belongs to a union, he or she should inform the union representative. If there is no union, the patient may contact OSHA or discuss the situation with the employer.

If the patient is a union member and agrees, the physician can contact the union, which may assist in hazard investigation, identify and warn other workers potentially affected by the hazard, and pressure the employer to take corrective action if it is unwilling to do so. The union can also help the patient to obtain any available benefits. The patient can sometimes identify appropriate contacts, such as shop stewards, members of the union's health and safety or workers' compensation committees, an occupational health specialist employed by the union at the local or national level, or an official of the union local.

Committees on Occupational Safety and Health (COSH), coalitions of labor, health, and legal professionals and community and environmental activists working to prevent job-related illness and injury, may be able to help with both diagnosis and followup of an occupational disease. These groups provide education and technical assistance nationwide on a range of topics, including the health effects of specific hazards, control measures, how to use government agencies, and the legal rights of disabled workers.

Obligation to Notify the Employer

When treating an occupational injury or illness, healthcare providers will often be required to report to government agencies, health departments, or insurance carriers. As part of that reporting process, the employer should also be notified. When there is imminent danger to coworkers or the public health, the employer should also be contacted to correct the exposure situation.

Obligations to Notify the Government

States may have laws that require direct physician reporting of occupational disease. If management is uncooperative despite notification that a hazardous situation exists, OSHA should be contacted, with the patient's consent. In addition to the federal agencies specifically empowered to protect worker health and safety, physicians may contact the state or local health department, which may initiate action or may refer the problem to one of the federal agencies. Many states also require physicians to report any occupational injury or illness to the Workers' Compensation carrier.

Obligation to Inform Colleagues and the Public

It has happened that an individual primary care physician or specialist was the first to suspect a link between a workplace exposure and a serious health problem. This is likely to recur in the future, especially if the physician practices in a small town or industrial area or provides health care to worker groups through a company or union. Armed with an increased index of suspicion and the occupational history, the physician may be able to alert workers and companies and prevent the occurrence of a major health problem. Even if the physician chooses not to be involved in subsequent investigation or research, it is important that information about suspected problems and hazards be made available to workers and employers in similar industrial settings, government agencies, healthcare professionals, and, perhaps, the public at large. Case reports in the medical literature, at medical meetings, or through the media can be very helpful in this regard.

SUMMARY

Industrial, workplace, and environmental exposures represent a different kind of challenge to primary care and emergency department physicians. Patients often present as a diagnostic dilemma, or with common symptoms that do not respond to the usual medical treatment. The challenge for the nonoccupational health professional is to correctly establish and treat the condition. This chapter offers a simple approach to all patients that will aid in the diagnosis and treatment of occupational and environmental diseases. This approach utilizes additional questions applied to the medical history and access to printed and electronic information resources. Exposures to these materials also have public health implications. Physicians who make the diagnosis of an occupationally or environmentally related disease have an obligation to prevent further injury. They should work with employee groups, employers, and government agencies to identify the toxic agent and prevent the development of disease in other potentially exposed individuals.

REFERENCES

Core Occupational Health Resources

1. Hathaway GJ, Proctor NH, Hughes JP, Fischman ML: Proctor and Hughes' Chemical Hazards in the Workplace, 4th ed. New York, John Wiley & Sons, 1996. Classic text addresses 542 chemicals likely to be encountered in various work settings.
2. Stellman JM: International Labour Organization: Encyclopaedia of Occupational Health and Safety, 4th ed., Geneva Switzerland 1998. This four-volume reference provides encyclopedic information on oc-
cupational hazards, the injuries and diseases associated with them, and preventive measures. Often the best place to begin research for those who know nothing about workers' exposures except their industry type. Also a good source for information about institutions and organizations active in occupational health and safety.
3. Last JM, Wallace RB, eds: Maxcy-Rosenau-Last Public Health and Preventive Medicine, 14th ed. Stamford, CT, Appleton & Lange, 1998. The basic textbook of public health—encompasses the essential knowledge about public health and preventive measures.
4. Wald P, Stave G: Physical and Biological Hazards in the Workplace. 2nd Edition New York, John Wiley & Sons, 2002. Major reference on health risks posed by physical and biologic hazards in the workplace. Designed as a companion to *Proctor and Hughes' Chemical Hazards in the Workplace*. Offers occupational information on how to control, diagnose, and treat conditions caused by exposure to every biologic and physical agent encountered in the workplace.

Additional Readings

5. Burgess WA: Recognition of Health Hazards in Industry: A Review of Materials and Processes, 2nd ed. New York, John Wiley & Sons, 1995. Excellent descriptions of industrial processes and general types of exposures.
6. Clayton GD, Clayton FE, eds: Patty's Industrial Hygiene and Toxicology, 4th ed. New York, John Wiley & Sons, 1995 (8 volumes). Excellent reference on occupational health and general toxicological data.
7. Gosselin RE, Smith RP, Hodge HC: Clinical Toxicology of Commercial Products, 5th ed. Baltimore, Williams & Wilkins, 1984. Useful as a first step for identifying trade name products and their ingredients, addresses and telephone numbers of companies, and estimates of relative toxicities of various chemicals.
8. Key MM: Occupational Diseases: A Guide to Their Recognition. Washington, DC, US Department of Health, Education, and Welfare, 1977. DHEW publ. no. (NIOSH) 79–116. Helpful in identifying chemicals associated with various occupations and routes of entry; not comprehensive.
9. Lewis RJ: Hazardous Chemicals Desk Reference, 4th ed. New York, Van Nostrand Reinhold, 1996. A compendium of over 20,000 chemicals, including specific health hazards, chemical and physical properties, relevant regulations, and more. A good first book to use if you know the specific chemical(s).
10. Magos L: Three cases of methylmercury intoxication which eluded correct diagnosis. Arch Toxicol 1998;72:701–705. Case report on which the clinical vignette of this chapter is based.
11. Rom WN, ed: Environmental and Occupational Medicine, 3rd ed. Philadelphia, Lippincott-Raven, 1998. Excellent general textbook on occupational medicine. Not comprehensive for many specific chemicals, but excellent discussions of pathophysiologic mechanisms.
12. Sullivan JB, Krieger GR: Hazardous Materials Toxicology: Clinical Principles in Environmental Health. Baltimore, Williams & Wilkins, 1992. Excellent reference with sections on basic science and clinical principles of hazardous materials toxicology, organ system toxicity with principles of immediate treatment and evaluation, specific hazardous substances and general industries, and regulatory, health, and safety aspects of hazardous materials.
13. Zenz C, ed: Occupational Medicine Principles and Practice, 3rd ed. Chicago, Mosby–Year Book, 1994. Broad, detailed textbook overview of occupational health issues.

CHAPTER 93

HAZMAT INCIDENT RESPONSE WITH PRE- AND INTERHOSPITAL CARE OF THE POISONED PATIENT

Frank G. Walter / Neal E. Flomenbaum

PART I: HAZMAT INCIDENT RESPONSE

A hazardous material can be defined as any substance (solid, liquid, or gas) capable of harming people, property, or the environment; therefore, the list of hazardous materials is understandably large.[15,17] Paracelcus (1493–1541), the father of modern toxicology and pharmacology, expressed this eloquently: "Everything is a poison, there is nothing which is not. Only the dose differentiates a poison from a remedy."

A hazardous materials emergency is an uncontrolled or unexpected release of a hazardous material. Hazmat incident response is an area of special expertise within the field of clinical toxicology. In general, hazmat incident response focuses on poisoning care in the prehospital setting, prepares for multicasualty incidents, and emphasizes patient decontamination to treat the patient and to prevent contamination of healthcare providers. Although hazmat response focuses on these distinctions, general poisoning treatment principles are the same for hazmat response as they are for care of the patient who has overdosed, ie, therapeutically intervening to modify toxicodynamics and toxicokinetics by altering absorption, administering antidotes, providing basic supportive care, changing catabolism, distributing the poison differently, and enhancing elimination, if possible. In other words, the general principles of toxicology apply regardless of whether a patient is at a hazmat incident or in the prehospital, interhospital, or inpatient setting. Although patient-care resources vary among these treatment settings, the fundamental principles of patient care remain the same.

Because the number of hazardous materials is so large, it is efficient to group hazardous materials according to their toxicological characteristics. Various classification systems have been devised. The International Hazard Classification System (IHCS) is the most commonly used (Table 93–1).[13,74] Individual hazmat studies commonly utilize their own classification systems, emphasizing the toxicodynamic effects of hazardous materials such as systemic asphyxiants or highlighting individual chemicals such as ammonia or chlorine or general classes of chemicals such as acids, bases, or volatile organic compounds.[15,17,42,79]

The Epidemiology of Hazmat Incidents

Although the concepts regarding hazardous materials toxicology are centuries old, the systematic study of hazmat epidemiology only began in recent decades. Because the United States Department of Transportation (DOT) regulates transportation of hazardous materials, it has been collecting data on hazmat incidents since 1971. Recent data indicate that in the United States the number of incidents has increased from 13,900 in 1996 to 17,501 in 1999 while the number of deaths has diminished from 120 in 1996 to 7 in 1999.[73,79]

For decades, the vast majority of hazmat incidents were thought to occur during transportation because only the DOT collected, published, and promulgated data regarding hazmat incidents that occur during transportation. In the late 1980s medical science began to focus on the epidemiology of hazmat incidents. To date, there are fewer than 20 hazmat epidemiology articles in peer-reviewed medical journals.[7,9,10,25,27,30–33,39–41,63,68,80] Nevertheless, data from these articles and other US government sources indicate that the majority of hazmat incidents actually occur at fixed facilities rather than during transportation.[1]

The most commonly encountered substances at hazmat incidents vary from one locale to another and are predominately determined by the major industries in a particular area.[79,80] For example, pesticides are the most commonly encountered class of hazardous materials in Fresno County, whose major industry is agribusiness. Although most hazmat incidents involve only one hazardous material, more than one hazardous material can be encountered at a given incident. One study described 107 hazmat incidents involving a total of 156 materials.[79,80]

The vast majority of consequential hazmat incidents are caused by gases, vapors, or aerosols. In one study, four of the five most commonly encountered individual chemicals were ammonia, phosphine, sulfur oxides, and hydrogen sulfide.[79,80] The important implication for decontamination is that gases do not usually secondarily contaminate people because they do not adhere to patients. Therefore, patients exposed only to gases generally do not require skin decontamination to prevent secondary contamination, and much greater efficiency is possible in patient care at gas, vapor, and aerosol hazmat incidents. Inhalation is the most common route of exposure at hazmat incidents and was the route of exposure at 73% of the hazmat incidents, accounting for 76% of the exposed patients described in one study.[15,17,79]

The vast majority of hazmat incidents do not generate patients. Of 19,042 hazmat incidents, only 1692 incidents (9%) produced patients.[42,79] For this reason, the predominant role of the paramedic is providing pre- and postexposure monitoring and care for hazmat entry team members rather than providing care for victims of hazmat incidents.[12,79]

On the other hand, most patient-producing hazmat incidents are multicasualty incidents. For example, in the previously cited study, the 1692 patient-producing incidents generated 7756 patients.[42,79] Most hazmat patients do not require hospital admission. Of the 7756 total patients in the previously cited study, 68% were transported to and treated at a hospital but were not admitted; 14%

TABLE 93–1. International Hazard Classification System

Class 1: Explosives	**Class 5: Oxidizers and organic peroxides**
Division 1.1: Mass explosion hazard	Division 5.1: Oxidizers
Division 1.2: Projection hazard	Division 5.2: Organic peroxides
Division 1.3: Predominantly a fire hazard	
Division 1.4: No significant blast hazard	**Class 6: Poisonous materials and infectious substances**
Division 1.5: Very insensitive explosives	Division 6.1: Poison materials
Division 1.6: Extremely insensitive detonating articles	Division 6.2: Infectious substances
Class 2: Gases	**Class 7: Radioactive substances**
Division 2.1: Flammable gases	
Division 2.2: Nonflammable compressed gases	**Class 8: Corrosive materials**
Division 2.3: Poisonous gases	
Division 2.4: Corrosive gases (Canada)	**Class 9: Miscellaneous hazardous materials**
Class 3: Flammable/combustible liquids	
Class 4: Flammable solids	
Division 4.1: Flammable solid	
Division 4.2: Spontaneously combustible materials	
Division 4.3: Dangerous when wet materials	

were treated on scene but were not transported; 7% were transported to a hospital but were only observed and not treated; 6% were transported to, treated at, and admitted to a hospital; and 5% were seen at their physicians' offices within 24 hours of the hazmat incident.[42,79]

Hazmat incidents can result in fatalities as well as injuries. In one study with 1692 patient-producing hazmat incidents, 61 incidents (4%) caused 83 deaths. The 83 deaths in 7756 patients represent a fatality rate of about 1%. Among the 83 total fatalities, 76% were employees, 19% were the general public, and 5% were rescue personnel responding to the hazmat incident. The most commonly reported causes of death were trauma (65%), thermal burns (16%), respiratory tract injury (10%), chemical burns (6%), and other causes (3%). The most commonly encountered hazardous materials reported at fatal hazmat incidents were ammonia, hydrogen chloride, and nitrogen fertilizer; nitrogen fertilizer caused deaths by explosions. Rescue personnel and healthcare providers must focus on the whole patient and not just poisoning because hazmat victims can also have injuries caused by vehicular crashes, explosions, or thermal burns.[42,79]

Emergency personnel and equipment can become contaminated at hazmat incidents. For example, in one study, contamination occurred to one ambulance that drove through a puddle of liquid organic phosphorus pesticides that had spilled from a crashed exterminator truck. This ambulance was responding to a call for a "motor vehicle crash."[79,80] This illustrates the principle that emergency responders must always be careful because any motor vehicle crash or fire can be an unrecognized hazmat incident.

Hazardous Materials and Hazmat Response

Chemical Names and Numbers. Chemical compounds may be known by several names, including the chemical, common, generic, or brand (proprietary) name.[11,13] For example, methanol or methyl alcohol (chemical names) may also be called wood alcohol. Brand names of methyl alcohol include Sterno and Colonial Spirit. A chemical may be the sole substance in a given hazardous material or one of several compounds in a mixture.

The Chemical Abstracts Service (CAS) of the American Chemical Society (ACS) numbers chemicals to overcome the confusion regarding multiple names for a single chemical. The CAS assigns a unique CAS registry number (CAS#) to atoms, molecules, and mixtures. For example, the CAS# of methanol is 67–56–1.[50] These numbers provide a unique identification for chemicals as well as a means for crosschecking chemical names. Identifying a chemical by name and CAS# is critical because one must be as specific as possible about the hazardous material in question. Trade or brand names can be misleading. The material safety data sheet (MSDS) describing a product usually lists the chemical name, the CAS#, and the brand name.[51] If at all possible, hazmat responders must precisely identify the material in question or serious management errors can occur.

Vehicular Placarding: UN Numbers, NA Numbers, and PIN. Substances in each hazard class of the International Hazard Classification System (Table 93–1) are assigned four-digit identification numbers, which are known as United Nations (UN), North American (NA), or Product Identification Numbers (PIN) and are displayed on characteristic vehicular placards. This system is used by the US DOT in the *North American Emergency Response Guidebook*.[74] The IHCS is limited in predicting the potential health hazards of a substance. Chemicals are assigned by their most dangerous physical characteristic, eg, explosiveness or flammability. Other potential hazards of an agent, such as its ability to cause cancer or birth defects, are not considered. This system provides very little guidance in treating poisonings caused by hazardous materials.

National Fire Protection Association 704 System for Fixed Facility Placarding. Fixed facilities such as hospitals or laboratories use a placarding system that is different from the vehicular placarding system. The National Fire Protection Association (NFPA) 704 system is used at most fixed facilities.[59] The NFPA system uses a diamond-shaped sign that is divided into four color-coded quadrants; red, yellow, white, and blue. This system gives hazmat responders information about the flammability, reactivity, health effects, and also other information, such as the water reactivity, oxidizing activity, or radioactivity.

The red quadrant on top indicates flammability. The blue quadrant on the left indicates health hazard. The yellow quadrant on the right indicates reactivity. The white quadrant on the bottom is for other information, such as OXY for an oxidizing product, W for a product that has unusual reactivity with water, and the standard radioactive symbol for radioactive substances.

Numbers in the red, blue, and yellow quadrants indicate the degree of hazard: numbers range from 0, which is minimal, to 4, which is severe and indicate specific levels of hazard.

Like all placarding systems, this one also has limitations. It does not name the specific hazardous substances in the facility and gives no information about the quantities or locations of the materials.

Substance Identification. Once a hazardous materials emergency has been recognized, responders must know what the material is and its potential health effects. Obviously, exact identification is desirable but not always possible. Information with regard to the site of the hazmat incident, such as the type of business, laboratory, or vehicle, allows hazmat responders to safely search for and identify essential placards or documents. Fixed facility placards, vehicular placards, MSDSs, bills of lading, shipping documents, inventory sheets, verbal information from employees and management, are potential sources of information.

CHEMTREC is a service of the Chemical Manufacturers Association. It has information about shippers, products, and manufacturers. CHEMTREC can be reached at 1–800–424–9300.[19] The internet address for CHEMTREC is *http://www.cmahq.com/ cmawebsite.nsf/pages/chemtrec*. CHEMTREC provides information at no charge, 24 hours a day. Details of an incident are relayed to the shipper's or manufacturer's 24-hour emergency contact, and they, in turn, are linked to hazmat incident responders. Technical data are available on handling the substance(s) involved, including the physical characteristics, transportation, and disposal.

A regional poison center is a valuable source of information. Other information sources include local and state health departments, the American Conference of Governmental and Industrial Hygienists (ACGIH), the Occupational Safety and Health Administration (OSHA), National Institutes of Occupational Safety and Health (NIOSH), Agency for Toxic Substances and Disease Registry (ASTDR), and the Centers for Disease Control and Prevention (CDC).[1,4,5,50,55,62]

If the name of the substance is known before arrival at the scene, then research can begin en route with reviews of the physical, chemical, and toxicologic properties of the material. If the chemical is not known before arrival at the scene, efforts to obtain this information should begin as soon as safely possible. Responder safety is a priority.

Even if the exact identity of the toxic material is not known, hazmat responders may be able to classify the hazardous material into one of several major toxicologic classes by identifying a hazmat toxidrome that allows them to reasonably treat the patient and protect themselves and others; for example, do patients have irritation of the mucous membranes and upper airway caused by a highly water-soluble irritant gas? Do the patients exhibit signs of asphyxia with major central nervous system and/or cardiopulmonary signs and symptoms? Do patients exhibit signs of cholinergic excess caused by organic phosphorus compounds or carbamate poisoning? Do patients exhibit chemical burns compatible with corrosives? Do patients have the odor of solvents with signs of CNS depression and cardiac irritability, compatible with exposure to hydrocarbons or halogenated hydrocarbons?

Also, even when the exact identity of the hazardous material is not known, what is usually known is the physical state of the material, (ie, solid, liquid, or gas). Airborne toxicants potentially mean many more victims. Airborne toxicants include not only gases and vapors but also the liquid suspensions, fog, and mists and the solid suspensions smoke, fumes, and dusts.

State. The physical state of a material determines how it will spread through the environment and gives clues to the potential route(s) of exposure for the material.

Unless moved by physical means such as wind, ventilation systems or people, solids will usually stay in one area. Solids can cause exposures by inhalation of dusts, by ingestion, or rarely by absorption through skin and mucous membranes. Solids that sublime, that is change directly from a solid into a gas without passing through the liquid state, can give off vapors that can cause airborne exposure. Only two commonly encountered solids sublime, dry ice and naphthalene. A vapor is defined as a gaseous dispersion of the molecules of a substance that is normally a liquid or a solid at standard temperature and pressure (STP), i.e., $0°C$ ($32°F = 273°K$) and 1 atm (760 torr = 760 mm Hg = 14.7 psi).

Uncontained liquids will spread over surfaces and flow downhill. Liquids can evaporate, creating a vapor hazard. As noted, hazardous materials in a gaseous form pose the greatest exposure risk.

Primary and Secondary Contamination. The state of matter will also help healthcare providers determine whether the hazardous material presents a significant risk of secondary contamination and whether decontamination of the skin and mucous membranes is necessary.

Primary contamination is defined as contamination of people or equipment caused by direct contact with the initial release of a hazardous material by direct contact at its source of release. Primary contamination can occur whether the hazardous material is a solid, a liquid, or a gas.

Secondary contamination is defined as contamination of healthcare personnel or equipment caused by direct contact with a patient or equipment covered with adherent solids or liquids that have been removed from the source of the hazardous material spill. Secondary contamination generally occurs only with solids or liquids. Patients or equipment covered with adherent solid or liquid hazardous materials must be decontaminated before transportation, to prevent downstream contamination of healthcare providers and equipment. Patients who have been exposed only to gases generally do not require skin decontamination. An exception would be a patient whose sweaty skin was exposed to a highly water-soluble irritant gas such as ammonia that dissolves in sweat to produce corrosive ammonium hydroxide. In this case, the primary purpose of decontamination is to prevent or treat the patient's chemical burns caused by the caustic action of aqueous ammonium hydroxide on perspiring skin rather than preventing secondary contamination of rescuers.

Aerosols are airborne toxicants that are not gases. Aerosols are suspensions of solids or liquids in air, such as solid dusts or liquid mists, that can cover victims with these adherent solids or liquids, which can effect secondary contamination. These patients do require decontamination to prevent secondary contamination.

Water Solubility. The water solubility of a hazardous material determines whether water alone is sufficient for skin decontamination or whether a detergent must also be used. The general rule regarding solubility is that "Like dissolves like." In other words, a polar solvent, such as water, will dissolve polar substances such as salts and sugars. For example, the herbicide paraquat is actually a salt, paraquat dichloride, that is miscible in water. Therefore, if a patient's skin is contaminated with paraquat, copious water irrigation is sufficient for skin decontamination. A mild liquid detergent is acceptable but is not necessary. On the other hand, a nonpolar solvent, such as toluene, is not water-soluble and is immiscible. Therefore, if a patient's skin is contaminated with toluene, water irrigation alone may be insufficient for decontamination, and a mild liquid detergent is also necessary.

Vapor Pressure. The vapor pressure (VP) is useful to estimate whether enough of a solid or liquid will be released in the gaseous state to pose an inhalation risk. VP is defined essentially as the quantity of the gaseous state overlying an evaporating liquid or a subliming solid. The lower the VP, the less likely the chemical will volatilize and generate a respirable gas. Conversely, the higher the VP of a chemical, the more likely it will volatilize or generate a respirable gas. A chemical with a higher VP poses a greater inhalation risk than does a chemical with a lower VP. Water has a VP of approximately 20 mm Hg at 70°F (21°C), and acetone has a VP of 250 mm Hg at the same temperature. Therefore, acetone evaporates more rapidly than water and poses more of an inhalation risk. Standard reference texts (*Merck Index, 2000 Emergency Response Guidebook*) list vapor pressures for commonly encountered chemicals.

Hazmat Scene Control Zones. Scene management is a fundamental feature at a hazmat incident. It is almost always necessary to isolate the scene, deny access to the public and the media, and limit access to emergency response personnel in order to prevent needless contamination. Three scene control zones are typically used and are described by "temperature," "color," or "explanatory terminology."(Table 93–2 and Fig. 93–1). NIOSH[55] and the Environmental Protection Agency (EPA) utilize the temperature terminology system.

The *hot zone* is the area immediately surrounding a hazardous materials incident. It extends far enough to prevent the primary contamination of people and materials outside this zone. Primary contamination can occur to those who enter this zone. In general, evacuation, but no decontamination or patient care, is carried out in this zone.

The *warm zone* is the area surrounding the hot zone and contains the decontamination or access corridor where victims, the

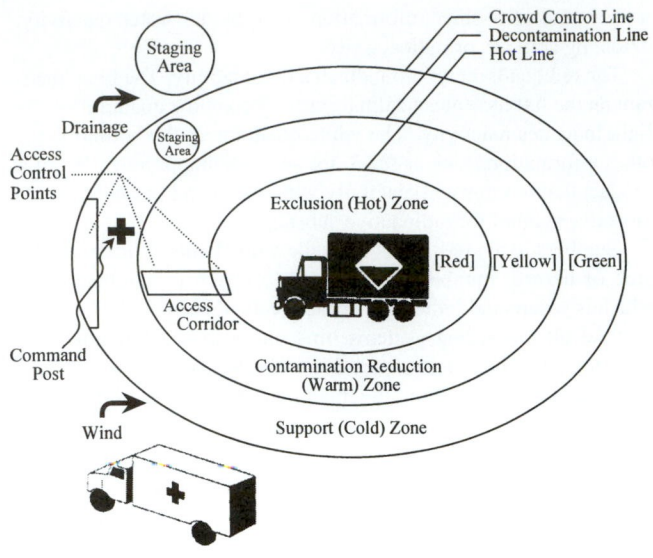

Figure 93–1. NIOSH/OSHA recommended control zones. (Modified from ATSDR guidelines).

hazmat entry team members, and their equipment are decontaminated. It includes two control points for the access corridor. In general, the only victim care in this area before any necessary skin decontamination, is opening the airway, cervical spine control, and placement on a backboard.

The *cold zone* is the area beyond the warm zone. Contaminated victims and hazmat responders must be decontaminated before entering this area from the warm zone. Equipment and personnel are not expected to become contaminated in this zone. This is the area where resources are assembled to support the hazmat emergency response. The incident command center is usually located in the cold zone, and definitive patient care is conducted here. This zone includes the primary survey and resuscitation with management of airway (with cervical spine control), breathing, circulation, disability, and exposure with evaluation for toxicity and trauma (ABCDE). Definitive care also includes antidotal treatment for specific poisonings.

Personal Protective Equipment

A critical goal of hazmat emergency responders is protecting themselves as well as the public. Safeguarding hazmat responders includes wearing appropriate personal protective equipment (PPE) to (1) prevent exposure to the hazard and (2) prevent injury to the wearer from incorrect use of or malfunction of the PPE equipment.

PPE can create significant health hazards, including loss of cooling by evaporation, heat stress, physical stress, psychological stress, impaired vision, impaired mobility, and impaired communication. Because of these risks, individuals involved in hazmat emergency response must be trained regarding the appropriate use, decontamination, maintenance, and storage of PPE. This training includes instruction regarding the risk of permeation, penetration, and degradation of PPE. PPE with a self-contained breathing apparatus (SCBA) has a fixed supply of air that significantly limits

TABLE 93–2. The Nomenclatures of the Hazmat Control Zones

Temperature Terminology System[a]	Color Terminology System	Explanatory Terminology System
Hot zone	Red zone	Exclusion or restricted zone
Warm zone	Yellow zone	Decontamination or contamination reduction zone
Cold zone	Green zone	Support zone

[a]NIOSH, EPA. Adapted with permission from the Advanced Hazmat Life Support Provider Mannual, 2nd ed. Tucson, AZ, Arizona Board of Regents, 2000.

the amount of time the wearer can operate in the hot zone, usually about 20 minutes.

Levels of Protection.   The EPA defines four levels of protection for PPE, levels A (highest) through D (lowest). The different levels of PPE are designed to provide a choice of PPE, depending on the hazards at a specific hazmat incident (Table 93–3).

Level A provides the highest level of both respiratory and skin (clothing) protection and provides vapor protection to the respiratory tract, mucous membranes, and the skin. This level of PPE is airtight, and the breathing apparatus must be worn under the suit.

Level B provides the highest level of respiratory protection but less skin protection. Level B provides skin splash protection by using chemical-resistant clothing. It does not provide skin vapor protection but does provide respiratory tract vapor protection

Level C protection should be used when the type of airborne substance is known, when its concentration can be measured, when the criteria for using air-purifying respirators are met, and when skin and eye exposures are unlikely. Level C provides skin splash protection, the same as level B; however, level C has a lower level of respiratory protection than either level A or B.

Level D is basically a regular work uniform. It should not be worn when significant chemical respiratory or skin hazards exist. It provides no respiratory protection and minimal skin protection. Level D was specifically developed to show *what not to wear* for chemical protection.

PPE Respiratory Protection.   Personnel must be fit-tested before using any respirator. A tiny space between the edge of the respirator and the face of the hazmat responder could permit exposure to an airborne hazard. Contact lenses cannot be worn with any respiratory protective equipment. Corrective eyeglass lenses must be mounted inside the face mask of the PPE.

Level A PPE mandates use of a self-contained breathing apparatus. A SCBA is composed of a face piece connected by a hose to a compressed air source. Open-circuit SCBAs, most often used in emergency response, provide clean air from a cylinder to the wearer, who exhales into the atmosphere. In the open-circuit, positive-pressure SCBA, air is supplied to the wearer from a cylinder and supplied to the face piece under positive pressure. Thus, a higher air pressure is maintained inside the face piece than outside. This affords the SCBA wearer the highest level of protection

against airborne hazards because any leakage will force air out of the face piece and not allow airborne hazards to enter against the higher pressure within the face piece. Disadvantages of SCBA include its bulkiness, heaviness, and a limited time period of respiratory protection because of the limited amount of air in the tank.

A supplied-air respirator (SAR) may be used in level B PPE and differs from SCBA in that air is supplied through a line that is connected to a source located away from the contaminated area. Only positive-pressure SARs are recommended for hazmat use. One major advantage of SARs over SCBA is that they allow an individual to work for a longer period. However, a hazmat worker must stay connected to the SAR and cannot leave the contaminated area by a different exit.

An air-purifying respirator (APR) may be used in level C PPE and allows breathing of ambient air after inhalation through a specific purifying canister or filter. There are three basic types of APRs: chemical cartridge, disposable, and powered-air. Although APRs afford the wearer increased mobility, they can be used only where there is sufficient oxygen in the ambient air. The chemical cartridges/canisters purify the air by filtration, adsorption, and/or absorption. Filters may also be used in combination with cartridges to provide increased protection from particulates such as asbestos.

Hazmat Incident Response Rules and Standards

OSHA and NFPA have developed, respectively, rules and guidelines regarding hazmat incident response. OSHA rules are mandated as law and must be followed. Meeting NFPA guidelines will ensure OSHA compliance.

The Superfund Amendments and Reauthorization Act of 1986, known as SARA, required OSHA to develop and implement standards to protect employees responding to hazardous materials emergencies. This resulted in the "Hazardous Waste Operations and Emergency Response" standard, 29 CFR 1910.120, or HAZWOPER.[75]

NFPA 471, "Recommended Practice for Responding to Hazardous Materials Incidents," outlines the following tactical objectives: incident response planning, communication procedures, response levels, site safety, control zones, personal protective equipment, incident mitigation, decontamination, and medical monitoring.[52]

NFPA 472, "Standard on Professional Competence of Responders to Hazardous Materials Incidents," helps define the minimum skills, knowledge, and standards for training outlined in HAZWOPER for the following three types of responders.[53]

First Responder at the Awareness Level.   First responders at the awareness level during the course of their normal duties could be first on the scene at an emergency incident involving hazardous material. They are expected to recognize the presence of hazardous materials, protect themselves, secure the area, and call for better trained personnel. They must take a safe position and keep other people from entering the area. They must recognize that the level of mitigation exceeds their training and call for a hazmat response team. Most emergency medical technician (EMT) basic curricula include this level of first responder training.

First Responder at the Operational Level.   These individuals are trained in all competencies of the awareness level and are addi-

TABLE 93–3.   Personal Protective Equipment

	Protects Respiratory System From:			Protects Skin and Eyes From:	
Level[a]	Select Vapors and Aerosols	Gases, Vapors, and Aerosols	Oxygen-Deficient Atmospheres	Liquids and Solids	Gases and Vapors
D					
C	+			+	
B	+	+	+	+	
A		+	+	+	+

[a]Definitions: level A, a self-contained breathing apparatus (SCBA) worn under a vapor-protective, fully encapsulated, airtight, chemical-resistant suit; level B, a positive-pressure supplied-air respirator with an escape SCBA worn under a hooded, splash protective, chemical-resistant suit; level C, an air-purifying respirator worn with a hooded, splash protective, chemical-resistant suit; level D: regular work clothing (offers no protection).

tionally trained to protect nearby persons, the environment, or exposed property from the effects of hazmat releases. Operational level certified individuals are expected to assume a defensive posture, to control the release from a safe distance, and to keep the hazardous material from spreading. Operational level individuals are trained to perform absorption of liquids, diking of liquids to contain the spill, vapor suppression, and vapor dispersion. They do not operate within the hot zone.

Hazardous Materials Technician.
Hazardous materials technicians respond to hazmat releases, or potential releases, for the purpose of controlling the release. They are trained in the use of chemical-resistant suits, air-monitoring equipment, mitigation techniques, and the interpretation of physical properties of hazardous materials. Technicians are capable of containing an incident, making safe entry into a hazardous environment, determining the appropriate course of action, victim rescue, and cleaning up or neutralizing the incident in order to return the property to a safe and usable status, if possible. These individuals are trained to operate within the hot zone to mitigate the incident. This certification level includes knowledge of hazardous material chemistry, air-monitoring equipment, tools used within the hot zone, and more.

NFPA 473, "Standard for Competencies for EMS Personnel Responding to Hazardous Materials Incidents," identifies the competencies of emergency medical personnel who may be required to respond to hazmat incidents for medical support of hazmat team members, or for triage, treatment, and transportation of patients. NFPA 473 defines the difference between EMS/HM level I responders and EMS/HM level II responders. HM is an abbreviation for hazmat.[54]

EMS/HM Level I Responders.
EMS/HM level I responders are personnel who, in the course of their normal activities, may provide patient care activities in the cold zone at hazmat incidents. This normally includes EMS personnel outside the fire department. EMS/HM level I responders shall provide care only to those individuals who no longer pose a significant risk of secondary contamination to others. EMS/HM level I responders are trained to the first responder awareness level.

EMS/HM Level II Responders.
EMS/HM level II responders are personnel who, in the course of their normal activities, may provide patient care activities in the warm zone at hazmat incidents. EMS/HM level II responders are able to provide care to those individuals who still pose a significant risk of secondary contamination. EMS/HM level II responders are also able to coordinate EMS activities at hazmat incidents and provide medical support for the other hazmat response personnel. EMS/HM level II responders are trained to the first responder operational level.

Prehospital Hazmat Emergency Response Team Composition, Organization, and Responsibilities

Basic Hazmat (BH) Components

- Awareness level responders
- Operational level responders
- Hazardous materials technicians

Advanced Hazmat Components
Advanced Hazmat Providers.
Paramedics who complete an Advanced Hazmat Life Support (AHLS) course are trained in the recognition of signs and symptoms caused by exposure to hazardous materials. They are also trained to deliver antidotal therapy to victims of hazmat poisonings, as approved by state and local protocols.

The inclusion of such training into a department's hazmat response team is beneficial, not only for the needs of the public but also to protect hazmat technicians who make entry into hazardous atmospheres. Protection of hazmat team members should be the primary responsibility of AHLS paramedics. Ideally, entry into hazardous atmospheres should not be performed, unless an AHLS paramedic is on scene, with resuscitative equipment in place, including a drug box containing approved antidotes for specific hazardous materials.

Medical Control.
Obtaining medical control should begin early in the development of the hazmat team. Incidents involving hazardous materials can have far-reaching community implications. Involving a physician with board preparation and/or board certification in medical toxicology is imperative. The ideal medical director for a hazardous materials team should be board certified in medical toxicology and should be familiar with the operations and logistics of functioning in the prehospital environment. This physician should be consulted in all aspects of planning for a hazmat response. In addition to developing training curricula and treatment plans for toxic exposures, this physician can work with emergency responders and hospitals to help integrate emergency personnel into the incident command structure and assist with the logistics of decontamination and hospital preparedness for victims of hazmat incidents.

On-line, direct medical control plays an important role in caring for hazmat victims. Contact with medical control should be established as soon as possible after deciding that hot zone entry is necessary. Communication with the physician should include all pertinent information about the involved materials and any special medical conditions of the entry crew. This prealert notification allows the physician and hospital staff to be prepared to institute contingency plans when patients are identified who may require transport to a receiving facility.

Medical control should also include consultation with a regional poison control center, if possible. Field personnel should be familiar with how to access information through the poison center. Medical toxicologists should be available at the poison center. Similarly, the poison center should be familiar with the level of training of responding EMS personnel. This relationship will be valuable in the analysis of unknown substances, in developing decontamination procedures, and for treating hazmat patients.

Hazmat Incident Command System (ICS)/Incident Management System (IMS).[6,20,44,48,49]
An ICS/IMS must be used at all hazmat incidents. Standard Operating Procedures (SOPs) need to specify who will assume hazmat incident command (IC), what the responsibilities of the hazmat incident commander are, when IC will be required, and who will report to the incident commander. The *hazmat safety officer* should be a hazmat technician, is responsible for the safety of all personnel within the hazmat sector, and has the authority to stop any unsafe operation. *Hazmat research personnel* ensure that information about the hazardous material involved in

the incident is retrieved and available (Table 93–4). This information should include physical properties, isolation distances, incompatibilities, signs and symptoms of exposure, BHLS and AHLS treatment, protective clothing required, and cleanup techniques. *Hazmat decontamination personnel* should have completed the operational level of training. SOPs should address when, where, and by whom decontamination should be established, including the minimum number of personnel needed, and what level of personal protection will be required for the decontamination crew. *Hazmat entry team and backup team* personnel must be hazmat technicians. SOPs should include the type of communication equipment that is required and what hand signals are to be used should the communication equipment fail. The SOP should also include a preentry medical evaluation form that should be completed on each entry team member and backup team member before entry, after decon, and 10 minutes after decontamination. The exclusion criteria for entry must be on this form and available to all team members (Table 93–5).

The primary responsibility of the *prehospital hazmat medical sector* is the protection of the hazmat entry team personnel. This is accomplished by researching and recording clinically pertinent information about the hazardous material (Table 93–4), remaining available on scene for medical treatment, and assessing individuals before entry into, and on exit from, a hazardous environment. Documentation of each assessment should be recorded on a prepared form and compared to the exclusion criteria defined by NFPA 471 (Table 93–4). A position in the hazmat medical sector should be held by individuals trained as AHLS paramedics, preferably with EMS/HM level II responder competency and ideally with hazmat technician level competency.

Patient Care Responsibilities of the Prehospital Decontamination Team and the Hazmat Entry Team.

Hazmat responders should identify the entry and exit areas by controlling points for the access corridor (decontamination corridor) from the hot zone, through the warm zone, to the cold zone (Fig. 93–1). This corridor should be upwind, uphill, and upstream from the hot zone, if possible. Hazmat entry team members should remove victims from the contaminated hot zone and deliver patients to the inner control point of the access (decontamination) corridor (Fig. 93–1). Hazmat decontamination team members decontaminate patients in the decontamination (access) corridor of the contamination reduction (warm) zone (Fig. 93–1). After decontamination, hazmat responders deliver patients to paramedics in the cold zone (Fig. 93–1).

Patient Care Responsibilities of EMS Paramedics at Hazmat Incidents.

EMS paramedics who are not part of the hazmat team should report to the incident staging area and await direction from the incident commander. They should approach the site from upwind, uphill, and upstream, if possible.

EMS paramedics should remain in the cold zone until properly protected hazmat incident responders arrive, decontaminate, and deliver patients to them for further triage. Then, EMS paramedics should evaluate each patient, direct patients without complaints to the occupant staging area, and take patients with complaints to the patient staging area. An EMS paramedic should stay with the patients in the occupant staging area to continually reevaluate these asymptomatic victims and transfer them to the patient staging area if they do become symptomatic. Patients leaving the occupant staging area should receive instructions regarding potential signs

and symptoms that may develop that will necessitate their subsequent evaluation at a healthcare facility.

Initial EMS patient care takes place in the cold zone's patient staging area, including medical management of hazmat victims. Decontamination should not be necessary because EMS paramedics in the cold zone should care only for decontaminated patients or patients who did not have skin contamination.

Transportation of patients from the hazmat incident is ultimately under the control of the incident commander but is usually delegated to the prehospital hazmat medical sector and EMS paramedics in consultation with a base hospital physician. In general, no victim with skin contamination should be transported from the hazmat site without being properly decontaminated. Before transportation, EMS should notify the base hospital of the number of victims being transported, as well as their toxicological history, patient assessments, and treatment rendered. The base hospital physician may have additional orders, either before or after consultation with the poison control center and/or a medical toxicologist. If a patient is to be transported to a hospital other than the base hospital, the receiving hospital should be contacted.

Emergency Department Responsibilities for Hazmat Victims

In general, hospitals and emergency departments do not have adequate decontamination equipment, personal protective equipment, fit testing, or training in the safe use of personal protective equipment. Therefore, it is critical that hospitals be involved with community hazmat planning and ensure that hazmat victims are decontaminated in the field before delivery to the hospital. In addition, the hospital should have a preestablished protocol by which hazmat response teams will respond to the hospital to decontaminate patients who arrive at the hospital before decontamination. In general, hazmat patients who require skin decontamination should be denied entry to the emergency department until decontaminated by an appropriately trained and equipped hazmat response team, unless the emergency department attending physician allows the patient to enter after carefully assessing the risks and benefits to the contaminated patient, the other patients in the emergency department, and the emergency department healthcare personnel.

If a hospital chooses to have its own hazmat response team, then the hospital must comply with all OSHA and EPA regulations that apply to prehospital hazmat response teams. This is usually an impractical solution for hospitals. Therefore, it is essential that the hospital prospectively arrange for prehospital hazmat teams to respond to the hospital when a contaminated patient presents to the hospital. This requires development of ongoing relationships between the hospital and prehospital hazmat EMS providers before a hazmat incident occurs.

Role of the Emergency Physician.

The ED physician should:

- Provide prehospital medical control as the base hospital emergency physician, if possible.
- Activate the hospital's disaster plan, if indicated.
- Contact the poison control center and/or medical toxicologist or, alternatively, call the hospital's chemical spill coordinator or the hospital's radiation control personnel if the substance is believed to be radioactive.
- Decide what procedures should be used in the field for decontamination in conjunction with the poison control center and/or medical toxicologist.

TABLE 93–4. Hazmat Incident Response AHLS Paramedic Worksheet

- ❏ Research hazardous material information (use 3 references) and contact poison center
- ❏ Contact most appropriate base hospital
- ❏ Preentry medical evaluation on entry team and backup teams
- ❏ Brief entry and backup teams on signs and symptoms of exposure
- ❏ During entry, be available for immediate treatment and/or transport, following emergency decontamination.
- ❏ Postentry medical evaluation (immediate and 10 minutes postentry, if possible)
- ❏ After incident, update hospital on incident termination

Chemical name: _____ **Synonyms:** _____

Physical Properties	Routes of Exposure	Hazard Class	
❏ Solid IDLH: _____	❏ Inhalation	❏ Corrosive	❏ Poison
❏ Liquid VP: _____	❏ Absorption	❏ Explosive	❏ Other:
❏ Gas BP: _____	❏ Ingestion	❏ Flammable gas	_____
FP: _____		❏ Flammable solid UN#: _____	
Solubility: _____		❏ Oxidizer CAS#: _____	

Toxicology

- ❏ Irritant gas
- ❏ Simple asphyxiant
- ❏ Systemic asphyxiant
    - ❏ Carbon monoxide
    - ❏ Cyanide
    - ❏ Methemoglobin inducer
    - ❏ Sulfide
- ❏ Cholinesterase inhibitor
    - ❏ Carbamate
    - ❏ Organic phosphorus compound
- ❏ Caustic
    - ❏ Acid
    - ❏ Alkali
- ❏ Hydrocarbon or halogenated hydrocarbon
- ❏ Other: _____

Signs and Symptoms

Skin	Respiratory	Cardiovascular	Nervous System
❏ Irritation	❏ Irritation	❏ Tachydysrhythmias	❏ Excitation
❏ Chemical burns	❏ Laryngeal spasm	❏ Bradydysrhythmias	❏ Seizures
❏ Thermal burns	❏ Bronchospasm	❏ Angina	❏ Depression
❏ Fasciculations	❏ Bronchorrhea	❏ Rales	
❏ Diaphoresis	❏ Depression		Other
Eyes	❏ Hypoxia		❏ Emesis
❏ Constriction / Miosis	❏ Rales		❏ Salivation
❏ Dilation / Mydriasis			❏ Diarrhea
❏ Irritation			❏ Urination
❏ Lacrimation			

Treatment

Decon	Breathing	Cardiovascular	Nervous System
	❏ Oxygen	❏ Monitor	❏ Benzodiazepine for seizures
Airway	❏ Bag valve ventilation	❏ IV	
❏ Suction	❏ β-Adrenergic agonist	❏ ACLS guidelines	Antidote: _____
❏ Intubate		❏ Fluids	
		❏ Vasopressors	Other: _____
		❏ CPR	

Modified with permission from The Advanced Hazmat Life Support Provider Manual, 2nd ed. Tucson AZ, Arizona Board of Regents, 2000.

- ■ Advise prehospital EMS personnel on precautions and adequate decontamination procedures.
- ■ Decide if field decontamination procedures are adequate with the help of the poison control center and/or medical toxicologist.
- ■ Meet the ambulance and decontaminated patients outside of the ED and reassess for the adequacy of decontamination before patient entry into the ED.
- ■ Call an appropriate level trauma alert if the patient has physical injuries.
- ■ Decide if and how a decontamination room should be used, if necessary, and if available.

- ■ Decide if an additional decontamination area should be prepared outside the ED and, if so, establish the external unit.[3,14,16,21,22,24,29,34,37,43,64,67,71]

Role of the Emergency Charge Nurse. The ED charge nurse should:

- ■ Ensure that a contaminated patient does not walk into the ED without being decontaminated.
- ■ Deny ED entry in consultation with the attending emergency physician if a patient with skin contamination has not been decontaminated before arrival in the ED, and if necessary, con-

TABLE 93–5. Hazmat Entry Team Member Preentry Exclusion Criteria

Respiratory rate >24 per minute
Pulse >70% of the maximum heart rate for age;
   eg, age 20; 140 beats/min; age 50; 120 beats/min
Blood pressure Diastolic >105 mm Hg
Temperature <97.0°F or >99.5°F (<36°C or >37.5°C)
Skin Dermatitis
Recent medical history Nausea, vomiting, diarrhea, fever, upper respiratory infection, heat illness, or substantial alcohol intake within past 72 hours; new prescription medications taken within past 2 weeks or nonprescription medications taken within past 72 hours; any alcohol within past 6 hours; pregnancy

Modified with permission from the Advanced Hazmat Life Support Provider Manual 2nd ed. Tucson, AZ, Arizona Board of Regents, 2000.

tact dispatch to send a hazmat response team to the ED while the patient waits outside the ED in an area of limited patient traffic.

■ Notify hospital security to provide ED security and deny entry of contaminated patients unless the attending emergency physician makes a conscious decision to allow entry after considering the risks and benefits.

■ Notify the chemical spill coordinator, the ED director, and the clinical supervisor, who will notify the on-call administrator.

■ Review current ED status and staffing and assign personnel to care for all ED patients.

■ Provide liaison to hospital security, the administrator on call, and the chemical spill coordinator.

■ Notify public affairs.

Additional recommendations for the care of contaminated hazmat patients in emergency departments are excerpted from the *Annals of Emergency Medicine* and used here with permission:[16]

No medical consensus exists for the minimum level of personal protection required for hospital decontamination. This is especially true regarding respiratory protection, which is only necessary when toxic vapors are at concentrations high enough to cause potentially harmful effects to staff. After clothing removal, a contaminated patient poses minimal inhalation risk when decontamination is performed outside the ED. However, if a patient is placed in a poorly ventilated treatment room (enclosed space), personnel without respiratory protection could have symptoms from inhalation of off-gassing vapors from clothing, skin, or vomitus. Selecting the appropriate protective equipment depends on the specific hazardous substance identified. Surgical masks never provide adequate protection from toxic vapors.[16]

Legal requirements do apply to hospital-based decontamination. All EDs incorporated in an emergency response plan for hazardous materials incidents through Local Emergency Planning Committees, an agreement with a facility or hazardous waste site, or other means, must meet OSHA requirements [29 CFR 1910.120(q)] for both training and response to hazardous materials, because it is likely they will be faced with chemically exposed patients without previous decontamination at some time. Under these regulations, emergency medical personnel who would decontaminate victims exposed to a hazardous substance should be trained

at a minimum to the first-responder operations level. . . For response to an unknown hazard, OSHA regulations require level B protection, which includes a positive-pressure self-contained breathing apparatus and splash-protective chemical resistant clothing. However, these regulations should not be interpreted to require the use of this equipment for treatment of contaminated patients in all hospitals. Use of self-contained breathing apparatus can itself pose significant problems to ED staff. These hazards include increased weight, improper use of the equipment, problems with donning and doffing, and decreased dexterity. Other options include having the patients decontaminate themselves if they are capable, designating a local fire department hazardous materials teams to assist in or perform the decontamination, or proceeding with decontamination with less than level B protection if assistance is not available within a suitable time interval based on the patient's condition. Hospitals frequently receiving contaminated casualties or in high-risk areas may need to consider additional training and equipment, such as specialized chemical-resistant clothing and respirators.[16]

Medical Management of Hazmat Victims

Decontamination. Decontamination has two important functions: altering absorption for the patient and preventing secondary contamination of others. Primary goals at any hazmat incident are protecting emergency responders, preventing secondary contamination, and decreasing morbidity and mortality of hazmat victims.[6,12,16,18,28,38,45–47,70,77]

Exposure solely to gases, such as simple asphyxiants, generally requires no skin or mucous membrane decontamination to prevent secondary contamination of others. However, exposure to highly water-soluble irritant gases, such as ammonia, can cause skin and mucous membrane irritation and chemical burns that are treated with copious water irrigation. This effort of decontamination treats the patient rather than prevents secondary contamination of healthcare providers.

When indicated by the presence of adherent solids or liquids on a patient, skin decontamination should be performed in the field, in the decontamination zone. This is a two-step procedure. First remove all clothing, jewelry, and shoes. Bag and tag these possessions. The patient's possessions should be left at the scene, stored, and may need to be disposed of as hazardous waste. Any adherent solid particles should be brushed away from the patient. Gently blot away any obvious adherent liquid. Step two is meticulous washing with large quantities of water. Also use a mild liquid detergent if the adherent solids or liquids are not water-soluble or if the identity of the material is unknown. Most decontamination solutions are made for equipment, not people. Do not use these potentially irritating solutions on people. Pay close attention to all exposed skin and in particular the skin folds, the axillae, the genital area, and the feet. Use luke-warm water with gentle water pressure to reduce the risk of hypothermia. Apply water systematically from head to toe, protecting the patient's airway.

Exposed, symptomatic eyes should be continuously irrigated with water throughout the patient contact, including transport, if possible. Remember to check for and remove contact lenses. Use of Morgan therapeutic lenses is the most efficient method to decontaminate a patient's eyes, but this requires using an ocular topical anesthetic such as proparacaine.

Primary Survey and Resuscitation: The Basics. In general, the primary patient assessment and resuscitation are performed only after any necessary skin decontamination in the warm zone. The only two procedures that are commonly performed before any necessary skin decontamination are opening the patient's airway and spine precautions. Common sense dictates that if liquid or solid contamination involves only the patient's eyes or a small body part, such as a hand, then supportive care may be performed while decontamination is in progress. This procedure will also depend on the toxicity of the hazardous material.

The primary survey and resuscitation is described by the mnemonic *A, B, C, D, E:* Airway with cervical spine control, if necessary, Breathing; Circulation, Disability (nervous system), Exposure with environmental control.

Hazmat Patient Assessment. Hazmat patient assessment includes a history and physical examination. History is guided by the *AMPLE* mnemonic: Allergies, Medications, Past medical history, Last normal menstrual period, Last tetanus shot, Last meal, and Events.

Determine the events that led up to the hazmat incident. Who was involved in the hazmat incident? Are there other patients who need to be searched for and rescued? What is the exact identity of the hazardous material? Is there more than one hazardous material? What was the route of exposure? Where did the hazmat incident occur? Was there a confined–space exposure? When did the hazmat incident occur? How long was the exposure? How and why did the hazmat incident occur? Was there an explosion? Was there a fire? Is this hazmat incident an act of terrorism?

Secondary Survey. After the primary survey and resuscitation, hazmat patient assessment involves a secondary survey. This hazmat secondary survey focuses on identifying poisoning complications, recognizing preexistent problems that have the potential for exacerbation, assessing for accompanying trauma or burns, and recognizing toxic syndromes (*toxidromes*). There are five fundamental hazmat toxidromes or *hazidromes:* the irritant gas toxidrome, the asphyxiant toxidrome, the cholinergic toxidrome, the corrosive toxidrome, and the hydrocarbon and halogenated hydrocarbon toxidrome (Table 93–6).

The hazmat patient assessment secondary survey also includes determining whether the patient has complications from poisoning. These complications can involve derangements of the Airway, Breathing, Cardiovascular system, Disability (the nervous system), or the organs of Elimination (the liver and kidneys).

For example, the respiratory system (Airway and Breathing) can react in only a limited number of ways to various insults. The upper airway can become obstructed from edema caused by thermal or chemical burns. Ventilatory insufficiency can be caused by loss of central nervous system respiratory drive or by neuromuscular blockade with muscular weakness or paralysis caused by an organic phosphorus compound or carbamate poisoning. Aspiration pneumonitis can be caused by emesis with an unprotected airway. Acute lung injury (ALI) can be caused by direct damage to the alveolar-capillary membrane because of the local toxic effects of poorly water-soluble irritant gases such as phosgene and nitrogen dioxide, or ALI can be caused by other insults such as prolonged hypoxia or hypoperfusion.

Patient assessment emphasizes that we must treat the patient, not the poison. Knowing what the patient was exposed to does not necessarily mean that the patient was poisoned. Although knowledge about the poison is important, knowledge about the patient's condition, derived from the primary survey and continual reassessments, is even more important. Even if the patient has been poisoned, preservation of the patient's vital functions with a primary survey and resuscitation, ie, basic supportive care, is the cornerstone of treatment, taking precedent over administering any antidote.

Poisoning Treatment Paradigm. The poisoning treatment paradigm (Alter absorption, Antidote administration, Basics, Change catabolism, Distribute differently, and Enhance elimination) is an important AHLS mnemonic (*A, B, C, D, E*).[79]

Altering absorption (decontamination) is the cornerstone of toxicologic treatment. Hazmat antidotes are limited in number (Table 93–7). Basics, ie, the primary survey and resuscitation, are fundamental to the care of all patients, including hazmat victims. Poisonings caused by some hazardous materials can be treated effectively by changing their catabolism, distributing them differently, or enhancing their elimination. An example of changing catabolism is the antidote sodium thiosulfate accelerating the catabolism of highly toxic cyanide to its relatively nontoxic metabolite thiocyanate. An example of enhancing elimination is ventilating with 100% oxygen to enhance exhalation of carbon monoxide. Many inhaled toxicants, including gases such as carbon monoxide, are eliminated by exhalation. All the antidotes discussed are found in great detail in the appropriate Antidotes in Depth elsewhere in the text.

PART II: PREHOSPITAL AND INTERHOSPITAL CONSIDERATIONS

Whether a patient with a toxicologic emergency is one of many from a hazmat incident or, more typically, is the sole victim of a single exposure, once that patient is in the care of the EMTs and paramedics, the prehospital issues are, for the most part, the same. As noted in the beginning of this chapter, the vast majority of hazmat incidents do not generate patients, and when they do, usually there are only a few victims.

Because paramedics and EMTs are capable of providing high-quality care for critically ill patients, the facilities may be able to utilize EMTs and paramedics to transfer seriously ill victims of carbon monoxide poisoning to hyperbaric oxygen facilities, victims of envenomations to antivenom treatment centers, and victims of drug overdoses and poisonings to designated poison treatment centers and other hospitals capable of providing necessary hemodialysis and/or hemoperfusion. Appropriate pre- and interhospital care of the poisoned or overdosed patients begins with a knowledge of those aspects of management described in detail in Chapters 3, 31, and 95. Unfortunately, there is a dearth of sound scientific information regarding management of poisonings and overdoses in the prehospital setting, and many of the recommendations that follow have been extrapolated from similar situations that arise in the hospital setting.

Personal Danger to EMTs and Paramedics

When hazmat incidents occur, the danger to rescue personnel is often recognized immediately, and the series of protective measures detailed earlier in this chapter will generally protect the

TABLE 93–6. Primary Hazmat Toxidromes or Hazidromes

Hazidrome	Typical Toxicants	Predominant Route of Exposure	Pathophysiology Effects	Site of Toxicity
Irritant gas: High water-solublity	Ammonia, formaldehyde, hydrogen chloride, sulfur dioxide	Inhalation	Irritant and corrosive local effects; readily dissolves in the water of exposed mucous membranes and the upper airway	**A**irway
Irritant gas: Intermediate water-solubility	Chlorine	Inhalation	Irritant and corrosive local effects; dissolves in the water of exposed mucous membranes and the upper and lower airways	**A**irway, **B**reathing
Irritant gas: Poor water-solublity	Phosgene, nitrogen dioxide	Inhalation	Irritant and corrosive local effects by slowly dissolving in the water of the alveolar-capillary membrane of the lung	**B**reathing
Asphyxiant: Simple	Carbon dioxide, methane, propane	Inhalation	Displacement of oxygen from the ambient atmosphere	**C**ardiovascular, **D**isability
Asphyxiant: Systemic (chemical)	Isobutyl nitrite, carbon monoxide, hydrogen cyanide, hydrogen sulfide, hydrogen azide	Inhalation	Interferes with oxygen transportation and/or utilization	**C**ardiovascular, **D**isability
Caustic	Acids (hydrochloric, nitric, sulfuric) Alkalis (ammonium, potassium hydroxide, or sodium)	Skin and mucous membranes	Irritant and corrosive local effects	**A**irway, **C**ardiovascular
Cholinergic	Organic phosphorus pesticides, carbamate insecticides	Skin	Excess acetylcholine accumulation at both muscarinic and nicotinic receptors in the peripheral and central nervous system	**D**isability
Cholinergic	Organic phosphorus nerve agents	Inhalation and/or skin		**D**isability
Hydrocarbon and halogenated hydrocarbons	Chloroform, gasoline, propane, toluene	Inhalation	Inhalation causes lethargy to coma and cardiac irritability	**C**ardiovascular **D**isability

Modified with permission from the Advanced Hazmat Life Support Provider Manual, 2nd ed. Tucson, AZ, Arizona Board of Regents, 2000.

EMT or paramedic from subsequent primary or secondary exposure and illness. Much more problematic, however, is the solitary exposure victim. Victims of deliberate poisonings and patients who have taken drug overdoses with suicidal intent are often unable or unwilling to describe accurately the extent of the ingestion or exposure (Chaps. 3 and 31). Conversely, after a suicide "gesture" the patient may deliberately exaggerate the nature of the overdose or exposure or suggest that there is a widespread danger to others.

When dealing with an actual or possible source of danger, EMTs and paramedics must protect themselves from exposure to poisons or inhalation of toxic chemicals and fumes by using appropriate protective equipment and providing adequate ventilation within enclosed places suspected of containing high concentrations of toxic gases. Many toxic gases are colorless and odorless, and some chemicals (eg, organic phosphorus compounds) can be absorbed through intact skin. Paramedics and EMTs must also be aware of the danger of mouth-to-mouth resuscitation for patients suspected of having cyanide poisoning.[8]

Overdose victims who are conscious or who have an altered level of consciousness other than coma present other difficulties in the prehospital setting. They may be combative, placing themselves and paramedics or EMTs at risk, or they may be unwilling to accept medical care, particularly transport to the hospital. Prehospital care providers must maintain their objectivity and compassion and not allow these factors to alter acceptable standards of care such that the patient is placed at greater risk.

As with all patient interactions, care must be taken to avoid blood and body fluid contamination. Patients using illicit drugs intravenously are especially prone to blood-borne infections (HIV and hepatitis), and great care must be taken to avoid contamination during treatment and handling of drug paraphernalia.

Initial Prehospital Management of a Poisoned or Overdosed Patient. Prehospital personnel should be mindful that the patient's condition may deteriorate rapidly and unpredictably. For an unconscious patient, definitive control of the airway with endotracheal intubation and establishment of an IV line should be considered early in the management. A properly secured airway not only ensures adequate ventilation and oxygenation but may limit further aspiration of gastric contents. Indications for the use of $D_{50}W$, thiamine, naloxone, and oxygen in a patient with an altered level of consciousness are generally consistent with their use in the ED as described in Chapters 3 and 31. However, the value of the empiric use of naloxone and $D_{50}W$ in the prehospital setting has been questioned in two retrospective studies; the findings are summarized in the antidote section below.[35,36]

The Role of the EMT or Paramedic in Establishing a Diagnosis of Poisoning or Overdose

One of the most important functions an EMT or paramedic can perform in managing a patient with a toxicologic emergency is to evaluate the patient's environment to the extent permitted by the

TABLE 93–7. Hazmat Antidotes

Antidote in Depth Citation	Antidote	Poisoning	Common Adult Doses[a]	Common Pediatric Doses
See p 1353	Atropine	Organic phosphorus compounds, carbamates, nerve agents	1–2 mg IV bolus; titrate with repeated doses.	0.02–0.04 mg/kg IV bolus, never less than 0.1 mg, titrate with repeated doses
See p 1341	Calcium gluconate	Systemic hydrofluoric acid or fluoride poisoning	10–20 mL of 10% solution (1–2 amps). IV slowly; repeat doses may be required.	0.2–0.3 mL of 10% solution/kg IV slowly; repeat doses may be required
See p 1341	Calcium gluconate	Hydrofluoric acid skin burns	Topical application of 2.5 to 10% topical gel or solution	Topical application
See p 1341	Calcium chloride	Systemic hydrofluoric acid or fluoride poisoning	5–10 mL of 10% solution (0.5–1 amp) IV slowly; repeat doses may be required	0.1–0.2 mL of 10% solution/kg IV slowly; repeat doses may be required
See p 1511	Cyanide antidote kit: amyl nitrite	Cyanide, nitriles	By inhalation	By inhalation
See p 1511	Cyanide antidote kit: sodium nitrite	Cyanide, nitriles	10 mL of 3% solution (1 amp) slow IV bolus, over 5 minutes	0.12–0.33 mL/kg of 3% solution slow IV bolus over 5 minutes, up to a maximum dose of 15 mg/kg in a nonanemic child
See p 1511	Cyanide antidote kit: sodium thiosulfate	Cyanide, nitriles	50 mL of 25% solution (1 amp) slow IV bolus	1.65 mL/kg slow IV bolus of 25% solution up to a maximum of 50 mL (1 amp)
See p 1450	Methylene blue	Methemoglobin-forming compounds	1–2 mg/kg (0.1–0.2 mL/kg of 1% solution) slow IV bolus over 5 minutes; repeat doses may be required	1–2 mg/kg (0.1–0.2 mL/kg of 1% solution) slow IV bolus over 5 minutes; repeat doses may be required
See p 1492	Oxygen	Simple asphyxiants, systemic asphyxiants, methemoglobin-forming compounds, carbon monoxide, cyanides, azides, hydrozoic acid, hydrogen sulfide	100%, by inhalation	100%, by inhalation
See p 1361	Pralidoxime (2-PAM)	Organic phosphorus nerve agents	1–2 g slow IV infusion, over 10 minutes, then 500 mg/h continuous IV infusion	20–40 mg/kg slow IV infusion over 10 minutes, then 10–20 mg/kg/h continuous IV infusion
See p 667	Pyridoxine	Hydrazines	25 mg/kg IV	25 mg/kg IV

[a]These are commonly used doses for hazmat poisonings. Specific doses for a given patient must always be determined by the treating clinician. See other chapters and specifically the individual Antidotes in Depth for additional information including indications, contraindications, and complications of each agent.
Modified with permission from the Advanced Hazmat Life Support Provider Manual, 2nd ed. Tucson, AZ, Arizona Board of Regents, 2000.

patient's condition. For example, an elderly patient brought in unconscious from home may be suffering from hypoglycemia, hyperosmolar coma, diabetic ketoacidosis, sepsis, poisoning, overdose, intoxication, etc. However, if the EMT notices an unvented space heater in the corner of the room and reports this finding to the emergency physician, the diagnosis of carbon monoxide (CO) poisoning can be pursued expeditiously. This consideration is especially important because oxygen administration en route may begin to treat the signs and symptoms before the patient is examined in the ED, thereby potentially obscuring the etiology of the patient's initial altered consciousness. Reporting the presence of the space heater to the local health department or EPA will allow appropriate personnel to seek out and eliminate the CO source before others die from the exposure.

In addition to noting empty pill bottles, suicide notes, or illicit drug paraphernalia found with a patient, prehospital personnel should be aware of any unusual smells, sources of toxic gases, and evidence of toxic chemicals in the patient's environment. Chemicals in the workplace, for example, may present a difficult diagnostic challenge that is made easier if the EMT notes the few *specific* chemicals that are available.

Prehospital evaluation and care should include transport to the ED of containers (labeled or not), pills and pill bottles, and any possible ingested plant material for definitive identification. Some prehospital personnel carry "patient belongings" bags in the ambulance for this purpose. If possible, an animal at the scene, which may be either a source or a victim of poisoning, should be restrained or contained and transported later by appropriate personnel such as the ASPCA.

Finally, recognition of the possibility of concomitant trauma to the victim is essential for appropriate and timely management. Many overdose patients also become victims of blunt or penetrating trauma. Conversely, many trauma victims are also inebriated or overdosed on medications or drugs.

Gastric Decontamination in the Prehospital Setting

No method of gastric decontamination has been adequately proven to alter morbidity or mortality.[2] Therefore, routine use of gastric decontamination is no longer a standard of care, and its use in selected oral ingestions should be carefully considered and justified.[2]

Administration of syrup of ipecac to alert patients after a recent oral ingestion may be considered. In some types of poisoning, gastric emptying (most typically by emesis) may be possible only early in the clinical course, before the resultant toxicity precludes such intervention, as in colchicine or a heavy metal poisoning. Especially when transport time is long, therefore, syrup of ipecac may have to be administered at home as directed by a regional poison center or by prehospital personnel if it is to be administered at all. Arguments against prehospital administration of syrup of ipecac include (1) that a patient who starts vomiting en route to the hospital may be difficult to position properly, and (2) that controlling the airway in the back of a moving ambulance may be difficult, with the added danger that the patient may lose the gag reflex before vomiting. Orogastric lavage, which may be an appropriate alternative form of gastric emptying, has not gained widespread use in the prehospital setting.

Prehospital administration of activated charcoal (AC) may offer a relatively safe and attractive alternative to both emesis and lavage. In an area where ambulance transport time was relatively short (about 10–12 minutes on average), the authors of one pilot study were able to demonstrate that prehospital, AC could be administered in an average of 5.0 minutes from the first encounter with paramedics versus 51.4 minutes when AC was delayed until arrival in the ED.[23] In another retrospective review of prehospital charts of adults with the diagnosis of "drug overdose," gastrointestinal decontamination was initiated with ipecac in only 6 of 361 (2%) patients. No patient received AC despite a median transport time of 25 minutes. The median time to administration of AC in the ED was 82 minutes.[82] Even when no form of gastric decontamination is offered in the prehospital setting, ambulance transportation to the ED by itself appears to result in decreased time to gastric decontamination. In a retrospective review of 167 overdose patients receiving gastric lavage or activated charcoal, the median interval from presentation to gastric decontamination for the 105 patients who arrived by ambulance was 55 minutes compared to 73 minutes for the nonambulance patients.[83] The authors concluded that although ambulance-transported overdose patients waited a shorter time than nonambulance patients for gastrointestinal decontamination, the delay was unacceptably long in either case. The findings of this study support the argument that some form of gastrointestinal decontamination should be initiated prehospital.

It is virtually impossible to design a protocol that takes into consideration all of the factors relevant to the very large number of substances that may be involved in an overdose or poisoning. In addition, variations in transport time in different regions of the country (eg, urban vs rural settings) may make gastric emptying essential or lifesaving in one case and unnecessary or dangerous in another case involving the same drug or toxin.

For these reasons, EMTs and paramedics must be able to contact a physician located in a hospital ED, regional poison center, or base station telemetry unit to tailor options in gastric decontamina-

tion or gastric emptying to the individual patient. The various methods of gastric emptying and indications and contraindications for their use are described in Chapter 31. Specific issues regarding gastric decontamination are thoroughly discussed in Chapter 5.

The Role of Antidotal Therapy in Prehospital Care: Recommendations for Specific Antidotes that EMTs and Paramedics Should Carry

The list of antidotes available to hospital-based care providers is quite extensive when compared to lists of medications that paramedics typically carry in their drug boxes or vehicles (see Tables 3–1 and 93–8). Several considerations must be addressed before an antidote is made available for use in the prehospital setting: (1) the vast majority of poisonings and overdoses require care directed by clinical presentation as opposed to care for a known or presumed drug or toxin (Chaps. 3 and 31); (2) there are space limitations in the prehospital setting, restricting the total number of medications and the amount of equipment that can be carried; (3) antidotes that are rarely used may have to be restocked, often at considerable cost, to comply with manufacturers' expiration dates, loss of potency, deterioration to harmless or toxic substances (eg, the cyanide antidote kit); (4) medications that must be refrigerated or prepared (mixed) for each shift are impractical; (5) antidotes used inappropriately may be extremely toxic or lethal to a patient (eg, the cyanide antidote kit). Some prehospital care systems address this last issue by providing only nontoxic or relatively nontoxic antidotes, or the nontoxic *component(s)* of

TABLE 93–8. Medications Commonly Carried by Paramedics that Can Also Be Used as Antidotes[a,b]

Medication	Antidotal Use
Atropine	β-Adrenergic antagonist, calcium channel blocker, and cardiac glycoside (digoxin) overdoses; muscarinic mushroom (*Clitocybe, Inocybe*) poisoning; organic phosphorus and carbamate insecticide poisoning
Benzodiazepines[c]	Stimulants
Calcium chloride	Calcium channel blocker overdose (causing hypotension and bradydysrhythmias), hydrofluoric acid
Diphenhydramine	Extrapyramidal reactions from antipsychotics or antiemetics
Glucagon	β-Adrenergic antagonists, calcium channel blocker overdoses
Oxygen	Carbon monoxide, cyanide, hydrogen sulfide poisoning
Sodium bicarbonate	(1) Cyanide, methanol, ethylene glycol (reversal of metabolic acidosis) (2) Salicylates, chlorpropamide, phenobarbital, formic acid, chlorphenoxyherbicides (enhanced elimination) (3) Cyclic antidepressants, quinine, carbamazepine, type IA and IC antidysrhythmics, cocaine, some phenothiazines (reversal of type IA ECG effects)

[a]Use of medications outside of protocols may not be permissible in some areas, even with on-line medical control.
[b]Table does not include medications such as $D_{50}W$, thiamine and naloxone primarily intended to be used as standard component of overdose management antidotes for an altered level of consciousness.
[c]Usually administered with $D_{50}W$ and oxygen to avoid masking hypoglycemia and hypoxia.

multistep antidotes such as only the sodium thiosulfate from the cyanide antidote kit.

Few organized attempts to study the use of antidotes in the prehospital setting have been conducted to date, and virtually all of the studies that have been published are retrospective analyses.[2–4,12,23,25,36,69,84] One such study investigating the safety of the prehospital use of 0.4 to 0.8 mg of naloxone in 813 patients found it to be a safe component of paramedic treatment protocols for patients with an acute loss of consciousness.[84] However, another retrospective study of the empiric use of naloxone by paramedics in 730 patients with acute alterations in mental status found that selective administration based on the presence of pinpoint pupils, bradypnea, or circumstantial evidence of drug use correctly identified "narcotized" patients with a sensitivity of 92% and a specificity of 76%. The authors concluded that implementing a screening strategy for naloxone use based on these historical and physical findings could reduce naloxone administration by 75% while achieving cost savings, faster prehospital care, and fewer iatrogenic effects of naloxone.[35] Interestingly, these same authors reviewed 340 records retrospectively in an attempt to identify a subset of prehospital patients at risk for hypoglycemia by utilizing the clinical findings of tachycardia, diaphoresis, and a history of diabetes. In stark contrast to the results of their naloxone study, they found that only 76% of hypoglycemic patients were identified, and with a specificity of only 54%[36]. Thus, the prehospital use of hypertonic dextrose could be reduced by only 46%, and this would have the effect of withholding it from 25% of hypoglycemic patients. In marked contrast to their conclusions regarding naloxone, the authors concluded here that selective use of $D_{50}W$ for AMS would be feasible only with concomitant field use of a rapid, accurate test of serum glucose.[36]

Uncommon or unusual poisonings present additional problems in the use of antidotes in the prehospital setting. One way of dealing with uncommon poisonings is to have protocols, treatments, and antidotes readily available for use after an identified index case or cases indicate the possibility of a large number of exposures. Examples of such poisonings may be found in the hazmat portion of this chapter and include CO and cyanide exposures as well as lethal drugs or combinations that may affect a particular population, such as sudden widespread availability of fentanyl, unexpectedly potent opioids, or opioid substitutes and combinations.

Finally, EMTs and paramedics should be mindful that almost all prehospital care protocols are sign- or symptom-driven; few, if any, ambulances routinely carry all available specific antidotes to treat all potential poisonings. Moreover, even when an antidote (such as glucagon) is available because the medication is also used in other ALS protocols, its dosage as an antidote may differ (see Table 93–7).[56–58] For these reasons, rather than applying a series of protocols over a prolonged period of time to treat a variety of signs and symptoms, EMTs and paramedics should initiate early telemetry contact with a base station physician, and a rational decision should be made regarding any further treatment or immediate transport of the patient to a facility where a specific antidote is available.

The Optimal Position for Transporting a Poisoned or Overdosed Patient

In one attempt to identify the optimal transport position for a poisoned or overdosed patient, volunteers were given 80 mg/kg of acetaminophen to simulate an overdose, and five different (stationary) body positions commonly used in prehospital and emergency department settings were examined over a 2-hour period.[76] Although the difference did not reach statistical significance, initial drug absorption was lowest in the left lateral decubitus position, a position that also offers advantages in preventing aspiration, enhancing oropharyngeal drainage, and maximizing patient observation in an ambulance.[76]

The Role of the EMT or Paramedic in Transferring a Poisoned or Overdosed Patient for Definitive Care

Certain poisonings and overdoses require specific treatments not available at a community hospital or not available soon enough to help a particular patient (Table 93–9). Emergency physicians must sometimes weigh the benefits and risks of transferring ill, poisoned, or overdosed patients to tertiary care centers. In general, a patient presenting with a toxicologic emergency should be moved to another facility only if the primary hospital does not have the necessary therapy and if there is no acceptable alternative treatment available.

Hyperbaric Oxygen for Carbon Monoxide Poisoning. Criteria for determining which patients may benefit from hyperbaric oxygen treatment (HBO) are discussed in detail in Chapter 97. A CO poisoning victim should be provided with 100% oxygen while being transported to a hyperbaric chamber; assisted ventilation should be provided to any patient who is not breathing spontaneously. A physician or paramedic able to administer advanced cardiac life support should accompany the patient. Attention to the patient's ongoing cardiorespiratory needs is critical.

The safety of transferring CO-poisoned patients for HBO was addressed in a 10-year retrospective study of 297 consecutive CO-poisoned patients requiring HBO.[69] The authors concluded that CO-induced cardiac or respiratory arrests, myocardial infarctions, and worsening mental status are not likely to occur during transport to the hyperbaric chamber if they did not occur before the decision to perform HBO, and, therefore, transfer need not be deferred for fear of these occurrences. However, dysrhythmias, hypotension, seizures, agitation, and emesis as well as repeat cardiac arrests and near arrests can occur; therefore, complete prepared-

TABLE 93–9. **Patients with Poisoning or Overdose Who May Require Transfer to Special Treatment Centers**

Poisoning/Overdose	Type of Care
Carbon monoxide (high levels and/or serious clinical sequelae)	Hyperbaric oxygen
Snake or spider venom	Antivenom treatment
Lithium, salicylates, theophylline, methanol, or ethylene glycol	Hemodialysis and/or hemoperfusion
Acetaminophen (with significant hepatic damage)	Hepatic transplantation
Myocardial depressants (massive amounts that cannot be metabolized or dialyzed or otherwise treated, such as lidocaine, calcium channel blockers)	Cardiopulmonary bypass
Infants with serious poisonings or drug overdoses from a variety of sources	Neonatal and pediatric intensive care unit

ness for cardiac resuscitation, airway control, and volume expansion during transport was recommended.[69]

Transfer principles for referral to a hyperbaric treatment center are outlined in Tables 93–10 and 97–2.

Hemoperfusion and/or Hemodialysis.   Transferring a patient to a facility capable of hemodialysis or hemoperfusion is most commonly required for poisoning with methanol or ethylene glycol and serious overdoses of lithium, salicylates, or theophylline (Chaps. 33, 39, 61, and 66). All initial treatment should be instituted before, and continued during, interhospital transport. Patients sick enough to require hemodialysis or hemoperfusion should ideally be transported in an advanced life-support ambulance and with an accompanying physician.

Antivenom Treatment Centers for Envenomations.   Because envenomations are relatively rare and may be extremely serious or lethal, victims may require transportation to a specialty center for treatment. Table 93–11 outlines the New York City snake bite protocol, which includes a section on patient transport.

Legal Considerations in Transferring Poisoned or Overdosed Patients

Incorrect interpretation of the United States Federal EMTALA and COBRA legislation[72] adopted and implemented to prevent inappropriate transfers of indigent patients (patient dumping) may hinder or prevent transporting a patient who, though medically "unstable," may nevertheless require specialized treatment or facilities. Nothing in the legislation precludes such a transfer provided that: (1) the treatment is considered necessary; that is, the benefits of the transfer outweigh the risks; (2) the sending and receiving institutions are in agreement regarding the necessity of the transfer and the medical care being provided to accomplish it; (3) the transfer is effected in accordance with accepted medical practice; and (4) the transfer is not for economic reasons.

As with any patient transfer between institutions, care must be taken to ensure that before transport the patient has been medically stabilized as much as possible within the time constraints dictated by the nature of the exposure. With respect to the level of care during transport, a physician accompanying a patient would be ideal, but in most situations properly trained and qualified paramedics

TABLE 93–10.   Suggested Protocol for Transferring a Patient to Hyperbaric Treatment

A physician at the sending facility must perform a basic physical examination and laboratory assessment including:

    History (past medical history, medications, complaints)
    COHb (in carbon monoxide cases)
    Chest radiograph
    Electrocardiogram
    Blood tests—chemistry profile, toxicology tests (if applicable)
    Pregnancy test (for women of childbearing age)
    Neurologic examination (including mental status exam)
    Formal ENT examination for smoke inhalation, noting any indicators of respiratory involvement including stridor, hoarseness, carbonaceous sputum, and singed nasal hairs
    Any patient requiring transfer for hyperbaric treatment is best considered unstable; therefore, the sending institution should consider the need for physician accompaniment when indicated.

TABLE 93–11.   Snakebite Protocol for New York City

Identification of snake

    Record verbal description of snake, time of bite, description of wound(s), and signs and symptoms of envenomation.
    If snake is identified as poisonous or symptoms warrant proceed with first-aid measures and transportation.
    If snake is identified as nonpoisonous, treat as any other animal bite

First-aid measures for poisonous snakebite to be instituted by EMS or other trained medical personnel

    DO NOT EMPLOY TOURNIQUET, CUT AND SUCTION, OR CRYOTHERAPY
    If snake has been identified as an elapid (cobra, mamba, coral snake, sea snake, krait, tiger snake, taipan), apply an Ace bandage on the affected extremity, encompassing the wound(s) and extending up the entire extremity.
    Do not apply an Ace bandage if the snake has been identified as a crotaline (rattlesnake, copperhead, cottonmouth, fer-de-lance, puff adder, Gaboon viper).
    Splint the affected extremity to decrease mobility in all bites.
    Begin a large-bore IV in an unaffected extremity and start an infusion of 0.9% sodium chloride or lactated Ringer solution.
    Transport immediately.

EMS or 911

    Ambulance unit should have a trained paramedic, capable of intubation and CPR if necessary, when transferring a patient from another hospital.
    Helicopter transport is available through EMS (or 911) if deemed necessary
    Receiving hospital ED must be informed of estimated time of arrival and method of transportation.

and vehicles equipped to provide advanced life support may be acceptable, especially if the alternative (ie, not transporting the patient) would probably result in morbidity or mortality.

SUMMARY

The use of $D_{50}W$, thiamine, naloxone, oxygen, activated charcoal, possibly syrup of ipecac or orogastric lavage, and benzodiazepines, as well as many other therapeutic modalities discussed elsewhere in this text, are also applicable to prehospital management. There are, however, certain unique and important considerations for the prehospital setting:

- Initial management should incorporate concern for and elimination of any possible risk to rescue personnel at the scene.
- Without compromising patient care, paramedics and EMTs should try to note and collect evidence at the scene that may be essential to establish a definitive diagnosis.
- Specific antidotes must be used appropriately; conversely the lack of availability of other antidotes (antivenom) or treatment (HBO) at particular hospitals must be considered in deciding the best time for subsequent transport or rapid evacuation to a specialized treatment facility.
- Appropriate use of paramedics or EMTs and well-equipped vehicles will facilitate safe transport of poisoned or overdosed patients to specialty or tertiary care centers.

Pitfalls to avoid in providing prehospital care to victims of poisonings or overdoses include these:

■ Not recognizing or acting on index cases to prevent further exposures or deaths: the opportunity to prevent large-scale hazmat incidents.

■ Relying on sign- or symptom-driven standing protocols to treat a patient for a prolonged period of time or using standard advanced-life-support dosages of medications when only a larger dose of medication or a specific antidote, not available at the scene, will save the patient.

ACKNOWLEDGMENTS

Theodore I. Benzer contributed to this chapter in a previous edition.

REFERENCES

1. Agency for Toxic Substances and Disease Registry: Web page: *www.atsdr.cdc.gov*

2. American Academy of Clinical Toxicology (AACT) and the European Association of Poison Centres and Clinical Toxicologists (EAPCCT): AACT-EAPCCT position statement on gastrointestinal decontamination. J Toxicol Clin Toxicol 1997;35:695–762.

3. American College of Emergency Physicians. Clinical policy for the initial approach to patients presenting with acute toxic ingestion or dermal or inhalation exposure. Ann Emerg Med 1999;33:735–761.

4. American Conference of Governmental Industrial Hygienists (ACGIH): 1996 TLVs and BEIs: Threshold Limit Values and Biological Exposure Indices. Cincinnati, OH, ACGIH; 1996.

5. American Conference of Governmental Insustrial Hygienists: Web page: *www.acgih.org.*

6. Bates G, Criss E, Spaite D: Prehospital organization—medical control of hazardous materials incidents. In: Sullivan JB, Kreiger GR, eds: Clinical Environmental Health and Hazardous Materials Toxicology, 2nd ed. Philadelphia, Williams & Williams, 1992: 355–364.

7. Bertazzi PA: Industrial disasters and epidemiology. A review of recent experiences. Scand J Work Environ Health 1989;15:85–100.

8. Berumen U Jr: Dog poisons man. JAMA. 1983;249:353.

9. Binder S. Deaths, injuries, and evacuations from acute hazardous materials releases. Am J Public Health 1989;79:1042–1044.

10. Binder S, Bonzo S: Acute hazardous materials release. Am J Public Health 1989;79:1681.

11. Borak J, Callan M, Abbott W: Hazardous Materials Exposures. Englewood Cliffs, NJ: Brady Publications; 1991.

12. Bronstein AC: Medical management of hazmat victims. In Walter FG, Klein R, Thomas RG, eds: Advanced Hazmat Life Support Provider Manual, 2nd ed. Tucson, AZ, Arizona Board of Regents, 2000:49–65.

13. Bronstein AC, Currance PL: Emergency Care for Hazardous Materials Exposure, 2nd ed. St. Louis: Mosby-Year Book; 1994.

14. Burgess JL, Blackmon GM, Brodkin CA, Robertson WO: Hospital preparedness for hazardous materials incidents and treatment of contaminated patients. West J Med 1997;167:387–391.

15. Burgess JL, Keifer MC, Barnhart S, et al: Hazardous materials exposure information service: development, analysis, and medical implications. Ann Emerg Med. 1997;29:248–254.

16. Burgess JL, Kirk M, Borron SW, Cisek J: Emergency department hazardous materials protocol for contaminated patients. Ann Emerg Med. 1999;34:205–212. Comments in: Ann Emerg Med 1999;34(2): 223–225.

17. Burgess JL, Pappas GP, Robertson WO. Hazardous materials incidents: the Washington Poison Center experience and approach to exposure assessment. J Occup Environ Med. 1997;39:760–766.

18. Cancio LC: Chemical casualty decontamination by medical platoons in the 82d Airborne Division. Mil Med 1993;158:1–5. Comment in: Mil Med 1993;158:A6–A7.

19. CHEMTREC. Web page: *www.cmahq.com.* Available by phone: 1–800–424–9300

20. Christen H, Maniscalco P: The EMS Incident Management System. Upper Saddle River, NJ, Prentice Hall, 1998:1–15.

21. Cone DC, Davidson SJ: Hazardous materials preparedness in the emergency department. Prehosp Emerg Care 1997;1:85–90.

22. Cox RD. Decontamination and management of hazardous materials exposure victims in the emergency department. Ann Emerg Med 1994;23:761–770.

23. Crockett R, Krishel SJ, Manoguerra A, et al. Prehospital use of activated charcoal: a pilot study. J Emerg Med 1996;14:335–338.

24. Domestic Preparedness Program, Defense Against Weapons of Mass Destruction: Technician-Hospital Provider Course Manual. Aberdeen, MD, US Army CBDCOM, Domestic Preparedness Office; 1997.

25. el Sanadi N, Grove C, Takacs M, et al: A hospital-based, hazardous materials decontamination and treatment unit: utilization patterns over a nine-month period. Prehospital Disaster Med 1993;8:337–340.

26. Furtado MC, Walter FG, Klein R: Personal protective equipment and decontamination. In: Walter FG, Klein R, Thomas RG, eds: Advanced Hazmat Life Support Provider Manual, 2nd ed. Tucson, AZ, Arizona Board of Regents, 2000:67–79.

27. Geller RJ, Singleton KL, Tarantino ML, et al: Nosocomial poisoning associated with emergency department treatment of organophosphate toxicity - Georgia, 2000. MMWR 2001;51:1156–1158.

28. Gold MB, Bongiovanni R, Scharf BA, Gresham VC, Woodward CL: Hypochlorite solution as a decontaminant in sulfur mustard contaminated skin defects in the euthymic hairless guinea pig. Drug Chem Toxicol 1994;17:499–527.

29. Gough AR, Markus K: Hazardous materials protections in ED practice: laws and logistics. J Emerg Nurs 1989;15:477–480.

30. Hall HI, Dhara VR, Kaye WE, Price-Green P: Public health consequences of hazardous substance releases. Toxicol Ind Health 1996;12: 289–293.

31. Hall HI, Dhara VR, Kaye WE, Price-Green P: Surveillance of hazardous substance releases and related health effects. Arch Environ Health 1994;49:45–48.

32. Hall HI, Dhara VR, Price-Green PA, Kaye WE: Surveillance for emergency events involving hazardous substances—United States, 1990–1992. MMWR 1994;43:1–6.

33. Hall HI, Haugh GS, Price-Green PA, et al: Risk factors for hazardous substance releases that result in injuries and evacuations: data from 9 states. Am J Public Health 1996;86:855–857.

34. Hall SK: Management of chemical disaster victims. J Toxicol Clin Toxicol 1995;33:609–616.

35. Hoffman JR, Schriger DL, Luo JS: The empiric use of naloxone in patients with altered mental status: a reappraisal. Ann Emerg Med 1991;20:246–252.

36. Hoffman JR, Schriger DL, Votey SR, Luo JS. The empiric use of hypertonic dextrose in patients with altered mental status: A reappraisal. Ann Emerg Med 1992;21:20–24.

37. Huff JS: Lessons learned from hazardous materials incidents. Emerg Care Q 1991;7:17–22.

38. Hurst C: Decontamination. In: Zatchuk R, ed: Textbook of Military Medicine. Washington, DC, Borden Institute, US Dept of Army, Surgeon General, 1997:351–359.

39. Kales SN, Castro MJ, Christiani DC: Epidemiology of hazardous materials responses by Massachusetts district HAZMAT teams. J Occup Environ Med 1996;38:394–400.

40. Kales SN, Polyhronopoulos GN, Castro MJ, et al: Injuries caused by hazardous materials accidents. Ann Emerg Med 1997;30:598–603.

41. Kales SN, Polyhronopoulos GN, Castro MJ, Goldman RH, Christiani DC: Mechanisms of and facility types involved in hazardous materials incidents. Environ Health Perspect 1997;105:998–1001.

42. Kaye W. Hazardous substances emergency events surveillance 1993–1996. Presented at North American Congress of Clinical Toxicology, Orlando, FL, 1998.

43. Kirk MA, Cisek J, Rose SR: Emergency department response to hazardous materials incidents. Emerg Med Clin North Am 1994;12: 461–481.

44. Klein R, Criss EA: Establishing and organizing a hazmat response team. In: Walter FG, Klein R, Thomas RG, eds: Advanced Hazmat Life Support Provider Manual, 2nd ed. Tucson, AZ, Arizona Board of Regents, 2000:125–177.

45. Lavoie FW, Coomes T, Cisek JE, Fulkerson L: Emergency department external decontamination for hazardous chemical exposure. Vet Hum Toxicol 1992;34:61–64.

46. Leonard LG, Scheulen JJ, Munster AM: Chemical burns: effect of prompt first aid. J Trauma 1982;22:420–423.

47. Leonard RB: Hazardous materials accidents: Initial scene assessment and patient care. Aviat Space Environ Med 1993;64:546–551.

48. Levitin HW, Siegelson HJ: Hazardous materials. Disaster medical planning and response. Emerg Med Clin North Am 1996;14:327–348.

49. Londorf D: Hospital application of the incident management system. Prehosp Disaster Med 1995;10:184–188.

50. Ludwig H: NIOSH Pocket Guide to Chemical Hazards. Washington, DC, US Government Printing Office for the US Department of Health and Human Services (DHHS) and the National Institute of Occupational Safety and Health (NIOSH), 1994.

51. MSDS SEARCH. Web page: *www.msdssearch.com/DBlinks.*

52. National Fire Protection Association (NFPA) Technical Committee on Hazardous Materials Response Personnel: NFPA 471, Recommended Practice for Responding to Hazardous Materials Incidents. Quincy, Massuchessetts. NFPA, 1997.

53. National Fire Protection Association (NFPA) Technical Committee on Hazardous Materials Response Personnel: NFPA 472, Standard on Professional Competence of Responders to Hazardous Materials Incidents. Quincy, Massachussetts. NFPA, 1997.

54. National Fire Protection Association (NFPA) Technical Committee on Hazardous Materials Response Personnel: NFPA 473, Standard for Competencies for EMS Personnel Responding to Hazardous Materials Incidents. Quincy, Massachussetts. NFPA, 1997.

55. National Institute of Occupational Safety and Health Web page: *www.cdc.gov/niosh.*

56. Nelson L: What to do when drug poisoning causes hypotension. J Crit Illness 1996;11:88–92.

57. Nelson L, Hoffman RS: Effective strategies for drug induced bradycardia and heart block. J Crit Illness 1994;9:916–930.

58. Nelson L, Hoffman RS: What to do when drug poisoning causes tachycardia. J Crit Illness 1994;9:831–842.

59. NFPA: Web page: *www.nfpa.org.* Notes available by phone: 1–800–344–3555.

60. Noll G, Hildebrand M, Yvorra J: Personal protective clothing and equipment. In: Daly P, ed: Hazardous Materials, Stillwater, Fire Protection Publications, Oklahoma State University, 1995:285–322.

61. Olson KR: Hazmat-o-phobia. Why aren't hospitals ready for chemical accidents? West J Med 1998;168:32–33.

62. OSHA: Web page: *www.osha.gov.* Notes available by phone: 1–202–693–1999.

63. Phelps AM, Morris P, Giguere M: Emergency events involving hazardous substances in North Carolina, 1993–1994. NC Med J 1998;59:120–122.

64. Pons P, Dart RC: Chemical incidents in the emergency department: If and when. Ann Emerg Med 1999;34:223–225. Comment in: Ann Emerg Med 1999;34:205–209.

65. PPE specifically for biologic agents: Chemical and Biological Terrorism; Research and Development to Improve Civilian Medical Response. Washington, DC, National Academy Press, 1999:41–42.

66. Rubin JN: Roles and responsibilities of medical personnel at hazardous materials incidents. Semicond Saf Assoc J 1998;12:25–30.

67. Shapira Y, Bar Y, Berkenstadt H, et al: Outline of hospital organization for a chemical warfare attack. Isr J Med Sci 1991;27:616–622.

68. Shaw GM, Windham GC, Leonard A, Neutra RR: Characteristics of hazardous material spills from reporting systems in California. Am J Public Health 1986;76:540–543.

69. Sloan EP, Murphy DG, Hart R, et al: Complications and protocol considerations in carbon monoxide-poisoned patients who require hyperbaric oxygen therapy: Report from a ten-year experience. Ann Emerg Med 1989;18:629–634. Comments in: Ann Emerg Med 1990;19:1356–1357.

70. Sullivan F, Wang R, Jenouri I: Principles and protocols for prevention, evaluation, and management of exposure to hazardous materials. Emerg Med Rep 1998;19:21–32.

71. Tur-Kaspa I, Lev EI, Hendler I, Siebner R, Shapira Y, Shemer J: Preparing hospitals for toxicological mass casualties events. Crit Care Med 1999;27:1004–1008. Comments in: Crit Care Med 1999;27:873–874.

72. United States Public Law 99–272. 9121 and 42 USC 1395 DD: cc (a) 1 (1).

73. US Department of Trasportation: Web page: *www.dot.gov.*

74. US Department of Transportation (DOT), Transport Canada (TC), Secretariat of Communications and Transportation of Mexico (SCT): 2000 North American Emergency Response Guidebook, 2nd ed. Washington, DC, DOT, TC, SCT, 2000.

75. US Government: Title 29, Code of Federal Regulations. 1986:Parts 1910.120.

76. Vance MV, Selden BS, Clark RF: Optimal patient position for transport and initial management of toxic ingestions. Ann Emerg Med. 1992;21:243–246.

77. Waldron RL 2d, Danielson RA, Shultz HE, Eckert DE, Hendricks KO: Radiation decontamination unit for the community hospital. Am J Roentgenol 1981;136:977–981.

78. Walter FG: Envenomations. American College of Emergency Physicians, Dallas, 1995.

79. Walter FG, Bronstein AC: Hazardous materials epidemiology: Hazmat happens. In: Walter FG, Klein R, Thomas RG, ed. Advanced Hazmat Life Support Provider Manual. 2nd ed. Tucson, AZ. Arizona Board of Regents, 2000:3–20. 16:114–116.

80. Walter FG, Dedolph R, Kallsen G, et al. Hazardous materials incidents: A one-year retrospective review in central California. Prehospital and Disaster Medicine 1992;7:151–156.

81. Walter FG, Fernandez MC, Haddad LM. North American venomous snakebite. In Haddad LM, Shannon MW, Winchester JF, ed. Clinical Management of Poisoning and Drug Overdose. 3rd ed. Philadelphia WB Saunders, 1998:333–352.

82. Wax PM, Cobaugh DJ. Prehospital gastrointestinal decontamination of toxic ingestions: A missed opportunity. Am J Emerg Med 1998;16:114–116.

83. Wolsey BA, McKinney PE: Does transportation by ambulance decrease time to gastrointestinal decontamination after overdose? Ann Emerg Med. 2000;35:579–584.

84. Yealy DM, Paris PM, Kaplan RM, et al: The safety of prehospital naloxone administration by paramedics. Ann Emerg Med 1990;19:902–905.

Dennis Price

Methemoglobin (Met Hb)
Normal level: 1%, slightly higher in infants
Action level: 20%: Asymptomatic patient
                  10–20%: Symptomatic patient
Values greater than or equal to the action level usually necessitate clinical intervention. Values less than this level may necessitate intervention based on the clinical condition of the patient.

A 27-year-old man was brought to the Emergency Department (ED) by ambulance with a complaint of shortness of breath. The patient had a history of acquired immunodeficiency syndrome (AIDS), complicated by *Candida* esophagitis and two episodes of *Pneumocystis carinii* pneumonia. His medical regimen included zidovudine and dapsone. The patient said that he had recently become depressed over the death of a close friend and took "all of his medications" in a suicide attempt 3 hours before arrival. He vomited once at home and began getting short of breath about 2 to 3 hours later.

On physical examination, the patient appeared cachectic and acutely short of breath. His vital signs were: blood pressure 90/40 mm Hg, pulse 140 beats/min, respiratory rate 40 breaths/min, rectal temperature 100.2°F (37.9°C). A pulse oximeter indicated 88% saturation on room air. The skin was diaphoretic with old track marks. Examination was remarkable for perioral cyanosis. His neck was supple and without jugular venous distention. The chest was clear to auscultation with good airflow. Cardiac examination revealed a tachycardia with normal S_1 and S_2 heart sounds and a grade 1/6 systolic ejection murmur heard best at the left lower sternal border. The abdomen was nontender with good bowel sounds and no hepatomegaly. Examination of extremities revealed no clubbing or edema, but the nail beds were markedly cyanotic. His neurologic examination was normal. A 100% nonrebreathing oxygen mask was applied, and the patient was attached to a cardiac monitor. An intravenous (IV) line was inserted, and blood samples were obtained for a complete blood count, electrolytes, BUN, glucose, and acetaminophen level. After a few minutes of oxygen therapy, the patient's heart rate decreased to 128 beats/min, but he was still cyanotic and tachypneic, and the pulse oximeter continued to indicate 86 to 88% oxygen saturation. Arterial blood gas analysis was obtained while the patient was receiving supplemental oxygen, but the house officer thought that it might be a venous specimen because it was so darkly colored. The results were: pH 7.34, P_{CO_2} 30 mm Hg, P_{O_2} 400 mm Hg calculated oxygen saturation 99%. The patient was given 60 g of activated charcoal in a slurry of water and 50 mL of 70% sorbitol orally.

The electrocardiogram (ECG) showed a sinus tachycardia with normal axis, intervals, ST segments, and T waves. The chest radiograph was normal. A serum acetaminophen level was zero. All other laboratory test results were unremarkable. Cooximetry of an arterial specimen revealed: total hemoglobin 8.4 g/dL, oxyhemoglobin 64%, methemoglobin 33%, deoxyhemoglobin 1%, carboxyhemoglobin 2%.

The patient received 60 mg of methylene blue (0.1 mL/kg of 1% solution) IV over 20 minutes. Pulse oximetry indicated a drop to 73 to 75% for several minutes with no change in his clinical symptoms. About 40 minutes after the methylene blue infusion, the patient was less cyanotic, and a repeat methemoglobin level was 6%. Three hours later he was again short of breath and cyanotic, and his methemoglobin had risen to 24%. Another 60 mg of methylene blue was infused and led to an improvement in his color and tachypnea within 20 minutes. His repeat methemoglobin level was 4%.

Over the first 24 hours, the patient required a total of three doses of methylene blue therapy. His hemoglobin subsequently fell to 6.2 g/dL, and he was transfused with 2 units of packed red blood cells. While in the hospital, the patient was evaluated by a psychiatrist and enrolled in an AIDS support group. The patient was discharged 6 days after admission with a hemoglobin of 9.7 g/dL and normal cooximetry values.

INTRODUCTION

Biologic systems constantly need to protect themselves from oxidants in order to survive. Cellular components such as enzyme systems and structural elements become oxidized spontaneously and have increased rates of oxidation when exposed to exogenous oxidants. When hemoglobin becomes oxidized, it forms methemoglobin. This occurs when the iron atom in hemoglobin loses one electron to an oxidant, and the ferrous (Fe^{2+}) state of iron is transformed into the ferric (Fe^{3+}) state.

Some oxidation of hemoglobin occurs normally during oxygen transport, and this oxidation is increased in the presence of some hereditary conditions; however, oxidizing compounds from the environment and drugs are the major source of oxidant stress to the individual. Although it is typically not life threatening, methemoglobinemia may produce symptoms because of cellular hypoxia and should be considered in a complete differential diagnosis of the cyanotic patient with no apparent cardiovascular cause. Methylene blue, an exogenous electron carrier, will reduce oxidized hemoglobin.

HISTORY AND EPIDEMIOLOGY

Physicians became aware of methemoglobin in the latter half of the 19th century. Methemoglobin was first described by Felix Hoppe-Seyler in 1864.[25] He was a physiologic chemist who studied blood in the laboratory. Subsequently, in 1891, a case of drug-induced methemoglobinemia that resolved on its own was described.[53] In the late 1930s methemoglobinemia was recognized as a predictable adverse effect of the use of sulfanilamide, and the use of methylene blue was recommended to treat the ensuing cyanosis.[34] Concurrent use of methylene blue was also recommended by some authors when these drugs were utilized.[82] In 1948 an enzyme defect was reported in twin brothers that caused cyanosis in the absence of cardiopulmonary disease; the cyanosis responded to ascorbic acid therapy.[27] In the past half-century, the biochemistry, genetic predisposition, and treatment modalities for methemoglobinemia were greatly elucidated. Computerized searches today produce thousands of articles dealing with methemoglobin.

Methemoglobinemia can be hereditary or acquired. The hereditary types are exceedingly rare, with only several hundred cases reported to date in the literature.[5,36,48,49,67] Even acquired methemoglobinemia, although more common than hereditary methemoglobinemia, occurs only infrequently. This is in part because of increased federal regulation of industrial manufacturing methods and food processing,[62] major historic causes of acquired methemoglobinemia, and in part because of the limited clinical manifestations at the lower methemoglobin concentrations. The AAPCC data annually show fewer than 100 uses of methylene blue as an antidote (Chap. 116 and page 1752).

ETIOLOGIES

Nitrates and nitrites are powerful oxidizing agents that represent two of the most common methemoglobin-forming compounds. Sources of nitrates and nitrites include drinking well water, food, industrial compounds, and pharmaceuticals. The contamination of drinking water occurs mainly with nitrates because nitrite is easily oxidized to nitrate in the environment. Nitrates are very soluble and easily contaminate shallow rural wells by way of the runoff of water containing nitrogen-based fertilizers and nitrogenous waste from animal and human sources. Foods such as cauliflower, carrots, spinach, and broccoli have high nitrate content, and nitrates enter the food chain as preservatives in meat products such as hot dogs and sausage.[1,2,13]

The oxidation reaction of nitrates that occurs in vivo and in vitro is complex and poorly understood. Ingested nitrates are reduced to nitrites by bacteria in the intestinal tract (especially in infants) and can then be absorbed, ultimately leading to methemoglobin production. This conversion is not essential, however, because nitrates themselves can oxidize hemoglobin.[23,32,76]

In the past, nitrates were a too common cause for well water contamination, and infant fatalities were associated with methemoglobinemia.[15,51] A number of reports from the Midwest United States demonstrated the problems of poorly constructed shallow wells that permit contamination by surface waters containing chemicals, pesticides, fertilizers, and microorganisms.[54] In several South Dakota studies, 20 to 50% of wells contained both coliform bacteria and water that exceeded the Environmental Protection Agency (EPA) standards for permissible quantities of nitrogen as nitrates (10 ppm or 10 mg/L).[40] In New York State, 419 wells from rural farms demonstrated elevated levels of nitrogen compounds, and 15.7% were found to have nitrate levels greater than 10 mg/L.[26]

Nitroglycerin (glyceryl trinitrate) and organic nitrates are more effectively absorbed through mucous membranes and intact skin than from the gastrointestinal (GI) tract. The onset of action is also more rapid, and the total effect is much greater, through the former.[16,20,64] Aromatic amino and nitro compounds may indirectly produce methemoglobin. These agents do not form methemoglobin in vitro and are therefore assumed to do so by chemical conversion to some extremely active in vivo intermediate compounds.[10,77]

Methemoglobin and carboxyhemoglobin levels are found in victims of fires and automobile exhaust fume poisoning.[7,38,41,46,73] Heat-induced hemoglobin denaturation in burn patients and the inhalation of nitrogen oxides from smoke inhalation are suggested to be causative factors for methemoglobin formation.

Topical anesthetics such a prilocaine and benzocaine regularly produce methemoglobinemia.[30,44,59] These agents are ubiquitous and are found in the various topical and local anesthetics used for medical procedures.

Because of its use by AIDS patients, dapsone is increasingly implicated as a cause of methemoglobinemia. Cases of prolonged methemoglobinemia from dapsone ingestion have been reported and are related to its long half-life and the methemoglobin-forming potential of its metabolites.[19]

The bladder anesthetic pyridium (phenazopyridine) is another commonly reported oxidizing agent.[14,21,29,56,74] Other causes of methemoglobinemia are listed in Table 94–1.

HEMOGLOBIN PHYSIOLOGY AND METHEMOGLOBIN

Hemoglobin consists of four polypeptide chains noncovalently attracted to one another. Each of these subunits carries one heme molecule deep within the structure. The polypeptide chain protects the iron moiety of the heme molecule from inappropriate oxidation (Fig. 94–1).

The iron is held in position by six coordination bonds. Four of these bonds are between iron and the nitrogen atoms of the protoporphyrin ring, with the fifth and sixth bond sites lying above and below the protoporphyrin plane. The fifth site is occupied by histidine of the polypeptide chain. Changes in the amino acid sequence of the polypeptide chain, as occur in hemoglobin M, influence this protective "pocket," allowing easier iron oxidation (Fig. 94–2). This process is referred to as hemoglobin autooxidation. The sixth coordination site is where most of the activity within hemoglobin occurs. Oxygen transport occurs here, and this site is altered with formation of methemoglobin or carbon monoxide poisoning (Fig. 94–3). It is at this site that an electron is lost to toxic oxidants transforming iron from its ferrous to its ferric form, producing oxidized hemoglobin: methemoglobin.

Hemoglobin will transport an oxygen molecule only when its iron atom is in the reduced ferrous state (Fe^{2+}). During oxygen transport the iron atom actually transfers an electron to oxygen, thus transporting oxygen as a superoxide charged particle $Fe^{3+}O_2$. When oxygen is released, the ferrous state is restored, and hemoglobin is ready to accept another oxygen molecule. Interestingly, a

TABLE 94–1. Common Etiologies of Methemoglobinemia

Hereditary
Hemoglobin M
NADH methemoglobin reductase deficiency
  (homozygote and heterozygote)

Acquired
A. Medications
    Amyl nitrite
    Benzocaine
    Dapsone
    Lidocaine
    Nitroglycerin
    Nitroprusside
    Phenacetin
    Phenazopyridine
    Prilocaine (local anesthetic)
    Quinones (chloroquine, primaquine)
    Sulfonamides (sulfanilamide, sulfathiazide, sulfapyridine,
      sulfamethoxazole)

B. Chemical agents
    Aniline dye derivatives (shoe dyes, marking inks)
    Butyl nitrite
    Chlorobenzene
    Fires (heat-induced denaturation)
    Food adulterated with nitrites
    Food high in nitrates
    Isobutyl nitrite
    Naphthalene
    Nitrophenol
    Nitrous gases (seen in arc welders)
    Silver nitrate
    Trinitrotoluene
    Well water (nitrates)

Pediatric
  Reduced NADH methemoglobin reductase activity in infants (< 4 months)
  Associated with low birth weight, prematurity, dehydration, acidosis,
    diarrhea, and hyperchloremia

small percentage of oxygen is released from hemoglobin with its shared electron (forming superoxide O_2^-) and leaving iron oxidized. This sixth coordination site becomes occupied by a water molecule. This abnormal unloading of oxygen contributes to the steady-state level of methemoglobin of approximately 1% found in normal individuals. In summary, the differences between hemoglobin and methemoglobin are subtle and involve only a small part of the hemoglobin molecule but make methemoglobin incapable of oxygen transport.

METHEMOGLOBIN PHYSIOLOGY AND KINETICS

Because of the spontaneous and environmentally induced oxidation of hemoglobin, the erythrocyte has developed multiple mechanisms to maintain the normal level of methemoglobin at less than 1%.[8] All of these systems donate an electron to the oxidized iron atom. The half-life of methemoglobin acutely formed as a result of exposure to oxidants is between 1 and 3 hours.[39,52] If there is continuous adsorption of the oxidant, or if the metabolites of the oxi-

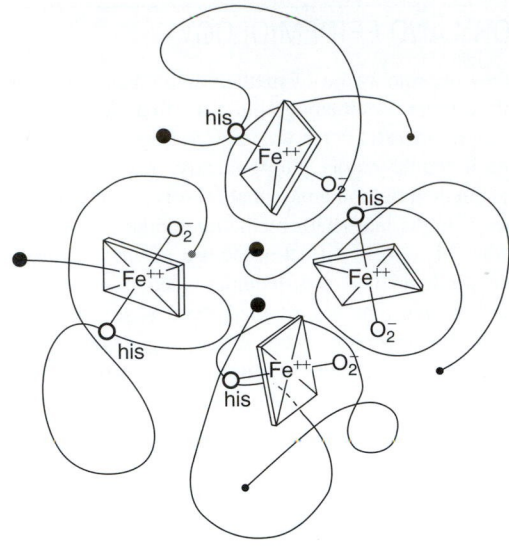

Figure 94–1. The hemoglobin molecule is symbolically represented with its heme center being surrounded by the globin portion of the molecule.

dant are themselves oxidants, then the half-life of methemoglobin will be prolonged.

Quantitatively the most important reductive system requires nicotinamide adenine dinucleotide (NADH), which is generated in the Embden Meyerhof glycolytic pathway (Fig. 94–4). This electron donor, along with the enzyme NADH methemoglobin reductase, reduces the oxidized ferric (Fe^{3+}) iron or heme to the more functionally favorable ferrous (Fe^{2+}) iron state. There are numerous cases of hereditary deficiencies of the enzyme NADH methemoglobin reductase.[36,49,67] Homozygotes for this enzyme deficiency usually have methemoglobin levels of 10 to 50% under normal conditions without any clinical provocations, whereas heterozygotes do not ordinarily demonstrate methemoglobinemia except when subject to oxidant stresses. Additionally, because this enzyme system lacks full activity until about 4 months of age, infants are more susceptible than adults to oxidizing stresses.[57,84]

Oxidized iron can be reduced nonenzymatically using ascorbic acid and reduced glutathione as electron donors, but this method is much slower and quantitatively less important under normal circumstances.

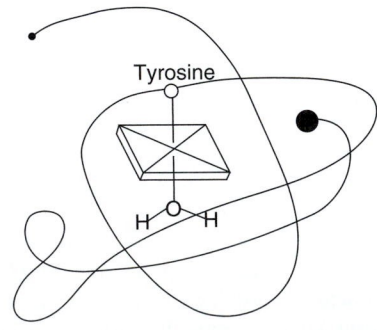

Figure 94–2. Hemoglobin M occurs when histidine is replaced by tyrosine in the amino acid sequence of the polypeptide chain. Hemoglobin M is more easily autooxidized (as shown) to methemoglobin.

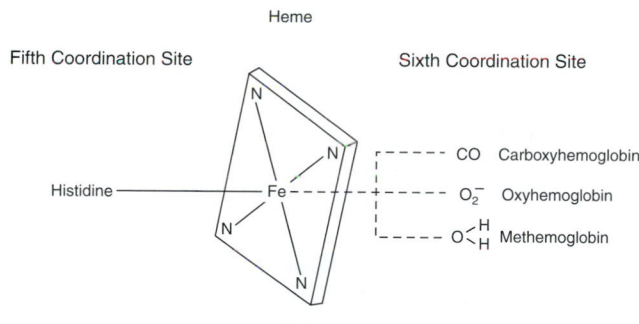

Heme

Fifth Coordination Site

Sixth Coordination Site

Histidine

CO Carboxyhemoglobin

O_2^- Oxyhemoglobin

$O\!\!<^H_H$ Methemoglobin

Figure 94–3. The heme molecule is depicted with its bonding sites. Oxyhemoglobin, carboxyhemoglobin, and methemoglobin all involve the sixth coordination bonding site of iron.

Within the red cell there is another enzyme system for reducing oxidized iron that is dependent on the nicotinamide-adenine dinucleotide phosphate (NADPH) generated in the hexose monophosphate shunt pathway (Fig. 94–5). This NADPH reduces only a small percentage of methemoglobin under normal circumstances, whereas the NADH-dependent methemoglobin reductase system plays the major role. Because of its relatively minor role in methemoglobin reduction, patients with a deficiency of NADPH methemoglobin reductase do not exhibit methemoglobinemia under normal circumstances.[72]

When the NADPH methemoglobin reductase system is provided with an exogenous electron carrier such as methylene blue, this system is accelerated to reduce oxidized hemoglobin.[23] Methylene blue is reduced to leukomethylene blue by NADPH-dependent methemoglobin reductase, using NADPH as the electron donor; leukomethylene blue directly reduces the heme iron (see Antidotes in Depth: Methylene Blue).

CLINICAL MANIFESTATIONS

The clinical manifestations of methemoglobinemia are related to impaired oxygen delivery to the tissue. The manifestations of toxicity of acquired methemoglobinemia are usually more severe than those produced by a corresponding degree of anemia. This discordance occurs because methemoglobin not only decreases the available oxygen carrying capacity but also increases the affinity of the

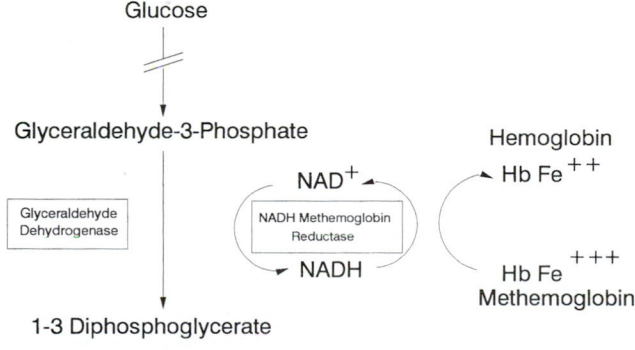

Glucose

Glyceraldehyde-3-Phosphate

Hemoglobin

Hb Fe^{++}

Glyceraldehyde Dehydrogenase

NAD^+

NADH Methemoglobin Reductase

NADH

Hb Fe^{+++} Methemoglobin

1-3 Diphosphoglycerate

Figure 94–4. The role of glycolysis in the Embden-Meyerhof pathway in the reduction of methemoglobin.

unaltered hemoglobin for oxygen. This shifts the oxygen hemoglobin dissociation curve to the left, which further impairs oxygen delivery.[16] This effect is attributed to the formation of heme compounds intermediate between normal reduced hemoglobin (all four iron atoms are ferrous) and methemoglobin, in which one or more of the iron moieties are in the ferric state.[5,17] The degree to which this high-oxygen-affinity hemoglobin reduces oxygen delivery to the tissue from arterial blood is unclear because the work was done at partial pressures of oxygen found in venous blood.[17]

Because the symptomatology associated with methemoglobinemia is related to impaired oxygen delivery to the tissue, concurrent diseases such as congestive heart failure, chronic obstructive pulmonary disease, or pneumonia may greatly increase the clinical effects of methemoglobinemia. Anemia has profound effects as well (see Fig. 94–6). Predictions of symptoms and recommendations for therapy are based on methemoglobin concentrations in previously healthy individuals with normal hemoglobin levels.

Cyanosis is a consistent physical finding in methemoglobinemia. Cyanosis occurs when just 1.5 g/dL of methemoglobin is present. This represents only a 10% conversion of hemoglobin to methemoglobin if the baseline hemoglobin is 15 g/dL. In contrast, it takes 5 g/dL of deoxyhemoglobin (which represents 33% of hemoglobin) in the deoxygenated form to produce the same degree of cyanosis. Sulfhemoglobin, another darkly pigmented hemoglobin, also produces a detectable bluish color when its level is only 0.5 g/dL (this represents only 3% of hemoglobin converted to sulfhemoglobin). In summary, a wide range of levels of pigment produce the same degree of cyanosis.

In previously healthy individuals, methemoglobin concentrations of 10 to 20% usually result in cyanosis without apparent adverse clinical manifestations. At 20 to 50% methemoglobin concentration, dizziness, fatigue, headache, and exertional dyspnea may develop. At about 50% methemoglobin, lethargy and stupor usually appear; and the lethal concentration is probably greater than 70% (Table 94–2).

The cyanosis associated with methemoglobinemia is generalized, being both peripheral and central. Patients often appear in less distress or less ill than patients with cyanosis secondary to cardiopulmonary causes.

Some patients may have a mixed etiology for their cyanosis, such as cardiopulmonary-induced hypoxia together with methemoglobinemia. The blood oxygen-carrying capacity in such situations may be drastically reduced (Fig. 94–6; see Chap. 20 for a discussion of O_2 content of blood).

Symptomatology of methemoglobinemia is determined not only by the absolute concentration of methemoglobin but also by its rates of formation and elimination. Levels of methemoglobin that may be clinically benign when caused by hereditary defects or maintained chronically are likely to produce more severe signs when acutely acquired. Healthy subjects lack the compensatory mechanisms that develop over a lifetime in individuals with hereditary compromise, such as erythrocytosis and increased 2,3-diphosphoglyceric acid.

Certain compounds characteristically produce prolonged methemoglobinemia. For instance, dapsone has a very long half-life in overdose situations.[18,19] Aniline and numerous toxic metabolites of aniline are capable of oxidizing hemoglobin. In the presence of renal failure, drugs such as phenazopyridine (Pyridium) are slowly eliminated and cause prolonged methemoglobinemia.

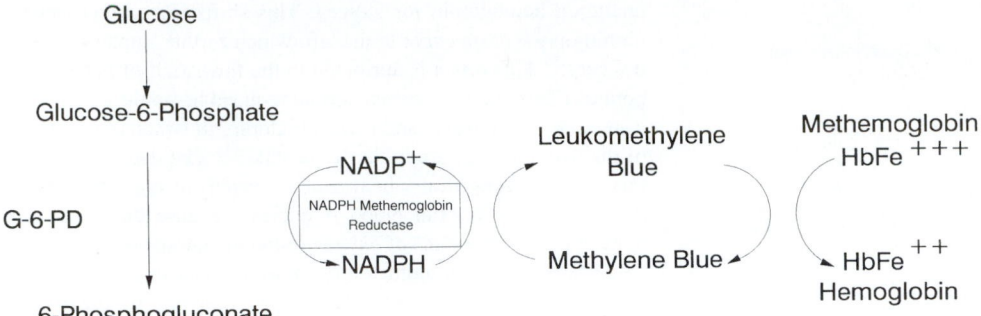

Figure 94–5. The role of hexose monophosphate shunt in the reduction of methemoglobin by methylene blue.

Some compounds producing oxidant stress may have associated toxicities unrelated to the development of methemoglobinemia, such as seizures caused by benzocaine and lidocaine or hypotension caused by nitrates.[61]

DIAGNOSTIC TESTING

For those individuals in whom methemoglobinemia is suspected, a source for the oxidant stress should be sought. Arterial blood gas sampling may reveal blood with a characteristic chocolate brown color. The arterial P_{O_2} should be normal reflecting the adequacy of pulmonary function to deliver dissolved oxygen to the blood. However, the arterial P_{O_2} does not measure the more important physiologic parameter, the hemoglobin oxygen saturation (Sa_{O_2}) or content of the blood. When the partial pressure of oxygen is known, and oxyhemoglobin and deoxyhemoglobin are the only species of hemoglobin, oxygen saturation can be calculated accurately from the arterial blood gas. If, however, other hemoglobins are present, such as methemoglobin, sulfhemoglobin, or carboxyhemoglobin, then the fractional saturation of the hemoglobin must be determined by the cooximeter.

The cooximeter is a spectrophotometer that identifies the absorptive characteristics of several hemoglobin species at different wavelengths. Because oxyhemoglobin, deoxyhemoglobin, methemoglobin, and carboxyhemoglobin all have different absorptions at the different measuring points of the cooximeter, their proportions and concentrations can be determined. Some newer instru-

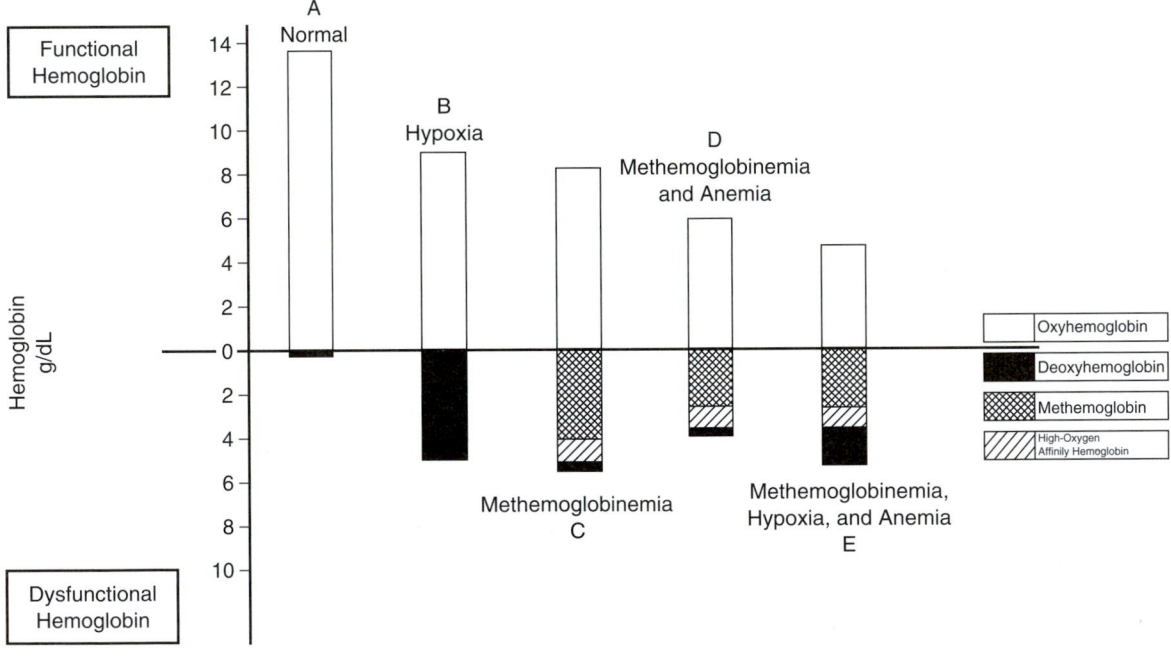

Figure 94–6. Clinical manifestations of methemoglobinemia depend on the level of methemoglobin as well as host factors such as preexisting disease, anemia, and hypoxemia. Five examples of arterial blood gas analyses are presented. **A.** Blood gas from a normal individual with 14 g/dL of hemoglobin. Almost all hemoglobin is saturated with oxygen. **B.** Blood gas from a patient with cardiopulmonary disease producing cyanosis in which only 9 g/dL of hemoglobin is capable of oxygen transport. **C.** Methemoglobin concentration of 28% in an otherwise normal individual will reduce hemoglobin available for oxygen transport to less than 9 g/dL (approximately 4 g/dL of methemoglobin and 1.3 g/dL of high-oxygen-affinity hemoglobin because of the left shift of the oxyhemoglobin dissociation curve). **D.** The same degree of methemoglobin as in **C** but in a patient with a hemoglobin of 10 g/dL. Only 6 g/dL of hemoglobin would be capable of oxygen transport. **E.** Methemoglobinemia and anemia to the same degree as **D** but in a hypoxic patient.

TABLE 94–2. Signs and Symptoms Typically Associated with Methemoglobin Concentrations in Healthy Patients with Normal Hemoglobin Concentrations

Methemoglobin Concentration (%)	Signs and Symptoms
1–<3 (Normal)	None
3–15	Possibly none
	Slate gray cutaneous coloration
	Pulse oximeter will read low SaO_2
15–20	Cyanosis
	Chocolate brown blood
20–50	Dyspnea
	Exercise intolerance
	Headache
	Fatigue
	Dizziness, syncope
	Weakness
50–70	Tachypnea
	Metabolic acidosis
	Dysrhythmias
	Seizures
	CNS depression
	Coma
>70	Grave hypoxic symptoms
	Death

ments have expanded the spectrum at which they read and are also able to read fetal hemoglobin and sulfhemoglobin.[22,86]

The pulse oximeter applied to a patient's finger at the bedside was developed to estimate oxygen saturation trends in critically ill patients. The device takes advantage of the unique absorptive characteristics of oxyhemoglobin and deoxyhemoglobin and the different concentrations of these two hemoglobin species during different phases of the pulse. Each manufacturer has calibrated its oximeter using volunteers breathing progressively hypoxic gas mixtures.[68,75,81] In other words, the oxygen saturation values displayed by the pulse oximeter are derived from comparison with these experimentally derived tables.

Methemoglobin interferes with pulse oximetry in a complicated fashion. Like the cooximeter, the pulse oximeter reads absorbance of light at wavelengths of 660 nm and 940 nm, which are chosen to efficiently separate oxyhemoglobin and deoxyhemoglobin. However, methemoglobin absorption at these wavelengths is greater than that of either oxyhemoglobin or deoxyhemoglobin.[3,60] Therefore, when methemoglobin is present, tables that do not take into account the presence of methemoglobin are inaccurate. The degree of inaccuracy is unique for each brand of instrument.

In the dog model, the pulse oximeter oxygen saturation (SaO_2) values drop with increasing methemoglobin levels. This fall in (SaO_2) is not exactly proportional to the fraction of methemoglobin, however, as the pulse oximeter overestimates the level of real oxygen saturation. For example, in the case when the methemoglobin level measured in the blood using a cooximeter was 20%, the pulse oximeter indicated an SaO_2 of 90%. However, as the methemoglobin concentration approached 30%, the pulse oximeter saturation values approached 85% and then leveled off regardless of how high the methemoglobin level increased.[3,80]

From our experience and that of others,[30,79] much lower levels of oxygen saturation (SaO_2) than 85% can occur by pulse oximetry when methemoglobin levels rise above 30%. These differences result from variations in the way different model pulse oximeters deal with methemoglobin interference. The clinician, therefore, needs to understand both how the particular pulse oximeter in use handles methemoglobin and that cooximetry determination is needed when methemoglobinemia is suspected.

The pulse oximeter reading in patients with methemoglobinemia may not be accurate, but it may be helpful when it is compared with that of the arterial blood gas: if there is a difference between the *measured* oxyhemoglobin of the pulse oximeter (SaO_2) and the *calculated* oxyhemoglobin of the arterial blood gas (PO_2), then a "saturation gap" exists. The calculated PO_2 will be greater than the measured SaO_2 if methemoglobin is present (Table 94–3).

Hyperlipidemia also interferes with accurate cooximetry determination. Triglyceride levels above 500 mg/dL cause the instrument to indicate falsely elevated methemoglobin levels. When triglycerides are present, lipemic serum should be washed free of this interfering substance in order to evaluate for methemoglobinemia.[55,78]

Methylene blue causes a transient decrease in the pulse oximetry reading because of its blue color and excellent absorption at 660 mm.[45,47,83]

ACQUIRED METHEMOGLOBINEMIA AND INFANCY

Infants are more susceptible to methemoglobinemia than adults. An infant's NADH methemoglobin reductase is not fully active until 4 to 6 months of age.[61] Infants who are bottle-fed may be exposed to nitrates and nitrites in well water, and additionally, infants have a relatively large body surface area, making adsorption of oxidants more of a threat to them than adults.

Methemoglobinemia of unknown origin is often reported in infants.[66,71,85] The patients are usually ill for other reasons such as dehydration, acidosis, diarrhea, and hyperchloremia with an associated methemoglobinemia.[31] These infants can have methemoglobin levels in the 20 to 67% range with severe consequences. Most of these patients are very young (under 6 months), and many are small for their age.[37]

METHEMOGLOBINEMIA AND HEMOLYSIS

The enzyme defect responsible for oxidant-induced hemolysis is glucose-6-phosphate dehydrogenase deficiency. A review of hemolysis shortly after the discovery of this enzyme defect addressed the confusion regarding the relationship of hemolysis and methemoglobinemia.[6] The review, which stressed the distinctness of these disease entities, was reaffirmed in 1991 (E. Beutler, personal communication).

Confusion persists today for a number of reasons. Both hemolysis and methemoglobinemia are caused by oxidant stress, and hemolysis can occur following episodes of methemoglobinemia. Additionally, certain erythrocyte protective mechanisms against oxidants (NADPH production) are the same in two disorders. Furthermore, methylene blue treatment of methemoglobin is reported to produce hemolysis,[28,35] although it is not clear if the methylene blue or the oxidant ingested contributes to the methemoglobinemia.

TABLE 94–3.   Hemoglobin Oxygenation Analysis

Measuring Device	Source	What is Measured	How Are Data Expressed?	Benefits	Pitfalls	Insight
Blood gas analyzer	Blood	Partial pressure of dissolved oxygen in whole blood	Po_2	Also gives information about pH and Pco_2	Calculates Sao_2 from the partial pressure of oxygen in serum; inaccurate if forms of Hb other than OxyHb and DeoxyHb are present	If gap exists between ABG and pulse oximeter, an abnormal Hb form may exist
Cooximeter	Blood	Directly measures absorptive charateristics of oxyhemoglobin, deoxyhemoglobin, methemoglobin, carboxyhemoglobin at different wavelength bands in whole blood	Sao_2 % MethHb, %CoHb, %OxyHb, %DeoxyHb	Measures hemoglobin species directly	Provides data on hemoglobin only; most instruments will not measure sulfhemoglobin, HbM, and some other forms of Hb	Most accurate method to determine oxygen content of blood
Pulse oximeter	Monitor	Absorptive characteristics of oxyhemoglobin in pulsatile blood assuming the presence of only Oxy- and Deoxyhemoglobin in vivo	% Oxy Hb	Moment-to-moment bedside data	Inaccurate data if interfering substances are present: methemoglobin, sulfhemoglobin, carboxyhemoglobin, methylene blue	Maximum depression 75–85% regardless of how much methemoglobin is present

However, oxidants damage the erythrocyte at different locations in the two disease entities. Hemolysis occurs when oxidants damage the erythrocyte by acting directly as electron acceptors or through the formation of hydrogen peroxide or other oxidizing free radicals. Oxidants forming irreversible bonds with sulfhydryl groups of hemoglobin cause denaturation and precipitation of the protein. These precipitates are sufficient quantitatively to form Heinz bodies within the red cell. Cells with large numbers of Heinz bodies are removed by the reticuloendothelial system, producing hemolysis. Alternatively, some oxidants can destroy the erythrocyte membrane directly, causing non–Heinz body hemolysis. Methemoglobinemia does not necessarily progress to hemolysis if unchecked.

Numerous cases describe the occurrence of hemolysis following methemoglobinemia, although most poisonings with these compounds do not in fact manifest both types of toxicity. This is reported with dapsone,[18,19,58] phenazopyridine (Pyridium),[14,21,29,56,74] amyl nitrite,[11] and aniline.[33,40,50] These instances of combined occurrences may represent the incidental toxicity of an oxidizing agent or represent the depletion of all cellular defenses against oxidants. Currently it is not possible to predict when hemolysis will follow methemoglobinemia with any level of certainty; however, clearly there is an increased incremental risk.

Another source of confusion concerning hemolysis and methemoglobinemia is that reduced glutathione (GSH) is required to protect against both. Erythrocytes are able to withstand hemolytic oxidant damage as long as they can maintain adequate levels of reduced glutathione, the principal cellular antioxidant. Glutathione is maintained in its reduced form by using NADPH as its reducing agent. Cells with reduced capacity to produce NADPH (ie, eryth-rocytes of patients with G-6-PD deficiency or cells with depleted reduced glutathione/NADPH) are thus susceptible to hemolysis. In the presence of methemoglobinemia, reduced glutathione plays a minor role as a reducing agent, but NADPH is necessary for successful antidotal therapy. This codependence on the reducing power of NADPH generated by the hexose monophosphate shunt links the two disorders. Competition for NADPH by oxidized glutathione and exogenously administered methylene blue is postulated to be the cause of methylene blue–induced hemolysis, ie, competitive inhibition of glutathione reduction. The clinical importance of this phenomenon is uncertain. It may be easier to consider hemolysis and methemoglobin formation as subclasses of disorders of oxidant stress. They should be considered separate clinical entities sharing limited characteristics.

MANAGEMENT

For most patients with mild methemoglobinemia, no therapy is necessary other than withdrawal of the offending agent and oxygen administration, as reduction of the methemoglobin will occur by means of intact normal reconversion mechanisms (NADH methemoglobin reductase). In the clinical setting, continued absorption, prolonged half-life, and toxic intermediate metabolites may prolong methemoglobinemia. Patients should be examined carefully for signs of physiologic stress related to decreased oxygen delivery to the tissue (Fig. 94–7). Obviously, changes in mental status, such as stupor or lethargy, or ischemic chest pain necessitates immediate treatment, but subtle changes in behavior or inattentiveness also may be signs of global hypoxia and should

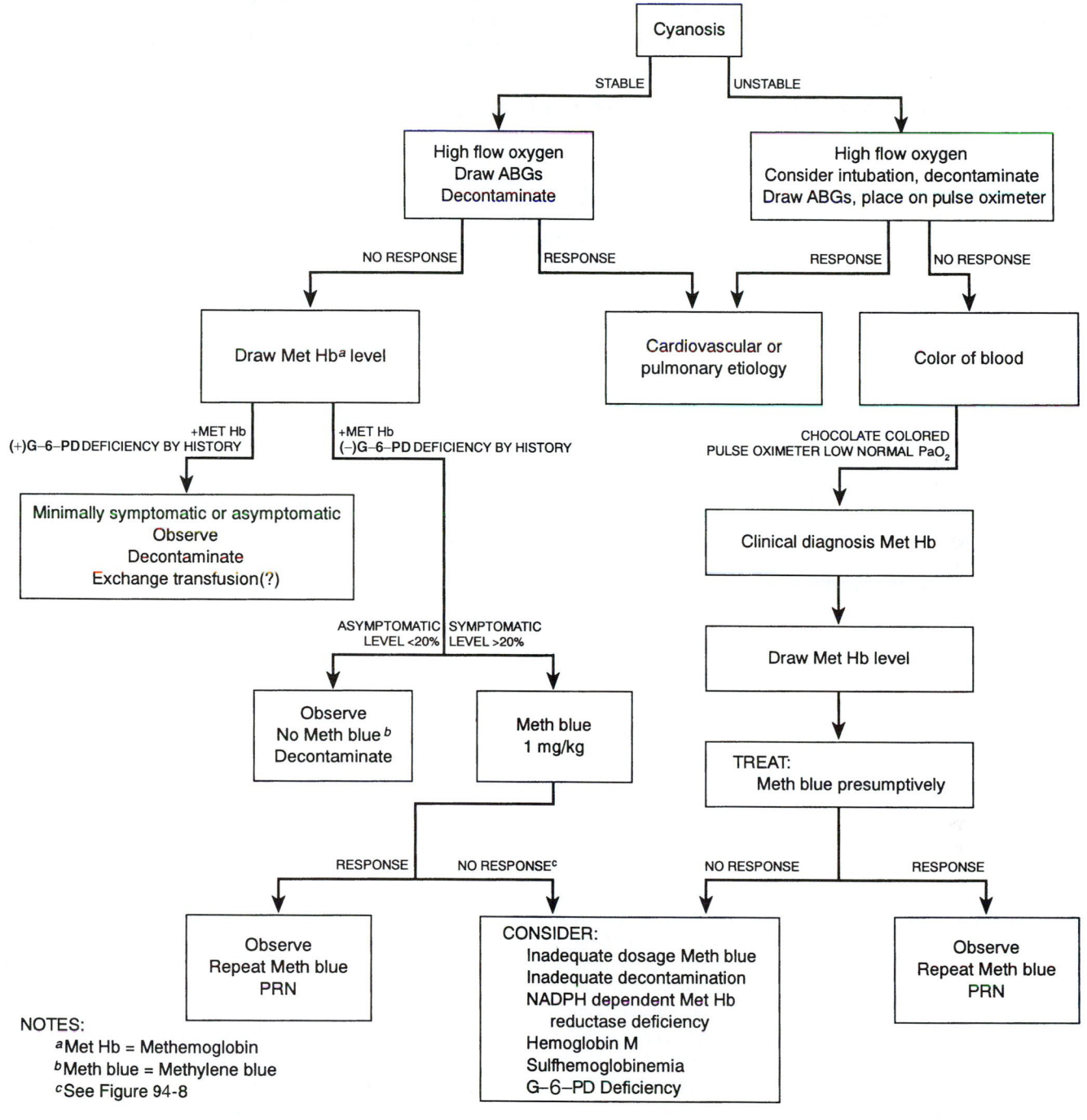

Figure 94–7. Toxicologic assessment of the cyanotic patient.

be treated as well. Abnormal vital signs, such as tachycardia and tachypnea, thought to be caused by tissue hypoxia or the functional anemia of methemoglobinemia, should also be treated aggressively. Patients who develop lactic acidosis or ischemic ECG changes should be treated as well. A methemoglobin level alone is generally not an adequate indication of need for therapy.

The most widely accepted treatment of methemoglobinemia is the administration of methylene blue, 1 to 2 mg/kg body weight as a 1% solution, infused IV over 5 minutes. This is 0.1 to 0.2 mL/kg of a 1% solution. The 5-minute infusion helps prevent painful

local responses from rapid infusion. When a painful reaction occurs, it can be minimized by flushing the IV rapidly with at least 15 to 30 mL of fluid following the infusion. Improvement should be noted within 1 hour of methylene blue administration. If cyanosis has not disappeared within 1 hour of the infusion, a second dose should be given, and other factors considered (Fig. 94–8).

The use of methylene blue in patients with G-6-PD deficiency is controversial. Deficiency of this enzyme is estimated to be present in 200 million people worldwide. Its incidence in the United States is highest among African Americans (11%).[4] For this rea-

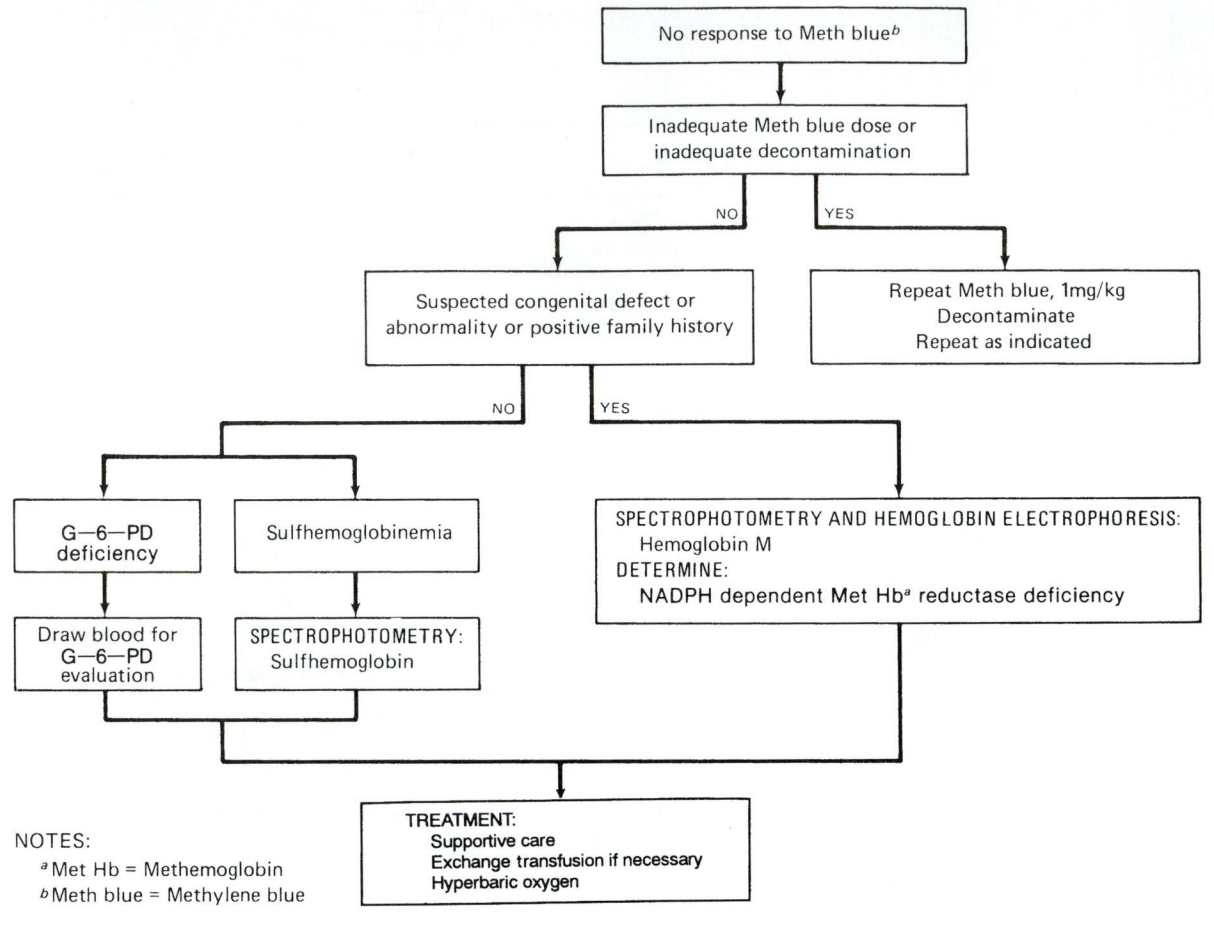

Figure 94–8.   Management algorithm for patients with suspected methemoglobinemia unresponsive to initial therapy.

son, G-6-PD–deficient patients have been excluded from most treatment protocols because methylene blue is a mild oxidant and case reports have suggested methylene blue's toxicity. However, because of the lack of immediate availability of the test for G-6-PD deficiency, most patients with no known history of G-6-PD deficiency who need treatment receive methylene blue therapy before their G-6-PD status is known. Although many patients with G-6-PD deficiency have undoubtedly been treated unknowingly, few case reports of toxicity have actually been reported.

Methylene blue itself is an oxidant, but in an assessment of the hemolytic potency of varied drugs, methylene blue in doses of 390 to 780 mg proved to be only a moderate hemolytic agent.[43] Even the authors of the review most frequently cited as a rationale for withholding methylene blue treatment were unsure that the methylene blue that had been given to their G-6-PD–deficient patient produced hemolysis;[70] the dose of methylene blue was small in the patient under study, and the patient had taken other agents capable of producing hemolysis. Patients with G-6-PD deficiency have variable activity of the enzyme and manifest different levels of disease in response to oxidant stress. For all of these reasons, the judicious use of methylene blue is warranted in most of these patients, with G-6-PD deficiency and symptomatic methemoglobinemia.

If methylene blue treatment fails to significantly relieve the methemoglobinemia, a number of possibilities should be consid-

ered. The cause of the oxidant stress may not have been identified and adequately removed, allowing for continuing oxidation. In such situations, decontamination of the gut (emesis, lavage, activated charcoal, or possibly whole-bowel irrigation) and skin cleansing must be assured. Additional doses of methylene blue are also indicated.

Theoretically, exchange transfusion or hyperbaric oxygen may be beneficial when methylene blue is ineffective. Both interventions are time consuming and costly, but hyperbaric oxygen offers the alternative of allowing the dissolved oxygen time to protect the patient while the body reduces methemoglobin. Ascorbic acid has no place in the management of acquired methemoglobinemia because the rate at which it reduces methemoglobin is considerably slower than that of the normal intrinsic mechanisms.[9] Methylene blue has no therapeutic effect on sulfhemoglobinemia.[65]

DAPSONE

The treatment of dapsone deserves special consideration because of the frequency in which it is seen in overdose situations and its tendency to produce prolonged methemoglobinemia. The N-hydroxylation of dapsone to its hydroxylamine metabolite by a cytochrome P450–mediated reaction is in part responsible for methemoglobin formation both in therapeutic and overdose situations. Both the parent compound and it metabolites are oxidants. Cimetidine is an inhibitor of this metabolic pathway and reduces methemoglobin levels during therapeutic dosing.[69] In overdose situations, cimetidine may exert some protective effects as well and should be given.

SULFHEMOGLOBIN

Sulfhemoglobin is a darkly colored hemoglobin with a sulfur atom incorporated into the heme molecule but not attached to iron. The exact location of the sulfur atom in the porphyrin ring is unclear. Sulfhemoglobin is a darker pigment than methemoglobin, producing cyanosis when only 0.5 g/dL of blood is affected. The cyanosis produced is similar to that produced by methemoglobinemia. It is characterized in the laboratory by its spectrophotometric appearance and its lack of reaction when cyanide is added to the mixture. The methemoglobin absorption peak is eliminated by the addition of cyanide. However, this is not routinely done in clinical laboratory practice, and the diagnosis is often made by the failure to improve with methylene blue. In the laboratory, isoelectric focusing techniques further define the substance.

Sulfhemoglobin is an extremely stable compound that is eliminated only when the red blood cell is removed naturally from circulation. Although the oxygen-carrying capacity of hemoglobin is reduced by sulfhemoglobinemia, unlike methemoglobinemia there is a decreased affinity for oxygen in the remaining "unaltered" hemoglobin. This makes oxygen more available to the tissues. The oxyhemoglobin dissociation curve is shifted to the right (see Fig. 20–2). This phenomenon, fortunately, reduces the clinical effect of sulfhemoglobin at the tissue level.

Sulfhemoglobin can be produced experimentally in vitro by the action of hydrogen sulfide on hemoglobin and was produced in dogs fed elemental sulfur.[49] A number of drugs induce sulfhemoglobin in humans, including acetanilid, phenacetin, nitrates, trinitrotoluene, and sulfur compounds. Most of the drugs that produce methemoglobinemia have been reported in various degrees to produce sulfhemoglobinemia. Sulfhemoglobinemia is also recognized in individuals with chronic constipation and those who purge.[49] Table 94–4 lists some differences between methemoglobin and sulfhemoglobin.

Sulfhemoglobinemia usually requires no therapy other than the withdrawal of the offending agent. It also appears that patients come to the attention of clinicians earlier because sulfhemoglobinemia produces greater cyanosis than methemoglobinemia at a lower sulfhemoglobin level. There is no antidote for sulfhemoglobinemia because it is an irreversible chemical bond that occurs within the hemoglobin molecule. Exchange transfusion would lower sulfhemoglobin levels, but this approach is usually unnecessary.

SUMMARY

Oxidation of hemoglobin is a rare but treatable etiology of cyanosis. In the absence of findings of cardiopulmonary disease, cyanosis from methemoglobinemia is likely. The diagnosis is confirmed by cooximetry evaluation of blood. When treatment is clinically indicated, methylene blue is the treatment of choice. The source of oxidant stress should be sought and eliminated.

TABLE 94–4.   Differences Between Methemoglobin and Sulfhemoglobin

	Methemoglobin	Sulfhemoglobin
Definition	Commonly accepted: hemoglobin with an oxidized heme moiety	Less well understood: hemoglobin with sulfur attached through an oxidative reaction
Clinical appearance	Cyanosis, may appear ill	Cyanosis, appears less ill at a comparable degree
Spectrophotometric characteristics	Peak absorption at 570 and 620 mm	Peak absorption at 520 and 626 mm
Reversible by antidote	Yes	No
Level necessary to detect cyanosis	1.5 g/dL	0.5 g/dL
Etiologies	See Table 94–1	Similar to methemoglobin, an oxidant and a source of sulfur needed to produce sulfhemoglobin
Diagnosis	Cooximetry	Cyanide added to blood in laboratory will completely eliminate methemoglobin, but not sulfhemoglobin; some newer cooximeters measure directly
Effects on oxyhemoglobin dissociation curve	Decreased oxygen-carrying capacity, shifts curve to left with impaired O₂ delivery to tissues	Decreased oxygen-carrying capacity, shifts curve to right, improving O₂ delivery to tissue
Response to treatment	Very good	Eliminated only with RBC natural turnover, no specific treatment

REFERENCES

1. Bacon R: Nitrate preserved sausage meat causes an unusual food poisoning incident. Commun Dis Rep CDR Rev 1997;7:R45–R47.
2. Bakshi SP, Fahey JL, Pierce LE: Sausage cyanosis-acquired methemoglobinemic nitrite poisoning. N Engl J Med 1967;277:1072.
3. Barker SJ, Tremper KK, Hyatt J: Effects of methemoglobinemia on pulse oximetry and mixed venous oximetry. Anesthesiology 1989;70:112–117.
4. Beutler E: Glucose-6-phosphate dehydrogenase deficiency. N Engl J Med 1991;324:169–174.
5. Beutler E: Methemoglobinemia and other causes of cyanosis. In: Beutler E, Lichtman MA, Coller BS, Kipps TJ, eds: William's Hematology, 5th ed. New York, McGraw-Hill, 1995, pp. 654–663.
6. Beutler E: The hemolytic effect of primaquine and related compounds: A review. J Hematol 1959;14:103–139.
7. Birky M, Malek D, Paabo M: Study of biological samples obtained from victims of MGM Grand Hotel fire. J Anal Toxicol 1983;7:265–271.
8. Bodansky O: Methemoglobinemia and methemoglobin producing compounds. Pharmacol Rev 1951;3:144–196.
9. Bolyai JZ, Smith RP, Gray CT: Ascorbic acid and chemically induced methemoglobinemias. Toxicol Appl Pharmacol 1972;21:176–185.
10. Bower PJ, Peterson JN: Methemoglobinemia after sodium nitroprusside therapy. N Engl J Med 1975;293:865.

11. Brandes JC, Bufill JA, Pisciotta AV: Amyl nitrite-induced hemolytic anemia. Am J Med 1989;86:252–254.

12. Caprari P, Bozzi A, Ferroni L, et al: Membrane alterations in G6PD- and PK-deficient erythrocytes exposed to oxidizing agents. Biol Med Metab Biol 1991;45:16–27.

13. Chan TY: Food-borne nitrates and nitrites as a cause of methemoglobinemia. Southeast Asian J Trop Med Public Health 1996;27:189–192.

14. Cohen BL, Bovasso GJ: Acquired methemoglobinemia and hemolytic anemia following excessive Pyridium (phenazopyridine hydrochloride) ingestion. Clin Pediatr 1971;10:537–540.

15. Comly HH: Cyanosis in infants caused by nitrates in well water. JAMA 1945;129:112–116.

16. Craun GF, Greathouse DG, Gunderson DH: Methemoglobin levels in young children consuming high nitrate well water in the United States. Int J Epidemiol 1981;10:309–317.

17. Darling RC, Roughton FJW: The effect of methemoglobin on the equilibrium between oxygen and hemoglobin. Am J Physiol 1942;137:56–66.

18. Dawson AH, Whyte IM: Management of dapsone poisoning complicated by methemoglobinemia. Med Toxicol Adverse Drug Exp 1989;4:387–392.

19. Elonen E, Neuvonen PJ, Halmekoski J, Mattila MJ: Acute dapsone intoxication: A case with prolonged symptoms. Clin Toxicol 1979;14:79–85.

20. Fibuch EE, Cecil WT, Reed WA: Methemoglobinemia associated with organic nitrate therapy. Anesth Analg 1979;58:521–523.

21. Fincher ME, Campbell HT: Methemoglobinemia and hemolytic anemia after phenazopyridine hydrochloride (Pyridium) administration in end-stage renal disease. South Med J 1989;82:372–374.

22. Fogh-Andersen N, Siggarrad-Andersen O, Lundsgaard FC, Wimberly PD: Diode-array spectrophotometry for simultaneous measurement of hemoglobin pigments. Clin Chim Acta 1987;166:283–289.

23. Fung H: Pharmacokinetic determinants of nitrate action. Am J Med 1984;76:22–27.

24. Gaetani GD, Parker JC, Kirkman HN: Intracellular restraint: A new basis for the limitation in response to oxidative stress in human erythrocytes containing low-activity variants of glucose-6-phosphate dehydrogenase. Proc Natl Acad Sci USA 1974;9:3584–3587.

25. Garrison FH: An Introduction to the History of Medicine, 4th ed. Philadelphia and London, WB Saunders, 1929, pp. 566–567.

26. Gelberg KH, Church L, Casey G, et al: Nitrate levels in drinking water in rural New York State. Environ Res 1999;80:34–40.

27. Gibson QH: The reduction of methaemoglobin in red blood cells and studies on the causes of ideopathic methemoglobin. Biochem J 1948;42:13.

28. Goldstein BD: Exacerbation of dapsone-induced Heinz body hemolytic anemia following treatment with methylene blue. Am J Med Sci 1974;267:291–297.

29. Greenberg MS, Wong H: Methemoglobinemia and Heinz body hemolytic anemia due to phenazopyridine hydrochloride. N Engl J Med 1964;271:431–435.

30. Gupta PM, Lala DS, Arsura E: Benzocaine-induced methemoglobinemia. South Med J 2000;93:83–86.

31. Hanukoglo A, Danon PN: Endogenous methemoglobinemia associated with diarrheal disease in infancy. J Pediatr Gastroenterol Nutr 1996;23:1–7.

32. Harris JC, Rumack BH, Peterson RG, McGuire BM: Methemoglobinemia resulting from absorption of nitrates. JAMA 1979;242:2869–2871.

33. Harrison MR: Toxic methemoglobinemia: A case of acute nitrobenzene and aniline poisoning tested with exchange transfusion. Anaesthesia 1977;32:270–272.

34. Hartman AF, Perley AM, Barnett HL: A study of some of the physiological effects of sulfanilamide. II. Methemoglobin formation and its control. J Clin Invest 1938;17:699–710.

35. Harvey JW, Keitt AS: Studies of the efficacy and potential hazards of methylene blue therapy in aniline-induced methemoglobinemia. Br J Haematol 1983;54:29–41.

36. Hegesh E, Hegesh J, Kaftory A: Congenital methemoglobinemia with a deficiency of cytochrome b5. N Engl J Med: 1985;314:757–761.

37. Hjelt K, Lund JT, Scherling B, et al: Methemoglobinemia among neonates in a neonatal intensive care unit. Acta Paediatr 1995;84:365–370.

38. Hoffman RS, Sauter D: Methemoglobinemia resulting from smoke inhalation. Vet Hum Toxicol 1989;31:40–42.

39. Horne MK, Waterman MR, Simon LM, Garriott JC, Foerster EH: Methemoglobinemia from sniffing butyl nitrite. Ann Intern Med 1979;91:417–418.

40. Johnson CJ, Bonrud PA, Dosch TL, et al: Fatal outcome of methemoglobinemia in an infant. JAMA 1987;257:2796–2797.

41. Katsumata Y, Aoki M, Oya M, et al: Simultaneous determination of carboxyhemoglobin and methemoglobin in victims of carbon monoxide poisoning. J Forensic Sci 1980;25:546–549.

42. Kearney TE, Manoguerra AS, Dunford JV: Chemically induced methemoglobinemia from aniline poisoning. West J Med 1984;140:282–286.

43. Kellermeyer RW, Tarlov AR, Brewer GJ, et al: Hemolytic effect of therapeutic drugs: clinical considerations of the primaquine-type hemolysis. JAMA 1962;180:128–134.

44. Khan NA, Kruse JA: Methemoglobinemia induced by topical anesthesia: a case report and review. Am J Med Sci 1999;318:415–418.

45. Kirlangitis JJ, Middaugh RE, Zablocki A, Rodriquez F: False indication of arterial oxygen desaturation and methemoglobinemia following injection of methylene blue in urological surgery. Mil Med 1990;155:260–262.

46. Laney RF, Hoffman RS: Methemoglobinemia secondary to automobile exhaust fumes. Am J Emerg Med 1992;10:426–428.

47. Larsen VH, Freudendal-Pedersen A, Fogh-Andersen NF: The influence of patent blue V on pulse oximetry and haemoximetry. Acta Anesthesiol Scand 1995;39:53–55.

48. Lehman H, Huntsman RG, Cosey R, et al: Hemoglobinopathies associated with unstable hemoglobin. In: Williams JW, Beutler E, Erslev AJ, Lichtman MA, eds: Hematology, 4th ed. New York, McGraw-Hill, 1995, pp. 650–654.

49. Leroux A, Junien C, Kaplan JC, Bamberger J: Generalized deficiency of cytochrome b5 reductase in congenital methemoglobinemia with mental retardation. Nature 1975;258:619–620.

50. Lubash GD, Phillips RE, Shields JD, Bonsnes RW: Acute aniline poisoning treated by hemodialysis. Arch Intern Med 1964;114:530–532.

51. Lukens JN: The legacy of well water methemoglobinemia. JAMA 1987;257:2793–2795.

52. Machabert R, Testud F, Descotes J: Methaemoglobinemia due to amyl nitrite inhalation: a case report. Hum Exp Toxicol 1994;13:313–314.

53. Mansouri A, Lurie AA: Concise review: methemoglobinemia. Am J Hematol 1993;42:7–12.

54. Methemoglobinemia in an infant—Wisconsin. MMWR 1993;42:217–219.

55. Murray KM, Meth B: Methemoglobin, medline, and hyperlipemia. Crit Care Med 1987;15:797–798.

56. Nathan DM, Siegel AJ, Bunn F: Acute methemoglobinemia and hemolytic anemia with phenazopyridine. Arch Intern Med 1977;137:1636–1638.

57. Nathan GD, Oski FA: Hematology of Infancy and Childhood, 4th ed. Philadelphia, WB Saunders, 1993, pp. 698–731.

58. Neuvonen PJ, Elonen E, Haapanen EJ: Acute dapsone intoxication: Clinical findings and effect of oral charcoal and hemodialysis on dapsone elimination. Acta Med Scand 1983;214:215–220.

59. Nguyen SI, Cabrales RE, Bashour CA, et al: Benzocaine induced methemoglobinemia. Anesth Analg 2000;90:369–371.

60. Nijland R, Jongsma HW, Nijhuis JG, et al: Notes on the apparent discordance of pulse oximetry and multiwavelength hemoglobin photometry. Acta Anaesthesiol Scand 1995;107:49–52.

61. Nilsson A, Engberg G, Henneberg S, et al: Inverse relationship between age-dependent erythrocyte activity of methaemoglobin reductase and prilocaine-induced methaemoglobinemia during infancy. Br J Anaesth 1990;64:72–76.

62. Nitzan M, Volovitz B, Topper E: Infantile methemoglobinemia caused by food additives. Clin Toxicol 1979;15:273–280.

63. Odonohue WJ, Moss LM, Angelillo VA: Acute methemoglobinemia induced by topical benzocaine and lidocaine. Arch Intern Med 1980; 140:1508–1509.

64. Paris PM, Kaplan RM, Steward RD, Weiss LD: Methemoglobin levels following sublingual nitoglycerin in human volunteers. Ann Emerg Med 1986;15:171–173.

65. Park CM, Nagel RL: Sulfhemoglobinemia: Clinical and molecular aspects. N Engl J Med 1984;310:1579–1584.

66. Pollack ES, Pollack CV: Incidence of subclinical methemoglobinemia in infants with diarrhea. Ann Emerg Med 1994;24:652–656.

67. Prchal JT, Borgese N, Moore MR, et al: Congenital methemoglobinemia due to methemoglobin reductase deficiency in two unrelated American black families. Am J Med 1990;89:516–522.

68. Ralston AC, Webb RK, Runchiman WB: Potential errors in pulse oximetry. Anaesthesia 1991;46:291–295.

69. Rhodes LE, Tingle MD, Park BK, et al: Cimetidine improves the therapeutic/toxic ratio of dapsone in patients on chronic dapsone therapy. Br J Dermatol 1995;132:257–262.

70. Rosen PJ, Johnson C, Mcgehee WG, Beutler E: Failure of methylene blue treatment in toxic methemoglobinemia. Ann Intern Med 1971; 76:83–86.

71. Sager S, Garyson GH, Feig SA: Methemoglobinemia associated with acidosis of probable renal origin. J Pediatr 1995;126:59–61.

72. Sass MD, Caruso CJ, Farhangi M: TPNH-methemoglobin reductase deficiency: A new red-cell enzyme defect. J Lab Clin Med 1967; 5:760–767.

73. Schwerd W, Schulz E: Carboxyhemoglobin and methemoglobin findings in burnt bodies. Forensic Sci Int 1978;12:233–235.

74. Sharon M, Puente G, Cohen LB: Phenazopyridine (Pyridium) poisoning: possible toxicity of methylene blue administration in renal failure. Mt Sinai J Med 1986;3:280–282.

75. Sinex JE: Pulse oximetry: principles and limitations. Am J Emerg Med 1999;17:59–66.

76. Smith ER, Smiseth IK, Maryari D, et al: Mechanism of action of nitrates. Am J Med 1984;76:14–22.

77. Smith R, Olson M: Drug-induced methemoglobinemia. Semin Hematol 1973;10:253–268.

78. Spurzem JR, Bonchat HW, Shigeoka JW: Factitious methemoglobinemia caused by hyperlipemia. Chest 1984;88:84–86.

79. Totapally BR, Nolan B, Zureikat G, Inove S: An unusual case of methemoglobinemia in infancy. Am J Emerg Med 1998;16:723–724.

80. Tremper KK, Barker SJ: Using pulse oximetry when dyshemoglobin levels are high. J Crit Illness 1988;11:103–107.

81. Watcha MF, Connor MT, Hing AV: Pulse oximetry in methemoglobinemia: Am J Dis Child 1989;143:845–847.

82. Wendel WB: The control of methemoglobinemia with methylene blue. J Clin Invest 1939;18:179–185.

83. White CD, Weiss LD: Varying presentations of methemoglobinemia: two cases. J Emerg Med 1991;9:45–49.

84. Wintrobe MM, Lee GR: Wintrobe's Clinical Hematology, 10th ed. Lee GR, ed. Baltimore, Williams & Wilkins, 1999, pp. 1046–1055.

85. Yano SS, Danish EH, Hsia YE: Transient methemoglobinemia with acidosis in infants. J Pediatr 1982;100:415–418.

86. Zijlstra WG, Buursma A, Zwart A: Performance of an automated six-wavelength photometer (Radiometer OSM3) for routine measurement of hemoglobin derivatives. Clin Chem 1988;34:149–152.

ANTIDOTES IN DEPTH

Methylene Blue
Mary Ann Howland

Methylene blue is an extremely effective antidote for toxin-induced methemoglobinemia. Recently, other actions of methylene blue including inhibition of nitric oxide and guanylate cylase and inhibition of the generation of oxygen free radicals were discovered. These effects are being used to explain methylene blue's beneficial effects in the hepatopulmonary syndrome, modulation of streptozocin-induced insulin deficiency, and the reduction of the development of surgery-induced peritoneal adhesions.[13,14,18,34]

Methylene blue was initially recommended for use as an intestinal and urinary antiseptic and subsequently recognized as a weak antimalarial agent.[17] In 1933, Williams and Challis successfully used methylene blue to treat aniline-induced methemoglobinemia.[43]

Methylene blue is tetramethyl thionine chloride,[17] which as an electron acceptor is reduced to an elector donor status in the presence of NADPH and NADPH methemoglobin reductase to leukomethylene blue (see Fig. 94–5). Leukomethylene blue then becomes available to reduce methemoglobin to hemoglobin.[9,17] In the presence of methylene blue, methemoglobin reduction via this NADPH pathway is dramatically increased (four to five times in dogs), making methylene blue the treatment of choice for methemoglobinemia.

Spectrophotometric assays have been used to study the pharmacokinetics of methylene blue and leukomethylene blue.[9] Methylene blue has a pK_a close to −1, making it completely ionized in the GI tract.[10] Administration of 10 mg of methylene blue in capsule form to seven volunteers demonstrated good oral absorption, with an average urinary recovery of 74%.[10] The majority of the methylene blue was excreted as a salt complex of leukomethylene blue, whereas the remainder was excreted as the parent product.[10] Previous animal experiments suggest that methylene blue is poorly absorbed orally.

In a canine model, intravenous administration of increasing doses of methylene blue led to two divergent pharmacokinetic interpretations: a nonlinear single-compartment model and a classic linear two-compartment open model (volume of distribution 0.22–0.87 L/kg; plasma clearance 1.98–2.65 L/kg/h).[11]

Reports of the apparent paradoxic ability of methylene blue to induce methemoglobinemia suggest an equilibrium between the ability of methylene blue to oxidize hemoglobin directly to methemoglobin and the ability of methylene blue (through the NADPH and NADPH methemoglobin reductase pathway and leukomethylene blue production) to reduce methemoglobin to hemoglobin.[4,5] Methylene blue does not produce methemoglobin at doses of 1 to 2 mg/kg. The equilibrium seems to favor the reducing properties of methylene blue unless excessively large doses of methylene blue are given[3,16,42] or the NADPH methemoglobin reductase system is abnormal. This equilibrium constant may vary substantially, as 20 mg/kg IV in dogs and 65 mg/kg intraperitoneally in rats failed to produce methemoglobinemia.[37]

In the earliest studies, 50 to 100 mL of a 1% concentration of methylene blue was used intravenously to evaluate volunteers[27] and treat patients with aniline dye–induced methemoglobinemia.[43] Methemoglobin levels measured when symptoms were most pronounced were found to be approximately 1.0 g/dL (0.4–8.3% of total hemoglobin) and unlikely to be solely responsible for the adverse effects demonstrated. Other consequential adverse effects included shortness of breath, tachypnea, chest discomfort, burning sensation of the mouth and stomach, initial bluish-tinged skin and mucous membranes, paresthesias, restlessness, apprehension, tremors, nausea and vomiting, dysuria, and excitation. Urine and vomitus had a blue color. This experience led to the recommendation to avoid doses in excess of 7 mg/kg.

Methylene blue doses of 1 to 2 mg/kg IV or 65 to 130 mg orally every 4 hours reversed sulfanilamide-induced methemoglobinemia.[19,41] With these regimens a very rapid fall in methemoglobin occurred with a disappearance of cyanosis. Later investigations confirmed the effectiveness and safety of IV doses of 1 to 2 mg/kg of methylene blue in reversing the methemoglobinemia produced by sulfanilamide,[40] aniline dye,[12] and silver nitrate, among other agents.[38]

In high doses, methylene blue can also induce an acute hemolytic anemia in the absence or presence of methemoglobinemia.[16,25] In dose–response studies in G-6-PD–deficient homozygous African American men, daily doses with hemolytic potential were 390 to 780 mg (5.5–11 mg/kg) of methylene blue.[24] This was comparable to 15 mg of primaquine base.[24] Because of the sensitivity of neonates (HbF and diminished NADH reductase) to these risks, the smallest effective dose should be employed.[21,25] Because oxidizing agents can independently result in chemical-induced Heinz body hemolytic anemia, the contribution of methylene blue is often difficult to elucidate.[23]

Methylene blue is suggested to be ineffective in reversing methemoglobinemia in patients with G-6-PD deficiency[33] because the G-6-PD in the hexose monophosphate shunt is essential for the generation of NADPH. Without NADPH, methylene blue cannot act as a reducing agent in the transformation of methemoglobin to oxyhemoglobin. However, G-6-PD deficiency is an X-linked hereditary deficiency with more than 400 variants. The red cells containing the more common G-6-PD A⁻ variant found in 11% of African Americans retain 10% residual activity, mostly in younger erythrocytes and reticulocytes. The enzyme is barely detectable in those of Mediterranean descent who have inherited the defect. Therefore, it is impossible to predict before the use of methylene blue who will or will not respond and to what extent. Currently it appears that most individuals have adequate G-6-PD and do not express deficiency states in absolute but only in relative terms. This variable expression of their deficiency allows an effective response to most oxidant stresses.

A risk-to-benefit ratio must be determined when methylene blue is administered to achieve methemoglobin reversal. However, when therapeutic doses of methylene blue fail to have an impact on the methemoglobin level, the possibility of G-6-PD deficiency should be considered. Further doses of methylene blue should not be administered in these cases because the risk of methylene blue-induced hemolysis exists in the absence of any potential benefit. In these cases, exchange transfusion and hyperbaric oxygen are potential alternatives (Chap. 94). Theoretically normal cells might convert methylene blue to leukomethylene blue, and the leukomethylene blue might diffuse into G-6-PD–deficient cells and achieve methemoglobin reduction to hemoglobin.[2] Before it is assumed that G-6-PD deficiency is responsible for continued methemoglobin levels in spite of the administration of methyelene blue, continued toxin absorption and/or continued methemoglobin production must always be excluded.

Methylene blue is a dye. It will alter pulse oximeter readings.[6] Large doses may interfere with a clinician's ability to detect a decrease in cyanosis, and therefore, repeat cooximeter readings and arterial blood gas analysis should be used in conjunction with clinical findings. Methylene blue will cause the urine to turn a bluish-green and may cause dysuria, although it may also be prescibed for dysuria.[30] Methylene blue is quite irritating and exceedingly painful; even without extravasation it may cause local tissue damage.[31] Subcutaneous and intrathecal administration are contraindicated.[31] After IV access was unobtainable, intraosseous administration of 0.3 mL of a 1% solution (1 mg/kg) over 3 to 5 minutes into the anterior tibia of a 6-week-old infant was well tolerated.[20,29]

Intraamniotic injection of methylene blue may result in a number of different adverse effects, including infants born with skin dyed blue, leading to inaccurate pulse oximetry readings, methemoglobin, hemolysis, phototoxic skin reactions, or intestinal obstruction.[6,20,22,25,28,31] One infant exposed in utero at 5½ weeks was born normal.[22]

When there is continued absorption or slow elimination of the xenobiotic producing the methemoglobinemia, repetitive dosing of methylene blue may be required in conjunction with efforts to decontaminate the GI tract and perhaps stop the formation of the methemoglobin-inducing metabolite with the use of inhibitors of drug metabolism such as cimetidine.[7,32] A continuous IV infusion of methylene blue at 0.1 mg/kg/h or 3 to 7 mg/h in a concentration of 0.05% in normal saline has been used.[1,36] However, this method of administration has not yet been adequately studied.

Methylene blue is indicated when patients are symptomatic from methemoglobinemia. This usually occurs at methemoglobin levels greater than 20% but may occur at lower levels in anemic patients or those with cardiovascular, pulmonary, or central nervous system compromise. Judicious use of methylene blue is warranted in patients with questionable levels of G-6-PD deficiency. Very large doses of methylene blue may produce methemoglobinemia or a hemolytic anemia in the absence of a G-6-PD deficiency, but this is extremely rare at doses of 1 to 2 mg/kg IV. Methylene blue is ineffective in treating other entities such as sulfhemoglobinemia (Chap. 94).

In summary, methylene blue is a very effective reducer of xenobiotic-induced methemoglobinemia. When used in the proper dose, adverse reactions are limited, and the onset of action is rapid. Repeat doses are often required when methemoglobin-producing drugs such as dapsone with a long duration of effect are ingested. In most cases, doses of 1 to 2 mg/kg IV given over 5 minutes, followed immediately by a 15- to 30-mL fluid flush to minimize local pain is both effective and relatively safe. In neonates doses of 0.3–1 mg/kg are often effective.[21] The onset of action is quite rapid, with effects usually seen within 30 minutes. Methylene blue is available in 10-mL 1% ampules containing 10 mg/mL.

REFERENCES

1. Berlin G, Brodin B, Hilden J, Martensson J: Acute dapsone intoxication. A case treated with continuous infusion of methylene blue, forced diuresis and plasma exchange. J Toxicol Clin Toxicol 1984–1985; 22:537–548.
2. Beutler E, Baluda M: Methemoglobin reduction: studies of the interaction between cell populations and of the role of methylene blue. Blood 1963;22:323–333.
3. Blass N, Fung D: Dyed but not dead—methylene blue overdose. Anesthesiology 1976;45:458–459.
4. Bodansky O: Methemoglobinemia and methemoglobin-producing compounds. Pharmacol Rev 1951;3:144–196.
5. Bodansky O: Mechanism of action of methylene blue in treatment of methemoglobinemia. JAMA 1950;142:923.
6. Coleman MD, Coleman NA: Drug-induced methaemoglobinemia. Drug Safety 1996;14:394–405.
7. Coleman MD, Rhodes LA, Scott AK, et al: The use of cimetidine to reduce dapsone-dependent methemoglobinemia in dermatitis herpetiformis patients. Br J Clin Pharmacol 1992;34:244–249.
8. Crooks J: Haemolytic jaundice in a neonate after intra-amniotic injection of methylene blue. Arch Dis Child 1982;57:872–886.
9. DiSanto AR, Wagner JG: Pharmacokinetics of highly ionized drugs. I: Methylene blue—whole blood, urine and tissue assays. J Pharm Sci 1972;61:598–602.
10. DiSanto AR, Wagner JG: Pharmacokinetics of highly ionized drugs. II: Methylene blue—absorption, metabolism and excretion in man and dog after oral absorption. J Pharm Sci 1972;61:1086–1090.
11. DiSanto AR, Wagner JG: Pharmacokinetics of highly ionized drugs. III: Methylene blue—blood levels in the dog and tissue levels in the rat following intravenous administration. J Pharm Sci 1972;61: 1090–1094.
12. Etteldorf JN: Methylene blue in the treatment of methemoglobinemia in premature infants caused by marking ink. J Pediatr 1951;38:24–27.
13. Fallon MB: Methylene blue and cirrhosis: pathophysiologic insights, therapeutic dilemmas. Ann Intern Med 2000;133:738–740.
14. Galili Y, Ben-Abraham R, Rabau M, et al: Reduction of surgery-induced peritoneal adhesions by methylene blue. Am J Surg 1998;175: 30–32.
15. Geiger JC: Cyanide poisoning in San Francisco. JAMA 1932;99: 1944–1945.
16. Goluboff N, Wheaton R: Methylene blue-induced cyanosis and acute hemolytic anemia complicating the treatment of methemoglobinemia. J Pediatr 1961;58:86–89.
17. Goodman LS, Gilman A: The Pharmacological Basis of Therapeutics. New York, Macmillan, 1941, p. 869.
18. Haluzik M, Neduidkova J, Skrha J: Endocrine Research 1999;25: 163–171.
19. Harman A, Perley A, Barnett H: A study of some of the physiological effects of sulfanilamide. II: Methemoglobin formation and its control. J Clin Invest 1938;17:699–710.
20. Herman M, Chyka P, Butler A, Rieger S: Methylene blue by intraosseous infusion for methemoglobinemia. Ann Emerg Med 1999; 33:111–113.
21. Hjelt K, Lund JT, Scherling B, et al: Methemoglobinemia among neonates in a neonatal intensive care unit. Acta Pediatr 1995;84: 365–370.
22. Katz Z, Lancet M: Inadvertent intrauterine injection of methylene blue in early pregnancy. N Engl J Med 1981;304:1427.
23. Kearney T, Manoguerra A, Dunford JV: Chemically induced methemoglobinemia from aniline poisoning. West J Med 1984;140: 282–286.
24. Kellermeyer RW, Tarlov A, Brewer G, et al: Hemolytic effect of therapeutic drugs. JAMA 1962;180:128–134.
25. Kirsch I, Cohen M: Heinz body hemolytic anemia from the use of methylene blue in neonates. J Pediatr 1980;96:276–278.

26. McEnerney JK, McEnerney LN: Unfavorable neonatal outcome after intra-amniotic injection of methylene blue. Obstet Gynecol 1983;61: 35S–37S.

27. Nadler JE, Green M, Rosenbaum A: Intravenous injection of methylene blue in man with reference to its toxic symptoms and effect on the electrocardiogram. Am J Med Sci 1934;188:15–21.

28. Nicolini U, Monni G: Intestinal obstruction in babies exposed in utero to methylene blue. Lancet 1990;336:1258–1259.

29. Orlowski JP, Porembka DT, Gallagher JM, et al: Comparison study of intraosseous, central intravenous, and perpheral intravenous infusions of emergency drugs. Am J Dis Child 1990;144:112–117.

30. Prischl F, Hofinger I, Kramar R: Fever, shivering . . . and blue urine. Nephrol Dial Transplant 1999;14:2245–2246.

31. Raimer S, Quevedo E, Johnston R: Dye rashes. Cutis 1999;63: 103–106.

32. Rhodes LE, Tingle MD, Park BK, et al: Cimetidine improves the therapeutic/toxic ratio of dapsone in patients on chronic dapsone therapy. Br J Dermatol 1995;132:257–262.

33. Rosen PJ, Johnson C, McGehee WG, Beutler E: Failure of methylene blue treatment in toxic methemoglobinemia. Ann Intern Med 1971; 76:83–86.

34. Schenk P, Madl C, Rezaie-Majd S, et al: Methylene blue improves hepatopulmonary syndrome. Ann Intern Med 2000;133:701–706.

35. Serota FT, Bernbaum JC, Schwartz E: The methylene blue baby. Lancet 1979;2:1142–1143.

36. Southgate HJ, Masterson R: Lessons to be learned: A case study approach. Prolonged methemoglobinemia due to inadvertent dapsone poisoning; treatment with methylene blue and exchange transfusion. J Royal Soc Promotion Health 1999;119:52–55.

37. Stossel TP, Jennings RB: Failure of methylene blue to produce methemoglobinemia in vivo. Am J Clin Pathol 1966;45:600–604.

38. Strauch B, Buch W, Grey W, et al: Successful treatment of methemoglobinemia secondary to silver nitrate therapy. N Engl J Med 1969; 281:257–258.

39. Troche BI: The methylene blue baby. N Engl J Med 1989;320: 1756–1757.

40. Wendel WB: The control of methemoglobinemia with methylene blue. J Clin Invest 1939;18:179–185.

41. Wendel WB: Use of methylene blue in methemoglobinemia from sulfanilamide poisoning. JAMA 1937;109:1216.

42. Whitwam JG, Taylor AR, White JM: Potential hazard of methylene blue. Anesthesiology 1979;34:181–182.

43. Williams JR, Challis FE: Methylene blue as an antidote for aniline dye poisoning. J Lab Clin Med 1933;19:166–171.

44. Yiu P, Robin J, Pattison CW: Reversal of refractory hypotension with single dose methylene blue after coronary artery bypass surgery. J Thorac Cardiovasc Surg 1999;118:195–196.

SIMPLE ASPHYXIANTS AND PULMONARY IRRITANTS

Lewis S. Nelson

On a daily basis our bodies are exposed to a variety of potentially damaging external influences. Although most organs remain relatively protected from such influence, the skin and respiratory tract, by their nature, maintain constant contact with the external environment. At rest, the respiratory tract encounters nearly 3000 L of air during a typical 8-hour workday, and even mild exertion can triple the volume inhaled. Several critical mechanisms exist within the respiratory system to prevent or minimize toxicity from without and allow humans to breathe safely in what potentially is a hostile environment. Although these efficient mechanisms provide substantial protection under normal circumstances, they may be overburdened occasionally. Additionally, the lungs are also a common portal of entry for systemic toxins that have no pulmonary effects; the best examples of these are lead (Chap. 80), carbon monoxide (Chap. 97), and cyanide (Chap. 98).

The respiratory tract, as discussed in Chapter 20, performs several important physiologic functions. Its most important role involves the transfer of oxygen to hemoglobin across the pulmonary endothelium. This facilitates oxygen distribution throughout the body to permit effective cellular respiration. Diverse toxins may act at unique points in this distribution pathway to produce tissue hypoxia. For example, toxins such as opioids or paralytic agents may induce hypoventilation, whereas carbon monoxide or methemoglobin inducers may prevent binding of oxygen to hemoglobin. Certain toxins prevent adequate oxygenation of hemoglobin at the level of pulmonary gas exchange. Two mechanistically distinct groups of agents are capable of interfering with gas exchange: simple asphyxiants and pulmonary irritants. Impairment of transpulmonary oxygen diffusion, regardless of the etiology, reduces the oxygen content of the blood and can result in tissue hypoxia.

SIMPLE ASPHYXIANTS

Case 1 A 50-year-old medical researcher was discovered dead in a small refrigerated room that contained 15 new 10-cubic-inch blocks of dry ice. The dry ice was stored in the refrigerator (4°C, 39.2°F) at approximately 9 AM on the day of the scientist's death. The researcher was last seen at approximately noon, suggesting that at least 3 hours had elapsed between the initial dry ice storage and his first exposure. Scene analysis suggested that at the time of his death the decedent was crouching several inches from the ground to store samples in a container. There were no signs of struggle, and the decedent had no history of psychiatric disorders, recent personal crises, or medical illnesses.

Postmortem examination of the decedent was unrevealing, as was the toxicologic evaluation. A blood P_{CO_2} was not performed because of its well–described rapid postmortem rise. In order to confirm the cause of death, the conditions at the time of the event were reproduced using the same cold room. Air was sampled serially at several heights; the O_2 concentration fell and the CO_2 concentration rose within 20 minutes and peaked by 3 hours. The FIO_2, 3 hours after dry ice storage, was 13.6%, and the CO_2 concentration was 27.6%, both at a height of 9 inches. Concentrations of 20 to 30% (200,000–300,000 ppm) CO_2 are associated with the rapid development of unconsciousness and death. Additionally, the temperature of the room had fallen to −15°C (5°F). Thus, it appears that even at the cold temperatures of the cold room, sublimation of dry ice progresses rapidly.

Pathophysiology

Simple asphyxiants displace oxygen from ambient air, thereby reducing the fraction of oxygen in air, or FIO_2, below 21%, resulting in a fall of the partial pressure of oxygen. The partial pressure is a measure of the oxygen contribution to the total inspired air and is based on both the FIO_2 and the barometric pressure. For example, because the ambient pressure at sea level (less water vapor, 47 mm Hg) is 713 mm Hg, and the percentage of oxygen is 21%, the partial pressure of oxygen is 150 mm Hg. Under these typical conditions, the FIO_2 is a suitable surrogate for the partial pressure of oxygen. However, this relationship is not applicable at other barometric pressures. For example, at the summit of a mountain, the reduced barometric pressure results in a fall in the partial pressure of oxygen despite a near normal FIO_2. This reduced partial pressure may be insufficient to allow an adequate oxygen saturation, and supplemental oxygen becomes necessary. As barometric pressure falls, exposure to simple asphyxiant gases may further reduce the oxygen partial pressure to life-threatening levels. Conversely, underwater divers could, in theory, reduce their FIO_2 to less than 21% by adding simple asphyxiant gases, such as helium, to their breathing mixture and still maintain adequate oxygenation. This is because the elevated barometric pressure raises the partial pressure of oxygen to normal levels despite the addition of an asphyxiant gas. However, systemically poisonous gases that entered the breathing mixture would have a magnified effect, given their increased partial pressure at depth.

In general, simple asphyxiants have no pharmacologic activity. For this reason, exceedingly high ambient concentrations of these gases are necessary to produce asphyxia. Asphyxiation occurs when one is working in confined spaces or with extremely concentrated forms of the simple asphyxiants. The widespread use of liquefied gas, which expands several hundred-fold on depressurization or warming, accounts for a substantial number of workplace injuries.[105,152]

Clinical Manifestations

A patient exposed to any simple asphyxiant gas will develop characteristic symptoms of hypoxia (Table 95–1), which are directly related to the partial pressure of the gas in the air or, more correctly, to the reduction in ambient oxygen partial pressure.[105] Cardiovascular and central nervous system complications of simple asphyxiants predominate, as they are the organ systems with the greatest oxygen requirements, but as hypoxemia becomes severe, multi-system organ failure and death may occur.[32]

Under most circumstances, however, carbon dioxide exchange is not impaired, and hypercapnia does not occur. Because dyspnea develops more rapidly from hypercapnia than hypoxemia, the breathlessness associated with physical asphyxiation does not develop until severe hypoxemia intervenes.[68,96] Thus, as likely occurred in the above case, victims may succumb to hypoxemia without the development of the expected warning symptoms.

Specific Agents

Noble Gases: Helium, Neon, Argon, Xenon.
Noble gases, stored almost exclusively in the compressed form, are employed in numerous industrial and medical roles. Argon is predominantly used as a shielding gas during welding operations, and neon is utilized in lighting manufacture. Xenon, in its radioactive gaseous form, finds diagnostic medical applications in ventilation–perfusion scans. Helium has the lowest molecular weight and is the smallest member of the noble gas family of elements. Because of its lower lipid solubility, helium is used by underwater divers to replace nitrogen to prevent nitrogen narcosis at depth (see Nitrogen). Even at diving gas mixtures of 50% helium, divers suffer no adverse effects as long as a normal partial pressure of oxygen is maintained in the mixture. The fact that helium has a lower density than nitrogen results in a lower viscosity, or a marked decrease in flow resistance. This property of helium is the basis for its use in patients with increased airway resistance, such as asthmatics, and also faciliitates breathing by divers at depth, where the volume of air inspired per breath is severalfold greater than that at sea level. Similarly, helium's low viscosity has led to its utilization as an inflation gas for an intraaortic balloon, where rapid inflation and deflation is critical. All noble gases, when compressed, form cryogenic liquids, which expand rapidly to their gas phase on decompression. The liberation of these agents in closed spaces may result in asphyxiation or freezing injuries. Xenon has unique anesthetic properties because of its high lipid solubility; the other noble gases have no direct toxicity.

Short-Chain Aliphatic Hydrocarbon Gases: Methane, Ethane, Propane, Butane.
Methane (CH_4) has no direct toxicity, and animals can breathe a mixture of 80% methane and 20% oxygen without manifesting hypoxic symptoms because their FIO_2, and thus their oxyhemoglobin saturation, is essentially normal. Methane, also known as natural gas and "swamp gas," may be present in high ambient concentrations in bogs of decaying organic matter. In addition, compressed natural gas is now employed as an alternative fuel for automotive use. Methane exposure is an occupational hazard for miners, who have historically carried canaries into their workplace as an "early warning" sign for the presence of toxic gases or oxygen deficiency. Theoretically, the higher metabolic and respiratory rates of small animals (and children) make them more rapidly susceptible to gas exposures.

Methane is odorless and undetectable without sophisticated equipment.[21] For this reason, natural gas is intentionally adulterated with a small concentration of ethyl mercaptan, a stenching agent, which is responsible for the well-recognized sulfur odor of natural gas. Cooking with natural gas may lead to increased respiratory symptoms and pulmonary dysfunction.[71] However, methane itself is unlikely to be the etiology because its combustion is generally complete, and ambient levels are negligible. It is likely that exposure to nitrogen dioxide, one of the products of methane's combustion in air (70% nitrogen), is the explanation for these symptoms.

Ethane (C_2H_6) is an odorless gas with similar characteristics to methane that is occasionally implicated as a simple asphyxiant. It is also a component of natural gas and is used as a refrigerant. Propane (C_3H_8) is widely used in compressed, liquefied form both as an industrial and domestic fuel and as an industrial solvent. Butane (C_4H_{10}) is also a prevalent fuel and solvent. Deliberate butane inhalational from cigarette lighters for recreational purposes is associated with myocardial infarction[4] and cerebral damage,[51] predominantly in adolescents (Chap. 86).

Carbon Dioxide (CO_2)
Introduction. Although not a simple asphyxiant gas by definition because it produces physiologic effects, carbon dioxide closely resembles simple asphyxiants from a toxicologic viewpoint. Carbon dioxide gas has many practical industrial uses such as the production of carbonation in soft drinks and use as a shielding gas during welding. Carbon dioxide is widely used as a fire extinguisher, the basis of which is its ability to safely displace oxygen from the local environment. Dry ice, the frozen form of carbon dioxide, is an extremely cold substance ($-78.5°C$, $-141.3°F$) that undergoes conversion from solid to gas without liquefaction, a process known as sublimation. Profound poisoning may occur when dry ice is allowed to sublimate in a closed space, such as the cabin of a car[154] or, as in our case, in a cold storage room at 4°C (39.2°F). The large-scale emission of carbon dioxide from Lake Nyos, a carbonated volcanic crater lake in Cameroon, West Africa, resulted in nearly 2000 human and many more livestock deaths (Chap. 2).[81] In this disaster, simple asphyxiation was likely because medical evaluation of both survivors and fatalities demonstrated neither signs of cutaneous or pulmonary irritation

TABLE 95–1. Clinical Findings Associated with a Reduction of Inspired Oxygen

FIO_2[a,b] (%)	Symptoms/Signs
16–12	Tachypnea, hyperpnea (resultant hypocapnia), tachycardia, reduced attention and alertness, euphoria, headache, mild incoordination
14–10	Altered judgment, incoordination, muscular fatigue, cyanosis
10–6	Nausea, vomiting, lethargy, air hunger, severe incoordination, coma
< 6	Gasping respiration, seizure, coma, death

[a]At sea level barometric pressure (760 mm Hg); appropriate adjustments must be made for altitude and depth exposures.
[b]Normal FIO_2 is 21%.

nor toxicologic abnormalities.[165] Furthermore, inadvertent connection of respirable gas hoses to carbon dioxide sources has occurred in both industrial[68] and medical[72] settings. This is, fortunately, uncommon because of the mandated use of engineering controls to prevent the incorrect connection of hose and source terminals.

Pharmacology/Pathophysiology. Carbon dioxide, an end-product of normal human metabolism, dissolves in the plasma and is in equilibrium with carbonic acid (H_2CO_3). Dissolved carbon dioxide, measured as the P_{CO_2}, is primarily responsible for our respiratory drive, and the P_{CO_2} is tightly controlled by the central nervous system through the regulation of breathing. For this reason, exogenous carbon dioxide, combined with oxygen, was used medically as a respiratory stimulant in neonates. Under normal conditions, ambient air contains approximately 0.03% CO_2. When ambient concentrations rise above this level, uptake of carbon dioxide occurs, which stimulates respiration further, increasing the uptake of ambient carbon dioxide. Accordingly, closed anesthesia systems use scrubbers containing sodium hydroxide to chemically eliminate exhaled carbon dioxide. Failure of the scrubber system results in increasing depth of anesthesia from hypercapnia-induced hyperventilation.

Clinical Manifestations. Carbon dioxide produces both acute and subacute poisoning syndromes. The latter occurs during hypoventilation, when a patient fails to eliminate endogenous carbon dioxide, develops hypercapnia, and typically presents with gradual somnolence. This may be linked to respiratory failure, as in the case of emphysema or opioid poisoning, or may be iatrogenic, as during permissive hypercapnia.[84] Alternatively, intense carbon dioxide exposure may produce rapid and lethal poisoning. However, unlike other simple asphyxiants, experimental models of acute carbon dioxide poisoning in which the FiO_2 has been maintained at normal levels demonstrate that central nervous and respiratory systems manifestations occur within seconds.[70] This suggests that CO_2 is not solely a simple asphyxiant but also possesses a potential for systemic effects.

Nitrogen (N₂) Gas

Introduction. Although nitrogen, like carbon dioxide, may produce clinical effects independently of hypoxemia, most poisonings are characterized by the manifestations of the simple asphyxiants. Nitrogen gas is used as a carrier gas for chromatography, as a fertilizer, as a cryogenic agent for surgery, and extensively in manufacturing. However, poisoning by nitrogen gas is uncommon but may occur following the rapid evaporation of the liquid.[78]

Clinical Manifestations. Inadvertent connection of air-line respirator hoses to nitrogen and other inert gas sources results in acute asphyxiation, with unconsciousness in about 12 seconds[68],[105, 152] and death shortly thereafter. More indolent inhalational poisoning by nitrogen is characterized by impairment of intellectual function and judgment, giddiness, and euphoria, with more severely poisoned patients manifesting lethargy or coma.[45] Systemic absorption is not rapid, however, and prolonged, high-level exposure is required for poisoning. Nitrogen poisoning, also known as nitrogen narcosis, occurs in underwater divers while breathing air, which contains 70% nitrogen. It has been called "rapture of the deep" (*l'ivresse des grandes profondeurs*) and has unfortunately led to many deaths in the subaquatic environment. The underlying

mechanism of nitrogen narcosis is unknown, but the simple structure and relatively high lipophilicity of nitrogen suggests a mechanism similar to that of the anesthetic gases.[7, 45] To avoid nitrogen narcosis, less lipid-soluble inert gases such as hydrogen or helium are generally substituted for nitrogen. Substitution with oxygen, although intuitively logical, is not acceptable because of the risk of oxygen toxicity (see oxygen).

Dermal exposure to liquid nitrogen produces frostbite because of its extremely cold temperature.[89] Rarely, bubbles introduced through the skin may embolize through the vascular system and impair organ blood flow.[41]

Treatment

Treatment for all patients poisoned by simple asphyxiants begins with immediate removal from exposure and ventilatory assistance. Provision of supplemental oxygen is preferable, but room air usually suffices; hyperbaric oxygen therapy is unnecessary. Restoration of oxygenation, through spontaneous or mechanical ventilation occurs after only several breaths. Support of vital functions is the mainstay of therapy but is generally unnecessary following a brief exposure.

PULMONARY IRRITANTS

Case 2 In an attempt to clean a grimy bathtub in a newly purchased house, a 37-year-old woman mixed several over-the-counter cleaning products inlcuding bleach and toilet bowl cleaner. Seconds after the mixture had been created, an acrid cloud of green-tinted gas filled the room. The woman was able to escape the fumes rapidly but quickly began feeling pain in her eyes and throat. She remained at home for a half an hour but her symptoms progressed. She arrived in the emergency department with significant dyspnea, cough, and diffuse chest discomfort.

Her vital signs were: BP 120/85 mm Hg, pulse 120 beats/min, respiratory rate 32 breaths/min, and oral temperature 99°F (37.2°C). A pulse oximeter revealed a saturation of 83% on room air, and she was placed on 2 L nasal oxygen. Pertinent findings on her physical examination included teary, red eyes with normal vision. Her oropharyngeal mucosa was unremarkable, although she was salivating. She had no stridor, hoarseness, or dysphagia. Her lung examination demonstrated bilateral rales, and her heart sounds were normal. An arterial blood gas measurement yielded pH 7.50, P_{CO_2} 25 mm Hg, and P_{O_2} 50 mm Hg on 2 L of oxygen by nasal cannula. She was placed on a non-rebreather oxygen face mask, and her oxygen saturation climbed to 94%. Her electrocardiogram showed sinus tachycardia. The portable chest radiograph showed significant bilateral alveolar filling with a normal-sized heart.

She received one dose of nebulized dilute sodium bicarbonate and several doses of albuterol and was admitted to the ICU for observation. Over the next 24 hours her symptoms and abnormal pulmonary findings resolved, and she was discharged. On followup at 2 weeks, she was asymptomatic with a normal physical examination.

Introduction

The irritant gases are a heterogeneous group of chemicals that produce toxic effects via a final common pathway: the destruction of the integrity of the mucosal barrier of the respiratory tract (Table 95–2).

TABLE 95–2. Characteristics of Common Respiratory Irritants

Gas	Source/Exposure	Detection Threshold (ppm)	STEL or Ceiling[a]	IDLH[b] (ppm)
Ammonia	Fertilizer, refrigeration, synthetic fiber synthesis	5	35	300
Cadmium oxide fumes	Welding	Odorless	NA	9 mg/m³ (as Cd)
Carbon dioxide	Exhaust, dry ice sublimation		30,000	40,000
Chlorine	Water disinfection, pulp and paper industry	0.3	1	10
Copper oxide fumes	Welding		NA	100 mg/m³ (as Cu)
Ethylene oxide	Sterilant		5	800
Formaldehyde	Chemical disinfection	0.8	2	20
Hydrogen chloride	Chemical	1–5	5	50
Hydrogen fluoride	Glass etching, semiconductor		6	30 (as F)
Hydrogen sulfide	Petroleum industry, sewer, manure pits	0.025	20	100
Mercury vapor	Electrical equipment; thermometers; catalyst; dental fillings; metal extraction; heating or vacuuming elemental mercury		0.1 mg/m³	10 mg/m³
Methyl bromide	Fumigant		20	250
Nickel carbonyl	Nickel purification, nickel coating, catalyst		NA	2 (as N)
Nitrogen dioxide	Chemical synthesis; combustion emission	0.12	5	20
Ozone	Disinfectant; produced by high-voltage electrical equipment	0.05	0.1	5
Phosgene	Chemical synthesis; combustion of chlorinated compounds	0.5	0.2	2
Phosphine	Fumigant; semiconductors	2	1	50
Propane	Liquefied propane gas	Odorless		2,100
Sulfur dioxide	Environmental exhaust	1	5	100
Zinc chloride fumes	Artificial smoke (outdated)		2 mg/m³	50 mg/m³
Zinc oxide fumes	Welding	Odorless	10 mg/m³	500 mg/m³

[a]Short-term exposure limits or ceiling, given as OSHA PELs (if available) or NIOSH RELs
[b]Immediately dangerous to life and health: NIOSH, revised 1995 (documentation for each IDLH is available at *http://www.cdc.gov/niosh/idlh/idlhintr.html.*)
From: NIOSH Pocket Guide to Chemical Hazards; on-line version at http://www.cdc.gov/niosh/npg/pgdstart.html.

Pathophysiology

Pathologically, irritant chemicals damage both the more prevalent type I pneumocytes and the surfactant-producing type II pneumocytes.[85] Neutrophil influx, recruited in response to macrophage-derived inflammatory cytokines such as tumor necrosis factor-α, releases toxic mediators that disrupt the integrity of the capillary endothelial cells.[99,132] This host defense reponse results in accumulation of cellular debris and plasma exudate in the alveolar sacs, producing the characteristic clinical findings of acute lung injury (ALI; see below). Interestingly, the specific mechanisms by which the irritant gases damage the pulmonary endothelial and epithelial cells vary. Many irritant gases require dissolution in the lung water to liberate the ultimate toxicant, which is often an acid, as occurs when hydrogen chloride gas produces hydrochloric acid. The exact mechanism by which acids damage cells and induce an inflammatory response remains uncertain. Oxidation of intracellular proteins may result in rapid cytoskeletal shortening creating spaces between endothelial cells and allowing fluid movement into the alveolar spaces.[158] Other gases, such as oxygen, induce pulmonary damage solely through free-radical-mediated oxidative stress on the cellular membranes. Several gases, of which nitrogen dioxide and chlorine are characteristic, produce both acid and free radical oxidants. Furthermore, other respirable poisons, such as metals, induce respiratory tract effects through these and other mechanisms. Because the precise toxicologic and pathophysiologic effects vary widely depending on the physicochemical properties of the toxin, these are covered more completely in the discussions of the specific agents.

By virtue of its use as a war agent, phosgene has received more investigation than most other acid-forming irritant gases. In fact, much of our current understanding of irritant gas poisoning derives from the study of phosgene toxicity. Although the specific mechanisms of toxicity of the other acid-forming agents remains poorly defined, it is likely that they injure through a similar process. The liberated acids react with functional groups on epithelial and endothelial cell membranes and, via cellular messengers, result in a complex systemic inflammatory response. Phosgene stimulates the synthesis of lipoxygenase-derived leukotrienes. Leukotrienes are important chemotactic factors for neutrophils, which accumulate, liberate oxidants, and produce acute lung injury (ALI).[69] Acute lung injury may be prevented in rabbits by tomelukast, a leukotriene receptor antagonist,[56] and by methylprednisolone, which blocks leukotriene synthesis, although neither agent offers post-exposure benefit.[56] Ibuprofen, an inhibitor of the arachidonic acid cascade, and agents capable of reducing neutrophil influx, such as colchicine and cyclophosphamide, reduce lung injury and mortality in mice when administered shortly following phosgene exposure.[50,145] Intratracheal DBcAMP, a cAMP analogue, and other cAMP amplifiers, such as terbutaline or aminophylline, inhibit the release of leukotrienes and reduce toxicity.[77,146] Intratracheal *N*-acetylcysteine (NAC), administered 45 minutes post-exposure to phosgene-poisoned rabbits, decreases the formation of leukotrienes by an undefined means and limits the development of pulmonary edema.[144] Presumably administration via nebulization would prove similarly effective. Intravenous administration of NAC to patients with mild to moderate ALI, none of whom had phosgene-induced pulmonary damage, improved systemic oxygenation and reduced the need for ventilatory support.[153] However, the progression to pulmonary failure was not altered. Because damage to the lung had already occurred, the observed benefit of NAC may be related to improved hemodynamic function rather than an antioxidant effect.[59] (see Antidotes in Depth: *N*-Acetylcysteine)

Free radicals are highly reactive molecular derivatives, typically from oxygen or nitrogen, that bind to and destroy tissue near their site of generation. Through the initiation of a lipid peroxidative cascade, free radicals destroy lipid membranes and inhibit energy production through the electron transport chain (Chap. 12). Products of lipid peroxidation and cellular damage initiate neutrophilic influx, presumably in an immunologic attempt to combat a pathogen. Ironically, free radicals generated by the invading inflammatory cells contribute to the pulmonary damage. Fortunately, the lung has antioxidant systems, both enzymatic (eg, superoxide dismutase, glutathione peroxidase, catalase) and nonenzymatic (eg, glutathione, ascorbate), that detoxify virtually all free radicals present in the lung.[126] However, the oxidant burden imposed by oxidant gases can overwhelm these detoxifying systems and produce cellular damage.

Clinical Manifestations

Regardless of the mechanism by which the mucosa is damaged, the clinical presentations of patients exposed to irritant gases are similar. Those exposed to agents that result in irritation within seconds generally develop mucosal injury limited to the upper respiratory tract. The rapid onset of symptoms is usually a sufficient signal to escape the exposure. Patients may present with oral, nasal, and pharyngeal pain in addition to drooling, mucosal edema, cough, or stridor.[156] Conjunctival irritation or chemosis, as well as dermatologic irritation, is often noted because concomitant ocular and cutaneous exposure to the gaseous agent is usually unavoidable. Agents that are less rapidly irritating may not provide an adequate signal of their presence and not prompt expeditious escape. Prolonged breathing thus allows entry of the toxic gas further into the bronchopulmonary system, where delayed toxic effects may subsequently be noted. Tracheobronchitis, bronchiolitis, bronchospasm, and pulmonary edema are typical inflammatory responses of this anatomic region and represent the spectrum of acute lower respiratory tract injury.

Experimental models assessing the water solubility of a gas to predict the location of its associated lesions have largely agreed with the clinical data.[79] Exceptions to this relationship of an agent and its expected toxicity are, however, common. For example, in situations where escape from ongoing exposure is prevented, patients may develop lower respiratory tract injury following prolonged exposure to acutely irritating gases. Alternatively, rapid onset of upper respiratory irritation may be noted in patients following exposure to concentrated agents that are generally associated with delayed symptomatology. Exposure to exceedingly high concentrations of any gas may produce hypoxemia analogous to that resulting from exposure to a simple asphyxiant gas.

The most characteristic and worrisome clinical manifestation of irritant gas exposure is "acute lung injury," a syndrome formerly described as non-cardiogenic pulmonary edema.[8] ALI consists of the clinical, radiographic, and physiologic abnormalities caused by pulmonary inflammation and alveolar filling that must be both acute in onset and not attributable solely to pulmonary capillary hypertension as occurs in patients with congestive heart failure.[8] The most severe manifestation of ALI is the acute respiratory distress syndrome (ARDS). The criteria for the diagnosis of ARDS is based on the ratio of the partial pressure of dissolved oxygen (PaO_2) to the inspired oxygen fraction (FIO_2).[8] That is, patients with an appropriate history and clinical presentation for ALI with a PaO_2/FIO_2 ratio < 200 meet the definition of ARDS. Importantly, positive end-expiratory pressure (PEEP) is not part of the oxygenation criteria (Chap. 20). Both ALI and ARDS are nonspecific syndromes resulting from diverse physiologic insults such as sepsis or trauma. Patients with ALI may present with dyspnea, chest tightness, chest pain, cough, frothy sputum, wheezing or rales, and arterial hypoxemia. Typical radiographic abnormalities include bilateral pulmonary infiltrates with an alveolar filling pattern and a normal cardiac silhouette differentiating this syndrome from congestive heart failure.

Specific Agents

Acid- or Base-Forming Gases

Highly Water-Soluble Agents

Ammonia (NH_3). Ammonia is a common industrial and household chemical used in the synthesis of plastics and explosives, as a fertilizer, a refrigerant, and a cleaning agent. The odor is characteristic and may effectively act as a warning of exposure and stimulus to avoid further exposure. Its dissolution in water to form ammonium hydroxide (NH_4OH), a base, rapidly produces severe upper airway irritation. Patients with exposures to highly concentrated gas or exposure for prolonged duration may develop tracheobronchial or pulmonary inflammation. Experimental inhalation of nebulized high-dose ammonia causes ALI manifested by a fall in oxygen saturation and a rise in airway pressure within 2 minutes of initiation.[149] Corroborating this, when a bomb fragment pierced an ammonia-carrying condenser pipe in a converted brewery cellar serving as a World War II bomb shelter, those patients closest to the source suffered ALI with a mortality rate of 63%.[22]

Chloramines. This series of chlorinated nitrogenous compounds (Fig. 95–1) includes monochloramine (NH_2Cl) and dichloramine ($NHCl_2$). The chloramines are most commonly generated by the admixture of ammonia with sodium hypochlorite (NaOCl) bleach, often in an inappropriate effort to potentiate the individual cleaning powers.[46,119] Interestingly, the addition of bleach to septic systems may result in liberation of the chloramines following its reaction with urinary nitrogenous compounds.[106] On dissolution of the chloramines in the epithelial lining fluid, hypochlorous acid, ammonia, and oxygen-radicals are generated, all of which act as

A. $3NaOCl^- + 2NH_3 \rightarrow NH_2Cl + NHCl_2 + 3NaOH$

B. $NH_2Cl + H_2O \rightarrow HOCl + NH_3 \uparrow$

         $HOCl \rightarrow HCl + \{O\}$

Figure 95–1. Chloramine chemistry. **A.** Sodium hypochlorite (bleach) plus ammonia form mono- and dichloramine. **B.** Chloramine dissolves in water to liberate hypochlorous acid, hydrochloric acid, ammonia, and nascent oxygen, an oxidant.

irritants. Although less water soluble than ammonia, the chloramines typically promptly result in symptoms. Because these initial symptoms are often mild, however, they may not prompt immediate escape, resulting in prolonged or recurrent exposure.[133]

Hydrogen Chloride (HCl). The largest and most important use of hydrogen chloride gas is in the production of hydrochloric acid. Dissolution of hydrogen chloride gas in lung water after inhalation similarly produces hydrochloric acid.[19,125] Pyrolysis of polyvinylchloride, a plastic commonly used in pipe fabrication, generates HCl and is an occupational hazard of firefighters.[117] By adsorbing to respirable carbonaceous particles generated in the fire, HCl may be deposited at the alveolar level and produce pulmonary toxicity.

Hydrogen Fluoride (HF). Hydrogen fluoride and its aqueous form, hydrofluoric acid, are used in the gasoline, glassware, building renovation, and semiconductor industry. Hydrogen fluoride gas dissolves in epithelial lining fluid to form a weak acid, hydrofluoric acid. The intact HF molecule is the predominant form in solution, and few free hydronium ions are liberated. Low-dose inhalational exposures may result in irritant symptoms,[171] and large exposures may cause bronchial and pulmonary parenchymal destruction.[16] Death following inhalation may be from acute lung injury but is usually related to systemic fluoride poisoning independent of the route of exposure because of calcium binding and subsequent hypocalcemia and hyperkalemia.[167]

Patients with inhalational exposure to hydrogen fluoride should have frequent electrocardiographic evaluations and correction of serum electrolytes. The administration of nebulized 2.5% calcium gluconate should be considered in order to limit systemic fluoride absorption (made as 1.5 mL 10% calcium gluconate + 4.5 mL normal saline or water).[87] Nebulized calcium, by binding fluoride ion locally, may prevent fluoride-induced cellular and systemic toxicity. Systemic calcium salts should be administered as needed to correct hypocalcemia (Chap. 87 and Antidote in Depth: Calcium).

Sulfur Dioxide/Sulfuric Acid (SO_2/H_2SO_4). Sulfur dioxide has multiple industrial applications and is a by-product found in smelting and oil refining. It may also be generated by the inadvertent mixing of chemicals, such as an acid with sodium bisulfite ($NaHSO_3$). Sulfur dioxide is highly water soluble and has a characteristic pungent odor that provides warning of its presence at concentrations well below those that are irritating. In the presence of catalytic metals (Fe, Mn), environmental sulfur dioxide is readily converted to sulfurous acid, H_2SO_3, within water droplets. Atmospheric sulfur dioxide and H_2SO_4 have severe health consequences; during the London Fog incident in 1952, 4000 deaths occurred primarily from respiratory causes.[93] Exposure to atmospheric sulfur dioxide results in a dose-related bronchospasm, which is most pronounced and difficult to treat in asthmatic patients and the likely cause of death during the London Fog. Sulfurous acid is a major environmental concern and the cause of "acid rain." Inhalation of sulfurous acid or dissolution of sulfur dioxide in epithelial lining fluid produces typical pathologic and clinical findings associated with ALI.[134] Large acute exposure to either produces the expected acute irritant response of both the upper and lower respiratory tract,[24] and pulmonary dysfunction (see RADS reactive airways dysfunction syndrome) may persist for several years.[127]

Intermediate Water-Soluble Agents

Chlorine (Cl_2). Chlorine gas is a valuable oxidizing agent with varied industrial uses, and occupational exposure is common. Chlorine gas was used by both the French and the Germans in World War I as a chemical warfare agent (Chap. 100).[42] Although chlorine gas is not generally available for use in the home, domestic exposure to chlorine gas is common. The admixture of an acid to household bleach (ie, sodium hypochlorite) liberates chlorine gas (Fig. 95–2).[60] Because the anionic component of the acid is not involved in the reaction, combining hypochlorite with virtually any acid, such as phosphoric, hydrochloric, or sulfuric acid, may result in the release of chlorine gas. As such, inappropriate mixing of cleaning agents is the cause of most non-occupational exposures.[112] Rare patients have intentionally generated chlorine gas in this manner for purportedly "pleasurable" purposes.[128] Concentrated chlorine gas may be generated when aging swimming pool chlorination tablets, such as calcium hypochlorite [$Ca(OCl)_2$] or trichloro-*s*-triazinetrione (TST), decompose.[97,173] Furthermore, the inadvertent mixture of $Ca(OCl)_2$ and TST results in excessive chlorine gas generation and may be explosive.[97] Acute Cl_2 toxicity may occur when compressed chlorine gas is used for the direct chlorination of public swimming pools[164] or drinking water systems.[44] Occasional mass poisoning may occur during industrial or transportation incidents.[74]

The odor threshold for Cl_2 is low, but it may be difficult to distinguish toxic from permissible air levels until toxicity is manifest. The intermediate solubility characteristics of Cl_2 result in only mild initial symptoms following moderate exposure and permit a substantial time delay, typically several hours, before the development of clinical symptoms. chlorine dissolution in the lung water generates HCl and hypochlorous (HClO) acids. The hypochlorous acid rapidly degenerates into HCl and nascent oxygen (O^-). The unpaired nascent oxygen atom produces additional pulmonary damage by initiating a free-radical oxidative cascade. Although the majority of life-threatening Cl_2 poisonings follow acute, large exposures, chronic low-level exposure or sequential moderate poisonings are associated with increased bronchial responsiveness.[49,124]

Hydrogen sulfide (H_2S). Hydrogen sulfide exposures occur most frequently in the petroleum-refining industry,[20] although poisoning occurs in asphalt, synthetic rubber, and nylon industries workers and rarely in hospital workers using acid to clean drains clogged with plaster of paris sludge.[122] Hydrogen sulfide is present in natural sources such as volcanic emission, in caves, and in sulfur springs, and it is also a decay product of organic material found in sewers or manure pits.[118] Hydrogen sulfide, as well as hydrogen fluoride and phosphine, are differentiated from the other irritant gases by their abilities to produce significant systemic toxicity. Hydrogen sulfide inhibits mitochondrial respiration in a fashion similar to that of cyanide (Chap. 98).

$$\text{A} \quad HCl + HOCl \rightarrow Cl_2[\uparrow] + H_2O$$
$$\text{B} \quad Cl_2 + H_2O \rightarrow 2HCl + \{O\}$$
$$Cl_2 + H_2O \rightarrow HCl + HOCl$$

Figure 95–2. Chlorine chemistry. **A.** Formation of chlorine gas from the acidification of hypochlorite (bleach). **B.** Dissolution of chlorine in mucosal water to generate both hydrochloric and hypochlorous acids (HCl and HOCl) and oxidants {O}.

H_2S has the distinctive odor of "rotten eggs," which, although helpful in diagnosis, is not specific for this agent. Despite a sensitive odor threshold of several parts per billion,[131] rapid olfactory fatigue ensues, providing a misperception that the exposure and its attendant risk have diminished. At low and moderate levels (up to 500 ppm), upper respiratory tract mucosal irritation occurs and is the principal toxicity.[155] In a large series of acutely exposed patients ALI was evident in 20%.[20] The rapidity of the occurrence of death in patients exposed to high levels of H_2S makes it likely that either simple asphyxiation or cytochrome oxidase inhibition is causal in most cases. In the aforementioned series of sulfide poisonings, 10 of the 14 deaths occurred before arrival at the hospital.[20]

Poorly Water-Soluble Agents

Phosgene (Carbonyl Chloride, $COCl_2$).[42] During World War I, phosgene was an important weapon of mass destruction that produced countless deaths (Chap. 100). Currently, phosgene is employed in the synthesis of various organic compounds, such as isocyanates, and it occasionally produces poisoning. It is also a by-product of heating or combustion of various chlorinated organic compounds.[150]

Exposure to phosgene may initially produce limited manifestations but can result in acute mucosal irritation following intense exposure. In fact, the pleasant odor of fresh hay, rather than prompting escape, may ironically promote deep and prolonged breathing of the toxic gas. The most consequential clinical effect related to phosgene exposure is delayed-onset ALI. Because of the accumulation of a significant alveolar burden of phosgene, symptoms are generally severe once they occur. The delay in onset may be nearly a day, so prolonged observation of patients thought to be phosgene poisoned is warranted. The mechanism of phosgene toxicity is dependent on the dissolution of the gas into the epithelial lining fluid with the resultant liberation of hydrochloric acid and reactive oxygen species.

Oxidant Gases. Rather than acidic or alkaline metabolites, free radicals mediate the pulmonary toxicity of certain irritant gases. However, the clinical distinction between acid- or alkali-forming agents and oxidant gases is quite difficult, although it may ultimately prove therapeutically relevant.

Oxygen (O_2). Oxygen toxicity is uncommon in the workplace but, ironically, is common in hospitalized patients. Although O_2 may produce central nervous system and retinal toxicity, pulmonary damage is more common. On the basis of several clinical studies, it appears that humans can tolerate 100% O_2 at sea level for up to 48 hours without significant acute pulmonary damage.[35] Under hyperbaric conditions (2.0 atmospheres absolute), such as during compressed-air diving or while inside a pressurized hyperbaric chamber, oxygen toxicity may develop within 3–6 hours.[27] Delayed pulmonary fibrosis, presumably from healing of subclinical injury, may develop, however, in patients breathing lower concentrations of O_2 at sea level for shorter periods of time.[28]

Although it may appear paradoxical that O_2, an essential molecule, may be deleterious at elevated concentrations, it is not. In mitochondria, O_2 plays a critical role as the ultimate acceptor for electrons completing the electron transport chain. It is this same potent oxidizing activity that allows O_2 to remove electrons from other compounds generating the reactive oxygen intermediates.[142]

Generation of reactive oxygen species, including superoxide (O_2^-), hydroxyl radical (OH·), hydrogen peroxide (HOOH), and singlet oxygen (O·),[140,142] produces cellular necrosis[76] and increases pulmonary capillary permeability.[170] Experimental prevention of these effects by the administration of either parenteral NAC,[143] a chemical antioxidant, or superoxide dismutase, an enzymatic antioxidant,[160,172] suggests that the mechanism of toxicity relates to the oxidant, or electrophilic, effects of these reactive oxygen species (Chap. 12). Although several other agents have shown promise in preventing oxygen-mediated toxicity, none has yet proven to be therapeutic for patients already manifesting pulmonary toxicity. In the future, magnetic resonance imaging enhanced by a gadolinium derivative[15] or the measurement of urinary *o*-tyrosine, a marker for hydroxyl radical generation,[94] may allow early diagnosis and quantitation of endothelium damage in patients at risk for iatrogenic pulmonary oxygen toxicity. These techniques may ultimately prove useful for patients exposed to other pulmonary irritants and may help guide the evaluation of potential therapeutic modalities. Currently, techniques to prevent pulmonary oxygen toxicity emphasize reduction of the inspired oxygen concentration with the use of positive end–expiratory pressure ventilation, although this approach failed to prove beneficial in at least one clinical trial.[121]

Oxides of Nitrogen (NO_x). Oxides of nitrogen are a series of variably oxidized nitrogenous compounds.[47] The most important substances included in this series are the stable free radicals nitrogen dioxide (NO_2), and nitric oxide (NO) as well as nitrogen tetroxide (dinitrogen tetroxide, N_2O_4), nitrogen trioxide (N_2O_3), and nitrous oxide (N_2O). The oxides of nitrogen have limited value in industrial operations, although they may be generated during welding and brazing. NO_2, in addition to hydrogen cyanide, is produced in the pyrolysis of nitrocellulose, which is a substantial component of radiographic film. For example, fire in the radiology department of the Cleveland Clinic in 1929 resulted in 125 casualties, virtually all of whom died of cyanide or nitrogen dioxide gas poisoning.[53] Nitrogen dioxide toxicity can occur when the gas is generated by the propane-driven ice-cleaning machines used in indoor ice skating rinks with poor ventilation.[90] Military exposure to high levels of NO_2 may occur during closed-space fires, as in submarines.[98] Nitrogen dioxide is also the cause of "Silo-filler's disease," in which the toxic gas generated during the decomposition of silage accumulates within the silo shortly after grain storage[39] (Chap. 111). Before ventilation, such high concentrations may accumulate in the silo that entrance produces asphyxiation from the depletion of oxygen. Additionally, substantial quantities of NO_2 remaining after incomplete ventilation may produce the delayed-onset pulmonary toxicity characteristic of the silo filler's disease. Chronic indoor exposure to NO_2,[71] generated during cooking, or outdoor exposure to photochemical smog,[141] of which the oxides of nitrogen are a component, may predispose to the development or exacerbation of chronic lung diseases.[161]

The various oxides of nitrogen may directly oxidize respiratory tract cellular membranes but more typically generate reactive nitrogen intermediates, or radicals, such as peroxynitrite ($ONOO^-$) which subsequently damage the pulmonary epithelial cells.[163] In addition to generating oxidant cascades, dissolution in the respiratory tract water generates nitric acid (HNO_3) and nitric oxide (NO), which produce injury consistent with other inhaled acids. In fact, inhalation of HNO_3 produces the same clinical syndrome.[57] Antioxidants afford significant protection to human endothelial cells exposed to NO_2, implying an important role for free radicals in the toxicology of these agents.[159]

Nitric oxide, an endogenous compound important as a neurotransmitter and vasorelaxant, is used clinically as exogenous inhalational therapy for pulmonary hypertension and ALI. In patients with ARDS, low-level inhaled nitric oxide (~60 ppb) improves oxygenation[137] but has not yet been demonstrated to improve outcome.[33] Nitric oxide is less soluble in the epithelial lining fluid than the other oxides of nitrogen and, although protective at low dose, produces irritant effects following large exposures.[169] Its pulmonary oxidative toxicity, the manifestations of which are typical of the oxidant gases, is substantially enhanced by conversion to reactive nitrogen intermediates such as $ONOO^-$.[6] This radical selectively interacts with tyrosine to produce nitrotyrosine, which may subsequently serve as a marker for oxidant damage.[58] Nitric oxide may be absorbed from the lung and is rapidly bound by hemoglobin to form nitrosylhemoglobin (NOHb) and subsequently methemoglobin.

Ozone (O_3).   Ozone is abundant in the stratospheric region found between 5–31 miles above the planet. Ozone is formed by the action of ultraviolet light on oxygen molecules and thus reduces the amount of solar ultraviolet irradiation reaching Earth.[88] The high ozone concentration at this altitude may occasionally cause symptoms in occupants of high flying planes.[130] Ozone is another important component of photochemical smog and, as such, contributes to chronic lung disease.[91] It is produced in significant quantities by welding and high-voltage electrical equipment and in more moderate doses by photocopying machines and laser printers. Because of its high electronegativity (only fluorine is higher), ozone is one of the most potent oxidizing agents available. For this reason it is used as a bleaching agent, particularly as an alternative to chlorine in water purification and sewage treatment.

The pulmonary toxicity associated with ozone is primarily a result of its high reactivity toward unsaturated fatty acids and amino acids with a sulfhydryl functional group.[162] Ozonation and free radical damage to the lipid component of the membrane initiates an inflammatory cascade, with resultant influx of inflammatory cells.[82,132] Increased permeability of the pulmonary epithelium results in alveolar filling from the transudation of proteins and fluids characteristic of acute lung injury. Antioxidant agents, such as vitamin E, that react preferentially with free radicals before membrane damage occurs prevent or limit the pulmonary toxicity of ozone.[135]

Miscellaneous Irritant Gases

Methylisocyanate.   Methylisocyanate (MIC, Fig. 95–3) is one of a series of compounds sharing a similar isocyanate (N=C=O) moiety. Toluene diisocyanate (TDI) and diphenylmethane diisocyanate (MDI) are important chemicals in the polymer industry. In Bhopal, India in 1984, an inadvertent release of MIC resulted in immediate and persistent respiratory symptoms[75] in approximately 200,000 local inhabitants with approximately 2500 deaths.[104] ALI was evident both clinically[107] and radiographically. MIC is a significantly more potent respiratory irritant than the other regularly

used isocyanate derivatives[43] such as TDI (see occupational asthma). Cyanide poisoning does not occur, and empiric antidotal therapy is not indicated.

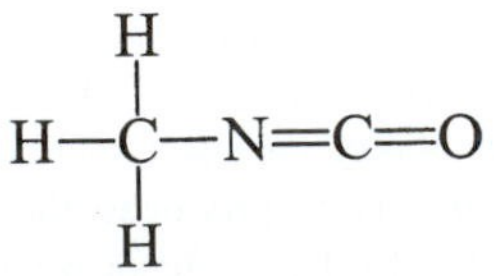

Riot Control Agents: Capsaicin, CS, and CN.   Historically, riot control agents (Fig. 95–4), or Mace, consisted primarily of chloroacetophenone (CN) or chlorobenzylidenemalononitrile (CS). Both are white solids that are dispersed as an aerosol. This is generally accomplished through mixture with a pyrotechnic agent as a grenade or with a volatile organic solvent in a personal protection canister. Because the delivery systems of these agents are both of limited sophistication and subject to prevailing environmental conditions, dosing is unpredictable, and unintended self-poisoning common. After low-level exposure, ocular discomfort and lacrimation alone are expected, accounting for their common appellation: "tear gas." The effects are transient, and complete recovery is typical within 30 minutes, although long-lasting pulmonary effects may occur[138] (see Asthma and Reactive Airways Dysfunction Syndrome, RADS). Closed-space or close-range exposure may produce significant ocular toxicity,[52] dermal burns, laryngospasm, ALI, or death. Because of their high potential for severe toxicity, CN and CS were replaced for civilian use by oleoresin capsicum, also known as pepper spray or pepper mace. Although capsaicin, its active component, is considerably less toxic, pneumonitis[10] and death,[151] unfortunately, still occur.

These riot control agents invoke the release of substance P, a neuropeptide involved with the transmission of pain impulses.[66] Substance P also induces neurogenic inflammation, which, in the lung, results in pulmonary edema and bronchoconstriction (see section on RADS). In addition, the severe pulmonary toxicity of CS and CN is likely related to their ability to alkylate tissues in a manner similar to mustard agents.[30]

Current therapy for inhalation of capsaicin, or of any tear gas, is primarily supportive. Extracorporeal membrane oxygenation has been utilized in children to maintain oxygenation in the presence of severe pulmonary toxicity.[10] Substance P antagonists,

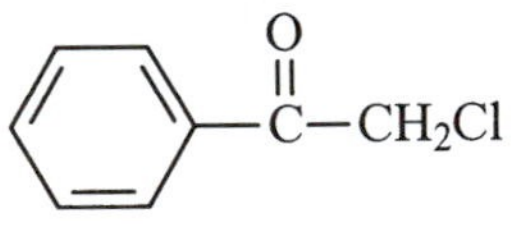

Choroacetophenone, CN

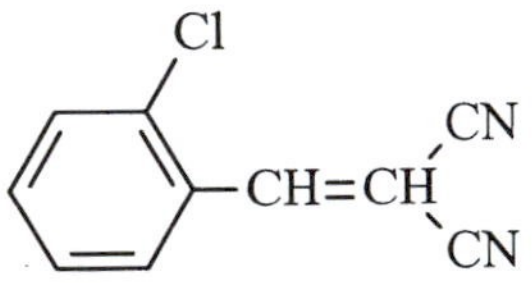

Chlorobenzylidenemalononitrile, CS

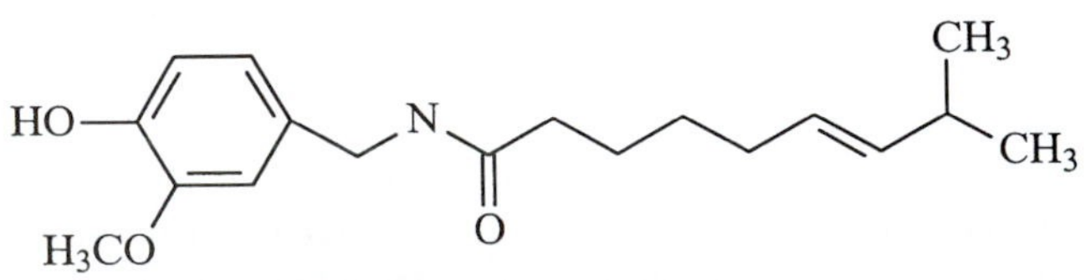

Capsaicin, OC

Figure 95–4.   Riot control agents.

Figure 95–3.   Methylisocyanate.

which are currently not available for clinical use, show promise in experimental models.[113]

Metal Pneumonitis. Acute inhalational exposures to certain metal compounds produce clinical effects identical to the aforementioned chemical irritants. For example, zinc chloride ($ZnCl_2$) fume[64] was formerly used as artificial smoke because of its dense white character and an aqueous solution is still used as a soldering flux. Cadmium oxide (CdO) is generated during the burning of cadmium metal in an oxygen-containing environment as occurs during smelting or welding. The refining of nickel using carbon monoxide (Mond process) produces nickel carbonyl [$Ni(CO)_4$], a volatile pulmonary oxidant.[147] Inhalation of volatilized elemental mercury,[109] which occurs during the vaccuuming of mercury spills or home extracting of precious metals, may be noxious. Although at sufficient concentration many of these metal exposures produce warning symptoms, severe toxicity may occur even at undetectable concentrations. The mechanism of toxicity may relate to overwhelming oxidant stress or inactivation of natural antioxidant systems.[174] Patients with metal-induced pneumonitis present with chest tightness, cough, fever, and signs consistent with ALI. Metal pneumonitis is distinguishable from other causes of ALI only by history or, retrospectively, by finding elevated serum or urine metal levels.[3] In particular, metal pneumonitis should be differentiated from the more common and substantially less consequential metal fume fever (see below). In addition to standard supportive measures, patients with acute metal-induced pneumonitis should be hospitalized and receive corticosteroids. Chelation therapy has no documented benefit for the treatment of ALI but should be used based on conventional indications. Nebulized NAC may potentially act as both an antioxidant and a chelator, but documentation of any beneficial effect remains elusive.[92]

Management

Standard and Supportive Measures.
Management of patients with acute respiratory tract injury begins with meticulous support of airway patency, bronchial and pulmonary secretions, and oxygenation. Although various theoretical and experimental treatment modalities have been proposed, supportive care remains the mainstay of therapy. Supplemental oxygen, bronchodilators, and airway suctioning should be used if clinically indicated. Nitrovasodilators, diuretics, and morphine have little role in the management of ARDS, although low-dose morphine may prove beneficial as an anxiolytic agent.[123] Corticosteroid therapy, designed to reduce the inflammatory host defense response, frequently improves surrogate markers of pulmonary damage[101,102] such as oxygenation status but generally offers little outcome enhancement in patients with ARDS.[9] Importantly, most studies of ARDS involve predominantly septic or traumatized patients, with few patients suffering from inhalational poisoning. Because the inflammatory response initiated by bacterial endotoxin differs from that caused by irritant gases,[86] the applicability of these studies to the treatment of poisoned individuals is limited. There is an interesting report of simultaneous, equivalent chlorine exposure in two sisters with improved outcome in the sister who received steroid treatment.[25] Most available research evaluates parenterally administered corticosteroid, although a single animal model demonstrates a beneficial effect of nebulized beclomethasone following acute chlorine poisoning.[55] However, a human pretreatment model of inhaled budesonide fails to document a substantive alteration of the effects

of ozone inhalation.[115] Additionally, ketoconazole, an antifungal with antiinflammatory effects,[2] and nonsteroidal antiinflammatory agents, such as ibuprofen,[145] variably improve experimental lung function or mortality in patients with acute lung injury of various non-toxicological etiologies and have little current role in the therapeutic armamentarium. Furthermore, most of the aforementioned studies assess acute outcome and not long-term effects in survivors. Because corticosteroids experimentally reduce the late fibroproliferative phase during lung recovery, they may ultimately prove beneficial.[100] Overall, there is little reason to suspect any specific benefit of corticosteroids and other antiinflammatory agents in most poisoned patients. However, because most studies demonstrate some benefit and little identifiable risk, corticosteroid use appropriately remains routine and based largely on local practices.

The clinical similarities among patients with irritant gas exposure and other etiologies of acute lung injury suggest that similar management principles should be applied. Positive end-expiratory pressure (PEEP) and inverse-ratio ventilation are successful in enhancing the oxygenation of patients with ARDS of various etiologies.[110] Lower-tidal-volume mechanical ventilation, using 6 mL/kg and plateau pressures of 30 cm of water, produced lower mortality and less need for mechanical ventilation than traditional volume ventilation with 12 mL/kg.[1] Although not specifically evaluated in any of these studies, there are sound theoretical reasons to believe that all of these modalities should improve oxygenation in poisoned patients as well.[129] Although it is always important to reduce the inspired concentration of oxygen to below 50% as rapidly as possible, patients poisoned by irritant gases may be even more susceptible to oxygen toxicity as a result of depletion of endogenous antioxidant barriers.[120]

Neutralization Therapy.
A therapy unique to several of the acid- or base-forming irritant gases is chemical neutralization. Although contraindicated in acid or alkali injury of the gastrointestinal tract, the large surface area of the lung and the relatively small amount of toxin present allow dissipation of the heat and gas generated during neutralization. Case studies suggest that nebulized 2% sodium bicarbonate may be beneficial in patients poisoned by acid-forming irritant gases.[164] The vast majority of these cases involve chlorine gas exposure, and most patients received other symptomatic therapies as well.[13] Although there appears to be no specific benefit for patients exposed to chloramine, nebulized bicarbonate therapy appears to be safe.[119] It is important to note that an adequately controlled, prospective evaluation of bicarbonate therapy in poisoned patients for either safety or efficacy has not yet been attempted. Any sodium bicarbonate solution utilized should be sufficiently diluted to prevent irritation. Typically, 1 mL of 7.5% or 8.4% sodium bicarbonate solution is added to 3 mL of sterile water (resulting in an approximately 2% solution for nebulization).

In addition, it remains uncertain whether nebulized sodium bicarbonate therapy alters the natural course of irritant-induced pulmonary damage. The fact that many irritants produce concomitant oxidant injury suggests that it may not. Nebulized 4% sodium bicarbonate administered to chlorine-poisoned sheep improved oxygenation but failed to decrease mortality rates.[26] Therefore, patients receiving nebulized bicarbonate therapy require observation beyond the time of symptom resolution. Neutralizing agents, such as Tris buffer (trishydroxymethylaminomethane, THAM) and methenamine (hexamethylenetetramine, HMT) are no longer utilized, although there are indications that they may be efficacious.[37] Because the administration of neutralizing agents for alkaline irritants such as ammonia, has not been attempted, they should not be utilized at this time.

Antioxidants. Antioxidant agents include reducing agents, such as NAC, free-radical scavengers, such as vitamin E, and enzymes, such as superoxide dismutase. Although the concept of treating pulmonary oxidant stress with antioxidants or free-radical scavangers is intriguing, most currently available evidence suggests that these agents offer negligible benefit.[108] The rapid onset of the self-perpetuating destructive effects initiated by redox reactions may hinder any post-exposure therapy. This interpretation is supported by pretreatment models in which antioxidants are effective at preventing or at least limiting the pathologic effects. Utilization of these and other newer agents targeted against inflammatory mediators or the oxidative cascade are in the earliest investigative stages.

Advanced Pharmacological Therapy

Perfluorocarbon Partial Liquid Ventilation Partial liquid ventilation involves the intrapulmonary adminstration of perfluorocarbons, which are inert liquids with low surface tension and excellent oxgyen-carrying capacity. Studies in patients with non—chemically -induced ARDS suggest that exfoliated tissue, and presumably persistent toxin, may be effectively lavaged from the bronchopulmonary tree by this method.[63] This approach may ultimately prove important because bronchopulmonary decontamination is otherwise anatomically difficult. In addition, partial liquid ventilation improves oxygenation in experimental models [31,62] as well as in humans with ARDS.[62] Perfluorocarbons, administered intravenously as hemoglobin substitutes, are eliminated via the lungs. Following acid aspiration, systemic perfluorocarbons attenuate lung injury through an undefined, though probably immunomodulatory, mechanism.[114] In the future this may prove to be a highly useful therapy, but, because of its limited availablity and high cost, it is currently suitable only for an academic or research setting.

Exogenous Surfactant. Several other recent developments may prove useful in the general management of patients with ARDS. Surfactant replacement therapy initially received attention as a treatment for patients with ARDS because of its beneficial effects in infant respiratory distress syndrome.[73] Surfactant therapy may be beneficial in patients with ARDS because their surfactant levels are diminished. This decrease results from both destruction of surfactant-producing pneumocytes and alteration of the structure and function of existing surfactant by protein exudates.[54] Although several experimental and clinical studies [166,168] suggested the safety and efficacy of surfactant therapy in patients with ARDS, large randomized, controlled clinical trials fail to show a benefit.[4] However, these studies generally involved patients with sepsis-related ARDS, and most of these patients died of septic complications, not of pulmonary failure. Thus, the inability to show a beneficial effect may not adequately reflect the potential of surfactant in irritant gas–induced ARDS. In fact, a promising model of oxygen-induced lung injury in primates noted a beneficial effect of aerosolized surfactant.[67]

OTHER INHALATIONAL PULMONARY TOXINS

A particulate, or dust, is a solid dispersed in a gas. Dust respresents a substantial source of occupational particulate exposure and is an important cause of acute pulmonary toxic syndromes. A respirable particulate must have an appropriately small size (generally <10 μm) and aerodynamic proportions to enter the terminal respiratory tree. Nonrespirable particulates, also called nuisance dusts, are trapped by the upper airways and are not generally thought to cause pulmonary damage. However, recent insight into long-term high-level exposure to nuisance dusts suggests that they may alter mucociliary clearance and accumulate in the lung.[61,111] In distinction from the irritant gases, there is no unifying toxic mechanism among the respirable particulates. Many of the particulate diseases, such as asbestos exposure and its sequelae, are chronic in nature; only the acute or subacute syndromes are discussed here.

Inorganic Dust Exposure

Silicosis is a range of pulmonary diseases associated with inhalation of crystalline silica (SiO_2), or quartz. It typically occurs in workers involved in occupations where rock or granite is pulverized, including mining, quarry work, or sandblasting. Although typically a chronic disease, intense subacute exposure may produce acute silicosis in a few weeks and death within 2 years. The mechanism of toxicity probably relates to the relentless inflammatory response generated by the pulmonary macrophages. These cells engulf these indigestable particles and are destroyed, releasing their lytic enzymes and oxidative products locally within the pulmonary parenchyma. Patients present with dyspnea, cor pulmonale, restrictive lung findings, and classic radiographic findings. Treatment is limited and includes steroids and supportive care.

Silica combined with other minerals are referred to as silicates, the most important of which include asbestos and talc. Talc, or magnesium silicate $[(Mg_3Si_4)O_{10}(OH)_2]$, is widely used in industry, but its home use has been curtailed over the past two decades because of unfortunate cases of severe pulmonary injury. Much of the toxicity of talc is related to free silica or asbestos contamination. Improvement following acute massive exposure may be accompanied by progressive pulmonary fibrosis.

Organic Dusts

Inhalation of dusts from cotton or similar natural fibers, usually during the refinement of cotton fibers (byssinosis), produces chest tightness, dyspnea, and fever that typically begin within 3 to 4 hours of exposure. Symptoms often resolve during the work week but return following a weekend hiatus.[139] Byssinosis is probably caused by an endotoxin present on the cotton and is not immunologic in nature. A similar syndrome is "grain fever," which is caused by a respirable compound associated with grain dust, as occurs during harvesting, milling, or transporting.

Hypersensitivity Pneumonitis

Hypersensitivity pneumonitis, also known as extrinsic allergic alveolitis, represents the final common pathway for many different organic dust exposures. The name attached to the individual syndrome typically identifies the associated occupation or substrate. For example, "bagassosis" is the term associated with sugar cane (bagasse), and "farmer's lung" is the term associated with moldy hay, although both are caused by thermophilic Actinomycetes. When associated with puffball mushroom spores (*Lycoperdon* sp.), the syndrome is called "Lycoperdonosis" (see Mushrooms, Chap. 76), and when caused by bird droppings, it is called "bird fancier's lung." The implicated allergen is capable of depositing in the pulmonary parenchyma and eliciting a cell mediated (type IV) immunological response (see Immunologic Principles, Chap. 15). The clinical findings include fever, chills, and dyspnea beginning 4 to -8 hours following exposure. The chest radiograph, although usually normal, may reveal diffuse or discrete infiltrates. Progressive disease is associated with a honeycombing pattern on the radiograph and a restrictive lung disease pattern on formal pulmonary function testing. Treatment includes corticosteroids and avoidance of the antigen.

Metal Fume Fever/Polymer Fume Fever

Metal fume fever is a recurrent influenza-like syndrome that develops several hours following exposure to metal oxide fumes generated during welding, galvanizing, or smelting. Although most symptoms of metal fume fever are similar to those expected with irritant gas exposures (dyspnea, cough, chest pain), the presence of fever, typically between 38° and 39°C (100.4–102.2°F), distinguishes the syndromes[11]. In addition, patients may experience headache, metallic taste, myalgias, and chills.[12] Direct pulmonary toxicity probably does not occur, and patients with metal fume fever generally have normal chest radiographs. Interestingly, acute tolerance develops so that repeat daily exposures produce progressively milder symptoms. However, the tolerance also disappears rapidly, and after a short work hiatus such as a weekend, the original intensity resumes;[136] this accounts for the designation "Monday morning fever." Many metal oxides are capable of eliciting this syndrome, but it is most frequently noted in patients who have welded galvanized steel, which contains zinc. Metal fume fever also occurs commonly after the high temperature welding of copper-containing compounds, accounting for the historical appellation "brass foundry workers ague." Serum and urine metal levels are not elevated after the acute event, although they may be chronically elevated from daily occupational exposure.[116]

The etiology of metal fume fever is still debated, but the syndrome has features suggestive of both an immunologic and a toxic etiology.[11] Antigen release with immunologic response appears to be responsible for the induction of symptoms. On subsequent exposure, pro-inflammatory cytokines, such as tumor necrosis factor-α, and various interleukins can be detected in bronchoalveolar lavage fluid.[83] However, because symptoms can occur with the patient's first exposure to fumes, a direct toxic effect on the respiratory mucosa presumably exists. As noted above, exposure to certain metal fumes, such as cadmium oxide or other zinc compounds, may produce direct toxic effects on the pulmonary parenchyma.

The management of patients with metal fume fever is supportive and includes analgesics and antipyretics. There is no specific antidote, and chelation therapy should not be instituted unless otherwise indicated. Patients with ALI are probably suffering from metal toxicity (eg, cadmium pneumonitis). The natural course of metal fume fever involves spontaneous resolution within 48 hours.

Persistent symptoms are rare and should prompt investigation for metal toxicity.

A remarkably similar syndrome occurs subsequent to inhaling pyrolysis products of fluorinated polymers (eg, Teflon), which is aptly termed "polymer fume fever."[148] Patients develop self-limited viral-illness-type symptoms several hours after exposure to the fumes. As with metal fumes, very large exposures to polymer fumes may result in direct pulmonary toxicity. Supportive care remains the therapy of choice.

Asthma and Reactive Airways Dysfunction Syndrome (RADS)

Asthma, or reversible airways disease, is a clinical syndrome that includes intermittent episodes of dyspnea, cough, chest pain or tightness, wheezes on auscultation, and measurable variations in expiratory airflow. Episodes are typically triggered by a chemical agent or physical stimulus and resolve over several hours with appropriate therapy. The underlying process is immunologic in most cases, with allergen-triggered release of inflammatory mediators causing bronchiolar smooth muscle contraction and subsequent inflammation. Because asthma affects 5- to 10% of the world's population, and the triggers are often nonspecific, it is not surprising that work-aggravated asthma is extremely common. The patients are previously sensitized, and the initial irritant exposure causes bronchospasm or similar symptoms. Thus, work-aggravated asthma is discovered early in the worker's employment, and a more appropriate workplace or occupation can be pursued.

Occupational asthma, or asthma occasioned by a workplace exposure to a sensitizing agent, accounts for perhaps 10% of all newly diagnosed asthma in adults. Casual exposure to one of the 250 or more known sensitizers[23] (Table 95–3) is usually associated with a latency period of weeks or months of exposure before symptom onset. Once symptoms begin, however, they recur consistently following reexposure to the inciting trigger agent. Occupational asthma with latency may be IgE-dependent, in which case it is identical to allergic asthma, or IgE-independent. The IgE-dependent form is most commonly associated with high-molecular-weight compounds (>5000 Da) or with certain haptenic low-molecular-weight agents (eg, acetic anhydride). The low-molecular-weight agents (eg, nickel, isocyanates) more typically cause

TABLE 95–3. Common Sensitizers Producing Occupational Asthma

Agent Class	Example of Sensitizer	Primary Risk Occupations
High-MW agents[a]		
Proteins	Crab shell	Seafood processors
Low-MW agents		
Acrylate	—	Adhesives, plastics
Glutaraldehyde	—	Health care workers
Isocyanates	Toluene diisocyanate	Polyurethane foam, automobile painters
Metals	Nickel sulfate	Nickel plating
Trimellitic anhydride	—	Chemical workers
Wood dust	Western red cedar (*Thuja plicata*)	Foresters, carpenters

[a]MW = molecular weight.

IgE-independent disease, which manifests as the delayed reaction pattern of cell-mediated, or type IV, hypersensitivity. Because, in either case, contact with a trigger may be difficult to avoid, reassignment or an outright occupational change may be required. Treatment for exacerbations is comparable to standard asthma therapy and includes bronchodilators and corticosteroids.

Acute exposure to irritant gas may result in the development of a persistent asthma-like syndrome[36] that has also been termed "reactive airways dysfunction syndrome" (RADS),[18, 5] "irritant-induced asthma",[157,17] or "occupational asthma without latency". Virtually every irritative inhalant is reported to cause this syndrome, and those not yet described are probably simply unrecognized. Although asthma is typically associated with massive inhalational exposure, occasional patients may be susceptible to low-level exposure.[80] RADS is often compared to occupational asthma because both are chemically induced disorders, most frequently occurring following chemical exposure in the workplace. However, in comparison with those who develop occupational asthma, patients who develop RADS have a lower incidence of atopy and are exposed to agents not typically considered to be immunologically sensitizing.[17] In addition, the airflow improvement with β_2-adrenergic agonist therapy is significantly better in patients with occupational asthma.[48] Bronchial biopsy performed in patients with RADS generally reveals a chronic inflammatory response.[18,48] RADS may have a neurogenic etiology,[14,29] as opposed to an immunologic origin, as in patients with occupational asthma, which may differentiate these clinically similar diseases on a mechanistic basis. Neurogenic inflammation results from increased vascular permeability, presumably secondary to release of substance P from unmyelinated sensory neurons (C-fibers).[38] Neurogenic inflammation is inhibited by substance P depletors such as capsaicin[95] and enhanced by substances that inhibit neutral endopeptidase, the enzyme responsible for the degradation of substance P.[103] The role of corticosteroids is undefined, but animal models suggest an antiinflammatory benefit.[34] Recovery may take months, with the delay related to either ongoing low-level exposures to endopeptidase inhibitors[40] or persistent irritation of impaired tissue by environmental irritants (ie, pollution).

SUMMARY

The overall quality of the air we breathe is becoming increasingly inferior, and fluctuations in environmental pollutants periodically cause epidemic disease. Although the spectrum of agents capable of causing pulmonary toxicity is large, the pathologic changes are rather limited. Gases that have little or no irritant potential or systemic toxicity cause simple asphyxiation, in which the ambient atmosphere has a diminished oxygen concentration. Parenchymal irritation and ALI follow exposure to acid-forming or free radical-generating gases and can progress in severely toxic patients to ARDS. RADS is described in patients following exposure to virtually all of the irritant gases. Treatment of all such exposures centers on supportive and respiratory care.

REFERENCES

1. The Acute Respiratory Distress Syndrome Network: Ventilation with lower tidal volumes compared with traditional tidal volumes for acute lung injury and the acute respiratory distress syndrome. N Engl J Med 2000;342:1301–1308.

2. The Acute Respiratory Distress Syndrome Network: Ketoconazole for early treatment of acute lung injury and acute respiratory distress syndrome: a randomized clinical trial. JAMA 2000;283:1995–2002.

3. Ando Y, Shibata E, Tsuchiyama F, Sakai S: Elevated urine cadmium concentrations in a patient with acute cadmium pneumonitis. Scand J Work Environ Health 1996;22:150–153.

4. Anzueto A, Baughman RP, Guntupalli KK, et al: Aerosolized surfactant in adults with sepsis-induced adult respiratory distress syndrome. N Engl J Med 1996;334:1417–1421.

5. Bardana EJ: Reactive airways dysfunction syndrome (RADS): guidelines for diagnosis and treatment and insight into prognosis. Ann Allergy Asthma Immunol 1999;83:583–586.

6. Beckman JS, Koppenol WH: Nitric oxide, superoxide and peroxynitrite: the good, the bad and the ugly. Am J Physiol 1996;271:C1424–C1437.

7. Bennett PB, Papahadjopoulos D, Bangham AD: The effect of raised pressure of inert gas on phospholipid membranes. Life Sci 1967;6:2527–2533.

8. Bernard GR, Artigas A, Brigham KL, et al, The American–European Consensus Conference on ARDS: Definitions, mechanisms, relevant outcomes, and clinical trial coordination. Am J Respir Crit Care Med 1994;149:818–824.

9. Bernard GR, Luce JM, Sprung CL, et al: High-dose corticosteroids in patients with the adult respiratory distress syndrome. N Engl J Med 1987;317:1565–1570.

10. Billmire DF, Vinocur C, Ginda M, et al: Pepper-spray-induced respiratory failure treated with extracorporeal membrane oxygenation. Pediatrics 1996;98:961–963.

11. Blanc P, Wong H, Bernstein MS, Boushey HA: An experimental human model of metal fume fever. Ann Intern Med 1991;114:930–936.

12. Blount BW: Two types of metal fume fever: Mild vs. serious: Mil Med 1990;155:372–377.

13. Bosse GM: Nebulized sodium bicarbonate in the treatment of chlorine gas inhalation. J Toxicol Clin Toxicol 1994;32:233–238.

14. Bozic CR, Lu B, Hopken UE, et al: Neurogenic amplification of immune complex inflammation. Science 1996;273:1722–1725.

15. Brasch RC, Berthezene Y, Vexler V, et al: Pulmonary oxygen toxicity: demonstration of abnormal capillary permeability using contrast-enhanced MRI. Pediatr Radiol 1993;23:495–500.

16. Braun J, Stoss H, Zober A: Intoxication following the inhalation of hydrogen fluoride. Arch Toxicol 1984;56:50–54.

17. Brooks SM, Hammad Y, Richards I, Giovinco-Barbas J, Jenkins K: The spectrum of irritant-induced asthma: Sudden and not-so-sudden onset and the role of allergy. Chest 1998;113:42–49.

18. Brooks SM, Weiss MA, Bernstein IL: Reactive airways dysfunction syndrome. Case reports of persistent asthma syndrome after high level irritant exposure. Chest 1985;88:376–384.

19. Burleigh-Flayer HK, Wong KL, Alarie Y: Evaluation of the pulmonary effects of HCl using CO_2 challenges in guinea pigs. Fund Appl Toxicol 1985;5:978–985.

20. Burnett WW, King EG, Grace M, Hall WF: Hydrogen sulfide poisoning: review of 5 years' experience. Can Med Assoc J 1977;117:1277–1280.

21. Byard RW: Methane. Death scene gas analysis in suspected methane asphyxia. Am J Forensic Med Pathol 1992;13:69–71.

22. Caplin M: Ammonia-gas poisoning. Forty-seven cases in a London shelter. Lancet 1941;2:95–96.

23. Chan-Yeung M, Malo JL: Aetiological agents in occupational asthma. Eur Respir J 1994;7:346–371.

24. Charan NB, Myers CG, Lakshminarayan S, Spencer TM: Pulmonary injuries associated with acute sulfur dioxide inhalation. Am Rev Respir Dis 1979;119:555–560.

25. Chester EH, Kaimal J, Payne CB, Kohn PM: Pulmonary injury following exposure to chlorine gas: Possible beneficial effects of steroid treatment. Chest 1977;72:247–250.

26. Chisholm CD, Singletary EM, Okerberg CV, Langlinais PC: Inhaled sodium bicarbonate for chlorine inhalation injuries [abstract]. Ann Emerg Med 1989;18:466.

27. Clark JM, Lambertsen CJ: Rate of development of pulmonary O_2 toxicity in man during O_2 breathing at 2.0 Atm abs. J Appl Physiol 1971;30:739–752.

28. Collins JF, Smith JD, Coalson JJ, et al: Variability of lung collagen amounts after prolonged support for respiratory failure. Chest 1984; 85:641–646.

29. Colten HR, Krause JE: Pulmonary inflammation—a balancing act. N Engl J Med 1997;336:1094–1096.

30. Cucinell SA, Swentzel KC, Biskup R, et al: Biochemical interactions and metabolic fate of riot control agents. Fed Proc 1971;30:86–91.

31. Curtis SE, Peek JT, Kelly DR: Partial liquid ventilation with perflubron improves arterial oxygenation in acute canine lung injury. J Appl Physiol 1993;75:2696–2702.

32. DeBehnke DJ, Hilander SJ, Dobler DW, et al: The hemodynamic and arterial blood gas response to asphyxiation: A canine model of pulseless electrical activity. Resuscitation 1995;30:169–175.

33. Dellinger RP, Zimmerman JL, Taylor RW, et al: Effects of inhaled nitric oxide in patients with acute respiratory distress syndrome: Results of a phase II trial. Crit Care Med 1998;26:15–23.

34. Demnati R, Fraser R, Martin JG, Plaa G, Malo JL: Effects of dexamethasone on functional and pathological changes in rat bronchi caused by high acute chlorine exposure. Toxicol Sci 1998;45:242–246.

35. Deneke SM, Fanburg BL: Normobaric oxygen toxicity of the lung. N Engl J Med 1980;303:76–86.

36. Deschamps D, Soler P, Rosenberg N, et al: Persistent asthma after inhalation of a mixture of sodium hypochlorite and hydrochloric acid. Chest 1994;105:1895–1896.

37. Diller WF: Medical phosgene problems and their possible solution. J Occup Med 1978;20:189–193.

38. Di Maria GU, Bellofiore S, Geppetti P: Regulation of airway neurogenic inflammation by neutral endopeptidase. Eur Respir J 1998;12:1454–1462.

39. Douglas WW, Hepper NGG, Colby TV: Silo-filler's disease. Mayo Clin Proc 1989;64:291–304.

40. Dusser DJ, Djokic TD, Borson DB, Nadel JA: Cigarette smoke induces bronchoconstrictor hyperresponsiveness to substance P and inactivates airway neutral endopeptidases in the guinea pig. Possible role of free radicals. J Clin Invest 1989;84:900–906.

41. Dwyer DM, Thorne AC, Healey JH, et al: Liquid nitrogen instillation can cause venous gas embolism. Anesthesiology 1990;73:179–181.

42. Eckert WG: Mass deaths by gas or chemical poisoning: a historical perspective. Am J Forensic Med Pathol 1991;12:119–125.

43. Ferguson JS, Schaper M, Stock MF, et al: Sensory and pulmonary irritation with exposure to methyl isocyanate. Toxicol Appl Pharmacol 1986;82:329–335.

44. Fleta J, Calvo C, Zuñiga M, et al: Intoxication of 76 children by chlorine gas. Hum Toxicol 1986;5:99–100.

45. Fowler B, Ackles KN, Porlier G: Effects of inert gas narcosis on behaviour—a critical review. Undersea Biomed Res 1985;12:369–402.

46. Gapany-Gapanavicius M, Molho M, Tirosh M: Chloramine-induced pneumonitis from mixing household cleaning agents. Br Med J 1982;285:1086.

47. Gaston B, Drazen JM, Loscalzo J, Stamler JS: The biology of nitrogen oxides in the airway. Am J Respir Crit Care Med 1994;149:538–551.

48. Gautrin D, Boulet LP, Boutet M, et al: Is reactive airways dysfunction syndrome a variant of occupational asthma? J Allergy Clin Immunol 1994;93:12–22.

49. Gautrin D, Leroyer C, Infante-Rivard C, et al: Longitudinal assessment of airway caliber and responsiveness in workers exposed to chlorine. Am J Respir Crit Care Med 1999;160:1232–1237.

50. Ghio AJ, Kennedy TP, Hatch GE, Tepper JS: Reduction of neutrophil influx diminishes lung injury and mortality following phosgene inhalation. J Appl Physiol 1991;71:657–665.

51. Gray MY, Lazarus JH: Butane inhalation and hemiparesis. J Toxicol Clin Toxicol 1993;31:483–485.

52. Gray PJ: Treating CS gas injuries to the eye: exposure at close range is particularly dangerous (letter). Br Med J 1995;311:871

53. Gregory KL, Malinoski VF, Sharp CR: Cleveland Clinic fire survivorship study, 1929–1965. Arch Environ Health 1969;18:508–515.

54. Gregory TJ, Longmore WJ, Moxley MA, et al: Surfactant chemical composition and biophysical activity in adult respiratory distress syndrome. J Clin Invest 1991;88:1976–1981.

55. Gunnarsson M, Walther SM, Seidal T, Lennquist S: Effects of inhalation of corticosteroids immediately after experimental chlorine gas lung injury. J Trauma 2000;48:101–107.

56. Guo YL, Kennedy TP, Michael JR, et al: Mechanism of phosgene-induced lung toxicity: Role of arachidonate mediators. J Appl Physiol 1990;69:1615–1622.

57. Hajela R, Janigan DT, Landrigan PL, et al: Fatal pulmonary edema due to nitric acid inhalation in three pulp-mill workers. Chest 1990;97:487–489.

58. Hallman M, Bry K, Turbow R, Waffarn F, Lappalainen U: Pulmonary toxicity associated with nitric oxide in term infants with severe respiratory failure. J Pediatr 1998;132:827–829.

59. Harrison PHM, Wendon JA, Grimson AES, et al: Improvement by acetylcysteine of haemodynamics and oxygen transport in fulminant hepatic failure. N Engl J Med 1991;324:1852–1857.

60. Hattis RP, Greer JR, Dietrich S, et al: Chlorine gas toxicity from mixture of bleach with other cleaning products—California. MMWR 1991;40;619–629.

61. Henderson RF, Barr ED, Cheng YS, et al: The effect of exposure pattern on the accumulation of particles and the response of the lung to inhaled particles. Fund Appl Toxicol 1992;19:367–374.

62. Hirschl RB, Tooley R, Parent A, et al: Improvement of gas exchange, pulmonary function, and acute lung injury with partial liquid ventilation: A study model in a setting of severe respiratory failure. Chest 1995;108:500–508.

63. Hirschl RB, Pranikoff T, Wise C, et al: Initial experience with partial liquid ventilation in adult patients with adult respiratory distress syndrome. JAMA 1996;275:383–389.

64. Hjortso E, Qvist J, Bud MI, et al: ARDS after accidental inhalation of zinc chloride smoke. Intens Care Med 1988;14:17–24.

65. Holmes PS: Pneumomediastinum associated with inhalation of white smoke. Mil Med 1999;164:751–752.

66. Holzer P: Capsaicin: cellular targets, mechanisms of action, and selectivity for thin sensory neurons. Physiol Rev 1991;43:143–201.

67. Huang YC, Caminiti SP, Fawcett TA, et al: Natural surfactant and hyperoxic lung injury in primates. I. Physiology and biochemistry. J Appl Physiol 1994;76:991–1001.

68. Hudnall JB, Suruda A, Campbell DL: Deaths involving air-line respirators connected to inert gas sources. Am Ind Hyg Assoc J 1993; 54:32–35.

69. Hyde DM, Miller LA, McDonald RJ, et al: Neutrophils enhance clearance of necrotic epithelial cells in ozone-induced lung injury in rhesus monkeys. Am J Physiol 1999;277:L1190–L1198.

70. Ikeda N, Takahashi H, Umetsu K, Suzuki T: The course of respiration and circulation in death by carbon dioxide poisoning. Forensic Sci Int 1989;41:93–99.

71. Jarvis D, Chinn S, Luczynska C, Burney P: Association of respiratory symptoms and lung function in young adults with use of domestic gas appliances. Lancet 1996;347:426–431.

72. Jawan B, Lee JH: Cardiac arrest caused by an incorrectly filled oxygen cylinder: A case report. Br J Anaesth 1990;64:749–751.

73. Jobe AH: Pulmonary surfactant therapy. N Engl J Med 1993;328:861–868.

74. Jones RN, Hughs JM, Glindmeyer H, Weill H: Lung function after acute chlorine exposure. Am Rev Respir Dis 1986;134:1190–1195.

75. Kamat SR, Patel MH, Kolhatkar VP, et al: Sequential respiratory changes in those exposed to the gas leak at Bhopal. Indian J Med Res 1987;86(Suppl):20–38.

76. Kazzaz JA, Xu J, Palaia TA, et al: Cellular oxygen toxicity. Oxidant injury without apoptosis. J Biol Chem 1996;271:15182–15186.

77. Kennedy TP, Michael JR, Hoidal JR, et al: Dibutyryl cAMP, aminophylline, and β-adrenergic agonists protect against pulmonary edema caused by phosgene. J Appl Physiol 1989;67:2542–2552.

78. Kernbach-Wighton G, Kijewski H, Schwanke P, Saur P, Sprung R: Clinical and morpological aspects of death due to liquid nitrogen. Int J Legal Med 1998;111:191–195.

79. Kimbell JS, Gross EA, Joyner DR, et al: Application of computational fluid dynamics to regional dosimetry of inhaled chemicals in the upper respiratory tract of the rat. Toxicol Appl Pharmacol 1993;121:253–263.

80. Kipen HM, Blume R, Hutt D: Asthma experience in an occupational and environmental medicine clinic: Low dose reactive airways dysfunction syndrome. J Occup Med 1994;36:1133–1137.

81. Kling GW, Clark MA, Compton HR, et al: The 1986 Lake Nyos gas disaster in Cameroon, West Africa. Science 1987;236:169–175.

82. Koren HS, Devlin RB, Graham DE: Ozone-induced inflammation in the lower airways of human subjects. Am Rev Respir Dis 1989;139:407–415.

83. Kuschner WG, D'Alessandro A, Wentermeyer SF, et al: Pulmonary responses to purified zinc oxide fume. J Invest Med 1995;43:371–378.

84. Laffey JG, Kavanagh BP: Carbon dioxide and the critically ill—too little of a good thing? Lancet 1999;354:1283–1286.

85. Laskin DL, Heck DE, Laskin JD: Role of inflammatory cytokines and nitric oxide in hepatic and pulmonary toxicity. Toxicol Lett 1998;102–103:289–293.

86. Lavnikova N, Prokhorova S, Lakhotia AV, Gordon R, Laskin DL: Distinct inflammatory responses of adherant vascular lung neutrophils to pulmonary irritants. J Inflammation 1998;48:56–66.

87. Lee DC, Wiley JF, Snyder JW: Treatment of inhalational exposure to hydrofluoric acid with nebulized calcium gluconate. J Occup Med 1993;35:470.

88. Lehmann P: The ozone hole. Med J Aust 1995;163:576–578.

89. Leu HJ, Clodius L: An unusual cause of gangrene: cold injury caused by liquid nitrogen. Schweiz Med Wochenschr 1989;119:192–195.

90. Levy JI, Lee K, Yanagisawa Y, Hutchinson P, Spengler JD. Determinants of nitrogen dioxide concentrations in indoor ice skating rinks. Am J Public Health 1998;88:1781–1786.

91. Lippmann M: Health effects of ozone: a critical review. J Air Pollut Control Assoc 1989;39:672–695.

92. Livardjani F, Ledig M, Kopp P, Dahlet M, Leroy M, Jaeger A: Lung and blood superoxide dismutase activity in mercury vapor exposed rats: Effect of N-acetylcysteine treatment. Toxicology 1991;66(3):289–295.

93. Logan WPD: Mortality in the London fog incident, 1952. Lancet 1953;1:336–339.

94. Lubec G, Widness JA, Hayde M, Menzel D, Pollak A: Hydroxyl radical generation in oxygen-treated infants. Pediatrics 1997;100:700–704.

95. Lundberg JM, Saria A: Capsaicin-induced desensitization of airway mucosa to cigarette smoke, mechanical and chemical irritants. Nature 1983;302:251–253.

96. Manning HL, Schwartzstein RM: Pathophysiology of dyspnea. N Engl J Med 1995;333:1547–1553.

97. Martinez TT, Long C: Explosion risk from swimming pool chlorinators and review of chlorine toxicity. J Toxicol Clin Toxicol 1995;33:349–354.

98. Mayorga MA: Overview of nitrogen dioxide effects on the lung with emphasis on military relevance. Toxicology 1994;89:175–192.

99. McDonald DM, Thurston G, Baluk P: Endothelial gaps as sites for plasma leakage in inflammation. Microcirculation 1999;6:7–22.

100. Meduri GU, Belenchia JM, Estes RJ, et al: Fibroproliferative phase of ARDS: Clinical findings and effects of corticosteroids. Chest 1991;100:943–952.

101. Meduri GU, Headley AS, Golden E, et al: Effect of prolonged methylprednisolone therapy in unresolving acute respiratory distress syndrome: A randomized controlled trial. JAMA 1998;280:159–165.

102. Meduri GU: Levels of evidence for the phamacologic effectiveness of prolonged methylprednisolone treatment in unresolving ARDS. Chest 1999;116:116S–118S.

103. Meggs WJ: RADS and RUDS—the toxic induction of asthma and rhinitis. J Toxicol Clin Toxicol 1994;32:487–501.

104. Mehta PS, Mehta AS, Mehta SJ, Makhijani AB: Bhopal tragedy's health effects: A review of methylisocyanate toxicity. JAMA 1990;264;2781–2787.

105. Miller TM, Mazur PO: Oxygen deficiency hazards associated with liquefied gas systems: Derivation of a program of controls. Am Ind Hyg Assoc J 1984;45:293–298.

106. Minami M, Katsumata M, Miyake K, et al: Dangerous mixture of household detergents in an old-style toilet: A case report with simulation experiments of the working environment and warning of potential hazard relevant to the general environment. Hum Exp Toxicol 1992;11:27–34.

107. Misra NP, Pathak R, Gaur KJBS, et al: Clinical profile of gas leak victims in acute phase after Bhopal episode. Indian J Med Res 1987;86(Suppl):11–19.

108. Morcillo EJ, Estrela J, Cortijo J: Oxidative stress and pulmonary inflammation: pharmacological invervention with antioxidants. Pharmacol Res 1999;40:393–404.

109. Moromisato DY, Anas NG, Goodman G: Mercury inhalation poisoning and acute lung injury in a child. Use of high-frequency oscillatory ventilation. Chest 1994;105:613–615.

110. Morris AH, Wallace CJ, Menlowe RL, et al: Randomized clinical trial of pressure-controlled inverse ratio ventilation and extracorporeal CO₂ removal for adult respiratory distress syndrome. Am J Respir Crit Care Med 1994;149:295–305.

111. Morrow PE. Dust overloading in the lungs: Update and appraisals. Toxicol Appl Pharmacol 1992;113:1–12.

112. Mrvos R, Dean BS, Krenzelok EP: Home exposures to chlorine/chloramine gas: Review of 216 cases. South Med J 1993;86:654–657.

113. Murai M, Morimoto H, Maeda Y, Fujii T: Effects of the tripeptide substance P antagonist, FR 113680, on airway constriction and airway edema induced by neurokinins in guinea-pigs. Eur J Pharmacol 1992;217:23–29.

114. Nader ND, Knight PR, Davidson BA, Safaee SS, Steinhorn DM: Systemic perfluorocarbons suppress the acute lung inflammation after gastric acid aspiration in rats. Anesth Analg 2000;90:356–361.

115. Nightingale JA, Rogers DF, Chung KF, Barnes PJ: No effect of inhaled budenoside on the response to inhaled ozone in normal subjects. Am J Respir Crit Care Med 2000;161:479–486.

116. Noel NE, Ruthman JC: Elevated serum zinc levels in metal fume fever. Am J Emerg Med 1988;6:609–610.

117. Orzel RA: Toxicologic aspects of firesmoke: Polymer pyrolysis and combustion. Occup Med 1993;8:415–429.

118. Osbern LN, Crapo RO: Dung lung: A report of toxic exposure to liquid manure. Ann Intern Med 1981;95:312–314.

119. Pascuzzi TA, Storrow AB: Mass casualties from acute inhalation of chlorine gas. Mil Med 1998;163:102–104.

120. Pelled B, Schechter Y, Alroy G, et al: Deleterious effects of oxygen at ambient and hyperbaric pressure in the treatment of nitrogen dioxide–poisoned mice. Am Rev Respir Dis 1973;108:1152–1157.

121. Pepe PE, Hudson LD, Carrico CJ: Early application of positive end-expiratory pressure in patients at risk of the adult respiratory distress syndrome. N Engl J Med 1984;311:281–286.

122. Peters JW: Hydrogen sulfide poisoning in a hospital setting. JAMA 1981;246:1588–1589.

123. Pino F, Puerta H, D'Apollo MD, et al: Effectiveness of morphine in non-cardiogenic pulmonary edema due to chlorine gas inhalation. Vet Hum Toxicol 1993;35:36.

124. Potts J: Factors associated with respiratory problems in swimmers. Sports Med 1996;21:256–261.

125. Promisloff RA, Lenchner GS, Cichelli AW: Reactive airway dysfunction syndrome in three police officers following a roadside chemical spill. Chest 1990;98:928–929.

126. Quinlan T, Spivak S, Mossman BT: Regulation of antioxidant enzymes in lung after oxidant injury. Environ Health Perspect 1994; 102:79–87.

127. Rabinovitch S, Greyson ND, Weiser W, et al: Clinical and laboratory features of acute sulfur dioxide inhalation poisoning: Two year follow up. Am Rev Respir Dis 1989;139:556–558.

128. Rafferty P: Voluntary chlorine inhalation: A new form of self-abuse? Br Med J 1980;281:1178–1179.

129. Ranieri VM, Suter PM, Tortorella C, et al: Effect of mechanical ventilation on inflammatory mediators in patients with acute respiratory distress syndrome: A randomized controlled trial. JAMA 1999;82: 54–61.

130. Reed D, Glasser S, Kaldor J: Ozone toxicity symptoms among flight attendants. Am J Ind Med 1980;1:43–54.

131. Reiffenstein RJ, Hulbert WC, Roth SH: Toxicology of hydrogen sulfide. Annu Rev Pharmacol Toxicol 1992;32:109–134.

132. Reinhart PG, Bassett DJ, Bhalla DK: The influence of polymorphonuclear leukocytes on altered pulmonary epithelial permeability during ozone exposure. Toxicology 1998;127:17–28.

133. Reisz GR, Gammon RS: Toxic pneumonitis from mixing household cleaners. Chest 1986;89:49–52

134. Riechelmann H, Maurer J, Kienast K, et al: Respiratory epithelium exposed to sulfur dioxide—functional and ultrastructural alterations. Laryngoscope 1995;105:295–299.

135. Roehm JN, Hadley JG, Menzel DB: The influence of vitamin E on the lung fatty acids of rats exposed to ozone. Arch Environ Health 1972;24:237–242.

136. Ross DS: Welder's metal fume fever. J Soc Occup Med 1974;24: 125–129.

137. Rossaint R, Falke KJ, Lopez F, et al: Inhaled nitric oxide for the adult respiratory distress syndrome. N Eng J Med 1993;328: 399–405.

138. Roth VS, Franzblau A: RADS after exposure to riot-control agent: A case report. J Occup Environ Med 1996;38:863–865.

139. Rylander R. Health effects of cotton dust exposures. Am J Ind Med 1990;17:39–45.

140. Ryrfeldt A, Bannenberg G, Moldeus P: Free radicals and lung disease. Br Med Bull 1993;49:588–603.

141. Samet JM, Utell MJ: The environment and the lung: Changing perspectives. JAMA 1991;266:670–675.

142. Sanders KA, Huecksteadt T, Xu P, Sturrock AB, Hoidal JR: Regulation of oxidant production in acute lung injury. Chest 1999;116: 56S–61S.

143. Sarnstrand B, Tunek A, Sjodin K, Hallberg A: Effects of N-acetylcysteine stereoisomers on oxygen-induced lung injury in rats. Chem Biol Interact 1995;94:157–164.

144. Sciuto AM, Strickland PT, Kennedy TP, Gurtner GH: Protective effects of N-acetylcysteine treatment after phosgene exposure in rabbits. Am J Respir Crit Care Med 1995;151:768–772.

145. Sciuto AM, Stotts RR, Hurt HH: Efficacy of ibuprofen and pentoxifylline in the treatment of phosgene-induced acute lung injury. J Appl Toxicol 1996;16:381–384.

146. Sciuto AM, Strickland PT, Kennedy TP, et al: Intratracheal administration of DBcAMP attenuates edema formation in phosgene-induced acute lung injury. J Appl Physiol 1996;80:149–157.

147. Shi Z. Nickel carbonyl: Toxicity and human health. Sci Total Environ 1994;148:293–298.

148. Shusterman DJ: Polymer fume fever and other fluorocarbon pyrolysis-related syndromes. Occup Med 1993;8:519–531.

149. Sjoblom E, Hojer J, Kulling PEJ, Stauffer K, Suneson A, Ludwigs U: A placebo-controlled experimental study of steroid inhalation therapy in ammonia-induced lung disease. J Toxicol Clin Toxicol 1999;37:59–67.

150. Snyder RW, Mishel HS, Christensen GC: Pulmonary toxicity following exposure to methylene chloride and its combustion product, phosgene. Chest 1992;101:860–861.

151. Steffee CH, Lantz PE, Flannagan LM, et al: Oleoresin capsicum (pepper) spray and "in custody deaths." Am J Forensic Med Pathol 1995;16:185–192.

152. Suruda A, Agnew J: Deaths from asphyxiation and poisoning at work in the United States, 1984–1986. Br J Ind Med 1989;46: 541–546.

153. Suter PM, Domenighetti G, Schaller MD, et al: N-Acetylcysteine enhances recovery from acute lung injury in man: A randomized, double-blind, placebo-controlled clinical study. Chest 1994;105: 190–194

154. Takaoka M, Morinaga K, Karakowa K, et al: A case report of acute carbon dioxide intoxication by dry ice. Jpn J Toxicol 1988;1:87–90.

155. Tanaka S, Fujimoto S, Tamagaki Y, et al: Bronchial injury and pulmonary edema caused by hydrogen sulfide poisoning. Am J Emerg Med 1999;17:427–429.

156. Tanen DA, Graeme KA, Raschke R: Severe lung injury after exposure to chloramine gas from household cleaners. N Engl J Med 1999;341:848–849.

157. Tarlo SM, Broder I: Irritant-induced occupational asthma. Chest 1989;96:297–300.

158. Tatsumi T, Fliss H: Hypochlorous acid and chloramines increase endothelial permeability: possible involvement of cellular zinc. Am J Physiol 1994;267:H1597–H1607.

159. Tu B, Wallin A, Moldeus P, Cotgreave I: The cytoprotective roles of ascorbate and glutathione against nitrogen dioxide toxicity in human endothelial cells. Toxicology 1995;98:125–136.

160. Turrens JF, Crapo JD, Freeman BA: Protection against oxygen toxicity by intravenous injection of liposome-entrapped catalase and superoxide dismutase. J Clin Invest 1984;73:87–95.

161. Tunnicliffe W, Burge P, Ayres J: Effect of domestic concentration of nitrogen dioxide on airway responsiveness to inhaled allergen in asthmatic patients. Lancet 1994;344:1733–1736.

162. Uppu RM, Cueto R, Squadrito GL, Pryor WA: What does ozone react with at the air/lung interface? Model studies using human red blood cell membranes. Arch Biochem Biophys 1995;319:257–266.

163. Velsor LW, Postlethwait EM: NO$_2$-induced generation of extracellular reactive oxygen is mediated by epithelial lining layer antioxidants. Am J Physiol 1997;273:L1265–1275.

164. Vinsel PJ: Treatment of acute chlorine gas inhalation with nebulized sodium bicarbonate. J Emerg Med 1990;8:327–329.

165. Wagner GN, Clark MA, Koenigsberg EJ, Decata SJ: Medical evaluation of the victims of the 1986 Lake Nyos disaster. J Forensic Sci 1988;33:899–909.

166. Walmrath D, Günther A, Ghofrani HA, et al: Bronchoscopic surfactant administration in patients with severe adult respiratory distress syndrome and sepsis. Am J Respir Crit Care Med 1996;154:57–62.

167. Watson AA, Oliver JS, Thorpe JW: Accidental death due to inhalation of hydrofluoric acid. Med Sci Law 1973;13:277–279.

168. Weg JG, Balk RA, Tharratt RS, et al: Safety and efficacy of an aerosolized surfactant in human sepsis-induced adult respiratory distress syndrome. JAMA 1994;272:1433–1438.

169. Weinberger B, Heck DE, Laskin DL, Laskin JD: Nitric oxide in the lung: therapeutic and cellular mechanisms of action. Pharmacol Ther 1999;84:401–411.

170. Weir KL, O'Gorman EN, Ross JA, et al: Lung capillary albumin leak in oxygen toxicity. A quantitative immunochemical study. Am J Respir Crit Care Med 1994;150:784–789.

171. Wing JS, Sanderson LM, Brender JD, Perrota DM, Beauchanp RA: Acute health effects in a community after release of hydrofluoric acid. Arch Environ Health 1991;46:155–160.

172. Wispe JR, Warner BB, Clark JC, et al: Human Mn-SOD in pulmonary epithelial cells of transgenic mice confers protection from oxygen injury. J Biol Chem 1993;267:23937–23941.

173. Wood BR, Colombo JL, Benson BE: Chlorine inhalation toxicity from vapors generated by swimming pool chlorinator tablets. Pediatrics 1987;79:428–430.

174. Yoshida M, Satoh M, Shimada A, Yasutake A, Sumi Y, Tohyama C: Pulmonary toxicity caused by acute exposure to mercury vapor is enhanced in metallothionein-null mice. Life Sci 1999;64:1861–1867.

Christopher P. Holstege / Mark A. Kirk

Firefighters discovered an unresponsive 39-year-old man in a smoke-filled room at an apartment building fire. At the scene, his initial vital signs were a palpable systolic blood pressure of 70 mm Hg; pulse 160 beats/min, and apnea. A large amount of soot was noted in the patient's upper airway during endotracheal intubation in the field. He was placed on 100% oxygen during transport. On arrival at the Emergency Department (ED), he was unresponsive to painful stimuli and had a palpable systolic blood pressure of 100 mm Hg. No evidence of head trauma or skin burns was noted. Pupils were equal and reactive to light. Intense conjunctival irritation and corneal burns were noted. He had singed nasal hairs and soot in his oropharynx. Carbonaceous material was suctioned from his endotracheal tube. Breath sounds were equal, with diffuse wheezes in all lung fields. He was placed on a ventilator with 100% oxygen and administered aerosolized albuterol. His blood pressure continued to improve with intravenous (IV) fluid therapy. He had no response to 2 mg of naloxone, 100 mg of thiamine, and 25 g of 50% dextrose IV.

His initial electrocardiogram (ECG) showed a sinus tachycardia without evidence of ischemia. Initial laboratory data revealed: WBC 14,000 cells/mm^3, hemoglobin 11.3 g/dL, sodium 141 mEq/L, potassium 3.5 mEq/L, chloride 111 mEq/L, bicarbonate 12 mEq/L, BUN 27 mg/dL, creatinine 0.7 mg/dL, and blood glucose 80 mg/dL. A blood lactate concentration was 14 mEq/L. Arterial blood gas analysis on 100% oxygen showed pH 7.17, P_{CO_2} 30 mm Hg, and P_{O_2} 150 mm Hg. Cooximeter measured a carboxyhemoglobin concentration of 38% and a methemoglobin concentration of 0.8%. A blood ethanol concentration was 179 mg/dL. A chest radiograph was unremarkable.

Because of his critical condition, the presence of metabolic acidosis and the possibility of cyanide poisoning, 12.5 g of sodium thiosulfate was given IV. The patient was taken to the intensive care unit, where mechanical ventilation and fluid resuscitation continued. He had no further significant hemodynamic instability. Within 4 hours of admission he received hyperbaric oxygen therapy. He had a progressive improvement in mental status and was awake 6 hours after admission. The patient had complete recovery with no neurologic deficits. Admission whole-blood cyanide concentration of 1.80 µg/mL (< 1 µg/mL normal) was reported 12 hours later.

INTRODUCTION

Smoke inhalation is the leading cause of death from fire. Smoke contains numerous toxins that are generated during combustion. Combustion, or pyrolysis, is the rapid decomposition or oxidation of a substance (fuel) by heat. This process generates flame (light),

heat, and smoke as combustion products. Smoke is a complex mixture of heated air, suspended solid and liquid particles, gases, fumes, aerosols, and vapors. Combustion products are difficult to predict in a fire; in fact, even the composition of smoke often is quite variable within the same fire environment.[9,31,97] Chemical composition of the fuel, oxygen availability, and temperature determine the combustion products.[49,116] Table 96–1 lists toxic combustion products of common fuels.[9,25,36,39,87,97,102,103,116] The variety of materials now used in our environment contributes to the broad spectrum of combustion products present in typical smoke.[25]

The association of smoke inhalation with burns produces a more serious systemic illness.[35,114,120,135] Burn victims with smoke inhalation injury have a higher morbidity and mortality than those with burns only; the incidence of acute respiratory failure is 61% versus 12%, respectively.[7,24,122,133,136] In addition, burn edema is accentuated, and nonburned tissue has increased vascular permeability when associated with smoke inhalation injuries.[34]

HISTORY AND EPIDEMIOLOGY

Disastrous fires are frequent reminders of the role of inhalation injuries in fire deaths.[31,66] Every 17 seconds a fire department responds to a fire somewhere in the United States. In 1999, the National Fire Protection Agency reported 3570 fire deaths and 21,875 fire injuries in the United States.[59] Compared with other countries, the United States has one of the highest fire death rates in the world.[77] An estimated 50 to 80% of these fire deaths are the result of smoke inhalation injuries rather than dermal burns or trauma.[13, 50, 87, 137]

Fire injuries can result from an array of inhaled toxic chemicals and/or thermal burns. Before 1942, toxic inhalation was considered unusual from dwelling fires. However, in that year a fire at the Cocoanut Grove Night Club in Boston proved that toxic gases may be generated in typical dwelling fires:

> The complications encountered were similar to those resulting from inhalation of certain war gases. From the experience of the Cocoanut Grove fire, we know that such pulmonary complications are to be found not solely in warfare, but may be encountered at any moment in civilian life.[96]

From 1955 to 1972, a threefold increase in death from inhalational injury was reported and was attributed to abundant use of newer synthetic materials for building and furnishings.[13] Despite improved firefighting resources, mass casualties from smoke in-

**TABLE 96–1.   Common Materials and Their
                Combustion Products**

Products	Combustion Products
Wool	Carbon monoxide, hydrogen chloride, phosgene, chlorine, cyanide
Silk	Sulfur dioxide, hydrogen sulfide, ammonia, cyanide
Nylon	Ammonia, cyanide
Wood, cotton, paper	Carbon monoxide, acrolein, acetaldehyde, formaldehyde, acetic acid, formic acid, methane
Petroleum products	Carbon monoxide, acrolein, acetic acid, formic acid
Polystyrene	Styrene
Acrylic	Acrolein, hydrogen chloride, carbon monoxide
Plastics	Cyanide, hydrogen chloride, aldehydes, ammonia, oxides of nitrogen (methemoglobinemia), phosgene, chlorine
Polyvinyl chloride	Carbon monoxide, hydrogen chloride, phosgene, chlorine
Polyurethane	Cyanide, isocyanates
Melamine resins	Ammonia, cyanide
Rubber	Hydrogen sulfide, sulfur dioxide
Sulfur-containing material	Sulfur dioxide
Nitrogen-containing material	Cyanide, isocyanates, oxides of nitrogen (methemoglobinemia)
Fluorinated resins	Hydrogen fluoride
Fire-retardant materials	Hydrogen chloride, hydrogen bromide

halation continue to be reported. On November 11, 2000, 170 deaths primarily from smoke inhalation occurred when a cable train carrying skiers caught fire in a tunnel in Austria. Most of the victims apparently managed to escape the burning train but were killed by "acrid smoke" as they tried to flee.[2]

PATHOPHYSIOLOGY

Toxic combustion products are classified into three categories: simple asphyxiants, irritant toxins, and chemical asphyxiants (Table 96–2). Simple asphyxiants (eg, carbon dioxide) exert a space-occupying effect, filling an enclosed space at the expense of oxygen.[31,36,112,135] In addition, combustion uses oxygen and can result in an oxygen-deprived environment.[31]

TABLE 96–2.   Toxic Combustion Products

Simple asphyxiants	Irritants
Carbon dioxide	High water-solubility
Methane	(upper airway injury)
Oxygen-deprived environment	Acrolein
	Sulfur dioxide
Chemical asphyxiants	Ammonia
Carbon monoxide	Hydrogen chloride
Hydrogen cyanide	Intermediate water-solubility
Hydrogen sulfide	(upper and lower respiratory injury)
Oxides of nitrogen	Chlorine
(Methemoglobinemia)	Isocyanates
	Poor water-solubility
	(pulmonary parenchymal injury)
	Oxides of nitrogen
	Phosgene

Irritant toxins are chemically reactive compounds that exert a local effect on the respiratory tract (Chap. 95). Acrolein is one of the most common irritant gases generated by fires.[72] High concentrations are measured in air samples from fire environments and in the blood of fire victims.[1,128] Acrolein penetrates cell membranes easily because it is lipid soluble. It then injures cells by denaturing intracellular proteins and nucleic acids.[40,137] Ammonia is generated when wool, silk, nylon, or synthetic resins are burned. It reacts with the mucosa to produce the alkaline agent ammonium hydroxide.[26,68] Sulfur dioxide, a combustion product of sulfur-containing material, is found in more than 50% of air samples from fires.[18] Sulfurous acid is a strong caustic that forms when sulfur dioxide reacts with the moisture of the respiratory mucosa. Polyvinyl chloride (PVC) is widely used in home and office furnishings, floor coverings, and electrical insulation; therefore, high concentrations of its combustion products, hydrogen chloride, chlorine, and phosgene, are present in many fires.[14,31,36,74] In the presence of mucosal water, chlorine generates hydrogen chloride and oxygen free radicals that cause an oxidative injury.[32] Phosgene produces delayed alveolar injury. Isocyanates, combustion products generated from upholstery, cause intense irritation of the upper and lower respiratory tract.

Inhalation of soot particles and aerosols enhance the exposure to irritant toxins in a fire environment. Combustion of organic material produces finely divided carbonaceous particulate matter (soot) suspended in hot air and gases. These particles are not just composed of carbon; organic acids, aldehydes, and reactive chemical radicals are adsorbed to their surfaces.[36,53,112,135] Soot adheres to the mucosa of the airways, allowing adsorbed irritant chemicals to react with the mucosal surface moisture. The deposition of these particles in the respiratory tract depends on their size, with those of 1 to 3 μm reaching the alveoli.[82] Experimental animals have markedly decreased lung injury when exposed to smoke filtered to remove particulates.[63] Sulfur dioxide is often found adsorbed onto the surface of carbonaceous particles, and the combustion of PVC generates a large amount of particulate-filled smoke coated with hydrogen chloride, chlorine, and phosgene.[18,36,74] Also, irritant gases can "piggyback" on aerosol droplets and alter the site of deposition of the gas.[51]

Water solubility is the most important chemical characteristic in determining the level of the respiratory tract injury. Caustic injury from water-soluble chemicals occurs in the upper airway and results in damage to mucosal cells and release of mediators of inflammation and oxygen free radicals.[17,83,102] This intense inflammatory response increases microvascular permeability and movement of fluid from the intravascular space into the tissues of the upper airway. The loosely attached underlying tissue of the supraglottic larynx, the usual site of edema, may become massively swollen.[55] An edematous upper airway may develop in minutes to hours and progress to occlude the upper airway completely.[105] Chemicals with low water solubility reach the lung parenchyma, where they react slowly to create a delayed toxic effect. In addition to water solubility, concentration of the substance inhaled, duration of exposure, particle size, respiratory rate, absence of protective reflexes, and preexisting disease influence the level of the respiratory tract injury.

Tracheobronchial injuries result from inhaled particulates and toxic gases causing increased airway resistance from intraluminal debris, airway mucosal edema, inspissated secretions, and bronchospasm. Toxic chemicals induce an intense inflammatory reaction secondary to caustic injury to mucosal cells.[24,73,123] Damaged cells release chemotactic factors that stimulate production of an exudate rich in protein and inflammatory cells.[130] This reaction eventually results in sloughing of the mucosa. Exudate, mucosal sloughing, and reactive bronchorrhea combine to create casts of the airways. In animal models and victims of smoke inhalation, casts block major airways, increasing airway resistance and preventing passage of oxygen to the alveoli.[24,123,130] Increased tracheobronchial vascular permeability causes interstitial edema of the airways and increased airway resistance. Bronchoconstriction and subsequent wheezing are caused by a response to mediators of inflammation, a reflex response to toxic mucosal injury.[47,126]

Toxic chemicals reaching the alveoli injure the lung parenchyma.[91] At autopsy, carbon particles are found in alveoli.[28] Caustics, proteolytic enzymes, free radicals, and mediators of inflammation all contribute to acute lung injury (ALI).[62,65,126,135] Pathophysiologic changes of ALI decrease lung compliance and bacterial defense, cause ventilation-perfusion mismatch and intrapulmonary shunt, and increase extravascular lung water and microvascular permeability.[24,41,126,130] Decreased lung compliance from atelectasis is produced when toxic chemicals deactivate pulmonary surfactant.[24,91,99,130] In animals, patchy atelectasis occurs rapidly after smoke is inspired.[24,91,130] In addition, ventilation-perfusion mismatch occurs when pulmonary blood flow is diverted by hypoxia and vasoactive mediators of inflammation.[69,70,90,126] Toxins further damage the normal pulmonary defense systems by impairing mucociliary clearance, altering alveolar macrophage function, and impairing phagocytosis of bacteria, which contribute to the subsequent development of pulmonary infections and sepsis.[10,11,38,52,104] The combination of inflammatory response and delayed toxic effects of some inhaled chemicals may explain the limited initial manifestations of parenchymal injury during the first 24 hours after smoke exposure.

Chemical asphyxiants exert toxic effects at tissues distant from the lung. Incomplete combustion of organic materials generates carbon monoxide, considered the most common serious acute hazard to victims of inhalation injury (Chap. 97).[12,31,128,137] Carbon monoxide prevents oxygen from binding to hemoglobin, creating a functional anemia. It also hinders the release of oxygen at the tissues by shifting the oxyhemoglobin dissociation curve to the left. Other mechanisms, such as lipid peroxidation, may contribute to the toxicity of carbon monoxide (Chap. 97).[118] Cyanide is produced from combustion of nitrogen-containing products such as plastics, melamine resins, polyurethanes, wool, silk, nylon, nitrocellulose, polyacrylonitriles, synthetic rubber, and paper.[97] High concentrations of cyanide are measured in air samples from fires, and elevated blood cyanide concentrations occur in both fire survivors and fire fatalities.[3,8,9,22,31,48,58,109,110,113,132] Cyanide has at least an additive, if not synergistic, effect in smoke inhalation toxicity (Chap. 98).[8,81,94,101,103] Nitrogen-containing materials also generate oxides of nitrogen, which are irritants and methemoglobin inducers (Chap. 94).

Depending on the fuel, other combustion products are generated that act by local irritation or systemic toxicity. Such compounds as metal oxides, hydrocarbons, hydrogen fluoride, and hydrogen bromide may contribute to toxicity. A variety of cyclic and straight-chained hydrocarbons may be measured in fire environments.[31] Benzene is detected from combustion of petroleum products and plastics.[128] Antimony, bromine, cadmium, chromium, cobalt, gold, iron, lead, and zinc are recovered in air samples taken during fires and from soot removed from the surface of the trachea and bronchi of fire victims.[12,31] Unusual fires at industrial sites, clandestine drug laboratories, transportation incidents, or natural disasters, such as volcanoes produce additional toxic inhalants.

CLINICAL MANIFESTATIONS

The primary clinical problem in the smoke inhalation victim is respiratory compromise. Obtaining a history from a patient with smoke inhalation may be difficult because of the individual's voice changes. Frankly hoarse speech may be heard. Speech may progressively worsen as the airways become increasingly edematous. Stridor may be audible. Acute respiratory arrest may develop as the upper airways become progressively narrow and then close. The patient may have difficulty managing airway secretions. Copious quantates of soot-containing sputum may be expectorated. Auscultation of their lungs may demonstrate rhonchi, rales, and/or wheezing. In severe bronchospasm, breath sounds may be virtually inaudible. Direct laryngoscopy may demonstrate soot accumulation, copious secretions, and edematous tissue. These factors may make visualization of the vocal cords difficult.

Smoke inhalation victims may develop acute mental status changes. These changes include agitation, confusion, or coma. Conjunctival injection, marked lacrimation, and blepharospasm may be seen on ophthalmologic examination. Tachycardia and tachypnea may be pronounced, and hypotension may occur with faint or no peripheral pulses noted.

DIAGNOSTIC TESTING

Because smoke inhalation injury causes pulmonary and airway damage, diagnostic studies should focus on assessing oxygenation and ventilation. Therefore, arterial blood gas (ABG) analysis, carboxyhemoglobin concentration, methemoglobin concentration, and chest radiography are the most important laboratory tests to obtain.

ABG analysis assesses both arterial oxygenation and alveolar ventilation. Serial measurements are helpful in identifying hypoxemia or ventilatory failure. The presence of metabolic acidosis may be an early clue to tissue hypoxia.

The accuracy of oxygen saturation measurement depends on the method used. Oxygen saturation calculated from an ABG analysis may be unreliable in the setting of carbon monoxide or cyanide poisoning, but measured oxygen saturation determined by cooximeter accurately reflects the percent saturation of oxygenated hemoglobin. Transcutaneous measurement of oxygen saturation is unreliable in the patient with smoke inhalation because it overestimates oxygen saturation in the presence of carboxyhemoglobin.[6,37,93,129]

An elevated carboxyhemoglobin concentration in a fire victim indicates substantial exposure to combustion products and a greater possibility of developing smoke inhalation toxicity.[23,136] Some clinical series suggest that carboxyhemoglobin elevation may be considered an index of cyanide poisoning because of a significant correlation between measured concentrations of the two toxins.[4,8,22,75,110] Unfortunately, postmortem studies do not support this correlation.[5,71] Carboxyhemoglobin concentration alone is a poor predictor of the severity of smoke inhalation because a low or nondetectable concentration does not exclude the possibility of developing inhalation injury.[79,111] Admission carboxyhemoglobin measurements are inaccurate predictors of peak concentrations.[80] Because elevated methemoglobin concentrations are reported in fire victims, they should also be assessed in the initial laboratory evaluation.[54,108] A cooximeter will provide an accurate methemoglobin measurement. Blood cyanide analysis is of little clinical use because it takes hours to obtain results. Therapy should never await laboratory confirmation of elevated blood cyanide. Accurate measurement depends on acquiring the sample soon after exposure because cyanide is rapidly eliminated from the blood following smoke inhalation.[8,61]

Lactic acidosis, common in patients with smoke inhalation, is the result of pulmonary dysfunction resulting in hypoxia, carbon monoxide poisoning, cyanide poisoning, and/or tissue hypoperfusion.[8,111] Hypoxia from any cause impairs aerobic metabolism and generates lactic acid.

A chest radiograph is most commonly normal in the early course of smoke inhalation and is an insensitive indicator of pulmonary injury.[23,100,134] Subtle findings within 24 hours of exposure include perivascular haziness, peribronchial cuffing, bronchial wall thickening, and subglottic edema.[67,115] Serial chest radiographs following a baseline study are extremely helpful in detecting pulmonary disease following smoke inhalation.[47] Widespread airways disease usually occurs more than 24 hours after inhalation injury and may represent acute lung injury, acute respiratory distress syndrome, aspiration, volume overload, infection, or cardiogenic pulmonary edema.[115]

Nuclear imaging and pulmonary function testing, although not readily available for initial evaluation, can detect pulmonary injury after smoke inhalation. Xenon ventilation studies can detect small airway and alveolar injury before radiographic changes occur.[47,84] Abnormal flow–volume curves can indicate early upper airway obstruction.[46] Abnormal spirometry, especially forced expiratory volume (FEV_1), detects early obstructive pulmonary defects of smoke inhalation, which may precede abnormalities of arterial blood gases or radiography.[47,85]

MANAGEMENT

Critical airway compromise may be present on arrival at the hospital or may develop suddenly or insidiously.[29,46,105] A major pitfall in managing a patient with smoke inhalation is failing to appreciate this potential for rapid deterioration. History and physical findings help to determine significant smoke exposure and the potential for clinical deterioration (Table 96–3). The clinical effects of smoke exposure and their appropriate treatment are described in Figure 96–1. Upper airway patency must be rapidly

TABLE 96–3. Factors that Suggest an Increased Risk of Smoke Inhalation Injury

History	Signs
Closed-space exposure	CNS depression
Loss of consciousness	Carbonaceous sputum
Entrapment	Edema of posterior pharynx
	Face or neck burns
Symptoms	Hoarseness
Respiratory distress	Singed nasal hairs
	Stridor

established. When obvious oropharyngeal burns are observed, upper airway injury is almost certain. If such obvious injuries are not present, the degree of injury may be underestimated.[46] Direct evaluation of the upper airway is essential in assessing patients at high risk for inhalation injury.[29,46,47,55] Fiberoptic endoscopy is the preferred method. When evidence of upper airway injury exists, early endotracheal intubation should be performed under controlled circumstances instead of waiting for the patient to decompensate. Indications for early intubation include coma, visible burns or edema of the oropharynx, stridor, or full-thickness circumferential neck burns.[7,46,47,105] Massive fluid resuscitation of the burned patient contributes to upper airway edema formation.[46,47,86,105] Therefore, early intubation may be necessary in the patient with dermal burns undergoing aggressive fluid management.[46]

Although inhaled β_2-adrenergic agonists are effective and considered the first line of therapy for acute reversible bronchoconstriction from asthma or chronic obstructive pulmonary disease (COPD), their efficacy has not been evaluated in patients with smoke inhalation.[15,76] However, pathophysiologic changes induced by irritant toxins in smoke are partially reversible, suggesting that β_2-adrenergic agonists will improve airflow obstruction.[56,78] The benefits of corticosteroids for smoke inhalation injury are not demonstrated in either clinical or animal studies.[89,106] Corticosteroids are effective in the management of refractory acute asthma but should be avoided in patients with burns and inhalation injury because mortality and infection rates are increased in these patients.[84]

Pathophysiologic changes in the lung may cause progressive hypoxia over hours to days. Treatment of progressive respiratory failure includes mechanical ventilation, continuous positive airway pressure, positive end-expiratory pressure, and vigorous clearing of pulmonary secretions.[88] Frequent airway suctioning, chest physiotherapy, and therapeutic bronchoscopy can clear inspissated secretions, plugs, and casts. Inhalation injury can progress to ALI. Experimental treatment includes the use of high-frequency ventilation, percutaneous arteriovenous carbon dioxide removal, perfluorocarbons, inhaled nitric oxide, extracorpeal membrane oxygenation, instillation of natural surfactant, and continuous infusion of heparin and deferoxamine-hetastarch complex for improving inhalation injury.[21,27,33,64,92,95,98]

Respiratory compromise and other conditions may not be caused by smoke inhalation but rather by trauma or underlying medical problems. Trauma from falls or explosions must be suspected and treatment begun simultaneously with treatment of burns and inhalation injury. Comatose patients should be considered to have other etiologies and should receive naloxone, thiamine, and hypertonic dextrose as indicated. Inhaled toxins such as carbon monoxide can directly cause altered mental status, but drug and ethanol intoxication contribute significantly to adult fire fatalities and injuries. Blood ethanol concentrations correlate with elevated concentrations of carbon monoxide and cyanide, implying that intoxication impairs escape and prolongs toxic smoke exposure.[5,12,87]

Toxins may injure the skin or mucous membranes in addition to the respiratory mucosa.[26] A chemical's duration of contact with tissue is one important factor in determining the extent of chemical injury to the skin and eyes. Rapid removal of soot from skin or eyes may prevent continued injury. The eyes should be evaluated for corneal burns caused by thermal or irritant chemical injury. Patients with signs of ocular irritation should have their eyes irri-

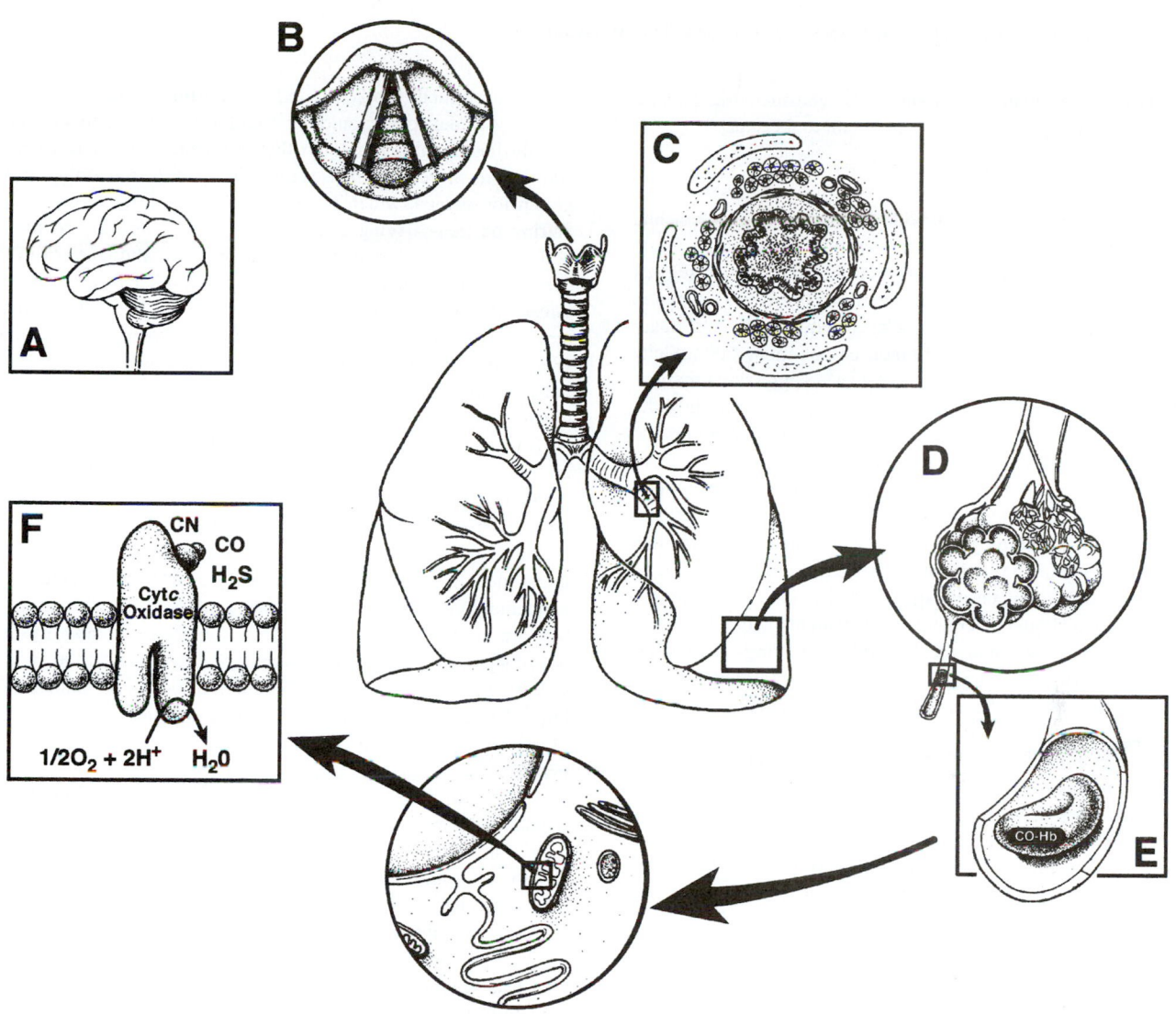

Pathophysiology	Signs and Symptoms	Management
A) Direct CNS toxic effects	Coma Hypoventilation	Oxygen; Secure unprotected airway
B) Upper airway edema	Hypoxemia; Respiratory distress Stridor Hoarse voice	Oxygen Direct visualization of vocal cords Endotracheal intubation

C) Bronchiolar airway obstruction
   Mucosal edema
   Intraluminal debris and casts
   Inspissated secretions
   Bronchospasm
	Respiratory distress
	Hypoxemia
	Wheezes
	Cough
	Increased peak airway pressures
		Oxygen
		Removal of debris and secretions
		   Chest physiotherapy
		   Frequent airway suctioning
		   Therapeutic bronchoscopy
		Inhaled beta-adrenergic agonists

D) Atelectasis Surfactant destruction Acute Lung Injury	Respiratory distress Hypoxemia Rales Chest radiographic changes	Oxygen Continuous positive airway pressure Mechanical ventilation Positive end expiratory pressure
E) Impaired oxygen carrying capacity (carbon monoxide or methemoglobinemia)	CNS depression or seizures Myocardial ischemia Dysrhythmias Metabolic acidosis	Oxygen Consider hyperbaric oxygen Consider methylene blue
F) Impaired oxygen use at tissues (cyanide, hydrogen sulfide, or carbon monoxide)	CNS depression or seizures Myocardial ischemia Dysrhythmias Metabolic acidosis	Oxygen Assure adequate tissue perfusion Consider treating suspected cyanide toxicity with sodium thiosulfate Consider hyperbaric oxygen

Figure 96–1. The final common pathway from all pathophysiologic changes that occur in smoke inhalation is hypoxia. All treatments should be focused on improving oxygen delivery and oxygen utilization.

gated. Dermal decontamination should be considered to prevent dermal burns from toxin-laden soot adherent to the skin.

Carbon Monoxide

The treatment for carbon monoxide poisoning is supplemental oxygen therapy, administered by a high-flow, tight-fitting mask, endotracheal tube, or hyperbaric oxygen therapy. Studies suggest that hyperbaric oxygen is superior to normobaric 100% oxygen in correcting toxicity and preventing delayed sequelae.[117,121,124] In addition, hyperbaric oxygen used to treat carbon monoxide toxicity decreases burn edema of the skin and airways, preserves marginally viable burn tissue, promotes wound closure, enhances host defenses, reduces extravascular lung water in pulmonary injury, and possibly treats methemoglobin or cyanide poisoning.[48,79]

Based on current literature, patients with low carboxyhemoglobin (COHb) concentrations and without a history of loss of consciousness, coma, neurologic findings, cardiovascular instability, or pregnancy are at low risk for significant sequelae and can be treated with 100% oxygen therapy.[119,131] If readily available, hyperbaric oxygen should be considered in patients with a history of loss of consciousness, coma, focal neurologic findings, pregnancy, or elevated COHb concentration (consider if greater than 25%).[119] Hyperbaric oxygen may be administered to patients only after life-threatening conditions such as associated trauma or hemodynamic instability have been treated and the patient's condition has stabilized. Controversy surrounds the lengthy transportation of critically ill patients to a facility solely for hyperbaric oxygen therapy. If a patient with major burns has associated inhalation injury, consultation with the burn center before transport to a hyperbaric oxygen facility is often necessary (Chap. 97 and Antidote in Depth: Hyperbaric Oxygen).

Cyanide

The amount of cyanide exposure and its contribution to the overall toxicity of a patient with smoke inhalation is not predictable. Cyanide toxicity causes agitation, coma, seizures, cardiovascular compromise, and metabolic acidosis. Other toxins and hypoxia may create similar signs and symptoms in the patient with smoke inhalation. Furthermore, no rapid laboratory test exists to confirm cyanide toxicity. Cyanide poisoning should be suspected in seriously ill patients with smoke inhalation. Only after life-support measures, including 100% oxygen therapy, are instituted should specific treatment for cyanide toxicity be considered.[8,81,94,101,102,110] Treatment options include supportive care alone, administration of all or part of the Cyanide Antidote Kit, and hyperbaric oxygen therapy. Patients have survived potentially lethal cyanide concentrations with just oxygen therapy and supportive care.[16,107] Hyperbaric oxygen has been suggested to improve the outcome of cyanide toxicity, although the data supporting its use alone are not convincing.[48,127] Currently, hyperbaric oxygen therapy is considered only an adjunct treatment for cyanide poisoning in the presence of concomitant carbon monoxide poisoning.[125]

The Cyanide Antidote Kit (amyl nitrite, sodium nitrite, and sodium thiosulfate) is the only antidote for cyanide poisoning available in the United States at the time of this writing. Amyl nitrite and sodium nitrite produce methemoglobinemia. Detoxification occurs when methemoglobin binds cyanide to form cyanomethemoglobin, but alternate mechanisms to methemoglobin formation are proposed. Sodium thiosulfate donates sulfur to the enzyme rhodanese, which converts cyanide to thiocyanate. Nitrite-induced methemoglobin and sodium thiosulfate work synergistically to detoxify cyanide.[19,20] Unfortunately, methemoglobin is a dysfunctional hemoglobin that is unable to carry oxygen; in addition, its presence increases the affinity of the remaining hemoglobin for oxygen, which prevents its release at the tissues.[30] Impairing oxygen-carrying capacity and oxygen delivery to tissues with nitrite-induced methemoglobinemia is a valid concern in the presence of tissue hypoxia from COHb and other factors. Sodium thiosulfate has few adverse side effects and can be safely administered to all patients seriously ill from smoke inhalation. Thus, when coma, seizures, cardiac dysrhythmias, hypotension, or metabolic acidosis are present, sodium thiosulfate alone should be given empirically.

Because cyanomethemoglobin is not measured as cyanide or methemoglobin by current clinical laboratory methods, there is a theoretical concern that formation of the cyanomethemoglobin complex may underestimate the total amount of impaired hemoglobin. Thus, the measured methemoblobin does not reflect true impairment in oxygen-carrying capacity. However, measured peak methemoglobin concentrations after a single dose of sodium nitrite are not well studied. Volunteers (obviously without cyanide poisoning) administered approximately one ampule (300 mg) of sodium nitrite generated concentrations of only 7% methemoglobin.[60] These concentrations are similar to the peak concentrations of only 9% measured in successfully treated cyanide-poisoned patients.[57]

In a small series of fire victims treated with sodium nitrite, methemoglobin concentrations peaked at 7.8 to 13.4% between 35 and 70 minutes after slow intravenous infusion.[61] Corresponding COHb concentrations decreased before peak methemoglobin concentrations had been reached. To the contrary, a case of hypotension and prolonged impairment of oxygen-carrying capacity in a smoke inhalation victim following the rapid infusion of sodium nitrite was reported.[42] Because the safety of nitrites has not been studied in a large population of concomitant cyanide and carbon monoxide poisoning and the effect of cyanomethemoglobin on oxygen-carrying capacity is not understood, it is reasonable to treat with thiosulfate alone initially and to reserve nitrite for refractory cases. If it is given, it should be in a clinical setting where COHb and methemoglobin can be measured rapidly.[102] In the presence of elevated concentrations of COHb, nitrite should be withheld. When hyperbaric oxygen therapy is available, sodium nitrite may be administered just before entrance into the hyperbaric chamber, if still clinically indicated, without concern of impairing oxygen-carrying capacity.[43] Hydroxycobalamin binds cyanide and is a safe and effective antidote.[8,44] It is not yet approved in the United States, but because of its apparent safety and efficacy, it can be given empirically to patients seriously ill with smoke inhalation, thus eliminating the need for nitrites (Chap. 98 and Antidotes in Depth: Cyanide).[8,44]

Methemoglobinemia

Although rarely reported in fire victims, methemoglobinemia can result from inhalation of certain toxic combustion products.[54,108] Elevated concentrations of methemoglobin in the presence of elevated COHb concentrations increase tissue hypoxia. In cases of smoke inhalation, initial treatment with oxygen and, if readily available, hyperbaric oxygen is best. Oxygen therapy alone should be effective for most cases. Methylene blue should be administered only in the presence of elevated methemoglobin concentrations (more than 20–30%) and/or serious symptoms.

Methemoglobinemia from smoke inhalation may be more common than is generally believed, going unrecognized because it is bound as cyanomethemoglobin and not measured. Combustion products producing methemoglobinemia may be protective against cyanide poisoning from smoke inhalation. Theoretically, methylene blue administered in the presence of cyanomethemoglobin could release free cyanide and potentially worsen toxicity.[45] The primary goal of therapy is to improve tissue oxygenation. With this in mind, methylene blue should not be withheld in situations where it is clinically indicated (Chap. 94 and Antidotes in Depth: Methlyene Blue).

SUMMARY

Smoke inhalation continues to contribute significantly to the morbidity and mortality of fire victims. A basic knowledge of the pathophysiology of smoke inhalation injury is imperative for clinicians caring for these patients. A spectrum of events is possible, from rapid upper airway occlusion to delayed pulmonary edema. Controversies in the care of these patients still exist, and further research is warranted. However, definitive therapies are available and should be considered in the care of the patients.

REFERENCES

1. Anderson RA, Cheng KN, Harland WA: The toxicology of fire deaths. Acta Med Leg Soc 1984;34:110–121.
2. Anonymous: Cable car fire kills about 170. Richmond Times-Dispatch. Richmond, 2000, November 12:A1.
3. Ansell M, Lewis FA: A review of cyanide concentrations found in human organs. J Forensic Med 1970;17:148–155.
4. Barillo DJ, Goode R, Esch V: Cyanide poisoning in victims of fire: Analysis of 364 cases and review of the literature. J Burn Care Rehabil 1994;15:46–57.
5. Barillo DJ, Goode R, Rush BF, et al: Lack of correlation between carboxyhemoglobin and cyanide in smoke inhalation. Current Surg 1986:421–423.
6. Barker SJ, Tremper KK: The effect of carbon monoxide inhalation on pulse oximetry and transcutaneous P_{O_2}. Anesthesiology 1987;66:677–679.
7. Bartlett RH, Niccole M, Tavis MJ, et al: Acute management of the upper airway in facial burns and smoke inhalation. Arch Surg 1976;111:744–749.
8. Baud FJ, Barriot P, Toffis V, et al: Elevated blood cyanide concentrations in victims of smoke inhalation. N Engl J Med 1991;325:1761–1766.
9. Becker CE: The role of cyanide in fires. Vet Hum Toxicol 1985;27:487–490.
10. Bidani A, Wang C, Heming T: Cotton smoke inhalation primes alveolar macrophages for tumor necrosis factor-alpha production and supresses macrophage antimicrobial activities. Lung 1998;176:325–336.
11. Bidani A, Wang CZ, Heming TA: Early effects of smoke inhalation on alveolar macrophage functions. Burns 1996;22:101–106.
12. Birky MM, Clarke FB: Inhalation of toxic products from fires. Bull NY Acad Med 1981;57:997–1013.
13. Bowes PC: Casualties attributed to toxic gas and smoke at fires: A survey of statistics. Med Sci Law 1976;16:104–110.
14. Brandt-Rauf PW, Fallon LF, Tarantini T: Health hazards of fire fighters: Exposure assessment. Br J Ind Med 1988;45:606–609.
15. Brenner BE: Bronchial asthma in adults: Presentation to the emergency department. Am J Emerg Med 1983;3:306–333.
16. Brivet F, Delfraissy JF, Duche M, et al: Acute cyanide poisoning: Recovery with nonspecific supportive therapy. Intensive Care Med 1983;9:33–35.
17. Cahalane M, Demling RH: Early respiratory abnormalities from smoke inhalation. JAMA 1984;251:771–773.
18. Charan NB, Meyers CG, Lakshminarayan S, et al: Pulmonary injuries associated with acute sulfur dioxide inhalation. Am Rev Respir Dis 1979;119:555–560.
19. Chen KK, Rose CL: Nitrite and thiosulfate in cyanide poisoning. JAMA 1952;149:113–119.
20. Chen KK, Rose CL, Clowes GH: Comparative values of several antidotes in cyanide poisoning. Am J Med Sci 1934;188:767–781.
21. Cioffi WG, deLemos RA, Coalson JJ, et al: Decreased pulmonary damage in primates with inhalation injury treated with high-frequency ventilation. Ann Surg 1993;218:328–337.
22. Clark CJ, Campbell D, Reid WH: Blood carboxyhaemoglobin and cyanide levels in fire survivors. Lancet 1981;1:1332–1335.
23. Clark WR, Bonaventura M, Meyers W: Smoke inhalation and airway management at a regional burn unit: 1974–1983. J Burn Care Rehabil 1989;10:52–62.
24. Clark WR, Nieman GF: Smoke inhalation. Burns 1988;14:473–494.
25. Clarke FB: Toxicity of combustion products: Current knowledge. Fire J 1983;77:84–101.
26. Close LG, Catlin FI, Cohn AM: Acute and chronic effects of ammonia burns of the respiratory tract. Arch Otolaryngol 1980;106:151–158.
27. Cox CS, Zwischenberger JB, Traber DL, et al: Heparin improves oxygenation and minimizes barotrauma after severe smoke inhalation in an ovine model. Surg Gynecol Obstet 1993;176:339–349.
28. Cox ME, Heslop BF, Kempton JJ, et al: The Dellwood fire. Br Med J 1955:942–946.
29. Crapo RO: Smoke-inhalation injuries. JAMA 1981;246:1694–1696.
30. Curry S: Methemoglobinemia. Ann Emerg Med 1982;11:214–221.
31. Davies JW: Toxic chemicals versus lung tissue—an aspect of inhalation injury revisited. J Burn Care Rehabil 1986;7:213–222.
32. Decker WJ, Koch HF: Chlorine poisoning at the swimming pool: An overlooked hazard. Clin Toxicol 1978;13:377–381.
33. Demling R, LaLonde C, Ikegami K: Fluid resuscitation with deferoxamine hetastarch complex attenuates the lung and systemic response to smoke inhalation. Surgery 1996;119:340–348.
34. Demling R, Lalonde C, Youn YK, et al: Effect of graded increases in smoke inhalation injury on the early systemic response to a body burn. Crit Care Med 1995;23:171–178.
35. Demling RH, Knox J, Youn Y, et al: Oxygen consumption early postburn becomes oxygen delivery dependent with the addition of smoke inhalation injury. J Trauma 1992;32:593–599.
36. Dyer RF, Esch VH: Polyvinyl chloride toxicity in fires: Hydrogen chloride toxicity in fire fighters. JAMA 1976;235:393–397.
37. Eisenkraft JB: Pulse oximeter desaturation due to methemoglobinemia. Anesthesiology 1988;68:279–282.
38. Fein A, Leff A, Hopewell PC: Pathophysiology and management of the complications resulting from fire and the inhaled products of combustion: Review of the literature. Crit Care Med 1980;8:94–98.
39. Guzzardi L: Toxic products of combustion. Topics Emerg Med 1985;7:45–51.
40. Hales CA, Barkin PW, Jung BW, et al: Synthetic smoke with acrolein but not HCl produces pulmonary edema. J Appl Physiol 1988;64:1121–1133.
41. Hales CA, Musto SW, Janssens S, et al: Smoke aldehyde component influences pulmonary edema. J Appl Physiol 1992;72:555–561.
42. Hall AH, Kulig KW, Rumack BH: Suspected cyanide poisoning in smoke inhalation: Complications of sodium nitrite therapy. J Toxicol Clin Exp 1989;9:3–9.
43. Hall AH, Kulig KW, Rumack BH: Toxic smoke inhalation (editorial). Am J Emerg Med 1989;7:121–122.

44. Hall AH, Rumack BH: Hydroxycobalamin/sodium thiosulfate as a cyanide antidote. J Emerg Med 1987;5:115–121.

45. Hall AH, Rumack BH: Increasing survival in acute cyanide poisoning. Emerg Med Rep 1988;9:129–136.

46. Haponik EF, Meyers DA, Munster AM, et al: Acute upper airway injury in burn patients. Am Rev Respir Dis 1987;135:360–366.

47. Haponik EF, Summer WR: Respiratory complications in burned patients: Diagnosis and management of inhalation injury. J Critical Care 1987;2:121–143.

48. Hart GB, Strauss MB, Lennon PA, et al: Treatment of smoke inhalation by hyperbaric oxygen. J Emerg Med 1985;3:211–215.

49. Hartzell GE: Overview of combustion toxicology. Toxicology 1996;115:7–23.

50. Harwood B, Hall JR: What kills in fires: Smoke inhalation or burns? Fire J 1989;84:29–34.

51. Henderson RF, Schlesinger RB: Symposium on the importance of combined exposures in inhalation toxicology. Fund Appl Toxicol 1989;12:1–11.

52. Herlihy JP, Vermeulen MW, Joseph PM, et al: Impaired alveolar macrophage function in smoke inhalation injury. J Cell Physiol 1995;163:1–8.

53. Hill IR: Particulate matter of smoke inhalation. Ann Acad Med Singapore 1993;22:119–123.

54. Hoffman RS, Sauter D: Methemoglobinemia resulting from smoke inhalation. Vet Hum Toxicol 1989;31:168–170.

55. Hunt JL, Agee RN, Pruitt BA: Fiberoptic bronchoscopy in acute inhalation injury. J Trauma 1975;15:641–649.

56. Jagoda A, Shepherd SM, Spevitz A, et al: Refractory asthma, Part 1: Epidemiology, pathophysiology, pharmacologic interventions. Ann Emerg Med 1997;29:262–274.

57. Johnson WS, Hall AH, Rumack BH: Cyanide poisoning successfully treated without 'therapeutic methemoglobin levels.' Am J Emerg Med 1989;7:437–440.

58. Jones J, Mcmullen MJ, Dougherty J: Toxic smoke inhalation: Cyanide poisoning in fire victims. Am J Emerg Med 1987;5:318–321.

59. Karter M: Fire loss in the United States during 1999. Quincy: National Fire Protection Association, 2000, pp. 1–40.

60. Kiese M, Weger N: Formation of ferrihaemoglobin with aminophenols in the human for the treatment of cyanide poisoning. Eur J Pharmacol 1969;7:97–105.

61. Kirk MA, Gerace R, Kulig KW: Cyanide and methemoglobin kinetics in smoke inhalation victims treated with the cyanide antidote kit. Ann Emerg Med 1993;22:1413–1418.

62. Laffon M, Pittet J-F, Modelska K, et al: Interleukin-8 mediates injury from smoke inhalation to both the lung endothelial and the alveolar epithelial barriers in rabbits. Am J Respir Crit Care Med 1999;160:1443–1449.

63. LaLonde C, Demling R, Brain J, et al: Smoke inhalation injury in sheep is caused by the particle phase, not the gas phase. J Appl Physiol 1994;77:15–22.

64. LaLonde C, Ikegami K, Demling R: Aerosolized deferoxamine prevents lung and systemic injury caused by smoke inhalation. J Appl Physiol 1994;77:2057–2064.

65. LaLonde C, Nayak U, Hennigan J, et al: Plasma catalase and glutathione levels are decreased in response to inhaltion injury. J Burn Care Rehabil 1997;18:515–519.

66. Layton TR, Elhauge ER: U.S. fire catastrophes of the 20th century. J Burn Care Rehabil 1982;3:21–28.

67. Lee MJ, O'Connell DJ: The plain chest radiograph after acute smoke inhalation. Clin Radiol 1988;39:33–37.

68. Levy DM, Divertie MB, Litzow TJ, et al: Ammonia burns of the face and respiratory tract. JAMA 1964;190:873–876.

69. Loick HM, Traber LD, Stothert JC, et al: Smoke inhalation causes a delayed increase in airway blood flow to primarily uninjured lung areas. Intensive Care Med 1995;21:326–333.

70. Loick HM, Traber LD, Tokyay R, et al: The effects of dopamine on pulmonary hemodynamics and tissue damage after inhalation injury in an ovine model. J Burn Care Rehabil 1992;13:305–315.

71. Lundquist P, Rammer L, Sorbo B: The role of hydrogen cyanide and carbon monoxide in fire casualties: A prospective study. Forensic Sci Int 1989;43:9–14.

72. Mahut B, Delacourt C, de Blic J, et al: Bronchiectasis in a child after acrolein inhalation. Chest 1993;104:1286–1287.

73. Mallory TB, Brickley WJ: Management of the Cocoanut Grove burns at Massachusetts General Hospital. Pathology: with special reference to the pulmonary lesions. Ann Surg 1943;117:865–884.

74. Markowitz JS, Gutterman EM, Schwartz S, et al: Acute health effects among firefighters exposed to a polyvinyl chloride (PVC) fire. Am J Epidemiol 1989;129:1023–1031.

75. Matsubara K, Akane A, Maseda C, et al: "First pass phenomenon" of inhaled gas in the fire victims. Forensic Sci Int 1990;46:203–208.

76. McFadden ER: Therapy for acute asthma. J Allergy Clin Immunol 1989;84:151–158.

77. McNeil DG: Why so many more Americans die in fires? New York Times, 1991, December 22:3.

78. Mellins RB, Park S: Respiratory complications of smoke inhalation in victims of fires. J Pediatr 1975;87:1–7.

79. Meyer GW, Hart GB, Strauss MB: Hyperbaric oxygen therapy for acute smoke inhalation injuries. Postgrad Med 1991;89:221–223.

80. Meyers RA, Britten JS: Are arterial blood gases of value in treatment decisions for carbon monoxide poisoning? Crit Care Med 1989;17:139–142.

81. Moore SJ, Ho IK, Hume AS: Severe hypoxia produced by concomitant intoxication with sublethal doses of carbon monoxide and cyanide. Toxicol Appl Pharmacol 1991;109:412–420.

82. Morgan WK: The respiratory effects of particles, vapours, and fumes. Am Ind Hyg Assoc J 1986;47:670–673.

83. Moritz AR, Henriques FC, McLean R: The effects of inhaled heat on the air passages and lungs: An experimental investigation. Am J Pathology 1945;21:311–331.

84. Moylan JA, Chan C: Inhalation injury—An increasing problem. Ann Surg 1977;188:34–37.

85. Musk AW, Smith TJ, Peters JM, et al: Pulmonary function in firefighters: Acute changes in ventilatory capacity and their correlates. Br J Ind Med 1979;36:29–34.

86. Navar PD, Saffle JR, Warden GD: Effect of inhalation injury on fluid requirements after thermal injury. Am J Surg 1985;150: 716–720.

87. Nelson GL: Regulatory aspects of fire toxicology. Toxicology 1987; 47:181–199.

88. Nieman GF, Clark WR, Goyette DA: Positive end expiratory pressure (PEEP) efficacy following wood smoke inhalation (abstract). Am Rev Respir Dis 1986;133:A347.

89. Nieman GF, Clark WR, Hakim T: Methylprednisolone does not protect the lung from inhalation injury. Burns 1991;17:384–390.

90. Nieman GF, Clark WR, Paskanik AM, et al: Unilateral smoke inhalation increases pulmonary blood flow to the injured lung. J Trauma 1994;36:617–623.

91. Nieman GF, Clark WR, Wax SD, et al: The effects of smoke inhalation on pulmonary surfactant. Ann Surg 1980;191:171–181.

92. Nieman GF, Paskanik AM, Fluck RR, et al: Comparison of exogenous surfactants in the treatment of wood smoke inhalation. Am J Respir Crit Care Med 1995;152:597–602.

93. Nijland R, Jongsma HW, Nijhuis JG, et al: Notes on the apparent discordance of pulse oximetry and multi-wavelength haemoglobin photometry. Acta Anaesthesiol Scand Suppl 1995;107:49–52.

94. Norris JC, Moore SJ, Hume AS: Synergistic lethality induced by the combination of carbon monoxide and cyanide. Toxicology 1986;40: 121–129.

95. Ogura H, Saitoh D, Johnson AA, et al: The effects of inhaled nitric oxide on pulmonary ventilation–perfusion matching following smoke inhalation injury. J Trauma 1994;37:893–898.

96. Oliver O: Management of the Cocoanut Grove burns at the Massachusetts General Hospital. Ann Surg 1943;117:801–802.

97. Orzel RA: Toxicologic aspects of firesmoke: Polymer pyrolysis and combustion. Occup Med 1993;8:414–429.

98. O'Toole G, Peek G, Jaffe W, et al: Extracorporeal membrane oxygenation in the treatment of inhalational injuries. Burns 1998;24:562–565.

99. Oulton MR, Janigan DT, MacDonald JM, et al: Effects of smoke inhalation on alveolar surfactant subtypes in mice. Am J Pathol 1994;145:941–950.

100. Peitzman AB, Shires GT, Teixidor HS, et al: Smoke inhalation injury: Evaluation of radiographic manifestations and pulmonary dysfunction. J Trauma 1989;29:1232–1239.

101. Pitt BR, Radford EP, Gurtner GH, et al: Interaction of carbon monoxide and cyanide on cerebral circulation and metabolism. Arch Environ Health 1979;34:354–355.

102. Prien T: Toxic smoke compounds and inhalation injury—a review. Burns 1988;14:451–460.

103. Purser DA, Woolley WD: Biological studies of combustion atmospheres. J Fire Sci 1983;1:118–144.

104. Riyami BM, Kinsella J, Pollok AJ, et al: Alveolar macrophage chemotaxis in fire victims with smoke inhalation and burns injury. Eur J Clin Invest 1991;21:485–489.

105. Robinson L, Miller RH: Smoke inhalation injuries. Am J Otolaryngol 1986;7:375–380.

106. Robinson NB, Hudson LD, Riem M, et al: Steroid therapy following isolated smoke inhalation injury. J Trauma 1982;22:876–879.

107. Saincher A, Swirsky N, Tenenbein M: Cyanide overdose: Survival with fatal blood concentration without antidotal therapy. J Emerg Med 1994;12:555–557.

108. Schwerd W, Schulz E: Carboxyhaemoglobin and methaemoglobin findings in burnt bodies. Forensic Sci Int 1978;12:233–235.

109. Shusterman D, Alexeeff G, Hargis C, et al: Predictors of carbon monoxide and hydrogen cyanide exposure in smoke inhalation patients. J Toxicol Clin Toxicol 1996;34:61–71.

110. Silverman SH, Purdue GF, Hunt JL, et al: Cyanide toxicity in burned patients. J Trauma 1988;28:171–176.

111. Sokal JA, Kralkowska E: The relationship between exposure duration, carboxyhemoglobin, blood glucose, pyruvate and lactate and the severity of intoxication in 39 cases of acute carbon monoxide poisoning in man. Arch.Toxicol. 1985:196–199.

112. Stone JP, Hazlett RN, Johnson JE, et al: The transport of hydrogen chloride by soot from burning polyvinyl chloride. J Fire Flammability 1973;4:42–51.

113. Symington IS, Anderson RA, Oliver JS, et al: Cyanide exposures in fires. Lancet 1978;2:90–92.

114. Tasaki O, Goodwin C, Saitoh D, et al: Effects of burns on inhalational injury. J Trauma Inj Inf Crit Care 1997;43:603–607.

115. Teixidor HS, Rubin E, Novick GS, et al: Smoke inhalation: Radiologic manifestations. Radiology 1983;149:383–387.

116. Terrill JB, Montgomery RR, Reinhardt CF: Toxic gases from fires. Science 1978;200:1343–1347.

117. Thom SR: Antagonism of carbon monoxide–mediated brain lipid peroxidation by hyperbaric oxygen. Toxicol Appl Pharmacol 1990;105:340–344.

118. Thom SR: Carbon monoxide mediated brain lipid peroxidation in the rat. J Appl Physiol 1990;63:997–1003.

119. Thom SR, Keim LW: Carbon monoxide poisoning: A review of epidemiology, pathophysiology, clinical findings, and treatment options including hyperbaric oxygen. J Toxicol Clin Toxicol 1989;27:141–156.

120. Thom SR, Mendiguren I, Van Winkle T, et al: Smoke inhalation with a concurrent systemic stress results in lung alveolar injury. Am J Respir Crit Care Med 1994;149:220–226.

121. Thom SR, Taber RL, Mendiguren II, et al: Delayed neuropsychologic sequelae after carbon monoxide poisoning: Prevention by treatment with hyperbaric oxygen. Ann Emerg Med 1995;25:474–480.

122. Thompson PB, Herdon DN, Traber DL, et al: Effects on mortality of inhalation injury. J Trauma 1986;26:163–165.

123. Thorning DR, Howard ML, Hudson LD, et al: Pulmonary responses to smoke inhalation: Morphologic changes in rabbits exposed to pine wood smoke. Hum Pathol 1982;13:355–364.

124. Tomaszewski CA, Rudy J, Rosenberg N, et al: Prevention of neurologic sequelae from carbon monoxide by hyperbaric oxygen in rats (abstract). Neurology 1992;42:196.

125. Tomaszewski CA, Thom SR: Use of hyperbaric oxygen in toxicology. Emerg Med Clin North Am 1994;12:437–459.

126. Traber DL, Linares HA, Herndon DN: The pathophysiology of inhalation injury—a review. Burns 1988;14:357–364.

127. Trapp WG: Massive cyanide poisoning with recovery: A boxing-day story. Can Med Assoc J 1970;102:517.

128. Treitman RD, Burgess WA, Gold A: Air contaminants encountered by firefighters. Am Ind Hyg Assoc J 1980;41:796–802.

129. Tremper KK, Barker SJ: Using pulse oximetry when dyshemoglobin levels are high. J Crit Illness 1988;3:103–107.

130. Wang CZ, Li A, Yang ZC: The pathophysiology of carbon monoxide poisoning and acute respiratory failure in a sheep model with smoke inhalation injury. Chest 1990;97:736–742.

131. Weiss LD, Van Meter KW: The applications of hyperbaric oxygen therapy in emergency medicine. Am J Emerg Med 1992;10:558–568.

132. Wetherell HR: The occurrence of cyanide in the blood of fire victims. J Forensic Sci 1966;11:167–173.

133. Witten ML, Quan SF, Sobonya RE, et al: New developments in the pathogenesis of smoke inhalation-induced pulmonary edema. West J Med 1988;148:33–36.

134. Wittram C, Kenny JB: The admission chest radiograph after acute inhalation injury and burns. Br J Radiol 1994;67:751–754.

135. Youn Y, Lalonde C, Demling R: Oxidants and the pathophysiology of burn and smoke inhalation injury. Free Radic Biol Med 1992;12:409–415.

136. Zawacki BE, Jung RC, Joyce J, et al: Smoke, burns, and the natural history of inhalation injury in fire victims: A correlation of experimental and clinical data. Ann Surg 1977;185:100–110.

137. Zikria BA, Ferrer JM, Floch HF. The chemical factors contributing to pulmonary damage in "smoke poisoning". Surgery 1972;71:704–709.

CHAPTER 97 CARBON MONOXIDE

Christian Tomaszewski

Carbon Monoxide (CO)

MW	=	28.01 daltons
Gas density	=	0.968 (air = 1.0)
Carboxyhemoglobin levels		
Nonsmokers	=	1–2%
Smokers	=	5–10%
Action level	=	>10%
TLV–TWA	=	50 ppm

Values greater than or equal to the action level usually necessitate clinical intervention. Values less than this level may necessitate intervention based on the clinical condition of the patient.

A 35-year-old woman was found sitting outside of a warehouse. Her boss stated that she had been operating a forklift in an enclosed building all morning. She came stumbling out complaining of dizziness and headaches. Coworkers in an adjoining building also complained of mild headache. After collapsing outside, she regained consciousness immediately but still appeared confused to coworkers. Prehospital personnel started an IV of 0.9% sodium chloride and placed her on 100% oxygen at the scene before transport.

On arrival at the ED, the patient was still somewhat drowsy, oriented only to person and place, and complaining of a severe headache. Initial vital signs were: blood pressure 92/58 mm Hg, pulse 112 beats/min, respirations 26 breaths/min, and rectal temperature 100°F (38°C). Examination of the head revealed midsize reactive pupils with a supple neck. Chest examination revealed clear lungs with a regular tachycardia. Neurologic examination revealed good strength and sensation bilaterally with normal reflexes. The patient refused to stand because of weakness and dizziness. The boss arrived and stated that the patient was probably suffering from the flu or food poisoning. Several other employees had been complaining of similar symptoms all week. This was not surprising because the local health department had reported record cases of influenza A that season.

The patient was placed on a cardiac monitor and 100% oxygen by nonrebreather face mask. A fingerstick bedside blood glucose was 80 mg/dL. As the physician obtained a blood specimen for carboxyhemoglobin determination, the patient then related that she had been having palpitations and mild chest pain. An ECG was ordered.

Laboratory results finally returned. The ECG revealed normal sinus rhythm without ischemic changes. Arterial blood gas results were: pH 7.32, Pco_2 32 mm Hg, Po_2 124 mm Hg. Later a carboxyhemoglobin level of 18% returned. Further questioning of EMS personnel revealed that patient transport was delayed, and the patient was on 100% oxygen for at least 30 minutes before the blood drawing in the emergency department.

After 2 hours on 100% oxygen, the patient remained somewhat drowsy and still complained of a severe headache. On brief mental status examination the patient was still amnestic for the events that occurred and was oriented only to person and place. She could apparently remember only two out of three objects at 5 minutes. In addition, when standing she still had problems walking a straight line heel to toe. The health care worker decided to consult a local poison center to see if further neurologic evaluation was warranted. After discussing the case with the poison center, the health care worker felt that she should transfer the patient to the nearest hyperbaric facility for further treatment.

The patient was transferred by helicopter, requiring less than one hour to reach the hyperbaric center. On arrival she was fully alert and mentioned her concern for HBO treatment when in fact she might be pregnant. A urine pregnancy test was promptly done, testing positive. After being explained the risks and benefits of the procedure, she decided to proceed with HBO treatment. After one dive, her symptoms improved, but 4 hours later she still complained of a mild headache. A second HBO treatment was recommended by the hyperbaric staff 6 hours after her initial treatment. She refused, stating that she was severely claustrophobic and refused to reenter the confines of the monoplace unit.

On the subsequent day the patient felt much better. A bedside mini–mental status examination revealed good attention and memory. A more formal neuropsychological battery revealed no deficiencies. She returned to work in 3 days. At 3-week followup, she reported no untoward symptoms. Seven months later she gave birth to an apparently normal infant boy.

The onset of headache and dizziness, especially with involvement of coworkers, strongly suggested an airborne toxin. With poor air circulation, there could be a buildup of various air pollutants, microbial agents, and allergens that could result in sick building syndrome. Although patients suffering from sick building syndrome often have a headache, this is usually accompanied by irritation of the airways and mucous membranes, which would occur with CO poisoning.[18] The forklift was a likely culprit for an exposure in this case. Propane, the typical fuel of indoor forklifts, is an asphyxiant and at low doses can cause euphoria[232] (Chap. 95). However, the accompanying mercaptans would have alerted workers to a dangerous leak. Nitrogen dioxide, an occasional combustion product of propane, can cause delayed respiratory symptoms but does not typically cause headache.[89] The most likely gas exposure responsible for these symptoms is CO.

For optimal performance propane-powered forklifts are typically adjusted to produce no less than 10,000 ppm CO in exhaust and in fact average more than 30,000 ppm.[60] In an enclosed warehouse, with poor ventilation, CO levels could exceed toxic levels within an hour at this rate of production. Workers, as in the case example, would succumb to its toxic effects without warning because CO is a clear, odorless, nonirritating gas.

INTRODUCTION

Carbon monoxide (CO) is the leading cause of poisoning morbidity and mortality in the United States. A comprehensive review of death certificate data compiled by the National Center for Health Statistics shows an average of 5613 deaths each year (1979–1988) from CO poisoning.[34] More recent estimates show at least 2100 unintentional poisonings each year in the United States.[236] A more significant problem may be the morbidity associated with this poisoning. One source has estimated that approximately 10,000 people seek medical attention or lose at least 1 day of normal activity because of CO toxicity each year.[178] The most serious complication of this poisoning is persistent or delayed neurologic dysfunction in 14 to 40% of discharged patients.[144,190] These numbers may underestimate the real problem because many more patients may be treated and released for a myriad of complaints when in reality they have unrecognized CO poisoning.

EPIDEMIOLOGY

Although CO is found naturally in the body as a by-product of hemoglobin degradation, it reaches toxic concentrations following inhalation or by absorption and metabolism following exposure to methylene chloride.[35] External sources of CO include incomplete combustion of any carbonaceous fossil fuel. In a 10-year review of CO-related deaths, over half of unintentional deaths were caused by motor vehicle exhaust.[34] Occupants of motor vehicles are not the only victims of exhaust gases. Carbon monoxide poisoning is also reported in children riding in the back of pickup trucks.[83] Workers also become symptomatic from use of propane-powered equipment indoors such as forklifts[57,61] and ice skating rink resurfacers.[102] Even occupants of boats are not immune to this insidious toxin.[187]

In the past 10 years, unintentional CO exposures from nonvehicular sources have resulted in an average of 500 deaths per year in the United States.[34] Predominantly, these have involved the burning of charcoal, wood, or natural gas for heating and cooking.[41,62,64,82] Furnaces for heating are often the culprits, especially when the flue is blocked.[15,76,88] Gas kitchen stoves are an important source of CO in indigent populations with marginal heating systems.[193] In fact, the use of gas stoves for supplemental heat is predictive of high COHb levels in patients with headache and dizziness.[86]

Fires are another important source of CO exposure. In the past 10 years, CO was listed as the cause of or major contributor to 15,523 fire deaths.[34] Carbon monoxide is considered to be the most common hazard to smoke inhalation victims.[15,46,185,220] Exposure to smoke that may include cyanide, another by-product of fire combustion, can result in morbidity and mortality greater than that predicted by the amount of CO exposure alone[13] (Chaps. 96 and 98).

PHARMACOLOGY

CO has a molecular mass of 28.01 daltons. It has a gas density 0.968 relative to air. CO is found naturally in the body as a by-product of heme degradation.[35] As a gas, CO appears to be a neu-

ronal messenger by virtue of the fact that as a gas it can diffuse and signal adjacent cells.[9] Heme oxygenase, the responsible enzyme, is primarily found in the liver and spleen, to break down old blood. But a second form is in the brain, where once CO is produced it can behave like nitric oxide (NO), binding to guanylate cyclase and thereby increasing cGMP levels.[128] Although low endogenous levels are physiologic, excessive concentrations of CO from exogenous sources may be problematic because CO persists much longer than NO.[73]

PHARMACOKINETICS AND TOXICOKINETICS

Carbon monoxide is readily absorbed after inhalation. The Coburn-Forster-Kane (CFK) model allows the prediction of COHb levels based on exposure history.[37] This model has been simplified to allow estimation of the equilibrium based on the ambient concentration of CO in ppm: $COHb (\%) = 100/[1 + (643.3/ppm\ CO)]$.[216] This assumes that the individual weighs 70 kg and is not anemic. With exponential uptake, it may take more than 4 hours for equilibrium to be attained. Meanwhile, endogenous production of CO is not factored in because its contribution to COHb is only 2%.

Once absorbed, CO is carried in the blood, primarily bound to hemoglobin. The Haldane ratio states that CO has approximately a 200 to 250 times greater affinity than oxygen for hemoglobin.[25] Therefore, CO is primarily confined to the blood compartment, but eventually up to 15% of total CO body stores are taken up by tissue, primarily bound to myoglobin.[36] The dissolved CO concentration in the serum, therefore, may better reflect the ultimate potential for poisoning, as it is available for diffusion into all tissue compartments, including the brain.[123]

Elimination of CO, like absorption, from the blood can be modeled mathematically, using the CFK model. The equation predicts a half-life of 252 minutes.[37] In actual volunteer studies, means of 249 and 320 minutes have been found.[155,161] With 100% oxygen, these half-lives can be reduced significantly to means of 47, 78, and 80 minutes in studies of volunteers who attain COHb levels of 10 to 12%.[155,161,199] Two series of patients poisoned with CO showed actual mean half-lives of 74 and 131 minutes when treated with 100% oxygen.[19,230]

Methylene chloride, a paint-stripping agent, is another source of CO. It is readily absorbed through the skin or by inhalation and is metabolized in the liver to CO.[196] After a delay of 8 hours or longer, peak levels of COHb can range from 10 to 50%.[59,115,122,171] Because of ongoing production of CO, the apparent COHb half-life is prolonged to 13 hours.[169] COHb levels after methylene chloride exposure appear to be proportional to the concentration and duration of exposure.[185]

PATHOPHYSIOLOGY

CO's most obvious effect is binding to hemoglobin, rendering it incapable of delivering oxygen to the cells, because as previously stated, the affinity for hemoglobin is 200 to 250 times greater than that of oxygen.[54] Therefore, in spite of adequate partial pressures of oxygen in blood (PO_2), there is decreased arterial oxygen content. Further insult occurs because CO causes a leftward shift of the oxyhemoglobin dissociation curve, thus decreasing the offloading of oxygen from hemoglobin to tissue.[174] This may result in part from a decrease in erythrocyte 2,3-diphosphoglycerate concentration.[7,215] The net effect of all these processes is the decreased ability of oxygen to be carried by the bloodstream and released to cells.

Carbon monoxide toxicity cannot be attributed solely to COHb-mediated hypoxia.[170] Neither clinical effects nor the phenomena of delayed neurologic deficits can be completely predicted by the extent of binding between hemoglobin and CO.[140,149,191,210] Furthermore, it does not explain why negligible levels of COHb (4–5%) can result in cognitive impairment.[119] An early study showed that dogs breathing 13% CO died within an hour with COHb levels 54 to 90%; however, exchange transfusion of this same blood into healthy dogs caused no untoward effects.[71] Comparable levels of anemia also lacked adverse effects. The conclusion was that inherent to CO toxicity is its delivery to target organs such as the brain and heart.[70,71]

The delivery of CO intracellularly and its binding to heme proteins other than hemoglobin may also account for its toxicity. Ten to 15% of the total body store of CO is extravascular.[36] Some of this CO may be interfering with cellular respiration by binding to mitochondrial cytochrome oxidase, as occurs in vitro.[8,26] Initial studies show that this binding is especially exaggerated under conditions of hypoxia and hypotension.[20]

Inactivation of cytochrome oxidase may be only an initial part of the cascade of events resulting in an ischemic reperfusion injury to the brain after CO poisoning. During recovery from the initial poisoning, white blood cells are attracted to and adhere to the damaged brain microvasculature.[212] This attraction may be partly attributable to endothelial changes from initial cytochrome oxidase dysfunction, mediated primarily through the free radical nitric oxide.[98,204] Carbon monoxide displaces nitric oxide from platelets that in turn form peroxynitrites, even stronger inactivators of cytochrome oxidase.[212] Multiple animal studies show that nitric oxide is ultimately responsible for much of the endothelial damage from CO, which can be blocked by nitric oxide synthase inhibitors.[208,211,214] After the leukocytes attach to the damaged endothelium, they release proteases that convert xanthine dehydrogenase to xanthine oxidase, an enzyme that promotes formation of oxygen free radicals.[202] The end result of this process is delayed lipid peroxidation of the brain, as demonstrated in a rat model.[201]

CO neuronal damage may not be a simple matter of cytochrome oxidase inactivation accompanied by ischemic-reperfusion injury. In addition, glutamate increases in rat brains after CO poisoning.[239] Glutamate is an excitatory amino acid that can bind at N-methyl-D-aspartate (NMDA) receptors and cause intracellular calcium release, resulting in delayed neuronal cell death.[16] Blockade of NMDA receptors can prevent the neuronal death and learning deficits that accompany serious CO poisoning in a mouse.[99] Newer data suggest that ultimately CO neuronal cell death may be a form of apoptosis.[221] Rises in the glutamate in rat brain in the first hour after severe CO poisoning are followed by a later rise in hydroxyl radicals.[162] Ultimately, at 1 to 3 weeks the animals show histologic evidence of both neuronal necrosis and apoptosis in the frontal cortex, globus pallidus, and cerebellum that are accompanied by deficits in learning and memory in a radial maze. The role of apoptosis has been confirmed in bovine pulmonary artery cells, where CO exposure is accompanied by activation of caspase-1, a protease implicated in delayed cell death.[207] Confirmatory evidence was provided in the same study in that both caspase-1 and nitric oxide synthase inhibitors blocked apoptosis. The end result

of all these cellular processes is brain injury within the basal ganglia and hippocampus, resulting in impaired learning.[205] Thus, animal models correlate well with what ultimately occurs in victims of serious CO poisoning, namely, the learning and memory deficits so common in persistent or delayed neurologic sequelae.

Myoglobin is another heme-protein that binds CO with an affinity about 60 times greater than that of oxygen.[38] A dog model demonstrates that this binding is enhanced under hypoxic conditions.[38] This binding may partially explain the myocardial impairment that occurs in both animal studies[43] and low-level exposures in patients with ischemic heart disease.[6] Isolated rat heart studies demonstrate that this toxic effect on the heart exists regardless of COHb formation.[27] The combination of COHb formation, which decreases oxygen-carrying capacity, and the production of reduced myoglobin in the heart, which decreases oxygen extraction, may explain the preterminal dysrhythmias seen in animal studies.[66] Volunteers, especially those with preexisting heart disease, develop an increase in life-threatening dysrhythmias and ischemic changes with low-level exposures (resulting in COHb levels up to 6%) during stress testing.[2,183]

Several recent studies suggest that CO effects on the cardiovascular system are necessary for ischemic reperfusion injury of the brain. Hypotension, essential for ischemic reperfusion injury, results from a combination of myocardial depression from carboxymyoglobin formation and vasodilation from cellular effects of CO. Carbon monoxide is a presumed neural messenger that activates guanylate cyclase, which in turn relaxes vascular smooth muscle.[224,226] Also, CO can act on platelets to displace nitric oxide, which in turn is also a potent vasodilator.[111,206] These factors contribute to the hypotension that occurs in animal experiments with high doses of CO toxicity.[69,78] Such an episode of hypotension may be represented clinically by the syncope or loss of consciousness that accompanies serious CO poisoning and portends a worse clinical outcome.[31,63,134] In the rhesus monkey, cerebral white matter lesions correlate better with decreases in blood pressure than with COHb level.[69,150] Lipid peroxidation of the brain in rats develops an hour after a CO exposure that has terminated in syncope and hypotension.[201] This delay is comparable to that necessary to produce mitochondrial destruction from oxidative stress in rats exposed to CO.[238] In a feline model, central nervous system damage comparable to that associated with CO can be reproduced only when hypoxia is accompanied by one interval of ischemia, confirming the ischemic-reperfusion model for central nervous system insult after CO poisoning.[151]

CLINICAL MANIFESTATIONS
Effects of Acute Exposure

The earliest symptoms associated with CO poisoning are often nonspecific and readily confused with other illnesses, typically viral syndromes[23] (Table 97–1). The initial symptom reported by volunteers within 4 hours of exposure to 200 ppm COHb levels (15–20%) is headache; shorter exposures at 500 ppm lead to nausea as well.[197,198] The incidence of CO poisoning in symptomatic patients presenting with flulike symptoms to emergency departments in the winter ranges from 3 to 24% in some series.[29,53,85,86] Because the typical presenting complaints are headache, dizziness, and nausea, and the most frequent exposures occur during winter, it is not surprising that influenza is the most common misdiagnosis.[53,76] Carbon monoxide poisoning is also frequently misdiag-

TABLE 97–1.   Clinical Manifestations of Carbon Monoxide Poisoning

Severity	Symptoms	Signs
Mild	Headache	Vomiting
	Nausea	
	Dizziness	
Moderate	Confusion	Tachypnea
	Chest pain	Tachycardia
	Dyspnea	Cognitive deficits
	Weakness	Ataxia
	Blurred vision	Myonecrosis
Severe	Chest pain	Coma
	Palpitations	Seizures
	Disorientation	Ventricular dysrhythmias
		Hypotension
		Myocardial ischemia

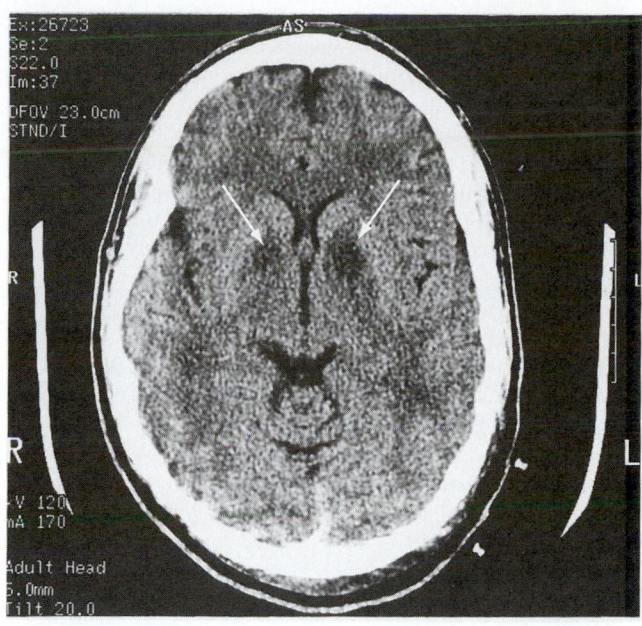

Figure 97–1. Computerized tomography of the brain showing bilateral lesions of the globus pallidus (lucent areas) in a patient with poor recovery from severe CO poisoning. (Courtesy of New York City Poison Center Fellowship in Medical Toxicology.)

nosed as food poisoning,[11] gastroenteritis,[64,93] and even colic in infants.[163] Children tend to show nonspecific symptoms, eg, nausea, headache, and vomiting, with CO poisoning, making the diagnosis equally difficult.[44]

Continued exposure to CO can lead to symptoms attributable to another extremely oxygen-dependent organ, the heart. Low-level exposures (COHb 2–4%) in volunteers with stable angina result in decreased exercise tolerance as well as signs and symptoms of myocardial ischemia.[2,3,5] At higher levels (COHb 6%) there is a greater frequency of premature ventricular contractions during exercise.[183] Myocardial infarction, life-threatening dysrhythmias, and cardiac arrest are commonly described in victims of CO poisoning.[4,127,179,188] In fact, acute mortality from CO is usually a result of ventricular dysrhythmias, probably predominantly caused by the accompanying hypoxia.[2,4,43,179]

The central nervous system is the most sensitive area to CO poisoning. Acutely, otherwise healthy patients may manifest headache, dizziness, and ataxia at COHb levels as low as 15 to 20%; with longer exposures, syncope, seizures, or coma can result.[23,90] Patients may present with symptoms of an acute stroke.[11,105] The EEG can show diffuse frontal slow-wave activity.[63,148] Within a day of exposures that result in coma, the CT scan can show decreased density in the central white matter and globus pallidus (Fig. 97–1).[186,217] Autopsies show involvement of other areas including the cerebral cortex, hippocampus, cerebellum, and substantia nigra.[116]

Metabolic changes may reflect CO's toxic effects better than any particular COHb level. Mild CO cases may be accompanied by respiratory alkalosis to compensate for the reduction in oxygen-carrying capacity and delivery.[130] Longer exposures with decreased levels of consciousness result in metabolic acidosis, from the lactate production that accompanies tissue hypoxia.[191] In fact, a series of 48 CO poisoned cases showed retrospectively that hydrogen ion concentration, rather than COHb level, was a better predictor of poor recovery during initial hospitalization.[223]

Although the brain and heart are the most sensitive, other organs may also manifest the effects of CO poisoning. One-fifth to one-third of severe CO cases, ie, those that required intubation, go on to develop cardiogenic pulmonary edema.[75,192] This does not appear to be a direct effect of CO. Studies of sheep with prolonged exposure to CO, resulting in COHb levels greater than 50%, showed no anatomic or physiologic change in lung function.[184] Al-

though myonecrosis and even compartment syndromes occur, patients rarely develop renal failure.[14,182] Retinal hemorrhages can develop with exposures greater than 12 hours.[48,105] Cherry-red skin coloration occurs only after excessive exposure (2–3% of cases referred to one hyperbaric center) and may represent a combination of CO-induced vasodilation with concomitant tissue ischemia.[144,172] Another classic but uncommon phenomenon is the development of cutaneous bullae following severe exposures.[144] These bullae are thought to be caused by a combination of pressure necrosis and possibly direct CO effects in the epidermis.[95,120]

Delayed Effects

The persistent or delayed effects of CO poisoning are varied and include dementia, amnestic syndromes, psychosis, parkinsonism, paralysis, chorea, cortical blindness, apraxia and agnosias, peripheral neuropathy, and incontinence.[65,121] The neurologic deterioration can be preceded by a lucid period of 2 to 40 days after the initial CO poisoning.[31] In patients admitted to an intensive care unit for severe CO toxicity and treated with 100% oxygen, 14% of survivors had permanent neurologic impairment.[111] In a Korean series of 2360 CO-poisoned patients, almost 3% continued to show memory failure or parkinsonian features 1 year postexposure.[31] In contrast, another series of 63 seriously poisoned patients showed memory impairment in 43% and deterioration of personality in 33% at 3-year followup.[190] Children have shown behavioral and educational difficulties after severe poisoning.[114] However, older patients (more than 30 years old) appear to be much more susceptible to developing delayed sequelae.[31] Most cases of delayed neurologic sequelae are associated with loss of consciousness in the acute phase of intoxication.[31,63,190]

Delayed neurologic sequelae probably involve lesions of the cerebral white matter and basal ganglia.[65] Weeks postexposure, autopsies show necrosis of the white matter, globus pallidus, cerebellum, and hippocampus.[63] Computerized tomography and MRI confirm the damage to the white matter and hippocampus.[94,150,186,217] Animal studies show that marked COHb alone cannot cause similar white-matter lesions; there must be an episode of hypotension.[69,151] The fact that the areas permanently damaged in serious CO poisoning cases are the areas with the poorest vascular supply in the brain is consistent with these animal findings.

Effects of Chronic Exposure

Often, patients will complain of persistent headaches and cognitive problems after long-term exposure to low levels of carbon monoxide. Unfortunately, to date, there are no controlled studies showing that such exposures, in the absence of a severe acute poisoning episode, result in any long-term sequelae. With continued exposure to low levels of CO, highway toll workers have trouble performing on parallel processing tasks.[101] Warehouse workers, chronically exposed to CO from propane combustion, have intermittent problems with headache, nausea, and lightheadedness.[57] However, unless there has been an episode of severe poisoning with acute deterioration, most workers go on to have resolution of their symptoms.[60] Without baseline testing before exposure, it is hard to definitely attribute one woman's permanent verbal memory, learning, and visual recall problems to long-term CO exposure. She had had ongoing headache, depression, and confusion from a 3-year exposure to CO at 180 ppm from a faulty furnace.[176] Although it is unclear that chronic exposure to low levels of CO can do any damage, healthcare providers still should be vigilant for symptomatic individuals in order to prevent continued or catastrophic outcomes.

DIAGNOSTIC TESTING

The most useful diagnostic test obtainable in a suspected CO poisoning is a COHb level. Normal levels of COHb range from 0 to 5%, with levels at the high range in neonates and patients with hemolytic anemia,[234] as carbon monoxide is a natural by-product of the breakdown of protoporphyrin to bilirubin.[35] Carboxyhemoglobin levels average 6% in one-pack-per-day smokers but can range as high as 10%.[195] Although high COHb levels confirm exposure to CO, particular levels are not necessarily predictive of symptoms or outcome. In fact, COHb can return to normal or be zero if the patient has been treated with oxygen before obtaining the blood test.[140,149,191]

The usual method for measuring COHb is with a CO-oximeter, which spectrophotometrically reads the percentage of total hemoglobin saturated with CO.[12,39] Traditionally, arterial blood is used for this determination; however, venous blood levels from a heparinized (lithium heparin tube) specimen are just as accurate.[219] Of note, refrigerated heparinized samples yield accurate carboxyhemoglobin levels for several weeks, making retrospective evaluations possible.[52] Bedside tests with ammonia or sodium hydroxide are unable to differentiate reliably various levels of COHb versus controls.[153] Breath-sampling methods may be used for screening patients; however, ethanol, a common cointoxicant, can falsely elevate breath levels unless an activated charcoal filter is used.[113,161,222] Because of the similarities in extinction coefficients, COHb is misinterpreted as oxyhemoglobin on pulse oximetry (Chap. 20).[10] The pulse oximetry reading overestimates oxyhemo-

globin by the approximate amount of carboxyhemoglobin present.[22,80]

Recently, some clinicians have begun to measure CO directly in blood samples, rather than carboxyhemoglobin.[123] This technique involves assaying CO directly with infrared spectrophotometry after it is extracted from the blood sample with a manometer.[138] Based on calculations, rather than true experimental data, the assumption has been made that for a patient with a normal hemoglobin, a CO concentration of 1 mmol/L corresponds to 11% COHb.[154] A simpler method to measure plasma CO content is to add a known solution of hemoglobin followed by sodium dithionite to form COHb.[30] The resulting COHb is measured spectrophotometrically, with the assumption that 1 mole of hemoglobin binds 4 moles of CO. Interestingly, in one study, plasma CO ranged 0.14 to 0.6 mg/L but was the same in smokers (average 4.6%COHb) and nonsmokers (average 1%).[30] At this time, further research is required to determine the clinical import of plasma CO content.

Additional laboratory tests may be useful in severe poisoning cases. An arterial blood gas will confirm the presence of metabolic acidosis, a complication of CO poisoning associated with neurologic sequelae and death.[117] This acidosis is presumably a reflection of high lactate, an index more reliable than COHb in determining severity of toxicity.[191] Unfortunately, arterial pH does not correlate with either COHb level or initial neurologic examination, making it a poor criterion for deciding the need for HBO treatment.[140] Mild elevations of CPK are common (ranging 20 to 1315 IU/L in one series of 65 cases), but severe rhabdomyolysis and its complications are also reported.[182] Cardiac monitoring and a 12-lead ECG are essential to document ischemia or dysrhythmias in symptomatic patients with preexisting coronary artery disease or severe exposure. Recently, it has been found that rats have early increases in glutathione released from erythrocytes, a potential marker for CO oxidative stress that could ultimately lead to brain injury.[209]

The problem with using COHb levels to base treatment is that there is a wide variation in clinical manifestations with identical COHb levels.[139,146] Furthermore, particular COHb levels are not predictive of symptoms or final outcome.[130,140,149,191] In a large prospective study of CO poisoning, COHb levels did not correlate with loss of consciousness and were not predictive of delayed neurologic sequelae.[168] Part of the problem is that admission COHb levels are inaccurate predictors of peak levels.[140] The use of nomograms to extrapolate to earlier levels has not been validated. Their credibility is also suspect because of the great variability in COHb half-lives and differences in treatment with oxygen.

Neuropsychological Testing

The extent of neurologic insult from CO can be assessed with a variety of tests. The most basic is documentation of a normal neurologic examination with a quick mini–mental status examination. A more sensitive indicator of the acute effects of CO on cortical function is a detailed neuropsychiatric test battery developed specifically for CO patients.[143] The advantages of such testing, which usually takes about 30 minutes, are that (1) it can reliably distinguish 79% of the time between CO-poisoned patients and controls, and (2) it shows improvement with appropriate HBO treatment.[132] Unfortunately, such testing shows a sensitivity of only 77% and specificity of 80% for CO poisoning.[173] There may be practice effects as well, if repeated testing is performed. The biggest problem with such neuropsychiatric testing is that it is unclear if deficits in the test during the acute CO poisoning are at all predictive of which patients will develop neurologic sequelae and therefore require HBO treatment.

Neuroimaging

Acute changes on CT scan of the brain have been seen within 12 hours of CO exposure that resulted in loss of consciousness.[103,135,147] Symmetric low-density areas in the region of the globus pallidus, putamen, and caudate nuclei frequently occur.[96,107,147] Although a normal initial CT usually predicts a favorable outcome, changes in the globus pallidus and subcortical white matter early within the first day after poisoning are associated with poor outcomes[135,165] (Fig. 97–1). In one series of 18 patients, a negative CT within a week of admission was associated with favorable outcome.[217] The use of contrast may enhance early isodense changes that may not be visible on initial CT scan.[237] MRI appears to be superior in detecting basal ganglia lesions.[94,104] Neuroimaging usually does not influence patient management and can be reserved for patients who show poor response or have an equivocal diagnosis.

The most promising area of neuroimaging after CO poisoning is in the area of assessment of regional cerebral perfusion. Single-photon emission computed tomography (SPECT) gauges regional blood flow noninvasively using an iodine or technetium tracer.[49] In one series of 13 patients with delayed neurologic sequelae, all cases showed patchy hypoperfusion throughout the cerebral cortex initially within 11 days of poisoning.[32] These changes in perfusion can occur as early as 1 day and primarily involve watershed regions such as the temporoparietooccipital area.[49] Xenon-enhanced computed tomography, which may be more readily available, appears to parallel perfusion changes seen on SPECT scanning.[181] Deficits on SPECT scanning appear to be associated with delayed neurologic sequelae.[33] Unfortunately, because of the scant availability of the procedure and the lack of comprehensive studies, SPECT scanning is not the definitive tool at this time for determining prognosis or need for HBO.

Positron emission tomography (PET) can be also be used for looking at regional blood flow as well as oxygen metabolism in the brain. In one series of severely CO-poisoned patients, PET examination after HBO treatment showed increased oxygen extraction and decreased blood flow in the frontal and temporal cortices.[50] Of note, patients with permanent deficits persisted in showing these abnormalities on PET scanning.[51] Although PET scanning cannot be used to predict outcome, abnormalities that persist on the scan usually indicate those patients with permanent neurologic sequelae.

To complement perfusion studies, EEG mapping was performed on CO-poisoned patients. Although initial studies show that many patients have regional EEG abnormalities after poisoning, it is undetermined if these are predictive of persistent or delayed neurologic problems.[49,55] EEG mapping may be discrepant relative to SPECT scanning because EEG preferentially shows subcortical lesions.[49]

MANAGEMENT

The mainstay of treatment is initial attention to the airway. One hundred percent oxygen should be provided as soon as possible by either nonrebreather face mask or endotracheal tube. The immediate effect of oxygen will be to enhance the dissociation of COHb.[174] In volunteers this reduces the half-life of COHb from a mean of 5 hours (range 2–7 hours) in room air to approximately 1 hour in 100% oxygen at normal atmospheric pressure.[155,161] Actual poisonings show a range in half-lives of 30 to 150 minutes when breathing 100% oxygen; the longer elimination half-lives appear to be most often associated with long, low-level exposures.[142] With oxygenation and intensive care treatment, hospital mortality rates for serious exposures range from 1 to 30%.[63,111]

Cardiac monitoring and intravenous access are necessary in any patient with consequential carbon monoxide poisoning. Hypotension can initially be treated with intravenous fluids; inotropic agents may also be necessary to treat any myocardial depression.[126] Standard ACLS protocols can be followed for the treatment of life-threatening dysrhythmias. Patients with depressed mental status should have a rapid blood glucose check. This should precede the administration of intravenous dextrose because of the theoretical potential for hyperglycemia-induced exacerbation of cerebral damage (see Antidotes in Depth: Dextrose).[159,166,167] However, animal studies of CO poisoning suggest that hypoglycemia can be deleterious as well.[156,158,160] Correction of any acidemia with bicarbonate is controversial and could result in further cell hypoxia secondary to a left shift of the oxyhemoglobin dissociation curve.

Hyperbaric Oxygen

Hyperbaric oxygen therapy appears to be the treatment of choice for patients with significant CO exposures.[81,149] One hundred percent oxygen at ambient pressure reduces the half-life of COHb to 40 minutes; at 2.5 atmospheres absolute, it is reduced to 20 minutes.[155,161,177] Actual CO-poisoned victims treated with HBO show half-lives ranging from 4 to 86 minutes.[142] Hyperbaric oxygen also increases the amount of dissolved oxygen by about 10 times, which is sufficient alone to supply cerebral needs.[16] But this is not the most important clinical issue because most patients have already been stabilized and have appreciably decreased carboxyhemoglobin levels just with ambient oxygen, even before using the chamber.

More importantly, in rats following loss of consciousness from CO exposure, hyperbaric, but not normobaric, oxygen therapy prevents brain lipid peroxidation.[200] This is because HBO appears to prevent ischemic reperfusion injury by a variety of mechanisms. First, in animal models HBO accelerates regeneration of inactivated cytochrome oxidase, which may be the initiating site for CO neuronal damage.[21] Second, HBO also prevents the subsequent leukocyte adherence to brain microvascular endothelium, a process essential for amplification of central nervous system damage from CO.[28,203] This may explain why HBO, but not 100% oxygen at atmospheric pressure, prevented delayed deficits in a learning and memory maze model.[218]

Clinical studies of the effectiveness of HBO in preventing neurologic damage from CO are not as convincing as basic science studies would suggest. In uncontrolled human clinical series, the incidence of persistent neuropsychiatric symptoms, including memory impairment, ranged from 12 to 43% in patients treated with 100% oxygen, and has been as low as 0 to 4% in patients treated with HBO.[75,130,145,149,190] The first randomized study of CO poisoning had over 300 patients and failed to show a benefit from HBO in patients who had no initial loss of consciousness.[168] Unfortunately, seriously ill patients were not randomized to surface pressure oxygen; they received either one or three treatments of HBO. Flaws in that study included significant delays to treatment and use of suboptimal pressure. A smaller ($n = 60$), more recent controlled study avoided some of these flaws and showed that HBO was able to decrease delayed neurologic sequelae from 23% to 0% in CO-poisoned patients without loss of consciousness.[213] However, all patients with syncope, a marker of serious poisoning, were excluded. A very small study ($n = 26$) of patients presenting with GCS > 12 after CO poisoning included almost half with loss of consciousness.[55] Randomization to HBO versus 100% normobaric oxygen resulted in decreased EEG abnormalities and less reduction in blood flow reactivity to acetazolamide at 3 weeks. Unfortunately, all of these studies failed to definitively study all CO poisoned patients, including those with syncope or coma.

The first randomized trial to really address the issue of HBO efficacy in seriously CO-poisoned patients was recently completed with 191 patients.[180] All CO-poisoned patients referred for HBO treatment were randomized to a minimum of three daily treatments of HBO (2.8 ATA for 60 minutes, 100 minutes total) or 100% oxygen (1.0 ATA for 100 minutes). Although the HBO group had a higher incidence of persistent neurologic sequelae at 1 month, there was no significant difference between the two groups; over two-thirds of each group had persistent problems. This study, although the largest controlled, randomized study to date, suffered from several flaws.[137] Fewer than half of the patients had followup at 1 month. Disproportionate numbers of suicide cases (about two-thirds) and drug toxicity (44%), with accompanying neuropsychological defects, could have confounded any beneficial effect from HBO. Finally, HBO treatment was delayed over 6 hours, making it much less likely to be effective.[75,168] In light of prior clinical and animal studies, it would be premature to reject HBO as an early viable treatment for serious CO poisoning. This is even truer because of the low risk of using HBO in CO poisoning.[188]

Indications for Hyperbaric Oxygen Therapy

Specific indications for HBO after acute CO poisoning are listed (Table 97–2), but these have not been prospectively evaluated. The patients most likely to benefit are those most at risk for persistent or delayed neurologic sequelae, such as patients presenting in coma.[75,108,189,235,240] Other potential markers for delayed neurologic sequelae include a history of syncope.[31,63,134,190] This may represent the episode of hypotension that is necessary for causing neuronal damage from CO-induced ischemic-reperfusion injury in animal models.[69,150] Patients with long exposures, or "soaking" periods, are also at greater risk for neurologic sequelae.[17,229] The

TABLE 97–2. Indications for Hyperbaric Oxygen Treatment in Carbon Monoxide Poisoning

Definite
  Loss of consciousness
  Seizures
  Coma
  Altered mental status

Relative
  Persistent neurologic symptoms after several hours of oxygen treatment
  Pregnancy
  Persistent cardiac ischemia
  Increased carboxyhemoglobin levels

presence of a significant metabolic acidosis may be a reliable marker for this.[117,191,223] Some authors advocate ongoing myocardial ischemia as an indication for HBO; however, in our experience, these patients usually already meet neurologic criteria for treatment (eg, loss of consciousness, ongoing mental status changes). Isolated cardiac ischemia, more importantly, deserves immediate proven myocardial salvaging therapy rather than delayed treatment with an unproven therapy such as HBO.

Some authors advocate treating all patients with COHb levels of 40% or greater with HBO.[97,141] Many HBO centers arbitrarily use a more conservative level of 25% as an indication for HBO. More important than actual level are patient history and examination. If the patient had loss of consciousness or significant neurologic symptoms (eg, coma, seizures, focal neurologic deficits, GCS < 15), he or she should be treated with HBO regardless of COHb levels. It is still unclear if mild neurologic symptoms (eg, confusion, headache, dizziness, visual blurring) or abnormal mental status testing on initial presentation is prognostic of delayed sequelae. These symptoms simply represent CO poisoning, which, at COHb levels approaching 20% in volunteers, can cause some temporary mental impairment.[118,197] Patients with these mild signs and symptoms deserve several hours of oxygen by nonrebreather face mask; then, if symptoms do not resolve, HBO can be considered. However, any delay in HBO may decrease its efficacy.[75]

Beyond good supportive care, all CO-poisoned patients require 100% oxygen as soon as possible. Hyperbaric oxygen may provide additional benefits, as outlined above. This might be especially useful in smoke-inhalation victims, to treat concomitant cyanide poisoning, chemical pneumonitis, and thermal burns.[84] Some authors recommend selective use of HBO because of cost and difficulties in transport if the primary facility lacks a chamber.[152] However, complications that may make such transfers and treatment unsafe are rare.[188] Although HBO cannot be recommended for every patient with CO poisoning, it is a relatively safe treatment that should be considered in all serious exposures. Fortunately, three-quarters of cases with delayed neurologic sequelae will resolve, albeit after several months.[31] It is our hope that completion of well-designed and scientifically controlled clinical studies will allow clarification of the indications for HBO.

Delayed Administration of Hyperbaric Oxygen. The optimal timing and number of HBO treatments for CO poisoning is unclear at this time. Patients treated later than 6 hours tend to fare worse in terms of delayed sequelae (30% vs 19%) and mortality (30% vs 14%).[75] One reason that this large randomized study may have failed to show any benefit from HBO is that patients were treated more than 6 hours after poisoning.[180] However, others suggest that late treatment may still be useful. Patients who have experienced unconsciousness from CO may benefit from an initial treatment of HBO as late as 6 hours postexposure, with no resulting neurologic sequelae.[146,240] In addition, patients who did not receive HBO initially and have already developed neuropsychological sequelae may have benefitted from HBO as late as 21 days postexposure.[145]

The problem with studies showing HBO benefits days after an acute poisoning, or after chronic poisoning, is that these cases are all anecdotal and lack controls. In fact, almost all cases of delayed neurologic sequelae resolve within 2 months in mild poisoning[213] and ~75% within 1 year in severe poisoning.[31] In fact, benefits in these delayed or chronic cases may simply represent the salutary effects of HBO. A preliminary study shows that HBO improves memory scores temporarily by over 50% in normal volunteers.[100]

Repeat Treatment With Hyperbaric Oxygen.   There are no studies to date that show that more than one HBO treatment is helpful in CO poisoning. However, this has still been advocated for patients who have persistent symptoms, particularly coma, after initial treatment.[47] In a nonrandomized retrospective study, CO-poisoned patients who received a second HBO treatment had a reduction in delayed neurologic sequelae from 55%, seen in comparable controls, to 18%.[74] However, prospective studies have failed to confirm any benefit from a repeated HBO treatment, and therefore, it cannot be recommended at this time.[168]

Treatment of Carbon Monoxide–Poisoned Pregnant Patients.
The management of CO exposure in the pregnant patient is difficult because of the potential adverse effects of both the toxin and its treatment. A literature review of all CO exposures during pregnancy revealed a high incidence of fetal central nervous system damage and stillbirth after severe maternal poisonings.[225] A series of three severely symptomatic patients who did not receive HBO had adverse fetal outcomes: two stillbirths and one case of cerebral palsy.[110] There have even been cases of limb malformations, cranial deformities, and a variety of mental disabilities in children poisoned in utero.[24,124] Although neurologic sequelae have been noted after severe acute exposures, a retrospective case-control study showed no association of CO exposure in the last trimester with low birth weight.[1]

Maternal COHb levels do not accurately reflect fetal hemoglobin or tissue levels.[40,45,72,129] In primate studies, a single CO exposure insufficient to cause clinical disease in a rhesus mother led to intrauterine hypoxia, fetal brain injury, and increased rates of fetal death.[67,68] In humans, minor exposures without loss of consciousness in the mother have resulted in poor fetal outcomes.[24,110] In one fetal loss case, the fetus had much higher levels than the peak COHb of 24% measured in the mother.[42] The problem is that CO absorption and elimination are slower in the fetal circulation than in the maternal circulation.[68,125] A mathematical model predicts that elimination of CO from the fetus takes 3.5 times longer than maternal CO elimination.[91]

Treatment of pregnant patients with HBO is not without theoretical risk. Animal studies show conflicting results on the effects of HBO on fetal development.[225] Some studies have shown that HBO causes developmental abnormalities in the central nervous, cardiovascular, and pulmonary systems of the fetus.[133] This is in marked contrast to the extensive Russian experience, where hundreds of pregnant women were treated with HBO, apparently without significant perinatal complications and with improvement in fetal/maternal status for their underlying conditions (eg, toxemia, anemia, diabetes).[136] Cases in this country where HBO was used for CO poisoning have resulted in normal infants at birth.[56,92,110,225]

There currently is no scientific validation for an absolute level at which to dive a pregnant patient for CO exposure. Arbitrarily, COHb levels greater than 20% are defined as an indication to dive a pregnant patient regardless of symptoms.[225] Pregnant patients should not be treated any differently if they meet criteria for HBO that have already been mentioned (see Table 97–2). Additional criteria would include any signs of fetal distress, such as abnormal fetal heart rate. Elevated levels of COHb (>15%), especially with a symptomatic mother, warrant HBO if locally available. This will facilitate more efficient treatment of the mother because of the necessity for prolonged oxygen therapy in pregnant patients, in the face of uncertain fetal COHb levels.

Treatment of CO Poisoning in Children.   It has been suggested that children are most sensitive to the effects of carbon monoxide because of their increased metabolic rate.[44] Epidemiologic studies suggest that pediatric patients can become symptomatic at COHb levels less that 10%, lower than is commonly expected in adults.[109] The other problem is that these cases may have unusual presentations. Most pediatric patients manifest nausea, headache, or lethargy.[44] An isolated seizure or vomiting may be the only manifestation of CO toxicity in an infant or child.[90]

In drawing COHb levels in infants, clinicians must be aware of two confounding factors. First, many CO-oximeters can give falsely elevated COHb levels, in proportion to the amount of fetal hemoglobin present.[227] Second, carbon monoxide is produced during breakdown of protoporphyrin to bilirubin. Therefore, infants can normally have high levels of COHb, >3%, and even higher in the presence of kernicterus.[194,228] Thus, before it is assumed that an elevated COHb level implies CO poisoning in an infant, the contribution of jaundice and fetal hemoglobin must be considered in the final analysis.

Although children may be more susceptible to acute toxicity with CO, their long-term outcomes appear to be more favorable than adults. In a series of 2360 serious CO cases, all incidences of delayed neurologic sequelae were in adults aged over 30 years.[31] Two pediatric series of CO poisoning show an incidence of delayed neurologic sequelae of approximately 10% after severe CO poisoning.[106,131] This low incidence, in patients treated only with 100% normal-pressure oxygen treatment, has been used as an argument to avoid HBO.[131] However, there still is a real risk of such sequelae, and HBO has been used successfully to prevent such sequelae.[175] If the use of surface-pressure oxygen is selected to treat a pediatric case, it is comforting to know that the COHb half-life is approximately 44 minutes, which is comparable to that in adults.[109]

Other Neuroprotective Treatments

A variety of neuroprotective agents have been tested in animal models. They are targeted primarily at preventing the delayed neurologic sequelae associated with serious CO poisoning. One of the simplest treatments tested is insulin. Hyperglycemia has been shown to exacerbate neuronal injury from stroke as well as in arrest situations, and in CO poisoning of rodents, it is associated with worse neurologic outcome.[159] However, insulin, independent of its glucose-lowering effect, appears to be protective after ischemia.[79] In rodent studies, improved neurologic outcome, as measured by locomotor activity, occurs after CO poisoning treated with insulin.[233] In light of these findings, it is reasonable to aggressively treat documented hyperglycemia with insulin in serious CO poisoning cases.

Many neuroprotective agents involve blockage of excitatory amino acids, such as glutamate, that are implicated in neuronal cell death after CO poisoning. Pretreatment of mice with dizocilpine (MK-801), which blocks the action of glutamate at *N*-methyl-D-aspartate receptors, ameliorates learning, memory, and hippocampal deficits with CO poisoning.[99] Ketamine, a glutamate antagonist as well, decreases mortality of rats poisoned with CO after carotid ligation.[157] Use of related drugs, although promising, awaits further animal testing because of potential adverse effects.

Other modalities have been tested in preventing neuronal damage from CO without much success. Hypothermia, rather than being beneficial, actually increases mortality in animals.[160,164] Allopurinol has been tested to prevent formation of free radicals through xanthine oxidase. This drug, when given as pretreatment, prevents lipid peroxidation mediated by xanthine oxidase in CO poisoning.[202] This strategy has not been promising because of the necessity for pretreatment.

Prevention of Carbon Monoxide Exposures

Early diagnosis will prevent much of the associated morbidity and mortality associated with CO poisoning, especially in unintentional exposures. The increased quality of home carbon monoxide–detecting devices will allow personal intervention in the prevention of exposure.[112] Routine laboratory screening of emergency department patients during the winter is not very efficacious in diagnosing unsuspected CO poisoning; the yield is less than 1% when patients are tested in whom the diagnosis of CO exposure was already excluded by history.[87,222] Instead, selecting patients with CO-related complaints, such as headache, dizziness, or nausea, increases the yield to 5 to 11%.[77,222] During winter, risk factors such as gas heating or symptomatic cohabitants in patients with influenza symptoms (eg, headache, dizziness, nausea) will be the most useful method for deciding when to obtain COHb levels on potential cases.[85,86,88]

The issue of symptomatic cohabitants is especially important from a preventive standpoint. Alerting other cohabitants to this danger and effecting evacuation may prevent needless deaths.[231] Most communities have multiple resources for on-site evaluation. Usually the local fire department or utility company can either check home appliances or measure ambient CO levels with portable monitoring equipment. Current workplace standards for ambient CO exposures are 35 ppm for a 1-hour limit and 9 ppm for an 8-hour limit.[58] There is a ceiling limit of 200 ppm (measured over a 15-minute period). Just a 4-hour exposure to 100 ppm of CO can result in COHb greater than 10% with symptoms.[161] Until rescue personnel arrive, natural-gas-fueled appliances should be turned off and the area evacuated, leaving all windows and doors open.

SUMMARY

Unintentional exposures to CO can easily be misdiagnosed. Carbon monoxide should also be suspected in any patient with coma, acidosis, or signs of cardiac ischemia that may be attributable to suicide. Fire victims, in addition to airway problems and potential cyanide toxicity, may succumb to CO toxicity.[13] The mainstay of treatment in all these cases is good supportive care with early oxygenation to increase the elimination of CO. Because of the overwhelming clinical successes with HBO and its limited risks, early use of this treatment modality in severe exposures is encouraged. Discussion with a poison control center or hyperbaric facility will help in identifying those patients most likely to benefit from such treatment.

REFERENCES

1. Alderman BW, Baron AE, Savitz DA: Maternal exposure to neighborhood carbon monoxide and risk of low birth weight. Public Health Rep 1987;102:410–414.
2. Allred EN, Bleecker ER, Chaitman BR, et al: Short-term effects of carbon monoxide exposure on the exercise performance of subjects with coronary artery disease. N Engl J Med 1989;321:1426–1432.
3. Anderson EW, Andelman RJ, Strauch JM, et al: Effect of low-level carbon monoxide exposure on onset and duration of angina pectoris. A study in ten patients with ischemic heart disease. Ann Intern Med 1973;79:46–50.
4. Anderson RF, Allensworth DC, DeGroot WJ: Myocardial toxicity from carbon monoxide poisoning. Ann Intern Med 1967;67:1172–1182.
5. Aronow W, Isbell MW: Carbon monoxide effect on exercise-induced angina pectoris. Ann Intern Med 1973;79:392–395.
6. Aronow WS, Cassidy J, Vangrow JS, et al: Effect of cigarette smoking and breathing carbon monoxide on cardiovascular hemodynamics in anginal patients. Circulation 1974;50:340–347.
7. Astrup P: Intraerythrocyte 2,3-diphosphoglycerate and carbon monoxide exposure. Ann NY Acad Sci 1970;174:252–254.
8. Ball EG, Strittmatter CF, Cooper O: The reaction of cytochrome oxidase with carbon monoxide. J Biol Chem 1951;193:635–647.
9. Baringa M: Carbon monoxide: Killer to brain messenger in one step. Science 1993;259:309.
10. Barker SJ, Tremper KK: The effect of carbon monoxide inhalation on pulse oximetry and transcutaneous P_{O_2}. Anesthesiology 1987;66:677–679.
11. Barret L, Canel V, Faure J: Carbon monoxide poisoning, a diagnosis frequently overlooked. J Toxicol Clin Toxicol 1985;23:309–313.
12. Barrows GH, Thomas BB, Short CS, et al: A simple carbon monoxide screening method on hemoglobin absorbance ratios [abstract]. Am J Clin Pathol 1986;85:387.
13. Baud FJ, Barriot P, Toffis V, et al: Elevated blood cyanide concentrations in victims of smoke inhalation. N Engl J Med 1991;325:1761–1766.
14. Bessoudo R, Gray J: Carbon monoxide poisoning and nonoliguric renal failure. Can Med Assoc J 1978;119:41–44.
15. Birky MM, Clarke FB: Inhalation of toxic products from fires. Bull NY Acad Med 1981;57:997–1013.
16. Boerema I, Meyne I, Brummelkamp WH, et al: Life without blood. Arch Chir Neer 1959;11:70–83.
17. Bogusz M, Cholewa L, Pach J, et al: A comparison of two types of acute carbon monoxide poisoning. Arch Toxicol 1975;33:141–149.
18. Bourbeau J, Brisson C, Allaire S: Prevalence of sick building syndrome symptoms in office workers before and after being exposed to a building with an improved ventilation system. Occup Environ Med 1996;53:204–210.
19. Britten JS, Myers RAM: Effects of hyperbaric treatment on carbon monoxide elimination in humans. Undersea Biomed Res 1985;12:431.
20. Brown SD, Piantadosi CA: In vivo binding of carbon monoxide to cytochrome oxidase in rat brain. J Appl Physiol 1990;68:604–610.
21. Brown SD, Piantadosi CA: Recovery of energy metabolism in rat brain after carbon monoxide hypoxia. Ann Neurol 1992;89:666–672.
22. Buckley RG, Aks SE, Eshom JL, et al: The pulse oximetry gap in carbon monoxide intoxication. Ann Emerg Med 1994;24:252–255.
23. Burney RE, Wu S-C: Mass carbon monoxide poisoning: Clinical effects and results of treatment in 184 victims. Ann Emerg Med 1982;11:394.
24. Caravati EM, Adams CJ, Joyce SM, et al: Fetal toxicity associated with maternal carbon monoxide poisoning. Ann Emerg Med 1988;17:714–717.
25. Caugher WS: Carbon monoxide bonding in hemeproteins. Ann NY Acad Sci 1970;174:148–153.
26. Chance BC, Erecinska M, Wagner M: Mitochondrial responses to carbon monoxide. Ann NY Acad Sci 1970;174:193–203.
27. Chen KC, McGrath JJ: Response of the isolated heart to carbon monoxide and nitrogen anoxia. Toxicol Appl Pharmacol 1985;81:363–370.

28. Chen Q, Banick PD, Thom SR: Functional inhibition of rat polymorphonuclear leukocyte B2 integrins by hyperbaric oxygen is associated with impaired cGMP synthesis. J Pharmacol Exp Ther 1996; 276:929–933.

29. Chisolm CD, Reilly J, Berejan B: Carboxyhemoglobin levels in patients with headache [abstract]. Ann Emerg Med 1986;16:497.

30. Chlamers AH: Simple, sensitive measurement of carbon monoxide in plasma. Clin Chem 1991;37(8):1442–1445.

31. Choi HS: Delayed neurological sequelae in carbon monoxide intoxication. Arch.Neurol 1983;40:433–435.

32. Choi IS, Kim SK, Lee SS, Choi YC: Evaluation of outcome of delayed neurologic sequelae after carbon monoxide poisoning by technetium-99m hexamethylproplylene amine oxime brain single photon emission computed tomography. Eur Neurol 1995;35: 137–142.

33. Choi IS, Lee MS, Lee YJ, et al: Technetium-99m HM-PAO SPECT in patients with delayed neurologic sequelae after carbon monoxide poisoning. J Korean Med Sci 1992;7:11–18.

34. Cobb N, Etzel RA: Unintentional carbon monoxide-related deaths in the United States, 1979 through 1988. JAMA 1991;266:659–663.

35. Coburn RF: Endogenous carbon monoxide production. N Engl J Med 1970;282:207–209.

36. Coburn RF: The carbon monoxide body stores. Ann NY Acad Sci 1970;174:11–22.

37. Coburn RF, Forster RE, Kane PB: Considerations of the physiological variables that determine the blood carboxyhemoglobin concentration in man. J Clin Invest 1965;44:1899–1910.

38. Coburn RF, Mayers LB: Myoglobin oxygen tension determines from measurements of carboxyhemoglobin in skeletal muscle. Am J Physiol 1971;220:66–74.

39. Commins BT, Lawther PJ: A sensitive method for the determination of carboxyhemoglobin in a finger prick sample of blood. Br J Ind Med 1965;22:139–143.

40. Copel JA, Bowen F, Bolognese RJ: Carbon monoxide intoxication in early pregnancy. Obstet Gynecol 1982;59:26s–28s.

41. Cox BD, Wichelow MJ: Carbon monoxide levels in the breath of smokers and nonsmokers: Effect of home heating systems. J Epidemiol Community Health 1985;39:75–78.

42. Cramer CR: Fetal death due to accidental maternal carbon monoxide poisoning. J Toxicol Clin Toxicol 1982;19:297

43. Cramlet SH, Erickson HH, Gorman HA: Ventricular function following carbon monoxide exposure. J Appl Physiol 1975;39: 482–486.

44. Crocker PJ, Walker JS: Pediatric carbon monoxide toxicity. J Emerg Med 1985;3:443–448.

45. Curtis GW, Alger EJ, McDay AJ, et al: The transplacental diffusion of carbon monoxide. Arch Pathol Lab Med 1955;59:677–690.

46. Davies JWL: Toxic chemicals versus lung tissue—an aspect of inhalation injury revisited. J Burn Care Rehabil 1986;7:213–222.

47. Dean BS, Verdile VP, Krenzelok EP: Coma reversal with cerebral dysfunction recovery after repetitive hyperbaric oxygen therapy for severe carbon monoxide poisoning. Am J Emerg Med 1993;11: 616–618.

48. Dempsey LC, O'Donnell JJ, Hoff JT: Carbon monoxide retinopathy. Am J Ophthalmol 1976;82:692–693.

49. Denays R, Makhoul E, Dachy B, et al: Electroencephalographic mapping and ^{99m}Tc HMPAO single-photon emission computed tomography in carbon monoxide poisoning. Ann Emerg Med 1994; 24:947–952.

50. DeReuck J, Decoo D, Lemahieu I, et al: A positron emission tomography study of patients with acute carbon monoxide poisoning treated by hyperbaric oxygen. J Neurol 1993;240:430–434.

51. DeReuck J, Van Aken J, Decoo D, et al: Delayed neurological deterioration following acute carbon monoxide poisoning: comparison of clinical outcome, neuroimaging and positron emission tomography findings. Cerebrovasc Dis 1991;1:273–290.

52. Diaz JE, Roberts JR: Carboxyhemoglobin after blood storage. Ann Emerg Med 1997;30:239–240.

53. Dolan MC, Haltom TL, Barrows GH, et al: Carboxyhemoglobin levels in patients with flu-like symptoms. Ann Emerg Med 1987;16: 782–786.

54. Douglas CG, Haldane JS, Haldane JBS: The laws of combustion of hemoglobin with carbon monoxide and oxygen. J Physiol 1912;44: 275–304.

55. Ducasse JL, Celsis P, Marc-Vergnes JP: Non-comatose patients with acute carbon monoxide poisoning: Hyperbaric or normobaric oxygenation. Undersea Hyperbaric Med 1995;22:9–15.

56. Elkharrat D, Faphael JC, Korach JM, et al: Acute carbon monoxide intoxication and hyperbaric oxygen in pregnancy. Intens Care Med 1991;17:289–292.

57. Ely EW, Moorehead B, Haponik EF: Warehouse workers' headache: Emergency evaluation and management of 30 patients with carbon monoxide poisoning. Am J Med 1995;98:145–155.

58. Environmental Protection Agency: Air Quality Criteria for Carbon Monoxide. EPA 600 8/90/045. Research Triangle Park, NC, Environmental Criteria and Assessment Office, Office of Health and Environmental Assessment (GENERIC)., 1997.

59. Fagin J, Bradley J, Williams D: Carbon monoxide poisoning secondary to inhaling methylene chloride. Br Med J 1980;281:1461.

60. Fawcett TA, Moon RE, Fracica PJ, et al: Warehouse workers' headache: carbon monoxide poisoning from propane-fueled forklifts. J Occup Med 1992;34:12–15.

61. Fort L, Griggs P: Carbon monoxide poisoning in North Carolina. NC Med J 1987;48:317–321.

62. Foutch RG, Henrichs W: Carbon monoxide poisoning at high altitudes. Am J Emerg Med 1988;6:596–598.

63. Garland H, Pearce J: Neurological complications of carbon monoxide poisoning. Q J Med 1967;36:445–455.

64. Gasman JD, Varon J, Gardner JP: Carbon monoxide poisoning. West J Med 1990;153:656–657.

65. Ginsberg MD: Carbon monoxide intoxication: Clinical features, neuropathology, and mechanisms of injury. J Toxicol Clin Toxicol 1985;23:281–288.

66. Ginsberg MD, Myers RAM: Experimental carbon monoxide encephalopathy in the primate. I. Physiologic and metabolic aspects. Arch Neurol 1974;30:202–208.

67. Ginsberg MD, Myers RE: Fetal brain damage following maternal carbon monoxide intoxication: An experimental study. Acta Obstet Gynecol Scand 1974;53:309–317.

68. Ginsberg MD, Myers RE: Fetal brain injury after maternal carbon monoxide intoxication: Clinical and neuropathologic aspects. Neurology 1976;26:15–23.

69. Ginsberg MD, Myers RE, McDonaugh BF: Experimental carbon monoxide encephalopathy in the primate. II. Clinical aspects, neuropathology and physiologic correlation. Arch Neurol 1974;30: 209–216.

70. Goldbaum LR, Orellano T, Dergal E: Mechanism of the toxic action of carbon monoxide. Ann Clin Lab Science 1976;6:372–376.

71. Goldbaum LR, Ramirez RG, Absalon KB: XIII. What is the mechanism of carbon monoxide toxicity? Aviat Space Environ Med 1975; 46:1289–1291.

72. Goldstein DP: Carbon monoxide poisoning in pregnancy. Am J Obstet Gynecol 1965;92:526–528.

73. Gorman DF: Carbon monoxide: From toxic poison to brain messenger. S Pac Underwater Med Soc J 1995;25:77

74. Gorman DF, Clayton D, Gilligan JE, et al: A longitudinal study of 100 consecutive admissions for carbon monoxide poisoning to the Royal Adelaide Hospital. Anaesth Intens Care 1992;20:311–316.

75. Goulon M, Barios A, Raphin M, et al: Carbon monoxide poisoning and acute anoxia due to breathing coal gas and hydrocarbons. Ann Med Interne 1969;120:335–349.

76. Grace TW, Platt FW: Subacute carbon monoxide poisoning: another great imitator. JAMA 1981;246:1698–1700.

77. Greene C, Lumpkin JR, Baker FJI: Association between unsuspected carbon monoxide exposure and headache [abstract]. Ann Emerg Med 1983;12:244–245.

78. Halebian B, Robinson N, Barie P, et al: Whole body oxygen utilization during acute carbon monoxide poisoning and isocapneic nitrogen hypoxia. J Trauma 1986;26:110–117.

79. Hamilton MG, Trammer BI, Auer RN: Insulin reduction of cerebral infarction due to transient focal ischemia. J Neurosurg 1996;84: 146–148.

80. Hampson NB: Pulse oximetry in severe carbon monoxide poisoning. Chest 1998;114:1036–1041.

81. Hampson NB: Hyperbaric Oxygen Therapy:1999 Committee Report. Kensington, MD, Undersea and Hyperbaric Medical Society; 1999, p. 1.

82. Hampson NB, Kramer CC, Dunford RG, et al: Carbon monoxide poisoning from indoor burning of charcoal briquets. JAMA 1994; 271:52–53.

83. Hampson NB, Norkool DM: Carbon monoxide poisoning in children riding in the back of pickup trucks. JAMA 1992;267:538–540.

84. Hart GB, Strauss MB, Lennon PA, et al: Treatment of smoke inhalation by hyperbaric oxygen. J Emerg Med 1985;3:211–215.

85. Heckerling PS: Occult carbon monoxide poisoning: a cause of winter headache. Am J Emerg Med 1987;5:201–204.

86. Heckerling PS, Leiken JB, Maturen A, et al: Predictors of occult carbon monoxide poisoning in patients with headache and dizziness. Ann Intern Med 1987;107:174–176.

87. Heckerling PS, Leiken JB, Maturen A, et al: Screening hospital admissions from the emergency department for occult carbon monoxide poisoning. Am J Emerg Med 1990;8:301–304.

88. Heckerling PS, Leikin JB, Maturen A: Occult carbon monoxide poisoning: validation of a prediction model. Am J Med 1988;84: 251–256.

89. Hedberg K, Hedberg CW, Iber C, et al: An outbreak of nitrogen dioxide-induced respiratory illness among ice hockey players. JAMA 1990;263:3024–3025.

90. Herman LY: Carbon monoxide poisoning presenting as an isolated seizure. J Emerg Med 1998;16:429–432.

91. Hill EP, Hill JR, Power GG, et al: Carbon monoxide exchanges between the human fetus and mother: A mathematical model. Am J Physiol 1977;232:H311–H323

92. Hollander DI, Nagey DA, Welch R, et al: Hyperbaric oxygen therapy for the treatment of acute carbon monoxide poisoning in pregnancy: a case report. J Reprod Med 1987;32:615–617.

93. Hopkinson JM, Pearce PJ, Oliver JS: Carbon monoxide poisoning mimicking gastroenteritis. Br Med J 1980;281:214–215.

94. Horowitz AL, Kaplan R, Sarpel G: Carbon monoxide toxicity: MR imaging in the brain. Radiology 1987;162:787–788.

95. Howse AJG, Seddon H: Ischemic contracture of muscle associated with carbon monoxide CO and barb poisoning. Br Med J 1966; 1:192–195.

96. Ikeda T, Kondo T, Mogami H, et al: Computerized tomography in cases of acute carbon monoxide poisoning. Med J Osaka Univ 1978;29:253–262.

97. Ilano AL, Raffine TA: Management of carbon monoxide poisoning. Chest 1990;97:165–169.

98. Ischiropoulos H, Beers MF, Ohnishi ST, et al: Nitric oxide production and perivascular tyrosine nitration in brain after carbon monoxide poisoning in the rat. J Clin Invest 1996;97:2260–2267.

99. Ishimaru H, Katoh A, Suzuki H, Fukuta T, Kameyama T, Nabeshima T: Effects of N-methyl-D-aspartate receptor antagonists on carbon monoxide-induced brain damage in mice. J Pharmacol Exp Ther 1992;261:349–352.

100. Jackson WR: Hyperbaric oxygenation effects on the cognitive function of memory. Undersea Biomed Res 1992;19 (Suppl):62.

101. Johnson BL, Cohen A, Struble R, et al: Field evaluation of carbon monoxide exposed toll collectors (HEW Publication No. (NIOSH) 74–126). In: Xintaras C, Johnson BL, deGroot I, eds: Behavioral Toxicology: Early Detection of Occupational Hazards. Washington, DC, US Government Printing Office, 1974, pp. 306–328.

102. Johnson EJ, Moran JC, Paine SC, et al: Abatement of toxic levels of CO in Seattle skating rinks. Am J Public Health 1975;65:1087–1090.

103. Jones JS, Lagasse J, Zimmerman G: Computed tomographic findings after acute carbon monoxide poisoning. Am J Emerg Med 1994; 12:448–451.

104. Kanaya N, Imaizumi H, Nakayama M, et al: The utility of MRI in acute stage of carbon monoxide poisoning. Intens Care Med 1992; 18:371–372.

105. Kelley JS, Sophocleus GJ: Retinal hemorrhages in subacute carbon monoxide poisoning: exposure in homes with blocked furnace flues. JAMA 1978;239:1515–1517.

106. Kim JK, Coe CJ: Clinical study on carbon monoxide in children. Yonsei Med J 1987;28:266

107. Kim KS, Weinberg PE, Suh JH, et al: Acute carbon monoxide poisoning: computed tomography of the brain. Am J Neuroradiol 1980; 1:399–402.

108. Kindwall EP: Carbon monoxide poisoning treated with hyperbaric oxygen. Respir Ther 1975;5:29–33.

109. Klasner AE, Smith SR, Thompson MW, Scalzo AJ: Carbon monoxide mass exposure in a pediatric population. Acad Emerg Med 1998;5:992–996.

110. Koren G, Sharav T, Pastuszak A, et al: A multicenter, prospective study of fetal outcome following accidental carbon monoxide poisoning in pregnancy. Reprod Toxicol 1991;5:397–403.

111. Krantz T, Thisted B, Strom J, et al: Acute carbon monoxide poisoning. Acta Anaesthesiol Scand 1988;32:278–282.

112. Krenzelok EP, Roth R, Full R: Carbon monoxide . . . the silent killer with an audible solution. Am J Emerg Med 1996;14:484–486.

113. Kurt TL, Anderson RJ, Weed WG: Rapid estimation of carboxyhemoglobin by breath sampling in an emergency setting. Vet Hum Toxicol 1990;32:227–229.

114. Lacey DJ: Neurologic sequelae of acute carbon monoxide poisoning. Am J Dis Child 1981;135:145–147.

115. Langehennig PL, Seeler RA, Berman E: Paint removers and carboxyhemoglobin. N Engl J Med 1976;295:1137.

116. Lapresle J, Fardeau M: The central nervous system and carbon monoxide: II. Anatomical study of brain lesions following intoxication with carbon monoxide (22 cases). Prog Brain Res 1976;24: 31–74.

117. Larkin JM, Brahos GJ, Moylan JA: Treatment of carbon monoxide poisoning: Prognostic factors. J Trauma 1976;16:111–114.

118. Laties V: Carbon monoxide and behavior. Arch Neurol 1980;167: 68–72.

119. Laties V, Merigan WH: Behavioral effects of carbon monoxide on animals and man. Annu Rev Pharmacol Toxicol 1979;19:357–392.

120. Leavell UW, Farley CH, McIntyre JS: Cutaneous changes in a patient with CO poisoning. Arch Dermatol 1969;99:429–433.

121. Lee MS, Marsden CD: Neurological sequelae following carbon monoxide poisoning clinical course and outcome according to the clinical types and brain computed tomography scan findings. Move Dis 1996;9:550–558.

122. Leiken JB, Kaufman D, Lipscomb JW, et al: Methylene chloride report of 5 exposures and 2 deaths. Am J Emerg Med 1990;8: 534–537.

123. Levasseur L, Galliot–Guilley M, Richter F, et al: Effects of mode of inhalation of carbon monoxide and of normobaric oxgyen administration on carbon monoxide elimination from the blood. Hum Exp Toxicol 1996;15:898–903.

124. Longo LD: The biologic effects of carbon monoxide on the pregnant woman, fetus and newborn infant. Am J Obstet Gynecol 1977;129: 69–103.

125. Longo LD, Hill EP: Carbon monoxide uptake and elimination in fetal and maternal sheep. Am J Physiol 1977;232:H324–H330.

126. Lowe-Ponsford FL, Henry JA: Clinical aspects of carbon monoxide poisoning. Adv Drug React Acute Poisoning Rev 1989;8:217–240.

127. Marius-Nunex AL: Myocardial infarction with normal coronary arteries after acute exposure to carbon monoxide. Chest 1990;97: 491–494.

128. Marks GS, Brien JF, Nakatsu K, et al: Does carbon monoxide have a physiological function? Trends Pharmacol Sci 1991;12:185.

129. Martland HS, Martland HS Jr: Placental barrier in carbon monoxide, barbiturate, and radium poisoning. Am J Surg 1950;80:270–279.

130. Mathieu D, Nolf M, Durocher A, et al: Acute carbon monoxide poisoning: risk of late sequelae and treatment by hyperbaric oxygen. J Toxicol Clin Toxicol 1985;23:315–324.

131. Meert KL, Heidemann SM, Sarnaik AP: Outcome of children with carbon monoxide poisoning treated with normobaric oxygen. J Trauma 1998;44:149–154.

132. Messier LD, Myers RAM: A neuropsychological screening battery for emergency assessment of carbon monoxide poisoned patients. J Clin Psychol 1991;47:675–684.

133. Miller PD, Telford ID, Haas GR: Effect of hyperbaric oxygen on cardiogenesis in the rat. Biol Neonate 1971;17:44–52.

134. Min SK: A brain syndrome associated with delayed neuropsychiatric sequelae following acute carbon monoxide intoxication. Acta Psychiatr Scand 1986;73:80–86.

135. Miura T, Mitomo M, Kawai R, et al: CT of the brain in acute carbon monoxide intoxication: characteristic features and prognosis. Am J Neuroradiol 1985;6:739–742.

136. Molzhaninov EV, Chaika VK, Domanova AI, et al: Experience and prospects of using hyperbaric oxygenation in obstetrics. In: Proceedings of the Seventh International Congress on Hyperbaric Medicine, Moscow, 1981. Moscow, Nauka, 1983, pp. 139–141.

137. Moon RE, DeLong E: Hyperbaric oxygen for carbon monoxide poisoning: are currently recommmended regimens effective? Med J Aust 1999;170:197–199.

138. Moureu H, Chavin P, Truffert L, et al: Nouvelle micomethode pour la determination rapide et precise de l'oxycarbonemie par absorption selective dans l'infrarouge. Arch Mal Professionnelles 1957;18:116–124.

139. Myers RAM: Carbon monoxide poisoning. J Emerg Med 1984;1:245–248.

140. Myers RAM, Britten JS: Are arterial blood gases of value in treatment decisions for carbon monoxide poisoning? Crit Care Med 1989;17:139–142.

141. Myers RAM, Goldman B: Planning an effective strategy for carbon monoxide poisoning. Emerg Med Rep 1987;8:193–200.

142. Myers RAM, Jones DW, Britten JS: Carbon monoxide half life [abstract]. Proceedings of the VIII International Congress on Hyperbaric Medicine, Long Beach, CA, 1987, p. 263.

143. Myers RAM, Mitchell JT, Cowley RA: Psychometric testing and carbon monoxide poisoning. Disaster Med 1983;1:279–281.

144. Myers RAM, Snyder S, Majerus TC: Cutaneous blisters and CO poisoning. Ann Emerg Med 1985;14:603–606.

145. Myers RAM, Snyder SK, Emhoff TA: Subacute sequelae of carbon monoxide poisoning. Ann Emerg Med 1985;14:1163–1167.

146. Myers RAM, Snyder SK, Linberg S, et al: Value of hyperbaric oxygen in suspected carbon monoxide poisoning. JAMA 1981;246:2478–2480.

147. Nardizzi LR: Computerized tomographic correlate of carbon monoxide poisoning. Arch Neurol 1979;36:38–39.

148. Neufeld MY, Swanson JW, Klass DW: Localized EEG abnormalities in acute carbon monoxide poisoning. Arch Neurol 1981;38:524–527.

149. Norkool DM, Kirkpatrick JN: Treatment of acute carbon monoxide poisoning with hyperbaric oxygen: A review of 115 cases. Ann Emerg Med 1985;14:1168–1171.

150. Okeda R, Funata N, Takano T, et al: The pathogenesis of carbon monoxide encephalopathy in the acute phase—physiological and morphological conditions. Acta Neuropathol 1981;54:1–10.

151. Okeda R, Funata N, Takano T, et al: Comparative study on pathogenesis of selective cerebral lesions in carbon monoxide poisoning and nitrogen hypoxia in cats. Acta Neuropathol 1982;56:265–272.

152. Olson KR: Carbon monoxide poisoning: mechanisms, presentation, and controversies in management. J Emerg Med 1984;1:233–243.

153. Otten EJ, Rosenberg J, Tasset JT: An evaluation of carboxyhemoglobin spot tests. Ann Emerg Med 1985;14:850–852.

154. Pace N, Consolazio F, White WA, et al: Formulation of the principal factors affecting the rate of uptake of carbon monoxide by man. Am J Physiol 1946;147:352–359.

155. Pace N, Stajman E, Walker EL: Acceleration of carbon monoxide elimination in man by high pressure oxygen. Science 1950;111:652–654.

156. Penney DG: Acute carbon monoxide poisoning in an animal model: the effects of altered glucose on morbidity and mortality. Toxicology 1993;80:85–101.

157. Penney DG, Chen K: NMDA receptor-blocker ketamine protects during acute carbon monoxide poisoning, while calcium blocker verapamil does not. J Appl Toxicol 1996;16:297–304.

158. Penney DG, Helfman CC, Dunbar JC, et al: Acute severe carbon monoxide exposure in the rat: effects of hyperglycemia and hypoglycemia on mortality, recovery, and neurological deficit. Can J Physiol 1991;69:1168–1177.

159. Penney DG, Helfman CC, Hull JA, et al: Elevated blood glucose is associated with poor outcome in the carbon-monoxide-poisoned rat. Toxicol Lett 1990;54:287–298.

160. Penney DG, Sharma P, Sutariya BB, et al: Development of hypoglycemia is associated with death during carbon monoxide poisoning. J Crit Care 1990;5:169–179.

161. Peterson JE, Stewart RD: Absorption and elimination of carbon monoxide by inactive young men. Arch Environ Health 1970;21:165–171.

162. Piantadosi CA, Zhang J, Levin ED, et al: Apoptosis and delayed neuronal damage after carbon monoxide poisoning in the rat. Exp Neurol 1997;147:103–114.

163. Piatt JP, Kaplan AM, Bond GR, et al: Occult carbon monoxide poisoning in an infant. Pediatr Emerg Care 1990;6:21–23.

164. Pierce EC, Zacharias A, Alday JM: Carbon monoxide poisoning: experimental hypothermic and hyperbaric studies. Surgery 1972;72:229

165. Pracyk JB, Stolp BW, Fife CE, et al: Brain computerized tomography after hyperbaric oxygen therapy for carbon monoxide poisoning. Undersea Hyperbaric Med 1995;22:1–7.

166. Pulsinelli WA, Levy DE, Sigsbee B, et al: Increased damage after ischemic stroke in patients with hyperglycemia with or without established diabetes mellitus. Am J Med 1983;74:540–544.

167. Pulsinelli WA, Waldman S, Rawlinson D, et al: Moderate hyperglycemia augments ischemic brain damage: a neuropathologic study in the rat. Neurology 1982;32:1239–1246.

168. Raphael JC, Elkharrat D, Jars-Guincestre MC, et al: Trial of normobaric and hyperbaric oxygen for acute carbon monoxide intoxication. Lancet 1989;2:414–419.

169. Ratney RS, Wegman DH, Elkins HB: In vivo conversion of methylene chloride to carbon monoxide. Arch Environ Health 1974;28:223–236.

170. Raybourn MS, Cork C, Schimmerling W, et al: An in vitro electrophysiological assessment of the direct cellular toxicity of carbon monoxide. Toxicol Appl Pharmacol 1978;46:769–779.

171. Rioux JP, Myers RAM: Hyperbaric oxygen for methylene chloride poisoning: report on two cases. Ann Emerg Med 1989;18:691–695.

172. Riser D, Bonsch A, Schneider B: Should coroners be able to reconize unintentional carbon-monoxide related deaths immediately at the death scene? J Forensic Sci 1995;40:596–598.

173. Rottman SJ: Carbon monoxide screening in the ED. Am J Emerg Med 1991;9:204–205.

174. Roughton FJW, Darling RC: The effect of carbon monoxide on the hemoglobin dissociation curve. Am J Physiol 1944;141:17–31.

175. Rudge FW: Carbon monoxide poisoning in infants: treatment with hyperbaric oxygen. South Med J 1993;86:334–337.

176. Ryan C: Memory disturbances following chronic, low-level carbon monoxide exposure. Arch Clin Neuropsychol 1990;5:59–67.

177. Sasaki T: One-half clearance time of carbon monoxide hemoglobin in blood during hyperbaric oxygen therapy. Bull Tokyo Med Dent Univ 1975;22:63–77.

178. Schaplowsky AF, Oglesbay FB, Morrison JH, et al: Carbon monoxide contamination of the living environment: a national survey of home air and children's blood. J Environ Health 1974;36: 569–573.

179. Scharf SM, Thames MD, Sasrgent RK: Transmural myocardial infarction after exposure to carbon monoxide in coronary-artery disease. N Engl J Med 1974;291:85–86.

180. Scheinkestel CD, Bailey M, Myles PS, et al: Hyperbaric or normobaric oxygen for acute carbon monoxide poisoning: a randomized controlled clinical trial. Med J Aust 1999;170:203–210.

181. Sesay M, Bidabe AM, Guyot M, et al: Regional cerebral blood flow measurements with Xenon-Ct in the prediction of delayed encephalopathy after carbon monoxide intoxication. Acta Neurol Scand [Suppl] 1996;166:22–27.

182. Shapiro AB, Maturen A, Herman G, et al: Carbon monoxide and myonecrosis: a prospective study. Vet Hum Toxicol 1989;31: 136–137.

183. Sheps DS, Herbst MC, Hinderliter AL, et al: Production of arrhythmias by elevated carboxyhemoglobin in patients with coronary artery disease. Ann Intern Med 1990;113:343–351.

184. Shimazeu T, Ikeuchi H, Hubbard GB, et al: Smoke inhalation injury and the effect of carbon monoxide in the sheep model. J Trauma 1990;30:170–175.

185. Shusterman D, Alexeeff G, Hargis C, et al: Predictors of carbon monoxide and hydrogen cyanide exposure in smoke inhalation patients. J Toxicol Clin Toxicol 1996;34:61–71.

186. Silver DAT, Cross M, Fox B, Paxton RM: Computed tomography of the brain in acute carbon monoxide poisoning. Clin Radiol 1996; 51:480–483.

187. Silvers SM, Hampson NB: Carbon monoxide poisoning among recreational boaters. JAMA 1995;274:1614–1616.

188. Sloan EP, Murphy DG, Hart R, et al: Complications and protocol considerations in carbon monoxide-poisoned patients who require hyperbaric oxygen therapy: report from a ten-year experience. Ann Emerg Med 1989;18:629–634.

189. Smith GI, Sharp GR: Treatment of carbon monoxide poisoning with oxygen under pressure. Lancet 1960;2:905–906.

190. Smith JS, Brandon S: Morbidity from acute carbon monoxide poisoning at 3 years following. Br Med J 1973;1:318–321.

191. Sokal JA, Kralkowska E: The relationship between exposure duration, carboxyhemoglobin, blood glucose, pyruvate and lactate and the severity of intoxication in 39 cases of acute carbon monoxide poisoning in man. Arch Toxicol 1985;57:196–199.

192. Sone S, Higashihara T, Kotake T, et al: Pulmonary manifestations in acute carbon monoxide poisoning. Am J Roentgenol 1974;120: 865–871.

193. Sterling TD, Sterling E: Carbon monoxide levels in kitchens and homes with gas cookers. J Air Pollut Control Assoc 1979;29: 238–241.

194. Stevenson DK, Vreman HJ: Carbon monoxide and bilirubin production in neonates. Pediatrics 1997;100:252–254.

195. Stewart R, Baretta ED, Platte LR, et al: Carboxyhemoglobin levels in American blood donors. JAMA 1974;229:1187–1195.

196. Stewart RD: Paint remover hazard. JAMA 1976;235:398–401.

197. Stewart RD, Peterson JE, Baretta ED, et al: Experimental human exposure to carbon monoxide. Arch Environ Health 1970;21:154–164.

198. Stewart RD, Peterson JE, Fisher TN, et al: Experimental human exposure to high concentrations of carbon monoxide. Arch Environ Health 1973;26:1–7.

199. Takeuchi A, Vesely A, Rucker J, et al: A simple "new" method to accelerate clearance of carbon monoxide. Am J Respir Crit Care Med 2000;161:1816–1819.

200. Thom SR: Antagonism of carbon monoxide-mediated brain lipid peroxidation by hyperbaric oxygen. Toxicol Appl Pharmacol 1990; 105:340–344.

201. Thom SR: Carbon monoxide–mediated brain lipid peroxidation in the rat. J Appl Physiol 1990;68:997–1003.

202. Thom SR: Dehydrogenase conversion to oxidase and lipid peroxidation in brain after carbon monoxide poisoning. J Appl Physiol 1992; 73:1584–1589.

203. Thom SR: Functional inhibition of leukocyte B₂ integrins by hyperbaric oxygen in carbon monoxide-mediated brain injury in rats. Toxicol Appl Pharmacol 1993b;123:248–256.

204. Thom SR: Leukocytes in carbon monoxide-mediated brain oxidative injury. Toxicol Appl Pharmacol 1993a;123:234–247.

205. Thom SR: Learning dysfunction and metabolic defects in globus pallidus and hippocampus after CO poisoning in a rat model [abstract]. Undersea Hyperbaric Med 1997;23(suppl):20.

206. Thom SR, Fisher D, Xu YA, et al: Role of nitric oxide-derived oxidants in vascular injury from carbon monoxide in the rat. Am J Physiol 1999;276:H984–H992.

207. Thom SR, Fisher D, Xu YA, et al: Adaptive responses and apoptosis in endothelial cells exposed to carbon monoxide. Proc Natl Acad Sci 2000;97:1305–1310.

208. Thom SR, Ischiropoulos H: Mechanism of oxidative stress from low levels of carbon monoxide. Res Rep Health Effects Inst 1997;80: 1–19.

209. Thom SR, Kang M, Fisher D, Ischiropoulos H: Release of glutathione from erythrocytes and other markers of oxidative stress in carbon monoxide poisoning. J Appl Physiol 1997;82:1424–1432.

210. Thom SR, Keim LW: Carbon monoxide poisoning: a review of epidemiology, pathophysiology, clinical findings, and treatment options including hyperbaric oxygen therapy. J Toxicol Clin Toxicol 1989; 27:141–156.

211. Thom SR, Ohnishi ST, Fisher D, et al: Pulmonary vascular stress from carbon monoxide. Toxicol Appl Pharmacol 1999;154:12–19.

212. Thom SR, Ohnishi ST, Ischiropoulos H: Nitric oxide release by platelets inhibits neutrophil B2 integrin function following acute carbon monoxide poisoning. Toxicol Appl Pharmacol 1994;128: 105–110.

213. Thom SR, Taber RL, Mendiguren I, Clark JM, Hardy KR, Fisher AB: Delayed neuropsychological sequelae after carbon monoxide CO poisoning: prevention by treatment with hyperbaric oxygen. Ann Emerg Med 1995;25:474–480.

214. Thom SR, Xu YA, Ischiropoulos H: Vascular endothelial cells generate peroxynitrite in response to carbon monoxide exposure. Chem Res Toxicol 1997;10:1023–1031.

215. Thomas MF, Penney DG: Hematologic responses to carbon monoxide and altitude: a comparative study. J Appl Physiol 1977;43:365

216. Tikuisis P: Modeling the uptake and elimination of carbon monoxide. In: Penney DG, ed: Carbon Monoxide. Boca Raton, CRC Press, 1996, pp. 69–86.

217. Tom T, Abedon S, Clark RI, Wong W: Neuroimaging characteristics in carbon monoxide toxicity. J Neuroimag 1996;6:161–166.

218. Tomaszewski C, Rosenberg N, Wathen J, et al: Prevention of neurological sequelae from carbon monoxide by hyperbaric oxygen in rats [abstract]. Neurology 1992;42(Suppl 3):196.

219. Touger M, Gallagher EJ, Tyrell J: Relationship between venous and arterial carboxyhemoglobin levels in patients with suspected carbon monoxide poisoning. Ann Emerg Med 1995;25:481–483.

220. Treitman RD, Burgess WA, Gold A: Air contaminants encountered by firefighters. Am Ind Hyg Assoc J 1980;41:796–802.

221. Turcanu V, Dhouib M, Gendrault JL, et al: Carbon monoxide induces murine thymocyte apoptosis by a free radical-mediated mechanism. Cell Biol Toxicol 1998;14:47–54.

222. Turnbull TL, Hart RG, Strange GR, et al: Emergency department screening for unsuspected carbon monoxide exposure. Ann Emerg Med 1988;17:478–483.

223. Turner M, Esaw M, Clark RJ: Carbon monoxide poisoning treated with hyperbaric oxygen: metabolic acidosis as a predictor of treatment requirements [abstract]. J Accid Emerg Med 1999;16:96–98.

224. Utz J, Ullrich V: Carbon monoxide relaxes ileal smooth muscle through activation of guanylate cyclase. Biochem Pharmacol 1991; 41:1195–1201.

225. Van Hoesen KB, Camporesi EM, Moon RE, et al: Should hyperbaric oxygen be used to treat the pregnant patient for acute carbon monoxide poisoning? A case report and literature review. JAMA 1989; 261:1039–1043.

226. Verma A, Hirsch DJ, Glatt CE, et al: Carbon monoxide: a putative neural messenger. Science 1993;259:381–384.

227. Vreman HJ, Ronquillo RB, Ariagno RL, et al: Interference of fetal hemoglobin with the spectrophotometric measurement of carboxyhemoglobin. Clin Chem 1988;34:975–977.

228. Vreman HJ, Stevenson DK: Carboxyhemoglobin determined in neonatal blood with a co-oximeter unaffected by fetal oxyhemoglobin. Clin Chem 1994;40:1522–1527.

229. Wasowaski J, Myslack Z, Graczyk M, et al: An attempt at comparing the results of carboxyhemoglobin level in blood and gasometric determination in capillary blood in cases of carbon monoxide poisoning when treatment began at the place of accident. Anaesth Resusc Intens Ther 1976;4:245–249.

230. Weaver LK, Larson-Lohr V, Howe S, et al: Carboxyhemoglobin (COHb) half-life (t$_{1/2}$) in carbon monoxide poisoned patients treated with normobaric oxygen or HBO—an interim report. Undersea Hyperbaric Med 1994;21:13

231. Wharton M, Bistowish JM, Hutcheson RH: Fatal carbon monoxide poisoning at a motel. JAMA 2001;261:1177–1178.

232. Wheeler MG, Rozycki AA, Smith RP: Recreational propane inhalation in an adolescent male. J Toxicol Clin Toxicol 1992;30:135–139.

233. White SR, Penney DG: Initial study: Effects of insulin and glucose treatment on nuerologic outcome after CO poisoning. Ann Emerg Med 1994;23:606–607.

234. Wright GR, Shephard RJ: Physiological effects of carbon monoxide. Int Rev Physiol 1979;20:311–368.

235. Yee LM, Brandon GK: Successful reversal of presumed carbon monoxide-induced semicoma. Aviat Space Environ Med 1983;54: 641–643.

236. Yoon SS, MacDonald SC, Parrish RG: Deaths from unintentional carbon monoxide poisoning and potential for prevention with carbon monoxide detectors. JAMA 1998;279:685–687.

237. Zeiss J, Brinker R: Role of contrast enhancement in cerebral CT of carbon monoxide poisoning. J Comput Assist Tomogr 1988;12: 341–343.

238. Zhang J, Piantadosi CA: Mitochondrial oxidative stress after carbon monoxide hypoxia in the rat brain. J Clin Invest 1992;90:1193–1199.

239. Zhang J, Piantadosi CA: Nitric oxide mediates excitotoxicity induced by carbon monoxide poisining in rat brain [abstract]. Undersea Hyperbaric Med 1995;22:16–16.

240. Ziser A, Shupak A, Halpern P, et al: Delayed hyperbaric oxygen treatment for acute carbon monoxide poisoning. BMJ 1984; 289:960.

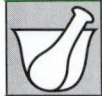

ANTIDOTES IN DEPTH

Hyperbaric Oxygen
Stephen R. Thom

Hyperbaric oxygen (HBO) therapy is a treatment modality in which a person breathes 100% O_2 while exposed to increased atmospheric pressure in a specialized chamber. Treatments are typically conducted at pressures 2 to 3 times higher than normal atmospheric pressure (1 atmosphere = 14.7 psi), or 2 to 3 atmospheres absolute (ATA). The hyperbaric chamber, per se, is not the therapeutic agent. Oxygen is the therapeutic drug, and the chamber serves as a dosing device. Hyperbaric oxygen treatment can be delivered in either a mono- or multiplace hyperbaric chamber. Monoplace chambers, which accommodate only a single patient, are pressurized with pure oxygen. Larger walk-in, or multiplace, chambers accommodate two or more patients as well as support staff for hands-on patient care. These chambers are pressurized with air while patients breathe pure oxygen via mask, head tent, or endotracheal tube. Portable "chambers" made of synthetic textile materials capable of withstanding pressures of 2 ATA can also be inflated with gas, typically air. The current use of these portable chambers has been for emergency treatment of high-altitude sickness, although they have been investigated for HBO use in remote or wilderness situations.[47,52,88,101]

In 1967, an international scientific organization, the Undersea and Hyperbaric Medical Society (UHMS), was founded to foster the exchange of data on the physiology of diving and hyperbaric medicine. The UHMS publishes a biannual report, "Hyperbaric Oxygen Therapy: A Committee Report," which outlines current knowledge and lists those conditions for which HBO is considered to be an effective treatment.[43] In toxicology, HBO is most commonly used for treatment of carbon monoxide (CO) poisoning. Hyperbaric oxygen therapy can also be considered for managing life-threatening poisonings from cyanide (CN^-), hydrogen sulfide (H_2S), or carbon tetrachloride (CCl_4) and in patients with methemoglobinemia. Management of patients with diverse poisonings of greater rarity have been investigated experimentally.[110]

Therapeutic mechanisms of action for HBO are based on elevation of both hydrostatic pressure and the partial pressure of oxygen. All perfused tissues are subjected to elevated partial pressures of oxygen in association with HBO exposure. Because, under normal environmental conditions, hemoglobin is virtually saturated with oxygen on passage through the pulmonary microvasculature, the primary effect of HBO is to increase dissolved oxygen content of plasma. Application of each additional atmosphere of oxygen increases the dissolved oxygen concentration in the plasma by 2.2 mL O_2/dL (vol%) (Chap. 20). Elevation of the hydrostatic pressure causes a reduction in the volume of gas according to Boyle's law. This action has direct relevance to pathologic conditions where gas bubbles are present in the body, such as arterial gas embolism and decompression sickness. In fact, HBO therapy was recently used successfully in an unusual case of cerebral gas embolism resulting from unintentional ingestion of a large amount of hydrogen peroxide.[71]

There is now ample evidence that reactive species of oxygen and nitrogen are second messengers in vivo and that they serve to signal a variety of cellular response (Fig. 97–2). Pharmacologic actions linked to reactive species and the resulting cellular signaling cascades are an active focus of investigation with regard to mechanisms of action of HBO. In animal studies, HBO is beneficial in the treatment of various forms of reperfusion injury.[11,36,37,40,54,75,86,91,95,103,107,113,122,124] These results initially appear paradoxical given the fact that HBO is expected to accelerate production of reactive oxygen species, which commonly contribute to reperfusion injuries. Interactions between circulating neutrophils and endothelial cells in the reperfused vascular bed are a major part of the reperfusion pathologic cascade. Methods to impede adherence between neutrophils and reperfused endothelium are frequently beneficial in experimental models of reperfusion injury.[115] For example, inhibition of the membrane-bound neutrophil β_2 integrin adhesion molecules and their intercellular adhesion molecule (ICAM) endothelial counterreceptors is typically achieved by infusing monoclonal antibodies. Hyperbaric oxygen can diminish injuries associated with a number of pathologic processes characterized by oxidative stress because HBO inhibits β_2 integrin-dependent neutrophil adhesion.[103,109,113,124] In fact, HBO exhibits efficacy over a broader period of time pre- and postinjury than monoclonal antibody infusions, and HBO is not associated with immunocompromise, as noted following the use of anti–β_2 integrin infusions.[67,77,103]

The affinity of CO for heme proteins is well known, and formation of carboxyhemoglobin (COHb) is a recognized effect of CO exposure. An elevated COHb can precipitate tissue hypoxia, and this stress appears to be responsible for fatalities, cardiac injuries, and the acute neurologic abnormalities that develop in approximately 14 % of survivors of serious CO poisoning.[2,29,33] However, both clinical and animal studies have failed to establish a correlation between elevated COHb levels and delayed neurologic injuries.[23,44,72,103] In experimental CO poisoning, endothelial changes mediated by the free radical nitric oxide are a prerequisite for neutrophil adherence to the cerebral microvasculature.[44] Activated leukocytes incite a cascade of biochemical and cellular processes that lead to oxidative injury. Brain injury is demonstrated as impaired glucose metabolism in the basal ganglia and hippocampus and as impaired learning.[106,110] Hyperbaric oxygen inhibits experimental brain injury by inhibiting β_2 integrin-dependent leukocyte adhesion.[103] Neutrophils from humans exposed to hyperbaric oxygen exhibit the same diminished adherence as those in animals.[104]

Use of supplemental oxygen is a cornerstone to the treatment of CO poisoning.[51] Since 1960, hyperbaric oxygen has been used with increasing frequency for severe CO poisoning, as clinical recovery appeared to be improved beyond that expected with ambient-pressure oxygen therapy.[34,64,72] However, no definition is established for staging the severity of CO poisoning. Therefore, it remains difficult to evaluate patients in a prospective manner or compare the efficacy of different treatments. Some centers propose using psychometric screening tests to identify patients with subtle neurologic compromise and as a method to stratify patients

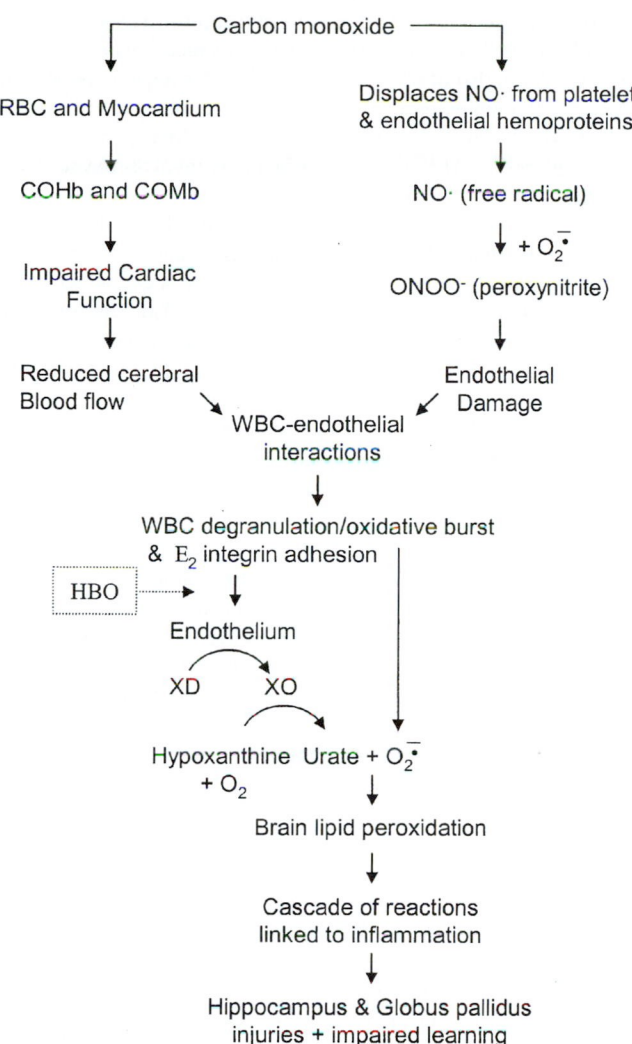

Figure 97–2.   Cascade of events as identified in rat model of CO poisoning.[44,103,106,110] COHb = carboxyhemoglobin; COMb = carboxymyoglobin; XD = xanthine dehydrogenase; XO = xanthine oxidase; NO• = free radical nitric oxide.

for treatment. However, when examined in a prospective study, abnormalities during the initial screening did not correlate with development of delayed sequelae.[105]

The first prospective clinical trial involving HBO therapy failed to find it superior to ambient-pressure treatment.[81] This study has been criticized because the authors used a low oxygen partial pressure (2 ATA) versus the more usual protocols with 2.5 to 3 ATA and because nearly half of all patients received hyperbaric treatments more than 6 hours after they were discovered.[15] In 1969, a retrospective study indicated that HBO reduced mortality and morbidity only if administered within 6 hours after CO poisoning.[35] HBO has been found effective in several prospective investigations: In one trial involving mildly to moderately poisoned patients, 23 % of patients (7 of 30) treated with ambient-pressure oxygen developed neurologic sequelae, whereas no patients (0 of 30; *p* < .05) treated with HBO (2.8 ATA) developed

sequelae.[105] In another prospective, randomized trial, 26 patients were hospitalized within 2 hours of discovery and were equally divided between two treatment groups: ambient-pressure oxygen, or 2.5-ATA O_2.[30] Three weeks later patients treated with HBO had significantly fewer abnormalities on electroencephalogram, and SPECT scans showed that cerebral vessels had nearly normal reactivity to carbon dioxide, in contrast to diminished reactivity in patients treated with ambient-pressure oxygen.

The fourth prospective trial investigating hyperbaric oxygen therapy for CO poisoning involved 191 patients and reported no benefit from relatively unorthodox administration of hyperbaric versus ambient-pressure oxygen therapy that extended over 3 days.[85] Concerns with this study include a mean delay to treatment of 7.5 hours, and only 46% of patients who entered the study were assessed to evaluate delayed neurologic sequelae. An adequate fraction of the population was studied to make comparisons with regard to the incidence of acute neurologic abnormalities, and no significant difference was found between treatment groups. Controversy exists, however, over the validity of the conclusion because 67% of the study population had attempted suicide, and the evaluation was performed with an arbitrary set of psychometric tests influenced by depression. Therefore, it is unclear whether abnormalities ascribed to CO may have been secondary to underlying, preexisting pathology. Furthermore, comatose patients accounted for 53% of the study group, and 44% of patients had taken additional poisons, but no specific information on these cases was provided to assess whether central nervous system insults may have been caused by factors other than CO.

A recent reevaluation of the subset of patients in this study who were presumed to be suffering from mild CO poisoning once again presents the dilemma of patient selection criteria. These reconstructed data were examined to assess the difference in incidence of acute or persistent neurologic sequelae between the two treatment groups.[50] Those treated with HBO had a significantly lower incidence of sequelae than did those treated with ambient-pressure oxygen. Finally, in as yet the largest prospective, randomized trial, which involved 575 patients, the incidence of delayed neurologic sequelae was lower among noncomatose patients who had suffered transient unconsciousness when treated with hyperbaric oxygen versus ambient-pressure oxygen therapy.[65] Because most patients with sequelae resolved their symptoms spontaneously over a period of 6 months, the benefit of HBO treatment has been discussed in terms of reducing the incidence and duration of functional disabilities caused by CO poisoning.

This study[65] and a recent double blind randomized trial[119a] have demonstrated that HBO therapy reduces cognitive sequelae after acute CO poisoning. The most recent study[119a] was performed with 152 patients treated three times at 6–12 hour intervals with HBO or normobaric O_2 inside a hyperbaric chamber. Interim analysis was conducted at 50, 100, and 150 patients, with a goal of 200 patients. The trial was stopped after the third interim analysis because HBO was found to be efficacious (*p* = 0.007 for the difference in cognitive sequelae between groups). There were 144 patients who had complete neuropsychological data at all follow up time points. Among these patients, 24% of the group treated with HBO had cognitive sequelae compared to 43.1% of the normobaric O_2-treated group (*p* = 0.014). Post hoc subgroup analysis showed that HBO reduced cognitive sequelae in patients with any of the following: loss of consciousness, COHb ≥25%, age ≥50 years, or a base excess <−2 mEq/L.

The mechanisms of action for HBO therapy in CO poisoning may include hastened dissociation of CO from hemoglobin and from cytochrome oxidase and temporary inhibition of leukocyte β_2 integrin adhesion molecules to blunt the cascade of vascular injury.[16,31,76,103] Clinical indications for HBO in CO poisoning are reviewed in greater detail in Chapter 97 and specifically Table 97–2.

Support for use of HBO comes from the studies outlined above and from nine nonrandomized comparative studies.[34,35,42,55,64,66,72,73,83] Studies that have failed to find benefit to treatment have consistently suffered from serious methodologic shortcomings. There is a legitimate concern over the lack of reliable methods to assess the severity of poisoning. Whether this problem leads to over-, or underutilization of HBO is not clear. Therefore, pending the results from additional studies, use of HBO in CO-poisoned patients who have suffered loss of consciousness during CO exposure, or who have a neurologic abnormality on clinical examination, continues to be advocated. Important caveats regarding HBO include the observation that treatment efficacy may diminish if treatment is delayed for more than 6 hours after poisoning.[35] There also is discussion in the literature that patient outcome may be improved if more than a single treatment is administered.[34]

Methylene chloride (CH_2Cl_2) is an organic solvent used commercially in aerosol sprays and as a paint stripper. It is readily absorbed through the skin or by inhalation and metabolized by the cytochrome P450 oxidase system to yield CO.[97] This process is slow, and peak COHb levels of 10 to 50% may not be reached for 8 hours or more.[22,32,48,56,62,97] Methylene chloride toxicity can have many of the same acute manifestations as CO poisoning.[94] Acute signs and symptoms are attributable to the direct effects of this solvent on the central nervous system and to concomitant hypoxia. Effects that are present after 1 hour or more, especially if the COHb level is elevated, may be partially caused by CO toxicity. Treatment with HBO in this setting has been reported.[41,84]

Carbon monoxide (CO) and cyanide (CN^-) poisonings can occur together in victims of smoke inhalation.[3,4,6,7,8,10,28,53,68, 89,90,100,117,120] Experimental evidence suggests that these agents can produce synergistic toxicity.[5,70,74,76,78] Toxicity from CN^- stems from binding to cytochrome aa_3 and inhibiting oxidative phosphorylation.[107] Animal studies demonstrate that ambient-pressure 100% O_2 can enhance protection from CN^- toxicity[87] and also enhance CN^- metabolism to thiocyanate when thiosulfate is used concomitantly.[13] Hyperbaric oxygen may have direct effects to reduce CN^- toxicity[27,45,46,92,102] or to augment antidote treatments.[20,87,119] However, not all animal studies have found HBO to improve outcome,[118] and clinical experience regarding CN^- treatment with HBO is sparse. In a series of smoke-inhalation victims with both toxic CO and CN^- levels who received both HBO and treatment for CN^- involving sodium nitrite and sodium thiosulfate, four of five patients survived without apparent neurologic damage.[39] The results with HBO in clinical cases of isolated CN^- poisonings refractory to standard antidote treatment (sodium nitrite plus sodium thiosulfate) have been equivocal. One case showed dramatic improvement,[111] but another was without response.[59] Further research in this area is necessary. Because CN^- is among the most lethal poisons, and toxicity is rapid, standard antidotal therapy for isolated CN^- poisoning is of primary importance. Hyperbaric oxygen may be an adjunct to be considered in refractory cases (Chap. 98).

Hydrogen sulfide (H_2S) binds to cytochrome aa_3 and impairs oxidative phosphorylation. Hence, one of its mechanisms of toxicity is similar to that of CN^-, although it is more readily dissociated from cytochrome oxidase by O_2.[98] Clinical manifestations of toxicity are similar to those with CO and CN^-.[98] Management of patients with serious H_2S poisoning principally involves oxygenation and cardiovascular support as well as consideration of sodium nitrite.[38] In animals, HBO may be more effective than sodium nitrite in preventing mortality.[12] There are several instances where HBO has appeared to be beneficial.[19,94,121] Relatively late treatment with HBO, 10 hours or more after poisoning, has also been reported beneficial in some[114] but not all cases.[1] There are no definitive data regarding use of HBO in H_2S poisoning, but it should be considered in refractory cases.

Carbon tetrachloride (CCl_4) hepatotoxicity may be diminished by HBO. Mortality was decreased in a number of animal studies,[9,18,60,69,82] and there are several case reports of patients surviving potentially lethal ingestions with HBO therapy.[57,96,112,123] HBO appears to inhibit the mixed-function oxidase system responsible for conversion of CCl_4 to hepatotoxic free radicals.[17,63] Because there are no proven antidotes for CCl_4 poisoning, HBO should be considered with potentially severe CCl_4 exposures. However, there may be a delicate balance between those oxidative processes that are therapeutic and those that mediate hepatotoxicity.[14] Therefore, when HBO is being considered, it should be instituted before the onset of liver function abnormalities.

When arranging for treatment with HBO, probably the first consideration must be the logistic requirements for transporting a patient to a hyperbaric facility. From a review of 297 consecutive CO-poisoned patients, it was concluded that transfer need not be deferred because of a concern over cardiac or respiratory arrest, myocardial infarction, or deterioration in mental status if these events had not occurred before transfer.[93] Intensive care support for pediatric cases is also achievable.[49,116] An additional consideration is the potential adverse effects of HBO per se, which are usually mild, self-limited, and also relatively rare. However, the risks must always be considered in any therapeutic setting. Preexisting conditions that require evaluation for possible management before HBO is initiated include claustrophobia, sinus congestion, and patients with scarred or noncompliant structures in the middle ear such as those found in otosclerosis.[51] Middle ear barotrauma from eustachian tube dysfunction may occur in up to 2% of patients and is relatively easily managed by oral decongestants or, rarely, by tympanostomy tubes.[99] Transient nearsightedness, thought to be related to lenticular changes from oxygen, occurs in association with protracted treatment courses not typically used for toxins. These eye changes are found when treatments span weeks in approximately 33% of patients over age 50. They resolve between 3 and 6 weeks after treatments cease.[51] There are no notable pulmonary oxygen toxicity risks with standard therapeutic protocols because the duration of exposure is usually kept to less than 2 hours.[25,80,108] However, approximately one in 10,000 patients may sustain central nervous system oxygen toxicity, which is manifested as a grand mal seizure. If mechanical trauma can be avoided during the convulsion, there are no residual effects.[25] A physiologic effect of hyperoxygenation is vasoconstriction. This causes negligible changes in blood pressure because of a small (about 10%) decrease in cardiac output, principally as a result of vagal stimulation with a reduction in heart rate.[79] Previous exposure to the chemotherapeutic agent bleomycin is considered a relatively strong contraindication to HBO. Bleomycin may exacerbate pulmonary oxygen toxicity.[26,58] Therefore, on a case-by-case basis, careful consideration of this risk must be weighed against the potential benefits of HBO. The only well-recognized absolute contraindication for HBO therapy is an unvented pneumothorax because of the obvious risk of exacerbating this condition while in the hyperbaric chamber and especially on decompression. Additional theoretical concerns include the risk of fire in an environment with elevated concentrations of oxygen and the risk of rapid decompression, should a mechanical malfunction occur in the hyperbaric chamber. A matter that must be evaluated on a case-by-case basis is the need for hands-on critical care of patients. This matter is sometimes quite important, for example, in smoke inhalation victims who require frequent tracheal suctioning because of airways injuries. In this case, use of a large, multiplace hyperbaric chamber where medical attendants can stand next to a patient may be advantageous.

In conclusion, the mechanisms of action and efficacy of HBO in toxicology continue to be investigated. Some research findings are provocative because they highlight the fact that traditional assessments of mechanisms for toxicity of some agents are incomplete. Questions persist on many issues. More work is required to discern those cases where clear benefit arises with HBO treatment and to define the constraints that may limit its efficacious use.

REFERENCES

1. Al-Mahasneh QM, Cohle SD, Haas E: Lack of response to hyperbaric oxygen in a fatal case of hydrogen sulfide poisoning [abstract]. Vet Hum Toxicol 1989;31:353.
2. Anderson EW, Andelman RJ, Strauch JM: Effects of low-level carbon monoxide exposure on onset and duration of angina pectoris. Ann Intern Med 1973;79:46–50.
3. Anderson RA, Thomson I, Harland WA: The importance of cyanide and organic nitriles in fire fatalities. Fire Materials 1979;3:91–99.
4. Anderson RA, Harland WA: Fire deaths in the Glasgow area. III. The role of hydrogen cyanide. Med Sci Law 1982;22:35–40.
5. Ballantyne B: Hydrogen cyanide as a product of combustion and a factor in morbidity and mortality from fires. In: Ballantyne B, Marrs T, eds: Clinical and Experimental Toxicology of Cyanides. Bristol, UK, John Wright, 1987, pp. 248–291.
6. Barillo DJ, Goode R, Rush BF, et al: Lack of correlation between carboxyhemoglobin and cyanide in smoke inhalation injury. Curr Surg 1986;46:421–423.
7. Barillo DJ, Goode R, Esch V: Cyanide poisoning in victims of fire: analysis of 364 cases and review of the literature. J Burn Care Rehabil 1994;15:46–57.
8. Baud FJ, Barriot P, Toffis V, et al: Elevated blood cyanide concentrations in victims of smoke inhalation. N Engl J Med 1991;325:1761–1766.
9. Bernacchi A, Myers R, Trump BF, Margello L: Protection of hepatocytes with hyperoxia against carbon tetrachloride induced injury. Toxicol Pathol 1984;12:315–323.
10. Birky MM, Paabo M, Brown JE: Correlation of autopsy data and materials in the Tennessee jail fire. Fire Safety J 1979;2:17–22.
11. Bitterman H, Cohen L: Effects of hyperbaric oxygen in circulatory shock induced by splanchnic artery occlusion and reperfusion in rats. Can J Physiol Pharmacol 1989;67:1033–1037.
12. Bitterman N, Talmi Y, Lerman A: The effect of hyperbaric oxygen on acute experimental sulfide poisoning in the rat. Toxicol Appl Pharmacol 1986;84:325–328.
13. Breen PH, Isserles SA, Westley J, et al: Effect of oxygen and sodium thiosulfate during combined carbon monoxide and cyanide poisoning. Toxicol Appl Pharmacol 1995;134:229–234.
14. Brent JA, Rumack BH: Role of free radicals in toxic hepatic injury: I. Free radical biochemistry. J Toxicol Clin Toxicol 1993;31: 173–196.
15. Brown SD, Piantadosi CA: Hyperbaric oxygen for carbon monoxide poisoning. Lancet 1989;1:1032–1033.
16. Brown SD, Piantadosi CA: Reversal of carbon monoxide-cytochrome C oxidase binding by hyperbaric oxygen in vivo. Adv Exp Biol Med 1989;248:747–754.
17. Burk RF, Lane JM, Patel K: Relationship of oxygen and glutathione in protection against carbon tetrachloride-induced hepatic microsomal lipid peroxidation and covalent binding in the rat. J Clin Invest 1984; 74:1996–2001.
18. Burk RF, Reiter R, Land JM: Hyperbaric oxygen protection against carbon tetrachloride hepatotoxicity in the rat: Association with altered metabolism. Gastroenterology 1986;90:812–818.
19. Burnett WW, King EG, Grace M: Hydrogen sulfide poisoning: review of 5 years' experience. Can Med Assoc J 1977;117:1277–1280.
20. Burrows GE, Way JL: Cyanide intoxication in sheep: Therapeutic value of oxygen or cobalt. Am J Vet Res 1977;38:223–227.
21. Chance B, Erecinska M, Wagner M: Mitochondrial responses to carbon monoxide toxicity. Ann NY Acad Sci 1970;174:193–204.
22. Chang YL, Yang CC, Deng JF, et al: Diverse manifestations of oral methylene chloride poisoning: report of 6 cases. J Toxicol Clin Toxicol 1999;37:497–504.
23. Choi S: Delayed neurologic sequelae in carbon monoxide intoxication. Arch Neurol 1983;40:433–435.
24. Clark CJ, Campbell D, Reid WH: Blood carboxyhaemoglobin and cyanide levels in fire survivors. Lancet 1981;1:1332–1335.
25. Clark JM: Oxygen toxicity. In: Bennett PB, Elliott DH, eds: The Physiology and Medicine of Diving, 4th ed. Philadelphia, WB Saunders, 1993, pp. 121–169.
26. Comis RL: Bleomycin pulmonary toxicity: Current status and future directions. Semin Oncol 1992;19:64–70.
27. Cope C: The importance of oxygen in the treatment of cyanide poisoning. JAMA 1961;175:1061–1064.
28. Copeland AR: Accidental fire deaths: the 5-year Metropolitan Dade County experience from 1979 to 1983. Z Rechtsmed 1985;94:71–79.
29. Cramlet SH, Erickson HH, Gorman HA: Ventricular function following acute carbon monoxide exposure. J Appl Physiol 1975;39: 482–486.
30. Ducasse JL, Celsis P, Marc-Vergnes JP: Non-comatose patients with acute carbon monoxide poisoning: hyperbaric or normobaric oxygenation? Undersea Hyperbaric Med 1995;22:9–15.
31. End E, Long CW: Oxygen under pressure in carbon monoxide poisoning. J Ind Hyg Toxicol 1942;24:302–306.
32. Fagin J, Bradley J, Williams D: Carbon monoxide poisoning secondary to inhaling methylene chloride. Br Med J 1980;281:1461.
33. Ginsberg MD, Myers RE: Experimental carbon monoxide encephalopathy in the primate. I. Physiologic and metabolic aspects. Arch Neurol 1974;30:202–208.
34. Gorman DF, Clayton D, Gilligan JE, Webb RK: A longitudinal study of 100 consecutive admissions for carbon monoxide poisoning to the Royal Adelaide Hospital. Anaesth Intens Care 1992;20:311–316.
35. Goulon M, Barois A, Rapin M, et al: Carbon monoxide poisoning and acute anoxia due to breathing coal gas and hydrocarbons. Ann Med Interne 1969;120:335–349. (English translation in J Hyperbaric Med 1986;1:23–41.)
36. Haapaniemi T, Nylander G, Sirsjo A, et al: Hyperbaric oxygen reduces ischemia-induced skeletal muscle injury. Plast Reconstr Surg 1996;97:602–609.
37. Haapaniemi T, Sirsjo A, Nylander G, et al: Hyperbaric oxygen treatment attenuates glutathione depletion and improves metabolic restitution in postischemic skeletal muscle. Free Radical Res 1995;23: 91–101.

38. Hall AH, Rumack BH: Hydrogen sulfide poisoning: An antidotal role for sodium nitrite? Vet Hum Toxicol 1997;39:152–154.

39. Hart GB, Strauss MB, Lennon PA, Whitcraft DD: Treatment of smoke inhalation by hyperbaric oxygen. J Emerg Med 1985;3: 211–215.

40. Horn PC, Webster DA, Amin HM, et al: The effect of hyperbaric oxygen on medial collateral ligament healing in a rat model. Clin Orthop Rel Res 1999;360:238–242.

41. Horowitz BZ: Carboxyhemoglobinemia caused by inhalation of methylene chloride. Am J Emerg Med 1986;4:48–51.

42. Hsu LH, Wang JH: Treatment of carbon monoxide poisoning with hyperbaric oxygen. Chinese Med J 1996;58:407–413.

43. Hyperbaric Oxygen Therapy: A Committee Report. Bethesda, MD, Undersea and Hyperbaric Medical Society, 1999, pp. 1–82.

44. Ischiropoulos H, Beers MF, Ohnishi ST, et al: Nitric oxide production and perivascular tyrosine nitration in brain after carbon monoxide poisoning in the rat. J Clin Invest 1996;97:2260–2267.

45. Isom GE, Way JL: Effect of oxygen on cyanide intoxication. VI. Reactivation of cyanide inhibited glucose metabolism. J Pharmacol Exp Ther 1974;189:235–243.

46. Ivanov KP: The effect of elevated oxygen pressure on animals poisoned with potassium cyanide. Pharmacol Toxicol 1959;22: 476–479.

47. Jay GD, Tetz DJ, Hartigan LF, et al: Portable hyperbaric oxygen therapy in the emergency department with a modified Gamow bag. Ann Emerg Med 1995;26:707–711.

48. Kaufman D, Lipscomb JW, Leikin JB: Methylene chloride report of 5 exposures and 2 deaths. Vet Hum Toxicol 1989;31:352.

49. Keenan HT, Bratton SL, Norkool DM, et al: Delivery of hyperbaric oxygen therapy to critically ill, mechanically ventilated children. J Crit Care 1998;13:7–12.

50. Kehat I, Shupak A: Letter. Undersea Hyperbaric Med 2000;27:47.

51. Kindwall EP, ed: Hyperbaric Medicine Practice. Flagstaff, AZ, Best Publishing, 1994.

52. King SJ, Greenbee RR: Successful use of the Gamow hyperbaric bag in the treatment of altitude illness at Mt. Everest. J Wilderness Med 1990;1:193–202.

53. Kirk MA, Gerace R, Kulig KW: Cyanide and methemoglobin kinetics in smoke inhalation victims treated with the cyanide antidote kit. Ann Emerg Med 1993;22:1413–1418.

54. Krakovsky M, Rogatsky G, Zarchin N, et al: Effect of hyperbaric oxygen therapy on survival after global cerebral ischemia in rats. Surg Neurol 1998;49:412–416.

55. Lamy M, Hauguet M: Fifty patients with carbon monoxide intoxication treated with hyperbaric oxygen therapy. Acta Anaesthesiol Belg 1969;1:49–53.

56. Langehennig PL, Seeler RA, Berman E: Paint removers and carboxyhemoglobin. N Engl J Med 1976;295:1137.

57. Larcan A, Lambert H: Current epidemiological, clinical, biological, and therapeutic aspects of acute carbon monoxide intoxication. Bull Acad Natl Med (Paris) 1981;165:471.

58. Lazo JS, Sebati SM, Schellens JH: Bleomycin. Cancer Chemother Biol Respir Modifiers 1996;16:39–47.

59. Litovitz TL, Larkin RF, Myers RAM: Cyanide poisoning treated with hyperbaric oxygen. Am J Emerg Med 1983;1:94–101.

60. Lowe-Ponsford FL, Henry JA: Clinical aspects of carbon monoxide poisoning. Adv Drug React Acute Poisoning Rev 1989;8:217–240.

61. Lundquist P, Lennart R, Sorbo B: The role of hydrogen cyanide and carbon monoxide in fire casualities: A prospective study. Forensic Sci Int 1989;43:9–14.

62. Mahmud M, Kales SN: Methylene chloride poisoning in a cabinet worker. Environ Health Perspect 1999;107:769–772.

63. Marzella L, Muhvich K, Myers RAM: Effect of hyperoxia on liver necrosis induced by hepatotoxins. Virchows Arch 1986;51:497–507.

64. Mathieu D, Nolf M, Durocher A, et al: Acute carbon monoxide poisoning risk of late sequelae and treatment by hyperbaric oxygen. J Toxicol Clin Toxicol 1985;23:315–324.

65. Mathieu D, Wattel F, Mathieu-Nolf M, et al: Randomized prospective study comparing the effect of HBO versus 12 hours NBO in non-comatose CO poisoned patients. Undersea Hyperbaric Med. 1996;23 (Suppl):7.

66. Meyer A: Experimentelle erfahrungen uber die kohlenoxydverguftung des zentralnervens systems. Z Ges Neurol Psychiatr 1928;112: 187–212.

67. Mileski WJ, Sikes P, Atiles L, et al: Inhibition of leukocyte adherence and susceptibility to infection. J Surg Res 1993;54:349–354.

68. Mohler SR: Air crash survival: injuries and evaluation of toxic hazards. Aviat Space Environ Med 1975;46:86–88.

69. Montani S, Perret C: Oxygenation hyperbare dans l'intoxication experimentale au tetrachlorure de carbon. Rev Fr Etudes Clin Biol 1967;12:274–278.

70. Moore SJ, Norris JC, Walsh DA, Hume AS: Antidotal use of methemoglobin forming cyanide antagonists in concurrent carbon monoxide/cyanide intoxication. J Pharmacol Exp Ther 1987;242: 70–73.

71. Mullins ME, Beltran JT: Acute cerebral gas embolism from hydrogen peroxide ingestion successfully treated with hyperbaric oxygen. J Toxicol Clin Toxicol 1998;36:253–256.

72. Myers RAM, Snyder SK, Emhoff TA: Subacute sequelae of carbon monoxide poisoning. Ann Emerg Med 1985;14:1163–1167.

73. Norkool DM, Kirkpatrick JN: Treatment of acute carbon monoxide poisoning with hyperbaric oxygen: a review of 115 cases. Ann Emerg Med 1985;14:1168–1171.

74. Norris JC, Moore SJ, Hume AS: Synergistic lethality induced by the combination of carbon monoxide and cyanide. Toxicology 1986;40: 121–129.

75. Nylander G, Nordstrom H, Lewis D, Larsson J: Metabolic effects of hyperbaric oxygen in postischemic muscle. Plast Reconstruct Surg 1987;79:91–97.

76. Pace N, Strajman E, Walker EL: Acceleration of carbon monoxide elimination in man by high pressure oxygen. Science 1950;111: 652–654.

77. Park MK, Muhvich KH, Myers RAM, et al: Effects of hyperbaric oxygen in infectious diseases: Basic mechanisms. In: Kindwall EP, ed: Hyperbaric Medicine Practice. Flagstaff, AZ, Best, 1994, pp. 141–172.

78. Pitt BR, Radford EP, Gurtner GH, Traystman RJ: Interaction of carbon monoxide and cyanide on cerebral circulation and metabolism. Arch Environ Health 1979;34:354–359.

79. Plewes JL, Farhi LE: Peripheral circulatory responses to acute hyperoxia. Undersea Biomed Res 1983;10:123–129.

80. Pott F, Westergaard P, Mortensen J, Jansen EC: Hyperbaric oxygen treatment and pulmonary function. Undersea Hyper Med 1999;26: 225–228.

81. Raphael JC, Elkharrat D, Guincestre MCJ, et al: Trial of normobaric and hyperbaric oxygen for acute carbon monoxide intoxication. Lancet 1989;2:414–419.

82. Rapin M, Got C, Le Gall JR: Effect de l'oxygene hyperbare sur la toxicite tetrachlorure de carbone chez le rat. Rev Fr Etudes Clin Biol 1967;12:594–599.

83. Roche L, Bertoye A, Vincent P: Comparison de deux groupes de vingt intoxications oxycarbonees traitees par oxygene normobare et hyperbare. Lyon Med 1968;49:1483–1499.

84. Rudge FW: Treatment of methylene chloride induced carbon monoxide poisoning with hyperbaric oxygen. Mil Med 1990;155: 570–572.

85. Scheinkestel CD, Bailey M, Myles PS, et al: Hyperbaric or normobaric oxygen for acute carbon monoxide: a randomized controlled clinical trial. Med J Aust 1999;170:203–210.

86. Shandling AH, Ellestad MH, Hart GB, et al: Hyperbaric oxygen and thrombolysis in myocardial infarction: the HOT MI pilot study. Am Heart J 1997;134:544–550.

87. Sheehy M, Way JL: Effect of oxygen on cyanide intoxication: III. Mithridate. J Pharmacol Exp Ther 1968;161:163–168.

88. Shimada H, Morita T, Kunimoto F, Saito S: Immediate application of hyperbaric oxygen therapy using a newly devised transportable chamber. Am J Emerg Med. 1996;14:412–415.

89. Shusterman D, Alexeeff G, Hargis C, et al: Predictors of carbon monoxide and hydrogen cyanide exposure in smoke inhalation patients. J Toxicol Clin Toxicol 1996;34:61–71.

90. Silverman SH, Purdue GF, Hunt JL, et al: Cyanide toxicity in burned patients. J Trauma 1988;28:171–176.

91. Sirsjo A, Lehr HA, Nolte D, et al: Hyperbaric oxygen treatment enhances the recovery of blood flow and functional capillary density in postischemic striated muscle. Circ Shock 1993;40:9–13.

92. Skene WG, Norman JN, Smith G: Effect of hyperbaric oxygen in cyanide poisoning. In: Brown IW, Cox B, eds: Proceedings of the Third International Congress on Hyperbaric Medicine. Washington, DC, National Academy of Sciences, National Research Council, 1966, pp. 705–710.

93. Sloan EP, Murphy DG, Hart R, et al: Complications and protocol considerations in carbon monoxide-poisoned patients who require hyperbaric oxygen therapy: report from a ten-year experience. Ann Emerg Med 1989;18:629–634.

94. Smilkstein MJ, Bronstein AC, Pickett HM: Hyperbaric oxygen therapy for severe hydrogen sulfide poisoning. J Emerg Med 1985;3: 27–30.

95. Stavitsky Y, Shandling AH, Ellestad MH, et al: Hyperbaric oxygen and thrombolysis in myocardial infarction: the "HOT MI" randomized multicenter study. Cardiology 1998;90:131–136.

96. Stewart RD, Boettner EA, Southworth RR: Acute carbon tetrachloride intoxication. JAMA 1963;183:994–997.

97. Stewart RD, Hake CL: Paint remover hazard. JAMA 1976;235: 398–401.

98. Stine RJ, Slosberg B, Beacham BE: Hydrogen sulfide intoxication. Ann Intern Med 1976;85:756–758.

99. Stone JA, Loar H, Rudge FW: An eleven year review of hyperbaric oxygenation in a military clinical setting. Undersea Biomed Res 1991;18(Suppl):80.

100. Symington IS, Anderson RA, Thomson I, et al: Cyanide exposure in fires. Lancet 1978;2:91–92.

101. Taber RL: Protocols for the use of a portable hyperbaric chamber for the treatment of high altitude disorders. J Wilderness Med 1990;1: 181–192.

102. Takano T, Miyazaki Y, Nashimoto I, Kobayashi K: Effect of hyperbaric oxygen on cyanide intoxication: In situ changes in intracellular oxidation reduction. Undersea Biomed Res 1980;7:191–197.

103. Thom SR: Functional inhibition of leukocyte β2 integrins by hyperbaric oxygen in carbon monoxide-mediated brain injury in rats. Toxicol Appl Pharmacol 1993;123:248–256.

104. Thom SR, Mendiguren I, Hardy KR, et al: Inhibition of human neutrophil β2 integrin-dependent adherence by hyperbaric oxygen. Am J Physiol 1997;272:770–771.

105. Thom SR, Taber RL, Mendiguren II, et al: Delayed neuropsychologic sequelae after carbon monoxide poisoning: prevention by treatment with hyperbaric oxygen. Ann Emerg Med 1995;25:474–480.

106. Thom SR: Learning dysfunction and metabolic defects in globus pallidus and hippocampus after CO poisoning in a rat model. Undersea Hyperbaric Med 1997;23(Suppl):20.

107. Thomas MP, Brown LA, Sponseller DR, et al: Myocardial infarct size reduction by the synergistic effect of hyperbaric oxygen and recombinant tissue plasminogen activator. Am Heart J 1990;120: 791–800.

108. Thorsen E, Aanderud L, Aasen TB: Effects of a standard hyperbaric oxygen treatment protocol on pulmonary function. Eur Respir J 1998;12:1442–1445.

109. Tjarnstrom J, Wikstrom T, Bagge U, et al: Effects of hyperbaric oxygen treatment on neutrophil activation and pulmonary sequestration in intestinal ischemia-reperfusion in rats. Eur Surg Res 1999;31: 147–154.

110. Tomaszewski CA, Thom SR: Use of hyperbaric oxygen in toxicology. Emerg Med Clin North Am 1994;12:437–459.

111. Trapp WG, Lepawsky M: 100% survival in five life-threatening acute cyanide poisoning victims treated by a therapeutic spectrum including hyperbaric oxygen. Paper presented at the First European Conference on Hyperbaric Medicine, Amsterdam, 1983.

112. Truss CD, Killenberg PG: Treatment of carbon tetrachloride poisoning with hyperbaric oxygen. Gastroenterology 1982;82:767–769.

113. Ueno S, Tanabe G, Kihara K, et al: Early post operative hyperbaric oxygen therapy modifies neutrophile activation. Hepatogastroenterology 1999;46:1798–1799.

114. Vicas I, Fortin S, Uptigrove OF: Hydrogen sulfide exposure treated with hyperbaric oxygen [abstract]. Vet Hum Toxicol 1989;31:353.

115. Virkhaus RB, Lucchesi R, Simpson PJ, et al: The role of adhesion molecules in cardiovascular pharmacology: meeting review. J Pharmacol Exp Ther 1995;273:569–575.

116. Waisman D, Shupak A, Weisz G, et al: Hyperbaric oxygen therapy in the pediatric patient: the experience of the Israel Naval Medical Institute. Pediatrics 1998;102:E53.

117. Way JL: Cyanide intoxication and its mechanism of antagonism. Annu Rev Pharmacol Toxicol 1984;24:451–481.

118. Way JL, End E, Sheehy MH, et al: Effect of oxygen on cyanide intoxication. Toxicol Appl Pharmacol 1972;22:415–421.

119. Way JL, Gibbon SL, Sheehy M: Effect of oxygen on cyanide intoxication. I. Prophylactic protection. J Pharmacol Exp Ther 1966;13: 381–382.

119a. Weaver LK, Hopkins RO, Chan KJ, et al: Outcome of acute carbon monoxide poisoning treated with hyperbaric or normobaric oxygen (abstract). Undersea Hyp Med 2001;28(Suppl): 15.

120. Wetherill HR: The occurrence of cyanide in the blood of fire victims. J Forensic Sci 1966;11:167–173.

121. Whitcraft DD, Bailey TD, Hart GB: Hydrogen sulfide poisoning treated with hyperbaric oxygen. J Emerg Med 1985;3:23–25.

122. Wong HP, Zamboni WA, Stephenson LL: Effect of hyperbaric oxygen on skeletal muscle necrosis following primary and secondary ischemia in a rat model. Surg Forum 1996;47:705–707.

123. Zamboni WA, Roth AC, Russell RC, et al: Morphologic analysis of the microcirculation during reperfusion of ischemic skeletal muscle and the effect of hyperbaric oxygen. Plast Reconstruct Surg 1993: 1110–1123.

124. Zearbaugh C, Gorman DF, Gilligan JE: Carbon tetrachloride/chloroform poisoning: Case studies of hyperbaric oxygen in the treatment of lethal dose ingestion. Undersea Biomed Res 1988;15:44.

CHAPTER 98 CYANIDE AND HYDROGEN SULFIDE

William Kerns II / Gary Isom / Mark A. Kirk

Cyanide

MW:	=	26.02 daltons
Whole blood:	=	<1 µg/mL
	=	38.5 µmol/L

Airborn

Immediately fatal	=	270 ppm
Life threatening	=	110 ppm > 30 min

Hydrogen Sulfide

MW:	=	34.08 daltons
Airborne concentrations:		
Odor threshold	=	0.02–0.13 ppm
Olfactory fatigue	=	100–150 ppm
Immediately fatal	=	700 ppm

Values greater than or equal to the action level usually necessitate clinical intervention. Values less than this level may necessitate intervention based on the clinical condition of the patient.

CYANIDE POISONING

Case 1 A previously healthy 19-year-old woman arrived at the Emergency Department (ED) in coma, apneic, and hypotensive. Her boyfriend accompanied her and stated that she began retching immediately after drinking from a refrigerated, open seltzer bottle. The boyfriend attempted to taste the seltzer, but the patient knocked it from his hand. She soon collapsed, and EMS was summoned.

Paramedics intubated the patient because of apnea. Prehospital vital signs included a blood pressure 110 mm Hg by palpation and a pulse of 110 beats/min. No odors or unusual findings were noted in their apartment. Medics brought the seltzer bottle to the hospital.

Initial survey in the ED revealed a comatose (GCS 5) woman with a blood pressure of 90 mm Hg by palpation and a pulse of 74 beats/min. A detailed physical examination was remarkable for dilated and sluggish pupils, roving ocular movements, occasional nonpurposeful movement, and bilateral decorticate posturing. The remainder of the examination was normal.

There was no response to intravenous naloxone (0.8 mg) or dextrose (25 g). Blood pressure improved to 130 mm Hg after 1500 mL 0.9% saline bolus. Activated charcoal was instilled via a nasogastric tube.

Diagnostic studies included an ECG, which revealed nonspecific S-T changes. Arterial blood gas showed pH 7.01, P_{CO_2} 21 mm Hg, and P_{O_2} 575 mm Hg on 100% oxygen. Electrolytes were normal except for a serum bicarbonate of 8.9 mEq/L. Glucose was 276 mg/dL (after dextrose bolus). Computed tomography of the head was normal.

On further questioning, the boyfriend stated that he tasted the seltzer and that it was "bitter." He complained of transient nausea en route to the hospital. With this additional information, cyanide was suspected, and the patient received 100 mEq sodium bicarbon-ate intravenously and the cyanide antidote kit, including 12.5 g sodium thiosulfate and 300 mg sodium nitrite. Follow-up arterial blood gas analysis and cooximetry 30 minutes later demonstrated improvement in pH to 7.17 with a methemoglobin level of 9.5%. A second bolus of sodium thiosulfate and sodium nitrite was then given at one-half the initial dose. Over the next 12 hours, the metabolic acidosis resolved.

Additional diagnostic studies revealed a lactate of 10 mmol/L (obtained before treatment with cyanide antidotes). Serum acetaminophen, salicylate, toxic alcohol, and urine drugs of abuse screen were negative.

When the parents of the patient arrived at the hospital, they claimed that the boyfriend was abusive to their daughter on numerous occasions. The police determined that the boyfriend worked at a jewelry manufacturing company and had ready access to cyanide-containing reagents. The boyfriend was arrested on suspicion of attempted homicide, and the seltzer bottle, when analyzed, revealed a "high" concentration of cyanide.

The remainder of the patient's acute course was uneventful. At 5-month followup, however, the patient complained of difficulty with memory and stiffness of her limbs. The physical examination revealed generalized bradykinetic movements consistent with secondary parkinsonism.

History and Epidemiology

Use and misuse of cyanide-containing compounds has justifiably given it a reputation as one of the more toxic agents known. Scheele, the Swedish chemist who first identified cyanide in 1782, was one of its first victims; he was reported to have died from acute hydrogen cyanide poisoning in 1786. Since that time, cyanide has been responsible for an extensive number of poisonings in a variety of settings including chemical warfare, suicides, murders, occupational exposures, judicial executions, and environmental exposures.

Napoleon III was the first to employ hydrogen cyanide as a chemical warfare agent. During World Wars I and II, the gas was used on the battlefield by both sides. Hydrogen cyanide in the form of Zyklon B was also used as a genocidal agent by the Germans during World War II.

Suicides represent the most common cyanide exposure according to the American Association of Poison Control Center (AAPCC) TESS data (Chap. 116 and p. 1752). They frequently involve chemists or technicians working in laboratories where cyanide salts are common reagents.[24,32,48,49,72,86,134] Potassium cyanide was used in the 1978 Jonestown mass suicide in which over 900 people died.

Occupational exposures to cyanide occur because many industrial processes utilize cyanide reagents, including electroplating, metal refining, photography, and fumigation. Fortunately, despite the potential hazard, deaths from occupational exposures are rare. In 1988 workers mistakenly used hydrogen chloride instead of sodium hypochlorite to clean an electroplating vat containing zinc cyanide sludge. The resulting release of cyanide gas killed five workers.[87]

Because cyanide salts are readily available, they are used in intentional poisonings, in which they may be disguised as consumer products. Such incidents include seven deaths resulting from consumption of cyanide-tainted acetaminophen in 1982[29] and a death from a cyanide-laced decongestant in 1991.[68] Not surprisingly, intentional food tampering also occurs. In 1988, contaminated yogurt resulted in severe toxicity.[92] In 1989 the Department of Agriculture found traces of cyanide in fruit imported from Chile after a terrorist threat led to an inspection.[57]

The combustion of many materials such as wool, silk, synthetic rubber, polyurethane, and nitrocellulose releases cyanide. Thus, there is the threat of cyanide poisoning from fires and smoke inhalation.[14,89,108,118]

Ingestion of cyanogenic chemicals represents another source of exposure. Cyanogenic chemicals liberate cyanide during their metabolism. Acetonitrile, a clinically relevant cyanogen, is itself relatively nontoxic, but biotransformation via cytochrome P450 forms a cyanohydrin that readily breaks down to an aldehyde and cyanide (see Fig. 98–1) Unintentional poisoning of children with acetonitrile-based artificial-nail remover was first reported in 1988.[39,53,83,88] Symptoms caused by acetonitrile are similar to those of cyanide ion poisoning. However, onset was delayed (range 3–24 hours) because of the time required for biotransformation from parent compound to toxic metabolite. Other nitriles, such as proprionitrile, resulted in cyanide poisoning.[23]

Many plants contain cyanogenic compounds including the *Prunus* species, the pitted fruits—apricots, bitter almond, cherry, and peaches. The pits contain the glucoside amygdalin, D-mandelonitrile-β-d-glucoside, which, when ingested, is biotransformed by intestinal β-d-glucosidase to glucose, aldehyde, and cyanide (see Fig. 98–1). Cases of cyanide poisoning occur following ingestion of apricot seeds and laetrile (a purported antineoplastic agent).[60,61] Cassava (*Manihot*), a tuber containing two cyanogens, linamarin and lotaustralin, similarly releases cyanide. This is of little consequence in the United States, but cassava is a staple, inexpensive food source in certain developing countries. Although fermentation techniques remove cyanide, improper preparation results in cyanide poisoning.[3,7,31]

Iatrogenic cyanide poisoning may occur during nitroprusside administration. Sodium nitroprusside is a potent vasodilator used to reduce blood pressure and afterload. One disadvantage of nitro-

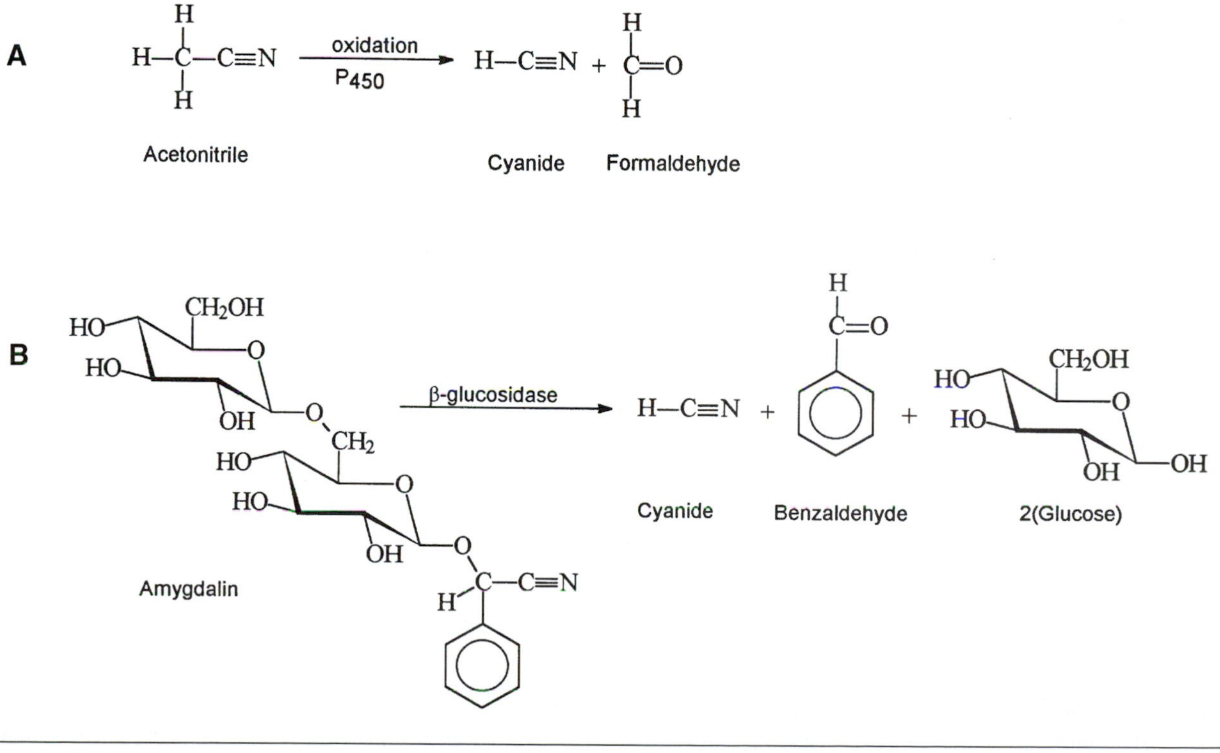

Figure 98–1. Biotransformation of cyanogens (a) acetonitrile and (b) amygdalin to cyanide.

prusside is the in vivo release of cyanide. Each nitroprusside molecule contains five cyanide molecules. If thiosulfate stores are depleted, as in the malnourished or postoperative patient, cyanide may accumulate even with therapeutic nitroprusside infusion rates (2–10 μg/kg/min). Manifestations appear within hours to days of initiating nitroprusside and include altered mental status, acidosis, or tachyphylaxis. Concurrent administration of thiosulfate[44,113] or hydroxocobalamin with nitroprusside may prevent toxicity.

Pharmacology

The dose required to produce toxicity is dependent on the form of cyanide (gas or salt), the duration, and the route of exposure. However, cyanide is an extremely potent toxin with small exposures leading to symptoms. An oral lethal dose of KCN is approximately 200 mg. An airborne concentration of 270 ppm HCN may be immediately fatal, and exposures over 110 ppm for longer than 30 minutes are generally considered life-threatening. The TLV for hydrogen cyanide is 10 ppm during an 8-hour day.

Acute toxicity occurs through a variety of routes, including inhalation, ingestion, dermal, and parenteral. In industrial poisoning, it is not uncommon that exposure occurs through multiple routes.[26,119] HCN, a gas under standard temperature and pressure, readily crosses membranes because it has a low molecular weight (27 Da) and is non-ionized. After absorption and dissolution in blood, cyanide exists in equilibrium as the anion and undissociated HCN. HCN is a weak acid with a pK_a of 9.21. Therefore, at physiologic pH 7.4, the compound exists primarily as HCN. Rapid diffusion across alveolar membranes followed by direct distribution to target organs accounts for the rapid lethality associated with HCN inhalation. Oral exposure causes a slightly longer time to death (20 min) compared to parenteral exposure (5 min) as demonstrated in animal models.[10]

Pharmacokinetics and Toxicokinetics

Cyanide is eliminated from the body by multiple pathways. A small portion (1–2%) is lost through the lungs by exhalation as HCN. A number of minor pathways of metabolism (less than 15% of total) account for cyanide elimination including conversion to 2-aminothiazoline-4-carboxylic acid, incorporation into the one-carbon metabolic pool, or combination with hydroxycobalamin to form cyanocobalamin.

The major route for detoxification of cyanide is the enzymatic conversion to thiocyanate. Two sulfur transferase enzymes, rhodanese (thiosulfate-cyanide sulfurtransferase) and β-mercaptopyruvate-cyanide sulfurtransferase, catalyze this reaction. The primary pathway for metabolism is thought to be rhodanese, which is widely distributed throughout the body with the highest concentration in the liver. This enzyme catalyzes the transfer of a sulfane sulfur from a sulfur donor (such as thiosulfate) to cyanide to form thiocyanate. In acute poisoning, the limiting factor in cyanide detoxification by rhodanese is the availability of adequate quantities of sulfur donors. The endogenous stores of sulfur are rapidly depleted, and cyanide metabolism slows. Hence, sodium thiosulfate's efficacy as an antidote stems from its acceleration of the metabolic inactivation of cyanide. This is a favorable reaction in that the sulfation of cyanide is essentially irreversible, and the sulfation product, thiocyanate, has little inherent toxicity.

Thiocyanate is eliminated in urine. Urinary thiocyanate levels are markers of cyanide exposure. However, caution should be used in interpreting urinary thiocyanate levels because heavy smoking will increase urinary concentrations and can be misinterpreted.

There are limited human data regarding the cyanide elimination half-life. Elimination appears to follow first-order kinetics,[79] although it varies widely in reports from 1.2 to 66 hours.[14,54,59,79] Disparity in values may result from the number of samples used to perform calculations and effects of antidotal treatment.

Pathophysiology

Cyanide is a nonspecific inhibitor of enzymes, including succinic acid dehydrogenase, superoxide dismutase, carbonic anhydrase, cytochrome oxidase, and many others.[10,141] Of these, the interaction of cyanide and cytochrome oxidase is best understood and perhaps the most important toxicologically. Cyanide inhibition of other enzymes may underlie some of the symptoms of chronic exposures and delayed symptoms associated with acute exposure.

Cytochrome oxidase is an iron-containing metalloenzyme essential for oxidative phosphorylation and, hence, aerobic energy production. It functions in the electron transport chain within mitochondria, converting catabolic products of glucose into adenosine triphosphate (ATP). Cyanide induces cellular hypoxia by inhibiting cytochrome oxidase at the cytochrome a_3 portion of the electron transport chain (see Fig. 98–2). Hydrogen ions that normally would have combined with oxygen at the terminal end of the chain are no longer incorporated. Thus, despite sufficient oxygen supply, oxygen cannot be utilized, and ATP molecules are no longer formed. Unincorporated hydrogen ions accumulate, leading to acidemia.

Hyperlactemia occurs following cyanide poisoning because of failure of aerobic energy metabolism. During aerobic conditions, when the electron transport chain is functional, lactate is converted to pyruvate by mitochondrial lactate dehydrogenase. In this process, lactate donates hydrogen moieties that reduce nicotinamide adenine dinucleotide (NAD) to NADH. Pyruvate then enters the tricarboxylic acid cycle with resulting ATP formation. When cytochrome a_3 within the electron transport chain is inhibited by cyanide, there is a relative paucity of NAD and predominance of NADH, favoring the reverse reaction; ie, pyruvate is converted to lactate.[14,22,53,54,68,80,83,117,119]

Central nervous system injury occurs via several mechanisms, including impaired oxygen utilization, oxidant stress, and enhanced release of excitatory neurotransmitters. Cranial imaging from survivors of cyanide poisoning reveals that injury occurs in the most oxygen-sensitive area of the brain, the basal ganglia.[20,27,48,115,116] The dopaminergic neurons of this brain area appear to be sensitive to cyanide and are the neurons that most readily undergo degeneration following massive, acute intoxications or repeated exposures.

Cyanide causes direct neurotoxicity by inducing cellular oxidative stress.[71] The exact mechanism is undefined, but it may occur through inhibition of antioxidant enzymes such as catalase, glutathione dehydrogenase, glutathione reductase, or superoxide dismutase.[5] Cyanide-induced lipid peroxidation displays tissue specificity. Lipid peroxidation occurs to the greatest extent in the brain, whereas the liver and heart display no generation of reactive oxygen species following experimental cyanide exposure.[6] The tissue specificity explains the predominance of neurologic findings in patients with cyanide poisoning.

There is also compelling evidence that excitatory amino acids, such as glutamate, mediate cyanide neurotoxicity. Glutamate stim-

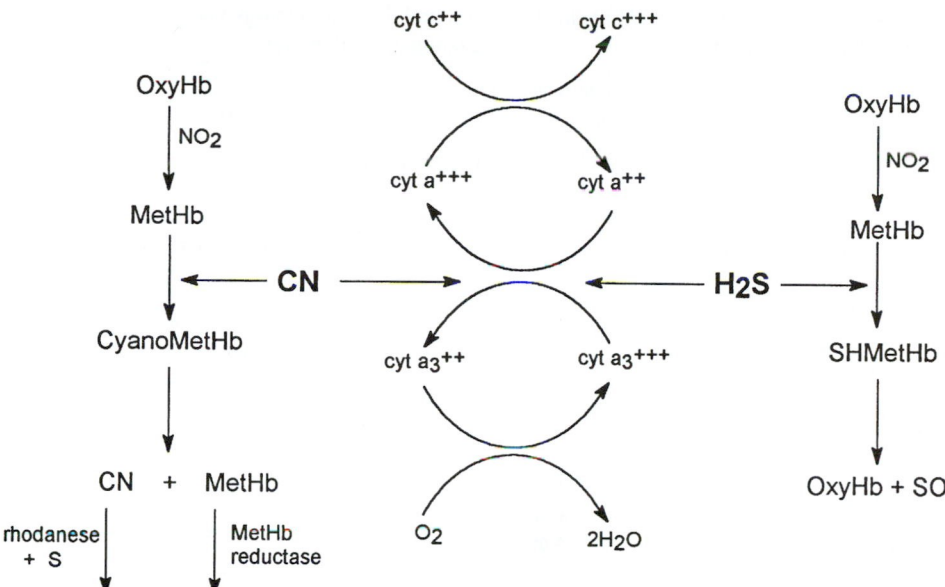

Figure 98–2. Pathway of cyanide and hydrogen sulfide toxicity and detoxification.

ulation of N-methyl-D-aspartate (NMDA) receptors results in calcium and sodium entry into the cytosol of neurons. Cyanide releases glutamate, directly stimulates NMDA receptors,[105,106] and augments cytosolic calcium release by excitatory amino acids. Ultimately, excess calcium results in cell death. Experimental studies demonstrate that NMDA inhibitors, such as dextrophan and dizocilpine, attenuate cyanide histopathology and lethality.[65,138]

Sulfurtransferase metabolism via rhodanese is crucial for detoxification. However, the aforementioned cyanide-induced metabolic derangement may decrease enzyme detoxification. Lowered ATP, reactive oxygen species, and increased cytosolic calcium stimulate protein kinase C activity that in turn inactivates rhodanese.[90] Conversely, NMDA and protein-kinase inhibitors increase detoxification.[90,91,109]

Acute Clinical Manifestations The amount of cyanide, chronicity of exposure, route of exposure, and premorbid condition of the individual influence onset and severity of illness. A critical combination of these factors overwhelms endogenous detoxification pathways, leading to illness. There is no reliable pathognomonic symptom or toxidrome associated with acute cyanide poisoning. Clinical manifestations reflect dysfunction of oxygen-sensitive organs, with central nervous and cardiovascular findings predominating. The time to onset of symptoms is rapid with inorganic and gaseous forms—usually in minutes. Symptoms occur hours later following poisoning with cyanogens because of their biotransformation requirements. The bitter almond odor associated with cyanide poisoning is not uniformly present and, when present, is detectable by only 60% of the population (Chap. 28).

Central nervous system signs and symptoms are typical of progressive hypoxia and include headache, anxiety, agitation, confusion, lethargy, convulsions, and coma. A centrally mediated tachypnea occurs initially, followed by bradypnea.

The cardiovascular responses to cyanide are complex. Studies of isolated heart preparation and intact animal models show that the principal cardiac insult is progressive failure, with slowing of rate and loss of contractile force as a result of ATP depletion. Sev-

eral reflex mechanisms, including catecholamine release and central vasomotor activity, may modulate myocardial performance and vascular response in patients with cyanide poisoning. In laboratory investigations, there is a brief period of increased inotropy caused by reflex compensatory mechanisms just before myocardial depression. Clinically, there may be an initial bradycardia and hypertension, followed by hypotension with reflex tachycardia, but the terminal event is consistently bradycardia and hypotension. Ventricular dysrhythmias do not appear to be an important factor.

Both cardiogenic pulmonary edema and acute lung injury are found at necropsy.[39,49,54,80,117] Postulated causes of acute lung injury in cyanide poisoning include neurogenic or membrane leak from direct cellular toxicity.

Gastrointestinal symptoms occur following ingestion of inorganic cyanide and cyanogens and include abdominal pain, nausea, and vomiting.[3,39,53,54,74,83,88,92,117] These symptoms are caused by hemorrhagic gastritis identified on necropsy and are thought to be secondary to the corrosive nature of cyanide salts.[49]

Cutaneous manifestations may vary. Traditionally, a cherry-red skin color is described as a result of increased venous hemoglobin oxygen saturation, which results from decreased utilization of oxygen at the tissue level.[32,119] This phenomenon may be more evident on funduscopic examination, where veins and arteries may appear similar in color. Despite the inference in the name, cyanide does not directly cause cyanosis. The occurrence of cyanosis in some cases is likely secondary to shock.[86,134,145]

Chronic Clinical Manifestations Survivors of serious, acute poisoning may develop delayed neurologic sequelae.[20,27,40,48,55,95,115,116] Parkinsonian symptoms, including dystonia, dysarthria, rigidity, and bradykinesia, are most common. Symptoms typically develop over weeks to months, but subtle findings can be present within a few days. Cranial computerized tomography and magnetic resonance imaging consistently reveal basal ganglia (globus pallidus, putamen, and hippocampus) damage, with radiologic changes appearing several weeks after onset of symptoms. The extrapyramidal manifestations may progress or resolve. Response to pharmacotherapy with antiparkinsonian agents is generally disappointing. It is unclear if delayed manifestations result from direct cellular injury or secondary hypoxia.

Chronic, low-level exposure to cyanide may result in insidious syndromes, including tobacco amblyopia, tropical ataxic neuropathy, and Leber hereditary neuropathy.

Tobacco amblyopia is a progressive loss of visual function occurring almost exclusively in male smokers. Affected smokers have lower plasma cyanocobalamin and thiocyanate levels than unaffected smoking counterparts, suggesting a reduced ability to detoxify cyanide. Cessation of smoking and administration of hydroxocobalamin often reverses symptoms.

Tropical ataxic neuropathy is a demyelinating disease associated with cassava consumption. Neurologic manifestations include paresthesias, sensory ataxia, optic atrophy, and sensorineural hearing loss. Concomitant dermatitis and glossitis suggest an association of high dietary cassava and low vitamin B_{12} intake. Elevated thiocyanate levels in affected individuals further implicate cyanide as the etiology. Removal of dietary cassava and institution of vitamin B_{12} therapy alleviates symptoms.

Leber hereditary optic atrophy, a condition of subacute visual failure affecting men, is thought to be caused by rhodanese deficiency.[50,147]

Diagnostic Testing

Because of nonspecific symptoms and delay in laboratory confirmation, the clinician must rely on historical circumstances and some initial findings to raise suspicion of cyanide poisoning and institute therapy (see Table 98–1).

The bitter almond odor of HCN can be detected by 60% of the population.[82] The threshold for those persons who can sense the odor is estimated to be 1 to 5 ppm concentration in air. It should be stressed that even at high toxic concentrations, some individuals cannot smell hydrogen cyanide. Also, the action of cyanide is so rapid that detection of the odor may occur too late to prevent severe toxicity. Hence, detection of cyanide should not be dependent on the characteristic odor.

Laboratory findings suggestive of cyanide poisoning reflect the known metabolic abnormalities including metabolic acidosis, elevated lactate, and increased anion gap. However, similar findings may occur following hydrogen sulfide, sodium azide, ethylene glycol, methanol, and other acid-generating toxins.

Elevated venous oxygen saturation results from reduced tissue extraction.[60,72,93] A venous oxygen saturation greater than 90% from superior vena cava or pulmonary artery blood indicates decreased oxygen utilization. This is not specific for cyanide and could represent cellular poisoning from other agents such as carbon monoxide, hydrogen sulfide, or sodium azide.

Cyanide results in nonspecific electrocardiographic findings. There is initial bradycardia, followed by transient tachycardia, and then recurrent life-threatening bradycardia. A myocardial injury pattern or AV conduction blocks may also occur.

Blood cyanide determination can confirm toxicity, but this determination is not available in a sufficiently rapid manner to affect initial treatment. Whole blood or serum is usually analyzed. In mammals, including primates, whole-blood levels are twice serum levels[9] as a result of cyanide sequestration in red blood cells.[136] Background whole-blood levels in nonsmokers range between 0.02 and 0.5 μg/mL.[11,54,61,89] Higher blood levels suggest toxicity. Detecting urinary cyanide is difficult, and urinary thiocyanate is a

TABLE 98–1. Cyanide Poisoning: Emergency Management Guidelines

When to suspect cyanide
Sudden collapse of laboratory or industrial worker
Fire victim with coma or acidosis
Suicide or unexplained coma or acidosis
Ingestion of artificial nail remover
Ingestion of seeds or pits from *Prunus* species
ICU patient with altered mental status, acidosis, and tachyphylaxis to nitroprusside

Supportive care
Control airway, ventilate, and give 100% oxygen
Crystalloids and vasopressors for hypotension
Administer $NaHCO_3$; titrate according to ABG and serum HCO_3

Antidote
Amyl nitrite pearls are included in the kit for prehospital use. For hospital management, sodium nitrite is the preferred methemoglobin inducer and is given in lieu of the pearls.
Give sodium nitrite ($NaNO_2$) as a 3% solution over 2–4 minutes IV:
    Adult dose: 10 mL (300 mg)
    Pediatric dose: See Table 98–2
Caution: Monitor blood pressure frequently and treat hypotension by slowing infusion rate and giving crystalloids and vasopressors. Obtain methemoglobin level 30 minutes after dose and consider possible excessive methemoglobin formation if patient deteriorates during therapy.
Give sodium thiosulfate (NaS_2O_3) as a 25% solution IV:
    Adult dose: 50 mL (12.5 g)
    Pediatric dose: 1.65 mL/kg

Decontamination
Protect health care provider from contamination
Cutaneous: carefully remove all clothing and flush the skin
Ingestion: lavage with a large-bore orogastric tube and instill 1 g/kg activated charcoal

Laboratory
Arterial blood gas
Electrolytes and glucose
Blood lactate
Whole-blood cyanide concentration (for later confirmation only)
Consider a central venous blood gas

more readily detectable and useful marker of cyanide exposure. Plasma thiocyanate levels are of little value in assessing patients with acute poisoning, as there is little correlation with symptoms.

Management

Because cyanide poisoning is rare, it is easy to overlook the diagnosis unless there is an obvious history of exposure. Thus, the most critical step in treatment is considering the diagnosis in high-risk situations (see Table 98–1) and initiating empiric therapy with 100% oxygen and the cyanide antidote kit, which contains nitrites and thiosulfate. Both thiosulfate and nitrite have antidotal efficacy when given alone in animal models of cyanide poisoning but even greater benefit when their use is combined.[41] Thiosulfate donates the sulfur atoms that are necessary for rhodanese-mediated cyanide biotransformation to thiocyanate. The mechanism of nitrite is less clear. Traditional rationale relies on the ability of nitrite to generate methemoglobin. Because cyanide has a higher affinity for methemoglobin than cytochrome a_3, cytochrome oxidase function is restored. However, other mechanisms such as improved hepatic blood flow or nitric oxide formation are alternate explanations (see Antidote in Depth: Cyanide Antidotes). Oxygen is also critical for cyanide treatment, enhancing the antidotal effect of nitrite and thiosulfate.[36]

The initial care (see Table 98–1) of the cyanide-poisoned patient begins by directing attention to airway patency, ventilatory support, and oxygenation. Establish intravenous access and obtain blood samples for renal function, glucose, and electrolyte determinations. A whole-blood cyanide level may be obtained for later confirmation of exposure. An arterial blood gas and serum lactate level will help assess the acid-base status. Initiation of crystalloid and a vasopressor infusion for hypotension is warranted.

Decontamination of the cyanide-poisoned patient occurs concurrently with initial resuscitation. Exposure to cyanide may take place by multiple routes including ingestion, inhalation, dermal, or parenteral. The route of exposure determines which decontamination technique to employ. No matter which decontamination modality is used, always protect the health care provider from potential contamination by utilizing protective devices such as water-impervious gowns, gloves, and eyewear. For patients with cutaneous exposure, remove clothing and flush the skin with water. Particular attention should be given to open wounds because CN^- or HCN is readily absorbed through abraded skin. For inhalation exposure, removal from the area of exposure is critical. First responders should exercise extreme caution when entering potentially hazardous areas such as chemical plants and laboratories where a previously healthy person is "found down." Following oral exposure, orogastric lavage may prevent further cyanide absorption, although absorption is rapid. Instillation of activated charcoal is often considered ineffective because of low binding of cyanide (1 g activated charcoal adsorbs 35 mg cyanide).[4] However, a potentially lethal oral dose of cyanide is a few hundred milligrams. This amount of cyanide is within the adsorptive capacity of a 1 g/kg dose of activated charcoal. Additionally, prophylactic charcoal administration improved survival in animals given LD_{100} doses of KCN.[84] Based on the potential benefits and minimal risks, activated charcoal administration is advocated.

Administer the cyanide antidote kit as soon as cyanide poisoning is suspected (see Tables 98–1 and 98–2). The kit contains nitrite and sodium thiosulfate. The nitrite component is found in two forms: amyl nitrite and sodium nitrite. Amyl nitrite is contained within glass pearls that are crushed and intermittently inhaled or intermittently introduced into the ventilator system to initiate methemoglobin formation. The amyl nitrite pearls are reserved for

TABLE 98–2.   Cyanide Mangement: Pediatric Nitrite Guidelines[a]

Hemoglobin (g)	NaNO$_2$ (mg/kg)	3% NaNO$_2$ solution (mL/kg)
7.0	5.8	0.19
8.0	6.6	0.22
9.0	7.5	0.25
10.0	8.3	0.27
11.0	9.1	0.30
12.0	10.0	0.33
13.0	10.8	0.36
14.0	11.6	0.39

[a]Pediatric thiosulfate dose: 1.65 mL/kg of 25% solution. Adapted, with permission, from Berlin CM: The treatment of cyanide poisoning in children. Pediatrics 1976;46:793–796.

instances in which intravenous access is delayed or not possible. Intravenous sodium nitrite is preferred and is supplied as a 10 mL volume of a 3% solution (300 mg). The goal of intravenous nitrite therapy has been to achieve a methemoglobin level of 20 to 30%. This level is not based on cyanide treatment data but represents the maximum tolerated concentration without adverse symptoms from methemoglobin in a healthy individual. Clinical response is reported at lower methemoglobin levels, 3.6 to 9.2%. These reports are not conclusive, as levels are not typically drawn serially, and peak levels may be misrepresented. Also, methemoglobin levels do not include cyanomethemoglobin. Therefore, lower than expected methemoglobin concentrations may represent indirect evidence of cyanide poisoning.

Adverse effects of nitrites include excessive methemoglobin formation and, because of potent vasodilation, hypotension and tachycardia. Avoiding rapid infusion, monitoring blood pressure, and adhering to dosing guidelines will limit adverse effects. Because of excessive methemoglobinemia during nitrite treatment, pediatric dosing guidelines were developed.[18] Based on the premise that nitrite oxidizes hemoglobin on a mole-for-mole basis, doses were calculated for various hemoglobin concentrations (Table 98–2). These values are useful if the patient is known to be anemic. However, when giving nitrite empirically, treat based on a presumed 12-g hemoglobin concentration. Do not delay treatment while awaiting a hemoglobin measurement.

Sodium thiosulfate is the second component of the cyanide antidote kit. It is supplied as 50 mL of a 25% solution. It is a substrate for a reaction that is essentially irreversible, converting a highly toxic entity to a relatively harmless compound. (Thiocyanate does, however, have its own toxicity in the presence of renal failure, including abdominal pain, vomiting, rash, and central nervous system dysfunction.)[44] There are no adverse reactions to thiosulfate itself. The pediatric dose of thiosulfate is adjusted for weight.

Acidemia should be treated with adequate ventilation and sodium bicarbonate administration based on arterial blood pH and serum bicarbonate determination.

Patients who do not survive cyanide poisoning are suitable organ donors. Heart, liver, kidney, pancreas, cornea, skin, and bone were successfully transplanted following cyanide poisoning.[34,63,85,128]

Other Therapies.   Although the cyanide kit is the mainstay of antidotal therapy in the United States, other treatments are currently used abroad. In Europe, 4-dimethylaminophenol (4-DMAP), rather than sodium nitrite, is the oxidizing agent of choice. It generates methemoglobin more rapidly than sodium nitrite, with peak methemoglobin concentrations at 5 minutes after 4-DMAP rather than 30 minutes following sodium nitrite. The dose of 4-DMAP is 3 mg/kg and is coadministered with thiosulfate. As with sodium nitrite, its major adverse effect is excessive methemoglobin formation.

Hydroxocobalamin, a vitamin B_{12} precursor, is also employed in Europe for acute and chronic cyanide poisoning.[24] Hydroxocobalamin is a metalloprotein with a central cobalt atom that chelates cyanide, forming cyanocobalamin (vitamin B_{12}). Cyanocobalamin is eliminated in the urine or releases the cyanide moiety at a rate sufficient to allow detoxification by rhodanese. For this reason, thiosulfate is coadministered with hydroxocobalamin. One molecule of hydroxocobalamin binds one molecule of cyanide, yielding a molecular weight binding ratio of 50:1. Four grams of hydroxocobalamin is the standard initial dose and is expected to bind 200 mg of cyanide. The dose may be repeated in cases of massive poisoning. Typically, 8 g of thiosulfate is coadministered. Hydroxocobalamin has few adverse effects, which include allergic reaction and a reddening of the skin.[33,62] There are no hemodynamic or cardiodynamic adverse effects.[17,114]

Cobalt in the form of dicobalt edetate has been used as a cyanide chelator, but serious adverse effects limit its usefulness. These include hypotension, cardiac dysrhythmias, decreased cerebral blood flow, and angioedema.[31,101]

Stroma-free methemoglobin, oxidized hemoglobin from which the cell membrane has been removed, is an investigational agent. It attenuates lethality and prevents hemodynamic changes in animal models.[30,129,130] The advantage to this treatment lies in providing exogenous methemoglobin to bind cyanide without compromising oxygen-carrying capacity of native hemoglobin. Removal of the cell membrane eliminates antigenicity.

α-Ketoglutaric acid is another investigational antidote. Its molecular configuration renders it amenable to nucleophilic binding of cyanide. Pretreatment with α-ketoglutarate reduced lethality and increased sodium thiosulfate efficacy in animal studies.[21,47,69,102] The advantage to α-ketoglutarate is direct binding of cyanide without generation of methemoglobin.

Hyperbaric oxygen (HBO) has been used in cyanide treatment, often with dramatic clinical improvement.[46,49,54,86,116,117,131] However, these patients received multiple therapies during resuscitation, so improvement cannot be attributed to HBO alone. Experimental data regarding HBO are contradictory. In a murine model, survival increased with 100% oxygen at 2 atm compared to normobaric oxygen. However, combined HBO and nitrite/thiosulfate did not confer additional protection compared to normobaric oxygen and nitrite/thiosulfate. Currently, the Undersea and Hyperbaric Medical Society supports hyperbaric therapy for cyanide poisoning when complicated by coincident carbon monoxide intoxication.[144] Until further studies clearly demonstrate the efficacy of hyperbaric therapy for isolated cyanide, it should not supplant the combination of normobaric oxygen, nitrite, and thiosulfate.

HYDROGEN SULFIDE POISONING

Case 2 A 23-year-old man entered an empty petroleum storage tank to perform repairs. He rapidly collapsed and fell unconscious. Two coworkers attempted a rescue, but both collapsed immediately after entering the tank. Firefighters wearing self-contained breathing apparatus entered the tank and removed all three victims. Both of the would-be rescuers regained consciousness after removal from the tank. The first worker to collapse was removed and noted to be cyanotic, with minimal respiratory effort. When paramedics arrived on the scene, he was immediately intubated.

He arrived in the Emergency Department intubated, receiving 100% oxygen by assisted ventilation. He had shallow spontaneous respirations and responded only to deep painful stimuli. Vital signs were: blood pressure 110/72 mm Hg, pulse 140 beats/min, respiratory rate 34 breaths/min, and rectal temperature 102°F (38.4°C). Pertinent findings on physical examination included dilated pupils, marked conjunctival injection, and diffuse rales in both lung fields.

Laboratory data showed an ABG with pH 7.21, Pco_2 30 mm Hg, Po_2 48 mm Hg, and calculated bicarbonate 11 mEq/L. The carboxyhemoglobin level was 1.5%. A serum lactate was 10.5 mEq/L. The electrocardiogram showed a sinus tachycardia with normal inter-

vals and axis. Chest radiograph showed diffuse alveolar infiltrates and a normal-sized heart.

The patient was placed on a ventilator with 100% oxygen and positive end-expiratory pressure of 10 cm H_2O. Over the next hour, his oxygenation improved, and his Po_2 was 335 mm Hg. He rapidly required less ventilatory support. The lactic acidosis resolved over the next 8 hours. His neurologic status slowly improved over the next 20 hours, at which point he appeared alert and would follow commands. Following extubation, a repeat neurologic examination was normal. Followup 1 week later did not show any adverse effects. Air samples from the tank, taken the day after the exposure, revealed: hydrogen sulfide 880 ppm, methane 420 ppm, carbon dioxide 400 ppm, carbon monoxide 50 ppm, and oxygen 18%.

History and Epidemiology

Hydrogen sulfide (H_2S) toxicity is not common. The AAPCC TESS reported only 1370 exposures in 1998. Only 400 of these exposures required evaluation at a health care facility, fewer than 200 reported moderate or major effects, and only three deaths occurred. From 1983 to 1992, the AAPCC database reported 5563 exposures and 29 deaths attributed to hydrogen sulfide.[125] US Occupational Safety and Health Administration (OSHA) records show 80 occupationally related fatalities between 1984 and 1994.[51] Hydrogen sulfide's rapid and deadly onset of clinical effects have been termed the "slaughterhouse sledgehammer effect." Poisoned workers are "knocked-down," most frequently in an agricultural or industrial event. Numerous case reports describe multiple victims in these events. Would-be rescuers often become victims when they attempt a rescue in an environment with high concentrations of hydrogen sulfide.[45,78,99,103,125] In the OSHA data, 25% of fatalities involved rescuers.[51]

Hydrogen sulfide is also implicated in environmental disasters. In 1950, 22 people died and 320 were hospitalized in Poza Rica, Mexico, when a local natural gas facility inadvertently released hydrogen sulfide into the air.[94] Hydrogen sulfide claimed nine lives when a sour gas well failed, releasing a cloud of the poisonous gas into the Denver City, Texas community in 1975.[13]

Hydrogen sulfide is produced naturally by bacterial decomposition of proteins and is used or produced in many industrial activities. Industrial sources of hydrogen sulfide include pulp paper mills, heavy-water production, the leather industry, petroleum distillation and refining, roofing asphalt tanks, vulcanizing of rubber, viscose rayon production, and coke manufacturing from coal.[35,66,103,123,135] It is a major industrial hazard in oil and gas production, particularly in sour gas fields (natural gas containing sulfur). Decay of sulfur-containing products, such as fish, sewage, and manure, also produces hydrogen sulfide. Several farm workers and rescuers have died from exposure to hydrogen sulfide generated in liquid manure pits.[99,103] Natural sources are volcanoes, caves, sulfur springs, and underground deposits of natural gas.[45,66,111]

Pharmacology

Hydrogen sulfide is a colorless gas, more dense than air, with an irritating odor of "rotten eggs." It is highly lipid soluble, a property that allows easy penetration of biologic membranes. Systemic absorption usually occurs through inhalation, and it is rapidly distributed to tissues.[111] The tissues most sensitive to hydrogen sulfide are those with high oxygen demand. Hydrogen sulfide's systemic toxicity results from its potent inhibition of cytochrome oxidase, thereby interrupting oxidative phosphorylation.[12,124] Hydrogen sulfide binds to the ferric (Fe^{3+}) moiety of cytochrome a$_3$ oxidase complex with a higher affinity than cyanide[121] (see Fig. 98–2). The resulting inhibition of oxidative phosphorylation produces cellular hypoxia and anaerobic metabolism.[121] In addition to producing cellular hypoxia, hydrogen sulfide causes potassium channel–mediated hyperpolarization of neurons and potentiates other neuronal inhibitory mechanisms. It also alters brain neurotransmitter content and release.[2,111] A proposed mechanism of death is poisoning of the brainstem respiratory center through selective uptake by lipophilic white matter in this region.[139]

In addition to systemic effects, hydrogen sulfide produces intense dermal irritation. It reacts with the moisture on the surface of mucous membranes to form sodium sulfide, which produces the irritant chemical effect. Despite skin irritation, it has little dermal absorption.

Toxicokinetics

The major pathways of hydrogen sulfide detoxification are enzymatic and nonenzymatic oxidation of sulfides and sulfur to thiosulfate and polysulfides.[25] Other pathways, such as methylation to dimethyl sulfide and conversion to sulfite or sulfate by oxidized glutathione, may also play a role in detoxification and elimination.[15] Hydrogen sulfide binds to metalloproteins such as heme proteins. It is a detoxification pathway when it binds to endogenously produced methemoglobin to form sulfmethemoglobin. However, binding to heme proteins such as cytochrome oxidase is its major mechanism of toxicity. Only small amounts of sulfide are excreted in urine or exhaled into the air. Sulfhemoglobin is not found in significant concentrations in the blood of animals or fatally poisoned humans.[123]

Clinical Manifestations

Acute Manifestations. The primary target organs of hydrogen sulfide poisoning are those of the central nervous system and respiratory system. The clinical findings reported in two large series are shown in Table 98–3.[8,35] The intensity of exposure likely accounts for the diverse clinical findings in the reports. A distinct dose response to hydrogen sulfide is identified. The odor threshold is between 0.02 and 0.13 ppm, and it has a strong, intense odor at 20 to 30 ppm. Mild mucous membrane irritation occurs at 50 to 100 ppm, and olfactory fatigue or paralysis occurs at 100 to 150 ppm. Thus, the ability to perceive the odor is rapidly extinguished because of olfactory nerve paralysis at higher levels. Prolonged exposure can occur when the extinction of odor recognition is misinterpreted as dissipation of the gas. Strong irritation of the upper respiratory tract and eyes, as well as pulmonary edema, occurs at 200 to 300 ppm. At greater than 500 ppm, H$_2$S produces systemic effects. Rapid unconsciousness and cardiopulmonary arrest occur at concentrations greater than 700 ppm.[15,111]

Symptoms of mucous membrane irritation occur early and at low levels of exposure. Mucous membrane irritation of the eye produces keratoconjunctivitis. If exposure persists, damage of the epithelial cells will produce reversible corneal ulcerations ("gas eye") and, rarely, irreversible corneal scarring.[97] The irritant effects of the respiratory tract include rhinitis, bronchitis, and pulmonary edema.[8,35]

Neurologic manifestations are common and may be severe. In one series, 75% of 221 patients with acute hydrogen sulfide exposure lost consciousness at the site of exposure.[35] In acute, massive exposures, rapid loss of consciousness ("knockdown") results from paralysis of the respiratory center of the brain.[96,124] If the patient is removed from the exposure rapidly, recovery may be prompt and complete. Secondary neurologic effects can result from hypoxia secondary to respiratory compromise.[15,111] Neurologic outcome can be quite variable, ranging from no neurologic impairment to permanent sequelae. Delayed neuropsychiatric sequelae have occurred after acute exposures.[35,38,66,77,125,126,132,133,140] Most evidence suggests that the early rapid CNS effects are direct neurotoxic effects of hydrogen sulfide, whereas the permanent neurologic sequelae result from hypoxia secondary to respiratory insufficiency.[15,96,97,111] Reported neuropsychiatric changes include memory failure (amnestic syndrome), lack of insight, disorientation, delirium, and dementia.[140] Neurosensory abnormalities include transient hearing impairment, vision loss, and anosmia. Motor symptoms are likely caused by injury of the basal ganglia and result in ataxia, position/intention tremor, and muscle rigidity.[132] Common neuropathologic findings observed on CT scan and at autopsy are subcortical white matter demyelination and globus pallidus degeneration.[52,133]

Acute exposures affect other organ systems. Myocardial hypoxia or direct toxic effects of hydrogen sulfide on cardiac tissue may cause cardiac dysrhythmias, myocardial ischemia, or myocardial infarction.[56] Because unresponsiveness is rapid, trauma from falls should not be overlooked.[8]

Chronic Manifestations. Most data about chronic, low-level exposures to hydrogen sulfide come from oil and gas industry workers. Mucous membrane irritation seems to be the most prominent problem in patients with low-level exposures. Workers report nasal, pharyngeal, and eye irritation, fatigue, headache, dizziness, and poor memory with low-level, chronic exposures. In one series, one-third of viscous rayon workers left their jobs because of persistent eye irritation ("spinner's eye"). The chronic irritating effects of hydrogen sulfide were thought to be the cause of reduced lung volumes observed in sewer workers.[112] Volunteer studies have not demonstrated significant cardiovascular effects at low-level exposures (<10 ppm).[19] The liver, kidneys, and endocrine system are unaffected. No studies demonstrate increased incidences of cancer with low-level exposures.[42]

Rapid loss of consciousness after a high-level exposure ("knockdown") was a well known and, amazingly, accepted part of the workplace in the gas and oil industry for many years.[64]

TABLE 98–3. Hydrogen Sulfide Poisoning: Clinical Manifestations

When to suspect hydrogen sulfide poisoning
- Person rapidly loses consciousness ("knocked down")
- Rotten eggs odor
- Rescue from enclosed space, such as sewer or manure pit
- Multiple victims with sudden death syndrome
- Cardiac arrest in previously healthy worker at work site

System	Signs and Symptoms
Cardiovascular	Chest pain, bradycardia
Central nervous	Headache, weakness, dysequilibrium, convulsions, coma
Gastrointestinal	Pharyngitis, nausea, vomiting
Ophthalmic	Conjunctivitis
Pulmonary	Dyspnea, cyanosis, hemoptysis, rales

Some workers experienced repeated "knockdowns," and these workers reported an increased incidence of respiratory diseases and cognitive deficits. Clearly, single or repeated high-level exposures resulting in unconsciousness can cause serious cognitive dysfunction. Case series suggest that protracted low-level exposures may cause subtle changes measurable by only the most sensitive neuropsychiatric tests.[38,76]

Epidemiologic data regarding the effects of low-level environmental exposures to hydrogen sulfide are somewhat clouded in populations exposed to complex pollution mixtures. Other malodorous sulfur compounds such as methyl mercaptan and methyl sulfide are generated as by-products of pulp mills. Study populations exposed to this complex mixture of pollutants demonstrate a dose-related increase in nasal symptoms, cough, nausea, and vomiting.[42]

Hydrogen sulfide's strong odor at low levels can magnify irritant effects by triggering a strong psychological response.[99] Hydrogen sulfide has been the alleged source of mass psychogenic illness cases.[99] Clinical, epidemiologic, and toxicologic analyses suggested that 943 cases of illness in Jerusalem were caused by the odor of low concentrations of hydrogen sulfide gas. The most frequent associated symptoms are headaches, faintness, dizziness, nausea, chest tightness, difficulty breathing (hyperventilation), irritation of eyes, nose, and throat, weakness, and extremity numbness.[28] Mild to moderate hydrogen sulfide toxicity produces nonspecific signs and symptoms that could closely mimic psychogenic illness. Attempting to identify true toxicity from a powerful emotional reaction can be extremely difficult. Therefore, symptomatic patients need to be assessed for toxicity even when mass psychogenic illness is suspected.

Diagnostic Testing

Because there is no rapid method of detection that is of clinical diagnostic use, management decisions must be made based on history, clinical presentation, and diagnostic tests that infer hydrogen sulfide's presence. Circumstances surrounding the patient's illness will often be the best evidence for suspecting hydrogen sulfide poisoning (see Table 98–3). At the bedside, the smell of rotten eggs on clothing or emanating from the blood, exhaled air, or gastric secretions suggests hydrogen sulfide exposure.[67] In addition, blackening of copper and silver coins in a patient's pocket or darkening of jewelry are clues to exposure. Paper impregnated with lead acetate changes color when exposed to hydrogen sulfide and is used to detect its presence in the patient's exhaled air but is not rapidly available.[42]

Specific tests for laboratory confirmation of hydrogen sulfide exposure are not readily available in clinical laboratories. Therefore, the presence of hydrogen sulfide is best confirmed by directly measuring the gas in the environment. It can be detected in atmospheric air samples by monitoring devices such as colorimetric tubes or toxin-specific air-sampling devices. Many emergency response teams investigate the toxic environment of a hazardous materials incident with detection devices that measure hydrogen sulfide by electrochemical sensors.

In acute poisoning, readily available diagnostic tests that are biomarkers of hydrogen sulfide poisoning may be useful but nonspecific. An arterial blood gas analysis would demonstrate metabolic acidosis and normal oxygen saturation unless pulmonary edema was present. Metabolic acidosis reflected by elevated serum lactate concentrations is expected but not specific for hy-

drogen sulfide poisoning. Hydrogen sulfide, like cyanide, decreases oxygen consumption and is reflected as an elevated mixed venous oxygen measurement. Because sulfhemoglobin is not typically generated in patients with hydrogen sulfide poisoning, an oxygen saturation gap is not expected.[123]

After serious injury from hydrogen sulfide, diagnostic testing for neurologic structure and function may show abnormalities for weeks or months. Brain MRI and CT demonstrate structural changes such as globus pallidus degeneration and subcortical white matter demyelination. Neuropsychological testing after serious hydrogen sulfide poisoning demonstrates specific abnormalities in cortical functions such as concentration, attention, verbal abstraction, and short-term retention. SPECT/PET brain scans define neurotoxin-induced lesions that correlate well with clinical neuropsychological testing.[38]

Clinical laboratory tests may be useful for confirming exposure but are not readily available for clinical decision making in an acute exposure. In biologic specimens, sulfide ions can be measured by microdiffusion isolation with colorimetry determination, an ion-selective electrode, ion-interaction reversed-phase HPLC, or extractive alkylation with GC/MS.[75,78,98,111] Whole-blood sulfide levels greater than 0.05 mg/L are considered abnormal. Reliable measurements are ensured only if the level is obtained within 2 hours after the exposure and analyzed immediately.[111] In acute exposures, blood and urine thiosulfate levels may be reflective of exposure, and urinary thiosulfate excretion is used to monitor chronic low-level exposure in the workplace.[75]

In postmortem investigations, sulfide levels may be useful, but their use requires rapid sample collection because sulfide concentrations rise with tissue decomposition.[111] In addition to blood sulfide levels, sulfide and thiosulfate levels are found at their highest concentrations in lung and brain.[75,98] At autopsy, a greenish discoloration of the gray matter, viscera, and bronchial secretions may be noted.[75]

Management

Hydrogen sulfide poisoning should be suspected whenever a person is found unconscious in an enclosed space, especially if the odor of rotten eggs is noted. No rescuer should enter until proper self-contained breathing apparatus (SCBA) is available. Unintentional exposure can lead to injuries and even death in well-meaning rescuers without proper protective equipment. There are numerous cases of multiple rescuers injured in an attempt to remove one victim from an environment with high concentrations of hydrogen sulfide.[45,51,78,99,103,125]

The initial treatment (Table 98–4) is immediate removal of the victim from the contaminated area into a fresh-air environment. Administer high-flow oxygen as soon as possible. Optimal supportive care and advanced cardiac life support have the greatest influence on the patient's outcome. Because death is rapid from inhalation of hydrogen sulfide, limited human cases are reported in the literature. Most patients have significant delays before receiving treatment. Therefore, specific treatments and antidotal therapies do not show definitive improvement in patient outcome.

Most animal studies and human case reports suggest that oxygen therapy is beneficial for hydrogen sulfide poisoning.[16,25,110,124] In rats, HBO was more effective than normobaric oxygen, nitrite, or sham treatment in preventing mortality from sulfide poisoning.[25] Studies showing benefit of HBO for cyanide toxicity have led to the use of HBO in hydrogen sulfide poisoning. Case reports

TABLE 98–4. Hydrogen Sulfide Poisoning: Emergency Management

Supportive care
  Prehospital
    Attempt rescue only if using SCBA
    Move victim to fresh air
    Administer 100% oxygen
    During extrication, consider traumatic injuries from falls
    Apply ACLS protocols as indicated
  Emergency department
    Maximize ventilation and oxygenation
    Consider PEEP for pulmonary edema
    Treat acidosis based on arterial pH and serum bicarbonate analysis
    Administer crystalloid and vasopressors for hypotension

Antidote
  Give sodium nitrite (3% NaNO$_2$) IV over 2–4 minutes
    Adult dose: 10 mL (300 mg)
    Pediatric dose: see Table 98–2
  Caution:
    Monitor blood pressure frequently
    Obtain methemoglobin level 30 minutes after dose
  Consider HBO if immediately available

suggest that HBO is beneficial.[12,146] Proposed mechanisms for oxygen's beneficial effects are competitive reactivation of oxidative phosphorylation by inhibiting hydrogen sulfide–cytochrome binding, enhanced detoxification by catalyzing oxidation of sulfides and sulfur, and improved oxygenation in the presence of pulmonary edema.[16,120] All patients suspected of hydrogen sulfide poisoning should receive supplemental oxygen and HBO when readily available. Because data on the efficacy of HBO are limited, it is not necessary to transfer the patient solely for HBO therapy.

The similarities in the toxic mechanism between hydrogen sulfide and cyanide created an interest in the use of nitrite-induced methemoglobin as an antidote. Methemoglobin protects animals from toxicity of hydrogen sulfide poisoning in both pretreatment and postexposure models.[25,121–123] Nitrite-generated methemoglobin acts as a scavenger of sulfide. Hydrogen sulfide's affinity for methemoglobin is greater than that for cytochrome oxidase.[121] When hydrogen sulfide binds to methemoglobin, it forms sulfmethemoglobin.[16] Because hydrogen sulfide poisoning is rare, no studies exist to evaluate the clinical outcomes of patients treated with sodium nitrite. Animal studies suggest that nitrite must be given within minutes of exposure to ensure effectiveness.[16] However, several human case reports showed rapid return of normal sensorium when nitrites were administered soon after exposure.[66,107,126] Patients with suspected hydrogen sulfide poisoning with altered mental status, coma, hypotension, or dysrhythmias should probably receive sodium nitrite by slow infusion. Sodium thiosulfate is of no benefit in the treatment of hydrogen sulfide poisoning because it is a biotransformation product.

Treatment of patients with hydrogen sulfide poisoning requires optimal supportive care. Treatments and antidotes beyond supportive care are not of proven clinical benefit. Because hydrogen sulfide toxicity is severe, and case reports suggest the occurrence of delayed sequelae, the potential benefits of nitrite therapy and HBO should be considered for seriously ill patients exposed to hydrogen sulfide. Use of these therapies occurs after optimum supportive care has been ensured.

SUMMARY

Both cyanide and hydrogen sulfide are high-risk industrial agents. Industrial precautions are essential to limit worker risk. Cyanide is of great concern with regard to homicide and suicide. There are particular metabolic risks and concerns with regard to exposure of both agents, as both agents bind specifically to the ferric moiety of the cytochrome a$_3$ oxidase complex. Odor recognition is dangerous and not a definitive approach to diagnosis. The laboratory evaluation is not usually useful in diagnosis.

Decontamination, removal from the site of exposure, and oxygen are essential. The controversies over the ideal therapeutic gestures for these agents is substantial, and extensive research continues.

REFERENCES

1. ACGIH: Threshold limit values and biological exposure indices for 1990–1991. ACGIH,1990.
2. Abe K, Kimura H: The possible role of hydrogen sulfide as an endogenous neuromodulator. J Neurosci 1996;16:1066–1071.
3. Akintonwa A, Tunwashe OL: Fatal cyanide poisoning from cassava-based meal. Hum Exp Toxicol 1992;11:47–49.
4. Andersen AH: Experimental studies on the pharmacology of activated charcoal. I. Adsorption power of charcoal in aqueous solutions. Acta Pharmacol 1946;2:69–78.
5. Ardelt BK, Borowitz JL, Isom GE: Brian lipid peroxidation and antioxidant protective mechanisms following acute cyanide intoxication. Toxicol 1989;56:147–154.
6. Ardelt BK, Borowitz JL, Maduh EU, Swain SL, Isom GE: Cyanide-induced lipid peroxidation in different organs: Subcellular distribution and hydroperoxide generation in neuronal cells. Toxicol 1994;89:127–137.
7. Aregheore EM, Agunbiade BS: The toxic effects of cassava (*Manihout esculenta* grantz) diets on humans. Vet Hum Toxicol 1991;33:274–275.
8. Arnold IM, Dufresne RM, Alleyne BC: Health implications of occupational exposures to hydrogen sulfide. J Occup Med 1985;27:373–376.
9. Ballantyne B: Artifacts in the definition of toxicity by cyanides and cyanogens. Fundam Appl Toxicol 1983;3:400–408.
10. Ballantyne B: Toxicology of cyanides. In: Ballantyne B, Marrs TC, eds: Clinical and Experimental Toxicology of Cyanides. Bristol, UK, IOP Publishers, 1987, p. 42.
11. Baselt RC: Disposition of Toxic Drugs and Chemicals in Man, 5th ed. Foster City, CA, Chemical Toxicology Institute, 2000.
12. Baskin SI: The cardiac effects of cyanide. In: Baskin SI, ed: Principles of Cardiac Toxicology. Boca Raton, CRC Press, 1991, pp. 419–430.
13. Morris J: The Brimstone Battles: Death came from a cloud: A silent killer took 9 lives in 1975. Could it happen again? Houston Chronicle (Special Report), *HoustonChronicle.com,* 2000.
14. Baud FJ, Barriot P, Toffis V, et al: Elevated blood cyanide concentrations in victims of smoke inhalation. N Engl J Med 1991;325:1761–1766.
15. Beauchamp RO, Bus JS, Popp JA: A critical review of the literature on hydrogen sulfide toxicity. Crit Rev Toxicol 1984;13:25–97.
16. Beck JF, Bradbury CM, Connors AJ: Nitrite as an antidote for acute hydrogen sulfide toxicity? Am J Ind Hyg 1981;42:805–809.
17. Beregi JP, Riou B, Lecarpentier Y: Effects of hydroxocobalamin on rat cardiac papillary muscle. Intensive Care Med 1991;17:175–177.
18. Berlin CM: The treatment of cyanide poisoning in children. Pediatrics 1976;46:793–796.

19. Bhambani Y, Burnham R, Snydmiller G: Effects of 10 ppm hydrogen sulfide inhalation in exercising men and women. J Occup Environ Med 1997;39:122–129.

20. Bhatt MH, Obeso JA, Marsden CD: The time course of post-anoxic akinetic-rigid and dystonic syndromes. Neurology 1993;43:314–317.

21. Bhattacharya R, Vijayaraghavan R: Cyanide intoxication in mice through different routes and its prophylaxis by α-ketoglutarate. Biomed Environ Sci 1991;4:452–459.

22. Binder L, Frederickson L: Poisoning in laboratory personnel and health care professionals. Am J Emerg Med 1991;9:11–15.

23. Bismuth C, Baud FJ, Djeghout H, Astier A, Aubriot D: Cyanide poisoning from proprionitrile exposure. J Emerg Med 1987;5:191–195.

24. Bismuth C, Baud FJ, Pontal G: Hydroxocobalamin in chronic cyanide poisoning. J Toxicol Clin Exp 1988;8:35–38.

25. Bitterman N, Talmi Y, Lerman A: The effect of hyperbaric oxygen on acute experimental sulfide poisoning in the rat. Toxicol Appl Pharmacol 1986;84:325–328.

26. Blanc P, Hogan M, Mallin K, Hryhorczuk D, Hessl S, Bernard B: Cyanide intoxication among silver-reclaiming workers. JAMA 1997;253:367–371.

27. Borgohain R, Singh AK, Radhakrishna H, Chalapathi Rao V, Mohandas S: Delayed onset generalised dystonia after cyanide poisoning. Clin Neurol Neurosurg 1995;97:213–215.

28. Boxer P: Occupational mass psychogenic illness. J Occup Med 1985;27:867–870.

29. Brahams D: Medicine and the law: "Sudafed" capsules poisoned with cyanide. Lancet 1991;337:968.

30. Breen PH, Isserles SA, Tabac E, Roizen MF, Taitelman UZ: Protective effect of stroma-free methemoglobin during cyanide poisoning in dogs. Anesthesiology 1996;85:558–564.

31. Brian MJ: Case reports: Cyanide poisoning in children in Goroka. Papua New Guinea Med J 1990;33:151–153.

32. Brivet F, Delfraissy JF, Bertrand P, Dormont J: Case reports: Acute cyanide poisoning—Recovery with nonspecific supportive care. Intensive Care Med 1983;9:33–35.

33. Brouard A, Blaisot B, Bismuth C: Hydroxocobalamin in cyanide poisoning. J Toxicol Clin Exp 1987;7:155–168.

34. Brown PWG, Buckels JWC, Jain AB, McMaster P: Successful cadaveric renal transplantation from a donor who died of cyanide poisoning. Br Med J 1987;294:1325.

35. Burnett WW, King EG, Grace M: Hydrogen sulfide poisoning: Review of 5 years' experience. Can Med Assoc J 1977;117:1277–1280.

36. Burrows GE, Way JL: Cyanide intoxication in sheep: The therapeutic value of oxygen or cobalt. Am J Vet Res 1977;38:223–227.

37. Cai Z, McCaslin PP: Selective effects of cyanide (100 mM) on the excitatory amino acid–induced elevation of intracellular calcium levels in neuronal culture. Neurochem Res 1992;17:803–808.

38. Callender T, Morrow L, Subramanian K, Duhon D, Ristov M: Three-dimensional brain metabolic imaging in patients with toxic encephalopathy. Environ Res 1993;60:295–319.

39. Caravati EM, Litovitz TL: Pediatric cyanide intoxication from an acetonitrile-containing cosmetic. JAMA 1988;260:3470–3473.

40. Carella F, Grassi MP, Savoiardo M, Contri P, Rapuzzi B, Mangoni A: Dystonic-parkinsonian syndrome after cyanide poisoning: Clinical and MRI findings. J Neurol Neurosurg Psychiatry 1988;51:1345–1348.

41. Chen KK, Rose CL: Nitrite and thiosulfate therapy in cyanide poisoning. JAMA 1952;149:113–119.

42. Chou S, Bitter P, Longstreth J: Toxicologic profile for hydrogen sulfide. Agency for Toxic Substances and Disease Registry. Atlanta: US Department of Health and Human Services, 1999.

43. Cottrell JE, Casthely P, Brodie JD, Patel K, Klein A, Turndorf H: Prevention of nitroprusside-induced cyanide toxicity with hydroxocobalamin. N Engl J Med 1978;298:809–811.

44. Curry SC, Arnold-Capell P: Toxic effects of drugs used in the ICU: Nitroprusside, nitroglycerin, and angiotensin-converting enzyme. Crit Care Clin North Am 1991;7:555–581.

45. Deng JF, Chang SC: Hydrogen sulfide poisoning in hot springs resevoir cleaning: Two case reports. Am J Ind Hyg 1987;11:447–451.

46. DiNapoli J, Hall AH, Drake R, Rumack BH: Cyanide and arsenic poisoning by intravenous injection. Ann Emerg Med 1989;18:308–311.

47. Dulaney MD, Brumley M, Willis JT, Hume AS: Protection against cyanide toxicity by oral α-ketoglutaric acid. Vet Hum Toxicol 1991;33:571–575.

48. Feldman JM, Feldman MD: Sequelae of attempted suicide by cyanide ingestion: A case report. Int J Psychiatry Med 1990;20:173–179.

49. Fernando GCA, Busuttil A: Cyanide ingestion: Case studies of four suicides. J Forensic Med Pathol 1991;12:241–246.

50. Freeman AG: Optic neuropathy and chronic cyanide intoxication: A review. J R Soc Med 1988;81:103–106.

51. Fuller DC, Suruda AJ: Occupationally related hydrogen sulfide deaths in the United States from 1984 to 1994. J Occup Environ Med 2000;42:939–942.

52. Gaitonde UB, Sellar RJ: Long term exposure to hydrogen sulphide producing subacute encephalopathy. Br Med J 1987;294:614.

53. Geller RJ, Ekins BR, Iknoian RC: Cyanide toxicity from acetonitrile-containing false nail remover. Am J Emerg Med 1991;9:268–270.

54. Graham DL, Laman D, Theodore J, Robin ED: Acute cyanide poisoning complicated by lactic acidosis and pulmonary edema. Arch Intern Med 1977;137:1051–1055.

55. Grandas F, Artieda J, Obeso JA: Brief report: Clinical and CT scan findings in a case of cyanide intoxication. Mov Disord 1989;4:188–193.

56. Gregorakos L, Dimopoulos G, Liberi S: Hydrogen sulfide poisoning: Management and complications. Angiology 1995;46:1123–1131.

57. Grigg B, Modeland V: The cyanide scare: A tale of two grapes. FDA Consumer 1989;July–Aug:7–11.

58. Guidotti TL: Occupational exposure to hydrogen sulfide in the sour gas industry: Some unresolved issues. Int Arch Occup Environ Health 1994;66:153–160.

59. Hall AH, Doutre WH, Kulig KW, Rumack BH: Nitrite/thiosulfate treated acute cyanide poisoning: Estimated kinetics after antidote. Clin Toxicol 1987;25:121–133.

60. Hall AH, Linden CH, Kulig KW, Rumack BH: Cyanide poisoning from laetrile ingestion: Role of nitrite therapy. Pediatrics 1986;78:269–272.

61. Hall AH, Rumack BH: Clinical toxicology of cyanide. Ann Emerg Med 1987;15:1067–1074.

62. Hall AH, Rumack BH: Hydroxocobalamin/sodium thiosulfate as a cyanide antidote. J Emerg Med 1987;5:115–121.

63. Hantson P, Mahieu P, Hassoun A, Otte J: Outcome following organ removal from poisoned donors in brain death status. J Toxicol Clin Toxicol 1995;33:709–712.

64. Hessel P, Herbert F, Melenka L, Yoshida K, Nakaza M: Lung health in relation to hydrogen sulfide exposure in oil and gas workers in Alberta, Canada. Am J Ind Med 1997;31:554–557.

65. Himori N, Tanaka Y, Kurasawa M, et al: Dextrorphan attenuates the behavioral consequences of ischemia and the biochemical consequences of anoxia: Possible role of N-methyl-d-aspartate receptor antagonism and ATP replenishing action in its cerebroprotecting profile. Psychopharmacology 1993;11:153–162.

66. Hoidal CR, Hall AH, Robinson MD: Hydrogen sulfide poisoning from toxic inhalations of roofing asphalt fumes. Ann Emerg Med 1986;15:826–830.

67. Horowitz BK, Marquardt K, Swenson E: Calcium polysulfide overdose: A report of two cases. J Toxicol Clin Toxicol 1997;35:299–303.

68. Howard J, Pouw TH, Arnold J, Logan B, Kobayashi JM, Davis J: Cyanide poisonings associated with over-the-counter medication—Washington state, 1991. Morbidity and Mortality Weekly Report 1991;40:161, 167–168.

69. Hume AS, Mozingo JR, McIntyre JB, Ho IK: Antidotal efficacy of alpha-ketoglutaric acid and sodium thiosulfate in cyanide poisoning. J Toxicol Clin Toxicol 1995;33:721–724.

70. Ivanov KP: The effect of elevated oxygen pressure on animals poisoned with potassium cyanide. Pharmacol Toxicol 1959;22:476–479.

71. Johnson JD, Conroy WG, Burris KD, Isom GE: Peroxidation of brain lipids following cyanide intoxication in mice. Toxicology 1987;46:21–28.

72. Johnson RP, Mellors JW: Arteriolization of venous blood gases: A clue to the diagnosis of cyanide poisoning. J Emerg Med 1988;6:401–404.

73. Johnson WS, Hall AH, Rumack BH: Cyanide poisoning successfully treated without "therapeutic methemoglobin levels." Am J Emerg Med 1989;7:437–440.

74. Jones AW, Lofgren A, Eklund A: Two fatalities from ingestion of acetonitrile: Limited specificity of analysis by headspace gas chromatography. J Anal Toxicol 1992;16:104–106.

75. Kage S, Takekawa K, Kurosaki K, Imamura T, Kudo K: The usefulness of thiosulfate as an indicator of hydrogen sulfide poisoning: Three cases. J Legal Med 1997;110:220–222.

76. Kilburn K, Warshaw R: Hydrogen sulfide and reduced-sulfur gases adversely affect neurophysiological functions. Toxicol Ind Health 1995;11:185–197.

77. Kilburn KH: Case report: Profound neurobehavioral deficits in an oil field worker overcome by hydrogen sulfide. Am J Med Sci 1993;303:301–305.

78. Kimura K, Hasegawa M, Matsubara K: A fatal disaster case based on exposure to hydrogen sulfide concentration at the scene. Forensic Sci Int 1994;66:111–116.

79. Kirk MA, Gerace R, Kulig KW: Cyanide and methemoglobin kinetics in smoke inhalation victims treated with the cyanide antidote kit. Ann Emerg Med 1993;22:1413–1418.

80. Krieg A, Saxena K: Cyanide poisoning from metal cleaning solutions. Ann Emerg Med 1987;16:582–584.

81. Kruszyna R, Kruszyna H, Smith RP: Comparison of hydroxylamine, 4-dimethylaminophenol and nitrite protection against cyanide poisoning in mice. Arch Toxicol 1982;49:191–202.

82. Kurt TL: Chemical asphyxiants. In: Rom WN, ed: Environmental and Occupational Medicine. Boston, Little, Brown, 1992, pp. 539–549.

83. Kurt TL, Day LC, Reed WG, Gandy W: Cyanide poisoning from glue-on nail remover. Am J Emerg Med 1991;9:271–272.

84. Lambert RJ, Kindler BL, Schaeffer DJ: The efficacy of superactivated charcoal in treating rats exposed to a lethal dose of potassium cyanide. Ann Emerg Med 1988;17:595–598.

85. Litovitz TL, Felberg L, White S, Klein-Schwartz W: 1995 annual report of the American Association of Poison Control Centers toxic exposure surveillance system. Am J Emerg Med 1996;14:487–537.

86. Litovitz TL, Larkin RF, Myers RAM: Cyanide poisoning treated with hyperbaric oxygen. Am J Emerg Med 1983;1:94–101.

87. Litovitz TL, Schmitz BF, Holm KC: 1988 annual report of the American Association of Poison Control Centers national data collection system. Am J Emerg Med 1989;7:495–545.

88. Losek JD, Rock AL, Boldt RR: Cyanide poisoning from a cosmetic nail remover. Pediatrics 1991;88:337–340.

89. Lundquist P, Rammer L, Sorbo B: The role of hydrogen cyanide and carbon monoxide in fire casualties: A prospective study. Forensic Sci Int 1989;43:9–12.

90. Maduh EU, Baskin SI: Protein kinase C modulation of rhodanese-catalyzed conversion of cyanide to thiocyanate. Res Commun Mol Pathol Pharmacol 1994;86:155–173.

91. Maduh EU, Neally EW, Song H, Wang PC, Baskin SI: A protein kinase C inhibitor attenuates cyanide toxicity in vivo. Toxicology 1995;100:129–137.

92. Marcus SJ: American Association Poison Control Centers (AAPCC) Alert 1988;Jan 4.

93. Martin-Bermudez R, Maestre-Romero A, Goni-Belzunegui MV, Bautista-Lorite A, Arenas-Cabrera C: Venous blood arteriolization and multiple organ failure after cyanide poisoning. Intensive Care Med 1997;23:1286.

94. McCabe L, Clayton G: Air pollution by hydrogen sulfide in Poza Rica, Mexico. An evaluation of the incident of Nov 24, 1950. Arch Ind Hyg Occup Med 1952;6:199–213.

95. Messing B, Storch B: Computer tomography and magnetic resonance imaging in cyanide poisoning. Eur Arch Psychiatry Neurol Sci 1988;237:139–143.

96. Milby T, Baselt R: Hydrogen sulfide poisoning: Clarification of some controversial issues. Am J Ind Med 1999;35:192–195.

97. Milby TH: Hydrogen sulfide intoxication. Occup Health 1961;Dec 11:431–437.

98. Mitchell T, Savage J, Gould D: High-performance liquid chromatography detection of sulfide in tissues from sulfide-treated mice. J Appl Toxicol 1993;13:389–394.

99. MMWR: Leads from the MMWR: Acute illness epidemic West Bank-Jerusalem. JAMA 1983;249:2617–2620.

100. Moore SJ, Norris JC, Walsh DA, Hume AS: Antidotal use of methemoglobin forming cyanide antagonists in concurrent carbon monoxide/cyanide intoxication. J Pharmacol Exp Ther 1987;242:70–73.

101. Nagler J, Provoost RA, Parizel G: Hydrogen cyanide poisoning: Treatment with cobalt EDTA. J Occup Med 1978;20:414–416.

102. Norris JC, Utley WA, Hume AS: Mechanism of antagonizing cyanide-induced lethality by α-ketoglutaric acid. Toxicology 1990;62:275–283.

103. Osbern LN, Crapo RO: A report of toxic exposure to liquid manure. Arch Intern Med 1981;95:312–314.

104. Patel MN, Ardelt BK, Yim GKW, Isom GE: Cyanide induces Ca^{2+}-dependent and -independent release of glutamate from mouse brain slices. Neurosci Lett 1991;131:42–44.

105. Patel MN, Peoples RW, Yim GKW, Isom GE: Enhancement of NMDA-mediated responses by cyanide. Neurochem Res 1994;19:1319–1323.

106. Patel MN, Yim GKW, Isom GE: N-methyl-d-aspartate receptors mediate cyanide-induced toxicity in hippocampal cultures. Neurotoxicology 1993;14:35–40.

107. Peters JW: Hydrogen sulfide poisoning in a hospital setting. JAMA 1981;246:1588–1589.

108. Pitt BR, Radford EP, Gurtner GH, Traystman RJ: Interaction of carbon monoxide and cyanide on cerebral circulation and metabolism. Arch Environ Health 1979;34:354–359.

109. Rathinavelu A, Sun P, Borowitz JL, Isom GE: Cyanide induces protein kinase C translocation: Blockade by NMDA antagonists. J Biochem Toxicol 1994;9:235–240.

110. Ravizza A, Carugo D, Cerchiari EL: The treatment of hydrogen sulfide intoxication: Oxygen versus nitrites. Vet Hum Toxicol 1982;24:241–242.

111. Reiffenstein RJ, Hulbert WC, Rother SH: Toxicology of hydrogen sulfide. Annu Rev Pharmacol Toxicol 1992;32:109–134.

112. Richardson D: Respiratory effects of chronic hydrogen sulfide exposure. Am J Ind Med 1995;28:99–108.

113. Rindone JP, Sloane EP: Cyanide toxicity from sodium nitroprusside: Risks and management. Ann Pharmacother 1992;26:515–519.

114. Riou B, Gerard JL, La Rochelle CD, Bourdon R, Guidicelli JF: Hemodynamic effects of hydroxocobalamin in conscious dogs. Anesthesiology 1991;74:552–558.

115. Rosenberg NL, Myers JA, Martin WWR: Cyanide-induced parkinsonism: Clinical, MRI, and 6-fluorodopa PET studies. Neurology 1989;39:142–144.

116. Rosenow F, Herholz K, Lanfermann H, et al: Neurological sequelae of cyanide intoxication—The patterns of clinical, magnetic resonance imaging, and positron emission tomography findings. Ann Neurol 1995;38:825–828.

117. Shragg TA, Albertson TE, Fisher CJ: Cyanide poisoning after bitter almond ingestion. West J Med 1982;139:65–69.

118. Silverman SH, Purdue GF, Hunt JL, Bost RO: Cyanide toxicity in burned patients. J Trauma 1988;28:171–176.

119. Singh BM, Coles N, Lewis P, Braithwaite RA, Nattrass M, FitzGerald MG: The metabolic effects of fatal cyanide poisoning. Postgrad Med J 1989;65:923–925.

120. Smilkstein MJ, Bronstein AC, Pickett HM: Hyperbaric oxygen therapy for severe hydrogen sulfide poisoning. J Emerg Med 1985;3:27–30.

121. Smith L, Kruszyna H, Smith RP: The effect of methemoglobin on the inhibition of cytochrome c oxidase by cyanide, sulfide, or azide. Biochem Pharmacol 1977;26:2247–2250.

122. Smith RP, Gosselin RE: Current concepts about the treatment of selected poisonings: nitrite, cyanide, barium, and quinidine. Annu Rev Pharmacol Toxicol 1976;16:189–199.

123. Smith RP, Gosselin RE: Hydrogen sulfide poisoning. J Occup Med 1979;21:93–97.

124. Smith RP, Kruszyna R, Kruszyna H: Management of acute sulfide poisoning. Arch Environ Health 1976;31:166–169.

125. Snyder JW, Safir EF, Summerville GP: Occupational fatality and persistent neurological sequelae after mass exposure to hydrogen sulfide. Am J Emerg Med 1995;13:199–203.

126. Stine RJ, Slosberg B, Beacham BE: Hydrogen sulfide intoxication: A case report and discussion of treatment. Ann Intern Med 1976;85:756–758.

127. Suchard JR, Wallace KL, Gerkin RD: Acute cyanide toxicity caused by apricot kernel ingestion. Ann Emerg Med 1998;32:742–744.

128. Swanson-Biearman B, Krenzelok EP, Snyder JW, Unkle DW, Nathan HM, Yang SL: Successful donation and transplantation of multiple organs from a victim of cyanide poisoning. J Toxicol Clin Toxicol 1993;31:95–99.

129. Ten Eyck RP, Schaerdel AD, Ottinger WE: Comparison of nitrite treatment and stroma-free methemoglobin solution as antidotes for cyanide poisoning in a rat model. J Toxicol Clin Toxicol 1985;23:477–487.

130. Ten Eyck RP, Schaerdel AD, Ottinger WE: Stroma-free methemoglobin solution: An effective antidote for cyanide poisoning. Am J Emerg Med 1985;3:519–523.

131. Trapp WG: Massive cyanide poisoning with recovery: A Boxing Day story. Can Med Assoc J 1970;102:517.

132. Tveldt B, Edland A, Skyberg K: Delayed neuropsychiatric sequelae after acute hydrogen sulfide poisoning: Affection of motor function, memory, vision, and hearing. Acta Neurol Scand 1991;84:348–351.

133. Tveldt B, Skyberg K, Aaserud O: Brain damage caused by hydrogen sulfide: A follow-up study of six patients. Am J Ind Med 1991;20:91–101.

134. Van Heijst ANP, Douze JMC, Van Kesteren RG, Van Bergen JAEM, Van Dijk A: Therapeutic problems in cyanide poisoning. J Toxicol Clin Toxicol 1987;25:383–398.

135. Vanhoorne M, Rouck A, Bacquer D: Epidemiological study of eye irritation by hydrogen sulphide and/or carbon disulphide in viscose rayon workers. Ann Occup Hyg 1995;39:307–315.

136. Vesey CJ, Wilson J: Red cell cyanide. J Pharm Pharmacol 1978;30:20–26.

137. Vick JA, Froehlich H: Treatment of cyanide poisoning. Mil Med 1991;156:330–339.

138. Vornov JJ, Tasker RJ, Coyle JT: Delayed protection by MK-801 and tetrodotoxin in a rat organotypic hippocampal culture model of ischemia. Stroke 1994;25:457–465.

139. Warenycia MW, Goodwin LR, Beneshin CG: Acute hydrogen sulfide poisoning: Demonstration of selective uptake of sulfide by the brainstem by measurement of brain sulfide levels. Biochem Pharmacol 1989;38:973–981.

140. Wasch HH, Estrin WJ, Yip P: Prolongation of P-300 latency associated with hydrogen sulfide poisoning. Arch Neurol 1989;46:902–904.

141. Way JL: Cyanide intoxication and its mechanism of antagonism. Annu Rev Pharmacol Toxicol 1984;24:451–481.

142. Way JL, End E, Sheehy MH, et al: Effect of oxygen on cyanide intoxication. IV. Hyperbaric oxygen. Toxicol Appl Pharmacol 1972;22:415–421.

143. Weger NP: Treatment of cyanide poisoning with 4-dimethyl-aminophenol (DMAP): experimental and clinical overview. Middle East J Anesthesiol 1990;10:389–412.

144. Weiss LD, Van Meter KW: The applications of hyperbaric oxygen therapy in emergency medicine. Am J Emerg Med 1992;10:558–569.

145. Wessen DE, Foley R, Sabatini S, Wharton J, Kapusnik J, Kurtzman NA: Treatment of acute cyanide intoxication with hemodialysis. Am J Nephrol 1985;5:121–126.

146. Whitcraft DD, Bailey TD, Hart GB: Hydrogen sulfide poisoning treated with hyperbaric oxygen. J Emerg Med 1985;3:23–25.

147. Wilson J: Cyanide in human disease: A review of clinical and laboratory evidence. Fundam Appl Toxicol 1983;3:397–399.

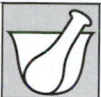

ANTIDOTES IN DEPTH

Cyanide Antidotes
William Kerns II

In addition to decontamination, airway management, high-flow oxygen, and sodium bicarbonate, the standard treatment for cyanide poisoning in the United States is the administration of the cyanide antidote kit. Because of the swift action of cyanide, successful treatment is dependent on preparedness and timely delivery of specific antidotes. A kit was designed to provide all necessary components for rapid treatment. The main components of the kit are the specific antidotes amyl nitrite, sodium nitrite, and thiosulfate. The kit also contains a nasogastric tube intended for gastric lavage in cases of ingestion and supplies for parenteral drug administration. Decontamination of cyanide-poisoned patients is covered in detail in the main part of Chapter 98. This discussion focuses on the pharmacologic aspect of the specific antidotes in the kit.

MECHANISM OF ACTION OF NITRITES AND THIOSULFATE

The cyanide antidotes act by separate and synergistic mechanisms: nitrites via induction of cyanide binding to hemoglobin, and thiosulfate via biotransformation of cyanide.

Animal studies clearly demonstrate that nitrites antagonize the toxic effects of cyanide. For example, in awake canines poisoned with subcutaneous NaCN injection and then treated with inhaled amyl nitrite or intravenous sodium nitrite, both nitrite forms increased the LD_{50} fourfold.[13,15] However, the exact mechanism by which nitrite exerts its antagonistic effect has not been fully elucidated. The most widely suggested mechanism involves nitrite-induced oxidation of hemoglobin to methemoglobin. Methemoglobin contains a ferric iron (Fe^{3+}) that competes effectively with the ferric iron in cytochrome a_3 for cyanide ions. Cyanmethemoglobin is formed, and mitochondrial respiration is restored. Several investigations support this mechanism. In one study, cyanmethemoglobin was detected in cyanide-poisoned canines following nitrite therapy.[13] In another study, methemoglobin restored cytochrome oxidase activity in isolated enzyme preparations that were inhibited by cyanide.[1,40]

However, there are data that do not support methemoglobin formation as the mode by which nitrites work. For example, in experimental studies, methemoglobin formation lags behind resolution of toxicity.[47] Additionally, nitrites antagonize cyanide despite pretreatment with methylene blue to prevent methemoglobin formation.[24]

Other data suggest that an alternate mechanism of action may underlie nitrite therapy. One such mechanism may be nitrite-induced vasodilation and enhanced hepatic and other organ blood flow. This occurs as nitrites undergo denitration with subsequent release of nitric oxide, an effective vasodilator. Vasodilation increases blood flow to organs rich in the enzyme rhodanese, such as the liver, enhancing cyanide detoxification.[45] Experiments with other vasodilators such as isosorbide dinitrate or chlorpromazine demonstrate similar benefit.[29,43]

Thiosulfate, the second component of the kit, by itself antagonizes cyanide toxicity. In a canine model, thiosulfate treatment protected against three lethal doses of sodium cyanide.[15] Thiosulfate works by supplying sulfur for sulfurtransferase-mediated biotransformation of cyanide to thiocyanate (SCN). A sulfurtransferase enzyme, such as rhodanese, must be present for detoxification.[26] In a canine model of parenteral NaCN poisoning, thiosulfate infusion increased cyanide biotransformation by 30-fold compared to controls.[44]

By acting through separate mechanisms, nitrite and thiosulfate are synergistic in their ability to antagonize cyanide. Nitrites and thiosulfate independently protected against four and three lethal doses of cyanide, respectively, but their combined administration increased protection to 13 times the lethal dose.[15] Addition of oxygen to these two antidotes further increases survival.[12] For these reasons, the current strategy for the management of cyanide poisoning includes oxygen, nitrites, and thiosulfate whenever possible.

ADMINISTRATION

Amyl nitrite is a temporizing measure, used only until intravenous access is obtained. The glass ampules are crushed and intermittently inhaled by the patient (30 seconds on, 30 seconds off). This assumes that the patient breathes spontaneously. Administration of amyl nitrite in the apneic patient requires some creativity. One suggested mode of delivery is to place the crushed amyl nitrite ampule in an aerosol chamber inserted into the outflow tract of an ambu-bag or mechanical ventilator. Administration can be controlled via oxygen tubing connected directly to the aerosol chamber, independent of the oxygen supply to the ambu-bag. In this way, amyl nitrite is administered in an intermittent fashion (30 seconds on, 30 seconds off), and the patient receives continuous high-flow oxygen.

Intravenous sodium nitrite is preferred over inhaled amyl nitrite. The initial adult dose is 300 mg (10 mL of a 3% solution), given over 2 to 4 minutes.[14] In children, the dose is 0.33 mL/kg (10 mg/kg) of the 3% solution, assuming adequate hemoglobin is present. Because nitrite oxidizes hemoglobin on a mole-per-mole basis, anemic patients are at risk for excessive methemoglobin formation and require less nitrite (see Table 98–2). A bedside hemoglobin measurement may be useful to guide nitrite therapy. However, if rapid hemoglobin assessment is not available, children are assumed to have a hemoglobin of 12 g/dL.

Thiosulfate is supplied as 12.5 g in a 25% solution (50 mL). The adult dose is 12.5 g, and the pediatric dose 1.65 mL/kg.

In cases in which the patient does not improve or develops recurrent cyanide toxicity, a second dose of the antidotes may be required. Because thiosulfate is nontoxic, a repeat dose poses no risk. However, additional sodium nitrite may result in an adverse effect. Unfortunately, there are no data to guide the amount or timing of a second nitrite dose. Some authors suggest one-half the initial dose to avoid excessive methemoglobin formation,[3,6] but the original developer of the cyanide kit recommends repeating the dose in full.[13] One approach is to reassess the patient 30 minutes after initiating therapy, including pH and methemoglobin levels. A methemoglobin measurement at 30 minutes should represent its peak level.[27,28] For patients with persistent symptoms, acidemia, and less than 10% methemoglobin, the full dose of sodium nitrite can be repeated. If the methemoglobin is greater than 10%, one-half the original dose seems prudent.

ADVERSE DRUG EFFECTS

Adverse effects of nitrite therapy are predictable based on pharmacologic properties and include hypotension and excessive methemoglobinemia.

In volunteers given 4 mg/kg intravenous sodium nitrite, the systolic blood pressure fell almost 20 mm Hg, and all but one experienced orthostatic symptoms.[27] If hypotension occurs, slow the infusion rate and start crystalloid and/or vasopressors as needed.

Most patients tolerate methemoglobin formation without difficulty. In cases of drug-induced methemoglobin, levels less than 30% typically do not produce symptoms unless the patient has an underlying illness that interferes with oxygen delivery such as anemia, cardiovascular disease, or pulmonary disease.[16] Nitrite administration in antidotal doses rarely produces levels approaching 30%. In healthy subjects, 400 mg and 600 mg intravenous sodium nitrite produced 10 and 17% methemoglobin, respectively.[13] In another study of healthy subjects, 4 mg/kg intravenous sodium nitrite produced peak methemoglobin levels of 7% 30 minutes after injection.[27] In clinical case reports of cyanide poisoning, nitrite therapy results in similar methemoglobin levels. In a series of adult fire victims with both cyanide and carbon monoxide poisoning, methemoglobin peaked at 50 minutes and ranged in values from 7.9 to 13.4%.[28] All but one of these adult patients received a single dose of nitrite. Sodium nitrite (300 mg) therapy for cyanide poisoning from apricot kernel ingestion in an adult woman produced an initial methemoglobin of 7.3%. The patient received an additional 150 mg sodium nitrite 5 hours later for persistent acidosis and developed a subsequent methemoglobin level of 10.3%.[42] Methemoglobin peaked at 20% 1 hour after a single nitrite dose for bitter almond–induced cyanide poisoning in an elderly woman.[39] Cyanide cases in which patients develop symptomatic methemoglobinemia after nitrites are rare but occur. A suicidal patient awoke after a second full dose of sodium nitrite but became cyanotic and complained of dyspnea. His methemoglobin level was 58%.[46] One fatality directly attributable to methemoglobin appears in the pediatric literature. A 17-month-old child ingested what was later determined to be a nontoxic amount of cyanide-containing reagent. He received two doses of nitrite totaling 28 mg/kg (recommended total dose for nonanemic child 15 mg/kg). The patient developed vomiting, apnea, seizures, and then cardiopulmonary arrest in temporal relationship to the nitrite.[6]

Thiosulfate is a very safe antidote with minimal direct adverse reactions. In one volunteer study, 12.5 g of thiosulfate infused over 20 minutes resulted in nausea, vomiting, burning at the injection site, and localized muscle cramping.[21] Thiocyanate, the renally eliminated cyanide detoxification product, is also relatively harmless. Toxicity from thiocyanate occurs, but usually in association with prolonged nitroprusside therapy in the ICU setting, especially when the patient has renal dysfunction.[18] Manifestations of thiocyanate toxicity include hypotension, abdominal pain, rashes, nausea, vomiting, and altered mental status. Thiocyanate toxicity is not expected from one or two doses of thiosulfate for acute cyanide poisoning.

INDICATIONS

The rapid onset of cyanide toxicity and lack of a distinct toxidrome necessitates empiric therapy, often based only on historical circumstances or suspicion inferred from initial clinical data. Historical situations include the sudden collapse of a laboratory or industrial worker who has access to cyanide reagents, suicide or unexplained coma and acidosis, ingestion of artificial nail remover, or ingestion of seeds from *Prunus* sp. Also, consider cyanide poisoning in the ICU patient receiving nitroprusside who develops symptoms of cyanide poisoning such as altered mental status, tachyphylaxis, acidemia, decreased oxygen consumption, or increased venous oxygen content. When suspicion is high, treat with oxygen, sodium bicarbonate, and both components of the kit. When suspicion is lower, administer oxygen, bicarbonate, and only the thiosulfate.

There are several conditions in which only one of the components of the antidote kit is indicated, including smoke inhalation, prevention of nitroprusside toxicity, and hydrogen sulfide toxicity.

Cyanide poisoning occurs in victims of fire and smoke inhalation when there has been combustion of nitrogenous substances.[5] Although thiosulfate can be given safely to these patients to treat cyanide poisoning, the use of nitrites is controversial. The concern with regard to nitrites lies in critically reducing the fraction of normal hemoglobin during methemoglobin formation when other abnormal hemoglobins, (sulfhemoglobin, carboxyhemoglobin, and methemoglobin) are often present as a result of airborne toxins from the smoke. Unfortunately, there are limited data regarding this specific situation. In a small series of fire victims with confirmed cyanide and carbon monoxide toxicity, peak carboxyhemoglobin and methemoglobin levels did not coincide. The highest carboxyhemoglobin levels (mean 26%, range 5–38%) were detected at presentation and rapidly decreased with a mean elimination half-life of 51 minutes. Peak methemoglobin levels (mean 10.5%, range 7.9–13.4%) were measured between 35 and 70 minutes into the patient's resuscitation.[28] However, cyanmethemoglobin levels were not measured in this series, and the clinical impact of this abnormal hemoglobin is unknown. For this reason, it is prudent to give only thiosulfate during initial resuscitation and to reserve nitrite use for fire victims with refractory altered mental status and acidemia. Measurement of hemoglobin, carboxyhemoglobin, and methemoglobin will help guide therapy.

Thiosulfate administration is suggested during nitroprusside infusion to prevent cyanide toxicity. In a canine model, prophylactic thiosulfate reduced red cell and plasma cyanide as well as preventing lactate accumulation.[30] Prophylactic thiosulfate also reduced cyanide buildup in humans receiving nitroprusside during cardiovascular surgery.[35] The recommended dose of thiosulfate is 1 g for every 100 mg of sodium nitroprusside.[18,35]

The nitrite portion of the kit is indicated in hydrogen sulfide poisoning. Hydrogen sulfide has cytotoxicity similar to cyanide, inhibiting cytochrome oxidase and impairing normal mitochondrial respiration. Methemoglobin competes with cytochrome for sulfide, forming sulfmethemoglobin. In isolated cytochrome preparations inhibited by sulfide, the addition of methemoglobin restored enzyme activity. Human experience with nitrite for hydrogen sulfide is limited to case reports. These cases describe improved sensorium following nitrite treatment.[23,33,41] Dosing guidelines are the same as for cyanide treatment. Thiosulfate treatment is not necessary, as sulfation is not a pathway of hydrogen sulfide detoxification.

HYDROXOCOBALAMIN

Pharmacology

Chelation is another viable treatment modality for cyanide poisoning. The best-studied chelators contain cobalt, which complexes with cyanide to form cobaltocyanides. In animal models, cobalt compounds increased the LD_{50} of cyanide.[20] Two notable cobalt compounds, dicobalt edetate and hydroxocobalamin, are used in human poisoning. Although an effective chelator,[20] dicobalt edetate has significant adverse effects, including angioedema, hypotension, dysrhythmias, and impaired cerebral blood flow, that limit its clinical usefulness.[9,32] Hydroxocobalamin (a vitamin B_{12} precursor) is a cobalt-centered metalloprotein that avidly complexes cyanide on a one-to-one molar ratio, forming cyanocobalamin (vitamin B_{12}). Hydroxocobalamin chelates intracellular cyanide. Rescue therapy with hydroxocobalamin in cyanide-poisoned animals reversed myocardial depression,[36] restored spontaneous breathing,[34] and, most importantly, improved survival.[31,34]

Adverse Drug Reactions

Hydroxocobalamin is in general a safe antidote. Allergic reaction is the most serious adverse event.[11,22] However, the most common reaction is transient reddening of the skin, tears, and urine.[11,17,19,22] In smokers given hydroxocobalamin, all subjects experienced skin reddening that resolved by 48-hour followup.[21] In smoke inhalation victims, red urine was observed for up to 1 week following hydroxocobalamin.[25]

From a cardiovascular standpoint, hydroxocobalamin is a safer chelating agent than dicobalt edetate. It lacks myocardial toxicity.[5,37,38] Hypertension was noted in volunteers, the highest of which was 205/123 mm Hg.[21] However, subjects did not develop any symptoms or end organ manifestations, and blood pressure elevation resolved within 48 hours.

Last, hydroxocobalamin interferes with common laboratory testing, including bilirubin, aspartate aminotransferase, creatinine, chloride, magnesium, and iron.[19,21] The interference is likely related to the red color of hydroxocobalamin, which hinders colorimetric analytic techniques.

Indications and Dosage

The majority of clinical experience with hydroxocobalamin comes from France, where it has been used successfully to treat acute cyanide, acetonitrile, and proprionitrile poisoning.[7,11,22] Hydroxocobalamin has also been used to treat chronic illness related to cyanide such as Leber's hereditary optic atrophy and tobacco amblyopia.[8] Hydroxocobalamin may also prevent cyanide toxicity associated with sodium nitroprusside infusion,[17,48] although thiosulfate is more readily available in the United States[22] and is less expensive.[18,35,48] The suggested dose for acute cyanide poisoning is 4 g intravenously. Coadministration of 8 g of thiosulfate is thought to act synergistically, reducing the required amount of hydroxocobalamin.[22]

REFERENCES

1. Albaum HG, Tepperman J, Bodansky O: A spectrophotometric study of the competition of methemoglobin and cytochrome oxidase for cyanide in vitro. J Biol Chem 1946;163:641–647.
2. Astier A, Baud FJ: Complexation of intracellular cyanide by hydroxocobalamin using a human cellular model. Hum Exp Toxicol 1996;15:19–25.
3. Baskin SI, Horowitz AM, Neally EW: The antidotal action of sodium nitrite and sodium thiosulfate against cyanide poisoning. J Clin Pharmacol 1992;32:368–375.
4. Baud FJ, Barriot P, Toffis V, et al: Elevated blood cyanide concentrations in victims of smoke inhalation. N Engl J Med 1991;325:1761–1766.
5. Beregi JP, Riou B, Lecarpentier Y: Effects of hydroxocobalamin on rat cardiac papillary muscle. Intensive Care Med 1991;17:175–177.
6. Berlin CM: The treatment of cyanide poisoning in children. Pediatrics 1976;46:793–796.
7. Bismuth C, Baud FJ, Djeghout H, et al: Cyanide poisoning from proprionitrile exposure. J Emerg Med 1987;5:191–195.
8. Bismuth C, Baud FJ, Pontal G: Hydroxocobalamin in chronic cyanide poisoning. J Toxicol Clin Exp1988;8:35–38.
9. Brian MJ: Case reports: Cyanide poisoning in children in Goroka. Papau New Guinea Med J 1990;33:151–153.
10. Brink NG, Kuehl FA, Folkers K: Vitamin B_{12}: The identification of vitamin B_{12} as a cyano-cobalt coordination complex. Science 1950;112:354.
11. Brouard A, Blaisot B, Bismuth C: Hydroxocobalamin in cyanide poisoning. J Toxicol Clin Exp 1988;7:155–168.
12. Burrows GE, Way JL: Cyanide intoxication in sheep: The therapeutic value of oxygen or cobalt. Am J Vet Res 1977;38:223–227.
13. Chen KK, Rose CL: Nitrite and thiosulfate therapy in cyanide poisoning. JAMA 1952;149:113–119.
14. Chen KK, Rose CL: Treatment of acute cyanide poisoning. JAMA 1956;162:1154–1155.
15. Chen KK, Rose CL, Clowes GHA: Methylene blue, nitrites, and sodium thiosulphate against cyanide poisoning. Proc Soc Exp Biol Med 1933;31:250–251.
16. Coleman MD, Coleman NA: Drug-induced methaemoglobinaemia: Treatment issues. Drug Saf 1996;14:394–405.
17. Cottrell JE, Casthely P, Brodie JD, et al: Prevention of nitroprusside-induced cyanide toxicity with hydroxocobalamin. N Engl J Med 1978;298:809–811.
18. Curry SC, Arnold-Capell P: Toxic effects of drugs used in the ICU: Nitroprusside, nitroglycerin, and angiotensin-converting enzyme. Crit Care Clin North Am 1991;7:555–581.
19. Curry SC, Connor DA, Raschke RA: Effect of the cyanide antidote hydroxocobalamin on commonly ordered serum chemistry studies. Ann Emerg Med 1994;24:65–67.
20. Evans CL: Cobalt compounds as antidotes for hydrocyanic acid. Br J Pharmacol 1964;23:455–475.
21. Forsyth JC, Mueller PD, Becker CE, et al: Hydroxocobalamin as a cyanide antidote: Safety, efficacy and pharmacokinetics in heavily smoking normal volunteers. J Toxicol Clin Toxicol 1993;31:277–294.
22. Hall AH, Rumack BH: Hydroxocobalamin/sodium thiosulfate as a cyanide antidote. J Emerg Med 1987;5:115–121.
23. Hoidal CR, Hall AH, Robinson MD: Hydrogen sulfide poisoning from toxic inhalations of roofing asphalt fumes. Ann Emerg Med 1986;15:826–830.
24. Holmes RK, Way JL: Mechanism of cyanide antagonism by sodium nitrite. Pharmacologist 1982;24:182.
25. Houeto P, Borron SW, Sandouk P, et al: Pharmacokinetics of hydroxocobalamin in smoke inhalation victims. J Toxicol Clin Toxicol 1996;34:397–404.
26. Isom GE, Way JL: Effects of oxygen on antagonism of cyanide intoxication: Cytochrome oxidase, in vitro. Toxicol Appl Pharmacol 1984;74:57–62.

27. Kiese M, Weger NP: Formation of ferrihemoglobin with aminophenols in the human for the treatment of cyanide poisoning. Eur J Pharmacol 1969;7:97–105.

28. Kirk MA, Gerace R, Kulig KW: Cyanide and methemoglobin kinetics in smoke inhalation victims treated with the cyanide antidote kit. Ann Emerg Med 1993;22:1413–1418.

29. Kong A, Shen A, Burrows GE, et al: Effect of chlorpromazine on cyanide intoxication. Toxicol Appl Pharmacol 1983;71:407–413.

30. Krapez JR, Vesey CJ, Cole PV: Effects of cyanide antidotes used with sodium nitroprusside infusions: Sodium thiosulphate and hydroxocobalamin given prophylactically to dogs. Br J Anaesth 1981;53: 793–803.

31. Mushett CW, Kelley KL, Boxer GE, Rickards JC: Antidotal efficacy of vitamin B12a (hydroxo-cobalamin) in experimental cyanide poisoning. Proc Soc Exp Biol Med 1952;81:234–237.

32. Nagler J, Provoost RA, Parizel G: Hydrogen cyanide poisoning: Treatment with cobalt EDTA. J Occup Med 1978;20·414–416.

33. Peters JW: Hydrogen sulfide poisoning in a hospital setting. JAMA 1981;246:1588–1589.

34. Posner MA, Tobey RE, McElroy H: Hydroxocobalamin therapy of cyanide intoxication in guinea pigs. Anesthesiology 1976;44: 157–160.

35. Rindone JP, Sloane EP: Cyanide toxicity from sodium nitroprusside: Risks and management. Ann Pharmacother 1992;26:515–519.

36. Riou B, Baud FJ, Astier A, Barriot P, Lecarpentier Y: In vitro demonstration of the antidotal efficacy of hydroxocobalamin in cyanide poisoning. J Neurosurg Anesthesiol 1990;2:296–304.

37. Riou B, Berdeaux A, Pussard E, Guidicelli JF: Comparison of the hemodynamic effects of hydroxocobalamin and cobalt edetate at equipotent cyanide antidotal doses in conscious dogs. Intensive Care Med 1993;19:26–32.

38. Riou B, Gerard JL, La Rochelle CD, et al: Hemodynamic effects of hydroxocobalamin in conscious dogs. Anesthesiology 1991;74: 552–558.

39. Shragg TA, Albertson TE, Fisher CJ: Cyanide poisoning after bitter almond ingestion. West J Med 1982;139:65–69.

40. Smith L, Kruszyna H, Smith RP: The effect of methemoglobin on the inhibition of cytochrome c oxidase by cyanide, sulfide, or azide. Biochem Pharmacol 1977;26:2247–2250.

41. Stine RJ, Slosberg B, Beacham BE: Hydrogen sulfide intoxication: A case report and discussion of treatment. Ann Intern Med 1976;85: 756–758.

42. Suchard JR, Wallace KL, Gerkin RD: Acute cyanide toxicity caused by apricot kernel ingestion. Ann Emerg Med 1998;32:742–744.

43. Sun P, Borowitz JL, Kanthasamy AG, et al: Antagonism of cyanide toxicity by isosorbide dinitrate: Possible role of nitric oxide. Toxicol 1995;104:105–111.

44. Sylvester D, Hayton WL, Morgan RL, Way JL: Effects of thiosulfate on cyanide kinetics in dogs. Toxicol Appl Pharmacol 1983;69: 265–271.

45. Tamulinas CB, Nizamani S, Myers M: The effect of blood flow on cyanide metabolism in the isolated perfused rat liver. Fed Proc 1985; 44:1796.

46. Van Heijst ANP, Douze JMC, Van Kesteren RG, et al: Therapeutic problems in cyanide poisoning. J Toxicol Clin Toxicol 1987;25: 383–398.

47. Way JL: Cyanide intoxication and its mechanism of antagonism. Annu Rev Pharmacol Toxicol 1984;24:451–481.

48. Zerbe NF, Wagner KJ: Use of vitamin B12 in the treatment and prevention of nitroprusside-induced cyanide toxicity. Crit Care Med 1993;21:465–467.

CHAPTER 99 RADIATION

Joseph Rella

A 16-year-old boy broke open an exit sign, and the liquid contents spilled on his clothing. Shortly thereafter he discovered a radioactive caution sticker on the back of the frame. Concerned that their son would become radioactive, his parents called the paramedics. On arrival to the hospital, the radiation safety officer was notified. The patient was stripped of his clothing, which was collected, and his skin was washed with lukewarm water and soap. The patient's vital signs and clinical examination were normal. A portable dosimeter measured 28 µCi of radioactivity in the boy's urine from the isotope tritium (^{3}H), the radioactive source in the exit sign. Intravenous crystalloid fluids were administered to increase urine output, and the patient remained asymptomatic. He was discharged from the hospital the next day. Routine blood work remained normal several days later; however, long-term outcome and genotoxicity remain to be evaluated.

INTRODUCTION

Over the last century, radiation injuries and the nature of radiation itself have been vigorously studied as a result of the expanding uses and prevalence of radiation in our society. Today, radionuclides are used for a wide variety of purposes ranging from detecting smoke to powering spacecraft. Although useful, radionuclides can present a danger to humans chiefly through the particles they emit during the process of radioactive decay. This ionizing radiation may cause injury to cellular structures and molecules, such as DNA, and may result in mutations, neoplasms, or cell death. The particles of radiation, their sources, and the mechanisms by which they pose a health risk are the subjects of the following discussion.

HISTORICAL EXPOSURES

Radiation as a toxin became a concern for scientists only a year following the discovery of x-rays by Wilhelm Roentgen in 1895.[62] Thomas Edison conducted thousands of experiments using an x-ray generator of his own design. He reported corneal injuries in several of his workers in 1896. Eight years later, Clarence Dally, one of Edison's most dependable assistants, became the first radiation-related death in the United States.[19]

Physicians quickly recognized this new tool and began to manufacture x-ray machines to help diagnose various illnesses. Very closely following the development of x-rays that appeared to reveal the inner structure of objects, the British army developed and used mobile x-ray machines to find bullets and shrapnel in wounded soldiers in the Sudan.

However, over the next 10 to 15 years, radioactive substances also found their way into society as objects of fascination and as a means of alternative medical therapies. Energetically marketed as cure-alls, products such as the Revigator and Radithor enticed people to drink water charged with radon or radium. These products ushered in 20 years of health products using radioactive materials.[38,39]

In 1915, the British Roentgen Society, recognizing the potential hazards of radiation, proposed standards for radiation protection of workers, which included shielding, restricted work hours, and medical examinations. However, no dose limits were in effect because dose quantitation and measurement were unavailable.

The opening of the Radium Luminous Materials Corporation in Orange, New Jersey in 1917 represented the first of several companies to profit from the novelty and popularity of radium's bluish glow. In an industry that eventually employed over 4000 workers, nearly all of whom were female, the radium was hand-painted onto watch and instrument dials. These young women were instructed to obtain a fine tip on their paintbrushes using a technique called "lip pointing," which meant using their lips and tongues to shape their paintbrushes. Unaware of the danger, some of these women also painted their nails, lips, and eyelids with the radioactive paint. By 1927, about 100 of these women died from osteosarcoma, brain tumors, and developed other noncancerous lesions of the mouth, all related to radium exposure.[40,48]

The only wartime use of a nuclear bomb occurred in August 1945 when the United States dropped two bombs, Little Boy and Fat Man, on Hiroshima and Nagasaki, Japan, respectively.[17] Little Boy used a uranium core and liberated energy equivalent to 12,500 tons of TNT. Fat Man used a plutonium core and liberated an energy equivalent to 20,000 tons of TNT. Estimates of dead and injured for both cities are well over 200,000.[23] Most of the deaths were from the bomb blast, but many thousands died from acute radiation syndrome (ARS) and radiation-induced cancers. In addition to the people of those cities who were victims of the bombs, at least 20,000 men and women from Britain, Australia, New Zealand, and India who formed the British Commonwealth Occupation Forces (BCOF) were also exposed to residual radiation as they were involved in security and clean-up tasks. There are even records of Australian soldiers playing football on the flattened hypocenter of Hiroshima.[53,54] Since that time there have been thousands of nuclear bomb tests around the world in the atmosphere, underground, and underwater.

With the beginning of the nuclear age also came criticality events of varying kinds where individuals were exposed to large amounts of radiation. Criticality refers to the chain reaction of fissionable atoms that results in the release of energy. It is the basic operating principle behind fission bombs and nuclear reactors and is an efficient means of generating energy. Two criticality events occurred in Los Alamos in 1945 during experiments in which scientists performed what was called "tickling the dragon." In the 1940s determining the amount of fissionable material necessary to precipitate a chain reaction was less of a calculation and more trial and error. Harry Daghlian and Louis Slotin, two scientists involved in the development of the first atomic bomb, were to bring subcritical amounts of fissionable material together to see if a reaction would occur. Both men died of ARS following exposure to high levels of radiation released during these experiments. Since 1945, there have been numerous criticality events, the most recent occurring in Tokaimura, Japan in 1999. In this instance, workers making fuel for nuclear reactors allowed too much uranium to enter an improper container. The critical event that resulted killed one worker and caused the evacuation of all the people living within 350 meters of the manufacturing plant.

During the early 1950s, radiologists utilized a thorium-containing contrast agent called Thoratrast. During that time when imaging modalities were limited, the α-emitting thorium dioxide provided critical medical information. Unfortunately, thorium was discovered to accumulate in hepatic tissue and to have a very slow elimination rate. Cases of thorium-induced hepatic carcinomas and angiosarcomas led to its eventual discontinuance.

Although many nuclear reactor incidents occur around the world, the most serious occurred at Chernobyl in Ukraine in 1986. In this instance, a series of errors led to a fire at the reactor core, several explosions, and a meltdown of the reactor. Over the first 10 days following the incident, a cloud spread to the Baltic States, Scandinavia, and Europe carrying radioactive material, predominantly ^{131}I and ^{137}Cs. In addition to the 31 people who died in the first few weeks following the event of ARS, nearly 250 others in the surrounding area were hospitalized, and an unknown number suffered other long-term sequelae.[18,21,33]

Not all radiation events occur at nuclear facilities. In September 1987 in Goiânia, Brazil, two men scavenged the contents of an abandoned medical clinic and unwittingly opened a source of ^{137}Cs. As in the early part of the century, the fascinating bluish glow contributed to many radiation exposures, some of them quite extensive. In the end, the government monitored approximately 113,000 individuals and found nearly 250 individuals who were contaminated.[44]

THE PRINCIPLES OF RADIOACTIVITY

Particles of Radiation

A 15th century word, radiation is defined as energy sent out in the form of waves or particles. Although considered by physicists as outdated and inaccurate, the particle-wave theory remains a useful model by which to understand the toxicologic aspects of radiation.

Photons are massless particles that travel at the speed of light and mediate electromagnetic radiation. Depending on the energy of the particles, and therefore their wavelength, the radiation has different names. Radiation having the lowest energy and the longest wavelength are called radio waves. As photons become more energetic and have shorter wavelengths, they are called, sequentially, microwaves, heat or infrared, visible light, and ultraviolet. γ and x-rays have greater energy than ultraviolet and can penetrate deeply into the body, which makes them useful for radi-

ation therapy. X-rays and γ rays are similar except that x-rays consist of a spectrum of different wavelengths, whereas γ rays have a fixed value specific to the radioactive material from which they radiate. Because of their small size and high energy, γ radiation and x-rays can penetrate several feet of insulating concrete.

β *particles* are also called electrons. They are emitted during β-decay from an unstable radionuclide, which is an atom that disintegrates by emitting a particle, electromagnetic radiation or both. Positrons, positively charged electrons, may also be emitted during decay processes. High-energy electrons have less penetration than gamma radiation but may still pass several centimeters into human skin.[71] β particles cause health problems chiefly through incorporation, which occurs when a radionuclide is inhaled, ingested, or deposited on a wound, thus gaining direct access to body tissues.[4]

α *particles* are helium nuclei (two protons and two neutrons) stripped of their electrons. These relatively massive particles are emitted during α decay. These particles are the most easily shielded of the emitted particles mentioned and are stopped by a piece of paper or clothing. Like β particles, α particles principally cause health effects only when they are incorporated.

Neutrons are primarily released from nuclear fission, although high-energy photon beams used in radiotherapy may also produce them. The natural decay of radionuclides does not include emission of neutrons. This is mainly a health hazard for workers in a nuclear power facility or victims of a nuclear explosion. Unique among the particles of radioactivity, when neutrons are stopped or captured they can cause a previously stable atom to become radioactive. This is the principle behind radioactive fallout.

Cosmic rays complete the group of various kinds of radiation to which an individual may be exposed. Cosmic rays are streams of electrons, protons, and α particles thought to emanate from stars and supernovas. They rain down on the earth from all directions only to give up their energy as they strike the nuclei of oxygen and nitrogen in the upper reaches of the earth's atmosphere. By the time it reaches the earth, the energy of cosmic radiation is reduced by several orders of magnitude. Traveling or living at altitude where the atmosphere shields relatively less cosmic radiation naturally means greater exposure to cosmic rays but in general is not considered a toxicologic threat to humans.

Ionizing Radiation versus Nonionizing Radiation

Ionizing radiation refers to any radiation with sufficient energy to disrupt an atom or molecule with which it impacts. In this interaction, an electron is removed or some other decay process occurs, leaving behind a changed atom. Depending on the specifics of the interaction, these atoms may now be charged, ionized, or highly reactive free radicals. Hydroxyl free radicals, formed by ionizing water, are responsible for biochemical lesions that are the foundation of radiation toxicity (Chap. 12).

The space between collisions of ionizing radiation and their target molecules vary with the particle type and its energy. For example, because of its large size, collisions along the path of an α particle are clustered together, limiting its ability to penetrate tissue. By comparison, collisions along the path of γ rays are spread out, increasing their ability to penetrate tissue. It is this ability to penetrate tissue and transfer energy that accounts for the relative dangers of the forms of radiation and tissue susceptibility. The rate at which ionizing radiation transfers its energy to target molecules is called the linear energy transfer (LET), which is expressed in kiloelectron volts per micrometer (keV/µm; Table 99–1).

For a source of radiation to pose a threat to tissue, the ionizing particle must be placed in close proximity to where it can do its damage. High-energy photons penetrate deeply and so pose a similar risk whether they come from an external source or from an incorporated source. α and β particles have much more limited tissue penetration. In general, radionuclides that radiate these particles must first be incorporated to pose a threat to tissue because clothing and skin usually offer a sufficient barrier.

Nonionizing radiation spans a wide spectrum of electromagnetic radiation frequencies. Generally, nonionizing radiation consists of relatively low-energy photons and is used safely in cell phone and television signal transmission, radar, microwaves, and magnetic fields that emanate from high-voltage electricity and metal detectors. Although these are all considered radiation in that they are all energies released from a source, these photons lack the necessary energy required to cause ionization and cellular damage. However, damage to tissue may occur through the production of heat, as with microwaves.

There has been extensive investigation into the potentially harmful effects of these extremely low-frequency electromagnetic fields (EMF) in recent years. Among the investigated sources of EMF are cell phones, magnetic resonance imaging (MRI), ultraviolet (UV) rays, ultrasound, and high-voltage electric wiring. Although the literature is replete with experimental studies of many kinds, the results often suffer from poor design, complicated confounders, and a general lack of reproducibility. With the exception of the association between UV light (sunlight) and melanoma, the experimental literature concerning health risks from nonionizing radiation leaves the answers poorly defined.[56, 66]

Radioactive Decay

Many atomic nuclei are unstable despite the nuclear forces that hold them together. In 1900, Marie Curie discovered that unstable nuclei decay or transform into more stable nuclei (daughters) via the emission of various particles or energy. Radioactive decay occurs through five mechanisms: emission of γ rays, α particles, β particles, or positrons, or capture of an electron (see above). It is

the emission of these various particles that makes radioactive decay dangerous to humans because these particles form ionizing radiation.

The half-life ($t_{1/2}$), a term first utilized by Ernest Rutherford in 1904, is the period of time it takes for a radioisotope to lose half of its radioactivity. Every radioisotope has a characteristic half-life. Some isotopes exist for millionths of a second, and others last billions of years. In every case, the activities of radioactive isotopes diminish exponentially with time. The equation $R = R_0 e^{-\lambda t}$ describes radioactive decay, where R is the activity, R_0 is initial activity, t is time, and λ is the decay constant. Each radioisotope has its own decay constant (Table 99–1).

Radiation Units of Measure

The amount of radiation to which an object is exposed, that is, the amount emitted from a source that falls on an object, is given in units called roentgens (R). A roentgen is a unit for measuring the quantity of x-ray or γ radiation by measuring the amount of ionization produced in air. It may be loosely defined as the amount of x-radiation that produces one electrostatic unit of charge in one cubic centimeter of air at standard temperature and pressure. As an example, an individual standing at a given distance from the x-ray–generating tube of a particular x-ray machine is exposed, on the skin, to a particular number of roentgens of x-rays.

Not all roentgens to which an individual is exposed pose a risk for cellular damage. Much of the radiation passes through the body and does not cause harm. Only the fraction of that given number of roentgens that is absorbed by the tissue has a probability of causing cellular damage. The unit that describes absorbed radiation is the rad (radiation absorbed dose), which corresponds to an absorption of energy in any medium of 100 ergs/g [an erg is the unit of energy in the centimeter-gram-second (cgs) scale]. The units of the International System (SI), first introduced in the 1970s, have largely replaced the older units of the cgs. The gray (Gy) is the corresponding SI unit to the rad and is equivalent to 100 rads.

Not all radiations produce the same effects at the tissue level. For example, a given number of grays of x-rays produce less cellular damage than the same number of grays of α particles when all other conditions are equal. To predict the degree of damage that radiation of any type may cause, other units of measure are needed to normalize the different potencies in terms of their risk. The rem (roentgen equivalent man, in cgs) and the sievert (Sv, in SI) are the units that allow this calculation. These units are useful for comparing the effects of different radiations or evaluating the danger of a mixture of radiations, such as in radioactive decay, where some isotopes emit more than one kind of radiation at a time (eg, β and γ). In defining rem, x-rays are the standard radiation for comparison. One rem may be defined as the dose of radiation that produces damage equivalent to one rad of x-rays (or 0.01 Sv). Thus, for x-rays, one Sv is equivalent to 100 rem. To perform the normalization, the dose in grays is multiplied by a relative biologic effectiveness-dependent quality factor (Q). This factor Q multiplies the amount of radiation by 1 for x-rays and β particles, 2 for α particles, and by 5 or more for neutron radiation. Thus, 1 Sv is equivalent to 1 Gy of x-rays. As a very coarse reference point, a regular chest x-ray imparts about 20 to 40 mrem or 0.2 to 0.4 mSv to an individual, but it must be remembered that this radiation dose is delivered very quickly to a limited portion of the body and is quite different from a similar amount delivered over a

TABLE 99–1. Physical Properties of Radioisotopes

Isotope	Half-Life	Mode of Decay	Decay Energy (MeV)[a]
^{47}Ca	4.53 days	β$^-$	1.979
^{14}C	5730 years	β$^-$	0.156
^{51}Cr	27.8 days	Electron capture	0.752
^{57}Co	270 days	Electron capture	0.837
^{67}Cu	61.8 hours	β$^-$	0.576
^{3}H	12.26 years	β$^-$	0.02
^{123}I	13.3 hours	Electron capture	1.4
^{131}I	8 days	β$^-$	0.970
^{40}K	1.28×10^9 years	β$^-$/β$^+$ electron capture	1.35/l.505
^{32}P	14.3 days	β$^-$	1.710
^{222}Rn	3.8 days	α	5.587
^{85}Sr	64 days	Electron capture	1.11
^{201}Tl	73 hours	Electron capture	0.41
^{238}U	4.51×10^9 years	α	4.268
^{133}Xe	5.27 days	β$^-$	0.427

[a]Energy is given in mega-electron volts.

longer period of time to a worker through an occupational exposure.

In 1910, the curie (Ci) became the unit defining the activity of radioactive decay. One curie equals 3.7×10^{10} disintegrations per second based on the decay of 1 g of radium. The SI unit is the becquerel (Bq), named for Antoine Henri Becquerel, who first reported invisible emanations from naturally occurring minerals that fogged photographic plates in 1896. One becquerel is equivalent to one disintegration per second (thus, 1 Ci is equivalent to 3.7×10^{10} Bq). This number corresponds to an amount of radioactivity in a source. For example, following the Chernobyl incident, 1.2×10^7 TBq (terabecquerel, 1.2×10^{19} disintegrations per second) of radioactive material was released into the atmosphere. By comparison, the men who removed the source of ^{137}Cs in Goiânia found 50.9 TBq (50.9×10^{12}) of cesium. A thallium stress test utilizes 111×10^6 Bq (3 mCi) of ^{201}Tl, and the average indoor concentration of ^{222}Rn in the United States is 55 Bq/m^3.

Irradiation versus Contamination versus Incorporation

An object that is irradiated is exposed to ionizing radiation. This type of exposure includes handling radioactive isotopes, medical diagnostic imaging modalities such as x-ray machines and CT scanners, and rare exposures to criticality events. These sources of ionizing radiation can generate high-energy photons, which penetrate tissue well and have the potential to cause tissue damage. A whole-body irradiation is one in which the entire body is exposed at once, whereas more commonly shielding devices, such as lead aprons, and collimation techniques limit the amount of exposed tissue to the intended target. The risk of tissue damage depends on the total amount of radiation and the tissue type itself because different tissue types have their own intrinsic resistance to radiation damage. An irradiated object does not become radioactive itself (unless exposed by neutrons), and although it may suffer from the effects of the radiation, it does not become a radiation hazard.

Contamination occurs when a radioactive substance covers an object completely or in part. Several examples include a laboratory worker who unintentionally spills a radioactive nuclide on his or her clothes or skin or a victim of an industrial spill whose skin and clothes are soiled by a substance containing a radioactive nuclide. In these similar cases, the source of radiation is the nuclide undergoing its normal decay process, and the individual is exposed to particles such as those mentioned in Table 99–1. The risk for tissue damage is usually quite low, assuming that the contamination is detected and appropriate measures for decontamination are instituted.

Incorporation is a third type of potential exposure. When an individual is exposed via inhalation, ingestion, intravenous administration, or percutaneously, radionuclides that are normally stopped by the skin may be absorbed and concentrated into tissue. This principle is utilized in many diagnostic and therapeutic procedures such as bone scans, gallium scans, liver and spleen scans, and strontium-89 therapy. However, depending on the dose and type of radionuclide used, incorporation may lead to tissue damage, as was the situation for many people following the event at Chernobyl. In this instance, the release of particulate radiation contaminated with ^{131}I gained access to tissues, resulting in an increase in thyroid cancer among children and adolescents in the most contaminated regions of Ukraine and Belarus.[5,31,68]

EPIDEMIOLOGY

Everyone is exposed to radiation in one form or another each day. The various sources and quantities of ionizing radiation Americans are exposed to on an annual basis are presented in Table 99–2. There are naturally occurring sources of radiation in the earth's crust that make the largest annual contribution to man's radiation exposure, and man-made sources of radiation, which make a relatively smaller contribution to our average annual exposure.

Exposures to man-made sources of radiation are not required to be reported and in general do not result in significant morbidity. However, the AAPCC TESS reports 191 exposures to radioactive isotopes in 1998, of which 166 (87%) were unintentional, and 15 (8%) involved children under 6 years of age. No deaths were reported (p. 1752 and Chap. 116).

Natural Sources of Radiation

A wide variety of natural sources expose humans on a daily basis to ionizing radiation. In the United States the estimated annual dose equivalent of radiation is 3.6 mSv, and natural sources contribute about 80% of that annual dose.[8,19] Terrestrial sources of radiation originate from radionuclides in the earth's crust that move into the air and water. These primordial radionuclides, so named because their physical half-lives are comparable to the age of the earth, include uranium, actinium, and thorium. Geographic areas vary with regard to the content of these radionuclides.

Radon, a radioactive noble gas, accounts for most of the human exposure to radiation from natural sources. This gas, a natural decay product of uranium and thorium, enters homes and other buildings from the building materials themselves or through microscopic cracks in the building's structures. Radon poses a risk to humans via inhalation and exposure to the lung tissue and is associated with an increased incidence of lung cancer.[50] This risk of lung cancer is further increased for heavy smokers who additionally expose their lungs to 200 mSv from ^{210}Po (a radon daughter) that is naturally found in tobacco smoke. Areas of New York, New Jersey, and Pennsylvania, called the Reading Prong, have particu-

TABLE 99–2. Average Annual Amount of Ionizing Radiation Received in the United States

Source	Dose[a]	
	mSv[b]	%
Natural	2.94	82
Radon[c]	2.0	55
Cosmic	0.27	8
Terrestrial	0.28	8
Internal	0.39	11
Man-made	0.63	18
X-ray diagnosis	0.39	11
Nuclear medicine	0.14	4
Consumer products	0.10	3
Occupational	<0.01	<0.3
Total	**3.6**	**100**

[a]All doses are averages and contain some variability within the measurement.
[b]mSv = millisieverts.
[c]Average effective dose to bronchial epithelium alone.

larly high levels of radon as a result of a richer concentration in the earth's crust of primordial radionuclides that liberate radon. The Environmental Protection Agency has recommended household level intervention when radon levels exceed 147 Bq/m^3 (4 pCi/L). Individuals can test their own homes for radon with either short-term (less than 90 days) or long-term (greater than 90 days) commercially available measurement devices.

The second largest natural source of radiation originates from ingested radionuclides, of which ^{40}K, a naturally occurring isotope, is the most abundant. Together with other primordial radionuclides in our diet, this source of internal radiation accounts for about 12% of the annual dose of absorbed radiation.

Man-Made Sources

As mentioned earlier, man-made sources of radiation can be found in many consumer products and in many different types of industry (Table 99–3). The National Council on Radiation Protection and Measurements (NCRP) estimates the annual number of workers exposed to radiation to be nearly a million.[19] On average, those occupations with the highest exposures (about 12 mSv/yr) are uranium miners, nuclear power operators, and sailors in close proximity to nuclear reactors. Those with lesser additional exposures (about 1–2 mSv/yr) include physicians, x-ray technologists, nuclear fuel processing workers, and workers in other industries that use radionuclides.

Medical occupational exposure principally includes physicians, nurses, and x-ray technologists, who receive an additional annual effective dose of about 1 mSv. This dose can range up to 17 mSv with certain techniques such as fluoroscopy but are only partial body exposures because of the appropriate use of lead aprons and other protective barriers. Medical procedures also account for substantial annual exposure to man-made radiation for patients. In 1989, the NCRP estimated the annual number of various diagnostic procedures involving radiation in the United States to exceed 250 million. Medical sources of exposure to patients account for about 0.5 mSv or 15% of the average annual exposure.

Exposures have been studied in emergency physicians, orthopedists, and interventional cardiologists.[20,30,69,72] Each of these fields utilizes different modalities of radiation, which pose different risks to the individual performing the procedure. Two studies examining exposure to physicians assisting in cervical spine x-rays found the calculated whole-body exposure ranged up to 0.027 mSv per procedure, or 0.75% of the estimated annual dose equivalent of radiation in the United States.[30,72] This exposure annualized over a year neared the NCRP upper limits of safety and might be exceeded if the number of procedures were to increase. Two other studies examined physician exposure to radiation by fluoroscopy used in interventional cardiology and orthopedic procedures. These doses ranged from 0.05 to 0.3 mSv per procedure. In each of these four studies, appropriate shielding was used, and dosimeters measured individual areas of exposed body parts such as extremities and the head. Radiation was undetectable beneath a lead apron. Estimated whole-body exposures to these procedures were considered not to exceed the limits established by OSHA of 50 mSv per year. Although the likelihood of exceeding established radiation limits is low regardless of the procedure, and even assuming a reasonable increase in the number of procedures performed, appropriate shielding and safety training are emphasized to minimize the risk of exposure.

TABLE 99–3. Uses of Radioisotopes

Americium-241	Used in smoke detectors, measure lead levels in paint, steel, and paper production
Cadmium-109	Analyze metal alloys
Calcium-47	Biomedical research of cell function and bone formation
Californium-252	Inspect luggage for explosives, gauge moisture content of soil and silo materials
Carbon-14	Pharmaceutical research, radiometric dating
Cesium-137	Measure dosages of radioactive pharmaceuticals, oil industry to measure flow in pipelines
Chromium-51	Red blood cell survival studies
Cobalt-57	Nuclear medicine
Copper-67	Chemotherapy
Curium-244	Mining industry
Iodine-123	Diagnosis of thyroid disorders
Iodine-129	Used to check some radioactivity counters in in vitro diagnostic testing laboratories
Iodine-131	Treatment of thyroid disorders
Iridium-192	Test the integrity of pipeline welds, boilers, and aircraft parts
Iron-55	Analyze electroplating solutions
Krypton-85	Indicator lights, textile industry
Nickel-63	Detect explosives, voltage regulators, surge protectors
Phosphorus-32	Molecular biology and genetics research
Plutonium-238	Power source for NASA spacecraft
Polonium-210	Photographic film production
Promethium-147	Thermostats, textile industry
Radium-226	Lightning rods
Selenium-75	Protein studies
Sodium-24	Industrial pipelines integrity
Strontium-85	Study bone formation and metabolism
Technetium-99m	Nuclear medicine
Thallium-204	Measures pollutant levels, textile industry
Thoriated tungsten	Electric arc welding
Thorium-229	Fluorescent lights
Thorium-230	Coloring and fluorescence in colored glazes and glassware
Tritium	Basic science and pharmaceutical studies, for self-luminous signs, luminous dials, gauges, and wrist watches; luminous paint
Uranium-234	Dental fixtures
Uranium-235	Fuel for nuclear power plants and naval nuclear propulsion systems, fluorescent glassware, colored glazes, and wall tiles
Xenon-133	Nuclear medicine

Various medical scans utilize radioactive nuclides to study various disease processes, some of which are noted in Table 99–4. Other radionuclides utilized in medical diagnostics include indium-111, gallium-67, and chromium-51. Other scientific research utilizes tritium (^{3}H) and phosphorus-32. These nuclides decay through β-particle capture or emission. In general, unintentional topical exposure to these radionuclides in this setting is not considered hazardous because skin and clothing provide adequate barriers against the poorly penetrating particles emitted. In the case of unintentional incorporation, it is highly unlikely that the amount infused will be sufficient to cause a serious health risk.

Depleted uranium (DU) is used by the military of the United States and several other governments as an alloy for tank-killer projectiles. ^{235}U is extracted from naturally occurring uranium, re-

TABLE 99–4. Nuclear Medicine Procedures: The Type and Amount of Radionuclide

Test	Radionuclide	Amount
Whole-body bone scan	^{99}Tc	25 mCi
Radionuclide cerebral angiogram	^{99}Tc-DTPA	15 mCi
Cardiac ejection scan (MUGA)	TcO$_4$	20 mCi
DISIDA/hepatobiliary scan	^{99}Tc-DISIDA	5 mCi
Ventilation/perfusion scan	^{133}Xe/^{99}Tc-MAA	10 mCi/4 mCi
Thyroid scan	^{123}I	200 μCi
Myocardial perfusion scan (exercise)	^{201}Tl/^{99}Tc-sestamibi	3 mCi/20 mCi
Strontium-89 therapy	^{89}Sr	4 mCi
Venogram	Tc-pertechnetate	20 mCi

ducing the overall radioactivity by about 40%. The ^{238}U that remains is called "depleted." Munitions made of this alloy, which is favored because of its density, are fired at extremely high velocities to penetrate the target armor. Exposure to α radiation emitted from ^{238}U is considered a negligible radiation hazard, although currently many studies are investigating the potential link between DU and the incidence of leukemias, other cancers, and birth defects.[3,7,11,14,28,42,43,45,46,49]

EXPOSURE LIMITS

The various agencies involved in regulating radiation exposures to both workers and the public include the Occupational Safety and Health Administration (OSHA), the Nuclear Regulatory Commission (NRC), and the Department of Transportation. The NRC has established "Standards for Protection against Radiation," which regulates radiation exposures using a twofold system of dose limitation: doses to individuals shall not exceed limits established by the NRC, and all exposures shall be kept as low as reasonably achievable (ALARA). The total effective dose equivalent may not exceed 50 mSv/yr to reduce the risk of stochastic effects (see the following discussion on stochastic vs deterministic injury). The dose to the fetus of a pregnant radiation worker may not exceed 5 mSv over 9 months and should not substantially exceed 0.5 mSv in any one month, although this amount is not carefully defined.[27, 57]

PATHOPHYSIOLOGY

Ionizing radiation causes both direct and indirect damage to tissue, where the cell's radiosensitivity is directly related to its rate of proliferation and inversely related to its degree of differentiation.[52] Directly, radiation impacts on the target molecule and causes damage. If the target molecule is DNA, a mutation may arise, which may then result in alteration of a germ line, development of a neoplasm, or cell death. The risk of these consequences, however, is low because of the relative paucity of DNA within a cell and the even smaller percentage of active DNA within a given cell.

Indirectly, radiation impacts a molecule and creates a reactive species, which may chemically react with organic molecules in cells, altering their structure or function. These radiation-induced ions are quite unstable, however, and usually convert to free radicals. Most importantly, radiation may impact a water molecule, which is in great abundance, to generate a hydroxyl radical (OH•).[19] The hydroxyl radical diffuses only a short distance

through the tissue because of its highly reactive nature and itself causes molecular damage (Chap. 12).

Direct damage predominates with high-LET radiations (see above), whereas indirect damage predominates with low-LET radiations.[19] Although any molecule may be damaged in a variety of ways that may lead to cell injury of varying severity, double-stranded breaks in DNA are the type of damage most likely to cause chromosomal aberrations or cell death.[32] Thousands of these types of lesions occur daily in the human body from natural radiation.

For this reason, there are several mechanisms that protect and repair damage that may result from either direct or indirect means of radiation damage. It is estimated that up to 90% of all chromosomal breaks heal by adhesion in a process known as "restitution." All that is required for DNA to heal is oxygen and time, which forms the basis for fractionated radiation therapy. Because many types of cancer repair their damage less efficiently than do normal cells, radiation damage will accumulate in cancer cells during radiation therapy, and more cancer cells are killed. Sulfhydryl-containing molecules, such as glutathione, and other scavengers provide protection against free radicals. These molecules react with free radicals and inactivate them quickly, thus limiting the damage they can cause. Following a large radiation exposure, however, both restitution and the protection provided by free radical scavengers may be overwhelmed, and damage may occur.

STOCHASTIC VERSUS DETERMINISTIC EFFECTS OF RADIATION

The radiation damage just described has two consequential results: it kills cells or it alters cells and causes cancer. Injuries that do not require a threshold limit to be exceeded include mutagenic and carcinogenic changes to individual cells where DNA is the critical target. This is the stochastic effect of radiation. Theoretically, there is no dose of radiation too small to have the potential of causing cancer in an exposed individual.[9] Current theories suggest that a single dose of radiation causes a change in the genome that potentially alters the structure of a protooncogene, control of an oncogene, or activates oncogenic viruses in hosts.[22] These effects may take several months to years to manifest.

Whereas the stochastic effects of radiation may follow less severe exposures, such as prolonged exposure to radon gas, the deterministic effects of radiation usually follow a large whole-body exposure, such as a Chernobyl- or Tokaimura-type event. In terms of cell death, a relatively large number of cells of an organ system must be killed before an effect becomes clinically evident. This number of killed cells constitutes a threshold limit that must be exceeded, and this is what is known as the deterministic or nonstochastic effects of radiation. The ARS is an important example of the deterministic effects of radiation (see below).

ACUTE RADIATION SYNDROME

The Army Medical Corps first described the acute radiation syndrome in 1946 when victims of the explosions at Hiroshima and Nagasaki were admitted for treatment at Osaka University Hospital.[34] Understanding the features of ARS is essential for managing a patient who is exposed to a large whole-body irradiation, generally considered to be 2 Sv (500 times the average annual exposure) or more. In many cases, a reliable estimate of the radiation dose is difficult, thus making it more practical to focus on the clinical features of radiation injury and their prognostic utility.

The acute radiation syndrome involves a sequence of events that varies with the severity of the exposure.[16] Generally, more severe exposures lead to more rapid onset of symptoms and more severe clinical features. There are four classic clinical stages described, which begin with the early prodromal stage of nausea and vomiting. These symptoms begin anywhere from minutes to hours postexposure and may last a few hours to a few days. Although the time to onset postexposure is inversely proportional to the dose received, the duration of the prodromal phase is directly proportional to the dose. That is, the greater the dose received, the more rapid the onset of symptoms, and the longer the duration, except in cases where death follows rapidly.[52] Except following the highest doses of radiation, symptoms usually subside within hours, and patients generally recover. The second, or latent stage begins at this time and may last from several days to weeks. During this period, the patient may feel well and have no other clinically apparent difficulties. The duration of this stage is inversely related to dose. The third stage usually begins in the third to fifth week after exposure with severe gastrointestinal disturbances, abdominal pain, fever, bleeding, infection, and epilation. The various systems failures that are responsible for the third stage are described below. The fourth stage is recovery and may last weeks to months before it is completed.

These four stages describe the clinical manifestations that may be observed as a result of massive exposure, but the various systems of the body manifest their own injuries, which constitute several subsyndromes.[16] These subsyndromes are not mutually exclusive of one another and may overlap as cell death or damage progresses. The CNS syndrome describes the manifestations of injury to the central nervous system following massive irradiation. This syndrome, following exposure to radiation doses of about 15 Sv or greater, is characterized by rapid or immediate onset of pyrexia, ataxia, loss of motor control, apathy, lethargy, and seizures, resulting from free radical–induced massive cell death and cerebral edema. Historically, the occurrence of hypotension and dysrhythmias was considered to be part of a neurovascular syndrome. However, a cardiovascular (CV) syndrome may be a more accurate term, deriving from autopsy evidence of myocardial necrosis following massive radiation exposure. Once these subsyndromes are manifest, they may never resolve.[13,16,52,58]

The gastrointestinal (GI) syndrome may begin following an exposure to about 5 Sv or more where there is gastrointestinal mucosal cell injury and death. Symptoms include anorexia, nausea and vomiting, and diarrhea. As the mucosal lining is sloughed, there may be persistent bloody diarrhea, hypersecretion of cellular fluids into the lumen, and a loss of peristalsis, which may progress to abdominal distension and dehydration. Destruction of the mucosal lining allows for colonization by enteric organisms and sepsis.

The hematologic changes that occur following an exposure to about 1 to 5 Sv are called the hematopoietic syndrome. Hematopoietic stem cells are highly radiosensitive, in contrast to the more mature erythrocytes and platelets. Lymphocytes are also radiosensitive and can die quickly from cell lysis following an exposure. This contrasts with granulocytes, which endure radiation better. In addition to stem cell death and white cell depletion with immunodeficiency, platelets are consumed in gingival and gastrointestinal microhemorrhages. The main effect of radiation-induced hematopoietic syndrome is pancytopenia leading to death from sepsis complicated by hemorrhage. A lymphocyte nadir typically occurs 8 to 30 days postexposure, with higher doses achieving earlier nadir.[15]

The pulmonary system is not spared injury from irradiation. Pneumonitis may occur within 1 to 3 months following a dose of 6 to 10 Sv. This may lead to respiratory failure, pulmonary fibrosis, or cor pulmonale months or years later.

DOSE ESTIMATION AND PROGNOSIS

Determining the dose received by an individual who was irradiated is important in providing appropriate therapy and establishing a prognosis. However, estimating the dose received is difficult for a number of reasons, such as the absence of a radiation-monitoring device, exposure to radiation of mixed form (such as γ and neutron radiation), and partial shielding of various body parts.[58] In cases of whole-body irradiation, it is the ARS itself that allows for an estimate of the radiation dose received. The onset of symptoms and their severity provide a rough idea of the severity of the exposure, although evaluating the white blood cell count makes a more accurate estimate.[52]

As previously mentioned, the hematopoietic syndrome manifests as a fall in the lymphocyte count. This presents a relatively accurate estimate of dose received up to about 3 Sv. At higher doses of radiation, lymphocytes tend to lyse in great numbers. Peripheral granulocytes do not lyse to the same extent as lymphocytes and are therefore more reliable in estimating radiation dose than lymphocytes at doses greater than 3 Sv. If the absolute lymphocyte count is greater than 1200/mm^3 at 48 hours, the patient is unlikely to have received a fatal dose. If at 48 hours the lymphocyte count is as low as 300 to 1200/mm^3, a fatal dose may have been received, and this indicates the need for more aggressive supportive measures. The severity of thrombocytopenia and reticulocytopenia may also indicate the severity of the radiation dose. Additional radiation dose estimators include the presence and number of dicentric chromosomes in blood and bone marrow.[1,51]

Those patients receiving 5 to 20 Sv may survive if they receive optimal supportive care. This dose may be received from a criticality event, such as at Tokaimura, or from severe events such as at Chernobyl. After the Tokaimura event, one worker who received 17 Sv died 3 months after his exposure. At Chernobyl, 20 of 21 workers who were exposed to radiation in the 6 to 16 Sv range expired despite receiving intensive supportive care, while 7 of 21 who were exposed to 4 to 6 Sv died. Survival is inversely proportional to the radiation dose absorbed, and even the relatively radioresistant cell types can be killed by high amounts of radiation. For these reasons, 20 Sv or more of acutely absorbed radiation is considered supralethal.[61] CNS and CV syndromes can begin almost immediately, and death, which for triage purposes should be considered inevitable, will likely occur within 24 to 48 hours, before the other subsyndromes of ARS occur.

Within the group exposed to 5 to 20 Sv, depending on the dose received, there may be milder forms of CNS and CV syndromes that last for a longer time. A severe GI syndrome in which high fever and persistent hematochezia are present suggests a poor prognosis. This syndrome may overlap with a severe form of hematopoietic syndrome in which damage to bone marrow stem cells is so severe that bone marrow function may not recover for weeks or months. These patients will likely require bone marrow transplantation as well as multiple transfusions of platelets and red blood cells, optimal supportive care, and infection control to survive.

Patients exposed to radiation in the range of 2 to 5 Sv will likely survive with medical care. Although the median lethal dose of radiation for humans is estimated to be 4.5 Sv, the manifestations of ARS will be similar to those noted above but will likely be delayed and less severe. Many patients will survive without bone marrow transplantation if supportive care optimizes fluid and electrolyte replacement and controls bleeding and infection.

Survival is expected for those patients acutely exposed to less than 2 Sv with little medical intervention necessary. Mild forms of GI and hematopoietic syndromes may occur in delayed fashion compared to more severe exposures.

CARCINOGENESIS

There are good data to support that radiation increases the incidence of various cancers in humans. One of the most important sources of these data is life-span studies of atomic bomb survivors in Japan.[12] This group of people is extensively studied over the last half-century, and although the relative risks assigned to specific cancers are modified over the years and subject to interpretation, there is a general agreement that the incidences of leukemia (except CLL), female breast carcinoma, and thyroid cancer increase following a sufficient exposure.[22,29,53,60,63,64] Because of technical and logistic difficulties in performing appropriate studies, there is difficulty in estimating the cancer risk from exposure to low-dose radiation. This risk is largely extrapolated from models of high-dose exposures.[12] These cancers usually do not appear until years after the exposure. For those exposed while they are young, the excess incidence of cancer occurs only when they are at the age when those cancers otherwise appear in the unirradiated population.[19]

Pulmonary exposure to radon has been studied extensively in the last few years. Both uranium miners and household residents in areas such as New Jersey and Sweden, with excessive radon exposure, are at increased risk for developing lung cancer from exposure to radon gas. A cohort of nonsmoking uranium miners showed a 12-fold increased risk of lung cancer over controls, which is similar to the estimates of the increased risk of lung cancer caused by radiation exposure in atomic bomb survivors.[8, 55] Radon exposure in the residence is also associated with an increased risk of lung cancer and may be related to its concentration in the air as well as duration of exposure.[47,59] The increased risk of lung cancer from exposure to radon gas is modified by concurrent cigarette smoking, which may have a multiplicative effect rather than an additive effect.[47]

COMMONLY ENCOUNTERED RADIONUCLIDES

Most exposures that come to medical attention are not large, whole-body irradiations but are rather small spills in the laboratory or inadvertent exposures from one of many products that are commercially available. With the notable exception of a well-known case of massive americium contamination, the vast majority of these types of cases are not reported.[15,67]

■ *Americium* (symbol Am, atomic number 95, and atomic weight 243) Americium was discovered in 1946 in Chicago during the Manhattan Project. Its most stable isotope, americium-243, has a half-life of over 7500 years, although [241]Am, with a half-life of 470 years, was the first isotope to be isolated. It decays by α activity and γ emissions and will accumulate in bone if incorporated.[36] It is used to test machinery integrity, glass thickness, and in smoke detectors, where it ionizes the air between two electrodes and generates an electric current that soot may impede. α particles from these detectors are easily absorbed within a few centimeters of the surrounding air and pose little risk. One gram of americium oxide provides enough americium for more than 5000 smoke detectors. Potentially useful chelators include diethylenetriaminepentaacetic acid (DTPA) and linear tetrahydroxypyridinone (LIHOPO).

■ *Cesium* (symbol Cs, atomic number 55, and atomic weight 132) Bunsen discovered Cs spectroscopically in 1860. It decays by β activity and γ emissions and tends to follow the potassium cycle in nature, providing a whole-body dose if incorporated. It is used as a radiation source in radiation therapy and as a radionuclide source for atomic clocks. Potential chelators include Prussian blue and its several derivatives.[10,35]

■ *Iodine* (symbol I, atomic number 53, and atomic weight 126.9) Courtois discovered iodine in 1811. There are 23 isotopes of iodine; [127]I is the only stable one. [125]I is used in thyroid studies and decays by γ emissions. [131]I is used in metastatic surveys and decays by β activity and γ emissions. These isotopes will accumulate in thyroid tissue if incorporated and can cause local damage to thyroid tissue; however, the patient does not pose a danger to other humans because of this source of γ radiation. Prophylactic treatment with iodine may limit thyroid incorporation in the event of a large exposure.

■ *Phosphorus* (symbol P, atomic number 15, and atomic weight 30) Phosphorus was discovered in 1669 by Brand. [32]P has a half-life of 14 days and decays by β activity. The maximum range of decay particles in air is 20 feet, and in tissue, $^1/_3$ inch. For soluble ^{32}P compounds bone receives approximately 20% of the dose following ingestion or inhalation. Shielding for ^{32}P and other β emitters should be made of material with atomic numbers of less than 13 (aluminum) to reduce the generation of Bremsstrahlung x-rays (braking radiation), electromagnetic radiation produced by the rapid change of velocity of a fast moving particle as it approaches an atomic nucleus and is deflected.

■ *Radon* (symbol Rn, atomic number 86, and atomic weights range from 204 to −224) Discovered in 1900 by Dorn, it was first called *radium emanation,* then *niton,* and finally radon in 1923. Radon is the heaviest noble gas. Radon is the decay product of radium as well as a decay product of thorium and actinium, where it is also called thoron and actinon, respectively. [222]Rn decays by α activity and γ emissions. Exposure of radon gas to the pulmonary epithelium is associated with an increased incidence of lung cancer in both uranium miners and in those who dwell in residences with increased levels of radon. Damage to bronchial epithelium results from radon's α emissions as well as radiation from radon daughters that precipitate as solids and remain in the lungs. Good enclosed space ventilation, abstinence from cigarette smoking, and monitoring of radon levels will help to minimize this risk.

■ *Technetium* (symbol Tc, atomic number 43, and atomic weight 98.9) Discovered in 1937, it was the first element to be produced artificially. Tc does not exist in terrestrial materials but does seem to exist literally among the stars. [99]Tc is used in testicular, bone, and thyroid scans and has a half-life of 6 days. Tc decays by β activity and γ emission.

- *Thallium* (symbol Tl, atomic number 81, and atomic weight 204) Crookes discovered thallium spectroscopically in 1861. [201]Tl is used in cardiology, has a half-life of 73 hours, and decays by electron capture and gamma emission. Chelation is with Prussian blue (Chap. 83).
- *Tritium* is an isotope of hydrogen whose nucleus contains one proton and two neutrons, and its symbol is ^{3}H.[71] Tritium decays by β activity and is used in basic science research as a radioactive label, as well as for luminous dials. Tritium has a half-life of 12.25 years, and it tends to follow the water cycle in humans, providing a whole-body dose if incorporated. However, its biological half-life is 10 to 12 days, which can be decreased by increasing urine output, greatly limiting its potential toxicity.
- *Xenon* (symbol Xe, atomic number 54, and atomic weight 131) Ramsay and Travers discovered Xe in 1898. There are 31 isotopes of Xe, 22 of which are unstable. [133]Xe is used in ventilation/perfusion scans. Its half-life is 5.27 days, and it decays by β activity and γ emission.

EMERGENCY MANAGEMENT

When one or more patients who have been exposed to massive irradiation present to the emergency department (ED), attention must first be paid to the more conventional injuries that may also be present.[52] In a mass casualty setting, a triage center may be established to make a prehospital assessment. Many times radiation exposures occur with fires or explosions, and patients may have burns, smoke inhalation injuries, or traumatic injuries. Most survivable radiation injuries require prompt treatment but are not life threatening in the first few hours postevent. Thus, there is time to determine if the nature of the exposure was an irradiation or contamination by a radionuclide. Routine considerations of airway, breathing, and circulation take priority for these patients as with all others. If a patient should require surgery, the Armed Forces Radiobiology Research Institute (AFRRI) recommends that surgery proceed immediately because of the delayed and impaired wound healing associated with irradiated tissue.

Other smaller-scale exposures to radiation still require at least a brief evaluation for burns and trauma, depending on the circumstances surrounding the nature of the exposure. Calls to the poison center from a residence require referral to emergency services for an expert evaluation of the level of contamination of the site and appropriate decontamination measures. Exposures in the laboratory or nuclear medicine suites require referral to the radiation safety officer in the building for a similar evaluation.

Decontamination

Patients exposed to radionuclides may be contaminated with radioactive material either externally or internally or both. Historically no medical personnel have ever developed ARS through exposure to a contaminated patient, although caution must be exercised when performing decontamination to minimize exposure to care providers. Unless there is active ongoing radiation, many authors recommend decontamination at the site of exposure to minimize the spread of radioactive materials.[52] All clothing should

be removed, and patients should be thoroughly washed in soap and water. Solutions used successfully in the past have included green soap, phosphate-based detergents, and chelating agents such as EDTA and DTPA.[58] This can remove up to 95% of radioactive material from the patient. Open wounds should be scrubbed to minimize the risk of internal contamination. A portable dosimeter may assist in external decontamination. If the patient was exposed to neutron radiation such as from a nuclear reactor, blood samples testing for induced [24]Na by γ-spectrophotometric analysis may help as an additional indicator of total dose received. Collected emesis and feces may also be analyzed, if desired, to help estimate total body dose. All clothing and liquid used to decontaminate must be collected and be clearly marked as radioactive waste. Obviously, there should be no eating, drinking, or smoking at the scene of decontamination.

For patients with smaller exposures to radionuclides, such as laboratory workers, decontamination is often the only management technique required to limit injury. Portable dosimeters will identify contaminated areas, which may be sealed off to limit spread of exposure, especially if the radionuclide is in gaseous form. As with larger exposures, contaminated clothing must be removed and collected. Contaminated skin must be washed with lukewarm soap and water, repeatedly if needed, with care taken not to abrade the skin and risk inadvertent incorporation. Washing may also be guided by a portable dosimeter. The cesium-exposed patients in Goiânia received repeated baths in warm water and neutral soap over the first 2 days of their hospitalization, as did the Hanford americium patient whose skin was contaminated with nearly 200 GBq of [241]Am.[67] If the patient is still contaminated after repeated washing, many recommend using a cream hand cleaner that contains no abrasives. The palms and soles of the Goiânia patients that were heavily contaminated were treated with titanium dioxide mixed with hydrated lanolin.[44]

In evaluating an area where a spill of radioactive material has occurred, a judgment must be made regarding the severity of the incident so that appropriate steps are taken. If a major incident has occurred involving large amounts of radioactive material, a large contaminated area, airborne radioactivity, or spread of radiation outside an authorized area, many academic centers recommend evacuation, notification of the radiation safety officer in an institutional setting, and calling local or regional emergency response. Minor incidents involve small amounts of radioactive material where the individual knows how to clean the site, has appropriate decontamination material on hand, and can clean the area in a reasonably short time. Several different decontaminating agents are commercially available from general stores and many scientific suppliers. These agents come in the form of concentrated detergents or foaming sprays where a small spill is quickly wiped clean and disposed of in an appropriate container.

Medical Management of ARS

In the ED, after airway and breathing have been managed appropriately, intravenous (IV) access should be established. As with thermal burns, peripheral IVs are more prone to infection, and central venous access is recommended. Fluid replacement may begin with crystalloid solution where the rate will be modified by recorded inputs and outputs and assessment of surface area burns if any.

Emergency management of emesis and pain may be difficult in those patients who received a high dose of radiation. Many types of antiemetics are used to control an irradiated patient's vomiting. The 5-HT antagonists ondansetron and granisetron are particularly effective in this setting. Mild pain may be managed with acetaminophen, but nonsteroidal antiinflammatory medications are not recommended, as they may exacerbate gastric bleeding in a patient for whom bleeding may soon become difficult to control. Morphine is recommended for the management of more severe pain, which may develop within a few hours after the injury from burns, mucositis, and other complications. As with burn patients, prophylactic use of antibiotics is not recommended.

In the ED it is important to obtain blood samples for baseline lymphocyte count and for blood typing. As was mentioned earlier, the degrees of lymphopenia and granulocytopenia within the first 24 to 48 hours postexposure are important for estimating the dose and directing therapy. Blood typing early is important because the patient may require transfusions of red blood cells and platelets. Use of irradiated cells is recommended to avoid graft-versus-host disease.

For patients who survive the acute period, sepsis is the leading cause of death. To maximize survival, patients with a severe radiation exposure should be treated as other severely burned or immunocompromised patients regarding their risk of infection. Rigorous attention must be paid to the proper use of H_2 antagonists, antibiotics, antifungals, antivirals, and cultures of body fluids.

Special Management Techniques

Some patients may require supportive measures to boost their immune system and decrease the risk of infection.[52] Colony-stimulating factors have been used to stimulate blood cell growth by increasing the rate of stem-cell division, accelerating the maturation process, or by the release of immature forms into the peripheral circulation. Colony-stimulating factors were used successfully at Goiânia and decreased the period of leukocyte depression while raising the nadir. Stimulating factors are more effective when given soon after the exposure.

Following Chernobyl, 13 patients received bone marrow transplantation (BMT) for hematopoietic support until the irradiated bone marrow could recover.[1,52] Unlike patients who undergo bone marrow suppression for clinical reasons, patients involved in a radiation exposure may have incomplete exposure and are usually partially shielded, which may allow for survival of some stem cells. Eleven of these BMT patients at Chernobyl died, complicating the interpretation of the efficacy of transplantation. Bone marrow transplantation does not change the mortality risk from the other subsyndromes of ARS. The ability of BMT to improve the clinical course of an irradiated patient depends on how likely the patient was to die from hematopoietic syndrome alone. This remains a controversial mode of treatment for irradiated patients.

Probiotics is the introduction of selective nonpathogenic strains of *Lactobacillus* and Bifidobacteria into the gastrointestinal tract to suppress the number of pathogens.[52] Experimentally, this technique increases survival in canine and rodent models. Probiotics was also used in Chernobyl on three men whose survival time was prolonged, although not statistically, when compared respectively to case controls.

Incorporation of radionuclides presents a challenge to the treating physicians where the goal is removal of an internal store of the radioactive material. Experimentally, beagle dogs treated with DTPA showed decreased incidences of bone cancer when exposed

to ^{241}Am. These dogs were injected with 11 kBq/kg and were potentially exposed to up to 5 Gy during the course of the experiment.[37] Both Ca-DTPA and Zn-DTPA are approved for human use for decontamination of transuranium elements. The calcium salt is the treatment of choice for early decontamination, whereas the zinc salt is used preferentially for long-term treatment.[11] Rat experiments with LIHOPO demonstrate decreased retention of plutonium and uranium even after incorporation into bone.[11,70]

Prussian blue, ferric ferrocyanide, absorbs cesium ions and is used in fission product recovery. Experimentally, ferric ferrocyanide is used to reduce the incorporation of cesium into animals and was used to treat 37 patients exposed to cesium in Goiânia, Brazil.[35] In that group, elimination of cesium followed first-order kinetics and was enhanced by up to 35% by doses up to 10 g per day in adults. Orally administered Prussian blue derivatives (soluble $K_3Fe[Fe(CN)_6]$ and insoluble $Fe_4[Fe(CN)_6]_3$) prevented the oral absorption of cesium in rats, pigs, and humans, and no toxic effects were reported.[10]

PREGNANCY AND RADIATION

In the normal course of events, uncertainty exists regarding the normal viability of the fertilized ovum, and there is a naturally high rate of embryo loss during the early weeks of pregnancy. When exposure to radiation is possible, pregnant women exhibit extreme concern over its potential teratogenic effects, even though maternal exposures to less than 0.05 Sv is considered not to be teratogenic.[2,24] Unfortunately, there is little direct information concerning the effects of radiation in early human pregnancy. Experimental data using rats and mice show increased mortality rates both in vitro and in vivo following irradiation as well as a dose-response curve that depicts incremental increases in radiation dose corresponding to increasingly greater effects in causing malformations.[65] Experimental human data from the 1930s show increased lethality and induction of abortion when pregnant women were exposed to 3.6 Sv and 5 Sv for a therapeutic abortion by x-ray.[26,41]

The most important sources of information concerning the teratogenic effects of fetal irradiation are the survivors of the nuclear bomb blasts of World War II. The three principal risks to a fetus following radiation exposure are congenital abnormalities, severe mental retardation, and the late development of a neoplasm. The embryo is at particular risk because of its rapid development, and there are several periods of particular sensitivity so that irradiation at specific times is associated with increased risk of specific problems. Roughly speaking, uterine absorption of 0.2 to 0.5 Sv during the first week postconception (PC) risks lethality, during the second to seventh weeks PC risks congenital abnormalities and growth retardation, and during the 8th to 15th weeks PC risks mental retardation. After the 15th week PC, these complications tend not to be as prevalent but are demonstrated.[65]

Accurate specification of the risks from fetal doses is difficult, especially at doses less than 0.2 Sv. Different models consider dose-response relationships for developmental complications and cancer development as linear or linear-quadratic, and with or without a threshold limit. A risk of congenital abnormalities of 5% following exposure to 0.2 Sv compares to a widely accepted average incidence for congenital abnormality of 6% for newborns throughout the world.[65] Patients receiving various diagnostic procedures in the hospital may be exposed to these doses.[25] Clearly, pregnant women who are exposed to radiation are at risk for a fetal complication, although that risk may be difficult to quantify at the low doses expected with routine radiologic procedures.[6] Consideration should always be given to the potential maternal benefit of the radiologic procedure as well as the potential risk to the fetus.[57]

SUMMARY

The danger of ionizing radiation to humans is through the disruption of cellular structure and function. Cell death and mutagenesis are the destructive consequences of an exposure to radiation. Fortunately, large exposures of radiation to the general population are rare outside of the setting of an armed conflict, and most contaminations that occur are small and easily controlled.

In general, recognition of the exposure and thorough decontamination are the critical steps to minimizing the potential toxicity of an exposure. Careful attention to storage of radioactive waste and contaminated materials and good supportive care are usually all that are required to care for most patients.

REFERENCES

1. Baranov A, Gale RP, Guskova A, et al: Bone marrow transplantation after the Chernobyl nuclear accident. N Engl J Med 1989;321: 205–212.
2. Bentur Y, Horlatsch N, Koren G: Exposure to ionizing radiation during pregnancy: perception of teratogenic risk and outcome. Teratology 1991;43:109–112.
3. Birchard K: Does Iraq's depleted uranium pose a health risk? Lancet 1998;351:657.
4. Blattmann H: Radiation physics. Experientia 1989;45:2–5.
5. Broga DW, Gilbert MA: A review of three incidents involving the release of ^{125}I from seeds interstitially implanted within the prostate gland. Health Phys 1983;45:593–597.
6. Castronovo FP: Teratogen update: Radiation and Chernobyl. Teratology 1999;60:100–106.
7. Clancy T: Armored Cav: A Guided Tour of an Armored Cavalry Regiment. New York, Berkley Publishing Group, 1994.
8. Clarke RH, Southwood TRE: Risks from ionizing radiation. Nature 1989;338:197–198.
9. Cohen BL: A test of the linear–no threshold theory of radiation carcinogenesis. Environ Res 1990;53:193–220.
10. Dresow B, Nielsen P, Fischer R, Pfau AA, Heinrich HH: In vivo binding of radiocesium by two forms of Prussian blue and by ammonium iron hexacyanoferrate. Clin Toxicol 1993;31:563–569.
11. Durakovic A: Medical effects of internal contamination with uranium. Croat Med J 1999;40:49–66.
12. Fabrikant JI: The carcinogenic risks of low-LET and high-LET ionizing radiations. J Radiat Res 1991;32:143–164.
13. Fanger H, Lushbaugh CC: Radiation death from cardiovascular shock following a criticality accident. Arch Pathol 1967;83:446–460.
14. Fetter S, von Hippl FN: The hazard posed by depleted uranium munitions. Sci Glob Security 1999;8:125–161.
15. Filipy RE, Toohey RE, Kathren RL, Dietert SE: Deterministic effects of ^{241}Am exposure in the Hanford americium accident case. Health Phys 1995;69:338–345.
16. Finch SC: Acute radiation syndrome. JAMA 1987;258:664–667.
17. Forrow L, Sidel VW: Medicine and nuclear war. JAMA 1998; 280:456–461.
18. Franic Z, Lokobauer N, Marovic G: Radioactive contamination of cistern waters along the Croatian coast of the Adriatic sea by ^{90}Sr. Health Phys 1999;77:62–66.
19. Fry RJ, Fry SA: Health effects of ionizing radiation. Med Clin North Am 1990;74:475–488.
20. Fuchs M, Schmid A, Eiteljörge T, Modler M, Stürmer KM: Exposure of the surgeon to radiation during surgery. Int Orthop 1998;22: 153–156.
21. Golosov VN, Walling DE, Panin ED, et al: The spatial variability of Chernobyl-derived ^{137}Cs inventories in a small agricultural drainage basin in central Russia. Appl Radiat Isot 1999;51:341–352.
22. Gross L: Oncogenic effects of ionizing radiation. Ann NY Acad Sci 1985;459:255–257.
23. Groves LM: Now It Can Be Told. New York, Da Capo, 1983.
24. Haigh F, Given-Wilson R: Current working practices during pregnancy in British radiologists. Clin Radiol 1991;44:108–112.
25. Harding LK: Pregnancy and ionizing radiation. Br Med J 1993; 306:146–147.
26. Harris W: Therapeutic abortion produced by the roentgen ray. Am J Roentgenol 1932;27:415–419.
27. Hart GC: Diagnostic medical exposures to ionizing radiation during pregnancy. Nucl Med Commun 1994;15:403–404.
28. Hooper FJ, Squibb KS, Siegel EL, McPhaul K, Keogh JP: Elevated urine uranium excretion by soldiers with retained uranium shrapnel. Health Phys 1999;77:512–519.
29. Hoshi M, Matsuura M, Hayakawa N, Ito C, Kamada N: Estimation of radiation doses for atomic-bomb survivors in the Hiroshima University registry. Health Phys 1996;70:735–740.
30. Ingegno M, Nahabedian M, Tominaga GT, Scannell G, Waxman K: Radiation exposure from cervical spine radiographs. Am J Emerg Med 1994;12:15–16.
31. Jacob P, Kenigsberg Y, Zvonova I, et al: Childhood exposure due to the Chernobyl accident and thyroid cancer risk in contaminated areas of Belarus and Russia. Br J Cancer 1999;80:1461–1469.
32. Jaspers NG, Zdzienicka MZ: Inhibition of DNA synthesis by ionization radiation. Methods Mol Biol 1999;113:535–542.
33. Jonsson B, Forseth T, Ugedal O: Chernobyl radioactivity persists in fish. Nature 1999;400:417.
34. Keller Col. PD: A clinical syndrome following exposure to atomic bomb explosions. JAMA 1946;131:504–506 (reprinted: JAMA 1987;258:661–663).
35. Lipsztein JL, Bertelli L, Oliveira CA, Dantas BM: Studies of Cs retention in the human body related to body parameters and Prussian blue administration. Health Phys 1991;60:57–61.
36. Lloyd RD, Taylor GN, Angus W, Miller SC: Soft tissue tumors in beagles injected with ^{241}Am citrate. Health Phys 1995;68:225–233.
37. Lloyd RD, Taylor GN, Mays CW: ^{241}Am removal by DTPA vs. occurrence of skeletal malignancy. Health Phys 1998;75:640–645.
38. Macklis RM, Bellerive MR, Humm JL: The radiotoxicology of radithor. Analysis of an early case of iatrogenic poisoning by a radioactive patent medicine. JAMA 1990;264:619–621.
39. Macklis RM: The great radium scandal. Sci Am 1993;269:94–99.
40. Martland HS: Occupational poisoning in manufacture of luminous watch dials. JAMA 1929;92:466–473.
41. Mayer M, Harris W, Wimpfheimer S: Therapeutic abortion by means of x-ray. Am J Obstet Gynecol 1936;32:945–957.
42. McDiarmid MA, Hooper FJ, Squibb K, McPhaul K: The utility of spot collection for urinary uranium determinations in depleted uranium exposed Gulf War veterans. Health Phys 1999;77:261–264.
43. McDiarmid MA, Keogh JP, Hooper FJ, et al: Health effects of depleted uranium on exposed Gulf War veterans. Environ Res 2000;82:168–180.
44. Oliveira AR, Hunt JG, Valverde NJL, Brandão-Mello CE, Farina R: Medical and related aspects of the Goiânia accident: an overview. Health Phys 1991;60:17–24.
45. Pellmar TC, Fuciarelli AF, Ejnik JW, et al: Distribution of uranium in rats implanted with depleted uranium pellets. Toxicol Sci 1999;49: 29–39.
46. Pellmar TC, Keyser DO, Emery C, Hogan JB: Electrophysiological changes in hippocampal slices isolated from rats embedded with depleted uranium fragments. Neurotoxicology 1999;20:785–792.
47. Pershagen G, Åkerblom G, Axelson O, et al: Residential radon exposure and lung cancer in Sweden. N Engl J Med 1994;330:159–164.

48. Polednak AP, Stehney AF, Rowland RE: Mortality among women first employed before 1930 in the US radium dial-painting industry. Am J Epidemiol 1978;107:179–195.
49. Priest ND: Toxicity of depleted uranium. Lancet 2001;357:244–245.
50. Prime D: Exposure to radon decay product in dwellings. J R Soc Health 1987;107:228–230.
51. Ramalho AT, Nascimento AC, Littlefield LG, Natarajan AT, Sasaki MS: Frequency of chromosomal aberrations in a subject accidentally exposed to ^{137}Cs in the Goiânia (Brazil) radiation accident: intercomparison among four laboratories. Mutat Res 1991;252:157–160.
52. Reeves GI: Radiation injuries. Crit Care Clin 1999;2:457–473.
53. Roff SR: Mortality and morbidity of members of the British Nuclear Tests Veterans Association and the New Zealand Tests Veterans Association and their families. Med Confl Surviv 1999;15(Suppl 1): 1–51.
54. Roff SR: Residual radiation in Hiroshima and Nagasaki. Lancet 1996;348:620.
55. Roscoe RJ, Steenland K, Halperin WE, Beaumont JJ, Waxweiler RJ: Lung cancer mortality among nonsmoking uranium miners exposed to radon daughters. JAMA 1989;262:629–633.
56. Rothman KJ, Loughlin JE, Funch DP, Dreyer NA: Overall mortality of cellular telephone customers. Epidemiology 1996;7:303–305.
57. Russell JG: Pregnancy and ionizing radiation. Br Med J 1992; 305:1172–1173.
58. Saenger EL: Radiation accidents. Ann Emerg Med 1986;15: 1061–1066.
59. Schoenberg JB, Klotz JB, Wilcox HB, et al: Case-control study of residential radon and lung cancer among New Jersey women. Cancer Res 1990;50:6520–6524.
60. Shimizu Y, Mabuchi K, Preston DL, Shigematsu I: Mortality study of atomic-bomb survivors: implications for assessment of radiation accidents. World Health Stat Q 1996;49:35–39.
61. Shipman TL: Acute radiation death resulting from an accidental nuclear critical excursion. J Occup Med (Spec Suppl) 1961;3:146–192.
62. Spiers FW: A note on Roentgen's x-ray absorption measurements in 1895. Br J Radiol 1986;59:1109–1110.
63. Stewart A: Detecting the health risks of radiation. Med Confl Surviv 1999;15:138–148.
64. Stewart AM, Kneale GW: A-bomb survivors: Reassessment of the radiation hazard. Med Confl Surviv 1999;15:47–57.
65. Stovall M, Blackwell CR, Cundiff J, et al: Fetal dose from radiotherapy with photon beams: report of AAPM radiation therapy committee task group no. 36. Med Phys 1995;22:63–83.
66. Tintinalli JE, Krause G, Gursel E: Microwave radiation injury. Ann Emerg Med 1983;12:645–647.
67. Toohey RE, Kathren RL: Overview and dosimetry of the Hanford americium accident case. Health Phys 1995;69:310–317.
68. Tronko MD, Bogdanova TI, Komissarenko IV, et al: Thyroid carcinoma in children and adolescents in Ukraine after the Chernobyl nuclear accident. Cancer 1999;86:149–156.
69. Vañó E, González L, Guibelalde E, Fernández JM, Ten JI: Radiation exposure to medical staff in interventional and cardiac radiology. Br J Radiol 1998;71:954–960.
70. Volf V, Burgada R, Raymond KN, Durbin PW: Chelation therapy by DFO–HOPO and 3,4,3-LIHOPO for injected Pu-238 and Am-241 in the rat: effect of dosage, time, and mode of chelate administration. Int J Radiat Biol 1996;70:765–772.
71. Wang B, Takeda H, Gao WM, et al: Induction of apoptosis by beta radiation from tritium compounds in mouse embryonic brain cells. Health Phys 1999;77:16–23.
72. Weiss EL, Singer CM, Benedict SH, Baraff LJ: Physician exposure to ionizing radiation during trauma resuscitation: a prospective clinical study. Ann Emerg Med 1990;19:134–138.

CHAPTER 100 CHEMICAL AND BIOLOGIC WEAPONS

Jeffrey R. Suchard

Case 1   On March 20, 1995, during peak morning commuter traffic, a religiously motivated terrorist cult released sarin in the Tokyo subway system. Cult members concealed the nerve agent in plastic bags wrapped in newspaper, which they placed on five subway car floors and punctured with umbrellas before leaving the trains. Fifteen subway stations were filled with a noxious substance, resulting in a mass casualty event.[134,138,139] Initial reports suggested an explosion with consequent toxic gas release, and preparations were made to receive victims with burns, blast and inhalation injuries, and carbon monoxide exposure. The first ambulatory victims reached local hospitals one-half hour after the chemical release with complaints of eye pain and dim vision. Ambulances began arriving 15 minutes later. Victims denied any explosion and reported instead that people abruptly began collapsing in the subway stations.[138] St. Luke's International Hospital received the largest number of victims, about 500 patients within the first hour, mostly arriving by private vehicle or on foot.[137,138] Nearly 2 hours after the event, the fire department reported that the causative material was acetonitrile and that victims were suffering from cyanide toxicity.[138] Medical teams noted, instead, symptoms more consistent with a cholinergic toxidrome. Mildly affected victims had ocular complaints related to miosis, rhinorrhea, and mild headache. Moderately ill victims also had dyspnea, vomiting, muscle fasciculations, and weakness. The most critical victims had seizures, coma, and respiratory or cardiac arrest.[134] Serum cholinesterase levels were severely depressed in the sickest patients. Sarin was confirmed as the causative agent 3 hours after its release.[138] A total of 5510 people sought medical attention at more than 200 hospitals and clinics in the Tokyo area.[174] The majority of patients were either minimally affected, and were discharged home after a short observation period, or had no demonstrable toxicity. One thousand fifty patients were at least moderately ill. Eight fatalities occurred the first day, later increasing to 12.[208] A survey conducted 4 years after the terrorist attack revealed that a majority of victim respondents have persistent physical and psychological complaints.[203]

Case 2   On March 10, 1998, employees at a collection agency in Phoenix, Arizona opened an envelope containing a payment for $53.99, some granular material, and a threatening note. The letter read, "You S.O.B.!!!! You have just been exposed to anthrax spores prepare to die . . . you better have a coffin ready . . . Also a standard pestelence *(sic)* has been put on you and your family. . . ."[181] After a 911 call, police and a fire department hazmat team responded to the scene. Little useful information was immediately available regarding what kind of decontamination or treatment would be necessary, leading the potentially exposed employees to believe they were destined to a rapidly fatal illness. Nine employees and one police officer were quarantined, and several nearby businesses were evacuated while a decontamination shower was constructed at the scene.[182] The local media learned of the evolving story, resulting in a television broadcast that revealed a nude victim. The victims were transported to a local hospital ED, where they were examined, advised to return if they developed flulike symptoms, and given prescriptions for ciprofloxacin. However, their clothes, wallets, and purses were still in quarantine, making it difficult for the victims to fill these potentially life-saving prescriptions. The perpetrator was easily discovered from return address information accompanying the payment. He was indicted 2 days after the anthrax scare on charges of mailing threatening communications and the threatened use of weapons of mass destruction. If convicted, the perpetrator may face up to 5 years in prison or a $250,000 fine for the first charge and up to life imprisonment for the second. Within 4 days, bacteriologic testing of the envelope and letter confirmed the absence of *Bacillus anthracis;* the granular material was believed to be salt and pepper.[94,181]

INTRODUCTION

Recent years have witnessed an enormous resurgence of interest in chemical and biologic weapons (CBW). Although "unconventional" warfare has been practiced since antiquity, it was not until the 20th century that such weapons have been manufactured and utilized on a mass scale (Table 100–1). Additional concern about CBW arises from their appeal to terrorist groups. Biologic weapons in particular are viewed as a "poor man's atomic bomb," in that the technology and financial outlay required to produce them are much less than for nuclear weapons, although the potential morbidity and mortality remain high.

Chemical weapons clearly fall within the purview of medical toxicology, as they are specifically designed to produce adverse effects in humans. Some agents generally considered nonlethal, such as tear gas and pepper spray, fit this definition and are also discussed in this chapter, but smoke- and flame-producing military munitions are not. Biologic weapons bridge the gap between infectious disease, epidemiology, and toxicology. Although key differences exist between biologic and chemical warfare agents, they share many characteristics, including intent of use, dispersion methods, and defensive measures (Table 100–2). Furthermore, many biologic warfare agents exert their effects through microorganism-derived toxins or are purified toxins themselves.

TABLE 100–1. Unconventional Weapons: Definitions and Acronyms

Chemical warfare	Intentional use of weapons designed to kill, injure, or incapacitate on the basis of toxic or noxious chemical properties
Biologic warfare	Intentional use of microorganisms or toxins derived from living organisms to cause death, disability, or damage in humans, animals, or plants
Terrorism	The unlawful use of force against persons or property to intimidate or coerce a government, the civilian population, or any segment thereof, in furtherance of political or social objectives
CW	Chemical warfare or chemical weapon
BW	Biological warfare or biologic weapon
CBW	Chemical and/or biologic warfare, or weapons
NBC	Nuclear, biologic and/or chemical; usually in reference to weapons
WMD	Weapons of mass destruction; nuclear, radiologic, chemical, and/or biologic weapons intended to produce mass casualties

HISTORY

The first well-documented use of chemical weapons occurred in 429 BC when Spartans besieging Athenian cities burned pitch-soaked wood and brimstone to produce sulfurous clouds.[56] Chemical weapons were sporadically used, or their use considered, up through the 19th century, and in 1854 the British Lord Playfair even suggested that asphyxiating enemy soldiers with poison gases was more humane than killing them with conventional weapons.[114]

Large-scale chemical warfare began in World War I. On April 22, 1915, the Germans released chlorine from compressed gas cylinders near Ypres, Belgium. A cloud of chlorine gas drifted over Allied lines, killing hundreds and forcing 15,000 troops to retreat. The Germans had not anticipated such impressive effectiveness and were unable to fully exploit their tactical advantage.[56,114,178] Both sides rapidly escalated the use of toxic gases, released from cylinders or artillery shells, including various pulmonary irritants, lacrimators, arsenicals, and cyanides.

The Germans first used sulfur mustard on July 12, 1917, again near Ypres. The first mustard attack alone caused over 20,000 casualties and presented new problems.[56,114,178] Unlike prior war gases, mustard was persistent in the environment and vesicated the skin in addition to injuring the lungs and mucous membranes. The Allies soon responded in kind. Sulfur mustard was unequaled in its ability to incapacitate opponents.[19] Injuries far outweighed fatalities, tying up manpower and resources to care for the wounded. About 2 to 3% of 120,000 British WWI sulfur mustard casualties died, but only 30% of the survivors could be released from the hospital within 30 days.[115]

Only one major CW event occurred during World War II. On December 2, 1943, German planes bombed Allied ships in Bari, Italy. The SS *John Harvey* was destroyed, releasing the contents of 2000 mustard bombs into the harbor, which caused over 600 Allied military and an unknown number of civilian casualties.[19,114,178]

Germany began producing nerve agents just before World War II. Tabun was developed in 1936 by Gerhard Schrader when conducting insecticide research for IG Farbenindustrie.[69,174] Tabun was abandoned as an insecticide because of its overwhelming human toxicity and was instead reported to the government, as mandated for all discoveries of potential military importance.

TABLE 100–2. Chemical versus Biologic Weapons: Comparison and Contrast

Similarities
  Agents most effectively dispersed in aerosol or vapor forms
  Delivery systems frequently similar
  Movement of agents highly subject to wind and weather conditions
  Appropriate personal protective equipment prevents illness

Differences	Chemical weapons	Biologic weapons
• Rate at which attack results in illness	Rapid, usually minutes to hours	Delayed, usually days to weeks

• Identifying release	Easier because of
	  Rapid effects
	  Possible chemical odor
	  Commercially available chemical detectors
		Harder because of
		  Delayed effects
		  Lack of color, odor, or taste
		  Lack of real-time detectors

• Agent persistence	Variable
	  Liquids semipersistent to persistent
	  Gases nonpersistent
		Generally nonpersistent; most BW degraded by sunlight, heat, desiccation (exception, anthrax spores)

• Victim distribution	Near and downwind from release point	Victims may be widely dispersed by time disease is apparent
• First responders	EMTs, hazmat teams, firefighters, law enforcement officers	Emergency physicians and nurses, primary care practitioners, infectious disease physicians, epidemiologists, public health officials, hospital administrators, laboratory experts (but may be same as CW if release is identified immediately)
• Decontamination	Critically important in most cases	Not needed in delayed presentations; less important for acute exposures
• Medical treatment	Chemical antidotes, supportive care	Vaccines, antibiotics, supportive care
• Patient isolation	Unnecessary after adequate decontamination	Crucial for easily communicable diseases (eg, smallpox, pneumonic plague); however, many BW agents are not easily transmissible

Adapted from Henderson DA: The looming threat of bioterrorism. Science 1999;283:1279–1282.

Sarin was synthesized in 1938 and named after its developers: Schrader, Ambrose, Rudringer, and Van der Linde.[69] Between 10,000 and 30,000 tons of tabun and 5 to 10 tons of sarin were produced during World War II. Soman was synthesized in 1944, but no large-scale production facilities were developed. When the Allies discovered these nerve agents at the end of the war, code names were designated based on the order of their development. Tabun was called GA (the letter *G* standing for German), sarin was GB, and soman was GD. There was no "GC" agent because that code already stood for gonorrhea.[69]

In 1952, the British synthesized an even more potent nerve agent when searching for a DDT replacement. This substance was given to the United States for military development and was named VX, with the letter *V* presumably standing for venom. A VX leak killed 6000 sheep near a military base in Skull Valley, Utah in 1968.[69,99,174] Egypt is believed to have used riot-control agents, mustard, and possibly nerve agents in the Yemen War of 1963–1967. The United States used defoliants and riot-control agents in Vietnam and Laos, claiming that these were not forbidden by the Geneva Protocol, which the United States finally ratified in 1975. Iraq used sulfur mustard, tabun, and soman during its war with Iran and may have also used cyanide against the Kurds.[76,96,114,178]

More recently, terrorist groups have begun to employ chemical weapons. Sarin was released twice by the Aum Shinrikyo cult in Japan. The first release occurred in Matsumoto in 1994, killing seven and injuring over 600.[122,135] A more highly publicized sarin attack occurred in the Tokyo subway system in 1995, killing 12 and resulting in over 5000 persons seeking medical attention.[171] Cult members have also used VX in assassinations.[118,121,130,192]

Biologic warfare (BW) has ancient roots. Missile weapons poisoned with natural toxins have been used as early as 18,000 years ago (Chap. 1). Recent excavation of an Egyptian tomb, circa 2100 BC, yielded arrows coated with cardiac glycosides and paralytic toxins.[125] The first recorded, but probably apocryphal, use of BW appears in the Old Testament. Chapters 4 through 6 of the first book of Samuel describe how the Philistines were stricken with bubonic plague after capturing the Ark of the Covenant from the Israelites in battle.

More reliable accounts of ancient biologic warfare also occurred. Around 600 BC, the Athenians used hellebore, and the Assyrians used ergot alkaloids, to poison enemy water supplies.[113] In 200 BC, the Carthaginian general Maharbal tainted wine consumed by rebel African forces with the anticholinergic herb mandragora and then ambushed the intoxicated troops. In 184 BC, Hannibal ordered earthen pots filled with "serpents of every kind" hurled onto enemy ships, thereby winning the naval battle of Eurymedon against King Eumenes of Pergamon.[42,82,178] In 67 BC, King Mithridates VI of Pontus was retreating from the Roman general Pompey near Trebizond, modern northeast Turkey. At the advice of a physician-counselor, Mithridates maneuvered Pompey's troops into a region where the honey was contaminated with grayanotoxins from rhododendron nectar. The Romans ate the poisoned honey and were effectively ambushed.[87,154]

From AD 1344 to 1346, the Tartars besieged the Genoan trade city of Kaffa on the Black Sea coast. When the Tartars began to die of bubonic plague, the dead bodies were hurled over the battlements. Within the city, plague forced the Genoans to flee, and they then disseminated the disease to other trade ports and eventually to the rest of Europe, causing the Black Death.[34] In 1763, Sir Jeffrey Amherst, the commander of British forces during the French and Indian War, instituted a policy of spreading smallpox to Native Americans by giving them contaminated blankets and handkerchiefs.[28,145]

During World War I, Germany was the only combatant nation with an active BW program. German agents infected Allied livestock with anthrax and glanders.[204] Eighty years after its capture, viable spores were found in a German device to disseminate anthrax.[148]

Shiro Ishii, a Japanese army doctor, headed an active BW program throughout Japan's war with China and World War II.[57,202] Several centers were founded, the most famous being Unit 731 in Manchuria, where human experimentation on POWs and imprisoned civilians took place. Several field trials on Chinese civilians and Russian troops also took place. The Soviets, Germany, France, Britain, and Canada all started BW research facilities in the period between the World Wars.

The United States' BW research program began in 1941, and its main facility was founded at Camp Detrick, Maryland. Fort Detrick, as it is now known, remains the home of the United States Army Medical Research Institute of Infectious Diseases (USAMRIID). Anthrax and botulinum toxin were the foci of weapons development; it has been estimated that the United States could have manufactured 1,000,000 anthrax bombs and 275,000 botulinum bombs by 1945 had full-scale production been implemented.[14]

The British BW program was established in 1940 at Porton Down, but most of the field testing of anthrax occurred on Gruinard Island off the northern coast of Scotland.[120] In 1979, the soil was still found to be contaminated with viable anthrax spores.[98] The island was decontaminated with 5% formaldehyde in sea water, and was passed as safe by the British government in 1988.[3]

During the Cold War, the US military maintained active research into biologic weapons, including field trials with bacterial simulants. In 1950, ships in San Francisco harbor released aerosols of *Serratia marcesans* and other simulants, which resulted in a minor outbreak of *Serratia* sepsis. In 1966, lightbulbs filled with *Bacillus subtilis* var *globigii* were dropped in the New York City subway system, confirming the hypothesis that the piston-like action of the subway trains would rapidly disperse the bacterial aerosol throughout the city.[28,120,145,153] In London in 1978, the Bulgarian exile Georgi Markov was assassinated by a tiny metal pellet fired from a gun designed to appear like an umbrella. He was thought to have died from sepsis until the pellet was found at autopsy.[31,83] Since the fall of the Soviet Union, it has been confirmed that the KGB used umbrella guns firing ricin pellets to assassinate Markov and others. In 1979, an outbreak of human anthrax with at least 66 fatalities occurred in the Russian city of Sverdlovsk. Soviet officials first blamed the outbreak on gastrointestinal anthrax from a shipment of contaminated meat.[103] Autopsies showed death from inhalational anthrax, and epidemiologic investigation showed that nearly all cases occurred downwind from a military facility. These data are consistent only with a release of aerosolized anthrax, which has since been confirmed by Russian authorities.[116] In the late 1970s and early 1980s, many reports from Southeast Asia and Afghanistan claimed that Soviet-supported troops were using a biologic weapon known as yellow rain.[58,100,180] Some samples of yellow rain contained tricothecene mycotoxins, although controversy remains as to whether this represents intentional biologic warfare or a naturally occurring phenomenon.[128,159]

During the recent Gulf War there was concern about Saddam Hussein's weapons of mass destruction.[84] The Iraqis had an active

BW research program, investigating at least five bacteria, one fungus, five viruses, four toxins, simulants, and various dispersion methods.[160,210] They produced and weaponized thousands of liters of anthrax spores, botulinum toxin, and aflatoxin into bombs and as payloads for SCUD missiles.

Biologic terrorism is now recognized as a growing public health concern.[30,61,62,106,169,184] In 1984, a large outbreak of salmonellosis was traced to intentional contamination of restaurant salad bars by the Rajneeshee cult in Oregon.[191] The Aum Shinrikyo cult investigated cholera and Q fever, unsuccessfully released anthrax spores and botulinum toxin, and even sent members to Africa to obtain the Ebola virus.[13,140] Even the mere threat of biologic agent release can temporarily terrorize a city. The end of the 1990s saw a huge increase in anthrax threats, none of which were proven true.[26,193] Even naturally occurring disease outbreaks can give rise to concern for biological terrorism. In 1999, an outbreak of West Nile–like virus encephalitis in New York, with fifty human cases, was investigated as a potential BW agent release,[149] as was a case of brucellosis acquired under suspicious circumstances.[26a]

GENERAL CONSIDERATIONS

Nerve Gas, Mustard Gas, Poison Gas: What are War Gases?

The term "war gas" is generally a misnomer. Sulfur mustard and nerve agents are liquids at normal temperatures and pressures, and riot-control agents are solids. However, these weapons are most efficiently dispersed as aerosols. Some CW agents, such as chlorine, phosgene, and hydrogen cyanide, are truly gases.

Liquid chemical weapons have a certain degree of volatility and may evaporate into poisonous gases. Volatility is inversely related to persistence, the tendency to remain in the environment. Persistent agents such as sulfur mustard or VX can contaminate an area for prolonged periods. The toxic hazard from semipersistent agents such as sarin or nonpersistent agents such as hydrogen cyanide dissipates more rapidly. Persistent agents pose greater hazards to first responders and other healthcare providers.[18,114] Victims exposed to CW gases will not require as rigorous decontamination because the hazard will dissipate by the time they reach medical care.

CBW aerosols and CW gases and vapors are highly subject to local atmospheric conditions. Less dispersion occurs with inversion layers and in the absence of strong wind, as typically occurs at night or in the early morning. Enclosed spaces are also ideal, preventing wind dispersion and even simple dilution. Except for hydrogen cyanide, CW gases and vapors are all denser than air and will pool in low-lying areas.

CW dispersion in enclosed, low-lying spaces was utilized in the Tokyo subway sarin attack. The number of fatalities could have been much higher had the nerve agent been aerosolized instead of simply allowed to evaporate. Photos from the attack show severely affected or deceased victims in very close proximity to mildly affected, ambulatory individuals.[198] Presumably, sarin concentrations decreased with distance from the source, and only a few victims were actually contaminated with liquid. After removal from high-concentration areas, the victims' bodies posed less threat to bystanders because of dilution and improved ventilation. Even so, some healthcare providers were secondarily exposed, as the victims were not disrobed before entering the hospitals. Up to

46% of hospital staff in areas with poor ventilation reported symptoms consistent with acute poisoning. Fortunately, all these secondary exposures were mild.[131,134,138] About one-third of rescue workers in the 1994 Matsumoto sarin incident also developed mild toxicity. Rescuers arriving at the scene later were less likely to develop symptoms.[124]

Preparation for CBW Incidents

A rational medical response to CBW agent events differs from the common response to isolated toxicologic incidents. Eckstein[39] proposed some new "rules of engagement" for modern CBW terrorism. Healthcare providers must learn new material related to unconventional weapons. Fortunately, a multimillion-dollar Domestic Preparedness Program was funded in 1996 by the Nunn-Lugar-Domenici initiative for WMD defense.[133] Medical providers in 120 major US cities are receiving training in the recognition and treatment of chemical and biologic casualties.[39,41]

Healthcare providers must protect themselves and their facilities first, or ultimately no one will receive care. New medicolegal and ethical considerations will arise in CBW mass-casualty events that are otherwise infrequently seen. Triage in disaster medicine includes separating patients into an "expectant" category (ie, the expected outcome is death). The greatest good for the greatest number of victims may preclude heroic interventions in a few critical patients. Charges of negligence may later arise regarding delays in treatment or failure to diagnose subtle signs of disease, even if such actions were unavoidable at the time.

The responses to chemical and biologic weapons will also differ.[62] Chemical weapons produce almost immediate effects, making a "scene" or "hot zone" evident. The first responders for a chemical event will be fire and police authorities, hazmat teams, and EMS. With biologic weapons, the victims will not present for care at the same time in the same place. BW event first responders will be local and distant emergency departments and primary care offices. Many BW agents initially produce nonspecific symptoms of diseases rarely or never seen in common practice. Inhalational anthrax and pneumonic plague, for example, could easily be misdiagnosed as influenza or acute bronchitis. Providers on the new front lines need to be educated regarding the expected signs, symptoms, and clinical courses of BW agents.[150,200] Only if potential BW victims are identified and aggressively treated early after exposure (within the first 24 to 48 hours) can mortality be decreased and, in cases of smallpox or plague, secondary or tertiary cases prevented.[41]

Even with increasing awareness and education, many physicians remain inadequately prepared. Only 53% of surveyed emergency medicine residencies included training in BW issues, and more than 70% rated themselves as less than adequate or very poor in recognizing BW casualties.[142] There is currently no standard curriculum for training emergency physicians about the health hazards related to nuclear, biological, and chemical (NBC) weapons, although progress in this regard is under way.[41,142] Critical care specialists, too, are recognizing their lack of preparation for chemical mass-casualty incidents.[86]

In preparation for the 1996 Olympic Games in Atlanta, a multidisciplinary task force was assembled to detect, identify, and respond to any CBW threat or release of toxic industrial chemicals.[168] Efforts included stockpiling antibiotics and antidotes, training first-responders, enhanced surveillance, and augmenting clinical capabilities. The group correctly suspected that the most likely terrorist event was use of conventional explosives; nevertheless, samples from the Centennial Park explosion were rapidly obtained to rule out dissemination of any CBW agent. Such an intense response to the threat of CBW terrorism would be difficult to maintain for extended periods.

Recommendations for more sustained health care facility domestic preparedness include improved training to recognize CBW mass casualty events, efforts to protect healthcare providers, and establishing decontamination and triage protocols.[97] Specific recommendations are listed in Table 100–3. Several issues remain unclear, such as the optimal choice of personal protective equipment, determining who needs decontamination, and what is to be done with wastewater produced by mass decontamination.[97]

Communication is always a key issue in disaster management. Preestablished lines of communication and command should be implemented.[150] Outside agencies should also be alerted to CBW incidents, which in the United States should include at a minimum the Federal Bureau of Investigation and the CDC (Table 100–4).[81] On a tactical level, communication can be severely impaired by personal protective gear, which points out the need for loudspeakers or some other form of public address.[97,194]

How Do BW Incidents Differ from Naturally Occurring Outbreaks?

Because the clinical effects of bioweapons are delayed, and the symptoms may be insidious, it may be difficult to differentiate occult BW releases from naturally occurring disease outbreaks. Several epidemiologic criteria have been proposed to aid in such determinations,[127,205] many of which should be present in a BW incident (see Table 100–5).

A ploy to avoid early detection would be to release an endemic infection (or a disease that mimics endemic infection) during its season of peak incidence. In some areas of the United States, for example, a few cases of bubonic plague would not attract notice;

TABLE 100–4.   CBW Phone Numbers/Contacts

CDC Emergency Preparedness and Response Branch
(770) 488-7100
   For advice, or to report a suspected or actual event

CDC Bioterrorism Preparedness and Response Activity
(404) 639-0385

FBI Weapons of Mass Destruction Operations Unit
(202) 324-6928
(202) 324-3000 (Public Relations)

Department of Justice Domestic Preparedness National Response Hotline
(800) 424-8802
   To report a suspected or actual event

CB HelpLine
(800) 368-6498
   Nonemergent planning and information source for civilian emergency responders

CB HotLine
(800) 424-8802
   For chemical and biologic weapons emergencies

US Army Medical Research Institute of Infectious Disease (USAMRIID) Hotline
(888) 872-7443 (USA-RIID)
   To assist in BW threat assessment, diagnosis, and treatment issues

Commander, USAMRIID
(301) 619-2833 (Phone)
(301) 619-4625 (Fax)
   For information on diagnostics, medical management, and vaccines

that is, until dozens or hundreds of cases were identified. An outbreak of inhalational anthrax during the influenza season may similarly be hidden among patients with identical early symptoms until unusually high mortality was evident. By the time the BW outbreak was recognized, the perpetrators could have disposed of any physical evidence and fled the area. On the other hand, even a single case of smallpox (anywhere in the world), Ebola virus infection, or Congo-Crimean hemorrhagic fever (in nonendemic areas) would immediately raise suspicion of a BW attack.

Decontamination

Decontamination serves two functions: (1) to prevent further absorption and spread of a noxious substance on a given casualty and (2) to prevent spread to other persons. Decontamination is critical for most chemical weapons exposures but is less crucial for biologic agents. Victims of an occult BW agent release will not present for medical care until they become symptomatic, usually several days later, when decontamination will make no difference. Also, CW agents can be dispersed as liquids, which are more amenable to decontamination than gases or aerosols and are more likely to spread on a person or between persons.

Chemical Weapons Decontamination.   Exposure to chemical agents mandates rapid and thorough decontamination. Agents that are exclusively gases at normal temperatures and pressures (eg,

TABLE 100–3.   Recommendations for Healthcare Facility Response to CBW Incidents

- Immediate access to personal protective equipment (PPE) for healthcare providers
- Decontamination facilities that can be made operational within 2 to 3 minutes
- Provision of food, water, and psychological support for staff, who may be required to perform for extended periods
- Triage of victims into those able to decontaminate themselves (decreasing the workload for healthcare providers) and those requiring assistance
- A brief sign-in process where patients are assigned numbers and given identically numbered plastic bags to contain their clothing and valuables
- Decontamination facilities allowing for simultaneous use by multiple persons and that provide some measure of visual privacy
- Secondary triage to separate persons requiring immediate medical treatment from those with minor or no apparent injuries who are sent to a holding area for observation
- Providing victims with written information regarding the agent involved, potential short- and long-term effects, recommended treatment, stress reactions, and possible avenues for further assistance
- Careful handling of information released to the media to prevent conflicting or erroneous reports
- Instituting postexposure surveillance studies

TABLE 100–5. Epidemiologic Clues Suggesting Bioweapons Release

- Large epidemic with unusually high morbidity and/or mortality
- Epidemic curve (number of cases versus time) showing an "explosion" of cases, reflecting a point source in time rather than insidious onset
- Tight geographic localization of cases, especially downwind of potential release site
- Predominance of respiratory tract symptoms because most BW agents are contracted by aerosol inhalation
- Simultaneous outbreaks of multiple unusual diseases
- Immunosuppressed and elderly persons more susceptible
- Nonendemic infection ("impossible epidemiology")
- Unseasonal time for endemic infection
- Organisms with unusual antimicrobial resistance patterns, reflecting BW genetic engineering
- Animal casualties from same disease outbreak
- Absence of normal zoonotic disease host
- Low attack rates among persons incidentally working in areas with filtered air supplies or closed ventilation systems, using HEPA masks, or remaining indoors during outdoor exposures
- Delivery vehicle or munitions discovered
- Law enforcement or military intelligence information
- Claim of BW release by belligerent force

chlorine, phosgene, or hydrogen cyanide), however, require only removing the victim from the area of exposure as a means of decontamination. Vapor exposures are also terminated by leaving the area and may require no skin decontamination of victims.[114] Japanese experience with sarin suggests that clothing should be removed from victims of nerve agent vapor exposure and isolated in plastic bags, and this probably holds true also for mustard vapor. If vapor is the only source of exposure, skin decontamination will not be necessary,[172] but clothing must still be removed.

CW agents dispersed as liquids present the greatest need for decontamination. Because nerve agents are highly potent and have rapid onset of effects, it is unlikely that any victims with significant dermal contamination will survive to reach medical care.[172] Liquid-contaminated clothing must be removed, and if able, victims should remove their own clothing.

Nerve agents are hydrolyzed and inactivated by solutions that release chlorine or solutions that are sufficiently alkaline. To avoid potential dermal and mucous membrane injury, a 1:10 dilution of household bleach in water (producing a 0.5% sodium hypochlorite solution) is currently recommended, not only for nerve agents but also for sulfur mustard and many biological agents.[97,110,174] Alternatives include regular soap and water or copious water alone. Rapid decontamination is more important than the solution used because 15 to 20 minutes is necessary for hypochlorite solutions to inactivate chemical agents.[97] Care should be taken to clean the hair, intertriginous areas, axillae, and groin.[174]

Decontamination after sulfur mustard exposure is more problematic than for nerve agents. First, it is more likely that significantly contaminated victims will survive to reach medical care, and they may remain asymptomatic for several hours. Also, the biochemical damage becomes irreversible long before symptoms develop. Decontamination within 1 to 2 minutes is the only effective means of limiting tissue damage from mustard.[176] The actual means of mustard decontamination, however, are identical to those for nerve agents. Victims must be disrobed and thoroughly showered. Dilute hypochlorite solutions (eg, 0.5% sodium

hypochlorite, a 1:10 dilution of household bleach) have been advocated to inactivate mustard, but copious water irrigation will also suffice.[114] Symptomatic victims of mustard exposure should still be decontaminated, even though it is unlikely to benefit that particular casualty, to prevent the spread of agent to others.[176] Lewisite and phosgene oxime must also be decontaminated quickly, although they produce immediate symptoms, making it more likely that victims will present promptly when decontamination is most effective.

Water irrigation is generally recommended for riot control agent exposures because hypochlorite solutions may exacerbate skin lesions.[114] Inadequately decontaminated patients exposed to lacrimator agents can produce secondary cases among healthcare providers, so any contaminated clothing should be removed and isolated.

Biologic Weapons Decontamination. BW agents are most effectively dispersed by aerosol. Shortly after a known or suspected release of bioaerosols, decontamination is a minor concern. Aerosols sized appropriately to reach the lower respiratory tract (<5 μm particles) produce little surface contamination. Simple clothing removal eliminates a high proportion of deposited particles, and subsequent showering with soap and water is expected to remove 99.99% of any remaining organisms on the skin.[81] Thus, decontamination after BW aerosol exposure (if needed at all) is achieved through disrobing and showering with soap and water, which can even occur at the victims' homes, thereby reducing strain on disaster response manpower and materiel in multiple-victim exposures.[41,62,81,150] Any gross, visible evidence of skin exposure to biologic agents is decontaminated by thorough irrigation, sterilizing the skin with a sporocidal/bactericidal solution (eg, 0.5% sodium hypochlorite), and a final water rinse.[81,150] With occult bioweapons releases, where victims will not present until late after exposure, decontamination will not be helpful and will only delay care.

Other Decontamination Issues. Anthrax spores are difficult to destroy by common decontamination methods. BCTP (bicomponent triton tri-*n*-butyl phosphate) is an antimicrobial nonionic nanoemulsion of oil, water, and laboratory detergents that is nontoxic to humans but can destroy anthrax spores, other bacteria, and viruses.[5,186] Aqueous foams containing the enzyme organophosphorus hydrolase are effective in environmental decontamination of nerve agents.[92,93]

Significant issues remain regarding decontamination measures. The number of people requiring decontamination may easily outstrip capacity. In a simulation of sarin and sulfur mustard decontamination, the maximum capacity was 16 patients per hour.[190] Incidents with hundreds or thousands of victims may need to rely on communal showers. Decontamination wastewater should ideally be contained and treated, but few facilities have the capability or funds to do this. Wastewater may, however, be a minor issue. In BW incidents there is only a temporary risk because of rapid environmental degradation, whereas in large-scale CW events the wastewater poses only a small percentage of the total environmental impact.[97]

What Is the Risk of CBW Agent Exposure?

The actual release of CBW agents is characterized as a low-probability, high-consequence event.[18,150] Potential sources for civilian exposure include terrorist attacks, inadvertent releases from domestic stockpiles, direct military attacks, and industrial accidents. Terrorists may sabotage military or industrial stockpiles or directly attack the populace. Experience has shown that physicians are much more likely to encounter hoaxes,[26] isolated cases,[156] or limited incidents with a modest number of casualties.[1,191] Riot control agents are exceptions, in that treating tear gas and pepper spray victims is a routine occurrence in many urban emergency departments.

Technical and organizational obstacles decrease the chance of major CBW terrorist events. Obtaining or producing chemical or biologic weapons, although simpler than for nuclear weapons, is only part of the process. Effective dissemination is difficult if the goal is to maximize the casualties. Proper milling of biologic agents to produce stable, respirable aerosols requires technical sophistication probably only attainable with governmental research support.[85,184] Illustrating this point are the ineffectiveness of the Aum Shinrikyo's BW releases and the limited number of sarin fatalities despite tremendous funds available to support these attacks.[140] Low-technology attacks such as food contamination, poisoning of livestock, and enclosed-space weapons dispersal appear more likely to occur than attacks resulting in hundreds, thousands, or millions of casualties.[184] Smaller attacks, or merely threatening use of CBW agents, may be more desirable if they exert the same political influence.

Nevertheless, even inefficiently dispersed agents of sufficient toxicity can produce multiple casualties and terrorize the populace, as occurred in the Matsumoto and Tokyo sarin attacks. Impact estimates of efficiently dispersed BW agents are alarming. Fifty kilograms of anthrax spores disseminated along a 2-km line upwind of one-half million people would be expected to kill 95,000 and incapacitate another 125,000 people: nearly a 50% casualty rate.[40] The societal economic impact of bioterrorist attacks range from $477.7 per 100,000 persons exposed for brucellosis to $26.2 billion per 100,000 exposed for anthrax.[79]

The chemical agents most likely to be used militarily appear to be sulfur mustard and the nerve agents. A "low-tech" terrorist attack could involve releasing industrial chemicals, such as chlorine, phosgene, or ammonia gas. Although the list of potential BW agents is long, only a handful of pathogens have credible risk of producing public health disasters, thus overwhelming healthcare resources, causing high mortality, widespread panic, and massive disruption of commerce.[85] Topping this list are anthrax, smallpox, and plague, followed by botulinum toxin, hemorrhagic fever viruses, and tularemia.

Psychological Effects

The threat or actual use of CBW presents unique psychologic stressors. Even among trained persons, a CBW-contaminated environment will produce high stress through the necessity of wearing protective gear, potential exposure to agents, high workload intensity, and interactions with the dead and dying. About 10 to 20% of participants in military training exercises, where no chance of actual exposure exists, experience moderate to severe psychological symptoms.[54] Disorders of mood, cognition, and behavior will be common among exposed or potentially exposed victims as a result of the uncertainty, fear, and panic that may accompany a CBW incident, even a hoax. The psychological casualties will probably outnumber victims requiring medical treatment. Civilians without adequate training are likely to confuse somaticized

symptoms with true exposure. Medical resources may easily be overwhelmed unless triage can identify those who will benefit most from appropriate counseling, education, and psychological support. Psychiatrists should be enlisted in plans to manage CBW incidents for their expertise in treating anxiety, fear, panic, somatization, and grief.[35,68]

Experience with actual or threatened exposures to CBW agents have borne out these concerns. In Israel during the Gulf War, anxiety-related somatic reactions to missile attacks were reported in 18 to 38% of persons surveyed,[24] and over 500 people sought medical attention in emergency departments for anxiety.[10] Among 5510 people seeking medical attention after the Tokyo subway sarin release, only about 25% were hospitalized.[171] Some of the "victims" presented days or even weeks after the incident,[134,139] apparently feeling unwell and thinking they had been exposed.[208]

Uncontrolled release of information may compound terror and increase psychological casualties. Imagine the influx of patients resulting from a news report suggesting that anyone with dizziness or nausea be checked for nerve agent toxicity, or that fever and cough indicate infection with anthrax.

The Israeli Experience during the Gulf War

Israel as a country is probably best prepared for CBW disasters. In late 1990, the civilian population was supplied with rubber masks, atropine syringes, and Fuller's earth decontamination powder.[10] Major Israeli hospitals conduct chemical mass-casualty practice drills every 3 to 5 years.[194] These drills identified several key lessons, including designating specific hospitals for chemical casualties, blocking hospital access to a single guarded entrance to prevent internal contamination, and extending nurses' authority to initiate treatment by established protocols. The Israeli plan provides two tiers of triage. The first triage occurs outside the hospital by protected medical personnel who perform only life-saving interventions, such as intubation, hemorrhage control, and antidotal therapy. Patients are then decontaminated and enter the hospital. Patients are then triaged again to separate areas according to severity of illness, where dedicated healthcare teams provide the appropriate interventions.[164,194]

Thirty-nine ballistic missiles with conventional warheads were launched against Israel in early 1991, with only six missiles causing direct casualties. Many more "injuries" resulted from CBW defensive measures and psychological stress than from trauma. Out of 1060 injuries reported from emergency departments during this time period, 234 persons were directly wounded in explosions (most injuries were minor), and there were only two fatalities from trauma.[10,77] Over 200 people presented for medical evaluation after self-injection of atropine, a few requiring admission to the hospital.[6,10,77] About 540 people sought care for acute anxiety reactions. Some suffocated from improperly used gas masks, fell and injured themselves when rushing to rooms sealed against CBW agents, or were poisoned by carbon monoxide in these airtight rooms.[2,10,77] Increased rates of myocardial infarction and cerebrovascular accidents were observed.[10] No obstetric complications occurred among women wearing gas masks during labor and delivery.[10,43]

Some innovations devised during the Gulf War crisis included using neonatal incubators as CW protective devices[44] and respirator systems to ventilate multiple victims from a single machine.[60] A survey of hospital staff members found that only 42% would report for duty following a CW attack.[165]

CHEMICAL WEAPONS

Nerve Agents

Physical Characteristics and Toxicity. Nerve agents (Fig. 100–1) are extremely potent organic phosphorus cholinesterase inhibitors and are the most toxic of the known chemical weapons.[114] For example, sarin is 1000-fold more potent in vitro than the pesticide parathion.[172] Aerosol doses causing 50% human mortality (LCt_{50}) range from 400 mg-min/m^3 for tabun down to 10 mg-min/m^3 for VX, compared to 2500 to 5000 mg-min/m^3 for hydrogen cyanide. Dermal exposure LD_{50}s for nerve agents range from 1700 mg for sarin down to only 6 to 10 mg for VX.[114,172] Pure nerve agents are clear and colorless. Tabun has a faint fruity odor, and soman has been variably described as smelling sweet, musty, fruity, spicy, nutty, or like camphor. Subjects exposed to sarin and VX have been unable to describe the odor.[99,172] The G-agents tabun (GA), sarin (GB), and soman (GD) are volatile and present a significant vapor hazard. Sarin is the most volatile, only slightly less so than water. VX is an oily liquid with low volatility and higher environmental persistence.[99,114,172] Other G- and V-agents have been developed but are not discussed here in detail.

Pathophysiology. The pathophysiology of nerve agents is essentially identical to that of organic phosphorus insecticides (Chap. 88), differing only in terms of potency and physical characteristics of the toxins. The resultant toxidrome includes muscarinic (salivation, lacrimation, urination, defecation, GI cramping, and emesis, or SLUDGE syndrome) and nicotinic (muscle fasciculation, weakness, paralysis) signs as well as central effects (loss of consciousness, seizures, respiratory depression).[69,170,174]

Clinical Effects. Nerve agent vapor exposures produce rapid effects, within seconds to minutes, whereas the effects from liquid exposure may be delayed as the agent is absorbed through the skin.[110,172] Vapor or aerosol exposures have historically been more common, whether through experiments or from unintentional releases in the laboratory[170] or in terrorist attacks.[122,139] Aerosol or vapor exposure initially affects the eyes, nose, and respiratory tract. Miosis is common, resulting from direct contact of the nerve agent with the eye, and may persist for several weeks.[170,174] Other ocular effects include conjunctival injection and blurring and dimming of the vision. Dim vision is often ascribed to pupillary constriction, but central neural mechanisms also play a role.[172] Ciliary spasm produces ocular pain, headache, nausea, and vomiting, often exacerbated by near-vision accommodation.[69] Rhinorrhea, airway secretions, bronchoconstriction, and dyspnea occur with increasing exposures. With a large vapor exposure, one or two breaths may produce loss of consciousness within seconds, followed by seizures, paralysis, and apnea within minutes.[110]

Nerve agents permeate ordinary clothing, allowing for percutaneous absorption and rendering patients potential hazards for healthcare personnel until properly decontaminated.[55] Mild dermal exposure produces localized sweating and muscle fasciculations after an asymptomatic period lasting up to 18 hours. Moderate skin exposure also produces systemic effects with nausea, vomiting, diarrhea, and generalized weakness. Substantial dermal contamination will produce earlier and more severe symptoms, often with abrupt onset. Severe toxicity from any route causes loss of consciousness, seizures, generalized fasciculations, flaccid paralysis, apnea, and/or incontinence.[114,172,174] Cardiovascular effects are less predictable, as either bradycardia (muscarinic) or tachycardia (nicotinic) may occur.[110] Subtle CNS effects may continue for weeks but typically resolve if no anoxic brain injury occurred. Neither delayed peripheral neuropathy nor the intermediate syndrome has been described in humans exposed to nerve agents.[174,175]

What Has Been Learned from the Japanese Sarin Incidents?

Ocular effects were most common after sarin vapor exposure, with

Military Designation	Common Name	Proper Name	Chemical Formula
GA	Tabun	Ethyl-N,N-dimethylphosphoramidocyanidate	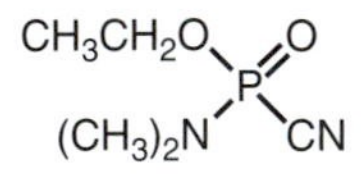 CH_3CH_2O, $(CH_3)_2N$ — P(=O) — CN
GB	Sarin	Isopropyl-methylphosphonofluoridate	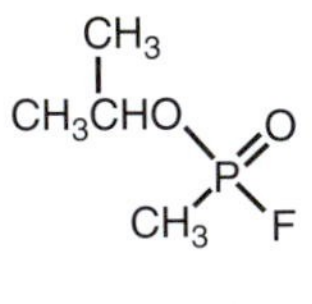 CH_3CHO (with CH_3), CH_3 — P(=O) — F
GD	Soman	Pinacolyl-methylphosphonofluoridate (1,2,2-trimethylpropyl-methylphosphonofluoridate)	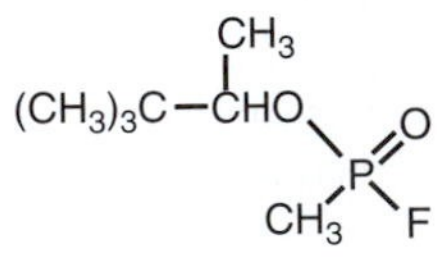 $(CH_3)_3C$—CHO (with CH_3), CH_3 — P(=O) — F
VX	-	O-Ethyl-S-[2-(diisopropylamino)ethyl]-methylphosphonothiolate	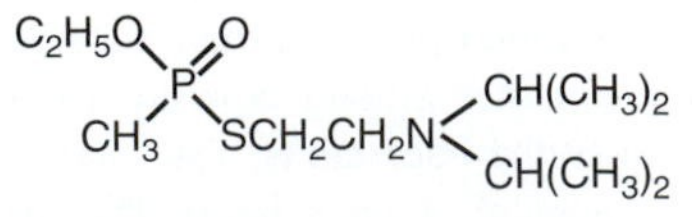 C_2H_5O, CH_3 — P(=O) — SCH_2CH_2N $< \begin{matrix} CH(CH_3)_2 \\ CH(CH_3)_2 \end{matrix}$

Figure 100–1 Nerve agents.

miosis (89 to 99% of symptomatic victims), eye pain, dim vision, and decreased visual acuity.[69,139] Other common complaints were cough, throat tightness, nausea, headache, dizziness, chest discomfort, and abdominal cramping.[104,187] Among 111 patients admitted to one hospital, the most common presenting signs and symptoms were miosis (99%), headache (74.8%), dyspnea (63.1%), nausea (60.4%), eye pain (45.0%), blurred vision (39.6%), dim vision (37.8%), and weakness (36.9%).[134,139] Excessive secretions were less common, with rhinorrhea seen in about one-quarter of patients admitted at one hospital,[139] and in none of 58 patients at another.[187] Tachycardia and hypertension were more common than bradycardia.[129,187] Reversible coronary vasospasm was reported in one severely affected patient.[78] Five mildly affected pregnant patients were admitted for observation, and all had healthy babies without complication, the first one born 3 weeks after the incident.[134,136,139] Secondary exposures occurred among EMTs and hospital personnel in both the Tokyo[104,131,134] and Matsumoto[122,124] incidents, apparently from evaporation of nerve agent that had condensed on the primary victims' clothing. Followup studies show persistent neurologic, neurobehavioral, and electrocardiographic changes,[161,209] although these studies are limited by small numbers and great potential for introducing bias. Psychological sequelae included acute stress reactions in one-third of admitted patients[139] and posttraumatic stress disorder.[203,209]

What is the Treatment for Victims of Nerve Agent Exposure?

Decontamination. Decontamination is crucial to treating nerve agent toxicity. In critically ill patients, antidotal treatment may be necessary before or during the decontamination process; but generally, decontamination should occur before other treatment is instituted.

Atropine Atropine is the standard anticholinergic antidote for the muscarinic effects of nerve agents.[38] Atropine does not reverse nicotinic effects but does have some central effects and may thus assist in halting seizure activity.[69,99,172]

Atropine is administered parenterally, either by the intravenous (IV) or intramuscular (IM) route, and the dose is determined by titration to effect. The standard dose determined by the American military is 2 mg, an amount expected to produce substantial benefit in reversing nerve agent toxicity but one that should be tolerated by an unpoisoned individual unintentionally receiving the drug.[172] Current recommendations place the minimum initial dose of atropine in adults at 2 mg; dosing in children begins at 0.02 mg/kg, with a minimum of 0.1 mg. Severely intoxicated patients receive an initial dose of 5 to 6 mg.[69,172] Repeat doses are given every 2 to 5 minutes until resolution of muscarinic signs of toxicity. Therapeutic endpoints are drying of respiratory secretions and resolution of bronchoconstriction, bradycardia, and/or seizures (if initially present). Reversal of miosis or development of tachycardia is not a reliable marker to guide atropine therapy.[69] The total amount of atropine necessary to treat nerve agent poisoning is often much less than required for organic phosphorus insecticide toxicity of a similar degree. Typically, less than 20 mg is required in the first 24 hours, even in severe cases.[69,172,174] Fewer than 20% of moderately ill patients admitted at one hospital for sarin poisoning in Tokyo required more than 2 mg atropine.[139]

American troops in the Gulf War were issued three MARK I kits for immediate field treatment of nerve agent poisoning. Each kit contains two autoinjectors: an AtroPen containing 2 mg of atropine in 0.7 mL diluent, and a ComboPen containing 600 mg of

2-PAM in 2 mL diluent (Survival Technology, Rockville, MD).[172] These autoinjectors permit rapid IM injections of antidote through protective clothing and are given in the lateral thigh.[38] Treatment algorithms guided the number of MARK I kits to administer. In general, conscious casualties not in severe distress self-administer 1 kit (2 mg atropine), moderate to severe cases receive 3 kits (6 mg atropine) initially, and all receive additional doses as necessary every 5 to 10 minutes.[38,114,172]

Because most nerve agent victims would likely result from aerosol or vapor exposure to the respiratory tract, aerosolized atropine sulfate was temporarily approved by the FDA as an investigational new drug (IND) during the Gulf War.[141] Atropine need not be given solely for ocular effects, which are likely to be present in otherwise unaffected or mildly affected vapor exposure casualties. Although miosis is a sensitive marker of exposure,[132] it is poorly responsive to parenteral atropine,[134] even in high doses.[172] Atropine eyedrops reversed miosis[187] and complaints of dim vision[129] in patients exposed to sarin vapor. In one report, however, all five patients discontinued the drops because of photophobia and loss of accommodation, claiming that their ability to focus was better before the atropine drops,[129] probably as a result of the "pinhole" effect.

Healthy persons receiving 2-mg doses of atropine experience dry mouth, dry skin, mydriasis, paralysis of accommodation, and a pulse rate increase of about 35 beats per minute. Most effects resolve within 4 to 6 hours except for visual blurring, which lasts up to 24 hours. Decreased sweating carries significant risk for heat-related injury, especially among individuals exerting themselves in hot environments and possibly wearing airtight protective gear.[172] In Israel during the Gulf War, many persons presented for medical evaluation after inadvertent autoinjection of atropine, although very few required admission.[6,10]

In a mass casualty incident, a hospital's intravenous atropine supplies may be rapidly depleted. Alternative sources include atropine from ambulances, opthhalmic and veterinary preparations, or substituting glycopyrrolate.[69]

Oximes. Oximes are nucleophilic compounds that reactivate organic phosphorus-inhibited cholinesterase enzymes by removing the dialkylphosphoryl moiety. The only oxime approved in the Unites States by the FDA is pralidoxime (pyridine-2-aldoxime) chloride, or 2-PAM, a monopyridinium compound. Other pralidoxime salts are used elsewhere, such as the methanesulfonate salt of pralidoxime (P2S) in the United Kingdom and 2-PAM methiodide in Japan, as well as the bispyridinium compounds trimedoxime (TMB4) and obidoxime (Toxogonin) in other European countries.[99,139,172] Oximes should be given in conjunction with atropine, as they are not particularly effective in reversing muscarinic effects when given alone. Oximes are the only nerve agent antidotes that can reverse the neuromuscular nicotinic effects of fasciculations, weakness, and flaccid paralysis.

Oximes are effective only if administered before irreversible dealkylation, or "aging," of the organic phosphorus-cholinesterase complex occurs. Soman (GD) has an aging half-life of 2 to 6 minutes in humans.[37] It is unlikely that soman-poisoned victims will reach medical care early enough for oxime therapy to be of great benefit. For comparison, tabun (GA) has an aging half-life of about 14 hours, sarin (GB) 3 to 5 hours, and VX 48 hours.[37] Pralidoxime is effective against sarin and VX in animal studies but not against tabun because of ineffective nucleophilic attack against that particular agent. Obidoxime also is effective against sarin but not against tabun.[99]

The bispyridinium Hagedorn (H-series) oximes, particularly HI-6 and HLö-7, have been studied in a military context.[99] HI-6 appears beneficial against soman (possibly through direct pharmacologic action and/or reactivation of aged soman-inhibited ChE) but is not very effective against tabun. HLö-7 has reactivating activity for both soman- and tabun-inhibited ChE and may thus represent a universal oxime antidote for nerve agents. Administration of HI-6 and HLö-7 by autoinjector is difficult because they are not stable in aqueous solution.

For more details about pralidoxime administration, dosing, and side effects, see Antidotes in Depth: Pralidoxime. The ComboPen autoinjector in MARK I kits contains 600 mg pralidoxime, which produces a therapeutic maximal plasma concentration of 6.5 μg/mL.[172] When possible, however, pralidoxime is optimally administered IV. Repeat pralidoxime dosing or continuous infusions is less likely to be needed for nerve agents than for organic phosphorus insecticides because severe effects are shorter-lived in properly decontaminated patients.[69]

Anticonvulsants.   Severe nerve agent toxicity rapidly induces convulsions, which persist for a few minutes until the onset of flaccid paralysis. Diazepam has beneficial effects beyond other anticonvulsants and simple GABA$_A$ channel agonism, including effects on choline transport across the blood-brain barrier and acetylcholine turnover.[99] Current American military doctrine is to administer 10 mg diazepam IM by ComboPen autoinjector at the onset of severe toxicity whether seizures are present or not. Thus, whenever three MARK I kits are used, a victim is given diazepam as well. Additional autoinjectors are given by medical personnel as necessary for seizures.[114] If intravenous access is feasible, IV diazepam in 5-mg doses every 15 minutes (up to 15 mg) is recommended.[99]

Pyridostigmine Pretreatment.   The first large-scale use of pyridostigmine as a pretreatment for nerve agent toxicity occurred during Operation Desert Storm.[80] Pyridostigmine is a carbamate acetylcholinesterase inhibitor that is freely and rapidly reversible, whereas nerve agent inhibition is permanent once "aging" occurs. Toxicity from rapidly aging nerve agents such as soman (GD) can probably not be reversed by standard oxime therapy in realistic clinical situations. Almost paradoxically, then, a carbamate can occupy cholinesterase, blocking access of nerve agent to the active site, and thereby protect the enzyme from permanent inhibition. Following nerve agent exposure, pyridostigmine is rapidly hydrolyzed from acetylcholinesterase and can also be easily displaced by oximes, regenerating functional enzyme. Between 20 and 40% cholinesterase inhibition is desired to protect against nerve agents.[38] Sixty milligrams of pyridostigmine bromide reduces cholinesterase activity by 28.4% in healthy individuals. Asthmatics taking 30-mg doses had a mean 24.3% reduction in cholinesterase activity without significant reductions in respiratory function or response to inhaled atropine.[147] In animal studies, pyridostigmine confers a benefit against soman and tabun but not against sarin or VX.[37,38] Also, it must be recognized that pyridostigmine is not an antidote but is instead a pretreatment adjunct that greatly enhances atropine and oxime efficacy.[55,174]

American troops in the Gulf War took 30 mg pyridostigmine bromide orally every 8 hours when under threat of nerve agent attack. Cholinergic side effects, mostly gastrointestinal, were com-

mon but rarely required treatment or discontinuing therapy.[80] Israeli soldiers taking the same dose also reported a range of mostly cholinergic symptoms but also a high incidence (71.4%) of dry mouth, which may be more related to environmental and psychological stresses.[166] Nine Israeli patients were hospitalized during the Gulf War for acute pyridostigmine overdoses.[4] All patients recovered fully, including one who self-treated with atropine autoinjectors and presented with anticholinergic toxicity and another who suffered cardiac arrest, apparently from coingesting 4000 mg propranolol.

Other Nerve Agent Therapies.   Calcium channel blockers are effective against soman toxicity in animal models. Other areas of research include prophylactic anticholinergic agents, NMDA-channel antagonists, administration of exogenous cholinesterase (to bind nerve agent) or carboxylesterase (to degrade nerve agent), and monoclonal antibodies against nerve agents.[38,47,99,152]

Vesicants

Vesicants are agents that cause blistering of skin and mucous membranes (Fig. 100–2).

Sulfur Mustard.   Sulfur mustard is bis(2-chloroethyl) sulfide, a vesicant alkylating compound similar to the nitrogen mustards as used in chemotherapy. Nineteenth-century scientists described the compound as smelling like mustard, tasting like garlic, and causing blistering of the skin on contact. Sulfur mustard is known by many names. The Allies of World War I called it Hun Stoffe (German Stuff), abbreviated as HS and later as just H. Distilled, nearly pure mustard is designated HD. The French called it Yperite, after the site where it was first used, and the Germans called it LOST after the two chemists who suggested its use as a chemical weapon, *Lo*mmel and *St*einkopf. It was also called "yellow cross" after the markings on German artillery shells filled with mustard.[19,32,115,176] Mustard was used by the Italians and Japanese in the 1930s, by Egypt in the 1960s, and by Iraq against Iran in the 1980s.[11,114] Some Iranian mustard casualties were treated in Europe, producing a number of recent reports on treatment.[66,126,189] Nonbattlefield exposures have also occurred among Baltic Sea fishermen recovering corroding shells dumped after WWII [1,189] and persons unearthing shells from old battlefields.[156,176]

Physical Characteristics.   Sulfur mustard is a yellow to brown oily liquid with an odor resembling mustard, garlic, or horseradish. Mustard has relatively low volatility and high environmental persistence. Nonetheless, most historical mustard casualties occurred from vapor exposure, a danger that increases in warmer climates. Mustard vapor is 5.4 times denser than air. Mustard freezes at 13.9°C (57°F), so it is sometimes mixed with other substances, including such CW agents as chloropicrin or Lewisite, to reduce the freezing point and allow dispersion as a liquid.[32,114,176]

Pathophysiology.   Sulfur mustard toxicity occurs through several mechanisms. First, mustard is an alkylating agent. Mustard spontaneously undergoes intramolecular cyclization to form a highly-reactive sulfonium ion that alkylates sulfhydryl (-SH) and amino (-NH$_2$) groups (Fig. 100–3).[19,32,114,176] The most important acute toxic manifestation is indirect inhibition of glycolysis. Sulfur mustard rapidly alkylates and crosslinks purine bases in nucleic acids. DNA repair mechanisms are activated, depleting NAD$^+$, which in

Military Designation	Name(s)	Chemical Formula
H, HD	**Sulfur mustard** *bis*-(2-Chloroethyl) sulfide 2,2′-Dichloroethyl sulfide	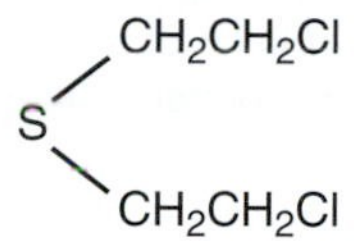 $S \begin{cases} CH_2CH_2Cl \\ CH_2CH_2Cl \end{cases}$
L	**Lewisite** 2-Chlorovinyldichloroarsine β-Chlorovinyldichloroarsine	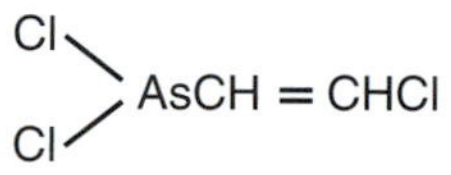 $\begin{matrix} Cl \\ Cl \end{matrix} AsCH=CHCl$
CX	**Phosgene oxime** Dichloroformoxime	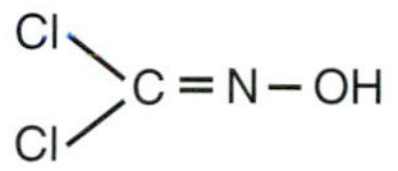 $\begin{matrix} Cl \\ Cl \end{matrix} C=N-OH$

Figure 100–2   Vesicants.

turn inhibits glycolysis and ultimately leads to cellular necrosis from ATP depletion.[19] Mustard also depletes glutathione, leading to loss of protection against oxidant stress, dysregulation of calcium homeostasis, and further inactivation of sulfhydryl-containing enzymes.[176] Mustard is also a weak cholinergic agonist.[114,176]

Clinical Effects.   The organs most commonly affected by mustard are the eyes, skin, and respiratory tract. During WWI, 80 to 90% of American mustard casualties had skin lesions, 86% had ocular involvement, and 75% had airway injury. Iranian soldiers treated in Europe had more airway (95%) and ocular injuries (92%), versus 83% with skin lesions, because of the more extensive vaporization in the warm environment.[19,176] Incapacitation may be severe in terms of number of lost man-days, time for le-

sions to heal, and increased risk of infection. In contrast, mortality is rather low. In WWI, only 2 to 3% of British mustard casualties and fewer than 2% of American casualties died. Fatality rates of 3 to 4% were reported from the Iran-Iraq War.[19,115] Most deaths occur several days after exposure, from either respiratory failure, secondary bacterial pneumonia, or bone marrow suppression.

Dermal exposure produces dose-related injury. After a latent period of 4 to 12 hours, victims develop erythema that may progress to vesicle and/or bulla formation and skin necrosis. Warm, moist, and thin skin is at increased risk of mustard injury, including the perineum, scrotum, axillae, antecubital fossae, and neck. The vesicle fluid does not contain mustard because all chemical reactions are complete within a few minutes.[115] If decontamination is not performed immediately after exposure, injury

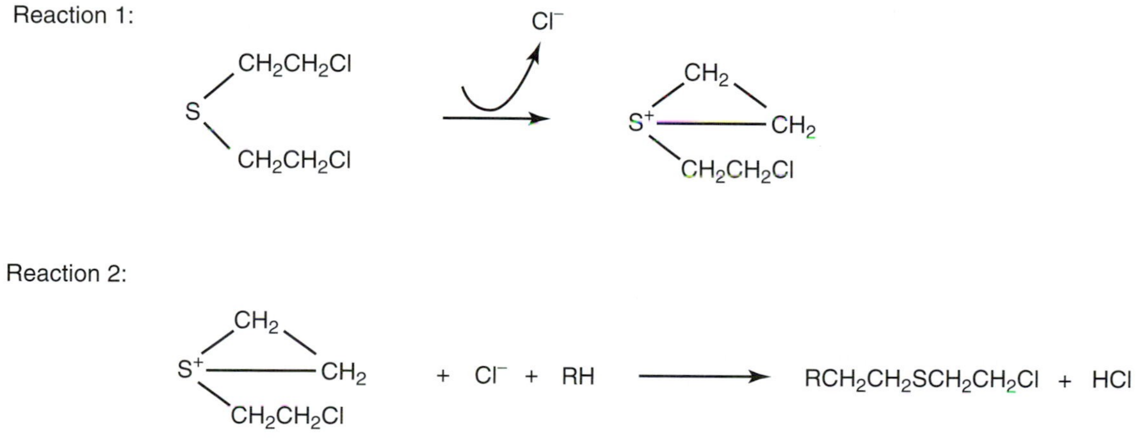

Reaction 1:

$S \begin{cases} CH_2CH_2Cl \\ CH_2CH_2Cl \end{cases} \longrightarrow \begin{matrix} CH_2 \\ S^+ \!-\!\!-\!\!- CH_2 \\ CH_2CH_2Cl \end{matrix} + Cl^-$

Reaction 2:

$\begin{matrix} CH_2 \\ S^+ \!-\!\!-\!\!- CH_2 \\ CH_2CH_2Cl \end{matrix} + Cl^- + RH \longrightarrow RCH_2CH_2SCH_2CH_2Cl + HCl$

Reaction 1 = Cyclization (produces highly reactive ethylenesulfonium ion).

Reaction 2 = Alkylation.

A second round of cyclization and alkylation crosslinks cellular macromolecules.

Figure 100–3   Mechanism of sulfur mustard toxicity.

can not be prevented. Later decontamination may, however, limit the severity of lesions and further spread of the agent. Skin exposure to vapor typically results in first- or second- degree burns, whereas liquid exposure may result in full-thickness burns.[176] Mustard easily penetrates normal clothing and uniforms, and many soldiers received gluteal, perineal, and scrotal burns from sitting on contaminated objects. Other dermal effects include changes in pigmentation, increased incidence of melanocytic nevi and cherry angiomas, and chronic neuropathic symptoms in mustard-burned areas.[32,46,176,189]

Latency of several hours also occurs following ocular and respiratory tract exposures. Ocular effects include pain, miosis, photophobia, lacrimation, blurred vision, blepharospasm, and corneal damage. Permanent blindness is rare, with recovery generally within a few weeks. Inhalation of mustard results in a chemical tracheobronchitis. Hoarseness, cough, sore throat, and chest pressure are common initial complaints. Bronchospasm and obstruction from sloughed membranes occur in more serious cases, but lung parenchymal damage occurs only in the most severe inhalational exposures. Productive cough associated with fever and leukocytosis is not uncommon 12 to 24 hours after exposure and represents a sterile bronchitis or pneumonitis. Nausea and vomiting are common within the first few hours. High-dose exposures may also cause bone marrow suppression.[19,32,114,176]

Various long-term sequelae have been associated with sulfur mustard. Factory workers chronically exposed to mustard have increased risk for respiratory tract carcinomas, although no clear association exists for battlefield exposures. A delayed keratitis, sometimes many years after ocular exposure, may also occur, as well as skin changes noted above.[175]

Treatment. Decontamination is essential in treating the sulfur mustard casualty, even among asymptomatic victims. Further treatment is largely supportive and symptomatic. Military recommendations are to keep skin lesions clean and to treat with topical antibiotics. Small blisters (<1 cm) need not be debrided, but larger bullae should be unroofed. Fluid losses tend to be less than for thermal burns. Skin healing can take weeks to months, although skin grafting is rarely necessary. Ocular injuries usually heal completely with routine chemical burn care. Severe eye injuries may require topical mydriatics, anesthetics, and petroleum jelly to prevent formation of lid synechiae. Respiratory tract injuries are treated with antitussives, inhaled bronchodilators, mucolytics, and oxygen supplementation as needed. Antibiotics should be reserved until confirmation of a bacterial pathogen. Early intubation should be considered for severe airway involvement to assist in ventilation, provide positive airway pressures, and facilitate brochoscopic removal of pseudomembranes and debris.[19,114,176] Several antiinflammatory and sulfhydryl-scavenging agents have shown benefit in animals as prophylactic therapy (or if given immediately after exposure), but there are no data to support their use after injury has occurred.[176]

Lewisite. Lewisite (2-chlorovinyldichloroarsine) was developed to avoid some shortcomings in the use of sulfur mustard in World War I. It was difficult to stage attacks across mustard-contaminated ground, and a less persistent alternative was desired. US Army Captain W. L. Lewis isolated this chemical in pure form in 1918. Lewisite was never used in combat because the first shipment was en route to Europe when the war ended, and it was intentionally destroyed at sea. British Anti-Lewisite (BAL, or dimercaprol) was developed as a specific antidotal agent and remains in use for chelation of arsenic and other heavy metals.[99,176]

Pure Lewisite is an oily, colorless liquid. Impure preparations are colored from amber to blue-black to black and have the odor of geraniums. Lewisite is more volatile than mustard and is easily hydrolyzed by water and by alkaline solutions such as sodium hypochlorite. These properties increase safety for offensive battlefield use but make maintaining a potent vapor concentration difficult.

Lewisite toxicity is similar to that of sulfur mustard, resulting in dermal and mucous membrane damage, with conjunctivitis, airway injury and vesiculation. An important clinical distinction is that Lewisite is immediately painful, whereas initial contact with mustard is not. Other differences are faster onset of inflammatory response and healing of lesions from Lewisite, less secondary infection of Lewisite lesions, and less subsequent pigmentation changes.[176] The mechanisms of Lewisite toxicity are not completely known but appear to involve glutathione depletion and arsenical interaction with enzyme sulfhydryl groups. Nevertheless, Lewisite toxicity is qualitatively and quantitatively different from that of the arsenic it contains. Treatment consists of decontamination with copious water and/or dilute hypochlorite solution, supportive care, and BAL. BAL is given parenterally for systemic toxicity and is also used topically for dermal or ocular injuries. Alternative heavy metal chelators that may be used as Lewisite antidotes include DMPS and DMSA.[99]

Phosgene Oxime. Although classified as a vesicant, phosgene oxime (dichloroformoxime, or CX) does not cause vesication of the skin. CX is more properly an urticant or "nettle" agent, in that it produces erythema, wheals, and urticaria likened to stinging nettles. Phosgene oxime produces immediate irritation of the skin and mucous membranes. CX has never been used in battle, and little is known about its effects on humans.[114,176]

Cyanides (Blood Agents)

Several cyanides have been used as chemical weapons. During World War I, the French used hydrogen cyanide (HCN) and cyanogen chloride (CNCl), designated as agents AC and CK, respectively, without great success; the Austrians introduced cyanogen bromide (CNBr). Cyanide weapons are relatively ineffective because of rapid dispersion and their "all or nothing" biologic activity. An exposed individual either rapidly succumbs to cyanide toxicity or will rapidly recover with minimal sequelae. Mass casualty events from cyanide CW agents have been reported during the Iran-Iraq War and from Iraq's suppression of the Kurds.[12,114]

The cyanides have been called "blood agents" based on the understanding early in the 20th century that they were carried in the blood to exert systemic toxicity, whereas the other known CW agents produced local effects. This term is now antiquated because sulfur mustard and nerve agents can be carried in the blood and because the target of cyanide toxicity is cellular respiration in the mitochondria. The clinical effects and treatment of cyanide toxicity are covered elsewhere (Chap. 98 and Antidotes In Depth: Cyanide Antidotes) and do not differ significantly if used as a weapon. Hydrocyanic acid gas persists for only a few minutes in the atmosphere because it is lighter than air and rapidly disperses. Cyanogen chloride additionally causes ocular and respiratory tract irritation and can produce delayed pulmonary edema in victims who are not rapidly killed.[12,114]

Pulmonary Agents

Both chlorine (agent CL) and phosgene (agent CG) were used as war gases in World War I. Chlorine, phosgene, various organohalides, and nitrogen oxides belong to a group of toxic chemicals designated "pulmonary agents" because they can all induce delayed pulmonary edema from increased alveolar-capillary membrane permeability.[99,114,196] Although pulmonary agents have not been used militarily since 1918, the risk of chlorine and phosgene exposure remains because of their extensive use in industry or possibly as a terrorist weapons. See Chapter 95 for clinical details, as the remainder of this section highlights military issues regarding these agents.

When released on the battlefield, chlorine forms a yellow-green cloud with a distinct, pungent odor. Phosgene is either colorless or seen as a white cloud as a result of atmospheric hydrolysis. Phosgene smells like grass, sweet newly mown hay, or corn, or like moldy hay. Although sulfur mustard was known as the "king of war gases,"[19] phosgene accounted for about 85% of all WWI deaths from chemical weapons.[99] Phosgene produces injury by hydrolysis in the lungs to hydrochloric acid and by forming diamides that crosslink cell components (Fig. 100–4). Battlefield exposure triggers cough, chest discomfort, dyspnea, lacrimation, and the peculiar complaint that smoking tobacco produces an objectionable taste. High-level exposures may produce acute lung injury within 2 to 6 hours. WWI phosgene fatalities developed a mushroom-shaped efflux of pink foam at their mouths from pulmonary edema fluid. Prolonged observation after phosgene exposure is the rule, as some casualties have initially appeared well and have been discharged, only to return in severe respiratory distress a few hours later.[99,114,196]

Riot Control Agents

Riot control agents (Fig. 100–5) are intentionally nonlethal compounds that temporarily disable exposed individuals through intense irritation of exposed mucous membranes and skin. These compounds are also known as lacrimators, irritants, harassing agents, and human repellents but are most commonly called "tear

A.

B.

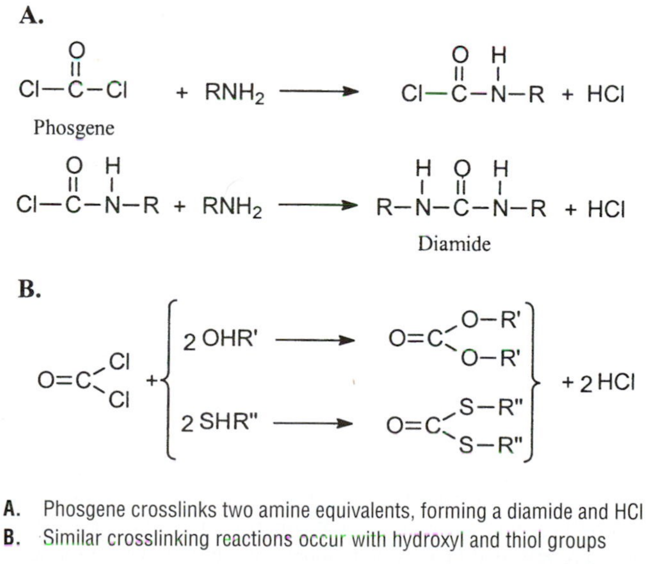

A. Phosgene crosslinks two amine equivalents, forming a diamide and HCl
B. Similar crosslinking reactions occur with hydroxyl and thiol groups

Figure 100–4   Proposed mechanisms of phosgene toxicity.

gas."[71] Common characteristics include rapid onset of effects within seconds to minutes, relatively brief duration once exposure has ceased and the victim has been decontaminated, and a high safety ratio (lethal dose vs effective dose).[99,114,173]

CN (chloroacetophenone) has been widely used since WWI. CN is the active ingredient in the Chemical Mace® brand nonlethal weapon originally produced in 1965 by the General Ordinance Equipment Company, later a division of Smith & Wesson.[185] CS (*o*-chlorobenzilidene malononitrile) has largely replaced CN because of its higher potency, lower toxicity, and improved chemical stability.[71,88,173] When used for crowd control, both CN and CS are disseminated as aerosols or as smoke from incendiary devices. Exposed persons develop burning irritation of the eyes, progressing to conjunctival injection, lacrimation, photophobia, and blepharospasm. Mucous membranes of the upper aerodigestive tracts can also be involved. Inhalation causes chest tightness, cough, sneezing, and increased secretions. Dermal exposure may cause a burning sensation, erythema, or vesiculation, depending on the dose. Victims generally remove themselves from the offensive environment and recover within 15 to 30 minutes. Most deaths related to riot control agents occur from respiratory tract complications in closed-space exposures where exiting the area is impossible.[99,114,173]

Personal protective devices dispensing lacrimator substances also cause chemical injuries in peacetime. Law enforcement agencies and private citizens may have access to products containing CS, CN, and/or OC (oleoresin capsicum, or pepper spray). OC is the essential oil derived from pepper plants (*Capsicum anuum* species) which contains capsaicin (trans-8-methyl-*N*-vanillyl-6-noneamide), a naturally occurring lacrimator. Capsaicin activates heat-dependent nociceptors, explaining why exposures are experienced as "hot."[25] Severe respiratory tract injuries and fatalities are occasionally reported from exposures to these devices.[15,183,197,207]

Chloropicrin (trichloronitromethane or nitrochloroform) is another lacrimator previously used as a CW agent that occasionally causes human toxicity through its use as a fumigant and soil insecticide.[146,188] DM (10-chloro-5,10-dihydrodiphenarsazine, or diphenylaminearsine) is a vomiting agent. Clinical effects are delayed for several minutes, by which time the victim may have absorbed a significant amount. In addition to upper respiratory and ocular irritation, DM causes more prolonged systemic effects with headache, malaise, nausea, and vomiting.[114,173]

The primary treatment for all riot control agents is removal from exposure. Contaminated clothing should be removed and placed in airtight bags to prevent secondary exposures.[88] Skin irrigation with copious cold water is used for significant dermal exposures.[16,88,91] Symptomatic treatments, such as topical ophthalmic anesthetics, nebulized bronchdilators, or oral antihistamines and corticosteroids, are indicated as appropriate in more severely affected victims.[16] Capsaicin-induced dermatitis has been treated variably with immersion in water or oil, vinegar, bleach, lidocaine gel, and topical antacid suspensions.[65,75,185,206] Cold water produces earlier symptomatic relief, but oil immersion has longer-lasting benefit.[75]

Incapacitating Agents

3-Quinuclidinyl benzilate (BZ or QNB; Fig. 100–6) is an antimuscarinic compound most likely to be used as an incapacitating CW agent. BZ is 25-fold more potent centrally than atropine, with an ID_{50} of about 0.5 mg. Clinical effects are characteristic for anti-

Military Designation	Name(s)	Chemical Formula
CN	1-Chloroacetophenone 2-Chloroacetophenone 2-Chloro-1-phenylethanone Tear gas Chemical mace	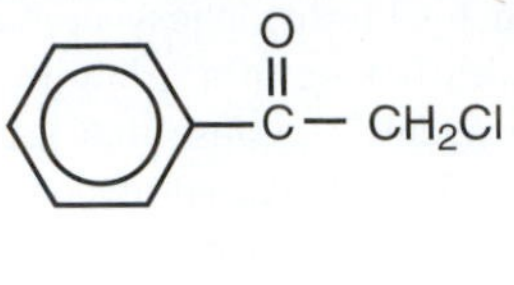
CS	o-Chlorobenzylidene malononitrile 2-Chlorobenzalmalononitrile Tear gas	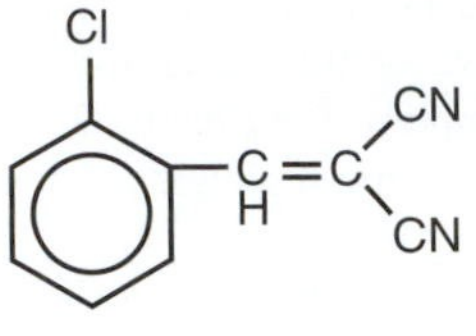
DM	Adamsite 10-chloro-5,10-dihydrophenarsazine Diphenylaminechlorarsine Vomiting gas	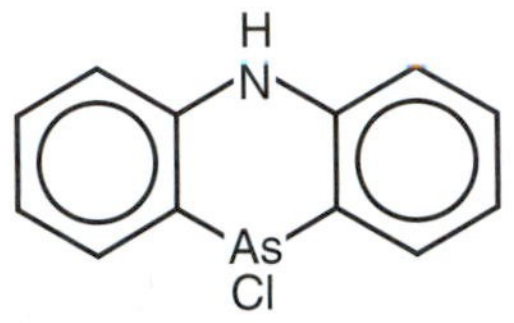
OC	Capsaicin trans-8-Methyl-N-vanillyl-6-noneamide Oleoresin capsicum Pepper spray	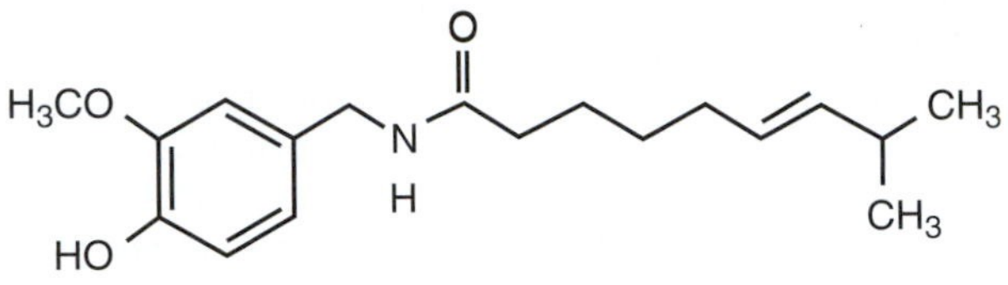

Figure 100–5   Riot control agents.

cholinergics, with drowsiness, poor coordination, slowing of thought processes, and progression to delirium. BZ takes at least an hour to produce initial manifestations, peaks at 8 hours, continues to incapacitate for 24 hours, and takes 2 to 3 days to fully resolve (Table 100–6).[82] During the recent Balkan wars, Yugoslavian forces had access to several chemical weapons, including CS, mustard, sarin, and BZ.[119] Allegations were made that Bosnian Serbs used BZ against civilians, who reported hallucinations associated with attacks by artillery shells emitting smoke. Although CW exposure can not be completely excluded, the hallucinations can be ascribed to exhaustion and multiple physical and psychological stressors.[59,167] Lysergic acid diethylamide (LSD) has also been investigated as an incapacitating agent.

BIOLOGIC WEAPONS

Biologic warfare agents fall into three main categories: bacteria, viruses, and toxins. Bacteria and viruses are living organisms and will reproduce in suitably exposed victims, although only a few are transmissible from person to person. With the notable exceptions of pneumonic plague, smallpox, and viral hemorrhagic fevers, BW victims should not be contagion risks if standard universal precautions are employed. Some authorities consider biologic toxin weapons as chemical agents because they are not themselves living organisms. For instance, capsaicin is discussed in this chapter among the chemical weapons because its effects mimic those of artificially manufactured lacrimators. Toxin weapons are considered here, as elsewhere, to be biologic weapons because they are derived from living organisms. Also, many bacterial BW agents exert their effects through toxins they elaborate.

All the agents discussed here have been investigated as or manufactured into weapons. Space in a toxicology (as opposed to infectious disease) text does not permit in-depth review of all BW agents, so summaries of clinical effects, diagnostic modalities, prophylaxis, and treatment regimens and additional information of toxicologic interest are found in Table 100–7.

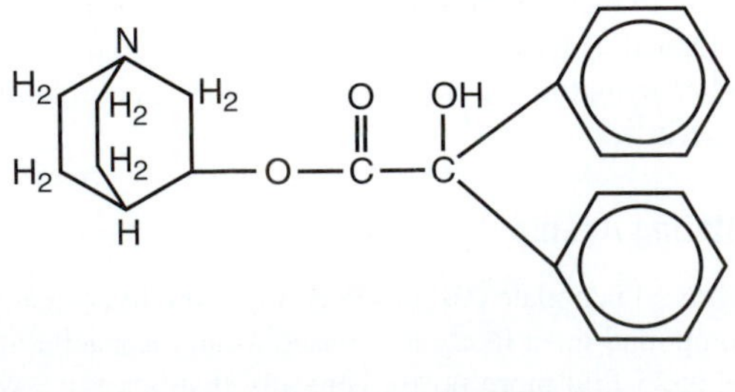

The 2001 Bioterrorist Anthrax Outbreak

Starting on September 27, 2001, a 63-year-old Florida man developed malaise, fatigue, fever, chills, anorexia, and sweats. He was admitted to the hospital, October 2nd, after presenting with additional complaints of nausea, vomiting, and confusion. Chest radiography showed cardiomegaly, a left perihilar infiltrate, small left pleural effusion, and a prominent superior mediastinum. Lumbar puncture revealed hemorrhagic meningitis with many gram-positive bacilli. *Bacillus anthracis* was isolated from the cerebrospinal fluid after only 7 hours incubation and from blood cultures within

Figure 100–6   Incapacitating agent BZ (3-quinuclidinyl benzilate, QNB).

TABLE 100-6. Chemical Weapons Toxidromes

Chemical Weapon	Onset	Eyes	Upper Airways and Mucous Membranes	Lungs	Skin	CNS	GI Tract	Other
					Organ System			
Nerve agents Tabun (GA), Sarin (GB), Soman (GD), VX								
Aerosol/vapor (mild/ moderate exposure)	Rapid (sec-min)	Miosis, eye pain, dim or blurred vision	Rhinorrhea, ↑ secretions	Dyspnea, cough, wheezing, bronchorrhea	—	Headache	Nausea, vomiting, abdominal cramps	—
Dermal exposure (mild/moderate exposure)	Delayed (min-h)	—	—	—	Localized sweating	—	Nausea, vomiting, diarrhea, cramping	Subjective weakness, local muscle fasciculations
Severe exposure (any route)	As above (by route)	Miosis	↑ Secretions	Apnea	—	Sudden collapse, seizures	Incontinence	Generalized fasciculations, weakness, flaccid paralysis
Vesicants								
Sulfur mustard (H, HD)	Delayed (h)	Conjunctivitis, pain, blurred vision, blindness (temporary)	Irritation, hoarseness, barky cough, sinus tenderness, tracheobronchitis	(More severe exposures) productive cough, pseudomembrane formation, airway obstruction	Erythema, vesicles, bullae, with necrosis	—	Nausea, vomiting	Bone marrow suppression (in severe exposures)
Lewisite (L)	Immediate irritation Delayed vesication	Pain, blepharo- spasm, conjunctivitis, lid edema	(Same as sulfur mustard)	(Same as sulfur mustard)	Erythema, vesicles	—	—	Shock (in severe exposures)
Phosgene oxime (CX)	Immediate irritation Delayed urtication	Pain, corneal damage	Irritation	Acute lung injury	Pain, blanching, erythema, urticaria necrosis	—	—	—
Pulmonary agents								
Phosgene (CG) and chlorine (CL)	Immediate irritation Delayed acute lung injury	Irritation	Irritation, stridor (chlorine)	Dyspnea, cough, acute lung injury	—	—	—	Chlorine effects more rapid than phosgene
Cyanides								
Hydrogen cyanide (AC)	Rapid (sec-min)	—	—	Hyperpnea then apnea	—	Anxiety, agita- tion, sudden collapse, seizures	—	—
Cyanogen chloride (CK)	Rapid (sec-min)	Irritation	Irritation	Hyperpnea then apnea	—	Anxiety, agita- tion, sudden collapse, seizures	—	—

(continued)

TABLE 100-6. Chemical Weapons Toxidromes (*continued*)

Chemical Weapon	Onset	Eyes	Upper Airways and Mucous Membranes	Lungs	Skin	CNS	GI Tract	Other
					Organ System			
Riot control agents								
Lacrimators (CN, CS) Capsaicin (OC)	Immediate	Pain, lacrimation, blepharospasm, conjunctivitis	Irritation	Cough, chest pain	Burning pain, erythema, vesiculation (severe exposures)	Anxiety	Nausea, retching (may occur with CN/CS)	—
Adamsite (DM)	Rapid (min)	Irritation	Irritation, sneezing	Cough, chest pain	—	Headache	Nausea, vomiting, abdominal cramps	—
Incapacitating agents								
3-Quinuclidinyl benzilate (BZ)	Delayed (h)	Mydriasis	Dry mouth	—	—	Anticholinergic delirium	—	—

TABLE 100–7.   Biologic Warfare Agents Summary

Bacteria

Anthrax (*Bacillus anthracis*)

Clinical syndromes

Inhalational anthrax is likely from BW aerosol release following inhalation of spores. One- to 6-days (maximum 8 weeks) incubation period, then fever, malaise, cough, extreme weakness, and mild chest discomfort. Progresses to dyspnea, stridor, diaphoresis, cyanosis, and shock. Fatality rate >80% if untreated with death occurring within 24–36 hours of severe symptoms. Spores enter chest lymphatics, germinate in lymph nodes, and cause hemorrhagic mediastinitis, septicemia, and meningitis. Also known as woolsorters' disease because of strong occupational association.

Cutaneous anthrax results from inoculation of spores through broken skin and accounts for 95% of naturally occurring human anthrax cases. Black eschar forms with significant surrounding edema; 10–20% mortality if untreated; death is rare with antibiotic therapy.

Gastrointestinal anthrax is unlikely to occur from BW release

Diagnostic tests: Chest radiograph (CXR) with widened mediastinum; blood Gram stain and culture

Drug therapy: Efficacy for inhalation anthrax once symptoms develop is unpredictable

Ciprofloxacin 400 mg IV q8–12h and other fluoroquinolones

Doxycycline 200 mg IV, then 100 mg IV q8–12h

PCN 2 million U IV q2h, plus streptomycin 30 mg/kg IM qd (or gentamicin) and other agents to offer multidrug therapy.

Chemoprophylaxis: Give along with vaccine until exposure excluded; if exposure occurred, continue antibiotics for 4 wk if vaccine available, and for 8 wk if vaccine not available; ciprofloxacin 500 mg PO bid or doxycycline 100 mg PO bid

Vaccine: Licensed vaccine given at 0, 2, 4 wk and 6, 12, 18 mo; annual booster for at-risk populations

Precautions: Standard; inhalation anthrax is not transmissible; dermal lesions potentially transmissible by contact with broken skin

Additional notes: *Bacillus anthracis* produces three toxins: protective antigen (PA), edema factor, and lethal factor. PA facilitates endocytosis of the other two toxins and is so named because antibodies against it protect the subject from the other two toxins. Anthrax vaccine adsorbed (AVA, Bioport Corporation) is made from an avirulent, nonencapsulated strain that produces PA. AVA has been determined to be safe and effective. Most side effects are localized, minor, and self-limited, similar to other routine vaccinations; systemic reactions are rare. Edema factor is a calmodulin-dependent adenylate cyclase. Increased intracellular cAMP upsets water homeostasis, leading to massive edema and impaired neutrophil function. Lethal factor is a zinc metalloprotease that stimulates macrophages to release TNF-α and IL-1β, contributing to death in systemic anthrax infections. Undue concern has arisen regarding the safety of anthrax vaccination, fueled by uncertainty about the etiology of Gulf War syndrome, possible violations of informed consent among military personnel who received drugs and vaccines against other CBW agents, and misinformative Internet websites. Several service members have been punished or discharged in highly publicized refusals to accept vaccinations against anthrax.

References[8,9,22,26,27,29,36,50,52,53,73,108,111,113,123,143,144,151,157,158,162,211]

Plague (*Yersinia pestis*)

Clinical syndromes

Pneumonic plague may occur from BW release or inhaling respiratory droplets from infected individuals. After 2–3 days of incubation, pneumonia develops with fever, chills, cough, headache, hemoptysis, and the appearance of systemic toxicity. Cases rapidly develop dyspnea, stridor, cyanosis, respiratory failure, and cardiovascular collapse, sometimes with a bleeding diasthesis.

Bubonic plague occurs from the bite of infected fleas, which may occur naturally in endemic areas or from intentional release. After 2–10 days of incubation, patients develop fever, malaise, and painful adenopathy (buboes). Some patients progress to septicemia and/or pneumonic plague.

Diagnostic tests: CXR with pulmonary infiltrates. "Safety-pin" coccobacilli on Gram stain. Leukocytosis with left shift. Organism cultured from blood, sputum, or bubo aspirate.

Drug therapy:

Streptomycin 30 mg/kg IM/d divided bid for 10 days or gentamicin 5 mg/kg IM or IV qd for 10 days.

Doxycycline 200 mg IV, then 100 mg IV q 12h for 10–14 days

Chemoprophylaxis:

Tetracycline 500 mg PO qid for 7 days

Doxycycline 100 mg PO q 12h for 7 days

Vaccine: An old whole-cell vaccine is no longer available and was not effective against aerosol. A new vaccine against pneumonic plague is under development.

Precautions: Pneumonic plague is highly contagious; droplet precautions (respiratory isolation) until patient treated with antibiotics for 3 days. Standard precautions otherwise.

References[50,72,107–109,112,113]

Brucellosis (*Brucella* spp.)

Clinical syndrome:

Nonspecific febrile illness, with chills and malaise after 5–60 days (or longer) incubation.

Pulmonary symptoms expected from BW release.

Diagnostic tests: Serology, culture.

Drug therapy: Doxycycline 200 mg/d PO, plus rifampin 600–900 mg/d PO for 6 weeks

Chemoprophylaxis: Doxycycline 200 mg/d PO, plus Rifampin 600–900 mg/d PO for 3 weeks

Vaccine: No human vaccine

Precautions: Standard

References[50,70,112]

Cholera (*Vibrio cholerae*)

Clinical syndrome: **Secretory diarrhea;** 1 to 5-day incubation, then vomiting, abdominal distension and pain, little or no fever, progressing to profuse, watery diarrhea, which may exceed 5–10 L/d.

(continued)

TABLE 100–7. Biologic Warfare Agents Summary (continued)

Cholera (*Vibrio cholerae*) (*continued*)
Diagnostic tests: "Rice-water" stools, stool microscopy with few or no RBCs or WBCs
Drug therapy: Shortens course of diarrhea; 3 days PO antibiotic therapy
  Ciprofloxacin 500 mg bid, erythromycin 500 mg q6h, tetracycline 500 mg q6h, or doxycycline 300 mg q12h
Chemoprophylaxis: NA
Vaccine: Licensed vaccine, but provides only short-lived and incomplete protection
Precautions: Standard; fecal-oral transmission
Additional notes: Cholera produces enterotoxins resulting in massive secretory diarrhea. Not an ideal BW agent. Must be ingested instead of inhaled.
  Routine water chlorination kills most cholera bacteria.
References[50,113]

Q Fever (*Coxiella burnetti*)
Clinical syndrome: **Pulmonary syndrome or nonspecific febrile illness.** 10 to 40-day incubation, then fever, headache, fatigue, and malaise lasting 2 days
  to 2 wk. Cough and pleuritic chest pain common; incapacitating but rarely fatal.
Diagnostic tests: Serology, CXR with patchy infiltrates in 50% (even without pulmonary symptoms)
Drug therapy: Tetracycline 500 mg PO q6h for 5–7 days or doxycycline 100 mg PO q12h for 5–7 days
Chemoprophylaxis: Tetracycline or doxycycline starting 8–12 days postexposure for 5 days
Vaccine: IND vaccine
Precautions: Standard
Additional notes: *Coxiella burnetti* can persist on inanimate objects for weeks to months and can cause clinical disease with inhalation of a single
  organism.
References[21,50,113]

Tularemia (*Francisella tularensis*)
Clinical syndromes
  Typhoidal tularemia is expected from BW aerosol release; 2 to 10-day incubation, then fever, prostration, weight loss, cough, and chest discomfort
  Ulceroglandular tularemia occurs more commonly in naturally acquired cases. Local skin ulcer with regional lymphadenopathy, fever, chills, headache,
    and malaise
Diagnostic tests: Serology, culture, CXR with infiltrates, mediastinal lymphadenopathy, or effusions
Drug therapy: Streptomycin 30 mg/kg/d divided bid for 10–14 days or gentamicin 3–5 mg/kg/day for 10–14 days
Chemoprophylaxis: Doxycycline 100 mg PO q12h for 14 days or tetracycline PO 2g/d for 14 days
Vaccine: IND vaccine
Precautions: Standard
References[45,50,112,113]

Viruses
Smallpox (Variola)
Clinical syndrome: **Fever and rash.** 12 to 14-day incubation, then malaise, fever, rigors, vomiting, headache, backache. Rash follows 2–3 days later, with
    macules that progess to papules, vesicles, and pustules, which ultimately scab over. Skin lesions develop synchronously with centrifugal distribution
    (differentiating them from varicella lesions, which otherwise appear identical), most prominent on face and extremities; 30% mortality rate in unvacci-
    nated populations
Diagnostic tests: ELISA, PCR, virus isolation from pharyngeal swabs or scab material
Drug therapy: None proven; cidofovir and ribavarin effective in vitro
Chemoprophylaxis: Immediate vaccination or varicella immune globulin within a few days of exposure
Vaccine: Licensed calf-lymph vaccine; IND cell-culture vaccine
Precautions: Airborne and contact precautions. Highly contagious, often with 10–20 secondary cases per index case. Quarantine exposed persons (even if
    asymptomatic) for 17 days, and all patients until lesions scab over.
Additional Notes: Smallpox certified by WHO as eradicated in 1980, with only remaining variola stocks at CDC in Atlanta and Russian State Research Cen-
    ter of Virology and Biotechnology (VECTOR) in Koltsovo, Novosibirsk Region. Planned destruction of remaining *Variola* in 1999 delayed because of the
    potential for antiviral research and concern for unintentional or intentional release. Currently believed that North Korea and Iraq also have *Variola* stocks.
    Many previously vaccinated individuals no longer protected. Remaining amount of vaccine inadequate should *Variola* release occur.
References[17,23,50,63,64,89,90,105,112,113,163]

Venezuelan equine encephalitis
Clinical syndrome: **Encephalitis.** 2 to 6-day incubation, then malaise, fever, rigors, photophobia, myalgias. Incapacitating, but rarely fatal; full recovery
    takes 1–2 wk
Diagnostic tests: Leukopenia with lymphocytopenia, serology, virus isolation from serum or throat swab
Drug therapy: NA
Chemoprophylaxis: NA
Vaccine: IND vaccine
Precautions: Standard (theoretical transmission from respiratory droplet nuclei)
References[50,113,179]

Viral hemorrhagic fevers (VHFs; Lassa fever, Dengue, yellow fever, Crimean-Congo hemorrhagic fever, Marburg, Ebola, and Hanta viruses)
Clinical syndrome: **Fever, shock, hemorrhage.** Variable incubation (4–21 days), then fever, malaise, prostration, and increased vascular permeability
    that may result in bleeding complications. Extent of renal, hepatic, and hematologic involvement varies with infectious agent.

(continued)

TABLE 100–7.   Biologic Warfare Agents Summary (*continued*)

Viral hemorrhagic Fevers (continued)
  Diagnostic tests: Serology, viral isolation
  Drug therapy: Ribavarin for some VHFs
  Chemoprophylaxis: NA
  Vaccine: IND vaccines for some
  Precautions: Contact precautions
  References[50,74,113]

Toxins
  Botulinum toxin
    Clinical syndrome: **Unexplained paralysis/death.** 1 to 5-day incubation, followed by multiple bulbar nerve palsies with symmetric descending paralysis
      (Chap. 75). BW release may be aerosol or contamination of food/water.
    Diagnostic tests: Ag-ELISA, Ex vivo mouse studies
    Drug therapy: Licensed CDC trivalent equine antitoxin for serotypes A, B, E; IND heptavalent equine despeciated antitoxin fragments [F(ab ′)$_2$] for serotypes
      A–G
    Chemoprophylaxis: NA
    Vaccine: IND pentavalent toxoid for serotypes A–E
    Precautions: Standard
    Additional notes: Botulinum toxin is 15,000 times more potent than VX nerve agent. Developed as bioweapon in WWII and more recently by Iraq and ter-
      rorist groups. May have been used in the 1942 assassination of Gestapo chief Reinhard Heydrich.
      References[33,48,50,113,117,140,160,177,210]

  Ricin
    Clinical syndromes
      Pulmonary syndrome if aerosol inhaled. Weakness, fever, cough, respiratory distress, hypoxia, pulmonary edema. May incapacitate or kill within 36–72
        hours depending on dose.
      "Septicemic" syndrome with parenteral exposure; fever, elevated WBC count, shock
    Diagnostic tests: ELISA, serology
    Drug therapy: NA
    Chemoprophylaxis: NA
    Vaccine: None (investigational toxoid developed for animals)
    Precautions: Standard
    Additional notes: Ricin is one of the most toxic and easily produced plant toxins, derived from the castor bean plant *Ricinus communis* (Chap. 78).
      Investigated as a BW agent by the US military in WWI. Never used in battle but has been used in politically motivated assassinations. Inhibits protein
      synthesis at the ribosome.
      References[31,49,50,83,113,178]

  Staphylococcal enterotoxin B (SEB)
    Clinical syndromes:
      Pulmonary syndrome if aerosol inhaled; 3–12 hours incubation, then fever, chills, headache, myalgias, cough, chest pain. Fever persists 2–5 days,
        cough for up to 4 weeks. Incapacitating but rarely fatal.
      Gastrointestinal syndrome if ingested. Identical to staphylococcal food poisoning (Chap. 74)
    Diagnostic tests: Ag- or Ab-ELISA, serology, abnormal CXR in severe inhalation cases
    Drug therapy: NA
    Chemoprophylaxis: NA
    Vaccine: None
    Precautions: Standard
    Additional notes: SEB is a "superantigen" that induces profound activation of the immune system, even in minute quantities.
      References[50,113,135]

  Tricothecene mycotoxins
    Clinical syndromes:
      Inflammation, injury, and necrosis of exposed skin, mucous membranes, and airways; resembles vesicant CW exposure, a dermally active bioweapon.
      Alimentary toxic aleukia if ingested; gastroenteritis, fever, chills, bone marrow suppression, and secondary sepsis; resembles acute radiation poisoning
    Diagnostic tests: Isolation of toxin (or metabolites) from biologic or environmental samples
    Drug therapy: NA
    Chemoprophylaxis: NA
    Vaccine: None
    Precautions: Standard
    Additional notes: Tricothecene mycotoxins (Fig. 100–7) are produced by filamentous fungi (molds) or various genera, including *Fusarium, Myrote-
      cium, Trichoderma,* and *Stachybotrys.* Tricothecene toxins are unusual among potential BW agents because toxicity can occur with exposure to intact
      skin. They are potent inhibitors of protein synthesis in eukaryotic cells, particularly in rapidly proliferating tissues. Exposure to any mucosal surface re-
      sults in severe irritation. Dermal exposure can produce inflammatory lesions lasting for 1 to 2 weeks, vesiculation, and death in higher doses.
        Several reports from the 1970s and 1980s suggested that Soviet-supported forces were using tricothecene mycotoxins, particularly the toxin T-2, as
      BW agents. Aerosol and droplet clouds called "yellow rain" were associated with mass casuality incidents in Afghanistan, Laos, and Kampuchea.

(*continued*)

TABLE 100–7. Biologic Warfare Agents Summary *(continued)*

Tricothene mycotoxins (continued)
  Alimentary toxic aleukia
    Additional notes:
        Yellow rain attacks were also reported in the Iran-Iraq War. Such attacks would involve multiple routes of exposure, with skin deposition predominating. Early symptoms included nausea, vomiting, weakness, dizziness, and ataxia. Diarrhea would ensue, first watery then bloody. Within 3–12 hours victims would develop dyspnea, cough, chest pain, sore mouths, bleeding gums, epistaxis, and hematemesis.

        Evidence that tricothecene mycotoxins were used as BW agents was mostly circumstantial. Although T-2 toxin was found in victims' blood and urine, it was also found in samples from unexposed individuals, probably from baseline ingestion of contaminated foods. Environmental samples containing yellow rain droplets inconsistently contained mycotoxins. Eyewitness accounts of yellow rain attacks varied widely (including various descriptions of the alleged agent's color), and, despite the large number of such attacks, no contaminated ordinance or dispersal device was ever recovered. It was also discovered that yellow rain droplets were comprised mostly of pollen grains. Supporters of the yellow rain as BW theory retorted that pollen grains are an ideal size to act as aerosol biotoxin carriers. However, the pollen in yellow rain samples did not contain protein, similar to pollen that has been digested by bees. Further, the distribution of pollen species found in yellow rain was indistinguishable from the contents of Asian honeybee feces, and mass bee defecation resulting in showers of yellow droplets has been observed.

        The yellow rain as bee feces theory assumes that any mass casualty incidents were from endemic disease outbreaks, other CBW agents not yet identified, or a combination of both. Not explained by the bee feces theory is the presence of polyethylene glycol in some yellow rain samples. Whether yellow rain was intentional biologic warfare or a completely natural phenomenon, it remains that tricothecene mycotoxins could potentially be used as effective, dermally active BW agents.
        References[20,50,58,67,100–102,113,128,155,159,180,199,201]

---

24 hours. The patient had progressive clinical deterioration and died on hospital day number 4.[74a]

On October 4th, the Centers for Disease Control released a public health message regarding this case, which initially appeared to be an isolated, perhaps naturally-occurring sporadic event; another case of anthrax had been reported in Texas earlier the same year.[26b] Nevertheless, the rarity of inhalational anthrax (especially outside of a high-risk occupation), combined with increased suspicion in the wake of events on September 11, 2001, led to intense investigation of a potential bioterrorist event. Within days, epidemiologic investigation suggested workplace exposure to anthrax spores, and personnel working in the same building were started on prophylactic ciprofloxacin.[26c] By October 12th, a case of cutaneous anthrax was reported from New York in association with a suspicious letter opened on September 25th.[26d] Anthrax cases and environmental contamination were also soon detected in Washington, DC and in association with a New Jersey postal facility. Public response included misuse and hoarding of antibiotics, purchasing gas masks (often with inappropriate filtering mechanisms for biological weapons), numerous false alarms related to miscellaneous powdery substances, and copycat hoaxes. By November 7, 2001, a total of 22 cases of anthrax were reported: 10 inhalational (4 of these were fatal) and 23 cutaneous (7 confirmed and 5 suspected) cases.[26e] While the overall morbidity and mortality from this bioterrorist event were relatively low, the overall impact was high. Several hundred postal and other facilities were

tested for *B. anthracis* spore contamination, and public health authority-recommended antibiotic prophylaxis was initiated for approximately 32,000 persons.[26e] Additional indirect costs and effects are more difficult to quantify, including the number of persons self-initiating antibiotic treatment without an evident indication, lost production and wages, environmental and biologic sample testing, decontamination efforts, and an international sense of unease.

Although investigation of this outbreak is still ongoing while this section is being written, several important lessons regarding BW preparedness can be gleaned. Estimates of tens of thousands of deaths from an anthrax attack[79] depend on efficient BW agent dispersion. The military-style goal of anthrax as a "Weapon of Mass Destruction" is probably out of reach for a lone madman or even most terrorist organizations; however, the technically easier anthrax letter has clearly proven itself to be a "Weapon of Mass Disruption". As predicted, the psychological impact far exceeded the actual medical emergency, and it also appears to remain true that events with a modest number of medical patients are more likely than true mass-casualty BW incidents. On the other hand, prior assumptions regarding the clinical aspects of anthrax were not as reliable. The mortality rate among the 10 cases of inhalational anthrax was 40%, considerably lower than expected and probably due to improved supportive care and a wider choice of antibiotics compared to historical controls. Presentation with fulminant illness (sepsis) still appears to be predictive of a fatal outcome, yet

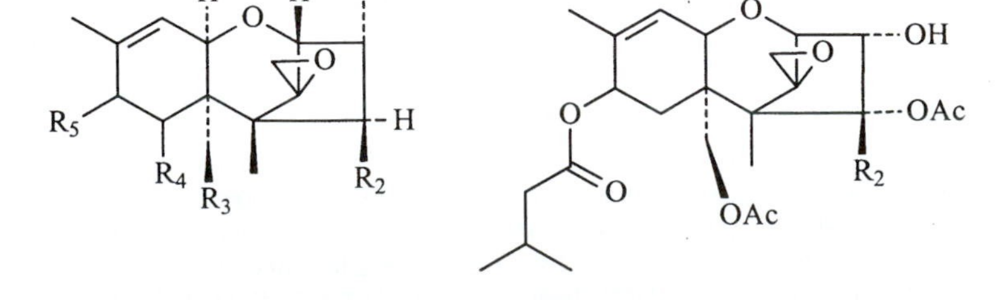

Figure 100–7 Tricothecene mycotoxins. A. Tetracyclic tricothecene nucleus B. T-2 toxin.

the initial phase of illness does not necessarily lead to death if treated with appropriate antibiotics.[74a] Pleural effusions were the most common radiographic abnormality rather than a widened mediastinum, and pulmonary parenchymal infiltrates were seen in seven patients, whereas earlier teaching had been that pneumonia does not commonly occur with inhalation anthrax.[52,73,74a,113]

SUMMARY

Unconventional weapons of mass destruction continue to pose a threat to public safety. Chemical and biologic weapons releases are considered more likely to occur than nuclear weapons incidents, as CBW agents utilize resources subject to less governmental control and require less sophisticated technology and financial outlay than nuclear weapons. CBW agents are appealing to terrorist groups because the impact in terms of death, disability, economic losses, and panic remain high. The psychological impact of CBW terrorism may well exceed that for conventional or nuclear weapons. Although the probability of incidents resulting in widespread public health disasters appears low, the anthrax terrorist events of 2001 demonstrate that the consequences are high, and that substantial preparations must be made in advance. Smaller CBW incidents, unintentional releases, and hoaxes have occurred and will probably continue to occur. Toxicologists and associated healthcare professionals occupy a unique position to impact preparedness and response through familiarity with chemical hazards and biologic toxins.

REFERENCES

1. Aasted A, Darre E, Wulf HC: Mustard gas: Clinical, toxicological, and mutagenic aspects based on modern experience. Ann Plast Surg 1987;19:330–333.
2. Adir Y, Bitterman H, Kol S, Melamed Y: Hyperbaric oxygen treatment for carbon monoxide intoxication acquired in the sealed room during the Persian Gulf war. Isr J Med Sci 1991;27:669–673.
3. Aldhous P: Gruinard Island handed back. Nature 1990;344:801.
4. Almog S, Winkler E, Amitai Y, et al: Acute pyridostigmine overdose: A report of nine cases. Isr J Med Sci 1991;27:659–663.
5. Alper J: From the bioweapons trenches, new tools for battling microbes. Science 1999;284:1754–1755.
6. Amitai Y, Almog S, Singer R, et al: Atropine poisoning in children during the Persian Gulf crisis: A national survey in Israel. JAMA 1992;268:630–632.
7. Associated Press: Report: 3 nations hide deadly virus. Arizona Republic, June 13, 1999, p. A9.
8. Associated Press: Air Force major faces court-martial rather than take anthrax vaccine. LA Times, January 8, 2000, p. A17.
9. Bair J: Marine loses in court over anthrax shots. LA Times, December 4, 1999, p. A14.
10. Barach P, Rivkind A, Israeli A, et al: Emergency preparedness and response in Israel during the Gulf War. Ann Emerg Med 1998;32:224–233.
11. Barranco VP: Mustard gas and the dermatologist. Int J Dermatol 1991;30:684–686.
12. Baskin SI, Brewer TG: Cyanide poisoning. In: Sidell FR, Takafuji ET, Franz DR, eds: Medical Aspects of Chemical and Biological Warfare. Washington DC, Office of the Surgeon General, 1997, pp. 271–286.
13. Beardsley T: Facing an ill wind: The U.S. gears up to deal with biological terrorism. Sci Am 1999;280:19–20.
14. Bernstein BJ: The birth of the US biological-warfare program. Sci Am 1987;256(6):116–121.
15. Billmire DF, Vinocur C, Ginda M, et al: Pepper-spray-induced respiratory failure treated with extracorporeal membrane oxygenation. Pediatrics 1996;98:961–963.
16. Blaho K, Winbery S: "Safety" of chemical batons. Lancet 1998;352:1633.
17. Breman JG, Henderson DA: Poxvirus dilemmas—monkeypox, smallpox, and biologic terrorism. N Engl J Med 1998;339:556–559.
18. Brennan RJ, Waeckerle JF, Sharp TW, Lillibridge SR: Chemical warfare agents: Emergency medical and emergency public health issues. Ann Emerg Med 1999;34:191–204.
19. Borak J, Sidell FR: Agents of chemical warfare: Sulfur mustard. Ann Emerg Med 1992;21:303–308.
20. Budiansky S: Is yellow rain simply bees' natural excreta? Nature 1983;303:3.
21. Byrne WR: Q fever. In: Sidell FR, Takafuji ET, Franz DR, eds: Medical Aspects of Chemical and Biological Warfare. Washington DC, Office of the Surgeon General, 1997, pp. 523–537.
22. Cairney R: Antivaccine advocates line up to support airman. Can Med Assoc J 1999;160:883.
23. Capps L, Vermund SH, Johnsen C: Smallpox and biological warfare: The case for abandoning vaccination of military personnel. Am J Public Health 1986;76:1229–1231.
24. Carmell A, Liberman N, Mevorach L: Anxiety-related somatic reactions during missile attacks. Isr J Med Sci 1991;27:677–680.
25. Caterina MJ, Schumacher MA, Tominaga M, et al: The capsaicin receptor: a heat-activated ion channel in the pain pathway. Nature 1997;389:816–824.
26. Centers for Disease Control and Prevention: Bioterrorism alleging use of anthrax and interim guidelines for management—United States, 1998. MMWR 1999;48:69–74.
26a. Centers for Disease Control and Prevention: Suspected brucellosis case prompts investigation of possible bioterrorism-related activity—New Hampshire and Massachusetts, 1999. MMWR 2000;49:509–512.
26b. Centers for Disease Control and Prevention: Public health message regarding anthrax case. October 4, 2001. Available from: URL: *http://www.bt.cdc.gov/DocumentsApp/Anthrax/10042001Forida/04Oct01.asp.* Accessed Oct 24, 2001.
26c. Centers for Disease Control and Prevention: Update: Public health message regarding Florida anthrax case. October 7, 2001. Available from: URL: *http://www.bt.cdc.gov/DocumentsApp/Anthrax/10072001Florida/07Oct01.asp.* Accessed Oct 24, 2001.
26d. Centers for Disease Control and Prevention: Update: Public health message regarding anthrax. October 12, 2001. Available from: URL: *http://www.bt.cdc.gov/DocumentsApp/Anthrax/10122001Florida/10122001Message.asp.* Accessed Oct 24, 2001.
26e. Centers for Disease Control and Prevention: Update: Investigation of bioterrorism-related anthrax and adverse events from antimicrobial prophylaxis. MMWR 2001;50:973–976.
27. Centers for Disease Control and Prevention: Surveillance for adverse events associated with anthrax vaccination—U.S. Department of Defense, 1998–2000. MMWR 2000;49:341–345.
28. Christopher GW, Cieslak TJ, Pavlin JA, Eitzen EM: Biological warfare. A historical perspective. JAMA 1997;278:412–417.
29. Cieslak TJ, Eitzen EM: Clinical and epidemiologic principles of anthrax. Emerg Infect Dis 1999;5:552–555.
30. Cole LA: The specter of biological weapons. Sci Am 1996;275(6):60–65.
31. Crompton R, Gall D: Georgi Markov—Death in a pellet. Med Leg J 1980;48(2):51–62.
32. Dacre JC, Goldman M: Toxicology and pharmacology of the chemical warfare agent sulfur mustard. Pharmacol Rev 1996;48:289–326.
33. Davis RA: The assassination of Reinhard Heydrich. Surg Gynecol Obstet 1971;August:304–318.
34. Derbes VJ: De Mussis and the great plague of 1348: A forgotten episode of bacteriological warfare. JAMA 1966;196:179–182.

35. DiGiovanni C: Domestic terrorism with chemical or biological agents: Psychiatric aspects. Am J Psychiatry 1999;156:1500–1505.

36. Dixon TC, Meselson M, Guillemin J, Hanna PC: Anthrax. N Engl J Med 1999;314:815–826.

37. Dunn MA, Hackley BE, Sidell FR: Pretreatment for nerve agent exposure. In: Sidell FR, Takafuji ET, Franz DR, eds: Medical Aspects of Chemical and Biological Warfare. Washington DC, Office of the Surgeon General, 1997, pp. 181–196.

38. Dunn MA, Sidell FR: Progress in medical defense against nerve agents. JAMA 1989;262:649–652.

39. Eckstein M: The medical response to modern terrorism: Why the "rules of engagement" have changed. Ann Emerg Med 1999;34:219–221.

40. Eitzen EM: Use of biological weapons. In: Sidell FR, Takafuji ET, Franz DR, eds: Medical Aspects of Chemical and Biological Warfare. Washington DC, Office of the Surgeon General, 1997, pp. 437–450.

41. Eitzen EM: Education is the key to defense against bioterrorism. Ann Emerg Med 1999;34:221–223.

42. Eitzen EM, Takafuji ET: Historical overview of biological warfare. In: Sidell FR, Takafuji ET, Franz DR, eds: Medical Aspects of Chemical and Biological Warfare. Washington DC, Office of the Surgeon General, 1997, pp. 415–423.

43. Elchalal U, Lurie S, Goldshmit C, et al: Delivery with gas mask during missile attack. Lancet 1991;337:242.

44. Epstein Y, Linder N, Lubin D, et al: The incubator as a chemical warfare protective device in neonatal intensive care units. Isr J Med Sci 1991;27:648–651.

45. Evans ME, Friedlander AM: Tularemia. In: Sidell FR, Takafuji ET, Franz DR, eds: Medical Aspects of Chemical and Biological Warfare. Washington DC, Office of the Surgeon General, 1997, pp. 503–512.

46. Firooz A, Komeili A, Dowlati Y: Eruptive melanocytic nevi and cherry angiomas secondary to sulfur mustard gas. J Am Acad Dermatol 1999;40:646–647.

47. Fischetti M: Gas vaccine: Bioengineered immunization could shield against nerve gas. Sci Am 1991;264(4):153.

48. Franz DR: Defense against toxin weapons. In: Sidell FR, Takafuji ET, Franz DR, eds: Medical Aspects of Chemical and Biological Warfare. Washington DC, Office of the Surgeon General, 1997, pp. 603–619.

49. Franz DR, Jaax NK: Ricin toxin. In: Sidell FR, Takafuji ET, Franz DR, eds: Medical Aspects of Chemical and Biological Warfare. Washington DC, Office of the Surgeon General, 1997, pp. 631–642.

50. Franz DR, Jahrling PB, Friedlander AM, et al: Clinical recognition and management of patients exposed to biological warfare agents. JAMA 1997;278:399–411.

51. Franz DR, Parrott CD, Takafuji ET: The U.S. biological warfare and biological defense programs. In: Sidell FR, Takafuji ET, Franz DR, eds: Medical Aspects of Chemical and Biological Warfare. Washington DC, Office of the Surgeon General, 1997, pp. 425–436.

52. Friedlander AM: Anthrax. In: Sidell FR, Takafuji ET, Franz DR, eds: Medical Aspects of Chemical and Biological Warfare. Washington DC, Office of the Surgeon General, 1997, pp. 467–478.

53. Friedlander AM, Pittman PR, Parker GW: Anthrax vaccine: Evidence for safety and efficacy against inhalational anthrax. JAMA 1999;282:2104–2106.

54. Fullerton CS, Ursano RJ: Behavioral and psychological responses to chemical and biological warfare. Mil Med 1990;155:54–59.

55. Gunderson CH, Lehmann CR, Sidell FR, Habbari B: Nerve agents: A review. Neurology 1992;42:946–950.

56. Haller JS: Gas warfare: Military-medical responsiveness of the allies in the great war, 1914–1918. NY State J Med 1990;90:499–510.

57. Harris S: Japanese biological warfare research on humans: A case study of microbiology and ethics. Ann NY Acad Sci 1992;666:21–52.

58. Harruff RC: Chemical-biological warfare in Asia. JAMA 1983;250:497–498.

59. Hay A: Surviving the impossible: the long march from Srebrenica. An investigation of the possible use of chemical warfare agents. Med Conflict Survival 1998;14:120–155.

60. Heller O, Aldar Y, Vosk M, Shemer J: An argument for equipping civilian hospitals with a multiple respirator system for a chemical warfare mass casualty situation. Isr J Med Sci 1991;27:652–655.

61. Henderson DA: Bioterrorism as a public health threat. Emerg Infect Dis 1998;4:488–492.

62. Henderson DA: The looming threat of bioterrorism. Science 1999;283:1279–1282.

63. Henderson DA: Smallpox: Clinical and epidemiologic features. Emerg Infect Dis 1999;5:537–539.

64. Henderson DA, Inglesby TV, Bartlett JG, et al: Smallpox as a biological weapon: Medical and public health management. JAMA 1999;281:2127–2137.'

65. Herman LM, Kindschu MW, Shallash AJ: Treatment of mace dermatitis with topical antacid suspension. Am J Emerg Med 1998;16:613–614.

66. Heyndrickx A, Heyndrickx B: Management of war gas injuries. Lancet 1990;336:1248–1249.

67. Holden C: "Unequivocal" evidence of Soviet toxin use. Science 1982;216:154–155.

68. Holloway HC, Norwood AE, Fullerton CS, et al: The threat of biological weapons: Prophylaxis and mitigation of psychological and social consequences. JAMA 1997;278:425–427.

69. Holstege CP, Kirk M, Sidell FR: Chemical warfare nerve agent poisoning. Crit Care Clin 1997;13:923–942.

70. Hoover DL, Friedlander AM: Brucellosis. In: Sidell FR, Takafuji ET, Franz DR, eds: Medical Aspects of Chemical and Biological Warfare. Washington DC, Office of the Surgeon General, 1997, pp. 513–521.

71. Hu H, Fine J, Epstein P, et al: Tear gas—harassing agent or toxic chemical weapon? JAMA 1989;262:660–663.

72. Inglesby TV, Dennis DT, Henderson DA, et al: Plague as a biological weapon: Medical and public health management. JAMA 2000;283:2281–2290.

73. Inglesby TV, Henderson DA, Bartlett JG, et al: Anthrax as a biological weapon: Medical and public health management. JAMA 1999;281:1735–1745.

74. Jahrling PB: Viral hemorrhagic fevers. In: Sidell FR, Takafuji ET, Franz DR, eds: Medical Aspects of Chemical and Biological Warfare. Washington DC, Office of the Surgeon General, 1997, pp. 591–602.

74a. Jernigan JA, Stephens DS, Ashford DA, et al: Bioterrorism-related inhalational anthrax: The first 10 cases reported in the United States. Emerg Infect Dis [serial online]2001;7(6). Available from: URL: *http://www.cdc.gov/ncidod/EID/eid.htm.* Accessed Nov 13, 2001.

75. Jones LA, Tandberg D, Troutman WG: Household treatment for "chile burns" of the hands. J Toxicol Clin Toxicol 1987;25:483–491.

76. Kadivar H, Adams SC: Treatment of chemical and biological warfare injuries: Insights derived from the 1984 Iraqi attack on Majnoon Island. Mil Med 1991;156:171–177.

77. Karsenty E, Shemer J, Alsech I, et al: Medical aspects of the Iraqi missile attacks on Israel. Isr J Med Sci 1991;27:603–607.

78. Kato T, Yoshimoto N, Sawano M, Hamabe Y: Coronary vasospasm in a patient suffering from sarin poisoning. Am J Emerg Med 2000;18:113–114.

79. Kaufmann AF, Meltzer MI, Schmid GP: The economic impact of a bioterrorist attack: Are prevention and postattack intervention programs justifiable? Emerg Infect Dis 1997;3:83–94.

80. Keeler JR, Hurst CG, Dunn MA: Pyridostigmine used as a nerve agent pretreatment under wartime conditions. JAMA 1991;266:693–695.

81. Keim M, Kaufmann AF: Principles for emergency response to bioterrorism. Ann Emerg Med 1999;34:177–182.

82. Ketchum JS, Sidell FR: Incapacitating agents. In: Sidell FR, Takafuji ET, Franz DR, eds: Medical Aspects of Chemical and Biological

Warfare. Washington DC: Office of the Surgeon General, 1997, pp. 287–305.

83. Knight B: Ricin—a potent homicidal poison. Br Med J 1979 Feb 3; 1(6159):350–351.

84. Knudson GB: Operation Desert Shield: Medical aspects of weapons of mass destruction. Mil Med 1991;156:267–271.

85. Kortepeter MG, Parker GW: Potential biological weapons threats. Emerg Infect Dis 1999;5:523–527.

86. Kvetan V: Critical care medicine, terrorism, and disasters: Are we ready? Crit Care Med 1999;27:873–874.

87. Lampe KF: Rhododendrons, mountain laurel, and mad honey. JAMA 1988;259:2009.

88. Lancet: "Safety" of chemical batons. 1998;352:159.

89. Lancet: Is smallpox history? 1999;353:1539.

90. LeDuc JW, Becher J: Current status of smallpox vaccine. Emerg Infect Dis 1999;5:593–594.

91. Lee BH, Knopp R, Richardson ML: Treatment of exposure to chemical personal protection agents. Ann Emerg Med 1984;13:487–488.

92. LeJeune KE, Dravis BC, Yang F, et al: Fighting nerve agent chemical weapons with enzyme technology. Ann NY Acad Sci 1998;864: 153–170.

93. LeJeune KE, Wild JR, Russel AJ: Nerve agents degraded by enzymatic foams. Nature 1998;395:27–28.

94. Leonard C: Letter threatening anthrax called hoax. Arizona Republic, Phoenix AZ. March 14, 1998, B1.

95. Lesho E, Dorsey D, Bunner D: Feces, dead horses, and fleas—Evolution of the hostile use of biological agents. West J Med 1998; 168:512–516.

96. Macilwain C: Study proves Iraq used nerve gas. Nature 1993;363:3.

97. Macintyre AG, Christopher GW, Eitzen E, et al: Weapons of mass destruction events with contaminated casualties: Effective planning for health care facilities. JAMA 2000;283:242–249.

98. Manchee RJ, Broster MG, Melling BJ, et al: *Bacillus anthracis* on Gruinard Island. Nature 1981;294:254–255.

99. Marrs TC, Maynard RL, Sidell FR: Chemical Warfare Agents. Toxicology and Treatment. Chichester, John Wiley Sons, 1996.

100. Marshall E: The Soviet elephant grass theory. Science 1982;217:32.

101. Marshall E: A cloudburst of yellow rain reports. Science 1982;218: 1202–1203.

102. Marshall E: Yellow rain evidence slowly whittled away. Science 1986;233:18–19.

103. Marshall E: Sverdlovsk: Anthrax capital? Science 1988;240: 383–385.

104. Masuda N, Takatsu M, Morinari H, Ozawa T: Sarin poisoning in Tokyo subway. Lancet 1995;345:1446.

105. McClain DJ: Smallpox. In: Sidell FR, Takafuji ET, Franz DR, eds: Medical Aspects of Chemical and Biological Warfare. Washington DC, Office of the Surgeon General, 1997, pp. 539–559.

106. McDade JE, Franz D: Bioterrorism as a public health threat. Emerg Infect Dis 1998;4:493–494.

107. McEvedy C: The bubonic plague. Sci Am 1988;258(2):118–123.

108. McGovern TW, Christopher GW, Eitzen EM: Cutaneous manifestations of biological warfare and related threat agents. Arch Dermatol 1999;135:311–322.

109. McGovern TW, Friedlander AM: Plague. In: Sidell FR, Takafuji ET, Franz DR, eds: Medical Aspects of Chemical and Biological Warfare. Washington DC, Office of the Surgeon General, 1997, pp. 479–502.

110. Med Lett Drugs Ther: Treatment of nerve gas poisoning. Med Lett 1995;37(948):43–44.

111. Med Lett Drugs Ther: Anthrax vaccine. Med Lett 1998;40(1026): 52–53.

112. Med Lett Drugs Ther: Drugs and vaccines against biological weapons. Med Lett 1999;41(1046):15–16.

113. Medical Management of Biological Casualties, 2nd ed. Fort Detrick, MD, US Army Medical Research Institute of Infectious Diseases, 1996.

114. Medical Management of Chemical Casualties, 2nd ed.. Aberdeen Proving Ground, MD, Chemical Casualty Care Office, US Army Medical Research Institute of Chemical Defense, 1995.

115. Mellor SG, Rice P, Cooper GJ: Vesicant burns. Br J Plast Surg 1991; 44:434–437.

116. Meselson M, Guillemin J, Hugh-Jones M, et al: The Sverdlovsk anthrax outbreak of 1979. Science 1994;266:1202–1208.

117. Middlebrook JL, Franz DR: Botulinum toxins. In: Sidell FR, Takafuji ET, Franz DR, eds: Medical Aspects of Chemical and Biological Warfare. Washington DC, Office of the Surgeon General, 1997, pp. 643–654.

118. Miki A, Katagi M, Tsuchihashi H, Yamashita M: Determination of alkylmethylphosphonic acids, the main metabolites of organophosphorus nerve agents, in biofluids by gas chromatography–mass spectroscopy and liquid-liquid-solid-phase-transfer-catalyzed pentafluorobenzylation. J Anal Tox 1999;23:86–93.

119. Miller J: U.S. watching for chemical weapons use. Arizona Republic, Phoenix AZ, April 16, 1999 p. A13.

120. Mobley JA: Biological warfare in the twentieth century: Lessons from the past, challenges for the future. Mil Med 1995;160:547.

121. Morimoto F, Shimazu T, Yoshioka T: Intoxication of VX in humans. Am J Emerg Med 1999:17:493–494.

122. Morita H, Yanagisawa N, Nakajima T, et al: Sarin poisoning in Matsumoto, Japan. Lancet 1995;346:290–293.

123. Morris K: US military face punishment for refusing anthrax vaccine. Lancet 1999;353:130.

124. Nakajima T, Sato S, Morita H, Yanagisawa N: Sarin poisoning of a rescue team in the Matsumoto sarin incident in Japan. Occup Environ Med 1997;54:697–701.

125. Neuwinger HD: African ethnobotany—Poisons and drugs: chemistry, pharmacology, toxicology. HerbalGram 1998;43:64–67.

126. Newman-Taylor AJ, Morris AJR: Experience with mustard gas casualties. Lancet 1991;337:242.

127. Noah DL, Sobel AL, Ostroff SM, Kildew JA: Biological warfare training: Infectious disease outbreak differentiation criteria. Mil Med 1998;163:198–201.

128. Nowicke JW, Meselson M: Yellow rain—a palynological analysis. Nature 1984;309:205–206.

129. Nozaki H, Aikawa N: Sarin poisoning in Tokyo subway. Lancet 1995;345:1446–1447.

130. Nozaki H, Aikawa N, Fujishima S, et al: A case of VX poisoning and the difference from sarin. Lancet 1995;346:698–699.

131. Nozaki H, Hori S, Shinozawa Y, et al: Secondary exposure of medical staff to sarin vapor in the emergency room. Intensive Care Med 1995;21:1032–1035.

132. Nozaki H, Hori S, Shinozawa Y, et al: Relationship between pupil size and acetylcholinesterase activity in patients exposed to sarin vapor. Intensive Care Med 1997;23:1005–1007.

133. Nunn-Lugar-Domenici Amendment to the FY 97 Defense Authorization Act, Pub L No. 104–201, Title XIV: Defense Against Weapons of Mass Destruction, Subtitle A: Domestic Preparedness. US Congress; June 27, 1996.

134. Ohbu S, Yamashina A, Takasu N, et al: Sarin poisoning on Tokyo subway. South Med J 1997;90:587–593.

135. Okudera H, Morita H, Iwashita T, et al: Unexpected nerve gas exposure in the city of Matsumoto: Report of rescue activity in the first sarin gas terrorism. Am J Emerg Med 1997;15:527–528.

136. Okumura T: Organophosphate poisoning in pregnancy. Ann Emerg Med 1997;29:299.

137. Okumura T, Suzuki K, Fukuda A, et al: The Tokyo subway sarin attack: Disaster management, part 1: Community emergency response. Acad Emerg Med 1998;5:613–617.

138. Okumura T, Suzuki K, Fukuda A, et al: The Tokyo subway sarin attack: Disaster management, part 2: Hospital response. Acad Emerg Med 1998;5:618–624.

139. Okumura T, Takasu N, Ishimatsu S, et al: Report of 640 Victims of the Tokyo subway sarin attack. Ann Emerg Med 1996;28:129–135.

140. Olson KB: Aum Shinrikyo: Once and future threat? Emerg Infect Dis 1999;5:513–516.

141. Orma PS, Middleton RK: Aerosolized atropine as an antidote to nerve gas. Ann Pharmacother 1992;26:937–938.

142. Pesik N, Keim M, Sampson TR: Do US emergency medicine residency programs provide adequate training for bioterrorism? Ann Emerg Med 1999;34:173–176.

143. Petosa C, Collier RJ, Klimpel KR: Crystal structure of the anthrax toxin protective antigen. Nature 1997;385:833–838.

144. Pile JC, Malone JD, Eitzen EM, et al: Anthrax as a potential biological warfare agent. Arch Intern Med 1998;158:429–434.

145. Poupard JA, Miller LA: History of biological warfare: Catapults to capsomeres. Ann NY Acad Sci 1992;666:9–20.

146. Prudhomme JC, Bhatia R, Nutik JM, Shusterman DJ: Chest wall pain and possible rhabdomyolysis after chloropicrin exposure. J Occup Environ Med 1999;41:17–22.

147. Ram Z, Molcho M, Danon YL, et al: The effect of pyridostigmine on respiratory function in healthy and asthmatic volunteers. Isr J Med Sci 1991;27:664–668.

148. Redmond C, Pearce MJ, Manchee RJ, Berdal BP: Deadly relic of the Great War. Nature 1998;393:747–748.

149. Reuters: N.Y. outbreak not work of terrorists, experts say. LA Times, October 12, 1999, p. A21.

150. Richards CF, Burstein JL, Waeckerle JF, Hutson HR: Emergency physicians and biological terrorism. Ann Emerg Med 1999;34:183–190.

151. Richter P: U.S. sailors being punished for refusing anthrax vaccine. Arizona Republic, Phoenix AZ. March 12, 1999, p. A6.

152. Rickett DJ, Glenn JF, Houston WE: Medical defense against nerve agents: New direction. Mil Med 1987;152:35–41.

153. Robertson AG, Robertson LJ: From asps to allegations: Biological warfare in history. Mil Med 1995;160:369–373.

154. Root-Bernstein RS: Infectious terrorism. Atlantic Monthly 1991;267 (5):44–50.

155. Rosen JD: Yellow rain. Science 1983;221:698.

156. Ruhl CM, Park SJ, Danisa O, et al: A serious skin sulfur mustard burn from an artillery shell. J Emerg Med 1994;12:159–166.

157. Russell PK: Vaccines in civilian defense against bioterrorism. Emerg Infect Dis 1999;5:531–533.

158. Schofer JM: Violations of informed consent during war. JAMA 1999;281:1657.

159. Seeley TD, Nowicke JW, Meselson M, et al: Yellow rain. Sci Am 1985;253(3):128–137.

160. Seelos C: Lessons from Iraq on bioweapons. Nature 1999;398:187–188.

161. Sekijima Y, Morita H, Yanagisawa N: Follow-up of sarin poisoning in Matsumoto. Ann Intern Med 1997;127:1042.

162. Shafazand S, Doyle R, Ruoss S, et al: Inhalational anthrax. Epidemiology, diagnosis, and management. Chest 1999;116:1369–1376.

163. Shalala DE: Smallpox: Setting the research agenda. Science 1999;285:1011.

164. Shapira Y, Bar Y, Berkenstadt H, et al: Outline of hospital organization for a chemical warfare attack. Isr J Med Sci 1991;27:616–622.

165. Shapira Y, Marganitt B, Roziner I, et al: Willingness of staff to report to their hospital duties following an unconventional missile attack: A state-wide survey. Isr J Med Sci 1991;27:704–711.

166. Sharabi Y, Danon YL, Berkenstadt H, et al: Survey of symptoms following intake of pyridostigmine during the Persian Gulf war. Isr J Med Sci 1991;27:656–658.

167. Sharp D: Alleged chemical warfare in Bosnia conflict. Lancet 1998;351:1500.

168. Sharp TW, Brennan RJ, Keim M, et al: Medical preparedness for a terrorist incident involving chemical or biological agents during the 1996 Atlanta Olympic Games. Ann Emerg Med 1998;32:214–223.

169. Sidel VW: Weapons of mass destruction: The greatest threat to public health. JAMA 1989;262:680–682.

170. Sidell FR: Clinical effects of organophosphorus cholinesterase inhibitors. J Appl Toxicol 1994;14:111–113.

171. Sidell FR: Chemical agent terrorism. Ann Emerg Med 1996;28:223–224.

172. Sidell FR: Nerve agents. In: Sidell FR, Takafuji ET, Franz DR, eds: Medical Aspects of Chemical and Biological Warfare. Washington DC, Office of the Surgeon General, 1997, pp. 129–179.

173. Sidell FR: Riot control agents. In: Sidell FR, Takafuji ET, Franz DR, eds: Medical Aspects of Chemical and Biological Warfare. Washington DC, Office of the Surgeon General, 1997, pp. 307–324.

174. Sidell FR, Borak J: Chemical warfare agents: II. Nerve agents. Ann Emerg Med 1992;21:865–871.

175. Sidell FR, Hurst CG: Long-term health effects of nerve agents and mustard. In: Sidell FR, Takafuji ET, Franz DR, eds: Medical Aspects of Chemical and Biological Warfare. Washington DC, Office of the Surgeon General, 1997, pp. 229–246.

176. Sidell FR, Urbanetti JS, Smith WJ, Hurst CG: Vesicants. In: Sidell FR, Takafuji ET, Franz DR, eds: Medical Aspects of Chemical and Biological Warfare. Washington DC, Office of the Surgeon General, 1997, pp. 197–228.

177. Simpson LL: The origin, structure, and pharmacological activity of botulinum toxin. Pharmacol Rev 1981;33:155–188.

178. Smart JK: History of chemical and biological warfare: An American perspective. In: Sidell FR, Takafuji ET, Franz DR, eds: Medical Aspects of Chemical and Biological Warfare. Washington DC, Office of the Surgeon General, 1997, pp. 9–86.

179. Smith JF, Davis K, Hart MK, et al: Viral encephalitides. In: Sidell FR, Takafuji ET, Franz DR, eds: Medical Aspects of Chemical and Biological Warfare. Washington DC, Office of the Surgeon General, 1997, pp. 561–589.

180. Spyker MS, Spyker DA: Yellow rain: Chemical warfare in southeast Asia and Afghanistan. Vet Hum Toxicol 1983;25:335–340.

181. Steckner S: Arrest in anthrax threat. Arizona Republic, Phoenix AZ. March 12, 1998, p. B1.

182. Steckner S, Miller E: Anthrax threat probably hoax. Arizona Republic, Phoenix AZ. March 11, 1998, p. B1.

183. Steffee CH, Lantz PE, Flannagan LM, et al: Oleoresin capsicum (pepper) spray and "in-custody deaths." Am J Forensic Med Pathol 1995;16:185–192.

184. Stern J: The prospect of domestic bioterrorism. Emerg Infect Dis 1999;5:517–522.

185. Suchard JR: Treatment of capsaicin (Mace?) dermatitis. Am J Emerg Med 1999;17:210–211.

186. Susman E: New substance deactivates anthrax spores. Emerg Med News 1998;20(12):34.

187. Suzuki T, Morita H, Ono K, et al: Sarin poisoning in Tokyo subway. Lancet 1995;345:980.

188. TeSlaa G, Kaiser M, Biederman L, Stowe CM: Chloropicrin toxicity involving animal and human exposure. Vet Hum Toxicol 1986;28:323–324.

189. Thomsen AB, Eriksen J, Smidt-Nielsen K: Chronic neuropathic symptoms after exposure to mustard gas: A long-term investigation. J Am Acad Dermatol 1998;39:187–190.

190. Törngren S, Persson SA, Ljungquist A, et al: Personal decontamination after exposure to simulated liquid phase contaminants: functional assessment of a new unit. J Toxicol Clin Toxicol 1998;36:567–573.

191. Török TJ, Tauxe RV, Wise RP, et al: A large community outbreak of salmonellosis caused by intentional contamination of restaurant salad bars. JAMA 1997;278:389–395.

192. Tsuchihashi H, Katagi M, Nishikawa M, Tatsuno M: Idenitification of metabolites of nerve agent VX in serum collected from a victim. J Anal Toxicol 1998;22:383–388.

193. Tucker JB: Historical trends related to bioterrorism: An empirical analysis. Emerg Infect Dis 1999;5:498–504.

194. Tur-Kaspa I, Lev EI, Hendler I, et al: Preparing hospitals for toxicological mass casualties events. Crit Care Med 1999;27:1004–1008.

195. Ulrich RG, Sidell S, Taylor TJ, et al: Staphylococcal enterotoxin B and related pyrogenic toxins. In: : Sidell FR, Takafuji ET, Franz DR, eds: Medical Aspects of Chemical and Biological Warfare. Washington DC, Office of the Surgeon General, 1997, pp. 621–630.

196. Urbanetti JS: Toxic inhalational injury. In: Sidell FR, Takafuji ET, Franz DR, eds: Medical Aspects of Chemical and Biological Warfare. Washington DC, Office of the Surgeon General, 1997, pp. 247–270.

197. Vaca FE, Myers JH, Langdorf M: Delayed pulmonary edema and bronchospasm after accidental lacrimator exposure. Am J Emerg Med 1996;14:402–405.

198. Van Biema D: Prophet of poison. Time 1995(April 3);145(14): 26–33.

199. Wade N: Yellow rain and the cloud of chemical war. Science 1981; 214:1008–1009.

200. Waeckerle JF: Domestic preparedness for events involving weapons of mass destruction. JAMA 2000;283:252–254.

201. Wannemacher RW, Wiener SL: Trichothecene mycotoxins. In: Sidell FR, Takafuji ET, Franz DR, eds: Medical Aspects of Chemical and Biological Warfare. Washington DC, Office of the Surgeon General, 1997, pp. 655–676.

202. Watts J: Japan taken to court over germ-warfare allegations. Lancet 1999;351:657.

203. Watts J: Tokyo terrorist attack: Effects still felt 4 years on. Lancet 1999;353:569.

204. Wheelis M: First shots fired in biological warfare. Nature 1998;395: 213.

205. Wiener SL: Strategies of biowarfare defense. Mil Med 1987;152: 25–28.

206. Williams SR, Clark RF, Dunford JV: Contact dermatitis associated with capsaicin: Hunan hand syndrome. Ann Emerg Med 1995;25: 713–715.

207. Winograd HL: Acute croup in an older child: An unusual toxic origin. Clin Pediatr 1977;16:884–887.

208. Woodall J: Tokyo subway gas attack. Lancet 1997;350:296.

209. Yokoyama K, Araki S, Murata K, et al: Chronic neurobehavioral and central and autonomic nervous system effects of Tokyo subway sarin poisoning. J Physiol (Paris) 1998;92:317–323.

210. Zilinskas RA: Iraq's biological weapons: The past as future? JAMA 1997;278:418–424.

211. Zoon KC: Vaccines, pharmaceutical products, and bioterrorism: Challenges for the U.S. Food and Drug Administration. Emerg Infect Dis 1999;5:534–536.

K. TOXIC ENVENOMATIONS

CHAPTER 101 SNAKES AND OTHER REPTILES

James R. Roberts / Edward J. Otten

Case 1 A 25-year-old man exploring the mountains of Virginia was bitten on the toe by an unidentified snake when he was rock-climbing in bare feet. He did not hear a rattle and only caught a glimpse of the copper-colored snake as it crawled away. Within 10 minutes he noted mild swelling and discomfort around a single puncture wound on the top of the fourth toe.

Within 1 hour the man developed moderate throbbing pain in the entire foot, associated with paresthesias. At 2 hours a hemorrhagic blister developed at the bite site. The swelling had progressed to the dorsum of the ankle, but he had no systemic symptoms. A friend drove him to a local hospital. No specific first aid was administered. The swelling did not progress past the ankle, and there was no nausea, vomiting, diaphoresis, dizziness, or systemic weakness. The vital signs, a CBC, and coagulation profile were normal. The patient reported only mild pain of the foot.

Because of progression of local symptoms and lack of definitive identification of the snake, the patient was admitted to the hospital. Antivenom was obtained but not administered. The foot demonstrated moderate pain and stiffness; edema reached the lower leg at 24 hours but did not progress further. No systemic symptoms developed, and the laboratory profile remained normal. Minor surgical debridement of a small area of skin slough on the toe was required. The patient was discharged after 48 hours to continue extremity elevation, and outpatient physical therapy was arranged. After 10 days of a progressive decrease in swelling, the patient had full use of the foot with only minor stiffness. Within 3 weeks the stiffness had disappeared completely.

Case 2 A 6-year-old girl was bitten on the left ankle by a 2-foot snake in her backyard. The snake was not positively identified, but rattlesnakes (western diamondback) were known to frequent the area. The child's father reported that she complained of severe pain in the leg within 30 seconds of the bite. Within 5 minutes she became weak and diaphoretic and vomited. She appeared pale and became agitated and disoriented.

The child was immediately taken to the hospital but became more lethargic en route. No first aid was administered. By the time she arrived at the hospital (transportation time of 25 minutes), the child's face and lips were swollen, and generalized muscle fasciculations were noted. The initial vital signs were palpable blood pressure 40 mm Hg, pulse 150 beats/min, shallow respirations at 38 breaths/min, and temperature 97°F (36.1°C). The patient was slightly cyanotic and obtunded. The entire lower leg was swollen, and two small puncture wounds were evident over the medial malleolus of the ankle, in the area of the saphenous vein. Arterial blood gas analysis revealed the following: pH 7.12, P_{CO_2} 20 mm Hg, and P_{O_2} 130 mm Hg (while breathing oxygen at 4 L/min).

Initial therapy consisted of the placement of a thigh tourniquet to impede lymphatic flow and the rapid infusion of lactated Ringer solution. Blood was drawn for a CBC, BUN, creatinine, electrolytes, type and crossmatch, and clotting studies, including fibrinogen level. A Foley catheter was inserted, and gross hematuria was noted.

The child was immediately skin-tested for sensitivity to horse serum. Within 3 minutes erythema developed at the skin test site. Although sensitivity to antivenom was suggested by the reaction, the consensus of the treating physician and a toxicology consultant was that the benefits of antivenom outweighed the risks. The decision was made to treat aggressively with antivenom. To ameliorate allergic reactions, 125 mg of methylprednisolone plus 25 mg of diphenhydramine were given IV. An infusion of 1 mg epinephrine in 1 L of 0.9% sodium chloride solution saline was prepared but not initially given. Broad-spectrum antibiotics and tetanus prophylaxis were given.

After fluid administration (30 mL/kg over 30 minutes), the blood pressure was measured at 85/50 mm Hg. With continuous ECG monitoring, crotaline polyvalent antivenom (Wyeth Laboratories) was administered by slow IV push at a rate of 1 vial (diluted 1:10 with 0.9% NaCl solution) over 2 minutes. During administration of the second vial, the child's blood pressure became unobtainable but quickly responded to titration of the epinephrine infusion, increasing the rate of the crystalloid infusion, and stopping the antivenom. Subsequent vials of antivenom were infused more slowly (each vial over 5 minutes), and the hypotension did not return. A total of 15 vials of antivenom was given over 2 hours. This depleted the city's entire supply of antivenom, and additional vials could not be located. The tourniquet was removed without sequelae after the antivenom had been administered. The epinephrine infusion was not required after the initial hypotensive episode, but a transient episode of urticaria responded to an additional 25 mg of diphenhydramine IV. Significant initial laboratory values included PT 25 seconds (control 12 seconds), PTT 65 seconds (control 25 seconds), fibrinogen 60 mg/dL (normal 170–410 mg/dL), platelet count 15,000/mm³, and leukocyte count 28,800/mm³. The hemoglobin/hematocrit, electrolytes, BUN, and creatinine were normal.

The child's clinical condition improved greatly over the next 8 hours. Her pulse and respirations slowed, her consciousness improved, and her blood pressure stabilized at 95/40 mm Hg. The gross hematuria cleared after the infusion of 4 units of fresh frozen plasma and 6 units of platelet concentrate. Except for a moderate thrombocytopenia that persisted for 6 days, the coagulopathy resolved in 48 hours, and no other bleeding complications were noted. The swelling about the face decreased, but she developed increased edema and hemorrhagic blisters at the site of the bite. The peripheral pulses remained intact. The entire leg swelled to about twice its normal size, but there was no objective evidence for a compartment syndrome, and gradually the edema abated.

Minor surgical debridement was required at the site of the bite. One week after therapy the child developed a low-grade fever and generalized urticaria and malaise, interpreted as serum sickness. The symptoms responded to oral prednisone and diphenhydramine, and the child eventually recovered without sequelae.

EPIDEMIOLOGY

Incidence of Venomous Snakebites in the United States

Venomous snakes are found throughout the United States, except Maine, Alaska, and Hawaii. They are common in the Appalachian states and in southern and western states but rare in New England and the northern states. There are approximately 6000 to 8000 venomous snakebites per year, and many thousands more from nonvenomous species. Mortality from snakebite is considered to be quite rare in the United States, with estimates ranging from 5 to 15 deaths per year.[34,58] Exact statistics are lacking, but mortality rates can be significantly higher in other countries. There may be as many as 27,000 rattlesnake bites and 100 fatalities per year in Mexico,[18] and thousands of deaths per year in some underdeveloped locales of India, Burma, and African countries.

Because snakes hibernate in the winter, most bites in the United States occur between May and October. Snakes may bite at night, but the most common time for envenomation is from 2 to 6 PM.[90] Coral snakes are particularly known for their nocturnal habits. The majority of bites occur in the extremities, but bites to the face and tongue have been reported when snakes are purposefully held near the body. The striking range of a snake is approximately one-half its length.

Children, intoxicated individuals (mostly men), snake handlers, and collectors are frequent victims. Over half of the bites occur while the individual is purposely handling a known venomous snake. There is a significant market for many illegal and dangerous reptiles, and a surprising number of individuals keep and sell venomous snakes as pets. Many specimens are exotic and highly toxic species from other countries. Some religious groups in the mid- and southeastern states handle poisonous snakes (usually rattlesnakes) as a routine ceremonial practice (see *Acts* 28:4 and *Mark* 16:17–18), and envenomation is common.

Identification of a Venomous Snake

Of the 120 species of snakes native to North America, approximately 30 species are dangerous (Table 101–1). Most of these venomous snakes are members of the Viperidae (subfamily Crotalineae), which includes the rattlesnakes (*Crotalus* and *Sistrurus*), copperheads, and semiaquatic water moccasins. These three snakes are also called pit vipers because of the presence of a pit-like depression of the skin behind the nostril that contains a heat-sensing organ. The other family of venomous snakes native to the United States is the Elapidae, which includes the coral snakes.

TABLE 101–1. Scientific and Common Names of Some Medically Important Venomous Snakes of North America

Scientific Name	Common Name
Crotalinae: Pit Vipers	
Agkistrodon contortrix contortrix	Southern copperhead
Agkistrodon contortrix laticinctus	Broad-banded copperhead
Agkistrodon contortrix mokason	Northern copperhead
Agkistrodon piscivorus conanti	Florida cottonmouth
Agkistrodon piscivorus piscivorus	Eastern cottonmouth
Agkistrodon piscivorus leucostoma	Western cottonmouth
Bothrops lanceolatus	Fer-de-lance
Rattlesnakes	
Crotalus adamanteus	Eastern diamondback
Crotalus atrox	Western diamondback
Crotalus cerastes cerastes	Mojave Desert sidewinder
Crotalus cerastes cercobombus	Sonoran Desert sidewinder
Crotalus horridus horridus	Timber
Crotalus horridus atricaudatus	Canebrake
Crotalus molossus	Northern black tailed
Crotalus ruber ruber	Red diamond
Crotalus scutulatus scutulatus	Mojave
Crotalus viridis cerberus	Arizona black
Crotalus viridis helleri	Southern Pacific
Crotalus viridis lutosus	Great Basin
Crotalus viridis nuntius	Hopi
Crotalus viridis oreganus	Northern Pacific
Crotalus viridis viridis	Prairie
Sistrurus catenatus catenatus	Eastern massasauga
Sistrurus catenatus edwardsi	Desert massasauga
Sistrurus catenatus tergeminus	Western massasauga
Sistrurus millarius millarius	Carolina pigmy
Elapidae: Coral Snakes	
Micruroides euryxanthus	Sonoran
Micrurus fulvius fulvius	Eastern
Micrurus fulvius tenere	Texas

Exact identification of a snake is often not possible unless the victim brings the offending reptile to the hospital. Ideally, the snake should be captured and killed, but this is usually impossible, delays transport, and poses an additional threat to the victim or prehospital personnel. Because of the excitement generated by the bite, the victim's identification of the snake may not be accurate. Identifying a snake by its color or markings is difficult for the novice. Knowledge of the indigenous venomous snakes is often helpful to medical personnel. Snake handlers and owners of pet snakes usually know the exact species responsible for the bite, but some are reluctant to offer specific information out of fear of prosecution or confiscation of the illegal snake by authorities.

Rattlesnakes have rattles that are occasionally heard before a strike. Water moccasins have a distinct white mouth (cotton mouth) and white buccal mucosa. The undersurface of pit vipers has a single row of plates or scales, as opposed to the double row found on nonvenomous varieties. The venomous snakes in the United States usually have a triangular-shaped head, vertically elliptical pupils (except the coral snakes, which have round pupils, like nonvenomous snakes), and easily identifiable fangs (Fig. 101–1). Fangs are paired, needlelike structures that inject venom. Rattlesnakes have the longest fangs, reaching 3 to 4 cm. Fangs retract on a hingelike mechanism into the roof of the mouth. In addi-

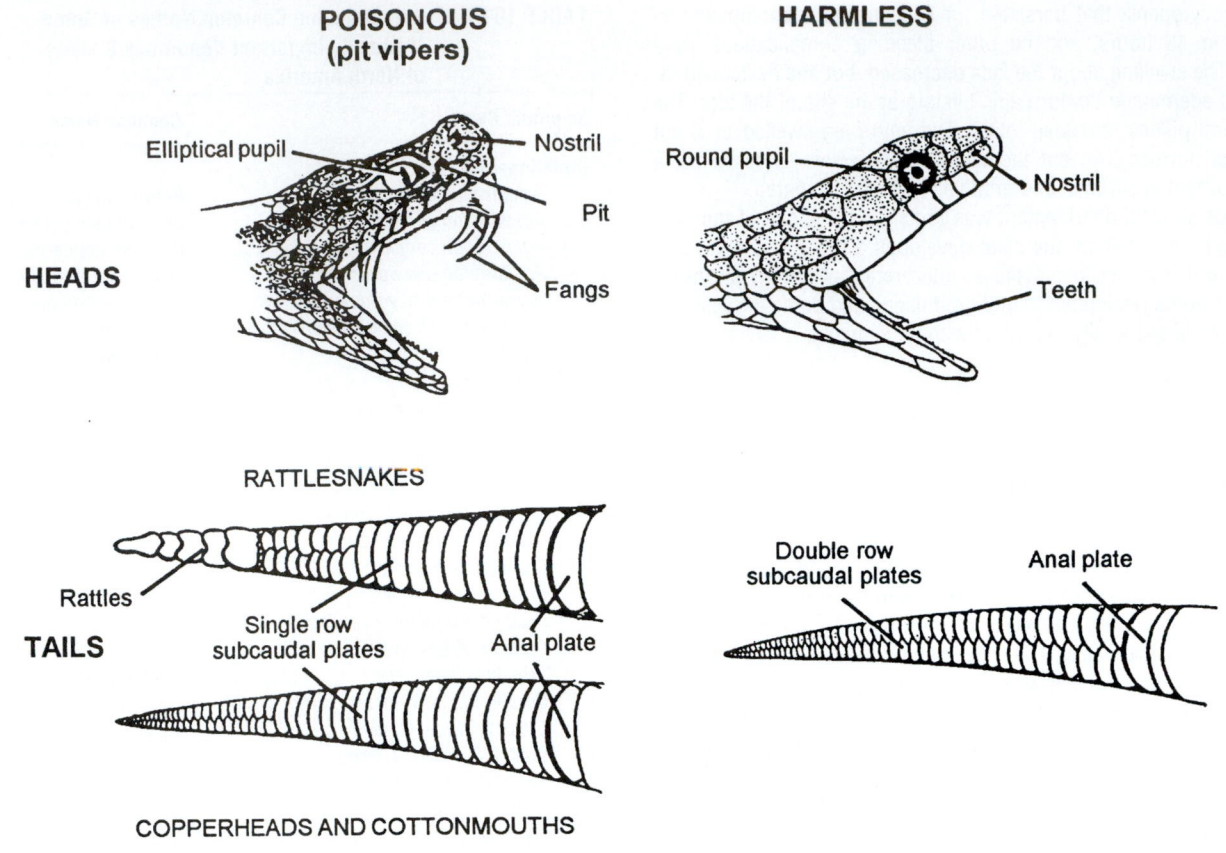

Figure 101–1 Features of pit vipers and harmless snakes. *(Modified and reprinted with permission from Parrish HM, Carr CA: Bites by copperheads in the United States. JAMA 1967;201:927.)*

tion to fangs, venomous snakes also have rows of small teeth. An adult snake usually has two fangs, but fangs may be single or multiple.

The fangs of coral snakes are much smaller (1 to 3 mm) than those of the rattlesnakes, and discrete fang marks may not be obvious after envenomation. There appears to be a curious propensity of coral snakes to hang on to a victim or "chew" for a few seconds, and a history of this activity may help identify a coral snakebite when the offending reptile cannot be located. Removal of a coral snake from the skin has been likened to separating pieces of Velcro. Coral snakes have easily identifiable red, yellow, and black bands along the length of the body. Coral snakes and the similarly colored nonpoisonous scarlet king snake are often confused. In one report of 39 victims of coral snake bites, nine patients were envenomated because they erroneously believed they were dealing with the nonpoisonous scarlet king snake.[55] The coral and king snakes can be distinguished by the spacing of their colored rings and color of the head. Coral snakes have black snouts, whereas king snakes have red snouts. Both species have red, yellow, and black rings, but in different sequences: The red and yellow rings touch in the coral snake but in king snakes are separated by black rings ("Red on yellow kills a fellow, red on black, venom lack").

About 60% of reported venomous bites from reptiles native to the United States are rattlesnake bites.[83] Tissue destruction from rattlesnake venom may be quite significant, resulting in amputation or permanent disability (Fig. 101–2). About 40% of bites are

from the copperheads and water moccasins, and fewer than 1% from the docile coral snake.[68,77]

Characteristics of a Venomous Snakebite

The severity and clinical manifestations of envenomation depend on a number of factors, including numbers of strikes, depth of envenomation, size of the snake, potency and amount of venom injected, size and underlying health of the victim, and location of the bite.[60,71] Larger snakes generally inject more venom, but the potency is species-variable. Children and small adults, as well as those with underlying medical conditions (diabetes, cardiovascular disease) may be more seriously affected by envenomation.[69] Envenomation usually occurs in subcutaneous tissues, and less commonly in muscle. In one report, distal crotaline bites on the digits tended to have less severe clinical manifestations than did bites proximal to the interphalangeal joints.[66]

Systemic absorption occurs as a result of lymphatic and venous drainage of the envenomated sites. As a general rule, the distance between fang marks on the skin is equal to approximately the depth of the bite, but this guideline is quite variable and has limited clinical significance. Intravenous envenomation may occur, resulting in the rapid development of life-threatening complications.[26] Airway obstruction necessitating tracheal intubation has been reported after a rattlesnake bite to the face and tongue.[31] One rather bizarre observation is that individuals may be envenomated by rattlesnakes thought to be dead, even up to 60 minutes after de-

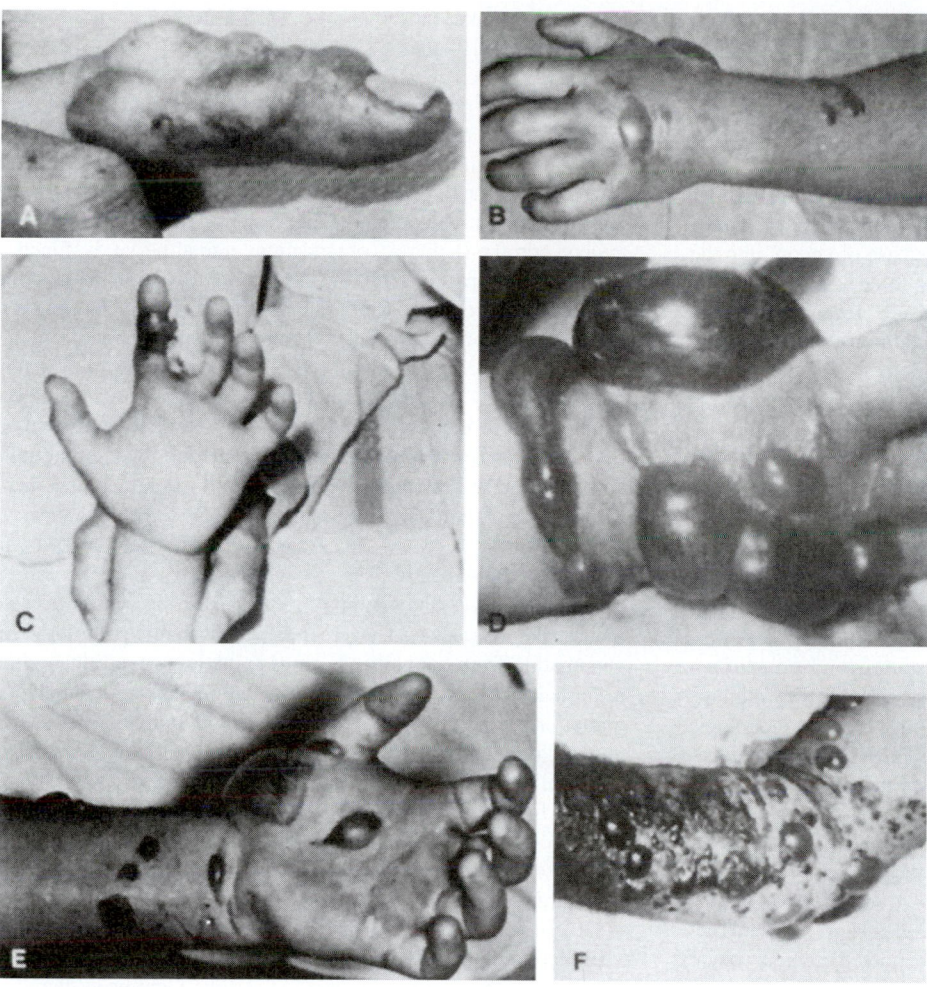

Figure 101–2 (**A**) Bullae filled with serous fluid 12 hours following a bite by *Crotalus atrox*. (**B**) Bullae 12 hours following a bite by an unknown rattlesnake. (**C**) Bullae containing serosanguineous fluid 24 hours following a bite by *Crotalus adamanteus*. (**D**) Bullae containing serosanguineous fluid 36 hours following a bite by *Crotalus viridis helleri*. (**E**) Bullae containing blood and serosanguineous fluid 36 hours following a bite by *Crotalus viridis oreganus*. (**F**) Bullae containing blood and serosanguineous fluid 72 hours following a bite by *Crotalus horridus*. (Reprinted with permission from Russell FE: Snake Venom Poisoning. Philadelphia, JB Lippincott, 1980, p. 296.)

capitation. This is likely due to persistent reflexes in the venom apparatus.[84]

Pit vipers produce a characteristic bite when they strike, and distinct fang marks can usually be identified. The small delicate fangs of coral snakes may not produce easily identifiable fang marks. Fang marks may be single, double, and occasionally multiple. Although most snakes have two fangs, the exact number of fang marks may vary because of glancing blows and/or multiple strikes. Protection by clothing or shoes can alter classical findings. The bites of rodents, lizards, and even thorn or cactus injuries can be mistaken for the bite of a poisonous snake.

PHARMACOLOGY OF VENOM

It is difficult to attribute specific pathology or pathophysiology to particular components of snake venom. Crotaline venom is a complex heterogeneous solution and suspension of various proteins, peptides, lipids, carbohydrates, and enzymes and contains RNAse and DNAse, kinins, leukotrienes, histamine, phospholipase, serotonin, hyaluronidase, acetylcholinesterase, collagenase, and metallic ions.[51,52] It has been referred to as a "mosaic of antigens." Numerous unidentified proteolytic enzymes, procoagulants and anticoagulants, cardiotoxins, hemotoxins, and neurotoxins abound in crotaline venom, making it very complex to analyze. Snake venom can simultaneously damage tissue directly, affect blood vessels and cellular elements of blood, and alter the myoneural junction and nerve transmission. Toxic components of snake venom exhibit their pathology at varying times, and some of the variation in clinical manifestations of envenomation result not only from the specific properties of the venom but from differences in absorption rates and ability to permeate membranes and tissues. In addition, the content and potency of venom in any given snake vary with size, age, diet, climate, time of year, and possible crossbreeding between different species. Coral snake venom consists of a number of unidentified neurotoxins with curarelike effects that produce systemic neurotoxicity as opposed to local tissue injury.

Venom is both circulating and tissue fixed. Circulating venom is more readily neutralized by antivenom, whereas the effects of tissue-fixed venom are more difficult to counteract. This likely accounts for the clinical observation that antivenom corrects systemic dysfunction and coagulopathy but does little to reverse local pathology. Antivenom may halt progression of further edema, hemorrhage, and soft tissue swelling, but once these conditions are present, it is unlikely that antivenom will rapidly reverse pathology at the site of envenomation.

PATHOPHYSIOLOGY AND CLINICAL MANIFESTATIONS

Crotaline Envenomation

Local Reactions. Crotaline (pit viper) venom is usually injected only into the subcutaneous tissue, although deeper, intramuscular (subfascial) envenomation may rarely occur. Not every bite from a venomous snake, however, results in the release of venom into the victim. So-called dry bites may occur in up to 20% of strikes,[56] although it is our experience that a true "dry bite" from a rattlesnake is quite rare. Repeat strikes may result in additional envenomation because the snake's entire supply of venom is not usually exhausted with the first attack. About 25 to 75% of stored venom is discharged following a rattlesnake bite, and the entire supply is replenished in 3 to 4 weeks.[77]

It is usually not difficult to identify serious crotaline envenomation (Fig. 101–3). Symptoms may range from mild to severe, but the initial benign presentation of a pit viper bite may be very misleading [50](Tables 101–2 and 101–3). Generally, within minutes after significant envenomation from a pit viper, the area around the bite becomes swollen. Pain, often severe, quickly develops. Within minutes to hours, ecchymosis, blistering, and signs of tissue necrosis may be evident both proximal and distal to the bite. The patient may describe numbness, tingling, or other neurologic symptoms around the bite. Edema may progress to involve an entire extremity within a few hours, and systemic symptoms may develop. The local reaction to pit viper envenomation results from altered blood vessel permeability and direct necrosis of the tissue caused by the venom. Additional tissue damage can result from the effects of ischemia, swelling, and rarely secondary infection. In addition to local myonecrosis, generalized severe rhabdomyolysis in the absence of impressive muscular swelling may occur. This finding is considered characteristic following envenomation

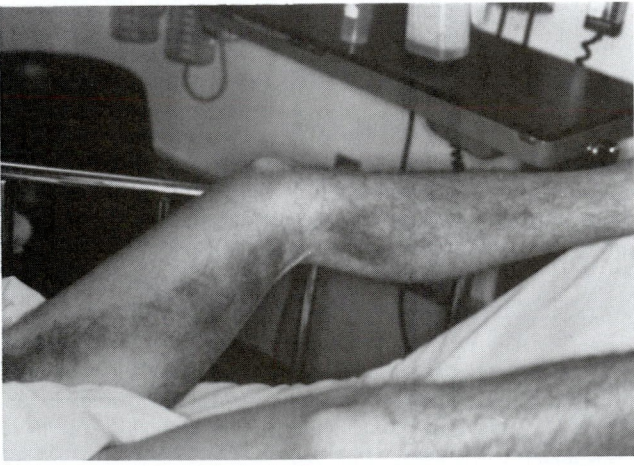

Figure 101–3 This patient's ascending subcutaneous hemorrhagic ecchymosis developed within 8 hours of a copperhead bite to the foot. The ecchymosis follows the course of lymphatic or venous drainage. Only minor discomfort was noted, and there was no coagulopathy. The actual cause is unknown, but this is an example of the hemorrhagic diathesis produced by crotaline envenomation. *(Reproduced with permission from Roberts JR, Greenberg MI: Ascending hemorrhagic signs after a bite from a copperhead. N Engl J Med 1997;336:1262–1263.)*

of the canebrake rattlesnake (*Crotalus horridus atricaudatus*) found in the Gulf Atlantic states.[12]

Local reaction to all rattlesnake venom is usually quite pronounced, but a potential exception to this is envenomation from the Mojave rattlesnake (*Crotalus scutulatus*), a pit viper found in Arizona and other southwestern states. Envenomation from the Mojave rattlesnake may not always produce immediate, severe local symptoms. The potent venom can produce a systemic neurotoxic syndrome (lethargy, obtundation, cranial nerve dysfunction, and respiratory paralysis) in the absence of significant local symptoms, requiring extreme caution in prognosticating lack of envenomation or when treating an apparently "benign" bite from this snake.[53] Mojave venom, unlike the venom of other rattlesnakes, does not usually produce a significant coagulopathy.[17] An unusual combination of neurologic and hematologic toxicity and local tissue injury has been reported after envenomation by a Southern Pacific rattlesnake.[13] Crotamine, a neurotoxic protein found in the venom of the South American rattlesnake (*Crotalus durissus terrificus*), typically produces analgesia at the bite location and contains potent opioid activity. [62]

Compared with the venom of rattlesnakes, the venom of water moccasins produces less-severe local and systemic pathology. Envenomation from copperheads tends to be less severe than either rattlesnake or water moccasin envenomation. Copperhead envenomation often results in only minimal edema and pain and usually requires only conservative local treatment.[89] Although the soft tissue swelling from a copperhead bite may be significant, envenomation from this snake does not usually cause a coagulopathy, systemic symptoms, or extensive tissue destruction. We have been unable to find a report of a lethal copperhead bite in the medical literature.

It is difficult to quantify crotaline envenomation initially. Envenomation is a dynamic and ever-changing process that can rapidly or unpredictably progress to serious local or systemic involvement. It may require a number of hours for the full extent of envenomation to become evident. On rare occasions symptoms may appear to be resolving, only to return minutes to hours later with greater intensity. If local symptomatology is initially ameliorated or arrested by antivenom therapy, there may be a recurrence of the swelling when antivenom levels drop hours later. As a general rule, however, it may be assumed that if no symptoms develop within 6 to 8 hours, envenomation from a North American pit viper (other than Mojave rattlesnake) has not occurred (dry bite).

Systemic Signs. Most bites from pit vipers that occur on the extremities are limited to local or regional pathology, but systemic symptoms of life-threatening proportions may develop (Table 101–3). When venom is injected subcutaneously, it travels by lymphatic and superficial venous channels and spreads rather slowly to reach the general circulation. It generally requires a number of hours for subcutaneous envenomation to produce systemic symptoms, but this timetable is quite variable, with symptoms occasionally occurring quite rapidly even with subcutaneous envenomation. Intravascular envenomation produces significant systemic symptoms in a matter of minutes.[26] Direct blood envenomation is probably quite rare, but this, in addition to the unusual case of overt anaphylaxis, may account for the majority of fatalities. Bites to the head and neck may also be more dangerous than extremity bites because of the rapid absorption of venom from these highly vascular areas and because of airway compromise.

TABLE 101–2.   Evaluation and Treatment of Crotaline Envenomation

Extent of Envenomation	Clinical Observations	Antivenom Recommendation[a]	Other Treatment	Disposition
None	Fang marks may be seen, but there are no local or systemic manifestations after 6–8 hours of observation.	None	Local wound care Tetanus prophylaxis Value of prophylactic antibiotic unknown	Discharge with followup after 6–8 hours of observation[b]
Minimal	Minor local swelling and discomfort. No systemic symptoms, normal laboratory findings. No blisters, ecchymoses, or necrosis. No progression after 6 hours of observation.	None	Same as above	Same as above
Moderate	Progression of swelling beyond area of bite. Moderate to severe pain. Petechiae and ecchymosis of bite area. Minor systemic symptoms, such as anxiety, nausea, tingling, may be seen. Minor laboratory value abnormalities may be noted.	5–10 vials, depending on severity	Tetanus prophylaxis Broad-spectrum antibiotics Cardiac and vital sign monitoring IV fluids Analgesics Assess for compartment syndrome, debridement as necessary Follow laboratory abnormalities	Admit for observation to monitored unit
Severe	Marked progressive swelling and pain, early blisters, ecchymoses, and necrosis. Systemic symptoms such as vomiting, fasciculations, weakness, tachycardia, hypotension, incontinence, epistaxis, hematuria, coagulopathy, hemolysis, renal failure, or cardiopulmonary arrest.	10–40 vials	Tetanus prophylaxis, prophylactic antibiotics, cardiac and vital sign monitoring, IV fluids, analgesics, vasopressors, oxygen, monitor coagulopathy, assess for compartment syndrome, debridement as necessary	Admit to intensive care unit

[a]The dosing regimen refers to the Wyeth polyvalent crotalid antivenin.
[b]Admit all patients with bites from a Mojave rattlesnake because of potential for delayed toxicity.

Rarely, respiratory compromise from airway obstruction or bronchospasm can be a direct consequence of crotaline envenomation.

Systemic signs of pit viper envenomation are varied. Some symptoms may result from fear, pain, or anxiety alone. In mild cases the patient may manifest nonspecific weakness, malaise, nausea, and restlessness. More severe envenomation produces confusion, abdominal pain, vomiting, sweating, dyspnea, tachycardia, blurred vision, salivation, and an unusual or metallic taste in the mouth. Severe envenomation may induce a coagulopathy characterized by spontaneous epistaxis, hematuria, proteinuria, or disseminated intravascular coagulation (DIC). Neurologic symptoms, such as fasciculations, slurred speech, and seizures, may occur. Rarely, crotaline envenomation (Mojave rattlesnake and possibly the Southern Pacific rattlesnake) may produce cranial nerve dysfunction, dysphagia, dysphonia, paresthesias, and respiratory paralysis.[13] Mojave toxin A, responsible for neurotoxicity of the Mojave rattlesnake, is believed to act at presynaptic terminals of the neuromuscular junction by inhibiting acetylcholine release. Although crotaline venom may be directly nephrotoxic, renal failure is probably secondary to hemoglobinuria, myoglobinuria, or cardiovascular collapse. Multisystem failure, predominantly cardiac arrest or ARDS, may be the end result of severe envenomation.[21]

Significant crotaline envenomation may produce complex but rather dramatic hematologic abnormalities, usually a combination of hypoprothrombinemia, thrombocytopenia, fibrinolysis, and hypofibrinogenemia. Venom affects the blood coagulation pathway,

endothelial cells, and platelets[3,9,76,82] (see Fig. 101–3). *Crotalus atrox* venom, for example, can render human blood uncoagulable. Isolated intravascular hemolysis, characterized by a Coombs-positive hemolytic anemia without a significant coagulopathy, has been described following the bite of a Hopi rattlesnake (*Crotalus viridus nuntius*).[32] A routine coagulation profile should be obtained following envenomation by a crotaline (and repeated in 4–12 hours). A significant coagulopathy, especially thrombocytopenia, may be present with a paucity of other systemic effects. Laboratory abnormalities, including prolonged PT and PTT, are frequently seen, and changes in red blood cell morphology, decreased platelet count and function, and bleeding tendencies have been well described. Elevation in the D-dimer activity (range 500–4000 ng/mL) may occur. Coagulopathy is attributed to a complex variety of anticoagulants, procoagulants, fibrinolysin, and hemorrhagins in crotaline venom (see Table 101–4). Overall, crotaline venom has a thrombinlike effect, but specific hematologic effects are species-dependent. No single venom contains all of the identified hemostatically active components, and some portions of snake venom may have therapeutic uses as anticoagulants or platelet receptor (GPIIb/IIIa) antagonists. Thrombocytopenia ($<150,000/mm^3$) is a common finding following envenomation from most species of rattlesnakes.[3] It appears to be especially common, and often severe, following the bite of the timber rattlesnake (*Crotalus horridus horridus*), the rattlesnake inhabiting the Appalachian mountains of the eastern United States.[3] Significant thrombocytopenia can occur in the absence of elevations in

TABLE 101–3. Signs and Symptoms of Rattlesnake Envenomation (N = 100)

Sign or Symptom	Percent
Fang marks	100
Swelling and edema	74
Pain	65
Ecchymosis	51
Vesiculations	40
Changes in pulse rate	60
Weakness	72
Sweating and/or chills	64
Numbness or tingling of tongue and mouth or scalp or feet	63
Faintness or dizziness	57
Nausea, vomiting, or both	48
Blood pressure changes	46
Change in body temperature	31
Swelling of regional lymph nodes	40
Fasciculations	41
Increased clotting time	39
Sphering of red blood cells (spherocytes)	18
Tingling or numbness of affected part	42
Necrosis	27
Respiratory rate changes	40
Decreased hemoglobin	37
Abnormal electrocardiogram	26
Cyanosis	16
Hematemesis, hematuria, or melena	15
Glycosuria	20
Proteinuria	16
Unconsciousness	12
Thirst	34
Increased salivation	20
Swollen eyelids	2
Retinal hemorrhage	2
Blurring of vision	12
Convulsions	1
Muscle contractions	6
Increased platelets	4
Decreased platelets	42

Adapted, with permission, from Russell FE: *Snake Venom Poisoning.* Philadelphia, JB Lippincott, 1980, p. 281.

TABLE 101–4. General Hemostatic Characteristics of Snake Venom

Enzymes that clot fibrinogen
Enzymes that degrade fibrinogen
Plasminogen activators
Prothrombin activators
Factor V activators
Factor X activators
Anticoagulant activities including inhibitors of prothrombinase complex formation, inhibitors of thrombin, phospholipases, and protein C activators
Enzymes with hemorrhagic activity
Enzymes that degrade plasma serine proteinase inhibitors
Platelet aggregation inducers including direct-acting enzymes, direct-acting nonenzymatic components, and agents that require a cofactor
Platelet aggregation inhibitors including: α-fibrinogenases, 5′-nucleotidases, phospholipases, and disintegrins

From Markland FS: *Snake venoms and the hemostatic system.* Toxicon 1998;36:1749–1800.

prothrombin times or partial thromboplastin times. The protein crotalocytin that is found in timber rattlesnake venom causes platelet aggregation and is thought to be at least partially responsible for the thrombocytopenia. Platelet consumption at the site of envenomation may occur.[82] Patients may experience spontaneous epistaxis, hematuria, or hematemesis. An initial drop in fibrinogen levels (to near zero) and platelet count (in the 10,000–50,000/mm³ range) frequently occur after moderate to severe crotaline envenomation. Following the trend in these laboratory parameters is an important way to assess the progression or reversal of systemic envenomation.

A major difficulty in objectively grading the severity of crotaline envenomation and following its progress is that no scoring system readily fits the vagaries of envenomation. Most patients exhibit only a subset of all of the possible consequences, so all, some, or none of the anticipated signs and symptoms may develop in any given individual. In addition, some of the characteristics of envenomation (nausea, tachycardia, restlessness, tachypnea) may be related to fear and not to envenomation. A validated severity score for the objective assessment of crotaline envenomation has been developed and holds promise as a standardization tool for research and clinical evaluation.[24]

Anaphylaxis Rarely, patients bitten by crotalines may experience classic anaphylaxis from the venom itself that can complicate evaluation or mimic a severe systemic reaction to venom. In one report a man developed pruritus and shortness of breath accompanied by hypotension, generalized urticaria, and wheezes immediately following a rattlesnake bite.[46] The symptoms quickly responded to standard treatment for anaphylaxis (epinephrine, antihistamines, and corticosteroids). The patient had been bitten previously and may have been sensitized at that time. Snake handlers may be sensitized through inhalation or skin contact and develop IgE antibodies to venom. Antivenom is not indicated for the treatment of anaphylaxis, but differentiating anaphylaxis from envenomation is often clinically difficult. The presence of pruritus and urticaria or wheezing, uncommon with envenomation, should suggest anaphylaxis.[12]

Recurrence Phenomena of Crotaline Envenomation There are sparse data on the details concerning the natural history of crotaline envenomation following initial treatment with traditional antivenoms. Studies assessing the efficacy and safety of ovine Fab antivenom have, however, shed interesting light on the clinical course of victims of crotaline envenomation treated with this new antivenom. Definite recurrent local and coagulopathic effects, in the form of worsening of symptoms after initial clinical improvement, are described.[5,81] The recurrence phenomena are attributed to the interrelated kinetics and dynamics of venom and antivenom. Simply stated, Fab antivenom has a clinical half-life shorter than that of venom, and once tissue injury and coagulation deficits have been halted or corrected, there may be a worsening of tissue injury and coagulaopthies unless additional antivenom is administered. This may result in greater tissue injury and a risk of hemorrhage. Of particular concern is coagulopathy recurrences that are manifested days to weeks after hospital discharge. The exact clinical significance of this observation, and need for clinical intervention, are uncertain and may be predominately theoretical. However, during the first 24 hours of treatment, additional antivenom may be warranted if the recurrence phenomena are consequential. Currently the most reasonable way to address possible delayed recurrent effects of crotaline envenomation, especially coagulopathy and issues concerning subsequent surgical procedures and trauma, would be careful followup after hospital discharge. This concern has not been extended to coral snake envenomation [see discussion in Antidotes in Depth: Antivenom (Crotalid and Elapid)].

Elapid Envenomation

The severe local reaction to crotaline envenomation is in contrast with the usually minor pain and clinically unimpressive local reactions that occur with a coral snake bite. However, lack of local symptoms does not signify that serious envenomation has not occurred. It is difficult to judge initially which patients bitten by coral snakes will develop symptoms. About 75% of patients bitten by a coral snake are subsequently determined to have been envenomated.[55] Coral snake envenomation may be manifested by serious systemic reactions with little symptomatology at the actual site of envenomation even after an asymptomatic period of up to 12 hours. The venom of the eastern coral snake (*Micrurus fulvius*) is probably more potent than that of the Sonoran coral snake (*Micruroides euryxanthus*) or the Texas coral snake *(Micrurus tenere).*

Systemic Effects. The systemic effects of elapid envenomation are characteristically delayed for a number of hours (Table 101–5). One report described a patient who had an asymptomatic period of 13 hours followed by a sudden and precipitous deterioration severe enough to require ventilatory support.[56] The neurologic abnormalities noted included slurred speech, paresthesias, ptosis, diplopia, dysphagia, stridor, muscle weakness, fasciculations, and respiratory paralysis.[56] Coral snake envenomation results in fewer cardiovascular effects than crotaline envenomation; the major immediate cause of death is respiratory arrest. Pulmonary aspiration is a common sequela in the subacute phase. Patients can develop total-body paralysis that may last 3 to 5 days and take weeks to resolve completely. With respiratory support, however, the paralysis is completely reversible. Primary cardiac arrest and cardiac dysrhythmias are rare, even in severely envenomated patients.

TABLE 101–5. Signs and Symptoms of Envenomation by the Eastern Coral Snake (*Micrurus Fulvius*) (*N* = 20)

Sign or Symptom	Percent
Fang marks	85
Local swelling	40
Paresthesias	35
Nausea	30
Vomiting	25
Euphoria	15
Weakness	15
Dizziness	10
Diplopia	10
Dyspnea	10
Diaphoresis	10
Muscle tenderness	10
Fasciculations	5
Confusion	5

Reprinted, with permission, from Kitchens CS, Van Mierop LHS: *Envenomation by the eastern coral snake (Micrurus fulvius): A study of 39 victims.* JAMA 1987;258:1615.

The benign local effect of coral snake envenomation can be misleading and mistakenly be equated with a dry bite. Because it is difficult to judge initially which patients are envenomated, any patient with coral snake exposure with fang marks or other evidence of skin penetration requires at least 24 hours of observation. Clinical deterioration may be totally unexpected and progress rapidly. Coral snake envenomation can be fatal, but with supportive care and antivenom therapy, patients usually recover completely. In one series, 6 of 39 patients required intubation and ventilation, but none died or suffered tissue loss or permanent neurologic sequelae.[56]

MANAGEMENT OF POISONOUS SNAKEBITE

Objectives for Treatment of Patients with Envenomation

The specific treatment of a patient with a snakebite is controversial, and the literature contains confusing and contradictory recommendations. Folklore and home remedies abound. The benign natural history of many bites undoubtedly has accounted for many "miraculous cures" from such unlikely interventions as ethanol, electric shocks, carbolic acid, strychnine, cauterization, and cryotherapy. Many accepted treatment plans are based on anecdotal or biased information with conclusions drawn from animal studies or uncontrolled case reports. There are no universally accepted standards of care for many aspects of treatment.[90] Many authors tend to be staunch advocates of their particular regimens and unwilling to accept a less rigid approach. The initial objectives are to determine the identity of the offending snake and presence or absence of envenomation, to provide basic supportive therapy, to treat the local and systemic effects of envenomation, and to limit or repair tissue loss and/or functional disability (see Table 101–2).

Two distinct therapeutic approaches are promulgated. One recommends primarily antivenom therapy, whereas the other advocates primarily a surgical approach with an emphasis on surgical debridement and early fasciotomy. Some advocate a very conservative approach that eschews both routine surgery and antivenom, citing a lack of serious morbidity in patients given symptomatic treatment and supportive care after snakebite.[8,59] A combination of medical therapy (mainly supportive care and possibly antivenom) and conservative surgical treatment (mainly debridement of devitalized tissue), individualized for each patient, will likely provide the best results. In general, the more rapidly treatment is instituted, the better the final outcome, but no specific standard of care exists for the institution of various interventions.

Observation of Asymptomatic Patients

All patients reporting a history of snakebite from North American Crotalines should be observed for 6 to 8 hours after the bite if the skin is broken and the offending snake cannot be positively identified as nonpoisonous. If the patient has been bitten by an exotic or non-native snake, it would be prudent to extend the period of observation to 12–24 hours. Fang marks can be quite subtle and initially mistaken for scratches or teeth marks. Although most poisonous snakebites declare their presence by the development of significant symptomatology within a few minutes of the bite, delayed toxicity or resolution of symptoms with a serious recurrence hours later may rarely occur.[39] Delayed symptomatology has been specifically noted after the bite of coral snakes and the Mojave rattlesnake; patients possibly bitten by these snakes should be observed for 24 hours regardless of symptoms. The initial presentation of other pit viper bites may be misleading, and significant worsening of a seemingly benign bite may occur as long as 8 hours after presentation,[50] but such cases are quite unusual. A prudent and conservative approach would be to observe all victims of possible crotaline bites for at least 6 to 8 hours after the bite and admit those with systemic symptoms at any time postenvenomation or those with progressive local symptoms. Restlessness, anxiety, abdominal pain, nausea, and tachycardia are nonspecific symptoms but could signal systemic envenomation, and they should not be routinely dismissed as being a result of fear or anxiety. Any patient bitten by a mamba, cobra, krait, Puff Adder or other unidentified non-native snake should be admitted for observation since the pharmacology of the venom of these snakes is complex and not well characterized.

Initial Treatment for Stable Snakebite Victims

No first aid measures or specific field treatment has been proven to positively affect the outcome from a crotaline envenomation. Undue importance has been placed on the immediate prehospital care of patients with snake bites, and some therapies are clearly detrimental. When the patient is not in extremis, and medical attention is available within a few hours, the prudent approach is a conservative one. The excitement or hysteria generated by a possible poisonous snakebite compels some caregivers to intervene quickly, often irrationally, and with unproven or harmful procedures. It is common to confuse treatment priorities and create additional morbidity with hurried or ill-conceived attempts to stop or limit "certain death" or amputation. In reality, both death and amputation are quite rare if proper medical attention is available within a few hours. Most morbidity stems from delayed treatment, either because of inaction on the patient's part (often related to alcohol intoxication) or because of inaccessible medical care. Prehospital care should generally be limited to immobilization of the patient and rapid transport to a medical facility. Physical activity, such as walking, and elevation of an extremity should be avoided because these maneuvers may hasten systemic absorption of venom.

Initial Treatment of Unstable Snakbite Victims

A possible exception to the dictum of conservative nonintervention in the field can be invoked if deterioration is immediate, the victim is more than 3 to 4 hours from medical care, and significant envenomation is certain. If there are immediate symptoms of severe envenomation, the traditional tourniquet or incision and suction may have some value and can be considered. These procedures should not be done routinely in the field and should be considered only when significant envenomation is certain. Unfortunately, this determination is often a difficult or retrospective clinical decision for most laypersons and many physicians, so there is considerable opportunity for errors in judgment.

Tourniquet/Constriction Band

Although an extremity tourniquet will decrease distal-to-systemic egress of venom, the true value of any intervention designed to limit the systemic absorption of venom is uncertain. Although this has not been studied prospectively, retrospective data fail to demonstrate a benefit in reducing the severity of envenomation with tourniquet application following crotaline bites.[1] A standard of care is impossible to determine because of lack of scientific proof that limiting absorption is clinically helpful and by confusion of anecdotal reports that are uncontrolled and do not consider different species and degrees of envenomation. Also there is no standardization of technique, such as amount of pressure applied or length of tourniquet application. Suggested techniques include a simple thin tourniquet, a broad band, or wrapping an entire extremity with a compression device.

As a conservative temporizing recommendation for extremity envenomation, a wide (2–4 cm) constricting band loosely applied to limit lymphatic (but not venous) flow may be placed a few inches proximal to the bite. Although this has the theoretical disadvantage of concentrating venom in the extremity and increasing local necrosis, a device that decreases systemic absorption of venom may be beneficial in instances where systemic signs and symptoms are rapidly occurring.

The specific effect of a tourniquet on the course of envenomation in humans is unknown, but animal studies suggest a possible benefit. A porcine model using *Crotalus atrox* (western diamondback rattlesnake) venom demonstrated that a constriction band tourniquet placed immediately after experimental envenomation and maintained in place for 4 hours was effective in reducing systemic venom absorption from an extremity without increasing local swelling and local tissue injury.[10] When a blood pressure cuff was maintained to 45 mm Hg, the maximum plasma concentration of venom was reduced by 25%, and total venom absorption was reduced by 33%. This model also demonstrated that removal of the constriction band 4 hours postenvenomation did not result in a significant surge in plasma venom concentration. A sudden worsening of symptoms has been reported, however, after tourniquet removal in patients with crotaline envenomations.[44,51] Therefore, antivenom should be given before tourniquet removal to decrease toxicity from sudden systemic absorption of pooled venom. In the absence of antivenom therapy, the band should remain in place for a few hours, but pressures should be checked and the constriction loosened or moved proximally if it becomes too tight as a result of swelling.

The difficulties of laypersons applying and monitoring a properly applied tourniquet are easy to appreciate. If a tourniquet is used in the field, a reasonable guide would be to wrap it as tight as a compression bandage would be applied for a sprained ankle, and combine the compression with immobilization. There is some evidence that a broad, firm, constrictive wrap (elastic bandage) placed over the bitten area and encircling the entire immobilized limb offers advantage over the traditional tourniquet. This wrapping procedure (the Sutherland wrap) is intended to collapse lymphatics and superficial veins to retard venom uptake and is controversial but suggested as beneficial in the treatment of nonnecrotizing elapid snakebites in Australia.[72,91] In a human volunteer study simulating intradermal and subcutaneous envenomation using labeled radiotracer, immediately wrapping an entire extremity with a rolled elastic bandage to a pressure of 50 to 70 mm Hg significantly increased transit time from periphery to the systemic circulation.[48] The benefit of this technique for the more necrotizing bite of a crotaline or for coral snake envenomations in the United States is unclear.

Thus, the suggested constriction band is not a true tourniquet; if it is applied properly, a finger may be easily placed between the band and the skin. A tourniquet that occludes venous or arterial flow is contraindicated and may compound the initial insult by increasing edema and aggravating ischemia.

Incision and Suction

Under field circumstances, when serious envenomation is certain, the envenomated tissue may be incised and suction applied in an effort to extract venom. Alternatively, suction may be applied without skin incision, via the puncture wounds themselves. Suction is of theoretical value only within the first 5 to 30 minutes after the bite and is generally considered only after severe envenomation by a rattlesnake when medical care is hours away. Other crotalines (copperheads and water moccasins) and coral snakes do not warrant this aggressive therapy.

Two parallel incisions, 0.5 to 1 cm long traversing the fang marks, should be made just deep enough to penetrate the subcutaneous fat (intramuscular envenomation is rare). Care should be taken to avoid tendons, blood vessels, or nerves, and incisions parallel to the long axis of the extremity are preferred. Cross-hatch or cruciate incisions should not be made because they offer no additional value and may increase scarring or predispose to skin necrosis. Continuous suction is applied for 20 to 30 minutes. The value of mouth suction is unproved; it can introduce bacteria and is not recommended by the authors. Swallowed venom is likely not harmful because venom is not absorbed through the intact oral mucosa; however, local oral injury is possible if venom contaminates open lesions on the buccal mucosa.

In a single anecdotal report, orolingual edema (lips and tongue) with airway compromise severe enough to prompt fiberoptic assisted nasotracheal intubation has been attributed to the direct mucosal absorption of the venom of a Canebrake rattlesnake. In this case the envenomated person incised a recent bite on his finger and sucked out the venom. No break in the mucosa of the oral cavity was identified.[54a]

It is estimated that even under ideal circumstances, incision and ideally applied suction will remove less than 20 to 30% of injected venom. Although it has theoretical benefit, neither a definite decrease in morbidity and mortality nor a mitigation of the severity of local or systemic symptoms is documented with incision and suction.[67] Some authorities believe that such surgical therapy is never indicated as first aid treatment, but theoretically the rare patient may experience minimal benefit. We discourage any form or incision and suction for first aid treatment, but cases should be individualized and clinical judgment carefully applied.

There may be some value to a commercially available plunger-type suction device (The Extractor, Sawyer Products, Long Beach, CA) that can generate up to 1 Atm of negative pressure when placed over nonincised puncture wounds to extract venom.[4] Animal models addressing this intervention give conflicting results. In one study this device removed up to 37% of radiolabeled venom when applied for 3 minutes immediately after venom injection. In another, no benefit of negative-pressure venom extraction was found, and additional injury was possible from the device. Like incision and suction, venom extractors are currently unproved therapy.[11,29,30,72,79] Simple suction cups supplied in first aid kits are worthless.

It should be stressed that tourniquets, incision and suction, and vacuum extraction should not be considered if the patient can rapidly reach a hospital or if there are no definite signs of serious envenomation. Minor pain or swelling is not an indication for

zealous field treatment. Furthermore, these treatments are never a substitute for rapid transport, in-hospital evaluation, or antivenom therapy. The bitten area should not be placed in ice, as cryotherapy is not effective in neutralizing venom and may compound the initial injury.[63] Minor cooling may be of some value and is not harmful, but such recommendations are difficult to quantify and can be misinterpreted by the lay public.

Immediate In-Hospital Therapy

The initial in-hospital approach to a victim of a poisonous snakebite follows standard accepted guidelines for stabilization and assessment of any patient with a potentially serious medical problem.[64] A complete medical history, including current tetanus immunization status and sensitivity to medication and horse serum, should be obtained. Patients may be shown pictures of local snakes to make specific identification, but mistakes are common. A careful description of the bite and the extent of the local pathology should be documented, including measuring the diameter of the extremity and noting the extent of edema by marking the skin with a pen to help recognize progression of the envenomation. This evaluation should be repeated as required by the clinical condition. A comprehensive physical examination should be done, with emphasis on vital signs, cardiorespiratory and neurologic status, neurovascular status of the extremity, and evaluation for evidence of bleeding (in the stool, gums, or urine). A baseline complete blood count (CBC), electrolytes, urinalysis, BUN, glucose, INR and partial thromboplastin times (PTT), fibrinogen level, and platelet count should be obtained initially and repeated in 4 to 8 hours. Because venom may interfere with typing and crossmatching procedures, additional blood should be drawn because a future transfusion may be required.

Pain and anxiety should be alleviated. Tetanus prophylaxis should be addressed, and antibiotics are utilized by some authors, although supportive evidence for antibiotic use is limited. Initially the extremity should be immobilized in a well-padded splint and kept at or below heart level until it is certain that there is no systemic envenomation (see Table 101–2). If the patient remains stable, the extremity should be elevated to decrease edema. Ice should not be applied, and incision and suction or the use of a tourniquet are not indicated at this juncture. If the patient is discharged, a followup visit should be arranged in 48 to 72 hours.

Victims of proven copperhead bites should be observed for 4 to 6 hours and evaluated for signs of systemic involvement, the development of coagulation abnormalities, or progression of the local pathology. The length of observation and extent of evaluation for known copperhead bites should be individualized. In the absence of progression of local symptoms and the lack of any systemic symptoms, observation for a few hours may be sufficient. In many instances the entire care of a patient with a minimal copperhead envenomation can be accomplished in the emergency department, but a conservative approach is advised. Hospitalization, if only for further observation, would be prudent for the unreliable patient or if there are questions as to the identification of the snake or progression of symptoms. Testing for sensitivity to horse serum is not advised.[83]

Antivenom Therapy

Antivenom therapy is discussed in detail in Antidotes in Depth: Antivenom (Crotalid and Elapid) at the end of this chapter. Once a victim of a poisonous snakebite has been identified, the availability of antivenom of should be determined, and attempts made to obtain adequate supplies. Currently it may be impossible to obtain Wyeth Crotalid antivenom because of a nationwide shortage. In January 2001, Wyeth announced intention to eventually discontinue production of North American coral snake antivenom and crotalid polyvalent antivenom but to continue producing enough product to satisfy demand until an alternative source is identified. The availability of Fab crotaline antivenom is also problematic at this time.

Surgical Therapy

Surgery is not a concern in the treatment of coral snakebites, and similarly, copperhead and water moccasin bites rarely require surgical intervention except for delayed local debridement. There is, however, historical controversy as to the role of surgery to treat patients who are envenomated by rattlesnakes. Some authors have advocated extensive early debridement, surgical excision of envenomated tissue, and the liberal use of fasciotomy to decompress an extremity.[49,59,89] A compartment syndrome cannot be reliably diagnosed in envenomated extremities without directly measuring compartment pressures. Envenomation may mimic a compartment syndrome by producing distal paresthesias, tense soft tissue swelling, pain on passive stretch of muscles within a compartment, and muscular weakness. However, because subfascial envenomation is uncommon, much of the impressive edema produced by envenomation does not occur in compartmentalized areas. Although there is little doubt that some crotaline bites may eventually require some surgical debridement or even skin grafting, the initial routine use of tissue excision, fasciotomy, or "exploration and debridement" is not recommended.[40] It is unlikely that excising tissue will halt the envenomation process significantly. With the development of techniques to monitor compartment pressures, indications for fasciotomy should be rare and only based on objective data. Using noninvasive vascular arterial studies and skin temperature determinations in patients with rattlesnake envenomation, one report demonstrated that pulsatile arterial blood flow to an envenomated extremity actually increased after envenomation, even distal to the site of envenomation.[20] Skin temperatures also usually increased, but a decrease in skin temperature was associated with vascular insufficiency. One patient in their series developed an arterial embolism, necessitating embolectomy. The authors concluded that increased tissue pressures are not severe enough to cause ischemia to an extremity in most patients bitten by a rattlesnake if antivenom and supportive care are given, and those at risk for ischemia can be identified by noninvasive techniques.

Surgical debridement of necrotic tissue and hemorrhagic blebs and blisters is usually done between the third and sixth day after envenomation. Physical therapy should be instituted early to ameliorate joint stiffness and decrease swelling.

Blood Products

A minor bleeding diathesis as defined by alterations in platelet count, PT/PTT, fibrin split products, and fibrinogen levels is common with crotaline envenomation, and all victims of crotaline envenomation should be evaluated for a coagulopathy, even in the absence of severe symptoms.[26,69] Coral snake venom does not alter coagulation. Crotaline-induced coagulopathy usually resolves spontaneously or is corrected with antivenom therapy, but occasionally fresh frozen plasma, cryoprecipitate, packed red blood cells, or platelet transfusions are required. Thrombocytopenia fol-

lowing rattlesnake envenomation may be difficult, or impossible, to totally correct with platelet transfusions or with large amounts of antivenom. The initial elevation of platelet counts that occurs following platelet transfusion or antivenom administration tends to be transient (lasting only 12–24 hours), and thrombocytopenia may persist for days to weeks after normalization of other coagulation parameters. The significance of prolonged thrombocytopenia in the absence of bleeding complications is uncertain. In the absence of bleeding, thrombocytopenia may be a benign self-limiting disorder that is best tolerated and closely followed in lieu of repeated platelet transfusions or additional antivenom administration.[75] The decision to administer blood products should be based on clinical condition, trend of clotting parameters, and other standard criteria for the treatment of coagulopathies.[9] Criteria for the use of blood products appear to be quite arbitrary in clinical practice. It is recommended that blood products be used only if antivenom is ineffective, and component therapy be used for specific conditions. In general, blood products should be administered if coagulation abnormalities continue to be unstable after antivenom use or if active bleeding occurs. Minor oozing or microscopic hematuria can frequently be treated with antivenom alone. Persistent thrombocytopenia, as an isolated finding, probably does not require aggressive threatment.[75] Hypofibrinogenemia alone is generally not associated with clinically significant bleeding and may not need to be corrected.

The specific mechanism by which antivenom reverses the coagulopathy is unknown, but crotaline antivenom appears to decrease platelet aggregation in vitro. Fibrinogen levels, and PT/PTT parameters are positively affected by antivenom. Heparin does not appear to correct the coagulopathy associated with crotaline envenomation. Monitoring trends in the coagulation profile is one objective way of assessing the seriousness of envenomation and the response to antivenom therapy. Some patients given the equine polyvalent antivenom demonstrate conversion to a positive direct Coombs antibody screen, and this finding should not necessarily be taken as evidence of likely hemolysis.

Antibiotics

The incidence of wound infection following crotaline envenomation is quite low. In one report only 1 in 33 patients not treated with prophylactic antibiotics following a rattlesnake bite developed evidence of a wound infection, prompting the authors to conclude that routine prophylactic antibiotics are not warranted.[16] It would be difficult to cover the multiple gram-positive and gram-negative organisms that could potentially cause infection after envenomation, and some authors eschew their prophylactic use. No benefit has been proven for routine antibiotic use following minor bites, or from the bites of nonvenomous species. However, infection is often difficult to differentiate from envenomation, and the short-term use of broad-spectrum antibiotics for patients with serious bites is intuitively reasonable.[16] A first-generation cephalosporin or a penicillinase-resistant penicillin should suffice. The mouths of snakes harbor various aerobic and anaerobic bacteria (Fig. 101–4).[36] *Mycobacterium* infection has been reported following snakebite.[45] Tetanus prophylaxis should be administered, and hyperimmune tetanus antitoxin given if there is inadequate primary immunization or if the history is uncertain. Antibiotics are potentially beneficial if treatment included an unsterile incision, especially if mouth suction was used.

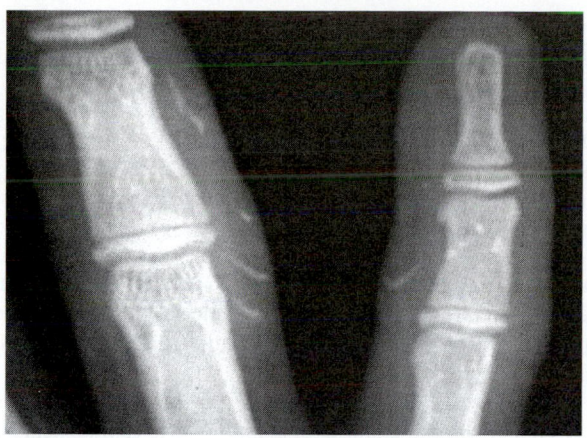

Figure 101–4 Significant local morbidity can result from the bite of non-venomous snakes. This 10-year-old boy was bitten on the hand by a large albino python. After removal of the snake, the boy complained of persistent pain, redness, and swelling. The radiograph demonstrates retained teeth in the soft tissues. Following a short hospitalization for intravenous antibiotics, the child recovered without sequelae. (Courtesy of the Toxicology Fellowship of the New York City Poison Center.)

Other Considerations

There is no rationale for the use of corticosteroids or antihistamines in the routine treatment of patients with snakebite, but they are used to combat the rare case of anaphylaxis from exposure to venom or the more common acute and delayed allergic reactions to antivenom. Corticosteroids may be detrimental to local tissue in the early stages of envenomation.[19] Cardiovascular collapse is a life-threatening consequence of severe systemic envenomation and should be treated aggressively with large amounts of antivenom, invasive monitoring, and standard intensive care techniques.[21] Vasopressors may be required, and respiratory compromise should be anticipated in severe cases. Because of sudden and unpredictable respiratory paralysis associated with coral snake envenomation, tracheal intubation should be considered at the first sign of bulbar paralysis. Any patient given antivenom or with significant envenomation should be observed in an intensive care unit.

There are several reports of a beneficial effect of high-voltage electric shock treatment for poisonous snakebites, but this approach is unproved and cannot be recommended.[25,38] Multiple treatments with hyperbaric oxygen suggest that enhanced healing of myonecrosis may occur in mice injected with *Crotalus atrox* venom. There was no effect on the edema associated with envenomation in one study, and the beneficial effect was dose-dependent, and up to 10 treatments (1 to 1.5 hours at 2 to 2.75 Atm) were given.[54] The mechanism of action is not known but is speculated to be related to enhanced tissue oxygenation. The effects of hyperbaric oxygen therapy of poisonous snakebites in humans is unknown; its use should be considered experimental at this time.

Nonvenomous Snakebites

There are approximately 50,000 snakebites annually in the United States, and most (90–95%) are from nonvenomous snakes.[34] Most snakes in the United States are nonvenomous, and the majority are

of the Colubrid family, which are generally considered harmless to humans. However, several authors have reported toxic secretions from Duvernoy glands in many common species, including the hognose snake, garter snake, parrot snake, banded water snake, and ringneck snake.[37,65,86] Although no deaths have been reported, some victims developed coagulopathies and local edema and hemorrhage that could be confused with early crotaline envenomation.[63] There is no antivenom available to treat bites from these snakes, and serious complications from nonvenomous snakebites are extremely rare.

Although Colubrids do not possess true fangs, some species, such as the common wandering garter snake (*Thamnophis* sp.), have elongated and grooved posterior maxillary teeth (a primitive rear fang) that can penetrate the skin and deliver irritating saliva into the victim via a chewing motion. Some clinicians believe that the presence of teeth marks at the bite excludes the possibility that the bite was made by a venomous snake. Although it is true that fang marks are absent following nonvenomous snakebites, venomous snakes do have teeth, and abrasions or teethmarks may occur in conjunction with a venomous bite. This fact, along with the possibility that snakes heretofore considered nonvenomous may be dangerous, should make the clinician more cautious in diagnosing a nonvenomous bite based entirely on the presence of teeth marks.

When there is no sign of envenomation after an appropriate period of observation following a suspected nonpoisonous snakebite, attention should be focused on the basic principles of wound care. Incision and suction, excision, and wide debridement are obviously unnecessary in such bites. The wound should be treated as a contaminated puncture wound, as it may contain foreign material, especially broken teeth. Any foreign material should be removed, and an appropriate dressing applied. Certain large snakes of the Biodae family (not seen in the United States, except as pets or in zoologic gardens), including boas, pythons, and anacondas, may present a special problem because the force of contraction of their jaws may be great enough to cause severe tissue contusion or fractures and retained teeth (Fig. 101–4). These reptiles also have numerous large, brittle teeth that commonly are broken off and lodged in the wound when the bitten part is forcibly extricated from the snake's mouth. Usually radiographs of the bitten area are needed to exclude fracture or foreign body.

The morbidity associated with a nonvenomous snakebite is from the rare case of bony injury and wound infection. Some authors recommend antibiotics for nonvenomous snakebites, but their routine cannot be supported. In one report no infections followed nonpoisonous snakebites in 72 patients bitten by a variety of nonpoisonous snakes indigenous to New England and imported boa constrictors and pythons.[88] Although *Clostridium tetani* has not been isolated from the mouths of snakes, the ubiquitous nature of this organism requires prophylaxis following the recommended approach for a contaminated wound. A cogent argument can be made for administering prophylactic antibiotics in nonvenomous snakebites if tooth fragments are retained or if there is significant soft tissue contusion. A first-generation cephalosporin or anti-staphylococcal penicillin given for 7 to 10 days should be adequate. Outpatient therapy is appropriate; the patient should be instructed with regard to wound care and to seek medical care if signs of infection occur. Minor abrasions from nonvenomous snakes require only local wound care and tetanus prophylaxis. Delayed infection should prompt an investigation for a retained foreign body, especially a tooth fragment.[42]

Special Considerations for the Management of Pregnant Patients with Snakebites

There is scant information available on the effects of poisonous snakebites during pregnancy. If envenomation is significant, fetal morbidity, mortality, or normal delivery may occur. Three of the four pregnant women bitten by crotalines in one report delivered normal infants, but one woman suffered a spontaneous abortion within 24 hours. The mechanism of injury to the fetus from envenomation includes uterine artery hypotension and subsequent hypoxia, hemorrhagic complications such as abruptio placentae, or uterine contractions initiated by venom.[70]

Intracranial hemorrhage and death in an infant born at 34 weeks of gestation was reported in a woman envenomated by a copperhead during the 28th week of her pregnancy.[28] At the time of the bite she was given antivenom and developed hypotension, which was treated with large doses of epinephrine. It is suggested that the α-adrenergic effects of epinephrine on the uterine artery, coupled with maternal hypotension, contributed more to the fetal demise than the direct effects of venom. As in each case of snakebite, it is prudent to evaluate the need for antivenom carefully during pregnancy and to administer it only when envenomation is significant and the benefits of antivenom outweigh the possible risks from allergic reactions. Fetal monitoring should be routine following poisonous snakebite.

Repeated Exposure to Snake Venom

Handlers and collectors are at risk for multiple bites over their careers, and questions have been raised about possible immunity. No evidence was established that immunity develops as a result of repeated envenomation in one report of 14 patients with two or more bites.[71] Victims of repeat bites may actually be at greater risk for anaphylaxis because of a prior sensitization and the development of IgE antibodies to venom.

Exotic Snakebite

About 3% of poisonous snakebites in the United States are from nonnative species.[2,7,35] Many such snakes are owned by collectors, illegally imported, or stolen from zoos or pet stores. However, private individuals may easily purchase a plethora of vipers, cobras, and adders by mail or at reptile shows. There is surprisingly little regulation on the sale or ownership of exotic snakes in the United States. Exotic venomous snakes pose a particularly difficult problem in both diagnosis and management. Many victims are collectors or researchers who can identify the offending snake. However, because of fear of legal retribution, some owners of exotic snakes can be quite vague about the circumstances or origin of their envenomation. If they cannot provide identification, the local zoo, regional poison center, or herpetology society may be helpful. Once the snake is identified, the antivenom must be obtained. This is always a formidable task and often impossible, but local zoos, poison centers, or collectors may have the antivenom. Some poison centers, some zoos, and The American Association of Zoological Parks and Aquariums (301–562–0777) maintains the *Antivenom Index,* a listing of currently available antivenoms for exotic snakes, but these resources are limited in their ability to deliver many antivenoms. Bites from many nonnative elapidae snakes, such as mambas, kraits, cobras, and several Australian species, are associated with high morbidity and mortality rates. Approximately one-third of bites from the king cobra are fatal.[35]

Bites from these snakes may not display early local or systemic signs (Table 101–2); therefore, the grading system developed for North American pit vipers is not helpful. Although local tissue destruction and edema may develop, classically it is the neurologic signs, such as ptosis, dysphagia, muscular weakness, paresis, ophthalmoplegia, and respiratory failure, that are noted, often at a delayed or advanced stage. Cobra envenomation usually produces significant local toxicity, and these snakes are the only elapids whose venom possesses hemorrhagic activity. Enzyme-linked immunosorbent assay (ELISA) techniques may be used to identify specific venom antigens in suspected exotic snakebites. This technique is not currently available in the United States but is used in Africa, Asia, and Australia.

Guidelines for the administration of antivenom for exotic snakes are vague and empiric. In addition, there is little standardization of the antivenom; antivenoms for the same snake vary by manufacturer. Because exotic snakes are generally quite poisonous, if fang marks are present, envenomation is strongly suspected, the snake has been identified, and the specific antivenom has been obtained, many physicians believe that it is logical to proceed with antivenom administration empirically. Antivenom is administered according to the package insert. Generally four to five vials are administered under the same guidelines given for crotaline antivenom. If the antivenom cannot be obtained, then supportive care and close in-hospital observation may be all that is possible. Local incision and suction are best avoided. Compression immobilization of an entire extremity with an elastic bandage (the Sutherland wrap) for the bite of some elapids (eg, sea snakes, kraits, cobras, and brown snakes) experimentally decreases the movement of elapid snake venom from the bite site to the systemic circulation and may be useful when antivenom is not available. This intervention, when it does not delay transport to medical care, has been recommended for bites from exotic elapids.[91] Crotalineae Polyvalent Antivenom (Wyeth), commonly used for North American pit vipers, is ineffective for the bites of elapid snakes but is active against South American pit vipers, such as the bushmaster, cascabel, and fer-de-lance. Coral snake antivenom is active only against the eastern North American coral snake and is not effective against the western, Mexican, or South American species. It is prudent to obtain expert assistance in managing any exotic snakebite, but in reality, this is usually quite difficult.

One report documents rather dramatic reversal of the neurotoxic effects of a monocellate cobra (*Naja kaouthia*) bite following the intravenous administration of the anticholinesterase neostigmine methyl sulfate (0.5 mg every 20 minutes for four doses).[33] The major neurotoxin from this snake is believed to resemble curare, causing a postsynaptic blockade of nicotinic neuromuscular receptor sites. The neurotoxicity from sea snakes and other elapids has been experimentally reversed with neostigmine.[80] Edrophonium chloride (10 mg administered intravenously with 0.5 mg of atropine) has also been suggested.

Other Poisonous Reptiles in the United States

In North America there are two indigenous species of venomous lizards that belong to the order Squamata, the same order as venomous snakes: the Gila monster (*Heloderma suspectum*) and the beaded lizard (*Heloderma horridum*). These lizards are found primarily in the desert areas of Arizona, southwestern Utah, southern Nevada, New Mexico, California, and Mexico. They are large, slow-moving, nocturnal thick-bodied lizards that are prized by collectors and hobbyists. Adults are 30 to 40 cm long and are generally shy creatures, so bites are relatively rare, usually unintentional or secondary to handling. Gila monsters are known for their forceful bite and propensity to hang on tenaciously during a bite and may be difficult to disengage. Some rather innovative anecdotal techniques have been developed to remove a Gila monster from an extremity, including the use of chisels, screwdrivers, and crowbars, pouring gasoline or ammonia into the lizard's mouth, or holding a flame to the animals jaw. Teeth may break off in the wound.

Gila monster venom is complex, containing components similar to those of snake venoms, including numerous enzymes, hyaluronidase, phospholipase A, kallikrein, and serotonin.[41,78,85] Helothermine is the suspected toxin. Their venom delivery systems are not as efficient as those of poisonous snakes and consists of venom glands and grooved teeth, rather than fangs. Dry bites often occur because of the ineffective mechanism of delivery. Following skin puncture and venom release, the victim experiences local tenderness and soft tissue swelling, pain, and edema; there are occasional reports of anaphylactic reactions, hypotension, angioedema of lip, tongue, and throat, respiratory depression, coagulopathy, and myocardial infarction.[73,74] Significant tissue destruction is unusual, but maceration may occur, and a cyanosis or blue discoloration is noted about the wound. There is no antivenom available against lizard venom. Treatment consists of avoiding overaggressive local treatment and providing supportive care and wound care. Serious morbidity from lizard bites is unusual. The characteristics of the beaded lizard are similar, but their bites are less commonly confronted clinically.

Other Venomous or Poisonous Animals

It was generally believed that there are poisonous or venomous members of all classes of animal except birds. Recent discoveries in New Guinea, however, have added birds to the list.[27,47] Three avian *Pitohui* species have been found to contain homobatrachotoxin, a poison very similar to that in poison dart frogs of South America. Like the frogs, the *Pitohui* birds are conspicuous and brightly colored. There is little information available concerning the toxicity of these birds.

Several species of mammals contain venomous members. For example, the male Australian duckbilled platypus (*Ornithorhynchus anatinus*) has a hollow spur that may inject venom, and the Cuban insectivore (*Solendon paradoxes*) and North American short-tailed shrew both secrete venom from the maxillary glands and bite with the lower incisors. Envenomations from mammals are quite rare, and little is known about the specific clinical toxicity from these creatures.

Several species of amphibians, frogs, toads (*Anura*), newts, and salamanders (*Urodela*) can secrete toxins through their skins, which may be a defensive repellant or alarm mechanism.[6,15,22,23,43] These creatures are not truly venomous, for they have no specific mechanism for delivering the toxin. Most cases of toxicity involve children or pets ingesting the animals. The best-known examples are the Colombian poison dart frogs (*Phyllobates* and *Atelopus*), which secrete the toxins zetekitoxin, tetrodotoxin, and batrachotoxin.[67] Batrachotoxin irreversibly activates (depolarizes) the sodium channel and is 250 times more toxic than curare in mice. Newts of the genus *Taricha* contain the irreversible sodium channel blocking agent tetrodotoxin in their skin and internal organs. Their toxicity would be expected to be similar to that occurring

with puffer fish (fugu) poisoning. Ingestion of a newt has potential adverse consequences. Treatment is supportive. The East Coast species is less toxic than the West Coast variety, the Oregon rough-skinned newt (*Taricha granulosa*). Salamanders of the genus *Salamandra* contain a very potent CNS toxin, salamandarin. Large exposures could theoretically produce neurotoxicity.

Toad species of the genus *Bufo* have been abused by a curious technique of licking their skin, which contains a number of toxic substances, including biogenic amines (serotonin), steroids, and polypeptides. An LSD-like high is reported, but there is considerable folklore and confusion on the exact effects.[61] Toxicity is reported following toad licking, toad mouthing, ingestion of toads, and eating toad soup. Salivation, seizures, and cardiac dysrhythmias have been reported with ingestion of toxin from *Bufo alvarius*, the Colorado River toad. The cane toad (*Bufo marinus*) is less toxic. Bufotalin, a cardioactive steroid toxin (bufadienolide) derived from this toad, has a chemical structure very similar to that of digoxin (Chaps. 48 and 77 for further details).

SUMMARY

Numerous critical decisions challenge the physician faced with a patient who has possibly been bitten by a poisonous snake. The first, and often most difficult, basic questions to address are whether or not the patient was actually bitten by a snake and, if so, has envenomation occurred. When these basic questions remain unanswered, nonintervention, observation, and watchful waiting are most prudent. Unfortunately, patients are frequently unable or unwilling to supply important information concerning the offending reptile, and an intuitive clinical approach is the only alternative. In general, a conservative approach is advocated. Because this is an uncommon scenario, it is prudent to seek help from local experts or poison centers. Phone advice, however, is often difficult to obtain, and treating a snakebite over the phone is a challenge to any consultant. Most clinicians have little or no experience with a poisonous snakebite, and even many toxicologists have limited experience. No physician practicing in the United States has significant experience with exotic snakebites. To complicate matters further, there is little consensus and no definitive standard of care established for many aspects of snakebite care.

Likely the most pressing clinical issues surround local care, surgical intervention, and decisions concerning the use and amount of antivenom. These issues have been addressed in detail in the preceding discussion. In general, surgical intervention should be very conservative, yet a compartment syndrome, albeit rare, should be treated aggressively. Minimally symptomatic patients should receive minimal intervention, but severely envenomated patients require aggressive care. Determining exactly where a patient fits in this continuum may be quite difficult.

REFERENCES

1. Amaral CF, Campolina D, Dias MB, et al: Tourniquet ineffectiveness to reduce the severity of envenomation after *Crotalus durissus* snake bite. Toxicon 1998;36:805–808.
2. Bey TA, Boyer L, Walter FG, et al: Exotic snakebite: Envenomation by an African puff adder. J Emerg Med 1997;15:827–831.
3. Bond GR, Burkhart KK: Thrombocytopenia following timber rattlesnake envenomation. Ann Emerg Med 1997;30:40–44.

4. Bornstein AD, Russell FE, Sullivan JB: Negative pressure suction in field treatment of rattlesnake bite. Vet Hum Toxicol 1985;25: 297–299.

5. Boyer LV, Seifert SA, Cain JS: Recurrence phenomena after immunoglobulin therapy for snake envenomations: Part 2. Guidelines for clinical management with Crotaline Fab antivenom. Ann Emerg Med 2001;37:196–210.

6. Bradley SG, Klika LJ: A fatal poisoning from the Oregon rough skinned newt (Taricha granulosa). JAMA 1981;246:247.

7. Britt A, Burkhart KK: Naja naja cobra bite. Am J Emerg Med 1997; 15:529–531.

8. Burch JM, Agarwal R, Mattox KL, et al: The treatment of crotaline envenomation without antivenom. J Trauma 1988;28:35–43.

9. Burgess JL, Dart RC: Snake venom coagulopathy: Use and abuse of blood products in the treatment of pit viper envenomation. Ann Emerg Med 1991;20:795–780.

10. Burgess JL, Dart RC, Egen NB, et al: Effects of constriction bands on rattlesnake venom absorption: A pharmacokinetic study. Ann Emerg Med 1992;1:1068–1093.

11. Bush SP, Hegewald KG, Green SM, et al: Effects of a negative pressure venom extraction device (Extractor) on local tissue injury after artificial rattlesnake envenomation in a porcine model. Wild Environ Med 2000;11:180–188.

12. Bush SP, Jansen PW: Severe rattlesnake envenomation with anaphylaxis and rhabdomyolysis. Ann Emerg Med;1995;25:845–848.

13. Bush SP, Siedenburg E: Neurotoxicity associated with suspected Southern Pacific rattlesnake envenomation. Wild Environ Med 1999; 10:247–249.

14. Carroll RR, Hall EL, Kitchens CS: Canebrake rattlesnake envenomation. Ann Emerg Med 1997;30:45–48.

15. Chadwick JB: New England's venomous mammals. N Engl J Med 1969;281:274.

16. Clark RF, Selden, BS, Furbee B: The incidence of wound infection following crotaline envenomation. J Emerg Med 1993;11:583–586.

17. Corrigan JJ, Jeter MA: Mojave rattlesnake (Crotalus scutulatus scutulatus) venom: In vitro effect on platelets, fibrinolysis, and fibrinogen clotting. Vet Hum Toxicol 1990;32:439–441.

18. Cruz NS, Alvarez RG: Rattlesnake bite complications in 19 children. Pediatr Emerg Care 1994;10:30–33.

19. Cunningham ER, Sabback MS, Smith RM, et al: Snakebite: Role of corticosteroids as immediate therapy in an animal model. Am Surg 1979;45:757–759.

20. Curry SC, Kraner JC, Kunkel DB, et al: Noninvasive vascular studies in management of rattlesnake envenomation to extremities. Ann Emerg Med 1985;4:1081–1084.

21. Curry SC, Kunkel DB: Death from a rattlesnake bite. Am J Emerg Med 1985;3:227–235.

22. Daly JW: Biologically active alkaloids from poison frogs (Denodrobatidae). Toxin Rev 1982;1:33.

23. Daly JW, Myers CW, Whittaker N: Further classification of skin alkaloids from neotropical poison from Denodrobatidae, with a general survey of toxic/noxious substances in the amphibia. Toxicon 1987;25: 1023–1095.

24. Dart RC, Hurlbut KM, Garcia R, Bkoren J: Validation of severity score for the assessment of crotaline snakebite. Ann Emerg Med 1996;27:321–326.

25. Dart RC, Lindsey D, Schulman A: Snakebites and shocks [letter]. Ann Emerg Med 1988;17:1262.

26. Davidson TM: Intravenous rattlesnake envenomation. West J Med 1988;148:45–47.

27. Dumbacher JP, Beehler BM, Spande TF, et al: Homobatrachotoxin in the genus Pitohui: Chemical defense in birds? Science 1992;258: 799–801.

28. Entman SS, Moise KJ: Anaphylaxis in pregnancy. South Med J 1984; 77:402.

29. Forgey WE: More on snake-venom and insect venom extractors [letter]. N Engl J Med 1993;328:516.

30. Gellert GA: Snake-venom and insect-venom extractors: An unproved therapy [letter]. N Engl J Med 1992;327:1322.

31. Gerkin R, Sergent K, Curry SC: Life-threatening airway obstruction from rattlesnake bite to the tongue. Ann Emerg Med 1987;16: 813–816.

32. Gibly RL, Nowlin SW, Berg RA: Intravascular hemolysis associated with North American crotaline envenomation. J Toxicol Clin Toxicol 1998;36:337–343.

33. Gold BS: Neostigmine for the treatment of neurotoxicity following envenomation by the Asiatic cobra. Ann Emerg Med 1996;28:87–89.

34. Gold BS, Barish RA: Venomous snakebites: current concepts in diagnosis, treatment and management. Emerg Med Clin North Am 1992; 10:249–267.

35. Gold BS, Pyle P: Successful treatment of neurotoxic king cobra envenomation in Myrtle Beach, South Carolina. Ann Emerg Med 1998; 32:736–738.

36. Goldstein EJ, Citron DM, Gonzalez H, et al: Bacteriology of rattlesnake venom and implications for therapy. J Infect Dis 1979;14: 818–821.

37. Gomez HF, Davis M, Phillips S, McKinney P, Brent J: Human envenomation from a wandering garter snake. Ann Emerg Med 1994;23: 1117–1118.

38. Guderian RH, MacKenzie CK, Williams JF: High voltage shock treatment for snakebite [letter]. Lancet 1986;2:229.

39. Guisto JA: Severe toxicity from crotaline envenomation after early resolution of symptoms. Ann Emerg Med 1995;26:387–389.

40. Hall EL: Role of surgical intervention in the management of crotaline snake envenomation. Ann Emerg Med 2001;37:175–180.

41. Hendon RA, Tu AT: Biochemical characterization of the lizard toxin gilatoxin. Biochemistry 1981;20:3517–3522.

42. Herman RS: Nonvenomous snakebite. Ann Emerg Med 1988;17: 1262–1263.

43. Hitt M, Ettinger DD: Toad toxicity. N Engl J Med 1986;314: 1517–1518.

44. Ho M, Warrell DA, Looareesuwan S, et al: Clinical significance of venom antigen levels in patients envenomated by the Malaysian pit viper. Am J Trop Med Hyg 1986;35:579–587.

45. Hofer M, Hirschel B, Kirschner P, et al: Disseminated osteomyelitis from Mycobacterium ulcerans after a snakebite. N Engl J Med 1993; 328:1007–1009.

46. Hogan DE, Dire DJ: Anaphylactic shock secondary to rattlesnake bite. Ann Emerg Med 1990;19:814–816.

47. Holloway M: Pitohui: The colorful bird that looks better than it tastes. Sci Am 1993;258:20–22.

48. Howarth DA, Southee AE, Whyte IM: Lymphatic flow rates and firstaid in simulated peripheral snake or spider envenomation. Med J Aust 1994;161:695–699.

49. Huang TT, Lynch JB, Larson DL, et al: The use of excisional therapy in the management of snakebite. Ann Surg 1974;179:598–607.

50. Hurlbut KM, Dart RC, Spaite D: Reliability of clinical presentation for predicting significant pit viper envenomation. Ann Emerg Med 1988;12:438.

51. Iyaniwura TT: Snake venom constituents: biochemistry and toxicology, Part 1. Vet Hum Toxicol 1991;33:468–474.

52. Iyaniwura TT: Snake venom constituents: biochemistry and toxicology, Part 2. Vet Hum Toxicol 1991;33:475–480.

53. Jansen PW, Perkin RM, VanStralen D: Mojave rattlesnake envenomation: Prolonged neurotoxicity and rhabdomyolysis. Ann Emerg Med 1992;21:322–325.

54. Kelly JJ, Sadeghani K, Gottlieb SF, et al: Reduction of rattlesnake-venom-induced myonecrosis in mice by hyperbaric oxygen therapy. J Emerg Med 1991;9:1–7.

54a. Kerns W, Tomaszewski C: Airway obstruction following canebrake rattlesnake envenomation. J Emerg Med 2001;20:377–380.

55. Kitchens CS, Van Mierop LHS: Envenomation by the eastern coral snake (Micrurus fulvius fulvius). JAMA 1987;258:1615–1618.

56. Kunkel DB, Curry SC, Vance MV, Ryan PJ: Reptile envenomations. J Toxicol Clin Toxicol 1983–84;21:503–526.

57. Kwan T, Paiusco AD, Kohl L: Digitalis toxicity caused by toad venom. Chest 1992;102:949–950.

58. Langley RL, Morrow WE: Deaths resulting from animal attacks in the United States. Wild Environ Med 1997;8:8–16.

59. Lawrence WT, Giannopoulos A, Hansen A: Pitviper bites: Rational management in locals in which copperheads and cottonmouths predominate. Ann Plast Surg 1996;36:276–285.

60. Lewis JV, Portera CA: Rattlesnake bite of the face: Case report and review of the literature. Am Surg 1994;60:681–682.

61. Lyttly T, Goldstein D, Gartz J: Bufo toads and bufotenine: Fact and fiction surrounding an alleged psychedelic. J Psychoactive Drugs 1996;28:267–281.

62. Mancin AC, Soares AM, Andriao-Escarso SH, et al: The analgesic activity of crotamine, a neurotoxin from Crotalus durissus venom. Toxicon 1998;36:1927–1937.

63. McCollough N, Gennaro J: Evaluation of venomous snakebite in the southern United States. J Fla Med Assoc 1963;49:959–967.

64. McKinney PE: Out-of-hospital and interhospital management of Crotaline snakebite. Ann Emerg Med 2000;37:168–174.

65. McKinstry DM: Evidence of toxic saliva in some colubrid snakes of the United States. Toxicon 1978;16:523–534.

66. Moss ST, Bogan G, Dart RC, et al: Association of rattlesnake bite location with severity of clinical manifestations. Ann Emerg Med 1997;30:58–61.

67. Myers CW, Daly JW: Dart-poison frogs. Sci Am 1983;248:96–105.

68. Parrish HM: Incidence of treated snakebites in the United States. Public Health Rep 1966;81:269–276.

69. Parrish HM, Goldner JC, Silbert SL: Comparison between snakebites in children and adults. Pediatrics 1965;36:251.

70. Parrish HM, Khan MS: Snakebite during pregnancy. Report of four cases. Obstet Gynecol 1966;27:468–471.

71. Parrish HM, Pollard CB: Effects of repeated poisonous snakebites in man. Am J Med Sci 1959;237, 277–286.

72. Peam J, Morrison J, Charles N, et al: First aid for snakebite. Med J Aust 1981;2:293–295.

73. Placentine J, Curry SC, Ryan PJ: Life-threatening anaphylaxis following Gila monster bite. Ann Emerg Med 1986;15:147–149.

74. Preston CA: Hypotension, myocardial infarction, and coagulopathy following Gila monster bite. J Emerg Med 1989;7:38–40.

75. Rao RB, Palmer M, Touger M: Thrombocytopenia after rattlesnake envenomation. Ann Emerg Med 1998;31:139–141.

76. Roberts JR, Greenberg JI: Ascending hemorrhagic signs after a bite from a copperhead. N Engl J Med 1997;336:1262–1263.

77. Russell FE: Snake Venom Poisoning. Philadelphia, JB Lippincott, 1980.

78. Russell FE, Bogert CM: Gila monster: Its biology, venom and bite—a review. Toxicon 1981;19:341–359.

79. Russell FE, Emery JA: Incision and suction following injection of rattlesnake venom. Am J Med Sci 1961;241:160–161.

80. Sakai A, Junsuke T, Mamoru V: Efficacy of anticholinesterase against paralysis caused by postsynaptic neurotoxic snake venom [abstract]. Ann Emerg Med 1995;26:712–713.

81. Seifert SA, Boyer LV: Recurrence phenomena after immunoglobulin therapy for snake envenomations: Part 1. Pharmacokinetics and pharmacodynamics of immunoglobulin antivenoms and related antibodies. Ann Emerg Med 2001;37:189–195.

82. Simon TL, Grace TG: Envenomation coagulopathy in wounds from pit vipers. N Engl J Med 1981;305:443–447.

83. Spaite D, Dart R, Sullivan JB: Skin testing in cases of possible crotaline envenomations. Ann Emerg Med 1988;7:105–106.

84. Suchard JR, LoVecchio F: Envenomations by rattlesnakes thought to be dead. N Engl J Med 1999;340:1930.

85. Tu AT: Handbook of Natural Toxins, Vol. 5. New York, Marcel Dekker, 1991, pp. 755–776.

86. Vest DK: Toxic Duvernoy's secretions of the wandering garter snake *Thaminophis elegans vagrans*. Toxicon 1981;19:831–839.

87. Watt CH, Genarro JF: Pit vipers in south Georgia and north Florida. Trans South Surg Assoc 1965;77:378–386.

88. Weed HG: Nonvenomous snakebite in Massachusetts: Prophylactic antibiotics are unnecessary. Ann Emerg Med 1993;22:220–224.

89. Whitley RE: Conservative treatment of copperhead snakebites without antivenom. J Trauma 1996;41:219–221.

90. Wingert WA, Chan L: Rattlesnake bites in southern California and rationale for recommended treatment. West J Med 1988;148:37–43.

91. Winkel KD, Hawdon GM, Levick N: Pressure immobilization for neurotoxic snake bites. Ann Emerg Med 1999;34:294–295.

ANTIDOTES IN DEPTH

Antivenom (Crotaline and Elapid)

James R. Roberts / Edward J. Otten

The relative safety and efficacy of antivenoms has been demonstrated for the treatment of poisonous snakebite from reptiles found outside the United States.[15,20] No large-scale controlled human trials have demonstrated a consistent decrease in morbidity or mortality with standard equine polyvalent crotaline antivenom therapy used to treat envenomation secondary to snakes found in the United States. In addition, no rigorous risk/benefit analysis of antivenom is available. Snake venom produces reversible effects (multiorgan dysfunction and coagulopathy) and largely irreversible effects (local soft tissue injury). Preliminary data from clinical studies of a new ovine-derived Fab antivenom developed for use against venomous snakes in the United States suggests that antivenom therapy does indeed control or lessen progression of, but does not significantly reverse, local swelling and tissue injury secondary to crotaline envenomation. This antivenom reverses, but may not totally eliminate, systemic effects, including venom-induced coagulopathy.[4,8,17] Therefore, we consider, as do most authorities, antivenom to be a mainstay in the treatment of serious poisonous snakebites. Some clinicians, however, eschew its use entirely, preferring surgical therapy and/or supportive care.[13,22]

Those who advocate antivenom use promulgate that antivenom ameliorates tissue injury and general systemic toxicity and reverses coagulopathies from snake venom, primarily referencing data from nonnative species and animal studies, small uncontrolled series, and anecdotal human case reports. Antivenom is thought to "neutralize" systemic and tissue-fixed venom by a yet unknown mechanism. The potential for antivenom to reverse venom-induced coagulopathy seems to be the most reasonable justification for aggressive antivenom administration. However, some components of venom-induced coagulopathy, especially thrombocytopenia and neurologic effects of some rattlesnakes, may be resistant to antivenom therapy.[3,6,21] Opponents of routine antivenom use emphasize the significant potential for hypersensitivity reactions and lack of scientific proof substantiating a change in morbidity and mortality in humans. Antivenom will no doubt continue to be the subject of debate for some time. However, based on current knowledge and clinical evidence, our opinion is that antivenom is the treatment of choice in cases of serious envenomation where there is evidence of systemic effects and coagulopathy. Because antivenom is derived from animals inoculated with venom from only a few snakes, it is likely that only a portion of the venom-induced pathology will be neutralized by current products. Mild to moderate local tissue injury that remains stable or is only minimally progressive, in the absence of systemic dysfunction or coagulopathy, is not an absolute indication for antivenom therapy. Although this is a controversial area, and each case must be individualized, such local pathology is not likely to be reversed with antivenom, and the risk/benefit analysis does not support routine antivenom use. Additional study is required to define more precisely the role of new antivenoms and to unravel the vagaries of dosing.

Historically, two types of antivenom have been available to treat snakebites in the United States: crotaline and coral snake antivenom. Both are derived from horse serum. Recently a third type of antivenom has been made commercially available. It is a refined crotaline antivenom (CroFab, Protherics, Savage Laboratories) derived from sheep serum and formulated more specifically for the crotalines found in the United States. This product holds promise as an effective and less allergenic alternative to currently available horse serum products.[7] If clinical experience validates very positive early clinical trials, this new antivenom may replace the current polyvalent crotaline antivenom; however, current experience is too limited to provide definitive guidance to the practicing clinician.

Numerous antivenoms exist for bites from exotic or foreign snakes, but they have limited availability, are difficult to obtain, and are rarely used. Because the products that are currently available are primarily derived from horse serum products, this discussion focuses on the clinical use and specifics of administration of this type of antivenom. However, in January 2001, Wyeth-Ayerst announced that it intends to eventually halt production of equine-based antivenom for coral snakes and crotalines. The company has stated that it will produce enough antivenom to satisfy demand for several years until an alternate source is identified. However, at the time of this writing, all types of antivenom used for the treatment of crotaline envenomation are in very short supply, and adequate amounts of antivenom may not be available to most hospitals.

There are no specific standards concerning the amount of antivenom that should be routinely stocked in hospital pharmacies. Most hospitals that do not treat snakebite patients on a regular basis do not stock any antivenom but rely on networks for obtaining it when the need arises; however, this is always problematic. With the current supply problems, it is unrealistic to expect that large supplies of antivenom can be obtained on short notice. The announcement concerning the planned discontinuation of all equine-based antivenoms by Wyeth leaves many practical issues unsettled at the current time. It is suggested that hospitals with such needs contact the manufacturers, Wyeth Pharmaceuticals and Protherics (Altana, division of Savage) Laboratories, on an as-needed basis (current nationwide phone numbers can be found in the *Physician's Desk Reference*).

CROTALINE POLYVALENT ANTIVENOM (EQUINE ORIGIN)

Crotaline polyvalent antivenom (Antivenin Crotalidae Polyvalent, Wyeth-Ayerst) is active against the venom of rattlesnakes (*Crotalus, Sistrurus*), water moccasins, copperheads (*Agkistrodon*), some South American pit vipers, and some Asian snakes. It is not effective for bites of exotic snakes, such as cobras and other elapididae. Antivenom is a refined and concentrated preparation of equine serum immunoglobulins (IgG) formulated into a freeze-dried powder to be reconstituted before use. It is a suspension of various venom-neutralizing antibodies prepared from the serum of horses that are gradually hyperimmunized against the venom of a specific cadre of pit vipers found in the Western hemisphere: *Crotalus adamanteus* (eastern diamondback rattlesnake), *Crotalus atrox* (western diamondback rattlesnake), *Crotalus durrisus terrificus* (tropical rattlesnake), and *Bothrops atrox* (fer-de-lance). These crotalines share many of the common antigens found in pit viper venom throughout the world, so the polyvalent antivenom is presumed effective against a number of species, including all pit vipers found in the United States. Even though the polyvalent antivenom is not derived from copperheads or other crotalines, such as the Mojave rattlesnake, Pacific rattlesnake, and timber rattlesnake, it is commonly administered following severe envenomation from these species.[3] Antivenom may be less effective against these snakes, and it has been suggested that the neurotoxicity from the Mojave rattlesnake may be resistant to crotaline polyvalent antivenom.[6] Crotaline polyvalent antivenom is given to ameliorate the effects of local and systemic envenomation by pit vipers, and it is thought by some clinicians to be lifesaving. A minority of authors consider the risk/benefit of antivenom to be unacceptable and argue against its use under all circumstances. Animal studies document a decrease in mortality and amount of tissue necrosis when antivenom is given immediately after envenomation. A delay in treatment of even a few hours lessens the beneficial effects of antivenom in animal models. Case reports and anecdotal evidence support the concept that antivenom will lessen the progression of local tissue injury and halt or reverse, at least temporarily, systemic effects, including most coagulation defects.

When indicated, antivenom should be given as soon as possible to neutralize circulating and tissue-fixed venom. However, it is impossible to define the exact benefit of any specific time line, and the value of late administration is impossible to quantify. Delay of antivenom administration for a few hours is unlikely to result in a significant change in morbidity or mortality in the majority of cases. Crotaline antivenom should not be given "prophylactically" to patients with minimal symptoms or to those who demonstrate no evidence of envenomation. It is prudent, however, routinely to obtain adequate supplies of antivenom for possible use should the subsequent development of symptoms warrant treatment. It is our experience that most bites from large rattlesnakes will progress to an extent that antivenom is required and that copperhead envenomation rarely, if ever, mandates antivenom administration. Some authors recommend the use of prophylactic antivenom in all cases of proven bites from the Mojave rattlesnake because local symptomatology may not precede systemic symptoms. The severity of envenomation by water moccasins lies somewhere between that of the relatively benign copperhead and the more destructive rattlesnake.

Because it is a horse serum product, antivenom use entails a significant incidence of immediate and delayed hypersensitivity reactions,[10] including minor cutaneous hypersensitivity (urticaria), anaphylaxis, anaphylactoid reactions, and serum sickness. As the dose or rapidity of administration of antivenom is increased, the incidence of acute and delayed hypersensitivity reactions also increases. Because the ammonium sulfate precipitation process currently used to prepare antivenom is inefficient, the serum contains unwanted contaminants in the form of extraneous heterologous proteins such as albumin, α- and β-globulins, and IgM in addition

to the venom-specific IgG. These contaminants are largely responsible for the allergic properties of antivenom.

Anaphylactic reactions result from the presence of circulating IgE antibodies to horse protein in the recipient's blood and from direct degranulation and histamine release from mast cells or basophils by horse proteins. Serum sickness is caused by the delayed production of antibodies by the recipient following the infusion of a relatively large dose of foreign protein (antigen excess reaction). Serum sickness often develops a few days to weeks after the administration of horse serum and is virtually certain to occur if more than four to five vials of horse serum–derived antivenom are given. Fortunately, serum sickness is generally mild, easily treated, and not associated with significant chronic sequelae, although rarely immune-complex vasculitis, myocarditis, neuritis, and glomerulonephritis are noted. There are few data on the exact incidence of allergic reactions, but some form of hypersensitivity occurs in 20 to 40% of patients receiving antivenom[11] (see Table 101–6). The majority of patients given antivenom will experience urticaria as the only acute adverse reaction.

Technique of Administration

Before antivenom is administered, the patient should be asked about previous antivenom exposure or allergies. Sensitivity to medications or tetanus toxoid are not contraindications to the use of antivenom. The use of skin testing for sensitivity to horse serum is controversial, and we do not recommend its use before antivenom administration. Skin testing is an unreliable predictor of either immediate or delayed hypersensitivity reactions. Both false-positive (about 50%) and false-negative (about 20%) skin tests are encountered.

At this time there is no standard of care with regard to the issue of skin testing or the use of antivenom based on the results of skin

TABLE 101–6. Complications of Crotalidae Antivenom Therapy

Snake involved[a]	
Eastern diamondback rattlesnake	10
Cottonmouth (moccasin)	10
Copperhead	2
Unidentified	18
Number of patients treated with antivenom	26 (66%)
Average number of vials of antivenom	19.5 (range 1–119)
Incidence of immediate allergic reactions	23% (6 patients)
Cutaneous symptoms only	3 patients
Systemic reaction	3 patients
Incidence of immediate hypersensitivity	
Positive skin test	67% (4 of 6)
Negative skin test	10% (2 of 20)
Incidence of delayed reactions (serum sickness)	50% (10 of 20)
Symptoms of serum sickness	
Rash, pruritus, urticaria	100%
Fever or malaise	30%
Arthralgias	10%
Lymphadenopathy	10%
Peripheral neuritis	None
Renal failure	None

[a]Not all treated with antivenom.
Based on a retrospective study of 26 patients with crotalidae snake bites treated with antivenin. Data from Jurkovich GJ, Luterman A, McCullar K: *Complication of Crotalidae antivenin therapy.* J Trauma 1988;28:1032–1037.

testing. Because some authors advocate its use, we discuss the technique. Skin testing is usually done with plain horse serum provided with the antivenom by the manufacturer; more clinical information may be gleaned if skin testing is done with the actual reconstituted antivenom, although this is not standardized. The skin test is accomplished with 0.01 to 0.02 mL of serum injected intradermally (not subcutaneously) in the volar forearm, with a 0.9% sodium chloride solution control. A positive test is defined by the development of erythema, edema, wheal formation, or intense itching at the site within 15 to 30 minutes. Testing may be done with a 1:10 dilution of horse serum or antivenom (reconstituted and then also diluted 1:10). In one report six patients had a positive skin test, but only four developed an immediate reaction to antivenom.[11] Of 20 patients with a negative skin test, two (10%) developed immediate hypersensitivity. It may be intuitively tempting to skin test all patients who potentially may require antivenom, but skin testing should be considered only if the decision has been made to administer antivenom. Patients should not be "prophylactically" tested for horse serum allergy because the skin test may sensitize the individual to future use of horse serum products, a particular problem in snake collectors and handlers at risk for subsequent bites.

Significant allergic reactions have been reported following skin testing, emphasizing that this procedure is not innocuous.[19] Although fatal anaphylaxis secondary to antivenom administration has been suggested in some reviews, we have been unable to find a single documented death directly related to antivenom therapy. In life- or limb-threatening situations the administration of antivenom to patients with a positive skin test or known allergy to horse serum is warranted.[14,16] Antivenom administration may be continued in selected cases of serious envenomation even in the presence of an allergic reaction. In such cases, where the skin test is positive or a reaction develops during administration of antivenom, the prophylactic or concomitant use of corticosteroids, epinephrine, and antihistamines has alleviated most of the allergic symptoms. Treatment should entail both the use of H_1 and H_2 antihistaminic receptor blockade (with 1 mg/kg diphenhydramine IV and 300 mg cimetidine or 50 mg ranitidine IV). In one study the cutaneous and systemic signs and symptoms of immediate hypersensitivity were all effectively treated with antihistamines and epinephrine, with no adverse sequelae.[11] Slowing the rate of infusion of the antivenom or increasing the dilution frequently lessens the severity of the allergic reaction (Chap. 101). There is no practical way to desensitize patients to antivenom.

The routine pretreatment of all patients who receive antivenom is controversial. Because urticaria is the most common immediate hypersensitivity reaction, we believe it is intuitively reasonable to pretreat all patients with antihistamines. However, many authors reserve H_1- and H_2-blocking antihistamines (diphenhydramine, 0.5–1 mg/kg IV, alone or in combination with cimetidine, 300 mg every 6 hours) and corticosteroids (methylprednisolone, 1–2 mg/kg IV) for patients with a positive skin test or for those who develop a reaction during the infusion. The value of corticosteroids for the treatment of acute allergic reactions is probably limited. Anaphylaxis usually requires the cautious use of subcutaneous epinephrine (0.3–0.5 mg every 20 minutes in adults, repeated three times if needed) or an IV infusion of epinephrine (1 mg in 1 L of 0.9% sodium chloride solution, titrated to effect) in addition to other standard supportive measures. One report described the simultaneous use of antivenom and an epinephrine in-

fusion in a severely envenomated patient who displayed allergy to horse serum.[14]

One problem with current polyvalent antivenom is that it is difficult to reconstitute, requiring approximately 1 hour to prepare. Reconstituted antivenom should be diluted to 1:10 to 1:100 in 0.9% sodium chloride solution and given IV. It is not given intramuscularly or directly into the area of the bite. Intraarterial administration of antivenom has been investigated in animal models envenomated with *Crotalus atrox* venom. The intraarterial route is experimental and offers no clear benefit over intravenous administration.[1] Antivenom is initially infused slowly (25–50 mL/h), but the rate of infusion may be cautiously increased in the absence of allergic reactions. If antivenom is well tolerated, subsequent vials can be diluted 1:2 or 1:4 with 0.9% sodium chloride solution. An infusion rate of 2 to 10 vials/h is a general guideline, but data are lacking on the ideal protocol. In critical situations, multiple vials of crotaline antivenom have been safely given by bolus injection.[5] Antivenom should be given with constant observation of the clinical status and vital signs and with the patient on a cardiac monitor in an area where cardiopulmonary resuscitation is possible.

Recommendations for the amount of polyvalent antivenom required for an envenomation are vague and varied and subject to much debate (see Table 101–2). Children usually require more antivenom per body weight than adults, but there is no standard dose of antivenom.[5] Because of the unpredictable progression of envenomation, and the worsening of clinical symptoms following initial improvement (recurrence phenomena), it is often difficult initially to estimate the total amount of antivenom required.[4,17] What initially appears to be a minor bite may progress over a period of hours to become a severe local or even a systemic envenomation.

Patients with mild symptomatology should not be given antivenom. There is no justification for infusions of one or two vials in minor cases. At least 5 to 10 vials of antivenom are generally recommended initially for both adults and children in cases of moderate envenomation, but up to 30 to 40 vials may be required in cases of severe systemic envenomation. There are reports of patients safely receiving more than 100 vials, but such massive doses are unusual.[5] The initial dose of antivenom should be given as soon as possible but administered cautiously to limit reactions from rapid infusion. Anecdotally, antivenom may reverse some of the venom-induced coagulopathy even if given more than 24 hours after the bite, negating the need for blood products traditionally administered for coagulation defects. Although most reports document a favorable effect of antivenom on PT/PTT values, platelet counts are less favorably affected. Thrombocytopenia may not respond to antivenom administration, or a significant rebound may be noted in a few days. In some cases, a coagulopathy may return or persist for days to weeks. In the specific case of proven rattlesnake bite, we advocate the initial use of five vials of polyvalent antivenom in all instances where symptoms are rapidly progressive or initially severe. This is because in our experience, once symptoms begin to progress rapidly, they usually continue, and to the extent that antivenom is warranted, early treatment is likely to be more effective than late administration.

In contrast to rattlesnake bites, studies have reported that antivenom was required in only 12% of bites from copperheads and water moccasins.[21,22] Table 101–2 presents guidelines for estimating the degree of envenomation and the need for antivenom based on symptoms, but it is stressed that each case must be individualized, and repeat clinical examinations are needed to assess the true extent of envenomation. One problem with attempting to guide antivenom use by a grading system is that the severity of the coagulopathies seen following snakebites do not always correlate with objective signs of envenomation. In general, all of the antivenom should be given over the first 24 hours. Although its efficacy after 24 hours has been questioned, antivenom is advised in severe poisonings even after this time, especially if a coagulopathy persists. All patients who receive antivenom should be hospitalized for at least 24 hours. Discharged patients should have a followup visit and evaluation for coagulopathy within 7 to 10 days. Those who initially have a significant coagulopathy are more at risk for recurrent abnormal coagulation tests, although the significance of a persistent asymptomatic thrombocytopenia, or the need for treatment, is unknown. Theoretically such patients are at risk for trauma or surgery until the coagulopathy has completely resolved.

There is approximately a 50% chance of developing serum sickness within 3 to 20 days of antivenom administration, especially if more than five vials are administered. The frequency of serum sickness is directly related to the number of vials of antivenom that was administered. If more than 30 vials are given, serum sickness can be routinely expected. The development of serum sickness cannot be predicted on the basis of a positive or negative skin test for horse serum sensitivity. Mild cases of serum sickness consist of urticaria, pruritus, and mild systemic symptoms, such as malaise. Occasionally arthralgias, lymphadenopathy, and fever may develop. Immune-complex glomerulonephritis, neuritis, vasculitis, and myocarditis rarely occur. The syndrome of serum sickness after antivenom use has not been well characterized or studied, but it is usually neither serious nor associated with chronic sequelae.[10] Symptoms last for about a week, but may be fleeting or present for up to 3 weeks. Most patients respond favorably to antihistamines or systemic corticosteroids. There is a trend toward the routine prophylactic use of corticosteroids or antihistamines to prevent serum sickness, but controlled trials are lacking. Because antihistamines and short-term steroid regimens are safe, their prophylactic use can be considered following large doses of antivenom.

ELAPID ANTIVENOM (EQUINE ORIGIN)

An antivenom of equine origin is available to treat envenomation by the Eastern coral snake (*Micrurus fulvius fulvius*) and Texas coral snake (*Micrurus fulvius tenere*), but none is available against the venom of the less virulent Arizona (Sonoran, *Micruroides euryxanthus*) coral snake or coral snakes found in Mexico, Central America, or South America. Deaths have not been reported after the bite of the Sonoran coral snake. In contrast to the recommendation to withhold crotaline polyvalent antivenom unless signs of significant envenomation are evident, coral snake antivenom is recommended prophylactically in any symptomatic patient and in asymptomatic cases where it is assumed or proven that the patient was bitten by a coral snake.[12] Following the bite of a coral snake, there may be little objective evidence to suggest envenomation for a number of hours, but systemic symptoms can develop insidiously. Therefore, at least three to five vials of coral snake antivenom are given initially and repeated on the basis of the clinical condition. The caveats for the administration of crotaline antivenom (skin testing, rate of infusion, treatment of reactions) apply to coral snake antivenom, except that usually less antivenom

is required for coral snakes. Up to 10 vials may be administered, but dosing recommendations are vague.

ALTERNATIVES TO EQUINE-DERIVED ANTIVENOM

Some of the clinical problems currently associated with the administration of equine-based antivenom may be eliminated by the development of alternative sources for neutralizing antibodies.[2,7,9] Less antigenic antivenoms can be produced by techniques such as an affinity purification process designed to concentrate venom-specific proteins and eliminate the unwanted and immunogenic extraneous proteins present in current equine-derived antivenoms. Techniques have been developed to generate highly refined, purified, and potent antivenoms derived from sheep and chickens. Ovine and possibly avian antivenoms are expected to be safer and more economical than equine antivenoms.

Fab Antivenom (Ovine Origin)

A crotaline antivenom (CroFab, Protherics and Savage Laboratories), derived from sheep and produced using the Fab technique, is now FDA approved, but supplies are limited. The manufacturing process includes isolation of specific antibody fragments of IgG (Fab and Fab$_2$) by papain digestion of isolated IgG antibodies to eliminate the Fc portion of the immunoglobulin, affinity purification, and lyophilization. The Fab fragments have a smaller molecular weight, are potentially less immunogenic, and may have increased tissue penetration compared to whole IgG. CroFab polyvalent ovine-derived antivenom is obtained by inoculating sheep with the venom of the eastern and western diamondback rattlesnake, the cottonmouth, and the Mojave rattlesnake. This makes this new product theoretically more potent against the snakes found in the United States, and it may prove to be a superior product by ameliorating adverse reactions and widening the therapeutic profile. One report does anecdotally suggest that the CroFab product has superior activity against the neurotoxicity of the Mojave rattlesnake.[7] The local manifestations of copperhead envenomation have been successfully treated with CroFab. In preliminary studies, the severe acute or chronic hypersensitivity reactions associated with horse serum products was significantly reduced (but not eliminated), but clinical experience is very minimal. Only 42 patients have been enrolled in clinical trials at the time of the writing. Minor urticaria, rash, bronchospasm, and pruritis have been associated with this product.

The pharmacokinetics and pharmacodynamics of Fab antivenom differ from those of other antivenoms, and there is an apparent mismatch between effective duration of Fab antivenom and venom-induced local and systemic pathology.[17] The duration of action of the CroFab antivenom appears to be less than that of traditional equine-derived polyvalent antivenom. The elimination half-life is 12 to 23 hours and is less than that of the pathologic effects of venom, so periodic or repeat dosing is required to combat the recently described recurrence phenomena identified in early clinical trials[4] (see discussion on recurrence phenomena in Chap. 101). Currently, dosing guidelines are unclear and require further clarification, but guidelines call for initial control of symptoms, usually with four to eight vials, with repeat scheduled dosing every 2 hours with two vials, for 18 to 24 hours of dosing. In some instances of severe envenomation, much higher doses may be required.

Prospective data on Fab antivenom have generated for the first time important information on the clinical effect of antivenom. The use of a clinical severity-of-illness scale has demonstrated for the first time that antivenom will decrease dysfunction in the central nervous system and the gastrointestinal and cardiovascular systems and will correct coagulopathies associated with envenomation from snakes native to the United States.[8] In an animal lethality model, the new antivenom was five times more potent than traditional antivenom against 14 different crotaline snake venoms. However, the progression of local tissue injury was ameliorated but not significantly reversed, suggesting that, once developed, ecchymosis, edema, and local cell injury secondary to crotaline venom are essentially irreversible. Although initial clinical trials are quite promising, and the antivenom appears effective in halting progression of many aspects of crotaline envenomation while minimizing allergic reactions, clinical experience with this new antivenom is too limited to allow definitive recommendations. Given the fact that crotalid Polyvalent antivenom from Wyeth may not be available in the future, CroFab may be the only available antivenom for North American Crotalines.

REFERENCES

1. Bania TC, Bernstein SL, Baron BJ, et al: Intraarterial vs intravenous administration of antivenin for the treatment of Crotalideae atrox envenomation. A pilot study. Acad Emerg Med 1998;5:894–898.

2. Bogdan GM, McKinney P, Porter RS, et al: Clinical efficacy of two dosing regimens of affinity purified, mixed monospecific Crotaline antivenom Ovine Fab (CroFab) [abstract]. Ann Emerg Med 1997;4:518.

3. Bond GR, Burkhart KK: Thrombocytopenia following timber rattlesnake envenomation. Ann Emerg Med 1997;30:40–44.

4. Boyer LV, Seifert SA, Cain JS: Recurrence phenomena after immunoglobulin therapy for snake envenomations: Part 2. Guidelines for clinical management with Crotaline Fab antivenom. Ann Emerg Med 2001;37:196–210.

5. Buntain WL: Successful venomous snakebite neutralization with massive antivenom infusion in a child. J Trauma 1983;23:1012–1014.

6. Burgess JL, Dart TC: Snake venom coagulopathy: Use and abuse of blood products in the treatment of pit viper envenomation. Ann Emerg Med 1991;20;795–801.

7. Clark RF, Williams SR, Nordt SP, et al: Successful treatment of Crotaline-induced neurotoxicity with a new polyspecific Crotaline Fab antivenom. Ann Emerg Med 1997;30:54–57.

8. Dart RC, McNally J: Efficacy, safety, and use of snake antivenom in the United States. Ann Emerg Med 2001;37:181–188.

9. Dart RC, Seifert SA, Carroll L, et al: Affinity-purified, mixed monospecific Crotaline antivenom Ovine Fab for the treatment of Crotaline venom poisoning. Ann Emerg Med 1997;30:33–39.

10. Howland MA, Smilkstein MJ: Primer on immunology with applications to toxicology. Contemp Manage Crit Care 1991;1:109–145.

11. Jurkovich GJ, Luterman A, McCullar K, et al: Complications of Crotalineae antivenom therapy. J Trauma 1988;28:1032–1037.

12. Kitchen CS, Mierop LHS: Envenomation by the Eastern coral snake (*Micrurus fulvius fulvius*). JAMA 1987;258:1615–1618.

13. Lawrence WT, Giannopoulos A, Hansen A: Pit viper bites: Rational management in locales in which copperheads and cottonmouths predominate. Ann Plast Surg 1996;36:276–285.

14. Loprinzi CL, Hennessee J, Tamsky L, et al: Snake antivenom administration in a patient allergic to horse serum. South Med J 1983;76:501–502.

15. Otero-Patino R, Cardoso JL, Higashi HG, et al: A radomized, blinded, comparative trial of one pepsin-digested and two whole IgG antivenoms for *Bothrops* snake bites in Uraba, Colombia. The Regional Group on Antivenom Therapy Research. Am J Trop Med Hyg 1998;8:183–189.

16. Otten EJ, McKimm D: Venomous snakebite in a patient allergic to horse serum. Ann Emerg Med 1983;12:624–627.

17. Seifert SA, Boyer LV: Recurrence phenomena after immunoglobulin therapy for snake envenomations: Part 1. Pharmacokinetics and pharmacodynamics of immunoglobulin antivenoms and related antibodies. Ann Emerg Med 2001;37:189–195.

18. Seifert SA, Boyer LV, Dart RC, et al: Relationship of venom effects to venom antigen and antivenom serum concentrations in a patient with *Crotalus atrox* envenomation treated with a Fab antivenom. Ann Emerg Med 1997;30:49–53.

19. Spaite D, Dart R, Sullivan JB: Skin testing in cases of possible crotaline envenomations. Ann Emerg Med 1988;17:105–106.

20. Warrell DA, Looareesuwan S, Theakson DG, et al: Randomized comparative trials of three monospecific antivenoms for bites by the Malaysian pit viper in Southern Thailand: Clinical and laboratory correlations. Am J Trop Med Hyg 1986;35:1235–1237.

21. White RR, Weber RA: Poisonous snakebite in central Texas: Possible indications for antivenom treatment. Ann Surg 1991;213:466–471.

22. Whitley RE: Conservative treatment of copperhead snakebites without antivenom. J Trauma 1996;41:219–221.

In-Hei Hahn / Neal A. Lewin

A 24-year-old man presented to the emergency department (ED) with a chief complaint of a "bite" on his right hand that occurred several hours previously. He was unpacking crates of vegetables in his grocery store when he initially felt the bite on his hand. Within 2 hours it became painful and blistered. He had seen several small brown spiders in the bottom of the empty crates. His vital signs were: blood pressure 130/80 mm Hg, pulse 74 beats/min, respiration 12 breaths/min, and temperature 100°F (37.2°C). The only remarkable finding was a painful blister surrounded by erythema on the dorsal aspect of his right thumb. The lesion was cleaned with soap and water. Two hours later, the wound became slightly ulcerated and painful. Based on the history and physical findings, the presumptive diagnosis of a local cutaneous reaction to a brown recluse spider bite was made. The patient was shown a picture of the suspected spider and identified the brown recluse as his presumed attacker. The patient was to be followed by a dermatologist as an outpatient. He was told to return if systemic symptoms developed.

INTRODUCTION

Most clinicians regard bites and stings as inconsequential and more of a nuisance than a threat to life. However, many serious diseases are arthropod-borne, such as encephalitis, Rocky Mountain spotted fever (RMSF), human ehrlichiosis, babesiosis, and Lyme disease. Some spiders and ticks produce neurotoxic venoms that can produce painful lesions, systemic disease, or paralysis. This chapter highlights the significant clinical syndromes produced by bites or stings from the phylum Arthropoda, specifically the classes Arachnida (spiders, scorpions, and ticks) and Insecta (bees, wasps, hornets, and ants) (Table 102–1). Infectious diseases transmitted by arthropods are not discussed in this chapter.

Arthropoda is the largest phylum in the animal kingdom, with at least 1.5 million species identified and half a million yet to be classified and includes more species than all other phyla combined (Fig. 102–1).[3] Arthropoda means "joint-footed" in Latin and describes their jointed bodies and legs connected to a chitinous exoskelelton.[3] The majority of arthropods, fortunately, are benign and beneficial; others are dangerous as a result of their ability to cause envenomation, physical trauma, anaphylaxis to sensitizing antigens, foreign body reactions, or contact dermatitis while also serving as vectors for other disease-causing organisms.[113,115] Araneism or arachnidism is the result of the envenomation caused by a spider bite. "Bites" are different from "stings." Bites are defined as purposeful biting from the oral pole by species for either catching prey or blood feeding and not inadvertent biting by plant-feeding species.[41,104] "Stings" occur from a modified ovipositor at the aboral pole that is no longer able to function in egg-laying. Stinging behavior is typically used for defense. Most spiders are venomous, which enables them to secure, neutralize, and assist in digestion of their prey, but they are not aggressive toward humans unless provoked.

Spiders can also be divided into categories based on whether they pursue their prey as hunters or trappers. Trappers snare their prey by spinning webs, feed, and enshrine excess victims in a cocoon for a later feast. Although capable of producing silk, hunters do not spin such intricate webs and forage or lie in wait for their insect prey.

The order of spiders (Araneae) differs from other members of the class because of various anatomic differences best assessed by an entomologist. Simplistically, the arachnids have four pairs of legs whereas insects have three pairs. The arachnid's body is divided into cephalothorax, pedicle, unsegmented abdomen, and 3 or 4 pairs of spinnerets from which silk is spun. Two pedipalps are attached anteriorly on the cephalothorax on either side of their chelicerae (jaws) and are used for sensation. Spiders have eight eyes but are quite myopic. Prey is localized by touch as they land in the spider's web. All spiders are venomous (except for the family *Uloboridae*) and use their venom to kill or immobilize their prey. However, the chelicerae of many species are too short to penetrate human skin. The remaining species of medical importance include the widow spiders (*Lactrodectus* spp.), the violin spiders (*Loxosceles* spp.), and the hobo spider (*Tegenaria agrestis*) in the United States. In Australia, the funnel web spider (*Atrax robustis*) can cause serious illness and death. In South America, the Brazilian huntsmen (*Phoneutria fera*) and arantia armedeira (*Phoneutria nigriventer*) are also threats to humans.

HISTORY AND EPIDEMIOLOGY

Since the time of Aristotole, spiders and their webs were used for medicinal purposes. Special preparations were concocted to cure a fantastic array of ailments including earache, running of the eyes, "wounds in the joints," warts, gout, asthma, "spasmodic complaints of females," chronic hysteria, cough, rheumatic affections for the head, and stopping the flow of blood.[122]

The *Latrodectus* species has an infamous history as a medical problem, hence the name *mactans*, which means "murderer" in Latin.[95] Hysteria regarding spider bites peaked during the 17th century in a region of Italy known as Taranto. The syndrome tarantism characterized by lethargy, stupor, and a restless compulsion to walk or dance was blamed on the *Lycosa tarantula*, a spi-

TABLE 102–1.   Insects and Other Arthropods That Bite, Sting, or Nettle Humans

Arthropod	Description
Honeybee (*Apis mellifera*)	Hairy, yellowish brown with black markings
Bumblebee and carpenter bee (*Bombus* spp. and *Xylocopa* spp.)	Hairy, but larger than honeybees and colored black and yellow
Vespids (yellow jackets, hornets, paper wasps)	Short-waisted, robust black and yellow or white combination
Schecoids (thread-waisted wasps)	Threadlike waist
Nettling caterpillars (browntail, Io, hag, and buck moths, saddleback and puss caterpillars)	Caterpillar-shaped
Southern fire ant (*Solenopsis* spp.)	Ant-shaped
Spiders (*Arachnida*) black widow, brown recluse	Body with two regions, cephalothorax and abdomen; eight legs
Scorpions (*Centruroides*)	Eight-legged, crablike, stinger at the tip of the abdomen; pedipalps (pincers) highly developed (not a true insect)
Centipedes (*Chilopoda*)	Elongated, wormlike, with many jointed segments and legs; one pair of poison fangs behind head

der that would pounce on its prey like a wolf. Deaths were associated with these outbreaks. Dancing the rapid tarantella to music was the presumed remedy. The real culprit involved in this epidemic was the *Latrodectus tredecimguttatus*.[95] Other epidemics of arachnidism occurred in Spain 1833 and 1841.[75] In North America, there was a rise of spider exposures during the late 1920s, Rome reported large numbers in 1953, and Yugoslavia reported a large number of cases between 1948 and 1953.[17,75] These epidemics may be related to actual reporting biases as well as climatic variations.[95] Spider bites are more numerous in warmer months, presumably because both spiders and humans are more active at that time of the year.

Approximately 200 species of spiders are associated with significant envenomations.[105,106] Eighteen genera of North America

spiders produce poisonings that require clinical intervention (Table 102–2). In one series of 600 suspected spider bites, 80% were determined to be caused by arthropods other than spiders, such as ticks, bugs, mites, fleas, lepidopterous insects, flies, beetles, water bugs, and *Hymenoptera*. Ten percent of the presumed bites were actually manifestations of other nonarthropod disorders.[105,106]

From 1995 to 2000, there were an average of 22,000 spider exposures, 50,000 insect exposures, and no more than three fatalities reported per year, and these were caused by hymenoptera and loxosceles exposures (see p. 1752 and Chap. 116). In most cases, mortality is rare if supportive care is available and the health care provider addresses the severe pain and associated catecholamine release, which may affect the very young, the elderly, and those with underlying cardiopulmonary disease.

BLACK WIDOW SPIDER (*LATRODECTUS MACTANS;* HOURGLASS SPIDER)

There are five species of widow spiders in the United States: *Latrodectus mactans* (black widow), *Latrodectus hesperus* (western black widow), *Latrodectus variolus* (found in New England, Canada, south to Florida, and west to eastern Texas, Oklahoma, and Kansas)*, Latrodectus bishopi* (brown widow of the south), and *Latrodectus geometricus* (brown widow or brown button spider). Dangerous widow spiders in other parts of the world include *L. geometricus*, *L. mactans tredecimguttatus* (European widow spider of southern Europe), *L. mactans hasselti* (red-back spider found in Australia, Japan, and India), and *L. mactans cinctus* in South Africa. These spiders live in temperate and tropical latitudes in stone walls, crevices, woodpiles, outhouses, barns, stables, and rubbish piles. They molt multiple times and can change colors as a result. The ventral markings on the abdomen are species specific, and the classic red hourglass-shaped marking is noted in only the *Latrodectus mactans*. Other species may have variations on their ventral surface, such as triangles and spots. The female *Latrodectus mactans* is typically shiny, jet black, large (8–10 mm), with a rounded abdomen and a red hourglass mark on its ventral surface. Her larger size and ability to penetrate human skin with her fangs

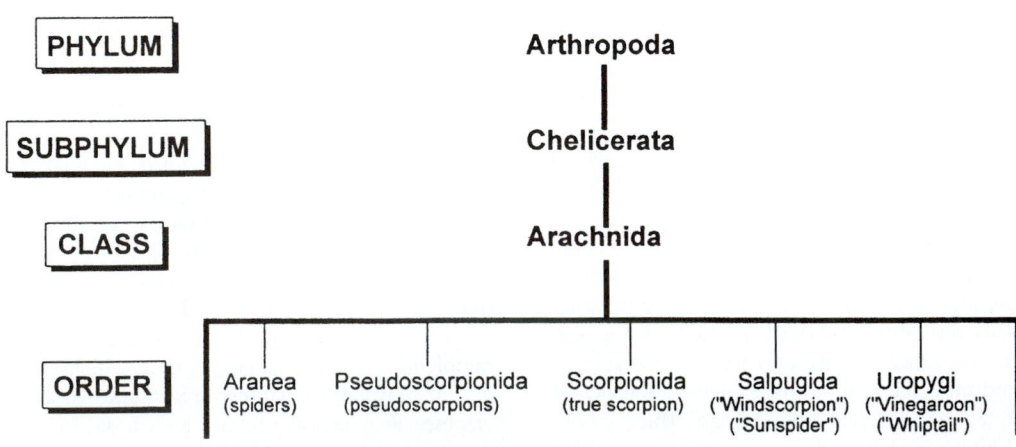

Figure 102–1   Taxonomy of the phylum Arthropoda. *(Reprinted with permission from Allen C: Arachnid envenomations. Emerg Clin North Am 1992;10:270.)*

TABLE 102–2.   North American Spiders of Medical Importance

Genus	Common Name
Araneus sp.[a]	Orb weaver
Argiope aurantia[a]	Orange argiope
Bothriocyrtum sp.	Trap door spider
Chiracanthium sp.[a]	Running spider
Drassodes sp.	Gnaphosid spider
Heteropoda sp.	Huntsman spider
Latrodectus sp.	Widow spider
Liocranoides sp.[a]	Running spider
Loxosceles sp.[a]	Brown, violin, or recluse spider
Lycosa sp.[a]	Wolf spider
Misumenoides sp.	Crab spider
Neoscona sp.[a]	Orb weaver
Peucetia varidans	Green lynx spider
Phidippus sp.[a]	Jumping spider
Rheostica (Aphonopelma) sp.	Tarantula
Steatoda grossa	False black widow spider
Tegenaria agrestis[a]	Hobo spider
Ummidia sp.	Trap door spider

[a]Associated with necrotic lesions.

makes her more venomous and toxic than the male, which is smaller and lighter in color, with a more elongated abdomen and fangs that are usually too short to envenomate humans (Table 102–3). Black widow females are trappers and inhabit large untidy irregularly shaped webs. Webs are placed in or close to the ground and in secluded, dimly lit areas that can trap flying insects such as the outdoor privy, barns, sheds, and garages.[3] The bite from the *Latrodectus mactans* may produce *latrodectism*, a constellation of signs and symptoms resulting from systemic toxicity.

Pathophysiology

The neurotoxic venom produces symptoms usually within minutes to several hours. This venom is more potent on a volume-per-volume basis than that of a pit viper and contains six active components with molecular weights of 5000 to 130,000 Da.[3] The six components are α-latrotoxin (α-LTX), five latroinsectotoxins (α-, β-, γ-, δ-, and ε-LITs) affecting insects, and latrocrustatoxin (α-LCT) active only for crustaceans.[47] α-LTX binds with nanomolar affinity to specific presynaptic receptors, neurexin I-α and calcium-independent receptor for α-latrotoxin (CIRL), otherwise known as *latrophilin*,[15,50,57] triggering a cascade of events: sustained opening of nonspecific cation channels, a massive influx of calcium, and a dramatic exocytosis of the synaptic vesicles with the release of neurotransmitters such as acetylcholine and norepinephrine.[3,88]

The toxic effects of α-LTX are complex, as suggested by the presence of two structurally and functionally different types of receptors. Type I or calcium-dependent receptors are represented by neurexin I-α, a neuronal glycoprotein.[88] Neurexin I-α receptors are neuron-specific cell membrane proteins with one transmembrane domain and the extracellular region typical for cell adhesion molecules otherwise known as ankyrins.[71] Ankyrins constitute a family of proteins that coordinate interactions between various integral membrane proteins and cytoskeletal elements.[47] Neurexin I-α is not required for the excitotoxic action of α-LTX. Neurexin I-α–deficient mice were created and were still susceptible to α-

LTX via stimulation of the CIRL receptor.[38] These type II receptors bind to α-LTX independently of Ca^{2+} in the extracellular medium. CIRL is a neuronal receptor that belongs to the family of seven-transmembrane-domain G-protein-coupled receptors. CIRL is thought to be coupled to phospholipase C, resulting in subsequent phosphoinositide metabolism.[15,65] CIRL-1 and CIRL-3 are high-affinity neuronal receptors. CIRL-2 has 14 times less affinity to α-LTX than CIRL-1 but is expressed ubiquitously, specifically in placenta, kidney, spleen, ovary, heart, lung, as well as brain.[57] Although the nervous system is the primary target for α-LTX, the cells from other tissues are also susceptible to the α-LTX because of the presence of CIRL-2.[57]

Clinical Manifestations

Widow spiders usually bite on unintentional skin contact, although one patient developed lactrodectism following the intentional intravenous injection of a crushed whole black widow spider.[22] A sharp pain typically described as a pinprick occurs as the victim is bitten, and a pair of red spots may evolve at the site. The local reaction is limited, such as a small wheal-and-flare reaction, which is often associated with a halo (Table 102–4). The effects from the bite spread by continuity. For example, if one is bitten on the hand, the pain will progress up the arm to the elbow, shoulder, and then toward the trunk during systemic poisoning. Typically a briefer time to symptom onset denotes severe envenomation. Several signs and symptoms are described with the bite of the female black widow spider.

Hypertoxic myopathic syndrome of latrodectism involves muscle cramps and typically presents 15 minutes to an hour following the bite, initially occurring at the site of the bite, but it may later involve rigidity of other skeletal muscles, particularly muscles of the chest, abdomen, and face. The pain increases over time and occurs in waves that may cause the patient to writhe. Large muscle groups are affected first, although fine muscle fasciculations are also noted. Classically, severe abdominal wall spasm occurs and may be confused with a surgical abdomen, especially in children who cannot relate the history with the initial bite.[22] Muscle pain often subsides within a few hours but may recur for several days. Transient muscle weakness and spasms may persist for weeks to months.

Additional clinical findings include "*facies latrodectismica,*" which describes the sweating, contorted, grimaced face associated with blepharitis, conjuctivitis, rhinitis, cheilitis, and trismus of the masseters.[75] A fear of death, *pavor mortis*, has also been described.[75] Nausea, weakness, hyperesthesias, ptosis, hyperreflexia, seizures, tremor, arthralgias, restlessness, bronchorrhea, vomiting, priapism, urinary retention, salivation, diaphoresis, and increased cerebrospinal fluid pressure are also noted.[3] Presumably this wide array of signs and symptoms is caused by the cholinergic and sympathomimetic actions of the released neurotransmitters.

Life-threatening complications include hypertension, reported in up to 31% of the cases, that may progress to severe hypertension.[22,28,81] Several postulated mechanisms of this hypertension are activation of the vasomotor centers of the brainstem and spinal medulla as well as the massive release of norepinephrine from the adrenal glands and peripheral nerve endings, resulting in vasoconstriction.[31,55] Shock, coma, or paralysis of the respiratory musculature with secondary respiratory arrest may occur. Death has been reported, secondary to seizures and respiratory compromise. The highest-risk groups are infants, elderly, chronically ill, and preg-

TABLE 102–3. Brown Recluse and Black Widow Spiders: Comparative Characteristics

	Brown Recluse (*Loxosceles*)	Black Widow (*Latrodectus*)
Description	Female brown, 6–20 mm, violin-shaped mark on dorsum of cephalothorax; female greater toxicity than male	Female jet black, 8–10 mm, red hourglass mark on ventral surface; female greater toxicity than male
Major venom component	Sphingomyelinase D	α-Latrotoxin
Pathophysiology of envenomation	Vascular injury, dermonecrosis, hemolysis	Lymphatic, hematogenous spread Neurotoxicity
Epidemiology	Bites more common in warmer months N. America (southern and western states): *L. reclusa* S. America: *L. laeta, L. gaucho* Europe: *L. rufescens* Africa (Southern): *L. parrami, L. spiniceps, L. pillosa, L. bergeri* Asia/Australia: rare	Bites more common in warmer months in subtropical and temperate areas; perennial in tropics N. America: *L. mactans, L. hesperus, L. geometricus* Europe: *L. tredecimGuttatus* Africa (southern): *L. indistinctus* Australia: *L. hasselti* Asia/S. America: rare

Clinical effects	Cutaneous
	  Initial (0–2 hours after bite): painless, erythema, edema
	  2–8 hours hemorrhagic, ulcerates, painful
	  1 wk: eschar
	  Months: healing
		Cutaneous
		  Initial (5 min–1 hour after bite): local pain
		  1–2 hours: puncture marks
		  1/2 to several hours: regional lymph nodes swollen, central blanching at bite site with surrounding erythema
		CVS: initial tachycardia followed by bradycardia, dysrhythmias, initial hypotension followed by hypertension
		GI: nausea, vomiting, mimic acute abdomen

	Hematologic
	Methemoglobinemia, hemolysis, thrombocytopenia, DIC
		Hematologic: leukocytosis
		Metabolic
		  Hyperglycemia (transient)
		  Urinary VMA (increased)
		Musculoskeletal: hypertonia, abdominal rigidity, "facies latrodectismica"
		Neurologic
		  CNS: psychosis, hallucinations, visual disturbance, seizures
		  PNS: pain at the site
		  ANS: increase in all secretions; sweating, salivation, lacrimation, diarrhea, bronchorrhea, mydriasis, miosis, priapism, and ejaculation

	Renal: renal failure, secondary to hemolysis	Renal: glomerulonephritis, oliguria, anuria Respiratory: bronchoconstriction, pulmonary edema
Treatment	1. Analgesia 2. Wound care 3. Dapsone (?) 4. Hyperbaric oxygen (?) 5. Antivenom (?) not available universally 6. Corticosteroids (?)	1. Analgesia 2. Calcium gluconate (?) 3. Muscle relaxants 4. Antivenom

nant women. Extreme restlessness occurs, and recovery usually ensues within 24 to 48 hours, but symptoms may last several days with more severe envenomations.

Diagnostic Testing

Laboratory data are generally not helpful in managing or predicting outcome. According to one study, the most common findings include leukocytosis and increased creatine phosphokinase and lactate dehydrogenase levels.[28] There is currently no specific laboratory assay capable of confirming latrodectism.

Management

Treatment involves establishing an airway and supporting respiration and circulation if indicated. Wound evaluation and local wound care including tetanus prophylaxis are essential.[130] The routine use of antibiotics is not recommended.

Pain management is a substantial component of patient care and will depend on the degree of symptomatology. One grading system used divides the severity of the envenomation into three categories.[28] Grade 1 envenomations range from having no symptoms to local pain at the envenomation site with normal vital signs. A grade 2 envenomation involves muscular pain at the site with migration of the pain to the trunk, diaphoresis at the bite site, and normal vital signs. Grade 3 envenomations include the grade 2 symptoms and abnormal vital signs, nausea, vomiting, and headache. Under this grading system, a grade 1 envenomation may require only cold packs and orally administered nonsteroidal antiinflammatory agents. Grade 2 and 3 envenomations will probably require intravenous opioids and benzodiazepines to control

TABLE 102–4. Signs and Symptoms of Latrodectism

Local
  Pain at bite site, erythema, edema, urticaria, piloerection
  Limb pain, local adenopathy

Systemic (general)
  Facies latrodectismica: sweaty, flushed, blepharoconjunctivitis, grimaced
  Pavor mortis (fear of death)
  Priapism
  Salivation
  Urinary retention
  Vomiting

Neuromuscular
  Muscle cramps: thighs, abdomen, chest
  Muscle rigidity, fibrillation, contractions, tremor

Cardiopulmonary
  Bronchorrhea
  Hypertension, tachycardia

Laboratory
  Leukocytosis, hyperglycemia, elevated creatinine phosphokinase

pain and muscle spasm. Traditionally, 10 mL of 10% calcium gluconate solution was given intravenously (IV) to decrease cramping. It was infused over 10 minutes and repeated at 30 minutes. A retrospective chart review of 163 patients envenomated by the black widow concluded that calcium gluconate was ineffective for pain relief compared with a combination of IV opioids (morphine sulfate or meperidine) and benzodiazepines (diazepam or lorazepam).[28] Another study found greater neurotransmitter release when extracellular calcium concentrations were increased, suggesting that the administration of calcium is irrational in patients suffering from latrodectism.[102] Calcium's mechanisms of action remain unknown, and its efficacy is anecdotal; therefore, we do not recommend calcium administration for pain management. Methocarbamol is a centrally acting muscle relaxant. The mechanism of action in humans has not been established but may be related to general central nervous system depression. Methocarbamol is not considered as effective as benzodiazepines. A benzodiazepine, such as diazepam, is more effective for controlling muscle spasms and also achieves sedation, anxiolysis, and amnesia. Because the use of antivenom may result in anaphylaxis and serum sickness, management should include primarily supportive care including opioids and benzodiazepines for controlling pain and muscle spasms.

Latrodectus antivenom is rapidly effective and curative. In the United States, the antivenom formulation is effective for all species but is available as a crude hyperimmune horse serum and may cause anaphylaxis and serum sickness. The morbidity of latrodectism is high with pain, cramping, and autonomic disturbances, but mortality is low. Hence, there is controversy over when to administer the black widow antivenom. The antivenom can be administered for severe reactions such as hypertensive crisis, intractable pain, or to high-risk patients such as pregnant women suffering from a threatened abortion.[95] The use of antivenom should probably not be considered for patients unless systemic symptoms are present, otherwise designated as grade 3, because of the risk for anaphylaxis or anaphylactoid reactions.[28] The usual dose is one to two vials diluted in 50 to 100 mL of 5%

dextrose or 0.9% NaCl solution, and the combination is infused over 1 hour [see Antidotes in Depth: Antivenom (Scorpion and Spider)]. Skin testing may identify a highly allergic individual but does not eliminate the occurrence of hypersensitivity reactions; therefore, we do not recommend skin testing. Pretreatment with histamine H₁ or H₂ blockers and epinephrine may be beneficial in preventing histamine release and/or anaphylaxis, but their efficacy is unproven. Patients with allergies to horse serum products and those who have received antivenom or horse serum products are at risk for IgE-mediated hypersensitivity reactions. Prevention consists of destroying the spider and taking precautions in the areas spiders inhabit. Creosote can be sprayed in outdoor areas every 3 months. When working in high-risk areas, gloves, heavy garments buttoned at the wrists and collars, and shoes should be worn.

In Australia, there is a purified equine-derived IgG-Fab₂ fragment antivenom (AV) for the red-back spider (RBS, *Latrodectus hasselti*). A recent study has shown that RBS-AV prevents latrodectism in mice envenomated with other widow spider venoms from the United States and Europe.[45] The red-back spider antivenom (CSL, Melbourne, Australia) is given as first-line therapy for patients presenting with any distressing signs or symptoms in Australia. Since its introduction in 1956, there have been no deaths, and the incidence of mild allergic reactions to RBS-AV is reported as 0.54% in 2144 uses.[119] This antivenom may have a future role in black widow spider envenomations in the United States.

BROWN RECLUSE SPIDER (*LOXOSCELES RECLUSA*; VIOLIN OR FIDDLEBACK SPIDER)

The *Loxosceles reclusa* was confirmed to cause necrotic arachnidism in 1957, although reports of systemic symptoms following brown spider bites appeared since 1872.[5] This spider has a brown violin-shaped mark on the dorsum of the cephalothorax, three pairs of eyes arranged in a semicircle on top of the head, and legs that are five times as long as the body. It is small (6–20 mm long) and gray to orange or reddish brown. *Loxosceles* spiders weave irregular white, flocculent adhesive webs that line their retreats.[36] Spiders in the genus Loxosceles have a worldwide distribution. In the United States, other species of this genus, which include *L. rufescens, L. deserta, L devia,* and *L. arizonica,* are prominent in the Southwest. They are hunter spiders, living in dark areas (woodpiles, rocks, basements), and their foraging is nocturnal. They are not aggressive but will bite if antagonized (Table 102–3). These spiders are resilient and can survive up to 6 months without water or food and tolerate temperatures from 8 to 43°C (46.4–109.4°F). They can live up to 2 years.[41] In common with the black widow spider, the female is more dangerous than the male and bites only when provoked.

Pathophysiology

The venom is cytotoxic; purification techniques have identified eight subcomponents, including various enzymes, such as hyaluronidase, deoxyribonuclease, ribonuclease, alkaline phosphatase, lipase, and sphingomyelinase-D.[67] The two main constituents of the venom are sphingomyelinase-D and hyaluronidase. Hyaluronidase is a spreading factor that facilitates the venom's ability to spread and penetrate tissue but does not induce lesion development.[67] Sphingomyelinase-D, with a molecular weight of 32,000 Da, is the primary constituent of the venom that causes necrosis and hemolysis. Sphingomyelinase-D causes human platelets to release serotonin and red blood cells to release hemoglobin.[67] Sphingomyelinase also reacts with sphingomyelin in the red blood cell membrane to release choline and N-acylsphingosine phosphate and to trigger a chain reaction releasing inflammatory mediators such as thromboxanes, leukotrienes, prostaglandins, and neutrophils that leads to vessel thrombosis, tissue ischemia, and skin loss.[67]

An early study in experimental animals describes the pathogenesis of the skin lesion requiring polymorphonuclear leukocytes and complement infiltration of blood vessels at the bite site with resultant blood vessel injury as the pathologic basis for skin loss.[112] They demonstrated early perivascular collections of PMNs with hemorrhage and edema progressing into intravascular clotting. Coagulation and vascular occlusion of the microcirculation occur, leading ultimately to necrosis.

Clinical Manifestations

From spring to autumn is the peak time for envenomation. Most victims are bitten in the morning. The clinical spectrum of loxoscelism can be divided into three major categories, varying from local cutaneous reaction to systemic loxoscelism. The first category includes bites that have very little if any venom injected, and there may be a small erythematous papule that becomes firm before healing and is associated with a localized urticarial response. In the second category, the bite undergoes a cytotoxic reaction. The bite, which may be initially painless or have a stinging sensation, blisters, bleeds, and then ulcerates 2 to 8 hours later (Table 102–3). The lesion may increase in diameter, with demarcation of central hemorrhagic vesiculation, sinking, and violaceous necrosis, surrounding ischemic blanching of skin, and outer erythema and induration over 1 to 3 days, otherwise known as the "red, white, and blue" reaction.[62,133] Necrosis of the central blister occurs in 3 to 4 days with eschar formation occurring between 5 and 7 days. After 7 to 14 days, the wound becomes indurated, and the eschar falls off, leaving an ulceration that heals by secondary intention. Local necrosis is more extensive over fatty areas (thighs, buttocks, and abdomen).[131] The size of the ulcer will determine the time for healing. Large lesions up to 30 cm may take 4 months or more to heal. A distinguishing sign of a brown recluse bite is the tendency of the lesion to extend downward, "flowing downhill" in a gravitation-dependent manner and becoming asymmetric, which is rare and separates it from most other arthropod bites.[41] The direction of the lesion is dependent on the victim's position while the vessel damage was produced.

Systemic loxoscelism, which is not predicted by the extent of cutaneous reaction, is the third category and occurs 24 to 72 hours after the bite. The young are particularly susceptible. The clinical manifestations of loxoscelism include fever, chills, weakness, edema, nausea, vomiting, arthralgias, petechial eruptions, convulsions, and hemolysis that can lead to hemoglobinemia, hemoglobinuria, renal failure, and death. Disseminated intravascular coagulation may also occur. Severe intravascular hemolysis associated with a brown recluse spider bite leading to death has been reported.[132]

Another extremely unusual presentation of loxoscelism is upper airway obstruction. This life-threatening complication was recently reported in a child who was bitten on his neck and subsequently developed progressive cervical soft tissue edema with airway obstruction and dermatonecrosis 40 hours later.[43] There has been one other report of stridor and respiratory distress following a brown recluse envenomation of the ear, and although the presentation is rare, respiratory compromise should be considered when an envenomation occurs near the airway.[40]

Diagnostic Testing

Bites from other spiders can become necrotic wounds, such as *Chiracanthium* (sac spider), *Phidippus* (jumping spider), *Argiope* (orb weaver), and *Tegenaria* (northwestern brown spider), and are often the actual culprits when the brown recluse is mistakenly blamed; therefore, definitive diagnosis is achieved only when the spider is positively identified. There is no routine laboratory test for loxoscelism. There are several techniques presently used for research that are not available for clinical application. The lymphocyte transformation test measures lymphocytes of a previously envenomated patient that have undergone blast transformation when exposed to Loxosceles venom. The lymphocytes will incorporate thymidine into the nucleoprotein to provide a quantitative response.[4] A passive hemagglutination inhibition test (PHAI) has been developed in guinea pigs. The PHAI assay is based on the property of certain brown recluse spider venom components to spontaneously adsorb to formalin-treated erythrocyte membranes and on the ability of the BRS venom to inhibit the antiserum-induced agglutination of venom-coated red blood cells.[10] The test is 90% sensitive and 100% specific as long as 3 days following venom injection and may prove to be useful for early diagnosis of a brown recluse spider envenomation.[10] Also, an enzyme immunoassay specific for the *Loxosceles* venom has been developed and used to confirm the presence of venom 4 days postenvenomation.[78] The drawbacks of using a skin biopsy are that the procedure is invasive and can cause further scarring with an increased potential for infection, and it has not been proven to diagnose early envenomations, before the development of dermatonecrosis. Another ELISA for the detection of venom antigens has been developed and correctly discriminated the mice inoculated with antigens of *Loxosceles intermidia* venom. The ELISA, immunoassay, and antivenom may become useful early diagnostic tools if envenomation can be proven early, especially before the development of the purplish discoloration and blister formation that usually progress to cutaneous necrosis.[26] There is currently no universally accepted or available laboratory test to aid in the diagnosis of *Loxosceles* envenomation.

Laboratory data may be remarkable for hemolysis, hemoglobinuria, and hematuria. A coagulopathy may be present with laboratory data significant for elevated fibrin split products, decreased fibrinogen levels, and a positive D-dimer assay. Other tests may show increases in PT and PTT, leukocytosis (up to 20,000–30,000 cells/mm^3), spherocytosis, Coombs-positive hemolytic anemia, thrombocytopenia, or abnormal renal and liver function tests.[3,7,36,104,105,106,130]

Treatment

Local treatment of the lesion is controversial. The most prudent management of the dermonecrotic lesion is cleansing, immobilization, tetanus prophylaxis, analgesics, and antipruritics as warranted (Table 102–5).[3,36,127,130] Early excision or intralesional injection of corticosteroids appears unwarranted; however, correc-

TABLE 102–5. Management of Brown Recluse Spider Bite

General wound care
Clean
Tetanus prophylaxis as indicated
Immobilize and elevate bitten extremity
Apply cool compresses; avoid local heat

Local wound care
Serial observations
Natural healing by granulation
Delayed primary closure
Delayed secondary closure with skin graft
Gauze packing, if applicable

Systemic
Antipruritic/antianxiety and/or analgesic agents
Antibiotics for secondary bacterial infection
(?) Polymorphonuclear white blood cell inhibitors: dapsone, colchicine
Antivenom (experimental)
(?) Hyperbaric oxygen

Laboratory
Culture
Gram stain
Biopsy to determine etiology of lesion
G-6-PD level if dapsone therapy elected

Modified, with permission, from Wasserman GS: *Wound care of spider and snake envenomations.* Ann Emerg Med 1988;17:1333.

tive surgery can be done several weeks after adequate tissue demarcation has occurred. One case series utilized curettage of the lesion to remove necrotic and indurated tissue from the lesion to remove any continuing action of the lytic enzymes on the surrounding tissue with positive results.[53] These patients had wound healing without further necrosis and minimal scarring. Electric shock delivered via stun guns was not found to be useful in a guinea pig envenomation model.[10] Cyproheptadine, a serotonin antagonist, was not beneficial in a rabbit model.[90] A randomized control study evaluating the efficacy of topical nitroglycerin for envenomated rabbits showed no difference in preventing skin necrosis and suggested the possibility of increased systemic toxicity.[70] Antibiotics should be used to treat cutaneous or systemic infection but should not be used prophylactically. The early use of dapsone in patients who develop a central purplish bleb or vesicle within the first 6 to 8 hours may inhibit local infiltration of the wound by polymorphonuclear leukocytes.[62] The dosage recommended is 100 mg twice a day for 2 weeks.[98] However, prospective trials with large numbers of patients are lacking. One study compared erythromycin and dapsone therapy, erythromycin and antivenom therapy, and erythromycin, dapsone, and antivenom therapy.[99] Although the treatment groups were very small, all groups showed wound healing at about 20 days. The use of dapsone in the management of a local lesion should be considered an experimental treatment because it has not been validated by controlled randomized clinical trials; therefore, dapsone use cannot be recommended at this time. Hepatitis,[101] methemoglobinemia, and hemolysis (Chap. 94) are associated with the use of dapsone. If dapsone therapy is utilized, a baseline glucose-6-phosphate dehydrogenase and weekly complete blood counts should be performed.

A recent animal study evaluated the effects on the size of skin lesions induced by *Loxosceles* envenomation of treatment with hy-

perbaric oxygen therapy (HBO), dapsone, and HBO and dapsone.[51] Unfortunately, the study design was limited and could find only a 100% difference in treatment groups. It was concluded that there was no clinically significant change in necrosis or induration from these treatment modalities. Further evaluation of these interventions remains appropriate. Another study using hyperbaric oxygen in the treatment of *Loxosceles*-induced necrotic lesions revealed no clinical improvement in the size of the lesion; however, the histology of the lesions improved. Whether this is of value in humans is yet to be determined.[117]

The use of 1.2 mg of colchicine, a leukocyte inhibitor, followed at 2-hour intervals with 0.6 mg for 2 days, then 0.6 mg every 4 hours for an additional 2 days has been recommended, but this treatment has substantial potential toxicity.[105,106]

Rabbit-derived intradermal anti-*Loxosceles* Fab (α-Loxd) fragments attenuated the dermonecrotic inflammation of rabbits injected with *L. deserta* venom in a time-dependent fashion.[42] At time zero after envenomation, the lesion development was blocked. One and 4 hours after envenomation, the α-Loxd Fab antivenom continued to suppress the lesion areas, although the longer the treatment was delayed, the smaller the difference was between treatment and control lesion areas. At 8 and 12 hours, there was no difference in lesion size. The typical 24-hour delay in lesion development makes the diagnosis difficult, and the antivenom would be useless if administered so late in the clinical course. The use of antivenom would be facilitated if the spider were caught and positively identified or another test could be used to positively identify a *Loxosceles* envenomation. Currently this antivenom is not available for commercial use. Patients manifesting systemic loxoscelism or those with expanding necrotic lesions should be admitted to the hospital. All patients should be monitored for evidence of hemolysis, renal failure, or coagulopathy. If hemoglobinuria ensues, increased IV fluids and urinary alkalinization may be used in an attempt to prevent acute renal failure. Hemolysis, if significant, can be treated with transfusions. Patients with a coagulopathy should be monitored with serial CBC, platelet count, PT, PTT, fibrin-split products, and fibrinogen. Disseminated intravascular coagulopathy may require treatment, based on severity.

HOBO SPIDER (*TEGENARIA AGRESTIS*, OTHERWISE KNOWN AS NORTHWESTERN BROWN SPIDER AND WALCKENAER SPIDER)

Healthcare providers should consider the hobo spider, formerly called the "aggressive house spider" as part of the differential for necrotic arachnidism.[84] The hobo spider is native to Europe and was introduced to the northwestern United States (Washington, Oregon, Idaho) in the 1920s or 1930s.[129] These spiders build webs within woodpiles, crawl spaces, basements, and moist areas. They are brown with gray markings and 7 to 14 mm in length. They are most abundant in the midsummer through the fall. They bite if provoked or threatened. *Tegenaria agrestis* is likely to be responsible for the majority of the "presumed brown recluse spider bites" in the Northwest and presents with similar clinical symptomatology, including "gravitational drift" in envenomated rabbits. Unlike the black widow and brown recluse spiders, the hobo males are more venomous than the females.

Pathophysiology

The toxin has been fractionated with three peptides identified as having potent insecticidal activity and no discernible effects in mammalian in vivo assays.[58] The peptide toxins, TaITX-1, -2, and -3, exhibit potent insecticidal properties by acting directly in the insect central nervous system and not at the neuromuscular junction.[58] Clinically, insects envenomated with *T. agrestis* venom and the insecticidal toxins purified from it developed a slowly evolving spastic paralysis. Currently little is known about the toxin and its mechanism of action in humans.

Clinical Manifestations

The local effects of the hobo spider's envenomation are similar to those of the brown recluse. The initial bite is painless. Induration may appear in 30 minutes, surrounded by an area of expanding erythema; a blister ensues in 15 to 35 hours, and rupture of these lesions creates an eschar-covered necrotic ulcer in 50% of cases.[128] Sloughing occurs, and healing with a scar can take from 45 days up to 3 years. Common symptoms associated with the bite are headache, weakness, and lethargy.[128] Systemic symptoms occur consisting of nausea, vomiting, fatigue, memory loss, and visual impairment. Serious outcomes have been reported, including aplastic anemia, intractable vomiting, a profuse secretory diarrhea, and death.[84]

Diagnostic Testing

There is no specific laboratory assay confirming envenomation with the *Tegenaria agrestis* spider.

Treatment

Treatment emphasizes local wound care and tetanus prophylaxis, although systemic corticosteroids for hematologic complications may be of value. Surgical graft repair for severe ulcerative lesions may be warranted when there is no additional necrosis.[84]

TARANTULAS

Tarantulas, ancestors to the true spider, belong to the family Theraphosidae (hairy mygalomorphs).[109] There are more than 1500 species, with approximately 40 species found in the deserts of western United States. Because of their great size and reputation, tarantulas are often feared. They are popular as pets and can be found all over the United States. The life span of the female can exceed 15 to 20 years. They have poor eyesight and detect their victims by vibrations.

Their venom has relatively minor effects except for a few tropical species. Tarantulas bite when provoked or roughly handled. Four genera of tarantulas (*Lasiodora, Grammastola, Acanthoscurria,* and *Brachypelma*) possess urticating hairs that are released in self-defense by rubbing their hind legs against their abdomen rapidly to create a small cloud.[41] There are four different types of hairs. Type 1 are found on tarantulas in the United States and do not penetrate the human skin. Type 2 hairs are incorporated into the silk web retreat but are not thrown off by the spider. Type 3 hairs can penetrate up to 2 mm into human skin, and type 4 hairs belong to the South American *Grammastola* spider and cause severe respiratory inflammation. These hairs cause intense inflammation that may remain pruritic for weeks.

Pathophysiology

Tarantula venom, specifically the venoms of *Dugesiella henzi* (Arkansas tarantula) and members of the genus *Aphonopelma* (Arizona tarantula) has been shown to contain hyaluronidase, nucleotides (adenosine triphosphate, adenosine diphosphate, and adenosine monophosphate), and polyamines (spermine, spermidine, putrescine, and cadaverine) that are used for digesting their prey from the inside out.[23,60,109] The role for spermine is unclear, but hyaluronidase is a spreading factor allowing more rapid entrance of venom toxin through destruction of connective tissue and intercellular matrix. ATP potentiates death in mice exposed to the *Dugesiella hentzi* venom and lowers the LD_{50} in comparison to venom without ATP.[25] Both venoms cause skeletal muscle necrosis when injected intraperitoneally into mice.[87] The primary injury results in rupture of the plasma membrane followed by the inability of mitochondria and sarcoplasmic reticulum to maintain normal levels of calcium in the cytoplasm, leading to cell death. *Dugesiella* venom is necrotoxic and similar to sea snake venom.[68] *Aphonopelma* venom is similar to scorpion venom in composition and clinical effects.

Clinical Manifestation

Urticating hairs provoke local histamine reactions in humans and are especially irritating to the eyes, skin, and respiratory tract. Inflammation can occur at all levels from conjunctiva to retina, and an allergic rhinitis may also develop if the hairs are inhaled.[60] Ophthalmia nodosa, a granulomatous nodular reaction to vegetable or insect hairs, has been reported with casual handling of tarantulas.[12,13] Other eye findings may include spines in the corneal stroma, anterior chamber inflammation, and migration into the retina. Bites also range from being painless to producing a deep throbbing pain that may last several hours without any inflammatory component, although fever has been associated even in the absence of infection, suggesting a direct pyretic action of the venom. Rarely, bites can also create a local histamine response, and hypersensitive individuals could have a more severe reaction.[41]

Treatment

Treatment is largely supportive. Cool compresses and analgesics should be given as needed. All bites should receive local wound care, including tetanus prophylaxis if necessary. If the hairs are barbed, as in some species, they can be removed by using adhesive or cellophane tape followed by compresses or irrigation with 0.9% sodium chloride solution. If the hairs are located in the eye, then surgical removal may be required, followed by medical management of inflammation. Urticarial reactions should be treated with oral antihistamines and topical or systemic corticosteroids.

SCORPIONS

Scorpions are invertebrate arthropods that have existed for longer than 400 million years.[29] Of the 650 known living species, most of the lethal species are in the Buthidae family. The genera of the family Buthidae include *Centruroides, Tityus, Leuirus, Androctonus, Buthus,* and *Parabuthus*.[29] Unlike most spiders, scorpions envenomate humans by stinging rather than biting. Their five-segmented tail contains a bulbous segment called the telson, which contains the venom apparatus. Fortunately, these members of the class Arachnida rarely cause mortality in victims older than 6 years.[100] According to AAPCC data from 1995 through 2000, there have been roughly 11,000 to 14,000 scorpion exposures in the United States, and no deaths reported (see p. 1752 and Chap. 116). These stings occur predominantly in the southwestern United States. The poisonous scorpions in the United States are *Centruroides gertschii* and, most important, *Centruroides exilicauda,* previously called *Centruroides sculpturatus Ewing* (bark scorpion). In general, scorpions sting only if disturbed.

Pathophysiology

Components of scorpion venom are complex and species-specific, those of the family Buthidae being most harmful to humans.[48,94,100] The venom is thermostable and consists of phospholipase, acetyl-cholinesterase, hyaluronidase, serotonin, and neurotoxins. Venom of the *Centruroides exilicauda* is primarily neurotoxic. Four neurotoxins designated toxins I through IV have been isolated from the *C. exilicauda.* These toxins target excitable membranes, especially at the neuromuscular junction, by opening sodium channels, resulting in repetitive depolarization of nerves in both sympathetic and parasympathetic nervous systems, and cause prolonged action potentials.[100] Depolarization causes increased calcium permeability at the presynaptic terminal and causes acetylcholine release. The effects of the toxin also include catecholamine release from adrenergic neurons, increased neurotransmitter release, catecholamine release from the adrenal gland, catecholamine-induced cardiac hypoxia, and action at the juxtaglomerular apparatus, causing increased renin secretion.[100]

Clinical Manifestations

All scorpions in the United States, except for the *C. exilicauda,* produce a local reaction consisting of erythema, tingling or burning, and occasionally discoloration and necrosis without tissue sloughing (Table 102–6). *Centruroides exilicauda* stings produce local paresthesias and pain that can be accentuated by tapping over the envenomated area (tap test), with no local skin evidence of envenomation.[31,100] Symptoms begin immediately after envenomation, progress to maximum severity in 5 hours, and may persist for up to 30 hours.[29,100] Both adrenergic and cholinergic symptoms occur: hypertension, tachycardia, seizures, hyperglycemia, and salivation, lacrimation, urination, defecation, and emesis, respectively. Other symptoms reported include pharyngeal spasm, muscular fasciculations, abdominal cramps, oliguria, pulmonary edema, and respiratory collapse (Table 102–6). Scorpions from the genus *Tityus* from Brazil and Trinidad have caused pancreatitis. Venoms of *Buthus* and *Parabuthus* of India and Africa possess phospholipase A, which may cause gastrointestinal (GI) and pulmonary hemorrhages and a disseminated intravascular coagulopathy.

Treatment

Because most envenomations produce no severe effects, local wound care including tetanus prophylaxis is usually all that is warranted. In young children or patients who manifest severe toxicity, hospitalization may be required. Treatment emphasizes support of the airway, breathing, and circulation. Corticosteroids, antihistamines, and calcium have been administered without any benefit.[31]

TABLE 102–6. **Envenomation Gradation for *Centruroides Exilicauda* (Bark Scorpions)**

Grade	Signs and Symptoms
I	Site of envenomation Pain and/or paresthesias Positive "tap test" (severe pain increase with touch or percussion)
II	As in grade I Pain and paresthesias remote from sting site (eg, paresthesias moving up an extremity, perioral "numbness")
III	One of the following: Somatic skeletal neuromuscular dysfunction: jerking of extremity(ies), restlessness, severe involuntary shaking and jerking, which may be mistaken for seizures Cranial nerve dysfunction: blurred vision, wandering eye movements, hypersalivation, trouble swallowing, tongue fasciculation, upper airway dysfunction, slurred speech
IV	Both cranial nerve and somatic skeletal neuromuscular dysfunction

Modified, with permission, from Curry SC, Vance MV, Ryan PJ, et al: *Envenomation by the scorpion Centruroides sculpturatus.* J Toxicol Clin Toxicol 1983–1984; 21:417–448; Allen C: *Arachnid envenomations.* Emerg Med Clin North Am 1992;10:276.

The severity of the envenomation dictates the need to use antivenin versus supportive care and pain management with opioids and benzodiazepines. One grading system suggests using antivenin for severe grade III and grade IV envenomations, which include somatic and/or cranial nerve dysfunction (Table 102–6).[31] A goat serum–derived antivenom is available in Arizona and has been used successfully in a limited number of severe cases.[18] This approach is not universally accepted. Proponents believe antivenom may resolve symptoms sooner, but opponents cite serum sickness as a substantial concern [see Antidotes in Depth: Antivenom (Scorpion and Spider)].[18]

A retrospective chart review of children younger than 10 years of age who experienced severe *Centruroides* scorpion envenomation found that anti-*Centruroides* antivenom resulted in rapid resolution of all symptoms in all 12 patients treated.[18] Of those treated with antivenom, 58% had a delayed rash or serum sickness.

Scorpion envenomation can be prevented by wearing shoes when walking, particularly at night, because of the nocturnal nature of the scorpions. Shoes, sleeping bag, and tent should be shaken out before use. Cracks and crevices should be filled, woodpiles and rubbish piles eliminated, and insecticides used in infested areas. The bark scorpion (*C. exilicauda*), which is fluorescent, can be demonstrated in the dark using a Wood's lamp.

TICKS

There are three families of ticks recognized in the world: (1) *Ixodidae* (hard ticks), (2) *Argasidae* (soft ticks), and (3) *Nuttalliellidae* (a small little known group that has characteristics of both hard and soft ticks). The terms "hard" and "soft" refer to the presence of a dorsal scutum or "plate" in the *Ixodidae* and is absent in the *Argasidae,* which are characteristically soft and leathery. Both types have clinical importance. Sexual dimorphism exists in the *Ixodidae* but not in the *Argasidae. Ixodidae* females are capable of enormous expansion up to 50 times their weight in fluid and blood.[37] All of the major tick-borne diseases in North America are transmitted by ixodid ticks, except for relapsing fever. The discussion below focuses on tick paralysis and not on any of the infectious diseases associated with tick bites. In 1912, Todd described a progressive ascending flaccid paralysis after bites from ticks.[124] In North America, human cases of tick paralysis are caused by *Dermacentor andersoni, Dermacentor variabilis, Amblyomma americanum, Amblyomma maculatum,* and *Ixodes scapularis.*

Pathophysiology

Venom secreted from the salivary glands during the blood meal is thought to cause the paralysis. The mechanism of action is not completely understood. Paralysis is caused by a neurotoxin, also called "ixovotoxin,"[1] that inhibits the release of acetylcholine at the neuromuscular junction.[83] Electrophysiology measurements in humans demonstrate motor- and sensory-nerve conduction slowing and reduction in muscle action potential amplitude without defects in neuromuscular transmission.[27,83]

Clinical Manifestations

Usually the tick must remain on the person for 5 to 6 days. Ticks typically attach to the scalp but can be found on any part of the body, including the ear canals and anus. Children, particularly girls, are most often affected as their long hair may limit the ability to find an imbedded tick. Initially patients may experience paresthesias, lower extremity weakness, mild diarrhea, followed by absent or decreased deep tendon reflexes, and an ascending generalized weakness that can progress to bulbar structures involving speech, swallowing, and facial expression develops within 24 to 48 hours. If the tick is not removed, respiratory weakness can lead to hypoventilation, lethargy, coma, and death. The differential diagnosis includes Guillain-Barré syndrome, poliomyelitis, botulism, transverse myelitis, and spinal cord lesions. The cerebrospinal fluid remains normal, and the rate of progression is rapid, unlike Guillain-Barré syndrome and poliomyelitis.[33,110]

Treatment

The most important aspect of treatment is to consider tick paralysis in any patient with ascending paralysis. Other than removal of the entire tick, which is curative, treatment is entirely supportive. Symptoms should improve within several hours after tick removal.

Preventing tick bites includes wearing protective clothing and spraying clothes with insect repellant. DEET repels ticks but does not kill them. Permanone is a new tick repellant, an aerosol spray for use on clothing, that contains permethrin which kills ticks on contact.[64] According to one study, permethrin in concentrations of 0.036 to 2.276 mg/m² induces 90 to 100% mortality as well as 100% effectiveness for 1 month and a decrease in effectiveness to 52% after the first washing.[64] Close inspection of all body parts and scalp is important. Proper removal of the tick is important; otherwise, infection or incomplete tick removal may occur. The tick should be grasped as close to the skin surface as possible with blunt curved forceps, tweezers, or gloved hands. Steady pressure without crushing the body should be used because any expressed fluid may infect the patient. After tick removal, the site should be disinfected. Traditional methods using petroleum jelly, topical lidocaine, fingernail polish, isopropyl alcohol, or a hot match head

are ineffective and/or may induce the tick to salivate or regurgitate into the wound.[85]

HYMENOPTERA: BEES, WASPS, HORNETS, YELLOW JACKETS, AND ANTS

Within the order Hymenoptera, there are three families of clinical significance: Apidae (honeybees and bumblebees), Vespidae (yellow jackets, hornets, and wasps), and Formicidae (fire ants). Insects of this subclass (Fig. 102–2) are of great medical importance because stings can cause acute toxic and allergic reactions that can be fatal (Table 102–7). An event that has caused significant economic and health issues is the introduction of the African honeybee to Brazil because it was thought that they were more efficient honey producers. They have migrated toward the southern border of the United States. Unfortunately, they produce less honey and pose a greater threat to humans. African bees are characterized by large populations, frequent swarming, nonstop flights of at least 20 km, and a tendency toward mass attack with little provocation.[79]

Apis mellifera and *Bombus* species (honeybees and bumblebees) build nests away from humans and are passive unless disturbed. *Apidae* can sting only once because the stinger is a modified ovipositor that resides in the abdomen. The structure is barbed and has a venom sac attached. Once the stinger embeds into the skin, the stinger disembowels the Apid. Vespids, on the other hand, are more aggressive, build nests in trees, under awnings, and yellow jackets inhabit the ground. Also, they have fewer barbs and are able to sting multiple times.[41]

Pathophysiology

Several allergens (Table 102–8) and pharmacologically active compounds have been found in honeybee venom. The three major venom proteins for the honeybee are melittin, phospholipase A, and hyaluronidase.[69] Other proteins include apamin, acid phosphatase, and other unidentified proteins. Phospholipase A_2 represents the major antigen/allergen in bee venom.[16]

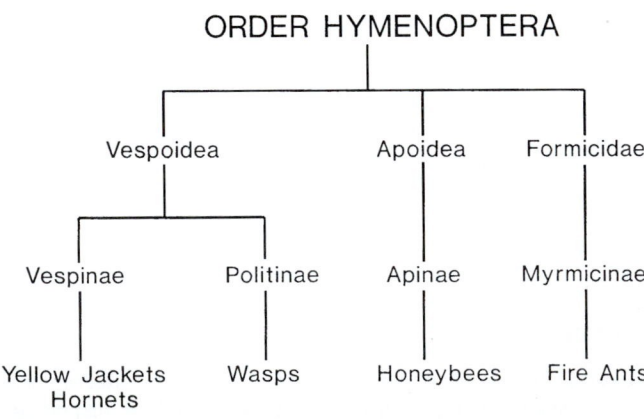

Figure 102–2 Taxonomy of Hymenoptera. (*Reproduced with permission from Sinkinson CA, French RS, Graft DF, eds: Individualizing therapy for Hymenoptera stings. Emerg Med Rep 1990;11:134.*)

TABLE 102–7.   Classification of Reactions to Hymenoptera Sting

Reaction	Clinical Presentations
Local	
Minimal	Localized pain, pruritus, swelling
	Lesion <5 cm
	Duration several hours
Large	Localized pain and pruritus
	Contiguous swelling and erythema
	Lesion >5 cm
	Duration 1–3 days
Systemic	
Minimal	Localized pain, pruritus, swelling
	Distant and diffuse urticaria, angioedema, pruritus, and/or erythema; conjunctivitis
	Abdominal pain, nausea, diarrhea
Severe	Dermatologic
	Local: pain, pruritus, and swelling
	Distant: urticaria, angioedema, pruritus, and/or erythema
	Gastrointestinal
	Nausea, abdominal pain, diarrhea
	Respiratory
	Nasal congestion, rhinorrhea, hoarseness, bronchospasm, stridor, tachypnea, dyspnea, cough, wheezing
	Cardiovascular
	Tachycardia, hypotension, dysrhythmias, myocardial infarction
	Miscellaneous
	Seizures, feeling of impending doom, uterine contractions

Reprinted, with permission, from Sinkinson CA, French RS, Graft DF, eds: *Individualizing therapy for hymenoptera stings.* Emerg Med Rep 1990;11:134.

TABLE 102–8.   Composition of Hymenoptera Venom

Vespid (wasps, hornets, yellow jackets)
Biogenic amines (diverse)
Phospholipase A, phospholipase B
Hyaluronidase
Antigen 5
Acid phosphatase
Mast cell degranulating peptide
Kinin

Apids (honeybees)
Biogenic amines (diverse)
Phospholipase A, phospholipase B (?)
Hyaluronidase
Acid phosphatase
Minimine
Mellitin
Apamin
Mast cell degranulating peptide

Formicids (fire ants)
Biogenic amines (diverse)
Phospholipase
Hyaluronidase
Unidentified others
Piperidines

Modified, with permission, after Sinkinson CA, French RS, Graft DF, eds: *Individualizing therapy for hymenoptera stings.* Emerg Med Rep 1990;11:134; King TP, Valentine MD: *Allergens of hymenoptera venoms.* Clin Rev Allergy 1987;5:137; Stablein JJ, Lockey RF: *Adverse reactions to ant stings.* Clin Rev Allergy 1987;5:161.

Melittin is the principal component of honeybee venom and acts as a detergent to disrupt the cell membrane and liberate potassium and biogenic amines.[8] Histamine release by bee venom appears to be largely mediated by a mast cell degranulation peptide. Apamin is a neurotoxin that acts on the spinal cord. Adolapin inhibits prostaglandin synthase and has antiinflammatory properties that might account for its use in arthritic therapy.[111] Phospholipase A and hyaluronidase are the chief enzymes in bee venom.

The vespid venoms contain three major proteins that serve as allergens and a wide array of vasoactive peptides and amines.[69] The intense pain following stings by vespids is largely caused by serotonin, acetylcholine, and wasp kinins. Antigen 5 is the major allergen in vespid venom.[80] Its biologic function is unknown. Mastoparans are similar in action to the mast cell degranulation peptide but weaker.[8] One study found that phospholipase A may be responsible for inducing coagulation abnormalities.[89]

Clinical Manifestations

Normally, the honeybee sting is manifested as localized edema without a systemic reaction. Rarely, a sting in the oropharynx can produce airway compromise. Toxic reactions occur with multiple stings (more than 500 stings are described as possibly fatal)[41] and include GI symptoms, headache, fever, syncope, and, rarely, rhabdomyolysis, renal failure, and seizures. Bronchospasm and urticaria are typically absent. This type of toxic reaction is not an IgE-mediated response as are anaphylactic reactions.

Anaphylaxis is IgE-mediated. The IgE antibodies attach to tissue mast cells and basophils in individuals who have been previously sensitized to the venom. These cells are then activated, allowing for the progression of the cascade reaction of increased vasoactive substances, such as leukotrienes, eosinophil chemotactic factor-A (ECF-A), and histamine (Chap. 15). An anaphylactic reaction is not dependent on the number of stings. Patients who are allergic to hymenoptera venom will develop a wheal-and-flare reaction at the site of the inoculum; the shorter the interval between the sting and onset of systemic symptoms, the more likely the reaction will be severe. Fatalities can occur within several minutes; even initially mild symptoms may be followed by a fulminant course. Generalized urticaria, throat and chest tightness, stridor, fever, chills, and cardiovascular collapse can ensue.

Treatment

Application of ice at the site is usually sufficient to halt discomfort. The stinger should be removed by scraping with a credit card or scalpel, as opposed to pulling, which may release additional retained venom. General supportive care is indicated. Death may ensue if the anaphylactic reaction is not managed properly and expeditiously. Treatment consists of immediate airway and circulatory support, with fluid resuscitation in an attempt to reverse hypotension. For adult patients, subcutaneous epinephrine (0.3–0.5 mg), or intravenous infusion at 20–50 mg/min; 1 mg in 1 LNS, infused at a rate of 20–50 mL/min titrated to effect should be used. For pediatric patients, the dose of epinephrine SC is 0.01 mg/kg up to 0.3 mg. The infusion rate for infants and children should start at 0.025 mL/kg/min, not to exceed 0.375 mL/kg/min.[9]

β_2-Selective inhaled agonists such as albuterol may be used to relieve bronchospasm not relieved with epinephrine. Diphenhydramine (1 mg/kg up to 50 mg) or corticosteroids may be necessary, but these medications are secondarily important to the immediate airway and cardiopulmonary support with fluids, epinephrine, and vasopressors. A delayed reaction, characterized by fever, malaise, headache, polyarthralgias, and lymphadenopathy, may first appear 1 to 2 weeks after the sting. Unless specifically suggested, the distant bite may be forgotten, and the diagnosis of a delayed reaction missed.[2,76]

Prevention, especially in the allergic person, includes avoiding bright clothing, flowers, scented deodorants and shampoos, perfumes, and barefoot walks outdoors. An emergency kit containing a prefilled spring-loaded epinephrine syringe (EpiPen® delivers 0.3 mg, EpiPen Jr® delivers 0.15 mg) with careful instructions from a physician as well as an antihistamine (diphenhydramine) and an emergency alert card or tag should be carried or worn by the sensitized individual. Commercial preparations of venom from the honeybee, yellow jacket, white-faced hornet, yellow hornet, and wasp can be used for diagnosis and immunotherapy for patients with life-threatening reactions to stings. Several authors have discussed the indications and safety of immunotherapy.[69,134]

FIRE ANTS

There are native fire ants in the United States, but the imported fire ants *Solenopsis invicta* and *Solenopsis richteri* are the significant pests and have no natural enemies. *Solenopsis invicta*, the most aggressive species, now infests 13 southern states.[114] The migration of fire ants is limited by freezing temperatures in the winter. Fire ants are named for the burning pain inflicted after exposure. The imported fire ant attacks with little warning. Firmly grasping the skin with its mandibles, the fire ant arches its back, inserts its 0.5- to 1.0-mm stinger extruding from their abdomen into the flesh, and injects venom from the attached sac. Pivoting at the head, the fire ant injects an average of seven or eight stings in a circular pattern. Unlike bees and wasps, fire ants introduce their venom slowly, over seconds to minutes, and the onset of pain is delayed and necrosis can occur at the site.[114]

Pathophysiology

Unlike the venoms of wasps, bees, and hornets that contain mostly aqueous proteins, the imported fire ant venom is 95% alkaloid, with a small aqueous fraction that contains soluble proteins.[74] Of the alkaloids, 99% is a 2,6-disubstituted piperidine that has hemolytic, antibacterial, insecticidal, and cytotoxic properties. These alkaloids do not cause allergic reactions but produce a pustule and pain. The aqueous portion of the venom contains the allergenic activity of fire ant venom, *Sol i* I through IV.[52,114] The proteins identified in the venom include a phospholipase, a hyaluronidase, and the enzyme *N*-acetyl-β-glucosaminidase.[32,114]

Clinical Manifestations

There are three categories suggested to categorize the reactions for the imported fire ant: local, large local, and systemic.[113] Local reactions occur in nonallergenic individuals. Large local reactions are defined as painful, pruritic swelling at least 5 cm in diameter and are contiguous with the sting site. Systemic reactions involve signs and symptoms remote from the sting site. The sting initially forms a wheal that burns and itches at the site; several hours later clear vesicles develop, and pustules are noted within 12 hours. In 24 hours, the pustules umbilicate on an erythematous base. Late cutaneous allergic reactions can occur in some persons who experience indurated pruritic lumps at the site of subsequent stings.[32] Large reactions may lead to enough tissue edema that may compromise blood flow to an extremity. Anaphylaxis occurs in 0.6 to 6% of persons who have been stung.[114] Often, healing occurs with scarring in 10 to 14 days.

Diagnosis

Clinical clues such as the pustule developing at the sting site 24 hours later, species identification, and history may help to identify fire ant exposure. There are no laboratory assays to determine exposure. Fire ant allergy can be determined by correlating the clinical manifestation of fire ant sting reactions with imported fire ant–specific IgE determined by skin testing or RAST.

Treatment

Local reactions require cold compresses and cleansing with soap and water. Some authors recommend topical or injected lidocaine with or without 1:100,000 epinephrine and topical vinegar and salt mixtures to decrease pain at the site of the bite and sting.[54,76] Topical application of aluminum sulfate and papain is not effective for reducing pain or pruritus.[21,103] Large local reactions can be treated with oral corticosteroids, antihistamines, and analgesics. Secondary infections should be treated with antibiotics. Systemic reactions should be treated with subcutaneous epinephrine (0.3–0.5 mL of 1:1000) or intravenous epinephrine if shock or cardiac arrest ensues (see page 1583 and Table 15–7). Immunotherapy may be considered for patients known to have a history of anaphylaxis after imported fire ant stings and evidence on skin testing of IgE responses to fire ants. Of 65 patients treated with immunotherapy, 47 (72%) were stung inadvertently; after treatment, only one patient developed anaphylaxis. In a control group who elected not to undergo immunotherapy, six patients received inadvertent stings, and all six had anaphylaxis.[56]

BUTTERFLIES, MOTHS, AND CATERPILLARS

Butterflies and moths are insects of the order *Lepidoptera*. One family of butterflies and nine families of moths have a caterpillar stage that is clinically important. Caterpillar, which means "hairy cat" in Latin, is the larval stage. The puss caterpillar (*Megalopyge opercularis*) undergoes five or six instars (molts) before reaching maturity. Other names are woolly/hairy worm, wooly slug, opossum bug, tree asp, Italian asp, and little perrito in Spanish.[116] The puss caterpillar is considered the most toxic of the caterpillars in the United States. The spines are yellowish with black tips, and the hairs vary in colors ranging from pale yellow and gray to brown.[14] The spines contain an urticarial poison.

Pathophysiology

The toxin is contained within the hollow spine, not the hairs, and is poorly understood. It is believed that the toxin is produced by specialized basal cells and is passively transmitted to the victim by touch. The toxin may be a protein or a substance that conjugates with proteins.[35]

Clinical Manifestations

The sting is painful, and white or red papules may appear. The classic gridlike pattern develops within 2 to 3 hours of contact. The following symptoms may occur: nausea, vomiting, fever, headache, restlessness, tachycardia, hypotension, urticaria, seizures, and even radiating lymphadenitis and regional adenopathy.[92]

Treatment

Treatment should be immediate, with removal of the embedded spines using cellophane tape and application of ice. Strong analgesics such as morphine may be tried. If muscle cramps develop, benzodiazepines should be administered. One study recommended the use of 10% calcium gluconate, 10 mL administered IV, which provided pain relief.[77] Topical corticosteroids can be used to decrease local inflammation. Antihistamines such as diphenhydramine (25–50 mg for adults and 1 mg/kg, maximum 50 mg, in children) may be used to relieve pruritus and urticaria.[77,92]

BLISTER BEETLES

Blister beetles, found in the eastern United States, southern Europe, Africa, and Asia, are from the order Coeloptera, family Meloidae. *Epicauta vittata* is the most common of over 200 blister beetles identified in the United States.[59] When the beetle senses danger, it exudes cantharidin by filling its breathing tubes with air, closing its breathing pores, and building up body fluid pressure until fluid is pushed out through one or more leg joints.[41] Cantharidin is a potent blistering agent found throughout all 10 stages of the blister beetle's life.[24] The male biosynthesizes 17 mg of the toxin, approximately 10% of his live weight, whereas the female loses most of her reserves as she ages. But in the wild, the female repeatedly acquires cantharidin as copulatory gifts from her mates.[24] Cantharidin, known popularly as "Spanish fly," takes its name from the Mediterranean beetle *Cantharis vesicatoria* and has been used for millennia as a sexual stimulant. The aphrodisiac properties are related to cantharidin's ability to cause vascular engorgement and inflammation of the genitourinary tract, hence the reports of priapism and pelvic organ engorgement.[123] Cantharidin has been used for the treatment of bladder and kidney infections, stones, stranguria (bladder spasm), and various venereal diseases.[59] In the last century, cantharidin was commonly used for the treatment of pleurisy, pneumonia, arthritis, neuralgias, and various dermatitides. The only medical preparation available for medical purposes today is a 1% topical solution for wart removal.[30]

Cantharidin poisoning has been reported by cutaneous exposure,[20] unintentional inoculation,[93] and inadvertent ingestion of the beetle itself.[121] There have been fewer than 30 cases of Spanish fly poisoning since 1900.[59]

Pathophysiology

Cantharidin is a natural defensive toxicant produced by blister beetles and shares a structural similarity with the herbicide endothall. Cantharidin inhibits the activity of protein phosphatases types 1 and 2A, which may alter endothelial permeability by enhancing the phosphorylation state of endothelial regulatory proteins, resulting in elevated albumin flux. Hence, the barrier function was altered.[63] Because cantharidin circulates bound to albumin and is renally excreted, enhanced permeability of albumin may be responsible for cantharidin's systemic effects, which lead to diffuse injury of the vascular endothelium and resulting blistering, hemorrhage, and inflammation.

Clinical Manifestations

The clinical effects can mostly be attributed to the irritative effects on the exposed organ systems. The secretions cause an urticarial dermatitis that is manifested several hours later by burns, blisters, or vesiculobullae.[20] Symptoms may be immediate or delayed over several hours. In addition to the local effects, cantharidin can be absorbed through the lipid bilayer of the epidermis and cause systemic toxicity with diaphoresis, tachycardia, hematuria, and oliguria from an extensive dermal exposure.[123] If the periorbital region is contaminated, edema and blistering can also evolve. Eye findings from direct contact with the beetle or hand contamination may result in decreased vision, pain, lacrimation, corneal ulcerations, filamentary keratitis, and anterior uveitis.[93] When ingested, severe GI disturbances and hematuria can occur, described primarily from cantharidin toxicosis in horses.[96] Initial patient complaints may include burning of the oropharynx, dysphagia, abdominal cramping, vomiting, hematemesis followed by lower GI tract hematochezia, and tenesmus.[86] Although equids develop cantharidin toxicosis from their diet, there is one case of an inadvertent blister beetle ingestion by a child who thought it was the edible *Eulepida mashona* or white grub and developed hematuria and abdominal cramping.[121] The genitourinary effects include dysuria, urinary frequency, hematuria, proteinuria, and renal impairment. Most symptoms resolved over several weeks. However, death has been reported from renal failure with acute tubular necrosis.[123] Most human exposures involve inadvertent contact with the beetle or its secretions, resulting in a dermatitis, keratoconjunctivitis, and periorbital edema secondary to hand-eye involvement, also called "the Nairobi Eye."[93]

Diagnostic Testing

Cantharidin toxicosis has been identified for equine and ruminant exposures by screening urine and gastric contents with high-performance liquid chromatography and gas chromatography/mass spectrometry.[96,97] This method has not been utilized for clinical practice.

Treatment

Treatment is largely supportive. Wound care and tetanus status should be assessed. For keratoconjunctivitis, consult an ophthalmologist early in the clinical course and start the patient on topical corticosteroids (prednisolone 0.125%), mydriatics (cyclopentolate 1%), and antibiotics (ciprofloxacin 0.3%).

SUMMARY

Healthcare providers should have an extensive knowledge regarding bites and stings by arthropods and arachnids to enable them to recognize local and systemic reactions. The treatment of arthropod-borne disease rarely entails the use of antivenoms. Proper hygiene to prevent secondary infections, avoiding contact with arthropods, decreasing the arthropod population mechanically and/or chemically, and the use of repellents are important measures to decrease morbidity from arthropods. The patient should bring the arthropod to the hospital if possible to facilitate identification, and every attempt should be made to describe the evolution of the bite to assist in the differential diagnosis.

REFERENCES

1. Abbott KH: Tick paralysis: A review. Proc Mayo Clin 1943;18: 59–64.

2. Abramowicz M, ed: Insect venoms. Med Lett Drug Ther 1983;25: 53–54.

3. Allen C: Arachnid envenomations. Emerg Med Clin North Am 1992;10:269–298.

4. Anderson PC: What's new in loxoscelism? Mo Med 1973;70; 711–718.

5. Atkins JA, Wingo CW, Soderman WA: Probable cause of necrotic spider bite in the midwest. Science 1957;126:73.

6. Baba A, Cooper JR: The action of black widow spider venom on cholinergic mechanisms in synapatosomes. J Neurochem 1980;34: 1369–1379.

7. Babcock JL, Marmer DJ, Steele RW: Immunotoxicology of brown recluse spider venom. Toxicon 1986;24:783–790.

8. Banks BEC: The composition of Hymenoptera venoms with particular reference to venom of the honey bee. In: Kornalik F, Mebs D, eds: Proceedings of the 7th European Symposium on Animal Plant and Microbial Toxins, Prague, 1986, p. 41.

9. Barach EM, Nowak RM, Lee TG, Tomlanovich MC. Epinephrine for the treatment of anaphylactic shock. JAMA 1984;251:2118.

10. Barrett SM, Romine-Jenkins M, Blick KE: Passive hemagglutination inhibition test for diagnosis of brown recluse spider bite envenomation. Clin Chem 1993;39:2104–2107.

11. Barrett SM, Romine-Jenkins M, Fisher DE: Dapsone or electric shock therapy of brown recluse spider envenomation? Ann Emerg Med 1994;24:21–25.

12. Belyea DA, Tuman DC, Ward TP, Babonis TR: The red eye revisited: ophthalmia nodosa due to tarantula hairs. South Med J 1998; 91:565–567.

13. Bernardino CR, Rapuano C: Ophthalmia nodosa caused by casual handling of a tarantula. CLAO 2000;26:111–112.

14. Bishopp FC: The puss caterpillar and the effects of its sting on man. Washington, DC, US Department of Agriculture, 1923, Department Circular 288:1–14.

15. Bittner MA: Alpha-latrotoxin and its receptors CIRL (latrophilin) and neurexin I-α mediate effects on secretion through multiple mechanisms. Biochimie 2000;82:447–452.

16. Blaser K, Carballido J, Faith A, et al: Determinants and mechanisms of human immune responses to bee venom phospholipase A₂. Int Arch Allergy Immunol 1998;117:1–10.

17. Bogen E: Arachnidism, a study in spider poisoning. JAMA 1926; 86:1894–1896.

18. Bond GR: Antivenin administration for Centruroides scorpion sting risks and benefits. Ann Emerg Med 1992;21:788–791.

19. Boyer-Hassen LV, McNally JT: Spider bites. In: Auerbach PS, ed: Wilderness Medicine: Management of Wilderness and Environmental Emergencies. St.Louis, CV Mosby, 1995, pp. 769–786.

20. Browne SG: Cantharidin poisoning due to a blister beetle. Br Med J 1960;2:1290–1291.

21. Bruce S, Tschen EH, Smith EB: Topical aluminum sulfate for fire ant stings. Int J Dermatol 1984;23:211.

22. Bush SP, Naftel J, Farstad D: Injection of a whole black widow spider. Ann Emerg Med 1996;27:532–534.

23. Cabbiness SG, Gehrke CW, Kuo KC, et al. Polyamines in some tarantula venoms. Toxicon 1980;18:681–683.

24. Carrel JE, McCairel MH, Slagle AJ, et al: Cantharidin production in the blister beetle. Experientia 1993;49:171–174.

25. Chan TK, Geren CR, Howell DE, Odell GV: Adenosine triphosphate in tarantula spider venoms and its synergistic effect with the venom toxin. Toxicon 1975;13:61–63.

26. Chavez-Olortegui C, Zanetti VC, Ferreira AP, et al. Elisa for the detection of venom antigens in experimental and clinical envenoming by Loxosceles intermedia spiders. Toxicon 1998;36:563–569.

27. Cherington M, Snyder RD: Tick paralysis: Neurophysiologic studies. N Engl J Med 1968;278:95–97.

28. Clark RF, Wethem-Kestner S, Vance MV, Gerkin R: Clinical presentation and treatment of black widow spider envenomation: A review of 163 cases. Ann Emerg Med 1992;21:782–787.

29. Connor DA, Seldon BS: Scorpion envenomation. In: Auerbach PS, ed: Wilderness Medicine: Management of Wilderness and Environmental Emergencies. St.Louis, CV Mosby, 1995, pp. 831–842.

30. Coskey RJ: Treatment of plantar warts in children with a salicylic acid-podophyllin-cantharidin product. Pediatr Dermatol 1984;2: 71–73.

31. Curry S: Black widow spider envenomation. In: Harwood A, Linden C, Luten R, et al, eds: The Clinical Practice of Emergency Medicine. Philadelphia, JB Lippincott, 1991, pp. 617–619.

32. DeShazo RD, Butcher BT, Banks WA: Reactions to the stings of the imported fire ants. N Engl J Med 1990;327:462–466.

33. Felz MW, Smith CD, Swift TR: A six year old girl with tick paralysis. N Engl J Med 2000;342:90–94.

34. Finkelstein A, Rubin L, Tzen M: Black widow spider venom: effect of purified toxin on lipid bilayer membranes. Science 1976;193: 1009–1011.

35. Foot NC: Pathology of the dermatitis caused by Megalopyge opercularis, a Texas caterpillar. J Exp Med 1922;35:737–753.

36. Gendron BP: Loxosceles reclusa envenomation. Am J Emerg Med 1990;8:51–54.

37. Gentile, DA. Tick-borne diseases. In: Auerbach PS, ed: Wilderness Medicine: Management of Wilderness and Environmental Emergencies. St. Louis, CV Mosby, 1995, pp.787–812.

38. Geppert M, Khvotchev M, Krasnoperov V, et al: Neurexin Iα is a major α-latrotoxin receptor that cooperates in a α-latrotoxin action. J Biol Chem 1998;273:1705–1710.

39. Gertsch WJ: American Spiders, 2nd ed. New York, Van Nostrand Reinhold, 1979.

40. Ginsburg CM, Weinburg AG: Hemolytic anemia and multiorgan failure associated with a localized cutaneous lesion. J Pediatr 1988;112: 496–500.

41. Goddard J. Physician's Guide to Arthropods of Medical Importance, 3rd ed. 2000, pp. 37–38.

42. Gomez, HF, Miller MJ, Trachy JW, Marks RM, Warren JS: Intradermal anti-loxosceles Fab fragments attenuate dermonecrotic arachnidism. Acad Emerg Med 1999;6:1195–1202.

43. Goto CS, Abramo TJ, Ginsburg CM: Upper airway obstruction caused by brown recluse spider envenomization of the neck. Am J Emerg Med 1996;14:660–662.

44. Grattan-Smith PJ, Morris JG, Johnston HM, et al: Clinical and neurophysiological features of tick paralysis. Brain 1997;120: 1975–1987.

45. Graudins A, Padula M, Broady K, Nicholson GM: Red-back spider (Latrodectus hasselti) antivenom prevents the toxicity of widow spider venoms. Ann Emerg Med 2001;37:154–160.

46. Gray RR: Getting to know funnel-webs. Aust Nat Hist 1981;20: 256–258.

47. Grishin EV: Black widow spider toxins: The present and the future. Toxicon 1998;36:1693–1701.

48. Gueron M, Reuben I, Sofer S: The cardiovascular system after scorpion envenomation: A review. J Toxicol Clin Toxicol 1992;30: 215–258.

49. Gueron M, Sofer S: Vasodilators and calcium channel blocking agents as treatment of cardiovascular manifestations of human scorpion envenomation. Toxicon 1990;28:127–128.

50. Henkel AW, Sankaranarayan S: Mechanism of alpha-latrotoxin action. Cell Tissue Res 1999;296:229–233.

51. Hobbs GD, Anderson AR, Greene TJ, Yealy DM: Comparison of hyperbaric oxygen and dapsone therapy for *Loxosceles* envenomation. Acad Emerg Med 1996;3:758–761.

52. Hoffman DR: Allergens in Hymenoptera venom. XVII. Allergenic components of *Solenopsis invicta* (imported fire ant) venom. J Allergy Clin Immunol 1983;80:300–306.

53. Hollabaugh RS, Fernandes ET: Management of the brown recluse spider bite. J Pediatr Surg1989;24:126–127.

54. Horen WP: Insect and scorpion stings. JAMA 1972;221:894–898.

55. Hunt DW: The bites and stings of summer. Part 2. Spider bites. Emerg Med Services Mag 1986;June:75–81.

56. Hylander RD, Ortiz AA, Freeman TM, Martin ME: Imported fire ant immunotherapy: effectiveness of whole body extracts [abstract]. J Allergy Clin Immunol 1989;83:232.

57. Ichtchenko K, Bittner MA, Krasnoperov V, et al: A novel ubiquitously expressed alpha-latrotoxin receptor is a member of the CIRL family of G-protein-coupled receptors. J Biol Chem 1999; 26;274: 5491–5498.

58. Johnson JH, Bloomquist JR, Krapcho KJ, et al: Novel insecticidal peptides from *Tegenaria agrestis* spider venom may have a direct effect on the insect central nervous system. Arch Insect Biochem Physiol 1998;38:19–31.

59. Karras DJ, Farrell SE, Harrigan RA, Henretig FM, Gealt LG: Poisoning from "Spanish fly" (cantharidin). Am J Emerg Med 1996;14: 478–483.

60. Kelley TD, Wasserman G: The dangers of pet tarantulas: Experience of the Marseilles poison centre. J Toxicol Clin Toxicol. 1998;36: 55–56.

61. Key GF: A comparison of calcium gluconate and methocarbamol (Robaxin) in the treatment of latrodectism (black widow spider envenomation). Am J Trop Med Hyg 1981;30:273.

62. King LE, Rees RS: Dapsone treatment of a brown recluse bite. JAMA 1983;648.

63. Knapp J, Boknik P, Luss I, et al: The protein phosphatase inhibitor cantharidin alters vascular endothelial cell permeability. J Pharmacol Exp Ther 1999:289:1480–1486.

64. Kocisova A, Para L: Possibilities of long-term protection against blood-sucking insects and ticks. Cent Eur J Public Health 1999;7(1): 27–30.

65. Krasnoperov VB, Bittner MA, Brevis R, et al. α-Latarotoxin stimulates exocytosis by the interaction with a neuronal G-protein-coupled receptor. Neuron 1997;18:925–937.

66. Kunkel DB: The sting of the arthropod. Emerg Med 1996;28: 137–141.

67. Kurpiewski G, Forrester LJ, Barrett JT, et al: Platelet aggregation and sphingomyelinase-D activity of a purified toxin from the venom of LR. Biochem Biophys 1981;18;467–476.

68. Lee CK, Chan TK, Ward BC, Howell DE, Odell GV: The purification and characterization of a necrotoxin from tarantula, *Dugesiella hentzi* (Girard), venom. Arch Biochem Biophys 1974 Sep;164(1): 341–350.

69. Lichtenstein LM, Valentine MD, Sobotka AK: Insect allergy: The state of the art. J Allergy Clin Immunol 1979;64:5–12.

70. Lowry BP, Bradfield JF, Carroll RG, et al: A controlled trial of topical nitroglycerin in a New Zealand white rabbit model of brown recluse spider envenomation. Ann Emerg Med 2001;37: 161–165.

71. Lux SE, John KM, Bennet V: Analysis of cDNA for human erthrocyte ankyrin indicates a repeated structure with homology to tissue-differentiation and cell-cycle control proteins. Nature 1990; 344:36–42.

72. Macchiavello A: Cutaneous arachnidism experimentally produced with the glandular poison of *L laeta*. PR J Public Health Trop Med 1947;23:266–279.

73. Macchiavello A: Cutaneous arachnidism or gangrenous spot in Chile. PR J Public Health Trop Med 1947;22:425–466.

74. Mac Connell JG, Blum MS, Buren WF, et al: Fire ant venoms: chemotaxonomic correlations with alkaloidal compositions. Toxicon 1976;14:69–78.

75. Maretic Z, Stanic N: The health problem of arachnidism. Bull WHO 1954;11:1007–1022.

76. Marshall TK: Wasp and bee stings. Practitioner 1957;178:712–722.

77. Micks DW. Clinical effects of the sting of "puss caterpillar" on man. Texas Rep Biol Med 1952;10:399–405.

78. Miller MJ, Gomez HF, Snider RJ, et al: Detection of *Loxosceles* venom in lesional hair shafts and skin: application of a specific immunoassay to identify dermonecrotic arachnidism. Am J Emerg Med 2000;18:626–628.

79. Minton SA, Bechtel HB: Arthropod envenomation and parasitism. In: Auerbach PS, ed: Wilderness Medicine: Management of Wilderness and Environmental Emergencies. St.Louis, CV Mosby, 1995, pp. 742–768.

80. Monsalve RI, Lu G, King TP: Expressions of recombinant venom allergen, antigen 5 of yellow jacket (*Vespula vulgaris*) and paper wasp (*Polistes annularis*), in bacteria or yeast. Protein Exp Purif 1999; 16(3):410–416.

81. Moss HS, Binder LS: A retrospective review of black widow spider envenomation. Ann Emerg Med 1987;16:188–191.

82. Muller GJ: Black and brown widow spider bites in South Africa. S Afr Med J 1993;83:399–405.

83. Murnaghan MF: Site and mechanism of tick paralysis. Science 1960;131:418–419.

84. Necrotic arachnidism—Pacific Northwest 1988–1995. MMWR 1996;45:433–436.

85. Needham GR: Evaluation of five popular methods for tick removal. Pediatrics 1985;75:997–1002.

86. Oaks WW, DiTunno DJ, Magnani T, et al: Cantharidin poisoning. Arch Intern Med 1960;105:574–582.

87. Ownby CL, Odell GV: Pathogenesis of skeletal muscle necrosis induced by tarantula venom. Exp Mol Pathol 1983;38(3):283–296.

88. Petrenko AG, Kovalenko VA, Shamotienko OG, et al: Isolation and properties of the α-latrotoxin receptor. EMBO J 1990;9:2023–2027.

89. Petroianu G, Liu J, Helfrich U, Maleck W, Rufer R: Phospholipase A₂-induced coagulation abnormalities after bee sting. Am J Emerg Med 2000;18:22–27.

90. Phillips S, Kohn M, Baker D, et al: Therapy of brown spider envenomation: A controlled trial of hyperbaric oxygen, dapsone therapy, and cyproheptadine. Ann Emerg Med 1995;25:363–368.

91. Picotti GB, Bondiolotti GP, Meldolesi J: Peripheral catecholamines release by alpha-latrotoxin in the rat. Arch Pharmacol 1982;320:224.

92. Pinson RT, Morgan JA: Envenomation by the puss caterpillar (*Megalopyge opercularis*). Ann Emerg Med 1991;20:562–564.

93. Poole TRG: Blister beetle periorbital dermatitis and keratoconjunctivitis in Tanzania. Eye 1988;12:883–885.

94. Rachesky IJ, Banner W, Dansky J, et al: Treatments for *Centruroides exilicauda* envenomation. Am J Dis Child 1984;138: 1136–1139.

95. Rauber A: Black widow spider bites. J Toxicol Clin Toxicol 1984; 21:473.

96. Ray AC, Kyle AL, Murphy MJ, Reagor JC: Etiologic agents, incidence, and improved diagnostic methods of cantharidin toxicosis in horses. Am J Vet Res 1989;50:187–191.

97. Ray AC, Post LO, Hurst JM, Edwards WC, Reagor JC: Evaluation of an analytical method for the diagnosis of cantharidin toxicosis due to ingestion of blister beetles (*Epicauta lemniscata*) by horses and sheep. Am J Vet Res 1989;41:932–933.

98. Rees RS, Altenbern DP, Lynch JB, et al: Brown recluse spider bites: A comparison of early surgical excision versus dapsone and delayed surgical excision. Ann Surg 1985;202:659–663.

99. Rees R, Campbell D, Rieger E, et al: The diagnosis and treatment of brown recluse spider bites. Ann Emerg Med 1987;16:945–949.

100. Rimza ME, Zimmerman DR: Scorpion envenomation. Pediatrics 1980;66:298–301.

101. Robertson FM, Olsen SB, Jackson MR: Dapsone hepatitis following treatment of a brown recluse spider bite. Compl Surg 1992;33–35.

102. Rosenthal L, Sacchetti D, Madeddu L, Meldoles J: Mode of action of α-latrotoxin: role of divalent cations in Ca^{2+}-dependent and Ca^{2+}-independent effects mediated by the toxin. Mol Pharmacol 1990;38:917–923.

103. Ross EV, Badame AJ, Dale SE: Meat tenderizer in the acute treatment of imported fire ant stings. J Am Acad Dermatol 1987;16:1189–1192.

104. Russell FE: Arachnid envenomations. Emerg Med Services 1991;20;16–24.

105. Russell FE: Venomous animal injuries. Curr Prob Pediatr 1973;3:1–47.

106. Russell FE, Gertsch WJ: Arthropod bites. Toxicon 1983;21:337–339.

107. Russell FE, Marcus P, Streng JA: Black widow spider envenomation during pregnancy—report of a case. Toxicon 1979;17:188.

108. Schanbacher FL, Lee CK, Wilson IB, et al: Composition and properties of tarantula *Dugesiella henzi* (Girard) venom. Toxicon 1973;11:21–29.

109. Schanbacher FL, Lee CK, Wilson IR, et al: Purification and characterization of tarantula *Dugesiella henzi* venom hyaluronidase. Comp Biochem Physiol 1973;44:389–396.

110. Schaumburg HH, Herskovitz S: The weak child—a cautionary tale. N Engl J Med 2000;342:127–129.

111. Schkenderov S, Koburova K: Adolapin—a newly isolated analgetic and anti-inflammatory polypeptide from bee venom. Toxicon 1982;20:317–321.

112. Smith CW, Micks DW: The role of polymorphonuclear leukocytes in the lesion caused by the venom of the brown spider, *Loxosceles reclusa*. Lab Invest 1970;22:90–93.

113. Stafford CT, Hoffman DR, Rhoades RB: Allergy to imported fire ants. South Med J 1989;82:1520–1527.

114. Stafford CT: Hypersensitivity to fire ant venom. Ann Allergy Asthma Immunol 1996;77:87–99.

115. Stewart C, Roberge R, Lawler H, eds: Emergency management of arachnid envenomations: Spider bites and scorpion stings. Emerg Med Rep 1993;14:75–82.

116. Stipetic ME, Rosen PB, Borys DJ: A retrospective analysis of 96 "asp" (*Megalopyge opercularis*) envenomations in central Texas during 1996. J Toxicol Clin Toxicol 1999;37:457–462.

117. Strain GM, Snider TG, Tedford B, et al: Hyperbaric oxygen effects on brown recluse spider (*Loxosceles reclusa*) envenomation in rabbits. Toxicon 1991;29:989–996.

118. Sutherland SK: Treatment of arachnid poisoning in Australia. Aust Fam Physician 1990;19:50–61.

119. Sutherland SK, Trinca JC: Survey of 2144 cases of red-back spider bites. Med J Aust 1978;2:620–623.

120. Szeto TH, Wang XH, Smith R, et al: Isolation of a funnel-web spider polypeptide with homology to mamba intestinal toxin 1 and the embryonic head inducer Dickkopf-1. Toxicon 2000;38:429–442.

121. Tagwireyi D, Ball DE, Loga PJ, Moyo S: Cantharidin poisoning due to "blister beetle" ingestion. Toxicon 2000;38:1865–1869.

122. Thorp RW, Woodson WD: Black Widow, America's Most Poisonous Spider. Chapel Hill, North Carolina Press, 1945.

123. Till JS, Majmudar BN: Cantharidin poisoning. South Med J 1981;74:444–447.

124. Todd JL: Tick bite in British Columbia. Can Med Assoc J 1912;2:1118–1119.

125. Toewe CH: Bug bites and stings. Am Fam Physician 1980;21:90–95.

126. Trestrail JH: Poisonous spiders and spider bite poisonings: Bites and stings of poisonous insects. Unpublished monograph.

127. Verheyden CN: Snakebite and spider bite. Hosp Physician 1988;24:21–32.

128. Vest DK: Envenomation by *Tegenaria agrestis* (Walckenaer) spiders. Toxicon 1987;25:221.

129. Vest DK: Necrotic arachnidism in the northwestern United States and its probable relationship to *Tegenaria agrestis* (Walckenaer) spiders. Toxicon 1987;25:175.

130. Wasserman G: Wound care of spider and snake envenomations. Ann Emerg Med 1988;17:1331–1335.

131. Wasserman GS, Kunkel D: Venomous bites and stings. J Toxicol Clin Toxicol 1984;21:417–502.

132. Williams ST, Khare VK, Johnston GA, et al: Severe intravascular hemolysis associated with brown recluse spider envenomation. Am J Clin Pathol 1995;104:463–467.

133. Yarbrough BE: Current treatment of brown recluse spider bites. Curr Concepts Wound Care 1987;10:4–6.

134. Youlten LJ, Atkinson BA, Lee TH: The incidence and nature of adverse reactions to injection immunotherapy in bee and wasp venom allergy. Clin Exp Allergy 1995;25:159–165.

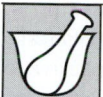 ## ANTIDOTES IN DEPTH

Antivenom (Scorpion and Spider)
Jeffrey N. Bernstein

Antivenom for spiders and scorpions is prepared by immunizing animals with venom and then collecting the immune serum for administration. Monkeys, horses, goats, sheep, chicken, and rabbits have been used as sources of antivenom. The animals are placed on an immunization schedule to allow production of immunoglobulins, mostly specific IgG. Optimal antibody production typically takes about 6 weeks. The choice of animal used to make an immune serum is more often dictated by the availability of a species, financial considerations, and tradition than by scientific modeling. Although manufacturers may state that a specific animal gives a "cleaner" (ie, less immunogenic) product, no studies have compared immune sera of different animals for human compatability or tolerance.

The terms *antivenom* and *antivenin* have been used interchangeably. Wyeth, the maker of Crotalid and Micrurus antivenom, and Merck and Co., the makers of Latrodectus antivenom, have adopted *antivenin* as part of the brand name for their products. Brand name recognition of the term antivenin has largely been responsible for the use of this term in place of antivenom. Except where it refers to a specific brand name, the term antivenom is used in this Antidote in Depth and throughout this textbook.

The exact identity of the species of arachnid that attacks its victim is rarely known in the clinical setting. A specimen of the spider or scorpion is not usually available. The species is usually inferred from geographic distribution. For example, black widow envenomations that occur in southern Arizona are presumed to be from *Latrodectus hesperus* rather than *L. mactans*. Occasionally, stings or bites have resulted from scorpions or spiders in imported oriental rugs and fruit. The clinician must also be aware that professional and amateur entomologists may be exposed to bites or stings from exotic species, although, in these instances, the genus of the arachnid, or even the common name, is often known.

CENTRUROIDES EXILICAUDA

Centruroides species is the only scorpion of medical importance in the United States. It is indigenous to the desert southwest of Arizona but has been reported to inhabit Texas, New Mexico, California, and Nevada as well.[5] Occasionally, envenomations occur in nonindigenous areas of the country from "stowaway" scorpions in the luggage of travelers.[21]

The two poison centers in Arizona receive between 2000 and 3000 calls annually for scorpion envenomations. At one time the mortality from scorpion envenomation in this country was twice as high as that of all other venomous animals combined.[14] Although the incidence remains high, no deaths associated with the toxic effects of scorpion venom have been reported for more than 35 years. One recent death, however, of a 62-year-old woman, was likely secondary to an anaphylactic reaction to scorpion venom.[12] The low incidence of fatalities is attributable to the development of pediatric intensive care and better methods of supportive care as well as the use of antivenom.

Antivenom for this species of scorpion was produced in Mexico, in horses, as early as the 1930s.[6] In 1947, antivenom was produced from rabbits and cats immunized with *C. sculpturatus* and *C. gertschi*.[18] The Antivenom Production Laboratory at Arizona State University (APL-ASU) began producing antivenom to *C. sculpturatus* in goats in 1965, and this product continues to be the antivenom in use for treatment of scorpion stings in Arizona. Currently, production of the APL-ASU antivenom has ceased, and it is estimated that the current repository of antivenom should last until the year 2004. Because no FDA approval exists for this product, its use is restricted to the state of Arizona, where it is supplied free of charge to hospitals for compassionate use. Its transport across state lines is prohibited.

Efficacy of the APL-ASU antivenom is demonstrated in both animals and humans.[2,3,6] In a study of 15 children below age 11 years, 12 patients receiving antivenom had resolution of neurologic, respiratory, and cardiovascular symptoms within 3 hours of initiating therapy. In those patients who did not receive antivenom therapy, symptoms lasted 15 to 24 hours.[10]

A prospective evaluation of the incidence of immediate and delayed hypersensitivity to *Centruroides* antivenom found the incidence of immediate hypersenitivity to be 3.4%, much lower than previously reported.[3,10] The incidence of delayed allergic reaction or serum sickness was 61%, which was consistent with previous reports.

In view of the limited mortality from envenomation and the risk of serious immediate hypersensitivity or serum sickness from the administration of antivenom, there is rarely, if ever, an absolute indication for administration of scorpion antivenom. Administration of antivenom is, therefore, reserved for patients with the most severe scorpion envenomations, typically in children under age 6. A four-level severity grading of scorpion envenomation has been described (see Table 102–6).[6] Administration of antivenom is recommended for patients with grades III or IV systemic toxicity. It should be noted, however, that these same symptoms can also be successfully managed in an intensive care setting with aggressive airway management, monitoring, and benzodiazepine infusions. Geographic and financial factors also may favor the administration of antivenom. Transport times to hospitals equipped for appropriate pediatric intensive care in the southwest desert are often long and, in addition, may require costly air transportation. The ability to administer an effective antidote in a remote emergency department may limit expense or delay in achieving appropriate care. The decision to administer antivenom should be based on an analysis of the potential risks and benefits. Before administration of antivenom, an appropriate allergy history should be taken. A history of allergy to antiserum or to animal products is not a contraindication to antivenom administration; however, patients or their guardians should be cautioned of possible adverse reactions. Informed consent should be obtained.

Scorpion antivenom was formerly supplied as lyophilized serum and may occasionally be found in hospitals in this form. Currently it is shipped from APL-ASU to the hospital as fresh immune serum. Each vial contains 5 mL of serum for intravenous use over 15 to 30 minutes. Experience with crotaline antivenom, however, suggests that more dilute concentrations given over a longer time period may be better tolerated by patients and may produce fewer acute allergic reactions. More severely envenomated patients will require faster infusion rates. Acute or delayed allergic reactions occur in approximately 3.4 to 85% of patients receiving antivenom therapy.[3,6,10]

Serum sickness, or type III hypersensitivity, may occur in as many as 61 to 85% of patients.[6,10] Experience with crotaline antivenom suggests that the risk of serum sickness is directly correlated with the number of vials of antivenom received. Serum sickness typically occurs within 2 weeks of antivenom administration.

The Mexico-Pharma Polyvalent Scorpion Antivenom may also be effective against North American *Centruroides* stings; however, there is no known reliable repository of this antivenom in the United States.[1] Although antibody fragments (Fab) were developed from immune goat serum for the treatment of *Centruroides*, they are not commercially available.[2] Recently, Orphan Pharmaceutical U.S. (OPUS) together with Bioclon received orphan drug status from the FDA for their product Alacramyn, an Fab$_2$. Bioclon, is a Mexican-based company that has substantial but unpublished clinical experience with the use of Fab$_2$ for treatment of Mexican *Centruroides*. A listing of scorpion antivenoms available throughout the world is presented in Table 102–9.[20] Individual patient risk factors such as known sensitivity to antivenom or specific animal products and allergy to conventional medications should be considered in the decision to utilize any of these antivenom products.

LATRODECTUS SPECIES (L. MACTANS, L. HESPERUS, L. BISHOPI, L. GEOMETRICUS)

The administration of the black widow spider antivenom is also controversial. Although black widow envenomation is associated with severe muscle pain and cramping and autonomic distur-

bances,[4,9] mortality is low. Indications for antivenom administration include severe muscle cramping, hypertension, diaphoresis, nausea, vomiting, and respiratory difficulty that is unresponsive to other therapy (Chap. 102). Pregnancy is also suggested as a possible indication for antivenom administration.[17] Symptomatic treatment can almost always be accomplished with muscle relaxants and opioids individually or in combination. Some authors believe that antivenom has too high a risk-to-benefit ratio to justify its use.[16] In selected patients, however, the use of antivenom may reduce pain and suffering, shorten the course of the envenomation, and reduce or eliminate the need for hospitalization.

Antivenin (Merck and Co.) for black widow venom (*Latrodectus mactans*) is made by immunizing horses. Each vial of antivenin contains 6000 antivenin units standardized by biologic assay in mice. Because the venoms of *Latrodectus* species are virtually identical by immunologic and electrophoretic mechanisms, *Latrodectus mactans*–derived antivenom is presumed to be effective in other species of *Latrodectus* as well.[11] A recent shortage of antivenin (Merck and Co.) prompted the discovery that antivenom against *Latrodectus hasseltii*, the redback spider of Australia, also neutralizes venom of *Latrodectus mactans* in a mouse model.[7] In a review of 163 cases of *Latrodectus* envenomation (presumed *Latrodectus hesperus*), antivenom reduced the duration of symptoms from a mean of 22 hours to a mean of 9 hours. Symptoms usually subside within 1 to 3 hours of administration of the antivenom. Hospital admission rate fell from 52% in those who were managed with opioids and muscle relaxants to 12% in those patients receiving antivenom.[4] Delayed administration of antivenom is also effective, even when given as late as 90 hours after envenomation.[13,19]

Dosage of *antivenin* (Merck and Co.) is usually the contents of one reconstituted vial (2.5 mL) diluted in 50 mL of saline for intravenous administration. Black widow antivenom can also be given IM; however, this route carries the disadvantage of slower, more erratic absorption, less control over the rate of administration, and the inability to stop administration of the drug should an allergic reaction occur. For these reasons, the intramuscular route is not recommended.

Despite the apparent efficacy of antivenom, the decision to give horse serum for a disease with limited mortality is of great

TABLE 102–9. **Antivenoms Available Worldwide**

Scorpion	Antivenin
Androctonus	France—Pasteur Merieux antiscorption venom serum
Buthotus	Iran—scorpion antivenom
Buthus occitanus	France—Pasteur Merieux antiscorpion venom serum
	Germany—Twyford scorpion
Buthus gibbosusbrulla	Turkey—anti-scorpion antivenom
Centruroides (elegans, limpidus, noxius, suffusus)	Mexico—Pharma polyvalent scorpion antivenom
Euscorpius (carpathicus, italicus)	Turkey—anti-scorpion antivenom
Leiurus quinquestreatus	France—Pasteur Merieux antiscorpion antivenom
	Israel—Leiurus quinquestriatus
	Turkey—anti-scorpion antivenom
Mesobuthus eupeus	Iran—scorpion antivenom
Odontobuthus doriae	Iran—scorpion antivenom
Parabuthus species	South African—scorpion antivenom
Scorpio maurus	Iran—scorpion antivenom
	Turkey—anti-scorpion antivenom

Reprinted, with permission, from Theakston RDG, Warrell DA: *Antivenoms: a list of hyperimmune sera currently available for the treatment of envenoming by bites and stings.* Toxicon 1991;29:1419–1470.

concern. Death from bronchospasm and anaphylaxis is reported as a complication of antivenom administration, as is serum sickness.[4] Black widow antivenom is listed as a Pregnancy Category C agent.

LOXOSCELES SPP. (L. RECLUSA, L. LAETA, L. REFUSCENS, L. ARIZONICA, L. UNICOLOR)

Envenomation by the brown recluse spider, *Loxosceles reclusa,* although low in mortality, is a significant source of morbidity, particularly in the southeast United States. Antivenom to *L. reclusa* was produced in rabbits. Antivenom is effective if given before the onset of necrosis, usually within the first 24 to 48 hours.[15] Anti-*Loxosceles* Fab blocks dermonecrosis in a rabbit model, but only if given within 4 hours of envenomation.[8] Comparisons, however, do not reveal significant differences between dapsone- and antivenom-treated animals[15] and suggest that a combination may be the best therapy.[5] No commercially available antivenom exists for the treatment of *Loxosceles* envenomation.

SUMMARY

Controversy exists over the indication for antivenom administration in both spider and scorpion envenomations. Consideration should be given to the known efficacy of the antivenom, the relative morbidity and mortality of the disease, the risk of giving a foreign immune serum, the level of available supportive care, the cost of supportive care, and the cost of obtaining or importing antivenom.

REFERENCES

1. Antivenom Index. The American Zoo and Aquarium Association and The American Association of Poison Control Centers, 1994.
2. Bernstein JN, Dart RC, Garcia R, et al: Efficacy of antiscorpion (*Centruroides exilicauda*) Fab in a mouse model [abstract]. Vet Hum Toxicol 1994;36:346.
3. Bond RG: Antivenin administration for *Centruroides* scorpion sting: risks and benefits. Ann Emerg Med 1992;21:788–791.
4. Clark RF, Werthern-Kestner S, Vance MV, Gerkin R: Clinical presentation and treatment of black widow spider envenomation: a review of 163 cases. Ann Emerg Med 1992;21:782–787.
5. Cole HP 3rd, Wesley RE, King LE Jr: Brown recluse spider envenomation of the eyelid: An animal model. Ophthalm Plastic Reconstruct Surg 1995;11:153–164.
6. Curry SC, Vance MV, Ryan PJ, et al: Envenomation by the scorpion *Centruroides sculpturatus.* J Toxicol Clin Toxicol 1983–1984;21:417–449.
7. Daly FFS, Hill RE, Bogdan GM, Dart RC: Neutralization of *Latrodectus hesperus* venom by antivenom raised against *Latrodectus hasseltii* in a murine model [abstract]. Ann Emerg Med 2000;35:S57
8. Gomez HF, Miller MJ, Trach JW, et al: Intradermal anti-loxosceles Fab fragments attenuate dermonecrotic arachnidism. Acad Emerg Med 1999;6:1195–1202.
9. Kobernick M: Black widow spider bite. Am Fam Physician 1984;29:241–245.
10. LoVecchio F, Welch S, Klemens J, et al: Incidence of immediate and delayed hypersensitivity to *Centruroides* antivenom. Ann Emerg Med 1999;34:615–619.
11. McCrone JD, Netzcoff ML: An immunological and electrophoretical comparison of the venoms of the North American *Latrodectus* spiders. Toxicon 1965;3:107–110.
12. McNally J, Arizona Poison and Drug Information Center, personal communication.
13. O'Malley, Dart RC, Kuffner EF: Successful treatment of latrodectism with antivenin after 90 hours [correspondence]. N Engl J Med 1999;340:657.
14. Rachesky IJ, Banner W, Dansky J, Tong T: Treatments for *Centruroides exilicauda* envenomation. Am J Dis Child 1984;138:1136–1139.
15. Rees R, Campbell D, Rieger E, King LE: The diagnosis and treatment of brown recluse spider bites. Ann Emerg Med 1987;16:945–949.
16. Robertson WO: Black widow spider case. Am J Emerg Med 1997;15:211.
17. Russell FE, Marcus P, Streng JA: Black widow spider envenomation during pregnancy. Toxicon 1979;17:188–189.
18. Schnur L, Schnur P: A case of allergy to scorpion antivenin. Ariz Med 1968;25:413–414.
19. Suntorntham S, Roberts JR, Nilsen GJ: Dramatic clinical response to the delayed administration of black widow spider antivenom. Ann Emerg Med 1994;24:1198–1199.
20. Theakston RDG, Warrell DA: Antivenoms: A list of hyperimmune sera currently available for the treatment of envenoming by bites and stings. Toxicon 1991;29:1419–1470.
21. Trestrail JH: Scorpion envenomation in Michigan: Three cases of toxic encounters with poisonous stow-aways. Vet Hum Toxicol 1981;23:8–11.

CHAPTER 103 MARINE ENVENOMATIONS

Richard S. Weisman

A 28-year-old man was stung on the lateral surface of his right hand by a lionfish when he reached into his tropical fish aquarium to adjust the aerator. Within seconds he experienced severe pain and swelling of his hand. On route to the hospital the patient applied an ice pack. In the emergency department he was awake, alert, and in considerable distress. His vital signs were: blood pressure 150/90 mm Hg, pulse 110 beats/min, respiratory rate 18 breaths/min, and temperature 98.6°F (37°C) (orally).

There were three small linear puncture marks, approximately 8 mm apart, on the lateral surface of the patient's right hand. The hand was swollen and erythematous with a normal neurovascular examination.

The hand was immersed in water that had been heated to 110°F (43.3°C). This resulted in pain relief within 5 minutes. The pain recurred, however, when the water cooled to room temperature. The patient received a diphtheria-tetanus toxoid vaccination and was discharged 4 hours after arrival. No systemic signs had developed, and his pain was significantly relieved. He was instructed to take ibuprofen, 400 mg every 6 hours, for pain and to have his hand examined by his private physician the next day.

HISTORY AND EPIDEMIOLOGY

During the last quarter of the 20th century, sport diving and other water-related activities became increasingly popular, resulting in a significant increase in the incidence of marine envenomations.[45] Worldwide, there are an estimated 40,000 to 50,000 marine envenomations each year.[50] Internationally, marine envenomations are recognized as a significant risk for swimmers in open-water athletic events.[26] For athletes swimming off the coast of Australia, these are a significant cause of mortality.[20] Table 103–1 lists the most common etiologies of painful marine envenomations, along with characteristic symptoms and therapy. The healthcare provider must be prepared to care for patients with a variety of marine-related maladies ranging from dermatitis to life-threatening allergic reactions, trauma, and envenomations.[4,10]

The marine organisms that are capable of causing harm to humans can be divided into the vertebrates and invertebrates, some of which are swimmers and some nonswimmers. Because of their strength and mobility, the vertebrates are capable of inflicting more structural damage than the often passive invertebrates. However, the potential morbidity and even mortality that can result from contact with venomous and nonvenomous invertebrates should not be underestimated.

Among the most frequently reported vertebrate envenomations are those caused by stingrays, catfish, scorpionfish (Scorpaenidae), and leatherjacks.[57] In the United States, most Scorpaenidae stings reported to poison centers are the result of lionfish exposures in home aquaria.[40] The stingray (class: Chondrichthyes; order: Rajiformes) is responsible for approximately 1800 envenomations each year, primarily along the west coast of the United States.[3]

Among the invertebrates, the coelenterates, echinoderms, annelid worms, and mollusks are recognized as frequent causes of marine envenomations.[57] The Coelenterata are responsible for more marine envenomations than any other phylum.[36]

GENERAL PATHOPHYSIOLOGY

Many creatures of the sea have improved their odds of surviving the natural evolutionary process by developing elaborate apparatuses both to deliver venom to their prey and to limit the risk of falling victim to their predators. These venoms are typically complex mixtures of high-molecular-weight proteins and low-molecular-weight compounds containing histamine, bradykinin, and indole derivatives.[29,33,39,54,62,64] They produce pain, degranulate mast cells, interfere with cellular transport and metabolism, disrupt neuronal transmission, and cause myocardial depression.[4]

Vertebrates

Stingray Eleven different species of rays are found in US coastal waters.[48] Stingrays can often be distinguished from other fish by having gills exclusively located on the ventral surfaces of their bodies.[29] The stingray is armed with a tail barb that will reflexively impact on anything with which it comes in to contact. Stingrays tend to burrow into the sand, where divers may unintentionally step on them. The long serrated spines on the dorsum of the stingray's tail can easily penetrate human flesh and produce a deep, jagged laceration, most commonly on a lower extremity.[52] Severe trauma may occur without envenomation. Although uncommon, fatalities have been attributed to stingrays, with chest injuries, exsanguination, and tetanus.[19] More common extremity injuries result in deep ulcers at the wound site and secondary bacterial infections.[8]

The venom isolated from the stingray contains a mixture of phosphodiesterase, 5'-nucleotidase, and serotonin.[28] When stingray venom is experimentally administered to animals, it causes peripheral vasoconstriction, bradycardia, conduction abnormalities, respiratory depression, ataxia, and seizures.[54]

TABLE 103–1. Organisms Responsible for Painful Marine Envenomations

Organism	Common Signs/Symptoms	Treatment

Pterois
  Lionfish
  Turkeyfish
  Zebrafish
  Tigerfish
  Scorpionfish
	Pain, swelling	Warm water, analgesics, digital block

Synanceja Stonefish	Pain, swelling, hypotension, dysrhythmias	Warm water, analgesics, digital block, antivenom
Trachinus Weeverfish	Pain, swelling, nausea, edema vomiting, diaphoresis, hypotension seizures, dysrhythmias	Analgesics, digital block

Dasyatis
  urolophus
  Stingray
	Pain, deep ulcerated wound, muscle cramping, weakness, hypotension, syncope, dysrhythmias, seizures	Warm water, analgesics, antibiotics

Sea snakes
  Enhydrina
    schistosa
  Hydrophis
    ornatus
  H. cyanocinctus
  Lapemis
    hardwickii
  Pelamis platurus
  Thalassophina
    viperina
  Aipysurus laevis
	Pain, swelling, neuropathies, paralysis, respiratory failure, myonecrosis, renal failure	Analgesics, IV hydration, antivenom

Coelenterata
  Jellyfish
  Sea anemones
  Corals
  Hydroids
	Pain, burning, urticaria lymphadenopathy, anaphylaxis	5% acetic acid, remove tentacles, papain tenderizer, analgesics, antihistamines

Physalia
  Portuguese
    man-of-war
	Pain, burning, urticaria lymphadenopathy, anaphylaxis	5% acetic acid, remove tentacles, papain tenderizer, analgesics, antihistamines

Millepora Fire coral	Pain, burning, urticaria, intense pruritis	5% acetic acid, remove tentacles, corticosteroids

Acanthaster
  Crown of thorns
Diadema
  Sea urchins
	Pain, erythema, nausea, vomiting, syncope, ataxia, paresthesias, muscle cramps, respiratory distress	Warm water, surgical removal of spines, analgesia

The wound will often initially appear cyanotic or dusky and subsequently becomes erythematous, hemorrhagic, and then necrotic.[8] The pain is usually out of proportion to the amount of visible tissue injury. Most human victims experience severe pain and burning, which may intensify for several hours after the sting. When systemic effects occur, they may include muscle cramping, weakness, tremor, syncope, hypotension, cardiovascular collapse, convulsions, and paralysis.

Treatment of stingray stings consists of thorough wound cleansing and debridement, tetanus prophylaxis, irrigation of the wound to remove as much venom as possible, and treatment of infection should it develop. The bacterial flora that has been cultured from marine animals, sea water, and ocean sediment is diverse. Antibiotic therapy should address infections by *Vibrio* species in general and *Vibrio vulnificus* specifically.[34,37] A third-generation cephalosporin is generally considered to be appropriate.[47] Pain control may be achieved by immersing the affected limb in hot water 110 to 115°F (43.3–46.1°C), but systemic analgesia may also be required.

Scorpaenidae The Scorpaenidae (class Osteichthyes; order Perciformes) are the most common vertebrates that sting humans. The most dangerous members of the Scorpaenidae family, *Pterois* (lionfish, turkeyfish, zebrafish, tigerfish, scorpionfish) and *Synanceja horrida* (stonefish), are almost exclusively found in the Gulf of Mexico and Pacific and Indian oceans.

Within the Scorpaenidae family, the stonefish (*Synanceja horrida*) is most likely to be responsible for serious injury.[63] Their venom glands are located near the tips of their spines, which is ideal for delivering large amounts of venom. This camouflaged fish can be found in coral reefs or among the algae. Unlike most of the other venomous fish, the stonefish prefers to attack humans rather than to swim away.

The major component of venom from the stonefish (*Synanceja verrucosa*) is verrucotoxin, a high-molecular-weight (150,000 Da), heat-labile, antigenic, nondialyzable protein.[64] In addition, the stonefish venom contains norepinephrine, dopamine, and tryptophan,[23] which may be responsible for the observed cardiotoxicity.[22] Stonustoxin, which is also isolated from the stonefish (*Synanceja horrida*), results in significant hypotension, which is mediated through activation of the nitric oxide pathway.[27] In addition stonustoxin has a widely studied cytolytic effect in animal studies. The hemolytic activity of stonustoxin is secondary to pore formation in the cell membrane.[15,38,66] An experimental monoclonal antibody against stonustoxin demonstrates hematoprotective effects in mice.[67] The stonefish venom appears to be directly myotoxic. The pain caused by the envenomation is so excruciating that it may cause a diver to lose consciousness. The pain will continue to intensify for several hours after the initial sting. Other localized symptoms from scorpaenid envenomations may include erythema and ecchymosis, induration, hyperesthesia, anesthesia or dysesthesia of the affected limb, and, subsequently, lymphadenopathy. Early systemic manifestations include nausea, vomiting, diaphoresis, dyspnea, hypotension, and syncope. More severe systemic manifestations may occur in patients with more significant envenomations and can include cardiac dysrhythmias, conduction abnormalities, myocardial ischemia, pulmonary edema, convulsions, and paralysis.[29]

Lionfish are among the most beautiful of reef fish; their long curved dorsal spines are ornately covered with a lacy tissue that allows them to corner their prey before suddenly lunging. Lionfish do not normally attack humans unless they become cornered without an escape route. When attacking, they erect their dorsal, anal, and pectoral spines and make quick thrusting jabs at their pray (or an intruder).

The venom glands of the lionfish (*Pterois* species) are smaller than the glands of the stonefish (*Synanceja* species). The *Pterois* venom consists of a complex mixture of inflammatory mediators including prostaglandin $F_{2\alpha}$, thromboxane B_2, and prostaglandin E_2.[6] Victims experience severe burning pain and swelling within seconds of contact with the spines. The serious cardiovascular effects that may result from stonefish envenomations are less commonly observed after lionfish envenomation.

The weeverfish (order: Perciformes; family: Trachinidae) inhabits the muddy- or sandy-bottomed bays within the temperate zones of the eastern Atlantic Ocean, Mediterranean Sea, and European coastal waters.[30] The relatively small fish (10–50 cm) often burrows into the ocean bottom, leaving only its head visible. Most envenomations occur when a diver or fisherman steps on the fish. The fish has sharp dorsal and opercular spines that are capable of penetrating a leather boot. Venom-containing glandular tissue surrounds the spines in a thin integumentary sheath.[13]

The venom of the weeverfish, which has not been completely characterized, consists of several peptides, high-molecular-weight proteins, mucopolysaccharides, serotonin, epinephrine, norepinephrine, and histamine.[53] Following envenomation, the victim will experience a burning or crushing pain that increases in intensity as it spreads through the limb. The wound site appears edematous, erythematous, and ecchymotic. The edema may involve the entire affected limb and may persist for months after the sting.[30] The systemic manifestations that occur with weeverfish envenomations include headache, fever, chills, nausea, vomiting, diaphoresis, hypotension, seizures, and cardiac dysrhythmias.[13]

The intensity of pain experienced by victims of Scorpaenidae envenomations can be extremely variable and probably reflects both the amount of venom injected and the depth of the injury. Treatment for Scorpaenidae envenomations should include soaking the affected limb in water heated to 110 to 115°F (43.3–46.1°C). If the patient fails to improve within minutes after placement of the limb in warm water, an oral analgesic will be needed. Mild to moderate pain will respond to an oral or parenteral nonsteroidal antiinflammatory drug, but severe pain should be treated with a parenteral opioid analgesic. The administration of a digital nerve block with 0.25% bupivacaine was successfully used in a patient with refractory pain.[24] If spines or barbs have broken off in the envenomated tissue, they must be removed. This can often be accomplished with forceps and a magnifying lens. Tetanus immune status should evaluated, and antibiotics should be considered as above. Blisters that form at the site of the envenomation should be surgically excised. The fluid aspirated from blisters following a lionfish envenomation contains high concentrations of prostaglandins $F_{2\alpha}$ and E_2 and thromboxane B_2. An antivenom is available from the health services departments of most of the major aquaria throughout the United States. The antivenom is most often required for victims of stonefish envenomations in whom life-threatening systemic toxicity has developed or is developing.

Sea Snakes There are more than 50 species of sea snakes, the most common reptile found in the ocean. Sea snakes are found in the Pacific and Indian oceans, commonly along the coast of Southeast Asia, the Malay Archipelago, and the Persian Gulf, and account for approximately 150 deaths each year.[19] There are no sea snakes in the Atlantic Ocean or Caribbean Sea. All species of sea snakes are toxic, and seven are reportedly fatal to man.[3] These include: *Astrotia stokesii, Enhydrina schistosa, Hydrophis ornatus* and *H. cyanocinctus, Lapemis hardwickii, Pelamus platurus,* and *Thalassophina viperina.* Most of the snakes range from 3 to 4 feet in length, but some may be considerably longer.[46]

The majority of sea snake bites do not result in envenomation because the snake's fangs are short and easily dislodged.[21] In one review, a 90% incidence of dry bites was reported.[19] The venom is a peripheral neurotoxin that alters sodium and chloride permeability without affecting the Na^+-K^+-ATPase pump.[25] Phospholipases, nerve growth factor, capillary permeability factor, anticomplement-active factor, acetylcholinesterase, hyaluronidase, leucine aminopeptidase, 5′-nucleotidase, and several hemolytic and myotoxic compounds have also been identified in the venom.[3] Animal studies of olive sea snake venom demonstrate nephrotoxicity in mice.[56]

The symptoms that follow a sea snake envenomation typically occur in the absence of a local reaction. Commonly, 3 to 6 hours after envenomation the patient develops both cranial and peripheral neurologic abnormalities including paralysis and respiratory failure, myonecrosis, myoglobinuria, and renal failure.[46] The olive sea snake (*Aipysurus laevis*) differs from others in that its venom is primarily myopathic, although it also causes paralysis and respiratory failure.[21]

The treatment of sea snake envenomations is similar to the care of terrestrial snake bites (see Chap. 101). Emphasis should be placed on stabilization of the patient's vital signs. Pulmonary and renal function must be carefully monitored. With any evidence of an envenomation, polyvalent sea snake antivenom should be administered (Commonwealth Serum Laboratories, Melbourne, Australia). This equine-derived immunoglobulin is prepared against two of the more common sea snake venoms, *Enhydrina schistosa* and *Notechis scutatis*.[9] However, it is believed to have activity against most of the other sea snake venoms as well.

Invertebrates

Coelenterata (Jellyfish, Sea Anemones, Corals, and Hydroids)

There are approximately 9000 species in the phylum Coelenterata, of which several hundred are dangerous to man. The phylum is characterized by a unique gastrovascular cavity that has a single opening for both digestion and circulation. Most of the marine life within this phylum contain stinging structures called nematocysts (cnidocytes). These poisonous dartlike structures are tightly coiled and enclosed within their venom sacs. Following external contact, the nematocysts are shot out of their containment sacs, injecting their venom as they penetrate the flesh of their prey. In general, the nematocyst venom is a complex mixture containing bradykinin, hemolysin, serotonin, histamine, prostaglandins, adenosine triphosphatase, nucleotidases, hyaluronidase, alkaline and acid proteases, alkaline and acid phosphatases, phosphodiesterases, fibrinolysin, leucine aminopeptidase, RNase, and DNase.[12] Nematocysts extracted from the sea nettle jellyfish contains large amounts of leukotriene B_4, which, with a corresponding high neutrophil chemotactic activity, is responsible for the local wheals at the sting site.[16] The jellyfish also produces polypeptides that are highly toxic to human hepatocytes.[14] Isolated jellyfish tissue free of nematocysts has cytolytic and hemolytic effects in vitro.[1] The sea anemone (*Actinia equina*) produces equinatoxin II, which also demonstrates cytolytic properties.[2,43]

Jellyfish travel in groups called smucks, which may contain more than a thousand individual jellyfish. The jellyfish has long tentacles that hang down from an air-filled pneumatophore. The tentacles contain hundreds of thousands of nematocysts, each containing a small amount of venom. Most of the members of this family are capable of incapacitating small fish or other marine life, but to humans they typically cause only a painful sting. Subsequently, a severe burning sensation followed by erythematous or violaceous lesions and regional lymph node involvement occur. More significant envenomations may lead to ulceration with a delayed healing phase. Anaphylactoid reactions manifested by bronchospasm, dysrhythmias, hypotension, and cardiovascular collapse can occur. Erythema nodosum and arthralgias are also reported.[5]

The Portuguese man-of-war (*Physalia*) is a well-known, pale-blue, bell-shaped inhabitant of the waters along the Florida coast in both the Atlantic Ocean and the Gulf of Mexico.[59] The Portuguese man-of-war is most commonly found close to shore between July and September following severe tropical storms. Tentacles of the Portuguese man-of-war may trail as far as 10 feet behind the body. The almost invisible tentacles contain nematocysts that can release a neurotoxic venom capable of causing excruciating pain. Subsequently, linear red papules and large erythematous welts develop. Envenomations may be accompanied by nausea, vomiting, myalgia, headache, chills, respiratory distress, and cardiovascular collapse.[36] When multiple stings are inflicted on the victim, death may ensue. Tentacles dislodged in turbulent water may remain capable of discharging nematocysts for a significant time after detachment.

The sea wasp or box jellyfish (*Chironex fleckeri*) is the most venomous and deadly of all stinging marine life. It is found predominantly in the Australian and Southeast Asian waters but can also be found in the open ocean.[58] The sea wasp, like the Portuguese man-of-war, often rides the current of the tide. Each box jellyfish carries enough venom to kill several adults. At least 72 fatalities have been attributed to the box jellyfish in waters off the coast of Australia and Southeast Asia.[19,65] The overall fatality rate for envenomation is estimated to approach 20%. The sting from a sea wasp may result in hypotension, profound muscle spasm, respiratory paralysis, and cardiac arrest. Death has occurred within 30 seconds of envenomation.[32]

A single strategy can be used for the management of most nematocyst envenomations. If nematocysts are still present on the surface of the skin, they should be inactivated with a 5% solution of acetic acid (vinegar). Following inactivation, nematocysts are best removed by applying shaving cream to the area, then shaving the site with the dull edge of a knife or the edge of a credit card. Health care providers should wear gloves to prevent being stung by any nematocysts remaining on the victim's skin. The shaving cream surrounds the nematocysts during the scraping process preventing recontact with the patient and facilitating removal.

However, for *Chrysaora quinquecirrha* (American sea nettle), *Pelagia noctiluca* (little mauve stinger jellyfish), and *Cyanea captillata* (hair or "lion's mane" jellyfish), application of vinegar may precipitate firing of the nematocyst. In these species a slurry of baking soda should be applied for 10 minutes. It has been suggested that fresh water or alcohol (isopropanol or ethanol) should be avoided, as both may cause a discharge of the nematocysts already present on the skin surface. Alcohols do not destroy or deactivate nematocysts and are therefore not recommended. Knowing when *Chrysaora quinquecirrha*, *Pelagia noctiluca*, and *Cyanea captillata* are responsible for an envenomation requires a knowledge of the local fauna. Unfortunately, these species are often not recognized to be present in a region until several patients have failed to improve or have worsened with the use of 5% acetic acid.

Papain (meat tenderizer) may be effective in destroying any remaining nematocysts.[41] If tentacles remain attached to the skin, shaving cream, baking soda, or flour may be applied over the tentacles. After a few minutes, a dull knife or any available firm object (such as the side of a credit card) should be scraped across the skin to carefully dislodge the nematocysts. Fresh water should never be used to flush the affected areas, as a change in osmotic pressure can cause all of the remaining inactivated stinging cells to discharge.

If the wound has a high risk of secondary infection, the patient should be treated with a third-generation cephalosporin.[47] Patients should receive tetanus prophylaxis based on their previous immunization history. Pruritus may respond well to antihistamines or corticosteroids.

A sheep-derived *Chironex* antivenom is available for victims of sea wasp envenomations (Commonwealth Serum Laboratory, Australia). This antivenom is best administered intravenously (one ampule, 20,000 units, diluted 1:5 to 1:10 in isotonic crystalloid) over a 5-minute period[39] and may be readministered every 2 hours until there is no further progression of symptoms. Antivenom has proven efficacy in preventing acute pain and cardiovascular symptoms.

The larvae of the jellyfish *Linuche unguiculata* are capable of causing an atopic dermatitis after they become attached to the fibers of bathing attire.[61] This is called seabather's eruption or sea lice and is commonly reported between March and June along the southeast coast of Florida. Symptoms usually resolve spontaneously hours to days after the development of a pruritic, erythematous maculopapular rash, limited to areas covered by swim suits.

The fire coral (*Millepora*) is not a true coral but a close relative of the fresh water *Hydra* containing very powerful and deeply penetrating nematocysts with a very toxic venom. Fire coral, frequently identified incorrectly as seaweed, is most commonly found in shallow tropical waters. Contact with the fire coral may result in an immediate burning or stinging pain, urticaria, and intense pruritis.[3] The wheals may take several weeks to resolve and may leave a hyperpigmented scar. Treatment of fire coral envenomation should consist of immediate irrigation with seawater followed by rinsing with either a 5% acetic acid solution or isopropanol. Systemic corticosteroids have been used for treating the rash if it persists.[3]

Sponges and Cone Shells Sponges belong to the phylum Porifera. They contain the protein spongin, which gives sponges their elastic and porous properties. Some sponges contain tiny calcium carbonate and silica spicules, which can lead to itching when exposed to the skin. Certain sponges such as the fire sponge, red sponge, and bun sponge also contain toxins within their coating. Sponges can easily penetrate skin by using their calcium carbonate and silica spicules. Exposures can lead to painful edematous eruptions within minutes after contact. Pain and paresthesias may also be present and in certain cases may persist for weeks to months. The marine sponge (*Tethya lyncurium*) also contains a pore-forming protein, termed *Tethya* hemolysin, which rapidly lyses erythrocytes[44] and alters intracellular adenosine triphosphate (ATP) production.[43] Treatment of sponge exposures usually requires only the removal of spicules with adhesive tape or the edge of a credit card. Supportive care with an oral analgesic and diphenhydramine is often sufficient.

The cone snails comprise perhaps the largest known genus (*Conus*) of marine animals in existence, numbering approximately 500 species. This snail is a nocturnal predatory carnivore, with a potent neurotoxin. It has an ejectable tooth on the end of a long flexible proboscis.[31] It attacks its prey (or humans) by sinking its venomous tooth deep into its victim's flesh. Their venom contains conotoxins, which selectively target multiple specific ion channels in vitro.[17,62] Approximately 100 conotoxin genetic sequences have been documented, which represent a mere 0.2% of the estimated library size. This constitutes a potentially limitless resource of pharmacotherapy.[35] Multiple clinical applications are currently being studied, including animal studies that demonstrate potential implications for treatment of central nervous system disorders.[49] In fact, ziconotide, a conotoxin derivative, is currently being used experimentally to treat neuropathic pain.

Signs and symptoms developing from the poorly characterized venom include local pain, a burning sensation, numbness, ischemia, and paresthesias. Distal manifestations include paresthesias of the lips and tongue, aphonia, dysphagia, blurred vision, coma, and cardiovascular collapse. Although at least 15 deaths are cited in one review,[19] in most instances, symptoms do not progress beyond local manifestations and resolve in 6 to 8 hours.

Toxic Octopi   The giant monster octopus prefers to avoid humans when possible. However, when provoked, this sea creature mounts an effective attack. The octopus has a distinct venom delivery system consisting of two sets of salivary glands that will release venom from a powerful parrotlike beak.

The blue-ringed octopus (*Hapalochlaena maculosus*) contains the potent neurotoxin tetrodotoxin (see Chaps. 10 and 74) as well as at least eight other neuroactive amines.[20] Symptoms from an envenomation may include local pain, a burning sensation, numbness, and ischemia, while paresthesias may extend from the wound site to involve the lips and tongue. Aphonia, dysphagia, blurred vision, coma, and cardiovascular collapse may ensue. Fatality is typically described when small children handle the octopus outside of the water.[19] Sodium channel blockade during neuronal activation is responsible for hypotension and respiratory failure.

The treatment of a blue-ringed octopus envenomation is symptomatic and supportive. Support of respiration, blood pressure, and pulse must be assured. The use of a direct-acting vasopressor such as norepinephrine or phenylephrine may be needed to maintain blood pressure.[13]

Crown of thorns   A careless brush with the crown of thorns (*Acanthaster planci*) can produce many deep and painful puncture wounds and occasionally, nausea, vomiting, and muscular paralysis. The venom is composed of toxic saponins with hemolytic and anticoagulant effects and histaminelike substances.[60] Therapy is primarily symptomatic and supportive, utilizing immersion of the affected body part in hot water (110–115°F, 43.3–46.1°C) and the administration of oral analgesics for pain relief.[52]

Sea Urchins   Many nonvenomous sea urchins have very long, sharp, and brittle calcium carbonate spines that easily penetrate flesh and tend to snap off, leaving a barbed foreign body behind. The spines of the urchin (*Diadema*) can be as long as a foot and can easily advance deep into muscle and joint spaces, resulting in tissue destruction, pain, and infection.

Many species of sea urchin have venom glands located both at the ends of their spines and in pedicellariae, which are fanglike jaws located at the ends of flexible stalks used to gather food. The victim of a venomous sting will experience intense pain, erythema, and swelling. The venom is believed to be composed of steroid glycosides, hemolysins, proteases, serotonin, and cholinergiclike substances. Partial paralysis of the affected extremity has been reported with some species. Rarely, systemic symptoms may develop, including nausea, syncope, paresthesias, ataxia, muscle cramps, weakness, and respiratory distress.[7] There is no universally accepted treatment for sea urchin spine puncture wounds. Submerging the affected area in hot water (110–115°F, 43.3–46.1°C) seems to be helpful for pain relief. The decision to remove embedded spines should be based on their location, evident infection, or persistent pain. Removal should be attempted only after radiographic localization and may necessitate use of an operating microscope.[39]

SUMMARY

Healthcare providers should become familiar with the toxic marine life found in their geographic region. Although marine envenomations rarely result in severe morbidity, hundreds of painful envenomations may occur each day at coastal locations during certain seasons of the year. Understanding the clinical course and effective therapies for envenomations or contact can often help reduce anxiety and painful consequences.

REFERENCES

1. Allavena A, Mariottini GL, Carli AM, et al: In vitro evaluation of the cytotoxic, hemolytic and clastogenic activities of Rhizostoma pulmo toxin(s). Toxicon 1998;36:933–936.
2. Anderluh G, Barlic A, Potrich C: Lysine 77 is a key residue in aggregation of equinatoxin II, a pore-forming toxin from sea anemone *Actinia equina*. J Membr Biol 2000;173:47–55.
3. Auerbach PS: Marine envenomations. In: Auerbach PS, ed: Wilderness Medicine: Management of Wilderness and Environmental Emergencies, 3rd ed. New York, Macmillan, 1995, pp. 1327–1374.
4. Auerbach PS: Marine envenomations. N Eng J Med 1991;325: 486–493.
5. Auerbach PS, Hays JT: Erythema nodosum following a jellyfish sting. J Emerg Med 1987;5:487–491.
6. Auerbach PS, McKinnney HE, Rees RS, Heggers JP: Analysis of vesicle fluid following the sting of the lionfish *Pterois volitans*. Toxicon 1987;25:1350–1353.
7. Baden HP, Burnett JW: Injuries from sea urchins. South Med J 1977;23:459–460.
8. Bars P: Wound necrosis caused by the venom of stingrays. Med J Aust 1984;141:854–855.
9. Baxter EH, Gallichio HA: Protection against sea snake envenomation: Comparative potency of four antivenins. Toxicon 1976;14:347–355.
10. Brown CK, Shepherd SM: Marine trauma, envenomations and intoxications. Emerg Med Clin North Am 1992;10:385–408.
11. Burnett HW, Burnett JW: Prolonged blurred vision following coelenterate envenomation. Toxicon 1990;28:731–733.
12. Burnett JW, Calton GJ: The chemistry and toxicology of some venomous pelagic coelenterates. Toxicon 1977;15:177–196.
13. Cain D: Weeverfish sting: An unusual problem. Br Med J 1983; 287:406.
14. Cao CJ, Eldefrawi ME, Eldefrawi AT, et al: Toxicity of sea nettle toxin to human hepatocytes and the protective effects of phosphorylating and alkylating agents. Toxicon 1998;36:269–281.

15. Chen D, Kini RM, Yuen R, et al: Hemolytic activity of stonustoxin from stonefish venom: pore formation and the role of cationic amino acid residues. Biochem J 1997;325:685–691.

16. Czarnetzki BM, Thiele T, Rosenbach T: Evidence for leukotrienes in animal venoms. J Allergy Clin Immunol 1990;85:505–509.

17. Favreau P, Le Gall F, Benoit E: A review on conotoxins targeting ion channels and acetylcholine receptors of vertebrate neuromuscular junction. Acta Physiol Pharmacol Ther Latinoam 1999;49:257–267.

18. Fenner PJ: Dangers in the ocean: The traveler and marine envenomation. J Travel Med 1998;5:135–141.

19. Fenner PJ: Marine envenomation: An update—A presentation on the current status of marine envenomation first aid and medical treatments. Emerg Med 2000;12:295–302.

20. Flachsenberger WA: Respiratory failure and lethal hypotension due to blue-ringed octopus and tetrodotoxin envenomations observed and counteracted in animal models. J Toxicol Clin Toxicol 1987;24:485–502.

21. Fulde GWO, Smith F: Sea snake envenomation at Bondi. Med J Aust 1984;141:44–45.

22. Garnier, P, Sauviat MP, Goudey-Perriere F, et al: Cardiotoxicity of verrucotoxin, a protein isolated from the venom of Synanceia verrucosa. Toxicon 1997;35:47–55.

23. Garnier P, Grosclaude JM, Goudey-Perriere, et al: Presence of norepinephrine and other biogenic amines in stonefish venom. J Chromatogr B Biomed Appl 1996;685:364–369.

24. Garyfallou GT, Madden JF: Lionfish envenomation. Ann Emerg Med 1996;28:456–457.

25. Gerencser GA, Loo SY: Effect of Laticauda semifasciata (sea snake) venom on sodium transport across frog skin. Comp Biochem Physiol 1982;72A:727–730.

26. Gerrard DF: Aquatic sports injuries and rehabilitation: Open water swimming. Clin Sports Med 1999;18:337–349.

27. Ghadessy FJ, Chen D, Kini RM, et al: Stonustoxin is a novel lethal factor from stonefish venom. cDNA cloning and characterization. J Biol Chem 1996;271:25575–25581.

28. Halstead BW: Current status of marine toxicology—An overview. Colton, CA, International Biotoxicological Center, World Life Research Institute, 1980.

29. Halstead BW: Poisonous and Venomous Marine Animals of the World. Princeton, NJ, Darwin Press, 1978, pp. 1–135.

30. Halstead BW, Modglin FR: Weeverfish stings and venom apparatus of weever (Trachinus). Z Tropenmed Parasitol 1958;9:129.

31. Hinegardner RT: The venom apparatus of the cone shell. Hawaii Med J 1958;17:533–536.

32. Holmes JL: Marine stingers in far North Queensland. Aust J Dermatol 1996;37:23–26.

33. Hopkins BJ, Hodgson WC: Enzyme and biochemical studies of stonefish and soldierfish venoms. Toxicon 1998;36:791–793.

34. Johnson JM Becker SF, McFarland LM: Vibrio vulnificus: Man and the sea. JAMA 1985;253:2850–2853.

35. Jones RM, Bulaj G: Conotoxins—new vistas for peptide therapeutics. Curr Pharm Des 2000;6:1249–1285.

36. Kaufman MB: Portuguese man-of-war envenomation. Pediatr Emerg Care 1992;8:27–28.

37. Kelly MT, McCormick WF. Acute bacterial myositis caused by Vibrio vulnificus. JAMA 1981;246:72–73.

38. Khoo HE, Chen D, Yuen R: Role of free thiol groups in the biological activities of stonustoxin, a lethal factor from stonefish venom. Toxicon 1998;36:469–476.

39. Kizer KW: Marine envenomations. J Toxicol Clin Toxicol 1984;21:527–555.

40. Kizer KW, McKinney HE, Auerbach PS: Scorpaenidae envenomation: A five-year poison center experience. JAMA 1985;253:807–810.

41. Loder JS: Treatment of jellyfish stings. JAMA 1973;226:1228.

42. Lorenz B, Batel R, Bachinski N, et al: Purification and characterization of two exopolyphosphatases from the marine sponge Tethya lyncurium. Biochim Biophys Acta 1995;1245:17–28.

43. Malovrh P, Barlic A, Podlesek Z, et al: Structure–function studies of tryptophan mutants of equinatoxin II, a sea anemone pore-forming protein. Biochem J 2000;346:223–232.

44. Mangel A, Leitao JM, Batel R, et al: Purification and characterization of a pore-forming protein from the marine sponge Tethya lyncurium. Eur J Biochem 1992;210:499–507.

45. McGoldrick J, Marx JA: Marine envenomations. J Emerg Med 1992;10:71–77.

46. Mercer HP, McGill JJ, Ibraham RA: Envenomation by sea snake in Queensland. Med J Aust 1981;1:130–132.

47. Morris JG, Tenney J: Antibiotic therapy for Vibrio vulnificus infection. JAMA 1985;253:1121–1122.

48. Mullaney PJ: Treatment of sting ray wounds. Clin Toxicol 1970;3:613–615.

49. Olivera BM, Cruz LJ, Yoshikami D: Effects of Conus peptides on the behavior of mice. Curr Opin Neurobiol 1999;9:772–777.

50. Otten EJ: Venomous animal injuries. In: Rosen P, ed: Emergency Medicine: Concepts and Clinical Practice, 3rd ed. St. Louis: Mosby-Year Book, 1992.

51. Patel MR, Wells S: Lionfish envenomation of the hand. J Hand Surg 1993;18:523–525.

52. Roscoe MD: Cutaneous manifestations of marine animal injuries, including diagnosis and treatment. Cutis 1977;19:507–510.

53. Russell FE: Weeverfish sting: The last word. Br Med J 1983;287:981–982.

54. Russell FE: Comparative pharmacology of some animal toxins. Fed Proc 1967;26:1206–1218.

55. Russell FE: Stingray injuries. Public Health Rep 1959;74:855–859.

56. Ryan S, Yong J: The nephrotoxicity of fractionated components of Aipysurus laevis venom. Exp Toxicol Pathol 1997;49:47–55.

57. Schwartz S: Venemous marine animals of Florida: morphology, behavior, health hazards. J Fla Med Assoc 1997;84:433–440.

58. Southcott RV: Studies on Australian Cubomedusae, including a new genus and species apparently harmful to man. Aust J Marine Freshw Res 1956;7:254.

59. Stein MR, Marrachini JV, Rothschild NE: Fatal Portuguese man-of-war (Physalia physalis) envenomation. Ann Emerg Med 1989;18:312–315.

60. Taira E, Tananara N, Fanatsu M: Studies on the toxin in the spines of the starfish Acanthaster planci. 1. Isolation and properties of the toxin found in spines. Sci Bull Coll Agr Univ Ryukus 1975;22:203–212.

61. Tomchik RS, Russell MT, Szmant AM, Black NA: Clinical perspectives on seabather's eruption, also known as sea lice. JAMA 1993;269:1669–1672.

62. Utkin IN, Kasheverov IE, Tsetlin VI: α-Neurotoxins and α-conotoxins—nicotinic cholinoreceptor blockers. Bioorg Khim 1999;25:805–810.

63. Wiener S: Observations on the venom of the stonefish (Synanceja trachynis). Med J Aust 1959;2:260–265.

64. Wiener S: The production and assay of stone-fish antivenene. Med J Aust 1959;4:715–719.

65. Williamson JA, LeRay LE, Wohlfahrt M, Fenner PJ: Acute envenomation by box jellyfish (Chironex fleckeri). Med J Aust 1989;141:851–853.

66. Yew WS, Khoo HE: The role of tryptophan residues in the hemolytic activity of stonustoxin, a lethal factor from stonefish venom. Biochimie 2000;82:251–257.

67. Yuen R, Cai B, Khoo HE: Production and characterization of monoclonal antibodies against stonustoxin from Synaceja horrida. Toxicon 1995;33:1557–1564.

II. SPECIAL POPULATIONS

CHAPTER **104** ## USE OF THE INTENSIVE CARE UNIT FOR POISONED PATIENTS

Mark A. Kirk

Over the past several decades, the intensive care unit (ICU) has improved survival from many serious conditions. This is the direct result of the ability to continuously monitor physiologic parameters, pay meticulous attention to supportive care, and use the most modern medical technology and treatment. Most critically ill poisoned patients have acutely reversible conditions that will clearly benefit from intensive care intervention.[88]

Unlike many diseases managed in the ICU, toxicologic emergencies do not have a well-recognized clinical course or predictable complications. More than almost any other disease managed in the ICU, uncertainties typify toxicologic emergencies. A patient's history is often unreliable with regard to the kind of poison ingested, time of ingestion, and amount ingested. The poison may have unknown or unpredictable toxic effects. The therapies, antidotes, and complications of acute poisoning may be unfamiliar to the ICU staff. These uncertainties challenge healthcare providers and influence decisions about admitting patients to the ICU.

Often a patient will be admitted to the ICU, not for intervention but for observation and monitoring.[111] Of the 10.8 million reported poison exposures from 1995 to 1999, only 5% had toxic effects serious enough to be admitted to the hospital (see p. 1752 and Chap. 116). In addition, fewer than 25% of those hospitalized required specific treatments or antidotes other than GI decontamination.[11,63,111] Many physicians elect to observe poisoned patients in an ICU in anticipation of possible delayed, unrecognized life-threatening toxicity. The ICU provides necessary monitoring and individual nursing care that can help in the early recognition of developing toxicity. Intensive care units allow healthcare providers the best opportunity to minimize morbidity and decrease mortality. However, ICU care is very expensive and has contributed significantly to the escalation of healthcare costs.

The ICU admission guidelines presented in this chapter are intended to encourage effective use of ICU resources without compromising patient care. Effective guidelines must consider the unique characteristics of a toxin, the capabilities of the hospital, and all realistic alternatives for managing and observing poisoned patients without compromising care. Current medical literature allows us to develop only very general guidelines. Future clinical studies addressing the use of healthcare resources for the poisoned patient will allow refinement of these guidelines. Although it is impossible to be all-inclusive, this chapter provides a decision-making strategy for most toxins discussed in this text.

CRITERIA FOR ICU ADMISSION

Overcrowded ICUs and escalating healthcare costs have been incentives to develop severity-of-illness models that predict the benefits of ICU care. The Acute Physiology and Chronic Health Evaluation (APACHE II/III), the Mortality Probability Model (MPM II), the Simplified Acute Physiology Score (SAPS II), and the Pediatric Risk of Mortality (PRISM II/III) are widely studied and generally accepted severity-of-illness models that score certain physiologic parameters and other factors in order to estimate risks and predict outcomes.[52,104] These models are most effective for stratifying risks in clinical research trials and comparing quality of care among ICUs. Clinical studies to validate such scoring systems included patients with a variety of medical and surgical conditions. No study exclusively investigated patients with overdoses or included large numbers of overdose patients. Clinical outcome predictors used in these scoring systems, such as neurologic outcome following cardiac arrest, are not reliable in the poisoned patient.[27,85] Severe poisoning may clinically mimic brain death yet have complete neurologic recovery.[4,78,82,107,110] In addition, many toxicologic emergencies occur in young patients who are free of underlying chronic diseases. This increases the likelihood of surviving significant insults such as prolonged hypotension or hypoxia. Despite negative predictors of outcome, aggressive resuscitation efforts are justified for the subgroup of patients who are poisoned. Specifically, prolonged cardiac resuscitation should be provided for the victim of a cardiac arrest resulting from cyclic antidepressant overdoses, β-adrenergic antagonists, calcium channel blockers, or severe hypothermia.[29,49,69,77,95]

Few studies have evaluated the use of the ICU for poisoned patients.[11,27,43,46,48,50,56,99,102] Prospective studies have focused on mortality rates, use of resources, or types of toxins ingested, whereas others, mostly retrospective, have focused on a single toxin. These studies included relatively small study populations.

A set of criteria was established to determine whether initial clinical assessment could identify those poisoned patients at risk of developing serious toxicity, thus needing ICU admission.[11] The specific toxin ingested was not considered in defining risks. Criteria defining high-risk patients were need for intubation, unresponsiveness to verbal stimuli, seizures, P_{CO_2} >45 mm Hg, systolic blood pressure <80 mm Hg, QRS duration >0.12 seconds, or any cardiac rhythm except normal sinus rhythm, sinus tachycardia, or sinus bradycardia. Patients were classified as low risk when none of the above criteria were present in the emergency department (ED). Retrospectively, 209 cases were analyzed using the above parameters. The most commonly ingested drugs in both the high- and low-risk groups were barbiturates, benzodiazepines, cyclic antidepressants, ethanol, opioids, phenothiazines, and salycilates. None of the 151 patients considered low risk developed complications or required ICU interventions after admission. Of the 58 patients deemed high risk, 35 required ICU interventions such as intubation, treatment of dysrhythmias, treatment of seizures, intravenous vasopressors, or hemodialysis/hemoperfusion. Seven patients developed high-risk complications such as hypoxia, respiratory failure, hypotension, or seizures after admission, but all had other high-risk criteria in the ED. Although the authors concluded that the clinical course of poisoned patients can be predicted during the initial 2 to 3 hours of observation, toxins with delayed or prolonged toxic effects, such as sustained-release products, lithium, and oral hypoglycemic agents, were not prominent in their study population.

In this study population, 70% of the low-risk patients were admitted to the ICU for observation. Because none of these patients developed complications or required ICU intervention, the authors postulated that applying these criteria would have eliminated 50% of the ICU days without compromising care. The limitations of this study are its retrospective design, relatively small study population, and limited variety of toxin exposures. However, it does suggest that with some clinical judgment, many poisoned patients will not require ICU admission.

Ideally, clinical indicators for ICU care should be established for each toxin. Universal criteria cannot be applied to all poisoned patients because of the unique clinical course of some toxins. Until more specific predictors of outcome are developed for individual toxins, nothing will be more useful than experience and good clinical judgment in predicting who may benefit from ICU admission. At present, withholding ICU care from poisoned patients based solely on a nonspecific "score" will not result in significant cost savings in the ICU but may increase the risk of morbidity and mortality.[17,54,104]

END-ORGAN TOXICITY AS BASIS FOR ICU ADMISSION

It seems reasonable to assume that a patient's signs and symptoms can be used to decide the need for ICU admission. The presence of certain signs, symptoms, or abnormal diagnostic tests requires ICU observation or intervention, whatever the toxic exposure. This approach is most consistent with the philosophy of "treating the patient and not the poison" and may prove most helpful for patients with polydrug ingestions.

Central nervous system (CNS) manifestations are common to many poisonings. Toxin-induced acute delirium or coma often requires ICU admission because these findings will not resolve quickly. Any comatose or delirious patient without an identifiable

cause requires continued investigation in the ICU. Toxin-induced status epilepticus is best managed in the ICU.

A poisoned patient with any signs of respiratory compromise needs ICU admission. Toxins may act by several different mechanisms to produce respiratory compromise. For example, organic phosphorus insecticide poisoning compromises respiratory status by CNS depression, respiratory muscle weakness, and copious pulmonary secretions. In addition, ICU admission is required when impaired oxygen-carrying capacity or tissue hypoxia is evident from poisons such as hydrogen sulfide, cyanide, carbon monoxide, or methemoglobin inducers.

Toxins cause cardiac dysrhythmias, hypotension, hypertension, and ischemia. Any evidence of cardiovascular toxicity requires that the patient be admitted to the ICU. Toxin-induced chest pain can be caused by myocardial ischemia from cocaine or carbon monoxide exposure and should be treated with the same sense of urgency and caution as those suspected of having a myocardial infarction from any other etiology. Persistent, toxin-induced hypertension, especially with associated headache or chest pain, also requires ICU intervention.

Gastrointestinal symptoms, particularly vomiting and diarrhea, are an early manifestation of poisoning by many toxins. When symptoms are severe and persistent, significant fluid and electrolyte losses can occur. For example, a patient with a serious iron ingestion can have a GI mucosal injury, leading to vomiting, diarrhea, profound volume loss, and significant hypotension. Hepatotoxicity from poisoning or overdose usually occurs days after toxin exposure. If hepatotoxicity is evident at the time of admission (especially with hepatic encephalopathy), ICU management is suggested.

Renal toxicity may be a direct toxic effect or a complication of other toxic manifestations, such as hypotension or rhabdomyolysis. Severe toxin-induced metabolic acidosis is best managed in an ICU. Metabolic acidosis is an important clue to the presence of toxins such as ethylene glycol, methanol, and salicylates. Investigation into the cause of an unexplained acidosis should be pursued in the ICU. Persistent or refractory hypoglycemia, resulting from an oral hypoglycemic, insulin overdose, or other toxins, is also best managed in an ICU. In addition, severe toxin-induced alterations in temperature regulation or electrolyte disturbances merit close monitoring and intervention in the ICU.

The complications of chemical burns of the skin are similar to those of thermal burns. The injured dermis may be unable to prevent significant fluid losses, regulate core body temperature, and prevent infection. Besides these complications, systemic toxic effects may occur through dermal absorption. As little as 2.5% body surface area exposure to concentrated hydrofluoric acid has resulted in hypocalcemia and death.[103]

Diagnostic tests such as routine laboratory analysis, electrocardiography, and radiography are used as indicators of end-organ toxicity. Diagnostic tests may demonstrate definite end-organ toxicity or provide early warning signs of impending serious toxic effects. These diagnostic tests may suggest the need for aggressive management or more careful monitoring. Elevated serum levels of some drugs indicate that serious toxicity is likely. Although diagnostic tests are extremely useful for deciding about using the ICU, relatively few patients should be admitted to the ICU based on the results of a single diagnostic test.

End-organ toxicity is the most important reason to admit poisoned patients to the ICU. However, restricting ICU admission to those with only end-organ toxicity is inadequate. Minimally symptomatic or asymptomatic patients may require ICU admission because other factors must be considered.

ADDITIONAL INFORMATION INFLUENCING ICU ADMISSION OF THE POISONED PATIENT

In addition to end-organ toxicity, the toxin, its treatment, and specific patient characteristics should influence ICU admission decisions.

Toxin Characteristics as Basis for ICU Admission

Both the known and unknown about a toxin will assist with ICU admission decisions. Some toxins have proven their ability to cause harm or death to humans. Well-described, expected toxic effects assist in early recognition of poisoning. For other toxins, the consequences after human exposure are not yet reported.

ICU admission is always warranted for patients with expected serious toxic effects from an ingested poison. This is especially true for those toxins known to be deadly, such as calcium channel blockers, cocaine, cyanide, cyclic antidepressants, and salicylates. For example, patients with salicylate poisoning who develop respiratory distress or significant metabolic derangements require close attention and aggressive treatment available only in the ICU.

Indicators of toxicity should be identified for individual toxins so that high-risk patients may be closely monitored and aggressively treated. Because they are some of the most common and potentially lethal overdoses reported, cyclic antidepressants have been studied in great detail to determine indicators of toxicity and safe disposition.[2,14,15,28,50,74,80,105] They have accounted for up to 25% of drug overdoses admitted to adult ICUs, yet many admissions have been for trivial overdoses.[21] Research efforts have focused on identifying those patients at risk for serious toxicity. These studies suggest that patients may be safely discharged if they remain asymptomatic for a 6-hour observation period after presentation.[2,15,34,50,79,105] Prolonged QRS duration on a 12-lead ECG is predictive of serious complications such as seizures and dysrhythmias.[5,74,108] Any patient manifesting persistent tachycardia, ECG abnormalities (including QRS ≥0.10 seconds), hypotension, anticholinergic signs, or neurologic symptoms requires ICU monitoring.[15,34] Unlike cyclic antidepressants, most toxins do not have such extensive literature to define high-risk patients.

The natural history of some toxins is unknown. New pharmaceutical and industrial products are introduced each year with little data on toxic exposure doses or human health effects. Sometimes animal studies provide the only known toxicologic data, or preclinical trials for new drugs may have excluded the populations at risk, such as infants, children, or the elderly. In these cases, the clinician must often make therapeutic decisions and anticipate potential toxicity with little or no reliable data. Because early recognition of serious toxicity could prevent an adverse outcome, expectant observation may be the only rational approach. For example, multiple suicidal and unintentional ingestions followed the introduction of fluoxetine. Because, at that time, clinicians lacked experience treating overdoses of this drug and had no data regarding the natural course and toxic dose, many patients were admitted to the ICU to observe for toxic effects. Now that clinicians have experience with this drug and studies are available demonstrating

few severe manifestations, ICU resources are seldom needed to treat such patients.[8,16,97]

Failure to appreciate the potential for serious, delayed toxic effects is a major pitfall in managing poisoned patients. An asymptomatic patient may be a "time bomb" with the potential to deteriorate rapidly. Delayed or continued absorption, slow tissue distribution, interference with cellular function, production of toxic metabolites, or depletion of target organ reserve capacity are causes of delayed onset of clinical effects.[9]

Certain toxins prolong GI absorption, delaying onset of toxicity. Opioids and the anticholinergic drugs, such as cyclic antidepressants and antihistamines, will delay gastric emptying and prolong drug absorption.[14] In children, Lomotil (atropine and diphenoxylate) can produce delayed and prolonged coma from slowed GI motility.[67] Salicylates produce pylorospasm, which delays gastric emptying.[7] Iron, meprobamate, salicylates, theophylline, and verapamil may form gastric bezoars, producing prolonged GI absorption.[3,57,76,90,98]

Sustained-release preparations and enteric coatings enhance patient compliance but, in overdose, may delay absorption and in turn delay the onset of toxicity.[22,71] Published cases of overdoses with sustained-release theophylline, sustained-release verapamil, and enteric-coated aspirin report delayed onset of toxicity (more than 16 hours), and peak serum levels were measured more than 24 hours after ingestion.[7,87,96,109]

Common sustained-release preparations of toxicologic importance include β-adrenergic antagonists, calcium channel blockers, lithium, phenylpropanolamine, potassium, and theophylline.[71] Serial drug level measurements are necessary to verify peaks and ensure decreasing levels. Serial levels may show the benefits of GI decontamination or warn of increasing potential for serious toxic effects. When serum levels are unobtainable, admission and observation are required for many sustained-release and enteric-coated overdoses. In addition, smuggling ("body-packing") or hiding ("body stuffing") contraband drugs in the GI tract has resulted in delayed onset of serious toxicity from ruptured bags.[68,86]

Clinical effects may be delayed when toxicity depends on alteration of enzyme functions, cellular reproduction, or metabolic function. Toxicity of monoamine oxidase inhibitors (MAOI) may not be apparent for more than 12 hours after an overdose but then may progress rapidly to cardiovascular collapse.[62] Because of the delay in onset of severe toxicity, even if the patient is asymptomatic, a history of MAOI ingestion mandates ICU monitoring for 24 hours. The GI toxicity of colchicine may resolve within hours of ingestion with apparent recovery, only to have multisystem organ failure occur 24 to 72 hours later.[6] When there is potential for serious delayed toxicity, the patient may need prolonged close monitoring.

Physiologic Monitoring and Specialized Treatment as Requirements for ICU Admission

The ICU setting offers the most highly skilled staff and modern technology available to manage complex medical problems. Also, it provides a nurse-to-patient ratio that allows for frequent or continuous monitoring of basic physiologic parameters. Invasive monitoring is routinely used in the ICU and is beneficial to some poisoned patients. Hemodynamic parameters are valuable for the patient with hypotension, intravascular volume depletion, or respiratory failure from acute lung injury (ALI). Intraarterial monitoring provides a more accurate and continuous record of actual blood pressure in a patient with cardiovascular compromise. A pulmonary artery catheter assists fluid and inotropic therapy for patients with ALI and toxin-induced cardiogenic pulmonary edema. Both invasive and noninvasive measurements of vital signs, neurologic status, and intake/output measurements, along with continuous cardiac monitoring, make possible early detection of toxicity, recognition of conditions needing active intervention, and prevention of complications.

Most critically ill poisoned patients have acute reversible conditions requiring supportive care measures (ie, ventilator support, vasopressor support, and close monitoring) that ICUs are most equipped to provide. Most often, supportive care measures improve the outcome of critically ill poisoned patients more than antidotes and specialized treatments. The mortality for patients with barbiturate overdoses dropped from 20% in the 1930s to less than 2% in the 1950s.[18] This significant decrease in mortality was attributed to therapy that focused on supportive care measures such as maintaining a patent airway, preventing hypoxia with the administration of oxygen, and treatment of shock. A study published in 1987 reported a good outcome in most of 103 critically ill overdosed patients treated with only mechanical ventilation, vasopressor support, and careful monitoring.[27] In a pediatric study, only 19 of 105 patients admitted to the ICU required specialized treatment beyond mechanical ventilation and careful monitoring.[56]

With few exceptions, antidotes and specific treatments should be administered in the ICU setting. Although possibly lifesaving, these treatments may have inherent risks. For example, antivenom administration for rattlesnake envenomations may cause anaphylaxis, and rapid intravenous infusion of deferoxamine for iron poisoning may cause hypotension. Because these treatments may be unfamiliar to staff and have their own inherent risks, the ICU is the most prudent environment to monitor such treatments.

In toxicologic emergencies, a familiar medication may be an antidotal therapy that requires doses that far exceed conventional regimens or indications that deviate from common treatment protocols. High doses of atropine (hundreds of milligrams) may be necessary for the treatment of organic phosphorus insecticide poisoning.[25,39,60] Very high doses of epinephrine may be necessary to overcome receptor antagonism from β-adrenergic antagonists. Intravenous calcium, which is no longer a routine part of advanced cardiac life support (ACLS) protocols, is commonly used to reverse toxicity from calcium channel blockers[83] and (by intraarterial infusion) from hydrofluoric acid burns of the extremities.[106] Sodium bicarbonate as a bolus and infusion is the treatment of choice for cyclic antidepressant and type IA antidysrhythmic agent cardiac toxicity.[79,94] Instead of the usual first-line vasopressor, dopamine, direct vasopressors such as norepinephrine or phenylephrine may be more appropriate for the treatment of toxin-induced hypotension. Some drugs are administered in unconventional doses, whereas other familiar drugs should be avoided in treating toxic emergencies. For example, type IA antidysrhythmic agents, such as procainamide and quinidine, must not be used in patients with overdoses of cardiac sodium channel antagonists, such as cyclic antidepressants, phenothiazines, and propoxyphene.

A false sense of security can result when an antidote reverses toxicity but has a shorter duration of effect than the toxin. An example is a patient, comatose from an opioid overdose, who responds to naloxone, awakens, and refuses further treatment. Toxicity may recur when naloxone's short duration of effect allows opioid toxicity to recur. These patients must be closely observed for the possible need to readminister the antidote.

Extracorporeal methods of eliminating toxins, such as hemodialysis or hemoperfusion, are best performed in the ICU. Invasive procedures such as extracorporeal membrane oxygenation, cardiopulmonary bypass, and intraaortic balloon pump–assisted perfusion have been used successfully in resuscitating critically ill poisoned patients.[19,30,37,44,47,49,58,59,75,93]

Patient Factors as Criteria for ICU Admission

Preexisting medical conditions increase a patient's risk for developing toxicity. Many elderly patients have chronic medical problems and do not tolerate major physiologic stressors without significant compromise. For example, a patient with underlying cardiac disease may develop severe myocardial ischemia from a modest carbon monoxide exposure. An elderly or infirmed patient with chronic salicylism is more likely to have major respiratory and CNS complications than a younger or healthier patient.[1] Conditions that alter drug metabolism or elimination, such as renal or hepatic disease, may prolong toxicity or produce toxicity after lesser amounts are ingested.

Patients with physical dependency on ethanol, benzodiazepines, or barbiturates may be admitted to the hospital for acute withdrawal or, during hospitalization, go through a period of abstinence that results in an acute withdrawal syndrome.[35] Withdrawal from ethanol and sedative-hypnotics can have serious consequences and complications. ICU management may be necessary because large doses of medications with respiratory depressant effects may be required to treat acute withdrawal from these agents.

Eighty percent of recognized suicide attempts involve an overdose of medications.[73] Acute complications of poisoning make it difficult to adequately assess suicidal risks. Patients have an increased rate of suicide following discharge from an ICU for drug overdose.[99] Until suicidal risks are adequately assessed, it must be assumed that an overdosed patient needs close observation. Institutions differ on monitoring policies for suicidal patients not on a psychiatric unit. The ultimate goal of treatment for any suicidal patient is to provide a maximally safe environment. In many hospitals, the ICU is the safest place, but also the most expensive place, to observe a patient with suicidal risks until it is medically safe to transfer the patient to the psychiatric service.

COMPLICATIONS THAT PROLONG ICU CARE

Poisoning produces both anticipated and unanticipated complications that can prolong ICU care and decrease survival. Serious complications of poisoning include pulmonary compromise, rhabdomyolysis, compartment syndrome, and anoxic brain injury. Complications such as acute renal or fulminant hepatic failure may also prolong an ICU course.

Pulmonary compromise following toxic exposures often develops after several hours or days in the ICU. Pulmonary complications following a toxic exposure include aspiration pneumonitis, ALI, and adult respiratory distress syndrome (ARDS). Aspiration of gastric contents is a common complication following poisoning, especially when a patient's mental status is altered and protective airway reflexes are lost.[40,51,92] In a series of 185 barbiturate overdoses, the incidence of pulmonary aspiration increased with the depth of coma.[40] Poisoned patients may aspirate spontaneously while lying unresponsive before being discovered, from stomach dilation secondary to bag-valve-mask ventilation, from GI decontamination procedures such as orogastric lavage, or during insertion of endotracheal or nasogastric tubes.[55,70,81] Loss of airway protective reflexes allows liquid gastric contents to enter the lungs and cause a pulmonary parenchymal inflammatory reaction and a subsequent ventilation–perfusion mismatch.[13] Pulmonary aspiration results in an increased risk of secondary bacterial invasion of the lungs, prolonged hypoxemia, and progression to ARDS. The mortality of aspiration pneumonitis is reported to be as high as 30 to 60%.[13,23]

ALI/ARDS results from either a direct cellular toxic effect or a microvascular injury to the lung. Central neurogenic mechanisms may be responsible for some drug-induced ALI. Carbon monoxide, chlorine, cyclic antidepressants, nitrogen oxides, opioids, organic phosphorus insecticides, phosgene, salicylates, and sedative-hypnotics are reported to produce ALI.[26,31,33,45,89,92,101] Frequently invasive hemodynamic monitoring and other ICU interventions are necessary to manage this complex condition, which can progress to ARDS. Additionally, toxic inhalation, shock, respiratory failure, and sepsis are complications of poisonings that may lead to ARDS, which has a mortality as high as 50%.[10,32,72] Its treatment requires expertise and technology that are best provided in an ICU.

Drug- and toxin-induced rhabdomyolysis represents skeletal muscle injury with resultant leak of myocyte contents into the plasma.[20,36,53] It may be caused by direct toxic injury to muscle cells, pressure necrosis, or excessive energy expenditure from severe agitation, seizures, or hyperthermia. Barbiturates, carbon monoxide, doxylamine and cocaine are toxins that frequently produce rhabdomyolysis.[20] Acute renal failure, dysrhythmias from electrolyte disturbances, and disseminated intravascular coagulation complicate this condition. Ensuring adequate urine output and closely monitoring laboratory tests may prevent serious complications.

Rhabdomyolysis may not always be generalized muscle injury but can be a local injury within a fascial compartment.[20,65] Compartment syndrome is the increased pressure within a fascial compartment that compromises distal blood flow. Irreversible muscle damage may occur within 6 to 12 hours. The comatose poisoned patient may develop compartment syndrome after lying on an extremity. Commonly, compartments in the hand, arm, forearm, buttocks, thigh, or leg are involved. Establishing the diagnosis requires close examination of all compartments, reassessment, serial creatinine phosphokinase (CPK) levels, and early surgical consultation for evidence of ischemia.

Poisoning causes global cerebral anoxia from prolonged shock, respiratory failure, or direct toxic/metabolic effects. Distinguishing anoxic cerebral injury from reversible encephalopathy can be difficult in poisoned patients. Coma and loss of brainstem reflexes after prolonged severe cerebral hypoxia indicates a poor prognosis.[61] In contrast, patients with reversible encephalopathy can have profound CNS depression that mimics brain death, yet recover fully.[4,78,82,107,110] As mentioned previously, clinical predictors of outcome may be unreliable when applied to poisoned patients; therefore, the diagnosis of brain death should be made cautiously. Often, cerebral edema is a secondary effect of global cerebral anoxia, although some toxins have direct cellular effects. Cerebral edema can be a complication of acetaminophen-induced fulminant hepatic failure and the result of direct neuronal injury from salicylate and lead poisoning.[64,84,100] Aggressive ICU care is necessary to treat toxin-induced cerebral injuries.

CRITERIA FOR SAFE DISPOSITION FROM THE ICU

Once the acute toxic effects have resolved, most patients are safe to transfer out of the ICU. Patients with cyclic antidepressant overdoses have been studied to determine when it is safe to discontinue monitoring. Concerns arose from case reports of patients developing sudden death as late as several days following a cyclic antidepressant overdose.[14,66,91] In most cases, delayed complications developed in the setting of continued toxicity evidenced by lethargy or sinus tachycardia. More recent studies demonstrate that dysrhythmias do not occur after signs of toxicity have resolved (ie, CNS and cardiac manifestations).[15,38,79] Current recommendations based on these studies suggest cardiac monitoring for an additional 24 hours after normalization of ECG and resolution of other signs of continued toxicity.[94] This additional period of monitoring should occur after discontinuation of all specific forms of therapy, such as serum alkalinization. Most toxins have not received the attention given to cyclic antidepressants; therefore, pending further research and experience, clinical judgment is the only basis for deciding when to discharge a patient from the ICU.

The same issues previously mentioned may be pitfalls to a patient's safe discharge from an ICU. Continued GI absorption must be terminated before discharge from the ICU because it may cause prolonged or worsening clinical effects. Carefully consider discharge decisions about patients exposed to toxins with serious delayed clinical effects, such as colchicine. Also, be mindful that the duration of action of the toxin may be longer than the duration of action of the specific treatment or antidote.

Finally, the patient's suicidal intent must be considered before transfer to a less closely monitored hospital unit. Transfer from the ICU should be delayed pending assessment of suicide risk or other important psychosocial issues. Early involvement of psychiatric services, chemical dependency counseling, and social services can expedite ICU disposition. Disposition and treatment options can be considered at a time when the patient is still medically unstable by interviewing family, friends, and outpatient counselors.

ALTERNATIVES TO ICU ADMISSION

Often, placing patients in the ICU solely for observation is not an effective use of this expensive resource. Until further clinical studies are available to define those patients at risk, many poisoned patients will be admitted to the ICU for observation. When information about the toxin, the patient, and the capabilities of the medical unit are all considered, many patients can be safely observed outside the ICU. Some considerations to assist with disposition decisions are presented in Table 104–1.

Alternatives to the ICU include a medical floor bed, an intermediate care unit, a telemetry-monitored bed, a medical psychiatric unit, or an ED observation unit. Capabilities for managing poisoned patients may vary considerably between institutions and in different types of patient care areas. It is essential to understand the capabilities of the unit where a patient is being considered for admission. If the nursing staff is unfamiliar with the potential for rapid deterioration of the patient, or the staffing pattern does not allow for close observation, the results could be disastrous. For example, it is unrealistic to expect a nurse to manage intravenous fluids, record hourly intake and output measurements, record fre-

TABLE 104–1.   Considerations for Intensive Care Admission

Toxin characteristics

  Does the ingested toxin have known serious sequelae (eg, cyclic antide-
    pressant cardiotoxicity)?

  Can the patient deteriorate rapidly from its toxic effects?

  Is the onset of toxicity likely to be delayed (eg, sustained-release prep-
    aration, slowed GI motility, or delayed toxic effects)?

  Does the toxin have cardiac effects that will require cardiac monitoring?

  Is the amount ingested a potentially serious or potentially lethal dose?

  Is the required or planned therapy unconventional (eg, large doses of
    atropine for treating overdoses of organic phosphorus insecticides)?

  Does the therapy have potentially serious adverse effects?

  Is there significant risk of the unknown?

  Is there insufficient literature to describe the potential human toxic
    effects?

  Are potentially serious coingestants likely (must take into account the
    reliability of the history)?

Patient characteristics

  Does the patient have any signs of serious end-organ toxicity?

  Is there progression of the end-organ effects?

  Are laboratory data suggestive of serious toxicity?

  Are serum drug concentrations rising?

  Is the patient a high risk for complications requiring ICU intervention?

    Seizures

    Unresponsive to verbal stimuli

    Level of consciousness impaired to the point of potential airway
      compromise

    P_{CO_2} >45 mm Hg

    Systolic blood pressure <80 mm Hg

    Cardiac dysrhythmias

    Prolonged ECG complexes and intervals (QRS duration ≥0.10 seconds;
      QT prolongation)

  Does the patient have preexisting medical conditions that could predis-
    pose to complications?

    Chronic alcohol or drug dependence

    Chronic liver disease

    Chronic renal failure or insufficiency

    Heart disease

    Pregnancy

  Is the patient suicidal?

Assessing the capabilities of the inpatient unit/observation unit

  Does the admitting team (attending, house staff, students) appreciate
    the potential seriousness of a toxicologic emergency?

  Is the nursing staff:

    Familiar with this toxicologic emergency?

    Familiar with the potential for serious complications?

  Is the staffing adequate to monitor the patient?

    What is the ratio of nurses to patients?

    Are time-consuming nursing activities required? (eg, hourly urine pH
      assessments or whole-bowel irrigation)

  Can a safe environment be provided for a suicidal patient?

    Can a patient have suicide precautions and monitoring with a medical
      floor bed?

    Can a one-to-one observer be present in the room with the patient?

    Can the patient be restrained?

quent vital signs, and check hourly urine pH measurements for a salicylate-poisoned patient while caring for eight other patients. Emergency department observation may be an alternative for observing and treating selected poisoned patients.[24,42] Nearly one-third of EDs in the United States currently have emergency department observation units.[12,41] Many are capable of frequent monitoring of vital signs, continuous cardiac monitoring, and maintaining a safe environment for suicidal patients.[12,41] Patients

with a low risk of serious toxicity or life-threatening complications who require only observation may be ideal candidates for ED observation units.

Clinicians can make educated decisions regarding observation outside of the ICU when toxins have a well-defined toxicity profile. For example, acetaminophen toxicity has a well-known clinical course and an effective antidote. Toxicity develops slowly over several days. Antidote administration does not require special ICU care, and conversely, the ICU can offer little to prevent hepatotoxicity. Most patients with an acetaminophen overdose can be treated outside of the ICU, providing suicide risks can be monitored and regular administration of the antidote ensured.

Many poisoned patients use ICU resources because of suicidal risks. Other than the ICU, many hospitals cannot provide an alternative for observing a high-risk suicidal patient. Less costly alternatives are available, but they must assure a safe environment for suicidal patients. An ED observation unit, an intermediate care unit, a medical psychiatric unit, or a one-on-one observer can safely observe these patients.

Future studies must define prognostic factors for poisoning complications. Patients can then be stratified into high-risk or low-risk groups. The limitations of current studies prevent generalizing the results to individual patients or certain subgroups. Unfortunately, many current clinical guidelines now being used to ration care may be based on poorly tested models with no scientific basis and may be motivated by financial concerns. Guidelines should be based on sound evidence so that they can provide the best care with less intensive use of health care resources.

SUMMARY

Acute poisoning challenges medical and nursing staff because of its unpredictable clinical course and unfamiliar therapies. Poisoned patients are especially challenging because their clinical history is incomplete and the medical literature is often limited. These unknowns create many uncertainties in management. Because the ICU offers the highest level of skilled staff and modern technology available, most seriously poisoned patients should be admitted there. Whether this is clinically justified or is an effective use of resources for a given patient is always an issue because admission of the poisoned patient continues to be based mostly on clinical judgment and the best available information.

REFERENCES

1. Anderson R, Potts D, Gabow P, et al: Unrecognized adult salicylate
   intoxication. Ann Intern Med 1976;85:745–748.

2. Banahan B, Schelkun P: Tricyclic antidepressant overdose: Conservative management in a community hospital with cost-saving implications. J Emerg Med 1990;8:451–454.

3. Bernstein G, Jehle D, Bernaski E, et al: Failure of gastric emptying
   and charcoal administration in fatal sustained-release theophylline
   overdose: Pharmacobezoar formation. Ann Emerg Med 1992;21:
   1388–1390.

4. Bird T, Plum F: Recovery from barbiturate overdose coma with a
   prolonged isoelectric electroencephalogram. Neurology 1968;18:
   456–460.

5. Boehnert M, Lovejoy F: Value of the QRS duration vs the serum
   drug level in predicting seizures and ventricular arrhythmias after an
   acute overdose of tricyclic antidepressants. N Engl J Med 1985;313:
   474–479.

6. Boehnert M, McGuigan M: Colchicine. Clin Toxicol Rev 1983;5:1.

7. Bogacz K, Caldron P: Enteric-coated aspirin bezoar: Elevation of serum salicylate level by barium study. Am J Med 1987;83:783–786.

8. Borys D, Setzer S, Ling L, et al: Acute fluoxetine overdose: A report of 234 cases. Am J Emerg Med 1992;10:115–120.

9. Bosse GM, Matyunas NJ: Delayed toxidromes. J Emerg Med 1999; 17:679–690.

10. Bresler M, Sternbach G: The adult respiratory distress syndrome. Emerg Med Clin North Am 1989;7:419–430.

11. Brett A, Rothchild N, Gray R, et al: Predicting the clinical course in intentional drug overdose. Arch Intern Med 1987;147:133–137.

12. Brillman J, Mathers-Dunbar L, Graff L, et al: Management of observation units. Ann Emerg Med 1995;25:823–830.

13. Bynum L, Pierce A: Pulmonary aspiration of gastric contents. Am Rev Respir Dis 1976;114:1129–1136.

14. Callaham M: Admission criteria for tricyclic antidepressant ingestion. West J Med 1982;137:425–429.

15. Callaham M, Kassel D: Epidemiology of fatal tricyclic antidepressant ingestion: Implications for management. Ann Emerg Med 1985; 14:1–9.

16. Chiang W, Ford M, Wax P: Prospective evaluation of fluoxetine ingestions [Abstract]. Vet Hum Toxicol 1990;32:348.

17. Civetta J: Setting objectives: Perspectives for care. In: Civetta JM, Taylor RW, Kirby RR, eds: Critical Care, 2. Philadelphia, JB Lippincott, 1992, pp. 13–23.

18. Clemmesen C, Nilsson E: Therapeutic trends in the treatment of barbiturate poisoning: The Scandinavian method. Clin Pharmacol Ther 1961;2:220–229.

19. Corkeron MA, van Heerden PV, Newman SM, et al: Extracorporeal circulatory support in near-fatal flecainide overdose. Anaesth Intens Care 1999;27:405–408.

20. Curry S, Chang D, Connor D: Drug- and toxin-induced rhabdomyolysis. Ann Emerg Med 1989;18:1068–1084.

21. Dec W: Tricyclic antidepressants in the intensive care. J Intens Care Med 1990;5:69.

22. Dederich R, Szefler S, Green E: Intrasubject variation in sustained release theophylline absorption. J Allergy Clin Immun 1981;67: 465–471.

23. Dines D, Titus J, Sessler A: Aspiration pneumonitis. Mayo Clin Proc 1970;45:347–360.

24. Dribben W, Welch J, Dunn D, et al: The utilization of emergency department observation units for the poisoned patient [abstract]. J Toxicol Clin Toxicol 1999;37:586.

25. Du Toit P, Muller F, Van Tonder W, et al: Experience with the intensive care management of organophosphate insecticide poisoning. S Afr Med J 1981;60:227–229.

26. Duberstein J, Kaufman D: A clinical study of an epidemic of heroin intoxication and heroin-induced pulmonary edema. Am J Med 1971; 51:704–707.

27. Elk J, Linton D, Potgieter P: Treatment of acute self-poisoning in a respiratory intensive care unit. S Afr Med J 1987;72:532–534.

28. Emerman CL, Connors AF, Burma GM: Level of consciousness as a predictor of complications following tricyclic overdose. Ann Emerg Med 1987;16:326–330.

29. Evans JS, Oram MP: Neurological recovery after prolonged verapamil-induced cardiac arrest. Anaesth Intens Care 1999;27:653–655.

30. Fell R, Gunning A, Bardhan K, et al: Severe hypothermia as a result of barbiturate overdose complicated by cardiac arrest. Lancet 1968; 392–394.

31. Fisher C, Albertson T, Foulke G: Salicylate-induced pulmonary edema: Clinical characteristics in children. Am J Emerg Med 1985; 3:33–37.

32. Fowler A, Hamman R, Zerbe G, et al: Adult respiratory distress syndrome: Prognosis after onset. Am Rev Respir Dis 1985;132: 472–478.

33. Frand U, Shim C, Williams M: Heroin-induced pulmonary edema. Ann Intern Med 1972;77:29–35.

34. Frommer D, Kulig K, Marx J, et al: Tricyclic antidepressant overdose. JAMA 1987;257:521–526.

35. Fruensgaard K: Withdrawal psychosis: A study of 30 consecutive cases. Acta Psych Scand 1976;53:105–118.

36. Gabow P, Kaehny W, Kelleher S: The spectrum of rhabdomyolysis. Medicine 1982;61:141–151.

37. Gillard P, Laurent M: Dextropropoxyphene-induced cardiogenic shock: treatment with intra-aortic balloon pump and milrinone [letter]. Intensive Care Med 1999;25:335.

38. Goldberg R, Capone R, Hunt J: Cardiac complications following tricyclic antidepressant overdose. JAMA 1985;254:1772–1775.

39. Golsousidis H, Kokkas V: Use of 19,590 mg of atropine during 24 days of treatment after a case of unusually severe parathion poisoning. Human Toxicol 1985;4:339–340.

40. Goodman J, Bischel M, Wagers P, et al: Barbiturate intoxication: Morbidity and mortality. West J Med 1976;124:179–186.

41. Graff L, Zun L, Leikin J, et al: Emergency department observation beds improve patient care: Society for Academic Emergency Medicine debate. Ann Emerg Med 1992;21:967–975.

42. Gummin D, Butler J, Roberts R, et al: Utilization of an emergency department observation unit for acute intoxications (abstract). J Toxicol Clin Toxicol 1999;37:586.

43. Gunawardana RH, Abeywarna C: Intensive care utilisation following attempted suicide through self-poisoning. Ceylon Med J 1997;42: 18–20.

44. Hart L, Cobaugh D, Dean B, et al: Successful use of extracorporeal membrane oxygenation (ECMO) in the treatment of refractory respiratory failure secondary to hydrocarbon aspiration (Abstract). Vet Hum Toxicol 1991;33:361.

45. Heffner J, Sahn S: Salicylate-induced pulmonary edema. Ann Intern Med 1981;95:405–409.

46. Henderson A, Wright M, Pond SM: Experience with 732 acute overdose patients admitted to an intensive care unit over six years. Med J Aust 1993;158:28–30.

47. Hendren W, Schieber R, Garrettson L: Extracorporeal bypass for the treatment of verapamil poisoning. Ann Emerg Med 1989;18: 984–987.

48. Heyman EN, LoCastro DE, Gouse LH, et al: Intentional drug overdose: Predictors of clinical course in the intensive care unit. Heart Lung 1996;25:246–252.

49. Holzer M, Sterz F, Schoerkhuber W, et al: Successful resuscitation of a verapamil-intoxicated patient with percutaneous cardiopulmonary bypass. Crit Care Med 1999;27:2818–2823.

50. Hulten BA, Adams R, Askenasi R, et al: Predicting severity of tricyclic antidepressant overdose. J Toxicol Clin Toxicol 1992;30: 161–170.

51. Jay S, Johanson W, Pierce A: Respiratory complications of overdose with sedative drugs. Am Rev Resp Dis 1975;112:591–598.

52. Knaus W, Draper E, Wagner D, et al: APACHE II: A severity of disease classification system. Crit Care Med 1985;13:818–829.

53. Koppel C: Clinical features, pathogenesis and management of drug-induced rhabdomyolysis. Med Toxicol 1989;4:108–126.

54. Kruse J, Thill-Baharozian M, Carlson R: Comparison of clinical assessment with APACHE II for predicting mortality risk in patients admitted to a medical intensive care unit. JAMA 1988;260: 1739–1742.

55. Kulig K, Bar-Or D, Cantrill S, et al: Management of acutely poisoned patients without gastric emptying. Ann Emerg Med 1985;14: 562–567.

56. Lacroix J, Gaudreault P, Gauthier M: Admission to a pediatric intensive care unit for poisoning: A review of 105 cases. Crit Care Med 1989;17:748–750.

57. Landsman I, Bricker J, Reid B, et al: Emergency gastrotomy: Treatment of choice for iron bezoar. J Pediatr Surg 1987;22:184–185.

58. Lane AS, Woodward AC, Goldman MR: Massive propranolol overdose poorly responsive to pharmacologic therapy: Use of the intra-aortic balloon pump. Ann Emerg Med 1987;16:1381–1383.

59. Larkin GL, Graeber GM, Hollingsed MJ: Experimental amitriptyline poisoning: treatment of severe cardiovascular toxicity with cardiopulmonary bypass. Ann Emerg Med 1994;23:480–486.

60. LeBlanc F, Benson B, Gilg A: A severe organophosphate poisoning requiring the use of an atropine drip. J Toxicol Clin Toxicol 1986; 24:69–76.

61. Levy DE, Bates D, Caronna JJ, et al: Prognosis in nontraumatic coma. Ann Intern Med 1981;94:293–301.

62. Linden C, Rumack B, Strehlke C: Monoamine oxidase inhibitor overdose. Ann Emerg Med 1984;13:1137–1144.

63. Litovitz TL, Klein-Schwartz W, White S, et al: 1999 annual report of the American Association of Poison Control Centers Toxic Exposure Surveillance System. Am J Emerg Med 2000;18:517–574.

64. Manton WI, Kirkpatrick JB, Cook JP: Does the choroid plexus really protect the brain from lead? Lancet 1984;2:351.

65. Matsen FA: Compartment syndrome: A unified concept. Clin Orthop 1975;113:8–14.

66. McAlpine S, Calabro J, Robinson M, et al: Late death in tricyclic antidepressant overdose revisited. Ann Emerg Med 1986;15: 1349–1352.

67. McCarron M, Challoner K, Thompson G: Diphenoxylate-atropine (Lomotil) overdose in children: An update (Report of eight cases and review of the literature). Pediatrics 1991;87:694–700.

68. McCarron M, Wood J: The cocaine body packer syndrome. JAMA 1983;250:1417–1420.

69. McVey FK, Corke CF: Extracorporeal circulation in the management of massive propranolol overdose [see comments]. Anaesthesia 1991;46:744–746.

70. Merigian K, Woodard M, Hedges J, et al: Prospective evaluation of gastric emptying in the self-poisoned patient. Am J Emerg Med 1990;8:479–483.

71. Minocha A, Spyker D: Acute overdose with sustained release drug formulations. Med Toxicol 1986;1:300–307.

72. Montgomery A, Stager M, Carrico C, et al: Causes of mortality in patients with the adult respiratory distress syndrome. Am Rev Respir Dis 1985;132:485–489.

73. Murphy G, Wetzel R: Family history of suicidal behavior among suicide attempters. J Nerv Ment Dis 1982;170:86–90.

74. Niemann J, Bessen H, Rothstein R, et al: Electrocardiographic criteria for tricyclic antidepressant cardiotoxicity. Am J Cardiol 1986;57: 1154–1159.

75. Noble J, Kennedy D, Latimer R, et al: Massive lignocaine overdose during cardiopulmonary bypass. Br J Anesthes 1984;56:1439–1441.

76. North D: Meprobamate and bezoar formation [letter]. Ann Emerg Med 1987;16:472–473.

77. Orr D, Bramble M: Tricyclic antidepressant poisoning and prolonged external cardiac massage during asystole. Br Med J 1981; 283:1107–1108.

78. Ostermann ME, Young B, Sibbald WJ, et al: Coma mimicking brain death following baclofen overdose. Intensive Care Med 2000;26: 1144–1146.

79. Pentel P, Benowitz N: Tricyclic antidepressant poisoning: Management of arrhythmias. Med Toxicol 1986;1:101–121.

80. Pentel P, Sioris L: Incidence of late arrhythmias following tricyclic antidepressant overdose. J Toxicol Clin Toxicol 1981;18:543–548.

81. Pond SM, Lewis-Driver DJ, Williams GM, et al: Gastric emptying in acute overdose: A prospective randomised controlled trial. Med J Aust 1995;163:345–349.

82. Powner D: Drug-associated isoelectric EEGs. A hazard in brain death certification. JAMA 1976;236:1123.

83. Ramoska E, Spiller H, Winter H, et al: A one-year evaluation of calcium channel blocker overdoses: Toxicity and treatment. Ann Emerg Med 1993;22:196–200.

84. Reed JR, Palmisano PA: Central nervous system salicylate. Clin Toxicol 1975;8:623–631.

85. Rinaldo J, Snyder J: Survival database: Central nervous system injury. Am Rev Respir Dis 1989;140:S25–S27.

86. Roberts J, Price D, Goldfrank L: The body stuffer syndrome: A clandestine form of drug overdose. Am J Emerg Med 1986;4:22–27.

87. Robertson N: Fatal overdose from sustained-release theophylline preparation. Ann Emerg Med 1985;14:154–158.

88. Ron A, Aronne L, Kalb P, et al: The therapeutic efficacy of critical care units. Arch Intern Med 1989;149:338–341.

89. Rorison D, McPherson S: Acute toxic inhalations. Emerg Med Clin North Am 1992;10:409–435.

90. Schwartz H: Acute meprobamate poisoning with gastrotomy and removal of a drug-containing mass. N Engl J Med 1976;295: 1177–1178.

91. Sedal L, Korman M, Williams P, et al: Overdosage of tricyclic antidepressants: A report of two deaths and a prospective study of 24 patients. Med J Aust 1972;2:74–79.

92. Shannon M, Lovejoy F: Pulmonary complications of severe tricyclic antidepressant ingestion. J Toxicol Clin Toxicol 1987;25:443–461.

93. Shub C, Gau G, Sidell P, et al: The management of acute quinidine intoxication. Chest 1978;73:173–178.

94. Smilkstein M: Reviewing cyclic antidepressant cardiotoxicity: Wheat and chaff. J Emerg Med 1990;8:645–648.

95. Southall D, Kilpatrick S: Imipramine poisoning: Survival of a child after prolonged cardiac massage. Br Med J 1974;4:508.

96. Spiller H, Meyers A, Ziemba T, et al: Delayed onset of cardiac arrhythmias from sustained-release verapamil. Ann Emerg Med 1991; 20:201–203.

97. Spiller H, Morse S: Fluoxetine ingestion: A one year retrospective study. Vet Hum Toxicol 1990;32:153–155.

98. Sporer K, Manning J: Massive ingestion of sustained-release verapamil with a concretion and bowel infarction. Ann Emerg Med 1993; 22:603–605.

99. Strom J, Thisted B, Krantz T, et al: Self-poisoning treated in an ICU: Drug pattern, acute mortality and short term survival. Acta Anaesthesiol Scand 1986;30:148–153.

100. Sutherland LR, Muller P, Lewis DR: Massive cerebral edema associated with fulminant hepatic failure in acetaminophen overdose. Am J Gastroenterol 1981;76:446–448.

101. Tafuri J, Roberts J: Organophosphate poisoning. Ann Emerg Med 1987;16:193–202.

102. Tay SY, Tai DY, Seow E, et al: Patients admitted to an intensive care unit for poisoning. Ann Acad Med Singapore 1998;27:347–352.

103. Tepperman P: Fatality due to acute systemic fluoride poisoning following a hydrofluoric acid skin burn. J Occup Med 1980;22: 691–692.

104. Teres D: Current directions in severity modeling: Limitations leading to a new definition of a high-performance intensive care unit. In: Irwin RS, Cerra FB, Rippe JM, eds: Intensive Care Medicine, 4th ed. Philadelphia, Lippincott-Raven, 1999, pp. 2470–2481.

105. Tokarski G, Young M: Criteria for admitting patients with tricyclic antidepressant overdose. J Emerg Med 1988;6:121–124.

106. Vance M, Curry S, Kunkel D, et al: Digital hydrofluoric acid burns: Treatment with intraarterial calcium infusion. Ann Emerg Med 1986;15:890–896.

107. White A: Overdose of tricyclic antidepressants associated with absent brain-stem reflexes. Can Med Assoc J 1988;139:133–134.

108. Wolfe T, Caravati E, Rollins D: Terminal 40-ms frontal plane QRS axis as a marker for tricyclic antidepressant overdose. Ann Emerg Med 1989;18:348–351.

109. Wortzman D, Grunfeld A: Delayed absorption following enteric-coated aspirin overdose. Ann Emerg Med 1987;16:434–436.

110. Yang K, Dantzker D: Reversible brain death: A manifestation of amitriptyline overdose. Chest 1991;99:1037–1038.

111. Zimmerman J, Knaus W, Judson J, et al: Patient selection for intensive care: A comparison of New Zealand and United States hospitals. Crit Care Med 1988;16:318–326.

CHAPTER 105 REPRODUCTIVE AND PERINATAL PRINCIPLES

Jeffrey S. Fine

Reproductive and perinatal principles in toxicology derive from many areas of basic science and are applied to many aspects of clinical practice. This chapter reviews several principles of reproductive medicine that have implications for toxicology—the physiology of pregnancy and placental drug transfer, the effects of chemical substances on the developing fetus and the neonate, and the management of overdose in pregnant woman.

One of the most dramatic effects of exposure to a toxin during pregnancy is the birth of a child with congenital malformations. Teratology, the study of birth defects, has classically been concerned with the study of physical malformations. A broader view of teratology includes "developmental" teratogens—agents that induce structural malformations, metabolic or physiologic dysfunction, or psychological or behavioral alterations or deficits in the offspring, either at or after birth.[205] Only 4 to 6% of birth defects are related to known pharmaceutic agents or occupational and environmental exposures.[28,205]

Reproductive effects of toxins may occur before conception. Female germ cells are formed in utero; adverse effects from xenobiotic (foreign substance) exposure can theoretically occur from the time of a woman's own intrauterine development to the end of her reproductive years. An example of a drug that had both teratogenic and reproductive effects in the same individual is diethylstilbestrol (DES), which caused vaginal and/or cervical adenocarcinoma in some women exposed in utero and also had effects on fertility and pregnancy outcome.[14,20]

Men generally receive less attention with respect to reproductive risks. Male gametes are formed after puberty; only from that time on are they susceptible to toxic injury. An example of a toxin affecting male reproduction is dibromochloropropane, which reduces spermatogenesis and, consequently, fertility. In general, little is known about the contribution of the sperm to teratogenesis.

Occupational exposures to reproductive toxins are potentially important but often poorly defined. It has been estimated that there are 20 million women of reproductive age in the workforce.[181] Although approximately 90,000 chemicals are used commercially in the United States, only 2200 industrial and pharmaceutic agents have been specifically evaluated for reproductive toxicity. Many agents have teratogenic effects when tested in animal models, but relatively few well-defined human teratogens have been identified.[211] Thus, most tested chemicals do not appear to present a human teratogenic risk, but most chemicals have not been tested. Some of the presumed safe chemicals may have other reproductive, nonteratogenic toxicity. Several excellent reviews are available.[171,205,250]

Another type of toxic exposure for a pregnant woman is the intentional overdose. Although a drug taken in overdose may have direct toxicity for the fetus, the acute toxicity to the fetus frequently results from maternal pulmonary and/or hemodynamic compromise such as hypoxia or shock.

Toxic exposures before and during pregnancy can have effects throughout gestation and may extend into and beyond the newborn period. In addition, the effects of drug administration in the perinatal period (up to 4 weeks of age) and the special case of drug delivery to an infant via the breast milk deserve special consideration.

PHYSIOLOGIC CHANGES DURING PREGNANCY THAT AFFECT DRUG DISTRIBUTION

Many physical and physiologic changes that occur during pregnancy affect both absorption and distribution of drugs in the pregnant woman and consequently affect the amount of drug delivered to the fetus.[95,155]

During pregnancy there is delayed gastric emptying, decreased gastrointestinal (GI) motility, and increased transit time through the GI tract. These changes result in delayed but more complete GI absorption of drugs and, consequently, lower peak plasma concentrations. Because blood flow to the skin and mucous membranes is increased, absorption from dermal exposure may be increased. Similarly, absorption of inhaled agents may be increased because of increased tidal volume and decreased residual lung volume.

An increased free drug concentration in the pregnant woman may be caused by several factors such as decreased plasma albumin, increased binding competition, and decreased hepatic biotransformation during the later stages of pregnancy. Fat stores increase during the early stages of pregnancy; free fatty acids are released during the later stages and, with them, drugs that may have accumulated in the lipid compartment. The increased concentration of free fatty acids can compete with circulating free drug for binding sites on albumin.

Other factors may lead to decreased free drug concentrations. Early in pregnancy, increased fat stores as well as the increased plasma and extracellular fluid volume will lead to a greater volume of distribution. Increased renal blood flow and glomerular filtration may result in increased renal elimination.

Cardiac output increases throughout pregnancy, with the placenta receiving a gradually increasing proportion of total blood volume. Drug delivery to the placenta may therefore increase over the course of pregnancy.

These processes interact dynamically, and it is difficult to predict their net effect. The concentrations of many drugs such as lithium, gentamicin, and carbamazepine decrease during pregnancy even if the administered dose is not changed.[117]

Though this is not specifically related to the physiologic changes occurring during pregnancy, the fetus may be exposed to drugs and chemicals that accumulated in adipose tissue before pregnancy. For example, typical retinoid malformations were seen in a baby born to a woman whose pregnancy began 1 year after she discontinued use of the drug etretinate (retinoic acid).[124]

TOXIN EXPOSURE IN PREGNANT WOMEN

Prescribed and over-the-counter medications, alcohol, caffeine, nicotine, drugs of abuse, and chemicals in the workplace are all sources of xenobiotic exposure to pregnant women. Between 30 and 80% of pregnant women take medication some time during pregnancy, primarily analgesics, antipyretics, antimicrobials, and antiemetics as well as vitamins, caffeine, ethanol, and nicotine.[22,24,35,47,56,196,197] Some pregnant women use medications to treat chronic disease; others use medications unknowingly before the determination of pregnancy.

Pharmaceutical manufacturers categorize medications according to their potential benefits and risks for a pregnant woman and the fetus according to standards promulgated by the US Food and Drug Administration (FDA) (Table 105–1).[233] Classification systems similar to that of the FDA have been developed in Sweden and Australia.[5,187,203] The US system has been criticized for being too conservative.[74] Both systems have been criticized for conveying an impression of a hierarchy of harmful effects; for example, in the US system, that a category C drug is worse than a category B drug in pregnancy.[74,187] US FDA category C is the default for drugs about which there is little or no specific information available and for which the risk is unknown.

Agents classified as US FDA category X and category D drugs are listed in Tables 105–2 and 105–3, respectively. Some of these agents are known or suspected human teratogens and are more fully described in Table 105–4. Manufacturers may label certain drugs as category X even when there is only limited information associating an agent with any adverse fetal or neonatal effects. Certain agents with D ratings may cause problems only at certain times during pregnancy. Even drugs that are category D or X drugs may have a very low risk of teratogenicity or other adverse effect, and exposure to these agents, even during the first trimester, may not be a sufficient indication to terminate a pregnancy. Specific current information on individual drugs and toxins can be obtained from local and regional teratogen information services.[75,119] Motherrisk is a Canadian program that uses specific drug information to advise women about the actual risk of a particular drug or toxin to them in a current or planned pregnancy[172] (Chap. 16).

Although most women are concerned about the teratogenic effects of medications, in utero exposure to therapeutic medications can have other pharmacologic effects on the newborn infant such as hyperbilirubinemia or withdrawal reactions (see below).[23,30]

Estimates of substance use in pregnancy vary tremendously depending on the geographic location, practice environment, patient population, and drug-screening method.[41,126] In a 1992 national sample screened by verbal report and urine drug screen, 5.5% of women used some substance at some time during pregnancy.[164]

TABLE 105–1.   FDA Use-in-Pregnancy Ratings

Category	Risk to Human Fetus	Example	FDA Terminology
A	No known risk	Multiple vitamins	***Controlled studies show no risk.*** Adequate, well-controlled studies in pregnant women have failed to demonstrate risk to the fetus.
B	No known risk	Acetaminophen, penicillin	***No evidence of risk in humans.*** Either animal findings show risk but human findings do not, or, if no adequate human studies have been done, animal findings show no risk.
C	Possible risk	Albuterol	***Risk cannot be ruled out.*** No human studies and no animal studies show risk. However, potential benefits may justify the potential risk.
D	Known risk, but benefit may outweigh risk	Tetracycline	***Positive evidence of risk.*** Investigational or postmarketing data show risk to the fetus. Nevertheless, potential benefits may outweigh the potential risk.
X	Known risk, but risk significantly outweighs benefit	Isotretinoin	***Contraindicated in pregnancy.*** Studies in animals or humans or investigational or postmarketing reports have shown fetal risk that clearly outweighs any possible benefit to the patient.

Based on Federal Register 1979;44:37434–37467.

This survey found that 20% of pregnant women smoked, 20% drank ethanol, and 3% used marijuana. Only 0.5% of pregnant women used cocaine, 0.1% used methadone, and fewer than 0.1% used heroin. There is evidence that women tend to decrease their exposure to medications and substances once they know they are pregnant.[25,99,103]

PLACENTAL REGULATION OF XENOBIOTIC TRANSFER TO THE FETUS

With respect to the transfer of chemicals from mother to fetus, the placenta functions like other lipoprotein membranes. Most xenobiotics enter the fetal circulation by passive diffusion down a concentration gradient across the placental membranes. The characteristics of a substance that favor this passive diffusion are low molecular weight, lipid solubility, neutral polarity, and low protein binding.[166] Polar molecules and ions may be transported through interstitial pores.[230]

TABLE 105–2. Use-in-Pregnancy Category X Drugs[a]

Antineoplastic agents (aminopterin, leuprolide)[b]

Benzodiazepines (temazepam, quazepam, triazolam, flurazepam)[b]
   Possible neonatal withdrawal after maternal use, may cause cleft palate[59]
   Temazepam—possible interaction with diphenhydramine leading to a stillbirth
   Quazepam—minor anomalies in fetal mice

Chenodiol—hepatotoxicity, hemorrhagic adrenal necrosis, interstitial renal hemorrhage in primates exposed in utero

Cholesterol-lowering agents (ie, lovastatin)—teratogenic in rodents at high doses; reports of birth defects with human exposures during first trimester

Danazol—may cause female pseudohermaphroditism

Ergotamine—possible maternal hypertension or decreased uterine blood flow

Estrogens—possible increased risk of congenital malformations

Ethanol—see Table 105–4

Iodine-(iodinated glycerol, iodine^{-127}, iodine^{-133})[b]—may cause neonatal hypothyroidism or goiter

Menadione—see Table 105–4

Mifepristone—abortifacient

Misoprostol—see Table 105–4

Progestogens (norethindrone, norethynodrel, norgestrel, oral contraceptives)

Quinine—malformations associated with use of toxic doses as abortifacient; also thrombocytopenic purpura and hemolysis in a G6PD-deficient infant

Retinoids (etretinate, isotretinoin, vitamin A)—see Table 105–4

Ribavirin—teratogenic or embryolethal in animal species

Vaccines (MMR, smallpox)—small risk of congenital rubella or other fetal viral syndromes; fetal death has been associated with smallpox vaccination

---

[a]Category assigned by manufacturer. Some of these agents are recognized human teratogens (see Table 105–4). Comments are included for agents not listed in Table 105–4. For current information on individual agents, additions, and changes, please consult current drug references such as the Physician's Desk Reference or individual package inserts.

[b]Other agents in this drug class carry category D ratings (see Table 105–3).

Data adapted from Briggs GG, Freeman RK, Yaffe SJ: Drugs in Pregnancy and Lactation: A Reference Guide to Fetal and Neonatal Risk, 5th ed. Baltimore, Williams & Wilkins, 1998.

Xenobiotics with a molecular weight greater than 1000 Da do not diffuse passively across the placenta, and this characteristic is used to therapeutic advantage. For example, warfarin (MW 1000 Da) easily crosses the placenta and causes specific fetal malformations.[235] However, heparin (MW 20,000 Da), which is too large to cross the placenta, is not teratogenic and is consequently the preferred anticoagulant during pregnancy. Most drugs have molecular weights between 250 and 400 Da and easily cross the placenta.

Thiopental is highly lipid soluble and crosses the placenta rapidly. Fetal plasma levels reach maternal levels within a few minutes. Muscle relaxants such as vecuronium are more polar and cross the placenta slowly.[61]

Although the state of ionization is a limiting factor for diffusion, some highly charged compounds can diffuse across the placenta. Valproic acid ($pK_a = 4.7$) is nearly completely ionized at physiologic pH, yet there is rapid equilibration across the placental membrane. The small amount of drug that exists in the nonionized form rapidly crosses the placenta; as equilibrium is reestablished, a new small amount of nonionized drug becomes available for diffusion.[165]

Fetal blood pH changes during gestation. Embryonic intracellular pH is high relative to the pregnant woman. During this developmental stage, weak acids will diffuse across the placenta to the embryo and remain there because of "ion trapping." Many teratogens such as valproic acid, trimethadione, phenytoin, thalidomide, warfarin, and isotretinoin are weak acids. Although ion trapping does not explain the mechanism of teratogenesis, it may explain how the embryo accumulates the toxin. Late in gestation the fetal blood is 0.10 to 0.15 pH units more acidic than the mother's, which may permit weakly basic drugs to concentrate in the fetus during this period.[166]

The relative concentrations of protein binding sites in the pregnant woman and fetus also have an impact on the extent of drug transfer to the fetus.[166] As maternal free fatty acid concentrations increase near term, these fatty acids can displace drugs such as valproic acid or diazepam from maternal protein binding sites and make more free drug available for transfer to the fetus. Fetal albumin levels increase during gestation and exceed maternal albumin concentrations by term. Because the fetus does not have high levels of free fatty acids to compete for protein binding sites, these sites are available for binding the drugs. At birth, when neonatal free fatty acid levels increase two- to threefold, they displace stored drug from the binding protein. In the cases of valproic acid and diazepam, the elevated levels of free drug have been shown to have adverse effects on the newborn infant.[80,100,165,180]

The placenta may also affect drug presentation to the fetus by ion trapping and drug metabolism. The placenta blocks the transfer of some positively charged ions such as cadmium and mercury[89] and may even accumulate them. This barrier does not protect the fetus, however, because these heavy metal ions interfere with normal placental function and may lead to placental necrosis and subsequent fetal death.[158]

The placenta contains drug-metabolizing enzymes capable of performing both phase I and phase II reactions (Chaps. 11 and 14). However, the concentration of biotransforming enzymes in the placenta is significantly lower than that in the liver, and it is unlikely that the level of enzymatic activity is protective for the fetus. Moreover, the fetus may be exposed to reactive intermediates that form during these processes. However, glutathione may also be present in the placenta and detoxify some of these reactive intermediates.[106]

Placental transfer of drugs can have a positive effect when it provides fetal therapy. For example, if a fetus is found to have supraventricular tachycardia or atrial flutter, digoxin can be given to the mother to treat the baby.[193]

EFFECTS OF XENOBIOTIC AGENTS ON THE DEVELOPING ORGANISM

One of the basic premises of teratogenicity is that the particular toxic effects of a drug are determined by the organism's stage of development.[29,207] The fertilized ovum is thought to be resistant to toxic insult before implantation.[29] However, drugs and chemicals in the fallopian or uterine secretions may prevent implantation of the embryo. Drug exposure leading to cell loss or chromosomal abnormalities may also lead to a spontaneous abortion, possibly even before pregnancy has been detected. If the preimplantation embryo survives a toxic exposure, the functional cells usually pro-

TABLE 105–3.   Use-in-Pregnancy Category D Drugs[a]

Drug Category/Class/Agent	Known or Presumed Effect
Aminoglycosides	Eighth nerve damage, hearing loss.
Amiodarone	Contains iodine and may cause neonatal goiter.
Angiotensin-converting enzyme inhibitors	See Table 105–4.
Anticonvulsants (aminoglutethimide, barbiturates, carbamazepine, oxazolidinediones, phensuximide, phenytoin, valproic acid)	See Table 105–4. There are case reports of malformations with phensuximide. Aminoglutethimide has been associated with virilization.
Antidepressants (amitryptiline, butryptiline, clomipramine, dibenzepin, dothiepin, imipramine, iprindole, nortryptiline, opipramol)	Occasional reports of malformations, antidepressant toxicity or withdrawal, and urinary retention. Seizures associated with clomipramine. Desipramine is category C.
Antineoplastic agents	This group includes multiple agents with different effects. Not all agents are definitely toxic during pregnancy, but there is concern for chromosomal damage and immunosuppression with these agents.
Antithyroid (carbimazole, methimazole, propylthiouracil)	Possible aplasia cutis (carbimazole, methimazole) and other malformations, neonatal hypothyroidism and goiter.
Aspirin	Maternal effects: anemia, antepartum/postpartum hemorrhage, prolonged gestation, prolonged labor. May be beneficial in pregnancy-induced hypertension. Infant effects: hemorrhage; high doses may lead to intrauterine growth retardation and increased perinatal mortality.
Atenolol	Can cause IUGR, related to total dose and duration. Maternal therapy near term may lead to fetal/neonatal bradycardia. Other β-adrenergic receptor antagonists may cause similar effects.
Azathioprine	Limb reduction defects in rabbits. Sporadic human anomalies or neonatal immunodeficiency.
Carbarsone	Contains arsenic, which has caused fetal fatalities.
Colchicine	Teratogenic and embryocidal in mice and rabbits.
Cortisone	Reports of malformations, concern about neonatal adrenal hyperplasia or insufficiency.
Coumarin derivatives/warfarin	Table 105–4.
Diuretics (thiazides, ethacrynic acid, potassium sparing)	First trimester use may be associated with malformations. Possible hypoglycemia, thrombocytopenia, hyponatremia, hypokalemia. Concerns about the thiazide diuretics have been extended to other classes of diuretics.
Iodine-containing compounds	Hypothyroidism and goiter.
Lithium	See Table 105–4.
Methylene blue	Intraamniotic injection—methemoglobinemia, staining of fetal skin
Nonsteroidal antiinflammatory agents	These agents generally carry a category B designation, but there is concern when they are used for more than 48 hours or after 34 weeks of gestation. Closure of ductus arteriosus with pulmonary hypertension, oligohydramnios. Most information based on indomethacin. Adverse maternal effect observed when used with β-adrenergic antagonists.
Opioid analgesics/antagonists	These agents generally carry a category B designation, but use near delivery may lead to respiratory depression; antagonists may precipitate fetal or neonatal opioid withdrawal.
Penicillamine	See Table 105–4.
Progestogens (ethisterone, ethynodiol, hydroxyprogesterone, medroxyprogesterone)	Possible association with cardiovascular malformations, hypospadias. Masculinization of the female infant.
Sedative-hypnotic agents (barbiturates, benzodiazepines, meprobamate)	Possible malformations, neonatal sedation or withdrawal; barbiturates have been associated with hemorrhagic disease; benzodiazepines have been associated with floppy infant syndrome and cleft lip or palate.[59]
Sulfonamides and sulfa analogues	Use near term may lead to neonatal jaundice.
Sulfonylureas (acetohexamide, chlorpropamide, tolazamide, tolbutamide)	Poor control of diabetes mellitus in pregnancy. Use near term is associated with prolonged neonatal hypoglycemia.
Sympathomimetic agents (levarterenol, metaraminol)	Possible maternal hypertension, decreased uterine blood flow.
Tetracyclines	See Table 105–4.
Vitamin D and analogues	See Table 105–4.

[a]Category assigned by manufacturer. Some of these agents are recognized human teratogens (see Table 105–4). Comments are included for agents not listed in Table 105–4. For current information on individual agents, additions, and changes, please consult current drug references such as the Physician's Desk Reference or individual package inserts.
Data adapted from Briggs GG, Freeman RK, Yaffe SJ: Drugs in Pregnancy and Lactation: A Reference Guide to Fetal and Neonatal Risk, 5th ed. Baltimore, Williams & Wilkins, 1998.

ceed to normal development.[207] Teratogens that act in such a manner elicit an "all-or-none response": the exposed embryo will either die or go on to normal development.

Teratogens generally behave according to a dose–response curve; as the dose of the teratogen increases, the magnitude of the effect increases. For example, in animal experiments, more members of a litter will be malformed when the dose of a teratogen is increased, or in the case of an "all or none" response, more members of a litter may die. However, the dose–response effect does not generally mean that a higher dose will cause worse malformations than a lower dose. Strictly, teratogenic effects are those that occur at doses that do not cause maternal toxicity because maternal toxicity itself might be responsible for an observed adverse or teratogenic effect on the developing organism.

TABLE 105–4. Human Teratogens

Agent	Reported Effects	Comments
Androgens	Masculinization of female embryo: clitoromegaly with or without fusion of labia minora	Effects are dose dependent: stimulates growth and differentiation of sex-steroid receptor-containing tissue.
Angiotensin-converting enzyme inhibitors (ie, enalapril)	Fetal/neonatal death, prematurity, oligohydramnios, neonatal anuria, IUGR, secondary skull hypoplasia, limb contractures, pulmonary hypoplasia	Does not interfere with organogenesis. Small risk of effects related to chronic fetal hypotension during second/third trimester. If in use during early pregnancy, can be switched during first trimester.[28]
Alkylating agents (busulfan, chlorambucil, cyclophosphamide, mechlorethamine)	Growth retardation, cleft palate, microphthalmia, hypoplastic ovaries, cloudy corneas, renal agenesis, malformations of digits, cardiac defects, other anomalies	10–50% malformation rate, depending on which drug. Cyclophosphamide-induced damage requires cytochrome P450 monoxidase activation. Metabolite interacts with DNA, resulting in cell death.
Antimetabolites (aminopterin, (azauridine, cytarabine, 5-FU, 6-MP, methotrexate)	Hydro/microcephaly, meningoencephalocele, anencephaly, abnormal cranial ossification, cerebral hypoplasia, growth retardation, eye, ear, and nose malformations, cleft palate, malformed extremities/fingers, reduction in derivatives of first branchial arch	These folate antagonists inhibit dihydrofolate reductase, resulting in cell death. Depending on specific agent, 7–75% rate of malformation.[238]
Carbamazepine	Upslanting palpebral fissures, epicanthal folds, short nose with long philtrum, fingernail hypoplasia, developmental delay, neural tube defects (NTD).	Mechanism may involve an epoxide intermediate. Risk unquantified but may be significant for minor anomalies; 1% risk for NTD.[105]
Carbon monoxide	Cerebral atrophy, mental retardation, microcephaly, convulsions, spastic disorders, intrauterine death	With severe maternal poisoning, high risk for neurological sequelae; no increased risk in mild unintentional exposures.
Cocaine	IUGR, microcephaly, neurobehavioral abnormalities, vascular disruptive phenomenon (limb amputation, cerebral infarction, visceral/urinary tract abnormalities)	Vascular disruptive effects caused by decreased uterine blood flow and fetal vascular effects from first trimester through the end of pregnancy. Risk for major disruptive effects is low.
Coumarins	Fetal warfarin syndrome: nasal hypoplasia, chondrodysplasia punctata, branchydactyly, skull defects, abnormal ears, malformed eyes, CNS malformations, microcephaly, hydrocephalus, skeletal deformities, mental retardation, spasticity	10–25% risk of malformation for first-trimester exposure, 3% risk of hemorrhage, 8% risk of stillbirth. Bleeding is an unlikely explanation for effects produced in the first trimester. CNS defects may occur during second and third trimesters and may be related to bleeding.[104,237]
Diethylstilbesterol (DES)	Female offspring: vaginal adenosis, clear cell carcinoma, irregular menses, reduced pregnancy rates, increased rate of preterm deliveries, increased perinatal mortality and spontaneous abortion. Male offspring: epididymal cysts, cryptorchidism, hypogonadism, diminished spermatogenesis.	DES stimulates estrogen receptor-containing tissue and may cause misplaced genital tissue with propensity to develop cancer. 40–70% risk of morphologic changes in vaginal epithelium. Risk of adenocarcinoma approximately 1/1000 for exposure before the 18th week. Most children exposed to DES in utero can conceive and deliver normal children.
Ethanol	Fetal alcohol syndrome (FAS): pre/postnatal growth retardation, mental retardation, fine motor dysfunction, hyperactivity, microcephaly, maxillary hypoplasia, short palpebral fissures, hypoplastic philtrum, thinned upper lips, joint, digit anomalies.	Other effects: increased incidence of spontaneous abortion, premature delivery, and stillbirth; neonatal withdrawal. Effects may be direct cytotoxic effects of ethanol or acetaldehyde and/or indirect effects of alcoholism and other substance/tobacco use. FAS in 10–40% of offspring of alcoholic women consuming above 2 g/kg/d (6 oz/d) ethanol over the first trimester. Fetal alcohol effects at lower doses. There may be a threshold for effects, but a safe dose has not been identified.[218]
Iodine	Thyroid hypoplasia after the eighth week of development	High doses of radioisotopes can produce cell death and mitotic delay. Tissue- and organ-specific damage is dependent on the specific radioisotope, dose, distribution, metabolism, and localization.
Lead	Lower scores on developmental tests	Higher risk when maternal lead is >10 μg/dL.
Lithium carbonate	Possible increased risk of Ebstein anomaly	Low risk.
Methyl mercury, mercuric sulfide	Normal appearance at birth; cerebral palsy-like syndrome after several months; microcephaly, mental retardation, cerebellar symptoms, eye/dental anomalies.	Inhibit enzymes, particularly those with sulfhydryl groups. 13 of 220 babies born following the Minamata Bay exposure had severe disease. Mothers of affected babies ingested 9–27 ppm mercury; greater risk with ingestion at 6–8 months of gestation. In acute poisoning, the fetus is 4–10 times more sensitive than an adult. Pathologically there are atrophy and hypoplasia of the brain cortex and abnormalities in cytoarchitecture.[89,243]
Misoprostol	Vascular disruptive phenomena such as limb reduction defects; moebius syndrome.	Prostaglandin analogue. Effects occur after the period of early organogenesis

TABLE 105–4.   Human Teratogens (continued)

Agent	Reported Effects	Comments
Oxazolidine-2,4-diones (trimethadione, paramethadione)	Fetal trimethadione syndrome; V-shaped eyebrows, low-set ears with anteriorly folded helix, high arched palate, irregular teeth, CNS anomalies, severe developmental delay, cardiovascular, genitourinary, and other anomalies	83% risk of at least one major malformation with any exposure; 32% die. Characteristic facial features are associated with chronic exposure.
Polychlorinated biphenyls	Cola-colored children; pigmentation of gums, nails, and groin; hypoplastic, deformed nails; IUGR; abnormal skull calcifications	Cytotoxic agent. Body residue can affect subsequent offspring for up to 4 years after exposure. Most cases followed high consumption of PCB-contaminated rice oil; 4–20% of offspring were affected.
Penicillamine	Cutis laxa, hyperflexibility of joints	Copper chelator: copper deficiency inhibits collagen synthesis/maturation. Few case reports; low risk.
Phenytoin	Fetal hydantoin syndrome; microcephaly, mental retardation, cleft lip/palate, hypoplastic nails/phalanages, characteristic facies—low nasal bridge, inner epicanthal folds, ptosis, strabismus, hypertelorism, low-set ears, wide mouth	Phenytoin has a direct effect on cell membranes and folate and vitamin K metabolism. Epoxide intermediate postulated as teratogenic agent. Effects seen with chronic exposure. 5–10% risk of typical syndrome, 30% risk of partial syndrome. Risk is confounded by those associated with epilepsy itself and use of other agents.[88]
Progestins	Masculinization of female embryo	Stimulates or interferes with sex-steroid receptor-containing tissue. Effects only after exposure to high doses of some testosterone-derived progestins. Doses in current oral contraceptives do not cause these effects.
Radiation, ionizing	Microcephaly, mental retardation, eye anomalies, growth retardation, visceral malformations	Significant doses of radiation from diagnostic or therapeutic sources produce cell death and mitotic delay. There is no measurable risk with x-ray exposures of 5 rads or less at any stage of pregnancy.[14]
Retinoids (isotretinoin, etretinate, high-dose vitamin A)	Spontaneous abortions, micro/hydrocephalus, deformities of cranium, ears, face, heart, limbs, liver	Retinoids can cause direct cytotoxicity and alter programmed cell death. Neural crest cells are particularly sensitive. For isotretinoin, 38% risk of malformations; 80% are CNS malformations. Effects have been associated with vitamin A doses of 25,000–100,000 U/d. Exposures below 10,000 U/d present no risk to fetus. Topical retinoids are not considered a reproductive risk.[225]
Smoking	Placental lesions, IUGR, increased perinatal mortality, increased risk of SIDS[73,123,213,244]	Effects related to a combination of vasoconstriction (nicotine effect), hypoxia secondary to hypoperfusion, CO, and CN, and altered development of neurons and neural pathways.[201,216]
Streptomycin	Hearing deficiency	Rare reports. A low-risk phenomenon that could be associated with long-duration maternal therapy during pregnancy.
Tetracycline	Yellow, gray-brown, or brown staining of deciduous teeth, hypoplastic tooth enamel	Effects seen from 4 months of gestation on because tetracyclines have to interact with calcified tissue. Effects in 50% of fetuses exposed to tetracycline; 12.5% exposed to oxytetracycline.
Thalidomide	Limb phocomelia, amelia, hypoplasia, congenital heart defects, renal malformations, cryptorchidism, abducens paralysis, deafness, microtia, anotia	Approximately 20% risk when exposure to drug occurs during days 34–50 of gestation.
Valproic Acid	Lumbosacral spina bifida with meningomyelocele; CNS defects, microcephaly, cardiac defects. narrow face with high forehead, epicanthal folds, broad low nasal bridge with short nose, long philtrum with a thin vermilion border, long thin fingers and toes.	Risk for spina bifida is approximately 1%, but the risk for dysmorphic facies may be greater. The mechanism of teratogenicity is unknown. Possible explanations include interference with glutathione, folate, or zinc metabolism, or regulation of intracellular pH. Risk is confounded by those associated with epilepsy itself or use of other agents.
Vitamin D	Possible association with supravalvular aortic stenosis, elfin facies, and mental retardation	Large doses of vitamin D may disrupt cellular calcium regulation. Genetic susceptibility may play a role.

Adapted from: Koren G, Nulman I: Teratogenic drugs and chemicals in humans. In: Koren G, ed: Maternal–Fetal Toxicology: A Clinician's Guide, 2nd ed. New York, Marcel Dekker, 1994; and Brent RL: The application of the principles of toxicology and teratology in evaluating the risks of new drugs for the treatment of drug addiction in women of reproductive age. NIDA Res Monogr 1995;149:132–181.

Organogenesis occurs during the embryonic stage between days 18 and 60 of gestation. Most gross malformations are determined before day 36, although genitourinary and craniofacial anomalies occur later.[29] The period of susceptibility to teratogenic effects varies for each organ system (Fig. 105–1). For instance, the palate has a very short period of sensitivity, lasting approximately 3 weeks, whereas the central nervous system (CNS) remains susceptible throughout gestation.

Theoretically, knowing the exact time of teratogen exposure during gestation should allow prediction of a teratogenic effect; this is true in animal models, where dose and time can be strictly controlled. It is also true for thalidomide, where different limb anomalies are related to exposures on different days.[207] In most clinical situations, relating teratogenicity to a particular drug exposure is difficult because drugs are generally administered intermittently or chronically, and also it is often difficult to determine the exact time of exposure relative to conception.

During the fetal period, formed organs continue their cellular differentiation and grow to functional maturity. Exposure to toxic agents such as cigarettes during this period generally leads to growth retardation. Teratogenic malformations or death may still occur as a result of disruption or destruction of growing organs, as has been the result of exposure to the angiotensin-converting enzyme inhibitors during the second and third trimesters.[17]

Another concern during the fetal period is the initiation of carcinogenesis (see Chap. 16). Significant cellular replication and proliferation lead to a dramatic growth in size of the organism. At the same time, when the fetus is exposed to xenobiotic agents, development of biotransformation systems may expose the organism to reactive metabolites that might initiate tumor formation. Some tumors, such as neuroblastoma, appear early in postnatal life, suggesting a prenatal origin. In pregnant rats given ethylnitrosourea during the embryonic period, lethal or teratogenic effects occur.[182] If ethylnitrosourea is administered during the fetal period, there is an increased incidence of tumors in the offspring. Clear-cell vaginal and cervical adenocarcinomas are seen in the offspring of women exposed to diethylstilbesterol during pregnancy.[20]

MECHANISMS OF TERATOGENESIS

Cytotoxicity is one mechanism of teratogenesis and is the characteristic result of exposure to alkylating or antineoplastic agents. Aminopterin, for example, inhibits dihydrofolate reductase activity and leads to suppression of mitosis and cell death. If exposure to a cytotoxic agent occurs very early in development, the embryo may die, whereas sublethal exposure during organogenesis may result in maldevelopment of particular structures. There is evidence that following cell death, the remaining cells in an affected region may try to repair the damage caused by the missing cellular elements. This "restorative growth" may lead to uncoordinated growth and exacerbate the original malformation.

In the case of the cytotoxic agents, the mechanism of action is understood, although it is not always clear why particular agents affect particular structures. With other agents, the structural effects have a clearer relationship to the site of action. For instance, when

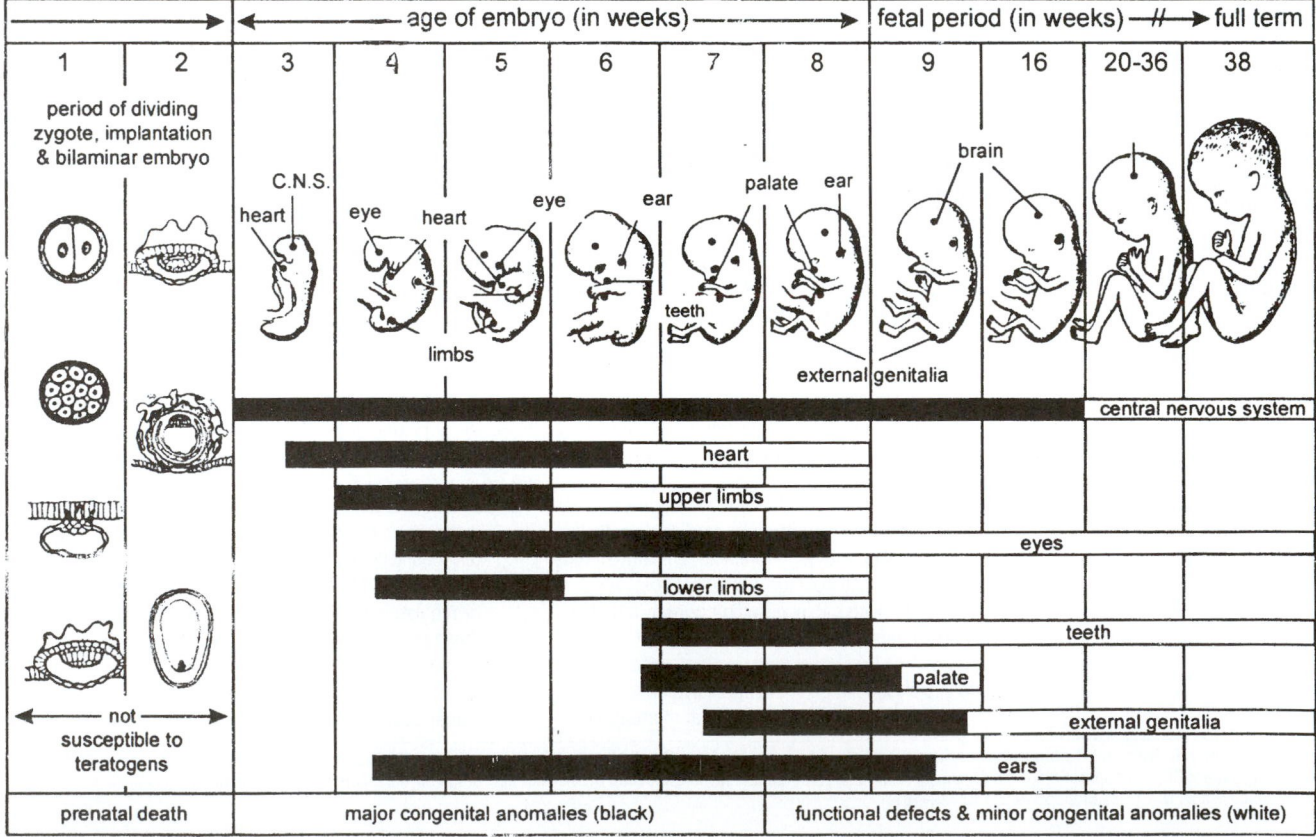

Figure 105–1.   Critical periods of fetal development. *(Modified with permission from Moore KL, Persaud TVN: The Developing Human: Clinically Oriented Embryology, 5th ed. Philadelphia: Saunders, 1993).*

glucocorticoids are administered in large doses to experimental animals during the period of organogenesis, malformations of the palate occur. Glucocorticoid receptors are found in high concentrations in the palate of the developing embryo.[176]

Caloric deficiency is not considered teratogenic during the period of organogenesis. However, specific nutritional or vitamin deficiencies can be teratogenic; an increased incidence of neural tube defects is seen with folate deficiency.[135] Ethanol affects the fetus both directly and indirectly. The craniofacial malformations seen in the fetal alcohol syndrome probably result from ethanol effects during the period of organogenesis. Growth retardation may represent direct effects on fetal growth or indirect effects resulting from maternal nutritional deficiencies.

MANAGEMENT OF ACUTE POISONING IN THE PREGNANT WOMAN

Suicide and suicide attempts during pregnancy are uncommon. Each year a small number of women die during pregnancy or the postpartum period; 1 to 5% of these pregnancy-related deaths may be the result of suicide. Between 2 and 12% of women who attempt or commit suicide may be pregnant.[113,173,246] Reported reasons for these suicide attempts include loss of a lover, economic crisis, prior loss of children, and unwanted pregnancy and desire for an abortion.[52,133,246] In one series, 12% of ingestions were attempts to terminate pregnancy[173] (Chap. 30).

Medication ingestion is a common method of attempting suicide during pregnancy. Analgesics, vitamins, iron, antibiotics, and psychotropic medications account for 50 to 79% of the reported ingestions by pregnant women.[173,177] These agents are frequently prescribed for and used by pregnant women.

Managing any acute overdose during pregnancy always raises several questions. Is the general management different? Do altered metabolism and pharmacokinetics increase (or decrease) the woman's risk of morbidity or mortality from a drug overdose? Is the fetus at risk of poisoning from a maternal overdose? Is there a teratogenic risk to the fetus from an acute drug overdose or poisoning? Is the use of antidotes contraindicated or modified? When should a potentially viable fetus be emergently delivered to prevent toxicity? When should abortion be recommended?

Physiologic changes during pregnancy affect pharmacokinetics, and drugs taken in overdose have altered pharmacokinetics. In any significant overdose during pregnancy, pregnancy-related alterations in pharmacokinetics are not likely to protect the woman from significant morbidity or mortality.

Although a single high-dose exposure to a drug during the period of organogenesis might mimic an experimental model to induce teratogenesis, most drugs commonly ingested in overdose do not induce physical deformities. Ethanol and many of the anticonvulsant agents are teratogenic and may be ingested in toxic doses, but their teratogenicity is probably related to chronic exposure. Acute acetaminophen intoxication in the first trimester may lead to an increased risk of spontaneous abortion,[185] suggesting a teratogenic effect similar to the all-or-none response described earlier. There is, for example, a report of multiple severe congenital malformations in the stillborn fetus of a woman who overdosed on isoniazid during the 12th week of pregnancy.[130] However, because the background incidence of congenital malformations is 3 to 6%, it is almost impossible to determine for a single case whether a particular drug exposure is the etiology of any observed malformations.[53] It is very unlikely that possible teratogenesis would ever lead to a recommendation for abortion after an acute overdose.

In general, any condition that leads to a severe metabolic derangement in the pregnant woman is likely to have an adverse impact on the developing fetus. As a general approach, the management of overdose in a pregnant woman should follow the principles outlined in Chap. 3 and 31, with close attention paid to the airway, oxygenation, and hemodynamic stability. The use of naloxone and dextrose has not been specifically assessed in pregnancy but should be guided by the same considerations raised in managing a nonpregnant patient with alterations in respiratory or neurologic function. Opioid-induced respiratory failure in a pregnant woman will lead to fetal hypoxia and adverse effects; opioid withdrawal in a pregnant woman, whether induced by abstinence or the use of naloxone, may potentially lead to adverse effects on the fetus or the pregnancy. Evaluation of the benefits and risks of the use of naloxone for an opioid-poisoned woman in respiratory distress or coma suggests that reduced morbidity for both mother and fetus may be achieved by the use of carefully titrated doses of naloxone to minimize the likelihood of maternal withdrawal (see Chap. 62 and Antidotes in Depth: Opioid Antagonists).

Gastroinestinal decontamination is frequently a part of the early management of acute poisoning in the nonpregnant patient. Pregnancy is considered a relative contraindication to the use of syrup of ipecac because vomiting increases both intrathoracic and intraabdominal pressure; therefore, gastric lavage is a more appropriate method of gastric emptying for the pregnant patient shortly after a life-threatening ingestion. The usual concerns about protecting the airway apply to the pregnant patient as well.

There is no specific contraindication to the use of activated charcoal in a pregnant woman. There may be a specific role for whole-bowel irrigation in the treatment of iron overdose in pregnancy (see below).

In considering the use of antidotes, the primary concern should be for the health of the pregnant woman. Almost all antidotal agents are categorized as FDA pregnancy-risk category C; that is, there is little information to guide their use. Ethanol is classified as category D (positive evidence of risk), although this is related to chronic use throughout pregnancy, not as an antidote. Pyridoxine and thiamine are category A drugs; N-acetylcysteine, magnesium, glucagon, and naloxone are category B drugs.

Thus far, there are no reports of adverse effects on the fetus from antidotal treatment of a poisoned pregnant woman. Conversely, in at least in one case, withholding deferoxamine therapy may have contributed to the death of both a woman and her fetus.[145,224] In the hypothetical case of a pregnant woman poisoned with a toxic alcohol, we would support the use of ethanol until hemodialysis can be performed, although thus far there are no data to predict specific outcome. Currently the physician will need to weigh the short-term toxicity of high ethanol levels against the unknown risk of fomepizole.

ACETAMINOPHEN

Acetaminophen is the most common analgesic agent used during pregnancy and is one of the most common agents ingested in overdose during pregnancy.[152,185] There are two published series as well as a number of individual reports totaling more than 100 cases of acute acetaminophen overdose during all trimesters of pregnancy. In the two large series representing 112 acute and chronic overdoses, 33 patients had acetaminophen levels in the toxic range.[152,185] These studies, in addition to the case reports described below, demonstrate that most pregnant women recover from an acetaminophen ingestion without adverse effects to themselves or their babies.

In the two large series of acetaminophen overdose during pregnancy,[152,185] 8 of 28 women who overdosed in the first trimester and continued their pregnancy experienced spontaneous abortions, most within 2 weeks of the ingestion. Five of the 8 women had toxic acetaminophen levels; one woman received N-acetylcysteine (NAC) within 8 hours, and four received NAC between 12 and 17 hours. In one of these cases there was both maternal and fetal death. Five patients with toxic acetaminophen levels and 14 with nontoxic levels delivered healthy term newborns. Ten women had elective terminations of pregnancy.

The two large series include 32 second-trimester acute overdoses.[152,185] Two women who had nontoxic acetaminophen levels had spontaneous abortions—one had symptoms of a threatened abortion several days before the overdose, and the second was assaulted the day before the overdose and aborted the day after. Six women with toxic acetaminophen levels delivered full-term healthy infants, 19 women with nontoxic levels delivered full-term babies, and one woman with a nontoxic level delivered a premature infant 2 months following the overdose. Four women had elective terminations of pregnancy.

There are three case reports of women with acute overdoses in the second trimester. One woman who overdosed at 15.5 weeks of gestation had a toxic acetaminophen level, was treated with intravenous NAC beginning 20 hours after the ingestion, and developed hepatotoxicity. She had a spontaneous rupture of membranes at 31 weeks and delivered a "healthy" male infant at 32 weeks.[138] One woman who overdosed at 16 weeks had a toxic acetaminophen level, was treated with NAC within 8 hours, and did not develop hepatotoxicity.[190] She delivered a normal female infant at term. One woman overdosed at 20 weeks, received intravenous NAC starting some time between 8 and 18 hours after ingestion, and developed hepatotoxicity. She had labor induced at 41 weeks because of weight loss and delivered a male infant.[222] The infant was irritable and developed hyperbilirubinemia, both of which resolved after phototherapy.

The two large series described above included 39 third-trimester overdoses.[152,185] Twelve women had toxic acetaminophen levels; eight delivered healthy term infants, two women who had no evidence of hepatotoxicity delivered "normal" premature infants 2 days after the overdose, one woman with hepatotoxicity delivered a moderately ill premature infant at 32 weeks of gestation, and one woman with severe hepatotoxicity delivered a stillborn infant with hepatic necrosis at 33 weeks of gestation (Table 105–5). Twenty-seven women had nontoxic acetaminophen levels; two delivered premature infants (one of whom had respiratory distress), and 25 delivered full-term infants. Of these full-term infants, one developed a withdrawal syndrome, one developed pyloric stenosis, and three had physical anomalies. Altogether, in these two series, 6 of 39 women with third-trimester overdoses had premature delivery, usually within 2 to 3 days of the overdose.

In addition to the large series described, there are eight case reports of third-trimester acetaminophen overdoses (Table 105–5). Three additional women, two with an acute and one with a chronic third trimester overdose, are briefly described with toxic aceta-

minophen levels who were treated with NAC and who delivered healthy infants while receiving NAC.[95]

There are also several case reports of adverse pregnancy outcome in the setting of chronic use of acetaminophen or acute overdose in addition to other chronic substance use.[39,95,121,140,185] It is difficult to interpret these reports with respect to specific acetaminophen effect because of the confounders of chronic disease, chronic use, or use of additional medications or substances.

Acetaminophen is an FDA use-in-pregnancy category B drug; at recommended doses it is considered safe for use during pregnancy. However, in overdose, it may put the developing organism at risk. As the third-trimester cases described above demonstrate, acetaminophen crosses the placenta to reach the developing fetus. The clinical series[152,185] suggest that there may be some increased risk of spontaneous abortion after overdose during the first trimester. There is also a question about whether overdose during the first trimester can lead to late sequelae, for instance, premature labor.

Some experimental work may help to explain early pregnancy loss after overdose. Acetaminophen prevented the development of preimplantation (two-cell stage) mouse embryos in culture, an effect that was not associated with alterations in glutathione concentrations,[127] and acetaminophen also led to abnormal neuropore development in cultured rat embryos.[221] These data suggest that acetaminophen may be directly toxic to the immature organism. However, other work reported that similar embryotoxic effects were associated with reductions in glutathione concentrations[242] and that N-acetyl-p-benzoquinoneimine (NAPQI) produced nonspecific toxicity when added to the rat embryo culture medium.[221]

The fetal liver has some ability to metabolize acetaminophen to a reactive intermediate in vitro. P450 activity was detected in intact hepatocytes as well as microsomal fractions isolated from the livers of fetuses aborted between 18 and 23 weeks of gestation.[192] Fetal P450 activity was only 10% of the activity of hepatocytes isolated from adults without cerebral activity selected as kidney donors; fetal P450 activity increased with increasing gestational age. In two clinical cases, cysteine and mercapturate conjugates were identified in newborns exposed to acetaminophen in utero, suggesting the fetus'/newborn's ability to metabolize acetaminophen through the P450 system. These data suggest that the fetus in utero and the neonate can generate a toxic metabolite; the clinical cases suggest that the fetal liver is susceptible to injury.

This P450 activity has not been further characterized. However, CYP2E1, one of the cytochromes responsible for acetaminophen metabolism, is present in human fetal tissues as early as 16 weeks of gestation.[157] CYP3A4 and CYP2E1 are also involved in acetaminophen metabolism but are not present in fetal liver. CYP3A7 is a functional fetal form of the CYP3 family, but its metabolic activity with respect to acetaminophen has not been studied.[86]

The most difficult questions relate to management of overdose during the third trimester. Can acetaminophen overdose lead to premature labor even if a pregnant woman does not have a toxic level or develop hepatotoxicity? Should a woman be emergently delivered following overdose? Does NAC treatment of the mother help the fetus? What is the appropriate treatment of a neonate exposed to acetaminophen in utero?

The clinical cases may help with at least the last two questions (see Table 105–5). Five women, all less than 36 weeks of gesta-

TABLE 105–5. Reported Cases of Third-Trimester Acetaminophen Overdoses

Gestational Age (Weeks)	Maternal		Infant		Comment	Ref
	APAP Level (μg/mL) (time[a])	AST Peak (IU/L) (time[a])	APAP Level (μg/mL) (time[a])	Hepato-toxicity (Yes/No)		
27	0 (36 h)	1226 (36 h)	ND	No	C/S for fetal distress. Infant: mild respiratory distress syndrome	76
27–28	56 (16 h)	6226 (96 h)	ND	Yes	Ingestion over 24 h. No fetal movements at presentation. PO NAC started 20 h. Induced labor 4 d. Infant: stillborn with diffuse hepatic necrosis. Hepatic APAP 250 μg/g.	85
29	160 (10 h)	4300 (50 h)	76 (16 h, cord)	No	Ingestion of aspirin, caffeine, and quinine, followed 17 h later by APAP. Presented in labor. Treated with oral methionine. Spont delivery 16 h. Infant: moderate hyaline membrane disease. Peak AST – 86 (cord).	129
32	448 (12 h)	5269 (48 h)	0 (84 h, cord)	No	Four whole-blood exchange transfusions. Discharge home at 54 d of life. Died at 106 d, no apparent cause. IV NAC started 12 h. Induced delivery at 84 h. Infant: transient hypoglycemia, mild respiratory distress, mild jaundice. Peak AST 56 (day 1 of life).	153, 195
33	135 (28 h)	6237 (66 h)	330 (3 d,cord)	Yes	Oral NAC 12 h. Fetal death 2 d, spont delivery 3 d. Infant: stillborn with diffuse hepatic necrosis.	185
36	280 (3–4 h)	Normal	217 (6–7 h, cord)	No	Ingestion of APAP, ethanol, barbiturates. Elective C/S 6–7 h. Infant: double volume exchange transfusion at 18 h. Discharge at 40 d, "cot death" at 157 d.	189
36	200 (5 h)	25 (24 h)	ND	No	PO NAC (? time). Infant: spont delivery 6 weeks after ingestion. Normal neonatal course.	36
38	216 (4 h)	Normal	13 (17 h, cord)	No	NAC (? route). Infant: normal neonatal course.	120, 199
"Term"	147 (9 h)	28 (9 h)	133 (9 h, 4 h of life)	No	Infant INR = 3 at 4 h of life. IV NAC. No problems. AST 86 at 4 h of life.	12
Term?	89 (11 h)	326 (35 h)	144 (11 h, 4 h of life)	No	Mother presented in labor at 6 h. Infant received IV NAC at 4 h of life. AST 55 at 4 h of life.	202

[a]Time after maternal ingestion.

Abbreviations: APAP = acetaminophen; C/S = cesarean section; IV = intravenous; NAC = *N*-acetylcysteine; ND = not done or not reported; PO = oral; Post = postingestion; Spont = spontaneous; h = hours; d = days; Apgars (when reported) are 1 minute and 5 minutes.

tion, developed hepatotoxicity. Two infants died in utero with evidence of severe hepatotoxicity, although what effect in utero postmortem changes may have had on serum acetaminophen levels or liver pathology is unclear. The other three infants experienced problems associated with prematurity but did not develop obvious hepatotoxicity. One of these three had an exchange transfusion, and this one had an unexplained death at 3 months of age. Four women, all at more than 36 weeks of gestation, did not develop hepatotoxicity. One infant had an exchange transfusion and did not develop hepatotoxicity but died a "cot death" at 5 months of age. One infant received IV NAC and had a transient elevation of AST and PT. Two infants were not treated; both did well, although one had a transient elevation of AST.

Severe maternal hepatoxicity associated with any signs of fetal distress is an indication of urgent delivery. Although a fetus with prolonged exposure to acetaminophen in utero is at risk of developing severe hepatotoxicity, not all at-risk infants will be affected. What role gestational age, maternal disease state, or other maternal factors may play is unknown. There are insufficient case data to suggest that acetaminophen overdose per se is an indication for urgent delivery. Although there are insufficient data, there may be an indication for urgent delivery when the acetaminophen level is in the toxic range even though hepatotoxicity has not yet developed.[227] Significant acetaminophen overdose with or without hepatotoxicity may precipitate premature spontaneous labor, and even women with nontoxic levels may be at a slightly increased risk.

In two cases exchange transfusion was employed to treat the exposed neonate. In both cases the acetaminophen metabolic half-life was prolonged, and in neither case was this affected by the transfusion. Interestingly, these two infants had unexplained deaths at several months of age. There is insufficient information on which to base a recommendation regarding exchange transfusion as therapy for prenatal exposure.

The pregnant woman with acute toxic acetaminophen ingestion should be treated with *N*-acetylcysteine (see Chap. 32 and Antidotes in Depth: *N*-Acetylcysteine). This therapy is to treat the mother. Although maternal hepatoxicity or delayed NAC therapy may be associated with fetal toxicity,[185] there is insufficient information to indicate that prevention of maternal toxicity will prevent fetal toxicity in either the first or the third trimester. NAC was found in cord blood after administration to four mothers before delivery,[95] although NAC did not cross the sheep placenta in vivo[209] or the perfused human placenta in vitro.[99] Even if NAC does cross the placenta, whether it prevents fetal hepatotoxicity is unknown because not all exposed fetuses develop hepatotoxicity.

Four third-trimester cases are presented where the mothers overdosed at or after 36 weeks of gestation and did not develop hepatotoxicity, and the infants did well. One of these infants received NAC. There are anecdotal reports of infants who received NAC postnatally and did well. Current theory suggests that infants and young children are less likely to develop hepatoxicity after acetaminophen overdose than teenagers or adults because of immature P450 activity and increased sulfation activity. It is intriguing to consider that this metabolic protection might extend to the newborn exposed to acetaminophen in utero. It also makes it difficult to know to what extent postnatal NAC therapy for the prenatally exposed newborn might prevent toxicity. Although there are no reported cases, it would seem that the premature newborn exposed in utero would be the best candidate for postnatal NAC therapy.

IRON

Iron is another common ingestant during pregnancy; maternal toxicity is generally greater than fetal toxicity. In two reported cases, normal babies were delivered although the mothers died.[169,183] In another case, the mother had severe iron toxicity with acidosis, shock, renal failure, and disseminated intravascular coagulation but was not treated with deferoxamine because of concerns about its teratogenic risks. Instead, the mother received an exchange transfusion followed 45 minutes later by a spontaneous abortion of the 16-week fetus.[145,224] Neonatal and cord blood iron levels were not elevated. In several cases, pregnant women who had signs and symptoms of iron poisoning and elevated serum iron levels were treated with deferoxamine and subsequently delivered normal babies.[21,111,122,178,206,232]

Although the placenta transports iron to the fetus efficiently,[159] it also blocks the transfer of large quantities of iron. In a sheep model of iron poisoning, only a small amount of iron was transferred across the placenta despite significantly elevated serum iron levels.[51]

Deferoxamine is an effective antidote for iron poisoning (see Chap. 36 and Antidotes in Depth: Deferoxamine), but it is reported to be an animal teratogen that causes skeletal deformities and abnormalities of ossification (FDA class C pregnancy risk). A recent animal model observed similar effects, but only with doses of deferoxamine that caused maternal toxicity.[26] Experimentally, in sheep, little transfer of deferoxamine across the placenta was demonstrated;[51] therefore, the reported fetal effects may be secondary to chelation of essential nutrients (such as trace metals) on the maternal side of the placenta.[227]

In clinical case reports of iron overdose for which deferoxamine was used, there have been no adverse effects on the fetus, although most have been second-[111,206] or third-trimester poisonings.[21,111,122,169,178,232] There is one case series of 49 patients with iron poisoning during pregnancy—few exhibited any clinical toxicity other than vomiting and diarrhea; 25 received deferoxamine, most by the oral route.[153] One woman with a first-trimester overdose, eight women with second-trimester overdoses, and 12 women with third-trimester overdoses were treated with deferoxamine and subsequently delivered full-term infants; one whose mother overdosed at 30 weeks of gestation had webbed fingers on one hand. One woman overdosed at 20 weeks, had minimal clinical toxicity, received deferoxamine, and delivered a 2.5-kg male infant at 34 weeks. One woman with a first-trimester overdose and two women with second-trimester overdoses elected to terminate their pregnancies.

Further support for the safe use of deferoxamine in pregnancy is the experience with its use for pregnant women with thalassemia. Deferoxamine has been administered to them as part of the therapy for posttransfusion iron overload without adverse effects.[215]

Deferoxamine is probably safe for use in pregnant women. Considering the potentially fatal nature of severe iron poisoning, deferoxamine should be administered when signs and symptoms indicate significant poisoning.

Iron overdose may be one of the few specific indications for whole-bowel irrigation because iron is not adsorbed to activated charcoal (see Antidotes in Depth: Activated Charcoal). A case report demonstrated elimination of pill fragments following treatment of a pregnant woman with whole-bowel irrigation.[234]

CARBON MONOXIDE

Carbon monoxide is the leading cause of poisoning fatalities in the United States. In contrast to iron and most other drugs and toxins, when pregnant women are exposed to carbon monoxide, the fetus may be at greater risk of toxicity than the woman is herself. There are reports of both the mother and fetus dying, the mother surviving but the fetus dying, and both the mother and fetus surviving but with adverse neonatal outcome, primarily brain damage resembling that seen following severe cerebral ischemia.[37,50,116,136,146,161,168,249] Similar clinical effects have also been observed in animal models.[60,81,137]

The case literature suggests increased risk of poor fetal outcome with clinically severe maternal poisoning or significantly elevated carboxyhemoglobin levels.[116,168] Women with minimal symptoms and/or low levels of carboxyhemoglobin have a low risk of fetal toxicity,[116] but a lower limit of exposure without effect has not been specifically defined.

In animal models, under physiologic conditions, the fetus has a carboxyhemoglobin concentration 10 to 15% higher than the mother. After exposure to carbon monoxide, the fetus achieves peak carboxyhemoglobin levels 58% higher than those achieved by the mother at steady state, and the time to peak level is also delayed compared to the mother. Similarly, the elimination of carbon monoxide occurs more slowly in the fetus than in the mother.[91,136,137] One case report describes such a phenomenon: after 1 hour of supplemental oxygen, the maternal carboxyhemoglobin was 7%, and the fetal carboxyhemoglobin was 61% at the time of death in utero.[65]

Carbon monoxide leads to fetal hypoxia by several mechanisms: (1) maternal carboxyhemoglobin leads to a decrease in the oxygen content of maternal blood, and therefore, less oxygen is delivered across the placenta to the fetus, which normally has an arterial PO_2 of only 20 to 30 mm Hg; (2) fetal carboxyhemoglobin causes a decrease in fetal PO_2; (3) carbon monoxide shifts the oxyhemoglobin dissociation curve to the left and decreases the release of oxygen to the fetal tissues (an exacerbation of the physiologic left shift found with normal fetal hemoglobin); and (4) carbon monoxide may inhibit cytochrome oxidase or other mitochondrial functions.[136,137,174]

The treatment for severe carbon monoxide poisoning is hyperbaric oxygen therapy (HBO) (see Chap. 97 and Antidotes in Depth: Hyperbaric Oxygen). Questions have been raised about the use of HBO in pregnant women because animal models have suggested adverse effects of HBO on the embryo or fetus.[70,156,204,226] The applicability of the animal models to humans is difficult to assess; many of the animal models employed hyperbaric conditions of greater pressures and duration than those clinically employed for humans.

HBO has been used therapeutically for carbon monoxide poisoning in pregnancy with good results reported, although there are limited data on the long-term followup of the children.[32,69,77,92,116,235] One large series reported 44 women who were exposed to carbon monoxide during pregnancy and were treated with hyperbaric oxygen regardless of clinical severity or gestational age—33 had term births, one had a premature delivery 22 weeks after HBO during an episode of maternal fever, two had spontaneous miscarriages (one 12 hours after severe poisoning and one 15 days after mild poisoning), one delivered a child with Down syndrome, one had an elective abortion, and six were lost to

followup.[66] Unfortunately, details regarding trimester of exposure, maternal carboxyhemoglobin level, and severity of symptoms are not available, and it is therefore difficult to interpret the reported outcomes. Although HBO appears safe for pregnant women and seems to present little risk to the fetus, it is not clear whether HBO prevents carbon monoxide–related fetal toxicity for those at risk. Carbon monoxide can have a severe impact on fetal health and development, and, as noted above, the maternal carboxyhemoglobin level may not accurately reflect the fetal carboxyhemoglobin level. Hyperbaric oxygen should therefore be considered for any pregnant woman exposed to carbon monoxide, especially for a woman with an elevated carboxyhemoglobin level or any evidence of fetal distress. If hyperbaric oxygen therapy is not available, 100% oxygen should be administered to the mother for a period of time five times longer than the time needed for the maternal carboxyhemoglobin to return to the normal range.

SUBSTANCE USE IN PREGNANCY

One of the most complex areas of toxicology deals with issues of substance use during pregnancy and its effects on the woman, on the pregnancy itself, and on fetal and postnatal development. This section is a review of some of the important aspects of this topic.

Clinical research in the area of substance use in pregnancy is very difficult to perform. With the increased use of cocaine during the latter half of the 1980s and 1990s, there was great interest in determining the effects of cocaine use during pregnancy. As research in this area progresses, many of the critical methodologic issues related to substance use research have also been highlighted.[71,97,131,167,252]

Substance-using women often have multiple risk factors for adverse pregnancy outcomes such as low socioeconomic status, polysubstance use, ethanol and cigarette use, sexually transmitted diseases, AIDS, malnutrition, and lack of prenatal care. Lack of prenatal care is highly correlated with premature birth, and smoking is associated with spontaneous abortion, growth retardation, and sudden infant death syndrome (SIDS).[109,244] Other factors not specifically related to substance use such as age, race, gravidity, and prior pregnancies also have an effect on pregnancy outcome. Each of these factors represents a significant potential confounding variable when the effects of a particular agent such as cocaine or marijuana are evaluated during pregnancy and must be controlled for in research design. Many of these factors are also significant confounders in evaluation of postnatal growth and development.

There may be bias in the selection of study subjects. For example, if all the patients are selected from an inner-city hospital obstetric service, there is potential for overestimating the effects of the substance being studied. If cohorts are followed over a long period of time, study subjects are frequently lost to followup. Are the ones who continue more motivated, or do they have more problems that need attention?

Categorizing patients into substance use groups is difficult. Self-reporting of substance use is frequently unreliable or inaccurate, and making determinations about the nature, frequency, quantity (dose), or timing (with respect to gestation) of drug use is difficult. Because substance users frequently use multiple substances, it may be difficult to categorize subjects into particular drug-use groups, and patients using different drugs may therefore be grouped together. In fact, there may be no actual drug-free control groups.

When urine drug screens are used to identify drug users, there is a high probability of false negatives because drug screens reflect only recent use. This factor is particularly important because drug use tends to decrease later in pregnancy, and a negative urine drug screen in the third trimester or at delivery may fail to identify a woman who was using drugs early in pregnancy. Testing for drugs in hair or meconium may improve the accuracy of the analysis with regard to the entire pregnancy.[118,132]

Another bias involves selection of infants who are exposed to substances. Evaluating newborn who are "at risk," show signs of "withdrawal," or have positive urine drug screens will miss some exposed infants. When research concerns the neurobehavioral development of children exposed in utero to substances, it is important that the examiners performing the evaluation be blinded to the infants' drug exposure category.

Finally, there may be a bias against publishing research that shows a negative or "not significant" effect.[115]

Ethanol

Ethanol use during pregnancy produces a constellation of fetal effects. The most severe effects are seen in the fetal alcohol syndrome (FAS), characterized by intrauterine or postnatal growth retardation, mental retardation or behavioral abnormalities, and facial dysmorphogenesis, particularly microcephaly, short palpebral fissures, epicanthal folds, maxillary hypoplasia, cleft palate, hypoplastic philtrum, and micrognathia.[104]

Differential expression of the syndrome may reflect the effects of different ethanol doses at critical periods specific for particular effects. The craniofacial anomalies probably represent teratogenic effects during organogenesis, whereas some central nervous system abnormalities and growth retardation may result from adverse effects later in gestation. Incomplete expression of fetal alcohol syndrome such as neurobehavioral abnormalities in the absence of the facial features are termed fetal alcohol effects. In an attempt to formalize diagnostic criteria for fetal alcohol syndrome and alcohol-related effects, the Institute of Medicine has proposed some additional descriptors—alcohol-related birth defects and alcohol-related neurodevelopmental disorder.[223]

The fully expressed syndrome may be related to consumption of the equivalent of 2 to 3 ounces of 100% ethanol (four to six "standard" drinks of hard liquor) per day throughout pregnancy,[218] although binge drinking (at least five standard drinks per occasion) with a significantly elevated peak blood ethanol concentration may be more important.[82] Approximately 20% of women consume some ethanol during pregnancy;[164] only 1 to 2% consume four or more drinks each day.

The incidence of FAS is 0.5 to 3 per 1000 live births; 4% of women who drink heavily may give birth to children with FAS.[3] This means that several hundred children with fetal alcohol syndrome and several thousand with fetal alcohol effects will be born each year; ethanol use is considered the leading preventable cause of mental retardation in this country.[223] Although the primary determinant of fetal alcohol syndrome or effects is the level of maternal ethanol consumption, there is some evidence that paternal ethanol exposure may play a contributing role.[2]

Other effects of ethanol use during pregnancy may include an increased incidence of spontaneous abortion, premature deliveries, and stillbirths,[48,134] neonatal ethanol withdrawal,[75] and possibly carcinogenesis.[112] Infants may be irritable or hypertonic and may have problems with habituation and arousal. Long-term behavioral and intellectual effects include decreased IQ, learning disability, memory deficits, speech and language disorders, hyperactivity, and dysfunctional behavior in school.[149]

The mechanisms of ethanol-induced teratogenesis have not been fully elucidated.[16,87] Much of the work in animals has focused on the developing nervous system, where alcohol adversely affects nerve cell growth, differentiation, and migration, particularly in areas of the neocortex, hippocampus, sensory nucleus, and cerebellum.[64,84] Ethanol or its metabolite acetaldehyde may be directly toxic, or ethanol may disturb the regulatory balance of trophic neurotransmitters in sensitive regions.[245] One model proposes that sociobehavioral risk factors, such as drinking behavior, smoking behavior, low socioeconomic status, and cultural/ethnic influences create provocative biologic conditions such as high peak blood ethanol levels, circulating tobacco constituents, and undernutrition. These provocative factors exacerbate fetal vulnerability to ethanol-related hypoxia and free radical–induced cell damage.[4]

Opioids

Opioid addiction remains a significant cause of both maternal and neonatal morbidity. Approximately 0.2% of pregnant women may use heroin or methadone, and up to 75,000 babies per year may be exposed to opioids in utero.[164] Pregnant opioid users are at increased risk for many medical complications of pregnancy such as hepatitis, sepsis, endocarditis, sexually transmitted diseases, and AIDS and may be at increased risk for obstetric complications such as miscarriage, premature delivery, or stillbirth.[71,83] Some of the obstetric complications may be related to associated risk factors in addition to the opioid use.

The most common effect of maternal opioid use is on fetal growth.[83,252] There is an increased incidence of low birth weight in babies born to opioid-using mothers compared to controls, and the effect is greater for heroin than for methadone. Women who receive low-dose methadone and good prenatal care have birth outcomes similar to nonusers but still are at increased risk for pregnancy-related complications.[71]

The most significant acute neonatal complication of opioid use during pregnancy is the neonatal withdrawal syndrome (NWS), characterized by hyperirritability, gastrointestinal dysfunction, respiratory distress, and vague autonomic symptoms including yawning, sneezing, mottling, and fever.[48] Myoclonic jerks or seizures may also signify neurologic irritability. Withdrawing infants are recognizable by their extreme jitteriness despite efforts at consolation; ecchymoses and contusions may be found on the tips of their fingers or toes as a result of trauma from striking the sides of the bassinet. The features of NWS are detailed in Table 105–6. From 60 to 90% of opioid-exposed offspring will show some signs of withdrawal.[71]

Some of the manifestations of the neonatal withdrawal syndrome may be caused by enhanced α-adrenergic activity in the locus ceruleus. Firing of neurons in this region of the brain leads to such NWS-like behaviors as wakefulness and tremors—effects that are inhibited by opioid agonists. Chronic opioid administration leads to tolerance as well as an increased number of α_2-adrenergic receptors. Presumably, withdrawal of opioids causes increased stimulation of a large number of receptors in this region, leading to clinical signs of withdrawal.

TABLE 105–6.   Signs and Symptoms of Neonatal Opioid Withdrawal

Neurologic excitability	Gastrointestinal dysfunction
Exaggerated Moro reflex	Dehydration
Frequent yawning and sneezing	Diarrhea
High-pitched crying	Poor feeding
Hyperactive deep tendon reflexes	Poor weight gain
Increased muscle tone	Uncoordinated and constant
Increased wakefulness	sucking
Irritability	Vomiting
Seizures	Autonomic signs
Tremors	Fever
	Increased sweating
	Mottling
	Nasal stuffiness
	Temperature instability

From the Committee on Drugs: Neonatal drug withdrawal. Pediatrics 1998;101:1079–1118. Used with permission.

Opioid withdrawal symptoms typically occur within 2 weeks of birth. Heroin withdrawal usually occurs within the first 24 hours; however, methadone withdrawal may be delayed because it has a larger volume of distribution and slower metabolism in the neonate, and therefore an increased half-life. Methadone withdrawal occurs when the plasma level falls below 0.06 μg/mL.[193] The onset and severity of symptoms may be related to whether heroin, methadone, or both were used, how much was used chronically, how much was used near the time of delivery, the character of the labor, whether analgesic or anesthetic agents were used, and the maturity, nutrition, and medical condition of the neonate.[55] Acute neonatal withdrawal symptoms generally last from days to weeks, but some symptoms may persist for months.[48]

From 5 to 7% of babies showing signs of withdrawal experience seizures, generally by 10 days after birth.[90] Seizures may be more likely after methadone withdrawal than after heroin withdrawal.[251] These seizures do not necessarily imply an underlying chronic seizure disorder; in one small study, children who had withdrawal seizures were normal at 1-year followup.[58]

Treatment of withdrawal begins with provision of a comforting environment: swaddling or tightly wrapping the infant, minimal handling or stimulation, and demand feeding. More severe symptoms may require pharmacologic therapy. One way of determining the need for therapy is to use a severity-scoring scale. In general, babies who are extremely irritable, have feeding difficulties, diarrhea, or significant tremors, or are crying continuously are candidates for pharmacologic therapy.[48,110]

Opioid agonists such as morphine, methadone, tincture of opium and paregoric; and sedative-hypnotic agents such as diazepam and phenobarbital have been used to treat withdrawal symptoms.[48,110] Tincture of opium diluted to a final dose of 0.4 mg/mL of morphine equivalent may be the preferred agent because it is a pure opioid agonist and the formulation has no additives. However, there are few well-controlled trials evaluating the relative efficacy of the different agents.[228]

Opioid agonists may be more effective at preventing withdrawal seizures from heroin or methadone than phenobarbital or diazepam.[90,104] However, sedative-hypnotic agents are commonly used by heroin users or adults maintained on methadone, and sedative-hypnotic withdrawal seizures may contribute to the overall abstinence symptomatology. In this setting there may be a role for phenobarbital. Because oral administration of phenobarbital may delay achieving a therapeutic level, parenteral administration may be required.

Infants of opioid-using mothers are at increased risk for SIDS compared to controls.[105,107] The relative risk is 3.6 for methadone and 2.3 for heroin. The mechanism may be related to a decreased medullary responsiveness to CO_2, or the effect may be related to some condition of the postnatal environment.[105,236]

Although young children born to opioid users do not seem to have significant differences in behavior compared to controls, older children have increased learning problems and school dysfunction particularly related to behavior difficulties.[252]

Cocaine

Approximately 1% of pregnant women in the United States use cocaine some time during their pregnancy.[164] The rate may be as high as 15% in certain populations,[54] and it is estimated that more than 100,000 infants born in the United States each year may be exposed to cocaine in utero.[41] The consequences of cocaine use during pregnancy have been extensively reviewed.[94,97,175]

The most commonly reported obstetric complications of gestational cocaine use are abruptio placentae, premature delivery, and intrauterine growth retardation. Significant perinatal problems include seizures, cerebral infarctions, and other CNS effects.[45,175] A metaanalysis of studies published before 1989 concluded that adverse effects on head circumference, gestational age, and birth weight that had been attributed to the maternal use of cocaine during pregnancy were related to polysubstance use, but not necessarily to cocaine.[139] In this analysis, no increased risk of abruptio placentae was demonstrated. However, later work, which tried to control for polysubstance use although not always for smoking or ethanol use, suggested that there were significant effects of gestational cocaine use on intrauterine growth and prematurity.[114,175,220] The incidence of abruptio placentae may also be significant when related to acute use.[212] It seems that good prenatal care can mitigate many of the adverse effects of cocaine.[141,184,252]

Significant congenital malformations have been reported among some infants who were exposed to cocaine in utero, specifically genitourinary malformations, cardiovascular malformations, and limb-reduction defects.[34,75] In one large population-based study, there was no increase in the incidence of malformations.[147]

Animal models have also identified teratogenic effects of in utero cocaine exposure. Decreased maternal and fetal weight gain and an increased frequency of fetal resorption were demonstrated in rats;[68] sporadic physical anomalies have also been observed.[46] Teratogenic effects similar to those observed in humans were reported in mice: bony defects of the skull, cryptorchidism, hydronephrosis, ileal atresia, cardiac defects, limb deformities, and eye abnormalities.[72,142,143,154] Cocaine caused hemorrhage, edema, and subsequently limb-reduction defects in rats when administered during midgestation in the postorganogenic period.[240]

The perinatal effects of cocaine are probably mediated through a vascular mechanism. Cocaine administration to the pregnant ewe causes increased uterine vascular resistance, decreased uterine blood flow, increased fetal heart rate and arterial blood pressure, and decreased fetal P_{O_2} and O_2 content.[10,247] Similar effects have been seen in rats.[170] Fetal hypoxia may cause rupture of fetal blood vessels and infarction in developing organ systems such as the genitourinary system[44,154,217] or the CNS.[40,57,241] Hyperthermia or direct effects of cocaine in the fetus may exacerbate these effects.[27] Limb-reduction defects similar to those attributed to cocaine have been produced after mechanical clamping of the uterine vessels.[27,239] A developing concept is that following vasospasm and ischemia, reperfusion occurs with the generation of oxygen free radicals and subsequent injury.[247,248]

Despite the reported malformations and a possible mechanism, neither the human epidemiology nor the effects observed in animal models suggest a specific teratogenic syndrome. The risk of a significant malformation from prenatal cocaine exposure is low, but the effect, if one occurs, may be severe.[29,60,75]

One of the greatest concerns about prenatal cocaine exposure has been the potential adverse effect on the developing child, and this has been one of the most intensive areas of epidemiologic research. The most common findings in early infancy are lability of state and autonomic regulation, decreased alertness and orientation, and abnormal reflexes, tone, and motor maturity; however, many studies show no effect.[70] For some children these effects may manifest in later infancy as difficulty with information processing and learning. However, preliminary evidence suggests that for school-age children, any observed cognitive deficits may be more related to the home environment than to prenatal cocaine exposure, even for those children who showed some of the typical neonatal behaviors.[43,231] Nonetheless, there is also evidence of impairments in modulating attention and impulsivity, which makes handling unfamiliar, complex, and stressful tasks more difficult,[150] and these effects are also observed in animal models of prenatal cocaine exposure.[62,219]

The mechanism of neurotoxicity has not been specifically elucidated. As described above for many of the maternal and fetal physical defects, cocaine may have direct toxicity, or effects may be mediated through hypoxia or oxygen free radicals. Because cocaine interferes with neurotransmitter reuptake, it is likely that cocaine also disrupts normal neural ontogeny by interfering with the trophic functions of neurotransmitters on the developing brain.[144,151]

BREAST-FEEDING

In the United States, breast-feeding is the recommended method of infant nutrition because it offers nutritional, immunologic, and psychological benefits. Many women use prescription and nonprescription medications while breast-feeding and are concerned about the possible ill effects on the infant of these medications in the breast milk. This concern extends to the possible exposure of the infant to occupational and environmental chemicals via breast milk.[191] The response to many of these concerns can be determined by the answer to the question: "Does the risk to an infant from a chemical exposure via breast milk exceed the benefit of being breast-fed?"[128]

Pharmacokinetic factors determine the amount of drug available for transfer from maternal plasma into breast milk; only free drug can traverse the mammary alveolar membrane. Most drugs are transported by passive diffusion. A few drugs, such as ethanol and lithium, are transported through aqueous-filled pores. The factors that determine how well a chemical diffuses across the membrane are similar to those for other biologic membranes such as the placenta: molecular weight, lipid solubility, and degree of ionization.

Large-molecular-weight compounds, such as heparin or insulin, will not pass into breast milk. Lipid solubility is important not only for diffusion but for drug accumulation in breast milk be-cause milk is rich in fat, especially milk that is produced in the postcolostral period (3–4 days postpartum). With a pH near 7.0, breast milk is slightly more acidic than plasma. Therefore, in plasma, weak acids exist largely as ionized molecules and cannot be easily transported into milk. On the other hand, weak bases exist largely as nonionized molecules in the plasma and are available for transport into milk. Once in the breast milk, ionization of the weak base occurs, and the chemical is concentrated as a result of ion trapping. In other words, weak bases may concentrate in breast milk. Sulfacetamide (pK_a 5.4, a weak acid) has a concentration in plasma 10 times that in breast milk, whereas sulfanilamide (pK_a 10.4, a weak base) is found in equal concentrations in both plasma and breast milk.[128]

The net effect of these physiologic processes is expressed in the milk/plasma (M/P) drug ratio. Drugs with higher M/P ratios have relatively greater concentrations in breast milk. The M/P ratio does not reflect the actual concentration of a drug in the breast milk and a drug with a high M/P ratio is not necessarily found at high concentration in the breast milk. Morphine has an M/P ratio of 2.46 (is concentrated in milk), but only 0.4% of a maternal dose is excreted into the breast milk.[9] In general, for most pharmaceuticals, about 1 to 2% of the maternally administered dose is presented to the infant in breast milk.[128]

The M/P ratio has several limitations. It does not take into account differences in drug concentration that may result from (1) repeat or chronic dosing, (2) breast-feeding at different times relative to maternal drug dosing, (3) differences in milk production during the day or even during a particular breast-feeding session, (4) the time postpartum (days, weeks, or months) when the measurement is made, and (5) maternal disease.

A spot breast milk drug concentration or a concentration estimate based on the M/P ratio allows an estimation of the quantity of drug to which an infant is exposed, assuming a constant breast-milk concentration:

$$\text{infant dose} = \text{breast-milk concentration} \times \text{amount consumed}$$

The effect of this dose on the infant depends on the bioavailability of drug in breast milk, the pharmacokinetic parameters that determine drug levels in the infant, and the infant's receptor sensitivity to the drug. These parameters are often different in neonates than in adults and may lead to drug accumulation; generally, absorption is greater, but metabolism and clearance are reduced. These effects are exaggerated in premature infants.[179,188] Nonetheless, the amount of most drugs delivered to infants in breast milk is adequately metabolized and eliminated.[188]

Many of the considerations above are theoretical. Published guidelines on the advisability of breast-feeding during periods of maternal drug therapy are generally based on the expected effects of full doses in the infant or on case reports of adverse occurrences. For this reason, the number or specifically contraindicated drugs is quite small.[8]

In its published guidelines, the American Academy of Pediatrics discourages substance use during the breast-feeding period because of direct effects on the baby as well as detrimental effects on the physical and emotional health of the mother and on the caregiving environment. Although ethanol is not specifically contraindicated for the breast-feeding mother, adverse effects in the infant are noted with maternal consumption of large amounts.[8]

The American Academy of Pediatrics (AAP) recommends the temporary cessation of breast-feeding when the mother is exposed to metronidazole, an in vitro mutagen, and certain radiopharmaceuticals, specifically isotopes of copper, gallium, indium, iodine, sodium, and technetium. In these cases breast milk can be collected and stored before medication use for later feeding to the baby. Breast-feeding is resumed when the milk is no longer radioactive, generally 1 to 3 days for most of the isotopes mentioned except gallium, in which radioactivity may be present for 2 weeks. Metronidazole may be administered as a single 2-g dose, allowing breast-feeding to be discontinued for only 12 to 24 hours.[128]

Although there are few data demonstrating specific effects, the AAP suggests caution with regard to breast-feeding while using sedative-hypnotic, antidepressant, and antipsychotic medications. These medications modulate neurotransmitters in the central nervous system, which may adversely effect the developing nervous system.

For most drugs a risk-benefit analysis must be made. For example, lithium is transferred in breast-milk and may lead to measurable, though sub-therapeutic, serum levels in the breast-fed infant. The effects of this small dose are unknown, however many practitioners feel that the benefit of treating a mother's bipolar illness outweighs the potential risk to the infant.[208] Similarly, the breast-fed infant of a woman who smokes is exposed to nicotine and other tobacco constituents both by inhalation and via breast milk. Although this child may be at increased risk for respiratory illness as a result of exposure to tobacco smoke, some of the risk may be reduced by breast feeding.[8,186]

Many drugs, foods, and environmental agents that have been found in breast milk and some of their effects are listed in Table 105–7. In addition to the effects listed, there may be a small increased risk of carcinogenicity associated with exposure to some environmental agents through breast milk.[191]

In most cases, women do not need to stop breast-feeding while using pharmaceutic agents. However, "compatibility" with breast-feeding is generally based on the lack of reported adverse effects, which may reflect limited clinical experience with a particular drug in breast-feeding patients. Therefore, in the setting of limited information, exposure to a drug through breast-milk should be regarded as a small potential risk, and the infant should receive appropriate medical follow-up. Not all "compatible" drugs are safe in all situations. For instance, phenobarbital can produce CNS depression in an infant if the mother's serum level is in the high therapeutic or supratherapeutic range, which often occurs while dosage adjustments are being made. Such a level may or may not produce CNS depression in the mother. Nalidixic acid, nitrofurantoin, sulfapyridine, and sulfisoxazole, although generally safe, can cause hemolysis in a breast-fed infant with glucose-6-phosphate dehydrogenase deficiency.

Decisions on breast-feeding should be made with the informed involvement of the woman, her physicians, and, when necessary, a consultant with special expertise in this field. Guidelines may be obtained from several sources.[18,30,128,172]

TOXICOLOGIC PROBLEMS IN THE NEONATE

It has been estimated that approximately 8% of all medication doses administered in neonatal intensive care units (NICU) may be up to 10 times greater or 10 times less than the dose ordered.[162] As many as 30% of newborns in NICUs may sustain adverse drug reactions, some of which may be life-threatening or fatal.[9] Physio-

logic differences between adults and newborn infants affect drug absorption, distribution, and metabolism;[163,179] these pharmacokinetic differences account for some cases of drug toxicity seen in the newborn infant.

Gastrointestinal (GI) absorption of drugs in the neonate is generally slower than in adults.[163,179] this delay may be related to decreased gastric acid secretion, decreased gastric emptying and transit time, and decreased pancreatic enzyme activity. The GI environment of the newborn and young infant may allow the growth of *Clostridium botulinum* and the subsequent development of infantile botulism (Chap. 75). Infantile botulism has been reported in infants several weeks of age.[96,229]

Although it is uncommon, cutaneous absorption of drugs may be a route of toxic exposure in the newborn.[65,200] Aniline dyes used for marking diapers are absorbed, causing methemoglobinemia,[200] and contaminated diapers were responsible for one epidemic of mercury poisoning.[13] The absorption of hexachlorophene antiseptic wash has led to neurotoxicity with marked vacuolization of myelin seen microscopically.[125,148,214] Antiseptic ethanol has caused hemorrhagic necrosis of the skin of some premature infants. Iodine antiseptics have led to hypothyroidism in mature newborns.[38] An increased potential for absorption and toxicity has followed the dermal application of corticosteroids[78,198] and boric acid[63] in children with cutaneous disorders.

Other routes of exposure have led to clinical poisoning. Aspirated talcum powder has been responsible for several deaths.[31,160] Inhalation of mercury from incubator thermometers may be a potential risk,[7] and death has been reported following the ophthalmic instillation of cyclopentolate hydrochloride.[15]

Because of differences in total body water and fat compared to the adult, the distribution of absorbed drugs may differ in neonates. Water represents 80% of body weight in a full-term baby compared to 60% in an adult. About 20% of a term baby's body weight is fat compared to only 3% in a premature baby. The increased volume of water means that the volume of distribution for some water-soluble drugs, such as theophylline or phenobarbital, is increased.

Protein binding of drugs is to a smaller extent in newborns than in adults: the serum concentration of proteins is lower, there are fewer receptor sites that become saturated at lower drug concentrations, and binding sites have decreased binding affinity.[179] Protein binding has potential relevance with respect to bilirubin, an endogenous metabolite that at very high concentrations can cause kernicterus; bilirubin competes with exogenously administered drugs for protein binding sites. In vitro, certain drugs such as sulfonamides and ceftriaxone displace bilirubin from protein receptor sites; this may potentially increase the risk of kernicterus, although this has not been clinically demonstrated. Conversely, bilirubin may itself displace other drugs such as phenobarbital or phenytoin, leading to increased plasma drug levels.

Newborn infants have decreased hepatic metabolic capacity compared to adults, and this may lead to drug toxicity. For instance, the newborn has limited ability to oxidize drugs, so theophylline is metabolized primarily to the active metabolite caffeine instead of methylxanthine and 1,3-dimethyluric acid, which are the primary inactive metabolites in the adult. In addition, immaturity of the P450 system leads to increased elimination half-lives of drugs such as phenytoin, phenobarbital, and theophylline.

Two syndromes related to immature metabolic function have been described. The "gasping-baby syndrome," characterized by gasping respirations, metabolic acidosis, hypotension, central ner-

TABLE 105–7. Drugs, Foods, and Environmental Agents That Have Been Associated with Effects on some Nursing Infants

Drug	Effect
	Use with Caution
5-Aminosalicylic acid	Diarrhea
Acebutolol, atenolol, nadolol, sotalol, timolol	Hypotension, bradycardia, tachypnea, cyanosis
Amiodarone	Possible hypothyroidism
Aspirin	Metabolic acidosis; may affect platelet function; rash
Bromocriptine	Suppresses lactation.
Chloramphenicol	Potential risk for aplastic anemia or gray-baby syndrome.[128]
Chlorpromazine	Galactorrhea in mother; drowsiness and lethargy in infant, decline in developmental scores.
Cimetidine	Possible antiandrogenic effects[128]
Clemastine	Drowsiness, irritability, refusal to feed, highpitched cry, meningismus
Clofazimine	Possible increased skin pigmentation
Cyclophosphamide, cyclosporine, doxorubicin, methotrexate	Neutropenia, thrombocytopenia, possible immune suppression, unknown effect on growth or association with carcinogenesis.
Ergotamine	Vomiting, diarrhea, seizures. May inhibit prolactin secretion and lactation.
Fluoxetine	Colic, irritability, feeding and sleep disorders, slow weight gain
Haloperidol	Decline in developmental scores
Lamotrigine	Potential therapeutic serum concentrations in infant
Lithium	Subtherapeutic levels in infant
Metronidazole, tinidazole	In vitro mutagen
Phenindione	Risk of hemorrhage.
Phenobarbital	Sedation in exposed infants, withdrawal after weaning from phenobarbital-containing milk, methemoglobinemia
Primidone	Sedation, feeding problems
Sulfapyridine, sulfisoxazole	Caution in infant with jaundice or G-6-PD deficiency and ill, stressed, or premature infant
Sulfasalazine	Bloody diarrhea
Tetracycline	May cause staining of infant teeth after prolonged maternal use.[128]
Thiouracil, methimazole	May cause thyroid suppression and goiter.[128]
	Use is compatible with breast-feeding despite known effect
Ethanol	Large doses: decreased milk ejection reflex. Infant: drowsiness, diaphoresis, decreased growth and weight gain
Bendroflumethazide	Supresses lactation
Caffeine	Irritability, poor sleeping pattern (no effect with usual amount of caffeinated beverages)
Carbimazole	Goiter
Chloral hydrate	Sleepiness
Chlorthalidone	Excreted slowly
Contraceptive pills with estrogen/ progesterone	Rare breast enlargement; decrease in milk production and protein content (not confirmed in several studies)
Danthron	Increased bowel activity
Dexbrompheniramine maleate with d-isoephedrine	Crying, irritability, poor sleeping pattern
Estradiol	Withdrawal vaginal bleeding
Indomethacin	Seizure
Iodine topical	Odor of iodine on infant's skin
Iodine, iodides	Goiter
Methyprylon	Drowsiness
Nalidixic acid	Hemolysis in infant with G-6-PD-deficiency
Nitrofurantoin	Hemolysis in infant with G-6-PD-deficiency
Phenytoin	Methemoglobinemia
Theophylline	Irritability
	Food and environmental agents
Aspartame	Caution if mother has phenylketonuria
Chocolate (theobromine)	Irritability or increased bowel activity if mother consumes large amounts
Fava beans	Hemolysis in infant with G-6-PD deficiency
Hexachlorobenzene	Skin rash, diarrhea, vomiting, dark urine, neurotoxicity, death
Lead	Possible neurotoxicity
Methylmercury, mercury	Possible neurodevelopmental toxicity
Polyhalogenated biphenyls	Lack of endurance, hypotonia, sullen expressionless facies
Silicone	Esophageal dysmotility
Tetrachloroethylene	Obstructive jaundice, dark urine
Vegetarian diet	Vitamin B_{12} deficiency

Adapted from The transfer of drugs and other chemicals into human milk. American Academy of Pediatrics Committee on Drugs. Pediatrics 2001;108:776–789. Used with permission.

vous system depression, convulsions, renal failure, and occasionally death, has been attributed to high concentrations of benzyl alcohol and benzoic acid in the plasma of affected infants.[6,33,79] Benzyl alcohol, a bacteriostatic agent, was added to intravenous flush solutions and accumulated in newborns after repetitive doses. The high concentrations of benzoic acid could not be further metabolized to hippuric acid by the immature liver. Immature glucuronidation in the neonate is responsible for the "gray-baby syndrome" following high doses of chloramphenicol[93] (see Chaps. 46 and 106).

The umbilical vessels are a common site of vascular access in sick neonates. Because blood drains into the portal vein, it is possible that IV medications experience a "first-pass" effect, although whether this route of drug administration affects drug metabolism or clearance has not been well studied. Most renal functions, including glomerular filtration rate and tubular secretion, are relatively immature at birth;[101] a newborn's glomerular filtration rate is approximately 30% of that of an adult. Drugs such as aminoglycoside antibiotics and digoxin are excreted unchanged by the kidney and therefore depend on glomerular filtration for clearance. Dosing of these agents in the newborn must account for these differences.

Very little information is available to guide the clinician in the management of drug poisoning in the newborn infant. Cutaneous absorption is probably already complete by the time toxicity is noted, although further exposure may be prevented. Gastrointestinal decontamination is not generally performed in neonates; syrup of ipecac is contraindicated, and the neonate may be at increased risk of fluid, electrolyte, and thermoregulatory problems following gastric lavage or the use of cathartic agents. Multiple-dose activated charcoal has been used in a 1.4-kg 2-week-old premature infant to treat theophylline poisoning.[210] Hemodialysis, hemoperfusion, and exchange transfusion have been used in neonates to treat drug toxicity (see Chaps. 6 and 106).

SUMMARY

The use of medications and chemicals in the pregnant or breastfeeding woman is a complex area of medical practice and presents the clinician with potentially difficult management decisions. The previous discussion has highlighted some of the important principles of drug effects in both the pregnant woman and the fetus. Appropriate management of many of the potential problems will be facilitated by the coordinated efforts of obstetricians, perinatologists, neonatologists, pediatricians, and toxicologists.

REFERENCES

1. Abel EL, Sokol RJ: Incidence of fetal alcohol syndrome and impact of FAS-related anomalies. Drug Alcohol Depend 1987;19:51–70.
2. Abel EL: Paternal exposure to alcohol. In: Sonderegger TB, ed: Perinatal Substance Abuse: Research Findings and Clinical Implications. Baltimore, The Johns Hopkins University Press, 1992, pp. 132–160.
3. Abel EL: An update on incidence of FAS: FAS is not an equal opportunity birth defect. Neurotoxicol Teratol 1995; 17:437–443.
4. Abel EL, Hannigan JH: Maternal risk factors in fetal alcohol syndrome: Provocative and permissive influences. Neurotoxicol Teratol 1995;17:445–462.
5. Addis A, Sharabi S, Bonati M: Risk classification systems for drug use during pregnancy: are they a reliable source of information? Drug Safety 2000;23:246–253.
6. American Academy of Pediatrics: Benzyl alcohol: Toxic agent in neonatal units. Pediatrics 1983;72:356–358.
7. American Academy of Pediatrics: Mercury vapor contamination of infant incubators: A potential hazard. Pediatrics 1984;67:637.
8. American Academy of Pediatrics Committee on Drugs: The transfer of drugs and other chemicals into human milk. Pediatrics 2001;108:776–789.
9. Aranda JV, Portuguez-Malavasi A, Collinge JM, et al: Epidemiology of adverse drug reactions in the newborn. Dev Pharmacol Ther 1982;5:173–184.
10. Arbeille P, Maulik D, Salihagic A, et al: Effect of long-term cocaine administration to pregnant ewes on fetal hemodynamics, oxygenation, and growth. Obstet Gynecol 1997;5:795–802.
11. Atkinson HC, Begg EJ, Darlow BA: Drugs in human milk: Clinical pharmacokinetics considerations. Clin Pharmacokinet 1988;14:217–240.
12. Maw M, Dhawan A, Baker AJ, Mielli-Vergani G: Neonatal paracetamol poisoning. Arch Dis Child Fetal Neonatal Ed 1999;81:F78.
13. Banzaw TM: Mercury poisoning in Argentine babies linked to diapers. Pediatrics 1981;67:637.
14. Barnes AB, Colton T, Gundersen J, et al: Fertility and outcome of pregnancy in women exposed in utero to diethylstilbestrol. N Engl J Med 1980;302:609–613.
15. Bauser CR, Trottier MCT, Stern L: Systemic cyclopentolate (Cyclogyl) toxicity in the newborn infant. J Pediatr 1973;82:501.
16. Becker HC, Diaz-Granados JL, Randall CL: Teratogenic actions of ethanol in the mouse: a minireview. Pharmacol Biochem Behav 196;55:501–513.
17. Beckman DA, Brent RL: Teratogenesis: Alcohol, angiotensin-converting-enzyme inhibitors, and cocaine. Curr Opin Obstet Gynecol 1990;2:236–245.
18. Bennett PN, ed: Drugs and Human Lactation, 2nd ed. Amsterdam, Elsevier, 1996.
19. Bentur Y: Ionizing and nonionizing radiation in pregnancy. In: Koren G, ed: Maternal–Fetal Toxicology: A Clinician's guide, 2nd ed. New York; Marcel Dekker, 1994, pp. 515–574.
20. Bibbo M, Gill WB, Azizi F, et al: Follow-up study of male and female offspring of DES-exposed mothers. Obstet Gynecol 1977;49:1–8.
21. Blanc P, Hryhorczuk D, Danel I: Deferoxamine treatment of acute iron intoxication in pregnancy. Obstet Gynecol 1984;64:12S–14S.
22. Bologa M, Koren G, Fassos FF, McGuigan M, Rieder MJ: Drugs and chemicals most commonly used by pregnant women. In: Koren G, ed: Maternal–Fetal toxicology: A Clinician's Guide, 2nd ed. New York, Marcel Dekker, 1994, pp. 89–117.
23. Bologa M, ul Qamar I, Laila W, Koren G: Direct drug toxicity to the fetus. In: Koren G, ed: Maternal–Fetal toxicology: A Clinician's Guide, 2nd ed. New York, Marcel Dekker, 1994, pp. 267–300.
24. Bonati M, Bortolus R, Marchetti F, et al: Drug use in pregnancy: An overview of epidemiological (drug utilization) studies. Eur J Clin Pharmacol 1990;38:325–328.
25. Bonati M, Fellin G: Changes in smoking and drinking behaviour before and during pregnancy in Italian mothers: Implications for public health intervention. Int J Epidemiol 1991;20:927–932.
26. Bosque MA, Domingo JL, Corbella J: Assessment of the developmental toxicity of deferoxamine in mice. Arch Toxicol 1995;69:467–471.
27. Brent RL: Relationship between uterine vascular clamping, vascular disruption syndrome, and cocaine teratogenicity. Teratology 1990;41:757–760.
28. Brent RL, Beckman DA: Angiotensin-converting enzyme inhibitors, an embryopathic class of drugs with unique properties: information for clinical teratology counselors. Teratology 1991;43:543–546.

29. Brent RL: The application of the principles of toxicology and teratology in evaluating the risks of new drugs for the treatment of drug addiction in women of reproductive age. NIDA Res Monogr 1995;149: 130–179.

30. Briggs GG, Freeman RK, Yaffe SJ: Drugs in Pregnancy and Lactation, 5th ed. Baltimore, Williams & Wilkins, 1998.

31. Brouillette F, Weber ML: Massive aspiration of talcum powder by an infant. Can Med Assoc J 1978;122:354–355.

32. Brown DB, Mueller GL, Golich FC: Hyperbaric oxygen treatment for carbon monoxide poisoning in pregnancy: A case report. Aviat Space Environ Med 1992;63:1011–1014.

33. Brown WJ, Buist NR, Cory-Gipson HT, et al: Fatal benzyl alcohol poisoning in a neonatal intensive care unit. Lancet 1982;1:1250.

34. Buehler BA, Conover B, Andres RL: Teratogenic potential of cocaine. Semin Perinatol 1996;20:93–98.

35. Buitendijk S, Bracken MB: Medication in early pregnancy: prevalence of use and relationship to maternal characteristics. Am J Obstet Gynecol 1991;167:33–40.

36. Byer AJ, Trayler TR, Semmer JR. Acetaminophen over-dose in the third trimester of pregnancy. JAMA 1982;247:3114–3115.

37. Caravati EM, Adams CJ, Joyce SM, Schafer NC: Fetal toxicity associated with maternal carbon monoxide poisoning. Ann Emerg Med 1988;17:714–717.

38. Chabrolle JP, Rosier A: Goiter and hypothyroidism in the newborn after cutaneous absorption of iodine. Arch Dis Child 1978;53: 495–498.

39. Char V, Chandra R, Fletcher AB, Avery GB: Polyhydramnios and neonatal renal failure: a possible association with maternal acetaminophen ingestion. J Pediatr 1975;86:138.

40. Chasnoff IJ, Bussey ME, Salvich R, Stack CM: Perinatal cerebral infarction and maternal cocaine use. J Pediatr 1986;111:456–459.

41. Chasnoff I: Drug use and women: Establishing a standard of care. Ann NY Acad Sci 1989;562:208–210.

42. Chasnoff IJ, Landress HJ, Barrett ME: The prevalence of illicit-drug or alcohol use during pregnancy and discrepancies in mandatory reporting in Pinellas County, Florida. N Engl J Med 1990;322: 1202–1206.

43. Chasnoff IJ, Anson A, Hatcher R, Stenson H, Iaukea K, Randolph LA: Prenatal exposure to cocaine and other drugs. Ann NY Acad Sci 1998;846:314–328.

44. Chavez GF, Mulinare J, Cordero JF: Maternal cocaine use during early pregnancy as a risk factor for congenital anomalies. JAMA 1989;262:795–798.

45. Chiroboga CA: Neurological correlates of fetal cocaine exposure. Ann NY Acad Sci 1998;846:109–125.

46. Church MW, Dintcheff BA, Gessner P. Dose-dependent consequences of cocaine on pregnancy outcome in the Long-Evans rat. Neurotoxicol Teratol 1988;10:51–58.

47. Collaborative Group on Drug Use in Pregnancy: Medication during pregnancy: an intercontinental cooperative study. Int J Gynaecol Obstet 1992;39:187–196.

48. Committee on Drugs: Neonatal drug withdrawal. Pediatrics 1998; 101:1079–1088.

49. Coustan D: Nonprescription drugs and alcohol: Abuse and effects in pregnancy. In: Reece EA, Hobbins JC, Mahoney MJ, Petrie RH, eds: Medicine of the Fetus and Mother. Philadelphia, JB Lippincott, 1992, pp. 317–327.

50. Cramer CR: Fetal death due to accidental maternal carbon monoxide poisoning. J Toxicol Clin Toxicol 1982;19:297–301.

51. Curry S, Bond GR, Rashke R, et al: An ovine model of maternal iron poisoning in pregnancy. Ann Emerg Med 1990;19:632–638.

52. Czeizel A, Lendvay A: Attempted suicide and pregnancy. Am J Obstet Gynecol 1988;158:1084–1085.

53. Czeizel ARE, Tomcsik M, Timar L: Teratologic evaluation of 180 infants born to mothers who attempted suicide by drugs during pregnancy. Obstet Gynecol 1997;90:195–201.

54. Day NL, Cottreau CM, Richardson GA: The epidemiology of alcohol, marijuana, and cocaine use among women of child bearing age and pregnant women. Clin Obstet Gynecol 1993;36:232–245.

55. Desmond MM, Wilson GS: Neonatal abstinence syndrome: Recognition and diagnosis. Addict Dis 1975;2:112–121.

56. De Vigan C, de Walle HEK, Cordier S, et al: Therapeutic drug use during pregnancy: a comparison in four European countries. J Clin Epidemiol 1999;52:977–982.

57. Dixon SD, Bejar R: Echoencephalographic findings in neonates associated with maternal cocaine and metamphetamine use: Incidence and clinical correlates. J Pediatr 1989;118:770–778.

58. Doberczak TM, Shanzer S, Cutler R, et al: One-year followup of infants with abstinence-associates seizures. Arch Neurol 1988;45: 649–653.

59. Dolovich LR, Addis A, Vaillancourt JMR, Power JDB, Koren G, Einarson TR: Benzodiazepine use in pregnancy and major malformations or oral cleft: meta-analysis of cohort and case-control studies. BMJ 1998;317:839–843.

60. Dominick MA, Carson TL: Effects of carbon monoxide exposure on pregnant sows and their fetuses. Am J Vet Res 1983;44:35–40.

61. Douglas MJ: Perinatal physiology and pharmacology. In: Norris MC, ed: Obstetric Anesthesia. Philadelphia, JB Lippincott, 1993.

62. Dow-Edwards D: Comparability of human and animal studies of developmental cocaine exposure. NIDA Res Monogr 1996;164: 146–174.

63. Ducey J, Brooke D: Transcutaneous absorption of boric acid. Pediatrics 1973;43:644–651.

64. Eckardt MJ, File SE, Gessa GL, et al: Effects of moderate alcohol consumption on the central nervous system. Alcohol Clin Exp Res 1998;22:998–1040.

65. Elhassani HB: Neonatal poisoning: Causes, manifestations, prevention, and management. South Med J 1986;79:1535–1543.

66. Elkharrat D, Raphael JC, Korach JM, et al: Acute carbon monoxide intoxication and hyperbaric oxygen in pregnancy. Intensive Care Med 1991;17:282–292.

67. Eyler FD, Behnke M: Early development of infants exposed to drugs prenatally. Clin Perinatol 1999;26:107–150.

68. Fantel AG, MacPhail BJ: The teratogenicity of cocaine. Teratology 1982;26:17–19.

69. Farrow JR, Davis GJ, Toy TM, et al: Fetal death due to nonlethal maternal carbon monoxide poisoning. J Forensic Sci 1990;35: 1448–1452.

70. Ferm VH: Teratogenic effects of hyperbaric oxygen. Proc Soc Exp Biol Med 1964;90:854–858.

71. Finnegan LP, Kandall SR: Maternal and neonatal effects of alcohol and drugs. In: Lowinson JH, Ruiz P, Millman RB, Langrod JG, eds: Substance Abuse: A Comprehensive Textbook, 2nd ed. Baltimore, Williams & Wilkins, 1992, pp. 628–656.

72. Finnell RH, Toloyan S, van Waes M, Kalivas PW: Preliminary evidence for a cocaine-induced embryopathy in mice. Toxicol Appl Pharmacol 1990;103:228–237.

73. Fried PA: Prenatal exposure to tobacco and marijuana: effects during pregnancy, infancy, and early childhood. Clin Obstet Gynecol 1993; 36:319–337.

74. Friedman JM: Report of the Teratology Society Public Affairs Committee symposium on FDA classification of drugs. Teratology 1993; 48:5–6.

75. Friedman JM, Polifka JE: Teratogenic Effects of Drugs: A Resource for Clinicians (TERIS), 2nd ed. Baltimore, The Johns Hopkins University Press, 2000. *http://depts.washington.edu/~terisweb/teris/.*

76. Friedman S, Gatti M, Baker T: Cesarean section after maternal acetaminophen overdose. Anesth Analg 1993;77:632–634.

77. Gabrielli A, Layon AJ, Gallagher TJ: Carbon monoxide intoxication during pregnancy: A case presentation and pathophysiologic discussion with emphasis on molecular mechanisms. J Clin Anesth 1995;7: 82–87.

78. Gemme G, Ruffa G, Bonioli E, et al: Cushing's syndrome due to topical administration of corticosteroids. Am J Dis Child 1984;138: 987–988.

79. Gershanik J, Boecler B, Ensley H, et al: The gasping syndrome and benzyl alcohol poisoning. N Engl J Med 1982;307:1384–1388.

80. Gillberg C: "Floppy infant syndrome" and maternal diazepam [letter]. Lancet 1977;2:244.

81. Ginsberg MD, Myers RE: Fetal brain injury after maternal carbon monoxide intoxication. Neurology 1976;26:15–23.

82. Gladstone J, Nulman I, Koren G: Reproductive risks of binge drinking during pregnancy. Reprod Toxicol 1996;10:3–13.

83. Glantz JC, Woods JR: Cocaine, heroin, and phencyclidine: Obstetric perspectives. Clin Obstet gynecol 1993;36:279–301.

84. Guerri C: Neuroanatomical and neurophysiological mechanisms involved in central nervous system dysfunctions induced by prenatal alcohol exposure. Alcohol Clin Exp Res 1998;22:304–312.

85. Haibach H, Akhter JE, Muscato MS, et al: Acetaminophen overdose with fetal demise. Am J Clin Pathol 1984;82:240–242.

86. Hakkola J, Tanaka E, Pelkonen O: Developmental expression of cytochrome P450 enzymes in human liver. Pharmacol Toxicol 1998; 82:209–217.

87. Hannigan JH: What research with animals is telling us about alcohol-related neurodevelopmental disorder. Pharmacol Biochem Behav 1996;55:489–499.

88. Hanson JW: Teratogen update: Fetal hydantoin effects. Teratology 1986;33:349–353.

89. Harada M: Congenital Minamata disease: Intrauterine methylmercury poisoning. Teratology 1986;125–126.

90. Herzlinger RA, Kandall SR, Vaughan HG: Neonatal seizures associated with narcotic withdrawal. J Pediatr 1977;91:638–641.

91. Hill EP, Hill JR, Power GG, Longo LD: Carbon monoxide exchanges between the human fetus and mother: A mathematical model. Am J Physiol 1977;232:H311–H323.

92. Hollander DI, Nagey DA, Welsch R, et al: Hyperbaric oxygen therapy for the treatment of acute carbon monoxide poisoning in pregnancy. J Reprod Med 1987;32:615–617.

93. Holt D, Harvey D, Hurley R: Chloramphenicol toxicity. Adverse Drug React Toxicol Rev 1993;12:83–95.

94. Holtzman C, Paneth N: Maternal cocaine use during pregnancy and perinatal outcomes. Epidemiol Rev 1994;16:315–334.

95. Horowitz RS, Dart R, Jarvie DR, Bearer CF, Gupta U: Placental transfer of *N*-acetylcysteine following human maternal acetaminophen toxicity. J Toxicol Clin Toxicol 1997;35:447–451.

96. Hurst DL, Marsh WW: Early severe infantile botulism. J Pediatr 1993;124:909–911.

97. Hutchings DE: The puzzle of cocaine's effects following maternal use during pregnancy: Are there reconcilable differences? Neurotoxicol Teratol 1993;15:281–286.

98. Hytten FE: Physiologic changes in the mother related to drug handling. In: Krauer B, Krauer F, Hytten F, del Pozo E, eds: Drugs in Pregnancy. Orlando, Academic Press, 1984, pp. 7–17.

99. Ihlen BM, Amundsen A, Sande HA, Daae L: Changes in the use of intoxicants after onset of pregnancy. Br J Addict 1990;85: 1627–1631.

100. Jager-Roman E, Deichl A, Jakob S, et al: Fetal growth, major malformations, and minor anomalies in infants born to women receiving valproic acid. J Pediatr 1986;111:997–1004.

101. John EG, Guignard JP: Development of renal excretion of drugs during ontogeny. In: Polin RA, Fox WW, eds: Fetal and Neonatal Physiology. Philadelphia, WB Saunders, 1992, pp. 153–159.

102. Johnson D, Simone C, Koren G: Transfer of *N*-acetylcysteine by the human placenta. Vet Hum Toxicol 1993;35:365.

103. Johnson SF, McCarter RJ, Ferencz C: Changes in alcohol, cigarette, and recreational drug use during pregnancy: Implications for intervention. Am J Epidemiol 1987;126:695–702.

104. Jones KL: Smith's Recognizable Patterns of Human Malformation, 5th ed. Philadelphia, WB Saunders, 1997.

105. Jones KL, Lacro RV, Johnson KA, Adams J: Pattern of malformations in the children of women treated with carbamazepine during pregnancy. N Engl J Med 1989;320:1661–1666.

106. Juchau MR, Rettie AE: The metabolic role of the placenta. In: Fabro S, Scialli AR, eds: Drug and Chemical Action in Pregnancy. New York, Marcel Dekker, 1986, pp. 153–169.

107. Kandall SR, Doberczak TM, Mauer KR, Strashun RH, Korts DC: Opiate v CNS depressant therapy in neonatal drug abstinence syndrome. Am J Dis Child 1983;137:378–382.

108. Kandall SR, Gaines J: Maternal substance use and subsequent sudden infant death syndrome (SIDS) in offspring. Neurotoxicol Teratol 1991;13:235–240.

109. Kandall SR, Gaines J, Habel L, et al: Relationship of maternal substance abuse to subsequent sudden infant death syndrome in offspring. J Pediatr 1993;125:120–126.

110. Kandall SR: Treatment strategies for drug-exposed neonates. Clin Perinatol 1999;26:231–243.

111. Khoury S, Odeh M, Oettinger M: Deferoxamine treatment for acute iron intoxication in pregnancy. Acta Obstet Gynecol Scand 1995; 74:756–757.

112. Kiess W, Linderkamp O, Hadorn HB, Haas R: Fetal alcohol syndrome and malignant disease. Eur J Pediatr 1984;143:160–161.

113. Kleiner GJ, Greston WM: Suicide during pregnancy. In: Cherry SH, Merkatz IR, eds: Complications of Pregnancy: Medical, Surgical, Gynecologic, Psychosocial, and Perinatal, 4th ed. Baltimore, Williams & Wilkins, 1991, pp. 269–289.

114. Kliegman RM, Madura D, Kiwi R, et al: Relation of maternal cocaine use to the risk of prematurity and low birth weight. J Pediatr 1994;124:751–756.

115. Koren G, Graham K, Shear H, et al: Bias against the null hypothesis: the reproductive hazards of cocaine. Lancet 1989;1: 1440–1442.

116. Koren G, Sharav T, Pastuszak A, et al: A multicenter, prospective study of fetal outcome following accidental carbon monoxide poisoning in pregnancy. Reprod toxicol 1991;5:397–403.

117. Koren G: Changes in drug disposition in pregnancy and their clinical implication. In: Koren G, ed: Maternal–Fetal Toxicology: A Clinician's Guide, 2nd ed. New York, Marcel Dekkeer, 1994, pp. 3–14.

118. Koren G: Measurement of drugs in neonatal hair: A window to fetal exposure. Forensic Sci Int 1995;70:77–82.

119. Koren G, Pastuszak A, Ito S: Drug therapy: drugs in pregnancy. N Engl J Med 1998;338:1128–1137.

120. Kumar A, Goel KM, Rae MD: Paracetamol overdose in children. Scottish Med J 1990;35:106–107.

121. Kurzel RB: Can acetaminophen excess result in maternal and fetal toxicity? South Med J 1990;83:953–955.

122. Lacoste H, Goyert GL, Goldman LS, et al: Acute iron intoxication in pregnancy. Obstet Gynecol 1992;80:500–501.

123. Lambers DS, Clark KE: The maternal and physiologic effects of nicotine. Semin Perinatol 1996;20:115–126.

124. Lammer EJ: A phenocopy of the retinoic acid embryopathy following maternal use of etretinate that ended one year before conception. Teratology 1988;37:472.

125. Lampert PW, O'Brian JS, Garrett R: Hexachlorophene encephalopathy. Acta Neuropathol 1973;23:326–333.

126. Land DB, Kushner R: Drug abuse during pregnancy in an inner-city hospital: Prevalence and patterns. J Am Osteopath Assoc 1990;90: 421–426.

127. Laub DN, Elmagbari NO, Elmagbari NM, Hausburg MA, Gardiner CS: Effects of acetaminophen on preimplantation embryo glutathione concentration and development in vivo and in vitro. Toxicol Sci 2000;56:150–155.

128. Lawrence RA: Drugs in breast milk. In: Lawrence RA, Lawrence RM: Breastfeeding: A guide for the Medical Professional, 5th ed. St. Louis, CV Mosby, 1999, pp. 351–393, 744–867.

129. Lederman S, Fysh WJ, Tredger M, et al: Neonatal paracetamol poisoning: Treatment by exchange transfusion. Arch Dis Child 1983; 58:631–633.

130. Lenke RR, Turkel SB, Monsen R: Severe fetal deformities associated with ingestion of excessive isoniazid in early pregnancy. Acta Obstet Gynecol Scand 1985;64:281–282.

131. Lester BM, LaGrasse L, Freier K, Brunner S: Studies of cocaine-exposed human infants. NIDA Research Monograph 1995;149: 175–209.

132. Lester BM: The Maternal Lifestyles Study. Ann NY Acad Sci 1998;846:297–305.

133. Lester D, Beck AT: Attempted suicide and pregnancy. Am J Obstet Gynecol 1988;158:1084–1085.

134. Little BB, Snell LM, Gilstrap LC: Alcohol use during pregnancy and maternal alcoholism. In: Gilstrap LC, Little BB, eds: Drugs and Pregnancy. New York, Elsevier, 1992, pp. 367–374.

135. Locksmith GJ, Duff P: Preventing neural tube defects: the importance of periconceptional folic acid supplements. Obstet Gynecol 1998;91:1027–1034.

136. Longo LD: The biological effects of carbon monoxide on the pregnant woman, fetus and newborn infant. Am J Obstet Gynecol 1977; 129:69–103.

137. Longo LD, Hill EP: Carbon monoxide uptake and elimination in fetal and maternal sheep. Am J Physiol 1977;232:H324–H330.

138. Ludmir J, Main DM, Landon MB, Gabbe SG: Maternal acetaminophen overdose at 15 weeks of gestation. Obstet Gynecol 1986; 67:750–751.

139. Lutiget B, Graham K, Einarson TR, Koren G: Relationship between gestational cocaine use and pregnancy outcome: A meta-analysis. Teratology 1991;44:405–414.

140. Maalouf EF, Battin M, Counsell SJ, Rutherford MA, Manzure AY: Arthrogryposis multiplex congenital and bilateral mid-brain infarction following maternal overdose of coproxamol. Eur J Paediatr Neurol 1997;5/6:183–186.

141. MacGregor SN, Keith LG, Bachicha JA, et al: Cocaine abuse during pregnancy: correlation between prenatal care and perinatal outcome. Obstet Gynecol 1989;74:882–885.

142. Mahalik MP, Gautieri RF, Mann DE: Teratogenic potential of cocaine hydrochloride in CF-1 mice. J Pharm Sci 1980;69:703–706.

143. Mahalik MP, Hitner HW: Antagonism of cocaine-induced fetal anomalies by prazosin and diltiazem in mice. Reprod Toxicol 1992; 6:161–169.

144. Malanga CJ, Kosofsky BE: Mechanisms of action of drugs of abuse on the developing fetal brain. Clin Perinatol 1999;26:17–37.

145. Manoguerra AS: Iron poisoning, report of a fatal case in an adult. Am J Hosp Pharm 1976;33:1088–1090.

146. Margulies JL: Acute carbon monoxide poisoning during pregnancy. Am J Emerg Med 1986;4:516–519.

147. Martin ML, Khoury MJ, Cordero JF: Trends in rates of multiple vascular disruption defects, Atlanta, 1968–1989. Teratology 1992;45: 647–653.

148. Martin-Boyer G, Lebretton R, Toga M, et al: Outbreak of accidental hexachlorophene poisoning in France. Lancet 1982;1:91–95.

149. Mattson SN, Riley EP: A review of the neurobehavioral deficits in children with fetal alcohol syndrome or prenatal exposure to alcohol. Alcohol Clin Exp Res 1998;22:279–294.

150. Mayes LC, Grillon C, Granger R, Schottenfeld R: Regulation of arousal and attention in preschool children exposed to cocaine prenatally. Ann NY Acad Sci 1998;846:126–145.

151. Mayes LC: Developing brain and in utero cocaine exposure: effects on neural ontogeny. Dev Psychopathol 1999;11:685–714.

152. McElhatton PR, Sullivan FM, Volans GN, Fitzpatrick R: Paracetamol poisoning in pregnancy: An analysis of the outcomes of cases referred to the teratology information service of the national poisons information service. Hum Exp Toxicol 1990;9:147–153.

153. McElhatton PR, Roberts JC, Sullivan FM: The consequences of iron overdose and its treatment with desferrioxamine in pregnancy. Hum Exp Toxicol 1991;10:251–259.

154. Mehanny SZ, Abdel-Rahman MS, Ahmed YY: Teratogenic effect of cocaine and diazepam in CF-1 mice. Teratology 1991;43:11–17.

155. Metcalfe J, Stock M, Barron D: Maternal physiology during pregnancy. In: Knobil E, Neill J, eds: The Physiology of Reproduction. New York, Raven Press, 1988, pp. 2147–2197.

156. Miller PD, Telford IR, Haas GF: Effect of hyperbaric oxygen on cardiogenesis in the rat. Biol Neonate 1971;17:44–52.

157. Miller MS, Juchau MR, Guengerich FP, Nebert DW, Raucy JL: Drug metabolic enzymes in developmental toxicology. Fund Appl Toxicol 1996;34:165–175.

158. Miller RK: Placental transfer and function: The interface for drugs and chemicals in the conceptus. In: Fabro S, Scialli AR, eds: Drug and Chemical Action in Pregnancy. New York, Marcel Dekker, 1986, pp. 123–152.

159. Moriss FH, Boyd RDH: Placental transport. In: Knobil E, Neill JD, eds: The Physiology of Reproduction, vol. 2. New York, Raven Press, 1988, p. 2083.

160. Motomatsu K, Adachi H, Uno T: Two infant deaths after inhaling baby powder. Chest 1979;75:448–450.

161. Muller GL, Graham S: Intrauterine death of the fetus due to accidental maternal carbon monoxide poisoning in pregnancy. Reprod Toxicol 1991;5:397–403.

162. Murphy MG, Turner BS: Pharmacology in neonatal care. In: Merenstein GB, Gardner SL, eds: Handbook of Neonatal Intensive Care. St Louis, CV Mosby, 1989, p. 146.

163. Nagourney BA, Aranda JV: Physiologic differences of clinical significance. In: Polin RA, Fox WW, eds: Fetal and Neonatal Physiology. Philadelphia, WB Saunders, 1992, pp. 169–177.

164. National Institute of Drug Abuse: National Pregnancy & Health Survey: Drug Use Among Women Delivering Livebirths: 1992. Rockville, MD, National Institutes of Health, 1996.

165. Nau H, Helge H, Luck W: Valproic acid in the perinatal period: Decreased maternal serum protein binding results in fetal accumulation and neonatal displacement of the drug and some metabolites. J Pediatr 1984;104:627–634.

166. Nau H: Physicochemical and structural properties regulating placental drug transfer. In: Polin RA, Fox WW, eds: Fetal and Neonatal Physiology, vol. 1. Philadelphia, WB Saunders, 1992, pp. 130–141.

167. Neuspiel DR: Behavior in cocaine-exposed infants and children: Association versus causality. Drug Alcohol Depend 1994;36:101–107.

168. Norman CA, Halton DM: Is carbon monoxide a workplace teratogen? A review and evaluation of the literature. Ann Occup Hyg 1990;34:335–347.

169. Olenmark M, Biber B, Dottori O, Rybo G: Fatal iron intoxication in late pregnancy. J Toxicol Clin Toxicol 1987;25:347–359.

170. Patel TG, Laungani RG, Grose EA, Dow-Edwards DL: Cocaine decreases uteroplacental blood flow in the rat. Neurotoxicol Teratol 1999;21:559–565.

171. Paul M, ed: Occupational and Environmental Reproductive Hazards: A Gude for Clinicians. Baltimore, Williams & Wilkins, 1993.

172. Pellegrini EM, Koren G: Motherrisk I: A new model for counseling in reproductive toxicology. In: Koren G, ed: Maternal–Fetal Toxicology: A Clinician's guide, 2nd ed. New York, Marcel Dekker, 1994, pp. 707–725. http://www.motherisk.org/.

173. Perrone J, Hoffman RS: Toxic ingestions in pregnancy: Abortifacient use in a case series of pregnant overdose patients. Acad Emerg Med 1997;4:206–209.

174. Piantadosi CA: Carbon monoxide, oxygen transport, and oxygen metabolism. J Hyperbaric Med 1987;2:27–44.

175. Plessinger MA, Woods JR: Cocaine in pregnancy: recent data on maternal and fetal risks. Obstet Gynecol Clin North Am 1998;25: 99–119.

176. Pratt R, Salomon DS: Biochemical basis for the teratogenic effects of glucocorticoids. In: Juchau MR, ed: The Biochemical Basis of Chemical Teratogenesis. New York, Elsevier/North-Holland, 1981, pp. 179–199.

177. Rayburn W, Aronow R, DeLancey B, Hogan MJ: Drug overdose during pregnancy: An overview from a metropolitan poison control center. Obstet Gynecol 1984;64:611–614.

178. Rayburn WF, Donn SM, Wulf ME: Iron overdose during pregnancy. Successful therapy with deferoxamine. Am J Obstet Gynecol 1983; 149:717–718.

179. Reed MD, Besunder JB: Developmental pharmacology: Ontogenic basis of drug disposition. Pediatr Clin North Am 1989;36: 1053–1074.

180. Rementeria JL, Bhatt K: Withdrawal symptoms in neonates from intrauterine exposure to diazepam. J Pediatr 1977;90:123–126.

181. Reproductive Health Hazards in the Workplace. Office of Technology Assessment. Washington DC, Congress of the United States, 1985.

182. Rice JM, Donovan PJ, Anderson LM: Mutagenesis and carcinogenesis. In: Fabro S, Scialli AR, eds: Drug and Chemical Action in Pregnancy. New York, Marcel Dekker, 1986, pp. 205–236.

183. Richards R, Brooks SHE: Ferrous sulphate poisoning in pregnancy with afibrogenaemia as a complication. West Indian Med J 1966;15: 134–140.

184. Richardson GA, Day NL: Maternal and neonatal effects of moderate cocaine use during pregnancy. Neurotoxicol Teratol 1991;13: 455–460.

185. Riggs BS, Bronstein AC, Kulig K, et al: Acute acetaminophen overdose during pregnancy. Obstet Gynecol 1989;74:247–253.

186. Riordan J: Drugs and breastfeeding. In: Riordan J, Auerbach KG, eds: Breastfeeding and Human Lactation, 2nd ed. Sudbury, Jones and Bartlett, 1999, pp. 163–219.

187. Ritchie H, Bolton, P: The Australian categorization of risk of drug use in pregnancy. Aust Fam Physician 2000;29:237–241.

188. Rivera-Calimlim L: The significance of drugs in breast milk: Pharmacokinetic considerations. Clin Perinatol 1987;14:51–70.

189. Roberts I, Robonson MJ, Mughal MZ, et al: Paracetamol metabolites in the neonate following maternal overdose. Br J Clin Pharmacol 1984;18:201–206.

190. Robertson RG, van Cleave BL, Collins JJ: Acetaminophen overdose in the second trimester of pregnancy. J Fam Pract 1986;23:267–268.

191. Rogan WJ: Breastfeeding in the workplace. Occup Med 1986;1: 411–413.

192. Rollins DE, von Bahr C, Glaumann H, et al: Acetaminophen: Potentially toxic metabolite formed by human fetal and adult liver microsomes and isolated fetal liver cells. Science 1979;205: 1414–1416.

193. Rosen TS, Pippenger CE: Pharmacologic observations on the neonatal withdrawal syndrome. J Pediatr 1984;88:1044–1048.

194. Rosenberg AA, Galan HL: Fetal drug therapy. Pediatr Clin North Am 1997;44:113–135.

195. Rosevear SK, Hope PL: Favourable neonatal outcome following maternal paracetamol overdose and severe fetal distress. Br J Obstet Gynaecol 1989;96:491–493.

196. Rubin JD, Ferencz C, Loffredo C: Use of prescription and non-prescription drugs in pregnancy. J Clin Epidemiol 1993;46:581–589.

197. Rubin PC, Craig GF, Gavin K, Summer D: Prospective survey of use of therapeutic drugs, alcohol, and cigarettes during pregnancy. Br Med J 1986;292:81–83.

198. Ruiz-Maldonado R, Zapta G, Tamayo L, et al: Cushing's syndrome after topical application of corticosteroids. Am J Dis Child 1982; 138:274–275.

199. Ruthnum P, Goel KM: ABC of poisoning: Paracetamol. Br Med J 1984;289:1538–1559.

200. Rutter N: Percutaneous drug absorption in the newborn: Hazards and uses. Clin Perinatol 1987;14:911–930.

201. Salafia C, Shiverick K: Cigarette smoking and pregnancy II: Vascular effects. Placenta 1999;20:273–279.

202. Sancewicz-Pach K, Chmiest W, Lichota E: Suicidal paracetamol poisoning of a pregnant woman just before delivery. Przeglad Lekarski 1999;56:459–462.

203. Sannerstedt R, Lundborg P, Bengt R, et al: Drugs during pregnancy: An issue of risk classification and information to prescribers. Drug Safety 1996;14:69–77.

204. Sapunar D, Saraga-Babic M, Peruzovic M, Marusic M: Effects of hyperbaric oxygen on rat embryos. Biol Neonate 1993;63:360–369.

205. Schardein JL: Chemically Induced Birth Defects. New York, Marcel Dekker, 1985.

206. Schauben JL, Augenstein WL, Cox J, Sato R: Iron poisoning: report of three cases and a review of therapeutic intervention. J Emerg Med 1990;8:309–319.

207. Scialli AR, Fabro S: The stage dependence of reproductive toxicology. In: Fabro S, Scialli AR, eds: Drug and Chemical Action in Pregnancy. New York, Marcel Dekker, 1986, pp. 191–204.

208. Schou M: Lithium treatment during pregnancy, delivery, and lactation: an update. J Clin Psychiatry 1990;51:410–413.

209. Selden BS, Curry SC, Clark RF, et al: Transplacental transport of *N*-acetylcysteine in an ovine model. Ann Emerg Med 1991;20: 1069–1072.

210. Shannon M, Amitai Y, Lovejoy FH: Multiple dose activated charcoal for theophylline poisoning in young infants. Pediatrics 1987;80: 368–370.

211. Shepard TH: Catalog of Teratogenic Agents. Baltimore, The Johns Hopkins University Press, 1992, p. xiii.

212. Shiono PH, Klebanoff MA, Nugent RP, et al: The impact of cocaine and marijuana on low birth weight and preterm birth: A multicenter study. Am J Obstet Gynecol 1995;174:19–27.

213. Shiverick KT, Salafia C: Cigarette smoking and pregnancy I: Ovarian, uterine, and placental effects. Placenta 1999;20:265–272.

214. Shuman RM, Leach RW, Alvord EC: Neurotoxicity of hexachlorophene in humans. Arch Neurol 1975;32:320.

215. Singer ST, Vichinsky EP: Deferoxamine treatment during pregnancy; is it harmful? Am J Hematol 1999;60:24–26.

216. Slotkin TA: Fetal nicotine or cocaine exposure: which one is worse? J Pharmacol Exp Ther 1998;285:931–945.

217. Slutsker L: Risks associated with cocaine use during pregnancy. Obstet Gynecol 1992;79:778–789.

218. Sokol RJ, Abel EL: risk factors for alcohol-related birth defects: threshold, susceptibility, and prevention. In: Sonderegger TB, ed: Perinatal Substance Abuse: Research Findings and Clinical Implications. Baltimore, The Johns Hopkins University Press, 1992, pp. 90–103.

219. Spear LP, Campbell J, Snyder K, Silveri M, Katovic N: Animal behavior models. Increased sensitivity to stressors and other environmental experiences after prenatal cocaine exposure. Ann NY Acad Sci 1998;846:76–88.

220. Sprauve ME, Lindsay MK, Herbert S, Graves W: Adverse perinatal outcome in parturients who use crack cocaine. Obstet Gynecol 1997; 89:674–678.

221. Stark KL, Lww QP, Namkung MJ, Harris CH, Juchau MR: Dysmorphogenesis elicited by microinjected acetaminophen analogs and metabolites in rat embryos cultured in vitro. J Pharmacol Exp Ther 1990;255:74–82.

222. Stokes IM: Paracetamol overdose in the second trimester of pregnancy. Br J Obstet gynaecol 1984;91:286–288.

223. Stratton K, Howe C, Battaglia FC, eds: Committee to Study Fetal Alcohol Syndrome, Institute of Medicine: Fetal Alcohol Syndrome: Diagnosis, Epidemiology, Prevention, and Treatment. Washington, DC, National Academy Press, 1996.

224. Strom RL, Schiller P, Seeds AF, ten Bensel R: Fatal poisoning in a pregnant female. Minn Med 1976;59:483–489.

225. Teelman K: Retinoids: Toxicology and teratogenicity to date. Pharmacol Ther 1989;40:29–43.

226. Telford IR, Miller PD, Haas GF: Hyperbaric oxygen causes fetal wastage in rats. Lancet 1969;2:220–221.

227. Tenenbein M: Poisoning in pregnancy. In: Koren G, ed: Maternal–Fetal Toxicology: A Clinician's Guide. New York, Marcel Dekker, 1990, pp. 89–114.

228. Theis JGW, Selby P, Ikizler Y, Koren G: Current management of the neonatal abstinence syndrome: a critical analysis of the evidence. Boil Neonate 1997;71:345–356.

229. Thilo EH, Townsend SF, Deacon J: Infant botulism at 1 week of age: Report of two cases. Pediatrics 1993;92:151–153.

230. Thornburg KL, Faber JJ: Transfer of hydrophilic molecules by placenta and yolk sac of the guinea pig. Am J Physiol 1977;233:C114–C126.

231. Tronick EZ, Beeghly M: Prenatal cocaine exposure, child development, and the compromising effects of cumulative risk. Clin Perinatol 1999;26:151–171.

232. Turk J, Aks S, Ampuero F, Hryhorczuk D: Successful therapy of iron intoxication in pregnancy with intravenous deferoxamine and whole bowel irrigation. Vet Hum Toxicol 1993;35:441–444.

233. US Food and Drug Administration: Labeling and prescription drug advertising: content and format for labeling for human prescription drugs. Fed Register 1979;44:37434–37467.

234. Van Amedyne KJ, Tenenbein M: Whole bowel irrigation during pregnancy. Am J Obstet Gynecol 1989;162:646–647.

235. Van Hoesen KB, Camporesi EM, Moon RE, et al: Should hyperbaric oxygen be used to treat the pregnant patient for acute carbon monoxide poisoning? A case report and literature review. JAMA 1989;261:1039–1043.

236. Ward SLD, Keens TG: Prenatal substance abuse. Clin Perinatol 1992;19:849–860.

237. Warkany J: Warfarin embryopathy. Teratology 1976;14:205–210.

238. Warkany J: Aminopterin and methotrexate: Folic acid deficiency. Teratology 1978;17:353–358.

239. Webster WS, Lipson AH, Brown-Woodman PDC: Uterine trauma and limb defects. Teratology 1987;35:253–260.

240. Webster WS, Brown-Woodman PDC: Cocaine as a cause of congenital malformations of vascular origin: Experimental evidence in the rat. Teratology 1990;41:689–697.

241. Webster WS, Brown-Woodman PDC, Lipson AH, Ritchie HE: Fetal brain damage in the rat following prenatal exposure to cocaine. Neurotoxicol Teratol 1991;13:621–626.

242. Weeks BS, Gamache P, Klein N, Hinson JA, Bruno M, Khairallah E: Acetaminophen toxicity to cultured rat embryos. Teratog Carcinog Mutagen 1990;10:361–371.

243. Weiss B, Doherty RA: Methylmercury poisoning. Teratology 1975;12:311–313.

244. Werler MM: Teratogen update: smoking and reproductive outcomes. Teratology 1997;55:382–388.

245. West JR, Chen WA, Pantazis NJ: Fetal alcohol syndrome: The vulnerability of the developing brain and possible mechanisms of damage. Metab Brain Dis 1994;9:291–322.

246. Whitlock FA, Edwards JE: Pregnancy and attempted suicide. Compr Pyschiatry 1968;9:1–12.

247. Woods JR: Maternal and transplacental effects of cocaine. Ann NY Acad Sci 1998;846·1–11.

248. Woods JR, Plessinger MA, Fantel A: An introduction to reactive oxygen species and their possible roles in substance abuse. Obstet Gynecol Clin North Am 1998;25:221–236.

249. Woody RC, Brewster MA: Telencephalic dysgenesis associated with presumptive maternal carbon monoxide intoxication in the first trimester of pregnancy. J Toxicol Clin toxicol 1990;28:467–475.

250. Working PK, ed: Toxicology of the Male and Female Reproductive Systems. New York Hemisphere, 1989.

251. Zelson C, Rubio E, Wasserman E: Neonatal narcotic addiction: 10-year observation. Pediatrics 1971;48:181–189.

252. Zuckerman B, Frank D, Brown E: Overview of the effects of abuse and drugs on pregnancy and offspring. NIDA Res Monogr 1995;149:16–38.

106 PEDIATRIC PRINCIPLES

Jeffrey S. Fine

Because calls to poison centers regarding child exposures to potential toxins are more frequent than those for any other age group, and because poisoning is a significant cause of pediatric injury morbidity, pediatricians have been active in helping to establish and promote the field of medical toxicology as well as regional poison control centers. Although the basic approach to the medical management of toxicologic problems outlined in Chapters 3 and 31 is generally applicable to children as well as adults, there are issues such as abuse by poisoning that are of particular concern to children when special considerations may be appropriate. This chapter provides a pediatric perspective on the application of toxicologic principles.

EPIDEMIOLOGY

In order to gain a perspective on the problem of pediatric poisoning, it is necessary to understand the magnitude of the problem. When assessing the impact of a particular type of injury such as poisoning, epidemiologists examine a number of parameters to measure the effects, such as exposure, morbidity, mortality, and cost. All of these parameters are difficult to measure accurately. One of the important sources for information on the extent and effects of poisoning exposures is the American Association of Poison Control Centers (AAPCC). Each year the AAPCC compiles standardized data collected from poison centers throughout the United States; the 1999 annual review includes information submitted by 64 poison centers. In the following discussion, comments on AAPCC data refer to cumulative information from the last five published reports covering the years 1995 to 1999. (See Chap. 116 and p. 1752 for a detailed discussion of the AAPCC database.)

The AAPCC reports approximately 1.5 million potentially toxic exposures per year for children and adolescents aged 0 to 19, and these pediatric exposures represent 67% of the reported poisoning exposures for all age groups. Children under the age of 6 account for 79% of all reported pediatric exposures; children between 6 and 12 account for 10%, and adolescents 13 to 19 account for 11%. Children under the age of 6 account for 53% of all reported pediatric and adult poisoning exposures. Girls represent 46% of the reported poisoning exposures among young children and 56% of the reported exposures among adolescents.

Ninety-nine percent of the AAPCC reported poisoning exposures in children under 6 years of age are unintentional. In contrast, only 53% of the reported adolescent poisoning exposures are unintentional, whereas 43% are intentional, mostly the result of suicide attempts. This high frequency of suicidal intent has also been reported by others.[112] The remaining 4% of adolescent expo-

sures have miscellaneous causes such as adverse drug reactions or are unknown. These differences in the reason for exposure between young children and adolescents are specifically reflected in the outcomes of these exposures (discussed below).

Approximately 10,000 exposures each year are classified as adverse drug reactions. These reports account for approximately 0.3% of exposures in young children and approximately 2% of exposures in older children and adolescents.

Table 106–1 shows the leading causes of reported exposures in children and adolescents. According to the AAPCC, approximately 55% of reported pediatric exposures in children are to nonpharmaceutic agents, substances that are commonly found around the house such as cleaning agents, cosmetics, plants, hydrocarbons, and insecticides; whereas approximately 45% are to pharmaceutic agents. Table 106–1 lists the most common *reported* exposures, but these agents are not necessarily the ones that cause the most serious morbidity and mortality (see Table 106–2).

For children under the age of 6 months, poisoning is unusual but may result from the inadvertent administration of an incorrect drug or drug dose by a parent,[48] intentional administration of a drug by a parent or sibling,[13,38] or passive exposure, for instance to the smoke of "crack cocaine."[12] Any poisoning in a child under 1 year of age should be carefully evaluated for possible child abuse or neglect.[13]

Several characteristics associated with ingestions in toddlers differentiate them from ingestions in adolescents or adults: (1) they are without suicidal intent; (2) there is usually only one substance involved; (3) the substances are usually nontoxic; (4) the amount is usually small; and (5) children usually present for evaluation soon after the ingestion. As many as 30% of children who experience one ingestion will experience a repeat ingestion.[72] Children who ingest poisons may also be at risk for other types of injuries.[10,42]

The peak age for childhood poisoning is between 1 and 3 years.[26] Unintentional ingestion is unusual after age 5, although it may reflect mistaken consumption of a substance from a mislabeled container.[21] Between the ages of 5 and 9, poisoning may be a reflection of intrafamilial stress or suicidal intent. After age 9 and through adolescence, overdose or poisoning frequently results either from a suicidal gesture or attempt or from an adverse effect while seeking drug-induced euphoria. Unintentional poisonings are largely preventable (Chap. 116).

Because many children are exposed to nontoxic substances or to nontoxic amounts of toxic substances, it is not surprising that the relative number of children and adolescents who are reported to suffer significant morbidity is small (Table 106–3). However, because there are millions of exposures each year, the number of

TABLE 106–1. Average Annual Exposures Reported to the AAPCC (1995–1999)[a]

Age <6 Years		Age 6–19 Years	
Category	**Number of Exposures**	**Category**	**Number of Exposures**
Cosmetics/personal care products	144,380	Analgesics	46,103
Cleaning substances	115,632	Bites/envenomations	20,470
Analgesics	88,435	Cleaning substances	19,233
Plants	80,456	Cough/cold preparations	18,337
Cough/cold preparations	68,482	Cosmetics/personal care products	17,594
Foreign bodies	66,505	Foreign bodies	15,557
Topical agents	55,265	Plants	15,208
Antimicrobials	38,403	Stimulants/street drugs	13,800
GI preparations	35,985	Antidepressants	12,677
Vitamins	33,378	Food products/poisoning	12,120

[a]See page 1752 and Chap. 116 for references and discussion.

children reported by the AAPCC who suffer at least moderate effects is approximately 60,000 per year. Sixty percent of these seriously poisoned children are adolescents. Although the AAPCC is not the only source for epidemiologic data, there is little detailed information available anywhere on poisoning morbidity. Estimates of the rate of emergency department visits for poisoning and overdose are approximately 300 to 650 per 100,000 for children under 5 and 360 per 100,000 for adolescents.[26,44,47,109] The Centers for Disease Control estimate that approximately 100,000 children are seen in emergency departments each year for poisoning-related injuries, and 20,000 are hospitalized.[27] Reported rates of hospitalization for young children range from 40 to 170 per 100,000.[28,44,93,112]

Following exposure to drugs or poisons, adolescents are more frequently hospitalized than children. Suicidal adolescents may suffer serious toxicity more frequently than children after unintentional ingestions, although some adolescents may be admitted primarily for psychiatric evaluation. The peak age for hospitalizing young children exposed to drugs or poisons is between 1 and 3, reflecting the peak age of exposure. Hospitalized children under the age of 2 are more commonly exposed to nonpharmaceutical substances, whereas children over the age of two and adolescents are more commonly exposed to pharmaceuticals.[44,112]

Although the AAPCC reports outcome related to age, it does not generally stratify outcome with regard to age and substance. In one earlier multi-year review, the AAPCC reported those agents

TABLE 106–2. Agents Responsible for Significant Pediatric Poisoning Morbidity and Mortality[a]

	<6 Years Old[a]				13–17 Years Old[b]	
	Reported Major Effects[c]		**Reported Deaths**		**Reported Deaths[d]**	
Category	**Number**	**%[e]**	**Number**	**%[e]**	**Number**	**%[e]**
Cleaning agents/chemicals	277	12	6	6	3	1
Cardiovascular agents	182	8	5	5	17	7
Hydrocarbons	168	7	17	16	53	23
Sedative hypnotic agents	153	7	1	1	3	1
Antidepressants	125	6	5	5	37	15
Insecticides/pesticides	122	5	6	6	1	.4
Analgesic agents	119	5	14	13	47	20
Anticonvulsants	106	5	3	3	4	2
Bites/envenomations	100	4	1	1	0	0
Stimulants/street drugs	84	4	6	6	31	13
Iron	85	4	7	6	0	0
Carbon monoxide	42	2	22	20	5	3
Alcohols	52	2	4	4	10	4
Theophylline	38	2	1	1	2	1
Total for listed substances	1653	73	98	90	213	93
Totals reported	2270		109		230	

[a]Data from Litovitz T, Manoguerra A: Comparison of pediatric poisoning hazards: an analysis of 3.8 million exposure incidents. Pediatrics 1992;89:999–1006.
[b]Data from AAPCC 1995–1999, See Chapter 116 and page 1752 for references and discussion.
[c]Major effect = life-threatening signs and symptoms.
[d]No specific outcome effects for this age group are reported, and therefore, the number of major effects cannot be calculated.
[e]Not all reported substances are listed and therefore columns do not add up to 100%.

TABLE 106–3. **Outcome of Reported Pediatric Exposures (1991–1995)[a]**

Age (years)	Effects (% of reported exposures)[b]			
	Minor or none	Moderate	Major	Death
0–5	98.01	1.86	0.12	0.004
6–12	93.78	5.86	0.35	0.009
13–19	83.23	15.25	1.47	0.05
All children and adolescents 0–19	95.65	4.01	0.32	0.01

[a]See page 1752 and Chap. 116 for references and discussion.
[b]Minor = minimal signs and symptoms, often not requiring therapy; moderate = more pronounced, prolonged, or systemic signs and symptoms, often requiring therapy; major = life-threatening signs and symptoms.

causing the greatest number of major and fatal effects in children less than 6 years old.[74] The agents that cause significant morbidity and mortality are listed in Table 106–2. Other reports of hospitalized patients describe a similar distribution of agents causing significant morbidity, but with some differences.[28,31,32,122] In Australia, for instance, quinine, digoxin, and eucalyptus oil were significant causes of hospitalization, whereas in India, kerosene was the leading cause of poisoning hospitalizations.[24,54,82]

Poison-related deaths represent approximately 2.5% of annual childhood and adolescent deaths from unintentional injury.[84] The AAPCC reported 369 child and adolescent deaths from 1995 to 1999; these deaths represent 9.5% of the reported poisoning fatalities for all age groups. Thirty-one percent were children aged 0 to 5, 8% were children 6 to 12, and 61% were adolescents 13 to 19 years old.

The number of children under age 5 dying from poisons is extremely low. The AAPCC reports 25 per year on average between 1983 and 1999—a 95% decrease from a high of 456 in 1959.[26] This dramatic decrease in poisoning mortality may be the result of improved poisoning prevention (for example, child-resistant closures) and improved medical care, or may reflect a decrease in reporting (discussed later). Fifty percent of the childhood fatalities result from unintentional ingestions, 23% are from carbon monoxide poisoning, and 11% are caused by therapeutic medication errors; the remaining 16% have miscellaneous causes.

Although the AAPCC data provide a remarkable amount of epidemiologic information, there are questions about accuracy.[56,57,117] The most serious concern is that many significant poisonings may not be reported to poison centers. For instance, physicians managing "common" toxicologic problems may not feel the need for the assistance of a local or regional poison center and may not feel compelled to participate in the reporting process (Chap. 116). Therapeutic misadventures may also go unreported. In Rhode Island, only 45 of 369 poisoning deaths were reported to the regional poison center.[71] In comparison to the AAPCC, the National Center for Health Statistics reported that from 1995 to 1998, the last year for which information is available, there were 170 poison-related deaths for children under 5 years old, 169 for children aged 5 to 14, and 878 for adolescents aged 15 to 19.[88] For the same years, the AAPCC reported 90 deaths for children under 6, 22 for children 6 to 12, and 172 for adolescents 13 to19 years of age.

The most notable difference between the toxins listed in Table 106–2 and earlier studies is that salicylates are no longer a leading cause of reported poisoning morbidity and mortality.[33,37] This change may be related to both federal regulations requiring child-resistant closures as well as the decreased use of aspirin following the recognition of its association with Reye syndrome in children[15,60,83,94] (Chap. 33).

There are some significant etiologic differences in Table 106–2 between children and adolescents, particularly with regard to the lethality of agents. The leading three categories/agents for children are fumes (carbon monoxide), hydrocarbons, and analgesic agents, which account for 49% of all reported poisoning deaths. The top three categories for adolescents are hydrocarbons, antidepressants (almost exclusively tricyclic antidepressants), and analgesic agents (41% salicylates, 39% acetaminophen, 20% opioids), accounting for 58% of reported poisoning deaths. Importantly, the hydrocarbon deaths in children generally result from unintentional aspiration, but almost all the hydrocarbon deaths in adolescents were related to abuse of inhaled hydrocarbons such as trichloroethane or chlorofluorocarbons. Forty-seven percent of AAPCC-reported adolescent deaths are deemed suicides, and 34% are related to substance abuse; 6% are unintentional, and 10% have unknown causes.

Poisoning also has an economic cost. For one 3-month period, 21 children who ingested medications were hospitalized for a total of 39 days altogether at a cost of $95,000.[65] Charges for hospitalization may be approximately $5000 per child.[122] In a large economic analysis of the cost of injury in the United States, the lifetime cost was $495 per child and $10,839 per adolescent or young adult injured by poisoning.[93]

BEHAVIORAL, ENVIRONMENTAL, AND PHYSICAL ISSUES

A simplistic approach to childhood poisonings is that unobserved toddlers exploring their environment inadvertently ingest toxins. This approach ignores the complex interaction of factors that may lead to pediatric ingestions.

One approach to understanding injury causation utilizes an infectious diseaselike model in which host, agent, and environment are identified.[55] In the case of poisoning, the host is the child or adolescent, the agent is the particular toxin, and the environment is usually the home. This approach to injury prevention considers intervention with respect to these three factors during three time periods relative to injury occurrence: the preinjury, injury, and postinjury phases. The postinjury phase is mainly concerned with the medical management of a poisoning once it has occurred and is the focus of much of the rest of this textbook. Considering these factors allows us to focus on several aspects of poisoning, although it is often difficult to examine any single factor independently, and the relative contribution of these factors has not been well defined.

With regard to the agent, that is the toxin itself, there are a number of issues that affect the preinjury and injury phases. Ideally, pharmaceutic and nonpharmaceutic substances would have beneficial or useful effects without potential toxicity. Practically, however, there may be ways to reduce the toxicity of available agents. Less toxic rodenticides such as warfarin have replaced many more toxic types such as thallium or sodium monofluoroacetate. Nontoxic paradichlorobenzene mothballs have largely replaced toxic camphor-containing mothballs.

Denatonium benzoate (Bitrex), an aversive bittering agent, is added to some liquid chemicals such as windshield washer fluid or antifreeze, with the expectation that this will prevent unintentional poisoning.[61] Some trials have shown that older children respond negatively to these agents but that younger children may ingest one to two teaspoons of a substance before responding to the bitter flavor.[16,102] This is an important consideration because even this small an amount of a substance such as methanol may be toxic (see below). The utility of this agent in poison prevention is largely unstudied.[95]

The problem of unintentional ingestions is compounded by poison "look-alikes," pharmaceutic or toxic substances that resemble candy or food products.[46] Some common examples are ferrous sulfate tablets that look like M&M candies, prenatal vitamins that resemble Good and Plenty candies, and fuel oils that come in cans that resemble soft drink containers. Many shampoos and dishwashing detergents are given lemon or strawberry scents and have pictures of fruits on the labels. Children are not always capable of distinguishing nontoxic candies, fruits, and sodas from poison "look-alikes" and may be attracted to bright colors, pleasant smells, and appealing packages. Eliminating these "look-alikes" might prevent many unintentional ingestions.

Probably the most significant change to the physical aspect of the toxin itself has been packaging of pharmaceuticals and some other toxic substances with child-resistant closures mandated by the Poison Prevention Packaging Act of 1972 (Chap. 116). This legislation is credited with a significant reduction in morbidity and mortality related to poisoning from aspirin and other regulated products, although this finding has been challenged.[94,113] Child-resistant closures were also shown to reduce the number of toxic exposures to kerosene in South Africa.[67]

Nonetheless, problems with child-resistant closures include pharmaceuticals being dispensed in nonresistant containers, resistant containers not being properly closed, and medicines being out of the resistant container for use.[25,104] Seventy percent of toxic pharmaceuticals may be in non-child-resistant or in improperly functioning child-resistant containers. Several studies have identified poor functioning of the closures when there is sticky liquid or pill residue around the top of the container or screw threads.[62,65,121]

Although child-resistant containers are a significant deterrent to unintentional ingestions in toddlers, they are not completely effective, and even without the problems noted, some children can open them. A sense of security associated with these closures may lead some parents to be less compulsive with regard to safe storage. It has been recommended that for a few pharmaceuticals associated with a large number of significant poisonings (iron or antidepressant agents), a double barrier be instituted, such as a unit dose dispenser within a child-resistant container.[65]

A discussion of containers and storage naturally leads to consideration of the environment, which is particularly important in the preinjury and the injury phases. About 80% of childhood phrmaceutical ingestions occur at home; the remainder occur at the homes of grandparents, other relatives, and friends. The medicine usually belongs either to the child or to the mother, although a significant number of medications both at home and away from home belong to a grandparent.[62,73] Grandparents, other relatives, or family friends without children regularly around the home may not receive or keep medications in child-resistant containers and may not be attentive to safe-storage recommendations.

Medications are frequently kept in the kitchen or bedroom while they are being used.[62,121] In the kitchen, medications are in the refrigerator, on the table, or on the counter, and in the bedroom, medications are on a dresser or bedside table. A mother's purse is another location in which to find medications. In general, there are not significant differences in the storage practices in the homes of children who ingest and those who do not ingest medicines, so storage practices alone cannot predict the likelihood of childhood poisoning.[106,121]

One important caveat relates to the storage of nonpharmaceutic substances, particularly those in liquid form. Toxic materials should not be transferred to familiar containers such as food jars or wine or soda bottles for storage. Both children and adults have been exposed to poisons such as sodium hydroxide or potassium cyanide stored in bottles in the refrigerator.[110]

Childhood and adolescence are times of tremendous growth and development.[123] Some of these physical and social changes place children and teenagers at increased risk for poisonings. By 7 months of age an infant sitting up can pivot in order to grab an object; by 9 to 10 months of age most infants can creep and crawl; by 15 months of age most toddlers are walking quite competently and eagerly exploring. Between 9 and 12 months of age a child is developing a skillful pincer grasp with the thumb and forefinger that allows him or her to pick up small objects. Throughout this period, one of the child's primary sensory experiences is sucking on or gumming objects that are placed in the mouth.

The combination of three developmental skills—the ability to move around the home and go beyond the immediate view of a guardian, the ability to pick up and manipulate small objects, and the tendency of children to put things in their mouths—places them at risk for both foreign body aspiration and toxic ingestions. In addition, the fact that infants crawl and that children younger than 2 are just becoming comfortable moving around in an upright position explains why they are more likely to ingest common household substances. Pharmaceutic products stored in cabinets are generally out of reach of these young children, although a 1-year-old sitting on a bed or standing near a bedside table would be able to grab something off that table.

As children develop socially, they desire to become more like their parents, and they tend to imitate behaviors, such as taking medicine or using mouthwash. Children are taught that medicine is good for them when they are sick. Many children's medicines are sweetened and flavored to make them more palatable, and in fact, many parents encourage their children to take medicines by telling them "it tastes like candy." Children have also been observed "making tea" from plants or "making pizza" with mushrooms from the yard.[21]

As children become more mobile, agile, and curious, toxic substances that were previously outside their reach now become accessible, even when stored in some difficult-to-reach places. There is some evidence to suggest that parents underestimate the developmental skills of their children.[42] We should also reconsider the meaning of the term "unintentional" with respect to childhood poisoning: the toddler quite purposefully intends to get to a pill and eat it, but the subsequent injury is unintentional.

We have tried to explain some of the reasons why a child wants to ingest a pill: because it is there, it looks like candy or food, the parent takes pills, and taking medicine is considered good for health. These reasons may not be sufficient to explain why a child does something that he or she knows should not be done. One other aspect of childhood poisoning that must be considered is the interaction between the child's temperament and his or her social environment.

Many authors have tried to identify psychosocial predictors for childhood poisoning in general and repeat poisoning in particular.[17,45,64,105] As many as 30% of children may have repeat episodes of ingestions, frequently of the same substance. Certain risk factors have been identified for single and repeated episodes of childhood poisoning, such as hyperactivity, impulsive risk-taking behavior, rebelliousness, or negativistic attitude. Other factors seem to be associated more with the parents, such as medical illness, depression, or social isolation. Finally, a stressful environment or major social problem may also be a contributing factor.[103,105] It is not difficult to imagine a situation where a parent is depressed, cannot give adequate attention to a demanding child, and uses antidepressant medication that is kept at the bedside. In a bid for attention or as an expression of anger or frustration, the child ingests some of the parent's medicine.

HISTORY OF THE INGESTION

The appropriate management of any poisoned patient is influenced by the history of the exposure. Parents or guardians who are not abusing children will generally provide information to the extent they are able. As a rule, in the case of children, the substance and time of ingestion are known, although the number of pills or the volume of liquid ingested may be inaccurate. Clues to the amount ingested are the number of pills or volume of liquid in a bottle before and after an ingestion, the number of pills set out on the night table, or the area of a spot of liquid after a spill. When symptoms are suggestive of poisoning but the history is inadequate, remember to try to get information about possible exposure outside of the home, such as with a babysitter, grandparent, friend, or other relative. About 15% of childhood poisonings occur outside the home.[62,90]

Suicidal adolescents may be unreliable when relating the history of an ingestion. When caring for these patients, the clinician must utilize the history provided but should remain skeptical about the reported type and number of agents ingested as well as the time of ingestion.

In cases in which a child may be the victim of abuse or intentionally poisoned by a caretaker, the healthcare provider must insure that (1) the history of the poisoning remains consistent over time and between those people providing the details of the event, (2) the child's clinical presentation is consistent with the history of the poisoning, and (3) the reported actions are consistent with the child's developmental level.

GASTROINTESTINAL DECONTAMINATION

Chapter 5 is devoted to a complete discussion of gastrointestinal decontamination. This section reiterates and emphasizes only a few important points.

As previously described, children frequently ingest small quantities of single agents. For most of these ingestions gastric emptying is unnecessary. Some examples of nontoxic ingestions are eating a crayon or the leaf of a jade plant, licking the cap of a household bleach container, or swallowing two adult-strength acetaminophen tablets.

Orogastric lavage is generally the preferred method of gastric emptying when indicated for most serious ingestions. Even small children can generally tolerate orogastric lavage with a large-bore 28F or 34F tube. However the smaller "large-bore" tubes may not

be effective for removing large pills or fragments from the stomach of a small child. In order to use orogastric lavage safely in a child with a diminished gag reflex or in one who is comatose, the trachea should be intubated to protect the airway.

Administration of syrup of ipecac to poisoned patients was, until recently, considered a primary emergency intervention. However, the AAPCC reports that the use of syrup of ipecac for case management declined from 13% in 1983 to only 1% 1999. Nonetheless, there may still be a limited role for the use of syrup of ipecac in the management of particular cases—for an ingestion of (1) a massive amount of a slow-release product with onset of effects and toxicity that will be delayed for several hours, (2) tablets that are too large to pass through an orogastric tube, or (3) medications with only limited adsorption to activated charcoal (see Chap. 5 and Antidotes in Depth: Syrup of Ipecac).

One special pediatric consideration is the use of syrup of ipecac at home. The American Academy of Pediatrics, the American College of Emergency Physicians, and the American Medical Association, as well as some pediatric toxicologists, advocate having a one-ounce bottle of syrup of ipecac at home for administration after advice from a regional poison control center.[2-5,92]

An attempt was made to examine the potential benefit of the use of syrup of ipecac at home by studying children under 5 years of age who had ingested acetaminophen.[6] Although all measured levels were nontoxic, patients who received syrup of ipecac had peak acetaminophen levels that were lower than expected based on the reported dose, and the effect was greater if the syrup of ipecac was administered at home. The difficulty with this study is that what the *actual* peak levels would have been without treatment is unknown, and therefore, the extent of the actual treatment effect is unknown. Also, whether the effect would have been the same if the quantity ingested were enough to produce a toxic level is unknown.

When syrup of ipecac is administered at home, it can be given within an hour of the ingestion, the optimal time for its use, and vomiting would be expected to occur within 20 to 30 minutes. For a patient who would subsequently be evaluated in the emergency department, this might be beneficial. However, the patients considered appropriate for syrup of ipecac at home are usually those children with ingestions deemed not likely to result in significant poisoning and who can remain at home. These patients are not likely to benefit from the administration of syrup of ipecac, at home or elsewhere, and can probably remain home without any therapy at all. The utility of syrup of ipecac to prevent serious poisoning morbidity remains unproven.

Activated charcoal is one of the current mainstays of poison treatment.[7,31] Children generally will not drink activated charcoal willingly. Some children can be coaxed to do so if the activated charcoal is disguised in a baby bottle or soft drink container or sweetened with juice or sorbitol.[119] A nasogastric tube may have to be inserted to administer activated charcoal. This can be a small-bore tube because it is not intended for lavage, although the smaller the bore, the more difficult it will be to administer the thick mixture of activated charcoal. Placement of the tube, the presence of activated charcoal in the stomach, the effects of the toxin, or the previous use of syrup of ipecac may all make the child vomit. Aspiration of activated charcoal or stomach contents is a risk. For activated charcoal to be used safely in a patient who is comatose and does not have a gag reflex, the trachea should be intubated, and the airway protected. Even activated charcoal alone is unnecessary for a nontoxic ingestion.

Activated charcoal is available for home use.[68] Administration of activated charcoal at home or by prehospital personnel allows for administration significantly earlier than can be achieved at the time of arrival in the emergency department.[34] Although it would seem to have potential benefit as home therapy, activated charcoal is unpalatable, difficult to administer, quite messy, and not always available, and as a result has not yet achieved widespread use.[87] Whether the earlier administration of activated charcoal would affect outcome is also unknown. If activated charcoal should replace syrup of ipecac for home therapy, it will require a substantial reeducation effort on the part of pediatricians and toxicologists.

METHODS OF ENHANCED ELIMINATION

For consequential poisoning with toxins such as methanol, ethylene glycol, salicylates, lithium, and theophylline, either hemodialysis or charcoal hemoperfusion is the optimal technique to enhance elimination, depending on the particular toxin. These techniques can be performed on newborns or small infants in specially equipped centers with dedicated personnel.[21,68] The primary limiting factor is the ability to obtain vascular access.[14,41,86,111] However, even large centers that routinely do pediatric hemodialysis may not be able to manage the very small infant.

Exchange transfusion is a technique which is occasionally used to enhance drug elimination. This technique might be applicable in cases where multiple-dose activated charcoal cannot be administered, the toxin is poorly adsorbed to charcoal, or access to specialized pediatric hemodialysis or hemoperfusion is not readily available. Exchange transfusion has been used successfully for poisoning by salicylates[40,76] and theophylline.[11,89,100] Another drug for which exchange transfusion may be the treatment of choice is chloral hydrate.[8] This agent is still widely used as a sedative-hypnotic agent for children undergoing diagnostic studies such as computed tomography (CT) scans. Chloral hydrate toxicity is mediated in great part through one of its metabolites, trichloroethanol. For a small child who receives a supratherapeutic dose and manifests toxicity, exchange transfusion may be a therapeutic alternative if hemodialysis is unavailable.

AGENTS THAT MAY BE TOXIC OR FATAL IN SMALL QUANTITIES

When children ingest small quantities of toxic substances, they potentially ingest large doses relative to their small size.[66,70] There are a number of substances that may cause significant toxicity or even death with as little as one pill or one teaspoonful. These substances are listed in Table 106–4.

AGENTS THAT MAY HAVE DELAYED TOXICITY IN CHILDREN

There are several agents that warrant particular concern because their effects may be significantly delayed. Classic examples are atropine/diphenoxylate (Lomotil)[18,36,78] and oral hypoglycemic agents such as chlorpropamide.[53,91] Both of these agents have been

TABLE 106–4. Substances That Can Cause Severe Toxicity to an Infant after a Small Dose

Antihistamines
Benzocaine
β-Adrenergic antagonists (sustained release)
Calcium channel blockers (sustained release)
Camphor
Clonidine
Diphenoxylate/atropine (Lomotil)
Methanol/ethylene glycol
Methylsalicylate
Opioids (methadone, codeine)
Phenothiazines
Quinine/chloroquine
Theophylline
Tricyclic antidepressants

reported to cause serious morbidity with initial symptoms or recurrence of symptoms as late as 24 hours after ingestion.

Children who have ingested or may have ingested these medications should be admitted for observation and monitoring even if they are asymptomatic because effects may not become apparent for 24 hours. With the advent of new slow-release formulations of calcium channel blockers and β-adrenergic antagonists, concern for delayed toxicity has been extended to other drugs.

AGENTS THAT HAVE UNUSUAL OR IDIOSYNCRATIC REACTIONS IN CHILDREN

Benzyl Alcohol: Gasping Syndrome

Benzyl alcohol is a preservative added to liquid pharmaceutical preparations; for small-volume medications administered to adults, the benzyl alcohol additive is quite safe (Chap. 56). At toxic doses, benzyl alcohol can cause respiratory failure, vasodilation, hypotension, convulsions, and paralysis. Intravenous flush solutions containing benzyl alcohol were implicated as the cause of the "gasping syndrome" in sick newborns; severe metabolic acidosis, encephalopathy, respiratory depression, and gasping.[1] The association was made when infants with this syndrome were found to have elevated levels of benzoic acid and hippuric acid, metabolites of benzyl alcohol.[22,49] Benzyl alcohol is metabolized by the conjugation of benzoic acid with glycine to form hippuric acid. This pathway may not be functional in premature infants. Benzyl alcohol administration has also been associated with kernicterus and intraventricular hemorrhage in premature infants.[58,63]

Although benzyl alcohol has been removed from many medications used in neonates, there are still preparations containing this agent.[118]

Imidazolines/Clonidine: CNS Effects

Imidazoline agents such as tetrahydrozoline, oxymetazoline, xylometazoline, and naphazoline are nonprescription sympathomimetic agents used as nasal decongestants and conjunctival vasoconstrictors (Chap. 35). Clonidine is an imidazoline derivative used as an antihypertensive agent (Chap. 51). In small children, these agents can cause central nervous system depression, respiratory depression, bradycardia, miosis, and hypotension.[9,75,120] The presumed mechanism of action is through stimulation of central α_2-adrenergic receptors. Although naloxone has been reported to reverse some of the CNS effects of clonidine, there are no reports of its successful use with the other imidazoline agents (Chap. 51).

Ethanol: Hypoglycemia

Ethanol is the primary component of alcoholic beverages as well as a major constituent of many liquid preparations such as mouthwash, vanilla flavoring, and perfume. Besides the well-known sedative-hypnotic effects, ethanol intoxication in children is associated with hypoglycemia.[69,114] Ethanol-induced hypoglycemia may cause seizures and may exacerbate the other CNS effects induced by ethanol intoxication. The mechanism of hypoglycemia is presumed to be related to the fasting state induced by depressed consciousness in the young child with limited glycogen stores. Whether the metabolism of ethanol is specifically related to the development of hypoglycemia is unknown. There does not seem to be a blood alcohol level threshold for the development of hypoglycemia, which has been seen with blood alcohol levels as low as 20 mg/dL[35] (Chaps. 40 and 64).

Chloramphenicol: Gray Baby Syndrome

Chloramphenicol is a broad-spectrum antibiotic that has been used in pediatrics because of its activity against *Haemophilus influenzae*. Its use in the United States has largely been replaced by other antibiotics because of the association with aplastic anemia. When administered at high doses, chloramphenicol can produce the "gray baby syndrome"—abdominal distension, vomiting, metabolic acidosis, progressive pallid cyanosis, irregular respirations, hypothermia, hypotension, and vasomotor collapse. Although these effects are seen primarily in premature newborn infants, they can also be seen in older children and adults (Chap. 46).

Gray baby syndrome is associated with serum concentrations greater than 100 mg/L. Increased chloramphenicol levels may result from (1) inadequate conjugation of chloramphenicol with glucuronic acid because of inadequate activity of glucuronyl transferase in the newborn liver and (2) decreased renal elimination of unconjugated chloramphenicol. The exact mechanism of toxicity is unknown; there has been speculation that free radicals produced during the metabolism of chloramphenicol may interfere with mitochondrial function.[59]

PROBLEMS WITH DRUG DOSING AND ADMINISTRATION

Because children are small, they generally require smaller amounts of drugs to achieve therapeutic plasma levels, even when the dosing requirement per kilogram is greater than for an adult. Therefore, children are particularly susceptible to therapeutic errors in drug dosing. The AAPCC reports that almost 11% of the poisoning deaths in children for 1995 through 1999 were related to therapeutic medication error or misuse.

Dosing and drug administration errors take many forms:

1. The wrong drug is administered. In one nursery, an epidemic mimicking neonatal sepsis was caused when racemic epinephrine was inadvertently administered instead of vitamin E because both drugs were manufactured by the same company, distributed in nearly identical bottles, and stored near each other inside the nursery refrigerator.[107]

2. A drug dose is calculated incorrectly.[23,85,99] A 1-kg premature infant required sedation for a diagnostic study. A high dose of chloral hydrate, 100 mg/kg, was calculated to be 1 g (1000 mg) instead of 100 mg. The child had a cardiopulmonary arrest and died.

3. A drug dose is calculated correctly but written illegibly or transcribed incorrectly. When drugs require milligram-per-kilogram dosing, it is easy to make decimal mistakes in the calculation or in the transcription. Clearly written orders and prescriptions are essential.

4. A drug dose is calculated and ordered correctly, but the wrong dosage form is dispensed. Acetaminophen suppositories (120 mg) were ordered for a toddler, but adult-strength suppositories (650 mg) were distributed and administered every 4 hours. The child developed hepatotoxicity requiring hospitalization and therapy (Chap. 32).

5. A drug dose is correctly calculated, formulated, and dispensed, but the wrong dose is administered to the child.

Somewhat different errors can occur when drugs are administered intravenously:

6. Medications may be infused at an incorrect rate, either by miscalculation or through illegibility. This can be avoided by writing out the order in longhand, for example, "five milliliters per hour to deliver five milligrams per kilogram per hour."

7. Intravenous medications may be administered as a bolus rather than a slow infusion. Phenytoin, which has a recommended administration rate in adults of no more than 50 mg/min, should be infused at a rate of no more than 1 mg/kg/min in a child.

8. A drug meant to be administered by one route is given by another. In one case, paraldehyde was administered through an umbilical artery catheter with subsequent development of gangrene of the lower extremities and by death.[51]

INTENTIONAL POISONING AND CHILD ABUSE

Intentional poisoning of children is an unusual though significant form of child abuse. There are several types of intentional poisoning, some of which define pathologic characteristics of the caretaker: (1) undifferentiated child abuse, neglect, or impulsive acts under stress; (2) factitious illness (Münchausen syndrome by proxy); (3) overt parental psychosis; (4) altruistic motivation or bizarre childrearing practices; and (5) the Medea complex, or the vengeful killing of a child out of spite for one's spouse.[13,108]

Intentional poisoning is rarely suspected unless the patient dies and an autopsy is performed, a wide-ranging drug screen is ordered, or the history is bizarre enough to raise suspicions. In many cases where children were later found to be poisoned, the initial diagnoses were sepsis, meningitis, seizures, intracranial hemorrhage, gastroenteritis, apnea, apparent life-threatening events, or metabolic derangements.[13] In addition to many pharmaceutic agents, salt, pepper, water, caffeine, ethylene glycol, herbs, plants, and traditional remedies have been used to poison children.[13,39] Although the death rate from unintentional poisoning in childhood is much less than 1%, the death rate from inflicted poisoning may be as high as 20 to 30%.[13,39,108]

Intentional poisoning may be associated with other abuse; approximately 20% of poisoned children may have evidence of physical abuse.[13,39] Of children presenting to the emergency department after presumed unintentional poisoning, 36% had previous emergency department visits for trauma, 7% for poisoning, 6% for both trauma and poisoning, and 1.4% for failure to thrive. At the time of the visit, only 7% were evaluated for possible abuse, and 2.7% were considered neglected.[96] These data do not prove an association between poisoning and physical trauma; however, in some children, repeat episodes of trauma and/or poisoning may be a manifestation of significant intrafamilial stress. Healthcare providers must remain vigilant to the possibility that a presumed unintentional poisoning may have been inflicted, especially in the setting of a repeat ingestion or when there have been previous evaluations for trauma.

Substance abuse by a parent or guardian may play a role in unintentional or intentional poisoning of children. Children have been intoxicated with cocaine by passive inhalation[12] as well as through breast milk.[29] Children have been given doses of methadone mixed in orange juice to quiet them down.[37] There are reports of babysitters blowing marijuana smoke into babies' faces to "get them high" or quiet them down.[13]

Factitious illness (Münchausen syndrome by proxy, MSBP) is a condition in which a parent, usually the mother, fabricates a history of a nonexistent disease in a child or creates the signs and symptoms of disease in a child.[80,81,97] This is usually a manifestation of the parent's complex psychiatric illness, which may include Münchausen syndrome itself.[19,52] There may be only a fine line separating MSBP from an intentional poisoning with intent to harm or kill a child. Regardless of the specific intent, this condition is considered a form of child abuse.

A child's fabricated illness can lead to multiple medical evaluations by multiple physicians, frequent hospitalizations, unnecessary surgery and diagnostic testing, unnecessary prescribing and administration of medication, and occasionally, the death of the child. Administration of exogenous drugs is frequently the mechanism of creating a particular set of signs and symptoms. Agents that have been used to create factitious illness include analgesics, antidepressants, insulin, syrup of ipecac, Lomotil, phenothiazines, sedative-hypnotics, warfarin, phenolphthalein, and hydrocarbons.[98] Several warning signals are outlined in Table 106–5 that may suggest a diagnosis of MSBP.

In one illustrative case of MSBP,[50] a 29-month-old boy with a previous history of appendectomy was hospitalized multiple times for vomiting, diarrhea, and dehydration. Evaluation included multiple laboratory evaluations of blood and stool, a gastric pH probe, CT, MRI, endoscopy, and upper GI series. At the fourth admission a small bowel obstruction was identified, and the child had lysis of adhesions. Nonetheless, symptoms recurred every 2 to 4 months, necessitating hospitalization. The child failed to thrive and required a nasoduodenal tube for feeding, which frequently became dislodged. The child went on to have a jejunostomy tube and a permanent central venous catheter placed. Eighteen months after his initial presentation, the child presented in congestive heart failure with evidence of cardiomyopathy. A urine screen identified emetine and cephaline, components of syrup of ipecac. The child recovered, was removed from his home to protective custody, and remained asymptomatic while receiving a regular diet.

TABLE 106–5. Factitious Illness (Münchausen Syndrome) by Proxy: Suggestive Characteristics in Clinical Situations

1. A persistent or recurrent illness that cannot be explained.
2. The history of disease or results of diagnostic tests are inconsistent with the general health and appearance of the child.
3. The signs and symptoms cause the clinician to remark that "I've never seen anything like this before!"
4. The signs and symptoms do not occur when the child is separated from the parent.
5. The parent is particularly attentive and refuses to leave the child's bedside even for a few minutes.
6. The parent develops particularly close relations with hospital staff.
7. The parent seems less worried about the child's condition than the physician.
8. Treatments are not tolerated—intravenous lines fall out frequently; prescribed medications lead to vomiting.
9. The proposed diagnosis is a very rare disease.
10. "Seizures" are unwitnessed by medical staff and reportedly do not respond to any treatment.
11. The parent has a complicated medical or psychiatric history.
12. The parent is or was associated with the healthcare field.

Adapted, with permission, from Meadow R: Münchausen syndrome by proxy. Arch Dis Child 1982;57:92–98.

Siblings of children being poisoned may also suffer or have suffered from factitious illness. In addition, there is grave psychiatric illness that is manifested by the victim, the parents, and the siblings.[20,79]

Child abuse or neglect is part of the differential diagnosis in any case of childhood poisoning. Intentional poisoning should be considered for (1) any medical case with a confusing presentation, history, or symptomatology; (2) any child with multiple presentations for a rare or unexplained medical condition; (3) any child who presents with apnea or an apparent life-threatening event; (4) "ingestions" in a child under 6 to 9 months of age; (5) massive ingestions by small children; (6) intoxications with substances to which a child could or would not have access; (7) ingestion of multiple substances by a small child; (8) "accidental ingestions" in the school-age child who is at low risk for unintentional ingestions; (9) a repeat ingestion; or (10) a history of previous trauma.

These considerations of child abuse notwithstanding, rare diseases do occur. One child's rare inherited metabolic disorder, methyl malonic acidemia, was misdiagnosed as ethylene glycol poisoning because the chromatographic appearance of the metabolite propionic acid was similar to that of ethylene glycol.[101]

SUMMARY

Children are frequently exposed to potentially toxic agents; fortunately, most childhood exposures are ingestions of nonpoisonous materials or small nontoxic quantities of potentially toxic agents. When a child sustains a significant toxic exposure, management follows general toxicologic principles. Although most childhood exposures are unintentional, the clinician should be alert to the possibility of the intentional poisoning of a child with pharmaceutic or household agents.

The normal development of children puts them at risk for unintentional ingestions. A chaotic home environment or a disorganized social structure may compound these risks. Children's small size puts them at increased risk for medication dosing and dispensing errors, and their immature metabolic processes may lead to unexpected toxicity from pharmaceutical agents.

As toxicologists, we should encourage parents to provide as safe a home environment as possible to prevent unintentional ingestions, and we must encourage practitioners to exercise special vigilance when administering medications to children.

REFERENCES

1. American Academy of Pediatrics: Benzyl alcohol: Toxic agent in neonatal units. Pediatrics 1983;72:356–358.
2. American Academy of Pediatrics: Protect your child . . . prevent poisoning. *http://www.aap.org/family/poistipp.htm*
3. American College of Emergency Physicians: How to childproof your home. *http://www.acep.org/library/index.cfm/id/275.htm*
4. American College of Emergency Physicians: How to protect your child from poison. *http://www.acep.org/library/index.cfm/id/194.htm*
5. American Medical Association: PolicyFinder H-60.998: Ipecac as a household poison emetic. *http://www.ama-assn.org/apps/pf_online/ pf_online?f_n=browse&doc=policyfiles/HOD/H-60.998.HTM*
6. Amitai Y, Mitchell AA, McGuigan MA, Lovejoy FH: Ipecac-induced emesis and reduction of plasma concentrations of drugs following accidental overdose in children. Pediatrics 1987;80: 364–367.
7. Anonymous: Position statement and practice guidelines on the use of multi-dose activated charcoal in the treatment of acute poisoning. American Academy of Clinical Toxicology; European Association of Poisons Centres and Clinical Toxicologists. J Toxicol Clin Toxicol 1999;37:731–751.
8. Anyebuno MA, Rosenfeld CR: Chloral hydrate toxicity in a term infant. Dev Pharmacol Ther 1991;17:116–120.
9. Bamshad MJ, Wasserman GS: Pediatric clonidine intoxications. Vet Hum Toxicol 1990;32:220–223.
10. Baraff LJ, Guterman JJ, Bayer MJ: The relationship of poison center contact and injury in children 2 to 6 years old. Ann Emerg Med 1992;21:153–157.
11. Barazarte V, Rodriguez Z, Ceballos S, et al: Exchange transfusion in a case of severe theophylline poisoning. Vet Hum Toxicol 1992; 34:524.
12. Bateman DA, Heagarty MD: Passive freebase cocaine ("crack") inhalation by infants and toddlers. Am J Dis Child 1989;143:25–27.
13. Bays J: Child abuse by poisoning. In: Reece R, ed: Child Abuse: Medical Diagnosis and Management. Philadelphia, Lea & Febiger, 1994, pp. 69–106.
14. Bebeukelear MM, Batisky, DL, Melber SL: Acute hemodialysis in children. In: Henrich WL, ed: Principles and Practice of Dialysis, 2nd ed. Williams & Wilkins, 1999, pp. 534–548.
15. Belay ED, Bresee JS, Holman RC, Khan AS, Shahriari A, Schonberger LB: Reye's syndrome in the United States from 1981 through 1997. N Engl J Med 1999;340:1377–1382.
16. Berning CK, Griffith JF, Wild JE: Research on the effectiveness of denatonium benzoate as a deterrent to liquid detergent ingestion by children. Fund Appl Toxicol 1982;2:44–48.
17. Bithoney WG, Snyder J, Michalek J, Newberger EH: Childhood ingestions as symptoms of family distress. Am J Dis Child 1985; 139:456–459.
18. Block SM, Dansky R, Davis MD: Lomotil poisoning in children: Two case reports. S Afr Med J 1977;51:553–554.
19. Bools CN, Neale BA, Meadow SR: Münchausen syndrome by proxy: A study of psychopathology. Child Abuse Neglect 1994;18:773–788.
20. Bools CN, Neale BA, Meadow SR: Co-morbidity associated with fabricated illness (Münchausen syndrome by proxy). Arch Dis Child 1992;67:77–79.
21. Brayden RM, MacClean WE, Bonfiglio JF, Altemeier W: Behavioral antecedents of pediatric poisonings. Clin Pediatr 1993;32: 30–35.
22. Brown WJ, Buist NR, Cory-Gipson HT, et al: Fatal benzyl alcohol poisoning in a neonatal intensive care unit. Lancet 1982;1:1250.
23. Caldwell NA, Hughes DK: How to decrease errors in dose. J Pediatr 2000;137:142.
24. Campbell D, Oates RK: Childhood poisoning—A changing profile with scope for prevention. Med J Aust 1992;156:238–240.
25. Centers for Disease Control: Unintentional ingestions of prescription drugs in children under five years old. MMWR 1987;36:124–126.
26. Centers for Disease Control: Update: Childhood poisoning—United States. MMWR 1985;34:117–118.
27. Centers for Disease Control: Unintentional poisoning among young children—United States. MMWR 1983;32:529–531.
28. Chan TYK, Chan AYW, Pang CW: Epidemiology of poisoning in the new territories south of Hong Kong. Hum Exp Toxicol 1997;16: 204–207.
29. Chasnoff IA, Lewis DE, Squires L: Cocaine intoxication in a breast-fed infant. Pediatrics 1987;80:836–838.
30. Chavers BM, Kjellstrand CM, Wiegand C, et al: Techniques for use of charcoal hemoperfusion in infants: Experience in two patients. Kidney Int 1980;18:386–389.
31. Chyka PA, Seger D: Position statement: single-dose activated charcoal. American Academy of Clinical Toxicology; European Association of Poisons Centres and Clinical Toxicologists. J Toxicol Clin Toxicol 1997;35:721–741.
32. Clarke A, Walton WW: Effect of safety packaging on aspirin ingestion by children. Pediatrics 1979;63:687–693.
33. Craft AW: Circumstances surrounding deaths from accidental poisoning 1974–80. Arch Dis Child 1983;58:544–546.
34. Crockett R, Krishel SJ, Manoguerra A, Williams SR, Clark RF: Prehospital use of activated charcoal: a pilot study. J Emerg Med 1996; 14:335–338.
35. Cummins LH: Hypoglycemia and convulsions in children following alcohol ingestion. J Pediatr 1961;58:23–26.
36. Cutler EA, Barrett GA, Craven PW, Cramblett HG: Delayed cardiopulmonary arrest after Lomotil ingestion. Pediatrics 1980;65: 157–158.
37. Deeths TM, Breeden JT: Poisoning in children—A statistical study of 1,057 cases. J Pediatr 1971; 78:299–305.
38. Densen-Gerber J: The forensic pathology of drug-related child abuse. Leg Med Annu 1978;135–148.
39. Dine MS, McGovern ME: Intentional poisoning of children—An overlooked category of child abuse: Report of seven cases and review of the literature. Pediatrics 1982;70:32–35.
40. Done AK, Otterness LJ: Exchange transfusion in the treatment of oil of wintergreen (methyl salicylate) poisoning. J Pediatr 1956;18: 80–85.
41. Donckerwolcke RA, Bunchman TE: Hemodialysis in infants and small children. Pediatr Nephrol 1994;8:103–106.
42. Eriksson M, Larsson G, Winbladh B, Zetterstrom R: Accidental poisoning in pre-school children in the Stockholm area. Acta Paediatr Scand 1979;275(Suppl):96–101.
43. Fazen LE, Lovejoy FH, Crone RK: Acute poisoning in a children's hospital: A 2-year experience. Pediatrics 1986;77:144–151.
44. Ferguson J, Sellar C, Goldacre MJ: Some epidemiological observations on medicinal and non-medicinal poisoning in preschool children. J Epidemiol Commun Health 1992;46:207–210.
45. Flagler SL, Wright L: Recurrent poisoning in children: A review. J Pediatr Psych 1987;12:631–641.
46. Flomenbaum NE, Howland MAH, Weissman R: Pretty poison. Emerg Med 1986;4:69–84.

47. Gallagher SS, Finison K, Guyer B, Goodenough S: The incidence of injuries among 87000 Massachusetts children and adolescents: Results of the 1980–81 statewide childhood injury prevention program surveillance system. Am J Public Health 1984;74:1340–1347.

48. Gaudreault P, McCormick MA, Lacouture PG, Lovejoy FH: Poison exposures and use of ipecac in children less than 1 year old. Ann Emerg Med 1986;15:808–810.

49. Gershanik J, Boecler B, Ensley H, et al: The gasping syndrome and benzyl alcohol poisoning. N Engl J Med 1982; 307:1384–1388.

50. Goebel J, Gremse DA, Artman M: Cardiomyopathy from ipecac administration in Münchausen syndrome by proxy. Pediatrics 1993;92:601–603.

51. Gooch WM, Kennedy J, Banner W, McGuire HJ: Generalized arterial and venous thrombosis following intra-arterial paraldehyde. Clin Toxicol 1979;15:39–44.

52. Gray J, Bentovim A: Illness induction syndrome: I. A series of 41 children from 37 families identified at the Great Ormond Street Hospital for Children NHS Trust. Child Abuse Neglect 1996;20: 655–673.

53. Greenberg B, Weihl C, Hug G: Chlorpropamide poisoning. Pediatrics 1968;41:145–147.

54. Gupta S, Govil YC, Misra PK, Nath R, Srivastava KL: Trends in poisoning in children: experience at a large referral teaching hospital. Natl Med J India 1998;11:166–168.

55. Haddon W: Advances in the epidemiology of injuries as a basis for public policy. Pub Health Rep 1980;95:411–421.

56. Hamilton RJ, Goldfrank LR: Poison center data and the Pollyanna phenomenon. J Toxicol Clin Toxicol 1997;35:21–23.

57. Harchelroad F, Clark RF, Dean B, Krenzelok EP: Treated vs toxic exposures: discrepancies between a poison control center and a member hospital. Vet Hum Toxicol 1990;32:156–159.

58. Hiller JL, Benda GI, Rahatzad M, et al: Benzyl alcohol toxicity: Impact on mortality and intraventricular hemorrhage among very low birth weight infants. Pediatrics 1986;77:500–506.

59. Holt D, Harvey D, Hurley R: Chloramphenicol toxicity. Adverse Drug React Toxicol Rev 1993;12:83–95.

60. Hurwitz ES: Reye's syndrome. Epidemiol Rev 1989;11:249–253.

61. Jackson MH, Payne HA: Bittering agents: Their potential application in reducing ingestions of engine coolants and windshield wash. Vet Hum Toxicol 1995;37:323–326.

62. Jacobson BJ, Rock AR, Cohn MS, et al: Accidental ingestions of oral prescription drugs: A multicenter survey. Am J Public Health 1989;79:853–856.

63. Jardine DS, Rogers K: Relationships of benzyl alcohol to kernicterus, intraventricular hemorrhage, and mortality in preterm infants. Pediatrics 1989;83:153–160.

64. Jones J: The child accident repeater. Clin Pediatr 1980;19:284–288.

65. King WD, Palmisano PA: Ingestion of prescription drugs by children: An epidemiologic study. South Med J 1989;82:1468–1471.

66. Koren GK: Medications which can kill a toddler with one tablet or teaspoon. J Toxicol Clin Toxicol 1993;31:407–413.

67. Krug A, Ellis JB, Hay IY, et al: The impact of child-resistant containers on the incidence of parafin (kerosene) ingestion in children. S Afr Med J 1994;84:730–734.

68. Lamminpaa A, Vilska J, Hoppu K: Medical charcoal for a child's poisoning at home: Availability and success of administration in Finland. Hum Exp Toxicol 1993;12:29–32.

69. Leung AK: Ethyl alcohol ingestion in children. A 15-year review. Clin Pediatr 1986;25:617–619.

70. Liebelt EL, Shannon MW: Small doses, big problems: A selected review of highly toxic common medications. Pediatr Emerg Care 1993;9:292–297.

71. Linakis JG, Frederick KA: Poisoning deaths not reported to the regional poison control center. Ann Emerg Med 1993;22:1822–1828.

72. Litovitz TL, Flagler SL, Manoguerra AS, et al: Recurrent poisoning among pediatric poisoning victims. Med Toxicol Adverse Drug Exp 1989;4:381–386.

73. Litovitz TL, Klein-Schwartz W, Veltri JC, Manoguerra AS: Prescription drug ingestions in children: Whose drug? Vet Hum Toxicol 1986;28:14–15.

74. Litovitz T, Manoguerra A: Comparison of pediatric poisoning hazards: An analysis of 3.8 million exposure incidents. Pediatrics 1992;89:999–1006.

75. Mahieu LM, Rooman RP, Goosens E: Imidazoline intoxication in children. Eur J Pediatr 1993;152:944–946.

76. Manikian A, Stone S, Hamilton R, et al: Exchange transfusion as an alternative to hemodialysis in severe infant salicylism [abstract]. J Toxicol Clin Toxicol 1996;34:585.

77. Mauer SM, Chavers BM, Kjellstrand CM: Treatment of an infant with severe chloramphenicol intoxication using charcoal-column hemoperfusion. J Pediatr 1980;96:136–139.

78. McCarron MM, Challoner KR, Thompson GA: Diphenoxylate-atropine (Lomotil) overdose in children: An update (report of eight cases and review of the literature). Pediatrics 1991;87:694–700.

79. McGuire TL, Feldman KW: Psychologic morbidity of children subjected to Münchausen syndrome by proxy. Pediatrics 1989;83: 289–292.

80. Meadow R: Münchausen syndrome by proxy. Arch Dis Child 1982; 57:92–98.

81. Meadow R: Münchausen syndrome by proxy: The hinterland of child abuse. Lancet 1977;2:343–345.

82. Mehta A, Kasla RR, Bavdekar SB, Hathi GS, Joshi SY: Acute poisonings in children. J Ind Med Soc 1996;94:219–220.

83. Monto AS: The disappearance of Reye's syndrome: a public health triumph. N Engl J Med 1999;340:1423–1424.

84. National Safety Council: Accident Facts, 1996 Edition. Itasca, IL, National Safety Council, 1996.

85. Nelson LS, Gordon PE, Simmons MD, Goldberg WL, Howland MA, Hoffman RS: The benefit of house officer education on proper medication dose calculation and ordering. Acad Emerg Med 2000;7(11): 1311–1316.

86. Nevins TE, Mauer SM: Infant hemodialysis. In: Nissenson AR, Fine RN, eds: Dialysis Therapy, 2nd ed. Philadelphia, Hanley and Belfus, Inc, 1993, pp. 349–353.

87. Nordt SP, Manoguerra A, Williams SR, Clark RF: The availability of activated charcoal and ipecac for home use. Vet Hum Toxicol 1999;41:247–248.

88. Office of Analysis and Epidemiology, National Center for Health Statistics, Centers for Disease Control: Compressed Mortality File. *http://wonder.cdc.gov/*

89. Osborn HH, Henry G, Wax P, et al: Theophylline toxicity in a premature neonate—Elimination kinetics of exchange transfusion. J Toxicol Clin Toxicol 1993;31:639–644.

90. Polakoff JM, Lacouture PG, Lovejoy FH: The environment away from home as a source of potential poisoning. Am J Dis Child 1984; 138:1014–1017.

91. Quadrani DA, Spiller HA, Widder P: Five year retrospective evaluation of sulfonylurea ingestion in children. J Toxicol Clin Toxicol 1996;34:267–270.

92. Quang LS, Woolf AD: Past, present, and future role of ipecac syrup. Curr Opin Pediatr 2000;12:153–162.

93. Rice DP, MacKenzie EJ, Jones AS, et al: Cost of Injury in the United States: A Report to Congress. San Francisco, Institute for Health and Aging, University of California; and Injury Prevention Center, Johns Hopkins University, 1989.

94. Rodgers GB: The safety effects of child-resistant packaging for oral prescription drugs: two decades of experience. JAMA 1996;275: 1661–1665.

95. Rodger GC, Tenenbein M: The role of aversive bittering agents in the prevention of pediatric poisonings. Pediatrics 1994;93:68–69.

96. Rodgers GC, Baird J: Association between childhood poisoning and trauma and child abuse and neglect. Unpublished data cited in Bays J: Child abuse by poisoning. In: Reece R, ed: Child Abuse: Medical

Diagnosis and Management. Philadelphia, Lea & Febiger, 1994, pp. 69–106.

97. Rosenberg DA: Münchausen syndrome by proxy. In: Reece R, ed: Child Abuse: Medical Diagnosis and Management. Philadelphia, Lea & Febiger, 1994, pp. 266–278.

98. Rosenberg DA: Web of deceit: A literature review of Münchausen syndrome by proxy. Child Abuse Negl 1987; 11:547–563.

99. Rowe C. Koren T. Koren G: Errors by paediatric residents in calculating drug doses. Arch Dis Child 1998;79:56–58.

100. Shannon M, Wernovsky G, Morris C: Exchange transfusion in the treatment of severe theophylline poisoning. Pediatrics 1992;89: 145–147.

101. Shoemaker JD, Lynch RE, Hoffman JW, Sly WS: Misidentification of proprionic acid as ethylene glycol in a patient with methylmalonic acidemia. J Pediatr 1992;120:417–421.

102. Siebert JR, Frude N: Bittering agents in the prevention of accidental poisoning: children's reactions to denatonium benzoate (Bitrex). Arch Emerg Med 1991;8:1–7.

103. Siebert R: Stress in families of children who have ingested poisons. BMJ 1975;3:87–89.

104. Slagle MA, Chyka PA: Pharmacists use of safety caps on refilled prescriptions. Am Pharm 1994;NS34:37–40

105. Sobel R: The psychiatric implications of accidental poisoning in childhood. Pediatr Clin North Am 1970:17:653–685.

106. Sobel R: Traditional safety measures and accidental poisoning in childhood. Pediatrics 1969;44:811–816.

107. Solomon SL, Ford-Jones EL, Baker WM, et al: Medication errors with inhalant epinephrine mimicking an epidemic of neonatal sepsis. N Engl J Med 1984;310:166–170.

108. Tenenbein M: Pediatric toxicology: Current controversies and recent advances. Curr Probl Pediatr 1986;16:192–233.

109. Thomas SHL, Bevan L, Bhattacharyva, et al: Presentation of poisoned patients to accident and emergency departments in the north of England. Hum Exp Toxicol 1996;15:466–470.

110. Thompson JN: Corrosive esophageal injuries: A study of nine cases of concurrent accidental caustic ingestion. Laryngoscope 1987;97: 1060–1068.

111. Tolman IJ, Done GA: Hemodialysis of the neonate weighing less than 4 kg. ANNA J 1989;16:421–424.

112. Trinkoff AM, Baker SP: Poisoning hospitalizations and deaths from solids and liquids among children and teenagers. Am J Public Health 1986;76:657–660.

113. Viscusi WK: Consumer behavior and the safety effects of product safety regulation. J Law Econ 1985;28:527–554.

114. Vogel C, Caraccio T, Mofenson H, Hart S: Alcohol intoxication in young children. J Toxicol Clin Toxicol 1995;33:25–33.

115. Walton WW: An evaluation of the posion prevention packaging act. Pediatrics 1982; 69:363–370.

116. Wax PM, Cobaugh DJ: Prehospital gastrointestinal decontamination of toxic ingestions: a missed opportunity. Am J Emerg Med 1998; 16:114–116.

117. Weisman RS, Goldfrank LR: Poison center numbers. J Toxicol Clin Toxicol 1991;29:553–557.

118. Weissman DB, Jackson SH, Heicher DA, Rockoff MA: Benzyl alcohol administration in neonates. Anesth Analg 1990;70:673–674.

119. West L: Innovative approaches to the administration of activated charcoal in pediatric toxic ingestions. Pediatr Nurs 1997;23: 616–619.

120. Wiley JF, Wiley CC, Torrey SB, Henretig FM: Clonidine poisoning in young children. J Pediatr 1990:116:654–658.

121. Wiseman HM, Guest K, Murray VSG, et al: Accidental poisoning in childhood: A muticentre survey. 2. The role of packaging in accidents involving medications. Hum Toxicol 1987;6:303–314.

122. Woolf A, Wieler J, Greenes D: Costs of poison-related hospitalizations at an urban teaching hospital for children. Arch Pediatr Adolesc Med 1997;151:719–723.

123. Zuckerman BS, Duby JC: Developmental approach to injury prevention. Pediatr Clin North Am 1985;32:17–29.

Judith C. Ahronheim / Mary Ann Howland

The US population is aging steadily: Those older than 65 years of age comprise not only an increasing proportion of the population at large (12%) but an increasing proportion of patients seen in medical practices. Patients older than 65 years of age account for 43% of emergency department visits and 48% of all critical care admissions from emergency departments.[49]

Although the elderly account for only a small minority of toxicologic exposures, once exposed they have the highest mortality rate. For example, people aged 60 and older accounted for only 3.8% of toxicologic exposures in 1998 but for 23% of deaths (see Chap. 116 and p. 1752 for a complete review of poison center data).

There are several possible reasons for this vulnerability. First, there is a lack of recognition of drug toxicity in the elderly.[3] Because of pharmacokinetic and pharmacodynamic changes in late life, which are discussed later, a medication dose thought to be therapeutic may produce an unexpectedly serious effect. The presentation of toxicity may be atypical. Falls, a common presentation of disease in the elderly, may be the presenting sign of drug toxicity; if the patient is cognitively impaired and the fall is unwitnessed, the immediate consequences of the fall may be adequately addressed without recognizing its cause.[30,43,45] Drug overdose can also result in focal neurologic deficits that may be attributed solely to structural cerebrovascular or cardiovascular disease, without identifying the toxicologic etiology.[54] The drugs most commonly responsible for toxicity in the elderly are listed in Table 107–1.

The presentation of drug toxicity may be delayed in the elderly. Drugs with a long half-life may not reach a steady state and hence achieve peak action until many days after the prescription is written and the drug therapy is initiated. In one case, a 78-year-old woman received a prescription for the hypnotic flurazepam (Dalmane). She experienced no apparent adverse effects initially, but after taking the drug nightly for a week, she developed slurred speech and weakness, which resolved within a few days of stopping the drug. In some older patients, the active metabolite of flurazepam, desalkylflurazepam, has a half-life of up to 100 hours or longer, which requires days to achieve a steady state. When peak effects are delayed in this way drug toxicity can easily be mistaken for non-drug-related illness.

SUICIDE AND INTENTIONAL POISONINGS

The risk of suicide by all methods increases steadily with age, particularly among white men.[38,42] Although data for individual ethnic groups are sparse, white men have a substantially higher risk of suicide than their same-age cohorts among the African Ameri-

can population.[38,41,42] Death by suicide is more common among men than among women, but women are responsible for more suicide attempts. The male-to-female ratio of suicide attempts narrows with increasing age, so that in the oldest age groups men attempt suicide slightly more often than women, when all methods of attempted suicide are considered[21] (Chap. 114).

Although firearms are the most frequent means of death by suicide and far outpace suicides by drug overdose among men over 65 (73% vs 3%), among women drug overdose is nearly as frequent a cause of death as firearms, each accounting for about 25% of successful suicides. When death by inhalation is included, poison exposure surpasses gunshot wounds as a cause of death among elderly women.[38] Drug overdose is commonly utilized in suicide attempts by the elderly of both sexes.[21]

Within the elderly group, the pattern of medications responsible for suicidal deaths may be changing, as safer serotonin reuptake inhibitors (SSRIs) are increasingly prescribed for depression instead of tricyclic antidepressants (TCAs) which are more likely to be lethal in overdose.[10] In Sweden, the relative fatality ratio for benzodiazepines was reported to be correspondingly increasing. Overdose of benzodiazepines is rarely fatal unless it is accompanied by alcohol or another toxic ingestion or occurs in the presence of serious medical problems. However, when all deaths from benzodiazepines are examined, they probably occur more often in older adults.[16]

UNINTENTIONAL POISONING AND ADVERSE DRUG EVENTS

It is difficult to distinguish poisoning from adverse drug events (ADEs) in the geriatric population. Compared to younger adults, the elderly are at increased risk of unintentional poisoning as well as other drug events. An ADE is defined as "an injury resulting from medical intervention related to a drug."[5] This definition encompasses events that result from both inappropriate use of medications, such as a prescribing error, and from appropriate use. Life-threatening reactions may occur with therapeutic doses; examples include the serotonin syndrome and the neuroleptic malignant syndrome. The serotonin syndrome occurs most commonly when two or more drugs that increase serotonin activity are used concurrently.[32] The elderly are at enhanced risk of drug interactions because of the increased numbers of medications used simultaneously.[58]

The serotonin syndrome and neuroleptic malignant syndrome are relatively unpredictable and may occur at all ages. However, other severe ADEs are more likely to occur among the elderly and

TABLE 107–1. Drugs Most Commonly Responsible for Toxicity in the Elderly[a]

Analgesics
    Acetaminophen
    Opioids
    Salicylates and other NSAIDs
Anticholinergics
Anticoagulants
Antidepressants
Antipsychotics
Cardiovascular medications
    β-Adrenergic antagonists
    Calcium channel blockers
    Digoxin
Magnesium-containing antacids/laxatives
Sedative-hypnotics
Theophylline

[a]Polypharmacy increases toxicity as a result of diverse drug–drug interactions.

are potentially avoidable if patients are carefully monitored. Examples include severe bleeding as a result of nonsteroidal anti-inflammatory agents (NSAID gastropathy), metformin-induced lactic acidosis, and prolonged hypoglycemia from sulfonylureas.[39,52,53]

Although reported poisoning exposures among the elderly are much less frequent than among other age groups, the incidence of ADEs increases steadily with age.[7,34] Moreover, when they occur, they are more likely to be serious. Serious ADEs are defined as those resulting in death, hospitalization, prolongation of hospitalization, or permanent or serious disability and are most prevalent among people 85 years of age and older.[7]

PHARMACOKINETIC FACTORS

Age-related pharmacokinetic changes occur in the elderly. The most important and consistent pharmacokinetic change that occurs with aging is a decrease in renal function. Glomerular filtration rate (GFR) declines, on the average, by 50% between the ages of 30 and 80 years.[14,48] The GFR cannot be accurately predicted by serum creatinine because muscle mass, the source of serum creatinine, declines with age, and therefore in late life, serum creatinine may not be elevated even when the GFR is significantly impaired.

Because it is impractical and often difficult to measure 24-hour creatinine clearance before instituting therapy with a needed, renally excreted drug, clinicians commonly estimate creatinine clearance using age-adjusted formulas or nomograms. The frequently applied Cockcroft-Gault formula, derived from clinical experience in hospitalized patients, is fairly predictive of renal function when renal function is stable.[11] However, age-related declines in GFR are not universal, and data from longitudinal studies suggest that as many as one-third of the elderly do not experience this age-related decline.[36] Moreover, predictive formulas could overestimate actual creatinine clearance in chronically ill, debilitated elderly by as much as 20%.[17] For all of these reasons, it is difficult to accurately predict the renal elimination of drugs or drug metabolites in the elderly. A practical solution is to assume that renal function has declined and to exercise particular caution when prescribing maintenance doses of drugs with a narrow thera-

peutic-to-toxic ratio (Table 107–2). Failure to do so is an important cause of toxicity.[35]

With advancing age, there are changes in hepatic function as well. Liver mass decreases with an associated decrease in hepatic blood flow,[61] which results in decreased efficiency of drug removal by hepatic extraction. Enzymatic processes are often unpredictable,[29] and there is considerable controversy over the extent to which advanced age alters the ability of drugs to undergo hepatic metabolism, particularly oxidative processes.[51] Hepatic conjugation does not decline significantly with age, so drugs such as temazepam and oxazepam that are metabolized by these processes do not have a prolonged elimination half-life. In contrast, because hepatic oxidative enzyme activity may decline, drugs such as diazepam and flurazepam that are metabolized by that system are eliminated more slowly.[24] Recognition and study of subfamilies and subtypes of cytochrome P450 enzymes have revealed that activity of some isoenzymes declines with age, whereas that of others does not.

Unlike conjugated metabolites, which tend to be inactive, products of oxidative metabolism are often active. Because these active metabolites are generally excreted by the kidney, the presence of active drug may be markedly prolonged, as demonstrated by the patient who developed flurazepam toxicity a week after beginning the drug. Other changes in enzyme systems may occur in late life. For example, a decline in gastric alcohol dehydrogenase leads to increased peak effect of ethanol in the elderly.[46] Decline in this enzyme is attributed to the increased incidence of gastric atrophy with age. Whether age-related changes occur in metabolic enzymes that are present in many organ systems, such as intestine, brain, and kidney, and what impact such changes have on drug disposition, are likely to become active areas of research.

Because age-related alterations in enzyme activity are not associated with any clinical signs or easily recognized laboratory abnormalities, it is impossible to predict a particular patient's ability to eliminate a hepatically metabolized drug. The following factors contribute to this inability to predict metabolism: the age-indepen-

TABLE 107–2. Drugs with Narrow Therapeutic-to-toxic Ratio and Potential for Accumulation in the Presence of Diminished Renal Function

Antimicrobial agents
    Aminoglycosides
    Imipenem
    Pyrazinamide
    Vancomycin
Benzodiazepines with active metabolites
    Chlordiazepoxide
    Clorazepate
    Diazepam
    Flurazepam
    Halazepam
Digoxin
Lithium
Meperidine (active metabolite is normeperidine)
Metformin
Procainamide (active metabolite N-acetyl procainamide)
Salicylates
Sulfonylureas with active metabolites
    Chlorpropamide
    Acetohexamide

dent genetic variability in hepatic metabolism, the ability of microsomal oxidative enzymes to be induced or inhibited by many exogenous substances, and the possibility that advanced age may affect the inducibility or inhibition of one or more enzymes in this system. Comorbidities and coadministered drugs are additional complicating factors. Because of these uncertainties, caution must be paid to particular drugs such as those shown in Table 107–3.

Age-related alterations in body composition can affect drug disposition in later life (see Table 107–4). For example, lean muscle mass declines and the fat-to-lean ratio increases with advancing age.[44] Thus, highly lipid-soluble drugs tend to have an increased volume of distribution (Vd). As a result, there may be a delay before steady state is reached, and peak effect and toxicity may occur later than expected. This mechanism may be an additional reason drugs such as diazepam and flurazepam have prolonged half-lives in otherwise healthy elderly patients. In contrast to lipid-soluble drugs, hydrophilic substances, such as ethanol, have a smaller Vd; this may account in part for the more rapid and more pronounced peak effect of ethanol in the elderly.

Protein synthesis declines with age.[47] Although serum albumin remains in the normal range in the healthy elderly,[9] patients in this age group are probably more likely to experience a rapid decrease in albumin levels when there is acute or chronic illness or when protein intake does not keep up with demand.[62] A decline in serum protein increases the free or active fraction of drugs that are otherwise highly protein-bound. Free drug is able to travel more readily to the liver and kidney for metabolism or excretion, so a gradual change in the serum protein level is unlikely to lead to a change in the patient's response to the drug. However, these changes may be clinically important for interpreting serum levels of highly bound drugs. Clinical laboratories typically measure total (free plus bound) levels of drug. Because most drug is bound, the reported value reflects mostly bound drug. Thus, the total drug concentration may be in the therapeutic range even though the unbound fraction (which is responsible for drug action) is elevated. Phenytoin, which is highly bound to albumin, serves as an illustrative example. If the serum level of phenytoin is reported as subtherapeutic, the physician might order a dose increase even though the free fraction of phenytoin actually is in the therapeutic range. With a dose increase, the free or active fraction of the drug may increase to toxic levels.

Basic drugs are not bound to albumin but to α_1-acid glycoprotein (AAG), an acute-phase reactant that tends to increase rather than decrease with age.[1] However, the increase attributed to age is most likely related to underlying disease. These unpredictable changes would be expected to have the reverse effect on the ratio of bound to unbound drug in any laboratory report.[55] The correlation between clinical effect and free drug levels requires further study because there may be complex factors involved, including alterations in Vd and specific tissue concentrations.

The contribution of gastrointestinal absorption to drug toxicity is unknown. Absorption declines modestly, if at all, with advancing age. However, age-related changes in the gastric mucosa may account for enzymatic changes, as demonstrated in the case of alcohol dehydrogenase, noted above.

PHARMACODYNAMIC FACTORS

Pharmacodynamic factors may also affect a patient's response to a particular drug. In general, age-related physiologic changes in target or nontarget organs lead to increased sensitivity to a given drug, although sensitivity to some drugs may also be decreased. For example, there is evidence that β-adrenergic receptor sensitivity declines with aging, leading to a diminished response to both β-adrenergic agonists and antagonists.[12,59] However, it is likely that most elderly respond normally to drugs of this category[20] in terms of therapeutic response, adverse effects, and toxicity.

The observation of enhanced sensitivity to drugs[25] is probably related to altered pharmacokinetics in many, if not most, cases. Proving that enhanced sensitivity is related to altered pharmacodynamics would require demonstrating that the concentration of drug at the tissue site was not increased as the result of diminished elimination.[18] However, regardless of the mechanism, it is important for practical purposes to recognize that the response to a given drug might be altered in specific ways among the elderly. These altered responses are probably caused less by chronologic aging and more by an increased prevalence of disease in an aged population.[25] Examples of pathophysiologic changes frequently seen among the elderly that are unmasked by medications are given in Table 107–5.

RISK FACTORS FOR ADVERSE EVENTS

The likelihood of experiencing an ADE increases with the increasing number of drugs prescribed for a patient.[37] Geriatric patients take more prescription and nonprescription drugs than any patient group.[7] A complicated drug regimen reduces adherence, increases medication errors, and increases the risk of clinically important drug interactions. Among hospitalized patients, approximately 7% of adverse drug reactions occur as a consequence of drug–drug interactions; and in a chronic disease hospital, as many as 22% are reportedly caused by these interactions.[6]

Concurrent disease in target or nontarget organs may also alter the patient's sensitivity to a drug,[27] resulting in a serious ADE even when the patient is given a standard or previously used dose of the drug. Coexistent disease is often subclinical, and the patient's enhanced sensitivity may not be anticipated. A patient with subclinical Alzheimer disease whose cognitive function is overtly normal may acutely develop delirium or symptoms of dementia when given drugs that do not ordinarily have this effect. Delirium

TABLE 107–3.   Drugs Whose Bioaccumulation is Dependent on Hepatic Function[a]

High Extraction	Oxidation
Imipramine	Chlordiazepoxide
Labetalol	Diazepam
Lidocaine	Quinidine
Meperidine	Theophylline
Metoprolol	Thioridazine
Morphine	Triazolam
Nifedipine	
Nortriptyline	
Propoxyphene	
Propranolol	
Verapamil	

[a]Drugs with a high hepatic extraction will have increased serum levels when hepatic perfusion decreases; bioaccumulation also occurs when hepatic oxidative functions deteriorate.

TABLE 107–4. Special Pharmacokinetic Considerations in the Elderly

	Young	Elderly	Consideration
Fat (% of body weight)	15	30 (↑)	↑ V_d for drugs distributing to fat (diazepam, amitriptyline, lidocaine)
Intracellular water (% body weight)	42	30 (↓)	↓ V_d for water-soluble drugs
Muscle (% of body weight)	17	12 (↓)	↓ V_d for drugs distributing into lean tissue (digoxin, acetaminophen, caffeine, ethanol)
Albumin (g/dL)	4	↓ With acute or chronic illness	↑ Free levels of drugs >90% bound to albumin, especially in overdose; interpretation of serum concentration altered
α-Acid glycoprotein	Normal	↑ With acute or chronic illness	Affects distribution of basic drugs
Liver	Normal	↓ Size ↓ Hepatic blood flow ↓ In oxidation (phase 1 reactions)	Liver enzymes not predictive; drugs with high extraction (propranolol, triazolam) may increase; drug accumulation (diazepam)
Kidney	Normal	↓ GFR ↓ Renal blood flow ↓ Tubular secretion	Accumulation (lithium, aminoglycosides, N-acetyl procainamide, ACE inhibitors, cimetidine)

Modified, with permission, from Mayersohn M: Special pharmacokinetic considerations in the elderly. In: Evans WE, Schentag JJ, Justo WJ, eds: Applied Pharmacokinetics Principles of Therapeutic Drug Monitoring 3rd ed. Vancouver, Applied Therapeutics, 1992, pp. 1–43; and Fox FJ, Auestad A: Geriatric emergency clinical pharmacology. Emerg Med Clin North Am 1990;8:221–239.

is a medical emergency and an important cause of emergency department visits among the elderly.[27]

Another contributing factor is physician lack of knowledge about principles of geriatric therapeutics.[19] In one recent series of hospitalized patients, failure to consider advanced age was the most common factor associated with clinically important prescribing errors, and inattention to abnormal renal function was the second most important.[35] Inattention to risk factors can lead to significant morbidity or mortality—for example, metformin, a biguanide oral hypoglycemic agent, may produce life-threatening lactic acidosis in the presence of renal insufficiency.[28] Compounding the problem of lack of knowledge is the fact that new drugs are often inadequately studied in the elderly[50,57] (see Chap. 117 for further details). Reactions occurring in a small percentage of patients in a special subgroup can easily be missed during the initial investigations. Even when a substantial number of subjects older than 60 years are studied, much smaller proportions of patients older than 70 may be included in clinical trials.[2] Thus, the adults at highest risk for many forms of drug toxicity are those least often studied. Subjects undergoing drug testing are generally young adults and disease-free, so pharmacokinetic profiles do not reflect patterns of drug disposition that are characteristic of geriatric patients. Pharmacokinetic testing may be limited to a one-time dose, and frequently the evaluation takes place over a short period of time. On the average, approximately five half-lives of a drug are necessary to achieve steady-state drug levels. Therefore, a drug with a half-life of 24 hours may not reach a steady state for 5 days, and in the presence of prolonged elimination associated with age-related factors, a steady state may not be reached for substantially longer. As a result, even if the elderly are included in a drug trial, the ultimate effect of that drug might not be noted during testing intervals that are frequently designed for a younger population.

Morbidity and mortality occurring in elderly patients as a result of specific drugs might be avoided if the responsible drugs were studied under the predictably high-risk conditions typically present in the elderly. For example, benoxaprofen, a long-acting nonsteroidal antiinflammatory agent, was responsible for several elderly patient deaths from cholestatic jaundice. The jaundice and other serious dose-related toxicities from the drug were recognized only belatedly. Another example is the antibiotic temafloxacin. Temafloxacin was available for only 3 months before it was withdrawn following three reported deaths and more than 300 cases of

TABLE 107–5. Pathophysiologic Disorders Exacerbated by Drugs in the Elderly

Disorder	Drug	Possible Outcome
ADH secretion (increased)	Chlorpropamide; many others	Hyponatremia
Androgenic hormones (male) decreased	Digoxin; spironolactone	Gynecomastia
Baroreceptor dysfunction, venous insufficiency	Diuretics; cyclic antidepressants; methyldopa	Orthostatic hypotension
Bladder dysfunction	Diuretics	Incontinence
Dementia	Many	Confusion
Gastritis (atrophic)	NSAIDs, salicylates	Gastric hemorrhage
Immobility; cathartic bowel	Anticholinergics, opioids	Constipation
Nodal disease (sinus or AV)	Digoxin; verapamil; diltiazem; β-adrenergic antagonists	Bradycardia
Parkinson disease	Metoclopramide; antipsychotics	Parkinsonian symptoms
Prostatic hyperplasia	Anticholinergics; tricyclic antidepressants, disopyramide	Urinary retention
Thermoregulation	Phenothiazines	Hypo- or hyperthermia
Venous insufficiency	Dihydropyridine-type calcium channel blockers	Edema

Modified, with permission, from Ahronheim JC: Handbook of Prescribing Medications for Geriatric Patients. Boston, Little, Brown, 1992, p. 3.

hypoglycemia, many of which occurred in elderly patients with diminished renal function. Other adverse effects noted with this drug included hemolytic anemia and hypersensitivity reactions associated with respiratory distress.

If pharmacokinetic studies identify vulnerable subgroups, safe maximum doses could be recommended for specific populations at risk, theoretically limiting the risk for these individuals.[4] As a result of these problems, the Food and Drug Administration (FDA) now requires sponsors of new drug applications to present effectiveness and safety data for important demographic subgroups, including the elderly, in their FDA submission data.[15]

Drugs involved in serious drug interactions such as digoxin, warfarin, and diuretics are commonly prescribed in the elderly population. This situation is complicated by the fact that elderly patients often have multisystem disease and may visit several physicians, who prescribe medications without specific knowledge of, or attention to, the remainder of the patient's drug regimen, thereby increasing the risk of inappropriate drug combinations.[56] For example, a urologist prescribed trimethoprim-sulfamethoxazole for a patient receiving warfarin, which had previously been prescribed by her internist; this produced a drug–drug interaction that increased warfarin sensitivity and led to a life-threatening intestinal hemorrhage. In another case, an ophthalmologist prescribed acetazolamide for a patient taking hydrochlorothiazide that had previously been prescribed by her primary care physician for systemic hypertension, with a resultant drug–drug interaction consisting of hypokalemia, weakness, falling, and injury.

Herbal preparations also may interact with prescription medications.[22,40] The use of herbal preparations has increased substantially in recent years, particularly among patients with illnesses that afflict the elderly such as cancer and depression. Very few patients voluntarily report use of these or other nonprescribed therapies to their physicians, and too often the physician fails to inquire specifically about such "alternative" or "complementary" therapies. Drug interactions involving herbals also occur with nonprescription preparations such as dextromethorphan, a common component of cough medicine, and St. John's wort (hypericum), a heavily promoted herbal remedy for depression.[33] Combinations of herbals and SSRIs have been reported to cause serotonin syndrome.[8,22] Poisonings and other problems related to herbal preparations are discussed further in Chapter 77.

The use of nonprescription pharmaceuticals may cause further problems. For example, excessive use of magnesium-containing preparations may cause severe toxicity, often in older individuals. Impaired renal clearance or gastrointestinal motility, and medical comorbidities are just three risk factors that potentiate magnesium toxicity in the elderly. The source of magnesium in these cases may include the cathartics magnesium hydroxide ("milk of magnesia") and magnesium citrate, antacid preparations, and magnesium sulfate (Epsom salts).[23]

Outdated and discontinued drugs are an additional problem for the elderly who often retain products in their homes for decades. In one case, a suicidal 70-year-old woman presented to the emergency department with abdominal cramps, melena, and hematemesis several hours after ingesting purple oblong tablets. These tablets contained mercuric chloride, a topical antiseptic last used commonly over 50 years ago. In other cases, patients continue to obtain prescriptions for the same drug year after year. One example is meprobamate, a sedative-hypnotic that is still widely available but far less often prescribed today than the benzodiazepines. Unlike benzodiazepines, meprobamate manifests signifi-

cant drug interactions and has a narrower therapeutic-to-toxic ratio. Patients may be unwilling to change, or the physician may continue to renew the prescription without sufficiently reevaluating the patient. One 90-year-old woman who presented with heart block had been taking digoxin 0.25 mg daily for many years without a clear indication. Although her BUN and creatinine were normal, her digoxin level was elevated. A dose that might have been appropriate previously had become excessive for her current ability to eliminate the drug. Advancing unappreciated cardiac disease may have made her more sensitive to the drug as well.

Other age-related factors may increase the risk of unintentional poisonings in geriatric patients: impaired vision, hearing, and memory may lead to misunderstanding or the inability to follow directions concerning the use of prescription and nonprescription drugs. Dementia is an important risk factor in unintentional poisonings. In addition to cognitive impairment, patients with dementia sometimes exhibit abnormal feeding behaviors, including ingestion of inappropriate substances. In one case, a 74-year-old woman with Alzheimer disease ingested a glassful of ceramic glaze during an art class in the nursing home where she lived. That substance contained 30% lead oxide, a soluble lead salt that resulted in an acute lead level of 80 mg/dL. In a published case,[60] an 88-year-old woman with dementia ingested 10 ounces of a cleaning solution containing pine oil and isopropyl alcohol (Pine-Sol) that had been left unattended during house cleaning. The patient developed a depressed level of consciousness and respiratory compromise. Although unintentional toxin ingestion is rarely fatal, in this case the ingestion of the reportedly pleasant tasting pine oil eventually led to cardiorespiratory complications and this patient's death.[60]

In another case, an 88-year-old man with dementia developed deep stupor from ingestion of medications belonging to his daughter, with whom he lived. The daughter had a chronic pain syndrome and was using a variety of medications including a long-acting morphine preparation (Oramorph SR 60 mg) and diazepam (Valium 10 mg). The patient had a tendency to wander and put food as well as nonfood substances in his mouth and had ingested some of these medications during his unsupervised wandering.

TOXICOLOGIC MANAGEMENT CONSIDERATIONS FOR THE GERIATRIC PATIENT

Management decisions must be made with the foregoing principles in mind. Gastrointestinal decontamination should proceed as in younger patients. Because constipation is a more frequent problem in the elderly, when multiple-dose activated charcoal is indicated, particular attention must be paid to gastrointestinal function and motility. Cathartics or whole-bowel irrigation may be more frequently indicated in this patient population to prevent concretions or desorption. The specific precautions and contraindications in the basic management of gastrointestinal decontamination detailed in Chapter 31 are particularly pertinent for the geriatric population.

The presence of clinical or subclinical heart failure or renal failure may increase the risk of fluid overload when sodium bicarbonate is used. In the elderly, hemodialysis or hemoperfusion may be indicated earlier in cases of lithium or theophylline poisoning, where elimination may be hampered by a decreased creatinine clearance or reduced endogenous clearance, respectively.

A problem that may go unrecognized in geriatric patients is the development of drug withdrawal symptoms. Because elderly patients are typically not perceived as drug abusers, the physician may not be aware of the chronic use of prescribed benzodiazepines or opioid analgesics and consequently might fail to consider the possibility of drug withdrawal when unanticipated complications occur during the hospitalization. When a patient's general condition appears to be improving but then unexpectedly deteriorates, the individual should always be evaluated for the possibility of sedative-hypnotic or opioid withdrawal and managed accordingly.

Strategies to limit unintentional toxic exposures in elderly patients with cognitive or sensory impairment should be similar to those employed in young children, who are at high risk for ingesting toxic substances or pharmaceuticals prescribed for others in the household. The strategies should include the removal of potentially dangerous substances and unnecessary drugs from the elderly patient's environment. The physician should request that the patient or caregiver bring all medications to the office and then limit the number of pills dispensed. It may be necessary to limit medications such as antidepressants to a one-week supply or to choose alternative medications with a better therapeutic ratio. Administration and control of the medications may of necessity become the responsibility of the caregiver rather than the patient.

ADMISSION CRITERIA

When geriatric patients are evaluated in the emergency department for poisonings or serious ADEs, the need for hospital admission should be guided by concerns about the patient's frailty weighed carefully against the known hazards of hospitalization for the elderly.[13]

The physician should be particularly alert to certain situations that might mandate admission: elder abuse or neglect, unresolved acute mental status change, inadequate home care, unexplained falls or overdose of medications with prolonged durations of action.

When there is concern that the established caregivers at home are abusing the patient, the patient will require further observation, removal from the environment, and hospitalization, if necessary. Signs of actual physical abuse may be more obvious than signs of neglect.[31] Vulnerable elderly who are physically disabled or cognitively impaired may be brought to the hospital because of presumed illness, but the source of the problem may actually be the caregiver. The caregiver, frequently a family member, may be depleting the patient's funds for personal use, which may include the purchase of illicit drugs. Patients may become ill because funds were diverted from the purchase of food or because the patient's prescription drugs were sold on the street. More direct abuse may take the form of intentional poisoning of the patient by overdose of the patient's own prescription drugs.

Unresolved acute mental status change may require close observation and hospitalization. Elderly patients who are confused or unable to walk are sometimes mistakenly assumed to be chronically impaired. However, incomplete explanation of an altered mental status or physical impairment should prompt careful inquiry into the patient's baseline functional status. Functional deterioration should not be assumed to be age related. Many very

elderly patients are cognitively normal, physically robust, and independent in all activities of daily living. Inability to walk or the manifestation of pain on weight bearing, especially when pain is in the hip, in the presence of a negative radiograph may suggest that there is an occult fracture that will be revealed only with a bone scan or MRI.

Overdose with long-acting agents requires careful monitoring. Because duration of action of certain drugs may be markedly prolonged among geriatric patients, a higher degree of vigilance is required. A classic example is associated with the use of the sulfonylurea chlorpropamide, which has a half-life of 24 to 72 hours or more and can cause protracted hypoglycemia. Hypoglycemia leading to serious morbidity or death is an important drug-related problem among the elderly and occurs with virtually all sulfonylurea agents,[52] although the duration of hypoglycemia may vary.

SUMMARY

Older patients may account for only a small fraction of poisoning victims, but when poisoned, they have the highest mortality rate. More importantly, the elderly are much more likely to experience serious adverse drug events as a consequence of appropriate or inappropriate use of medications. Attention to risk factors is essential in this vulnerable population. Important risk factors include pharmacokinetic and pharmacodynamic changes; the presence of overt or subclinical disease, including dementia; patient and physician error; suicide risk; complex therapeutic drug regimens; and a general lack of knowledge about the principles of geriatric prescribing.

REFERENCES

1. Abernethy DR, Kerzner L: Age effects on alpha-1-acid glycoprotein concentration and imipramine plasma protein binding. J Am Geriatr Soc 1984;32:705–708.
2. Abrams WB: Food and Drug Administration (FDA) guidelines for the study of drugs in elderly patients: An industry perspective. In: Inclusion of Elderly Individuals in Clinical Trials: Cardiovascular Disease and Cardiovascular Therapy as a Model. Kansas City, Marion Merrell Dow, 1993, pp. 213–217.
3. Anderson R, Potts D, Gabow P, et al: Unrecognized adult salicylate intoxication. Ann Intern Med 1976;85:745–748.
4. Bateman DN, Chaplin S: Adverse reactions. BMJ 1988;2 96:761–764.
5. Bates DW, Cullen DJ, Laird N: Incidence of adverse drug events and potential adverse drug events. Implications for prevention. JAMA 1995;274:29–34.
6. Boston Collaborative Drug Surveillance Program: Adverse drug interactions. JAMA 1972;220:1238–1239.
7. Burke LB, Jolson H. Goetsch R, et al: Geriatric drug use and adverse drug event reporting in 1990: A descriptive analysis of the two national data bases. Annu Rev Gerontol Geriatr 1992;12:1–28.
8. Callaway JC, Grob CS: Ayahuasca preparations and serotonin reuptake inhibitors: A potential combination for severe adverse interactions. J Psychoactive Drugs 1998;30:367–369.
9. Campion EW, deLabry LO, Glynn RJ: The effect of age on serum albumin in healthy males: Report from the normative aging study. J Gerontol 1988;43:M18–M20.
10. Carlsten A, Waern M, Allebeck P: Suicides by drug poisoning among the elderly in Sweden 1969–1996. Soc Psychiatry Psychiatr Epidemiol 1999;34:609–614.

11. Cockcroft DW, Gault M: Prediction of creatinine clearance from serum creatinine. Nephron 1976;16:31–41.

12. Connolly MJ, Crowley JJ, Charan NB, et al: Impaired bronchodilator response to albuterol in healthy elderly men and women. Chest 1995;108:401–406.

13. Creditor MC: Hazards of hospitalization of the elderly. Ann Intern Med 1993;118:219–223.

14. Davies DF, Shock NW: Age changes in glomerular filtration rate: Effective renal plasma flow and tubular excretory capacity in adult males. J Clin Invest 1950;29:496–507.

15. Department of Health and Human Services, Food and Drug Administration: Investigational new drug applications and new drug applications. Federal Register 1998;63:6854–6862.

16. Drummer OH, Ranson DL: Sudden death and benzodiazepines. Am J Forensic Med Pathol 1996;17:336–342.

17. Drusano GL, Muncie HL, Hoopes JM, et al: Commonly used methods of estimating creatinine clearance are inadequate for elderly debilitated nursing home patients. J Am Geriatr Soc 1988;36:437–441.

18. Feely J, Coakley D: Altered pharmacodynamics in the elderly. Clin Geriatr Med 1990;6:269–283.

19. Ferry ME, Lamy PP, Becker LA: Physicians' lack of knowledge of prescribing for the elderly: A study in primary care physicians in Pennsylvania. J Am Geriatr Soc 1985;33:616–625.

20. Fitzergald JD: Age-related effects of beta blockers and hypertension. J Cardiovasc Pharmacol 1988;12:S83–S92.

21. Frierson RL: Suicide attempts by the old and the very old. Arch Intern Med 1991;151:141–144.

22. Fugh-Berman A: Herb–drug interactions. Lancet 2000;355:134–138.

23. Fung MC, Weintraub M, Bowen DL: Hypermagnesemia: Elderly over-the-counter drug users at risk. Arch Family Med 1995;4:718–723.

24. Greenblatt DJ, Divoll M, Harmatz JS, et al: Kinetics and clinical effects of flurazepam in young and elderly noninsomniacs. Clin Pharmacol Ther 1981;30:475–486.

25. Gurwitz JH, Avorn J: The ambiguous relation between aging and adverse drug reactions. Ann Intern Med 1991;114:956–966.

26. Hall RCW, Platt DE, Hall RC: Suicide risk assessment: A review of risk factors for suicide in 100 patients who made severe suicide attempts. Psychosomatics 1999;40:18–27.

27. Johnson J: Delirium in the elderly. Emerg Med Clin North Am 1990;8:255–265.

28. Jurovich MR, Wooldridge JD, Force RW: Metformin-associated non-ketotic metabolic acidosis. Ann Pharmacother 1997;31:53–55.

29. Kinirons MT, Crome P: Clinical pharmacokinetics considerations in the elderly. An update. Clin Pharmacokinet 1997;33:302–312.

30. Kruse W: Problems and pitfalls in the use of benzodiazepines in the elderly. Drug Saf 1990;5:328–344.

31. Lachs M, Pillemer K: Abuse and neglect of elderly persons. N Engl J Med 1995;332:437–443.

32. Lane R, Baldwin D: Selective serotonin reuptake inhibitor-induced serotonin syndrome: A review. J Clin Psychopharmacol 1977;17:208–221.

33. Lanz MS, Buchalter E, Giambanco V: St. John's wort and antidepressant drug interactions in the elderly. J Geriatr Psychiatr Neurol 1999;12:7–10.

34. Leape LL, Brennan TA, Laird N, et al: The nature of adverse events in hospitalized patients. Results of the Harvard medical practice study II. N Engl J Med 1991;324:377–384.

35. Lesar TS, Briceland L, Stein DS: Factors related to errors in medication prescribing. JAMA 1997;277:312–317.

36. Lindeman R, Tobin J, Shock NW: Longitudinal studies on the rate of decline in renal function with age. J Am Geriatr Soc 1985;33:278–285.

37. May FE, Stewart RB, Cluff LE: Drug interactions and multiple drug administration. Clin Pharmacol Ther 1977;22:322–328.

38. Meehan PJ, Saltzman LE, Sattini RW: Suicides among older United States residents: Epidemiologic characteristics and trends. Am J Public Health 1991;81:1198–1200.

39. Meneilly GS, Cheung E, Tuokko H: Counterregulatory hormone responses to hypoglycemia in the elderly patient with diabetes. Diabetes 1994;43:403–410.

40. Miller LG: Herbal medicinals. Selected clinical considerations focusing on known or potential drug–herb interactions. Arch Intern Med 1998;158:2200–2211.

41. Monk M: Epidemiology of suicide. Epidemiol Rev 1987;9:51–59.

42. National Center for Health Statistics: Death rates for 72 selected causes, by 5-year age groups, race and sex. United States, 1994. Hyattsville, MD: Public Health Service, 1996.

43. Nelson R, Amin M: Falls in the elderly 1990. Emerg Med Clin North Am 1990;8:309–324.

44. Novak LP: Aging, total body potassium, fat-free mass, and cell mass in males and females between ages 18 and 85 years. J Gerontol 1972;27:428–443.

45. Olsky M, Murray J: Dizziness and fainting in the elderly. Emerg Med Clin North Am 1990;8:295–308.

46. Pozzato G, Moretti M, Franzin F, et al: Ethanol metabolism and aging: The role of "first pass metabolism" and gastric alcohol dehydrogenase activity. J Gerontol 1995;50A:B135–B141.

47. Rattan SI, Derventzi A, Clark BFC: Protein synthesis, posttranslational modifications, and aging. Ann NY Acad Sci 1992;663:48–62.

48. Rowe J, Andres R, Tobin J, et al: The effect of age on creatinine clearance in men: A cross-sectional and longitudinal study. J Gerontol 1976;31:155–163.

49. Sanders A: Geriatric Emergency Medicine Task Force: The care of the elderly in emergency departments: A report prepared by the Society for Academic Emergency Medicine. Lansing, MI, Geriatric Emergency Medicine Task Force, 1992.

50. Schwartz J, Temple R, Lemke J, et al: Drug testing in the elderly. Pharmacol Ther 1992;17:1715–1748.

51. Schwartz JB: Clinical pharmacology. In: Hazzard WR, Blass JP, Ettinger WH, et al, eds: Principles of Geriatric Medicine and Gerontology, 4th ed. New York, McGraw-Hill, 1999, pp. 303–311.

52. Shorr RI, Ray WA, Daugherty JR, et al: Individual sulfonylureas and serious hypoglycemia in older people. J Am Geriatr Soc 1996;44:751–755.

53. Seltzer HS: Drug-induced phyoglycemia. Endocrinol Metab Clin North Am 1989;18:163–183.

54. Svenson J: Obtundation in the elderly patient. Am J Emerg Med 1987;5:524–527.

55. Svensson CK, Woodruff MN, Baxter JR, et al: Free drug concentration monitoring in clinical practice: Rationale and current status. Clin Pharmacokinet 1986;11:450–469.

56. Tamblyn RM, McLeod PJ, Abramowitz M, Laprise R: Do too many cooks spoil the broth? Multiple physician involvement in medical management of elderly patients and potentially inappropriate drug combinations. Can Med Assoc J 1996;154:1177–1184.

57. US Food and Drug Administration Center for Drug Evaluation and Research: From test tube to patient: Improving health through human drugs. Rockville MD, FDA, 1999; http://fda.gov/cder.

58. Vestal RE, Cusack BJ: Pharmacology and aging. In: Schneider EL, Rowe JW, eds: Handbook of the Biology of Aging, 3rd ed. San Diego, Academic Press, 1990, pp. 349–383.

59. Vestal RE, Wood AJJ, Shand DG: Reduced beta-adrenoceptor sensitivity in the elderly. Clin Pharmacol Ther 1979;26:181–186.

60. Welker JA, Zaloga GP: Pine oil ingestion: A common cause of poisoning. Chest 1999;116:1822–1826.

61. Woodhouse KW, Wynne HA: Age-related changes in liver size and hepatic blood flow: The influence on drug metabolism in the elderly. Clin Pharmacokinet 1988;15:287–294.

62. Young VR: Amino acids and proteins in relation to the nutrition of elderly people. Age Ageing 1990;19:S10–S24.

CHAPTER 108

THE HIV-POSITIVE PATIENT

AIDS Pharmacology and Toxicology

Kevin Smothers / Neal A. Lewin

OVERVIEW AND EPIDEMIOLOGY

AIDS remains a leading cause of death of young adults. Worldwide, an estimated 16,000 persons become newly infected with HIV each day, and over 36 million people have been infected since its discovery, with approximately 22 million dying from the disease.[55] Fortunately, recent trends in the United States show a dramatic decrease in deaths from AIDS because of new aggressive antiviral treatment modalities and opportunistic infection prophylaxis. Since 1995, the annual death rate among persons with AIDS has precipitously declined.[20] The introduction of highly active antiretroviral therapy (HAART) and improved HIV plasma measurement has completely changed the management of HIV-infected patients. HIV infection is now managed as a chronic disease requiring expert knowledge of complex drug regimens and close monitoring for common side effects and development of symptomatic AIDS. There is at present no cure or vaccine. Consequently, clinicians are facing new toxicologic issues daily: the availability of new drugs (approved and unapproved) and multidrug regimens leading to overdoses; polypharmacologic interactions; and an array of toxidromes that require an in-depth understanding of the management of an intentional or unintentional overdose and the adverse effects of these therapies. As will become apparent from a review of the specific AIDS medications in this chapter, most of the known toxicity of these agents is related to their adverse effects and drug interactions.

In order to understand the effect of the antiviral agents, it is imperative to review the HIV-1 replication cycle and the potential points of inhibition by these drugs (Fig. 108–1). The first step in HIV-1 replication is the attachment of the virus envelope to specific host-cell receptors. The surface glycoprotein gp120 attaches to CD4 molecules on the cell surfaces of some lymphocytes and macrophages. Next, entry into the cells occurs, followed by transcription of the viral genome (viral RNA into proviral DNA) by reverse transcriptase. Integration with the host nucleus mediated by an integrase protein forms a provirus. Expression of the integrated provirus produces both spliced and unspliced mRNA transcripts that encode the regulatory and structural viral proteins. Finally, new virus particles assemble, and particles bud through the cell membrane as mature infectious HIV-1 virus.[49]

Understanding the reproduction cycle of HIV has led to the development of pharmacologic interventions to inhibit each stage of the cycle. Thus, drugs are now available to inhibit viral attachment, reverse transcription, protease, and the regulatory proteins (Fig. 108–1).[49]

HIV INFECTION AND TOXICOLOGY

Management of AIDS is complex and demanding. Patients and providers must constantly balance optimal suppression of viral replication and opportunistic infections with the knowledge that adverse drug reactions occur commonly and the treatment regimens are ever more consuming of time for daily activities. With treatment options limited, patients must choose to remain on medication that has caused a drug reaction, some of which were quite severe.[5] Unapproved therapies remain available through a network of buyers' clubs even with advances in HIV therapy.

In an effort to help seriously ill AIDS patients, the Food and Drug Administration (FDA) has made readily available many new medications to treat HIV-related problems through controlled expanded-access programs.[14] This novel approach to drug testing has shortened the time required to make potentially useful drugs available to patients.[14] Under these programs, HAART was developed with great success and has helped decrease the use of uncontrolled medications obtained through a network of buyers' clubs.

Nonetheless, use of alternative therapies by persons with HIV infection remains active and increases the adverse drug reactions and toxicity from AIDS treatment regimens (Table 108–1). Several of these agents are being used in their native herbal form by patients who are unaware of which herbs they are using but who believe that medicinal herbs are less toxic than traditional therapy[1] (see Chap. 77). In many circumstances, health care providers are unaware that patients are combining traditional and alternative therapies. Because of this, untested and unapproved agents are being used with only limited information about toxicity.

Patients with HIV infection take, on average, six to nine medications for the remainder of their lives, making the magnitude and extent of drug exposure in these patients substantial. Several reports show that adverse drug reactions are greatly increased with HIV infection.[26,48] Hypersensitivity reactions are encountered regularly. Dosing errors by patients with HIV dementia complex increase the risk of drug reactions and drug overdoses as well.

A recent study of 1450 HIV-infected patients with a CD4 count of 500 cells/mm^3 or less calculated adverse event rates from the use of AZT (ZDV), didanosine (ddI), zalcitabine (ddC), cotrimoxazole, and dapsone. The conclusions of the study were that the adverse events from these drugs were common, that serious events requiring hospitalization were rare, that adverse events rates increase progressively with a fall in CD4 count, and that race and gender may modify risk with several of these drugs (female > male with ddI and cotrimoxazole; white > black from cotrimoxazole).[71]

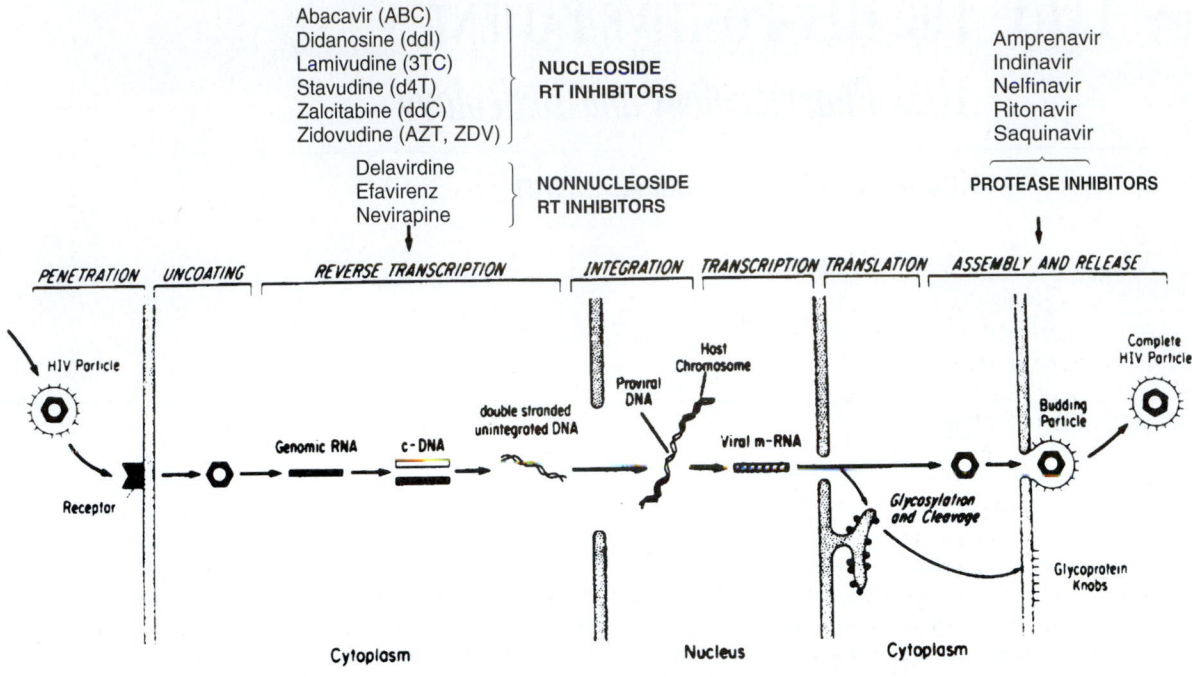

Figure 108–1. Summary of the replication cycle of HIV and potential points of inhibition by antiretroviral agents. *(Modified with permission from Threlkeld SC, Hirsch MS: Antiretroviral therapy: Current trends. In: Gold JWM, Telzak EE, White DA, eds: The Diagnosis and Management of the HIV-Infected Patient, part 1. Med Clin North Am 1996;80:1264. Previously published in Hirsch M, D'Aquila R: Drug therapy: Summary of HIV replication cycle and available antiretroviral agents. N Engl J Med 1993;328:1687. Massachusetts Medical Society.)*

Most individuals infected with HIV are also emotionally affected. They face a multitude of psychosocial stressors at all stages of their illness. Although there is a more optimistic overall prognosis with multidrug regimens, patients still must balance the constant frustration of living with a chronic relapsing disease. Depression remains common and often difficult to diagnose. The rate of suicide is significantly greater in persons with HIV infection than in the general population.[27] Although better treatment of the disease has decreased this risk, it is still seven times that of the general population.[87] In a study of military personnel, it was found that there was not a significantly increased risk of death from suicide in the months following being told of HIV results. It should be noted that this population was asymptomatic, whereas previous studies have evaluated patients with active disease.[31] The overall incidence of depression in HIV-infected patients is 7 to 10% and is particularly high immediately before and after HIV testing.[4] Organic brain disease (HIV dementia) is very common in AIDS, and because depression and dementia overlap, depression is unrecognized and untreated.[16] Polypharmaceutical toxic overdose is the suicide method most often chosen, which in turn may reflect the easy access to a large number of highly toxic medications prescribed during the course of the illness.

HIV INFECTION: DRUG METABOLISM AND ELIMINATION

HIV-infected individuals initially have normal hepatic and renal function and, therefore, normal drug metabolism and elimination. As noted previously, cells infected directly by HIV possess the CD4 receptor, allowing the gp120 portion of the HIV to bind, thereby permitting viral penetration into the cell.[45] Because intestinal, hepatic, renal, and biliary cells do not possess CD4 receptors, they are not directly affected by HIV, and patients with asymptomatic HIV infection usually maintain their ability to metabolize and eliminate drugs. However, persons with advanced HIV infection develop altered drug pharmacokinetics resulting from the many infections, immunologic factors, and drugs that alter hepatic and renal function. HIV-associated nephropathy (HIVAN) is a syndrome characterized by massive proteinuria, hematuria, azotemia, and unusual clinical renal pathologic features; the renal insufficiency created by this syndrome may alter drug elimi-

TABLE 108–1. **Alternative or Unproven Therapies for HIV/AIDS**

Acupuncture
Allicin
Anabolic steroids
Trichosanthin (compound Q)
DHEA (dehydroepiandrosterone)
Hypericin (St. John's wort)
Imuthiol/dithiocarb
Malaleuca
Marijuana
Massage therapy
N-Acetylcysteine (NAC)
Oral interferon-α
Ribavirin
Thalidomide
Vitamin C

nation.[77] HIVAN is seen in all risk groups for HIV infection: men who have sex with men (MSM), injection drug users (IDU), recipients of contaminated blood and blood products, and children born to infected mothers. The most common histopathology in HIVAN is focal and segmental glomerulosclerosis (FSGS).[45] Another cause of renal damage is electrolyte imbalance, which can result from the drugs used in HIV disease[86] (Table 108–2).

The incidence of enteropathy is high in HIV-infected patients, resulting in malabsorption of oral medications.[6,91] Diarrheal syndromes with malabsorption occur in more than half of AIDS patients during their lifetime, and bacteria, fungi, viruses, parasites, and drugs are implicated as causative.[96] There are several HIV-related causes of impairment of hepatic function that in turn may affect drug metabolism. Interestingly, glutathione, which is important for drug metabolism and detoxification as well as combating oxidative stress, is decreased in HIV-infected cells.[93] Some HIV-infected patients are slow acetylators of certain drugs;[62] numerous opportunistic infections and cancers seen in HIV-infected patients directly impair the function of the liver, and, most important, several of the treatments for HIV infection and AIDS are directly hepatotoxic and nephrotoxic. Finally, many drug–drug interactions alter metabolism (Tables 108–3 to 108–5).

SPECIFIC ANTIRETROVIRAL AGENTS

Inhibitors of Viral Attachment

A logical approach to block the replication cycle would be to interfere with the binding of surface gp120 to cell surface CD4 molecules. The use of recombinant soluble CD4 or immunoglobulins directed at viral epitopes (antigenic determinants) has been tried, but thus far, all pharmacologic agents in this category are strictly experimental. None is yet available, nor are any data on adverse effects of these experimental drugs available.[98]

Nucleoside Analogue Reverse Transcriptase Inhibitors

The nucleoside analogue reverse transcriptase inhibitors inhibit reverse transcription of viral RNA into proviral DNA. They are in-corporated into the growing DNA strand and prevent its further replication.[44] Nucleoside analogue reverse transcriptase inhibitors include zidovudine (AZT, ZDV), zalcitabine (ddC), didanosine (ddI), stavudine, lamivudine (3TC) and abacavir.

Zidovudine.   Zidovudine (AZT, ZDV; Retrovir) was the first licensed antiretroviral treatment for HIV infection in the United States. It is a deoxynucleoside analogue of thymidine. Cellular kinases convert zidovudine into its triphosphate form (AZTTP), which is the active intracellular compound. This triphosphate form competitively inhibits viral reverse transcriptase, thereby terminating viral DNA chain formation (see Fig. 108–1).

In therapeutic doses, zidovudine is rapidly absorbed from the gastrointestinal tract and reaches a peak serum concentration of 0.62 µg/mL in approximately 1 hour.[105] Zidovudine has a plasma half-life of 1.1 hours, and AZTTP has an intracellular half-life of 3 hours.[42] Zidovudine achieves high cerebrospinal fluid (CSF) concentrations (50% of plasma). It is metabolized principally in the liver by glucuronide conjugation and is subject to a first-pass effect, resulting in a bioavailability of approximately 60% of the ingested drug.[105] The metabolite (G-AZT) has no antiviral activity, although the glucuronidation process may be reversible, and G-AZT may be reconverted to AZT. Zidovudine and G-AZT are excreted almost exclusively by the kidneys, with a mean half-life of 1 hour.[57] Only 19% of the dose is recovered in the urine as parent drug,[42] strongly suggesting that metabolism is more important than renal clearance in the elimination of AZT. In patients with end-stage renal disease, the half-life of AZT is three times normal.[35] Consequently, dosage adjustments are required for both hepatic and renal dysfunction. Zidovudine is adsorbed by activated charcoal and is dialyzable.

The dose of AZT is 600 mg/day in equally divided doses every 8 or 12 hours. The most common adverse effects are nausea, vomiting, myalgias, fatigue, malaise, insomnia, and severe headaches.[40] Zidovudine causes or is associated with a multitude of neuropsychiatric reactions[4,23] such as mania, Wernicke encephalopathy, dementia, and seizures. It can cause a severe myopathy (polymyositislike syndrome) after prolonged use secondary to myocyte mitochondrial toxicity.[7,30] Acute hepatitis and nail dyschromia are also reported. Zidovudine has been associated with potentially fatal cases of lactic acidosis in patients with liver disease.[95] The majority of these effects are transient, occur only during therapy, and gradually diminish after the drug is discontinued and/or the dosage is reduced.

The major adverse effect of AZT is hematologic toxicity.[35,44] Anemia usually occurs after 4 to 6 weeks of therapy, and granulocytopenia develops after 6 to 8 weeks of therapy. Many patients require multiple blood transfusions and cytokine agents. Although macrocytosis usually appears early with the use of AZT, vitamin B_{12}, folate, and erythropoietin deficiencies are rarely identified.[100] Zidovudine does not cause GI blood loss. Anemia is usually caused by selective red cell aplasia or hypoplasia,[103] but bone marrow aplasia of all cell lines also occurs.[35] Although the bone marrow effects are usually reversible after discontinuing AZT, in some cases the marrow never or only partially recovers. Erythropoietin, granulocyte colony-stimulating factor (G-CSF), and granulocyte-macrophage colony-stimulating factor (GM-CSF), singly or in combination, greatly reduce the bone marrow toxicity associated with AZT.[39,69,76]

Certain drugs used in conjunction with AZT increase its toxicity (see Table 108–5). When AZT is used with ganciclovir or am-

TABLE 108–2.	Drug-Induced Electrolyte Disorders in HIV Disease
Disorder	**Drug**
Hyponatremia	Didanosine, itraconazole, TMP-SMX, zalcitabine
Hypokalemia	Amphotericin B, cidofovir, didanosine, foscarnet, itraconazole
Hypocalcemia	Amphotericin B, cidofovir, foscarnet, pentamidine
Hypoglycemia	Pentamidine, zalcitabine
Hypomagnesemia	Amphotericin B, foscarnet, pentamidine
Hypernatremia	Amphotericin B, foscarnet, pentamidine
Hyperkalemia	Pentamidine, TMP-SMX
Hypercalcemia	Foscarnet
Hyperglycemia	Abacavir, cidofovir, pentamidine, protease inhibitors, zalcitabine
Hyperuricemia	Didanosine, zalcitabine, zidovudine
Hypophosphatemia/ hyperphosphatemia	Foscarnet
Metabolic acidosis	Didanosine, stavudine, zalcitabine, zidovudine

TABLE 108–3.   Toxicity of Medications Used to Treat Patients with HIV Disease

Drug	Organ System	Signs, Symptoms, Laboratory
Antifungal therapy		
Amphotericin B (AmB)	Hematologic	Anemia, leukopenia, thrombocytopenia
	Renal	Azotemia,[a] renal tubular acidosis
	Miscellaneous	Fever, chills, rigors, vomiting, headache
Fluconazole (Diflucan)	Gastrointestinal	Anorexia, nausea, vomiting, hepatitis (rare)
Flucytosine (5-FC)	Hematologic	Bone marrow suppression[a]
Itraconazole (Sporanox)	Neurologic	Dizziness, headache, seizure (all rare)
	Miscellaneous	Rashes, anemia
Ketoconazole (Nizoral)	Gastrointestinal	Anorexia, nausea, vomiting
	Miscellaneous	Paresthesias, thrombocytopenia, hepatitis
Antimycobacterial therapy		
Azithromycin (Zithromax)	Gastrointestinal	Nausea, vomiting, diarrhea
	Miscellaneous	Hypoacusis (high doses), headache, dizziness
Clarithromycin (Biaxin)	Gastrointestinal	Nausea, vomiting, diarrhea
	Miscellaneous	Hypoacusis (high doses), headache, dizziness
Rifabutin (Mycobutin)	Gastrointestinal	Nausea,[a] vomiting,[a] diarrhea,[a] hepatotoxicity
	Hematologic	Mild neutropenia and thrombocytopenia
	Miscellaneous	Hypersensitivity reactions
Antiopportunistic therapy **(PCP, toxoplasmosis, cryptosporidiosis)**		
Atovaquone (Mepron)	Miscellaneous	Rashes, anemia, leukopenia, elevated AST and ALT
Dapsone	Gastrointestinal	Anorexia, nausea, vomiting, hepatitis
	Hematologic	Methemoglobinemia
	Neurologic	Headache, nervousness, insomnia, blurred vision, paresthesias, peripheral neuropathy, psychosis
	Dermatologic	Exfoliative dermatitis,[a] toxic epidermal necrolysis, erythema multiforme
	Miscellaneous	Sore throat, fever, pallor, malaise, myalgias
Paromomycin (Humatin)	Dermatologic	Rash
	Gastrointestinal	Nausea, vomiting, diarrhea
	Neurologic	Vertigo, headache
Pentamidine (Pentam) (IV)	Cardiovascular	Hypotension, dysrhythmias (torsades de pointes), phlebitis
	Dermatologic	Rash, Stevens-Johnson syndrome
	Endocrine	Hypoglycemia[a] (early) and hyperglycemia (late), hypocalcemia, hypokalemia
	Gastrointestinal	Anorexia, nausea, vomiting, metallic taste
	Hematologic	Leukopenia, thrombocytopenia
	Renal	Azotemia,[a] renal failure (rare)
Sulfadiazine	Dermatologic	Rash,[a] Stevens-Johnson syndrome,[a] toxic epidermal necrolysis,[a] erythema multiforme[a]
	Neurologic	Headaches, depression, hallucinations, ataxia, tremor
	Renal	Crystalluria, hematuria, proteinuria, nephrolithiasis
Sulfadoxine-pyrimethamine	Hematologic	Agranulocytosis, aplastic anemia, thrombocytopenia, leukopenia
TMP-SMX (Bactrim, Septra)	Dermatologic	Rash,[a] Stevens-Johnson syndrome,[a] toxic epidermal necrolysis,[a] erythema multiforme[a]
	Gastrointestinal	Nausea, vomiting, diarrhea, hepatitis
Antiretroviral drugs **Protease Inhibitors**		
All protease inhibitors	Endocrine	Abnormal fat distribution, "buffalo hump," central obesity, breast enlargement, cushingoid appearance, peripheral wasting
Amprenavir (Agenerase)	Gastrointestinal	Nausea, diarrhea
	Dermatologic	Rash, Stevens-Johnson[a]
	Neurologic	Headache
Indinavir (Crixivan)	Gastrointestinal	Increased indirect hyperbilirubinemia
	Genitourinary	Nephrolithiasis
Nelfinavir (Viracept)	Gastrointestinal	Diarrhea
Ritonavir (Norvir)	Gastrointestinal	Abdominal pain, altered taste
	Neurologic	Circumoral paresthesias
	Miscellaneous	Serum lipid abnormalities
Saquinavir (Invirase, Fortovase)	Gastrointestinal	Elevated AST and ALT, nausea, diarrhea
	Neurologic	Headache
Nucleoside analogue reverse transcriptase inhibitors		
Abacavir (ABC; Ziagen)	Gastrointestinal	Nausea
	Miscellaneous	Hypersensitivity reactions[a]

TABLE 108–3.   Toxicity of Medications Used to Treat Patients with HIV Disease (continued)

Drug	Organ System	Signs, Symptoms, Laboratory
Nucleoside analogue reverse transcriptase inhibitors		
Didanosine (Videx)	Gastrointestinal	Diarrhea, nausea, pancreatitis[a]
	Neurologic	Peripheral neuropathy,[a] headaches
	Miscellaneous	Hyperuricemia, rash, lactic acidosis
Lamivudine (3TC; Epivir)	Gastrointestinal	Abdominal pain
	Neurologic	Headache
	Miscellaneous	Cough, malaise, nasal symptoms
Stavudine (d4T; Zerit)	Neurologic	Peripheral neuropathy
	Miscellaneous	Lactic acidosis
Zalcitabine (ddC; Hivid)	Dermatologic	Cutaneous eruptions, nail changes, aphthous stomatitis
	Gastrointestinal	Diarrhea, nausea, pancreatitis[a]
	Hematologic	Leukopenia, thrombocytopenia
	Neurologic	Peripheral neuropathy,[a] headaches
	Miscellaneous	Fever, malaise, peripheral edema, arthralgias, lactic acidosis
Zidovudine (AZT, ZDV; Retrovir)	Dermatologic	Nail changes
	Hematologic	Anemia,[a] leukopenia,[a] thrombocytosis, macrocytosis
	Gastrointestinal	Nausea,[a] vomiting,[a] acute hepatitis
	Neurologic	Wernicke's encephalopathy, dementia, seizures, lethargy, nystagmus, insomnia, headache, mania, ataxia, polymyositis
	Miscellaneous	Lactic acidosis
Non–Nucleoside analogue reverse transcriptase inhibitors		
Delavirdine (Descriptor)	Dermatologic	Rash
	Gastrointestinal	Nausea, vomiting, diarrhea, elevated AST and ALT
	Neurologic	Headache, fatigue
Efavirenz (Sustiva)	Dermatologic	Rash, pruritus
	Gastrointestinal	Nausea, vomiting, diarrhea, dyspepsia, elevated AST and ALT
	Neurologic	Dizziness, headache, fatigue, insomnia
	Miscellaneous	Fever, increased sweating
Foscarnet (Foscavir) (DNA Polymerase inhibitor and NNRTI)	Dermatologic	Genital and oral ulcers, fixed drug eruptions (rare)
	Gastrointestinal	Nausea, vomiting
	Hematologic	Anemia (rare)
	Neurologic	Malaise, headaches, seizures, coma
	Renal	Azotemia,[a] renal failure, diabetes insipidus
	Miscellaneous	Hypocalcemia,[a] hypophosphatemia, hypokalemia, hypomagnesemia
Nevirapine (Viramune)	Dermatologic	Rash
	Gastrointestinal	Diarrhea, elevated AST and ALT
	Hematologic	Neutropenia
	Neurologic	Headache
	Miscellaneous	Fever
Ribavirin	Gastrointestinal	Nausea, vomiting, diarrhea
	Hematologic	Anemia (normochromic, normocytic), bone marrow suppression, aplastic anemia
	Neurologic	Fatigue, headache
Rifabutin	Gastrointestinal	Nausea,[a] vomiting,[a] diarrhea,[a] hepatotoxicity
	Hematologic	Mild neutropenia and thrombocytopenia
	Miscellaneous	Hypersensitivity reactions
Antiviral drugs		
Acyclovir (Zovirax)	Gastrointestinal	PO: Nausea, vomiting
	Neurologic	IV: Seizures, encephalopathy, coma, hallucinations
	Renal	IV: Crystalluria, acute tubular necrosis, renal failure
Cidofovir (Vistide)	Renal	Nephrotoxicity
Cytokines		
Erythropoietin	Cardiovascular	Hypertension
G-CSF	Hematologic	Thrombosis, phlebitis
GM-CSF	Miscellaneous	Fever, bone pain, myalgias, flushing
Ganciclovir (Cytovene)	Gastrointestinal	Nausea, vomiting, diarrhea, elevated AST and ALT
	Hematologic	Leukopenia,[a] anemia, thrombocytopenia
	Neurologic	Headache, dizziness, confusion, seizures
	Renal	Worsening of renal function[a]

(continued)

TABLE 108–3. Toxicity of Medications Used to Treat Patients with HIV Disease (continued)

Drug	Organ System	Signs, Symptoms, Laboratory
Herbs		
Compound Q	Neurologic	Delirium,[a] dementia,[a] coma,[a] paresis,[a] myalgia
	Miscellaneous	Hypersensitivity reactions, hypoglycemia, fever
	Dermatologic	Photosensitivity[a]
	Miscellaneous	MAO inhibitor[a]
Immunomodulators		
Ampligen	Miscellaneous	Flulike symptoms, flushing
Disulfiram (Antabuse)	Cardiovascular	Hypotension
With alcohol[b]	Gastrointestinal	Nausea, vomiting
	Neurologic	Confusion, headache
	Miscellaneous	Facial flushing, respiratory difficulty
Dithiocarb	Gastrointestinal	Metallic taste, GI upset, hepatotoxicity
Without alcohol[b]		
N-Acetylcysteine	Gastrointestinal	Nausea, vomiting
	Dermatologic	Rash
	Miscellaneous	Fever
Interferon-α	Cardiovascular	Ventricular tachydysrhythmias
(Roferon-A, Intron-A)	Gastrointestinal	Nausea, vomiting
	Hematologic	Bone marrow suppression
	Neurologic	Confusion, paresthesias
	Pulmonary	Interstitial, pneumonitis
	Miscellaneous	Fever, chills, malaise
Androgen therapy		
Fluoxymesterone	Gastrointestinal	Hepatic dysfunction
Nandrolone decanoate	Dermatologic	Hair Loss
(Deca Durabolin)		Rash with dermal preparations (patch)
		Acne
Oxymetholone	Metabolic	Lipid abnormalities
Oxandrolone	Metabolic	Lipid abnormalities
Stanozolol	Metabolic	Lipid abnormalities
Testosterone	Urologic	Increased prostate size
		Virilization
Treatment of cachexia		
Human growth hormone	Rheumatologic	Joint pain
(Somatotropin)	Gastrointestinal	Diarrhea
Dronabinol (THC)	Neurologic	Dizziness, confusion, sommolence
Thalidomide (Synovir)	Neurologic	Worsen preexisting neuritis
	Reproductive	Embryopathy—phocomelia
Megestrol (Megace)	Cardiovascular	Superior vena cava syndrome, fluid retention, CHF
	Endocrinologic	Glucose intolerance, Cushing syndrome
	Gastrointestinal	Vomiting
	Neurologic	Headache, depression

[a]Significant toxicity.
[b]Metabolic toxicity.

photericin B, bone marrow toxicity is greatly increased. Some drugs (acyclovir, α-interferon, dipyridamole) increase in vitro antiretroviral activity, whereas others (ribavirin, stavudine) decrease in vitro activity and should not be administered with AZT. Higher drug levels are achieved when AZT is combined with agents (aspirin, atovaquone, fluconazole, indomethacin, phenytoin, valproic acid, interferon, methadone, probenecid) that decrease metabolism through competitive demand for glucuronidation, and with others (probenecid, sulfadiazine, TMP-SMX) that decrease renal clearance through impaired tubular excretion, but this clinically is insignificant with appropriate monitoring and dosage adjustment. Rifampin and rifabutin clearly enhance zidovudine glucuronidation, which results in a drop in serum concentration and treatment

failure.[12] Lamivudine and ritonavir increase the concentration of AZT when used concomitantly.

Intentional AZT overdoses are occurring with increasing frequency. In the few case reports of AZT overdose, patients ingested 3.6 to 20.0 g of drug without any long-term sequelae.[50,70,75,84,92] Transient headache, nausea, lethargy, nystagmus, mild ataxia, seizure, or no symptoms at all are reported.[50,70,75,84,92] No short-term or long-term hematologic effects were identified at 6-week followup.[50,75] The lethal dose of AZT in humans has not been determined. All reported cases of AZT overdose to date were managed conservatively. Current recommendations for treatment of AZT overdose include activated charcoal in addition to other standard methods of managing an acute drug overdose.

TABLE 108–4.   Clinical Presentations Associated with Medications Used to Treat HIV Disease

Clinical Presentation	Drug[a]
Confusion	AZT, interferon-α, compound Q, acyclovir, ganciclovir
Cyanosis	Dapsone, primaquine
Fever	Compound Q, G-CSF, dapsone, amphotericin B, AZT, TMP-SMX, ddI, nevirapine
Flushing	Ampligen, disulfiram (with alcohol), G-CSF
Headache	AZT, ddC, ddI, foscarnet, ribavirin, disulfiram (with alcohol), sulfadiazine, itraconazole, amphotericin B, azithromycin, 3TC, interferon-α, saquinavir, indinavir
Hepatitis	AZT, dapsone, diflucan, ketoconazole, itraconazole, fluconazole
Pallor	AZT, interferon-α, ribavirin, TMP-SMX, dapsone, amphotericin B, 5-FC, foscarnet, ddC, ganciclovir
Peripheral neuropathy	AZT, ddC, ddI, dapsone, 3TC, stavudine, quinolones
Rash	Zalcitabine, didanosine, foscarnet, hypericin, NAC, disulfiram, G-CSF, TMP-SMX, sulfadiazine, dapsone, pentamidine, itraconazole, ribavirin, nevirapine, delavidine, thalidomide
Renal colic	Sulfadiazine, TMP-SMX, indinavir
Seizures	AZT, foscarnet, acyclovir, ganciclovir, INH, interferon-α

[a]AZT = zidovudine; ddC = zalcitabine; ddI = didanosine; G-CSF = growth colony-stimulating factor; NAC = *N*-acetylcysteine; TMP-SMX = Bactrim, Septra; 3TC = lamivudine

Zalcitabine.   Zalcitabine (ddC, dideoxycytidine; Hivid) is approximately 10 times more potent an inhibitor of HIV replication than AZT.[106] At present ddC is recommended for combination therapy with AZT. Zalcitabine undergoes intracellular conversion to its active form (dideoxycytidine triphosphate, ddCTP) in a manner similar to that of AZT. It is well absorbed in the GI tract, with an oral bioavailability of 70 to 80%, peak serum concentration of 0.5 µg/mL, and CSF concentration of approximately 20% of serum level.[45] The agent has a plasma half-life of approximately 1 to 2 hours and an intracellular half-life of 2 to 3 hours. It is eliminated mostly by renal clearance (70%).[106] Zalcitabine is adsorbed to activated charcoal and is probably dialyzable. The recommended dosage is 0.75 mg every 8 hours with AZT 200 mg every 8 hours.

Unlike zidovudine, ddC has little bone marrow toxicity.[106] Macrocytosis and anemia have not been encountered. Mild thrombocytopenia and leukopenia may develop.

Seventy-five percent of patients using ddC develop a transient symptom complex that appears to be a dose-related toxic effect, including cutaneous eruptions, fevers, malaise, headache, aphthous stomatitis, arthralgias, peripheral edema, nail changes, nausea, and diarrhea.[106] In most cases, these symptoms subside during therapy and do not necessitate discontinuing the drug. A severe sensory peripheral neuropathy, manifested by painful dysesthesias of the feet, develops in 30% of patients treated with ddC.[67,72,106] The neuropathy occurs relatively late, usually after more than 10 weeks of use, and gradually subsides after termination of therapy.[67,72,106] Although rare, pancreatitis, which may be fatal, has been reported in patients using ddC both alone and in combination with AZT.[67]

Several drugs cause adverse drug interactions when used with ddC (see Table 108–5). Agents with the potential to cause peripheral neuropathy and pancreatitis should be avoided, as should drugs such as amphotericin B and foscarnet, which decrease renal clearance of ddC and may potentiate toxicity. There are no reported cases of overdose with this agent. Conservative management with activated charcoal is appropriate.

Didanosine.   Didanosine (ddI, dideoxyinosine; Videx) has a mechanism of action similar to those of AZT and ddC. It is approved for use as a single agent or in combination therapy for HIV infection. Didanosine is converted intracellularly to its active form, dideoxyadenosine triphosphate (ddATP). Didanosine is very acid-labile and must be administered in a buffered form. It has an oral bioavailability of 23 to 40%, with peak plasma concentrations reached in 0.6 to 1.0 hour.[59] The mean plasma half-life of ddI is 1.5 hours,[59] and the intracellular half-life of ddATP is 12 to 24 hours.[2] Didanosine penetrates the CSF at 20% of the plasma concentration. The drug is metabolized by hepatic glucuronidation and renal clearance. The recommended dosage of ddI is 200 mg twice a day.

Didanosine has a toxicity profile similar to that of ddC. The principal adverse effects are diarrhea (34%), painful sensory peripheral neuropathy (34%)[72], and pancreatitis (9%)[59]. Pancreatitis may be fatal and is associated with a prior history of pancreatitis, advanced HIV disease, and concomitant use of other medications that affect the pancreas (see Table 108–5).[59] Pancreatitis should be considered whenever a patient taking ddI develops abdominal pain, nausea, and vomiting. Asymptomatic hyperuricemia is common with higher doses and probably reflects normal metabolic degradation of the drug.[59] Headaches, rashes, and elevated hepatic aminotransferases may occur.[59] Bone marrow toxicity is not encountered with ddI usage,[59] so white blood cells, platelets, and hemoglobin tend to increase during administration. Because ddI is administered in a buffered form, it should not be administered with other drugs that bind to buffer or require an acid environment for absorption (Table 108–5). Concomitant use of ddC, IV pentamidine, and ganciclovir increases the risk of pancreatitis. There are no reported cases of overdoses. Conservative management with activated charcoal and close monitoring for evidence of pancreatitis are indicated.

Stavudine.   Stavudine (2′,3′-didehydro-3′-deoxythmidine; d4T; Zerit) was approved for use in the United States in 1994. This nucleoside reverse transcriptase inhibitor is currently being used in patients intolerant to AZT, ddI, or ddC or if immunologic deterioration occurs on the regimens already outlined. Stavudine is well absorbed orally, and the usual dose is 40 mg twice a day. It is often given in combination with ddI or lamivudine. Concomitant use with AZT results in lower levels of stavudine. Apparently, zidovudine monophosphate inhibits intracellular phosphorylation of thymidine kinase, an important step in conversion of stavudine to its active drug. Its principal adverse reaction is peripheral neuropathy similar to ddI and ddC.[72] No reports of overdose appear in the literature.

Lamivudine.   Lamivudine (2′-deoxy-3′-thiacytidine; 3TC; Epivir) was approved for use in United States in 1995. This nucleoside reverse transcriptase inhibitor is used in combination with AZT. It is well absorbed orally and penetrates CSF similarly to ddI and ddC. The intracellular half-life is 10 to 15 hours. The dose is 150 mg

TABLE 108–5. HIV Drug Interactions

	Interacting Drugs	Effect	Comments
Antifungal drugs			
Amphotericin B (AmB)	AZT[a]	Bone marrow toxicity	Monitor CBC frequently.
	Flucytosine (5-FC)	Increased antifungal activity, increased bone marrow toxicity	Given as adjunct to AmB. Trials under way with 5-FC as adjunct to fluconazole and itraconazole. Monitor 5-FC levels weekly when used with AmB for cryptococcal meningitis. Monitor CBC.
	Nephrotoxic agents	Increased nephrotoxicity	Prehydration may reduce nephrotoxicity.
Fluconazole (Diflucan), itraconazole (Sporanox)	Hydrochlorothiazide	Decreased renal clearance of fluconazole	Coadministration results in approximately 40% increase in serum fluconazole concentrations. Clinical significance unknown.
	Phenytoin	Decreased phenytoin metabolism	Monitor phenytoin levels.
	Rifampin	Increased fluconazole metabolism	May explain apparent fluconazole failure. Increased dose of fluconazole may be required.
	Sulfonylureas	Increased hypoglycemia	Monitor blood glucose.
	Warfarin	Decreased warfarin metabolism	Monitor INR.
Flucytosine (5-FC)	Amphotericin B,[a] ganciclovir[a]	Increased bone marrow toxicity	Monitor 5-FC levels weekly when used with amphotericin B. Monitor CBC.
	Antacids	Decreased 5-FC absorption	Antacids should be taken at least 2 hours before 5-FC.
Ketoconazole (Nizoral)	Antacids, ddl, H$_2$ antagonists	Decreased ketoconazole bioavailability	Basic pH reduces ketoconazole absorption. Give ketoconazole 2 hours before antacids, ddl, or H$_2$ antagonists.
	Isoniazid	Increased ketoconazole metabolism	Higher doses of ketoconazole may be needed.
	Phenytoin	Altered metabolism	Coadministration may cause altered metabolism of one or both drugs. Monitor serum phenytoin.
	Warfarin	Warfarin is increased, probable inhibition of warfarin metabolism	Monitor patient and INR every 2 days. Adjust warfarin as needed.
Antimycobacterial therapy			
Azithromycin (Zithromax), clarithromycin (Biaxin)	Antacids	Decreased azithromycin absorption	Administer these drugs at least 2 h apart.
	AZT (see AZT)		
	Carbamazepine, theophylline, ergots, warfarin	Decreased metabolism of drugs listed in Interacting Drugs for clarithromycin	Increased serum concentration of drugs listed in Interacting Drugs. Monitor levels and INR. Avoid concomitant use with ergots.
Capreomycin	Nephrotoxic agents[a]	Increased nephrotoxic and/or ototoxic effects	Monitor BUN, serum creatinine, and capreomycin levels.
	Phenothiazines	Increased risk of respiratory paralysis	Monitor respiratory function closely; if signs of respiratory distress occur, discontinue medication.
Ciprofloxacin, norfloxacin, ofloxacin (quinolone group)	Antacids, ddl, iron supplements, sucralfate, zinc	Decreased quinolone group absorption	Quinolone group form chelate complexes, decreasing absorption. Patients should take quinolones and medications listed in column 2 at least 2 hours apart.
	Theophylline	Increased serum theophylline	Ciprofloxacin can decrease metabolic clearance of theophylline; ofloxacin and temafloxacin less likely to decrease clearance. Monitor theophylline levels.
	Foscarnet	Increased risk of seizures	Monitor for seizures.
	Warfarin	Increased INR	Decreased warfarin metabolism. Monitor INR.
Cycloserine	Isoniazid,[a] ethionamide[a]	Increased CNS toxicity	Use cycloserine with caution in patients on INH or ethionamide.
Ethambutol	Aluminum salts	Decreased ethambutol absorption	Avoid coadministration.
Ethionamide	Cycloserine[a]	Increased CNS toxicity	Use cycloserine with caution in patients on ethionamide.
Isoniazid (INH)	Acetaminophen, carbamazepine, phenytoin	Decreased acetaminophen, carbamazepine, and phenytoin metabolism	Monitor phenytoin and carbamazepine serum levels.
	Aluminum salts	Decreased INH absorption	INH should be taken 1 hour before antacids containing aluminum.
	Corticosteroids	Increased INH metabolism	High doses of INH may be required.
	Cycloserine[a]	Increased CNS toxicity	Use cycloserine with caution in patients on INH.
	Ketoconazole	Increased metabolism	See ketoconazole (antifungal).
	Phenytoin	Increased serum levels of phenytoin	Monitor serum levels, look for signs of phenytoin toxicity.

(continued)

TABLE 108–5.   HIV Drug Interactions (continued)

	Interacting Drug	Effect	Comments
	Rifampin	Altered INH metabolism	Coadministration may result in increased hepatotoxicity. Monitor liver enzymes.
	Sulfonylureas	Hyperglycemia	INH may lead to loss of glucose control in patients on sulfonyl-ureas. Monitor blood sugar.
Rifampin, rifabutin	Dapsone, flucona-zole, ketocona-zole, methadone, oral contracep-tives, steroids, AZT, sulfonyl-ureas	Increased metabolism of drugs listed in Interacting Drugs; rifampin may precipitate acute withdrawal when given with methadone	Rifampin and rifabutin, to a lesser extent, induce hepatic micro-somal enzymes (cytochrome P450). Patients may require higher doses of drugs listed in Interacting Drugs when co-administered with rifampin or rifabutin. Consider increasing methadone dose by 10 mg every 1–2 d starting the day rifampin is added. Some patients may require a 50% dose increase. Split dosing may help.
	β-Adrenergic antagonists	Decrease β-adrenergic antagonist pharmacologic effect because increased hepatic metabolism from enzyme induction by rifampin	Monitor therapeutic response of β-adrenergic antagonists—may need to increase dose of β antagonists.

Antiopportunistic therapy
(PCP and toxoplasmosis therapy)

	Interacting Drug	Effect	Comments
Atovaquone (Mepron)	Phenytoin	Possible increased phenytoin levels	Both drugs are highly protein-bound and may displace each other.
Clindamycin (Cleocin)	Kaolin-pectin	Decreased clindamycin absorption	Administer kaolin-pectin 2 hours before clindamycin. Anti-diarrheal agents should not be used with clindamycin until *C. difficile* has been excluded as the cause of diarrhea.
Dapsone	AZT (ZDV)	Increased bone marrow toxicity	Monitor CBC frequently.
	ddl	Decreased dapsone absorption	Administer dapsone and ddl at least 2 hours apart.
	Probenecid	May decrease dapsone clearance	Clinical significance may be small because only 5–15% of the dapsone is excreted in the urine.
	Pyrimethamine/primaquine	Increased risk of hemolysis	Monitor CBC.
	H₂ receptor antagonists	Increased dapsone plasma concen-tration	Consider decreasing dapsone dosing; avoid H₂ receptor an-tagonists.
	Rifampin	Increased dapsone clearance	Higher doses of dapsone may be necessary.
	Trimethoprim	Decreased TMP clearance	The plasma concentrations of both drugs are increased when they are used together. Consider reducing the TMP dose in patients with anemia.
Pentamidine (IV)	Foscarnet[a]	Severe hypocalcemia; may increase risk of nephrotoxicity	Strongly consider alternatives before combining these drugs. Pretherapy hydration may reduce nephrotoxicity.
Pyrimethamine	AZT	Possible increased bone marrow suppression	Increased bone marrow suppression may occur during initial pyrimethamine therapy for toxoplasmosis. Consider holding AZT when using maximum pyrimethamine doses during acute therapy. Give folinic acid with pyrimethamine.
	TMP-SMX	Anemia	See TMP-SMX entry below.
Sulfadiazine	Sulfonylureas	increased hypoglycemia	Sulfonamides may potentiate hypoglycemic effects by displacing these agents from their protein-binding sites. Monitor serum glucose.
	Warfarin	Increased prothrombin time	Sulfonamides may potentiate the effects of warfarin by displac-ing it from its binding sites. Monitor INR.
TMP-SMX (Bactrim, Septra)	Pyrimethamine	Megaloblastic anemia	Additive inhibition of dihydrofolate reductase. Use together in low dosages. Monitor serum iron. Give folinic acid with pyrimethamine.
	Warfarin	Increased prothrombin time	TMP-SMX inhibits warfarin metabolic clearance. Monitor INR.

Protease inhibitors

	Interacting Drug	Effect	Comments
Indinavir	Amiodarone	Increased concentration of amiodarone; decreases meta-bolism of amiodarone	Contraindication.
Saquinavir	Cisapride	Potential life-threatening dys-rhythmias, increased concen-tration of antihistamines, in-creased cardiotoxicity	Concurrent administration is contraindicated.
	Ketoconazole	increased levels of protease inhibitors	

(continued)

TABLE 108–5. HIV Drug Interactions (continued)

	Interacting Drug	Effect	Comments
	Norvir (Ritonavir)	Inhibits P450 enzymes	
	Rifampin	Decreased levels of protease inhibitors	
Antiretroviral drugs			
Ampligen	AZT	See AZT	
	IFN-α	See Interferon-α	
Didanosine (ddI; Videx)	Antacids	Bioavailability of ddI increases because of increased stomach pH	May be advantageous, must be monitored.
	Dapsone	Decreased dapsone absorption	Administer dapsone and ddI at least 2 hours apart.
	Ganciclovir	Possible increased risk of pancreatitis (dose related)	These drugs can be used together with caution.
	H₂ receptor antagonists	Decreased serum concentration of ddI and ranitidine	
	Itraconazole	Decreased itraconazole absorption	
	Indinavir	Therapeutic effect of indinavir is decreased, buffers in ddI decrease the absorption of indinavir	
	Ketoconazole	Decreased ketoconazole absorption	The buffered ddI tablets raise gastric pH to enhance ddI absorption. Ketoconazole requires an acidic pH for absorption and should be given 2 hours before ddI.
	Pentamidine,[a] (IV) ddC[a]	Increased risk of pancreatitis	IV pentamidine, ddC, and ddI cause pancreatitis; hold ddI during acute PCP treatment with pentamidine; unknown clinical significance in combination therapy with ddC and ddI.
	Quinolones, tetracyclines	Decreased quinolone/tetracycline absorption	Quinolones and tetracyclines bind to cations (Al³⁺, Mg²⁺) in ddI buffer, decreasing their bioavailability. These antibiotics should be taken at least 2 hours before ddI.
Foscarnet (Foscavir)	Ciprofloxacin (see Ciprofloxacin)	Increased risk of seizure	
	Nephrotoxic agents[a]	Increased nephrotoxicity	Up to 50% of patients on foscarnet develop nephrotoxicity. Avoid coadministration with other nephrotoxic drugs. If coadministration is required, monitor BUN and serum creatinine three times weekly.
	Pentamidine[a] (IV)	Hypocalcemia, nephrotoxicity	See Pentamidine under Antiopportunistic Therapy.
Interferon-α	Ampligen	Increased in vitro antiretroviral activity	Clinical significance unknown.
	AZT	See AZT	
Ribavirin	AZT	See AZT	
Rifabutin	See Rifampin/ rifabutin under antimycobacterial therapy		
Zidovudine (AZT, ZDV; Retrovir)	Acetaminophen, aspirin, NSAIDs	Decreased AZT metabolism, possible increased bone marrow toxicity	Although increased bone marrow toxicity has occurred rarely, acetaminophen can be given with AZT. A multicenter trial failed to support an association between anemia and ASA or NSAID use with AZT.
	Acyclovir	Increased in vitro antiretroviral activity	Clinical significance unknown. Reports of improved survival with AZT and acyclovir are unsubstantiated. There is a single case report of neurotoxicity in a patient taking both AZT and acyclovir. Most experts think these drugs can be given together safely.
	Amphotericin B[a], dapsone[a]	Increased bone marrow toxicity, may increase AZT toxicity	Monitor CBC frequently.
	Atovaquone (Mepron)	Increased AZT serum concentration; potential toxicity appears to decrease the glucuronidation of AZT	Monitor AZT during concomitant use with Mepron.
	Interferon-α	Increased in vitro antiretroviral activity, increased AZT-related bone marrow toxicity	
	Interferon β	Serum AZT levels may decrease glucuronidation of AZT	Monitor. Lower dose of AZT may be needed.

(continued)

TABLE 108–5. HIV Drug Interactions (continued)

	Interacting Drug	Effect	Comments
	Clarithromycin	Decreased/increased AZT serum concentration, altered rate of absorption of AZT (usually increases rate of absorption of AZT)	
	Dipyridamole	Increased in vitro antiretroviral activity	Clinical significance unknown.
	Ganciclovir[a]	Increased bone marrow toxicity (neutropenia)	AZT should be held during induction therapy with ganciclovir but can be reinstituted with caution during maintenance. Hematopoietic growth factors may be necessary to treat neutropenia.
	Lamivudine	Increased AZT serum concentration	
	Methadone	Decreased AZT metabolism	No recommendation for dose change in patients on AZT and methadone; monitor for AZT toxicity when methadone is started or after methadone dose is increased.
	Phenytoin	Increased or decreased phenytoin levels, may inhibit zidovudine glucuronidation and zidovudine clearance	Monitor phenytoin levels.
	Probenecid	Decreased AZT metabolism and clearance	Clinical significance is probably small because only 19% of AZT is excreted in the urine.
	Ribavirin	Decreased in vitro antiretroviral activity, hematologic toxicity	Clinical significance unknown.
	Ritonavir	Increased AZT serum concentration	
	Sulfadiazine/ pyrimethamine	Decreased AZT clearance, increased bone marrow toxicity	AZT's half-life may double in patients receiving both agents. Clinical significance unknown. Consider holding AZT during initial therapy for toxoplasmosis and restarting when maintenance begins. Give folinic acid with pyrimethamine.
	TMP-SMX (Bactrim, Septra)	Possible increased anemia, neutropenia	Anemia and neutropenia are more common when AZT and high-dose TMP-SMX are combined. Consider withholding AZT during acute therapy for PCP with high-dose TMP-SMX. AZT may be taken with low-dose TMP-SMX for PCP prophylaxis.
Zalcitabine (ddC; Hivid)	Amphotericin B,[a] foscarnet[a]	Decreased renal clearance of ddC, may increase risk of pancreatitis and peripheral neuropathy	Discontinue use of ddC before starting these drugs.
	Dapsone, disulfiram, ethionamide, INH, phenytoin, ribavirin	Possible increased peripheral neuropathy	These drugs alone are associated with peripheral neuropathy; therefore do not combine them with ddC.
	ddI,[a] IV pentamidine[a]	Increased pancreatitis	Do not use these drugs concomitantly with ddC.
	Probenecid	Increased risk of zalcitabine toxicity	Toxicity: peripheral neuropathy, pancreatitis, lactic acidosis, hepatomegaly, hepatic failure. Monitor patient for adverse effects of zalcitabine; if they occur, decrease zalcitabine dose.

Antiviral Drugs

	Interacting Drug	Effect	Comments
Acyclovir (Zovirax)	Interferon-α	Increased antiviral activity in vitro	Clinical significance unknown.
	AZT		See AZT (antiretroviral drugs).
	Probenecid	30% Decreased acyclovir clearance	Consider reducing acyclovir dose.
Ganciclovir (Cytovene)	Amphotericin B,[a] antineoplastic agents,[a] 5-FC	Increased bone marrow toxicity	These agents inhibit replication of rapidly dividing cells and so increase bone marrow toxicity. Monitor closely for anemia and neutropenia.
	AZT	Neutropenia	See Zidovudine under Antiretroviral Drugs.
	ddI	Pancreatitis	See ddI under Antiretroviral Drugs.
	Imipenem/cilastatin	Increased CNS toxicity	Seizures.
	Probenecid	Decreased ganciclovir clearance	Clinical significance unknown. Monitor CBC frequently.

Herbs

	Interacting Drug	Effect	Comments
Compound Q	Antiretrovirals	Increased CNS toxicity	Unknown phenomenon.
Hypericin	Sympathomimetics	Possible hypertensive crisis	Hypericin is a weak MAO inhibitor. Clinical significance is unknown. Avoid combining these drugs.

Immunomodulators

	Interacting Drug	Effect	Comments
Disulfiram (Antabuse)	Alcohol	Severe GI and CNS toxicity	Avoid concomitant use.
Dithiocarb	Phenytoin, INH, warfarin	Decreased metabolism of Interacting Drugs	Monitor phenytoin level and prothrombin. Observe for signs of INH toxicity.

(continued)

TABLE 108–5. HIV Drug Interactions (*continued*)

	Interacting Drug	Effect	Comments
Flagyl	Cisplatin	Increased toxicity of cisplatin	
Interferon-α	Cardiovascular	Ventricular tachydysrhythmias	
(Roferon-A, Intron-A)	Gastrointestinal	Nausea, vomiting	
	Hematologic	Bone marrow suppression	
	Neurologic	Confusion, paresthesias	
	Pulmonary	Interstitial pneumonitis	
	Miscellaneous	Fever, chills, malaise	
N-Acetylcysteine	Disulfiram (Antabuse)	Decreased effect of tetracyclines	Unregulated form in use may be toxic.
	Dithiocarb	Decreased effect of penicillin G	

aCombinations with serious toxicity. This list is not exhaustive, and continuous updating is essential.
Modified, with permission, from Amodio-Groton M, Currier J: HIV drug interactions. AIDS Clin Care 1992;4:25–29.
For additional up to date HIV drug interactions see: http://www.hivatis.org

twice daily. Lamivudine has no significant toxicity. There is a minor interaction with TMP-SMX resulting in higher levels of lamivudine. No reports of overdose appear in the literature.

Abacavir. Abacavir (ABC; Ziagen), a guanosine analogue, is the most potent nucleoside analogue available.[33] It is primarily given in combination with AZT and lamivudine in a dosage of 300 mg twice daily. It is well absorbed orally and eliminated by hepatic metabolism. Cytochrome P450 enzymes are not responsible; consequently, there are no reports of drug interactions. Gastrointestinal side effects are common but insignificant. The most significant and potentially fatal toxicity is severe hypersensitivity reaction occurring in the first weeks of therapy.[33] Patients present acutely ill with fever, fatigue, vomiting, and abdominal pain. A rash may or may not be present. Patients should never be restarted on abacavir if previous hypersensitivity was documented or even suspected. There are no reports of overdose in the literature.

Non–Nucleoside Analogue Reverse Transcriptase Inhibitors

Nevirapine. Nevirapine (Viramune), a nonnucleoside reverse transcriptase inhibitor, (NNRTI) is approved by the FDA for use in combination with other antiviral agents. The NNRTI drugs are chemically different from the presently available nucleoside analogue RT inhibitors. The NNRTIs bind directly to the RT enzyme, causing allosteric inhibition of enzyme function.[98] Although nevirapine is a potent inhibitor of HIV, development of resistance is common when it is used as a single agent. It has excellent bioavailability and is specific to HIV. It is highly protein bound and extensively metabolized by the liver; consequently, dialysis is unlikely to be of benefit in removing this drug. The typical dose is 200 mg twice daily. Hypersensitivity reactions are common, necessitating gradual dosage escalation to avoid the rash.[33] Rash in association with constitutional symptoms and oral lesions requires drug discontinuation. Nevirapine induces hepatic cytochrome P450 enzymes, resulting in adverse drug interaction with protease inhibitors.[33] Overdose with this agent has not been reported in the literature.

Efavirenz. Efavirenz (Sustiva) is another potent NNRTI when used in conjunction with multiple antiretroviral agents. It has a prolonged half-life, and dosing is 600 mg daily. Pharmacokinetics and toxicity are similar in many ways to nevirapine. Transient CNS symptoms (dizziness and dysphoria) occur with initial treatment but gradually resolve.

Delavirdine. Delavirdine (Rescriptor) is another NNRTI and similar in activity and toxicity to nevirapine. The dose is 400 mg three times a day. Unlike the other NNRTIs, delavirdine decreases cytochrome P450 activity, resulting in increased concentrations of drugs eliminated by these enzymes. This is especially significant with concomitant use of protease inhibitors.

Protease (Proteinase) Inhibitors

The viral protease (proteinase) enzyme is essential for viral replication.[41] Inhibition of the protease leads to defective viral particles (see Fig. 108–1). These nonnucleoside protease inhibitors are valuable because they prevent viral replication even in chronically infected cells and prevent cell-to-cell transmission of HIV. No intracellular processing of the drug is needed here, as is the case with the nucleoside analogue RT inhibitors by cellular kinases. They all are rapidly absorbed and highly protein bound with an excellent bioavailability. All are metabolized via the hepatic P450 cytochromes, which accounts for the many drug–drug interactions. The inactive metabolite is fecally excreted. Toxicity profiles are similar for all agents with some gastrointestinal symptoms and rash[41] (see Table 108–3). An interesting unexplained phenomenon seen with patients on protease inhibitors is the abnormal distribution of fat.[41] Over time, patients develop central obesity, "buffalo hump," breast enlargement, cushingoid appearance, and peripheral wasting. Insulin resistance with resultant diabetes mellitus and increased bleeding in hemophiliacs may occur. The greatest concern is to avoid coadministration with certain antihistamines (astemizole), dopamine antagonists (metoclopramide), ergot derivatives (dihydroergotamine), or prokinetic agents (cisapride) because of the increased incidence of life-threatening cardiac dysrhythmias (torsades de pointes); and it is contraindicated to use with certain sedatives (midazolam and triazolam) because oversedation and confusion occur commonly. The protease inhibitors currently available in the United States are saquinavir, ritonavir, indinavir, nelfinavir, and amprenavir.

Saquinavir. Saquinavir (Fortovase, Invirase) is synergistic with RT inhibitors. Headache and liver enzyme abnormalities may occur with this drug.[41] Currently this drug is approved only in combination with RT inhibitors.

Ritonavir. Ritonavir (Norvir) has greater oral bioavailability than does saquinavir. Common adverse effects are circumoral paresthesias, altered taste, and liver enzyme and lipid abnormalities.[41] A report of concomitant use with MDMA (ecstasy) was fatal, suggesting that ritonavir decreased elimination of MDMA through inhibition of the P450 cytochrome system, as this is the principal pathway by which MDMA is metabolized.[3,51]

Indinavir. Indinavir (Crixivan), like ritonavir, has good bioavailability. Additional adverse effects are increased indirect bilirubin and nephrolithiasis of crystallized indinavir in 2 to 5% of treated patients.[41] There is a report of a moderate overdose (6000 mg, with the usual dose being 800 mg) that produced transient gastrointestinal distress and peripheral neuropathy.[13] The patient was managed conservatively and suffered no lasting sequelae.

Nelfinavir. Nelfinavir (Viracept) is similar to other protease inhibitors. It is a newer well-tolerated agent that may be given twice daily.

Amprenavir. Amprenavir (Agenerase) is similar to other protease inhibitors. It is a newer agent that is given twice daily. Rare cases of severe Stevens-Johnson syndrome have been reported.

Immunomodulators

Ampligen. Ampligen is a mismatched double-stranded RNA molecule with antiviral and immune-modulatory properties.[18] Ampligen belongs to the hybridon class of drugs, which are oligonucleosides that are complementary sequences to portions of the HIV genome. They affect transcription and translation by competitively inhibiting viral RNA and messenger RNA[18] and by promoting the production of interferons. Ampligen is synergistic with AZT and IFN-α.[28] Ampligen may serve a role in combination therapy with other retroviral agents.

At present there is little information on the absorption, pharmacokinetics, metabolism, elimination, and toxicity of ampligen. In doses of 250 mg twice a week there are no reports of clinically significant toxicity.[28] Some patients may develop influenzalike symptoms and flushing.

Disulfiram and Dithiocarb. Dithiocarb (diethyldithiocarbamate, DTC; Imuthiol), the major metabolite of disulfiram (Antabuse), may bolster depressed immune functions in HIV-infected patients by unknown mechanisms.[52] Although no clinical trials have evaluated disulfiram, the same benefit as with DTC is postulated. The majority of patients use disulfiram because of its easy access. Some have obtained the raw chemical DTC and make DTC enteric-coated capsules or enemas.

The principal toxicity from disulfiram and DTC occurs with concomitant ethanol ingestion (disulfiram or "Antabuse" reactions). The interaction causes varying degrees of facial flushing, headache, nausea, vomiting, respiratory difficulty, weakness, blurred vision, hypotension, and altered mental status (see Chap. 65).

Disulfiram treatment without alcohol use may cause drowsiness, lethargy, metallic taste, and abdominal discomfort. On very rare occasions hepatotoxicity, peripheral neuropathy, psychosis, and dementia develop.

Interferon-α. Interferons are host cell-derived cytokines that possess broad-spectrum antiviral and immune-modulating activity. There are three classes: α, β, and γ. They inhibit viral transcription, translation, assembly, and release. They stimulate T-cell-mediated cytotoxicity, natural killer cell activity, macrophage functions, and antibody synthesis.[74] Parenteral preparations of recombinant interferon-α (IFN-α Roferon-A, Intron-A) are somewhat effective treatments for the early stages of AIDS-associated Kaposi's sarcoma.[60] Oral preparations have not been proven effective, although they are readily available as alternative therapies (see Table 108–1).

Bioavailability for oral preparations of interferon-α is very poor. After intramuscular or subcutaneous injection, peak serum concentrations are achieved in 4 to 8 hours. The elimination half-life is approximately 3 to 5 hours. Interferon-α penetrates the CSF poorly and is thought to be eliminated via the kidneys.

Parenterally administered IFN-α often produces adverse effects. Many patients experience transient fever, malaise, chills, and lymphopenia. Nausea, vomiting, paresthesias, confusion, and bone marrow suppression are also common. In a recent case report, intravenous IFN-α caused an acute interstitial pneumonitis in a patient being treated for a recurrent multifocal hemangioendothelioma. This patient had received radiotherapy before the interferon-α therapy, and it is known that IFN-α is a potent radiosensitizer. The mechanism of the pneumonitis is unknown, and treatment is stopping of the IFN-α and supportive care.[104] The hematologic effects are dose dependent and reversible. Reversible cardiac dysfunction is also reported.[36] The bone marrow toxicity of IFN-α is synergistic with that of AZT (see Table 108–5). Overdosage is usually self-limited and should be treated supportively.

N-Acetylcysteine. Patients with HIV infection have a deficiency of intracellular glutathione, and cysteine precursors such as N-acetylcysteine (NAC; Mucomyst) seem to correct for this.[1] Glutathione is important to the cell not only for clearing reactive oxygen intermediates produced during drug metabolism but also for combating oxidative stress induced by inflammatory cytokines, normal immune responses that stimulate HIV replication.[83] Tumor necrosis factor (TNF) levels are high in advanced HIV infection, and NAC blocks TNF. Because of the high cost of prescription N-acetylcysteine, buyers' clubs provide their own brand of NAC of unmeasured quality.

The pharmacokinetics of NAC are discussed in Chap. 32. There is little toxicity from use of the correct dose of the prescription drug. Some patients experience nausea and vomiting; rarely, fever and rash occur. Experience with the nonprescription form of NAC is limited.

Medicinal Herbs

Hypericin. Hypericin (pseudohypericin) is an anthraquinone dimer extracted from the plant *Hypericin triquetrifoltan* that has in vitro activity against HIV by either reverse transcriptase inhibition[85] or blockade of viral assembly or budding.[68] A herbal preparation (St. John's wort, a combination of several herbs) is available through buyers' clubs. The amount of active hypericin in this compound is low and of doubtful efficacy.

Very little is known about the pharmacokinetics of hypericin and St. John's wort. Photosensitization is the principal toxicity, and it can be severe. Moreover, patients are taking large doses of the herbal preparation while the full toxic effects remain unknown.

Hypericin's antiretroviral activity appears to be synergistic with AZT.[85] It is a mild monoamine oxidase inhibitor, and drug interactions with sympathomimetic agents are possible (see Table 108–5). For all of these reasons, this drug should not be used in combination with other drug treatments.

Trichosanthin. Trichosanthin (GLQ223) is derived from the Chinese plant *Trichosanthin kirilowii;* it exhibits potent inhibitory activity against HIV through inactivation of viral ribosomes and may be efficacious.[65] Extracts are fairly easy to obtain, and some patients are using these herbal preparations (known as compound Q). Trichosanthin has poor oral bioavailability and causes intense diarrhea when taken orally. It is therefore administered intramuscularly or intravenously.

The pharmacokinetics are unknown, but the toxicity profile is well reported.[56,99] Parenteral administration is often associated with severe neurotoxicity; approximately 24 to 72 hours after administration, some patients develop an acute encephalomyelitis manifested by fever, myalgia, paresis, delirium, dementia, and coma. This syndrome is more likely to develop when GLQ223–15 is used with other antiretroviral agents and is usually self-limiting and reversible. Hypersensitivity reactions ranging from rashes to anaphylaxis are common, and premedication with prostaglandin inhibitors is usually required.[64] Hypoglycemia also may occur.

Coma secondary to compound Q usually occurs less than 1 week after IV infusion. Whether combination therapy will result in delayed CNS toxicity has not been determined.

Antivirals

Acyclovir. Acyclovir (Zovirax) is a synthetic purine nucleoside analogue. It requires intracellular phosphorylation mediated by thymidine kinase to convert it to its active form, acyclovir triphosphate, which inhibits viral reverse transcriptase and thus terminates viral DNA synthesis. Acyclovir is used principally in the treatment of herpes simplex virus (HSV) and varicella-zoster virus (VZV) infections. Acyclovir is available in oral, IV, and topical preparations. It is poorly absorbed, with an oral bioavailability of approximately 15 to 30%.[34] Recommended oral doses achieve peak serum concentrations in 1.5 hours.[34] Excellent CSF concentrations (50% of serum) are achieved. It is eliminated, 90% unchanged, in the urine by glomerular filtration and tubular secretion. The half-life of acyclovir is 2.5 hours with normal renal function and 20 hours with end-stage renal disease. Acyclovir is adsorbed to activated charcoal and is dialyzable. The usual dosage is 200 to 800 mg orally five times daily or 10 to 12 mg/kg IV three times daily.

Acyclovir has a relatively low toxicity at recommended doses. The most common adverse reactions are nausea, vomiting, and headache. Intravenous use may cause acute renal dysfunction and encephalopathy. Rapid IV infusion can result in acyclovir crystalluria and subsequent acute tubular necrosis and renal failure. Renal deposition is easily preventable by slow infusion over 1 hour. Encephalopathy manifests as lethargy, confusion, hallucinations, delirium, tremors, seizures, and/or coma. It is encountered with high-dose administration and generally resolves with discontinuation of the drug.[34] Prolonged use has been reported to cause neutropenia and thrombocytopenia.[46] Probenecid decreases renal clearance of acyclovir, and acyclovir potentiates the in vitro antiviral effect of AZT. Because the toxicity from oral acyclovir is minimal, even in overdose, standard overdose management utilizing activated charcoal is recommended.

Ganciclovir. Ganciclovir (DHPG; Cytovene) is a nucleoside analogue used in the treatment of serious cytomegalovirus (CMV) infection. It is structurally similar to acyclovir but is 50 times more active against CMV.[97] Ganciclovir utilizes cellular kinases for conversion to its active triphosphate form, as CMV lacks the gene for thymidine kinase. Ganciclovir triphosphate acts to inhibit viral DNA replication.[37]

Ganciclovir is available orally, intravenously, intravitreally, and via a sustained-release intraocular device. The oral preparation is approved for prevention of CMV and advanced HSV infection, whereas all other preparations are for treatment of active CMV infection. With the usual IV dosage (5 mg/kg) the peak plasma levels are approximately 6 to 15 µg/mL, and the serum half-life is 2.9 hours.[37] The drug is excreted almost entirely unmetabolized by the kidneys.[37]

Toxicity frequently limits therapy with ganciclovir. Almost all patients using the drug experience some form of hematologic toxicity.[11,24] Leukopenia often necessitates lowering the dose. Anemia and thrombocytopenia are also common.[37] Azotemia is commonly seen and requires dosage adjustments. Nausea, vomiting, abnormal liver function tests, diarrhea, confusion, seizures, headaches, and dizziness are less frequent.[37]

Adverse reactions are dose dependent and exacerbated by renal dysfunction. The toxicity from ganciclovir is usually reversible with dosage reduction or discontinuance of the drug and supportive care. There are reports that the hematologic toxicity may be fatal.[37] Agents such as G-CSF and GM-CSF significantly decrease the hematologic toxicity of ganciclovir.

Cidofovir. Cidofovir (1,3-hydroxy-2-phosphonylmethoxypropylcytosine, HPMPC, Vistide) is a newer potent viral DNA polymerase inhibitor effective against ganciclovir-resistant CMV. It is administered intravenously and eliminated through glomerular filtration and renal tubular secretion. It must be administered with probenecid. Nephrotoxicity is common, dose dependent, and potentially life-threatening. Patients may experience fevers, headache, amnesia, anxiety, confusion, seizures, gastrointestinal upset, abnormal taste, cough, and neutropenia. Hemodialysis and probenecid should reduce plasma concentrations in the event of an overdose.

Foscarnet. Foscarnet (phosphonoformate; Foscavir), a pyrophosphate analogue, is a viral DNA polymerase inhibitor and NNRTI. It is active against a number of herpes viruses and retroviruses, but its greatest clinical use has been for resistant herpes simplex virus (HSV) infection and cytomegalovirus (CMV) retinitis. Foscarnet may prolong the lives of HIV-infected patients.[3] Rapid emergence of viral resistance has limited its usefulness in HIV infection. Foscarnet may have its greatest utility in combination with AZT, ddI, or ddC.[22]

Foscarnet is very poorly absorbed, with an oral bioavailability of 12 to 22%, and is poorly tolerated because of GI toxicity.[90] Consequently, IV administration is required to yield therapeutic concentrations of the drug. The plasma half-life is 3 hours, and it penetrates the CSF (13 to 68% of plasma).[89] Foscarnet is cleared principally by the kidneys (80%), with 20% deposited in bone. The recommended initial dose is 60 mg/kg IV every 8 hours for 2 to 3 weeks, followed by a 90 to 120 mg/kg per day maintenance dose. Foscarnet is dialyzable.

Renal toxicity is the major dose-limiting adverse effect. A decrease in creatinine clearance is common.[89] Nephrogenic diabetes insipidus[38] and acute renal failure[15] are reported. Common electrolyte abnormalities include hypocalcemia, hypophosphatemia, hypokalemia, and hypomagnesemia. Foscarnet should not be administered with IV pentamidine because of increased risk of hypocalcemia (see Table 108–5).

Fatigue, malaise, headache, nausea, and vomiting are common and are dose-related effects.[89] Severe neurotoxicity, with seizures and coma, is seen in about 10% of cases and is directly related to overdosage and electrolyte abnormalities. Genital and oral ulceration[43] and fixed drug eruptions[25] are rare adverse effects. Bone marrow toxicity, manifested by anemia, is rarely encountered.

Several cases of unintentional overdose have resulted in renal and neurotoxicity. The majority of patients were treated supportively with hydration and replacement of electrolyte deficiencies. Hemodialysis may be of benefit.

Ribavirin.   Ribavirin possesses broad-spectrum antiviral activity against many RNA and DNA viruses. It inhibits HIV replication at relatively high concentrations (50 μg/mL), levels at which it can interfere with host cell RNA and DNA synthesis.[32] At present, ribavirin is approved for use only in an aerosolized form (Virazole) for the treatment of respiratory syncytial virus infections. Although there is no evidence that oral ribavirin is clinically effective in HIV infection,[81] it remains available through buyers' clubs. Ribavirin's mechanism of action is poorly understood and differs depending on the class of virus.[29] This drug appears to inhibit viral protein production by inhibiting messenger RNA and viral-coded RNA polymerases.

Ribavirin is incompletely absorbed from the GI tract, with an oral bioavailability of 45%. In oral doses of 600 to 2400 mg it reaches peak serum concentrations (5.1 to 12.6 μmol/L) in 1.5 hours.[61] Significant CSF concentration can be achieved after prolonged administration.[28] The metabolism of ribavirin is incompletely understood. Ribavirin accumulates in RBCs and achieves concentrations approximately ninefold greater than that in the serum.[29] The drug is phosphorylated to triphosphate nucleotides, which are polar and become trapped in RBCs. Renal excretion accounts for approximately one-third of the drug's elimination.[29] The serum half-life is 9 hours, and the RBC half-life is 40 days.

Toxicity from ribavirin is dose dependent. Low-dose (600 mg/d) ribavirin is not associated with any toxicity, even in those who are very symptomatic with HIV infection.[74] In doses approaching 2400 mg/d, however, patients may experience nausea, vomiting, fatigue, and headache.[29] The most significant toxicity seen at these or higher doses is a normochromic, normocytic anemia caused by rapid extravascular RBC clearance.[32] Very high doses can result in bone marrow suppression with resultant aplastic anemia.[32] Ribavirin has antagonistic effects on HIV replication when used in conjunction with AZT.[61] Overdoses are best treated conservatively with supportive care.

Cytokines.   Erythropoietin (EPO; Epogen, Procrit), G-CSF (Leukine, Prokine), and GM-CSF (Neupogen) are recombinant glycoproteins that stimulate hematopoietic cell growth and maturation.[66] These agents are available only in parenteral forms and are well tolerated. Erythropoietin may cause hypertension and predisposes to increased thrombosis. Use of G-CSF is associated with fever, myalgia, flushing, and phlebitis as well as mild azotemia and elevated transaminases. Use of GM-CSF may cause bone pain.

AGENTS EFFECTIVE AGAINST OPPORTUNISTIC INFECTIONS

Pneumocystis carinii Pneumonia and Toxoplasmosis Therapy

Trimethoprim-Sulfamethoxazole   Trimethoprim-sulfamethoxazole (TMP-SMX, cotrimoxazole; Bactrim, Septra) is commonly used for the treatment and prophylaxis of *Pneumocystis carinii* pneumonia (PCP) and prophylaxis against toxoplasmosis.[17] It is well absorbed and reaches a peak serum concentration in 1 to 4 hours. Both components are protein bound (44 and 70%, respectively). TMP-SMX is metabolized in the liver through a number of pathways and excreted via the kidneys through both glomerular filtration and tubular secretion. The serum half-life is approximately 10 hours.

There is a high incidence of adverse reactions associated with the use of TMP-SMX in HIV-infected patients. Nausea and vomiting are almost unavoidable, and virtually all HIV-infected patients who use this drug experience some degree of hypersensitivity manifested by various rashes, fever, leukopenia, thrombocytopenia, myelosuppression, nephritis, and hepatitis. With high doses, TMP induces hyperkalemia through sodium channel inhibition in the distal tubule.[21] These adverse effects are dose dependent and usually do not require discontinuance of treatment.[5,63] Adverse neurologic reactions rarely occur but include headaches, depression, hallucination, focal seizures, ataxia, and tremor. General toxicologic management is indicated for TMP-SMX overdose. TMP-SMX increases AZT and lamivudine levels.

Sulfadoxine-Pyrimethamine.   Sulfadoxine-pyrimethamine (Fansidar) is sometimes used for PCP prophylaxis. The drug has a very prolonged half-life (7 to 9 days). Severe, potentially fatal, cutaneous reactions such as erythema multiforme, Stevens-Johnson syndrome,[73] and toxic epidermal necrolysis[78] have occurred.

Sulfadiazine, used to treat toxoplasmosis, may induce acute renal failure secondary to sulfadiazine crystalluria with stone formation. This condition is usually associated with dehydration, which is increasingly common in AIDS-related diarrheal conditions. Hypersensitivity reactions such as fever, rashes, and leukopenia are common.

Dapsone.   Dapsone, used for the treatment and prophylaxis of PCP and prevention of toxoplasmosis, is associated with a number of adverse effects. Anorexia, nausea, and vomiting frequently occur. Fever, rash, and a mononucleosislike syndrome may occur. Neurologic toxicity is manifested as headache, nervousness, insomnia, blurred vision, paresthesia, peripheral neuropathy, and psychosis. There are reports of eosinophilic pneumonia caused by dapsone.[54] Hemolytic anemia and methemoglobinemia are the major adverse effects of dapsone. Hemolysis occurs in the setting of glucose-6-phosphate dehydrogenase (G6PD) deficiency. Dapsone-induced methemoglobinemia is the most consequential toxicity in AIDS patients who are already compromised by anemia and hypoxemia.[80,88] Obtaining a methemoglobin level and CBC is mandatory. Treatment with standard GI decontamination with multiple-dose activated charcoal and methylene blue has been successful for methemoglobinemia (Chap. 31 and Antidotes in Depth: Methylene Blue).

Pentamidine. Pentamidine (Pentam) is frequently used for the treatment and prophylaxis of PCP. Toxic effects are common (approximately 50%).[8] The drug is administered parenterally and by aerosol. Inhaled pentamidine is well tolerated, although some patients develop bronchospasm, which responds well to bronchodilator agents. The vast majority of adverse effects are seen with parenteral usage.

Anorexia, nausea, metallic taste, orthostatic hypotension, hypoglycemia followed by hyperglycemia, hepatitis, dysrhythmias, azotemia, leukopenia, and thrombocytopenia are observed in various combinations in most patients.[8] Severe hypotension occurs when the drug is administered too rapidly. Torsades de pointes can occur, and therefore an ECG should be obtained before administration of pentamidine.[102] Hypoglycemia followed by hyperglycemia is the direct result of toxic injury to the insulin-producing pancreatic islet β cells.[8] This results in inappropriately high insulin levels and subsequent hypoglycemia. Several days to months later, diabetes mellitus develops. Severe hypocalcemia results from coadministration with foscarnet. Frequently there is a mild elevation in creatinine; rarely, renal failure ensues.

In a recent case report a patient received 40 times the prescribed dose of IV pentamidine as the result of a pharmacy mixing error. Severe hypotension persisted, and a pressor was necessary to maintain blood pressure. Charcoal hemoperfusion was performed over a 4-hour period. Pentamidine levels fell during hemoperfusion; however, reaccumulation occurred in the serum because of release of drug from tissue stores. The authors observed that the blood pressure stabilized during hemoperfusion, but they were uncertain as to the direct contribution of this modality to clinical improvement.[101]

Atovaquone. Atovaquone (Mepron) is another drug for treatment prophylaxis for PCP[53] and toxoplasmosis.[58] The oral bioavailability is low, but administration with food greatly increases absorption. It is highly protein bound (99%) and is recirculated in the enterohepatic system with eventual fecal excretion. None of the drug is excreted by the kidneys. Toxicity is limited to mild rashes, leukopenia, anemia, and elevated transaminases.

Antifungal Drugs

Amphotericin B. Amphotericin B (AmB; Fungizone) remains an important treatment for a number of serious systemic fungal infections. Unfortunately, its administration is associated with systemic toxicity.[9] During IV administration, fevers, chills, rigors, vomiting, and headaches often occur. Premedication with hydrocortisone, NSAIDs, and diphenhydramine greatly reduces these forms of toxicity. Renal impairment is the most significant adverse effect. Azotemia, observed in approximately 80% of cases,[9] is dose dependent and reversible with dosage reduction. A type I (distal) renal tubular acidosis may occur (Chap. 23). Amphotericin B should not be given with other nephrotoxic agents. Anemia secondary to reduced erythropoietin is common. Leukopenia and thrombocytopenia are rare. Concurrent administration with AZT results in greater bone marrow toxicity. Earlier preparations of amphotericin B were associated with ventricular fibrillation during infusion.

Flucytosine. Flucytosine (5-FC; Ancobon) is often used in conjunction with amphotericin B. The drug's principal toxicity is bone marrow suppression. Severe reversible leukopenia and anemia often limit use.

Ketoconazole. Ketoconazole (Nizoral) is an imidazole used in the treatment of mucocutaneous candidiasis and maintenance therapy for coccidioidomycosis and histoplasmosis. The drug is absorbed erratically (oral bioavailability is 75%). Absorption is impaired by antacids and H_2 blockers.[94] Ketoconazole has a short half-life (2 to 8 hours) and is highly protein bound (>90%).[94] Minimal CSF penetration limits its utility in CNS mycoses. The usual dose is 200 to 400 mg/d. Anorexia, nausea, and vomiting are the principal toxic reactions. Paresthesias, thrombocytopenia, and mild hepatitis may occur. Ketoconazole suppresses testosterone and cortisol synthesis. Isoniazid and rifampin increase ketoconazole metabolism. Ketoconazole decreases astemizole (Hismanal) metabolism, and coadministration may result in life-threatening dysrhythmias. Didanosine decreases the antifungal effect of ketoconazole. Ketoconazole increases the levels of saquinavir by threefold.

Fluconazole. Fluconazole (Diflucan) is a triazole used in the treatment of serious *Candida* infections and CNS mycoses (cryptococcosis and coccidioidomycosis). Fluconazole has a high oral bioavailability (>90%), long serum half-life (30 hours), low protein binding (12%), and excellent CSF penetration (60 to 80%).[10] Renal excretion accounts for more than 90% of the drug's metabolism; dosage adjustments are required in patients with renal disease.[10] The usual dose is 100 to 400 mg/d.

Fluconazole is minimally toxic with standard dosing. Gastrointestinal upset, rashes, dizziness, and headache are the most common adverse reactions.[82] Rare episodes of anemia, seizures, or hepatitis are reported, but they occur in patients with advanced HIV disease who were taking multiple drugs and resolve with discontinuation of fluconazole.[82]

Itraconazole. Itraconazole (Sporanox) is an oral triazole used in the treatment of serious non-CNS fungal infections (histoplasmosis, blastomycosis, and coccidioidomycosis). On an empty stomach, the drug has an oral bioavailability of 85%; it is highly protein bound (>90%).[94] Absorption is impaired by antacids and H_2 blockers. Itraconazole is metabolized in the liver to inactive metabolites. It is widely distributed in the body, with therapeutic tissue levels at sites of fungal infection.[94] The standard dosage is 100 to 400 mg/d. The toxic profile is similar to that of ketoconazole. Itraconazole interferes weakly with the cytochrome P450 (CYP3A4) enzyme system, so it will decrease the metabolism of cyclosporine, digoxin, astemizole, and terfenadine. Rifampin, phenytoin, and carbamazepine increase the elimination of itraconazole and may result in treatment failures.

Antimycobacterial Therapy

Rifabutin. Rifabutin (Mycobutin), a rifamycin S derivative, inhibits DNA-dependent RNA polymerase and is approved for prophylactic therapy for *Mycobacterium avium* complex (MAC) and is also used in combination therapy for MAC.

Rifabutin is well absorbed from the GI tract, with peak serum levels of 0.49 μg/mL occurring 4 hours after administration.[74] The serum half-life is 16 hours; the intracellular half-life is 10 times higher.[74] Rifabutin is principally eliminated in the bile, where enterohepatic circulation results in progressive deacetylation. One of the metabolites (25-deacetylrifabutin) retains the same biologic activity as the parent drug.[74] Rifabutin is adsorbed to activated charcoal and is dialyzable. The recommended dosage of rifabutin is 300 mg/d.

Rifabutin has a relatively mild toxicity profile. Gastrointestinal upset with nausea, vomiting, and diarrhea are common. Clinically insignificant hepatotoxicity is manifest by elevated aminotransferases, bilirubin, and alkaline phosphatase. Neutropenia and thrombocytopenia may occur. Various hypersensitivity reactions (rash and fever) are reported. Rifabutin stimulates cytochrome P450 microsomal enzymes, which may increase metabolism of certain drugs, especially drugs like AZT. Conversely, ritonavir causes elevation of rifabutin levels, resulting in toxicity[19] (see Table 108–5).

A patient who overdoses with rifabutin should be treated supportively. Induction of emesis is usually not necessary and may be contraindicated because of the frequency of vomiting associated with overdose. Intravenous hydration and activated charcoal are the standard of care. Hemodialysis and charcoal hemoperfusion might be useful in severe overdose where supportive therapy is not adequate.

Clarithromycin. Clarithromycin (Biaxin) is a macrolide analogue of erythromycin with broad-spectrum antimicrobial activity against MAC. It is used both for prophylaxis and in combination with other drugs in treatment of MAC. It is acid stable with an oral bioavailability of 85%.[47] The majority of the drug is metabolized by the liver to an active 14-hydroxyl metabolite. Approximately 20 to 30% of the drug is renally excreted unchanged. The parent compound and metabolite have serum half-lives of 2 to 6 hours and 2 to 9 hours, respectively.[47] The usual dose for MAC disease is 500 to 1000 mg twice a day. Clarithromycin is better tolerated than erythromycin, with less GI upset. Headache and dizziness occur rarely. Reversible dose-related hearing loss has occurred in patients treated for MAC infection. Clarithromycin, like all macrolide antibiotics except for azithromycin, inhibits cytochrome P450 hepatic metabolism and consequently decreases elimination of theophylline, carbamazepine, cyclosporine, warfarin, corticosteroids, and ergotamine. Combination with ergots may precipitate signs of ergotism (Chap. 45).

Azithromycin. Azithromycin (Zithromax) is another macrolide with a spectrum similar to that of clarithromycin. The oral bioavailability is 37%.[47] It has wide tissue distribution with very low serum concentrations and is extensively metabolized by the liver, with only 5% excreted unchanged by the kidneys.[47] The toxicity profile and drug interactions are unlike those of clarithromycin because it does not inhibit CYP3A4.

SUMMARY

As the HIV pandemic continues, new drugs are being formulated and used, mostly in combination. With the multiple-organ-system disease that HIV creates and with its effect on drug metabolism, many adverse and potentially fatal reactions have been reported. With recognition of various toxidromes and understanding management strategies, it is the hope that a decrease in morbidity and mortality will occur.

REFERENCES

1. Abrams DI: Alternative therapies. In: Sande MA, Volberding PA, eds: The Medical Management of AIDS, 6th ed. Philadelphia, WB Saunders, 1999, pp. 601–612.
2. Ahluwalia G, Johnson MA, Friedland A, et al: Cellular pharmacology of the anti-HIV agent 2,3-dideoxyadenosine [abstract]. In: Proceedings of the American Association of Cancer Research, New Orleans, May 1988, vol. 29. Baltimore, Waverly, 1988, p. 349.
3. AIDS Trials Group: Mortality in patients with the acquired immunodeficiency syndrome treated with either foscarnet or ganciclovir for cytomegalovirus retinitis. N Engl J Med 1992;326:213–220.
4. Atkinson JH, Capaldini L, Levine JF, et al: Dementia, depression and quality of life. Patient Care 1996;131–143.
5. Beall G, Sanwo M, Hussain H: Allergic disease in AIDS: Drug reactions and desensitization in AIDS, Immun Allergy Clin North Am 1997;17:319–338.
6. Berning SE, Huitt GA, Iseman MD, et al: Malabsorption of antituberculosis medication by a patient with AIDS. N Engl J Med 1992;327:1817–1818.
7. Besson LJ, Greene JB, Louie E, et al: Severe polymyositis-like syndrome associated with zidovudine therapy of AIDS and ARC [letter]. N Engl J Med 1988;318:708.
8. Bouchard P, Sai P, Reach G, et al: Diabetes mellitus following pentamidine-induced hypoglycemia in humans. Diabetes 1982;31:40–45.
9. Bowler WA, Oldfield EC III: New approaches to amphotericin B administration. Infect Med 1992;9:17–23.
10. Brammer KW, Farrow PR, Faulkner JK: Pharmacokinetics and tissue penetration of fluconazole in humans. Rev Infect Dis 1990;12(Suppl 3):S318–S326.
11. Buhles WC Jr, Mastre BJ, Tinker AJ, et al: Ganciclovir treatment of life- or sight-threatening cytomegalovirus infection: Experience in 314 immunocompromised patients. Rev Infect Dis 1988;10(Suppl 3):S495–S506.
12. Burger DM, Rege AB, Greenspan DL, et al: Pharmacokinetic interaction between rifampin and zidovudine. Antimicrob Agents Chemother 1993;37:1426.
13. Burkhart KK, Kemerer K, Donovan JW: Indinavir overdose. J Toxicol Clin Toxicol 1998;36:747.
14. Byar DP, Schoenfeld DA, Green SB, et al: Design considerations for AIDS trials. N Engl J Med 1990;323:1343–1348.
15. Cacoub P, Deray G, Baumelou A, et al: Acute renal failure induced by foscarnet: 4 cases. Clin Nephrol 1988;29:315–318.
16. Capaldini L: Psychosocial issues and psychiatric complications of HIV disease. In: Sande MA, Volberding PA, eds: The Medical Management of AIDS, 6th ed. Philadelphia, WB Saunders, 1999, pp. 241–263.
17. Carr A, Tindall B, Brew BS, et al: Low dose trimethoprim-sulfamethoxazole prophylaxis for toxoplasmic encephalitis in patients with AIDS. Ann Intern Med 1992;117:106–111.
18. Carter WA, Brodsky I, Pellegrino MG: Clinical, immunological, and virological effects of ampligen, a mismatched double stranded RNA, in patients with AIDS or AIDS-related complex. Lancet 1987;1:1286–1292.
19. Cato A III, Cavanaugh J, Shi H, et al: The effect of multiple doses of ritonavir on the pharmacokinetics of rifabutin. Clin Pharmacol Ther 1998;63:414–421.
20. Centers for Disease Control and Prevention: HIV/AIDS Surveillence Report; Mid-year 2000 Edition, Vol. 12, No. 1. MMWR 2000;46:861.
21. Choi MJ, Fernandez PC, Patnaik A, et al: Brief report: Trimethoprim-induced hyperkalemia in a patient with AIDS. N Engl J Med 1993;328:703–704.
22. Chow YK, Hirsch MS, Merril DP, et al: Use of evolutionary limitations of HIV-1 multidrug resistance to optimize therapy. Nature 1993;361:650–654.

23. Cohn J, Shapiro C, Keyes C, Smothers K: Neurologic disease associated with zidovudine [AZT (ZDV)] [abstract]. Presented at the 27th ICAAC, Washington, DC, 1987, p. 381.

24. Collaborative DHPG Treatment Study Group: Treatment of serious cytomegalovirus infections with 9-(1,3-dihydroxy-2-propoxymethyl) guanine in patients with AIDS and other immunodeficiencies. N Engl J Med 1986;314:801–805.

25. Connolly GM, Gazzard BG, Hawkins DA: Fixed drug eruption due to foscarnet. Genitour Med 1990;66:97–98.

26. Coopman SA, Johnson RA, Platt R: Cutaneous disease and drug reactions in HIV infection. N Engl J Med 1993;328:1670–1674.

27. Cote TR, Biggar RJ, Dannenberg AL: Risk of suicide among persons with AIDS. JAMA 1992;268:2066–2068.

28. Crumpacker KS, Bubley G, Hussey S, Connor J: Ribavirin enters cerebral spinal fluid. Lancet 1986;2:45–46.

29. Crumpacker KS, Heagy W, Bubley G, et al: Ribavirin treatment of the acquired immunodeficiency syndrome (AIDS) and acquired immunodeficiency syndrome–related complex (ARC). Ann Intern Med 1987;107:664–674.

30. Dalakas MC, Illa I, Pezeshkpour GH, et al: Mitochondrial myopathy caused by long-term zidovudine therapy. N Engl J Med 1990; 322:1098–1105.

31. Dannenberg AL, McNeil JG, Brundage JF, et al: Suicide and HIV infection mortality follow-up of 4147 HIV-seropositive military service applicants. JAMA 1996;276:1743–1746.

32. DeClerq E: Perspectives for the chemotherapy of AIDS. Anticancer 1987;7:1023–1038.

33. Deeks SG, Volberding PA: Antiretroviral therapy: In: Sande MA, Volberding PA, eds: The Medical Management of AIDS, 6th ed. Philadelphia, WB Saunders, 1999, pp. 97–115.

34. DeMiranda P, Blum MR: Pharmacokinetics of acyclovir after intravenous and oral administration. J Antimicrob Chemother 1983;12 (Suppl B):29–37.

35. DeRay G, Diquet B, Martinez F, et al: Pharmacokinetics of zidovudine in a patient on maintenance hemodialysis. N Engl J Med 1988; 319:1606–1607.

36. Deyton LR, Walker RE, Kovacs JA, et al: Reversible cardiac dysfunction associated with interferon alfa therapy in AIDS patients with Kaposi's sarcoma. N Engl J Med 1989;321:1246–1249.

37. Drew WL: Antiviral therapy of CMV infection. AIDS Reader 1993; 3:99–104.

38. Farese RV, Schambelan M, Hollander H, et al: Nephrogenic diabetes insipidus associated with foscarnet treatment of cytomegalovirus retinitis. Ann Intern Med 1990;112:955–956.

39. Fischl M, Galpin JE, Levine JD, et al: Recombinant human erythropoietin for patients with AIDS treated with zidovudine. N Engl J Med 1990;322:1488–1493.

40. Fischl MA, Parker CB, Pettinelli C, et al: A randomized controlled trial of a reduced dose of zidovudine in patients with acquired immunodeficiency syndrome. N Engl J Med 1990;323:1009–1014.

41. Flexner C: HIV-protease inhibitors. N Engl J Med 1998;338: 1281–1292.

42. Furman PA, Fyfe JA, St Clair MH, et al: Phosphorylation of 3′-azido-3′-deoxythymidine and selective interaction of the 5′-triphosphate with human immunodeficiency virus reverse transcriptase. Proc Natl Acad Sci USA 1986;83:8333–8337.

43. Gilquin J, Weiss L, Kazatchkine MD: Genital and oral erosions induced by foscarnet [letter]. Lancet 1990;1:287.

44. Gold JWM: The diagnosis and management of HIV infection. In: Gold JWM, Telzak EE, White DA, eds: The Diagnosis and Management of the HIV-Infected Patient, Part 1. Med Clin North Am 1996; 80:1283–1307.

45. Greene WC: The molecular biology of human immunodeficiency virus type I infection. N Engl J Med 1991;324:308–317.

46. Grella M, Ofosu JR, Klein BL: Prolonged oral acyclovir administration associated with neutropenia and thrombocytopenia. Am J Emerg Med 1998;16:396–398.

47. Guay DRP: Pharmacokinetic of new macrolides. Infect Med 1992;9 (Suppl A):9–13.

48. Harb GE, Jacobson MA: Human immunodeficiency virus (HIV) infection: Does it increase susceptibility to adverse drug reactions? Drug Saf 1993;9:1–8.

49. Hardy WD: The human immunodeficiency virus. In: Gold JWM, Telzak EE, White DA, eds: The diagnosis and management of the HIV-infected patient, part I. Med Clin North Am 1996;80: 1239–1263.

50. Hargreaves M, Fuller G, Costello C, Gazzard B: Zidovudine overdose [letter]. Lancet 1988;2:509.

51. Henry JA, Hill IR: Fatal interaction between ritonavir and MDMA. Lancet 1998;352:1751–1752.

52. Hersh EM: Dithiocarb sodium (diethyldithiocarbamate) therapy in patients with symptomatic HIV infection and AIDS. JAMA 1991; 265:1538–1544.

53. Hughes W, Leoung G, Kramer F: Comparison of atovaquone (566C80) with trimethoprim-sulfamethoxazole to treat Pneumocystis carinii pneumonia in patients with AIDS. N Engl J Med 1993;328: 1521–1527.

54. Jaffuel D, Lebel B, Hillaire-Buys D, et al: Drug points: Eosinophilic pneumonia induced by dapsone. BMJ 1998;317:181.

55. Jones LJ, DeCock KM, Jaffe HW: Current trends in the epidemiology of HIV/AIDS. In: Sande MA, Volberding PA, eds: The Medical Management of AIDS, 6th ed. Philadelphia, WB Saunders, 1999, pp. 3–22.

56. Kahn J, Kaplan L, Gambertoglio J, et al: A phase I study of GLQ223 in subjects with AIDS and ARC. Paper presented at the VI International Conference on AIDS, San Francisco, June, 1990.

57. Klecker RW, Collins JM, Yarchoan R, et al: Plasma and cerebrospinal fluid pharmacokinetics of 3′-azido-3′-deoxythymidine: A novel pyrimidine analog with potential application for the treatment of patients with AIDS and related diseases. Clin Pharmacol Ther 1987;41:407–412.

58. Kovacs JA: Efficacy of atovaquone in treatment of toxoplasmosis in patients with AIDS. Lancet 1992;2:637–638.

59. Lambert JS, Seidlin M, Reichman RC, et al: 2′,3′-dideoxyinosine (ddI) in patients with acquired immunodeficiency syndrome or AIDS-related complex: A phase I trial. N Engl J Med 1990;322: 1333–1340.

60. Lane HC, Kovacs JA, Feinberg J: Anti-retroviral effects of interferon-α in AIDS-associated Kaposi's sarcoma. Lancet 1988;2: 1218–1222.

61. Laskin OL, Longstreth JA, Hart CC, et al: Ribavirin disposition in high-risk patients for acquired immunodeficiency syndrome. Clin Pharmacol Ther 1987;41:546–555.

62. Lee BL, Moore L, Wilson M, et al: Increased prevalence of slow acetylator status in patients with the acquired immunodeficiency syndrome. Abstract presented at the 93rd annual meeting of the American Society of Clinical Pharmacology and Therapeutics, Orlando, March 1992, p. 183.

63. Masur H: Drug therapy: Prevention and treatment of Pneumocystis pneumonia. N Engl J Med 1992;327:1853–1860.

64. Mayer RA, Sergios PA, Coonan K, O'Brien L: Trichosanthin treatment of HIV-induced immune dysregulation. Eur J Clin Invest 1992;22:113–122.

65. McGrath MA, Hwang KM, Caldwell SE, et al: GLQ223: An inhibitor of human immunodeficiency virus replication in acutely and chronically infected cells of lymphocyte and mononuclear phagocytes lineage. Proc Natl Acad Sci USA 1989;86:2844–2848.

66. Mcphedran P: Using hematopoietic hormones in HIV disease. AIDS Clin Care 1992;4:43–44.

67. Meng TC, Fischl MA, Boota AH, et al: Combination therapy with zidovudine and dideoxycytidine in patients with advanced human immunodeficiency virus infection. Ann Intern Med 1992;116:13–20.

68. Meruelo D, Lavie G, Lavie G: Therapeutic agents with dramatic antiretroviral activity and little toxicity at effective doses: Aromatic

polyclic diones hypericin and pseudohypericin. Proc Natl Acad Sci USA 1988;85:5230–5234.

69. Miles SA, Mitsuya RT, Lee K, et al: Recombinant human granulocyte colony-stimulating factor increases circulating burst forming unit: Erythron and red blood cell production in patients with severe human immunodeficiency virus infection. Blood 1990;75:2137–2142.

70. Moore EC, Cohen F, Kauffman RE, Aravind MK: Zidovudine overdose in a child. N Engl J Med 1990;322:408–409.

71. Moore RD, Fortyana I, Keruly J, et al: Adverse events from drug therapy for human immunologic virus disease. Am J Med 1996;101:34–40.

72. Moyle GJ, Sadler M: Peripheral neuropathy with nucleoside antiretrovirals: risk factors, incidence and management. Drug Saf 1998;19:481–494.

73. Navin TR, Miller KD, Satriale RF, Lobel HO: Adverse reactions associated with pyrimethamine-sulfadoxine prophylaxis for *Pneumocystis carinii* infections in AIDS. Lancet 1985;1:1332.

74. Obrien RJ, Lyle MA, Snider DE Jr: Rifabutin (ansamycin LM 427): A new rifamycin-S derivative for the treatment of mycobacterial disease. Rev Infect Dis 1987;9:519–530.

75. Pickus OB: Overdose of zidovudine [letter]. N Engl J Med 1988;318:1206.

76. Pluda JM, Yarchoan R, Smith PD, et al: Subcutaneous recombinant granulocyte-macrophage colony-stimulating factor used as a single agent and in an alternating regimen with zidovudine in leukopenic patients with severe human immunodeficiency virus infection. Blood 1990;76:463–472.

77. Rao TK: Renal complications in HIV disease. Med Clin North Am 1996;80:1427–1451.

78. Raviglione MC, Dinan WA, Pablos-Mendez A, et al: Fatal toxic epidermal necrolysis during prophylaxis with pyrimethamine and sulfadoxine in a human immunodeficiency virus infected person. Arch Intern Med 1988;148:2683–2685.

79. Reines ED, Gross PA: Antiviral agents. Med Clin North Am 1988;72:691–715.

80. Reiter WM, Cimoch PJ: Dapsone-induced methemoglobinemia in a patient with *P. carinii* pneumonia and AIDS. N Engl J Med 1987;317:1741–1742.

81. Roberts RB, Jurica K, Meyer WA, et al: Phase I study of ribavirin in human immunodeficiency virus infected patients. J Infect Dis 1990;162:638–642.

82. Robinson PA, Knirsch AK, Joseph JA: Fluconazole for lifethreatening fungal infections in patients who cannot be treated with conventional antifungal agents. Rev Infect Dis 1990;12(Suppl 3):S349–S363.

83. Roederer M, Ela SW, Staal FJ, et al: *N*-Acetylcysteine: A new approach to anti-HIV therapy. AIDS Res Hum Retroviruses 1992;8:209–217.

84. Routy JP, Prajs E, Blanc AP, et al: Seizure after zidovudine overdose. Lancet 1989;1:184–185.

85. Schinazi RF, Chu CK, Babu JR, et al: Anthraquinones as a new class of antiviral agents against human immunodeficiency virus. Antiviral Res 1990;13:265–272.

86. Schoenfeld P: HIV infection and renal disease. AIDS Clin Care 1991;3:9–11.

87. Selwyn PA, Alcabes P, Hartel D, et al: Clinical manifestations and predictors of disease progression in drug users with human immunodeficiency virus infection. N Engl J Med 1992;327:1607–1703.

88. Sin DD: Dapsone- and primaquine-induced methemoglobinemia in HIV-infected individuals. J Acquir Immune Defic Syndr Hum Retroviral 1996;12:477–481.

89. Sjovall J, Bergdahl S, Movin G, et al: Pharmacokinetics of foscarnet and distribution to cerebrospinal fluid after intravenous infusion in patients with human immunodeficiency virus infection. Antimicrob Agents Chemother 1989;33:1023–1031.

90. Sjovall J, Karlson A, Ogenstad S, et al: Pharmacokinetics and absorption of foscarnet after intravenous and oral administration to patients with human immunodeficiency virus. Clin Pharmacol Ther 1988;44:65–73.

91. Smith PD: Gastrointestinal infections in AIDS. Ann Intern Med 1992;116:63–177.

92. Spear JB, Kessler HA, Lehrman SN, de Miranda P: Zidovudine overdosage. Ann Intern Med 1988;109:76–77.

93. Staal FJT, Ela SW, Roederer M, et al: Glutathione deficiency and human immunodeficiency virus infection. Lancet 1992;1:909–912.

94. Sugar AM, Stern JJ, Dupont B: Overview: Treatment of cryptococcal meningitis. Rev Infect Dis 1990;2(Suppl 3):S338–S348.

95. Sundar K, Suarez M, Banogon PE, et al: Zidovudine-induced fatal lactic acidosis and hepatic failure in patients with acquired immunodeficiency syndrome: Report of two patients and review of the literature. Crit Care Med 1997;25:1425.

96. Tanowitz HB, Simon D, Weiss L, et al: Gastrointestinal manifestations. In: Gold JWM, Telzak EE, White DA, eds: The Diagnosis and Management of the HIV-Infected Patient, part 1. Med Clin North Am 1996;80:1395–1414.

97. Tay-Kearney ML, Jabs DA: Ophthalmic complications of HIV infection. In: Gold JWM, Telzak EE, White DA, eds: The Diagnosis and Management of the HIV-Infected Patient, part 1. Med Clin North Am 1996;80:1471–1492.

98. Threlkeld SC, Hirsch MS: Antiviral therapy: The epidemiology of HIV and AIDS: Current trends. In: Gold JWM, Telzak EE, White DA, eds: The Diagnosis and Management of the HIV-Infected Patient, part 1. Med Clin North Am 1996;80:1263–1283.

99. Waites L, Levin AS, Starrett BA, et al: Trichosanthin treatment of HIV disease. Paper presented at the sixth international conference on AIDS, San Francisco, June 1990.

100. Walker RE, Parker RI, Kovacs JA, et al: Anemia and erythropoiesis in patients with acquired immunodeficiency syndrome (AIDS) and Kaposi sarcoma treated with zidovudine. Ann Intern Med 1988;108:372–376.

101. Watts RG, Conte SE, Zuilinden E, et al: Effect of charcoal hemoperfusion on clearance of pentamidine after accidental overdose. J Toxicol Clin Toxicol 1997;35:89–92.

102. Wharton JM, Demopulos PA, Goldschlager N: Torsades des pointes during administration of pentamidine isothionate. Am J Med 1986;83:571–576.

103. Whitley RJ, Gnann JW Jr: Acyclovir: A decade later. N Engl J Med 1992;327:782–789.

104. Wolf Y, Haddad R, Jossopov J, et al: Alpha interferon induced severe pneumonitis. J Toxicol Clin Toxicol 1997;35:113–114.

105. Yarchoan R, Klecker RW, Weinhold KJ, et al: Administration of 3′-azido-3′-deoxythymidine, an inhibitor of HTLV III/LAV replication, to patients with AIDS or AIDS-related complex. Lancet 1986;1:575–580.

106. Yarchoan R, Thomas RV, Allain JP, et al: Phase I studies of 2′,3′-dideoxycytidine in severe human immunodeficiency virus infection as a single agent and alternating with zidovudine (AZT). Lancet 1988;1:76–81.

This chapter focuses on the assessment and management of complications arising in substance users, unrelated to the direct effects of the drugs involved. Optimal medical and psychiatric care and the initiation of preventive strategies require the healthcare provider to have a thorough understanding of all aspects of the substance user's life. The following discussion focuses on the epidemiology of substance use and aims to provide a further understanding of the infectious, traumatic, psychiatric, and sociologic issues unique to the substance-using population.

DIAGNOSING SUBSTANCE DEPENDENCE/ABUSE DISORDERS

There are many substance users, and a certain percentage of them are drug dependent. In the most recent *Diagnostic and Statistical Manual of Mental Disorders* (DSM-IV), a diagnosis of substance dependence is based on the presence of at least three symptoms (from a list of seven) occurring at any time in a 12-month period (Table 109–1).[5] This modified concept of dependence stresses the impaired control of substance use and applies to a variety of substances that do not normally produce signs of physiologic dependence (eg, anticholinergics, nonsteroidal antiinflammatory agents).

Substance abuse implies a dangerous pattern of substance use and includes the inability to fulfill important roles (eg, neglect of children, absence from work), frequent use in physically hazardous environments (driving an automobile, operating a machine), recurrent substance-related legal problems, and continued use despite social problems caused or worsened by the effects of the substance.[5] Despite these rather clear definitions, there is still a great deal of controversy as to what constitutes drug use, dependence, and abuse.

The risk analysis for the single use of a drug is extensive and includes infection, injury, and end-organ toxicity such as stroke or myocardial ischemia. Individuals who use drugs multiple times have added risks that include such entities as dependence, prostitution, criminal activities such as theft and drug sales, violence, homelessness, and lost productivity. The societal implications of these behaviors are significant; it is estimated that 21% of tax dollars in New York City are spent on problems related to substance abuse.[16]

EPIDEMIOLOGY

It has been proposed that the proper theoretical construct should consider drug use as a communicable disease.[47,49] This is controversial, as the study of the frequency and distribution of drug use may be approached differently than that of an infectious disease or hypertension. The application of traditional epidemiologic concepts to the study of substance use should be done with great caution. The use of drugs may be prolonged, short-term, or episodic and may be associated with unique aspects of life style. Data collection can be difficult because there is no universally accepted point that separates "use" from "abuse." Reports of drug availability and the aggressiveness of law enforcement may vary greatly and give false impressions of the prevalence of substance use. For example, a brief visit by a clandestine chemist to a community may be followed by a sharp rise in the synthesis and use of a "designer drug."[30]

The limitations of epidemiologic data can be appreciated by an understanding of the methods and sources of data collection. Many different methods exist to define the epidemiology of substance abuse. The Drug Abuse Warning Network (DAWN), part of the federal agency SAMHSA, collects data on persons presenting to emergency departments aged 6 years and older.[90] In 1999, 488 hospitals participated in data collection. Data are collected by designated members of the emergency department or medical records staff based on the emergency department record and analytic drug detection. At each facility reporting data, a drug-related episode must meet all four of the following criteria:

1. The patient was treated in the hospital emergency department.
2. The presenting problem was directly related to drug use.
3. The case involved the use of an illegal drug or the use of a legal drug contrary to directions.
4. The patient's reason for taking the substance includes dependence, suicide attempt, and/or mind-altering effects.

The DAWN data provide useful information on trends in morbidity and mortality associated with illicit drugs, but the data must be interpreted with caution because only episodes in which a drug is part of the presenting problem are reported. For example, an increased reporting of cocaine could mean that more cocaine users with HIV-related infections are seeking medical care rather than that more persons are using cocaine. The analysis does not indicate the nature of the relationship between drug use and the presenting problem; which of the various drugs, if any, caused the episode; or if the patient was a naive or experienced substance user. Finally, there is concern that DAWN data may underreport drug-related episodes.[12] Critically ill patients may not provide a history of drug use in the emergency department, and analytic results are often not available until the patient has left the emergency department. Records generated outside of the emergency department are excluded from review. In summary, DAWN data are

TABLE 109–1. Substance Dependence Defined by at Least Three of the Following in a 12-Month Period

- Tolerance
- Withdrawal
- Administration in larger doses or over longer periods than originally intended
- Decreased control over usage
- Increased time investment in acquisition, use, or recovery from the substance
- Decreased participation in occupational, recreational, or social events
- Continued use despite social, psychological, or physical problems caused by the substance

Reprinted, with permission, from American Psychiatric Association: Diagnostic and Statistical Manual of Mental Disorders, 4th ed. Washington, DC, APA, 1994.

valuable, but the healthcare provider must understand their significant limitations (see Chap. 116 for further discussions).

The 1999 National Household Survey on Drug Abuse (NHSDA) surveyed 66,706 individuals aged 12 and older in households, noninstitutional group quarters (eg, shelters, rooming houses, dormitories), and civilians living on military bases.[91] This survey collected data on the time of last drug use and frequency of illicit drug use, opinions about drugs, problems associated with drug use, and drug abuse treatment experience. Demographic data were also collected including employment, education, income, general and mental health status, and access to health care. In 1999, a new sample design was initiated using an interactive, bilingual, computer-based questionnaire that allowed the sample size to be expanded almost fourfold from previous years and included both national and state assessments of substance use prevalence.

Other sources of data include information obtained from local and federal law enforcement agencies detailing trends in drug preferences, purity, and prices. Prescription audits establish the changes in prescribing patterns for a specific drug. Many communities perform independent local surveys to define attributes of the region that contribute to the area's incidence and prevalence of substance use.

The most recent data from the National Household Survey on Drug Abuse revealed that an estimated 14.8 million Americans (6.7% of the population 12 years of age and older) were current (in the month before the interview) illicit drug users. This is an approximately 40% decrease from 1979, which was the year with the highest recorded rate. Four percent of the 12-year-olds reported current drug use, with inhalants and nonmedical use of psychotherapeutics being most common. By age 14, the rate of current drug use increased to 9.2%, with marijuana being the dominant drug. In 1999, 10.9% of adolescents (12 to 17 years) were current users of illicit substances. Of the adolescents, 7.7% had used marijuana, and 5.3% had used some other illicit drug. The highest rates of drug use were among those individuals aged 18 to 20, with rare individuals using illicit drugs after age 50 years. Fifty-six percent of youth reported that obtaining marijuana was fairly or very easy, and 16% had been approached during the past 30 days by someone offering to sell them drugs.

Men have a higher rate of current illicit drug use than women (8.7 vs 4.9%). Among pregnant women, 3.4% reported the current use of illicit drugs, which was significantly lower than in age-matched nonpregnant women (8.1%). The rate of illicit drug use in metropolitan areas (7.1%) was higher than in rural areas (4.2%).

The rate of current illicit drug use for blacks (7.7%) remained higher than for whites (6.6%) and Hispanics (6.8%) in 1999. The rate was highest among the Native American/Inuit population (10.6%) and lowest among Asians (3.2%). Illicit drug use correlates with educational status, with those who had not completed high school having the highest rate of use (7.1%), while college graduates have the lowest rate of use (4.8%). In addition to education, current employment status predicts illicit drug use. In 1999, 16.5% of unemployed adults versus 6.5% of full-time employed adults used illicit drugs. The cause-and-effect relationship of all these data is unclear.

Approximately 30.2% of all Americans are currently smoking tobacco. Of the users, 25.8% smoked cigarettes, 5.5% smoked cigars, 3.4% used smokeless tobacco, and 1.1% smoked pipes. Up to age 20, current cigarette smoking rates increase by year of age from 2.2% at age 12 to 43.5% at age 20. After age 25, rates decline, reaching 22.5% in the 50 to 64 age group and 10.7% of people aged 65 and older. Native Americans and Inuits have the highest rate of tobacco usage, with 43.1% reporting the current use of at least one form of tobacco. The lowest current tobacco use rates were observed for Asians (18.6%). Current cigarette use is highly correlated with illicit drug use, and this association is strongest for adolescents. Men were more likely to report use of tobacco products. In general, the prevalence of cigarette smoking decreases with increasing levels of education.

In 1999, 47.3% of the population older than 12 years were current ethanol users, with 20.2% involved in binge drinking (five or more drinks at one occasion in the past month) and 5.6% classified as heavy users (five or more drinks per occasion on five or more days in the past month). About 29.4% of persons 12 to 20 years of age reported current use of alcohol. Of this underage group, 20.2% were binge drinkers, and 6% were heavy drinkers. Individuals between the ages of 18 and 25 years had the highest prevalence of binge and heavy drinking, with the peak rate occurring at age 21. Whites have the highest rate of current ethanol use, and Asians have the lowest. Men have greater representation in all categories of ethanol consumption. The level of alcohol use was strongly associated with illicit drug use. The rates of alcohol consumption also increased with increasing educational attainment and for full-time employment.

An evaluation of trends in the NHSDA data indicates that rates of marijuana use are currently increased relative to the 1980s and are approximately equal to rates seen in mid- to late 1970s. Of great concern is the doubling of the rate of heroin initiation in the age group 12 to 17. The annual number of new users of any form of cocaine increased by 45% between 1994 and 1999 with an over threefold increase in the age 12 to 17 group. The rate of new hallucinogen use has remained constant over the past several years but is markedly elevated from the 1980s. The rate of new inhalant use has more than doubled over the past 8 years. The rate of first use of methamphetamine among youths aged 12 to 17 rose significantly from 1990 to 1998, from 2.2 to 7.4 per 1000 potential new users.

DAWN data indicate that the four drugs mentioned most commonly in emergency department reports—alcohol-in-combination (35%), cocaine (30%), marijuana (16%), and heroin/morphine (15%)—were unchanged from the previous year. The majority of individuals indicated that smoking and sniffing heroin were the most common routes of administration, with only 37% ever having injected heroin by 1999. Compared to 1998, total drug-related emergency department episodes were stable for gender, race/ethnicity, and most age subgroups. Dependence and suicide were the most frequently cited motives for taking the drugs among the group of emergency department patients. Illicit drug mentions increased from 1990 to 1999 as follows: marijuana (455%), methamphetamine (100%), heroin (149%), and cocaine (110%). Among patients aged 35 and older, drug-related episodes increased 124% from 1990 to 1999, while the episodes in the other age groups increased less than 20%. Inhalants were not ranked in the 15 most-mentioned drugs for any age group.

MEDICAL PROBLEMS RELATED TO ADULTERANTS, CONTAMINANTS, DILUENTS, AND ROUTES OF ADMINISTRATION

In the clinical evaluation of patients who are using "street drugs," the presence of a variety of unknown chemicals should be presumed. Contaminants are by-products of the synthetic or preparatory process. Diluents are bulk-enhancing inactive substances that have similar physical properties (color, physical state, taste, odor) to the illicit drug and serve to decrease the quantity of active drug. Common diluents include any of the sugars (mannitol, inositol), cornstarch, flour, talc (magnesium silicate), and sodium bicarbonate. Adulterants are intentionally added pharmacologically active agents, and are chosen to provide either synergistic or antagonistic effects. An example of a synergistic adulterant would be the addition of phenobarbital to low-grade heroin to enhance the central nervous system (CNS) depression. Antagonistic adulteration would be illustrated by the addition of caffeine to heroin as an analeptic agent to diminish the depressant effects of heroin and enable more drug to be used.[87]

Common adulterants found in cocaine, heroin, and hallucinogens include any of the local anesthetics (lidocaine most commonly), caffeine, amphetamines, phencyclidine, lysergic acid diethylamide, and phenylpropanolamine.[32] Occasionally, substances are added for the purpose of inflicting physical harm (eg, strychnine, thallium). Data from crime laboratories indicates that many street drug sales involve illicit material with no mind-altering potential, sold for large sums of money to the unwary substance user. Of 614 alleged cocaine samples collected in Los Angeles County, cocaine was found to be totally absent in 19%, combined with stimulant substitutes in 23%, and found by itself in 58%. Fifty percent of the amphetamine samples lacked any of the alleged drug.[53] A more recent illustration of street drug impurities involves the adulteration of heroin with scopolamine.[41] Of the 241 patients who were available for this analysis, 55% presented with signs and symptoms of heroin intoxication. Interestingly, these patients became severely agitated with anticholinergic symptoms when naloxone was administered.

Clandestine drug laboratories may produce an undesired chemical as a result of a sloppy synthesis. In the early 1980s, "designer" chemists produced a formulation contaminated with 1-methyl-4-phenyl-1,2,3,6-tetrahydropyridine (MPTP) while attempting to synthesize an analogue of meperidine. This contaminant caused a rapidly developing, severe form of parkinsonism characterized by hypokinesia, rigidity, tremor, and fixed posture (see Chap. 62).[15,55]

The illegal synthesis of drugs can also be associated with potential exposures to metals, caustics, and solvents. These unintentional exposures occur during the synthetic process or by the injection of contaminated product. Methcathinone (CAT) is a synthetic amphetamine produced from ephedrine. In the synthesis, ephedrine is oxidized using sodium dichromate in an acid environment and then extracted using solvents. "Green cat" was sold at a reduced price and was contaminated with residual chromium salts, with the potential for chromium-induced multisystem organ failure.[30] Methamphetamine abuse was associated with an epidemic of lead poisoning when lead acetate was used in the synthetic process.[3,57] Law enforcement personnel consider all clandestine laboratories as harboring hazardous materials and proceed with great caution in their investigations.

Unique medical problems also occur in substance users related to the route of drug administration. Barotrauma occurs in individuals while smoking cocaine and nasally insufflating cocaine and other drugs. Patients will present with cough, chest pain, and dyspnea secondary to a pneumothorax, pneumomediastinum, or pneumopericardium. Barotrauma occurs secondary to an increased intraalveolar pressure generated by the deep inhalation followed by a Valsalva maneuver and the cough provoked by the drug and heated gases. Carbonaceous sputum is quite common in individuals smoking cocaine and is probably related to the inhalation of residue from the butane and alcohol used to ignite the drug.[40] Heroin overdose can also be associated with acute lung injury (ALI/ARDS) accompanied by fever and leukocytosis. ALI is most likely related to hypoxia and usually becomes clinically apparent within 6 hours of the toxicity but may be delayed up to 24 hours (see Chap. 95). Chronic exposure to starch, cotton fibers, and talc causes pulmonary granulomas when injected.[75] The chronic nasal application of cocaine commonly leads to epistaxis and septal perforation.

MEDICAL ILLNESS IN THE SUBSTANCE USER

The poisoned patient's clinical manifestations are often nonspecific and could represent acute medical, surgical, psychiatric, or combined processes.[20,21,72,73,86] A thorough history and physical examination are essential because the differential diagnosis is often extensive. Medical causes must be meticulously sought before a primary psychiatric disease can be diagnosed. A psychiatric diagnosis in a substance user must often be a diagnosis of exclusion. Drug-induced agitation or coma has an extensive differential diagnosis and involves many substances that may not be reported on routine urine and serum drug screens. Without a history, it is often impossible to distinguish between a primary medical event and a drug-induced event. Even then, the primary and secondary characteristics can simulate each other. It is best to admit the patient to a medical facility and provide close observation for either clinical resolution or worsening symptomatology. The healthcare provider must always assume the presence of concomitant trauma and thoroughly examine the patient for subtle injuries.

INFECTIOUS COMPLICATIONS

The diagnosis and management of the infected substance user can be complicated by the presence of multiple medical problems and the unique psychosocial aspects of the individual's life. Common difficulties are the lack of a clear history, malnutrition, poverty, homelessness, concomitant HIV-1 infection, noncompliance, and associated mental illness. Parenteral drug users often purchase "street" antibiotics at the time they obtain their drugs. One study demonstrated that 18% of intravenous drug users (IVDUs) had purchased antibiotics compared to only 5% of nonparenteral drug users.[59] The self-administration of antibiotics before hospital arrival can make the diagnosis of an infectious process very difficult. Frequent parenteral injections, colonization with resistant *Staphylococcus aureus,* and the self-administration of antibiotics are important considerations in the evaluation of infectious processes. The drug itself is usually not contaminated with the causative organism.[70]

Immunologic dysfunction is probably of minor importance in the pathogenesis of infection in drug users who are not infected with HIV. There is no evidence for an impaired humoral immunity in parenteral drug users. In fact, there is evidence of a polyclonal B-cell activation with IgM, the immunoglobulin most frequently elevated in IVDUs. Clinical examples of enhanced humoral response include a false-positive rheumatoid factor and Venereal Disease Research Laboratory (VDRL) test. Depressed cell-mediated immunity is, however, common in IVDUs. In vitro lymphocyte response to mitogens is diminished by the addition of methadone, and the delayed hypersensitivity skin test is commonly absent in heroin addicts. Altered populations and functioning of helper, suppressor, and natural killer cells are demonstrated in patients receiving methadone, but the clinical significance is uncertain. Clinical infections typical of T-cell dysfunction were uncommon in drug abusers before the advent of the HIV virus.[13,56] The influence of cocaine on the immune response is an area of active research, with data thus far suggesting an immunosuppressive effect of cocaine and its metabolites. Cocaine increases the risk of HIV infection in humans even when there is control for parenteral drug use. It is postulated that this increased susceptibility may be a result of decreased immune function in these patients.[22,23,54,77,79,98] Interestingly, cocaine has an antiviral effect in vitro by enhancing the secretion of interferon.[36]

Infection is the most common cause of death in hospitalized parenteral drug users. Infectious complications account for 60% of hospital admissions among IVDUs, and endocarditis is associated with 5 to 8% of these episodes.[59] It is estimated that two cases of endocarditis will occur per 1000 IVDUs per year.[59] Infective endocarditis implies infection of the endocardial surface of the heart and the physical presence of microorganisms in the lesion. Endocarditis is of great importance, given its high frequency of serious complications and significant mortality.

The initial history and physical examination are of limited value in diagnosing endocarditis in the febrile IVDU. Fever is nonspecific because it may be associated with bacterial, viral, fungal, or protozoan infections; reactions to injected drugs, adulterants, or contaminants; or of unknown origin. The presence of embolic phenomena and echocardiographically demonstrated vegetations are the most important predictors of endocarditis in febrile IVDUs. All IVDUs with a fever should be admitted for the evaluation of bacteremia and possible endocarditis.[95] The diagnosis of viral syndromes and other trivial illnesses cannot be established on the initial evaluation. Of all parenterally abused drugs, cocaine injection has the highest incidence of endocarditis.[18] Table 109–2 lists the common criteria adopted for the diagnosis of endocarditis in the IVDU.[95]

Endocarditis in the IVDU presents in a similar fashion to non–substance-using patients with a few exceptions. Important differences include a high incidence of right-sided endocarditis

TABLE 109–2.   Criteria for Diagnosis of Endocarditis in Parenteral Drug Users

1. Temperature greater than or equal to 38.0°C (100.4°F) with two positive blood cultures and vegetations on 2-D echocardiography.
2. Temperature greater than or equal to 38.0°C (100.4°F) with new vegetations seen on 2-D echocardiography with negative blood cultures (culture-negative endocarditis).
3. Positive blood cultures with new vegetations seen on 2-D echocardiography in absence of fever.
4. Temperature greater than 38.0°C (100.4°F), positive blood cultures, evidence of systemic embolization or valve regurgitation, but absence of vegetations on echocardiography.

Reprinted, with permission, from Weisse AB, Heller DR, Schimenti RJ, et al: The febrile parenteral drug abuser: A prospective study in 121 patients. Am J Med 1993;94: 274–280.

(tricuspid valve) and the absence of underlying structural heart disease in two-thirds of IVDUs with endocarditis.[94] Cardiac murmurs are noted in only 35% of IVDUs with proven endocarditis.[59] The distribution of valvular involvement in IVDUs with endocarditis is illustrated in Table 109–3.[60] A study of 74 intravenous opioid abusers with endocarditis found the following bacterial agents: *Staphylococcus aureus,* 61%[17]; streptococci, 16%; *Pseudomonas aeruginosa,* 14%; polymicrobial, 8%; and *Corynebacterium,* 1%.[59] S. aureus is of endogenous origin in the majority of cases, as it is infrequently isolated from street heroin or paraphernalia. Biventricular and multiple-valve disease occur more frequently with *Pseudomonas* infections. Left-sided endocarditis secondary to *P. aeruginosa* is often refractory to antibiotic therapy and has a mortality rate of 60%. Regional and transient variations occur (eg, *P. cepacia* for a few years in New York City), making it important that clinicians have knowledge of current epidemiologic trends unique to their institutions.

HIV infection predisposes the IVDU to unusual pathogens including *Corynebacterium species, Neisseria* species, *Salmonella* species, and fungal infections of the endocardium.[27,67,83] Parenteral drug abuse is the most common risk factor for recurrent native-valve endocarditis. Patients frequently survive the initial infection, with subsequent infections causing more significant cardiac complications (valvular dysfunction, myocardial abscess, and conduction blocks). A study of IVDUs with endocarditis and HIV infection demonstrated that HIV infection was not associated with a lower maximum temperature but was associated with a decreased white blood cell count.[84] A prospective cohort study of 292 consecutive IVDUs with endocarditis found that clinical outcome was generally similar according to HIV status but that a CD4 count less than 200 was a strong risk factor for mortality.[82]

All IVDUs who present with fever (>38°C, >100.4°F) should be admitted and have at least two blood samples obtained from different sites for aerobic, anaerobic, and fungal cultures (Fig.

TABLE 109–3.   Distribution of Valvular Involvement in Intravenous Drug Users with Endocarditis

Tricuspid valve alone or in combination	52%
Aortic valve alone	19%
Mitral valve alone	11%
Aortic and mitral valves together	13%

Reprinted, with permission, from Levine D, Sobel J: Infections in Intravenous Drug Abusers. New York, Oxford University Press, 1991.

109–1).[68,95] Empiric antibiotic therapy should consider the most common organisms and their antibiotic sensitivities in the geographic location. Initial coverage is usually directed against *S. aureus* using either nafcillin or vancomycin if methicillin-resistant organisms are common. The addition of an aminoglycoside provides synergy against *S. aureus* and may shorten the duration of therapy to 2 weeks in patients with right-sided endocarditis. Left-sided involvement mandates 6 weeks of intravenous antibiotic therapy. The typical aminoglycoside dosing used for synergy with *S. aureus* provides little effect against *Pseudomonas,* which requires large doses (8 mg/kg) for satisfactory activity. The initial use of an aminoglycoside to provide protection against gram-negative organisms is controversial. Enterococcal endocarditis is typically treated with a combination of vancomycin and gentamicin. Enterococci that develop gentamycin resistance are commonly treated with streptomycin, and resistance to vancomycin is treated with early surgical intervention, as there is no established antibiotic therapy. It is essential that antibiotic therapy is based on susceptibility data and that pharmacokinetic information is followed closely. Septic emboli are frequent after the initiation of antibiotic therapy. Vegetation size does not correlate with embolization; however, vegetations greater than 2 cm are associated with a 33% mortality versus a 1.3% mortality with vegetations less than than 2 cm.[21,60]

Skin and soft tissue infections represent the most common infectious etiologies requiring hospital admission (Fig. 109–2). Approximately one-third of IVDUs, particularly those who inject subcutaneously or intramuscularly, have soft tissue abscesses or cellulitis at any give time. Microbiologic contamination can occur at one of any steps, including production, mixing, dilution, or

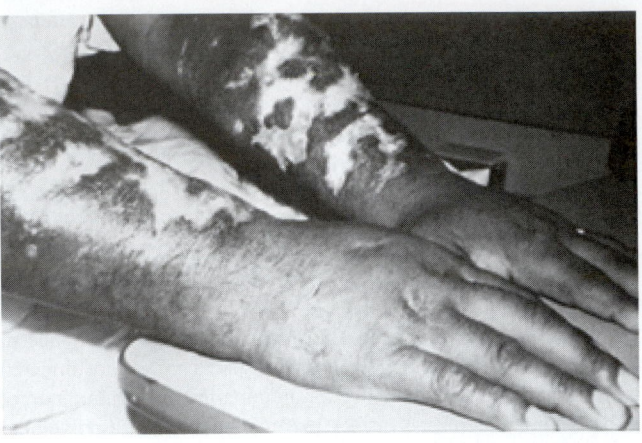

Figure 109–2 Markedly swollen hands with ulcerated cellulitic forearms in a chronic heroin user. The dorsum of each hand demonstrates nonpitting edema.

preparation of the drugs or at the time of injection through contaminated paraphernalia or skin. The infection may involve only a limited region of the epidermis and superficial dermis, as in "skin popping," or may extend into a more typical abscess, cellulitis, or necrotizing fasciitis. The infection may progress to involve the mediastinum, great vessels, muscle, or fascia and can lead to sepsis and death. Necrotizing fasciitis may present subtly with pain and hemodynamic instability disproportionate to the apparent diameter of the infected area. Great care must be maintained, as bullae, crepitance, and skin necrosis are late physical findings in necrotizing fasciitis. Imaging procedures such as ultrasound or computed tomography can help identify abscesses in the neck and groin if the diagnosis is uncertain. Vascular imaging before surgery is sometimes necessary if a pseudoaneurysm is suspected at the infected site (Fig. 109–3). Early antibiotic therapy and surgical drainage are essential.[9,21,60]

Suppurative thrombophlebitis is an inflammation of the vein wall caused by the presence of bacteria and is frequently associated with thrombosis. Fever, warmth, tenderness, swelling, and lymphadenopathy are common. Superficial and deep venous involvement may occur, depending on the injection site (Fig. 109–4). Recurrent injections can lead to deep venous thrombosis with the potential for pulmonary emboli. Antibiotic therapy should include a semisynthetic penicillin or vancomycin. Surgery is usually required. Anticoagulants are usually contraindicated because a clear benefit has not been established, and the IVDU is at great risk from complications related to anticoagulation.[21,60]

Mycotic aneurysms may occur as an isolated entity or accompany endocarditis. The femoral (most common) and neck vessels are the sites of mycotic aneurysms that occur directly during the injection of drugs. Frequent intravascular injections cause the formation of a perivascular hematoma that subsequently becomes infected by direct spread of cutaneous bacteria or overlying infections. These usually represent pseudoaneurysms, as only the vascular adventitia is involved. Involvement of the cerebral or abdominal vessels most commonly occurs during an episode of bacteremia with infection of the arterial vasa vasorum. Common clinical findings include fever, a painful pulsatile mass associated with a bruit or thrill, and ischemia distal to the mass. Early diagnosis before rupture is essential and commonly involves the use of

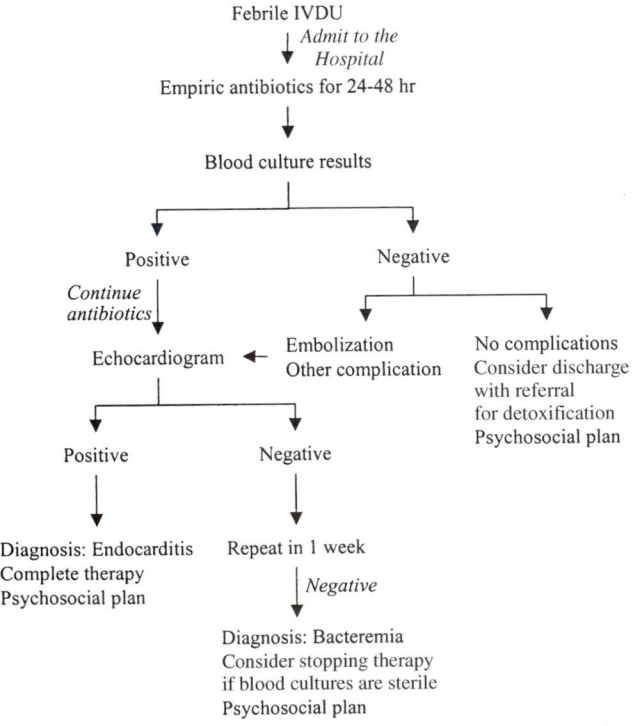

Febrile IVDU
↓ *Admit to the Hospital*
Empiric antibiotics for 24–48 hr
↓
Blood culture results
↓
Positive ——— Negative
Continue antibiotics
Echocardiogram ← Embolization / Other complication | No complications / Consider discharge with referral for detoxification / Psychosocial plan
↓
Positive ——— Negative
↓ ↓
Diagnosis: Endocarditis / Complete therapy / Psychosocial plan | Repeat in 1 week
↓ *Negative*
Diagnosis: Bacteremia / Consider stopping therapy if blood cultures are sterile / Psychosocial plan

Figure 109–1 Algorithm for the evaluation of the febrile intravenous drug user.

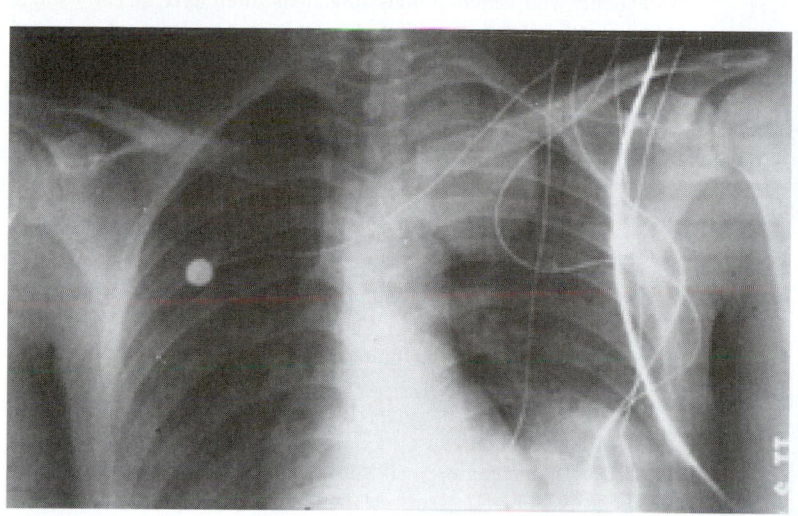
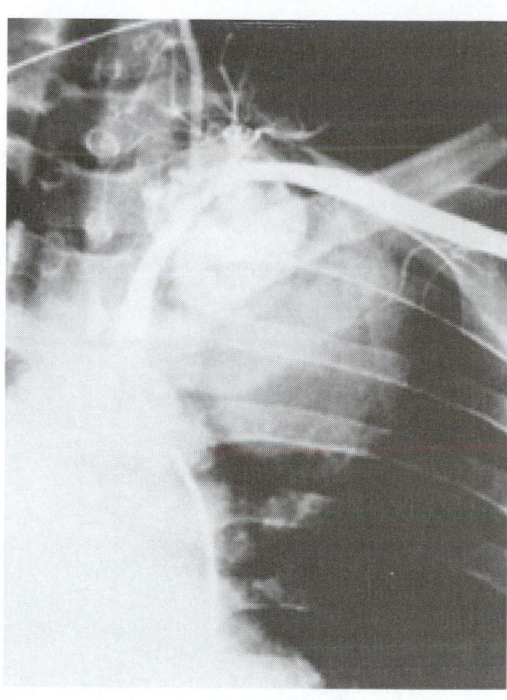

A   **B**

Figure 109–3 **A.** Chest radiograph of a young drug abuser who used the supraclavicular approach for heroin injection. The large mass in the left chest was thought to be a pseudoaneurysm. **B.** An arch aortogram performed on the patient revealed a large pseudoaneurysm and hematoma subsequent to an arterial tear during attempted injection. Surgical repair was performed. *(Courtesy of Richard Lefleur, Department of Radiology, Bellevue Hospital.)*

ultrasound or angiography. Needle aspiration and incisions must be avoided in inguinal or neck masses before imaging procedures, as clinical examination may be unreliable in detecting the presence of an aneurysm. Early surgical excision is usually required, as expansion and rupture are common.[21,60]

Viral hepatitis is very common in substance users and is acquired by parenteral drug administration and by sexual transmission. Virtually every form of viral hepatitis can be found in substance users with high prevalence and incidence rates. IVDUs account for 15% of acute hepatitis B infections. Data from the United States and Europe indicate that 25 to 50% of IVDUs have antibodies against hepatitis B surface antigen.[46,78,85] Approximately 5 to 12% of infected patients become hepatitis B surface antigen carriers with higher percentages among those who are also HIV infected. Ethanol abuse in combination with hepatitis B infection is associated with a more severe injury to the liver. Hepatitis B polymerase chain reaction testing of 681 syringes returned to a needle exchange program revealed a decline from 7.8% at the programs outset to 2.6% and an overall rate of 12.1% for Hepatitis C antibodies. The hepatitis D virus is a co-virus that requires the presence of hepatitis B for its replication. This virus occurs in 80% of chronic carriers of hepatitis B but is present in less than 10% of IVDUs who have serum antibodies to hepatitis B surface antigen. Patients are most commonly infected with hepatitis B before they acquire of hepatitis D. Simultaneous infection with both hepatitis B and D is uniquely common in IVDUs and will more likely result in fulminant hepatic failure.[58]

Hepatitis C (HCV) is the next emerging infectious disease (after HIV) to strike persons who inject drugs. HCV infection frequently occurs early in the time course of drug use, usually before the patient seeks help for drug problems. Of additional concern is the fact that approximately 80% of persons infected become chronic carriers. There is currently no vaccine for HCV, and the rapid mutation rate of the virus will make development difficult.[97] A recent study in the United States found 1.8% of unselected patients to have antibodies to hepatitis C, with people using illegal drugs or engaging in high-risk sexual behavior accounting for the majority of cases.[4] The incidence of hepatitis C among IVDUs is in excess of 70% in Amsterdam and Spain.[43] A study of 362 IVDUs in a Spanish prison found the prevalence of concomitant HBV-HCV to be 42.5%, and the HIV-HBV-HCV coinfection rate was 37.3%. The overall rate of a single virus infection was 13%. A case-control study of 2316 HCV-seropositive blood donors revealed intravenous drug abuse (odds ratio 50) and sex with an IVDU (odds ratio 6.3) to be strong risk factors for HCV among United States blood donors. In the United States, intravenous drug use currently accounts for 60% of HCV transmission, while sexual exposures account for 20%, and other known exposures (occupational, hemodialysis, household, perinatal) account for 10%. Blood transfusion rarely accounts for recently acquired HCV infections. July 1992 is when multiantigen anti-HCV tests to screen blood donors came into general use. Even among IVDUs who do not share needles, 54% of HCV infections may be attributed to cooker/cotton sharing.[39] Because 25% of patients infected with HCV will develop end-stage liver disease, it is a statistical certainty that a large number of drug users will develop cirrhosis. Even with antiviral therapy, the need for liver transplants will exceed the number of organs available in the very near future.[1,64]

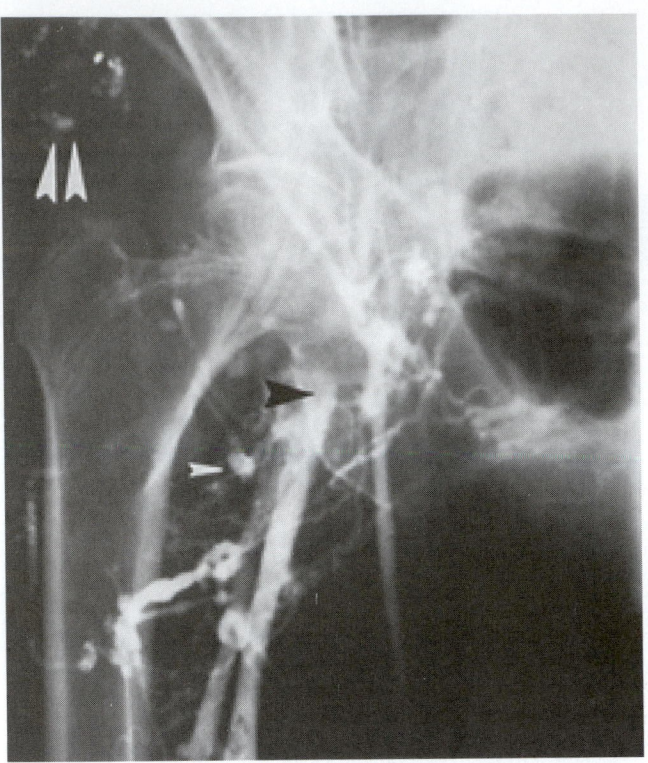

Figure 109–4 Venogram of a 50-year-old patient who routinely injected heroin into his groin. Occlusion of the femoral vein *(large arrow)* with diffuse aneurysmal dilation *(small arrow)* and extensive collaterals are shown. Incidental radiopaque materials are noted in the right buttock *(double arrow)*. By history, this represents either bismuth or arsenicals he received as antisyphilitic therapy. *(Courtesy of Richard Lefleur, Department of Radiology, New York University.)*

Splenic abscesses are common and may be multiple and small or singular and large. Common symptoms include fever, abdominal pain, left shoulder pain, and pleuritic chest pain. Physical examination may reveal splenomegaly, left upper quadrant tenderness, and left pleural effusion. Antibiotics with percutaneous drainage or splenectomy are the mainstays of therapy.[24]

Most lung infections result from the common respiratory pathogens that occur in community-acquired pneumonias. Opportunistic infections must be considered if the patient is HIV infected. Primary pulmonary infections must be distinguished from septic pulmonary emboli arising from endocarditis or extremity deep venous thrombosis. Lung abscesses are common and occur through aspiration, necrotizing pneumonia, or septic emboli. Tuberculosis is common even in the non-HIV-infected patient as a result of alcoholism, malnutrition, crowding, poor compliance with medical care, and coughing induced during the smoking and nasal insufflation of drug. Pneumonia is one of the most common infections in febrile substance users. The initial antibiotic therapy must be broad based before definitive cultures, and the healthcare provider must always consider the possibility of multiple processes affecting the lung simultaneously.[60]

Bone and joint infections are also common in parenteral drug users. The infection most commonly occurs during an episode of bacteremia but may also develop via the spread from contiguous foci. Most joint infections involve the knee, but other common

sites include the sternoclavicular, manubriosternal (Fig. 109–5), costochondral (almost pathognomonic for substance use), and sacroiliac joints. Vertebral osteomyelitis commonly involves the cervical and lumbosacral spine (see Fig. 8–12B) and may lead to epidural abscess formation with possible spinal cord compression. Patients with vertebral body infections often have an early subtle presentation, and a prompt diagnosis is based on a heightened awareness in a substance user with spine pain, fevers, and/or focal neurologic deficits. A diagnostic aspiration is essential in assessing skeletal infections, as there is commonly a discrepancy between organisms causing bone and joint infections and those isolated from the blood. Specific antimicrobial therapy for 4 to 6 weeks is essential, along with frequent arthrocentesis and debridement of necrotic bone as needed.[19] The rheumatologic manifestations of hepatitis B or hepatitis C and chronic amyloidosis associated with frequent parenteral drug use should also be considered in substance users with bone or joint pain.[48]

The evaluation of a substance user with neurologic findings is quite challenging and must involve both infectious and noninfectious etiologies. In the non-HIV-infected patient, endocarditis is the most common cause of CNS infection, which includes brain abscesses, meningitis, and subarachnoid hemorrhage from ruptured mycotic aneurysms. Mycotic aneurysms present with focal neurologic dysfunction as a result of the expanding aneurysm, or subarachnoid/intracerebral hemorrhage (see Fig. 8–24). Cerebral

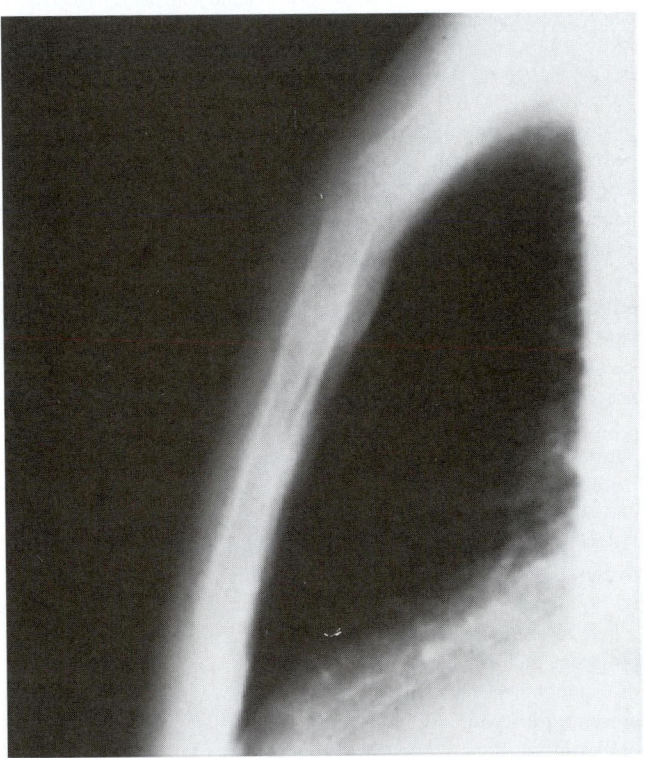

Figure 109–5 A patient with a manubriosternal osteomyelitis complicating IV drug use. He presented with chest pain and fever that developed over 2 weeks. The patient was treated with long-term antistaphylococcal penicillinase-resistant antibiotics. The manubriosternal region is also a characteristic site for osteomyelitis in parenteral drug users. *(Courtesy of the New York City Poison Center Toxicology Fellowship).*

abscesses usually result from emboli arising from the mitral or aortic valves. Cerebritis may have a viral etiology or be caused by excessive bacteremia associated with endocarditis.[60]

Currently, the incidence of sexually transmitted diseases (STDs) in substance users is increasing dramatically. Prostitution and sexual promiscuity are strongly related to drug use. The most important organisms include HIV, penicillinase-producing strains of *Neisseria gonorrhoeae, Treponema pallidum, Haemophilus ducreyi,* and *Chlamydia trachomatis.*[35] Approximately one-third of female IVDUs have a history of prostitution, and 60% of IVDUs report a history of an STD.[21,60] The common practice of exchanging sex (usually unprotected) for crack cocaine has dramatically increased the incidence of all sexually transmitted diseases. The risk of transmission of HIV infection in parenteral drug users via the sexual route is tremendous. A 1993 Centers for Disease Control study of male IVDUs with known HIV infection revealed that 28% reported having vaginal or anal sex without a condom during the preceding 30 days, and 23% admitted to trading sex for money. Thirty-two percent had not revealed their HIV status to all partners.[25] A study of an indigent group of emergency department patients who admitted to using cocaine once each week found a syphilis rate of 28%.[31] A study of 311 lower-risk patients entering residential drug treatment found the prevalence of sexually transmitted diseases to be as follows: *Chlamydia trachomatis* 2.3%; *Neisseria gonorrhoeae* 1.6%; trichomoniasis 43%; syphilis 6%.[6]

The healthcare provider must always consider the possibility of uncommon infections in the substance abuser. In the early 1970s, a group of patients acquired *Plasmodium vivax* in California by the sharing of needles.[33] Substance users risked quinine toxicity in the 1930s as the drug was added to heroin to help control malaria. The ease of travel to areas endemic with malaria makes this disease a consideration even in the United States. Historically, tetanus is the oldest infectious complication afflicting patients who use parenterally administered drugs. Tetanus and botulism must be considered in substance users, as *Clostridium* spp can grow well in facial sinuses (as with cocaine insufflation) or in extremities as a result of "skin popping" or compromised extremity perfusion.[7,96]

Bleach distribution and needle/syringe exchange programs were developed in an attempt to minimize the spread of infectious diseases and have been a subject of great controversy. The last 15 years have provided data demonstrating that these programs are generally effective in limiting the transmission of infectious diseases. The number of new programs has been increasing by about 20% per year. Approximately one-half of new HIV infections are a result of reuse and sharing of contaminated syringes. Results from several programs demonstrate a reduction in the transmission of hepatitis B, hepatitis C, and HIV.[11,14,28,38,43,51,63,89,93] The healthcare provider must understand the limitations of these programs and educate each IVDU, as drug sharing can play an important role in the social organization of the drug-using culture.[37] The HCV epidemic will provide society with a chance to learn from the HIV experience and institute appropriate preventive measures. Additional research is needed to maximize the availability of these resources and to integrate them into other needed health and social services for substance users.

The HIV epidemic remains a significant problem for injecting drug users. CDC data indicate that 22% of the new cases of HIV between July 1999 and June 2000 were in patients injecting drugs.[45] An encouraging recent study evaluated the HIV incidence

rate among IVDUs living in New York City between 1992 and 1997 and found the incidence to be low (0.7 per 100 person-years at risk) for a high-seropositivity population of patients.[29] The significant epidemic of HIV infection among IVDUs in New York City appears to be declining as demonstrated by this low incidence and declining prevalence. Data from the Centers for Disease Control indicate that the recent marked declines in AIDS incidence and deaths began in 1996 and continued into 1998. This is associated with the widespread use of combination antiretroviral therapies. These dramatic declines have slowed during the latter part of 1998 and 1999. In 1999, the incidence and death rates each quarter have stabilized. AIDS prevalence continued to rise in 1999, although the rate of increase has slowed.

TRAUMATIC COMPLICATIONS

Deaths in substance users may occur unrelated to the drug, as a result of an overdose of the drug, as a result of medical complications associated with the drug, or from drug-induced psychological responses that lead to trauma. Drug use increases both the incidence of trauma and the severity of each event. Numerous drugs such as alcohol, marijuana, cocaine, and benzodiazepines are all demonstrated to impair driving tasks.[52] Benzoylecgonine was detected in 27% of all New York City residents sustaining fatal injuries, and cocaine was detected in 18%. This study found that two-thirds of the deaths were not from acute toxicity but resulted from homicides, suicides, automobile collisions, and falls.[10,69] A study involving six regional trauma centers demonstrated that 40% of adult trauma patients had a positive blood alcohol content on admission.[88] A recent CDC report indicates that in 1997 and 1998, 38% of traffic fatalities were alcohol related.[2] A prospective study of patients at a level I trauma center found that 71% screened positive for alcohol or drugs and that cocaine and opioids represented 91% of positive drug screens.[26] Of 1118 patients admitted to a level I trauma center, 24% were currently alcohol dependent, and 18% were currently dependent on another drug. In a study of 450 trauma patients, 70% had positive blood ethanol and/or urine toxicology results, and victims of intentional trauma showed an even higher percentage of positive screens (80%).[65]

In a study of 231 injured patients aged 12 to 18 years, alcohol use was identified in 39%.[62,66] Toxicologic testing results from 1356 trauma patients aged 10 to 14 years revealed that 9% were positive for alcohol and/or other psychoactive drugs.[61] Even though the elderly have a lower incidence of drug-related trauma, 14% of drivers over age 60 were found to have the presence of ethanol in their blood.[44]

Numerous studies from burn centers demonstrate that substance use is commonly associated with thermal injury and that substance users have a greater percentage of burned body surface area, inhalation injury, and mortality.[42] Substance use is one of the most substantial risk factors for traumatic brain injury. Similar relationships exist between substance use and hypothermia fatalities, drownings, and spinal cord injuries.

A study of 634 patients admitted to a Chicago level I trauma center following trauma demonstrated that 45% were considered impaired with either alcohol or drugs.[74] Of the impaired group, only 17% were cited by police for driving under the influence. These data indicate the importance of close working relationships and dialogue between the healthcare provider and law enforcement to communicate possible mechanisms involved in the traumatic event.

The clinical evaluation of poisoned patients is difficult, and thus, more diagnostic testing is required to determine occult internal organ injury. Common examples include the need for a computed tomography evaluation of the brain and abdomen, as physical diagnosis is less reliable if the patient is intoxicated. Sympathomimetic agents may cause a tachycardia unrelated to blood loss, and the relative hypertension may mask hypovolemic shock. Long bone, pelvic, and cervical spine fractures may not be perceived as painful events, mandating a low threshold for obtaining radiographs.

Routine drug testing may be important to allow for an early diagnosis of substance use and the initiation of chemical dependence treatment. One study suggested that surgical services identified alcoholism in fewer than 25% of affected patients and addressed the problem in fewer than one-half of the patients detected. Chemical dependence consultation and referral for rehabilitation are critical to the management of these patients if prevention of further events is to be achieved. A number of authors suggest that patients are more amenable to a "critical intervention" and referral for rehabilitation in the posttraumatic period. Long-term survival may depend more on substance use rehabilitation than on initial trauma management.[34,76]

PSYCHIATRIC ILLNESS

Comorbidity implies the presence of two or more psychiatric disorders in the same patient. The National Institute of Mental Health's Epidemiologic Catchment Area Study remains a landmark study demonstrating the large percentage of substance users with a dual diagnosis. This study was conducted in the early 1980s and involved the interviews of more than 20,000 people in five communities in the United States. In this study, 76% of men and 65% of women demonstrated comorbidity (Table 109–4).[50,81] The consequences of substance use for patients include symptom exacerbation, increased hospitalization, medication noncompliance, disruptive behaviors, decreased social functioning, and higher rates of utilization of acute services leading to more costly care.

TABLE 109–4. Prevalence of Other Psychiatric Disorders among Men and Women Diagnosed as Having Drug Use Dependence Disorders

Specific Additional Diagnoses	Prevalence of Other Disorders	
	Men (%)	Women (%)
Alcohol use dependence	60	30
Antisocial personality disorder	22	10
Phobic disorders	19	29
Major depression	14	28
Dysthymia	9	12
Obsessive-compulsive disorder	6	9
Mania	5	7
Schizophrenia	5	8
Panic disorder	3	6

Reprinted, with permission, from Kandal DB: Epidemiological trends and implications for understanding the nature of addiction. In: O'Brien CP, Jaffe JH, eds: Addictive States. New York, Raven Press, 1992, pp. 23–40.

There is evidence to suggest that the integration of mental health and drug and alcohol services will result in improved detection, assessment, and management of comorbidity.[80]

Studies thus far describe the incidence of comorbidity, but they do not explain the reasons for the associations. It is uncertain whether the use of substances with mind-altering properties is an attempt at self-medication or whether mentally ill patients are less able to contend with the effects of substance use and thus are more likely to become dependent. The causal relationship between these disorders is complex, and further studies are necessary to determine whether substance use and abuse contribute to the risk of developing other psychiatric disorders or vice versa.

A reliable psychiatric diagnosis in substance users requires a 2-week period of abstinence to eliminate the potential for concurrent intoxication or withdrawal. Several important principles must be remembered when performing a psychiatric evaluation of a substance user. The medical assessment must always precede the psychiatric evaluation. In most patients with a presumed dual diagnosis, inpatient care is probably the best setting, and psychotropic medications are initiated only when spontaneous remission is not possible. Care must be given to identifying medical and drug-induced disease that may masquerade as psychiatric illnesses. Substance abusers are often unable to give reliable clinical information, and emphasis must be placed on analytic drug data from biologic specimens, physical examinations, laboratory testing, history from family and friends, past medical histories, and family psychiatric histories. In prescribing medication, avoid addictive agents once detoxification is accomplished, as these drugs may stimulate the cycle of euphoria and craving and thus jeopardize the recovery. Psychiatric and rehabilitative approaches are often conflicting in philosophy and must be carefully coordinated to optimize care.

SUMMARY

The optimal care of substance users is quite challenging and demands a thorough understanding of all aspects of their life style. The healthcare provider must approach these patients in a compassionate and nonjudgmental manner so as to gain their confidence and enhance the care rendered. It is essential to maintain knowledge of the current patterns of substance use and to understand the many medical, surgical, and psychiatric issues these patients face as a result of their drug use. Physicians are an integral part of a team of professionals that includes psychologists, home care nurses, social workers, substance abuse counselors, law enforcement personnel, clergy, and volunteers at shelters. In an era of cost containment, it is essential that each provider of healthcare maintain a focus on this important group of individuals and not allow financial pressures to alter appropriate decisions.

REFERENCES

1. Abraham HD, Degli-Esposti S, Marino L: Seroprevalence of hepatitis C in a sample of middle class substance abusers. J Addict Dis 1999; 18:77–87.
2. Alcohol involvement in fatal motor-vehicle crashes—United States, 1997–1998. MMWR 1999;38:1086–1087.
3. Allcott JV, Barnhart RA, Mooney LA: Acute lead poisoning in two users of illicit methamphetamine. JAMA 1987;258:510–511.

4. Alter MJ, Kruszon-Moran D, Nainan O, et al: The prevalence of hepatitis C virus infection in the United States, 1988–1994. N Engl J Med 1999;341:556–562.

5. American Psychiatric Association: Diagnostic and Statistical Manual of Mental Disorders, 4th ed. Washington, American Psychiatric Association, 1994.

6. Bachmann LH, Lewis I, Allen R, et al: Risk and prevalence of treatable sexually transmitted diseases at a Birmingham substance abuse treatment facility. Am J Public Health 2000;90:1615–1618.

7. Bardenheier B, Prevots D, Khetsuriani N, Wharton M: Tetanus surveillance—United States, 1995–1997. MMWR CDC Surveill Summ 1998;47:1–13.

8. Bayer BM, Mulroney SE, Hernandez MC, et al: Acute infusions of cocaine result in time- and dose-dependent effects on lymphocyte responses and corticosterone secretion in rats. Immunopharmacology 1995;29:19–28.

9. Binswanger IA, Kral AH, Bluthenthal RN, et al: High prevalence of abscesses and cellulitis among community-recruited injection drug users in San Francisco. Clin Infect Dis 2000;30:579–581.

10. Blanc PD, Saxena M, Olson KR: Drug detection and trauma cause—A case control study of fatal injuries. J Toxicol Clin Toxicol 1994;32:137–145.

11. Bluthenthal RN, Kral A, Gee L, et al: The effect of syringe exchange use on high-risk injection drug users: a cohort study. AIDS 2000;14:605–611.

12. Brookoff D, Campbell EA, Shaw LM: The underreporting of cocaine-related trauma: Drug abuse warning network reports versus hospital toxicology tests. Am J Public Health 1993;83:369–371.

13. Brown SM, Stimmel B, Taub R, et al: Immunologic dysfunction in heroin addicts. Arch Intern Med 1974;134:1001–1006.

14. Bruneau J, Lamothe F, Franco E, et al: High rates of HIV infection among injection drug users participating in needle exchange programs in Montreal: results of a cohort study. Am J Epidemiol 1997;146:994–1002.

15. Burns RS, Lewitt PA, Ebert MH, et al: The clinical syndrome of striatal dopamine deficiency: Parkinsonism induced by MPTP. N Engl J Med 1985;312:1418–1421.

16. Center on Addiction and Substance Abuse at Columbia University: Substance abuse and urban America: Its impact on an American city. New York, 1996.

17. Chambers HF, Korzeniowski OM, Sande MA: *Staphylococcus* aureus endocarditis: Clinical manifestations in addicts and nonaddicts. Medicine 1983;62:170–177.

18. Chambers HF, Morris DL, Tauber MG, Modin G: Cocaine use and the risk for endocarditis in intravenous drug abusers. Ann Intern Med 1987;106:833–836.

19. Chandrasekar PH, Narula A: Bone and joint infections in intravenous drug abusers. Rev Infect Dis 1986;8:904–910.

20. Cherubin CE: The medical sequelae of narcotic addiction. Ann Intern Med 1967;67:23–33.

21. Cherubin CE, Sapira JD: The medical complications of drug addiction and the medical assessment of the intravenous drug abuser: 25 years later. Ann Intern Med 1993;119:1017–1028.

22. Chiappelli F, Frost P, Manfrini E, et al: Cocaine blunts human CD4$^+$ cell activation. Immunopharmacology 1994;3:233–240.

23. Chiappelli F, Kung MA, Villanueva P, et al: Immunotoxicology of cocaethylene. Immunopharmacol Immunotoxicol 1995;2:399–417.

24. Chun C, Raff M, Varghese R, et al: Splenic abscess. Medicine 1980;59:50–65.

25. Continued sexual risk behavior among HIV-seropositive, drug-using men—1993. MMWR 1996;45:151–154.

26. Cornwell EE 3rd, Belzberg H, Velmahos G, et al: The prevalence and effects of alcohol and drug abuse on cohort-matched critically injured patients. Am Surg 1998;64:461–465.

27. Currie PF, Sutherland GR, Jacob AJ, et al: A review of endocarditis in acquired immunodeficiency syndrome and human immunodeficiency virus infection. Eur Heart J 1995;16:15–18.

28. Des Jarlais DC, Paone D, Friedman SR, et al: Regulating controversial programs for unpopular people: Methadone maintenance and syringe exchange programs. Am J Public Health 1995;85:1577–1584.

29. Des Jarlais DC, Marmor M, Friedman P, et al: HIV incidence among drug users in New York City, 1992–1997: evidence for a declining epidemic. Am J Public Health 2000;90:352–359.

30. Emerson TS, Cisek JE: Methcathinone: A Russian designer amphetamine infiltrates the rural midwest. Ann Emerg Med 1993;22:1897–1903.

31. Ernst AA, Martin DH: High syphilis rates among cocaine abusers identified in an emergency department. Sex Transm Dis 1992;20:66–69.

32. Fucci N, DeGiovanni N: Adulterants encountered in the illicit cocaine market. Forensic Sci Int 1998;95:247–252.

33. Friedman CT, Dover AS, Roberto RR, Kerns OA: A malaria epidemic among heroin addicts. Am J Trop Med Hyg 1973;22:302–307.

34. Fuller MG, Diamond DL, Jordan ML, Walters MC: The role of a substance abuse consultation team in a trauma center. J Stud Alcohol 1995;56:267–271.

35. Goldsmith M: Sex tied to drugs = STD spread. JAMA 1988;260:2009–2011.

36. Grattendick K, Jansen DB, Lefkowity DL, Lefkowitz SS: Cocaine causes increased type I interferon secretion by both L929 cells and murine macrophages. Clin Diagn Lab Immunol 2000;7:245–250.

37. Grund JP, Friedman SR, Stern LS, et al: Syringe-mediated drug sharing among injecting drug users: Patterns, social context, and implications for transmission of blood-borne pathogens. Soc Sci Med 1996;42:691–703.

38. Hagan H, Jarlais DC, Friedman SR, et al: Reduced risk of hepatitis B and hepatitis C among injection drug users in the Tacoma syringe exchange program. Am J Public Health 1995;85:1531–1537.

39. Hagan H, Thiede T, Weiss N, et al: Sharing of drug preparation equipment as a risk factor for hepatitis C. Am J Public Health 2001;91:42–46.

40. Haim DY, Lippman ML, Goldberg SK, Walkenstein MD: The pulmonary complications of crack cocaine: A comprehensive review. Chest 1995;107:233–240.

41. Hamilton RJ, Perrone J, Hoffman R, et al: A descriptive study of an epidemic of poisoning caused by heroin adulterated with scopolamine. J Toxicol Clin Toxicol 2000;38:597–608.

42. Haum A, Perbix W, Hack HJ, et al: Alcohol and drug abuse in burn patients. Burns 1995;21:194–199.

43. Heimer R, Khoshnood K, Jariwala-Freeman B, et al: Hepatitis in used syringes: The limits of sensitivity of techniques to detect hepatitis B virus DNA, hepatitis C virus RNA, and antibodies to HBV core and HCV antigens. J Infect Dis 1996;4:997–1000.

44. Higgins JP, Wright SW, Wrenn KD: Alcohol, the elderly, and motor vehicle crashes. Am J Emerg Med 1996;14:265–267.

45. HIV/AIDS Surveillance Report. Nation Center for HIV, STD, and TB Prevention. Midyear 2000 Edition.

46. Hoffman I, Stratton J, Lemon S, et al: Hepatitis B among parenteral drug abusers—North Carolina. JAMA 1986;256:1262–1269.

47. Hughes PH, Barker NW, Crawford MA, Jaffe JH: The natural history of a heroin epidemic. Am J Public Health 1972;62:995–1001.

48. Jacob H, Charytan C, Rascoff JH, et al: Amyloidosis secondary to drug abuse and chronic skin suppuration. Arch Intern Med 1978;138:1150–1151.

49. Jonas S: Heroin utilization: A communicable disease? NY State J Med 1972;72:1292–1299.

50. Kandal DB: Epidemiological trends and implications for understanding the nature of addiction. In: O'Brien CP, Jaffe JH, eds: Addictive States. New York, Raven Press, 1992, pp. 23–40.

51. Kaplan EH, Heimer R: HIV incidence among New Haven needle exchange participants: Updated estimates from syringe tracking and testing data. J Acquir Immune Defic Syndr Hum Retrovirol 1995;10:175–176.

52. Kirby JM, Maull K, Fain W: Comparability of alcohol and drug use in injured drivers. South Med J 1992;85:800–803.

53. Klatt EC, Montgomery S, Namiki T, et al: Misrepresentation of stimulant street drugs. A decade of experience in an analysis program. J Toxicol Clin Toxicol 1986;24:441–450.

54. Klein TW, Matsui K, Newton CA, et al: Cocaine suppresses proliferation of phytohemagglutinin-activated human peripheral blood T-cells. Int J Immunopharmacol 1993;1:77–86.

55. Langston JW, Ballard P, Tetrud JW, Irwin I: Chronic parkinsonism in humans due to a byproduct of meperidine analog synthesis. Science 1983;219:979–980.

56. Layon J, Idris A, Warzynski M, et al: Altered T lymphocyte subsets in hospitalized intravenous drug abusers. Arch Intern Med 1984;144: 1376–1380.

57. Lead poisoning associated with intravenous-methamphetamine use—Oregon, 1988. MMWR 1989;38:830–831.

58. Lettau L, McCarthy J, Smith M, et al: Outbreak of severe hepatitis due to delta and hepatitis B viruses in parenteral drug abusers and their contacts. N Engl J Med 1987;317:1256–1262.

59. Levine D, Crane L, Zervos M: Bacteremia in narcotic addicts at the Detroit Medical Center. II. Infectious endocarditis: A prospective comparative study. Rev Infect Dis 1986;8:374–396.

60. Levine D, Sobel J: Infections in Intravenous Drug Abusers. New York, Oxford University Press, 1991.

61. Li G, Chanmugam A, Rothman R, et al: Alcohol and other psychoactive drugs in trauma patients aged 10–14 years. Inj Prev 1999;5: 94–97.

62. Loiselle JM, Baker MD, Templeton JM, et al: Substance abuse in adolescent trauma. Ann Emerg Med 1993;22:1530–1534.

63. Lurie P, Drucker E: An opportunity lost: HIV infections associated with lack of a national needle-exchange programme in the USA. Lancet 1997;349:604–608.

64. MacDonald M, Wodak A, Dolan K, et al: Hepatitis C virus antibody prevalence among injecting drug users at selected needle and syringe programs in Australia, 1995–1997. Med J Aust 2000;172:57–61.

65. Madan AK, Yu K, Beech DJ: Alcohol and drug use in victims of life-threatening trauma. J Trauma 1999;47:568–571.

66. Mannenbach MS, Hargarten SW, Phelan MB: Alcohol use among injured patients aged 12 to 18 years. Acad Emerg Med 1997;4:40–44.

67. Manoff SB, Vlahov D, Somomon L, et al: Human immunodeficiency virus infection and infective endocarditis among injecting drug users. Epidemiology 1996;7:566–570.

68. Marantz PR, Linzer M, Feiner CJ, et al: Inability to predict diagnosis in febrile intravenous drug abusers. Ann Intern Med 1987;106: 823–828.

69. Marzuk PM, Tardiff K, Leon AC, et al: Fatal injuries after cocaine use as a leading cause of death among young adults in New York City. N Engl J Med 1995;332:1753–1757.

70. Moustoukas NM, Nichols RL, Smith JW, et al: Contaminated street heroin: Relationship to clinical infections. Arch Surg 1983;118: 746–749.

71. Netzer RO, Zollinger E, Seiler C, Cerny A: Infective endocarditis: clinical spectrum, presentation and outcome. An analysis of 212 cases 1980–1995. Heart 2000;84:25–30.

72. O'Connor PG, Samet JH, Stein MD: Management of hospitalized intravenous drug users: Role of the internist. Am J Med 1994;96: 551–558.

73. O'Connor PG, Selwyn PA, Schottenfeld RS: Medical care for injection-drug users with human immunodeficiency virus infection. N Engl J Med 1994;331:450–459.

74. Orsay EM, Doan-Wiggins L, Lewis R, et al: The impaired driver: Hospital and police detection of alcohol and other drugs of abuse in motor vehicle crashes. Ann Emerg Med 1994;24:51–55.

75. Pare JP, Cote G, Fraser RS: Long-term follow-up of drug abusers with intravenous talcosis. Am Rev Respir Dis 1989;139:233–241.

76. Parran TV, Weber E, Tasse J, et al: Mandatory toxicology testing and chemical dependence consultation follow-up in a level-one trauma center. J Trauma 1995;38:278–280.

77. Pellegrino T, Bayer BM: In vivo effects of cocaine on immune cell function. J Neuroimmunol 1998;83:139–147.

78. Piot P, Goilav C, Kegels E: Hepatitis B: Transmission by sexual contact and needle sharing. Vaccine 1990;8S:37–40

79. Pirozhkov SV, Watson RR, Chen GJ: Ethanol enhances immunosuppression induced by cocaine. Alcohol 1992;6:489–494.

80. RachBeisel J, Scott J, Dixon L: Co-occurring severe mental illness and substance use disorders: a review of recent research. Psychiatr Surv 1999;50:1427–1434.

81. Regier DA, Farmer ME, Rae DS, et al: Comorbidity of mental disorders with alcohol and other drug abuse: results from the Epidemiologic Catchment Area (ECA) study. JAMA 1990;264:2511–2518.

82. Ribera E, Miro J, Cortes E, et al: Influence of human immunodeficiency virus 1 infection and degree of immunosuppression in the clinical characteristics and outcome of infective endocarditis in intravenous drug users. Arch Intern Med 1998;158:2043–2050.

83. Rivera Del Rio JR, Flores R, Melendez J, et al: Profile of HIV patients with and without bacterial endocarditis. Cell Mol Biol 1997;43: 1153–1160.

84. Robinson DJ, Lazo MC, Davis T, Kufera J: Infective endocarditis in intravenous drug users: does HIV status alter the presenting temperature and white blood cell count? J Emerg Med 2000;19:5–11.

85. Rodriguez-Mendez M, Gonzalez-Quintela A, Aguilera A, Barrio E: Prevalence, patterns, and course of past hepatitis B virus infection in intravenous drug users with HIV-1 infection. Am J Gastroenterol 2000;95:1316–1322.

86. Selwyn PA: Illicit drug use revisited: What a long, strange trip it's been. Ann Intern Med 1993;119:1044–1045.

87. Shannon M: Clinical toxicity of cocaine adulterants. Ann Emerg Med 1988;17:1243–1247.

88. Soderstrom CA, Smith GS, Dischinger PC, et al: Psychoactive substance use disorders among seriously injured trauma center patients. JAMA 1997;277:1769–1774.

89. Strathdee SA, Patrick DM, Currie SL, et al: Needle exchange is not enough: lessons from the Vancouver injecting drug use study. AIDS 1997;11:59–65.

90. Substance Abuse and Mental Health Services Administration/Office of Applied Studies: 1999 Annual Emergency Department Data. August 2000. Department of Health and Human Services, Rockville, MD.

91. Substance Abuse and Mental Health Services Administration/Office of Applied Studies. 1999 National Household Survey on Drug Abuse. August 2000. Department of Health and Human Services, Rockville, MD.

92. Tortu S, Beardsley M, Deren S, et al: HIV infection and patterns of risk among women drug injectors and crack users in low and high sero-prevalence sites. AIDS Care 2000;12:65–76.

93. Vlahov D, Junge B: The role of needle exchange programs in HIV prevention. Public Health Rep 1998;113(Suppl 1):75–80.

94. Watanakunakorn C: Changing epidemiology and newer aspects of infective endocarditis. Adv Intern Med 1977;22:21–24.

95. Weisse AB, Heller DR, Schimenti RJ, et al: The febrile parenteral drug abuser: A prospective study in 121 patients. Am J Med 1993;94: 274–280.

96. Werner SB, Passaro D, McGee J, et al: Wound botulism in California, 1951–1998: Recent epidemic in heroin injectors. Clin Infect Dis 2000; 31:1018–1024.

97. Williams I: Epidemiology of hepatitis C in the United States. Am J Med 1999;107:2S–9S.

98. Xu W, Flick T, Mitchel J, et al: Cocaine effects on immunocompetent cells: an observation of in vitro cocaine exposure. Int J Imunopharmacol 1999;21:463–472.

CHAPTER 110 HEALTHCARE WORKERS

Michael I. Greenberg

The numbers and types of potential toxins that healthcare workers may be exposed to are as varied as the occupations and job categories that exist in a modern healthcare facility. Typically, the particular toxic hazards that a worker may be exposed to are related more to the immediate work environment within the healthcare facility such as the ICU, laboratory, or ambulance than to the job or profession itself (eg, nurse, physician, unit receptionist).

Although each category of healthcare worker may be exposed to toxins inherent to the performance of the specific duties required, it is important to remember that all healthcare workers also can be exposed to toxins that are generated or exist in areas proximate to their immediate work environment but that have nothing at all to do with the performance of their specific duties.

COMMON TOXIC EXPOSURES

Hospital and healthcare workers constitute the largest single group of employees in the United States today.[28,35] Job-related health and safety issues for these employees have not received appropriate attention until recently. Large numbers of people pass through hospitals each year as patients, visitors, vendors, delivery personnel, and so forth. Consequently, many people, beyond just those who work in the health care industry, may potentially be exposed to various toxic hazards within the hospital environment. Individuals employed in healthcare occupations can be exposed to a multitude of hazardous toxins and chemicals. Certain work areas as well as specific jobs within those areas in the hospital environment have specific toxic hazards commonly associated with them. Knowing which toxins may be associated with specific jobs will facilitate the formulation of a differential diagnosis list for each exposed patient. Table 110–1 lists the most common potential toxic hazards for workers in the healthcare industry. Table 110–2 cites the locations of greatest risk for exposure. These chemical hazards can be categorized as disinfectants, sterilizing agents, solvents, anesthetic agents, chemotherapeutic agents, latex-containing products, detergents, tissue fixatives, and chemical reagents. They may enter the body by dermal absorption, inhalation, ingestion, or unintentional needle stick, with the most common exposure routes being inhalation (through aerosolization) and skin absorption.

GLUTARALDEHYDE

Glutaraldehyde is a saturated dialdehyde compound that is recognized as both a disinfectant and as an effective chemical sterilant (see Chap. 84). Glutaraldehyde finds its most common use as a

disinfectant for medical equipment such as endoscopes, dialysis equipment, and anesthesia and respiratory therapy equipment.[42,71] In the hospital, glutaraldehyde is also commonly found in the histology laboratory, where it may be used as a tissue fixative. It is not corrosive to metal and will not damage glass, rubber, or plastic. It is frequently found in concentrated form but is usually employed as a dilute solution. Most studies suggest that 1.0% glutaraldehyde is the minimum effective concentration when the intended use is as a high-level disinfectant.[36,37] Although glutaraldehyde is commonly used as a 2% solution in hospitals, it may be found in formulations with concentrations as high as 50%.[71] The solution generally should not be used when the concentration is ≤1% glutaraldehyde.[37] As a result of evaporation, the concentration of glutaraldehyde baths and shelf solutions may change over time. The higher the concentration of the solution, the greater the volatility at room temperature, and consequently the higher the concentration of airborne chemical. The evaporation of glutaraldehyde is one way in which workers can become exposed to this chemical. Consequently, it is important to frequently monitor the concentration. Glutaraldehyde test kits are commercially available for the purpose of monitoring solution concentration.

The germicidal ability of glutaraldehyde results from the alkylation of sulfhydryl, hydroxyl, carboxyl, and amino groups within microbes interfering with RNA, DNA, and protein synthesis.[54] Glutaraldehyde-based solutions are widely used in hospitals, primarily because of their superior biocidal activity, efficacy in the presence of organic material, lack of corrosive effects on endoscopy and other equipment, and ability to prevent the coagulation of proteinaceous material on equipment. In aqueous solution this agent tends to be acidic but is not sporicidal in acidic media.[87] Only when the pH of the solution is increased to 7.5 to 8.0 does it regain sporicidal activity. However, at alkaline pH, polymerization of the glutaraldehyde molecules occurs, gradually blocking the active aldehyde sites of the glutaraldehyde molecules, which are resposible for the biocidal activity. The polymerization activity in alkaline solution effectively limits the shelf life of glutaraldehyde solutions to a maximum of 28 days.

Glutaraldehyde is chemically related to formaldehyde and, on exposure, can cause very similar adverse effects, including irritation of the eyes, respiratory tree, and skin. The irritant effects of glutaraldehyde are related to the pH of the solution, which tends to vary with the manufacturer. In addition, it can cause sensitization resulting in allergic contact dermatitis as well as new-onset asthma.[41] Exposure can also result in severe exacerbations of underlying asthma.[41] Inhalational exposure resulting in recurrent epistaxis has also been reported.[73] In addition, fetal toxicity has been identified in certain animal studies.[14]

TABLE 110–1. Chemical and Physical Hazards for Healthcare Workers

Chemical hazards
Disinfectants
    Isopropyl alcohol, iodine, povidone, chlorine, phenol
Sterilants
    Formaldehyde, glutaraldehyde, ethylene oxide (EtO)
Solvents
    Acetone, benzoin, ethanol
Anesthetic agents
    Nitrous oxide, enflurane, halothane, isoflurane
Chemotherapeutic agents
    Antineoplastic and cytotoxic drugs
Pharmaceuticals
    Pentamidine, ribavirin
Heavy metals
    Mercury
Detergents
Tissue fixatives
Laboratory reagents

Biomedical adhesives
    Methyl methacrylate

Physical hazards
Ionizing radiation
Nonionizing radiation
    Laser hazards
    Electrocautery smoke

Allergic sensitization hazards
Latex (as in latex gloves)
Lab animal allergy

TABLE 110–2. Toxic Hazards for Healthcare Workers by Location

Hospital-wide
Disinfectants
    Isopropyl alcohol, iodine, povidone, chlorine, phenol
Sterilants
    Formaldehyde, glutaraldehyde, ethylene oxide (EtO)
Solvents
    Acetone, benzoin, ethanol
Detergents
Ionizing radiation
Latex-containing materials

Operating rooms
Anesthetic agents
    Nitrous oxide, inhalational anesthetics
    Tissue fixatives, biomedical adhesives (methacrylates)
    Nonionizing radiation, laser hazards, electrocautery smoke

Pharmacy
Chemotherapeutic agents, pentamidine, ribavirin

Hospital clinical and research laboratories
Tissue fixative, laboratory chemicals and reagents, laboratory animal allergy

Outpatient/day hospital facilities
Chemotherapeutic agents, pentamidine, ribavirin

Hospital repair shops
Mercury, solvents

Healthcare workers may be exposed to glutaraldehyde vapors in several ways. When equipment is processed in poorly ventilated areas or in open immersion baths or after spills, evaporation of glutaraldehyde may occur, and ambient air levels may easily exceed recommended limits. Various work practice control measures may be helpful in these circumstances, including the use of exhaust hoods ducted to the outside, appropriate lids for immersion baths, and personal protective gloves (nitrile rubber, butyl rubber, polyethylene) and eye protection. In some cases, fitted half-face respirators with organic vapor filters or supplied-air respirators may be appropriate. Recently, automated machinery has come to market for endoscopic disinfection. The use of such equipment is very effective in limiting worker exposure. When exposure is probable, area dosimeters are available for measuring glutaraldehyde levels in the ambient air.

In addition to healthcare workers, both hospitalized and outpatients may be exposed to the toxic effects of glutaraldehyde in certain circumstances. For example, proctitis may result when residual glutaraldehyde solution contaminates the air-water channel of the equipment used for lower gastrointestinal endoscopy.[29] In a similar way, keratopathy can occur following the use of inadequately rinsed ophthalmic instruments following soaking in glutaraldehyde solution.[44]

Treatment for glutaraldehyde skin and inhalational exposures requires prompt removal from exposure. For skin exposures copious irrigation with water provides adequate decontamination. Severe inhalation exposures may require hospital admission for observation, supportive care, and treatment of bronchospasm.

FORMALDEHYDE

Formaldehyde, a gas at standard temperature and pressure, is used as a disinfectant and a sterilant in both its liquid and gaseous states. However, formaldehyde is generally found in the hospital setting as an aqueous solution known as formalin, which acts as a bactericide, tuberculocide, fungicide, virucide, and sporicide.[123] Formaldehyde acts by alkylating amino and sulfhydryl groups in proteins as well as the ring nitrogen atoms of purines.[54]

Formalin, the most commonly encountered solution, contains formaldehyde at a concentration of 37% in methanol and water and is used primarily as a fixative for histology specimens and as an embalming material. In addition, formaldehyde-containing solutions are sometimes used as disinfectants. The hospital autopsy room is probably the location that can be expected to demonstrate the highest air levels of formaldehyde gas and students may be similarly exposed during gross anatomy laboratory.[31] Significant exposure to formaldehyde occurs in renal transplant units when dialysis equipment is not thoroughly rinsed and tested for the presence of residual formaldehyde.[30] In other health-related venues, exposure may occur when formaldehyde is used in the preparation of viral vaccines, as an embalming agent, and for preserving anatomic specimens. In the past, formaldehyde was used as a sterilant for surgical instruments as well.

Following ingestion, formalin causes local corrosive injury in the gastrointestinal tract as metabolism of formaldehyde generates formic acid. Elevated formate levels can be associated with circulatory collapse, severe metabolic acidosis, and the development of acute renal failure. Intentional ingestions of formalin may result in death within a matter of hours.[80] However, if the patient survives for a period of 48 hours, recovery generally can be expected.[80]

The use of formaldehyde in the hospital is limited to some degree by its irritating fumes and obnoxious odor, which is manifest at rather low ambient levels (<1 ppm) (see Chap. 95). Inhalational exposure to low concentrations of formaldehyde initially results in mucous membrane irritation manifested as conjunctivitis and sore throat. This may be followed by the development of pulmonary irritation with coughing, shortness of breath, and difficulty breathing. However, repeat exposure to formaldehyde gas in patients who were suspected of having formaldehyde-related asthma failed to induce symptoms consistent with asthma such as wheezing and shortness of breath.[56] At high concentrations (50 to 100 ppm) of exposure, pulmonary edema and death are reported.[80] Although formaldehyde is a proven animal carcinogen, its carcinogenicity in humans is not certain. The specific concern involves the ability of formaldehyde to chemically react with hydrogen chloride to yield bis(chloromethyl)ether, a compound that is a known pulmonary carcinogen. There is no definitive scientific evidence linking formaldehyde to the development of chronic obstructive pulmonary disease in individuals who are chronically exposed. Several studies performed in both the United States and elsewhere suggest that formaldehyde may be a causative agent for either nasal or pulmonary cancers.[3,140]

MERCURY

Elemental mercury is widely encountered in hospital environments in various kinds of medical equipment and monitoring devices including sphygmomanometers, thermometers, and thermostats. When such equipment breaks, healthcare workers, patients, and visitors may be exposed to elemental mercury. Repairing biomedical equipment may also be a source of mercury spills. Mercury is also used as a tissue fixative in the histology laboratory. Dentists and oral surgeons can be occupationally exposed to the mercury used in dental amalgams.[49,115,119] In all of these cases, exposure is by inhalation because at room temperature mercury easily vaporizes and becomes airborne.

When heated and acutely inhaled, mercury vapor can cause direct respiratory damage in the form of corrosive bronchitis and potentially fatal interstitial pneumonitis. Chronic exposure to mercury results in primarily neurologic effects, which are discussed in Chap. 81.

ANTINEOPLASTIC AGENTS AND OTHER "HAZARDOUS DRUGS"

The American Society of Hospital Pharmacists defines "hazardous drugs" to include those that are known to be genotoxic, carcinogenic, teratogenic and/or able to impair fertility, and those that can cause serious organ or other toxic manifestations at low doses in animals or humans.[8] Table 110–3 lists some common drugs that are considered to be hazardous by these criteria.

The preparation, administration, and disposal of hazardous drugs may expose pharmacists, nurses, physicians, as well as other healthcare workers to these chemicals. The degree of absorption that may take place during work and the significance of these exposures are often difficult to characterize and quantify. Conse-

quently, it is difficult to set safe levels of exposure on the basis of current scientific information.[113] Nevertheless, it is essential to minimize human exposure to all hazardous drugs. Although monitoring the work environment for cytotoxic drugs can be problematic, measurable air levels of many of these agents can be detected when they are prepared outside of protective cabinets or hoods.[78] Elevated levels of fluorouracil and cyclophosphamide are found in these circumstances, implying the possibility of respiratory exposure to workers.[103,117] Cyclophosphamide is also demonstrated in measurable concentrations on surfaces of work areas,[91,117] implying the possibility of dermal exposure by workers. Nurses who handle cytotoxic drugs absorb these agents and demonstrate urinary mutagenicity, which increases during the course of the work week.[52,53] In addition, levels of urinary thioethers act as indirect markers of exposure to cytotoxic drugs and are elevated in healthcare workers who handle cytotoxic drugs when compared to controls.[72,74]

Although chemotherapeutic agents and other hazardous drugs may pose specific potential hazards to an individual, one important common denominator of concern is the potential for bone marrow suppression with the possible development of marrow aplasia and aplastic anemia.[10,131,137] In addition, many of these agents may have inherent carcinogenic potential of their own.[48,68–70,78,125,126,132] Obviously removal from exposure is the first essential step in treatment. However, a complete blood count should be monitored at regular intervals. No published guidelines are available for such monitoring, but the patient's psychological needs should be considered, and such monitoring is medically prudent as well as psychologically comforting. Referral to a specialist in occupational medicine is essential in such cases to arrange for medical monitoring.

TABLE 110–3.   Potentially Hazardous Drugs in the Workplace

Azathioprine	Ifosfamide
L-Asparaginase	Interferon-α
Bleomycin	Isotretinoin
Busulfan	Leuprolide
Carboplatin	Lomustine
Carmustine	Mechlorethamine
Chlorambucil	Melphalan
Chloramphenicol	Mercaptopurine
Chlorozotocin	Mitomycin
Cisplatin	Mitotane
Cyclophosphamide	Nafarelin
Cyclosporine	Pipobroman
Cytarabine	Plicamycin
Dacarbazine	Procarbazine
Dactinomycin	Ribavirin
Daunorubicin	Streptozotocin
Diethylstilbestrol	Tamoxifen
Doxorubicin	Testolactone
Estradiol	Thioguanine
Estramustine	Thiotepa
Etoposide	Uracil mustard
Floxuridine	Vidarabine
Fluorouracil	Vinblastine
Ganciclovir	Vincristine
Hydroxyurea	Zidovudine
Idarubicin	

REPRODUCTIVE HAZARDS

The potential reproductive risk of exposure to carcinogens must also be considered.[126,132] The agents that are generally considered to be significant reproductive risks for healthcare workers include agents that fall into the following categories: inhalational anesthetic gases, antineoplastics, sterilizing chemicals, tissue fixatives, aerosolized antivirals, and ionizing radiation.

Anesthetic Agents

The first report of adverse reproductive effects related to anesthetic agents appeared in the late 1960s. Subsequently, an increased rate of teratogenic events among anesthetists was reported,[12] and in 1971 an increase in unsuccessful pregnancies among nurse anesthetists and nurses working in the operating room was noted.[33] A 16.4% increased risk of birth defects among female nurse anesthetists who continued to work while pregnant, compared with those nurse anesthetists who did not, was also reported.[39] The American Society of Anesthesiologists completed a survey of anesthetists, operating room nurses, and operating room technicians with regard to work-related reproductive risks.[7] In this study of 50,000 individuals, the investigators discovered an increased (1.3- to 2.0-fold) risk of spontaneous miscarriage relative to controls. In addition, the number of congenital abnormalities noted in these individuals was approximately double that for the unexposed women. The risk of congenital abnormalities was noted to be 1.6 times greater for nurse anesthetists. The following discussion details the reproductive risks involved with exposure to two operating room gases.

Ethylene Oxide. Ethylene oxide (EtO) is one of the most significant reproductive hazards to which healthcare workers may be exposed. A gaseous chemical with an odor similar to that of ether, EtO finds its principal use in the hospital setting in the gas sterilization of medical and surgical equipment that cannot be safely sterilized by heat and moisture. It is important to note that currently, there is no acceptable substitute for EtO sterilization (ie, cold sterilization), and the continued use of EtO is essential for the control of nosocomial infections. Therefore, EtO continues to be widely used in hospitals around the world.

Hospital workers become exposed to EtO largely as the result of residual ethylene oxide gas that remains in and around sterilization equipment. When removed from the gas sterilizer, the material being sterilized may contain residual amounts of the gas as well. Proper gas sterilization techniques, therefore, require periods of thorough aeration in order to allow residual ethylene oxide to properly dissipate.

Inhalation provides the primary means for acute exposure to ethylene oxide.[17] At low concentrations, such an exposure results in irritation to mucous membranes. However, exposure to increasingly elevated concentrations of EtO can cause gastrointestinal symptoms including nausea, vomiting, and diarrhea as well as headache. Some exposed individuals describe an unusual but distinctly nonmetallic taste as well.[17] Following substantial acute exposures, central nervous system depression can occur.[17] Such exposures may be followed by delayed symptoms including weakness, malaise, and lack of coordination. Ethylene oxide exposure–associated central nervous system dysfunction is reported to involve deficits in cognition, memory, and psychomotor skills.[17] Cataracts may also occur following exposure to very high concentrations of EtO.[124] In addition, pulmonary edema and ECG abnor-

malities have been reported as late sequelae of EtO exposure.[124] Skin burns can result from dermal exposure to ethylene oxide–containing solutions, the severity and depth of which depend on the length of exposure and concentration of the ethylene oxide solution at issue.[127]

Ethylene oxide is classified as a human carcinogen even though its human carcinogenicity is highly controversial. EtO is, however, a proven genotoxic animal carcinogen.[22,64,116] In laboratory animals, EtO acts by alkylation of DNA and cellular proteins.[86] The Occupational Safety and Health Administration (OSHA) released formal standards concerning occupational exposure to ethylene oxide in 1984. These standards are based on animal and human data and indicate that exposures to EtO present a carcinogenic, mutagenic, reproductive, neurologic, and sensitization hazard to workers. This standard set the permissible exposure level (PEL) for ethylene oxide at 1.0 part per million (ppm), determined as an 8-hour time-weighted average air concentration. In addition, OSHA established an action level (AL) for EtO of 0.5 ppm determined as an 8-hour time-weighted average. In 1988, OSHA amended previously published standards by adding a short-term exposure limit (STEL) for EtO of 5.0 ppm, determined as a 15-minute time-weighted average. The promulgation of this short-term exposure standard serves to benefit exposed workers in hospitals as well as those in facilities involved in the commercial manufacture of this agent.

The exposure of healthcare workers to EtO can be thought of as consisting of essentially three distinct factors: personal practices, equipment conditions, and ventilation characteristics. On the basis of an analysis of these three components, each hospital and work site must determine the strategy it will use in developing a control program that will reduce ethylene oxide exposure to the limits addressed by OSHA standards.

There are several biologic markers for ethylene oxide exposure, including hemoglobin adducts and sister-chromatid exchanges. These markers are not demonstrated to be consistent indicators of genotoxicity or increased risk of disease. Nonetheless, these changes do appear to reflect exposure to ethylene oxide, although the application of these methods is not yet reflected in clinical practice.[48]

Nitrous Oxide. Physicians, veterinarians, and dentists and their assistants may be exposed to nitrous oxide (N_2O) during procedures in which this agent is used (see Chap. 53). The acute toxic effects of N_2O may also be of concern in the setting of substance abuse.[133]

Several animal studies raise concern about the potential for adverse health effects related to N_2O exposures. These studies generally reveal reproductive and developmental abnormalities in laboratory animals exposed to high concentrations of N_2O. Spontaneous abortions occurred in rats exposed to N_2O at concentrations ≥1000 ppm.[138,139] Published data by The National Institute of Occupational Safety and Health (NIOSH) indicate that concentrations of 1000 ppm can be found in hospital and dental operating facilities not utilizing waste gas scavenging systems.[101,102] In humans, observational studies demonstrate specific adverse effects following exposure to N_2O including a reduction in overall fertility.[122] In addition, an increase in the rate of spontaneous abortions was reported along with increases in neurologic, renal, and liver disease.[33] Female dental assistants exposed to N_2O for more than 5 hours per week had a significantly increased incidence of diminished fertility in comparison with unexposed female dental assistants.[122] Exposed individuals suffered a 59% decrease in ability to conceive during any given menstrual cycle compared with unexposed controls. When an effective gas-scavenging system was in place, however, the probability of conception was noted to be equal to that of the unexposed controls.[122]

N_2O often is the exclusive anesthesia drug used by dentists in their private offices. The problem with use in this setting is that exposures in private dental offices are more difficult to control than in other settings. NIOSH demonstrated exposures to N_2O as high as 300 ppm in hospital operating rooms and exposures higher than 1000 ppm of N_2O in dental operatories.[101] The extremely high levels found in dental offices occur despite the general use of gas-scavenging systems. In addition, control of N_2O escaping into the ambient air tends to be more difficult to control during dental procedures. Only the patient's nose is covered during dental anesthesia administration, as opposed to covering both the nose and mouth during other forms of surgery.

In 1977, NIOSH published a technical report entitled "Control of Occupational Exposure to N_2O in the Dental Operatory."[101,102] This report describes various methods for limiting the concentration of waste N_2O in this setting and notes that properly operating scavenging systems can reduce N_2O concentrations in the ambient air by as much as 70%.[92]

The potential medical problems attributable to N_2O exposure in dental medicine alone involve more than 400,000 individuals (dentists, dental assistants, and dental hygienists) involved in dentistry in the United States.[34] In addition, the American Dental Association (ADA) reported in 1983 that 35% of dentists used N_2O to control pain and anxiety in their patients.[6] The ADA 1991 Survey of Dental Practice indicated that 58% of dentists reported having N_2O anesthetic equipment, but only 64% of those practitioners also reported having a scavenging system.[6] The percentage of pediatric dentists using N_2O increased from 65% in 1980 to 88% in 1988.[45]

The fact that N_2O may adversely impact reproductive outcomes was first demonstrated in animal models. Several studies in humans have demonstrated adverse reproductive effects following exposure to nitrous oxide.[40,138,139]

OSHA does not currently have a standard for N_2O. In addition, there is currently no NIOSH recommended exposure limit intended to prevent adverse reproductive effects. However, NIOSH recommends an exposure limit of 25 ppm as a time-weighted average for N_2O, which is intended primarily to prevent decreases in mental performance, changes in audiovisual ability, and deterioration of manual dexterity of dental personnel who work with N_2O[101,102] (see Chap. 53).

The primary organization that has specifically addressed the protection of workers from the reproductive hazards of N_2O to date has been the American Conference of Governmental Industrial Hygienists (ACGIH), which has recommended a threshold limit value for N_2O of 50 ppm as an 8-hour TWA.[1,2] These guidelines state that "control to this level should prevent embryo-fetal toxicity in humans and significant decrements in human psychomotor and cognitive functions or other adverse health effects in exposed personnel."[1]

INHALATIONAL MEDICATIONS
Ribavirin

The treatment of respiratory syncytial virus in pediatric patients often involves the administration of antiviral agents delivered via

aerosol. When administered either via hood, oxygen tent, or nebulizer, significant amounts of these agents may escape into the ambient room air. Consequently, nurses, respiratory therapists, visitors, physicians, and occasionally others may be exposed. One of the most commonly used antiviral agents is the synthetic nucleoside ribavirin.[59,62] Ribavirin has not been conclusively shown to exert adverse reproductive effects in humans but is teratogenic in laboratory animals.[86] A recent study demonstrated that the typical in-hospital occupational exposure to ribavirin, even without the use of appropriate personal protective equipment, would not result in significant levels of ribavirin.[82] However, another study evaluated urine collected from respiratory therapists and nurses following the completion of their work shifts. Despite the use of high-efficiency respirators worn by all subjects, ribavirin was detected in the urine of 11 of the 17 individuals.[46] The urine levels of ribavirin were significantly higher for the nurses than for the respiratory therapists.[46] Hospital personnel should avoid exposure to ribavirin before and during pregnancy as well as during lactation.[142] Other potential adverse health effects referable to aerosolized ribavirin have included ocular irritation as well as contact lens damage.[47] The precise mechanism for the action of ribavirin is unknown; however, ribavirin may act as an analogue of guanosine.

Pentamidine

Another antiinfective agent administered via aerosol is pentamidine, previously commonly used to treat *Pneumocystis carinii* pneumonia. Just as with ribavirin, this mode of drug administration can result in exposure to various healthcare workers, patients, and visitors. One report indicated that the removal of the delivery nebulizer from the patient's mouth before it was turned off increased the ambient levels of pentamidine.[106] In addition, if the patient coughed, the levels of pentamidine in the air increased as well.[106] Another report documented the acute onset of bronchospasm in a nurse with no prior history of asthma immediately following the administration of aerosolized pentamidine to a patient.[103] Bronchospasm is also reported in patients receiving pentamidine treatments.[46]

Additional chronic effects of occupational pentamidine exposure are reported as well. One example of such chronic effects involves the case of a respiratory technician whose carbon monoxide diffusing capacity declined significantly during the time that he worked with pentamidine aerosols.[46] Pentamidine levels have been detected in the urine of those healthcare workers who are involved in the administration of pentamidine aerosol treatments.[95] This probably represents evidence of systemic absorption of pentamidine as a result of this type of inhalation exposure. However, 16 healthcare workers who administered aerosolized pentamidine while working were studied, and despite the fact that aerosolized pentamidine levels in the ambient air were documented to be elevated, no pentamidine was detected in the urine of any of these subjects. These investigators emphasize the importance of taking steps to minimize healthcare worker exposure to aerosolized pentamidine.[15]

RADIATION

Table 110–1 lists the most common toxic physical hazards found in the hospital and healthcare setting. Ionizing and nonionizing radiation represent important sources of exposure hazards for healthcare workers; a complete discussion of the biophysics of these hazards can be found in Chap. 99.

Ionizing Radiation

Healthcare workers may be exposed to ionizing radiation in essentially two ways. Exposure may occur as the result of random scatter from x-ray beams, especially from portable x-ray or fluoroscopy equipment used in the emergency department,[24] operating room, cardiac catheterization laboratories, intensive care units, or the radiology department. Exposure can also occur as the result of γ or β emissions from patients who are treated with radioactive implants or who are undergoing diagnostic nuclear medicine procedures. Almost any hospital staff member may be at risk of exposure from these sources, but some personnel (especially nurses) seem to be at greater risk. In a prospective study of radiation exposure in the emergency department, mean lapel and wrist dosimetry was measured during a 2-year period for emergency department personnel.[24,100] Emergency physicians demonstrated a lapel level that was approximately half that of radiology technicians. However, when wrist levels were compared, emergency physicians were found to have almost twice the exposure of radiology technicians. This may reflect direct physical involvement when, for example, small children require stress films of extremities. Another study of physician exposure to ionizing radiation during trauma resuscitation efforts revealed that significant radiation exposures can occur in this setting as well.[144] To obtain complete cervical spine radiography, healthcare workers may be asked to manually stabilize a patient's neck.[130] When radiographic procedures are done, the use of protective garments by healthcare workers should be considered mandatory. Personnel positioned more than several feet from the x-ray beam will generally experience relatively insignificant exposures.[60]

When an acute, unintentional radiation exposure takes place, the effects are usually local and superficial, resulting in erythroderma. More significant exposure may result in radiodermatitis. More serious effects from occupational exposure are distinctly rare. However, the degree of risk to healthcare workers is yet to be precisely determined. Only a few studies address the risk related to long-term, low-dose x-ray exposure.[9,21,141] However, several studies identify a high prevalence of cancer of the thyroid as well as the development of thyroid nodules resulting from occupational radiation exposure.[11] OSHA has promulgated a formal standard for ionizing radiation, limiting radiation exposure.[112]

Nonionizing Radiation

Lasers. Table 110–1 lists nonionizing radiation hazards that may be present in the healthcare work environment. One of the most common forms of nonionizing radiation is lasers. The term "laser" is an acronym for "Light Amplification by Stimulated Emission of Radiation." The energy is a specific form of light that is produced when energy of electrical origin interfaces with a solid, liquid, or gas medium. The resultant light is a single wavelength consisting of a parallel focused high-energy beam.

Several different types of lasers are currently available for medical use, including the Nd:Yag (neodymium:yttrium-aluminum-garnet) laser, the carbon dioxide laser, the argon laser, the dye laser, and the excimer laser.[88] Lasers can be used to incise or destroy tissue, depending on the unique physical properties of the laser beam.

When a concentrated laser beam destroys tissue, cell vaporization results and causes what is known as a "laser plume" of smoke, which is actually a complex mixture of steam, cellular debris, and smoke associated with a pungent, unpleasant odor. The odor can be so intense that the use of high-pressure extraction devices may be necessary to eliminate it from the area. Laser plume odor is noxious, and healthcare workers have been "overcome" by the this exposure.[145]

Inhalational exposure to the laser "plume" during operative procedures is also of concern. Studies have attempted to determine if pathogenic organisms or even viable cells might be disseminated during the production of a laser plume. Aerosols produced from laser-treated rodents contain intact cells in the laser plume, but these cells proved to be culture negative for pathogens.[88] Other investigators have recovered pathogenic bacteria from laser plume cultures.[88] These studies concluded that the laser plume could carry and disseminate pathogenic material during laser treatments. Nonetheless, there are no current recommendations addressing special precautions to be taken in this regard or regarding the advisability of pregnant individuals avoiding laser plumes. It is important to note that the smoke generated by electrocautery devices used to stop small amounts of local bleeding can also be harmful in ways similar to the laser plume.

Ocular toxicity from laser exposure is an important concern. A specific period of time, measured in maximal permissible exposure times (MPEs), determines the amount of time that the eye can be safely exposed to a laser beam. All personnel working around lasers must be thoroughly knowledgeable in the proper use of eye protection during laser operations. The acute ocular injury that may result from exposure to a laser beam may be ameliorated by proper eye protective devices, although there may be ocular damage from long-term laser exposure with or without proper eye protection. Macular damage may occur in ophthalmologists exposed to laser beams during operative conditions over the course of many years.[145] Several recommendations, established specifically for healthcare workers, describe steps to be taken to provide protection of the eyes from laser injury.[43]

An additional concern with regard to lasers is the potential for the development of an explosive hazard during use. Explosions have occurred when lasers caused the ignition of either anesthetic gases or bowel gases.[43] In one case report, a 41-year-old patient with carcinoma of the larynx was seriously injured when a laser ignited the patient's endotracheal tube, causing severe laryngeal and tracheal burns.[43]

Ultraviolet Light Radiation. Ultraviolet light radiation (UVLR) is a form of nonionizing radiation that may represent a health hazard to certain healthcare workers. This form of radiation ranges in wavelength from 200 to 400 nm.

Three specific "regions" exist within the UVLR spectrum that are the focus of most concern. UVLR in the "A" region (UV-A) is reported to be the most important factor in the development of cataracts following exposure, whereas UV-B is generally considered the most dangerous of the UVLR exposures. UV-C, on the other hand, is considered to be the most benign of this form of radiation and has germicidal properties only. Consequently, UV-C is often used as a means of food and air sterilization. UV-C light sources can be found at entryways to operating room areas in the hospital as well as in the food service areas. To date, no firm scientific evidence has been reported to implicate UV-C radiation as a source for health problems in exposed individuals.

ALLERGENS

PHARMACEUTICALS

Pharmaceuticals may present a significant risk to healthcare workers as a result of acute or chronic low-dosage exposure. As previously discussed, chemotherapeutic agents are an example; others include certain antibiotics and such proteolytic enzymes as pancreatic extracts and papain. Most pharmaceuticals are hazardous primarily by inhalational exposure and primary pulmonary toxicity. The pulmonary hazards more commonly occur where pharmaceuticals are manufactured. However, healthcare workers who administer and/or prepare these agents are also at risk of developing either asthma or other allergic manifestations. Preparations involving drugs that generate dusts are a particular problem. Even the simple act of counting pills can produce small amounts of powder that may aerosolize and sensitize an individual.

Another specific material of concern is psyllium, which is often found as a constituent in bulk laxatives. Psyllium is implicated in the sensitization of exposed workers and is associated with the development of occupationally related asthma.[55] The problem is probably more common in chronic care facilities, where the use of laxatives is widespread. In one study, as many as 18% of healthcare workers reported allergic reactions while handling psyllium.[58] The reactions varied from mild mucosal irritation to respiratory compromise. Psyllium challenge testing to evaluate sensitization of personnel working in chronic care institutions[85] found the prevalence of asthmatic symptoms to be similar to that found in workers manufacturing psyllium.

Other forms of testing of workers for possible sensitization to various inhaled drugs and allergens are inefficient and may not be accurate prognostically. Assays to measure specific hazardous drug levels or their metabolites in blood and urine and tests measuring urine mutagenicity or cytogenetic changes are difficult to perform and of uncertain significance. Because the use of these inhalational materials may be episodic, poorly documented, and difficult to quantify, control of the problem is difficult. Preventive measures depend on adequate measures to reduce exposure and many hospitals have instituted the use of "biologic safety cabinets" (BSCS) and built-in vertical air flow systems, which are widely used in the preparation of hazardous drugs. Several agencies including OSHA and the American Society of Hospital Pharmacists have published guidelines for the proper handling of these agents.[8,110]

METHACRYLATE COMPOUNDS

Methacrylate-containing compounds are widely used in orthopedic surgery and in dental procedures as biologic adhesives. In order to create the adhesive, a liquid and a powder constituent are mixed together. During the mixing process, healthcare workers may be exposed to the components.

Upper respiratory irritation and contact dermatitis, allergic as well as irritant-type dermatitis, may follow acute exposure to methacrylate compounds.[38,121] Sensitization to methacrylate dusts repeatedly has resulted in the development of asthma[16] in dental assistants and several dental patients.[4] Allergic conjunctivitis associated with occupational exposure to methacrylate is also reported.[51] The appropriate use of exhaust systems in conjunction with adequate ventilation can help to limit the possibility of significant exposures.

LATEX ALLERGY

Approximately 2% of the general population may be affected by mild to severe allergic reactions to latex.[5] Frequency of exposure may be a factor. For example, up to 50% of children who have spina bifida reportedly experienced severe latex reactions.[79] Such children may be sensitized by frequent bladder catheterizations using rubber tubing and by individuals wearing latex gloves. Three percent of all hospital workers experience immediate-type hypersensitivity to latex, and as many as 10% of operating room nurses may react to rubber in this way.[146,147] Approximately 5% of workers involved in the manufacturing of surgical gloves and in the rubber industry also may develop an immediate-type hypersensitivity to rubber.[147]

Latex is the milk-like sappy material that emanates from the rubber tree *Hevea brasiliensis.* Adverse reactions to natural rubber products were first reported in the early 1930s and were attributed to the many compounding agents that may be added during production.[5] In fact, the hand dermatitis that occurs in reaction to latex gloves is usually caused by a delayed (type IV) hypersensitivity reaction to thiurams or other additives rather than to the latex itself.[135] Since evidence for immunoglobulin (Ig) E–mediated (type I) reactions to protein antigens in latex itself were first documented some 15 years ago, the incidence of such reactions has increased dramatically. Implementation of "universal precautions" against infectious diseases is the major reason for this increase.[5] However, in addition to the substantial increase in the use of latex gloves by healthcare workers in order to avoid infection, the apparent antigenicity of latex products has increased as a result of changes in manufacturing process designed to increase production.[136] Although the amount of antigen present in latex gloves tends to be highly variable, factors that lower the amount of allergen in these gloves include leaching and steam sterilization. Studies have identified different possible antigens in latex. Although the cornstarch used in latex gloves is nonallergenic,[147] latex particles can be adsorbed by the starch and become aerosolized, thus increasing the possibility of airborne exposure.

The clinical presentation of latex allergy can be highly variable. The most common presenting symptoms are localized urticaria or simple dermatitis. However, systemic symptoms including generalized urticaria, rhinitis, asthma, and anaphylaxis can develop.[5]

Sensitization is largely dependent on two specific factors: the amount of antigen in the product and the form of exposure. The most serious reactions attributable to latex result from parenteral or mucosal contact.[147] Specific examples of such exposures include those that occur intraoperatively or during barium enemas, genitourinary catheterization, and dental procedures.

IgE-mediated reactions to latex product exposure on the job have been recognized since 1988. Recent surveys indicate that 10 to 17% of all hospital personnel, 7.4% of surgeons, and 5.2 to 10.7% of operating room staff are sensitive to latex.[146]

The diagnosis of IgE-mediated allergy typically is confirmed by skin prick or radioallergosorbent testing (RAST). However, the interpretation of these tests for latex sensitivity can be problematic, as there are currently no standardized commercial extracts for skin testing available in the United States. Older RAST methods had only a 60 to 65% sensitivity, whereas newer tests have a somewhat higher sensitivity.[75]

The first and simplest approach to testing is to apply the rubber material to the skin and then wait approximately 30 minutes to see if any skin reaction or other symptoms occur. Another approach is the so-called "prick test," in which a drop of fluid containing the presumed allergen is applied to the surface of the skin at the site of a needle prick or a series of superficial skin abrasions. Although these types of tests tend to be the most sensitive for determining allergy to rubber, they may potentially trigger life-threatening reactions. Consequently, it is extremely important to have appropriate resuscitation equipment and drugs (including the means for airway control) readily available to treat possible anaphylactic reactions and also to have physicians in attendance capable of providing advanced cardiac life support, should that become necessary.

In order to prevent occupational exposure of healthcare workers, nonlatex, low antigen–containing, powder-free gloves and latex substitutes for nonglove products must be utilized. A future goal involves the production of rubber products for hospital use that have no or only very minimal allergenicity.

Another important issue to consider is the accuracy of labeling of rubber products. The removal of antioxidants and the accelerant previously used in the vulcanization process was thought to have made rubber gloves "safe for rubber-allergic persons."[136] Although gloves manufactured in this way are labeled as protective for latex-allergic individuals, this is true for people who have only delayed-type hypersensitivity dermatitis, leading to simple scaling and blisters of their hands and not to the much more serious immediate-type hypersensitivity. This point is illustrated by the report of a cardiac catheterization nurse who developed periorbital swelling and pharyngeal edema following exposure to latex in gloves that were supposedly "nonallergenic." Within approximately 90 minutes following exposure to this "safe" product, this individual required epinephrine and intravenous corticosteroid therapy.[105]

Gloves have historically been used to protect people from various hazards found in their work environment. Rubber gloves can, however, represent a substantial toxic hazard for some workers and may possibly be lethal for those with immediate-type hypersensitivity to latex. In the hospital setting, where so many individuals rely on latex gloves, a periodic review of workers' skin reactions to exposure to rubber products is important. However, as illustrated above, it is important to be aware that workers' sensitivities to rubber products may have manifestations other than simple dermal manifestations, and workers who complain of mucosal irritation, difficulty breathing, or upper airway irritation should be evaluated promptly.

When a sensitized individual is continually exposed to latex, increased sensitivity occurs with the possibility of developing permanent and potentially life-threatening respiratory sequelae. As many as 15 to 17% of healthcare workers are sensitized to latex and ultimately develop occupational asthma.[5,81] Because there is no cure for latex-related allergy, avoidance of exposure is the most important means for preventing an allergic reaction to latex. It is important to remember that latex reactions can be minimized through early diagnosis.

Currently, there are no published guidelines for the establishment of a latex-safe environment. However, it is clear that those individuals who manifest findings consistent with anaphylaxis must be permanently removed from such exposure.[128]

Further, it is unlikely that a rubber glove proven to be completely safe will be developed for individuals who have immediate-type hypersensitivity in the near future. In some instances, vinyl gloves may be a reasonable substitute; however, they offer no protection against environmental (airborne) contamination.

One recent study indicated that approximately 25% of medical personnel had demonstrable hand contamination with bacteria when wearing vinyl gloves, whereas only approximately 2% had hand contamination when wearing rubber-containing gloves.[105] Consequently, the use of vinyl gloves corrects the potential for exposure to one serious toxin while exposing the worker to significant risks for pathogen exposure.

Some workers may attempt to protect their hands using a vinyl glove covered by a rubber glove. This approach to "double gloving" may give the worker sufficient protection from bacterial contamination, but there is still the possibility of continued latex sensitization, airborne contamination, and possible anaphylaxis. Table 110–4 lists some of the measures that can be taken to implement a latex-safe environment for healthcare workers.

OTHER SENSITIZING ALLERGENS

Large numbers of healthcare workers and those working in related fields such as pharmaceutical developments may be exposed to animal-derived allergenic materials on a regular basis. These individuals may develop what has come to be known as laboratory animal allergy (LAA), a clinical syndrome characterized by rhinitis, upper airway inflammation, and occasionally bronchospasm. It is important to note that the majority of workers suffering from LAA report symptoms associated with rhinitis and upper airway symptoms as opposed to asthmatic symptoms.[50]

LAA involves the development of a hypersensitivity reaction in association with dermal or inhalational exposure to animal allergens. LAA is an IgE-mediated reaction affecting approximately 30% of workers exposed to lab animals.[50] Exposure to animal urine and saliva seems to be an especially powerful inciting agent for the development of LAA. Although specific risk factors for the development of LAA are not well defined, several studies address this question. Surprisingly, a history of atopy was not found to increase the risk of LAA in some studies.[118] However, atopy is indeed an associated risk factor in other studies.[81,118] One study found a history of allergic symptoms in 168 of 364 animal handlers.[98] There is also controversy with regard to the ability of skin prick and RAST tests to detect LAA.

To control exposure for workers, systematic surveillance for the presence of airborne allergens may be useful. One study demonstrated a strong correlation between airborne rat urinary allergen and the symptoms of LAA.[99] In another study of over 500 animal handlers, almost 25% of workers reported LAA symptoms, with a substantial percentage of those reporting the need to cease working as a result of the severity of their LAA-related symptoms.[50] The latter study was unable to demonstrate a salutary effect of the use of personal protective equipment. However, this study recommends using dustless animal bedding, reducing the use of animal bedding materials, and using local exhaust ventila-

TABLE 110–4. Creating a Latex-Safe Environment

1. Glove education for all employees.
2. Comprehensive employee health histories, updated periodically, including history of food sensitivity.
3. Do not rely on "hypoallergenic" claims.
4. Replace latex nosepieces and rubber dental dams.
5. Create latex-safe crash carts.
6. Clean and maintain all air ducts and filters.
7. Remove all powdered gloves as the ultimate protective strategy.

tion (hoods) when cleaning animal cages in order to minimize the aerosolizing of allergens. For workers who have not developed asthma, respiratory protective devices are recommended. In 58% of workers suffering from LAA, the use of PPE was reported to improve symptoms.[20] Investigators point out that the expense of more rigorous exposure prevention is justified by the savings from decreased time lost from work.

SELF-POISONING

Healthcare workers have relatively easy access to a wide variety of drugs, toxic laboratory chemicals, and other toxic materials. Consequently, it might be expected that intentional self-poisoning with these substances is a problem. In addition, many healthcare workers have knowledge regarding the effects of these drugs and toxins. The literature supports the claim that healthcare personnel utilize different substances in suicidal gestures than does the general public: barbiturates, potassium, insulin, carbon monoxide, cyanide, azides, and methemoglobin-forming chemicals may be more commonly used in suicidal attempts by healthcare personnel.[18] This should be kept in mind when treating a healthcare worker for an unknown overdose or poisoning.

HAZARDOUS LABORATORY CHEMICALS AND REAGENTS

A multitude of potentially dangerous chemicals and reagents are present in various hospital locations. These materials are found in the greatest types and quantities in the hospital, clinical, and research laboratory facilities. In order to address some of the unique dangers of the laboratory workplace, OSHA has promulgated a standard for occupational exposures to hazardous chemicals in clinical and academic laboratories.[107]

In general, most of these materials fall into the category of either weak or strong acids or bases or organic solvents. Toxicity from exposure to these substances is generally represented by skin burns as a result of unintentional dermal exposures. On occasion, intentional ingestions occur and result in injury consistent with the substance ingested. The pathophysiology and treatment of these injuries are dealt with elsewhere in this book.

One specific laboratory chemical of special concern is sodium azide. This chemical is widely available in hospitals and thus is of concern because of its availability as a toxicant. Sodium azide is often found as a component chemical in the fluid used to dilute blood samples before autoanalyzer analysis. In addition, sodium azide can be found as a constituent of one of the buffering reagents used in testing for the presence of hepatitis antigen.[120] Sodium azide exerts its toxic effects within the mitochondria, where it interferes with energy transfer by mediating the uncoupling of oxidative phosphorylation. In addition, the enzymes catalase and cytochrome oxidase are specifically inhibited by sodium azide. The precise mechanisms responsible for the toxicity of sodium azide have not been fully elucidated.

Clinically, sodium azide poisoning may result in a wide range of effects including many in the central nervous system such as seizures, hyporeflexia, coma, and headache. In addition, nausea, vomiting, diarrhea, and hypotension resulting from vascular smooth muscle relaxation have been reported. Death may follow, and at autopsy pulmonary, cerebral, and myocardial edema with myocardial necrosis all have been reported.[77]

The treatment of sodium azide poisoning is primarily aimed at providing symptomatic relief and cardiovascular support. Because clinical deterioration may be delayed, intensive care monitoring should be considered for a minimum of 72 hours.

HAZARDOUS CHEMICALS AND DRUG SPILLS

Written policies addressing the management of both small and large spills in the health care setting. Small spills are considered to involve less than 5 mL of material, whereas large spills are defined as involving more than 5 mL of material. Of special concern are those spills involving hazardous drugs (known human mutagens, carcinogens, teratogens, or reproductive toxicants or those known to be acutely toxic to an organ system). In addition, investigational drugs should be handled as hazardous drugs unless reliable information to the contrary can be verified.

All spills should be cleaned up as quickly as possible by trained personnel wearing double latex gloves, gowns, and eye protection. NIOSH-approved respirators should be worn if airborne or aerosol exposure is likely. Liquids should be wiped with absorbent gauze pads, and solids wiped with wet absorbent gauze. The spill area should then be cleaned three times with a detergent solution and rinsed copiously with water. The spread of large spills (greater than 5 mL) should be limited by applying absorbent sheets or spill control pads. If dusts or powders are involved, damp cloth coverings should be used.

Spill kits should be available in areas prone to spills. These kits should generally contain splash goggles, gloves, low-permeability gowns, various absorbent materials, "sharps" containers, scoops to collect glass fragments, and special waste disposal bags. These kits may be preprepared by hospital personnel, or commercially prepared kits may be purchased.

SUBSTANCE ABUSE

The legal and ethical questions surrounding potential substance use and abuse by healthcare workers are complex. Medical and sociological literature that discusses this subject tends to be contradictory and confusing. Much of the recent data is generated by anonymous surveys, usually with relatively low response rates. These surveys are often confounded by reporting bias and nonresponse bias. Nonetheless some of the reports describing these surveys are informative.

The belief that physicians are more likely than others to have substance abuse problems is a longstanding one despite the lack of firm evidence. In the 1960s, reports indicated that physicians were 100 times more likely than the general population to become dependent on "narcotic" drugs or opioids.[94] However, during the 1980s it was recognized that the true prevalence of alcohol and/or drug use among physicians had not been well defined.[19,26,134] Most studies at that time involved only very small sample sizes and did not utilize currently accepted methods of epidemiologic analysis. More recent data based on survey methodologies appear to provide a more reliable basis for making projections.[57]

Although frequent reports claim that one in 10 physicians is likely to become dependent on drugs or alcohol in the course of his or her career, the data supporting this are not clear.[143] Since the mid-1980s there have been two major surveys of drug use among US physicians. A survey of 500 practicing physicians in New England with a 70% response rate reported overall levels of drug use that were comparable to those of the general population.[89] Although substantial numbers of physicians had used drugs "recreationally" or for self treatment, most such use was experimental or occasional. In a later report on alcohol use data from the same survey, 2% of physicians reportedly had a current drinking problem, and 3% had been treated for alcohol-related problems.[10] The authors concluded that "physicians were no more likely to abuse substances nonmedically than were other professionals."[90]

More recently, a survey of 9600 US physicians, with a response rate of 59%, found that physicians were less likely to use tobacco and illicit substances than were members of the general population, but were more likely to use alcohol and to self-treat with prescription medications such as codeine and benzodiazepines.[65] In this study respondents were asked whether they had "ever abused or been dependent on" alcohol or other drugs. Combining alcohol and other drugs, 7.9% answered this question positively. In surveys of the general population, using data collected from diagnostic surveys rather than self-reports, the lifetime risk of any substance use disorder has been estimated to range from 13% to 26%.[23,63,76]

A survey of 824 physicians defined "impairment" as meeting any one of a number of criteria such as having received treatment, answering yes to two or more CAGE questions, or acknowledgment that drug use had affected professional functioning.[83] Respondents were divided into medical specialists, surgeons, and anesthesiologists. Overall, from 14.4 to 19.9% of these groups met the definition of impairment. However, the authors do not report the numbers meeting the individual criteria for impairment, and the data showing drug use are reported separately for impaired and nonimpaired groups. In addition, the reported drug use data are for any lifetime use only. The longitudinal Johns Hopkins Precursors Study reported that, among 1014 male physicians, the prevalence of alcohol abuse was 12.9%.[129] The staff of a California teaching hospital were surveyed using the SMAST (the 13-item Short Michigan Alcoholism Screening Test).[129,114] A total of 569 questionnaires were sent, and a response rate of less than 50% was obtained. They reported that 4% of respondents were classified as alcoholic, and 10% were classified as possibly alcoholic.

Only limited data are available regarding medical students and resident physicians. In a recent self-reported survey among resident physicians, the use of psychoactive substances was generally lower than among similar age groups in the general population, although as was the case for their older colleagues, the use of benzodiazepines was greater, with self-treatment generally being cited as the reason for such use.[66] A study of former anesthesiology residents has reported lower lifetime use of marijuana and cocaine among this group than among other groups of residents, suggesting possible self-selection for drug use and specialty, but in all cases, the use of these drugs was lower among residents than among similarly aged groups in the general population.[84]

The epidemiology of substance abuse in medical students is less clear. In a survey of 2046 (with a 67% response rate) senior students at 23 medical schools, lower rates of substance use were reported for most drugs compared to similar age groups in the general population.[13] However, for some drugs, namely alcohol, sedative hypnotics, and psychedelic agents other than LSD, the usage rates were somewhat higher among the students. The data further

indicate that, except for sedative hypnotics, the use of which did increase after entry into medical school, patterns of drug use are generally established before beginning medical education. In a study of alcohol in one medical school, use by students tended to decline over the students' careers in school, but as many as 18% were alcohol abusers (using research diagnostic criteria) during the first 2 years of medical education.[32]

Among physicians in treatment for problems with alcohol and other drugs, anesthesiologists, psychiatrists, and family practitioners have been reported to be overrepresented.[25,57,114,134] However, the pattern of specialty representation differs widely among reports and there are many treatment programs that do not report overrepresentation of particular specialties. Also, because of the differences among treatment programs in their attractiveness to, or recruitment of, particular specialties, these data cannot be taken to indicate differences among specialties in the prevalence of problems associated with alcohol and other drugs. In a recent study no differences were noted among anesthesiologists, medical specialists, and surgeons in the numbers who met their criteria for impairment.[83] Psychiatrists were also most likely to report all types of drug use and current self-treatment in a survey of drug use among New England physicians.[89] Several surveys of drug use patterns among resident physicians have reported higher levels of use of specific drugs in some specialties including psychiatry, anesthesia, surgery, and emergency medicine.[27,67,97] However, these studies reported small numbers of respondents, and patterns across specialties could not be reliably measured.

SUMMARY

Many of the chemical and physical hazards to healthcare professionals are regulated by the Occupational Safety and Health Administration. The broadest level of OSHA communication is the so-called Hazard Communication Standard,[112] which requires all employers to inform their employees of the specific chemical hazards involved in their jobs. In the healthcare setting, this standard includes the preparation of drugs and medicines by pharmacists and nurses. In addition, this standard requires that employees be provided with written information in the form of the Material Safety Data Sheets describing the chemical hazards to which they may be exposed on the job.[61]

In addition, strict and enforceable OSHA "standards" for several chemical hazards such as formaldehyde[109] and ethylene oxide[111] have been promulgated. "Guidelines" expressing OSHA's opinion about the proper handling of certain specific hazards are also issued. Although not carrying the force of an OSHA standard, these guidelines are meant to disseminate information and to engender voluntary compliance. An example of such a guideline is the 1986 "Safe Handling of Anticancer or Cytotoxic Drugs," which describes the need for proper engineering controls when cytotoxic agents are handled in the healthcare setting.[108]

Important OSHA regulations govern employer reporting requirements to OSHA with regard to workplace injuries and/or deaths. Previously promulgated regulations have been expanded to require the reporting of work-related incidents resulting in the death of an employee or the inpatient hospitalization of three or more employees. In addition, the regulation requires the employer to report such incidents to OSHA by either written or verbal communication within 8 hours after the employer learns of an event.

These regulations apply to workers in the healthcare industries as well as generally to other industries in the United States.

REFERENCES

1. American Conference of Governmental Industrial Hygienists: 1994 Threshold Limit Values for Chemical Substances and Physical Agents and Biological Exposure Indices. Cincinnati, ACGIH, 1993.
2. American Conference of Governmental Industrial Hygienists: Documentation of the Threshold Limit Values and Biological Exposure Indices, 6th ed. Cincinnati, ACGIH, 1992, pp. 1134–1138.
3. Acheson ED, Barnes HR, Gardner MJ, et al: Formaldehyde in the British chemical industry. Lancet 1984;1:611–616.
4. Agner T, Menne T: Sensitization to acrylates in a dental patient. Contact Dermatitis 1994;30:249–250.
5. Altman LC: Occupational exposure to latex. West J Med 1995;163:369–370.
6. American Dental Association: The 1991 Survey of Dental Practice: General Characteristics of Dentists. Chicago, American Dental Association, 1992.
7. American Society of Anesthesiology Ad Hoc Committee on the Effect of Trace Anesthetics on the Health of Operating Room Personnel: Occupational Disease among operating room personnel: A national study. Anesthesiology 1974;41:321–340.
8. American Society of Hospital Pharmacists: ASHP technical assistance bulletin on handling cytotoxic and hazardous drugs. Am J Hosp Pharm 1990;47:1033–1049.
9. Anderson M, Engholm G, Ennow K, et al: Cancer risk among staff at two radiotherapy departments in Denmark. Br J Radiol 1991;64:455–460.
10. Anderson RW, Puckett WH, Dana WJ, et al: Risk of handling injectable antineoplastic agents. Am J Hosp Pharm 1982;39: 1881–1887.
11. Antonelli A, Silvano G, Bianchi F: Risk of thyroid nodules in subjects occupationally exposed to radiation: A cross sectional study. Occup Environ Med 1995;52:500–504.
12. Askrog V, Harvald B: Teratogenic effects of inhalational anesthetics. Nordisk Med 1970;83:498–500.
13. Baldwin DC, Hughs PH, Conard SE, et al: Substance use among senior medical students: A survey of 23 medical schools. JAMA 1991;265:2074–2078.
14. Ballantyne B: Toxicology of Glutaraldehyde. Review of Studies and Human Health Effects. Danbury, CT, Union Carbide, 1995.
15. Balmes JR, Estacio PL, Quinlan P, et al: Respiratory effects of occupational exposure to aerosolized pentamidine. J Occup Environ Med 1995;37:145–150.
16. Bardana EJ: Occupational asthma and related respiratory disorders. Dis Month 1995(Mar);41:141–200.
17. Bihari V, Srivastava AK, Gupta BN: Occupational health hazards among operating room personnel exposed to anesthetic gases: A review. J Environ Pathol Toxicol Oncol 1994;13:213–219.
18. Binder L, Fredrickson L: Poisonings in laboratory personnel and health care professionals. Am J Emerg Med 1991;9:11–15.
19. Bissell L, Haberman PW: Alcoholism in the Professions. New York, Oxford University Press, 1984.
20. Bland SM, Levine MS, Wilson PD, et al: Occupational allergy to laboratory animals: An epidemiologic study. J Occup Med 1986;28:1151–1157.
21. Boice JD, Mandel JS, Doody MM, et al: Health survey of radiologic technologists. Cancer 1992;69:586–598.
22. Bolt HM: Quantification of endogenous carcinogens. The ethylene oxide paradox. Biochem Pharmacol 1996;52:1–59.
23. Bourdon KH, Rae DS, Locke BZ, et al: Estimating the prevalence of mental disorders in US adults from the epidemiologic catchment area survey. Public Health Rep 1992;107:663–668.
24. Braun BJ, Skiendzielewski JJ: Radiation exposure of emergency physicians. Ann Emerg Med 1982;11:535–540.
25. Brooke D, Edwards G, Taylor C: Addiction as an occupational hazard: 144 doctors with drug and alcohol problems. Br J Addict 1991;86:1011–1016.
26. Brewster JM: Prevalence of alcohol and other drug problems among physicians. JAMA 1986;255:1913–1920.
27. Bunch WH, Dvonch VM, Storr CL, et al: The stresses of the surgical residency. J Surg Res 1992;53:268–271.
28. Bureau of Labor Statistics: Outlook 2000. Washington, DC, US Department of Labor, Bureau of Labor Statistics, Bulletin 2352, 1990, pp. 51, 54.
29. Castelli M, Qizilbash A, Seaton T: Post-colonoscopy proctitis. Am J Gastroenterol 1986;81:887.
30. Centers for Disease Control. Formaldehyde exposure in a gross anatomy laboratory-Colorado. MMWR 1983;31:698–700.
31. Centers for Disease Control. Occupational exposure to formaldehyde in dialysis units. MMWR 1986;35:399–401.
32. Clark DC, Eckenfels EJ, Daugherty SR, et al: Alcohol use patterns through medical school. JAMA 1987;257:2921–2926.
33. Cohen EN, Beliville JW, Brown BW: Anesthesia, pregnancy, and miscarriage: A study of operating room nurses and anesthetists. Anesthesiology 1971;35:343–347.
34. Cohen EN, Gift HC, Brown BW, et al: Occupational disease in dentistry and chronic exposure to trace anesthetic gases. J Am Dent Assoc 1980;101:21–31.
35. Cohen JH: Occupational stress among nurse executives. Nurse Admin Q 1989;13:41–46.
36. Cole EC, Rutala WA, Nessen L, et al: Effect of methodology, dilution, and exposure time on the tuberculocidal activity of glutaraldehyde-based disinfectants. Appl Environ Microbiol 1990;56: 1813–1817.
37. Collins FM, Montalbine V: Mycobactericidal activity of glutaraldehyde solutions. J Clin Microbiol 1976;4:408–412.
38. Conde-Salazar L, Guimaraens D, Romero CV: Occupational allergic contact dermatitis from anaerobic acrylic sealants. Contact Dermatitis 1988;18:129–132.
39. Corbett TN, Cornell RG, Endres IL, et al: Birth effects among children of nurse anesthetists. Anesthesiology 1974;41:341–344.
40. Corbett TH, Cornell RG, Endres JL, Millard RI: Effects of low concentrations of nitrous oxide on rat pregnancy. Anesthesiology 1973;39:299–301.
41. Corrado OJ, Osman J, Davies RJ: Asthma and rhinitis after exposure to glutaraldehyde in endoscopy units. Hum Toxicol 1986;5:325–327.
42. Cowan RE, Manning AP, Ayliffe GA, et al: Aldehyde disinfectants and health in endoscopy units. Gut 1993;34:1641–1645.
43. Cozine K, Rosenbaum LM, Rosenbaum SH: Laser induced endotracheal tube fire. Anesthesiology 1981;55:583–585.
44. Dailey JR, Parnes RE, Aminlari A: Glutaraldehyde keratopathy. Am J Ophthalmol 1993;115:256–258.
45. Davis MJ: Conscious sedation practices in pediatric dentistry: A survey of members of the American Board of Pediatric Dentistry College of Diplomates. Pediatr Dent 1988;10:328–329.
46. Decker JA, Seitz TA, Shults RA, et al: Occupational exposures to aerosolized pharmaceuticals and control strategies. Scand J Work Environ Health 1992;18(Suppl 2):100–102.
47. Diamond SA, Dupuis LL: Contact lens damage due to ribavirin exposure. Drug Intell Clin Pharm 1989;23:425–428.
48. Dumont D: Risques encourus par les personnels soignants manipulant des cytostatiques. Arch Mal Prof 1989;50:1209–1253.
49. Echeverria D, Heyer NJ, Martin MD, et al: Behavioral effect of low level exposure to elemental mercury among dentists. Neurotoxicol Teratol 1995;17:161–189.
50. Eggleston PA, Wood RA: Management of allergies to animals. Allergy Proc 1992;13:289–292.
51. Estlander T, Kanerva L, Kari O, et al: Occupational conjunctivitis associated with type IV allergy to methacrylate. Allergy 1996;51: 56–59.
52. Falck K, Grohn P, Sorsa M, et al: Mutagenicity in urine of nurses handling cytostatic drugs. Lancet 1979;1:1250–1251.

53. Falck K, Sorsa M, Vainio H: Use of the bacterial fluctation test to detect mutagenicity in urine of nurses handling cytostatic drugs. Mutat Res 1981;85:236–237.

54. Favero MS, Bond WW: Chemical disinfection of medical and surgical materials. In: Block SS, ed: Disinfection, Sterilization and Preservation, 4th ed. Philadelphia, Lea & Febiger, 1968, pp. 617–641.

55. Freeman GL: Psyllium hypersensitivity. Ann Allergy 1994;73: 490–492.

56. Frigas E, Filley WV, Feed CE: Bronchial challenge with formaldehyde gas: Lack of bronchoconstriction in 13 patients suspected of having formaldehyde induced asthma. Mayo Clin Proc 1984;59: 295–299.

57. Gallegos KV, Lubin BH, Bowers C, et al: Relapse and recovery: Five to ten year follow up study of chemically dependent physicians: The Georgia experience. Md Med J 1992;41:315–319.

58. Gillespie BF, Rathburn FJ: Adverse effects of psyllium. Can Med Assoc J 1994;146:16–17.

59. Gladu JM, Ecobichon DJ: Evaluation of exposure of health care personnel to ribavirin. J Toxicol Environ Health 1989;28:1–12.

60. Grazer RE, Meislin HW, Westerman BR, et al: Exposure to ionizing radiation in the emergency department from commonly performed portable radiographs. Ann Emerg Med 1987;16:417–420.

61. Greenberg MI, Cone DC, Roberts JR: The material safety data sheet: A useful resource for the emergency physician. Ann Emerg Med 1996;27:347–352.

62. Harrison R, Bellows J, Rempel D, et al: Assessing exposures of health care personnel to aerosols of ribavirin. MMWR 1988;37: 560–563.

63. Helzer JE, Burnam A, McEvoy LT: Alcohol abuse and dependence. In: Robins LN, Regier DA, eds: Psychiatric Disorders in America: The Epidemiologic Catchment Area Study. New York, The Free Press, 1991, pp. 81–115..

64. Hopkins J: The carcinogenic potential of ethylene oxide. Food Chem Toxicol 1994;32:191–193.

65. Hughes PH, Brandenburg N, Baldwin D, et al: Prevalence of substance use amomng US physicians. JAMA 1992;267:2333–2339.

66. Hughes PH, Conard SE, Baldwin DC, et al: Resident physician substance use in the United States. JAMA 1991;265:2069–2073.

67. Hughes PH, Baldwin DC, Sheehan DV, et al: Resident physician substance use by specialty. Am J Psychiatry 1992;149:1348–1354.

68. International Agency for Research on Cancer: IARC Monographs on the Evaluation of the Carcinogenic Risk to Humans, Vol. 50. Pharmaceutical Drugs. Lyon, France, IARC, 1990.

69. International Agency for Research on Cancer: IARC Monographs on the Evaluation of the Carcinogenic Risk to Humans, Suppl 7. Overall Evaluations of Carcinogenicity: An Updating of IARC Monographs Vols. 1 to 42. Lyon, France, IARC, 1987.

70. International Agency for Research on Cancer: IARC Monographs on the Evaluation of the Carcinogenic Risk to Humans, Vol. 26. Some Antineoplastic and Immunosuppressive Agents. Lyon, France, IARC, 1981.

71. Jackuck SJ, Bound CL, Steel J: Occupational hazard in hospital staff exposed to 2% glutaraldehyde in an endoscopy unit. J Soc Occup Med 1989;39:69–71.

72. Jagun O, Ryan M, Waldron HA: Urinary thioether excretion in nurses handling cytotoxic drugs. Lancet 1982;1:443–444.

73. Janardhanan R: Endoscopist's nose. Gastrointest Endosc 1986;32: 247.

74. Karakaya AE, Burgaz S, Bayhan A: The significance of urinary thioethers as indicators of exposure to alkylating agents. Arch Toxicol 1989;13(Suppl):117–119.

75. Kelly KJ, Kurup VP, Reijula KE, Fink JN: The diagnosis of natural rubber latex allergy. J Allergy Clin lmmunol 1994;93:813–816.

76. Kessler RC, McGonagle KA, Zhao S, et al: Lifetime and 12 month prevalence of DSM-III-R psychiatric disorders in the United States. Arch Gen Psychiatry 1994;51:8–19.

77. Klein-Schwartz W, Gorman RL, Oderda GM, et al: Three fatal sodium azide poisonings. Med Toxicol Adverse Drug Exp 1989;4: 219–227.

78. Kolmodin-Hedman B. Hartvig P. Sorsa M, et al: Occupational handling of cytostatic drugs. Arch Toxicol 1983;54:25–33.

79. Konz KR, Chia JK, Kurup VP, et al: Comparison of latex hypersensitivity among patients with neurologic defects. J Allergy Clin Immunol 1995;95:950–954.

80. Koppel C, Baudisch H, Schneider V, et al: Suicidal ingestion of formalin with fatal complications. Intensive Care Med 1990;16: 212–214.

81. Lemiere C, Charpin D, Vervloet D: Is atopy a risk factor of occupational asthma? Rev Mal Respir 1995;12:231–239.

82. Linn WS, Gong H, Anderson KR, et al: Exposures of health-care workers to ribavirin aerosol: A pharmacokinetics study. Arch Environ Health 1995;50:445–451.

83. Lutsky I, Hopwood M, Abram SE, et al: Use of psychoactive substances in three medical specialties: Anesthesia, medicine and surgery. Can J Anaesth 1994;41:561–567.

84. Lutsky I, Abram SE, Jacobson GR, et al: Substance abuse by anesthesia residents. Acad Med 1991;66:164–166.

85. Maio JL, Cartier A, L'Archeveque J, et al: Prevalence of occupational asthma and immunologic sensitivity to psyllium among health personnel in chronic care hospitals. Am Rev Respir Dis 1990;142: 1359–1366.

86. Marczynski B, Marek W, Baur X: Ethylene oxide as a major factor in DNA and RNA evolution. Med Hypotheses 1995;44:97–100.

87. Masferrer R, Marquez R: Comparison of two activated glutaraldehyde solutions: Cidex and Sonacide. Respir Care 1977;22:257–262.

88. Matthews J, Newsome SW, Walters NP: Aerobiology of irradiation with carbon dioxide laser. J Hosp Infect 1985;6:230–233.

89. McAuliffe WE, Rohman M, Santangelo S, et al: Psychoactive drug use among practicing physicians and medical students. N Engl J Med 1986;315:805–810.

90. McAuliffe WE, Rohman M, Breer P, et al: Alcohol use and abuse in random samples of physicians and medical students. Am J Public Health 191;81:177–182.

91. McDevitt JJ, Lees P, McDiarmid MA: Exposure of hospital pharmacists and nurses to antineoplastic agents. J Occup Med 1993;43: 1942–1945.

92. McGlothlin JD, Jensen PA, Cooper TC, et al: In-Depth Survey Report: Control of Anesthetic Gases in Dental Operatories at University of California at San Francisco Oral Surgical Dental Clinic, San Francisco, CA. Cincinnati, Department of Health and Human Services, Centers for Disease Control, National Institute for Occupational Safety and Health, report no. ECTB 166B-12b, 1990.

93. Minami M, Katsumata M, Miyake K, et al: Dangerous mixture of household detergents in an old-style toilet: A case report with simulation experiments of the working environment and warning of potential hazard relevant to the general environment. Hum Exp Toxicol 1992;11:27–34.

94. Modlin HC, Montes A: Narcotic addiction in physicians. Am J Psychiatry 1964;121:358–363.

95. Montgomery AB, Corkery KJ, Brunette ER, et al: Occupational exposure to aerosolized pentamidine. Chest 1990;98:386–388.

96. Mrvos R, Dean BS, Krenzelok EP: Home exposures to chlorine/chloramine gas: Review of 216 cases. South Med J 1993; 86:654–657.

97. Myers T, Weiss E: Substance use by interns and residents: Analysis of personal, social and professional differences. Br J Addiction 1987;82:1091–1099.

98. Newill CA, Eggleston PA, Prenger VL, et al: Prospective study of occupational asthma to laboratory animal allergens: Stability of airway responsiveness to methacholine challenge for one year. J Allergy Clin Immunol 1995;95:707–715.

99. Nieuwenhuijsen MJ, Gordon S, Harris JM, et al: Variation in rat urinary aeroallergen levels explained by differences in site, task, and exposure group. Ann Occup Hyg 1995;39:819–825.

100. National Institute for Occupational Safety and Health: Health Hazard Evaluation Report: Hennepin County Medical Center, Minneapolis, MS. Cincinnati, US Department of Health and Human Services, Public Health Service, Centers for Disease Control, HETA 84BO46Bl584, 1985.

101. National Institute for Occupational Safety and Health: Control of Occupational Exposure to N_2O in the Dental Operatory. Cincinnati, US Department of Health, Education, and Welfare, Public Health Service, Centers for Disease Control, DHEW (NIOSH) pub. no. 77Bl7l, 1977.

102. National Institute for Occupational Safety and Health: Criteria for a Recommended Standard: Occupational Exposure to Waste Anesthetic Gas and Vapors. Cincinnati, US Department of Health, Education, and Welfare, Public Health Service, Centers for Disease Control, DHEW (NIOSH) pub. no. 77B–140, 1977.

103. Neal AD, Wadden RA, Chiou WL: Exposure of hospital workers to airborne antineoplastic agents. Am J Hosp Pharm 1983;40:597–601.

104. Norback D: Skin and respiratory symptoms from exposure to glutaraldehyde in medical services. Scand J Work Environ Health 1988;14:366–371.

105. Olsen RJ, Lynch P, Coyle MB, et al: Examination gloves as barriers to hand contamination in clinical practice. JAMA 1993;270:350–353.

106. O'Riordan TG, Smaldone GC: Exposure of health care workers to aerosolized pentamidine. Chest 1992;101:1494–1499.

107. OSHA Regulations (Standards 29 CFR) 1910.1450. Occupational Exposure to Hazardous Chemical in Laboratories, 1990.

108. OSHA Instruction. PUB 8–1.1 Guidelines for Cytotoxic (Antineoplastic) Drugs, 1986.

109. OSHA Regulations (Standards 29 CFR) 1910.1048. Occupational Exposure to Formaldehyde, 1992.

110. OSHA Regulations (Standards 29 CFR) 1910.1003–13. Carcinogens, 1997.

111. OSHA Regulations (Standards 29 CFR) 1910.1047. Ethylene oxide, 1997.

112. OSHA Regulations (Standards 29 CFR) 1910.90. Hazard Communication Standard, 1997.

113. OSHA Technical Manual, Section VI, Chapter 2. Controlling exposure to hazardous drugs, 1994.

114. Pelton C, Ikeda RM: The California physicians diversion program's experience with recovering anesthesiologists. J Psychoactive Drugs 1991;23:427–431.

115. Pohl L, Bergman M: The dentist's exposure to elemental mercury vapor during clinical work with amalgams. Acta Odontol Scand 1995;53:44–81.

116. Preston RJ, Fennell TR, Leber AP, et al: Reconsideration of the genetic risk assessment for ethylene oxide exposures. Environ Mol Mutagen 1995;26:189–202.

117. Pyy L, Sorsa M, Hakala E: Ambient monitoring of cyclophosphamide in manufacture and hospitals. Am Ind Hyg Assoc J 1988;49:314–317.

118. Renstrom A, Malmberg P, Larsson K, et al: Prospective study of laboratory animals allergy: Factors predisposing to sensitization and development of allergic symptoms. Allergy 1994;49:548–552.

119. Ritchie KA, MacDonald EB, Hammersley R, et al: A pilot study of the effects of low level exposure to mercury on the health of dental surgeons. Occup Environ Med 1995;52:813–817.

120. Roberts RJ, Simmons A, Barrett DA: Accidental exposure to sodium azide. Am J Clin Pathol 1974;61:879–880.

121. Romaquera C, Vilaplana J, Grimalt F: Contact sensitization to methacrylate in a limb prosthesis. Contact Dermatitis 1989;21:125.

122. Rowland AS, Baird DD, Weinberg CR, et al: Reduced fertility among women employed as dental assistants exposed to high levels of nitrous oxide. N Engl J Med 1992;327:993–997.

123. Rubbo SD, Gardener JF, Webb RL: Biocidal activities of glutaraldehyde and related compounds. J Appl Bacteriol 1967;30:78–87.

124. Sass-Kortsak AM, Purdham JT, Bozek PR, et al: Exposure of hospital operating room personnel to potentially harmful environmental agents. Am Ind Hyg Assoc J 1992;53:203–209.

125. Schmahl D, Kaldor JM: Carcinogenicity of Alkylating Cytostatic Drugs. IARC scientific publications, no. 78. Lyon, France, International Agency for Research on Cancer, 1986.

126. Selevan SG, Lindbohm ML, Hornung RW, et al: A study of occupational exposure to antineoplastic drugs and fetal loss in nurses. N Engl J Med 1985;313:1173–1178.

127. Sexton RJ, Henson EV: Experimental ethylene oxide human skin injuries. Arch Ind Hyg Occup Med 1990;2:549–564.

128. Shepherd GM: Safe use of latex rubber [letter]. Ann Intern Med 1995;23:234–235.

129. Siegel BJ, Fitzgerald FT: A survey on the prevalence of alcoholism among the faculty and house staff of an academic teaching hospital. West J Med 1988;148:593–595.

130. Singer CM, Baraff LJ, Benedict SH, et al: Exposure of emergency medicine personnel to ionizing radiation during cervical spine radiography. Ann Emerg Med 1989;18:822–825.

131. Skov T: Handling antineoplastic drugs in the European Community countries. Eur J Cancer Prev 1993;2:43–46.

132. Stucker I, Caillard JF, Collin R, et al: Risk of spontaneous abortion among nurses handling antineoplastic drugs. Scand J Work Environ Health 1991;16:102–107.

133. Suruda AJ, McGlothlin JD: Fatal abuse of nitrous oxide in the workplace. J Occup Med 1990;32:682–684.

134. Talbott GD, Gallegos KV, Wilson PO, et al: The Medical Association of Georgia's impaired physicians program: Review of the first 100 physicians: analysis of specialty. JAMA 1987;257:2927–2930.

135. Tomazic VJ, Withrow TJ, Hamilton RG: Characterization of the allergens in latex protein extracts. J Allergy Clin Immunol 1995;96:635–642.

136. Turjanmaa K: Allergy to natural rubber latex: A growing problem. Ann Med 1994;26:297–300.

137. Valanis B, Vollmer WM, Labuhn K, et al: Antineoplastic drug handling protection after OSHA guidelines. J Occup Environ Med 1992;34:149–155.

138. Vicira E, Cleaton-Jones JP, Austin JC, et al: Effects of low concentrations of nitrous oxide on rat fetuses. Anesth Analg 1980;59: 175–177.

139. Vieira E: Effect of the chronic administration of nitrous oxide 0.5% to gravid rats. Br J Anaesthesiol 1979;51:283–287.

140. Vaughan TL, Stewart PA, Teschke K, et al: Occupational exposure to formaldehyde and wood dust and nasopharyngeal cardinoma. Occup Environ Med 2000;57:376–384.

141. Wang JX, Inskip PD, Boice JD, et al: Cancer incidence among medical diagnostic x-ray workers in China, 1950 to 1985. Cancer 1990; 45:889–955.

142. Waskin H: Toxicology of antimicrobial aerosols: A review of aerosolized ribavirin and pentamidine. Respir Care 1992;36: 1026–1036.

143. Webster TG: Problems of drug addiction and alcoholism among physicians. In: Scheiber SC, Doyle BB, eds: The Impaired Physician. New York, Plenum Press, 1983, pp. 27–38.

144. Weiss EL, Singer CM, Benedict SH, et al: Physician exposure to ionizing radiation during trauma resuscitation: A prospective clinical study. Ann Emerg Med 1990;19:134–138.

145. Wenig BL, Stenson KM, Wenig BM, et al: Effects of plume produced by the Nd:YAG laser and electrocautery on the respiratory system. Lasers Surg Med 1993;13:242–245.

146. Wolf BL: Anaphylactic reaction to latex gloves. N Engl J Med 1993; 329:278–280.

147. Yassin MS, Lierl MB, Fischer TJ, et al: Latex allergy in hospital employees. Ann Allergy 1994;72:245–249.

CHAPTER 111 FARM TOXICOLOGY

William J. Meggs / Ricky L. Langley / Paul A. James

A 20-year-old farmer and talented mechanic who could repair automobiles, trucks, tractors, and farm machinery helped a neighboring farmer store peanut vines for use as animal feed. He had reasons to believe that the vines were sprayed with a pesticide for spider mites. The operation involved bailing and compressing the vines. The dust was so thick that he "could not see the tractor." Before this day, he was in excellent health, had no medical problems, did not smoke or drink, and was taking no medications. That night he broke out in a rash, his tongue swelled, he developed a headache, and he became short of breath. He developed a cough productive of "blackish brown dirtlike material." He saw a physician for the problems that week and was treated for "bronchitis" with no improvement. He attempted to have the peanut greens analyzed for the incriminated miticide, which was not approved for use on peanuts. His neighbor destroyed the greens and told him the greens had been analyzed and there was no pesticide on them but refused to produce a report.

Over the next weeks he continued to be ill and did not respond to treatment for bronchitis. He was referred to a pulmonologist, who diagnosed chemically induced asthma, or "RADS." Over the next years, he had a series of exacerbations of his respiratory disease requiring multiple courses of prednisone. His tolerance of respiratory irritants was extremely low, with exacerbations of his asthma from exposures to smoke, dusts, and fumes.

Five years after the exposure, he developed a flulike syndrome with fever, aches and pains, fatigue, chills, night sweats, cough, and dyspnea, while being tapered off prednisone for asthma. Treatment for bronchitis and influenza were ineffective. Tests for Rocky Mountain spotted fever, Lyme disease, and infectious mononucleosis were negative. Arthritis and musculoskeletal symptoms continued, with a waxing and waning course. The next year, he was referred to NIH, where an extensive evaluation excluded rheumatoid arthritis, systemic lupus erythematosus, AIDS, and cancer. A diagnosis of fibromyalgia was given. Asthma remained severe and required treatment with corticosteroid, anticholinergic, and β-adrenergic agonist inhalers supplemented by courses of prednisone.

After 10 years, attempts to continue working were abandoned. He suffered from chronic fatigue, chronic musculoskeletal pain, asthma, and an intolerance of chemical fumes that prevented his continuing with mechanical work. His wife had a career and supported the family.

INTRODUCTION

Contemporary farming methods rely heavily on agricultural chemicals, which can be toxic to farmers and their families, rural resi-

dents, and visitors. Table 111–1 summarizes a study of mortality and morbidity from agricultural chemical poisonings in the United States.[35] Of the approximately 330,000 exposures to agricultural chemicals reported to poison centers from 1985 to 1990, there were over 25,000 hospitalizations. Suicidal intent occurred in 2.3% of the exposures, approximately two-thirds of the deaths, and over 17% of the hospitalizations. Organic phosphorus pesticide poisonings led all other categories associated with hospitalizations and death. Paraquat, diquat, chlorophenoxy compounds, chlorinated hydrocarbons, carbamates, strychnine, arsenic, and anticoagulants were also associated with deaths. Although this data analysis demonstrated the importance of suicides associated with agricultural chemicals, unintentional poisonings can also be lethal and account for 77% of the hospitalizations.

The evaluation of unexplained illnesses should always include a history of environmental and occupational exposures. Nonspecific symptoms or illness involving multiple organ systems should raise the specter of poisoning. Clinicians caring for patients from rural areas should know of the hazards of agricultural chemicals (Table 111–2). Education can prevent poisonings, and physicians should take an active role in discussing potential hazards with their patients.

Chronic illness developing after acute chemical exposure to a wide variety of substances occurs in a number of settings, including agricultural work. Chronic asthma and rhinitis can be induced by acute, subacute, and chronic exposures to dusts, smoke, and fumes. Reactive polyarthritis is associated with inhalant exposures to a chemical irritant,[64] and is a syndrome with many features similar to irritable bowel syndrome.[39] Exposures to organic phosphorus pesticides and solvents are associated with chronic encephalopathy and neuropsychiatric disability.[48] Gulf war soldiers had remarkable chemical exposures, and many believe that chemical exposures led to some of the disabilities associated with service in the Gulf War. An intolerance of chemicals is found in a high percentage of patients in these settings.

Asthma can develop after an acute exposure to dusts, smoke, and fumes and is termed reactive airways dysfunction syndrome (RADS). Though the original description required one single exposure to a chemical irritant, it is now recognized that asthma can develop after chronic or subacute exposures.[9] An upper airway analogue of RADS, termed reactive upper-airways dysfunction syndrome (RUDS), also is recognized.[42] Like the majority of patients with rhinitis and asthma, individuals with asthma induced by exposure to respiratory irritants have an intolerance to chemical irritants, including the products of combustion, perfumes and fragrances, cleaning products, and solvents. Many cases of chemically induced asthma are severe, difficult to treat, and disabling.

TABLE 111–1. Summary of Exposures, Hospitalizations, and Deaths Associated with Farm Chemicals by Method or Intent, United States, 1985–1990

	Unintentional (%)	Intentional (%)	Unknown (%)	Totals
Exposures	327,599 (96.9)	7,848 (2.3)	2,723 (0.8)	338,170
Hospitalizations	19,753 (77.7)	4,458 (17.5)	1,207 (4.7)	25,418
Deaths	97 (28.4)	217 (63.6)	27 (7.9)	341

Adapted from Klein-Schwartz W, Smith GS: Agricultural and horticultural chemical poisonings: Mortality and morbidity in the United States. Ann Emerg Med 1997; 29: 232–238.

PULMONARY DISEASES

Occupational asthma is one of the many pulmonary diseases associated with farm work. Pulmonary diseases associated with agricultural exposures are listed in Table 111–3. The relative risk of occupationally attributed asthma is higher among agricultural workers than white collar and service occupations.[7] A Swedish study found that asthma in a farm population increased from 5.3%

TABLE 111–2. Common Toxins Encountered in Rural Areas

Pesticides
Ascaricides
Fungicides
Herbicides
Insecticides
Rodenticides

Asphyxiants
Butane, propane (bottled gas)
Carbon dioxide (grain elevators, silos)
Hydrogen sulfide (septic tanks, liquid manure tanks)
Methane (decaying organic matter, compost)

Hydrocarbons
Gasoline
Hydraulic fluid
Kerosene
Motor oils

Plant toxins resulting in dermatoses
Crop dermatitis (celery, cucumber, limes)
Flowering plants—pyrethrins
Poison ivy, oak, and sumac
Tobacco (cutaneous absorption of nicotine)

Envenomations
Insects
Reptiles

Inorganic chemicals
Ammonia
Carbon monoxide
Nitrogen
Nitrous oxide
Phosphorus
Potash

to 9.8% from 1984 to 1996, with the storage mite being an important allergen.[36] Asthma varies greatly among different types of farm activities.[34] Involvement with animal production increases a farmer's risk of asthma by a 6.3 odds ratio. A combination of working in animal production, smoking, and a positive family history results in an odds ratio of 8.1.[43] Farmers are exposed to animals, plants, and chemicals that can provoke bronchospasm by diverse mechanisms. Animal danders, urine, saliva, and fecal proteins can be antigenic. Contact with horses, cows, sheep, and household pets can result in hypersensitivity reactions. Some farmers with asthma develop IgE to the grain storage mite (*Glycyphagus destructor*) as demonstrated by RAST testing.[30] Citrus red mite (*Panonychus citri*) has recently been identified as the most common sensitizing allergen of asthma and rhinitis in citrus farmers.[33] Exposure to a wide variety of food antigens can trigger allergic asthma in farmers, although workers who process foods are more susceptible than farmers. Pyrethrins, which are pesticides derived from chrysanthemums, can cause allergic asthma.

Pesticides can be absorbed by inhalation, ingestion, or through dermal contact. Unintentional poisoning primarily occurs via dermal absorption. Respiratory symptoms can occur with exposure to organic phosphorus compounds, carbamates, and chlorinated hydrocarbons[16,54] (see Chaps. 88 and 89). Pesticides can affect breathing via several mechanisms: (1) they may act as irritants causing bronchospasm, (2) they may cause respiratory failure from weakness of the muscles of respiration, (3) they may cause depression of the respiratory drive center, and (4) they may cause pulmonary edema. The parasympathetic stimulation seen in organic phosphorus and carbamate poisoning can directly cause bronchospasm.

Anhydrous ammonia is a respiratory irritant that at high doses may cause pulmonary edema.[55] Ammonia, which is frequently used as a fertilizer, reacts with water to form ammonium hydroxide, a strong alkali. Most individuals who are exposed recover without sequelae, although bronchiolitis obliterans occurs after exposure. Fumigants, such as methyl bromide and carbon disulfide, can cause pulmonary edema if inhaled.[55] Certain fungicides containing arsenic may lead to the development of lung cancer.

Pulmonary fibrosis is reported primarily from the ingestion, not inhalation, of paraquat. The pulmonary damage appears to be dose related. Systemic and pulmonary poisoning may also occur from dermal absorption. Both type I and II alveolar epithelial cells accumulate paraquat. The destruction of these alveolar cells occurs followed by infiltration with inflammatory cells and hemorrhage. Subsequently, proliferation of fibroblasts occurs, leading to the development of fibrosis, which may impair gas exchange. Dinitrophenols, which uncouple oxidative phosphorylation, can cause malaise, headache, thirst, hyperthermia, dyspnea, and respiratory failure.[55] These compounds can be absorbed through the skin.

Chlorine-containing cleaning agents can act as upper airway respiratory irritants and may cause pulmonary parenchymal damage if the exposure is prolonged. Certain veterinary antibiotics can act as sensitizers, and farmers may develop asthma from these compounds.

Silo filler's disease results from exposure to nitrogen dioxide (NO_2) in silos. Ensilage is the process in which green crops are preserved in silos after cutting to be fed to livestock during the winter.[51] Once in storage, nitrates in the plants are oxidized to nitrogen dioxide and nitrogen tetroxide. This process starts shortly after filling of the silo and continues for several weeks. If a farmer

TABLE 111–3. Pulmonary Diseases Associated with Toxins on the Farm

Disease	Exposure	Onset	Symptoms	Chest radiograph
Silo filler's disease (chemical alveolitis)	Silo gas (NO_2)	Immediate to days	Cough, dyspnea	Diffuse alveolar edema or miliary pattern
Farmer's lung (hypersensitivity pneumonitis)	Moldy hay, silage, bedding	4–8 hours	Cough, dyspnea, flulike symptoms	Diffuse nodular, patchy consolidation
Mycotoxicosis	Moldy dust	Hours	Flulike symptoms	Usually normal
Grain fever	Grain dust	Immediate to hours	Cough, flulike symptoms	Normal
Occupational asthma	Animal and plant proteins, chemicals	Immediate to hours	Bronchospasm, bronchorrhea, cough	Normal or hyperinflation

enters a recently filled silo that has not been properly ventilated, a reddish-brown haze about the silage that has a bleach-like odor may be noted. This haze actually represents the presence of nitrogen oxides in gaseous form.

Nitrogen dioxide is a mild irritant, and the farmers may be exposed for several minutes, allowing the gas to penetrate deep within the lungs. The nitrogen dioxide reacts with water in the airways to form nitrous (NHO_2) and nitric acids (NHO_3), resulting in a chemical pneumonitis and pulmonary edema. Depending on the degree of exposure, symptoms may present as a mild tracheobronchitis and cough or may be more severe with pulmonary edema and pneumonitis, which may prove fatal.[47,51] In some case series, fatality rates were 30%. It is not unusual for severe symptoms to present hours after exposure. Initially, patients may present with cough, shortness of breath, chest pain, nausea, vomiting, and cyanosis. If the exposure was prolonged and the concentration of nitrogen oxides was high, then pulmonary edema may rapidly develop. Patients should be admitted to the hospital and treated with a course of corticosteroids and oxygen if necessary. Because nitrates may be formed from nitrogen dioxide, methemoglobinemia may also occur (see Chap. 94).

If patients recover, they may pass into a latent phase of apparent improvement, which lasts for 2 to 6 weeks. The patient may suddenly relapse with dyspnea, cough, fever, and pulmonary edema. This relapse represents a fibrotic, obliterative lesion of the terminal airways termed *bronchiolitis obliterans*. Patients with bronchiolitis obliterans may have airway obstruction and reduced carbon monoxide diffusion capacity. The chest radiograph may show small opacities similar to the pattern seen with miliary tuberculosis or confluent opacities similar to pulmonary edema. Corticosteroids are beneficial and usually result in recovery without long-term pulmonary dysfunction. Pulmonary fibrosis occurs in untreated cases.

HEALTH EFFECTS OF AGRICULTURAL DUSTS

The agricultural environment is usually very dusty. Agricultural operations are the third leading cause of particulate air pollution in the United States. Agricultural dust can be either organic or inorganic, depending on the source.[14] Inorganic dust arises from rock or soil and is relatively benign, acting mainly as a mild irritant.

Occasionally, cases of silicosis may develop from plowing sandy soils.[56] Organic dusts are derived from plant or animal products and are more biologically active. This type of dust may consist of the following: animal dander, hair, feathers, urine and feces, insects or mites or their bodily components, bacteria, endotoxin, fungal spores or hyphae, mycotoxins, pollen grains, feed grains, hay, silage, and other plant products.

Grain dust contains organic and inorganic particles. The mixture is variable, depending on the type of grain, where and under what conditions it is grown, and methods of harvest, storage, and processing. Thus, certain grains, such as durum wheat and barley, are more irritating than others; and health problems increase as moisture content and resultant spoilage increase.

Biologic effects of grain dust may include an acute respiratory inflammatory response such as nasal stuffiness, rhinorrhea, sore throat, acute bronchitis, asthma, chronic bronchitis, acute febrile syndrome, hypersensitivity pneumonitis, and eye and skin irritation.[16] Possible etiologic agents in grain dust, which may account for asthma, include sensitivity to grain weevils.[5] Febrile reactions may be caused by endotoxins, which are lipopolysaccharides of gram-negative bacterial cell walls.[49] Bronchitis may be caused by proteolytic enzymes produced by microbes or the total dust load. Symptoms of bronchitis are greatest in workers exposed to environments where the total dust load is greater than 5 mg per cubic meter. These levels can be exceeded during unloading operations.

DIFFERENTIAL DIAGNOSIS OF ORGANIC RESPIRATORY DUST DISEASE IN AGRICULTURAL WORKERS

Agricultural dust is a complex mixture of animal and plant materials. The biologic activity of the dust varies depending on local environmental conditions, such as temperature, humidity, state of decomposition, product source, and concentration of the dust. Agricultural workers who smoke tend to have more frequent symptoms. Several distinctive symptoms are associated with organic dust inhalation.[16,54] These include hypersensitivity pneumonitis, organic dust toxic syndrome, and occupational asthma. Because these symptoms are frequently associated with grain crops, silo filler's disease must also be considered in the differential diagnosis.

The time course of symptoms, the characteristics of the symptoms, pulmonary function test results, including carbon monoxide diffusion capacity, arterial blood gas analysis, and chest roentgenogram are important diagnostic considerations. Bronchial alveolar lavage and pulmonary biopsy are occasionally useful.

Organic dust toxic syndrome is much more common than hypersensitivity pneumonitis.[16] Prevalence estimates suggest that <8% of exposed individuals will develop hypersensitivity pneumonitis, and 30 to 40% of exposed individuals may develop organic dust toxic syndrome. Several individuals exposed to moldy straw or hay may develop organic dust toxic syndrome, but only one or two members of an exposed group may develop hypersensitivity pneumonitis.[8,16] Antibodies are frequently elevated in patients with hypersensitivity pneumonitis.[19] The demonstration of antibodies to *Micropolyspora faeni* or *Thermoactinomyces* is evidence of exposure with a host reaction but has poor predictive value for the risk of development of symptoms. Antibodies are not detected in the organic dust toxic syndrome. There appear to be no long-term sequelae associated with organic dust toxic syndrome; however, restrictive lung disease may develop if a patient with hypersensitivity pneumonitis continues to have dust exposure. If avoidance of dust exposure is not possible, then agricultural workers should use tight-fitting dust masks or respirators. If symptoms persist, it may be necessary to avoid potential agricultural work that would involve exposure to organic dust.

RESPIRATORY HAZARDS OF ANIMAL CONFINEMENT FACILITIES

Confinement buildings are facilities where a large number of animals are raised in small, enclosed spaces. The buildings are equipped with systems for temperature, humidity, feeding, watering, and ventilation control. Close to one million persons are occupationally exposed to poultry, swine, and cattle in confinement facilities in the United States.

Respiratory hazards arise from organic dust and toxic gas exposures.[15] Organic dusts are primarily from dried fecal material and feed grains. Toxic gases arise from urine and fecal degradation, incomplete combustion of fuels, and animal respiration. Over 40 different gases have been identified, but hydrogen sulfide, ammonia, methane, carbon dioxide, and carbon monoxide are most commonly noted.

Ammonia and hydrogen sulfide can be adsorbed to dust particles that are inhaled. Bacteria and endotoxins can also be inhaled. Workers can develop symptoms within minutes of entering the confinement facility.[16,54] Symptoms of cough, runny nose, scratchy throat, eye irritation, chest tightness, wheezing, and dyspnea may occur and usually subside within 24 to 48 hours of exposure. As with other chronic organic dust exposures, smokers are more likely to be affected.

Fatal exposures from high concentrations of toxic gases are reported. Deaths occurring in manure pits are associated with high methane or hydrogen sulfide concentrations. Ambient hydrogen sulfide levels may reach 400 to 500 ppm. At these levels, unconsciousness, convulsions, and sudden death may rapidly occur. Workers entering closed spaces or those containing manure should wear self-contained breathing apparatus. The individual should wear a lifeline and should have an observer outside the tank with rescue equipment at all times.

SKIN DISEASE OF FARMERS ASSOCIATED WITH CHEMICALS

Irritant and allergic contact dermatitis can result from a number of agents on the farm, and farming has the highest incidence of occupational skin disease. In California in 1979, 6.1 cases of occupational skin disease occurred per 1000 farm workers per year versus 1.59 cases per 1000 workers per year for all industries.[40] Plant and animal products accounted for 63% of the cases, with poison oak (see Chap. 78) accounting for 48% of the cases. Other plants including weeds and flowers, leather, hides, fur, feathers, lumber, and wood products less commonly cause dermatitis.

Agricultural chemicals cause 20% of cases, and a recent review cited approximately 75 farm chemicals that are known to cause dermatitis.[2] Fungicides and herbicides are the most common chemical sensitizers, accounting for more than half of the cases in the California study.[40] Edible food products can also cause dermatitis, with fruits and nuts causing over half of the cases associated with edible food products.[40] Vegetables grown without the use of pesticides are also associated with contact dermatitis.[1] The animal feed preservative propionic acid is associated with acute irritant contact dermatitis.[27] Contact dermatitis associated with photosensitivity occurs by exposure to alantolactone in chrysanthemum farming.[38] Careful history and testing may be required to distinguish the cause of dermatitis in an individual case, as both the herbicide on the plant and the plant itself may be etiologic. Contact pemphigus is associated with the chlorinated hydrocarbon pesticide dihydrodiphenyltrichlorethane. The proposed mechanism is that systemic absorption after the topical contact is responsible for the alteration of skin structure and activation of immunologic mechanisms leading to blister formation and acantholysis.[65]

Sensitization often follows an exposure only to a concentrated solution, but once a worker is sensitized, minute exposures can cause inflammation. Dilutions of one part per million can produce a positive patch test response in sensitized individuals.[28,44]

Skin infections must be considered in the differential diagnosis of dermatitis in farm workers, and zoonotic skin diseases are common. A number of *Trichophyton* and *Microsporium* species have nonhuman hosts including cattle, dogs, horses, sheep, pigs, and wildlife (deer and moose). Infections in humans can be more severe than those from anthrophilic species. In severe cases, pustular folliculitis and hair loss on exposed areas of the arms, head, and trunk is reported.[3]

A number of studies indicate that farmers have an increased risk of melanoma and other skin cancers that most likely relates to their increased exposure to ultraviolet radiation from sunlight.[6]

CHEMICAL HAZARDS OF GREENHOUSE WORKERS

Greenhouses are used to grow flowers, shrubs, and vegetables. Use of greenhouses can extend the growing season and allow seedlings to develop before the soil is warm enough for planting. The enclosed environment of greenhouses could potentially lead to exposures of workers to higher levels of toxic chemicals and plant materials than other agricultural environments. Health effects found among greenhouse workers include irritant reactions, asthma, and dermatitis.[29]

FOOD CROP TOXICITY

Green tobacco sickness is an occupational illness of farm workers associated with skin contact to wet green tobacco. In 1992 and 1993 NIOSH (National Institute of Occupational Safety and Health) studies, 10 and 14 cases per 1000 tobacco workers, respectively, required medical care, and of these, 25% had to be hospitalized with 4% in the intensive care unit. Children under 16 years of age represented 9% of cases. As many as 50% of tobacco workers are affected to some extent. Dermal absorption of nicotine is the etiology; it is demonstrated that increased urinary levels of nicotine and conicotine correlated with symptoms.[22] Severity is affected by clothing, hydration status, and previous exposures including smoking history. Symptoms of dizziness, headache, nausea, and vomiting resolve with hydration, antiemetics, and observation. Avoiding dermal contact with green tobacco, particularly when wet, prevents the illness.

CHEMICAL EYE INJURIES

Exposure of the eyes of farmers to numerous chemical agents can result in injury. Anhydrous ammonia, which is used as a fertilizer, causes severe eye injury and blindness.[26] Injury occurs rapidly because of the high solubility of ammonia and is typical of an alkaline injury. Irrigation of exposed eyes should be started immediately after exposure and continued until the pH of the tears normalizes when checked 15 minutes after the termination of irrigation. Irrigation with many liters of normal saline over hours may be required.[10] Pesticides such as malathion are chemical irritants to eyes and skin, as are their organic solvents and inert ingredients. Protective goggles should always be worn while working with anhydrous ammonia, pesticides, and other liquids (see Chap. 27).

TOXIC BITES AND ENVENOMATIONS

Farmers work outdoors and are exposed to venomous nonfarm animals (see Table 111–4).[25] There are no data on occupational risk of envenomation to farmers in the United States. A retrospective review of 40 consecutive snakebite victims in Brazil found that all 40 were farm laborers, and 35 of the 40 were bitten on the lower extremities.[4] Each year in the United States, thousands of individuals are bitten or stung by toxic or venomous animals,[46] and approximately 50 deaths per year are reported.[50,66] Numerous visits to the emergency department and millions of dollars are spent on treatment each year for severe reactions or injuries after an animal bite or sting.[23]

There are 20 venomous snakes in the United States (see Chap. 101). An estimated 8000 venomous snakebites occur each year in the United States, with 10 to 15 deaths reported. Venomous snakes are found in all the lower 48 states, with the highest census of snakebites occurring in the southern states. Most snakebites occur from April to October, when farmers in most regions are planting and harvesting crops. Farmers, like others in the outdoors, should wear shoes and trousers and watch where they step or place their hands. They should also be aware that snakes frequently are found in shaded areas of barns or under equipment during hot summer months.

Stings are the most frequently reported adverse events involving insects, and 0.5 to 5% of the population may develop anaphy-

TABLE 111–4. Common Animals that Bite, Envenomate, or Cause Allergic Reactions in Agricultural Workers

I. **Reptiles**
  A. **Snakes** (see Chap. 101)
    1. Crotalinae—pit vipers
      a. Rattlesnakes
      b. Copperheads, cottonmouth moccasins
    2. Elapidae—coral snakes
      a. Eastern coral
      b. Arizona coral
II. **Arthropods** (see Chap. 102)
  A. **Insects**
    1. Hymenoptera
      a. Ants
      b. Wasps
      c. Hornets
      d. Bees
      e. Yellow jackets
    2. Diptera
      a. Biting flies
      b. Mosquitoes
    3. Siphonaptera
      a. Fleas
    4. Hemiptera
      a. Bed bugs
      b. Cone nose bugs
    5. Lepidoptera
      a. Butterflies
      b. Moths
  B. **Arachnids**
    1. Araneae
      a. Black widow spider
      b. Brown recluse spider
      c. Other spiders
    2. Scorpions
      a. Bark scorpion
      b. Other scorpions
    3. Acari
      a. Ticks
      b. Mites
  C. **Centipedes**
    1. Giant desert centipede

laxis after a sting[67] (see Chap. 102). In the United States, 30 to 40 deaths per year are caused by insect stings. Bees, wasps, hornets, and fire ants of the order Hymenoptera are primarily responsible for anaphylactic reactions, although other insects may rarely cause anaplylaxis. Venom immunotherapy is extremely effective prophylaxis in individuals with a positive clinical history and positive skin test results. Farmers with a history of anaphylaxis after envenomation should be given emergency treatment kits (Ana-Kit® or Epi-Pen®) to accompany them when in danger of exposure and should be referred to an allergist for desensitization.

Another animal that can envenomate farmers or agricultural workers is the scorpion. Most cases in the United States occur in the Southwest. The bark scorpion is the most venomous in the United States. It frequently hides under rocks or wood piles. Both sympathetic and parasympathetic nervous system manifestations may occur after a sting. Respiratory compromise is generally the most significant side effect following envenomation and is more common in infants and young children.

Numerous other animals may cause painful or itchy bites or contribute to exacerbation of allergies, but fortunately, they rarely cause severe health problems in the United States.

SUBACUTE AND CHRONIC ORGANIC PHOSPHORUS COMPOUND POISONING

Farm workers share with rural residents living by fields, pesticide-manufacturing plant workers, and exterminators the potential for chronic exposures to organic phosphorus pesticides. The clinical manifestations reported with chronic exposures differ from those following acute exposures (see Chap. 88). A study of exposed orchard sprayers found headache to be the most common complaint, followed by nausea, weakness or fatigue, and chest tightness. Symptoms of abdominal pain, vertigo or incoordination, vomiting, perspiration, cough, vision disturbance, loss of appetite, dyspnea, nasal discharge, miosis, and wheezing were also reported.[61]

Neuropsychiatric deficits and paralysis can occur from both chronic and acute exposures to organic phosphorus compounds. Neuropsychiatric disability has been verified in controlled studies[52,53,58] and found to correlate with measures of the severity of acute poisoning.[58] Persistent peripheral neuropathy has also been described, with decreased finger and toe vibrotactile sensitivity.[58] A study of farm workers who suffered a single acute poisoning found that poisoned workers performed poorly relative to matched controls on all neuropsychological tests, including verbal and visual attention, visual memory, visuomotor speed, sequencing and problem solving, motor steadiness, and dexterity.[52] A literature review found a consistent picture of impaired vigilance and reduced concentration, reduced information processing and psychomotor speed, memory deficit, linguistic disturbances, depression, anxiety, and irritability.[17]

A controlled study of sheep farmers with chronic exposure to organic phosphorus pesticides in sheep dip found significantly worse performance on tests to assess sustained attention and speed of information processing relative to controls, as well as "vulnerability to psychiatric disorder" as determined by a questionnaire. Short-term memory and learning testing was not affected in this study.[59] Peripheral neuropathy was documented in chronically exposed workers in India,[18] and elevated tactile and vibratory thresholds were recognized in exposed workers relative to controls.[41]

Paralysis is reported as a complication of organic phosphorus poisoning. Delayed bilateral recurrent laryngeal nerve paralysis occurred 25 to 35 days after poisoning with chlorpyrifos, parathion, and methamidophos.[13] Chronic fatigue[11] and chemical sensitivity[44,62] can occur.

Occasionally patients present with devastating neurotoxicity that is out of proportion to their histories of exposure to an organic phosphorus compound. Recent studies have revealed genetic variations in the ability to detoxify organic phosphorus compounds. Many organophosphorothioate insecticides are detoxified by bioactivation of the parent compound by the cytochrome P450 systems followed by hydrolysis of the resulting oxygenated metabolite (oxon) by serum and liver paraoxonases (PON1). Examples include malathion, which is metabolized to malaoxon, parathion, which is metabolized to paraoxon, and chlorpyrifos, which is metabolized to chlorpyrifos oxon. These oxons are then degraded by paraoxonase. Polymorphisms in human populations greatly change the rate of hydrolysis of compounds such as paraoxon. Studies of normal mice injected with purified PON1 and of PON1 knockout mice support the hypothesis that differential sensitivity to these compounds can result from genetic variations in metabolism through the P450/PON1 pathway.[20]

PREVENTION OF FARM POISONINGS

The farm presents unique challenges for prevention of poisonings (Table 111–5). Education is the most important component of a prevention program,[35] and it must focus on populations at risk, including small children and their families. Topics to be emphasized

TABLE 111–5. The Prevention of Farm Poisonings

- Safety programs for farmers
- Proper protective clothing when using toxic chemicals
- Closed-system product and equipment designs
- Strict adherence to pesticide labels
- Reduced use of toxins by improved agricultural biotechnology and integrated pest management
- Improved rural health access to primary care physicians trained in agricultural medicine
- Emphasis on safety
- Proper cleaning and disposal of containers
- Water source for immediate decontamination

in safety education include the use of protective clothing, respirators, and other equipment. Using appropriate equipment for applying pesticides, strict adherence to pesticide labels, knowledge of reentry times after spraying, and first aid for exposures to agrichemicals should be emphasized. Understanding the indications for using a pesticide and utilizing only those needed are important components of safety that begin before a product is purchased. Pesticide labels are important legal documents, and farmers should be educated to read them carefully several times before use of the pesticide.

Protective clothing should be used by those working with chemicals, but expense and the discomfort of bulky clothing on hot summer days may limit its use. Understanding risks can increase compliance with recommendations for wearing protective clothing. Research into affordable, comfortable protective clothing is ongoing. Farmers must know that contaminated protective clothing can be a source of pesticide poisoning, even after repeated laundering.[12] Powered dust respirators have been shown to prevent asthma in farmers with allergic asthma to occupational antigens.[63]

Mixing and loading of pesticides are particularly dangerous because concentrated solutions are handled. Equipment design with closed systems can decrease exposure. Minimizing the use of toxic chemicals is a strategy that can reduce poisoning while limiting adverse environmental effects. Integrated Pest Management, an agricultural program that emphasizes surveillance rather than routine applications of pesticides, has great potential to reduce the use of toxic chemicals in agriculture. Bioengineered strains of plants may require less pesticide and indirectly reduce toxic hazards in the future. An improved rural health care system with access to primary care physicians who are aware of farm toxicology is also needed.

Educating farmers and their families about first aid may be life saving in emergency situations because farms are often far from medical facilities. Farm workers must know decontamination techniques. Rescuers must recognize that the clothing, bronchial secretions, skin, blood, and urine of victims of organic phosphorus compound poisoning can poison others secondarily, and rescuers must therefore protect themselves.

HIGH-RISK GROUPS FOR FARM POISONINGS

Populations at risk for poisonings from agricultural chemicals may be divided into occupational and nonoccupational groups. Poisonings occur in workers at increased risk of exposure. These include handlers of pesticides: mixers, loaders, and applicators, flaggers for aerial sprayers, and harvesters of recently sprayed produce. Migrant workers may camp near recently sprayed fields and have language barriers that further complicate evacuation and possibly increase risk.

Another population that is at high risk for farm poisonings is children, especially those under 10 years old.[57] Because they are smaller, a similar exposure will have a greater effect than in the case of an adult. Children are curious by nature, willing to explore exciting tastes and smells on the farm. They wear minimal clothing in the summer, affording limited protection from skin absorption. The skin of children is more absorbent with a larger surface area per unit weight. The tendency of small children to place things in their mouths increases the risk of ingestion. The case of a 1-year-old who was severely poisoned after hugging his father who was wearing clothing contaminated with parathion illustrates the particular vulnerability of farm children.[57] Carbon monoxide poisoning of children riding in the back of pick-up trucks is reported.[24] Tractor exhaust can be a source of carbon monoxide poisoning; farm workers riding behind a tractor on a two-seat tobacco setter have suffered carbon monoxide poisoning.[60] Farm families generally drink well water, and contamination of ground water with nitrates from fertilizers has led to methemoglobinemia (see Chap. 94). Infants are especially vulnerable, and fatalities are reported in this age group.[32,37]

TRANSPORTATION CONCERNS IN RURAL AREAS

Exposures to farm chemicals often occur in isolated areas distant from medical resources. First aid and decontamination supplies may not be readily available. Transportation is often by farm vehicles, and decontamination is readily forgotten, even by knowledgeable personnel. Transportation without decontamination at the scene prolongs exposure and places healthcare personnel at risk for illness. This may have dire consequences for helicopter transport.[31] Agrichemical exposures are sometimes complicated by major trauma, which further diverts attention from necessary decontamination. The chemicals at the scene should always be identified and communicated to the receiving hospital. Table 111–6 outlines the important considerations for transporting poisoned farm workers.

TABLE 111–6. Considerations for Transportation of Poisoned Farm Victims

- Avoid contamination and poisoning of rescuers
- Maintain ABCs
- Initiate decontamination
  Remove victim from source of exposure
  Remove any contaminated clothing
  Irrigate and wash with soap and water profusely
- Identify source of chemical exposure; collect label if available
- Optimize transporation, using helicopter transport if possible
- Healthcare personnel should wear protective clothing
- Means of transportation should reflect severity of injury to patient and health risk to transport team

INFORMATION RESOURCES ON FARM POISONINGS

Healthcare providers are usually unaware of the resources available to farmers. The state Cooperative Extension Service is a resource for farmers and farm families. Restricted-use pesticides require a trained and licensed applicator who has undergone training for handling such compounds. Unfortunately, although a license is necessary to purchase a restricted use pesticide, the licensee may have a farm laborer apply the chemical without adequate supervision.

County agricultural extension agents are a useful resource, and these agents often make recommendations to farmers regarding options for pest control. The 4H clubs provide education in health and safety to farm children. Chemical companies are another resource, especially if the chemical product is known by the clinician. Chemtrac® is one toll-free number (800–424–9300) available to farmers to assist with questions of toxicity.

Rural healthcare providers are another resource. These practitioners often may have backgrounds in agriculture and should have more experience than their urban colleagues in addressing health problems associated with farm chemicals. Primary physicians for farmers and farm laborers can play a vital role in educating farmers about prevention. Unfortunately, this practice is not often emphasized in medical education.

Regional poison control centers are the premier resource for assistance with poisonings. These centers are most effectively utilized if the chemical agent is known. Algorithms for patient treatment are succinct and up to date. Emergency medical personnel are another resource for farmers. In rural areas, lay health personnel are capable of immediate responses and should be trained to minimize poisoning by initiating early decontamination.

On the Internet, information on the safe use of pesticides can be found in the 2000 *North Carolina Agricultural Chemicals Manual* at *http://ipmwww.ncsu.edu/agchem/agchem.html*. The Applied Agricultural Chemicals site at *http://www.inform. umd. edu:8080//EdRes/Topic/AgriEnv/ndd/occsafe/APPLIED_AGRI-CULTURAL_CHEMICALS.html* also has valuable information. The Agricultural Consumer and Environmental Sciences Library at *http://www.library.uiuc.edu/agx/chemistry/cheminfo.htm* provides an extensive bibliography on agricultural chemicals and associated hazards. The Australian National Health and Medical Research Council maintains a site on aerial spraying at *http://www.health.gov.au/nhmrc/publicat/fullhtml/dp4.htm*. The University of California Cooperative Extension service maintains a site on hazardous environmental chemicals in the environment at *http://ace.orst.edu/info/extoxnet/newsletters/n61_86.htm*.

SUMMARY

The risks associated with farming are diverse. They represent many environmental, chemical, botanical, and zoological possibilities. Careful analysis of the pesticides, pests, crops, and local flora and fauna must be considered to care for these diverse risks. An increased interest in improved occupational health and safety has led to the development of the science and epidemiology of farm-related toxicology.

REFERENCES

1. Aberer W: Occupational dermatitis from organically grown parsnip *(Pastinaca sativa L.)*. Contact Dermatitis 1992;26:62.

2. Abrams K, Hogan DJ, Maibach HI: Pesticide-related dermatoses in agricultural workers. In: Cordes DH, Rea DF, eds: Health Hazards of Farmers. State Art Rev Occup Med1991;6:463–492.

3. Armstrong KR, Post, K: The role of farm animals in the control of zoonotic skin diseases in man. In: Dosman JA, Crockfort DW, eds: Principles of Health and Safety in Agriculture. Boca Raton, CRC Press, 1989, pp. 288–291.

4. Barraviera B, Bonjorno JC Jr, Arkaki D, et al: A retrospective study of 40 victims of crotalus snake bites. Analysis of the hepatic necrosis observed in one patient. Rev Soc Bras Med Trop 1989;22:5–12.

5. Blainey AD, Topping MP, Ollier S, et al: Allergic respiratory disease in grain workers: the role of storage mites. J. Allergy Clin Immunol 1989;84:296–303.

6. Blair A, Zahm SH: Cancer among farmers. In: Cordes DH, Rea DF, eds: Health Hazards of Farmers. State Art Rev Occup Med 1991;6:335–354.

7. Blanc P: Occupational asthma in a national disability survey. Chest 1987;92:613–617.

8. Brinton WT, Vastbinder EE, Greene JW, et al: An outbreak of organic dust toxic syndrome in a college fraternity. JAMA 1987;258:1210–1212.

9. Brooks SM, Weiss MA, Bernstein IL: Reactive airways dysfunction syndrome (RADS): Peristent asthma syndrome after high level irritant exposure. Chest 1985;88:376–384.

10. Clark R: Occular emergencies. In: Tintinalli JE, Krome RL, Ruiz E: Emergency Medicine: A Comprehensive Study Guide. New York, McGraw-Hill, 1992, p. 834.

11. Corrigan PM, McDonald S, Brown A, et al: Neurasthenic fatigue, chemical sensitivity, and GABAa receptor toxins. Medical Hyp 1994;265:195–200.

12. Council on Scientific Affairs, American Medical Association: Biotechnology and the American agricultural industry. JAMA 1991;265:1429–1436.

13. De Silva HJ, Sanmuganathan PS, Senanayake N: Isolated bilateral recurrent laryngeal nerve paralysis: A delayed complication of organophosphorus poisoning. Hum Exp Toxicol 1994;13:171–173.

14. Donham KJ: Hazardous agents in agricultural dusts and methods of evaluation. Am J Ind Med 1986;10:205–220.

15. Donham KJ: Relationships of air quality and productivity in intensive swine housing. Agri-Practice 1989;10:15–26.

16. do Pico GA: Hazardous exposure and lung disease among farm workers. Clin Chest Med 1992;13:311–328.

17. Ecobichon DJ, Joy RM: Pesticides and Neurological Disease, 2nd ed. Boca Raton, CRC Press, 1994.

18. Ernest K, Thomas M, Paulose M, et al: Delayed effect of exposure to organophosphorus compounds. Indian J Med Res 1995;101:81–84.

19. Fink JN: Hypersensitivity pneumonitis. Clin Chest Med 1992;13:303–309.

20. Furlong CE, Li WF, Richter RJ, et al: Genetic and temporal determinants of pesticide sensitivity: Role of paraoxonase (PON1). Neurotoxicology. 2000;21:91–100.

21. Ghosh SK, Saiyed HN, Gokani VN, Thakker MU: Occupational health problems among workers handling Virginia tobacco. Int Arch Occup Environ Health 1986;58:47–52.

22. Ghosh SE, Gokani VN, Parikh JR, et al: Protection against "green symptoms" from tobacco in Indian harvesters: A preliminary intervention study. Arch Environ Health 1987;42:121–124.

23. Goldstein EJC: Bite wounds and infection. Clin Infect Dis 1992;14:633–640.

24. Hampson NB, Norkool DM: Carbon monoxide poisoning in children riding in the back of pickup trucks. JAMA 1992;267:538–540.

25. Hassen LB: Reptile and arthropod environments. In: Cordes DH, Rea DF, eds: Occupational Medicine: State of the Art Reviews, vol. 6. Philadelphia, Henly & Belfus, 1991, pp. 447–461.

26. Helmers S, Top FH, Knapp LW: Ammonia injuries in agriculture. J Iowa Med Soc 1971;36:271–280.

27. Henschel R, Agathos M, Breit R: Acute irritant contact dermatitis from propionic acid used in animal feed preservation. Contact Dermatitis. 1999;40:328.

28. Hogan DJ, Lane PR: Allergic contact dermatitis to a herbicide (barban). Can Med Assoc J 1986;132:285–300.

29. Illing HP: Is working in greenhouses healthy? Evidence concerning the toxic risks that might affect greenhouse workers. Occup Med 1997;47:281–293.

30. Iverson M, Dahl R: Allergy to storage mites in asthmatic patients and its relation to damp housing conditions. Allergy 1990;45:81–85.

31. James PA, St Clair MB: Agrichemicals complicating emergency helicopter transport of a farm worker. J Agromed 1994;1:21–27.

32. Johnson CJ, Bonrud PA, Dosch TL, et al: Fatal outcome of methemoglobinemia in an infant. JAMA 1987;257:2796–2797.

33. Kim YK, Son JW, Kim HY, et al: Citrus red mite *(Panonychus citri)* is the most common sensitizing allergy of asthma and rhinitis in citrus farmers. Clin Exp Allergy 1999;29:1102–1109.

34. Kimbell-Dunn M, Bradshaw L, Slater T, et al: Asthma and allergy in New Zealand farmers. Am J Indust Med 1999;35:51–57.

35. Klein-Schwartz W, Smith GS: Agricultural and horticultural chemical poisonings: Mortality and morbidity in the United States. Ann Emerg Med 1997;29:232–238.

36. Kronqvist M, Johansson E, Pershagen G, et al: Increasing prevalence of asthma over 12 years among dairy farmers on Gotland, Sweden: storage mites remain dominant allergens. Clin Exp Allergy 1999;29:35–41.

37. Kross BC, Ayebo AD, Fuorrtes LJ: Methemoglobinemia: Nitrate toxicity in rural American. Am Fam Physician 1992;46:183–188.

38. Kuno Y, Kawabe Y, Sakakibara S: Allergic contact dermatitis associated with photosensitivity, from alantolactone in a chrysanthemum farmer. Contact Dermatitis 1999;40:224–225.

39. Lieberman AD, Craven MR: Reactive intestinal dysfunction syndrome (RIDS) caused by chemical exposures. Arch Environ Health 1998;53:354–358.

40. Mathias CGT: Epidemiology of occupational skin disease in agriculture. In: Dosman JA, Crockfort DW, eds: Principles of Health and Safety in Agriculture. Boca Raton, CRC Press, 1989, pp. 285–287.

41. McConnell R, Keifer M, Rosenstock L: Elevated quantitative vibrotactile threshold among workers previously poisoned with methamidophos and other organophosphate pesticides. Am J Indust Med 1994;25:325–334.

42. Meggs WJ, Elsheik T, Metzger WJ, et al: Nasal pathology and ultrastructure in patients with chronic airway inflammation (RADS and RUDS) following an irritant exposure. J Toxicol Clin Toxicol 1996;34:383–396.

43. Melbostad E, Eduard W, Magnus P: Determinants of asthma in a farming population. Scand J Work Environ Health 1998;24:262–269.

44. Milby TH, Epstein WL: Allergic contact sensitivity to malathion. Arch Environ Health 1964;9:434–437.

45. Miller CS, Mitzel HC: Chemical sensitivity attributed to pesticide exposure versus remodeling. Arch Environ Health 1995;50:119–129.

46. Moore RM, Zehmer RB, Moulthrop JI, Parker RK: Surveillance of animal-bite cases in the United States, 1971–1972. Arch Environ Health 1977;32:267–270.

47. Morgan WK, Seaton A: Occupational Lung Diseases, 2nd ed. Philadelphia, WB Saunders, 1984.

48. Morrow LA, Ryan CM, Hodgson MJ: Alterations in cognitive and psychological functioning after organic solvent exposure. J Occup Med 1990;32:444–450.

49. Olenchock SA, May JJ, Pratt DS, et al: Endotoxins in the agricultural environment. Am J Indust Med 1986;10:325–327.

50. Parish HM: Analysis of 460 fatalities from venomous animals in the United States. Am J Med Sci 1963;245:129–141.

51. Parkes WR: Occupational Lung Disorders, 2nd ed. London, Butterworths, 1982.

52. Rosenstock L, Keifer M, Daniell W, et al: Chronic central nervous system effects of acute organophosphate pesticide intoxication. Lancet 1991;338:223–227.

53. Savage E, Keefe T, Mounce L, et al: Chronic neurological sequela of acute organophosphate pesticide poisoning. Arch Environ Health 1988;43:38–45.

54. Schenker M, Ferguson T, Gamsky T: Respiratory risks associated with agriculture. In: Cordes DH, Rea DF, eds: Occupational Medicine: State of the Art Reviews, vol. 6. Philadelphia, Hanley & Belfus, 1991, pp. 415–428.

55. Shaver CS, Tong T: Chemical hazards to agricultural workers. In: Cordes DH, Rea DF, eds. Health Hazards of Farmers. State Art Rev Occup Med 1991;6:391–413.

56. Sherman RP, Barman ML, Abraham JL: Silicate pneumoconiosis of farm workers. Lab Invest 1979;140:576–582.

57. Shuman SH, Caldwell ST, Whitlock NH, Brittain JA: Etiology of hospitalized pesticide poisonings in South Carolina, 1979–1982. J South Carolina Med Soc 1986;36:73–77.

58. Steenland K, Jenkins B, Ames RG, et al: Chronic neurological sequela to organophosphate pesticide poisoning. Am J Public Health 1994;84:731–736.

59. Stephens R, Spurgeon A, Calvert IA, et al: Neuropsychological effects of long-term exposure to organophosphates in sheep dip. Lancet 1995;345:1135–1139.

60. Struttman TW, Brandt V, Scjheerer A, et al: Outdoor carbon monoxide poisoning attributed to tractor exhaust—Kentucky, 1997. MMWR 1997;46:1224–1227.

61. Sumerford WT, Hayes WJ Jr, Johnson JM: Cholinesterase response and symptomatology from exposure to organic phosphorus insectides. AMA Arch Ind Hyg Occup Med 1953;7:383.

62. Tabershaw IR, Cooper WC: Sequelae of acute organic phosphate poisoning. J Occup Med 1966;8:5–19.

63. Taivainen AI, Tukiainen HO, Terho EO, Husman KR: Powered dust respirator helmets in the prevention of occupational asthma among farmers. Scand J Work Environ Health. 1998;24:503–507.

64. Tilsted D, Hansen AM, Rasmussen K: Formaldehyde in the occupational environment. A possible cause of chemically induced reactive arthritis. Ugeskr Laeger 1996;158:4525–4527.

65. Tsankov N, Kazandjieva J, Gantcheva M: Contact pemphigus induced by dihydrodiphenyltrichlorethane. Eur J Dermatol. 1998;8:442–443.

66. Warpinski JR, Bush RK: Stinging insect allergy. J Wilderness Med 1990;1:249–257.

67. Valentine MD: anaphylaxis and stinging insect hypersensitivity. JAMA 1992;268:2830–2833.

Susi U. Vassallo

The desire to improve athletic performance by pharmacologic manipulation is an ageless pursuit. The word "doping" comes from the Dutch word "doop," a viscous opium juice used by the ancient Greeks.[29] According to the International Olympic Committee (IOC), doping is defined as "the administration of or use by a competing athlete of any substance foreign to the body or of any physiological substance taken in abnormal quantity or taken by an abnormal route of entry into the body with the sole intention of increasing, in an artificial manner, his/her performance in competition."[228] In spite of the prohibition of doping, many athletes admit that they would use a banned substance to win if they would not be caught.[17]

There are several ways to classify doping for the purposes of study. Some categorize agents according to the expected effect of the drug. For example, some substances increase muscle mass, others decrease recovery time, increase energy, or mask the presence of other drugs. However, one drug may have several expected effects. For example, diuretics may be used to mask the presence of other agents by forcing their excretion or may be used to reduce weight. Clenbuterol is an anabolic agent but is also a stimulant because of its β_2-adrenergic agonist effects. Bromontan is another stimulant but is used as a masking agent. Depending on the substance, it is used before competition to improve future performance or during competition to improve immediate results.[29]

The International Olympic Committee divides doping into three categories: prohibited substances, prohibited methods, and restricted drugs[229] (Table 112-1).

HISTORY AND EPIDEMIOLOGY

The International Olympic Committee (IOC) began testing for drugs during the 1968 Olympic games. Subsequently, many prominent athletes were sanctioned and even stripped of their Olympic medals as a result of testing positive for banned substances. In the XXVII Olympiad in Sydney, Australia, four gold medals were reissued to other athletes based on the results of drug testing.[228] Many world-class sporting events have been marred by the controversy surrounding the systematic use of performance-enhancing drugs by the participating athletes. The prevalence of performance-enhancing drugs among athletes of all ages and abilities is far more serious from a public health perspective than the highly publicized cases involving a few world-class athletes. In fact, one-third of the needles and syringes exchanged in a needle exchange program in Wales were employed for the use of anabolic steroids.[165] Infection has resulted from the sharing of needles for intravenous vitamin complex injection. Three Brazilian soccer players from the same club contracted hepatitis C as a result of the parenteral injection of vitamins minutes before game time[161] (see Chap. 109).

The majority of studies on the epidemiology of performance-enhancing substances have investigated anabolic steroid use. It is estimated that there are one million current or former androgenic steroid users in the United States alone.[231] Studies of high school students document that 6.6% of male seniors have used anabolic steroids, and 35% of these individuals were not involved in organized athletics.[34] Others find rates of androgenic steroid use in adolescent athletes from 3% to 19%.[7,113,124,177,226] The National Collegiate Athletic Association (NCAA) reported that 4% of all college athletes use androgenic steroids, but the rate of use was much higher in certain groups. The reported use of anabolic steroids in college football players is 20 to 30%.[66] The Drug Enforcement Agency (DEA) reported that 30 to 50% of both androgenic anabolic steroids and human growth hormone sold illegally are misrepresentations, increasing the potential for untoward effects.[230]

Sudden unexpected death in young athletes is uncommon. The use of performance-enhancing drugs is linked to an epidemic number of deaths in certain groups of competitors. The incidence is estimated to be one to two cases per 200,000 athletes per year.[72] Between 1983 and 1988, there were fewer than 60 reported cases of sudden cardiac death among high school athletes, approximately 12 per year in the United States.[148] Excluding trauma, cardiac death is the most frequent cause of sports-related death in young athletes.[142] There is speculation that the use of erythropoietin, introduced into Europe in 1987, may have contributed to the large number of deaths in young endurance athletes over the next few years.[217] Eighteen young elite cyclists from Belgium and The Netherlands died.[73,166] Over a period of 3 years, from 1989 to 1992, seven young elite Swedish orienteers died suddenly. All had been training within the same geographic area. With about 200 orienteers qualified on the international elite level, this corresponds to an annual mortality rate of 1%.[93,144,223] No cardiac abnormalities associated with sudden unexpected death in athletes, such as hypertrophic cardiomyopathy or valvular disease, were found.[148]

ANABOLIC AGENTS

Androgenic Steroids

Androgenic anabolic steroids (AAS) increase muscle mass and lean body weight and cause nitrogen retention.[153] "Anabolic" means tissue building. "Androgenic" means masculinizing. The

TABLE 112–1. Prohibited Classes of Substances and Prohibited Methods

I. **Prohibited classes**
  A. **Stimulants**
      Albuterol (salbutamol)*
      Amphetamines
      Bromantan
      Caffeine
      Cocaine
      Ephedrine
      Terbutaline*
  B. **Narcotics**
      Buprenorphine
      Heroin
      Methadone
      Morphine
      Pentazocine
      Pethidine
  C. **Anabolic agents**
      1. **Anabolic-androgenic steroids**
          Androstenediol
          Androstenedione
          Dehydroepiandrosterone (DHEA)
          Dihydrotestosterone
          Nandrolone
          Oxandrolone
          Stanozolol
          Testosterone (T:E ratio >6; see text)
      2. **β₂-Adrenergic agonists**
          Clenbuterol
          Salmeterol
          Terbutaline
  D. **Diuretics**
      Acetazolamide
      Furosemide
      Mannitol
      Spironolactone
      Triamterene
  E. **Peptide hormones, mimetics, and analogues**
      1. Chorionic gonadotropin in men
      2. Corticotropins
      3. Erythropoietin
      4. Growth hormone
      5. Insulin*
      6. Insulin-like growth factor
      7. Pituitary and synthetic gonadotropins
II. **Prohibited methods**
  A. Blood doping
  B. Administering artificial oxygen carriers or plasma expanders
  C. Pharmacologic, chemical, and physical manipulation
III. **Classes of prohibited substances in certain circumstances**
  A. β-Adrenergic antagonists
  B. Cannabinoids
  C. Ethanol
  D. Glucocorticosteroids*
  E. Local anesthetics*

*May be permitted with appropriate documentation.
Modified from www.olympic.org (International Olympic Committee, 2000).

androgenic effects of steroids are responsible for male appearance and secondary sexual characteristics such as increased growth of body hair and deepening of the voice in both men and women. Testosterone, the prototypic anabolic androgenic steroid, is the treatment of choice for hypogonadism in men and other disorders such as delayed puberty in boys, aplastic anemia, Fanconi's ane-

mia, or endometriosis. Normal therapeutic dosing includes testosterone enanthate and testosterone cypionate for hypogonadism in doses of 200 mg every 10 to 14 days.[14]

In the 1970s and 1980s, the Federal regulation of anabolic steroids was under the direction of the Food and Drug Administration. Anabolic steroids were required to be prescribed by physicians but were not scheduled according to the Controlled Substances Act. Because of increasing media reports on the use of anabolic steroids in sports, particularly by high school students and amateur athletes, Congress enacted the The Anabolic Steroids Control Act of 1990, which amended the Controlled Substances Act and classified anabolic steroids as Schedule III, alongside, among others, amphetamines, phencyclidine, and lysergic acid. (Schedule III means that a drug has a currently accepted medical use in treatment in the United States and has less potential for abuse than the drugs in Schedule I or II.) Nevertheless, anabolic steroids are still available illicitly through the US mail and over the Internet from international marketers, veterinary pharmaceutical companies, and some legitimate United States manufacturers (Table 112–2). The US Food and Drug Administration estimates that the sale of illicit AAS amounts to $300 to $500 million annually.[50]

Pharmacology

The Leydig cells of the testis produce 95% of endogenous male testosterone, and the remainder comes from the adrenal glands. Normally 4 to 10 mg of testosterone and 1 to 3 mg of androstenedione are produced daily in men. Women secrete small amounts of testosterone daily from their ovaries and adrenal glands, about 0.04 to 0.12 mg, as well as 2 to 4 mg of androstenedione.[205]

Testosterone is degraded rapidly in the liver. Therefore, in order to create a substance that is useful clinically, testosterone is esterified at the 17-hydroxy position, forming a hydrophobic compound that is released gradually from an oily vehicle.[14] Most of these esters of testosterone must be injected intramuscularly to avoid extensive first-pass hepatic metabolism associated with oral administration.[14] The alternative to esterification at the 17-hydroxy position is to alkylate the position. Alkylated androgens

TABLE 112–2. Commonly Encountered Anabolic Steroids on the Illicit Market

Generic Name	Trade Name
Boldenone	Equipoise
Ethylestrenol	Maxibolin
Fluoxymesterone	Halotestin
Methandriol	
Methandrostenolone	Dianabol
Nandrolone decanoate	Durabolin or DecaDurabolin
Oxandrolone	Anavar
Oxymetholone	Anadrol
Stanozolol	Winstrol
Testosterone enanthate	Testoviron or Delatestryl
Testosterone propionate	Testex
Trenbolone	Finajet

Adapted from www.usdoj.gov/dea/concern/steroids.htm (US Drug Enforcement Agency, 2001).

may be administered orally because they are more resistant to hepatic metabolism. Alkylated androgens account for more of the complications associated with anabolic androgenic steroid use because they are most commonly used by athletes.[14]

Administration

About 50% of AAS are used orally, and of the 50% of users who inject intramuscularly, about one-quarter of these share needles.[67,158] Unlike clinical dosing regimens, which consist of fixed doses at regular intervals, AAS are typically used in cycles by athletes.[14] Cycling refers to the use of anabolic steroids at regularly recurring time intervals. For example, the athlete may use steroids for 2 months and then go for 2 months without steroid use. Cycling is based on athletes' individual preferences and not on any validated protocol. Cycles average between 6 to 8 weeks. "Stacking" implies combining use of several steroids at one time, often involving both oral and intramuscular administration. Most athletes use an average of five different steroids at one time, to avoid "plateauing," or developing tolerance, to any one drug. Doses are frequently hundreds of times therapeutic recommendations.[2,225] "Pyramiding" implies starting the anabolic steroid at a low dose, increasing to many times the normal dose, and then tapering once again. Fat-soluble steroids may require several months to be totally excreted, whereas water-soluble steroids may require only 2 days to 2 weeks to be cleared by the kidney. Therefore, water-soluble testosterone esters became important for "bridging therapy." Bridging refers to the practice of halting the administration of long-lasting alkylated testosterone formulations in time for them to clear from the urine and using injections of testosterone esters to replace the orally administered alkylated formulations. This strategy was well documented to have been used by the East German swimmers. In a review of the subject, the practices of the former German Democratic Republic are reported, based on extensive research of previously classified records.[79] Clearance profiles for testosterone congeners were determined for each athlete. In general, the daily injection of testosterone esters was used when the alkylated testosterone derivatives needed to be stopped to avoid detection. These daily injections of testosterone propionate would be halted at 4 to 5 days before competition. Testosterone to epitestosterone values (T:E) were ascertained on departure to a sporting event. Under normal conditions this ratio should approximate 1:1, since both steroids are released endogenously in this ratio. In these urine samples, a few days before the 1989 European Swimming Championships, four female swimmers (winners of 10 Olympic gold medals) had T:E ratios >6. Officials involved in doping were sure that values would decrease to acceptable levels in time for the event, based on the science of the athlete's clearance of testosterone esters. Later, preparations of epitestosterone propionate were prepared for injection to bring the T:E ratio back to the acceptable level of <6.[79]

Clinical Manifestations of AAS

These are summarized in Table 112–3.

Musculoskeletal There is no question that, when combined with strength training, supraphysiologic doses of testosterone increase muscle strength and size.[24] The most common musculoskeletal complications of steroid use are tendon and ligament rupture.[80,104,128,133]

TABLE 112–3. Side Effects of Anabolic Steroids

Musculoskeletal	Sterility
Tendon and ligament rupture	Prostatic carcinoma
Premature epiphyseal closure	Masculinization of female athletes
Radial nerve palsy	Renal
Hepatic	Wilms tumor
Elevated enzymes	Renal cell carcinoma
Peliosis hepatis	Psychiatric
Hepatocellular carcinoma	Aggressiveness
Cholangiocellular carcinoma	Irritability
Infection	Psychosis
Cutaneous abscess	Delirium
Candida albicans endophthalmitis	Withdrawal
HIV	Cardiovascular
Hepatitis B and C	Hypertension
Dermatologic	Carotid artery occlusion
Acne	Myocardial infarction
Keloids	Sudden death
Seborrheic furunculosis	Cerebrovascular accident
Striae	Poststeroid balance disorder
Endocrine	Decreased HDL
Gynecomastia	Increased platelet aggregation
Testicular atrophy	Pulmonary embolus

Hepatic Hepatic subcapsular hematoma with hemorrhage has been reported.[194] Peliosis hepatis, a condition of blood-filled sinuses in the liver,[15,221] occurs most commonly with alkylated androgens and may not improve when the androgens are stopped. This condition is not associated with the dose or duration of treatment.[14,110,201]

Infection Local complications from injection include infected joints,[76] cutaneous abscess,[143,180] and *Candida albicans* endophthalmitis.[224] Injection of steroids with contaminated needles has transmitted infectious diseases such as HIV and hepatitis B and C.[158,179,181,196,199] One individual developed severe chickenpox after prolonged use of AAS.[111]

Dermatologic Cutaneous side effects are common and include keloid formation, sebaceous cysts, comedones, seborrheic furunculosis, folliculitis, and striae.[195] Acne is associated with steroid use and is sometimes referred to as "gymnasium acne."[48,169] A common triad of acne, striae, and gynecomastia occurs. The production of sebum is an androgen-dependent process, and dihydrotestosterone is active in sebaceous glands.[14]

Endocrine Gynecomastia occurs commonly and results from the conversion of testosterone to estradiol in peripheral tissues. Two categories of antiestrogens are available to block the unwanted feminizing side effects of the androgenic steroids. These include the aromatase inhibitors, such as anastrozole and aminoglutethimide, and the estrogen receptor blockers, such as clomid and tamoxifen.

In contrast, cyproterone acetate is a chlorinated progesterone derivative that inhibits 5α-reductase. It blocks the conversion of testosterone to dihydrotestosterone and subsequently enhances its conversion to estradiol (Fig. 112–1). Its antiandrogen activity is used to block the formation of secondary sex characteristics in

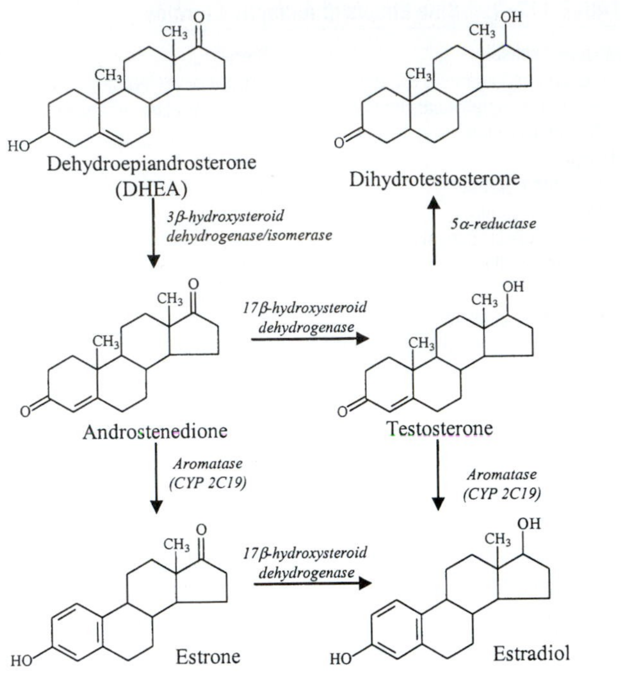

Figure 112–1 The metabolic pathways of DHEA.

young female gymnasts. It is reported to cause hepatotoxicity in some cases.[14,84,89]

Cardiovascular Cardiac complications include acute myocardial infarction and sudden cardiac arrest.[9,78,102,108,136,138,150] Autopsy examination of the heart may reveal biventricular hypertrophy, extensive myocardial fibrosis, and contraction band necrosis. Myofibrillar disorganization and hypertrophy of the interventricular septum and left ventricle are present.[136] Intense training and use of AAS impair diastolic function by increasing the thickness of the left ventricular wall. Animal models and in vitro myocardial cell studies show similar pathologic changes.[58,122,151,207,213] In addition to direct myocardial injury, vasospasm or thrombosis may occur.[151] Alkylated androgens lower HDL-cholesterol and may increase platelet aggregation.[2,78] Thromboembolic events such as pulmonary embolus have been reported.[64,86] CNS events such as stroke,[119,120,198] carotid arterial occlusion,[127] and poststeroid balance disorder may occur.[27]

Neuropsychiatric Withdrawal symptoms from anabolic steroids include decreased libido, fatigue, and myalgias.[118,232] Distractability, depression or mania, delirium, irritability, insomnia, hostility, anxiety, mood lability and aggressiveness ("roid rage") may occur.[19,82,173,174,206] Choreiform movements are reported after treatment with steroids.[209] These neuropsychiatric effects do not appear to be associated with differences in plasma steroid concentrations.[206]

Cancer An association between the use of anabolic steroids and the development of cancer has been made in experimental animals.[186] Testicular and prostatic carcinoma are reported in more

frequent users of AAS.[77,85,184] Hepatocellular carcinoma,[112,160] peliosis hepatis, and cholangiocellular carcinoma also occur.[14,95] Wilms tumor and renal cell carcinoma have been reported in young AAS users.[33,175]

Dehydroepiandrosterone

Dehydroepiandrosterone (DHEA) is a precursor to testosterone (Fig. 112–1). It was banned by the FDA in 1996 but was subsequently marketed as a nutritional supplement and is available for purchase without a prescription.[205] DHEA is converted to androstenedione and then to testosterone by the enzyme 17β-hydroxysteroid dehydrogenase.[107,134,139] Administration of androstenedione in dosages of 300 mg/day increases testosterone and estradiol concentrations in some men and women.[131] Women with adrenal insufficiency given DHEA replacement in a dose of 50 mg orally once daily for 4 months demonstrated increases in serum levels of DHEA, androstenedione, testosterone, and dihydrotestosterone. Serum total and high-density cholesterol concentrations simultaneously decreased. Some women experienced androgenic side effects including greasy skin, acne, and increased growth of body hair.[12] Sense of well-being and sexuality increased after 4 months of treatment.[12] This improvement has been reported in normal men and women as well.[155,156] The neuropsychiatric effects of DHEA have been demonstrated in animals. Increased hypothalamic serotonin, anxiolytic effects, antagonism at the γ-aminobutyric acid (GABA$_A$) receptor, and agonism of the N-methyl-D-aspartate (NMDA) receptor are demonstrated.[12,140,152]

OTHER ANABOLIC AGENTS
Clenbuterol

Clenbuterol is a β$_2$-adrenergic agonist shown to decrease fat deposition and to prevent protein breakdown in animal models.[8] Clenbuterol increases the glycolytic capacity of muscle and causes hypertrophy, enhancing the growth of fast twitch fibers.[141,234] β$_2$-adrenergic receptors are found in skeletal muscle and may mediate the anabolic effect of this class of drugs.[45] Clenbuterol is also a potent "nutrient-partitioning agent," meaning it is able to increase the amount of muscle and decrease the amount of fat produced per pound of feed given to cattle and other animals.[81,183] Other β$_2$-adrenergic agonists such as oral albuterol have similar anabolic properties; however, the half-life of oral albuterol is much shorter, making it less attractive as an anabolic agent.[154] The half-life of clenbuterol is about 27 hours, whereas that of oral albuterol is 3 to 6 hours.[105b] The long half-life and greater anabolic potency when compared to other β-adrenergic agonists place clenbuterol at the center of the controversy regarding the acceptability of using β-adrenergic agonists for athletes. It is recognized that some athletes have asthma, and a ban on β-adrenergic agonists must be weighed against the medical necessity of this class of drugs. Oral use of β$_2$-adrenergic agonists is banned, but inhalational use of the β$_2$-adrenergic agonists is allowed with a letter from a physician.[229] Inhalational use of β$_2$-adrenergic agonists has not been demonstrated to share the anabolic properties associated with parenteral or oral use.[60,202,217] Athletes typically use doses of 60 to 100 µg/d of clenbuterol, and in some cases as much as 600 µg/d.

PEPTIDES AND GLYCOPROTEIN HORMONES

Creatine

Creatine is a nitrogenous amino acid synthesized naturally by the liver, kidneys, and pancreas. In its phosphorylated form it is involved in the resynthesis of adenosine triphosphate (ATP) from adenosine diphosphate (ADP). Supplemental creatine may act similarly.[204] Because ATP is the immediate source of energy for muscle contraction, creatine is used by athletes to increase energy during short, high-intensity exercise. It is estimated that 2.5 million kilograms of creatine were consumed in the past year.[1] Exceptional athletes have admitted to using creatine as part of their training nutritional regimen, leading to interest by athletes at all levels. Numerous studies demonstrate improved performance with creatine supplementation.[26,35,100,149]

Creatine is found in skeletal muscle as well as heart, brain, and kidney. Two-thirds of creatine is stored primarily in the phosphorylated form (PCr), and the remainder as free creatine (Cr).[16] Consuming carbohydrates with creatine supplements increases total creatine and PCr stores in skeletal muscle.[97] This is why creatine is marketed in combination with carbohydrate. Human endogenous production is 1 g of creatine per day, and normal diets containing meat and fish result in another 1 to 2 g per day as dietary intake. One to two grams of creatine are eliminated daily by irreversible conversion to creatinine.[219]

Creatine supplementation is most commonly accomplished with creatine monohydrate. A dose of 20 to 25 g/d can increase the skeletal muscle total creatine concentration by 20%.[35,97,99,109] Therefore, the suggested regimen is an oral loading dose of 20 g per day for the first week, followed by approximately 2 to 5 g/d maintenance. When dosing is by weight, the recommended dose is 0.3 g/kg/d loading dose and 0.03 g/kg/d maintenance.[99,109] Many athletes exceed this dose. Because skeletal muscle has a saturation limit of creatine of 150 to 160 mmol/kg, the philosophy of "more is better" may not hold true under these circumstances.[115,116] Athletes may use creatine for 4 weeks, then stop for an unspecified period before starting again. Creatine costs about $9/d during the loading phase and $5/d during maintenance.

One adverse effect of creatine supplementation is weight gain. It is thought that this primarily represents water retention.[99,149,216] However, there is evidence that net protein increase is partially responsible for the weight gain with the long-term use of creatine.[116] Diarrhea was the most commonly reported side effect of creatine use in one study of 52 male college athletes. Muscle cramping, weight gain, and dehydration were the other complaints, although many subjects had no complaints at all.[115] Creatine supplementation increases urinary creatine and creatinine excretion[99] and may increase plasma creatinine concentrations slightly.[1] Long- and short-term creatine supplementation did not affect renal function adversely.[171,172] Elevations of creatinine are observed in individuals with large muscle mass or increased meat intake without creatine supplementation.[1] One patient is reported in the literature who developed interstitial nephritis that improved with the cessation of creatine use. He had been taking 5 g/d for 4 weeks. It was unknown if the ingestion of creatine caused the nephritis.[125] In another report a young man with focal segmental glomerular sclerosis developed an elevation in creatinine and decreased glomerular filtration rate (GFR) when creatine supplementation

was begun. The values returned to baseline on cessation of creatine supplementation.[176] The possibility of developing decreased renal function is a theoretical concern. Ingestion of large amounts of creatine may result in formation of the carcinogenic substance *N*-nitrososarcosine, which has been shown to induce esophageal cancer in rats.[10,11]

Human Growth Hormone

Human growth hormone (hGH) is an anabolic peptide hormone secreted by the anterior pituitary gland. It causes its anabolic effect by stimulating protein synthesis and by increasing growth and muscle mass in children. The FDA approved hGH in 1996 for treatment of cachexia in patients with acquired immunodeficiency syndrome. It is commonly used for children with growth hormone deficiency in daily doses of 5 to 26 μg/kg body weight.[214] Growth hormone is used by athletes for its anabolic potential and is particularly attractive because laboratory detection is difficult. Recombinant human growth hormone (rhGH) was found in the belongings of Chinese swimmers at the 1998 World Swimming Championships and in the Tour de France cycling event in 1998, suggesting the use of hGH by elite athletes.[220] In one survey, 12% of people in gyms used hGH for body building.[75] In another survey of adolescents, 5% of 10th grade boys had used hGH. Recombinant human growth hormone has been available since 1984 and costs $3000/month for therapeutic doses. Pituitary-derived hGH may be sold as recombinant growth hormone on the black market.

Growth hormone secretion is stimulated by growth hormone-releasing hormone and is inhibited by somatostatin. Human growth hormone is released in a pulsatile manner, mainly during sleep. Exercise stimulates its release, and more intense exercise causes proportionately more hGH release.[28,55,205] Amino acids such as ornithine, L-arginine, tryptophan, and L-lysine increase hGH through an unknown mechanism and are often ingested for this purpose.[55,101,205] γ-hydroxybutyrate and its congeners are purported to affect the release of hGH by inducing sleep.

Growth hormone receptors occur in many tissues, including the liver. Binding of hGH to hepatic receptors causes the secretion of insulin-like growth factor 1 (IGF-1), which has potent anabolic effects and is the mediator responsible for many of the actions of hGH. Human growth hormone stimulates protein synthesis and tissue growth by nitrogen retention and increased movement of amino acids into tissue. The effects on increasing muscle mass and size are well proven in growth hormone–deficient individuals, but studies do not support a resultant increase in strength related to this increase in muscle size.[46,137] Human growth hormone improves muscle and cardiac function, increases red cell mass and oxygen-carrying capacity, stimulates lipolysis, normalizes serum lipid concentrations, and decreases subcutaneous fat. It also improves mood and sense of well-being.[46,54,103,190,214]

Musculoskeletal Effects Human growth hormone administration may cause myalgias, arthralgias, and edema.[214] The effects of hGH on skeletal growth depend on the age of the user. In preadolescence, too much hGH may cause increased bony growth and gigantism.

Endocrine Growth hormone may cause glucose intolerance and hyperglycemia. In adults, excess hGH may cause acromegaly.

Cutaneous Skin changes occur, such as increased melanocytic nevi and changes in skin texture.[168,170]

Cardiovascular Lipid profiles may be adversely affected. High-density lipoproteins (HDLs) are decreased, a change associated with increased risk of coronary artery disease.[235]

Infection Because it must be given parenterally, there is a risk of transmission of infection.[137] The black market sale of cadaveric human pituitary-derived growth hormone carried with it a risk of Creutzfeldt-Jakob disease.[63]

Cancer Long-term users of hGH may be at increased risk of prostate cancer because of the complications associated with IGF-1.[94]

Insulin-like Growth Factor 1

IGF-1 is a peptide chain structurally related to insulin. IGF-1 is approved for the clinical treatment of dwarfism and insulin resistance. Children with antibodies to recombinant growth hormone may respond to IGF-1. Because of its newness, not much is known about the use of IGF-1 by athletes. In one group of 189 weight lifters, 14.3% had taken what they believed to be IGF-1, 85% had heard of it, and most said they would consider using it in the future.[163] There are few studies on the efficacy of IGF-1 in improving the conditioning of athletes. IGF-1 is attractive to female athletes, as it does not cause virilization.[205]

IGF-1 is produced in the liver and many other cell types. A recombinant form is available.[188] Human growth hormone is the primary stimulus for the release of IGF-1, although insulin and nutrition play a role.[188] The effects of growth hormone are primarily mediated by IGF-1. IGF-1 binds principally to the type 1 IGF receptor, which has 40% homology with the insulin receptor and a similar tyrosine kinase subunit.[208] IGF-1 also binds to insulin receptors; however, it has only 1% of the affinity of insulin for the insulin receptor. IGF-1 increases glucose utilization by causing the movement of glucose into cells, increasing amino acid uptake, and stimulating protein synthesis.

The actions of IGF-1 can be classified as either anabolic or insulin-like.[188] Both growth hormone and DHEA are known to increase IGF-1 levels.[155] IGF-1 must be administered parenterally, and it is as expensive as growth hormone. One published regimen for use calls for 30 μg/d for 1 month or 50 μg/d on training days after consumption of a large carbohydrate meal.[163]

Side effects are similar to those associated with the use of growth hormone, and acromegaly may occur. Other effects include headache, jaw pain, edema, and effects on lipid profiles. A potentially serious side effect of IGF is hypoglycemia. High endogenous plasma IGF levels are associated with an increased risk for prostate cancer.[43]

Insulin

Insulin is used by body builders for its anabolic properties. It has been described in "muscle magazines" as "the most powerful anabolic hormone on the planet."[123] Of 20 self-identified anabolic androgenic steroid users in one gym, five (25%) reported insulin use to increase muscle mass.[182] None had any medical reason to use insulin. They had injected insulin from 20 to 60 times over the 6

months preceding the study.[182] Their practice was to inject 10 units of regular insulin and then eat sugary foods after injection.

Insulin inhibits proteolysis and promotes growth by stimulating movement of glucose and amino acids into muscle and fat cells. It increases the synthesis of glycogen, fatty acids, and proteins[57] (see Chap. 26).

Two cases of hypoglycemia have been reported in body builders using insulin. One patient used 80 units of regular insulin in both thighs every hour over a 3- to 4-hour period while simultaneously eating large amounts of carbohydrates on each of the previous two days. On the day of presentation he had injected 320 units of regular insulin over the previous 4 hours, but he had not eaten. The patient had a seizure at the gym and arrived comatose in the emergency department. The serum glucose was 18 mg/dL.[178] Another young bodybuilder developed grave posthypoglycemic encephalopathy following the use of intravenous insulin.[71]

Human Chorionic Gonadotropin

Human chorionic gonadotropin (hCG) is a glycoprotein that stimulates testicular steroidogenesis in men. In women, hCG is secreted by the placenta during pregnancy. Human chorionic gonadotropin may be used by male athletes to prevent testicular atrophy during and after androgen administration.[121] Analysis of hCG in 740 urinary specimens of male athletes revealed abnormal concentrations in 21 individuals. This prompted the IOC ban on the use of hCG in 1987.[31,51] Presently it is not possible to distinguish exogenous hCG administration from hCG production in early pregnancy, and female urine samples are not tested.[121]

Very small amounts of hCG are measured in normal men and nonpregnant women.[121] At this time, measurement is by immunoenzymatic assay. The decision limit, the concentration at which the test is considered positive, is set at 5 IU/mL in the urine. Trophoblastic tumors and nontrophoblastic tumors can increase hCG levels, and this must be considered in the evaluation of an elevated urinary hCG.[62]

Although administration of hCG causes an increase in the total testosterone produced, the testosterone to epitestosterone ratio remains the same because epitestosterone production is also stimulated.

OXYGEN TRANSPORT

Erythropoietin

Erythropoietin (EPO) induces erythropoiesis by a receptor-mediated mechanism that stimulates stem cells to develop into mature red blood cells. EPO increases maximal oxygen uptake by 6 to 7%, an effect that lasts approximately 2 weeks after rHuEPO administration is completed.[69] EPO increases exercise capacity and hematocrit values and is used by athletes, often with additional iron supplementation, for these purposes.[13,130,147,162] EPO has been available since 1988 as a human recombinant product (rHuEPO). Although it has been on the International Olympic Committee's list of banned drugs since 1990, it is particularly difficult to detect (see Laboratory Detection).[229]

Increases in hematocrit subsequent to erythropoietin use are believed to have contributed to the deaths of a number of competitive cyclists in Europe between 1987 and 1990. Nineteen Belgian and Dutch cyclists died of uncertain causes suspected to be related to EPO.[68] The 1998 Tour de France was marred by the discovery of widespread erythropoietin use by several different cycling teams.

EPO is secreted primarily by the kidney, although some is produced by other tissues, including the liver. The mean half-life of EPO is 4.5 hours following IV administration and 25 hours after subcutaneous administration.[83,189] In dialysis patients, a typical dose is approximately 50 units/kg body weight, three times a week.[105] Erythropoietin enhances endothelial activation and platelet reactivity and increases the systolic blood pressure during submaximal exercise.[21,203] These effects, in addition to the increase in hematocrit, increase the risk for thromboembolic events, hypertension, and hyperviscosity syndromes.[21,146,162] There is preliminary evidence that abuse of rHuEPO might pose a risk of decreased endogenous erythropoietin production and subsequent depression of reticulocytosis and anemia.[38,162]

An erythropoietin overdose occurred in a patient who self-administered 10,000 units/d for an unknown period of time as a result of a dosing error. The patient presented to the hospital confused, with plethoric facies, blackened toes, decreased pulses, and a hematocrit of 72%. Emergent erythropheresis was performed and resulted in rapid reduction of the hematocrit and improvement in the patient's condition.[233] Another report of deliberate daily self-administration of an unknown dose of rHuEPO resulted in a hematocrit of 70%. The patient was treated emergently with phlebotomy and intravenous hydration and improved.[32]

Perfluorocarbons

Perfluorocarbons (PFCs) are synthetic oxygen-carrying compounds that may be used as red blood cell substitutes. These liquids, composed of eight to ten carbon atoms where fluorine substitutes for hydrogen, are excellent solvents for gases.[96] In 1966, it was shown that mice could survive when fully submerged in perfluorocarbons infused with oxygen.[47] PFCs are attractive to some athletes compared to red blood cell transfusions, as perfluorocarbons are without risk of infectious contaminants, have a shelf life greater than 1 year, require no crossmatching, are stable at room temperature, and do not increase the viscosity of blood. Several cyclists have been hospitalized for illnesses that were possibly associated with PFC use. Symptoms included transient back pain, malaise, flushing, and fever of several hours duration.[96] Dose-related thrombocytopenia is transient and occurs 3 to 4 days after administration.[200]

PFCs increase vascular tone, and this may cause hypertension. Both systemic and pulmonary vascular resistance are increased.[96] Intravenous infusion of these emulsions results in a liquid bolus that can cause cardiac arrest.[210]

Because perfluorocarbons are perceived by the immune system as foreign substances, they are rapidly cleared by the reticuloendothelial system. The plasma half-life is about 12 hours. PFCs accumulate in the liver and spleen and are slowly transported to the lung. Over a period of months to years, the PFCs are eliminated unchanged in the expired air.[210]

Autotransfusion

The infusion of autologous or heterologous blood for the purpose of increasing the hematocrit is known as blood doping. Blood dop-

ing was used in the Olympic Games as early as 1972 by a Finnish steeplechaser. During subsequent summer and winter Olympics, distance runners, cyclists, and skiers acknowledged their use of this practice. The US cycling team admitted to using blood transfusions in the 1984 Olympics. Subsequently, the International Olympic Committee banned the practice.

Blood doping has been shown to be beneficial in endurance athletes. Infusion of 400 mL of packed red blood cells (PRBCs) into distance runners increased the total red blood cell (RBC) concentration and decreased the time required for a 10-km race by 69 seconds.[30] Blood doping is also shown to increase the speed of the performance of cross-country skiers.[22] The preparatory technique involves the removal of 1000 mL of blood, the immediate replacement of plasma volume, and the freezing and storage of the RBCs. After 5 to 6 weeks, the time needed to return to normocythemia, reinfusion of frozen RBCs resulted in an increased hemoglobin concentration from 45% to 49%, a 5% increase in oxygen utilization, and increased endurance capacity.[92] Removal of 800 mL of blood resulted in a 30% reduced work time during running. Reinfusion of the packed red cells resulted overnight in an increase in maximal work time of 23% and an increased maximal oxygen uptake by 9%. This correlated well with the change in hemoglobin (Hb) concentration.[70]

There is a similarity between blood doping and altitude acclimatization, and the benefits are similar. Endurance athletes living at sea level are at a disadvantage in their training when compared to athletes training at high altitudes. One problem with altitude training is that exercise capacity is reduced, and the intensity of the training is decreased until acclimitization occurs. This offsets some of the beneficial effects of altitude training. Many athletes avoid this by "living high and training low" or by training in an oxygen-rich environment while acclimatizing to the altitude. A 10% increase in hemoglobin caused by altitude acclimatization resulted in an increase of 6% in maximal oxygen uptake and 25% increase in endurance capacity on return to sea level.[92,106]

STIMULANTS

Caffeine

Caffeine is a central nervous system stimulant resulting in a feeling of decreased fatigue (see Chap. 39). Caffeine increases endurance performance.[74,164] This may occur through several different mechanisms including increased calcium permeability in the sarcoplasmic reticulum and enhanced contractility of muscle, phosphodiesterase inhibition and subsequent increased cyclic nucleotides, and adenosine blockade leading to blood vessel dilation and inhibited lipolysis.[74,90] The IOC urinary caffeine concentration limit is 12 μg/mL urine. Caffeine-containing herbal products, tablets, or drinks could result in elevated urinary concentrations. For example, a level resulting in disqualification could occur by drinking eight cups of coffee, each containing 100 mg of caffeine, about 2 to 3 hours before competing.

Amphetamines

The beneficial effects of amphetamines in sports result from their ability to mask fatigue and pain.[60] Initial studies done in soldiers showed they could march longer and ignore pain when taking amphetamines.[212] In one study in college students, resting and maximal heart rate, strength, acceleration, and anaerobic capacity increased. However, although the perception of fatigue decreased, lactic acid continued to accumulate, and maximal oxygen consumption remained the same.[44] Other studies have shown no significant effects on exercise performance[117] (see Chap. 68).

Sodium Bicarbonate

Sodium bicarbonate loading, known as "soda loading," has a long history of use in horse racing.[18] Sodium bicarbonate buffers the lactic acidosis caused by exercise, thereby delaying fatigue and enhancing performance.[90]

During high-intensity exercise, metabolism becomes anaerobic, and lactic acid is produced. Several studies demonstrated improved performance in running with the ingestion of sodium bicarbonate 2 to 3 hours before competition.[49,187] The study dose was 0.2 to 0.3 g/kg body weight of sodium bicarbonate. The effects of sodium bicarbonate are greatest in exercise lasting longer than 4 minutes because anaerobic metabolism contributes more to total energy production, and energy from aerobic metabolism becomes less.[90,91]

Side effects of bicarbonate loading include diarrhea, abdominal pain, and the possibility of hypernatremia.[90]

Diuretics

The IOC bans diuretic use.[229] Diuretics are used in sports in which the athlete must achieve a certain weight to compete in discrete weight classes. In addition to weight loss, body builders find that diuretic use gives greater definition to the physique as the skin draws tightly around the muscles.[3] Diuretics also dilute the urine and are used to make it more difficult to detect other banned drugs.[37,61] Diuretic use in a body builder caused hypokalemia and hypotension[3] (see Chap. 51).

Nutritional Supplements

In a survey of advertisements for food, there were 89 companies selling products as nutritional supplements in 12 different health and body-building magazines. There were 311 products, 235 unique ingredients, and 914 instances where ingredients were mentioned.[167] Only 75% of the products listed the ingredients. In spite of extensive literature searches by the authors, no information could be found for 58% of the ingredients.[167] Amino acids were the most frequently mentioned ingredient, and the most frequent advertising claim was for muscle growth. Many instances of unusual ingredients were found, such as levodopa and glandular material. Plant and insect steroids were included in 9% of the advertised products. On analysis, 22% of the products contained none of the ingredients listed in their advertisements, and one product contained 10 mg of folic acid, 25 times the recommended daily allowance. Because of the lack of regulation of these supplements by the FDA, the inflated advertising claims of the companies, and the misconceptions about what the supplements will do for the user, this billion dollar industry deserves further attention.[4,52,167] Disqualification from competition has resulted from instances in which supposedly benign herbal products contained undeclared substances such as ephedra, rendering urine testing positive. In addition to ephedrine, caffeine, corticosteroids, diuretics, and methyltestosterone have all been found undeclared in some products.[185]

MISCELLANEOUS AGENTS

Chromium Picolinate

Chromium acts as a cofactor to enhance the action of insulin.[98] It is found naturally in meats, grains, raisins, apples, and mushrooms.[204] It is sold as chromium picolinate because picolinic acid is thought to enhance chromium absorption.[204] In people who are chromium deficient, supplementation with chromium results in increased glycogen synthesis and glucose tolerance. Studies have not shown an increase in strength nor a change in body composition or glucose metabolism when chromium is administered in a controlled fashion.[6,56,114,135] Anemia may result from chromium picolinate doses greater that 200 μg/d.[52] A 24-year-old body builder developed rhabdomyolysis after ingesting 1200 μg of chromium picolinate, 6 to 24 times the daily manufacturer-recommended dose of 50 to 200 μg, over 48 hours.[145] Renal failure developed in one patient taking chromium picolinate, 600 μg/d for 6 weeks for weight reduction, about 12 to 45 times the usual intake of dietary chromium or three times the supplementation dose.[222] Another individual taking 1200 to 2400 μg/d of chromium picolinate for the previous 4 months for weight loss presented with renal failure, liver dysfunction, anemia, thrombocytopenia, and hemolysis. Chromium plasma concentrations were two to three times normal. Other causes of the abnormalities were excluded, and laboratory parameters improved with the cessation of chromium ingestion.[42]

Others

L-Carnitine, choline, boron, inosine, and magnesium have all been used by athletes in attempts to enhance performance. None of these supplements has been shown to improve performance, and no serious side effects are reported.[204]

ENVIRONMENTAL HAZARDS

In addition to the potential toxicity of performance-enhancing substances, athletes are subject to toxicity from their environment. Carbon monoxide exposures have occurred in indoor motor arenas from activities such as motorcross car races and monster truck pulls. Indoor arenas have elevated carbon monoxide (CO) levels during competitions. Ice rinks may have high levels of carbon monoxide from ice resurfacers, commonly known as Zambonis, after the inventor.[5,39,126] Ice skaters and hockey players as well as spectators have suffered CO exposure by this route. Oxides of nitrogen, particularly nitrogen dioxide, are additional products of incomplete combustion of fossil fuels.[40,132] Severe exposures to oxides of nitrogen may result in pulmonary toxicity[23] (see Chap. 95).

Swimmers, water polo players, and divers training in indoor pools may suffer from chlorine exposure, including erosion of tooth enamel, known as swimmer's erosion, dermatitis, and conjunctivitis.[41,59]

Elevated lead levels may occurr in athletes such as marathoners, triathletes, and cyclists who train in urban settings particularly near roadways.[159]. Unleaded gasoline has lowered the environmental lead risk. Biathletes and other shooters or persons training at indoor firing ranges are at risk for lead exposure from lead bullets.[211]

LABORATORY DETECTION OF PERFORMANCE-ENHANCING SUBSTANCES

Enormous amounts of energy and money are expended to determine the presence or absence of performance-enhancing substances. The World Anti-Doping Agency (WADA),[229] established in 1999, implemented a worldwide testing program before the XXVII Olympiad in Sydney, Australia, in which 2846 tests were conducted on athletes from 82 countries in 27 different sports. Unannounced out-of-competition testing was performed for the first time at an Olympic event and began two weeks before the start of the games. The first combined blood and urine test for the use of erythropoietin (EPO) was introduced in Sydney and represented the first use of blood sampling for the detection of previously undetectable performance-enhancing drugs. This test was targeted at the sports at high risk of EPO use, primarily endurance events. For the first time, teams of independent observers were involved in monitoring all aspects of the testing process.[229]

Analysis of samples on the international level is accomplished by just a few accredited laboratories. Certain classes of substances are prohibited, as well as any agents related to that class. The majority of tests are done on urine, with careful procedural requirements regarding handling of samples.

On arrival at the testing laboratory, the sample is checked for integrity, including the code, seal, visual appearance, density, and pH. Registration of the sample is completed, and the sample is divided into two aliquots, A and B. All testing is done on aliquot A, and any positive results are confirmed on aliquot B. Sample preparation is difficult and time consuming.

Capillary gas chromatography is the most important technique used in laboratories today in doping control. This method has detected a number of new agents in recent years, such as the stimulant bromantan at the XXVI Olympiad in Atlanta. Gas chromatography is typically combined with mass spectrometry for detection of the majority of substances.[157]

Analysis of the urine by gas chromatography mass spectrophotometry is the current standard for the detection of anabolic steroids.[36] Attention must be paid to proper storage of specimens, sometimes difficult in out-of-competition testing, as bacterial metabolism may increase urinary steroid concentrations.[25,65]

Detection of exogenously administered peptide hormones is difficult because of the structural similarity to the endogenous substance. Research continues in this area, as evidenced by the recent report using monoclonal antibodies to detect administration of recombinant human growth hormone.[227] Erythropoietin is directly measured by a monoclonal antierythropoietin antibody test that does not distinguish between endogenously produced and exogenously administered (recombinant) erythropoietin (rHuEPO). Therefore, indirect methods of detecting EPO use have been employed, such as the measurement of the hematocrit.

Some sports governing bodies, such as the International Cycling Federation and the International Skiing Federation, have chosen a hematocrit of 50% in men and 47% in women as the action level above which an athlete may be disqualified for presumed erythropoietin use. However, there is great variation among athletes in normal hematocrit values. Several studies have shown that hematocrits above the action values of 50% in men and 47% in women, are common in athletes. From 3 to 6% of athletes who did not use EPO had hematocrits >50%.[215] Of those athletes living and training at altitudes between 2000 and 3000 meters above sea level, 20.5% had hematocrit values exceeding 50%.[215] Other studies confirm the increased hematocrits of athletes training at altitudes from 1000 to 6000 meters.[20,215,192,193]

Although many endurance athletes may have increased blood volume, the hematocrit may be lowered because of the increased plasma volume, which exceeds the red blood cell volume. This dilutional pseudoanemia is sometimes called "sports anemia."[197] Additionally, hematocrit measurements are affected by hydration status, upright versus supine posture, nutrition, and change almost 3% with diurnal variation.[191] Because of natural variation between individuals, postural effects, and the ease of manipulation through saline infusion, the indirect detection of EPO use by measurement of hematocrit is fraught with potential for error.[162]

The ratio between serum soluble transferrin receptors (sTfr) and ferritin (ftn) has been studied as an indirect method of detection of EPO use. Soluble transferrin receptor is released from red blood cell progenitors. EPO stimulates erythropoiesis and causes an increase in sTfr and a decrease in ferritin.[88] People with other causes of polycythemia or accelerated erythropoiesis could also exhibit increased ratios and be falsely accused of EPO use. An increased hematocrit with a soluble transferrin receptor above 10 µg/mL and a ratio of sTfr/serum proteins above 153 has been proposed as an indirect measurement of EPO use.[13]

Erythropoietin has some fibrinolytic activity, and urine total fibrin and fibrinogen degradation products have been proposed, but are currently not well studied, as indirect markers of EPO use.[87]

A combination of multiple indirect markers of altered erythropoiesis was recently used in the XXVII Olympiad in Sydney, Australia, to detect rHuEPO use.[162] Current EPO use is known as the "ON model," and recent use but no longer using EPO is known as the "OFF model." Five variables predicted current rHuEPO use: the reticulocyte count, serum erythropoietin, soluble transferrin receptor, hematocrit, and the percentage of macrocytes. A combination of three variables including hematocrit, reticulocyte count, and the measurement of serum EPO, was the best mechanism for detecting recent rHuEPO use.[162]

An immunoblotting procedure, which takes advantage of the different charges on the natural and rHuEPO isoforms, is now under study. By isoelectric focusing, this technique obtains an image of EPO patterns in the urine.[129]

Confounding Agents

Some agents are available for the sole purpose of interfering with urine testing. Examples of these include urine additives such as "Klear," which is 90% methanol, and edible substances such as goldenseal tea, which produces colored urine.[29] The masking agents prohibited by the International Olympic Committee include bromantan, diuretics, epitestosterone, and probenecid.[229] Probenecid blocks the urinary excretion of the glucuronide conjugates of steroids. A number of urine samples were found to contain probenicid at the 1987 Pan American Games, and it was subsequently banned by the IOC.[53,218]

SUMMARY

The primary reason for drug testing in sports is to maintain the integrity and fairness of athletic events. The greatest supporters of drug testing in sport are the athletes themselves.[37] Drug testing attempts to assure a level playing field and create an environment whereby the athletes' abilities are tested, not their creativity or willingness to risk their health by using performance-enhancing substances.

REFERENCES

1. American College of Sports Medicine: The use of anabolic-androgenic steroids in sports. Med Sci Sports Exerc 1987;19:534–539.

2. Alen M, Reinila M, Vihko R: Response of serum hormones to androgen administration in power athletes. Med Sci Sports Exerc 1985; 17:354–359.

3. al-Zaki T, Taibot-Stern J: A bodybuilder with diuretic abuse presenting with symptomatic hypotension and hyperkalemia. Am J Emerg Med 1996;14:96–98.

4. Amos RJ: Adolescents' beliefs about and reasons for using vitamin/mineral supplements. J Am Diet Assoc 1987;87:1063–1065.

5. Anderson DE: Problems created for ice arenas by engine exhaust. Am Ind Hyg Assoc J 1971;32:790–801.

6. Anderson RA, Bryden NA, Polansky MM, Deuster PA: Exercise effects on chromium excretion of trained and untrained men consuming a constant diet. J Appl Physiol 1988;64:249–252.

7. Anderson WA, Albrecht MA, McKeag DB, et al: A national survey of alcohol and drug use by college athletes. Phys Sports Med 1991; 19:91.

8. Anonymous: Muscling in on clenbuterol. Lancet 1992;340:403.

9. Appleby M, Fisher M, Martin M: Myocardial infarction, hyperkalaemia and ventricular tachycardia in a young male body-builder. Int J Cardiol 1994;44:171–174.

10. Archer MC: Use of oral creatine to enhance athletic performance and its potential side effects. Clin J Sport Med 1999;9:119.

11. Archer MC, Clark SD, Thilly JE, Tannenbaum SR: Environmental nitroso compounds: reaction of nitrite with creatine and creatinine. Science 1971;174:1341–1343.

12. Arlt W, Callies F, van Vlijmen JC, et al: Dehydroepiandrosterone replacement in women with adrenal insufficiency. N Engl J Med 1999; 341:1013–1020.

13. Audran M, Gareau R, Matecki S, et al: Effects of erythropoietin administration in training athletes and possible indirect detection in doping control. Med Sci Sports Exerc 1999;31:639–645.

14. Bagatell CJ, Bremner WJ: Androgens in men—uses and abuses. N Engl J Med 1996;334:707–714.

15. Bagheri SA, Boyer JL: Peliosis hepatis associated with androgenic-anabolic steroid therapy. A severe form of hepatic injury. Ann Intern Med 1974;81:610–618.

16. Balsom PD, Soderlund K, Ekblom B: Creatine in humans with special reference to creatine supplementation. Sports Med 1994;18:268–280.

17. Bamberger M: Over the edge. Sports Illustrated 1997;86:60.

18. Ban BD: Sodium bicarbonate: speed catalyst or just plain baking soda. J Am Vet Med Assoc 1994;204:1300–1302.

19. Barker S: Oxymethalone and aggression. Br J Psychiatry 1987;151: 564.

20. Beard JL, Haas JD, Tufts D, et al: Iron deficiency anemia and steady-state work performance at high altitude. J Appl Physiol 1988; 64:1878–1884.

21. Berglund B, Ekblom B: Effect of recombinant human erythropoietin treatment on blood pressure and some haematological parameters in healthy men. J Intern Med 1991;229:125–130.

22. Berglund B, Hemmingson P: Effect of reinfusion of autologous blood on exercise performance in cross-country skiers. Int J Sports Med 1987;8:231–233.

23. Berglund M, Braback L, Bylin G, et al: Personal NO2 exposure monitoring shows high exposure among ice-skating schoolchildren. Arch Environ Health 1994;49:17–24.

24. Bhasin S, Storer TW, Berman N, et al: The effects of supraphysiologic doses of testosterone on muscle size and strength in normal men. N Engl J Med 1996;335:1–7.

25. Bilton RF: Microbial production of testosterone. Lancet 1995;345: 1186–1187.

26. Birch R, Noble D, Greenhaff PL: The influence of dietary creatine supplementation on performance during repeated bouts of maximal isokinetic cycling in man. Eur J Appl Physiol Occup Physiol 1994; 69:268–276.

27. Bochnia M, Medras M, Pospiech L, Jaworska M: Poststeroid balance disorder—a case report in a body builder. Int J Sports Med 1999;20: 407–409.

28. Borer KT: The effects of exercise on growth. Sports Med 1995;20: 375–397.

29. Bowers LD: Athletic drug testing. Clin Sports Med 1998;17: 299–318.

30. Brien AJ, Simon TL: The effects of red blood cell infusion on 10-km race time. JAMA 1987;257:2761–2765.

31. Brooks RV, Collyer SP, Kieman AT, et al: HCG doping in sport and methods for its detection. In: Belloti P, Benzi G, Ljungqvist, eds: Official Proceedings of the Second International Athletic Federation World Symposium on Doping in Sport, London, International Athletic Federation (IAF) 1990, pp. 37–45.

32. Brown KR, Carter W Jr, Lombardi GE: Recombinant erythropoietin overdose. Am J Emerg Med 1993;11:619–621.

33. Bryden AA, Rothwell PJ, O'Reilly PH: Anabolic steroid abuse and renal-cell carcinoma. Lancet 1995;346:1306–1307.

34. Buckley WE, Yesalis CE 3rd, Friedl KE, et al: Estimated prevalence of anabolic steroid use among male high school seniors. JAMA 1988;260:3441–3445.

35. Casey A, Constantin-Teodosiu D, Howell S, et al: Creatine ingestion favorably affects performance and muscle metabolism during maximal exercise in humans. Am J Physiol 1996;271:E31–E37.

36. Catlin DH, Cowan D, Donike M, et al: Testing urine for drugs. Ann Biol Clin (Paris) 1992;50:359–366.

37. Catlin DH, Hatton CK: Use and abuse of anabolic and other drugs for athletic enhancement. Adv Intern Med 1991;36:399–424.

38. Cazzola M: A global strategy for prevention and detection of blood doping with erythropoietin and related drugs. Haematologica 2000; 85:561–563.

39. CDC: Carbon monoxide levels during indoor sporting events—Cincinnati, 1992–1993. MMWR 1994;43:21–23.

40. CDC: Nitrogen dioxide and carbon monoxide intoxication in an indoor ice arena—Wisconsin, 1992. MMWR 1992;41:383–385.

41. Centerwall BS, Armstrong CW, Funkhouser LS, Elzay RP: Erosion of dental enamel among competitive swimmers at a gas-chlorinated swimming pool. Am J Epidemiol 1986;123:641–647.

42. Cerulli J, Grabe DW, Gauthier I, et al: Chromium picolinate toxicity. Ann Pharmacother 1998;32:428–431.

43. Chan JM, Stampfer MJ, Giovannucci E, et al: Plasma insulin-like growth factor-I and prostate cancer risk: a prospective study. Science 1998;279:563–566.

44. Chandler JV, Blair SN: The effect of amphetamines on selected physiological components related to athletic success. Med Sci Sports Exerc 1980;12:65–69.

45. Choo JJ, Horan MA, Little RA, Rothwell NJ: Anabolic effects of clenbuterol on skeletal muscle are mediated by beta 2-adrenoceptor activation. Am J Physiol 1992;263:E50–E56.

46. Christ DM, Peake GT, Egan PA, et al: Body compostition response to exogenous GH during training in highly conditioned adults. J Appl Physiol 1988;65:579–584.

47. Clark LC Jr, Gollan F: Survival of mammals breathing organic liquids equilibrated with oxygen at atmospheric pressure. Science 1966;152:1755–1756.

48. Collins P, Cotterill JA: Gymnasium acne. Clin Exp Dermatol 1995; 20:509.

49. Costill DL, Verstappen F, Kuipers H, et al: Acid-base balance during repeated bouts of exercise: influence of HCO3. Int J Sports Med 1984;5:228–231.

50. Council on Scientific Affairs: Drug abuse in athletes. Anabolic steroids and human growth hormone. JAMA 1988;259:1703–1705.

51. Cowan DA, Kicman AT, Walker CJ, Wheeler MJ: Effect of administration of human chorionic gonadotrophin on criteria used to assess testosterone administration in athletes. J Endocrinol 1991;131:147–154.

52. Cowart VS: Dietary supplements: Alternatives to anabolic steroids? Physician Sports Med 1992;20:189–198.

53. Cowart VS: Drug testing programs face snags and legal challenges. Physician Sports Med 1988;16:165–173.

54. Cuneo RC, Salomon F, Wiles CM, et al: Growth hormone treatment in growth hormone-deficient adults. I. Effects on muscle mass and strength. J Appl Physiol 1991;70:688–694.

55. Cuttler L: The regulation of growth hormone secretion. Endocrinol Metab Clin North Am 1996;25:541–571.

56. Davis JM, Welsh RS, Alerson NA: Effects of carbohydrate and chromium ingestion during intermittent high-intensity exercise to fatigue. Int J Sport Nutr Exerc Metab 2000;10:476–485.

57. Dawson RT, Harrison MW: Use of insulin as an anabolic agent. Br J Sports Med 1997;31:259.

58. De Piccoli B, Giada F, Benettin A, et al: Anabolic steroid use in body builders: an echocardiographic study of left ventricle morphology and function. Int J Sports Med 1991;12:408–412.

59. Decker WJ, Koch HF: Chlorine poisoning at the swimming pool: an overlooked hazard. Clin Toxicol 1978;13:377–381.

60. Dekhuijzen PN, Machiels HA, Heunks LM, et al: Athletes and doping: effects of drugs on the respiratory system. Thorax 1999;54:1041–1046.

61. Delbeke FT, Debackere M: The influence of diuretics on the excretion and metabolism of doping agents—V. Dimefline. J Pharm Biomed Anal 1991;9:23–28.

62. Delbeke FT, Van Eenoo P, De Backer P: Detection of human chorionic gonadotrophin misuse in sports. Int J Sports Med 1998;19:287–290.

63. Deyssig R, Frisch H: Self-administration of cadaveric growth hormone in power athletes. Lancet 1993;341:768–769.

64. Dickerman RD, McConathy WJ, Schaller F, Zachariah NY: Cardiovascular complications and anabolic steroids. Eur Heart J 1996;17:1912.

65. Donike M, Geyer H, Gotzmann A: Recent advances in doping analysis (3). Koln, Sport und Buch Straub, 1996, pp. 95–113.

66. Duda M: NCAA: Only 4% of athletes used steroids. Physician Sports Med 1985;13:30.

67. DuRant RH, Rickert VI, Ashworth CS, et al: Use of multiple drugs among adolescents who use anabolic steroids. N Engl J Med 1993;328:922–926.

68. Eicher ER: Better dead than second. J Lab Clin Med 1992;120:359–360.

69. Ekblom B, Berglund B: Effect of erythropoietin administration on maximal aerobic power. Scand J Med Sci Sports 1991;1:88–93.

70. Ekblom B, Goldbarg AN, Gullbring B: Response to exercise after blood loss and reinfusion. J Appl Physiol 1972;33:175–180.

71. Elkin SL, Brady S, Williams IP: Bodybuilders find it easy to obtain insulin to help them in training. BMJ 1997;314:1280.

72. Epstein SE, Maron BJ: Sudden death and the competitive athlete: perspectives on preparticipation screening studies. J Am Coll Cardiol 1986;7:220–230.

73. Escher S, Maierhofer WJ: Erythropoietin and endurance: A recipe for disaster. Your Patient Fitness 1992;6:15.

74. Essig D, Costill DL, Van Handel PJ: Effects of caffeine ingestion on utilization of muscle glycogen and lipid during leg ergometer cycling. Int J Sports Med 1980;1:86–90.

75. Evans NA: Gym and tonic: a profile of 100 male steroid users. Br J Sports Med 1997;31:54–58.

76. Evans NA: Local complications of self administered anabolic steroid injections. Br J Sports Med 1997;31:349–350.

77. Falk H, Thomas LB, Popper H, Ishak KG: Hepatic angiosarcoma associated with androgenic-anabolic steroids. Lancet 1979;2:1120–1123.

78. Ferenchick G, Schwartz D, Ball M, Schwartz K: Androgenic-anabolic steroid abuse and platelet aggregation: a pilot study in weight lifters. Am J Med Sci 1992;303:78–82.

79. Franke WW, Berendonk B: Hormonal doping and androgenization of athletes: a secret program of the German Democratic Republic government. Clin Chem 1997;43:1262–1279.

80. Freeman BJ, Rooker GD: Spontaneous rupture of the anterior cruciate ligament after anabolic steroids. Br J Sports Med 1995;29:274–275.

81. Freidl KE, Moore RJ: Clenbuterol, ma huang, caffeine, L-carnitine, and growth hormone releasers. Natl Strength Condition Assoc 1992;14:35.

82. Freinhar JP, Alvarez W: Androgen-induced hypomania. J Clin Psychiatry 1985;46:354–355.

83. Fried W, Johnson C, Heller P: Observations on regulation of erythropoiesis during prolonged periods of hypoxia. Blood 1970;36:607–616.

84. Friedman G, Lamoureux E, Sherker AH: Fatal fulminant hepatic failure due to cyproterone acetate. Dig Dis Sci 1999;44:1362–1363.

85. Froehner M, Fischer R, Leike S, et al: Intratesticular leiomyosarcoma in a young man after high dose doping with Oral-Turinabol: A case report. Cancer 1999;86:1571–1575.

86. Gaede JT, Montine TJ: Massive pulmonary embolus and anabolic steroid abuse. JAMA 1992;267:2328–2329.

87. Gareau R, Brisson GR, Chenard C, et al: Total fibrin and fibrinogen degradation products in urine: a possible probe to detect illicit users of the physical-performance enhancer erythropoietin? Horm Res 1995;44:189–192.

88. Gareau R, Gagnon MG, Thellend C, et al: Transferrin soluble receptor: a possible probe for detection of erythropoietin abuse by athletes. Horm Metab Res 1994;26:311–312.

89. Garty BZ, Dinari G, Gellvan A, Kauli R: Cirrhosis in a child with hypothalamic syndrome and central precocious puberty treated with cyproterone acetate. Eur J Pediatr 1999;158:367–370.

90. Ghaphery NA: Performance-enhancing drugs. Orthop Clin North Am 1995;26:433–442.

91. Gledhill N: Bicarbonate ingestion and anaerobic performance. Sports Med 1984;1:177–180.

92. Gledhill N: Blood doping and related issues: a brief review. Med Sci Sports Exerc 1982;14:183–189.

93. Gnarpe H, Gnarpe J: Increasing prevalence of specific antibodies to Chlamydia pneumoniae in Sweden. Lancet 1993;341:381.

94. Goldberg M: Dehydroepiandrosterone, insulin-like growth factor-I, and prostate cancer. Ann Intern Med 1998;129:587–588.

95. Goldman B: Liver carcinoma in an athlete taking anabolic steroids. J Am Osteopath Assoc 1985;85:56.

96. Goodnough LT, Scott MG, Monk TG: Oxygen carriers as blood substitutes. Past, present, and future. Clin Orthop 1998;85:89–100.

97. Green AL, Hultman E, Macdonald IA, et al: Carbohydrate ingestion augments skeletal muscle creatine accumulation during creatine supplementation in humans. Am J Physiol 1996;271:E821–E826.

98. Hallmark MA, Reynolds TH, DeSouza CA, et al: Effects of chromium and resistive training on muscle strength and body composition. Med Sci Sports Exerc 1996;28:139–144.

99. Harris RC, Soderlund K, Hultman E: Elevation of creatine in resting and exercised muscle of normal subjects by creatine supplementation. Clin Sci (Colch) 1992;83:367–374.

100. Harris RC, Viru M, Greenhaff PL, Hultman E: The effect of oral creatine supplementation on running performance during maximal short term exercise in man. J Physiol 1993;467:74P.

101. Haupt HA: Anabolic steroids and growth hormone. Am J Sports Med 1993;21:468–474.

102. Hausmann R, Hammer S, Betz P: Performance enhancing drugs (doping agents) and sudden death—a case report and review of the literature. Int J Legal Med 1998;111:261–264.

103. Healy ML, Russell-Jones D: Growth hormone and sport: abuse, potential benefits, and difficulties in detection. Br J Sports Med 1997; 31:267–268.

104. Hill JA, Suker JR, Sachs K, Brigham C: The athletic polydrug abuse phenomenon. A case report. Am J Sports Med 1983;11:269–271.

105. Hillman RS: Hematopoietic agents: Growth factors, minerals and vitamins. In: Hardman JG, Limbird LE, eds: Goodman and Gilman's The Pharmacological Basis of Therapeutics, 10th ed. New York, McGraw Hill, 2001, pp. 1487–1517.

105b. Hoffman RJ, Hoffman RS, Freyberg CL, Poppenga RH, Nelson LS: Clenbuterol ingestion causing prolonged tachycardia, hypokalemia, and hypophosphatemia with confirmation by quantitative levels. J Toxicol Clin Toxicol 2001;39:339–344.

106. Horstman D, Weiskopf R, Jackson R, et al: The influence of polycythemia induced by four week sojourn at 4300 meters on sea level work capacity. In: Landry F, Orban WAR, eds: Exercise Physiology. Miami, Symposia Specialists, 1978, pp. 533–539.

107. Horton R, Tait JF: Androstenedione production and interconversion rates measured in peripheral blood and studies on the possible site of its conversion to testosterone. J Clin Invest 1966;45:301–313.

108. Huie MJ: An acute myocardial infarction occurring in an anabolic steroid user. Med Sci Sports Exerc 1994;26:408–413.

109. Hultman E, Soderlund K, Timmons JA, et al: Muscle creatine loading in men. J Appl Physiol 1996;81:232–237.

110. Ishak KG, Zimmerman HJ: Hepatotoxic effects of the anabolic/androgenic steroids. Semin Liver Dis 1987;7:230–236.

111. Johnson AS, Jones M, Morgan-Capner P, et al: Severe chickenpox in anabolic steroid user. Lancet 1995;345:1447–1448.

112. Johnson FL, Lerner KG, Siegel M, et al: Association of androgenic-anabolic steroid therapy with development of hepatocellular carcinoma. Lancet 1972;2:1273–1276.

113. Johnson MD: Anabolic steroid use in adolescent athletes. Pediatr Clin North Am 1990;37:1111–1123.

114. Joseph LJ, Farrell PA, Davey SL, et al: Effect of resistance training with or without chromium picolinate supplementation on glucose metabolism in older men and women. Metabolism 1999;48:546–553.

115. Juhn MS, O'Kane JW, Vinci DM: Oral creatine supplementation in male collegiate athletes: a survey of dosing habits and side effects. J Am Diet Assoc 1999;99:593–595.

116. Juhn MS, Tarnopolsky M: Oral creatine supplementation and athletic performance: a critical review. Clin J Sport Med 1998;8: 286–297.

117. Karpovich PV: Effect of amphetamine sulfate on athletic performance. JAMA 1959;170:558–561.

118. Kashkin KB, Kleber HD: Hooked on hormones? An anabolic steroid addiction hypothesis. JAMA 1989;262:3166–3170.

119. Kennedy MC: Anabolic steroid abuse and toxicology. Aust NZ J Med 1992;22:374–381.

120. Kennedy MC, Corrigan AB, Pilbeam ST: Myocardial infarction and cerebral haemorrhage in a young body builder taking anabolic steroids. Aust NZ J Med 1993;23:713.

121. Kicman AT, Brooks RV, Cowan DA: Human chorionic gonadotrophin and sport. Br J Sports Med 1991;25:73–80.

122. Kinson GA, Layberry RA, Hebert B: Influences of anabolic androgens on cardiac growth and metabolism in the rat. Can J Physiol Pharmacol 1991;69:1698–1704.

123. Kneller B: Exogenous insulin. Musclemag Int 1996;171:24–34.

124. Korkia P: Use of anabolic steroids has been reported by 9% of men attending gymnasiums. BMJ 1996;313:1009.

125. Koshy KM, Griswold E, Schneeberger EE: Interstitial nephritis in a patient taking creatine. N Engl J Med 1999;340:814–815.

126. Kuffner E: Athletes. In: Greenberg MI, ed: Occupational, Industrial and Environmental Toxicology. St Louis, CV Mosby, 1997, pp. 19–28.

127. Laroche GP: Steroid anabolic drugs and arterial complications in an athlete—a case history. Angiology 1990;41:964–969.

128. Laseter JT, Russell JA: Anabolic steroid-induced tendon pathology: a review of the literature. Med Sci Sports Exerc 1991;23:1–3.

129. Lasne F, de Ceaurriz J: Recombinant erythropoietin in urine. Nature 2000;405:635.

130. Lavoie C, Diguet A, Milot M, Gareau R: Erythropoietin (rHuEPO) doping: Effects of exercise on anaerobic metabolism in rats. Int J Sports Med 1998;19:281–286.

131. Leder BZ, Longcope C, Catlin DH, et al: Oral androstenedione administration and serum testosterone concentrations in young men. JAMA 2000;283:779–782.

132. Levy JI, Lee K, Yanagisawa Y, et al: Determinants of nitrogen dioxide concentrations in indoor ice skating rinks. Am J Public Health 1998;88:1781–1786.

133. Liow RY, Tavares S: Bilateral rupture of the quadriceps tendon associated with anabolic steroids. Br J Sports Med 1995;29:77–79.

134. Longcope C, Kato T, Horton R: Conversion of blood androgens to estrogens in normal adult men and women. J Clin Invest 1969;48: 2191–2201.

135. Lukaski HC, Bolonchuk WW, Siders WA, Milne DB: Chromium supplementation and resistance training: Effects on body composition, strength, and trace element status of men. Am J Clin Nutr 1996;63:954–965.

136. Luke JL, Farb A, Virmani R, Sample RH: Sudden cardiac death during exercise in a weight lifter using anabolic androgenic steroids: pathological and toxicological findings. J Forensic Sci 1990;35: 1441–1447.

137. Macintyre JG: Growth hormone and athletes. Sports Med 1987; 4:129–142.

138. Madea B, Grellner W: Long-term cardiovascular effects of anabolic steroids. Lancet 1998;352:33.

139. Mahesh VB, Greenblatt RB: The in vivo conversion of dehydroepiandrosterone and androstenedione to testosterone in the human. Acta Endocrinol 1962;41:400–406.

140. Majewska MD, Demirgoren S, Spivak CE, London ED: The neurosteroid dehydroepiandrosterone sulfate is an allosteric antagonist of the GABAA receptor. Brain Res 1990;526:143–146.

141. Maltin CA, Delday MI, Reeds PJ: The effect of a growth promoting drug, clenbuterol, on fiber frequency and area in hind limb muscles from young male rats. Biosci Rep 1986;6:293–299.

142. Maron BJ, Epstein SE, Roberts WC: Causes of sudden death in competitive athletes. J Am Coll Cardiol 1986;7:204–214.

143. Maropis C, Yesalis CE: Intramuscular abscess: another anabolic steroid danger. Physician Sports Med 1994;22:105–110.

144. Marshall A: Mystery death of orienteers. The Independent, November 15, 1992.

145. Martin WR, Fuller RE: Suspected chromium picolinate-induced rhabdomyolysis. Pharmacotherapy 1998;18:860–862.

146. Maschio G: Erythropoietin and systemic hypertension. Nephrol Dial Transplant 1995;10(Suppl 2):74–79.

147. Mayer G, Thum J, Cada EM, et al: Working capacity is increased following recombinant human erythropoietin treatment. Kidney Int 1988;34:525–528.

148. McCaffrey FM, Braden DS, Strong WB: Sudden cardiac death in young athletes. A review. Am J Dis Child 1991;145:177–183.

149. McNaughton LR, Dalton B, Tarr J: The effects of creatine supplementation on high-intensity exercise performance in elite performers. Eur J Appl Physiol Occup Physiol 1998;78:236–240.

150. McNutt RA, Ferenchick GS, Kirlin PC, Hamlin NJ: Acute myocardial infarction in a 22-year-old world class weight lifter using anabolic steroids. Am J Cardiol 1988;62:164.

151. Melchert RB, Herron TJ, Welder AA: The effect of anabolic-androgenic steroids on primary myocardial cell cultures. Med Sci Sports Exerc 1992;24:206–212.

152. Melchior CL, Ritzmann RF: Dehydroepiandrosterone is an anxiolytic in mice on the plus maze. Pharmacol Biochem Behav 1994; 47:437–441.

153. Mooradian AD, Morley JE, Korenman SG: Biological actions of androgens. Endocr Rev 1987;8:1–28.

154. Moore NG, Pegg GG, Sillence MN: Anabolic effects of the beta 2-adrenoceptor agonist salmeterol are dependent on route of administration. Am J Physiol 1994;267:E475–E484.

155. Morales AJ, Haubrich RH, Hwang JY, et al: The effect of six months treatment with a 100 mg daily dose of dehydroepiandrosterone (DHEA) on circulating sex steroids, body composition and muscle strength in age-advanced men and women. Clin Endocrinol (Oxf) 1998; 49:421–432.

156. Morales AJ, Nolan JJ, Nelson JC, Yen SS: Effects of replacement dose of dehydroepiandrosterone in men and women of advancing age. J Clin Endocrinol Metab 1994;78:1360–1367.

157. Muller RK, Grosse J, Thieme D, et al: Introduction to the application of capillary gas chromatography of performance-enhancing drugs in doping control. J Chromatogr A 1999;843:275–285.

158. Nemechek PM: Anabolic steroid users—another potential risk group for HIV infection. N Engl J Med 1991;325:357.

159. Orlando P, Perdelli F, Gallelli G, et al: Increased blood lead levels in runners training in urban areas. Arch Environ Health 1994;49: 200–203.

160. Overly WL, Dankoff JA, Wang BK, Singh UD: Androgens and hepatocellular carcinoma in an athlete. Ann Intern Med 1984;100: 158–159.

161. Parana R, Lyra L, Trepo C: Intravenous vitamin complexes used in sporting activities and transmission of HCV in Brazil. Am J Gastroenterol 1999;94:857–858.

162. Parisotto R, Gore CJ, Emslie KR, et al: A novel method utilising markers of altered erythropoiesis for the detection of recombinant human erythropoietin abuse in athletes. Haematologica 2000;85: 564–572.

163. Parry DA: Insulin-like growth factor 1(IGF 1). A new generation of performance enhancement by athletes. J Performance Enhancing Drugs 1996;1:48–51.

164. Pasman WJ, van Baak MA, Jeukendrup AE, de Haan A: The effect of different dosages of caffeine on endurance performance time. Int J Sports Med 1995;16:225–230.

165. Pates R, Temple D: The Use of Anabolic Steroids in Wales. Cardiff, Wales: Welsh Committee on Drug Misuse, 1992.

166. Pena N: Lethal injection. Bicycling 1991;32:80–81.

167. Philen RM, Ortiz DI, Auerbach SB, Falk H: Survey of advertising for nutritional supplements in health and bodybuilding magazines. JAMA 1992;268:1008–1011.

168. Pierad GE, Estrada A, Nikkels AR, et al: Growth and phenotypic modifications induced in melanocytic nevi during growth hormone therapy. J Cutan 1991;18:384.

169. Pierard GE: [Image of the month. Gymnasium acne: a fulminant doping acne]. Rev Med Liege 1998;53:441–443.

170. Pierard-Franchimont C, Henry F, Crielaard JM, Pierard GE: Mechanical properties of skin in recombinant human growth factor abusers among adult bodybuilders. Dermatology 1996;192: 389–392.

171. Poortmans JR, Auquier H, Renaut V, et al: Effect of short-term creatine supplementation on renal responses in men. Eur J Appl Physiol Occup Physiol 1997;76:566–567.

172. Poortmans JR, Francaux M: Long-term oral creatine supplementation does not impair renal function in healthy athletes. Med Sci Sports Exerc 1999;31:1108–1110.

173. Pope HG Jr, Katz DL: Affective and psychotic symptoms associated with anabolic steroid use. Am J Psychiatry 1988;145:487–490.

174. Pope HG Jr, Katz DL: Psychiatric and medical effects of anabolic-androgenic steroid use. A controlled study of 160 athletes. Arch Gen Psychiatry 1994;51:375–382.

175. Prat J, Gray GF, Stolley PD, Coleman JW: Wilms tumor in an adult associated with androgen abuse. JAMA 1977;237:2322–2323.

176. Pritchard NR, Kalra PA: Renal dysfunction accompanying oral creatine supplements. Lancet 1998;351:1252–1253.

177. Radakovich J, Broderick P, Pickell G: Rate of anabolic-androgenic steroid use among students in junior high school. J Am Board Fam Pract 1993;6:341–345.

178. Reverter JL, Tural C, Rosell A, et al: Self-induced insulin hypoglycemia in a bodybuilder. Arch Intern Med 1994;154:225–226.

179. Rich JD, Dickinson BP, Feller A, et al: The infectious complications of anabolic-androgenic steroid injection. Int J Sports Med 1999;20: 563–566.

180. Rich JD, Dickinson BP, Flanigan TP, Valone SE: Abscess related to anabolic-androgenic steroid injection. Med Sci Sports Exerc 1999; 31:207–209.

181. Rich JD, Dickinson BP, Merriman NA, Flanigan TP: Hepatitis C virus infection related to anabolic-androgenic steroid injection in a recreational weight lifter. Am J Gastroenterol 1998;93:1598.

182. Rich JD, Dickinson BP, Merriman NA, Thule PM: Insulin use by bodybuilders. JAMA 1998;279:1613.

183. Ricks CA, Dalrymple RH, Baker PK, Ingle DL: Use of a beta-agonist to alter fat and muscle deposition in steers. J Anim Sci 1984; 59:1247–1255.

184. Roberts JT, Essenhigh DM: Adenocarcinoma of prostate in 40-year-old body-builder. Lancet 1986;2:742.

185. Ros JJ, Pelders MG, De Smet PA: A case of positive doping associated with a botanical food supplement. Pharm World Sci 1999;21: 44–46.

186. Rosner F, Khan MT: Renal cell carcinoma following prolonged testosterone therapy. Arch Intern Med 1992;152:426, 429.

187. Rupp JC, Bartels RL, Zuelzer W, et al: Effect of sodium bicarbonate ingestion on blood and muscle pH and exercise performance. Med Sci Sports Exerc 1983;15:115.

188. Russell-Jones DL, Umpleby M: Protein anabolic action of insulin, growth hormone and insulin-like growth factor I. Eur J Endocrinol 1996;135:631–642.

189. Salmonson T, Danielson BG, Wikstrom B: The pharmacokinetics of recombinant human erythropoietin after intravenous and subcutaneous administration to healthy subjects. Br J Clin Pharmacol 1990; 29:709–713.

190. Salomon F, Cuneo RC, Hesp R, Sonksen PH: The effects of treatment with recombinant human growth hormone on body composition and metabolism in adults with growth hormone deficiency. N Engl J Med 1989;321:1797–1803.

191. Schmidt W, Biermann B, Winchenbach P, et al: How valid is the determination of hematocrit values to detect blood manipulations? Int J Sports Med 2000;21:133–138.

192. Schmidt W, Dahners HW, Correa R, et al: Blood gas transport properties in endurance-trained athletes living at different altitudes. Int J Sports Med 1990;11:15–21.

193. Schmidt W, Spielvogel H, Eckardt KU, et al: Effects of chronic hypoxia and exercise on plasma erythropoietin in high-altitude residents. J Appl Physiol 1993;74:1874–1878.

194. Schumacher J, Muller G, Klotz KF: Large hepatic hematoma and intraabdominal hemorrhage associated with abuse of anabolic steroids. N Engl J Med 1999;340:1123–1124.

195. Scott MJ Jr, Scott MJ 3rd, Scott AM: Linear keloids resulting from abuse of anabolic androgenic steroid drugs. Cutis 1994;53:41–43.

196. Scott MJ, Scott MJ Jr: HIV infection associated with injections of anabolic steroids. JAMA 1989;262:207–208.

197. Shaskey DJ, Green GA: Sports hematology. Sports Med 2000;1: 27–38.

198. Shiozawa Z, Tsunoda S, Noda A, et al: Cerebral hemorrhagic infarction associated with anabolic steroid therapy for hypoplastic anemia. Angiology 1986;37:725–730.

199. Sklarek HM, Mantovani RP, Erens E, et al: AIDS in a bodybuilder using anabolic steroids. N Engl J Med 1984;311:1701.

200. Smith DJ, Lane TA: Effect of a high concentration perfluorocarbon emulsion on platelet function. Biomater Artif Cells Immobilization Biotechnol 1992;20:1045–1049.

201. Soe KL, Soe M, Gluud C: Liver pathology associated with the use of anabolic-androgenic steroids. Liver 1992;12:73–79.

202. Spann C, Winter ME: Effect of clenbuterol on athletic performance. Ann Pharmacother 1995;29:75–77.

203. Stohlawetz PJ, Dzirlo L, Hergovich N, et al: Effects of erythropoietin on platelet reactivity and thrombopoiesis in humans. Blood 2000;95:2983–2989.

204. Stricker PR: Other ergogenic agents. Clin Sports Med 1998;17:283–297.

205. Sturmi JE, Diorio DJ: Anabolic agents. Clin Sports Med 1998;17:261–282.

206. Su TP, Pagliaro M, Schmidt PJ, et al: Neuropsychiatric effects of anabolic steroids in male normal volunteers. JAMA 1993;269:2760–2764.

207. Takala TE, Ramo P, Kiviluoma K, et al: Effects of training and anabolic steroids on collagen synthesis in dog heart. Eur J Appl Physiol Occup Physiol 1991;62:1–6.

208. Thissen JP, Ketelslegers JM, Underwood LE: Nutritional regulation of the insulin-like growth factors. Endocr Rev 1994;15:80–101.

209. Tilzey A, Heptonstall J, Hamblin T: Toxic confusional state and choreiform movements after treatment with anabolic steroids. Br Med J (Clin Res Ed) 1981;283:349–350.

210. Tremper KK: Perfluorochemical "blood substitutes." Anesthesiology 1999;91:1185–1187.

211. Tripathi RK, Sherertz PC, Llewellyn GC, et al: Reducing exposures to airborne lead in a covered, outdoor firing range by using totally copper-jacketed bullets. Am Ind Hyg Assoc J 1990;51:28–31.

212. Tyler DB: The effect of amphetamine sulfate and some barbiturates on the fatigue produced by prolonged wakefulness. Am J Physiol 1947;150:243–262.

213. Urhausen A, Holpes R, Kindermann W: One- and two-dimensional echocardiography in bodybuilders using anabolic steroids. Eur J Appl Physiol Occup Physiol 1989;58:633–640.

214. Vance ML, Mauras N: Growth hormone therapy in adults and children. N Engl J Med 1999;341:1206–1216.

215. Vergouwen PC, Collee T, Marx JJ: Haematocrit in elite athletes. Int J Sports Med 1999;20:538–541.

216. Volek JS, Kraemer WJ: Creatine supplementation: Its effect on human muscular performance and body composition. J Strength Condition Res1996;10:200–210.

217. Wadler GI: Drug use update. Med Clin North Am 1994;78:439–455.

218. Wagner JC, Ulrich LR, McKean DC, Blankenbaker RG: Pharmaceutical services at the Tenth Pan American Games. Am J Hosp Pharm 1989;46:2023–2027.

219. Walker JB: Creatine: biosynthesis, regulation, and function. Adv Enzymol Rel Areas Mol Biol 1979;50:177–242.

220. Wallace JD, Cuneo RC, Baxter R, et al: Responses of the growth hormone (GH) and insulin-like growth factor axis to exercise, GH administration, and GH withdrawal in trained adult males: a potential test for GH abuse in sport. J Clin Endocrinol Metab 1999;84:3591–3601.

221. Walter E, Mockel J: Images in clinical medicine. Peliosis hepatis. N Engl J Med 1997;337:1603.

222. Wasser WG, Feldman NS, D'Agati VD: Chronic renal failure after ingestion of over-the-counter chromium picolinate. Ann Intern Med 1997;126:410.

223. Wesslen L, Pahlson C, Friman G, et al: Myocarditis caused by *Chlamydia pneumoniae* (TWAR) and sudden unexpected death in a Swedish elite orienteer. Lancet 1992;340:427–428.

224. Widder RA, Bartz-Schmidt KU, Geyer H, et al: Candida albicans endophthalmitis after anabolic steroid abuse. Lancet 1995;345:330–331.

225. Wilson JD. Androgen abuse by athletes. Endocr Rev 1988;9:181–199.

226. Windsor R, Dumitru D: Prevalence of anabolic steroid use by male and female adolescents. Med Sci Sports Exerc 1989;21:494–497.

227. Wu Z, Bidlingmaier M, Dall R, Strasburger CJ: Detection of doping with human growth hormone. Lancet 1999;353:895.

228. *www.asda.org.au:* Australian Sports Drug Agency, 1999.

229. *www.olympic.org:* International Olympic Committee, 2000.

230. *www.usdoj.gov/dea/concern/steroids.htm:* US Drug Enforcement Agency, 2001.

231. Yesalis CE, Kennedy NJ, Kopstein AN, Bahrke MS: Anabolic-androgenic steroid use in the United States. JAMA 1993;270:1217–1221.

232. Yesalis CE, Streit AL, Vicary JR, et al: Anabolic steroid use: indications of habituation among adolescents. J Drug Educ 1989;19:103–116.

233. Zelman G, Howland MA, Nelson LS, Hoffman RS: Erythropoietin overdose treated with emergency erythropheresis. J Toxicol Clin Toxicol 1999;37:602–603.

234. Zeman RJ, Ludemann R, Easton TG, Etlinger JD: Slow to fast alterations in skeletal muscle fibers caused by clenbuterol, a beta 2-receptor agonist. Am J Physiol 1988;254:E726–E732.

235. Zuliani U, Bernardini B, Catapano A, et al: Effects of anabolic steroids, testosterone, and HGH on blood lipids and echocardiographic parameters in body builders. Int J Sports Med 1989;10:62–66.

III. PREVENTIVE, PSYCHOSOCIAL, NURSING, EPIDEMIOLOGIC, RESEARCH, AND LEGAL PERSPECTIVES

CHAPTER **113** PSYCHOSOCIAL PRINCIPLES IN ASSESSMENT AND INTERVENTION

Frances A. Gautieri / Kenneth O. Brambill

THE HEALTHCARE ENVIRONMENT

Healthcare systems in the United States have become larger and more complex as multiple partnerships are formed that expand the scope of services and help to achieve operational efficiencies through consolidation of functions. A parallel emphasis on decentralization of primary care programs seeks to increase access for patients at the community level and encourages development of new resources and joint planning with community-based organizations.

To address quality of care concerns in a healthcare environment characterized by large and extended networks, regulatory standards place increasing emphasis on ensuring that services are provided within a comprehensive, reliable, and functional continuum of care. Objectives include clear, appropriate, and effective communication and coordination at each level of care and especially at the transfer points in the process as patients move through multiple settings, assessment of continuing care needs, and provision for all necessary referrals and transfers to aftercare services.[18]

The key position of emergency departments within healthcare networks places responsibility and offers opportunity to initiate well-coordinated care management with particular attention to continuity and followup. Integrated healthcare systems are made up of many organizations, settings, and levels of care. They include formal and informal linkages to community-based health, mental health, substance abuse treatment, and social service agencies, all of which interact with emergency department interdisciplinary teams in their management of toxicologic emergencies.

Even with the highest levels of clinical and technologic expertise applied in the diagnosis and treatment of poisoned or overdosed patients, successful outcomes may be compromised by inadequacies in aftercare and followup. Therefore, it is important for emergency departments to identify and cultivate appropriate referral resources for a wide range of continuing-care services. The emergence of integrated systems with their emphasis on collaboration among healthcare and community service agencies has improved information and referral processes and supports shared objectives that include promotion of primary care, effective case management, and continuity among multiple providers in various settings.[7] In addition to the clinical and quality-of-care reasons for coordination and collaboration between healthcare providers and community agencies, financing factors related to managed care and other cost containment trends also support the need for integration of services.[19]

Obstacles to continuity and followup because of gaps in service and access barriers related to lack of coverage persist to varying degrees in all communities despite improvements in delivery systems. This reality presents an ongoing challenge to healthcare providers. Emergency departments may consider these to be opportunities to take initiative in developing specialized resources, working proactively to identify and highlight unmet needs, and advocating for adequate funding and access for the uninsured to continuing care services, in order to support the goal of achieving a comprehensive continuum of care.

HISTORICAL PERSPECTIVE

The importance of understanding the social and community context for medical conditions and larger public health problems has been recognized in the United States for over 100 years. The rationale for a psychosocial approach in healthcare began to emerge clearly in the first decade of the 20th century as the medical profession perceived the negative and pathogenic conditions in poor, densely populated urban areas and the correlation with the major public health issues of the time. The growing awareness of the linkage between social factors and serious health problems led to the introduction of social service workers as an extension of the hospital into the community, first in 1905 at Massachusetts General Hospital in Boston and then in 1906 at Bellevue Hospital in

New York City.[12] These early outreach workers began to make home visits, educate patients and families about health and nutrition, and offer supportive counseling and concrete services to provide for basic human needs of food, clothing, and shelter in order to improve compliance with medical recommendations and attempt to ameliorate unhealthy conditions in the environment. Their reports about the conditions in which patients were living helped to heighten awareness about social problems and gain support for public health initiatives.[26]

This early emphasis on the environment or social context as a determinant of pathologic conditions was later refined to incorporate the influence of psychological factors. The term "psychosocial" came to reflect the dynamic interaction of internal and external aspects of a person's life, personality, and milieu—the person in his or her situation.[16] Emotions, feelings, developmental factors, individual coping patterns, family background, cultural differences, and socioeconomic factors came to be recognized as significant variables in patient response to illness or injury.

The importance of addressing the psychosocial needs of patients in healthcare settings was well accepted so that by 1930, there were more than 1000 hospital-based social service departments in the United States.[9] Professional social workers are present today in all areas of healthcare. The scope of their practice paralleled the growth of medical specialization while adhering to the basic generic principles of the psychosocial evaluation, planning, and intervention process. In the new healthcare environment of integrated networks and closer working relationships with community agencies, social workers may develop, implement, and facilitate the linkages necessary for continuing care and coordination of services.

THE PSYCHOSOCIAL APPROACH IN EMERGENCY MEDICINE

Psychosocial factors are significant in the evaluation and treatment of patients with toxicologic emergencies. The patient's personal history, current situation, patterns of coping, and other psychosocial variables can be essential in understanding what precipitated the emergency event and can affect treatment and continuing care planning, case management, outcome potential, and options for prevention.

With the development of comprehensive emergency services in the 1970s, the multidisciplinary healthcare model was adopted. Many emergency departments incorporated social work as part of the basic interdisciplinary team to assist in the assessment and management of acute medical and psychiatric conditions. The liaison or emergency psychiatrist and the social worker became part of the crisis intervention team needed to care for the patient who was poisoned. Emergency medicine as a specialty area of practice has grown rapidly.[19] There has been a concomitant movement toward on-site social work coverage for emergency service patients rather than on-call consultation. Many large urban hospitals have moved toward 24-hour coverage by social work staff. The availability of social workers on site in emergency departments has contributed to professional credibility, enhanced team functioning, and improved services for patients and families.[17] Social workers are able to engage families and other collateral sources to identify and assess potential support systems, to assist patients in obtaining concrete services, and to make effective referrals for continuing

care. However, in those settings where social workers are not part of the healthcare team, the responsibility for addressing psychosocial needs rests with the attending physician and may be assigned to another discipline based on the particular staffing structure.

The increased focus on emergency services is related to the major public health and social welfare problems that continue to escalate in volume and severity and are manifested daily by patients who appear in emergency departments. There is increased public awareness that poverty, homelessness, drug and alcohol use, family breakdown, child abuse and neglect, and violence are phenomena that affect all communities. Transformation of these broad social issues into acute medical or psychiatric problems as well as personal and family crises occurs in hospital emergency departments across the country, in cities, suburbs, small towns, and even rural areas, where the patient may present with an overdose, in withdrawal, as a sexual assault victim who was drugged by the perpetrator in a social setting, or perhaps as a case of a seemingly unintentional pediatric ingestion.

SUBSTANCE USE AND SOCIAL DYSFUNCTION

The adult substance user may be dysfunctional in one or several areas of his or her life.[15] Substance abuse is often accompanied by difficulties in holding a job, maintaining personal relationships, and carrying out family and child-care responsibilities. It is common in hospital emergency departments to see patients from widely different backgrounds for whom alcohol or drug use has precipitated a crisis. Examples of this diversity might include a wealthy businessman with family supports and solid community ties who fell while intoxicated and suffered a fracture but sees himself as a social drinker and denies any problem with alcohol; a battered housewife, depressed and frightened, who took an overdose of barbiturates in a desperate effort to obtain relief from an intolerable situation; and an undomiciled man, a veteran with no current source of income, long estranged from family and friends, who has fallen into polydrug use that masks long-standing depression. In each of these examples attention to the psychosocial factors is critical to comprehensive case evaluation and differential treatment planning.

Social problems are often interrelated. For example, drug or alcohol use or abuse by caregivers is clearly associated with a high risk of child abuse and neglect.[5,23] Among women, childhood sexual abuse and domestic violence correlate with increased incidence of substance abuse.[14] Maternal drug involvement frequently leads to placement of children.[3] Conversely, the fear of losing their children often prevents women from acknowledging substance problems and obtaining needed services.[2] It is also known that drug and alcohol use among adolescents and suicidal attempts in this age group usually reflect long-standing family problems and may indicate abuse and neglect, including sexual abuse.[22] Among homeless adolescents and those who develop patterns of running away from families or group homes, the pervasiveness of alcohol and drug use is a significant factor.[28]

As the ability to identify child abuse and neglect improves, it becomes increasingly obvious that childhood incidents, including ingestions, are often correlated with neglect by their caregivers and exacerbated by extraordinary family stress related to marital problems, joblessness, dislocation, and homelessness. Psychosocial assessment has become an important component in the comprehensive evaluation of patients with toxicologic emergencies and may even be required under state-mandated child protection laws in cases where there is any suspicion that a child's ingestion or an adolescent's drug use, alcohol intoxication, or suicide attempt might be related to abuse or neglect by a parent or guardian.

The need to recognize indicators of substance use in adolescents cannot be overstated, and screening for drug use should be considered in all medical emergencies including trauma.[24] The overdose of an adult who has young children in his or her care raises serious questions about whether his or her drug use has caused a situation in which children are, have been, or could be endangered or neglected. Also, factors related to ethnic and cultural variables, and the particular needs of the elderly, the undomiciled, and other special populations, must be recognized and applied in assessment, treatment, and continuing care planning.[11]

The relationship between substance use and maternal/child health problems has become evident.[10] There is urgent need to develop standardized protocols for the identification of drug use in pregnancy and to intervene expeditiously to improve outcomes for both women and their infants. Women of childbearing age who appear in emergency departments with substance-related conditions require meticulous attention, continuity of care, and active followup. Encounters with the healthcare system in emergencies provide the opportunity for pregnant drug-involved women to access many other services. This is accomplished most effectively through the assistance of social work staff who are in a unique position at the interface between the hospital and the community. They are able to address clinical as well as personal concrete needs such as food, clothing, financial aid, and emergency shelter and to help patients negotiate complex social systems.[6]

THE EMERGENCY DEPARTMENT CONTACT: OPPORTUNITY FOR INTERVENTION

The hospital emergency department is usually the first point of entry into the healthcare system for substance users. Often they are assessed, treated, and released to the same environment in which their drug-taking behavior is supported and reinforced, only to return repeatedly to the emergency department with more evidence of debilitation and dysfunctional behavior. A comprehensive psychosocial approach, including early patient identification and intervention, is a prerequisite for a positive outcome for these apparently intractable, complex, and multicausal cases. Opportunities to intervene should not be lost; the patient's contact with ED staff offers the hope and possibility of breaking the cycle of drug and/or alcohol abuse.[1] Staff should not be deterred by the fact that success rarely occurs following initial contact but rather depends on a gradual, incremental process that includes ready access to a community service network, a flexible case management approach, and active followup.

CONSIDERATIONS IN EMERGENCY CARE OF SUBSTANCE USERS

The taking of a comprehensive substance use and alcohol history is of paramount importance in an emergency department because the visit often provides an excellent opportunity for a therapeutic

intervention. Patients who have alcohol use problems remain in the hospital longer than the nonproblem drinkers.[20] The numbers of emergency department visits associated with heroin and cocaine use tend to ebb and flow, depending on the extent of problems experienced among the newest or heaviest users.[27] However, frequently someone who has suffered injury or assault simultaneous to intoxication or oversedation has never had the opportunity for a healthcare professional to help him or her examine personal behavior and to focus on the psychosocial consequences, health issues, and treatment options related to chemical dependence. This becomes even more important when, as is sometimes the case, demographic data and psychosocial history had to be obtained from a family member or other collateral source because of incapacitation of the patient. Because information relating to drug and alcohol use carries a social stigma, interviewees often construct elaborate defenses and will invariably deny the existence of a problem. In these instances, if the interviewer has a reasonable suspicion that there is substance involvement, it is wise to offer intervention, referral resources, and counseling as a matter of course. Very frequently if the physician does not provide information about drinking behavior, it may not be obtained or pursued by the treatment team.[21] It is important for the patient to receive clear, unambiguous information from sensitive, empathic, and credible healthcare providers about the physical and social consequences of drug and alcohol consumption.[4] The emergency episode presents an opportunity for focused education and counseling that has potential for motivating the patient toward change.

Social workers who practice case finding are frequently looked to as confidants by substance users for whom they provide supportive counseling. They should not ignore anecdotal information provided during their interactions with active users about the stressors involved in that person's daily activities, around drug procurement, differential quality of available street drugs, obstacles to rehabilitation, and any new drug-taking trends that could pose health problems for the general patient population in the community.

Substance users also confront the risk of HIV. It has been widely recognized that sharing of unsterile injecting paraphernalia while using illicit substances is a principal cause of AIDS. Moreover, many cocaine users claim that cocaine is an aphrodisiac.[13] This causes chronic smokers of crack-cocaine in particular to engage in sexual practices for pay and/or pleasure, frequently ignoring the need for safety precautions to prevent AIDS and other sexually transmitted diseases. This activity is believed to be the leading cause of AIDS among women and heterosexual men and, through sex, can lead to infection of others such as spouses and unborn children. It is therefore important to augment screening and counseling about substance and alcohol use with information about AIDS and to offer referrals for HIV testing and, where possible, arrange pretest counseling within the emergency department as rapidly as possible for those who request to be tested.

THE ASSESSMENT PROCESS

Any patient who has taken an overdose of a medication, whether prescribed or not, alcohol, or illicit substance or has ingested a poison, whether or not he or she manifests suicidal ideation, requires interdisciplinary assessment, support, and preliminary intervention in the emergency services setting. Decisions about psychiatric consultation, evaluation, and treatment follow medical stabilization. However, the social worker may be needed from the point of triage to determine whether there are family or child welfare issues that require immediate attention. For example, if the patient is an unaccompanied child or adolescent, or if the patient is a parent of young children for whom care must be arranged, efforts must be initiated promptly to reach responsible family members or to seek assistance from appropriate child welfare agencies.

Patients with toxicologic emergencies are, by definition, high risk, based on accepted psychosocial indices (Table 113–1). The psychosocial evaluation process is fluid and multifaceted (Table 113–2). Psychosocial assessments can be initiated through interviewing of collateral sources before a patient is physically able to respond. Delay in obtaining psychosocial information can have serious consequences, as in cases where an overdosed adult patient may have small children who were left unattended.

Psychosocial assessment includes clinical observation and interviewing of the patient and accompanying family members or friends; it may also involve contact with health or social service agencies to which the patient may be known. In cases involving young children, nonverbal modalities using play or drawings may be helpful after the situation is medically stabilized. Observation of interactions between the child and parent or caregiver and the responses of family members to the emergency can be helpful in understanding family dynamics. Assessment efforts are enhanced when therapeutic rapport can be established early in the contact. It is essential to adopt a sensitive, empathic approach in which the social worker clearly explains why personal and family information is needed.

In evaluating an adult patient who has overdosed or is in withdrawal from a toxin, it is important to elicit information with regard to the toxin in the patient's history of drug and alcohol use and any involvement with substance abuse treatment programs, including detoxification, methadone maintenance, and drug-free modalities. Contact with current treatment programs can be very helpful in coordinating the case and should be encouraged, especially in arranging discharge plans. It is also important to differentiate, early in the contact, the adult with no children from the adult with minor children in his or her care. The psychosocial needs of an isolated, undomiciled, middle-aged man are very different from those of a pregnant 24-year-old woman on methadone maintenance with two preschool children. In the latter example, the social worker's immediate focus must be on the needs of the children, pending medical stabilization of their mother. If the children are present, they should be evaluated. If they are not present, their whereabouts should be determined. Any indication that they

TABLE 113–1. Screening Guide for High-Risk Emergency Department Patients

Psychosocial assessment is required whenever the case involves:
- Drugs or alcohol
- Suspicion of child abuse or neglect
- Domestic violence or other crime
- Suggestion of suicidal intent
- Psychiatric history
- Mental retardation or developmental disability
- Physical handicap, including vision or hearing impairment
- Frail or elderly
- Medical conditions with home care needs
- Patient with minor children
- Homelessness

TABLE 113–2. Psychosocial Evaluation Process

Assessment
Perform clinical observation/evaluation
Interview patient and collaterals
Obtain information on family history and current situation
Evaluate minor children for immediate needs
Establish drug and alcohol profile, including past treatment attempts
Identify potential family and community support

Interdisciplinary
Develop medical and psychosocial diagnosis

Collaboration
Plan for intervention based on differential case needs: medical or psychiatric admission, referral for detoxification, report to Child Protective Services

Implementation
Coordinate case
Facilitate intervention plan and advocate for services as needed
Refer to community agencies
Provide concrete services: food, clothing, financial assistance, transportation
Perform crisis counseling
Follow up
Establish case management and followup plan, either directly or via community agency

may have been left unattended requires immediate contact with local child protection authorities. In any event, the social worker's assessment must consider the impact of the woman's drug involvement on her ability to care for the children, her judgment in arranging adequate alternate child care with relatives or friends, and her own medical, counseling, and supportive service needs. The social worker should explore the family and community resources available to the patient, consult with the clinical staff of the woman's methadone treatment program, consider whether the case comes under state-mandated child protection reporting procedures, and develop a coordinated treatment plan that addresses prenatal needs in addition to a followup related to the patient's drug-induced emergency and the child welfare issues.

CASE EXAMPLES

The following cases support the efficacy of prompt psychosocial assessment as an integral part of comprehensive medical care.

Patient 1 A 2-year-old boy required admission for treatment following ingestion of antidepressant medication that had been prescribed for his paternal grandmother, with whom he lived. Social work assessment initiated in the emergency service revealed a troubled family, including an absent, drug-addicted natural mother; an inconsistently involved natural father with a history of drug use and incarcerations; the paternal grandmother; a paternal uncle; and an older sibling of the patient. Interviews with the grandmother and uncle initially suggested an unintentional ingestion by an active toddler with appropriate response by the family and prompt accessing of emergency medical care. Further exploration revealed a prior admission to another hospital, also ostensibly for the child's ingestion of the grandmother's medication. This raised concerns about the adequacy of supervision in the household and need for further evaluation to develop a safe discharge plan. The case was coordinated with Child Protective Services (CPS), and a discharge plan was developed that included home visits, parenting education for the grandmother, followup medical care for the child, and consultation with the grandmother's mental health provider as needed. It was determined that CPS would carry primary responsibility for case management.

Patient 2 A 14-year-old boy ingested acetaminophen and other nonprescription drugs in an apparent suicidal gesture. Initial psychosocial assessment elicited a history of family problems and sexual identity issues. The youngster was admitted for observation and further exploration of family, school, and other potential support systems. It became clear that the one stable person in the patient's life was his maternal grandmother. She was caring and supportive but unable to manage the boy's behavior or understand his mood swings. Both the patient and his grandmother agreed to recommendations for followup psychotherapy and family counseling in the adolescent mental health clinic. Interdisciplinary collaboration among three hospital units—the emergency department, the in patient service, and the outpatient clinic—made it possible to develop and implement a prompt, appropriate, and safe discharge plan.

Patient 3 A 77-year-old man was brought to the emergency department (ED) by his home health attendant after falling at home. He was immobilized on a board, unable to move his extremities, and had suffered trauma to his right eye as well as minor contusions. Medical examination revealed that the patient had a biliary tract shunt and that he suffered from cirrhosis of the liver. It was also noted that he had been drinking alcohol, was disoriented, and was somewhat agitated. The patient was admitted to the alcohol detoxification unit under close medical supervision. Psychosocial assessment initiated in the ED showed the patient to be a retired hospital worker who lived with his wife and had adult children and grandchildren and a large extended family, all of whom were very supportive. His medical condition had deteriorated following gallbladder surgery, which led to the need for a home health aide for 12 hours per day, 7 days a week. The social worker noted during hospital visits that the patient presided over his family in a patriarchal, often dictatorial manner and gave direction to everyone with whom he came in contact. He had been a vital, active person before the illnesses, which now had him confined to a wheelchair, increasingly dependent on his wife and home health aide, which he strongly resented. They were not always able to keep him away from alcohol despite its potential life-threatening impact on him in his deteriorated physical state. Prompt, effective collaboration between ED and alcoholism service teams led to appropriate care that addressed the medical, emotional, and substance abuse needs of this alcohol-dependent elderly man with depressive features whose strengths included a stable support network and health benefits. On discharge, he was referred to the hospital's alcohol aftercare treatment program and to the geriatric clinic for coordinated medical and psychiatric followup. A case conference was held with the home health agency to point out the need for vigilance because of the patient's propensity to sneak a drink of beer, and support was given to the family to reinforce the need to keep the patient engaged in pursuits not related to drinking.

Patient 4 A 41-year-old single unemployed man was admitted to hospital through the ED after falling out of bed following a long bout of alcohol bingeing. He was discovered on the floor by his brother, with whom he lived. The severity of his withdrawal required intensive care before he could be safely transferred to the alcohol detoxification unit. On arrival on the ward, the patient stated that he had not slept in 72 hours. He constantly paced the hallways, was very tremulous, and had to be patiently counseled against leaving prematurely. Psychosocial assessment showed the patient to be the eldest of three siblings who began alcohol consumption at age 9 and was drinking problematically by age 13. During adolescence, he was sent to a psychiatrist because of his intractable drinking problem. Nonetheless, he managed to complete high school and held restaurant jobs, the most recent one being 10 years before this hospital admission. The patient subsisted through the largesse of his brother, had Medicaid coverage, and had been involved in episodic outpatient alcohol treatment. On admission he was drinking 3 pints or more of vodka daily as well as several 16-ounce bottles of beer. The clinical impression was that of a 41-year-old, docile, chronic alcoholic, possibly with incipient organic brain damage as a result of long-term alcohol abuse. When medically cleared for discharge, he refused to await placement in a short-term rehabilitation program; therefore, the plan was adjusted for the patient to receive outpatient services with an active case management approach at a hospital-based alcoholism clinic.

Patient 5 A 26-year-old woman was brought to emergency services after exposure to numerous substances including heroin, cocaine, marijuana, and alcohol. From psychosocial assessment initiated in the ED, it was determined that she was also suffering from childhood sexual abuse that had occurred within the family and from current domestic violence, the result of her relationship with an abusive boyfriend. Medical problems included persistent anemia, asthma, and developmental disability. She was admitted to an inpatient unit for mentally ill chemical abusers (MICA). Relevant history included that the patient was the youngest of five siblings and lived primarily with her dysfunctional family. She received Supplemental Security Income and Medicaid. She became involved with illicit drugs at an early age and would frequently sleep in the homes of friends who also used drugs. She met her current boyfriend, a heavy user of alcohol and other drugs, when they both attended a sheltered workshop. He began battering her almost immediately, threatened her with weapons, and in some instances injured her so badly she required medical attention, and he was placed under arrest. Several orders of protection were issued for him through the courts. The patient stated she ingested the overdose in her effort of "trying to forget," that she also tried using crack but "it made my heart beat too fast." During the course of her treatment on the substance abuse unit, she repeatedly stated that on discharge she wished to continue her relationship with her boyfriend but wanted him to cease his battering behavior. The ED and MICA unit teams worked closely with the hospital's domestic violence coordinator in the treatment and continuing care planning for this vulnerable patient with limited functioning, numerous medical complaints, in an abusive relationship, and periodically experiencing suicidal depression and repressed rage partly from signs and symptoms of posttraumatic stress disorder. Coordinated efforts on discharge included followup case management to obtain housing with supportive services, substance abuse and mental health counseling, and attempts to engage the boyfriend in order to prevent further domestic violence. Subsequent threats by the boyfriend resulted in his incarceration as a result of the advocacy provided by the domestic violence coordinator who functioned as the primary case manager.

The patient responded well to the clinical and supportive services and showed signs of generally improved functioning.

Good psychosocial assessments form a basis for more effective case management, especially where treatment depends on referral to community agencies for services such as drug or alcohol treatment, family counseling, child welfare services, emergency financial assistance, shelter, or home healthcare. Emergency departments that have formal or informal relationships with community service providers are better able to assure continuity of care. Regularly updated resource lists with clear referral guidelines are invaluable (Table 113–3).

THE ROLE OF THE EMERGENCY DEPARTMENT IN THE CONTINUUM OF CARE

The effectiveness of a hospital ED is measured by how well individual cases are evaluated, treated, and managed and to what extent communication and coordination are maintained with other settings and organizations in the community that provide for continuing healthcare and social service needs. Efficacy is enhanced when the ED recognizes its strategic position in the continuum of care, seeks to develop and cultivate working relationships with a wide range of other providers, and makes reasonable efforts to formulate, implement, and follow up on continuing care plans.

The morbidity of substance abuse and its relationship to AIDS, the widespread use of drugs and alcohol at all levels of society, including women of childbearing age, the nationwide increase in neglect, maltreatment, and physical and sexual abuse of children, adolescent suicide, domestic violence, and the problems of homelessness are markers everywhere of severe societal distress. Changes in public policy and planning related to these issues are affecting delivery of services to ED patients. Eligibility restrictions on medical and financial assistance deriving from the 1996 Personal Responsibility and Work Opportunity Reconciliation Act, commonly referred to as *welfare reform*, have exacerbated access problems for continuing care services including substance abuse treatment and resulted in more barriers to the goal of a comprehensive continuum of care.[25] The challenge must be met by informed advocacy through awareness and involvement by emergency department staff at many levels beyond the care of the individual patient.

Even the best emergency care is limited in efficacy if resources for ongoing treatment and supportive services are nonexistent or inadequate. The individual who is homeless and drug dependent and must wait weeks or months for entry into an inpatient or outpatient drug treatment program will inevitably continue maladaptive behaviors, which might include the risk of HIV transmission to sexual partners and those sharing needles. Current experience demonstrates the benefit to patients of providing HIV counseling and education in the ED, which is often the sole healthcare resource for this significant group of high-risk patients. The ED encounter presents an opportunity for the patient and the healthcare provider to interact at a higher level of mutual advantage and to the benefit of the community. Addressing the needs of the whole person may interrupt patterns of repeated emergencies. The strategic importance of the ED should not be underestimated in developing effective approaches to current social and public health problems.

TABLE 113–3. Emergency Department Basic Resource Guide

Develop resource list and referral protocols for the following:
- Drug and alcohol treatment services for all modalities and levels of care: detoxification, sobering up, therapeutic communities, other residential programs, methadone maintenance, drug-free outpatient clinics, 12-step programs
- Mental health programs
- Family services agencies
- Child protective and voluntary child welfare services
- Crime victims services
- Shelters and emergency housing
- Concrete services: food, clothing, financial assistance, transportation
- Legal and advocacy services

REFERENCES

1. Abbott AA, ed: Alcohol, Tobacco, and Other Drugs: Challenging Myths, Assessing Theories, Individualizing Interventions. Washington, NASW Press, 2000.
2. Abbott AA: A feminist approach to substance abuse treatment and service delivery. Soc Work Health Care 1994;19:67–83.
3. Azzi-Lessing L, Olsen LJ: Substance abuse-affected families in the child welfare system: New challenges, new alliances. Soc Work 1996; 41:15–23.
4. Barber J: Working with resistant drug abusers. Soc Work 1995; 40:17–23.
5. Bays J: Substance abuse and child abuse: The impact of addiction on the child. Pediatr Clin North Am 1990;37:881–904.
6. Berger C: Cocaine and pregnancy: A challenge for health care providers. Health Soc Work 1990;15:310–316.
7. Berkman B: The emerging health care world: Implications for social work practice and education. Soc Work 1996;41:541–551.
8. Blending Perspectives and Building Common Ground. A Report to Congress on Substance Abuse and Child Protection. US Department of Health and Human Services. Washington, DC, US Government Printing Office, 1999.
9. Carlton TO: Clinical Social Work in Health Settings. New York, Springer, 1984, p. 4.
10. Chasnoff IJ, Schnoll SH: Consequences of cocaine and other drug use in pregnancy. In: Washton AM, Gold MS, eds: Cocaine: A Clinician's Handbook. New York, Guilford Press, 1987, pp. 241–251.
11. Dodgen CE, Shea WM: Substance Use Disorders. Assessment and Treatment. New York, Academic Press, 2000.
12. Friedlander WA: Social work in medical and psychiatric settings. In: Introduction to Social Welfare. Englewood Cliffs, NJ, Prentice-Hall, 1961, pp. 389–395.
13. Gold MS: Cocaine (and crack): Clinical aspects. In: Lowinson JH, Ruiz P, Millman RB, eds: Substance Abuse: A Comprehensive Textbook. Baltimore, Williams & Wilkins, 1992, p. 211.
14. Goldberg ME: Substance abusing women: False stereotypes and real needs. Soc Work 1995;40:789–798.
15. Herrington RE, Jacobson GR, Benzer DG, eds: Alcohol and Drug Abuse Handbook. St Louis, WH Green, 1987, pp. 259–260.
16. Hollis F: Casework: A Psychosocial Therapy. New York, Random House, 1965, Chapters 1, 10.
17. Johnson LC, Schwartz CL, Tate DS: Health care and social welfare. In: Social Welfare: A Response to Human Need. Boston, Allyn & Bacon, 1997.
18. Joint Commission on Accreditation of Health Care Organizations: 1999 Comprehensive Accreditation Manual for Hospitals, Update November 2000 Continuum of Care CC-1 to CC-8, Oakbrook Terrace, IL.

19. Linking Substance Abuse Treatment and Domestic Violence Services: A Guide for Administrators. Based on Treatment Improvement Protocol (TIP)25. Substance Abuse and Mental Health Services Administration; Center for Substance Abuse Treatment. DHHS Publication No.(SMA)00–3391. Washington, DC, US Government Printing Office, 2000.

20. McCusker J, Cherubin E, Zimberg S: Prevalence of alcoholism in general municipal hospital population. NY State J Med 1971;71: 751–754.

21. Niles BL, McCrady BS: Detection of alcohol problems in a hospital setting. J Addict Behav 1991;16:223–233.

22. Riggs S, Alario AG, McHorney C: Health risk behaviors and attempted suicide in adolescents who report prior maltreatment. Pediatrics 1990;116:815–821.

23. Rittner B, Dozier CD: Effects of court ordered substance abuse treatment in Child Protective Services cases. Social Work 2000;45: 131–140.

24. Screening and Assessing Adolescents for Substance Use Disorders. Treatment Improvement Protocol (TIP) Series 31. Substance Abuse and Mental Health Services Administration; Center for Substance Abuse Treatment. DHHS Publication No. (SMA) 99–3382. Washington, DC, US Government Printing Office, 1999.

25. Soskis CW: Social Work in the Emergency Room. New York, Springer, 1985, pp. 1–11.

26. Starr J: Hospital City. New York, Crown, 1957, pp. 185–193.

27. Treaster JB: Emergency hospital visits rise among drug abusers. New York Times, April 23, 1993.

28. Wyman JR: Drug Abuse Among Runaway and Homeless Youth Calls for Focused Outreach Solutions. NIDA Notes Volume 12, No. 5. September/October 1997. US DHHS, National Institutes of Health. NIH Publication No. 97–3478.

CHAPTER 114 PSYCHIATRIC PRINCIPLES

Michael H. Allen / Brett R. Goldberg / Wendy Rives (deceased) /
Mark R. Serper

Psychiatric problems may be the cause or the effect of many toxicology presentations. Suicide attempts and aggressive behaviors are commonly associated with intoxications and can be uniquely difficult to assess and manage. These patients are often viewed as either totally voluntary and deliberate or totally "out of control" and irrational. The truth is usually more complex, with some aspects occurring within the patient's awareness and control and other aspects either unknown or overwhelming to the patient. This chapter attempts to present schemas for understanding suicide and violence in ways that allow the physician to adopt the appropriate role of diagnostician and medical decision maker.

SUICIDE

Self-destructive behavior is among the most common and challenging emergency department (ED) presentations. In 1997, the National Center for Injury Prevention and Control (NCIPC) reported that there were only 7529 intentional poisoning deaths in the United States, but the National Center for Health Statistics (NCHS) has reported that self-inflicted injuries accounted for an average of 221,000 ED visits per year from 1992 through 1995, of which 128,000 were intentional poisonings.[11] Even so, only a fraction of suicides and suicide attempts ever come to attention. A recent population-based estimate of the 12-month prevalence of suicide attempts was 0.7%, suggesting that perhaps 10 times more attempts occur than present to EDs.[19] This does not even include many behaviors such as the predictable but "unintentional" overdoses that accompany the hopelessness and carelessness of the late stages of addiction.

Despite the high numbers affected, suicide has only recently been recognized as a major public health problem by the US Surgeon General. The overall rate of about 12/100,000 population per year has remained strikingly consistent for the past 50 years. The rate has declined for the younger elderly population while increasing for children and adolescents. Suicide is now the third leading killer of young people. Suicides, though clearly underreported, significantly outnumber homicides.

Identification of the acutely suicidal patient places an extreme burden on the physician to intervene and prevent deaths. Suicidal ideation is quite common. One recent survey estimates a 12-month incidence of suicidal ideation at 5.6%, representing some 10.5 million people.[19] Suicidal crises are heterogeneous, with suicide the final outcome of many possible psychiatric conditions and social circumstances. Self-poisoning or deliberate overdosing is a common method of attempting suicide, but this must also be differentiated from unintentional overdose, particularly in the young, the

mentally retarded, the confused elderly, and the chronic drug-abusing patient. This distinction is rendered even more complex by the possibility that suicidal ideation may be deliberately concealed.

In general, though, it is relatively easy to detect individuals at risk. The challenge is determining which of those of among the 128,000 intentional overdoses are seriously suicidal. Failure to do so has been associated with some of the largest damage awards in emergency medicine.

Much is known about the risk of suicide for various groups over time, but little can be said with certainty about individual patients at particular points in time. There is no typical suicidal patient who may be routinely hospitalized. There is no clinically useful test or rating scale. One investigator was able to prospectively identify almost all of those who ultimately died by suicide (97% sensitivity) but only at the cost of overpredicting suicide by almost half (56% specificity).[55] However, there is also no patient in distress for whom the risk of suicide is so remote that it need not be considered. Assessment of the potentially suicidal patient is a highly individualized exercise in clinical judgment.

Self-Poisoning

Suicide is usually discussed in terms of attempts and completions. When the term "suicide" is used alone, it refers to completed suicide. The two are considered separately because those who attempt and those who complete suicide appear to constitute different groups. Those who attempt suicide are more commonly younger women with personality disorders, and self-poisoning is common in this group. Those who complete suicide, however, are more commonly older men with major depression or alcoholism, and they typically use more violent methods. In 1997, 72% of suicides were white men, and 58% of suicides involved a firearm.[11]

The methods preferred by women have shifted over time. Self-poisoning was a very common method of suicide in the 1960s and 1970s, but it has since decreased, perhaps in part because of changing prescription practices and in part because of other social changes. In 1970, 47.9% of female suicides were by poisoning compared to 34.6% in 1993. In 1993, women, like men, were most frequently the victims of self-inflicted gunshot wounds (41.9%).[11] Antidepressant medications have been the most common drugs implicated in suicide because of their toxicity and frequent use in the populations at risk. This decline in self-poisoning may be related to decreased use of more lethal medications such as barbiturates and monoamine oxidase inhibitors.[18] Data from the Drug Abuse Warning Network suggest that newer antidepressants are significantly safer in overdose. While the risk of an attempt is roughly similar, the risk of death is 8.5 times greater with desipramine than fluoxetine.[37] When benzodiazepines were more tightly regulated in New York State, there was again a shift to somewhat more consequential overdoses with more dangerous nontriplicate prescription drugs.[35]

Psychiatric Management of Self-Poisoning

Table 114–1 depicts a case of suspected self-poisoning from the starting point of prehospital care through the completion of a comprehensive assessment and treatment planning. The upper row describes the evolving clinical course of the patient while the middle row shows the progression of emergency care provided to the patient. The bottom row lists specific diagnostic and treatment goals that should be completed at various points in the patient's care.

Focused Psychiatric Assessment

At a relatively early point in the patient's course, a focused psychiatric assessment may be needed to address specific clinical concerns that can arise at this stage. Thorough psychiatric consultation is possible only when a patient is no longer intoxicated or otherwise acutely medically compromised. The determination that the patient has improved cannot be established on the basis of blood levels but should be approached clinically. Psychiatric examination must be postponed until signs of intoxication such as somnolence, slurred speech, and ataxia are no longer present. There are several reasons for this approach.

First, the physician should not unequivocally attribute altered mental status to intoxication until signs of intoxication have passed and cognitive functions have returned to normal. Until that time, other medical conditions that might coexist with, or masquerade as, intoxication cannot be excluded. Second, the patient's cognitive functioning will be too impaired by the drugs and/or alcohol to provide critical historical details reliably. Third, much of what the patient reports will be ephemeral, caused by the predictable temporary effects on mood of the substances ingested.

Focused assessment may be necessary to ascertain elopement risk or decisional capacity. Subacute residual CNS effects of ingestions—confusion, fatigue, and fear—can dispose patients to wandering or flight. Additionally, the patient's intentions remain unclear at this point; the question of unintentional versus intentional ingestion cannot be completely resolved. For these reasons, a high level of supervision should be maintained, and patients should not be allowed to leave until assessment has been done of their mental status. Depending on the physical plant and personnel, it may be sufficient to place the patient in an open area in the direct line of sight of nursing staff. If such an arrangement is not possible, or the patient is agitated and disruptive, it may be necessary to separate the patient from the general population. Under these circumstances, an individual aide should be assigned to observe the patient. Some form of restraint may be necessary to prevent further injury.

In general, patients are presumed competent and must consent to treatment, but the issue of decisional capacity frequently arises at this point. Patients may request their discharge, refuse care, or become aggressive. Aggression may arise from lingering effects of toxic ingestions, severe anxiety, fear, anger at the loss of autonomy, or the discomfort of unpleasant procedures. Although patients may respond to verbal limit setting and repeated explanations of their care, they may also require sedation, restraint, and involuntary treatment. This chapter later discusses management of the violent patient. Patients are not allowed to make poor healthcare decisions if their ability to weigh the risks and benefits of the proposed care is limited by cognitive deficits or mental illness. In the setting of intoxication, appropriate care may be provided under the doctrine of implied consent.

The emergency exception to the doctrine of informed consent may also apply in circumstances where self-injury is suspected. The emergency exception permits forcible detention, restraint, medication over objection, and necessary medical care until psychiatric assessment can be accomplished. After the management of the immediate medical emergency and resolution of intoxication, suspected self-injury is sufficient evidence of impaired decisional capacity for the emergency physician to hold a patient for further psychiatric assessment. The emergency physician should note the patient's objections in the record and indicate the basis for the determination of diminished capacity.

After the self-poisoned patient is stabilized, there may be a need for a more thorough assessment of decisional capacity; psychiatric consultation may be useful at this stage to help document the degree of impairment, determine the etiology, and predict the likely course.

TABLE 114–1. Case Presentation

	Case	Evolution			Disposition
Patient course	Patient found in the community. Unresponsive	Patient monitored in the ED. Vital signs stable. Still unresponsive	Patient lethargic but following commands Answers simple questions	Patient fully awake and alert.	Evaluation complete
Treatment course	Prehospital	Triage Medical assessment	Observation and monitoring	Formal psychiatric evaluation	Treatment planning
Physician course	Patient identification Search for prescription drugs, drug paraphernalia Assessment of cardiac and respiratory functions	Orogastric lavage, activated charcoal Diagnostic testing (blood studies, ECG, toxicology) Contact collateral sources for history. Prior records	Focused psychiatric assessment: elopement, aggressive behavior, decisional capacity, addressing confidentiality, and immediate suicide risk.	Comprehensive psychiatric assessment: diagnostic interviewing, risk factors, future risk.	Treatments: medication, hospitalization, substance abuse, crisis intervention, family therapy

Immediate Risk. After these safety considerations have been addressed, the aim of the focused psychiatric assessment moves toward a determination of immediate suicide risk. This examination should answer the following questions:

1. What is the patient's attitude toward life-saving care?
2. What are the patient's current wishes with regard to living or dying?
3. What are the patient's thoughts about his or her rescue and likely recovery?

These questions can only be answered in the course of a frank discussion between the patient and the emergency physician. Do not be concerned about "provoking" further self-injurious impulses with this vital discussion; many patients will be relieved that the caregiver is speaking directly about their distress.

Reliability and Confidentiality. Mention should be made here about the difficult issues of reliability and confidentiality with regard to gathering history. Evasiveness, lack of detail, inconsistency, and improbability taken together suggest an unreliable history. It is appropriate to confront the patient with the implausible aspects of the history provided and offer an opportunity to provide more useful information. This is often successful, although subsequent reports are, of course, equally suspect.

The most important step from the standpoint of both clinical care and risk management is to locate other sources of information to clarify the patient's situation. A careful review of any previous records is critical. Any pattern to a patient's presentations such as increasing frequency, more aggravated behavior, or disheveled appearance should be noted.

Collateral contacts are another important source of information, though the level of involvement, sophistication, and reliability of the collaterals must also be taken into account. The mere fact that a person is a patient at a hospital is not considered confidential, and hence, the ED may make contacts that are limited to soliciting information without specific consent. An effort should be made to obtain consent for any broader discussion with family, friends, or other treaters. The patient may express concern about the ED staff contacting a family member or counselor. Any information to be imparted to third parties can be negotiated in advance with the patient. The patient may restrict consent to receiving information only and may withhold consent to impart certain information. More caution is indicated in contacting an employer. Although disclosing information about the patient without his or her consent is a breach of confidentiality, a physician may do so in the interest of protecting the patient.[5]

Comprehensive Psychiatric Assessment

The comprehensive psychiatric assessment includes a characterization of the suicidal ideation present, exploration of certain so-called risk factors, and the formulation of a diagnostic impression. These three elements help to determine the attendant risk and guide treatment planning.

Stress Vulnerability Model. The best understanding of suicide at this time is that it results from intrinsic vulnerability factors interacting with extrinsic circumstances. Intrinsic vulnerability may be conferred by a variety of traits such as impulsivity or conditions such as depression, anxiety, and hopelessness. Extrinsic factors include stressful life events, access to lethal means, and a host of other factors, positive and negative.

Characterization of Suicidal Ideation. The core of the suicide risk assessment is a detailed discussion of the patient's suicidal thoughts and urges. This must be included in every mental status examination. It is important to establish rapport and introduce the topic in an appropriate context in order to improve the patient's candor. This requires significant time and skillful interviewing, for which there is no substitute. This approach will enhance the therapeutic quality of the interview as well as its reliability. For example, almost everyone has had some period in life when he or she was discouraged. The clinician may spend a few moments talking with the patient about the point in life when he or she was most disheartened. This is done by asking the patient if he or she has been feeling "down" lately; and then, if the patient has, by asking if this is the worst the patient has ever felt. If the patient denies recent depression altogether or indicates that this is not the worst, it is helpful, for several reasons, to ask the patient to describe the point in his or her life when the patient felt worst, which may or may not be the current episode. Depression fluctuates a great deal, and characterizing the worst period assures that a prior history of major depression will not be overlooked.

At some point, the physician might ask if, during that worst period in the patient's life, the patient ever felt that perhaps things would never get better (hopelessness), that he or she could not go on (helplessness), or perhaps that he or she would be better off dead (passive suicidal ideation). If failing others was involved in the patient's demoralization (guilt), the physician might ask if the patient felt at any time as if others would be better off without him or her. These are common thoughts that most people can endorse without much difficulty and lay the groundwork for discussing more troublesome ideas in the suicidal spectrum. Ultimately, the patient must be asked directly if he or she has ever felt like "killing" himself or herself (active suicidal ideation). Nothing else will do. The more generic form, "hurting" himself or herself, which might seem to cover more, is in fact confusing to patients—even those who wish to die do not usually consciously intend to be hurt in the process. The latter is more typical of multiple suicide attempters than suicide completers.

For those patients who have felt like killing themselves at some point, the next step in this scenario might be to establish how the patient is currently and to compare this to a prior episode(s). One dimension to assess is the progression from passive to active suicidal ideation. Suicidal feelings may take the form of a relatively inchoate wish to die, perhaps from a fatal disease or injury, and then proceed to consideration of various active means of hastening death. Planning might range from fleeting thoughts or images of a variety of methods from which the patient recoils to a more detailed consideration of a particular, realistic method of choice to serious planning concerning acquisition of the means, and so-called last acts. At some point the patient goes beyond thinking to acting by hoarding pills or completing his or her will. An astute family member may observe a series of odd conversations including phone calls to distant friends and family members as the suicidal individual begins to implement the plan with a series of vague farewells. In psychological autopsy studies, approximately 50 to 70% of completed suicides gave some warning of their intention; 30 to 40% of completed suicides disclosed a direct and specific intent to kill themselves.[7,58]

Other dimensions to assess include frequency, urgency, chronicity, reactivity to positive and negative external events, and subjective distress. A schema for the detailed characterization of suicidal ideation appears in Table 114–2.

The communication of suicidal ideas either directly or indirectly should not be misconstrued as a "cry for help" and hence evidence of lower risk. Communication is probably related to the degree of preoccupation with morbid thoughts and to personality characteristics that dispose individuals to revealing their thoughts to various degrees.[38]

Multiaxial Diagnosis. Diagnostic assessment also weighs heavily in the overall risk analysis, as there is a group of treatable psychiatric disorders associated with a high risk of suicide. Psychological autopsy studies in the United States and Europe over the years have consistently revealed major psychiatric illness to be a factor in suicide, present in 93% of adult suicide cases by some reports.[56,59] This is also true of those who make medically serious attempts.[8] In particular, prospective cohort studies and retrospective case control investigations have revealed clinical depression to dramatically increase suicide risk.[13,31,48] For affective disorders, factors correlated with acute suicidality have included current depression, severe anxiety, anhedonia, panic, insomnia, ambivalence, and acute alcohol abuse. Responsibility for child care is inversely correlated with risk, suggesting a protective effect.[23]

After affective disorders, chronic alcoholism is the most commonly reported disorder, present in about 20% of cases. Moreover, alcoholic patients who also suffer from periodic episodes of depression are at more risk for suicide than patients who present with either disorder separately. As a result, any assessment conducted on patients with a substance abuse history must include an examination of symptoms of major depression.[23]

Schizophrenic patients are also at increased risk for suicide compared to the general population. Approximately 10% of schizophrenic patients will commit suicide.[13] Additionally, between 5 and 18% of patients with severe borderline personality disorder (especially patients who are comorbid for depression) ultimately kill themselves.[25,64] The odds of suicide attendant to various conditions are shown in Fig. 114–1.[36]

The ability to treat the two conditions most strongly associated with suicide—major affective disorder and alcoholism—suggests that most suicides are preventable. Indeed, a suicide prevention program directed at general practitioners in Sweden was able to demonstrate prevention based on the detection and treatment of depression.[57] The possibility of preventing suicide necessitates a comprehensive psychiatric assessment to identify contributory psychiatric disorders.

Risk Factors. A complete assessment should also include an examination of risk factors. Factors have been identified empirically that place groups of individuals at high risk for suicide. Although this level of prediction is actuarial and reflective of groups rather than individuals, knowledge of these risk factors is important.[45]

Although not specifically predictive, suicide is statistically more common in men than women and in whites than in nonwhites. Younger black men, however, have approximately the same suicide rate as white men the same age. Suicide rates for both black and white adolescents (15 to 19 years of age) have been increasing. In contrast, suicide rates in the elderly have decreased threefold since 1940 but still occur in disproportionately high numbers.[68]

Previous suicide attempts are an obvious risk factor. However, those who attempt suicide appear to be a somewhat different group demographically and diagnostically. Parasuicidal behavior is more common in 25- to 44-year-olds than in the elderly, and more common in women than men. Existing data also indicate that nonfatal suicide attempters are equally prevalent across racial and ethnic groups.[22,49] Most individuals who kill themselves seem to do so on the first attempt. Although that suicide attempt is still the strongest predictor of suicidal outcome, only about 1 in 10 attempters is ultimately successful.[32,55] Multiple attempters also appear to have higher risk than those who make a single attempt.[29] Medically serious attempts may be a better marker of risk. Those who make serious attempts tend to share with completers a higher rate of serious mental illness.[8]

A number of avenues of inquiry suggest that violent attempts are associated with a persistent deficiency in brain serotonin levels. Impulsive types of aggression, for example, have been linked to serotonergic dysfunction in prefrontal cortical regions of the brain.[20] This deficiency has been measured in postmortem brains and spinal fluid of suicide victims and survivors of violent attempts compared to nonviolent attempters and other patients. Serotonergic deficiencies persist during periods of acute psychi-

TABLE 114–2. Characterization of Suicidal Ideation

Dimension	Benign	Intermediate	Malignant
Onset	None	Chronic, stable	New or fluctuating
Frequency	Occasional	Daily	Constant
Pesistence	Fleeting thoughts	Persistent thoughts	Preoccupation
Urgency	Disinterested	Engaged	Intense
Complexity	Simple	Some detail	Elaborate
Activity	Passive ideas	Plans without action	Action
Emotional response	Death repellent	Ambivalent	Death desirable
Circumstances	Victim identifies one clear precipitant	Several complex contributory stressors	Either noncontributory or overwhelming stressors
Alternatives	Some, realistic	Few, problematic	Seems hopeless
Insight	Recognizes remediable psychologic problem	Overvalued ideas present, temporarily reassured	Morbid delusions present, reassurance impossible
Intent	Opposed to suicide	Suicide acceptable but prefers to live	Resolutely suicidal

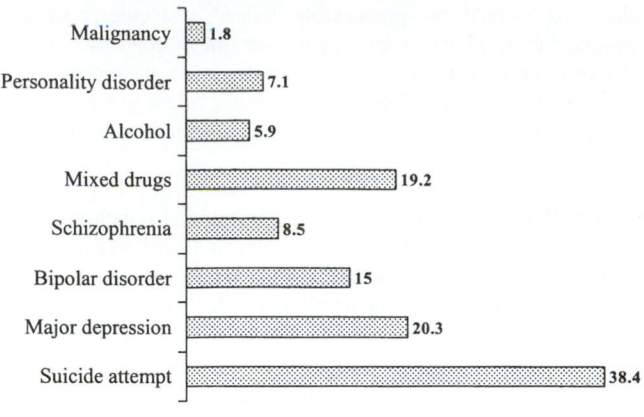

Figure 114–1. Increased likelihood of suicide for various conditions. *(Data from Inskip HM, Harris EC, Barraclough B: Lifetime risk of suicide for affective disorder, alcoholism and schizophrenia. Br J Psychiatry 1998; 172:35–37.)*

atric illness as well as remission. Relatedly, low levels of serum cholesterol have also been associated with increased risk for violent suicidal behavior and aggression towards others.[30] Low serum cholesterol level may interfere with serotonergic functioning and may also serve as a marker for future violent behavior. Unfortunately, these finding have not yet developed into a clinical tool.

Hopelessness has also received a significant amount of study as a potential predictor of suicide. However, hopelessness appears to have high sensitivity but low specificity.[9] Identifying hopelessness as a problem also suggests possible interventions.

Ultimately, most persons belonging to a high-risk group do not commit suicide, and some individuals with no apparent risk factors do. Many risk factors are not modifiable. This type of information, then, weighs most heavily in the assessment in the absence of other more specific data, early in the hospital course, or in the case of the uncooperative or hostile patient. The best foundation for treatment planning and clinical decision making is direct examination and clinical diagnosis.

Treatment

Following the comprehensive psychiatric assessment, the next step is deciding on treatment alternatives. Any patient who has made a suicide attempt must be considered to be at risk, and some further intervention is warranted. The risk of a subsequent lethal attempt is approximately 1% per year over the first 10 years. The risk is highest in the first 1 month to 1 year.

The treatment alternatives available will depend on the psychiatric sophistication of the staff available to the ED at any given time. The following section describes the commonly used interventions in the emergency department; they can be used singly or in combination.

Medications can be used acutely in the treatment of severe anxiety or psychosis; however, in the case of antidepressants, a period of weeks is required for therapeutic effect, so their immediate use is not indicated in the ED. In fact, there are concerns about prescribing medications with relatively high potential for lethality in overdose, such as tricyclic antidepressants and monoamine oxidase inhibitors, to persons who have recently attempted suicide. However, newer antidepressants, and particularly the selective

serotonin reuptake inhibitors (SSRIs), can be used as first-line drugs for treatment of most depressions, and they are relatively safe in overdose. A marked drop in the number of deaths per million antidepressant prescriptions was observed between 1970 and 1974 in Europe.[34] Nonetheless, the initiation of antidepressant therapy by the nonpsychiatric physician is not recommended unless a tight linkage can be made between discharge and immediate (within days) aftercare by either a community outreach team or a crisis clinic.

Patients with depressive disorders may suffer from significant anxiety; also, patients with overwhelming situational stressors (job loss, new financial hardship, bereavement or divorce) may have episodic anxiety or insomnia. The prescription of a short course of a benzodiazepine may provide significant relief to the patient in crisis.

After the patient's immediate symptoms have been treated in the emergency department, the next treatment decision is determining the setting in which further treatment may safely be provided. Not all patients with suicidal ideation or even significant attempts necessarily require hospitalization, and there is still a substantial stigma attached to psychiatric hospitalization. In general, it should be the treatment used if less restrictive measures cannot insure the patient's safety. If significant doubt exists about the safety of outpatient treatment, the patient should be held in the ED for further evaluation, admitted to a general hospital with close nursing supervision, or admitted to a psychiatric unit. "Holding beds" now available in some larger psychiatric emergency services are ideal for this purpose. Some localities may also have crisis outreach services that follow the patient after discharge from the ED and improve appropriate monitoring and continuity of care.

Patients most likely to respond to interventions in the ED are individuals who until recently have been stable but who, as a result of some external event, find their way of life threatened. This results in a painful state of anxiety and the mobilization of some combination of adaptive and maladaptive coping strategies. Finally, a second event, the precipitant, intensifies the anxiety to the point that the patient cannot tolerate it and is thrown into crisis. The patient then feels desperate and may be completely immobilized or vulnerable to various strong impulses including the impulse to run away, strike out at someone else, or kill himself or herself. Reality testing is preserved, and no major psychiatric syndrome is present. The patient accurately perceives his or her situation, understands that the current reaction is a psychological problem, and is highly motivated to obtain help. The crisis may last for a matter of hours or weeks before the ED presentation and will ultimately resolve. Such patients respond well to crisis intervention and may actually undergo some positive development in the course of treatment.

By contrast, patients whose condition has been deteriorating for some time in the absence of significant stressors, and who appear on examination to be suffering from severe depressive symptoms, are unlikely to benefit rapidly from supportive techniques. If such patients present with suicidal ideation or attempts, it will be difficult, though not impossible, to manage them outside the hospital.

Outpatient settings have the advantage of maintaining the patient's functioning as much as possible. Work and child care responsibilities, financial obligations, and social relationships are not disrupted. Unnecessary regression is halted. The patient is able to assume more responsibility for his or her outcome, and independence helps preserve self-esteem. These individuals remain closer to and more engaged with the people and situations with which they must learn to cope. Their morale may be rapidly improved by the combination of support, planning, and modest early treatment successes.

In some cases, though, these same factors may be disadvantageous. Routine tasks may seem overwhelming. High levels of conflict may render major relationships at least temporarily unworkable. Inpatient settings offer the advantage of respite, high levels of structure, more intensive professional and peer support, constant supervision, and usually, more rapid pharmacologic and psychosocial intervention. The physical plant also reduces, though it cannot eliminate, the possible means of suicide.

The choice of inpatient or outpatient setting will depend on the balance of strengths and weaknesses of the patient, the involvement and competence of family or friends, the availability of a therapist in the community, and the ongoing stresses in the patient's life. This decision is best made by a psychiatrist after performing his or her own examination. Many facilities will not have a psychiatrist available much of the time. However, a trained mental health professional should be on call to every emergency department. This may be a psychiatric social worker, nurse clinician, or psychologist supervised on a regular basis by a psychiatrist or with a psychiatric consultant available by phone. When such services are not available, it is appropriate to detain patients in the ED until a practitioner with specific competence is available or to transfer the patient to another facility for evaluation. Every state has laws that provide for the involuntary commitment of the mentally ill under circumstances that vary from state to state. Any acute, deliberate self-injurious behavior would generally qualify. Chronic, repetitive dangerous behavior that is not "deliberate," such as frequent unintentional opioid or sedative-hypnotic overdoses, warrant careful evaluation; but in the absence of psychiatric illness, involuntary treatment is usually not an option. The practitioner should be familiar with the criteria for commitment and the classes of healthcare providers so empowered under state law.

There are other treatment interventions that can be provided in the emergency setting; these include crisis intervention, substance abuse counseling, and family therapy. A single session in the ED may be sufficient to defuse a crisis or to spur the drug-abusing patient to seek help; alternatively, the intervention may be begun in the ED and continued in another setting.

Crisis intervention is a brief, highly focused therapy that seeks to deconstruct how a crisis occurred, with an eye toward examining the patient's role. Often, patients have distorted perceptions of the crisis, and a gentle "correction" of catastrophic thinking can be extremely helpful. (Here is an example. Patient: "I'm going to be broke and unemployed the rest of my life." Physician: "How did you get your last job?" Patient: "Well, I interviewed a couple of times." Physician: "So people have hired you in the past, right?") The crisis is presented to the patient as an unfortunate and perhaps tragic experience that he or she can overcome. Ideally, the patient should have a relief of symptoms and learn how crises may be avoided in the future. This intervention will likely fail for patients with severe depression because of the presence of profound hopelessness. It is best utilized for patients who give a history of high functioning just prior to the crisis.

Substance abuse treatment is ultimately an intermediate- (weeks to months) to long-term (months to years) intervention. However, there are powerful initial steps that the emergency physician can take. Chief among these is confronting the patient about the medical consequences of substance use. This can take the form of discussion only, or the physician can invite the patient to examine clinical laboratory results or view remarkable clinician/diagnostic findings (hepatomegaly, repeated fractures from falls, increased liver enzymes or evidence of "silent" past myocardial infarction). There is little to be lost from a respectful but blunt confrontation of the patient's deterioration, and he or she may listen to a physician rather than family or friends. Peer counseling is particularly useful in addictive disorders; if possible, patients should be referred to community 12-step programs such as Alcoholics Anonymous. Family therapy can occur as a series of sessions over the long term or can be useful in the emergency setting to defuse a crisis, reinstate social supports for the patient, or educate families about mental illness. It is most important to respect a patient's request as to the level of family involvement; it may often occur in the emergency setting that patients are either too angry or ashamed to confront their families. At this point, it is prudent to defer and to assure the family that the patient is safe and that you will keep them informed as confidentiality and discretion allow.

VIOLENCE

The violent patient also presents unique challenges to the emergency physician. Violent patients are difficult to treat, and they tend to elicit strong negative reactions in ED personnel. In one study of violence in the ED, directors of residency programs in emergency medicine were surveyed as to the frequency of verbal threats, physical attacks, and the presence of weaponry in the area. Of the 127 institutions, 74.7% of the residency directors responded; 41 (32%) reported receiving at least one verbal threat each day; moreover, 23 (18%) reported that weapons were displayed as a threat at least once each month. Fifty-five program directors (43%) noted that a physical attack on medical staff occurred at least once a month.[41] In a second study, the authors conducted a retrospective review of university police log records and ED staff incident reports to examine the problem of violence in the ED setting. Almost 75% of the incidents occurred during the evening or night. Of the 686 episodes of violence in this study, more than 25% required physical restraint or removal from the premises; additionally, it was found that the police responded to the ED nearly twice daily.[54] These studies underscore the need for timely identification of the violent patient as well as appropriate management for this diagnostically heterogeneous group. The assessment and management of the violent patient should include provisions for patient and staff safety as well as a thorough search for the cause of violent behavior. This section addresses the differential diagnosis of violent behavior, the pharmacotherapy of aggressive and/or agitated behavior, and the use of seclusion and restraint. It also provides an overview of potential risk factors for violent behavior.

Stress-Vulnerability Model of Aggression

As with suicide, there are many and varied causes of violent behavior, some more social and some more medical in nature. It is most helpful to think of violence as the outcome of a dynamic interaction among numerous factors both intrinsic and extrinsic to the individual, some of which promote and some of which ameliorate the potential for violent behavior at any given moment. This is a stress-vulnerability model. Education may provide alternatives to violence, but delirium may cause an otherwise nonviolent person to misinterpret healthcare efforts. Their education is of no benefit in the delirious state. Hence, they become violent under circumstances that would not normally be sufficient to provoke a violent outburst. Some patients, on the other hand, come from cultures in which violence is viewed positively, and these patients require little stress or provocation before responding violently.

In the ED, likely medical sources of vulnerability include metabolic derangements, drug and/or alcohol intoxication, withdrawal syndromes, seizure disorders, head trauma, psychotic states, and personality disorders. Additionally, patients with severe pain, delirium, or extreme anxiety can respond to the efforts of emergency personnel with resistance, hostility, or frank aggression.

Prediction

Research on risk factors for community violence may not apply to the prediction of inpatient violence. Some researchers have postulated that violence committed outside the hospital may not be predictive of inpatient violence and that hospital violence may result from the interaction of patients with specific factors found in the hospital environment.[33] However, other studies support the notion that the best predictor of future violence is still past violence.[63, 53] Adding to the confusion of the issue, a study conducted in Germany examined the violence potential of nearly 18,000 inpatients:[63] 8.3% of incoming patients had a history of previous violence, but only 2.7% of inpatients in their study actually committed a violent act in the hospital. Even if prior violence is a good predictor of future violence, it is not a perfect predictor. Other factors, such as mental illness and substance abuse, need to be examined in order to make meaningful predictions of inpatient violence for each individual case.

One study found that the most common types of hospital violence were incidents of aggression against objects in the hospital (56.7%), violence directed against the hospital staff (27.8%), and violence directed against other patients (14.4%).[62] In this study, men were not found to be committing significantly greater incidents of violence than women. Other studies concur that male patients are not necessarily more of a risk for inpatient violence than female inpatients. For example, another study examining inpatient violence found that close to half of the violent incidents were committed by female patients.[39] Furthermore, they found that the number of violence-related injuries committed by male and female inpatients was almost proportional to the ratio of male and female inpatients on the unit. They concluded that gender should not be considered a risk factor for inpatient violence. Long hospitalization was not considered a factor predictive of violence for the majority of inpatients. As with outpatient violence, the correlation of violence with younger age appears to hold true in the inpatient setting.[53, 62]

Substance Use

The association between substance use and violence is well established. Alcohol is found in the offender, the victim, or both in one-half to two-thirds of homicides and serious assaults.[17] Substance abuse is seldom the sole cause, but it may contribute to violence in a number of ways. The direct pharmacologic effects include disinhibition and misinterpretation, suspiciousness, or paranoia. Psy-chological effects of substance use include cultural expectations of appropriate behavior under the influence and the ability to excuse or disavow inappropriate behavior that occurs while intoxicated. Substance use then interacts with other physiologic, cognitive, psychological, situational, and cultural factors including any mental illness. A tripartite model has been described: (1) systemic violence related to drug distribution, (2) economic compulsive violence associated with the criminal activity necessary to sustain a drug habit, and (3) psychopharmacologic violence resulting from the direct effects of the particular drug or toxin.[28]

Mental Illness

The relationship between mental illness and violence is also complex. Efforts made to destigmatize mental illness have confused the issue, but it seems clear that mental illness is associated with a greater risk for violence. In one large epidemiologic study, the prevalence of violence for those with no disorder was 2%. Schizophrenia was associated with an 8% rate of violent behavior, and other mental disorders were all similar at approximately 12%. But of all respondents reporting violent behaviors, 42% had a substance use disorder. Substance use more than tripled the rate of violence for schizophrenics. For various reasons, mental illness appears to reduce the threshold for aggression, and the more comorbid conditions present, the greater the risk.[65]

For whatever reason, researchers are consistently finding a greater prevalence of personality disorders among violent inpatients than nonviolent inpatients.[50] However, antisocial personality is the condition most strongly associated with both substance abuse and aggression. In one study, when the history of juvenile deviance was controlled, alcohol—the drug most commonly associated with violence—accounted for only 2% of the violent behavior.

In conclusion, some aggressive behavior is attributable to the direct pharmacologic effects of substances but probably represents a modest fraction. Substances are also a part of the setting of violent behavior in the community, a coincidental part of the life style of violent individuals; and both substance use and violence are related to common underlying characteristics such as character disorder.

Medication Noncompliance

Many research studies currently list medication noncompliance as a risk factor for violence that is as serious as substance use or mental illness. One study associated medication noncompliance and substance use with increased violence risk in the mentally ill.[67] They suggest that medication noncompliance may lead to self-medicating through the use of illicit substances, and substance use may lead to further medication noncompliance. These two factors together may then have the effect of increasing violence for the mentally ill. This study also suggested that low insight into their illness can be associated with greater violence. However, they found that poor insight was correlated with substance use and medication noncompliance, so it is unclear if poor insight is truly predictive. Other studies have replicated these findings.[66] Patients entering the ED who did not adhere to their medications as outpatients may be more of a risk for inpatient violence. Furthermore, inpatients who refuse to adhere to medication prescribed in the hospital also are more of a risk for violence, especially when comorbid with substance abuse disorders.

Additional Factors in Violent Behavior

Many of the factors correlated with aggression are easy to observe and monitor in the hospital. However, some additional factors that influence violent behavior may not be as easy to detect. For example, one study examining violent behavior found that most violent incidents in the hospital occur on Mondays and Fridays, with very few on the weekends.[40] They pointed out that this finding reflected findings of violence research in the general population and postulated that the explanation for the inpatient violence is the same as that for the general population. Mondays and Fridays have special significance in the workweek, and weekends are usually less stressful. This finding illustrates the point that seemingly minor social stressors can be as conducive to violent behavior as any other factor.

Furthermore, researchers have postulated a seasonal variation of violence.[16] They reported finding an increase in the frequency of assaults by inpatients during the winter months and hypothesized that increased population density, cold temperature, and less sunlight during the day could account for the increased violence. This finding is in contrast to the literature on outpatient violence, which has reported greater incidence of violence during the hot months.[6] However, this same review conceded that any extreme temperature could evoke aggressive feelings and frustration. A third study examined temperature and violence and found that more aggressive acts occur during the summer months, both in the hospital and in the community.[24] They cited several explanations, one of which was that the high rate of staff turnover, as vacations are taken, disrupts the social networks the patients have established, evoking aggressive feelings.

Although it is unclear whether the cold can provoke aggression as much as it has been established that heat can, it does seem clear that overcrowding and social stressors can lead to violent behavior. If the effects of temperature and social stressors (eg, holidays) correlate so drastically with violence in the community, it is likely that such effects would have even more impact when comorbid with severe mental illness, substance use, or any of the other risk factors of aggression. Physicians would be wise to keep that in mind when dealing with potentially dangerous inpatients.

Assessment

The comprehensive evaluation of the violent patient should include a complete physical examination. The examination may reveal the underlying cause of the violent behavior as well as insuring the treatment of any secondary patient injuries. Laboratory analysis of blood chemistry, a complete blood count, and diagnostic imaging as guided by the examination and available clinical history may also be helpful.

Illicit drug and alcohol use often present with symptoms of violence. Acute intoxication with cocaine can produce extreme psychomotor agitation, delirium, and transient psychosis characterized by paranoia and hallucinations; a clinically indistinguishable syndrome can be seen following the ingestion of amphetamines. Phencyclidine intoxication is manifested by assaultiveness, muscle rigidity, dysarthria, nystagmus, autonomic instability, and ataxia. Alcohol intoxication is characterized by typical signs of cerebellar dysfunction (slurred speech, gait ataxia, and incoordination); however, persons who are intoxicated are also at risk for violent behavior. Cannabis does not typically produce violent or aggressive behavior; however, paranoia can occur with intoxication and can secondarily promote reactions of extreme fear associated with distorted perception; the same can be said for intoxication with LSD and psilocybin, particularly in the naive user.

Withdrawal syndromes from specific drugs can also promote aggressive behavior as a consequence of physical discomfort or anticipatory anxiety. Opioid withdrawal is characterized by myalgias, rhinorrhea, and piloerection; alcohol, benzodiazepines, and barbiturates share a common syndrome of autonomic hyperreactivity and subsequent delirium. Patients suffering from any of these signs and symptoms may become aggressive, verbally abusive, or threatening. Prompt recognition of these syndromes and immediate treatment can prevent some aggressive outbursts. Because drug use is often concealed, is difficult to ascertain on clinical grounds, and frequently contributes to violent behavior, urine toxicologic studies may be useful to enhance the understanding and long-range treatment of some patients.

Delirium can be a cause of aggression. Patients are often suddenly confused, frightened, or frankly psychotic as a result of impaired perception. Patients may require sedation or restraint in order to prevent injury; some guidelines for this are presented in the next section.

Although persons suffering from psychotic disorders are not generally aggressive, there are aspects of the psychotic state that place patients at risk for aggressive behavior. Paranoid ideation can serve to promote misperceptions of impending bodily harm ("They're trying to kill me"), sexual victimization ("Men and women are raping me"), and humiliation ("Everyone is laughing at me"). It follows that these fearful perceptions might provoke violent reactions in a patient. Hallucinations can cause aggression, either as a result of command hallucinations or in reaction to the anxiety and irritation that patients experience with loud or persistent "voices." Persons with either borderline or antisocial personality disorder are at risk for violent acting-out as a result of poor impulse control.

Violence risk has also been associated with cognitive dysfunction. Both acute mental illness and chronic substance use can result in neurologic impairment. Psychiatric patients with compromised cognitive abilities such as impaired attention, memory, or executive functioning (ie, reasoning and planning) have been found to be at increased risk for violence.[61] Patients presenting with cognitive impairment may also be at increased risk for committing acts of violence in the ED.

Treatment

The acute pharmacotherapy of violent behavior is directed simply at reducing the level of arousal. A recent review of this issue proposed a model for the efficient use of medication for the control of episodic as opposed to chronic agitation and aggression.[3] In this model, agitation and violent outbursts are viewed as transient disturbances of the usual treatment relationship between the physician and patient. Pharmacotherapy and seclusion or restraint are to be used only as needed to restore that relationship, for the benefit of the patient as well as other members of the milieu. The restoration of the treatment relationship is necessary in order to take measures to understand and deal with the cause of the agitation, with the input and consent of the patient, thus preventing future incidents. For this reason, sleep is considered an undesirable use of medication. Sleep delays rather than promotes assessment, may further frighten or anger the patient, and does not even guarantee elimination of the agitated state on awakening.

As aggression derives from varied and multiple etiologies, it follows that there is much debate about the specific sedative used, the route of administration, and the dosing interval. Studies examining the treatment of aggression and/or agitation have included such diverse populations as schizophrenics, acutely intoxicated patients (alcohol), trauma patients, postoperative patients, patients in alcohol withdrawal, and patients with presumed personality disorders. Treatment settings for these studies included psychiatric inpatient units, intensive care units, and the ED.[1,14,42–44] An excellent review examined a number of these studies and found that both benzodiazepines and antipsychotics afforded relief of agitation and aggression.[21]

It seems, however, that there are specific clinical situations when benzodiazepines and neuroleptics might be preferentially used. Haloperidol has been safely used in the treatment of agitation and aggression in patients with psychoses, alcohol intoxication, and delirium.[2,14,42,43] The drug can be administered orally, intravenously, or intramuscularly; dosing intervals range from 30 minutes to 2 hours. The usual regimen is 5 mg haloperidol given every 30 to 60 minutes; most patients respond after 1 to 3 doses. The dose of haloperidol needed to achieve sedation rarely exceeds a total of 50 mg.

Benzodiazepines are also quite effective for tranquilization; their use has been examined in patients with psychoses, stimulant intoxication, and postoperative agitation.[1,26,46,47] Lorazepam 1 to 2 mg may be given orally or parenterally and repeated at 30- or 60-minute intervals, respectively, until the patient is calm. Because diazepam is poorly absorbed from intramuscular sites, the preferred route of administration is intravenous or oral. Diazepam may be given as 5 to 10 mg IV with repeat dosing as needed; concerns about respiratory depression mandate careful observation of patients receiving tranquilization with these agents. Diazepam may have a unique role in the treatment of agitation secondary to cocaine intoxication, as seizures may emerge in this syndrome (see Chap. 67). Antipsychotics, particularly low-potency antipsychotics, are known to lower seizure threshold in animals, so their use for patients with cocaine intoxication may be limited. Studies have examined the use of combinations of lorazepam with antipsychotics in patients with psychiatric illness and delirium; it appears that the combination of benzodiazepine and antipsychotics afforded relief of psychotic symptoms while allowing for a reduced dose of antipsychotic medications.[2,15,60]

Physical Restraint

Seclusion and restraint are also used in the treatment of violent behavior. Seclusion can help to diminish environmental stimuli and thereby reduce hyperreactivity; it is not commonly used in the medical ED, so its use is not discussed in great detail here. However, a few reminders are worthwhile to mention: as seclusion is defined by a condition of very limited interactive and environmental cues, it is not indicated for patients with unstable medical conditions, delirium, dementia, self-injurious behavior (cutting, head banging), or who are suffering extrapyramidal reactions to antipsychotic medication.[4] Restraint is used to prevent patient and staff injury. All facilities should have clear written policy guidelines for restraint that address monitoring, provisions for patient comfort, and documentation. (Chap. 115)

Training

Finally, it has been shown that training in the management of aggression helps to reduce violence and injuries through the early identification of impending episodes of violence, use of verbal techniques to defuse incidents, and appropriate physical techniques to minimize injuries in those that occur. It behooves the healthcare provider to maintain his or her skills through training and to advocate for continuing medical education on this topic at the workplace.[12]

SUMMARY

Both violent and suicidal behavior in the ED may be the cause or the effect of many toxicologic presentations. Patients presenting with suicidal or aggressive behavior pose unique problems for the clinician who must make appropriate assessment and management decisions. Identifying risk factors for suicide and aggression can aid the clinician in employing preventive or early intervention strategies in the ED. Important risk factors for both suicidal and violent behavior include past history of the behavior, comorbid mental illness, substance intoxication, and young age groups. Mental status examination for suicidality should focus on extrinsic factors such as current ideation, intent, lethality of plan, current life stressors, as well as intrinsic vulnerability factors such as comorbid mental illness, feelings of hopelessness, and impulsivity. In terms of violence risk assessment, substance intoxication, mental illness and psychiatric medication noncompliance, alone or in combination, are robust predictors of aggressive behavior in the ED and other inpatient settings. Early detection and rapid intervention for patients at risk for suicide or violence is, to date, the best means for preventing injury or death.

ACKNOWLEDGMENT

Cherie Elfenbein contributed to this chapter in a previous edition.

REFERENCES

1. Abel RM, Reis RL: Intravenous diazepam for sedation following cardiac operations: Clinical and hemodynamic assessments. Anesth Analg 1971;50:244–248.
2. Adams F: Neuropsychiatric evaluation and treatment of delirium in the critically ill cancer patient. Cancer Bull 1984;36:156–160.
3. Allen MH: Managing the agitated psychotic patient: A reappraisal of the evidence. J Clin Psychiatry 2000;61(Suppl 14):11–20.
4. American Psychiatric Association: Clinician Safety. Task Force report no. 33. Washington, DC, American Psychiatric Association,1992.
5. American Psychiatric Association: The Principles of Medical Ethics with Annotations Especially Applicable to Psychiatry. Washington, DC, American Psychiatric Association, 1989.
6. Anderson CA: Temperature and aggression: ubiquitous effects of heat on occurrence of human violence. Psychol Bull 1989;106:74–96.
7. Barraclough B, Bunch J, Nelson B, Sainsbury P: A hundred cases of suicide: Clinical aspects. Br J Psychiatry 1974;125:355–373.
8. Beautrais AL, Joyce PR, Mulder RT, et al: Prevalence and comorbidity of mental disorders in persons making serious suicide attempts: a case control study. Am J Psychiatry 1996;153:1009–1014.
9. Beck A, Steer R, Kovacs M, Garrison B: Hopelessness and eventual suicide: a 10-year prospective study of patients hospitalized with suicidal ideation. Am J Psychiatry 1985;142:559–563.

10. Bick PA, Hannah AL: Intramuscular lorazepam to restrain violent patients [letter]. Lancet 1986;1:206.

11. Burt C, Fingerhut L: Injury visits to hospital emergency departments: United States, 1992–1995. Vital Health Statistics 1998;13(131). Washington, DC, National Center for Health Statistics, 1998.

12. Carmel H, Hunter M: Compliance with training in managing assaultive behavior and injuries from inpatient violence. Hosp Commun Psychiatry 1990;41:558–560.

13. Clayton PJ: Suicide. Psychiatr Clin North Am 1985;8:203–214.

14. Clinton JE, Sterner S, Steimachers Z, Ruiz E: Haloperidol for sedation of disruptive emergency patients. Ann Emerg Med 1987;16:319–322.

15. Cohen S, Khan A, Johnson S: Pharmacological management of manic psychosis in an unlocked setting. J Clin Psychopharmacol 1987;7:261–264.

16. Coldwell JB, Naismith LJ: Violent incidents in special hospitals. Br J Psychiatry 1989;154:270.

17. Collins JJ, Schlenger WE: Acute and chronic effects of alcohol use on violence. J Stud Alcohol 1988;49:516–522.

18. Crome P: The toxicity of drugs used for suicide. Acta Psychiatr Scand 1993;371(Suppl):33–37.

19. Crosby AE, Cheltenham MP, Sacks, JJ: Incidence of suicidal ideation and behavior in the United States. Suicide Life Threat Behav 1999;29:131–140.

20. Davidson RJ, Putnam, KM, Larson CL: Dysfunction in the neural circuitry of emotion regulation: A possible prelude to violence. Science 2000;289:591–594.

21. Dubin W: Rapid tranquilization: Antipsychotics or benzodiazepines? J Clin Psychiatry 1988;49(Suppl 12):5–12.

22. Fawcett J, Clark DC, Busch KA: Assessing and treating the patient at risk for suicide. Psychiatr Ann 1993;23:244–255.

23. Fawcett J, Scheftner WA, Fogg L, et al: Time-related predictors of suicide in major affective disorder. Am J Psychiatry 1990;144:923–926.

24. Flannery RB, Penk WE: Cyclical variations in psychiatric patient-to-staff assaults: Preliminary inquiry. Psychol Rep 1993;72:642.

25. Frances A, Blumenthal S: Personality as a predictor of youthful suicide. In: Risk Factors for Youth Suicide. Report of the Secretary's Task Force on Youth Suicide, Vol. 2. Alcohol, Drug Abuse, and Mental Health Administration. DHHS pub. No. (ADM) 89–1624. Washington, DC, US Government Printing Office, 1989, pp. 160–171.

26. Garza-Trevino E, Hollister LE, Overall JE, Alexander WF: Efficacy of combinations of intramuscular antipsychotics and sedative-hypnotics for control of psychotic agitation. Am J Psychiatry 1989;146:1598–1601.

27. Goldfrank LR, Hoffman RS: The cardiovascular effects of cocaine. Ann Emerg Med 1991;20:165–175.

28. Goldstein PJ: The drugs–violence nexus: A tripartite conceptual framework. J Drug Issues 1986;15:493–506.

29. Goldstein R., Black D, Nasrallah,A, Winokur G: The prediction of suicide, Sensitivity, specificity, and predictive value of a multivariate model applied to suicide among 1906 patients with affective disorders. Arch Gen Psychiatry 1991;48:418–422.

30. Golomb BA, Stattin H, Mednick S: Low cholesterol and violent crime. J Psychiatry Res 2000;34:301–309.

31. Hagnell O, Lanke J, Rorsman B: Suicide rates in the Lundby study: Mental illness as a risk factor for suicide. Neuropsychobiology 1981;7:248–253.

32. Harris EC, Barraclough B: Suicide as an outcome for mental disorders: A meta-analysis. Br J Psychiatry 1997;170:205–227.

33. Hassan SD, Sobel RN: Violence in the community as a predictor of violence in the hospital. Psychiatr Serv 2001;52:240–241.

34. Henry JA: A fatal toxicity index for antidepressant poisoning. Acta Psychiatr Scand 1989;354:37–45.

35. Hoffman RS, Wipfler MG, Maddaloni MA, Weisman RS: The effect of the triplicate benzodiazepine prescription regulation on sedative-hypnotic overdoses. NY State J Med 1991;91:436–439.

36. Inskip HM, Harris EC, Barraclough B: Lifetime risk of suicide for affective disorder, alcoholism and schizophrenia. Br J Psychiatry1998;172:35–37.

37. Kapur S, Mieczkowski T, Mann JJ: Antidepressant medications and the relative risk of suicide attempt and suicide. JAMA 1992;268:3441–3445.

38. Kovacs M, Beck A, Weissman A: The communication of suicidal intent. Arch Gen Psychiatry 1976;33:198–201.

39. Lam JN, McNiel DE, Binder RL: The relationship between patients' gender and violence leading to injuries. Psychiatr Serv 2000;51:1167–1170.

40. Larkin E, Murtagh S, Jones S: A preliminary study of violent incidents in a special hospital (Rampton). Br J Psychiatry 1988;153:226–231.

41. Lavoie F, Carter G, Danzi D, Berg R: Emergency department violence in United States teaching hospitals. Ann Emerg Med 1988;17:1227–1233.

42. Lenehan G, Gastfriend DR, Stetler C: Use of haloperidol in the management of agitated or violent, alcohol-intoxicated patients in the emergency department: A pilot study. J Emerg Nurs 1985;11:72–79.

43. Lerner Y, Lwow E, Levitin A, Belmaker R: Acute high-dose parenteral haloperidol treatment of psychosis. Am J Psychiatry 1979;136:1061–1064.

44. McClish A, Andrew D, Tetreault L: Intravenous diazepam for psychiatric reactions following open heart surgery. Can Anaesth Soc J 1968;15:63–79.

45. Meehl PE: Psychodiagnosis: Selected Papers. Minneapolis, University of Minnesota Press, 1973.

46. Modell JG: Further experience and observations with lorazepam in the management of behavioral agitation [letter]. J Clin Psychopharmacol 1986;6:385–387.

47. Modell JG, Lenox RH, Weiner S: Inpatient clinical trial of lorazepam for the management of manic agitation. J Clin Psychopharmacol 1985;5:109–113.

48. Monk M: Epidemiology of suicide. Epidemiol Rev 1987;9:51–69.

49. Moscicki EK, O'Carroll P, Rae DS, et al: Suicide attempts in the Epidemiologic Catchment Area Study. Yale J Biol Med 1988;61:259–268.

50. National Center for Injury Prevention and Control: Suicide in the United States. *http://www.cdc.gov/ncipc/factsheets/suifacts.htm*.

51. Nolan KA, Volavka J, Mohr P, et al: Psychopathy and violent behavior among patients with schizophrenia or schizoaffective disorder. Psychiatr Serv 1999;50:787–792.

52. Nutter DO, Massumi RA: Diazepam in cardioversion. N Engl J Med 1965;273:650–651.

53. Owen C, Tarantello C, Jones M, et al: Violence and aggression in psychiatric units. Psychiatr Serv 1998;49:1452–1457.

54. Pane G, Winiarski A, Salness K: Aggression directed toward emergency department staff at a university teaching hospital. Ann Emerg Med 1991;20:283–286.

55. Pokorny AD: Prediction of suicide in psychiatric patients. Arch Gen Psychiatry 1983;40:249–257.

56. Rich CL, Young D, Fowler RC: San Diego suicide study, I: Young vs. old subjects. Arch Gen Psychiatry 1986;43:577–582.

57. Rihmer Z, Rutz W, Pihlgren H: Depression and suicide on Gotland: An intensive study of all suicides before and after a depression-training programme for general practitioners. J Affect Disord 1995;35:147–152.

58. Robins E, Gassner S, Kayes J, et al: The communication of suicidal intent: A study of 134 consecutive cases of successful (completed) suicide. Am J Psychiatry 1959;115:724–733.

59. Robins E, Murphy GE, Wilkinson RH, et al: Some clinical considerations in the prevention of suicide based on a study of 134 successful suicides. Am J Public Health 1959;49:888–889.

60. Salzman C, Green A, Rodriguez-Villa F, et al: Benzodiazepines combined with neuroleptics for management of severe disruptive behavior. Psychosomatics 1986;27(Suppl):17–21.

61. Serper M, Bergman AJ, Copersino ML, Chou J, Richarme D, Cancro R: Learning and memory impairment in cocaine dependent and co-morbid schizophrenic patients. Psychiatry Res 2000;93:21–32.

62. Soliman AE-D, Reza H: Risk factors and correlates of violence among acutely ill adult psychiatric inpatients. Psychiatr Serv 2001;52: 75–80.

63. Spiessl H, Krischker S, Cording C: Aggression in the psychiatric hospital. A psychiatric basic documentation based 6-year study of 17,943 inpatient admissions. Psychiatr Prax 1998;25:227–230.

64. Stone MH: The course of borderline personality disorder. In: Tasman A, Hales RE, Frances AJ, eds: Review of Psychiatry, Vol. 8. Washington, DC, American Psychiatric Press, 1987, pp. 103–122.

65. Swanson J, Holzer C, Ganju V, Jono R: Violence and psychiaric disorder in the community: Evidence from the Epidemiologic Catchment Area Survey. Hosp Commun Psychiatry 1990;41:761–770.

66. Swanson JW, Swartz MS, Borum R, et al: Involuntary out-patient commitment and reduction of violent behavior in persons with severe mental illness. Br J Psychiatry 2000;176:324–331.

67. Swartz MS, Swanson JW, Hiday VA, et al: Violence and severe mental illness: the effects of substance abuse and nonadherence to medication. Am J Psychiatry 1998;155:226–231.

68. US Department of Commerce: Statistical Abstracts of the United States, 116th ed. Washington, DC, US Government Printing Office, 1996.

CHAPTER 115 NURSING PRINCIPLES

Susan Callaghan-Montella / Barbara E. Soppet

Management of the poisoned patient requires an integrated response on the part of healthcare providers of all disciplines. This chapter offers specific considerations with regard to general nursing management and a detailed approach to patient evaluation. The discussion is not intended to be specific only to nurses, nor does it assume that the nurse's role in care is limited to these points. The collaborative roles of all emergency care providers consistently overlap, and it is this spontaneous team response that is essential for successful resuscitation. The necessity of professional collaboration is particularly evident in the areas of assessment, physical findings, toxidrome identification, and in the implementation of all aspects of standard medical management (see Chap. 3 and 31).

The optimal approach to the poisoned patient, as a nursing process, is assessment, planning, implementation, and evaluation. However, as in the medical management of the poisoned or overdosed patient (Chap. 3 and 31), the customary sequence of evaluation must sometimes be altered to address each particular clinical situation. With respect to the patient with an altered level of consciousness, even before the full assessment is performed, the airway must be stabilized, the cervical spine protected, and supplemental oxygen, dextrose, thiamine, and naloxone must be administered as indicated. In the case of a severely agitated patient who is breathing but combative, physical and chemical restraints to assure patient and staff safety may preclude a full patient assessment. Only after immediate life-threatening issues are addressed can the formal nursing process begin. If the patient arrives in the emergency department (ED) awake, alert, and oriented, the standardized clinical approach should be initiated immediately (Table 115–1).

TRIAGE: INITIAL ASSESSMENT OF THE PATIENT

Often, the first healthcare professional to evaluate a patient in the ED is the triage nurse. Information crucial to diagnosis and treatment may be available only at this early encounter, before the patient's consciousness becomes altered as a result of a central nervous system (CNS) depressant. An astute, inquisitive, and intuitive triage assessment often results in initiation of the necessary therapy and avoidance of subsequent mortality and morbidity.

The triage (from the French "to sort") nurse separates the emergent and urgent patients from the nonurgent and establishes the priority of care. In doing this, the nurse must perform another vital function, which is to sort out critical information that may identify a particular toxic syndrome, thus allowing for more timely

intervention. The practitioner's ability to obtain and use the vital signs, together with the information provided to the examiner's senses of sight, touch, and smell, can provide valuable clues to the nature of an ingestion.

The first priority of the triage nurse is to initiate a primary survey and identify any immediate life-threatening problems necessitating treatment. Immediate airway management with appropriate attention to the possibility of head/cervical spine injury must be accomplished before assessment proceeds. Once airway, breathing, bleeding, and circulation are assessed and stabilized (see "General Acute Management" later in this chapter, Chap. 3 and 31, and Fig. 3–1), the next task is to establish the database necessary for ongoing management of the patient. The questions that need to be asked as part of patient assessment and the sequence of delivery of care are covered in the next sections.

Who Is This Patient?

The patient's age, sex, general appearance, hygiene, mental status, physical findings, and social, family, and medical history all will assist in the development of a differential diagnosis, the development of a priority assessment, and the preparation of a plan of care.

Unfortunately, in poisoned patients, a history is not always readily available. Often the patient is unaccompanied and unable to offer details of his or her illness. Hence, prehospital teams become potential sources of very valuable data: Were there family, friends, or neighbors present? Was any important information secured from this source? What relevant prehospital clinical data are available? What was the condition at the scene? Was there a suicide note? Were there any signs of ingestion—pill bottles, "syringes," tablets, capsules, or bottles or containers that might contain or have contained a toxin? Remember that the label may not reflect the substance that was actually in the bottle. The need to initiate therapy rapidly often precludes waiting for laboratory results. Changes in level of consciousness, associated with pupillary findings and vital signs, may assist the nurse in the recognition of a toxidrome (see Chap. 17 and Table 17–2).

If the patient has ingested a toxic substance, what drug or substance was taken? Is there any characteristic odor that might indicate a specific ingestion or clinical condition? The odor of vomitus, sweat, and urine, as well as the color and quality of stool, can be diagnostic. Are there characteristic physical signs? The ingestion of multiple substances may have toxicologic effects. Is alcohol responsible for the patient's condition? Has it been ingested in addition to other substances, and can it potentiate their effects? Were any remedies initiated by the family or friends? Are there

TABLE 115–1. Standard Emergency Department Nursing Care Plan for the Poisoned Adult Patient

Assessment

  Objective: Triage examination (categorize patient's emergency)
    Check Airway: Is it open and clear? Can patient speak, cough? Are there obvious signs of head or neck trauma?
      Breathing: Presence or absence, rate, rhythm, abnormal breath sounds?
      Circulation: Assess pulse, blood pressure, skin color and temperature, capillary refill, cutaneous moisture.
    Neurologic status: Level of consciousness, pupils, movement of extremities, gag reflex.
    General appearance: Dress, body size, tissue turgor, cleanliness, wounds, bruises, marks on skin, odor on breath.

  Subjective: Brief History (from patient if alert and/or obtain details from those accompanying patient)
    Chief complaint
    Name of substance taken
    Route of administration
    Amount taken
    Time taken
    Time of onset of symptoms
    Past medical history
    Maintenance medications
    Allergies, risk factors
    Prehospital treatment initiated at the scene by EMS personnel.

Intervention (see Fig. 3–1)

  Administer oxygen via nasal cannula or face mask (if patient is breathing), or initiate respirations with pocket mask or bag valve-mask with 100% oxygen
    (if patient is not breathing)
  If pulse absent, proceed with appropriate resuscitation care plan; remove all clothing
  Stabilize cervical spine as appropriate
  Insert oral or nasal airway as necessary
  Clear patient's secretions with suction if necessary
  Check equipment for proper functioning; assist physician with intubation
  Request chest radiograph
  Obtain vital signs, including rectal temperature; attach the patient to a cardiac monitor and pulse oximeter
  Initiate IV therapy using a macrodrip initially and D_5W or 0.9% sodium chloride solution
  Draw blood for serum glucose, CBC, BUN, electrolytes, ABGs, and appropriate toxicology testing; test blood with glucose indicator strip; β-HCG testing if
    appropriate
  Obtain 12-lead ECG
  Prepare naloxone first and then $D_{50}W$ and thiamine for administration
  Rapidly evaluate patient's response, neurologic status, and vital signs
  Evaluate the need for physical restraint if patients's mental status is altered and/or he is a danger to himself or others

  If patient is conscious
    Check gag reflex
    Prepare to administer activated charcoal if appropriate
    Have functional suction unit available
    Keep the patient in an open, observable area

  If patient is unconscious
    Protect airway with intubation, when indicated
    Prepare for orogastric lavage with orogastric tube, if appropriate (Chaps. 3 and 31)
    Following lavage, administer activated charcoal and a cathartic
    Consider need for a specific antidote.

Evaluation: Monitor

  Vital signs, include a repeat temperature
  Cardiac monitoring, pulse oximetry; 12-lead ECG
  Rapid head-to-toe assessment
  Response to emetic (if given) or orogastric lavage and cathartic
  Oral and IV fluids given (input)
  Urine amount (output)
  Emotional status: evaluate the need for psychiatric consultation and/or social service assessment if patient is stable.
  Prepare patient for admission to hospital or continued observation; notify family and friends in accordance with patient wishes.
  If patient is discharged, after medical and psychiatric clearance, provide patient (and family if appropriate) with discharge instructions and followup care;
    ensure, through feedback, that instructions are understood.

any clinical conditions, other than a toxic ingestion, that might present in this fashion, and, if so, how must immediate management be altered? What additional tests are necessary to evaluate the patient? If alcohol is present as a suspect or confounding substance, a blood alcohol level may be indicated.

Reporting to the poison center offers the potential for a discussion with experts and provides for clinical followup in cases of toxic ingestions. Collaboration with these specialists will improve immediate patient management and clinical followup. The poison control staff's awareness of new trends and "fad" drugs can assist clinicians in the initial understanding and management.

Where Did the Exposure Occur?

Is the time of the exposure known? Was the patient at home, alone, at a social gathering or at work? Was the ingestion taken in a secluded or hidden place? Such information may reveal whether there was a purpose to the patient's exposure. Was it an intentional or unintentional exposure? A toxic ingestion taken in a secluded hotel room should suggest the possibility of a suicide attempt, which would necessitate additional clinical interventions, both acute and long term. A positive pregnancy test in a patient of childbearing age may be a determining factor in decisions about specific supportive measures. Is a pregnancy responsible for the ED presentation, or is it a coincidental finding? Does the pregnancy contraindicate any otherwise routine therapies?

When Did the Exposure Occur?

It is necessary to determine how much time has elapsed since the exposure and how much of the drug can be expected to be absorbed. These factors affect general management (eg, activated charcoal or orogastric lavage followed by activated charcoal) as well as decisions regarding toxin-specific antidotes or tertiary care procedures (eg, hemoperfusion and hemodialysis).

The time of year and climatic conditions must be appreciated, especially in the case of patients found on the street. Environmental conditions can rapidly alter thermoregulation in the drug-overdosed patient. Hypothermia or hyperthermia requires a comprehensive care plan. The need for a core temperature is therefore an integral part of admission vital signs. If the patient's temperature is at either extreme of a traditional thermometer, and there is a suspicion of hypothermia or hyperthermia, or the patient is agitated or uncooperative, an indwelling temperature device that can monitor the extremes of temperature of 60 to 120°F (15.5 to 48.9°C) should be used. Both hypothermia and hyperthermia may cause an altered mental status and may prevent a response or signs of a response to appropriate therapeutics. In addition, the patient's temperature may provide clues to the possibility of a preexisting or concomitant disease process that must be considered in developing a plan of care.

How Did This Emergency Occur?

What route of exposure was used? Was it intentional or unintentional and a result of ignorance or impaired judgment? Was this event a manifestation of chronic abuse? What implements were used? Were any other substances taken that might potentiate the effects of the toxic substances?

Any patient presenting with an altered mental status that compromises airway and circulation should be triaged as emergent and afforded prompt attention.

GENERAL ACUTE MANAGEMENT: PLANNING AND INTERVENTION

The nursing and medical roles in this phase of care are quite similar and interdependent, and thus, the nurse should be reasonably comfortable with the recognition of common toxic syndromes so as to anticipate tasks of care and facilitate their delivery. The nurse must coordinate the patient's immediate physical care as it relates to immediate survival as well as overall well-being (Tables 115–1 and 115–2). Priority must be given to life-threatening aspects. Assessment, plan implementation/intervention, and evaluation may, therefore, be applied in a systematic manner to both immediate and ongoing therapeutic considerations. (Nursing care interventions for emergency management: a quick reference tool, may be found in Table 115–3.)

As in the case of any resuscitative measure, adequacy of the patient's airway is clearly the first therapeutic consideration. Patients with suspected toxic exposures who enter the hospital with respiratory depression initially require assisted ventilation. The American Heart Association's guidelines suggest that a mouth-to-mask equipped with one-way valve, or bag valve mask techniques be used to minimize any possibility of infectious disease contamination. Whenever possible, two people should be present, one controlling ventilation with the bag and the other maintaining head position and face-mask seal. An oxygen reservoir and 100% oxygen should be attached to the bag. In cases in which respiratory arrest occurs and intubation is necessary, 100% oxygen with tidal volumes of 10 to 15 mL/kg should be delivered. In the event that respiratory arrest occurs in a patient with opioid toxicity, naloxone must be used judiciously. In these cases aggressive airway control may be preferred to the rapid reversal of respiratory depression with naloxone. Vomiting, which also occurs with this reversal, poses the further risk of aspiration in a patient with CNS depression. Insertion of an oropharyngeal airway and aggressive airway management with mouth-to-mask or bag valve mask devices may be all that is required until an improved level of consciousness is achieved. In the event that naloxone *is* used, the doses should be given in 0.05-mg increments to avoid the complications of rapid reversal in a patient where airway control is necessary. For pa-

TABLE 115–2. Examples of Nursing Diagnosis in Toxicologic Emergencies

Airway clearance (ineffective)
Aspiration
Body temperature (altered)
Bowel elimination (altered)
Breathing pattern (ineffective)
Cardiac output (decreased)
Coping ineffective
Fear
Gas exchange (impaired)
Hypothermia/hyperthermia
Infection
Injury
Poisoning
Self-esteem disturbance
Sensory perceptual alteration
Tissue perfusion (altered)
Violence
Volume deficit (fluid)

TABLE 115–3. **Alphabetic Tool in the Assessment and Stabilization of the Poisoned Patient with a Toxicologic Emergency**

<u>A</u>irway and <u>A</u>ntidote	Control airway using C-spine precautions as needed
	Consider need for immediate and specific antidote by history or examination eg, naloxone, cyanide antidote kit, removal and/or irrigation of noxious topical agents).
<u>B</u>reathing and <u>B</u>ehavior control	Place on O$_2$ mask (bag valve mask as needed)
	Does mental status/behavior require physical restraint/chemical restraint or antidotal care?
	Are there any contraindications?
<u>C</u>irculation and <u>C</u>oma antidotes	Check pulse; start CPR if absent
	Start IV
	Place on cardiac monitor and pulse oximetry
	Administer D$_{50}$W, thiamine, and naloxone only if indicated
<u>D</u>rug elimination	Decontaminate; emesis or orogastric lavage if indicated
	Administer activated charcoal and cathartic as needed
	Continue irrigation to achieve topical decontamination
	Consider specific antidote, if not already initiated
<u>E</u>xpose, <u>E</u>xamine, <u>E</u>valuate	Perform a quick examination after completely undressing the patient
<u>F</u>luid management	Is the patient in need of a fluid bolus?
	Are there any specific intravenous infusions that should be initiated (eg, naloxone or sodium bicarbonate)?
<u>G</u>et vital signs and tests	Obtain a complete set of vital signs including a core temperature to exclude hypothermia/hyperthermia
	Obtain routine blood work, U/A; consider blood and urine for toxicology testing
	Obtain ABG, ECG, chest radiograph
	Consider other radiographs or tests that may be needed to exclude other injury or complications (eg, C-spine radiograph, head CT, carboxyhemoglobin level)
<u>H</u>ead-to-toe and <u>H</u>istory	Look for hidden clues; do a complete and thorough reevaluation of the patient
	Obtain a detailed history from ambulance personnel and/or significant others
<u>I</u>nitiate consultation	Contact psychiatric or social service consults; consider other specialty consultation as necessary

tients who do not require intubation, oral airways are tolerated only by unconscious patients lacking a gag reflex. Nasal airways should be used in conscious patients who require an airway but have an intact gag reflex.

For a conscious but lethargic patient who needs only supplemental oxygen, many types of airway adjuncts are available. It is important not to confuse the nonrebreathing mask, delivering 95 to 100% oxygen, with the rebreather mask, which delivers an FIO$_2$ of only 50 to 60%. Awareness of the idiosyncrasies of various types of Venturi masks and the manufacturer's recommendations for assembly eliminates unnecessary confusion under emergent circumstances. Some patients may tolerate nasal cannulas better than face masks because they are less confining, but "mouth breathers" fare better clinically with masks. When a nurse receives a patient who is intubated and being ventilated via bag valve mask, tube placement and the presence of breath sounds should be verified. Reassessment includes vital signs, pulse oximetry, level of consciousness, cardiovascular and neurologic status, and the approach to maintaining adequate circulation. Respiratory therapy should be notified to provide ongoing ventilatory support and continuous monitoring of ventilation–perfusion adequacy.

The patient must then be undressed completely, and a rapid head-to-toe assessment performed. The presence of a gag reflex, speech quality, recall of events, and emotional state are evaluated. Pupil size and reactivity, extraocular movements, and the presence of nystagmus, tremors, weakness, paralysis, and paresthesias should be noted as well as any other physical findings.

Prompt attention to the "ABCs" is standard emergency procedure. Ongoing reassessment yields valuable data, which provide clues to the presence of particular toxins, the need for emergent intervention, and the likelihood of complications. After immediate lifesaving measures and a secondary assessment have been completed, a 12-lead electrocardiogram (ECG) should be done to search for dysrhythmias and/or conduction abnormalities. Cardiac monitoring in the poisoned or overdosed patient is essential, with monitor rate alarms set and functioning. Cardiac rate and function as part of a toxidrome can offer valuable clues to the identification of the substance. The presence of a cardiac dysrhythmia in and of itself may indicate the presence of a particular substance, or it may assist in the management of a concomitant problem or complication. For instance, heroin could certainly be responsible for a patient's near respiratory arrest, but one would not expect a tachydysrhythmia without suspecting other concomitant drug use or complications, such as dehydration, aspiration pneumonitis, endocarditis, or a mixed heroin-cocaine overdose. Cocaine is often associated with atrial and ventricular dysrhythmias as well as acute myocardial infarctions, but any of these findings are suggestive not diagnostic. This information, when correlated with additional data, helps provide the information for nursing diagnosis and ongoing plan of care.

When frequent blood pressure evaluation is necessary, an external blood pressure monitor or arterial line should be considered. Once an IV has been established and fluid replacement initiated, specific management may necessitate IV medication administration. Many nurses develop shortcuts in the calculation of IV fluid infusion time and flow rates. Some emergency departments continue to use preprinted, readily accessible IV "drip tickets" in the ED for drugs that are frequently infused intravenously. These precalculated dose charts also serve as markers on the IV bottles, but infusion pumps that automatically calculate and deliver doses in a predetermined time frame are ideal for use in a busy ED. Any drip used for hemodynamic support or antidotal therapy should utilize an infusion pump for delivery.

If thiamine, 50% dextrose, and naloxone are administered intravenously, documentation of the patient's response to therapy and anticipation of the need for further interventions and complications of care become the priorities of the nurse. A patient with a depressed level of consciousness secondary to hypoglycemia or opioid overdose may respond rapidly to the antidotes $D_{50}W$ and naloxone, respectively, whereas a patient with Wernicke's encephalopathy will have an immediate biochemical benefit and a delayed clinical response to thiamine. When and how the patient responds, as well as the duration of the response, yield clues to the etiology of the obtundation and thus to further management strategies. If the only etiology is an injected opioid, then an immediate response to naloxone is anticipated, varying in intensity from slow, appropriate movement to violent thrashing, associated with retching and coughing. If the patient has been intubated, the nurse must be alert to these possibilities to prevent tube dislocation or self-inflicted injury by the patient, and if the patient is not intubated prevention of aspiration is essential. The nurse then reevaluates any change in status to determine whether additional therapies are appropriate or whether previous interventions may be discontinued (Table 115–4). In the event that an IV line is not readily accessible, naloxone, as well as atropine, epinephrine, and lidocaine, can be administered via the endotracheal tube. Though an intravenous route is preferable, each of these agents is well absorbed from the tracheobronchial tree.

The presence of persistent CNS alteration requires attention to the possibility that toxic substances present in the gastrointestinal (GI) tract may require evacuation or adsorption to prevent further toxin absorption. Coexisting illnesses or injuries can also complicate management decisions. Consideration must be given to whether additional diagnostic studies, such as a head CT, might provide further information significant for the treatment plan. Ongoing neurologic assessment is essential.

Activated charcoal is administered by mouth in the conscious, intact patient or via the nasogastric or orogastric tube in the patient who is unable to take medications by mouth or in any patient without an intact gag reflex. Naloxone, if indicated, may be administered in bolus doses or as a continuous infusion. The nursing considerations for the most common antidotes used in the emergency setting are presented in Table 115–4. A more in-depth discussion of these agents is presented in the individual Antidotes in Depth as well as throughout the text.

Orogastric lavage is described in detail in Chap. 31 and Table 31–1. The goal is to create a siphon effect and ensure uninterrupted flow. A large enough age appropriate orogastric tube with multiple distal and lateral openings should be used. Nasogastric tubes are not adequate for overdose management (except liquids). After passage of the orogastric tube, these patients are placed in the left lateral decubitus position for administration of 0.9% NaCl solutions, drainage, and subsequent administration of activated charcoal.

Lavage tubes are now available with special ports to permit a more efficient, cleaner method of medication administration,

which is especially desirable for giving activated charcoal. Lavage tubes with preestablished bite blocks are also available if preferred. Patients who are alert and have an intact gag reflex may choose to drink the activated charcoal. Because activated charcoal is unattractive in appearance, some clinicians prefer to administer it to the patient in an opaque cup (or prepackaged opaque plastic bottle) with an opaque flexible straw. When a cup is used, it should be held away from the patient to conceal the appearance. A washcloth should be provided to wipe the patient's face when the emergency situation has passed, as activated charcoal will transiently discolor the skin. (For dosing of activated charcoal, see Chap. 31 and Table 31–2.)

Magnesium or sorbitol cathartics, although rarely indicated (see Chap. 31 and Table 31–3), may be given simultaneously with activated charcoal, and administered orally or via an orogastric or nasogastric tube. The nurse should be prepared to handle the resultant diarrhea with a bedpan and wash basin. Should the patient be discharged soon after cathartic administration, he or she should be advised to expect copious black diarrhea because of the rapid transit of activated charcoal.

During gastric decontamination, the role of the nurse includes the continuous monitoring and reassessment of the patient's clinical status, anticipating changes that might occur in response to or in spite of therapy. Verification of the initial placement of the orogastric tube as well as continued patency and accuracy of placement is essential to avoid aspiration. In lavaging children and agitated patients, additional assistance may be necessary to minimize trauma during insertion and to avoid complications that might result from the tube being dislodged from the esophagus. In general, agitated patients should not be lavaged before sedation to limit the potential trauma to the patients' upper airway and GI tract. In cases in which the patient is obtunded, endotracheal intubation may offer protection of the airway and prevent aspiration from tube displacement or posttherapy vomiting.

Even the patient with a normal level of consciousness requires continuous monitoring of vital signs and ventilatory status. Serial neurologic and pulmonary evaluation must be done and documented. Patients who are combative must be prevented from terminating any essential aspect of care prematurely.

If the patient can understand and is willing to accept a reasonable explanation for the discomfort associated with therapy, reassurance and explanation may be all that are necessary to achieve patient compliance. On the other hand, patients who are disoriented or refuse to accept a reasonable explanation for essential therapy must be protected from potential risks associated with unplanned withdrawal of therapy. It is essential that a patient whose impaired capacity to make a decision is secondary to a toxicologic effect (hypoxia, hypoglycemia, etc) not be permitted to terminate care, as it would be likely to adversely affect outcome.

Although standard precautions should be used for all patients, it is important to emphasize the measures necessary to avoid contamination from the poisoned patient. Parenteral drug use is known to be associated with a risk for both HIV infection and hepatitis. Alcohol and drug use are known to increase the risk for tuberculosis. Healthcare workers may also risk danger from exposure to toxic topical substances when decontaminating a patient (see Chap. 93 and 110).

For these reasons, the resuscitation team should apply gowns, gloves, masks, and protective eyewear before approaching the patient. Needleless devices and needles with shields or retraction devices should be used whenever possible for both drug adminis-

TABLE 115–4. Antidotes for Toxicologic Management

Antidote: **Antivenoms**

Toxin: Snake and spider envenomations

Action

Complexation and inhibition of target toxin.

Nursing considerations

Beware: High incidence of hypersensitivity reactions including urticaria, anaphylaxis, and serum sickness. Allergic reaction development is directly proportional to rate, amount, and allergenicity (ie, horse vs human) of antivenom administered. Keep diphenhydramine, epinephrine, and corticosteroids readily available. Get a good history of allergies and previous antivenom exposure. Skin testing for sensitivity before administration is controversial. Antivenom is given slowly intravenously. Initial vial should be diluted 1:10–1:100 in 0.9% sodium chloride and administered at approximately 50 mL/h. In the absence of an allergic reaction, subsequent vials may be reconstituted 1:2 or 1:4, and infusion rates may be judiciously increased and titrated to patient response/reaction. The process of reconstitution is time consuming, and the availability of the antivenom is restricted. Be sure to consider this time constraint and plan early for timely utilization.

Antidote: **Atropine**

Toxin: Acetylcholinesterase inhibitors (organic phosphorus pesticides and carbamate insecticides)

Action

Antagonist to acetylcholine; blocks muscarinic and CNS manifestations.

Nursing considerations

If patient is placed on a drip, use 20-mL vials. Hundreds of milligrams may be used in massive poisoning. Maximal oxygenation should be achieved before atropine administration to avoid risk of ventricular tachydysrhythmias associated with atropine. This may not be achievable, however, without atropine, when copious secretions and bronchospasm are present. Tachycardia is not a contraindication (may be caused by hypoxia and autonomic stimulation). Heart rate may actually slow as oxygenation improves, although increases of 10–20 beats/min are not uncommon. Has no effect on skeletal muscle weakness or paralysis. Pupillary dilation is an early response and is not a therapeutic endpoint. Glycopyrrolate (Robinul) may be substituted for atropine if the patient shows signs of CNS atropine toxicity (ie, agitation, hallucinations).

Antidote: **Calcium chloride, calcium gluconate**

Toxin: Ethylene glycol

Action

Combats systemic hypocalcemia caused when metabolism of ethylene glycol produces oxalic acid, which combines with calcium and precipitates in the brain, kidneys, etc.

Nursing considerations

Calcuim chloride is never given intramuscularly or subcutaneously. Parenteral use is IV only. Avoid extravasation of calcium preparations. Calcium gluconate is preferred. Administer slowly—rapid infusion causes vasodilation, nausea/vomiting, dysrhythmias, bradycardia, syncope, a shortened QT interval on ECG, and may cause cardiac arrest. Place patient on cardiac monitor. Monitor patient's vital signs.

Antidote: **Calcium chloride, calcium gluconate**

Toxin: Hydrofluoric acid

Action

Combats tissue destruction and hypocalcemia caused by complexation of fluoride with calcium.

Nursing considerations

Intravenous calcium considerations are as noted under ethylene glycol. For hydrofluoric dermal burns, infiltration of the affected tisssues with calcium gluconate is recommended until pain subsides. Recurrence of pain may indicate the need for additional subcutaneous or intraarterial dosing of calcium gluconate. Topical treatment of hydrofluoric acid burns is accomplished by the mixing of calcium with K-Y jelly to make a calcium paste, which is applied to the affected area. Burns of the hand may be treated by filling a surgical glove with the paste and placing it on the hand.

Antidote: **Cyanide antidote kit (amyl nitrite pearls, 3% sodium nitrite, and 25% sodium thiosulfate)**

Toxin: Cyanide

Action

Nitrite-induced methemoglobin binds with cyanide to make cyanomethemoglobin. With the addition of thiosulfate and the enzyme rhodanese, the cyanomethemoglobin is converted to methemoglobin and thiocyanate, the latter being excreted in the urine.

Nursing considerations

Check expiration dates of kit components (amyl nitrite has shortest shelf life). Sodium nitrite intravenously is preferable to the amyl nitrite for immediate use. For adults, 10 mL of a 3% sodium nitrite solution is administered intravenously, followed by 50 mL of 25% aqueous solution of sodium thiosulfate in the same line. Amyl nitrite pearls are used as an immediate measure until the IV insertion necessary for sodium nitrite. The pearls are crushed into a piece of gauze and inhaled. If IV insertion is delayed, a new amyl nitrite pearl should be used every 3 minutes because of rapid dissipation. In the case of an unconscious patient, the amyl nitrite–soaked gauze is placed in the reservoir of the bag valve mask. Maintain airway control, watch for nitrite-induced hypotension, and continue appropriate supportive therapy. Have vasopressors available. Creation of thiocyanate in the presence of renal failure may cause abdominal pain, vomiting, and CNS dysfunction, but would be rare after one or two doses. Pulse oximetry is unreliable as a measurement because of the creation of methemoglobin. Administration of 100% oxygen treats patient hypoxia and potentiates the action of antidotes. Check the package insert for dosing of nitrites in children and for those with anemia. In unclear cases, or where coexisting carboxyhemoglobinemia is suspected, thiosulfate can be administered alone without nitrites. Cyanide poisoning may be a complication of nitroprusside administration.

TABLE 115–4. Antidotes for Toxicologic Management (continued)

Antidote: **Deferoxamine**

Toxin: Iron

Action

Chelates excessive iron.

Nursing considerations

Dosing may be IM or IV depending on degree of toxicity. Severe toxicity requires intravenous dosing at 15 mg/kg/h reconstituted in D_5W, lactated Ringer solution, or normal saline to a usual maximum of 6–8 g/d. Dosing should continue as long as the patient is ill, urine remains red-orange color, but not longer than 24–36 hours. Monitor vital signs. High doses and rapid rates of infusion can cause hypotension; hypersensitivity can manifest as urticaria. Prolonged use of intravenous form may contribute to ARDS. Intramuscular dosing causes pain and induration at site. Rotate sites of injection; reconstitute until completely dissolved with 2 mL sterile water. Solution will remain stable for 1 week at room temperature. Oral dose is not FDA approved and is not recommended.

Antidote: **Dextrose**

Toxin: Hypoglycemic agents, ethanol

Action

Increase glucose availability for utilization

Nursing considerations

Should be considered for any patient with altered mental status. Whenever possible rapid bedside glucose level determination should be done. $D_{50}W$ is available in 50- to 100-mL prefilled syringes (25 g per 50 mL); a large volume and viscous, often messy, and difficult (slow) to administer. Children require more dilute solutions; 20–25% concentrations. All individuals should be given doses of 0.5–1 g/kg.

Antidote: **Digibind (digoxin-specific antibody fragments)**

Toxin: Digoxin

Action

Binds digoxin, digitoxin, and other plant or animal derived digoxinlike cardioactive steroids, effectively reducing the amount of free drug available in the circulation and allowing for excretion in the urine.

Nursing considerations

Dosing of antibodies depends on ingested dose and total body load. Each vial (38 mg) will bind 0.5 mg of digoxin. The required amount is reconstituted with 4 mL of sterile water as a bolus dose intravenously or, in more stable clinical situations, administered over 30 minutes. Children require additional dilution. Use immediately or within 4 hours if refrigerated. Monitor vital signs and cardiac rhythm! Until free digoxin levels decrease, patients may manifest nausea, vomiting, and dizziness. Cardiac abnormalities include SA node block, ventricular dysrhythmias, bradycardias, and/or ventricular tachycardias caused by reentrant excitation. Observe for potential (but rare) allergic reactions and hypokalemia.

Antidote: **Dimercaprol (British antilewisite, BAL)**

Toxin: Arsenic, lead, mercury

Action

Heavy metal chelator

Nursing considerations

Contact of drug with skin may cause reactions, and therefore, this drug must be administered by *deep* IM injection. May cause pain or abscess at injection site; rotate sites. Prolonged use of BAL may cause chelation of essential trace metals—limit use to 5-day courses. Maintaining alkaline urine may protect kidney from damage; monitor I&O. Has many adverse affects including hypertension, fever, diaphoresis, nausea, vomiting, headaches, salivation and lacrimation, and burning feeling of lips, mouth, and throat. Avoid in patients with peanut allergy (formulated in peanut oil) and G-6-PD deficiency (may cause hemolysis).

Antidote: **Fomepizole**

Toxin: Ethylene glycol, methanol

Action

Blocks alcohol dehydrogenase (ADH), which metabolizes ethylene glycol and methanol to toxic metabolites. This enzymatic blockade by fomepizole prevents the formation of the toxic metabolites responsible for patient morbidity and mortality.

Nursing considerations

Give 15 mg/kg over 30 minutes then 10mg/kg every 12 hours for 48 hours, followed by 15 mg/kg every 12 hours until ethylene glycol and methanol levels approximate zero. Fomepizole may be used as sole therapy or in conjunction with hemodialysis. If used in conjunction with hemodialysis, 15 mg/kg should be given q4h because hemodialysis eliminates the antidote as well as the toxin. Therapy should be initiated immediatedly on diagnosis. Headache, nausea, and dizziness may occur during treatment After mixing, fomepizole can be refrigerated, but room temperature storage is acceptable. Do not store undiluted in refrigerator, as undiluted fomepizole must be passively warmed in order to facilitate dilution. If refrigerated, reconstituted solution is stable for 48 hours.

(continued)

TABLE 115–4. Antidotes for Toxicologic Management (continued)

Antidote: **Glucagon**

Toxin: β-Adrenergic antagonists, calcium channel blockers

Action

Glucagon is a polypeptide hormone that stimulates the mobilization of glycogen to increase glucose levels and by increasing cyclic AMP levels in the heart. This latter action causes an increase in the inotropic and chronotropic activity of the heart, antagonizing β-adrenergic antagonist and calcium channel blocker effects on the heart.

Nursing considerations

Glucagon is packaged as a powder to be reconstituted. An initial bolus dose of 50 μg/kg of glucagon is recommended and infused over 1 minute. Additional bolus or infusion doses may be necessary. Watch for hypersensitivity, generalized allergic reactions. Nausea and vomiting can occur. Monitor cardiac status and vital signs for changes induced by inotropic and chronotropic effects. Glucagon may induce hyperglycemia and/or hypokalemia. Check electrolytes and watch for ECG changes or problems related to electrolyte shifts.

Antidote: **Methylene blue**

Toxin: Methemoglobin

Action

Methylene blue is reduced to leukomethylene, which in turn reduces methemoglobin to hemoglobin. The presence of methylene blue enhances the reduction of methemoglobin and makes it the treatment of choice.

Nursing considerations

Methemoglobin has a greater affinity for oxygen than hemoglobin and does not allow dissociation of oxygen to the tissue. Pulse oximetry is helpful in detection but is not a true measure of clinical status. Although oxygen saturation will register below normal, it often does not reflect severely toxic levels. The oxygen saturation will fall to approximately 85% but not continue to fall despite additional rise in methemoglobin levels. Arterial oxygen levels of blood gases (Po_2) are normal. Blood gases reflect measurements of partial pressure, not oxygen-carrying capacity. Do not depend on ABGs to detect hypoxemia. Do not rely on pulse oximetry to convey severity of symptoms. Give methylene blue 1% solution as soon as possible at 1–2 mg/kg, which for a 70-kg person is 70–140 mg or 7–14 mL of the 1% solution. This should be given slowly intravenously over 5 minutes. Pain at the site of infusion can be minimized with slow infusion and by following with a flush of saline. The patient's urine will become greenish blue. Pulse oximetry measurement will fall abruptly and then should improve.

Antidote: ***N*-Acetylcysteine (NAC, Mucomyst)**

Toxin: Acetaminophen

Action

Detoxifies metabolite (enhances glutathione synthesis) early and mediates inflammatory response late (>24h) after ingestion.

Nursing considerations

Unpleasant odor. Shold be diluted to a 5% concentration from a 20% solution by mixing 1 part 20% NAC solution and 3 parts diluent (ie, water, fruit juice, or carbonated beverage). Must be used within 1 hour of dilution. After opening, can be stored in refrigerator for 96 hours. Repeat dose if vomiting occurs within 1 hour of administration. May try antiemetic (metoclopramide or a serotonin antagonist such as ondansetron) or NG tube for persistent vomiting. If repeat dose of activated charcoal is indicated for a coingestant, separate by at least 1–2 hours. Although not FDA approved, the oral dose can be administered as IV *N*-acetylcysteine in extreme cases (see dosing schedule in Chap. 32).

Antidote: **Naloxone**

Toxin: Opioids

Action

Competes with opioids at the receptor sites; reverses respiratory depressant effects and improves blood pressure and CNS manifestations.

Nursing considerations

Patients withdrawing from opioids exhibit nausea, vomiting, agitation, restlessness, diaphoresis, abdominal pain, and piloerection. Careful attention must be paid to issues of airway protection and patient safety. Concentrations of naloxone may vary with manufacturer. Available also in neonatal concentration, but this preparation has no use in the ED for treatment of drug overdoses. Prepackaged bolus doses containing 2 mg facilitate rapid titration from 0.05 to 2.0 mg in opioid-dependent patients and is an appropriate dose for the management of the suspected opioid overdose.

Antidote: **Octreotide**

Toxin: Oral hypoglycemic agents

Action

Suppresses the release of endogenous insulin stores. It is especially useful in treating hypoglycemia caused by agents that stimulate the release of endogenous insulin such as the sulfonylureas.

Nursing considerations

May be given subcutaneously or intravenously. For subcutaneous administration, 50 μg every 6 hours is recommended for adults. Children's dose of 4–5 μg/kg/d (up to 50 μg) should be administered in divided doses every 6 hours. Subcutaneous administration sites should be rotated. For intravenous administration, dilute octreotide in sterile 0.9% NaCl or dextrose and infuse over 15–30 minutes or administer IV bolus over 3 minutes. Patients may experience stinging at the IV site, which rarely lasts more than 15 minutes. Gastrointestinal symptoms include nausea, abdominal pain, and diarrhea. Octreotide should be refrigerated for prolonged storage but it is stable at room temperature for 14 days as long as it is protected from light. Octreotide should be administered at room temperature. Refrigerated ampules should be passively rewarmed before administration.

(continued)

TABLE 115–4. **Antidotes for Toxicologic Management (continued)**

Antidote: **Physostigmine salicylate**

Toxin: Anticholinergics (eg, antihistamines, atropine, scopolamine, and some plants and mushrooms)

Action

Reverses coma, seizures, and severe myoclonic and choreoathetoid activity from anticholinergic agents.

Nursing considerations

Use only clear, colorless solutions. IM route is unacceptable because of erratic absorption. Establish airway, ventilation, and hemodynamic stabilization first. Patient should have a narrow QRS complex on both ECG and current monitor strip. Excessive use or too rapid administration may cause SLUDGE, bronchorrhea, seizures, bradycardia, and respiratory depression. Have atropine on hand, equal to one-half the dose of physostigmine given, to reverse cholinergic activity.

Antidote: **Pralidoxime chloride (2-PAM-chloride, Protopam)**

Toxin: Acetylcholinesterase inhibitors (organic phosphorus pesticides and carbamate insecticides)

Action

Restores acetylcholinesterase activity and detoxifies remaining organic phosphorus molecules.

Nursing considerations

Protect the airway! After regaining consciousness, patients may become agitated. Transient dizziness and blurred vision may be related to the rate of infusion. Avoid rapid IV bolus; respiratory and cardiac arrest may occur. Reduce rate or stop infusion if hypotension occurs. Rarely used alone. Works synergistically with atropine. Avoid dermal contact with the patient to avoid pesticide self-contamination. Wash all dermal areas exposed to pesticides with copious amounts of water. Wear protective clothing (gloves, gown). Dispose of contaminated clothing and leather.

Antidote: **Sodium bicarbonate**

Toxin: Amantadine, carbamazepine, chlorphenoxy herbicides, chlorpropamide, cocaine, encainide, flecainide, methotrexate, phenobarbital, phenothiazines, procainamide, propoxyphene, quinidine, salicylates, and tricyclic antidepressants

Action

By reversing Na channel blockade $NaHCO_3$ treats the widened QRS seen on ECG in amantadine, carbamazepime, cocaine, encainide, flecainide, phenothiazines, procainamide, propoxyphene, quinidine, salicylates, and tricyclic antidepressants. For chlorphenoxy herbicides, chlorpropamide, formic acid derived from methanol, methotrexate, phenobarbital, and salicylates, alkalinization facilitates ion trapping and enhances urinary elimination of these drugs.

Nursing considerations

Give 1–2 mEq/kg of sodium bicarbonate as a bolus. Place two or three ampules (88–132 mEq) of sodium bicarbonate in 1 L of D_5W. IV should run at 1.5–2 times the maintenance fluid range (alkalinizes serum and urine). Alkalemia, hypokalemia, and decreased ionized calcium occur with bicarbonate therapy. Monitor pH (blood and urine) and electrolytes closely and replace as needed. Maintain serum pH between 7.50 and 7.55. Maintain urine pH at 7.5–8.0. Observe patient's neurologic status. Hyperosmolarity, hypernatremia, and paradoxic CSF acidosis may occur. Give patients supplemental oxygen to decrease tissue hypoxia. Sodium bicarbonate causes precipitation of calcium salts and may inactivate catecholamines. Use separate IV access.

Antidote: **Thiamine hydrochloride**

Toxin: Alcohol, alcoholism/malnutrition

Action

Facilitates aerobic metabolism of glucose to produce ATP; links glycolysis to the Krebs cycle. Also has a role in maintaining normal neuronal conduction.

Nursing considerations

Given in conjunction with $D_{50}W$ to treat or to avoid development of Wernicke encephalopathy in adults and adolescents. Thiamine is not routinely administered to children unless they are malnourished.

Antidote: **Vitamin K₁ (mephyton, aquamephyton)**

Toxin: Anticoagulants (warfarin, superwarfarins)

Action

Required for blood clotting; reverses anticoagulant deficiency and is indicated for long-term control of bleeding due to vitamin K deficiency.

Nursing considerations

Unless a patient is critically ill, give by other means than IV route; IV route may cause anaphylactoid reaction and in rare instances death. Dilute only in D_5W, 0.9% NaCl or D_5 0.9% NaCl, or D_5NS preservative-free solutions and infuse slowly to decrease risk of anaphylactoid reactions. Use oral preparations for long-term care. Restrict volume of SC doses to 5 mL per site. Avoid IM administration to avoid hematoma formation. Onset of action is slow, even following IV administration.

(continued)

tration and any arterial or venous puncture. Irrigation and lavage equipment with splashguards should be considered.

RESTRAINING THE AGITATED PATIENT

Increased public awareness of patient's rights and a heightened sensitivity toward the appropriate use of restraints have been promoted by HCFA, JCAHO, and other credentialing bodies. Their efforts have led to the development of specific restraint and seclusion guidelines that became effective January 1, 2001, which urge all practitioners to make every effort to avoid unnecessary restraint use. The standards do support the emergency use of chemical and physical restraints to prevent a patient from harming her- or himself or others. In these cases, the patient must be a danger to himself or another and not aware of his illness or the ramifications of his actions. Restraints, physical or chemical, may never be used as a method of coercion, threat, or restriction of a competent patient's wishes, even if the ultimate outcome might be adverse.

Overdosed or poisoned patients who have an altered level of consciousness, who become agitated and uncooperative, or who exhibit violent behavior as a result of poisoning often require the application of physical restraints until their condition stabilizes and they are capable of understanding the value of essential interventions (see Chap. 118). All efforts at verbal reassurance, using staff members who may have developed a rapport with the patient, must be employed. If this fails, and the impaired patient continues to refuse and thwart important care, physical restraint may be necessary as a primary therapy or until chemical restraint can be administered safely. Basic patient care objectives are to protect the patient from self-injury and to protect others from injury by the patient. Restraints should be used only when there is absolutely no other alternative, and the least restrictive method that assures safety should be employed. The decision to physically restrain a patient must be made only after all other attempts at calming the patient have failed and there is a true threat to patient (pulling out an intravenous line or endotracheal tube) or staff safety. A conscientious humane interaction may help to defuse a potentially volatile situation, allowing the patient to maintain some control in his or her care. A skilled interviewer must recognize the patient's feelings of powerlessness, fear, misunderstanding, and, in some cases, embarrassment or anger. Identifying these feelings while describing your understanding of the patient's personal needs and offering to provide information to allay the patient's concerns are often helpful.

If the patient continues to pose a threat to himself or herself or others, the clinician must impose limits and inform the patient that such behavior cannot be tolerated. It may be suggested that the patient's inability to maintain a peaceful and cooperative demeanor may necessitate the summoning of "a specially trained crisis group" that will assist in regaining control. At this point, sometimes the mere presence of an organized group of individuals will help the patient rethink his or her behavior and reestablish self-control. If all of these measures fail, and physical restraint becomes necessary, clear, objective documentation of the events leading to physical restraint must be entered in the chart. Knowledge of certain toxidromes will alert the clinician to substances that increase the likelihood for violent behavior. The patient's medical condition, including alertness, orientation, and thought process, should be noted, along with a detailed description of the measures used to secure the patient's cooperation before the application of physical restraints. A physician's written order must be present on the chart. In an emergency situation a verbal order may be acceptable as an interim measure. However, a physician (or licensed practitioner) must evaluate the patient and write an order for the physical restraint within 1 hour of the initiation of the intervention. Less restrictive methods such as mittens should be considered, and the approach documented as inappropriate or ineffective, before limb or chemical restraints are used. Because all inappropriate patients" have the right to be free from restraints of any form that are not medically necessary or are used as a means of coercion, discipline, convenience, or retaliation,..." practitioners must document the absolute need, all prior less restrictive attempts, and an ongoing assessment to achieve release of restraint in the continuing nursing care.

Clinical staff and security personnel expected to participate as members of the restraint team should be given formal training in technique and philosophy. This preparation allows for clear definition and understanding of roles and responsibilities before mobilization for crisis intervention. A team approach to the application of restraints, with a team leader in control, is essential. If possible, a team of five staff members should be gathered. Each of the first four is responsible for securing one extremity, while the fifth, who assumes the role of leader, is positioned at the patient's head. The team leader's role is critical and should be assumed by the staff member most experienced in crisis intervention techniques and restraint application.

In approaching the patient requiring restraint, it is important to ensure that all potentially dangerous items such as keys, shoes, pens, pins, and stethoscopes are removed from the patient's immediate accessibility. The team leader should secure the patient's head by grasping the forehead with one hand and securing the chin with the other (Fig. 115–1). This immobilizes the patient's head, minimizing the leverage he or she gains by lifting the head, shoulders, and chest. The leader should speak calmly to the patient, explaining the necessity for the procedure and requesting the patient's help.

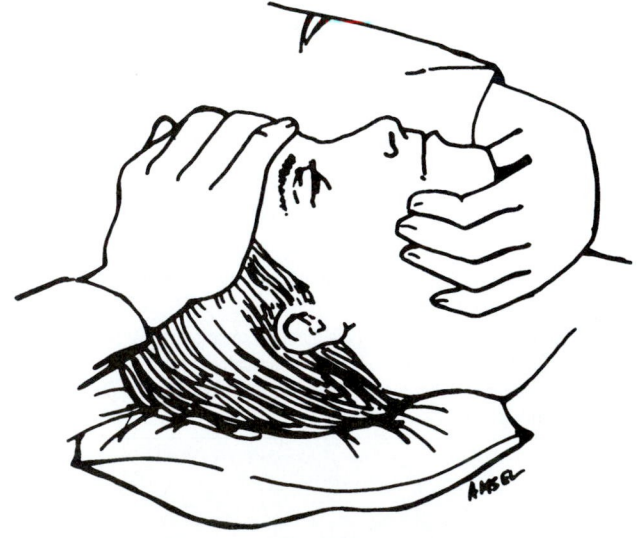

Figure 115–1.   Appropriate approach by the team leader to secure the patient's head by grasping the forehead with one hand and securing the chin with the other. (Universal precautions should be utilized at all times.)

The other members must be agile, clear as to strategy, and firm in their approach. The team members' strength is not as important as proper hand placement and technique. The limb should be grasped securely, with one hand just above the joint and one hand immediately below, so as to immobilize elbows and knees in extension, thus restricting movement (Fig. 115–2). Pressure directly on the joint should be avoided, as it is painful, may cause injury, and will initiate a response from the patient that may inhibit successful restraint. The restraints should be applied sequentially, starting with the upper extremities, so that the other limbs remain well immobilized while each is being restrained. The lower extremities are bound together to create three-point restraint. Initiating restraint with the arms prevents the patient from attempting to vault off the stretcher with only his or her feet restrained and potentially incurring head and facial trauma. If a sixth team member is available, he or she may apply the restraints while the others continue to secure the limbs. Otherwise, the team leader should identify which limb to restrain and direct specific team members to assist each other. The team leader should take note of any individual who is unable to control his or her assigned limb, necessitating additional assistance. Throughout this effort, the team leader should constantly reassure the patient in a calm, firm manner and maintain a secure hold on the patient's head and chin.

Many institutions continue to use metal or leather restraints. These restraints increase the risk of injury to a patient's extremities, particularly in an emergency situation. Although some institutions prefer to use lamb's wool and roller gauze, in the setting of the ED, this method is acceptable only as an interim measure, as this form of restraint is not secure enough to sustain continued, safe control of the agitated patient. The use of cloth restraints with padded centers allows for both flexibility and security without patient injury. A hitch knot[1] should be slipped over the extremity, but direct pressure should not be placed over any joint (Fig. 115–3). The ends of each restraint should be securely fastened to a nonmovable part of the stretcher with a slip knot, which allows rapid removal of the restraint if necessary. The loose ends of each restraint must be tucked under the mattress, well out of reach of the patient (Fig. 115–4).

After the restraints are secured (Fig. 115–5), each limb should be checked for discoloration and any compromise of pulse and capillary refill. The clinician must be able to place two fingers easily under the restraint, assuring that circulation is not impaired. At no time should the patient's face, mouth, or neck be covered or restrained in any manner under any circumstances. In addition, restraint of the chest is not recommended, as it may impair respirations.

The patient should be told why the restraints were applied and what change in behavior is expected to allow him or her to regain independent responsibility and minimize the length of time that the restraints are required.

Once the environment is made safer for the patient and staff, chemical restraint should be considered. Patients under the influence of drugs and/or alcohol are often incapable of making critical decisions and controlling behavior. Chemical restraint with the use of intravenous benzodiazepines in situations where these agents are not contraindicated will help reestablish a calm, safe environment and minimize the complications of tachycardia and hyperthermia associated with hyperactivity (see Chap. 67 and 72).

A note should be made in the patient's chart that three-point restraints were applied because of a specific patient behavior. The patient's initial response to the intervention and current condition must be noted. Continued observation must then be part of the care plan. The restraints should be checked on a periodic basis to assure that the patient remains protected, that essential clinical needs are being met, and that circulation and pulse remain intact. Each periodic reassessment requires documentation to validate the need for continued physical restraint and why the therapy cannot as yet be terminated.

Patients presenting with altered levels of consciousness often arrive with concomitant trauma, compartment syndromes, and/or decubiti secondary to their prior immobility. Accurate observation and intervention to prevent further injury are essential, especially in cases where restraint may further immobilize the patient. The documentation of preexistent conditions will prevent misallocation of responsibility.

A restraint flow sheet should be developed to satisfy documentation requirements and to serve as a clinical reminder to fulfill the patients' basic personal needs at regular intervals. A regularly scheduled systematic retrospective review of the data with corrective recommendations should be part of the ED's Quality Performance Program.

If data secured during treatment suggest any suspicion of self-destructive or suicidal behavior, the patient should be placed on a 1:1 suicide watch until further psychiatric evaluation can be accomplished. This level of care requires that the individual be placed under the direct observation of one staff member, who then documents on an hourly basis (at a minimum) the patient's behavior, comments, and actions. A full psychiatric evaluation should be

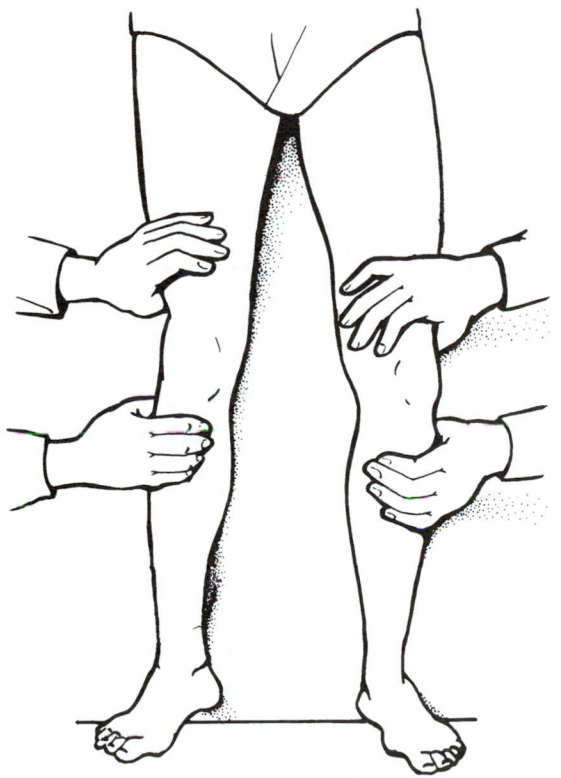

Figure 115–2. Appropriate approach to limb restraint, using one hand just proximal and one hand just distal to the joint. This immobilizes both elbows and knees in extension and effectively restricts movement. (Universal precautions should be utilized at all times.)

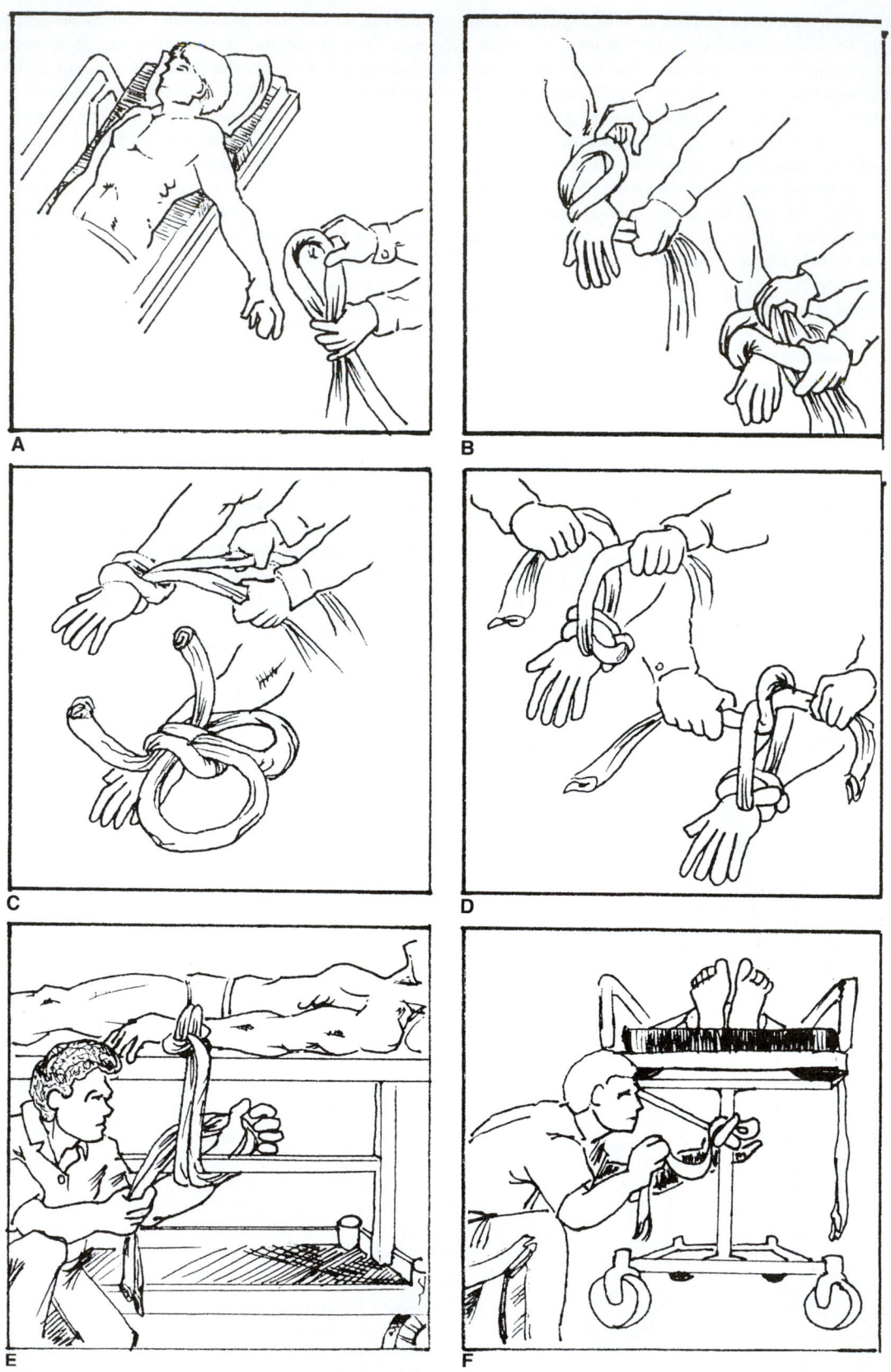

Figure 115–3. Restraints must have a padded center. A hitch knot is slipped over the extremity. The sequence of securing the extremity applies no direct pressure over the joint. (Universal precautions should be utilized at all times.)

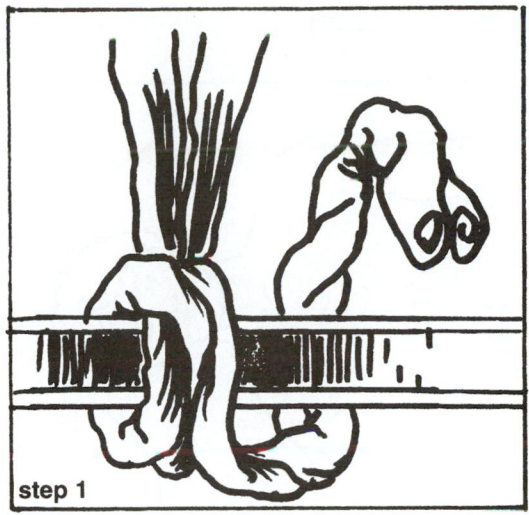

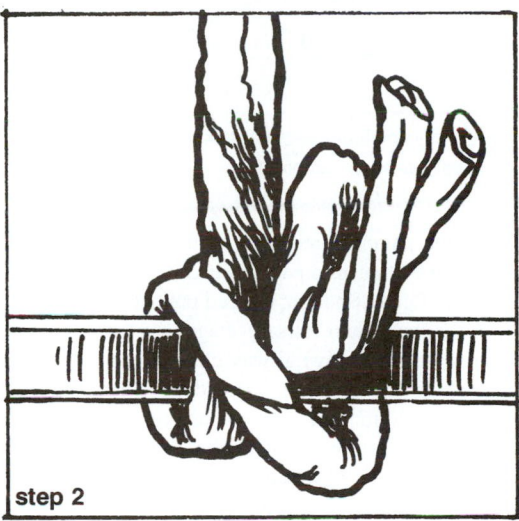

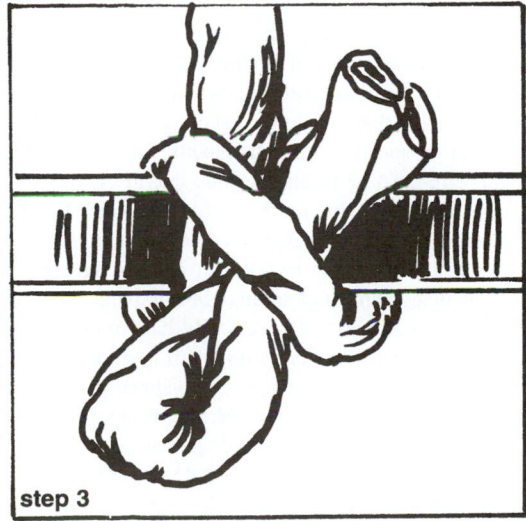

Figure 115–4. The technique for applying a slip knot. The ends of the restraint are securely fastened to a nonmovable part of the stretcher with a slip knot so that rapid removal can be accomplished. All loose ends must be tucked under the mattress, out of the patient's reach.

done as soon as the patient is alert and cooperative enough to answer questions and discuss the events leading up to hospitalization (see Chap. 114). Removal of the patient's clothing and property and dressing the patient in a hospital gown may also act as a deterrent to patient elopement.

DISPOSITION: ACUTE AND LONG TERM

Continued reassessment of the patient's condition yields information that will constitute the nursing documentation of the patient's ongoing status and ultimate disposition. The nurse must begin planning for disposition at a very early stage in the patient's care. Immediately following the acute phase of intervention, attention must be given to notification of the individual's family. In the case of a patient who is responsible for the care of children, careful consideration must be made as to the children's safety and welfare. In the case of a substance-using parent, the social services staff must be notified to assure an immediate home assessment and followup after patient hospitalization (see Chap. 113). The patient's property must be secured and protected, even if the patient is not admitted. Caution must be exercised while undressing patients. Searching pockets and property may result in exposure to dangerous items such as needles, syringes, knives, razor blades, and drugs, which pose a threat to staff safety. Gloves should always be worn, and dangerous items should be turned over to security personnel.

Familiarity with the pattern of toxicologic symptoms allows the nurse to suspect a likely toxin. Consideration of the clinical manifestations of the particular substance(s) allows the nurse to anticipate not only ongoing care needs but also those that will affect the patient at the time of discharge.

Patients not requiring medical admission to the hospital must be alert and communicative before psychiatric consultation is recommended. Referral sources for rehabilitation of substance users should be available. Finally, clear, concise, specific discharge instructions must be given to the patient. Details of these instructions must be noted, and a signature indicating patient understanding must be entered on the chart. In many cases, duplicate instruction sheets are used to minimize omissions and standardize the individual effort. A copy is given to the patient for reference on discharge, and a signed copy attached to the permanent record. This level of documentation is particularly important in verifying the patient's capacity to understand, especially in a previously impaired patient. This documentation is important not only from a medical-legal point of view but also from a quality management perspective.

DISCHARGE INSTRUCTIONS

Each patient to be discharged should have individualized instructions. Considerations when giving the instructions include the patient's level of comprehension from a healthcare, cultural, and linguistic perspective. The same level of understanding is necessary of the caregiver's level of comprehension, if the patient's care is to be entrusted to another. Social factors such as whether the patient has a home, whether the patient is pregnant, whether the patient is responsible for living children, and, if so, whether he or she is able to provide necessary care, must be considered in the discharge plan. Before release from the institution, the patient must

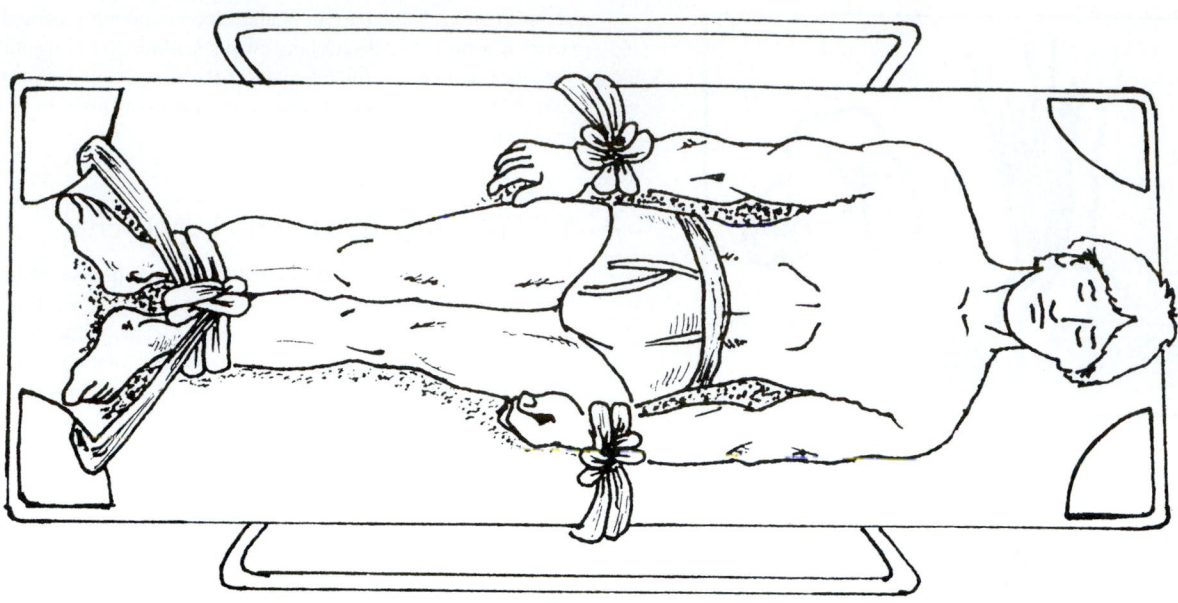

Figure 115–5.   When the restraints are secured, each limb must be checked for discoloration and any compromise of pulse and capillary refill. The clinician must be able to place two fingers under the restraint. The patient's face, mouth, and neck must not be covered or restrained.

be provided with clothing appropriate for the weather through family contact or, in some institutions, through the support of social services. Instruction with regard to poison prevention must be given both verbally and in written format. This is paramount, especially in cases where poisoning was unintentional. Followup must be arranged and stressed with the patient and caregiver. Hospital-based performance improvement assurance mechanisms for recall must be in place and readily activated in the event that the patient fails to follow up as instructed. All teaching issues should be rediscussed with the patient at the time of discharge. Questions addressed during an earlier phase of treatment, when the patient may have had an altered sensorium, must be readdressed to assure understanding. Psychiatric consultation is essential before discharge in any case where personal destructive behavior is suspected. In cases of drug or alcohol abuse, referral should be available for outpatient drug or alcohol treatment; it should be recommended, and its utilization facilitated.

DOCUMENTATION

Staffing deficiencies, particularly in EDs, have made ongoing documentation extremely difficult, especially when patients remain many hours before a final disposition. The use of checklists optimizes continued periodic documentation and minimizes the need for extensive, detailed notes.

EVALUATION OF THE POISONED PATIENT AND THE QUALITY OF CARE RENDERED

The evaluation of care entails an appraisal not only of the nursing care received by the patient but also of the overall quality of care. The assessment of the patient's physical and emotional status and

evaluation of the patient's response to the nursing care plan are measured in terms of desired patient outcomes, based on an established standard of care. Specific desired patient outcomes can also be based on the individual nursing diagnoses (see Table 115–2). For a diagnosis of ineffective airway clearance, the expected outcome of effective gas exchange would be evidenced by a Po_2 value greater than 80 mm Hg on room air, for example. In altered tissue perfusion, the presence of strong palpable pulses demonstrates adequate circulatory function. Ongoing reassessment of the patient's vital signs and neurologic status is essential to evaluate the patient's response to therapy.

The second part of the process, evaluation of the overall quality of care, is an assessment of the nurse's adherence to the care plan and to the nursing standard of care. Regulatory agencies mandate that written care plans and measurable nursing standards be developed and that adherence to the established standard be documented in both prospective and retrospective audits. To meet this requirement, care must be taken to ensure that the standard of care is meaningful and reasonable for the staff nurse. Once the standard guidelines have been established, an evaluation tool should be generated to test whether or not the set criteria have been met. This quality management program may be complex.

Emergency patients do not necessarily have a clearly defined diagnosis. Many patients present with an array of complaints, and others are unable to give any history. A poisoned patient may initially have to be placed into a more generic category such as "altered mental status," until a specific diagnosis is confirmed. This problem-oriented approach may necessitate multiple interventions to define the appropriate management strategy.

The ED is always an environment with unpredictable demands. Few options are available such as ambulance diversion, or supplemental staff to bring order out of chaos when overcrowding occurs. The variation in occupancy of the ED as well as patient acuity greatly affects the quality and thoroughness of patient care given. When a care plan or standard is established, it must be flex-

NURSING CHART AUDIT
EMERGENCY DEPARTMENT TREATMENT—ADULT
GENERAL ADULT TREATMENT

PRIORITIES AND EXAMINATION
- ☐ Checked patient for ABCs
- ☐ Cleared airway and ventilated with BVM if not breathing or severe respiratory depression
- ☐ C-spine immobilzed if indicated
- ☐ ET tube inserted if CNS depression makes it tolerable
- ☐ Nasal O_2 if patient is awake but lethargic
- ☐ IV established
- ☐ History (from patient, family, friends) obtained if possible

- ☐ Nursing assessment performed - head to toe
  1. Vital signs (BP _____ P _____ RR _____ T _____)
  2. Neurologic check: verbal and motor response, pupils
  3. Evidence of head trauma
  4. Odor of breath
  5. Neck evaluation for tenderness, trauma, venous distension, tracheal position
  6. Chest evaluation—breath sounds, chest rise, sign of injury
  7. Abdominal evaluation—appearance, tenderness, bowel sounds and masses
  8. Extremities—movement, sensation, color, pulses, skin temperature, capillary refill, puncture marks, scars, deformities
- ☐ Bloods drawn for CBC, electrolytes, glucose, toxicology tests, and ABGs
- ☐ Urine obtained for toxicology screen (rare use)

IMMEDIATE TREATMENT
- ☐ Orders written by MD and signed by RN
- ☐ 100 mL of $D_{50}W$ IV
- ☐ Naloxone 0.05–2.0 mg IV (given first if opioid suspected)

- ☐ Thiamine 100 mg IV
- ☐ Seizures controlled with diazepam/other agents if indicated

REMOVING INGESTANTS (when indicated)
- ☐ Ipecac 30 mL followed by several glasses of water (unless contraindicated) for awake patient (rare use)

- ☐ Cuffed endotracheal intubation followed by lavage with saline via orogastric tube if patient is obtunded, comatose, or lacks a gag reflex

ADSORPTION OF INGESTANTS AFTER (OR IN PLACE OF) EMESIS OR LAVAGE
- ☐ Oral activated charcoal. 1.0 g/kg or 10 x the amount of drug, if quanity known (whichever is greater)

CATHARSIS
- ☐ Sorbitol 70%, 50 mL: magnesium citrate, 10 oz. or magnesium sulfate 30 g, if indicated

- ☐ SPECIFIC ANTIDOTES INDICATED AND GIVEN?

- ☐ INTAKE MONITORED–IV, PO, NG?

- ☐ OUTPUT MONITORED–URINE, EMESIS (LAVAGE), STOOL?

CONSULTATION
- ☐ Psychiatry called
- ☐ Social services called
- ☐ Poison Center called
- ☐ Medical toxicologist called

DISPOSITION
- ☐ Treated and released in <24 h
- ☐ Treated and released in >24 h
- ☐ Transferred to psychiatric unit
- ☐ Admitted
- ☐ Other

FOLLOW-UP PLAN
- ☐ Medical
- ☐ Psychiatric
- ☐ Social Services

DISCHARGE INSTRUCTIONS—IF INDICATED
- ☐ Specific instructions documented
- ☐ Documentation of patient understanding

COMMENTS

CHART NUMBER _____ DATE OF VISIT _____

Figure 115–6. Example of a retrospective chart audit.

ible enough to be useful and valid whether the ED is peaceful or exceedingly busy, and it must be independent of the patient's severity of illness.

Many patient interventions must be accomplished in a relatively brief period of time. Outcome is often measured by an analysis of short-term goals. In many hospitals, however, admitted patients may be delayed for prolonged periods of time in the ED or kept in observation units. Under these circumstances, newly developed distinct standards may become appropriate.

Because emergent patients continually arrive without warning, achieving a standard such as the measurement of vital signs every 4 hours becomes a difficult task. However, a standard should not simply be monitored. A mechanism must also be established whereby noncompliance can be addressed and corrective actions implemented. Once corrective actions are initiated, their effectiveness must also be evaluated. Not only must standards be flexible and measurable, but also the personnel responsible for initiating corrective actions must have the ultimate authority with the staff for interpreting and implementing the standard in the plan of care.

Finally, the principles of the standardized care plan (suggested in Table 115–1) must be routinely assessed and reevaluated. This audit analyzes both the conscious and unconscious patient in a sin-gle plan. We believe that the standard quality management project should be as simple as possible without compromising standards. This allows staff participation in the project to be less tedious while serving as a positive personal learning experience.

By use of this chart audit, a threshold for performance can be established. Any value falling below this threshold requires further evaluation because the established standard of care is not as yet achieved. Specific objective criteria should be developed for each problematic area; the data collected can then be evaluated, and corrective action initiated. Constant reevaluation should continue until the threshold is met. Figure 115–6 is suggested as an objective retrospective chart audit.

ACKNOWLEDGMENT

The graphics for this chapter were done by William P. Callaghan.

REFERENCE

1. Cassidy J: The Klutz Book of Knots: How to tie the world's 25 most useful hitches, ties, wraps, and knots. Palo Alto, CA: Klutz Press, 1989.

CHAPTER 116 POISON INFORMATION CENTERS AND POISON EPIDEMIOLOGY

Robert S. Hoffman

HISTORY

In 1950, the American Academy of Pediatrics created a Committee on Accident Prevention in order to explore methods to reduce injuries in young children. A subsequent survey by that committee demonstrated that injuries resulting from unintentional poisoning were a significant cause of childhood morbidity. Simultaneously came the realizations that a source of reliable information on the active ingredients of common household agents was lacking and that there were few accepted methods for treating poisoned patients. In response to this void, the first poison information center was created in Chicago in 1953.[53] Although initially designed to provide information to healthcare providers, both the popularity and the success of this center stimulated a poison information center movement, which rapidly spread across the country. The myriad of new poison information centers not only offered product content information to healthcare providers but also began to offer first aid and prevention information to members of the community.

Approximately 40 years have passed, and in that short time, countless achievements have been realized by a relatively small group of remarkably altruistic individuals. Many of these legislative and educational accomplishments, which are chronicled in Chapter 1, have directly reduced the incidence and severity of poisoning in all age groups.[52,56,58] Concurrently, the number, configuration, and specific role of poison information centers has shifted in response to public and professional needs.[21,61] Regional centers are staffed by highly trained and certified health professionals who are assisted by extensive information systems. Support is provided by 24-hour access to board-certified medical toxicologists and consultants from all disciplines of medicine as well as from industry.

The poison information center of today is charged with many of the same mandates as the original centers. These responsibilities include maintaining a database, providing information to public and health professionals, collecting epidemiologic data on the incidence and severity of poisoning, preventing unnecessary hospitalizations following exposure, and educating healthcare professionals on the diagnosis and treatment of poisoning. This chapter explores some of these critical roles and offers a vision of the future.

MAINTAINING A DATABASE ON PRODUCT CONTENTS AND POISON MANAGEMENT

The first toxicology database created in the United States was a set of cumbersome 5" × 8" index cards produced in the 1950s by the United States National Clearinghouse of Poison Control Centers.[53] When it grew to include more than 16,000 cards, the sheer volume of space required to store this information, as well as the extensive time it took to hand-search through these cards, created the necessity of a central repository, such as a poison information center. The quantity of information continued to grow in concert with a rapid expansion of information technology, and the unwieldy index card database was privatized and transformed into microfiche. Even though this source was substantially smaller, specialized equipment was still required, and searching remained time consuming. Numerous encyclopedic and clinical textbooks were written to supplement the database and provide resources for the office or the bedside. With the growth of the computer age and the Internet, the product known as Poisindex took hold as the major source of data on the contents of innumerable household and industrial products, drugs, and plant and animal toxins. Poisindex also provides unified management strategies for many potentially toxic exposures.

With this evolution of information technology, poison information centers are no longer perceived as the sole guardians of toxicology information. Although these services are still essential for the public at large, and those professionals away from their computers, a predictable decline in poison center utilization has paralleled this growth in availability of information. A 1991 study in Utah demonstrated that 82.6% of emergency physicians who had Poisindex available in their institution often did not consult the poison information center.[9] A similar 1994 New York State study suggested that 76% of physicians who had Poisindex in their emergency departments perceived that this decreased their own use of their poison information center.[59]

Superficially, it might seem that this is an acceptable trend in that it allows poison information centers to be more available to those individuals who do not have access to the information. However, this practice not only undermines the efforts of poison infor-

1747

mation centers to gather epidemiologic data (see below), it also creates an understanding gap. In other words, the interpretation of the data may be more essential than the data itself. For example, some commonly used sources of toxicology information such as the *Physicians' Desk Reference (PDR)* and material safety data sheets (MSDS) occasionally provide information that is frankly inaccurate, potentially misleading, or significantly limited.[25,50] There may be similar limitations with regard to wider access to Poisindex. For example, consider the case of a clinician caring for a lethargic child whose only medication is Zantac syrup. After the other causes of altered mental status have been excluded, the clinician considers drug toxicity. Consultation with references suggests that altered consciousness would not be expected with use of this medication. However, a certified poison information specialist at a regional poison center recognized the potential for drug error and had the physician review the syrup bottle in question and call the pharmacy where the drug was provided. Although the prescription was written for Zantac (ranitidine), the bottle actually contained Zyrtec syrup (cetirizine).

Thus, although originally designed as providers of information, poison information centers must now be considered valued consultants, with staff who not only provide content information but also interpret clinical material and link both to appropriate management strategies. This goal is achieved only through rigorous training and certification criteria designed to provide a valued interaction with healthcare professionals.[2] Another illustrative example of the value of poison information centers can be drawn from the use of flumazenil for benzodiazepine overdose (see Chap. 63). Although it may easily be determined by anyone capable of using an index that flumazenil is an antidote for benzodiazepine overdoses, many subtle characteristics of the patient or the overdose often contraindicate its use. A prospective study determined that when flumazenil was used before consultation with the poison information center, it was used despite the presence of contraindications in 10/14 (71%) cases, resulting in one serious adverse event.[8] In the study mentioned earlier, although physicians with access to Poisindex were less likely to call the poison information center, 86.7% still felt that using the poison information center to gain access to a physician toxicologist was a valued resource.[9] Current efforts are under way to link poison information centers with centers for poison treatment (CPT), which are healthcare facilities that can provide both bedside consultation and unique diagnostic and therapeutic interventions for a subset of patients with severe or complex poisoning.[1] Preliminary data suggest that direct bedside consultation and care help reduce length of hospital stay and healthcare costs.[15]

COLLECTING POISON EPIDEMIOLOGY DATA

Recent data demonstrate that poisoning is the third leading cause of injury-related fatalities, ranking behind motor vehicle crash and firearm use.[22] Understanding the evolving trends in poisoning is essential to the development of enhanced surveillance, prevention, and education programs designed to reduce unintentional poisoning. Although data can be analyzed from numerous sources such as death certificates, hospital discharge coding records, and poison information centers, it is essential to recognize the biases that are inherent in each of these reports (see Chap. 120). Because not all

significant poisoning results in either hospitalization or fatality, data from poison information centers appear to offer a unique perspective.

Unfortunately, the term "poisoning" is often defined differently and therefore may be confusing. For the purposes of this text, "poisoning" is any exposure to a drug, toxin, chemical, or naturally occurring substance that results in injury. Yet the data collected and disseminated by poison information centers is limited to exposures.[38–47] Many exposures are of no consequence because of the properties of the substance involved, the magnitude or duration of the exposure, or confusion about whether an actual exposure has occurred; therefore, data collected by poison information centers are inherently flawed.

The situation is further confounded by multiple biases that are introduced by the reporting process itself. To begin with, reporting is voluntary. Because the majority of calls concern self-reported data that come from the home and are never subsequently confirmed, large statistical errors can be introduced into the database. A significant percentage of existing data may actually represent potential or possible exposures. Also, current events, hoaxes, and media awareness campaigns all may influence self-reporting rates. Additionally, in order to report, a caller must have a telephone and probably speak English. Although telecommunications devices for the hearing impaired and translation services exist, they are rarely used.

When hospitals report to the poison center, a comparison of the hospital chart with the poison center record shows good agreement.[30] Unfortunately, a reporting bias similar to that described above is well recognized with regard to professional utilization of poison information centers and has been called the "Pollyanna phenomenon."[26] For example, in the spring of 1995, poison centers in the northeast United States began to receive numerous reports of severe psychomotor agitation and other manifestations of anticholinergic syndrome in heroin users. In the beginning, most of these calls were for help in establishing a diagnosis, determining possible etiologic agents, and questions regarding treatment with physostigmine.[27] Although the epidemic continued for many months, once the media announced that the heroin supply was tainted with scopolamine, and clinicians became familiar with the indications and administration of physostigmine, calls began to taper off. Stated simply, healthcare professionals are less likely to call the poison information center regarding issues with which they are familiar, are of little clinical consequence, or are not recognized as being related to a poison. Thus, a bias is introduced that results in overreporting of new and serious events and underreporting of the familiar or very common, the extremely rare and unrecognized, and the inconsequential. Numerous comparisons support this contention.

Fatal Poisoning

A 4-year study compared deaths from poisoning reported to the Rhode Island Medical Examiner with those reported to the area poison information center.[37] Not surprisingly, the Medical Examiner reported many more deaths: 369 compared to 45 reported by the poison information center. Although the majority of the cases not reported to the poison information center were victims who died at home, were pronounced dead on arrival to the hospital, or those in whom poisoning was not suspected until the postmortem analysis, 79 unreported fatalities were admitted to the hospital with a suspected poisoning. In 10 of these cases, the authors concluded that a toxicology consultation might have altered the outcome. Examples of interventions that, if recommended and performed, might have resulted in a more favorable outcome included the proper use of antidotes such as naloxone, *N*-acetylcysteine for acetaminophen poisoning, the cyanide antidote kit, sodium bicarbonate for a tricyclic antidepressant overdose, and hyperbaric oxygen for carbon monoxide as well as hemoperfusion for a theophylline overdose and hemodialysis for a lithium overdose. Similarly, when medical examiner data were analyzed in Massachusetts, over 47% of poison fatalities had not been reported to the poison information center.[55] Similarly, a California study evaluating 358 poisoning fatalities reported to the medical examiner showed that only 10 poison center fatalities had been reported over a similar time period, demonstrating a similar reporting gap.[4] Once again in this study, whereas the majority of underreporting was with respect to prehospital deaths (68%), only 5 of 113 hospital patients who ultimately died were reported to the poison information center. Additionally, a cross-sectional comparison of national mortality with poison information center data for agricultural chemical poisoning demonstrated a similar trend of underreporting of fatalities to poison information centers.[34] Finally, when data for an entire year from the National Center for Health Statistics (NCHS) were compared to the same 1 year of data from the American Association of Poison Control Centers (AAPCC) Toxic Exposure Surveillance System (TESS), it was apparent that TESS captured only about 5% of annual poison fatalities.[29] It is logical to assume that similar barriers exist to reporting nonfatal poisonings.

Nonfatal Poisoning

An early outreach study in Massachusetts determined that hospitals geographically close to a poison information center reported their cases almost twice as often as hospitals remotely located (46% vs 27% of total cases).[10] Additionally, the authors noted that private physicians were less likely to report cases than residents in training. A 1-year retrospective review demonstrated that only 26% (123/470) of poisoned patients who were treated in a particular emergency department were reported to the poison information center.[28] Interestingly, only 3% of inhalational exposures were reported, compared with 95% of cyclic antidepressant ingestions. The authors also noted, as suggested above, that reporting decreased when exposures tended to cluster. Finally, in the physician survey study cited earlier, physicians reported that they would "almost never" contact the poison information center for asymptomatic exposures (62.9%), chronic toxicity (50.4%), or simply for the purposes of reporting to the database (90.2%).[9]

Occupational Exposures

Toxin exposure is an all too common event at the workplace. As a result of the long-recognized association between occupational exposure and illness, a number of federal and state government-funded agencies, such as NIOSH, OSHA, and ATSDR, exist to prevent occupational illness, educate the public, and to collect data on exposures to occupational toxins. Legislation provides for mandatory reporting in some instances and offers workers job protection for voluntary reporting. Poison information centers also provide information on occupational exposures and collect data. Once again, there are discrepancies between poison information data and the data collected by governmental agencies. A 6-month survey in California noted that only 15.9% of the occupational cases reported to the poison information center were captured by a state reporting system.[6] These cases tended to underrepresent dermatitis, the most common occupational toxicologic illness. A followup study by the same authors demonstrated that over a third of calls came directly from the individual, 70% of whom were unaware of the link between their occupation and their symptoms.[5] Although these data suggest that poison information centers can provide a valuable service for occupational exposures, one author expressed concern, noting in a followup study that the poison information center failed to identify an average of 12 people per workplace who were also potentially exposed in addition to the index case.[7]

Adverse Drug Events

Recent data suggest that a striking number of adverse drug events (ADEs) occur each year in the United States, with many resulting in death.[13,36] The ease of 24-hour telephone access, combined with the ability to consult with a health professional, make poison information centers ideal resources for reporting of ADEs.[14] Yet, over 76% of physicians surveyed stated that they would "almost never" contact the poison information center regarding adverse drug reactions.[9] Moreover, 30/56 (53.6%) poison information centers surveyed stated that they had not submitted any of their ADE data to the Food and Drug Administration's MedWatch program.[12] Many of the other centers reported only partial compliance with the MedWatch system.

Drugs of Abuse

Poison information centers also collect data on exposures to drugs of abuse. These data consist largely of calls for information from the concerned public and reports of overdose requiring healthcare intervention. Although ethanol and tobacco are the most common substances used in society, these cases are rarely reflected in poison information data, with the exception of unintentional exposures in children. In fact, because most substance abuse does not result in immediate interactions with the healthcare system, other databases such as the NIDA Household Survey might better reflect substance abuse trends.[17] Yet even this database has significant limitations.[3,24] However, because poison information centers are more focused on immediate healthcare effects of exposures, it could be argued that only those cases where healthcare interaction is required are of value in the database. Whereas poison information center data is collected passively, the Drug Abuse Warning Network (DAWN) provides an active surveillance system of a sample of hospital visits and deaths that relate to substance abuse. Unfortunately, because DAWN data uses hospital chart "mentions," which are infrequently validated, the data have been significantly criticized.[57] As such, it is clear that none of these three systems accurately encompasses the scope of the substance abuse problem.

Data Summary

With the current limitations of the TESS data, it should be clear that neither the numerator nor the denominator of poisoning can be easily appreciated. Analysis of these data for trends may be more useful because the inherent biases involved in TESS reporting are probably consistent over many years. Efforts should be directed to encourage reporting by such enhanced access methods as Web-based forms, direct laboratory interfaces, etc. Additional resources should be directed at improved case definitions (distinguishing asymptomatic exposure from poisoning) and integration with other essential databases such as MedWatch and the NCHS.

Despite its limitations, TESS data have significant utility. It is often an *exposure* rather than an actual *poisoning* that provides the impetus for contact with healthcare. For those exposures that are unlikely to be consequential, the poison information center can intervene to prevent potentially harmful attempts at home decontamination and costly unnecessary visits to healthcare providers. For those exposures that may result in poisoning, the time immediately following exposure is ideal moment to initiate first aid measures designed to prevent or lessen the severity of poisoning. Thus, the cost, benefits, and efficacy of poison information centers especially with regard to home calls must be measured in terms of exposures and not poisonings (see below).

PREVENTING UNNECESSARY HOSPITALIZATIONS FOLLOWING EXPOSURE

When visits to pediatric emergency departments for acute poisoning were analyzed, one study demonstrated that 95% of parents had not contacted the poison information center before coming to the hospital.[11] Sixty-four percent of those children required no hospital services. In contrast, when parents called the poison information center first, fewer than 1% subsequently went to the hospital. When 589 callers to one poison information center were surveyed, 464 (79%) stated that they would have utilized the emergency care system if the poison information center was unavailable.[32] TESS data confirm that approximately 75% of exposures that originate outside of healthcare facilities can be safely managed on site with limited telephone followup (TESS). Suggesting simple techniques or reassurance can successfully reduce hospital visits, although it should be remembered than in many of these cases, only a potential exposure occurred. Unfortunately, many barriers prevent a person from calling a poison center, including a lack of familiarity, intellectual and cultural factors, language difficulties, and confidentiality concerns. Also, recent survey data demonstrate the additional barriers of caregiver comfort with the hands-on contact provided by the healthcare system and a concern over implications of child abuse or neglect when reporting to agencies with governmental ties.[54]

The national average cost to the poison information center for a single human exposure call is less than $35.[61] A federally funded study concluded that in 1 year, poison information centers reduced the number of patients who were treated and not hospitalized by 350,000 and reduced hospitalizations by an additional 40,000 patients.[49] Each call to a poison information center prevented at least $175 in subsequent medical costs, providing strong theoretical evidence to support the cost efficacy of poison information centers. In fact, two natural experiments support these calculations: In 1988, Louisiana closed its state-sponsored poison information center. During the year that followed, the cost of emergency medical services for poisoning in Louisiana increased by more than $1.4 million. This additional expenditure represented a greater than threefold increase above the operating cost of that center.[33] Similarly, because of financial disputes in California, direct access to the San Francisco poison information center was electronically restricted for one major county, with a recording referring callers instead to the 911 system for assistance.[51] The result of each

blocked call was to increase healthcare costs by approximately $33. Moreover, these calculations do not account for unmeasured benefits to society from poison information center interventions such as reduced waiting times for ambulances and hospital treatments because of lower volumes, money saved by the prevention or reduction of injury from early intervention, or lives saved by enhancing access to or utilization of the healthcare system for seriously poisoned patients.

PROVIDING EDUCATION FOR THE PUBLIC AND HEALTH PROFESSIONALS

Poison center staff work closely with physicians, community health educators, community support groups, and parent-teacher associations to develop poison prevention activities.[48] Common strategies advocated to prevent poisoning are listed in Table 116–1. Poison information centers are also actively involved in enhancing training programs for paramedics,[20] medical students,[31] pharmacy students,[16] and resident physicians[16,60] and form an integral part of postgraduate training programs in medical toxicology fellowships.

As stated previously, there is an inherent risk in both enhanced public and professional education programs. Currently, decreased telephone utilization of the poison information center could equally be the result of a decrease in the incidence of exposure or poisoning or an enhanced understanding of the prevention, diagnosis, and treatment of poisoning. Although education should never be viewed as detrimental, programs must include an emphasis on the continued use of poison information centers to ensure access to current information in a rapidly changing discipline. In actuality, as a result of the ongoing analysis of incoming calls, the knowledge base has the potential to change as rapidly as the calls are reported. Thus, additional emphasis should be applied to routine utilization of the poison information center as a public health tool to improve the accuracy of epidemiologic data. Reporting of rare or suspected events can serve as sentinel efforts that help

TABLE 116–1.   Common Strategies Advocated to Help Prevent Poisoning

All medications and toxic substances should be kept in their original containers. Food and drink containers should never be used for the excess of a toxic substance.

Never store toxic substances in unlocked cabinets under the sink.

Apply locks to medicine cabinets that are within reach. In the absence of a lock, the more toxic medications and pharmaceuticals should be stored on the highest shelves.

Medications should never be left in the glove compartment of the family car.

Parents should buy or accept medication only if it is in a child-resistant container.

Medication should be considered as medicine, not a plaything and certainly not candy.

Adults should not take their medications in front of children. This will limit exposure to drug-taking role models that may become objects of imitative behavior.

Unused portions of prescription medications should be discarded by flushing down the toilet at the completion of drug therapy.

Syrup of ipecac and activated charcoal should be readily available in the home for use if directed by a poison information specialist or physician.

It should be anticipated that about 10% of children who have ingested a poison will do so again within a year.

identify consequential adverse drug events long before normal postmarketing surveillance tools identify areas of concern.

DEVELOPMENT OF PUBLIC HEALTH INITIATIVES

The early public health efforts of poison information centers focused on attempts to alter product concentration and to enhance product labeling and packaging. These clearly beneficial endeavors still continue. However, current events have also increased poison center activities in preparedness for disasters resulting from nuclear, biologic, and chemical terrorism.[23,35] The need for 24-hour rapid access to centralized information, existing data entry and retrieval systems, and links to experts in medical toxicology and emergency medicine helps to place poison information centers in critical roles in both local and national initiatives. Early contributions have included development of triage and treatment protocols and assessments of antidote supplies.[18,19]

TABLE 116–2. **Goals for Improving Poisoning Epidemiology Data**

Removal of barriers to reporting
  Multiple methods of reporting
    Telephone
    Facsimile
    Internet based or e-mail
    Communications devices for the hearing impaired
    Rapid access to translation services
    Standard mail
  Uniform access to a single toll-free number
  Enhanced awareness of the public health role of poison information
    centers
  Enhanced education of caregivers and healthcare professionals
  Public health legislation requiring professional reporting of exposures
Distinguishing potential exposures form actual exposures
  Create category for unconfirmed exposures
  Divide confirmed exposures by certainty
    Confirmed by history
    Confirmed by physical examination
    Confirmed by quantitative and qualitative laboratory analysis
Integration with other databases
  Utilization of standardized data collection instrument (include ICD codes,
    for example)
  Interact with data from
    Hospital and commercial laboratories
    Pharmacy ADE reports
    Hospital discharges
    Public health departments
      Such as with lead screening programs
    Fire departments and hazardous materials responders
    Industry
    Workplace exposures
    Death certificates
    Drug abuse monitoring systems
Provide real-time analysis
  Enhance speed of data collection and reporting
  Analyze data as it is reported, to identify emerging trends
  Mandate use of proper epidemiologic and statistical analyses of data
Provide rapid and regular feedback to primary reporters
Issue timely analyses and reports

SUMMARY

Poison information centers provide unique benefits to society. Public education efforts help reduce the likelihood of exposure. Provision of first aid advice helps to diminish the consequences of a poisoning once an exposure has occurred. Reassurance and proper first aid help to curtail unnecessary utilization of expensive healthcare. Interactions with healthcare professionals streamline the care of poisoned patients and improve access to toxicologically specific antidotes and the services of medical toxicologists. Data on exposures are used effectively to create legislation to further limit poisoning by altering contents or improving packaging or labeling.

Goals for the continued success of poison information centers must include providing uniform ease of access for the entire country through a single toll-free number, maintaining a uniformly high quality of service, and working to improve the accuracy of the TESS database. Poison information centers must publicize the need for reporting all poisonings including ADEs and strive to develop real-time systems of active surveillance. Finally, TESS reporting must be integrated with other databases so that the true numerator and denominator of poisoning can be understood and so that a concerted response to poisoning and poison prevention can be made. These and other initiatives are summarized in Table 116–2.

ACKNOWLEDGMENT

Richard S. Weisman, PharmD, contributed to Table 116–1 in the previous edition of this book.

REFERENCES

1. American Academy of Clinical Toxicology: Facility assessment guidelines for regional toxicology treatment centers. J Toxicol Clin Toxicol 1993;31:211–217.
2. American Association of Poison Control Centers: Criteria for certification as a regional poison control center, October 1991. Vet Hum Toxicol 1978;20:117–118.
3. Biemer PP, Witt M: Repeated measures estimation of measurement bias for self-reported drug use with applications to the National Household Survey on Drug Abuse. NIDA Res Monogr 1997;167: 439–476.
4. Blanc PD, Kearney TE, Olson KR: Underreporting of fatal cases to a regional poison control center. West J Med 1995;162:505–509.
5. Blanc PD, Maizlish N, Hiatt P, Olson KR, Rempel D: Occupational illness and poison control centers. Referral patterns and service needs. West J Med 1990;152:181–184.
6. Blanc PD, Olson KR: Occupationally related illness reported to a regional poison control center. Am J Public Health 1986;76:1303–1307.
7. Bresnitz EA: Poison Control Center follow-up of occupational disease. Am J Public Health 1990;80:711–712.
8. Burda T, Leikin JB, Fischbein C, et al: Emergency department use of flumazenil prior to poison center consultation. Vet Hum Toxicol 1997;39:245–247.
9. Caravati EM, McElwee NE: Use of clinical toxicology resources by emergency physicians and its impact on poison control centers. Ann Emerg Med 1991;20:147–150.
10. Chafee-Bahamon C, Caplan DL, Lovejoy FH: Patterns in hospitals' use of a regional poison information center. Am J Public Health 1983; 73:396–400.
11. Chafee-Bahamon C, Lovejoy FH: Effectiveness of a regional poison center in reducing excess emergency room visits for children's poisonings. Pediatrics 1983;72:164–169.

12. Chyka PA, McCommon SW: Reporting of adverse drug reactions by poison control centers in the US. Drug Safety 2000;23:87–93.

13. Chyka PA: How many deaths occur annually from adverse drug reactions in the United States. Am J Med 2000;109:122–130.

14. Chyka PA: Role of US poison centers in adverse drug reactions monitoring. Vet Hum Toxicol 1999;41:400–402.

15. Clark RF, Williams SR, Nordt SP, Pearigen PD, Deutsch R: Resource-use analysis of a medical toxicology consultation service. Ann Emerg Med 1998;31:705–709.

16. Cobaugh DJ, Goetz CM, Lopez GP, et al: Assessment of learning by emergency medicine residents and pharmacy students participating in a poison center clerkship. Vet Hum Toxicol 1997;39:173–175.

17. Crider RA: Heroin incidence: a trend comparison between National Household Survey data and indicator data. NIDA Res Monogr 1985;57:125–140.

18. Dart RC, Goldfrank LR, Chyka PA, et al: Combined evidence-based literature analysis and consensus guidelines for stocking of emergency antidotes in the United States. Ann Emerg Med 2000;36:126–132.

19. Dart RC, Stark Y, Fulton B, et al: Insufficient stocking of poisoning antidotes in hospital pharmacies. JAMA 1996;276:1508–1510.

20. Davis CO, Cobaugh DJ, Leahey NF, Wax PM: Toxicology training of paramedic students in the United States. Am J Emerg Med 1999;17:138–140.

21. Felberg L, Litovitz TL, Morgan J: State of the nation's poison centers: 1995 American Association of Poison Control Centers Survey of US Poison Centers. Vet Hum Toxicol 1996;38:445–453.

22. Fingerhut LA, Cox CS: Poisoning mortality, 1985–1995. Public Health Rep 1998;113:218–233.

23. Geller RJ, Lopez GP: Poison center planning for mass gatherings: The Georgia Poison Center experience with the 1996 Centennial Olympic Games. J Toxicol Clin Toxicol 1999;37:315–319.

24. Gfroerer J, Lessler J, Parsley T: Studies of nonresponse and measurement error in the national household survey on drug abuse. NIDA Res Monogr 1997;167:273–295.

25. Greenberg MI, Cone DC, Roberts JR: Material safety data sheet: A useful resource for the emergency physician. Ann Emerg Med 1996;27:347–352.

26. Hamilton RJ, Goldfrank LR: Poison center data and the Pollyanna phenomenon. J Toxicol Clin Toxicol 1997;35:21–23.

27. Hamilton RJ, Perrone J, Hoffman RS, et al: A descriptive study of an epidemic of poisoning caused by heroin adulterated with scopolamine. J Toxicol Clin Toxicol 2000;38:597–608.

28. Harchelroad F, Clark RF, Dean B, Krenzelok EP: Treated vs reported toxic exposures: Discrepancies between a poison control center and a member hospital. Vet Hum Toxicol 1990;32:156–159.

29. Hoppe-Roberts JM, Lloyd LM, Chyka PA: Poisoning mortality in the United States: Comparison of national mortality statistics and poison control center reports. Ann Emerg Med 2000;35:440–448.

30. Hoyt BT, Rasmussen R, Giffin S, Smilkstein MJ: Poison center data accuracy: A comparison of rural hospital chart data with the TESS database. Acad Emerg Med 1999;6:851–855.

31. Jordan JK, Dean BS, Krenzelok EP: Poison center rotation for health science students. Vet Hum Toxicol 1987;29:174–175.

32. Kearney TE, Olson KR, Bero LA, et al: Healthcare cost effects of public use of a regional poison control center. West J Med 1995;162:499–504.

33. King WD, Palmisano PA: Poison control centers: Can their value be measured? South Med J 1991;84:722–726.

34. Klein-Schwartz W, Smith GS: Agricultural and horticultural chemical poisonings: Mortality and morbidity in the United States. Ann Emerg Med 1997;29:232–238.

35. Krenzelok EP, Allswede MP, Mrvos R: The poison center role in biological and chemical terrorism. Vet Hum Toxicol 2000;45:297–300.

36. Lazarou J, Pomeranz BH, Corey PN: Incidence of adverse drug reactions in hospitalized patients: A meta-analysis of prospective studies. JAMA 1998;279:1200–1205.

37. Linakis JG, Frederick KA: Poisoning deaths not reported to the regional poison control center. Ann Emerg Med 1993;22:42–48.

38. Litovitz TL, Bailey KM, Schmitz BF, et al: 1990 Annual report of the American Association of Poison Control Centers National Data Collection System. Am J Emerg Med 1991;9:461–509.

39. Litovitz TL, Clark LR, Soloway RA: 1993 Annual report of the American Association of Poison Control Centers Toxic Exposure Surveillance System. Am J Emerg Med 1994;12:546–584.

40. Litovitz TL, Felberg L, Soloway RA, et al: 1994 Annual report of the American Association of Poison Control Centers Toxic Exposure Surveillance System. Am J Emerg Med 1995;13:551–597.

41. Litovitz TL, Felberg L, White S, et al: 1995 Annual report of the American Association of Poison Control Centers Toxic Exposure Surveillance System. Am J Emerg Med 1996;14:487–537.

42. Litovitz TL, Holm KC, Bailey KM, Schmitz BF: 1991 Annual report of the American Association of Poison Control Centers National Data Collection System. Am J Emerg Med 1992;10:452–505.

43. Litovitz TL, Holm KC, Clancy C, et al: 1992 Annual report of the American Association of Poison Control Centers Toxic Exposure Surveillance System. Am J Emerg Med 1993;11:494–555.

44. Litovitz TL, Klein-Schwartz W, Caravati EM, et al: 1998 Annual report of the American Association of Poison Control Centers Toxic Exposure Surveillance System. Am J Emerg Med 1999;17:435–487.

45. Litovitz TL, Klein-Schwartz W, Dyer KS, et al: 1997 Annual report of the American Association of Poison Control Centers Toxic Exposure Surveillance System. Am J Emerg Med 1998;16:443–497.

46. Litovitz TL, Klein-Schwartz W, White S, et al: 1999 Annual report of the American Association of Poison Control Centers Toxic Exposure Surveillance System. Am J Emerg Med 2000;18:517–574.

47. Litovitz TL, Smilkstein M, Felberg L, et al: 1996 Annual report of the American Association of Poison Control Centers Toxic Exposure Surveillance System. Am J Emerg Med 1997;15:447–500.

48. Lovejoy FH, Robertson WO, Woolf AD: Poison centers, poison prevention and the pediatrician. Pediatrics 1994;94:220–224.

49. Miller TR, Lestina DC: Costs of poisoning in the United States and savings from poison control centers: A benefit-cost analysis. Ann Emerg Med. 1997;29:239–245.

50. Mullen WH, Anderson IB, Kim SY, et al: Incorrect overdose management advice in the Physicians' Desk Reference. Ann Emerg Med 1997;29:255–261.

51. Phillips KA, Homan RK, Hiatt PH, et al: The costs and outcomes of restricting public access to poison centers. Results from a natural experiment. Med Care 1998;36:271–280.

52. Rodgers GB: The safety effects of child-resistant packaging for oral prescription drugs: Two decades of experience. JAMA 1996;275:1661–1665.

53. Scherz RG, Robertson WO: The history of poison control centers in the United States. Clin Toxicol 1978;12:291–296.

54. Schwartz L, Howland MA, Mercurio-Zappala M, Hoffman R: The use of focus groups to plan poison prevention programs [abstract]. J Toxicol Clin Toxicol 2000;38:558.

55. Soslow AR, Woolf AD: Reliability of data sources for poisoning deaths in Massachusetts. Am J Emerg Med 1992;10:124–127.

56. Temple AR: Testing of child-resistant containers. Clin Toxicol 1978;12:35–66.

57. Ungerleider JT, Lundberg GD, Sunshine I, Walberg CB: DAWN: Drug Abuse Warning Network or data about worthless numbers? J Anal Toxicol 1980;4:269–271.

58. Waltar WW: An evaluation of the poison prevention packaging act. Pediatrics 1982;69:363–370.

59. Wax PM, Rodewald L, Lawrence R: The arrival of the ED-based POISINDEX: Perceived impact on poison control center use. Am J Emerg Med 1994;12:537–540.

60. Wolf LR, Hamilton GC: Objectives to direct the training of emergency medicine residents of off-service rotations: Toxicology. J Emerg Med. 1994;12:391–405.

61. Youniss J, Litovitz T, Vilanueva P: Characterization of US poison centers: A 1998 survey conducted by the American Association of Poison Control Centers. Vet Hum Toxicol 2000;42:43–53.

CHAPTER 117 ADVERSE DRUG EVENTS

Louis R. Cantilena, Jr.

Case A 39-year-old woman was brought to the Emergency Department (ED) after several episodes of syncope. These episodes began approximately 2 days before admission and were accompanied by a witnessed 4- to 5-second loss of consciousness with spontaneous recovery. There were no postictal symptoms or loss of bowel or bladder sphincter control associated with these episodes. At least one episode occurred when the patient was lying down and was preceded by palpitations, dyspnea, and diaphoresis. There was no prior history of trauma and no history of cardiac or neurologic illness. The patient denied suicidal ideation or intentions, dieting, or use of nonprescription or dietary supplement products.

Ten days earlier, terfenadine, 60 mg twice daily, and cefaclor, 250 mg three times daily, had been prescribed for the treatment of recurrent sinusitis. On the eighth day of this combined therapy, the patient began taking ketoconazole, 200 mg twice daily, left over from an old prescription for vaginitis. The patient had experienced past episodes of yeast vaginitis, usually in this same setting of prolonged antibiotic therapy. There was no family history of cardiac disease. The patient had a normal electrocardiogram approximately 15 years before this admission. Other medications included medroxyprogesterone acetate, 2.5 mg per day for 10 days of the patient's menstrual cycle.

In the ED, the patient's vital signs were: blood pressure 106/72 (without orthostatic changes); pulse regular, 88 beats per minute; respiratory rate 16/min; and oral temperature was 37.2°C (99°F). The physical examination was entirely normal. An electrocardiogram was remarkable for a corrected QT interval of 655 milliseconds, prominent T-U waves throughout the precordial leads, and nonspecific ST-T–wave abnormalities. The remainder of the laboratory examination was within normal limits.

All medications were discontinued, and the patient was admitted to the telemetry unit for observation. Approximately 10 hours after admission, the patient experienced paroxysmal episodes of palpitations and dyspnea and a near syncopal episode identical to the one she had experienced before admission. Figure 117–1 shows the recording from her telemetry monitor, indicating torsades de pointes. The patient spontaneously recovered from this episode and remained in the hospital for approximately 5 days, during which time her QT interval gradually returned to normal. A full cardiac evaluation including echocardiogram and exercise stress testing was normal. Following discharge, outpatient 24-hour Holter monitoring revealed no abnormalities. The patient's plasma from the time of admission was subsequently analyzed for unmetabolized terfenadine and its primary metabolite. These results revealed a markedly increased concentration of parent terfenadine, which is normally not found in patients taking this antihistamine.[28]

This patient presented in December 1989 at a military hospital in the Washington, DC area. A consultation service in clinical pharmacology and medical toxicology played a vital role in establishing the diagnosis of an adverse drug event caused a drug-drug interaction with terfenadine and ketoconazole. The drug terfenadine (Seldane) was approved for marketing in 1985 and was widely regarded as a safe, nonsedating antihistamine. At the time this case occurred, the drug was the eighth most frequently prescribed drug in the United States. The possibility of making this drug available without prescription was being discussed in the pharmaceutical press at the time. The drug was widely regarded as safe and had been marketed for nearly 6 years, with millions of dosages taken worldwide.

The availability of a medical subspecialty with expertise in drug-induced disease and knowledge of drug metabolism proved to be an important component of the case of terfenadine. In 1989 the drug label for terfenadine mentioned the possibility of torsades de pointes occurring only in the setting of overdose with the antihistamine. The potential for life-threatening drug interactions with terfenadine was unrecognized at that time. Subsequently, the Food and Drug Administration (FDA) funded prospective research that demonstrated a significant drug-drug interaction involving terfenadine and inhibitors of the cytochrome P450 3A (CYP3A) system.[17, 18] Several years later, the FDA announced their intention to withdraw terfenadine from the marketplace, citing the risk of dangerous drug-drug interactions, which had caused several deaths, as the primary reason.[12] The manufacturer voluntarily withdrew Seldane from the market before final regulatory action could be taken. This case is an example of the discovery of a serious, life-threatening adverse drug event (based on a drug-drug interaction) found during the postapproval period for a widely used drug. Terfenadine proved to be the first of several agents that would eventually be withdrawn from the United States market because of potentially lethal drug-drug interactions resulting in cardiac dysrhythmias. After the terfenadine withdrawal, the close attention paid by the FDA to drug effects on cardiac repolarization may make this particular drug-drug interaction problem less likely to occur in the future, but the approval of every drug or medical device carries with it some potential risk.[14] The FDA and the drug industry must always rely on postmarketing surveillance for further safety data regarding the toxicity of an agent after approval. There are systems in place to monitor postapproval drug safety that are intended to detect instances where the safety profile of an approved agent may appear to be different after marketing. Individual pharmaceutical manufacturers are responsible for monitoring the safety of their products and reporting to the FDA, on a

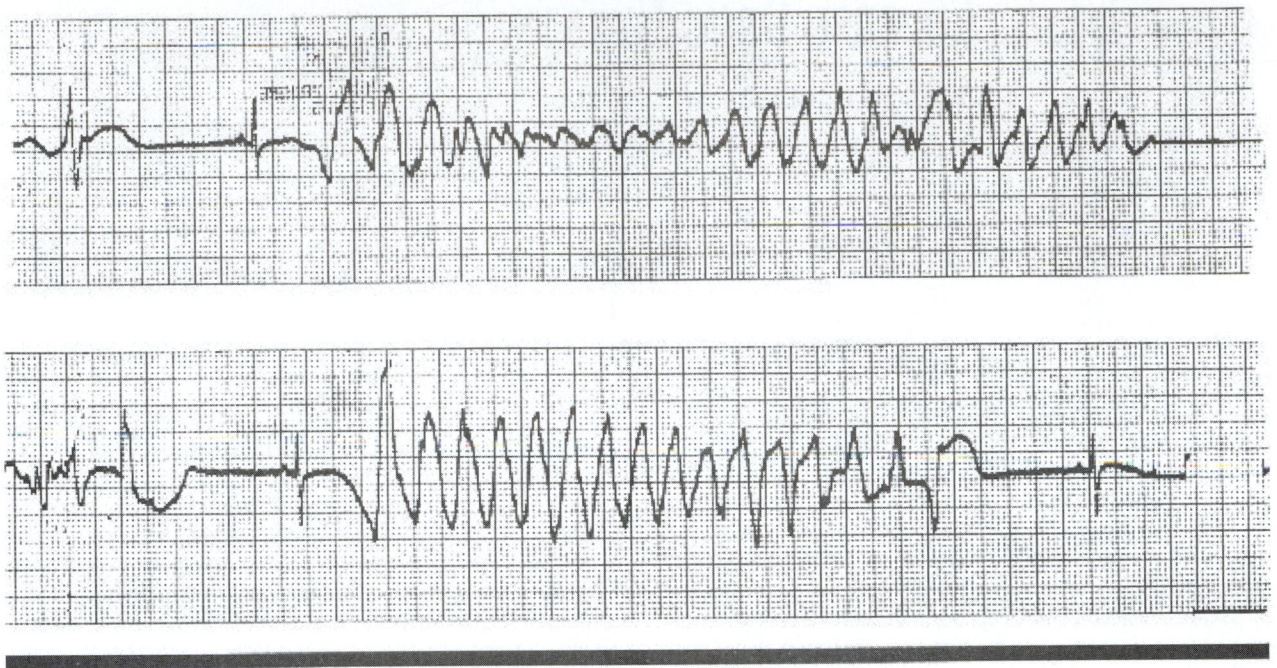

Figure 117–1. Telemetry recording from the patient taking terfenadine and ketoconazole showing torsades de pointes. *(From Monahan BP, Ferguson CL, Kil-leavy ES, et al: Torsades de pointes occurring in association with terfenadine use. JAMA 1990;264:2788–2790, with permission.)*

regular basis, any adverse events that were reported to them. The FDA's postmarketing surveillance for all medical products is another system in place to monitor drug and medical device safety. Health professionals contribute to ongoing passive surveillance of drug safety. This chapter focuses on drug-induced disease resulting from adverse drug events (ADEs) caused by both inherent drug toxicity and medical therapeutic errors. The topics covered in this chapter include a brief overview of the process for drug approval currently in place in the United States, a discussion about the diagnosis of drug-induced disease, medical errors as a cause of drug-induced disease, and the role of the medical toxicologist in the discovery, reporting, and prevention of ADEs.

HISTORY OF THE UNITED STATES DRUG APPROVAL PROCESS

Today in the United States, approvals of new therapeutic agents are occurring at an unprecedented rate. The evolution of the system that currently exists for review of drug applications and approval of new therapeutic agents is the result of significant recent changes in the US drug law. Initially, the drug law evolution was closely linked to a series of medical product disasters that occurred during the 20th century in the United States. Before 1900, there was no legal requirement for a company to test a product for safety or efficacy or even to make valid claims in the drug label. Products such as aspirin containing heroin were sold as cough syrup. Wine with cocaine was marketed to enhance sales of the alcoholic beverage. Further, there was no requirement for systematic testing of products to determine purity or the presence of possible adulterants in product formulations. The Food and Drug Act of

1906 required drugs to meet a standard for strength and purity. The burden of proof, however, was placed on the FDA to show that the drug was incorrectly labeled or that the advertising or label was false or misleading.

The Federal Food, Drug and Cosmetic Act of 1938 resulted from a tragedy in which more than 100 patients (mostly children) died from poisoning by an excipient of an oral solution of sulfanilamide. A pharmaceutical company, in an attempt to improve the palatability of a sulfanilamide product for pediatric formulations, introduced the solvent diethylene glycol into the formulation. Diethylene glycol is similar to ethylene glycol, and both produce a sweet-tasting but deadly ingestant. Only after almost a full year of marketing were cases of renal failure and death reported in sufficient numbers to alert authorities to the extremely toxic nature of the product. Ensuing congressional hearings resulted in passage of the Food Drug and Cosmetic Act of 1938. This law required companies (1) to list the ingredients of the product on the product label and (2) to provide the known risks concerning use of the product to physicians or pharmacists, (3) made illegal the misbranding of food or medical products, and (4) for the first time required companies to test their products for safety before being sold. Drugs already marketed before 1938 were exempt from the requirement (see Chap. 1).

The next significant chapter in the history of FDA regulatory law occurred during the 1960s. An application for the approval of α-N-phthalylglutaramide (Thalidomide), a sedative that had already been marketed in Europe, was submitted to the Food and Drug Administration. The sedative drug apparently did not affect respiration, had a rapid onset and short duration of action, did not cause a morning-after effect, and was inexpensive. A medical reviewer at the FDA (Dr. F. Kelsey) delayed approval by asking the sponsor to clarify several issues in the reportedly poorly organized new drug application (NDA). The delay in US approval turned out to be fortuitous because, in the interim, an article that linked an unusual teratogenic effect of phocomelia to exposure to this agent appeared in the European medical literature. Congressional hearings were again held in the United States, and the Kefauver-Harris act of 1968 became law. This law required a manufacturer or sponsor to (1) file an investigational new drug application (IND) before beginning a clinical study with a drug in humans, (2) demonstrate that the drug was effective for the condition that it was being marketed to treat, and (3) provide adequate directions for safe usage of the drug. Moreover, the act did not exempt drugs that were already on the market. Thus, the evolution of the legal requirements for proving drug safety and efficacy in the United States are closely linked to the occurrence or near-occurrence of significant drug-induced disease.

Subsequent US laws that affect the FDA's review and approval of products include (1) the Orphan Drug Act of 1983, which provides financial incentives to drug manufacturers to develop drugs for the treatment of rare diseases and conditions (see http://www.fda.gov/orphan/designat/recent.htm for a list of drugs that have been approved under the Orphan Drug Act.); (2) The Prescription Drug User Fee Act of 1992, which required manufacturers to pay user fees to the Federal Government for new drug applications and supplements, enabling the FDA to hire additional reviewers to accelerate the review process so that reviews are performed under the user fee category on a shortened timetable than the average review period before the legislation; (3) Section 112 of the Food and Drug Administration Modernization Act of 1997, which allowed for an accelerated drug approval process for agents to treat life-threatening illnesses such as AIDS and cancer if the agent had the potential to address medical needs unmet by currently available drugs. Many of the accelerated drug approval programs rely on efficacy results based on a surrogate marker that is known to be linked to the ultimate indication for the drug. For ex-

ample, the protease inhibitors were shown to reduce HIV viral load for the treatment of AIDS and were approved based on the accelerated track with confirmatory clinical trials under way that ultimately showed an increased survival.

Has the accelerated drug approval process led to an increase in the need to withdraw unsafe medications?[14,32,38] Figure 117–2 shows the number of FDA drug approvals for new molecular entities (NME) per year from 1993 to 1999 as well as the median approval time and the FDA review time for drug products for corresponding years. Both the median approval time and review times have decreased during this 6-year period despite an increase in the number of NMEs approved during this time period. The number of safety-based withdrawals of NME drugs is shown in Fig. 117–3 by 5-year approval periods and as percentages of the approved-drug cohort that was withdrawn. This figure suggests that althoughwhile the number of NMEs approved as new drugs in the United States is increasing per year, the percentage of NMEs withdrawn for safety reasons has been relatively stable, with the exception of drugs approved between 1985 and 1989, which showed that 4.4% of the drugs approved in these 4 years were eventually withdrawn. Interestingly, it was during that same time period that terfenadine and astemizole were approved for marketing. However, it is possible that in some cases there may be as much as a 10- to 15-year lag in the postmarketing detection system (ie, MedWatch) for rare or difficult to diagnose ADEs. Time may yet show that the recent drug approval cohorts have not reached their peak for detection. The next several years will ultimately determine whether or not there is an association between the increased rate for drug approval and the rate of safety-related drug withdrawals. Other issues such as gender effects on ADEs also require closer examination. A recent General Accounting Office report dated January 19, 2001 *(http://www.gao.gov)* has highlighted the fact that 8 of 10 drugs recently withdrawn from the US market posed greater health risks to women than to men.

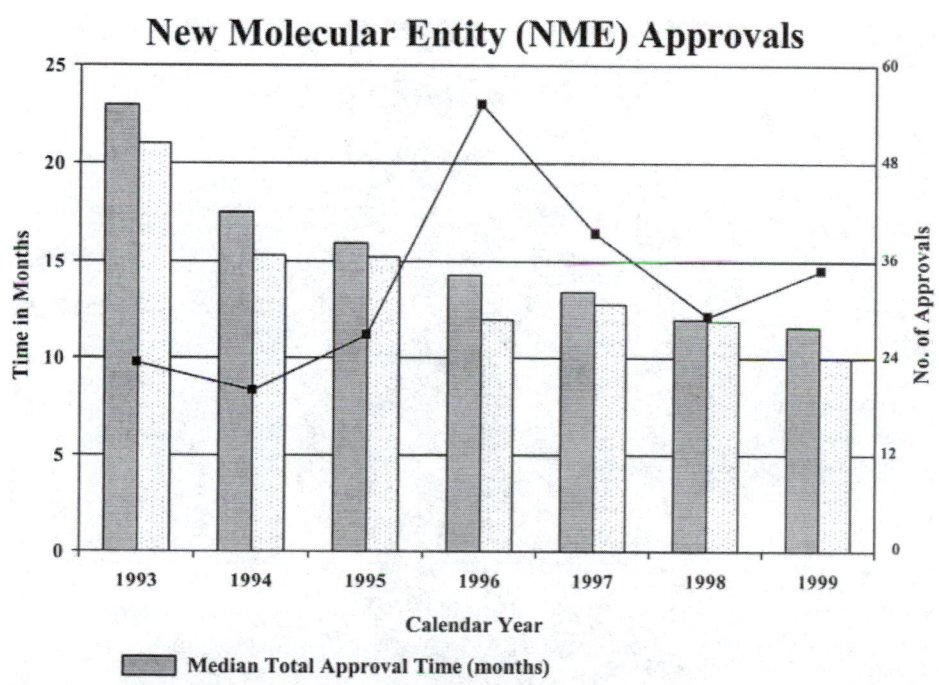

New Molecular Entity (NME) Approvals

- ▨ **Median Total Approval Time (months)**
- ▢ **Median Total FDA Review Time (months)**
- ▪━▪ **Number of NMEs Approved**

Figure 117–2. Yearly new molecular entity (NME) US approvals by FDA and median approval and review time for 1993 through 1999. (From www.fda.gov.)

Safety-Based NME Withdrawals
(Based on Year of Approval)

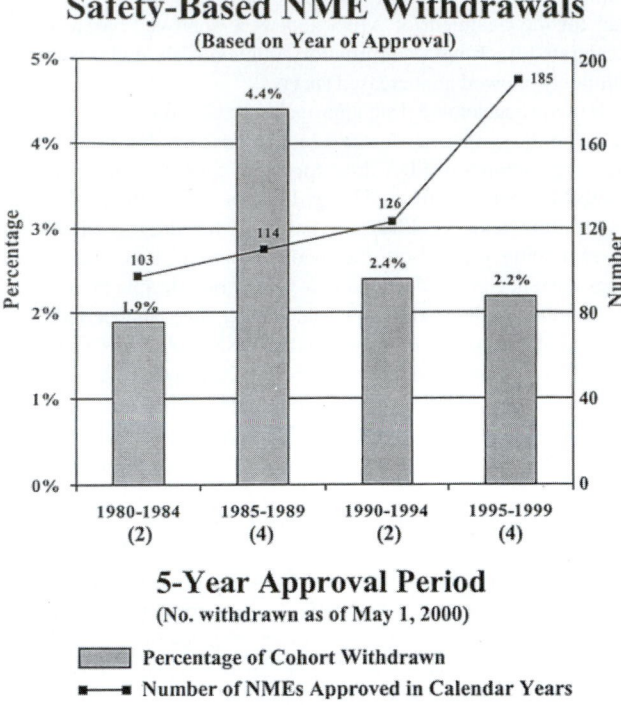

5-Year Approval Period
(No. withdrawn as of May 1, 2000)

■ Percentage of Cohort Withdrawn
■—■ Number of NMEs Approved in Calendar Years

Figure 117–3. The number and percentage of approved drugs withdrawn from the US market for safety reasons by 5-year periods. (From www.fda.gov.)

THE DRUG DEVELOPMENT PROCESS

A schematic overview of the process for drug development of a NME is shown in Fig. 117–4. The process begins with the preclinical evaluation of the candidate drug. During this evaluation, toxicologic testing is performed in more than one animal species as well as other testing including stability of the product, manufacturing methods, purity, and carcinogenicity. Dose-response relationships in animal models and in vitro receptor binding or surrogate marker effects are often determined at this time in the program. Also, this is the time when many manufacturers determine the drug's metabolism in animal and in vitro human systems. Following this preclinical testing, the sponsor submits an IND application to the FDA for approval to initiate human testing. This application contains all relevant data concerning animal and in vitro toxicology testing, product manufacturing and purity, and a protocol for utilizing the drug in initial human investigation. Within 30 days, the FDA must review the application and either allow the proposed human study to proceed or inform the sponsor that additional data or preclinical work is required before clinical testing of the candidate drug can begin.

The clinical study of new medications is divided into four basic phases. Phase 1 clinical testing involves a relatively small number of subjects with the primary aim of determining the safety and toxicity of the drug. Many Phase 1 studies will also determine the human pharmacokinetics of the drug. Phase 1 studies are normally conducted in 20 to 100 healthy volunteer subjects with the notable exception of Phase 1 studies for cancer chemotherapeutic agents, which only enroll patients with cancer.

Phase 2 clinical testing is designed to determine the potential efficacy of the drug product in humans and sometimes explores the range of effective drug dosages. In this phase, approximately 100 to 300 subjects are studied. In Phase 2 clinical trials, subjects generally have the diseases for which the drug is intended or are capable of demonstrating the appropriate, validated, biologic surrogate marker to indicate response to the drug.

Phase 3 clinical drug studies usually involve large-scale clinical trials in the actual population for which the drug is intended to be used. Typically, this phase of a drug's development will involve testing a treatment cohort of several hundred to several thousand patients who have the target disease, depending on both the prevalence of the disease and effectiveness of the drug. The primary goal of Phase 3 studies is to determine the safety and efficacy of the candidate drug in the actual patient population it will be used in, under conditions close to the anticipated medical use. A candidate drug completing Phase 1, 2, and 3 can thus be approved for marketing after study in only 2000 to 4000 patients. In the setting of a fast-track approval or under the Orphan Drug regulations, substantially fewer patients will receive the drug before its approval for marketing.

After the FDA approves a drug for marketing, Phase 4 clinical studies are initiated. Phase 4 studies may be marketing-type studies comparing the new drug to a competitor. However, enhancement of safety information is the primary goal of most Phase 4 studies. The methods by which Phase 4 safety studies are conducted are primarily observational and epidemiologic studies. Main sources of data for the postapproval monitoring of the safety of a drug are the spontaneous reports gathered by both the pharmaceutical manufacturer and FDA. The fields of pharmacovigilance and pharmacoepidemiology are typically employed in the conduct of Phase 4 studies.[27] Until 1993, the FDA utilized the spontaneous reporting system (SRS) to gather information regarding ADEs occurring in patients using the approved drug. In 1993, this system

New Drug Application (NDA) Timeline

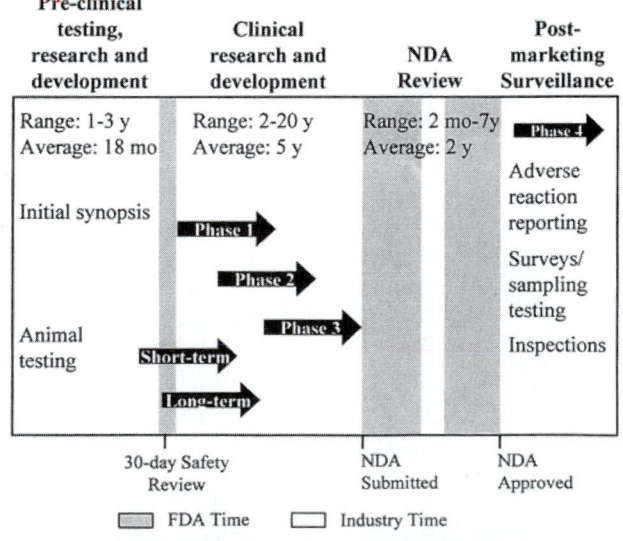

Figure 117–4. Schematic representation of new drug development. (From www.fda.gov.)

was renamed and promoted as the MedWatch system.[20] This system relies on spontaneous reports by healthcare professionals or patients regarding the occurrence of deleterious effects associated with the use of a medical product. The primary goals of the MedWatch system are (1) to increase awareness of drug- and device-induced disease; (2) to clarify what should (and should not) be reported to the agency; (3) to make it easier to report adverse effects by creating a single system for health professionals to use in reporting adverse events and product problems to the agency; and (4) to provide regular feedback to the health care community about safety issues involving medical products.[26] Currently, the MedWatch program is supported by over 140 organizations, representing health professionals and industry, that have agreed to be MedWatch Partners to help achieve these goals.

Medical product manufacturers that are regulated by the FDA are required to report adverse events occurring in association with the use of their products. Healthcare professionals are encouraged (but not required) to report ADEs. An adverse event is any undesirable experience associated with the use of a medical product in a patient. The MedWatch system has tried to make reporting by healthcare providers easier. A MedWatch report can be made by either facsimile, telephone, mail, or Internet. Establishing causality for a specific medical product is not required before submission of a MedWatch report. The FDA is primarily interested in the report of a serious adverse event, whether or not a causal relationship is established. An event is *serious* and should be reported when the patient outcome is one of the following:

1. Death, and the death is suspected to be a direct result of the adverse event.
2. Life-threatening, if the patient was considered to be at substantial risk of dying at the time of the adverse event or the use or continued use of the product would result in the patient's death. (Examples include gastrointestinal hemorrhage, bone marrow suppression, pacemaker failure, and infusion pump failure that permits uncontrolled free flow and results in excessive drug dosing.)
3. Hospitalization (initial or prolonged) if admission to the hospital or prolongation of a hospital stay resulted from the adverse event. (Examples include anaphylaxis, pseudomembranous colitis, or bleeding causing or prolonging hospitalization.)
4. Disability, if the adverse event resulted in a significant, persistent, or permanent change, impairment, damage, or disruption in the patient's body function/structure, physical activities, or quality of life. (Examples include cerebrovascular accident caused by drug-induced coagulopathy, toxicity, and peripheral neuropathy.)
5. Congenital anomaly, if there are suspicions that exposure to a medical product before conception or during pregnancy resulted in an adverse effect on the child. (Examples include vaginal cancer in female offspring from diethylstilbestrol during pregnancy or limb malformations in the offspring from thalidomide use during pregnancy.)
6. Requires intervention to prevent permanent impairment or damage if use of a medical product is suspected to result in a condition requiring medical or surgical intervention to preclude permanent impairment or damage to a patient. (Examples include acetaminophen overdose-induced hepatotoxicity requiring treatment with *N*-acetylcysteine to prevent permanent damage, burns from radiation equipment requiring drug

therapy, or breakage of an orthopedic screw requiring replacement of hardware to prevent malunion of a fractured long bone.)[26]

Physician reports are given priority for review by the FDA in the MedWatch system. A well-documented case of a serious adverse event is a significant and useful contribution to the MedWatch system. The medical toxicologist may be the first person to encounter a patient with a serious ADE in the ED or may be one of the first consultants called to see a patient with a suspected serious drug-induced disease. Reports of serious ADEs to the FDA or to the manufacturer can evolve into an epidemiologically detectable signal that can catalyze subsequent, more detailed investigations (examples of cases where this has occurred are provided later in this chapter).

Reporting serious ADEs has periodically been encouraged by various healthcare groups in conjunction with the FDA. With the introduction of the MedWatch system and MedWatch partner programs, medical societies and organizations such as the American Medical Association, the American College of Medical Toxicology, and the American Academy of Pediatrics have encouraged their members to report to the MedWatch system. As a requirement for accreditation, the Joint Commission on Accreditation of Healthcare Organizations mandates hospitals to collect, analyze, and report significant and unexpected ADEs to the FDA.

The primary limitation of the MedWatch system and, in fact, of most Phase 4 drug studies is the exclusive reliance on spontaneous reporting of adverse events. Significant underreporting is known to occur in such systems. Current estimates are that fewer than 10% of ADEs are reported.[15,29,31] The true incidence of the reported ADE is almost never obtainable because the denominator, which is the number of actual exposures to the drug, is rarely accurately known. Despite these limitations, the MedWatch system is capable of detecting significant adverse events. The relatively small number of patients or subjects exposed to the drug before approval (Phases 1–3) is one reason why relatively uncommon ADEs are not detected until the postapproval marketing phase. For example, in order to detect an uncommon adverse event occurring in approximately 1 of 5000 individuals exposed to a drug with 95% probability that the ADE resulted from exposure to that drug, approximately 15,000 patients would have to be exposed to the drug.[25] In a balanced (equal numbers of drug and placebo recipients) placebo-controlled clinical trial, 30,000 subjects would need to be enrolled. Premarketing clinical studies (Phase 1, 2, and 3) may not be able to detect rare ADEs, ADEs that are incorrectly diagnosed, or ADEs that result from a drug interaction that may not have been tested in the development program. An example of a rare ADE not detected until postmarketing involves the drug felbamate, which was approved by the FDA in September 1993 and subsequently found to be associated with aplastic anemia during postmarketing surveillance. Felbamate-induced aplastic anemia had not been detected during the drug development program for the agent. By July 1994, nine cases had been reported from an estimated 100,000 patients exposed to felbamate in the United States. Most of the aplastic anemia cases occurred in patients who had taken the drug for less than 1 year. The nine cases represented an approximate 50-fold increase in aplastic anemia over the expected rate with the very low background rate of two to five cases per million per previous year,[1,34] allowing the FDA to attribute this rare condition to exposure to felbamate.

Attributing a serious ADE to a drug solely from MedWatch reports occurs uncommonly. A primary role of the MedWatch system is to generate a "hypothesis" for a potential association of an ADE with a specific drug.

An example of this "hypothesis generation" function of Med-Watch is the question of whether phenylpropanolamine (PPA) causes hemorrhagic stroke in patients using nonprescription diet suppressants or cough and cold preparations containing PPA. In the early 1990s, the Spontaneous Reporting System (SRS, now MedWatch) detected a potential association of hemorrhagic stroke and nonprescription use of PPA. An industry-sponsored prospective, case-controlled study resulted, to determine if such an association existed. The multicenter study demonstrated that an association did exist, especially for women ages 18 to 49. The Nonprescription Drug Advisory Committee (NDAC) of FDA reviewed this study and the associated MedWatch data in the fall of 2000 and decided that the evidence supported such an association. Consequently, the idea of removing PPA from the market was considered and then implemented. Although the entire process of signal identification from MedWatch to presentation of results from the prospective epidemiologic study required nearly a decade for PPA, the process demonstrates the value of the hypothesis-generating ability of the MedWatch system.

ESTABLISHING THE DIAGNOSIS OF DRUG-INDUCED DISEASE

The recognition and diagnosis of a drug-induced disease, or an ADE, is an essential skill for practitioners, including medical toxicologists and clinical pharmacologists. The diagnosis of an ADE is typically made as a result of a systematic medical evaluation. One approach to making the diagnosis of drug-induced disease involves consideration of six related questions concerning the patient's clinical presentation, as shown in Table 117–1.

The first question concerns the timing of the onset of the adverse event in relationship to the reported exposure to the drug. Perhaps because of publicity or word of mouth, ADEs are sometimes reported to the FDA MedWatch system even when the onset of the adverse event occurs before the first exposure to the suspect drug. A careful reconstruction of the time course of drug exposure and onset of adverse effects is extremely important in assessing causality. The time course differs considerably for different adverse clinical events. An anaphylactic reaction to a drug occurs within minutes of exposure, whereas renal insufficiency caused by a drug is not likely to be clinically detectable for up to several days after the exposure. A drug that causes cancer (a carcinogen) may not produce a clinically detectable effect for decades. Establishing a time course is an essential first step in the process of making the diagnosis of drug-induced disease.

TABLE 117–1. Considerations When Establishing the Diagnosis of an Adverse Drug Event (ADE)

- Was the timing of the adverse event appropriate relative to the exposure to the drug?
- Has the suspected ADE effect been reported before?
- Is there evidence of excessive exposure to the drug?
- Are there other more likely etiologies reponsible for the suspected ADE?
- What is the patient's response to withdrawal or cessation (dechallenge) of the drug?
- What is the patient's response to rechallenge?

The second question is whether or not this adverse effect has been reported previously for the suspect drug. An adverse drug effect that occurs commonly is likely to be known before the approval of the drug and is therefore usually found on the drug label. For example, respiratory depression and mental status changes were well known before the approval of fentanyl, an opioid agonist. Less common ADEs for drugs that have been on the market for a period of time are sometimes reported in the literature, included in various medical databases, and in some cases will appear in a revised drug label for the medical product. Previous reports linking the observed adverse effect to drug exposure are very helpful to the toxicologist trying to establish a significant level of probability for causality in the setting of an ADE.

However, in the setting of a newly approved drug or a previously unreported possible ADE, neither previous reports, the medical literature, nor the drug label will help establish causality. In this setting, the clinician must rely more on what is known of the pharmacology, the pharmacokinetics, and the anticipated pharmacodynamics of the suspect drug as well as the timing of the appearance and observed time course of the adverse event. It is important to put "drug-induced disease" in the differential diagnosis for the patient presenting for medical care. Someone has to be the first to report what is ultimately recognized as an adverse effect for every drug or toxin. Appropriate vigilance for the possibility of a new ADE significantly increases the probability that a finding can be made early after introduction of a new drug to prevent more widespread drug-induced morbidity or mortality.

"Is there evidence of excess exposure to the drug?" The majority of ADEs that occur are predictable on the basis of the known pharmacology of the specific drug. Such ADEs are referred to as "type A" ADEs.[8] For example, antihistamines such as diphenhydramine are known to cause significant anticholinergic effects. When a patient presents with mental status changes and clinical findings consistent with the anticholinergic toxidrome after significant exposure to an antihistamine-containing product, the observed effects are consistent with an ADE attributable to the antihistamine. Occasionally, proof of drug excess can come from measurement of the drug substance in plasma. In the case of the patient with a history of manic-depressive illness, who exhibits hyperreflexia and tremors, the measurement of an elevated lithium plasma concentration supports the diagnosis of lithium toxicity or an ADE attributable to lithium. In either case, knowing the pharmacology of the drug is important for establishing the diagnosis of an ADE.

When an ADE is caused by an allergic mechanism or another mechanism unrelated to dose of the drug, ie, a "type B" ADE, evidence of drug excess usually does not contribute to the diagnosis. In this setting, other factors such as allergy history or pharmacogenetic background are weighed more heavily to support the diagnosis of an ADE.

The next issue to address in considering possible causality is whether there are other more likely etiologies that could be responsible for the observed effects. Although it is important to be appropriately vigilant for possible adverse drug effects, it is equally important not to miss an alternative cause for the patient's condition. There are certain clinical settings in which establishing an ADE becomes a diagnosis by exclusion. For example, in the case of persistent fever, the assignment of the diagnosis "drug fever" should not be made until a complete search for infectious causes has excluded this etiology.

Another factor to consider in contemplating a diagnosis of ADE is "What is the patient's response to cessation of a suspect drug (dechallenge)?" In this case, the pharmacokinetics of the agent and the timing of resolution of the specific condition must be carefully considered. In some instances, the resolution of a "type A" ADE closely follows the pharmacokinetics of the suspect agent. For example, in the case of acute ethanol intoxication, central nervous system effects resolve in association with decreasing plasma concentrations of ethanol. However, confounding this approach is the case of a penicillin rash, which may develop within 1 or 2 days of starting the medication but may take several days to weeks to completely resolve. In this case of a "type B" ADE, the resolution of the condition (rash) occurs over a much longer time period than would be predicted by the pharmacokinetics of the agent. When a suspected ADE resolves after discontinuation of exposure to the offending agent, along a predictable time course, then the result of this "dechallenge" would support the diagnosis of ADE.

Last, the clinician may have the opportunity or need to rechallenge the patient with the suspect agent. If the rechallenge results in the identical response or effect, then this would be considered strong evidence to support a causal relationship for the suspect agent and the adverse event. In the setting of a serious or life-threatening adverse event, it is too dangerous to perform a rechallenge with the suspect drug, in which case the response to rechallenge will not be known. In this setting, the weight of evidence previously discussed will then be the only factor available to assign the probability of causality.

EXAMPLES OF DRUG WITHDRAWALS FROM THE UNITED STATES MARKET

When concern for the safety of a particular drug no longer suggests an acceptable risk–benefit relationship for continued availability of a drug product, the FDA begins a defined process to remove the drug from the market. Table 117–2 contains a compilation of products that have been withdrawn or removed from the market in the United States for reasons of safety or efficacy. The manufacturers have voluntarily withdrawn the majority of the drugs listed in Table 117–2 from the United States market. Only very rarely has the FDA itself actually removed a drug from the market. One example where the FDA did act is the drug phenformin, which was removed by the FDA after due process was completed. More typically, the manufacturer removes the drug from the market after notification by the Food and Drug Administration that regulatory action is being initiated against their product. For several of the products listed in Table 117–2, the pharmaceutical manufacturer filed suit against the Food and Drug Administration to fight or delay the planned regulatory action against the product. The manufacturer's legal action generally prolongs the time the product remains on the market because the drug usually continues to be sold while the legal proceedings and appeals proceed through the courts. Several of the more recent drug withdrawals in the United States are discussed as examples.

Over the last several years, three types of ADE have been of particular concern as a result of unexpected drug safety issues discovered during the postmarketing phase for a drug product. These are (1) prolongation of the QT interval, (2) significant drug-drug

interactions, and (3) hepatotoxicity. Each of these safety issues is represented below by a recent drug withdrawal.

Prolongation of the QT Interval

Three recent drug withdrawals exemplified a serious drug safety issue with an agent found to prolong the QT interval when administered alone or as the result of increasing plasma concentrations of the drug as a result of inhibition of its metabolism by other medications. The three examples in this category are terfenadine (Seldane), astemizole (Hismanal), and cisapride (Propulsid).

Clinical studies with terfenadine began in the early 1970s. The investigational new drug application was filed with the Food and Drug Administration in 1972. Clinical studies were completed in the drug development package by 1983, and the new drug application was submitted to the FDA at that time. After 26 months of review, terfenadine was approved for marketing in the United States in 1985. The case presented in the beginning of this chapter was in fact the initial indication of a serious drug-drug interaction and led to a subsequent prospective FDA-funded clinical investigation to establish the interaction. Significant labeling changes, the addition of a "black box" warning in the drug label, and a series of "Dear Doctor" letters highlighting this new safety issue were initiated in 1992. In 1998, the drug was voluntarily withdrawn from the market by the sponsor, coincident with FDA approval of fexofenadine, a noncardiotoxic metabolite of terfenadine, marketed as an extended-release combination with pseudoephedrine (Allegra-D™).[11] The terfenadine case pointed out for the first time the potential for noncardiovascular drugs to cause potent or fatal cardiotoxic effects subsequent to a drug-drug interaction.

Astemizole (Hismanal™), another antihistamine, was approved by the FDA in 1988. In the late 1980s and early 1990s, postmarketing reports from the FDA Spontaneous Reporting System (SRS) pointed out cardiac-related ADEs similar to those associated with terfenadine. The SRS and other reports again suggested an association between either excessive doses of astemizole or its administration in combination with inhibitors of its metabolism and deleterious cardiac repolarization effects leading to increased risk for cardiac dysrhythmias, particularly torsades de pointes. In the mid 1990s, "Dear Doctor" letters were sent to prescribers in the United States. A significant modification of the drug label to include a "black box" warning for these newly discovered, potentially fatal drug-drug interactions was made. In June 1999, the FDA announced that the sponsor was voluntarily withdrawing astemizole from the market.[10] There are substantial parallels between terfenadine and astemizole. Both agents are nonsedating antihistamine compounds that are metabolized by cytochrome P450 (CYP3A) and alter cardiac repolarization to produce prolongation of the QT interval, leading to cardiac dysrhythmias, torsades de pointes, and sudden death.

The most recent voluntary drug withdrawal resulting from altered cardiac repolarization and increased risk of cardiac dysrhythmia involved cisapride (Propulsid™). By December 31, 1999, cisapride was associated with 341 reports of cardiac dysrhythmias including 80 fatalities. The mechanism for the prodysrhythmic effect is less well documented for cisapride than for astemizole and terfenadine, but the drug is believed to alter cardiac repolarization, possibly through a potassium channel mechanism, and inhibition of cisapride metabolism increases the risk for dysrhythmia and death. Administration of cisapride with inhibitors of CYP3A such

TABLE 117–2. List of Drug Products Withdrawn or Removed from the Market for Reasons of Safety and Effectiveness

Name of Drug	Year of Introduction	Month and Year of Withdrawal	Reason for Withdrawal
Adenosine phosphate	1933	1973 (FDA)	Formerly marketed as a component of Adeno for injection, Adco for injection, and other drug products, it was determined to be neither safe nor effective for its intended uses as a vasodilator and an antiinflammatory agent.
Adrenal cortex	1937	January 1978 (FDA)	The low level of corticosteroids found in adrenal cortex injection and adrenal cortex extract were determined to present a substantial risk of undertreatment of serious conditions such as adrenal cortical insufficiency, burns, and hypoglycemia. The FDA determined that adrenal cortex for injection and adrenal cortex extract represented a significant potential hazard and directed the removal of these drug products.
Alosetron hydrochloride	February 2000 (FDA)	November 2000	Reported cases of intestinal damage resulting from reduced blood flow to the intestine (ischemic colitis) and severely obstructed or ruptured bowels.
Aminopyrine	1964 (NDA)	October 1977 (NDA)	Aminopyrine caused agranulocytosis, a condition characterized by a decrease in the number of certain white blood cells and lesions on the mucous membrane and skin. Some of the cases of agranulocytosis were fatal.
Astemizole	December 1988 (FDA)	Voluntarily withdrawn June 1999	Because of low prescription usage and the availability of other agents with fewer propensities for drug interactions, Janssen Pharmaceutica discontinued this agent from manufacture.
Azaribine		Approval of NDA withdrawn June 1977	The use of azaribine, formerly marketed as Triazure tablets, was associated with very serious thromboembolic events.
Benoxaprofen		Voluntarily withdrawn August 1982	Formerly marketed as Oraflex tablets, was associated with fatal cholestatic jaundice among other serious adverse reactions.
Bithionol		Approval of NDA withdrawn October 1967	Formerly marketed as an active ingredient in various topical drug products, it was shown to be a potent photosensitizer with the potential to cause serious skin disorders.
Bromfenac sodium	July 1997 (FDA)	Voluntarily withdrawn June 1998	Formerly marketed as Duract capsules, it was associated with fatal hepatic failure.
Butamben		Approval of NDA withdrawn August 1964	Formerly marketed as Efocaine, it was associated with severe adverse reactions such as severe tissue slough and transverse myelitis.
Camphorated oil		1982 (FDA)	Products containing camphorated oil were associated with poisoning in infants and young children following unintentional ingestion.
Carbetapentane citrate		Approval of NDA withdrawn November 1972	Formerly marketed as Candette Cough Jel, it was determined not to be safe because the inexact methods of measuring the gel by consumers were potentially dangerous.
Casein, iodinated		October 1964	Formerly marketed as a component of Neo-Barine, it was associated with thyrotoxic side effects.
Chlorhexidine gluconate	1976 (FDA)	Early 1984 (FDA)	Formulated for use as a patient preoperative skin preparation. Chlorhexidine gluconate topical tincture 0.5%, formerly marketed as Hibitane, was associated with chemical and thermal burns when used as a patient preoperative skin preparation.
Chlormadinone acetate		March 1972 (FDA)	Formerly marketed as a component of the combination drug products Estalor-21 and C-Quens tablets, it was associated with the development of mammary tumors in dogs.
Chloroform	1831?	1976 (FDA)	National Cancer Institute studies demonstrated that chloroform is carcinogenic in animals.
Cisapride monohydrate	July 1993	July 2000	Marketed as Propulsid, its primary health risk was torsades de pointes. Propulsid remains minimally available on a patient-by-patient basis for those with severely debilitating conditions.
Cobalt		1967 (FDA)	All drug products containing cobalt salts (except radioactive forms of cobalt and its salts and cobalamin and its derivatives). FDA found that cobalt salts were not safe or effective for treatment of iron-deficiency anemia. The toxic effects of cobalt salts include liver damage, claudication, and myocardial damage.
Dexfenfluramine hydrochloride	April 1996 (FDA)	September 1997	Formerly marketed as Redux capsules, it was associated with valvular heart disease.
Diamthazole dihydrochloride		July 1977	Formerly marketed as Asterol ointment, powder, and tincture, was associated with neurotoxicity.
Dibromsalan		1975 (FDA)	Formerly marketed in a number of drug products, largely antibacterial soaps, as an antimicrobial, preservative, or for other purposes; was, with other halogenated salicylanilides listed in this table, found to be a potent photosensitizer capable of causing disabling skin disorders.

(continued)

TABLE 117–2. List of Drug Products Withdrawn or Removed from the Market for Reasons of Safety and Effectiveness (continued)

Name of Drug	Year of Introduction	Month and Year of Withdrawal	Reason for Withdrawal
Diethylstilbestrol	1941 (FDA)	February 1975 (FDA)	All oral and parenteral drug products containing 25 mg or more of diethylstilbestrol per unit dose. Diethylstilbestrol, marketed in various tablet and parenteral drug products, was associated with adenocarcinoma of the vagina in the offspring of the patient when used in early pregnancy.
Dihydrostreptomycin sulfate		July 1970 (FDA)	Formerly marketed in several parenteral drug products, it was associated with ototoxicity.
Dipyrone		June 1977 (FDA)	Formerly marketed as Dimethone tablets and injection, Protemp oral liquid, and other drug products; it was associated with potentially fatal agranulocytosis.
Encainide hydrochloride	December 1986 (FDA)	December 1991	Formerly marketed as Enkaid capsules, it was associated with increased death rates in patients who had asymptomatic heart rhythm abnormalities after a recent heart attack.
Fenfluramine hydrochloride	1973	September 1997 (FDA)	Formerly marketed as Pondimin tablets, it was associated with valvular heart disease.
Flosequinan		July 1993	Formerly marketed as Manoplax tablets, it was the subject of a study that indicated the drug had adverse effects on survival and that beneficial effects on the symptoms of heart failure did not last beyond the first 3 months of therapy. After the first 3 months of therapy, patients on the drug had a higher rate of hospitalization than patients taking a placebo.
Gelatin	1682?	April 1978 (FDA)	Gelatin for intravenous use, formerly marketed as Knox Special Gelatine Solution Intravenous-6 percent, was found not to be suitable as a plasma expander because the drug caused increased blood viscosity, reduced blood clotting, and prolonged bleeding time.
Glycerol, iodinated		April 1993 (FDA)	Formerly marketed as Iodur Elixir and other drug products, it was found to have carcinogenic potential.
Gonadotropin, chorionic	1939 (FDA)	July 1972	Chorionic gonadotropins of animal origins, formerly marketed as Synapoidin Steri-Vial, were shown to produce allergic reactions.
Grepafloxacin hydrochloride	November 1997	November 1999	Formerly marketed as Raxar, this antibiotic drug was withdrawn because of its primary health risk relating to torsades de pointes.
Mepazine		May 1970	Formerly marketed as Pacatal tablets, and mepazine acetate, formerly marketed as Pacatal for injection, was associated with granulocytopenia, agranulocytosis, paralytic ileus, urinary retention, seizures, hypotension, and jaundice.
Metabromsalan		1975 (FDA)	Formerly marketed in a number of drug products, largely antibacterial soaps, as an antimicrobial, preservative, or for other purposes, was, with other halogenated salicylanilides listed in this table, found to be a potent photosensitizer capable of causing disabling skin disorders.
Methamphetamine hydrochloride	1943 (FDA)	March (1973)	Formerly marketed as Methedrine injection and Drinalfa injection and used as an adjunct treatment for weight reduction, it was found to have a history of serious abuse and a severe risk of dependence.
Methapyrilene		June 1979	Formerly marketed in many drug products, it was shown to be a potent carcinogen.
Methopholine		March 1965	Formerly marketed as Versidyne tablets, it was associated with ophthalmic changes and corneal opacities in dogs.
Mibefradil dihydrochloride	June 1997	June 1998	Formerly marketed as Posicor tablets, it was associated with potentially harmful interactions with other drugs. Mibefradil dihydrochloride reduced the activity of certain liver enzymes that are important in helping the body eliminate many other drugs. Inhibiting these enzymes can cause some of these drugs to accumulate to dangerous levels in the body.
Neomycin sulfate	1952 (FDA)	January 1989 (FDA)	Parenteral neomycin sulfate was found to present toxicity problems when used to irrigate wounds and was found not to be acceptable for the treatment of urinary tract infections because of the availability of newer, safer antibiotics that were as effective as, or more effective than, parenteral neomycin sulfate.
Nitrofurazone	1945 (FDA)	December 1974 June 1975	All drug products containing nitrofurazone (except topical drug products formulated for dermatologic application). Nitrofurazone, formerly marketed in nasal drops, otic drops, and vaginal suppositories, was associated with mammary neoplasia in rats.
Nomifensine maleate		January 1986 (FDA)	Formerly marketed as Merital capsules; it was associated with an increased incidence of hemolytic anemia.
Oxyphenisatin		March 1973	Oxyphenisatin, formerly marketed in Lavema Compound Solution and Lavema Enema Powder; it was associated with hepatitis and jaundice.
Oxyphenisatin acetate		February 1972	Formerly marketed in Dialose Plus capsules, Noloc capsules, and other drug products; it was associated with hepatitis and jaundice.

(continued)

TABLE 117–2. List of Drug Products Withdrawn or Removed from the Market for Reasons of Safety and Effectiveness (continued)

Name of Drug	Year of Introduction	Month and Year of Withdrawal	Reason for Withdrawal
Phenacetin		November 1983	Formerly marketed in A.P.C. with Butalbital tablets and capsules and other drug products, was associated with a high potential for harm to the kidneys and the possibility of hemolytic anemia and methemoglobinemia resulting from abuse.
Phenformin hydrochloride		November 1978 (FDA)	Formerly marketed as D.B.I. tablets, Meltrol-50 capsules, and other drug products; it was associated with lactic acidosis.
Pipamazine		July 1969	Formerly marketed as Mornidine tablets and injection; it was associated with hepatic lesions.
Potassium arsenite	April 1980 (FDA)	Voluntarily withdrawn	Formerly marketed as Fowler's Solution (oral); it was toxic and highly carcinogenic.
Potassium chloride		July 1977 and April 1992	All solid oral dosage form drug products containing potassium chloride that supply 100 mg or more of potassium per dosage unit (except for controlled-release dosage forms and those products formulated for preparation of solution before ingestion). Concentrated solid oral dosage forms of potassium salt were associated with small bowel lesions.
Povidone	1986 (FDA)	April 1978	All intravenous drug products containing povidone. Povidone, marketed as Polyvinylpyrrolidone in Normal Saline, was found to be unsafe for use as a plasma expander in the emergency treatment of shock because povidone accumulates in the body and may cause storage disease with the formation of granulomas. Povidone also interferes with blood coagulation, hemostasis, and blood typing and crossmatching.
Reserpine	1953 (FDA)	May 1977	All oral dosage form drug products containing more than 1 mg of reserpine. Reserpine, marketed as Reserpoid tablets, Rau-Sed tablets, and other drug products for the treatment of hypertension and psychiatric disorders, were associated with a greater frequency and severity of adverse effects in strengths greater than 1 mg.
Sparteine sulfate		August 1979	Formerly marketed as Spartocin injection and Tocosamine sterile solution, it was found to have unpredictable effects and was associated with tetanic uterine contractions and obstetric complications.
Sulfadimethoxine		March 1966	Formerly marketed in Madricidin capsules, it was associated with Stevens-Johnson syndrome and fatalities.
Sulfathiazole		September 1970	All drug products containing sulfathiazole (except those formulated for vaginal use). Sulfathiazole, formerly marketed in Tresamide tablets and several other brands of tablets, was associated with renal complications, rash, fever, blood dyscrasias, and liver damage.
Suprofen	1988 (FDA)	May 1987	All drug products containing suprofen (except ophthalmic solutions). Suprofen, formerly marketed as Suprol capsules, was associated with flank pain syndrome.
Sweet spirits of nitre		1980 (FDA)	Also known as spirit of nitre, spirit of nitrous ether, and ethyl nitrite spirit; it was associated with methemoglobinemia in infants.
Temafloxacin hydrochloride		September 1997	Formerly marketed as Omniflox tablets, it was associated with hypoglycemia in elderly patients as well as a constellation of multisystem organ involvement characterized by hemolytic anemia, frequently associated with renal failure, markedly abnormal liver tests, and coagulopathy.
Terfenadine	May 1985 (FDA)	February 1998 (FDA)	Formerly marketed in Seldane and Seldane-D tablets, it was associated with serious heart problems when used concurrently with certain drugs, including certain antibiotics and antifungals.
3,3′,4′,5-Tetrachloro-salicylanilide		1975 (FDA)	Formerly marketed in a number of drug products, largely antibacterial soaps, as an antimicrobial, preservative, or for other purposes; it was, with other halogenated salicylanilides listed in this table, found to be a potent photosensitizer capable of causing disabling skin disorders.
Tetracycline	1953 (FDA)		All liquid oral drug products formulated for pediatric use containing tetracycline in a concentration greater than 25 mg/mL. Concentrated tetracycline was associated with temporary inhibition of bone growth, permanent staining of the teeth, and enamel hypoplasia in children.
Ticrynafen		May 1996	Formerly marketed as Selacryn tablets, it was associated with liver toxicity.
Tribromsalan		1975 (FDA)	Formerly marketed in a number of drug products, largely antibacterial soaps, as an antimicrobial, preservative, or for other purposes; it was, with other halogenated salicylanilides listed in this table, found to be a potent photosensitizer capable of causing disabling skin disorders.

(continued)

TABLE 117–2. List of Drug Products Withdrawn or Removed from the Market for Reasons of Safety and Effectiveness (continued)

Name of Drug	Year of Introduction	Month and Year of Withdrawal	Reason for Withdrawal
Trichloroethane		1977 (FDA)	All aerosol drug products intended for inhalation containing trichloroethane. Trichloroethane is potentially toxic to the cardiovascular system and was associated with deaths from misuse or abuse.
Troglitazone	January 1997	March 2000	Formerly marketed as Rezulin, a widely used diabetic drug; it was withdrawn because of its apparent cause of liver failure.
Urethane		March 1977	Urethane (also known as urethan and ethyl carbamate), formerly marketed as an inactive ingredient in Profenil injection, was determined to be carcinogenic.
Vinyl chloride		1974 (FDA)	All aerosol drug products containing vinyl chloride. The inhalation of vinyl chloride is associated with acute toxicity manifested by dizziness, headache, disorientation, and unconsciousness.
Zirconium		1977 (FDA)	Formerly used in several aerosol drug products as an antiperspirant, it was associated with human skin granulomas and toxic effects in the lungs and other internal organs of test animals.
Zomepirac sodium		March 1983	Formerly marketed as Zomax tablets, it was associated with fatal and near-fatal anaphylactoid reactions.

as clarithromycin results in prolongation of the QTc (QT interval corrected for heart rate) interval on the surface electrocardiogram.[33] Despite several modifications in the drug label to enhance the warnings for the product, reports of significant cardiotoxicity continued. In March 2000, the manufacturer agreed to stop marketing this agent as of July 2000.[9] Unlike the voluntary withdrawals of astemizole and terfenadine, the sponsor was able to retain the ability to make cisapride available to patients who meet specific clinical eligibility criteria for a limited-access protocol. It is unclear at this point whether or not this agent will eventually be completely withdrawn from the US market.

Clinically Significant Drug-Drug Interactions

The cases of terfenadine, astemizole, and cisapride emphasize both the potential for a drug to alter cardiac repolarization as an ADE and also the importance of understanding the metabolism of a drug and the potential consequences of an alteration of the metabolism of that drug.

An example of a drug recently withdrawn from the US market because of postmarketing discovery of a plethora of drug-drug interactions is mibefradil (Posicor™). Mibefradil is a calcium channel blocker chemically unlike other available calcium channel blockers. The drug was approved by the FDA for the treatment of patients with hypertension and chronic stable angina. Clinical research in the United States drug development program began in 1992 with filing of the investigational new drug application with the FDA. The 4-year clinical program concluded with submission of the new drug application in 1996. After 15 months of review, the FDA approved mibefradil for marketing in 1997. At the time mibefradil was approved, information regarding its inhibition of hepatic enzymes of the P-450 system were known and printed on the drug label. The initial labeling for mibefradil specifically listed three drug-drug interactions: astemizole, cisapride, and terfenadine. Inhibition of CYP3A by mibefradil was known to cause accumulation of parent (unmetabolized) drug in the case of these three drugs, leading to an increased risk for cardiac dysrhythmias. During the 1 year that mibefradil was marketed, information began to accumulate regarding drug-drug interactions with many other agents as well. As the in vitro and in vivo drug interaction data continued to accumulate for mibefradil, the FDA made label-

ing changes and issued a public warning for these potential drug interactions within 5 months of its initial approval. In addition, the sponsor distributed a letter to healthcare professionals warning of drug-drug interactions. In the face of a growing and significant list of drug-drug interactions, and a 3-year international study demonstrating no clinical benefit of mibefradil over placebo for congestive heart failure, the FDA initiated regulatory action. In an unprecedented step for a drug with numerous drug interactions, the FDA then requested that it be withdrawn from the market approximately 1 year after it was approved. The FDA felt that the diversity of drug-drug interactions could not be addressed by standard drug label instructions and additional public warnings.

Drugs That Cause Hepatotoxicity

Another category of ADE of concern recently is those agents that cause hepatotoxicity. In June, 1998, the manufacturer of the nonsteroidal antiinflammatory drug (NSAID) bromfenac sodium (Duract™) withdrew this agent from the US market. Clinical trials with bromfenac began in the United States in 1984 with filing of the investigational new drug application. The new drug application was submitted for review to the FDA in 1994 and after 28 months of review was approved in 1997. The drug was introduced into the United States market later that same year but withdrawn approximately 11 months later after postmarketing discovery of significant hepatotoxicity. Although no cases of serious liver injury had apparently been reported during premarketing clinical trials, after introduction to the market a higher incidence of liver enzyme elevation was found in patients who were being treated with the agent. Postapproval exposure of patients to bromfenac was generally for longer time periods than those for which subjects in the clinical trials were treated. Because of a preapproval concern by the FDA that long-term exposure to bromfenac could cause hepatotoxicity, bromfenac labeling specified that the product was to be used for 10 days or less. This dosing limitation appeared to be in conflict with the initial approved drug indication for treatment of a chronic condition (eg, osteoarthritis). Information concerning elevated liver enzymes was actually included in the original product labeling. The postmarketing surveillance of this product identified rare cases of hepatitis and liver failure, including some patients who required liver transplantation, among those using the drug for more than the 10 days specified on the label. In February 1998, approximately 6 months after approval for marketing, the FDA amended the drug label for bromfenac sodium with a special "black box" warning indicating that the drug should not be taken for more than 10 days and emphasizing the risk of severe hepatitis and liver failure. The label change was done in conjunction with a required "Dear Doctor" letter to prescribers informing them of this labeling change. Nonetheless, severe injury and death from long-term use of bromfenac sodium continued to be reported, and ultimately, the sponsor agreed to voluntarily withdraw bromfenac sodium from the market. The withdrawal of bromfenac sodium raised several important questions concerning interpretation of "safety laboratories," such as liver enzymes during the drug development program, and also raised questions concerning the effectiveness of drug labeling.

Another example of a drug recently withdrawn for safety concerns related to hepatotoxicity is the oral hypoglycemic agent troglitazone (Rezulin™). Although it was approved in the mid-1990s, severe liver toxicity was detected by postmarketing surveillance for troglitazone beginning in 1997. Increasingly serious labeling changes and warnings to prescribers recommending close monitoring of liver function tests in patients taking troglitazone were issued over the next 2 years. In March 1999, an FDA advisory committee reviewed the status of troglitazone and its risk of liver toxicity and recommended continued marketing of this drug in patients with type II diabetes who were not well controlled by other drugs. When two newer agents for type II diabetes, rosiglitazone and pioglitazone, became available, the FDA concluded that the risk profile for troglitazone was significantly worse than these newer agents and then asked the manufacturer of troglitazone to remove the drug from the market.[16] Analogous to the example with mibefradil, this FDA-initiated drug withdrawal was based on a change in the risk-benefit profile for the specific agent in light of new safety information discovered during the postapproval phase for the drug.

One voluntary withdrawal of two separate drugs used in combination serves as an example of the discovery and publicizing of an unusual adverse event occurring years after individual drug approval but after a significant increase in the prescription use of the combination product. The drug fenfluramine was approved in 1973 after an FDA review period of 75 months. Clinical investigation of a similar agent, dexfenfluramine, began in 1991 in the United States with approval of its IND. The new drug application for this product was filed in 1993, and after 35 months of review the drug was approved for marketing in 1996. A significant increase in prescription use of a combination product of fenfluramine with phentermine (referred to as "fen-phen") began to occur in the 1990s when clinical data suggested that this drug combination was effective in a weight loss program.[35–37] Dexfenfluramine was approved for weight loss as a single agent for up to 1 year of use. Use of the fen-phen drug combination, however, was never fully approved by the FDA and was therefore considered an "off-label usage" of the product. The number of prescriptions for the drug combination soared in the mid-1990s. In July 1997, research from the Mayo Clinic reported 24 cases[7] of an unusual form of cardiac valvular disease causing aortic and mitral regurgitation in patients using the fen-phen combination. The publicity surrounding the potential linkage of this drug combination to an unusual adverse event led to a significant increase in reports of possible adverse events associated with this drug combination. The FDA issued a public health advisory and initiated fur-

ther epidemiologic studies in order to ascertain its prevalence. The FDA also encouraged echocardiographic studies of valvular diseases in patients taking fenfluramine or dexfenfluramine either alone or in combination with phentermine. Although at the onset neither the FDA, the product manufacturers, nor the medical community expected valvular lesions to be associated with either fenfluramine or dexfenfluramine, the epidemiologic evidence suggested a possible association, leading the FDA to conclude that these agents should be removed from the US market. The potential association of valvular heart disease with these agents is an example of the use of a case-control study to explore a possible causal relationship between drug exposure and an ADE. In this case, it is unclear what the strength of the MedWatch signal was for the possible association of cardiac valvular disease with exposure to the fen-phen combination. If the association between cardiac valvular lesions and exposure to the drug combination or components of the combination is ultimately proven to be true, however, this would serve as an example of elucidation of a rare, unexpected ADE as the result of a dramatic increase in the number of exposed patients utilizing a product.

ADVERSE DRUG EVENTS CAUSED BY MEDICAL ERRORS

Medical therapy results in unintended injury to an estimated 1.3 million people in the United States annually.[23] The incidence of adverse drug events (ADEs) has been studied within both the inpatient and outpatient settings. Primarily because of the availability of data, the inpatient setting is more extensively studied. Depending on the method utilized for detection of ADEs, studies have reported an ADE rate of between 2.0 and 6.5 per 100 medical and 100 surgical admissions in certain inpatient settings.[3,6] When the upper rate of 6.5% is extrapolated to all hospitalized patients in the United States, the estimated cost incurred as a result of ADEs is a staggering $5.6 million per year for a single 700-bed teaching hospital.[4] Half of this $5.6 million, or $2.8 million, was considered a result of *preventable* ADEs.[4] A preventable ADE is one that would not have happened if an error in prescription, dispensing, or drug administration had not occurred.

The method for data acquisition can influence the observed rate for studies examining ADEs.[30] Automated, computer-based systems generally do not detect as many errors as are found by manual review of hospital charts by a healthcare professional. The number of medications being administered to an inpatient correlates with the potential for the occurrence of ADEs.[2] The risk for medication-related errors in the pediatric population has also been studied.[22] A rate of nearly five medication errors for every 1000 medication orders is reported in the pediatric inpatient setting.[13] The financial impact of all ADEs occurring in the inpatient setting is estimated at approximately $2 billion per year in the United States.[4,5] In these estimates, costs that are included are those resulting from an increased hospital length of stay and increased patient morbidity. Costs not included in the estimate are the costs to the healthcare system for malpractice claims or the costs to the patient or healthcare systems incurred after discharge from the hospital. The costs of outpatient drug-induced patient morbidity are also estimated to be considerable in the United States.[19]

Preventable adverse medical events (not just ADEs) are estimated to be the eighth leading cause of death in the United States.

If this extrapolation is accurate, then deaths from preventable adverse medical events exceed deaths from motor vehicle crashes or AIDS in the United States.

A significant number of preventable ADEs result from medical errors. A recent Institute of Medicine report has drawn attention to the large number of medical errors occurring in the United States. In the setting of a tertiary-care teaching hospital, the overall medication error rate was estimated to be 3.13 errors for each 1000 orders written for inpatients. More than one-half of these errors were judged to be significant.[24] Medication-related errors are a large and important subset of overall medical errors in that the vast majority of medication-related errors are preventable. The incidence of medication-related errors as a cause of death may be increasing in the United States.[21]

Recommendations of the Institute of Medicine report include the following:

1. The Congress should create a Center for Patient Safety within the agency of Health Care Research and Quality to set national goals for patient safety, to investigate causes and seek remedies for errors, and to educate.
2. A nationwide mandatory reporting system should be established to provide for the collection of standardized information about adverse events that result in death or serious harm.
3. The development of a voluntary reporting effort should be encouraged by the Center for Patient Safety.
4. The Congress should pass legislation to extend peer review protection to data related to patient safety and quality improvement that are collected and analyzed by healthcare organizations for internal use or shared with others solely for the purposes of improving safety and quality.
5. Performance standards and expectations for healthcare organizations should focus greater attention on patient safety.
6. Performance standards and expectations for health professionals should focus greater attention on patient safety.
7. The Food and Drug Administration should increase attention to the safe use of drugs in both pre- and postmarketing processes through the following actions: developing standards for the design of drug packaging and labeling that will maximize safety in use; requiring pharmaceutical companies to test (using FDA-approved methods) proposed drug names to identify and remedy potential sound-alike and look-alike confusion with existing drug names; and working with physicians, pharmacists, consumers, and others to establish appropriate responses to problems identified through postmarketing surveillance, especially for concerns that are perceived to require immediate response to protect safety of patients.
8. Healthcare organizations and the professionals that affiliate with them should make continuously improved patient safety a declared and serious aim by establishing patient safety programs with defined executive responsibility.
9. Healthcare organizations should implement proven medication safety practices.

The committee writing the Institute of Medicine report stated that they recognized that no single activity or recommendation would provide a solution to the medical error problem; however, they suggested that a combination of the activities proposed in the recommendations will provide a roadmap or starting point for a safer healthcare system.[21]

THE ROLE OF THE CLINICAL TOXICOLOGIST IN THE DETECTION AND PREVENTION OF ADVERSE DRUG EVENTS

Clinical toxicologists include healthcare professionals, such as physicians, pharmacists, and nurses, with a focus on the recognition and treatment of drug- and/or toxin-induced disease. Medical toxicologists are physicians who have recieved subspeciality training in clinical toxicology. Clinical paharmacists are generally Doctors of Pharmacy (PharmD) with comparable advanced training. Clinical toxicologists occupy an important role in ADE detection and prevention. There are at least three main areas in which the clinical toxicologist can have significant beneficial impact. These areas include patient care, education, and administrative functions. In patient care, it is common for the medical toxicologist to be the first medical specialist called to see a patient with a potential ADE. As a result, clinical toxicology occupies an important position as sentinel for drug-induced disease. Maintenance of clinical skills and appropriate continuing education is essential, especially in the area of newly approved therapeutic agents or newly recognized ADEs caused by older approved therapeutic agents. Maintenance of a current knowledge base in the area of therapeutics enhances the ability of the clinical toxicologist to diagnose drug-induced disease. Perhaps more than any other medical specialty, clinical toxicologists are likely to include a thorough medication history that also includes nonprescription products, herbal products, and so-called nutraceutical dietary supplements. As stated previously, obtaining a history for drug exposure is an essential component in attributing an observed adverse medical event to a specific drug product. The clinical toxicologist's involvement in the clinical arena, especially in settings where the initial diagnosis of ADEs can be made, serves to provide an important role model: the clinical toxicologist is an educator in the specialty to promote the detection and prevention of ADEs.

Medical toxicologists occupy many different roles in clinical practice in the United States. An obvious role for the medical toxicologist is as educator in the academic setting of a medical school and affiliated teaching hospitals. Here, the academic toxicologist can champion the inclusion of education in therapeutics in the curriculum for medical school students and residents-in-training and take an active role in the implementation of the instruction. Assuring that the curriculum in therapeutics includes recognition and prevention of ADEs and medical errors that lead to ADEs could have a significant beneficial impact on the ultimate outcome of the education process toward reduction of preventable ADEs. In addition to making sure that quality information is presented in the curriculum for trainees, the medical toxicologist can often create a special teaching opportunity for this type of education by establishing an elective experience or in some instances a required clinical experience in the curriculum for training in therapeutics. Participation in a quality learning experience can significantly impact on the graduates' knowledge of and attitudes toward therapeutics and risk reduction in the practice of medicine. Although the Institute of Medicine report discussed earlier did not focus on education initiatives in its main recommendations for reduction of medical errors in United States, it seems logical that education be considered one of the major tools to prevent medical errors with therapeutic agents. Education can intervene at the point of initiation by adding emphasis on therapeutics during the education process for writers of the prescription. Surveys of medical errors involving therapeutic agents show that a lack of specific drug knowledge is a common cause of preventable medical errors involving medication.[22]

In the private practice setting, the medical toxicologist sometimes has an opportunity to educate fellows in training in the medical specialty as well as peers who call on them for consultations. In these settings, a consistent approach to the patient that includes the listing of drug-induced disease, drug excess, or potential drug-drug interactions to explain an unexpected drug response can provide an example for one's medical colleagues.

The administrative functions that the clinical toxicologist can perform could also beneficially impact on enhancing detection and prevention of ADEs. The main administrative functions that fall into this category include the reporting of ADEs and hospital or health organization committee service (for example, the pharmacy and therapeutics committee).

ADEs are known to be significantly underreported in the United States.[15,29,31] Reporting ADEs at the local (hospital) and national level (MedWatch) has been a priority and has been made less difficult administratively. Despite efforts to encourage filing of ADE reports, the overall reporting rates do not appear to have changed significantly. A well-documented, complete report to MedWatch made by a healthcare professional is given priority review by the Food and Drug Administration. The MedWatch system encourages reporting of serious adverse events by all practitioners. Because the clinical toxicologist is likely to encounter a significant number of drug-induced disease cases from a diagnostic standpoint, practitioners of the specialty can make a significant impact on ADE reporting. Clinical toxicologists and their trainees should always submit an adverse event report locally for appropriate cases they encounter. Hospitals generally do not mandate or request that the reported event be "serious" as a requirement. The FDA's MedWatch system asks that reported events be serious in nature. Manual review of reports and database checks are performed by FDA, and duplicative reporting is accounted for when noted. In addition to reporting of the ADE, the clinical toxicologist should promote publication of case reports of all new adverse events or adverse events occurring with newly approved products. Such publication often stimulates appropriate reporting of ADEs from other practitioners.

Service on hospital or healthcare organization committees is another important opportunity for clinical toxicologists to impact on the drug-induced disease problem. Whenever possible, clinical toxicologists should participate in the local hospital pharmacy and therapeutics committee. Often these committees have ADE-monitoring subcommittees where the expertise of the medical toxicologist in diagnosing drug-induced disease could prove beneficial to the organization. These committees systematically analyze trends in ADEs and occasionally recommend various interventions for the medical pharmacy, or nursing staff to reduce the potential risk for ADEs. These interventions include a targeted educational program, system modifications to reduce error risk, or limitation of a specific drug usage by certain components of the organization. Another committee where the toxicologist can have an impact on ADEs and medical error prevention is the quality assurance committee of the hospital or healthcare organization. Careful analysis of medical errors or ADE reports brought to the quality assurance committee can often reveal significant trends that are sometimes amenable to educational initiatives or systematic improvements in process. Again, the medical toxicologist can play an important

role on the committee as a practitioner of clinical medicine with specialized expertise in the potentially harmful effects of drugs.

SUMMARY

Drug-induced disease is common in both inpatient and outpatient settings in the practice of medicine. The resulting ADEs have a significant impact on patient mortality and morbidity in addition to producing a significant burden on the healthcare system. ADEs caused by newly approved drugs and ADEs resulting from a previously unrecognized association with therapeutic agents with a long marketing history continue to be a significant cause of mortality and morbidity. The medical toxicology specialty is well positioned to have a beneficial impact toward recognition and prevention of ADEs and medical errors. Early recognition of drug-induced disease by the medical toxicologist can benefit the individual patient in many cases and may lead to prevention of further patient harm by prompt ADE reporting to local authorities and, if appropriate, to the FDA. The rapidly expanding number of approved therapeutic agents requires that the medical toxicologist and other practitioners have a strong continuing education commitment to reduce the risk for ADEs and medication errors. Local and national-level involvement by the specialty of medical toxicology to design and implement programs and activities aimed at decreasing the medical error rate and the occurrence of preventable ADEs should benefit patients and, by extension, society.

REFERENCES

1. Alter BP: Bone marrow failure disorders. Mt Sinai J Med 1991; 58:521–534.
2. Bates DW, Cullen DJ, Laird NM, et al: Incidence of adverse drug events and potential adverse drug events: Implications for prevention. JAMA 1995;274:29–34.
3. Bates DW, Leape LL, Petrychi S: Incidence and prevention of adverse drug events in hospitalized adults. J Gen Intern Med 1993;8:289–294.
4. Bates DW, Spell N, Cullen DJ, et al: The costs of adverse drug events in hospitalized patients. JAMA 1997;277:307–311.
5. Classen DC, Pestonik SL, Evans R, et al: Adverse drug events in hospitalized patients: Excess length of stay, extra costs and attributable mortality. JAMA 1997;277:301–306.
6. Classen DC, Pestonik SL, Stanley L, et al: Computerized surveillance of adverse drug events in hospital patients. JAMA 1991;266: 2847–2851.
7. Connolly HM, Crary JL, McGoon MD, et al: Valvular heart disease associated with fenfluramine-phentermine. N Engl J Med 1997;337: 581–588.
8. Edwards IR, Aronson JK: Adverse drug reactions: Definitions, diagnosis and management. Lancet 2000;356:1255–1259.
9. FDA Talk Paper: "Janssen pharmaceutical stops marketing cisapride in the US," March 23, 2000.
10. FDA Talk Paper: "Janssen pharmaceutical announces the withdrawal of Hismanal from the market," June 21, 1999.z
11. FDA Talk Paper: "FDA approves Allegra-D manufactured to withdraw Seldane from marketplace," December 29, 1997.
12. FDA Talk Paper: "FDA Proposes to Withdraw Seldane Approval," January 13, 1997.
13. Folli HL, Poole RL, Benitz WE, et al: Medication error prevention by clinical pharmacies in two children's hospitals. Pediatrics 1987;79: 718–722.
14. Friedman MA, Woodcock J, Lumpkin MM, et al: The safety of newly approved medicines. Do recent market removals mean there is a problem? JAMA 1999;281:1728–1734.

15. Griffin JP, Weber JC: Voluntary systems of adverse reaction reporting. Part II. Adverse Drug React Acute Poisoning Rev 1986;5:23–55.

16. HHS News, P00–8, "Rezulin to be Withdrawn from the Market," March 21, 2000.

17. Honig PK, Woosley RL, Zamani K, et al: Changes in the pharmacokinetics and electrocardiographic pharmacodynamics of terfenadine with concomitant administration of erythromycin. Clin Pharmacol Ther 1992;52:231–238.

18. Honig PK, Wortham DC, Zamani K, et al: Terfenadine-ketoconazole interaction study, pharmacokinetic and electrocardiographic consequences. JAMA 1993;269:1513–1518.

19. Johnson JA, Bootman JL: Drug-related morbidity and mortality: A cost-of-illness model. Arch Intern Med 1995;155:1949–1956.

20. Kessler DA: Introducing MEDWatch: a new approach to reporting medications and device adverse effects and product problems. JAMA 1993;269:2765–2768.

21. Kohn LT, Corrigan JM, Donaldson MS: To Err Is Human: Building a Safer Health System. Washington, DC, Committee on Quality of Health Care in America, Institute of Medicine, 2000.

22. Koren G, Haslam R: Pediatric medication errors: predicting and preventing tenfold disasters. J Clin Pharmacol 1994;34:1043–1045.

23. Leape LL, Bates DW, Cullen DJ: Systems analysis of adverse drug events. JAMA 1995;274:35–43.

24. Lesar TS, Briceland L, Stein DS: Factors related to errors in medication prescribing. JAMA 1997;277:312–317.

25. Lewis JA: Post-marketing surveillance: how many patients? Trends Pharmacol Sci 1981;2:93.

26. MedWatch Web site: *http://www.fda.gov/medwatch/partner.htm.*

27. Meyboom RHB, Egberts ACG, Gribnau FWJ, Hekster YA: Pharmacovigilance in perspective. Drug Safety 1999;21:429–447.

28. Monahan BP, Ferguson CL, Killeavy ES, et al: Torsades de pointes occurring in association with terfenadine use. JAMA 1990;264:2788–2790.

29. Moride Y, Harambaru F, Requejo AA, Bejaud B: Underreporting of adverse drug reactions in general practice. Br J Clin Pharmacol 1997;43:177–181.

30. O'Neill RT: Some FDA perspectives on data monitoring in clinical trials in drug development. Stat Med (England) 1993;12:601–608; discussions 609–614.

31. Rogers AS, Israel E, Smith CR, et al: Physician knowledge, attitudes and behavior related to reporting adverse drug events. Arch Intern Med 1988;148:1596–1600.

32. Schwartz J: Is FDA too quick to clear drugs? Growing recalls, side-effect risks raise questions. Washington Post, A01, March 23, 1999.

33. van Haarst AD, van't Klooster GA, van Gerven JM, et al: The influence of cisapride and clarithromycin on QT intervals in healthy volunteers Clin Pharmacol Ther 1998;64:542–546.

34. Wallace Laboratories: Express telegram to physicians. Cranbury, NJ: Wallace Laboratories, August 1, 1994.

35. Weintraub M, Sundaresan PR, Madan M, et al: Long-term weight control study (weeks 0–34): The enhancement of behavior modification, caloric restriction, and exercise by fenfluramine plus phentermine versus placebo. Clin Pharmacol Ther 1992;51:586–594.

36. Weintraub M, Sundaresan PR, Schuster B, et al. Long-term weight control study (weeks 34–104): An open-label study of continuous fenfluramine plus phentermine versus targeted intermittent medication as adjuncts to behavior modification, caloric restriction, and exercise. Clin Pharmacol Ther 1992;51:595–601.

37. Weintraub M. Long-term weight control: The National Heart, Lung, and Blood Institute–funded multimodal intervention study. Clin Pharmacol Ther 1992;51:581–585.

38. Wood AJJ: The safety of new medicines: The importance of asking the right questions. JAMA 1999;281:1753.

Walter LeStrange / Kevin Porter

The use of emergency services has increased dramatically since the early 1970s, and along with it the number of toxicologic emergencies has increased steadily and continues to rise today. This chapter is concerned primarily with the medical-legal management of patients who present to an emergency department (ED) with an organic impairment, that is, a relatively recent deterioration in the level of cognitive or behavioral function caused by the effects of drugs or alcohol. A secondary component of this chapter addresses the legal dilemmas associated with the social and ethical issues that emergency practitioners routinely face.

Patients who are experiencing toxicologic emergencies require immediate care yet are often unable to give consent because their impaired consciousness prevents them from making decisions. Treating patients who present with an acute organic impairment manifested by confusion and irrational, or even dangerous, behavior is extremely difficult. Emergency physicians must recognize the medical-legal problems created when the impaired patient refuses treatment or admission to the hospital and insists on leaving against medical advice. No clear guidelines are available to the physician confronted with such a toxicologic emergency. There is no nationally recognized standard of law relating to these issues; instead, the relevant laws vary from state to state. The emergency physician must become familiar with the legal requirements of informed consent and the essential management necessary to avoid liability for negligence and abandonment. Of particular concern are the risk management and liability issues that relate to the patient who attempts to leave the ED while impaired. The legal requirements of informed consent in emergency settings, the duty to treat, medical malpractice, battery, and negligence are examined here, and guidelines based on generally accepted common law principles, as well as New York State case law and statutes, are suggested for developing appropriate patient care plans and departmental policies.

INFORMED CONSENT

A patient who understands the risks and benefits of medical treatment is afforded a legally enforceable right to accept or refuse any treatment that is proposed, by reference to constitutionally protected rights of privacy and control of one's body. When a determination is made that a patient is capable of consenting to or refusing treatment, the law requires that adequate information be disclosed to patients so that they may comprehend (1) the potential risks and benefits associated with receiving the treatment recommended, in order to make an informed consent to treatment; (2) the potential risks of not receiving treatment, in order to make an informed refusal; and (3) possible alternative treatments and their potential risks. Personal autonomy and self-determination are the two basic principles that provide the foundation for the modern doctrine of informed consent, which requires the practitioner "to

disclose to the patient such alternatives thereto and the reasonably foreseeable risks and benefits involved as a reasonable medical, dental, or pediatric practitioner under similar circumstances would have disclosed, in a manner permitting the patient to make a knowledgeable evaluation."[18]

An early landmark case in the evolution of the doctrine of informed consent to treatment is *Schloendorff v Society of New York Hospital* (1914),[21] which upheld the right of individuals to self-determination and, therefore, the right to consent to or refuse any proposed treatment. The "emergency doctrine" was first enunciated in the *Schloendorff* decision to address aspects of the doctrine of informed consent that are problematic when patients are deemed not capable of participating in the consent process. Justice Cardozo's decision in *Schloendorff* stated:

> Every human being of adult years and sound mind has a right to determine what shall be done with his own body and a surgeon who performs an operation without his patient's consent commits an assault, for which he is liable in damages, except in cases of emergency where the patient is unconscious and where it is necessary to operate before consent can be obtained.[21]

In the matter of *Storar* (1981), the Court of Appeals held the right of a competent individual to refuse medical assistance as a matter of law in New York.[6] Section 2504 of the New York State Public Health Law gives physicians the authority to treat patients without consent if "the person is in immediate need of medical attention and an attempt to secure consent would result in delay of treatment which would increase the risk to the person's life or health."[17] As currently formulated, Section 2504 is interpreted to apply under special circumstances. Exceptions to idealized informed consent and the right to refuse treatment include the cases of minors and victims of emergencies for whom delays in treatment while consent is being obtained would seriously compromise the patient's clinical condition.[1]

The New York State Public Health Law provides basic guidelines describing the extent of disclosure requirements for a patient. However, disclosure of pertinent information is frequently not possible in the provision of emergency care to the organically impaired patient who has limited or no decision-making capacity.

Often the physician's well-intended efforts to communicate treatment information to the impaired patient prove ineffectual and present the practitioner with a medical-legal dilemma. The physician is unable to discuss in a legally meaningful way the implication of the proposed treatment with the impaired patient; however, there is a duty to treat patients who present with the potential for permanent disability or life-threatening conditions. In these situations, consent on the part of the impaired patient is considered to be implied, and emergency treatment should be provided. Support for this view of implied consent is a general tenet of tort law.[16] Implied consent is manifest by patient action and determined by the emergency nature of the patient's condition and capacity to consent.

PATIENT REFUSAL AND IMPLIED CONSENT

Patient 1 A 34-year-old man was brought to the ED alert and oriented after ingesting 40 to 50 aspirin tablets (325 mg each). He was fully cognizant of the physician's intent to treat him and initially refused treatment. However, very soon after arrival, his level of consciousness deteriorated and the physician initiated emergency management, including the use of restraints to allow orogastric lavage to be performed with limited patient resistance.

This case raises two important issues. First, the practitioner must question whether or not the patient, although "alert and oriented," is initially capable of making a decision for himself. Given the history of abnormal behavior manifested by an apparent deliberate overdose ingestion, a reasonable argument could be made that the patient's judgment is so impaired that his initial refusal of treatment should not be honored. This conclusion must be supported by specific documentation in the medical record of the nature of the ingestion, specific statements suggesting suicidal ideations or attempts (if any), and the patient's statements and behavior. Where available, a written psychiatric consultation should be obtained. If psychiatric consultation is not immediately available, the emergency physician should use whatever mental health resources are available (eg, social worker) to assist in evaluating the suicidal intention of the patient.

Second, this case illustrates how the doctrine of implied consent can be applied to a difficult clinical situation. Patients who present with an altered consciousness are presumed under law to have consented to necessary treatment. The law further assumes that the patient would have consented to the indicated treatment if conscious and able to communicate with his physician. The 34-year-old man in this case developed an altered level of consciousness and required immediate intervention, potentially to save his life. By using the legal assumptions in the doctrine of implied consent, the emergency physician is able lawfully to intervene on the patient's behalf without any consequential risk of potential liability for assault and battery.

Documentation describing the patient's altered level of consciousness would be particularly critical in support of the physician's determination that the patient's condition was emergent and justified the physician's invocation of a specific duty to treat the patient that arises under the law of implied consent.

If the facts of this case are altered slightly, a more complex ethical and legal problem may confront the physician. Assume that the same patient was witnessed to have ingested these pills, remains fully cognizant with no observable deterioration, adamantly refuses any medical intervention, and desires to leave the ED. What course of action should the emergency physician follow? The ethical issue is whether a person has the right to commit suicide under any and all circumstances. The legal issue is whether, after you determine that in a particular situation the patient should not be allowed to commit suicide, you have the legal right to intervene. Under such circumstances, a strong argument can neverthe-

less be made mandating immediate patient care intervention. The medical record should document any statements or actions by the patient suggesting impaired judgment. Further, an accurate and detailed description of this attempt at suicide should be recorded, and the source of this information (family, police, friends) noted in the ED record. If the patient persists in his refusal to accept intervention, the application of physical restraints may be necessary and should be considered, with these actions performed in a timely manner. Such a patient could also benefit from psychiatric consultation, and the hospital chaplain might be utilized as an additional resource in this situation.

After restraints are applied correctly (Chap. 115), all appropriate medical interventions can be initiated. To obtain maximal legal protection, the emergency physician must document the reasons for intervention in the specific factual manner described.

FORCIBLE RESTRAINT OF THE IMPAIRED PATIENT

Patient 2 A 31-year-old woman who reportedly injected heroin was brought to the ED by emergency medical service (EMS) and became apneic within a few seconds of arrival. On administration of 2 mg of naloxone IV, the patient regained consciousness and demanded immediate release. The patient was fully alert and oriented, with no evidence of hypoxia or other clinical signs to suggest impaired judgment at this particular time. Routine evaluation of the patient's belongings revealed a small glassine envelope of white powder.

The right of a hospital to retain and physically restrain a person who has an altered level of consciousness for evaluation and emergency intervention is generally well supported by states and case law.[4] This case represents a frequent problem that arises when a patient is brought to an ED in an obviously incapacitated or dangerously unstable clinical condition as a result of ingestion of pharmacologic or toxicologic agents and who, after partial recovery, demands to be released from the hospital. In most states, legal precedents for such a situation have yet to be formally established by either written statutes or reported case law. However, reasonably clear guidelines for the management of such impaired patients have evolved from legal precedents governing appropriate medical assessment, from risk management considerations, and from the predictability of patient injury in the event of premature discharge.

A staff decision to allow a treated or partially treated patient with a drug overdose who subsequently becomes alert to return to the community must be based on a medical assessment encompassing a number of factors. The initial concern is the patient's capacity to comprehend. Before the patient can be permitted to leave the hospital, a determination would have to be made that the patient is capable of understanding the information presented and has neither a medical nor a psychiatric problem preventing her from making a voluntary decision.

In the case of patient 2, such an assessment cannot be limited to an evaluation of the patient's statements at the time she is oriented and "apparently capable" only because of the administration of naloxone. In a situation such as this, patients may appear to be alert, demand to be released from the ED, and may even be willing to sign the leaving "Against Medical Advice" ("AMA") or refusal of medical assistance (RMA) waiver that is included as part of many ED records. Under these circumstances, it must be determined whether the ED staff has a legal duty to prevent such an individual from leaving before the patient's toxic metabolic condition is resolved.

Common ED practice and sound legal principles suggest that both the hospital and its staff have a duty to prevent such a person from leaving if the duration of the effect of the involved drugs or toxins is characteristically longer than that expected of the antidote. Patient 2 was brought to the ED in a comatose state after the injection of heroin. Naloxone treatment rendered her temporarily awake and alert. She should not be allowed to leave on demand because the emergency physician can predict with reasonable medical certainty that recurrence of coma or apnea will happen to the patient in the near future. (see Antidotes in Depth: Opioid Antagonists).

In other words, if this patient is permitted to leave, her life or health will be placed at significant risk. Such a person could collapse while driving an automobile or lose consciousness in a location where no medical attention is available. A physician who makes a judgment that such an event is probable or likely has a duty to inform the individual of the life-threatening nature of the condition and then to retain, with physical restraints if necessary, the patient in the hospital until "medically cleared."

Liability in this situation is further reduced when the chart substantiates the medical judgment that was the basis for the decision to use restraints and to retain the patient. Such documentation should specifically note the likely relapse of the patient into a symptomatic state and should further state that such an occurrence could place the patient and others in a life-threatening situation.

When such documentation is clearly entered on the medical record, legal challenge to the decision to restrain the patient has very limited chance of success. Sound risk management principles support treatment and detainment rather than premature release of the patient. Conversely, prematurely releasing a seriously intoxicated patient exposes both the physician and the hospital to a claim of negligence on the grounds of failure to foresee a likely and harmful event.

RISK MANAGEMENT CONSIDERATION AND DOCUMENTATION

Patient 3

6:05 PM. A 28-year-old woman was brought to the ED by the police. The police believed she might be a "bodypacker" (an individual who swallows drugs to avoid arrest and prosecution).

6:10 PM. The triage nurse helped the patient onto a stretcher and brought her to the treatment area. The physician was summoned to see the patient. Her vital signs at that time were: blood pressure 130/70 mm Hg; pulse 78 beats/min; respiratory rate 24 breaths/min; temperature 36.7°C (98°F).

As the physician initiated the examination, the patient became combative and uncooperative. The physician verbally ordered that the patient be restrained. The patient was given 40% oxygen via face mask, cardiac monitoring was begun, and an intravenous line was started with D_5W at 125 mL/h; a bolus of 100 mL of $D_{50}W$ and 100 mg of thiamine were then administered IV. Orogastric lavage was then performed, and 50 g of activated charcoal were administered.

7:10 PM. The patient's vital signs were: blood pressure 120/70 mm Hg; pulse 82 beats/min; respiratory rate 24 breaths/min. The patient was noted to be stable and transferred to the observation unit. Oxygen and cardiac monitoring were discontinued. No further orders were written, and the patient remained restrained.

11:15 PM. The vital signs were blood pressure 110/60 mm Hg; pulse 92 beats/min; respiratory rate 18 breaths/min. A nurse's note stated that the patient was resting comfortably.

11:50 PM. The initial physician completed his shift and was replaced at midnight by another physician. The first physician informed his replacement that the patient was stable and resting in the holding area.

4:20 AM. The patient was found unresponsive, with agonal respirations. She was hypotensive and had no palpable radial pulse. She felt very hot to the touch and had a rectal temperature of 108°F (42.2°C). Resuscitative efforts were initiated but unsuccessful.

4:50 AM. The patient was pronounced dead.

Several important risk management questions frequently arise in medical malpractice litigation involving the ED. To prove that a case constitutes medical malpractice, a plaintiff's attorney must show clear and convincing evidence of a departure from good practice by the physician. The attorney must further demonstrate that the negligent act or omission by the physician proximately caused the patient's injury. Courts have held that where "there is substantial probability that the [defendant physician's] negligent conduct caused the resulting injury, that sufficient evidence has been developed against [the] physician."[25]

The problem issues covered by an improperly documented ED record are numerous, but they can be minimized if the practitioner is cognizant of risk management principles. When the attorney for the patient (plaintiff's attorney) introduces evidence to prove a case, the central document in the medical malpractice trial is likely to be the ED record. Thus, every entry in that record is scrutinized with great care by both parties (plaintiff and defendants), and the importance of completing it with knowledge of risk management implications should be a concern for all emergency physicians.

The emergency physician is required to write a medical record that will amply support the basis for the medical judgments exercised. When a physician chooses to write only a summary statement on the ED record without noting supporting clinical data or patient history, claims alleging failure to diagnose will be extremely difficult, if not impossible, to defend. One of the basic elements of the defense in a medical malpractice case is that the physician's judgment was appropriate, given the clinical facts and the patient's history available at that time. Therefore, emergency physicians who do not record supporting clinical data and history deprive themselves of a strong "medical judgment" defense.

Inappropriate entries or markings on the medical record can weaken the defense in a liability case. For example, in attempting to correct an error in entering a Po_2 value, if the emergency physician or nurse totally obliterates the number, an attorney representing a patient may suggest to the jury that the obliteration was done intentionally to conceal clinical data harmful to the position of the defense. If a physician must correct a prior entry made on the ED record, the preferable method is to draw a single line through the value or word to be changed and insert the correct information directly above and to initial the correction. Dating the correction also precludes potential difficult questions in a courtroom setting. By following these suggestions, the emergency physician avoids any accusations that he or she intentionally concealed an error in judgment (Fig. 118–1).

A frequent claim is that the patient was abandoned or improperly monitored. For patient 3, although the chart appears to document repeated vital signs at appropriate intervals, no temperature is included after the first set until the patient is moribund; nor is any mention made again of the continued use of restraints, the patient's continued need for these restraints, or any adverse effects developing from the use of the restraints. Quality assurance reviews of ED records very often demonstrate inadequate charting by physicians and nurses monitoring patients who remain on the ED for prolonged periods of time (longer than 8 hours). Under any circumstances, a lapse of documentation of the patient's clinical condition for 4 hours or more after the initial physician and nursing assessment creates a potential risk management problem. In a lawsuit the plaintiff's attorney would undoubtedly use such a record to develop the theory that no care whatsoever was given to the patient during this time interval and that the patient was abandoned.

Monitoring notations in the patient's record are considered inadequate when they offer no insight into the patient's clinical status. Thus, any monitoring note for a patient who must be retained in the ED for a lengthy period of evaluation, observation, or until an inpatient bed becomes available must include specific clinical data and observations (laboratory results, radiographic findings, hemodynamic changes, and infusion of medications and solutions). All of these deficiencies would undoubtedly be noticed and highlighted at trial by a plaintiff's expert, who frequently is a physician board-certified in emergency medicine and/or medical toxicology.

Any documentation supporting the restraint of an impaired patient against his will must include a clinical description to support such a forcible impediment to the patient's right to liberty and freedom of movement. Such a clinical description should specifically describe any manifestation of agitation and uncooperative behavior. The record should refer to the specific uncooperative acts of the patient and, most importantly, should comment on the difficulties in providing care to the patient because of the patient's actions. If such documentation is present, a theory of negligence against the emergency physician for inappropriate restraints would be virtually impossible to sustain.

Physicians who order restraints for patients in the ED need to exercise extreme caution in the language used to describe such patients. A judgmental physician's note stating that a patient is "a chronic drunk and obnoxious" could undermine the support for the use of restraints. Poorly written physician notes can become an issue in a medical malpractice action, with the plaintiff's attorney focusing on the derogatory nature of such a statement and suggesting a less-than-caring attitude by the doctor toward the patient. A plaintiff's appeal criticizing the ethical and social consciousness of the physician could very likely be seized on by a jury and result in a punitive verdict against the physician. As a general rule, all healthcare professionals should depict a compassionate and professional manner by describing patient behavior and life styles in objective and concrete terms. An alternative and more appropriate description of a patient comparable to the one above would note that the patient had a "history of alcohol abuse and was uncooperative and combative."

To summarize, a well-documented ED record consistent with the accepted risk management principles set forth is the best course for the emergency physician managing a difficult overdose situation where legal principles may appear to present problems in providing proper medical management.

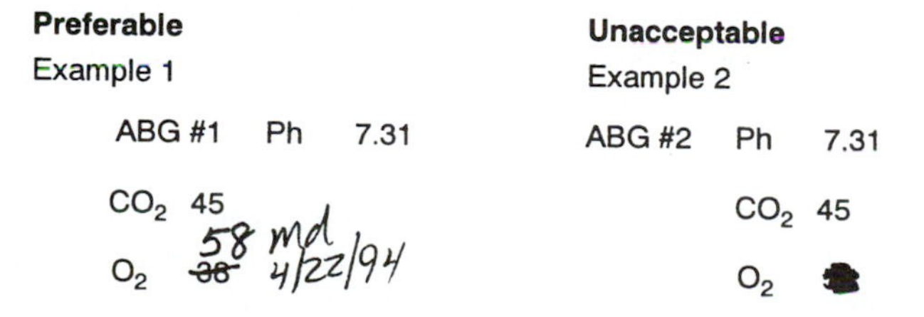

BLOOD ALCOHOL AND EVIDENCE COLLECTION

Patient 4 A 41-year-old male automobile driver was brought to the ED from a motor vehicle crash in which two other motorists were killed. The patient had no physical injuries and was brought to the hospital because he refused an alcohol breath analysis at the scene. On arrival, he was alert and oriented, responded appropriately to all commands, and demonstrated a normal gait and motor function.

The police officers who accompanied the patient informed the ED staff that he was suspected of driving while intoxicated and might be charged with vehicular homicide. The officers then requested that the emergency physician draw a blood specimen to determine blood alcohol concentration. The patient refused to allow ED staff to draw blood for an alcohol determination.

(1) Can blood be drawn against a patient's will? (2) If the blood is drawn under these circumstances, can the physician be accused by the patient of assault and battery? (3) Do law officers have the right to demand that ED staff obtain specimens against a patient's will? (4) Could a specimen for blood alcohol concentration be obtained from an obtunded patient, ie, without consent? What are the legal implications? (5) When a specimen is obtained for legal proceedings, what is the appropriate chain for evidence collection?

Several of the questions raised by this case involve constitutional issues of significant magnitude. Defendants in criminal trials have claimed that a compulsory blood test obtained under circumstances similar to those above violates the Fifth Amendment privilege against self-incrimination and infringes on the constitutionally protected concerns for human dignity and privacy, as expressed in the Fourth Amendment. However, in 1966, in *Schmerber v California,*[22] in a case involving "an apparently inebriated driver," the Supreme Court of the United States ruled that blood may be taken from a patient against his or her will if done in the context of a lawful arrest. The decision in *Schmerber* is extremely important in that it recognizes society's judgment that blood tests do not constitute an unduly extensive imposition on an individual's personal privacy and bodily integrity. In explaining its decision, the Court stated:

Preferable	Unacceptable
Example 1	Example 2

Example 1
ABG #1   Ph   7.31
CO₂ 45
O₂   ~~88~~ 58 *md 4/22/94*

Example 2
ABG #2   Ph   7.31
CO₂ 45
O₂   ■

Figure 118–1. Examples of the preferred and an unacceptable procedures for correcting an error in the medical record.

In the case of a conscious individual, a chemical test can be administered since he is deemed to have given his consent when he used the highway. It is not necessary that a person be given the opportunity to revoke his consent. The only reason the opportunity is given is to eliminate the need for the use of force by police officers if an individual in a drunken state should refuse to submit to the test.[23]

In order to ensure compliance with constitutional standards set forth in *Schmerber,* the states have tailored laws and regulations governing the seizure of blood for the purpose of blood alcohol testing, broadly requiring that the procedure be (1) done in a reasonable, medically approved manner, (2) be incident to a lawful arrest, and (3) be based on the belief that the arrestee is intoxicated. State laws and regulations governing chemical testing for drunk driving generally reflect the strong public interest in protecting the public from potentially dangerous drunk drivers while providing a measure of protection for the physical well-being of the suspected drunk driver.

Generally, under state implied consent laws, a person is deemed to have given consent to a chemical test by operating a motor vehicle on a public thoroughfare.[24] However, a conscious person is usually given an opportunity to withdraw his or her consent to obtaining a blood sample to avoid the dangerous and volatile situation that can arise with the need for the use of physical force by the police in order to obtain a blood sample.[13] Numerous states, including New York and California, allow a patient to refuse a blood alcohol test in circumstances similar to those involving patient 4.

However, in order to protect the public from the dangers of drunk drivers, such a refusal to submit to a blood test would probably result in a suspension of the person's driving privileges. In New York State, for example, the person would be informed by the arresting police officer that his license to drive will be immediately suspended if he refuses to undergo a blood alcohol test, and, in fact, if the person still refuses to submit to the test after being so warned, his license is immediately suspended. The person is then entitled to a hearing concerning the suspension of his license within a period of 15 days and could face revocation of his license for a minimum of 6 months.[24] Perhaps the most serious consequence of refusing to submit to a blood test is that such refusal is admissible at a subsequent criminal trial as evidence of consciousness of guilt.[12] This statutory approach is similar to the law in many states including California.[24]

Notwithstanding the relatively standardized approach followed in New York and California, it is critically important that the ED staff be familiar with the specific requirements of the law in the state where the crash takes place. For example, Illinois and Texas both authorize a blood test on an individual such as patient 4 regardless of the patient's expressed will or refusal.

Illinois law governing the administration of blood alcohol tests contains a statutory approach substantially similar to that of New York. However, in a case where a law enforcement officer has probable cause to believe that the individual is under the influence of alcohol and that a motor vehicle driven by, or in actual physical control of, the individual has caused the death of another or injuries to another consisting of severe bleeding wounds, distorted extremities, or injuries requiring an injured party to be carried from the scene, the law enforcement official is authorized to order an involuntary blood test be performed on that individual responsible.[15] Texas law governing the administration of blood alcohol

tests is very similar to that of Illinois. Texas authorizes an involuntary blood test to be performed on an individual in a case where a law enforcement officer has probable cause to believe that the individual was driving while intoxicated, was involved in a vehicular crash as a result of driving while intoxicated, and that a person has died or will die as a direct result of the accident.[24]

Although state laws clearly reflect the interest in protecting people from the danger of death or injury inflicted by drunk drivers, procedural requirements governing the actual withdrawal of blood are concerned with the physical well-being of the person suspected of drunk driving and with adherence to a "chain of evidence" approach. As a general rule, the healthcare professional personally supervising the blood drawing should first make a medical judgment that drawing blood does not put the person at risk.[11]

In determining whether to comply with the request of a law officer to draw blood for legal purposes, the staff should also consider the possibility of being held amenable to suit. In most states, if the patient consented to a blood test or was unable to refuse consent, any action alleging assault and battery would be unsuccessful. Furthermore, states have statutory provisions that protect those who are authorized to collect blood from liability under these circumstances.

In Illinois, "a person authorized to collect blood . . . cannot be held civilly liable for damages when the person, in good faith, withdraws blood . . . for evidentiary purposes under this Code, upon the request of a law enforcement officer, unless the act is performed in a willful and wanton matter."[24] Willful and wanton within the meaning of this section is described in the code as "a course of action that shows an actual or deliberate intention to cause harm or which, if not intentional, shows an utter indifference to or conscious disregard for the health or safety of another."[24] At least one court in Illinois has held that a staff member's forcible restraint of a patient's arm was not willful and wanton.[20]

In Texas, a person authorized to collect a blood sample or the hospital where the blood sample is taken cannot be held liable for damages for complying with the request of a police officer to take a blood sample if the sample was taken according to recognized medical procedures. However, Texas law does not relieve a person from liability for negligence in the taking of a blood sample.[24]

In New York, a person entitled to draw blood for the purposes of determining the alcohol content therein cannot be sued or held liable for any act or omission while drawing blood at the request of a police officer. However, a patient who may have a cause of action for an act or omission in the course of having his or her blood withdrawn may maintain an action and recover against the state, and the state can then bring an action against the person entitled to draw blood or the hospital employing such person in order to recover the amount awarded the patient.[24]

In California, the legislature has recognized two conditions that specifically exempt persons from blood tests under the implied consent law and that must be addressed by anyone entitled to draw blood for such testing. The California Vehicle Code specifically provides that persons afflicted with hemophilia or using a prescribed anticoagulant for a heart condition are exempt from a blood test,[24] although this is not a medical standard, as blood drawing is performed routinely to assess the success of anticoagulation.

Finally, anyone entitled to draw blood for legal reasons should be familiar with and comply with statutory guidelines and/or regulations describing the specific procedures to be followed in the withdrawal of blood from a patient suspected of driving while intoxicated. Generally, to admit the results of a blood test into evidence, the prosecution must show that the blood sample was (1) tested by a scientific method acceptable in state court, (2) actually drawn from the suspect, and (3) handled throughout utilizing a proper chain of custody. Compliance with respective state laws and/or state administrative regulations will not only protect against an allegation that the specimen was obtained in a manner deviant from recognized medical procedures but will also further the interests of justice by ensuring the admissibility of a specimen in a later criminal proceeding.

In New York, the Vehicle and Traffic Law Section and the New York Code of Rules and Regulations govern methods and procedures for the collection of blood samples. In New York State, only a physician, RN, or RPA may withdraw blood for blood alcohol analysis, or, if acting under the direction and supervision of a physician, a medical laboratory technician, medical technologist, an employee of a clinical laboratory including a phlebotomist, medical laboratory technician, or medical technologist who is competent and acting under the general supervision of a lab director and the personal supervision and direction of a physician. The physician need not physically be present but must authorize the taking of a sample.[14] The New York Code of Rules and Regulations also prohibits the use of alcohol or phenol as an antiseptic on the area of skin from which the blood is to be withdrawn and describes the type of equipment that is to be used: either a sterile dry needle into a vacuum container containing a solid anticoagulant or a sterile dry needle and syringe, and the sample must be deposited into a clean container containing a solid anticoagulant, which container shall then be capped or stoppered and identified.[23]

Similarly, the Illinois Vehicle Code and regulations promulgated by the Illinois Department of Public Health, set forth in the Illinois Administrative Code, provide procedural steps for the withdrawal of blood samples for chemical analysis of alcohol or drug content.[5] The Code provides that the blood sample should be collected in the presence of the arresting officer by a physician authorized to practice medicine, a registered nurse, or other qualified person trained in venipuncture and acting under the direction of a licensed physician. The Code also describes the appropriate equipment to be used in the collection of blood samples. Specifically, the Code calls for the collection of two tubes of blood and provides that the skin in the area in which the blood is to be collected should not be cleaned with alcohol or another volatile organic substance.[5] In addition to providing a procedure for the withdrawal of blood, the Illinois Administrative Code contains protocol for the labeling of the blood samples and delivery to a laboratory certified by the Department of Health. The Illinois Vehicle Code and Illinois Administrative Code also call for the blood to be tested to determine the concentration of alcohol and/or drugs present by a laboratory method acceptable in a court of law.

In Texas, under the Transportation Code, when a person submits to a blood test at the request of a law enforcement officer, only a physician, qualified technician, chemist, registered professional nurse, or licensed vocational nurse may withdraw blood for the purpose of determining alcoholic content, and the specimen must be obtained in a sanitary place.[24]

In California, the California Vehicle Code specifically provides a list of persons authorized to withdraw blood, and the California Code of Regulations outlines the specific procedures for the taking of a blood specimen.[24]

Because the situations described above inevitably occur in EDs everywhere, all emergency physicians should review with hospital counsel the local state laws and regulations governing blood alcohol testing at the request of a law enforcement official, particularly when beginning a new position in a different hospital or state. The laws and regulations vary from state to state and are the subject of frequent restructuring and amendment. The examples provided in this discussion are aimed at illustrating the source of law and some of the approaches to blood alcohol testing in the case of a person suspected of drunk driving.

EVIDENCE COLLECTION

Once the blood specimen is obtained, another significant medical-legal task confronts the staff: compliance with the chain of evidence, which can eliminate the risk of nonadmissibility of a specimen in a later criminal proceeding. In cases where laboratory results are likely to be used in a court of law regarding criminal conduct, it is essential to establish the appropriate chain of evidence and to process the laboratory specimens in a meticulous fashion. This result may or may not support a charge of driving while intoxicated.

First, the specimen must be obtained in full view of a witness. Second, if the hospital laboratory is used to analyze the specimen, the laboratory should be alerted that the specimen is likely to become evidence in a criminal trial. Accordingly, every processing step for that specimen, beginning with the act of collection, each individual test done on the specimen, and transport to and from the laboratory must be documented with the name of the person performing the task. The "chain of evidence" requires that each step in the processing and transport of the specimen be documented without a break in the custody of the specimen. These same requirements apply to specimens for analyses (such as toxicologic testing) sent to an outside laboratory. To ensure the chain of custody from the hospital to the outside laboratory, at the minimum, prudent practice would suggest sending the specimens in a clearly labeled package and obtaining a receipt from the laboratory.

Some practitioners have questioned the legality of blood alcohol concentrations when these tests are drawn for another purpose. For example, in a seriously traumatized victim a blood alcohol concentration may be drawn to diagnose or exclude a cause of an altered level of consciousness and altered level of perception. In these cases, the legality of the laboratory value obtained can be questioned. It should be noted that the entire medical record can be introduced as evidence if it is deemed relevant by the court. However, without a chain of evidence, an attorney can challenge the validity of a blood alcohol concentration.

Furthermore, the outside laboratory should be called before delivery of the specimen and instructed to document each step in the performance of the required test. Usually, the police department will sign for and assume responsibility for all such specimens taken to an outside laboratory.

DISCHARGING PATIENTS WITH ELEVATED BLOOD ALCOHOL LEVELS

Currently in most jurisdictions the legal limit of a blood alcohol concentration (BAC) is 80 mg/dL. Because some number is required to provide an objective standard for the law, this guideline may be appropriate to assess legal blood alcohol concentrations, but it is not accurate to determine clinical intoxication or impairment. Patients who chronically abuse alcohol may have baseline alcohol concentrations several times the legal level, yet do not appear to be clinically impaired or intoxicated. Although such patients would be considered legally intoxicated, they do not act this way. Blood alcohol concentrations alone should not be used as the criterion for delaying discharge of such patients from the ED. However, if the patient is known to be operating a motor vehicle, assistance should be obtained from family, friend, or taxi to limit the patient's use of the motor vehicle.

The decision to discharge a patient with a high BAC who is clinically unimpaired should be based on sound clinical grounds. To minimize the liability associated with this decision, the physician should carefully document the patient's condition. The patient's motor function and ability to reason should be tested, and the results documented. A detailed discharge summary must document results that reflect the patient's competency. It is also advised that the physician counsel and caution the patient regarding the health implications of the elevated blood alcohol concentration and risk to self and others in the operation of any type of motor vehicle and document that this advice was given. The physician should initiate the social and psychological support necessary for the patient to seek alcohol detoxification. Following these recommendations minimizes the legal liability of the emergency physician and hospital: the potential for any litigation to be successful is significantly reduced on the grounds of comparative negligence.

RISK MANAGEMENT CONSIDERATIONS FOR PATIENT TRIAGE, DISCHARGE, AND TRANSFER

Patient 5 A 26-year-old male injection drug user (IDU) was brought to the ED after falling in the street and bumping his head. The odor of alcohol was noted on the patient's breath. He was alert and oriented and denied any loss of consciousness. The patient was evaluated by the triage nurse and then by an emergency physician. A complete physical examination, including a detailed neurologic examination, was performed. The entire examination was normal, and the patient was released.

Essential Components of Triage That Minimize Potential Risk Management Problems

Beginning with the initial contact at triage, medical personnel must be extremely observant in evaluating the victim of a head injury. This task is more difficult and more important if the patient has potentially abused illicit drugs, alcohol, or medications. The assessment should be initiated by obtaining a past medical history, including medical problems, allergies, and immunizations. The history of alcohol or substance abuse (acute and chronic) should also be obtained to determine the potential impact on the patient's clinical presentation, particularly neurologic findings.

The chief complaint should be solicited and documented in the patient's words. A subjective interpretation of a patient's complaints, particularly in this setting, should be avoided; similarly, a presumptive diagnosis should not be made. Sound medical and legal principles governing triage establish that the nurse and physician must objectively describe findings based on observations and assessment. If the patient was brought by ambulance, the

report of prehospital personnel should be incorporated into the triage notes. In situations similar to that of patient 5, careful assessment and documentation of mental status is critical because the history offered (IDU) and the clinical findings (odor of alcohol) are highly suggestive of acute and chronic substance abuse.

The final component of triage is assessing and recording vital signs. Vital signs should be documented in the appropriate area of the chart, and the time should be noted accordingly. For patients not immediately triaged to a patient care area, vital signs must be retaken at fixed intervals. At these times, patients should also be reassessed, and any change in the clinical condition should be noted. If any deterioration or suspicion of significant changes in the patient's condition occurs, the patient may need to be recategorized and "up-triaged." Patients may also improve, and recategorization may occur for this reason as well.

A three-category triage system classifies patients as emergent (any life-threatening condition, must be evaluated immediately); urgent (less acute, not life-threatening but may become life-threatening); or nonurgent (no immediate threat) in order to determine the priority of care (Chap. 115).[8]

Occasionally, the triage professional needs to provide treatment to the emergent patient (eg, oxygen therapy, hemorrhage control, insertion of an airway). In this instance, documentation of emergency interventions and their outcome is required. Careful documentation of immediate interventions provides important information essential to ongoing emergency care and may also be valuable in the defense of a civil lawsuit.

Reducing the Legal Risks Associated with Patient Discharge

Detailed criteria for release from an ED serve to protect patients from injury following premature discharge and also to reduce the health care provider's risk of liability. Such criteria are particularly important for a patient whose mental status might be impaired from alcohol or drug abuse. Sample criteria include giving the patient and/or family members written discharge instructions. Advise the patient to return to the ED if any abnormal symptoms appear or reappear and describe any activities to perform and/or avoid at home (eg, rest, elevation, and ice). Verbal instructions should include followup information regarding prescriptions (eg, adverse effects, impact on driving, medicating schedule) and emphasize the goal of sobriety and desirability of detoxification. Documentation that such written and verbal instructions were given to the patient and that the patient understood them is essential. The patient's signature, with date and time, should be obtained to indicate that the patient received discharge instructions. However, in cases of head injury and/or intoxication, if discharge is recommended, and the patient is accompanied by family or friends the accompanying individuals should also sign the chart, indicating that instructions were understood. The chart should clearly state the relationship of the family member or friend to the patient.

Finally, in any situation in which the ED staff suspect that drugs were utilized, social services, substance use counseling, and/or psychiatric consultation is useful and strongly recommended. Whether the intoxication was a conscious intentional act or unintentional, psychiatric consultation is indicated to ensure safe risk management practices. By doing this, the emergency physician will obtain another objective professional assessment of the patient's ability to make basic decisions about his or her care and to plan for future behavior modification.

Potential Legal Liabilities Associated with Patient Transfer and Refusal to Treat

"Patient dumping" increased dramatically as a phenomenon in the 1980s. Patient dumping occurs when a hospital that is capable of providing emergency medical care to a particular patient turns the individual away because of the patient's inability to pay. Congress enacted the Consolidated Omnibus Budget Reconciliation Act (COBRA), which encompassed the Emergency Medicine Treatment and Active Labor Act (EMTALA), in 1985. This statute was intended to create significant penalties for hospitals and physicians who discharge patients solely for financial reasons.

The statute also focuses on patient transfers from EDs to other institutions. It states that "if an individual patient has an emergency medical condition that has not been stabilized, it is unlawful to transfer the patient unless a number of conditions are met." These conditions are as follows:

1. The physician must certify in writing the professional opinion that the anticipated medical benefits of transfer outweigh the risks.
2. If capable, the patient must consent to the transfer.
3. The sending hospital must assure adequate medical treatment during the transfer to minimize the risks to the patient or fetus.
4. The receiving facility must be notified before the transfer, agree to accept the patient, and have the capability to treat the patient.
5. Adequate medical information, such as a copy of the medical records and/or a well-prepared interinstitutional transfer form, must accompany the patient.

Sanctions under EMTALA can be severe. A physician who authorizes an inappropriate transfer is subject to fines of up to $50,000 for each violation. If such an action is found to be "gross and flagrant," the physician could be excluded from the Medicare and state Medicaid programs. An institution held responsible for a pattern of inappropriate transfers could be suspended or terminated from the Medicare program for violating any EMTALA requirement.[7] Therefore, the guidelines concerning documentation of triage decisions, discharge, and transfer must be followed without any deviation to ensure that the acts of an individual will not lead to any institutional or individual liability.

LEGAL CONSIDERATIONS FOR POISON CENTERS AND INFORMATION SPECIALISTS

Patient 6 The local poison center received a call from concerned parents regarding the acute ingestion of a full bottle of liquid acetaminophen by their child. The parents were advised by an information specialist to administer 30 mL of syrup of ipecac to induce vomiting. Three days later the baby lapsed into coma, and the parents called the 911 emergency number. An ambulance arrived and transported the child to the local hospital. The child suffered irreversible liver damage. Action was subsequently brought against the local poison center, alleging inappropriate advice and failure to recommend transport to a hospital.

Telephone Contact with a Poison Information Specialist

As a general rule, any physician who decides to treat a patient enters into a physician–patient relationship that creates well-established legal duties. Courts have ruled that the physician–patient encounter need not be a face-to-face interaction to have legal consequences. For example, the absence of physical contact between a physician and patient as in the practice of radiology and pathology does not preclude a patient from asserting that a duty of care exists.[2] More particularly, and quite relevant to the practice of a poison center, a New York State court ruled that an initial telephone call from a patient to a physician can be sufficient basis to hold that physician responsible for inappropriate advice or a significant error in judgment.[10] Given the legal precedents previously stated, it is eminently clear that patient contact with a poison information specialist is a sufficient foundation for a subsequent legal action if inappropriate advice was given. In this case, a medical toxicologist could criticize the advice given to the parents. In particular, the recommendation apparently failed to include a directive to seek immediate emergency assistance. The advice to give the child syrup of ipecac was appropriate, but the failure to recommend emergency transport rendered the totality of the advice given substandard and less than the applicable duty of care.

Standards of Care Applicable to Poison Information Specialists

Any discussion of the standard of care to which a poison information specialist should be held would be misleading without mentioning several operational aspects of most poison centers. The specialists are required to have rapid and accurate access to a standard information resource system, such as Poisindex, a computerized information source that is updated quarterly and contains both basic information and recommendations to deal with most encountered toxic exposures. Advice that differs significantly from an existing protocol or standard of care will be subject to critical review in a civil lawsuit. If a patient were to bring an action, the negligence theory against the poison center might rely particularly on deviations from the standard recommendations.

It would be inaccurate to suggest, however, that the duty of care owed by a poison information specialist can be measured only by how closely the advice given compares with the standard resources. Frequently, a specialist may encounter situations that cannot be managed in accordance with an information system alone, and the poison information specialist should seek counsel from a doctor of pharmacy or physician consultant working with the poison center. If this were to occur, any subsequent legal proceeding would also review carefully the content of the input given by the consultant as to its accuracy and appropriateness to the underlying toxicologic problem.

Practices of Regional Poison Centers that Can Reduce Potential Liabilities

Clearly there are some inherent risks of potential liability for a poison center. To minimize such risk and the risk of civil actions against a poison center, quality assurance and risk management programs should be a regular function. Usually regional poison centers practice this routinely. Daily physician audits or monitoring of the advice given by poison information specialists should be done. Such interactions enhance care and ensure patient safety for the individual and establish a higher general standard.

The medical toxicologists and clinical pharmacists responsible for supervising the poison information specialist must be able to adequately assess the competence and capabilities of the staff and to make recommendations, take corrective actions, and provide suggestions for improvement to involved members.

Both individual case audits and departmental committee review of complicated toxic ingestions should be addressed, evaluating the quality of poison information specialist documentation. The medical toxicologist must assess the adequacy of the patient history obtained and should pay particular attention to the written documentation of advice given. In the event of a lawsuit, the most likely area of dispute will be what was actually said to the patient.

In a case similar to that of patient 6, a patient might be told by the poison center to seek immediate emergency help from a physician or ambulance service but choose not to follow this advice, with poor outcome or disastrous consequences. The failure of the poison information specialist to document such advice meticulously could lead to a significant credibility issue in subsequent litigation. If the patient's lawyer knew that such specific documentation were lacking, then a likely claim in the lawsuit would be that the advice was not actually given.

IMPLICATIONS OF LIVING WILLS, DO-NOT-RESUSCITATE ORDERS, ADVANCED DIRECTIVES, AND PHYSICIAN-ASSISTED SUICIDE FOR PATIENTS WITH DRUG OVERDOSE OR TOXIC INGESTION

Patient 7 A 75-year-old unresponsive man was brought to the ED by EMS. He reportedly had ingested a large quantity of phenobarbital. The patient was well known to the medical center staff and had been previously diagnosed as having metastatic prostate cancer. The ED staff suspected that the patient had completed a living will and explicitly requested that no advanced life support and resuscitation be utilized.

On arrival in the ED, the patient was hypotensive with a blood pressure of 80/40 mm Hg, a pulse of 80 with normal sinus rhythm, a respiratory rate of 4 breaths/min, and a rectal temperature of 96°F (35.6°C). Naloxone, dextrose, and thiamine were immediately administered with no response; an endotracheal tube was then inserted, and ventilation with 100% oxygen was provided. Orogastric lavage was performed, and activated charcoal was instilled before removal of the lavage hose. Despite the administration of 2 L of lactated Ringer solution, his systolic blood pressure remained at 80 mm Hg, and a dopamine infusion was started. Neurologic examination at the time revealed fixed and dilated pupils with absent corneal and oculocephalic reflexes. The patient was transferred to the MICU for further management.

(1) Should this patient be resuscitated? (2) What is the implication of a living will for a patient who has intentionally ingested a drug overdose? Advanced directives, a living will, or a healthcare proxy (a document that transfers to an agent the right to make life-and-death decisions for an impaired patient) are considered to be legally binding when a patient presents with symptoms from a naturally occurring disease process. It is not the intent of any state to use these documents to assist a patient who has attempted to commit suicide. (Revisions of state law have been established in Oregon.) Such a view would be considered violative of public policy.

A decision in this instance cannot be made simply by reference to the patient's intentions as individually expressed in a living will or by the designated agent in the healthcare proxy. The regulatory authorities in most states (living will and healthcare proxy statutes are regulated by state health departments) would probably indicate that the patient should be resuscitated in this situation because of society's position that a physician should not assist in a suicide attempt.

In view of the current debate in the medical, legal, and ethical literature with regard to euthanasia in controlled and state-approved circumstances, the approach to this hypothetical case may very well be different in different locations in the future. This area of law and ethics is evolving at a rapid and variable pace throughout the individual states. The issues regarding physician-assisted suicide and the circumstances under which it is permissible were left ambiguous by a 1997 United States Supreme Court decision. Ethicists have taken strong positions on both sides of this controversial issue, and a clear understanding of the controlling law in this area remains to be elucidated. Accordingly, this is an issue that ED practitioners will have to monitor closely as individual state governments and health departments create regulations. One of the arguments asserted by those in the medical community supporting physician-assisted suicide is that patients experiencing extreme suffering with no possible amelioration by medical means are a protected class and should be granted equal protection under the constitution. Whether or not this view will prevail is highly uncertain at this time. EDs should routinely incorporate discussions of these issues into their educational programs.

INTOXICATION AND PATIENT CONFIDENTIALITY

Patient 8 A 52-year-old man was seen by his general practitioner during his lunch hour for the complaint of recurring headaches. The patient was the local school bus driver in a small rural community. The physician believed that the patient was intoxicated and noted the odor of alcohol on his breath. The patient was well known and respected throughout the community. The physician confronted the patient with his suspicion, and the patient adamantly denied alcohol use. The physician requested permission to draw blood tests, including a blood alcohol level. The patient refused and threatened to sue the physician if he reported his suspicions.

(1) Would the release of information regarding the physician's suspicions constitute a violation of patient confidentiality? (2) Do the facts of this case present a public policy exception to the patient's rights of confidentiality in light of the general societal need to protect the safety of passengers and children?

This case presents a dilemma that occasionally confronts every practitioner. As a first point it must be emphasized that any release of patient information to an individual or agency not involved in the patient's care (school authority or supervisors) would clearly be a technical violation of the normal patient confidentiality requirements. However, the facts in any particular case may create an exception to the normal rules governing the release of patient information. In this case, a convincing and compelling argument could be made that public policy mandates practitioners to advise school authorities of the bus driver's potentially intoxicated condition. This position could be taken in the interest of preserving life and safety of children who might ride on his bus at a time when he became impaired.

If the bus driver chooses to bring a lawsuit against the practitioner and hospital on the grounds that he had lost his job because of the unauthorized release of medical information, such a case could be well defended with the public policy arguments just given. There is little likelihood of success of such a lawsuit. These principles would apply to any scenario involving an individual who is responsible for public safety (eg, train conductor, airline pilot, police officer).

A more complicated situation arises if the patient does not appear to be intoxicated but the physician smells the odor of alcohol on the patient's breath. In this case the physician may be less willing to report his or her suspicion because of the seriousness of the accusation and the degree of uncertainty regarding the extent of alcohol use. Despite this dilemma, the highest ethical standards suggest that the physician has a duty to protect society and to report any suspicions to the appropriate authority.

IMPLICATIONS FOR EMANCIPATED MINORS, CHILD ABUSE AND NEGLECT, AND THE UNBORN FETUS

Patient 9   A 17-year-old woman presented to the ED for altered mental status. Physical examination revealed an obviously pregnant young woman with a blood pressure of 150/100 mm Hg, pulse of 140 beats/min, respiratory rate of 30 breaths/min, and rectal temperature of 101°F (38.3°C). Her skin was diaphoretic, and her pupils were 6 to 7 mm and reactive to light. The remainder of her evaluation was unremarkable except for a 28-week size uterus with strong fetal heart tones. After receiving 20 mg of Valium IV, the patient's vital signs normalized, and she admitted to frequent crack cocaine use. She had no prenatal care and was not married. Her 2-year-old child was brought in from home by the police for evaluation.

The ED received a telephone call from the patient's grandmother (the legal guardian) inquiring about her condition. The patient indicated that she did not want her grandmother to know about her admission or pregnancy.

(1) Can the physician accept the patient's wishes not to inform the grandmother of her medical condition? (2) Is the patient an emancipated minor capable of making her own consent for treatment? (3) What is the responsibility of the ED staff when confronted with a patient who refuses to obtain needed social service help for his or her child? (4) Can the hospital and the ED staff compel this patient to go for routine prenatal care in the obstetric clinic?

Many states have guidelines that protect the confidentiality of adolescent patients seeking obstetric and gynecologic healthcare. Despite the wishes of this young patient to keep her status confidential, a delicate balance must be considered when the emer-

gency physician is confronted with an impaired adolescent who is pregnant or who is the mother of a small child. In the case above, societal concerns and sound hospital policy suggest that the grandmother should be fully informed of the patient's medical condition. There are several reasons for this conclusion, and one controlling factor in this decision is the state's interest in insuring the protection of a small child. When balanced against this overriding ethical concern, the patient's desire for confidentiality cannot be met.

The legal doctrine of emancipated minor varies somewhat in different states, but the general definition is consistent and quite similar throughout the United States: If an adolescent patient lives apart from her parental home and is pregnant, then such a grouping of factual elements would constitute emancipated minor status in virtually all states. If this patient was not impaired by cocaine or some other drug or substance of abuse, then she would have a legal right to make decisions about her healthcare in all respects. However, her ingestion of crack cocaine permitted the ED staff to treat her despite her protestations because of her present inability to fully comprehend the implications of her actions. As noted in Chap. 114, the patient's impairment must be documented as to specific clinical symptoms.

Statutes in all states require the ED staff (often as a mandated reporter) to inform the designated state authorities when child abuse or neglect is suspected. The 2-year-old in the above case should not be permitted to leave the ED under the care of this young patient/mother because the expanded definition of neglect in most state statutes would preclude disposition at this stage of care. The appropriate course of action for the ED staff includes the provision of maximum support for this potentially imperiled child.

A social worker should assist with an assessment of the home situation. It is often beneficial if the social worker (a child abuse specialist) speaks to the state authorities in addition to the ED staff. In this example, a possible resolution that is minimally disruptive to the child's well-being might be placement with the grandmother. This should be done only with the approval if the state child abuse authority.

If the hospital and ED staff seek to compel this patient obtain outpatient care in the obstetric clinic, some form of court intervention would have to be sought. As a rule, the courts have been reluctant to compel care of the fetus on the grounds of abuse and neglect despite behavior by the mother harmful to the prospects for the child. However, a case plan that includes close followup of the adolescent mother's condition by an in-hospital child abuse interdisciplinary team in conjunction with a child welfare agency that has jurisdictional responsibility for the adolescent's care is probably the optimal method to achieve a coordinated solution to this difficult ethical and medical problem. There are times when a court order is not effective and a more appropriate solution may be the intervention of a child welfare agency.

HEALTH INSURANCE AS A BARRIER TO DRUG AND ALCOHOL SCREENING IN TRAUMA PATIENTS

Patient 10   A 25-year-old unrestrained man was involved in a motor vehicle crash and was ejected from the automobile. He was brought to the ED via EMS immobilized and intubated. He had signs of head trauma, was responsive to verbal commands, had no sensory or motor response from the neck down, and had minimal shoulder shrug. Radiographs revealed a C5–6 fracture. It is likely that the patient has suffered a permanent spinal injury and will require long term hospitalization and rehabilitative care.

This crash occurred in a state where insurance companies are not required to reimburse claims when alcohol or drugs are involved. By statute a majority of US states do not consider the insurer liable for any loss sustained or contracted in consequence of an insured person who is intoxicated or under the influence of any controlled substance unless prescribed by a physician.[9,19] In the past year, this hospital has had three claims for extensive hospitalization and numerous procedures denied for trauma patients on these grounds. The ED did not have a policy requiring blood and alcohol levels on all trauma patients, and therefore the ED physician followed the administrator's advice and did not obtain the indicated blood alcohol levels.

Studies repeatedly demonstrate that 40 to 50% of all patients admitted to level I trauma centers have positive blood alcohol levels at the time of injury. No-fault insurance has a maximum allowable coverage in the range of $50,000.00. For this patient, it is likely that $50,000.00 would be exhausted in the first month of care, and then the patient's standard health insurance would be applied to the extended hospital stay. (1) Does insurance law allow insurance companies to refuse benefits to trauma patients who are legally intoxicated or have ingested an illegal substance? (2) What are the legal and ethical implications for physicians if they adhere to administrative directives and fail to take blood alcohol levels when clinically indicated? (3) If the medical record has been subpoenaed, can the patient cite "patient confidentiality" and avoid a release of his medical record?

Because most states permit insurance companies to refuse benefits to trauma patients for injuries that involve the patient's use of alcohol or controlled substances, concerns about the effect of screening for alcohol and narcotics on insurance coverage are valid.[19] Thus, the trauma victim who presents in the ED not only may pose a challenge in terms of medical management but also may create an administrative dilemma that encompasses legal, ethical, and professional concerns. Such policies can influence institutional and physician behavior and lead to administrative directives or mandates requiring that the emergency physician not take a blood alcohol level even though such a test is clinically indicated.

Further, although federal confidentiality regulations protect clinical records of patients participating in drug and alcohol abuse programs, there are no such barriers to disclosure in the case of the ED patient who is both impaired and a trauma victim. Information about acute and chronic alcohol use is gathered as a part of the history taken at the time of the ED admission, and it is appropriate for the ED staff to seek such information to determine its effect on treatment and outcome. Under such conditions, the information obtained would be exempt from the special federally created laws regarding patient confidentiality.

In regard to this legal and ethical dilemma for the practitioner, several comments may help the emergency physician provide appropriate care to this patient. The ED physician's first duty is to the patient and not to a vague, off-the-record administrative directive that does not have a basis in institutional policy and procedure. Further, such a policy would not be deemed consistent with good and accepted department medical practice, nor would it be

sanctioned by applicable law. An emergency physician who chooses not to draw a clinically indicated blood alcohol level to protect hospital reimbursement would likely be deemed unethical by the state licensing board. Additionally, if such a fact pattern were presented under a theory of medical malpractice, it is likely that a plaintiff's attorney would have little difficulty in obtaining an expert with board certification in emergency medicine or medical toxicology who would criticize such action.

A number of questionable or illegal "creative" administrative procedures have been offered to prevent disqualification of impaired trauma patients from insurance coverage. One such administrative mechanism involves obtaining blood alcohol levels on a "John Doe" basis, allowing the practitioner to utilize the clinical data without recording a level in the patient's record. This is a dangerous practice for a number of reasons. A subsequent provider of care in the same hospital may not be aware of the "John Doe" practice and therefore may not take into consideration the elevated blood alcohol in the subsequent care and treatment. Further, any attempt to obtain reimbursement for treatment could subject the hospital and perhaps the physicians involved to charges of fraud and/or filing of a false claim. For these reasons, such a procedure cannot be recommended.

THE JEHOVAH'S WITNESS REFUSAL TO ACCEPT TREATMENT

A comprehensive review of medical-legal issues must always include a discussion of the care of the patient who is also a Jehovah's Witness. Although religious and legal issues rarely are relevant in toxicologic emergencies, the rights of a patient who is also a Jehovah's Witness is a subject worthy of a detailed discussion. This analysis may allow for a thoughtful review of toxicologic issues. The most common problems involving a patient who is a Jehovah's Witness is the patient's refusal to receive transfusions of any blood or blood products regardless of the indications. Three variations of this scenario have been discussed in legal briefs:

1. A conscious patient who understands the risks and benefits of medical treatment requires emergency transfusions. The patient refuses all transfusions and risks death as a consequence.
2. An unconscious patient arrives in an ED and requires emergency blood transfusions to sustain life. Family members accompanying the patient inform the staff that the patient is a Jehovah's Witness, and they refuse to consent to any blood transfusions.
3. The parents of a child requiring emergency transfusions to sustain life refuse to allow blood to be given to their child on the grounds of religious beliefs.

A serious legal and ethical dilemma occurs when an individual who understands the risks and benefits of medical treatment refuses the treatment necessary to save his or her life. Numerous case decisions have involved this issue. The courts generally agree that a competent individual has a constitutional right to refuse medical treatment. Refusal to accept life-saving treatments, or in this case blood transfusions, is supported by the fact that every individual is entitled to bodily integrity and privacy. In fact, in the landmark case of *Fosmire v Nicoleau*, New York's highest court, the State Court of Appeals, ruled definitively that the state's interest in preserving an individual's life cannot override the individual's right to refuse life-saving medical treatments.[3] This constitutional right is not specific to any particular religious belief.

The courts have had to struggle with the question of how to deal with the parent of a small child who is refusing blood transfusions for himself or herself. In such cases, the court has generally decided that the rights of the parent (patient) must be protected even though the individual has responsibility for minors or children. In most cases, the individual's right to refuse treatment is protected under the First Amendment if it is linked to a religious objection or, in the absence of a religious objection, may be linked to the fundamental right of privacy for everyone.

One of the most difficult situations created by patients who are Jehovah's Witnesses arises when the patient is unconscious and requires emergency blood transfusions, and accompanying family members refuse to sign consent for transfusions. Under these circumstances the physician must immediately determine whether the patient's illness is emergent (life threatening), urgent, or nonurgent (not life threatening). In emergent cases, particularly when there is inadequate time to make a detailed assessment, the physician has a duty to treat the patient immediately. This premise is the same as the principle of implied consent discussed with respect to patient 7. Immediate action rarely creates any significant liability, whereas delays and deliberations followed by negative outcomes can carry enormous liability. If the case is not emergent, the emergency physician should verify the family's request, provided that this delay will not jeopardize the patient's condition. The family should be given an opportunity to provide clear and convincing evidence that the patient would have refused transfusions or other medical interventions.

The most difficult situation of all arises in cases of minors or children whose competent guardian or parent refuses to allow medical treatment for the child. In such a case, virtually all states invoke the parens patriae doctrine, which permits the state to protect its citizens who are unable to protect themselves. This doctrine has been upheld in many cases by not allowing Jehovah's Witness patients to refuse the transfusion of blood products into their children. The emergency physician must be mindful of several communication issues when administering transfusions to a child in such circumstances: The parents or guardians must be told that a transfusion is anticipated and that the hospital will proceed on the basis of state law. A progress note must be entered into the chart documenting the time of transfusion, the medical necessity of the transfusion, and the details of conversation(s) with the parents; obtaining a court order to administer blood transfusions to a child in a life-threatening circumstance is not required and therefore must not delay emergency treatment.

An emergency physician who is confronted with a life-threatening refusal of blood products by a patient who is also a Jehovah's Witness should work very closely with the risk management staff of the hospital. Legal advice should always be sought when possible to ensure that all risk management concerns are addressed.

SUMMARY

The risk management and legal issues of an active emergency department have implications for many patients. The ability of providers to function responsibly is dependent on an understanding of these ever-evolving principles. Those patients whose consciousness is abnormal because of a toxin represent an acute complex medicolegal emergency. A well-organized hospital is dependent on a close working relationship among the legal, risk management, and medical personnel. Only in this manner can they learn, cooperate, and meet the needs of the ever-evolving clinical dilemmas they confront.

ACKNOWLEDGMENT

To Mr. Frank Sanotoro, who assisted in the research for parts of this chapter.

REFERENCES

1. Borak J, Veilleux S: Informed consent in emergency settings. Ann Emerg Med 1984;13:731–735.
2. *Capuano v Jacobs*, 33 A.D., 2d. 743, 305 N.Y. State, 2d 837 (1960).
3. *Fosmire v Nicoleau*, A.D., 2d. 876, 551 N.Y. State (1990).
4. *Gonzalez v State*, 110 A.D., 2d. 810, 488 N.Y. 2d. 231, 67 N.Y. 2d. 647 (1985).
5. Illinois Administrative Code 77, Chapter 1, subchapter f, Section 510.110.
6. *In the Matter of Storar*, 52 N.Y. 2d 363, 377 (1981).
7. Krugh T: Medical COBRA: The federal anti-dumping act. For the Defense 1992;June:14–16.
8. New York City Health and Hospitals Corporation, Bellevue Hospital Center: Policy and Procedure Manual for Emergency Services, 1993.
9. New York Insurance Law §3216 (d) (2) (K); California Insurance Code §10369.12; 215 Illinois Consolidated Statutes 5/357.25.
10. *O'Neil v Montefiore Hospital*, 11 A.D., 2d 132, 202 N.Y. State, 2d 436 (1960).
11. *People v Ebner*, 195 A.D.2d 1006, 600 N.Y.S.2d 569 (4th Dept 1993); but see *People v Moser*, 70 N.Y.2d 476, 522 N.Y.S.2d 497, 517 N.E.2d 212 (1987).
12. *People v Ferrara*, 158 Misc. 2d 671, 602 N.Y. (Richmond Cty 1993); *People v Rosado*, 158 Misc. 2d 50, 600 N.Y.S. 2d 624 (Bronx Cty 1993).
13. In New York, *People v Kates*, 53 N.Y.2d 590, 444 N.Y.S.2d 446, 428 N.E.2d 852 (1981); In California, see *Hughey v Department of Motor Vehicles*, 1 Cal.Rptr.2d 115, 235 Cal.App.3d 752 (App. 3 Dist. 1991).
14. *People v Olmstead*, 649 N.Y.S.2d 624 (4th Dep't 1996).
15. *People v Ruppel*, 303 Ill. App.3d 885,237 Ill. Dec. 21, 708 N.E.2d 824 (4 Dist. 1999); 625 ILCS 5/11–501.2 (c) (2) (3).
16. Prosser WL: The Law of Torts. St Paul, West, 1984.
17. Public Health Law Section 2504(4). McKinney's Consolidated Laws of New York Annotated book 44, public health law sections 2100–3399. St. Paul, West, 1985.
18. Public Health Law, Section 2805 (d) (1). McKinney's Consolidated Laws of New York Annotated, book 44, public health saw sections 2100–3399. St. Paul, West, 1985.
19. Rivara FP, Tollefson S, Tesh E, Gentilello LM, Screening trauma patients for alcohol problems: are insurance companies barriers? J Trauma 2000;48:115–118.
20. *Ruppel v Ramseyer*, 33 F.Supp. 720 (C.D.Ill. 1999)
21. *Schloendorff v Society of New York Hospital*, 211 N.Y. 125, 105 N.E. 92, 93 (1914).
22. *Schmerber v California*, 384 US 757, 16L ed 2d. 908, 86 Sct 1826 (1966).
23. Title 10 of the New York Code of Rules and Regulations Section 59.2.
24. In New York, under the Vehicle and Traffic Law, "any person who operates a motor vehicle is considered to have consented to a chemical test of breath, blood, urine or saliva for the purpose of determining alcoholic and/or drug content, provided that such test is administered

at the direction of a police officer." N.Y. Vehicle and Traffic Law §1194 (McKinney's Consolidated Laws of New York, Annotated, book 62A, vehicle and traffic law sections 600ff St. Paul, West, 1996). In Illinois, under the Illinois Vehicle Code, "Any person who drives or is actual physical control of a motor vehicle upon the public highways of this State shall be deemed to have given consent . . . to a chemical test or tests of blood, breath, or urine for the purposes of determining the content of alcohol . . ." 625 ILCS 5/11–501.1. In Texas, under the Transportation Code, "if a person is arrested for an offense arising out of acts alleged to have been committed while the person was operating a motor vehicle in a public place . . . while intoxicated,

the person is deemed to have consented . . . to submit to the taking of one or more specimens of the person's breath or blood for analysis to determine the alcohol concentration. . .Tex. Transportation Code Ann. § 724 (Vernon 1991). In California, under the Vehicle Code, "any person who drives a motor vehicle is deemed to have given his or her consent to chemical testing of his or her blood or urine for the purpose of determining the alcoholic content of his or her blood. . ." Cal. Vehicle Code §23612 (West 1996).

25. *Vialva v City of New York,* 118 A.D., 2d. 701, 499 N.Y. 2d. 977 (2nd Dept. 1986).

CHAPTER 119 POSTMORTEM TOXICOLOGY

Rama B. Rao / Mark Flomenbaum

Postmortem toxicology assists in understanding the physiologic and biochemical effects of a xenobiotic at the time of death. A pathologist initiates the first investigative step by collecting specific fluid and tissue samples at autopsy. Several variables may cause quantitative changes in xenobiotic concentrations from the time of death to the time of autopsy. In addition, other artifacts may affect the interpretation of the clinical effects of the xenobiotic identified.

The identification and understanding of xenobiotic-related deaths has significant public health consequences. The forensic pathologist may be the first to identify and report critical information regarding rare fatal drug reactions, medication errors, or rapidly fatal epidemics associated with illicit drug use. As in the case of occupational and environmental xenobiotic-related fatalities, interventions can be implemented to prevent subsequent morbidity and mortality. In addition, the pathologist describes gross and microscopic autopsy findings that may elucidate mechanisms of xenobiotic toxicity, enhancing knowledge that may affect clinical practice.

Using multiple sources of information (Table 119–1), forensic pathologists attempt to establish cause and manner of death. *Cause of death* is the physiologic agent or event necessary for death to occur. For example, the presence of cyanide in the toxicologic evaluation may be sufficient to establish cardiorespiratory arrest from cyanide poisoning. *Manner of death* distinguishes natural from nonnatural deaths. Nonnatural deaths, depending on the jurisdiction, can be divided into several categories (Table 119–2). With the identification of cyanide, the manner of death cannot be considered natural. The medical examiner must make the best determination of the manner of death based on available evidence.[79,85]

The consequences of *manner of death* are far reaching. Homicide necessitates involvement of law enforcement officials for further investigation. Cases deemed suicide not only impact survivors psychologically but also may nullify life-insurance payments, whereas a case deemed an accident may have a double-indemnity insurance clause. Liability suits in workplace disasters may be similarly affected if illicit drugs are identified in the postmortem specimens of involved workers.

Postmortem toxicology can be used in other investigations as well. For example, when carboxyhemoglobin is identified in the human remains of airplane crashes, a cabin fire before descent is more probable than a fire on impact. This type of postmortem analysis is useful in reconstruction of events leading to the crash.[5,44,50]

Techniques for detecting certain compounds in postmortem tissue were developed in the early 19th century and generally focused on identifying heavy metals as a cause of death in homicides.[34,58,60,75,78,79] As the field of forensic pathology developed, laboratory technology progressed rapidly, allowing for more refined qualitative and quantitative identification of xenobiotics. The interpretation of postmortem xenobiotic concentrations, however, is an evolving field. This chapter reviews factors affecting xenobiotic concentrations identified on autopsy and discusses subsequent models for interpreting postmortem toxicologic reports.[31,33,38–40,46,54,62,65]

THE TOXICOLOGIC INVESTIGATION

Ordinarily, toxicologic samples are collected as part of a complete autopsy. In the hospital, when a death is assumed to be from natural causes, the hospital pathologist may perform an autopsy with consent of the family.

The medicolegal autopsy, however, is performed in a medical examiner's office by a forensic pathologist. These autopsies are done in cases in which the manner of death is either unknown or other than natural. When consent for a complete autopsy is not obtained from the family, and the medical examiner decides that a full autopsy may not be necessary, only fluid samples are obtained for analysis.

The sampling of fluid and tissue may be obtained minutes to years after death. The postmortem interval, defined by the state of bodily decomposition, can vary depending on environmental conditions such as ambient temperature, humidity, and immersion under water.[51] Samples may be collected during advanced stages of decomposition or even after embalming or in exhumed bodies.[4,35,61]

DECOMPOSITION AND POSTMORTEM BIOCHEMICAL CHANGES

In the first stage of decomposition, *autolysis,* endogenous enzymes are released, and mechanisms maintaining cellular integrity fail.[45] Chemicals move across leaky membranes down relative concentration gradients. Glycolysis continues in red blood cells until glucose is depleted, and lactate is produced. Ultimately, intracellular ions and proteins are released into the blood, and tissue and blood acidemia develops (see Table 119–3).[79]

The next stage of decomposition, *putrefaction,* involves digestion of tissue by bacterial organisms. Typically these bacteria originate in the bowel or respiratory system. Later other organisms may be introduced by insects or other external sources. As the pu-

TABLE 119–1. Artifacts and Information Affecting Postmortem Toxicologic Interpretation

Xenobiotic dependent
Pharmacokinetic considerations
 State of absorption/distribution at time of death
 Postmortem redistribution
 Postmortem metabolism
Pharmacodynamic considerations
 Expected clinical effects
 Synergistic interactions
Postmortem xenobiotic stability during
 Putrefaction
 Preservation
Previously published tissue concentrations

Decedent dependent
Comorbid conditions
Tolerance
Pharmacogenetic differences

Autopsy Dependent
Postmortem interval (state of decomposition)
Undiagnosed conditions
Sample specimens
Sample sites
Handling and preservation

Other
Laboratory techniques
Evidence at scene
Chain of custody

TABLE 119–3. Normal Postmortem Biochemical Changes[23,53,79]

Increased	Decreased	Stable	Variable
Amino acids	Cl^-	BUN/Cr (vitreous)	Lipids
Ammonia	Glucose	Cholinesterases	T_3
Ca^{2+}	Na^+	Cortisol (serum)	
Epinephrine	pH	Proteins (serum)	
Hepatic enzymes	T_4	Sulfates	
Insulin (esp. right heart blood)			
K^+			
Mg^{2+}			

Intracavitary spaces may be injected with preserving substances, and solid organs may or may not be removed (Table 119–4).[36,37]

SAMPLES USED FOR TOXICOLOGIC ANALYSIS

Ideally, bodies in the early postmortem interval have several commonly used tissues for toxicologic sampling[19,30,42,47,64] (Table 119–5).

Blood

Intravascular blood is a common source for toxicologic examination. Unlike antemortem specimens that usually report plasma concentrations, cell lysis after death precludes this distinction, and "blood" concentrations are reported.

Other sources of blood may be available to the forensic pathologist. Occasionally, extravasated blood identified at autopsy is collected for analysis. In cases where there is a prolonged hospitalization between the exposure and death, antemortem samples may be useful and can be obtained from hospital blood banks or laboratories.

Vitreous Humor

Another source commonly used for sampling is the vitreous humor.[13,18,20] Because of the relatively avascular nature of the fluid, the vitreous humor is well protected from the early decompositional changes that typically occur in blood. Certain physiologic markers such as renal function and specific electrolyte concentrations can be reliably approximated from vitreous humor samples for up to 3 or 4 days in refrigerated bodies. Potassium concentrations are less reliable. The aqueous content of the vitreous is higher than that of blood and may affect partitioning of certain water-soluble xenobiotics.

trefactive process progresses, gases may form, causing foul odors and bloating.[79]

If death occurs in a very warm, dry climate, such as a desert or comparably arid environment, the body may proceed to desiccate so rapidly that putrefactive changes may not occur. The result, *mummification,* produces a lightweight cadaver with a tight, dry skin enveloping a prominent bony skeleton.[79]

If the environment is very cold and hypoxic, such as at great depths under water, putrefaction will be slowed. Anoxic decomposition of fatty tissues occurs, forming a white, cheesy material known as *adipocere.*

Another phase of decomposition, *anthropophagia,* occurs in unprotected postmortem environments where insects or other animals feed on the tissue remnants.[79]

Most morgue refrigerators achieve low enough temperatures to prevent the postmortem interval from progressing. Another factor that may alter or interfere with the natural decompositional changes is embalming. This process preserves dead tissues and can be performed by a variety of techniques. Typically, blood is drained through large vessel pumps, and a substance is injected intravascularly to perfuse and preserve the face and/or other tissues.

TABLE 119–2. Categories of Manner of Death

Natural
Nonnatural
 Homicide
 Suicide
 Accident
 Therapeutic Complication[a]
 Undetermined

[a]Not all jurisdictions recognize therapeutic complication as a manner of death.

TABLE 119–4. Some Historical Constituents of Embalming Fluid[a]

Calcium oxalate	Methanol
Ethanol	Methylsalicylate
Formalin	Phenol
Glutaraldehyde	Quarternary ammonium compounds
Isopropanol	Sodium benzoate
Metals	Thyme

[a]Some, like ethanol and metals are banned for use as preservatives.

TABLE 119–5. Sampling Sites[13,18,20,30,42,79]

Routine	Less routine	Uncommon
Bile	Bone	Antemortem blood
Blood	CSF	Extravasated blood
Brain	Fat	Extravasated fluid
Liver	Hair	Casket fluid
Stomach contents	Kidneys	Insect larvae
Urine	Lungs	Pupae casings
Vitreous humor	Muscle	Soil
	Nails	
	Skin	

Urine

Urine may be available at autopsy and can reveal renally eliminated substances or their metabolites. Because the bladder serves as a reservoir in which metabolism is unlikely to occur, the drugs and their concentrations obtained at autopsy may reflect antemortem concentrations.

Gastric Contents

The contents of the stomach are inspected grossly for color and for presence or absence of pill fragments, food particles, activated charcoal, or other foreign materials. Typically xenobiotic gastric concentrations are reported as milligrams of substance per gram of total gastric contents.

Several factors may affect the gastric contents identified on autopsy. Xenobiotic-induced pylorospasm, diminished intestinal motility, or decreased splanchnic blood flow may all decrease gastric emptying.

Solid Organs and Other Sources

Xenobiotic concentrations in solid organs are usually reported as milligrams of substance per kilogram of homogenized tissue. Other sources of sampling such as hair and nails are typically used for thiol-avid agents such as metals. Rarely, tracheal aspirates of gases can be analyzed to confirm inhalational exposures.

Other Samples

When the body is embalmed, remaining organs, muscle tissue, or the embalming fluid may be utilized for analysis. Soil samples may be obtained in exhumed bodies. In putrefied and anthropophagized bodies, fluids, and potentially insect parts can be analyzed. Entomotoxicology is the science of examining anthropophagic insects at various stages of development to increase information regarding the decedent's death.[32,49] Entomotoxicologists take samples of the insects and can extrapolate, by stage of life, environmental conditions, and season, the approximate time of death. The species *Caliphoridae,* or bluebottle fly, is attracted to unprotected remains by a very fine scent that develops within hours of death. The adult fly lays eggs on mucosal surfaces or open wounds in the flesh. Once the eggs hatch, the larvae feed on the decomposing tissue. Larval samples can be examined for the presence of toxins, but these must be collected and preserved immediately, as the larvae can continue to metabolize certain xenobiotics if they are allowed to remain alive. In another phase of life, the larvae undergo pupation, secreting a substance that encloses

them into pupal casings. These casings are often found in the soil beneath the body. Some toxins have been identified in the casings even after the adult fly has emerged[68] (Table 119–6).

INTERPRETATION OF POSTMORTEM TOXICOLOGIC RESULTS

Once fluid and tissue samples are collected and analyzed for the presence of xenobiotics, the process of interpreting the results begins. This complex task attempts to account for the clinical effects of a xenobiotic at the time of death. Integration of this information allows the forensic pathologist to establish cause and/or manner of death or assists in deciding if the xenobiotic was contributory to death. Multiple confounding variables can affect the sample concentrations of xenobiotics from the time of death to that of the autopsy (Table 119–1).

Artifacts Relating to the Xenobiotic

Postmortem Redistribution Xenobiotic blood concentration may be higher at autopsy than at the time of death if the agent undergoes significant postmortem redistribution.[43,84,90] This occurs most often in substances with large volumes of distribution, where postmortem decomposition results in release of intracellular xenobiotic into the extracellular compartment.[67] For example, digoxin may be released from tissue into the blood as autolysis progresses, resulting in a higher blood concentration at autopsy than at the time of death. If the potential for postmortem redistribution artifact is not considered, xenobiotic concentrations obtained at autopsy may be misinterpreted as supratherapeutic or toxic, and the cause of death may be inappropriately attributed to the identified agent (see Table 119–7, part A).

Less commonly, xenobiotic concentration may fall secondary to postmortem metabolism. For example after death, blood cholinesterases, which are stable in postmortem tissue, continue to degrade cocaine. Unless blood is collected immediately at the time of death in tubes containing enzyme inhibitors such as sodium fluoride, the concentration of cocaine will fall and not accurately reflect the concentration of the drug at the time the decedent expired[48,56,82] (see Table 119–7, part B).

When information is available regarding postmortem redistribution or metabolism, it should be considered and the toxicologic results should be interpreted accordingly.

State of Absorption and Distribution As in the case of the living, the state of absorption, distribution, and other toxicokinetic principles at the time of death affect the sampling concentration. In the case of a xenobiotic with minimal postmortem metabolism or redistribution, the phase of absorption is suggested by the relative quantity of xenobiotic in different fluids and solid organs. For ex-

TABLE 119–6. Xenobiotics Identified in Larvae/Pupal Casings[32,49,68,79]

Benzoylecgonine	Morphine
Cocaine	Nortriptyline
Heroin	Oxazepam
Malathion	Phenobarbital
Mercury	Triazolam
Methamphetamine	

TABLE 119–7. **Examples of Postmortem Xenobiotic Concentration Changes**[43,48,56,67,82,84,90]

A. Increased
    Digoxin because of redistribution
    Amitriptyline because of it large V_d
    Ethanol during putrefaction

B. Decreased
    Cocaine because of postmortem metabolism
    Glucose because of postmortem red cell consumption

ample, a high concentration of xenobiotic and pill fragments in the gastric contents, with progressively lower concentrations in the liver, blood, vitreous, and brain, suggests an early phase of absorption. When a xenobiotic is administered orally and the tissue concentration is highest in the liver, the relationship suggests a postabsorption, but predistribution concentration. A concentration found to be highest in the urine suggests that the xenobiotic was in an elimination phase at the time of death. Although this approach has it limitations, it may be important for correlating the state of absorption and the expected clinical course of the xenobiotic.

Xenobiotic Stability Xenobiotic stability refers to the ability of an agent to maintain its molecular integrity despite changes in the cellular and chemical environment during storage, the addition of preservatives, or with decomposition.[3,10,12,73,80,87–89] Putrefaction causes degradation of some xenobiotics. Xenobiotics resistant to this process are "stable." One study assessing this potential postmortem artifact analyzed homogenized liver tissue infused with various concentrations of xenobiotics.[80] The samples were allowed to putrefy outdoors, and sequential sampling of xenobiotic concentrations was performed. The xenobiotics that decreased in concentration as putrefaction progressed were considered "labile," whereas samples with a constant concentration were stable (Table 119–8). The authors proposed that the chemical moieties of a xenobiotic determine its stability. For example, labile agents share the molecular configuration of an oxygen-nitrogen bond, thiono groups (C=S, P=S), or aminophenols. Chemical structures enhancing stability include single-bonded sulfur groups, carbon-oxygen and carbon-nitrogen bonds, as well as sulfur-oxygen and hydrogen-nitrogen bonds. Although not explicitly studied in otherwise intact, putrefying bodies, a less stable xenobiotic may be recovered in a lower concentration than the actual concentration at the time of death. This artifact must be considered when information regarding xenobiotic stability is available.

Xenobiotic Chemical Interactions In some cases, artifact may result from a chemical interaction with a xenobiotic added during the postmortem period, such as embalming fluid.[29] A study of xenobiotic-spiked blood and formalin in test tubes described the formation of amitriptyline through methylation of nortriptyline.[22] In this situation the identication of amitriptyline, which was not present at the time of death, would confuse interpretation of the toxicologic findings. Where such chemical interactions are described in the literature, the postmortem xenobiotic concentrations should be interpreted accordingly (Table 119–8).

Expected Clinical Effects of the Xenobiotic In order for a fatality to be attributed to a xenobiotic, the expected clinical course of a particular xenobiotic exposure should be consistent with the au-

topsy findings. What are the implications, for example, if a person is found dead 90 minutes after last being seen, and a large concentration of acetaminophen is identified in both the gastric contents and blood? Although suicidal intent (manner) may be supported by this finding, the rapid nature of the death is inconsistent with the clinical course typically associated with acetaminophen overdose. Thus, another cause of death must be sought.

Interpretation of postmortem toxicology must also incorporate clinically relevant consequences of xenobiotic interactions. For example, the combined ingestion of phenobarbital and ethanol can cause fatal respiratory depression. Although neither may be fatal by absolute concentrations alone, their clinical synergy potentially alters interpretation of the toxicologic findings.

Artifacts Relating to Autopsy

The Role of Autopsy In many xenobiotic-related deaths the findings are nonspecific.[86] In some cases, the autopsy reveals confirmatory or supportive findings, such as hepatic necrosis in a decedent with a history of acetaminophen overdose. Large numbers of pills on gross inspection of the stomach may corroborate intent. The autopsy may reveal other findings such as coronary artery narrowing, chronic hypertension, renal abnormalities, or a clinically silent myocardial injury. Such information may be useful to assess the significance and potential impact of a xenobiotic in a patient with previously undiagnosed conditions. In other cases, the absence of a chronic condition may be strongly suggestive of a xenobiotic-related death. For example, a decedent with an autopsy finding of aortic dissection in the absence of chronic hypertensive findings may suggest a xenobiotic-induced hypertensive crisis such as from cocaine.

During putrefaction, bacteria cause fermentation of endogenous carbohydrates, resulting in ethanol formation. In decedents without gross evidence of putrefaction, especially those in cool, dry environments, endogenous ethanol production is minimal.[14,15] With a more advanced postmortem interval or an environment more conducive to ethanol production, the distinction between endogenous and exogenous sources of ethanol becomes more difficult. Multiple sample sites become useful in making the distinction.[81]

Antemortem Physiologic Considerations Inherent to the Body

The clinical response to a xenobiotic may be affected by acquired and inherited physiologic conditions that are not identified on autopsy. Tolerance, an acquired condition in which higher and higher xenobiotic concentrations are required to produce a given clinical effect, is an important consideration. Respiratory depression and death from methadone, for example, may be easily diagnosed in an opioid-naive individual with a history of methadone exposure and methadone-positive postmortem samples. However, the methadone concentrations in a patient who chronically uses methadone may not produce the same outcome. Unfortunately, there are no biochemical, or histologic markers on autopsy that can be used to predict clinically dangerous xenobiotic concentrations in tolerant individuals. Assessment of tolerance in death, as in life, ultimately depends on other information and the best judgment of the investigator.

The other important consideration is ability to metabolize certain agents, particularly through specific hepatic enzyme pathways. Some acquired states of enhanced enzyme induction or inhibition may affect the predicted antemortem concentrations of agents such as phenobarbital.

Alternatively, there is genetic variability in the expression of certain metabolic enzymes. For example, pharmacogenetic differences in metabolic enzymes, such as CYP2D6, predisposed some individuals to fatal hypotension from the inability to metabolize debrisoquine. Such distinctions are not routinely identifiable on autopsy.[24]

Handling of the Body

After death, the handling of the body can result in the development of artifacts.[72,74] In one reported case methanol was detected in the vitreous humor of a decedent, postembalming.[9] The methanol was subsequently traced to a spray cleanser that likely settled on the surface of open eyes during washing of the body.

In the United States, preservatives containing certain metals are currently banned for use in embalming. When these xenobiotics are added during the postmortem period, they can interfere with the interpretation of metal concentrations present before death. Formalin may also affect stability or quantitative identification of some xenobiotics (Table 119–8). When necessary, an

TABLE 119–8. Xenobiotic Stability and Laboratory Recovery[10,12,22,27,73,79,80,87]

- Quantitative recovery affected by preservatives
  As, Pb, Hg, Cu, Ag
  Cyanide
  Carbon monoxide
  Ethchlorvynol
  Nortriptyline (converted to amitriptyline in fixatives)

- Chemical stability in formalin

Stable	Labile
Succinylcholine	Desipramine
Phenobarbital	
Diazepam	
Phenytoin (30 days)	

- Chemical stability in putrefying liver

Stable	Labile
Acetaminophen	o,p-Aminophenols
Amitriptyline	Chlordiazepoxide
Barbiturates	Chlorpromazine
Chloroform	Clonazepam
Clemastine	Malathion
Dextropropoxyphene	Metronidazole
Diazepam	Nitrofurazone
Doxepin	Nitrazepam
Flurazepam	p-Nitrophenol
Glutethemide	Obidoxime
Hydrochlorothiazide	Perphenazine
Imipramine	Trifluoperazine
Lorazepam	
Methaqualone	
Morphine	
Nicotine	
Paraquat	
Pentachlorophenol	
Quinine	
Strychnine	
Vegetable alkaloids	

analysis of embalming fluid used by the mortician can determine the potential for postmortem contamination.[16] Similarly, in exhumed bodies, soil samples from above and below the body must be obtained to ensure that the soil contents did not leach into postmortem tissue.

Artifacts Related to Sampling Sites

Site-specific differences in postmortem xenobiotic blood concentrations are common.[28] For example, blood drawn from femoral vessels may have a low glucose because of postmortem glycolysis, but the glucose concentration of blood removed from the right heart chambers may be high as a result of release of liver glycogen stores. Such differences in xenobiotic sampling are also reported; therefore, the individual interpreting the toxicologic report must know the exact site sampled.[17,47] Ideally more than one site is available for comparison. Multiple samples may not routinely be obtained if the history and autopsy strongly suggest a nontoxicologic cause of death. The comparison of concentrations in different sites may reveal important information regarding state of xenobiotic absorption at the time of death, and acute versus chronic exposure.[6–8,17,21,25,41,52,56,63,64,66,67,69–71,76,77,81,83]

What is the meaning of the xenobiotic concentration if a patient who takes digoxin daily for paroxysmal atrial fibrillation is found dead 1 hour after his last dose? At autopsy the following day, the postmortem right heart blood digoxin concentration was 5.6 ng/mL. This high blood concentration may reflect either the early state of absorption or postmortem redistribution of digoxin. Alternatively, the individual may have suffered death from chronic digoxin toxicity. Sampling another site, such as the vitreous humor, becomes important to make the distinction. The vitreous concentration will likely reflect the chronic concentration of digoxin as it equilibrates with blood over a period of hours after ingestion. If the vitreous humor concentration is 0.9 ng/mL, and the creatinine is 0.8 mg/dL, it is unlikely that chronic digoxin toxicity was responsible for the patient's death.

Other Sample Sites Extravasated intracranial blood is unlikely in most cases to undergo metabolism before or after death. These clots serve as useful samples in patients with a prolonged survival period following an exposure. Furthermore, when compared to intravascular blood, samples from intracranial clots may assist in analyzing the sequence of events preceding death. For example, a woman with a past history of suicide attempts, on fluoxetine, complained of a headache while preparing invitations for her husband's surprise party. She was found dead on her bed with an empty bottle of oxycodone. On autopsy, seven oxycodone tablets were found in her stomach. There was evidence of chronic hypertensive disease, never previously diagnosed, and a large intracranial subarachnoid hemorrhage. Although the husband did not believe she was suicidal at the time, the life insurance company refused to disburse funds on the grounds that her death might have been a suicide. Subsequent toxicology of the extravasated, intracranial blood revealed the presence of fluoxetine and undetectable concentrations of oxycodone. With this information the medical examiner was able to certify the cause of death as subarachnoid hemorrhage secondary to chronic hypertensive disease, and the manner of death as natural. The gastric contents were interpreted as an attempt by the patient to relieve the associated headache. The insurance company was subsequently satisfied, and the life insurance policy was honored.

Blood in the abdominal or thoracic cavities is less useful, as it may be contaminated by bacteria or other substances that may affect xenobiotic stability.

Other Considerations

Published therapeutic, toxic, and fatal postmortem concentrations are available to aid in interpretation of postmortem specimens.[2,55] The conditions associated with these reported concentrations are not necessarily comparable with those of a particular case under investigation. Thus, these resources are valuable but should be used mainly as guidelines and not absolute values defining fatal toxic concentrations.

After postmortem concentrations have been obtained, some authors suggest using the standard formula (Concentration = Dose/V_d) and solving for the dose the patient potentially ingested. This formula applies to antemortem therapeutic dosing regimens following drug absorption and distribution. Comparable conditions may not be present in fatal poisonings. Thus, attempts to define whether a xenobiotic is associated with a therapeutic or intentional overdose should be made within the substantial limitations discussed above.

Other Limitations

Although there are generalized standards of practice in forensic investigations, specimen collection and laboratory methodology may vary.[1] Some xenobiotic concentrations may be falsely elevated or depressed depending on chosen methodology.[57] Laboratory toxicology techniques go beyond the scope of this chapter, but these variables must also be given consideration in postmortem toxicologic interpretations. Just as during life, other limits may include availability of information relating to the scene of death and the handling of specimens through a proper legal chain of custody.

SUMMARY

In order to interpret postmortem toxicological reports effectively, it is essential to understand potential biochemical changes and the artifacts that affect postmortem sampling. Unfortunately, there is no single resource that systematically correlates xenobiotic blood and tissue concentrations, as postmortem decomposition and complexity vary. Hence, postmortem toxicology is an evolving field that may only permit the most likely truth associated with the xenobiotic identified and the circumstances in question.[11,26,59]

Research and development will depend on the collaboration among the physicians caring for the patients at the time of death, as well as forensic pathologists, and medical toxicologists.

REFERENCES

1. Andollo W: Quality assurance in postmortem toxicology. In: Karch SB, ed: Drug Abuse Handbook. Boca Raton, CRC Press, 1998, pp. 953–969.
2. Baselt RC, ed: Disposition of Toxic Drugs and Chemicals in Man, 5th ed. Foster City, Chemical Toxicology Institute, 2000.
3. Battah AH, Hadidi KA: Stability of trihexyphenidyl in stored blood and urine specimens. Int J Legal Med 1998;111:111–114.
4. Berryman HE, Bass WM, Symes SA, Smith OC: Recognition of cemetery remains in the forensic setting. J Forensic Sci 1991;36: 230–237.
5. Blackmore DJ: Aircraft accident toxicology: UK experience 1967–1972. Aerospace Med 1974;45:987–994.
6. Bonnichsen R, Gerrtinger P, Maehly AC: Toxicological data on phenothiazine drugs in autopsy cases. J Legal Med 1970;67:158–169.
7. Briglia EJ, Bidanset JH, Dal Cortivo LA: The distribution of ethanol in postmortem blood specimens. J Forensic Sci 1993;38:1019–1021.
8. Caplan YH, Levine B: Vitreous humor in the evaluation of postmortem blood ethanol concentrations. J Anal Toxicol 1990;14: 305–307.
9. Caughlin J: An unusual source for postmortem findings of methyl ethyl ketone and methanol in two homicide victims. Forensic Sci Int 1994;67:27–31.
10. Chace DH, Goldbaum LR, Lappas NT: Factors affecting the loss of carbon monoxide from stored blood samples. J Anal Toxicol 1986;10: 181–189.
11. Chamberlain RT: Role of the clinical toxicologist in court. Clin Chem 1996;42:1337–1341.
12. Chikasue F, Yashiki T, Kojima T: Cyanide distribution in five fatal cyanide poisonings and the effect of storage conditions on cyanide concentration in tissue. Forensic Sci Int 1988;38:173–183.
13. Choo-Kang E, McKoy C, Escoffery C: Vitreous humor analytes in assessing the postmortem interval and the antemortem clinical status. West Med J 1983;32:23–26.
14. Clark MA, Jones JW: Studies on putrefactive ethanol production. I: Lack of spontaneous ethanol production in intact human bodies. J Anal Toxicol 1982;27:366–371.
15. Coe JI, Sherman RE: Comparative study of postmortem vitreous humor and blood alcohol. J Forensic Sci 1970;15:185–190.
16. Coe JI: Comparative postmortem chemistries of vitreous humor before and after embalming. J Forensic Sci 1976;21:583–586.
17. Coe JI: Postmortem chemistry of blood, cerebrospinal fluid, and vitreous humor. Legal Med Ann 1977;76:55–92.
18. Coe JI: Use of chemical determinations on vitreous humor in forensic pathology. J Forensic Sci 1972;17:541–546.
19. Craig PH: Standard procedures for sampling—a pathologist's prospective view. Clin Toxicol 1979;15:597–603.
20. Daae LN, Teige B, Svaar H: Determination of glucose in human vitreous humor. J Legal Med 1978;80:287–290.
21. Davis GL: Postmortem alcohol analyses of general aviation pilot fatalities, Armed Forces Institute of Pathology 1962–1967. Aerospace Med 1973;44:80–83.
22. Dettling RJ, Briglia EJ, Dal Cortivo LA, Bidanset JH: The production of amitriptyline from nortriptyline in formaldehyde-containing solutions. J Anal Toxicol 1990;14:325–326.
23. Devgun MS, Dunbar JA: Post-mortem estimation of gamma-glutamyl transferase in vitreous humor and its association with chronic abuse of alcohol and road-traffic deaths. Forensic Sci Int 1985;28:179–180.
24. Druid H, Holmgren P, Carlsson B, Ahlner J: Cytochrome P450 2D6 (CYP2D6) genotyping on postmortem blood as a supplementary tool for interpretation of forensic toxicological results. Forensic Sci Int 1999;99:25–34.
25. Druid H, Holmgren P: A compilation of fatal and control concentrations of drugs in postmortem femoral blood. J Forensic Sci 1997; 42:79–87.
26. Ernst MF, Poklis A, Gantner GE: Evaluation of medicolegal investigators' suspicions and positive toxicology findings in 100 drug deaths. J Anal Toxicol 1982;27:61–65.
27. Falconer B, Moller M: The determination of carbon monoxide in blood treated with formaldehyde. J Legal Med 1971;68:17–19.
28. Felby S, Olsen J: Comparative studies of postmortem barbiturate and meprobamate in vitreous humor, blood and liver. J Forensic Sci 1969;14:507–514.
29. Fomey RB, Carroll FT, Nordgren IK, et al: Extraction, identification and quantitation of succinylcholine in embalmed tissue. J Anal Toxicol 1982;6:115–119.
30. Forrest AR: Obtaining samples at post mortem examination for toxicological and biochemical analyses. J Clin Pathol 1993;46:292–296.

31. Garriott JC: Interpretive toxicology. Clin Lab Med 1983;3:367–384.
32. Goff ML, Lord WD: Entomotoxicology. A new area for forensic investigation. Am J Forensic Med Pathol 1994;15:51–57.
33. Goldman P, Ingelfinger JA: Completeness of toxicological analyses. JAMA 1980;243:2030–2031.
34. Goulding R: Poisoning as a fine art. Med Legal J 1978;46:6–17.
35. Grellner W, Glenewinkel F: Exhumations: synopsis of morphologic findings in relation to the postmortem interval. Survey on a 20-year the literature. Forensic Sci Int 1997;90:139–159.
36. Halmai J: Common thyme (*Thymus vulgaris*) as employed for the embalming. Ther Hungarica 1972;20:162–165.
37. Hanzlick R: Embalming, body preparation, burial, and disinterment. Pathology 1994;15:122–131.
38. Hearn WL, Keran EE, Wei H, Hime G: Site dependent postmortem changes in blood cocaine concentrations. J Forensic Sci 1991;36:673–684.
39. Hearn WL, Walls HC: Introduction to postmortem toxicology. In: Karch SB, ed: Drug Abuse Handbook. Boca Raton, CRC Press, 1998, pp. 863–873.
40. Hearn WL, Walls HC: Common methods in postmortem toxicology. In: Karch SB, ed: Drug Abuse Handbook. Boca Raton, CRC Press, 1998, pp. 890–926.
41. Hearn WL, Walls HC: Strategies for postmortem toxicological investigation. In: Karch SB, ed: Drug abuse handbook. Boca Raton, CRC Press, 1998, pp. 926–953.
42. Helper BR, Isenschmid DS: Specimen selection, collection, preservation, and security. In: Karch SB, ed: Drug Abuse Handbook. Boca Raton, CRC Press, 1998, pp. 873–889.
43. Hilberg T, Rogde S, Morland J: Postmortem drug redistribution—human cases related to results in experimental animals. J Forensic Sci 1999;44:3–9.
44. Hill IR: Toxicological findings in fatal aircraft accidents in the United Kingdom. Am J Forensic Med Pathol 1986;7:322–326.
45. Iwasa Y, Onaya T: Postmortem changes in the level of calcium pump triphosphatase in rat heart sarcoplasmic reticulum. Forensic Sci Int 1988;39:13–22.
46. Jones GR: Interpretation of postmortem drug levels. In: Karch SB, ed: Drug Abuse Handbook. Boca Raton, CRC Press,1998, pp. 970–985.
47. Jones GR, Pounder DJ: Site dependence of drug concentrations in postmortem blood—a case study. J Anal Toxicol 1987;11:186–190.
48. Karch SB: Introduction to the forensic pathology of cocaine. Am J Forensic Med Pathol 1991;12:126–131.
49. Kintz P, Tracqui A, Ludes B, et al: Fly larvae and their relevance in forensic toxicology. Am J Forensic Med Pathol 1990;11:63–65.
50. Klette K, Levine B, Springate C, Smith ML: Toxicological findings in military aircraft fatalities from 1986–1990. Forensic Sci Int 1992;53:143–148.
51. Krompecher T: Experimental evaluation of rigor mortis. v. Effect of various temperatures on the evolution of rigor. Forensic Sci Int 1981;17:19–26.
52. Kunsman GW, Rodriguez R, Rodriguez P: Fluvoxamine distribution in postmortem cases. Am J Forensic Med Pathol 1999;20:78–83.
53. Langford AM, Taylor KK, Pounder DJ: Drug concentration in selected skeletal muscles. J Forensic Sci 1998;43:22–27.
54. Levine BS, Smiith ML, Froede RC: Postmortem forensic toxicology. Clin Lab Med 1990;10:571–589.
55. Lewin JF, Pannell LK, Wilkinson LF: Computer storage of toxicology methods and postmortem drug determinations. Forensic Sci Int 1983;23:225–232.
56. Logan BK, Smirnow D, Gullberg RG: Lack of predictable site-dependent differences and time-dependent changes in postmortem concentrations of cocaine, benzoylecgonine, and cocaethylene in humans. J Anal Toxicol 1997;20:23–31.
57. Long C, Crifasi J, Maginn D, et al: Comparison of analytical methods in the determination of two venlafaxine fatalities. J Anal Toxicol 1997;21:166–169.
58. Mellen PF, Bouvieer EC: Nineteenth-century Massachusetts coroner inquests. Am J Forensic Med Pathol 1996;17:207–210.
59. Messite J, Stellman SD: Accuracy of death certificate completion. JAMA 1996;275:794–796.
60. Niyogi SK: Historic development of forensic toxicology in America up to 1978. Am J Forensic Med Pathol 1980;1:249–264.
61. Oxley DW: Examination of the exhumed body and embalming artifacts. Med Legal Bull 1984;33:1–7.
62. Peat MA: Advances in forensic toxicology. Clin Lab Med 1998;18:263–278.
63. Peclet C, Picotte P, Iobin F: The use of vitreous humor levels of glucose, lactic acid and blood levels of acetone to establish antemortem hyperglycemia in diabetics. Forensic Sci Int 1994;65:1–6
64. Pla A, Hernandez AF, Gil F, et al: A fatal case of oral ingestion of methanol. Distribution in postmortem tissues and fluids including pericardial fluid and vitreous humor. Forensic Sci Int 1991;49: 193–196.
65. Polson CJ, Gee DJ, Knight B: The Essentials of Forensic Medicine, 4th ed. Oxford, Pergamon Press, 1985, pp. 3–39.
66. Pounder DJ, Carson DO, Johnston K, Orihara Y: Electrolyte concentration differences between left and right vitreous humor samples. J Forensic Sci 1998;43:604–607.
67. Pounder DJ, Davies JI: Zopiclone poisoning: tissue distribution and potential for postmortem diffusion. Forensic Sci Int 1994;65:177–183.
68. Pounder DJ: Forensic entomo-toxicology. Forensic Sci Soc 1991;31:469–472.
69. Prouty RW, Anderson WH: A comparison of postmortem heart blood and femoral blood ethyl alcohol concentrations. J Anal Toxicol 1987;11:191–197.
70. Prouty RW, Anderson WH: The forensic science implications of site and temporal influences on postmortem blood-drug concentrations. J Forensic Sci 1990;35:243–270.
71. Ritz S, Harding P, Martz W: Measurement of digitalis-glycoside levels in ocular tissues. Int J Legal Med 1992;105:155–159.
72. Rivers RL: Embalming artifacts. J Forensic Sci 1978;23:531–535.
73. Robertson MD, Drummer OR: Stability of nitrobenzodiazepines in postmortem blood. J Forensic Sci 1998;43:5–8.
74. Rohrig TP: Comparison of fentanyl concentrations in unembalmed and embalmed liver samples. J Anal Toxicol 1998;22:253.
75. Rosenfeld L: Alfred Swaine Taylor (1806–1880), pioneer toxicologist—and a slight case of murder. Clin Chem 1985;31:1235–1236.
76. Schonheyder RC, Renriques U: Postmortem blood cultures. Evaluation of separate sampling of blood from the right and left cardiac ventricle. APMIS 1997;105:76–78.
77. Schoning P, Strafuss AC: Analysis of postmortem canine blood, cerebrospinal fluid, and vitreous humor. Am J Vet Res 1981;42:1447–1449.
78. Smith PW, Lacefield DJ, Crane CR: Toxicological findings in aircraft accident investigation. Aerospace Med 1970;41:760–762.
79. Spitz WU, ed: Spitz's and Fischers Medicolegal Investigation of Death. Springfield, IL, Charles C Thomas, 1993.
80. Stevens HM: The stability of some drugs and poisons in putrefying human liver tissues. J Forensic Sci Soc 1984;24:577–589.
81. Stone BE, Rooney PA: A study using body fluids to determine blood alcohol. J Anal Toxicol 1984;8:95–96.
82. Tardiff K, Gross E, Wu J, et al: Analysis of cocaine positive fatalities. J Forensic Sci 1989;34:53–63.
83. Vermeulen T: Distribution of paroxetine in three postmortem cases. J Anal Toxicol 1998;22:541–544.
84. Vorpahl TE, Coe JI: Correlation of antemortem and postmortem digoxin levels. J Forensic Sci 1978;23:329–334.
85. Wetli CV: Investigation of drug-related deaths—an overview. Am J Forensic Med Pathol 1984;5:111–120.
86. Winek CL, Wahba WW: The role of trauma in postmortem blood alcohol determination. Forensic Sci Int 1995;74:213–214.
87. Winek CL, Esposito FM, Cinicola DP: The stability of several compounds in formalin fixed tissues and formalin-blood solutions. Forensic Sci Int 1990;44:159–168.

88. Winek CL, Wahba WW, Rozin L, Winek CL Jr: Determination of ethchlorvinyl in body tissues and fluids after embalmment. Forensic Sci Int 1988;37:161–166.

89. Winek CL, Zaveri NR, Wahba WW: The study of tricyclic antidepressants in formalin fixed human liver and formalin solutions. Forensic Sci Int 1993;61:175–183.

90. Worm K, Dragsholt C, Simonsen K, Kringsholm B: Citalopram concentrations in samples from autopsies and living persons. Int J Legal Med 1998;111:188–190.

CHAPTER 120 PRINCIPLES OF EPIDEMIOLOGY AND RESEARCH DESIGN

Kevin C. Osterhoudt

In 1963 Reye and Johnson described series of patients with encephalopathy and fatty degeneration of the liver.[22,34] Further anecdotal observation of similar patients allowed the development of a hypothesis that aspirin may be an etiologic factor in Reye syndrome.[13] Given such a common exposure as salicylate therapy and such a rare disease as Reye syndrome, how would researchers investigate whether an association between salicylate and Reye syndrome truly exists?

In 1976 a case series suggested that enteral erythromycin given to neonates might predispose to infantile hypertrophic pyloric stenosis.[35] How might this association be confirmed given that pyloric stenosis typically occurs in approximately one of every 500 infants, but intake of erythromycin is unusual among this group?

Gastric emptying has a long tradition as a method of gastrointestinal decontamination to treat patients after acute oral overdose. Hyperbaric oxygen therapy (HBO) is considered as a therapy to prevent delayed neurologic sequelae from carbon monoxide (CO) poisoning. How can it be determined if these treatments actually offer a patient benefit?

Advances in clinical medicine are usually achieved through a typical scientific method. First, astute clinicians make interesting observations. These observations lead to the generation of hypotheses. Research questions are analyzed with epidemiologic investigation, and initial studies are examined with methodologic scrutiny. Initial analytic techniques are improved, and confirmatory studies are performed. Ultimately, models relating cause to effect are formulated.

The field of medical toxicology is rapidly transitioning from a descriptive discipline to one of rigorous scientific exploration. New associations between toxins and diseases are being explored every year. Recent high-profile associations include those between silicone breast implants and connective tissue diseases, and insecticide exposure and childhood cancer. An understanding of basic principles of research design and epidemiology is required to interpret published studies and to lay the groundwork for future investigation in toxicology.

EPIDEMIOLOGIC TECHNIQUES AVAILABLE TO INVESTIGATE CLINICAL PROBLEMS

Different study formats are listed in Table 120–1.

Observational Design: Descriptive

A staggering array of poisons and venoms are able to injure people, necessitating reliance of toxicologists on good descriptive data regarding toxic outcomes. The Toxic Exposure Surveillance System (TESS) of the American Association of Poison Control Centers now has a database of over 27 million human poison exposure cases.[24] Descriptive case reporting serves a valuable purpose in describing the characteristics of a medical condition or procedure and remains a fundamental tool of epidemiologic investigation. A *case report* is a clinical description of a single patient or procedure with respect to a situation. Case reports are most useful for hypothesis generation. However, single case reports are not generalizable, as the reported situation may be atypical. A number of case reports can be grouped, on the basis of similarities, into a *case series*. Case series can be used to characterize an illness or syndrome, but without a control group they are severely limited in proving cause and effect. In the now classic paper, Reye described 21 children with encephalopathy and fatty degeneration of the liver that characterized the syndrome that now bears his name.[34] Further descriptive data collection suggested that use of aspirin might be associated with Reye syndrome (RS),[13] but analytic study would be required to support that hypothesis. Published annual reports of TESS data state that their descriptive data are meant to "identify hazards early, focus prevention education, guide clinical research, and direct training."[24] In these roles, descriptive data are often underappreciated.

Cross-sectional studies assess a population for the presence or absence of an exposure and condition simultaneously. Such data often provide estimates of *prevalence*—the fraction of individuals in a population sharing a characteristic or condition at a point in time. These studies, particularly helpful in public health planning, have been extremely useful in monitoring common environmental exposures, such as childhood lead poisoning, or population-wide drug use, such as occurs with tobacco, marijuana, and alcohol. The United States National Health and Nutrition Examination Survey investigations demonstrated that the percentage of children with blood lead levels >10 µg/dL decreased from 88.2% to 4.4% between 1976 and 1991, with the highest rates of plumbism among African American, low-income, or urban children.[4] An *analysis of secular trends* is a study type that compares changes in illness over time or geography to changes in risk factors. These analyses often lend circumstantial support to a hypothesis; however, because of the ecological nature of their design, individual data on risk factors are not available to allow exclusion of alternative hypotheses also consistent with the data. A prime example of an analysis of secular trends is Arrowsmith's finding that reports of RS declined between 1980 and 1985, coincident with a fall in sales of, or physician recommendations of, children's aspirin products.[2] This investigation added further confirmation to the etiologic role of aspirin in the development of Reye syndrome but could not exclude alternative hypotheses such as a change in viral epidemic patterns.

TABLE 120–1.   Types of Epidemiologic Study Designs[a]

Experimental
   Clinical trial
Observational: Analytic
   Cohort
   Case-control
Observational: Descriptive
   Analysis of secular trends
   Cross-sectional
   Case series
   Case report

[a]Study designs are listed in descending order from the design that offers the best epidemiologic evidence for association to that which offers the least.

Observational Design: Analytical

Hypotheses generated by theoretical reasoning or anecdotal association require analytic testing. Case-control studies and cohort studies are analytic techniques that utilize observational data, and each technique has its own advantages and disadvantages (Table 120–2). *Case-control studies* compare affected, treated, or diseased patients (cases) to nonaffected patients (controls) and look for a difference in prior risk factors or exposures (Fig. 120–1A). Because subjects are recruited into the study based on prior presence or absence of a particular outcome, case-control studies are always retrospective in nature. They are especially useful when the outcome being studied is rare, and they enable the investigation of any number of potential etiologies for a single disease.

RS is an illness well suited to case-control study. The incidence of RS peaked in the United States in the mid 1970s, and clustered together with viral epidemics of influenza A, influenza B, and varicella. Based on anecdotal observations in a series of patients, a hypothesis was formulated that salicylate may be an etiologic factor in RS.[13] Other putative contributory factors were also proposed, including viral infections, aflatoxin, pesticides, antiemetic drugs, and valproate. Exposures to salicylate were common in the 1970s, but the incidence of RS was less than 10 cases per million persons under age of 18 years. In the epidemiologic investigation that served as a foundation for decades of research to follow, seven children diagnosed with RS were compared to 16 control children who were matched on the basis of age, gender, time, and viral symptoms.[37] Families were interviewed regarding the types and quantities of medications taken by the children. Salicylates were the only exposure found to be statistically different

TABLE 120–2.   Advantages of Case-Control versus Cohort Study Designs

Case-control study
   Smaller sample required when outcome is rare
   Reduced bias in outcome data
   Can study many exposures simultaneously
   Allows estimation of relative risk
   May obviate need for long followup period
Cohort study
   Provides more robust evidence of association
   Reduced bias in exposure data
   Can study many outcomes simultaneously
   Allows direct calculation of incidence
   Allows direct calculation of relative risk

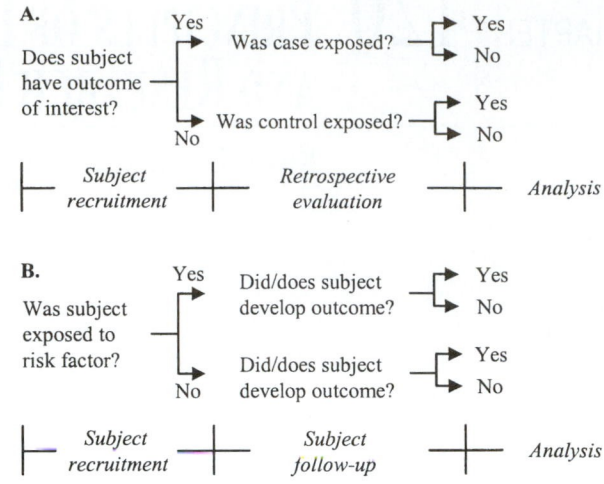

Figure 120–1.   A. Schematic representation of the **case-control study design.** Subjects with an outcome or condition of interest are selected, along with control subjects, and then are evaluated for previous exposure to a risk factor of interest. **B.** Schematic representation of the **cohort study design.** Subjects are recruited based on the presence or absence of a risk factor or exposure, then followed to see if they develop an outcome.

between cases and controls, and this became the first case-control study to identify increased odds of developing RS after aspirin therapy. Larger subsequent case control studies added confirmatory evidence to the association between salicylate use and RS.[15,21,40]

Cohort studies compare patients with certain risk factors or exposures to those patients without the exposure, then follow these cohorts to see which subjects develop the outcome of interest (Fig. 120–1B). In this respect, they allow the comparison of *incidence* (the number of new outcomes occurring within a population initially free of disease over a period of time) between populations who share an exposure and populations who do not. They may be retrospective or prospective and enable the study of any number of outcomes from a single exposure. They are particularly well suited to investigations in which the outcome of interest is relatively common. In circumstances when an outcome of interest is very uncommon, such as the case with RS, the large number of study subjects required might make a cohort study impractical. A suggested association between oral erythromycin administration to newborn infants and increased risk of idiopathic hypertrophic pyloric stenosis, which typically affects up to three individuals per 1000 live births, remained unstudied until a 1999 cohort study. Investigators studied a patient population in which 157 out of 282 infants born at a hospital in a 2-month period were treated with erythromycin prophylaxis because of a pertussis exposure.[18] Investigators separated these patients into cohorts based on exposure to erythromycin and looked at the differences of pyloric stenosis rates between the two groups. Neonates treated with erythromycin were found to be at significantly greater risk of pyloric stenosis than untreated controls. Perhaps the most famous and ambitious cohort study was the Framingham Heart Study in which 5209 residents of Framingham, MA, aged 30 to 62 years have been followed for over 50 years. This study provided a useful tool for studying the incidence of lung cancer, stroke, and cardiovascular disease in those exposed to cigarette smoke[11] and other toxins.

Experimental Design

Experimental studies are those in which the treatment, risk factor, or exposure of interest can be controlled by the investigator to study differences in outcome between the groups (Fig. 120–2). The prototype is the randomized, blinded, controlled clinical trial. Among epidemiologic study types, these provide the most convincing demonstration of causality. Clinical trials are used to measure the *efficacy* (the treatment effect within a controlled experimental setting) of treatment regimens and to draw inferences about the *effectiveness* of a treatment applied to the general population. Unfortunately, interventional studies are the most complex to perform, and several questions must be addressed by investigators before performing a clinical trial (Table 120–3). Human clinical trials have been especially difficult to apply to the practice of toxicology. Indeed, between 1992 and 1996, one author found only three such randomized clinical trials.[38] Characteristics of poisoned patients, which hamper attempts at clinical trials, are listed in Table 120–4. Volunteer studies, using nontoxic drugs or subtoxic drug doses, are often used to circumvent many of the problems in controlling human poisoning studies; but it is typically difficult to apply results from these studies to the actual physiology of toxic overdose.

Perhaps the best way to demonstrate an etiologic association between salicylate use and RS would be to perform a randomized, double-blinded, controlled clinical trial. Patients with influenza and fever could be randomly treated with salicylate or placebo, and the incidence of RS in both treatment groups could be determined. However, with such a strong association noted from case-control studies, and with suitable alternative antipyretic medications available, such a study would be unethical. As toxicologists strive to find evidence for, or against, the traditions of clinical practice, several important clinical trials have been published. Among them are many important examples and lessons in epidemiologic study design.

One trial attempted to evaluate whether or not corticosteroids might be beneficial in preventing esophageal strictures secondary to circumferential caustic injury of the esophagus.[1] Because of the inherent difficulty in recruiting eligible patients from a single institution, only 60 patients with esophageal injury were recruited over an 18-year period. These patients were randomized to therapy with or without corticosteroids and followed for the development of stricture. Ten of the 31 patients treated with corticosteroids developed strictures in comparison to 11 of 29 control patients. The authors concluded that there was no apparent benefit from the use of corticosteroids to treat children who have ingested a caustic

TABLE 120–3.   Considerations in Designing a Clinical Trial

What is the question of interest?
What is the target patient population?
How will the safety of subjects be assured?
What is a suitable control group?
How will outcomes be measured?
What difference in outcomes between groups is considered important?
What is the analysis plan?
How many subjects will be required?
How will randomization and blinding be achieved and maintained?
How long a followup period will be required?
How will loss of study subjects be handled?
How will treatment compliance be evaluated?

substance. A second study challenged our notions of gastrointestinal decontamination and randomized 876 acutely poisoned patients with respect to gastric emptying procedures.[32] Outcomes measured were clinical course, length of hospital stay, and complications. The investigators concluded that gastric emptying did not provide additional therapeutic benefit beyond that of antidotal activated charcoal. A third representative study demonstrated benefit from hyperbaric oxygen therapy with regard to the prevention of delayed neurologic sequelae after carbon monoxide poisoning.[39] Sixty patients with acute carbon monoxide poisoning were randomized to either ambient pressure or hyperbaric oxygen, then followed for the occurrence of neurologic dysfunction. The conclusions of each of the three aforementioned studies have encountered tremendous academic dissection and debate. Certain concerns with the methodology and analysis of these studies are examined later in this chapter to illustrate epidemiologic concepts. Additionally, each of these studies is described in more detail in the relevant chapters of this text (Chap. 87, 5, and 97, respectively).

MEASURES USED TO QUANTIFY THE STRENGTH OF AN EPIDEMIOLOGIC ASSOCIATION

The objective of analytic studies is to define and quantify the degree of statistical dependence between an exposure and an outcome. Such associations are ideally represented by the relative risk of developing an outcome if exposed in comparison to being unexposed. Thus, the *relative risk* can be defined as the incidence of

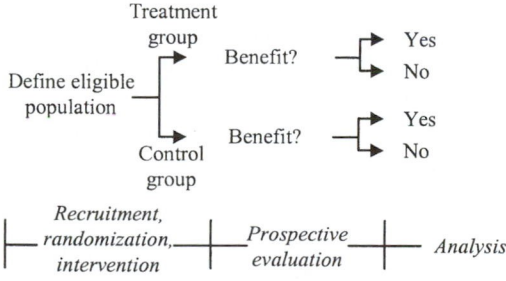

Figure 120–2.   Schematic representation of the design of a randomized clinical trial.

TABLE 120–4.   Difficulties in Applying Clinical Trials to Human Poisoning

It is unethical to intentionally "poison" subjects.
Poisoned patients represent a broad spectrum of demographic patterns.
A wide variety of poisons exist.
Exposures to any single poison are usually limited.
A limited number of poisoned patients are available at any one study site.
Uncertainty often exists as to type, quantity, and timing of most poison exposures.
Poisoning typically results in a relatively short course of illness.

OUTCOME

Figure 120–3. Use of a 2 × 2 table to calculate or estimate relative risk from analytic studies. In cohort studies, study subjects are selected on the basis of exposure. In case-control studies, subjects are selected on the basis of outcome. The letters a, b, c, and d represent the number of subjects either exposed or unexposed to a "risk factor" or treatment, with or without the outcome of interest. The odds ratio estimates the relative risk if the outcome of interest is rare.

Cohort Study

$$\text{Relative Risk} = \frac{a}{a+b} \Big/ \frac{c}{c+d}$$

Case Control Study

$$\text{Odds Ratio} = ad/bc$$

outcome in exposed individuals compared to the incidence of outcome in unexposed individuals. The relative risk can be calculated directly from cohort or interventional studies. However, in a case-control study, an investigator chooses the numbers of cases and controls to be studied, so true incidence data are not obtained. In case-control studies an *odds ratio* can be calculated, and the odds ratio will provide an estimate for relative risk in situations where the outcome is rare, such as when the outcome occurs in fewer than 10% of exposed individuals. The calculation of relative risk or odds ratio from analytic studies is demonstrated in Fig. 120–3.

A relative risk of 1.0 signifies that an outcome is equally likely to occur whether an individual is exposed or not and implies that no association exists between the exposure and the outcome. A relative risk approaching 0 suggests that an exposure is a marker of protection with regard to the outcome, and a relative risk approaching infinity suggests the exposure predicts a tendency toward the outcome. In the previously described case-control investigation of the link between salicylate use and RS, all of the seven case subjects had used aspirin compared to only 8 of 16 controls.[37] The odds ratio calculated from these data approaches infinity and suggests a strong association between exposure and outcome. In the described clinical trial of therapeutic corticosteroids (the "exposure") in the prevention of esophageal strictures (the "outcome"), 10 of 31 treated patients developed strictures compared to 11 of 29 untreated patients.[1] This relative risk calculation approximates 1 and seemingly demonstrates little benefit from corticosteroid therapy.

MEASURES USED TO QUANTIFY THE SIGNIFICANCE OF AN EPIDEMIOLOGIC ASSOCIATION

Analytic studies are performed to test hypotheses, typically that an exposure is associated with an outcome. The presence of such association in any given study has a number of possible explanations, as detailed in Table 120–5. The goal of statistical analysis is to determine the degree to which chance can be excluded as the true reason the results of the study were obtained. By convention,

statistical analysis typically tests the *null hypothesis*—the hypothesis that there is no association between exposure and outcome.

Because analytic studies involve only a sample of the total population, they contain two types of inherent error. *Type I error,* also referred to as alpha (α) error, is the likelihood that an investigator may conclude that an association exists when none truly does. *Type II error,* or beta (β) error, is the possibility that an investigator will be unable to find an association when one is really present. The most commonly reported measures of type I error in published toxicologic studies are the *p*-value and the confidence interval (CI). Statistical significance has customarily, but not necessarily, been defined as having less than a 1 in 20 chance of conducting a false-positive study. Therefore, a type I error of less than 5%, which corresponds to a *p*-value of less than 0.05, is usually deemed "statistically significant."

Perhaps a more informative description of the significance of an association is provided through the CI. The CI not only provides a test of statistical significance, it also offers information pertaining to the degree (and possible range) of differences observed. In an unbiased study, the 95% CI provides a range between which, if the study could be repeated an infinite number of times, the observed magnitude of effect would lie 95% of the time. One study reported it noteworthy that no toddlers ingesting one or two calcium channel antagonists became seriously ill, but a subsequent analysis of the CI around this small set of data demonstrated

TABLE 120–5. Types of Associations between Exposures and Outcomes That May Be Found with a Clinical Study

No Association	The outcome is independent of exposure.
Artifactual Association	
Chance	The association demonstrated by the study resulted from random error.
Bias	Systematic error in the study led to the noted association.
Indirect Association	The association is real, but not truly cause and effect (confounding).
Causal Association	The outcome is dependent on the exposure.

that the true incidence could be as high as 18%.[30] A CI around a relative risk or odds ratio is not statistically significant if it includes 1.0, and the narrower the CI the more precise the estimate of the magnitude of effect.

The likelihood that a study will find a difference if one truly exists is termed statistical *power* and relates to the likelihood of a false-negative study (type II error). Power is usually artificially set by an investigator before a study is performed and is typically set at 80% or 90% to practically limit the number of study subjects needed. Considerations applicable to choice of sample size are found in Table 120–6. The sample size of a study is determined by the frequency of the exposure and outcome within the study population, the strength of association deemed clinically relevant, and the amount of error deemed acceptable in the study. Because power is often set relatively low, it is difficult to state that an association does not exist. It is more proper to state that a study was unable to reject the null hypothesis to find an association. In the ongoing controversy regarding the utility of hyperbaric oxygen in the treatment of acute carbon monoxide poisoning, three randomized studies have alleged benefit,[9,26,39] and two have not.[33, 36] Conventional parameters for statistical significance suggest that, if unbiased, the positive studies met a bigger burden of evidence than did the negative studies.

DIFFERENTIATION BETWEEN CLINICAL SIGNIFICANCE AND STATISTICAL SIGNIFICANCE

The finding of a low *p*-value indicates a statistically high level of confidence that a difference between study groups exists but offers no indication that the difference is clinically important. The interpretation of statistical versus clinical significance is often facilitated through calculation of confidence intervals. Small actual differences between two groups can become statistically significant if large numbers of subjects are studied. Likewise, impressive associations of cause and effect can seem trivial if few subjects are in a study. The clinical significance of an association is left to the judgment of the individual interpreting a study. Ideally, a working definition of clinical significance is developed before a study is performed.

In the noted study of corticosteroids and corrosive injury of the esophagus, 64% of control subjects required esophageal replacement versus 40% of treated subjects.[1] The investigators' calcula-

tion of the *p*-value for this comparison is greater than 0.05. Many would interpret a reduction in esophageal replacement by approximately one-third to be potentially clinically important, yet it is unlikely that this study had statistical power to find such an association. Likewise, in a study suggesting no benefit from gastric emptying after acute overdose, when patients presenting within 1 hour of overdose were examined, 15 % of treated patients showed improvement versus 4% of controls.[32] Again, statistical significance was not achieved, but the clinical significance of these data is subject to speculation.

METHODOLOGIC PROBLEMS FOUND WITHIN CLINICAL STUDIES

Calculation of a *p*-value or confidence interval does nothing to assess the adequacy of study design. These measures are used to quantify the influence of random error, or chance, on research findings. Clinical research involving patients is particularly susceptible to *bias*, which can be defined as systematic error in the collection or interpretation of data. Because such error can lead to an inappropriate estimate of the association between an exposure and an outcome, careful evaluation of potential biases affecting a clinical study is of paramount importance.

Selection bias refers to error introduced into a study by the manner in which subjects are selected for inclusion in the study. This type of bias is most problematic for retrospective studies in which exposures and outcomes have both occurred at the time of subject recruitment. Selection bias may be introduced into a prospective clinical tudy if the study fails to enroll potential subjects, or if potential subjects refuse to participate, on a systematic basis. Selection bias may even influence the results of clinical trials. In the 1995 trial that found no difference in outcome between acutely poisoned patients treated with gastric emptying and patients from whom gastric emptying was withheld, all patients presenting to the emergency department after acute overdose were enrolled.[32] Because most patients with poisoning exposure are likely to do well with minimal support,[24] selection of patients on this basis might be expected to bias this study to find no effect. Reasoning suggests that the patients most likely to benefit from gastric emptying are those with life-threatening toxic ingestion presenting within the first hour after overdose. As mentioned previously, subgroup review of the results of this paper suggests clinical benefit within this group of patients, but without conclusive power.

Information bias refers to error introduced into a study as a result of systematic differences in the quality of data obtained between exposed and unexposed groups, or between those with and without the outcome of interest. Several distinct types of information bias may exist. Affected and nonaffected individuals may have differential memories with regard to exposures, so recall bias is a concern in retrospective studies. The potential for *recall bias* is frequently cited as criticism of early retrospective case-control studies of aspirin as an etiologic factor for RS, in which families were asked to recollect their children's aspirin use history. Critics suggest that the parents of children affected by RS might be more vigorous in their recall of exposures than the parents of unaffected children. Similarly, *interviewer bias* may occur if study personnel differ in how they solicit, record, or interpret information as a result of knowledge of the subjects' status with regard to exposures

TABLE 120–6.   Considerations in Choice of Sample Size

	Sample Size	
	Large	**Small**
Pros	• Able to detect associations of small magnitude • Less susceptible to some biases • More robust analysis	• Less work and less cost
Cons	• More work and more cost	• Might not detect associations of small magnitude • More susceptible to biases associated with patient differences

or outcomes. Prospective studies may be troubled by loss to followup, especially if subjects are lost from the study for reasons relating to either exposure or outcome (such as when subjects withdraw from a study because they are feeling better, or are "lost" because they die). *Misclassification bias* occurs when investigators incorrectly categorize subjects with respect to exposure or outcome. In a retrospective study of 378 children regarding the predictability of caustic esophageal injury from clinical signs and symptoms, it was found that 10 of 80 asymptomatic children had significant burns.[12] There is a possibility that these "asymptomatic" children were misclassified because of lack of rigorous written documentation of symptoms or signs within the medical charts.

Bias is best minimized through careful study design. It is important to precisely define the study question and the population at risk and to carefully define rigorous inclusion and exclusion criteria. The outcome should also be defined precisely. During data acquisition the best way to reduce bias may be to keep study personnel gathering exposure data blinded to outcome, and vice versa. Often, it may also be advisable to keep study subjects unaware of their status within a study to the extent that it is ethical (thus, "double-blinded"—neither investigators nor subjects are aware of the subjects' status within a study). Use of placebos or "sham treatments" is a way to facilitate blinding. One of the strongest criticisms of a 1995 trial of HBO for the prevention of delayed neurologic syndromes after CO poisoning[39] has been the failure to blind patients and investigators to the treatment in question.[28] It is inevitable that some degree of potential bias will be present in any clinical study. Such bias should be reviewed in analysis, and estimations of its magnitude and direction (bias toward or away from rejection of the null hypothesis) should be considered.

Unlike selection and information biases, which are errors introduced into studies primarily by the investigators or subjects, confounding is a special type of problem that may occur within a study as a result of interrelationships between the exposure of interest and another exposure. *Confounding* is a bias wherein an observed association is not a product of cause and effect but instead results from linking of the exposure of interest to another associated exposure. Studies pertaining to adverse effects of drugs of abuse are especially prone to confounding by variables such as concomitant caffeine use, alcohol use, tobacco use, nutritional deficiency, and/or psychiatric illness. Analytic studies may restrict characteristics of enrolled subjects or match subject characteristics between comparison groups in an effort to reduce confounding. Accordingly, it has been suggested that future studies on delayed neuropsychiatric syndromes after CO intoxication control for potential confounding from depression and cyanide exposure.[25] Randomization is an important method to assure that unsuspected confounding factors are equally distributed between treatment groups within interventional studies. During data analysis, confounding can often be controlled through stratification of data into subgroups or through multivariate analysis techniques.

BIASES INHERENT IN STUDIES USING THE AAPCC DATABASE

The Toxic Exposures Surveillance System database of the American Association of Poison Control Centers (AAPCC) is an ambitious effort to catalog and describe the epidemiology of poisoning

in the United States and Canada. These data serve to help identify new poisoning epidemics, focus prevention and education efforts, guide demographic and economic poisoning analyses, and guide implementation of public health policies. It is a desirable goal to use this database in defining the scope of toxicity for particular poisons and as a clinical research tool. In this regard, it is important to understand the biases inherent in the current database.

It has been suggested that selection bias might exist within poison center data if poisoning is unrecognized as a cause of illness or if a caregiver has no questions pertaining to the management of a recognized poisoning.[16] Indeed, a survey of 170 emergency physicians in Utah found that 53% admitted to utilizing a poison center for symptomatic acute overdoses, and only 10% contacted poison centers for the purposes of reporting cases to the national database.[8] Such selection might result in a bias of poison center data toward more severe cases. On the other end of the spectrum, investigation has found selection bias in poison center data suggesting that fatal poisonings may be severely underrepresented.[19] Another study of poison center utilization found that one emergency department reported 95% of cyclic antidepressant overdoses, 33% of venomous snakebites, and only 3% of inhalation exposures.[17]

Knowledge of information bias within TESS data is less well characterized. Phone interviews of callers, many under duress, by poison center personnel is certain to be subject to recall and interviewer bias. A comparison of rural hospital chart data to the TESS database demonstrated deficiencies in poison center reporting and in clinical information transfer to the TESS database.[20] Loss to followup remains a problem for many poison centers, and misclassification of poisonings by caregivers inadequately trained in diagnostic toxicology remains an enigma.

Despite the large volume of descriptive poisoning data available, it has proven difficult to derive valid, clinically useful conclusions from either the TESS database or from published case reports.[5] One suggested means through which to minimize information bias in descriptive toxicology is through the use of improved data collection charts.[6] Other researchers have found it useful in clinical studies to transform poison center data collection from a passive to an active process through use of specific research instruments.[27] Further efforts are required to reduce and to quantify the impact of selection, interviewer, recall, misclassification, and information biases within poison center data to optimize the value of this important resource.

EVIDENTIARY CRITERIA USED TO LINK CAUSE AND EFFECT

As was illustrated in Table 120–5, association of an exposure to an illness does not necessarily equate to cause and effect. In assessing causation it must be determined if bias is present in the selection or measurement of exposure or outcome. If a study is unbiased, the role of chance in the occurrence of the observed association must be explored. If an association is unbiased, unlikely to result from random error, and is not subject to confounding, then assumptions regarding to causation can be derived. Table 120–7 provides a list of evidentiary criteria that are often used to support causation.

Many toxicologists deem clinical trials indicating a lack of benefit from gastric emptying, or indicating a therapeutic benefit

TABLE 120–7. **Criteria Supporting Causation**

Study design	Was the association demonstrated in a well-designed study?
Temporality	Does the cause precede the effect?
Strength	What degree of relative risk was demonstrated in the analysis?
Dose response	Does an increased presence of risk factor correlate to greater or more frequent effect?
Consistency	Does the cause and effect hold true in different studies, locations, and populations?
Plausibility	Is the association in accordance with current scientific knowledge?
Specificity	Does the effect occur without the cause in question, or vice versa?

of hyperbaric oxygen therapy for carbon monoxide intoxication, unconvincing because of the degree of bias present in all relevant published clinical trials. Study design flaws such as bias and confounding are problematic for any epidemiologic study, and after decades of investigation, they still raise skepticism regarding the causative role of salicylate in RS. A wealth of evidence exists to support an etiologic relationship for salicylate with regard to RS. Salicylate administration in the prodromal phase of a viral illness was temporally related to the development of RS. The strength of association, as measured by the odds ratio from case-control studies, was enormous in epidemiologic terms. A study by a US Public Health Service Task Force determined that the adjusted odds ratio for an increased risk for RS if exposed to salicylate in the prodromal illness was 40.[21] Because of the rare nature of RS, this measure approximates that salicylate-exposed individuals were at 40 times greater risk of developing RS than those not exposed to salicylate. Concerns of bias in early analytic studies were addressed in further studies,[10] and the association between salicylate use and RS was consistent in refined analysis. Data from a number of studies suggested a dose-response correlation between salicylate use and RS.[21,37] Finally, the association was consistent throughout different studies performed in different populations. After reviewing the strong epidemiologic evidence linking salicylate use to RS, in 1986 the United States Food and Drug Administration required labeling of aspirin warning of the possible association. Further evidence supporting the results of earlier case-control studies was the observation that the incidence of RS has fallen dramatically in apparent parallel to a decline in salicylate use.[3,14]

However, in clinical toxicology it is virtually impossible to prove causal relationships beyond any doubt. The goal is to build empiric evidence so that associations can be confirmed or refuted with conviction. To some physicians the link between salicylate therapy and RS remains a matter of debate. A recent review of 49 cases of diagnosed RS in Australia found that most of the cases were able to be reclassified as other medical conditions such as inborn errors of metabolism.[29] Advances in medical technology, and a lack of absolute diagnostic criteria that could be applied to all possible RS patients, suggest that significant misclassification bias exists in most of the early RS research. Additionally, it has been suggested that antigenic shift within influenza B and varicella viruses may be an uncontrolled confounding variable in RS research.[23] Despite these dissenting views, the overwhelming majority of evidence suggests that the association between salicylate therapy and development of RS is an important one. Of note, aspirin was taken by millions, and yet the peak incidence of RS was

less than 10 cases per million. It remains unsolved whether salicylate use can cause RS in physiologically normal children with viral illness or, perhaps, whether there exists an unidentified metabolic abnormality that may place a specialized population at risk.

EVALUATION OF DIAGNOSTIC TESTS AND CRITERIA

In clinical practice it is often useful to have a test, which may be a laboratory result or clinical paradigm, to help arrive at a diagnosis or predict an outcome. For instance, historical questionnaires, capillary blood lead levels, and venous blood lead levels might all be used to identify children at risk of neurocognitive injury from plumbism.[7] However, each of these approaches is likely to have certain disadvantages in terms of effort, cost, discomfort, and/or accuracy. Targeting lead evaluation and therapy at children on the basis of exposure history is expected to be easy and inexpensive, but may not identify some children with significant poisoning; thus, the test may be susceptible to being falsely negative. Capillary blood testing is more costly and uncomfortable and may be susceptible to false-positive test results because of environmental lead dust present on fingertips. The possibility of false-positive or false-negative results must be considered with any diagnostic test (Fig. 120–4).

The utility of diagnostic testing is often described in terms of sensitivity, specificity, predictive value of a positive test (PPV),

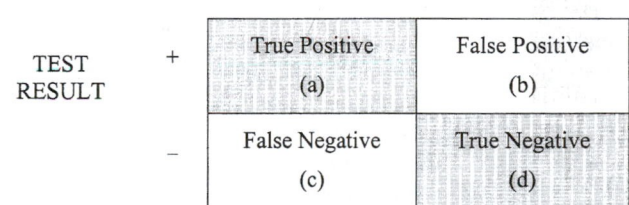

$$\text{Sensitivity} = \frac{a}{a+c} = \frac{\text{True Positives}}{\text{True Positives} + \text{False Negatives}}$$

$$\text{Specificity} = \frac{d}{b+d} = \frac{\text{True Negatives}}{\text{False Positives} + \text{True Negatives}}$$

$$\text{PPV} = \frac{a}{a+b} = \frac{\text{True Positives}}{\text{True Positives} + \text{False Positives}}$$

$$\text{NPV} = \frac{d}{c+d} = \frac{\text{True Negatives}}{\text{False Negatives} + \text{True Negatives}}$$

PPV= Positive predictive value
NPV= Negative predictive value

Figure 120–4. Possible results of diagnostic testing and the statistical characteristics used to describe the utility of diagnostic tests. The letters a, b, c, and d represent the numbers of tested individuals with or without the affliction of interest.

and predictive value of a negative test (NPV). A cross-sectional design is often utilized to study diagnostic tests, as we seek to determine the prevalence of positive tests among the diseased (*sensitivity*), and the prevalence of negative tests among the healthy (*specificity*). A perfect test would be highly sensitive and specific, but this is seldom possible in clinical toxicology. A highly sensitive test is often used in screening programs because they rarely lead to false-negative diagnoses. Specific tests are typically used to "rule-in" a diagnosis, as they rarely yield false-positive results. Whereas sensitivity and specificity are inherent properties of a diagnostic test applied to a given population; the probability of disease, based on the results of a test, is highly dependent on the prevalence of disease within the population being tested. The PPV is the probability of having disease in a patient with a positive test; the NPV is the probability of not having disease when the test result is negative.

A number of studies have tried to examine the utility of vomiting, leukocytosis, hyperglycemia, total iron-binding capacity, and radiographic findings in predicting toxicity after acute iron overdose. In a retrospective assessment of 40 patients with oral iron overdose, vomiting was found to predict a serum iron level above 300 μg/dL with a sensitivity of 84%, specificity of 50%, NPV of 44%, and PPV of 87%.[31] This suggested that the presence of vomiting should raise concern for iron toxicity but that the lack of vomiting was not particularly reassuring. The calculation of the sensitivity, specificity, PPV, and NPV are illustrated in Fig. 120–4. It is important to remember that these calculations, too, are subject to bias and that these calculations are best presented with confidence intervals.

SUMMARY

Clinical toxicology has embraced the vision of incorporating "evidence-based, or literature-based, medicine" into practice. Randomized clinical trials, though a noble goal, are rare and have proven difficult to perform within the discipline. As toxicologists move beyond descriptive data reporting, there remains great potential for scientific advancement in the field of toxicology via observational, hypothesis-testing, clinical research.

Clinical investigators are charged with the imperative to perform studies based on sound epidemiologic principles. All studies, by nature of population sampling, are at the mercy of chance, but such random error can be quantified using statistical techniques. Systematic error (bias) can be limited, but not entirely excluded, through careful study design. Clinicians interpreting published toxicologic research need to thoroughly evaluate a study's research objectives, design, data acquisition, analysis, and conclusions before applying the results to patient care (Table 120–8). Future epidemiologic investigation should allow more valid conclusions to be drawn regarding the associations between exposures and outcomes, or regarding the value of treatments for poisonings, discussed in the preceding chapters of this text.

Galen, an influential physician from the second century, remarked of his clinical trial, "All who drink of this remedy recover in a short time, except those whom it does not help, who all die. Therefore, it is obvious that it fails only in incurable cases." Unfortunately, error in contemporary clinical investigation of poisoning tends to be more insidious than the error in logic in Galen's conclusion, and skillful scrutiny of published research remains an important endeavor.

TABLE 120–8.   Questions to Consider when Evaluating a Study

Research objectives
What is the study question?
What is the studied population?
Study design
What type of study was performed?
How were subjects recruited and enrolled?
Why were subjects excluded?
What was the nature of the comparison group?
Data accrual
How were the data collected?
Are the exposures and outcomes clearly defined?
Are the observations reliable and reproducible?
Was randomization and/or blinding used?
Were subjects lost to followup?
Analysis
Are the results statistically significant?
Are the results clinically significant?
Are potential confounding variables controlled?
Was the study powered to detect important differences?
Conclusions
Are the conclusions justified by data?

ACKNOWLEDGMENTS

The author is grateful to Dennis Durbin, MD, MSCE, for his guidance in the preparation of this chapter. Eddy A. Brenitz, MD, authored this chapter in the previous edition.

REFERENCES

1. Anderson KD, Rouse TM, Randolph JG: A controlled trial of corticosteroids in children with corrosive injury of the esophagus. N Engl J Med 1992;323:637–640.
2. Arrowsmith JB, Kennedy DL, Kuritsky JN, et al: National pattern of aspirin use and Reye's syndrome reporting, United States, 1980 to 1985. Pediatrics 1987;79:858–863.
3. Belay ED, Bresee JS, Holman RC, et al: Reye's syndrome in the United States from 1981 through 1997. N Engl J Med 1999;340:1377–1382.
4. Brody DJ, Pirkle JL, Kramer RA, et al: Blood lead levels in the US population: Phase 1 of the third Health and Nutrition Examination Survey (NHANES III, 1988–1991). JAMA 1994;272:277–283.
5. Buckley NA, Smith AJ: Evidence based medicine in toxicology: Where is the evidence? Lancet 1996;347:1167–1169.
6. Buckley NA, Whyte IM, Dawson AH, et al: Preformatted admission charts for poisoning admissions facilitate clinical assessment and research. Ann Emerg Med 1999;34:476–482.
7. Campbell C, Osterhoudt KC: Prevention of childhood lead poisoning. Curr Opin Pediatr 2000;12:428–437.
8. Caravati EM, McElwee NE: Use of clinical toxicology resources by emergency physicians and its impact on poison control centers. Ann Emerg Med 1991;20:147–150.
9. Ducasse JL, Celsis P, Marc-Vergnes JP: Non-comatose patients with acute carbon monoxide poisoning: Hyperbaric or normobaric oxygen. Undersea Hyperbar Med 1995;22:9–15.
10. Forsyth BW, Horwitz RI, Acampora D, et al: New epidemiologic evidence confirming that bias does not explain the aspirin/Reye's syndrome association. JAMA 1989;261:2517–2524.
11. Freund KM, Belanger AJ, D'Agostino RB, et al: The health risks of smoking. The Framingham Study: 34 years of follow-up. Ann Epidemiol 1993;3:417–424.

12. Gaudreault P, Parent M, McGuigan MA, et al: Predictability of esophageal injury from signs and symptoms: a study of caustic ingestion in 378 children. Pediatrics 1983;71:767–770.

13. Giles HM: Encephalopathy and fatty degeneration of the viscera. Lancet 1965;1:1075.

14. Hall SM, Lynn R: Reye's syndrome [letter]. N Engl J Med 1999; 341:845.

15. Halpin TJ, Holtzhauer FJ, Campbell RJ, et al: Reye's Syndrome and Medication Use. JAMA 1982;248: 687–691.

16. Hamilton RJ, Goldfrank LR: Poison center data and the Pollyanna phenomenon. J Toxicol Clin Toxicol 1998;35:21–23.

17. Harchelroad F, Clark RF, Dean B, et al: Treated vs. reported toxic exposures: discrepancies between a poison control center and a member hospital. Vet Hum Toxicol 1990;32:156–159.

18. Honein MA, Paulozzi LJ, Himelright IM, et al: Infantile hypertrophic pyloric stenosis after pertussis prophylaxis with erythromycin; a case review and cohort study. Lancet 1999;354:2101–2105.

19. Hoppe-Roberts JM, Lloyd LM, Chyka P: Poisoning mortality in the United States: Comparison of national mortality statistics and poison control center reports. Ann Emerg Med 2000;35:440–448.

20. Hoyt BT, Rasmussen R, Giffin S, et al: Poison center data accuracy: A comparison of rural hospital chart data with TESS database. Acad Emerg Med 1999;6:851–855.

21. Hurwitz ES, Barret MJ, Bregman D, et al: Public health service study of Reye's syndrome and medications: Report of the main study. N Engl J Med 1987;257:1905–1911.

22. Johnson GM, Scurletis TD, Carrol NB: A study of sixteen fatal cases of encephalitis-like disease in North Carolina children. NC Med J 1963;24:464–473.

23. Johnson GM: Reye's syndrome [letter]: N Engl J Med 1999;341:846.

24. Litovitz TL, Klein-Schwartz W, White S, et al: 1999 Annual Report of the American Association of Poison Control Centers Toxic Exposures Surveillance System. Am J Emerg Med 2000;18:517–574.

25. Martin JD, Osterhoudt KC, Thom SR: Recognition and management of carbon monoxide poisoning in children. Clin Pediatr Emerg Med 2000;1:244–250.

26. Mathieu D, Wattel F, Mathieu-Nolf M, et al: Randomized prospective study comparing the effect of HBO versus 12 hours NBO in non-comatose CO poisoned patients. Undersea Hyperbar Med [Suppl] 1996; 23:7.

27. McFee RB, Caraccio TR, Mofensen HC: The granny syndrome and medication access as significant causes of unintentional pediatric poisoning [abstract]. J Toxicol Clin Toxicol 1999;37:593.

28. Olson KR, Seger D: Hyperbaric oxygen for carbon monoxide poisoning: does it really work? Ann Emerg Med 1995;25:535–537.

29. Orlowski JP: Whatever happened to Reye's syndrome? Did it ever really exist? Crit Care Med 1999;27:1582–1587.

30. Osterhoudt KC, Henretig FM: How much confidence that calcium channel blockers are safe? [letter] Vet Hum Toxicol 1998;40:239.

31. Palatnick W, Tenenbein M: Leukocytosis, hyperglycemia, vomiting, and positive x-rays are not indications of severe iron overdose in adults. Am J Emerg Med 1996;14:454–455.

32. Pond SM, Lewis-Driver DJ, Williams GM, et al: Gastric emptying in acute overdose: A prospective randomised controlled trial. Med J Aust 1995;163:345–349.

33. Raphael JC, Elkharrat D, Jars-Guineestre MC, et al: Trial of normobaric and hyperbaric oxygen for acute carbon monoxide intoxication. Lancet 1989;2:414–419.

34. Reye RDK, Morgan G, Baral J: Encephalopathy and fatty degeneration of the viscera: A disease entity in childhood. Lancet 1963; 2:749–752.

35. San Filippo JA: Infantile hypertrophic pyloric stenosis related to ingestion of erythomycin estolate: a report of five cases. J Pediatr Surg 1976;11:177–180.

36. Scheinkestel CD, Bailey M, Myles PS, et al: Hyperbaric or normobaric oxygen for acute carbon monoxide poisoning: A randomised controlled clinical trial. Med J Aust 1999;170:203–210.

37. Starko KM, Ray CG, Dominguez LB, et al: Reye's syndrome and salicylate use. Pediatrics 1980;66:859–864.

38. Tenenbein M: Good reasons to publish in Clinical Toxicology. J Toxicol Clin Toxicol 1998;36:137–138.

39. Thom SR, Taber RL, Mendiguren II, et al: Delayed neuropsychologic sequelae after carbon monoxide poisoning: Prevention by treatment with hyperbaric oxygen. Ann Emerg Med 1995;25:474–480.

40. Waldman RJ, Hall WN, McGee H, et al: Aspirin as a risk factor in Reye's syndrome. JAMA 1982;247:3089–3094.

STUDY GUIDE: CASE STUDIES FROM THE TOXICOLOGY CONSULTATION SERVICE

CASE STUDIES WITH QUESTIONS

Case 1

A 28-year-old man presented to the hospital complaining of uncontrollable twitching of his extremities. He had a long history of uncomplicated intranasal heroin use and denied intravenous (IV) drug use, other substance abuse, or medical or surgical problems. He noted that he had recently changed his supplier of heroin. On examination he was found to be well developed, well nourished, and obviously uncomfortable. His vital signs were: blood pressure, 138/84 mm Hg; pulse, 110 beats/min; respiratory rate, 24 breaths/min; and rectal temperature, 99°F (37.2°C). Physical examination was normal except for the neurologic assessment. He was awake, alert, and fully oriented. His limbs showed irregular and bilateral spontaneous contractions, and their activity increased while he was examined. His mental status remained unchanged during these movements. Strength and sensation were within normal limits, and reflexes were brisk. Chvostek and Trousseau signs were negative.

The patient was attached to a cardiac monitor, and an IV line was inserted. Blood was sent for a complete blood count (CBC), serum electrolytes, glucose, calcium, magnesium, and creatine phosphokinase. A urinalysis was also requested. An electrocardiogram (ECG) showed a normal sinus rhythm with normal axis and intervals and a motion artifact.

1. What is the differential diagnosis of this patient's disorder?
2. What is the most likely toxin?
3. How are the clinical effects of this toxin manifested?
4. How should the patient with this clinical presentation be evaluated and treated?

Case 2

A 39-year-old man presented to the hospital complaining of feeling weak and tired and noted that his skin and eyes had turned yellow. He had a history of hepatitis B and alcohol abuse but was otherwise well until about 7 months earlier, when he was found to be Purified Protein Derivative-positive and to have an abnormal chest radiograph. At that time he was started on isoniazid, rifampin, and pyrazinamide for what was presumed to be active tuberculosis. About 4 weeks before presentation he began to notice a change in skin color and stopped his medications. He presented to the emergency department (ED) with worsening symptoms and progressive weakness.

Physical examination was notable for scleral and dermal icterus, lethargy with intact orientation, and asterixis. Laboratory analysis showed an aspartate aminotransferase (AST) and alanine aminotransferase (ALT) of 166 and 518 IU/L, respectively, a total bilirubin of 21 mg/dL, a prothrombin time (PT) of 21.7 seconds, and a glucose of 62 mg/dL. He was admitted to the hospital with a diagnosis of hepatic failure with an encephalopathy. His treatment consisted of lactulose, dextrose infusion, dietary control, and N-acetylcysteine. Despite aggressive care, his bilirubin continued to rise, his coagulopathy worsened, and his mental status deteriorated. The patient was evaluated for possible liver transplantation but was thought to be a poor candidate because of his history of alcoholism and the fact that he was positive for hepatitis B surface antigen. The patient died. His postmortem evaluation was thought to be consistent with fulminant isoniazid (INH) hepatotoxicity in the presence of alcoholic and viral liver disease (Fig. CS–1).

1. What is the incidence of INH hepatitis? What are the risk factors?
2. Is the metabolism of INH related to the risk of hepatotoxicity?
3. Can toxin-induced hepatitis be differentiated from viral and other causes of hepatic injury?
4. Why did this patient receive N-acetylcysteine?
5. How frequently should patients receiving INH be evaluated to prevent severe hepatotoxicity?

Case 3

A 16-year-old girl with a history of epilepsy who had recently become pregnant ingested a large quantity of unknown medications in a suicide attempt. She was brought to the hospital in status epilepticus. Although the patient was given a benzodiazepine, she continued to seize. A 15 mg/kg loading dose of phenytoin was given, but intermittent seizures persisted. A continuous infusion of a short-acting barbiturate was initiated, and her motor activity normalized. A bedside electroencephalogram (EEG) revealed electrical evidence of seizure activity, although no overt motor activity was noted concomitantly. Hypotension developed over a period of several hours and continued despite the administration of vasopressor agents. The patient died.

1. What is the differential diagnosis of drug-induced seizures?
2. What is the mechanism by which this particular toxin produces status epilepticus?
3. How should the patient in this case have been managed?
4. What antidotes, if any, should be used in the management of a patient with status epilepticus?

Case 4

A 20-month-old girl unintentionally ingested an unknown amount of a home hair permanent product. She presented to the ED with several episodes of vomiting. Physical examination revealed a child in apparent good health; she was crying and intermittently vomiting. Vital signs were normal, as was the remainder of the examination. The patient had no oropharyngeal lesions on direct inspection.

An IV line was inserted, and the patient received a 10 mL/kg bolus of 0.9% sodium chloride solution followed by a mainte-

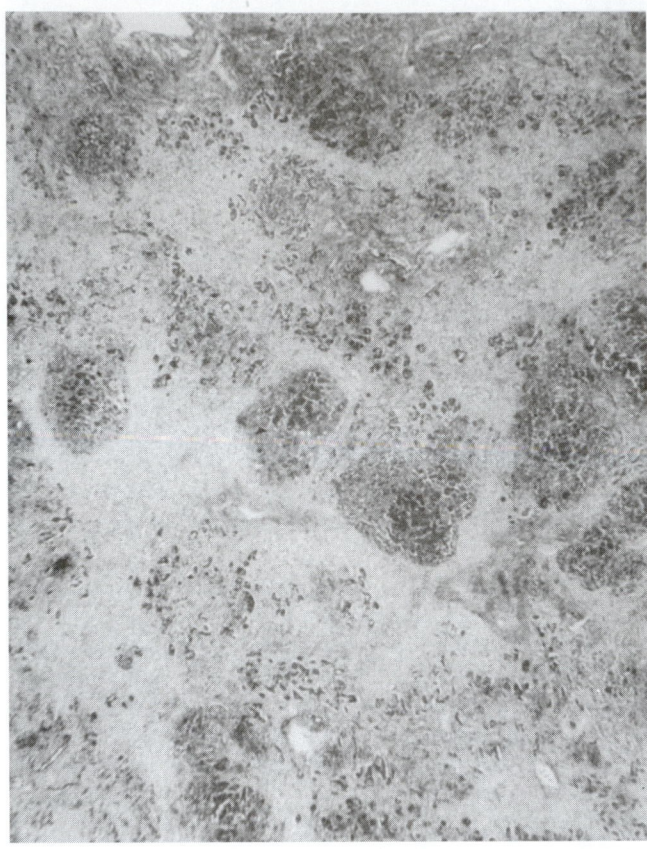

Figure CS–1 Postmortem histology of the patient's liver demonstrating fulminant hepatic failure with a nearly complete loss of hepatic architecture. Additional evidence for alcoholic liver disease and chronic viral hepatitis was noted.

nance infusion. A CBC and serum electrolytes were sent and later returned as normal. Chest and abdominal radiographs were unremarkable. Her vomiting stopped, and she was able to eat and drink normally. Although fluid resuscitation was given, her creatinine rose from 0.6 to 1.2 mg/dL on the second day and to 1.9 mg/dL on day 3. No other abnormalities were noted.

1. What agents are commonly found in hair care products?
2. What are the toxicities of these agents?
3. Is any other therapy required? Are there any specific antidotes?

Case 5

A 26-year-old woman received an anonymous box of candy in the mail. She ate a single piece, gave another piece to a friend, and two other people shared a third piece of candy. Within the first 24 hours of the ingestion, two patients experienced some gastrointestinal upset and had a few loose bowel movements, one patient noted constipation, and the other patient had no gastrointestinal complaints. All four patients noted pleuritic chest pain. At about 24 hours after ingestion all four patients developed numbness of the hands and feet, which progressed in severity over the next day such that the painful paresthesias limited walking in two patients. These symptoms were most pronounced in the two patients who ingested whole candies. Their pain became so severe as to confine

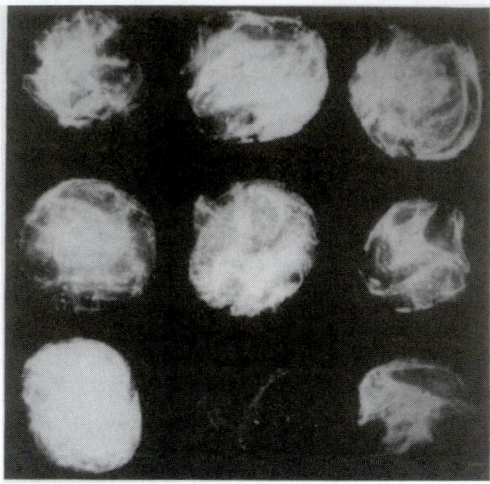

Figure CS–2 Radiographs of the remaining 9 of 12 candies revealed their heavy-metal content. The lack of uniform distribution of radiopaque material was highly suggestive of a handmade preparation. (Courtesy of the Medical Toxicology Fellowship of the New York City Poison Control Center.)

them to strict bed rest, requiring continuous infusion of morphine for pain control. Physical examination and laboratory evaluation, including CBC and differential, electrolytes, blood, urea, nitrogen (BUN), and glucose, were all unremarkable. Urinalysis showed trace proteinuria in the two most severely ill patients. The ECG demonstrated a sinus tachycardia with U waves and nonspecific T-wave morphology. Because of the atypical nature of both the patient's complaints and the candies (e.g. their weight and shape) a radiograph was obtained (Fig. CS-2). On the fifth day after ingestion, hypertension and tachycardia developed in the two more severely affected patients. Hair loss was noted on the sixth day and progressed to total alopecia during the second to third week.

1. What is the differential diagnosis of this illness, and what clinical findings suggest a specific toxin?
2. How does this toxin produce its toxicity?
3. What are the clinical stages of this poisoning?
4. Once considered, how is the diagnosis confirmed?
5. What are the treatment options for this poisoning?

Case 6

A 25-year-old presented to the ED complaining of a pruritic rash most prominent on his arms and legs. The patient knew of no allergies and had never had a similar rash. The rash began earlier in the day and was not associated with the introduction of any new medications, soaps, or foods. The patient stated that he had just returned from a two-day family camping trip during which time he went swimming in a lake. Examination of the rash revealed linear vesicles on an erythematous and mildly edematous base with marked excoriation. The rash was most prominent on his distal upper and lower extremities but was also present on his left neck and left buttock.

1. What is the differential diagnosis of this patient's rash?
2. What is phytophotodermatitis?
3. What is allergic contact dermatitis?
4. What is the therapy?

Case 7

A 79-year-old man was brought to the hospital complaining of malaise, anorexia, nausea, urinary frequency, shortness of breath, and worsening lethargy, all of 5 days' duration. He had a history of coronary artery disease and diabetes mellitus and was being treated with a β-adrenergic antagonist, a diuretic, a nitrate, and an oral hypoglycemic agent. The patient was well until about 1 week before the hospitalization, when he developed the onset of a cough and sore throat. A private physician was consulted, and an antibiotic was prescribed, but the patient never took the medicine.

The patient was ill-appearing and in obvious discomfort. His vital signs were: blood pressure, 90/50 mm Hg; pulse, 44 beats/min; respiration, deep at 26 breaths/min; and temperature, 94°F (34.4°C). The only positive findings on examination included right upper quadrant tenderness with guarding, decreased bowel sounds, and stool that tested trace positive for occult blood.

Laboratory data were as follows: ABG on a nasal cannula at 2 L/min; pH, 7.04; P_{CO_2}, 15 mm Hg; P_{O_2}, 115 mm Hg. The sodium was 132 mEq/L; potassium, 7.8 mEq/L; chloride, 91 mEq/L; bicarbonate, 6 mEq/L; BUN, 116 mg/dL; creatinine, 4.9 mg/dL; and glucose, 193 mg/dL. Urine analysis was trace positive for ketones, but without glucose.

Adjunctive laboratory studies were performed. A urine ferric chloride test was negative, and no urinary crystals or fluorescence was noted. Similarly, the serum calcium was normal. A serum lactate was determined to be 10.7 mEq/L. A repeat lactate concentration, drawn about 1 hour later, was 17.2 mEq/L.

Because of the abdominal pain, guaiac-positive stools, hypotension, and lactic acidosis in an elderly diabetic, the diagnosis of ischemic bowel was considered. A minilaparotomy was performed, and a visual inspection of the bowel as well as chemical analysis of the peritoneal fluid were thought to be normal.

1. What are the acid–base abnormalities?
2. What is the differential diagnosis?
3. How can the differential diagnosis be narrowed clinically?
4. What therapy is required?

Case 8

A 22-year-old man ate pizza and presented to the emergency department with tonic-clonic movements of all of his extremities that were described by the primary care provider as status epilepticus. The patient was awake throughout these periods. Initial vital signs were: blood pressure, 130/80 mm Hg; pulse, 105 beats/min; respirations, 20/min; rectal temperature 102.5°F (39.2°C). Physical examination was notable for pupils that were 4 mm in size, equal, round, and reactive to light. Skin was diaphoretic. Auscultation of the chest, heart, and abdomen was normal. Neurologic examination revealed an anxious man who was oriented to time, place, and person. Coarse uncontrollable movements of all extremities were noted. Reflexes were brisk and symmetric, and plantar flexion was present. The patient was treated with diazepam, phenobarbital, and phenytoin, after which he was noted to be stuporous, but with normal muscle tone. The only history available from friends was that the patient had had a "cold" recently.

1. What is the differential diagnosis of tonic-clonic movements in a patient with a normal mental status?

2. What is the experimental and physiologic basis for this patient's movement disorder?
3. What therapies are indicated for this patient?

Case 9

A 91-year-old woman with a history of glaucoma treated with acetazolamide and atrial fibrillation controlled with digoxin complained of chest pain, left-sided headache, and palpitations during dinner. Later that night, the family noted that she was confused and called an ambulance. On arrival at the hospital the patient was found to be lethargic and disoriented and afebrile. Her vital signs were: blood pressure, 128/78 mm Hg; pulse, 110 beats/min and irregular; respiratory rate, 20 breaths/min. She was noted to be diaphoretic and to have a right-sided facial droop, right-sided hemiparesis, and bilateral plantar extension.

1. What emergent therapy is required?
2. What are the risks of failing to identify this clinical problem?
3. How are these patients best managed?

Case 10

A 5-week-old child was admitted to the hospital for evaluation of neonatal sepsis. Following blood and urine cultures and a lumbar puncture, the child was started on an antibiotic regimen that included intravenous gentamicin. The child inadvertently received 10 times the recommended dose of IV gentamicin.

1. What are the most common calculation errors that occur in neonates?
2. How can these errors be prevented?
3. What toxicity can be expected from this error?
4. Are any special treatments indicated for patients with aminoglycoside toxicity?

Case 11

A 42-year-old woman with a history of IV drug use was admitted to the hospital with seizures and coma secondary to end-stage renal failure. Her admission laboratory studies were remarkable for a BUN of 140 mg/dL; creatinine, 10.8 mg/dL; potassium, 7.9 mEq/L; and bicarbonate, 4 mEq/L. ECG demonstrated severe hyperkalemic changes (Fig. CS–3). Immediate therapy consisted of intravenous calcium, insulin and dextrose, and sodium bicarbonate. The patient was intubated and given diazepam for her seizures. Peritoneal dialysis (PD) was begun because of poor vascular access.

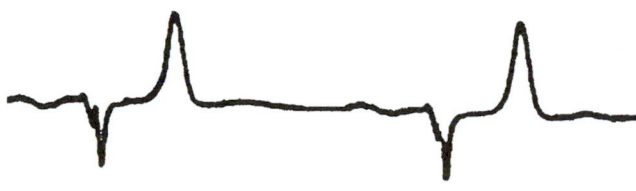

Figure CS–3 Electrocardiographic (ECG) findings of hyperkalemia. The initial ECG shows tall peaked T waves, a prolonged QRS complex, ST segment depression, a prolonged PR interval, and flattening of the P wave. As toxicity progresses, the P wave is lost, and the QRS complex widens. Ultimately, a sine-wave pattern can develop.

After 24 to 48 hours of PD she was extubated as her electrolyte status began to improve (BUN, 98 mg/dL; creatinine, 6.1 mg/dL; potassium, 4.0 mEq/L). Inadvertently, she was then dialyzed with 2 L of Uromatic (an irrigation solution containing 1.5 g of glycine/100 mL, used for urologic procedures) instead of standard PD solution. Subsequently, the patient had several more seizures, which were controlled with diazepam.

1. What toxicity would be expected from this agent?
2. What therapy is required?

Case 12

A 10-year-old boy suffered a midshaft femur fracture. Before external fixation he was given 30 mL of 2% lidocaine for a femoral block and another 10 mL with epinephrine subcutaneously for insertion of a tibial pin. He weighed 30 kg. Within 20 to 25 minutes he developed seizures, which did not respond to intravenous diazepam (5 mg) or to intravenous lorazepam (5 mg). General anesthesia was induced with IV methohexital, and the child was intubated. During induction of anesthesia the seizures stopped. The child subsequently had a transient episode of hypotension that responded rapidly to a fluid challenge. His ECG was within normal limits. Over the course of the next several hours he began to have spontaneous movements, then withdrew to pain, and slowly regained a normal mental status. The boy was extubated about 8 hours later and had a complete neurologic recovery.

1. What is the differential diagnosis?
2. What are the clinical consequences of this type of poisoning?
3. What is the treatment of this poisoning?
4. Is there a role in this case for the laboratory determination of serum drug levels?

Case 13

A 40-year-old man was found unresponsive in his car. The paramedics noted that he was apneic, with a sweet smell on his breath, as they intubated him. When he arrived in the ED the patient was hypotensive with a palpable blood pressure of 80 mm Hg and a tachycardia of 140 beats/min, with no spontaneous respirations and a rectal temperature of 97.6°F (36.4°C). His pupils were dilated to 6 mm and were sluggishly reactive to light. Neurologic examination showed deep coma with intact corneal reflexes.

The blood pressure failed to respond to an IV bolus of fluid, and the patient was started on dopamine. Almost immediately after the dopamine infusion was started he had a run of ventricular tachycardia (Fig. CS–4) that responded to electrical cardioversion. The rate of his dopamine drip was reduced. Following 2 to 3 hours of fluid resuscitation, his blood pressure returned to normal, and the dopamine infusion was discontinued. Eighteen hours later he was awake and alert. Abnormal liver enzymes were noted.

1. Do these findings suggest an overdose? If so, of what?
2. What are the mechanisms responsible for the cardiovascular and hepatic toxicities in this patient?
3. What tests could help confirm the diagnosis?
4. What specific treatment issues should be considered?

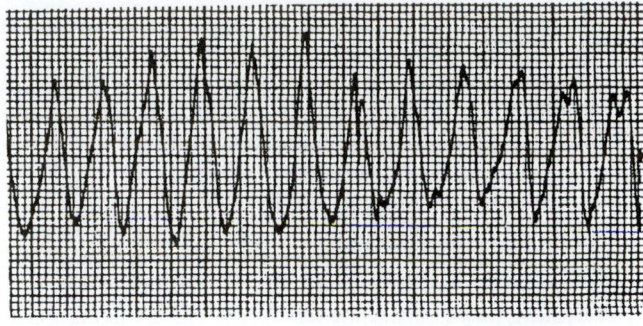

Figure CS–4 Rhythm strip from the patient demonstrating a regular wide-complex dysrhythmia felt to be consistent with ventricular tachycardia.

Case 14

A 62-year-old Asian man was bitten on the thumb by an unknown animal while playing Frisbee on a cool October morning in Central Park (New York City). He presented to the ED 2 hours later complaining of pain and swelling of his hand. The patient's entire hand and distal forearm were swollen, tender, tense, and warm. He had pain on passive extension of his fingers, normal sensation in his fingers, and both an adequate radial pulse and capillary refill. There were two "fang" marks noted at the bite site, both of which oozed serosanguineous fluid. Two hours later, the swelling progressed to his shoulder.

1. Is this patient's history consistent with the available epidemiologic data?
2. What are the complications of snake envenomation?
3. How should the patient be assessed for a compartment syndrome?

Case 15

An 84-year-old woman made a stew with milkweed (*Asclepias speciosa*) and presented to the hospital with vomiting. After questioning she noted that the milkweed appeared to differ from the usual plants she ate. Her vital signs were: blood pressure, 160/70 mm Hg; pulse, 80 beats/min; respiratory rate, 14 breaths/min; and temperature, 98°F (36.7°C). The remainder of her physical examination was unremarkable. CBC, serum electrolytes, BUN, and glucose were all within normal limits, and an ECG showed normal sinus rhythm with normal intervals.

The initial impression was that the patient had ingested a gastrointestinal irritant or was suffering from bacterial food poisoning. Intravenous rehydration was initiated, and the patient was given a dose of 60 g of oral activated charcoal. She vomited several more times. Over the next 12 hours she developed first-degree heart block (PR interval of 0.26 seconds) and a bradycardia of 50 beats/min, which fell to 20 beats/min during emesis.

1. What group of toxins is the most likely cause of this patient's poisoning?
2. What are the clinical manifestations produced by these poisons?
3. Are any routine laboratory tests useful to assist with this diagnosis?

4. What other evaluations will assist in establishing this diagnosis?
5. What treatment is indicated?

Case 16

An 18-year-old healthy female student who was taking part in a physiology laboratory experiment ingested about 1 L of a "buffered saline solution." Immediately thereafter she complained of headache and nausea and had a syncopal episode. Emergency medical services was contacted, and the patient was brought to the ED. On arrival, her vital signs were: blood pressure, 150/90 mm Hg; pulse, 110 beats/min; respiratory rate, 22 breaths/min; and rectal temperature, 98.6°F (37.0°C). Her physical examination was reported as unremarkable. She was evaluated for syncope, given the diagnosis of psychosomatic illness, and discharged. Twenty-four hours later she presented to a second hospital complaining of shortness of breath and was found to have congestive heart failure. She was transferred to the intensive care unit of a third institution and died 12 hours later.

1. What substances are commonly available in laboratories that could cause these symptoms?
2. By what mechanism does the implicated toxin produce its toxicity?
3. What therapy is required?
4. Are there any special risks to the medical personnel caring for the patient?

Case 17

A 49-year-old woman was referred to the ED by her private physician for evaluation of abnormal laboratory findings. The patient was recently diagnosed with gout after having presented with pain in her left great toe. At that time she was given colchicine, with total relief of her symptoms. On return home, her physician obtained the following laboratory studies: uric acid, 18 mg/dL; BUN, 100 mg/dL; creatinine, 2.8 mg/dL; and serum bicarbonate, 34 mEq/L. Her physician told her to stop the colchicine, drink water, and go to the hospital.

In the ED, the woman was described as thin, in no distress, and appearing slightly dehydrated. Her mouth and mucous membranes were dry. Her vital signs were: blood pressure, 114/70 mm Hg; pulse, 64 beats/min; respiration, 18 breaths/min; and rectal temperature, 98.0°F (36.7°C). With orthostatic testing her blood pressure fell to 100/60 mm Hg, and her pulse rose to 88 beats/min.

1. What is the acid–base abnormality, and what are the most common causes?
2. What toxins cause gout or arthritic symptoms?
3. What other adverse effects are associated with this class of toxin?
4. What therapy is required?

Case 18

A 45-year-old woman presented to the hospital complaining of persistent right great toe pain, abdominal pain, malaise, nausea, vomiting, and 25 episodes of diarrhea over the previous day. She had a history of gout, for which she had been given colchicine (0.6 mg) in the past with relief. Beginning almost 3 days before presentation, she began to take her colchicine for recurrent great toe pain. She took two tablets every 1 to 2 hours for a total of 50 to 60 mg, without relief. On presentation she was concerned that she was having so much abdominal discomfort that she was unable to take her colchicine. Her past medical history was remarkable for asthma, gout, hypertension, and renal insufficiency.

Her vital signs were: blood pressure, 170/80 mm Hg; pulse, 86 beats/min; respirations, 12 breaths/min; and temperature, 100.4°F (38.0°C). There were no orthostatic changes in her vital signs. The remainder of the examination was unremarkable.

1. What is colchicine, and why is it used?
2. What are the signs and symptoms of colchicine toxicity?
3. What immediate therapy is required? 4. What other therapies are available or under investigation?

Case 19

A 27-year-old man was found unresponsive at the international airport. When emergency medical services arrived, they found a well-developed man in respiratory distress. His vital signs were: blood pressure, 90 mm Hg by palpation; pulse, 78 beats/min; and respirations, 4 breaths/min. His skin was cool and moist, and his pupils were pinpoint.

The medics administered high-flow oxygen, started an IV line, and gave 2 mg of naloxone, 50 g of dextrose, and 100 mg of thiamine IV with a transient response. Another 2 mg of naloxone was given IV en route to the hospital, again with some improvement in mental status and respirations. On arrival at the ED the patient was lethargic but arousable to deep stimulation. His vital signs were: blood pressure, 110/70 mm Hg; pulse, 84 beats/min; respiratory rate, 6 breaths/min; and rectal temperature, 97.0°F (36.1°C). A pulse oximeter read 100% saturation on high-flow oxygen. His skin was cool, and the only abnormal finding on physical examination was the persistence of pinpoint pupils.

1. What happened?
2. What immediate diagnostic and therapeutic interventions are required?
3. How can the diagnosis be established?
4. What is the role of gastrointestinal decontamination?

Case 20

A 49-year-old unresponsive woman was brought to the ED. She had been smoking crack cocaine the day before admission. When her mother found her disoriented and having profuse diarrhea, she called an ambulance.

On arrival in the ED the woman was unresponsive, with no palpable blood pressure or pulse, spontaneous respirations of 8 breaths/min, and a rectal temperature of 99.0°F (37.2°C). She was immediately intubated, given 100% oxygen, and placed on a cardiac monitor, which showed a sinus tachycardia at 140 beats/min. Two large-bore IV lines were inserted, and lactated Ringer's solution was infused wide open. After several liters of fluid her blood pressure rose to 100 mm Hg by palpation.

After resuscitation she regained her mental status and complained of diffuse abdominal pain. Physical examination was notable for a distended abdomen with decreased bowel sounds and stool that was positive for occult blood. Radiographs demonstrated dilated loops of bowel.

1. What are the gastrointestinal manifestations of cocaine use?
2. What therapy is required?
3. What other toxins are associated with bowel ischemia or infarction?

Case 21

A 47-year-old man with a history of schizophrenia presented to the emergency department complaining of thirst. On examination he was noted to be diaphoretic, tachycardic (120 beats/min), tachypneic (28 breaths/min) with hyperpnea, with a temperature of 100.3°F (37.9°C) and a blood pressure of 100/80 mm Hg. When asked about medication use, the patient stated that he has been taking several aspirin tablets per day for the last several days.

1. What is the differential diagnosis?
2. What toxicologic syndrome is present?
3. What diagnostic tests are useful?
4. What therapy is indicated?

Case 22

A 60-year-old woman with a history of inflammatory bowel disease, lower gastrointestinal bleeding, and multiple lower extremity deep venous thromboses was admitted to the hospital with increased swelling of her right leg. A computed tomography (CT) scan showed a clot extending above her Greenfield filter. A second filter was inserted, and the patient was started on warfarin. A few days later, a large lesion was noted on her thigh and was said to resemble a burn. Later the lesion became necrotic and required extensive debridement.

1. What is the mechanism of action of warfarin?
2. What is the purple toe syndrome?
3. What is the skin lesion?

Case 23

A 36-year-old man came to the hospital complaining of eye pain and blurry vision after an unintentional splash of hydrofluoric acid (HF) into his right eye while at work. The patient was a healthy man who was employed by a construction company. His job was to clean the rust from some equipment. Although he knew he was supposed to wear safety glasses, an apron, and gloves while working with the acid, he was in a hurry and forgot his glasses. Immediately after the event, he flushed his eye for 20 minutes with tepid water. The pain persisted, and when he noted difficulty seeing, he came to the hospital. He denied any other exposure to HF.

Physical examination revealed an uncomfortable man with normal vital signs. Visual acuity was 20/20 in his left eye but only 20/100 in his right eye. His right lid was slightly reddened and swollen, there was a moderate degree of blepharospasm, and his conjunctivae were injected but without chemosis. A topical anesthetic was administered to allow a more complete examination. When his pain and spasm resolved, a slit lamp examination was performed and demonstrated multiple shallow punctate areas of fluorescein uptake without other abnormalities.

1. What is HF, and what is it used for?
2. What is the treatment for HF burns of the skin?
3. What is the treatment for HF burns of the eye?

Case 24

A 34-year-old recently discharged male Marine officer arrived at the ED via EMS in coma 3 hours after ingesting a bottle of pills and ethanol in a suicide attempt. He was unresponsive, and his vital signs were normal except for a heart rate of 110/min. Physical examination revealed mydriasis, a nonfocal neurologic exam, and absence of an identifiable toxicologic syndrome. His pulse oximeter was 99%, and his fingerstick glucose was 110 mg/dL. Laboratory testing, including serum chemistry and arterial blood gas analysis, was normal except for an ethanol level of 120 mg/dL. An electrocardiogram exhibited sinus tachycardia with a QRS duration of 110 milliseconds. Three hours following admission, the patient fully awakened and stated that he could neither see nor hear, although he seemed only minimally concerned by this predicament. Repeat ocular examination revealed that he had no light perception, and his pupils were 6 to 7 mm in diameter with minimal reactivity to light. Examination of his globe, extraocular movements, and retina were normal; optikokinetic nystagmus was absent. Auditory testing confirmed that he was unable to hear.

1. What are the toxicologic causes of blindness?
2. What are the toxicologic causes of hearing loss?
3. What is the most likely cause in this patient?
4. What therapeutic approach is appropriate?

Case 25a

A 10-year-old boy was brought to the hospital complaining of dysphagia and epigastric pain. He had essentially no past medical history other than a severe pollen allergy. On further review he revealed that he was recently started on Claritin. Physical examination revealed a well-developed boy who was somewhat uncomfortable. Vital signs were remarkable only for a slight tachycardia. Examination of the oropharynx was normal. Endoscopy revealed circular small erosions of his distal esophagus and stomach. The patient was treated with antacids and a clear liquid diet, and his symptoms resolved.

Case 25b

A 56-year-old woman presented to the hospital complaining of the inability to straighten her head, her eyes, and her tongue. She had a history of asthma, for which she normally took an inhaled β-adrenergic agonist alone. She was well until about 1 week earlier, when she was hospitalized for an exacerbation of her asthma. During her admission she received a parenteral antibiotic and corticosteroids. No other medications were given. After 4 days in the hospital, she was discharged on her inhaled β agonist and a prednisone taper.

The emergency department staff recognized that she had a dystonic reaction and gave her 50 mg of diphenhydramine intravenously over about 1 minute. Within 5 minutes all of her symptoms resolved, and she felt well.

1. What do these two cases have in common?
2. How did these atypical reactions occur?
3. Why do these events happen? How can they be prevented?

Case 26

A healthy suburban husband and wife presented to the hospital complaining of severe gastrointestinal distress. The couple and their two children had no significant medical problems and no history of occupational or environmental exposure to toxins. All members of the family were well until the day of admission, when the wife prepared a meal that consisted of some meat and wild mushrooms that she had picked from a neighbor's lawn. Although all four members of the family shared the meal, only the husband and wife ate the mushrooms. Everyone thought that the meal tasted fine and had no complaints until about 5 or 6 hours later, when the husband and wife began to experience nausea and vomiting, followed shortly thereafter by severe watery diarrhea. The children remained asymptomatic. When these symptoms became intolerable, they sought medical care.

On presentation to the hospital, both adults appeared ill and had vomiting and diarrhea. Their vital signs were notable for a resting tachycardia and orthostatic hypotension. They were afebrile and had otherwise normal physical examinations. Intravenous antiemetics were administered and hydration was begun.

1. What is the differential diagnosis for this illness?
2. How is the diagnosis confirmed?
3. What is the pathophysiology of this poisoning?
4. What treatment is indicated?

Case 27

A 41-year-old man with a history of alcohol and Xanax abuse ran out of his Xanax and began medicating himself with a chemical that he had saved from a chemistry laboratory some 20 years earlier. The patient presented to the hospital 1 month later with confusion and hallucinations. His initial vital signs were: blood pressure, 120/70 mm Hg; heart rate, 120 beats/min; respirations, 18 breaths/min; temperature, 98.6°F (37°C). His pupils were small and reactive, his skin was normal and without diaphoresis, and his bowel sounds were normal. Initial laboratory values were reported as: sodium 144 mEq/L, potassium 4.6 mEq/L, chloride "interfering substance," bicarbonate 31 mEq/L, BUN 7 mg/dL, Cr 1.0 mg/dL, Glu 114 mg/dL. The patient was admitted to psychiatry with a diagnosis of psychosis.

During a 3-day admission on psychiatry, the patient's condition deteriorated. He became comatose and required intubation. At that time, his laboratory values were: sodium 144 mEq/L, potassium 4.2 mEq/L, chloride 161 mEq/L, bicarbonate 26 mEq/L, BUN 12 mg/dL, Cr 1.1 mg/dL, Glu 164 mg/dL.

1. What general differential diagnosis should be considered?
2. What is the differential diagnosis of a low or negative anion gap?
3. What is the cause of the patient's dramatically elevated chloride?
4. What is the treatment for this patient?

Case 28

Three male co-workers at a dye manufacturing plant inadvertently mixed two chemicals. One employee, not wearing his respirator, was immediately overcome and collapsed. A second employee removed his respirator to call for help and also succumbed. The third employee fled the area to seek help, leaving his respirator in place. The two collapsed employees were safely evacuated by appropriately protected rescuers. EMS arrived and intubated both patients, who were apneic. A weak carotid pulse of 110 to 120 beats/min was obtained in both patients, and an ECG monitor

recorded a sinus tachycardia en route to the emergency department.

On arrival in the emergency department, the physical examinations of both patients were remarkably similar. Vital signs on one patient revealed a blood pressure of 170/108 mm Hg, heart rate of 120 beats/min, mechanical ventilation on an FIO_2 100% at 24/min, and a temperature of 99°F. Head and neck were atraumatic with 3-mm pupils and pink mucous membranes. Heart and lung examination was significant for clear breath sounds without wheezing or rales. The skin color was normal, without cutaneous burns, and was well perfused. A carboxyhemoglobin level was 4%, and arterial blood gas (ABG) on 100% was pH 7.37; PCO_2, 32 mm Hg; and PO_2, 242 mm Hg. The chest radiograph was negative.

1. What is the differential diagnosis for these patients' symptoms?
2. How does this exposure typically occur?
3. What are the expected clinical effects following exposure to this toxin?
4. What treatment is indicated?

Case 29

A 37-year-old woman ingested 30 sleeping pills in an apparent suicide attempt. She was brought to the emergency department via EMS approximately 1 hour after ingestion. Her initial vital signs were: blood pressure, 130/80 mm Hg; pulse, 100 beats/min; respirations, 12 breaths/min; and she was afebrile. Her physical examination was significant for marked depression of her mental status, normal pupillary function, and normal neurologic findings. As part of the routine evaluation, dextrose (25 g), naloxone (2 mg), and 10 L of vasal oxygen, were given. The patient's mental status continued to deteriorate, and she was intubated for airway protection. Orogastric lavage was performed with a 40-F tube, and activated charcoal was given. A pulse oximeter read 100% saturation, and a cardiac monitor revealed frequent multifocal premature ventricular beats and runs of nonsustained ventricular tachycardia (Fig. CS–5).

1. What sleep-inducing agents are available?
2. What are the clinical manifestations of poisoning by these agents?
3. Is there a role for empiric flumazenil administration?

Case 30

A 40-year-old woman was found unresponsive shortly after locking herself in the bathroom. Her husband found a suicide note and three syringes by her left arm, two of which were empty. EMS was summoned and found a lethargic woman, breathing spontaneously, with blood pressure 110 mm Hg by palpation and heart rate 80 to 90 beats/min. The patient was transported to the hospital along with the syringes. En route, a fingerstick revealed a glucose of 80 mg/dL, and the patient was given 50% dextrose (25 g) and 2 mg naloxone without improvement in her mental status. In the emergency department the patient was noted to be more arousable, with similar vital signs. Physical examination was significant for a slight contusion to her forehead and evidence of tongue biting. Pupils were 4 mm and reactive, and no toxidrome was identified. Her mental status gradually improved and was most consistent with a postictal period. The first electrocardiogram was interpreted as a sinus rhythm at 80 beats/min without evidence of axis devia-

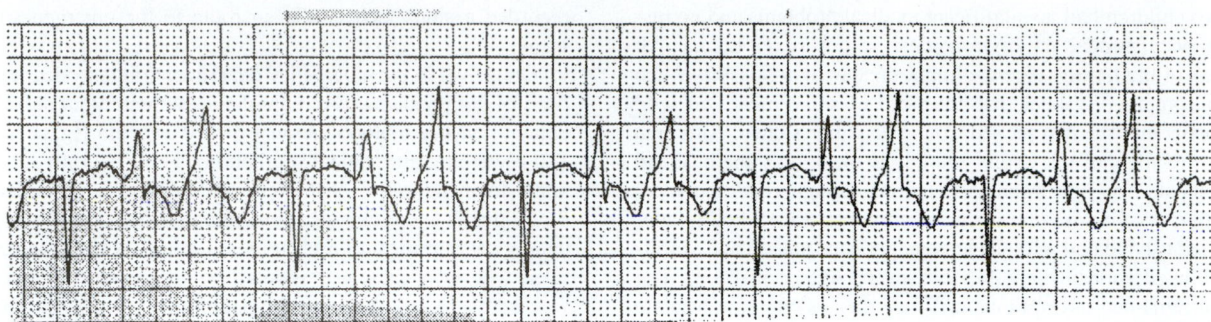

Figure CS–5   A lead II rhythm strip from the patient demonstrating ventricular ectopy of varying morphology. The patient also had short runs of ventricular tachycardia.

tion or widened intervals. Laboratory analysis was significant for an arterial blood gas with a pH of 7.29, P_{CO_2} of 40 mm Hg, and a P_{O_2} of 70 mm Hg, consistent with a metabolic acidosis. Subsequent arterial blood gases revealed rapid resolution of the acidosis. Electrolytes were normal. Serum and urine drug screens were negative for opioids, barbiturates, phencyclidine, aspirin, cyclic antidepressants, and acetaminophen. A serum ethanol level was also negative. The patient's sensorium cleared completely, and she had a normal mental status within a couple of hours; however, she would not elaborate on the substance she injected. The three syringes were sent to the laboratory for analysis.

1. What is the differential diagnosis for this exposure?
2. What are the manifestations of this poisoning?
3. What is the treatment?

Case 31

An 18-year-old man, recently immigrated from the Dominican Republic, presented to the hospital 1 hour after ingesting a granular rodenticide imported from his home country. He stated that the product was unavailable in this country. He complained of mild abdominal pain, appeared uncomfortable, and had vomited at least once. His vital signs were notable for a heart rate of 130 per minute, a normal blood pressure, and a respiratory rate of 30 per minute. On physical examination the patient had moist skin and mucous membranes, and his pupils were 1 mm in diameter. In addition, the patient was slightly lethargic with a normal mental status. The remainder of the neurologic examination was normal. Over the next hour, the patient developed pulmonary edema and required intubation.

1. What is the differential diagnosis of "rat poison" ingestion?
2. How does this type of poison work?
3. What is the treatment for patients poisoned by these agents?

Case 32

A 27-year-old woman who had used a herbal medication for 2 weeks to promote menstruation stopped the herb and sought medical care when she developed nausea, vomiting, and diarrhea. In the emergency department her vital signs were normal, and she was otherwise well. The patient was found to have jaundice, right upper quadrant tenderness, and an AST of 2000 IU, an ALT of 2000 IU, an LDH of 4000 IU, and a PT of 18 seconds. Acetami-

nophen was undetectable in her serum, and her urine pregnancy test was qualitatively positive.

1. What toxins may have caused this patient's hepatotoxicity?
2. Why is the history of herbal medicine important?
3. What herbal medications are used to treat female reproductive problems?

Case 33

A 52-year-old man presented to a Florida hospital emergency department complaining of nausea, vomiting, and leg weakness. The patient was well until 30 minutes after he ate a meal that included two fish he had caught that morning. The fish smelled and tasted normal. Initially he noted nausea, and this was followed shortly by several episodes of emesis and difficulty in standing and walking. His girlfriend, who had eaten a similar meal with the exception of the fish, remained asymptomatic. The patient was very ill-appearing, complaining of extreme fatigue and weakness. His vital signs included a blood pressure of 110/70 mm Hg, a heart rate of 120 beats/min, a respiratory rate of 12 breaths/min and labored, and a temperature of 97.7°F (36.5°C). His physical examination was remarkable for significant motor weakness throughout, including his respiratory muscles. During the first 30 minutes in the department, the patient's blood pressure fell to 85/60 mm Hg, and his respiratory status worsened. He received fluids and was orotracheally intubated, and ventilation was assisted with a good response. Within 1 hour of intubation the patient was completely flaccid and unresponsive.

1. What is the differential diagnosis for this illness?
2. What common marine illnesses present with neurologic symptoms?
3. What is the treatment for this patient's poisoning?

Case 34

A 35-year-old man presented to the hospital stating he ingested 1 pint of antifreeze. He had no significant past medical history and was asymptomatic. Vital signs were remarkable for tachycardia at 105 beats/min. Otherwise, the physical examination was negative. The first laboratory tests received were a measured serum osmolality of 365 mOsm/kg and an ethanol level of 0 mg/dL. The BUN and blood glucose levels were normal.

1. What is the differential diagnosis for an increased osmolar gap?
2. What chemicals may be in antifreeze?
3. How do patients with this poisoning typically present?
4. How is the causative agent predicted?
5. What is the therapy?

Case 35

A 22-year-old man was brought to the hospital by ambulance. His family said that they had found him at home confused, sweaty, and vomiting. A suicide note found at his side indicated that he had ingested as many as sixty 200-mg sustained-release theophylline pills approximately 3 hours earlier. On arrival at the emergency department he was noted to be confused and diaphoretic, with a blood pressure of 70/50 mm Hg, a pulse of 120 beats/min, a respiratory rate of 30 breaths/min, and a temperature of 98.6°F (37°C). The patient was lavaged with a large-bore orogastric tube and given activated charcoal (1 g/kg in a slurry of water with 70 mL of 70% sorbitol solution). A large-bore intravenous line was started, and bloods were sent for a complete blood count, electrolytes, and glucose, theophylline, and acetaminophen levels. The patient was given a bolus of lactated Ringer solution, and his blood pressure increased to 90/50 mm Hg.

Suddenly the patient seized and was noted to be in a regular supraventricular tachycardia at a rate of 150 beats/min (Fig. CS–6). The patient was intubated and treated with diazepam, phenytoin, pancuronium, and lidocaine. His blood pressure rose to 150/100 mm Hg, and his pulse remained at 150 beats/min.

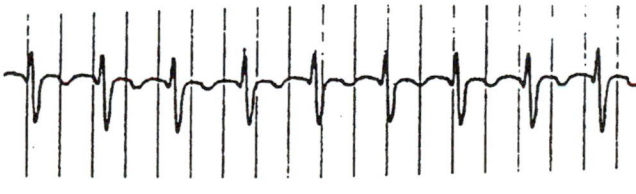

Figure CS–6 Rhythm strip from the patient demonstrating a regular narrow-complex rhythm characteristic of supraventricular tachycardia (SVT).

A nephrology consultation was obtained to facilitate immediate extracorporeal drug removal. At that time the first theophylline level was reported as 148 mg/mL. The patient was begun on a regimen of multiple-dose activated charcoal (1 g/kg/h), and plans for hemodialysis were made.

1. What are the major manifestations of acute theophylline toxicity?
2. What is the treatment of patients with acute theophylline overdoses?
3. Which patients qualify for extracorporeal drug removal?

Case 36

A 50-year-old medical researcher was discovered dead in a refrigerated room (8 ft wide × 14 ft deep × 8 ft high; 896 ft³) that contained 15 new blocks (10 inches × 10 inches × 10 inches) of dry

ice. The dry ice had been stored in the refrigerator (4°C, 39.2°F) at approximately 9 AM that day to reduce sublimation. The researcher was last seen at approximately noon, indicating that at least 3 hours had elapsed between storage and exposure. There were no signs of struggle, and the victim had no history of psychiatric disorders, recent personal crises, or medical illnesses.

1. What is "dry ice"? What is its toxicity?
2. What is asphyxiation?
3. In what other settings may this type of poisoning occur?
4. What is the treatment?

Case 37

A 60-year-old man with a history of untreated hypertension presented to the ED complaining of chest pain. The diagnosis of aortic dissection was confirmed, and the patient was started on nitroprusside and esmolol to control his blood pressure, which on presentation was 220/130 mm Hg. Because his aortic dissection was distal, medical rather than surgical management was provided, and his blood pressure was reduced to 170/80 mm Hg while he received 200 μg/min of a nitroprusside infusion. Two days later, in the ICU, the patient became confused, although his level of consciousness was normal. His arterial blood pH was 7.35, his P_{CO_2} was 37 mm Hg, his lactate level was minimally elevated, and his renal function was modestly abnormal.

1. What toxicities are associated with nitroprusside?
2. How does thiocyanate poisoning differ from cyanide poisoning?
3. How are patients with cyanide and thiocyanate poisoning managed?

Case 38

A 22-year-old man with no past medical history was brought to the ED after falling in the bathroom. His roommates reported that the patient had had a seizure, although it is unclear if the fall was the cause of his seizure or a sequela. The previous night the patient went to a dance club, where he had "had a few drinks" and may have used recreational drugs. His vital signs in the ED were normal, and he was awake but lethargic. An electrocardiogram, pulse oximeter, fingerstick glucose, and head CT were normal. The patient's laboratory values revealed a serum sodium of 120 mEq/L, a serum osmolality of 245 mOsm/L, and a urine osmolality of 491 mOsm/L. The patient inadvertently received 2 L of intravenous 0.9% NaCl, and his sodium fell to 107. Infusion of 1 cc/kg of 3% hypertonic saline improved his serum sodium and mental status.

1. What are the possible etiologies of this patient's seizure?
2. How should patients with drug-induced seizures be managed?
3. What is specific about the management of this patient's seizure?

Case 39

A 35-year-old man and his son mixed water into a plastic container of pool shock (a granular substance used to prepare a swimming pool for its first annual use) and reclosed the lid tightly. After several seconds, the container exploded, covering the man in a cloud of green smoke. He rapidly noted a burning in his eyes and throat and came to the ED for evaluation. On arrival, he had erythematous mucosal surfaces of his mouth and eyes and had a raspy voice. No stridor was present, and his lungs were clear. His vital signs were all normal; his oxygen saturation by pulse oximetry was 92% on room air.

1. What are irritant gases? How do they cause injury?
2. How can the type and extent of damage in patients exposed to irritant gases be predicted?
3. What is the evaluation and management strategy?

STUDY GUIDE: ANSWERS TO CASE STUDY QUESTIONS

Case 1

1. The patient had uncontrollable twitching of all extremities. Although a seizure disorder should be considered, it is extremely unlikely that a patient would have bilateral seizurelike activity and retain a normal mental status. Although a partial motor seizure (twitching of one extremity) is often associated with a normal mental status, when seizures cross the midline, consciousness is usually lost. Another cause of twitching could include electrolyte abnormalities. Either hypocalcemia or hypomagnesemia could produce these symptoms, but this patient's serum calcium and magnesium were both normal. Muscle fasciculations are seen with neuromuscular blocking agents, some snake and arthropod envenomations, and organic phosphorus agent toxicity. This patient's strength was normal, and he had none of the other signs or symptoms associated with these toxins. Myoclonus can result from muscle fatigue, anticholinergic agents, lithium, chlorinated hydrocarbons, or cocaine. Again, however, the patient had no other findings associated with these exposures. The most likely diagnosis is strychnine toxicity, the etiology of which would be the patient's new supply of heroin.

2. Strychnine is extracted from the seeds of the Indian tree *Strychnos nux vomica*. It has been used for centuries as a stimulant, an aphrodisiac, and, more recently (but no longer), as a rodenticide. Although strychnine poisoning is relatively rare, as many as 100 cases are reported annually. The alkaloid is an odorless white powder with a bitter taste that resembles that of heroin or quinine. It is rapidly and almost completely absorbed from the gastrointestinal or nasal mucosa and by all parenteral routes. Absorption does not occur, however, through intact skin. The toxin is quite potent, with an estimated human lethal dose of 5 to 8 mg/kg. Case reports note symptoms in adult patients who have been exposed to as little as 0.5 to 1.0 mg/kg.

Once absorbed, strychnine impairs resting inhibitory muscle tone by decreasing the ability of glycine to bind postsynaptically (refer to Fig. 10–12). Because glycine receptors are located for the most part in the spinal cord, the loss of inhibition produces motor, but not cognitive, disturbances. Although strychnine toxicity is usually said to produce seizures, these are more likely to be motor events that resemble seizures; patients often have a normal mental status and no postictal period. Because glycine receptors are present throughout the central nervous system (CNS) but decrease rostrally, higher brain functions may occasionally become impaired.

3. Within 15 to 20 minutes of exposure, patients begin to show signs of excitation. Early signs include nausea, fear, and apprehension. This is usually followed rapidly by myoclonus, hyper-

reflexia, and "seizures." These muscle events are characteristically described as episodic, involving largely extensor muscles, and are exacerbated by stimuli. Opisthotonos and the classic risus sardonicus are described. These events are all predictable from an understanding of glycine inhibitory physiology. When extensor muscles are stimulated, the normal response is for glycine to inhibit function of the flexor groups. The reverse is also true. This pharmacologic action prevents simultaneous contraction of both the flexor and extensor groups. Thus, in the presence of strychnine toxicity, the motor activity is often tonic (as opposed to tonic-clonic), with the direction of contraction favoring the strongest muscles in each group. Because extensor muscles are used to maintain posture, the extensors of the neck, back, and legs are often stronger than their corresponding flexors, and they contract.

Complications of strychnine toxicity include hyperthermia, rhabdomyolysis, and hypoventilation from the inability to move the muscles of respiration. This latter effect has been associated with fatalities.

4. Although laboratory confirmation of strychnine exposure (with either blood or urine specimens) is routinely available from reference laboratories, concentrations correlate poorly with either signs and symptoms or prognosis. Furthermore, analysis is rarely available on an immediate basis. Treatment is usually based on history, suspicion, and suggestive clinical findings.

The principles of management include airway protection, temperature control, prevention of absorption, reduction of muscle spasms, and prevention of secondary complications by maintaining good urine output. Although phenobarbital was used successfully in the past, benzodiazepines have become the therapeutic agents of choice. These agents function by increasing γ-aminobutyric acid (GABA) activity. γ-Aminobutyric acid is the other major inhibitory neurotransmitter in the CNS. Patients who fail to respond to benzodiazepines or barbiturates should be treated with neuromuscular blockade. Activated charcoal is useful, as its ability to adsorb strychnine in vitro has been well described. Volume resuscitation and rapid cooling may be required for severe cases. Finally, some authors have suggested the use of forced diuresis, potassium permanganate, peritoneal dialysis (PD), and urinary acidification. These techniques do not substantially increase strychnine elimination (forced diuresis and PD), have intrinsic toxicities (potassium permanganate), and may increase the risk of renal failure secondary to rhabdomyolysis (acidification). Most patients will have resolution of symptoms within 24 hours.

This patient was treated with diazepam and IV fluids and did well. He supplied a sample of his heroin, which was found to contain strychnine and no opioid whatsoever. This substitution, called a "death hit" on the street, is usually reserved for a client in poor standing.

SUGGESTED READINGS

Chapter 10, Neurotransmitter Principles.

Chapter 90, Rodenticides.

Anon. Case Records of the Massachusetts General Hospital. Case 12–2001. A 16-year old boy with an altered mental status and muscle rigidity. N Engl J Med 2001;344:1232–1239.

Anderson AH: Experimental studies on the pharmacology of activated charcoal: III. Adsorption from gastrointestinal contents. Acta Pharmacol 1948;4:275–284.

Boyd RE, Brennan PT, Deng JF, et al: Strychnine poisoning: Recovery from profound lactic acidosis, hyperthermia, and rhabdomyolysis. Am J Med 1983;74:507–512.

Case 2

1. Although the incidence of isoniazid (INH)-induced hepatotoxicity is dependent on the population investigated, a general rule of thumb is that about 10% of patients taking INH will have some chemical evidence of hepatic involvement (clinically asymptomatic with liver enzyme abnormalities); 10% of these patients (or 1%) will develop clinical evidence of hepatitis (anorexia, jaundice, right upper quadrant pain); and, if not discontinued, 10% of these patients (or 0.1% of all patients) will develop fulminant hepatic failure, potentially leading to death. In 1970, more than 2000 Capitol Hill employees converted their PPD status as a result of close exposure to a patient or several patients with active tuberculosis (Garibaldi). A total of 2321 employees were started on isoniazid prophylaxis. Although the incidence of chemical hepatitis is unknown, clinical evidence of hepatitis developed in 19 employees (0.08%), and two died of fulminant hepatic failure (0.09%). About half of the employees (9 of 19) became symptomatic within 60 days of the initiation of therapy, and all who developed symptoms did so within 6 months of initiation of therapy. The risk of hepatitis is almost doubled in alcoholics (33%) when compared to nonalcoholics (17%), and age greater than 35 years increases the risk almost 2.5-fold (27% vs 11%) (Dickinson). However, the risk appears to be lower when close monitoring and early intervention are performed (Nolan). Pediatric patients are relatively protected from hepatotoxicity. In children receiving INH prophylaxis, 7% (39 of 564) of patients had some elevation of liver enzymes, and only one had an AST greater than 100 IU/L (Nakajo).

2. One of the major pathways for the metabolism of INH is through acetylation to form acetylisoniazid. This acetylation is genetically determined, such that patients may be classified as either fast or slow acetylators (refer to Fig. 43–2). More than 90% of Asian Americans are rapid acetylators, whereas about 55% of African and white Americans are slow acetylators. Because one of the metabolites produced by acetylation was thought to be hepatotoxic, for many years it was generally accepted that fast acetylators were at increased risk of hepatotoxicity. However, detailed investigations demonstrate that acetylation status is not a risk factor for hepatotoxicity (Dickinson; Gurumurthy). This does not mean that metabolism is not important. Isoniazid is also metabolized by the cytochrome P450 system to form a hepatotoxic metabolite. Concomitant use of drugs that induce P450 activity (notably rifampin, ethanol, and oral contraceptives) increase the risk for hepatotoxicity.

3. Classic toxin-induced hepatic injury from acetaminophen or carbon tetrachloride produces massive centrilobular necrosis. Damage occurs primarily in this area because the cells surrounding the terminal hepatic vein are relatively oxygen-deprived and thus most sensitive to toxin-induced stresses. This is in contradistinction to classic viral hepatitis, which largely involves the periportal areas. Distinct histology is associated with chronic ethanol abuse. Liver enzyme abnormalities can be used to help differentiate acute alcoholic hepatitis from toxin-induced or viral hepatitis. Ethanol toxicity usually results in an AST that is twice the alanine aminotransferase (ALT), and the total elevation is rarely greater than 1000 IU/L. In acute toxic hepatitis, such as might result from an acetaminophen overdose, the AST and ALT are approximately equal, and the patient is not considered to be hepatotoxic until the values are greater than 1000 IU/L because lower values are rarely associated with symptoms. In fact, aminotransferase values in excess of 10,000 are commonly noted. In isoniazid hepatotoxicity the total aminotransferase elevations may reach the thousands, but the histology often has evidence of injury to both the terminal hepatic and periportal areas (Black).

4. Although this patient had no history or clinical evidence of acetaminophen poisoning, patients with hepatic failure of all etiologies may benefit from the administration of N-acetylcysteine (NAC) because of its ability to increase oxygen delivery, increase cardiac index, decrease systemic vascular resistance, and increase oxygen extraction (Harrison). The mechanisms for these effects are unclear.

5. Isoniazid prophylaxis should be started only when clinically indicated. Patients must be thoroughly educated to identify early symptoms of hepatotoxicity. In addition, they should be instructed to seek immediate attention if these signs and symptoms occur. Finally, high-risk patients should have biweekly monitoring of liver function tests at least during the first 6 months of therapy.

SUGGESTED READINGS

Chapter 14, Hepatic Principles

Chapter 43, Antituberculous Agents

Antidotes in Depth: N-Acetylcysteine

Black M, Mitchel JR, Zimmerman HJ, et al: Isoniazid-associated hepatitis in 114 patients. Gastroenterology 1975;69:289–301.

Dickinson DS, Bailey WC, Hirschowitz B, et al: Risk factors for isoniazid (INH)-induced liver dysfunction. J Clin Gastroenterol 1981;3:271–279.

Garibaldi RA, Drusin RE, Ferebee SH, Gregg MD: Isoniazid-associated hepatitis: Report of an outbreak. Am Rev Respir Dis 1972;106:357–365.

Gurumurthy P, Krishnamurthy MS, Nazareth O, et al: Lack of relationship between hepatic toxicity and acetylator phenotype in three thousand South Indian patients during treatment with isoniazid for tuberculosis. Am Rev Respir Dis 1984;129:58–61.

Harrison PM, Wendon JA, Gimson AES, et al: Improvement by acetylcysteine of hemodynamics and oxygen transport in fulminant hepatic failure. N Engl J Med 1991;324:1852–1857.

Nakajo MM, Rao M, Steiner P: Incidence of hepatotoxicity in children receiving isoniazid chemoprophylaxis. Pediatr Infect Dis 1989;8:649–650.

Nolan CM, Goldberg SV, Buskin SE: Hepatotoxicity associated with isoniazid preventive therapy: A 7-year survey from a public health tuberculosis clinic. JAMA 1999;281:1014–1018.

Case 3

1. The differential diagnosis of drug-induced seizures is quite long but should include common causes such as cocaine, cyclic antidepressants, theophylline, carbon monoxide, ethanol and sedative-hypnotic withdrawal, camphor, organophosphates, carbamazepine, lithium, hypoglycemic agents (sulfonylureas and insulin), β-adrenergic antagonists, type I antidysrhythmics, and isoniazid. Less common agents, such as gyramitrin-containing mushrooms, propoxyphene, MAO inhibitors, phenothiazines, lead, caffeine, cyanide, and agents that produce methemoglobinemia, should also be considered. True status epilepticus is uncommon and is more suggestive of toxicity from cocaine, theophylline, isoniazid, carbamazepine, or chlorinated hydrocarbons.

Subsequent history determined that the patient had been recently diagnosed as having a positive PPD and was started on isoniazid. A large number of her INH tablets had been ingested during her suicide attempt.

2. Isoniazid-induced seizures result from a depletion of GABA, which is one of the major inhibitory neurotransmitters and thus may be considered a natural anticonvulsant. Glutamic acid serves as an immediate precursor of GABA, and the conversion of glutamic acid to GABA is facilitated by a pyridoxine-dependent enzyme L-glutamic acid decarboxylase (GAD). Isoniazid interferes with this conversion of glutamic acid to GABA by at least three different mechanisms (refer to Fig. 43–3): (1) Isoniazid directly combines with pyridoxine to result in enhanced urinary elimination. (2) To be active, pyridoxine must be converted to pyridoxal 5′-phosphate by the enzyme pyridoxine phosphokinase. This enzyme is inhibited by isoniazid. (3) Isoniazid itself inhibits GAD. When GABA is reduced below a critical threshold, seizures result (Wood).

Isoniazid also inhibits other enzyme systems, including lactate dehydrogenase. This enzyme uses nicotinamide adenine dinucleotide (NAD) to interconvert lactate and pyruvate. By interfering with this conversion, any lactate formed (as occurs during seizures) might persist longer than expected. This may account for the clinical data that suggest that the acidosis formed during INH toxicity is "resistant" to therapy, but this has not been studied.

3. Emesis, coma, and seizures usually occur within 1 to 3 hours after a significant overdose. Although gastrointestinal decontamination is indicated, syrup of ipecac–induced emesis is contraindicated in patients with INH overdose. Orogastric lavage and activated charcoal seem to be the safest approach. Seizures should initially be treated with standard doses of a benzodiazepine (preferably diazepam or lorazepam). When ingestion of isoniazid is suspected, IV pyridoxine (vitamin B_6) should be administered as soon as possible. For INH ingestions of known quantity, it is generally recommended that pyridoxine be administered on a gram-for-gram basis. For patients in whom the quantity ingested is unknown, a dose of 5 g of pyridoxine can be administered to adults. Whether the amount ingested is known or not, the first dose of pyridoxine should never exceed 5 g in an adult or 70 mg/kg in children (Wason).

At higher initial or total doses, pyridoxine itself may cause neurologic toxicity. Acute effects include incoordination, ataxia, seizures, and death (in animals). Chronic exposure to high doses of pyridoxine causes a peripheral sensory neuropathy, which may not resolve completely after the medication is discontinued (Schaumberg).

In animal studies the anticonvulsant effects of pyridoxine were synergistic with diazepam (Chin). Thus, during the pyridoxine infusion, repeat doses of benzodiazepines should be administered. Pyridoxine may also be efficacious in reversing persistent coma caused by INH overdose (Brent).

Finally, in cases of severe intoxication, both hemodialysis and hemoperfusion have been reported to be successful at enhancing INH elimination but would rarely be indicated.

4. Given the frequency of tuberculosis in some populations, it may be resonable to give to any patient who presents with status epilepticus an empiric dose of pyridoxine (Shah). This decision depends in part on the clinician's individual patient population. Although seizures are common following overdose, status epilepticus is less common. Administering pyridoxine at a dose of 70 mg/kg or less is generally thought to be safe and may be effective in INH or monomethylhydrazine overdose. When seizures are refractory to benzodiazepines, an empiric trial of pyridoxine (and another dose of benzodiazepine) may be beneficial. When a history of intentional drug overdose is available, more liberal criteria for the administration of pyridoxine may be warranted. The New York City Health Department recently estimated that more than 1 million New Yorkers are PPD-positive. As tuberculosis continues in epidemic proportions in New York City and elsewhere, INH overdoses are likely to occur. A 10-fold increase in INH overdoses has occurred in New York City over the last few years.

SUGGESTED READING

Chapter 43, Antituberculous Agents.

Antidotes in Depth: Pyridoxine.

Brent J, Nguyen V, Kulig K, et al: Reversal of prolonged isoniazid-induced coma by pyridoxine. Arch Intern Med 1990;150:1751–1753.

Chin L, Sievers ML, Laird HE, et al: Evaluation of diazepam and pyridoxine as antidotes to isoniazid intoxication in rats and dogs. Toxicol Appl Pharmacol 1978;45:713–722.

Schaumberg H, Kaplan J, Widenbank A, et al: Sensory neuropathy from pyridoxine abuse: A megavitamin syndrome. N Engl J Med 1983;309:445–448.

Shah BR, Santucci K, Sinert R, Steiner P: Acute isoniazid neurotoxicity in an urban hospital. Pediatrics 1995;95:700–704.

Wason S, Lacouture PG, Lovejoy FH: Single high-dose pyridoxine treatment for isoniazid overdose. JAMA 1981;246:1102–1104.

Wood JD, Peesker SJ: A correlation between changes in GABA metabolism and isonicotinic acid hydrazide-induced seizures. Brain Res 1972;45:489–498.

Case 4

1. Although many hair products have similar names and uses, their ingredients may be quite varied. Initially, we must distinguish between hair or permanent relaxers and neutralizers. Relaxers usually contain an alkaline caustic (dilute sodium hydroxide or thioglycolate), whereas the neutralizers may contain bromates.

2. Nausea, vomiting, or oropharyngeal irritation may be the first symptoms to occur following an ingestion of either a caustic or bromate. If a caustic was ingested, drooling, stridor, and signs of gastrointestinal perforation or bleeding may develop. However, distinctly different delayed symptoms may result from bromate poisoning, specifically hearing loss and renal insufficiency. More commonly, skin reactions, including severe contact dermatitis, occur with topical exposure to bromates.

3. Initial therapy for patients with bromate ingestion consists of dilution and fluid and electrolyte resuscitation. Esophagoscopy is indicated if signs or symptoms of significant gastrointestinal burns are present. Sodium thiosulfate theoretically may act as an antidote by converting bromate to less toxic bromide. Most patients with small unintentional ingestions of this type of product do well with conservative therapy alone. In severe cases hemodialysis may be required, depending on the severity of renal insufficiency. This case was later confirmed as a bromate ingestion when the parents returned home to obtain the product container. The parents were given poison prevention education.

No gross auditory deficits were noted, but testing in a child of this age is not very precise. Over the next several days her creatinine level returned to normal, and she was discharged.

SUGGESTED READINGS

Chapter 87, Caustics and Batteries.

De Vriese A, Vanholder R, Lameire N: Severe acute renal failure due to bromate intoxication: report of a case and discussion of management guidelines based on a review of the literature. Nephrol Dial Transplant 1997;12:204–209.

Lue JN, Johnson CE, Edwards DL: Bromate poisoning from ingestion of professional hair-care neutralizer. Clin Pharmacol 1988;7:66–70.

McElwee NE, Kearney TE: Sodium thiosulfate unproven as bromate antidote [letter]. Clin Pharmacol 1988;7:570.

Case 5

1. The most dramatic finding in these patients was the presence of a rapidly developing, isolated, severely painful sensory peripheral neuropathy. Many agents are associated with the production of a peripheral neuropathy, including solvents, organic phosphorus compounds, heavy metals, isoniazid, ethanol, and mitotic inhibitors. When eventual multisystem involvement is added (gastrointestinal, cardiovascular, and renal), the diagnosis of heavy metal poisoning becomes more likely. Among the heavy metals, thallium is the most likely diagnosis because of the unique nature of the neurologic symptoms. The presence of both severe painful neuropathy and alopecia is essentially diagnostic of thallotoxicosis. Further evidence comes from the lack of hematologic toxicity, which is fairly common with other heavy metal exposures.

Thallium was first isolated in 1861 by Crookes. Its name is derived from the Greek, *thallus,* which means "budding twig," because the color of sulfur ores containing thallium is suggestive of young vegetation. Most thallium salts are colorless and odorless powders. In the late 19th century thallium sulfate was used to treat syphilis, gonorrhea, tuberculosis, and tinea corporis. Thallium salts were subsequently widely available as rodenticides until 1965, when their use was prohibited because of the risk of toxicity in humans and domestic animals. Thallium is still used in the semiconductor and optical industries and in very small quantities in medical diagnostics (in its radioactive form). Although it is more difficult to obtain since its over-the-counter sale was prohibited, thallium salts are still available through most chemical supply

houses because of the vast commercial and research applications for these compounds. Recent reports of thallium toxicity concentrate on its use as a homicidal and suicidal agent, as unintentional exposures have almost been eliminated.

2. Thallium salts most commonly enter the body by ingestion. Inhalation and insufflation of dust and dermal absorption are also reported. Experimentally, both the IV and SC routes produce toxicity as well. Although human data demonstrate some variability, many authors suggest that in adults fatality often results from ingestions of about 1 g of thallium salts (or 12 mg/kg in children). Because thallium distributes to most cells in the body, its volume of distribution is quite large, approximately 5 L/kg. Cellular absorption seems to be analogous to that of potassium, possibly accounting for the ECG changes noted in these patients and the theoretical role of potassium diuresis in the treatment strategy (see below). Once absorbed, thallium binds to sulfhydryl groups of diverse enzyme systems. In various experimental models inhibition of Na^+-K^+-ATPase, oxidative phosphorylation, the Krebs cycle, and monoamine oxidase have all been described. The elimination of thallium is slow, possibly as the result of enterohepatic circulation, with reported half-lives on the order of 1 to 5 days. The majority of elimination is fecal, and a small amount is renal.

3. The clinical stages of thallium intoxication are well defined (Lovejoy). Within the first 3 to 4 hours of exposure gastrointestinal symptoms predominate. Although nausea and diarrhea are common, many reports have documented constipation, which is often refractory to cathartics. Within several hours to several days after exposure patients begin to manifest neurologic symptoms consisting of painful peripheral neuropathy, altered mental status, seizures, and respiratory dysfunction. A motor component may accompany the sensory neuropathy. Simultaneously (or within a few days following the onset of neurologic symptoms), patients may enter a phase of autonomic instability, consisting of hypertension, tachycardia, salivation, and fever. During this stage myocardial failure may occur. Alopecia is the most reliable finding and usually begins within 2 weeks of exposure. Late findings consist of residual neurologic dysfunction, Mee lines, and dry skin.

4. In addition to history and physical examination, the diagnosis of thallium intoxication is usually confirmed by laboratory determination of thallium in the urine. Normal (nonexposed) patients have urinary thallium concentrations less than 5 ng/mL (5 μg/L). Generally, urine concentrations greater than this value or whole-blood concentrations greater than 30 μg/dL are consistent with exposure. In addition, examination of the hair roots has been demonstrated to show hyperpigmentation in about 95% of cases studied later than 4 days after exposure. Finally, thallium salts are radiopaque, so abdominal radiographs, or in this case radiographs of the candy, may be helpful.

The two more severely poisoned patients described had thallium spot urines obtained on day 2 of poisoning of 10,837 and 9569 μg/L, respectively.

5. Because of a paucity of both human and controlled animal data, there is little consensus on treatment. Gastrointestinal decontamination is indicated before the onset of vomiting and diarrhea, or at a later stage if radiopaque material is seen in the gastrointestinal tract. Thallium is adsorbed to activated charcoal in vitro, and there is a potential role for multiple-dose activated charcoal because of the enterohepatic circulation. Although forced potassium diuresis increases urinary clearance and decreases the half-life substantially, it is also associated with a transient exacerbation of neurologic symptoms (seen in all four patients described) because potassium increases CNS thallium concentrations while mobilizing thallium from other compartments. This is analogous to using $CaNa_2$ ethelenediaminetetraacetic acid (EDTA) alone for the treatment of severe lead intoxication. Prussian blue, which is not an FDA-approved antidote, may bind thallium in the gastrointestinal tract and supply potassium for enhanced urinary elimination as it exchanges potassium for thallium. Diverse chelators have been used with variable results. British anti-Lewisite (BAL) and $CaNa_2$ EDTA are not effective. Dithiocarb and the use of penicillamine without Prussian blue may exacerbate symptoms, as they redistribute thallium into the CNS. Although standard hemodialysis has little efficacy because of thallium's large volume of distribution, the combination of hemodialysis and hemoperfusion or hemoperfusion alone seems to be more beneficial than hemodialysis alone at enhancing elimination. Although only limited data are available, early coma, respiratory arrest, and cardiovascular instability appear associated with mortality.

These patients were all treated with activated charcoal and forced potassium diuresis. Prussian blue and hemodialysis were used only in the two sicker patients. Their symptoms, except for the alopecia, resolved over 2 to 3 weeks. Hair regrowth usually takes substantially longer.

SUGGESTED READINGS

Chapter 83, Thallium.
Chamberlain PH, Stavinoha WB, Davis H, et al: Thallium poisoning. Pediatrics 1958;22:1170–1182.
Hoffman RS, Stringer JA, Feinberg RS, et al: Comparative efficacy of thallium adsorption by activated charcoal, Prussian blue, and sodium polystyrene sulfonate. J Toxicol Clin Toxicol 1999;37:833–837.
Moeschlin S: Thallium poisoning. Clin Toxicol 1980;17:133–146.
Nordentoft T, Andersen EB, Mogensen PH: Initial sensorimotor and delayed autonomic neuropathy in acute thallium poisoning. Neurotoxicology 1998;19:421–426.

Case 6

1. The patient's history permits the exclusion of most common allergens, and the history of a recent camping trip suggests several different exposures. Nontoxicologic etiologies should be considered, particularly herpes zoster, scabies, or Lyme borelliosis. Arthropods, such as caterpillars, or insects may result in vesicular lesions, but rarely do they manifest in a linear pattern. The patient went swimming in a lake and could have "swimmer's itch," a dermatitis involving exposed areas of the body caused by *Schistosoma cercaride*, a free-swimming parasitic flatworm found in fresh water. However, this rash is typically diffuse and not linear. Because he did not swim in the ocean, he should not have seabather's eruption caused by larvae of "thimble jellyfish" *(Linuche unguiculata)*. This rash is usually localized to areas covered by a bathing suit, where the larvae are trapped and cause localized irritation. The symptoms often worsen on bathing as a result of osmotically activated discharge of the larval nematocysts. Unfortunately, the causative organisms of seabather's eruption are often inappropriately called "sea lice," which are true crustacean fish parasites; this may potentially lead to the inappropriate application of a pediculocide.

2. The patient's close contact with foliage is highly suggestive of exposure to plant toxins. There are many dermatologic manifestations of plant exposure, but the most common are allergic contact dermatitis and phototoxicity. Phototoxic reactions are caused by the presence of furocoumarins, notably psoralen, which cause exaggerated dermal injury following exposure to ultraviolet light. The Umbilliferae family consists of several psoralen-containing plants such as Queen Anne's lace, wild parsnip, and celery. Phytophototoxicity also occurs in gardeners using a hand-held nylon fiber weed cutter, as plant fragments containing psoralen are thrown toward the patient, accounting for the appellation "weed wacker dermatitis." Although psoralen is used therapeutically as a photosensitizer in the treatment of psoriasis (ie, PUVA therapy [pulsed ultraviolet actinotherapy]), uncontrolled exposure may result in bullous dermatitis analogous to a severe sunburn. Phototoxic reactions require not only exposure of moist skin to plant parts but also sun exposure, and when they result from direct dermal contact with the plant, the lesions that result are typically streaky and known as dermatitis bullosa striata pratensis. The presence of lesions in presumably covered areas such as the buttocks excludes phytophotodermatitis.

3. Allergic contact dermatitis caused by plants is a very common occupational disorder but is also seen frequently in campers, home gardeners, flower recipients, and perfume wearers. By far the most common type of allergic contact phytodermatitis is rhus dermatitis, caused by the various species of the family Anacardiaceae and the genus *Toxicodendron*. Rhus dermatitis, familiarly known as poison ivy or poison oak, appears as an edematous vesicular eruption in a telltale streaky pattern. The streaks result because the resin is applied while brushing against an implicated plant or spread manually by scratching while resin is lodged beneath the fingernails.

The agent responsible for poison ivy is urushiol, which is actually a collection of several different catechol derivatives with long and variably saturated hydrocarbon side chains (poison ivy is predominantly pentadecylcatechol). This agent is metabolized to a quinone that attacks a skin protein, probably keratin. Acting as a hapten, the urushiol alters this protein, causing the immune system to initiate an immune response against the altered protein following the first exposure. Subsequent exposure induces an amnestic response, typically of the type IV delayed hypersensitivity. Hypersensitivity to urushiol occurs in over half the people in the United States, suggesting prior exposure, and as many as 85% of patients are capable of being sensitized.

Allergic contact phytodermatitis is also produced by other plant toxins, notably the sesquiterpene lactones found in the Compositae family. This family includes chrysanthemum, feverfew, and dandelions. The dermatitis caused by these plants may appear similarly to poison ivy but is generally diffuse, not linear.

4. Clothing is the most effective prevention, but patients must be cautious when removing and washing clothes to avoid transfer of the resin to their skin. Similarly, because the resin is difficult to remove, particularly from beneath the fingernails, delayed exposure may occur. Soap and water may work best, but ethanol or isopropanol is often recommended. If the resin is washed off the skin within 10 minutes of exposure, it may be possible to avoid dermatitis. An effective barrier cream containing an organoclay, bentoquatam (IvyBlock®; quarternium-18 bentonite), was recently approved by the FDA.

Treatment of mild dermatitis can include a soothing agent such as Domeboro solution (aluminum acetate) or a lubricating agent such as petrolatum. It is probably best to avoid drying antipruritic lotions such as calamine except for weeping lesions. Potent topical corticosteroids can be considered for moderate lesions or for severe pruritis, but only mild agents such as hydrocortisone 1% should be used on the face or genitals. Systemic steroids are rarely indicated and are used only for patients with severe dermatitis; they should be continued for at least 2 weeks to avoid rebound dermatitis. Systemic antipruritics such as diphenhydramine may be helpful, but topical versions are sensitizing and should be avoided. Patients with severe rhus dermatitis who cannot avoid exposure (eg, occupational contact) may be candidates for oral hyposensitization therapy. This is performed by administering orally incrementally larger doses of urushiol, which over time transiently suppresses the immunologic response if the patient is dermally exposed to rhus.

SUGGESTED READINGS

Chapter 78, Plants.

Fisher AA: Poison ivy/oak dermatitis. Part I: Prevention: soap and water, topical barriers, hyposensitization. Cutis 1996;57:384–386.

Hjorth N, Roed-Petersen J, Thomsen K: Airborne contact dermatitis from Compositae oleoresins simulating photodermatitis. Br J Dermatol 1976;95:613–619.

Marks JG, Trautlein JJ, Epstein WL, et al: Oral hyposensitization to poison ivy and poison oak. Arch Dermatol 1987;123:476–478.

Marks JG Jr, Fowler JF Jr, Sheretz EF, et al: Prevention of poison ivy and poison oak allergic contact dermatitis by quaternium-18 bentonite. J Am Acad Dermatol 1995;33:212–216.

McGovern TW, LaWarre SR, Brunette C: Is it, or isn't it? Poison ivy look-alikes. Am J Contact Dermatol 2000;11:104–110.

Reynolds NJ, Burton JL, Bradfield JWB, Matthews CAN: Weed wacker dermatitis. Arch Dermatol 1991;127:1419–1420.

Case 7

1. The terminology of acid–base disorders often leads to confusion and error. The following definitions provide an appropriate frame of reference. The terms *acidosis* and *alkalosis* refer to processes. By definition a patient is said to have:

- A *metabolic acidosis* if the serum bicarbonate (HCO_3) is less than 24 mEq/L
- A *metabolic alkalosis* if the serum HCO_3 is more than 24 mEq/L
- A *respiratory acidosis* if the partial pressure of carbon dioxide (PCO_2) is greater than 40 mm Hg
- A *respiratory alkalosis* if the PCO_2 is less than 40 mm Hg

Any combination of acidoses and alkaloses can be present in any one patient at any given time. The terms *acidemia* and *alkalemia* refer only to the net pH of blood (acidemia being less than 7.40 and alkalemia being greater than 7.40). These terms do not describe the process or processes that led to the alteration in pH.

The patient had a primary metabolic acidosis with compensatory respiratory alkalosis with a net acidemia. The metabolic

acidosis is of the high-anion-gap variety (anion gap = 35). The anion gap is calculated as follows: anion gap = [sodium] − {[chloride] + [bicarbonate]}. If increased, it represents the presence of an unmeasured anion, usually an organic acid (eg, lactic acid) but occasionally an inorganic acid (eg, SO_4^{2-}).

2. Many people use different memory aids to help recall the differential diagnosis of a high-anion-gap metabolic acidosis, the most popular of which is the acronym MUDPIES: methanol, uremia, diabetic ketoacidosis (and other ketoacidoses), paraldehyde and phenformin (and metformin), ischemia (meaning all causes of lactate), isoniazid, and iron, ethylene glycol, and salicylates and solvents (such as toluene). Others use MUDPILES, in which the L represents lactate.

The best way to diagnose a metabolic disorder is via the history, physical examination, and simple laboratory tests. Is there a history of ingestion, alcoholism, or poorly controlled diabetes? In the absence of seizures, metabolic acidosis from INH should not occur. Iron poisoning should be accompanied by vomiting, and paraldehyde has a distinct odor. Visual symptoms often accompany methanol poisoning, and auditory symptoms (tinnitus) often accompany salicylate toxicity.

The serum electrolytes and ABG (arterial blood gas) not only define the problem but also give some specific clues to the etiology. Uremia and hyperglycemia are immediately evident. Renal insufficiency and hypocalcemia may occur with ethylene glycol intoxication. In addition, some simple urine tests may be very useful. The absence of ketones will help exclude ketoacidosis (although not definitively), a ferric chloride test will confirm salicylate ingestion, and oxalate crystals and fluorescence may be noted in ethylene glycol intoxication. Finally, a serum lactate concentration is very helpful. With the toxic alcohols, uremia, ketoacidosis, salicylates and solvents, organic acids other than lactate cause the majority of the acidosis. Thus, a high lactate concentration, specifically one that can account for the majority of the anion gap, can help exclude these agents from the differential diagnosis.

3. In the absence of visual symptoms and a history, methanol intoxication seems unlikely but cannot be excluded. Although the BUN and creatinine are elevated, the acidosis seems out of proportion to this elevation making uremic acidosis an unlikely cause. Diabetic ketoacidosis usually has more than trace ketones with a higher serum glucose, but, again, this cannot be excluded. There was no odor of paraldehyde. Without vomiting or seizure activity, iron and INH toxicity become less likely. With the low blood pressure and low temperature, causes of lactic acidosis (such as sepsis) should be considered. The renal insufficiency and acidosis may be explained by ethylene glycol toxicity.

Phenformin is an oral hypoglycemic of the biguanide class that was available in the United States until 1976. When phenformin was widely used, the incidence of life-threatening lactic acidosis was estimated at 1/4000 patients. Today, only metformin is available in the United States. Although severe metabolic acidosis is substantially less common with metformin, cases remain common given the drug's wide use. Their exact mechanism of action is unknown, but biguanides are thought to moderate blood glucose by reducing hepatic glucose release and increasing insulin receptor sensitivity. It may impair oxidative metabolism, and this later effect, which increases anaerobic glycolysis, may be responsible for the consequent metabolic acidosis. In addition, the biguanides are thought to be potent negative inotropes such that cardiac output is reduced (increasing lactate production) and glomerular filtration is decreased (inhibiting clearance of organic acids).

Renal insufficiency seems to be a major risk factor for biguanide toxicity (Misbin). This probably relates to impaired drug elimination. In animal models, significant lactic acidemia does not occur unless the animal is nephrectomized. Similarly, hepatic dysfunction increases the risk of toxicity both through impaired drug clearance and from decreased lactate metabolism. Other contributing factors include increased dosing (as in this patient) and concurrent illnesses that may result in a lactic acidosis (sepsis, myocardial infarction).

Further history revealed that this diabetic patient was taking phenformin, which he had obtained in Italy. When he developed polyuria and symptoms of a respiratory infection, he began to take increasing doses.

4. Gastrointestinal decontamination is indicated only in a recent acute oral overdose. Intravascular volume resuscitation is almost always required because of increased insensible losses. Correction of the pH with bicarbonate is often needed to prevent the pH from falling below 7.10 and is probably helpful as long as ventilation is adequate and volume overload does not occur. Many patients like this one are ketonuric. This ketoacidosis probably results from fatty acid degradation secondary to poor glucose utilization. Insulin (and glucose if necessary) can reverse this process, eliminating one cause of the patient's acidosis. In addition, it has been suggested that insulin partially reverses the inhibition of pyruvate dehydrogenase, allowing more rapid lactate degradation as it is shunted back to pyruvate. Although hemodialysis will not effectively remove phenformin or metformin, it can correct fluid and electrolyte abnormalities while allowing large volumes of bicarbonate administration, if necessary.

This patient received insulin and glucose and 15 ampules (>650 mEq) of sodium bicarbonate and was hemodialyzed twice. Over the course of 2 days his hemodynamic status stabilized, and his lactic acid concentration fell to 1.2 mEq/L. He was ultimately discharged from the hospital.

SUGGESTED READINGS

Chapter 24, Fluid, Electrolyte, and Acid–Base Principles.

Chapter 40, Antidiabetic and Hypoglycemic Agents.

Fulop M, Hoberman HD: Phenformin-associated metabolic acidosis. Diabetes 1976;25:292–296.

Gan SC, Barr J, Arieff AI, Pearl RG: Biguanide-associated lactic acidosis. Arch Intern Med 1992;152:2333–2336.

Kwong SC, Brubacher J: Phenformin and lactic acidosis: A case report and review. J Emerg Med 1998;16:881–886.

Lalau JD, Race JM: Metformin and lactic acidosis in diabetic humans. Diabetes Obes Metab 2000;2:131–137.

Misbin RI: Phenformin-associated lactic acidosis: Pathogenesis and treatment. Ann Intern Med 1977;87:591–595.

Stang M, Wysowski DK, Butler-Jones D: Incidence of lactic acidosis in metformin users. Diabetes Care 1999;22:925–927.

Case 8

1. Although this patient was originally described as having status epilepticus, it is important to remember that although seizures can occur with a normal mental status, global cerebral dysfunction causing bilateral motor movements must be associated with a change in consciousness. Thus, partial complex status epilepticus is not a concern here because of the bilateral motor movements and intact mental status. Fever, muscle rigidity, and an intact consciousness should always raise the possibility of strychnine toxicity or tetanus. Because these two disorders interfere with glycine-induced inhibitory tone in the spinal cord, mental status is normal until hypoventilation, acidemia, or hyperthermia becomes severe. Other considerations include fasciculations possibly induced by sympathomimetics (amphetamine and cocaine), cholinergic agents, black widow spider envenomation, or metal poisoning (arsenic, mercury, manganese), to name a few. Again, many of these disorders are associated with specific physical findings or impaired consciousness. Finally, myoclonus, which commonly results from exposure to tricyclic antidepressants, anticholinergics, bismuth, and DDT, should be considered.

A clue to potentially limit this differential diagnosis is the history of a cold. Common nonprescription cold remedies include sympathomimetics, antihistamines, anticholinergics, and dextromethorphan. The hyperthermia, muscle activity, and absence of other findings are suggestive of the serotonin syndrome, which can be the result of an interaction between dextromethorphan and a serotonin agonist.

The serotonin syndrome commonly results from the concomitant exposure to two agents that increase serotonin (5-HT) (see Fig. 10–8). These compounds can prevent neuronal degradation (MAO [monoamine oxidase] inhibitors), prevent reuptake (selective serotonin reuptake inhibitors, (tricyclic antidepressants) TCAs, meperidine, dextromethorphan), or increase serotonin synthesis (tryptophan). The resulting syndrome can be characterized by at least three of the following clinical criteria: altered mental status, agitation, myoclonus, hyperreflexia, fever, shivering, diaphoresis, ataxia, and diarrhea (Sporer). These symptoms should be present in association with exposure to serotonin agonists and in the absence of other causes of fever and altered mental status such as rapid increases in neuroleptic dosing.

Serotonin syndrome can begin very rapidly, within minutes of exposure, and if minimal may last only several hours. Severe cases can result in fatality, usually resulting from substantial elevations in body temperature, seizures, respiratory failure, and disseminated intravascular coagulation.

Further history revealed that the patient was taking Nardil (an MAO inhibitor).

2. The serotonin syndrome can be reproduced in animal models with a variety of combinations of agents that increase synaptic serotonin. Early animal studies using tryptophan and an MAO inhibitor were able to produce characteristic findings such as tremor, rigidity, and forepaw treading (Green). Nonspecific serotonin (5-HT$_1$ and 5-HT$_2$) antagonists such as cyproheptadine and methysergide attenuated these effects. Further delineation of the exact neurochemical mechanism for serotonin syndrome came from investigations with selective serotonin antagonists. More recent evidence suggests that stimulation of the 5-HT$_{1A}$ receptor may be the more important mechanism for generation of the serotonin syndrome, and 5-HT$_2$ receptor agonism plays a lesser role.

3. Initial therapy always begins with stabilization of the airway, breathing, and circulation. Next, attention should be paid to life-threatening elevations in body temperature. Patients with severe hyperthermia should be cooled rapidly with mist and fan or by submersion in iced water. The addition of a benzodiazepine is essential to prevent muscle activity, which contributers to hyperthermia (Brown). If muscular activity persists despite sedation, nondepolarizing neuromuscular blockade may be beneficial. There is no known specific advantage to dantrolene in this situation and its use for this indication should be rare.

Additionally, many experimental therapies have been tried with limited anecdotal success. Two patients were successfully treated with propranolol (Sporer). Although β-adrenergic antagonist therapy is usually contraindicated in patients with agitated delirium and hyperthermia (cocaine, alcohol withdrawal), propranolol has antagonistic properties at the 5-HT$_{1A}$ receptor. Similarly, cyproheptadine and methysergide have been used with limited success (Brown; Sporer). Although all these therapies are promising, they remain experimental and should therefore be used only with extreme caution.

Once control of muscle activity and body temperature have been achieved, the patient should receive intensive supportive care. Oral activated charcoal can be given if the ingestion was recent. Fluids should be administered in order to maintain a urine output of 3 mL/kg/h if there is a risk of myoglobinuric renal failure. Finally, electrolyte abnormalities should be evaluated and corrected. When the diagnosis is unclear, blood cultures, a CT scan of the head, and lumbar puncture may be indicated in addition to antibiotics.

Most patients who are diagnosed and treated promptly respond to therapy with rapid restoration of body temperature, muscle tone, and mental status.

SUGGESTED READINGS

Chapter 58, Serotonin Reuptake Inhibitors and Atypical Antidepressants

Chapter 60, Monoamine Oxidase Inhibitors

Brown TM, Skop BP: Pathophysiology and management of the serotonin syndrome. Ann Pharmacother 1996;30:527–533.

Green AR, Grahame-Smith DG: The role of brain dopamine in the hyperactivity syndrome produced by increased 5-HT synthesis in rats. Neuropharmacol 1974;13:949–959.

Radomski JW, Dursun SM, Reveley MA, et al: An exploratory approach to the serotonin syndrome: an update of clinical phenomenology and revised diagnostic criteria. Med Hypotheses 2000;55:218–224.

Sporer KA: The serotonin syndrome. Implicated drugs, pathophysiology and management. Drug Safety 1995;13:94–104.

Sternbach H: The serotonin syndrome. Am J Psychiatry 1991;148:705–713.

Yamada J, Sugimoto Y, Horisaka K: The evidence for the involvement of the 5HT$_{1A}$ receptor in 5-HT syndrome induced in mice by tryptamine. Jpn J Pharmacol 1989;51:421–425.

Case 9

1. The patient was administered high flow oxygen and attached to a cardiac monitor, an IV was started, blood specimens were obtained, and she was given 2 mg of naloxone, 25 g of dextrose, and 100 mg of thiamine. Following dextrose administration the patient promptly regained consciousness, and her hemiparesis resolved. When further history was obtained, the patient recalled that her acetazolamide prescription was recently refilled and that the pills appeared to differ from previous pills. Inspection of the pills revealed that she was given acetohexamide instead of acetazolamide (Dymelor instead of Diamox). Similar medication errors

have resulted in a number of severe injuries (Fig. CS–7). Ultimately, the laboratory reported her serum glucose concentration as 22 mg/dL. Hypoglycemia is a common cause of presentation to the ED. In a 12-month period during 1980 and 1981, 125 cases were recorded at Harlem Hospital (Malouf). Of these, only three patients (2.4%) presented with hemiparesis. Although other series report on a number of hypoglycemic patients presenting with focal neurologic deficits, neither the total patient pool nor the time taken to collect these patients is given (Seibert; Wallis). Thus, for lack of better demographic data, it seems safe to say that although hemiparesis and other focal findings resulting from hypoglycemia have been well described, they seem to occur in a minority (probably <10%) of cases.

2. The complications associated with unrecognized hypoglycemia are related in part to its etiology and in part to its duration and severity. The multiple etiologies encompassing severe diseases such as fulminant hepatic failure as well as relatively benign etiologies such as a missed meal in a diabetic patient on insulin create confusion in the literature with regard to outcome. For example, although the emergency department study done at Harlem Hospital (Malouf) reported an 11% mortality in the study group, only one death (0.8%) was directly attributed to hypoglycemia. Four survivors (3.2%), however, suffered from residual neurologic deficits. For comparison, 137 episodes of hypoglycemia noted in 94 inpatients resulted in an overall mortality of 27% (Fischer).

The treatment of hypoglycemia is quite simple—administer dextrose—but there was concern that the antidote is not entirely benign (Browning). Specifically, in animal models hyperglycemia clearly exacerbates ischemic brain injury. It is believed that this occurs as a result of the ischemic tissue's inability to oxidize glucose effectively. Anaerobic metabolism takes over, and local concentrations of lactic acid rise, increasing the damage. It is important to note that these studies use chronic hyperglycemia models, and no correlation with a single transient elevation in glucose (as results from a bolus of D$_{50}$W) has been made.

3. The solution to this problem would be to create a rapid means of detecting hypoglycemia. Although glucose reagent test strips are available for this purpose, it is clear that even in the best of

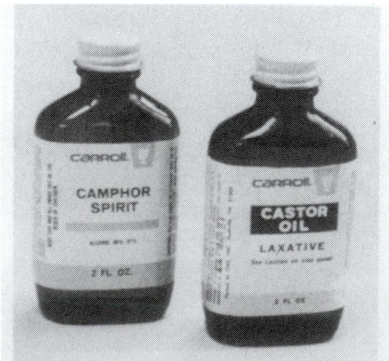

Figure CS–7 An example of look-alike camphor spirit and castor oil preparations. Camphorated oil is no longer available. Problems continually arise from other look-alike and sound-alike labeling or preparations.

studies sensitivity for detecting *numerical* hypoglycemia falls short of 100% (Lavery). Further confusion results from the realization that *clinical* hypoglycemia can exist in the absence of numerical hypoglycemia, especially in poorly controlled diabetic patients (Boyle).

Ultimately, we are left with the question of how to create a rational treatment strategy for patients with altered mental status. The majority of hypoglycemic patients do not present with focal findings, and most patients with ischemic cerebral vascular accidents (CVAs) do not present with coma. Those patients with ischemic CVAs who present with coma have either critical lesions which involve the reticular activating system or massive cerebral injury. Both of these events should have discernible associated findings and carry such poor prognoses that the added theoretical risk of giving dextrose seems minimal. It seems reasonable and safe to give dextrose to patients at either end of the altered mental status spectrum (mild confusion or disorientation and dense coma). When left with the small percentage of patients who have focality, it may be appropriate to use a glucose reagent test strip because this will confirm hypoglycemia in more than 90% of hypoglycemic patients.

By this reasoning, in a theoretical population of 1000 hypoglycemic patients, assuming a 10% incidence of focality (which seems high), 900 patients without focality should simply receive dextrose. Of the remaining 100 patients at least 90 would be correctly identified as hypoglycemic by reagent test strips. The remaining 10 patients (1%) are left to the clinician's perception of these issues.

It seems inappropriate to abandon the routine administration of $D_{50}W$ to patients with altered mental status. Simple reliance on reagent test strips may miss a significant percentage of patients with numerical hypoglycemia and an even greater percentage of patients with clinical hypoglycemia. It seems more logical to combine clinical and laboratory skills to modify the approach in a very small and select group of patients.

SUGGESTED READINGS

Chapter 3, Principles of Managing the Poisoned or Overdosed Patient: An Overview.

Chapter 31, Managing the Symptomatic Patient with a Possible Toxic Exposure.

Chapter 40, Antidiabetic and Hypoglycemic Agents.

Antidotes in Depth: Dextrose.

Boyle PJ, Schwartz NS, Shah SD, et al: Plasma glucose concentrations at the onset of hypoglycemic symptoms in patients with poorly controlled diabetes and in nondiabetics. N Engl J Med 1988;318: 1487–1492.

Browning RG, Olson DW, Stueven HA, Mateer JR: 50% dextrose: Antidote or toxin? Ann Emerg Med 1990;19:683–687.

Fischer KF, Lees JA, Newman JH: Hypoglycemia in hospitalized patients: Causes and outcomes. N Engl J Med 1986;315:1245–1250.

Lavery RF, Allegra JR, Cody RP, et al: A prospective evaluation of glucose reagent teststrips in the prehospital setting. Am J Emerg Med 1991;9:304–308.

Malouf R, Brust JC: Hypoglycemia: Causes, neurological manifestations, and outcome. Ann Neurol 1985;17:421–430.

Seibert DG: Reversible decerebrate posturing secondary to hypoglycemia. Am J Med 1985;78:1036–1037.

Wallis WE, Donaldson I, Scott RS, Wilson J: Hypoglycemia masquerading as cerebrovascular disease (hypoglycemic hemiplegia). Ann Neurol 1985;18:510–512.

Case 10

1. Although drug administration errors such as giving a drug to the wrong patient frequently occur in the care of adults and children, many poison center calls are generated by either prescribing or dispensing errors relating to the misuse of decimal points. Unfortunately, because many pediatric drugs require dose-per-kilogram calculations, mathematical errors can arise. This usually creates errors in factors of 10: the patient receives 10, 100, or 1000 times the dose required. There may be comparable errors of 1/10, 1/100, and so on that go unnoticed as toxicologic errors but are attributed to "therapeutic failures."

2. One of the more sensible approaches seems to be as follows: when ordering a drug write the dose, then in parentheses how the dose was calculated—5 mg of gentamicin (1 mg/kg). This would allow pharmacists and nurses to check the order easily. Also, when decimal points are required, they should always be preceded by 0(s)—.5 mg may get read as 5 mg; 0.5 mg is less likely to be misinterpreted. Another approach that may be safer is spelling out the dosage adjacent to the number such as "five milligrams" (5 mg) or "five tenths of one milligram" (0.5 mg).

3. Aminoglycoside ototoxicity and nephrotoxicity are both well described and appear to correlate better with trough than with peak levels. This may reflect saturation of drug uptake by these organs, limiting toxicity during peaks but allowing continual uptake during periods that trough levels remain elevated. Other risk factors seem to include advanced age, volume depletion, underlying renal disease, and concomitant use of nephrotoxic agents. In general, single overdoses of aminoglycosides are well tolerated and rarely cause toxicity in patients with normal renal function. In fact, most recommended dosing regimens for aminoglycosides involve large, extended-interval dosing to attain high peak levels and assure a prolonged trough. However, in the presence of renal impairment or repeated administration of excessive doses, significant toxicity may occur.

4. Although gentamicin can be removed by hemodialysis, this procedure is quite difficult in a small child. Complexation with ticarcillin or carbenicillin seems to be a safe and efficacious alternative to hemodialysis in adults. Forty-eight hours of ticarcillin therapy removed 50% more aminoglycoside by complexation than two 4-hour treatments of hemodialysis in the same period (Schentag). Consider exchange transfusion in neonates with renal failure in whom the aminoglycoside levels are predicted to remain toxic for more than 1 to 2 weeks.

This patient never developed renal impairment and was discharged from the hospital a few days later.

SUGGESTED READING

Chapter 46, Antibiotics.

Chapter 106, Pediatric Principles.

Chapter 117, Adverse Drug Events.

Cote CJ, Karl HW, Notterman DA, et al: Adverse sedation events in pediatrics: Analysis of medications used for sedation. Pediatrics 2000;106: 633–644.

Fisman DN, Kaye KM: Once-daily dosing of aminoglycoside antibiotics. Infect Dis Clin North Am 2000;14:475–487.

Lesar TS, Briceland L, Stein DS: Factors related to errors in medication prescribing. JAMA 1997;277:312–317.

Nelson LS, Gordon PE, Simmons MD, et al: The benefit of houseofficer education on proper medication dose calculation and ordering. Acad Emerg Med 2000;7:1311–1316.

Ross LM, Wallace J, Paton JY: Medication errors in a paediatric teaching hospital in the UK: five years operational experience. Arch Dis Child 2000;83:492–497.

Schentag JJ, Simons GW, Schultz RW, et al: Complexation versus hemodialysis to reduce elevated aminoglycoside serum concentrations. Pharmacotherapy 1984;4:374–380.

Case 11

1. The inadvertent infusion of 2 L of glycine solution (1.5 g/dL) into the peritoneal cavity produced findings similar to those of transurethral prostatectomy (TURP) syndrome, which occurs when large volumes of a glycine-containing solution are absorbed through the prostatic venous plexus. Toxicity is produced in two ways. The absorption of large volumes of low-osmolality (200 mOsm/L) hypotonic fluid produces a dilutional hyponatremia. This patient's sodium dropped from her previous concentration of 138 mEq/L to 117 mEq/L within 1 hour. In addition, in some patients, glycine (NH_2CH_2COOH) is metabolized to ammonia, resulting in as much as a 10-fold increase in ammonia concentrations. Coma, seizures, and transient blindness are described.

2. In the absence of life-threatening complications, and in the presence of normal renal function, fluid and electrolyte abnormalities rapidly correct. In patients with normal hepatic and renal function, ammonia metabolism also usually occurs rapidly. In the setting of life-threatening hyponatremia, patients can be treated with either diuresis (because this condition results from free water excess) or hypertonic (3%) saline if indicated.

This patient received rapid exchanges of peritoneal dialysis with a high-glucose-containing solution (which removes free water), and sodium correction occurred within 2 days. Her neurologic evaluation at the end of this time showed no deficits.

SUGGESTED READINGS

Chapter 24, Fluid, Electrolyte, and Acid–Base Principles.

Gravenstein D: Transurethral resection of the prostate (TURP) syndrome: A review of the pathophysiology and management. Anesth Analg. 1997;84:438–446.

Hahn RG: Blood ammonia concentrations resulting from absorption of irrigating fluid containing glycine and ethanol during transurethral resection of the prostate. Scand J Urol Nephrol 1991;25:115–119.

Hoekstra PT: Transurethral prostatic resection syndrome. J Urol 1983;130: 706–707.

Case 12

1. The differential diagnosis in this case is limited to three entities: lidocaine overdose, epinephrine overdose, or anaphylactic/anaphylactoid reactions. The development of systemic effects following lidocaine administration is dependent on both the dose delivered and the route of its administration. For this reason, a maximum dose of 3 mg/kg is usually recommended for IV administration. Because of slowed and incomplete absorption, subcutaneous (SC) doses can be increased to 3 to 5 mg/kg. The addition of small amounts of epinephrine to lidocaine further limits absorption, allowing for as much as 7 mg/kg of lidocaine to be safely infiltrated SC. Standard lidocaine with epinephrine solutions contain epinephrine in a 1:100,000 dilution, which means that 100 mL of anesthetic will contain 1.0 mg of epinephrine. The use of very large-dose subcutaneous lidocaine with epinephrine is currently advocated as a means of local anesthesia during tumescent liposuction. In this procedure, approximately 50 mg/kg of lidocaine plus epinephrine is infiltrated into the subcutaneous fat, and a trocar is repeatedly inserted to suction out the adipose tissue. Although this procedure exceeds the common dose limitations, the majority of the lidocaine is removed during the defatting process. However, deaths have been reported and appear to be caused by the excessive lidocaine dosing during this procedure. Lidocaine is absorbed orally but undergoes extensive first-pass hepatic metabolism.

True allergy to any local anesthetic is uncommon, accounting for only 1 to 2% of all adverse reactions to these agents. Allergy to the ester group of agents (which were not administered in this case) is more common than to the amides because of the allergenic metabolite *para*-aminobenzoic acid (PABA), which is formed from the degradation of these compounds. In addition, several common manifestations of severe allergic reactions (urticaria, angioedema, and bronchospasm) were absent. Lidocaine is an amide, as are bupivacaine, prilocaine, and etidocaine and mepivacaine. In general, patients with a known allergy to an ester should be given an amide, whereas patients allergic to an amide may receive another amide or an ester. One easy way to recall which group these agents belong to is to note their spellings. Common amides are spelled with two *i*'s, whereas common esters (cocaine, tetracaine, procaine, chloroprocaine) have only a single *i* (see Table 55–1).

This child received a total of 40 mL of 2% lidocaine. The term 2% means that 2 g of lidocaine are in every 100 mL of solution, or 20 mg of lidocaine are in every milliliter of solution. Thus, the total dose given was 800 mg in a 30-kg child, or about 27 mg/kg. This dose exceeds the suggested recommendation.

2. The major manifestations of lidocaine toxicity are limited to two end organs, the CNS and the heart. When the serum lidocaine concentration slowly increases, as during infusion or following subcutaneous overdose, CNS toxicity manifests initially as agitation, lightheadedness, muscle twitching, or anxiety. This can be followed by seizure activity. Higher levels or rapidly rising levels, as following bolus administration, produce CNS depression, seizure, and apnea. Cardiovascular toxicity is always preceded by CNS signs. Mild cardiovascular toxicity includes tachycardia and hypertension. More severe manifestations include hypotension, bradycardia, and eventual cardiovascular collapse.

Continuous infusion, old age, congestive heart failure, and hepatic dysfunction all enhance the potential for toxicity in that metabolism is impaired. When inadvertently injected IV, the presence of epinephrine may exacerbate both CNS and cardiovascular toxicity. Three hundred milligrams of lidocaine or 30 mL of a 1% solution with 1:100,000 epinephrine would also contain 0.3 mg of epinephrine. When given by rapid IV bolus, this dose of epinephrine might independently induce dysrhythmias. In animal models, acidemia and hypoxia enhance cardiac toxicity. As both acidemia and hypoxia commonly result from seizures, this helps explain why CNS toxicity often precedes cardiovascular toxicity and emphasizes the need for rapid control of both seizure activity and ventilation.

3. Because lidocaine has a very short distribution half-life (about 8 minutes), most patients with bolus lidocaine manifest transient toxicity. Thus, the goal should be to terminate seizure activity while maintaining oxygenation and perfusion (cardiopulmonary resusitation [CPR]). In general, a benzodiazepine is an adequate first choice for seizures, followed by a rapid-acting barbiturate, as illustrated in this case. Sodium channel blocking agents (such as the type IA and IC antidysrhythmic agents) should be avoided, and although sodium bicarbonate may be a theoretically attractive antidote, its role remains undefined. Although patients are reported to survive massive overdoses of lidocaine with the use of pacemakers and cardiopulmonary bypass (Noble), these techniques are usually not indicated because of lidocaine's short duration of toxicity. Sustained external chest compression, allowing time for drug distribution and metabolism, may be needed for asystolic patients. This approach must be distinguished from that necessary for other, longer-acting local anesthetics (eg, bupivacaine), where cardiopulmonary bypass may be considered the treatment of choice for patients with severe poisoning.

4. In general, lidocaine concentrations correlate quite well with toxicity. Therapeutic IV administration (ie, for dysrhythmia suppression) typically produces concentrations on the order of 1.5 to 3.5 mg/mL, and periodic measurement is important to prevent toxicity. Minor CNS symptoms often occur at 4 to 5 mg/mL, and seizures appear at concentrations above 8 to 10 mg/mL. Higher values are associated with coma, apnea, and cardiovascular collapse. Although useful for therapeutic drug monitoring, determination of serum lidocaine concentrations has little clinical utility in patients with acute overdose other than to document the exposure.

SUGGESTED READINGS

Chapter 52, Antidysrhythmic Agents.

Chapter 53, Inhalational Anesthetics.

De Jong RH, Ronfeld RA, De Rosa RA: Cardiovascular effect of convulsant and supraconvulsant doses of amide local anesthetics. Anesth Analg 1982;61:3–9.

Finkelstein F, Kreeft J: Massive lidocaine poisoning [letter]. N Engl J Med 1979;310:50.

Noble J, Kennedy DJ, Latimer RD, et al: Massive lignocaine overdose during cardiopulmonary bypass: Successful treatment with cardiac pacing. Br J Anaesth 1984;56:1439–1441.

Rao RB, Ely SF, Hoffman RS: Deaths related to liposuction. N Engl J Med 1999;340:1471–1475.

Thomas RD, Behbehani MM, Coyle DE, Denson DD: Cardiovascular toxicity of local anesthetics. Anesth Analg 1986;65:444–450.

Case 13

1. The presence of deep coma, apnea, intact corneal reflexes, and a nonfocal neurologic examination suggests a toxic-metabolic cause of coma. The overall constellation of signs and symptoms—CNS and respiratory depression, sweet odor, ventricular irritability, hypotension, and delayed liver toxicity—is highly suggestive of intoxication with a chlorinated hydrocarbon. In any case, an assessment of the patient's serum glucose, oxygen saturation, electrocardiogram, and, based on the circumstances, a carboxyhemoglobin level, should be part of his initial management.

In fact, the history (obtained retrospectively) was that this dentist had ingested a bottle of chloroform he used for cleaning his instruments.

Chloroform ($CHCl_3$) was first used as an anesthetic agent in 1847. The first death from chloroform anesthesia, secondary to respiratory depression in a healthy 15-year-old, was reported in 1848. Chloroform was used extensively throughout the 20th century, but its use was eventually discontinued because of its potential for cardiovascular and hepatic toxicity as well as its carcinogenicity. Other chlorinated hydrocarbons, such as carbon tetrachloride or perchlorethylene, produce similar clinical effects.

2. Chloroform produces hypotension by two mechanisms: direct myocardial depression and loss of vasomotor tone. Also, like the other halogenated hydrocarbons, chloroform sensitizes the myocardium to both endogenous and exogenous catecholamines. Thus, ventricular dysrhythmias occur either spontaneously or consequent to the use of a catecholamine (eg, dopamine, as in this case) to treat chloroform-induced hypotension.

Chloroform produces fatty infiltration and centrilobular necrosis of the liver similar to that produced by carbon tetrachloride. The mechanism of hepatotoxicity is thought to resemble acetaminophen hepatotoxicity in that the production of a toxic metabolite by the cytochrome P450 system is required before the onset of toxicity. Numerous studies using P450 inhibitors and inducers have confirmed this association. As with the case of acetaminophen poisoning, a potential role for glutathione depletion is described. Similarly, abnormalities in liver enzymes peak at 72 to 96 hours after a chloroform exposure.

3. In addition to the history and physical examination, chloroform concentrations can be obtained and do correlate with toxicity. However, most laboratories cannot perform this assay in the time required for the results to be clinically relevant. Also, when blood specimens are allowed to sit, even in sealed tubes, the chloroform goes into the gaseous space (ie, head space) above the blood. Thus, analysis of blood alone, without a specimen of the gas above it, may be misleading. A useful clinical pearl is that many halogenated hydrocarbons are radiopaque. Thus, the presence of "contrast material" in the gastrointestinal tract may be noted, or the upright abdominal radiograph may show a "double-bubble sign," representing the interfaces between air and gastric contents and hydrocarbon and gastric contents.

4. Although gastrointestinal decontamination is probably indicated after chloroform ingestion, the toxin is rapidly absorbed, and the utility of decontamination would be expected to be limited with delayed presentations. Activated charcoal is of limited value in patients with isolated chloroform ingestions. Good supportive care consisting of airway management and hemodynamic support is the mainstay of initial therapy. Catecholamines should be used with extreme caution because of the risk of inducing malignant dysrhythmias. There may be a theoretical benefit from the use of P450 inhibitors (eg, cimetidine), *N*-acetylcysteine, and hyperbaric oxygen alone and in combination with each other.

Reported ingestions are rare. In 1859, Dr. Glover (a chloroform expert) ingested about 5 oz. He was incoherent, pale, and diaphoretic and subsequently became comatose and died. In 1903 there were 47 cases with 19 fatalities reported, many from delayed hepatotoxicity.

SUGGESTED READINGS

Chapter 8, Diagnostic Imaging in Toxicology.

Chapter 14, Hepatic Principles.

Chapter 21, Cardiovascular Principles.

Chapter 86, Hydrocarbons.

Dally S, Garnier R, Bismuth C: Diagnosis of chlorinated hydrocarbon poisoning by x-ray examination. BMJ 1987;44:424–425.

Ekstrom T, Hogberg J: Chloroform-induced glutathione depletion and toxicity in freshly isolated hepatocytes. Biochem Pharmacol 1980;29:3059–3065.

Piersol GM: Fatal poisoning following the ingestion of chloroform. Med Clin North Am 1933;17:587–601.

Schroeder HG: Acute and delayed chloroform poisoning. Br J Anesth 1965;37:972–975.

Sipes RG, Krishna G, Gillette JR: Bioactivation of carbon tetrachloride, chloroform and bromotrichloromethane: Role of cytochrome P450. Life Sci 1977;20:1541–1548.

Thorpe CM, Spence AA: Clinical evidence for delayed chloroform poisoning. Br J Anaesth 1997;79:402–409.

Case 14

1. The patient's history is both typical and atypical for venomous snakebites. Snakes are poikilothermic, which means that their body temperature conforms to that of their environment. Cool weather reduces a snake's activity and makes snakebite very uncommon in the nonsummer months in the United States (Parrish). Most unintentional snakebites occur on the foot and ankle as a snake is startled by a victim; bites on the hand occur most commonly when the victim is attempting to handle a snake. This patient's bite on his hand is, however, consistent with his story. Snakebites are more common in male patients, accounting for 90% of bite victims in some studies. As in the case of most injuries, snakebites are commonly associated with ethanol use by the victim. This patient did not appear intoxicated.

The description of this patient's wound leaves little doubt as to its origin. Few animals produce the characteristic fang marks associated with snakebite. Of indigenous United States snakes, only the pit vipers (ie, Crotalinae subfamily or Crotalidae family) have fangs capable of producing these marks (see Fig. 101–1). The slow drainage of bloody fluid from the wound and the extremely rapid progression of the swelling to involve the proximal arm are consistent with envenomation by a native Crotaline species (see Table 101–2).

However, not all snakebites that occur in the United States are done by indigenous snakes. Importers and collectors of venomous snakes continually attempt to illegally import such animals for use as culinary delicacies, medicinal agents, and religious symbols as well as for other personal reasons. Because the variety and clinical toxicity of venomous snakes worldwide are extensive, and exotic snakebite wounds are often indistinguishable from those of native US snakes, the possibility that this patient was envenomated by an exotic snake is significant.

2. The clinical presentation of patients bitten by North American pit vipers includes both local and systemic effects. Local tissue necrosis and skin sloughing account for the major morbidity. The most pronounced systemic effects of North American Crotaline venoms are hematologic and include coagulopathy and thrombocytopenia. Although these hematologic effects may be associated with hemorrhage, this remains uncommon despite dramatic laboratory abnormalities. The Mojave rattlesnake is unique among North American Crotalines in that its venom is neurotoxic, and its victims may die from respiratory muscle paralysis.

The tissue effects of Crotaline venom are caused by several histotoxic components including hyaluronidase, collagenase, and metalloproteinase. These compounds directly damage tissue and produce localized swelling by initiating a cascade of proinflammatory mediators. The degree and rate of progression of the swelling are broadly related to the envenoming species of Crotaline. For example, copperhead bites *(A. contortrix)* typically produce only mild tissue effects, whereas the venom of true rattlesnakes (eg, *C. durrissus*) is more aggressive (exceptions abound, however).

3. Although tissue necrosis from Crotaline envenomation is painful and disfiguring, there is currently no suitable treatment other than impeccable wound care and, occasionally, antivenom. Functional impairment following healing is uncommon, however, and limb loss is even less so. The development of compartment syndrome, nevertheless, substantially increases the risk of disability or limb loss. A compartment syndrome results from increased pressure within the unexpandable spaces confined by the fascia of limbs. The skin surrounding the involved compartment is tense and warm, and the patients suffer severe pain in the affected part. Vascular compromise to the distal extremity and its sequelae are the major morbidities associated with compartment syndrome. The presence of a compartment syndrome is confirmed by direct measurement of the compartment pressures using a percutaneous needle apparatus. Although the clinical findings associated with Crotaline snakebite resemble those of a compartment syndrome, the compartment pressures of snakebite victims generally remain normal or are only slightly elevated (Mars). Because the fangs of most North American Crotalines are typically not long enough to enter these relatively deep spaces, the venom is typically deposited in the subcutaneous tissue. Thus, direct pressure measurement is critical before surgical compartment decompression is attempted.

Several authors still recommend the routine use of surgical compartment release, or fasciotomy, for the majority of snakebite victims with extremity swelling (Glass). However, there are little experimental or clinical data to support this practice (Russell). Subcutaneous injections of rattlesnake venom into the hind limbs of dogs did not produce elevated compartment pressures, whereas direct injection into the compartment was associated with dramatic elevations (Garfin). No appropriate controlled clinical study evaluating the need for or benefit of fasciotomy has been performed to date. In fact, most of the literature concerning routine fasciotomy is published as personal commentaries or uncontrolled case series. For these reasons, most toxicologists question the need for empiric fasciotomy, although it seems reasonable to perform a fasciotomy if the pressures are documented to be dangerously elevated (Roberts). Furthermore, there are both experimental (Garfin) and clinical evidence (Tunget-Johnson) that the early initiation of appropriate antivenom therapy may be beneficial. CroFab, an antibody fragment, may ultimately replace the Wyeth Polyvalent Crotalid antivenin and it is likely that this new agent will prove as beneficial as the current. Because fasciotomy is disfiguring and perhaps detrimental (Stewart), it seems reasonable to attempt a trial of antivenom before fasciotomy. The consequences of a delay to fasciotomy are unknown, but a window of several hours certainly exists before irreversible ischemic damage occurs.

The patient was unwavering in his account of the event despite the clinician's persistent concern as to the dubious nature of the patient's history. Elevated compartment pressures of 50 mm Hg were identified by direct measurement in the patient's hand and arm. Because the envenomating species was unknown but likely a member of the pit viper subfamily, and because the swelling was extensive, five vials of Polyvalent Crotalid Antivenin (Wyeth) were empirically administered. Because this antivenom has unknown, if any, utility against snakebites other than North American pit vipers, a fasciotomy was performed to relieve the elevated compartment pressures. Had the antibody fragment formulation been available, that would have been a suitable substitute, although substantially higher in cost for the drug (though perhaps less costly in overall costs). Two days after surgery, following coaxing by his son, the patient admitted that he was a purveyor of snakes for their meat. He acknowledged that his bite was inflicted at his home by a Western Diamondback rattlesnake (C. atrox). This is the largest of the North American Crotaline species and one of the few whose fangs are capable of entering the deep fascial compartments. Thus, both antivenom and probably fasciotomy were appropriate.

SUGGESTED READINGS

Chapter 101, Snakes and Other Reptiles.

Antidote in depth: Antivenom (Crotaline and Elapid).

Garfin SR, Castilonia RR, Mubarak SJ, et al: Rattlesnake bites and surgical decompression: Results using a laboratory model. Toxicon 1984; 22:177–182.

Glass TG: Early debridement in pit viper bites. JAMA 1976;235: 2513–2516.

Mars M, Hadley GP, Aitchison JM: Direct intracompartmental pressure measurement in the management of snakebites in children. S Afr Med J 1991;80:227–228.

Parrish HM, Carr CA: Bites by copperheads *(Ancistrodon contortrix)* in the United States. JAMA 1967;201:927–932.

Roberts RS, Csencsitz TA, Heard CW: Upper extremity compartment syndromes following pit viper envenomation. Clin Orthop 1985;193: 184–188.

Rosen PB, Leiva JI, Ross CP: Delayed antivenom treatment for a patient after envenomation by *Crotalus atrox*. Ann Emerg Med. 2000;35(1): 86–88.

Russell FE, Carlson RW, Wainschel J, Osborne AH. Snake venom poisoning in the United States: Experience with 550 cases. JAMA 1975;233: 341–344.

Stewart RM, Page CP, Schwesinger WH, et al: Antivenin and fasciotomy/debridement in the treatment of severe rattlesnake bites. Am J Surg 1989;158:543–547.

Tunget-Johnson CL, Pearigen PD, McDermott MJ, Gillingham BL: Resolution of elevated compartment pressures after rattlesnake envenomation with antivenin [abstract]. J Toxicol Clin Toxicol 1998;36: 458–459.

Case 15

1. Cardiac glycosides contain a group of C_{23} or C_{24} steroidal glycosides, found in both the plant and animal kingdoms. In animals, cardiac glycosides are limited to a few toad species, such as *Bufo marinus,* and in the plant kingdom most are found in the angiosperms. Foxglove *(Digitalis purpurea)* is the source of digoxin

and digitoxin. Many other plants contain cardiac glycosides, including Oleander *(Nerium oleander,* containing oleandrin and digitalinum), lily-of-the-valley *(Convallaria majalis,* containing convallatoxin), and red squill *(Urginea maritima,* which contains scilliroside). In this case, dogbane *(Apocynum cannabinum)* is known to contain the cardiac glycoside strophanthidin. The plant that the patient consumed is shown in Fig. CS–8.

2. Few cases of toxicity from glycosides other than digitalis have been reported, and most seem to follow a fairly consistent pattern. Vomiting is usually the initial complaint, occurring within minutes to hours of ingestion. Diaphoresis is often noted. Patients rapidly progress to a variety of bradydysrhythmias (especially high degrees of heart block) and/or ventricular tachydysrhythmias or ventricular fibrillation.

3. The only fairly consistent laboratory abnormality is an elevated serum potassium, which marks the degree of poisoning of the Na^+-K^+-ATPase pump by the drug. When potassium cannot be pumped back into cells during repolarization, its serum concentration rises. Thus, in the presence of acute digoxin poisoning, potassium serves as an excellent predictor of severity. In one series of cases of digoxin toxicity, a serum potassium concentration greater than 5.5 mEq/L (in the absence of hemolysis or renal failure) was *always* associated with fatality, whereas a potassium concentration less than 5.0 mEq/L was *always* associated with survival (Bismuth). Note that these data were obtained before the use of digoxin-specific Fab and that the outcome with this therapy is improved. Although it is unclear whether these criteria apply to ingestions of other cardiac glycosides, an elevated potassium concentration in these patients should be of concern as well. In reported cases of severe oleander poisoning, one patient had a normal potassium, and in the other it was elevated (Haynes; Shumaik).

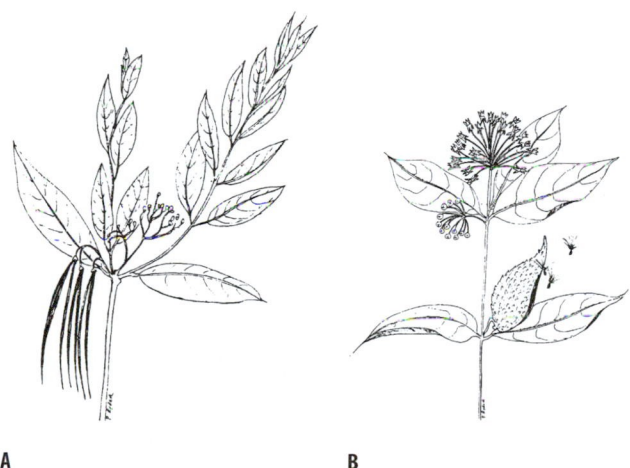

A **B**

Figure CS–8 Line drawings of the two plants in question. **A.** *Apocynum cannabinum,* commonly known as dogbane. **B.** *Asclepias speciosa,* commonly known as milkweed. *(Drawings courtesy of Pamela Ryder, Nurse Practitioner.)*

4. Diagnosis always begins with a history of exposure. The regional poison center or the botanic gardens may be helpful for species identification and determination of cardiac glycoside content. The ECG and serum potassium concentration may help define the extent of toxicity. Finally, a serum digoxin concentration should be obtained; if it is positive, at least three possibilities should be considered: the patient is taking digoxin, an endogenous digoxinlike immunoreactive substance (DLIS) is present, or a cardiac glycoside that cross-reacts with the digoxin assay is present. Although neonates, patients with renal failure, and pregnant women have measurable DLISs, these substances are not associated with toxicity. Also, with DLISs, digoxin concentrations rarely exceed 1 to 2 ng/mL. We assume that many (if not most) cardiac glycosides will cross-react with conventional digoxin assays, but it is unclear to what extent and what the implications of a particular concentration would be. Currently, a positive digoxin concentration serves only to confirm the exposure to a cardiac glycoside. Unfortunately, a negative digoxin concentration, particularly with highly specific digoxin assays, does not exclude the possibility of cardiac glycoside exposure.

5. Routine initial methods of gastrointestinal decontamination should be attempted. Specific treatment should be based on clinical symptoms, ECG abnormalities, and, possibly, serum potassium concentration. As in this case, digoxin-specific Fab has been used successfully to treat toxicity from other cardiac glycosides (Brubacher; Clark; Shumaik). Because these Fab are very specific for digoxin, the extent of their cross-reactivity with other cardiac glycosides is unknown. It is reasonable to begin with 5 to 10 vials of Digibind and administer additional doses liberally because an animal model suggests that larger doses of Fab may be required for nondigoxin cardiac glycosides (Clark). After ingestion of a nondigoxin cardiac glycoside, the "apparent" serum digoxin concentration should not be used to guide the dose of Fab, as different values may be achieved with different assays and the relative affinity of the Fab has not be defined. Thus, all Fab dosing in patients with nondigoxin cardiac glycoside poisoning should be determined on empiric grounds.

The bradycardia and heart block were suggestive of cardiac glycoside toxicity. Repeat serum electrolytes were within normal limits, but a serum digoxin concentration was reported as 4.61 ng/mL. The patient was given five vials of digoxin-specific Fab (Digibind) and had rapid resolution of ECG abnormalities. After the Digibind was administered, her digoxin concentration was reported to be 180 ng/mL. Consultation with a botanist identified the plant as a member of the dogbane family (Apocynum cannabinum).

SUGGESTED READINGS

Chapter 48, Cardiac Glycosides.
Antidotes in Depth: Digoxin-Specific Antibody Fragments (Fab).
Chapter 78, Plants.
Bismuth C, Gaultier M, Conso F, et al: Hyperkalemia in acute digitalis poisoning: Prognostic significance and therapeutic implications. Clin Toxicol 1973;6:153–162.
Brubacher J, Bruno R, Kaplan L, et al: Cross reactivity of monoclonal digoxin assays with cardioactive steroids. J Toxicol Clin Toxicol 1996;34:628.
Brubacher JR, Hoffman RS, Kile T: Toad venom poisoning: Failure of a monoclonal digoxin immunoassay to cross-react with the cardioactive steroids. J Toxicol Clin Toxicol 1996;34:529–530.
Brubacher JR, Ravikumar PR, Bania T, et al: Treatment of toad venom poisoning with digoxin-specific Fab fragments. Chest 1996;110:1282–1288.
Clark RF, Selden BS, Curry SC: Digoxin-specific Fab fragments in the treatment of oleander toxicity in a canine model. Ann Emerg Med 1991;20:1073–1077.
Eddleston M, Rajapakse S, Rajakanthan, et al: Anti-digoxin Fab fragments in cardiotoxicity induced by ingestion of yellow oleander: a randomised controlled trial. Lancet 2000;355:967–972.
Shumaik GM, Wu AU, Ping AC: Oleander poisoning: Treatment with digoxin-specific Fab antibody fragments. Ann Emerg Med 1988;17:732–735.

Case 16

1. The spectrum of substances that are available in laboratories is extensive and depends on the type of research that is performed in the laboratory. The class of substances most commonly implicated in such poisoning are the organic solvents such as methanol. Other widely available poisons include metal salts, cyanide, detergents, acids, and alkali. This unfortunate student drank a solution containing sodium azide (NaN_3), a potent cellular poison occasionally added to buffered solutions as an antimicrobial agent. Sodium azide also reacts violently with water to generate nitrogen gas. Its most common use today is for inflating automobile airbags.

2. Sodium azide is a direct vasodilator, producing dizziness and syncope shortly after large exposures. In addition, azide can interfere with mitochondrial phosphorylation, cytochrome oxidase, and several other enzyme systems in a manner that is poorly understood but thought to be similar to the mechanisms of cyanide toxicity (refer to Fig. 13–2). Large ingestions result in the rapid onset of gastrointestinal symptoms, hypotension, and seizures, with progression to multiorgan system failure over hours to days. With smaller ingestions, however, initial symptoms may be delayed for several hours.

The toxin is extremely potent, with immediate symptoms reported from ingestions of 40 to 80 mg. The human LD_{50} has been estimated at 35 mg/kg. Death is common with ingestions of gram amounts.

3. Because of the significant mortality associated with sodium azide ingestions, aggressive gastrointestinal decontamination with lavage and activated charcoal is indicated. Some clinicians have performed hemodialysis, with little success. Others have suggested the administration of the available cyanide antidote kit, containing sodium nitrite and sodium thiosulfate, because of a similarity between cyanide and sodium azide. However, experience with this therapy is largely unsuccessful. At present, supportive therapy seems to be all that can be offered.

4. When sodium azide is mixed with acids, hydrazoic acid (HN_3) is liberated. This volatile compound has the same toxicity as sodium azide. Thus, when exposed to the hydrazoic acid gas from the stomach (where sodium azide has combined with stomach acid) following regurgitation, belching, or insertion of nasogastric or orogastric tubes, rescuers and emergency medical staff have been reported to develop symptoms consistent with sodium azide toxicity (Senecal). Adequate ventilation and awareness of this problem are required for all healthcare workers.

SUGGESTED READINGS

Chapter 98, Cyanide and Hydrogen Sulfide.

Antidotes in Depth: Cyanide Antidotes.

Emmett EA, Ricking JA: Fatal self-administration of sodium azide. Ann Intern Med 1975;83:224–226.

Klein-Schwartz W, Gorman RL, Oderda GM, et al: Three fatal sodium azide poisonings. Med Toxicol Adverse Drug Exp 1989;4:219–227.

Senecal PE, Dyer JE, Osterloh JD, Olson KR: Toxic volatile hydrazoic acid (HN₃) from contact of sodium azide (NaN₃) with acids. Vet Hum Toxicol 1991;33:364.

Trout D, Esswein EJ, Hales T, et al: Exposures and health effects: an evaluation of workers at a sodium azide production plant. Am J Indust Med 1996;30:343–350.

Case 17

1. The patient had a significant metabolic alkalosis. The most common causes for this include protracted vomiting and nasogastric suctioning, diuretics, dehydration, and exogenous base administration (see Table 24–5). The patient's history excluded vomiting and nasogastric suctioning. In addition, the elevated BUN suggested that the mechanism was a contraction alkalosis, eliminating exogenous base administration from the diagnosis.

2. The classic toxin-induced gout is saturnine gout, resulting from lead poisoning. Gout is also reported with diuretic use. Arthritic syndromes may result from drug-induced lupuslike syndromes (etiologies: procainamide and hydralazine) and immune complex phenomena (eg, serum sickness following snake or spider antivenom administration). Multiple other agents, such as gold salt therapy, are associated with arthralgias. The most likely diagnosis in this case is diuretic abuse. Although diuretic-induced gout is uncommon, diuretic use and abuse are common causes of contraction alkalosis.

Further questioning revealed that the patient had a long history of self-administration of furosemide (as much as 400 mg/day) for what she described as bloating.

3. Excessive diuresis may also produce volume depletion, which manifested in this case as orthostatic hypotension, increased blood viscosity, and altered drug pharmacokinetics. Excessive use may also result in abnormalities of sodium, potassium (ie, hypokalemia), or calcium and vitamin deficiency, particularly from loss of thiamine, folate, or ascorbic acid.

4. The only therapy required was rehydration, discontinuation of the diuretic, and patient counseling. The first two are the easiest, but the latter is often refractory to psychiatric counseling. Ultimately her uric acid returned to normal, and she had no further episodes of gout.

SUGGESTED READINGS

Chapter 24, Fluid, Electrolyte, and Acid–Base Principles.

Chapter 80, Lead.

Constant J: Pearls and pitfalls in the use and abuse of diuretics for chronic congestive heart failure. Cardiology 1999;92:156–161.

Prichard BN, Owens CW, Woolf AS: Adverse reaction to diuretics. Eur Heart J 1992;13(Suppl G):96–103.

Scott JT, Higgens CS: Diuretic induced gout: a multifactorial condition. Ann Rheum Dis 1992;51:259–261.

Case 18

1. Colchicine is an alkaloid commonly derived from two plants: the autumn crocus *(Colchicum autumnale)* and the glory lily *(Gloriosa superba)*. Despite its long history of use as a poison and its well-appreciated gastrointestinal side effects, it is still used for the treatment of acute gout; for prophylaxis in gout, familial Mediterranean fever, amyloidosis, and biliary cirrhosis; and in certain dermatologic disorders. Tablets are available in 0.5 mg and 0.6 mg strengths as well as in an intravenous preparation (0.5 mg/mL). The maximum intravenous dose for patients with acute gouty arthritis is 4 mg.

The drug binds to intracelluar microtubules and prevents their polymerization. Because polymerization is most importantly involved in cell division, metaphase arrest occurs. Although this does not destroy the cells themselves, it prevents cellular multiplication and tissue renewal. Those cells with the highest rate of propagation, such as the gastrointestinal mucosal cells, are affected earliest and most severely. Cells that require microtubular function for other purposes, such as axons and cardiac conductive tissue, in which microtubules transport nutrients and organelles, manifest delayed dysfunction. This mechanism of action and much of the clinical toxicity of colchicine are shared by the vinca alkaloids, podophyllotoxin, and griseofulvin.

2. The initial manifestations of colchicine toxicity invariably include gastrointestinal symptoms. In fact, approximately 80% of patients taking therapeutic doses of colchicine have gastrointestinal complaints. Nausea, vomiting, and diarrhea may be so severe as to cause hemodynamic compromise. Abnormalities of the peripheral smear such as leukocytosis and the presence of immature forms may also be noted. This reflects interference with cell division and release of progenitor cells.

The second phase occurs 2 to 7 days after ingestion and may consist of sudden cardiac death. This can occur without warning, even after a period of many hours during which the patient appears clinically well. The presumed mechanism is a lack of myocardial cellular energy from impaired microtubule function. Myelosuppression, presenting as leukopenia or its sequelae, is common following severe poisoning. Over the subsequent week, if the patients survive, they may develop alopecia, rebound leukocytosis, and myoneuropathy.

Following single acute ingestions of colchicine, excellent prognostic criteria are available. In one study, patients with ingestions less than 0.5 mg/kg suffered at most gastrointestinal distress, whereas those who ingested between 0.5 and 0.8 mg/kg frequently developed myelosuppression and had a 10% fatality rate (Gaultier). In the same study, those who ingested more than 0.8 mg/kg died of cardiovascular collapse within about 72 hours of their ingestion. Those who do not manifest gastrointestinal symptoms by 12 hours are unlikely to develop consequential poisoning.

3. Patients who ingest colchicine require aggressive gastrointestinal decontamination including orogastric lavage (if early) and multiple-dose activated charcoal. Volume resuscitation is required to prevent hemodynamic compromise and maintain renal perfusion to improve elimination; about 20% of the drug is normally

eliminated unchanged in the urine. The remainder undergoes hepatic deacetylation followed by biliary elimination. Supportive care and intensive care unit observation are required during the second phase of toxicity.

Colchicine has a moderately large volume of distribution (2.2 L/kg) and is about 50% protein bound. These factors limit any potential role for hemodialysis. Similarly, exchange transfusion and peritoneal dialysis have been used without success. Although hemoperfusion may be more effective at removing colchicine from the blood, data on its clinical efficacy are lacking.

This patient was morbidly obese, so her 50- to 60-mg ingestion was less than 0.8 mg/kg. Her hospital course was complicated by worsening renal insufficiency (creatinine rose to 8.0 mg/dL), but she was ultimately discharged in a stable medical condition.

4. The use of granulocyte colony-stimulating factor (GCSF) may speed the return of bone marrow function, thus reducing the likelihood of sepsis. Without its use, return of bone marrow function, if possible, generally occurs over 1 to 2 weeks. In France, anticolchicine antibodies were successful in a patient with severe poisoning who survived despite presenting in cardiogenic shock 36 hours after a 60-mg (0.96 mg/kg) colchicine ingestion (Baud). This goat-derived antibody preparation is not available in the United States.

SUGGESTED READINGS

Chapter 47, Antineoplastic Agents.

Baud FJ, Sabouraud A, Vicaut E, et al: Brief report: Treatment of severe colchicine overdose with colchicine-specific Fab fragments. N Engl J Med 1995;339:642–645.

Bismuth C, Gaultier M, Canso F: Aplasie medullaire après intoxication aigue à la colchicine. Nouv Presse Med 1977;6:1625–1629.

Gaultier M, Kanfer A, Bismuth C, et al: Données actuelles sur l'intoxication par la colchicine à propos de 23 observations. Ann Med Interne 1969;192:605–617.

Harris R, Marx G, Gillett M, et al: Colchicine-induced bone marrow suppression: Treatment with granulocyte colony-stimulating factor. J Emerg Med 2000;18:435–440.

Case 19

1. "Body packers" typically fast for 1 to 2 days and then ingest illicit drugs that are wrapped and sealed in condoms, plastic wrap, aluminum foil, or a variety of other materials with the intention of international smuggling. The body packer, also known as a mule or courier, often takes an agent to retard bowel function (such as loperamide) for the duration of the airplane flight. When they arrive at their destination, they pass the packets (sometimes with the assistance of enemas or cathartics) and deliver them to their final destination. Although most body packers likely know the quantity of packets they ingested, they may not be forthcoming with information. Although the true prevalence of body packing is undefined, 28 body packers were caught in 1 month in a busy airport (Lancashire).

The most concerning complication of body packing is drug toxicity if the contents leak from one or more packages. The most commonly involved substances are heroin or cocaine, but other substances including methylenedioxymethamphetamine (MDMA), phencyclidine, or marijuana may be implicated. Cocaine is the drug of greatest risk to the patient because of its high lethality in overdose and the lack of a truly effective antidote (as with naloxone when heroin is the contraband). Body packers may also develop symptoms of mechanical bowel obstruction. Packets may occasionally be inserted rectally or vaginally; drug absorption may occur through these mucosal surfaces.

The clinical findings in this patient suggested opioid poisoning.

2. Immediate therapy in this case consisted of a large bolus (2–10 mg) of naloxone IV, which confirmed opioid intoxication and reversed the CNS and respiratory depression. This should be followed with a continuous naloxone infusion at about two-thirds of the arousal dose and titrated to clinical response. The risk of withdrawal is minimal because the likelihood of preexisting opioid dependence in a mule is unlikely. In patients with cocaine poisoning, aggressive administration of benzodiazepines, external cooling, and immediate surgical removal of the remaining packets is indicated.

3. The possibility of body packing must be considered in patients with symptoms of cocaine or heroin poisoning or bowel obstruction who have recently arrived in the United States from other countries, particularly from South America. The plain abdominal radiograph is frequently positive but may be negative even in patients with a substantial number of packets (Hoffman; McCarron) (see Fig. 8–8). Determining the content of the packages in symptomatic patients is based on the history and physical examination. In asymptomatic patients, urine drug screening is frequently helpful, presumably because of either subclinical leakage or exposure at the initial location (as mentioned, personal drug use is unlikely).

4. We have developed the following algorithm for handling the problem (see Fig. 67–3). Mechanical obstruction is an indication for surgery because conservative therapy may allow time for packet rupture. Cocaine intoxication is also an indication for immediate operative removal of the contraband. Patients frequently require gastrotomy, enterotomy to clear the small bowel, and colostomy after clearing the large bowel. The rationale for immediate surgery with cocaine intoxication is based on the assumption that each packet contains many times the LD_{50} of cocaine.

Patients with symptomatic heroin poisoning should be treated with high-dose naloxone therapy. These patients and those who are asymptomatic following either cocaine or heroin ingestions should receive both activated charcoal and whole-bowel irrigation (WBI) with polyethylene glycol electrolyte lavage solution (PEG-ELS; Colyte or Golytely). The PEG-ELS is given by mouth or nasogastric tube at 2 L/h until the rectal effluent is clear. Activated charcoal can be given intermittently during the infusion as desired. If packets are visible, serial abdominal radiographs should be followed for both clearing of packets and the development of intestinal obstruction. As mentioned, surgery is indicated if obstruction occurs or symptoms of cocaine intoxication develop.

Other authors have suggested the use of bulk laxatives and mineral oil (Caruana; McCarron). The patient is then observed until the stool becomes free of packets. We believe these strategies are inadequate. Bulk laxatives and mineral oil act slowly, necessitating that patients remain in the ICU for many days. Of greater concern, dissolution of the plastic packaging by mineral oil has been reported. We find that WBI is safe and well tolerated and clears the gastrointestinal tract more rapidly than these other techniques, an effect that is presumably beneficial. In addition, WBI facilitates contrast radiography, and it may help prepare the bowel if emergent surgery is required.

The endpoint of therapy remains controversial. Observation for "packet-free" bowel movements is unsatisfactory because packets may get "hung up" during passage through the gastrointestinal tract. Similarly, the endpoint of therapy cannot be a negative plain radiograph because even large numbers of packets may not be visualized. Therefore, we recommend that a complete gastrointestinal series with oral contrast be obtained before discharge. CT scan may ultimately prove an adequate confirmatory test, but there are cases in which packets are not visualized by this test.

SUGGESTED READINGS

Chapter 62, Opioids.

Chapter 67, Cocaine.

Antidotes in Depth: Whole-Bowel Irrigation.

Caruana DS, Weinbach B, Goerg D, Gardner LB: Cocaine-packet ingestion: Diagnosis, management, and natural history. Ann Intern Med 1984;100:73–74.

Hahn I, Hoffman RS, Nelson LS: Contrast CT scan fails to detect the last heroin packet. J Toxicol Clin Toxicol 1999;37:644–645.

Hoffman RS, Smilkstein MJ, Goldfrank LR: Whole bowel irrigation and the cocaine body packer: A new approach to a common problem. Am J Emerg Med 1990;8:523–527.

Lancashire MJR, Legg PK, Lowe M, et al: Surgical aspects of international drug smuggling. Br Med J 1988;296:1035–1037.

McCarron MM, Wood JD: The cocaine "body packer" syndrome. JAMA 1983;250:1417–1420.

Olmedo RE, Hoffman RS, Nelson LS: Limitation of whole-bowel irrigation and laparotomy in a cocaine "body-packer." J Toxicol Clin Toxicol 1999;37:645.

Case 20

1. Intestinal ischemia or infarction following cocaine use occurs either as a result of direct local vasoconstriction (seen with packet leakage in "body packers") or as a manifestation of systemic vasoconstriction. Vasoconstriction has been reported with all forms of cocaine use, including one case of transplacental exposure. In addition, a syndrome consisting of acute abdominal pain associated with diarrhea and occult-blood-positive or grossly bloody stools ("cocaine colitis") has been reported. These patients are found to have superficial ulcerations and diffuse areas of hemorrhage and necrosis on direct examination of their bowel. Also, there seems to be an association between acute gastrointestinal perforation and crack cocaine use, presumably as a result of a small area of acute ischemia with subsequent tissue necrosis. Occasionally, cocaine may be contaminated with heavy metals, such as arsenic or thallium, which may produce severe gastrointestinal complaints.

2. Initial therapy should consist of volume resuscitation and restoration of fluid and electrolyte balance. The next step is to differentiate between reversible ischemia and irreversible infarction. Although this may be aided by the use of CT scan or angiography (Fig. CS–9), severely ill patients should have direct operative visualization. In the operating room, patients may be treated with warmed saline laparotomy pads (Nalbandian) or may require resection. Theoretically, patients could be treated with the direct intraarterial administration of an α-adrenergic antagonist such as phentolamine in the setting of cocaine-induced ischemia, although this has not been reported.

This patient went to the operating room because of persistent abdominal pain. The entire colon and rectum were found to be

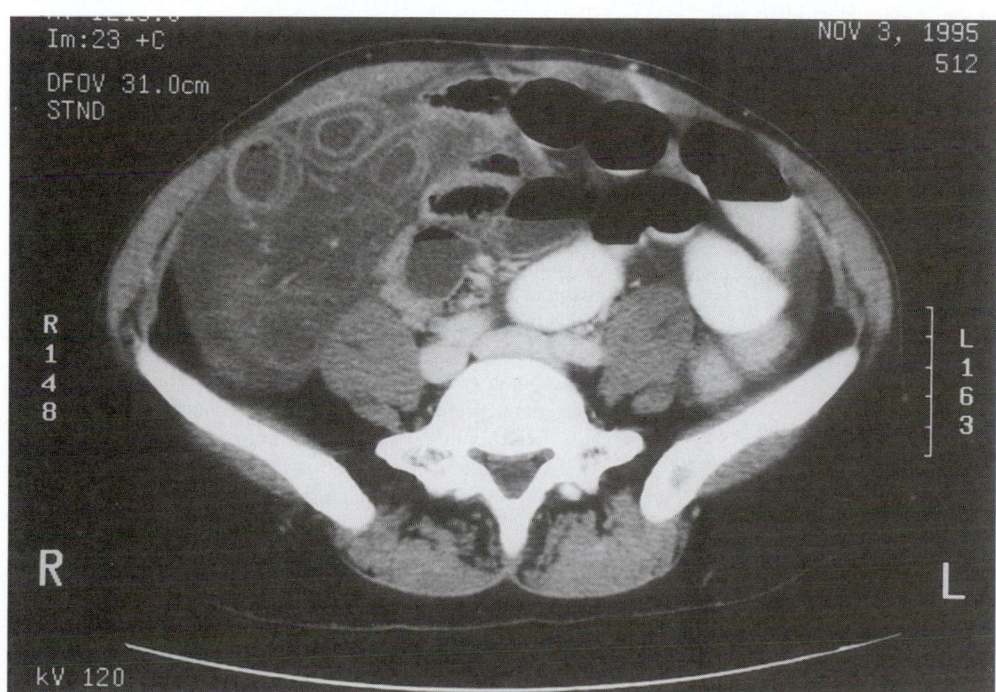

Figure CS–9 Computerized tomography (CT) scan in intestinal ischemia. The "target lesions" seen here demonstrating bowel wall edema can be associated with air in the bowel wall, air in the mesenteric veins, or air in the portal system. All CT findings occur late in the progression of this disorder, which often has to be diagnosed clinically. (*Courtesy of David T. Schwartz, MD, Department of Emergency Medicine, Bellevue Hospital Center, New York University School of Medicine.*)

necrotic, and she survived after the colon and rectum were removed.

3. The greatest number of cases of bowel ischemia and infarction associated with a drug seem to be related to digoxin therapy. Perhaps this is because patients taking digoxin tend to be elderly, have low flow states, and have disorders such as atrial fibrillation that predispose to embolization, rather than being a manifestation of digoxin therapy itself. In addition, any potent vasoconstrictor, such as ergots (Greene), could be expected to produce bowel ischemia, although these are rarely reported. Any agent that produces hypotension may place a susceptible patient at risk.

SUGGESTED READINGS

Chapter 67, Cocaine.

Endress C, Kling GA: Cocaine-induced small-bowel perforation. Am J Radiol 1990;154:1346–1347.

Greene FL, Ariyan S, Stansel HC: Mesenteric and peripheral vascular ischemia secondary to ergotism. Surgery 1977;81:176–179.

Lee HS, LaMaute HR, Pizzi WF, et al: Acute gastrointestinal perforations associated with use of crack. Ann Surg 1990;211:15–17.

Nalbandian H, Sheth N, Dietrich R, et al: Intestinal ischemia caused by cocaine ingestion: Report of two cases. Surgery 1985;97:374–376.

Telsey AM, Merrit A, Dixon SD: Cocaine exposure in a term neonate. Clin Pediatr 1988;27:547–550.

Case 21

1. This patient's vital sign abnormalities include tachypnea, tachycardia, and hyperthermia. In light of this patient's psychiatric history, consideration must be given to neuroleptic malignant syndrome and perhaps serotonin syndrome. Muscle rigidity and more significant hyperthermia typically occur in patients with these syndromes but may be mild or absent early in the course. Other causes not specific to schizophrenic patients include thyrotoxicosis (endogenous or exogenous), lithium poisoning, electrolyte abnormalities, and salicylate poisoning.

2. Hyperventilation that occurs with salicylate intoxication results both from salicylate's direct stimulatory effect on the central nervous system and in response to metabolic acidosis. It is important to remember that because hyperventilation can result from both tachypnea (ie, an elevated respiratory rate) and hyperpnea (ie, an increased tidal volume), the depth and rate of breathing must be observed. Tachycardia probably occurs in response to volume loss, acidosis, and hyperthermia. Salicylates uncouple oxidative phosphorylation. Thus, in severe poisoning, energy that was destined for adenosine triphosphate (ATP) synthesis is lost as heat. When hyperthermia is present, it is a grave sign.

Other findings on physical examination are relatively nonspecific until they are considered together as part of the salicylate "toxidrome." Diaphoresis is quite prominent. Although the exact mechanism is unknown, it may occur in response to the heat generated from uncoupling oxidative phosphorylation. Also, patients with acute ingestions may be actively vomiting or give a history of having vomited at home. Pupils, bowel sounds, muscle strength, and urinary function should all be normal. Rales suggest acute lung injury (ALI), another grave manifestation of toxicity. In severe salicylism altered mental status (possibly related to central nervous system hypoglycemia) may also be present.

Patients will often complain of the subjective feeling of shortness of breath. Problems with pulmonary gas exchange or ALI are present only with severe poisoning. Rather, it is the direct central respiratory stimulation that produces this perception. Dry mouth or thirst, as in this case, can be expected with the hyperventilation. Tinnitus or decreased auditory acuity results from salicylate's effect on the eighth cranial nerve. Although this finding can often occur near the upper limit of the therapeutic range, it is so uncommon with other exposures that it should always prompt a search for salicylates. Most other complaints, such as gastrointestinal discomfort, are nonspecific at best.

3. Although salicylate levels will be required to follow the patient's response to therapy and make decisions about extracorporeal drug removal, they have a long turnaround time and add little to the acute management unless they are very high or very low. Rapid diagnostic tests give more useful information. The arterial blood gas analysis is an excellent first test. In classic salicylism, the patient will have a respiratory alkalosis and a metabolic acidosis. The respiratory alkalosis develops first, from the central nervous system stimulation, and actually may appear as a pure respiratory alkalosis early on. Later, a multifactorial metabolic acidosis develops, and the patient's pH remains alkalemic but returns toward normal. In late or severe poisoning, the patient may be acidemic as a result of either overwhelming metabolic acidosis or respiratory failure.

The next rapid source of information is the urine. A ferric chloride test (1–2 drops of 10% $FeCl_3$ in 1 mL of urine turns purple in the presence of salicylates) is a highly sensitive and specific indicator of salicylates. Unfortunately, the test is only qualitative, so that it can not distinguish between salicylate exposure and salicylate toxicity. Urine pH is also useful. In early exposures alkaluria will be found in response to the respiratory alkalosis. The urine rapidly becomes acidic because of the excretion of salicylate and other organic acids, such that the most common findings are respiratory alkalosis and metabolic acidosis with alkalemia and aciduria. In addition to the pH, the presence of ketones in the urine is a sign of severe metabolic poisoning.

Electrolytes are another source of useful information. An anion gap metabolic acidosis will be present in patients with salicylism. Determining the renal function is essential because salicylates are eliminated in the urine. Patients with significant renal dysfunction are more likely to require extracorporeal drug removal. The potassium will have important implications for therapy (see below). Rarely, salicylates can produce hypoglycemia. In addition, low cerebrospinal fluid glucose has been documented even in the setting of a normal serum glucose. Thus, all fluids should contain dextrose.

Other laboratory tests are important but have less of an impact on management. Liver enzymes may be abnormal, as salicylate can cause liver toxicity. Coagulation times may be prolonged, either because of salicylate's effect on the liver or from a direct effect on vitamin K–dependent factors.

4. It is important to remember that in salicylate poisoning the respiratory alkalosis is protective. Abrupt decreases in respiratory rate, producing a respiratory acidosis, might be rapidly fatal (Berk). Thus, in patients who receive sedation or neuromuscular blockade or who develop respiratory failure (eg, from pulmonary or cerebral edema), it is essential to restore and maintain hyperventilation. This may require the use of ventilator settings that are considered excessive in most other situations.

Volume status is another important consideration. Salicylate elimination is partially dependent on glomecular filtration rate (GFR). Most poisoned patients are volume depleted. They have vomiting as part of their poisoning and will have diarrhea in response to the cathartic administration. Insensible losses are also higher than normal because of diaphoresis, hyperventilation, and hyperthermia. There is also an obligate diuresis that results from the water loss that must accompany salicylates and the organic acids as they are eliminated in the urine. Volume resuscitation is essential but should proceed cautiously because of the risk for ALI.

Gastrointestinal decontamination is more important here than with many other ingestions. Patients have the potential to ingest such large gram amounts that the use of activated charcoal alone may prove insufficient. In addition, aspirin is known to produce concretions and pylorospasm, two factors that increase the likelihood of drug recovery with orogastric lavage. When either the history is suggestive of a large ingestion or there are signs and symptoms of severe toxicity, orogastric lavage may be indicated even if the patient has had spontaneous emesis. This should always be followed by activated charcoal and a cathartic. Although recent studies have suggested that multiple-dose activated charcoal has a limited role in the postabsorptive phase of salicylate poisoning, it should still be used because of the potential for ongoing absorption as a result of concretions or incomplete decontamination.

Alkalinizing the urine enhances salicylate excretion by ion trapping (Temple). This can offer a substantial benefit in severely poisoned patients. The urine pH must be raised to at least 7.0, and preferably 7.5 to 8.0, to achieve optimal clearance. In fact, raising the pH from 5.0 to 6.5 offers very little benefit. Alkalinization can be accomplished with sodium bicarbonate infusion—a standard method might be to put three ampules (133 mEq) of sodium bicarbonate in 1 L of D_5W to run at twice maintenance. It is important to remember that hypokalemia will prevent successful alkalinization because of the $H^+–K^+$ exchange mechanism in the kidney. Also, extreme caution must be used in treating patients with early signs of ALI because alkalinization represents a significant salt and water load.

In patients with life-threatening toxicity, decontamination, activated charcoal, and urinary alkalinization may prove inadequate. Under these circumstances, extracorporeal drug removal is indicated. The choice of technique is between hemodialysis and charcoal hemoperfusion. Other techniques, such as peritoneal dialysis or CAVHD, are inferior and should not be considered. Although activated charcoal hemoperfusion is better at removing salicylate, hemodialysis is usually selected because of its added ability to correct the fluid and electrolyte abnormalities that occur with severe toxicity. Indications for hemodialysis include significant renal dysfunction, altered mental status, and ALI. In addition, patients with very high levels (100 mg/dL or greater) and those whose levels are rising despite other therapy should be considered candidates for hemodialysis.

Initial laboratory tests revealed a respiratory alkalosis and metabolic acidosis with signs of pulmonary compromise (pH 7.44, P_{CO_2} 28 mm Hg, P_{O_2} 70 mm Hg on room air). The urine had a pH of 5.0 with large ketones, and the ferric chloride test was positive. Electrolytes showed an anion gap of 17 with a creatinine of 1.5 mg/dL. The patient was given intravenous fluids, activated *charcoal by nasogastric tube, and sodium bicarbonate by infusion to alkalinize his urine. Because the chest radiograph was consistent with ALI, fluid administration was reduced, and nephrology was consulted to perform hemodialysis. The first salicylate level was reported as 76 mg/dL. The patient was intubated and hyperventilated for progressive respiratory failure. Hemodialysis was performed, the patient was extubated, and he recovered fully.*

SUGGESTED READINGS

Chapter 24, Fluid, Electrolyte, and Acid–Base Principles.

Chapter 33, Salicylates.

Anderson RJ, Potts DE, Gabow PA, et al: Unrecognized adult salicylate intoxication. Ann Intern Med 1976;85:745–748.

Berk WA, Anderson JC: Salicylate associated asystole: Report of two cases. Am J Med 1989;86:505–506.

Higgins RM, Connolly JO, Hendry BM: Alkalinization and hemodialysis in severe salicylate poisoning: Comparison of elimination techniques in the same patient. Clin Nephrol 1998;50:178–183.

Hill JB: Salicylate intoxication. N Engl J Med 1973;288:1110–1113.

Yip L, Dart RC, Gabow PA: Concepts and controversies in salicylate toxicity. Emerg Med Clin North Am 1994;12:351–364.

Case 22

1. Warfarin-induced coagulopathy results from a deficiency of coagulation factors II, VII, IX, and X. These factors (along with proteins S and C) must be activated in the liver by carboxylation of glutamic acid on their precursor proteins. This activation step is coupled to the oxidation of vitamin K and forms vitamin K 2,3-epoxide. This inactive form of vitamin K must be reduced back to its active form, vitamin K quinol, in order for activation to continue. Two steps in the reduction cycle are inhibited by warfarin (refer to Fig. 42–3). As a result, the body's stores of vitamin K rapidly decline, and coagulopathy ensues. Bleeding occurs commonly as an adverse effect of anticoagulation therapy. Some authors estimate that the risk for minor bleeding may be as high as 20% per year of therapy. Although less common, life-threatening bleeding may still occur in 5 to 7% of patients treated per year of therapy. Contributing factors such as drug interactions (cimetidine), concomitant medications (aspirin and ethanol), old age, and trauma all increase the risk of significant hemorrhage.

2. The purple toe syndrome is a relatively rare complication of warfarin administration that occurs predominantly in men, usually some time between the third and eighth week of therapy. The patient will present with painful purple lesions of the feet and toes (usually) or fingers (rarely) that blanch with pressure and do not seem to progress to necrotic lesions. Although the mechanism is unknown, many authors feel that the syndrome results from cholesterol microemboli that are shed from preexisting atheromatous plaques. The natural history of atherosclerotic plaques revolves around growth, ulceration, and then thrombosis at the site of ulceration secondary to loss of normal endothelial tissue. It is presumed that when ulceration occurs in the anticoagulated patient, thrombosis cannot occur. As a result, the exposed ulcer is able to release small emboli that drift downstream until they become lodged in capillaries. Because ulcerations are common on the descending aorta, lesions are expected in the lower extremities. Biopsies of involved digits, and rare cases of cholesterol emboli to other organs (eye and kidney), support this etiology. Although other authors suggest either a direct toxic effect of warfarin on capillaries or an intrinsic vasodilating effect, evidence for these mechanisms is lacking. Most patients will have gradual resolution of symptoms when anticoagulation is discontinued. Recurrent purple toe syndrome has occurred on rechallenge, but some experts suggest that the choice of a different anticoagulant, and a 1-year hiatus in anticoagulant therapy, will substantially reduce the incidence of repeated events.

3. In contrast to purple toe syndrome, warfarin skin necrosis usually occurs in women between their third and sixth day of therapy. A review states an overall incidence of between 0.01 and 0.1% for this disorder (Chan). Patients tend to be obese elderly women, and lesions tend to appear in high-pressure areas and those locations with a high subcutaneous fat content. Specifically, the buttocks, thighs, and breasts are the sites most commonly affected. Patients will often first notice pain at a small area of blistering or erythema. Over the next day, petechiae appear and coalesce into ecchymotic areas. Ultimately thrombosis develops in subcutaneous veins, and fat necrosis results. The lesion may extend deep into muscle and requires differentiation from necrotizing fasciitis or venous gangrene. All of these lesions may require extensive debridement or amputation.

Most cases of warfarin skin necrosis can be attributed to a relative deficiency of protein S and/or protein C. These factors are inhibitors of coagulation that are activated in the same vitamin K pathway as factors II, VII, IX, and X. The normal fluidity of the blood is maintained by a delicate balance between coagulation (the extrinsic and intrinsic cascades) and anticoagulation (proteins S and C and the fibrinolytic system). When warfarin is given to a patient with a relative deficiency of proteins S and C, the inhibition pathway is inactivated before the coagulation pathway, and coagulation proceeds unchecked. Interestingly, because protein S and C deficiencies are hypercoagulable conditions, patients will often present to health care with deep venous thrombosis or pulmonary embolus. Naturally most will be given warfarin. Because not all patients with warfarin skin necrosis have documented deficiencies of proteins S or C, other mechanisms of thrombosis such as trauma, malignancy, pregnancy, estrogen use, and infection have been invoked as contributors to skin necrosis.

Treatment of patients with warfarin skin necrosis has concentrated on restoring the balance between coagulation and inhibition. Patients can be given vitamin K_1 and fresh frozen plasma to reverse the warfarin and provide a source of exogenous proteins S and C. Heparin, corticosteroids, and vasodilators have also been administered. Most authors indicated that once a necrotic lesion occurs, tissue loss is inevitable. Local therapy with aggressive tissue debridement and wound repair may be indicated. Rechallenge with warfarin is considered inadvisable because the condition is likely to recur.

Over the next few days her lesion progressed over her entire thigh, and she ultimately required amputation of a necrotic lower extremity.

SUGGESTED READINGS

Chapter 42, Anticoagulants.
Chan YC, Valenti D, Mansfield AO, et al: Warfarin induced skin necrosis. Br J Surg 2000;87:266–272.

Feder W: "Purple toes": An uncommon sequela of oral coumarin drug therapy. Ann Intern Med 1961;55:911–917.
McGehee WG: Coumarin necrosis associated with hereditary protein C deficiency. Ann Intern Med 1984;101:59–60.
Nalbandian RM: Petechiae, ecchymoses and necrosis of skin induced by coumarin congeners. JAMA 1965;192:107–112.
Sallah S, Abdallah JM, Gagnon GA: Recurrent warfarin-induced skin necrosis in kindreds with protein S deficiency. Haemostasis 1998;28:25–30.
Sallah S, Thomas DP, Roberts HR: Warfarin and heparin-induced skin necrosis and the purple toe syndrome: infrequent complications of anticoagulant treatment. Thromb Haemostas 1997;78:785–790.

Case 23

1. Hydrofluoric acid (HF) is a simple mineral acid with unique properties that allow it to be used for rust and graffiti removal, for glass etching, and in the semiconductor industry. In spite of the fact that severe tissue injury occurs following even transient exposures, HF is a very weak acid. Because fluoride is the most electronegative anion, the dissociation constant for HF is very low (3.53×10^{-4}). This means that when compared to true strong acids such as HCl, an equimolar solution of HF produces about 1/1000 the number of available hydrogen ions.

Strong acids (those that are mostly dissociated into hydrogen ions) damage tissues by oxidation, as the hydrogen ions extract electrons. This occurs on the contact surface, and deep penetration is limited by the thick eschar that results from the burn. Because HF is a weak acid, it exists predominantly in an undissociated (uncharged) form that can penetrate into tissues. Once it is across cell membranes, dissociation begins. Because intracellular fluids are abundant with cations, the fluoride ion released from HF is able to form tight bonds and precipitate out of solution. This shifts the equilibrium, resulting in more production of both hydrogen and fluoride ions. As a result, tissues are injured both by the acid and from the loss of essential cations such as calcium and magnesium. Patients with significant injuries (greater than 2.5% body surface area burns from concentrated HF) may also demonstrate systemic toxicity in the form of metabolic acidosis, hyperkalemia, hypocalcemia, and hypomagnesemia. Ingestion of HF is particularly ominous (Kao).

2. Immediate first aid involves irrigation of the affected area to remove any excess HF. Although specialized commercial cationic irrigation solutions such as benzalkonium chloride are available, their efficacy is unproved. Usually, irrigation with cool water will suffice. The patient should be rapidly assessed for potential indicators of systemic toxicity (hypocalcemia, hyperkalemia, hypomagnesemia). Blood chemistries should be sent, but the best screening tools are the ECG and physical examination (Chvostek and Trousseau signs). If findings suggestive of systemic toxicity are noted, the patient should receive intravenous therapy directed at correcting these acid–base and electrolyte abnormalities. The next step is to supply exogenous cations with which fluoride can bind. Traditionally, this has involved the use of calcium salts. As a first step, a gel of calcium gluconate in sterile jelly can be purchased or prepared. This is then applied liberally to the affected skin with an occlusive dressing. We often use this modality for hand injuries, with an oversized surgical glove as the occlusive dressing. Involved tissue can either be infiltrated directly with calcium gluconate (never calcium chloride, as this is tissue toxic) or perfused via an arterial line. Some clinicians have also filled the venous system using tourniquet techniques similar to those used for regional anesthesia. The goal of these therapies is to provide pain relief, which is believed to signify termination of tissue destruction.

Unfortunately, controlled human trials comparing these techniques are not available, so that guidelines for their use must be empiric. Generally, the more invasive methods are reserved for either prolonged exposures or those exposures that result from high concentrations of HF and are clearly resulting in tissue destruction. Patients who present many hours after exposure with pain and no evidence of tissue injury can usually be treated fairly conservatively.

Recently, research has been directed at evaluating the role of intravenous magnesium therapy. One study compared direct infiltration of calcium gluconate to intravenous magnesium therapy in a rabbit model of HF injury (Cox). The magnesium group showed a significant decrease in burn size relative to the calcium group, with comparable rates of wound healing. A similar study in a rat model demonstrated that parenteral magnesium therapy protected against lethality and burn at least as well as calcium (Williams). Combined therapy with local calcium and systemic magnesium has not been evaluated. Although these studies are in no way conclusive, they suggest a benefit for intravenous magnesium. The dose and duration of therapy have yet to be elucidated.

3. Ocular exposures to HF are managed somewhat differently than skin exposures to HF or eye exposures to other acids or bases. Normally, prolonged irrigation of the eyes is felt to be beneficial following caustic exposure, and case reports document hours of irrigation following alkali exposures in an attempt to bring the conjunctival pH near normal. In a rabbit model of HF-induced ocular injury, repeated irrigations resulted in a sevenfold increase in corneal ulcerations (McCulley). These authors subsequently suggested that a single irrigation with 1 L of water or an isotonic solution of normal saline or magnesium chloride, given over about 30 minutes, was the most optimal therapy.

Although the use of calcium-containing solutions for irrigation or instillation seems attractive (based on analogy to skin injury), their role is still debated. Older studies, such as the one cited above, give fairly convincing evidence that calcium salts are irritating and increase the incidence of eye injury following HF exposure. Lately, this concept has once again come into question. One paper reported the use of 1% calcium gluconate eye drops in a patient with ocular exposure to 49% HF (Bentur). Although the patient suffered corneal injury, recovery was rapid and complete. Further work by the same author suggested that calcium gluconate irrigation was not advantageous compared to saline irrigation.

The patient was treated with a cycloplegic agent and topical antibiotic. He returned the next day for followup with an ophthalmologist. Repeat examination demonstrated 20/40 vision in the right eye, with complete resolution of lid edema and conjunctival injection. The small corneal defects were almost completely absent. One week later, his vision was 20/20, and the eye appeared normal.

SUGGESTED READINGS

Chapter 27, Ophthalmic Principles.
Chapter 87, Caustics and Batteries.

Beiran I, Miller B, Bentur Y: The efficacy of calcium gluconate in ocular hydrofluoric acid burns. Hum Exp Toxicol 1997;16:223–228.
Bentur Y, Tennenabum S, Yaffe Y, Halpert M: The role of calcium gluconate in the treatment of hydrofluoric acid eye burn. Ann Emerg Med 1993;22:1488–1490.
Cox RD: Evaluation of intravenous magnesium sulfate for the treatment of hydrofluoric acid burns. J Toxicol Clin Toxicol 1994;32:123–136.
Kao WF, Dart RC, Kuffner E, Bogdan G: Ingestion of low-concentration hydrofluoric acid: An insidious and potentially fatal poisoning. Ann Emerg Med 1999;34:35–41.
McCulley JP, Whiting DW, Petitt MG, Lauber SE: Hydrofluoric acid burns of the eye. J Occup Med 1983;25:447–450.
Williams JM: Intravenous magnesium in the treatment of hydrofluoric acid burns. Ann Emerg Med 1994;23:464–469.

Case 24

1. Many drugs and toxins are known to infrequently cause blindness. For example, vasodilators can reduce blood pressure to such an extent that ischemia of the occipital cortex occurs. However, hypotension-induced infarction is unlikely in a young patient presumably in good health but may be encountered in a more elderly patient. In addition, carbon monoxide and hydrogen sulfide may produce cortical blindness. In each of these situations the pupillary light reflex should be normal despite complete loss of vision because it does not require cortical input.

Methanol, a one-carbon alcohol, is perhaps the most common cause of toxin-induced acute visual loss. However, methanol must undergo metabolism to formic acid, a direct retinal toxin, and this conversion, mediated by alcohol dehydrogenase, is competitively blocked by ethanol or fomepizole. This patient's therapeutic ethanol level (>100 mg/dL) essentially eliminates consequential methanol poisoning unless the patient ingested ethanol following the development of methanol-induced blindness.

Agents such as cocaine and ergot alkaloids, which provoke diffuse vasospasm, can produce retinal ischemia and blindness. Visible retinal changes such as pallor or arterial vasoconstriction are expected in this situation. Alternatively, phencyclidine use is associated with "sun-gazers retinopathy" as a result of prolonged staring at the sun with subsequent ultraviolet damage to the retina. The "blind as a bat" associated with the anticholinergic toxidrome refers not to visual loss but to the loss of accommodation or near focus.

On extensive questioning, the patient reluctantly admitted to ingesting 30 tablets of quinine, 300 mg each, in a suicide attempt 3 to 4 hours before arriving in the ED.

2. Toxins may cause either irreversible or reversible hearing loss. The primarily reversible toxins include nonsteroidal antiinflammatory drugs (ibuprofen, naproxen, indomethacin, piroxicam), diuretics (furosemide, ethacrynic acid, acetazolamide, mannitol), antimicrobials (erythromycin, quinine), salicylates, and carbon monoxide. Those agents causing irreversible hearing loss include antimicrobials (aminoglycosides, vancomycin), antineoplastics (cisplatin, vincristine, vinblastine, bleomycin, nitrogen mustard), bromates, hydrocarbons (toluene, xylene, styrene), and heavy metals (arsenic, mercury).

This patient had no history of renal insufficiency or congestive heart failure, reducing the likelihood of diuretic exposure. The nonsteroidal antiinflammatory drugs (NSAIDs) and antimicrobials, however, are readily available.

3. Quinine is derived from the bark of the cinchona tree, the same tree from which aspirin is derived. It has a long history of use in herbal and homeopathic remedies and is still found in tonic water (about 2 mg/oz). It gained notoriety as a heroin adulterant because its bitter taste resembles that of heroin. It has only recently been removed from the market as a nonprescription remedy for leg cramps. It was also commonly used as an abortifacient, an agent that induces fetal miscarriage, often with disastrous results (Dannenberg). Quinine finds it widest use worldwide as an antimalarial agent, especially in regions where chloroquine resistance is endemic. This patient, a recently discharged Marine, had accumulated pills during his foreign service.

Quinine shares many properties with the two other agents derived from the cinchona tree. Like salicylates, quinine induces cinchonism, consisting of nausea, vomiting, tinnitus, dizziness, and headache. Like its optical isomer quinidine, quinine has cardiac effects analogous to the type IA antidysrhythmic agents, including impaired inotropy and myocardial electrical abnormalities (ie, QRS and QT prolongation). Unique to quinine, however, is its ability to produce blindness. Visual changes were initially thought to be secondary to retinal vasospasm and ischemia, and they were even reported to respond favorably to stellate ganglion blockade to relieve the vasospasm. This conception may, in fact, represent reporting bias because subsequent studies have not confirmed this benefit. Alternatively, quinine, or possibly a metabolite, is likely a direct retinal toxin (Bacon).

A large retrospective study of patients with acute quinine poisonings found that 42% had visual symptoms, 38% had tinnitus, 14% had altered mental status, and deep coma was present in 4%. Of those with visual symptoms, just over half had total blindness, which was permanent in about half of them. The risk of blindness was roughly correlated with quinine levels; patients with plasma quinine levels greater than 10 μg/mL at 10 hours postexposure are likely to suffer visual loss. However, there is currently little clinical utility for plasma quinine levels, as the test's availability and therapeutic interventions are limited.

4. The use of oral activated charcoal reduces the half-life of quinine in human volunteers with nontoxic ingestions. To enhance elimination of the drug once absorbed, forced diuresis proved better than hemodialysis, plasma exchange, or peritoneal dialysis for increasing clearance of drug. However, no investigation has ever shown that increasing clearance speeds recovery. Indeed, forced diuresis is a potentially dangerous procedure and almost never indicated. Although not adequately studied, the clinical value of charcoal hemoperfusion may surpass the above methods of enhancing elimination (Morgan). Although case reports suggest that stellate ganglion blockade is curative of the vasospasm and blindness, in a study of 34 treated cases it may have helped in only one. Fortunately, the visual changes generally resolve with supportive care.

The patient received several doses of oral activated charcoal. He was given intravenous saline at three times maintenance, and his urine pH remained below 7.5. He did not receive stellate ganglion blocks, nor was another method of enhanced elimination instituted. His electrocardiogram normalized over 12 hours, and his

vision improved over the subsequent 2 days without specific therapy. He was discharged to the psychiatry service.

SUGGESTED READINGS

Chapter 27, Ophthalmic Principles.

Chapter 28, Otolaryngologic Principles.

Boland ME, Roper SMB, Henry JA: Complications of quinine poisoning. Lancet 1985;1:384–385.

Dannenberg A, Dorman SF, Johnson J: Use of quinine for self-induced abortion. South Med J 1983;76:846–849.

Lockey D, Bateman DN: Effects of oral activated charcoal on quinine elimination. Br J Clin Pharmacol 1989;27:92–94.

Morgan MDL, Pusey CD, Rainford DJ, Robins-Cherry AM: The treatment of quinine poisoning with charcoal haemoperfusion. Postgrad Med J 1983;59:365–367.

Nordt SP, Clark RF: Acute blindness after severe quinine poisoning. Am J Emerg Med 1998;16:214–215.

Sabto J, Pierce RM, West RH, Gurr FW: Hemodialysis, peritoneal dialysis, plasmapheresis, and forced diuresis for the treatment of quinine overdose. Clin Nephrol 1981;16:264–268.

Smilkstein MJ, Kulig KW, Rumack BH: Acute toxic blindness: Unrecognized quinine poisoning. Ann Emerg Med. 1987;16:98–101.

Tridgell DE: Quinine-induced blindness during attempted heroin withdrawal. Med J Aust 1999;171:444,446.

Case 25

1. Both patients present with symptoms that are common but entirely inconsistent with their histories of exposure. Patient 25a appears to have ingested a caustic substance such as a strong acid or base. These findings would never be expected from Claritin ingestions. Patient 25b is suffering from a dystonic reaction. Dystonic reactions are common following neuroleptic or antiemetic therapy but, again, are not seen with corticosteroid administration. A careful review of patient 25b's hospital record failed to identify any potential cause for her dystonic reaction.

2. Patient 25a's medication prescription was reviewed. The bottle was properly labeled as Claritin, but the agent it contained had a very characteristic speckled appearance of Clinitest. Clinitest tablets contain copper sulfate, citric acid, sodium hydroxide, and sodium carbonate and are known for their ability to cause significant esophageal and gastric burns following ingestion of even a single tablet.

Patient 25b had a very similar problem. Her prescription bottle was properly labeled for a prednisone taper but contained Prolixin (fluphenazine). Fluphenazine has a well-established association with dystonic reactions.

3. Prescribing errors can occur at any point in the prescription process. The pharmacist must be able to read the prescription. Because many medications sound or are spelled similarly, illegible prescriptions are the most common cause of this error. Table CS–1 lists some of the more common prescribing errors that have resulted from poorly written prescriptions. Other errors occur because medications are stored on shelves in alphabetical order.

The best way to prevent this problem is by physicians taking responsibility for their prescription writing. Prescriptions should be clearly written or typed and should use the most recognizable

TABLE CS–1.   Common Prescription Errors

Intended Drug	Error	Intended Drug	Error
Acetohexamide	Acetazolamide	Lopid	Lorabid
Amiodarone	Amrinone	Lopid	Slobid
Atrovent	Alupent	Lortab	Lorabid
Betagan	Betagen	Lotensin	Loniten
Brevital	Brevibloc	Lotrimin	Lotrisone
Calcitrol	Calciferol	Lovastatin	Lotensin
Cefotan	Ceftin	Metoprolol	Misoprostol
Cefprozil	Cefazolin	Nifedipine	Nicardipine
Ceftazidime	Ceftizoxime	Nifedipine	Nimodipine
Cefzil	Ceftin	Norflex	Nofloxin
Celebrex	Celexa	Norvasc	Navan
Claritin	Clinitest	Oruvail	Elavil
Clinoril	Clozaril	Oruvail	Clinoril
Clonidine	Klonopin	Paxil	Taxol
Coumadin	Compazine	Paxil	Paclitaxel
Cyclobenzaprine	Cyproheptadine	Penicillamine	Penicillin
Cyclophosphamide	Cyclosporine	Pindolol	Parlodel
Cyclosporine	Cycloserine	Pitocin	Pitressin
Cytoxan	Cytotec	Plendil	Prinivil
Cytoxan	Cytosar	Prednisone	Prednisolone
Diazepam	Ditropan	Prednisone	Prolixin
Diamox	Dymelor	Premarin	Primaxin
Digoxin	Digitoxin	Prilosec	Prozac
Dolobid	Slobid	Propranolol	Propulsid
Doxepin	Doxycycline	Prozac	Proscar
Dynacirc	Dynapen	Quinidine	Quinine
Eldepryl	Enalapril	Retrovir	Ritonavir
Etidronate	Etretinate	Ridaura	Cardura
Feldene	Seldane	Rimantadine	Amantadine
Glipizide	Glyburide	Rimantadine	Ranitidine
Glucotrol	Glyburide	Reserpine	Respirdal
Hydromorphone	Morphine	Saquinavir	Sinequan
Hydroxyzine	Hydralazine	Slobid	Lopid
Imdur	K-Dur	Soma	Soma compound
Imferon	Interferon	Sulfasalazine	Sulfisoxazole
Inderal	Imdur	Terbutaline	Tetracycline
Inderal	Isordil	Symmetrel	Synthroid
Klonopin	Clonidine	Tagamet	Tegretol
Lamictal	Lomotil	Thiamine	Tenormin
Lanoxin	Lasix	Tobrex	Tobradex
Lanoxin	Lanoxin	Toradol	Torecan
Levoxine	Levoxine	Torsemide	Furosemide
Leucovorin	Leukeran	Vancenase	Vanceril
Levsin	Levoxin	Vincristine	Vinblastine
Librium	Librax	Xanax	Zantac
Lithostat	Lithobid	Xanax	Tenex
Lodine	Iodine	Zosyn	Zofran

Medication errors can result from similar sounding or spelling of medications. This
   risk is compounded when prescriptions are not clearly written.

name (generic vs proprietary) when appropriate. A clear explanation in the "Sig" section will also help this problem. If the prednisone taper said "Sig: one pill PO QD for asthma," rather than
"Sig: one pill PO QD," the pharmacist would have recognized the
inconsistency with Prolixin and questioned the prescription. The
same logic would apply to the Claritin prescription. Pharmacists
should not fill prescriptions that are incomplete or at all questionable. Finally, physicians should counsel their patients with regard
to any medication prescription. The patient should be told the
name of the medication and its indications, thus allowing for pa-

tient recognition to help limit adverse effects if the wrong medication is dispensed.

SUGGESTED READINGS

Chapter 117, Adverse Drug Events.
Ansari MZ, Collopy BT, Brosi JA: Errors in drug prescribing. J Qual Clin
   Pract 1995;15:183–190.
Johnson KB, Butta JK, Donohue PK, Glenn DJ: Discharging patients with
   prescriptions instead of medications: Sequelae in a teaching hospital.
   Pediatrics 1996;97:481–485.
Kaushal R, Bates DW, Landrigan C, et al: Medication errors and adverse
   drug events in pediatric inpatients. JAMA 2001;285:2114–2120.
Lesar TS, Briceland L, Stein DS: Factors related to errors in medication
   prescribing. JAMA 1997;277:312–317.
Ross LM, Wallace J, Paton JY: Medication errors in a paediatric teaching
   hospital in the UK: five years operational experience. Arch Dis Child
   2000;83:492–497.

Case 26

1. The differential diagnosis of the severe gastrointestinal distress in these two patients should include bacterial and viral gastroenteritis, food poisoning, toxic mushrooms, plant toxins, heavy
metals, organic phosphorus compounds, and exposures to cathartics. In the absence of a better history, exposure to cathartics and
heavy metals seems unlikely. Likewise, although exposures to
plants (eg, pokeweed) would be expected to produce very similar
clinical findings to those manifested in these patients, once again a
history of exposure is lacking. Similarly, whereas organic phosphorus insecticides often cause severe gastrointestinal symptoms,
in the absence of associated muscarinic (ie, salivation, lacrimation,
bronchorrhea, etc) or nicotinic (ie, muscle fasciculations and
weakness) findings, the diagnosis of organic phosphorus poisoning seems equally unlikely. If the patients' symptoms were attributable to food poisoning, the agent would have to be a preformed
toxin (*Staphylococcus* spp). However, because neither of the children is ill, and they ate the same meal except for the mushrooms, a
mushroom-related illness is immediately implicated.

Mushroom-related gastrointestinal distress is quite common
and can result from both relatively benign and life-threatening
mushroom toxins. The major discriminating factor is the time of
onset of the gastrointestinal symptoms. Mushrooms with nonspecific gastrointestinal toxins (eg, *Russula emetica*) produce nausea,
vomiting, and diarrhea within a few hours of ingestion. Muscarine-containing mushrooms (eg, *Inocybe napipes*) will produce
gastrointestinal symptoms as soon as 30 minutes after ingestion
(but like organic phosphorus exposure should have associated
muscarinic findings). Nausea and vomiting are both common in
patients exposed to hallucinogenic mushrooms (eg, *Psilocybe
cubensis*) and in patients who coingest alcohol with coprine-
containing mushrooms (*Coprinus atramentarius* through an An-
tabuselike reaction), but diarrhea is uncommon. Once again, these
symptoms present early after ingestion.

Delayed gastroenteritis (after 6 hours) is common after ingestion of monomethylhydrazine-containing mushrooms (eg, *Gyromitra esculenta*) and is often followed by seizures and hepatic
toxicity. Patients who ingest mushrooms containing orelline and
orellanine (eg, *Cortinarius orellanus*) similarly remain asymptomatic for at least 6 to 8 hours and then develop gastrointestinal

symptoms followed, in a number of days, by renal failure. Finally, hepatic failure and death from cyclopeptide-containing mushrooms (eg, *Amanita phalloides*) usually occurs several days after ingestion. The first sign of toxicity is gastrointestinal symptoms that occur no sooner than 6 hours postingestion.

If there has been an ingestion of a single kind of mushroom, the onset of symptoms can be used to discriminate between relatively benign and life-threatening exposures. Assessment of toxidromes (Antabuse reaction, muscarinic syndrome, hallucinations) will allow for a further subdivision of the type of ingestion based on clinical parameters. A problem that may arise, however, is that patients may simultaneously ingest different types of toxic mushrooms, creating a continuum of gastrointestinal symptoms.

2.   As illustrated above, clinical criteria are often sufficient to allow for the diagnosis of a specific type of ingestion. When additional evidence is required, analysis of the uneaten portion of the mushroom, or spores recovered from leftover food, emesis, or stool may be helpful. This analysis usually requires a trained mycologist because many mushroom species look similar, and specimens of the same species may look dissimilar at different stages of development (see Fig. 76–6).

In this case, the spores found in the patients' emesis were confirmed as having come from an Amanita (cyclopeptide-containing) mushroom.

3.   Cyclopeptides are large-molecular-weight compounds that interfere with protein synthesis by inhibiting RNA polymerase. As a result, the cells in organs with the highest replication rates are those most sensitive to cyclopeptide toxicity. These target organs include the gastrointestinal tract (especially the liver) and the kidneys. Within the liver classic centrilobular necrosis results, as those cells most sensitive to chemical stress die first. Clinically, patients develop signs of fulminant hepatic failure over the course of several days.

4.   Treatment of cyclopeptide toxicity is somewhat controversial. In some case series, fatality rates as high as 40 to 50% are reported. Initial therapy should begin with volume resuscitation and the administration of oral activated charcoal. In vitro evidence supports the use of activated charcoal, and repetitive dosing may be helpful because the toxin undergoes enterohepatic circulation. Multiple agents including thioctic acid, high-dose penicillin, silibinin, silymarin, cytochrome c, cimetidine, and *N*-acetylcysteine have all been used in experimental models. Human data regarding efficacy of these agents are generally inadequate, and many of these antidotes are not available. Anecdotal evidence is often presented in support of a role for charcoal hemoperfusion and plasmapheresis, but again, controlled data are lacking. Liver transplant has been used successfully in patients with fulminant liver failure.

SUGGESTED READINGS

Chapter 76, Mushrooms.

Becker CE, Tong TG, Boerner U: Diagnosis and treatment of *Amanita phalloides*-type mushroom poisoning: Use of thioctic acid. West J Med 1976;125:100–109.

Floersheim GL: Treatment of human amatoxin mushroom poisoning: Myths and advances in therapy. Med Toxicol 1987;2:1–9.

Jander S, Bischoff J, Woodcock BG: Plasmapheresis in the treatment of *Amanita phalloides* poisoning: II. A review and recommendations. Ther Apher 2000;4:308–312.

Nordt SP, Manoguerra A, Clark RF: 5-Year analysis of mushroom exposures in California. West J Med 2000;173:314–317.

Pinson CW, Daya MR, Benner KG, et al: Liver transplantation for severe *Amanita phalloides* mushroom poisoning. Am J Surg 1990;159:493–499.

Schneider SM, Borochovitz D, Krenzelok EP: Cimetidine protection against alpha amanitin hepatotoxicity in mice: A potential model for the treatment of *Amanita phalloides* poisoning. Ann Emerg Med 1987;16:1136–1140.

Wauters JP, Rossel C, Farquet JJ: *Amanita phalloides* poisoning treated by early charcoal hemoperfusion. Br Med J 1970;2:1465.

Case 27

1.   The history of running out of Xanax (alprazolam) should raise the possibility of sedative-hypnotic withdrawal. The findings of tachycardia and altered mental status are compatible with this diagnosis; however, withdrawal would also be expected to cause pupillary dilation, tremor, diaphoresis, fever, and hypertension, which the patient did not manifest. Furthermore, the time course is not right for withdrawal. Alprazolam has an intermediate half-life (12–15 hours), and the onset of withdrawal symptoms would not be expected to be delayed beyond several days to perhaps 1 week. Symptoms of ethanol withdrawal should also be present within the first few days of abstinence.

The patient's confusion and hallucinations could be caused by a broad variety of medical conditions. A careful medical evaluation to exclude CNS infection, head trauma, and metabolic derangements is mandatory. Acute intoxication with a hallucinogen could cause this clinical scenario. Sedative-hypnotic or ethanol intoxication may cause confusion, small pupils, and relatively normal vital signs, although hallucinations would be uncommon. Cocaine or amphetamines would be expected to cause more prominent sympathomimetic findings including diaphoresis, dilated pupils, marked agitation, and fever. Phencyclidine toxicity may present with relatively small pupils, but prominent nystagmus would be expected. Psychiatric illness could, of course, explain the patient's initial presentation but should be a diagnosis of exclusion.

Although it is rare today, bromism was a common diagnosis earlier this century. In the 1930s, between 3 and 7% of patients admitted to psychiatric hospitals were suffering from bromism, and some authors recommended routine bromide levels be sent on all psychiatric patients (Hanes). Characteristic findings of bromism in case series from this era included mental confusion, stupor, delusions, headache, hallucinations, nervousness, and weakness. A series of 400 cases of mild bromism found that the most common symptoms were headache, irritability, emotional instability, weakness, lethargy, slurred speech, irrelevant speech, delusions, disorientation, hallucinations, memory loss, and confusion. The "characteristic" acneiform eruption of bromism (also known as bromoderma) occurred in only 5 of 49 patients in one series and in 100 of 400 patients in another series (Sensenbach). The course of patients with bromism is often characterized by fluctuations in mental status. In a review of cases admitted to Boston City Hospital, Perkins wrote: "The course in these cases was characterized by pronounced, sudden and unpredictable ups and downs. These sudden changes were characteristic enough to suggest the diagnosis of bromidism *[sic]* in hitherto unsuspected cases" (Perkins).

Bromism, although rare, should be suspected in patients with altered mental status and the characteristic laboratory findings of a markedly elevated chloride and a low or negative anion gap. A 1990 survey of reference laboratories estimated that the incidence of bromism (arbitrarily defined as bromide concentration greater than 20 mmol/L) in the United States is now less than 100 cases per year (Bowers). Bromide-containing medications currently available include the rare use of bromide salts such as sodium bromide, potassium bromide, and ammonium bromide for treating refractory epilepsy or as sedatives. A few common medications also contain bromide as a "nonactive" ingredient. These include bromocriptine (Parlodel), dextromethorphan hydrobromide (Robitussin DM, Nyquil, Cheracol), pyridostigmine hydrobromide (Mestinon), and brompheniramine maleate (Drixoral, Dimetane, Bromarest). Bromism from these medications is not reported.

2. Remember that the anion gap, defined as anion gap = [sodium] − {[chloride] + [bicarbonate]}, is the difference between the measured cations and the measured anions. Equivalently, the anion gap could also be considered as the difference between the unmeasured anions and the unmeasured cations. With modern laboratory techniques, the normal range for the anion gap is 3 to 11 (Winter). An abnormally low anion gap will be caused by any condition resulting in increased unmeasured cations or decreased unmeasured anions. Causes of increased unmeasured cations include hypercalcemia, hypermagnesemia, hyperkalemia, high lithium levels, and multiple myeloma. Note that in all but the last of these cases, the cation can be easily measured, giving the correct diagnosis. Decreased unmeasured anions occurs with hypoalbuminemia. The anion gap will also be low if the chloride is falsely elevated. This occurs with bromide toxicity and might also be expected with iodide toxicity. Dilution of serum with water or normal saline (each of which has no unmeasured ions) will cause a decreased anion gap because the same number of unmeasured anions will be distributed in a greater volume of serum (Emmet).

3. Bromide may interfere with some standard laboratory tests for chloride, although this effect is much less pronounced now than it was in the past. The SMAC analyzer measures chloride by detecting the amount of thiocyanate released from mercuric thiocyanate. Bromide has a greater affinity for mercuric ion than chloride and therefore will displace more thiocyanate (Blume). The SMAC will measure an increase in chloride concentration of 1.6 mmol/L for each 1 mmol/L of bromide. Bromide will cause even greater interference with chloride in analyzers that use ion-specific channels. In these instruments each bromide molecule will be measured as 2.25 chloride molecules. Finally, chloride can be determined by a colorimetric technique. In this technique, each molecule of bromide will be counted as one molecule of chloride (Elin).

In some automated electrolyte analyzers, bromide will also interfere with bicarbonate determinations. This has been reported on several occasions with the Kodak Ektachem instrument. This machine uses an ion-selective channel for determining bicarbonate concentrations. Apparently bromide is able to cross this channel and cause a false elevation in measured bicarbonate. In one test, each 1 mEq/L of bromide falsely elevated the bicarbonate by about 2.5 mEq/L (Bowers). Kodak stopped marketing this machine in 1994.

4. Most patients suffering from bromide toxicity will recover with supportive care. Hydration with saline solutions will decrease the half-life of bromide from almost 2 weeks to about 3 days and is a useful addition to treatment. Forced diuresis with saline and loop diuretics has also been suggested. Although hemodialysis will reduce bromide's half-life to about 1 hour, especially in patients with renal dysfunction, it is rarely indicated in the absence of renal insufficiency except in the most severe cases.

Further history revealed that the patient had been taking sodium bromide for the preceding month. According to his diary he had taken up to 51 g on some days. Although this history had been available on admission, and a bromide level had been sent, the diagnosis of bromism was discounted or not considered. The patient was admitted to the intensive care unit, vigorously hydrated with 0.9% NaCl solution, and treated supportively. His mental status improved slowly over a period of 2 weeks, and he was extubated and regained consciousness. Serial bromide levels showed an initial level of 5481 mg/L (68.5 mmol/L), which dropped to 1355 mg/L (16.9 mmol/L) over a 2-week period. By the time the bromide level had dropped to 1355 mg/L, the patient was awake and oriented but not yet completely normal.

SUGGESTED READINGS

Chapter 24, Fluid, Electrolyte, and Acid–Base Principles.

Chapter 63, Sedative-Hypnotic Agents.

Blume RS, MacLowry JD, Wolff SM: Limitations of chloride determination in the diagnosis of bromism. N Engl J Med 1968;279:593–595.

Bowers GN, Onoroski M: Hyperchloremia and the incidence of bromism in 1990. Clin Chem 1990;36:1399–1403.

Elin RJ, Robertson EA, Johnson E: Bromide interferes with determination of chloride by each of four methods. Clin Chem 1981;27:778–779.

Emmet M, Narins RG: Clinical use of the anion gap. Medicine 1977;56:38–54.

Hanes FM, Yates A: An analysis of four hundred instances of bromide intoxication. South Med J 1938;31:667–671.

Matsufuji H, Hayashi T, Nishikawa M, et al: Bromide-induced pseudohyperchloridemia. Pediatr Neurol 2000;22:333.

Perkins HA: Bromide intoxication: Analysis of cases from a general hospital. Arch Intern Med 1950;85:783–794.

Sensenbach W: Bromide intoxication. JAMA 1944;125:769–772.

Winter SD, Pearson RJ, Gabow PA, et al: The fall in the serum anion gap. Arch Intern Med 1990;150:311–313.

Case 28

1. When presented with a scenario such as this, several toxins should come to mind immediately. Were the workers exposed to a simple asphyxiant such as carbon dioxide, methane, or nitrogen, which displace oxygen, thus inducing hypoxia? It is not likely that these agents were involved because the history is more consistent with a rapidly evolving toxicity, whereas hypoxia may take several minutes to develop. Asphyxiation often occurs in small chambers and enclosed spaces with limited ventilation, which was not the case here.

The ubiquitous poison carbon monoxide must also be considered as well as the chemical asphyxiants cyanide, hydrogen sulfide, and carbon disulfide. These later agents bind to cytochrome oxidase, blocking cellular respiration (refer to Fig. 13–2). Oxygen utilization is interrupted and cellular energy is rapidly depleted, causing cardiovascular collapse. Following resuscitation, cyanide causes a persistent metabolic acidosis, which mandates treatment with the Cyanide Antidote Kit (nitrites to induce a methemoglobinemia and thiosulfate to enhance cyanide detoxification). Removal from exposure and supportive care comprise the first-line therapy for hydrogen sulfide and carbon disulfide exposures, as their toxicities are usually rapidly reversible. A final consideration in this case is the irritant gases such as ammonia, nitrogen dioxide, or chlorine, which may rapidly induce pulmonary edema or bronchospasm. The patients' physical examination, chest radiographs, and arterial blood gases do not support these irritants as the cause of their collapse.

While general supportive measures were undertaken, the plant supervisor was contacted and revealed that the patients may have been exposed to hydrogen sulfide.

2. Hydrogen sulfide is a highly toxic colorless gas produced commonly during petroleum refining, during rayon manufacturing, and in the fishing and tanning industries. Natural sources of hydrogen sulfide include bacterial decomposition of sulfur in soil and decay of organic sulfur-containing products (sewers, manure, septic tanks). It is heavier than air, and many poisonings have occurred in tanks and wells where the gas concentrates at the bottom. Hydrogen sulfide does have the odor of rotten eggs, but olfactory fatigue occurs at higher concentrations of gas (>100 ppm), so most of the deadliest exposures occur without warning.

3. At lower levels of exposure, hydrogen sulfide is irritating to mucous membranes and conjunctivae. Increasing respiratory tract irritation occurs at higher levels, with pulmonary edema ultimately developing. At high levels, hydrogen sulfide inhibits cellular respiration by binding to cytochrome a_3 oxidase in the electron transport chain. This binding prevents oxidative phosphorylation from occurring, and thus, ATP cannot be generated, and cellular energy is depleted. The poisoned patient may suffer immediate collapse and imminent death if not removed from exposure. As was probably the case here, very brief exposure to more than 1000 ppm causes paralysis of respiration and collapse.

4. Hydrogen sulfide toxicity is often compared to cyanide poisoning because they both inhibit oxidative phosphorylation through the same mechanism. This has led to the suggestion that utilization of nitrites to induce a methemoglobinemia as in the Cyanide Antidote Kit would decrease the binding of hydrogen sulfide from cytochrome aa_3 as it does with cyanide. However, an important difference exists between cyanide and hydrogen sulfide toxicity. Cyanide binds tightly to the heme portion of cytochrome aa_3, and the induction of methemoglobinemia allows cyanomethemoglobin to be formed, thus freeing the cytochrome from the cyanide inhibition. Hydrogen sulfide binds more reversibly to the cytochrome complex, and thus, removal from exposure alone will decrease the binding of hydrogen sulfide so that further induction of methemoglobin is unnecessary and may be harmful. Methemoglobinemia, following a hypoxic insult, may further impair oxygen-carrying capacity and oxygen delivery to tissues and should be reserved for the moribund patient who has suffered a prolonged exposure. Thus, treatment in this patient following resuscitation is primarily oxygenation and ventilation.

Hyperbaric oxygen is another modality described for use in the hydrogen sulfide–poisoned patient. Increased tissue oxygen concentrations promote the binding of oxygen to cytochromes in place of sulfide–cytochrome binding. In addition, sulfide oxida-

tion to sulfates is enhanced in the presence of increased oxygen. Last, hyperbaric oxygen is an effective therapy used to minimize postanoxic tissue injury and increase oxygen delivery to marginally perfused regions. This is one of the proposed mechanisms of hyperbaric oxygen therapy following carbon monoxide exposure.

The two patients remained deeply obtunded and were transferred to the regional hyperbaric oxygen unit and received 100% oxygen at 2.8 ATA for 48 minutes. One patient awoke on emerging from the chamber and was extubated shortly afterwards. He had a full neurologic recovery and was discharged the following day. Unfortunately, the other patient (the one who collapsed first and thus had the longer exposure) remained in a state of postanoxic encephalopathy.

SUGGESTED READINGS

Chapter 98, Cyanide and Hydrogen Sulfide.
Milby TH, Baselt RC: Hydrogen sulfide poisoning: clarification of some controversial issues. Am J Indust Med 1999;35:192–195.
Ravizza AG, Carugo D, Cerchiari EL, et al: The treatment of hydrogen sulfide intoxication: Oxygen versus nitrites. Vet Hum Toxicol 1982;24:241–242.
Smilkstein MJ, Bronstein AC, Pickett HM, Rumack BH: Hyperbaric oxygen therapy for severe hydrogen sulfide poisoning. J Emerg Med 1985;3:27–30.
Smith RP, Kruszyna R, Kruszyna H: Management of acute sulfide poisoning. Arch Environ Health 1976;31:166–169.
Whitcraft DD, Bailey TD, Hart GB: Hydrogen sulfide poisoning treated with hyperbaric oxygen. J Emerg Med 1985;3:23–25.

Case 29

1. Most of the currently available nonprescription sleeping pills, or hypnotics, contain an antihistamine (H_1 receptor antagonist). The available agents, diphenhydramine, doxylamine, and pyrilamine, all have antimuscarinic effects. These effects would certainly be pronounced at doses that produce the degree of sedation seen in this patient. The other common nonprescription sleep aid is ethanol. At high doses, ethanol produces profound central nervous system (CNS) and respiratory depression. Patients may have an odor of alcohol, but this finding is neither sensitive nor specific for intoxication. Until 1989, the amino acid L-tryptophan was available without a prescription as a "natural" sleep aid. However, a contaminant in the production of this serotonin precursor was linked to the eosinophilia-myalgia syndrome and led to the removal of L-tryptophan from the market. It was recently replaced by L-hydroxytryptophan, a related molecule. Although the same contaminant that led to the withdrawal of L-tryptophan is present in L-hydroxytryptophan, there are no reports of eosinophilia-myalgia syndrome with L-hydroxytryptophan.

Barbiturates were widely used as prescribed hypnotics in the past, but because of their narrow therapeutic index (difference between therapeutic and toxic doses), they have fallen out of favor. Severe respiratory depression occurs in patients who overdose on barbiturates. This finding was not noted in this case. The barbiturates have been largely replaced by benzodiazepines, which produce no respiratory depression when ingested alone, even in overdose. Benzodiazepines work via a specific receptor, where they potentiate the effect of the inhibitory neurotransmitter GABA. Patients who overdose with benzodiazepines generally present with normal vital signs despite being deeply comatose. A new sleep agent, zolpidem (Ambien), is a nonbenzodiazepine agent that also works via the benzodiazepine receptor and produces similar clinical effects.

When dispensing of benzodiazepines in New York State changed to require a triplicate prescription form, there was a rise in the use and abuse of older sedative-hypnotic agents. This was presumably related either to the prescriber's perception of excessive governmental oversight or the laborious process required to complete a triplicate prescription. Meprobamate (Miltown, Equanil), widely used in the 1950s, produces CNS and respiratory depression similar to the barbiturates and may be associated with mild euphoria. It has a tendency to form concretions in the gastrointestinal tract, delaying complete absorption and producing a prolonged or cyclic coma. Glutethimide (Doriden) produces a toxidrome similar to the barbiturates but also manifests some mild anticholinergic effects. Ethchlorvynol (Placidyl) also produces a similar toxidrome, but it carries a distinctive odor similar to plastic. Chloral hydrate (Noctec) is a chlorinated hydrocarbon that is still favored by some pediatricians for procedural sedation. The chlorinated hydrocarbons are well known for their ability to sensitize the myocardium to catecholamines and produce dysrhythmias. The combination of deep coma and dysrhythmias, in the absence of hypoxia, should raise the suspicion of a chloral hydrate ingestion. New York State no longer requires triplicate prescribing but still monitors the prescribing of scheduled substances. The effect that this change will have on the prescribing habits of physicians remains to be seen.

2.   Chloral hydrate has been available for more than 100 years. Although it is directly sedating, it is so rapidly metabolized by alcohol dehydrogenase that only its metabolite, trichloroethanol, can be found in the blood. The trichloroethanol, which is responsible for the CNS and respiratory depression, is further metabolized to trichloroacetic acid or is glucuronidated and excreted. An interaction with ethanol forms the pharmacologic basis for the "Mickey Finn" or "knockout drops." By increasing the supply of the necessary reducing agent, NADH, ethanol metabolism enhances trichloroethanol production. In addition, ethanol inhibits the glucuronidation, and thus slows elimination, of trichloroethanol. Thus, higher trichloroethanol levels are maintained, with the expected result of enhanced toxicity.

Cases of chloral hydrate-induced ventricular dysrhythmias have been recognized for 50 years. Early therapeutic endeavors in these cases consisted of observation, or occasionally the use of lidocaine, which did not appear to be more successful therapeutically than observation alone. Procainamide is demonstrated it to be of little value in management. This may be related to the mechanism of enhanced dysrhythmia formation, which is believed to be a heightened sensitivity to catecholamines. This etiology is similar to dysrhythmogenesis produced by other halogenated hydrocarbons. For example, the general anesthetic agents, such as halothane, which capitalize on the CNS depressive abilities of the halogenated hydrocarbons, are known to produce ventricular dysrhythmias. During the act of abusing halogenated hydrocarbon solvents, patients have developed ventricular dysrhythmias and death, a phenomenon known as "sudden sniffing death." This effect is presumably caused by the outpouring of catecholamines, which further stimulates a myocardium made irritable by the solvent.

In the 1960s it was demonstrated that effective therapy of such dysrhythmias could be based on the underlying pathophysiology.

That is, if the myocardium is sensitive to catecholamines, an agent that reduces catecholamine binding could reduce the tendency for dysrhythmias. The agent first used was the β-adrenergic antagonist alprenolol, and several other β-adrenergic antagonists are also efficacious, including practolol and propranolol. On the basis of this hypothesis of toxicity, it is more easily understood why the class I antidysrhythmic agents were ineffective.

3.   Flumazenil is a competitive antagonist of benzodiazepines. In the setting of an isolated acute benzodiazepine overdose, significant morbidity is not expected. When benzodiazepines are combined with other sedatives such as ethanol, however, death may occur if timely supportive care is not instituted. Despite this, with appropriate supportive care, all such patients are expected to survive without morbidity. Therefore, the need to use flumazenil to reverse sedation in such a patient is questionable, especially given the potential pitfalls. If the patient is a chronic benzodiazepine user and has developed tolerance, abrupt reversal of the benzodiazepine may result in an acute withdrawal syndrome, which, like ethanol withdrawal, can result in altered consciousness, seizures, and death. Flumazenil would not be expected to have an effect in a patient with a pure chloral hydrate overdose. In addition, in the setting of a mixed benzodiazepine and chloral hydrate overdose, flumazenil has been reported to exacerbate ventricular dysrhythmias. This is probably a result of the catecholamine release secondary to acute benzodiazepine withdrawal.

This patient received lidocaine, 100 mg, with no response. Metoprolol was given with prompt resolution of all dysrhythmias. Gastric decontamination was performed, and the patient received activated charcoal. A pregnancy test and acetaminophen level were both negative. She remained stable for 24 hours and was discharged to the psychiatry service on day 2.

SUGGESTED READINGS

Chapter 63, Sedative-Hypnotic Agents.
Bowyer K, Glasser SP: Chloral hydrate overdose and cardiac arrhythmias. Chest 1980;77:232–235.
Cote CJ, Karl HW, Notterman DA, et al: Adverse sedation events in pediatrics: Analysis of medications used for sedation. Pediatrics 2000;106:633–644.
Graham SR, Day RO, Lee R, et al: Overdose with chloral hydrate: A pharmacologic and therapeutic review. Med J Aust 1988;149:686–688.
Gustafson A, Svensson SE, Ugander L: Cardiac arrhythmias in choral hydrate poisoning. Acta Med Can 1977;201:227–230.
Pershad J, Palmisano P, Nichols M: Chloral hydrate: the good and the bad. Pediatr Emerg Care. 1999;15:432–435.
Short TG, Maling T, Galletly DC: Ventricular arrhythmia precipitated by flumazenil. Br Med J 1988;296;1070–1071.

Case 30

1.   In generating the differential diagnosis of possible agents that could induce this scenario, it must be remembered that the patient has chosen a very serious route of administration and has probably also chosen an injectable agent that she felt to be lethal. In addition, she appears to have had a seizure but is now rapidly improving. If the potentially long list is limited to agents readily available, it shortens considerably: insulin, opioids, sedative-hypnotics, barbiturates, neuromuscular blocking agents, potassium chloride, lidocaine, and air embolus. Through varying postulated mechanisms of poor cerebral perfusion, it is possible that any of these agents could induce seizures. The first three agents mentioned can probably be excluded by her normal glucose and negative drug screen and failure to respond to naloxone; however, the use of a short-acting neuromuscular blocking agent such as succinylcholine to induce transient respiratory paralysis may be possible. Potassium chloride is an obvious consideration, as it has been implicated in multiple physician- or nurse-assisted suicides and is widely known as lethal. A transient dysrhythmia inducing a seizure that abated spontaneously as the potassium was redistributed intracellularly could be postulated. A third consideration would be lidocaine, which could also induce a seizure in high dose that would subsequently abate. Fortunately, all of these remaining possibilities simply required supportive care for the patient to do well.

The fluid of the third syringe was analyzed. It was colorless and odorless and noted to have a pH of 7.0, consistent with an injectable drug. Gas chromatography–mass spectrometry was completely negative for any organic substance; however, 1 to 2 mL injected intraperitoneally in a mouse caused collapse and death in 5 minutes. The remaining fluid in the syringe was taken to the hospital chemistry laboratory and analyzed. It had a potassium concentration of 2001.9 mEq/L and a chloride concentration of 2459 mEq/L, consistent with the available form of injectable KCl, which had 20 mEq/10 mL. As suspected, the gravity of her intentions was confirmed.

2. Potassium chloride, in intravenous administration, is of constant concern in hospital settings. Errors in infusion rate or concentration are well known to induce dysrhythmias, which may be fatal. It has often been implicated as the lethal modality utilized by the "Angel of Death" in hospital homicides of the terminally ill. Because 98% of body potassium is intracellular, transient extracellular hyperkalemia induces rapid toxicity before redistributing to intracellular stores. This transient hyperkalemia may be difficult to detect clinically in the living because redistribution is rapid and on postmortem because serum potassium routinely rises after death. It appeared that our patient may have been able to inject only some fraction of a lethal dose, resulting in a dysrhythmia, hypoperfusion, seizure, and then redistribution and recovery. In addition, the 25 g of dextrose given by the paramedics likely prompted insulin release and a further mechanism for uptake of the potassium load to intracellular stores.

In contrast, oral potassium overdoses have only rarely resulted in toxicity in patients with normal renal function. The sustained-release potassium preparations and the potassium "salt substitutes" have more often been implicated. In addition to routine management of the cardiovascular effects with calcium salts, insulin, dextrose, and sodium bicarbonate, further efforts must be directed at gastrointestinal decontamination to prevent further absorption.

Typical electrocardiographic findings progress with increasing potassium levels. Initially, "peaked" or tall T waves are seen in the chest leads. This can be followed by a shortened QT interval. At higher levels, the PR interval prolongs, and then the P waves disappear. Widening of the QRS complex and heart block occur shortly before the QRS joins the T wave in the characteristic "sine wave" pattern, which often degenerates into ventricular fibrillation and asystole.

3. Therapy for the cardiovascular toxicity of hyperkalemia should be initiated immediately with calcium salts. This tran-

siently antagonizes the effects of potassium on the myocardium but does not alter the serum potassium concentration. It should be followed by a glucose bolus with infusion and 5 to 10 units of regular insulin to increase potassium uptake into cells. Sodium bicarbonate therapy further shifts potassium intracellularly and may increase renal excretion of potassium. Potassium exchange resins such as sodium polystyrene sulfonate can be used both orally and rectally and are the only significant modality, excepting dialysis, to remove excess potassium from the body. These resins exchange potassium for sodium, and thus, serum electrolytes should be closely followed during therapy.

This patient recovered completely within the first 24 hours and was transferred for psychiatric evaluation.

SUGGESTED READINGS

Chapter 9, Electrocardiographic Principles.

Chapter 24, Fluid, Electrolyte, and Acid–Base Principles.

Cohen MR: Potassium chloride injection mix-up. Am J Hosp Pharm 1990; 47:2457–2458.

Saxena K: Clinical features and management of poisoning due to potassium chloride. Med Toxicol Adverse Drug Exp 1989;4:429–443.

Wetli CV, Davis JH: Fatal hyperkalemia from accidental overdose of potassium chloride. JAMA 1978;240:1339.

Case 31

1. In the United States, the commonly used rodenticides fall into two groups: anticoagulants and cholecalciferol. Anticoagulants, including coumadin, prevent activation of vitamin K–dependent clotting factors II, VII, IX, X. Following a latent period of at least 24 hours before the onset of significant coagulopathy, hemorrhagic complications such as intracranial hemorrhage may occur. Cholecalciferol causes the typical findings of hypercalcemia: confusion, weakness, hyporeflexia, and electrocardiographic changes.

In other countries, however, different agents are more commonly used as rodenticides. For example, in India, aluminum and zinc phosphides, which are both very highly toxic, are responsible for large numbers of suicides because of their easy availability and low cost. Phosphides, after liberation of phosphine gas, result in diffuse cellular poisoning, and patients manifest multisystem organ failure including pulmonary edema, seizures, and cardiac dysrhythmias. In many developing countries, cholinesterase inhibitors, such as organic phosphorus compounds and carbamates, are widely available as rodenticides because of their ease of production and low cost. Although not used as rodenticides in the United States, these same classes of chemicals are widely available here as various types of insecticides.

The patient stated that he had ingested Tres Pasitos, a rodenticide imported into this country from the Dominican Republic.

2. Acetylcholine (ACh), an excitatory neurotransmitter found in several organ systems of the body, is normally hydrolyzed by cholinesterases within the synapse (refer to Fig. 88–4). Inhibition of cholinesterases results in persistence of ACh and repetitive stimulation of the postsynaptic effector organ. Stimulation of muscarinic cholinergic receptors (M), found in various organs, results in salivation, lacrimation, urination, and diarrhea; the classic SLUD (salivation, lacrimation, urination, and defecation) findings. Also innervated by muscarinic receptors are the pupil (miosis), the heart (bradycardia), and the bronchi (bronchorrhea, bronchospasm). In reality, it is the effects of the last two systems that are the most life-threatening muscarinic effects. At the neuromuscular junction, nicotinic cholinergic receptor (N_M) stimulation results in muscle fasciculations and subsequent depolarizing blockade, an effect analogous to that occurring with succinylcholine. Finally, agonism of nicotinic cholinergic receptors (N_N) in the autonomic ganglia enhances sympathetic outflow with resultant hypertension, tachycardia, and mydriasis. Finally, in the central nervous system, ACh excess leads to diffuse cerebral dysfunction, producing anxiety, seizures, respiratory depression, and coma.

Because of the diverse functions of the cholinergic system, the clinical findings of cholinesterase inhibitor toxicity can be highly confusing. For example, direct parasympathetic stimulation to the heart produces bradycardia, whereas autonomic stimulation or bronchorrhea-induced hypoxia indirectly leads to tachycardia. Pupil size is also highly variable and results from interplay of the sympathetic and parasympathetic systems. The effects that predominate are difficult to predict but are related to the agent in question (lipid solubility, concentration, preference for various cholinesterase subtypes), route of administration, and individual patient variability.

3. Care of patients poisoned by organic phosphorus or carbamate agents is easily focused when one appreciates that death generally results from bronchorrhea-induced hypoxia or from respiratory failure secondary to neuromuscular blockade. Early intubation and management of pulmonary secretions are essential, as is assessment of oxygenation status. Both cutaneous and gastrointestinal decontamination are essential, with special precaution given to protect the caregiver, as dermal exposure or inhalation of the poison may lead to secondary toxicity. Patients with more than minimal symptoms, and certainly those with bronchorrhea or bradycardia, require antidotal therapy. This consists of both atropine and pralidoxime. Atropine, a competitive muscarinic antagonist, is utilized to eliminate continued respiratory secretions or to elevate heart rate. Rapidly escalating doses may be needed, starting with 1 mg in an adult. The clinical endpoint of atropinization is drying of respiratory secretions and improvement in oxygenation status. If any questions about the diagnosis existed before atropine therapy, failure of the patient to become anticholinergic after a standard dose of atropine (eg, dry, flushed skin, absent bowel sounds, mydriasis) should allay these concerns. Because respiratory paralysis is a result of nicotinic receptor overstimulation and atropine is effective only at muscarinic receptor sites, pralidoxime must be added in patients in whom concern for such complications exist. Pralidoxime, also known as 2-PAM, binds to the cholinesterase enzyme at a site distinct from the implicated cholinesterase inhibitor. Following a chemical interaction between the pralidoxime and the cholinesterase inhibitor, the product is released, allowing the cholinesterase enzyme to resume acetylcholine metabolism. Pralidoxime works directly on the enzyme, and it ameliorates toxicity at both muscarinic and nicotinic sites regardless of cholinergic receptor subtype. Any patient requiring more than a trial dose of atropine should receive pralidoxime. The initial dose of pralidoxime is 1 g intravenously over 15 to 30 minutes.

In the past, some have questioned the safety of pralidoxime in patients poisoned by carbamates. Because carbamates, unlike organic phosphorus compounds, undergo spontaneous hydrolysis

from cholinesterase, these authors feel that deliberate enzyme reactivation is unnecessary. In addition, one rodent model of carbamate (carbaryl) poisoning in which treatment included a different cholinesterase reactivator (obidoxime) suggests that the use of a cholinesterase reactivator alone, without atropine, may be dangerous. Another rodent model using pralidoxime in a lower equivalent dose than the former study could not reproduce these initial findings. This concern has no clinical relevance, as atropine should be used in all patients receiving pralidoxime. Importantly, because product identification is often inexact, and toxicity from the two agents cannot be differentiated clinically, the use of 2-PAM is generally indicated.

This patient received an initial 1-mg dose of atropine intravenously, which was doubled every 5 minutes. Resolution of the bronchorrhea occurred after the administration of 8 mg. He also received an initial 1-g bolus of pralidoxime intravenously, followed by an infusion of 500 mg per hour. Frequent readministration of atropine was required, and an infusion was initiated. Although atropine was initially effective at 6 mg per hour, the rate of infusion was increased to 9 mg per hour to prevent recurrent bronchorrhea. The patient remained on this regimen for approximately 5 days with frequent trials of atropine tapering. It was not until day 5 that the patient tolerated reduction in the dose, which was terminated over the next 36 hours. The total atropine dose received was approximately 1 g. Pralidoxime infusion continued for an additional 18 hours after the atropine was stopped and was then discontinued. Approximately 50 g of pralidoxime was infused over the patient's hospital course. The patient awoke on day 4 and was alert and oriented by day 5.

SUGGESTED READINGS

Chapter 90, Rodenticides.
Chapter 88, Insecticides: Organic Phosphorus Compounds, and Carbamates.
Antidotes in Depth: Pralidoxime.
Mercurio-Zappala M, Hack J, Salvador A, Hoffman RS: Carbaryl poisoning: 2-PAM or not 2-PAM. J Toxicol Clin Toxicol 1998;36:428.
Natoff IL, Reiff B: Effect of oximes on the acute toxicity of anticholinesterase carbamates. Toxicol Appl Pharmacol 1973;25:569–575.
Nelson LS, Hoffman RS, Rao R, et al: Poisonings associated with illegal use of aldicarb as a rodenticide—New York City, 1994–1997. MMWR 1997;46:961–963.

Case 32

1. The list of pharmaceuticals and chemicals that produce liver damage is exceedingly long. However, because of the acuity and severity of the patient's clinical presentation, most hepatotoxins can be eliminated. For example, alcohol-induced liver damage is uncommon in such a young person, and the magnitude of the liver enzyme elevation is inconsistent with this diagnosis. Similarly, patients with alcohol-induced hepatitis typically demonstrate AST elevations that are twice that of the ALT. The absence of acetaminophen in the serum, although it does not fully exclude acetaminophen-induced hepatotoxicity, certainly makes it less likely for that drug to be the cause. Iron salts, such as ferrous sulfate, are readily accessible for many women of childbearing age and may produce hepatotoxicity in overdose. However, hepatotoxicity is usually part of a syndrome of multiorgan system failure, which this patient does not manifest.

A large number of herbal medicines contain plant derivatives that are potentially hepatotoxic. Comfrey (*Symphytum officinale*), *Senecio*, and Jamaican Bush tea contain pyrrolizidine alkaloids, which are metabolized by the liver to compounds capable of alkylating cellular macromolecules. Reaction with endothelial cells in the hepatic vein results in chronic inflammation and subsequent fibrosis with sustained use that ultimately produces hepatic venooclusive disease. This syndrome is similar to the Budd-Chiari syndrome and may lead to hepatic failure. A constituent of germander *(Teucrium chamaedrys)* is metabolized to a reactive hepatotoxic metabolite. Recently, epidemic poisoning by germander occurred in France when capsules containing the concentrated extract were sold to facilitate weight loss. High-dose vitamin A capsules may produce swelling of the hepatic sinusoidal lining endothelial cells, causing hepatic failure. Many other herbals, such as chaparral and jin bu huan, have been associated with hepatic toxicity.

2. Despite the widespread use of herbal medicines in the United States, little scientific proof of their efficacy exists. When used in small amounts and on a short-term basis, most herbals are probably harmless. However, excessive dosing, drug interactions, and contamination or adulteration are common problems, primarily because the herbal industry is poorly regulated. Furthermore, many herbalists and alternative care providers treat empirically based on a patient's symptoms rather than on a specific diagnosis, as is standard in conventional medical practice. Although this form of therapy may at times appear effective, given the lack of formal scientific validation of many therapies, it remains unclear if their efficacy represents spontaneous resolution or actual cure.

3. Although this patient suggested that she used the herbal medication to "promote menstruation," this is often a euphemism for "inducing abortion." Pregnancy is a common cause of amenorrhea in women of childbearing age, and individual patients may at times not recognize the correlation. Several agents are available for legal use in the United States to induce abortion. Misoprostol (Cytotec, a prostaglandin analogue), methotrexate (an antimetabolite and embryocidal agent), and mifepristone (RU-486, a progesterone antagonist) are used alone or in combinations to terminate undesired intrauterine or ectopic pregnancies. Oral contraceptives are effective for emergency contraception if used shortly after unprotected intercourse. Quinine has a reputation as an abortifacient despite unproved efficacy and significant maternal toxicity.

Herbals have long been used as emmenagogues, or menstrual flow stimulators, and abortifacients. Because herbal medicines are easily obtained without a physician contact or prescription, herbal abortifacient and emmenagogue use remains common. Herbal abortifacients, like conventional drugs used for similar purposes, induce abortions through one of several different means. For example, they may initiate or enhance uterine contractions, arrest embryonic development, or interfere with the implantation environment. Patients who develop muscle weakness, fasciculations, and vomiting after consumption of an herbal abortifacient tea may be exposed to blue cohosh (*Caulophyllum thalictoides*). This herb contains methylcytisine, a nicotinic agonist similar to nicotine. Although most herbs are probably safe at small doses, their efficacy is based on anecdotal or historical evidence, and many have little scientific foundation.

Pennyroyal oil is the herbal abortifacient most highly associated with hepatotoxicity and the one taken by this patient. This oil, which is a derivative of either *Mentha pulegium* (European or Old World pennyroyal) or *Hedeoma pulegioides* (American pennyroyal), contains approximately 75% pulegone. Pulegone, a chemical with a pungent odor, is found in low concentrations in other mints such as spearmint and peppermint and is commercially available as a flavoring agent and insect repellent. Pulegone is metabolized by the liver and placenta to menthofuran, a reactive electrophilic compound. In a manner analogous to acetaminophen's metabolite NAPQI, menthofuran interacts with and destroys nearby cells, such as hepatocytes and placental cells. Because of the mechanistic similarity to acetaminophen, oral *N*-acetylcysteine use is suggested, although experimental or clinical proof of its benefit remains elusive. It is unclear whether pennyroyal oil is an effective abortifacient without simultaneously inducing maternal toxicity.

The patient was hospitalized following initiation of oral N-acetylcysteine. Over the next 3 days the patient's symptoms and liver enzyme abnormalities resolved. Her pregnancy spontaneously aborted.

SUGGESTED READINGS

Chapter 14, Hepatic Principles.
Chapter 30, Genitourinary Principles.
Chapter 77, Herbal Preparations.
Anderson IB, Mullen WH, Meeker JE, et al: Pennyroyal toxicity: measurement of toxic metabolites in two cases and review of the literature. Ann Intern Med 1996;124:726—734.
Brown PS: Female pills and the reputation of iron as an abortifacient. Med Histol 1977;21:291—304.
Rumack B, Sullivan J, Edell TA, Ferguson S: Fatality and illness associated with consumption of pennyroyal oil—Colorado. MMWR 1978; 27:511—513.

Case 33

1. The differential diagnosis of gastrointestinal distress followed shortly by neurologic impairment should include tetanus, botulism, organic phosphorus compound poisoning, ciguatera poisoning, shellfish poisoning, and tetrodotoxin poisoning. Because of the rapid progression (<l hour) of the motor weakness, both tetanus and botulism seem unlikely. In addition, no history of using any home-canned food was obtained. Likewise, although organic phosphorus compounds can produce severe gastrointestinal symptoms and nicotinic findings such as motor weakness and respiratory failure, the absence of prominent muscarinic signs such as salivation, lacrimation, bronchorrhea, and diarrhea makes organic phosphorus compound toxicity unlikely. The fact that the asymptomatic girlfriend ate a similar meal except for the fish implicates the fish as the source of the toxin.

2. Ciguatera poisoning, by far the most common form of fish-related toxicity, is caused by ingesting warm water reef fish. Hundreds of fish species can contain the toxin, but most cases involve ingestion of large carnivorous reef fish, particularly red snapper, barracuda, grouper, and sea bass. The toxin is produced by *Gambierdiscus toxicus*. This dinoflagellate is a primary food source for small reef fish, and the toxin is concentrated up the food chain from the smaller to the larger fish. Ciguatoxin is harmless to the fish, does not affect the appearance, odor, or taste of the meat, and is heat and acid stable. This toxin competitively inhibits the cal-

cium regulation of passive sodium channels, resulting in increased sodium permeability. Symptoms usually begin within 6 hours of ingesting the contaminated fish and are initially gastrointestinal, including nausea, vomiting, and watery diarrhea. These are followed by a constellation of bizarre neurologic symptoms that are almost exclusively sensory disturbances and include paresthesias, dysesthesias, numbness, tingling, and a sensation of loose teeth. The classic symptom of reversal of temperature discrimination in which cold objects are hot and vice versa appears to be merely a hyperesthesia or a dysesthesia. The patient's actual ability to discriminate hot versus cold remains intact. Symptoms usually resolve within 1 week, although in some individuals it may take months. Motor dysfunction from ciguatoxin is relatively uncommon, although myalgias, ataxia, weakness, and coma have all been reported. Treatment involves supportive care with particular attention to the patient's volume status. Mannitol has been reported to provide significant improvement in ciguatera poisoning, although its mechanism remains unknown.

Shellfish poisoning is caused by ingestion of mollusks such as mussels, clams, and oysters that have fed on a variety of dinoflagellates that produce various neurotoxins. Each dinoflagellate produces a specific toxin and clinical entity.

Ptychodiscus brevis, a dinoflagellate that is found primarily in the Caribbean and along the Florida coast, produces brevitoxin and causes neurotoxic shellfish poisoning. Brevitoxin is heat stable, and its mechanism of action involves increasing sodium channel permeability in peripheral axons. The clinical manifestations of neurotoxic shellfish poisoning typically present in 3 hours and resolve within 24 hours. These symptoms are very similar to those of ciguatera poisoning although typically not as severe. Respiratory tract irritation including conjunctivitis, rhinorrhea, and cough is another unique clinical manifestation involving *Ptychodiscus brevis* seen along coastal beaches during large dinoflagellate blooms. This mucosal irritation is caused by aerosolization of brevitoxin by the surf and improves on termination of exposure.

The *Protogonyaulax* dinoflagellates are found worldwide in temperate coastal waters including the Pacific Northwest and New England. These produce several neurotoxins including saxitoxin that are concentrated in the bivalve mollusks. Ingestion causes paralytic shellfish poisoning. Most cases occur during the summer or "non-R" months (May through August) when large diatomaceous blooms, often called red tides, occur. Although saxitoxin is also heat and acid stable, it differs from ciguatoxin and brevitoxin in that it inhibits sodium channel permeability in excitable membranes of peripheral nerves and muscle. The clinical manifestations of paralytic shellfish poisoning occur rapidly, usually within 30 minutes, and are primarily severe neurologic dysfunction. This may include paresthesias, headache, cranial nerve paralysis presenting as dysphonia, dysphagia, or diplopia, muscular weakness, and death secondary to respiratory failure. The motor weakness may persist for days to weeks. Gastrointestinal symptoms are less commonly noted. The diagnosis is clinical, and treatment is supportive.

In this patient the lack of any significant sensory complaints and the profound motor paralysis makes ciguatera toxicity unlikely. In addition, no history of ingesting any mollusk was obtained, making the diagnosis of shellfish poisoning equally doubtful.

Tetrodotoxin poisoning occurs primarily after ingesting a member of the family Tetraodontidea, which includes puffer fish (also known as blowfish, globe fish, balloon fish, or toadfish) and porcupine fish. Although the toxin has also been isolated from other animals, including certain North American newts *(Taricha granulosa)*, Central American frogs *(Atelopus* spp), and the Australian blue-ringed octopus *(Hapalochlaena maculosa)*, the majority of poisonings involve puffer fish ingestions. In Japan, puffer fish or *fugu* is a gourmet delicacy and requires special training and licensing to prepare. The greatest concentration of toxin is located in the gonads and liver.

Patients who ingest tetrodotoxin usually manifest toxicity relatively rapidly, within 3 hours and often within 15 to 30 minutes. Initially, patients may develop severe vomiting followed by paresthesias, lethargy, a floating sensation, and motor weakness. In severe cases, such as this one, rapid progression of ascending paralysis, respiratory failure, and hypotension occur. Many of these patients maintain their full cognitive function in the setting of total paralysis, creating a terrifying "locked in" syndrome.

Tetrodotoxin's cellular toxicity is quite complex; however, its primary mechanism is very similar to that of saxitoxin. It blocks fast sodium channels in peripheral axons and smooth muscle and thus inhibits conduction. In addition, it has direct effects on the medulla, producing profound emesis via the chemoreceptor trigger zone and respiratory depression.

3. Therapy is supportive with particular attention to airway and respiratory function as well as circulatory status. Orogastric lavage may be lifesaving if performed early, and activated charcoal may be beneficial. A few case reports suggest the efficacy of edrophonium or physostigmine for the reversal of the motor paralysis, although no clear benefit has ever been demonstrated. It is important to remember that symptoms resolve rapidly, usually over a few days, and that the prognosis is excellent for patients who survive the first 24 hours.

Further history revealed that the patient had eaten a blowfish. On his first hospital day he had profound hypertension (200/110 mm Hg) and tachycardia (120 beats/min) poorly responsive to nitroprusside but responsive to benzodiazepines with resultant normalization of his vital signs. Within 36 hours of presentation, his motor function improved rapidly, and after 72 hours he was extubated without difficulty. He was discharged home 7 days after the ingestion.

SUGGESTED READINGS

Chapter 74, Food Poisoning.

Chapter 103, Marine Envenomations.

Bagnus R, Kiberski T, Lauguer S: Clinical observations on 3009 cases of ciguatera (fish poisoning) in the South Pacific. Am J Trop Med Hyg 1979;28:1067–1073.

Cameron J, Capra MF: The basis of the paradoxical disturbance of temperature perception in ciguatera poisoning. J Toxicol Clin Toxicol 1993; 31:571–579.

Clark RF, Williams SR, Nordt SP, Manoguerra AS: A review of selected seafood poisonings. Undersea Hyperb Med 1999;26:175—184.

Lewis RJ: The changing face of ciguatera. Toxicon 2001;39:97—106.

Palafox NA, Jain LG, Pinano AZ, et al: Successful treatment of ciguatera fish poisoning with intravenous mannitol. JAMA 1988;259: 2740–2742.

Sims J, Ostman D: Puffer fish poisoning: Emergency diagnosis and management of mild human tetrodotoxication. Ann Emerg Med 1986;15: 1094–1098.

Case 34

1. The osmolar gap, or the difference between the calculated osmolarity and the measured osmolality, when used correctly provides substantial information, particularly shortly after the ingestion. However, proper interpretation is essential. The osmolar gap is essentially a comparison of the calculated and measured osmotic effects of the serum. Unfortunately, which of these values is higher in any given patient is unpredictable, and many normal patients, in fact, have negative osmolar gaps; the normal range is -14 to $+10$. Because the calculated osmolarity is defined as twice the serum sodium (multiplied by 2 because it is assumed that each positively charged sodium ion is associated with another negatively charged osmotically active particle) plus the molar sums of the glucose and BUN, this calculated value is not altered by the presence of any additional osmoles in the serum. However, any additional osmotically active molecules raise the measured osmolality so that the gap between measured and calculated osmolarity increases. Calculation using the molecular weight of ethylene glycol (62 g/mol) predicts that every 1 mOsm elevation in the osmol gap reflects a rise in the serum ethylene glycol level by 6.2 mg/dL (assuming that this is the only substance contributing to the gap). Importantly, charged molecules do not contribute to the osmol gap because they are offset by a reduction in similarly charged particles, predominantly bicarbonate. Therefore, as the uncharged ethylene glycol is metabolized to the charged acid derivatives, the osmolar gap falls. Fortunately, the anion gap concomitantly rises, allowing the diagnosis to be established.

The osmolar gap also rises in patients with various illnesses, such as sepsis, probably through accumulation of various unspecified, uncharged molecules. Thus, a moderately elevated osmolar gap, up to about 25 mOsm/L, in a clinically ill patient does not establish ethylene glycol or methanol poisoning unless the history is confirmatory. However, an extremely high osmol gap (greater than 75 mOsm/L) may be diagnostic, as no nontoxicologic clinical condition is likely to have this effect. Also, other causes of a high osmolar gap include hyperlipidemia, hyperproteinemia, mannitol infusion, alcoholic ketoacidosis, lactic acidosis, renal failure, and other alcohols (such as isopropanol).

With a measured osmolality of 365 mOsm/kg and a calculated osmolarity of 310 mOsm/L, this patient's osmolar gap was 55 mOsm, which is much larger than the upper limit of the range. A toxic effect of at least 45 mOsm is present, which could correspond with an ethanol level of 207 mg/dL, an ethylene glycol level of 279 mg/dL or a methanol level of 144 mg/dL. His ethanol level was measured as zero.

2. Most currently used radiator antifreezes contain ethylene glycol, a poorly volatile compound that, when added to water, raises its boiling point. Some radiator antifreezes now contain propylene glycol, a compound marketed as "environmentally friendly" or "nontoxic" antifreeze. Gasline antifreeze typically contains methanol, a highly volatile and easily combusted product.

3. Any alcohol can produce CNS depression; however, the degree to which each alcohol produces this effect varies according to its molecular size and arrangement. Generally, the greater the molecular weight of the alcohol, the greater is the CNS depression. For example, methanol will produce less CNS depression at a given serum concentration than ethanol or ethylene glycol.

The toxic manifestations of methanol and ethylene glycol such as acidosis, hypotension, end-organ damage, and death can be delayed. Ethylene glycol toxicity generally begins to manifest in 4 to 6 hours, whereas methanol toxicity can be delayed for up to 12 to 24 hours. Coingestion of ethanol will delay the manifestations of toxicity even further. It is important to recognize the possibility of toxicity early, before manifestations have occurred, because the goal of therapy is to prevent potentially irreversible organ damage.

Both methanol and ethylene glycol can cause acidosis through their metabolic by-products. Methanol is metabolized to formic acid, which, in addition to producing an acidosis, also damages the optic nerve. Ethylene glycol creates an acidosis largely through metabolism to glycolic acid and produces renal failure by metabolism to oxalate, which crystallizes as calcium oxalate in the renal tubules.

4. There are several quick and easy bedside tests that can be employed to differentiate toxic alcohols. These tests can prove extremely useful in many situations in which rapid alcohol concentrations cannot be obtained. Methanol toxicity can be assessed through questioning the patient about visual acuity. Typically, a patient with methanol intoxication may report snow field vision. Also, funduscopic examination of methanol-poisoned patients may show hyperemia of the optic disc and retinal edema.

Ethylene glycol toxicity can be assessed by examination of the patient's urine. The presence of calcium oxalate crystals or fluorescence of the urine may provide evidence for exposure.

Isopropanol can be identified because it is a unique alcohol that produces ketosis without acidosis and ketonuria without glycosuria.

5. Generally, patients with ethanol and isopropanol ingestions can be treated with supportive care with special attention to the airway. Methanol- or ethylene glycol–poisoned patients, however, require specific interventional therapy because of the propensity of these substances to cause severe and permanent organ damage.

The definitive therapy for patients toxic from ingestions of methanol or ethylene glycol is hemodialysis. All alcohols have small molecular weights, low lipophilicity, and low volumes of distribution and ionization, thus making them extremely amenable to extracorporeal removal. Hemodialysis is not without its risks, however, and a level documenting toxicity or clinical signs should be considered when deciding who should be dialyzed. Otherwise asymptomatic patients with methanol or ethylene glycol levels of 35 to 50 mg/dL require hemodialysis. The threshold for dialysis is higher than in the past because there is evidence that endogenous clearance following the administration of fomepizole may be a safe and effective alternative.

Ethanol or fomepizole therapy can be provided while awaiting or deciding on definitive therapy. Ethanol is metabolized by the enzyme alcohol dehydrogenase (ADH) preferentially over methanol or ethylene glycol. Fomepizole inhibits ADH. It is important to realize that it is the metabolic products and not the parent compounds that are responsible for systemic toxicity. An ethanol level of 100 to 150 mg/dL is desired and can be reached through a loading dose (orally or intravenously) of 0.8 g/kg of ethanol, followed by an hourly dose of 15% of the loading dose. Frequent ethanol concentrations should be obtained, and subsequent doses titrated to assure therapeutic levels and protect against toxicity. Ethanol is also removed through hemodialysis, and, therefore, the dose of ethanol should be increased by two to three times while the patient is being hemodialyzed.

Folic acid or folinic acid should be given to methanol-intoxicated patients to help increase metabolism of formic acid to a nontoxic metabolite. Similarly, thiamine and pyridoxine should be given to ethylene glycol–toxic patients.

Methanol is excreted almost exclusively through renal elimination. It could take weeks for a patient to eliminate enough methanol not to require hemodialysis; therefore, such a patient should be transferred to a facility that can perform hemodialysis as soon as possible. Ethylene glycol has an increased rate of renal elimination, and it may be possible in some circumstances, in a low degree of poisoning (level under 100 mg/dL in a patient with normal renal function), to keep the patient's ADH blocked by loading with ethanol or fomepizole for a few days until the ethylene glycol level falls.

Fomepizole (4-methylpyrazole) is an FDA-approved drug that, like ethanol, competes for alcohol dehydrogenase. Although it is expensive, the reduced nursing care (eg, intensive care unit if on ethanol), laboratory support (eg, serial ethanol levels), clinical effects (eg, ethanol intoxication), and side effects (eg, dilutional hyponatremia) probably make it cost neutral.

This patient was transferred to a facility providing hemodialysis, received hemodialysis within 6 hours of presentation, and had no adverse sequelae. An ethylene glycol level at an unknown point before hemodialysis was 240 mg/dL.

SUGGESTED READINGS

Chapter 24, Fluid, Electrolyte, and Acid–Base Principles.

Chapter 66, Toxic Alcohols.

Antidotes in Depth: Ethanol.

Brent J, McMartin K, Phillips S, et al: Fomepizole for the treatment of methanol poisoning. N Engl J Med 2001;344:424—429.

Brent J, McMartin K, Phillips S, et al: Fomepizole for the treatment of ethylene glycol poisoning. N Engl J Med 1999;340:832—838.

Hoffman RS, Smilkstein MJ, Howland MA, Goldfrank LR: Osmol gaps revisited: Normal values and limitations. J Toxicol Clin Toxicol 1993; 31:81–93.

Schelling JR, Howard RL, Winter SD, Linas SL: Increased osmolal gap in alcoholic ketoacidosis and lactic acidosis. Ann Intern Med 1990;113: 580–585.

Smithline N, Gardner KD: Gaps—anionic and osmolal. JAMA 1976;236: 1594–1597.

Winter ML, Ellis MD, Snodgrass WR: Urine fluorescence using a Wood's lamp to detect the antifreeze additive sodium fluorescein: A qualitative adjunctive test in suspected ethylene glycol ingestions. Ann Emerg Med 1990;19:663–667.

Case 35

1. Theophylline toxicity commonly begins with nausea and vomiting. The nausea and vomiting, although not life-threatening, are often quite significant in that they interfere with the administration of oral activated charcoal, which is considered to be the mainstay of initial therapy. As theophylline levels increase, sinus tachycardia usually occurs. Other supraventricular tachycardias and ventricular dysrhythmias also occur. Electrolyte abnormalities develop, largely as manifestations of catecholamine excess. Hypokalemia and hyperglycemia are the most common findings, although hypophosphatemia and hypomagnesemia as well as either hypo- or hypercalcemia have been reported. These electrolyte abnormalities may contribute to the dysrhythmogenesis. As theophylline intoxication becomes more severe, seizures appear and often herald the onset of life-threatening events. Finally, refractory hypotension and cardiovascular collapse are the most common causes of death.

The mechanism for many of these events relates to excess catecholaminergic stimulation. Theophylline increases circulating levels of both norepinephrine and epinephrine, predominantly the latter. This can increase the heart rate, produce electrolyte abnormalities, lower diastolic blood pressure (through β_2-adrenergic stimulation), and provoke dysrhythmias. Animal evidence supports this in that β-adrenergic antagonism abolishes most of these effects. In addition, at toxic doses, theophylline becomes a true inhibitor of phosphodiesterase, with the resultant increase in cyclic adenosine monophosphate (AMP) possibly contributing to hypotension through smooth muscle vasodilation. Finally, theophylline is also an adenosine antagonist. This effect has been associated with tachycardias and seizures.

2. Basic supportive care, with attention to airway, breathing, and circulation, takes precedent over routine poison management. Gastric decontamination is important in significant ingestions because patients will often take such large gram amounts of theophylline as to limit activated charcoal's efficacy. Although syrup of ipecac–induced emesis may be indicated very early on postingestion, it has the significant risk of interfering with the patient's ability to tolerate activated charcoal. Orogastric lavage is therefore generally preferred, although many sustained-release preparations are too large to pass through the lavage hose. Multiple-dose activated charcoal therapy is indicated for all ingestions of sustained-release theophylline products. When vomiting occurs, it can be controlled with an antiemetic. In general, metoclopramide is preferred because of its promotility mechanism and lack of effect on seizure threshold (seen with phenothiazine derivatives). When metoclopramide fails, ondansetron has been used with success. The first-line treatment for seizures is benzodiazepines. Experimental evidence supports the use of phenobarbital over phenytoin as a second-line agent. Neuromuscular blockade (as done in this case) may be necessary to control the motor manifestations but offers no protection against electrical status epilepticus. Supraventricular tachydysrhythmias may respond to calcium channel blockers or β-adrenergic antagonists. Ventricular dysrhythmias should be treated with lidocaine. The choice between these two agents usually depends on the patient's underlying medical condition, specifically on whether or not he or she has asthma. Hypotension should be initially treated with fluids, followed by a pure α-adrenergic agonist such as phenylephrine. When these steps fail, β-adrenergic antagonists have been used with success in animal models as well as some human case reports.

3. Both hemodialysis and hemoperfusion are useful for enhancing the elimination of theophylline. Hemoperfusion is superior, but many consultants are unfamiliar with this procedure and often opt for hemodialysis, which is an acceptable alternative. All patients with life-threatening manifestations of toxicity (seizures, hypotension, or unstable dysrhythmias) should have extracorporeal drug removal initiated. In addition, hemodialysis or hemoperfusion is indicated for those patients with high initial levels, those with rapidly rising levels, and all patients with levels above 90 mg/mL. It is important to remember that extracorporeal drug removal will have limited efficacy if gastrointestinal absorption continues. This underscores the need for adequate activated charcoal therapy and possibly suggests a role for whole-bowel irrigation in the most severely ill patients.

Hemodialysis was initiated, but the theophylline levels fell only to 126 µg/mL after the first therapy. Gastrointestinal decontamination was emphasized, and the patient had a second dialysis treatment, which lowered the level to 103 µg/mL. After the third dialysis treatment, the patient's theophylline level was 60 µg/mL, and his hemodynamic, acid–base, and neurologic status began to improve.

SUGGESTED READINGS

Chapter 6, Principles and Techniques Applied to Enhance Elimination of Toxic Compounds.

Chapter 39, Methylxanthines.

Biberstein MP, Ziegler MG, Ward DM: Use of beta-blockade and hemoperfusion for acute theophylline poisoning. West J Med 1984;141: 485–490.

Park GD, Spector R, Roberts RJ, et al: Use of hemoperfusion for the treatment of theophylline toxicity. Am J Med 1983;74:961–966.

Shannon MW: Comparative efficacy of hemodialysis and hemoperfusion in severe theophylline intoxication. Acad Emerg Med 1997;4:674—678.

Shannon M: Life-threatening events after theophylline overdose: a 10-year prospective analysis. Arch Intern Med 1999;159:989—994.

Vestal RE, Eiriksson CE Jr, Musser B, et al: Effect of intravenous aminophylline on plasma levels of catecholamines and related cardiovascular and metabolic responses in man. Circulation 1983;67:162–171.

Case 36

1. Dry ice is the solid form of carbonic acid, which under normal ambient conditions is gaseous carbon dioxide. Carbon dioxide gas is colorless, odorless, nonexplosive, and imparts an acidic taste at high concentrations because if dissolves in mucosal water to form carbonic acid. Carbon dioxide carried in the plasma (P_{CO_2}) is primarily responsible for our respiratory drive and the plasma P_{CO_2} is tightly controlled by the central nervous system through the regulation of breathing. For this reason, exogenous carbon dioxide, combined with oxygen, is used medically as a respiratory stimulant in neonates. Under normal conditions, ambient air contains approximately 0.03% CO_2. Dry ice is an extremely cold substance ($-78.5°C$) that undergoes conversion from solid to gas without liquefaction, a process known as sublimation.

Carbon dioxide may produce both acute and subacute toxicity. The latter occurs when a patient hypoventilates, fails to eliminate endogenous carbon dioxide, and develops hypercapnia. This may be secondary to respiratory failure (eg, COPD or opioid poisoning) or may be iatrogenic (eg, permissive hypercapnia) and is typically manifest as gradual somnolence. Alternatively, acute CO_2 toxicity produces immediate hypoxia or anoxia because of the physical ability of CO_2 to displace oxygen. That is, because at any given temperature and pressure a liter of air can contain only a certain number of particles, the sublimation of dry ice to CO_2 displaces the other components of ambient air, most importantly oxygen. Therefore, because the "toxicity" of simple asphyxiants does not involve deleterious effects of the gas itself, the clinical findings are largely proportional to the magnitude of the reduction in the fraction of inspired oxygen (FIO_2). Experimental models of acute CO_2 poisoning in which the FIO_2 has been maintained at normal levels have demonstrated that central nervous system and respiratory status deteriorate within seconds. This suggests that CO_2 is not simply a simple asphyxiant but rather that it has acute systemic effects as well. As in the disaster at Lake Nyos, a carbonated lake in Cameroon that released a massive cloud of CO_2 gas on the local community killing thousands, the patient in this case appeared to succumb extremely rapidly. This effect is typical of acute massive CO_2 exposure and is probably exacerbated by the reduced environmental FIO_2. Because there was no indication that the patient was trapped in the cold room or that another event had occurred (ie, myocardial infarction, seizure, etc) to prevent his fleeing, it appears most likely that the patient became incapacitated and subsequently asphyxiated. This is supported by the relatively high temperature in the cold room (4°C) compared to the dry ice and the poor ventilation of the room. Each block of dry ice, fully sublimated, will liberate enough carbon dioxide gas to approximately fill the entire room.

2. Asphyxiation is defined as illness caused by hypoxia. Hypoxic hypoxia is associated with a failure to oxygenate the blood. This may be result from mechanical causes such as choking or from the reduction of the oxygen content of breathable air. For example, death from suffocation by a plastic bag is caused by selective depletion of oxygen by rebreathing into the bag. Fire may deplete ambient oxygen and produce asphyxiation independently of the effects of smoke inhalation or carbon monoxide poisoning. Alternatively, at high altitude the reduced atmospheric pressure results in a reduced partial pressure of oxygen. Although the percentage of oxygen in air remains normal (ie, 21%), fewer molecules of oxygen are inspired with each breath, producing hypoxia. As in this case, displacement of breathable oxygen with another gas, or asphyxiation, is yet another example of hypoxic hypoxia.

However, not all asphyxiation results from hypoxemia. Because the delivery of oxygen relies primarily on hemoglobin, reduction in hemoglobin's ability to bind or release oxygen produces cellular asphyxiation. Thus, patients with carbon monoxide poisoning or severe anemia suffer tissue hypoxia from a marked reduction in the ability of hemoglobin to deliver oxygen (despite a normal PO_2). Alternatively, cyanide and carbon monoxide prevent the normal tissue utilization of oxygen through inhibition of mitochondrial oxidative phosphorylation. This cellular asphyxiation may also be lethal despite a normal PO_2.

3. Occupational exposure to carbon dioxide is widespread. It is used to carbonate soft drinks and as a shielding gas for welding. Carbon dioxide gas is produced by decomposition or fermentation of organic material. Asphyxiation by CO_2 has occurred in workers entering grain elevators, cargo ship holds, or brewery vats. Miners, understanding the risk of "black damp," in which carbonaceous material is oxidized to CO_2 (by oxygen, thus depleting it), lower candles or mice into caves before entering. Compressed carbon dioxide gas is used as a fire extinguisher because of its ability to safely displace oxygen from a fire environment. The use of this type of fire extinguisher in a closed space, such as an airplane or bank vault, may prove lethal. Dry ice is commonly used in the biomedical and frozen foods industries and is used to generate artificial smoke for stage productions. Previously, storage of dry ice in closed spaces such as submarines and automobiles has proven hazardous.

4. Removal from exposure and oxygenation provide the only specific therapy that is needed. Emergency supportive care, such as endotracheal intubation and hemodynamic support, should be used as clinically indicated. Central nervous system impairment is probably the most common effect and may be isolated or a component of multisystem organ failure. Long-term outcome in patients with mild to moderate poisoning, complications notwithstanding, is excellent.

On further scene investigation, it appeared that the external ventilation system was nonfunctional, although internal air movement within the refrigerator occurred via the cooling fan. The blocks of dry ice appeared grossly intact. Postmortem examination of the decedent was unrevealing, as was the toxicologic evaluation. A blood P_{CO_2} was not performed because of its well-described rapid postmortem rise. In order to confirm the cause of death, the conditions at the time of the event were reproduced exactly using the same cold room. Air was sampled serially at several heights; the O_2 concentration fell and the CO_2 concentration rose within 20 minutes and peaked by 3 hours. The FIO_2 3 hours after dry ice storage was 13.6%, and the CO_2 concentration was 27.6%, both at a height of 9 inches. Concentrations of 20 to 30% (200,000–300,000 ppm) CO_2 are associated with the rapid development of unconsciousness and death. Additionally, the temperature of the room had fallen to −15°C. Thus, it appears that even at the cold temperatures of the cold room, sublimation of dry ice progresses rapidly.

SUGGESTED READINGS

Chapter 95, Simple Asphyxiants and Pulmonary Irritants.

Baxter PJ, Kapila M, Mfonfu D: Lake Nyos disaster, Cameroon, 1986: the medical effects of large scale emission of carbon dioxide. BMJ 1989;298:1437.

Dalgaard JB, Deneker F, Fallentin B, et al: Fatal poisoning and other health hazards connected with industrial fishing. Br J Indust Med 1972;29:307—316.

Gibbons HL. Carbon dioxide hazards in general aviation. Aviat Space Environ Med 1977;48:261—263.

Ikeda N, Takahashi H, Umetsu K, Suzuki T: The course of respiration and circulation in death by carbon dioxide poisoning. Forensic Sci Int 1989;41:93—99.

Takaoka M, Morinaga K, Karakawa K, et al: A case report of acute carbon dioxide intoxication by dry ice. Jpn J Toxicol 1988;1:87—90.

Troisi FM: Delayed death caused by gassing in a silo containing green forage. Br J Indust Med 1957;14:56—58.

Case 37

1. Sodium nitroprusside contains an iron molecule coordinated with five cyanide and one nitric oxide molecules. It is the nitric oxide, formerly known as endothelial-derived relaxation factor (EDRF), that is responsible for the potent arterial and venous dilatory effects of this drug commonly used in critical care. The nitric oxide is released rapidly; the cyanide molecules are liberated gradually. In most patients, this release is slow enough that the endogenous detoxification mechanisms can eliminate the cyanide before it can interfere with cellular respiration. Those patients with poor nutritional status and patients receiving very rapid infusion rates may be unable to promptly detoxify the cyanide and poisoning ensues. Rarely, exposure of the photosensitive nitroprusside solution to sunlight may cleave cyanide prematurely, resulting in the actual intravenous administration of cyanide and resultant poisoning.

Cyanide is detoxified through high-affinity complexation with methemoglobin, which is normally present as 1 to 2% of the total hemoglobin. Additionally, nitroprusside itself may enhance the oxidation of hemoglobin to methemoglobin, ensuring a reliable detoxification mechanism. Regardless, the end product is the cyanomethemoglobin, a safe albeit non-oxygen-carrying form of hemoglobin. Subsequently, cyanide elimination involves the rhodanese-mediated transfer of sulfur directly to cyanide to form thiocyanate (SCN) or to cyanomethemoglobin, forming thiocyanate and regenerating methemoglobin. Thiocyanate is substantially less toxic than the cyanide and is eliminated slowly by the kidney ($t_{1/2} \sim$ 4 days). Thus, patients receiving large infusions of nitroprusside at a moderate rate do not develop cyanide poisoning but may develop thiocyanate toxicity, particularly if renal function is suboptimal.

2. Clinically cyanide and thiocyanate poisoning are similar, and their differentiation is often complicated, as in this case, by their common association with nitroprusside. When uncertainty exists, it is preferable to assume the diagnosis of cyanide poisoning given its more consequential effects. Patients with moderate degrees of either poisoning may present with malaise, headache, abdominal pain, altered mental status, and seizures. Importantly, those with cyanide poisoning also develop a metabolic acidosis with an elevated lactate, a critical finding representing the inhibition of oxidative metabolism.

The pharmacy and nursing records are often critical to determining the correct diagnosis. Patients who receive extremely rapid nitroprusside infusions (more than 1.5 mg/kg nitroprusside administered over a few hours or more than 4 µg/kg/min for more than 12 hours) may overwhelm the ability of rhodanese to metabolize cyanide. Those patients on prolonged infusions (>2 days) may exhaust the endogenous supply of sulfur donor (eg, thiosulfate). Interestingly, patients with renal failure may be less likely to develop cyanide poisoning because of the larger burdens of retained sulfur-containing substrates for rhodanese. However, as noted, in this same population, thiocyanate accumulates because its elimination is completely dependent on renal function.

The diagnosis of both cyanide and thiocyanate toxicity is usually established on clinical grounds alone because timely laboratory analysis is often impractical. If cyanide poisoning is suspected, the only routine laboratory test with diagnostic implications is the serum lactate level because it is typically above 10 mmol/L following acute poisoning. However, thiocyanate poisoning occurs in the absence of a lactate-associated metabolic acidosis but is often associated with renal insufficiency. Thiocyanate levels may be predictive of toxicity but not generally available in a clinically useful fashion.

3. Once the diagnosis of cyanide poisoning is seriously entertained, the patient should receive a standard dose (12.5 g in an adult) of intravenous sodium thiosulfate. This is the final part of the cyanide antidote kit and is notably benign. It may be utilized without administering the first two parts of the kit, amyl nitrite and sodium nitrite, respectively, which generate methemoglobin, a cyanide scavenger. Although potentially beneficial, their administration is not critical to antidotal function and often produces undesired effects such as hypotension and reduced oxygen delivery.

Because cyanide toxicity is predictable based on a rapid rate and long duration of infusion, patients in this situation should receive empiric therapy by the inclusion of sodium thiosulfate (5–10 g intravenously daily) in the infusion. Other non-FDA-approved antidotes, such as hydroxocobalamin, are used successfully in a similar prophylactic role. This latter antidote may be particularly beneficial in the patient with potential thiocyanate toxicity because it does not entail the conversion of cyanide to thiocyanate.

Thiocyanate toxicity, although of clinical concern, is not typically life threatening. Treatment is directed at reducing the formation of additional toxin by reducing the infusion rate or switching vasodilators. Hemodialysis is effective in patients with renal failure who develop thiocyanate toxicity.

The patient received 12.5 g of sodium thiosulfate, and his antihypertensive regimen was changed to labetolol with a modest improvement in his mental status. His serum cyanide level was undetectable, and his thiocyanate level was elevated.

SUGGESTED READINGS

Chapter 98, Cyanide and Hydrogen Sulfide.
Antidotes in Depth: Cyanide Antidotes.
Baud FJ, Barriot P, Toffis V, et al: Elevated blood cyanide concentrations in victims of smoke inhalation. N Engl J Med 1991;325:1761–1766.
Food and Drug Administration: New labeling for sodium nitroprusside emphasizes risk of cyanide toxicity. JAMA 1991;265:847.
Friedrich JA, Butterworth JF: Sodium nitroprusside: Twenty years and counting. Anesth Analg 1995;81:152–162.
Zerbe NF, Wagner BK: Use of vitamin B$_{12}$ in the treatment and prevention of nitroprusside-induced cyanide toxicity. Crit Care Med 1993;21:465–467.

Case 38

1. The differential diagnosis of a drug-induced seizure is lengthy, but this patient's history suggests that the prior night's events may be related. Nevertheless, common and treatable causes of seizure, such as hypoglycemia, must still be evaluated. In particular, ethanol-induced hypoglycemia, which occurs as a result of the alteration of the body's redox state during the metabolism of large amounts of ethanol, should be considered and assessed (see Chap. 64). Although profound ethanol intoxication is associated with seizures, such cases are uncommon. Ethanol withdrawal seizures, sometimes termed "rum fits," are common in an ED population but unlikely in a patient of this young age. Ethanol withdrawal seizures typically begin 12 to 24 hours following the patient's last drink and, although self-limited, are often treated with benzodiazepines to prevent the development of delirium tremens.

Many other drugs are commonly available at dance clubs, and several are prominently associated with seizures. The increasing use of heroin by a younger, club-going crowd is commensurate with the increasing purity of the available heroin and its capability for intranasal administration. Heroin or other opioids occasionally produce hypoxia-related seizures, which result from the profound respiratory depressant effects of these drugs. However, this patient's normal pulse oximetry and respiratory rate preclude heroin-induced hypoxia. γ-Hydroxybutyrate (GHB) and its precursors, γ-butyrolactone and butanediol, are used by dance club patrons as euphoriants and sedatives. Excessive dosing of GHB rapidly pro-

duces coma. Seizures occur occasionally, although their mechanism is not yet fully defined. However, GHB is very rapidly metabolized, and the clinical effects would not be expected to persist the following morning. Withdrawal from GHB and its congeners may also cause seizures. Ketamine, a dissociative anesthetic agent, is popular with a small segment of the club-going community. Its clinical effects, which are often described as dysphoric rather than euphoric, probably account for its relatively small, although growing, audience. It is likely that ketamine-induced seizures are rare because the drug has prominent anticonvulsant activity mediated by antagonism of the excitatory neurotransmitter glutamate at its NMDA receptor subtype.

Cocaine causes seizures, both through a direct pharmacologic means (sodium channel blockade) or by causing cerebrovascular ischemia or hemorrhage. Although cocaine is still widely available as a recreational agent, the patient's normal vital signs essentially eliminate acute cocaine toxicity as a diagnostic possibility. The intracranial complications require further evaluation. Methamphetamine similarly produces dramatic alterations in users' vital signs and is less frequently associated with seizures because it lacks the sodium channel effects of cocaine. Ecstasy, or methylenedioxymethamphetamine (MDMA), is an amphetamine derivative with a duration of effect of approximately 6 hours. It is widely used in dance clubs, during which time patrons dance continually until the euphoric effects of the drug subside. MDMA's effects are differentiated from those of methamphetamine by its specific potentiation of serotonergic neurotransmission, an effect that may also be the cause of MDMA-related seizures.

2. Seizures should be rapidly controlled to prevent the development of life-threatening complications such as hyperthermia, hypoxia, or rhabdomyolysis. Glucose and oxygen should be administered as needed. The optimal method for terminating an unrelenting seizure is the intravenous administration of a benzodiazepine, such as diazepam or lorazepam. Patients with suspected poisoning whose seizures remain refractory to the aforementioned interventions should receive intravenous pyridoxine, 5 g, for the possibility of isoniazid poisoning. Continuing seizure activity may require administration of a barbiturate (preferably a rapidly acting agent such as pentobarbital). Most drug-induced seizures will be controlled with these interventions, but rarely neuromuscular blockade will be required to prevent the development of life-threatening acidosis, rhabdomyolysis, or hyperthermia.

During or immediately following the termination of a seizure, patients should be assessed for hyperthermia and ventilatory status, and an attempt should be made to determine the etiology of the seizure. Most patients with new-onset seizures, without an identified reversible etiology, should have an assessment of their glucose and electrolytes in addition to a cranial CT. The specific need for these and other tests (such as a lead level) and the timing of these tests depend on the patient's clinical condition and related historical factors.

3. As a derivative of amphetamine, MDMA shares many of the parent's pharmacologic and clinical properties. Amphetamines enhance the release of biogenic amines (eg, norepinephrine, dopamine, serotonin) predominantly through the alteration of their presynaptic vesicular packaging. MDMA, however, is less active than methamphetamine at potentiating norepinephrine release and is associated with dramatically less autonomic stimulation. Importantly MDMA, perhaps because of its double-ring structure, has more pronounced effects on serotonin release than methamphetamine. Clinically, this translates into more profound psychedelic effects including distortions and illusions, but despite its categorization as a "hallucinogenic" amphetamine, MDMA does not produce overt hallucinations. Rather, it produces an elevation in the user's mood and sense of well-being. Psychotherapists have attempted to enhance their therapeutic relationship with patients through the use of MDMA as an "entactogen" or an "empathogen," meaning an agent that enhances introspection.

However, these attractive psychoactive serotonergic effects of MDMA are not without a price. In animal models and human subjects the habitual use of MDMA produces demonstrable neuronal toxicity that likely relates to the excitatory effects of serotonin. Although this effect is only beginning to be defined, chronic MDMA use risks this loss of serotonergic neurons with resultant alterations in cognition, mood, sleep, and memory. Each of these brain processes utilizes serotonin. The acute adverse effects include life-threatening hyperthermia and its sequelae, and this presentation may actually represent a form of the serotonin syndrome. Furthermore, and particularly relevant to this case, serotonin is the neurotransmitter intimately related to the regulation of antidiuretic hormone (ADH) release. In the setting of serotonin overabundance, excessive release of ADH may produce the syndrome of inappropriate ADH (SIADH), the most important consequence of which is hyponatremia. SIADH may be aggravated or masked by exercise (dancing)-induced loss of intravascular volume, which also causes ADH release and hampers the ability to differentiate SIADH from appropriate ADH release. Further, hyponatremia may be intensified by repletion of salt and water losses with water or other nonelectrolyte solutions. The management of SIADH must emphasize volume restriction because saline administration generally worsens the hyponatremia. In the presence of life-threatening complications of hyponatremia, such as status epilepticus, sufficient hypertonic saline to raise the serum sodium above 120 mEq/L is beneficial. In patients with volume depletion, repletion of intravascular volume with normal saline may be appropriate.

Based on his adverse response to normal saline, this patient likely had true SIADH with hyponatremia-related seizures.

SUGGESTED READINGS

Chapter 68, Amphetamines.

Greer G, Tolbert R: Subjective reports of the effects of MDMA in a clinical setting. J Psychoactive Drugs 1986;18:319–327.

Henry JA, Jeffreys KJ, Dawling S: Toxicity and deaths from 3,4-methylenedioxymethamphetamine ("ecstasy"). Lancet 1992;340:384–387.

Henry JA, Fallon JK, Kicman AT, et al: Low-dose MDMA ("ecstasy") induces vasopressin secretion. Lancet 1998;351:1784.

McCann UD, Szabo Z, Scheffel U: Positron emission tomographic evidence of toxic effect of MDMA ("ecstasy") on brain serotonin neurons in human beings. Lancet 1998;352:1433–1437.

Case 39

1. Gases may be irritant in nature through two distinct mechanisms. Certain chemicals, such as those used as tear gas, enhance the neuronal release of substance P, the neurotransmitter involved in the pain response. In conventional doses, the pain from these agents is accompanied by minimal visible changes in the surfaces they contact. Alternatively, irritant gases produce toxicity following their dissolution in mucosal water to form an acid or an alkali or by liberation a free radical. Once dissolved, these toxicologic mediators both activate pain or irritant receptors and directly injure the cell membranes of nearby tissue, producing clinical symptoms. In the eyes and oropharynx this manifests as pain, erythema, injection, or induration, and in the distal bronchopulmonary tree it causes capillary leak. The clinicopathologic syndrome associated with capillary leak is acute lung injury, which was formerly termed noncardiogenic pulmonary edema. Insight into the physicochemical nature of the irritant gas allows the prediction of the expected clinical findings.

2. In general, irritant gases fall into one of three categories, which differ based on the solubility of the chemical in water. Examples of agents that are highly irritating in low concentration include ammonia, hydrogen sulfide, hydrogen chloride, and chloramine gas. Chloramine is of interest not because of its extreme toxicity but because it is most commonly encountered as the result of an inadvertent household chemistry experiment. In a misguided attempt to "superclean" a surface, such as a toilet, ammonia and a hypochlorite containing product (eg, bleach) may be used in combination. The result of this mixture is the production of chloramine gas, which, in a closed space such as a typical bathroom, may produce an immediate irritant response prompting escape. Such highly irritant gases are said to have good warning properties because they produce burning in the eyes and throat immediately on exposure. More intense exposure as a result of either highly concentrated gas or inability to escape may result in dyspnea, stridor, bronchospasm, or upper airway obstruction.

Agents with poor water solubility are often nonirritating in moderate to high concentrations, and some agents in fact may be pleasant. Phosgene, the prototype, has an odor akin to "freshly mown hay" and was used effectively as a war gas because it lacked aversive qualities even at toxic doses. Because of their low solubility, patients exposed to such gases remain in the toxic environment, and the prolonged exposure allows the gas to reach the alveoli. On dissolution, irritation of both the upper and lower respiratory epithelium occurs, which may lead to acute lung injury. Other examples of poorly soluble gases include ozone and oxides of nitrogen such as nitrogen dioxide. Although initially asymptomatic, patients exposed to significant concentrations of these substances may develop pulmonary edema 12 to 16 hours following their exposure.

The agents with intermediate water solubility, of which chlorine is most representative, are irritating in high concentrations but may be quite tolerable at low levels. Very low-level exposure occurs poolside, and obviously no significant toxicity occurs. This patient, who was exposed to a high concentration of chlorine gas released from the pool shock container, which typically contains either concentrated calcium hypochlorite [$Ca(OCl)_2$] or trichloro-S-triazinetrione (TST), suffered rapid mucosal irritation. Because of the concentration of the gas, even with the brief exposure, the patient inhaled a sufficient quantity of gas to allow it to enter the bronchopulmonary tree. Chlorine releases both hydrochloric acid and reactive oxygen species, and both likely participate in the development of acute lung injury. In fact, the patient's chest radiograph revealed mild, diffuse, bilateral pulmonary infiltrates consistent with pulmonary edema.

3. Because upper airway swelling may be profound and lead to stridor and glottic occlusion, aggressive airway management is the rule. Direct visualization of the vocal cords and supraglottic area is indicated in symptomatic patients. Although orotracheal or nasotracheal intubation is preferred if needed, cricothyrotomy may become necessary. Although they are not well studied, corticosteroids should probably be used in patients with significant airway edema.

Pulmonary evaluation including serial physical examination, pulse oximetry or blood gas analysis, and radiography may be needed to adequately assess the extent of pulmonary damage. Supplemental oxygen should be used to prevent hypoxemia. Bronchospasm should be treated with β-adrenergic agonist nebulizers at standard doses. There is no current role for the routine use of corticosteroids as prophylaxis or treatment for acute lung injury, but their use in intractable bronchospasm is probably warranted.

Nebulized sodium bicarbonate has been shown to provide symptomatic relief in patients exposed to chlorine and is probably useful in all irritant gases that liberate acid. Through a neutralization reaction, the damaging effect of the acid is limited. Any heat or gas generated by this process should be readily dissipated by the bronchopulmonary system. Nebulized sodium bicarbonate should be used in concentrations less than 2%, which generally means about 4:1 dilution of standard 8% sodium bicarbonate. Note that although symptoms may improve, it remains undocumented that complications are reduced or that the natural history of the syndrome is altered. This is certainly of most concern following exposure to irritant gases, such as chlorine or ozone, that liberate

reactive oxygen species. Thus, patients who receive nebulized sodium bicarbonate should be observed for a prolonged period. Irritated eyes should receive copious irrigation with normal saline. Fluorescein staining may reveal corneal abrasions. Ophthalmologic consultation or followup is recommended if symptom resolution is not rapid.

Observation is required for all patients exposed to irritant gases. Those exposed to highly soluble agents may be safely discharged if they do not become symptomatic within 2 to 4 hours of exposure or after symptom resolution if prolonged or intense exposure did not occur. In such cases, delayed symptoms would not be expected. Admission is required for all symptomatic patients who were exposed to intermediate or poorly soluble gases because the extent of toxicity is unpredictable. History of exposure will determine the need for admission of patients exposed to intermediate or poorly soluble gases who are not initially symptomatic. If exposure is extensive, or the patient's ability to return if symptoms develop is not guaranteed, 24 hours of hospital observation with continuous pulse oximetry is warranted.

Despite significant findings of hypoxemia (ABG 7.47/30/65 on room air) and clinical and radiographic evidence of acute lung injury, the patient turned around rapidly and improved over the following 16 hours. The patient's dyspnea resolved by the morning, and although stridor did not develop, his throat irritation took 2 days to fully resolve. He was discharged the following day.

Study Questions for Goldfrank's Toxicologic Emergencies, Seventh Edition

CHAPTER 1

HISTORICAL PRINCIPLES AND PERSPECTIVES

1.1. *Toxicology* appears to be derived from the word *toxikon*. What does the word *toxikon* mean?

A. An evil curse
B. Death
C. Judicial punishment
D. Poisons of animal, vegetable, or mineral origin
E. The poison into which arrowheads are dipped

1.2. Which of the following was the poison of choice used by the ancient Greeks to execute criminals and dissidents?

A. Arsenic
B. Digitalis leaf
C. Hemlock
D. Heroin
E. Strychnine

1.3. Who is often credited with developing the concept of dose-response in toxicology?

A. Ambroise Paré
B. Galen
C. Maimonides
D. Paracelsus
E. Theodore Wormley

1.4. The author of *Traité des Poisons ou Toxicologie Générale* is often referred to as the father of modern toxicology. Who is this scientist?

A. Bonaventure Orfila
B. Claude Bernard
C. Richard Mead
D. Robert Christison
E. Theodore Wormley

1.5. In the late 19th century, which of the following was the drug of choice recommended for the treatment of opioid addiction?

A. Caffeine
B. Chloral hydrate
C. Cocaine
D. Heroin
E. Strychnine

1.6. The "poison squad" investigated

A. "Bad" street drugs
B. Chemicals in the workplace
C. Contaminated food
D. Environmental poisonings
E. Pharmaceutical disasters

1.7. Which of the following substances is detected by the Marsh test?

A. Arsenic
B. Chloroform
C. Cocaine
D. Mercury
E. Thallium

1.8. Poisonings from which of the following agents precipitated important federal regulatory legislation in the 1920s?

A. Caustics
B. Opioids
C. Pesticides
D. Petroleum distillates
E. Strychnine

1.9. Which of the following characteristics of early European poison centers was not a significant factor in the initial development of American poison centers?

A. Cataloging poison identification and treatment information
B. Data collection
C. Emphasis on prevention
D. Organization of toxicology treatment centers
E. Service to healthcare professionals

1.10. Which of the following was the focus of the much publicized Institute of Medicine report in 1999?

A. Cocaine epidemic
B. Emergency department staffing
C. Medical errors
D. Overproliferation of poison centers
E. Suicide

CHAPTER 2

TOXICOLOGIC PLAGUES AND DISASTERS IN HISTORY

2.1. In which city was a dense smog in 1952 thought responsible for 4000 excess deaths?

    A. London
    B. Mexico City
    C. New York City
    D. Paris
    E. Warsaw

2.2. A combination therapy used in obstetric anesthesia and known as "twilight sleep" refers to which of the following?

    A. Bromide and caffeine
    B. Bromide and chloral hydrate
    C. Chloral hydrate and ethanol
    D. Morphine and cocaine
    E. Morphine and scopolamine

2.3. What toxin was responsible for the 2500 deaths that occurred in Bhopal, India in 1984 after an explosion at a pesticide factory?

    A. Carbaryl
    B. DDT
    C. Hydrogen sulfide
    D. Methyl isocyanate
    E. Parathion

2.4. The use of Agent Orange during the Vietnam War created intense public health concern. Which chemical contaminant in this preparation has been the focus of attention?

    A. Anthrax
    B. Botulinum toxin
    C. Dioxin
    D. Mercury
    E. Sarin

2.5. The use of which of the following agents for the treatment of tinea infections caused needless morbidity and mortality during the 1930s?

    A. Cadmium
    B. Chromium
    C. Lead
    D. Mercury
    E. Thallium

2.6. The therapeutic use of Elixir of Sulfanilamide-Massengill was responsible for more than 100 deaths. Which diluent was responsible for these deaths?

    A. Benzyl alcohol
    B. Diethylene glycol
    C. Ethylene glycol
    D. Glycerol
    E. Propylene glycol

2.7. The eosinophilia-myalgia syndrome was associated with which of the following agents?

    A. Folate
    B. Melatonin
    C. Niacin
    D. Pyridoxine
    E. Tryptophan

2.8. Phossy jaw (mandibular necrosis) was associated with which of the following occupations?

    A. Felt hat makers
    B. Leather manufacturers
    C. Match makers
    D. Shipyard workers
    E. Synthetic dye makers

2.9. Which of the following chemicals is associated with an increased incidence of male infertility?

    A. Dibromochloropropane (DBCP)
    B. Diethylstilbestrol (DES)
    C. Diethyltin
    D. Dioxane
    E. Dioxin

2.10. A serious radiation incident occurred in 1987 in Brazil when 244 people were exposed to a radiation source found in a junkyard. The radiation was an isotope of which of the following elements?

    A. Cesium
    B. Iodine
    C. Plutonium
    D. Thallium
    E. Uranium

CHAPTER 5

TECHNIQUES USED TO PREVENT GASTROINTESTINAL ABSORPTION OF TOXIC COMPOUNDS

5.1. Which of the following is a proven effect of whole-bowel irrigation?

A. Decreased drug absorption after actual human poisoning
B. Clinical benefit after actual human poisoning
C. Decreased drug absorption in volunteer studies
D. Electrolyte disturbances following massive dosing
E. Interference with drug adsorption to activated charcoal in vivo

5.2. Which of the following is a proven effect of cathartics?

A. Decreased drug absorption after actual human overdose
B. Clinical benefit after actual human overdose
C. Decreased drug absorption in volunteer studies
D. Electrolyte disturbances after massive dosing
E. Interference with drug adsorption to activated charcoal

5.3. Which of the following cathartics is/are associated with life-threatening fluid and electrolyte disturbances?

A. Sodium sulfate
B. Sodium phosphate
C. Magnesium sulfate
D. Sorbitol
E. All of the above

5.4. Which of the following is the best guideline for an initial dose of activated charcoal?

A. 200 g
B. 100 g
C. 50 g
D. A 10:1 ratio, ie, 10 times the amount ingested, by history
E. 0.5–1.5 g/kg

5.5. Which of the following would be most completely adsorbed by 100 g of activated charcoal?

A. 100 tablets (325 mg) of aspirin
B. 100 sustained-release tablets (300 mg) of theophylline
C. 100 tablets (500 mg) of L-dopa
D. 100 mL of 30% ethanol
E. 1 g of potassium cyanide

5.6. Which of the following is true of activated charcoal and N-acetylcysteine interactions?

A. Activated charcoal adsorbs N-acetylcysteine in vitro but does not actually decrease bioavailability.
B. Activated charcoal adsorbs N-acetylcysteine and decreases its bioavailability, but probably not to a clinically significant degree.
C. A clinically significant decrease in N-acetylcysteine bioavailability by activated charcoal has been demonstrated, but this can be overcome by increasing N-acetylcysteine dosage.
D. The need to use activated charcoal and N-acetylcysteine concomitantly is an absolute indication for the use of IV NAC.
E. Well-controlled clinical studies have proven that the interaction between N-acetylcysteine and activated charcoal is of no significance.

5.7. Which of the following has/have been demonstrated in at least one study?

A. Emesis is more effective than orogastric lavage in preventing drug absorption.
B. Orogastric lavage is more effective than emesis in preventing drug absorption.
C. Orogastric lavage and emesis are equivalent in preventing drug absorption.
D. Activated charcoal is more effective than either emesis or orogastric lavage in preventing drug absorption.
E. All of the above

5.8. Which of the following has been adequately proven about emesis or orogastric lavage?

A. Both are clinically effective in most patients if done within 1 hour after an overdose.
B. Neither is clinically effective if performed more than 4 hours after an overdose.
C. Both are clinically effective at most times.
D. Neither is clinically effective at any time.
E. None of the above

5.9. Which of the following characteristics would make multiple-dose activated charcoal (MDAC) a more rational intervention?

A. The ingested agent is rapidly absorbed.
B. There is a highly effective antidote available.
C. The amount of drug ingested is 25 g.
D. It has been 4 hours since ingestion.
E. The ingested agent has a low intrinsic clearance and small V_d.

5.10. Multiple-dose activated charcoal does not increase the clearance of which of the following?

A. Phenobarbital
B. Phenytoin
C. Carbamazepine

D. Doxepin
E. Nortriptyline

CHAPTER 6

PRINCIPLES AND TECHNIQUES APPLIED TO ENHANCE ELIMINATION OF TOXIC COMPOUNDS

6.1. Alkalinization of the urine by administration of NaHCO$_3$ is likely to enhance the elimination of which of the following ?

A. Strong acids
B. Strong bases
C. Weak acids
D. Weak bases
E. Both weak acids and weak bases

6.2. Elimination by hemodialysis would not be expected to be useful for a compound with which of the following characteristics?

A. Low volume of distribution
B. High degree of protein binding
C. Low lipid solubility
D. Low molecular weight
E. Highly ionized at physiologic pH

6.3. Charcoal hemoperfusion may be preferable to hemodialysis in the case of toxins that exhibit

A. Large volumes of distribution
B. High degrees of protein binding
C. High lipid solubility
D. Low molecular weight
E. Neutral charge at physiologic pH

6.4. "Gastrointestinal dialysis" with multiple-dose activated charcoal may be effective for a toxin with which of the following characteristics?

A. Not absorbed by the intestine
B. High lipid solubility
C. Ingested with food
D. Diminished bowel motility
E. Low molecular weight

6.5. Which of the following characteristics of acetaminophen overdose makes hemoperfusion an undesirable treatment for overdoses?

A. High renal clearance
B. Lack of major morbidity
C. High volume of distribution

D. Efficacy of *N*-acetylcysteine (NAC)
E. Poor intestinal absorption

6.6. Continuous arteriovenous hemofiltration has the following advantage over conventional hemodialysis:

A. It may be better tolerated in hypotensive patients.
B. It achieves higher clearance rates.
C. It requires less monitoring and less staff.
D. It is indicated for a more varied range of toxins.
E. It can clear lipid-soluble toxins more rapidly.

6.7. Which of the following characteristics of paraquat diminish the efficacy of hemoperfusion for the clearance of the drug?

A. High molecular weight
B. High degree of protein binding
C. Tight binding to tissue sites
D. High volume of distribution
E. Nonpolar molecule

6.8. To which toxin does the following statement apply? Rebound of serum levels after hemodialysis as a result of equilibration from intracellular stores often requires repeat dialysis.

A. Ethylene glycol
B. Lithium
C. Salicylate
D. Theophylline
E. Ethanol

6.9. Removal of digoxin–antibody complexes from a patient with renal failure might best be accomplished by

A. Hemodialysis
B. Sorbent hemoperfusion
C. Continuous venovenous hemodiafiltration (CVVHD)
D. Plasmapheresis
E. Oral multiple-dose activated charcoal

6.10. Which statement most accurately describes the efficacy of peritoneal dialysis for the treatment of theophylline poisoning?

A. Complexity of the procedure precludes its practical use.
B. It can be done simultaneously, as a useful adjunct, with hemoperfusion.
C. Lack of hemodynamic effect makes it valuable for hypotensive patients.

D. It adds too little to clearance to ever be useful for seriously ill patients.

E. The peritoneum is impermeable to theophylline.

CHAPTER 7

LABORATORY PRINCIPLES AND TECHNIQUES FOR EVALUATION OF THE POISONED OR OVERDOSED PATIENT

7.1. Which laboratory technique is most commonly used to measure methanol and isopropanol?

A. Atomic absorption spectroscopy
B. Automated enzyme assay
C. Gas chromatography
D. Gas chromatography + mass spectrometry
E. Immunoassay

7.2. Which of the following laboratory measurements are not available as a point-of-care testing format?

A. Drugs of abuse in urine
B. Carbon monoxide
C. Blood lead
D. Digoxin
E. Tricyclic antidepressants

7.3. CLIA-88 requirements for moderately complex testing include which of the following?

A. Following manufacturer's instructions
B. Package insert must be available to all testing personnel
C. Biennial competency certification for all testing personnel
D. Controls must be run once a week
E. Entry of all results into laboratory computer

7.4. The gold standard for confirmation of drugs of abuse in urine is an analysis performed by which of the following?

A. Automated enzyme assay
B. Gas chromatography
C. Gas chromatography + mass spectrometry
D. Immunoassay
E. Thin-layer chromatography

7.5. Which statements about the analysis of drugs in body fluids are correct?

A. False-positive results are more common than false-negative results
B. Gas chromatography/mass spectroscopy should always be used, if available
C. A confirmed positive finding on a toxicology screen confirms the diagnosis of poisoning
D. The sensitivity of thin-layer chromatography is extremely high.
E. Immunoassays provide both high sensitivity and high specificity

7.6. Which laboratory methods does not use chemical modification to improve the detection or quantitation of drugs in body fluids?

A. Immunoassay
B. Gas chromatography
C. Mass spectroscopy
D. Thin-layer chromatography
E. Spectrophotometry

7.7. Concentrations of which of the following do not require knowledge of the time of ingestion or chronicity of exposure for proper interpretation?

A. Acetaminophen
B. Cocaine metabolites (benzoylecgonine)
C. Digoxin
D. Lithium
E. Theophylline

7.8. Which tests are likely to be readily available in the most hospital clinical laboratories?

A. Comprehensive toxicology screening
B. Drugs of abuse in urine (cocaine, opiates, amphetamines, cannabinoids, phencyclidine, benzodiazepines, barbiturates)
C. Heavy metals
D. Tricyclic antidepressants (quantitative)
E. "Volatile alcohols" (ethanol, methanol, isopropanol, acetone)

7.9. Comparable ethanol concentrations will be present in which pairs of specimens?

A. Serum and whole blood
B. Serum and urine
C. Serum and plasma
D. Serum and breath
E. Serum and saliva

7.10. Which types of tests are not regulated by CLIA-88?

A. Breath tests for ethanol and carbon monoxide
B. Salicylate and acetaminophen spot tests

C. Urine dipsticks

D. Visual examination of urine for fluorescein and oxalate crystals

E. Arterial blood gas

CHAPTER 8

DIAGNOSTIC IMAGING IN TOXICOLOGY

8.1. Which of the following hydrocarbons is the most radiopaque?

A. Methylene chloride

B. Methylbromide

C. Dichloromethane

D. Trichloroethylene

E. Carbon tetrachloride

8.2. Chronic exposure to which of the following may cause a decrease in bone density on radiographs?

A. Corticosteroids

B. Fluoride

C. Lithium carbonate

D. Calcium carbonate

E. Lead

8.3. Cerebellar atrophy can be noted on CT in patients who are exposed to which of the following?

A. Lithium carbonate

B. Cadmium

C. Manganese

D. Methylmercury

E. Magnesium

8.4. Bilateral basal ganglia lucencies have been associated with which of the following toxins?

A. Ethanol

B. Methanol

C. Manganese

D. Carbon dioxide

E. Vitamin A

8.5. Which of the following tablets or capsules would be expected to be most radiopaque in an overdosed patient?

A. Chloral hydrate

B. Trifluoperazine

C. Ferrous sulfate

D. Sustained-release verapamil

E. Enteric-coated aspirin

8.6. A welder developed respiratory symptoms several hours after working in a poorly ventilated workplace. Which of the following inhaled toxins could be responsible for coughing, wheezing, and diffuse airspace filling on chest film (acute lung injury)?

A. Carbon monoxide

B. Ozone

C. Nitrogen dioxide

D. Carbon dioxide

E. Zinc fumes

8.7. Which of the following agents could be responsible for diffuse intestinal distension (adynamic ileus) seen on an abdominal radiograph?

A. Amitriptyline

B. Oxycodone and acetaminophen

C. Cocaine

D. Ergotamine

E. All of the above

8.8. Abdominal radiographs are unlikely to be helpful in which of the following situations?

A. Abdominal pain after smoking crack cocaine

B. Bloody diarrhea in an 18-month-old child

C. Jaundice and coagulopathy occurring 3 days after an acetaminophen overdose

D. Suicidal ingestion of hydrochloric acid

E. A 27-year-old woman of Asian descent complaining of 3 weeks of abdominal cramping, anorexia, and constipation

8.9. The finding of a diffuse reticular or reticulonodular infiltrate on a chest radiograph is not associated with exposure to which of the following?

A. Nitrofurantion

B. Bleomycin

C. Nitrogen dioxide

D. Asbestos

E. Malathion

8.10. Chest radiographic abnormalities associated with procainamide administration include which of the following?

A. Hilar adenopathy

B. Diffuse patchy infiltrates

C. Fine reticular interstitial pattern

D. Pleural effusion

E. All of the above

CHAPTER 9

ELECTROCARDIOGRAPHIC PRINCIPLES

9.1. Bidirectional ventricular tachycardia is particularly characteristic of poisoning by what agent?

A. Diphenhydramine
B. Digoxin
C. Quinidine
D. Theophylline
E. Magnesium

9.2. Which of the following opioids can cause repolarization abnormalities in overdose patients?

A. Heroin
B. Morphine
C. Meperidine
D. Propoxyphene
E. Diphenoxylate

9.3. Prolongation of the QRS complex to greater than 100 milliseconds would not be expected with which of the following overdoses?

A. Thioridazine
B. Cyclic antidepressants
C. Amantadine
D. Omeprazole
E. Procainamide

9.4. The continuous cardiac monitor recording from a modified left chest lead is similar in appearance to which of the following leads from a 12-lead ECG recording?

A. aVF
B. V_1
C. Lead II
D. Leads I and III combined
E. V_6

9.5. Ventricular depolarization begins with depolarization and ends with the completion of repolarization. This period is defined by what portion of the ECG?

A. PR interval
B. QT interval
C. QRS complex
D. ST segment
E. P wave

9.6. All of the following ECG changes may be found in a patient with hypokalemia, except

A. ST elevation
B. Increased PR interval
C. Diminished or inverted T waves
D. Increased U-wave amplitude
E. QT prolongation

9.7. Exposure to hydrofluoric acid can cause life-threatening hypocalcemia. ECG changes consistent with this diagnosis include all of the following except

A. Prolonged ST segment
B. Unchanged T wave
C. Widened QRS complex
D. Increased QTc interval
E. Flattened P wave

9.8. A resident shows you an ECG revealing atrial fibrillation with a slow ventricular response. The patient's heart rate is 30 beats/min, and there are frequent premature ventricular contractions. Further questioning reveals that the patient has chronic atrial fibrillation and has the following medications in her purse: furosemide, digoxin, and nifedipine. She was brought to the ED by her granddaughter for the "flu," with nausea, vomiting, and dry chapped lips. Your initial working diagnosis should be

A. Pyloric stenosis
B. Digoxin toxicity
C. Calcium channel blocker toxicity
D. *Staphylococcus aureus* food poisoning
E. Depression

9.9. Which of the following conditions could increase the chances of torsades de pointes developing in a patient with hereditary long QT syndrome?

A. Hyperkalemia
B. Tachycardia
C. Hypermagnesemia
D. Bradycardia
E. Hypercalcemia

9.10. Ergot alkaloids are effective therapy for some migraine headaches. However, in ergot overdose, toxicity includes all of the following except

A. Coronary vasospasm
B. Valvular fibrosis and stenosis
C. Gangrene
D. Interstitial nephritis
E. Q waves on the ECG

CHAPTER 10

NEUROTRANSMITTER PRINCIPLES

10.1. Which one of the following receptors is an ion channel?

A. Nicotinic acetylcholine
B. $GABA_B$
C. α-Adrenergic
D. D_2 dopamine
E. A_1 adenosine

10.2. Which of the agents listed is thought to be responsible for self-termination of seizures?

    A. Serotonin
    B. Dopamine
    C. Adenosine
    D. Norepinephrine
    E. GABA

10.3. Following the ingestion of clonidine, which of the following receptors is thought to mediate CNS depression?

    A. β_2-Adrenergic
    B. Imidazoline
    C. $GABA_A$
    D. α_2-Adrenergic
    E. Acetylcholine muscarinic

10.4. Which one of the following agents causes the release of acetylcholine from nerve endings?

    A. Black widow spider venom
    B. Botulinum toxin
    C. Cocaine
    D. Clonidine
    E. Diphenhydramine

10.5. Which of the following neurotransmitters is antagonized by strychnine?

    A. Serotonin
    B. Glutamate
    C. Adenosine
    D. Dopamine
    E. Glycine

10.6. Which of the following agents antagonizes glutamate NMDA receptors?

    A. Phencyclidine
    B. Domoic acid
    C. Valproic acid
    D. Clozapine
    E. Cocaine

10.7. Which of the following agents inhibits dopamine-β-hydroxylase?

    A. Propranolol
    B. Disulfiram
    C. Clonidine
    D. Mescaline
    E. Chlorpromazine

10.8. Which of the following agents activates serotonin receptors to enhance gut motility?

    A. Cisapride
    B. Cyproheptadine
    C. Ondansetron

    D. Propranolol
    E. Sumatriptan

10.9. Which of the following agents antagonizes adenosine receptors?

    A. Theophylline
    B. Phenytoin
    C. Ethanol
    D. Diazepam
    E. MPTP

10.10. Which of the following agents produces seizures through antagonism at the $GABA_A$ receptor complex?

    A. Domoic acid
    B. Baclofen
    C. Penicillin
    D. Muscimol
    E. Carbamazepine

CHAPTER **11**

PHARMACOKINETIC AND TOXICOKINETIC PRINCIPLES

11.1. Which of the following factors may influence xenobiotic clearance?

    A. Age
    B. Enzyme induction or inhibition
    C. Gender
    D. Genetic phenotypes
    E. All of the above

11.2. If a 50-kg patient ingests 500 mg of ethanol and is found to have a peak ethanol level of 2 mg/dL (20 µg/mL), assuming 100% absorption and no metabolism, what is the volume of distribution for ethanol?

    A. 5 L/kg
    B. 25 L/kg
    C. 50 L/kg
    D. 0.5 L/kg
    E. 0.005 L/kg

11.3. The phase I oxidative process alcohol dehydrogenation occurs primarily in the

    A. Mitochondria
    B. Cytosol
    C. Colonic microflora
    D. Golgi apparatus
    E. Phospholipid membrane of the GI tract

11.4. Lithium is best described by a

    A. Zero-compartment model
    B. One-compartment model
    C. Two-compartment model
    D. Michaelis-Menten model
    E. Andover-Martin model

11.5. Xenobiotic distribution is affected by

    A. Active transport
    B. Ionization
    C. Lipid solubility
    D. Blood flow to the absorption site
    E. All of the above

11.6. A 3-year-old, 10-kg child ingests 10 mL of a 100% methanol solution. If the volume of distribution (V_d) for methanol is 0.6 L/kg, what is the predicted peak methanol level (assuming instantaneous distribution)?

    A. 16.7 mg/dL
    B. 167 mg/dL
    C. 167 mg/mL
    D. 1.67 mg/L
    E. 1.67 mg/dL

11.7. Phenytoin elimination is best characterized by which of the following processes?

    A. Michaelis-Menten kinetics
    B. Zero-order kinetics
    C. First-order kinetics
    D. Linear-order kinetics
    E. None of the above

11.8. A patient with an acetaminophen level of 150 mg/mL at 4 hours and a level of 37.5 mg/mL at 16 hours has an acetaminophen half-life of

    A. 2 hours
    B. 3 hours
    C. 4 hours
    D. 6 hours
    E. 12 hours

11.9. A 25-year-old, 60-kg man is taking 0.25 mg of digoxin each day to control his atrial fibrillation. Approximately 80% of the oral dose is absorbed. A steady-state digoxin level is 0.8 ng/mL. What is the patient's clearance of digoxin each day?

    A. 1100 ng/kg/d
    B. 2100 ng/kg/d
    C. 3100 ng/kg/d
    D. 4100 ng/kg/d
    E. 5100 ng/kg/d

11.10. Pharmacodynamics is a technique used to characterize

    A. Absorption across semipermeable membranes
    B. Distribution kinetics
    C. Concentration and clinical effects
    D. Metabolic rates and processes
    E. Elimination rates and processes

CHAPTER **12**

CHEMICAL PRINCIPLES

12.1. Which of the following is true about the elements?

    A. The periodic table is divided into metals and metalloids.
    B. All elements in a given period on the periodic table have similar chemical reactivity.
    C. Most of the elements represented on the periodic table are metals.
    D. The noble gases are so named because they are capable of reacting with all of the other elements.
    E. The alkali metals include chlorine and fluorine.

12.2. The transition metals are extremely important in the study of toxicology. Which one of the following statements is true?

    A. The elemental form of most transition metals is highly reactive and can be found only under special circumstances.
    B. The reactivity of transition metals is exploited by various physiologic enzyme systems.
    C. What makes the transition metals so important to toxicologists is that they form brightly colored salts.
    D. Chronic poisoning by transition metals cannot occur.
    E. Transition metals are incapable of accepting electrons, only donating them.

12.3. Which of the following is not a heavy metal?

    A. Mercury
    B. Thallium
    C. Lead
    D. Arsenic
    E. Bismuth

12.4. Which of the following regarding molecular bonding is correct?

    A. Bonds in which electrons are nearly equally shared are considered electrovalent.

B. The degree to which electrons are shared between elements is determined by the differences in the electronegativity of the elements.
C. When one mole of the ionic compound NaCl is dissolved in water one equivalent of NaCl is generated.
D. Most chemicals adsorb to activated charcoal via covalent bonds.
E. Truly symmetric bonds, such as between the chlorine atoms in Cl_2, are always polar.

12.5. Which of the following represents a toxicologically important reactive oxygen species?

A. CO
B. O_2
C. H_2O
D. OH•
E. O_6

12.6. Which of the following substances effects is mediated via redox chemistry?

A. Paraquat
B. Phenytoin
C. NaOH
D. Ba^{2+}
E. Hg^0

12.7. Methanol and isopropanol both contain the alcohol functional group. Which of the following statements is most accurate?

A. They have identical boiling points.
B. They have identical patterns of chemical reactivity.
C. They have similar physical and chemical properties.
D. They are metabolized at the same rate.
E. They have identical toxic effects.

12.8. The two stereoisomers $(-)$physostigmine and $(+)$physostigmine differ only in their three-dimensional orientation at one chiral center. Which of the following statements is true?

A. They have identical boiling points.
B. They have identical patterns of chemical reactivity, such as with acetylcholinesterase.
C. They have different structural formulas.
D. They are metabolized at the same rate.
E. They have identical toxic effects.

12.9. Which of the following is most accurate regarding nucleophiles and electrophiles?

A. Nucleophiles react most readily with other nucleophiles.

B. Electrophiles have a center or centers that are relatively electron deficient.
C. Nucleophiles are always radioactive.
D. Electrophiles are always negatively charged.
E. The term *electrophile* is synonymous with the term *free radical*.

12.10 Which of the following represents a nucleophile of importance to toxicologists?

A. Pb^{2+}
B. As^{3+}
C. NAPQI
D. Pralidoxime
E. 2,5-Hexanedione

CHAPTER **13**

BIOCHEMICAL PRINCIPLES

13.1. Which of the following is a phase I biotransformation reaction?

A. Sulfation
B. Glucuronidation
C. Carboxylation
D. Conjugation with glutathione
E. Transesterification

13.2. Which of the following undergoes hepatic metabolism to a toxic compound?

A. Paraquat
B. Cycasin
C. Salicylate
D. Bromobenzene
E. Cocaine

13.3. Which of the following toxins is associated with an uncoupling of oxidative phosphorylation?

A. Hydrogen sulfide
B. Sodium fluoroacetate
C. Dinitrophenol
D. Ricin
E. Carbon tetrachloride

13.4. Which of the following statements about biotransformation reactions is true?

A. The majority of the metabolites produced by phase I biotransformation of lipophilic toxins are water soluble and readily excretable.
B. Phase I biotransformation of a xenobiotic is always a mechanism for detoxification.

C. The metabolism of ethanol to acetaldehyde is a phase II reaction.

D. CYP2E1 has a higher K_m for ethanol than alcohol dehydrogenase, making it less likely to be involved in the metabolism of ethanol in most individuals.

E. Most phase I biotransformation enzymes are highly specific with regard to which substrates they act on.

13.5. Which of the following statements about phase II reactions is true?

A. Decreased availability of glutathione limits the rate of detoxification of both acetaminophen and bromobenzene.

B. Phase II reactions decrease the polarity of foreign compounds.

C. Phase II reactions are primarily oxidation-reduction reactions.

D. In many cases, the products of phase II biotransformation reactions are highly toxic.

E. Phase II enzymes result in addition of sulfhydryl, hydroxyl, or carboxyl groups to xenobiotics.

13.6. Which substance does not reduce the metabolic activity of CYP3A4?

A. Naringenin
B. Erythromycin
C. Ketoconazole
D. Phenytoin
E. Cimetidine

13.7. Which of the following drugs or toxins does not exert its toxic effects through inhibition of a specific enzyme?

A. Methotrexate
B. Ricin
C. MPTP
D. Sodium fluoroacetate
E. Coumadin

13.8. Which of the following agents is not known to exert its effects through a specific protein receptor?

A. Morphine
B. Atropine
C. Pancuronium
D. Mercury
E. Flumazenil

13.9. All of the following result in decreased cellular production of ATP except which drug or toxin?

A. Cyanide
B. Sodium fluoroacetate

C. Arsenic
D. Salicylates
E. Isoniazid

13.10. Which of the following agents causes injury at the site of its metabolic transformation?

A. Cyanide
B. Succinylcholine
C. Salicylate
D. Carbon tetrachloride
E. MPTP

CHAPTER **14**

HEPATIC PRINCIPLES

14.1. Which of the following statements about hepatotoxins is true?

A. The liver injury caused by most hepatotoxins is dose dependent.

B. Following ingestion of similar quantities of the mushroom *Amanita virosa*, some individuals may suffer severe effects while others remain asymptomatic.

C. Most hepatotoxins are idiosyncratic in that their effects cannot be predicted for any individual person.

D. Following exposure to halothane, acute hepatitis is extremely rare, occurring in fewer than 1/10,000 cases.

E. Because of the predominance of the portal circulation in the liver, only ingested toxins cause hepatotoxicity.

14.2. The toxic metabolite of acetaminophen is which of the following?

A. Benzquinolone
B. Benzidine
C. *N*-Mercaptophenetidin
D. *N*-Acetyl-*p*-benzoquinoneimine
E. Phenacetin

14.3. Which of the following statements is true?

A. Intrahepatic bile flow is a passive process, driven by secretion of large volumes of bile into the canaliculi.

B. Cholestasis rarely occurs in the absence of extensive hepatocellular injury.

C. Injury localized to the canalicular tight junctions results in hyperbilirubinemia because of bile leakage.

D. Small sulfated macromolecules are avidly taken up into an enterohepatic circulation.

E. Cholestasis is the most prominent early pathologic manifestation of vitamin A hepatotoxicity.

14.4. The localization of toxic hepatic injuries to specific zones of the liver may be related to which of the following?

A. Decreasing oxygen tension between the portal and central vein areas

B. Selective delivery of a toxin to the portal areas

C. Localization of specific biotransformation enzymes within the periportal or centrilobular areas

D. Regional decreased availability of substrates for phase II biotransformation reactions

E. All of the above

14.5. Which of the following statements regarding ethanol-induced liver disease is not correct?

A. An AST of 2000 IU/L is inconsistent with the diagnosis of acute ethanol-induced hepatitis.

B. The pathologic effects of amiodarone-induced hepatotoxicity are very similar to those of ethanol.

C. The AST is usually two to three times greater than the ALT.

D. Steatosis most likely occurs because of the altered oxidative capacity of the hepatocyte.

E. Alcoholic liver disease, in reality, is caused by thiamine deficiency.

14.6. Acute intraperitoneal hemorrhage is associated with hepatotoxicity caused by which of the following drugs?

A. Chlorpromazine
B. Anabolic steroids
C. Tetracycline
D. Isoniazid
E. Erythromycin

14.7. An AST of 5000 IU is consistent with hepatic injury caused by which of the following?

A. Acute extrahepatic obstruction of the common bile duct

B. Acute alcoholic hepatitis

C. Hepatotoxicity as a result of chronic treatment with methotrexate

D. Acute hepatic injury caused by acetaminophen toxicity

E. All of the above

14.8. The *Bacillus cereus* toxin induces a type of hepatic injury that is similar to all of the following except which?

A. Fialuridine
B. Reye syndrome
C. Acute fatty liver of pregnancy
D. Chlorpromazine
E. Zidovudine

14.9. Which biochemical marker is most predictive of the severity of liver injury in patients with acute hepatocellular necrosis?

A. Prothrombin time (INR)
B. AST
C. Serum bilirubin
D. Serum creatinine
E. Alkaline phosphatase

14.10. All of the following are true about hepatotoxicity caused by carbon tetrachloride except which statement?

A. It has been shown to be increased by the administration of oxygen.

B. It has been shown to be decreased by the administration of glutathione.

C. CCl_4 is metabolized by the ethanol-inducible CYP2E1.

D. Hepatocellular injury is initially localized to the zone 3, or centrilobular areas of the liver.

E. The most likely mechanism of hepatocellular injury is the initiation of lipid peroxidation by free radicals.

CHAPTER 15

IMMUNOLOGIC PRINCIPLES

15.1. Which of the following toxins is the poorest candidate for the development of antibody therapy?

A. Digoxin
B. Colchicine
C. Theophylline
D. Botulinum toxin
E. Tetanus toxin

15.2. The reactive airways dysfunction syndrome (RADS) is a chronic asthmalike condition associated with a single high-dose exposure to a respiratory irritant. Which of the following has been reported to induce RADS?

A. Toluene diisocyanate
B. Chlorine gas

C. Sulfur dioxide
D. Ethylene oxide
E. All of the above

15.3. Environmental adjuvants are substances that potentiate production of IgE in response to other substances. Which of the following is known to be such an adjuvant in experimental models?

A. Diesel exhaust particles
B. Ozone
C. Sulfur dioxide
D. Nitrogen dioxide
E. All of the above

15.4. An advantage of Fab fragments over whole antibody molecules in the immunotoxicotherapy of poisoning is

A. There is less risk of serum sickness.
B. There is less risk of anaphylaxis.
C. A smaller volume of antibody fragment is infused.
D. The volume of distribution of Fab fragments is greater than the volume of distribution of whole antibody.
E. All of the above

15.5. Selective IgA deficiency has been associated with which of the following pharmaceuticals?

A. Ticlopide
B. Aspirin
C. Hydrochlorothiazide
D. Phenytoin
E. Trimethoprim

15.6. Inhalation exposure to burning oil in Kuwait during the Persian Gulf War has been associated with

A. Systemic lupus erythematosus
B. Rheumatoid arthritis
C. Aplastic anemia
D. Testicular cancer
E. Parkinsonian syndrome

15.7. Systemic lupus erythematosus has not been associated with which of the following?

A. Procainamide
B. Hydralazine
C. Tartrazine
D. Hydrazine
E. Lidocaine

15.8. Penicillin induces autoimmune hemolytic anemia by

A. Altering the immune regulatory system that protects against self antigens
B. Molecular mimicry, in that the chemical structure of penicillin is so similar to antigens on the red blood cell surface that antibodies against penicillin will bind to red blood cells
C. Binding to red blood cells and producing an antibody against this bound penicillin
D. Directly damaging red cell membranes by the same mechanism by which it damages bacterial membranes
E. Binding to the first component of complement, thereby activating the complement cascade

15.9. A feature of the Spanish toxic oil syndrome was

A. Few people who were injured in this epidemic recovered.
B. Toxic induction of collagen vascular disease was most common in individuals with DR3 and DR4 HLA haplotypes associated with genetic susceptibility to the disease.
C. There were no hematologic abnormalities associated with this syndrome.
D. The etiologic agent in this syndrome was olive oil contaminated with heavy metals.
E. A hypersensitivity response to imported L-tryptophan.

15.10. Adverse effects reported in association with exposure to the dioxin TCDD (2,3,7,8-tetrachlorodibenzo-*p*-dioxin) include

A. An increase in cancer mortality and a decrease in cellular immune responses
B. An increase in cancer mortality but no effects on cellular immune responses
C. A decrease in cancer mortality but no effects on cellular immune responses
D. No effect on cancer mortality or cellular immune responses
E. An increase in cancer mortality and an increase in cellular immune responses

CHAPTER **16**

MUTAGENS, CARCINOGENS, AND TERATOGENS

16.1. Which of the following is not a recognized criterion for teratogenicity?

A. There should be biologic plausibility for the mechanism of action of the putative teratogenic agent.
B. There should be animal models of the exposure that mimic the effects in humans.

C. There should be quantitative proof of exposure with biologic markers.
D. There should be findings from epidemiologic studies showing that exposure produces an increase in the occurrence of specific phenotypic effects and a recognizable pattern of both major and minor malformations.
E. There should be a dose–response relationship that has been demonstrated in either animal models or human exposures.

16.2. Which of the following statements about smoking is true?

A. Mothers generally recall accurately the number of cigarettes they smoked during their pregnancy.
B. Maternal smoking has not been shown to have any neurobehavioral teratogenicity.
C. Blood nicotine levels accurately reflect the extent of chronic smoking.
D. Maternal smoking is associated with an increased rate of congenital malformations.
E. Infants of passive smokers are at risk of measurable exposure to cigarette smoke.

16.3. Which of the following outcomes has not been associated with maternal cigarette smoking?

A. Decreased birth weight
B. Congenital heart defects
C. Prematurity
D. Spontaneous abortions
E. Sudden infant death syndrome

16.4. Which of the following statements is not correct?

A. Mutagens produce alterations in DNA.
B. Mutations may occur in somatic and germ cells.
C. All mutagens are carcinogens.
D. The Ames test is a screen for mutagenicity.
E. Mutagenic activity cannot be predicted on the basis of chemical structure alone.

16.5. Which of the following agents is not a recognized human carcinogen?

A. Melphalan
B. Mercury
C. Cadmium
D. Diethylstilbestrol
E. Aflatoxin

16.6. Which statement regarding meconium is correct?

A. Drugs are present in meconium only after 26 weeks of gestation.
B. Meconium testing cannot be used for mass screening.
C. Meconium testing is less accurate than urine testing.
D. Meconium can only be used to detect cocaine and opioids.
E. Drugs are detectable in the first three meconium stools.

16.7. Which statement regarding prenatal exposure to methylmercury is false?

A. It is characterized by severe neurotoxicity.
B. First-trimester exposure is most critical.
C. Methylmercury achieves higher fetal than maternal concentrations.
D. Hair may be used to measure exposure in both mothers and infants.
E. Cord blood and maternal hair levels correlate well.

16.8. Which statement regarding prenatal lead exposure is false?

A. Prenatal lead exposure may result in neurodevelopmental toxicity.
B. Cord blood lead levels greater than 0.48 mmol/L are associated with low developmental scores at 6–24 months of age.
C. Prenatal lead exposure may result in obstetric complications such as spontaneous abortion, premature rupture of membranes, and preterm delivery.
D. There is poor correlation between maternal and cord blood lead levels.
E. Lead crosses the placenta by both active and passive transfer.

16.9. Which statement regarding hair is false?

A. Using hair analysis, it is not possible to differentiate systemic exposure and exposure by passive smoking of crack cocaine.
B. Hair can be used to estimate both maternal and fetal xenobiotic exposures.
C. Adult hair grows at a rate of approximately 1.5 cm per month
D. Maternal and fetal accumulation of cocaine and its metabolites follows a linear pattern.
E. Cocaine and its metabolites, including cocaethylene and benzoylecgonine, can be measured in hair.

16.10. Which of the following statements is false?

A. Nicotine and its metabolites accumulate in the amniotic fluid.

B. Amniocentesis is not commonly used as a routine investigation following xenobiotic exposure.

C. Specific fetal anomalies related to teratogenic exposures may be detected on ultrasound in the second trimester.

D. Following first-trimester retinoic acid use, neural tube defects have been demonstrated on midtrimester ultrasound.

E. Counseling regarding xenobiotic exposure may prevent unnecessary termination of pregnancy.

CHAPTER 17

VITAL SIGNS AND TOXIC SYNDROMES

17.1. Which of the following medications is likely to cause hypotension and tachycardia in overdose?

A. Clonidine
B. Digoxin
C. Morphine
D. Nifedipine
E. Nadolol

17.2. Which of the following can cause respiratory stimulation?

A. Opioids
B. Salicylates
C. Flunitrazepam
D. Propofol
E. Secobarbital

17.3. Which of the following agents is associated with hypertension?

A. Disulfiram/ethanol
B. Iron
C. Isopropanol
D. Lead
E. Organic phosphorus compounds

17.4. A bradycardia has been associated with which of the following ingestions?

A. Phenylpropanolamine
B. Iron
C. Isoniazid
D. Diphenhydramine
E. Phencyclidine

17.5. Chronic exposure to which of the following toxic inhalants may cause an increase in the incidence of hypertension?

A. Nitrates
B. Carbon disulfide
C. Carbon monoxide
D. Sulfur dioxide
E. Methane

17.6. Which of the following vital signs or physical findings permits the differentiation of opioid withdrawal from ethanol withdrawal?

A. Blood pressure
B. Pulse
C. Respiratory rate
D. Temperature
E. Pupil size

17.7. Which of the following vital signs or physical findings is most useful in the differentiation of adrenergic agent exposure from anticholinergic agent exposure?

A. Pulse
B. Temperature
C. Mental status
D. Pupil size
E. Peristaltism

17.8. In which of the following clinical situations would the patients' mental status be expected to be normal?

A. Adrenergic agent overdose
B. Anticholinergic agent overdose
C. Opioid agent overdose
D. Opioid agent withdrawal
E. Ethanol withdrawal

17.9. Which of the following agents is associated with life-threatening hyperthermia?

A. Arsenic
B. Botulism
C. Carbamazepine
D. Mercury
E. Phencyclidine

17.10. While treating a patient with cholinergic poisoning with atropine, which of the following is most important to monitor?

A. Blood pressure
B. Pulse
C. Respiratory rate
D. Temperature
E. Mental status

CHAPTER **18**

THERMOREGULATORY PRINCIPLES

18.1. In the central nervous system, thermosensitive neurons are located predominantly in which area?

   A. Posterior hypothalamus
   B. Substantia nigra
   C. Locus ceruleus
   D. Anterior hypothalamus
   E. Thalamus

18.2. Which of the following is the primary neurotransmitter causing stimulation of sweat glands?

   A. Norepinephrine
   B. Serotonin
   C. Acetylcholine
   D. Antidiuretic hormone
   E. Aldosterone

18.3. Which of the following is the main thermoregulatory response to cold in adult humans?

   A. Vasoconstriction
   B. Shivering
   C. Gluconeogenesis
   D. Mobilization of brown fat
   E. Piloerection

18.4. Which of the following best describes the classic electrocardiographic change associated with hypothermia?

   A. PR segment prolongation
   B. QT_c shortening
   C. Peaked T waves
   D. U waves
   E. J-point deflection

18.5. All of the following are part of the definition of heatstroke *except*

   A. Absence of sweating
   B. Temperature >106°F (41.1°C)
   C. Altered mental status
   D. Clear mental status
   E. Presence of sweating

18.6. All of the following drugs predispose to hyperthermia *except*

   A. Cocaine
   B. Antihistamines
   C. Lithium
   D. Cyclic antidepressants
   E. Organophosphates

18.7. Dantrolene sodium is the accepted treatment of choice in which condition?

   A. Exertional heatstroke
   B. Neuroleptic malignant syndrome
   C. Malignant hyperthermia
   D. Classical heatstroke
   E. Strychnine poisoning

18.8. All of the following may predispose to hypothermia *except*

   A. Thiamine deficiency
   B. Phenobarbital
   C. Hypoglycemia
   D. Carbon monoxide
   E. Salicylates

18.9. Which of the following is of greatest prognostic significance in hypothermia?

   A. Temperature 70–80°F (21–27°C)
   B. K^+ >10 meq/L
   C. Frostbite
   D. Unconsciousness
   E. Ethanol intoxication

18.10. Which of the following is not true regarding drug metabolism in hypothermia?

   A. Hepatic metabolism decreases.
   B. Renal clearance decreases.
   C. Glomerular filtration rate decreases.
   D. Volume of distribution increases.
   E. Neuromuscular blockade is prolonged.

CHAPTER **19**

NEUROLOGIC PRINCIPLES

19.1. Asymmetric (focal) neurologic findings can be found with which of the following overdoses?

   A. Amphetamine
   B. Diazepam
   C. Glyburide
   D. Haloperidol
   E. Phenytoin

19.2. Which of the following combinations of findings is most characteristic of coma caused by an overdose?

   A. Equal, reactive pupils with absent oculovestibular response
   B. Equal, reactive pupils with marked nystagmus in response to cold calorics

    C. Unequal, reactive pupils with flaccid right arm and leg

    D. Equal, nonreactive pupils with intact oculocephalic response

    E. Equal, reactive pupils with gaze palsy at rest, easily broken with oculocephalic maneuver

19.3. A young woman presents with normal pupils and bilateral papilledema. She is awake and alert, complaining of headache. She frequents health food stores and takes large quantities of multiple vitamins. Which of the following is the most likely etiology?

    A. Vitamin C

    B. Niacin

    C. Vitamin D

    D. Vitamin E

    E. Vitamin A

19.4. Through what mechanism does *Clostridium tetani* exert its effect on the CNS following initial infection?

    A. Blood-borne via *C. tetani* bacteremia

    B. Lymphatics

    C. Myelin sheath

    D. Axon

    E. Attachment of exotoxin to red blood cells

19.5. A pyridoxine overdose most commonly causes which of the following findings?

    A. Proximal weakness secondary to myopathy

    B. Marked atrophy caused by demyelination of peripheral nerve fibers

    C. Diffuse loss of reflexes secondary to an acute axonopathy

    D. Ataxia caused by sensory neuronopathy

    E. Autonomic instability caused by interference with transmission at the neuromuscular junction

19.6. Which of the following agents is most likely to produce permanent Parkinson disease?

    A. Droperidol (depot injection)

    B. Thioridazine

    C. Thiothixene

    D. Clozapine

    E. MPTP (1-methyl-4-phenyl-1,2,3,6-tetrahydropyridine)

19.7. Which of the following is an essential feature of delirium?

    A. Disorientation to place and time

    B. Stable level of consciousness

    C. Perceptual distortion

    D. Selectively impaired short-term memory loss

    E. Inattention

19.8. Asterixis is most reliably indicative of which of the following?

    A. Hepatic failure

    B. Overdose

    C. Postictal state

    D. Delirium

    E. Toxic metabolic encephalopathy

19.9. Which of the following is most likely to produce a kinetic tremor?

    A. Lithium

    B. Levodopa

    C. Phenothiazines

    D. Cocaine

    E. Hypomagnesemia

19.10. A patient being treated with increasing doses of antipsychotic agents for worsening "agitation" may actually be suffering from which of the following side effects of these medications?

    A. Tardive dyskinesia

    B. Tardive dystonia

    C. Parkinsonian tremor

    D. Chorea

    E. Akathisia

CHAPTER **20**

RESPIRATORY PRINCIPLES

20.1. Impaired ventilation as a result of chest wall rigidity is associated with which of the following toxins?

    A. Morphine

    B. Fentanyl

    C. Heroin

    D. Codeine

    E. Ethchlorvynol

20.2. Nebulized 2% sodium bicarbonate may be useful in patients exposed to which of the following pulmonary irritants?

    A. Nitrogen dioxide

    B. Chloracetophenone

    C. Chlorine

    D. Ammonia

    E. Ozone

20.3. Which of the following statements about monitoring parameters in patients with carbon monoxide poisoning is true?

A. The oxygen saturation from the arterial blood gas will be low, the P_{O_2} will be low, the pulse oximeter O_2 saturation will be low, and the oxygen saturation determined by the CO-oximeter will be low.

B. The oxygen saturation from the arterial blood gas analysis will be normal, the P_{O_2} will be normal, the pulse oximeter oxygen saturation will be low, and the oxygen saturation determined by the CO-oximeter will be low.

C. The oxygen saturation from the arterial blood gas will be normal, the P_{O_2} will be normal, the pulse oximeter O_2 saturation will be normal, and the oxygen saturation determined by the CO-oximeter will be low.

D. The oxygen saturation from the arterial blood gas will be low, the P_{O_2} will be normal, the pulse oximeter saturation will be low, and the oxygen saturation determined by the CO-oximeter will be low.

E. The oxygen saturation from the arterial blood gas will be low, the P_{O_2} will be normal, the pulse oximeter O_2 saturation will be low, and the oxygen saturation determined by the CO-oximeter will be low.

20.4. Which of the following gases is *not* a simple asphyxiant?

A. Carbon dioxide
B. Argon
C. Propane
D. Nitrogen
E. Nitrogen dioxide

20.5. Which of the following gases is *not* a chemical asphyxiant?

A. Cyanide
B. Hydrozoic acid
C. Hydrogen sulfide
D. Amyl nitrite
E. Chloracetophenone

20.6. Which of the following statements about monitoring parameters in patients with methemoglobinemia is true?

A. The oxygen saturation from the arterial blood gas will be low, the P_{O_2} will be low, the pulse oximeter O_2 saturation will be low, and the oxygen saturation determined by the CO-oximeter will be low.

B. The oxygen saturation from the arterial blood gas will be normal, the P_{O_2} will be normal, the pulse oximeter O_2 saturation will be low, and the oxygen saturation determined by the CO-oximeter will be low.

C. The oxygen saturation from the arterial blood gas will be normal, the P_{O_2} will be normal, the pulse oximeter O_2 saturation will be normal, and the oxygen saturation determined by the CO-oximeter will be low.

D. The oxygen saturation from the arterial blood gas will be low, the P_{O_2} will be normal, the pulse oximeter O_2 saturation will be low, and the oxygen saturation determined by the CO-oximeter will be low.

E. The oxygen saturation from the arterial blood gas will be low, the P_{O_2} will be normal, the pulse oximeter O_2 saturation will be low, and the oxygen saturation determined by the co-oximeter will be low.

20.7. Which of the following is not directly associated with the development of acute lung injury?

A. Phenobarbital overdose
B. Chlorine gas
C. Phosgene gas
D. Salicylate overdose
E. Heroin overdose

20.8. Which of the following mechanisms best explains the generation of opioid-induced acute lung injury?

A. Naloxone administration
B. Aspiration during a period of unconsciousness
C. Elevation of catecholamines produced by hypercapnia
D. Direct opioid-induced alterations in pulmonary capillary integrity
E. Acute myocardial dysfunction from high levels of opioid

20.9. The disasters at Lake Nyos and Lake Monoun in Cameroon resulted in over 1700 deaths by which toxin?

A. Carbon dioxide
B. Carbon monoxide
C. Cyanide
D. Hydrogen sulfide
E. Hydrogen chloride

20.10. Barotrauma (pneumothorax, pneumomediastinum, pneumopericardium) is associated with the use of all of the following drugs of abuse *except*

A. Intranasal cocaine
B. Smoking "crack" cocaine
C. Marijuana
D. Methlyenedioxymethamphetamine
E. Nitrous oxide

CHAPTER 21

CARDIOVASCULAR PRINCIPLES

21.1. Overdose of which of the following medications has caused torsades de pointes?

A. Diphenhydramine
B. Lidocaine
C. Terfenadine
D. Propoxyphene
E. Magnesium

21.2. Which of the following opioids can cause intraventricular conduction delays in overdose?

A. Heroin
B. Morphine
C. Meperidine
D. Propoxyphene
E. Diphenoxylate

21.3. Cardiac dysrhythmias from chloral hydrate and other halogenated hydrocarbons are believed to be caused by

A. Increased adrenergic release
B. Sensitization of the myocardium to catecholamines
C. AV conduction defects
D. Intraventricular conduction delays
E. Hypoxia

21.4. Prolongation of the QRS complex to greater than 100 msec would not be expected with which of the following overdoses?

A. Thioridazine
B. Amitriptyline
C. Amantadine
D. Omeprazole
E. Procainamide

21.5. Which of the following overdoses exposure does not cause bradycardia and hypotension?

A. Verapamil
B. Sotalol
C. Propoxyphene
D. Yohimbine
E. Magnesium

21.6. Overdoses of which of the following medications can cause hypotension that is refractory to therapy with intravenous dopamine?

A. Lithium
B. Amitriptyline
C. Ethchlorvynol
D. Phenobarbital
E. Propafenone

21.7. An increase in both blood pressure and pulse rate would be expected immediately following an overdose with which of the following?

A. Nifedipine
B. Phenylpropanolamine
C. Bretylium
D. Theophylline
E. Practolol

21.8. Which of the following toxic exposures would be least likely to cause intravascular volume depletion?

A. Theophylline
B. Iron
C. Cocaine
D. *Datura stramonium* (Jimson weed)
E. Organophosphates

21.9. Intraventricular conduction delay does not occur with which of the following antidysrhythmic drugs?

A. Lidocaine
B. Quinidine
C. Bretylium
D. Procainamide
E. Encainide

21.10. A decrease in blood pressure and a decrease in pulse rate would most commonly be expected to occur with which of the following overdoses?

A. Chlorpromazine
B. Amitriptyline
C. Glutethimide
D. Sotalol
E. Nifedipine

CHAPTER 22

GASTROINTESTINAL PRINCIPLES

22.1. Which of the following statements regarding the effects of caustics on the GI tract is true?

A. Acids cause a liquefactive necrosis of the mucosa.
B. Alkalis produce more damage to the gastric mucosa than to other parts of the GI tract.
C. Because the intragastric environment is already strongly acidic, strong acids are not likely to cause significant damage.
D. The acidemia following acid ingestion is typically non-anion-gap (normal anion gap) acidosis.
E. Caustic ingestions are associated with neoplasms years after the ingestion.

22.2. In the initial phase of acute radiation syndrome, vomiting that begins 2 hours after exposure indicates

A. A lethal exposure
B. Exposure to 100 rads (1Gy)
C. Exposure to over 600 rads (6Gy)
D. Exposure to over 2000 rads (20Gy)
E. An expected reaction to any degree of radiation exposure

22.3. Which of the following statements regarding the effects of alcohol on the GI tract is false?

A. Alcohol-induced lesions occur after acute ingestions at concentrations of 8% or higher.
B. Alcohol-induced erosive gastritis is a major cause of GI hemorrhage.
C. Alcohol decreases the secretion of gastric juices.
D. Alcohol increases gastric mucosal permeability.
E. Alcohol-induced diarrhea is partly due to decreased disaccharidase activity.

22.4. The major toxicity associated with eating oxalate-containing plants such as dumbcane (Dieffenbachia) is

A. Hypocalcemia
B. Renal failure
C. Pain and swelling of the mouth and tongue
D. Constipation
E. Peptic ulcers

22.5. Ingestion of which of the following caustic substances results in oral pain, ulcerations, pulmonary complications, and the formation of a pharyngeal pseudomembrane?

A. NaOH
B. Concentrated hydrochloric acid
C. Concentrated hydrofluoric acid
D. Paraquat
E. Ethanol in greater than 40% concentrations

22.6. Which of the following substances is associated with dry mouth?

A. Caustics
B. Carbamates
C. Tetrodotoxin
D. Anticholinergics
E. Obstruction caused by hastily swallowed drug packets

22.7. Which of the following substances does not cause diarrhea?

A. Colchicine
B. Mercuric chloride
C. Pokeweed
D. Phenothiazines
E. Toxic mushrooms

22.8. All of the following substances are associated with black stools except

A. Blood
B. Phenolphthalein
C. Senna
D. Bismuth subsalicylate
E. Iron

22.9. Which of the following statements about pancreatitis is false?

A. Acute pancreatitis may be differentiated from chronic pancreatitis by a lack of continuing inflammation, irreversible structural changes, and permanent impairment.
B. The toxin most commonly associated with chronic pancreatitis is ethanol.
C. Chronic obstructive pancreatitis is caused by pancreatic duct stenosis resulting from disruption of the duct during acute pancreatitis.
D. Alcoholic pancreatitis is accompanied by hypertriglyceridemia, small amounts of activated trypsin, and high concentrations of protein, zymogen, and trypsin inhibitors within the ducts.
E. Alcoholic pancreatitis histologically and clinically is considered a form of acute pancreatitis.

22.10. Which of the following drugs or toxins associated with pancreatitis significantly affects both the endocrine and exocrine pancreas?

A. Ethanol
B. Pentamidine
C. Estrogens
D. Androgens
E. Vacor

CHAPTER **23**

RENAL PRINCIPLES

23.1. Which of the following drugs is associated with myoglobinuric acute renal failure?

A. Mercuric chloride
B. Amphotericin
C. Amphetamine
D. Cisplatin
E. Acyclovir

23.2. A patient is brought to the emergency department having been found on the floor following a heroin overdose. Which of the following is not correct?

A. Intravenous normal saline may help prevent acute renal failure.
B. Intravenous injection of mannitol may help prevent acute renal failure.
C. Intravenous injection of furosemide may help prevent acute renal failure.
D. Alkalinization of the blood may cause tetany.
E. Alkalinization of the urine may prevent dissociation of hematin from the myoglobin molecule.

23.3. Which statement about acute interstitial nephritis is true?

A. Acute interstitial nephritis is clinically different from acute renal failure.
B. Acute interstitial nephritis caused by NSAIDs is often accompanied by the nephrotic syndrome.
C. Most patients with acute interstitial nephritis caused by β-lactam antibiotics have no signs of hypersensitivity.
D. The trimethoprim in co-trimoxazole prevents the interstitial nephritis associated with the sulfonamides.
E. Thiazides do not cause acute interstitial nephritis.

23.4. Which of the following causes nephrotic syndrome?

A. Bismuth
B. Cyclosporine
C. Cisplatin
D. Radiocontrast agents
E. Mercury

23.5. Which metal may cause chronic interstitial nephritis?

A. Uranium
B. Copper
C. Bismuth
D. Beryllium
E. Chromium

23.6. Which of the following may cause urinary tract obstruction?

A. Amitriptyline
B. Iodinated radiocontrast agents
C. Mitomycin C
D. Lithium
E. Cisplatin

23.7. Which of the following may cause prerenal failure?

A. Aspirin/phenacetin combinations
B. Carbon tetrachloride
C. Furosemide
D. Ampicillin
E. Tobramycin

23.8. Which of the following substances produces a metabolite that is nephrotoxic?

A. Gentamicin
B. Fenoprofen
C. Iodinated radiocontrast agents
D. Ethylene glycol
E. Mercuric chloride

23.9. Which of the following is not characteristic of analgesic nephropathy?

A. Eosinophiluria
B. Papillary necrosis
C. Chronic interstitial nephritis
D. History of gastric irritation
E. Methemoglobinemia

23.10. Which statement is true with regard to gentamicin nephropathy?

A. Oliguria is a common finding.
B. The lesion is in the distal convoluted tubule.
C. Smaller, more frequent doses decrease the injury.
D. Papillary necrosis is often seen.
E. Renal hypoperfusion worsens the toxicity.

CHAPTER **24**

FLUID, ELECTROLYTE, AND ACID-BASE PRINCIPLES

24.1. Which of the following does not cause a low anion gap?

A. Hypermagnesemia
B. Lithium toxicity
C. Bromism
D. Hypoalbuminemia
E. Metformin toxicity

24.2. Which of the following substances is associated with a high-anion-gap metabolic acidosis?

A. Inorganic sulfur
B. Digoxin
C. Nitrates
D. Organic mercury
E. Acetazolamide

24.3. All of the following agents have been associated with the syndrome of inappropriate antidiuretic hormone (SIADH) except

A. Selective serotonin reuptake inhibitors
B. MDMA
C. Sulfonylureas
D. Colchicine
E. Cisplatinum

24.4. All of the following agents have been associated with diabetes insipidus (DI) except

A. Propoxyphene
B. Methoxyflurane
C. Imipramine
D. Demeclocycline
E. Lithium

24.5. A 52-year-old man presents to the hospital with an anion-gap (24 mEq/L) metabolic acidosis and is found to have an osmolar gap of 15. Which of the following is the most likely diagnosis?

A. Methanol intoxication
B. Alcoholic ketoacidosis
C. Lactic acidosis
D. Renal failure
E. Any of the above

24.6. The boiling point elevation technique of measuring osmolality might be appropriate for determining the presence of which of the following compounds?

A. Ethanol
B. Methanol
C. Isopropanol
D. Ethylene glycol
E. Theophylline

24.7. Which of the following substances is associated with hyponatremia?

A. Glycyrrhizic acid
B. Sorbitol
C. Glycerol
D. Amphotericin
E. Foscarnet

24.8. All of the following agents cause hypokalemia except

A. Furosemide
B. Heparin
C. Theophylline
D. Toluene
E. Insulin

24.9. All of the following agents cause hyperkalemia except

A. Digoxin
B. Barium
C. Propranolol
D. Fluoride
E. Penicillin

24.10. All of the following agents are associated with hypomagnesemia except

A. Theophylline
B. Ethanol
C. Furosemide
D. Amphotericin
E. Lithium

CHAPTER **25**

HEMATOLOGIC PRINCIPLES

25.1. Neonates are at particular risk for hypoxic insult because

A. They are generally anemic.
B. The volume of distribution of many toxins is altered in neonates.
C. The persistence of fetal hemoglobin impairs oxygen unloading.
D. The tidal volume of neonates is much smaller.
E. The immature liver is less able to detoxify various toxins.

25.2. Which of the following is true of benzene?

A. The primary route of exposure is transcutaneous.
B. None of the metabolites are excreted in the urine.
C. Exposure may result in thrombocytosis.

D. Toxic metabolites are formed in the bone marrow.

E. Exposure may result in acute lymphocytic leukemia.

25.3. Chloramphenicol (CAP) toxicity is characterized by which of these statements?

A. The development of aplastic anemia is inevitable in all patients who develop anemia following exposure.

B. Aplastic anemia usually occurs within 5 months of exposure to CAP.

C. Toxicity to bone marrow is based on an immune mechanism.

D. Affected bone marrow cells are morphologically normal when viewed with an electron microscope.

E. Recovery following the onset of aplastic anemia occurs in about 25% of patients.

25.4. Which is true of an exposure to ionizing radiation?

A. Rapidly proliferating cells are at the greatest risk of injury.

B. A significant exposure will result in anemia almost immediately.

C. Inflammation is the most significant harmful effect.

D. One of the most sensitive indicators of an acute recent exposure is the platelet count.

E. It is not known to result in hematologic malignancies.

25.5. In the clinical course of aplastic anemia

A. Onset is fulminant.

B. Platelets are unaffected.

C. Most patients respond well to therapy.

D. Reticulocytosis is an important finding.

E. Death results from sepsis or hemorrhage.

25.6. The mature erythrocyte

A. Is 90% hemoglobin by dry weight

B. Carries on only aerobic metabolism

C. Has no mechanism to protect itself from oxidative attack

D. Can replace hemoglobin lost to senescence

E. Forms 2,3-diphosphoglycerate in the red cell before the loss of the red cell nucleus

25.7. Methemoglobin

A. Binds O_2 more tightly than hemoglobin

B. Is hemoglobin with the iron in the 3+ valence state

C. Shifts the oxyhemoglobin dissociation curve to the right

D. Normally constitutes about 8% of total hemoglobin

E. Is primarily reduced (in vivo) by ascorbic acid

25.8. Carbon monoxide

A. Shifts the oxyhemoglobin dissociation curve to the right

B. Has no effect on the unbinding of oxygen at tissue sites

C. Poisoning usually results from intentional exposures

D. Binds to the tissue cytochromes disrupting cellular respiration

E. Binding to hemoglobin is irreversible

25.9. In reference to G-6-PD deficiency

A. Women are more commonly affected than men.

B. Hemolysis may occur following exposure to strong reducing agents.

C. As red cells age, the activity of G-6-PD increases.

D. Measurement of G-6-PD activity is inaccurate following a hemolytic episode.

E. It is an autosomal dominant trait.

25.10. Acquired thrombocytopenia

A. Is most commonly mediated by direct toxicity

B. Has been reported following the use of quinine

C. Most commonly involves the IgA antibody

D. Usually occurs a week after reexposure to an inciting agent

E. Demonstrates an absence of megakaryocytes on bone marrow aspiration

CHAPTER **26**

ENDOCRINE PRINCIPLES

26.1. The CNS is particularly vulnerable to hypoglycemia because

A. It uses a greater amount of glucose than any other individual organ.

B. Brain cannot make use of free fatty acids as an energy substrate.

C. Confusion resulting from hypoglycemia may cause a delay in self-treatment.

D. Ketones cannot be used as an energy substrate in the initial phase of a hypoglycemic event.

E. All of the above

26.2. Which of the following agents acts by decreasing secretion of insulin from the pancreatic islet β cells?

A. Metformin
B. Troglitazone
C. Acarbose
D. Octreotide
E. Alanine

26.3. Which of the following statements about glucagon is correct?

A. Its secretion is enhanced by somatostatin.
B. It inhibits the enzyme phosphorylase, thereby enhancing the breakdown of glycogen.
C. It blocks the secretion of insulin for several hours after administration.
D. Its structure consists of a polypeptide that readily crosses cell membranes.
E. It is secreted in response to epinephrine, thereby enhancing gluconeogenesis.

26.4. Which of the following is correct with respect to hypoglycemia in diabetes?

A. Glucagon is likely to be ineffective as a treatment in non-insulin-dependent diabetes (NIDDM).
B. β-Adrenergic antagonists often worsen the patient's condition by causing hypokalemia.
C. Patients who are on metformin as monotherapy are particularly prone to hypoglycemia.
D. Observation of a patient who has sulfonamide-induced hypoglycemia is generally necessary for no more than 6 to 8 hours.
E. All of the above

26.5. Which of the following combination of circumstances may predispose to hypoglycemia?

A. Chronic insulin use in the setting of renal failure
B. Metformin use with glyburide administration
C. Alcohol intoxication with depleted glycogen stores
D. Pentamidine use in the setting of renal insufficiency
E. All of the above

26.6. Overdose with T_4 usually becomes clinically evident in what time period?

A. Several hours
B. 1 to 3 days
C. 1 week
D. 2 to 3 weeks
E. 1 month

26.7. Hypothyroidism occurs in approximately what percentage of patients on chronic lithium therapy?

A. 1.5%
B. 15%
C. 40%
D. 60%
E. 85%

26.8. Which of the following steroid hormone associations is incorrect?

A. Glucocorticoid excess, insulin resistance, hyperglycemia
B. Glucocorticoid hormone decrease, starvation, hypoglycemia
C. Hydrocortisone depletion, acute illness, hypotension
D. Glucocorticoid administration (acute), decrease in circulating neutrophils
E. Glucocorticoid excess, CNS excitability, acute psychosis

26.9. Which of the following effects are not commonly associated with anabolic steroid use?

A. Testicular atrophy
B. Decrease in LDL cholesterol
C. Decrease in sperm production
D. Hepatic malignancy
E. Gynecomastia

26.10. All of the following are usually irreversible effects of anabolic steroid use by women athletes, except for

A. Baldness
B. Deepening of the voice
C. Increase in facial hair
D. Clitoral hypertrophy
E. Amenorrhea

CHAPTER **27**

OPHTHALMIC PRINCIPLES

27.1. Which of the following is true of ocular irrigation after chemical exposures?

A. Use of a scleral shell irrigating device such as a Morgan lens should be avoided.
B. Outcome is poorer if water is used instead of other commercially available solutions.
C. Regardless of the exposure, irrigation should be continued for 2 hours.

D. Measurement of conjunctival pH may be an unreliable indicator of adequate irrigation.
E. Prolonged irrigation is important after severe alkali burns but not severe acid burns.

27.2. Which of the following pairings is correct regarding agent-specific ocular decontamination?

A. Phenol/PEG (polyethylene glycol) 400
B. Calcium hydroxide (lime)/EDTA
C. Hydrofluoric acid/calcium gluconate
D. Phosphorus/copper sulfate
E. All of the above

27.3. Which of the following may be indicated during the emergency management of severe alkali burns to the eye?

A. Emergency needle paracentesis of the anterior chamber
B. Topical corticosteroids
C. Topical ascorbate and citrate
D. Topical antibiotics
E. All of the above

27.4. Which of the following overdoses typically causes miosis?

A. Diazepam
B. Phenobarbital
C. Clonidine
D. LSD
E. Cocaine

27.5. Which of the following is true of the ocular toxicity of methanol?

A. Funduscopic abnormalities consistently precede visual changes.
B. The primary site of toxicity is the retina.
C. Toxicity is from formaldehyde, resulting from methanol metabolism.
D. Visual changes are consistently completely reversible.
E. Folate or folinic acid is not indicated once acidosis is evident.

27.6. Which of the following is true of the ocular toxicity of quinine?

A. It only occurs after massive, acute overdose.
B. It is caused by retinal vasoconstriction.
C. Full recovery of vision is expected, even after complete blindness.
D. It is well correlated to blood quinine concentration.
E. Funduscopic abnormalities consistently precede visual changes.

27.7. Which of the following contributes to the risk of systemic absorption and toxicity from eye drops?

A. Greater dose-to-body weight ratio in children
B. Preexisting conditions in the elderly
C. Lack of first-pass metabolism of drugs absorbed from the conjunctiva
D. Lack of familiarity with potential adverse effects
E. All of the above

27.8. Which of the following drugs may cause optic neuritis?

A. Amiodarone
B. Corticosteroids
C. Chloroquine
D. Ethambutol
E. Quinine

27.9. Which of the following characteristically causes vertical nystagmus?

A. Carbamazepine
B. Phenytoin
C. Phencyclidine
D. Ethanol
E. Diazepam

27.10. Which of the following is true of ocular effects of drug abuse?

A. Corneal defects have resulted from smoking "crack" cocaine.
B. Cocaine intoxication causes mydriasis.
C. Talc retinopathy occurs only after extensive intravenous drug use.
D. Miosis from opioids results from excessive pupillary constriction rather than inhibition of dilation.
E. All of the above

CHAPTER **28**

OTOLARYNGOLOGIC PRINCIPLES

28.1. Humans can normally detect sound in which of the following ranges?

A. 200 to 40,000 Hz
B. 100 to 40,000 Hz
C. 20 to 40,000 Hz
D. 20 to 20,000 Hz
E. 100 to 20,000 Hz

28.2. The odor of plastic or vinyl on a patient's breath may indicate an exposure to

A. Cyanide
B. Methyl salicylate
C. Turpentine
D. Ethchlorvynol
E. Nitrobenzene

28.3. Which of the following groups of patients is least likely to manifest tinnitus from salicylate toxicity?

A. Elderly
B. Men
C. Those with concomitant use of quinine
D. Children
E. Pregnant women

28.4. Which of the following agents is most likely to cause reversible hearing loss?

A. Cisplatin
B. Bromates
C. Arsenic
D. Quinine
E. Neomycin

28.5. In addition to stimulating the olfactory nerve, ammonia, acetone, and menthol also stimulate which other cranial nerve?

A. Facial
B. Trigeminal
C. Vagal
D. Hypoglossal
E. Glossopharyngeal

28.6. The stria vascularis of the cochlea may be susceptible to many toxins. Which of the following describes its major function?

A. Regenerates hair cells of the cochlea
B. Maintains the electrochemical gradient between the endolymph and the perilymph
C. Conducts neural transmission to the cochlear nucleus and the inferior colliculus
D. Secretes G proteins for the hair cells
E. Provides negative feedback for hair cell transmissions

28.7. Which of the following toxins demonstrates the concept of rapid olfactory fatigue at concentrations exceeding 100 to 150 ppm?

A. Carbon monoxide
B. Phosgene
C. Cyanide
D. Hydrogen sulfide
E. All of the above

28.8. Noise-induced hearing impairment is most likely demonstrated by the following:

A. Testing at the 3- to 6-kHz range
B. Testing at the 10- to 15-kHz range
C. Testing at the 15- to 20-kHz range
D. Testing above the 20-kHz range
E. Testing at any range

28.9. Which of the following substances is most likely to cause tinnitus in overdose?

A. Salicylates
B. Ibuprofen
C. Gentamicin
D. Haloperidol
E. Carbamazepine

28.10. ACE inhibitors cause taste dysfunction by which of the following mechanisms?

A. Inhibit adenylate cyclase at the stria vascularis
B. Antagonize calcium conduction
C. Decrease angiotensin II, an important protein for cochlear function
D. Angioedema
E. Chelate zinc at the taste receptors and the salivary proteins

CHAPTER **29**

DERMATOLOGIC PRINCIPLES

29.1. Which of the following plants can cause photodermatitis?

A. Bergamot orange
B. Wild carrot
C. Lime
D. Parsnip
E. All of the above

29.2. An acute irritant contact dermatitis on the face, groin, or axilla would best be treated by which of the following?

A. Low-potency corticosteroids
B. Medium-potency corticosteroids
C. High-potency corticosteroids
D. A corticosteroid ointment
E. Topical corticosteroids under occlusion

29.3. Which is not true of hydrofluoric acid burns?

A. Intense pain in the absence of significant findings may be present.

B. With concentrations of 70% or more, the appearance of physical findings may be delayed for hours.

C. Treatment includes soaking the affected area in iced solution of 25% magnesium sulfate or application of 10% calcium gluconate gel.

D. 5% calcium gluconate should be injected into the affected skin if there is persistent pain.

E. Hospitalization is recommended for burns larger than 5 cm^2 and for those with facial involvement.

29.4. Which topical medication most frequently causes allergic contact dermatitis?

A. Bacitracin
B. Anthralin
C. Silver sulfadiazine
D. Polymyxin
E. Neomycin

29.5. Which of the following does not result from latex hypersensitivity?

A. Angioedema
B. Asthma
C. Contact urticaria
D. Paronychia
E. Death

29.6. Which of the following plants does not cause dermatitis in persons allergic to poison ivy?

A. Ginkgo tree
B. Cashew
C. Mango
D. Japanese lacquer tree
E. Bergamot orange

29.7. What is the most significant factor that determines a chemical's percutaneous absorption?

A. Concentration
B. Molecular size
C. pH
D. Lipid solubility
E. Water solubility

29.8. Which of the following is a type of eczema?

A. Allergic contact dermatitis
B. Irritant contact dermatitis
C. Dyshidrosis
D. Atopic dermatitis
E. All of the above

29.9. Which epidermal cell is responsible for inducing allergic sensitization?

A. Langerhans cell
B. Merkel cell
C. Mast cell
D. Glomus cell
E. Melanocyte

29.10. The most likely drug to produce toxic epidermal necrolysis is

A. Bleomycin
B. Phenolphthalein
C. Allopurinol
D. Penicillamine
E. Ibuprofen

CHAPTER **30**

GENITOURINARY PRINCIPLES

30.1. Which of the following is a soil fumigant associated with testicular toxicity?

A. 1,2-Dibromo-3-chloropropane (DBCP)
B. Carbaryl
C. Yohimbine
D. Cantharidin
E. None of the above

30.2. The effects of yohimbine include which of the following?

A. Anticholinergic activity
B. α_1-Adrenergic antagonism
C. α_2-Adrenergic agonism
D. α_2-Adrenergic antagonism
E. β_2-Adrenergic agonism

30.3. Which of the following is not considered a toxic effect of Spanish fly?

A. Gastrointestinal bleeding
B. Hematuria
C. Oral pain
D. Seizures
E. Sinus tachycardia

30.4. A patient presents with hyperkalemia and bradycardia after the ingestion of an aphrodisiac agent. Which of the following treatments may be useful?

A. Calcium chloride
B. DMSA
C. Clonidine
D. Methylene blue
E. Digoxin-specific antibody fragments

30.5. Which of the following statements best describes the pharmacokinetics of nitrites?

A. Absorption occurs only after inhalation.
B. Excretion is completely renal.
C. A short half-life (seconds) is common.
D. Michaelis-Menten elimination kinetics occur.
E. None of the above

30.6. Which of the following abortifacients causes hepatotoxicity?

A. Black cohosh
B. Cantharidin
C. Pulegone
D. Trichosanthin
E. Mifepristone

30.7. All of the following statements about misoprostol are true, except

A. It is derived from *Cajanus cajun.*
B. It is a prostaglandin analogue.
C. It is used to treat gastric ulcers.
D. Abortion can occur with doses just above therapeutic.
E. It is commonly used as an abortifacient in Brazil.

30.8. All of the following have been used as an abortifacient, except

A. Pennyroyal oil
B. Quinine
C. Trichosanthins
D. Cimetidine
E. Mifepristone

30.9. Which of the following agents produces red urine?

A. Cascara
B. Senna
C. Beets
D. Carrots
E. Phenol

30.10. Which of the following is responsible for cyclophosphamide-induced hemorrhagic cystitis?

A. Pulegone
B. Acrolein
C. 1,2-Dibromo-3-chloropropane (DBCP)
D. Cantharidin
E. Trichosanthin

CHAPTER 31

MANAGING THE SYMPTOMATIC PATIENT WITH A POSSIBLE TOXIC EXPOSURE

31.1. A known opioid abuser is brought to the emergency department cyanotic, with a respiratory rate of 4 breaths/min. He is lethargic and combative. What is the first priority in his management?

A. Opening the airway and providing bag-valve-mask ventilation
B. Endotracheal intubation
C. 100% oxygen by nonrebreathing mask
D. Administration of naloxone IM or IV
E. Arterial blood gas

31.2. What is first-line therapy for a hypotensive patient with clear lungs and an unknown overdose?

A. Fluid challenge
B. Cardiac inotrope
C. Vasopressor
D. Whole blood
E. MAST trousers

31.3. Naloxone is indicated for administration in patients who

A. Exhibit symptoms of meperidine neurotoxicity
B. Develop nausea and vomiting following administration of morphine
C. Are comatose following a benzodiazepine overdose
D. Have respiratory depression of an unknown etiology
E. All of the above

31.4. Which of the following is least likely to cause a seizure in a patient who presents 1 hour after a suicide attempt?

A. Carbon monoxide
B. Isoniazid
C. Acetaminophen
D. Amitriptyline
E. Propoxyphene

31.5. A patient is brought to the emergency department comatose, presumably as a result of a toxic ingestion. Physical examination reveals a GCS of 3, bilaterally dilated pupils, and an otherwise nonfocal examination.

A. This patient will probably progress to brain death.

B. CNS trauma is unlikely given the nonfocal neurologic examination.
C. A brain CT is not indicated if a history of an ethanol ingestion is obtained.
D. The GCS is not useful for assessing changes in the neurologic status of patients with toxic-metabolic coma.
E. Complete recovery of patients with properly managed toxic-metabolic coma despite a low GCS is the rule rather than the exception.

31.6. A comatose patient has received initial stabilization of his airway, breathing, and circulation. The next consideration is

A. Administration of hypertonic dextrose, thiamine, naloxone, and oxygen
B. GI decontamination
C. CT of brain
D. Toxicology screen
E. Determination of serum electrolytes and anion gap

31.7. A patient presents with severe salicylism. Immediate consideration should be given to which of the following?

A. GI decontamination
B. Serum alkalinization
C. Urine alkalinization
D. Hemodialysis
E. All of the above

31.8. Which of the following is acceptable empiric therapy for a patient with an altered mental status?

A. Analeptics including physostigmine
B. Flumazenil
C. Forced diuresis
D. Urinary acidification
E. Thiamine

31.9. Which of the following statements is correct about poison management of a patient in her third trimester of pregnancy?

A. Sorbitol cannot be given with activated charcoal as it is contraindicated during pregnancy.
B. Shock is easier to identify in this patient than in a nonpregnant patient.
C. Hypotension may improve if the patient is turned to the right-lateral decubitus position.
D. Hyperbaric oxygen should be used at lower carboxyhemoglobin levels than with nonpregnant patients.
E. Naloxone should not be given, as there are limited data regarding its use in pregnancy.

31.10. A comatose patient presents with a rectal temperature of 106.2°F (41.2°C) and no additional history. How should the patient's fever be lowered?

A. He should be immersed in a tepid bath.
B. He should be rapidly and aggressively cooled to 101.5°F (38.6°C) either by using evaporative cooling or by immersion in an ice bath.
C. A towel soaked with rubbing alcohol should be placed on his forehead and his chest.
D. Rectal acetaminophen at a dose of 20 mg/kg should be administered.
E. Temperature should be monitored, and if it exceeds 107°F (41.7°C), the patient should be placed in an ice bath.

CHAPTER **32**

ACETAMINOPHEN

32.1. Which of the following is true of N-acetyl-p-benzoquinoneimine (NAPQI)?

A. It reacts readily with available electrophiles.
B. It is formed in the liver but not in other organs.
C. In the liver, it is mostly formed in Zone III.
D. It is formed after acetaminophen overdose but not after recommended dosing.
E. Glutathione stores must remain near normal to prevent toxicity.

32.2. Which of the following would theoretically increase the risk of acetaminophen toxicity after overdose?

A. Chronic use of cimetidine
B. Chronic use of ethanol and acute coingestion of ethanol
C. Acute coingestion of ethanol, without chronic ethanol use
D. Chronic use of ethanol without acute coingestion of ethanol
E. Acute coingestion of phenobarbital

32.3. Which of the following is not a reported cause of altered mental status in a patient who took a large acetaminophen overdose?

A. Metabolic inhibition by acetaminophen
B. Hypoglycemia
C. Cerebral edema
D. Opioid intoxication
E. Dehydration

32.4. Which of the following is true of *N*-acetylcysteine?

    A. It is a glutathione substitute but does not lead to increased glutathione supply.

    B. It is a glutathione substitute and prevents the formation *N*-acetyl-*p*-benzoquinoneimine.

    C. It decreases the capacity for sulfation of acetaminophen.

    D. If administered within 8 hours of an acute acetaminophen ingestion, it can prevent hepatic failure, regardless of the serum concentration of acetaminophen.

    E. It interferes with the acetaminophen assay.

32.5. Which of the following is true of acetaminophen overdose in pregnancy?

    A. *N*-Acetylcysteine does not cross the human placenta.

    B. The fetus is incapable of producing *N*-acetyl-*p*-benzoquinoneimine until late in the third trimester.

    C. *N*-Acetylcysteine has been proven to protect the fetus from serious toxicity.

    D. In every case in which maternal outcome has been good, fetal outcome has also been good.

    E. In nearly all cases, both maternal and fetal outcome has been good if *N*-acetylcysteine was used in a timely manner.

32.6. Which of the following best characterizes the lower acetaminophen nomogram line?

    A. Values above the line indicate that consequential hepatotoxicity is expected.

    B. In most cases, values even slightly below the line indicate that no further evaluation for acetaminophen toxicity is needed.

    C. A value below the line indicates that all subsequent values will also be below the line.

    D. It is an unsafe screening tool after overdose of extended-release acetaminophen.

    E. The line is both highly sensitive and highly specific as an indicator of risk.

32.7. Which of the following is true of acetaminophen exposure in patients less than 5 years old?

    A. They have increase capacity for sulfation, providing them with protection from acetaminophen-induced hepatic injury.

    B. They are less likely than adults to suffer toxicity related to repeated excessive dosing (chronic overdose).

    C. Acute febrile illness decreases the risk of acetaminophen-induced liver injury.

    D. The lower incidence of liver injury after acute acetaminophen exposure in these patients may be related to the amount of exposure, time to treatment, or decreased susceptibility.

    E. The acetaminophen nomogram does not apply to children.

32.8. Which of the following is true regarding renal injury after acetaminophen exposure?

    A. Hepatorenal syndrome is the only cause of acetaminophen induced renal injury.

    B. The incidence of renal injury is the same regardless of the degree of hepatic injury.

    C. Renal P450 metabolism of acetaminophen leads to the formation of *N*-acetyl-*p*-benzoquinoneimine.

    D. Pancreatic injury is more common than renal injury

    E. Renal injury cannot occur in the absence of hepatic injury.

32.9. Which of the following is true regarding the administration of activated charcoal after acetaminophen exposure?

    A. Activated charcoal does not interfere with the absorption of *N*-acetylcysteine.

    B. Activated charcoal does not decrease acetaminophen absorption.

    C. Interference with absorption of *N*-acetylcysteine is rarely a clinical concern.

    D. Multiple dose activated charcoal decreases the half-life of acetaminophen

    E. It may actually increase the absorption of acetaminophen

32.10. For which of the following cases is the acetaminophen nomogram not applicable?

    A. A patient who is comatose with a serum acetaminophen concentration of 20 mg/mL, and no history regarding the time of ingestion is available.

    B. A patient who presents with a history of single acute acetaminophen ingestion with a serum acetaminophen concentration of 20 mg/mL 28 hours after his ingestion.

    C. A patient who is taking 10 g of acetaminophen per day for 3 days, has a serum acetaminophen concentration of 50 mg/mL 4 hours after his last dose.

    D. A patient who gives a history of acute acetaminophen ingestion in a self-harm attempt presents with right upper quadrant tenderness with serum acetaminophen concentration of

30 mg/mL and an AST of 450 IU/mL 12 hours after his ingestion.

E. All of the above.

CHAPTER 33

SALICYLATES

33.1. The most typical acid-base pattern found a few hours after a significant acute salicylate ingestion by an adult with no other medical problems and using no other medications is

A. Acute respiratory alkalosis and alkalemia
B. Acute respiratory acidosis and acidemia
C. Acute respiratory alkalosis, metabolic acidosis and alkalemia
D. Acute respiratory alkalosis, metabolic acidosis and acidemia
E. Metabolic acidosis, compensatory respiratory alkalosis and acidemia

33.2. Which of the following statements best describes the effects of salicylate poisoning on glucose metabolism?

A. Most patients are hyperglycemic.
B. Most patients are hypoglycemic.
C. The CSF glucose level is consistent with the blood glucose level.
D. The rate of CSF glucose utilization exceeds the rate of supply even in the presence of a normal serum glucose.
E. The CSF glucose levels are consistently high, even when serum glucose is normal or low, and this accounts for many of the CNS manifestations of salicylate poisoning.

33.3. Which of the following statements regarding salicylate-induced induced acute lung injury is true?

A. It is increasingly likely to occur as the serum salicylate level rises beyond 50 mg/dL.
B. It is more likely to occur after an acute salicylate ingestion.
C. It reflects underlying cardiac disease, particularly CHF.
D. It has never been identified in children.
E. It almost always occurs in adults over 30 years of age.

33.4. Which of the following statements regarding salicylate pharmacokinetics is true?

A. Salicylate absorption from the stomach is negligible.

B. Salicylate absorption from the small bowel is negligible.
C. The dosage form of salicylates has a negligible effect on absorption.
D. After therapeutic doses, significant salicylate levels are achieved in 30 minutes and peak levels are achieved in an hour, except after an overdose, when peak levels may not be achieved for 4 to 6 hours or longer.
E. After an overdose, salicylate elimination is by first-order kinetics.

33.5. Which of the following statements regarding salicylate levels is true?

A. Except in rare instances, salicylate toxicity corresponds reliably with serum levels.
B. A falling serum salicylate level may indicate either increased clearance or decreased tissue distribution.
C. A serum salicylate level that is low or within the therapeutic range indicates that the patient can be managed appropriately without hemodialysis.
D. Peak serum salicylate levels may best be reflected by the CSF salicylate level.
E. Because CSF salicylate levels correlate poorly with toxicity, only serum salicylate levels should be used to determine treatment.

33.6. Which of the following signs and symptoms of salicylate poisoning always represents severe life-threatening toxicity?

A. Tinnitus rapidly followed by deafness
B. Vertigo
C. Lethargy
D. Markedly elevated temperatures
E. Hyperventilation, hyperactivity, and agitation

33.7. Which of the following statements regarding salicylate testing is true?

A. A bedside ferric chloride test indicates only salicylate use, not necessarily overdosage.
B. A false-negative ferric chloride test may occur if the urine used for testing was previously used for dipstick analysis with N-Multistix or Bili Labstix.
C. A positive urine ketone test means that the ferric chloride results are not reliable for salicylates.
D. As in the case of an acute acetaminophen overdose, an extremely high reported serum salicylate level unaccompanied by any clinical signs of toxicity mandates rapid, aggressive

treatment to eliminate the drug from the patient's body.

E. Ferric chloride testing is unreliable in patients with liver disease.

33.8. Which statement concerning salicylate elimination is true?

A. Forced diuresis is an effective way of eliminating salicylates, but not as effective as alkaline diuresis.

B. Because alkalinization of both the urine and blood is important, $NaHCO_3$ should be used.

C. Endotracheal intubation followed by hyperventilation is an effective alternative method of alkalinization for salicylate poisoning without the risk of hypernatremia or fluid overload from $NaHCO_3$ use.

D. Although a common complication of salicylate poisonings, hypokalemia does not interfere with urinary alkalinization.

E. Activated charcoal is ineffective in adsorbing salicylic acid.

33.9. All of the following are indications for hemodialysis for salicylate poisoning except

A. Severe fluid and electrolyte disturbances

B. High (>100 mg/dL) salicylate levels regardless of the blood pH

C. A patient who is unable to eliminate salicylates

D. An ill patient who has ingested moderate amounts of two or more dialyzable drugs

E. A patient who is experiencing deafness as a result of the overdose

33.10. Which of the following statistics regarding analgesics and salicylate poisoning is true?

A. Salicylate poisoning is the most common type of analgesic-related death reported to the American Association of Poison Control Centers (AAPCC).

B. The incidence of Reye syndrome continues to increase despite the decreased use of salicylates in children.

C. The FDA now prohibits the use of the same name for salicylate-containing products and for acetaminophen-containing products.

D. Methyl salicylate "liniments" and other externally applied salicylate products are not as toxic as ingested salicylates.

E. Analgesics are responsible for more deaths annually than any other product reported to the AAPCC.

CHAPTER **34**

NONSTEROIDAL AND OTHER ANTIINFLAMMATORY AGENTS

34.1. Which of the following pairs of nonsteroidal antiinflammatory (NSAID) agents are associated with the most serious toxicity?

A. Ibuprofen and naproxen

B. Meloxicam and phenylbutazone

C. Piroxicam and mefenamic acid

D. Indomethacin and piroxicam

E. Phenylbutazone and mefenamic acid

34.2. NSAIDs and corticosteroids differ in the mechanism of their antiinflammatory effects because of which of the following?

A. Only NSAIDs block production of prostaglandins.

B. NSAIDs are relatively more potent at the inhibition of cyclooxygenase I and II.

C. NSAIDs do not affect production of arachidonic acid.

D. NSAIDs do not affect production of leukotrienes.

E. NSAIDs promote thromboxanes preferentially to prostacyclins, making them better anticoagulants.

34.3. Which of the following statements is true with regard to the pharmacokinetics of the NSAIDs in overdose?

A. There is good evidence that the rate of absorption is significantly slower, resulting in delayed onset of toxicity.

B. The drugs are primarily excreted renally, and hepatic metabolism becomes unimportant.

C. The half-life stays similar to that seen with therapeutic doses.

D. The NSAIDs do not penetrate the blood-brain barrier.

E. The duration of toxicity is long because the NSAIDs bind irreversibly to COX-1 and COX-2 enzymes.

34.4. A patient presents with altered mental status, and a ferric chloride test performed at the bedside changes the color of the urine from yellow to a purple-brown. This indicates possible use of all of the following agents except for which one?

A. Salicylates

B. Phenothiazines

C. Phenylbutazone
D. Diflunisal
E. Anthraquinones

34.5. Aplastic anemia is most commonly associated with use of which of the following NSAIDs?

A. Sulindac
B. Phenylbutazone
C. Naproxen
D. Ketorolac
E. Ibuprofen

34.6. The following statements about the clinical effects resulting from the use of NSAIDs are true, except for which of the following?

A. Tinnitus indicates that the patient must also be using salicylates.
B. Aseptic meningitis has been reported in patients with or without autoimmune disorders.
C. Anaphylactoid reactions occur in up to 25% of adult asthmatics with nasal polyps and urticaria.
D. NSAIDs may enhance toxicity from digoxin, lithium, hypoglycemics, anticoagulants, or aminoglycosides.
E. Coma and metabolic acidosis commonly occur in patients with massive overdose of NSAIDs.

34.7. The following statements about the renal effects of NSAIDs are true, except for which of the following?

A. NSAIDs produce renal failure but not typically in patients who are otherwise normal.
B. NSAIDs account for approximately 15% of drug-induced renal failure.
C. NSAIDs have been reported to produce a variety of nephropathies including interstitial nephritis, nephrotic syndrome, and papillary necrosis.
D. NSAID use has been associated with hypokalemia.
E. NSAID effects at the kidney may enhance lithium, digoxin, and aminoglycoside toxicity and decrease effectiveness of antihypertensives such as ACE inhibitors, β-adrenergic antagonists, and diuretics.

34.8. Which of the following may be useful in treatment of the adverse affects of NSAIDs?

A. Cyclooxygenase II–selective agents
B. Misoprostol
C. Omeprazole
D. Leukotriene receptor antagonists
E. All of the above

34.9. Although salicylates are NSAIDs, the primary differences in management of patients with NSAID toxicity compared to salicylates is best described by which of the following?

A. Patients with NSAID toxicity benefit from hemodialysis but not urinary alkalinization.
B. NSAIDs are not adsorbed by activated charcoal.
C. Patients with NSAID toxicity benefit from urinary alkalinization but not hemodialysis.
D. Patients with NSAID toxicity necessitate early gastric lavage because the drug is not removed by hemodialysis.
E. Patients with NSAID toxicity benefit from neither hemodialysis nor urinary alkalinization.

34.10. Which of the following statements is correct with regard to overdoses of the COX-2–selective NSAIDs?

A. They are nontoxic.
B. They will likely produce toxicity similar to the other NSAIDs.
C. They have a greater likelihood of producing CNS toxicity.
D. They are more likely to produce gastrointestinal bleeding that the other NSAIDs.
E. The COX-2 selectivity is seen in overdoses.

CHAPTER **35**

ANTIHISTAMINES AND DECONGESTANTS

35.1. Which of the following H_2 antagonists significantly inhibit the cytochrome P450 oxidase system?

A. Nizatidine
B. Cimetidine
C. Famotidine
D. Ranitidine
E. Fexofenadine

35.2. Which of the following antihistamines has selective peripheral antihistamine activity?

A. Pheniramine
B. Clemastine
C. Methdilazine
D. Cetirizine
E. Meclizine

35.3. Which of the following isoenzymes of the cytochrome P450 oxidase system is responsible for most of the metabolism of astemizole?

A. CYP1A2
B. CYP2C9
C. CYP2E1
D. CYP2D6
E. CYP3A4

35.4. Diphenhydramine is acetylated most rapidly by which of the following groups of individuals?

A. Hispanics
B. American Indians
C. African Americans
D. Middle Easterners
E. Asians

35.5. Which of the following is *not* a clinical sign of progressive antihistamine toxicity?

A. Increasing delirium
B. Rising temperature
C. Faster heart rates
D. Falling respiratory rates
E. Increasing blood glucose levels

35.6. During the initial assessment of a patient who has ingested excessive amounts of OTC cold syrup containing antihistamine, which of the following investigations is essential?

A. Blood acetaminophen level
B. WBC differential
C. Cardiac enzymes
D. Urine specific gravity and protein
E. Stool occult blood testing

35.7. Which of the following decongestants would be most likely to cause hypertension and bradycardia?

A. Phenylpropanolamine
B. Pseudoephedrine
C. Terbutaline
D. Ephedrine
E. Isoephedrine

35.8. Which of the following imidazoline decongestants is a histamine H_2 agonist in addition to an α-adrenergic stimulant?

A. Xylometazoline
B. Naphazoline
C. Oxymetazoline
D. Tetrahydrozoline
E. Neumotazoline

35.9. An acute dystonic reaction can occur from which of the following antihistamines?

A. Fexofenadine
B. Doxylamine

C. Diphenhydramine
D. Meclizine
E. Hydroxyzine

35.10. Overdose of which of the following antihistamines has been associated with rhabdomyolysis?

A. Diphenhydramine
B. Brompheniramine
C. Doxylamine
D. Pyrilamine
E. Fexofenadine

CHAPTER **36**

IRON

36.1. A 20-month-old toddler is brought to the emergency department 30 minutes following potentially ingesting 100 mg/kg iron. An abdominal flat plate reveals multiple radiopaque iron fragments in the stomach. The patient is asymptomatic. Which of the following is the most rational first step in gastrointestinal decontamination?

A. Orogastric lavage with hypertonic phosphate
B. Syrup of ipecac
C. Orogastric lavage with deferoxamine
D. Orogastric lavage with normal saline
E. Whole-bowel irrigation with PEG-ELS

36.2. What is the second step in gastrointestinal decontamination for the patient in 36.1?

A. Consult surgery for emergent gastrotomy
B. Give activated charcoal, 1g/kg
C. Whole-bowel irrigation with PEG-ELS
D. Syrup of ipecac
E. Magnesium citrate by mouth

36.3. Following a significant iron ingestion, which of the following suggests that clinically consequential poisoning is not present?

A. The WBC is less than 15,000/mm^3
B. The serum glucose is less than 150 mg/dL
C. The total iron binding capacity (TIBC) is less than the serum iron level
D. The patient is asymptomatic for 6 hours in the ED
E. The serum potassium is normal

36.4. A 10-kg toddler ingests ten 325-mg tablets of ferrous sulfate. The poison center is contacted and must decide the significance of the patient's exposure. How much iron, in elemental form, did the child ingest?

A. 30 mg/kg
B. 10 mg/kg
C. 20 mg/kg
D. 65 mg/kg
E. 6.5 mg/kg

36.5. Which of the following is not an explanation for iron-induced metabolic acidosis?

A. Absorption of iron and transformation of ferrous to ferric state liberates an unbuffered proton
B. Iron is an acid, with a pK of 2.2
C. Iron disrupts oxidative phosphorylation
D. Iron decreases cardiac output, causing hypotension and poor tissue perfusion
E. Free iron is a vasodilator, causing hypotension and lactic acidosis

36.6. Which of the statements with regard to deferoxamine is correct?

A. Deferoxamine is readily synthesized in the laboratory.
B. Intravenous administration is the only acceptable route for deferoxamine.
C. The correct dose of deferoxamine is the molar equivalent of the amount of the iron ingested.
D. On a molar basis, one mole of deferoxamine binds one mole of iron.
E. Deferoxamine can remove iron from hemoglobin.

36.7. Management of iron poisoning in a patient who is 10 weeks pregnant and who has vomited 10 times should not include which of the following?

A. Fluid resuscitation
B. Whole bowel irrigation
C. Deferoxamine
D. Abdominal radiography
E. The monitoring of vital signs

36.8. Which of the following is not a potential consequence of short-term deferoxamine therapy?

A. Rate-related hypotension
B. *Yersinia* enterocolitis
C. Inability to follow serum iron levels
D. Ophthalmic toxicity
E. Acute lung injury

36.9. Deferoxamine administration can be stopped under which of the following circumstances?

A. The urine turns brownish-red

B. The TIBC exceeds the serum iron level
C. The WBC and glucose return to normal
D. The anion-gap acidosis resolves, and the patient appears well
E. Vomiting and diarrhea resolve

36.10. A 2-year-old was hospitalized and treated with intravenous deferoxamine for 2 days following a severe iron poisoning. His clinical improvement was dramatic, and he became asymptomatic. He once again developed a fever, followed by vomiting and diarrhea. Which of the following is a likely etiology?

A. An iron bezoar
B. *Yersinia enterocolitica* infection
C. Inadequate treatment with deferoxamine
D. *Clostridium difficile* infection
E. Reingestion of iron

CHAPTER **37**

VITAMINS

37.1. Which of the following statements about vitamin A is false?

A. It is a lipid-soluble vitamin.
B. β-Carotene is a precursor, which is rapidly converted to vitamin A.
C. Approximately 90% of the total vitamin A content of the mammalian body is stored in the liver, primarily as retinyl ester.
D. Hepatic reserves are often sufficient to prevent symptoms of vitamin A deficiency for several months.
E. In the retina, vitamin A is required for the regeneration of the photosensitive chromoprotein rhodopsin.

37.2. Which of the following descriptions of idiopathic intracranial hypertension is true?

A. It is pathognomonic for vitamin A toxicity
B. It can be present despite normal CSF opening pressures
C. It is best diagnosed with an MRI scan of the brain
D. It is invariably accompanied by focal neurologic findings but is essentially benign
E. Left untreated, it may lead to permanent visual loss.

37.3. Which of the following clinical findings is not consistent with vitamin A toxicity?

A. Prominent visual disturbances
B. Hepatosplenomegaly
C. Alopecia
D. Acrodynia
E. Abnormalities in bone growth

37.4. Hepatotoxicity from vitamin A is best described by which of the following?

A. Centrilobular necrosis
B. Periportal necrosis
C. Cirrhosis
D. Kupffer cell–mediated inflammation
E. Proliferation of bile ducts

37.5. Which of the following vitamins can interfere with coumadin therapy?

A. Vitamin B_6
B. Vitamin B_{12}
C. Vitamin C
D. Vitamin D
E. Vitamin E

37.6. Which of the following statements concerning vitamin B_6 is false?

A. It is a cofactor in GABA synthesis.
B. It is safe in single doses as high as 75 mg/kg/dose.
C. Even low-dose therapy, used chronically, can produce toxicity.
D. It is rapidly excreted.
E. It causes a proximal motor neuropathy.

37.7. Which one of the following descriptions of vitamin C is true?

A. It is a proven cold remedy
B. It is a uricosuric agent
C. It converts trivalent chromium to its less toxic hexavalent form
D. It can be given as an oral or intravenous dose after acute chromium exposure
E. It causes constipation at high doses

37.8. Which one of the following descriptions of vitamin D poisoning is true?

A. The patient's serum calcium is typically normal
B. Milk should contain vitamin D_2 because vitamin D_3 is more toxic
C. Vitamin D is a rapidly acting rodenticide.
D. Hematopoietic toxicity is common and may be severe.
E. Patients require cautious rehydration because of the risk of cardiac dysrhythmias.

37.9. Which one of the following descriptions of niacin flush is true?

A. It is rare.
B. It is readily prevented with aspirin.
C. It represents an anticholinergic side effect of the drug.
D. It occurs because of concomitant use of HMG-CoA reductase inhibitors.
E. It often precedes syncope.

37.10. Patients with niacin-induced hepatic toxicity have which of the following characteristics?

A. Are likely to develop the niacin flush syndrome
B. Have a liver biopsy demonstrating centrilobular necrosis
C. Are taking sustained-release niacin preparations
D. Are allergic to aspirin
E. Are alcohol dependent

CHAPTER **38**

DIETING AGENTS AND REGIMENS

38.1. Phentermine-fenfluramine ("phen-fen") was a combination diet regimen withdrawn from the market for association with which of the following pathologic entities?

A. Cerebral infarction
B. Mesenteric ischemia
C. Cardiac valvular regurgitation
D. Psychosis
E. Vasculitis

38.2. *Ma huang* or Chinese ephedra is a "herbal" supplement used to "increase energy" and "lose weight." This product is structurally and pharmacologically similar to which of the following drugs?

A. Caffeine
B. Cocaine
C. Amphetamine
D. Nicotine
E. Digoxin

38.3. "Starch blockers" or amylase inhibitors were promoted as diet aids that would prevent calorie absorption from ingested carbohydrates through inhibition of starch breakdown. This dieting approach was unsuccessful for which of the following reasons?

A. Adverse side effects, especially dry mouth
B. High cost
C. Inhibition of other vital enzymes led to hepato-toxicity
D. Amylase inhibition in vivo was clinically insignificant
E. Extensive muscle breakdown

38.4. Very low-calorie diets are associated with sudden death and which of the following cardiac abnormalities?

A. Atrial myxomas
B. Atrial fibrillation
C. First-degree AV block
D. Torsades de pointes
E. Ventricular fibrosis

38.5. Nonprescription phenylpropanolamine-containing appetite suppressants are no longer available because of risk of which of the following?

A. Mitral regurgitation
B. Hemorrhagic stroke
C. Primary pulmonary hypertension
D. Atrial fibrillation
E. Bradycardia

38.6. A 19-year-old woman develops headache and blurry vision following an overdose of phenylpropanolamine. Her pertinent vital data include a blood pressure of 180/115 mm Hg and a pulse of 58/min. An appropriate treatment for this patient might include which of the following?

A. Metoprolol
B. Ephedrine
C. Propranolol
D. Phentolamine
E. Diltiazem

38.7. Which of the following is the mechanism by which 2,4-dinitrophenol produces weight loss?

A. It blocks amylase and thus starch breakdown.
B. It prevents glucagon release.
C. It uncouples oxidative phosphorylation.
D. It increases insulin release.
E. It causes dysgeusia.

38.8. Cal-Ban 300 was a guar gum mixture used as a diet aid. Toxicity resulted from which of the following?

A. Dehydration
B. Constipation
C. Esophageal/intestinal obstruction
D. Hyperthermia
E. Nausea and bloating

38.9. Which one of following diet aids is not associated with primary pulmonary hypertension?

A. Fenfluramine
B. Aminorex
C. Dexfenfluramine
D. Phenylpropanolamine
E. Phenmetrazine

38.10. Patients with eating disorders may develop skeletal or cardiac myopathy as a result of chronic abuse of which of the following?

A. Syrup of ipecac
B. Laxatives
C. Diuretics
D. Anorexiants
E. Vitamin C

CHAPTER **39**

METHYLXANTHINES

39.1. Which of the following statements about the metabolism of caffeine is correct?

A. Caffeine is primarily eliminated by glomerular filtration.
B. In preterm infants, caffeine is metabolized in the liver to theophylline.
C. Caffeine's half-life is increased in smokers.
D. Caffeine induces microsomal enzyme activity.
E. Caffeine is primarily metabolized by hydroxylation.

39.2. Caffeine and theophylline exert physiologic effects at which of the following receptors?

A. Adenosine receptors
B. Muscarinic receptors
C. Nicotinic receptors
D. Dopaminergic receptors
E. Serotonergic receptors

39.3. Which of the following statements about caffeine toxicity is correct?

A. Cardiac toxicity is unreported with caffeine.
B. Side effects are not dose dependent.
C. Caffeine causes biphasic toxicity: anxiety followed by lethargy.
D. Tolerance to caffeine's stimulatory effects occurs after several years of chronic use.
E. Patients with hyperthyroidism are resistant to the stimulatory effects of caffeine.

39.4. Which of the following statements about caffeine and the gastrointestinal tract is correct?

A. Small doses of caffeine administered each day can cause gastric erosions in animals.
B. Caffeine can cause increased secretion of both pepsin and gastric acid.
C. Decaffeinated coffee can be used to prevent stomach injury in patients with ulcers.
D. Accumulated cyclic AMP causes an increase in secretions in the stomach.
E. Caffeine is a potent inhibitor of H_2 receptors in the stomach.

39.5. Which of the following statements regarding the possible side effects of caffeine is correct?

A. Caffeine decreases the force of contraction of muscle.
B. Caffeine increases the basal metabolic rate by 50%.
C. Caffeine has inconsistent effects on lipid profiles.
D. Effects of caffeine on pituitary function are not dose related.
E. Habitual caffeine ingestion is associated with increased bone density.

39.6. Which of the following is considered to be the most effective technique for increasing total body clearance of theophylline or caffeine?

A. Multiple-dose activated charcoal
B. Peritoneal dialysis
C. Charcoal hemoperfusion
D. Hemodialysis
E. Single-dose activated charcoal

39.7. Which of the following laboratory abnormalities occurs most often in patients with acute theophylline poisoning?

A. Hypokalemia
B. Respiratory acidosis
C. Hypoglycemia
D. Hyperchloremia
E. Hypernatremia

39.8. Which of the following toxicities is most likely to be observed in a patient with a theophylline level of 30 μg/mL following an acute ingestion?

A. Seizures and metabolic acidosis
B. Ventricular tachycardia
C. Coagulation disorders, bleeding, and hypotension
D. Nausea, vomiting, and sinus tachycardia
E. Hypotension and metabolic acidosis

39.9. Which of the following gastrointestinal decontamination techniques best reduces the absorption of theophylline and caffeine?

A. Emesis with syrup of ipecac
B. Gastric lavage
C. Activated charcoal
D. Cathartics
E. Whole-bowel irrigation

39.10. At therapeutic levels, theophylline exerts its primary pharmacologic effect by

A. Inhibiting the activity of acetylcholine on cyclic AMP
B. Stimulating β-adrenergic receptors in the lung
C. Inhibiting the activity of phosphodiesterase
D. Increasing intracellular concentrations of cyclic GMP
E. Antagonizing the activity of adenosine

CHAPTER **40**

ANTIDIABETIC AND HYPOGLYCEMIC AGENTS

40.1. Which of the following laboratory findings is diagnostic of an exogenous insulin overdose?

A. A persistent blood glucose level below 50 mg/dL
B. An α_1-glycoprotein level exceeding 3 mg/mL
C. A C-peptide level of less than 0.2 nmol/L
D. Insulin levels exceeding 6 mU/mL
E. Glucagon levels less than 15 mU/mL

40.2. Which of the following antidiabetic medications causes the highest incidence of iatrogenic hypoglycemia?

A. Glyburide
B. Rosiglitazone
C. Acetohexamide
D. Tolazamide
E. Phenformin

40.3. Which of the following fruits, when unripe, has been reported to depress blood glucose levels?

A. Kiwi
B. Grapefruit
C. Balsam pear
D. Ackee
E. Star

40.4. Which of the following might be caused by an oral hypoglycemic agent overdose?

A. Bronchoconstriction
B. Bradycardia
C. Hemiparesis
D. Miosis
E. Hypoactive bowel sounds

40.5. Which of the following is the most appropriate therapy for patients with recurrent hypoglycemia following a sulfonylurea overdose?

A. Dextrose then octreotide
B. Dextrose then diazoxide
C. Octreotide then streptozotocin
D. Dextrose then fructose
E. Octreotide is first-line therapy

40.6. Which of the following oral hypoglycemic medications has the longest duration of action?

A. Tolbutamide
B. Chlorpropamide
C. Glyburide
D. Tolazamide
E. Glipizide

40.7. The biguanide metformin differs from its predecessor phenformin because it has a lower incidence of which of the following?

A. Renal toxicity
B. Hepatic toxicity
C. Cardiac toxicity
D. Metabolic toxicity
E. Treatment failures

40.8. Which of the following is associated with significant hepatic toxicity?

A. Repaglinide
B. Troglitazone
C. Rosiglitazone
D. Pioglitazone
E. Acarbose

40.9. A young child is suspected to have ingested a single sulfonylurea tablet. Which of the following is true of the initial management?

A. Because the duration of action of most pills is short, brief observation should suffice.
B. Hospital admission is warranted in most cases.
C. Oral activated charcoal cannot adsorb sulfonylureas, so it should not be administered.
D. Measurement of serial drug levels may be useful to determine the appropriate observation period.
E. Prophylactic octreotide should be administered.

40.10. Which of the following oral hypoglycemic agents would be best for use in a patient with renal impairment?

A. Tolazamide
B. Metformin
C. Glyburide
D. Chlorpropamide
E. Glipizide

CHAPTER **41**

ANTICONVULSANTS

41.1. Which of the following statements with regard to phenytoin is false?

A. Intravenous administration of phenytoin is associated with a rate-related incidence of hemodynamic complications.
B. Serum phenytoin levels correlate with levels in the central nervous system.
C. Serum phenytoin levels >30 mg/L are associated with ataxia.
D. Phenytoin absorption following a single acute toxic ingestion is unpredictable.
E. Multiple-dose activated charcoal reduces the elimination half-life of intravenously administered phenytoin.

41.2. Which of the following statements with regard to carbamazepine is false?

A. Carbamazepine absorption following a single acute toxic ingestion is unpredictable.
B. Carbamazepine levels >40 mg/L are associated with coma.
C. QTc prolongation can result from carbamazepine overdose.
D. The carbamazepine 10,11-epoxide metabolite is not pharmacologically active.
E. Multiple-dose activated charcoal can reduce the enterohepatic circulation of carbamazepine.

41.3. Which of the following statements is false with regard to valproic acid?

A. Acute valproic acid overdose is associated with delayed thrombocytopenia.
B. Fatal valproic acid overdoses are associated with metabolic acidosis.
C. The incidence of fatal valproic acid–induced hepatotoxicity is greater in adults than children.

    D. The increasing importance of valproic acid in fatal overdose is likely related to the drug's increased use in the management of patients with mood disorders.

    E. Valproic acid is a structural analogue of the neurotransmitter γ-aminobutyric acid (GABA).

41.4. Which of the following is an indication for carnitine supplementation following acute valproic acid overdose?

    A. Seizure
    B. Metabolic acidosis
    C. Hyperammonemia
    D. Serum valproic acid level greater than twice therapeutic
    E. Cardiac dysrhythmia

41.5. Compared with adults, children who overdose with carbamazepine have an increased incidence of which of the following?

    A. Ileus
    B. Hypoglycemia
    C. Electrocardiographic abnormalities
    D. Choreoathetosis
    E. Hyponatremia

41.6. Which of the following anticonvulsants has a metabolite almost as active as the parent compound?

    A. Phenytoin
    B. Carbamazepine
    C. Gabapentin
    D. Vigabatrin
    E. Lamotrigine

41.7. All these drugs decrease phenytoin levels except which of the following?

    A. Gabapentin
    B. Theophylline
    C. Rifampin
    D. Phenobarbital
    E. Carbamazepine

41.8. Which of the following anticonvulsant drugs is associated with an increased incidence of agitation in overdose?

    A. Gabapentin
    B. Lamotrigine
    C. Felbamate
    D. Vigabatrin
    E. Topiramate

41.9. Which of the following anticonvulsants is not metabolized and entirely renally excreted?

    A. Phenytoin
    B. Lamotrigine
    C. Felbamate
    D. Vigabatrin
    E. Gabapentin

41.10. Which of the following statements is correct?

    A. Nonepileptic patients commonly seize following overdose with phenytoin, carbamazepine, or valproic acid.
    B. Patients with phenytoin ingestions are at substantial risk for cardiac dysrhythmias.
    C. Tremors are an uncommon occurrence following overdose.
    D. Vigabatrin is predictably associated with the serotonin syndrome.
    E. The anticonvulsant hypersensitivity syndrome is described following phenytoin, carbamazepine, and lamotrigine therapy only.

CHAPTER 42

ANTICOAGULANTS

42.1. In evaluating a child with a known single small unintentional ingestion of a long-acting anticoagulant rodenticide, which laboratory studies would be most appropriate?

    A. Obtain a PT (or INR) at baseline and 24 and 48 hours after exposure.
    B. Obtain a PT (or INR) at 24 and 48 hours after exposure.
    C. Obtain a PTT at baseline and 24 and 48 hours after exposure.
    D. Obtain a PTT at 24 and 48 hours after exposure.
    E. Obtain a factor V level immediately.

42.2. A patient has a 500-mL bag containing 50,000 units of heparin unintentionally infused instead of a fluid bolus. One hour after the mistake is discovered his PTT is reported as greater than 150 seconds. The patient is asymptomatic, with normal vital signs. Which therapy would be the most appropriate?

    A. Infuse protamine, 500 mg IV, and repeat the PTT.
    B. Infuse protamine, 250 mg IV, and repeat the PTT.

C. Exchange transfuse the patient; no repeat PTT is needed.

D. Give 2 units of FFP IV and repeat the PTT.

E. Observe the patient for bleeding and repeat the PTT.

42.3. A 70-year-old man with a metal valve in the aortic position becomes confused and unintentionally doubles his warfarin dose. He presents to the hospital 7 days later and is found to have weakness, tachycardia, orthostatic hypotension, and melena with a fall in hemoglobin of 2 g/dL. His INR is reported by the laboratory as 20. Which therapeutic regimen would be the most appropriate?

A. Intravenous vitamin K_1 given 10 mg at a time slowly, with repeat INR in 6 hours

B. Subcutaneous vitamin K_1 50 mg with a repeat INR in 6 hours

C. FFP 2 to 3 units as soon as available followed by subcutaneous vitamin K_1, 10 mg, followed by heparin to maintain therapeutic anticoagulation when bleeding stops

D. Whole blood

E. Observation

42.4. Which of the following is not a proposed reason for the prolonged action of long-acting anticoagulants?

A. The pellet form acts to delay and prolong absorption.

B. They are highly fat soluble and concentrated in the liver.

C. They are more potent inhibitors of vitamin K than warfarin.

D. They follow zero-order kinetics at doses ingested.

E. They are enterohepatically recirculated.

42.5. Which of the following statements is false with regard to warfarin pharmacology?

A. Cimetidine can decrease warfarin metabolism by inhibiting CYP3A4.

B. Allopurinol decreases anticoagulation by enhancing warfarin metabolism.

C. Warfarin is highly protein bound to albumin such that other albumin-bound drugs can prolong coagulation times by displacing warfarin.

D. Warfarin is a racemic mixture, with R warfarin being more active than S warfarin.

E. Warfarin inhibits both vitamin K 2,3-epoxide reductase and vitamin K quinone reductase.

42.6. Low-molecular-weight heparins differ from unfractionated (conventional) heparin in all of the following ways except

A. They have greater bioavailability.

B. They have targeted activity against factor X.

C. They achieve adequate anticoagulation with fixed dosing.

D. They are not monitored by the PTT.

E. They have a lower incidence of bleeding complications.

42.7. Which of the following statements about heparin-associated thrombocytopenia is false?

A. Is mild and transient, occurring in 25% of patients during the first few days of therapy

B. Is severe and occurs in about 1 to 5% of patients between the first and second weeks of therapy

C. Is caused by antibodies to heparin–platelet factor 4 complexes

D. Is produced by bone marrow depression

E. Is associated with the white clot syndrome

42.8. Venom of the North American rattlesnakes produces a severe coagulopathy by which of the following mechanisms?

A. Thrombin-like activity in venom activates the coagulation cascade.

B. Venom constituents inhibit vitamin K–dependent coagulation factors.

C. Venom binds to antithrombin III.

D. Venom directly inhibits factor VIII.

E. Venom inactivates platelets.

42.9. All of the following are true of hirudin except

A. It was originally detected in leech saliva.

B. It irreversibly blocks thrombin without the need for antithrombin III.

C. Platelet factor 4 is a natural inhibitor of hirudin.

D. It has a very small molecular weight and can directly enter clots.

E. It has a longer half-life and enhanced bioavailability than heparin.

42.10. Which of the following therapies may not be indicated in the early management of a patient with a large intentional ingestion of long-acting anticoagulants who presents with bleeding and a high INR?

A. Intravenous FFP for immediate control

B. Oral or subcutaneous vitamin K_1 therapy

C. Whole blood if the blood loss is severe and the patient is unstable

D. Phenobarbital to enhance elimination

E. Multiple-dose activated charcoal

CHAPTER **43**

ANTITUBERCULOUS AGENTS

43.1. Which of the following statements about rapid acetylators receiving isoniazid therapy is correct?

   A. They are at greater risk for hepatotoxicity and lower or equal risk for neurologic toxicity than are slow acetylators.

   B. They are at lower risk for neurologic toxicity and hepatotoxicity than are slow acetylators.

   C. They are at the same risk for hepatoxicity and lower risk for neurologic toxicity than are slow acetylators.

   D. They are at lower risk for hepatotoxicity and greater risk for neurologic toxicity than are slow acetylators.

   E. None of the above

43.2. Which of the following statements about hepatic toxicity from isoniazid is correct?

   A. About 20% of patients will show elevations in ALT with a 5% incidence of drug-induced liver disease.

   B. Almost all patients will have an elevation in liver enzymes with about a 10% incidence of liver disease.

   C. Most patients will have a transient elevation in liver function tests with about a 1% incidence of liver disease.

   D. Approximately 10% of patients will have an elevation in AST with about 1% of these patients going on to have clinical liver disease.

   E. None of the above

43.3. Which of the following adverse reactions has been associated with isoniazid therapy?

   A. Liver disease

   B. Systemic lupus erythematosus

   C. Arthritis

   D. Peripheral neuropathy

   E. All of the above

43.4. Which of the following statements about isoniazid is correct?

   A. Isoniazid stimulates the metabolism of phenytoin.

   B. Pyridoxine-dependent decarboxylation and transamination reactions are stimulated by isoniazid.

   C. Isoniazid therapy results in an accumulation of GABA in the central nervous system.

   D. The most frequent neurologic complication of isoniazid therapy is peripheral neuritis.

   E. None of the above

43.5. At what dose in an adult is ethambutol likely to cause optic neuropathy, visual hallucinations, abdominal pain, and confusion?

   A. 2 g

   B. 4 g

   C. 6 g

   D. 8 g

   E. 10 g

43.6. Usage of which of the following antituberculosis medications will make the urine orange-red?

   A. Isoniazid

   B. Ethambutol

   C. Rifampin

   D. Ethionamide

   E. Pyrazinamide

43.7. Which of the following statements about rifampin overdoses is correct?

   A. Cardiac dysrhythmias are common.

   B. The red discoloration of the skin can be partially removed by washing with soap and water.

   C. Rifampin is primarily eliminated by renal excretion of the parent compound.

   D. The half-life in overdose is greater than 20 hours.

   E. Rifampin should be removed by charcoal hemoperfusion if the patient becomes hypotensive.

43.8. Which of the following statements about treating isoniazid toxicity is correct?

   A. Diazepam may worsen isoniazid-induced seizures.

   B. Pyridoxine should be administered as a 5 to 10% solution, infused over 3 to 6 hours.

   C. If the amount of isoniazid ingested is known, pyridoxine should be given in a gram-for-gram dose.

   D. If the amount ingested is unknown, 50 g is the usual recommended dose in adults.

   E. Pyridoxine should be given slowly because of its fat solubility.

43.9. Which of the following signs and symptoms would be expected to occur with an isoniazid overdose?

   A. Hepatic failure

   B. Cardiac dysrhythmias

C. Seizures
D. Acute renal failure
E. Respiratory acidosis

43.10. Pyridoxine would not be effective as an antidote for which of the following poisonings?

A. Isoniazid (isonicotinic acid hydrazide)
B. *Gyromitra esculenta*
C. Phenelzine
D. Monomethylhydrazine
E. None of the above

CHAPTER **44**

ANTIMALARIAL AGENTS

44.1. Which of the following statements about quinine is correct?

A. Quinine is a structural analogue of acetylsalicylic acid.
B. It is a very safe and effective therapy for muscle cramps.
C. Intramuscular quinine administration is associated with an increased incidence of tetanus.
D. It remains the standard test for detecting covert heroin use.
E. Its major toxicity following overdose is renal failure.

44.2. Which of the following therapies is currently recommended for treating a patient with a quinine overdose?

A. Hemoperfusion
B. Multiple-dose activated charcoal
C. Stellate ganglion blockade
D. Forced acid diuresis
E. Peritoneal dialysis

44.3. In vitro experiments show that quinine has certain pharmacologic effects similar to which of the following classes of drugs?

A. Sulfonylureas
B. Thiazide diuretics
C. β-Adrenergic antagonists
D. Calcium channel blockers
E. Phenothiazines

44.4. Serum levels similar to those noted in poisonings do not cause toxicity in patients who are severely ill with malaria because of an increase in which of the following?

A. Hepatic clearance
B. Renal clearance
C. α_1-Glycoprotein
D. The volume of distribution
E. The number of sickle cells

44.5. Which of the following medications can be used to treat the cardiac toxicity from the cinchona alkaloids?

A. Propranolol
B. Disopyramide
C. Procainamide
D. Sodium bicarbonate
E. Bretylium

44.6. Which of the following antimalarial agents is a dihydrofolate reductase inhibitor?

A. Chloroquine
B. Dapsone
C. Halofantrine
D. Fansidar
E. Amodiaquine

44.7. Which of the following therapies is effective in the treatment of chloroquine toxicity?

A. Atropine and sodium bicarbonate
B. Pilocarpine and diphenhydramine
C. Corticosteroids
D. Diazepam and epinephrine
E. Sodium bicarbonate and quinidine

44.8. Which cardiovascular complication has been associated with mefloquine?

A. Prolonged PR interval
B. Increased platelet adhesion
C. Calcium channel blockade
D. Prolonged QTc
E. Third-degree heart block

44.9. Which is the most significant dose-related complication of halofantrine?

A. Hypoglycemia
B. Seizure
C. Torsades de pointes
D. Myocardial failure
E. Sleep disturbance

44.10. Which manifestation has been described in children receiving artemisinins?

A. Seizures
B. Dystonia
C. Facial diplegia
D. Blindness
E. Deafness

CHAPTER **45**

ANTIMIGRAINE AGENTS

45.1. Which of the following statements about the pharmacokinetics of ergotamine is correct?

A. Ergots are well absorbed by the oral route.
B. Ergots are eliminated unmetabolized in the urine.
C. The volume of distribution of the ergot alkaloids is 0.2 L/kg
D. The elimination half-life of the ergots is greater than 24 hours.
E. Rectal bioavailability is 20 times greater than oral.

45.2. Which of the following conditions may contraindicate the use of ergotamines?

A. Gout
B. Diabetes mellitus
C. Hypertension
D. Ulcerative colitis
E. Congestive heart failure

45.3. When were the ergotamine preparations introduced for the treatment of vascular headaches?

A. 1940s
B. 1950s
C. 1960s
D. 1970s
E. 1980s

45.4. Which of the following ergotamine preparations has been used in obstetric care to stimulate contraction of the uterus?

A. Ergonovine
B. Ergotamine
C. Ergocristine
D. Dihydroergotamine
E. Ergometrine

45.5. Which of the following medications should not be used to treat ergot-induced vasoconstriction?

A. Phentolamine
B. Captopril
C. Propranolol
D. Prazosin
E. Nifedipine

45.6. Following oral administration, peak ergotamine levels will occur at

A. 1 hour
B. 2 hours
C. 3 hours
D. 4 hours
E. 6 hours

45.7. Which of the following cardiac dysrhythmias would most likely be found in a patient with an exposure to ergot?

A. Sinus tachycardia
B. Sinus bradycardia
C. Atrioventricular block
D. Premature ventricular contractions
E. Ventricular tachycardia

45.8. Which of the following ergot medications would be most likely to cause retroperitoneal fibrosis?

A. Ergotamine
B. Ergonovine
C. Bromocriptine
D. Dihydroergotamine
E. Methysergide

45.9. Ergots were discovered when they were found to be contaminating

A. Peach trees
B. Rye grain
C. Corn
D. Tomato plants
E. Potato plants

45.10. The maximum quantity of ergotamine that should be taken daily and weekly is

A. 2 mg in 1 day, 6 mg in 1 week
B. 4 mg in 1 day, 20 mg in 1 week
C. 6 mg in 1 day, 10 mg in 1 week
D. 8 mg in 1 day, 16 mg in 1 week
E. 12 mg in 1 day, 24 mg in 1 week

CHAPTER **46**

ANTIBIOTICS

46.1. After an anaphylactic (IgE-mediated) reaction to penicillin, the risk for anaphylaxis to a cephalosporin is

A. Twice the general population risk (0.04%)
B. 10 times the general population risk (1%)
C. No increased risk
D. 50 times the general population risk (10%)
E. 1000 times the population risk (20%)

46.2. Risk factors that have been identified for imipenem-induced seizures include

   A. Pregnancy
   B. Cardiovascular disease
   C. Concurrent antibiotics
   D. Renal insufficiency
   E. Hepatic insufficiency

46.3. All of the following are risk factors for the development of aminoglycoside-induced nephrotoxicity except

   A. High trough levels
   B. Large total dose
   C. Genetic predisposition
   D. Presence of a renal infection
   E. Previous aminoglycoside therapy

46.4. Chloramphenicol overdose causes the following:

   A. Gastrointestinal upset only
   B. Seizures and gastrointestinal upset only
   C. Tinnitus, seizures, and gastrointestinal upset
   D. Gastrointestinal upset, metabolic acidosis, and cardiovascular collapse
   E. Acute hepatic failure

46.5. Risk factors for the development of "gray baby syndrome" include all of the following except

   A. Elevated serum chloramphenicol concentration
   B. Age 3 to 6 months
   C. Inability to excrete chloramphenicol
   D. High doses of chloramphenicol
   E. Inability to conjugate chloramphenicol

46.6. Toxic effects after fluoroquinolone exposure include all of the following except

   A. Renal failure
   B. Seizures
   C. Acute psychosis
   D. Hepatotoxicity
   E. Gastrointestinal upset

46.7. Erythromycin is involved in many drug interactions through its ability to inhibit

   A. CYP1A2
   B. CYP2D6
   C. CYP3A4
   D. CYP2D16
   E. CYP2D18

46.8. Risk factors for the development of the vancomycin-related "red man syndrome" include all of the following except

   A. Rapid infusion rates
   B. Increased concentrations
   C. Prior exposure
   D. Use of prophylactic techniques
   E. None; all are true

46.9. All of the following are considered to have drug interactions with ketoconazole except

   A. Terfenadine
   B. Cimetidine
   C. Astemizole
   D. Cisapride
   E. Verapamil

46.10. Which antibiotics have not been reported to cause seizures in humans or animals?

   A. Penicillins
   B. Cephalosporins
   C. Fluoroquinolones
   D. Aminoglycosides
   E. None of the above

CHAPTER **47**

ANTINEOPLASTIC AGENTS

47.1. Which of the following is the mechanism responsible for methotrexate-induced renal failure?

   A. Dihydrofolate reductase inhibition
   B. Thymidylate synthetase inhibition
   C. Precipitation of polyglutamate metabolites of methotrexate
   D. Precipitation of 7-hydroxy metabolites of methotrexate
   E. Deposition of immune complexes

47.2. Methotrexate inhibition of dihydrofolate reductase activity results in which of the following toxic manifestations?

   A. Bone marrow suppression
   B. Renal failure
   C. Seizures
   D. Hepatitis
   E. Peripheral neuropathy

47.3. The extravasation of which agent is associated with an increased incidence of tissue necrosis?

   A. Doxorubicin
   B. Methotrexate
   C. Carboplatin
   D. Bleomycin
   E. Cytarabine

47.4. The administration of repeat-dose activated charcoal increases the elimination of which agent?

A. Mechlorethamine
B. Vincristine
C. Doxorubicin
D. Carboplatin
E. Methotrexate

47.5. Inappropriate secretion of antidiuretic hormone (SIADH) is a toxic manifestation of which of the following agents?

A. Methotrexate
B. Cisplatin
C. Vincristine
D. Daunorubicin
E. Mitoxantrone

47.6. Which of the following cardiac manifestations is a dose-dependent response of doxorubicin?

A. Dysrhythmias
B. Repolarization abnormalities on the ECG
C. Pericarditis
D. Myocarditis
E. Cardiomyopathy

47.7. Color disturbance and high-frequency hearing loss are the toxic effects of which agent?

A. Methotrexate
B. Cisplatin
C. Daunorubicin
D. Vincristine
E. Cyclophosphamide

47.8. Which of the following has not been shown to lower the cerebrospinal fluid (CSF) methotrexate level after an intrathecal (IT) overdose?

A. CSF drainage
B. CSF perfusion
C. Intrathecal leucovorin
D. Intrathecal carboxypeptidase G class enzymes
E. CSF exchange

47.9. Which of the following is a factor associated with an increased incidence of extravasation during IV antineoplastic agent therapy?

A. Concentration of the antineoplastic agent
B. Placement of the IV over the dorsum of the hand
C. Use of antineoplastic agents with vesicant properties.
D. Administration by an inexperienced healthcare provider
E. Rate of infusion of the solution

47.10. Which of the following antineoplastic agents has MAOI activity?

A. Doxorubicin
B. Procarbazine
C. Carboplatin
D. Vinblastine
E. Chlorambucil

CHAPTER **48**

CARDIAC GLYCOSIDES

48.1. Which of the following statements about digoxin is correct?

A. Digoxin decreases cardiac excitability.
B. Digoxin decreases automaticity.
C. Digoxin increases cardiac refractoriness.
D. Digoxin decreases cardiac conduction velocity.
E. Digoxin increases atrioventricular conduction.

48.2. Which of the following statements about digoxin-specific Fab fragments is incorrect?

A. The antibodies are produced in sheep and then are enzymatically cleaved, separating the Fab and Fc fragments.
B. Digoxin-specific Fab fragments will correct digoxin-induced hyperkalemia.
C. Digoxin Fab fragments will reverse digoxin toxicity within minutes of administration.
D. Serum digoxin levels will increase dramatically following administration of the Fab fragments.
E. Patients with renal failure who receive digoxin-specific Fab require hemodialysis for removal of the antibody–antigen complex.

48.3. A potassium serum level of greater than _____ has been associated with a high probability of death in digoxin-poisoned patients.

A. 2.0 mEq/L
B. 2.5 mEq/L
C. 4.0 mEq/L
D. 4.5 mEq/L
E. 5.5 mEq/L

48.4. One of the early symptoms of digoxin toxicity is

A. Hypertension
B. Bradycardia
C. Wide QRS complex
D. Wide QTc interval
E. Atrial fibrillation

48.5. The elevation of serum potassium levels following toxic administration of digitalis has been attributed to

A. Acidemia
B. Increased gastrointestinal absorption
C. The inhibition of uptake of potassium by muscle
D. Increased renal tubular reabsorption
E. Inhibition of chloride channels

48.6. In a comparison of digoxin and digitoxin, which of the following statements is correct?

A. Digoxin is more highly bound to plasma proteins than is digitoxin.
B. Digitoxin is cleared by renal mechanisms only.
C. Digoxin is cleared primarily by the kidney.
D. Gastrointestinal absorption of digoxin is more complete than is that of digitoxin.
E. The duration of effect of digoxin is much greater than that of digitoxin.

48.7. Which of the following plants contains a cardiac glycoside with the ability to cause a digoxin-like poisoning?

A. Jimson weed
B. Lily of the valley
C. Yew
D. Bleeding heart
E. Glory lily

48.8. A 60-kg patient with with chronic digoxin toxicity (digoxin level 3 ng/mL), second-degree heart block, and a heart rate of 45 should receive how many vials of digoxin-specific Fab?

A. 1 vial
B. 2 vials
C. 5 vials
D. 10 vials
E. 15 vials

48.9. Which of the following therapeutic interventions is considered safest in the setting of acute digoxin toxicity?

A. Calcium gluconate
B. Quinidine
C. Verapamil
D. Lidocaine
E. Cardioversion

48.10. One standard vial of Digibind (containing 38 mg) will bind to how much digoxin?

A. 0.5 mg
B. 1.2 mg
C. 1.8 mg
D. 2.4 mg
E. 3 mg

CHAPTER **49**

β-ADRENERGIC ANTAGONISTS

49.1. Propranolol is more toxic than the other beta adrenergic antagonists. Which property is most responsible for this?

A. Potassium channel blockade causing prolonged QT interval and ventricular dysrhythmias.
B. Sodium channel blockade causing ventricular dysrhythmias and seizures.
C. Intrinsic sympathomimetic activity.
D. High lipid solubility.
E. Peripheral vasodilation resulting in profound hypotension.

49.2. What is unique about sotalol overdose?

A. Sodium channel blockade causing prolonged QT interval and predisposing to torsades de pointes.
B. Sodium channel blockade causing prolonged QRS duration and predisposing to ventricular dysrhythmias.
C. Potassium channel blockade causing prolonged QT interval and predisposing to torsades de pointes.
D. Potassium channel blockade causing prolonged QRS duration and predisposing to ventricular dysrhythmias.
E. Nitric oxide release resulting in peripheral vasodilation.

49.3. What features of β-adrenergic antagonist ingestion are most closely associated with a fatal outcome?

A. Ingestions of more than 1 g.
B. Ingestions of sustained-release products.
C. Ingestion of β-adrenergic antagonists with membrane-stabilizing effect.
D. Coingestion of other cardioactive toxins.
E. Ingestion of sotalol.

49.4. Which statement concerning the role of phosphodiesterase inhibitors (PDIs) in the management of β-adrenergic antagonist overdose is true?

A. PDIs typically increase the blood pressure without improving cardiac output.

B. PDIs have been shown in animal models to act in synergy with glucagon.

C. PDIs typically increase cardiac output without increasing blood pressure.

D. There is no evidence that PDIs are of benefit in β-adrenergic antagonist toxicity.

E. PDIs are easy to titrate because of a short half-life.

49.5. A 28-year-old previously healthy woman has taken 4 g of propranolol in a suicide attempt. Despite therapy with maximal doses of glucagon, high-dose insulin, epinephrine, isoproterenol, and milrinone, she remains profoundly hypotensive and bradycardic. Which of the following therapies is most indicated?

A. Hemodialysis.

B. Hemoperfusion.

C. High-dose calcium and atropine.

D. Ventricular pacing.

E. Intraaortic balloon pump.

49.6. A patient being treated for sotalol overdose suddenly develops ventricular tachycardia. Which management step is least likely to be effective?

A. Hypertonic sodium bicarbonate

B. Correction of hypomagnesemia

C. Overdrive pacing

D. Lidocaine

E. Cardioversion

49.7. Which of the following statements concerning the use of vasopressors in β-adrenergic antagonist toxicity is false?

A. Glucagon infusions may cause vomiting.

B. Epinephrine may cause hypertension.

C. Isoproterenol infusions may cause hypotension.

D. Norepinephrine may cause pulmonary edema.

E. Amrinone may cause hypertension.

49.8. Asymptomatic patients who have ingested a β-adrenergic antagonist require a period of observation. Which of the following minimum observation periods is true?

A. 4 hours for an atenolol overdose.

B. 6 hours for a propranolol overdose.

C. 9 hours for a sotalol overdose.

D. 12 hours for a sustained release metoprolol overdose.

E. 6 hours for an overdose of propranolol and diphenhydramine.

49.9. What agent, taken in overdose, is most likely to cause the following clinical scenario? The patient is conscious with the following vital signs: pulse 60/min and systolic blood pressure 60 mm Hg. Serum glucose is 300 mg/dL. The electrocardiogram shows a sinus rhythm with narrow complexes.

A. Propranolol

B. Digoxin

C. Diltiazem

D. Amitriptyline

E. Heroin

49.10. What agent, taken in overdose is most likely to cause the following clinical scenario? The patient is unconscious following a seizure and has the following vital signs: pulse 40/min; blood pressure 80/50 mm Hg; and respirations 12/min. Serum potassium is 5 mEq/L, and serum glucose is 60 mg/dL. The electrocardiogram shows sinus bradycardia with a QRS interval duration of 130 milliseconds.

A. Propranolol

B. Digoxin

C. Diltiazem

D. Amitriptyline

E. Heroin

CHAPTER **50**

CALCIUM CHANNEL BLOCKERS

50.1. In therapeutic dosing, which of the following channels do calcium channel blockers antagonize?

A. Voltage-sensitive L-type channels

B. Voltage-sensitive T-type channels

C. Receptor-activated S-type channels

D. Receptor-activated T-type channels

E. Naloxone-sensitive calcium channels

50.2. Which of the following proteins is involved in excitation/contraction coupling within the cardiac muscle cell?

A. Tropomyosin

B. Actin

C. Calmodulin

D. Myosin light-chain kinase

E. Myoglobin

50.3. Which of the following calcium channel blockers has the least affinity for myocardial tissue?

A. Verapamil
B. Diltiazem
C. Nifedipine
D. Bepridil
E. All have equal affinity for the myocardium

50.4. Following a calcium channel blocker overdose, which of the following findings is the patient unlikely to manifest?

A. Idioventricular junctional escape rhythm
B. Hypotension
C. Hyperglycemia
D. Acute lung injury
E. Seizures

50.5. A 50-year-old man presents 6 hours after ingesting 20 sustained release verapamil tablets. He is asymptomatic, and his physical examination is notable for a heart rate of 70 and a blood pressure of 130/85 mm Hg. Which of the following strategies for gastrointestinal decontamination is the most appropriate?

A. Emesis induced by syrup of ipecac, multiple-dose activated charcoal
B. Multiple-dose activated charcoal, whole-bowel irrigation
C. Orogastric lavage, whole-bowel irrigation
D. Multiple-dose activated charcoal alone
E. Orogastric lavage, single-dose activated charcoal

50.6. Which of the following therapeutic agents is correctly paired with its mechanism of action?

A. Calcium—enhances release of catecholamines
B. Glucagon—direct-acting β-adrenergic agonist
C. Dopamine—direct-acting β-adrenergic agonist
D. Amrinone—inhibits phosphodiesterase III
E. 4-Aminopyridine—causes release of insulin

50.7. Insulin is a current therapy for patients with calcium channel blocker poisoning. Which of the following is true of insulin therapy?

A. Insulin works by increasing central autonomic outflow.
B. Insulin therapy for calcium channel blocker poisoning should never be administered intravenously because of the risk of hypoglycemia.
C. Insulin should always be administered concomitantly with a norepinephrine infusion.
D. It is administered as a bolus of 0.1 U/kg of insulin and 25 to 50 g of dextrose followed by an infusion of 0.2 to 0.3 U/h of insulin and 0.5 g/kg/h of dextrose.

E. It is administered at the same dose as for patients with diabetic ketoacidosis.

50.8. Which of these descriptions of salvage therapy following pharmacotherapeutic failure is correct?

A. External pacemakers are almost always effective at capturing the myocardium.
B. Although internal pacemakers do not improve inotropy, they may be beneficial by raising the heart rate.
C. Intraaortic balloon pump therapy is a poor choice because of the potential need for its long-term use.
D. Hyperbaric oxygen therapy improves inotropy by raising the patient's oxygen carrying capacity.
E. Extracorporeal membrane oxygenation has produced excellent results in calcium channel blocker–poisoned patients.

50.9. A patient presents to the emergency department with profound hypotension and bradycardia following the overdose of his antihypertensive medications. By which of the following findings can calcium channel blocker or β-adrenergic antagonist overdose be differentiated?

A. Calcium channel blocker–poisoned patients are typically more profoundly bradycardic.
B. A high serum glucose is a reliable marker for calcium channel blocker poisoning.
C. A normal mental status in this patient would suggest calcium channel blocker poisoning.
D. Calcium channel blocker–poisoned patients should have an elevated serum calcium.
E. The electrocardiogram findings are completely different.

50.10. Which of the following dispositions is most appropriate for a 2-year-old child who ingested one or two diltiazem tablets 2 hours before assessment? The patient is asymptomatic and has a normal physical examination.

A. Close monitoring in the emergency department for 4 to 6 hours, and if the child remains clinically stable, discharge home with parents
B. Admission to the intensive care unit for continuous cardiac monitoring for 24 hours
C. Home management with close poison center contact
D. Admission to the pediatric ward for 24-hour observation
E. None of the above

CHAPTER **51**

MISCELLANEOUS ANTIHYPERTENSIVES

51.1. Angioedema is commonly associated with which of the following antihypertensive agents?

A. Clonidine
B. Hydralazine
C. Captopril
D. Reserpine
E. Bepredil

51.2. Naloxone may be an effective therapy for the reversal of clonidine poisoning. In which other antihypertensive agent poisoning may naloxone also be effective?

A. Prazosin
B. Angiotensin-converting enzyme inhibitors
C. Reserpine
D. Minoxidil
E. Verapamil

51.3. Clonidine exerts its hypotensive effect by acting as which of the following?

A. Central α_1 agonist
B. Central α_2 agonist
C. Central α_1 antagonist
D. Central α_2 antagonist
E. Peripheral α_1 agonist

51.4. Which of the following clinical findings is not expected in a patient with a large clonidine overdose?

A. Hypertension
B. Hypotension
C. Hypothermia
D. Miosis
E. Dysrhythmia

51.5. Which of the following agents is not considered, by physiologic effect, as being a sympatholytic agent?

A. Guanabenz
B. Terazosin
C. Guanethidine
D. Diazoxide
E. Trimethaphan

51.6. Concerning clonidine, which is theoretically correct?

A. Clonidine is a benzodiazepine.
B. Clonidine is metabolized primarily by the liver.
C. Yohimbine should be given to patients with clonidine overdose.
D. Clonidine is activated by demethylation to dopamine by monoamine oxidase.
E. Abrupt cessation of clonidine is associated with seizures.

51.7. A 56-year-old woman with a history of hypertension has just recovered from an episode of angioedema after beginning captopril for her hypertension. All of the following antihypertensive agents would be acceptable alternative medications except for which agent?

A. Atenolol
B. Fosinopril
C. Losartan
D. Diltiazem
E. All are acceptable

51.8. The mechanism of action of losartan is which of the following?

A. Peripheral α_1 antagonist
B. Angiotensin-converting enzyme inhibitor
C. Angiotensin II receptor antagonist
D. Direct vasodilator
E. Potassium-sparing diuretic

51.9. Which of the following antihypertensive agents and a potential adverse effect is incorrectly paired?

A. Diazoxide—hypoglycemia
B. Reserpine—depression
C. Hydralazine—lupuslike syndrome
D. Sodium nitroprusside—cyanide toxicity
E. Methyldopa—hemolytic anemia

51.10. Angioedema secondary to angiotensin-converting enzyme inhibitor use occurs after which of the following?

A. 1 to 2 days
B. 2 to 2 weeks
C. 1 to 2 months
D. 1 to 2 years
E. None of the above

CHAPTER **52**

ANTIDYSRHYTHMIC AGENTS

52.1. Conduction disturbances associated with flecainide, quinidine, and procainamide toxicity have been successfully treated with

A. Tocainide
B. Magnesium sulfate

C. Dobutamine
D. Sodium bicarbonate
E. Lidocaine

52.2. In the animal model of severe lidocaine toxicity, which therapeutic intervention has resulted in survival?

A. Cardiopulmonary resuscitation with or without mechanical chest compression
B. Charcoal hemoperfusion
C. Administration of magnesium sulfate followed by sodium bicarbonate
D. Administration of amiodarone
E. External pacing

52.3. Lidocaine is an aminoacyl amide that is a synthetic derivative of which of the following topical anesthetics?

A. Benzocaine
B. Cocaine
C. Tetracaine
D. Procaine
E. Dibucaine

52.4. If a patient with congestive heart failure (CHF) requires lidocaine for ventricular dysrhythmias, the pharmacokinetics will differ from a patient without CHF in what way?

A. CHF will decrease the hepatic clearance.
B. CHF will decrease the renal clearance.
C. CHF will increase the volume of distribution.
D. CHF will decrease the protein binding.
E. CHF will increase the fraction of ionized drug.

52.5. Which of the following statements about *N*-acetyl-procainamide (NAPA) is correct?

A. NAPA is a prodrug of procainamide.
B. NAPA plasma concentrations are not clinically relevant.
C. NAPA and procainamide can be removed by hemodialysis.
D. NAPA toxicity should be considered in patients who have a prolonged PR interval.
E. NAPA differs from procainamide because it does not cause drug-induced lupus erythematosus.

52.6. Which of the following is inconsistent with a diagnosis of quinidine overdose?

A. Torsades de pointes
B. Tachycardia
C. Hyperkalemia
D. Hypotension
E. Acute lung injury

52.7. If a patient with a tocainide overdose is alkalinized with intravenous sodium bicarbonate to a pH of 7.50, what alteration in pharmacokinetics can occur?

A. Increased clearance
B. Decreased clearance
C. Increased protein binding
D. Decreased protein binding
E. Increased volume of distribution

52.8. The primary difference between tocainide and lidocaine is that

A. Tocainide is highly protein bound.
B. Tocainide is ineffective for treating atrial dysrhythmias.
C. Tocainide's half-life is much shorter than that of lidocaine.
D. Tocainide is absorbed following oral administration.
E. Tocainide does not undergo extensive first-pass metabolism.

52.9. Marked QRS and PR interval changes associated with minimal QTc prolongation are noted with toxicity of which antidysrhythmic drug?

A. Quinidine
B. Procainamide
C. Flecainide
D. Lidocaine
E. Tocainide

52.10. Which of the following antidysrhythmics is a class IC analogue of lysergic acid with 5 to 10 times the antidysrhythmic potency of procainamide? The drug has been demonstrated to induce dysrhythmias and result in sudden cardiac death.

A. Propafenone
B. Bretylium
C. Encainide
D. Tocainide
E. Mexiletine

CHAPTER **53**

INHALATIONAL ANESTHETICS

53.1. Which clinical finding is not secondary to a direct toxic effect of nitrous oxide?

A. Megaloblastic anemia
B. Subacute combined degeneration of the spinal cord

C. Irreversible brain damage

D. Increased risk for spontaneous abortion

E. Reduced fertility

53.2. Which statement regarding abuse of halogenated volatile anesthetics is true?

A. Ingestion is associated with gastrointestinal symptoms but without hemodynamic or CNS findings because these agents are not well absorbed via the enteral route.

B. Hospital personnel have been involved in most reported cases.

C. Topical application to mucous membranes has not been associated with toxicity.

D. The acrid smell of halothane aids in making the diagnosis.

E. Tonic-clonic seizures usually occur.

53.3. Which of the following are risk factors for life-threatening hepatitis following halothane exposure?

A. Multiple exposures

B. Thin body habitus

C. Male gender

D. White race

E. Coadministration with other inhalational agents

53.4. Which of the following inhalational anesthetics is most associated with diabetes insipidus?

A. Halothane

B. Isoflurane

C. Methoxyflurane

D. Enflurane

E. Diethyl ether

53.5. Intraoperative carbon monoxide poisoning as a complication of closed-circuit anesthesia is most likely to occur when?

A. At the end of a long day of cases

B. At the end of a long week of cases

C. In the middle of the day

D. On the first case after a weekend

E. When soda lime is used instead of baralyme

CHAPTER **54**

NEUROMUSCULAR BLOCKING AGENTS

54.1. You are called to evaluate a patient with chronic renal failure who has persistent respiratory failure and quadriparesis 1 hour following a general anes-

thetic. Anesthesia was induced with O_2, N_2O, thiopental, fentanyl, and succinylcholine and maintained for the 4-hour procedure with O_2, N_2O, isoflurane, fentanyl, and rapacuronium infusion. Which of the following is the most likely cause of weakness?

A. Critical illness polyneuropathy

B. Rapacuronium metabolite

C. Acute necrotizing myopathy

D. Homozygous atypical plasma cholinesterase

E. Previously undiagnosed hepatic insufficiency

54.2. Which of the following is true with regard to critical illness polyneuropathy?

A. It is caused by residual nondepolarizing neuromuscular block.

B. It is associated with long-term nondepolarizing neuromuscular block.

C. It is associated with multiple organ failure.

D. It is caused by long-term glucocorticoid use.

E. It is irreversible.

54.3. Which of the following is correct with regard to succinylcholine?

A. It is appropriate for use in the emergency difficult pediatric airway.

B. It is eliminated primarily by the kidney.

C. It should not be used on the day of an acute spinal cord injury.

D. Neuromuscular block is augmented by pretreatment with a nondepolarizing neuromuscular blocker.

E. It can cause succinic acid intoxication.

54.4. Which of the following statements is correct?

A. Pancuronium causes tachycardia by blocking parasympathetic ganglia.

B. Chronic phenytoin therapy does not affect pancuronium metabolism.

C. Renal failure does not affect the duration of tubocurarine.

D. Chronic phenytoin therapy does not affect mivacurium metabolism.

E. When the ratio of the fourth to the first twitch on a supramaximal train of four electrical nerve stimuli is >0.7, the neuromuscular blocker effect is reversed enough so that a patient will not experience weakness.

54.5. Which of the following statements is correct with regard to general anesthesia?

A. The pupillary light reflex is unaffected while under general anesthesia, even when neuromuscular blockers are used.

B. Benzodiazepines before anesthesia decrease explicit recall following anesthesia.

C. The atracurium metabolite laudanosine can cause seizures in otherwise normal adults.

D. Pancuronium enhances morphine analgesia.

E. The incidence of awareness is increased when neuromuscular blockers are used.

54.6. Which of the following statements is correct with regard to malignant hyperthermia (MH) in adults?

A. Hyperpyrexia is an early sign of MH.

B. MH can be triggered by some nondepolarizing neuromuscular blockers.

C. Hyperkalemia and cardiac arrest can occur shortly after the onset of MH.

D. Like hyperthyroidism, MH is treated with β-adrenergic antagonists.

E. Tachycardia should be treated with IV calcium channel blockers.

54.7. Which of the following statements is correct with regard to succinylcholine-induced severe hyperkalemia?

A. It occurs in patients with renal failure.

B. It can occur following acute hemorrhagic shock.

C. It is prevented by pretreatment with a small dose of a nondepolarizing neuromuscular blocker.

D. It is prevented by pretreatment with a small dose of a depolarizing neuromuscular blocker.

E. It is caused by proliferation of presynaptic ACh receptors.

54.8. Pancuronium is the only commonly used NMB with which of the following characteristics?

A. It decreases heart rate and decreases arterial blood pressure.

B. It decreases heart rate and increases arterial blood pressure.

C. It increases heart rate and decreases arterial blood pressure.

D. It increases heart rate and increases arterial blood pressure.

E. It causes significant dose-dependent histamine release.

54.9. Sensitivity to pancuronium neuromuscular block is enhanced by which of the following?

A. Chronic phenytoin therapy

B. Long-term pancuronium therapy in a critically ill patient

C. Myasthenia gravis

D. Acute sepsis

E. Prior administration of neostigmine

54.10. Under which circumstance is the duration of succinylcholine effect more than doubled?

A. In hepatic insufficiency

B. Following chronic echothiophate eye drops

C. After systemic thermal burn injury

D. Following 2 units of fresh frozen plasma IV

E. When the dibucaine number is >70%

CHAPTER **55**

LOCAL ANESTHETICS

55.1. Which of the following statements regarding lidocaine toxicity is not correct?

A. Patients may develop seizures secondary to block of the cerebral inhibitory pathways.

B. Patients may develop coma secondary to block of cerebral excitatory pathways.

C. When lidocaine is used for nerve blocks, life-threatening toxicity does not occur.

D. Hypoxia and respiratory and metabolic acidosis all can increase the CNS and cardiovascular toxicity of lidocaine.

E. Toxic effects usually correlate with plasma concentrations.

55.2. Which of the following statements about the pharmacokinetics of local anesthetics is correct?

A. Only the ionized form can penetrate the nervous system.

B. The speed of onset is determined by the drug's pK_a.

C. The dose administered does not influence the time to onset of block.

D. Agents with greater protein binding have a shorter duration of effect.

E. Most of the local anesthetics are strong acids.

55.3. Which of the following is not a proposed mechanism of toxicity of the local anesthetic agents?

A. Uncoupling of oxidative phosphorylation

B. Sodium channel blockade

C. GABA antagonism

D. NMDA agonism

E. Altered sarcoplasmic release of calcium ions

55.4. Which of the following statements about local anesthetic allergies is correct?

A. Patients allergic to an amide agent could generally safely receive a preservative-free preparation of the same drug.
B. Allergy to local anesthetics is very common.
C. Most true local anesthetic allergies are to the amide agents.
D. Patients allergic to amide agents should never receive ester agents.
E. Patients allergic to one ester agent could safely receive a different ester agent.

55.5. Which of the following local anesthetics is an ester?

A. Cocaine
B. Mepivacaine
C. Bupivacaine
D. Lidocaine
E. Ropivacaine

55.6. Which of the following local anesthetic agents most frequently causes methemoglobinemia?

A. Lidocaine
B. Benzocaine
C. Cocaine
D. Prilocaine
E. Procaine

55.7. Following an inadvertent bolus of an excessive amount of lidocaine, which of the following should be expected to occur first?

A. Headache
B. Paralysis
C. Vomiting
D. Seizure
E. Asystole

55.8. A patient in the ICU on a lidocaine infusion for ventricular dysrhythmias is suspected of developing early lidocaine toxicity. What clinical findings did the healthcare provider likely notice to suggest this syndrome?

A. A plasma lidocaine level of 4 μg/mL
B. Hepatitis
C. Worsening ventricular tachycardia
D. Coma
E. Tremor

55.9. Which of the following statements regarding the treatment of local anesthetic poisoning is true?

A. The initial treatment for lidocaine toxicity is cardiopulmonary resuscitation.
B. The initial therapy for bupivacaine cardiotoxicity is lidocaine.

C. Regardless of the treatment adminstered, lidocaine poisoning is almost always fatal.
D. Hemodialysis, once the patient is stabilized, is highly efficacious in removing most local anesthetic agents.
E. The performance of CPR is not important in patients with bupivacaine poisoning.

55.10. Which of the following statements regarding lidocaine is correct?

A. Lidocaine is nontoxic orally because of poor bioavailability.
B. The metabolites of lidocaine, MEGX and GX, are pharmacologically inactive.
C. If lidocaine and prilocaine are combined, the lidocaine becomes able to penetrate skin.
D. Lidocaine is administered in doses up to 55 mg/kg during tumescent anesthesia.
E. Lidocaine routinely crossreacts with the cocaine drug-of-abuse assay.

CHAPTER **56**

PHARMACEUTIC ADDITIVES

56.1. Propylene glycol is metabolized hepatically by alcohol dehydrogenase to

A. Polyethylene glycol
B. Ethylene glycol
C. Lactate
D. Methanol
E. Oxalate

56.2. Polyethylene glycol 200 (PEG 200) has been associated with what organ toxicity?

A. Renal tubular necrosis
B. Acute pancreatitis
C. Central lobular hepatic necrosis
D. Cardiac myopathy
E. Pneumoconiosis

56.3. The "gasping" syndrome described in neonates is believed to result from

A. A decreased ability to metabolize benzyl alcohol
B. A decreased ability to metabolize benzoic acid
C. A glucose-6-phosphate dehydrogenase (G-6-PD) deficiency
D. Sterile water for injection
E. Methanol

56.4. Chlorobutanol has a chemical structure similar to that of

A. Trichloroethanol
B. Perchloroethylene
C. Vinyl chloride
D. Trifluoroperazine
E. Polyvinyl chloride

56.5. Thimerosal is a(n) _____ mercury compound widely employed as a pharmaceutical preservative.

A. Elemental
B. Organic
C. Inorganic
D. Pentavalent
E. Trivalent

56.6. Benzalkonium chloride is the most widely used _____ preservative in the United States.

A. Parenteral
B. Topical
C. Otic
D. Ophthalmic
E. Oral

56.7. The pharmaceutical additive(s) found most often in medications (except water) is/are

A. Glycerin
B. Thimerosal
C. Benzalkonium chloride
D. Phenol
E. Parabens

56.8. Acute renal failure from adulterated acetaminophen has been associated with which pharmaceutical additive?

A. Diethylene glycol
B. Polyethylene glycol
C. Benzyl alcohol
D. Propylene glycol
E. Sorbitol

56.9. Thrombocytopenia, hepatomegaly, renal dysfunction, and distal tubular crystal deposition were all manifested with what medication?

A. Sulfanilamide
B. Bacteriostatic water
C. Adulterated acetaminophen
D. E-Ferol
E. Thimerosal-containing vaccinations

56.10. Which hereditary syndrome predisposes patients to adverse effects from sorbitol?

A. Bruton disease
B. Turner syndrome
C. Tay-Sachs disease
D. Hurler syndrome
E. Hereditary fructose intolerance

CHAPTER **57**

CYCLIC ANTIDEPRESSANTS

57.1. Which of the following therapeutic interventions is the most effective in narrowing the QRS complex in patients with cyclic antidepressant toxicity?

A. Acetazolamide
B. Intravenous hypertonic saline
C. Intravenous hypertonic sodium bicarbonate
D. Hyperventilation
E. Intravenous lidocaine

57.2. Following a tricyclic antidepressant overdose, how soon after arrival in the emergency department will seizures, hypotension, or cardiac dysrhythmias occur?

A. 1 hour
B. 2 hours
C. 4 hours
D. 6 hours
E. 8 hours

57.3. Amoxapine differs from the other cyclic antidepressants in that it causes a higher incidence of which of the following in overdose?

A. Sinus tachycardia
B. Ventricular tachycardia
C. Respiratory depression
D. Seizures
E. Coma

57.4. Which of the following cyclic antidepressants causes a dose-related increase in systolic blood pressure?

A. Bupropion
B. Maprotiline
C. Trazodone
D. Venlafaxine
E. Amoxapine

57.5. Which of the following statements about the pharmacokinetics of the cyclic antidepressants is correct?

A. The volume of distribution is 2 to 5 L/kg.

B. The cyclic antidepressants are 60% protein bound.
C. They do not partition well into fat.
D. A very small percentage of the ingested dose is excreted unchanged in the urine.
E. The cyclic antidepressants bind to albumin.

57.6. Which of the following cyclic antidepressants is the most potent inhibitor of dopamine reuptake?

A. Amoxapine
B. Venlafaxine
C. Doxepin
D. Imipramine
E. Desipramine

57.7. Which of the following cyclic antidepressants does not inhibit the reuptake of either serotonin or norepinephrine?

A. Amitriptyline
B. Desipramine
C. Nortriptyline
D. Doxepin
E. Bupropion

57.8. Which of the following ECG changes is believed to be highly predictive of seizures and dysrhythmias in patients with first-generation tricyclic antidepressant toxicity?

A. Right bundle branch block
B. Prolonged PR interval
C. Decreased conduction velocity
D. A QRS complex >100 milliseconds
E. An S wave in leads I and aVL

57.9. Which of the following cyclic antidepressants has the most anticholinergic activity?

A. Amitriptyline
B. Doxepin
C. Fluoxetine
D. Maprotiline
E. Amoxapine

57.10. Which of the following antidysrhythmics can be safely used in patients with cyclic antidepressant toxicity?

A. Quinidine
B. Bretylium
C. Propranolol
D. Disopyramide
E. Lidocaine

CHAPTER 58

SEROTONIN REUPTAKE INHIBITORS AND ATYPICAL ANTIDEPRESSANTS

58.1. Which of the following is not a SSRI?

A. Paroxetine
B. Sertraline
C. Citalopram
D. Venlafaxine
E. Fluoxetine

58.2. Which finding on physical examination is seen more commonly in serotonin syndrome than in neuroleptic malignant syndrome?

A. Fever
B. Altered mental status
C. Hyperreflexia
D. Autonomic instability
E. Mydriasis

58.3. Serotonin syndrome involves overstimulation of which serotonin receptor?

A. 5-HT_1
B. 5-HT_2
C. 5-HT_3
D. 5-HT_4
E. 5-HT_5

58.4. SSRIs have been used to treat which of the following disorders?

A. Obesity
B. Attention deficit disorder
C. Dysrhythmias
D. Seizures
E. Hypersalivation

58.5. Which antidepressant does not inhibit the reuptake of serotonin?

A. Fluoxetine
B. Venlafaxine
C. Citalopram
D. Nefazodone
E. Mirtazapine

58.6. Which of the following effects has not been reported after an isolated overdose of SSRIs?

A. Seizures
B. Tachycardia
C. Mental status depression
D. Hyperthermia
E. Nausea and vomiting

58.7. Which therapy is not a treatment for serotonin syndrome?

   A. Antipyretics
   B. Active cooling
   C. Benzodiazepines
   D. Cyproheptadine
   E. Supportive care

58.8. SSRIs cause drug interactions by inhibiting which cytochrome P450 isoenzyme system?

   A. CYP2E1
   B. CYP2D6
   C. CYP1A2
   D. CYP3A4
   E. CYP2A10

58.9. Which of the following are requirements of the serotonin syndrome?

   A. Two dopaminergic drugs must be administered.
   B. Two serotonergic drugs must be administered.
   C. A serotonergic and a dopaminergic drug must be administered.
   D. A single serotonergic drug is administered.
   E. A single dopaminergic drug is administered.

58.10. The SSRI that is reported to cause seizures and dysrhythmias after overdose is

   A. Fluoxetine
   B. Sertraline
   C. Citalopram
   D. Nefazodone
   E. Mirtazapine

CHAPTER 59

ANTIPSYCHOTICS

59.1. A patient receiving chlorpromazine who is started on cimetidine may require a higher dose of chlorpromazine because

   A. Cimetidine increases the renal clearance of chlorpromazine.
   B. Chlorpromazine absorption is pH dependent.
   C. Chlorpromazine has substantial first-pass metabolism.
   D. Cimetidine increases the hepatic clearance of chlorpromazine.
   E. Cimetidine increases the distributive volume of chlorpromazine.

59.2. Optimum antipsychotic effects of the phenothiazines will not occur until the patient has received the medication for approximately

   A. 1 week
   B. 2 weeks
   C. 1 month
   D. 2 months
   E. 6 months

59.3. If a patient receiving thioxanthene or loxapine develops hyperthermia, muscle rigidity, autonomic dysfunction, and an altered level of consciousness, the patient is most likely experiencing

   A. An allergic reaction
   B. Tardive dyskinesia
   C. Drug toxicity from an excessive dose
   D. Neuroleptic malignant syndrome (NMS)
   E. An extrapyramidal reaction

59.4. If neuroleptic malignant syndrome (NMS) occurs, it is recommended to discontinue the antipsychotic, but if an antipsychotic is necessary, what should be done?

   A. If NMS occurs, no additional neuroleptics should be given.
   B. Treat with bromocriptine or dantrolene and restart therapy with the same neuroleptic.
   C. Discontinue the neuroleptic for 2 weeks and restart on another neuroleptic from a different class.
   D. Add benztropine to prevent the development of NMS.
   E. Add a benzodiazepine to prevent the development of NMS.

59.5. What is the most common extrapyramidal effect of antipsychotic therapy?

   A. Parkinsonism
   B. Dystonia
   C. Akathisia
   D. Tardive dyskinesia
   E. Malignant hyperthermia

59.6. What is the most serious central nervous system toxic effect of antipsychotic therapy?

   A. Parkinsonism
   B. Seizure disorders
   C. Akathisia
   D. Tardive dyskinesia
   E. Akinesia

59.7. Which treatment has been shown to be beneficial in tardive dyskinesia?

A. Cholinergic stimulation
B. Anticholinergics
C. Cyclobenzaprine
D. Clozapine
E. Lithium carbonate

59.8. Antipsychotics, when taken alone, are usually quite safe even when taken in significant overdose. The antipsychotic most frequently associated with causing death when taken as an overdose is

A. Haloperidol
B. Thioridazine
C. Chlorpromazine
D. Loxapine
E. Prochlorperazine

59.9. Which of the following dysrhythmias most commonly occurs in a patient with a mesoridazine overdose?

A. Bradycardia
B. Torsades de pointes
C. Increased QT and QRS intervals
D. Decreased PR interval
E. Atrial fibrillation

59.10. Phenothiazine metabolites are lipophilic and have large volumes of distribution. A qualitative analysis for phenothiazines in the urine from a patient who has taken a phenothiazine may remain positive for

A. 24 hours
B. 48 hours
C. 7 to 10 days
D. 21 days
E. Greater than 1 month

CHAPTER 60

MONOAMINE OXIDASE INHIBITORS

60.1. Which of the following is true regarding the MAO isozymes?

A. MAO-A is found only in the gastrointestinal tract.
B. The preferred substrate for MAO-A is serotonin.
C. MAO-B inhibition is responsible for tyramine sensitivity.
D. Selegiline is a selective MAO-A inhibitor.
E. All currently available MAO-A inhibitors are reversible, whereas the currently available MAO-B inhibitors are irreversible.

60.2. Severe hypertension in a MAO inhibitor–poisoned patient is best treated with the use of which of the following?

A. β-Adrenergic antagonists
B. α-Adrenergic antagonists
C. Calcium channel blockers
D. Labetalol
E. Nitroprusside

60.3. Monoamine oxidase metabolizes all of the following agents except for which one?

A. Dietary monoamines
B. Norepinephrine
C. Adenosine
D. Serotonin
E. Epinephrine

60.4. MAOI use results in which of the following?

A. Expanded storage pool of norepinephrine
B. Decreased urinary excretion of catecholamine
C. Decreased production of catecholamine
D. Increased production of 5-hydroxytryptamine
E. Increased secretion of catechols from the adrenal medulla

60.5. MAOI overdose may be best characterized by which of the following?

A. Delayed onset of symptoms
B. Hypothermia
C. Pinpoint pupils
D. Anticholinergic syndrome
E. Respiratory depression

60.6. Which of these drugs can safely be used with MAOIs without risking drug interactions?

A. Ephedrine
B. Phenylpropanolamine
C. Norepinephrine
D. Cocaine
E. Amphetamine

60.7. Tyramine may precipitate a hypertensive crisis in patients on MAOIs by which mechanism?

A. Inhibiting the metabolism of endogenous catecholamines
B. Direct binding to postsynaptic α receptors
C. Blockade of β-adrenergic receptors producing unopposed α-adrenergic effects
D. Release of stored norepinephrine
E. Blocks catechol-O-methyltransferase

60.8. Which drug may be given to a patient taking MAOIs without a potential interaction?

A. Albuterol
B. Meperidine
C. Fluoxetine
D. Barbiturates
E. Sulfonylureas

60.9. The serotonin syndrome can be avoided when using MAOIs in combination with which of the following agents?

A. Dextromethorphan
B. Imipramine
C. Clomipramine
D. Meperidine
E. Morphine

60.10. The newer MAOIs such as moclobemide are thought to be safer because of which of the following characteristics?

A. Reversible
B. Irreversible
C. MAO-A isoenzyme selective
D. MAO-B isoenzyme selective
E. Covalently bound to MAO

CHAPTER **61**

LITHIUM

61.1. In a patient with normal renal function, which is the least effective treatment for acute lithium poisoning?

A. Continuous arteriovenous hemofiltration (CAVH)
B. Hemodialysis
C. Peritoneal dialysis
D. Maximizing GFR
E. Continuous arterioarterial hemofiltration (CAAH)

61.2. Which of following concerning extracorporeal removal of lithium is not true?

A. The small size aids in its ability to be removed via hemodialysis.
B. Its small volume of distribution is similar to that of total body water at 0.6 to 0.9 L/kg.
C. Hemodialysis is a better modality than hemoperfusion for lithium removal because lithium does not bind well to charcoal.
D. It is well bound to proteins, especially albumin.
E. Its clearance via hemodialysis is mainly dependent on blood flow.

61.3. Which of the following is false?

A. Malignant cardiac disturbances are common in lithium toxicity.
B. Patients with lithium poisoning and mental status changes should undergo peritoneal dialysis immediately.
C. Patients with renal failure and lithium toxicity should be managed with aggressive decontamination and hemodialysis.
D. Cardiac changes such as ST and T wave changes may be noted in lithium toxicity and need not be treated aggressively.
E. Lithium is not bound to activated charcoal well.

61.4. All of the following statements regarding lithium clearance are true except

A. Patients who undergo hemodialysis will frequently develop a "rebound" and need to be redialyzed.
B. Hemodialysis effectively lowers both the serum and the central nervous system lithium concentration.
C. When trying to determine an accurate tissue level of lithium, the best time to check is 1 hour after dialysis.
D. An asymptomatic patient with a lithium level of 5.0 mEq/L should undergo dialysis.
E. A patient with chronic lithium poisoning and altered mental status should undergo hemodialysis.

61.5. The following pharmacokinetic statements regarding lithium are all true except

A. The volume of distribution is similar to total body water.
B. The vast majority is excreted by the kidneys.
C. Dehydration may lead to increase toxicity.
D. Lithium readily crosses cellular membranes of the kidney, liver, and CNS, leading to rapid onset of effects.
E. Lithium is rapidly absorbed and has a rapid peak serum level.

61.6. Which of the following statements regarding CAVH or CAAH is false?

A. They may be alternatives to hemodialysis in patients with lithium toxicity.
B. Their clearance per hour is less than that of hemodialysis.
C. Unlike hemodialysis, they do not demonstrate a "rebound" in lithium concentration.

D. They have the benefit of not requiring specialized personnel to perform.

E. They are better at preventing permanent neurologic deficits than hemodialysis.

61.7. Which of the following statements concerning decontamination and treatment of the acutely poisoned lithium patient is false?

A. Numerous studies in humans have shown sodium polystyrene sulfonate (SPS) to be beneficial in clearing lithium from the body.

B. Repeat doses of activated charcoal play no role in decontamination of patients poisoned with lithium.

C. Elimination of lithium can be increased by ensuring good GFR with a sodium-containing electrolyte solution.

D. Lithium is handled by the kidney in a manner similar to sodium.

E. Lithium's small size makes it amenable to hemodialysis.

61.8. All the following regarding lithium and its interactions are true except

A. Lithium shares the same valence as sodium and potassium.

B. It has an ionic radius that is similar to that of manganese.

C. Some of lithium's actions may involve the inhibition of inositol monophosphate.

D. cAMP function via norepinephrine is altered by lithium.

E. Lithium's interaction with numerous enzymes, neurotransmitters, and ions may explain its diverse actions.

61.9. Which statement regarding signs and symptoms of lithium toxicity is true?

A. Most patients will have nausea and vomiting after an acute ingestion.

B. Dehydration may play a significant role in toxicity with chronic overdose.

C. Subtle neurologic changes may be the presenting symptoms in a patient with chronic lithium toxicity.

D. Patients with acute toxicity usually develop dysarthria as the presenting neurologic finding.

E. Seizures are a sign of severe neurologic complications of lithium toxicity.

61.10. Lithium has not been used

A. To treat manic-depressive disorder

B. As a cell stimulator in neutropenic patients

C. As a prophylactic treatment for patients with muscle tension headaches

D. As a salt substitute in patients with hypertension

E. As a constituent of the soft drink 7-Up.

CHAPTER **62**

OPIOIDS

62.1. Which is not true concerning opioid receptors?

A. There may be an endogenous ligand that is identical to morphine.

B. Under the new system of opioid nomenclature, the opioid receptors are renamed OP.

C. The μ receptor is most closely associated with respiratory depression.

D. When stimulated, a κ receptor subtype ($κ_2$) may produce dysphoria.

E. All opioids bind to μ receptors better than they bind to κ receptors.

62.2. Which of the following is not true concerning the currently accepted or proven signal transduction mechanism through which opioid agonists produce their opioidlike clinical effects?

A. Some receptors inhibit adenylate cyclase activity through inhibitory G proteins.

B. Opioid receptors may enhance GABA binding on the chloride channel.

C. Several opioid agonists increase conductance through a potassium channel.

D. Closure of N-type calcium channels via a G protein is an accepted mechanism.

E. Any receptor subtype may utilize several different signal transduction mechanisms, depending on location.

62.3. Which statement is false regarding the clinical pharmacology and toxicology of opioid agonists?

A. Hypoventilation may result from hypopnea or bradypnea.

B. Support of ventilation and oxygenation is the primary mode of therapy.

C. It is not important to know the exact opioid agent to which the patient was exposed to provide adequate care.

D. The presence of small pupils in a person known to use illicit substances is sufficient evidence for opioid poisoning.

E. It is better to start with low doses of naloxone and proceed upward than to give a large initial dose.

62.4. Which of the following findings is not expected in patients following a suicidal opioid overdose?

    A. Altered mental status
    B. Respiratory depression
    C. Miosis
    D. Methemoglobinemia
    E. Abdominal distension

62.5. Which of these is not expected to occur in a patient with severe acute opioid toxicity after a single-agent opioid overdose?

    A. Seizures
    B. Apnea
    C. Pulmonary edema
    D. Cardiac dysrhythmias
    E. Acute hypertension

62.6. Which is true concerning naloxone?

    A. Naloxone is unconditionally safe and should be used liberally in patients with altered mental status regardless of historical or clinical factors.
    B. Because of enhanced receptor specificity, the dose of naloxone needed to reverse opioid intoxication may be higher in patients exposed to naturally occurring opiates than synthetic opioids.
    C. After administration of naloxone and reversal of opioid toxicity, the patient is considered cured and may be discharged home safely.
    D. Meperidine-induced seizures typically respond to naloxone.
    E. Naloxone may have a role in patients manifesting clonidine toxicity.

62.7. Concerning "body packers," which of the following is true?

    A. Body packers ingest illicit substances before arrest to avoid discovery of their drugs by police.
    B. It is usually impossible to differentiate cocaine body packers from heroin body packers without toxicology analysis.
    C. Patients may be asymptomatic for hours or days before developing toxicity.
    D. Opioid toxicity is an absolute indication for surgical removal of the packets.
    E. Patients not demonstrating toxicity should receive cascara or other potent irritant cathartics.

62.8. Which of the following is false concerning fentanyl and its analogues?

    A. Fentanyl and its illicit analogues are prevalent drugs of abuse among street users and physicians.
    B. Epidemic death rates in heroin abusers are occasionally related to fentanyl substitution.
    C. Fentanyl-induced rigidity may prevent adequate chest wall function.
    D. Fentanyl-induced seizures are probably better classified as a movement disorder.
    E. Fentanyl induces massive histamine release, which is commonly related to intraoperative death.

62.9. Which is false concerning the utilization of the laboratory?

    A. Naloxone, despite its structural similarity with morphine, does not crossreact with the morphine immunoassay.
    B. Fentanyl is often difficult to detect because of its high potency.
    C. Patients who eat poppy seeds may have positive assays for heroin.
    D. Patients who eat poppy seeds may have positive assays for morphine.
    E. Patients using therapeutic doses of codeine will have a positive morphine assay.

62. 10. Which of the following is true concerning methadone?

    A. Methadone poisoning is identical to that from other opioids except that the duration of effect of methadone is very prolonged.
    B. Acute, severe parkinsonian symptoms have resulted from MPTP (1-methyl-4-phenyl-1,2,3,6-tetrahydropyridine) contamination of illicit methadone synthesis.
    C. Patients are generally given high therapeutic doses of methadone to prevent withdrawal.
    D. *levo*-α-Acetylmethadol (LAAM, Orlaam) is a slightly shorter-acting opioid agent than methadone.
    E. Nalmefene is useful in the outpatient management of methadone-overdose patients.

CHAPTER **63**

SEDATIVE-HYPNOTIC AGENTS

63.1. Alkalinization of the urine with sodium bicarbonate will enhance urinary excretion of which of the following barbiturates?

    A. Amobarbital

B. Butabarbital
C. Secobarbital
D. Phenobarbital
E. Pentobarbital

63.2. The amount of drug that will be present in the blood compartment following an oral phenobarbital overdose depends on which of the following?

A. Rate constant of absorption
B. Volume of distribution
C. Quantity of drug ingested
D. Dissolution rate of the tablet
E. All of the above

63.3. Which of the following benzodiazepines has the shortest duration of action?

A. Triazolam
B. Diazepam
C. Oxazepam
D. Lorazepam
E. Alprazolam

63.4. Which of the following sedative-hypnotic agents is most likely to cause ventricular dysrhythmias?

A. Meprobamate
B. Ethchlorvynol
C. Glutethimide
D. Chloral hydrate
E. Methaqualone

63.5. Which of the following agents binds to benzodiazepine receptors and can be reversed with flumazenil?

A. Meprobamate
B. Ethchlorvynol
C. Glutethimide
D. Chloral hydrate
E. Zolpidem

63.6. Which of the following statements about bromides is correct?

A. Bromides interfere with the measurement of sodium.
B. The half-life of bromide may be as long as 12 days.
C. Bromide is eliminated primarily in the bile.
D. The administration of potassium will hasten the elimination of bromide.
E. Bromide tablets are radiopaque.

63.7. Anticholinergic symptomatology would be expected with which of the following sedative-hypnotics in overdose?

A. Ethchlorvynol
B. Glutethimide
C. Temazepam
D. Meprobamate
E. Clorazepate dipotassium

63.8. Which of the following statements about glutethimide is correct?

A. Elimination is primarily renal.
B. The half-life decreases in overdose.
C. An active metabolite may be responsible for the long duration of effects.
D. Toxicity is equivalent to that of the benzodiazepines.
E. Absorption is rapid and complete.

63.9. Which of the following statements about meprobamate is correct?

A. It is largely protein bound.
B. Volume of distribution is 0.75 L/kg.
C. Withdrawal symptoms respond well to methadone.
D. Elimination is primarily renal.
E. All of the above

63.10. Which of the following sedative-hypnotic agents would not result in a drug interaction in a patient concomitantly taking warfarin?

A. Chloral hydrate
B. Triazolam
C. Phenobarbital
D. Meprobamate
E. None of the above

CHAPTER **64**

ETHANOL

64.1. Which one of the following statements relating to ethanol metabolism is correct?

A. Acetate is converted to acetoacetate, which enters the Krebs (citric acid) cycle.
B. Gluconeogenesis is impaired by the conversion of pyruvate to lactate.
C. MEOS system (CYP2E1) is the main pathway for ethanol metabolism.
D. Oxidation of ethanol to acetaldehyde by ADH requires $NADP^+$.
E. Pyridoxine (vitamin B_6) is essential for the oxidation of acetaldehyde to acetate.

64.2. An 80-kg man ingests 100 mL of 80-proof whisky (V_d of 0.5 L/kg). Assuming instantaneous and complete absorption and no distribution or metabolism, what is the serum ethanol concentration?

A. 50 mg/dL.
B. 100 mg/dL.
C. 200 mg/dL.
D. 400 mg/dL.
E. 800 mg/dL.

64.3. Which one of the following is correct regarding alcoholic ketoacidosis (AKA)?

A. The serum lactate is generally negative.
B. Cellular redox state is low (reduced).
C. Nitroprusside test is strongly positive.
D. Normal anion metabolic acidosis.
E. Serum glucose exceeds 300 mg/dL (16.67 mmol/L).

64.4. Which one of the following occurs in the development of ethanol tolerance?

A. α-Amino-3-hydroxy-5-methyl-4-isoxazole propionate (AMPA) receptor up-regulation.
B. γ-Aminobutyric acid$_A$ (GABA$_A$) receptor up-regulation.
C. Kainate receptor up-regulation.
D. Metabotropic glutamate (mGluR) receptor up-regulation.
E. N-Methyl-D-aspartate (NMDA) receptor up-regulation.

64.5. Which one of the following is an essential cofactor for transketolase, pyruvate dehydrogenase, and α-ketoglutarate dehydrogenase?

A. Folate
B. Niacin
C. Pyridoxine
D. Riboflavin
E. Thiamine

64.6. Which one of the following is the major contributor to the increased anion gap metabolic acidosis in alcoholic ketoacidosis (AKA)?

A. Acetate.
B. Acetoacetate.
C. β-Hydroxybutyrate.
D. Lactate.
E. Pyruvate.

64.7. In a thiamine-deficient state, which one of the following is the rate-limiting step in the Krebs cycle?

A. Oxaloacetate to citrate.
B. Citrate to isocitrate.

C. Isocitrate to α-ketoglutarate.
D. α-Ketoglutarate to succinate.
E. Succinate to fumarate.

64.8. Which one of the following will most likely interact with ethanol to result in a disulfiramlike reaction?

A. Chloral hydrate.
B. Griseofulvin.
C. Isoniazid.
D. Niacin.
E. Ranitidine.

64.9. In which one of the following situations will the nitroprusside test be strongly positive?

A. Methanol intoxication.
B. Ethanol intoxication.
C. Ethylene glycol intoxication.
D. Isopropanol intoxication.
E. Phenol intoxication.

64.10. Which one of the following concerning ethanol ingestion is correct?

A. In certain people, cimetidine may result in mildly elevated ethanol levels.
B. Ethanol-induced hypoglycemia is more common in adults than children.
C. Fomepizole does not inhibit the metabolism of ethanol.
D. The facial flushing syndrome that occurs in some patients after ethanol ingestion is caused by an overactive ADH and an underactive aldehyde dehydrogenase.
E. Fortification of ethanol products with thiamine would eliminate Wernicke encephalopathy.

CHAPTER **65**

DISULFIRAM AND DISULFIRAMLIKE REACTIONS

65.1. In which one of the following industries would an occupational exposure to disulfiram most likely occur?

A. Dye manufacturing
B. Jewelry manufacturing
C. Plexiglas manufacturing
D. Rubber manufacturing
E. Wood manufacturing

65.2. Which one of the following enzymes is inhibited by disulfiram?

A. Alcohol dehydrogenase
B. Dopamine β-hydroxylase
C. Monoamine oxidase
D. Tryptophan 5-hydroxylase
E. Tyrosine hydroxylase

65.3. Why is the inhibitory effect of disulfiram on aldehyde dehydrogenase prolonged?

A. There are active metabolites.
B. Half-life of the parent compound that is longer than most drugs.
C. Irreversible inhibition of aldehyde dehydrogenase.
D. Large volume of distribution and slow release from tissue stores.
E. Prolonged enterohepatic circulation.

65.4. How long following cessation of disulfiram therapy are most patients at risk for a developing a disulfiram-ethanol reaction?

A. 24 hours
B. 1 to 2 days
C. 5 to 7 days
D. 1 to 2 weeks
E. 2 to 3 weeks

65.5. A patient exposed to which one of the following chemicals would be expected to develop a disulfiramlike reaction on exposure to ethanol?

A. Acrylamide
B. Calcium carbimide
C. Cobalt
D. Isopropyl alcohol
E. Nickel

65.6. Ingestion of which one of the following mushrooms would be expected to cause a disulfiramlike reaction on exposure to ethanol?

A. *Amanita pantherina*
B. *Chlorophyllum molybdites*
C. *Coprinus atramentarius*
D. *Cortinarius orellanus*
E. *Galerina autumnalis*

65.7. Which one of the following subfamilies of the cytochrome P450 mixed-function oxidase system does disulfiram predominantly inhibit?

A. CYP2E1
B. CYP2C9
C. CYP2D6
D. CYP3A4
E. CYP3E1

65.8 For which one of the following exposures would diethyldithiocarbamate, a disulfiram metabolite, be a potential antidote?

A. Elemental nickel
B. Nickel acetate tetrahydrate
C. Nickel-beryllium alloy
D. Nickel carbonate
E. Nickel carbonyl

65.9 Which one of the following is caused by chronic disulfiram therapy?

A. Decreased serum cholesterol
B. Decreased concentration of nickel in body fluids
C. Halitosis
D. Hypotension
E. Pancreatitis

65.10. Which of the following substrates is required by both alcohol dehydrogenase and aldehyde dehydrogenase?

A. ATP
B. GTP
C. NAD^+
D. $NADP^+$
E. Thiamine

CHAPTER **66**

TOXIC ALCOHOLS

66.1. Diagnostic clues that a patient may be poisoned with ethylene glycol (antifreeze) include which of the following?

A. Ketonuria
B. Fluorescent urine
C. Hypokalemia
D. Radiopaque density in stomach
E. Hyperemic optic discs

66.2. The retinal toxicity observed following methanol poisonings results from

A. Hyperosmolarity
B. Elevated lactic acid levels
C. Metabolism of methanol to formaldehyde
D. Metabolism of methanol to formic acid
E. Destruction of the retinal phospholipid membrane

66.3. Which of the following is considered to be an appropriate therapeutic intervention for a patient with ethylene glycol poisoning given IV ethanol who is unstable and is at a health care facility unable to perform hemodialysis?

A. Multiple-dose activated charcoal
B. Charcoal hemoperfusion
C. Forced alkaline diuresis
D. Peritoneal dialysis
E. Continuous arteriovenous hemofiltration

66.4. Ethylene glycol is metabolized to oxalic acid by which of the following enzymes?

A. Cytochrome P450 isozyme CYP3A4
B. Glutamic acid decarboxylase
C. Alcohol dehydrogenase
D. Pyruvic acid dehydrogenase
E. Reduced nicotinic acid dehydrogenase

66.5. Which of the following is characteristic of a severe isopropanol exposure?

A. Crystalluria
B. A high anion gap
C. Ocular toxicity
D. Ketonuria
E. Metabolic acidosis

66.6. Which of the following alcohols has the greatest percentage of renal clearance?

A. Ethanol
B. Methanol
C. Isopropanol
D. Ethylene glycol
E. Benzyl alcohol

66.7. Which of the following statements is correct about ethanol therapy for ethylene glycol or methanol overdoses?

A. Ethanol cannot be given orally.
B. The loading dose is 1.8 g ethanol/kg body weight.
C. The maintenance dose is usually 230 mg/kg/h.
D. Intravenous ethanol should be given as a 5 to 10% solution.
E. Ethanol therapy should result in a blood ethanol level of 50 mg/dL.

66.8. Which of the following substances has caused central nervous system toxicity, respiratory distress, hypotension, and renal and hepatic failure in the neonate?

A. Bacteriostatic sodium chloride
B. Propylene glycol (diluent)
C. Sterile water for injection
D. Ringer's lactate
E. Dextrose 10% solution

66.9. Which of the following electrocardiographic abnormalities may be found with an ethylene glycol overdose?

A. Long PR interval
B. Short QTc interval
C. Wide QRS complex
D. Long QTc interval
E. Peaked T waves

66.10. Calcium oxalate monohydrate crystals can be confused with which of the following crystals?

A. Sodium urate crystals
B. Struvite crystals
C. Calcium oxalate dihydrate crystals
D. Calcium pyrophosphate crystals
E. Hippurate crystals

CHAPTER **67**

COCAINE

67.1. In an animal model of cocaine toxicity, reversal of which of the following parameters is best associated with survival?

A. Hypertension
B. Tachycardia
C. Hyperthermia
D. Hyperventilation
E. Acidosis

67.2. Which of the following mechanisms explains cocaine-induced myocardial ischemia?

A. Increased myocardial oxygen demand from hypertension and tachycardia
B. Coronary artery spasm from α-adrenergic effects
C. Platelet aggregation and impaired thrombolysis
D. Increased atherogenesis
E. All of the above

67.3. A young man is brought to the hospital by customs agents because of suspected gastrointestinal drug smuggling. He has normal vital signs and a normal examination. Which of the following would be the most appropriate therapy?

A. Immediate surgical removal
B. Keeping the patient NPO in the ICU pending evaluation
C. Oral bulk laxative therapy in the ICU

D. Oral activated charcoal and whole-bowel irrigation
E. Single-dose activated charcoal without a cathartic

67.4. Genetically engineered mice that lack the dopamine reuptake pump have which of the following psychomotor responses to cocaine?

A. No response
B. A heightened initial response with shorter duration
C. A heightened initial response with longer duration
D. A normal response
E. An attenuated response with longer duration

67.5. Haloperidol is contraindicated following cocaine use for which of the following reasons?

A. It exacerbates seizures in animal models.
B. It increases lethality in animal models.
C. It may increase the risk of torsades de pointes.
D. It blocks presynaptic dopamine receptors, thus enhancing catecholamine effects.
E. All of the above

67.6. Which of the following therapies is contraindicated in a patient with cocaine-induced myocardial ischemia?

A. Nitroglycerin
B. Phentolamine
C. Metoprolol
D. Aspirin
E. Thrombolysis

67.7. Cocaine's direct effect on the heart is best described as that of a

A. Positive inotrope and chronotrope
B. Type IA and IC antidysrhythmic agent
C. Type II antidysrhythmic agent
D. Type IB antidysrhythmic agent
E. Type IV antidysrhythmic agent

67.8. Which of the following will not prolong the metabolism of cocaine?

A. Mivacurium
B. Succinylcholine
C. Pancuronium
D. Tetracaine
E. Bupivacaine

67.9. Which of the following is required to produce rhabdomyolysis in the setting of cocaine use?

A. Hyperthermia

B. Psychomotor agitation
C. Hypertension
D. Tachycardia
E. None of the above

67.10. Which of the following is not commonly found as a cocaine adulterant?

A. Starches
B. Thallium
C. Local anesthetics
D. Sympathomimetics
E. Sugars

CHAPTER **68**

AMPHETAMINES

68.1. Which of the following has been consistently demonstrated in animal models following the chronic administration of 3,4-methylenedioxymethamphetamine (MDMA)?

A. Basal ganglia damage
B. Diffuse white-matter atrophy
C. Serotonergic neuron damage
D. Neurofibrillary tangles
E. None of the above

68.2. Chronic use of diet medications such as fenfluramine has been associated with

A. Schizophrenia
B. Renal tubular acidosis
C. Acute dystonia
D. Primary pulmonary hypertension
E. Myocarditis

68.3. Intravenous methamphetamine use is associated with which of the following?

A. Lead toxicity
B. Thallium toxicity
C. Arsenic toxicity
D. Cobalt toxicity
E. Phosphine toxicity

68.4. Which of the following regarding "ice" is false?

A. It is more stereoisomerically pure than methamphetamine in the 1970s.
B. It has higher purity than methamphetamine in the 1970s.
C. It is a different salt form than methamphetamine in the 1970s.

D. It has larger macroscopic crystals than methamphetamine in the 1970s.

E. It is more likely to be synthesized from ephedrine than methamphetamine in the 1970s.

68.5. Necrotizing vasculitis from amphetamine use may affect the following organ system:

A. Central nervous system
B. Coronary arteries
C. Kidneys
D. Pancreas
E. All of the above

68.6. Which of the following statements concerning khat is false?

A. Adrenergic complications are less frequent than with amphetamine abuse.
B. The fresh leaves are less potent than the dried leaves.
C. Khat is commonly used in eastern and central Africa.
D. The primary active substance is cathinone.
E. Cathinone may be converted to cathine spontaneously.

68.7. Which of the following statements is false?

A. Neuroleptic agents such as haloperidol may be superior to diazepam in the treatment of amphetamine toxicity in animal models.
B. Benzodiazepines are not efficacious in the clinical management of amphetamine toxicity.
C. Benzodiazepines are more efficacious than neuroleptic agents in the management of ethanol withdrawal.
D. Benzodiazepines are more efficacious than neuroleptic agents in the management of acute cocaine toxicity.
E. Agitation from cocaine, amphetamine, phencyclidine, or ethanol withdrawal may be similar.

68.8. Acidification of the urine for amphetamine intoxication is not recommended because

A. Acidification will increase amphetamine elimination in the urine.
B. Acidification will decrease oxygen unloading to the tissues.
C. Acidification may cause a heatstrokelike syndrome.
D. Acidification will worsen hypokalemia.
E. Acidification will increase precipitation of myoglobin in the renal tubules.

68.9. Which of the following symptoms is not likely to be observed in a patient with amphetamine intoxication?

A. Urinary retention
B. Mydriasis
C. Tachycardia
D. Hypertension
E. Hyperthermia

68.10. Amphetamine toxicity is not expected to result in mortality from which of the following?

A. Intracranial hemorrhage
B. Dysrhythmias
C. Hypothermia
D. Aortic dissection
E. Agitation

CHAPTER **69**

PHENCYCLIDINE AND KETAMINE

69.1. Phencyclidine and ketamine antagonize the effects of glutamate at which receptor site?

A. GABA$_A$ receptor
B. Kainate receptor
C. Quisqualate receptor
D. N-Methyl-D-aspartate receptor
E. Postsynaptic glycine receptor

69.2. Which of the following clinical symptoms is not mediated by ketamine's effect on the NMDA receptor?

A. Analgesia
B. Anesthesia
C. Psychosis
D. Bronchodilation
E. Cognitive deficits

69.3. Which of the following statements about the clinical pharmacology of ketamine is incorrect?

A. Ketamine has approximately one tenth the potency of PCP.
B. Recovery time after a therapeutic intravenous dose averages 3 hours.
C. It is extensively metabolized by the cytochrome P450 liver isozymes.
D. Norketamine, a major metabolite, has one-third the anesthetic potency of ketamine.
E. The D(+)-isomer of ketamine is a more effective anesthetic.

69.4. Which of the following substances does not produce a false-positive test for phencyclidine?

A. PHP
B. PCE
C. Dextrorphan
D. Dextromethorphan
E. MDMA

69.5. Which neuropsychiatric disorder does PCP and ketamine intoxication most closely mimic?

A. Dementia
B. Depression
C. Schizophrenia
D. Mania
E. Obsessive-compulsive disorder

69.6. Which of the following is correct about the clinical presentation of a phencyclidine overdose?

A. Patients may have rotatory nystagmus.
B. Patients often have absent bowel sounds.
C. Patients often have dry mucous membranes.
D. There is often a metabolic alkalosis.
E. Cardiac dysrhythmias are common.

69.7. NMDA receptors modulate all of the following actions except

A. Appetite
B. Seizure activity
C. Cognition and memory
D. Neuronal development
E. Sensory perception

69.8. Animal models suggest that NMDA antagonists are protective in which disease processes?

A. Cerebrovascular accidents
B. Headache
C. Depression
D. Mania
E. Schizophrenia.

69.9. Which of the following statements about the clinical pharmacology of phencyclidine is correct?

A. It is not lipid soluble.
B. It is distributed primarily to extracellular fluid.
C. It is extensively protein bound.
D. Nine percent is excreted unchanged in the urine.
E. Renal excretion is increased with alkalinization.

69.10. Which of the following therapeutic interventions is effective in a patient with a phencyclidine overdose?

A. Emesis with syrup of ipecac
B. Activated charcoal
C. Gastric lavage
D. Sorbitol catharsis
E. Whole-bowel irrigation

CHAPTER **70**

LYSERGIC ACID DIETHYLAMIDE AND OTHER HALLUCINOGENS

70.1. Which of the following medications is the initial choice to treat anxiety and hypertension associated with hallucinogen use?

A. Propranolol
B. Phenylephrine
C. Diazepam
D. Labetalol
E. Haloperidol

70.2. Which of the following statements about hallucinations is true?

A. Hallucinogens alter and distort perception, thought, and mood.
B. Patients with drug-induced hallucinations cannot typically identify their surroundings.
C. The first use of hallucinogenic drugs was in the counterculture movements of the 1960s.
D. An illusion is identical to a hallucination but is not drug induced.
E. Because of their lack of sufficient prior life experiences, hallucinations cannot occur in children.

70.3. Which of the following best describes the role of the neurotransmitter serotonin in producing hallucinations?

A. Neuronal serotonin release is the primary mechanism by which LSD causes hallucinations.
B. The 5-HT$_2$ receptor subtype is responsible for hallucinations.
C. Antagonism of endogenous serotonin at several 5-HT receptor subtypes causes hallucinations.
D. Because of its role as a serotonin agonist, LSD is frequently implicated in the serotonin syndrome.
E. Although formerly believed to be serotonin mediated, most recent evidence suggests that acetylcholine agonism is the cause of the hallucinations.

70.4. Which of the following findings is a common physiologic response to hallucinogenic drugs?

A. Diarrhea
B. Tachycardia
C. Miosis
D. Hypothermia
E. Respiratory depression

70.5. Which one of these plants and mushrooms contains lysergic acid hydroxyethylamide?

A. *Datura stramonium*
B. *Ipomoea violacea*
C. *Lophophora williamsii*
D. *Amanita muscaria*
E. *Psilocybe cubenis*

70.6. Which of the following statements about lysergic acid diethylamide is true?

A. LSD has an easily recognized taste and smell.
B. LSD interferes with glucose utilization in the cerebral cortex
C. LSD is hepatically metabolized with an elimination half-life of about 2.5 hours
D. LSD is poorly absorbed by the gastrointestinal tract, which is why it must be smoked.
E. LSD remains legal in certain states.

70.7. Which of these structural classes is not a hallucinogen?

A. Lysergamides
B. Indolealkyamines
C. Methylxanthines
D. Phenylethylamine
E. Cannabinols

70.8. Which of the following statements about *Lophophora williamsii* is true?

A. Peyote *(Lophophora williamsii)* is a small black-brown spineless cactus.
B. Mescaline is the active hallucinogenic alkaloid.
C. Peyote buttons are aromatic and sweet.
D. There is delayed absorption of peyote from the GI tract.
E. The Native American Church is banned from peyote use.

70.9. Which of the following statements about hallucinogens is true?

A. Methylenedioxymethamphetamine (MDMA) produces clinical effects analogous to LSD.

B. *N,N*-Dimethyltryptamine (DMT) is a potent, long-acting hallucinogen with good gastrointestinal tract absorption.
C. Bufotenine is derived from *Bufo* sp., a large toad, and ingestion may be lethal.
D. Mescaline is found in *Lophophora williamsii*, the sea cucumber.
E. LSD still has several important clinical utilities.

70.10. Which of the following psychological parameters is affected by LSD?

A. Arousal
B. Emotion
C. Perception
D. Thought process
E. All of the above

CHAPTER **71**

MARIJUANA

71.1. Naturally occuring cannabinoid receptors are identified in association with which of the following?

A. Chronic marijuana users only
B. Normal humans and laboratory animals
C. Mice exposed to marijuana extract
D. Liver carcinoma
E. Pregnant women

71.2. Possible medical indications for marijuana include all of the following except which condition?

A. Glaucoma
B. Anorexia
C. Diabetes
D. Nausea
E. Asthma

71.3. Which of the following is the most psychoactive substance in marijuana?

A. Cannabidiol
B. Δ^9-Tetrahydrocannabinol
C. Cannabichromene
D. Dronabinol
E. Δ^6-Tricannabinol

71.4. Which of the following physical findings is not consistent with marijuana intoxication?

A. Conjunctival injection
B. Tachycardia
C. Lethargy

D. Nystagmus

E. Confusion

71.5. Which of the following is probably true of chronic marijuana usage?

A. Smokers develop medical problems similar to those of chronic cigarette smokers.

B. Female smokers have an increased incidence of breast cancer.

C. Male offspring of users have an increased incidence of learning disabilities.

D. Smokers have an increased risk for pulmonary embolus.

E. Men have increased sperm motility.

71.6. Which of the following is correct with respect to the detection of THC metabolites in urine?

A. Not routinely done on drug abuse screens

B. Confirmed by immunoassay techniques

C. Positive at levels of 5 ng/mL

D. Dependent on patterns of individual usage

E. Blocked by high levels of vitamin C

71.7. Common intentional adulterants to marijuana include which of the following?

A. MDMA and fentanyl

B. Propoxyphene and codeine

C. PCP and cocaine

D. Morphine and gluthethimide

E. Paraquat and diquat

71.8. Which of the following is true with regard to passive inhalation of marijuana?

A. Cannot cause a positive urine test

B. Cannot cause psychological responses

C. Can cause a positive screening test but negative confirmatory test

D. Consistently causes positive test results

E. Is not associated with physiologic responses

71.9. Prenatal use of marijuana can cause which of the following?

A. A withdrawal syndrome in the neonate

B. Complications similar to those associated with alcohol use

C. Consistent low birth weight

D. Neurobehavioral problems in the child

E. No measurable changes in male offspring

71.10. Which of the following is true with regard to the psychoactive compound in marijuana?

A. Concentrates in human breast milk and may be transferred to the newborn.

B. Does not have a specific receptor in the brain

C. Is excreted unchanged in the urine

D. Is distributed primarily in the body water

E. Is found in high concentration in the CSF

CHAPTER **72**

SUBSTANCE WITHDRAWAL

72.1. Which of the following increases mortality in patients with alcohol withdrawal?

A. Chlordiazepoxide

B. Dextrose-containing fluids

C. Chlorpromazine

D. Intravenous thiamine

E. Magnesium

72.2. Baclofen withdrawal and baclofen overdose share which of the following features?

A. Anxiety

B. Somnolence

C. Diaphoresis

D. Tremor

E. Seizures

72.3. Opioid withdrawal shares which of the following characteristics with ethanol withdrawal?

A. High rate of concurrent infections

B. Fever

C. Altered mental status

D. Tachycardia

E. High mortality rate

72.4. Which one of the following is true concerning alcohol withdrawal seizures?

A. They are usually partial complex in nature.

B. They are characteristically followed by a prolonged postictal phase.

C. More than a single seizure should suggest another diagnosis.

D. They are generally self-limited and do not require anticonvulsant therapy.

E. Always are accompanied by other signs of withdrawal.

72.5. Morbidity and mortality for alcohol withdrawal are *not* determined by which of the following?

A. Presence of concurrent illness

B. Occult infection

C. Ethanol level at the time of withdrawal

D. Subtherapeutic phenytoin levels

E. Volume status

72.6. Which one statement accurately characterizes patients with benzodiazepine withdrawal?

   A. Withdrawal occurs several days after cessation of benzodiazepines
   B. The patients typically do not respond to barbiturates
   C. They manifest seizures, miosis, tachycardia, piloerection, and agitation
   D. They always have concomitant thiamine deficiency
   E. Intravenous magnesium salts produces excellent symptom relief

72.7. Which one of the following regarding clonidine withdrawal is correct?

   A. It is more likely if doses greater than 1.2 mg/d are used
   B. It is best treated by therapy with a β-adrenergic antagonist
   C. It never includes CNS manifestations such as hallucinations or agitation
   D. It occurs most frequently following use of a clonidine patch
   E. Patients should be treated with naloxone

72.8. Which one of the following is false with regard to clonidine, naloxone, and opioids?

   A. Clonidine is used to treat opioid withdrawal.
   B. Naloxone is used to treat clonidine toxicity.
   C. Naloxone is used to treat opioid toxicity.
   D. Rapid detoxification programs use regimens that include both naloxone and clonidine.
   E. Opioids are used to treat clonidine withdrawal.

72.9. Which of the following is false with regard to opioid withdrawal seizures in neonates?

   A. They are associated with maternal methadone use.
   B. They are rarely associated with maternal heroin use.
   C. They never occur in adults.
   D. They do not occur for several weeks.
   E. They are best prevented with paregoric.

72.10. Which one of the following statements about γ-hydroxybutyrate withdrawal is correct?

   A. It is a phenomenon mediated by serotonin receptors.
   B. Patients should be treated with the pharmaceutical preparation sodium oxybate (γ-hydroxybutyrate).
   C. Is not generally a concern in those who use the drug exclusively at parties.

   D. It should not result from γ-butyrolactone abuse.
   E. It is treated with 1,4-butanediol in some experimental models.

CHAPTER **73**

NICOTINE AND TOBACCO PREPARATIONS

73.1. At "usual" doses achieved through smoking, nicotine can be expected to produce all of the following physiologic effects except

   A. Nausea
   B. Muscle tremor
   C. Increased lower esophageal sphincter tone
   D. Improved memory
   E. Increased neurohumoral production

73.2. Nicotine is least well absorbed from which site?

   A. Oral mucosa
   B. Lung
   C. Small intestine
   D. Skin
   E. Stomach

73.3. Which of the following statements about nicotine metabolism is most correct?

   A. 80 to 90% of a dose is excreted unchanged in urine.
   B. Excretion can be enhanced by urinary acidification.
   C. The volume of distribution is approximately 10 L/kg.
   D. The half-life of cotinine is 1 to 4 hours.
   E. Drugs metabolized by the P450 system have their metabolism induced by nicotine.

73.4. All the following can be early signs of acute nicotine poisoning except

   A. Erythema
   B. Hypertension
   C. Vomiting
   D. Seizures
   E. Atrial fibrillation

73.5. As nicotine poisoning progresses from the early phase to the late phase, which of the following changes is likely to occur?

   A. Muscle fasciculation to muscle paralysis
   B. CNS stimulation to CNS depression
   C. Tachycardia to bradycardia

D. Hypertension to hypotension
E. All of the above

73.6. Which of the following statements regarding the management of nicotine poisoning is the most appropriate?

A. Almost all exposures require immediate medical evaluation.
B. A serum level above 10 ng/mL predicts serious toxicity.
C. Mecamylamine is the best antidote for seizure control.
D. Syrup of ipecac should be used in pediatric cases only.
E. Fluid repletion and maintenance of hydration is preferable to urinary acidification as a method of enhancing elimination.

73.7. Which statement about tobacco sources is most correct?

A. Most cigarettes are manufactured from *Nicotiana rustica*.
B. Kreteks are derived from Indian tobacco.
C. Turkish tobacco is made from the *Lobelia inflata* plant.
D. Chewing tobacco is packaged in "twists" and "plugs."
E. Snuff is usually inhaled through the nose.

73.8. All the following nicotine-replacement therapies have been shown to reduce withdrawal symptoms except

A. Smokeless cigarettes
B. Exchange-resin gum
C. Transdermal patches
D. Nasal spray
E. Metered-dose oral inhalers

73.9. Which of the following is a manifestation of nicotine withdrawal?

A. Diarrhea
B. Depression
C. Increased heart rate
D. Muscle relaxation
E. Anorexia

73.10. Which statement about smoking-cessation treatment is correct?

A. Nicotine replacement therapy (NRT) eliminates craving for cigarettes.
B. NRT does not control weight gain.

C. Transdermal nicotine patches (TNP) are more effective than nicotine gum in producing abstinence.
D. NRT is not effective unless accompanied by a counseling or behavior modification program.
E. After 1 year the abstinence rate of TNP users is equivalent to the abstinence rate among spontaneous quitters.

CHAPTER **74**

FOOD POISONING

74.1. What toxin causes paralytic shellfish poisoning?

A. Brevitoxin
B. Saxitoxin
C. Domoic acid
D. Tetrodotoxin
E. Ciguatoxin

74.2. Which food poisoning has the highest fatality/case rate in the United States?

A. *C. botulinum*
B. Salmonella
C. Mushrooms
D. *E. coli* O157:H7
E. Scombroid

74.3. Which cause of food poisoning is not characterized by a rapid onset of symptoms after exposure (<12 hours)?

A. *Staphylococcus aureus*
B. *Bacillus cereus I*
C. Puffer fish/tetrodotoxin
D. *E. coli* O157:H7
E. Paralytic shellfish poisoning

74.4. Which symptom complex best matches the pattern for ciguatera food poisoning?

A. Abdominal pain, diarrhea, malaise, fatigue, diplopia, dysphagia, respiratory depression
B. Headache, flushing, chest pain, nausea, vomiting, occasionally bronchospasm and angioedema
C. Abdominal pain, nausea and vomiting followed by diarrhea
D. Abdominal pain, nausea, vomiting, diarrhea, temperature reversal, paresthesias
E. Paresthesias, numbness, dysphagia, dysarthria, headache, ataxia, vertigo, weakness

74.5. Which symptom complex best matches the pattern for staphylococcal food poisoning?

    A. Abdominal pain, diarrhea, malaise, fatigue, diplopia, dysphagia, respiratory depression

    B. Headache, flushing, chest pain, nausea, vomiting, occasionally bronchospasm and angioedema

    C. Abdominal pain, nausea, and vomiting followed by diarrhea

    D. Abdominal pain, nausea, vomiting, diarrhea, temperature reversal, paresthesias

    E. Paresthesias, numbness, dysphagia, dysarthria, headache, ataxia, vertigo, weakness

74.6. Which of the following food poisonings does not present with an anaphylaxislike picture?

    A. Tetrodotoxin

    B. Tartrazine

    C. Scombroid

    D. Metabisulfites

    E. Monosodium glutamate

74.7. What is the most common cause of food poisoning in the United States?

    A. Botulism

    B. Salmonella

    C. Mushrooms

    D. *E. coli* O157:H7

    E. Scombroid

74.8. Which mechanism of action describes the basis for the action of brevitoxin, the cause of neurotoxic shellfish poisoning?

    A. Histamine and anaphylaxis

    B. Obstruction of voltage-sensitive sodium channels

    C. Analogue of the neurotransmitter glutamic acid

    D. Stimulation of sodium flux through voltage-sensitive sodium channels

    E. Binding glycolipid (globotriaosylceramide) receptors, ribosomal inactivation, and cell death

74.9. Which mechanism of action describes the basis for the action of domoic acid, the cause of amnestic shellfish poisoning?

    A. Histamine and anaphylaxis

    B. Obstruction of voltage-sensitive sodium channels

    C. Analogue of the neurotransmitter glutamic acid

    D. Stimulation of sodium flux through voltage-sensitive sodium channels

    E. Binding glycolipid (globotriaosylceramide) receptors, ribosomal inactivation, and cell death

74.10. Match each food source with the correct organism or food poisoning toxin.

    A. Eggs   1. *Yersinia enterocolitica*

    B. Pork   2. Ciguatera

    C. Fried rice   3. *Salmonella* sp.

    D. Large fish   4. *E. coli* O157:H7

    E. Beef   5. *Bacillus cereus*

CHAPTER **75**

BOTULISM

75.1. Which are the cranial nerves most frequently affected in a patient with foodborne botulism?

    A. II, IV, VI, III, IX

    B. III, VI, IX, X, XI

    C. III, IV, V, VI, IX, X

    D. II, III, IV, V, VI, IX

    E. II, IV, IX, X, XI

75.2. Which of the following is a contraindication to the use of trivalent botulinum antitoxin?

    A. A history of anaphylaxis to this antitoxin

    B. A history of hypersensitivity to equine protein

    C. Pregnancy

    D. Previous treatment with human botulism immune globulin (BIG)

    E. Previous treatment with pentavalent botulinal toxoid (types A, B, C, D, and E)

75.3. Which of the following is considered to be a classic symptom of foodborne botulism?

    A. Psychomotor agitation

    B. Diarrhea

    C. Dementia

    D. Descending paralysis

    E. Fever

75.4. Which of the following foods has been implicated as the most common cause of infant botulism?

    A. Pears

    B. Formula

    C. Honey

    D. Green beans

    E. Carrots

75.5. Which of the following is considered to be an essential therapeutic modality for treating a patient with respiratory depression from botulism?

    A. Botulinal antitoxin
    B. Edrophonium chloride
    C. Penicillin
    D. Gastric lavage and saline catharsis
    E. Respiratory support

75.6. Which of the following is characteristic of the muscle and electromyographic findings in botulism?

    A. Brief, small, abundant motor unit action potentials.
    B. Abnormal axonal conduction
    C. Abnormal muscle enzymes
    D. Abnormal muscle contraction
    E. The lack of posttetanic facilitation

75.7. Which of the following is often found in patients with wound botulism but not foodborne botulism?

    A. Respiratory paralysis
    B. Fever
    C. Dysphagia
    D. Dysphonia
    E. Gastrointestinal symptoms

75.8. Which of the following is believed to be the mechanism of action of botulinum toxin?

    A. Inhibition of presynaptic acetylcholine release
    B. Destruction of the motor endplate
    C. Destruction of intrasynaptic acetylcholine
    D. Neuronal calcium channel blockade
    E. Nicotinic cholinergic receptor antagonism

75.9. Which of the following symptoms associated with botulism was reported to respond to therapy with guanidine?

    A. Ocular muscle function
    B. GI symptoms
    C. Respiratory function
    D. Skeletal muscle function
    E. Gag reflex

75.10. Which of the following conditions is most likely to be confused with the diagnosis of botulism?

    A. Mercury poisoning
    B. Lead poisoning
    C. *Shigella* food poisoning
    D. Guillain-Barré syndrome
    E. Clonidine poisoning

CHAPTER 76

MUSHROOMS

76.1. Muscimol, derived from *Amanita muscaria,* is a direct-acting agonist at which of the following receptor sites?

    A. Kainate receptor
    B. NMDA receptor
    C. Dopamine DA_1 receptor
    D. $GABA_A$ receptor
    E. Glycine receptor

76.2. Which of the following allows for differentiation of the toxicity associated with *Amanita smithiana* (AS) and *Cortinarius orellanus* (CO)?

    A. CO toxicity leads to renal failure.
    B. CO is also associated with hepatic toxicity.
    C. The toxin associated with AS is not identified.
    D. AS is associated with early GI toxicity.
    E. AS-induced renal dysfunction always recovers rapidly.

76.3. Which of the following mushrooms would be capable of causing seizures?

    A. *Amanita gemmata*
    B. *Clitocybe nebularis*
    C. *Gyromitra esculenta*
    D. *Cortinarius orellanus*
    E. *Paxillus involutus*

76.4. α-Amanitin causes toxicity at the cellular level by interfering with

    A. DNA transcriptase II
    B. RNA polymerase II
    C. RNA synthetase I
    D. DNA synthetase II
    E. DNA transcriptase I

76.5. Which of the following parts of a mushroom are often found immediately below the surface of the ground?

    A. Stipe
    B. Annulus
    C. Lamellae
    D. Volva
    E. Pileus

76.6. A person eats a meal containing freshly picked mushrooms. Several hours later, while relaxing with a glass of wine, the person experiences severe nausea and vomiting. Which mushroom did the person eat with dinner?

A. *Amanita muscaria*
B. *Clitocybe nebularis*
C. *Gyromitra esculenta*
D. *Cortinarius orellanus*
E. *Coprinus atramentarius*

76.7. A patient presents with complaints of diaphoresis, lacrimation, and salivation after eating a mushroom-containing meal. Physical examination reveals miosis and bradycardia. Ingestion of which of the following mushrooms causes this syndrome?

A. *Amanita gemmata*
B. *Clitocybe nebularis*
C. *Gyromitra esculenta*
D. *Cortinarius orellanus*
E. *Psilocybe cubensis*

76.8. Which of the following mushrooms is commonly sought for its hallucinogenic potential?

A. *Chlorophyllum molybdites*
B. *Clitocybe nebularis*
C. *Gyromitra esculenta*
D. *Cortinarius orellanus*
E. *Psilocybe cubensis*

76.9. Which of the following complications is associated with the use of thioctic acid treatment for *Amanita* mushroom poisoning?

A. Hypoglycemia
B. Hyperglycemia
C. Hypernatremia
D. Hypokalemia
E. Hypercalcemia

76.10. Which of the following mushrooms would be most likely to cause toxicity at approximately 5 to 10 hours after ingestion?

A. *Armillariella mellea*
B. *Clitocybe nebularis*
C. *Amanita muscaria*
D. *Gyromitra esculenta*
E. *Coprinus atramentarius*

CHAPTER **77**

HERBAL PREPARATIONS

77.1. Which of the following describes medicinals sold as "herbal preparations"?

A. Synthetic chemicals that are related to or derived from natural chemicals

B. A leafy plant without wooden stems
C. A mineral or animal preparation
D. A traditional remedy used to promote health
E. All of the above

77.2. Which statement concerning FDA regulations of herbal preparations is true?

A. The FDA approves marketing of those preparations that are proven safe and efficacious.
B. The FDA regulates marketing of herbal preparations to prevent misidentification, mislabeling, and misleading claims.
C. Herbal preparations are considered to be medications by the FDA.
D. Herbal preparations are considered to be dietary supplements by the FDA.
E. The FDA ensures that herbal preparations are manufactured according to federal standards of quality control.

77.3. Which of the following statements concerning the use of herbal preparations is true?

A. Herbal preparation use in the United States is greatest among persons of specific ethnic or cultural groups or those with a chronic disease.
B. Herbal preparation use in the United States is not associated with any known adverse effects.
C. Despite the popularity of herbals in the United States, western medications have displaced herbal preparation use worldwide.
D. The popular use of herbal preparations is a recent occurrence.
E. Herbal preparation sales in the United States are estimated at $100 million.

77.4. Which of the following statements concerning herbal preparations is true?

A. Most herbal preparations are safe.
B. Physicians should be discouraged from including a history of herbal preparation use when evaluating patients.
C. People who use herbal preparations are aware of the potential for toxic side effects.
D. Physicians are aware of the herbal preparation usage by their patients.
E. Patients should consult their herbal stores for information concerning toxic side effects of their herbal preparations.

77.5. Which of the following is a recommended treatment for aconite-induced tachydysrhythmias?

A. Sodium bicarbonate
B. Phenytoin
C. Lidocaine

D. Procainamide

E. Digoxin-specific Fab (Digibind®)

77.6. A male patient ingests the an herbal preparation intended to be applied topically as an aphrodesiac (Ch'an Su). He vomits several times and develops ventricular tachycardia. The definitive therapy for this patient is which of the following?

A. Sodium bicarbonate

B. Phenytoin

C. Lidocaine

D. Procainamide

E. Digoxin-specific Fab (Digibind®)

77.7. In an attempt to attain a "natural and legal high," a teenager ingests "herbal ecstasy." This product most likely contains which of the following?

A. Methylenedioxymethamphetamine (MDMA)

B. γ-Hydroxybutyrate

C. Ephedrine

D. Atropine and scopolamine

E. Mescaline

77.8. All of the following statements concerning betel nut (*Areca catechu*) are correct except for which one?

A. It is chewed by an estimated 200 million people for its euphoric effect.

B. The active ingredient is arecholine, a nicotinic agent.

C. Betel nut is also used as an asthma remedy.

D. Treatment of betel nut toxicity is supportive.

E. Long-term use is associated with leukoplakia and squamous cell carcinoma of the oral mucosa.

77.9. Which of the following toxicities is not associated with pyrrolizidine alkaloids?

A. Hepatic venoocclusive disease

B. Pulmonary hypertension

C. Cirrhosis

D. Hepatic carcinoma

E. Acute renal tubular necrosis

77.10. Which of the following statements concerning these common herbal preparations is false?

A. There is sufficient evidence that echinacea can prevent cancer.

B. Patients who are taking anticoagulants should avoid garlic because it contains an antiplatelet metabolite, ajoene.

C. Long-term use of ginseng is associated with "ginseng abuse syndrome," which consists of

hypertension, insomnia, anxiety, and morning diarrhea.

D. There is sufficient evidence that St. John's wort is beneficial as an antidepressant.

E. There is sufficient evidence that saw palmetto is an effective therapy for prostatic enlargement.

CHAPTER **78**

PLANTS

78.1. Which of the following is false with regard to common ornamental plants that contain raphides?

A. Their raphides act by a syringelike mechanism to release a bundle of needles.

B. Their injury can be associated with chemical as well as mechanical dermal injury.

C. The plants in the Aralia family, such as philodendron, pothos, and dieffenbachia, are common offenders.

D. The plants also include common holiday plants such as poinsettia and both the European and American mistletoes.

E. The raphides consist of oxalate crystals that can result in a range of pain from mild to severe after contact with skin or mucosa.

78.2. Which of the following statements concerning the relationship of the aconitine alkaloids and the cardiac glycosides is true?

A. They work through similar pharmacologic mechanisms.

B. The current digoxin assay can detect aconitine alkaloids.

C. The plants from which they derive belong to the same taxonomic family.

D. Both produce seizures following overdose.

E. They come from ornamental garden plants.

78.3. Ingestion of which of the following plants does not result in gastrointestinal symptoms?

A. Spider plant

B. Autumn crocus

C. Rosary pea plant

D. Mayapple plant

E. Pokeweed plant

78.4. A patient who chronically ingests plants that contain pyrrolizidine alkaloids may develop which one of the following syndromes?

A. Anticholinergic syndrome

B. Milk sickness syndrome
C. Hepatic venoocclusive syndrome
D. Neurolathrysm
E. Hallucinations

78.5. Neuropathy is induced by all of the following plants except which one?

A. Cassava *(Manihot esculenta)*
B. Grass pea *(Lathyrus sativus)*
C. Mayapple *(Podophyllum peltatum)*
D. Plantago *(Plantago lanceolata)*
E. Coyatillo or buckthorn *(Karwinskia humboldtiana)*

78.6. Hypoglycin in ackee fruit *(Blighia sapida)* is associated with which of the following symptoms?

A. Vomiting, brady- and tachydysrhythmias
B. Vomiting, hypoglycemia, and hepatoxicity
C. Photosensitivity reaction with discoloration and hyperkeratosis of the skin
D. Inhibition of cytochrome P450, drug interactions, and phototoxicity
E. Vomiting, hepatotoxicity, and encephalopathy

78.7. A patient who ingests which of the following plants may require hemodialysis?

A. Water hemlock *(Cicuta maculata)*
B. Rosary seed, castor bean *(Ricinis communis)*
C. Poison hemlock *(Conium maculata)*
D. Monkshood *(Aconitum napellus)*
E. Dock plant *(Rumex crispus)*

78.8. Phorbol esters are associated with which clinical consequence and plant?

A. Contact dermatitis, poinsettia and spurges *(Euphorbia* spp.)
B. Gastric carcinoma, bracken fern *(Pteridium* spp.)
C. Cholinergic symptoms, the calabar bean *(Physostigma venenosum)*
D. Nicotinic toxidrome, the blue cohosh plant *(Caulophyllum thalictroides)*
E. Hepatotoxicity, the pennyroyal plant *(Mentha pulegium, Hedeoma pulegioides)*

78.9. All of the following commonly reported plant ingestions are nontoxic except for which one?

A. African violet *(Saintpaulia* spp.)
B. Weeping fig tree *(Ficus benjamina)*
C. Jade plant *(Crassula* spp.)
D. Christmas cactus *(Schlumbergera bridgesii)*
E. Bittersweet nightshade *(Solanum dulcamara)*

78.10. Which of the following associations between consumption of large quantities of berries and symptoms is true?

A. Mistletoe and renal failure
B. Yew and cardiac toxicity
C. Holly and hallucinations
D. Pokeweed and spontaneous cerebral hemorrhage
E. Choke cherry and venoocclusive disease

CHAPTER **79**

ARSENIC

79.1. Which of the following diagnoses is least likely to be made in a patient with arsenic toxicity?

A. Thallium toxicity
B. Sepsis
C. Pharyngitis
D. Lead toxicity
E. Guillain-Barré syndrome

79.2. Which of the following symptoms are found with chronic but not with acute arsenic poisoning?

A. Nausea, vomiting, diarrhea
B. Palmoplantar keratoses
C. Hypotension
D. Encephalopathy
E. Dysrhythmias

79.3. Which arsenical species found in the urine would not be of concern?

A. Monomethylarsonic acid
B. As^{3+}
C. Arsenobetaine
D. As^{5+}
E. Dimethylarsinic acid

79.4. By which route is inorganic arsenic least absorbed?

A. Gastrointestinal
B. Mucous membranes
C. Respiratory
D. Parenteral
E. Dermal

79.5. Which of the following chelating agents is recommended for initial management of acute arsenical poisoning?

A. Deferoxamine
B. Dimercaprol
C. Succimer

    D. *N*-Acetylcysteine
    E. Penicillamine

79.6. All the following may be seen with subacute arsenic toxicity except

    A. Squamous cell carcinomas
    B. Alopecia
    C. Bone marrow depression
    D. Peripheral neuropathy
    E. Upper respiratory infection symptoms

79.7. The recommended dose of BAL (dimercaprol) to be administered every 4 hours in arsenic poisoning is

    A. 1 to 3 mg/kg IM
    B. 1 to 3 mg/kg IV
    C. 3 to 5 mg/kg IM
    D. 3 to 5 mg/kg IV
    E. Dose depends on urinary arsenic level

79.8. The primary pathophysiologic lesion produced by trivalent arsenic is

    A. Pyruvate dehydrogenase complex inhibition
    B. Inhibition of gluconeogenesis
    C. Depletion of glutathione
    D. Inhibition of thiolase
    E. Uncoupling of oxidative phosphorylation

79.9. All the following are potential sources of exposure to arsenic except

    A. Mining/smelting
    B. Herbal medications
    C. Well water
    D. Herbicides
    E. Broken thermometer

79.10. Which of the following malignancies has not been associated with chronic arsenic exposure?

    A. Bowen disease
    B. Lung
    C. Hepatic angiosarcoma
    D. Thyroid
    E. Bladder

CHAPTER 80

LEAD

80.1. The anemia of lead poisoning is in part caused by which of the following?

    A. Inhibition of vitamin B_{12}
    B. Decreased hemoglobin synthesis

    C. Increased release of immature RBCs
    D. A relative folate deficiency
    E. None of the above

80.2. The chronic form of lead poisoning may simulate which of the following?

    A. Carbamazepine toxicity
    B. Carbamate toxicity
    C. Diphenhydramine poisoning
    D. Sickle cell anemia
    E. None of the above

80.3. Treatment with British anti-Lewisite (BAL) is recommended for which of the following patients?

    A. A symptomatic patient with a lead level of 45 mg/dL
    B. An asymptomatic patient with a lead level of 25 mg/dL
    C. A patient without encephalopathy but symptoms of lead poisoning and a level of 75 mg/dL
    D. An asymptomatic patient with a lead level of 52 mg/dL
    E. None of the above

80.4. Which of the following may be a manifestation of severe lead poisoning?

    A. Metabolic acidosis
    B. Hypokalemia
    C. Cerebral edema
    D. Mydriasis
    E. Hepatic failure

80.5. Persons who may unknowingly be at risk for lead poisoning include which of the following?

    A. Copy machine operators
    B. Photographers
    C. Workers at battery-recycling plants
    D. Telephone operators
    E. All of the above

80.6. Which of the following statements about lead is correct?

    A. The major routes of entry into the body are the GI tract and the skin.
    B. Lead is present in trace quantities in virtually every food and beverage.
    C. Adults absorb a greater percentage of ingested lead than do children.
    D. Lead appears to concentrate in soft tissue.
    E. All of the above

80.7. At the biochemical level, lead interferes with the conversion of which of the following?

A. δ-Aminolevulinic acid to porphobilinogen
B. Porphobilinogen to uroporphyrinogen III
C. Uroporphyrinogen III to δ-aminolevulinic acid
D. Coproporphyrinogen to δ-aminolevulinic acid
E. None of the above

80.8. Chelation therapy of any kind is not recommended in patients with blood lead levels less than

A. 25 mg/dL
B. 35 mg/dL
C. 45 mg/dL
D. 50 mg/dL
E. 60 mg/dL

80.9. Which of the following chelating agents is considered to be the least toxic?

A. Calcium EDTA
B. Deferoxamine
C. Dimercaprol (BAL)
D. D-Penicillamine
E. Succimer

80.10. Which of the following statements about organic lead poisoning is correct?

A. It may result from sniffing leaded gasoline.
B. Leaded gasoline contains tetraethyl lead.
C. Symptoms may include irritability, nausea, vomiting, and anxiety.
D. Tremor, chorea, and convulsions can occur following exposure to tetraethyl lead.
E. All of the above

CHAPTER 81

MERCURY

81.1. Hematemesis is most closely associated with which of the following forms of mercury poisoning?

A. Elemental mercury
B. Methylmercury
C. Mercuric chloride
D. Mercurous chloride
E. Phenylmercury

81.2. Which of the following clinical presentations is most characteristic of chronic inorganic mercury intoxication?

A. Irritability, tremor, ataxia
B. Irritability, morbilliform rash, respiratory distress
C. Anorexia, tunnel vision, renal failure

D. Anorexia, respiratory distress, ataxia
E. Irritability, anorexia, hematochezia

81.3. A healthy 4-year-old ingested the contents of a mercury meat thermometer 6 hours ago. The most appropriate immediate management of this patient is

A. Administer activated charcoal and polyethylene glycol and admit for observation.
B. Administer activated charcoal and polyethylene glycol and discharge with followup instructions.
C. Proceed with usual anticipatory guidance appropriate for a 4-year-old child.
D. Administer DMSA orally at 10 mg/kg divided into three daily doses.
E. Administer BAL IM at 4 mg/kg every 4 hours until asymptomatic.

81.4. A 42-year-old photographer complains of visual difficulties, fatigue, anxiety, and inability to hold a camera steady for several weeks' duration. Which of the following occupational exposures is most likely to be responsible for his symptoms?

A. Nitric acid
B. Mercuric oxide
C. Silver nitrate
D. Sulfur dioxide
E. Formaldehyde

81.5. Which of the following statements is true regarding the pharmacokinetic properties of mercury?

A. Methylmercury is poorly absorbed in the gastrointestinal tract.
B. Inhalation is the most common route of mercuric chloride intoxication.
C. Absorbed elemental mercury is methylated to form methylmercury in the central nervous system.
D. Methoxyethylmercury is cleaved shortly after absorption to release the inorganic mercury ion.
E. The excretion of mercuric ions is predominantly fecal, with a total body half-life of 30 to 60 days.

81.6. Which of the following compounds is most likely to be associated with acute tubular necrosis?

A. Methylmercury
B. Phenylmercury
C. Elemental mercury
D. Ethylmercury
E. Mercuric chloride

81.7. Which of the following compounds has been most closely associated with the pathologic findings of atrophy of the calcarine cortex and granular cell layer of the cerebellum?

A. Elemental mercury
B. Mercurochrome
C. Calomel
D. Methylmercury
E. Cinnabar

81.8. Acrodynia is thought to occur as

A. A dose-dependent toxic effect of elemental mercury inhalation
B. A predictable consequence of dermal exposure to methylmercury
C. An idiosyncratic reaction to the use of methylmercury in teething children
D. A hypersensitivity reaction following exposure to mercury exposure
E. A catastrophic consequence of elemental mercury aspiration

81.9. The following is a true statement regarding mercury analysis:

A. Acceptable maximum blood and urine levels of mercury compounds have been established.
B. Toxic blood and urine levels of mercury compounds have been well established.
C. Analysis of hair for mercury provides an accurate predictor of total body inorganic mercury load.
D. Urine mercury levels are useful in confirming exposure and monitoring efficacy of therapy.
E. Stool analysis provides an accurate estimate of total body methylmercury load.

81.10. The following agent has shown the greatest efficacy in the chelation treatment of methylmercury intoxication:

A. Dimercaprol (BAL)
B. Dimercaptosuccinic acid (DMSA)
C. D-Penicillamine
D. Calcium EDTA
E. Deferoxamine

CHAPTER **82**

METALS

82.1. Choose the most correct description of the characteristic syndrome of bismuth poisoning?

A. Myoclonic encephalopathy
B. Parkinsonism
C. Wrist drop
D. Painful sensory neuropathy
E. Erethism

82.2. Bony fractures from bismuth poisoning

A. Are the result of high local tissue concentrations
B. Cause chronic limb deformities without chelation
C. Are likely caused by the movement disorder characterizing chronic bismuth encephalopathy
D. Are associated with non-healing cutaneous ulcerations
E. Have not been reported

82.3. Acute massive overdoses of colloidal bismuth subsalicylate typically result in

A. Renal compromise
B. Seizures
C. Encephalopathy
D. Diabetes insipidus
E. Diabetes mellitus

82.4. The most important part of managing the complications of chronic bismuth therapy is

A. Early recognition and cessation of bismuth dosing
B. Chelation with D-penicillamine
C. Hemodialysis with chelation
D. Saline diuresis to prevent concomitant renal failure and drug reabsorption
E. Use of *N*-acetylcysteine

82.5. Which of the following statements is correct?

A. The level of cadmium in the blood is usually a useful indicator of acute poisoning.
B. The elimination half-life of cadmium from the body is 7 to 30 days.
C. Calcium disodium EDTA is clinically useful for the removal of cadmium from the body, particularly the kidney.
D. There may be a threshold for cadmium toxicity in the kidney based on its limited capacity to synthesize metallothionein.
E. Cadmium poisoning is identical to that from mercury.

82.6. Four hours after performing welding operations on a bridge, a 29-year-old metal worker complains of shortness of breath, dry cough, and "flulike" symptoms. His physical examination and chest radiograph are unremarkable. Which of the following statements is the most correct?

A. A similar exposure tomorrow would likely result in worse symptoms.
B. The patient can be discharged only after a negative urine metal toxicology screen.
C. He should be observed and reevaluated for acute lung injury for 1 to 2 hours.
D. Hypersensitivity pneumonitis is the most likely diagnosis.
E. By morning the patient should be asymptomatic.

82.7. Which of the following statements is correct?

A. Brazing is similar to soldering except that the filler metal is heated to lower temperatures.
B. Brazing is used widely in the semiconductor industry.
C. Metal fumes are solid particles with a respirable diameter usually less than 1.0 mm.
D. Low-temperature metal-working operations such as soldering are of concern when they involve cadmium.
E. Flux agents are of little concern in welding operations because they are incinerated at the high temperatures that are employed.

82.8. Which of the following statements about copper is correct?

A. Acute inhalation of metallic copper filings causes metal fume fever.
B. Metallic copper ingestion by children is more consequential than by adults.
C. Most adults have an inadequate dietary intake of copper.
D. Only insoluble copper salts readily produce toxicity.
E. Despite the widespread use of copper metal, there are no commercial uses for copper salts.

82.9 Which of the following is true regarding the mechanism by which copper toxicity occurs?

A. Copper is an alkali metal and it produces a strongly basic solution in water.
B. Copper ions are potent inhibitors of oxidative phosphorylation.
C. Copper ions have a specific effect on the synthesis of myelin making copper a well-described neurotoxin.
D. Like iron ions, copper ions are involved with the generation of reactive oxygen species.
E. Deposition of copper in tissues produces a metallic interstitial fibrosis.

82.10 Which of the following antidotes is the most appropriate initial treatment for a patient with moderate or severe acute copper salt poisoning?

A. British anti-Lewisite (BAL) intramuscularly
B. British anti-Lewisite (BAL) intravenously
C. D-penicillamine orally
D. Succimer orally
E. Trientine

CHAPTER **83**

THALLIUM

83.1. Because of its ionic radius, thallium

A. Is poorly absorbed through the gastrointestinal tract
B. Accumulates in areas of high potassium concentration
C. Accumulates in bone
D. Is similar to sodium
E. Undergoes renal elimination similar to chlorine

83.2. In thallium poisoning, activated charcoal

A. Has no role in treating exposures, as small ions are not adsorbed to activated charcoal
B. Should be given to prevent absorption of potential coingestants
C. Has demonstrated limited adsorption binding in vitro but no clinical utility
D. Is indicated only in a single dose to prevent absorption of thallium
E. Should be given in multiple doses both to prevent absorption and to enhance elimination

83.3. The role of potassium administration in thallium poisoning is best described by which of the following statements?

A. Potassium administration enhances thallium elimination by competing for renal elimination.
B. Potassium administration enhances thallium elimination by liberating tissue stores of thallium.
C. Potassium administration enhances lethality of thallium in some animal models.
D. Potassium administration is associated with an exacerbation of neurologic symptoms in humans with thallium poisoning.
E. All of the above

83.4. Which of the following symptoms is not characteristic of acute thallium overdose?

A. Alopecia
B. Painful ascending neuropathy
C. Anemia
D. Diarrhea
E. Constipation

83.5. Which of the following statements is most correct regarding the role of extracorporeal removal of thallium poisoning?

A. Combined hemoperfusion and hemodialysis seem to provide clinically useful clearance rates.
B. Peritoneal dialysis is an acceptable choice, especially if the patient has renal failure.
C. A standard 4-hour run of hemodialysis will effectively remove a significant amount of thallium.
D. Continuous arterial hemofiltration (CAVH) has improved survival in animal models.
E. There is no role for extracorporeal removal in thallium poisoning.

83.6. Which of the following are/were accepted medicinal uses of thallium?

A. Syphilis
B. Tuberculosis
C. As a depilatory for ringworm
D. As a radioactive contrast agent
E. All of the above

83.7. Which of the following chelating agents has been demonstrated to improve survival or significantly enhance elimination in experimental models of thallium poisoning?

A. British anti-Lewisite (BAL)
B. Ethylene diamine tetraacetic acid (EDTA)
C. *N*-Acetylcysteine
D. D-Penicillamine
E. 2,3-Dimercaptosuccinic acid

83.8. Which of the following statements about Prussian blue is correct?

A. Oral Prussian blue is rapidly absorbed and binds thallium to enhance renal elimination.
B. Prussian blue exchanges potassium for thallium in the gastrointestinal tract to enhance fecal elimination of thallium.
C. Prussian blue enhances both renal and fecal elimination of thallium.
D. The major adverse effect of Prussian blue therapy is constipation, so it should be given with mannitol.

E. An FDA preparation of Prussian blue became available in the United States in 1997.

83.9. In the last 15 years, cases of thallium poisoning in the United States resulted from which of the following?

A. Intentional poisoning of a cocaine supply
B. Intentional poisoning of an MDMA supply
C. Unintentional exposure to thallium-containing rodenticides
D. Unintentional overdose with radiolabeled thallium for a cardiac scan
E. None of the above

83.10. All of the following statements about thallium poisoning in pregnancy are true except

A. Thallium is teratogenic in animal models.
B. Thallium exposure has resulted in fetal demise despite good maternal outcome.
C. Thallium exposure has resulted in normal fetal outcomes despite severe maternal poisoning.
D. Prussian blue is teratogenic and should not be used in pregnant patients with thallium toxicity.
E. Absence of fetal movements in utero have been attributed to thallium neurotoxicity.

CHAPTER **84**

ANTISEPTICS, DISINFECTANTS, AND STERILANTS

84.1. Which of the following agents is least likely to cause caustic injury of the GI tract?

A. Povidone-iodine
B. Iodide
C. Lugol solution
D. Molecular iodine
E. Tincture of iodine

84.2. Dermal exposure to which of the following antiseptics is associated with the development of vacuolar encephalopathy?

A. Chloroxylenol (Dettol®)
B. Cresol
C. Hexachlorophene (pHisoHex®)
D. Phenol
E. Sodium octylphenoxyethoxyethyl ether sulfonate (Phisoderm®)

84.3. Ingestion of which of the following cleaning agents is least likely to result in significant toxicity?

A.   Chlorhexidine
B.   Hydrogen peroxide
C.   Isopropanol
D.   Phenol
E.   Potassium permanganate

84.4. Methanol is a component of which of the following cleaning agents?

A.   Formalin
B.   Cresol
C.   Hexachlorophene
D.   Potassium permanganate
E.   Dakins solution

84.5. Low-molecular-weight polyethylene glycol has been proposed as a decontaminant for which of the following?

A.   Formaldehyde
B.   Iodine
C.   Iron
D.   Phenol
E.   Potassium permanganate

84.6. A patient presents with complaints of increasing tremor and slowing gait. Which of the following agents did the patient likely ingest?

A.   Boric acid
B.   Chlorates
C.   Formaldehyde
D.   Glutaraldehyde
E.   Potassium permanganate

84.7. Placing the patient in the Trendelenburg position may be useful after the ingestion of which of the following?

A.   Boric acid
B.   Chlorates
C.   Ethylene oxide
D.   Hydrogen peroxide
E.   Saturated solution of potassium iodide

84.8. Patients with boric acid poisoning typically display progression of involvement of which of the following organ systems?

A.   Dermal, CNS, renal, hepatic
B.   GI, CNS, hepatic, dermal
C.   GI, dermal, CNS, renal
D.   GI, pulmonary, CNS, renal
E.   Pulmonary, dermal, CNS, renal

84.9. Methylene blue may be relatively ineffective in treating chlorate-induced methemoglobinemia because

A.   Chlorate inactivates glucose-6-phosphate dehydrogenase.
B.   Chlorates are reducing agents.
C.   Chlorates inactivate NADPH methemoglobin reductase.
D.   An intact erythrocyte is necessary for methylene blue to be effective.
E.   Sodium thiosulfate is more effective.

84.10. Exposure to which of the following may increase the risk of cancer?

A.   Chlorhexidine
B.   Ethylene oxide
C.   Iodine
D.   Organic mercurials
E.   Phenol

CHAPTER 85

CAMPHOR AND MOTH REPELLENTS

85.1. The sale of which camphorated product is banned by the Food and Drug Administration?

A.   Camphor-containing products used on the mucous membranes
B.   Camphor-containing products used as muscle liniments
C.   Camphorated oil
D.   Camphorated spirits
E.   Paregoric

85.2 After the ingestion of a toxic dose of camphor, when are seizures likely to occur?

A.   5 minutes
B.   15 to 20 minutes
C.   1 to 2 hours
D.   2 to 4 hours
E.   As late as 24 hours after the ingestion

85.3. Which of the following tests can be used to differentiate naphthalene from paradichlorobenzene mothballs?

A.   Naphthalene is soluble in water, whereas paradichlorobenzene is not.
B.   Paradichlorobenzene will produce a green flame when burned, and naphthalene a yellow flame.
C.   Paradichlorobenzene is not soluble in ethanol, whereas naphthalene is.
D.   Paradichlorobenzene melts at a higher temperature than naphthalene.
E.   Naphthalene is more soluble in turpentine than paradichlorobenzene.

85.4. How can a mothball made of camphor be differentiated from mothballs made of either naphthalene or paradichlorobenzene?

   A. Place the mothball in water. Mothballs made of naphthalene or paradichlorobenzene will sink, whereas mothballs made of camphor will float.

   B. Feel the mothball. Mothballs made of naphthalene or paradichlorobenzene are more oily than mothballs made of camphor.

   C. Place the mothball in a saturated salt solution. Mothballs made of naphthalene and camphor will sink, whereas mothballs made of paradichlorobenzene will float.

   D. Place the mothball in chloroform. Mothballs made of camphor will cause an intense blue color change.

   E. X-ray the mothball. Mothballs made of camphor are more radiopaque than mothballs made of either naphthalene or paradichlorobenzene.

85.5. Following the ingestion of camphor by a child, which of the following is correct?

   A. Children should be referred for medical evaluation.

   B. Only children who develop overt toxicity need evaluation.

   C. Only children with glucose-6-phosphate dehydrogenase deficiency require evaluation.

   D. Only patients known to ingest more than 1 g of camphor should be sent to the emergency department.

   E. The odor of camphor on the breath suggests that serious poisoning has occurred.

85.6. Why are infants at increased risk of methemoglobinemia following exposure to naphthalene than adults?

   A. An infant has reduced NADH methemoglobin reductase activity.

   B. An infant has reduced glucose-6-phosphate dehydrogenase activity.

   C. An infant has lower glutathione stores.

   D. An infant metabolizes naphthalene differently.

   E. An infant absorbs more naphthalene from its gastrointestinal tract.

85.7. Which of the following is believed to be most responsible for causing naphthalene induced methemoglobinemia and hemolysis?

   A. α-Naphthol

   B. β-Naphthol

   C. α-Naphtholoquinone

   D. β-Naphtholoquinone

   E. Naphthalene, the parent compound

85.8. Which of the following is consistent with naphthalene-induced hemolysis?

   A. Elevated direct serum bilirubin

   B. Low serum haptoglobin

   C. Positive direct Coombs test

   D. Positive indirect Coombs test

   E. Normal peripheral blood smear with an abnormal bone marrow smear

85.9. Which of the following gastrointestinal decontamination procedures is contraindicated in patients with camphor ingestions?

   A. Emesis with syrup of ipecac

   B. Orogastric lavage

   C. Activated charcoal

   D. Cathartics

   E. Whole-bowel irrigation

85.10. Following chronic exposure to paradichlorobenzene, which of the following disorders is described?

   A. Peripheral neuropathies

   B. Hepatotoxicity

   C. Interstitial nephritis

   D. Tremor

   E. Seizures

CHAPTER 86

HYDROCARBONS

86.1. Which of the following physical properties of a hydrocarbon is considered most predictive of its pulmonary aspiration hazard?

   A. pH

   B. Oil/water partition coefficient

   C. Viscosity

   D. pK_a

   E. Molecular weight

86.2. Which of the following treatments is useful for hydrocarbon-induced pulmonary toxicity?

   A. Prophylactic antibiotics

   B. Mineral oil lavage

   C. Early corticosteroids

   D. Positive end-expiratory pressure

   E. Olive oil lavage

86.3. Sudden death associated with "huffing" of hydrocarbons is through what pathophysiologic mechanism?

A. Sudden pulmonary aspiration
B. Myocardial sensitization
C. Hypoxia with resultant myocardial ischemia
D. Myocarditis
E. All of the above

86.4. A 22-year-old chemical worker presents with progressive length-dependent peripheral neuropathy. Which of the following hydrocarbons is most likely etiologic?

A. Benzene
B. Toluene
C. Methyl *n*-butyl ketone (MBK)
D. Methyl ethyl ketone (MEK)
E. Kerosene

86.5 What is the mechanism responsible for the muscular weakness associated with toluene abuse?

A. Rhabdomyolysis
B. Metabolic acidosis
C. Hippuric acid accumulation
D. Hypokalemia
E. Dehydration

86.6. Which of the following best summarizes the role of gastric emptying after hydrocarbon ingestion?

A. Gastric emptying should be performed following any ingestion of hydrocarbon containing unknown additives.
B. Gastric emptying is most appropriate for agents with a low intratracheal LD_{50}.
C. Gastric emptying is performed to minimize risk of pneumonitis following GI absorption.
D. Gastric emptying should be reserved for any patient with an ingestion of aromatic hydrocarbon.
E. The risk of organ toxicity following the agent's gastrointestinal absorption outweighs the agent's aspiration risk.

86.7. Which of the following hydrocarbons is most likely to cause aspiration pneumonia?

A. Kerosene
B. Pine oil
C. Mineral oil
D. Motor oil
E. All of these hydrocarbons have the same risk.

86.8. Which of the following statements regarding the pulmonary complications seen with hydrocarbon toxicity is incorrect?

A. The pathophysiology is related to surfactant destruction.
B. Delayed formation of pneumatoceles occurs.
C. Erosion through the thin alveolar wall is common and produces a pneumothorax.
D. Right-sided radiographic findings are present in 75% of cases.
E. Pulmonary edema results from direct alveolar capillary damage.

86.9. Ingestion of which one of the following hydrocarbons presents a risk of carbon monoxide poisoning?

A. *n*-Hexane
B. Carbon tetrachloride
C. Methylene chloride
D. Mineral seal oil
E. Gasoline

86.10. A patient presents shortly after an intentional hydrocarbon ingestion. When does the patient need radiographic studies?

A. Immediately, and if normal, the patient may be discharged
B. Immediately if asymptomatic and again at 6 hours only if symptomatic
C. Only at 6 hours regardless of symptoms
D. Only at 6 hours if symptomatic
E. Only at 6 hours if hypoxic.

CHAPTER **87**

CAUSTICS AND BATTERIES

87.1. In vitro and animal models of dilutional therapy for caustic ingestions find all of the following except

A. There is local generation of heat.
B. There is minimal efficacy in attenuating caustic damage unless treatment is given within minutes of the exposure.
C. Dilutional therapy results in increased tissue damage on histologic inspection.
D. Cold milk may be best to attenuate the heat of dilution.
E. An increase in intraluminal pressure is only rarely found.

87.2. Neutralization therapy

A. Has no role in the management of caustic ingestions 30 minutes after the caustic exposure
B. Requires small volumes of neutralizing agent to attain physiologic pH

C. Is part of routine management early in the treatment of caustic ingestions
D. Has demonstrated increased tissue damage in animal models
E. Has not demonstrated an improvement in outcome in animal models

87.3. In caustic ingestions endoscopy is ideally performed

A. 24 hours after caustic exposure to allow for decreased inflammation
B. Within 12 hours of the exposure
C. Only after water-soluble contrast studies are negative
D. Between days 3 and 14 after the exposure
E. On all patients with a history of caustic exposure

87.4. Which of the following is true regarding the radiographic techniques described?

A. A normal contrast radiograph excludes perforations of the upper gastrointestinal tract.
B. The absence of free air under the diaphragm in noncontrast radiographs excludes a viscus perforation.
C. Pleural effusion on chest radiograph may indicate a perforation of the upper gastrointestinal tract.
D. Computed tomography (CT) of the chest is highly sensitive in detecting perforations.
E. Contrast radiography should be used to follow patients with grade I lesions.

87.5. Corticosteroid therapy

A. Should be employed in all patients before endoscopy
B. May have some benefit for patients with second-degree circumferential injuries
C. Is safest and most efficacious in patients with grade III injuries
D. May prevent perforations of the esophagus
E. Requires concomitant antibiotic therapy only in patients with fever or positive blood cultures

87.6. Antibiotic therapy

A. Should be employed in all patients with esophageal burns grade II and higher
B. Should be reserved only for patients with a ruptured viscus
C. Is demonstrated empirically to improve outcome in all patients with grade II or higher burns
D. Is recommended for patients treated with corticosteroids

E. Definitively decreases the incidence of stricture formation

87.7. Stricture for mation

A. Can be treated with corticosteroids
B. Presents within 24 hours of the caustic exposure
C. Requires dilation with a Foley balloon catheter
D. Is prevented by corticosteroid administration
E. Increases the risk of carcinoma in alkaline ingestions

87.8. Sodium hypochlorite ingestion

A. Requires serial arterial blood gases to monitor systemic toxicity
B. Rarely causes significant injuries in unintentional exposures
C. Causes delayed pain, mandating hospitalization for observation
D. Requires endoscopy in all patients with exposures
E. Responds well to acetic acid irrigation

87.9. Electrolyte and metabolic abnormalities found in patients with significant hydrofluoric acid exposures include all of the following except

A. Hyperkalemia
B. Hypermagnesemia
C. Hypocalcemia
D. Acidemia
E. Coagulopathy

87.10. Patients with hydrofluoric acid ingestion

A. Should have immediate nasogastric tube gastric aspiration
B. Have good outcomes when treated with oral magnesium citrate
C. Require emergent laparotomy, as these patients invariably suffer gastrointestinal perforations
D. Invariably present in ventricular fibrillation
E. Should be treated with activated charcoal to decrease mortality

CHAPTER **88**

INSECTICIDES: ORGANIC PHOSPHORUS COMPOUNDS AND CARBAMATES

88.1. Which of the following agents has been shown to reverse the neuromuscular junction acetylcholinesterase inhibition?

A. Atropine
B. Diazepam
C. Glycopyrrolate
D. Pralidoxime
E. Lorazepam

88.2. Which of the following is least likely to result from the various side groups attached to the active phosphate atom in the organic phosphorus compound?

A. Relative tightness of the binding to the cholinesterase
B. Time for endogenous hydrolysis of the organophosphate from the cholinesterase
C. Fat solubility of the organic phosphorus compound
D. Latency of symptom onset after exposure
E. Amount of nicotinic versus muscarinic cholinesterase inhibition

88.3. Signs and symptoms of cholinesterase inhibition can include all of the following except

A. Miosis
B. Mydriasis
C. Tachycardia
D. Bradycardia
E. Urinary retention

88.4. Systemic atropine for organic phosphorus compound poisoning will treat all of the following except

A. Bronchorrhea
B. Miosis
C. Muscle weakness
D. Diarrhea
E. Bronchoconstriction

88.5. Treatment with pralidoxime is not indicated in which of the following situations?

A. A patient 2 hours postexposure with respiratory distress and diarrhea
B. A patient 14 hours postexposure with miosis and blurred vision
C. A patient with diarrhea and muscle weakness presenting 3 days postexposure
D. A patient 30 minutes after skin splash exposure and complaining of local diaphoresis and chest tightness
E. A patient presenting 24 hours postexposure and complaining of trouble breathing

88.6. Which of the following medications is metabolized by plasma cholinesterase and may have enhanced

effects or toxicity in cholinesterase-inhibited patients?

A. Succinylcholine
B. Atropine
C. Lidocaine
D. Meperidine
E. Diazepam

88.7. A patient who has been exposed to an organic phosphorus compound and has a depressed cholinesterase level may not return to work until the level is greater than or equal to which percentage of normal?

A. 10%
B. 25%
C. 50%
D. 75%
E. 100%

88.8. Organic phosphorus compound-induced delayed neuropathy (OPIDN) has been associated with which of the following?

A. Neuropathic esterase depression greater than 70%
B. Acetylcholine depression greater than 50%
C. Immediate onset after exposure to organophosphates
D. Initial onset of muscle weakness within 24 to 48 hours after exposure to organophosphates
E. Response to pralidoxime

88.9. Pyridostigmine was chosen as a prophylactic agent for nerve-gas exposure during the Gulf War for all of the following reasons except

A. It passes the blood–brain barrier.
B. It will protect native acetylcholinesterase by initially binding to it then releasing.
C. It can be given orally rather than by injection.
D. Soldiers can function normally with 30% inhibition of cholinesterase.
E. It has a relatively short half-life.

88.10. Which of the following agents has not been implicated in the development of the intermediate syndrome?

A. Dimethoate
B. Malathion
C. Methamidofos
D. Diazinon
E. Carbaryl

CHAPTER **89**

INSECTICIDES: ORGANOCHLORINES, PYRETHRINS, DEET

89.1. Lindane causes seizures by binding to which of the following receptor sites in the brain?

   A. Serotonergic A_3 binding site
   B. Central dopaminergic receptors
   C. Glycinergic binding sites
   D. Ivermectin binding site on the chloride channel
   E. Picrotoxin binding site on the GABA receptor

89.2. Which of the following has not been associated with chronic exposure to chlordecone?

   A. Idiopathic intracranial hypertension
   B. Oligospermia
   C. Hyperthyroidism
   D. Aplastic anemia
   E. All of the above

89.3. Which of the following organochlorine pesticides is considered to have the least toxicity in animals?

   A. Mirex
   B. Aldrin
   C. Dieldrin
   D. Endosulfan
   E. Endrin

89.4. Which of the following toxic effects has been observed in children following overuse of *N,N*-diethyltoluamide (DEET)?

   A. Diarrhea
   B. Cardiac dysrhythmias
   C. Seizures
   D. Ataxia
   E. Anaphylaxis

89.5. Which of the following organochlorine pesticides is poorly absorbed dermally?

   A. DDT (dichorodiphenyltrichloroethane)
   B. Aldrin
   C. Dieldrin
   D. Endosulfan
   E. Endrin

89.6. Which of the following statements about DEET is correct?

   A. It is available to the consumer in concentrations ranging from 5 to 10%.
   B. It is often combined with pyrethroids.
   C. DEET is poorly absorbed through the skin.
   D. *N,N*-Diethyltoluamide and several active metabolites can be found in fat for up to 2 months following dermal application.
   E. The lower concentration products are not as effective as the higher concentration products.

89.7. DDT causes toxicity by binding to which of the following sites?

   A. Serotonergic A_3 binding site
   B. Sodium channel
   C. Glycinergic binding sites
   D. Ivermectin binding site on the chloride channel
   E. Picrotoxin binding site on the GABA receptor

89.8. Which of the following statements about chlorinated hydrocarbon pesticides is correct?

   A. They are potent stimulators of microsomal enzymes.
   B. They may alter the normal ascorbic acid and glucuronic acid pathways.
   C. They may enhance the metabolic breakdown of oral contraceptives.
   D. They may enhance the metabolism of anticonvulsants such as phenobarbital and phenytoin.
   E. All of the above

89.9. Which of the following statements is correct about DDT levels?

   A. Blood levels document exposure and are prognostic of long-term effects.
   B. Levels of DDT increase with age.
   C. DDT blood levels correlate with DDT urine levels.
   D. Symptoms of DDT toxicity have been shown to correlate with concentrations of DDT in both fat and blood.
   E. None of the above

89.10. Which of the following statements about pyrethroids is correct?

   A. They are extracted from geraniums.
   B. They are the active metabolites of piperonyl butoxide.
   C. Mammals demonstrate relatively little toxicity when exposed to these compounds.
   D. Most toxic effects involve the central nervous system.
   E. None of the above

CHAPTER **90**

RODENTICIDES

90.1. In evaluating the ingestion of an unknown rodenticide, which of the following correctly pairs a physical finding with its associated rodenticide?

  A. Hair loss—strychnine
  B. Opisthotonos—barium carbonate
  C. Garlic odor of stools—zinc phosphide
  D. "Smoking" vomitus and stools—yellow (white) phosphorus
  E. "Risus sardonicus"—thallium

90.2. Which statement regarding inorganic rodenticides (arsenic, thallium, yellow phosphorus, barium carbonate, zinc phosphide) and organic rodenticides (SMFA, ANTU, warfarin, red squill, strychnine, norbormide, Vacor) is true?

  A. All organic rodenticides are considered highly toxic.
  B. All organic rodenticides are considered moderately toxic.
  C. All inorganic rodenticides are considered highly toxic.
  D. All inorganic rodenticides are either highly or moderately toxic.
  E. Low-toxicity rodenticides may be found in both the organic and inorganic groups.

90.3. Which of the following rodenticides is considered "selective"?

  A. Yellow phosphorus
  B. SMFA
  C. Warfarin
  D. Norbormide
  E. Vacor

90.4. The toxicity of sodium monofluoroacetate (SMFA) is related to

  A. Its fluoride content
  B. Its interference with the Krebs cycle
  C. Its widespread availability to the public as well as commercial pest-control operators
  D. Its ability to be absorbed through unbroken skin
  E. Its hypertensive effects

90.5. Weakness plus gastrointestinal, neurologic, cardiovascular, and pulmonary dysfunction accompanied by a profound reduction in serum potassium characterizes poisoning by which of the following rodenticides?

  A. Strychnine

  B. Thallium
  C. α-Naphthylthiourea (ANTU)
  D. Barium carbonate
  E. Vacor (PNU)

90.6. Lethargy might be the only sign expected from repeated ingestions of which of the following rodenticides?

  A. Brodifacoum
  B. Bromethalin
  C. Cholecalciferol
  D. Strychnine
  E. Vacor

90.7. A rodenticide that may potentially cause cardiotoxicity characterized by atrioventricular block, ventricular irritability, and death as well as hyperkalemia, nausea, and vomiting is

  A. Strychnine
  B. Thallium
  C. Norbormide
  D. Red squill
  E. Bromethalin

90.8. A prolonged prothrombin time (INR) in a child with pica suggests which type of rodenticide ingestion?

  A. A single ingestion of ANTU earlier that day
  B. Repeated "nibbling" on cholecalciferol over a 2-week period
  C. A single ingestion of warfarin that day
  D. Two or three ingestions of bromethalin
  E. A single ingestion of 4-hydroxycoumarin (difenacoum) 2 days before

90.9. Based on known effects on rats, cats, and dogs, which of the following groups of physical findings are likely to occur after a human ingests bromethalin?

  A. Vomiting, gastrointestinal hemorrhage, hypotension
  B. Hematemesis, bloody stools, hypotension
  C. Congestive heart failure, dysrhythmias, sudden death
  D. Hypoxia from acute lung injury (ALI) and adult respiratory distress syndrome (ARDS)
  E. Tremors, focal motor seizures, decreased level of consciousness

90.10. Which of the following statistics regarding rodenticide ingestions between 1991 and 1995 is incorrect?

  A. There are between 15,000 and 17,000 exposures to rodenticides per year.

B. About 90% of rodenticide ingestions are by children less than 6 years of age.

C. There have been fewer than six reported deaths per year from rodenticides.

D. There are at least one and as many as five exposures to Vacor each year.

E. In 1995 for the first time, reported exposures to the nonwarfarin rodenticides cholecalciferol and bromethalin exceeded exposures to the warfarin-type rodenticides.

CHAPTER **91**

HERBICIDES

91.1. Which of the following describes the percent of herbicide active ingredients in the world total pesticide use of 5.7 billion pounds?

A. 10%
B. 25%
C. 40%
D. 60%
E. None of the above

91.2. The potentially toxic components in a typical herbicide formulation include which of the following?

A. The active ingredient only
B. The active ingredient and solvents only
C. The active ingredient and its organic solvent
D. The active ingredients, surfactants, and a variety of other adjuvants
E. The solvent only

91.3. Which of the following is correct with regard to the US Environmental Protection Agency?

A. It has no authority over inert ingredients in pesticides
B. It now requires the same battery of tests for all inert ingredients as for active ingredients
C. It is phasing out all inert ingredients with an unfavorable toxicity/use profile
D. It allows toxic inert ingredients to remain in pesticide formulations if they are "grandfathered" by having been introduced before 1977.
E. It is in the process of eliminating herbicide use altogether

91.4. The primary toxic hazard profile of airborne exposure to herbicide spray includes which of the following?

A. Systemic poisoning through the lungs from inhaled mist

B. Irritation to skin and upper respiratory tract
C. Systemic poisoning and contact allergy or minor skin irritation
D. Systemic poisoning from dermal absorption
E. Eye irritation

91.5. Which of the following is not characteristic of paraquat's toxic presentations?

A. Oral mucosa ulceration, diarrhea, total recovery without sequelae
B. Corrosive injury to the GI tract, acute tubular necrosis, delayed progressive pulmonary fibrosis
C. Corrosive injury to the GI tract, rapidly developing multiorgan failure, shock, and death
D. Cardiomyopathy following chronic inhalational exposure
E. Dermatitis and nail damage from skin contact

91.6. Which of the following is not one of paraquat's toxic mechanisms of action in the lung?

A. Active transport into the pneumocyte
B. Reduction-oxidation cycling that forms activated oxygen radicals and regenerates paraquat
C. Oxygen radical damage of cellular molecules resulting in cell damage, death, and inflammatory response
D. Proliferation of fibroblasts with collagen deposition and loss of alveolar integrity
E. Destruction of surfactant resulting in alveolar collapse

91.7. Which of the following therapies is associated with a better than 50% survival rate following the ingestion of a potentially fatal dose of paraquat?

A. Fuller's earth or activated charcoal within 2 hours
B. Continuous hemoperfusion until serum levels are undetectable
C. High-dose vitamin E and C plus lung irradiation
D. Extracorporeal membrane oxygenation and lung transplantation
E. There is no effective antidote

91.8. Which of the following is true with respect to diquat?

A. Is much less toxic than paraquat when comparing their LD_{50}.
B. Produces similar pulmonary effects as paraquat
C. Is not associated with life-threatening poisoning

D. Is not of the appropriate configuration to allow active transport in the lung
E. Cannot be obtained in the United States

91.9. For which of the following reasons does glyphosate itself have little human toxicity?

A. It undergoes extensive first-pass metabolism in the liver.
B. It is in a solution with a neutral pH.
C. It is less potent as an inhibitor of mammalian cholinesterase.
D. It interferes with a biosynthetic pathway not utilized in animals.
E. It cannot pass membranes because of its charge.

91.10. Glyphosate formulated with surfactant may cause surfactant-related systemic toxicity. When it is ingested in large amounts, which of the following does not occur?

A. Seizures unresponsive to anticonvulsant therapy.
B. Acute lung injury manifest as hypoxia or pulmonary edema.
C. Shock unresponsive to fluids and vasopressor amines
D. Hypotensive injury to kidneys, liver, and central nervous system
E. Oral and GI tract irritation, edema, and erosions

CHAPTER **92**

INDUSTRIAL POISONING: INFORMATION AND CONTROL

92.1. What is the preferred method of workplace hazard control?

A. Enclosure
B. Personal protective equipment
C. Shielding
D. Substitution
E. Ventilation

92.2. Which federal agency requires manufacturers to create material safety data sheets (MSDSs) for their products?

A. Department of Justice
B. Environmental Protection Agency
C. Equal Employment Opportunity Commission

D. National Institute of Occupational Safety and Health
E. Occupational Safety and Health Administration

92.3. The Hazardous Communication Standard (Haz-Com) was enacted as the national legislation on material safety data sheets, created as part of which authorizing legislation?

A. Americans with Disabilities Act
B. Occupational Safety and Health Act
C. Resource Conservation and Recovery Act
D. Superfund Amendments and Reauthorization Act
E. Toxic Substances Control Act

92.4. Emergency Planning and Community Right-to-Know Act was enacted as the national legislation on community safety, created as part of which authorizing legislation?

A. Americans with Disabilities Act
B. Occupational Safety and Health Act
C. Resource Conservation and Recovery Act
D. Superfund Amendments and Reauthorization Act
E. Toxic Substances Control Act

92.5. The Americans with Disabilities Act was established by Congress to prohibit discrimination on the basis of disability. The law specifically covers discrimination in which of the following areas?

A. Private accommodations and services
B. Private buildings
C. Private education
D. Private employment
E. Private services

92.6. According to the Occupational Safety and Health Act, who is responsible for providing a safe and healthy workplace?

A. Employer
B. Employer trade group
C. Local OSHA office
D. State Health Department
E. Union

92.7. Which of the following would be considered personal protective equipment?

A. Local exhaust ventilation
B. Positive-pressure respirator
C. Radiation dosimeter
D. Radiation shielding
E. Safety interlocks

92.8. Which of the following medical surveillance programs would be classified as primary prevention?

    A. Reviewing chest radiography for asbestos exposure
    B. Complete blood count for lead exposure
    C. Liver function for solvent exposure
    D. Renal function for toluene exposure
    E. Urine phenol for benzene exposure

92.9. The Toxic Substances Control Act requires manufactures to report which of the following events?

    A. Allegation of any adverse reactions
    B. Manufacturing of any amounts of a chemical
    C. Notification of suspicion of risk to nonhuman systems
    D. Postmarketing notification for new chemicals
    E. Reporting of health and safety studies

92.10. Which is the first step in workplace hazard control?

    A. Biologic monitoring
    B. Engineering controls
    C. Hazard assessment
    D. Industrial hygiene monitoring
    E. Medical surveillance

CHAPTER **93**

HAZMAT INCIDENT RESPONSE WITH PRE- AND INTERHOSPITAL CARE OF THE POISONED PATIENT

93.1. What is the primary objective at any hazardous materials release?

    A. Prevention of secondary contamination of responders
    B. The type of injuries to the victim(s)
    C. Triage of the victims
    D. Establishing the airway, breathing, and circulation
    E. None of the above

93.2. With the decontamination of critically ill victims, particular attention should be given to

    A. Skin folds
    B. Eyes
    C. Orifices
    D. Fingernails, toenails, and between toes
    E. All of the above

93.3. Which statement is true regarding the reactivity of hazardous materials with water?

    A. Reactivity with water of hazardous materials contaminating the body is usually not of clinical concern.
    B. Reactivity with water is important only if the hazardous material on the victim is visible to the naked eye.
    C. Flushing with water must be withheld pending consultation with a medical toxicologist.
    D. Dry wiping should be used when water reactivity is a concern.
    E. All of the above

93.4. Decontamination of victims exposed to radioactive materials involves which of the following considerations?

    A. Did incorporation occur?
    B. What type of radioactive exposure is it?
    C. Will neutralization be helpful?
    D. Will chelation be helpful?
    E. All of the above

93.5. The decontamination of a patient exposed to γ-radiation includes which of the following?

    A. Washing the patient with copious amounts of soap and water.
    B. Washing the patient with a low-toxicity organic solvent, such as amyl acetate.
    C. Placing the patient in a lead containment vessel to prevent secondary contamination.
    D. Avoiding direct exposure to the patient by wearing a lead apron.
    E. None of the above

93.6. Which of the following statements regarding personal protective gear is true?

    A. The typical garb available in the ED qualifies as level A protective clothing.
    B. Level B personal protective equipment is effective in situations with atmospheric contamination.
    C. Typical ED garb might qualify as level C protection.
    D. A firefighter typically wears level A protection for structural as well as chemical fires.
    E. None of the above

93.7. Which of the following statements is true with regard to the care of a contaminated victim?

    A. If and when a victim gets to the hospital, the issue of decontamination is moot because there is typically too little hazardous material remaining to be clinically significant for the medical practitioners.

B. The proper processing of most contaminated victims can be accomplished by simple administrative procedures and basic personal protective equipment.

C. If a contaminated victim arrives, the Hazardous Materials Team in the geographic region must be called before any medical treatment is considered.

D. All of the above

E. None of the above

93.8. Which of the following statements about a spill in which the wind is blowing from the north is correct?

A. People should be evacuated from the area to the west of the spill.

B. The command post should be established to the north of the spill.

C. Emergency equipment should approach the spill from the south.

D. An area of decontamination should be located to the south of the spill.

E. Emergency equipment leaving the scene of the spill should exit to the south.

93.9. Which of the following statements is correct?

A. The primary tenet of prehospital management in a hazardous materials release is immediate transport to the ED for treatment.

B. The clinical toxicity of the majority of hazardous materials releases is too complicated for management outside the ED.

C. The most common route of exposure at environmental releases is through inhalation.

D. Most hazardous materials incidents occur within 10 miles of a factory.

E. All of the above

93.10. Following acute whole-body irradiation with γ rays, all of the following are true except

A. At 25 rem, the prognosis is excellent, although chromosome aberrations have been reported.

B. Thrombocytopenia can occur in asymptomatic patients with exposure to 50 rem.

C. Acute radiation syndrome occurs within 24 hours of being exposed to 100 rem.

D. Exposure to >500 rem results in death within 2 weeks in most exposed persons.

E. Exposure to >5000 rem results in death and fulminant cardiovascular collapse within a 24- to 72-hour period.

CHAPTER **94**

METHEMOGLOBINEMIA

94.1. Which of the following compounds has a metabolite responsible for its toxicity?

A. Lidocaine

B. Benzocaine

C. Dapsone

D. Nitroglycerin

E. Nitrates

94.2. A 6-week-old infant presents with tachypnea, tachycardia, cyanosis, and fever. The infant becomes less cyanotic with oxygen therapy. Because the child lives on a farm, you analyze the arterial blood on a CO-oximeter and find a methemoglobin level of 7%. What would be the appropriate next step?

A. Consider methylene blue use because of the obvious stress that the infant is exhibiting.

B. Continue high-flow oxygen therapy because the infant responded well to the treatment and continue the workup for other causes of cyanosis.

C. Contact your nearest hyperbaric chamber.

D. Check the infant's G6PD level.

E. Place the infant on a monitor and evaluate the electrocardiogram.

94.3. Methemoglobinemia occurs when oxidant stress

A. Causes the globin portion of hemoglobin to change its configuration

B. Causes the porphyrin ring to destabilize

C. Causes the iron in the center of the porphyrin ring to lose an electron

D. Causes the denaturation of protein in the red cell membrane with subsequent hemolysis

E. Causes individuals with G6PD deficiency to undergo hemolysis

94.4. A cyanotic patient is brought to the emergency department from a house fire. Which of the following is least likely to be the cause of cyanosis?

A. Hypoxia from upper airway edema caused by thermal injury

B. Hypoxia from pulmonary injury caused by smoke inhalation

C. Hypoxia from carbon monoxide toxicity

D. Methemoglobinemia from inhaled smoke toxins

E. Hypoxia caused by bronchospasm

94.5. Which of the following has been associated with methemoglobinemia in young children?

A. Diaper ointments with tetracaine
B. Ingestion of naphthalene mothballs
C. High nitrate concentrations from well water
D. Diapers labeled with aniline dye
E. All of the above

94.6. Which of the following symptoms is expected to occur at a methemoglobin concentration of 15% in an otherwise healthy patient?

A. Shortness of breath at rest
B. Cyanosis
C. Dizziness and fatigue
D. Coma or asystole
E. Headache and confusion

94.7. Which of the following substances has been associated with the development of both methemoglobinemia and sulfhemoglobinemia?

A. Naphthalene
B. Metoclopramide
C. Thiazide diuretics
D. Lidocaine
E. Phenazopyridine

94.8. At what age do children develop full NADH methemoglobin reductase activity?

A. 2 months
B. 4 months
C. 6 months
D. 1 year
E. 2 years

94.9. Which amount of hemoglobin must exist in the Fe^{3+} state for a detectable cyanosis to be present?

A. 0.5 g/dL
B. 3 g/dL
C. 1.5 g/dL
D. 10 g/dL
E. None of the above

94.10. The red cell uses which of the following compounds as an electron donor to reduce methemoglobin and maintain the methemoglobin level at less than 1%?

A. NADH
B. NADPH
C. Ascorbic acid
D. Reduced glutathione
E. All of the above

CHAPTER 95

SIMPLE ASPHYXIANTS AND PULMONARY IRRITANTS

95.1. Which of the following statements is correct?

A. Acute lung injury (ALI) occurs commonly during myocardial infarctions (MI).
B. Development of ALI is commonly a preterminal event.
C. The diagnosis of the acute respiratory distress syndrome (ARDS) requires demonstration of extremely poor oxygenating ability in patients with an appropriate history.
D. ARDS is most commonly caused by inhalation of chlorine gas.
E. The increasing water solubility of a gas correlates directly with the potential of that gas to produce ALI.

95.2. Which is correct about simple asphyxiant gases?

A. Simple asphyxiants never produce measurable laboratory abnormalities.
B. Certain simple asphyxiant gases mediate physiologic changes in addition to hypoxia.
C. They vary in their ability to produce hypoxia.
D. Typical symptoms include shortness of breath and frothy, blood-tinged sputum.
E. It is impossible to succumb to simple asphyxiants outdoors.

95.3. The clinical presentation after exposure to a highly water-soluble irritant gas may include all of the following except

A. Drooling, cough, or stridor
B. Conjunctival and oropharyngeal mucosal erythema
C. Normal arterial blood gas measurement
D. Symptom onset delayed 24 hours
E. Improvement with nebulized 2% sodium bicarbonate

95.4. Which of the following concerning irritant gases is not correct?

A. Mixing sodium hypochlorite and ammonia may generate chloramine gas.
B. Burning plastic may liberate phosgene.
C. Silo-filler disease is related to excessive exposure to sulfur dioxide.
D. Burning nitrocellulose (radiographic film) is expected to generate nitrogen dioxide.
E. Inhalational hydrogen fluoride toxicity is predominantly related to its systemic absorption.

95.5. Reactive airways dysfunction syndrome (RADS) is unlikely after exposure to which toxic gas?

A. Helium
B. Chlorine
C. Methylisocyanate
D. Ammonia
E. Capsaicin

95.6. Management of patients with irritant gas exposure should include which of the following?

A. High-dose corticosteroid therapy to limit the immunologic response
B. Nebulized 8.4% sodium bicarbonate to neutralize the acid-forming gases
C. Hyperbaric oxygenation to limit hypoxic pulmonary damage
D. Supplemental oxygen only as necessary to maintain an adequate Po_2
E. Transtracheal instillation of surfactant

95.7. Which of the following describes phosgene?

A. Phosgene poisoning no longer occurs since its use as a war gas was banned by the Geneva Convention.
B. Prolonged exposure is unlikely because of its foul odor.
C. Dissolution in the mucosal water is rapid, but the onset of toxicity is delayed.
D. Once it has dissolved, the acidic products generate an influx of inflammatory cells.
E. Pulmonary toxicity can be completely averted with *N*-acetylcysteine (NAC).

95.8. Which of the following is used as a riot-control agent?

A. Cyanide
B. Methylisocyanate
C. Acrolein
D. Chloroacetophenone
E. Ozone

95.9. Which of the following statements best describes metal fume fever?

A. Direct pulmonary toxicity occurs, and serum metal levels are elevated.
B. It is a recurrent flulike syndrome that develops shortly after exposure to metal oxide fumes generated during welding, galvanizing, or smelting.
C. Exacerbation of symptoms during the workweek is typical.
D. The drug of choice in management is BAL.
E. Chest radiography during the episode usually reveals patchy pulmonary infiltrates.

95.10. All of the following describe toxic mechanisms of pulmonary irritants except

A. $NH_4^+ + HOCl \rightarrow H^+ + H_2O + NH_2Cl$
B. $Cl_2 + H_2O \rightarrow 2\,HCl + \{O\}$
C. $N_2 + 3\,H_2O \rightarrow H_2NO_3 + 2\,H_2$
D. $O_2 + Fe^{2+} \rightarrow Fe^{3+} + O_2^-$
E. $SO_2 + H_2O \rightarrow H_2SO_3$

CHAPTER **96**

SMOKE INHALATION

96.1. What percentage of fire-related deaths are from smoke inhalation?

A. Less than 10%
B. 10 to 30%
C. 50 to 80%
D. Greater than 90%
E. None of the above

96.2. Which of the following toxic gases is formed by combustion of plastics?

A. Styrene
B. Cyanide
C. Sulfur dioxide
D. Hydrogen fluoride
E. Hydrogen sulfide

96.3. Which of the following toxic gases is formed by the combustion of polyvinyl chloride?

A. Carbon monoxide
B. Hydrogen chloride
C. Phosgene
D. Chlorine
E. All of the above

96.4. Which of the following is the most important physical property of a toxin within smoke that determines the location of lung injury?

A. pH
B. Molecular weight
C. Particle size
D. Water solubility
E. Charge

96.5. Which of the following is not an irritant toxin?

A. Isocyanates
B. Ammonia
C. Acrolein
D. Cyanide
E. Chlorine

96.6. Which of the following is not a chemical asphyxiant?

  A. Cyanide
  B. Hydrogen sulfide
  C. Acrolein
  D. Carbon monoxide
  E. Oxides of nitrogen

96.7. Which of the following is not an indication for early endotracheal intubation in smoke inhalation victims?

  A. Coma
  B. Stridor
  C. Full-thickness circumferential neck burns
  D. Edematous oropharynx with carbonaceous sputum
  E. Wheezing

96.8. The level of the respiratory tract at which an irritant in smoke causes injury is dependent on which of the following?

  A. Water solubility of the toxin
  B. Concentration of the inhaled toxin
  C. Duration of exposure to the toxin
  D. Particle size of the toxin
  E. All of the above

96.9. Which of the following mechanisms does not increase airways resistance in the tracheobronchial tree following smoke inhalation?

  A. Intraluminal debris
  B. Bronchiolar mucosal edema
  C. Inspissated secretions
  D. Acute bronchospasm
  E. Thermal Injury

96.10. In the smoke inhalation victim, lactic acidosis may be caused by which of the following?

  A. Carbon monoxide
  B. Cyanide
  C. Hypoxemia
  D. Hypoperfusion
  E. All of the above

CHAPTER **97**

CARBON MONOXIDE

97.1. Carbon monoxide poisoning may occur from which of the following exposures?

  A. Propane

  B. Trichloroethylene
  C. Trichloroethane
  D. Methylene chloride
  E. All of the above

97.2. Which of the following is not true about carbon monoxide?

  A. It has an affinity of 200 to 250 times greater than oxygen for hemoglobin.
  B. It has an affinity 40 times greater than oxygen for myoglobin.
  C. It is a product of heme degradation.
  D. It binds to cytochrome oxidase.
  E. It causes a rightward shift in the oxyhemoglobin dissociation curve.

97.3. Which of the following can reliably be used to confirm CO exposure in an ethanol-inebriated patient before obtaining an arterial COHb level?

  A. Depression of pulse oximetry
  B. Cherry red discoloration of the skin
  C. Breath sampling for carbon monoxide concentration
  D. Oxygen saturation from arterial blood gas
  E. Venous carboxyhemoglobin level

97.4. Delayed or persistent neuropsychological sequelae after CO poisoning have included

  A. Memory and learning problems
  B. Cortical blindness
  C. Parkinsonism
  D. Incontinence
  E. All of the above

97.5. All of the following fetal outcomes have been associated with serious exposure to carbon monoxide during pregnancy *except*

  A. Stillbirth
  B. Mental retardation
  C. Cerebral palsy
  D. Normal infant
  E. Placental abruption

97.6. All of the following statements are true about carbon monoxide except

  A. It is more dense than air.
  B. It is nonirritating.
  C. It is colorless.
  D. It is odorless.
  E. It binds to myoglobin.

97.7. Which of the following is associated with central neurologic injury in animal models of CO poisoning?

A. Leukocyte adherence
B. Lysosomal degeneration
C. Hypertensive episode
D. Carboxyhemoglobin level no less than 50%
E. Decrease in cerebral adenosine

97.8. In addition to low densities in cerebral white matter, the other common abnormal area on magnetic resonance imaging (MRI) associated with severe CO poisoning and neurologic sequelae is the

A. Substantia nigra
B. Pineal gland
C. Hypothalamus
D. Globus pallidus
E. Cerebellum

97.9. The elimination half-life of carboxyhemoglobin with 100% oxygen at room pressure is closest to

A. 5 hours
B. 4 hours
C. 2 hours
D. 1 hour
E. 15 minutes

97.10. Which of the following is reliably associated with potential neuropsychological sequelae from carbon monoxide poisoning?

A. Syncope
B. Headache
C. COHb >20%
D. Metabolic alkalosis
E. None of the above

CHAPTER 98

CYANIDE AND HYDROGEN SULFIDE

98.1. The antidotal effect of nitrite in cyanide poisoning results in part from which of the following?

A. Formation of carboxyhemoglobin
B. Nitric oxide–induced vasodilation
C. Myocardial relaxation
D. Reduction in cerebrovascular autoregulation
E. Binding to cyanide and excretion of the complex

98.2. Adverse effects of nitrite administration include which of the following?

A. Rhabdomyolysis
B. Hair loss
C. Diminished P_{O_2}

D. Hypotension
E. Red, flushed skin

98.3. What is the most likely clinical manifestation following exposure to cyanide gas?

A. Ventricular tachycardia
B. Hematemesis
C. Convulsions
D. Abdominal pain
E. Cyanosis

98.4. Which of the following is not an accepted mechanism for cyanide toxicity?

A. Lipid peroxidation
B. Histotoxic hypoxia
C. NMDA receptor activation
D. Hypoxemia
E. Methemoglobinemia

98.5. A person survives severe cyanide poisoning, but over a period of several days the patient develops bradykinesia and a tremor. What area of the brain is likely to be abnormal on CT imaging of this patient?

A. Vermis of cerebellum
B. Basal ganglia
C. Reticular activating system
D. Frontal lobes of the cerebral cortex
E. Temporal lobes of the cerebral cortex

98.6. Which of the following physiological manifestations is consistent with cyanide poisoning?

A. Lowered central venous oxygen saturation
B. Nongap metabolic acidosis
C. Hypoglycemia
D. Hypophosphatemia
E. Elevated blood lactate

98.7. Which of the following is not a source of cyanide poisoning?

A. Incomplete combustion of nitrogen-containing organic compounds
B. Ingestion of nitriles
C. Apricot seed ingestion
D. Nitroprusside therapy
E. Burning of wood

98.8. Rescuers of hydrogen sulfide poisoning victims often become victims themselves because of olfactory fatigue and failure to smell the rotten egg odor. At what atmospheric concentration does olfactory fatigue occur?

A. 1 ppm
B. 10 ppm

C. 100 ppm
D. 1000 ppm
E. 10,000 ppm

98.9. Which of the following is not a common clinical manifestation of hydrogen sulfide poisoning?

A. Ocular pain
B. Diarrhea
C. Pulmonary edema
D. Respiratory paralysis
E. Metabolic acidosis

98.10. Which of the following is a source of hydrogen sulfide?

A. Decomposition of grain in silos
B. Incomplete combustion of silk
C. Combination of ammonia and hypochlorite
D. Sewer gas
E. Mercury refining

CHAPTER **99**

RADIATION

99.1. A criticality event occurs when which of the following occurs?

A. An individual receives a lethal amount of radiation
B. A mass casualty event occurs with radiation
C. A cell mutates into a neoplasm
D. A chain reaction of fissions occurs releasing nuclear energy
E. A critical number of cells die, and ARS begins

99.2. The amount of radiation exposed in the Goiânia incident was equivalent to which of the following?

A. A million times that administered for a thallium stress test
B. As much as exists in a smoke detector
C. Three times more than from a chest radiograph
D. A billion times that released after the Chernobyl incident
E. A thousand times less than that released following detonation of a fission bomb.

99.3. Cell phones, televisions, and metal detectors are not considered to be radiation hazards to humans because their signals consist of which of the following?

A. High-energy photons
B. Low-energy photons

C. High-energy electrons
D. Low-energy electrons
E. Low-energy α particles

99.4. Which of the following particles may cause an irradiated object to become radioactive?

A. α particle
B. β particle
C. Neutron
D. Photon
E. Positron

99.5. In general, radiosensitivity of cells varies according to which of the following relationships?

A. Directly with the rate of proliferation and directly with degree of differentiation
B. Directly with the rate of proliferation and inversely with degree of differentiation
C. Inversely with the rate of proliferation and directly with degree of differentiation
D. Inversely with the rate of proliferation and inversely with degree of differentiation
E. Independent of rate of proliferation or degree of differentiation

99.6. Which of the following is the most common effect when ionizing radiation enters cells?

A. Alter DNA
B. Ionize water
C. Form peroxides
D. Alter the structure of organic molecules
E. Alter RNA

99.7. Residential radon exposure is associated with which of the following malignancies?

A. Bone
B. Breast
C. Lung
D. Hematologic
E. Intestinal

99.8. Survivors of the atomic bomb blast in Nagasaki who had higher levels of radiation exposure tended to have which of the following?

A. A higher incidence of thyroid disease
B. A higher incidence of pancreatic carcinoma
C. A higher incidence of lung carcinoma
D. A higher incidence of osteogenic sarcoma
E. No significant increase in disease

99.9. Which of the following is true of children born to survivors of atomic bombings at Hiroshima and

Nagasaki who were not exposed to radiation in utero in comparison with a control population?

A. A higher incidence of leukemia
B. A higher incidence of thyroid disease
C. A higher incidence of mental retardation
D. A higher incidence of microcephaly
E. No discernible increase in disease

99.10. At which of the following doses is a single, whole-body irradiation likely to be immediately fatal?

A. 10 rad
B. 100 rad
C. 500 rad
D. 10 Gy
E. 100 Gy

CHAPTER **100**

CHEMICAL AND BIOLOGICAL WEAPONS

100.1. Which of the following chemical agents is least volatile and demonstrates the greatest environmental persistence?

A. Phosgene
B. Sarin
C. Soman
D. Tabun
E. VX

100.2. Which of the following produces painful skin vesicles within hours of contact?

A. Botulinum toxin
B. GD
C. Sulfur mustard
D. T-2 toxin
E. VX

100.3. High doses of atropine, sometimes in excess of 1000 mg, may be required to effectively treat the toxicity caused by which of the following?

A. Parathion
B. Sarin
C. Soman
D. Tabun
E. Phosgene

100.4. Inhalation of which of the following CBW agents is least likely to produce a pulmonary syndrome?

A. *Bacillus anthracis* spores
B. Botulinum toxin
C. *Coxiella burnetti*

D. Phosgene
E. *Yersinia pestis*

100.5. Treating victims exposed to which of the following CBW agents poses the greatest overall risk of contaminating healthcare facilities and personnel?

A. Anthrax spores
B. Sarin
C. Soman
D. Sulfur mustard
E. VX

100.6. A mass-casualty event where victims collapse with respiratory failure is least consistent with exposure to which of the following CBW agents?

A. Botulinum toxin
B. Cyanogen chloride
C. Lewisite
D. Tabun
E. VX

100.7. Complaints of eye pain, lacrimation, rhinorrhea, cough, nausea, and vomiting are least likely to occur from exposure to which of the following CBW agents?

A. Adamsite
B. Chloroacetophenone
C. Hydrogen cyanide
D. Sarin
E. Sulfur mustard

100.8. Which of the following CBW agents is not generally intended to be temporarily incapacitating?

A. Botulinum toxin
B. Capsaicin
C. Q fever
D. 3-Quinuclidinyl benzilate
E. Staphylococcal enterotoxin B

100.9. Soman toxicity would respond most favorably to treatment with which of the following agents/drugs?

A. 2,3-Dimercaprol
B. 4-Dimethylaminophenol
C. Pyridostigmine bromide
D. 3-Quinuclidinyl benzilate
E. Sodium nitrite

100.10. Which characteristic physical/chemical property is incorrectly associated with its corresponding CW agent(s)?

A. Density less than air—Hydrogen cyanide
B. Odor like garlic—Nerve agents

C. Odor like geraniums—Lewisite
D. Odor like hay—Phosgene
E. Volatility like water—Sarin

CHAPTER **101**

SNAKES AND OTHER REPTILES

101.1. Antivenom most consistently reverses what pathology in a Crotaline envenomation?

A. Pain at the bite site
B. Edema and ecchymosis at the bite site
C. Coagulopathy
D. Secondary infection
E. Seizures

101.2. A significant coagulopathy is most commonly associated with the bite of which of the following snakes?

A. Western diamondback rattlesnake
B. Sonoran coral snake
C. Mojave rattlesnake
D. Eastern coral snake
E. Black rat snake

101.3. The dose of equine-based Crotaline antivenom required to treat a pit viper bite

A. Is based on clinical presentation and response
B. Is initially two vials every 2 hours
. Is limited to 20 vials
D. Is based on the size of the snake
E. Is based on the number of fang marks

101.4. Which of the following abnormalities is most difficult to correct with antivenom?

A. Altered mental status
B. Thrombocytopenia
C. RBC hemolysis
D. Cardiovascular instability
E. Gastrointestinal dysfunction

101.5. Systemic effects of a western diamondback rattlesnake envenomation would most likely include

A. Headache and fever
B. Bloody diarrhea and abdominal cramps
C. Muscle fasciculations, nausea, and weakness
D. Confusion and diplopia
E. Seizures and bradycardia

101.6. Which of the following is true concerning local effects of eastern diamondback rattlesnake bites?

A. Pain is the most common symptom.
B. Tissue necrosis is common in copperhead bites.
C. Compartment syndrome occurs in 30% of bites.
D. Fangs commonly penetrate 2 to 4 cm.
E. Soft tissue swelling is maximum at 2 to 4 hours.

101.7. Allergic reactions to antivenom:

A. Do not occur in patients with negative skin tests
B. Are related to the number of vials given and rapidity of administration
C. Can be prevented by administering steroids
D. Are an absolute contraindication to its use
E. Are seen only in patients with prior antivenom exposure

101.8. Signs and symptoms of coral snake bite would most likely include

A. Significant swelling and pain
B. Early coagulopathy
C. Metallic taste and tongue edema
D. Diplopia and weakness
E. Chest pain and shortness of breath

101.9. Gila monster (*Heloderma suspectum)* bites

A. Are best treated with antivenin
B. Are associated with renal failure
C. Cause severe pain and moderate edema
D. Are commonly fatal
E. Are associated with a coagulopathy

101.10. A patient with a very serious systemic effects from a western diamondback rattlesnake bite is being given large doses of antivenom and develops dyspnea, hypotension, urticaria, and wheezing. What is the most appropriate next step?

A. Initially stop antivenom, treat for anaphylaxis, and restart antivenom
B. Send blood for type and crossmatch and administer platelets and cryoprecipitate
C. Stop antivenom altogether and proceed with surgical excision of envenomated tissue
D. Stop antivenom altogether and administer fluids, furosemide, high-dose steroids, and methotrexate
E. Increase antivenom and consider this a sign of ARDS and progressive envenomation

CHAPTER **102**

ARTHROPODS

102.1. Which of the following statements about black widow spider bites is correct?

   A. Only the male spider is capable of envenomating its victim.
   B. There is usually a severe local reaction.
   C. Severe muscle cramps, nausea, weakness, and tremor can develop within several hours.
   D. The antivenom should be administered to patients with mild to moderate symptoms.
   E. The spider can be identified by the violin markings on the spider's black abdomen.

102.2. Which of the following statements about the brown recluse spider is correct?

   A. Brown recluse bites occur year round in farm workers in most parts of the United States.
   B. The location of the bite is initially very painful.
   C. Within 1 hour the bite blisters and becomes necrotic.
   D. Antivenom should be administered at the first sign of tissue necrosis.
   E. The victim may develop fever, arthralgias, hemolysis, and DIC.

102.3. Which of the following statements about a sting from a *Centruroides* scorpion is correct?

   A. Stings occur predominantly in the northwestern United States.
   B. Mortality is approximately 25% in children.
   C. Mannitol relieves the intense muscle cramps.
   D. Victims may develop muscle fasciculations and cramps, seizures, renal failure, and cardiovascular collapse.
   E. None of the above

102.4. Which of the following statements about tick paralysis is correct?

   A. Improvement is often seen after the entire tick is removed from the skin.
   B. The tick must be on the skin for 2 to 3 hours before disease will develop.
   C. Absent deep tendon reflexes at 6 hours is characteristic.
   D. Calcium gluconate will effectively reverse muscle weakness.
   E. Boys get tick paralysis more commonly than girls.

102.5. Which of the following statements about hymenoptera stings is correct?

   A. The venoms produced by wasps, hornets, and yellow jackets are almost identical.
   B. Subcutaneous epinephrine 0.3 mL of 1:100,000 may be used to treat bronchospasm.
   C. A delayed reaction of fever, malaise, headache, polyarthritis, and lymphadenopathy may occur 1 to 2 days after a sting.
   D. Anaphylaxis associated with multiple bee stings is IgG mediated.
   E. Patients who have a history of severe reactions to bee stings should be provided a prefilled autoinjector syringe containing diphenhydramine 50 mg.

102.6. Which of the following statements about the funnel web spider is correct?

   A. The venom of the female spider is more toxic than that of the male spider.
   B. Envenomations can be treated effectively with cimetidine.
   C. They are found in Queensland, New South Wales, Tasmania, and Victoria.
   D. Fatalities have not been reported from this spider.
   E. The toxin of the funnel web spider is α-bungarotoxin.

102.7. Which of the following is not found in the venom of fire ants?

   A. Phospholipase
   B. Hyaluronidase
   C. *N*-Acetyl-β-glucosamidase
   D. Piperidine
   E. Cyanide

102.8. Which of the following arthropods is most likely to cause a necrotic lesion?

   A. *Apis mellifera*
   B. *Dugesiella henzi*
   C. *Atrax robusta*
   D. *Latrodectus mactans*
   E. *Tegenaria agrestis*

102.9. Which of the following is a true statement regarding an encounter with a tarantula?

   A. Most bite wounds are very painful and develop into large necrotic lesions.
   B. Hypotension is prominent and results from toxin-mediated myocardial dysfunction.

C. Eye exposure to urticating hairs is the predominant complaint.

D. An effective antivenom exists and is available through the zoo-venom network.

E. Myoglobinuric renal failure is the major concern following envenomation.

102.10. Which of the following may be the most beneficial therapeutic intervention for patients with severe pain from a black widow spider bite?

A. Loxosceles antivenom
B. Morphine
C. Calcium gluconate
D. Amitriptyline
E. Hyperbaric oxygen

CHAPTER 103

MARINE ENVENOMATIONS

103.1. Which of the following statements about Scorpaenidae envenomations is correct?

A. The lionfish will normally not attack man unless cornered.
B. The most common symptoms are nausea, vomiting, and diaphoresis.
C. The venom is a complex hemolytic toxin.
D. The lionfish is the most dangerous of the species.
E. Home aquarium injuries are a common cause of stonefish envenomations.

103.2. Which of the following Scorpaenidae envenomations would be most likely to be fatal?

A. Lionfish
B. Stonefish
C. Turkeyfish
D. Zebrafish
E. Tigerfish

103.3. An antivenom is available for which of the following aquatic envenomations?

A. Sea wasp
B. Stingray
C. Man-of-war jellyfish
D. Cone shell
E. Sea urchin

103.4. A patient who presents with a rash confined to the genital area 1 day after swimming in the ocean may have been exposed to which of the following?

A. Hydroids
B. Sea anemones
C. Box jellyfish
D. Fire coral
E. Thimble jellyfish

103.5. Which of the following fish have dorsal spines that are sharp enough and powerful enough to be thrust through a leather boot?

A. Stingray
B. Weeverfish
C. Lionfish
D. Starfish
E. Tigerfish

103.6. Which antibiotics should be selected for treating infected wounds from exposure to marine animals, sea water, and ocean sediment?

A. Aminoglycosides
B. Ampicillin
C. Third-generation cephalosporins
D. Fluoroquinolones
E. Chloramphenicol

103.7. Which of the following statements about the tentacles of the Portuguese man-of-war is correct?

A. They may be several hundred feet long.
B. Each man-of-war may have several hundred tentacles.
C. Once detached, tentacles are no longer capable of stinging.
D. The tentacles contain nematocysts that can deliver a neurotoxic venom.
E. They are found only in the Pacific Ocean.

103.8. Which of the following starfish is venomous?

A. Sea star
B. Ivory star
C. Crown-of-thorns
D. Flower star
E. Canterbury star

103.9. An envenomation from which of the following is most likely to result in the patient having spines embedded in the affected limb?

A. Stingray
B. Lionfish
C. Portuguese man-of-war
D. Sea urchin
E. Weeverfish

103.10. Which of the following statements about the venom isolated from the sea snake is correct?

A. It inhibits the reuptake of calcium into the sarcoplasmic reticulum.
B. It interferes with Na^+-K^+-ATPase activity.
C. It inhibits the slow calcium channels.
D. It causes direct stimulation of postsynaptic glycine receptors.
E. It alters both sodium and chloride permeability at peripheral nerve endings.

CHAPTER **104**

USE OF THE INTENSIVE CARE UNIT FOR POISONED PATIENTS

104.1. Which of the following criteria is *least* predictive of poor outcome when evaluating a poisoned patient?

A. Sinus tachycardia
B. P_{CO_2} greater than 45 mm Hg
C. Coma
D. QRS greater than 0.10 seconds
E. Systolic blood pressure less than 80 mm Hg

104.2. The skills and technology provided in the ICU are most beneficial for which of the following patients?

A. Patients with suicidal ideation
B. Asymptomatic patients needing extended observation only
C. Patients with serious end-organ toxicity
D. Asymptomatic patients with elevated serum concentrations of drugs such as phenytoin
E. Asymptomatic patients with ingestions of unknown toxins

104.3. Six hours following an overdose with a known ingestant, which of the following asymptomatic patients does not need admission to the ICU?

A. A patient with an overdose of sustained-release verapamil
B. A patient with an overdose of a newly released cardiac medication with no human overdoses previously reported in the medical literature
C. A patient with an overdose of aspirin with a rising serum salicylate concentrations
D. A patient with chronic renal failure who ingested digoxin
E. A patient with overdose of a tricyclic antidepressant

104.4. Which severity of illness scoring system most reliably predicts clinical outcome in poisoned patients?

A. Glasgow Coma Scale
B. Acute Physiology and Chronic Health Evaluation (APACHE II/III)
C. Mortality Probability Model (MPM II)
D. Simplified Acute Physiology Score (SAPS II)
E. No scoring system is reliable for predicting outcome of poisoned patients.

104.5. Which is *most* helpful in deciding to place a poisoned patient in the ICU?

A. A worst-case scenario history
B. Elevated serum drug level
C. Suspected ingestion of a toxin with an oral LD_{50} of 10 mg/kg in the rat
D. Signs of serious end-organ toxicity
E. Suicidal ideations

104.6. Which of the following complications following acute poisoning is *most* likely to be evident during the initial evaluation?

A. Loss of airway protective reflexes
B. Acute lung injury/adult respiratory distress syndrome
C. Brain death from anoxic brain injury
D. Acute renal failure from rhabdomyolysis
E. Fulminant hepatic failure from an acute acetaminophen overdose

104.7. A patient has phenytoin toxicity from chronic overmedication. He is alert, able to ambulate, and is not ataxic. He has prominent horizontal gaze nystagmus and a serum concentration of 35 mg/mL. What is the most appropriate disposition for this patient?

A. Admit to the ICU
B. Admit to the ward on telemetry
C. Discharge home
D. Discharge home if repeat serum concentration is not rising
E. Give additional phenytoin then discharge home

104.8. Patients with ingestion of which of the following are *least* likely to need an extended period of close monitoring following an overdose?

A. Sustained-release calcium channel blocker
B. Monoamine oxidase inhibitor
C. Fluoxetine
D. Colchicine
E. Sulfonylurea

104.9. In general, which of the following patients may not be safe for transfer from the ICU to an unmonitored medical floor bed?

  A. The patient whose signs of toxicity are resolving

  B. The patient who is medically stable but awaiting a psychiatric evaluation for suicidal ideations

  C. One in whom antidotal therapy is no longer required for treating acute toxicity

  D. A patient whose serum drug concentrations are declining and toxic effects are resolved

  E. A patient who ingested a sustained-release medication and has remained asymptomatic for 24 hours

104.10. In general, toxicologic emergencies challenge nursing/medical staff for which of the following reasons?

  A. The staff is frequently unfamiliar with the clinical effects and treatments.

  B. Most hospitalized poisoned patients require invasive procedures.

  C. Poisoned patients seldom require serial exams or close observation.

  D. Poisoned patients misuse valuable staff time because they are often asymptomatic and need only to be supervised until the psychiatrist is available.

  E. Hospitals do not have alternatives to the ICU for observing medically stable suicidal patients.

CHAPTER **105**

REPRODUCTIVE AND PERINATAL PRINCIPLES

105.1. Which of the following medications is most commonly ingested in overdose during pregnancy?

  A. Acetaminophen
  B. Diazepam
  C. Ferrous sulfate
  D. Ampicillin
  E. Salicylates

105.2. Which of the following medications is safe to administer during pregnancy?

  A. Tetracycline
  B. Ampicillin
  C. Valproic acid
  D. Warfarin
  E. Captopril

105.3. Which of the following signs and symptoms is associated with neonatal opioid withdrawal?

  A. Sleepiness
  B. Increased feeding
  C. Acidosis
  D. Hypotonia
  E. Diaphoresis

105.4. Which of the following antidotes is associated with teratogenicity in humans?

  A. Hyperbaric oxygen
  B. *N*-Acetylcysteine
  C. Deferoxamine
  D. Penicillamine
  E. Pralidoxime

105.5. Which of the following statements about the fetal alcohol syndrome is correct?

  A. After the first trimester, alcohol has not been shown to be teratogenic.

  B. At least 60 mL/day of absolute ethanol is necessary to cause fetal alcohol syndrome.

  C. Alcohol is second only to nicotine as the leading cause of birth defects.

  D. Neonatal alcohol withdrawal should be treated with tincture of opium.

  E. Children with fetal alcohol syndrome are generally large for gestational age.

105.6. Which of the following substances is associated with the lowest risk of an adverse effect if used during pregnancy?

  A. Caffeine
  B. Ethanol
  C. Nicotine
  D. Cocaine
  E. Isotretinoin

105.7. Which of the following statements about carbon monoxide poisoning during pregnancy is true?

  A. Peak maternal carboxyhemoglobin exceeds peak fetal carboxyhemoglobin.

  B. Lower fetal P_{O_2} diminishes the adverse effects of fetal carboxyhemoglobin.

  C. Therapy with 100% oxygen may be discontinued when the maternal carboxyhemoglobin returns to a normal level.

  D. Hyperbaric oxygen therapy should be administered for a period of time equal to twice the standard length of treatment.

  E. Fetal toxicity is generally greater than maternal toxicity.

105.8. Which of the following statement with regard to iron poisoning during pregnancy is true?

    A. Iron crosses the placenta by passive diffusion.
    B. Maternal toxicity exceeds fetal toxicity.
    C. The use of deferoxamine is contraindicated in pregnancy.
    D. Iron is the most commonly ingested pharmaceutic substance during pregnancy.
    E. The maternal serum iron level is directly correlated with fetal toxicity.

105.9. Which of the following anticonvulsants is *least* likely to be associated with congenital malformations?

    A. Carbamazepine
    B. Valproic acid
    C. Phenytoin
    D. Trimethadione
    E. Clonazepam

105.10. With respect to neonatal opioid withdrawal, which of the following is true?

    A. The onset of withdrawal from heroin is typically delayed compared to that from methadone.
    B. Withdrawal from methadone occurs when the plasma level falls below 10 mg/mL.
    C. Seizures are more common with heroin withdrawal than with methadone withdrawal.
    D. Paregoric is preferred to phenobarbital to prevent opioid withdrawal seizures.
    E. Withdrawal is felt to be modulated by serotonergic neurons in the locus ceruleus.

CHAPTER 106

PEDIATRIC PRINCIPLES

106.1. Which of the following descriptions is characteristic of poison exposure in a toddler?

    A. The intent is generally suicidal.
    B. Multiple substances are involved.
    C. Large quantities of ingested substances are involved.
    D. Inhalational exposures are common.
    E. Children present for evaluation soon after an ingestion is discovered.

106.2. Which of the following gastrointestinal decontamination techniques has been associated with the *least* fluid and electrolyte abnormalities in the pediatric patient?

    A. Magnesium sulfate
    B. Magnesium citrate
    C. Sorbitol
    D. Phosphosoda
    E. Polyethylene glycol

106.3. To which of the following substances are young children most commonly exposed?

    A. Plants
    B. Cosmetics and personal care products
    C. Analgesic agents
    D. Iron
    E. Hydrocarbons

106.4. Which of the following substances or category of substances is the leading cause of poisoning mortality in young children?

    A. Iron
    B. Hydrocarbons
    C. Carbon monoxide
    D. Antidepressant agents
    E. Cardiovascular agents

106.5. Which of the following may suggest factitious illness (Munchausen syndrome) by proxy?

    A. The parent remains aloof from hospital staff.
    B. Recurrent illness is associated with a well-recognized disease.
    C. Signs and symptoms occur when the child is separated from the parent.
    D. Prescribed medicines are poorly tolerated and frequently cause vomiting.
    E. The parent is relatively naive about the medical field.

106.6. Which of following is true about child-resistant containers?

    A. Child-resistant containers can prevent all children from opening them.
    B. Child-resistant containers are mandatory for the dispensing of all pharmaceuticals.
    C. Child-resistant containers are responsible for a significant decline in morbidity related to childhood poisoning.
    D. Children generally ingest medications contained in child-resistant containers.
    E. Child-resistant containers are designed to function even when pill dust or liquid residue sticks to cap or screw top.

106.7. Which of the following agents may be expected to have a significant delay (>12 hours) before the onset of symptoms?

A. Acetylsalicylate
B. Iron
C. Chloroquine
D. Glyburide
E. Isoniazid

106.8. Which of the following agents is correctly identified with its idiosyncratic reaction in small children?

A. Hexachlorophene—Cerebral edema
B. Propylene glycol—"Gasping" syndrome
C. Diethylene glycol—Hypoglycemia
D. Tetrahydrozoline—CNS depression
E. Acetaminophen—Renal tubular acidosis

106.9. The "gray baby" syndrome, which develops after high doses of chloramphenicol, is *not* associated with

A. Vomiting
B. Metabolic acidosis
C. Irregular respirations
D. Hyperthermia
E. Hypotension

106.10. Which of the following would increase the suspicion of child abuse in the setting of a childhood ingestion?

A. An 18-month-old child was observed to ingest two acetaminophen tablets from his mother's bedside table.
B. A 30-month-old child is found comatose on the living room floor the night after the parents 10th anniversary party.
C. A 16-month-old child ingests 10 iron sulfate pills that resemble candy.
D. A 12-month-old child swallows a small button battery that he finds on the floor of the living room.
E. A 6-month-old child ingests five aspirin tablets that she finds in the mother's purse.

CHAPTER 107

GERIATRIC PRINCIPLES

107.1 Which of the following is true when people over 65 years of age are compared to younger adults?

A. They account for a disproportionately high number of poisoning exposures.
B. They have a higher mortality rate following poisoning exposures.
C. They have a lower suicide rate.

D. They are less likely than other adults to be admitted to critical care units from emergency departments.
E. All of the above.

107.2. Facts about suicide in late life include all of the following *except* which statement?

A. Suicide rates among men increase significantly.
B. Suicide rates among women remain stable.
C. Firearms are the most common cause of completed suicides among men.
D. Firearms are the most common cause of completed suicides among women.
E. The male-to-female ratio of suicide attempts narrows with increasing age.

107.3. Risk factors for serious adverse drug events among the elderly include all of the following *except* which statement?

A. Enhanced pharmacodynamic effects of many substances
B. Complex regimens of prescription drugs
C. Federal restrictions regarding participation of elderly subjects in drug trials
D. Delayed appearance of toxicity for certain drugs
E. Coexisting occult disease

107.4. The presentation of toxicity in the elderly patient does not typically include which of the following?

A. Falls
B. Focal neurologic deficits
C. Memory loss
D. Agitation
E. Chest pain

107.5. Which of the following medications is not affected by an age-related decline in renal clearance?

A. Digoxin
B. Gentamicin
C. Lithium
D. Diazepam
E. Theophylline

107.6. Compared to younger adults, characteristics of alcohol metabolism that contribute to toxicity in the elderly include all the following *except* which statement?

A. Peak effect of alcohol occurs more rapidly.
B. Peak effect of alcohol is enhanced.
C. There is a decline in gastric alcohol dehydrogenase.

D. The half-life of alcohol is prolonged.

E. There is a smaller volume of distribution.

107.7. Which of the following medications will exhibit an age-related increase in the volume of distribution that will prolong the elimination half-life?

A. Salicylate

B. Acetaminophen

C. Lithium

D. Flurazepam

E. Ibuprofen

107.8. Which of the following antidotes must be used with caution in an elderly patient?

A. *N*-Acetylcysteine

B. Succimer

C. Deferoxamine

D. Polyvalent Crotalid antivenom

E. Sodium bicarbonate

107.9. Which of the following medications has a high hepatic extraction rate that may decline with age?

A. Lidocaine

B. Pentazocine

C. Propranolol

D. Tocainide

E. All of the above

107.10. Which of the following increases with age?

A. Intracellular water

B. Albumin production

C. Fat

D. Muscle

E. All of the above

CHAPTER **108**

THE HIV-POSITIVE PATIENT: AIDS PHARMACOLOGY AND TOXICOLOGY

108.1. Which of the following statements regarding lamivudine is correct?

A. Lamivudine was approved to be used against HIV/AIDS either as a single agent or as part of a combination therapy.

B. Adverse effects found with lamivudine are gastrointestinal irritation, headache, fatigue, and rash.

C. Lamivudine is a protease inhibitor.

D. Renal toxicity is the major dose-limiting effect of lamivudine.

E. Lamivudine does not penetrate into the central nervous system.

108.2. Zidovudine is an analogue of which of the following nucleosides?

A. Adenosine

B. Thymidine

C. Guanosine

D. Cytidine

E. None of the above

108.3. Which of the following statements regarding the adverse effects of zidovudine (AZT) is correct?

A. Side effects of AZT can include headache, nausea, and peripheral neuropathy as well as hematologic toxicity such as anemia.

B. When AZT is concurrently administered with ganciclovir or amphotericin B, the incidence of bone marrow toxicity is increased.

C. Microcytosis usually appears early with the use of AZT.

D. Gastrointestinal blood loss can be seen with AZT use.

E. Both A and B

108.4. Which of the following medications is likely to achieve the highest CSF penetration?

A. ddC

B. ddI

C. AZT

D. 3TC

E. d4T

108.5. Which of the following medications is a nonnucleoside reverse transcriptase inhibitor?

A. Invirase (saquinavir)

B. Crixivan (indinavir)

C. Epivir (lamivudine)

D. Viramune (nevirapine)

E. Norvir (ritonavir)

108.6. Which of the following statements about ganciclovir (Cytovene) is correct ?

A. Ganciclovir is used in the treatment of herpes simplex virus and varicella zoster virus.

B. Ganciclovir is eliminated by metabolic degradation in the liver.

C. Hematologic toxicity such as anemia, thrombocytopenia, and leukopenia is one of the main problems encountered with ganciclovir.

D. Ganciclovir can be administered orally, intramuscularly, and intravenously.

E. Ganciclovir is available only for parenteral administration.

108.7. Which of the following medication's primary activity in treating HIV is to inhibit viral protease?

A. Nevirapine
B. Indinavir
C. Delavirdine
D. Lamivudine
E. Ganciclovir

108.8. Which of the following is used for the prevention and treatment of *Pneumocystis carinii* pneumonia (PCP) as well as prophylactic agent against toxoplasmosis?

A. Pentamidine
B. Trimethoprim-sulfamethoxazole
C. Clarithromycin
D. Sulfadiazine
E. Ketocanzole

108.9. Alteration in blood glucose is one of the side effects of which of the following agents?

A. Ketoconazole
B. Atovaquone
C. Pentamidine
D. Dapsone
E. Cotrimoxasole

108.10. Which of the following statements is correct about amphotericin B and ketoconazole?

A. Amphotericin B is hepatotoxic, toxic to bone marrow, but rarely nephrotoxic.
B. Coadministration of ketoconazole with terfenadine may result in life-threatening dysrhythmias.
C. Amphotericin B, flucytosine, nizoral, sporanox, and clarithromycin can all be used for the treatment of fungal infection.
D. Ketoconazole is absorbed when given with agents such as antacids.
E. Patients should be pretreated with an antiemetic prior to receiving amphotericin B.

CHAPTER **109**

SUBSTANCE USERS

109.1. Which of the following is correct about endocarditis in the parenteral drug user?

A. Endocarditis is the most common infectious disease requiring hospital admission.
B. The absence of valvular vegetations on a transthoracic echocardiogram excludes the diagnosis of endocarditis.

C. Fewer than one-half of patients who ultimately have proven endocarditis have cardiac murmurs on hospital admission.
D. An intravenous drug user who presents with a temperature greater than 38°C (100.4°F) and a viral-like illness can be discharged home with close followup.
E. Left-sided endocarditis is more amenable to antibiotic therapy than right-sided disease.

109.2. Which of the following is correct concerning the purity of "street drugs"?

A. The sophistication of clandestine chemists is such that impurities are rarely if ever present.
B. The healthcare provider must always assume the presence of contaminants in samples injected by substance users.
C. Lidocaine is rarely added to cocaine before street sale, as the substance user would recognize its presence and not purchase additional samples.
D. Heavy metals are never found in "street drugs."
E. Law enforcement officers investigating a clandestine laboratory do not require special hazardous materials training, as the area is usually cleared of dangerous substances by the clandestine chemist.

109.3. Epidemiologic data indicate which of the following to be true?

A. Heroin-related episodes have decreased by 12% over the last 2 years.
B. Since 1990, marijuana-related episodes have increased 200%.
C. The Drug Abuse Warning Network collects data from the emergency department and the inpatient medical records.
D. Drug-related episodes as recorded by the Drug Abuse Warning Network pertain only to illicit drug use.
E. The rate of illicit drug use among youths fell in 1995 for the first time in 5 years.

109.4. Which of the following is true concerning the medical complications of substance use?

A. Early diagnosis of necrotizing fasciitis is easily made because of the presence of skin necrosis.
B. A groin abscess can be drained in the emergency department without angiography if there is no pulsation present.
C. Cotton or cigarette filters are rarely used today to filter material before injection.

D. The term "pocket shot" refers to the injection of drugs into the supraclavicular fossa in an attempt to hit the jugular, subclavian, or brachio-cephalic vein.

E. Intranasal heroin, as opposed to its intravenous administration, is substantially less addictive.

109.5. In the evaluation of the traumatized substance user, which of the following is correct?

A. A significant number of adolescents evaluated for trauma-related injuries have screens positive for alcohol or drugs of abuse.

B. Substance use in the elderly is never a cause of motor vehicle collisions.

C. The Drug Abuse Warning Network overreports drug-related trauma.

D. Substance use plays a role in thermal injury but not spinal cord injury.

E. Cocaine use was found in 70% of New York City residents who had fatal injuries.

109.6. Which of the following is correct concerning mental illness in the substance user?

A. Comorbidity is common in the substance-using population.

B. A reliable psychiatric diagnosis requires a 2-day period of abstinence to eliminate the potential for concurrent intoxication or withdrawal.

C. In patients with a dual diagnosis, outpatient care is preferable to inpatient therapy.

D. For many reasons, the psychiatric history provided by a substance user is generally accurate.

E. Substance use does not contribute to the risk of developing psychiatric disorders.

109.7. Which of the following is correct concerning substance users?

A. The vast majority of substance users meet the definition of substance abusers.

B. It is estimated that 5% of tax dollars in New York City cover substance use.

C. Substance abuse behaviors include recurrent substance-related legal problems and the inability to fulfill important roles.

D. A high school student who drives under the influence of alcohol would be labeled a drug abuser.

E. Substance dependence applies only to alcohol and illicit drug use.

109.8. Concerning infectious diseases in the substance user, which of the following is correct?

A. Tetanus cannot occur in substance users because immunizations are readily available.

B. Needle exchange and bleach treatment are not of benefit in the control of viral hepatitis.

C. Surgery is rarely indicated in the management of mycotic aneurysms, as antibiotics cause prompt resolution of the arterial pathology.

D. All intravenous drug users with a fever greater than 38°C (100.4°F) require hospital admission to exclude endocarditis.

E. Malaria has not been associated with parenteral drug use since the 1930s.

109.9. Concerning the medical care of substance users, which of the following is true?

A. Substance use is often unrecognized by physicians

B. The risk of pulmonary tuberculosis is low in substance users.

C. Crack has not been associated with an increased risk of sexually transmitted diseases.

D. The metabolism of methadone is not affected by other drugs.

E. The pharmacologic management of cocaine addiction is highly effective.

109.10. Concerning the evaluation of patients participating in injection drug use, which of the following is true?

A. Close living arrangements and malnutrition are the main causes of viral transmission in these patients.

B. Tap water is rarely used to dissolve drugs and rinse syringes.

C. Bleach must never be used to disinfect syringes before injection, as minute quantities remaining in the syringe will cause death in the injecting patient.

D. Access to sterile needles and syringes is restricted by laws requiring a prescription for their sale and drug-paraphernalia laws that make it illegal to possess any apparatus used in the administration of illegal drugs.

E. Household bleach is ineffective in killing the hepatitis B virus.

CHAPTER **110**

HEALTHCARE WORKERS

110.1. What is the minimum effective concentration for glutaraldehyde to be used as an effective disinfectant for hospital equipment?

A. 1%
B. 5%
C. 25%
D. 33%
E. 99%

110.2. Which of the following groups of patients have the highest incidence and prevalence of severe latex reactions?

A. Intubated patients
B. Patients with neuroblastomas
C. Children with congenital heart defects
D. Children with spina bifida
E. Patients with lupus erythematosus

110.3. Which of the following materials is implicated in the sensitization of exposed workers and associated with the development of occupationally related asthma, especially in chronic care facilities?

A. Latex
B. Vinyl
C. Mucomyst
D. Psyllium
E. Silver

110.4. Which group of physicians are most likely to report all types of self drug use and current self-treatment ?

A. Obstetricians
B. Surgeons
C. Family practitoners
D. Psychiatrists
E. Dermatologists

110.5. Hospital personnel should be encouraged to avoid workplace exposure to which drug before and during pregnancy as well as during lactation?

A. Acetaminophen
B. Ribavirin
C. ACE inhibitors
D. 100% oxygen
E. Thioethers

110.6. Formaldehyde is generally found in the hospital setting as an aqueous methanolic solution known as formalin. Formalin is an efficient agent against which of the following?

A. Spores
B. *Mycobacterium tuberculosis*
C. Viruses
D. Bacteria
E. All of the above

110.7. Laboratory animal allergy (LAA) is a clinical syndrome characterized by which of the following?

A. Rhinitis, upper airway inflammation, and occasionally bronchospasm
B. Rhinitis, uveitis, arthritis
C. Airway irritation, cough, sneezing
D. Shortness of breath, watery eyes, coryza
E. Rash, rhinitis, photophobia

110.8. Which of the following is correct with regard to resident physicians' use of psychoactive substances?

A. It is lower than among similar age groups in the general population.
B. It is the same as among similar age groups in the general population.
C. It is higher than among similar age groups in the general population.
D. This issue has yet to be studied.
E. There is no clinical problem.

110.9. The broadest level of OSHA communication is considered which of the following?

A. The Hazard Communication Standard
B. Community right-to know standard
C. SARA legislation
D. The Healthy Worker Act
E. HAZWOPER legislation

110.10. Which of the following ocular effects is associated with exposure to ethylene oxide?

A. Hyphema
B. Cataract formation
C. Conjunctivitis
D. Lid edema
E. Hordeolum formation

CHAPTER **111**

FARM TOXICOLOGY

111.1. Which of the following neurologic effects does not occur after organic phosphorus pesticide poisoning?

A. Alzheimer disease
B. Memory deficits
C. Depression
D. Paralysis
E. Peripheral neuropathy

111.2. Which class of pesticides is responsible for the most hospitalizations and deaths?

A. Gaseous fumigants
B. Organochlorine insecticides
C. Organic phosphorus insecticides
D. Herbicides
E. Long-acting anticoagulant rodenticides

111.3. Which one of the following is not a mechanism by which organic phosphorus pesticides alter respiration?

A. Bronchospasm
B. Bronchorrhea
C. Central depression of the respiratory drive
D. Acute lung injury
E. Weakness of respiratory muscles

111.4. Pulmonary fibrosis may theoretically result from each of the following routes of exposure to paraquat except which one?

A. Ingestion
B. Inhalation
C. Dermal absorption
D. Intraperitoneal
E. Intravenous

111.5. A farmer who enters an improperly aerated silo and develops pulmonary toxicity was exposed to which gas?

A. Nitrogen dioxide
B. Hydrogen chloride
C. Hydrogen cyanide
D. Phosgene
E. Endotoxin

111.6. Manure pit fatalities are caused by which toxin?

A. Methane
B. Carbon monoxide
C. Phosgene
D. Hydrogen sulfide
E. Ammonia

111.7. What is the most common cause of allergic contact dermatitis in farmers?

A. Latex
B. Carbamate insecticides
C. Animal dander
D. Poison ivy/oak
E. Fungicides

111.8. Clinical effects of grain dust exposure include which of the following?

A. Acute febrile reactions
B. Skin irritation
C. Hypersensitivity pneumonitis
D. Sore throat
E. Pneumonia

111.9. Integrated pest management emphasizes which of the following?

A. Annual crop rotation
B. Surveillance of the quality of pest damage and a measured response
C. Pesticide application pre- and postemergence
D. Use of only biologic agents for pest control
E. Introducing beneficial insects that kill harmful insects

111.10. Which chemical causes the most severe eye injuries in farmers?

A. Anhydrous ammonia
B. Carbamates
C. Gasoline
D. Hydraulic fluid
E. Grain dust

CHAPTER **112**

SPORTS TOXICOLOGY

112.1. The following is true about testosterone esters:

A. They must be given orally
B. They are best given early in the menstrual cycle
C. They are used as "bridging therapy"
D. They are not well detected by current laboratory methods
E. They cause most of the side effects seen in steroid users.

112.2. Plateauing, stacking, and cycling refer to the following:

A. Officially recognized Olympic sports
B. Methods of using androgenic anabolic steroids
C. Effects of growth hormone
D. Methods of using erythropoietin
E. Androgenic anabolic side effects

112.3. Which one of the following statements is true of clenbuterol?

A. It is the one drug of its class allowed by current Olympic Committee guidelines.
B. It is most often inhaled

C. It causes acne
D. It is a β-adrenergic agonist
E. It is a β-adrenergic antagonist

112.4. Which of the following drugs may be used as a masking agent?

A. Terbutaline
B. Furosemide
C. Creatine
D. Clenbuterol
E. Penicillin

112.5. Bromontan is best characterized as

A. β-Adrenergic antagonist
B. Androgenic anabolic steroid
C. Growth hormone antagonist
D. Masking agent
E. Diuretic

112.6. The following is true about alkylated anabolic androgenic steroids.

A. They must be injected intramuscularly to avoid detection
B. They may be administered orally
C. They have very few side effects because they are rarely used.
D. They are classified as "restricted except at doctors permisssion" by the IOC
E. Testosterone propionate is an alkylated androgen.

112.7. The following statement is true of creatine:

A. It may increase urinary creatinine excretion.
B. It causes weight loss.
C. Carbohydrate interferes with the absorption.
D. It is uncommonly used because of its exorbitant cost.
E. It causes "gymnasium acne."

112.8. A reported effect of insulinlike growth factor (IGF-1) is:

A. Hyperglycemia
B. Hypoglycemia
C. Virilization
D. Testicular atrophy
E. Weight loss

112.9. The following is true about perfluorocarbons:

A. They are difficult to use because crossmatching is required.
B. They increase the viscosity of blood
C. They are commonly contaminated with infectious materials

D. Dose-related thrombocytopenia is transient
E. They are perceived by the immune system as foreign substances

112.10. The following are true about chromium picolinate except:

A. It acts as a cofactor for insulin.
B. It is reported to cause anemia in high doses.
C. Renal insufficiency is a reported complication of use.
D. Carbohydrate is thought to enhance chromium absorption.
E. Its use is associated with increased risk of colon cancer.

CHAPTER **113**

PSYCHOSOCIAL PRINCIPLES IN ASSESSMENT AND INTERVENTION

113.1. Health care services in the United States are being reorganized into which of the following?

A. Large, monolithic institutions
B. Small family practice offices
C. Free-standing emergency and urgent care centers
D. Integrated health care networks
E. A national health system

113.2. Which is the term that best describes evaluation of the interaction of internal and external aspects of a person's life including familial and socioeconomic factors?

A. Paradigm of healthcare
B. Psychosocial assessment
C. Dysfunction and maladaptation scale
D. Developmental milestones
E. Ego function

113.3. The establishment of social work services in hospitals in the United States occurred during which time period?

A. 1855–1865
B. 1890–1900
C. 1900–1910
D. 1925–1935
E. 1945–1955

113.4. Which of the following was not a reason for the introduction of social service workers into hospitals?

A. Awareness of a correlation between social factors and serious health problems
B. To increase the use of inpatient hospital services
C. To make home visits to better understand the living situations of patients and families
D. To develop community resources to help meet the concrete needs of patients
E. To provide health education and supportive services

113.5. Why are obtaining a substantive alcohol and drug use history and providing referrals for substance abuse treatment as needed important in an emergency department?

A. Substance abuse is a leading cause of traffic injuries.
B. Most people drink socially.
C. Illegal drugs can sometimes include poisonous dilutants.
D. The patient may have never discussed this issue with a health professional.
E. Substances may cause hallucinations.

113.6. Substance abuse in women may be related to which of the following?

A. Socioeconomic level
B. Educational level
C. Marital status
D. Domestic violence
E. Region of residence

113.7. Drug use during pregnancy is best managed by which of the following?

A. The obstetrician or nurse/midwife
B. Admission to a detoxification program
C. Placing the mother in detention
D. Providing home health services
E. Early identification and coordination of prenatal care, drug treatment, parenting education, and social services

113.8. Which of the following is a key factor in the involvement of families with the child welfare system?

A. Number of children in the family
B. Ethnicity
C. Parental substance abuse
D. Living in urban areas
E. Educational level of parents

113.9. Which of the following is considered a major obstacle to the acknowledgment of drug or alcohol use by female substance users?

A. Difference in physiologic responses of women to substances
B. Mental illness among female substance abusers
C. Fear of the loss of their children
D. Risk of arrest and incarceration
E. Risk of losing public assistance

113.10. Which of the following is not a reason that social work services for substance users and other high-risk patients are needed in emergency departments?

A. To provide psychosocial assessments
B. To provide crisis intervention and counseling
C. To develop linkages with community agencies
D. To facilitate safe discharge plans and effective referrals for continuing care
E. To arrange for language interpreters

CHAPTER **114**

PSYCHIATRIC PRINCIPLES

114.1. Which of the following is the most common method for suicide in both sexes?

A. Drug overdose
B. Hanging
C. Deliberate gunshot wound
D. Carbon monoxide poisoning
E. Jumping from a height

114.2. What percentage of persons who complete suicide give some warning of their intention?

A. None
B. 10%
C. 25 to 33%
D. over 50%
E. over 90%

114.3. Major mental illness is found to be a factor in what percentage of adult suicides?

A. 5 to 10%
B. 33%
C. 50%
D. 75%
E. over 90%

114.4. Which of the following statements regarding the assessment of the suicidal patient is false?

A. The patient may require an individual aide for constant observation to prevent further self-injury.

B. Acute intoxication can interfere with the identification of underlying psychiatric illness.
C. Direct questions about suicidal ideation can cause the patient to become more impulsive and self-injurious.
D. Patients may require involuntary hospitalization.
E. The presence of depressive illness and/or alcoholism increases the risk of suicide.

114.5. Which of the following is true regarding the demographics of completed suicide?

A. Black men have a higher suicide rate than white men.
B. Adolescent suicide rates are declining in this country.
C. The suicide rate among white women is equivalent to that of black women.
D. Suicide is more common in men than in women.
E. The suicide rate in the United States has increased dramatically in the last decade.

114.6. All of the following agents are useful in the treatment of aggressive patients *except* which agent?

A. Diazepam
B. Lorazepam
C. Haloperidol
D. Phenobarbital
E. Droperidol

114.7. Which of the following lowers the seizure threshold?

A. Phenytoin
B. Secobarbital
C. Haloperidol
D. Alprazolam
E. Diazepam

114.8. Which of the following is not a useful intervention in the management of delirium?

A. Chemical sedation
B. Seclusion
C. Verbal reassurance
D. Restraint
E. Diagnostic testing to determine causation

114.9. When can confidentiality be breached by a physician?

A. The patient's employer needs to know a date of return to work.
B. The patient's family threatens to sue if information is not released.

C. The disclosure is in the interest of protecting the patient or other third party from further harm or decline.
D. The patient is a prominent person and law enforcement is making an inquiry.
E. The patient's case history is unique enough to warrant a published case report.

114.10. Which of the following are risk factors for suicide?

A. Male gender
B. Prior suicide attempts
C. Presence of alcoholism
D. Depressive illness
E. All of the above

CHAPTER **115**

NURSING PRINCIPLES

115.1. Which of the following is considered a function of triage?

A. Provide primary care
B. Sort acuity levels and identify the critically ill based on patient complaint and objective assessment
C. Do a total patient assessment
D. Administer all medications
E. Register the patient and secure insurance information

115.2. What is the initial intervention for a patient presenting unresponsive with pinpoint pupils, agonal respirations, and a fresh puncture wound at a venous site?

A. Naloxone
B. IV insertion
C. Utilization of a bag-valve-mask device with cervical spine stabilization and 100% oxygen
D. Cardiopulmonary resuscitation
E. None of the above

115.3. Which of the following is most important to administer to a combative patient who has an altered mental status and no focal findings?

A. Thiamine
B. $D_{50}W$
C. Oxygen
D. All of the above
E. None of the above

115.4. When a patient arrives with an unknown ingestion, which of the following should the nurse routinely do?

    A. Be alert to concomitant injuries
    B. Notify the poison center
    C. Use all five senses for clues to the nature of the ingestion
    D. Secure vital signs; initiate pulse oximetry
    E. All of the above

115.5. Which of the following are not functions of the poison center staff?

    A. Specialist advice regarding patient management
    B. Epidemiologic and research data
    C. Information about trends and fads in drug abuse
    D. Formal hospital staff education through didactic presentations
    E. All of the above

115.6. When inserting an orogastric tube for gastric lavage, which is the best position in which to place the patient?

    A. Left-lateral decubitus
    B. Supine
    C. Prone
    D. Standing
    E. High Fowler

115.7. Physical restraint should not be performed under which of these situations?

    A. In situations where the patient is a danger to himself or others
    B. If verbal reassurance and "limit setting" have failed to diminish patient behavior to a safe level
    C. In situations where the ingestion of a substance has impaired the patient's ability to understand the nature of his illness and his behavior thwarts necessary resusitative efforts
    D. All of the above
    E. None of the above

115.8. Pulse oximetry might not be helpful in assessing oxygenation in the patient with a toxic ingestion of which of the following chemicals?

    A. Cyanide
    B. Iron
    C. Cocaine
    D. Heroin
    E. β-Adrenergic antagonists

115.9. Which of the following statements regarding physical restraints is true?

    A. Should be leather or metal
    B. Should be padded, tied securely with a slip knot, with pulse checks performed for perfusion adequacy at least hourly
    C. Should be applied at no less than four points with legs separated, right upper and lower extremities restrained to the right side of the stretcher, left upper and lower extremities restrained to the left side of the stretcher
    D. Must be tied in a tight double knot for security
    E. Should be applied to the feet only

115.10. The specific treatment for a patient with a toxic serum level of acetaminophen is which of the following antidotes?

    A. Physostigmine
    B. Disulfiram
    C. *N*-Acetylcysteine
    D. Sodium thiosulfate
    E. Deferoxamine

CHAPTER **116**

POISON INFORMATION CENTERS AND POISON EPIDEMIOLOGY

116.1. Which of the following statements is most representative of the American Association of Poison Control Centers (AAPCC) Toxic Exposure Surveillance System (TESS) database?

    A. TESS data correlate well with fatal poisoning cases from medical examiners.
    B. TESS data correlate well with hospital discharge data for poisoning admission.
    C. TESS data correlate well with substance abuse data from the Drug Abuse Warning Network (DAWN).
    D. TESS data correlate well with occupational exposures reported to legislative authorities.
    E. None of the above

116.2. Appropriate use of the telephone services provided by poison centers has been demonstrated to do which of the following?

    A. Reduce mortality from childhood poisoning
    B. Reduce mortality from intentional adult exposures
    C. Prevent unnecessary utilization of health care services

D. Prevent recurrent poisoning in the home
E. Reduce morbidity following a known toxic exposure

116.3. Which of the following statements is true of poisoning epidemiology?

A. Poisoning is the third most frequent cause of injury-related fatalities
B. Poisoning is the third most frequent cause of fatalities.
C. Poisoning is the 10th most frequent cause of injury-related fatalities.
D. Poisoning is the 10th most frequent cause of fatalities.
E. Poisoning fatality is so uncommon that it is not listed in the top 10 causes of either all fatalities or injury-related fatalities.

116.4. In order for a substance to be classified as "nontoxic" which of the following factors is required?

A. The exposure must be unintentional.
B. The exposed individual must be free of symptoms.
C. The product must be absolutely identified.
D. Only a single product may be involved.
E. All of the above are correct.

116.5. The national average cost of a poison center responding to a single phone call is closest to which amount?

A. $3.50
B. $35.00
C. $350.00
D. $10.00
E. $100.00

CHAPTER **117**

ADVERSE DRUG EVENTS

117.1. Which of the following is not typically part of the drug development process before FDA approval?

A. Animal toxicology testing
B. Submission of an Investigation New Drug application to the FDA
C. Phase 1 testing in humans to prove the safety of the drug
D. Phase 3 testing to determine efficacy
E. Phase 5 testing to determine the best marketing strategy

117.2. MedWatch is the spontaneous reporting system developed by FDA. Which of the following are not among its goals?

A. To increase awareness of drug- and device-induced disease
B. To clarify what should (and should not) be reported to the agency
C. To provide a source of income for FDA
D. To make it easier to report adverse effects by creating a single system for health professionals to use in reporting adverse events and product problems to the agency
E. To provide regular feedback to the health care community about safety issues involving medical products

117.3. Which of the following is not generally considered in the recognition and diagnosis of drug-induced disease?

A. A temporal relationship
B. Prior reports of adverse effects
C. Biologic plausibility
D. Excessive exposure
E. Other likely causes

117.4. Which of the following is not a major cause of recall or withdrawal of drugs from the market in the United States?

A. Prolongation of the QTc interval
B. Hepatotoxicity
C. Contamination/adulteration
D. Drug-drug interactions
E. Carcinogenesis

117.5. Which of the following statement is correct about medical errors?

A. Medical errors, by definition, only occur to inpatients.
B. Preventable errors account for only a minority of all medical errors.
C. Most errors occur because healthcare providers are lazy
D. The Institute of Medicine report suggests that errors are a leading cause of death.
E. The only way to prevent errors is to computerize all medical care.

117.6. Which of the following qualities does not suggest that an adverse event is serious nor that the event requires reporting to MedWatch?

A. Death of a patient is suspected to be direct result of the event.
B. Disability resulted from the event.

C. Significant expense is required to rectify the event.

D. A congenital abnormality occurred resultant to exposure to a drug.

E. An antidote was administered following overdose in order to save the patient's life.

117.7. Which of the following statements regarding the current status of the FDA is correct?

A. The accelerated approval track has resulted in a substantially higher proportion of drug withdrawals due to safety issues.

B. The FDA provides incentives to companies that market drugs to treat rare diseases.

C. The FDA cannot charge manufacturers a fee for review of their new drug applications.

D. The FDA is powerless to regulate dietary supplements.

E. The FDA sponsors MedWatch, a mandatory reporting system, and has the authority to levy fines for failure to report.

117.8. Which of the following is not a benefit of having clinical toxicologists involved in the care of patients?

A. By observing for clusters or trends, they may identify drug-induced disease.

B. They take thorough medication and dietary supplement use histories.

C. They provide education concerning adverse medication events to other healthcare providers.

D. They prevent nearly all medication errors.

E. They work as or with administrators to identify potential problems early in their course.

117.9. Which of the following events in the history of federal drug regulation is correctly paired:

A. Food, Drug and Cosmetic Act, 1938: high incidence of allergy to sulfa antibiotics

B. Regulatory stance prevented adverse drug events: thalidomide

C. Aggressive drug removal strategy by the FDA: terfenadine

D. Institute of Medicine report: the importance of drug errors is overrated.

E. MedWatch: phase II drug trials.

117.10. Which of the following is a major limitation of the current MedWatch system?

A. It relies exclusively on spontaneous reporting.

B. It collects information only about the number of exposures ("denominator").

C. It covers both medications and devices, making its audience too broad.

D. It does not receive widespread support among medical organizations.

E. It cannot be a "hypothesis generating" system.

CHAPTER **118**

RISK MANAGEMENT AND LEGAL PRINCIPLES

118.1. What should the ED physician do when a patient suffering from drug-related impaired judgment refuses treatment and is aggressively trying to leave the ED?

A. Review the hospital policy on refusal of treatment

B. Allow the patient to leave the ED

C. Restrain the patient

D. Contact the Risk Management Department

E. Contact a family member

118.2. Which statement is not included in the definition of informed consent?

A. The patient must comprehend the risks and benefits associated with the treatment.

B. The patient must comprehend the risks of not receiving treatment.

C. The patient must comprehend even exceptionally rare risks of refusing therapy.

D. The patient must comprehend possible alternative treatments and their potential risks.

E. Personal autonomy and self-determination are two basic principles of informed consent.

118.3. Which of the following is not a correct action by an emergency physician when confronted with a patient who refuses critical medical care?

A. Contacting the psychiatric consultant.

B. Attempting to notify the patient's family.

C. Temporarily detaining the patient while inquiring about patient's understanding the necessity of treatment.

D. Agreeing to the patient's refusal of treatment without further inquiry.

E. Contact hospital security in the event that the patient becomes agitated.

118.4. Which of the following circumstances does not justify the forcible restraint of a patient?

A. A patient with severely impaired judgment because of drug ingestion who has a life-threatening medical complication

B. A chronic alcoholic patient who claims to have bumped his head, is alert and oriented, and does not want to wait to be seen

C. A patient with a heroin overdose who is resuscitated with naloxone and now has a normal mental status who demands to be released

D. A 60-year-old president of a major corporation who refuses immediate admission despite a suicide attempt with acetaminophen

E. A 16-year-old brought in by police for bizarre behavior who demands to be released

118.5. Which of the following is not necessary to prove a case of medical malpractice against an emergency physician?

A. A departure from accepted emergency department practice

B. A direct causal relationship between departure from care and injury

C. An inadequately documented medical record

D. A departure from the standard of care for the type of ED procedure involved

E. Negligent conduct that results in an injury

118.6. Which of the following does not represent poor medical record documentation from a risk management perspective?

A. Crossing out a hematocrit value with a magic marker

B. Inserting an accurate patient observation on the ED record 3 days after discharge without noting the time and date of entry

C. Describing with specificity the patient's angry facial expression

D. Describing with specificity the patient's symptoms and complaints

E. Physician notes that subjectively describe the patient's behavior

118.7. In which of the following scenarios should a "Do Not Resuscitate" request be honored?

A. A severely injured trauma victim whispers to a physician that he/she does not want resuscitation.

B. The mother of a 14-year-old child advises the emergency physician that her child suffering massive internal bleeding should not be resuscitated.

C. A nursing home patient with amyotrophic lateral sclerosis who has a properly prepared DNR order has an unexpected respiratory arrest while in the emergency department.

D. A 65-year-old patient presents to the emergency department in cardiac arrest. The daugh-

ter of the patient states that her father verbally expressed a desire not to be resuscitated.

E. The husband of a 40-year-old woman with a malignant brain tumor requests a DNR order for his wife.

118.8. The appropriate method by which to obtain an evidentiary blood specimen collection includes all of the following except which?

A. The specimen must be obtained in full view of a witness.

B. An obtunded suspect in a criminal investigation cannot have a blood specimen drawn until he/she is lucid and willing to consent to having his/her blood drawn.

C. Every person involved in the handling of the specimen must be identified.

D. Each step of the process and transport of the specimen must be documented without a break in the custody of the specimen.

E. Every individual who handles the specimen should sign the accompanying document.

118.9. In which of the following scenarios it is unacceptable to discharge a patient with an elevated blood alcohol level?

A. If a chronic alcoholic with a blood alcohol level above the legal limit is not impaired.

B. If a previously intoxicated patient is accompanied by family or friends.

C. If the patient is ambulatory, oriented, and unaccompanied.

D. If the patient is in the custody of law enforcement officials.

E. If the patient is known to the emergency department and is fully oriented, and transportation has been arranged to the patient's home.

118.10. When treating a patient who has abused illicit drugs, alcohol, or medications, sound risk management principles would not include which of the following?

A. A patient assessment that includes the past medical history, allergies, medications, and history of drug or alcohol abuse

B. The recording of vital signs

C. Documented discharge instructions that tell the patient which activities to avoid and what symptoms to look out for

D. Psychiatric consultation for patients suspected of suicidal intent or abusing medication

E. A subjective interpretation of the patient's complaint along with a presumptive diagnosis

CHAPTER **119**

POSTMORTEM TOXICOLOGY

119.1. Which of the following is not associated with a decrease in the measured postmortem xenobiotic blood concentrations from the time of death to the time of autopsy?

    A. Postmortem metabolism
    B. Xenobiotics with a large V_d
    C. Labile xenobiotics in putrefying tissue
    D. Glucose obtain in blood from the right femoral vein
    E. None of the above

119.2. Which of the following is most consistent with postmortem production of ethanol?

    A. A blood concentration of 0.4 mg/dL, and a vitreous concentration of 0.2 mg/dL, in a body without gross evidence of putrefaction
    B. A blood concentration of 0.2 mg/dL; a vitreous concentration of 0.2 mg/dL; and postmortem urine concentration of 0.1 mg/dl in a body without gross evidence of putrefaction
    C. A body with gross evidence of putrefactive changes with a blood ethanol concentration of 0.2 mg/dL
    D. A negative blood ethanol with a vitreous concentration of 0.2 mg/dL
    E. A negative blood ethanol with an aqueous concentration of 0.2 mg/dL.

119.3. Which one of the following represents a cause of death?

    A. Cardiorespiratory arrest secondary to carbon monoxide toxicity
    B. Suicide by exposure to carbon monoxide
    C. Homicide by strychnine poisoning
    D. Unintentional overdose of heroin
    E. Suicide by overdose of heroin

119.4. A sample of vitreous is obtained 2 days after death in a body in the early postmortem interval. The creatinine returns at 6.9 mg/dL, and the serum potassium at 7.5 mEq/L. Which of the following can be assumed?

    A. Cardiorespiratory arrest secondary to hyperkalemia
    B. Nothing, as creatinine and potassium are unreliable in the postmortem period
    C. The individual had some evidence of antemortem renal failure.

    D. Postmortem redistribution of creatinine and potassium
    E. A laboratory error

119.5. A larva identified on an exhumed body contains qualitative evidence of phenobarbital. What can be presumed?

    A. Phenobarbital is the cause of death
    B. Phenobarbital was present in the body before death
    C. Postmortem production of phenobarbital
    D. Phenobarbital must be a contaminant in the field
    E. Laboratory contamination

119.6. A body deposited directly into soil is discovered and exhumed. Arsenic is identified in the remains in the hair and nails. What can be safely presumed?

    A. Arsenic is the cause of death.
    B. The manner of death is suspicious for arsenic poisoning
    C. Nothing without further information
    D. Arsenic poisoning is the cause of death only if other causes can not be identified on autopsy
    E. None of the above

119.7. After a house fire, three badly burned bodies are found in the basement. Samples of right heart blood are available from only one body. It contains a carboxyhemoglobin concentration of 2%. What can be presumed?

    A. That all three died by cardiac arrest caused by the fire.
    B. Smoke inhalation killed the individual from whom the blood sample was obtained.
    C. Death of the individual with a carboxyhemoglobin concentration of 2% is suspicious for a cause of death different from the fire.
    D. Carbon monoxide is a by-product of postmortem hemoglobin metabolism.
    E. The patients were drunk before death.

119.8. A patient is found dead with a postmortem nortryptiline blood concentration of 500 ng/mL. What information can refute death from tricyclic antidepressant overdose?

    A. Gastric concentration of zero.
    B. Last therapeutic dose observed 90 minutes before death
    C. A body that has evidence of putrefaction
    D. All of the above
    E. None of the above

119.9. Which of the following body fluids is not typically useful for postmortem drug analysis?

   A. Vitreous humor
   B. Urine
   C. Feces
   D. Nails
   E. Lungs

119.10. Which of the following is true regarding the interpretation of postmortem drug levels?

   A. Analysis requires simple comparison of a tissue level to a nomogram of normal values.
   B. That analysis can be performed years after death suggests that proper tissue handling is rarely important.
   C. Nearly all drugs are stable in body fluid after death since metabolism ceases instantly.
   D. The clinical circumstances surrounding death and the patients clincal history are critical to proper interpretation.
   E. It is generally up to the primary care provider for the decedent to interpret the postmortem laboratory value.

CHAPTER **120**

PRINCIPLES OF EPIDEMIOLOGY AND RESEARCH DESIGN

120.1. In developing a questionnaire to use as a screening test to choose young children for targeted blood lead level testing, which of the following characteristics would be most desirable of the questionnaire?

   A. Elaborate testing procedures
   B. High cost
   C. High sensitivity
   D. Low specificity
   E. Susceptibility to information bias

120.2. The charts of children previously admitted to the hospital for possible tricyclic antidepressant ingestion were identified. Electrocardiographs from those patients suffering seizures were compared to those of an equal number of children without seizures in an effort to find electrocardiographic predictors of toxicity. This is an example of what type of study?

   A. Analysis of secular trends
   B. Case-control
   C. Case report
   D. Clinical trial
   E. Cohort study

120.3. A group of children with histories of tricyclic antidepressant (TCA) ingestion was compared to a group of control children with regard to electrocardiographic findings. An abnormal terminal 40-millisecond QRS vector between 120 and 270° (T40msecQRS) was found to have a sensitivity of 38% and a specificity of 74% of predicting TCA exposure. Based on this information, which of the following statements is most correct?

   A. Children had an abnormal T40msec QRS only if they actually overdosed on TCAs.
   B. The ECG has no value in the evaluation of pediatric TCA exposures.
   C. The high specificity excludes the presence of bias within the study.
   D. The majority of children with a history of TCA ingestion had a normal T40msec QRS.
   E. Seventy-four percent of normal children had an abnormal T40msec QRS.

120.4. Although case reports of deaths after verapamil overdoses exist, investigators find that 0 of 20 children with histories of verapamil ingestion became critically ill. Before concluding that pediatric verapamil overdoses are medically benign, which of the following would be most useful to examine in the study?

   A. Academic reputation of the senior author
   B. Confidence interval around the risk estimate
   C. Presence or absence of other ingested drugs among subjects
   D. Race of the enrolled study subjects
   E. Statistical significance of the result as reported by a *p*-value

120.5. Investigators construct a clinical trial to study the utility of hyperbaric oxygen in the prevention of delayed neurologic sequelae from carbon monoxide poisoning. Type I (α) error is set at 5%, and power is set by the investigators at 80%. The study fails to detect statistical difference between treated and untreated groups. Which of the following statements is most correct?

   A. A case-control study would be expected to provide more convincing evidence.
   B. Power calculations are best done after completion of a study.
   C. The low type I error minimized the influence of bias on the study.
   D. There is a 5% chance that the investigators failed to detect a true difference between treatment groups.
   E. There is a 20% chance that the investigators failed to detect a true difference between treatment groups.

120.6. In a retrospective study comparing physostigmine to diazepam for the treatment of anticholinergic delirium, the investigators search the medical records more vigorously to identify complications among the diazepam group than they do the physostigmine group. This is an example of what type of methodologic problem?

    A. Confounding
    B. Information bias
    C. Loss to follow-up
    D. Misclassification bias
    E. Selection bias

120.7. In a cohort study of coffee drinking it is found that coffee drinkers have a statistically significant increased rate of lung cancer. When controlled for cigarette smoking, coffee drinking no longer results in increased risk of lung cancer. In this study, cigarette smoking is an example of what epidemiologic phenomenon?

    A. Confounding
    B. Placebo effect
    C. Random variation
    D. Type I (α) error
    E. Type II (β) error

120.8. A study reports an odds ratio of 0.5. If the study is unbiased, this indicates which of the following?

    A. The results of the study are statistically significant.
    B. The risk of disease among those exposed is greater than the risk among those unexposed.
    C. The risk of disease among those unexposed is greater than the risk among those exposed.

    D. The study had a 5% chance of failing to find a significant result.
    E. The study had a 50% chance of finding a significant result.

120.9. The relationship between environmental lead exposure and systolic blood pressure is studied in a cohort study of 18,000 men. The mean SBP in lead-exposed subjects is 117 mm Hg, and the mean SBP in unexposed subjects is 119 mm Hg. This is found to be statistically significant with a p-value of 0.048. Which of the following conclusions is most accurate from this data?

    A. The large sample size likely allowed for statistical significance of this finding.
    B. Men exposed to lead should be treated with diuretics.
    C. The 95% confidence intervals around the two means overlap one another.
    D. No confounding variables exist with regards to this study.
    E. The statistical analysis was performed incorrectly.

120.10. A comparison of poison center data collected by medical examiners suggests that fewer than 10% of fatal poisonings are reported to poison centers. This is an example of which of the following?

    A. Confounding
    B. Effect modification
    C. Misclassification bias
    D. Placebo effect
    E. Selection bias

ANSWERS

CHAPTER **1**

HISTORICAL PRINCIPLES AND PERSPECTIVES

1.1. Answer: E   The term toxicology appears to be derived from two Greek terms: *toxikos* ("bow") and *toxikon* ("poison into which arrowheads are dipped"). Cave paintings of arrowheads and spearheads reveal that these weapons may have been crafted with small depressions at the end to hold poison.

American Heritage Dictionary, 2nd college ed. Boston, Houghton Mifflin, 1991.

1.2. Answer: C   Hemlock was the official poison used by the Greeks and was employed in the execution of Socrates.

Ober WB: Did Socrates die of hemlock poisoning? NY State Med J 1977;77:254–258.

1.3. Answer: D   Paracelsus' study on the dose-response relationship is usually considered the beginning of the scientific approach to toxicology. He was the first to emphasize the chemical nature of toxic agents. He underscored the need to differentiate between the therapeutic and toxic properties of chemicals when he stated in his Third Defense, "What is there that is not poison? All things are poison and nothing [is] without poison. Solely the dose determines that a thing is not a poison."

Deichmann WB, Henschler D, Holmstedt B, Keil G: What is there that is not poison? A study of the Third Defense by Paracelsus. Arch Toxicol 1986;58:207–213.

1.4. Answer: A   The French physician Bonaventure Orfila (1787–1853) has been called the father of modern toxicology. He emphasized toxicology as a distinct scientific discipline separate from clinical medicine and pharmacology. He was an early medical-legal expert and championed the use of chemical analysis and autopsy material as evidence to prove that a poisoning had taken place. His treatise, *Traité des Poisons ou Toxicologie Générale,* first published in 1814, went through five editions and was regarded as the foundation of experimental and forensic toxicology.

Orfila MP: Traité des Poisons. Paris, Chez Crochard, 1814.

1.5. Answer: C   During the later part of the 19th century, cocaine was enthusiastically recommended as a treatment for opioid addiction. In 1884, Sigmund Freud wrote *Uber Cocaine,* advocat-

ing cocaine as an opium and morphine addiction cure as well as a treatment for fatigue and hysteria.

Karch SB: The history of cocaine toxicity. Hum Pathol 1989;20:1037–1039.

1.6. Answer: C   In 1902, Dr. Harvey W. Wiley organized a "poison squad" that consisted of a group of volunteers who did self-experiments on food preservatives. Revelations from the "poison squad" as well as the publication of Upton Sinclair's muckraking novel *The Jungle,* exposing the lack of hygienic practices in the meat-packing industry, led to support for legislative intervention that resulted in the passing of the 1906 Pure Food and Drugs Act.

Anderson OE: Pioneer statute: The Pure Food and Drugs Act of 1906. J Public Law 1964;13:189–196.

1.7. Answer: A   The "Marsh test," which qualitatively tests for the presence of arsenic, was one of the first analytic tests used to detect the presence of a poison. Developed by James Marsh, this test was first used in a criminal case in 1839 during the trial of Marie Lefarge who was accused of using arsenic to murder her husband.

Smith S: Poisons and poisoners through the ages. Medico-Legal J 1952:20:153–167.

1.8. Answer: A   The Federal Caustic Poison Act of 1927 was the first federal legislation specifically addressing household poisoning. Spearheaded by the efforts of Dr. Chevalier Jackson, an otolaryngologist who showed that unintentional exposures to household caustic agents were an increasingly frequent cause of severe gastrointestinal burns, the Act mandated that lye- and acid-containing products clearly display a "poison" warning label.

Taylor HM: A preliminary survey of the effect which lye legislation has had on the incidence of esophageal stricture. Ann Otolaryngol Rhinol Laryngol 1935;44:1157–1158.

1.9. Answer: D   Unlike the poison center movement in the United States, the early European poison centers focused on the development of strong centralized toxicology treatment centers. One of the first inpatient treatment centers dedicated to the care of poisoned patients opened in Paris in the 1950s.

Govaerts M: Poison control in Europe. Pediatr Clin North Am 1970;17:729–739.

1.10. Answer: C   A 1999 Institute of Medicine (IOM) report suggested that 44,000 to 98,000 fatalities each year in the United States were the result of medical errors including many preventable medication errors. The IOM report focused on the fact that errors usually resulted from system faults and not solely from the carelessness of individuals.

Kohn LT, Corrigan J, Donaldson MS, eds: To Err Is Human: Building a Safer Health System. Washington, DC, National Academy Press, 2000.

CHAPTER **2**

TOXICOLOGIC PLAGUES
AND DISASTERS IN HISTORY

2.1. Answer: A   Air pollution is a source of toxic gases that has caused significant disease and death. A dense smog in London in 1952 was responsible for 4000 deaths. High levels of sulfur dioxide likely contributed to this outcome.

Logan WPD: Mortality in the London fog incident, 1952. Lancet 1953;1:336–338.

2.2. Answer: E   A morphine/scopolamine combination therapy known as "twilight sleep" was heavily used in obstetric anesthesia during the early 20th century. During the 1990s hundreds of cases of anticholinergic poisoning among heroin users presented to East Coast emergency departments. This outbreak of anticholinergic poisoning was attributed to the use of heroin mixed with scopolamine, a combination reminiscent of the twilight sleep regimen.

Pitcock CD, Clark RB: From Fanny to Fernand: The development of consumerism in pain control during the birth process. Am J Obstet Gynecol 1992;167:581–587.

2.3. Answer: D   A toxic gas leak at the Union Carbide pesticide plant in Bhopal, India, in 1984 resulted in one of the greatest civilian toxic disasters in modern history. An unintended exothermic reaction at this carbaryl-producing plant caused the release of over 24,000 kg of methyl isocyanate gas. This gas was quickly dispersed through the air over the densely populated area surrounding the factory, resulting in at least 2500 deaths and 200,000 injuries.

Varma DR, Guest I: The Bhopal accident and methyl isocyanate toxicity. J Toxicol Environ Health 1993;40:513–529.

2.4. Answer: C   Agent Orange was widely used as a defoliant during the Vietnam War. This herbicide consists of a mixture of 2,4,5-trichlorophenoxyacetic acid (2,4,5-T) and 2,4-dichlorophenoxyacetic acid (2,4-D) as well as small amounts of a contaminant, 2,3,7,8-tetrachlorodibenzo-*p*-dioxin (TCDD), better known as dioxin. Although a higher incidence of skin cancers has been found in veterans who handled Agent Orange, other possible dioxin-related adverse health effects such as cancer, birth defects, and hepatic dysfunction have not been observed. An increase in non-Hodgkin lymphoma among Vietnam veterans has occurred, but this is not clearly attributable to herbicidal exposure.

DeStefano F: Effects of Agent Orange exposure. JAMA 1995;273: 1494.

2.5. Answer: E   During the 1920s and 1930s dermatologists and other physicians prescribed thallium acetate, both as pills and a topical ointment (trade name Koremlu®), to remove infected hair. A 1934 study found 692 cases of thallium toxicity after oral and topical application and 31 deaths after oral use.

Munch JC: Human thallotoxicois. JAMA 1934;102:1929–1934.

2.6. Answer: B   In September and October 1937, more than 100 deaths were associated with the use of one of the early sulfa preparations, Elixir of Sulfanilamide-Massengill, which contained 72% diethylene glycol as the vehicle for drug delivery. Little was known about diethylene glycol toxicity at the time, and many cases of renal failure and death occurred. As a result of this catastrophe, animal drug testing was mandated by the Food, Drug, and Cosmetic Act of 1938 to avoid similar tragedies in the future. Unfortunately, diethylene glycol continues to be sporadically used in other countries as a medicinal diluent, resulting in additional deaths in South Africa (1969), India (1986), Nigeria (1990), Bangladesh (1990–1992), and Haiti (1996).

Geiling EHK, Cannon PR: Pathological effects of elixir of sulfanilamide (diethylene glycol) poisoning: A clinical and experimental correlation—final report. JAMA 1938;111:919–926.

2.7. Answer: E   In 1989–1990, eosinophilia-myalgia syndrome developed in more than 1500 people who had taken L-tryptophan. These patients presented with sclerodermalike features and eosinophilia. All affected patients had ingested tryptophan produced by a single manufacturer. This manufacturer had recently introduced a new process involving genetically altered bacteria to improve tryptophan production. A contaminant produced by this process has been suggested as the etiologic agent of this syndrome.

Vargas J, Uitto J, Jimenez SA: The cause and pathogenesis of the eosinophilia-myalgia syndrome. Ann Intern Med 1992;116: 140–147.

2.8. Answer: C   In the late 19th and early 20th centuries, an increased incidence of mandibular necrosis occurred among workers in the match-making industry. The use of yellow phosphorus in the production process was thought to be the etiologic agent of this disorder—hence, "phossy jaw."

Hughes JP, Baron R, Buckland DH, et al: Phosphorus necrosis of the jaw: A present day study. Br J Indust Med 1962;19:83–99.

2.9. Answer: A   In 1977, a study of Californian pesticide workers exposed to dibromochloropropane (DBCP) showed an increased incidence of male infertility.

Whorton MD, Krauss RM, Marshall S, Milby TH: Infertility in male pesticide workers. Lancet 1977;2:1259–1261.

2.10. Answer: A   In 1987 in Goiânia, Brazil, 244 people were exposed to cesium-137 when an abandoned radiotherapy unit was opened in a junkyard. One hundred four people showed evidence of internal contamination, 28 had local radiation injuries, and eight developed acute radiation syndrome. There were at least four deaths.

Oliveira AR, Hunt JG, Valverde NJL, et al: Medical and related aspects of the Goiânia accident: An overview. Health Phys 1991;60:17–24.

CHAPTER 5

TECHNIQUES USED TO PREVENT GASTROINTESTINAL ABSORPTION OF TOXIC COMPOUNDS

5.1. Answer: C WBI has decreased absorption in volunteer studies, but no proven effect in overdose has been shown yet. It has proven very safe, even after massive dosing, but theoretical concern has been raised because of in vitro interference with activated charcoal drug adsorption.

Hoffman RS, Smilkstein MJ, Goldfrank LR: Whole bowel irrigation and the cocaine body packer. Am J Emerg Med 1990;8: 523–527.

Makosiev F, Hoffman RS, Howland MA, Goldfrank LR: An in vitro evaluation of cocaine hydrochloride adsorption by activated charcoal and desorption upon addition of polyethylene glycol electrolyte lavage solution. J Toxicol Clin Toxicol 1993;31: 381–395.

Smith SW, Ling LJ, Halstenson CE: Whole bowel irrigation as a treatment for acute lithium overdose. Ann Emerg Med 1991;20: 536–539.

5.2. Answer: D There is no consistent proven benefit in either volunteers or poisoned patients. Severe and life-threatening fluid and electrolyte disturbances have occurred after repeated dosing of several cathartics.

Farley TA: Severe hypernatremic dehydration after use of an activated charcoal-sorbitol suspension. J Pediatr 1986;109:719–722.

5.3. Answer: E All cathartics are associated with fluid and electrolyte abnormalities

Farley TA: Severe hypernatremic dehydration after use of an activated charcoal-sorbitol suspension. J Pediatr 1986;109:719–722.

Martin R, Lisehora G, Braxton M, et al: Fatal poisoning from sodium phosphate enema: A case report and experimental study. JAMA 1987;257:2190–2192.

Smilkstein MJ, Steedle D, Kulig KW, et al: Magnesium levels after magnesium containing cathartics. J Toxicol Clin Toxicol 1988;26:51–65.

5.4. Answer: E The optimum dose of activated charcoal is the largest dose that can be safely tolerated, 0.5–1.5 g/kg. Two hundred grams exceeds any patient's tolerance. Fifty or 100 g might be appropriate but could be excessive in a child. The activated charcoal:drug ratio is a useful concept to be aware of when high-end dosing is needed and when initial dosing is inadequate, but it is not logical to use very small activated charcoal doses for small ingestions when a larger activated charcoal dose is well tolerated.

Olkkola KT: Effect of charcoal–drug ratio on antidotal efficacy of oral activated charcoal in man. Br J Clin Pharmacol 1985;19: 767–773.

5.5. Answer: E Using the concept of charcoal-to-drug ratio, it is evident that the amounts in A, B, and C would exceed the capacity of this charcoal dose. The same is true of the ethanol, but particularly because ethanol is so poorly adsorbed to activated charcoal. Cyanide is often considered not to be adsorbed to charcoal, but in fact it is, at a much lower affinity (1 g charcoal to 35 mg KCN). Despite the low affinity, a 100:1 charcoal-to-drug ratio would be more effective for cyanide than for any of the others listed.

Anderson AH: Experimental studies on the pharmacology of activated charcoal: I. Adsorption power of charcoal in aqueous solutions. Acta Pharmacol 1947;2:69–78.

Laass W: Therapy of acute oral poisonings by organic solvents: Treatment by activated charcoal in combination with laxatives. Arch Toxicol 1980;4(Suppl):406–409.

Neuvonen PJ, Olkkola KT: Effect of purgatives on antidotal efficacy of oral activated charcoal. Hum Toxicol 1986;5:255–263.

5.6. Answer: B When enough subjects are used, activated charcoal studies confirm NAC adsorption and decreased bioavailability. Indirect evidence, however, strongly suggests that the interaction is of no concern in most circumstances. Definitive studies have not been done, but there is no evidence that the efficacy of oral NAC is diminished when activated charcoal is used.

Ekins BR, Ford DC, Thompson MIB, et al: The effects of activated charcoal on N-acetylcysteine absorption in normal subjects. Am J Emerg Med 1987;5:483–487.

Spiller HA, Krenzelok EP, Grande GA, et al: A prospective evaluation of the effect of activated charcoal before oral N-acetylcysteine in acetaminophen overdose. Ann Emerg Med 1994;23: 519–523.

5.7. Answer: E Results of gastric emptying studies are highly methodology dependent, and each of the above results has been published. Importantly, the superiority of activated charcoal over gastric emptying has been fairly consistent.

Abdallah AH, Tye A: A comparison of the efficacy of emetic drugs and stomach lavage. Am J Dis Child 1967;113:571–575.

Boxer L, Anderson F, Rowe D: Comparison of ipecac-induced emesis with gastric lavage in the treatment of acute salicylate ingestion. J Pediatr 1969;74:800–803.

Corby D, Decker W, Moran M, et al: Clinical comparison of pharmacologic emetics in children. Pediatrics 1968;42:361–364.

Curtis RA, Barone J, Giacona N: Efficacy of ipecac and activated charcoal and cathartic: Prevention of salicylate absorption in a simulated overdose. Arch Intern Med 1984;144: 48–52.

Saetta JP, Quinton DN: Residual gastric content after gastric lavage and ipecacuanha induced emesis in self poisoned patients: An endoscopic study. J R Soc Med 1991;84:35–38.

5.8. Answer: E The only clear result is that, for most patients, gastric emptying is of no value. The only statistically significant benefit demonstrated has been among obtunded patients lavaged within 1 hour of ingestion. This, however, does not exclude benefit to later emptying in other subsets of patients not adequately studied.

Kulig KW, Bar-Or D, Cantrill SV, et al: Management of acutely poisoned patients without gastric emptying. Ann Emerg Med 1985;14:562–567.

Pond SM, Lewis-Driver DJ, Williams G, et al: Gastric emptying in acute overdose: A prospective randomised controlled trial. Med J Aust 1995;163:345–349.

5.9. Answer: E   The rate of absorption, time since ingestion, or amount ingested will not impact on the effectiveness of increased drug clearance by back-diffusion across the lumen of the GI tract. The availability of an effective antidote would make MDAC less logical. Medications with low intrinsic clearances have been found to be those most effectively cleared by MDAC.

Chyka PA: Multiple-dose activated charcoal and enhancement of systemic drug clearance: Summary of studies in animals and human volunteers. J Toxicol Clin Toxicol 1995;33:399–405.

5.10. Answer: D   Multiple-dose activated charcoal increases the clearance of phenobarbital, phenytoin, carbamazepine, and nortriptyline. Doxepin clearance did not increase significantly with MDAC.

Mowry JB, Furbee RB, Chyka PA: Poisoning. In: Chernow B, ed: The Pharmacologic Approach to the Critically Ill Patient, 3rd ed. Baltimore, Williams & Wilkins, 1994, pp. 978–980.

CHAPTER **6**

PRINCIPLES AND TECHNIQUES APPLIED TO ENHANCE ELIMINATION OF TOXIC COMPOUNDS

6.1. Answer: C   Weak acids, such as salicylates, dissociate in more alkaline urine. Weak bases, such as phencyclidine, dissociate in more acid urine. A weak acid or base is one that has a pK relatively close to neutral pH 7.0. Salicylates have a pK of about 3.5. Dissociation into ionized species (H^+ and salicylate, the anion) prevents reabsorption in the tubule and increases elimination in the urine. Strong acids and bases have low and high pKs, respectively, and will always be dissociated in body fluids so that manipulating urinary pH will have no effect on dissociation.

Morgan AG, Polak A: The excretion of salicylate in salicylate poisoning. Clin Sci 1971;41:475–484.

6.2. Answer: B   Hemodialysis removes solutes by diffusion from blood to dialysate across a semipermeable membrane. Molecules bound to plasma proteins, which are in general themselves too large to cross the membrane, will in turn not be dialyzed. Molecules with volumes of distribution larger than the volume of body water are bound to proteins or tissues or are soluble in nonaqueous phases, such as lipid, and are not diffusible. Diffusion is also limited with toxins of higher molecular weight. Molecular charge does not hinder successful dialysis.

Garella S: Extracorporeal techniques in the treatment of exogenous intoxications. Kidney Int 1988;33:735–754.

6.3. Answer: B   Charcoal hemoperfusion is more efficient than hemodialysis for compounds that are highly protein bound, such as theophylline. The affinity of many toxins for activated charcoal is great, and they may be avidly removed from their protein-binding sites. However, these proteins must be in the plasma. Like hemodialysis, charcoal hemoperfusion is not effective for toxins with large volumes of distribution (like lipid-soluble compounds such as tricyclic antidepressants). Affinity of activated charcoal is insignificant for many ions, while hemodialysis is useful for several substances with low molecular weight.

Garella S: Extracorporeal techniques in the treatment of exogenous intoxications. Kidney Int 1988;33:735–754.

6.4. Answer: E   Like hemodialysis, gastrointestinal dialysis is limited to toxins that cross the intestinal epithelial membrane. They must have relatively low molecular weight and low volumes of distribution (ie, not lipid soluble) to be accessible to the charcoal in the intestinal lumen while they are present in the plasma. This concept would not be applicable for toxins that are not absorbed by the intestine. Diminished bowel motility is a relative contraindication for administration of volumes of activated charcoal, often given with a cathartic such as sorbitol. Ingestion of a compound with food does not relate to the utility of the procedure.

Berg M, Berlinger W, Goldberg M, et al: Acceleration of the body clearance of phenobarbital by oral activated charcoal. N Engl J Med 1982;307:642–644.

6.5. Answer: D   Acetaminophen metabolism is almost all via hepatic pathways, and hepatic damage is potentially life threatening. The drug has a low molecular weight (151 Da). An oral dose of the drug is almost all absorbed, and the drug has a relatively low volume of distribution with only 25% protein bound. Despite these characteristics, which would lead to a prediction of significant clearance by hemoperfusion, the endogenous hepatic metabolism and the efficacy of the antidote, N-acetylcysteine, make hemoperfusion of no clear additional benefit. Furthermore, extracorporeal therapy such as hemoperfusion cannot remove toxic intrahepatic metabolites.

Winchester JF, Gelfand MC, Helliwell M, et al: Extracorporeal treatment of salicylate or acetaminophen poisoning—is there a role? Arch Intern Med 1981;141:370–374.

6.6. Answer: A   It may be better tolerated in hypotensive patients, but clearance rates are much lower. Because the therapy is continuous, there may be clinically significant clearance with time, but whether the clinical course is altered when clearance is achieved this slowly is not well established. The therapy requires high staffing rates as well as meticulous attention to fluid replacement and anticoagulation. As for hemodialysis, small volume of distribution and low lipid solubility are important limitations on the efficacy of continuous hemofiltration.

Golper TA, Bennett WM: Drug removal by continuous arteriovenous haemofiltration: A review of the evidence in poisoned patients. Med Toxicol 1988;3:341–349.

6.7. Answer: C Paraquat's relatively low volume of distribution and MW would appear to make it a toxin removable by extracorporeal therapy. Its degree of protein binding would not prevent its removal by charcoal hemoperfusion. However, its tight binding to tissue sites makes even hemoperfusion less than adequate. Although extraction ratios from serum are high, removal from binding sites in the lungs and other organs precludes effective treatment. It is possible that very early treatment is helpful.

Pond SM, Johnston SC, Schoof DD, et al: Repeated hemoperfusion and continuous arteriovenous hemofiltration in a paraquat poisoned patient. J Toxicol Clin Toxicol 1987;25:305–316.

6.8. Answer: B Lithium, with a very low MW, does have some intracellular distribution. Nonetheless, its removal by hemodialysis allows rapid equilibration from intracellular to extracellular volumes. Increases in serum levels may rebound within hours after cessation of dialysis and lead to an indication for repeat therapy. This intracellular distribution is much less for the other drugs or toxins listed.

Leblanc M, Raymond M, Bonnardeaux A, et al: Lithium poisoning treated by high-performance continuous arteriovenous and venovenous hemodiafiltration. Am J Kidney Dis 1996; 3:365–372.

6.9. Answer: D The size of the digoxin–Fab complex is too large for removal by any of the therapies listed except plasmapheresis. This treatment removes plasma and its constituents, and replaces it with fresh frozen plasma and/or albumin. Despite its efficacy, plasmapheresis is rarely indicated, as repeat administration of digoxin Fab usually suffices and is less expensive and simpler.

Rabetoy GM, Price CA, Findlay JWA, Sailstad JM: Treatment of digoxin intoxication in a renal failure patient with digoxin-specific antibody fragments and plasmapheresis. Am J Nephrol 1990;10: 518–521.

6.10. Answer: D Peritoneal dialysis has value in the management of chronic renal failure but rarely if ever in the case of intoxication. Although theophylline has a MW low enough to allow diffusion across the peritoneum, clearance rates are too slow, making it worthless for theophylline and other drugs or toxins. For hemodynamically unstable patients, this form of dialysis may be better tolerated, but such patients require high clearances if mortality is to be reduced, and this modality of dialysis does not offer such an effect.

Benowitz NL, Toffelmire EB: The use of hemodialysis and hemoperfusion in the treatment of theophylline intoxication. Semin Dial 1993;6:243–252.

CHAPTER **7**

LABORATORY PRINCIPLES AND TECHNIQUES FOR EVALUATION OF THE POISONED OR OVERDOSED PATIENT

7.1. Answer: C Gas chromatography (GC) typically separates, identifies, and quantifies methanol, acetone, ethanol, and isopropanol. These substances are sufficiently volatile to be present in easily measurable concentrations in the air (headspace) above a liquid specimen in a closed container. A portion of the headspace gases may be injected into a gas chromatograph for analysis. Alternatively, serum or plasma may be diluted in water and the diluted specimen directly injected into a packed column gas chromatograph. Laboratories that do not have GC equipment often measure serum ethanol by manual or automated spectrophotometric methods that use alcohol dehydrogenase, but methanol and isopropanol are poor substrates for alcohol dehydrogenase and therefore not readily measured by this technique.

Porter WH: Clinical toxicology. In: Burtis CA, Ashwood ER, eds: Tietz Textbook of Clinical Chemistry, 3rd ed. Philadelphia, WB Saunders, 1999, pp. 906–981.

7.2. Answer: D Several microparticle capture assays are available for drugs of abuse and tricyclic antidepressants in urine. Carbon monoxide may be measured in expired breath using a portable device. A hand-held anodic stripping device is available for measuring lead in whole blood. Digoxin concentrations are too low to be readily detected in microparticle capture formats.

Counter SA, Buchanan LH, Laurell G, Ortega F: Field screening of blood lead levels in remote Andean villages. Neurotoxicology 1998;19:871–877.

Middleton ET, Morice AH: Breath carbon monoxide as an indication of smoking habit. Chest 2000;117:758–763.

7.3. Answer: A Moderate-complexity testing must follow manufacturer's instructions, or it becomes high-complexity testing. A written procedure meeting the requirements of 42 CFR 493.1211 must be available to all testing personnel. Package inserts do not meet the requirements of 42 CFR 493.1211, paragraphs (b)(14) – (b)(16). Competency certification of testing personnel must take place at least annually. At least two levels of controls must be run on each day testing is done. All results must be permanently recorded in the medical record. It is not required that they be entered into the laboratory computer.

42 CFR 493. Code of Federal Regulations, Title 42, Volume 3, 10/2000. pp. 878–999. Accessed at http://www.phppo.cdc.gov/dls/clia/docs/42cfr49399.htm. Last accessed 2/15/01.

7.4. Answer: C NIDA guidelines for Federal workplace drug testing (now administered by SAMHSA) require quantitative confirmation by GC-MS of positive drug screening results before a verified positive test result can be reported. This standard has been widely adopted by other drug-testing laboratories.

Mandatory Guidelines for Federal Workplace Drug Testing. 53 FR 11979. Revised Sept. 1, 1994. Accessed at http://workplace.samhsa.gov/ORCResrc.nsf/f09f81ad4391c6698525688f0064e510/c65a6916e46834e485256976005278b7?OpenDocument. Last accessed 2/12/01.

7.5. Answer: E Proficiency testing data suggests that false-negative rates in toxicology testing are typically from 10 to 30%, while false positive rates are 0 to 10%. Gas chromatography-mass spectroscopy is relatively slow and expensive and constitutes overkill in many instances. Consistent clinical presentation provides adequate confirmation for most results of medical testing, particularly if done by immunoassays. Immunoassays have the sensitivity to detect nanomolar quantities, as in the case of digoxin assays, and also show excellent specificity when focused on a specific drug rather than a drug class. The sensitivity of thin-layer chromatography is typically around 0.5 to 1 mg/L, compared with 0.1 mg/L or less for other chromatographic approaches or immunoassays. Confirmed positives document the presence of a drug but do not necessarily establish the presence of clinical toxicity.

Osterloh JD: Utility and reliability of emergency toxicologic testing. Emerg Med Clin North Am 1990;8:693–723.

7.6. Answer: A Chemical derivatization reactions may be used to increase the volatility, and enhance the detectability of polar substances analyzed by gas chromatography. Most substances detected by thin-layer chromatography are visualized using various reagent dips or sprays. Spectrophotometric assays rely on a selective reaction with the target substance to create a light-absorbing compound.

Evenson MA: Spectrophometric Techniques In: Burtis CA, Ashwood ER, eds: Tietz Textbook of Clinical Chemistry, 3rd ed. Philadelphia, WB Saunders, 1999, pp. 75–93.

Ullman MD, Bowers LD, Burtis CA: Chromatography/mass spectroscopy. In: Burtis CA, Ashwood ER, eds: Tietz Textbook of Clinical Chemistry, 3rd ed. Philadelphia, WB Saunders, 1999, pp. 164–204.

7.7. Answer: B Acetaminophen and carbon monoxide have relatively short half-lives, with the result that the concentration measured at the time of presentation may substantially underestimate the seriousness of the exposure unless a correction for the time dependence of the concentration is undertaken. Digoxin and lithium both have prolonged distribution phases, and use of predistribution concentrations may lead to overestimation of eventual toxicity. Theophylline toxicity reflects time-integrated exposure, such that the same concentration is of much greater risk in a chronic overdose, relative to an acute one. The urinary assay for cocaine metabolites is qualitative and only suggests exposure.

Olson KR, Benowitz NL, Woo OF, Pond SM: Theophylline overdose: acute single ingestion versus chronic repeated overmedication. Am J Emerg Med 1985;3:386–394.

Sue YJ, Shannon M: Pharmacokinetics of drugs in overdose. Clin Pharmacokinet 1992;23:93–105.

7.8. Answer: B There are very few full-service toxicology laboratories. Tests for drugs of abuse in urine are available in multiple formats that are compatible with existing instrumentation in most clinical laboratories and are therefore widely available. Analysis for the other substances requires specialized skills and instrumentation.

College of American Pathologists Participant Summaries: Toxicology Survey Set T-B; Therapeutic Drug Monitoring (General) Survey Set Z-B; Urine Toxicology Survey Set UT-B; Serum Alcohol/Volatiles Survey Set AL2-B; Chemistry Survey Set C4-B. College of American Pathologists, 1999.

Wiley JF: Difficult diagnoses in toxicology. Poisons not detected by the comprehensive drug screen. Pediatr Clin North Am 1991;38:725–737.

7.9. Answer: C Alcohol is dissolved in the water of body fluids, and its concentration at equilibrium will be proportional to the water content. Serum and plasma both have a water content of 93% and will have comparable alcohol concentrations. Urine has higher water content, and alcohol concentrations are likewise higher by 5 to 7%. Additionally, the urine concentration will be determined by the average alcohol concentration in the serum over the time of formation, rather than the serum concentration at time of collection. This leads to a higher urine/serum ratio during times when alcohol concentration is declining. Although saliva has a higher water content than plasma, salivary concentrations are typically 4 to 6% lower than serum concentrations, presumably reflecting incomplete equilibration. Breath alcohol is measured in g/210 L of breath. The amount of alcohol in 210 L of breath is approximately equal to the amount in 100 mL of whole blood. Because of the lower water content of red cells, whole-blood alcohol concentration is about 13% lower than serum alcohol.

Caplan YH: Blood, urine and other fluid and tissue specimens for alcohol analysis. In: Garrott JC, ed: Medicolegal Aspects of Alcohol, 3rd ed. Tucson, Lawyers and Judges Publishing, 1996, pp. 137–150.

7.10. Answer: A Tests that are regulated by CLIA-88 are ones that involve the laboratory testing of human specimens. Breath tests are considered to be patient monitoring because no specimen is collected and are therefore exempt. Some testing of human specimens not affecting medical management decisions are exempted, including forensic testing, workplace drug testing by a NIDA-certified facility, and research testing where the results are not used for the "diagnosis, prevention, or treatment of any disease or impairment of, or the assessment of the health of individual patients."

42 CFR 493. Code of Federal Regulations, Title 42, Volume 3, 10/2000. pp. 878–999. Accessed at http://www.phppo.cdc.gov/dls/clia/docs/42cfr49399.htm. Last accessed 2/15/01.

CHAPTER **8**

DIAGNOSTIC IMAGING IN TOXICOLOGY

8.1. Answer: E Although knowing the atomic numbers of the constituent atoms in a molecule usually does not permit prediction of its radiopacity, for the simple molecules listed here, the one with the greatest number of chlorine atoms (atomic number 17) will be the most radiopaque. If a sufficient quantity of carbon tetrachloride is ingested, it may be visible in the stomach on an abdominal radiograph taken soon after the ingestion. It will most likely be visible on an upright film because layering of the hydrocarbon pool in the stomach can produce a sharp horizontal border.

Dally SL, Garnier R, Bismuth C: Diagnosis of chlorinated hydrocarbon poisoning by x-ray examination. Br J Indust Med 1987;44:424–425.

8.2. Answer: A Chronic corticosteroid use frequently causes osteoporosis. This can be complicated by insufficiency fractures, most commonly vertebral body compression fractures. Chronic glucocorticoid therapy is also associated with avascular necrosis, most frequently involving the femoral head and humeral head. The purported mechanism is increased fat deposition in the medullary cavity resulting in diminished blood flow. Avascular necrosis results in skeletal lucencies followed by reparative sclerosis and collapse. Other causes of avascular necrosis include alcoholism, sickle cell disease, Caisson disease (dysbarism), and trauma interrupting the skeletal blood supply. Fluorosis is associated with increased bone density. Lead intoxication causes transverse bands across the metaphysis in the immature skeleton.

Mankin HJ: Nontraumatic necrosis of bone (osteonecrosis). N Engl J Med 1992;326:1473–1479.

Neustadter LM, Weiss M: Medication-induced changes of bone. Semin Roentgenol 1995;30:88–95.

8.3. Answer: D Ingestion of toxic quantities of organic mercury, as can occur with contaminated foods, results in a variety of severe neurologic disorders including mental retardation, cortical blindness, and movement disorders. CT and MRI reveal atrophy of the cerebellum as well as the calcarine cerebral cortex. Chronic alcoholism and solvent vapor exposure also cause diffuse cerebral atrophy and cerebellar atrophy.

Davis LE, Kornfield M, Mooney HS, et al: Methylmercury poisoning: Long-term clinical radiological, toxicological, and pathological studies of an affected family. Ann Neurol 1994;35: 680–688.

Lexa FJ: Drug-induced disorders of the central nervous system. Semin Roentgenol 1995;30:7–18.

Warach SJ, Charness ME: Imaging the brain lesions of alcoholics. In: Greenberg JO, ed: Neuroimaging: A Companion to Adams and Victor's Principles of Neurology. New York, McGraw-Hill, 1995, pp. 503–515.

8.4. Answer: B The basal ganglia are especially susceptible to toxic and metabolic insult. Bilateral basal ganglia necrosis is seen following severe carbon monoxide, methanol, and cyanide poisoning as well as with hypotension, hypoxia, hypoglycemia, infectious encephalitis, and other disorders. The lesions of methanol poisoning involve the putamen, whereas carbon monoxide and cyanide involve the globus pallidus. Manganese deposits in the basal ganglia produce high-signal-intensity lesions on T_1-weighted MR imaging. Vitamin A is associated with pseudotumor cerebri in which the CT is normal or occasionally shows small ventricles.

Hantson P, Duprez T, Mahieu P: Neurotoxicity to the basal ganglia shown by magnetic resonance imaging (MRI) following poisoning by methanol and other substances. J Toxicol Clin Toxicol 1997;35:151–161.

Ho VB, Fitz CR, Chuang SH, Geyer CA: Bilateral basal ganglia lesions: Pediatric differential considerations. Radiographics 1993; 13:269–292.

8.5. Answer: C Although in vitro studies have found these listed tablets to have some degree of radiopacity relative to a uniform water bath, only iron is both sufficiently radiopaque and disintegrates slowly after ingestion to be visible on an abdominal radiograph in a patient with a suspected overdose. Radiographs can help confirm the diagnosis of iron tablet ingestion, quantify the amount ingested, and follow gastrointestinal decontamination.

However, iron preparations that are dissolved quickly or have a relatively low iron content may not be detectable radiographically.

O'Brien RP, McGeehan PA, Helmeczi AW, Dula DJ: Detectability of drug tablets and capsules by plain radiography. Am J Emerg Med 1986;4:302–312.

Savitt DL, Hawkins HH, Roberts JR: The radiopacity of ingested medications. Ann Emerg Med 1987;16:331–339.

8.6. Answer: C Delayed onset of diffuse pulmonary edema is characteristic of inhalation injury from a low-water-solubility irritant gas such as nitrogen dioxide and phosgene ($COCl_2$). The gas itself is nonirritating and so is inhaled without the victim's being aware of the toxic exposure. In the aqueous environment of the lung, nitrogen dioxide is converted into a highly irritating acid that is responsible for delayed onset of symptoms and radiographic findings. Nitrogen dioxide poisoning is also seen in agricultural workers (silo filler disease). Carbon monoxide and carbon dioxide are a chemical asphyxiant and a simple asphyxiant, respectively, which cause hypoxia without radiographic abnormalities. Metal fumes cause a delayed-onset influenzalike syndrome, usually without radiographic abnormalities.

Behrman AJ: Welders. In: Greenberg MI, Hamilton RJ, Phillips SD: Occupational, Industrial and Environmental Toxicology. St Louis, Mosby-Year Book, 1997, pp. 303–309.

Dee P, Armstrong P: Inhalational lung diseases. In: Armstrong P, Wilson AG, Dee P, Hansell DM, eds: Imaging of Diseases of the Chest, 2nd ed. St. Louis, Mosby-Year Book, 1995, pp. 426–460.

8.7 Answer: E Diffuse intestinal distension is characteristic of an adynamic ileus. Agents that inhibit intestinal motility, such as opioids and anticholinergic agents, can cause constipation and ileus. Adynamic ileus can also be caused by various intraperitoneal and systemic illnesses. Intestinal ischemia can cause a severe ileus. Ergotamine and cocaine can cause intestinal ischemia by inducing mesenteric vasospasm. An overdose of a calcium channel blocker such as verapamil or nifedipine can cause mesenteric ischemia as a result of hypotension and intestinal hypoperfusion.

Gatenby RA: The radiology of drug-induced disorders in the gastrointestinal tract. Semin Roentgenol 1995;30:62–76.

Wax PM: Intestinal infarction due to nifedipine overdose. J Toxicol Clin Toxicol 1995;33:725–728.

8.8. Answer: C Abdominal radiographs are unlikely to have any characteristic findings in a patient with liver failure caused by acetaminophen toxicity. Massive ascites can be detected; however, radiography offers no advantage over physical examination. Cocaine use is associated with intestinal infarction, which may show intramural gas on plain film, and with peptic ulcer perforation causing pneumoperitoneum (best seen on an upright chest radiograph). Gastric perforation and pneumoperitoneum can also be caused by a caustic ingestion with either acid or alkali. Although most disorders that cause bloody diarrhea do not have diagnostic radiographic findings, except occasionally intussusception, iron tablet ingestion could be detected radiographically in a child too young to give an accurate history. Radiopaque heavy metals are sometimes contained in traditional folk remedies and potions, and these may be visualized radiographically.

Cheng CLY, Svesko V: Acute pyloric perforation after prolonged crack smoking. Ann Emerg Med 1994;23:126–128.

Kulshrestha MK: Lead poisoning diagnosed by abdominal x-rays. J Toxicol Clin Toxicol 1996;34:107–108.

8.9. Answer: E   There are a very large number of causes of interstitial lung disease, and their radiographic appearance may be a fine or coarse reticular pattern or a reticulonodular pattern. Many of the disorders causing a reticular pattern can also cause multifocal ill-defined airspace filling. Hypersensitivity pneumonitis is a delayed-type allergic reaction to an ingested or inhaled allergen. Nitrofurantoin is the most commonly associated medication, and clinical signs generally begin 1 to 2 weeks into the course of therapy. Many cytotoxic chemotherapeutic agents cause direct pulmonary toxicity, resulting in interstitial lung disease that usually regresses with withdrawal of the offending medication. Bleomycin is one of the commonly associated agents. Nitrogen dioxide is a low-water-solubility irritant gas and is the cause of silo filler disease. In the initial phase, it causes diffuse airspace filling. However, after the acute episode resolves, after a delay of 2 to 3 weeks, a chronic interstitial lung disease known as *bronchiolitis obliterans* may ensue. This produces a fine nodular radiographic pattern. Asbestosis is a chronic interstitial lung disease causing a fine or coarse reticular radiographic pattern. The term asbestosis should not be applied to the calcified pleural plaques that are also associated with asbestos exposure. Malathion is an organophosphate insecticide whose muscarinic effects cause bronchorrhea. This produces diffuse, coalescent airspace filling. It is not associated with a reticular or nodular radiographic pattern.

Armstrong P, Wilson AG, Dee P, Hansell DM: Imaging of Diseases of the Chest, 2nd ed. St Louis, Mosby-Year Book, 1995, pp. 426–460, 461–483.

Fishman AP: Pulmonary Diseases and Disorders, 2nd ed. New York, McGraw-Hill, 1988, pp. 667–674, 793–811, 1465–1474.

8.10. Answer: D   Procainamide is a common cause of the drug-induced lupus syndrome. Pleural effusions are often the major clinical manifestation. Fever, myalgias, and arthralgias are also common. More serious systemic lupus involvement, such as renal or central nervous system disease, is uncommon. A pericardial effusion also occurs occasionally. Patchy infiltrates occur very rarely. Medication-induced hilar adenopathy is associated with phenytoin.

Fraser RO, Pare JAP, Pare PD, et al: Diagnosis of Diseases of the Chest, 3rd ed. Philadelphia, WB Saunders, 1991, pp. 2417–2479.

Miller WT: Pleural and mediastinal disorders related to drug use. Semin Roentgenol 1995;30:35–48.

CHAPTER **9**

ELECTROCARDIOGRAPHIC PRINCIPLES

9.1. Answer: B   Bidirectional ventricular tachycardia is particularly characteristic of severe digitalis toxicity and results from alterations of intraventricular conduction, junctional tachycardia with aberrant intraventricular conduction, or, on rare occasions, alternating ventricular pacemakers. The only other drug that is commonly associated with this dysrhythmia is aconitine, usually from traditional or alternative therapies. The electrocardiographic manifestations of acute and chronic cardiac glycoside poisoning are similar.

9.2. Answer: D   Repolarization is depicted on the ECG by the ST segment, the T wave, the QT interval, and the U wave. Propoxyphene causes blockade of the fast sodium channels and prolongation of the QT interval. In overdose patients, propoxyphene has been reported to cause seizures and dysrhythmias. Diphenoxylate is prescribed in combination with atropine for the symptomatic treatment of diarrhea. Both meperidine and the diphenoxylate and atropine combination have anticholinergic properties and cause tachycardia. Heroin and morphine decrease peripheral resistance but have no direct effect on repolarization.

Madfsen PS, Strom J, Reiz S: Acute propoxyphene poisoning in 222 consecutive cases. Acta Anaesth Scand 1984;28:661–665.

9.3. Answer: D   Thioridazine, the cyclic antidepressants, amantadine, and procainamide all cause blockade of the sodium channels and prolongation of the QRS complex. Omeprazole suppresses gastric secretion by specific inhibition of the sodium potassium ATPase enzyme system at the secretory surface of the gastric parietal cell. No cardiovascular toxicity has been reported, even following overdosage.

9.4. Answer: B   The recording from a modified left chest lead with the positive electrode in the V_1 position (lead MCL_1) is similar in appearance to a V_1 recording on a 12-lead ECG. This lead is commonly used in routine monitoring. A continuous cardiac monitor records from either lead MCL_1 or lead II (see Fig. 9–4). For lead MCL_1 the positive electrode is placed over the fourth intercostal space just to the right of the sternum. The negative electrode is placed at the second intercostal space, midline on the upper left chest, or on the outer third of the left clavicle. This lead visualizes ventricular activity well; however, lead II shows atrial activity, the P wave, much more clearly. Electrode placement for lead II has the positive electrode on the lower extreme left side of the left chest and the negative electrode on the second intercostal space in the midline of the upper right chest.

9.5. Answer: B   The QT interval spans from the beginning of the QRS complex to the terminus of the T wave (see Fig. 9–6).

9.6. Answer: A   The ECG findings consistent with hypokalemia include ST depression, not elevation, and a progressive decrease in the amplitude of the T wave (see Fig. 9–10). When the serum potassium decreases further, the amplitude of the U wave increases, and eventually the U and T waves fuse. The amplitude and duration of both the QRS complex and the P wave increase as the PR interval lengthens. Ventricular tachycardia, torsades de pointes, ventricular fibrillation, and asystole will eventually develop if proper therapy is not instituted.

9.7. Answer: C   The QT interval, not the QRS complex, may be widened. The most characteristic and reliable sign of hypocalcemia is a prolonged ST segment and increased QT interval (see Fig. 9–9). The T wave remains unchanged. The prolongation of the ST segment is approximately proportional to the decrease in ionized calcium.

9.8. Answer: B The electrocardiographic manifestations of digoxin toxicity are very variable. Ectopic rhythms appear as the first sign of poisoning in 10 to 15% of cases and may include non-paroxysmal junctional tachycardia, ventricular premature extrasystoles, ventricular flutter and fibrillation, atrial flutter and fibrillation, and bidirectional ventricular tachycardia. Conduction velocity is reduced in both myocardial and nodal tissue, resulting in an increased PR interval and AV block. Dehydration and calcium channel blockers both decrease the clearance of digoxin. An additional consideration is that the therapy for a calcium channel blocker overdose involves exogenous calcium administration. However, in a digoxin overdose additional calcium should be avoided. Intracellular calcium concentrations are already elevated, and the infusion of additional calcium could exacerbate the dysrhythmias.

9.9. Answer: D The hereditary long QT syndromes are typically considered adrenergic dependent because the torsades de pointes associated with them is generally triggered by adrenergic activation or enhancement of sympathetic nervous system tone. The acquired syndromes are referred to as pause dependent because the torsades de pointes associated with them generally occurs at slow heart rates or in response to short–long–short RR interval sequences. There is significant overlap between these two syndromes. Patients have variable susceptibility to prolongation of the QT interval by drugs and a variable response to a prolonged QT interval. Factors that contribute to the development of torsades de pointes include hypokalemia, hypomagnesemia, hypocalcemia, bradycardia, ischemia, and tissue hypoxia.

Splawski I, Timothy KW, Vincent GM, et al: Molecular basis of the long QT syndrome associated with deafness. N Engl J Med 1997;336:1562–1567.

Tan HL, Hou CJ, Lauer MR, Sung RJ: Electrophysiologic mechanisms of the long QT interval syndromes and torsades de pointes. Ann Intern Med 1995;122:701–714.

9.10. Answer: D The clinical effects of the ergot alkaloids are widespread. The mechanism of cardiovascular toxicity involves peripheral vasoconstriction, arteriolar constriction, and damage to the capillary endothelium. Valvular fibrosis with thickening and immobility has also been reported in patients following chronic use of ergotamines, although the mechanism is unclear. Evidence of myocardial injury and infarction occurs. Interstitial nephritis is not a common manifestation of toxicity in overdose.

Redfield MM, Nicholson WJ, Edwards WD, Tajik AJ: Valve disease associated with ergot alkaloid use: Echocardiographic and pathologic correlations. Ann Intern Med 1992;117:50–52.

CHAPTER **10**

NEUROTRANSMITTER PRINCIPLES

10.1. Answer: A Nicotinic receptors comprise portions of Na^+ channels. The other listed receptors are coupled to G proteins.

10.2. Answer: C Adenosine is released with excitatory neurotransmitters such as glutamate. Adenosine stimulates postsynaptic A_1 receptors to hyperpolarize the neuron and presynaptic A_1 receptors to inhibit Ca^{2+} influx and limit release of neurotransmitter.

Eldridge FL, Paydarfar D, Scott SC, Dowell RT: Role of endogenous adenosine in recurrent generalized seizures. Exp Neurol 1989;103:179–185.

10.3. Answer: D Stimulation of imidazoline receptors by clonidine contributes to hypotension and bradycardia. Clonidine's stimulation of α_2 receptors produces CNS depression as well as sympatholytic effects. Clonidine does not bind to the other listed receptors.

Dominiak P: Historic aspects in the identification of the I_1 receptor and the pharmacology of imidazolines. Cardiovasc Drugs Ther 1994;8(Suppl):21–26.

10.4. Answer: A Botulinum toxins prevent release of acetylcholine. Clonidine indirectly prevents acetylcholine release by stimulating presynaptic α_2 receptors on cholinergic nerve endings. Diphenhydramine blocks muscarinic acetylcholine receptors.

Baba A, Cooper JR: The action of black widow spider venom on cholinergic mechanisms in synaptosomes. J Neurochem 1980;34:1369–1379.

10.5. Answer: E Strychnine antagonizes the inhibitory effect of glycine at Cl^- channel glycine receptors. Strychnine has no major action on the other listed agents.

Betz H, Schmitt B, Becker CM, et al: The vertebrate glycine receptor protein. Biochem Soc Symp 1986;52:57–63.

10.6. Answer: A Phencyclidine binds within the NMDA Ca^{2+} channel to prevent calcium influx in response to glutamate binding. Domoic acid activates different glutamate receptors. Valproic acid, clozapine, and cocaine do not bind to glutamate receptors.

Thornberg SA, Saklad SR: A review of NMDA receptors and the phencyclidine model of schizophrenia. Pharmacotherapy 1996;16:82–93.

10.7. Answer: B Inhibition of this enzyme results in less norepinephrine release in response to nerve ending depolarization or actions of indirectly acting sympathomimetic agents.

Eneanya DI, Bianchine JR, Duran DO, Andresen BD: The actions and metabolic fate of disulfiram. Annu Rev Pharmacol Toxicol 1981;21:575–596.

10.8. Answer: A Cisapride activates $5-HT_4$ receptors to promote GI motility. Cyproheptadine, ondansetron, and propranolol block serotonin receptors. Sumatriptan activates $5-HT_1$ receptors, which do not affect GI motility.

Villalon CM, Terron JA, Ramirez-San Juan E, Saxena PR: 5-Hydroxytryptamine: Considerations about discovery, receptor classification and relevance to medical research. Arch Med Res 1995;26:331–344.

10.9. Answer: A Antagonism of A_1 and A_2 receptors by methylxanthines explains many of their toxic effects, including convulsions and increased adrenergic tone. Ethanol and diazepam prevent adenosine uptake, enhancing adenosine's actions.

Von Lubitz DK, Carter MF, Beenhakker M, et al: Adenosine: A prototherapeutic concept in neurodegeneration. Ann NY Acad Sci 1995;765:163–178.

10.10. Answer: C Penicillin appears to bind to the GABA binding site and within the Cl$^-$ channel to prevent Cl$^-$ influx in response to GABA. Baclofen binds to GABA$_B$ receptors. Domoic acid produces convulsions through actions at glutamate receptors. Muscimol activates GABA$_A$ receptors. Carbamazepine may produce convulsions through antagonism of adenosine receptors.

Fujimoto M, Munakata M, Akaike N: Dual mechanisms of GABA$_A$ response inhibition by β-lactam antibiotics in the pyramidal neurones of the rat cerebral cortex. Br J Pharmacol 1995; 116:3014–3020.

Tsuda A, Ito M, Kishi K, et al: Effect of penicillin on GABA-gated chloride ion influx. Neurochem Res 1994;19:1–4.

CHAPTER 11

PHARMACOKINETIC AND TOXICOKINETIC PRINCIPLES

11.1. Answer: E Factors that may influence xenobiotic elimination may include age, competition or inhibition of elimination processes, enzyme saturation, gender, genetics, and the physical and chemical properties of the xenobiotic.

11.2. Answer: D Volume of distribution (L/kg) is equal to dose divided by the peak plasma concentration. Dose is 500,000 mg. Peak concentration is 20 mg/mL. The distributive volume is 25,000 mL or $V_d = 0.5$ L/kg (see equation 11–6).

McCoy HG, Cipolle RJ, Ehlers SM, et al: Severe methanol poisoning: Application of a pharmacokinetic model for ethanol therapy and hemodialysis. Am J Med 1979;67:804–807.

11.3. Answer: B Alcohol dehydrogenase is primarily found in the cytosol of hepatic cells and in select extrahepatic metabolic cells.

11.4. Answer: C Lithium is best characterized by a two-compartment model. In a two-compartment model a xenobiotic is distributed instantaneously to a highly perfused central compartment and then is more slowly distributed to a peripheral (often intracellular) compartment.

Jaeger A, Sander P, Kopferschmitt J, et al: Toxicokinetics of lithium intoxication treated by hemodialysis. J Toxicol Clin Toxicol 1985;23:501–517.

11.5. Answer: E Distributive processes are affected by all of the factors than affect absorption plus many others, including degree of ionization, lipid solubility, active transport, and first-pass metabolism.

Gram TE: Drug absorption and distribution. In: Craig CR, Stitzel RE, eds: Modern Pharmacology with Clinical Applications. Boston, Little, Brown, 1997, pp. 13–24.

11.6. Answer: B The child ingested 10,000 mg of methanol. It will be distributed in 6000 mL. The predicted peak concentration is 1.67 mg/mL or 167 mg/dL (see equation 11–6).

Rowland M, Tozer TN: Clinical Pharmacokinetics Concepts & Applications, 2nd ed. Philadelphia, Lea & Febiger, 1989.

11.7. Answer: A Phenytoin is metabolized by enzymes that become saturated at concentrations just above the therapeutic range. As the dose increases, there is a disproportionate increase in plasma concentration. This is characteristic of Michaelis-Menten kinetics.

11.8. Answer: D Every 6 hours the patient's plasma acetaminophen level has fallen by 50%. Half-life is defined as the time required for a xenobiotic's concentration to decline by 50%. At 10 hours this patient's level can be predicted to have been 75 mg/mL and then at 16 hours 37.5 mg/mL.

Prescott LF, Roscoe P, Wright N: Plasma-paracetamol half-life and hepatic necrosis in patients with paracetamol overdosage. Lancet 1971;1:519–522.

11.9. Answer: D At steady state the amount of drug going into the system equals the amount of drug leaving the system. The amount of digoxin going into (and out of) the system is 80% of 0.25 mg or 200,000 ng/24 h. Clearance is the amount eliminated each day divided by the concentration at steady state (0.8 ng/mL). Cl = 250,000 ng/24 h (see equation 11–23). Clearance is conventionally reported as units/kg/time. Cl = 4166 ng/kg/d.

11.10. Answer: C Pharmacodynamics is the investigation of the relationship of drug concentration to clinical effects.

Woosley RL: Pharmacokinetics and pharmacodynamics of antiarrhythmic agents in patients with congestive heart failure. Am Heart J 1987;114:1280–1285.

CHAPTER 12

CHEMICAL PRINCIPLES

12.1. Answer C The periodic table is divided into metals and nonmetals, with a few metalloids in the transition zone. The majority of the represented elements are metals. Chemical reactivity trends down a group not along a period. Noble gases do not react with anything under conventional conditions but can be forced to react under extreme heat or pressure. Alkali metals include sodium and potassium; chlorine and fluorine are halogens (nonmetals)

12.2. Answer B Unlike alkali metals, whose metallic form is highly reactive, many transition metals, such as iron, zinc, copper, etc, are stable in their elemental (metallic) state. The active sites of many enzymes contain transition metals in their ionized form because of their high reactivity. The generation of free radicals is the most important toxicologic effect of transition metals, and although they often form impressive salts, this is inconsequential. Both acute and chronic poisoning may occur (eg, manganism, iron overload). Transition metals may attain several oxidation states by either gaining or losing electrons; in general they are positively charged and prefer to accept electrons.

12.3. Answer D Heavy metals have atomic masses greater than 200. Arsenic is neither "heavy" nor a metal; it is a metalloid, meaning that it has properties of both metals and nonmetals.

12.4. Answer B Electrovalent, or ionic, bonds involve one element's control over the shared electrons. When the bond is broken, one of the elements retains the electrons. More equal sharing of electrons occurs in covalent bonds, and the degree to which the electrons are attracted to one of the elements is determined by the element's electronegativity. Activated charcoal holds chemicals via Van der Waals and other noncovalent bonds.

12.5. Answer D OH• represents the hydroxyl radical. The remainder are not reactive oxygen species.

12.6. Answer A Paraquat undergoes redox cycling, which causes the release of reactive oxygen species. Phenytoin is a sodium channel blocker. Sodium hydroxide is an alkali, and barium salts mimic calcium in physiologic processes. Elemental mercury, Hg^0, is not chemically reactive.

12.7. Answer C Molecules with the same functional group, in general, have similar (although not identical) physical properties and chemical reactivity.

12.8. Answer A Optical isomers, such as ($-$) physostigmine and ($+$) physostigmine, have identical physical properties, such as boiling point. They differ in the way they interact with other three-dimensional structures such as the enzyme acetylcholinesterase. The ($-$) physostigmine isomer is biologically active, whereas the ($+$) physostigmine isomer is not.

12.9. Answer B Nucleophiles ("nucleus loving") have increased electron density, frequently in the form of a lone pair of electrons. Nucleophiles generally react with electrophiles ("electron loving"), which have a center or centers that is/are relatively electron deficient.

12.10. Answer D Pralidoxime, or 2-PAM, is a nucleophilic "antidote" used to reactivate cholinesterase enzyme that is occupied by an organic phosphorus compound. The other listed agents are important electrophiles.

CHAPTER 13

BIOCHEMICAL PRINCIPLES

13.1. Answer: C Sulfation, glucuronidation, and conjugation with glutathione are phase II reactions that occur after modification of the substrate by phase I reactions. Phase I reactions result in the addition of more reactive groups such as hydroxyl, amino, carboxyl, or sulfhydryl groups to lipophilic molecules.

Krishna DR, Klotz U: Extrahepatic metabolism of drugs in humans. Clin Pharmacokinet 1994;26:144–160.

13.2. Answer: D Bromobenzene, like acetaminophen, undergoes hepatic metabolism to a reactive metabolite that binds and injures hepatocytes. Paraquat is metabolized to a toxic metabolite by the lungs, causing in situ damage. Cycasin causes cancers in the colon, where it is metabolized to methoxymethanol. Neither salicylate nor cocaine requires metabolism to exert its toxic effects.

13.3. Answer: C Dinitrophenol toxicity is associated with severe hyperthermia related to uncoupling of ATP production.

Fosslien E. Mitochondrial medicine: Molecular pathology of defective oxidative phosphorylation. Ann Clin Lab Sci 2001;31: 25–67.

13.4. Answer: D Although phase I biotransformation increases the water solubility of many toxins, they remain relatively lipophilic and require phase II conjugation for excretion. Most of these enzymes are not highly selective, altering many different substrates within broad classes. The metabolism of ethanol to acetaldehyde is a phase I oxidation reaction. The higher K_m for ethanol of CYP2E1 makes alcohol dehydrogenase the primary enzyme for metabolizing ethanol in nontolerant persons.

Guegenrich FP: Catalytic selectivity of human cytochrome P450 enzymes: Relevance to drug metabolism and toxicity. Toxicol Lett 1994;70:133–138.

13.5. Answer: A Both acetaminophen and bromobenzene are metabolized by phase I reactions to highly reactive metabolites that may have significant toxicity when glutathione availability is limited. Phase II reactions are conjugation reactions that increase the polarity (and water solubility) and result in detoxification in most cases.

13.6. Answer: E Each of the substances reduces CYP3A4 activity. Erythromycin and fluconazole block the metabolism of terfenadine, increasing its cardiotoxicity. Grapefruit juice (naringenin) decreases the metabolism of dihydropyridine calcium channel blockers.

Peck CC, Temple R, Collins JM: Understanding consequences of concurrent therapies. JAMA 1993;269:1550–1552.

13.7. Answer: C MPTP does not affect toxicity through enzyme inhibition. All of the following agents block specific enzymes: Ricin: RNA polymerase; methotrexate: dihydrofolate reductase; warfarin: vitamin K 2,3-epoxide reductase; sodium fluoroacetate: aconitase.

13.8. Answer: D The toxicity of many metals, including mercury, is attributed to diffuse enzyme effects, most likely related to binding to the enzyme's sulfhydryl-containing moieties. All of the others exert their effects through interactions with specific protein receptors. Morphine: endorphin receptors; atropine: muscarinic receptors; pancuronium: nicotinic receptors; flumazenil: GABA receptors.

13.9. Answer: E Isoniazid inhibits the synthesis of pyridoxal 5′-phosphate, which results in a decrease in GABA production. All of the other agents inhibit cellular energy production: arsenic at the level of glycolysis, fluoroacetate at the level of the Krebs cycle, and cyanide and salicylates at the level of oxidative phosphorylation.

Fosslien E: Mitochondrial medicine—molecular pathology of defective oxidative phosphorylation. Ann Clin Lab Sci 2001;31: 25–67.

13.10. Answer: D Carbon tetrachloride causes in situ hepatic injury in the zone 3 areas of the liver, where it is metabolized. Of the others, only MPTP requires metabolic transformation to exert its toxicity, which occurs following transport of the metabolite into dopaminergic neurons and not at the site of its synthesis.

Brent JA, Rumack BH: Role of free radicals in toxic hepatic injury: II. Are free radicals the cause of toxin induced liver disease? J Toxicol Clin Toxicol 1993;31:173–196.

CHAPTER 14

HEPATIC PRINCIPLES

14.1. Answer: C The injury caused by the majority of hepatotoxins is related to characteristics of the injured individual subject and cannot be predicted before the injury. Less commonly, hepatotoxins produce predictable, dose-dependent injury in all subjects. These include such agents as acetaminophen, *Amanita* toxins, and carbon tetrachloride. Hepatitis caused by the direct hepatotoxic effects of halothane occurs in as many as 20% of exposed patients. Acute hepatic necrosis caused by an allergic mechanism is extremely rare. Liver injury may be caused by toxins delivered to the liver through inhalation and dermal absorption, as illustrated by industrial solvents associated with liver injury such as dimethylformamide, vinyl chloride, and carbon tetrachloride.

Lee WM: Drug-induced hepatotoxicity. N Engl J Med 1995;333: 1118–1127.

Neuberger J, Williams R: Halothane anesthesia and liver damage. Br Med J 1984;289:1136–1139.

14.2. Answer: D The metabolism of APAP illustrates the delicate balance that exists between detoxification and the production of injurious metabolites. In healthy adults taking therapeutic amounts of APAP, elimination occurs primarily through glucuronidation and secondarily through sulfation. Under normal circumstances less than 10% undergoes oxidative metabolism, resulting in the production of the electrophilic metabolite *N*-acetyl-*p*-benzoquinoneimine (NAPQI). In most cases NAPQI is rapidly detoxified by conjugation with glutathione. Excessive amounts of APAP overwhelm the pathways of sulfation and glucuronidation, resulting in increased synthesis of NAPQI, which reacts avidly with hepatocellular macromolecules if glutathione is not available.

14.3. Answer: C Intrahepatic bile flow has been shown to be an active, ATP-dependent process. Selective injury to the canaliculi by selective toxins, including injury to the tight junctions that separate the bile from the sinusoidal contents, leads to cholestasis in the absence of other evidence of cell injury. Large glucuronidated molecules are preferentially secreted into bile as substrates for the bile acid transport system. The most prominent early manifestation of vitamin A toxicity is accumulation of fat and swelling of the fat-storing, or Ito, cells.

Böhme M, Müller M, Leier I, et al: Cholestasis caused by inhibition of the adenosine triphosphate-dependent bile salt transporter in rat liver. Gastroenterology 1994;107:255–265.

14.4. Answer: E All of these mechanisms have been associated with localized injury by specific toxins.

14.5. Answer: E All of these statements are true. The AST and ALT rarely rise above 300 IU/L in alcohol-induced liver disease. The AST is usually greater than the ALT. Steatosis is related to metabolic dysfunction of the cell. Amiodarone produces a pathologic picture very similar to that of ethanol.

Lieber CS: Alcohol and the liver: 1994 update. Gastroenterology 1994;106:1085–1105.

14.6. Answer: B The anabolic steroids are associated with development of blood-filled cavities in the liver, a condition called peliosis hepatis. These may rupture, causing hemoperitoneum.

Bagheri SA, Boyer JL: Peliosis hepatis associated with androgenic-anabolic steroid therapy. Ann Intern Med 1974;81:610–618.

14.7. Answer: D The AST rarely rises above 1000 IU in cases of extrahepatic bile duct obstruction and rarely rises above 300 IU in hepatitis related to ethanol. Methotrexate causes indolent hepatitis leading to cirrhosis without dramatic elevations of hepatocellular enzymes. Acute massive hepatocellular injury by acetaminophen may cause very significant elevation of the AST.

Lee WM: Drug-induced hepatotoxicity. N Engl J Med 1995;333: 1118–1127.

14.8. Answer: D All of these toxins or conditions except chlorpromazine hepatotoxicity are associated with liver dysfunction secondary to failure of energy production by liver mitochondria. Chlorpromazine causes cholestasis.

Mahler H, Pasi A, Kramer JM, et al: Fulminant liver failure in association with the emetic toxin of *Bacillus cereus*. N Engl J Med 1997;336:1142–1148.

14.9. Answer: A The ability to make clotting factors is the best measurement of the functional capacity of the liver. Very high elevations of the bilirubin (>20 mg/dL) and the AST are consistent with extensive injury, but they are not useful predictors of functional capacity. Elevation of the creatinine also suggests serious injury. The alkaline phosphatase is not useful in predicting severity.

O'Grady JG, Tan KC, Williams R: Selection criteria and results of orthotopic liver transplantation in the UK. In: Williams R, Hughes

RD, eds: Acute Liver Failure. Improved Understanding and Better Therapy. London, Miter Press, 1991, pp. 77–80.

14.10. Answer: A   The presence of oxygen results in the production of a highly reactive metabolite that is rapidly cleared by binding to glutathione. In the absence of oxygen, a less reactive metabolite that does not readily bind glutathione leads to increased initiation of lipid peroxidation. Zone 3 injury by carbon tetrachloride is caused by the increased concentration of CYP2E1 in that area.

Burkhart KK, Hall AH, Gerace R, et al: Hyperbaric oxygen treatment for carbon tetrachloride poisoning. Drug Safety 1991;6: 332–338.

CHAPTER 15

IMMUNOLOGIC PRINCIPLES

15.1. Answer: C   One antibody molecule binds two molecules of toxin. Hence, sufficient antibody to neutralize the toxin can be delivered only for toxins that are lethal at concentrations in the nanogram-per-milliliter range. Because the lethal dose of theophylline is on the order of 100 mg/mL, it is not a good candidate for antibody therapy. Digoxin, colchicine, botulinum toxin, and tetanus toxin are all lethal at serum concentrations of 1 ng/mL or less and are hence excellent candidates for antibody therapy.

Scherrman JM, Terrien N, Urtizberea M, et al: Immunotoxicotherapy: present status and future trends. J Toxicol Clin Toxicol 1989; 27:1–35.

15.2. Answer: E   Exposure to a number of respiratory irritants has been associated with the inductions of RADS. In addition, toluene diisocyanate, ethylene oxide, chlorine, sulfur dioxide, ammonia, glacial acetic acid, smoke, and dust are associated with the induction of this asthma-like condition.

Brooks SM, Weiss MA, Bernstein IL: Reactive airways dysfunction syndrome (RADS): Persistent asthma syndrome after high level irritant exposure. Chest 1985;88:376–384.

15.3. Answer: E   Diesel exhaust particles, sulfur dioxide, ozone, sulfur dioxide, and nitrogen dioxide have all been demonstrated to potentiate production of IgE antibody to concomitantly administered proteins.

Matsumura Y: The effects of ozone, nitrogen dioxide, and sulfur dioxide on the experimentally induced allergic respiratory disorder in guinea pigs. I. The effects of sensitization with albumin through the airway. Am Rev Respir Dis 1970;102:430–437.

15.4. Answer: E   Fab fragments containing the variable region (antigen-binding site) are formed by papain cleavage of the antibody molecule, and the Fc portion of the molecule is discarded. The Fc portion of the molecule is implicated in both anaphylaxis and serum sickness, so there is less chance of these complications with the Fab fragment. The Fab fragment is approximately one-third the size of an antibody molecule, so it has a larger volume of distribution. A smaller amount of substance is required, so smaller infusion volumes can be used.

15.5. Answer: D   A number of case reports have linked phenytoin with a selective IgA deficiency, and in some cases this association has been verified by rechallenge with the drug. Selective IgA deficiency has also been observed in association with captopril and penicillamine.

Proesmans W, Jaeken J, Eeckels R: D-Penicillamine-induced IgA deficiency in Wilson's disease. Lancet 1976;2:804–805.

Talesnik E, Rivero SJ, Gonzalez B: Serum IgA deficiency induced by prolonged phenytoin treatment. Rev Invest Clin 1989;41: 331–335.

15.6. Answer: C   There are no reports of collagen vascular disease or cancer associated with exposure to burning oil in Kuwait during the Persian Gulf War. However, aplastic anemia has been observed.

Shem SC, Kumar R, Roberts IA: Aplastic anaemia after exposure to burning oil. Lancet 1995;346:183.

Stern MA, Eckman J, Otterman MK: Aplastic anemia after exposure to burning oil. N Engl J Med 1994;331:58.

15.7. Answer: E   In addition to reports of systemic lupus erythematosus associated with the pharmaceuticals hydralazine and procainamide, it has been associated with the yellow food coloring agent tartrazine and the laboratory chemical hydrazine. Lidocaine is not associated with systemic lupus.

Talmadge DW, Bice DE, Bloom JC, et al: Biologic Markers in Immunotoxicology. Washington DC, National Research Council, 1992, pp. 53–62.

15.8. Answer: C   Penicillin binds to red blood cells, and an antibody is produced against this bound penicillin. Methyldopa produces hemolytic anemia by disrupting the immune regulatory system that protects against self-antigens. Molecular mimicry, in that the chemical structure of a xenobiotic is so similar to antigens on the red blood cell surface that antibodies against the xenobiotic bind to red blood cells, is most commonly seen with infectious agents. Answers D and E are not known mechanisms of xenobiotic-induced hemolytic anemia.

Dell A, Antoine SM, Gaunt CJ, et al: Autoimmune determinants of rheumatic carditis: Localization of epitopes in human cardiac myosin. Eur Heart J 1991;12(Suppl D):155–162.

Tisch R, McDevitt H: Insulin dependent diabetes mellitus. Cell 1996;85:291–297.

15.9. Answer: B   The Spanish toxic oil syndrome occurred when approximately 100,000 inhabitants in and about Madrid consumed rapeseed oil contaminated with anilines. Approximately 20% of those exposed developed an acute illness, and about 1% developed a chronic disease with features of scleroderma and other collagen vascular diseases, including hematologic markers of these diseases. Those individuals who developed the chronic phase of the disease were more likely to have HLA haplotypes DR3 and DR4.

Kammuler ME, Bloksma N, Seinen W: Chemical-induced autoimmune reactions and Spanish toxic oil syndrome. Focus on hydantoins and related compounds. J Toxicol Clin Toxicol 1988;26: 157–174.

Noriega AR, Gomez-Reino J, Lopez-Encouentra A, et al: Toxic epidemic syndrome, Spain, 1981. Lancet 1982;2:697–702.

15.10. Answer: A Dioxins and furans may suppress cellular immunity in humans. The compound 2,3,7,8-tetrachlorodibenzo-*p*-dioxin (TCDD) suppresses T-helper cell function in exposed workers up to 20 years after exposure. Workers exposed to a mixture of phenoxy herbicides contaminated with dioxins and furans have increased total and respiratory cancer mortality relative to controls. An increased total cancer mortality, and in particular cancer mortality from digestive and respiratory cancers, was found in workers exposed to TCDD. This increase in cancer mortality may be secondary to impaired cellular immunity against tumors.

Ott MG, Zober A: Cause specific mortality and cancer incidence among employees exposed to 2,3,7,8-TCDD after a 1953 reactor accident. Occup Environ Med 1996;53:606–612.

Tonn T, Esser C, Schneider EM, et al: Persistence of decreased T-helper cell function in industrial workers 20 years after exposure to 2,3,7,8-tetrachlorodibenzo-*p*-dioxin. Environ Health Perspect 1996;104:422–426.

CHAPTER 16

MUTAGENS, CARCINOGENS, AND TERATOGENS

16.1. Answer: C Ideally there should be quantitative proof of exposure with measured biologic markers, but this is not one of Shepherd's criteria.

Shepherd TH: "Proof" of human teratogenicity. Teratology 1994; 50:97–98.

16.2. Answer: E Concentrations of both nicotine and cotinine have been shown to be significantly higher in the hair of both passive smokers and their infants than in control mother–infant pairs.

Eliopoulos C, Klein J, Phan MK, et al: Hair concentrations of nicotine and cotinine in women and their newborn infants. JAMA 1994;271:621–623.

16.3. Answer: B Maternal cigarette smoking has not been associated with congenital heart defects but has been associated with low birth weight, prematurity, increased spontaneous abortions, and SIDS.

Abel EL: Smoking and pregnancy. J Psychoactive Drug 1984;16: 327–328.

16.4. Answer: C Most carcinogens are mutagens, but not all mutagens are carcinogens.

Okey AB: Carcinogenesis and mutagenesis by xenobiotic chemicals. In: Kalant H, Roschlau WHE, eds: Principles of Medical Pharmacology, 5th ed. Toronto, Decker, 1989, pp. 632–643.

16.5. Answer: B Mercury is a teratogen but is not a recognized carcinogen.

Okey AB: Carcinogenesis and mutagenesis by xenobiotic chemicals. In: Kalant H, Roschlau WHE, eds: Principles of Medical Pharmacology, 5th ed. Toronto, Decker, 1989, pp. 632–643.

16.6. Answer: E Drugs may be detected in at least the first three meconium stools, although levels are often significantly decreased after the second stool and if there has been passage of meconium in utero.

Ostrea EM, Brady MJ, Parks PM, et al: Drug screening of meconium in infants of drug dependent mothers: An alternative to urine testing. J Pediatr 1989;115:474–477.

16.7. Answer: B Methylmercury is primarily a neurotoxin, and studies have shown that the nervous system is most vulnerable in later pregnancy (second and third trimesters) and in early postnatal life.

Grandjean P, Weithe P, Nielsen JB: Methylmercury: significance of intrauterine and postnatal exposures. Clin Chem 1994;40: 1395–1400.

Marsh DO, Clarkson TW, Cox C, et al: Fetal methylmercury poisoning, relationship between concentrations in single strand of maternal hair and child effects. Arch Neurol 1987;44:1017–1022.

Reynolds WA, Pitkin RM: Transplacental passage of methylmercury and its uptake by primate fetal tissues. Proc Soc Exp Biol Med 1975;148:523–536.

16.8. Answer: D Cord blood levels have been shown by many studies to correlate well with maternal blood lead levels.

Angell NF, Lavery JP: The relationship of blood lead levels to obstetric outcome. Am J Obstet Gynecol 1982;142:40–46.

Milman N, Christensen JM, Ibsen KK: Blood lead and erythrocyte zinc protoporphyrin in mothers and newborn infants. Eur J Pediatr 1988;147:71–73.

16.9. Answer: A Both cocaine and its metabolite benzoylecgonine are detectable in hair after known systemic exposure. Exposure via passive smoking results in external contamination, which is washable and thus able to be differentiated from systemic exposure.

Koren G, Klein J, Forman R, et al: Hair analysis of cocaine; differentiation between systemic exposure and external contamination. J Clin Pharmacol 1992;32:671–675.

16.10. Answer: D Valproic acid and carbamazepine are associated with an increased incidence of neural tube defects, and defects such as congenital cardiac defects and hydrocephalus have been demonstrated on midtrimester ultrasound following retinoic acid exposure.

Van Maldergem L, Jaumiaux E, Gillcrot Y: Morphological features of a cases of retinoic acid embryopathy. Prenat Diagn 1992; 12:699–701.

CHAPTER **17**

VITAL SIGNS AND TOXIC SYNDROMES

17.1. Answer: D Digoxin, nadolol, and morphine cause a brady-cardia in overdose. Clonidine can initially cause a tachycardia before a persistent bradycardia develops; however, the patient usually has an increase in blood pressure during the initial stimulatory phase. Nifedipine appears unique among the currently available calcium channel blocking agents in its ability to increase heart rate.

Weiner DA: Calcium channel blockers. Med Clin North Am 1988; 72:83–115.

17.2. Answer: B The opioids depress the respiratory rate by stimulation of the μ_2 receptors. Flunitrazepam, propofol, and secco-barbital are GABA agonists that produce central nervous system depression. The salicylates in overdose produce stimulation of the respiratory center, causing both tachypnea and hyperpnea.

Milhorn DE, Eldridge FL, Waldrop RG: Effects of salicylate and 2,4 dinitrophenol on respiration and metabolism. J Appl Physiol 1982;53:925–929.

17.3. Answer: D A disulfiram–ethanol interaction, iron, and iso-propanol poisoning can be associated with significant hypoten-sion. Organic phosphorus compound poisoning may result in mild hypotension. Increased blood pressure is one of the most sensitive markers of lead toxicity, and the association between the two has been significantly correlated in several studies.

Environmental Protection Agency: Supplement to the 1986 Air Quality Criteria for Lead. Addendum EPA/600/8–89/049A, Office of Health and Environmental Protection Assessment. Washington, DC, US Environmental Protection Agency, 1989, pp. A1–A67.

Pirkle JL, Schwartz J, Landis JR, Harlan WR: The relationship between blood lead levels and blood pressure and its cardiovascular risk implications. Am J Epidemiol 1985;121:246–258.

17.4. Answer: A Phencyclidine and diphenhydramine would be expected to cause a tachycardia in overdose. Iron and isoniazid either will not change heart rate or may cause an increase in heart rate as the patient becomes hypotensive or develops a metabolic acidosis. Phenylpropanolamine is a pure α-adrenergic agonist; as blood pressure increases, patients often will develop a reflex bradycardia.

Horowitz JD, Lang WJ, Howes LG: Hypertensive response induced by phenylpropanolamine in anorectic and decongestant preparations. Lancet 980;1:60–61.

17.5. Answer: B Chronic occupational exposure to carbon disul-fide has been suggested to cause an acceleration of atherosclerotic disease with an increase in both coronary artery disease and hyper-tension. Chronic exposure to sulfur dioxide causes an increase in chronic obstructive pulmonary disease and coronary artery disease. The nitrates can cause an increase in headaches and ortho-static hypotension, and chronic low-level exposure to carbon monoxide can cause an array of neuropsychiatric symptoms.

Partanen T: Coronary heart disease among workers exposed to carbon disulfide. Br J Indust Med 1970;27:313–325.

17.6. Answer: D The alcohol withdrawal syndrome is character-ized by tremulousness, tachycardia, tachypnea, hypertension, hy-perthermia, diaphoresis, and an altered level of consciousness. The opioid withdrawal syndrome is characterized by tachycardia, tachypnea, hypertension, a normal temperature, and anxiety with a normal level of consciousness.

Victor M, Adams RD: The effect of alcohol on the nervous system. Res Publ Assoc Res Nerv Ment Dis 1953;32:526–573.

17.7. Answer: E Adrenergic agent toxicity is typically mani-fested by hypertension, tachycardia, tachypnea, hyperthermia, an altered consciousness, and mydriasis. These findings may be noted in anticholinergic toxicity, although hypertension and tachypnea are not typically present. The major differences are the absence of peristalsis and diaphoresis and the presence of dry mucous membranes and urinary retention in anticholinergic poi-soning. In adrenergic poisoning, peristalsis and diaphoresis are present, and the mucous membranes are moist.

17.8. Answer: D Adrenergic, anticholinergic, and opioid agent overdoses typically are manifest by an altered level of conscious-ness. Opioid withdrawal is not associated with an altered level of consciousness but typically with anxiety. Ethanol withdrawal is associated with alcohol withdrawal seizures and an altered level of consciousness.

17.9. Answer: E Arsenic, botulism, and mercury are not typi-cally associated with thermoregulatory abnormalities early in the clinical course. Carbamazepine may be associated with hypother-mia. Phencyclidine poisoning typically results in hypertension, tachycardia, tachypnea, and hyperthermia. Diverse clinical mani-festations may occur depending on the dose taken or molecule used, but agitation and CNS stimulation with resultant hyperther-mia are common.

Barton CH, Sterling ML, Naziri ND: Phencyclidine intoxication: Clinical experience with 27 cases confirmed by urine assay. Ann Emerg Med 1981;10:243–246.

Barton CH, Sterling ML, Naziri ND: Rhabdomyolysis and acute renal failure associated with phencyclidine intoxication. Arch In-tern Med 1980;140:568–569.

Brecher M, Wang BW, Wong H, Morgan JP: Phencyclidine and violence: Clinical and legal issues. J Clin Psychopharmacol 1988; 8:397–401.

17.10. Answer: B The endpoint in anticholinergic treatment is clearing of the secretions from the tracheobronchial tree and dry-ing of most secretions. Although tachycardia is not a contraindica-tion to continued treatment, it is usually a good marker of success. Persistent tachycardia may suggest inadequate therapy or hypoxia.

DiKart WL, Kiestra SH, Sangster B: The use of atropine and oximes in organophosphate intoxication: A modified approach. J Toxicol Clin Toxicol 1988;26:199–208.

Koplovitz I, Mento R. Matthews C, et al: Dose-response effects of atropine and HI-6 treatment of organophosphorus poisoning in guinea pigs. Drug Chem Toxicol 1995;18:119–136.

CHAPTER 18

THERMOREGULATORY PRINCIPLES

18.1. Answer: D Thermosensitive neurons are located predominantly in the preoptic area of the anterior hypothalamus, although some are found in the posterior hypothalamus. Heating or cooling of the hypothalamus in conscious animals results in appropriate thermoregulatory responses.

Hensel H: Neural processes in thermoregulation. Physiol Rev 1973;53:948–1007.

18.2. Answer: C Sweat glands are controlled by sympathetic postganglionic nerve fibers that are cholinergic. Large amounts of acetylcholinesterase and a number of peptides are involved in neural transmission. Anticholinergic drugs impair sweat gland function and predispose to heat illness.

Hensel H: Neural processes in thermoregulation. Physiol Rev 1973;53:948–1007.

18.3. Answer: B Shivering is the main thermoregulatory response to cold in humans, except in neonates, where nonshivering thermogenesis prevails. Shivering is initiated in the posterior hypothalamus. Efferent stimuli from the posterior hypothalamus travel through the midbrain, pons, and lateral medullary reticular formation to the motor pathways of the tectospinal and rubrospinal tract, resulting in shivering. Heat produced without muscle contraction is nonshivering thermogenesis. Brown fat, the most important site of nonshivering thermogenesis, is found primarily in neonates.

Birzis L, Hemingway A: Descending brain stem connections controlling shivering in cat. J Neurophysiol 1956;19:37–43.

Bruck K: Non-shivering thermogenesis and brown adipose tissue in relation to age, and their integration in the thermoregulatory system. In: Lindberg O, ed: Brown Adipose Tissue. Amsterdam, Elsevier/North-Holland, 1970, pp. 117–154.

18.4. Answer: E A deflection occurring at the junction of the QRS and ST segment, now known as the Osborn wave, was first described in 1938. This J-point deflection is invariably found in the hypothermic patient when multiple electrocardiographic leads are obtained.

Emslie-Smith D: Accidental hypothermia: A common condition with a pathognomonic electrocardiogram. Lancet 1958;2: 492–495.

Osborn JJ: Experimental hypothermia: Respiratory and blood pH changes in relation to cardiac function. Am J Physiol 1953;175: 389–398.

Tomaszewski W: Changements électrocardiographiques observes chez un homme mort de froid. Arch Mal Coeur 1938;31:525–528.

Trevino A, Razi B, Beller BM: The characteristic electrocardiogram of accidental hypothermia. Arch Intern Med 1971;127: 470–472.

18.5. Answer: D Heatstroke is defined as a temperature >106°F (41.1°C) in the setting of mental status alteration. Although absence of sweating was once thought to comprise part of the definition of heatstroke, many patients with heatstroke have been noted on presentation to maintain the ability to sweat.

Malamud N, Haymaker W, Custer RP: Heatstroke: A clinicopathologic study of 125 fatal cases. Milit Surg 1946;99:397–444.

18.6. Answer: E Cocaine, antihistamines, lithium, and cyclic antidepressants predispose to hyperthermia. Organic phosphorus compound insecticides and other agents that cause cholinergic stimulation cause hypothermia by stimulation of inappropriate sweating and possibly through depression of the endogenous utilization of calorigenic substrates.

Maickel RP: Interaction of drugs with autonomic nervous function and thermoregulation. Fed Proc 1970;29:1973–1979.

18.7. Answer: C Dantrolene sodium is the preferred drug in the treatment of malignant hyperthermia. Dantrolene acts directly on skeletal muscle and either inhibits the release of calcium or increases calcium uptake through the sarcoplasmic reticulum. Dantrolene has not been demonstrated to improve outcome from heatstroke.

Bouchama A, Cafege A, Devol EB: Ineffectiveness of dantrolene sodium in the treatment of heatstroke. Crit Care Med 1991;19: 176–180.

Gronert GA: Controversies in malignant hyperthermia. Anesthesiology 1983;59:273–274.

18.8. Answer: E Thiamine deficiency, sepsis, hypoglycemia, and carbon monoxide poisoning predispose to hypothermia. Salicylates cause uncoupling of oxidative phosphorylation and predispose to hyperthermia.

Maickel RP: Interaction of drugs with autonomic nervous function and thermoregulation. Fed Proc 1970;29:1973–1979.

18.9. Answer: B Prolonged cardiorespiratory arrest and absolute temperature do not predict poor outcome. Profound hyperkalemia has been associated with the inability to successfully resuscitate severely hypothermic patients.

Althaus U, Aeberhard P, Schupbach P, et al: Management of profound accidental hypothermia with cardiorespiratory arrest. Ann Surg 1982;195:492–495.

Hauty MG, Esrig BC, Hill JG, Long WB: Prognostic factors in severe accidental hypothermia: Experiences from the Mt. Hood tragedy. J Trauma 1987;27:1107–1112.

18.10. Answer: D Volume of distribution has been shown to decrease in animals given gentamicin, lidocaine, and propranolol.

Koren G, Barker C, Bohn D, et al: Influence of hypothermia on the pharmacokinetics of gentamicin and theophylline in piglets. Crit Care Med 1985;13:844–847.

CHAPTER **19**

NEUROLOGIC PRINCIPLES

19.1. Answer: C   Although toxic-metabolic causes of altered consciousness are characterized by an absence of focality, hypoglycemia, caused in this case by glyburide, may sometimes present with asymmetric findings, suggesting a structural lesion, when in fact none is present. The pathophysiology is unknown.

Plum F, Posner J: The Diagnosis of Stupor and Coma, 3rd ed. Philadelphia, FA Davis, 1982, p. 220.

19.2. Answer: A   "Dissociated" nonfocal findings are the hallmark of toxic-metabolic alterations of mental status. Typically, these "dissociated" findings include a constellation of symmetric signs that are unlikely to be caused by structural disease because of the implausible anatomic requirements of such a lesion. Because another highly characteristic feature of toxic-metabolic coma is preservation of the pupillary light reflex, combining this intact reflex with a finding that suggests brainstem dysfunction, such as an absent oculovestibular response, would be difficult to explain anatomically and, therefore, is likely to be of toxic-metabolic origin.

19.3. Answer: E   Hypervitaminosis A may result in "pseudotumor" or benign intracranial hypertension, characterized by headache, papilledema, elevated intracranial pressure, and, if the macula becomes involved over time, some blurring of vision.

Bousser M: Benign intracranial hypertension and chronic hypervitaminosis Annu Rev Neurol (Paris) 1998;154:784–785.

19.4. Answer: D   Tetanus infection results in the formation of a neurotoxin that affects the neuromuscular junction, the sympathetic pathways, the spinal cord, and the brain. Tetanospasmin, the clinically important exotoxin of *Clostridium tetani,* travels from the point of entry, largely via the axon, to the CNS. There it blocks release of inhibitory neurotransmitters, thus producing disinhibited, widespread muscular spasm and autonomic instability.

19.5. Answer: D   Acute pyridoxine neuronopathy is caused by massive doses of pyridoxine, which disrupts the cellular metabolism of the dorsal root ganglion. The clinical picture is one of development of widespread sensory loss. Because the pathologic process involves only the dorsal root ganglion, motor function is unimpaired. Appendicular ataxia is marked and is a consequence of "sensory ataxia" rather than involvement of the cerebellum. In the chronic form, the prognosis in the few patients studied is poor, with persistent, incapacitating sensory ataxia. This is neither an axonopathy nor a demyelination (which are the other two principal forms of peripheral neuropathy) but is the prototypic neuronopathy. There is some autonomic instability in the acute form of the overdose, but it does not appear to be attributable to abnormalities at the neuromuscular junction.

Albin RL, Albers JW, Greenberg HS, et al: Acute sensory neuropathy-neuronopathy from pyridoxine overdose. Neurology 1987;37: 1729–1732.

19.6. Answer: E   Parkinson disease is characterized by tremor, rigidity, akinesia, and postural instability (TRAP). Drug-induced parkinsonism is caused by agents that either destroy cells in the substantia nigra, eg, 1-methyl-4-phenyl-1,2,3,6-tetrahydropyridine (MPTP) or, much more commonly, antagonize the effects of dopamine, either pre- or postsynaptically. The use of antipsychotic drugs is the most common reversible cause of parkinsonism. MPTP-induced parkinsonism has been reported almost exclusively in individuals using a synthetic opioid that contained MPTP. The syndrome differs from that of idiopathic Parkinson in its rapidity of onset. In most of the patients, the effects appear to be permanent.

19.7. Answer: E   Inattention is an essential feature of delirium. Memory is also frequently impaired, as is orientation. However, a delirious patient may not be completely disoriented to person, time, and place. Perceptual distortions, ie, hallucinations, are common in delirium but are not invariably present. Closely related to the lack of attention seen in delirium is a fluctuating level of consciousness, part of which entails the ill-defined characteristic "clouding of consciousness." Attention may sometimes be impaired in patients with psychiatric disease who are actively hallucinating or severely depressed but is far more characteristically diminished in patients with an organic confusional state.

19.8. Answer: E   Although asterixis was first described in patients with hepatic failure, it has since been described in association with a large number of toxic-metabolic encephalopathies, including intoxication with ethanol, anticonvulsants, tranquilizers, and sedative-hypnotics. It is also seen with renal failure, hyper- or hypoosmolar states, and ventilatory failure (probably secondary to acute hypercarbia). It has also been described in association with structural disease, but this is rare. These encephalopathies are typically accompanied by an alteration of mental status, although in mild cases the asterixis may be more prominent than the altered mental status. Asterixis can be classified along several different axes, based on the clinical picture, the presumed anatomic locus of the pathology in the nervous system, the neurotransmitters thought to mediate the movement disorder, or on the basis of the etiology of the asterixis. The most useful classification scheme in emergency medicine and toxicology is an etiologic one that focuses on the toxic-metabolic causes of asterixis.

Plum F, Posner J: The Diagnosis of Stupor and Coma, 3rd ed. Philadelphia, FA Davis, 1982, pp. 191–192.

19.9. Answer: A   Kinetic tremor is the preferred term for intention tremor and is distinct from the sustention tremor associated with excess sympathetic discharge or the resting tremor associated with Parkinson disease. Lithium is a common cause of tremor in which multiple mechanisms are probably involved. Although tremor is a frequent sign of toxicity, patients with therapeutic lithium levels may exhibit both a postural and kinetic tremor, which respond to dosage reduction. However, grossly irregular kinetic and resting tremor should be regarded as signs of severe toxicity until proved otherwise.

Van Putten T: Lithium-induced disabling tremor. Psychosomatics 1978;19:27–31.

19.10. Answer: E Akathisia is a form of involuntary motor restlessness that results in an inability to remain still for any sustained period. It is one of the most common of the extrapyramidal side effects of antipsychotics and typically occurs within 2 to 3 months of starting oral medication. Patients with akathisia do not manifest any particular movement and may often merely seem restless, making it easy to confuse this entity with psychotic agitation. Because this is a common and very troubling symptom to many patients, it is important to consider akathisia in the differential diagnosis of agitation in any patient on neuroleptics.

Braude WM, Barnes TR, Gore SM: Clinical characteristics of akathisia. A systematic investigation of acute psychiatric inpatient admissions. Br J Psychiatry 1983;143:139–150.

CHAPTER 20

RESPIRATORY PRINCIPLES

20.1. Answer: B Fentanyl is unique among all of the opioids, in that it has the ability to produce severe chest wall rigidity of a degree that can compromise ventilation. Although the exact mechanism for this effect is unknown, it is relieved by both naloxone and neuromuscular blocking agents.

Caspi J, Klausner JM, Safadi T, et al: Delayed respiratory depression following fentanyl anesthesia for cardiac surgery. Crit Care Med 1988;16:238–240.

Christian CM, Waller JL, Moldenhauer CC: Postoperative rigidity following fentanyl anesthesia. Anesthesiology 1983;58:275–277.

20.2. Answer: C Nebulized sodium bicarbonate provides relief from pain and cough in patients exposed to chlorine gas. This probably results from neutralization of hydrochloric acid that forms when chlorine gas dissolves in lung water. Although not studied, patients exposed to hydrogen chloride, sulfur dioxide, or other acid-forming gases may also be treated with dilute nebulized sodium bicarbonate.

Chisholm CD, Singletary EM, Okerberg CV, et al: Inhaled sodium bicarbonate therapy for chlorine inhalational injuries. Ann Emerg Med 1989;18;466.

20.3. Answer: C The formation of carboxyhemoglobin lowers the oxygen saturation of hemoglobin. Because this has no effect on pulmonary gas exchange, the Po_2 should be normal. Similarly, because the oxygen saturation of the arterial blood gas is defined by the Po_2, it should always relate to the Po_2 and will therefore be normal. The pulse oximeter misinterprets carboxyhemoglobin as oxyhemoglobin and therefore is also normal. Thus, the only way to establish the diagnosis of carbon monoxide poisoning is to test the specimen on a CO-oximeter, where the carboxyhemoglobin will be high and the oxygen saturation will be low.

Tremper KK, Barker SJ: Using pulse oximetry when dyshemoglobin levels are high. J Crit Illness 1988;3:103–107.

20.4. Answer: E Simple asphyxiants have no direct pulmonary or systemic toxicity. Nitrogen dioxide exposure, which can result

from exhaust of internal combustion engines, exposure to silage, and, in industry, is associated with respiratory irritation and the potential progression to bronchiolitis obliterans.

Milne JEH: Nitrogen dioxide inhalation and bronchiolitis obliterans: A review of the literature and report of a case. J Occup Med 1969;11:538–547.

20.5. Answer: E Cyanide, hydrozoic acid (a liberator of azide), and hydrogen sulfide all poison the cytochrome oxidase chain leading to anaerobic respiration and metabolic organ failure. Amyl nitrite is a potent methemoglobin inducer used in the treatment of cyanide poisoning. Chloracetophenone, commonly referred to as CN or mace, is a strong irritant gas that has no systemic toxicity.

Hu H, Fine J, Epstein P, et al: Tear gas: Harassing agent or toxic chemical weapon. JAMA 1989;262:660–663.

20.6. Answer: B The formation of methemoglobin lowers the oxygen saturation of hemoglobin. Because this has no effect on pulmonary gas exchange, the Po_2 should be normal. Similarly, because the oxygen saturation on the arterial blood gas is defined by the Po_2, it should always relate to the Po_2 and will therefore be normal. The pulse oximeter misinterprets methemoglobin as a mixture of both oxy- and deoxyhemoglobin such that the saturation measured by the pulse oximeter will be low, but will not directly correlate with the true methemoglobin level. In fact, the pulse oximeter tends to approach 85% saturation regardless of the methemoglobin level. Thus, the only way to establish the diagnosis of methemoglobinemia is to test the specimen on a CO-oximeter, where the methemoglobin will be high and the oxygen saturation will be low.

Tremper KK, Barker SJ: Using pulse oximetry when dyshemoglobin levels are high. J Crit Illness 1988;3:103–107.

20.7. Answer: A Noncardiogenic pulmonary edema results from exposure to many toxins, often with varied and unknown etiologies. Although it can result from barbiturate overdose, this would occur only following aspiration and thus would not be directly associated with the toxin.

Reed CR, Glauser FL: Drug-induced noncardiogenic pulmonary edema. Chest 1991;100:1120–1124.

20.8. Answer: C Recent experimental evidence in animals demonstrates that there is a profound increase in catecholamine levels associated with opioid-induced hypercapnia. This results in pulmonary edema following opioid overdose, especially when the opioid is reversed before correction of the hypercapnia. Hypoxia alone was insufficient to give the same effect. Although other models may be important, this study helps link opioid-induced noncardiogenic pulmonary edema to other causes of noncardiogenic pulmonary edema (such as neurogenic edema).

Mill CA, Flacke JW, Miller JD, et al: Cardiovascular effects of fentanyl reversed by naloxone at varying arterial carbon dioxide tensions in dogs. Anesth Analg 1988;67:730–736.

20.9. Answer: A These two disasters resulted from the massive release of carbon dioxide (a simple asphyxiant) from the depths of volcanic lakes. It was estimated that 250,000 tons of carbon dioxide were released by Lake Nyos alone. Because carbon dioxide is heavier than air, it then flowed down into low-lying valleys, where it killed humans and livestock merely by displacing oxygen.

Freeth KJ, Kay RLF: The Lake Nyos gas disaster. Nature 1987; 325:104–105.

Kling GW, Clark MA, Compton HR, et al: The 1986 Lake Nyos gas disaster in Cameroon, West Africa. Science 1987;236: 169–175.

20.10. Answer: D Barotrauma results from the deep inhalation and Valsalva maneuver that follows abuse of insufflated or inhaled toxins such as cocaine and marijuana and from a direct pressure injury resulting from high-pressure nitrous oxide canisters. It is not common following ingested toxins such as MDMA.

Birrer RB, Calderon J: Pneumothorax, pneumomediastinum, and pneumopericardium following Valsalva's maneuver during marijuana smoking. NY State J Med 1984;84:619–620.

Bush MN, Rubenstein R, Hoffman I, Bruno MS: Spontaneous pneumomediastinum as a consequence of cocaine use. NY State J Med 1984;84:618–619.

CHAPTER 21

CARDIOVASCULAR PRINCIPLES

21.1. Answer: C Terfenadine (but not its metabolites) blocks the potassium channels of the membrane to prolong the QT interval and predispose to development of torsades de pointes. Overdose of terfenadine may lead to toxic levels of the parent drug. Interference with metabolism of terfenadine by CYP3A4 (a member of the cytochrome P450 family) may also cause torsades de pointes.

Monahan BP, Ferguson CL, Killeavy ES, et al: Torsades de pointes occurring in association with terfenadine use. JAMA 1990;264:2788–2790.

21.2. Answer: D Propoxyphene is metabolized in the liver to norpropoxyphene, which has less analgesic effect, a much longer half-life, and local anesthetic properties similar to those of the class I antidysrhythmic agents. The marked QRS widening and dysrhythmias of propoxyphene toxicity may respond to sodium bicarbonate or lidocaine.

Stork CM, Redd JT, Fine K, Hoffman RS: Propoxyphene-induced wide QRS complex dysrhythmia responsive to sodium bicarbonate—a case report. J Toxicol Clin Toxicol 1995;33:179–183.

Whitcomb DC, Gilliam FR, Starmer CF, Grant AO: Marked QRS complex abnormalities and sodium channel blockade by propoxyphene reversed with lidocaine. J Clin Invest 1989;84: 1629–1636.

21.3. Answer: B The cardiovascular toxicity of chloral hydrate, inhalational anesthetics, and halogenated solvents (carbon tetrachloride) are believed to result from sensitization of the myocardium to catecholamine activity. Therefore, a β-adrenergic antagonist, such as propranolol, is the preferred antidysrhythmic agent for atrial or ventricular dysrhythmias.

Graham SR, Day RO, Lee R, Fulde GW: Overdose with chloral hydrate: A pharmacological and therapeutic review. Med J Aust 1988;149:686–688.

21.4. Answer: D Omeprazole (Prilosec) does not have any "quinidinelike" myocardial cell membrane activity. The other agents bind to either potassium or calcium channels during phase 2 of the action potential and prolong the QRS complexes.

Buckley NA, Whyte IM, Dawson AH: Cardiotoxicity more common in thioridazine overdose than with other neuroleptics. J Toxicol Clin Toxicol 1995;33:199–204.

Kim SY, Benowitz NL: Poisoning due to class IA antiarrhythmic drugs quinidine, procainamide, and disopyramide. Drug Safety 1990;5:393–420.

21.5. Answer: D Yohimbine is an α_2-adrenergic antagonist occasionally used in the treatment of impotence. The α_2-adrenergic receptors are primarily located on the presynaptic membrane and are "autoregulatory" receptors. Stimulating these receptors decreases the amount of norepinephrine released into the synapse. However, blocking these receptors leads to increased release of norepinephrine into the synapse. The expected adverse effects are tachycardia and hypertension.

Friesen K, Palatnick W, Tenenbein M: Benign course after massive ingestion of yohimbine. J Emerg Med 1993;11:287–288.

21.6. Answer: B Cyclic antidepressants cause norepinephrine depletion in nerve endings by increasing release and blocking reuptake. Agents (such as dopamine) that work primarily by increasing release of norepinephrine would be relatively ineffective in these toxic exposures. Phenylephrine or norepinephrine, which directly interact with the postsynaptic α receptors are more effective for treatment of the hypotension.

21.7. Answer: C Bretylium initially results in increased norepinephrine release from sympathetic neurons and inhibition of subsequent uptake. Bretylium can cause transient hypertension, tachycardia, and increased dysrhythmias through the norepinephrine release.

Leatham EW, Holt DW, McKenna WJ: Class III antiarrhythmics in overdose. Presenting features and management principles. Drug Safety 1993;9:450–462.

21.8. Answer: D Intravascular volume depletion in toxic exposures can occur through gastrointestinal losses (iron, theophylline), insensible losses, diaphoresis (cocaine, organic phosphorus compounds, theophylline), urinary losses (theophylline), interstitial redistribution (iron), and vascular dilatation (iron, theophylline). Jimson weed exposure causes the classic anticholinergic toxidrome of dry flushed skin, tachycardia, mydriasis, urinary retention, hallucinations, and decreased bowel sounds. However, the patients do not typically manifest intravascular volume depletion.

Gowdy JM: Stramonium intoxication: A review of symptomatology in 212 cases. JAMA 1972;221:585–587.

21.9. Answer: A Conduction delays are common with class IA, IC, and III antidysrhythmic agents. These agents affect the potassium or calcium channels during phase 2 of the action potential. The class IB agents, such as lidocaine, affect primarily the sodium channels during phase 0 and have little affect on the PR, QRS, or QT intervals.

Vaughan-Williams EM: Subgroups of class I antiarrhythmic drugs. Eur Heart J 1984;5:96–98.

21.10. Answer: D Sotalol is a class III antidysrhythmic agent that also has β-adrenergic antagonist properties. Overdose of class III antidysrhythmics prolongs the QT interval and leads to increased risk of dysrhythmias, including torsades de pointes. Overdose of sotalol may also present with features suggestive of β-adrenergic antagonist toxicity, including bradycardia and hypotension.

Reith DM, Dawson AH, Epid D, et al: Relative toxicity of beta blockers in overdose. J Toxicol Clin Toxicol 1996:34:273–278.

CHAPTER 22

GASTROINTESTINAL PRINCIPLES

22.1. Answer: E Both acid and alkali ingestions are linked to the development of squamous cell carcinomas of the esophagus and stomach, particularly at the gastroesophageal junction, many years after an ingestion. Alkalis cause liquefactive necrosis, allowing deep tissue penetration of the toxin. Acids produce damage to both the esophagus and stomach. The earlier belief that acids do not damage the esophagus likely relates to the aqueous form in which most acids are available. The metabolic acidosis is typically of the increased anion gap variety, and the serum lactate is elevated. It results primarily from tissue destruction and hypotension. Only in the case of hydrochloric acid, in which excessive chloride may be absorbed, is the acidosis initially of the normal anion gap type.

Appleqvist P, Salmo S: Lye corrosion carcinoma of the esophagus: a review of 63 cases. Cancer 1980;45:2655–2685.

Eaton H, Tennekoon GE: Squamous carcinoma of the stomach following corrosive acid burns. Br J Surg 1972;59:382–387.

Hopkins RA, Postlethwait RW: Caustic burns and carcinoma of the esophagus. Ann Surg 1981;194:146–148.

Kivrianta VK: Corrosion carcinoma of the esophagus. Acta Otolaryngol 1952;42:89–95.

Zargar SA, Kochhar R, Nagi B, et al: Ingestion of corrosive acids. Spectrum of injury to upper gastrointestinal tract and natural history. Gastroenterology 1989;97:702–707.

22.2. Answer: C Exposure to over 600 rads usually results in vomiting within 2 hours. Vomiting that occurs within minutes usually indicates a lethal exposure. Exposures to over 100 rads is associated with nausea and vomiting, and exposure to over 2000 rads can, in addition to causing GI symptoms within minutes, lead to death within 2 days.

Conklin JJ, Walker RL, Hirsch EF: Current concepts in the management of radiation injuries and associated trauma. Surg Gynecol Obstet 1985;156:809–826.

22.3. Answer: C Alcohol increases the secretion of gastric juices, reduces the transmucosal potential difference, allowing for back-diffusion of hydrogen ions, and increases mucosal permeability. Alcohol concentrations as low as 8% have been associated with GI lesions. In some series, alcohol-induced erosive gastritis, with or without concomitant use of salicylates, accounts for 45 to 90% of upper GI hemorrhages. Alcohol causes diarrhea for several reasons: decreased transit time, decreased pancreatic function, and decreased disaccharidase activity.

Geall MG, Phillips SF, Summerskill WHJ: Profile of gastric potential difference in man. Effects of aspirin, alcohol, bile, and endogenous acid. Gastroenterology 1970;58:437–443.

Nalin DR, Levine MM, Rhead J, et al: Cannabis, hydrochlorhydria and cholera. Lancet 1978;2:859–861.

22.4. Answer: C Oxalate-containing plants, particularly dumbcane, cause local irritation, which results in pain and edema of the mouth and tongue. On occasion, the effects may be severe enough to cause death. Probably because it is almost impossible to ingest significant amounts of oxalate-containing plants, systemic problems such as hypocalcemia and renal failure do not occur. Diarrhea, not constipation, may occur as the result of an ingestion. Peptic ulcers have not been described.

McIntire MS, Guest JR, Porterfield JF: Philodendron: An infant death. J Toxicol Clin Toxicol 1990;28:177–183.

22.5. Answer: D Paraquat ingestions result in lip, tongue, and pharyngeal pain and ulceration. Systemic complications include pulmonary edema, pneumothorax, hepatic and renal failure, dysrhythmias, shock, coma, and convulsions. A unique feature of paraquat is the formation of a pseudomembrane in the pharynx, said to resemble diphtheria. Of the other items listed, two—hydrofluoric acid and concentrated hydrochloric acid—are associated with severe systemic effects in addition to the local damage after acute ingestions, but none are associated with a pseudomembrane.

Stephens DS, Walker DH, Schaffer W, et al: Pseudodiphtheria. Ann Intern Med 1981;94:202–204.

22.6. Answer: D Anticholinergics typically cause dry mouth and decreased secretions, as does botulism. The opposite effect, ie, a cholinergic syndrome, including drooling and salivation, is caused by organic phosphorus compounds and carbamate insecticides and other anticholinesterases. Caustics and tetrodotoxin are also associated with drooling, as is partial obstruction from foreign bodies.

Nandi P, Ong GB: Foreign body in the esophagus: Review of 2,394 cases. Br J Surg 1978;65:5–9.

Torda TA, Sinclair E, Ulyatt DB: Puffer fish tetrodotoxin poisoning: Clinical record and suggested management. Med J Aust 1973;1:599–602.

22.7. Answer: D Phenothiazines are associated with constipation from pseudoobstruction. Colchicine, mercuric chloride, pokeweed, and toxic mushrooms are all commonly associated with diarrhea.

22.8. Answer: B Phenolphthalein in an alkaline medium is associated with pink stools. Phosphorus ingestion is associated with smoking stools with a garlic odor. Blood, of course, is associated not only with black, tarry stools (melena) but also with a stool positive for occult blood. Senna and bismuth subsalicylate (Pepto-Bismol) are associated with black stools but not stools positive for occult blood. Therapeutic doses of iron (as in vitamins) are associated with black, negative for occult blood stools, whereas iron poisoning from an iron tablet overdose is associated with gastrointestinal bleeding and, therefore, black (or red) stools positive for occult blood.

De Wolff FA, Edelbrock PM, deHaas EJM, Vermeg P: Experience with a screening method for laxative abuse. Hum Toxicol 1983; 2:385–389.

22.9. Answer: E Histologically, alcoholic pancreatitis is considered a form of chronic pancreatitis, but clinically, acute exacerbations are more typical of acute pancreatitis and treated as such. All of the other statements are true.

22.10. Answer: B The antibiotic pentamidine has been linked to pancreatitis characterized by abdominal pain and elevated amylase levels as well as to that characterized by hyperglycemia, diabetes, and hypoglycemia, particularly in patients with AIDS, who commonly use this medication. Ethanol and estrogens are more closely associated with acute and chronic (exocrine) pancreatitis, whereas androgens and Vacor predominantly affect the β cells in the islets of Langerhans.

Hauser L, Sheehan P, Simpkins H: Pancreatic pathology in pentamidine-induced diabetes in acquired immunodeficiency syndrome patients. Hum Pathol 1991;22:926–929.

Murphey SA, Josephs AS: Acute pancreatitis associated with pentamidine therapy. Arch Intern Med 1981;141:56–58.

CHAPTER 23

RENAL PRINCIPLES

23.1. Answer: C All of the other drugs can cause acute renal failure by direct toxicity.

Richards JR, Johnson EB, Stark RW, Derlet RW. Methamphetamine abuse and rhabdomyolysis in the ED: a 5-year study. Am J Emerg Med 1999;17:681–685.

23.2. Answer: E Early treatment with IV saline, bicarbonate, and mannitol may prevent tubular necrosis in rhabdomyolysis. However, primary renal failure may itself cause increased urinary myoglobin, detectable by dipstick.

Feinfeld DA, Briscoe AM, Nurse HM, et al: Myoglobinuria in chronic renal failure. Am J Kidney Dis 1986;8:111–114.

Ron D, Taitelman MD, Michaelson MD, et al: Prevention of acute renal failure in traumatic rhabdomyolysis. Arch Intern Med 1984; 144:277–280.

23.3. Answer: B Acute interstitial nephritis caused by NSAIDs is often accompanied by the nephrotic syndrome. Acute interstitial nephritis is a form of acute renal failure. The majority of patients with β-lactam-associated interstitial nephritis have at least one symptom of hypersensitivity. Thiazides are a cause of interstitial nephritis.

Sturmer T, Elseviers MM, De Broe ME: Nonsteroidal anti-inflammatory drugs and the kidney. Curr Opin Nephrol Hypertens 2001; 10:161–163.

23.4. Answer: E None of the other substances has ever been associated with nephrotic syndrome.

Becker CG, Becker EF, Maher JF, et al: Nephrotic syndrome after contact with mercury: A report of five cases, three after the use of ammoniated mercury ointment. Arch Intern Med 1962;110: 178–186.

23.5. Answer: D Beryllium is reported to cause chronic interstitial nephritis. None of the other metals has ever been reported to cause chronic interstitial nephritis. Uranium, bismuth, and chromium cause acute tubular necrosis.

Barnett RN, Brown DS, Cadorna CB, et al: Beryllium disease with death from renal failure. Conn Med 1961;25:142–147.

23.6. Answer: A The tricyclic antidepressants may cause acute neurogenic bladder. None of the other agents has ever been reported to cause urinary tract obstruction.

23.7. Answer: C Any diuretic may cause intravascular volume depletion. None of the other substances causes a primary decrease in renal perfusion. They are associated with intrinsic renal diseases. Aspirin/phenacetin causes chronic interstitial nephritis; carbon tetrachloride and tobramycin cause acute tubular necrosis, and ampicillin is associated with acute interstitial nephritis.

23.8. Answer: D The nephrotoxicity of ethylene glycol results from its metabolism to oxalic acid, which complexes with Ca^{2+} and deposits in the kidney. All of the other substances are nephrotoxic without being metabolized.

23.9. Answer: A Papillary necrosis follows the chronic interstitial inflammation of analgesic nephropathy; gastric irritation is caused by the aspirin component, and methemoglobinemia is related to chronic phenacetin toxicity. Eosinophiluria characterizes hypersensitivity reactions; analgesic nephropathy is a toxic reaction not caused by hypersensitivity.

23.10. Answer: E Renal hypoperfusion increases the toxicity of any nephrotoxin. The aminoglycosides cause nonoliguric acute renal failure; the lesion is primarily in the proximal tubule. Larger, less frequent dosing reduces the risk of renal injury, and papillary necrosis is not seen in aminoglycoside nephropathy.

DeBroe ME, Giuliano R, Verpooten G: Choice of drug and dosage regimen: Two important risk factors for aminoglycoside nephrotoxicity. Am J Med 1986;80:115–118.

Humes HD, Weinberg JM, Knauss TC: Clinical and pathophysiological effects of aminoglycoside toxicity. Am J Kidney Dis 1982; 2:5–29.

CHAPTER **24**

FLUID, ELECTROLYTE, AND ACID–BASE PRINCIPLES

24.1. Answer: E A low anion gap can result from an increase in unmeasured cations (magnesium or lithium) or a decrease in unmeasured anions (hypoalbuminemia). Bromide (like iodide) is falsely measured as chloride, producing a low (or even negative) anion gap. Metformin may increase lactic acid.

Gabow PA: Disorders associated with an altered anion gap. Kidney Int 1985;27:472–483.

Oh MS, Carroll HJ: Current concepts: the anion gap. N Engl J Med 1977;297:814–817.

24.2. Answer: A Inorganic sulfur has been reported to cause a high-anion-gap metabolic acidosis that is probably not related to the generation of hydrogen sulfide. It was felt to result from excess sulfate in a patient with renal dysfunction. Digoxin and organic mercury do not commonly cause acid–base abnormalities. Acetazolamide causes a low-anion-gap (nongap) metabolic acidosis, and excessive nitrates (NO_3) also potentially lower the anion gap because of an interference with the determination of chloride.

Schwartz SM, Carroll HM, Scharschmidt LA: Sublimed (inorganic) sulfur ingestion. A cause of life-threatening metabolic acidosis with a high anion gap. Arch Intern Med 1986;146: 1437–1438.

24.3. Answer: D All of the agents listed except for colchicine cause SIADH. Colchicine use is associated with the generation of diabetes insipidus (DI).

Vokes TJ, Robertson GL: Disorders of antidiuretic hormone. Endocrinol Metab Clin North Am 1988;17:281–299.

24.4. Answer: C All of the agents listed except for imipramine cause DI. Like most of the other antidepressants, imipramine is associated with SIADH.

Spigset O, Hedenmalm K: Hyponatremia and the syndrome of inappropriate antidiuretic hormone secretion (SIADH) induced by psychotropic drugs. Drug Safety 1995;12:209–225.

24.5 Answer: E In addition to the toxic alcohols (methanol and ethylene glycol), liver failure, renal failure, sepsis, shock, and the ketoacidoses are all associated with an elevated osmolality gap. This is one of the major limitations of using this test in patients with unknown causes of metabolic acidosis.

Inaba H, Hirasawa H, Mizuguchi T: Serum osmolality gap in postoperative patients in intensive care. Lancet 1987;1:1331–1335.

Schelling JR, Howard RL, Winter SD, et al: Increased osmolal gap in alcoholic ketoacidosis and lactic acidosis. Ann Intern Med 1990;113:580–582.

Sklar AH, Linas SL: The osmolal gap in renal failure. Ann Intern Med 1983;98:481–482.

24.6. Answer: D Only small-molecular-weight noncharged compounds substantially alter osmolality. Thus, an osmolality gap may be generated by ethanol, methanol, isopropanol, or ethylene glycol. The determination of osmolality is not useful in theophylline toxicity. The boiling point elevation technique uses the increase in the boiling point of serum to determine the osmolality. However, ethanol, isopropanol, and methanol boil at lower temperatures than serum (mostly water), and they do not alter the boiling point. They should be detected using the freezing point depression technique. Ethylene glycol has a very high boiling point and can be detected by the boiling point elevation technique.

Eisen TF, Lacouture PG, Woolf A: Serum osmolality in alcohol ingestions: Differences in availability among laboratories of teaching hospital, nonteaching hospital, and commercial facilities. Am J Emerg Med 1989;7:256–259.

24.7. Answer: A Glycyrrhizic acid (found in licorice) produces hyponatremia by having a mineralocorticoid effect. Amphotericin and foscarnet are associated with diabetes insipidus; sorbitol and glycerol produce hypernatremia largely through volume depletion.

Edwards CRW: Lessons from licorice. N Engl J Med 1991;325: 1242–1243.

Farese RV, Biglieri EG, Shackleton CHL: Licorice induced hypermineralocorticoidism. N Engl J Med 1991;325:1223–1227.

24.8. Answer: B Heparin produces hyperkalemia by suppression of aldosterone. Furosemide causes hypokalemia through its effect on the distal convoluted tubule of the kidney. Toluene is associated with a profound hypokalemia produced by a distal renal tubular acidosis. Theophylline and albuterol move potassium intracellularly through stimulation of the β-adrenergic receptor. Insulin is used for the treatment of hyperkalemia because it moves potassium intracellularly along with glucose.

Oster JR, Singer I, Fishman LM: Heparin-induced aldosterone suppression and hyperkalemia. Am J Med 1995;98:575–586.

24.9. Answer: B Soluble barium salts produce hypokalemia through prevention of potassium efflux. Digoxin and the other cardiac glycosides produce hyperkalemia by blocking Na^+-K^+-ATPase. β-Adrenergic antagonists (such as propranolol) produce hyperkalemia (in overdose) by preventing β-adrenergic–mediated potassium movement intracellularly. Fluoride appears to open potassium channels because its effects are blocked by quinidine. Penicillin is usually delivered as a potassium salt.

Wetherill SF, Guarino MJ, Cox RW: Acute renal failure associated with barium chloride poisoning. Ann Intern Med 1981;95: 187–188.

24.10. Answer: E Theophylline produces hypomagnesemia through activation of the β-adrenergic receptor. Ethanol is associated with renal magnesium wasting and poor gastrointestinal absorption. Furosemide and the other loop diuretics cause renal wasting of magnesium. Amphotericin produces a distal renal tubular acidosis. Lithium is associated with hypermagnesemia.

Brass EP, Thompson WL: Drug-induced electrolyte abnormalities. Med Toxicol 1982;24:207–228.

CHAPTER 25

HEMATOLOGIC PRINCIPLES

25.1. Answer: C Fetal hemoglobin has a greater affinity for oxygen than hemoglobin A. This confers an advantage in utero, as the fetus can compete effectively with maternal hemoglobin. It is a disadvantage after birth, as oxygen unloading at tissue sites may be impaired.

25.2. Answer: D Although transcutaneous absorption does occur, the most significant route of exposure is pulmonary. Benzene is metabolized by hepatic mixed-function oxidase. Phase I metabolites (phenol and hydroquinone) are substrates for phase II reactions (conjugation with sulfate and glucuronide). The products of phase II metabolism as well as *trans-trans*-muconic acid are excreted in the urine. The oxidative metabolites formed in the liver are transported by blood to the bone marrow, where a mixed-function oxidase produces metabolites toxic to the marrow. Thrombocytosis and acute lymphocytic leukemia are not described as consequences of benzene poisoning.

Ganousis LG, Goon D, Zyglewska T, et al: Cell-specific metabolism in mouse bone marrow stroma: Studies of activation and detoxification of benzene metabolism. Mol Pharmacol 1992; 42:1118–1125.

Schattenberg DG, Sillman WS, Gruntmeir JJ, et al: Peroxidase activity in murine and human hematopoietic cells: Potential relevance to benzene-induced toxicity. Mol Pharmacol 1994;46: 346–351.

Seaton MJ, Schlosser PM, Medinsky MA: In vitro conjugation of benzene metabolites by human liver: Potential influence of interindividual variability on benzene toxicity. Carcinogenesis 1995; 16:1519–1527.

25.3. Answer: B Two unrelated hematologic syndromes may develop after CAP exposure: anemia and aplastic anemia. Those with anemia generally recover following the cessation of CAP exposure, but aplastic anemia results in death. Electron microscopic abnormalities include disordered mitochondria and an increased density of the mitochondrial matrix.

Yunis AA: Chloramphenicol toxicity: induced bone marrow suspension. Semin Hematol 1973;10:225–234.

25.4. Answer: A Ionizing radiation directly damages cellular DNA, preventing cellular replication. It affects the most rapidly dividing cells. Cells that do not divide (mature red cells, neu-

trophils, and platelets) will be unaffected by an exposure but may not be replaced by bone marrow once they have lived out their normal life expectancy. Although inflammation is probably a significant effect of radiation exposure, direct damage to DNA is the most significant effect. Patients who survive an exposure are at increased risk of the development of hematologic malignancies.

Vicker MG, Bultmann H, Glade U, Hafker T: Ionizing radiation at low doses induces inflammatory reactions in human blood. Radiat Res 1991;128:251–257.

25.5. Answer: E Aplastic anemia is typically insidious in onset and affects the immature cellular elements first. The first manifestations are generally hemorrhage or anemia, and death follows the onset of hemorrhage or sepsis.

Moeschlin S, Speck B: Experimental studies on the mechanism of action of benzene on the bone marrow (radioautographic studies using ³H thymidine). Acta Hematol 1967;38:104–111.

Scott JL, Cartwright GF, Wintrobe MM: Acquired aplastic anemia: An analysis of 39 cases and review of the pertinent literature. Medicine 1959;38:119–172.

25.6. Answer: A The red cell's primary function is oxygen transport. It carries on aerobic and anaerobic respiration. The red cell has multiple enzymatic mechanisms to protect itself from oxidative attack, including NADH methemoglobin reductase and NADPH-dependent methemoglobin reductase. It produces 2,3-DPG as a by-product of aerobic respiration. As it lacks a nucleus, it cannot replace lost proteins.

25.7. Answer: B Methemoglobin is incapable of binding oxygen, so its presence may result in hypoxia. In addition, it shifts the oxyhemoglobin dissociation curve to the left so that oxygen is bound more tightly to hemoglobin. Normally, it makes up no more than 3% of blood and is reduced primarily by NADH-dependent methemoglobin reductase.

Darling RC, Roughton FJR: The effect of methemoglobin on the equilibrium between oxygen and hemoglobin. Am J Physiol 1942; 137:56–66.

25.8. Answer: D Carbon monoxide poisoning causes hypoxia both by displacing oxygen from hemoglobin and by shifting the oxyhemoglobin dissociation curve to the left. It produces cellular hypoxia by binding to tissue cytochrome oxidase. Carboxyhemoglobin has a shorter half-life in an oxygen-rich environment. Poisoning most commonly follows unintentional exposures.

25.9. Answer: D G-6-PD is encoded on the X chromosome, so it more commonly affects men than women. Hemolysis occurs following an exposure to an oxidizing agent. The activity of G-6-PD decreases as red cells age. The measurement of the activity of G-6-PD will not be accurate following an episode of hemolysis, as the cells with the least activity are hemolyzed selectively.

Herz F, Kaplan E, Scheye ES: Diagnosis of erythrocyte glucose-6-phosphate dehydrogenase deficiency in the Negro male despite hemolytic crisis. Blood 1970;35:90–93.

Kattamis CA: Glucose-6-phosphate dehydrogenase deficiency in female heterozygotes and the X-inactivation hypothesis. Acta Pediatr Scand 1967;172(Suppl):103–109.

25.10. Answer: B Acquired thrombocytopenia is usually immune mediated, with IgG most commonly implicated. Effects on the peripheral smear will be seen within 12 hours of reexposure to an inciting agent. Bone marrow aspiration will reveal normal or increased numbers of megakaryocytes.

Eisner EV, Shahidi NT: Immune thrombocytopenia due to a drug metabolite. N Engl J Med 1972;287:376–381.

CHAPTER 26

ENDOCRINE PRINCIPLES

26.1. Answer: E The brain is dependent on a constant supply of glucose. Because of a large ongoing demand for this substrate, the brain is also one of the earliest organs to manifest symptomatology.

Cortesao L, Saraiva AM, Guerreiro L: The endocrine pancreas. Acta Med Port 1995;8(Suppl 1):S47–S53.

Randle P, Hales C, Garland P, et al: The glucose fatty acid cycle. Its role in insulin sensitivity and the metabolic disturbances of diabetes mellitus. Lancet 1963;1:785–789.

26.2. Answer: D The agents listed are examples of substances that alter glucose metabolism. Metformin (a biguanide) and troglitazone (a thiazolidinedione) are drugs used in the treatment of diabetes that act by decreasing glucose production in the liver and increasing peripheral utilization. Acarbose is an α-glucosidase inhibitor that decreases absorption of glucose from dietary sources. Alanine is an amino acid that stimulates insulin secretion. Octreotide is a somatostatin analogue that blocks insulin secretion. It has a longer duration of action than its natural analogue, somatostatin, and has been used in the treatment of sulfonamide overdose.

Boyle PJ, Justice K, Krenz AJ, et al: Octreotide reverses hyperinsulinemia and prevents hypoglycemia induced by sulfonylurea overdoses. J Clin Endocrinol Metab 1993;76:752–756.

26.3. Answer: D Glucagon is a polypeptide hormone. It increases production of glucose by stimulating phosphorylase action, enhancing the breakdown of glycogen. It is secreted in response to hypoglycemia and epinephrine release. Glucagon itself will stimulate insulin release, which may contribute to its lack of efficacy in treatment of insulin-induced hypoglycemia in some circumstances. The secretion of both glucagon and insulin are blocked by somatostatin.

Rizza RA, Cryer PE, Gerich JE: Role of glucagon, catecholamines and growth hormone in human glucose counterregulation. Effect of somatostatin and combined alpha- and beta-adrenergic blockade on plasma glucose recovery and glucose flux rates after insulin-induced hypoglycemia. J Clin Invest 1979;64:62–71.

26.4. Answer: A NIDDM patients are more likely to have maximal glucagon effects before treatment; hence, they may not respond to this therapy. β-Adrenergic antagonists inhibit resuscitation of the patient by blocking the effect of epinephrine to restore blood sugar through gluconeogenesis. β-Adrenergic antagonists may also blunt the patient's early awareness of hypoglycemia as a result of the absence of tachycardia and other sympathetic manifestations.

26.5. Answer: E All are situations in which the patient is at increased risk of hypoglycemia. In the setting of renal failure both insulin use and pentamidine may result in hypoglycemia. Alcohol intoxication usually is not associated with this outcome, unless glycogen stores are previously depleted. Metformin (a biguanide) and troglitazone (a thiazolidinedione) do not cause hypoglycemia by themselves but can do so in combination with sulfonamides or insulin.

26.6. Answer: C T_3 is the metabolically more active thyroid agonist, and an overdose with this agent will be likely to cause symptoms in the first several days after an ingestion. The more commonly prescribed T_4 must first be converted to T_3 in order to act. These overdosed patients will usually not manifest symptoms until after the first week.

Golightly LK, Smolinske SC, Kulig KW, et al: Clinical effects of accidental levothyroxine ingestion in children. Am J Dis Child 1985;141:1025–2110.

26.7. Answer: B Lithium is commonly associated with hypothyroidism (5–15% of patients), and those who prescribe the drug or care for patients taking this agent should be aware of the association. It is commonly recommended that thyroid function tests be obtained on initiation of lithium therapy and at regular intervals thereafter.

Gittoes NJ, Franklyn JA: Drug-induced thyroid disorders. Drug Safety 1995;13:46–55.

26.8. Answer: D Glucocorticoid hormonal supplementation has a wide variety of effects when taken exogenously. An acute effect is demargination of polymorphonuclear leukocytes, raising the white blood count on routine testing. Of more clinical significance, patients may develop steroid psychosis from CNS excitation. Hyperglycemia frequently occurs with long-term administration. Depletion of hydrocortisone, a mineralocorticoid, is often associated with hypotension when the patient is stressed as with an acute illness.

Chrousos GP: The hypothalamic–pituitary–adrenal axis and immune-mediated inflammation. N Engl J Med 1995;332:1351–1362.

McMahon M, Gerich J, Rizza R: Effects of glucocorticoids on carbohydrate metabolism. Diabetes Metab Rev 1988;4:17–30.

26.9. Answer: B Anabolic agents can cause many deleterious effects, including those listed. An epidemic of use of these drugs exists in the United States, and clinicians should be aware of associated complications.

Hickson RC, Ball KL, Falduto MT: Adverse effects of anabolic steroids. Med Toxicol Adverse Drug Exp 1989;4:254–271.

26.10. Answer: E Amenorrhea and acne are usually completely reversed with cessation of use of anabolic steroids by women. The other effects are often irreversible.

CHAPTER 27

OPHTHALMIC PRINCIPLES

27.1. Answer: D Irrigating lenses do not increase injury and do improve consistency of irrigation. Water may be less comfortable, but there is no evidence that it is less effective. Severe acid and alkali burns should be irrigated for 2 hours or more, but most other agents require only brief irrigation. Limitations of paper strips, contamination by irrigation solutions, and failure of conjunctival pH to reflect anterior chamber pH are among the reasons that normal pH should be a necessary but not sufficient endpoint.

Herr RD, White GL, Bernshiel K, et al: Clinical comparison of ocular irrigation fluids following chemical injury. Am J Emerg Med 1991;9:228–231.

27.2. Answer: E PEG 400 may be superior to water, but marginally so, and never worth a delay in irrigation. EDTA on a cotton tip applicator can be used to remove residual lime after irrigation. Calcium gluconate drops have been used without evidence of benefit. Copper sulfate may inactivate residual reactive phosphorus particles.

Bentur Y, Tannenbaum S, Yaffe Y, Halpert M: The role of calcium gluconate in the treatment of hydrofluoric acid eye burn. Ann Emerg Med 1993;22:1488–1490.

Brown VKH, Box VL, Simpson BJ: Decontamination procedures for skin exposed to phenolic substances. Arch Environ Health 1975;30:1–6.

Rozenbaum D, Baruchin AM, Dafina Z: Chemical burns of the eye with special reference to alkali burns. Burns 1991;17: 136–140.

27.3. Answer: E Paracentesis and lavage may restore normal anterior chamber pH and reduce intraocular pressure. Short-course steroids are possibly of value; antibiotics are clearly indicated. Topical ascorbate restores depleted anterior chamber levels critical to normal healing; citrate binds elevated calcium and magnesium, which contribute to secondary injury.

27.4. Answer: C Central effects of clonidine decrease sympathetic output and cause miosis. Deep coma after diazepam or phenobarbital may be associated with miosis, but this is unusual and inconsistent. LSD and particularly cocaine result in mydriasis.

27.5. Answer: B Formate produced by methanol metabolism in the retina is the cause of ocular toxicity, which affects the retina primarily. Funduscopic examination is most often normal when visual symptoms first appear. When complete visual loss occurs even transiently, some residual visual loss is common following improvement. Folate or folinic acid speeds the breakdown of formate and prevents retinal folate depletion. The presence of acidosis indicates the need for folate or preferably folinic acid therapy.

Benton CD, Calhoun FP: The ocular effects of methyl alcohol poisoning: Report of a catastrophe involving 320 persons. Am J Ophthalmol 1953;36:1677–1685.

Garner CD, Lee EW, Terzo TS, et al: Role of retinal metabolism in methanol-induced retinal toxicity. J Toxicol Environ Health 1995;44:43–56.

27.6. Answer: D Quinine serum levels above 20 mg/mL within 10 hours of overdose consistently predict visual defects. Early funduscopic examination is often normal in the face of significant visual loss. The exact cause is unknown, but vasoconstriction has been excluded. Partial recovery is common after serious visual deficits. Less severe visual loss has occurred after quinine exposure in settings other than acute overdose.

Boland ME, Brennand Roper SM, Henry JA: Complications of quinine poisoning. Lancet 1985;1:384–385.

27.7. Answer: E All contribute to the risk of systemic absorption and toxicity from eye drops.

Hugues FC, Le Jeune C: Systemic and local tolerability of ophthalmic drug formulations. An update. Drug Safety 1993;8: 365–380.

27.8. Answer: D Amiodarone and chloroquine cause corneal deposits; steroids cause cataracts; quinine causes retinal abnormalities; ethambutol is the most important cause of optic neuritis.

27.9. Answer: C Each of the others causes nystagmus, which is almost always horizontal in character. Among them, however, only phencyclidine is typically associated with vertical nystagmus.

McCarron MM, Schulze BW, Thompson GA, et al: Acute phencyclidine toxicity: Incidence of clinical findings in 1,000 cases. Ann Emerg Med 1981;10:237–242.

27.10. Answer: E A "crack eye" is a multifactorial injury to the corneal epithelium; cocaine is a well-known sympathomimetic agent and mydriatic; talc retinopathy in some cases required the injection of thousands of tablets over a prolonged period; increased discharge of the central pupillary constrictor center has been documented.

Sachs R, Zagelbaum BM, Hersh PS: Corneal complications associated with the use of crack cocaine. Ophthalmology 1993;100: 181–191.

CHAPTER 28

OTOLARYNGOLOGIC PRINCIPLES

28.1. Answer: D Human speech is composed of sounds in the frequency of 250 to 3000 Hz; however, humans can normally detect sounds in the frequency range of 20 to 20,000 Hz.

Olishifski JB: Occupational hearing loss, noise, and hearing conservation. In: Zenz C, ed: Occupational Medicine: Principles and Practical Applications. Chicago, Year Book, 1988, pp. 274–323.

28.2. Answer: D A distinctive plastic or vinyl odor in the patient's breath or sweat may be appreciated in a patient with ethchlorvynol exposure. The odor may be diagnostic if the patient presents in a lethargic or comatose state.

Goldfrank LR, Weisman R, Flomenbaum N: Teaching the recognition of odors. Ann Emerg Med 1982;11:684–686.

28.3. Answer: A Tinnitus associated with salicylates usually begins at the high therapeutic or low toxic level (approximately 20–40 mg/dL). However, tinnitus may not be evident in elderly patients with hearing impairment despite significantly elevated salicylate concentrations.

Mongan E, Kelly P, Nies K, et al: Tinnitus as an indication of therapeutic serum salicylate levels. JAMA 1973;226:142–145.

28.4. Answer: D The primary mechanism of quinine-induced ototoxicity is related to prostaglandin inhibition. Quinine inhibits phospholipase A_2 enzyme, which converts phospholipids to arachidonic acid. Quinine also inhibits calcium channels that interact with prostaglandins. These effects tend to be reversible. All the other agents can cause loss of hair cells of the cochlea, causing mostly irreversible hearing loss.

Jung TTK, Rhee CK, Lee CS, et al: Ototoxicity of salicylate, nonsteroidal anti-inflammatory drugs, and quinine. Otolaryngol Clin North Am 1993;26:791–810.

Schacht J: Molecular mechanisms of drug-induced hearing loss. Hearing Res 1986;22:297–304.

28.5. Answer: B Primary odor detection is a function of the olfactory (I) nerve. For some irritant odors, such as ammonia and acetone, neurotransmission is conducted through the trigeminal (V) nerve.

Doty RL: A review of olfactory dysfunction in man. Am J Otolaryngol 1979;1:57–79.

Schneider BA: Anosmia: Verification and etiologies. Ann Otol 1972;81:272–277.

28.6. Answer: B The production of the cochlear fluids and the maintenance of the electrochemical gradient between the endolymph and the perilymph is a function of the stria vascularis. The stria vascularis contains a high concentration of oxidative enzymes, Na^+-K^+-ATPase, adenylate cyclase, and carbonic anhydrase, which may be susceptible to toxins. The cochlear fluids are critical to conduct sound waves to the hair cells, to provide nutrients and waste removal for the cells lining the cochlear duct, to control pressure distribution in the cochlea, and to maintain an electrochemical gradient for the function of the hair cells.

Huang MY, Schacht J: Drug-induced ototoxicity: pathogenesis and prevention. Med Toxicol 1989;4:452–467.

28.7. Answer: D Olfactory fatigue is the process of olfactory adaptation on exposure to a stimulus for a variable period of time, leading to temporal diminution of the smell. For example, hydrogen sulfide, a toxin that binds to cytochrome oxidase, is readily detectable as a distinct and offensive substance at the very low concentration of 0.025 ppm. At the higher and potentially toxic concentration of 50 ppm the odor is less offensive, and recognition may disappear after 2 to 15 minutes of exposure. At even higher concentrations, when toxicity is likely, the onset of olfactory fatigue is more rapid.

Reiffenstein RJ, Hulbert WC, Roth SH: Toxicology of hydrogen sulfide. Annu Rev Pharmacol Toxicol 1992;32:109–134.

28.8. Answer: A The section of the cochlea most at risk from loud noises is at the 9- to 13-mm region (the total length is 32 mm). This region is responsible for hearing at the 3 to 6 kHz range, corresponding to the typical noise-induced hearing-loss pattern. Even though human speech is composed of mostly low-frequency sounds, the ability to perceive higher-frequency sounds is extremely important in speech recognition. Because of this, the major impairment in patients with noise-induced hearing loss is an inability to discriminate speech, particularly from background noise.

Alberti PW: Occupational hearing loss. In: Ballenger JJ, ed: Diseases of the Nose, Throat, Ear, Head, and Neck, 14th ed. Philadelphia, Lea & Febiger, 1991, pp. 1053–1068.

28.9. Answer: A Although all of these medications have been associated with tinnitus, only salicylates will reliably produce tinnitus at toxic levels.

Seligmann H, Podoshin L, Ben-David J, et al: Drug-induced tinnitus and other hearing disorders. Drug Safety 1996;14:198–212.

28.10. Answer: E Angiotensin-converting enzyme (ACE) inhibitors such as captopril, enalapril, and lisinopril are among the most common medications that cause gustatory impairment, usually hypogeusia and dysgeusia. Because ACE inhibitors work by inhibiting zinc-dependent ACE, they also chelate zinc at taste receptors and salivary proteins, resulting in taste dysfunctions.

Henkin RI: Drug-induced taste and smell disorders. Incidence, mechanisms and management related primarily to treatment of sensory receptor dysfunction. Drug Safety 1994;11:318–377.

CHAPTER **29**

DERMATOLOGIC PRINCIPLES

29.1. Answer: E A number of plants leave chemicals on the skin that react with light, producing erythema, possible blistering, and pigmentation. *Rhus* dermatitis causes vesiculobullous allergic contact dermatitis.

Benezra C, Ducombs G, Sell Y, Fousserau J: Plant Contact Dermatitis. Toronto, Decker, and St. Louis, Mosby, 1985.

29.2. Answer: A Low-potency corticosteroid preparations should be used to treat steroid-responsive dermatitis on areas of thin skin, as on the face, or intertriginous skin, as in the groin and axilla. The risk of acneiform eruption, striae, telangiectasiae, petechiae, and atrophy increases with higher-potency corticosteroids and corticosteroids under occlusion. Ointments are messy and promote acneiform eruptions in areas with high concentrations of sebaceous glands.

Grevelink SA, Murrell DF, Olsen EA: Effectiveness of various barrier preparations in preventing and/or ameliorating experimentally produced toxicodendron dermatitis. J Am Acad Dermatol 1992;27:182–188.

Marks JG Jr, Fowler JF Jr, Sheretz EF, et al: Prevention of poison ivy and poison oak allergic contact dermatitis by quaternium-18 bentonite. J Am Acad Dermatol 1995;33:212–216

29.3. Answer: B All statements except B are true. Physical findings may be delayed for hours when the concentration of acid is less than 30%. With high concentrations, the symptoms are instantaneous.

Dunn BJ, MacKinnon MA, Knowlden NF, et al: Hydrofluoric acid dermal burns: An assessment of treatment efficacy using an experimental pig model. J Occup Med 1992;34:902–909.

29.4. Answer: E Neomycin is the most common cause of medication-related contact dermatitis. Bacitracin is the most common topical medication causing anaphylactic reactions.

Fisher AA: Contact Dermatitis, 4th ed. Baltimore, Williams & Wilkins, 1995.

29.5. Answer: D The symptoms of latex hypersensitivity range from mild-local to severe-systemic symptoms. With progressive latex contact, the symptoms usually worsen. Paronychia is an inflammation of the nail folds caused by skin disease such as eczema and psoriasis or by infections, especially *Candida albicans,* and *Staphylococcus aureus.*

Heese A, Van-Hintzenstern J, Peters KP, et al: Allergic and irritant reactions to rubber gloves in medical health services: Spectrum, diagnostic approach and therapy. J Am Acad Dermatol 1991;25:831–839.

29.6. Answer: E Bergamot orange contains furocoumarins, which cause a phototoxic dermatitis when the contaminated skin is exposed to ultraviolet light. The other plants are species of *Anacardiaciae* and contain urushiol, the chemical responsible for *Rhus* dermatitis.

29.7. Answer: D Although all these factors are significant, a chemical's lipid solubility has the greatest influence on absorption through the skin.

Wester RC, Maibach HI: In vivo percutaneous absorption: Critical factors in transdermal transport. In: Marzulli FN, Maibach HI, eds: Dermatoxicology, 4th ed. New York, Hemisphere, 1991, pp. 1–36.

29.8. Answer: E Eczemas are a group of inflammatory skin diseases with identical histopathologic features, which include a superficial perivascular infiltrate of mononuclear cells and intercellular epidermal edema. However, specific types of eczemas are recognized based on the causes and clinical appearances. Contact dermatitis may be produced by chemicals through allergy or irritancy. Atopic dermatitis is often associated with IgE immunoglobin–mediated inflammation and has a predominance for the nape of the neck and the antecubital and popliteal fossae, although any part of the body may be involved. These patients are particularly sensitive to chemical irritation. Dyshidrosis is characterized by vesicles in the palms, soles, and sides of the fingers, and the disease is exacerbated by irritation from frequent hand washing.

Shmunes E: The role of atopy in occupational skin diseases. Occup Med 1986;1:219–228.

29.9. Answer: A Langerhans cells are skin macrophages that present antigens that penetrate the epidermis to T lymphocytes, thus initiating the process of sensitization. Mycosis fungoides is a malignancy of Langerhans cells. Glomus cells form special arteriovenous shunts that regulate temperature on the skin and are most abundantly found on the hands, feet, ears, and center of the face. Glomus tumors occur as solitary or multiple small, purple, tender nodules and develop most commonly on the nail bed. Merkel cells are involved in touch reception and can lead to a carcinoma that usually presents as a single nodule on the head or extremities. Mast cells contain basophilic granules filled with histamine and other modulators of inflammation. Diseases in which the mast cells are involved include urticaria, immediate hypersensitivity reaction, pruritus, and mastocytosis.

Cohen SR, Samitz MH: Occupational skin disease. In: Moschella SL, Hurley HJ, eds: Dermatology. Philadelphia, WB Saunders, 1992, pp. 1871–1920.

29.10. Answer: C Although most drugs can produce a number of different skin reactions, frequently an individual drug is associated with a specific reaction. Patients treated with allopurinol have a higher risk of developing toxic epidermal necrolysis. Phenolphthalein is associated with fixed drug reactions. Bleomycin can cause a flagellate dermatitis with erythematous streaks that heal with pigmentation. Penicillamine has been linked to pemphigus-like bullous eruptions.

Bastuji-Garin S, Rzany B, Stern RS, et al: Clinical classification of cases of toxic epidermal necrolysis, Stevens-Johnson syndrome, and erythema multiforme. Arch Dermatol 1993;129:92–96.

CHAPTER **30**

GENITOURINARY PRINCIPLES

30.1. Answer: A DBCP exposure causes a decrease in spermatogenesis, which can be irreversible. In one series 7 of 10 men exposed had decreased or absent spermatogenic activity.

Teitelbaum DT. The toxicology of 1,2-dibromo-3-chloropropane (DBCP): a brief review. Int J Occup Environ Health 1999;5:122–126.

30.2. Answer: D Yohimbine is an α_2-adrenergic antagonist with cholinergic activity used to treat erectile dysfunction.

Owen JA, Nakatsu SL, Fenemore J, et al: The pharmacokinetics of yohimbine in man. Eur J Clin Pharmacol 1987;32:577–582.

30.3. Answer: D Cantharidin has vesicant activity and causes gastrointestinal hemorrhage, blister formation in the lower urinary tract, renal failure, vaginal bleeding, ECG changes, and DIC. Neurologic symptoms are rare.

Karras DJ, Farrell SE, Harrigan RA, et al: Poisoning from "Spanish fly" (cantharidin). Am J Emerg Med 1996;14:478–483.

30.4. Answer: E Steroids from the bufadienolide class (toad venom) are similar to digoxin in structure and presentation. Usefulness of digoxin-specific antibody fragments has been demonstrated in human and animal toxicity from bufotoxins.

Brubacher JR, Lachmanen D, Ravikumar PR, et al: Treatment of toad venom poisoning with digoxin-specfic Fab fragments. Chest 1996;110:1282–1288.

30.5. Answer: C Nitrites are absorbed via the skin, lungs, mucous membranes, and the GI tract. They are metabolized in the liver and excreted, partially unchanged, in the urine. The kinetics are first order with a half-life of 2 to 3 seconds.

Haverkos HW, Dougherty J: Health hazards of nitrite inhalants. Am J Med 1988;84:479–482.

30.6. Answer: C Pulegone, the ketone in pennyroyal oil, is a direct hepatotoxin, and fulminant hepatic failure can occur after ingestion of 2 oz of pennyroyal oil.

Bakerink JA, Gospe SM, Dimand RJ, et al: Multiple organ failure after ingestion of pennyroyal oil from herbal tea in two infants. Pediatrics 1996;98:944–947.

30.7. Answer: A Misoprostol is a synthetic prostaglandin analogue approved for prevention and treatment of gastric ulcers. It has been used extensively in Brazil as an abortifacient and can terminate pregnancy after small-dose exposures.

Davies NM, Longstreth J, Jamali F. Misoprostol therapeutics revisited. Pharmacotherapy 2001;21:60–73.

30.8. Answer: D Pennyroyal oil is hepatotoxic, quinine has oxytocic activity, and trichosanthins inhibit trophoblasts. All have been used as abortifacients. Mifepristone is an antiprogesterone agent used as a legal abortifacient in Europe.

Anderson IB, Mullen WH, Meeker JE, et al: Pennyroyal toxicity: measurement of toxic metabolite levels in two cases and review of the literature. Ann Intern Med 1996;124:726–34.

30.9. Answer: C Agents that produce red urine include: anthraquinones, beets, blackberries, eosin, erythrocytes, hemoglobin, myoglobin, rhubarb, rifampin.

Goldfrank LR, Osborn H: Rainbow urine. Hosp Physician 1978;3:22–26.

30.10. Answer: B Up to 46% of patients receiving cyclophosphamide develop hemorrhagic cystitis. Acrolein is a metabolite that damages the urothelium.

Droller MJ, Saral R, Santos G: Prevention of cyclophosphamide-induced hemorrhagic cystitis. Urology 1982;20:256–258.

CHAPTER **31**

MANAGING THE SYMPTOMATIC PATIENT WITH A POSSIBLE TOXIC EXPOSURE

31.1. Answer: A Opening the airway and ensuring oxygenation and ventilation are always the first priority and should never be delayed for labs or antidotes. In a hypoventilating or apneic patient, 100% oxygen is not effective. ET intubation can be performed more safely and less emergently after the patient has been oxygenated and ventilated.

31.2. Answer: A Multiple physiologic mechanisms exist for the hypotension seen after overdose and include decreased cardiac output relative to hypovolemia and decreased peripheral vascular resistance. Initial treatment is isotonic saline infusion. If hypotension or shock continues despite fluid challenge, then catheterization of the pulmonary artery and measurement of wedge pressure, venous oxygen saturation, and cardiac output are recommended to monitor subsequent fluid therapy and inotropic support.

31.3. Answer: D Naloxone reverses the respiratory depressant effect of all opioids. It does not reverse the effects of benzodiazapines. Meperidine neurotoxicity is caused by the metabolite normeperidine, which can cause CNS excitation and seizures. Administration of naloxone can increase toxicity by reversing the CNS depressant effects of the meperidine, allowing the excitatory effect of normeperidine to be unopposed.

31.4. Answer: C Seizures have been reported within 1 hour of an exposure to carbon monoxide, isoniazid, insulin, amitriptyline, and propoxyphene. Symptoms of acetaminophen overdose in the first 24 hours may include anorexia, pallor, nausea and vomiting and, following extremely large ingestions, may include coma and metabolic acidosis. Seizures have not been reported.

31.5. Answer: E Patients with overdoses of depressant drugs who reach the hospital alive and receive appropriate treatment have less than 5% mortality.

31.6. Answer: A After the primary survey has been completed, consideration should next be given to (1) hypertonic dextrose to diagnose, treat, or exclude hypoglycemia; (2) thiamine to prevent or treat Wernicke encephalopathy (not necessary in children); (3) naloxone for respiratory compromise or the possibility of opioid overdose; and (4) oxygen for treatment and prevention of hypoxia. Other investigations and therapies may be needed after these have been considered.

31.7. Answer: E Severe salicyclism should be treated aggressively. Indications for hemodialysis include renal failure, CNS impairment, pulmonary edema, hepatic dysfunction, severe acid–base disturbance despite appropriate treatment, clinical deterioration despite supportive care, and serum salicylate levels greater than 100 mg/dL.

Yip L, Dart R, Gabow P: Concepts and controversies in salicylate toxicity. Emerg Med Clin North Am. 1994;12:351–364.

31.8. Answer: E Patients with altered mental status as a result of Wernicke encephalopathy are suffering from thiamine deficiency.

The symptoms may be reversed with thiamine administration. The incidence of adverse reaction is exceedingly low. Analeptics such as amphetamines do not arouse a comatose patient reliably or predictably and may increase the risk of agitation. Administration of physostigmine in the absence of anticholinergic poisoning can cause a cholinergic reaction characterized by salivation, urination, defecation, and possibly severe bradycardia or asystole. Flumazenil is a competitive antagonist of benzodiazapines and can reverse the anxiolytic, anticonvulsant, sedative, and muscle relaxant effect of the benzodiazepines. It should not be administered for unknown overdoses, as it can cause withdrawal seizures in benzodiazapine-dependent patients and can lower the seizure threshold in patients with other overdoses. Forced diuresis has not been shown to be efficacious and can cause pulmonary and cerebral edema. Urinary acidification to enhance elimination of weak bases does not enhance removal of toxic compounds considerably, and complication from systemic acidosis and urine myoglobin precipitation can occur.

Cook CC, Hallwood PM, Thomson AD: B vitamin deficiency and neuropsychiatric syndromes in alcohol misuse. Alcohol Alcoholism 1998;33:317–336.

31.9. Answer: D Maternal carboxyhemoglobin levels do not accurately reflect fetal carboxyhemoglobin or tissue CO levels; therefore, any pregnant woman with symptoms or signs of carbon monoxide poisoning should receive HBO, regardless of maternal carboxyhemoglobin level. Sorbitol is not absorbed into the bloodstream, is not transferred across the placenta, and has no effects on the fetus. When considering the use of antidotes the primary concern should be for the health of the mother. Cardiac output and total blood volume increase throughout pregnancy; therefore, signs of shock may manifest later than they would in a woman who is not pregnant. Rolling a patient to her *left* (not right) side would remove vena caval compression from the gravid uterus, permitting more blood return to the heart.

Koren G, Sharav T, Pastuszak A, et al: A multicenter, prospective study of fetal outcome following accidental carbon monoxide poisoning in pregnancy. Reprod Toxicol 1991;5:397–403.

31.10. Answer: B Hyperthermia is associated with significant mortality regardless of etiology. Differential diagnosis of hyperthermia with mental status changes includes infectious diseases, heatstroke, seizures, thyroid storm, and effects of pharmaceuticals (anticholinergic syndrome, neuroleptic malignant syndrome, malignant hyperthermia, amphetamine toxicity). Rapid cooling results in improved outcomes in these patients. In heatstroke victims, cooling within 1 hour resulted in 5% mortality, but mortality rose to 18% when cooling required more than 1 hour. Dantrolene sodium should be administered for malignant hyperthermia.

CHAPTER 32

ACETAMINOPHEN

32.1. Answer: C NAPQI is itself an electrophile formed primarily in zone III (centrilobular) regions of liver (where most oxidative drug metabolism occurs) but also in the kidney and possibly other sites. It is always formed during acetaminophen metabolism but results in toxicity only when glutathione depletion is extensive (to <30% of normal in animal models).

Mitchell JR, Jollow DJ, Potter WZ, et al: Acetaminophen-induced hepatic necrosis. IV. Protective role of glutathione. J Pharmacol Exp Ther 1973;187:211–217.

32.2. Answer: D Chronic ethanol use theoretically increases risk of toxicity by inducing P450 but probably more importantly by depleting glutathione. Cimetidine is a P450 inhibitor, and acute ethanol ingestion a competitive P450 inhibitor; both would be expected to be protective. Acute phenobarbital has produced mixed effects in animal studies and is not known to be a significant factor.

Thummel KE, Slattery JT, Nelson SD, et al: Effect of ethanol on hepatotoxicity of acetaminophen in mice and on reactive metabolite formation by mouse and human liver microsomes. Toxicol Appl Pharmacol 1989;100:391–397.

Zimmerman HJ, Maddrey WC: Acetaminophen (paracetamol) hepatotoxicity with regular intake of alcohol: Analysis of instances of therapeutic misadventure. Hepatology 1995;22:767–773.

32.3. Answer: E In the first few hours after overdose, coingestion of opioids (combination acetaminophen-opioid products) is a common cause of altered mental status. Coma from a very high acetaminophen concentration can occur but is rare. Once liver dysfunction begins, hypoglycemia is common, and cerebral edema is one of the most common preterminal events of liver failure.

Anker AL, Smilkstein MJ: Acetaminophen: Concepts and controversies. Emerg Med Clin North Am 1994;12:335–349.

32.4. Answer: D There is no loss of efficacy if *N*-acetylcysteine (NAC) is given within 8 hours after ingestion. NAC can act as a glutathione substitute but also increases glutathione supply. NAC detoxifies *N*-acetyl-*p*-benzoquinoneimine but does not block its formation. NAC may increase the sulfation of acetaminophen.

Lauterburg BH, Corcoran GB, Mitchell JR: Mechanism of action of *N*-acetylcysteine in the protection against hepatotoxicity of acetaminophen in rats in vivo. J Clin Invest 1983;71:980–991.

Smilkstein MJ, Knapp GL, Kulig KW, Rumack BH: Efficacy of oral *N*-acetylcysteine in the treatment of acetaminophen overdose: Analysis of the national multicenter study (1976–1985). N Engl J Med 1988;319:1557–1562.

32.5. Answer: E The fetus is able to form NAPQI during most of pregnancy and is at risk for toxicity. Although NAC treatment has been followed by good outcome in nearly all cases, it is unclear whether NAC is effective in treating the fetus. Even though NAC fails to cross the placenta in experimental animal, it does cross the human placenta. However, good maternal outcome does not ensure fetal outcome.

Horowitz RS, Dart RC, Jarvie DR, et al: Placental transfer of *N*-acetylcysteine following human maternal acetaminophen toxicity. J Toxicol Clin Toxicol 1997;35:447–451.

Riggs BS, Bronstein AC, Kulig KW, et al: Acute acetaminophen overdose during pregnancy. Obstet Gynecol 1989;74:247–253.

32.6. Answer: B The original nomogram, based on a small number of patients, was 25% higher than the lower line and positioned to be highly sensitive to detect risk of AST or ALT increase, without regard to actual liver failure. Although 60% of those above the line may develop AST elevation if untreated, this reflects patients far above the line. Those immediately above the line have little risk of serious hepatotoxicity and almost no risk of hepatic failure or death. A value below the line excludes the need for further evaluation, despite the fact that subsequent acetaminophen measurements may be above the line in some patients. The reliability after extended-relief (ER) acetaminophen is controversial.

Bridger S, Henderson K, Glucksman E, et al: Deaths from low dose paracetamol poisoning. Br Med J 1998;316:1724–1725.

Prescott LF: Paracetamol overdosage: pharmacological considerations and management. Drugs 1983;25:290–314.

32.7. Answer: D When all cases with initial [APAP] above the treatment line are considered, the incidence of hepatotoxicity is lower in children under 5 years of age than in adults. However, these cases have not been stratified by both serum concentration of acetaminophen and time to treatment with N-acetylcysteine. This makes amount of exposure, delay to treatment, and decreased susceptibility all possible explanations for the lower incidence of hepatic injury. Although the fraction of acetaminophen metabolized by sulfation is increased in children, this does not necessarily confer decreased risk of NAPQI formation. The relative risk of chronic excessive dosing for children versus adults is not known, but children with acute febrile illnesses comprise one of the few groups in which toxicity after repeated excessive dosing has been described.

Day A, Abbott GD: Chronic paracetamol poisoning in children: a warning to health professionals. N Z Med J 1994;107:201.

Henretig FM, Selbst SM, Forrect C, et al: Repeated acetaminophen overdosing: Causing hepatotoxicity in children. Clin Pediatr, 1989;28:267–75.

Rumack BH: Acetaminophen overdose in young children: Treatment and effects of alcohol and other additional ingestants in 417 cases. Am J Dis Child 1984;138:428–433.

Tenenbein M: Why young children are resistant to acetaminophen poisoning. J Pediatr 2000;137:891–892.

32.8. Answer: C Renal P450 formation of N-acetyl-p-benzoquinoneimine is the likely cause of acute proximal renal tubular necrosis after acute overdose. Renal function abnormalities are rare overall but occur in as many as 25% of cases with significant hepatotoxicity and in more than 50% of those with hepatic failure. Pancreatic injury is rarely reported.

Hart SG, Beierschmitt WP, Wyand DS, Khairallah EA, Cohen SD: Acetaminophen nephrotoxicity in CD-1 mice. I. Evidence of a role for in situ activation in selective covalent binding and toxicity. Toxicol Appl Pharmacol 1994;126:267–275.

Prescott LF, Proudfoot AT, Cregeen RJ: Paracetamol-induced acute renal failure in the absence of fulminant liver damage. Br Med J 1982;284:421–422.

Wilkinson SP, Moodie H, Arroyo VA, et al: Frequency of renal impairment in paracetamol overdose compared with other causes of acute liver damage. J Clin Pharmacol 1977;30:220–224.

32.9. Answer: C Activated charcoal does appear to decrease acetaminophen absorption. It also absorbs N-acetylcysteine. There is no evidence that charcoal changes acetaminophen elimination. Because N-acetylcysteine is effective if given within 8 hours and activated charcoal is most effective if given early after ingestion, it is very rare that the administration of charcoal and N-acetylcysteine could not be separated by at least 2 hours.

Buckley NA, Whyte IM, O'Connell DL: Activated charcoal reduces the need for N-acetylcysteine treatment after acetaminophen (paracetamol) overdose. J Toxicol Clin Toxicol 1999;37:753–757.

Ekins B, Ford DC, Thompson MIB, et al: The effect of activated charcoal on N-acetylcysteine absorption in normal subjects. Am J Emerg Med 1987;5:483–487.

Spiller HA, Krenzelok EP, Grande GA, et al: A prospective evaluation of the effect of activated charcoal before oral N-acetylcysteine in acetaminophen overdose. Ann Emerg Med 1994;23:519–523.

32.10. Answer: E The acetaminophen nomogram applies to a single acute ingestion. In order to apply the nomogram, the time of the ingestion must be known, and an acetaminophen level must be obtained between 4 and 24 hours after ingestion. The nomogram cannot be used to rule out risk of hepatic injury after repeat excessive dosing (chronic overdose). In the rare circumstance when a patient has an acetaminophen concentration below the treatment line but has evidence of hepatic injury by physical and laboratory exam, reevaluation and treatment should be strongly considered.

Rumack BH, Peterson RG, Koch GG, et al: Acetaminophen overdose. 662 cases with evaluation of oral acetylcysteine treatment. Arch Intern Med 1981;141:380–385.

Smilkstein MJ, Douglas DR, Daya MR: Acetaminophen poisoning and liver function. N Engl J Med 1994;330:1310–1311.

Smilkstein MJ, Knapp GL, Kulig KW, et al: Efficacy of oral N-acetylcysteine in the treatment of acetaminophen overdose: Analysis of the national multicenter study (1976–1985). N Engl J Med 1988;319:1557–1562.

CHAPTER **33**

SALICYLATES

33.1. Answer: C Salicylates act directly on the respiratory center in the brainstem, causing hyperventilation and respiratory alkalosis. At the same time, salicylates, which are weak acids, interfere with the Krebs cycle, limit ATP production, generate lactate, and cause a ketoacidosis. Although the metabolic acidosis begins with the earliest stages of salicylate toxicity, the respiratory alkalosis predominates initially, leaving the patient with a respiratory alkalosis, metabolic acidosis, and alkalemia. An adult presenting with respiratory acidosis early after a salicylate overdose almost certainly is also using CNS depressants or is experiencing salicylate-induced acute lung injury. The combination of acute respiratory alkalosis, metabolic acidosis, and acidemia is an ominous finding indicating an immediately life-threatening salicylate overdose. Although it takes some time after ingestion for this pattern to develop in adults, children are said to present with these findings much earlier. Until ABG determinations became commonly available, and the precise combinations of pH and P_{CO_2} values for each of the primary disturbances were worked out, "respiratory alkalosis" was said to be the typical adult response in the early phase of salicylate poisoning. Even when metabolic acidosis predominates, the respiratory alkalosis is not merely compensatory.

Gabow PA, Anderson RJ, Pots DE, Schrier RW: Acid–base disturbances in the salicylate-intoxicated adult. Arch Intern Med 1978; 138:1481–1484.

Gaudreault P, Temple AR, Lovejoy FH: The relative severity of acute versus chronic salicylate poisoning in children: A clinical comparison. Pediatrics 1982;70:566–569.

Kaplan E, Kennedy J, David J: Effects of salicylate and other benzoates on oxidative enzymes of the tricarboxylic acid cycle in rat tissue homogenates. Arch Biochem Biophys 1954;51:47–61.

Tenney SM, Miller RM: The respiratory and circulatory action of salicylate. Am J Med 1955;19:498–508.

33.2. Answer: D   Despite a normal plasma glucose, CSF glucose fell by a third in salicylate-poisoned mice, indicating an excessive utilization of glucose in the CNS. For this reason, glucose supplementation probably is an important component in treating salicylate-poisoned patients even when serum salicylate levels are normal. Serum glucose levels may be low, normal, or high but do not correlate well with CSF glucose levels. As noted above, the CSF levels are typically lower than the plasma levels.

Thurston JH, Pollock PG, Warren SK, Jones EM: Reduced brain glucose with normal plasma glucose in salicylate poisoning. Clin Invest 1970;49:2139–2145.

33.3. Answer: E   Among the risks for developing salicylate-induced acute lung injury (ALI) are salicylate levels >30 mg/dL, age >30 years, cigarette smoking, chronic salicylate ingestion, and the presence of neurologic symptoms on admission. Although in one study the average salicylate level for those patients who developed salicylate-induced ALI was about 57 mg/dL, this was the average level also for patients in the study who did not develop salicylate-induced ALI. Salicylate-induced ALI is a form of ALI and does not reflect underlying cardiac disease. Treatment includes ventilation, oxygenation, hemodialysis, but not diuresis. Salicylate-induced ALI is identified as a distinct cause of ALI in children, although it rarely occurs in this age group.

Fisher CJ, Albertson TE, Foulke GE: Salicylate induced pulmonary edema. Clinical characteristics in children. Am J Emerg Med 1985;3:33–37.

Walters JS, Woodring JH, Stelling CG, et al: Salicylate-induced pulmonary edema. Radiology 1983;146:289–293.

33.4. Answer: D   Salicylate absorption is typically rapid, and peak levels are achieved quickly, except after an overdose. Salicylates are absorbed rapidly from the stomach, where the pK_a of salicylates (3.5) leaves about 50% in the ionized form. Salicylate absorption is less efficient in the small bowel but, because of the large surface area of the bowel, is effected there as well. Absorption is often influenced by the dosage form. As two of the five mechanisms for salicylate elimination become saturated by increasing concentrations of salicylate, elimination changes from first order to zero order.

Levy G: Clinical pharmacokinetics of salicylates. A reassessment. Br J Clin Pharmacol 1980;10:285S–290S.

33.5. Answer: D   A falling serum salicylate level does not always indicate success in eliminating salicylates from the body and may instead indicate redistribution into the body, tissues including the CSF, where most of the serious toxic effects occur. Redistribution, as opposed to elimination, is particularly likely to be the explanation for a decreasing salicylate level if the patient is concomitantly becoming increasingly acidemic. Except in narrowly defined circumstances such as a single acute ingestion, occurring more then 6 hours previously, in a patient whose blood pH is 7.4 or higher, the toxicity of salicylates correlates poorly with serum levels. A low or therapeutic salicylate level is not reassurance that the patient is not seriously poisoned unless a simultaneously obtained blood pH is in the alkalemic range and unless the salicylate level is a peak serum salicylate level. Concluding that a single level is a peak level is virtually impossible, even when the history seems to be reliable, and therefore, a repeat serum salicylate level several hours later will be necessary to resolve this issue. The CSF salicylate level correlates best with the peak serum salicylate level in part because it reequilibrates more slowly than the serum salicylate level. Although CSF salicylate levels undoubtedly correlate better with toxicity than do serum salicylate levels, CSF levels are impractical to obtain and consequently not particularly useful in managing patients.

Dugandzic RM, Tierney MG, Dickinson GE, et al: Evaluation of the validity of the Done nomogram in the management of acute salicylate intoxication. Ann Emerg Med 1989;18:1186–1190.

33.6. Answer: D   Markedly elevated temperatures with salicylate poisoning are thought to be the result of the uncoupling of oxidative phosphorylation and, in this circumstance, almost always represent a preterminal event. Deafness, with or without antecedent tinnitus, vertigo, lethargy, and other altered states of consciousness, except for coma and hyperventilation, are all associated with salicylism or salicylate poisoning at various stages following an acute ingestion and at various salicylate levels obtained after chronic ingestions. Coma is rare and generally occurs after massive ingestions (serum salicylate levels >100 mg/dL). Tragically, many of the signs and symptoms of salicylate poisoning may be mistaken for signs and symptoms of the condition for which salicylate was taken in the first place, prompting additional self-medication with disastrous consequences.

Miyahara JT, Karler R: Effect of salicylate on oxidative phosphorylation and respiration of mitochondrial fragments. Biochem J 1965;97:194–198.

33.7. Answer: A   The ferric chloride test utilizing several drops of $FeCl_3$ and 1 mL of urine will produce a purple color (positive test) hours after the ingestion of as few as one or two regular-strength aspirin tablets. Urine previously used for testing with N-Multistix or Bili Labstix sometimes yields a false-positive test.

A positive urine ketone test further supports the diagnosis of salicylate usage, reflecting the ketogenesis associated with salicylate use. Unlike an overdose of acetaminophen, exposures to toxic amounts of salicylates are usually accompanied by signs and symptoms of toxicity, although the signs may be confusing or unreliable at times. Conversely, initiating hemodialysis based only on a high salicylate level in the absence of any signs of toxicity has resulted in dialyzing patients with therapeutic, not toxic, levels. A large number of laboratories determine and sometimes report salicylate values as milligrams per liter, whereas most clinicians and toxicologists are accustomed to receiving and interpreting levels reported as milligrams per deciliter. A value of 15 mg/dL may be reported as 150 mg/L and could be mistakenly interpreted as a toxic level. There is no evidence that liver disease causes a false-positive or false-negative result.

Hahn IH, Chu J, Hoffman RS, Nelson LS: Errors in reporting salicylate levels. Acad Emerg Med 2000;7:1336–1337.

33.8. Answer: B The best way to alkalinize both the blood and urine is with NaHCO$_3$. Acetazolamide, which had been used in the past to achieve urinary alkalinization, causes acidemia and may exacerbate the systemic toxicity of salicylates. The renal excretion of salicylate depends much more on urine pH than on flow rate, and forced diuresis alone has never been demonstrated to be effective in eliminating salicylates. Respiratory alkalosis should not be considered a substitute for the metabolic alkalosis that results from NaHCO$_3$ administration because the latter can more effectively establish a gradient between the blood and CSF, favoring movement of salicylates to the blood. Moreover, intubating a patient with a serious salicylate overdose poses a particular risk to the patient, as few health care providers are skilled in insuring the required hyperventilation and hypocapnea for a salicylate-poisoned patient receiving mechanical ventilation. Hypokalemia must be corrected to achieve urinary alkalinization. One gram of activated charcoal can adsorb about 550 mg of salicylic acid in vitro and is moderately effective in vivo.

Heller I, Halevy J, Cohen S, et al: Significant metabolic acidosis induced by acetazolamide: Not a rare complication. Arch Intern Med 1985;145:1815–1817.

Levy G, Tsuchiya T: Effect of activated charcoal on aspirin absorption in man. Clin Pharmacol Ther 1972;13:317–322.

Prescott LF, Balali-Mood M, Critchley JA, et al: Diuresis or urinary alkalinization for salicylate poisoning. Br Med J 1982;285:1383–1386.

Vree TB, Van Ewuk-Beneken Kolmer EWJ, Verwey-Van Wissen CPWGM, Hekster YA: Effect of urinary pH on the pharmacokinetics of salicylate acid, with its glycine and glucuronide conjugates in human. Int J Clin Pharm Ther 1994;32:550–558.

33.9. Answer: E Hearing loss, with or without antecedent tinnitus, may be an early sign of salicylism or salicylate poisoning and not an indication of severity of the overdose. All of the other choices are indications for extracorporeal removal. Because hemodialysis (HD), but not hemoperfusion (HP), can correct fluid, electrolyte, and acid–base disorders, HD is the method of choice, although in some instances (such as mixed overdoses), a combination of HD and HP would be more effective.

Anderson RJ, Potts DE, Gabow PA, et al: Unrecognized adult salicylate intoxication. Ann Intern Med 1976;85:745–748.

Brien J: Ototoxicity associated with salicylates. Drug Safety 1993;9:143–148.

33.10. Answer: E On average, 240 analgesic-related deaths per year have been reported to the AAPCC, establishing analgesics as the category responsible for the greatest number of deaths each year. In addition, analgesics rank second only to cleaning substances among those medications or substances most frequently involved in human exposures. Among analgesic-related deaths, acetaminophen (alone or in combination) accounts for 50%, and aspirin (alone or in combination) accounts for 18%. The incidence of Reye syndrome as well as the use of aspirin in the pediatric population has decreased dramatically in the past decade. There are no restrictions placed on brand or product names of nonprescription medications, and consequently, the same name, "Bayer" or "Anacin," for example, may appear on a product containing salicylates, acetaminophen, both, or neither. Small amounts of salicylate-containing ointments and keratolytics can be lethal to small children when unintentionally ingested and extremely toxic even when applied externally.

Belay ED, Brasee JJ, Holman RL et al: Reye's syndrome in the United States from 1981 through 1997. N Engl J Med 1999; 340:1377–1382.

Brubacher JR, Hoffman RS: Salicylism from topical salicylates: Review of the literature. J Toxicol Clin Toxicol 1996;34:431–436.

CHAPTER 34

NONSTEROIDAL AND OTHER ANTIINFLAMMATORY AGENTS

34.1. Answer: E Although nonprescription agents such as the propionic acids, ibuprofen, and naproxen are probably used more frequently than prescription NSAIDs, phenylbutazone and mefenamic acid are the two agents most commonly associated with serious toxicity such as seizures or death.

34.2. Answer: C The major difference in the mechanism of NSAIDs and steroids is their site of inhibition. Steroids diminish production of phospholipase A$_2$ and arachidonic acid precursors used to make leukotrienes as well as prostacyclins, prostaglandins, and thromboxanes. NSAIDs act later in the cascade at the cyclooxygenase system, which generally allows increased production of leukotrienes (except perhaps indomethacin and diclofenac, which inhibit lipoxygenase enzymes in animals) by allowing buildup of arachidonic acid precursors.

Insel PA: Analgesic-antipyretic and antiinflammatory agents and drugs employed in the treatment of gout. In: Hardman JG, Limbird LE, Molinoff PB, et al, eds: Goodman & Gilman's The Pharmacological Basis of Therapeutics, 9th ed. New York, McGraw-Hill, 1996, pp. 617–657.

34.3 Answer: C   The data available at this time seem to indicate that the pharmacokinetics of the NSAIDs remains relatively constant. Renal excretion does increase with larger doses of naproxen, but hepatic metabolism still remains an important route of elimination.

Hall AH, Smolinkse SC, Conrad FL, et al: Ibuprofen overdose: 126 cases. Ann Emerg Med 1986;15:1308–1312.

Runkel R, Chaplin M, Savelium H, et al: Pharmacokinetics of naproxen overdoses. Clin Pharmacol Ther 1976;20:269–277.

34.4. Answer: E   Anthraquinone laxatives are associated with red discoloration of the urine when bicarbonate is added. All of the other agents have been reported to produce a color change to brown or purple when a few drops of ferric chloride are added to approximately 1 mL of urine.

Nordt SP: Diflunisal cross-reactivity with the Trinder method for salicylate determination. Ann Pharmacother 1996;30:1041–1042.

34.5. Answer: B   Aplastic anemia has been reported in therapeutic dosing of phenylbutazone, and although sale of this drug is now restricted, it is still available from other countries and in veterinary medicine. Though aplastic anemia has also been reported in patients using such agents as indomethacin and etodolac, these reports are rare.

34.6. Answer: A   Tinnitus has been reported following the use of a number of NSAIDs including nonprescription forms of ibuprofen and naproxen. Reports of tinnitus should prompt investigation of NSAID use if serum salicylate levels are low.

34.7. Answer: D   NSAIDs tend to cause hyperkalemia and salt and water retention problems in patients who have high angiotensin and low intravascular flow because of an underlying disease such as renal insufficiency, congestive heart failure, or cirrhosis of the liver. In otherwise compromised patients, NSAID-induced vasoconstriction may diminish clearance of drugs and counteract the beneficial effects of some antihypertensive agents.

Murray MD, Brater DC: Renal toxicity of the nonsteroidal antiinflammatory drugs. Annu Rev Pharmacol Toxicol 1993;34:435–465.

34.8. Answer: E H_2 receptor antagonists may have utility in trials designed to test their prevention of gastrointestinal bleeding from NSAID use. The agents listed have met with some success or are still experimental. For instance, leukotriene-receptor antagonists such as zileuton or the recently marketed zafirlukast may be useful in preventing anaphylactoid reactions in patients allergic to salicylates and NSAIDs.

Israel E, Fischer AR, Rosenberg MA, et al: The pivotal role of 5-lipoxygenase products in reaction of aspirin-sensitive asthmatics to aspirin. Am Rev Respir Dis 1993;148:1447–1451.

Singh G, Ramey DR, Morfeld D, et al: Gastrointestinal tract complications of nonsteroidal antiinflammatory drug treatment in rheumatoid arthritis. A prospective observational cohort study. Arch Intern Med 1996;156:1530–1536.

Zafirlukast for asthma. Med Lett 1996;38:111–112.

34.9. Answer: E   High protein binding limits any benefit from hemodialysis, and low renal elimination of unchanged drug prevents usefulness of urinary alkalinization in the setting of NSAID toxicity. Gastric lavage may be useful in overdose of the most toxic NSAID agents (phenylbutazone and mefenamic acid) but otherwise presents greater risk than benefit to the patient with toxicity from other agents.

Smolinske SC, Hall AH, Vandenberg SA, et al: Toxic effects of nonsteroidal anti-inflammatory drugs in overdose: An overview of recent evidence on clinical effects and dose-response relationships. Drug Safety 1990;5:252–274.

34.10. Answer: C   The COX-2 selective and preferential agents celecoxib, refocoxib, and meloxicam lose their selectivity at doses greater than those used therapeutically. There are currently no data available that suggest these agents will have either more or less toxicity than the other NSAIDs.

Lefkowith JB: Cyclooxygenase-2 specificity and its clinical implications. Am J Med 1999;106(5B):43S–50S.

CHAPTER **35**

ANTIHISTAMINES AND DECONGESTANTS

35.1. Answer: B   Cimetidine is the only H_2 antagonist to significantly inhibit the cytochrome oxidase pathways.

Martinez C, Albet C, Agundez JA, et al: Comparative in vitro and in vivo inhibition of cytochrome P450 CYP1A2, CYP2D6, and CYP3A by H_2-receptor antagonists. Clin Pharmacol Ther 1999;65:369–376.

35.2. Answer: D   Cetirizine binds much more selectively to peripheral H_1 receptors and has a decreased binding affinity to the cholinergic and α- and β-adrenergic receptor sites than do the other antihistamines. This results in fewer side effects and improved patient acceptability.

35.3. Answer: E   Terfenadine and astemizole are metabolized by the cytochrome P450 isoenzyme CYP3A4. This is important because medications such as erythromycin and ketoconazole are capable of inhibiting metabolism of terfenadine and astemizole.

35.4. Answer: E   Patients of Asian descent can acetylate diphenhydramine to a nontoxic metabolite twice as rapidly as patients of white descent, making the former much less sensitive to both the effects on psychomotor performance and the sedative effects.

Spector R, Choudhury AK, Chiang CK, et al: Diphenhydramine in Orientals and Caucasians. Clin Pharmacol Ther 1980;28:229–235.

35.5. Answer: E   Antihistamines in overdose should not cause hypoglycemia.

Ten Eick AP, Blumer JL, Reed MD: Safety of antihistamines in children. Drug Safety 2001;24:119–147.

35.6. Answer: A Many nonprescription cough and cold preparations contain acetaminophen as an active ingredient. Following an intentional ingestion, an acetaminophen level should be checked at 4 hours.

35.7. Answer: A Phenylpropanolamine is a pure α-adrenergic antagonist. It commonly causes a reflex bradycardia. The other medications have β-adrenergic activity and cause tachycardia.

Kernan WN, Viscoli CM, Brass LM, et al: Phenylpropanolamine and the risk of hemorrhagic stroke. N Engl J Med 2000;343: 1826–1832.

35.8. Answer: D Tetrahydrozoline is a histamine H_2 agonist in addition to an α-adrenergic stimulant. Stimulation of H_2 receptors increases the production of acid in the stomach.

Bousquet P, Feldman J: Drugs acting on imidazoline receptors: a review of their pharmacology, their use in blood pressure control and their potential interest in cardioprotection. Drugs 1999;58: 799–812.

35.9. Answer: C Diphenhydramine is usually considered to be the drug of choice for treating acute dystonic reactions. Paradoxically, it has been shown to be able to induce this same reaction.

Lavenstein BL, Cantor FK: Acute dystonia: An unusual reaction to diphenhydramine. JAMA 1976;236:291.

35.10. Answer: C Doxylamine in overdose has been found to cause rhabdomyolysis. This is a nontraumatic rhabdomyolysis and occurs in the absence of seizures or prolonged coma.

Mendoza FS, Atiba JO, Krensky AL, et al: Rhabdomyolysis complicating doxylamine overdose. Clin Pediatr 1987;26:595–597.

CHAPTER 36

IRON

36.1. Answer: B Orogastric lavage is expected to be of limited benefit because of the small tube size and stability of the iron tablets. Orogastric lavage with hypertonic phosphate is not effective and can cause hyperphosphatemia. Orogastric lavage with deferoxamine has been shown to increase toxicity because of increased levels of ferrioxamine. The administration of ipecac may allow the initiation of vomiting before that expected from the iron pills themselves.

36.2. Answer: C Whole-bowel irrigation is an effective modality in clearing the gut of ingested iron tablets. Activated charcoal binds poorly to iron. Emergent gastrotomy is rarely used in patients with massive ingestion of iron pills that are adherent to the gastrointestinal tract.

Foxford R, Goldfrank L: Gastrotomy: A surgical approach to iron overdose. Ann Emerg Med 1985;14:1223–1226.

Tenenbein M: Whole bowel irrigation in iron poisoning. J Pediatr 1987;111:142–145.

36.3. Answer: D Iron poisoning is a clinical diagnosis: patients who appear well with normal vital signs and no symptoms after 6 hours in the ED are unlikely to become ill. Although a WBC >15,000/mm³ and a serum glucose >150 mg/dL were associated with an iron level >300 μg/dL in pediatric patients, other patients with WBC <15,000/ mm³ and with serum glucose <150 mg/dL also had iron levels >300 μg/dL (Lacouture). The TIBC rises in iron poisoning, and many patients manifest iron poisoning with iron levels less than the TIBC.

Burkhart KK, Kulig KW, Hammond KB, et al: The rise in the total iron binding capacity after iron overdose. Ann Emerg Med 1991; 20:532–535.

Lacouture PG, Wason S, Temple AR, et al: Emergency assessment of severity in iron overdose by clinical and laboratory methods. J Pediatr 1981;99:89–91.

36.4. Answer: D Ferrous sulfate ($FeSO_4$) is 20% elemental iron by weight: 325 mg of $FeSO_4$ = 65 mg elemental Fe. Thus,

$$[10 \text{ tabs} \times 65 \text{ mg elemental iron} / \text{tab}] / 10 \text{ kg} = 65 \text{ mg} / \text{kg}$$

36.5. Answer: B Iron is not an acid. Metabolic acidosis results from (1) liberation of a proton during iron absorption, (2) iron inhibiting oxidative metabolism, (3) iron decreasing cardiac output, contributing to hypotension, and (4) free iron acting as a vasodilator, contributing to hypotension and tissue ischemia.

Reissman KR, Coleman TJ: Acute intestinal iron intoxication. II: Metabolic, respiratory and circulatory effects of absorbed iron salts. Blood 1955;10:46–51.

36.6. Answer: D Deferoxamine is derived from *Streptomyces pilosus* and is a very complex molecule, making synthesis difficult. When it is infused intravenously, deferoxamine levels are relatively constant and result in the greatest iron excretion, although all of the other routes have been used. Deferoxamine dosing is based on patient weight, not dose ingested. Because its molecular weight is more than 10 times that of iron, a molar equivalent dose is impractical. However, deferoxamine binds iron on a molar basis: 100 mg of deferoxamine binds 9 mg of iron. Deferoxamine removes only free iron and that located in low-affinity storage sites. It does not remove iron from transferrin or hemoglobin.

36.7. Answer: D Treatment of the iron-poisoned pregnant patient should follow all of the same treatment guidelines as for non-pregnant patients. Deferoxamine and whole-bowel irrigation have been used with good outcomes in pregnant women. Abdominal radiographs are relatively contraindicated in early pregnancy, and patients can be appropriately managed without them.

McElhatton PR, Roberts JC, Sullivan FM: The consequences of iron overdose and its treatment with desferrioxamine in pregnancy. Hum Exp Toxicol 1991;10:251–259.

36.8. Answer: D *Yersinia* superinfection has been reported to complicate the recovery of acutely iron-poisoned patients treated with deferoxamine. Acute lung injury (ie, pulmonary edema) is reported in the setting of deferoxamine therapy of four iron-poisoned patients and has raised concerns regarding total dose and duration of deferoxamine therapy. Hypotension is a common, rate-related adverse effect of intravenous therapy. Serum iron levels after deferoxamine therapy cannot be interpreted via RIA or colorimetric assays (ie, falsely low) but are normal when measured by atomic absorption. Ophthalmic toxicity occurs only with chronic therapy.

Tenenbein M, Kowalski S, Bowden DH, Adamson IYR: Pulmonary toxic effects of continuous desferrioxamine administration in acute iron poisoning. Lancet 1992;339:699–701.

36.9. Answer: D The excretion of ferrioxamine-chelated iron causes the reddish brown discoloration of the urine and is the expected finding in treatment with deferoxamine in iron-poisoned patients. Although much debate has centered on criteria for discontinuation of deferoxamine therapy in the iron-poisoned patient, most authors agree that when the patient looks well and the anion gap acidosis resolves, deferoxamine may be stopped.

Mills KC, Curry SC: Acute iron poisoning. Emerg Med Clin North Am 1994;12:397–413.

36.10. Answer: B *Yersinia* superinfection may complicate the recovery of acutely iron-poisoned patients treated with deferoxamine. Iron is a required growth factor for *Y. enterocolitica* although *Yersinia* spp lack the siderophore to solubilize iron and permit intracellular injury. Deferoxamine, a siderophore, fosters the growth of *Y. enterocolitica*.

Mofenson HC, Caraccio TR, Sharieff N: Iron sepsis: *Yersinia enterocolitica* septicemia possibly caused by an overdose of iron. N Engl J Med 1987;316:1092–1093.

CHAPTER 37

VITAMINS

37.1. Answer: B Carotenoids, including β-carotene, are very inefficiently converted to vitamin A. This makes them relatively safe dietary supplements.

Diplock A: Safety of antioxidant vitamins and beta-carotene. Am J Clin Nutr 1995;62:1510S–1516S.

37.2. Answer: E Idiopathic intracranial hypertension (IIH) must be diagnosed by lumbar puncture; the CSF is normal except that opening pressure is as high as 250 to 500 mm H_2O. In many patients, a CT or MRI scan should be performed in any patient with a headache to confirm that no mass effect is present, but this study alone is not diagnostic. IIH is not pathognomonic for vitamin A toxicity. Although vitamin A deficiency is most often associated with prominent visual disturbances, benign intracranial hypertension often manifests as headache with prominent visual disturbances such as diplopia (sixth cranial nerve palsy) and blurred vision (papillitis). In fact, visual impairment secondary to optic atrophy is often the only major long-term sequela of vitamin A toxicity. Focal findings should not occur.

Allain HJ, Weintraub M: Drug induced headache. Ration Drug Ther 1980;14:1–6.

37.3. Answer: D The skin change associated with vitamin A toxicity is desquamation. Acrodynia is actually a hypersensitivity reaction to mercury, not a poisoning. Hepatotoxicity is commonly noted.

Inkeles SB, Connor WE, Illingworth DR: Hepatic and dermatologic manifestations of chronic hypervitaminosis A in adults: Report of two cases. Am J Med 1986;80:491–496.

37.4. Answer: C Vitamin A hepatotoxicity is histologically defined as cirrhosis. Cirrhosis develops secondary to the proliferative effect vitamin A has on Ito cells. These cells deposit excessive amounts of collagen and result in scarring.

Kowalski TE, Falestiny M, Furth E, Malet PF: Vitamin A hepatotoxicity: A cautionary note regarding 25,000 IU supplements. Am J Med 1994;97:523–528.

37.5. Answer: E In animals, absorption of vitamin K is impaired by large doses of vitamin E. Coupled with the inhibitory effect vitamin E appears to have on the epoxidation of vitamin K to its active form, this means that excessive vitamin E supplementation may prolong prothrombin times in patients taking coumadin.

37.6. Answer: E Pyridoxine is rapidly excreted, and large doses are well tolerated unless they are one or two orders of magnitude above the therapeutic dose as an antidote (70 mg/kg). In contrast, doses as low as 200 mg/day have produced a toxic sensory neuropathy.

Schaumburg H, Kaplan J, Windebank A, et al: Sensory neuropathy from pyridoxine abuse: A new megavitamin syndrome. N Engl J Med 1983;309:445–448.

37.7. Answer: D Vitamin C is a useful oral or intravenous antidote for chromium toxicity. It converts hexavalent chromium to its less toxic trivalent form. Unfortunately, it holds little promise as a cold remedy. Large doses cause oxalaturia and diarrhea.

Korallus U, Harzdorf C, Lewalter J: Experimental basis for ascorbic acid therapy of poisoning by hexavalent chromium compounds. Int Arch Occup Environ Health 1984;53:247–256.

37.8. Answer: B Vitamin D toxicity manifests as nausea, vomiting, renal compromise, hypercalcemia, and hyperphosphatemia. The hematopoietic system is rarely affected.

Jacobus CH, Holick MF, Shao Q, et al: Hypervitaminosis D associated with drinking milk. N Engl J Med 1992;326:1173–1177.

Misselwitz J, Hesse V, Markestad T: Nephrocalcinosis, hypercalciuria and elevated serum levels of 1,25-dihydrovitamin D in children. Acta Paediatr Scand 1990;79:636–643.

37.9. Answer: B Niacin flush is mediated by the release of prostaglandin D_2 from a niacin-responsive cell in the skin. It does not result from a release of histamine. It can be prevented by taking 325 mg of aspirin 30 minutes before ingestion.

Whelan AM, Price SO, Fowler SF, Hainer BL: The effect of aspirin on niacin-induced cutaneous reactions. J Fam Pract 1992;34:165–168.

37.10. Answer: C Niacin-induced hepatitis appears to be more frequent and more severe among those with hyperlipidemias treated with sustained-release preparations than those receiving crystalline or immediate-release niacin. Hepatotoxicity is consistent with centrilobular cholestasis and parenchymal necrosis. These manifestations appear to be dose related and not a hypersensitivity response.

Rader JI, Calvert RJ, Hathcock JN: Hepatic toxicity of unmodified and time release preparations of niacin. Am J Med 1992;92:77–81.

CHAPTER 38

DIETING AGENTS AND REGIMENS

38.1. Answer: C Phentermine-fenfluramine is associated with valvular regurgitation, especially of the mitral and occasionally the aortic valve, as well as pulmonary hypertension.

Connolly HM, Crary JL, McGoon MD, et al: Valvular heart disease associated with fenfluramine-phentermine. N Engl J Med 1997;337:581–588.

38.2. Answer: C *Ma huang* and Chinese ephedra are synonymous with ephedrine, the sympathomimetic amine with structural and clinical properties similar to *d*-amphetamine. Ephedrine, in its various forms, is abused as a stimulant and sold over the counter as an unregulated "herbal" anorexiant. Many adverse events are reported, almost all of which result from its amphetaminelike properties.

Perrotta DM, Coody G, Culmo C: Adverse events associated with ephedrine-containing products—Texas, December 1993–September 1995. MMWR 1996;45:689–693.

38.3. Answer: D Popularized in the early 1980s, starch blockers appeared to be a scientific approach to weight loss. However, it was demonstrated that amylase secretion in vivo was only minimally inhibited and inadequate to alter calorie absorption.

Bo-Linn GW, Santa Ana CA, Morawski SG, Fordtran JS: Starch blockers—their effect on calorie absorption from a high-starch meal. N Engl J Med 1982;307:1413–1416.

38.4. Answer: D Torsades de pointes, ventricular tachycardia, ventricular fibrillation, and sudden death have all been reported with very low-calorie diets. Pathologic abnormalities found at autopsy include myocardial atrophy.

Singh BN, Gaarder TD, Kanegae T, et al: Liquid protein diets and torsade de pointes. JAMA 1978;240:115–9.

Sours HE, Frattali VP, Brand CD, et al: Sudden death associated with very low calorie weight reduction regimens. Am J Clin Nutr 1981;34:453–461.

38.5. Answer: B Although phenylpropanolamine was commonly found in the over-the-counter appetite suppressants for years, a case-control study described an associated increased risk of hemorrhagic stroke in women using this preparation. This paper, along with mounting case reports of similar problems, prompted an FDA recall of PPA products.

Kernan WN, Viscoli C, Brass LM, et al: Phenylpropanolamine and the risk of hemorrhagic stroke. N Engl J Med 2000;343:1826–1832.

38.6. Answer: D β-Adrenergic antagonists should be avoided in the management of hypertension secondary to mixed sympathomimetic agents (ie, α/β agonists) because of the risk of producing unopposed α agonism. A titratable α antagonist such as phentolamine provides effective control of blood pressure.

Ramoska E, Sacchetti AD: Propranolol-induced hypertension in treatment of cocaine intoxication. Ann Emerg Med 1985;14:112–113.

38.7. Answer: C 2,4-Dinitrophenol uncouples oxidative phosphorylation, preventing formation of ATP (calorie yield) from food sources. Unable to create high-energy bonds, this energy is dissipated as heat, resulting in hyperthermia. This effect proved consequential and precluded the effective use of this agent as a diet aid.

Cutting WC, Mehrtens HG, Tainter ML: Actions and uses of dinitrophenol. JAMA 1933;101:193–195.

Tainter ML, Cutting WC: Febrile, respiratory and some other actions of dinitrophenol. J Pharmacol Exp Ther 1933;48;410–429.

38.8. Answer: C Guar gum worked as a diet aid by absorbing water in the stomach and expanding, thus giving the sensation of satiety. Multiple reports of esophageal obstruction led to the removal of the product from the US market.

Lewis JH: Esophageal and small bowel obstruction from guar-gum containing diet pills: Analysis of 26 cases reported to the Food and Drug Administration. Am J Gastoenterol 1992;87:1424–1428.

38.9. Answer: D All of the others have been reported in association with primary pulmonary hypertension in a case-control study.

Abenhaim L, Moride Y, Brenot F, et al: Appetite suppressant drugs and the risk of primary pulmonary hypertension. N Engl J Med 1996;335:609–616.

38.10. Answer: A Patients with eating disorders abuse a wide range of medications in order to facilitate their obsession, including syrup of ipecac, laxatives, diuretics, and "diet pills" as well as cigarettes, cocaine, and amphetamines. Emetine toxicity, from chronic abuse of syrup of ipecac, may lead to cardiomyopathy. Although this is potentially reversible with discontinuation of ipecac, death from myocardial failure may occur.

Friedman EJ: Death from ipecac intoxication in a patient with anorexia nervosa. Am J Psychiatry. 1984;141:702–703.

Palmer EP, Guary AT: Reversible myopathy secondary to abuse of ipecac in patients with major eating disorders. N Engl J Med 1985;313:1457–1459.

CHAPTER **39**

METHYLXANTHINES

39.1. Answer: B In preterm infants, caffeine is converted significantly to theophylline. Only 5% of caffeine is recovered in the urine unchanged. The primary metabolic pathway is demethylation. Caffeine's half-life is decreased in smokers. Caffeine does not induce cytochrome metabolic enzymes.

39.2. Answer: A Caffeine and theophylline are both nonselective adenosine receptor antagonists.

Fredholm BB, Abbrocchio MP, Burnstock B, et al: VI. Nomenclature and classification of purinoceptors. Pharmacol Rev 1994;46: 143–156.

39.3. Answer: C Caffeine causes biphasic toxicity: anxiety, restlessness, tachycardia, tremor, irritability, tinnitus, and dysesthesias followed by lethargy and CNS depression.

Greden JF, Fontaine P, Lubetsky M, et al: Anxiety and depression associated with caffeinism among psychiatric inpatients. Psychiatry 1978;135:963–966.

39.4. Answer: B Caffeine stimulates pepsin and acid gastric secretion. Peptic ulcer disease as well as heartburn can be aggravated by caffeine ingestion. Decaffeinated coffee as well as regular coffee may contain other stimulants of acid secretion, such as essential oils. Caffeine is a potent stimulator of the H_2 receptor in the stomach.

Cohen A: Pathogenesis of coffee-induced gastrointestinal symptoms. N Engl J Med 1980;303:122–124.

39.5. Answer: C Effect of coffee on serum lipids and its effect on cardiovascular disease is controversial. Caffeine increases contraction of muscles and increases the basal metabolic rate by 10%. Habitual caffeine ingestion is associated with decreased bone density.

Wilson PWF, Garrison RJ, Kannel WB, et al: Is coffee consumption a contributor to cardiovascular disease? Arch Intern Med 1989;149:1169–1172.

39.6. Answer: C The estimated clearance of theophylline during charcoal hemoperfusion is 2.4 mL/kg/min. The clearance of theophylline with hemodialysis is 0.4 to 1.2 mL/kg/min. The clearance with multiple-dose activated charcoal is approximately 1 mL/kg/min, and the clearance of theophylline during peritoneal dialysis is 0.45 mL/kg/min.

Winchester JF, Gelfand MC, Knepshield JH, et al: Dialysis and hemoperfusion of poisons and drugs—update. Trans Am Soc Artif Intern Organs 1977;23:762–842.

39.7. Answer: A Patient's with acute theophylline toxicity will often be found to have a respiratory alkalosis, metabolic acidosis, hypokalemia, hyperglycemia, and leukocytosis.

Shannon MW, Lovejoy FH Jr: Hypokalemia after theophylline intoxication. The effects of acute vs chronic poisoning. Arch Intern Med 1989;149:2725–2729.

39.8. Answer: D Nausea, vomiting, and sinus tachycardia are the most common manifestations in patients with acute theophylline toxicity from an acute single ingestion as opposed to chronic repeated overmedication.

Olson KR, Benowitz NL, Woo OF, et al: Theophylline overdose: Acute single ingestion versus chronic repeated over-medication. Am J Emerg Med 1985;3:386–394.

39.9. Answer: C Only activated charcoal has been shown to be effective in reducing the absorption and subsequent area under the curve for theophylline. Both emesis and lavage failed to prevent drug absorption in a recent study. Similar effects would be expected for caffeine.

Minton N, Glucksman E, Henry JA: Prevention of drug absorption in simulated theophylline overdose. Hum Exp Toxicol 1995;14: 170–174.

39.10. Answer: E The primary pharmacologic effect of theophylline at therapeutic levels is to antagonize the activity of adenosine, which is believed to modulate histamine release and cause constriction of respiratory smooth muscles. Theophylline in high concentrations is known to increase the levels of circulating catecholamines and, in very high concentrations, to inhibit the activity of the enzyme phosphodiesterase, which is responsible for the metabolism of cyclic AMP.

Fredholm BB: Theophylline action on adenosine receptors. Eur J Respir Dis 1980;180(Suppl):29–36.

CHAPTER **40**

ANTIDIABETIC AND HYPOGLYCEMIC AGENTS

40.1. Answer: C A C-peptide level of less than 0.2 nmol/L is diagnostic of an exogenous insulin exposure. Endogenous insulin increases both insulin and C-peptide levels, as does administration of a sulfonylurea. None of the commercially available insulins contain C-peptide.

Bauman WA, Yalow RS: Hyperinsulinemic hypoglycemia: Differential diagnosis by determination of the species of circulatory insulin. JAMA 1984;252:2730–2734.

40.2. Answer: A Of the sulfonylureas, glyburide and chlorpropamide have been found to cause the highest incidence of hypoglycemia. As a class, the sulfonylureas were found to cause 63% of the cases of iatrogenic hypoglycemia.

Selzter HS: Severe drug induced hypoglycemia: A review. Compr Ther 1979;5:21–29.

40.3. Answer: D The unripe ackee fruit contains the toxin hypoglycin, which is capable of causing hypoglycemia.

CDC: Toxic hypoglycemic syndrome. Jamaica 1989–1991. MMWR 1992;41:53–55.

40.4. Answer: C The clinical presentation of hypoglycemia is varied and unpredictable. Hypoglycemia usually causes a hyperadrenergic state with tachycardia, tremor, and diaphoresis as well as findings of neuroglycopenia such as seizures, altered mental status, or focal neurologic syndromes. Bronchoconstriction, bradycardia, miosis, and hypoactive bowel sounds would be unusual.

Fischer KF, Lees JA, Newman JH: Hypoglycemia in hospitalized patients. N Engl J Med 1986;315:1245–1250.

40.5. Answer: A Following resolution of the hypoglyemia, octreotide is the current drug of choice and should be considered early in the management of sulfonylurea-related hypoglycemia that is refractory to or recurrent following dextrose administration. Diazoxide inhibits sulfonylurea-induced insulin release from islet β cells. However, hypotension may occur as a side effect, and the drug is not readily available. Streptozotocin, a drug that destroys pancreatic islet cells, is used to treat patients with insulinomas; however, it take hours to days to increase glucose levels and may result in permanent diabetes. Fructose will have no effect on increasing the blood glucose.

Boyle PJ, Justice K, Krentz, et al: Octreotide reverses hyperinsulinemia and prevents hypoglycemia induced sulfonylurea overdoses. J Clin Endrocrinol Metab 1993;76:752–756.

McLaughlin SA, Crandall CS, McKinney PE: Octreotide: An antidote for sulfonylurea-induced hypoglycemia. Ann Emerg Med 2000;36:133–138.

Palatnick W, Meatherall RC, Tenenbein M: Clinical spectrum of sulfonylurea overdose and experience with diazoxide therapy. Arch Intern Med 1991;151:1859–1862.

40.6. Answer: B Chlorpropamide has a duration of action of 24 to 72 hours, glipizide 16 to 24 hours, glyburide 18 to 24 hours, tolbutamide 6 to 12 hours, and tolazamide 16 to 24 hours.

Gerich JE: Oral hypoglycemic agents. N Engl J Med 1989;321: 1231–1245.

40.7. Answer: D Phenformin was withdrawn from the US market because of an unacceptably high incidence of severe lactic acidosis. The incidence of lactic acidosis from metformin has been reported to be 3 in 100,000.

Crofford OB: Metformin. N Engl J Med 1995;333:588–589.

40.8. Answer: B Troglitazone was withdrawn from the US market in 2000 because of liver toxicity, which developed in patients on therapeutic doses. Some cases were severe, requiring liver transplantation. Elevated aminotransferase levels have occurred in patients on acarbose, but most patients were asymptomatic, and resolution occurred after discontinuation of the drug.

Gitlin N, Julie NL, Spurr CL, et al: Two cases of severe clinical and histologic hepatotoxicity associated with troglitazone. Ann Intern Med 1998;129:36–38.

Hollander P: Safety of acarbose, an alpha-glucosidase inhibitor. Drugs 1992;21:20–24.

Neuschwander-Tetri BA, Isley WL, Oki JC, et al: Troglitazone-induced hepatic failure leading to liver transplantation. A case report. Ann Intern Med 1998;129:38–41.

40.9. Answer: B The onset of hypoglycemia is unpredictable and often delayed. Although not specifically studied, there is no reason to suspect that activated charcoal does not adsorb sulfonylureas. Serum sulfonylurea levels may be measured, but they are not clinically useful because of the long time needed for laboratory analysis.

CHAPTER **41**

ANTICONVULSANTS

40.10. Answer: C Approximately 50% of glyburide is eliminated by nonrenal clearance and is less affected by renal impairment than the other oral hypoglycemic agents. Patients with renal impairment should be carefully monitored while receiving any oral hypoglycemic agent. The primary risk factor for the development of metformin-induced metabolic acidosis is renal insufficiency, and metformin should not be used in this group.

41.1. Answer: B The incidence of hypotension and myocardial conduction defects following intravenous administration of phenytoin is 3.5%. CSF levels correlate more favorably with free phenytoin levels than total phenytoin levels because only the free drug can cross the blood-brain barrier. Routine phenytoin testing in most institutions measures total phenytoin, which includes free drug plus albumin-bound drug. Phenytoin levels >15 mg/L are associated with nystagmus, and levels >30 mg/L are associated with ataxia. A single loading dose of phenytoin results in therapeutic levels in only 46% of patients at 8 hours. MDAC reduces the $t_{1/2}$ of intravenously administered phenytoin from 44 to 22 hours.

Booker HE, Darcey B: Serum concentrations of free diphenylhydantoin and their relationship to clinical intoxication. Epilepsia 1973;14:177–184.

Earnest MP, Marx JA, Drury LR: Complications of intravenous phenytoin for acute treatment of seizures. JAMA 1983;249: 762–765.

41.2. Answer: D Carbamazepine is lipophilic and slowly absorbed. It also has some mild anticholinergic activity, which may delay its absorption as well. Carbamazepine levels >40 mg/L are associated with greater incidence of seizures, coma, and dysrhythmias. QTc prolongation was detected in 50% of carbamazepine overdose patients in one case series. MDAC reduces enterohepatic circulation of carbamazepine and should be recommended in severe overdoses and when levels are increasing.

Hojer J, Malmlund HO, Berg A: Clinical features in 28 consecutive cases of laboratory confirmed massive poisoning with carbamazepine alone. J Toxicol Clin Toxicol 1993;31:449–458.

41.3. Answer: C Leukopenia, thrombocytopenia, and anemia can occur 3 to 5 days following acute massive valproic acid ingestions. Metabolic acidosis and elevation of the serum lactate occur following acute massive valproic acid overdoses and is unrelated to hypotension. The incidence of fatal valproic acid–induced hepatic failure is 1/49,000 adults and 1/800 children. Although carbamazepine was responsible for 44% of fatalities secondary to ingestion of anticonvulsant agents in 1989, valproic acid was responsible for 89% in 1999. This likely relates to the widespread use of valproic acid as a mood-stabilizing drug.

Anderson GO, Ritland S: Life threatening intoxication with sodium valproate. J Toxicol Clin Toxicol 1995; 33:279–284.

41.4. Answer: C Hypocarnitinemia is associated with valproic acid therapy. The only proven benefit for carnitine supplementation is hyperammonemia.

Coulter DL, Allen RJ: Secondary hyperammonemia: A possible mechanism for valproate encephalopathy. Lancet 1980;1:1310.

Raskind JY, El-Chaar GM: The role of carnitine supplementation during valproic acid therapy. Ann Pharmacother 2000;34: 630–638.

41.5. Answer: D There is a higher incidence of dystonic reactions, seizures, and choreathetosis in children who overdose with carbamazepine. Hyponatremia is associated with chronic carbamazepine toxicity in adults. The other electrolyte abnormalities have not been associated with carbamazepine overdoses. Ileus is not associated with pediatric carbamazepine overdoses, although carbamazepine has mild anticholinergic activity.

Stremski ES, Brady W, Prasad K, et al: Pediatric carbamazepine intoxication. Ann Emerg Med 1995;25:624–630.

41.6. Answer: B Gabapentin, felbamate, lamotrigine, and phenytoin have no active metabolites. Carbamazepine 10,11-epoxide is a carbamazepine metabolite that is almost as active as the parent compound.

Dichter MA, Brodie MJ: New antiepileptic drugs. N Engl J Med 1996;334:1583–1590.

41.7. Answer: A Gabapentin has no documented interaction with other drugs. Theophylline, rifampin, and phenobarbital all decrease phenytoin levels through induction of the hepatic microsomal enzyme system. Carbamazepine enhances the hepatic metabolism of phenytoin and causes a well-documented decrease in phenytoin concentration.

41.8. Answer: D Mild lethargy is expected with gabapentin, felbamate, and lamotrigine. Lamotrigine is associated with de novo seizures in a toddler. Agitation and psychosis were the hallmarks of two of the four reported vigabatrin overdoses. There are no reports of topiramate overdose, but CNS depression would be expected following this type of ingestion.

Hopkins U, Shepherd G, Klein-Schwartz W, et al: Multicenter case series of gabapentin exposures [abstract]. J Toxicol Clin Toxicol 2000;38:575.

Buckley NA, Whyte IM, Dawson AH: Self poisoning with lamotrigine [letter]. Lancet 1993;342:1552–1553.

41.9. Answer: E Gabapentin is 100% renally excreted, and dose adjustments are necessary in patients with impaired renal function.

Vigabatrin is also largely renally excreted, felbamate is moderately excreted by the kidneys, and phenytoin and lamotrigine have negligible renal elimination.

41.10. Answer: E The anticonvulsant hypersensitivity syndrome is only associated with the aromatic anticonvulsants. Seizures are uncommon following phenytoin or valproic acid overdose in normal patients. Patients with phenytoin ingestion, no matter how large, do not develop cardiac dysrhythmias, unlike those receiving rapid intravenously administered phenytoin. Tremors are a frequent and important adverse effect of valproic acid therapy. Vigabatrin may cause psychosis acutely or chronically but does not interfere with serotonin systems.

Knowles SR, Shapiro LE, Shear NH: Anticonvulsant hypersensitivity syndrome: Incidence, prevention and management. Drug Safety 1999;21:489–501.

Rogvi-Hansen B, Gram L: Adverse effects of established and new antiepileptic drugs: An attempted comparison. Pharmacol Ther 1993;68:425–434.

CHAPTER **42**

ANTICOAGULANTS

42.1. Answer: B Long-acting anticoagulant rodenticides are structurally and biochemically similar to warfarin anticoagulants. As a result, they would be expected to produce changes in the PT (INR) early. The optimum timing of laboratory studies has been evaluated and determined to be 24 and 48 hours. If there is no suspicion of chronic exposure, baseline PT (INR) testing is not cost effective. Factor V is not activated by vitamin K, so it is abnormal only in patients with liver disease.

Smolinske SC, Scherger DL, Kearns PS, et al: Superwarfarin poisoning in children: a prospective study. Pediatrics 1989;84: 490–494.

42.2. Answer: E One milligram of protamine binds 100 units of heparin. Because protamine infusion is associated with anaphylaxis, it is indicated only for the reversal of consequential heparin overdose. Although the 50,000 units of heparin might lead to significant bleeding, it has a short half-life, and the patient is without symptoms. If reversal was required, excessive protamine might lead to worsening anticoagulation, so the protamine dose should be based on the amount of heparin remaining. Exchange transfusion and FFP have no role in adults with heparin overdose.

Holland CL, Singh AK, McMaster PRB, et al: Adverse reactions to protamine sulfate following cardiac surgery. Clin Cardiol 1984;7:157–162.

42.3. Answer: C Intravenous administration of vitamin K_1 has a slightly more rapid onset of action than subcutaneous administration but still requires many hours to normalize the INR. Clearly this patient is too sick for observation. Whole blood might be indicated if this were considered a life-threatening bleed. FFP will immediately correct the patient's coagulopathy and allow time for vitamin K_1 to have its effect. At that point, however, the patient will be at risk for embolic events and might require heparin.

Glover JJ: Conservative treatment of over anticoagulated patients. Chest 1995;108:987–990.

42.4. Answer: A Choices **B–E** highlight why long-acting anticoagulants are so dangerous. Clearly the pellet form has no role in this process and cannot explain the prolonged anticoagulation observed.

Leck JB, Park BK: A comparative study of the effect of warfarin and brodifacoum on the relationship between vitamin K_1 metabolism and clotting factor activity in warfarin-susceptible and warfarin-resistant rats. Biochem Pharmacol 1981;30:123–128.

Park BK, Leck JB: A comparison of vitamin K antagonism by warfarin, difenacoum, and brodifacoum in the rabbit. Biochem Pharmacol 1982;31:3535–3639.

42.5. Answer: B Allopurinol increases anticoagulation by increasing free drug levels of warfarin.

Majerus PW, Broze GJ, Miletich JP, Tollefsen DM: Anticoagulant, thrombolytic, and antiplatelet drugs. In: Hardman JG, Limbird LE, Molinoff PB, Ruddon RW, eds: Goodman & Gilman's The Pharmacological Basis of Therapeutics, 9th ed. New York, McGraw-Hill, 1996, pp. 1341–1359.

42.6. Answer: E Low-molecular-weight heparins have many of the same pharmacologic and toxicologic properties as conventional heparin. Choices **A–D** include some of the major differences between the two. Unfortunately, although these properties make administration and monitoring of low-molecular-weight heparins easier than with conventional heparin, they do not eliminate or even reduce the risk of bleeding complications.

Bounameaux H, Goldhaber SZ: Uses of low-molecular-weight heparin. Blood Rev 1995;9:213–219.

Green D, Hirsh J, Heit J, et al: Low molecular weight heparin: A critical analysis of clinical trials. Pharmacol Rev 1994;46:89–109.

42.7. Answer: D Heparin produces two forms of thrombocytopenia. The first is common, mild, and transient and results from platelet aggregation. The second results from IgG as discussed in choice **C**. This IgG activates platelets to produce the clot that has no fibrin (white clot). No bone marrow effects have been described.

Aster RH: Heparin-induced thrombocytopenia and thrombosis. N Engl J Med 1995;332:1374–1376.

42.8. Answer: A Venoms contain many components capable of producing severe coagulopathy. Thrombinlike activity converts fibrinogen to fibrin, producing a consumptive coagulopathy similar to DIC. Additional effects result from direct activation of factor X and the release of cell factors that begin coagulation.

Iyaniwura TT: Snake venom constituents: Biochemistry and toxicology, part 1. Vet Hum Toxicol 1991;33:468–480.

42.9. Answer: C Although originally obtained from leech saliva, hirudins used today are made by recombinant gene technology. Their low molecular weight, long half-life, and ability to directly block thrombin make them ideal anticoagulants, and they have been used as adjuncts to angioplasty. Unlike heparin, however, hirudins have no natural inhibitors (like platelet factor 4), so they can actually be used in patients with the severe form of heparin-associated thrombocytopenia.

Schiele F, Vuillemenot A, Mouhat T, et al: Anticoagulant therapy with recombinant hirudin in patients with thrombocytopenia induced by heparin. Presse Med 1996;25:757–760.

Serruys PW, Herrman JR, Simon R: A comparison of hirudin with heparin in the prevention of restenosis after coronary angioplasty. N Engl J Med 1995;333:757–763.

42.10. Answer: D For most patients with intentional ingestions of long-acting anticoagulants, oral or subcutaneous vitamin K_1 therapy will be sufficient. If rapid control of the coagulopathy is indicated, FFP can completely reverse the warfarinlike effect by supplying exogenous coagulation factors. However, FFP requires about 30 to 45 minutes to prepare, so whole blood would be indicated in patients who are very unstable. Because these agents are adsorbed to activated charcoal and enterohepatically recirculated, multiple-dose charcoal therapy is indicated. Phenobarbital has been shown to increase elimination in animals, but its sedating effects contraindicate its use.

Bachmann KA, Sullivan TJ: Dispositional and pharmacodynamic characteristics of brodifacoum in warfarin-sensitive rats. Pharmacology 1983;27:281–288.

Hoffman RS, Smilkstein MJ, Goldfrank LR: Evaluation of coagulation factor abnormalities in long-acting anticoagulant overdose. J Toxicol Clin Toxicol 1988;26:233–248.

Udall JA: Don't use the wrong vitamin K. West J Med 1970;112: 65–67.

CHAPTER **43**

ANTITUBERCULOUS AGENTS

43.1. Answer: C Although it was previously thought that rapid acetylators of INH were more predisposed to hepatotoxicity, this is not the case. Slow acetylators are more susceptible to the INH-induced peripheral neuritis.

Goel UC, Baja S, Gupta OP: Isoniazid-induced neuropathy in slow versus rapid acetylators. J Assoc Physicians India 1992;40: 671–672.

Gurumurthy P, Krishna Murthy MS, Nazareth O: Lack of relationship between hepatic toxicity and acetylator phenotype. Am Rev Respir Dis 1984;129:58–61.

43.2. Answer: D Approximately 10% of all patients maintained on INH will experience elevations in liver enzymes, and 10% of this group (1% overall) will develop liver disease.

Kozanoff DE, Snider DE, Caras GJ: Isoniazid hepatitis. Am Rev Respir Dis 1978;117:991–1001.

Nolan CM, Goldberg SV, Buskin SE. Hepatotoxicity associated with isoniazid preventive therapy: a 7-year survey from a public health tuberculosis clinic. JAMA 1999;281:1014–1018.

43.3. Answer: E   All these adverse reactions have been associated with INH.

Byrd RB, Nelson R, Elliot RC: Isoniazid toxicity. JAMA 1972; 220:1471–1473.

43.4. Answer: D   The most frequent neurologic complication of INH is peripheral neuritis. It is a distal sensory-motor neuropathy, is dose related, and is seen more often in slow acetylators and in those who are malnourished, alcoholic, uremic, or diabetic.

Goel UC, Baja S, Gupta OP, Dwiedi NC: Isoniazid-induced neuropathy in slow versus rapid acetylators. J Assoc Physicians India 1992;40:671–672.

43.5. Answer: E   In doses greater than 10 g/d ethambutol is likely to cause optic neuropathy, visual hallucinations, abdominal pain, and confusion.

Ducobu J, Dupont P, Laurent M: Acute isoniazid/ethambutol overdosage. Lancet 1982;1:632.

43.6. Answer: C   Rifampin can, in large doses, cause a characteristic orange-red staining of the tissues and urine (the red man syndrome).

Holdiness MR: A review of the redman syndrome. Med Toxicol Adverse Drug Exp 1989;4:444–451.

43.7. Answer: B   The red discoloration of the skin can be at least partially removed by scrubbing.

43.8. Answer: C   If the amount of isoniazid ingested is known, pyridoxine should be given in a gram-for-gram dose. If the amount is unknown, 70 mg/kg to a maximum of 5 g should be administered. This dose may be repeated if seizures recur or coma is prolonged.

Brown CV: Acute isoniazid poisoning. Am Rev Respir Dis 1972; 105:206–216.

43.9. Answer: C   Acute INH overdose classically presents as seizures, which are often refractory to conventional treatment.

Starke H, William S: Acute poisoning from overdose of isoniazid. Lancet 1976;83:406–408.

43.10. Answer: C   Phenelzine is the hydrazine analogue of phenylethylamine and acts as an MAO inhibitor. Pyridoxine will not reverse a poisoning with phenelzine.

George ME, Pinkerton MK, Bach C: Therapeutics of monomethylhydrazine intoxication. Toxicol Appl Pharmacol 1982;63: 201–208.

CHAPTER **44**

ANTIMALARIAL AGENTS

44.1. Answer: B   Quinine is an optical isomer of quinidine, although it is derived from the same tree *(Cinchona)* as salicin, a salicylic acid glycoside. Intramuscular and subcutaneous administration of quinine produces tissue necrosis. This was most prominent in the high incidence of tetanus mortality from both quinine-tainted heroin (Cherubin) and empiric malaria therapy in Vietnam (Yen). Although at one time quinine adulteration of heroin was so widespread that it was used as a marker for heroin use, the opioid assay is the current standard. Its most important toxicologic effect is blindness from direct retinal toxicity.

Cherubin CE: Urban tetanus. The epidemiologic aspects of tetanus in narcotic addicts in New York City. Arch Environ Health 1967; 14:802–808.

Yen LM, Dao LM, Day NP, et al: Role of quinine in the high mortality of intramuscular injection tetanus. Lancet 1994;344: 786–787.

44.2. Answer: B   Multiple doses of activated charcoal have been shown to improve the clearance of quinine. Hemoperfusion and peritoneal dialysis have not been shown to significantly improve clearance. Orogastric lavage is of limited value because of its rapid absorption. Forced acid diuresis may improve clearance but increases the risk of cardiac toxicity. Stellate ganglion nerve block was a previously recommended therapy for quinine-induced blindness.

Bateman DN, Blain PG, Woodhouse KW, et al: Pharmacokinetics and clinical toxicity of quinine overdosage: Lack of efficacy of techniques intended to enhance elimination. Q J Med 1985;54: 125–131.

Prescott LF, Hamilton AR, Heyworth R:. Treatment of quinine overdosage with repeated oral charcoal. Br J Clin Pharmacol 1989;27:95–97.

Sabto JK, Pierce RM, West RH, et al: Hemodialysis, peritoneal dialysis, plasmapheresis and forced diuresis for the treatment of quinine overdose. Clin Nephrol 1981;16:264–268.

44.3. Answer: A   In vitro experiments have shown that, similarly to the sulfonylureas, quinine can cause hypoglycemia by stimulating β cells in the pancreas to release insulin.

Henquin J: Quinine and the stimulus secretion coupling in pancreatic β cells: Glucose like effects on potassium permeability and insulin release. Endocrinology 1982;110:1325–1332.

44.4. Answer: C   Malaria may protect patients from quinine toxicity because it increases circulating levels of α_1 acid glycoprotein, the protein that binds 85 to 95% of serum quinine.

Silamut K, Molunto P, Ho M, et al: Alpha-1-glycoprotein (orosomucoid) and plasma protein binding of quinine in *Falciparum* malaria. Br J Clin Pharmacol 1991;32:311–315.

44.5. Answer: D Sodium bicarbonate can be safely used to treat conduction disturbances from quinine toxicity. All of the other choices will worsen intraventricular conduction delays.

Wasserman F, Brodsky L, Dick MM, et al: Successful treatment of quinidine and procainamide intoxication. N Engl J Med 1958; 259:797–802.

44.6. Answer: D Fansidar is a combination of pyrimethamine and sulfadoxine. Pyrimethamine is a dihydrofolate reductase inhibitor.

44.7. Answer: D Diazepam and epinephrine have been shown to reduce the mortality from chloroquine overdose when used in conjunction with early intubation and aggressive cardiovascular and neurologic support.

Riou B, Barriot P, Rimailho A, Baud FJ: Treatment of severe chloroquine poisoning. N Engl J Med 1988;318:1–7.

44.8. Answer: D Reports of torsades de pointes are rare, but the increase in QTc and risk of torsades de pointes are greater when mefloquine is used with quinine, chloroquine, or, most particularly, with halofantrine. With prophylactic use, neither the PR interval nor the QRS complex is prolonged, but the QT interval may be prolonged. Clinically insignificant bradycardia is common.

Nosten F, ter Kuile FO, Luxemburger C, et al: Cardiac effects of antimalarial treatment with halofantrine. Lancet 1993;341: 1054–1056.

44.9. Answer: C The primary toxicity in therapeutic and supratherapeutic doses is torsades de pointes and ventricular fibrillation associated with prolongation of the QTc. The QTc duration is related to serum concentration.

Touze JE, Keundjian BA, Viguier PIA, et al: Electrocardiographic changes and halofantrine plasma level during acute *falciparum* malaria. Am J Trop Med Hyg 1996;54:225–228.

44.10. Answer: A In children with cerebral malaria, a higher incidence of seizures and a delay to recovery from coma were noted in a comparison with quinine.

Boele van Hensbroek M, Onyiorah E, Jaffar E, et al: A trial of artemether or quinine in children with cerebral malaria. N Engl J Med 1996;335:65–75.

CHAPTER **45**

ANTIMIGRAINE AGENTS

45.1. Answer: E Rectal bioavailability is 20 times greater than via the oral route. The ergots are poorly absorbed by the oral route because they undergo extensive first-pass metabolism. The volume of distribution is 2 L/kg, and the half-life ranges from 90 to 360 minutes.

Ibraheem JJ, Palazzo L, Tfelt-Hansen P: Kinetics of ergotamine after intravenous and intramuscular administration of migraine sufferers. Eur J Clin Pharmacol 1982; 23:235–240.

Orton DA, Richardson RJ: Ergotamine absorption and toxicity. Postgrad Med J 1982;58:6–11.

45.2. Answer: C The ergot alkaloids are pure α-adrenergic agonists and can cause a significant increase in blood pressure.

Stumpf JL, Mitrzyk B: Management of orthostatic hypotension. Am J Hosp Pharm 1994;51:618–620.

45.3. Answer: B Although the ergot alkaloids have been used for obstetric purposes dating back to the early 1800s, they have been used to treat vascular headaches since about 1950.

Rall TW, Schleifer LS: Oxytocin, prostaglandins, ergot alkaloids and other tocolytic agents. In: Gilman AG, Rall TW, Nies AS, Taylor P, eds: Goodman & Gilman's The Pharmacological Basis of Therapeutics, 8th ed. New York, Macmillan, 1990, pp. 933–953.

45.4. Answer: A Ergonovine is used in obstetric practice because it stimulates uterine smooth muscle contraction. Ergonovine is also used during cardiac catheterization because of its ability to induce Prinzmetal angina.

Rall TW, Schleifer LS: Oxytocin, prostaglandins, ergot alkaloids and other tocolytic agents. In: Gilman AG, Rall TW, Nies AS, Taylor P, eds: Goodman & Gilman's The Pharmacological Basis of Therapeutics, 8th ed. New York, Macmillan, 1990, pp. 933–953.

45.5. Answer: C Propranolol is a β-adrenergic antagonist. Medications that are effective in reversing ergot-induced vasoconstriction are smooth muscle relaxants.

Carliner NH, Denune DP, Finch CS, Goldberg LI: Sodium nitroprusside treatment of ergotamine-induced peripheral ischemia. JAMA 1974;227:308–309.

Cobaugh DS: Prazosin treatment of ergotamine induced peripheral ischemia. JAMA 1980;244:1360.

Husum B, Metz P, Rasmussen JP, et al: Nitroglycerin infusion for ergotism. Lancet 1979;2:794–795.

O'Dell CW, Davis GB, Johnson AD, et al: Sodium nitroprusside in the treatment of ergotism. Radiology 1977;124:73–74.

Zimran A, Ofek B, Hershko C, et al: Treatment with captopril for peripheral ischemia induced by ergotamine. Br Med J 1984;288: 364.

45.6. Answer: B Peak ergotamine levels occur at approximately 2 hours after oral ingestion. Gastrointestinal decontamination will be most effective soon after the ingestion.

Orton DA, Richardson RJ: Ergotamine absorption and toxicity. Postgrad Med J 1982;58:6–11.

45.7. Answer: B Bradycardia is believed to be a reflex baroreceptor-mediated phenomenon associated with vasoconstriction, but a reduction in sympathetic tone, direct myocardial depression, and increased vagal activity may also be factors.

Peroutka SJ: Drugs effective in therapy of migrane. In: Hardman JG, Limbard LE, Molinoff PB, et al, eds: Goodman & Gilman's

The Pharmacological Basis of Therapeutics, 9th ed. New York, McGraw-Hill, 1996, pp. 491–496.

45.8. Answer: E   Methysergide can cause retroperitoneal fibrosis as well as pleuropericardial, endocardial, and endovascular fibrosis.

Bucci JA, Manoharan A: Methysergide-induced retroperitoneal fibrosis: Successful outcome and two new laboratory features. Mayo Clin Proc 1997;72:1148–1150.

45.9. Answer: B   The disease Holy Fire or St. Anthony's Fire caused ischemia and burning painful limbs. When people went to the shrine of St. Anthony, their symptoms would disappear because they were no longer eating contaminated grains.

Rall TW, Schleifer LS: Oxytocin, prostaglandins, ergot alkaloids and other tocolytic agents. In: Gilman AG, Rall TW, Nies AS, Taylor P, eds: Goodman & Gilman's The Pharmacological Basis of Therapeutics, 8th ed. New York, Macmillan, 1990, pp. 933–953.

45.10. Answer: C   Six milligrams is the maximum daily dose of ergotamine, and 10 mg the maximum weekly dose. Ergotism becomes more likely if this dose is exceeded.

Rall TW, Schleifer LS: Oxytocin, prostaglandins, ergot alkaloids and other tocolytic agents. In: Gilman AG, Rall TW, Nies AS, Taylor P, eds: Goodman & Gilman's The Pharmacological Basis of Therapeutics, 8th ed. New York, Macmillan, 1990, pp. 933–953.

CHAPTER 46

ANTIBIOTICS

46.1. Answer: A   The general population risk of anaphylaxis is 0.02%. The risk of anaphylaxis in patients with a previously documented penicillin-induced anaphylactic reaction is increased to 0.04%.

Anne S, Reisman RE: Risk of administering cephalosporin antibiotics to patients with history of penicillin allergy. Ann Allergy Asthma Immunol 1995;74:167–170.

46.2. Answer: D   Risk factors for seizures after imipenem use include central nervous system disease, prior seizure disorders, and abnormal renal function.

Pestotnik SL, Classen DC, Evans RS, et al: Prospective surveillance of imipenem/cilastatin use and associated seizures using a hospital information system. Ann Pharmacother 1993;27:497–501.

46.3. Answer: D   Other risk factors not mentioned include increased age, renal dysfunction, female gender, liver dysfunction, long duration of therapy, frequent doses, presence of other nephrotoxic drugs, and the presence of shock.

Appel GB: Aminoglycoside nephrotoxicity. Am J Med 1990;88 (Suppl 3C):16S–20S.

Moore RD, Smith CR, Lipsky JJ, et al: Risk factors for nephrotoxicity in patients treated with aminoglycosides. Ann Intern Med 1984;100:352–357.

46.4. Answer: D   The toxic symptoms caused after chloramphenicol overdose consist of nausea and vomiting followed in severe cases by metabolic acidosis and cardiovascular collapse.

Fripp RR, Carter MC, Werner JC: Cardiac function and acute chloramphenicol toxicity. J Pediatr 1983;103:487–490.

46.5. Answer: B   Risk factors include serum chloramphenicol concentrations >50 mg/mL resulting from high doses of chloramphenicol. Infants are predisposed to the "gray baby syndrome" because of an inability to conjugate chloramphenicol or to excrete unconjugated chloramphenicol in the urine.

Phelps SJ, Tsiu W, Barrett FF, et al: Chloramphenicol-induced cardiovascular collapse in an anephric patient. Pediatr Infect Dis J 1987;6:285–288.

46.6. Answer: D   Individual cases of acute ciprofloxacin overdose include gastrointestinal upset, renal failure, acute psychosis, and seizures.

Mulhall JP, Bergmann LS: Ciprofloxacin-induced acute psychosis. Urology 1995;46:102–103.

Rippelmeyer DJ, Synhavsky A: Ciprofloxacin and allergic interstitial nephritis [letter]. Ann Intern Med 1988;109:170.

Slavich IL, Gleffe RF, Haas EJ: Grand mal epileptic seizures during ciprofloxacin therapy. JAMA 1989;261:558–559.

46.7. Answer: C   Many clinically significant drug interactions described with erythromycin are attributed to its ability to inhibit, through inactivation, CYP3A4.

Danan G, Descatoire V, Pessayre D: Self-induction of erythromycin by its own transformation into a metabolite forming an inactive complex with reduced cytochrome P450. J Pharmacol Exp Ther 1989;250:746–751.

46.8. Answer: C   Tachyphylaxis to the "red man syndrome" develops in patients given multiple doses.

Wallace MR, Mascola JR, Oldfield EC 3d: Red man syndrome: Incidence, etiology and prophylaxis. J Infect Dis 1991;164:1180–1185.

46.9. Answer: B   Cimetidine is a cytochrome P450 inhibitor but does not interact directly with ketoconazole.

Hansten PD, Horn JR, Koda-Kimble MA, Young LY: A clinical perspective and analysis of current developments. In: Drug Interactions and Updates Quarterly. Vancouver, WA, Drug Interactions Newsletter, 1993, p. 905.

46.10. Answer: D   The main toxic effects attributed to the aminoglycosides consist of renal toxicity, ototoxicity, and neuromuscular toxicity. There are no human or animal trials that attribute proseizure activity to the aminoglycosides.

Grondahl TO, Langmoen IA: Epileptogenic effect of antibiotic drugs. J Neurosurg 1993;78:938–943.

Gutnick MJ, Van Duijn H, Citri N: Relative convulsant potencies of structural analogs of penicillin. Brain Res 1976;114:139–143.

CHAPTER 47

ANTINEOPLASTIC AGENTS

47.1. Answer: D The cause of nephrotoxicity is precipitation of methotrexate (MTX) and its 7-hydroxy metabolite in the renal tubular cells. Precipitates of MTX were identified in the kidney tissue of patients who died from MTX-induced renal toxicity. Salt- and water-depleted patients are most at risk for renal toxicity during high-dose therapy.

Abelson HI, Fosburg MT, Beardsley P, et al: Methotrexate induced renal impairment: Clinical studies and rescue from systemic toxicity with high dose leucovorin and thymidine. J Clin Oncol 1983;1:208–216.

Pitman SW, Parker LM, Tattersall MHN, et al: Clinical trial of high dose methotrexate with citrovorum factor—toxicological and therapeutic observations. Cancer Chemother Rep 1975;6:43–49.

47.2. Answer: A Methotrexate inhibits DNA synthesis at concentrations above 0.01 μM. The bone marrow and gastrointestinal mucosa are most susceptible to toxicity because they contain cells of high mitotic activity.

Stoller RG, Hande KR, Jacobs SA, et al: Use of plasma pharmacokinetics to predict and prevent methotrexate toxicity. N Engl J Med 1977;297:630–633.

47.3. Answer: A The antineoplastic agents with vesicant properties result in significant local tissue destruction because they can cause necrosis on contact. These agents include doxorubicin, daunorubicin, dactinomycin, epirubicin, idarubicin, mechlorethamine, mitomycin, mithramycin, and the vinca alkaloids. Doxorubicin extravasation is associated with tissue necrosis in 25% of cases. Although the other agents may cause tissue injury, they are less likely than the vesicants to do so.

San Angel F: Current controversies in chemotherapy administration. J Intraven Nurse 1995;18:16–22.

47.4. Answer: E Repeat-dose activated charcoal, in patients receiving MTX IV therapy, demonstrated a significant reduction in the area under the curve for MTX from 18 hours after dosing until the serum MTX level was lower than 0.01 μM. There are no known benefits of repetitive dosing of activated charcoal for the other agents.

Gadgil SD, Damle SR, Advani SH, et al: Effect of activated charcoal on the pharmacokinetics of high dose methotrexate. Cancer Treat Rep 1982;66:1169–1171.

47.5. Answer: C Vincristine stimulation of the hypothalamus may be responsible for the fever and SIADH noted in overdosed patients. Serum electrolytes should be monitored for 10 days following a course of therapy.

Rosenthal S, Kaufamn S: Vincristine neuropathy. Ann Intern Med 1974;81:733–737.

47.6. Answer: E The incidence of congestive cardiomyopathy associated with doxorubicin therapy is between 1 and 10% when the cumulative dose is less than 450 mg/m^2 and becomes greater than 20% when more than 550 mg/m^2 is administered.

von Hoff DD, Layard MY, Basa P, et al: Risk factors for doxorubicin induced congestive heart failure. Ann Intern Med 1979;91:710–717.

47.7. Answer: B Retinal and ototoxicity have been reported after high-dose cisplatin. The other agents are not associated with visual or auditory manifestations.

Chiuten D, Vogl SE, Kaplan BH, et al: Is there a cumulative or delayed toxicity from *cis*-diaminedichloroplatinum. Proc Am Assoc Cancer Res 1981;22:163–164.

Wilding G, Caruso R, Lawrence IS, et al: Retinal toxicity after high dose cisplatin therapy. J Clin Oncol 1985;3:1683–1689.

47.8. Answer: C CSF drainage, exchange, and perfusion are physical methods that have been shown to increase methotrexate (MTX) removal from the CSF. Carboxypeptidase-class enzymes administered IT will degrade MTX by cleaving MTX's terminal glutamate group. Leucovorin is a source of reduced folates that bypasses MTX inhibition of dihydrofolate reductase, which permits continued DNA/RNA synthesis. Leucovorin does not affect CSF MTX levels, and leucovorin, itself, may cause seizures and death when administered intrathecally.

Jardine LF, Ingram LC, Bleyer WA: Intrathecal leucovorin after intrathecal methotrexate overdose. J Pediatr Hematol Oncol 1996;18:302–304.

Marcaigh AS, Johnson MC, Smithson WA, et al: Successful treatment of intrathecal methotrexate overdose by using ventriculolumbar perfusion and intrathecal instillation of carboxypeptidase G2. Mayo Clin Proc 1996;71:161–165.

47.9. Answer: D Factors determining the outcome of an extravasational injury include the site of involvement and the chemical properties and concentration of the agent. Individuals inexperienced in the administration of antineoplastic agents can affect outcome by not taking appropriate actions before or after extravasation.

Ignoffo RJ, Friedman MA: Therapy of local toxicities caused by extravasation of cancer chemotherapeutic drugs. Cancer Treat Rev 1980;7:17–27.

47.10. Answer: B Procarbazine has disulfiram-like and monoamine oxidase inhibitory activity. Avoidance of ethanol and certain drugs and foods with high tyramine content is recommended.

Livingston MG, Livingston HM: Monoamine oxidase inhibitors. Drug Safety 1996;14:219–227.

CHAPTER 48

CARDIAC GLYCOSIDES

48.1. Answer: D   Digoxin decreases cardiac conduction velocity. Digoxin also decreases refractoriness and atrioventricular conduction. Digoxin increases automaticity by increasing myocardial excitability.

48.2. Answer: E   Patients with renal failure can be treated with digoxin-specific Fab without the need of extracorporeal removal of the complex. Free digoxin levels may gradually increase several days after administration if the complex is not renally cleared. If toxic symptoms reappear, the patient should be treated with additional digoxin Fab.

Warren SE, Fanestil DD: Digoxin overdose: Limitations of hemoperfusion–hemodialysis treatment. JAMA 1979;242:2100–2101.

48.3. Answer: E   Patients who had serum potassium levels greater than 5.5 mEq/L had a high probability of having a fatal outcome before the development of digoxin Fab.

Bismuth C, Gaultier M, Conso F, Efthymiou ML: Hyperkalemia in acute digitalis poisoning: Prognostic significance and therapeutic implications. Clin Toxicol 1973;6:153–162.

48.4. Answer: B   Bradycardia is usually one of the earliest symptoms of both acute and chronic digoxin toxicity. The AV block, hypotension, and most dysrhythmias appear later.

48.5. Answer: C   The primary cause of hyperkalemia in patients who have acute digoxin toxicity appears to be the inhibition of Na^+-K^+-ATPase, which inhibits the uptake of potassium into muscle.

Smith TW, Antman EM, Friedman PL, et al: Digitalis glycosides: Mechanisms and manifestations of toxicity. Prog Cardiovasc Dis 1984;27:21–41.

Woolf AD, Wenger T, Smith TW, Lovejoy FH: The use of digoxin-specific Fab fragments for severe digitalis intoxication in children. N Engl J Med 1992;326:1739–1744.

48.6. Answer: C   Digoxin is cleared primarily by the kidney and is dependent on intact renal function for drug elimination.

48.7. Answer: B   Lily of the valley *(Convallaria majalis)* contains a cardiac glycoside that, following a substantial exposure, will cause digoxinlike cardiac toxicity.

Hollman A: Plants and cardiac glycosides. Br Heart J 1985;54: 258–261.

48.8. Answer: B   This patient should receive just two vials of digoxin-specific Fab.

$$3 \, ng \, / \, mL \times 60 \, kg \, / \, 100 = 1.8 \, vials$$

Sinclair AJ, Hewick DS, Johnson PC, et al: Kinetics of digoxin and anti-digoxin antibody fragments during treatment of digoxin toxicity. Br J Clin Pharmacol 1989;28:352–356.

48.9. Answer: D   Lidocaine can be administered to treat ventricular dysrhythmias in patients who have digoxin toxicity. Intravenous calcium salts and cardioversion have been reported to cause asystole with digoxin toxicity. Quinidine and verapamil will inhibit drug elimination, and verapamil may worsen AV nodal conduction.

48.10. Answer: A   One vial (38 mg) will neutralize 0.5 mg of digoxin. If the quantity of digoxin acutely ingested is known, the amount of Digibind can be easily calculated using the assumption that 80% is available following ingestion.

Smith TW, Haber E, Yeatman L, Butler VP: Reversal of advanced digoxin intoxication with Fab fragments of digoxin-specific antibodies. N Engl J Med 1976;294:797–800.

CHAPTER 49

β-ADRENERGIC ANTAGONISTS

49.1. Answer: B   Propranolol is responsible for more deaths than any other β-adrenergic antagonist. This is both because it is more often ingested than the other agents and because of several properties that increase its toxicity. Propranolol is very lipid soluble, so it is rapidly absorbed and easily crosses the blood–brain barrier. Propranolol also has the most membrane-stabilizing effect of any of the β-adrenergic antagonists. This may result in seizures or ventricular dysrhythmias and is the most important explanation for propranolol's increased toxicity. Propranolol does not block potassium channels and has no intrinsic sympathomimetic activity and is not a peripheral vasodilator.

49.2. Answer: C   In addition to being a β-adrenergic antagonist, sotalol blocks delayed rectifier potassium channels. Sotalol overdoses are characterized by QT prolongation and often complicated by ventricular dysrhythmias, especially torsades de pointes.

49.3. Answer: D   The feature most predictive of fatality is a cardioactive coingestant. In pure β-adrenergic antagonist overdose, death is most likely in patients who ingested an agent with membrane-stabilizing activity such as propranolol.

49.4. Answer: C   Phosphodiesterase inhibitors increase cyclic AMP by preventing its breakdown. They have been shown beneficial in animal models of β-adrenergic antagonist overdose, although they do not have an additional benefit over glucagon. Phosphodiesterase inhibitors improve cardiac output but cause peripheral vasodilation that may prove harmful. They are difficult to titrate because of relatively long half-lives. For these reasons the phosphodiesterase inhibitors are third-line agents in β-adrenergic antagonist toxicity and should be used only in conjunction with pulmonary artery monitoring.

49.5. Answer: E   Patients who remain profoundly hypotensive and bradycardic will likely die of multiple organ failure. When medical treatment appears to be failing, it is important to consider invasive measures such as intraaortic balloon pump or extracorporeal circulation. These interventions will maintain perfusion while the toxin is being metabolized and may prove life saving. Hemodialysis and hemoperfusion will be almost impossible to perform in a profoundly hypotensive patient and would not be expected to be beneficial for agents such as propranolol that have large volumes of distribution. Calcium, atropine, and ventricular pacing could all be attempted, but in a patient who has failed therapy with glucagon and catecholamines, these interventions are almost certain to fail.

49.6. Answer: A Hypertonic sodium bicarbonate is probably of benefit for ventricular dysrhythmias caused by agents such as propranolol with a membrane-stabilizing effect. This treatment is unlikely to be of benefit for agents such as sotalol that prolong the QTc interval and cause torsades de pointes. Sotalol-induced dysrhythmias may respond to correction of hypokalemia or hypomagnesemia. Cardioversion may be indicated if the patient is unstable. Overdrive pacing and lidocaine have both been reported to be effective.

49.7. Answer: E Glucagon is the treatment of choice for most patients with β-adrenergic antagonist toxicity. Glucagon is relatively safe but may cause vomiting or hypertension. Catecholamine infusions are indicated in patients with severe β-adrenergic antagonist toxicity who have failed treatment with glucagon. It is likely that standard doses of catecholamines will not be effective, and clinicians must be prepared to use very high doses. Agents with strong α-adrenergic agonist effects such as epinephrine and norepinephrine may cause cardiac failure or severe hypertension from an unopposed α effect. Isoproterenol avoids this pitfall but may exacerbate hypotension through its vasodilating β2-adrenergic agonist effect. When catecholamine infusions are started, the patient must be monitored closely, and the clinician should be prepared to stop the infusion it there is evidence of deterioration. Whenever possible invasive hemodynamic or echocardiographic monitoring should be used. Phosphodiesterase inhibitors such as amrinone may be used when the preceding measures fail. These agents cause peripheral vasodilation and may cause hypotension.

49.8. Answer: B Patients who develop toxicity following regular-release β-adrenergic antagonist ingestion will do so within 6 hours. Patients who ingest sotalol often have delayed toxicity. These patients may be released from medical attention if their electrocardiogram remains normal after 12 hours of observation. Patients who have ingested a sustained-release product should be monitored for 24 hours. We also recommend longer periods of observation for patients who have coingested toxins such as opiates or anticholinergics that delay gastric emptying.

49.9. Answer: C Heroin and tricyclic antidepressants (such as amitriptyline) are excluded by the preserved mental status. A patient who took digoxin and had a sinus rhythm at 60/min would not be expected to be hypotensive. Propranolol toxicity would typically result in greater suppression of heart rate before the blood pressure dropped to 60 mm Hg. Furthermore, a patient this hypotensive after taking propranolol would typically be obtunded. Finally, of the agents listed above, only diltiazem would be expected to increase the glucose to this extent.

49.10. Answer: A All agents could cause seizures in the setting of cardiovascular collapse (diltiazem, digoxin) or respiratory arrest (heroin), but only amitriptyline and propranolol regularly cause seizures. Propranolol and amitriptyline are also the only agents with membrane-stabilizing effect to explain the prolonged QRS duration. Amitriptyline usually causes tachycardia in overdose, leaving propranolol as the most likely culprit. The slightly depressed glucose and slightly elevated potassium are also typical of propranolol overdose.

CHAPTER 50

CALCIUM CHANNEL BLOCKERS

50.1. Answer: A Calcium channel blockers antagonize the voltage-sensitive L-type calcium channels in both the myocardium and vascular smooth muscle. These channels are opened on cellular depolarization and allow influx of calcium to initiate muscular contraction.

Katz AM: Calcium channel diversity in the cardiovascular system. J Am Coll Cardiol 1996;28:522–529.

50.2. Answer: A When calcium enters the myocardial cell and is released from the sarcoplasmic reticulum, it binds troponin C, which causes a conformational change that displaces troponin and tropomyosin from the actin. This allows actin and myosin to bind, resulting in a contraction. Myosin light chain kinase is found only in smooth muscle cells and is activated by a calcium/calmodulin complex. There myosin light chain kinase activates myosin, allowing it to bind to actin, and a contraction occurs.

Ferrier GR, Howlett SE: Cardiac excitation–contraction coupling: Role of membrane potential in regulation of contraction. Am J Physiol Heart Circ Physiol 2001;280:H1928–1944.

50.3. Answer: C Verapamil has the greatest affinity for cardiac tissue, followed by diltiazem and bepridil. Nifedipine and the other dihydropyridines bind poorly to the myocardium. Because of this, in therapeutic dosing and often in overdose, dihydropyridines may cause reflex tachycardia instead of bradycardia as occurs following overdose with the other classes of calcium channel blockers.

Taira N: Differences in cardiovascular profile among calcium antagonists. Am J Cardiol 1987;59:24B–29B.

50.4. Answer: E Hypotension is the most common physiologic manifestation of calcium channel blocker toxicity. Alterations in conduction, including first-degree heart block, second-degree heart block, and junctional as well as ventricular escape rhythms, may be seen. Insulin release from the β islet cells is dependent on calcium influx via calcium channels; in CCB overdose, selectivity is lost, and this channel is antagonized. This impairs normal calcium influx, insulin release is reduced, and hyperglycemia ensues. Acute lung injury has been associated with calcium channel blocker poisoning. Although the mechanism is unknown, it may involve precapillary vasodilation, increased capillary pressures and transudates, and ultimately increased interstitial edema. That seizures are rare may reflect a neuroprotective effect of calcium channel blockers.

Schoffstall JM, Spivey WH, Gambone LM, Shaw RP, Sit SP: Effects of calcium channel blocker overdose-induced toxicity in the conscious dog. Ann Emerg Med 1991;20:1104–1108.

Devis G, Somers G, Van Obberghen E, Malaisse WJ: Calcium antagonists and islet function. I. Inhibition of insulin release by verapamil. Diabetes 1975;24:547–551.

50.5. Answer: B The rapidity with which aggressive whole-bowel irrigation clears the contents of the gastrointestinal tract likely makes it the most effective method of decontamination following overdose with sustained-release preparations. Syrup of ipecac is contraindicated because of the possibility of rapid clinical deterioration. Orogastric lavage should be strongly considered in all patients with potentially lethal ingestions, particularly if the patient presents early. However, given the large size of most sustained-release products, the benefit of orogastric lavage diminishes. Multiple doses of activated charcoal should be administered in all patients with ingestions of sustained-release products so that as the drug is released along the tablet's course through the gastrointestinal tract, activated charcoal is available to adsorb it and prevent systemic absorption.

Roberts D, Honcharik N, Sitar DS, Tenenbein M: Diltiazem overdose: Pharmacokinetics of diltiazem and its metabolites and effect of multiple dose charcoal therapy. J Toxicol Clin Toxicol 1991; 29:45–52.

50.6. Answer: D Amrinone is a potent phosphodiesterase III inhibitor that increases cyclic AMP levels by reducing its metabolism (see Fig. 50–4). Calcium acts by increasing the transcellular concentration gradient and improving calcium influx. Glucagon increases cyclic AMP levels by stimulating adenylate cyclase without activating the β-adrenergic receptor. 4-Aminopyridine inhibits the delayed potassium rectifying current, which prolongs nerve terminal depolarization, increases calcium influx, and results in more catecholamine release.

50.7. Answer: D High-dose insulin and euglycemic therapy have become significant advances. Indirect evidence suggests resultant increased calcium entry and increased myocardial utilization of carbohydrates.

Yuan TH, Kerns WP, Tomaszewski CA, et al: Insulin–glucose as adjunctive therapy for severe calcium channel antagonist poisoning. J Toxicol Clin Toxicol 1999;37:463–474.

50.8. Answer: B If myocardial depression is so severe that no pharmacologic agent is able to improve the patient's hemodynamic status, then invasive supportive measures are indicated. Intracardiac pacing, intraaortic balloon counterpulsation, and cardiopulmonary bypass have all been used successfully. Because poisoned patients generally require 12 to 48 hours of assistance while the calcium channel blocker is metabolized and eliminated, many of these invasive therapies are practical. Pacemakers do not capture very well because of the insensitivity of the poisoned myocardium, but if they do, they can increase tissue perfusion by raising the heart rate while not raising the contractility of the heart. Although there are no reports of extracorporeal membrane oxygenation (ECMO) use in this setting, it may be ideal because a patient can be supported for several days if needed.

Hendren WC, Schreiber RS, Garretson LK: Extracorporeal bypass for the treatment of verapamil poisoning. Ann Emerg Med 1989; 18:984–987.

50.9. Answer: B Neither the vital signs nor an electrocardiogram is particularly efficient at differentiating poisoning by the two agents. Some drugs, such as propranolol, prolong the duration of the QRS complex, but this action is not generalized among the drug class. Although the serum glucose is typically normal or high following calcium channel blocker poisoning, it may be high, low, or normal following β-adrenergic antagonist overdose. Perhaps because of a neuroprotective effect of many calcium channel blockers, patients often maintain a normal level of consciousness despite dramatic alterations in their vital signs.

50.10. Answer: B Although it is unclear what type of product formulation the child ingested, one must adopt the worst-case scenario and assume that these pills were a sustained-release formulation. In patients exposed to sustained-release calcium channel blockers, signs and symptoms of poisoning may be delayed 8 to 12 hours and may occur rapidly. Therefore, all children exposed to sustained-release products should be admitted to an intensive care setting and receive aggressive gastrointestinal decontamination including multiple doses of activated charcoal and whole-bowel irrigation.

Spiller HA, Meyers A, Ziemba T, Riley M: Delayed onset of cardiac arrhythmias from sustained-release verapamil. Ann Emerg Med 1991;20:201–203.

CHAPTER 51

MISCELLANEOUS ANTIHYPERTENSIVES

51.1. Answer: C Angiotensin-converting enzyme, in addition to metabolizing angiotensin I to angiotensin II, also metabolizes bradykinin. When inhibited, this increase in bradykinin results in vasodilation, increased interstitial fluid, and possibly angioedema or a persistent cough.

Israili ZH, Hall WD: Cough and angioneurotic edema associated with angiotensin-converting enzyme inhibitor therapy. Ann Intern Med 1992;117:234–242.

51.2. Answer: B Although naloxone is well known to be an effective "antidote" for clonidine poisoning, there is some evidence that it may also be effective in reversing the hypotensive effects of an ACE inhibitor overdose.

Millar JA, Sturani A, Rubin PC, Reid JL: Attenuation of the antihypertensive effect of captopril by the opioid receptor antagonist naloxone. Clin Exp Pharmacol Physiol 1983;10:253–259.

Varon J, Duncan SR: Naloxone reversal of hypotension due to captopril overdose. Ann Emerg Med 1991;20:1125–1127.

51.3. Answer: B Clonidine, as well as guanabenz, guanfacine, and methyldopa, exert their antihypertensive effect by acting as central α_2 agonists. This central α_2 agonism enhances the activity of inhibitory neurons in the vasoregulatory regions of the CNS, resulting in decreased sympathetic outflow from the brain. This sympathetic attenuation reduces heart rate, vascular tone, and ultimately blood pressure.

51.4. Answer: E Classic physical finding in a patient who is clonidine poisoned include CNS depression, bradycardia, hypotension, hypothermia, and miosis. Paradoxically, hypertension may be noted early in overdose, although it is caused by nonspecific peripheral α-adrenergic agonism and norepinephrine release. Typically this hypertension is limited, as the central sympatholytic effects become overwhelming and hypotension ensues. Dysrhythmias are uncommon, other than sinus bradycardia.

Anderson FJ, Hart GR, Crumpler CP, Lerman MJ: Clonidine overdose: Report of six cases and review of the literature. Ann Emerg Med 1981;10:107–112.

51.5. Answer: D Diazoxide is the only one of these agents that exerts its hypotensive effect by causing direct vasodilation. The other agents all indirectly produce hypotension by decreasing the effects of the sympathetic nervous system. Guanabenz is a centrally acting α₂ agonist, trimethaphan is a ganglionic blocker, guanethidine is a peripheral adrenergic neuron blocker, and terazosin is a peripherally-acting α₁ antagonist (see Table 51–1).

51.6. Answer: C Clonidine, an imidazoline, is itself an active compound that is eliminated primarily unchanged in the urine. Overdose produces a syndrome similar to opioid intoxication that is often successfully treated with naloxone. Yohimbine, an α₂ antagonist and pharmacologic converse of clonidine, is an attractive therapy although its use remains unstudied. Withdrawal of chronic therapy produces rebound hypertension.

51.7. Answer: B Although captopril, which contains a sulfhydryl moiety and is an active molecule, and fosinopril, which contains a phosphinate moiety and is a prodrug, are structurally different, there is no evidence that angioedema induced by ACE inhibitors is an allergic response. Rather, angioedema is caused by the mechanism of action of the class of drugs. Therefore, if a patient develops angioedema from one ACE inhibitor, the individual must be instructed that a similar event may occur if any other ACE inhibitor is used.

Orfan N, Patterson R, Dykewicz MS: Severe angioedema related to ACE inhibitor in patients with a history of idiopathic angioedema. JAMA 1990;264:1287–1290.

51.8. Answer: C Losartan antagonized the binding of angiotensin II to its receptors, resulting in decreased vasoconstriction and reduced sodium and water retention. Although similar to ACE inhibitors in that it reduces the effects of angiotensin II, losartan does not affect bradykinin metabolism, and angioedema and chronic cough would not be expected.

Triggle DJ: Angiotensin II receptor antagonism: Losartan—sites and mechanism of action. Clin Therapeutics 1995;17:1005–1030.

51.9. Answer: A Methyldopa treatment produces a 10% incidence of positive direct Coombs test, and hemolytic anemia can occur. Reserpine is a peripheral adrenergic neuron blocker that depletes catecholamines from nerve end terminals. Unfortunately, it can cross the blood–brain barrier, resulting in central cate-

cholamine depletion, and extrapyramidal symptoms, hallucinations, and particularly depression may occur. Hydralazine, in addition to procainamide, may cause an idiopathic lupuslike syndrome. Sodium nitroprusside is metabolized in erythrocytes to release both the vasodilator nitric oxide and cyanide. Diazoxide inhibits insulin release from the pancreatic islet cells and typically results in an elevated glucose.

51.10. Answer: E Although approximately one-third of cases of ACE inhibitor–associated angioedema occur in the first day, and one-third occur in the first few weeks of therapy, it is important to remember that this adverse event can occur at any time during therapy.

Slater EE, Merril DD, Guess HA, et al: Clinical profile of angioedema associated with angiotensin converting enzyme inhibition. JAMA 1988;260:967–970.

CHAPTER **52**

ANTIDYSRHYTHMIC AGENTS

52.1. Answer: D Sodium bicarbonate improves intraventricular conduction. It is believed that alkalinization reduces the binding of these antidysrhythmics to the fast sodium channels in the Purkinje fibers. The sodium alone is capable of improving conduction by increasing the extracellular concentration of the ion.

Kim SY, Benowitz, NL: Poisoning due to class IA antiarrhythmic drugs, quinidine, procainamide and disopyramide. Drug Safety 1990;5:393–420.

Salerno DM, Murakami MA, Johnston AA: Reversal of flecainide induced ventricular arrhythmia by hypertonic sodium bicarbonate in dogs. Am J Emerg Med 1995;13:285–293.

52.2. Answer: A In the animal model, severe lidocaine toxicity, including cardiac arrest after iatrogenic lidocaine overdose, was best treated with continued cardiopulmonary resuscitation with or without mechanical chest compression, cardiopulmonary bypass, or intraaortic balloon assist.

Freedman MD, Gal J, Freed CR: Extracorporeal pump assistance: novel treatment of acute lidocaine poisoning. Eur J Clin Pharmacol 1982;22:129–135.

52.3. Answer: B Lidocaine is a synthetic derivative of cocaine.

Amitai Y: Lidocaine. Clin Toxicol Rev 1985;8:1–2.

52.4. Answer: A Though CHF may alter the volume of distribution and protein binding of lidocaine, reduced hepatic perfusion is most significant. Lidocaine is a high-extraction-ratio drug, meaning its metabolism and clearance are highly dependent on hepatic blood flow. CHF may significantly reduce hepatic blood flow and drug clearance.

Prescott LF, Adjepon-Yamoah KK, Talbot RG: Impaired lidocaine metabolism in patients with myocardial infarction and cardiac failure. Br Med J 1976;1:939–941.

52.5. Answer: C NAPA and procainamide can be removed by hemodialysis, charcoal hemoperfusion, hemofiltration, and arteriovenous hemodiafiltration.

Atkinson AJ, Krumlovsky FA, Huang CM, et al: Hemodialysis for severe procainamide toxicity: Clinical and pharmacokinetic observations. Clin Pharmacol Ther 1976;20:585–592.

52.6. Answer: C Though many of the ECG manifestations of quinidine toxicity may mimic hyperkalemia, hyperkalemia is not typically described in these patients.

Shub G, Gan GT: Management of acute quinidine intoxication. Chest 1978;73:173–178.

52.7. Answer: B Urinary alkalinization with sodium bicarbonate decreases the clearance of tocainide.

Kreger RW, Hammil SC: New antiarrhythmic drugs: Tocainide, mexiletine, flecainide, encainide, amiodarone. Mayo Clin Proc 1987;62:1033–1050.

52.8. Answer: E Both tocainide and lidocaine are well absorbed following oral administration, and their clinical indications are identical. Tocainide differs from lidocaine in that it does not undergo extensive first-pass metabolism.

Kreger RW, Hammil SC: New antiarrhythmic drugs: Tocainide, mexiletine, flecainide, encainide, amiodarone. Mayo Clin Proc 1987;62:1033–1050.

52.9. Answer: C The marked QRS and PR interval changes associated with minimal QTc prolongation are noted with flecainide toxicity, in contrast to the more severe cardiotoxic ECG findings noted with the other antidysrhythmics, such as procainamide, tocainide, or quinidine.

Chung PKC, Tuso P: The electrocardiographic changes in a case of flecainide overdose. Conn Med 1990;54:183–185.

52.10. Answer: C Encainide is an analogue of lysergic acid with 5 to 10 times the antidysrhythmic potency of procainamide. In 1991 it was withdrawn from the market because of its prodysrhythmic effects and risk of sudden cardiac death.

Fish FA, Gillette PC, Benson DW Jr: Proarrhythmia, cardiac arrest and death in young patients receiving encainide and flecainide. J Am Coll Cardiol 1991;18:356–365.

Mortenson M, Bolon C, Kelley M, et al: Encainide overdose in an infant. Ann Emerg Med 1992;21:998–1001.

CHAPTER 53

INHALATIONAL ANESTHETICS

53.1. Answer: C Irreversible brain damage has been described with nitrous oxide abuse. However, this does not result from direct toxic effects but rather is secondary to asphyxia. Nitrous oxide interferes with the function of vitamin B_{12} and thereby can produce both megaloblastic anemia and subacute combined degeneration of the spinal cord. Women chronically exposed to trace levels of nitrous oxide have a two- to threefold increase in spontaneous abortion rates and have reduced fertility.

Nunn J: Clinical aspects of the interaction between nitrous oxide and vitamin B_{12}. Br J Anesth 1987;59:3–13.

53.2. Answer: B When ingested, the initial manifestations are gastrointestinal, but this is followed by CNS and cardiovascular effects as the drug is absorbed. Death has occurred following topical application of halothane to a "cold sore." Halothane has a distinct sweet/fruity odor. CNS depression rather than excitation (seizures) usually occurs.

Spencer J, Raasch F, Trefny F: Halothane abuse in hospital personnel. JAMA 1976;235:1034–1035.

53.3. Answer. A Life-threatening halothane hepatitis is felt to be immunologically mediated such that multiple exposures increase the risk of occurrence. Female gender and Hispanic ancestry are additional risk factors of unclear pathogenesis. Additionally, obesity probably increases risk through prolonging exposure from fat storage.

Touloukian J, Kaplowitz N: Halothane-induced hepatic disease. Semin Liver Dis 1981;1:134–142.

Vergani D, Tsantoulas D, Eddleston A, et al: Sensitization to halothane-altered liver components in severe hepatic necrosis after halothane anesthesia. Lancet 1978;2:801–803.

53.4. Answer: C Only methoxyflurane was commonly associated with diabetes insipidus. The toxicity appears to be associated with the total dose of anesthetic and the free fluoride concentration. Rare cases have been reported with enflurane as well.

Cousins M, Mazze R: Methoxyflurane nephrotoxicity: A study of dose-response in man. JAMA 1973;225:1611–1616.

Crandell W, Pappas S, MacDonald A: Nephrotoxicity associated with methoxyflurane anesthesia. Anesthesiology 1966;27:591–607.

53.5. Answer: D Lime is used in the closed circuit as an adsorbent for CO_2. When the lime becomes dry because of high flow rates of carrier gas, life-threatening levels of CO can be produced. These conditions are most likely to be generated when the circuit is not connected to patients for long periods of time, such as may occur after a weekend. Because of its lower concentration of potassium hydroxide, soda lime has a lower risk of producing CO.

Frink EJ, Nogami WM, Morgan SE, Salmon RC: High carboxyhemoglobin concentrations occur in swine during desflurane anesthesia in the presence of partially dried carbon dioxide absorbents, and literature review. Am J Dis Child 1981;135:628–630.

CHAPTER 54

NEUROMUSCULAR BLOCKING AGENTS

54.1. Answer: B Rapacuronium has an active metabolite, 3-OH-rapacuronium, which has 2.5 times the neuromuscular blocking potency of the parent drug and is eliminated by the kidney. Rapacuronium is contraindicated for drug infusion over 1 hour, especially in patients with renal failure, as this may lead to prolonged weakness. Critical illness polyneuropathy is associated with critical illness and is not an issue here. Acute necrotizing myopathy is a disease associated with long-term use of a neuromuscular blocker, typically a minimum of 2 days. Homozygous atypical cholinesterase may prolong the duration of succinylcholine up to about 4 hours, but this is rare (1:2500). Hepatic insufficiency slightly slows rapacuronium metabolism and is associated with reduced plasma cholinesterase levels. Usually liver failure has to be severe before the clinical duration of succinylcholine is significantly prolonged.

54.2. Answer: C   Multiple organ failure and sepsis are clearly associated with critical illness polyneuropathy, acute motor polyneuropathy, and acute myopathy of intensive care. Multiple organ failure may also slow hepatic, renal, and cholinesterase-mediated degradation of neuromuscular blockers. CIP is not associated with the use of nondepolarizing neuromuscular blockers, and recovery can be slow but generally does improve over time. Steroid myopathy is associated with corticosteroid use and does not require coexisting multiple organ failure or sepsis, although they may coexist.

54.3. Answer: A   Succinylcholine is contraindicated in routine pediatric cases but is appropriate for emergency use, especially with a potentially difficult airway. The drug is degraded in the plasma by plasma cholinesterase, and there is minimal elimination by the kidney. Sensitivity to hyperkalemia develops in the first few days, and it is safe to use in the first 24 hours after acute spinal cord injury. Neuromuscular blocking drugs do not cross the BBB. Succinic acid is an intermediate of the tricarboxylic acid cycle, and toxicity is not described with use of succinylcholine.

54.4. Answer: D   Chronic phenytoin or carbamazepine therapy accelerates hepatic drug metabolism, including the clearance of pancuronium and most other nondepolarizing neuromuscular blockers. Because of their organ-independent elimination, the clinical effect of atracurium and mivacurium is unaffected by hepatic enzyme induction. Pancuronium has an atropinelike affect and inhibits parasympathetic transmission at the cardiac muscarinic receptor. Tubocurarine is extensively eliminated by the kidney, and drug effect is substantially prolonged in renal failure. A TOF >0.7 is adequate to support a spontaneous airway and ventilation; however, at this degree of reversal, patients usually experience subjective weakness and diplopia.

54.5. Answer: E   The incidence of awareness is almost doubled when neuromuscular blockers are used during general anesthesia. Neuromuscular blockers by themselves do not block the pupillary light reflex; however, intravenous and inhalational agents blunt or block this reflex. A single dose of benzodiazepine before general anesthesia does not reduce the incidence of explicit awareness during general anesthesia. Laudanosine has been shown to lower the seizure threshold in dogs and may potentially contribute to seizures in a person with epilepsy, but it has never been shown to cause seizures in normal adults. Pancuronium and other neuromuscular blockers have no analgesic or sedative effect.

54.6. Answer: C   Hyperkalemia and cardiac arrest can occur early after the onset of an episode of MH. Hyperpyrexia is usually a late finding in MH. Succinylcholine, and not the nondepolarizing neuromuscular blockers, can trigger an episode of MH. The initial treatment of MH is removal of triggering agents and administration of dantrolene to correct the hypermetabolic state. β-Adrenergic antagonists can be used after dantrolene to treat tachycardia, but the tachycardia is secondary to hypermetabolism. Verapamil can cause myocardial depression, hyperkalemia and cardiac arrest. Calcium channel blockers are contraindicated for treating tachycardia associated with MH.

54.7. Answer: B   Succinylcholine-induced severe hyperkalemia has been reported to occur immediately following acute severe hemorrhagic shock. Patients with renal failure are no more likely to get hyperkalemia than those with normal renal function. The increment in plasma potassium observed following succinylcholine (typically about 0.5 mEq/L) is the same in persons with normal and abnormal renal function. Hyperkalemia after succinylcholine is not blunted by pretreatment with a nondepolarizing neuromuscular blocker. Following muscle or nerve injury, the proliferation of immature acetylcholine receptors on the muscle membrane, and not the presynaptic ACh receptors, leads to succinylcholine-induced hyperkalemia.

54.8. Answer: D   Pancuronium is the only commonly used nondepolarizing neuromuscular blocker that increases heart rate and arterial blood pressure; this is attributed to selective cardiac antimuscarinic (atropinelike) action, an indirect norepinephrine-releasing effect on postganglionic fibers, and block of presynaptic muscarinic receptors at the sympathetic nerve terminals. Pancuronium does not cause the release of histamine.

54.9. Answer: C   Myasthenia gravis greatly increases the sensitivity to nondepolarizing neuromuscular block. Chronic phenytoin accelerates the metabolism of pancuronium and shortens its duration. Long-term IV infusion of a nondepolarizing neuromuscular block induces resistance to subsequent administration of this drug. Acutely, sepsis is associated with resistance to nondepolarizing neuromuscular block. Neostigmine antagonizes the effects of nondepolarizing neuromuscular block.

54.10. Answer: B   The eye medication echothiophate is an organic phosphorus irreversible cholinesterase inhibitor that is systemically absorbed. Following chronic use there is near-total inhibition of cholinesterase, and there is significant prolongation of the effect of succinylcholine, which can last up to several hours. In hepatic insufficiency and following thermal burn injury, there is a mild decrease in plasma cholinesterase, but this usually causes only a mild increase in the duration of succinylcholine. Fresh frozen plasma contains plasma cholinesterase and increases the rate of succinylcholine degradation. A dibucaine number >70% indicates a normal plasma cholinesterase.

CHAPTER **55**

LOCAL ANESTHETICS

55.1. Answer: C   Life-threatening toxicity may occur when local anesthetics are used for nerve blocks. The mechanism is usually either unintentional direct intravascular injection (either intravenous or intraarterial) or relative overdose. At low toxic blood levels, excitatory CNS findings may be present, including shivering, tremors, and tonic-clonic seizures, all secondary to selective block of cortical cerebral inhibitory pathways. As the blood level rises further, both inhibitory and excitatory neurons are blocked, and generalized CNS depression ensues. Hypoxia and respiratory and metabolic acidosis have been reported to increase both the CNS and cardiovascular toxicity of local anesthetics. Toxic effects usually correlate with plasma lidocaine concentration.

Morishima H, Corvino B: Toxicity and distribution of lidocaine in nonasphyxiated and asphyxiated baboon fetuses. Anesthesiology 1981;54:182–186.

55.2. Answer: B Local anesthetics are weak bases. Because lipophilic, uncharged molecules more readily enter the neuron, drugs with a lower pK_a will have more uncharged molecules available at physiologic pH. Binding to neuronal proteins increases the duration of effect.

55.3. Answer: D NMDA receptor agonism is not a described mechanism of toxicity; all of the others are proved or proposed.

55.4. Answer: A Allergy to local anesthetics is rare and is generally to the ester class of drug. It is most likely a reaction to the common metabolite, PABA, so cross-sensitivity is common in this class. Amide allergy is rare and usually to the preservative methylparaben. Thus, preservative-free amides can be used in patients with "allergy" to amides.

55.5. Answer: A Cocaine is an ester. The currently available amide agents all have an "i" in the first four letters and two in the entire name.

55.6. Answer: B Although prilocaine, lidocaine, and tetracaine are reported to cause methemoglobinemia, benzocaine is the most frequent cause.

55.7. Answer: D Seizures usually precede cardiac arrest with lidocaine, although not all local anesthetic overdoses maintain this property. Paralysis does not occur, nor does headache.

55.8. Answer: E Although a lidocaine level of 4 μg/mL is supratherapeutic, it is slightly lower than the 5 to 9 μg/mL at which central nervous system effects typically manifest. Shivering and tremor are early findings, with lethargy, coma, seizures, and cardiovascular collapse developing as the plasma level rises.

55.9. Answer: A The treatment for lidocaine poisoning is primarily supportive care, including CPR, to allow the lidocaine to redistribute from the brain and heart. For longer-acting agents such as bupivacaine, lidocaine, phenytoin, bretylium, and bicarbonate have variable experimental success. Initial CPR is critical to allow drug redistribution and hepatic clearance, but prolonged CPR is suboptimal for bupivacaine poisoning because of the length of time required for drug clearance. Cardiopulmonary bypass may be superior in this situation.

55.10. Answer: D Even though lidocaine undergoes extensive first-pass hepatic metabolism, oral poisoning may occur. Lido-

caine's metabolites are active and may paradoxically reduce the efficacy of the parent compound through competition for binding sites. The eutectic mixture of lidocaine and prilocaine results in a compound that is able to penetrate the skin; neither agent can do so under normal circumstances. Tumescent anesthesia, used during liposuction, involves the adminstration of massive doses of lidocaine into the fat. Lidocaine does not crossreact with the cocaine assay, which detects benzoylecgonine, a structurally unrelated product.

CHAPTER **56**

PHARMACEUTICAL ADDITIVES

56.1. Answer: C Propylene glycol is metabolized by alcohol dehydrogenase to lactate and pyruvate and further broken down into carbon dioxide and water. The increased production of lactate may contribute to the metabolic acidosis that has been described with propylene glycol toxicity. Metabolic acidosis has been reported following the topical application of an antibiotic burn cream containing propylene glycol. Hyperosmolarity was also reported in these same patients.

Morshed KM, Jain SK, McMartin KE: Acute toxicity of propylene glycol: An assessment using cultured proximal tubule cells of human origin. Fundam Appl Toxicol 1994;23:38–43.

56.2. Answer: A Polyethylene glycol 200 appears to have the highest incidence of renal tubular necrosis. This is supported by studies in rats fed PEG 200 in their drinking water. A report of acute renal failure following the oral ingestion of the contents of a lava lamp containing PEG 200 has been described. Interestingly, the degree of toxicity appears to decrease as the molecular weight of the PEG increases. Polyethylene glycol 3350 electrolyte solutions are generally considered nontoxic even at very high dosages.

Smyth HF, Carpenter CP, Weil CS: The toxicology of the polyethylene glycols. J Am Pharmaceut Assoc 1950;39:349–354.

56.3. Answer: B Though the "gasping" syndrome was originally attributed to the immature metabolic capabilities of neonates, it was later found that neonates actually have an increased ability to metabolize benzyl alcohol to benzoic acid. Neonates have a glycine deficiency and therefore cannot further metabolize benzoic acid to hippuric acid. These neonates had been exposed to benzyl alcohol through medications reconstituted with bacteriostatic (not sterile water for injection) water preserved with benzyl alcohol.

Brown WJ, Buist WJ, Cory Gipson HT, et al: Fatal benzyl alcohol poisoning in a neonatal intensive care unit. Lancet 1982;1:1250.

Gershanik J, Boecler B, Ensley H, et al: The gasping syndrome and benzyl alcohol poisoning. N Engl J Med 1982;307:1384–1388.

56.4. Answer: A Chlorobutanol is closely related to trichloroethanol, the active metabolite of chloral hydrate. Chlorobutanol has resulted in central nervous system depression following acute poisonings. Chlorobutanol is a chlorinated hydrocarbon and may sensitize the myocardium to catecholamines, although no cases of ventricular dysrhythmias have been identified.

Borody T, Chinweah PM, Graham GG, et al: Chlorobutanol toxicity and dependence. Med J Aust 1979;1:288.

DeChristoforro R, Corden BJ, Hood JC, et al: High dose morphine complicated by chlorobutanol-somnolence. Ann Intern Med 1983; 98:335–336.

56.5. Answer: B Thimerosal is an organic mercuric compound widely used in vaccines, antivenins, immune globulins, and numerous other pharmaceuticals as a preservative. Thimerosal contains approximately 50% mercury by weight. Elevated mercury levels and several deaths have been attributed to thimerosal poisoning.

Pfab R, Mückter H, Roider G, et al: Clinical course of severe poisoning with thimerosal. J Toxicol Clin Toxicol 1996;34:453–460.

56.6. Answer: D Benzalkonium chloride (BAK) is a quaternary ammonium compound that is widely used in ophthalmic preparations. Although BAK is considered cytotoxic, it is the most effective ophthalmic preservative available based on its rapid onset of action, good tissue penetration, and long duration of activity.

Lemp MA, Zimmerman LE: Toxic endothelial degeneration in ocular surface disease treated with topical medications containing benzalkonium chloride. Am J Ophthamol 1988;105:670–673.

56.7. Answer: E The parabens. A survey conducted by the Food and Drug Administration identified the parabens as the second most commonly found ingredients in cosmetic formulations, with water being the most common. Because of the widespread exposure of humans to these agents, it is felt that the parabens have a relatively low order of toxicity, although they are associated with a higher incidence of allergic reactions than other pharmaceutic additives.

56.8. Answer: A Outbreaks of acute renal failure occurred in South Africa, Bangladesh, Nigeria, and Haiti when diethylene glycol was used to solubilize acetaminophen. One study identified diethylene glycol as the sole diluent in 19 of 69 foreign acetaminophen elixirs tested. Diethylene glycol poisoning presents initially with severe gastrointestinal symptoms. Hepatomegaly and acute renal failure generally follow. The majority of deaths have been attributed to the acute renal failure and lack of ability to perform hemodialysis. Unlike ethylene glycol poisoning, in which calcium oxalate crystal deposition is commonly seen and can be diagnostic, no oxalate crystals are seen in diethylene glycol poisoning. Diethylene glycol is not metabolized by alcohol dehydrogenase, and therefore, ethanol and 4-methylpyrazole may be ineffective.

Bowie MD, McKenzie D: Diethylene glycol poisoning in children. South Afr Med J 1972;46:931–934.

Calvery HO, Klumpp TG: The toxicity for human beings of diethylene glycol with sulfanilamide. South Med J 1939;32:1105–1109.

Hanif M, Mobarak MR, Ronan A: Fatal renal failure by diethylene glycol in paracetamol elixir: The Bangladesh epidemic. BMJ 1995;311:88–91.

56.9. Answer: D Thrombocytopenia, hepatomegaly, and renal dysfunction were all commonly described in the E-Ferol syndrome described in neonates. Oxalate-type crystals were identified in the distal renal tubules and collecting ducts, suggesting in vivo metabolism of ethylene oxide to ethylene glycol.

Alade SL, Brown RE, Paquet A: Polysorbate 80 and E-Ferol toxicity. Pediatrics 1986;77:593–597.

Martone WJ, Williams WW, Mortensen ML, et al: Illness with fatalities in premature infants: Association with intravenous vitamin E preparation, E-Ferol. Pediatrics 1986;78:591–600.

56.10. Answer: E Sorbitol is metabolized in the liver to fructose and glucose. There is a concern of potentially fatal toxicity for fructose-intolerant individuals receiving sorbitol-containing agents. There are several reports of patients with hereditary fructose intolerance dying following the parenteral infusion of sorbitol solutions.

Collins J: Time for fructose solutions to go. Lancet 1993;341:600.

Schulte MJ, Lenz W: Fatal sorbitol infusion in patient with fructose-sorbitol intolerance. Lancet 1977:2:188.

CHAPTER **57**

CYCLIC ANTIDEPRESSANTS

57.1. Answer: C Alkalinization of the blood to a pH of 7.45 to 7.50 with hypertonic sodium bicarbonate is more effective than the administration of hypertonic saline or hyperventilation. Acetazolamide would worsen toxicity by causing a loss of sodium bicarbonate in the urine. Lidocaine may be beneficial in treating ventricular dysrhythmias but has not been shown to reduce the duration of intraventricular conduction.

Bessen HA, Niemann JT, Haskell RJ, et al: Effect of respiratory alkalosis in tricyclic antidepressant overdose. West J Med 1983; 139:373–376.

Pentel PR, Benowitz NL: Tricyclic antidepressant poisoning—management of arrhythmias. Med Toxicol 1986;1:101–121.

57.2. Answer: A In a retrospective review of patients who presented to the emergency department with trivial signs of tricyclic antidepressant toxicity, more than one-half had a catastrophic deterioration within 1 hour.

Callaham M, Kassel D: Epidemiology of fatal tricyclic antidepressant ingestion: Implications for management. Ann Emerg Med 1985;14:1–9.

57.3. Answer: D The incidence of seizures with amoxapine is nine times greater than with the first-generation tricyclic antidepressants. The incidence of cardiac toxicity appears to be lower than with the other tricyclic antidepressants.

Litovitz TL, Troutman WG: Amoxapine overdose: Seizures and fatalities. JAMA 1983;250:1069–1071.

57.4. Answer: D Venlafaxine causes a dose-related increase in systolic blood pressure. It may be related to its ability to inhibit the reuptake of both norepinephrine and dopamine.

Cunningham LA, Borison RL, Carman JS: A comparison of venlafaxine, trazodone, and placebo in major depression. J Clin Psychopharmacol 1994;14:99–106.

57.5. Answer: D Less than 10% of the cyclic antidepressants is cleared by the kidneys. The volume of distribution is usually in the range of 10 to 50 L/kg. The protein binding is greater than 85%, with most of the drug binding to α_1-glycoprotein. The cyclic antidepressants are very lipophilic and are poorly water soluble.

57.6. Answer: B In comparison to other cyclic antidepressants, venlafaxine is a weaker inhibitor of both serotonin and norepinephrine reuptake but is a significantly more potent inhibitor of dopamine reuptake.

57.7. Answer: E Bupropion does not inhibit the reuptake of either serotonin or norepinephrine but is a weak inhibitor of the reuptake of dopamine.

57.8. Answer: D Seizures occurred in 30% of patients with QRS complexes >100 milliseconds, and dysrhythmias occurred in 50% of patients with QRS complexes >160 milliseconds. No patients were found to have these clinical manifestations if their QRS complexes were less than these values.

Boehnert M, Lovejoy FH Jr: Value of the QRS duration versus the serum drug level in predicting seizures and ventricular arrhythmias after an acute overdose of tricyclic antidepressants. N Engl J Med 1985;313:474–479.

57.9. Answer: A Amitriptyline has the greatest anticholinergic activity of the listed cyclic antidepressants. Clomipramine and trimipramine are the other antidepressants with potent anticholinergic activity. Doxepin, maprotiline, and amoxapine have significantly less activity, and fluoxetine (a selective serotonin-reuptake inhibitor) has no anticholinergic activity.

Burks JS, Walker JE, Rumack BH, et al: Tricyclic antidepressant poisoning: Reversal of coma, choreoathetosis and myoclonus by physostigmine. JAMA 1974;230:1405–1407.

57.10. Answer: E Lidocaine can be used to treat ventricular dysrhythmias in patients with cyclic antidepressant overdoses. All of the other antidysrhythmics tend to further slow intraventricular conduction and should be avoided.

CHAPTER 58

SEROTONIN REUPTAKE INHIBITORS AND ATYPICAL ANTIDEPRESSANTS

58.1. Answer: D Venlafaxine has the ability to inhibit the reuptake of serotonin but, in addition, inhibits the reuptake of norepinephrine and dopamine; thus, it is not considered a "SSRI."

58.2. Answer: C Both serotonin syndrome and neuroleptic malignant syndrome present with fever, altered mental status, and autonomic instability. Hyperreflexia is more commonly found with serotonin syndrome.

Sternbach H: The serotonin syndrome. Am J Psychiatry 1991; 148:705–713.

58.3. Answer: A Overstimulation of 5-HT_{1A} receptors was formally thought to be the inciting event causing serotonin syndrome. New data suggest involvement of the 5-HT_2 receptor.

Nisijima K: Potent serotonin $(5\text{-HT})_{2A}$ receptor antagonists completely prevent the development of hyperthermia in an animal model of the 5-HT syndrome. Brain Res 2001;890:23–31.

58.4. Answer: A In addition to depressive illness, SSRIs have been used in the treatment of many other disorders, including obesity and alcoholism.

Naranjo CA, Bremner KE: Clinical pharmacology of serotonin-altering medication for decreasing alcohol consumption. Alcohol Alcoholism 1993;2:221–229.

58.5. Answer: E Mirtazapine acts to increase neuronal serotonin through α_2-adrenergic antagonism.

deBoer T: The pharmacologic profile of mirtazapine. J Clin Psychiatry 1996;57(Suppl 4):19–25.

58.6. Answer: D SSRI overdoses commonly result in mental status depression and tachycardia, rarely in seizures, and have not yet been reported to cause hyperthermia.

Borys DJ, Setzer SC, Ling LJ, et al: Acute fluoxetine overdose: Report of 234 cases. Am J Emerg Med 1992;10;115–120.

58.7. Answer: A Because excess serotonergic activity is the cause of hyperthermia, antipyretics would not be expected to be useful. The other measures, however, serve to either acutely decrease temperature or block serotonergic activity, which may be useful.

Gerson SC, Baldessarini RJ: Motor effects of serotonin in the central nervous system. Life Sci 1980;27:1435–1451.

58.8. Answer: B The drug interactions caused by SSRIs are through inhibition of the activity of the CYP2D6 enzyme.

Rieseman C: Antidepressant drug interactions and the cytochrome P450 system: A critical appraisal. Pharmacotherapy 1995;15: 84S–99S.

58.9. Answer: B In general, two serotonergic drugs must be administered for the development of serotonin syndrome, although rare reports with a single agent are noted.

58.10. Answer: C A review of cases from Sweden found citalopram to cause seizures and wide QRS complex dysrhythmias after doses exceeding 60 mg were ingested. This risk necessitates close observation of these patients.

Personne M, Sjoberg G, Persson H: Citalopram overdose: Review of cases treated in Swedish hospitals. J Toxicol Clin Toxicol 1997; 35:237–240.

CHAPTER 59

ANTIPSYCHOTICS

59.1. Answer: B When patients in one study were placed on H_2 antagonists (ie, cimetidine, famotidine, nizatidine), steady-state plasma chlorpromazine levels decreased because of a change in gastrointestinal pH.

Howes CA, Pullar T, Sourindhrin I, et al: Reduced steady state plasma concentrations of chlorpromazine and indomethacin in patients receiving cimetidine. Eur J Clin Pharmacol 1983;24:99–102.

59.2. Answer: C Patients being treated with chlorpromazine for schizophrenia often will show improvement after the first week of therapy; however, optimal benefit of the medication at a particular dose will not be seen for 1 month.

May PRA, Van Putten T, Jenden DJ, et al: Chlorpromazine levels and the outcome of treatment in schizophrenic patients. Arch Gen Psychiatry 1981;38:202–207.

59.3. Answer: D Neuroleptic malignant syndrome was first described in 1968 and is characterized by hyperthermia, muscle rigidity, extrapyramidal effects, autonomic dysfunction, and altered consciousness.

Guze BH, Baxter JR: Neuroleptic malignant syndrome. N Engl J Med 1985;313:163–166.

59.4. Answer: C If antipsychotics are necessary, 1 to 2 weeks should elapse after symptoms resolve before they are reintroduced. The antipsychotic chosen should be from a different class than the one that precipitated the NMS and should have minimal extrapyramidal effects. The atypical antipsychotic clozapine is recommended.

Rosebush PI, Stewart T, Mazurek MF: The treatment of neuroleptic malignant syndrome: Are dantrolene and bromocriptine useful adjuncts to supportive care? Br J Psychiatry 1991;159:709–712.

59.5. Answer: A Parkinsonism occurs in 90% of susceptible patients within 72 days of initiation of therapy. It presents with shuffling gait, resting tremor, rigidity, pill rolling, and a masklike expression.

59.6. Answer: D The most serious CNS toxic effect of neuroleptic therapy is tardive dyskinesia. Once it occurs it is often permanent and at best shows minimal improvement.

59.7. Answer: A Cholinergic stimulation using an anticholinesterase (ie, physostigmine) may be beneficial in the amelioration of tardive dyskinesia.

59.8. Answer: B Deaths are rare and have been most frequently reported in cases associated with thioridazine and mesoridazine overdose or when antipsychotics are taken concomitantly in overdose with sympathomimetics, lithium, antihistamines, or cyclic antidepressants.

Baker PB, Merigian KS, Roberts JR, et al: Hyperthermia, hypertension, hypertonia and coma in a massive thioridazine overdose. Am J Emerg Med 1988;6:346–349.

59.9. Answer: C Thioridazine and mesoridazine typically increase QT, QRS, and PR intervals by inhibiting sodium channels.

Elkayam U, Frishman W: Cardiovascular effects of phenothiazines. Am Heart J 1980;100:397–401.

59.10. Answer: E The metabolites may be found in the urine up to 6 weeks after the last dose of parent compound is ingested. Following an overdose, urine may contain detectable quantities of phenothiazines for up to 3 months.

Curry SH, Davis JM, Janowsky DS, et al: Factors affecting chlorpromazine plasma levels in psychiatric patients. Arch Gen Psychiatry 1970;22:209–215.

CHAPTER 60

MONOAMINE OXIDASE INHIBITORS

60.1. Answer: B MAO-A is found in gut and brain, is sensitive to clorgyline, and has a preference for serotonin metabolism. All of the MAOIs with antidepressant effect inhibit MAO-A. MAO-B is found in platelets and brain, is sensitive to selegiline (Deprenyl), and prefers to metabolize dopamine. All currently available MAOIs are suicide inhibitors (irreversible).

60.2. Answer: E Because the patient's blood pressure may be unpredictable following an MAO inhibitor overdose, attempts to normalize the vital signs are most safely made with the use of a short-acting or reversible agent. Longer-acting antihypertensives may prove problematic if hypotension abruptly develops.

Linden CH, Rumack BH: Monoamine oxidase inhibitor overdose. Ann Emerg Med 1984;13:1137–1144.

60.3. Answer: C MAO metabolizes all biogenic amines, including the catecholamines (eg, norepinephrine) and serotonin. Hepatic MAO metabolizes the dietary monoamines, the most notorious of which is tyramine.

60.4. Answer: A MAO decreases intraneuronal degradation of norepinephrine, which results in an increased storage pool in the sympathetic nerve terminal.

60.5. Answer: A The onset of MAOI toxicity has been reported as late as 32 hours following ingestion. Agitation is characteristic, and pupils are not pinpoint but may be dilated. MAOIs have no anticholinergic effects and do not cause respiratory depression.

Linden CH, Rumack BH: Monoamine oxidase inhibitor overdose. Ann Emerg Med 1984;13:1137–1144.

60.6. Answer: C Interactions are likely to occur with the use of indirect-acting agents (those that release stored norepinephrine from the nerve terminal). The direct-acting agents (those that combine directly with postsynaptic receptors) such as norepinephrine, epinephrine, and isoproterenol are believed to be safe.

Livingston MG, Livingston HM: Monoamine oxidase inhibitors. An update on drug interactions. Drug Safety 1996;14:219–227.

60.7. Answer: D Tyramine, a monoamine derived from food, is an indirect-acting agent in that it causes the release of NE from storage vesicles. Normally it is inactivated in the liver and gut by MAO.

60.8. Answer: A The combination of MAOIs and meperidine or fluoxetine may result in the serotonin syndrome. The clinical effects of barbiturates, through P450 inhibition, and sulfonylureas, through enhanced insulin release, are potentiated when combined with certain MAOIs. Albuterol is a direct-acting adrenergic agent that can be given safely.

60.9. Answer: E Morphine sulfate is considered safe in patients on MAOIs. All of the other agents have been reported to precipitate the serotonin syndrome when used in patients on MAOIs.

Penn RG, Rogers KJ: Comparison of the effects of morphine, pethidine and pentazocine in rabbits pretreated with a monoamine oxidase inhibitor. Br J Pharmacol 1971;42:485–490.

60.10. Answer: A Moclobemide and the RIMAs are selective for MAO-A, but their increased safety is thought to result primarily from their competitive and reversible binding to MAO.

Hilton SE, Maradit H, Moller HJ: Serotonin syndrome and drug combinations: focus on MAOI and RIMA. Eur Arch Psychiatry Clin Neurosci 1997;247:113–119.

CHAPTER 61

LITHIUM

61.1. Answer: C Patients with normal renal function can eliminate lithium faster than peritoneal dialysis can if their GFR is maximized. Peritoneal dialysis can clear lithium only on the order of 10 to 15 mL/min, which is slightly less than the normally functioning kidney. CAAH and CAVH have reported values between 20 and 62 mL/min, whereas hemodialysis can achieve values greater than 100 mL/min and has been reported as high as 170 mL/min. Hemoperfusion plays no role because lithium does not bind to activated charcoal.

Hansen HE, Amdisen A: Lithium intoxication. Q J Med 1978;47:123–144.

Wilson JH, Donker AJ, van der Helm GK, et al: Peritoneal dialysis for lithium poisoning. Br Med J 1971;2:749–750.

61.2. Answer: D Lithium is an ideal drug for hemodialysis because it has a small volume of distribution, is a small molecule, and is not protein bound.

Blye E, Lorch J, Cartell S: Extracorporeal therapy in the treatment of intoxication. Am J Kidney Dis 1984;3:321–338.

61.3. Answer: B Patients who demonstrate toxicity from lithium that includes severe neurologic changes such as mental status changes should undergo extracorporeal removal in order to prevent permanent changes. Hemodialysis and not peritoneal dialysis is the treatment of choice. Peritoneal dialysis plays no role in treating lithium toxicity unless the patient is in renal failure, has a PD catheter already in place, and is awaiting hemodialysis.

Schou M: Long-lasting neurological sequelae after lithium intoxication. Acta Psychiatr Scand 1984;70:594–602.

61.4. Answer: B Patients who undergo hemodialysis frequently require repeat dialysis because of the "rebound" phenomenon. This rebound comes about as lithium equilibrates from the bone, brain, and other parts of the body. Unfortunately, HD clears only the serum and not the brain.

Jaeger A, Sauder P, Kopeferschmitt J, et al: When should dialysis be performed in lithium poisoning? A kinetic study in 14 cases of lithium poisoning. J Toxicol Clin Toxicol 1993;31:429–447.

61.5. Answer: D Although lithium is rapidly absorbed and has a quick onset to its peak serum level, it takes many hours for it to cross cellular membranes of the CNS, muscle, and bone, whereas it crosses into the kidneys and liver very rapidly. This accounts for the delay in neurologic signs and symptoms that these patients may experience.

Apte SN, Langston WJ: Permanent neurological deficits due to lithium toxicity. Ann Neurol 1983;13:452–455.

Frazer A, Mendel J, Secunda SK, et al: The prediction of brain lithium concentration from plasma or erythrocyte measure. J Psychiatr Res 1973;10:1–7.

61.6. Answer: E Although over time CAAH and CAVH can remove as much lithium as HD, it does take longer to accomplish this task. During this time, persistently increased levels of lithium may adversely affect the brain. Because HD removes the lithium faster, it may have a better opportunity to prevent permanent neurologic complications.

Ayuso Gatell A, Leon Regidor MA, Mestre Saura J, et al: Acute lithium poisoning: Treatment with continuous arteriovenous hemofiltration. Rev Clin Exp 1989;185:195–197.

Bellomo R, Kearly Y, Parkin G: Treatment of life threatening lithium toxicity with continuous arterio-venous hemodiafiltration. Crit Care Med 1991;19:836–837.

Schou M: Long-lasting neurological sequelae after lithium intoxication. Acta Psychiatr Scand 1984;70:594–602.

61.7. Answer: A Although numerous studies with SPS have been performed, they have almost all been in the animal model. Even though the possibility of lithium removal exists, the gastrointestinal (diarrhea) and electrolyte (hypokalemia) complications of high-dose SPS may prevent this from becoming a viable adjunct to current established therapy such as hemodialysis.

Gehrke JC, Watling SM, Gehrke CW, et al: In vivo binding of lithium using the cation exchange resin sodium polystyrene sulfonate. Am J Med 1996;14:37–38.

61.8. Answer: B Lithium's ionic radius is not similar to that of manganese. Lithium has a similar ionic radius to magnesium, and this similarity may explain how it alters some of magnesium's function. It may also serve as false transmitter for both potassium and sodium. These numerous interactions make it hard to define its exact mechanisms of action in the numerous disease processes for which it is used.

Atherton JC, Doyle A, Gee A, et al: Lithium clearance: Modification by the loop of Henle in man. J Physiol 1990;437:377–391.

Berridge MJ, Downes CP, Hanley RR: Neurological and development action of lithium. A unifying hypothesis. Cell 1989;59: 411–419.

Berridge MJ, Downes CP, Hanley RR: Lithium amplifies agonist-dependent phosphatidyl-inositol response in brain and salivary gland. Biochem J 1982;206:587–595.

61.9. Answer: D Fine tremor of the hands is a more common finding in patients who start to demonstrate neurologic effects from this agent. As toxicity progresses, changes in the reflexes (increased), irritability, and abnormal movements may be noted. Dysarthria is a more advanced symptom and is not consistently present.

Okusa MD, Jovita L, Crystal T: Clinical manifestations and mangement of acute lithium intoxication. Am J Med 1994;97: 383–389.

61.10. Answer: C One of the numerous uses for lithium is that of a prophylactic agent in patients with cluster headaches, not migraines. Although its mechanism is unknown, its interaction with serotonin may play some role in these patients.

Jaeger A, Sauder P, Kopeferschmitt J, et al: Toxicokinetics of lithium intoxication treated by hemodialysis. J Toxicol Clin Toxicol 1985;23:501–517.

CHAPTER 62

OPIOIDS

62.1. Answer: E Morphine has been identified in the brains of certain animals. The new opioid nomenclature renames the opioid receptors using the OP_x schema (eg, μ is now OP_3). The μ_2 receptor subtype produces respiratory depression. The κ_2 receptor is associated with psychotomimesis (dysphoria). Many of the agonist–antagonist agents bind to κ_1 or κ_3 better that they bind to μ receptors, accounting for their unusual clinical properties.

Dhawan BN, Cesselin F, Raghubir R, et al: Internation Union of Pharmacology. XII. Classification of opioid receptors. Pharmacol Rev 1996;48:567–592.

Donnerer J, Oka K, Brossi A, et al: Presence and formation of codeine and morphine in the rat. Proc Natl Acad Sci USA 1986; 83:4566–4567.

62.2. Answer: B Binding or enhancement of GABAergic neurotransmission has never been associated with opioid agents. The other mechanisms represent nonspecific inhibitory effects that have been demonstrated with each of the major opioid receptor subtypes.

Minami M, Satoh M: Molecular biology of the opioid receptors: Structures, functions and distributions. Neurosci Res 1995;23: 121–145.

62.3. Answer: D Hypoventilation may be related to either a decreased respiratory rate or a depressed tidal volume. Airway support is the mainstay of therapy; naloxone administration should not be performed until the patient is sufficiently stabilized by face-mask or endotracheal ventilation. The initial management of all opioid-poisoned patients is identical regardless of the agent. There are many causes of small pupils, and this finding is neither necessary nor sufficient for the diagnosis of opioid toxicity. Low-dose naloxone is generally efficacious and carries a lower risk of precipitating withdrawal.

Shook JE, Watkins WD, Camporesi EM: Differential roles of opioid receptors in respiration, respiratory disease, and opiate-induced respiratory depression. Am Rev Respir Dis 1990;142: 895–909.

62.4. Answer: D Altered mental status, respiratory depression, miosis, and depressed bowel function are the classic findings associated with opioid toxicity. Methemoglobinemia is not specifically associated with opioids.

Hoffman JR, Schriger DL, Luo JS: The empiric use of naloxone in patients with altered mental status: A reappraisal. Ann Emerg Med 1991;20:246–252.

62.5. Answer: E Apnea is a common manifestation of opioid toxicity. Noncardiogenic pulmonary edema is very common and may be subtle in presentation or dramatic. Several mechanisms for this entity have been proposed, and each has some clinical and experimental support. Certain agents, notably propoxyphene, may induce a wide-complex tachycardia. Seizures may be caused by opioid-induced hypoxia and are associated with tramadol or propoxyphene. Patients with chronic meperidine toxicity may also develop seizures. Although acute hypertension may be seen in patients using speedballs (combination of heroin with cocaine), it is not described after an isolated opioid exposure.

Luke JL, Levy ME: Heroin-related deaths—District of Columbia, 1980–1982. MMWR 1983;32:321–324.

Madsen PS, Strom J, Reiz S, et al: Acute propoxyphene self-poisoning in 222 consecutive patients. Acta Anesthesiol Scand 1984; 28:661–665.

62.6. Answer: E Although naloxone is quite safe, adverse outcomes may occur when it is used indiscriminately. For example, the vomiting associated with precipitated acute opioid withdrawal may cause pulmonary aspiration, especially in patients with other reasons for altered mental status. For unclear reasons, the synthetic opioids generally require higher doses of naloxone to reverse poisoning. Because the duration of effect of naloxone is shorter than those of many opioid agents, resedation and recurrence of respiratory depression may occur in patients discharged shortly after naloxone administration. At least 1 hour of observation, and preferably longer, should elapse between reversal and discharge. Meperidine-induced seizures are typically not responsive to naloxone. In fact, there is experimental evidence that naloxone may potentiate the seizures caused by meperidine, presumably by inhibiting an anticonvulsant effect of meperidine. Interestingly, propoxyphene-induced seizures may be prevented by naloxone. Because there is functional overlap between α_2 and μ receptors (ie, both receptors may be found on the same neuron and are coupled at a specific K^+ channel), clonidine-induced respiratory depression and altered mental status regularly respond to naloxone.

Smith DA, Leake L, Loflin JR, et al: Is admission after intravenous heroin overdose necessary? Ann Emerg Med 1992;21: 1326–1330.

Wiley JF, Wiley CC, Torrey SB, et al: Clonidine poisoning in young children. J Pediatr 1990;116:654–658.

62.7. Answer: C   Body packers are patients who ingest large numbers of multiply wrapped packages of concentrated cocaine or heroin in an attempt to transport illicit drugs from one country to another. Body stuffers hurriedly ingest unprotected drug to avoid police detection. Although generally asymptomatic, body packers are at risk for delayed and prolonged toxicity from packet leakage or rupture. Unlike patients body packing cocaine, in whom surgery is mandatory on development of symptoms, those with heroin packets can often be managed nonoperatively with continuous-infusion naloxone, activated charcoal, and whole-bowel irrigation. Irritant cathartics should be avoided because of the potential for bag rupture. Observation, however, must be performed by trained personnel, and airway support or naloxone must be rapidly available. Although rapid urine testing for drugs of abuse may assist in determining the packet content, the same information is usually obtained more quickly and reliably by asking the patient, determining the country of origin, or identifying toxidromes.

Goldfrank L, Weisman RS, Errick JK, et al: A dosing nomogram for continuous infusion intravenous naloxone. Ann Emerg Med 1986;15:566–570.

Utecht MJ, Facinelli Stone A, McCarron MM: Heroin body packers. J Emerg Med 1993;11:33–40.

62.8. Answer: E   Fentanyl is a common drug of abuse, and regional epidemics of heroin substitution with "superpotent" heroin occasionally produce a dramatic rise in heroin-related fatalities (eg, "China white"). It is also a substance of abuse among anesthesiologists. Fentanyl produces the least hypotension and the least elevation of plasma histamine levels of all the commonly used opioids. Death is typically related to chest wall rigidity, which may be antidopaminergic in nature. Although the ability of fentanyl to induce seizures remains controversial, EEG monitoring failed to demonstrate such activity. This activity may actually be myoclonus or another movement disorder.

Flacke JW, Flacke WE, Bloor BC, et al: Histamine release by four narcotics; a double blind study in humans. Anesth Analg 1987; 66:723–730.

Kram TC, Cooper DA, Allen AC: Behind the identification of China white. Anal Chem 1981;3:1379A–1386A.

Smith NT, Benthuysen JL, Bickford RG: Seizures during opioid anesthetic induction—are they opioid-induced rigidity? Anesthesiology 1989;71:852–862.

Ward CF, Ward GC, Saidman LJ: Drug abuse in anesthesia training programs. JAMA 1983;250:922–925.

62.9. Answer: C   Whether a similar drug is noted by the assay depends on the sensitivity and specificity of the assay used as well as the serum concentration of the agent. The opioid assay can differentiate naloxone and does not report a positive result. The metabolism of therapeutic doses of codeine to morphine will produce a positive morphine assay. Poppy seeds contain morphine, and elevated serum morphine levels are commonly noted. However, because humans cannot acetylate morphine, detection of 6-monoacetylmorphine, the substrate for the heroin assay and a metabolite of heroin, is unequivocal evidence for heroin use. The extremely small amounts of fentanyl present in blood (because of its high potency) make it very difficult to detect without sensitive assays.

Cone E, Dickerson S, Paul B, et al: Forensic drug testing for opiates. IV. Analytical sensitivity, specificity, and accuracy of commercial urine opiate immunoassays. J Anal Toxicol 1992;16: 72–78.

Kram TC, Cooper DA, Allen AC: Behind the identification of China white. Anal Chem 1981;3:1379A–1386A.

Mule SJ, Casella GA: Rendering the "poppy-seed defense" defenseless: Identification of 6-monoacetylmorphine in urine by gas chromatography/mass spectroscopy. Clin Chem 1988;34: 1427–1430.

62.10. Answer: A   Patients are generally given high therapeutic doses to prevent surreptitious illicit drug use. Excessive doses may produce toxicity identical to that of morphine with an important difference: the duration of effect of methadone is very prolonged (about 24 hours). Nalmefene does not have a sufficient duration of effect to prevent resedation in methadone-poisoned patients, and many patients require a continuous infusion of naloxone. Naltrexone has a longer duration than nalmefene but is unstudied for this indication. LAAM poisoning may prove even more problematic than methadone because its duration of effect is about 3 days. In 1982, several cases of acute, severe parkinsonian symptoms in intravenous drug users led to the discovery of MPTP (1-methyl-4-phenyl-1,2,3,6-tetrahydropyridine), an inadvertent product of synthesis of an illicit meperidine analogue.

Langston JW, Ballard, Tetrud JW, et al: Chronic parkinsonism in humans due to a product of meperidine-analog synthesis. Science 1983;219:979–980.

Predergast ML, Grella C, Perry SM, et al: *Levo*-alpha-acetylmethadol (LAAM): Clinical, research, and policy issues of a new pharmacotherapy for opioid addiction. J Psychoactive Drugs 1995;27:239–247.

Strain EC, Stitzer ML, Liebson IA, et al: Dose-response effects of methadone in the treatment of opioid dependence. Ann Intern Med 1993;119:23–27.

CHAPTER 63

SEDATIVE-HYPNOTIC AGENTS

63.1. Answer: D Alkalinization with sodium bicarbonate will enhance the urinary excretion of phenobarbital because it has a pK_a that is relatively lower than those of the other barbiturates.

Linton AL, Luke RG, Briggs JD: Methods of forced diuresis and its application in barbiturate poisoning. Lancet 1967;2:377–379.

63.2. Answer: E The amount of drug that will be present in the blood compartment depends on all these factors.

Hobbs WR, Rall TW, Verdoon TA: Hypnotic and sedatives; ethanol. In: Hardman JG, Limbird LE, Molinoff PB, et al, eds: Goodman & Gilman's The Pharmacological Basis of Therapeutics, 9th ed. New York, McGraw-Hill, 1996, pp. 373–376.

63.3. Answer: A Triazolam has the shortest half-life and no active metabolites.

Greenblatt DJ, Shader DR: Current status of benzodiazepines. N Engl J Med 1983;309:354–358.

63.4. Answer: D Cardiac dysrhythmias are the main cause of death in chloral hydrate overdoses.

King K, England JF: Chloral hydrate overdose. Med J Aust 1983; 2:260.

63.5. Answer: E Zolpidem is chemically unrelated to the benzodiazepines but binds to the same receptors in the brain and is reversed by flumazenil.

Salva P, Costa J: Clinical pharmacokinetics and pharmacodynamics of zolpidem. Clin Pharmacokinet 1995;29:142–153.

63.6. Answer: B The half-life of bromide is approximately 12 days, and it can accumulate if taken daily.

Vaiseman N, Koren G, Pencharz P: Pharmacokinetics of oral and intravenous bromide. J Toxicol Clin Toxicol 1986;24:403–413.

63.7. Answer: B Glutethimide has anticholinergic properties and can cause dry mouth, mydriasis, decreased GI motility, and CNS irritability.

Chazen JA, Garella S: Glutethimide intoxication. Arch Intern Med 1971;128:215–219.

63.8. Answer: C The metabolism of glutethimide results in several metabolites, some of which are biologically active and may contribute to its toxicity.

Curry SC, Hubbard JM, Gerkin R, et al: Lack of correlation between plasma 4-hydroxy glutethimide and severity of coma in acute glutethimide poisoning. Med Toxicol 1987;2:304–316.

Hansen AR, Kennedy KA, Ambre JA, Fischer LJ: Medical intelligence: Glutethimide poisoning. N Engl J Med 1975;292:250–252.

63.9. Answer: B Meprobamate is only 20% protein bound. It is metabolized in the liver, and there is no cross-tolerance with opioids. The volume of distribution of meprobamate is 0.75 L/kg.

Maddock RK, Blommer HA: Meprobamate overdosage. JAMA 1967;201:999–1003.

63.10. Answer: B Benzodiazepines such as triazolam generally do not interact with warfarin because they are weak inducers of the hepatic microsomal system.

Greenblatt DJ, Sellers EM, Shader RI: Drug disposition in old age. N Engl J Med 1982;306:1081–1088.

CHAPTER 64

ETHANOL

64.1. Answer: B Alcohol dehydrogenase (ADH) uses NAD^+ as a hydrogen acceptor to oxidize ethanol to acetaldehyde, which is further metabolized to acetate by aldehyde dehydrogenase (ALDH). Acetate is converted to acetylcoenzyme A, which enters the Krebs (citric acid) cycle and is metabolized to carbon dioxide and water. The ability of acetylcoenzyme A to enter the Krebs cycle is indirectly dependent on adequate thiamine stores. The metabolism of ethanol generates NADH and alters the redox (NAD^+/NADH) ratio, thereby forcing the conversion of pyruvate to lactate and preventing gluconeogenesis.

Hoffman RS, Goldfrank LR: Ethanol-associated metabolic disorders. Emerg Clin North Am 1989;7:943–961.

64.2. Answer: B Eighty-proof whisky contains 40% alcohol by volume; 40% ethanol is 40,000 mg of ethanol per 100 mL. Serum ethanol concentration (mg/dL) is equal to the amount of ethanol consumed divided by the volume of distribution (L/kg) of ethanol times the weight (kg) of the person. Thus, the serum ethanol concentration equals 40,000 mg divided by 500 mL/kg × 80 kg = 40,000 mg divided by 40,000 mL = 100 mg/dL.

64.3. Answer: B One of the hallmarks of alcoholic ketoacidosis (AKA) is a large anion gap metabolic acidosis. The pathophysiology of AKA involves an overwhelmingly low cellular redox state such that most of the acetoacetate is reduced to β-hydroxybutyrate. The nitroprusside test is used to detect the presence of ketones in serum and urine. The laboratory assay for ketones in a patient with AKA may be only mildly positive and substantially less than expected from the acid–base data because the nitroprusside reaction only detects molecules containing ketones such as acetone and acetoacetate and not β-hydroxybutyrate. The diagnostic criteria for AKA should include a recent history of alcohol intake with a relative or absolute decline in ethanol consumption 24 to 72 hours before presentation, a history of vomiting, a blood glucose level less than 300 mg/dL (16.7 mmol/L), and a metabolic acidosis for which other causes have been excluded by clinical observations or laboratory studies. Typically there is mild lactic acidosis in AKA as a result of volume depletion and conversion of pyruvate to lactate to regenerate NAD^+.

Fulop M: Alcoholic ketoacidosis. Endocrinol Metab Clin North Am 1993;22:209–219.

Soffer A, Hamburger S: Alcoholic ketoacidosis: A review of 30 cases. J Am Med Wom Assoc 1982;37:106–110.

64.4. Answer: E Animal studies indicate that the acute effects of ethanol are competitive inhibition of glycine's binding to the NMDA receptor and disruption of glutaminergic neurotransmission by inhibiting the response of the NMDA receptor. Persistent glycine antagonism and attenuation of glutaminergic neurotransmission by chronic ethanol exposure result in the compensatory up-regulation of NMDA receptors. Tolerance to ethanol results in enhanced EAA neurotransmission and NMDA receptor up-regulation, which appears to involve selective increases in NMDA R2B subunit levels and other molecular changes in specific brain loci. Abrupt withdrawal of ethanol thus produces a hyperexcitable state that leads to the ethanol withdrawal syndrome and excitotoxic neuronal death.

Tsai GE, Ragan P, Chang R, et al: Increased glutamatergic neurotransmission and oxidative stress after alcohol withdrawal. Am J Psychiatry 1998;155:726–732.

Tsai GE, Coyle JT: The role of glutamatergic neurotransmission in the pathophysiology of alcoholism. Annu Rev Med 1998;49:173–184.

Hu X-J, Ticku MK: Chronic ethanol treatment upregulates the NMDA receptor function and binding in mammalian cortical neurons. Brain Res Mol Brain Res 1995;30:347–356.

64.5. Answer: E Thiamine (vitamin B_1) is an essential cofactor for transketolase, pyruvate dehydrogenase, and α-ketoglutarate dehydrogenase.

Lavoie J, Butterworth RF: Reduced activities of thiamine-dependent enzymes in brains of alcoholics in the absence of Wernicke's encephalopathy. Alcohol Clin Exp Res 1995;19:1073–1077.

Butterworth RF, Kril JJ, Harper CG: Thiamine-dependent enzyme changes in the brains of alcoholics: relationship to the Wernicke-Korsakoff syndrome. Alcohol Clin Exp Res 1993;17:1084–1088.

64.6. Answer: C The anion gap in patients with AKA and DKA are very similar, with β-hydroxybutyrate being the primary anion contributor and lactate having a less consequential role. Ethanol metabolism generates NADH, resulting in an excess of reducing potential. This low redox state favors the conversion of pyruvate to lactate, diverting pyruvate from being a substrate for gluconeogenesis. To compensate for the lack of normal metabolic substrates, the body mobilizes fat from adipose tissue and increases fatty acid metabolism as an alternative source of energy. This response is mediated by a decrease in insulin and an increased secretion of glucagon, catecholamines, growth hormone, and cortisol. Fatty acid metabolism results in the formation of acetylcoenzyme A, which combines with the excess acetate that is generated from ethanol metabolism to form acetoacetate. Most of the acetoacetate is reduced to β-hydroxybutyrate because of the excess reducing potential or low redox state of the cell.

Fulop M, Hoberman HD: Diabetic ketoacidosis and alcoholic ketosis. Ann Intern Med 1979;91:796–797.

64.7. Answer: D Thiamine is an essential cofactor for α-ketoglutarate dehydrogenase. In a thiamine-deficient state, the rate-limiting step is the conversion of α-ketoglutarate to succinate.

64.8. Answer: B Drug–ethanol interactions resulting in a disulfiramlike reaction include carbamates, cephalosporins, chloramphenicol, chlorpropamide, coprinus mushroom, griseofluvin, metronidazole, nitrofurantoin, thiuram, and tolbutamide.

Fett DL, Vukov LF: An unusual case of severe grisofluvin–alcohol interaction. Ann Emerg Med 1994;24:95–97.

64.9. Answer: D The nitroprusside test is used to detect the presence of ketones in serum and urine. This laboratory assay for ketones in a patient with AKA may be only mildly positive and substantially less than expected from the acid–base status because the nitroprusside reaction detects only molecules containing ketones such as acetone and acetoacetate and not β-hydroxybutyrate. However, isopropanol is metabolized by the liver to acetone, and it will give a strongly positive nitroprusside test. On the other hand, metabolism of ethanol, ethylene glycol, methanol, and phenol does not result in significant amounts of ketones.

Fulop M: Alcoholic ketoacidosis. Endocrinol Metab Clin North Am 1993;22:209–219.

Fulop M, Hoberman HD: Diabetic ketoacidosis and alcoholic ketosis. Ann Intern Med 1979;91:796–797.

64.10. Answer: D Cimetidine inhibits ADH_3 or gastric ADH and results in minimal elevation in serum ethanol levels. Ethanol-induced hypoglycemia is arguably more common in children because of their reduced glycogen stores but is certainly not more common in adults. Fomepizole inhibits ADH and therefore reduces ethanol metabolism. Ethanol prevents thiamine absorption, so fortification is of limited value.

Hoffman RS, Goldfrank LR: Ethanol-associated metabolic disorders. Emerg Clin North Am 1989;7:943–961.

CHAPTER **65**

DISULFIRAM AND DISULFIRAMLIKE REACTIONS

65.1. Answer: D Chemicals structurally similar to disulfiram (tetraethylthiuram disulfide), including carbon disulfide, tetramethylthiuram disulfide (thiram), and tetramethylthiuram monosulfide, were recognized in the early 1900s as a cause for disulfiramlike reactions with ethanol. Many of these chemicals were used in the rubber industry as catalytic accelerators for the vulcanization process by which rubber is stabilized by the addition of sulfur. Workers exposed to these chemicals who then consumed ethanol developed symptoms of the disulfiram–ethanol reaction.

Williams EE: Effects of alcohol on workers with carbon disulfide. JAMA 1937;109:1472–1473.

65.2. Answer: B Disulfiram inhibits dopamine β-hydroxylase, an enzyme necessary for norepinephrine synthesis. This may account for a substantial part of its clinical toxicity.

65.3. Answer: C Disulfiram irreversibly inhibits aldehyde dehydrogenase. In order for acetaldehyde to be metabolized, new aldehyde dehydrogenase must be synthesized.

Vallari RC, Pietruszko R: Human aldehyde dehydrogenase: Mechanism of inhibition of disulfiram. Science 1982;216:637–639.

65.4. Answer: D Most patients remain at risk for a disulfiram–ethanol reaction for 1 to 2 weeks following cessation of disulfiram therapy. The duration of disulfiram's inhibition of aldehyde dehydrogenase is partially dependent on the dose ingested. A 500-mg dose functionally inhibits aldehyde dehydrogenase up to 3 to 4 days, a 1000-mg dose up to 5 to 6 days, and a 1500-mg dose up to 7 to 8 days. There are sustained-release disulfiram preparations. Following a subcutaneous dose of 2 g of disulfiram, a patient had an adverse reaction to oral ethanol at 21 days following the injection.

65.5. Answer: B Calcium carbimide (citrated calcium carbimide) is an aldehyde dehydrogenase inhibitor; along with disulfiram, this drug is also used in the management of alcoholism.

65.6. Answer: C Ingestion of ethanol following ingestion of various species of mushrooms can cause symptoms of a disulfiram–ethanol reaction. The classic mushroom species producing this reaction are the *Coprinus* mushrooms including *C. atramentarius, C. insignis, C. variegatus,* and *C. quadrifidus.* The metabolite of coprine, 1-aminocyclopropanol, inhibits aldehyde dehydrogenase activity in a similar fashion to disulfiram.

65.7. Answer: A Disulfiram is an inhibitor of cytochrome P450 2E1, the isozyme responsible for ethanol metabolism. Disulfiram does not inhibit cytochrome P450 2C9, 2C19, 2D6, or 3A4 activity.

Kharasch ED, Hankins DC, Jubert C, et al: Lack of single-dose disulfiram effect on cytochrome P-450 2C9, 2C19, 2D6, and 3A4 activities: Evidence for specificity toward P-450 2E1. Drug Metab Dispos 1999;27:717–723.

65.8. Answer: E Diethyldithiocarbamate, a disulfiram metabolite, is available as the chelator Dithiocarb. Although animal data and human case series suggest that diethyldithiocarbamate may be an effective chelator for the treatment of nickel carbonyl poisoning, no well-controlled human trial has evaluated this therapy. Because disulfiram increases nickel absorption in humans, it would be prudent to use diethyldithiocarbamate in the treatment of poisoning by the highly toxic chemical nickel carbonyl and not elemental or inorganic nickel poisoning.

Bradberry SM, Vale JA: Therapeutic review: Do diethyldithiocarbamate and disulfiram have a role in acute nickel carbonyl poisoning? J Toxicol Clin Toxicol 1999;37:259–264.

Sunderman FW: Use of sodium diethyldithiocarbamate in the treatment of nickel carbonyl poisoning. Ann Clin Lab Sci 1990; 20:12–21.

65.9. Answer: C Halitosis and skin odor described as having a sulfur or garlic smell is a common side effect of chronic disulfiram therapy. Disulfiram therapy increases concentrations of nickel in human body fluids. Disulfiram therapy can cause increased serum cholesterol.

Hopfer SM, Linden JV, Rezuke WN, et al: Increased nickel concentrations in body fluids of patients with chronic alcoholism during disulfiram therapy. Res Commun Chem Pathol Pharmacol 1987;55:101–109.

Major LF, Goyer PF: Effects of disulfiram and pyridoxine on serum cholesterol. Ann Intern Med 1978;88:53–56.

65.10. Answer: C NAD^+ is reduced to NADH during the oxidation of both ethanol and acetaldehyde using the enzymes alcohol dehydrogenase and aldehyde dehydrogenase, respectively.

Eneanya DI, Bianchine JR, Duran DO, et al: The actions and metabolic fate of disulfiram. Annu Rev Pharmacol Toxicol 1981; 21:575–596.

CHAPTER 66

TOXIC ALCOHOLS

66.1. Answer: B Patients who have ingested antifreeze often have a fluorescent urine because of fluorescein added to the product to aid in detecting radiator leaks.

Winter ML, Ellis MD, Snodgrass WR: Urine fluorescence using a Wood's lamp to detect the antifreeze additive sodium fluorescein: A qualitative adjunctive test in suspected ethylene glycol ingestions. Ann Emerg Med 1990;19:663–667.

66.2. Answer: D The retinal toxicity from methanol has been attributed to the metabolism of methanol to formic acid. Formate may inhibit the cytochrome oxidase chain, increasing lactate production and acidosis at the cellular level.

Sejersted OM: Formate concentrations in plasma from patients poisoned with methanol. Acta Med Scand 1983;213:105–110.

66.3. Answer: E Continuous arteriovenous hemofiltration is an effective alternative to hemodialysis in situations where hemodialysis cannot be performed.

Christiansson LK, Kaspersson KE, Kulling PEJ, Ovrebo S: Treatment of severe ethylene glycol intoxication with continuous arteriovenous hemofiltration dialysis. J Toxicol Clin Toxicol 1995;33: 267–270.

66.4. Answer: C Ethylene glycol is metabolized by alcohol dehydrogenase to oxalic acid.

Jacobsen D, Hewlett TP, Webb R, et al: Ethylene glycol intoxication: evaluation of kinetics and crystalluria. Am J Med 1988; 84:145–152.

66.5. Answer: D   The finding of ketones in the blood and urine in the absence of a metabolic acidosis, crystalluria, or an anion gap would be suggestive of an isopropanol ingestion.

Daniel DR, McAnalley BH, Garriott JC: Isopropyl alcohol metabolism after acute intoxication in humans. J Anal Toxicol 1981; 5:110–112.

66.6. Answer: D   Ethylene glycol has the highest degree of renal clearance of the listed alcohols. Good hydration alone will allow for clearance of ethylene glycol as long as renal function is maintained.

Cheng JT, Beysolow TD, Kaul B, et al: Clearance of ethylene glycol by kidneys and hemodialysis. J Toxicol Clin Toxicol 1987;25: 95–108.

66.7. Answer: D   Ethanol can be given as an intravenous infusion as a 5 to 10% solution. The loading dose is 0.8 g/kg, and the maintenance dose is 130 mg/kg/h. Ethanol can also be administered orally. The goal of therapy is to achieve a blood ethanol level of 100 to 150 mg/dL.

Noker PE, Eells JT, Tephly TR: Methanol toxicity: Treatment with folic acid and 5-formyltetrahydrofolic acid. Alcoholism Clin Exp Res 1980;4:378–383.

66.8. Answer: A   The administration of bacteriostatic sodium chloride, which contains benzyl alcohol, has been associated with causing central nervous system toxicity, respiratory distress, hypotension, and renal and hepatic failure in the neonate. Benzyl alcohol is metabolized to benzoic acid and hippuric acid.

Gershanik JJ, Boecler G, Ensley H, et al: The gasping syndrome and benzyl alcohol poisoning. N Engl J Med 1982;307: 1384–1388.

66.9. Answer: D   A prolonged QTc interval has been reported with ethylene glycol poisoning. This is a result of hypocalcemia from loss of calcium as insoluble calcium oxalate.

Catchings TT, Beamer WC, Lundy L: Adult respiratory distress syndrome secondary to ethylene glycol ingestion. Ann Emerg Med 1985;14:594–596.

66.10. Answer: A   Calcium oxalate monohydrate crystals are very similar in appearance to sodium urate crystals. They are often prism- or needlelike in shape.

Parry MF, Wallach R: Ethylene glycol poisoning. Am J Med 1974;57:143–150.

CHAPTER 67

COCAINE

67.1. Answer: C   When conscious dogs were given cocaine, all interventions that corrected hyperthermia (diazepam, cooling) improved survival. Interventions that corrected hypertension and tachycardia (propranolol) or acidosis (bicarbonate) tended to have no beneficial effect or even worsen toxicity. This experiment has

been replicated in other models and serves as the basis for current treatment regimens.

Catravas JD, Waters IW: Acute cocaine intoxication in the conscious dog: Studies on the mechanism of lethality. J Pharmacol Exp Ther 1981;217:350–356.

67.2. Answer: E   Cocaine produces myocardial ischemia by a variety of mechanisms. In addition to the mechanisms listed, rhythms that result in poor perfusion, dissection of the coronary arteries, and heightened receptor sensitivity during the withdrawal period have all been proposed as mechanisms of cocaine toxicity.

Hollander JE: Management of cocaine associated myocardial ischemia. N Engl J Med 1995;333:1267–1272.

67.3. Answer: D   Although comparative trials of interventions for body packers have not been performed, any approach to patients with large gastrointestinal quantities of cocaine must be both safe and rapid. Surgery is indicated only in the presence of symptoms of mechanical bowel obstruction. Observation alone and bulk laxative therapy act slowly and provide poorly defined endpoints. Although activated charcoal is useful for bags that may have ruptured, it offers little benefit with regard to reducing transport time. Thus, whole-bowel irrigation with intermittent activated charcoal is the preferred therapy.

Hoffman RS, Smilkstein MJ, Goldfrank LR: Whole bowel irrigation and the cocaine "bodypacker": A new approach to a common problem. Am J Emerg Med 1990;8:523–527.

67.4. Answer: A   The role of dopamine reuptake in cocaine toxicity was recently illustrated in a mouse experiment in which mice were genetically engineered to have either homozygous or heterozygous absence of the dopamine reuptake system. Homozygous mice had hyperlocomotion and poor weight gain and died at an early age but were insensitive to cocaine. This suggests that much of the psychomotor effects of cocaine result from the reuptake blockade of biogenic amines.

Giros B, Jaber M, Jones S, et al: Hyperlocomotion and indifference to cocaine and amphetamine in mice lacking the dopamine transporter. Nature 1996;379:606–612.

67.5. Answer: E   Although they have been used alone or in combination with benzodiazepines, no experimental evidence supports the use of drugs such as haloperidol or droperidol in cocaine toxicity. Several experimental models demonstrate the detrimental effects of blockade of the D_2 receptor. These drugs should be avoided.

Catravas JD, Waters IW: Acute cocaine intoxication in the conscious dog: Studies on the mechanism of lethality. J Pharmacol Exp Ther 1981;217:350–356.

Witkin JM, Godberg SR, Katz JL: Lethal effects of cocaine are reduced by the dopamine-1 receptor antagonist SCH 23390 but not by haloperidol. Life Sci 1989;44:1285–1291.

67.6. Answer: C   Both animal models and human investigations give evidence that strongly contraindicates the use of β-adrenergic antagonism in patients with cocaine toxicity. The resultant hypertension (from unopposed α-adrenergic tone) has been shown to exacerbate coronary vasospasm, raise diastolic blood pressure, and decrease survival. Theoretical, experimental, and clinical evidence supports the use of the other agents selected.

Guinn MM, Bedford JA, Wilson MC: Antagonism of intravenous cocaine lethality in nonhuman primates. Clin Toxicol 1980;16:499–508.

Lange RA, Cigarroa RG, Flores ED, et al: Potentiation of cocaine-induced coronary vasoconstriction by beta-adrenergic blockade. Ann Intern Med 1990;112:897–903.

Sand IC, Brody SL, Wrenn KD, Slovis CM: Experience with esmolol for the treatment of cocaine associated cardiovascular complications. Am J Emerg Med 1991;9:161–163.

67.7. Answer: B Numerous studies demonstrate that the direct effect of cocaine on the myocardium is blockade of phase 0 (rapid sodium influx) and phase 3 (delayed potassium rectifier) current, similar to the type IA and IC antidysrhythmic agents. This mechanism has important implications with regard to treatment of patients with cocaine-induced wide-complex dysrhythmias.

Bauman JL, Grawe JJ, Winecoff AP, Hariman RJ: Cocaine-related sudden cardiac death: A hypothesis correlating basic science and clinical observations. J Clin Pharmacol 1994;34:902–911.

Winecoff AP, Hariman RJ, Grawe JJ, et al: Reversal of the electrocardiographic effects of cocaine by lidocaine. Part 1. Comparison with sodium bicarbonate and quinidine. Pharmacotherapy 1994;14:698–703.

67.8. Answer: C A significant portion of cocaine is metabolized by plasma cholinesterase to form ecgonine methyl ester. All of the other ester anesthetics (such as choices **D** and **E**) and two of the neuromuscular blockers (choices **A** and **B**) are also metabolized by plasma cholinesterase. Competition could result in decreased metabolism of either or both.

Stewart DJ, Inaba T, Tang BK, Kalow W: Hydrolysis of cocaine in human plasma by cholinesterase. Life Sci 1977;20:1557–1564.

67.9. Answer: E Rhabdomyolysis typically occurs in the setting of acute cocaine toxicity that includes abnormal vital signs and psychomotor agitation. However, cocaine's direct vasospastic effects are sufficient to produce rhabdomyolysis in the absence of any of these findings.

Zamora-Quezada JC, Dinerman H, Stadecker MJ, Kelly JJ: Muscle and skin infarction after free-basing cocaine (crack). Ann Intern Med 1988;108:564–566.

67.10. Answer: B Agents that are used to adulterate cocaine have physical or pharmacologic properties that are similar to cocaine: white powders (starch, sugar, talc), sympathomimetics, and local anesthetics. Although thallium contamination has been reported, this is a rare event.

Insley BM, Grufferman S, Ayliffe HE: Thallium poisoning in cocaine users. Am J Emerg Med 1986;4:545–548.

Shannon MW: Clinical toxicity of cocaine adulterants. Ann Emerg Med 1988;17:1243–1247.

CHAPTER 68

AMPHETAMINES

68.1. Answer: C Chronic administration of MDMA causes permanent damage to serotonergic neurons in all animal models tested. These neurotoxic effects have not been well studied in humans. Indirect evidence of serotonergic effects includes the presence of lower levels of 5-hydroxyindoleacetic acid (5-HIAA) in the CSF of MDMA users than in controls. Clinical or histologic evidence of serotonergic neuron damage has not been reported in humans.

Molliver ME, Berger UV, Mamounas LA, et al: Neurotoxicity of MDMA and related compounds: Anatomic studies. Ann NY Acad Sci 1990;600:640–661.

Ricaurte GA, DeLanney LE, Irwin I, et al: Toxic effects of MDMA on central serotonergic neurons in the primate: Importance of route and frequency of drug administration. Brain Res 1988;446:165–168.

Ricaurte GA, Finnegan KF, Irwin I, et al: Aminergic metabolites in cerebrospinal fluid of humans previously exposed to MDMA: Preliminary observations. Ann NY Acad Sci 1990;600:699–710.

Schmidt CJ, Wu L, Lovenberg W: Methylenedioxymethamphetamine: A potentially neurotoxic amphetamine analogue. Eur J Pharmacol 1986;124:175–178.

68.2. Answer: D A case-controlled study substantiated the increased risk of primary pulmonary hypertension with amphetamine appetite-suppressant drugs, particularly with fenfluramine. The risk of pulmonary hypertension was increased 23-fold when the cumulative use of anorexic agents totaled more than 3 months. The exact cause of the pulmonary hypertension is unclear but is postulated to be related to serotonin's pulmonary vasoconstrictive effects.

Abenhaim L, Moride Y, Brenot F, et al: Appetite-suppressant drugs and the risk of primary pulmonary hypertension. N Engl J Med 1996;335:609–615.

Herve P, Launay J, Scrobohaci M, et al: Increased plasma serotonin in primary pulmonary hypertension. Am J Med 1995;99:249–254.

68.3. Answer: A Lead acetate may be used as a substrate for the synthesis of methamphetamine. Numerous cases of lead poisoning associated with methamphetamine abuse were reported in Oregon. Lead levels reported in these drug users were as high as 513 mg/dL, and some samples of illicit manufactured methamphetamine had lead contents as high as 60% by weight.

Allcott JV, Barnhart RA, Mooney LA: Acute lead poisoning in two users of illicit methamphetamine. JAMA 1987;258:510–511.

Chandler DB, Norton RL, Kauffman J, et al: Lead poisoning associated with intravenous methamphetamine use—Oregon, 1988. MMWR 1989;38:830–831.

68.4. Answer: C In the current epidemic, the chance of getting methamphetamine is much higher than in previous epidemics in the 1970s. "Ice" is typically greater than 80 to 90% pure and almost exclusively in the *dextro* isomer form, which has the most CNS activity. The ephedrine method, using pharmaceutical grade L-ephedrine, produces a product with few contaminants that is stereochemically pure. The production of the large crystal is possible by creating a supersaturated solution of methamphetamine hydrochloride.

Cho AK: Ice: A new dosage form of an old drug. Science 1990; 249:631–634.

Derlet RW, Heischober B: Methamphetamine. Stimulant of the 1990's? West J Med 1990;153:625–628.

68.5. Answer: E Necrotizing vasculitis is associated with amphetamine abuse, typically involving the small and medium-sized arteries. Progressive necrotizing arteritis can involve the central nervous, cardiovascular, gastrointestinal, and renal systems. Complications include cerebral infarction and hemorrhage, coronary disease, pancreatitis, and renal failure. The etiology of the arteritis remains unclear. Although various contaminants associated with parenteral drug abuse were postulated as potential etiologies, oral and IV amphetamine use in animal models is also associated with vasculitis, suggesting that this is a direct amphetamine effect.

Citron BP, Halpern M, McCarron MM, et al: Necrotizing angiitis associated with drug abuse. N Engl J Med 1970;283:1003–1011.

Rumbaugh CL, Bergeron RT, Scanlan RL, et al: Cerebral vascular changes secondary to amphetamine abuse in the experimental animal. Radiology 1971;101:345–351.

Rumbaugh CL, Fang HCH, Higgins RE, et al: Cerebral microvascular injury in experimental drug abuse. Invest Radiol 1976;11: 282–294.

68.6. Answer: B Khat, the fresh leaves and stems from the *Catha edulis* shrub, is one of the most commonly used drugs in eastern and central Africa and parts of the Arabian peninsula. Cathinone (benzylketoamphetamine), a more potent psychoactive compound, is the primary active agent. When the leaves and stems are dried, cathinone is converted to cathine (norpseudoephedrine), which is less potent.

Kalix P: Pharmacological properties of the stimulant khat. Pharmacol Ther 1990;48:397–416.

68.7. Answer: B In animal models, neuroleptic agents such as haloperidol appear to be superior to diazepam for the treatment of amphetamine toxicity. In clinical situations, diazepam appears to be very efficacious in the treatment of amphetamine toxicity. For treatment of cocaine toxicity, diazepam is superior to antipsychotic agents.

Derlet RW, Rice P, Horowitz BZ, Lord RV: Amphetamine toxicity: Experience with 127 cases. J Emerg Med 1989;7:157–161.

Derlet RW, Albertson TE, Rice P: Protection against *d*-amphetamine toxicity. Am J Emerg Med 1990;8:105–108.

Goldfrank LR, Hoffman RS: The cardiovascular effects of cocaine. Ann Emerg Med 1991;20:165–175.

68.8. Answer: E Rhabdomyolysis from amphetamine toxicity usually results from agitation and hyperthermia. Acidification of

the urine will increase the urinary elimination of amphetamine but result in the precipitation of ferrihemate in the renal tubules and increase the risk of acute renal failure. These complications outweigh any potential benefits.

Curry SC, Chang D, Connor D: Drug- and toxin-induced rhabdomyolysis. Ann Emerg Med 1989;18:1068–1084.

Davis JM, Kopin IJ, Lemberger L, et al: Effects of urinary pH on amphetamine metabolism. Ann NY Acad Sci 1971;179:493–501.

68.9. Answer: A Amphetamine is a sympathomimetic agent whose use may result in tachycardia, hypertension, mydriasis, diaphoresis, agitation, and hyperthermia. Urinary retention is one of the symptoms associated with an anticholinergic agent.

68.10. Answer: C Mortality from amphetamine intoxication usually results from agitation, hyperthermia, metabolic acidosis, rhabdomyolysis, dysrhythmias, and multiorgan failure. Intracranial hemorrhage may be secondary to vasculitis or to the increase in blood pressure. Similarly, aortic dissection may also be secondary to hypertension and tachycardia. Hypothermia is not a manifestion of amphetamine toxicity.

Jordan SC, Hampson F: Amphetamine poisoning associated with hyperpyrexia. Br J Med 1960;2:844.

Kalant H, Kalant OJ: Death in amphetamine users: Causes and rates. Can Med Assoc J 1975;112:299–304.

Kendrick WC, Hull AR, Knochel JP: Rhabdomyolysis and shock after intravenous amphetamine administration. Ann Intern Med 1977;86:381–387.

CHAPTER **69**

PHENCYCLIDINE AND KETAMINE

69.1. Answer: D Most studies demonstrate that PCP and ketamine bind with high affinity to sites located in the cortex and limbic structures of the brain. They block the *N*-methyl-D-aspartate (NMDA) receptors at serum concentrations encountered clinically.

Vincent JP, Kartalovski B, Geneste P, et al: Interaction of phencyclidine ("angel dust") with a specific receptor in rat brain membranes. Proc Natl Acad Sci USA 1979;76:4678–4682.

Zukin SR, Zukin RS: Specific [³H]phencyclidine binding in rat central nervous system. Proc Natl Acad Sci USA 1979;76: 5372–5376.

69.2. Answer: D The brochodilating effects of ketamine are produced via its ability to inhibit monoamine reuptake. All the others result from ketamine's inhibition of the NMDA receptor.

Jentsch JD, Roth RH. The neuropsychopharmacology of phencyclidine: From NMDA receptor hypofunction to the dopamine hypothesis of schizophrenia. Neuropsychopharmacology 1999;20: 201–225.

69.3. Answer: B Ketamine has approximately 1/10 the potency of PCP. Peak concentrations occur within 1 minute of IV administration and within 5 minutes of a 5 mg/kg IM injection. Ketamine distributes immediately into the CNS with the duration of its hypnotic and anesthetic effects resulting principally from its redistribution from the brain to other tissues. Recovery time averages 15 minutes for IV administration. Ketamine is extensively metabolized in the liver by the cytochrome P450 isozymes. The major pathway involves its *N*-demethylation to norketamine, a metabolite with one-third the anesthetic potency of ketamine. Commercially available preparations of ketamine contain equal concentrations of the two enantiomers. In a randomized double-blind evaluation of these two enantiomers on patients undergoing surgery, the D(+)-isomer of ketamine was a more effective anesthetic.

White PF, Way WL, Trevor AJ: Ketamine—Its pharmacology and therapeutic uses. Anesthesiology 1982;56:119–136

Zsigmond EK, Domino EF: Ketamine. Clinical pharmacology, pharmacokinetics and current clinical uses. Anesth Rev 1980;7: 13–33.

69.4. Answer: E   Molecules similar to PCP in structure cross-react with the PCP immunoassay. Some of the metabolites of PCP, such as PCE, PHP, TCP, and its pyrrolididine derivative, TCPy, cross-react with the immunoassay at concentrations 30 times higher than those utilized to detect PCP. Dextromethorphan and its metabolite dextrorphan also cross-react with Syva EMIT and TDx PCP immunoassays.

Warner A: Dextromethorphan: Analyte of the month. In: American Association of Clinical Chemistry: In Service Training and Continuing Education. 1993;14:27–28.

69.5. Answer: C   Data indicate that NMDA antagonists produce effects on behavior, sensation, and cognition that resemble aspects of endogenous psychoses, particularly schizophrenia. The behavioral abnormalities were first observed in studies in the late 1950s when PCP, administered to healthy volunteers, generated a form of organic psychosis that mimicked schizophrenia. When the drug was administered to schizophrenic patients, it uniformly intensified their primary symptoms of profound disorganization, some of these symptoms lasting for weeks.

Luby EG, Cohen BD, Rosenbaum G, et al: Study of a new schizophrenomimetic drug—Sernyl. AMA Arch Neurol Psychiatr 1959; 129:363–369.

Olney JW, Newcomer JW, Farber NB: NMDA receptor hypofunction model of schizophrenia. J Psych Res 1999;33:523–533.

69.6. Answer: A   Most toxins that cause CNS stimulation, including amphetamine and cocaine, cause mydriasis. PCP frequently causes miosis.

69.7. Answer: A   Neurologic, electroencephalographic, and pharmacologic testing demonstrates that PCP and ketamine cause diminution in all sensory modalities in a dose-dependent fashion. The NMDA receptor is also responsible for the development of the neuronal organization of the central nervous system.

69.8. Answer: E   The NMDA receptor is responsible for the development of the neuronal organization of the central nervous system. It is linked to hypoxic/ischemic brain injury by mediating

calcium influx, a final pathway in cell death. NMDA antagonists such as PCP are demonstrated to block hypoxic brain injury from stroke and trauma, and dementia. In a rat model of ischemic stroke, PCP had a protective effect on the brain, demonstrated by a decreased rate of seizure activity. Human trials fail to confirm this benefit.

Barone FC, Price WJ, Jakobsen S, et al: Pharmacological profile of a novel neuronal calcium channel blocker includes cerebral damage and neurological deficits in rat focal ischemia. Pharmacol Biochem Behav 1994;48:77–85.

69.9. Answer: D   Nine percent of phencyclidine is excreted unchanged in the urine. PCP is very lipophilic, it has a large volume of distribution, only about 65% is protein bound, and renal elimination is increased with urinary acidification.

Cook CE, Brine DR, Jeffcoat AR, et al: Phencyclidine disposition after intravenous and oral doses. Clin Pharmacol Ther 1982;31: 625–634.

69.10. Answer: B   Of the techniques commonly used for gastric decontamination, only activated charcoal is effective in the treatment of phencyclidine poisoning. Phencyclidine partitions into stomach acid, where activated charcoal has been shown to adsorb the phencyclidine, preventing absorption/reabsorption and increasing its nonrenal clearance.

Picchioni AL, Consroe PF: Activated charcoal: A phencyclidine antidote, or hog in dogs. N Engl J Med 1979;300:202.

Jackson EJ: Phencyclidine pharmacokinetics after a massive overdose. Ann Intern Med 1989;111:613–615.

CHAPTER **70**

LYSERGIC ACID DIETHYLAMIDE AND OTHER HALLUCINOGENS

70.1. Answer: C   Benzodiazepines remain the cornerstone of therapy, as the sedating effect will diminish both endogenous and exogenous sympathetic effects. A pure β-adrenergic antagonist is relatively contraindicated, as many hallucinogens have both α and β sympathetic effects. Unopposed α-adrenergic-mediated hypertension may develop from the use of a pure β antagonist or labetalol. Haloperidol may be useful in many patients but has several limitations, inlcuding the production of acute dystonic reactions and the potential for inadequate treatment if the hallucinations are caused by sedative-hypnotic or ethanol withdrawal.

Kulig K: LSD. Emerg Med Clin North Am 1990;8:551–558.

Miller PL, Gay GR, Ferris KC, Anderson S: Treatment of acute adverse psychedelic reactions: "I've tripped and I can't get down." J Psychoactive Drugs 1992;24:277–279.

70.2. Answer: A   An illusion is a mental impression that is derived from misinterpretation of an actual experience. A hallucination is a false perception that has no basis in the external environment. Both can be drug induced or result from other causes. Hallucinogens are a diverse group of drugs that cause hallucinations without clouding the patient's sensorium. Hallucinogens have been used for thousands of years by different cultures, largely for religious experiences. Hallucinations may occur in children.

Schultes RE, Hofmann A. Plants of the Gods. Rochester, VT: Healing Arts Press, 1992.

Strassman RJ: Hallucinogenic drugs in psychiatric research and treatment. J Nerv Ment Dis 1995;183:127–138.

70.3. Answer: B Serotonin (5-hydroxytryptamine) has many complex actions in the brain including the modulation of mood, cognition, personality, affect, appetite, motor function, sexual activity, temperature regulation, pain perception, and sleep induction. 5-HT$_2$ receptors are most closely implicated in hallucinations, although dopamine may play a role. The serotonin syndrome is caused by serotonin excess at the 5-HT$_1$ receptor subtype and is therefore unlikely to develop following the use of LSD.

Harrington MA, Zhong P, Garlow SJ, Ciarnello RD: Molecular biology of serotonin receptors. J Clin Psychiatry 1992;53(Suppl 10):8–27.

70.4. Answer: B Sympathomimetic effects are common and occur shortly after ingestion and often precede the hallucinogenic effects. Findings may include dilated pupils, tachycardia, hypertension, tachypnea, hyperthermia, diaphoresis, piloerection, dizziness, hyperactivity, ataxia, altered mental status, and coma.

70.5. Answer: B LSD or related compounds are found naturally in several species of morning glory or Hawaiian baby woodrose (*Rivea corymbosa* and *Ipomoea violacea,* respectively). Morning glory seeds contain lysergic acid hydroxyethylamide, which has 1/10 the hallucinogenic potency of LSD.

70.6. Answer: C LSD is a colorless, tasteless, odorless powder that is water soluble and is readily absorbed by the gastrointestinal tract. It has an elimination half-life of about 2.5 hours and is metabolized via the liver and excreted predominantly as a pharmacologically inactive compound. Only small amounts are eliminated unchanged in the urine. It does not alter glucose utilization in the brain.

70.7. Answer: C The major structural classes of hallucinogens are the lysergamides, indolealkylamines, phenylethylamines, and cannabinols. Lysergamides include LSD and lysergic acid hydroxyethylamide (ololiuqi). Psilocybin, *N,N*-dimethyltryptamine, and bufotenine are the major indolealkylamines. The most significant phenylethylamines include mescaline and amphetamine derivatives such as MDMA. Theophylline and caffeine are methylxanthines.

Abraham HD, Aldridge AM, Gogia P: The psychopharmacology of hallucinogens. Neuropsychopharmacology 1996;14:285–298.

70.8. Answer: B Peyote (*Lophophora williamsii*) is a small blue-green spineless cactus that grows in dry and rocky slopes throughout the southwestern United States and northern Mexico.

Peyote buttons are the round fleshy tops of the cactus, which have been sliced off and dried. Mescaline is the active hallucinogenic alkaloid found in the peyote cactus. Mescaline is absorbed rapidly from the gastrointestinal tract. The buttons are bitter tasting, and nausea, vomiting, and diaphoresis often precede the psychological effects.

Bullis RK: Swallowing the scroll: Legal implications of the recent supreme court peyote cases. J Psychoactive Drugs 1990;22:325–332.

Schwartz RH, Smith DE: Hallucinogenic mushrooms. Clin Pediatr 1988;27:70–73.

70.9. Answer: C DMT (*N,N*-dimethyltryptamine) is a potent short-acting hallucinogen that must be smoked, snorted, or administered parenterally. Toads of the genus *Bufo* have secretions that contain a complex mixture of cardiotoxins and hallucinogens such as bufotenine. Severe reactions and death have occurred from oral ingestion of the toad secretion. MDMA, or ecstasy, produces illusions, not hallucinations, and is therefore not similar to LSD. Mescaline derives from peyote (*Lophophora williamsii*), a small, brown, spineless cactus. LSD is a schedule I substance and has no clinical role.

70.10. Answer: E The psychological effects of LSD are dose related and include changes in arousal, emotion, perception, thought process, and self-image. The response to the drug is related to the person's mindset, emotions, or expectations at the time and can be altered by the group or setting. The person experiencing the effects of a hallucinogen is usually fully awake, alert, and oriented but confronted with diverse perceptual anomalies and varied sensations. The altered perceptual conditions typically last for 6 to 12 hours.

CHAPTER 71

MARIJUANA

71.1. Answer: B The naturally occurring endocannabinoids anandamide and 2-arachidonolylglycerol as well as cannabinoid receptors CB1 and CB2 have been identified in both humans and animals.

Ameri A. The effects of cannabinoids on the brain. Prog Neurobil 1999;58:315–348.

Axelrod J, Felder CC; Cannabinoid receptors and their endogenous agonist anadamide Neurochem Res 1998;23:575–581.

71.2. Answer: C There are no studies showing a positive effect of marijuana on diabetes. There have been a number of studies, limited by lack of a control or standard dose of marijuana, that show that marijuana may be efficacious in the treatment of asthma, glaucoma, nausea, and anorexia, especially that associated with AIDS.

Beal JE, Olson R, Laubenstein L, et al: Dronabinol as a treatment for anorexia associated with weight loss in patients with AIDS. J Pain Sympt Manag 1995;10:89–93.

Lane M, Vogel CL, Ferguson J, et al: Dronabinol and prochlorper-azine in combination for the treatment of cancer chemotherapy-induced nausea and vomiting. J Pain Sympt Manag 1991;6: 352–359.

71.3. Answer: B Δ^9-THC is used to establish the potency of cannabis products and is the primary psychoactive substance in marijuana. Over 400 compounds are identified, but most have lit-tle or no effect.

Hawks RL: The constituents of *Cannabis* and the disposition and metabolism of cannabinoids. In: Hawks RL:The Analysis of Cannabinoids in Biological Fluids. NIDA Research Monograph 42. Washington, DC, USDHHS, USGPO, 1982, pp. 125–317.

Joyce CRB, Curry SH: The Botany and Chemistry of Cannabis. London, J&A Churchill, 1970, pp. 1–60.

71.4. Answer: D Nystagmus is associated with phencyclidine intoxication, which may also cause acute behavioral changes. The pupillary findings associated with marijuana are variable and may show miosis or mydriasis. Conjunctival injection is the most com-mon ophthalmic finding.

Benowitz NL, Jones RT: Cardiovascular and metabolic considera-tions in prolonged cannabinoid administration in man. J Clin Phar-macol 1981;21:214–223.

Ohlsson A, Lingren JE, Wahlen A, et al: Plasma delta-9-tetrahy-drocannabinol concentrations and clinical effects after oral and in-travenous administration and smoking. Clin Pharmacol Ther 1980; 28:409–416.

71.5. Answer: A Chronic bronchitis, chronic cough, tracheo-bronchial histopathologic changes, and sputum production were similar in chronic marijuana and tobacco smokers. Carboxyhemo-globin levels and tar inhalation and retention were greater in mari-juana smokers than in tobacco smokers.

Tashkin DP, Coulson AH, Clark VA, et al: Respiratory symptoms and lung function in habitual heavy smokers of marijuana alone, smokers of marijuana and tobacco, smokers of tobacco alone and nonsmokers. Am Rev Respir Dis 1987;135:209–216.

Wu TC, Tashkin DP, Djahed B, Rose JE: Pulmonary hazards of smoking marijuana as compared with tobacco. N Engl J Med 1988;318:347–351.

71.6. Answer: D Immunoassay and GC-MS techniques in com-bination are very accurate at detecting THC in urine. Screening cutoff levels vary according to the user, and confirmation cutoff is 15 ng/mL, although levels as low as 2 ng/mL can be detected.

Ellis GM, Mann MA, Judson BA, et al: Excretion patterns of cannabinoid metabolites after last use in a group of chronic users. Clin Pharmacol Ther 1985;38:572–578.

Schwartz RH, Hawks RL: Laboratory detection of marijuana use. JAMA 1985;254:788–792.

71.7. Answer: C Drug users have become very creative in the mixing of various substances. Phencyclidine has been a common adulterant to enhance the hallucinations associated with marijuana and may be responsible for some of the bizarre reactions noted.

Other substances mixed with marijuana include heroin, malt liquor, formaldehyde, and alcohol.

Greenberg MI: Clues to toxic culprits can be found in the street drug lingo. Emerg Med News 1996;17:8–13.

71.8. Answer: D Passive inhalation of marijuana smoke has been a defense against a positive urine drug screen. Studies have shown that depending on the concentration of smoke in the area where it is inhaled and the amount of time the person is present, urine drug screens may be positive for days after exposure.

Chiang CN, Barnett G: Marijuana pharmacokinetics and pharma-codynamics. In: Redda KK, Walker CA, Barnett G, eds: Cocaine, Marijuana, Designer Drugs: Chemistry, Pharmacology, and Be-havior. Boca Raton, FL, CRC Press, 1989, pp. 113–126.

Cone EJ, Johnson RE, Darwin WD, et al: Passive inhalation of marijuana smoke: Urinalysis and room air levels of delta-9-tetrahydrocannabinol. J Anal Toxicol 1987;11:89–96.

71.9. Answer: D Pregnancy outcome studies of drug abuse are difficult to perform because of the many confounding variables in-cluding nutrition, prenatal care, tobacco usage, and alcohol and other drug usage. Birth weight varies between low and high de-pending on the amount of marijuana smoked. Most of the data do point to neurobehavioral disorders appearing at different develop-mental milestones starting around age 3 years.

Fried PA: Behavioral outcome in preschool and school-age chil-dren exposed prenatally to marijuana: A review and speculative interpretation. In: Wetherington CL, Smeriglio VL, Finnegan LP, eds: Behavioral Studies of Drug-Exposed Offspring: Methodolog-ical Issues in Human and Animal Research. NIDA Research Monograph 164. Washington, DC, USDHHS, USGPO, 1996, pp. 242–260.

Richardson GA, Day NL, McGauhey PJ: The impact of prenatal marijuana and cocaine use on the infant and child. Clin Obstet Gy-necol 1993;36:302–318.

71.10. Answer: A THC is hydrophobic and is stored in lipid tis-sue. The high fat content of breast milk makes it an ideal vehicle for storing and transporting THC. Exposure during the first post-partum month is associated with decreased motor development at 1 year.

Astley SJ, Little RE: Maternal marijuana use during lactation and infant development at one year. Neurotoxicol Teratol 1990;12: 161–168.

Perez-Reyes M, Wall ME: Presence of delta-9-tetrahydrocannabi-nol in human milk. N Engl J Med 1982;307:819–820.

CHAPTER 72

SUBSTANCE WITHDRAWAL

72.1. Answer: C Alcohol withdrawal treated with antipsy-chotics has a mortality of 6%. These drugs lower the seizure threshold, impair heat regulation, and fail to correct the neurologic origin of this disorder. Although magnesium is often used to treat alcohol withdrawal, it has no demonstrable benefit in alcohol withdrawal unless a magnesium deficiency is first identified. Thiamine is important for maintaining proper glucose metabolism.

Athen D: Comparative investigation of chlormethiazole and neuroleptic agents in the treatment of alcoholic delirium. Acta Psychiatr Scand [Suppl] 1986;329:167–170.

72.2. Answer: E Baclofen withdrawal and overdose can produce seizures. The mechanism is unclear but may relate to its role as a $GABA_B$ agonist. $GABA_B$ receptors function as both presynaptic autoreceptors and postsynaptic inhibitory receptors.

Ogata N: Pharmacology and physiology of $GABA_B$ receptors. Gen Pharmacol 1990;21:395–402.

72.3. Answer: D Tachycardia, mild hypertension, mild diaphoresis, and agitation are characteristics that the two withdrawal states share. Without intensive supportive care and benzodiazepines, ethanol withdrawal carries a high mortality rate. Opioid withdrawal can be treated on an outpatient basis in all but the rarest circumstances and is rarely associated with complications. Patients with uncomplicated opioid withdrawal should not have an altered mental status.

Victor M, Adams RD: The effect of alcohol on the nervous system. Res Publ Assoc Res Nerv Ment Dis 1953:32:526–533.

72.4. Answer: D Alcohol withdrawal seizures are usually brief, generalized tonic-clonic seizures with a short postictal period and often are the first and only sign of withdrawal.

Victor M, Adams RD: The effect of alcohol on the nervous system. Res Publ Assoc Res Nerv Ment Dis 1953:32:526–533.

72.5. Answer: D If the ethanol level at the time of withdrawal is elevated, the patient will typically experience a more severe withdrawal syndrome. Concurrent illness and occult infection also are markers for morbidity and mortality. Phenytoin does not prevent alcohol withdrawal seizures.

Rathlev N, D'Onofrio G, Fish SS, et al: The lack of efficacy of phenytoin in the prevention of recurrent alcohol-related seizures. Ann Emerg Med 1994;23:513–518.

Vinson DC, Menezes M: Admission alcohol level: A predictor of the course of alcohol withdrawal. J Fam Pract 1991;33:161–167.

72.6. Answer: C Benzodiazepine withdrawal can occur up to 10 to 14 days after cessation of drugs with active metabolites and is similar to alcohol withdrawal in its presentation. Thiamine and magnesium have little role unless a deficiency is first identified. Phenobarbital is an excellent choice for this condition.

Robinson GM, Sellers EM, Janacek E: Barbiturate and hypnosedative withdrawal by a multiple oral phenobarbital loading dose technique. Clin Pharmacol Ther 1981;30:71–76.

72.7. Answer: A As with most drugs that display a withdrawal syndrome, the higher the maintenance dose of clonidine, the more likely withdrawal will occur. In particular, doses above 1.2 mg/d are implicated. Hallucinations and agitation can occur. Withdrawal occurs less frequently following use of the patch because a

reservoir of drug in the skin remains for a period of time. β-Adrenergic antagonism will exacerbate the syndrome.

Reid JL, Wing LM, Dargie HJ, et al: Clonidine withdrawal in hypertension: changes in blood pressure and plasma and urinary noradrenaline. Lancet 1977;1:1171–1174.

72.8. Answer: E Opioids, clonidine, and naloxone share common sites in the locus ceruleus. This accounts for their usefulness in treating toxicity or withdrawal from one or the other. However, opioids are not used to treat clonidine withdrawal because hypertension and tachycardia are the life-threatening manifestations but do not respond to opioids.

Gold MS, Redmond DE Jr, Kleber HD: Clonidine blocks acute opiate withdrawal symptoms. Lancet 1978;2:599–601.

72.9. Answer: D In neonates, the usual adult opioid withdrawal symptoms are accompanied by mottling, fever, myoclonic jerks, and seizures. This latter symptom is characteristic of opioid withdrawal in neonates only and occurs in roughly 8% of children born to mothers on methadone maintenance and only 1% of those born to mothers who use heroin. Paregoric appears to be more effective than diazepam in controlling and preventing these seizures while preserving the suck reflex.

Herzlinger RA, Kandall SR, Vaughan HG Jr: Neonatal seizures associated with narcotic withdrawal. J Pediatr 1977;91:638–641.

72.10. Answer: C γ-Hydroxybutyrate (GHB) is a compound found in mammalian brain, and a metabolite of GABA. A withdrawal syndrome that resolves in 3 to 12 days has been reported that appears consistent with a mechanism similar to alcohol withdrawal, ie, adaptation to chronic use of the drug and physiologic derangements on withdrawal. Occasionally, symptoms can be severe and require high doses of benzodiazepines. Almost all reported cases are in patients using GHB for body building, and it is rare in club users. This likely relates to the need for continuous dosing in order for dependence to occur.

Craig K, Gomes HF, McManus JL, Bania TC: Severe gamma-hydroxybutyrate withdrawal: a case report and literature review. J Emerg Med 2000;18:65–70.

CHAPTER 73

NICOTINE AND TOBACCO PREPARATIONS

73.1. Answer: C Nicotine lessens lower esophageal sphincter pressure, causing gastroesophageal reflux. Even at low doses it can cause nausea, diarrhea, and tremor. It stimulates neurohumoral, catecholamine, endocrine, and exocrine glandular production and release, and it facilitates attention and memory while reducing irritability.

Benowitz NL: Pharmacologic aspects of cigarette smoking and nicotine addiction. N Engl J Med 1988;319:1318–1330.

73.2. Answer: E Nicotine, an alkaloid, is poorly absorbed in the acidic environment of the stomach and well absorbed in the alkaline environments of the mouth and small intestine. It is also absorbed in the lung (smoking) and through the skin (green-leaf tobacco sickness).

Jaffe JH: Drug addiction and drug abuse. In: Gilman AG, Rall TW, Nies AS, Taylor P, eds: Goodman & Gilman's The Pharmacological Basis of Therapeutics, 8th ed. New York, Pergamon Press, 1990, pp. 545–549.

73.3. Answer: B Because nicotine is a weak base, its excretion can be enhanced by urine acidification. Only 10 to 20% of a nicotine dose is eliminated unchanged in urine, while 80 to 90% is altered by liver metabolism. The half-life of nicotine is 1 to 4 hours, but the half-life of its principal metabolite, cotinine, is 19 hours. Nicotine is metabolized by the P448 system and does not affect the P450 pathway. Other elements of cigarette smoke are probably responsible for P450 induction.

Benowitz NL: Pharmacologic aspects of cigarette smoking and nicotine addiction. N Engl J Med 1988;319:1318–1330.

Jaffe JH: Drug addiction and drug abuse. In: Gilman AG, Rall TW, Nies AS, Taylor P, eds: Goodman & Gilman's The Pharmacological Basis of Therapeutics, 8th ed. New York, Pergamon Press, 1990, pp. 545–549.

73.4. Answer: A Acute nicotine poisoning is likely to cause pallor by vasoconstriction. Other cardiovascular signs include hypertension, tachycardia, and atrial fibrillation. GI disturbances are the most common signs of nicotine toxicity. Early neurologic effects include headache, confusion, and seizures.

Saxena K: Suicide plan by nicotine poisoning: A review of nicotine toxicity. Vet Hum Toxicol 1985;27:495–497.

73.5. Answer: E The usual sequence of events in significant exposures is cardiovascular and neuronal excitation followed by depression of these systems.

Obsert BB, McIntyre RA: Acute nicotine poisoning. Pediatrics 1953;11:338–340.

73.6. Answer: E Although acidification is likely to enhance urinary excretion, it is not advisable because of the risk of rhabdomyolysis occurring during the excitatory phase of poisoning. Most exposures occur in children and cause mild or no symptoms. Serious toxicity is predicted by levels greater than 50 ng/mL. Although mecamylamine and other compounds are competitive antagonists of nicotine, they have never been used to treat human overdoses. Because of the risk of seizures, syrup of ipecac should never be used in nicotine overdose.

Borys DJ, Seltzer SC, Ling LJ: CNS depression in an infant after the ingestion of tobacco: A case report. Vet Hum Toxicol 1988; 30:20–22.

73.7. Answer: D Chewing tobacco is bought in rope-like twists and bite-size cakes (plugs). Most cigarettes are made from *N. tabacum,* but "Turkish" cigarettes are made from *N. rustica,* a tobacco with higher nicotine content. Kreteks are made from a combination of tobacco and cloves, and "Indian" tobacco is made from *Lobelia inflata.* Although dry snuff is still sniffed in England, most snuff users place it in the mouth.

Kunkel DB: The toxic emergency: tobacco and friends. Emerg Med 1985;17:142–158.

73.8. Answer: A Smokeless cigarettes (aerosol rods) are no longer made because they failed to deliver a measurable dose of nicotine to the serum. Gum, patches, and most recently nasal spray have been introduced in the United States as smoking-cessation aids. The oral inhaler is available outside the United States.

Sepkovic DW, Colosimo SG, Axelrad CM, et al: The delivery and uptake of nicotine from an aerosol rod. Am J Public Health 1986;76:1343–1344.

73.9. Answer: B Nicotine withdrawal produces a general dysphoria, and antidepressants have been used in the treatment of this withdrawal. Withdrawal symptoms also include constipation, agitation, and increased appetite. Heart rate falls by an average of 9 beats/min because of reduced catecholamine levels.

Hughes JR, Higgins ST, Bickel WK: Nicotine withdrawal versus other drug withdrawal syndromes: Similarities and dissimilarities. Addiction 1994;89:1461–1470.

73.10. Answer: C A metaanalysis of nicotine-replacement therapies indicates that nicotine gum is probably the least effective. Transdermal nicotine patches produce abstinence at 1 year in at least 4% of users, when compared to cold turkey abstinence of 1%. They also reduce weight gain by an average of 4.4 kg. Cigarette craving is the most persistent symptom in smoking cessation and is not effectively controlled by nicotine replacement.

Silagy C, Mant D, Fowler G, Lodge M: The effectiveness of nicotine replacement therapies in smoking cessation. Online J Curr Clin Trials 1994; Doc 113.

CHAPTER 74

FOOD POISONING

74.1. Answer: B Saxitoxin is produced by the dinoflagellate *Protogonyaulax tamarensis,* which causes paralytic shellfish poisoning (PSP). The shellfish implicated are usually clams, oysters, mussels, and scallops. Neurologic symptoms predominate and include paresthesias and numbness of the mouth and extremities, a sensation of floating, headache, ataxia, vertigo, muscle weakness, paralysis, and cranial nerve dysfunction manifested by dysphagia, dysarthria, dysphonia, and transient blindness. Gastrointestinal symptoms are less common and include nausea, vomiting, abdominal pain, and diarrhea. Fatalities may occur from respiratory failure, usually within the first 12 hours after symptom onset.

Levin R: Paralytic shellfish toxins: Their origin, characteristics and methods of detection: A review. J Food Biochem 1991;15: 405–407.

74.2. Answer: A Over a 5-year period, 11 of 133 people with *C. botulinum* food poisoning died. This rate of death per case is 8 of 100, several times higher than the next two most lethal causes: shellfish (3/100) and *V. cholera* (2.9/100).

Bean NH, Goulding JS, Lao G, Angulo FJ: Surveillance for food-borne-disease outbreaks—United States, 1988–1992. MMWR 1996;45:1–55.

74.3. Answer: D   The average time between contact with infected food (hamburger) and symptoms was 5 days (range 1–21 days). Typical symptoms of the prodromal illness included bloody diarrhea. The other causes of food poisoning all have preformed toxin in the food source, and typical symptoms occur within a few hours after ingestion.

Brandt HR, Fouser LS, Watkins SL, et al: *Escherichia coli* O157:H7–associated hemolytic uremic syndrome after ingestion of contaminated hamburgers. J Pediatr 1994;125:519–526.

74.4. Answer: D   Symptoms of ciguatera intoxication include acute onset of diaphoresis; abdominal pain with cramps, nausea, vomiting, and a profuse watery diarrhea. Neurologic symptoms include headaches; a feeling of loose, painful teeth; dysesthesias and paresthesias; tingling, and numbness of the tongue, lips, throat, and perioral area. A striking manifestation is the reversal of temperature discrimination: hot substances feel cold or cold substances feel hot. Patients report that their extremities feel as if they are burning or feel extremely warm superficially but cold under the skin.

Bagnis R, Kubergki T, Laugier S: Clinical observations on 3,009 cases of ciguatera (fish poisoning) in the South Pacific. Am J Trop Med Hyg 1979;28:1067–1073.

Withers NW: Ciguatera fish poisoning. Annu Rev Med 1982;33:97–111.

74.5. Answer: C   Patients with staphylococcal food poisoning rarely have a significant temperature elevation, although 16% of cases had a subjective sense of fever. Abdominal pain, nausea followed by vomiting, and diarrhea dominate the clinical picture. Diarrhea does not occur in the absence of nausea and vomiting. The mean incubation period is 4.4 hours with a mean duration of illness of 20 hours.

The correct matches for all the stems are **A**, botulism; **B**, monosodium glutamate; **C**, *Staphylococcus;* **D**, ciguatera; **E**, paralytic shellfish poisoning.

Holmberg SD, Blake PA: Staphylococcal food poisoning in the United States: New facts and old misconceptions. JAMA 1984;251:487–489.

74.6. Answer: A   Tartrazine is a food additive found in yellow food coloring and may cause an anaphylaxislike picture when ingested. The same is true for metabisulfites, which are used to preserve food and may be found in wine, salad (bars), fruit juice, and canned shrimp. Ten percent of asthmatics react to metabisulfites with severe bronchospasm. Monosodium glutamate is a flavor enhancer that can cause burning, facial pressure, headache, flushing, chest pain, GI symptoms usually limited to nausea and vomiting, and, infrequently, life-threatening bronchospasm and angioedema. Scombroid is caused by histamine development in fish left unrefrigerated. Symptoms of numbness, tingling, or a burning sensation of the mouth, dysphagia, and headache develop. Of particular significance for scombroid poisoning is the development of flush characterized by an intense diffuse erythema of the face, neck, and upper torso. Rarely, pruritus, urticaria, angioedema, or bronchospasm is also seen.

Allen DH, Baker GJ: Chinese restaurant asthma. N Engl J Med 1981;305:1154–1155.

Kim R: Flushing syndrome due to mahimahi (scombroid fish) poisoning. Arch Dermatol 1979;115:963–964.

Settipane GA: The restaurant syndromes. Arch Intern Med 1986;146:2129–2130.

Squire EN: Angioedema and monosodium glutamate. Lancet 1987;1:988.

74.7. Answer: B   *Salmonella* accounted for more than 20,000 reported cases of food poisoning for a 5-year period, which was more than four times the number of cases of the next most common cause of food poisoning, *Shigella* spp. In descending order of frequency, common causes include: *Salmonella* spp. 21,000, *Shigella* spp. 4800, *Clostridia* spp. 3800; hepatitis A 2100; *Staphylococcus* spp. 1700; *Campylobacter* spp. 700; scombroid 500; *B. cereus* spp. 400; Norwalk virus 300; *E. coli* 250; trichinosis 190; *Giardia* 180; ciguatera 170; group A *Streptococcus* 130; *C. botulinum* 130; shellfish 65; *cholera* sp. 34; heavy metals 26; *V. parahaemolyticus* 20; mushrooms 18.

Bean NH, Goulding JS, Lao G, Angulo FJ: Surveillance for food-borne-disease outbreaks—United States, 1988–1992. MMWR 1996;45:1–55.

74.8. Answer: D   Brevitoxin, produced by *P. brevis,* is a lipid-soluble, heat-stable polyether ladder toxin. It stimulates sodium flux through the sodium channel of both nerve and muscle.

Asai S, Krzanowski JJ, Lockey R, et al: The site of action of *Ptychodiscus brevis* toxin within the parasympathetic axonal sodium channel H gate in airway smooth muscle. J Allergy Clin Immunol 1984;73:824–828.

Levin R: Paralytic shellfish toxins: Their origin, characteristics and methods of detection: a review. J Food Biochem 1991;15:405–407.

74.9. Answer: C   The etiologic agent of amnestic shellfish poisoning (ASP) is domoic acid, a structural analogue of glutamic and kainic acid, produced by the diatom *N. pungens.* ASP is characterized by GI symptoms of nausea, vomiting, abdominal cramps, and diarrhea and neurologic symptoms of memory loss and, less frequently, coma, seizures, hemiparesis, ophthalmoplegia, purposeless chewing, and grimacing. The mortality rate is 2%, with death most frequently occurring in older patients who suffer more severe neurologic symptoms. Ten percent of victims may suffer long-term anterograde memory deficits as well as motor and sensory neuropathy.

The correct matches are **A**, scombroid; **B**, tetrodotoxin and paralytic shellfish poisoning (saxitoxin); **C**, domoic acid, amnestic shellfish poisoning; **D**, brevitoxin (neurotoxic shellfish poisoning) and ciguatoxin; **E**, *E. coli* O157:H7 and hemolytic uremic syndrome.

Teitelbaum JS, Zatorre RJ, Carpenter S, et al: Neurologic sequelae of domoic acid intoxication due to ingestion of contaminated mussels. N Engl J Med 1990;322:1781–1787.

Perl TM, Bedard L, Kosatsky T, et al: An outbreak of toxic encephalopathy caused by eating mussels contaminated with domoic acid. N Engl J Med 1990;322:1775–1780.

74.10. The correct answers are: **A,** **3**; B, **1**; C, **5**; D, **2**; E, **4.**

Bagnis R, Kubergki T, Laugier S: Clinical observations on 3,009 cases of ciguatera (fish poisoning) in the South Pacific. Am J Trop Med Hyg 1979;28:1067–1073.

Brandt HR, Fouser LS, Watkins SL, et al: *Escherichia coli* O157:H7-associated hemolytic uremic syndrome after ingestion of contaminated hamburgers. J Pediatr 1994;125:519–526.

Centers of Disease Control and Prevention: *Bacillus cereus* food poisoning associated with fried rice at two child day care centers—Virginia 1993. JAMA 1994;271:1074.

Lee LA, Gerber AR, Lonsway DR, et al: *Yersinia enterocolitica* 0:3 infections in infants and children associated with the household preparation of chitterlings. N Engl J Med 1990;322:984–987.

St Louis ME, Morse DI, Potter ME, et al: The emergence of grade A eggs as a major source of *Salmonella* enteritis infections: New implications for the control of salmonellosis. JAMA 1988;259:2103–2107.

CHAPTER **75**

BOTULISM

75.1. Answer: B   The cranial nerves that are affected first are III, VI, IX, X, XI with diplopia, ptosis, blurred vision, and lateral rectus palsy. Neither the optic (II) or trigeminal (V) nerves are typically affected by botulinum toxin.

Terranova W, Palumbo JN, Breman JG: Ocular findings in botulism type B. JAMA 1979;241:475–477.

75.2. Answer: E   Because of the lethality of clinical botulism, the risks of hypersensitivity reactions, including anaphylaxis, are not considered contraindications to therapy. Pregnancy is also not considered a contraindication. Human botulism immune globulin has substantially fewer risks of hypersensitivity but is only effective for the initial treatment of an individual and, because it has long-lasting protective effect, prior treatment is not a contraindication for subsequent use of antitoxin. However, the pentavalent botulinum toxoid (A, B, C, D, and E), although only experimentally available for laboratory and military personnel, obviates the need for antitoxin following exposure to botulinum toxin.

Byrne MP, Smith LA. Development of vaccines for prevention of botulism. Biochimie 2000;82:955–966.

75.3. Answer: D   A descending symmetric paralysis is considered to be a classic finding in patients with foodborne botulism. An altered mental status should not be present unless the patient is or has been hypoxic, and the patient should be afebrile unless there is another cause for fever. Diarrhea is not present in many patients with botulism and is not useful in differentiating botulism from other foodborne disorders.

Terranova W, Palumbo JN, Breman JG: Ocular findings in botulism type B. JAMA 1979;241:475–477.

75.4. Answer: C   Honey is consistently found to contain *Clostridium* spores and has been implicated in at least 34% of the cases of infant botulism. Choices A, B, D, and E are possible, particularly if these foods are improperly canned; however, the illness would then be more consistent with foodborne botulism.

Midura TF. Update: Infant botulism. Clin Microbiol Rev 1996;9:119–125.

75.5. Answer: E   Respiratory support with intubation and ventilation will often be sufficient to allow the patient to survive the exposure. Botulinum antitoxin is not capable of reversing any respiratory depressant effects that precede the administration of the antitoxin. Edrophonium chloride will improve the clinical condition of the patient with myasthenia gravis but will only transiently improve the clinical condition of the patient with botulism. Penicillin and gastrointestinal decontamination are only of theoretical benefit.

Faich GA, Graebner RW, Sato S: Failure of guanidine therapy in botulism A. N Engl J Med 1971;285:773–776.

Tacket CO, Shandera WX, Mann JM, et al: Equine antitoxin use and other factors that predict outcome in type A foodborne botulism. Am J Med 1984;76:794–798.

75.6. Answer: A   The hallmark EMG findings in all forms of botulism are the presence of brief small abundant motor unit action potentials (BSAPs; or low-amplitude, short-duration potentials). Motor nerve conduction velocity remains normal because axon conduction is not affected. Primary muscle diseases also produce normal conduction velocity and a BSAP pattern, but in botulism serum levels of muscle enzymes and the muscle biopsies are normal. Posttetanic facilitation is noted in botulism as well as other entities such as Eaton Lambert and hypermagnesemia.

Valli G, Barbieri S, Scarlato G: Neurophysiological tests in human botulism. Electromyogr Clin Neurophysiol 1983;23:3–11.

75.7. Answer: B   Because the patient has an infected wound, a fever is often described. The presence of a fever is distinctly unusual in patients with foodborne botulism. Respiratory paralysis, dysphagia, and dysphonia are described with all forms of botulism. Gastrointestinal symptoms are found in many patients with foodborne botulism but are not found in patients with wound botulism.

Werner SB, Passaro D, McGee J, Schechter R, Vugia DJ: Wound botulism in California, 1951–1998: recent epidemic in heroin injectors. Clin Infect Dis 2000;31:1018–1024.

75.8. Answer: A   Botulinum antitoxin blocks the presynaptic calcium-dependent exocytosis of acetylcholine. Botulinum toxin has not been found to have any effect at motor endplates, nor does it alter the metabolic fate of acetylcholine. Although postsynaptic blockade appears to occur, it is caused by inhibition at the presynaptic level. Cholinesterase activity is not increased.

Humeau Y, Doussau F, Grant NJ, et al: How botulinum and tetanus neurotoxins block neurotransmitter release. Biochimie 2000;82:427–446.

75.9. Answer: A The most striking improvement reported following guanidine administration, 15 to 40 mg/kg/d, was an improvement in ocular function. Guanidine has been postulated to enhance acetylcholine release. Improvement in GI symptoms is not likely, and the drug can cause nausea and abdominal pain. Guanidine does not result in improvement in respiratory function. EMG studies have demonstrated slight improvement in skeletal muscle function.

Faich GA, Graebner RW, Sato S: Failure of guanidine therapy in botulism A. N Engl J Med 1971;285:773–776.

75.10. Answer: D When assessing a patient with descending paralysis, the Miller Fisher variant of the Guillain-Barré syndrome must be differentiated from botulism. This Guillain Barré variant also causes a descending paralysis. The distinction between the two entities is often made when protein is found in the cerebrospinal fluid of the patient with Guillain-Barré. None of the other choices would be expected to cause a descending paralysis. The gastrointestinal symptoms of both mercury and *Shigella* food poisoning are likely to be far more severe than those of botulism. Metallic material may be visible in the gastrointestinal tract with either lead or mercury poisoning. Clonidine overdose can cause respiratory compromise in children; however, the children typically start breathing following stimulation. Clonidine would also be expected to cause miosis, bradycardia, and hypotension, all of which would be unusual for a patient with botulism.

CHAPTER 76

MUSHROOMS

76.1. Answer: D Muscimol binds directly to the GABA$_A$ receptor, enhancing inward chloride ion currents. Ibotenic acid is decarboxylated to muscimol by the same process that decarboxylates glutamic acid to GABA. Both ibotenic acid and muscimol are found in mushrooms such as *Amanita muscaria*.

Olsen RW: The GABA postsynaptic membrane receptor–ionophore complex. Mol Cell Biochem 1981;39:261–279.

76.2. Answer: E Both *Amanita smithiana* (AS) and *Cortinarius orellanus* (CO) contain nephrotoxins. AS contains orelline and orellanine, and CO contains allenic norleucine. Neither toxic group is associated with hepatic compromise, but the *Amanita smithiana* does produce early (<3 h) gastrointestinal toxicity. Ingestion of either mushroom group may lead to renal compromise necessitating dialysis. Occasionally patients with CO-induced renal failure require long-term hemodialysis.

Schumacher T, Hoiland K: Mushroom poisoning caused by species of the genus *Cortinarius fries*. Arca Toxicol 1983;53:87–106.

Tulloss RE, Lindgren JE. *Amanita smithiana*—taxonomy, distribution and poisonings. Mycotaxon 1992;45:373–387.

76.3. Answer: C *Gyromitra esculenta* contains a toxin gyromitrin that, on hydrolysis, yields monomethylhydrazine. The hydrazine can react with pyridoxine, inhibiting GABA formation, which causes seizures. The mechanism of toxicity is felt to be identical to that of isoniazid.

Sotaniemi E, Hirvonen J, Isomaki H: Hydrazine toxicity in the human: Report of fatal cases. Ann Clin Res 1971;3:30–33.

76.4. Answer: B α-Amanitin causes toxicity at the cellular level by interfering with RNA polymerase II, which inhibits protein synthesis.

Sperti S, Montanaro L, Fiume L, Mattioli A: Dissociation constants of the complexes between RNA polymerase II and amanitins. Experientia 1973;29:33–34.

76.5. Answer: D The volva is often found just below ground level. This is important because it is the structure that helps distinguish *Amanita* spp. and several other toxic species from nontoxic mushrooms.

76.6. Answer: E *Coprinus atramentarius* contains coprine, the metabolite of which inhibits acetaldehyde dehydrogenase. Thus, following the ingestion of ethanol, acetaldehyde accumulates. This produces a characteristic "disulfiram" reaction consisting of nausea, vomiting, headache, flush, diaphoresis, tachycardia, and hypotension.

Carlson A, Henning P, Lindberg P, et al. On the disulfiram-like effect of coprine, the pharmacologically active principle of *Coprinus atramentarius*. Acta Pharmacol Toxicol 1978;42:292–297.

76.7. Answer: B *Clitocybe nebularis* can cause cholinergic symptoms of toxicity when ingested because it contains muscarine. Patients present with diaphoresis, miosis, bradycardia, hypersalivation, lacrimation, urination, and defecation. These effects can be reversed with the administration of atropine. Despite its name, *A. muscaria* contains little muscarine.

Carder CA, Wojciechlowski NJ, Skoutakis VA: Management of mushroom poisoning. Clin Toxicol Consult 1983;5:103–118.

76.8. Answer: E *Psilocybe cubensis*, or "magic mushrooms," can cause hallucinations if ingested or injected parenterally. These mushrooms contain psilocin and psilocybin, which are central serotonergic stimulants similar to LSD.

Curry SC, Rose MC: Intravenous mushroom poisoning. Ann Emerg Med 1985;14:900–902.

76.9. Answer: A Thioctic acid is not considered to be an effective antidote. Hypoglycemia is reported with the use of thioctic acid, although it is unclear if it is secondary to the drug or caused by hepatic failure.

Alleva FR: Thioctic acid and mushroom poisoning. Letter (followed by a comment by FC Bartter). Science 1975;187:216.

76.10. Answer: D *Gyromitra esculenta* would be most likely to cause toxicity at approximately 6 hours after ingestion. *Amanita muscaria* and *Clitocybe nebularis* would cause symptoms within 2 hours; *Armillariella mellea* is an edible nontoxic mushroom; and

Coprinus atramentarius would cause symptoms only after the consumption of alcohol.

Lampe, KF: Toxic fungi. Annu Rev Pharmacol Toxicol 1979;19: 85–104.

CHAPTER 77

HERBAL PREPARATIONS

77.1. Answer: E The definition of herbal preparation is unclear. The botanic definition of the term herb is specific for certain leafy plants without woody stems. However, herbal preparations often include nonherb plant materials, even animal and mineral products. Broadly, the term includes any "natural" or "traditional" remedy, but these terms are poorly defined. Many herbal preparations are used for their nonspecific adaptogenic properties and lack any disease-specific effects. Herbal preparations such as herbal stimulants and sedatives may contain active ingredients, but their intended use is without specific medicinal value.

77.2. Answer: D In 1994, Congress passed the Dietary Supplement and Health Education Act, which reduced the Food and Drug Administration's (FDA) oversight of products categorized as dietary supplements. This includes vitamins, minerals, herbals, amino acids, and any product that had been sold as a "supplement" before October 15, 1994. Herbal products can be marketed without any testing for efficacy or safety. The FDA must prove a herbal product is unsafe before it can be challenged. These products are manufactured without any federal standards of quality control, although good manufacturing standards are supposed to be promulgated. Although packaging claims to cure or prevent a specific disease are not permitted, claims detailing how a product affects the "body's structure or function" are acceptable. No FDA approval is required with regard to packaging or marketing.

Food and Drug Administration: Federal Register. Part II 21 CFR Part 101. Food labeling; Final Rule and Proposed Rules. December 28, 1995.

77.3. Answer: A Herbal preparation usage in the United States is increasing. Sales of herbal preparations in the US in 1999 were estimated at approximately $4 billion Although the prevalence of herbal preparation use in the United States may be higher among certain socioeconomic and cultural groups, herbal preparation use is not restricted to these groups. Herbal preparations continue to be the dominant form of healing in the developing world because of the high cost of "Western" medical treatment and the scarcity of "Western"-trained medical personnel. The World Health Organization estimates that 4 billion people, 80% of the world population, use herbal preparations for some aspect of primary health care. Peoples of all cultures have utilized herbal preparations to treat disease and to promote health since ancient times and perhaps prehistoric times.

77.4. Answer: A Most herbal preparations used in developed countries appear to be safe. In Hong Kong, herbal preparations accounted for 0.2% of hospital admissions despite their prevalence, 40 to 60% of the population. In the United Kingdom, a probable

association with exposure to herbals and toxicity was demonstrated in 32 cases out of 1070 inquiries. In a US ED study, 37% of respondents reported their physician was unaware of their herbal use. Many herbal stores are staffed by untrained personnel who may dispense incorrect medical advice and unfounded claims concerning their products.

Hung OL, Shih RD, Chiang WK, et al: Herbal preparation usage among urban emergency department patients. Acad Emerg Med 1997;4:209–213.

Perharic L, Shaw D, Colbridge M, et al: Toxicological problems resulting from exposure to traditional remedies and food supplements. Drug Safety 1994;11:285–294.

77.5. Answer: D Aconite (caowu and chuanwu) alkaloids are derived from the *Aconitum* plant. Aconite toxicity results from aconite alkaloids, including aconitine, mesaconitine, and hypoaconitine, which increase sodium influx through the sodium channel, delaying the final repolarization phase of the action potential and initiating premature excitation. Anecdotal case reports of aconite toxicity have suggested the use of amiodarone, flecainide, bretylium, and procainamide for tachydysrhythmias. Pharmacologic principles would suggest the use of a sodium channel blocker such as procainamide or flecainide. One case of aconite-induced refractory tachyarrhythmia was successfully managed with a ventricular assist device.

Tai YT, But PP-H, Young K, et al: Cardiotoxicity after accidental herb-induced aconite poisoning. Lancet 1992;340:1254–1256.

77.6. Answer: E Ch'an su is a traditional herbal remedy derived from the secretions of the parotid and sebaceous glands of a toad, *Bufo bufo gargarizans* or *Bufo melanosticus*. It is used as a topical anesthetic and cardiac medication. In New York City, it is also marketed as an aphrodisiac and is sold under names such as "Stone," "Love Stone," "Black Stone," and "Rock Hard." Ch'an su contains two groups of toxic compounds: cardioactive steroids consisting of bufadienolides, and bufotenine, a hallucinogenic compound. Digoxin-specific Fab (10 vials Digibind®) has been used to successfully treat ch'an su toxicity and should be empirically administered for any suspected case of ch'an su cardiotoxicity. Digoxin-specific Fab should also be empirically administered for toxicity associated with other herbal cardiac glycoside ingestions including oleander (*Nerium oleander*), squill (*Urginea maritima*), lily-of-the-valley (*Convallaria majalis*), and yellow oleander (*Thevetia peruviana*).

Brubacher JR, Ravikumar PR, Bania T, et al: Treatment of toad venom poisoning with digoxin-specific Fab fragments. Chest 1996;110:1282–1288.

77.7. Answer: C Herbal ecstasy contains ephedrine and is marketed as a natural stimulant. Reports of seizures, cardiovascular accidents, myocardial infarcts, and death are associated with its use. Ma-huang, Mormon tea, and squaw tea are common names for plants of the *Ephedra* genus that contain ephedrine.

CDC: Adverse events associated with ephedrine-containing products—Texas. MMWR 1996;45:689–693.

77.8. Answer: C Betel (*Areca catechu*) is chewed by an estimated 200 million people worldwide for its euphoric effect. The active ingredient is arecoline, a nicotinic agent and volatile alkaloid, which produces increased central acetylcholine. Arecoline is a bronchoconstrictor and may cause exacerbation of bronchospasm in asthmatic patients chewing betel nut.

Taylor RFH, Al-Jarad N, John LME, et al: Betel-nut chewing and asthma. Lancet 1992;330:1134–1136.

77.9. Answer: E Pyrrolizidine alkaloids are hepatotoxins found in many plant families. *Heliotropium* spp, *Senecio* spp, *Crotolaria* spp, and *Symphytum* spp are the most common sources of pyrrolizidine alkaloids. Conversion to the toxic, active principles probably occurs in vivo and probably involves metabolism in the liver to pyrroles, which serve as biologic alkylating agents. They cause hepatic venoocclusive disease, hepatomegaly, cirrhosis, and possibly hepatic carcinoma. Chronic low doses may cause pulmonary toxicity, resulting in pulmonary artery hypertension and right ventricular hypertrophy. Treatment of hepatic venoocclusive disease is supportive.

Huxtable RJ: Herbal teas and toxins: Novel aspects of pyrrolizidine poisoning in the United States. Perspect Biol Med 1980;24:1–14.

77.10. Answer: A Garlic is used as a traditional remedy for a host of infections and a treatment for hypertension, colic, and cancer. Side effects of garlic extracts have included contact dermatitis, gastroenteritis, nausea, and vomiting. Patients who are already taking anticoagulant medications should consume garlic with caution because of its antiplatelet metabolite, ajoene. Treatment remains supportive. Ginseng preparations have been used in China for the treatment of respiratory illnesses, gastrointestinal disorders, impotence, fatigue, and stress ("adaptogenic effect"). Its only recognized use in America is as an external demulcent. An estimated 6 million people regularly ingest ginseng in herbal teas or apply it as a cosmetic. Because of the lack of oversight in the health food industry, many ginseng products may not contain significant quantities of ginseng. In one study, 54 ginseng products were analyzed for ginseng. Sixty percent of those analyzed contained pharmacologically insignificant amounts of ginseng, and 25% contained no ginseng at all.

CHAPTER **78**

PLANTS

78.1. Answer: D Although poinsettia is in the Spurge (Euphorbiaceae) family, it does not produce a mechanical injury, but its milky sap may produce contact dermatitis. The mistletoes are in the mistletoe family (Loranthaceae or Viscaceae) and usually are responsible for gastrointestinal, not dermal, symptoms. The rest of the answers are true and pertain specifically to mechanical injury that can also be associated with introduction of chemical irritants depending on the species.

78.2. Answer: E Aconitine alkaloids are found in the ornamental plant monkshood, whereas foxglove, oleander, and lily-of-the-valley are examples of ornamental plants that contain cardiac glycosides. They are taxonomically unrelated. Their similar cardiac toxicity is achieved by different mechanisms: aconitine alkaloids activate sodium channels, and cardiac glycosides inactivate the sodium/potassium ATPase. Seizures are uncommon following poisoning with either agent.

78.3. Answer: A Despite its ominous name, the common household spider plant is nontoxic. Rosary pea (and Castor bean) contains a lectin that interferes with ribosomal RNA and protein processing in the gastrointestinal cells. Mayapple contains podophyllin, and Autumn crocus contains colchicine, both of which disturb microtubule processing and cellular mitosis. Pokeweed contains saponins that cause diarrhea.

78.4. Answer: C Pyrrolizidine alkaloids produce a venoocclusive syndrome resulting from proliferation of the intimal tissue of hepatic vasculature. In large, acute overdose they may produce centrilobular hepatic necrosis following their metabolism by the cytochrome P450 system in the liver. Hepatic congestion, ascites, and edema result from vascular occlusion. Patients may die, develop chronic cirrhosis and/or hepatic carcinoma, or recover completely. The pyrrolizidine alkaloids are transmitted in breast milk, but milk sickness refers to an illness transmitted through cow's milk after cows feed on white snakeroot *(Eupatorium rugosum)*. Neurolathyrism results from the ingestion of excitatory amino acids from certain plants.

Getahun H, Mekonnen A, TekleHaimanot R, et al: Epidemic of neurolathyrism in Ethiopia. Lancet 1999;354:306–307.

78.5. Answer: D Psyllium is contained in plantago plants and is a laxative bulking agent. All other plants listed produce peripheral neuropathy following acute (coyatillo or buckthorn and mayapple) or chronic ingestions (cassava and grass pea).

Spencer PS: Food toxins, AMPA receptors, and motor neuron diseases. Drug Metab Rev 1999;31:561–587.

78.6. Answer: B Hypoglycin A is responsible for "Jamaican vomiting sickness," which presents with vomiting, hypoglycemia, and hepatoxicity. Vomiting and brady- and tachydysrhythmias suggest cardiac glycosides or sodium channel effectors such as aconitine, veratradine, or grayanotoxins. St. John's wort results in photosensitivity. Pennyroyal oil with the ingredient pulegone and its metabolites results in hepatotoxicity.

78.7. Answer: A Water hemlock's cicutoxin is dialyzable, unlike coniine, ricin, or aconitine. Dock plant contains oxalates that may be responsible for renal calculi, a problem apparently more significant in animals than in humans.

78.8. Answer: A Phorbol esters are terpenoids found largely in the Euphorbiaceae or Spurge family. Not all plants with milky sap are spurges, but all spurges contain milky sap that causes various degrees of contact dermatitis and erosion of the gastrointestinal mucosa, depending on the species. Answer **B** is associated with ptaquiloside, **C** with physostigmine, **D** with *N*-methylcytosine, and **E** with pulegone.

78.9. Answer: E Ingestion of significant amounts of bittersweet nightshade or climbing nightshade alkaloids results in an anticholinergic syndrome. The other plants listed are nontoxic household plants.

78.10. Answer: B Yew berries (*Taxus* spp.) contain seeds that have sodium channel effects and produce brady- or tachydysrhythmias. The fleshy red aril is not toxic. Mistletoe, holly, and pokeweed are associated with gastrointestinal toxicity. Pokeweed ingestions can produce gastrointestinal, not cerebral, hemorrhage as well as leukocytosis. Significant chokecherry ingestions can result in cyanide toxicity. Venoocclusive disease is produced by pyrrolizidine alkaloids contained in over 350 plants, and comfrey or *Symphytum officinale* is probably the best known among these.

CHAPTER **79**

ARSENIC

79.1. Answer: D Lead toxicity produces a motor neuropathy that is not rapidly progressive and does not produce cardiovascular collapse. Arsenic and thallium toxicity share many common features, including gastrointestinal effects, a progressive neuropathy, which can be painful, and delayed alopecia. Mucous membrane irritation caused by oral ingestion of arsenic can mimic pharyngitis, whereas the multiorgan failure seen with acute arsenic toxicity can be misdiagnosed as sepsis.

Beckman KJ, Bauman JL, Pimental PA, et al: Arsenic-induced torsades de pointes. Crit Care Med 1991;19:290–291.

Bolliger CT, van Zijl P, Louw JA: Multiple organ failure with the adult respiratory distress syndrome in homicidal arsenic poisoning. Respiration 1992;59:57–61.

Heyman A, Pfeiffer JB, Willett RW: Peripheral neuropathy caused by arsenical intoxication: A study of 41 cases with observations on the effects of BAL (2,3-dimercaptopropanol). N Engl J Med 1956;254:401–409.

Le Quesne PM, McLeod J: Peripheral neuropathy following a single exposure to arsenic: Clinical course in four patients with electrophysiological and histological studies. J Neurol Sci 1977;32:437–451.

79.2. Answer: B These skin lesions have been detected in chronically exposed cases. Other skin manifestations include hypo- and hyperpigmentation, squamous cell carcinomas, and Bowen disease. All the other listed signs and symptoms are more typical of acute arsenic toxicity.

Cebrian ME, Albores A, Aguilar M, et al: Chronic arsenic poisoning in the north of Mexico. Hum Toxicol 1983;2:121–133.

Das D, Chatterjee A, Badal K, et al: Arsenic in ground water in six districts of West Bengal, India: The biggest arsenic calamity in the world. Part 2. Arsenic concentration in drinking water, hair, nails, urine, skin-scale and liver tissue (biopsy) of the affected people. Analyst 1995;120:917–924.

Tay CH, Seah CS: Arsenic poisoning from anti-asthmatic herbal preparations. Med J Aust 1975;2:424–428.

79.3. Answer: C Arsenobetaine is the most common form of arsenic found in seafood. It is excreted largely unchanged in the urine, producing arsenic levels as high as 1700 mg/L, but does not cause toxicity.

Arbouine MW, Wilson HK: The effect of seafood consumption on the assessment of occupational exposure to arsenic by urinary arsenic speciation measurements. J Trace Elem 1992;6:153–160.

79.4. Answer: E Intact skin provides a good barrier to inorganic arsenic absorption, although prolonged topical administration can irritate the skin, promoting systemic absorption. Better absorption occurs by all other routes mentioned, with inhaled arsenic particles being absorbed both via the lungs and by swallowed lung secretions.

Abernathy CO, Ohanian EV: Non-carcinogenic effects of inorganic arsenic. Environ Geochem Health 1992;14:35–41.

Robinson TJ: Arsenical polyneuropathy due to caustic arsenical paste. Br Med J 1975;3:139.

79.5. Answer: B Dimercaprol, a chelator, has been the standard therapy for inorganic arsenic toxicity and is the only chelator that can be administered parenterally to critically ill patients. Succimer (DMSA) is not FDA approved for arsenic chelation but has been used successfully in a few reported cases. Its role in treating critically ill patients remains to be defined. The effectiveness of penicillamine has never been proven, *N*-acetylcysteine remains an experimental therapy for arsenic toxicity, and deferoxamine is used to chelate iron.

Eagle H, Magnuson HJ: The systemic treatment of 227 cases of arsenic poisoning (encephalitis, dermatitis, blood dyscrasias, jaundice, fever) with 2,3-dimercaptopropanol (BAL). J Clin Invest 1946;25:420–441.

Lenz K, Hruby K, Drunl W, et al: 2,3-Dimercaptosuccinic acid in human arsenic poisoning. Arch Toxicol 1981;47:241–243.

79.6. Answer: A Squamous cell carcinomas are dermatologic cancers that develop after chronic exposure to arsenic. All the other manifestations have been reported in the weeks to months following an acute exposure.

Armstrong CW, Stroube RB, Rubio T, et al: Outbreak of fatal arsenic poisoning caused by contaminated drinking water. Arch Environ Health 1984;39:276–279.

Heyman A, Pfeiffer JB, Willett RW: Peripheral neuropathy caused by arsenical intoxication: A study of 41 cases with observations on the effects of BAL (2,3-dimercaptopropanol). N Engl J Med 1956;254:401–409.

Massey EW, Wold D, Heyman A: Arsenic: Homicidal intoxication. South Med J 1984;77:848–851.

Tay CH, Seah CS: Arsenic poisoning from anti-asthmatic herbal preparations. Med J Aust 1975;2:424–428.

79.7. Answer: C BAL, 3 to 5 mg/kg, is mixed in peanut oil and can be administered IM only.

Eagle H, Magnuson HJ: The systemic treatment of 227 cases of arsenic poisoning (encephalitis, dermatitis, blood dyscrasias, jaundice, fever) with 2,3-dimercaptopropanol (BAL). J Clin Invest 1946;25:420–441.

79.8. Answer: A   As^{3+} prevents the regeneration of lipoamide, a necessary cofactor in the conversion of pyruvate to acetylcoenzyme A. Arsenic^{5+} uncouples oxidative phosphorylation, and depletion of glutathione may potentiate As^{3+} toxicity. The inhibition of gluconeogenesis and thiolase are less important toxic effects of As^{3+}.

Buchet JP, Lauwerys R: Role of thiols in the in-vitro methylation of inorganic arsenic by rat liver cytosol. Biochem Pharmacol 1988;37:3149–3153.

Peters RA: I. Present state of knowledge of biochemical lesions induced by trivalent arsenical poisoning. Bull Johns Hopkins Hosp 1955;87:1–20.

Reichl F, Szinicz L, Kreppel H, et al: Effects of arsenic on carbohydrate metabolism after single or repeated injection in guinea pigs. Arch Toxicol 1988;62:473–475.

79.9. Answer: E   Thermometers contain elemental mercury. All others listed are potential sources or occupations for exposure.

Armstrong CW, Stroube RB, Rubio T, et al: Outbreak of fatal arsenic poisoning caused by contaminated drinking water. Arch Environ Health 1984;39:276–279.

Axelson O, Dahlgren E, Jansson CD, Rehnlund SO: Arsenic exposure and mortality: A case-referent study from a Swedish copper smelter. Br J Ind Med 1978;35:8–15.

Done AK, Peart AJ: Acute toxicities of arsenical herbicides. Clin Toxicol 1971;4:343–355.

79.10. Answer: D   All other malignancies listed have been associated with chronic arsenic exposure through either medicinal preparations, industrial or mining processes, or contaminated well water.

Bates MN, Smith SH, Hopenhayn-Rich C: Arsenic ingestion and internal cancers: A review. Am J Epidemiol 1992;135:462–476.

Bencko V, Symon K, Stalnik L, et al: Rate of malignant tumor mortality among coal burning power plant workers occupationally exposed to arsenic. J Hyg Epidemiol Microbiol Immunol 1980; 24:278–284.

Chen C, Chuang Y, Lin T, et al: Malignant neoplasms among residents of a Blackfoot disease-endemic area in Taiwan: High-arsenic artesian well water and cancers. Cancer Res 1985;45: 5895–5899.

Kasper ML, Schoenfield L, Strom RL, Theologides A: Hepatic angiosarcoma and bronchioloalveolar carcinoma induced by Fowler's solution. JAMA 1984;252:3407–3408.

CHAPTER **80**

LEAD

80.1. Answer: B   The major cause of anemia in lead poisoning is decreased hemoglobin synthesis. There is an increased production of red blood cells and increased release of reticulocytes to compensate for the decreased hemoglobin synthesis.

Agency for Toxic Substances and Disease Registry: The nature and extent of lead poisoning in children in the United States: a report to Congress. Atlanta, US Department of Health and Human Services, Public Health Service, DHHS report no. 99–2966, 1988.

80.2. Answer: D   Chronic low-level lead poisoning can simulate poliomyelitis, diphtheria, polyneuritis, and sickle cell anemia.

Nelson HS, Chisolm JJ: Lead toxicity masquerading as sickle cell crisis. Ann Emerg Med 1986;15:748–750.

80.3. Answer: C   Patients with blood levels of lead greater than 70 µg/dL or with clinical symptoms suggesting encephalopathy require inpatient chelation with intramuscular dimercaprol (BAL) at 300 to 450 mg/m^2/d and intravenous calcium EDTA at 1000 to 1500 mg/m^2/d.

Committee on Drugs: Treatment guidelines for lead exposure in children. Pediatrics 1995;96:155–160.

80.4. Answer: C   The patient with encephalopathy from lead poisoning may develop intractable seizures, cerebral edema, and coma with possible herniation.

Hagelmeyer CD, Moorhead JC, Horenblas L, Bayer MJ: Fatal lead encephalopathy following foreign body ingestion: Case report. J Emerg Med 1988;6:397–400.

80.5. Answer: C   Employees working in any metal-recycling plant are at risk for exposure to lead. Copy machine operators have exposures to ozone, photographers to silver, and telephone operators to excessive noise.

Baker EL, White RF, Pothier LJ, et al: Occupational lead neurotoxicity: Improvement in behavioural effects after reduction of exposure. Br J Ind Med 1985;42:507–516.

80.6. Answer: B   Lead is present in trace quantities in virtually every food and beverage that we utilize. Health foods have often been found to contain some of the highest concentrations of lead. As long as our ability to eliminate lead exceeds our exposure, lead levels will not rise into the range capable of causing illness. The major routes of entry into the body are by inhalation and ingestion. Children absorb a greater percentage of ingested lead than adults. Lead appears to concentrate in bone.

Crosby WH: Lead contaminated health food: The tip of an iceberg. JAMA 1977;238:1544.

80.7. Answer: A   Lead prevents the conversion of δ-aminolevulinic acid (ALA) to porphobilinogen and the conversion of coproporphyrinogen III to protoporphyrin IX by blocking the action of ALA dehydratase and coproporphyrinogen decarboxylase. This in turn causes ALA and coproporphyrin to accumulate in the urine, where they serve as "markers" for lead intoxication. Lead also blocks ferrochelatase from incorporating iron into protoporphyrin to form heme, which causes protoporphyrin to accumulate in the red blood cells. Lead also appears to inhibit the transport of iron across mitochondrial membranes in maturing normoblasts in the bone marrow, contributing to the accumulation of of protoporphyrin.

Chisolm JJ Jr, O'Hara DM: Lead Absorption in Children: Management Clinical and Environmental Aspects. Baltimore-Munich, Urban & Schwarzenberg, 1982, p. 229.

80.8. Answer: A Chelation therapy is not indicated in patients with blood lead levels less than 25 μg/dL although an environmental intervention should occur. Patients with blood lead levels of 25 to 45 μg/dL, need aggressive environmental intervention but should not routinely receive chelation therapy. The current recommended daily dose of succimer is 30 mg/kg/d for 5 days, followed by 20 mg/kg/d for 14 days. Children may need to be hospitalized for the initiation of therapy to monitor for adverse effects and initiate environmental abatement.

Committee on Drugs: Treatment guidelines for lead exposure in children. Pediatrics 1995;96:155–160.

80.9. Answer: E Succimer is considered to be the safest of the available chelating agents for lead poisoning. Mild gastrointestinal symptoms occur in about 12% of treated patients, generalized malaise in 5%, and elevated hepatic aminotransferases in about 4%.

Mann KV, Travers JD: Succimer an oral lead chelator. Clin Pharmacol 1991;10:914–922.

80.10. Answer: E All of the above statements about organic lead poisoning are correct.

Baselt RC, Cravey RH, eds: Tetraethyl lead. In: Disposition of Toxic Drugs and Chemicals in Man, 3rd ed. Littleton, MA, Yearbook Medical, 1989, pp. 778–779.

Bolanowska W, Piotrowski J, Garczynski H: Triethyl lead in the biological material in cases of acute tetraethyl poisoning. Arch Toxicol 1967;22:278–282.

CHAPTER **81**

MERCURY

81.1. Answer: C Caustic gastroenteritis is characteristic of the inorganic salts of mercury, in particular mercuric chloride. Mercurous chloride is less soluble and therefore less well absorbed than mercuric chloride.

Troen P, Kaufman SA, Katz KH: Mercuric bichloride poisoning. N Engl J Med 1951;244:459–463.

81.2. Answer: A This triad is characteristic of chronic or subacute inorganic mercury poisoning. Although anorexia, visual field constriction ("tunnel vision"), and acrodynia (morbilliform rash) are also findings in chronic inorganic mercury poisoning, respiratory distress, renal failure, and hematochezia are not.

Mortensen ME, Powell S, Sferra TJ: Elemental mercury poisoning in a household. MMWR 1990;39:424–425.

Taueg C, Sanfilippo DJ, Rowens B, et al: Acute and chronic poisoning from residential exposures to elemental mercury—Michigan, 1989–1990. J Toxicol Clin Toxicol 1992;30:63–67.

81.3. Answer: C The ingestion of elemental mercury by a healthy individual is without serious clinical consequences because of its poor gut absorption.

Magos L: Mercury. In: Seiler HG, Sigel H, eds: Handbook on Toxicity of Inorganic Compounds. New York, Marcel Dekker, 1988, pp. 419–436.

81.4. Answer: B Erethism, visual complaints, and tremor are characteristic complaints of chronic inorganic mercury poisoning.

Sunderman FW: Perils of mercury. Ann Clin Lab Sci 1988;18:89–101.

81.5. Answer: D Methoxyethylmercury, a long-chain alkyl organic compound, undergoes cleavage shortly following absorption to release the inorganic mercuric ion. Therefore, beyond absorption, this compound has clinical manifestations similar to the inorganic mercury compounds. Methylmercury is well absorbed from the gut (approximately 90%). The excretion of inorganic mercury is predominantly renal.

Klaassen C: Heavy metals and heavy-metal antagonists. In: Gilman AG, Rall TW, Nies AS, Taylor P, eds: Goodman & Gilman's The Pharmacological Basis of Therapeutics, 8th ed. New York, Pergamon Press, 1990, pp. 1592–1614.

Magos L: Mercury. In: Seiler HG, Sigel H, eds: Handbook on Toxicity of Inorganic Compounds. New York, Marcel Dekker, 1988, pp. 419–436.

81.6. Answer: E Mercuric chloride is the compound that, when ingested, leads to caustic gastroenteritis, hypovolemic shock, and acute tubular necrosis.

Troen P, Kaufman SA, Katz KH: Mercuric bichloride poisoning. N Engl J Med 1951;244:459–463.

81.7. Answer: D These characteristic pathologic findings in methylmercury poisoning manifest clinically as visual constriction and ataxia.

Takeuchi T: Pathology of Minamata disease. Acta Pathol Jpn 1982;32:73–99.

81.8. Answer: D Acrodynia is thought to be an idiosyncratic hypersensitivity reaction to the dermal application of inorganic mercury-containing preparations, particularly in children. Phenylmercury, an aryl organic mercury compound, behaves much like the inorganic compounds once absorbed because of the dissociation of the alkyl side chain from the mercuric ion.

Warkany J, Hubbard DM: Adverse mercurial reactions in the form of acrodynia and related conditions. Am J Dis Child 1951;81:335–373.

81.9. Answer: D Urine and blood mercury levels have not been well established to confirm or exclude toxicity. However, they may be useful to confirm exposure and to monitor treatment efficacy. There is some evidence that hair analysis may be similarly useful for analyzing exposure to organic mercury.

ATSDR: Toxicologic Profile for Mercury. Atlanta, USDHHS, 1992.

Suzuki T, Hongo T, Yoshinaga J, et al: The hair–organ relationship in mercury concentration in contemporary Japanese. Arch Environ Health 1993;48:221–229.

81.10. Answer: B The neurotoxicity of methylmercury is relatively resistant to treatment. DMSA was superior to penicillamine and DMPS in reducing brain mercury in mice poisoned with methylmercury.

Aaseth J, Friedheim EAH: Treatment of methyl mercury poisoning in mice with 2,3-dimercaptosuccinic acid and other complexing thiols. Acta Pharmacol Toxicol 1978;42:248–252.

CHAPTER 82

METALS

82.1. Answer: A Myoclonic encephalopathy is characteristic of bismuth poisoning. Parkinsonism results from manganese exposure. Wrist drop is characteristic of lead poisoning. Peripheral sensory neuropathy can be caused by many metals, but the most painful syndrome is that from thallium. Erethism is the characteristic personality change caused by mercury.

82.2. Answer: C Bismuth can localize to bone, and a retrospective review of arthropathies revealed that fractures occurred in patients with severe movement disorders.

82.3. Answer: A Acute overdoses most commonly cause renal compromise. Although one patient suffered myoclonus after acute overdose, there are no reports of encephalopathy from acute bismuth overdose.

82.4. Answer: A No single therapy with chelation or hemodialysis has been definitively proven to alter clinical outcome. Early recognition and withdrawal of chronic dosing often results in spontaneous recovery.

82.5. Answer: D The level of cadmium in the blood is usually not a useful indicator of acute poisoning. The elimination half-life of cadmium from the body is 7 to 30 years. Cadmium is bound by metallothionein primarily synthesized in the liver. The cadmium is distributed to the kidneys, where it is transported into renal tubular cells and bound again by metallothionein synthesized in the kidneys. It is felt that cadmium toxicity occurs when the ability of the kidneys to synthesize protective metallothionein is overwhelmed. There is histopathologic evidence of increased renal toxicity caused by cadmium in animals when calcium disodium EDTA is employed as a chelation agent.

82.6. Answer: D A urine metal toxicology screen is not typically helpful in acute inhalation exposures. In typical bridge repair metal-working operations, cadmium or other agents causing chemical pneumonitis and noncardiac pulmonary edema are not present. Metal fume fever is the most likely diagnosis, although not the only diagnosis. Hypersensitivity pneumonitis is a potential diagnosis because of birds nesting on bridges and exposure to avian fecal proteins. Acute lung injury from metal poisoning may not be evident within a short observation period, and the negative film and mild symptoms make this diagnosis unlikely. Metal fume fever generally resolves by the next day, and subsequent exposure produces less dramatic effects. After a hiatus, such as a weekend, tolerance is lost, and reexposure produces more pronounced symptoms.

Boyd G, McSharry CP, Banham SW, et al: A current view of pigeon fancier's lung. A model for pulmonary extrinsic allergic alveolitis. Clin Allergy 1982;12:53–59.

82.7. Answer: D Without proper ventilation, soldering produces air concentrations of cadmium that can cause fatal cadmium pneumonitis and noncardiogenic pulmonary edema. Brazing is properly classified as a welding operation because of the higher temperatures employed. Brazing is not widely used in the semiconductor industry. Metal fumes are typically solid particles in the 1.0- to 10.0-mm range, which is the optimal respirable range for deposition in the alveoli. The toxicity of flux agents must always be considered in the clinical evaluation of a metal worker.

Ando Y, Shibata E, Tsuchiyama F, Sakai S: Elevated urinary cadmium concentrations in a patient with acute cadmium pneumonitis. Scand J Work Environ Health 1996;22:150–153.

Blejer HP: Death due to cadmium oxide fumes. Ind Med Surg 1996;35:362–364.

Seidal K, Jorgensen N, Elinder CG, et al: Fatal cadmium-induced pneumonitis. Scand J Work Environ Health 1993;19:429–431.

82.8. Answer: B The daily requirement for copper ion of slightly more than 100 mg is easily met with normal nutrition. Metallic copper is essentially nontoxic, to both children and adults as are insoluble salts. Copper oxides produce metal fume fever.

82.9. Answer D. Copper is a transition metal and is thus highly reactive with water and oxygen. It generates reactive oxygen species which are the ultimate toxins. The remainder of the answers represent unlikely and undescribed effects.

82.10. Answer A. Because of the severe vomiting associated with copper salt poisoning, it is unlikely that oral medications would ever be appropriate. BAL can only be given via an intramuscular route since it is solubilized in oil. Trientine is useful for therapy of chronic copper poisoning, as in Wilson's disease.

CHAPTER 83

THALLIUM

83.1. Answer: B Thallium and potassium have similar ionic radii: 1.33 Å for potassium and 1.47 Å for thallium. As a result, thallium distributes into tissues similarly to potassium. This principle serves as the basis for the use of radiolabeled thallium for cardiac stress tests.

Mulkey JP, Oehme FW: A review of thallium toxicity. Vet Hum Toxicol 1993;35:445–453.

83.2. Answer: E Activated charcoal adsorbs thallium in vitro and should be used to prevent thallium absorption. Because thallium is enterohepatically recirculated, multiple doses of activated charcoal (MDAC) may be useful to enhance thallium elimination. In an animal model MDAC proved efficacious against thallium poisoning.

Hoffman RS, Stringer JA, Feinberg RS, Goldfrank LR: Comparative efficacy of thallium adsorption by activated charcoal, Prussian blue, and sodium polystyrene sulfonate. J Toxicol Clin Toxicol 1999;37:833–837.

Lund A: The effect of various substances on the excretion and the toxicity of thallium in the rat. Acta Pharmacol Toxicol 1956;12:260–268.

83.3. Answer: E All of the answers are true. Although potassium administration enhances thallium elimination by at least the two mechanisms described (choices **A** and **B**), it may redistribute thallium to the central nervous system. This is associated with an exacerbation of neurologic symptoms in humans and enhanced lethality in animal models.

Meggs WJ, Goldfrank LR, Hoffman RS: Effects of potassium in a murine model of thallium poisoning [abstract]. J Toxicol Clin Toxicol 1995;33:559. Papp JP, Gay PC, Dodson VN, Pollard HM: Potassium chloride treatment in thallotoxicosis. Ann Intern Med 1969;71:119–123.

83.4. Answer: C Alopecia and a painful ascending peripheral neuropathy are classic findings associated with thallium toxicity. Unlike most other metal salts, the gastrointestinal symptoms associated with thallium poisoning are mild and can include both diarrhea and constipation. Effects on hematopoiesis are not described.

Chamberlain PH, Stavinoha WB, Davis H, et al: Thallium poisoning. Pediatrics 1958;12:1170–1182.

Moeschlin S: Thallium poisoning. Clin Toxicol 1980;17:133–146.

83.5. Answer: A Combined hemodialysis and hemoperfusion may remove as much as 93 mg of thallium during a 3-hour run. This is at least three to four times more effective than hemodialysis and far superior to peritoneal dialysis. Neither hemodialysis alone nor peritoneal dialysis would be expected to remove enough thallium to justify their use based on associated risks. The use of CAVH or CAVHD has not been studied.

Aoyama H, Yoshida M, Yamamura Y: Acute poisoning by intentional ingestion of thallous malonate. Hum Toxicol 1986;5:389–392.

De Backer W, Zachee P, Verpooten GA, et al: Thallium intoxication treated with combined hemoperfusion–hemodialysis. Clin Toxicol 1982;19:259–264.

83.6. Answer: E All of the choices were accepted medicinal uses of thallium at one time. Because of severe toxicity and fatality, the only continued use of thallium is as a radioactive contrast agent. This technique uses only small amounts of thallium.

Lynche GR, Lond MB, Scovell JMS: The toxicology of thallium. Lancet 1930;12:1340–1344.

83.7. Answer: D Of all of the traditionally used chelating agents, only D-penicillamine has been shown to enhance the elimination of thallium in poisoned animals. Unfortunately, similar to potassium and sodium diethyldithiocarbamate (Dithiocarb), in doing so D-penicillamine redistributes thallium into vital organs. It should therefore not be used alone and may have some role when combined with Prussian blue.

Rios C, Monroy-Noyola A: D-Penicillamine and Prussian blue as antidotes against thallium intoxication in rats. Toxicology 1992;74:69–76.

83.8. Answer: B Prussian blue is poorly absorbed from the gastrointestinal tract. It functions as a cation exchange resin by donating a potassium ion for a thallium ion and subsequently forming a tight bond with thallium to enhance fecal elimination. No data support the contention that the potassium liberated by Prussian blue contributes to thallium elimination by enhancing renal clearance. Prussian blue neither constipates nor causes diarrhea. Mannitol is added to the therapeutic regimen because of the constipation often associated with thallium poisoning. Unfortunately, no FDA-approved Prussian blue product exists.

Heydlauf H: Ferric-cyanoferrate(II): An effective antidote in thallium poisoning. Eur J Pharmacol 1969;6:340–344.

Krazov J, Rios C, Altagracia M, et al.: Relationship between physiochemical properties of Prussian blue and its efficacy as antidote against thallium poisoning. J Appl Toxicol 1993;13:213–216.

83.9. Answer: A Three cases of thallium poisoning from contaminated cocaine were reported in 1986. Unintentional exposure to rodenticides should no longer occur because thallium-containing rodenticides have been banned in the United States for many years. The amount of thallium used for radiolabeled studies is so small that even a massive overdose would be unlikely to produce clinical signs or symptoms of toxicity.

Insley BM, Grufferman S, Ayliffe HE: Thallium poisoning in cocaine users. Am J Emerg Med 1986;4:545–548.

83.10. Answer: D Animal evidence supports the teratogenicity of thallium. Although some authors report normal births following thallium poisoning during pregnancy, clearly fetal demise and neonatal toxicity have also occurred. One author reported absent fetal movements and the subsequent birth of a normal child. Although not well studied, no evidence exists to support teratogenicity of Prussian blue. Therefore, it should be administered to pregnant women with thallium poisoning if indicated.

English JC: A case of thallium poisoning complicating pregnancy. Med J Aust 1954;1:780–782.

Moeschlin S: Thallium poisoning. Clin Toxicol 1980;17:133–146.

CHAPTER 84

ANTISEPTICS, DISINFECTANTS, AND STERILANTS

84.1. Answer: B   Iodine is much more toxic than iodide because of its propensity to cause significant local tissue injury. Although iodophors, such as povidone-iodine, have significantly less free iodine than tincture of iodine or Lugol solution, GI injury may still occur. Because iodide is not caustic, treatment of iodine ingestions includes conversion of iodine to the less toxic iodide. Benzalkonium chloride is a quaternary ammonium compound that has also been associated with caustic injuries.

Moore M: The ingestion of iodine as a method of attempted suicide. N Engl J Med 1938;219:383–388.

84.2. Answer: C   The bathing of premature infants with hexachlorophene (pHisoHex®) was associated with significant neurologic abnormalities including the development of vacuolar encephalopathy. No reports of significant toxicity from sodium octylphenoxyethoxyethyl ether sulfonate (Phisoderm®) can be found in the literature.

Martinez AJ, Boehm V, Hadfield MG: Acute hexachlorophene encephalopathy: Cliniconeuropathological correlation. Acta Neuropathol 1974;28:93–103.

84.3. Answer: A   Chlorhexidine is reported to have low toxicity, although few published cases of deliberate oral ingestion of chlorhexidine exist. Symptoms are usually mild, and gastrointestinal irritation is the most likely effect after oral ingestion. Chlorhexidine has poor enteral absorption.

Chan TY. Poisoning due to Savlon (cetrimide) liquid. Hum Exp Toxicol 1994;13:681–682.

84.4. Answer: A   Formalin consists of an aqueous solution of formaldehyde usually containing about 37% formaldehyde and 12 to 15% methanol. Although the methanol component of the formalin solution is readily absorbed and has resulted in methanol levels of 40 mg/dL, the rapid metabolism of formaldehyde to formic acid appears to be responsible for much of the acidosis.

Burkhart KK, Kulig KW: Formate levels following a formalin ingestion. Vet Hum Toxicol 1990;32:135–137.

84.5. Answer: D   Cutaneous decontamination of phenol with a low-molecular-weight polyethylene glycol solution was shown to decrease mortality, systemic effects, and dermal burns in a rat model. Although this study suggested that polyethylene glycol was superior to water as a decontamination agent, a subsequent study using a swine model could not demonstrate a difference between these two agents. Given the lack of definitive efficacy data, either low-molecular-weight polyethylene glycol (eg, PEG 300 or PEG 400), if it is readily available in the ED, or water is currently recommended for dermal irrigation and careful gastric decontamination.

Brown VK, Box VL, Simpson BJ: Decontamination procedures for skin exposed to phenolic substances. Arch Environ Health 1975;30:1–6.

84.6. Answer: E   Chronic ingestion of potassium permanganate may result in manganese poisoning, which causes an extrapyramidal syndrome similar to parkinsonism..

Holzgraefe M, Poser W, Kijewski H, Beuche W: Chronic enteral poisoning caused by potassium permanganate. J Toxicol Clin Toxicol 1986;24:235–244.

84.7. Answer: D   After hydrogen peroxide ingestion a careful examination should be performed to detect any evidence of gas formation. A chest radiograph may reveal gas in the cardiac chambers, mediastinum, or pleural space. Those with clinical or radiographic evidence of gas in the heart should be immediately placed in the Trendelenburg position to prevent gas from blocking the right ventricular outflow tract.

Christensen DW, Faught WE, Black RE, et al: Fatal oxygen embolization after hydrogen peroxide ingestion. Crit Care Med 1992;20:543–544.

84.8. Answer: C   Classic boric acid poisoning usually involves multiple exposures over a period of days. Gastrointestinal, dermal, CNS, and renal manifestations predominate. The initial symptoms—nausea, vomiting, diarrhea, and occasionally crampy abdominal pain—may be confused with an acute gastroenteritis. Following the onset of GI symptoms, many patients develop a characteristic intense generalized erythroderma ("boiled lobster" appearance). At about the time of the development of the erythroderma, patients, particularly young infants, may develop prominent signs of CNS irritability resembling meningeal irritation. Renal injury is common and is related to the renal elimination of this compound.

Wong LC, Heimbach MD, Truscott DR, Duncan BD: Boric acid poisoning: Report of 11 cases. Can Med Assoc J 1964;90:1018–1023.

84.9. Answer: A   Although methylene blue may be used in the treatment of symptomatic methemoglobinemia in an attempt to reduce methemoglobin to hemoglobin, its efficacy in the treatment of chlorate-induced methemoglobinemia may be limited compared to its efficacy in the treatment of other oxidant-induced methemoglobinemias. This may be a result of the inactivation by chlorates of glucose-6-phosphate dehydrogenase, an enzyme that is required for methylene blue's reduction of methemoglobin.

Steffen C, Wetzel E: Chlorate poisoning: mechanism of toxicity. Toxicology 1993;84:217–31.

84.10. Answer: B   Ethylene oxide acts as an alkylating agent, reacting with most cellular components including DNA and RNA. Retrospective studies have suggested a possible excess incidence of leukemia and gastric cancer in ethylene oxide–exposed workers. These studies have not been conclusive, and the carcinogenicity of ethylene oxide remains subject to debate.

Steenland K, Stayner L, Greife A, et al: Mortality among workers exposed to ethylene oxide. N Engl J Med 1991;324:1402–1407.

CHAPTER **85**

CAMPHOR AND MOTH REPELLENTS

85.1. Answer: C Camphorated oil and camphorated spirits contain varying concentrations of camphor. Historically, most camphorated oil was 20% w/w camphor with cottonseed oil, and most camphorated spirits contained 10% w/w camphor with isopropyl alcohol. Toxicity and death following ingestion of camphorated oil, which was commonly confused with castor oil and cod liver oil, prompted the FDA to ban the over-the-counter (OTC) sale of camphorated oil in the United States in 1983. Today, based on the 1983 FDA ruling, nonprescription camphor products may not contain greater than an 11% concentration of camphor. Camphorated oil, still used as an herbal remedy and muscle liniment, and products containing greater than 11% camphor can still be purchased legally outside of the United States.

85.2. Answer: B The seizures from camphor occur very soon after the ingestion, most commonly within 15 to 20 minutes.

85.3. Answer: B Paradichlorobenzene will produce a green flame when burned, naphthalene a yellow flame.

Winkler JV, Kulig K, Rumack BH: Mothball differentiation: naphthalene from paradichlorobenzene. Ann Emerg Med 1985;14: 30–32.

85.4. Answer: A The easiest way to differentiate camphor mothballs from naphthalene or paradichlorobenzene mothballs is to place the mothball in water. Mothballs made of naphthalene or paradichlorobenzene will sink, whereas mothballs made of camphor will float.

Koyama K, Yamashita M: A simple test for mothball component differentiation using water and a saturated solution of table salt: Its utilization for poison information service. Vet Hum Toxicol 1991; 33:425–427.

85.5. Answer: A As with most toxins, the toxic dose of camphor reported in the medical literature is highly variable. For this reason it is most reasonable to evaluate all patients in a medical setting. G-6-PD deficiency should not alter the management strategy. The odor of camphor is neither a sensitive nor a specific finding in predicting poisoning.

85.6. Answer: A Infants have reduced activity of NADH methemoglobin reductase (cytochrome b5 reductase), the enzyme responsible for the conversion of methemoglobin back to hemoglobin. There is no evidence that absorption or metabolism differs in infants.

85.7. Answer: A The oxidant stress responsible for naphthalene-induced hemolysis and methemoglobinemia is caused by the hepatic metabolites of naphthalene and not the parent compound. α-Naphthol is the metabolite that is predominantly responsible for naphthalene's hematologic toxicity.

Rieders F, Brieger H: Hemolytic action of naphthalene and its oxidation products. Pediatrics 1951;7:725–727.

85.8. Answer: B Naphthalene-induced hemolysis is similar in presentation to hemolysis from other toxins that cause oxidative stress. A decreased hemoglobin concentration and a decreased hematocrit are the hallmarks of hemolysis. Hyperbilirubinemia from hemolysis is characterized by an elevation of the indirect bilirubin (unconjugated bilirubin). The direct bilirubin (conjugated bilirubin) is normal unless the patient has hepatic or biliary dysfunction, which would not be expected with naphthalene. Serum haptoglobin is usually low because the haptoglobin–hemoglobin complex is cleared by the kidneys. Both the direct and indirect Coombs test are negative in naphthalene-induced hemolytic anemia. Lactate dehydrogenase is usually elevated. Gross or microscopic hemoglobinuria is confirmed by a urine dipstick that reacts strongly positive for hemoglobin with a paucity of red blood cells on microscopic examination. This should be differentiated from myoglobinemia by measuring the serum creatine phosphokinase, which will be elevated in patients with rhabdomyolysis and myoglobinuria.

Zuelzer WW, Apt L: Acute hemolytic anemia due to naphthalene poisoning: Clinical and experimental study. JAMA 1949;141: 185–190.

85.9. Answer: A The use of syrup of ipecac is contraindicated following camphor ingestions because of the risk of seizures. Gastric lavage, activated charcoal, cathartics, and whole-bowel irrigation could be used if appropriate. Most often activated charcoal or activated charcoal after cautious gastric lavage is all that would be necessary.

85.10. Answer: B Chronic exposure to paradichlorobenzene has been reported to cause hepatotoxicity in patients who were exposed to it where it was used as an insecticide.

Cotter LH: Paradichlorobenzene poisoning from insecticides. NY State J Med 1953;53:1690–1692.

CHAPTER **86**

HYDROCARBONS

86.1. Answer: C Substances with low viscosity (<60 SSU), low surface tension, and high volatility present higher aspiration risk. Viscosity is the tendency of a substance to resist flow, often measured in Saybolt Seconds Universal (SSU). Volatility is the tendency for a liquid to change from a liquid to a gas. Neither the pH nor pK_a of an agent significantly alter its aspiration risk. The oil/water partition coefficient influences distribution of hydrocarbon molecules into body tissues but does not independently influence aspiration risk. Although molecular weight does influence vapor pressure and thus the volatility of a compound, it is generally accepted that viscosity is the single property most closely related to aspiration hazard. At present, the European Community and the US Consumer Product Safety Commission stratify hydrocarbon aspiration hazard based solely on viscosity.

Gargas ML, Burgess RJ, Voisard DE, et al: Partition coefficients of low-molecular-weight volatile chemicals in various liquids and tissues. Toxicol Appl Pharmacol 1989;98:87–99.

Gerarde HW: Toxicological studies on hydrocarbons: IX. The aspiration hazard and toxicity of hydrocarbons and hydrocarbon mixtures. Arch Environ Health 1963;6:329–341.

86.2. Answer: D   Neither prophylactic antibiotics nor systemic corticosteroids have proven to be of benefit in animal or human studies of acute hydrocarbon aspiration. Their use remains controversial in the setting of hydrocarbon aspiration. Improved outcome with delayed corticosteroid therapy (5 to 10 days after onset of ARDS) has been reported. Olive oil and mineral oil lavage were advocated in the past as a means of increasing the viscosity of the resultant hydrocarbon mixture. Jet ventilation and positive end-expiratory pressure may be useful in patients who have severe pulmonary injuries.

Bysani GK, Rucoba RJ, Noah ZL: Treatment of hydrocarbon pneumonitis; high frequency jet ventilation as an alternative to extracorporeal membrane oxygenation. Chest 1994;106:300–303.

Marks MI, Chicoine L, Legere G, et al: Adrenocorticosteroid treatment of hydrocarbon pneumonia in children—a cooperative study. J Pediatr 1972;81:366–369.

86.3. Answer: B   Halogenated hydrocarbons sensitize the heart to endogenous catacholamines in animal models. Halogenated and possibly aromatic hydrocarbons can induce dysrhythmias and sudden death. The typical scenario of this occurrence is when sudden exertion occurs (eg, running) after significant hydrocarbon exposure, with a sudden surge of catacholamines. The mechanism appears to be sensitization of the myocardium to catecholamines. Successful treatment of dysrhythmias with β-adrenergic antagonists is reported.

Bass M: Sudden sniffing death. JAMA 1970;212:2075–2079.

Moritz F, de La Chapelle A, Bauer F, et al: Esmolol in the treatment of severe arrhythmia after acute trichloroethylene poisoning [letter]. Intens Care Med 2000;26:256.

86.4. Answer: C   Chronic exposure to a number of organic solvents (typically occupational) may be associated with peripheral neuropathy. Most notable is *n*-hexane, but other agents that can cause this include methyl *n*-butyl ketone and also trichloroethylene (particularly cranial neuropathies), carbon disulfide, acrylamide, ethylene oxide, and possibly toluene. Early case reports and series suggesting that toluene causes peripheral neuropathy have now come into question, as the toluene in these series may have been contaminated by *n*-hexane or MnBK. Methyl ethyl ketone (MEK) may exacerbate the neurotoxicity of *n*-hexane or MnBK, probably by interfering with metabolic pathways.

Graham DG: Neurotoxicants and the cytoskeleton. Curr Opin Neurol 1999;12:733–737.

Saida K, Mendell JR, Weiss HS: Peripheral nerve changes induced by methyl *n*-butyl ketone and potentiation by methyl ethyl ketone. J Neuropathol Exp Neurol 1976;35:207–225.

86.5. Answer: D   Toluene is metabolized to hippuric acid, the accumulation of which produces an anion-gap acidosis. Hippuric acid also produces a renal tubular acidosis resulting in hyperchloremia and hypokalemia. The muscle weakness is caused by profound hypokalemia. The findings resolve with replacement of potassium.

Kao KC, Tsai YH, Lin MC, et al: Hypokalemic muscular paralysis causing acute respiratory failure due to rhabdomyolysis with renal tubular acidosis in a chronic glue sniffer. J Toxicol Clin Toxicol 2000;38:679–681.

Batlle DC, Sabatini S, Kurtzman NA: On the mechanism of toluene-induced renal tubular acidosis. Nephron 1988;49:210–218.

86.6. Answer: E   Although this is an area of controversy, a strong argument can be made for gastric emptying following a toxic dose of a hydrocarbon with serious inherent toxicity. Gastric emptying should be avoided for hydrocarbons with high aspiration risk and little or no systemic toxicity.

Arena JM: Hydrocarbon poisoning—current management. Pediatr Ann 1987;16:879–883.

Mofenson HC, Greensher J: Controversies in the prevention and treatment of poisonings. Pediatr Ann 1977;6:717–725.

86.7. Answer: A   Because of its low viscosity, high volatility, and low surface tension, kerosene has the greatest risk.

Gerarde HW: Toxicological studies on hydrocarbons: IX. The aspiration hazard and toxicity of hydrocarbons and hydrocarbon mixtures. Arch Environ Health 1963;6:329–341.

86.8. Answer: C   All of these statements are consistent with hydrocarbon-induced pulmonary injury except that pneumothorax caused by pulmonary parenchymal destruction is rare.

86.9. Answer: C   Methylene chloride is metabolized in part to carbon monoxide.

Di Vincenzo GD, Kaplan CJ: Uptake, metabolism and elimination of methylene chloride vapors by humans. Toxicol Appl Pharmacol 1981;59:130–140.

86.10. Answer: C   Early x-rays may be prognostically indicated in patients who are severely symptomatic. In the asymptomatic patient, however, early radiography is unlikely to be cost effective. Radiographs performed immediately after hydrocarbon ingestion demonstrate low predictive value for the occurrence of aspiration pneumonitis. Patients observed for 6 hours after an ingestion, who demonstrate no abnormal pulmonary findings, have adequate oxygenation, are not tachypneic, and have a normal CXR after the observation period have a good prognosis with very low risk of subsequent deterioration.

Anas N, Namasonthi V, Ginsburg CM: Criteria for hospitalizing children who have ingested products containing hydrocarbon. JAMA 1981;246:840–843.

Wason S, Katona B: A review of symptoms, signs and laboratory findings predictive of hydrocarbon toxicity [abstract]. Vet Hum Toxicol 1987;29:492.

CHAPTER 87

CAUSTICS AND BATTERIES

87.1. Answer: C Dilutional therapy did not demonstrate increased damage, although efficacy was greatly diminished as the length of time following the caustic exposure increased.

Homan CS, Maitra SR, Lane BP, et al: Histopathological evaluation of the therapeutic efficacy of water or milk dilution for esophageal acid injury. Acad Emerg Med 1995;2:587–591.

Homan CS, Maitra SR, Lane BP, et al: Therapeutic effects of water and milk for acute alkali injury of the esophagus. Ann Emerg Med 1994;24:14–19.

87.2. Answer: E There are no data to support the routine use of neutralization. This technique may be potentially harmful.

Homan CS, Maitra SR, Lane BP, et al: Effective treatment for acute alkali injury to the esophagus using weak-acid neutralization therapy: An ex-vivo study. Acad Emerg Med 1995;2:952–958.

87.3. Answer: B Endoscopy is ideally performed within 12 hours of the exposure. No contrast studies are required before endoscopy. As wound healing occurs the tissues soften, and the risk of perforation from endoscopy is higher between 3 and 14 days.

Zargar SA, Kocchar R, Mehta S, Mehta SK: The role of fiberoptic endoscopy in the management of corrosive ingestion and modified endoscopic classification of burns. Gastrointest Endosc 1991;37:165–169.

87.4. Answer: C Pleural effusion may indicate perforation of the esophagus. Normal contrast radiographs can miss perforations. Absence of free air under the diaphragm does not rule out a viscus perforation. No large series of patients with caustic injuries has been evaluated by CT scan to determine sensitivity of this procedure. Contrast radiography is unnecessary in patients with grade I injuries because these do not progress to stricture formation.

Martel W: Radiologic features of esophagogastritis secondary to extremely caustic agents. Diagnost Radiol 1972;103:31–36.

Wu MH, Lai WW: Surgical management of extensive corrosive injuries of the alimentary tract. Surg Gynecol Obstet 1993;177:12–16.

87.5. Answer: B Corticosteroids may have some benefit in those patients with grade II circumferential injuries of the esophagus, although no study has been able to enroll enough patients to definitively demonstrate the utility of this agent. Corticosteroids may be harmful in patients with grade III injuries. If corticosteroids are employed, empiric therapy with antibiotics is mandatory to decrease the risk of overwhelming infection.

Anderson KD, Rouse TM, Randolph JG: A controlled trial of corticosteroids in children with corrosive injury of the esophagus. N Engl J Med 1990;323:637–640.

87.6. Answer: D No trials have demonstrated an improvement in outcome from empiric use of antibiotic therapy as treatment in caustic injury. The exception is that animals treated with corticosteroids had a decreased mortality when concomitantly placed on antibiotic therapy. Therefore, all patients placed on corticosteroids should be placed on antibiotics to decrease the risk of overwhelming infection.

Rosenberg N, Kunderman PJ, Vroman L, Moolten SE: Prevention of experimental esophageal stricture by cortisone II. Arch Surg 1953;66:593–598.

87.7. Answer: E Stricture formation usually occurs days to weeks after the exposure. Corticosteroids are not used in the treatment of strictures but rather for the possible prevention of stricture formation in grade II esophageal lesions. The risk of carcinoma is increased in survivors of lye ingestions who develop strictures.

Appelqvist P, Salmo M: Lye corrosion carcinoma of the esophagus: A review of 63 cases. Cancer 1980;45:2655–2658.

87.8. Answer: B Household bleach (sodium hypochlorite) rarely causes significant injury in unintentional exposures. Symptomatic patients or those with intentional ingestions should be evaluated as for other caustic agents.

Landau GD, Saunders WH: The effect of chlorine bleach on the esophagus. Arch Otolaryngol 1964;80:174–176.

87.9. Answer: B Life-threatening hydrofluoric acid exposure causes hypocalcemia, hypomagnesemia, hyperkalemia, acidemia, and coagulopathy, which is often seen on postmortem examination.

MacKinnon MA: Hydrofluoric acid burns. Dermatol Clin 1988;6:67–74.

87.10. Answer: A Intentional hydrofluoric acid ingestions are almost universally fatal. Rapid aspiration via nasogastric tube (NGT) may decrease systemic absorption, which is the primary cause of death in these patients. Oral administration of calcium or magnesium salts should follow NGT aspiration. Activated charcoal would not be expected to help.

Bost RO, Springfield A: Fatal hydrofluoric acid ingestion: a suicide case report. J Anal Toxicol 1995;19:535–536.

Menchel SM, Dunn WA: Hydrofluoric acid poisoning. Am J Forens Med Pathol 1984;5:245–248.

CHAPTER 88

INSECTICIDES: ORGANIC PHOSPHORUS COMPOUNDS AND CARBAMATES

88.1. Answer: D Pralidoxime will reverse the inhibition of acetylcholinesterase at the neuromuscular junction. Atropine and glycopyrrolate have no effect at nicotinic sites and are purely muscarinic agents. Atropine will cross the blood–brain barrier, whereas glycopyrrolate will not. Diazepam and lorazepam are GABA agonists.

DiKart WL, Kestra SH, Sangster B: The use of atropine and oximes in organophosphate intoxication: A modified approach. J Toxicol Clin Toxicol 1988;26:199–208.

88.2. Answer: E All of the choices except the last one will be affected by the side chains off the central phosphorus atom. Tightness of binding to cholinesterase is a function of charge distribution. Different side groups will alter charge distribution. Endogenous hydrolysis is affected by the ability of water to cleave the organic phosphorus molecule, another function of charge distribution. Fat solubility is affected by the number of hydrophilic and hydrophobic groups on the molecule, and latency of symptom onset is a direct effect of fat solubility.

88.3. Answer: E Stimulation of the cholinergic nervous system results in muscarinic and nicotinic hyperactivity. Miosis, bradycardia, diarrhea, and urination are the results of muscarinic overactivity. Mydriasis and tachycardia are from the nicotinic activity. Urinary retention is found with anticholinergic toxicity.

Tafuri J, Roberts J: Organophosphate poisoning. Ann Emerg Med 1987;16:193–202.

88.4. Answer: C Atropine will treat the muscarinic-induced signs and symptoms of cholinesterase toxicity. It will reverse bronchorrhea and bronchospasm, miosis, and diarrhea. It will not affect muscle strength.

88.5. Answer: B Pralidoxime therapy is indicated in all of the patients with systemic symptoms. With the exception of exposure to highly fat-soluble organic phosphorus compounds, the majority of patients who are toxic will have symptoms developing within 6 to 12 hours postexposure. The patient with isolated miosis 14 hours postexposure is showing localized symptoms and is unlikely to progress. The patient who is 3 days postexposure has systemic nicotinic symptoms, which may benefit from late pralidoxime therapy.

Lotti M: Treatment of acute organophosphate poisoning. Med J Aust 1991;154:51–55.

88.6. Answer: A Succinylcholine is metabolized via pseudocholinesterase (plasma cholinesterase) and will have a prolonged duration of action in an organic phosphorus compound–poisoned patient.

Nelson TC, Burritt MF: Pesticide poisoning: Succinylcholine induced apnea and pseudocholinesterase. Mayo Clin Proc 1986;61:750–755.

88.7. Answer: D Patients should not return to work until their cholinesterase activity level is 75% of normal or greater. Levels less than 10% are associated with severe toxicity. Patients with cholinesterase activity of 50% may appear normal but are still at significant risk for increased toxicity.

Coye MJ, Barnett PG, Midtling JE, et al: Clinical confirmation of organophosphate poisoning by serial cholinesterase analysis. Arch Intern Med 1987;147:438–442.

88.8. Answer: A OPIDN is a polyneuropathy occurring 1 to 3 weeks after exposure to certain organic phosphorus compounds. It is initially a sensory neuropathy that later develops accompanying motor loss. It is unrelated to acetylcholinesterase depression and pralidoxime therapy. NTE (neuropathic esterase) inhibition must be at least 70% before symptoms appear. It is an axonopathy.

Stuart LD, Oehme FW: Organophosphate delayed neurotoxicity: A neuromyelopathy of animals and man. Vet Hum Toxicol 1982;24:107–118.

88.9. Answer: A Pyridostigmine is a carbamate, which will not cross the blood–brain barrier. It will protect the acetylcholinesterase by binding about 30% of the active sites. In the doses used during the Gulf War, the acetylcholinesterase unbound spontaneously within 4 to 8 hours but may unbind more rapidly with oxime therapy. Pyridostigmine can be given orally.

Sidell FR, Borak J: Chemical warfare agents. II. Nerve agents. Ann Emerg Med 1992;21:865–871.

88.10. Answer: E All of the following are organic phosphorus compounds that have caused the IMS: dimethoate, malathion, methamidofos, diazinon, fenthion, parathion, and methylparathion. Carbaryl is a carbamate that has yet to be implicated in causing IMS.

DeBleecker J, Van Den Neucker K, Willems J: The intermediate syndrome in organophosphate poisoning. Presentation of a case and review of the literature. J Toxicol Clin Toxicol 1992;30:321–329.

CHAPTER **89**

INSECTICIDES: ORGANOCHLORINES, PYRETHRINS, DEET

89.1. Answer: E Lindane causes seizures by binding to the picrotoxin binding site on the GABA receptor. By binding to this site it inhibits chloride influx and inhibits the action of GABA causing seizures.

89.2. Answer: C Chronic exposure to chlordecone has been reported to cause idiopathic intracranial hypertension, oligospermia, and aplastic anemia. An association has not been established with hyperthyroidism.

Cohn WJ, Boylan JJ, Blanke RV, et al: Treatment of chlordecone (kepone) toxicity with cholestyramine. N Engl J Med 1978;98:243–248.

Rugman FP, Cosstick R: Aplastic anemia associated with organochlorine pesticide: Case reports and review of evidence. J Clin Pathol 1990;3:98–101.

89.3. Answer: A Dechlorane or mirex has the least toxicity of these organochlorine pesticides. Aldrin, dieldrin, endosulfan, and endrin are all highly toxic to man and other mammals.

Hayes WJ: Chlorinated hydrocarbon insecticides. In: Hayes WJ, Lawes ER, eds: Pesticides Studied in Man. Baltimore, Williams & Wilkins, 1991, pp. 731–868.

89.4. Answer: C Seizures have been reported with excessive dermal absorption and ingestion of DEET-containing products in children. The incidence of these severe reactions is greatest with the higher-concentration products.

Lipscomb JB, Kramer JE, Leiken JB: Seizures following a brief exposure to insect repellents *N,N*-diethyl-*n*-toluamide. Ann Emerg Med 1992;21:315–317.

Tenenbein M: Severe toxic reactions and death following ingestion of diethyltoluamide-containing insecticides. JAMA 1987;258:1509–1511.

89.5. Answer: A Dichorodiphenyltrichloroethane (DDT) is the least well absorbed organochlorine insecticide by the oral route. All of the others listed are very well absorbed through both an intact or a broken dermal barrier.

89.6. Answer: D *N,N*-Diethyltoluamide and several active metabolites can be found in fat for up to 2 months following dermal application. The currently formulated low-concentration products are of comparable efficacy to the high-concentration products.

Lurie AA, Glieberman SE, Tsizin YS: Pharmacokinetics of the insect repellent *N,N*-diethyltoluamide. Med Parasitol 1979;47:72–76.

89.7. Answer: B DDT causes toxicity by binding to sodium channels. DDT appears to act by lengthening the period of time in which the channel remains in its open configuration.

Tilson HA, Hong JS, Mactutus CF: Effects of 5,5-diphenylhydantoin (phenytoin) on neurobehavioral toxicity of organochlorine pesticides and permethrin. J Pharmacol Exp Ther 1985;233:285–289.

89.8. Answer: E Most organochlorine insecticides are capable of inducing hepatic microsomal enzymes. Alterations in the normal ascorbic acid and glucuronic acid metabolic pathways have also been reported.

Williams CH, Casterline JL: Effects on toxicity and on enzyme activity of the interactions between aldrin, chlordane, piperonyl butoxide and banol in rats. Proc Soc Exp Biol Med 1970;135:46–49.

89.9. Answer: B DDT blood levels document exposure but have no other clinical value. In a study of a community with a known exposure to DDT, levels were found to continue to increase with age, despite removal from the exposure.

Kriess K, Zack MM, Kimbrough RD, et al: Cross-sectional study of a community with exceptional exposure to DDT. JAMA 1981;245:1926–1930.

89.10. Answer: C Mammals demonstrate relatively little toxicity when exposed to pyrethroids. Most cases of toxicity associated with the pyrethrins are the result of hypersensitivity reactions.

Paton DL, Walker JS: Pyrethrin poisoning from commercial strength flea and tick spray. Am J Emerg Med 1988;6:232–235.

Wax PM, Hoffman RS: Fatality associated with inhalation of a pyrethrin shampoo. J Toxicol Clin Toxicol 1994;32:457–460.

CHAPTER **90**

RODENTICIDES

90.1. Answer: D Smoking vomitus and stools with a garliclike odor identify poisoning by yellow or white phosphorus. Opisthotonos and "risus sardonicus," which is trismus or facial grimacing, along with muscle twitching, extensor spasm, seizures, and medullary paralysis characterize strychnine poisoning. Hair loss is a late finding associated with thallium, and the odor associated with zinc phosphide is of rotten fish.

Simon FA, Pickering LK: Acute yellow phosphorus poisoning. JAMA 1976;235:1343–1366.

90.2. Answer: C According to the Federal Insecticide, Fungicide, and Rodenticide Act (FIFRA), those rodenticides with a single-dose LD_{50} of less than 50 mg/kg are considered highly toxic. All of the inorganic rodenticides fall into this category. Organic rodenticides such as SMFA, strychnine, and Vacor are highly toxic, whereas other organic rodenticides such as ANTU and cholecalciferol are considered moderately toxic, and norbormide, warfarin, and bromethalin are considered to be of low toxicity.

Federal Insecticide, Fungicide, and Rodenticide Act (FIFRA) *(http://www.epa.gov/pesticides/)*

90.3. Answer: D Norbormide is an irreversible smooth muscle constrictor that causes ischemic necrosis and death in rats but no other animals, presumably because it acts on a specific smooth muscle norbormide receptor found only in rats. All of the inorganic rodenticides such as yellow phosphorus along with organic rodenticides such as strychnine and SMFA are classified as "nonselective." When Vacor was first introduced on the market, it was erroneously thought to be selective for rodents. However, the selectivity misconception probably stemmed from the fact that the LD_{50} for Vacor varies widely from species to species in no particular logical sequence. In any event, the toxicity of Vacor is certainly not selective with respect to humans. Other selective rodenticides include α-naphthylthiourea (ANTU) and the cardiac glycoside red squill.

Bova S, Travis L, Debetto P, et al: Vasorelaxant properties of norbormide, a selective vasoconstrictor agent for the rat microvasculature. Br J Pharmacol 1996;117:1041–1046.

90.4. Answer: B Because SMFA interferes with the Krebs cycle, attempts have been made to provide a postblock substitute that could serve as an antidote. Thus far, glycerol monoacetate has been used successfully in this manner in monkeys. Also, attempts to inhibit the conversion of fluoroacetate to fluorocitrate have had limited experimental success. Unlike the case with hydrofluoric acid, the fluoride content of SMFA is not responsible for its catastrophic lethal effects. SMFA is available only to licensed pest-control operators and cannot be absorbed through unbroken skin. Recently a review of 38 exposures to SMFA over a 5-year period in Taiwan demonstrated that early hypotension is one of the most accurate prognostic indicators of mortality.

Chenoweth MB, Kandel A, Johnson LB, et al: Factors influencing fluoroacetate poisoning: Practice treatment with glycerol monoacetate. J Pharmacol Exp Ther 1951;102:31–49.

Chi CH, Chen KW, Chan SH, et al: Clinical presentation and prognostic factors in sodium monofluoroacetate intoxication. J Toxicol Clin Toxicol 1996;34:707–712.

90.5. Answer: D All of the features listed and possibly renal dysfunction characterize poisoning by the soluble (acetate, carbonate, chloride) but not insoluble (sulfate) forms of barium. No longer used as a rodenticide, but still available as a depilatory, (soluble) barium directly stimulates all types of muscle at the same time that it causes extracellular potassium to accumulate within the muscle cell, resulting in depolarization and paralysis. According to one investigator, the weakness appears to correlate better with the plasma barium concentration than with the serum potassium levels. Although strychnine, thallium, and Vacor are all associated with various types of neurologic dysfunction, none results in weakness and hypokalemia. ANTU probably acts by damaging lung capillaries and increasing permeability, resulting in pulmonary edema.

Phelan DM, Hagley SR, Guerin MD: Is hypokalemia the cause of paralysis in barium poisoning? Br Med J 1984;289:662.

Roza O, Berman LB: The pathophysiology of barium, hypokalemia and cardiovascular effects. J Pharmacol Exp Ther 1971;177:433–439.

90.6. Answer: C Cholecalciferol or vitamin D_3 is one of the newer commercial rodenticides currently in widespread use. Although data on human exposures are somewhat limited, there is reason to believe that repeated human ingestions would produce the signs and symptoms of hypercalcemia. Mild to moderate elevations in serum calcium result in lethargy and confusion. Although higher elevations of serum calcium can cause coma, ECG abnormalities (shortening of the QT interval), and ultimately death, no severe manifestations of hypercalcemia following cholecalciferol rodenticide ingestions have yet been described in humans. Brodifacoum, a long-acting anticoagulant, is not associated with alteration in mental status. Bromethalin, one of the newest rodenticides, might cause a decreased level of consciousness but not as a sole manifestation of toxicity: ataxia, focal motor seizures, and other signs of CNS stimulation would be expected to precede or accompany loss of consciousness. Strychnine is a highly toxic substance no longer used as a rodenticide that causes various types of CNS stimulation and pain until ultimately causing death by medullary paralysis. Vacor, another highly toxic rodenticide available in the 1970s, was associated with hyperglycemia, ketoacidosis, postural hypotension, and peripheral and autonomic neuropathies. Although coma (or death) might result secondarily, it would not be expected to be the sole manifestation of toxicity.

Jibani M, Hodges NH: Prolonged hypercalcemia after industrial exposure to vitamin D_3. Br Med J 1985;290:748–749.

Marsh R, Tunberg A: Characteristics of cholecalciferol: Rodent control—other options. Pest Control Technol 1986;14:43–45.

90.7. Answer: D Red squill, which is derived from the cabbage plant *Urginea maritima,* contains two potent cardioglycosides, scillaren A and B. It is said that following a human ingestion, the gastrointestinal manifestations including vomiting predominate, thus sparing the patient the potentially lethal cardiac sequelae. However, a human ingestion of two bulbs of the plant resulted in all of the manifestations of a massive cardiac glycoside ingestion, including death. Cardiac toxicity is not primarily associated with strychnine, thallium, or bromethalin. Although the same may also be said of norbormide, an irreversible smooth muscle constrictor in rats, recent work suggests that in the arteries of other mammals, norbormide may act as a calcium channel entry blocker.

Tuncock Y, Kozan O, Cowder C, et al: *Urginea maritima* (squill) toxicity. J Toxicol Clin Toxicol 1995;33:83–86.

90.8. Answer: E A single ingestion of a long-acting warfarin-type rodenticide more than 24 hours before presentation can produce a prolonged PT that may last for up to 7 weeks, necessitating treatment with vitamin K_1, fresh frozen plasma, and possibly even whole blood. A single ingestion of a "regular" or short-acting warfarin rodenticide will not cause any coagulation abnormalities, and, therefore, when the details of the ingestion are completely known, should not result in an aggressive diagnostic evaluation or treatment plan. Single small doses of ANTU are relatively harmless to humans, although massive amounts may result in pulmonary symptoms. Repeated doses of cholecalciferol or vitamin D_3 would be expected to produce hypercalcemia, and although very little is known about human ingestions of bromethalin, ingestions by cats and dogs result primarily in neurologic findings.

Lipton RA, Klass EM: Human ingestion of a "superwarfarin" rodenticide resulting in prolonged anticoagulant effect. JAMA 1984;252:3004–3005.

Routh CR, Triplett DA, Murphy MJ, et al: Superwarfarin ingestion and detection. Am J Hematol 1991;36:50–54.

90.9. Answer: E The physical findings associated with bromethalin ingestion in rats, cats, and dogs include ataxia, focal motor seizures, decerebrate posturing, decreased proprioception, depressed level of consciousness, and death. There is no reason to believe that similar neurologic findings would not occur in man. In fact, a recent abstract describes muscle tremors and myoclonic jerks with flexion of major muscle groups occurring after a (mixed) bromethalin ingestion. Although most of the other findings have been associated with one or more rodenticides, none has been associated with bromethalin.

Buller G, Heard J, Gorman S: Possible bromethalin-induced toxicity in a human: A case report. J Toxicol Clin Toxicol 1996;34:572.

Dorman DC, Zachary JF, Buck WB: Neuropathologic findings of bromethalin toxicosis in the cat. Vet Pathol 1992;29:138–144.

Dorman DC, Simon J, Harlin KA, et al: Diagnosis of bromethalin toxicosis in the dog. J Vet Diagn Invest 1990;2:123–128.

90.10. Answer: E Exposures to short- and long-acting warfarin-type rodenticides continued to represent the overwhelming majority of rodenticide exposures, and there is no reason to believe that this will change in the near future. Although Vacor was withdrawn from sale in 1979, one to five exposures, but no fatalities, have been reported each year through 1995.

CHAPTER 91

HERBICIDES

91.1. Answer: C The worldwide use of all pesticide active ingredients in 1997 is estimated to be 5.7 billion pounds. These are formulated with an equivalent poundage of adjuvant ingredients into approximately 17 billion pounds of commercial pesticide products. Herbicides, which are pesticidal agents directed specifically against plants, represent 40% of this total, or 2.25 billion pounds worldwide. The largest market segment for use is agronomic.

91.2. Answer: D It is a mistaken notion that the only item of toxicologic significance in a formulated pesticide is the active ingredient. Commercial formulations contain a variety of ingredients to allow storage, dilution with water, and application, and also assure effectiveness on the plant. Many types of formulations are possible, and the type of formulation will dictate the general composition. The majority of herbicidal active ingredients are water soluble, so it would be unusual to find an organic solvent. Nearly universal adjuvants are surfactants, either in the formulation itself or added to the tank mix before spraying

91.3. Answer: C The US EPA is carrying out a strategy on inert ingredients that first seeks to classify existing nonactive ingredients in registered pesticides according to toxicologic and environmental hazard and use profiles. The goal is to include only ingredients that are classified as "minimal risk." Newly introduced additives will have to demonstrate safety with data, but this will not be as burdensome as the data required for an active pesticide ingredient.

91.4. Answer: B In general, no matter what the identity of the herbicide active ingredient is, spray application is unlikely to deliver a systemically toxic dose because the pattern of droplet size that most sprayers deliver does not include many respirable particles of less than 10 μm. The larger droplets can be inhaled, but they remain in the nasopharynx or upper respiratory tract and cause self-limiting irritation. Likewise, the mist droplets can impact on the skin and cause minor skin irritation or contact allergy if the formulation contains a preservative, a degraded ethoxylated surfactant, or another agent to which the sprayer is allergic. Absorption through the skin of the generally water-soluble active ingredients is poor; systemic effects are not expected.

91.5. Answer: D Paraquat displays dose-related toxicity. Contact with paraquat can cause local injury to the skin and nail beds. Ingestion of <20 mg/kg often results in a poisoning injury restricted to the GI tract. Ingestion of 20 to 40 mg/kg places the person at risk for GI tract corrosion, acute renal failure, and delayed but progressive pulmonary fibrosis leading to death weeks after the ingestion. Ingestion of amounts greater than 40 mg/kg places the person at risk of fulminant toxicity resulting in GI corrosion,

perhaps with perforation of the esophagus, rapid onset of multiorgan failure, cardiovascular collapse, and death in 1 to 5 days.

91.6. Answer: E Paraquat's toxic effect on the lung results from a unique combination of physiologic effects that localize it and its role as an extremely potent free radical generator. Its structure is recognized by the polyamine transport mechanism into pneumocytes, where it accumulated against the concentration gradient with the plasma. It is reduced by an NADPH-dependent process to a free radical, which then immediately interacts with molecular oxygen, reforming the parent paraquat and forming a superoxide radical. The paraquat ion is thus recycled, which amplifies its toxic generation of radicals. The oxygen radicals react with lipids in cell membranes, proteins and DNA, causing injury and death of the cells. The inflammatory response initiates migration of fibroblasts, which extensively deposit collagen into the interstitium and alveolar spaces, causing obliteration of alveoli.

91.7. Answer: E Likelihood of fatality in paraquat poisoning is predicted by a nomogram of plasma concentration against time. An initial level exceeding 3 mg/L has been invariably fatal, irrespective of clinical interventions. Many modalities have been attempted clinically with no significant success in averting death once the progressive pulmonary fibrosis begins. Even lung transplantation, which has been successfully accomplished only once, fails to rescue the patient.

91.8. Answer: D Diquat and paraquat are of similar oral toxicity; the LD_{50} of diquat is the same order of magnitude as that of paraquat. Because it is not selectively taken into pneumocytes, as is paraquat, diquat's ability to injure the lung is much diminished in comparison. Ingestions of diquat are less common but have resulted in deaths. Diquat is readily available in gardening stores.

91.9. Answer: D Glyphosate is not metabolized but is rapidly excreted unchanged in the urine. Although it is only poorly absorbed, this is not the mechanism of its selective toxicity to plants. It does not inhibit acetylcholinesterase at all. In the plant glyphosate interferes with the enzyme enolpyruval shikimic acid phosphate synthetase, by which plants make aromatic amino acids as precursors to chlorophyll synthesis. Because this pathway does not exist in man, there is a dramatic selective toxicity to plants, leaving mammals unaffected. It has wide application as a herbicide, and therefore, the potential for exposure is likewise robust; restricted access does not account for little human toxicity.

91.10. Answer: A Reports of large-volume ingestions of formulated glyphosate occasionally causing serious toxicity and death prompted inquiry into the contribution of both glyphosate and surfactant into the clinical symptoms. The characteristic features in formulated glyphosate ingestions are shared by nearly all commercial formulations of pesticides and are seen most clearly when the active ingredient itself is of a relatively low order of toxicity. Surfactant effects include GI tract irritation, edema and erosions, lung injury manifested as mild to moderate hypoxemia and sometimes frank acute lung injury, hypotension that ultimately fails to respond to therapy, and some degree of dysfunction in the brain, liver, and kidneys caused by hypotension.

CHAPTER **92**

INDUSTRIAL POISONING: INFORMATION AND CONTROL

92.1. Answer: D   The correct answer is substitution because removing the hazard from the workplace and replacing it with a non-hazardous substance completely removes the exposure.

92.2. Answer: E   The correct answer is the Occupational Safety and Health Administration, which requires MSDSs to be produced as part of the Hazardous Communication Standard. This standard is the cornerstone for dissemination of information about the chemical components of each substance used in the workplace.

92.3. Answer: B   The correct answer is the Occupational Safety and Health Administration, which requires MSDSs to be produced as part of the Hazardous Communication Standard. The HCS requires employers to establish hazard communication programs to transmit information on the hazards of chemicals to their employees by means of labels on containers, material safety data sheets, and training programs. Implementation of these hazard communication programs will ensure that all employees have the "right to know" the hazards and identities of the chemicals they work with and will reduce the incidence of chemically related occupational illnesses and injuries.

92.4. Answer: D   The correct answer is the Superfund Amendments and Reauthorization Act. Emergency Planning and Community Right-to-Know Act was enacted by Congress as the national legislation on community safety. This law was designated to help local communities protect public health, safety, and the environment from chemical hazards. The law requires manufacturers to report the amount of toxic substances released each year (Toxic Release Inventory, TRI).

92.5. Answer: D   The correct answer is private employment. ADA was enacted by Congress to establish clear and comprehensive prohibition of discrimination on the basis of disability. The act specifically covers discrimination in the areas of (1) employment, (2) public services, (3) public accommodations and services operated by private entities, and (4) telecommunications.

92.6. Answer: A   The correct answer is the employer. The act specifically states that "each employer shall furnish to each of his employees employment and a place of employment which are free from recognized hazards that are causing or are likely to cause death or serious physical harm to his employees."

92.7. Answer: B   The correct answer is the positive-pressure respirator. The dosimeter is a monitoring device, and all of the others are engineering controls.

92.8. Answer: E   The correct answer is urine phenol for benzene exposure. Primary prevention requires monitoring of increased exposure before there is a health effect. All the other answers are examples of secondary prevention, where the test is monitoring a health effect from an exposure.

92.9. Answer: E   The correct answer is reporting of health and safety studies. The act requires reporting of those studies in addition to premanufacturing notification for new chemicals, allegation of significant adverse reactions, and notification of suspicion of substantial risk to health.

92.10. Answer: C   The correct answer is hazard assessment. Before any of the other processes can be carried out, health and safety professionals must know what hazards are present in the workplace and what are the potential exposures. Industrial hygiene monitoring would then be performed to determine the level of exposure. Engineering controls are then established to control the exposures, and industrial hygiene monitoring is continued to insure that the controls are operating effectively. Medical surveillance and/or biologic monitoring is used as a secondary control to determine that controls are operating effectively and that there are no other unsuspected exposure pathways that are not controlled.

CHAPTER **93**

HAZMAT INCIDENT RESPONSE WITH PRE- AND INTERHOSPITAL CARE OF THE POISONED PATIENT

93.1. Answer: A   Responders or medical practitioners are of no help if they themselves become victims. Therefore, the paramount concern at a hazardous materials release is prevention of significant secondary contamination so that rescue and medical treatment can occur.

ATSDR: Managing Hazardous Materials Incidents, vol 1: Emergency Medical Services—A Planning Guide for the Management of Contaminated Patients. Washington, DC, US Department of Health and Human Services, 1992.

93.2. Answer: E   Failure to decontaminate completely may result in increased morbidity and/or mortality but may be overlooked in severely injured victims.

Bronstein AC: Medical management of hazmat victims. In: Walter FG, Klein R, Thomas RG, ed: Advanced Hazmat Life Support Provider Manual, 2nd ed. Tucson, AZ, Arizona Board of Regents, 2000, pp. 49–65.

Leonard RB: Hazardous materials accidents: Initial scene assessment and patient care. Aviat Space Environ Med 1993;64: 546–551.

93.3. Answer: A   Water reactivity is a worksite safety concern because of explosions and fires when bulk amounts of certain chemicals come in contact with water. Decontamination of victims should not be delayed because of this concern. The flushing action of the water is very important in separating the hazardous materials from the skin or mucous membranes. Skin and mucous membranes already contain water and are reacting with the hazardous materials.

Bronstein AC: Medical management of hazmat victims. In: Walter FG, Klein R, Thomas RG, ed: Advanced Hazmat Life Support Provider Manual, 2nd ed. Tucson, AZ, Arizona Board of Regents, 2000, pp. 49–65.

93.4. Answer: E There are three types of exposures that may occur in a radioactive hazardous materials incident: irradiation, contamination, and incorporation. Specific therapeutic interventions may be helpful.

Waldron RL 2d, Danielson RA, Shultz HE, et al: Radiation decontamination unit for the community hospital. AJR Am J Roentgenol 1981;136:977–981.

93.5. Answer: E If there is no residual radioactive hazardous material on the victim, medical treatment can proceed without any special precautions.

Leonard RB, Ricks RC: Emergency department radiation, accident protocol. Ann Emerg Med 1980;9:462–470.

93.6. Answer: E Typical ED garb in the era of universal blood-borne pathogen precautions is designed to protect against splashes and sprays. There is an assumption of no risk of dermal or mucous-membrane absorption from air contamination. However, the typical ED garb has virtually no protective rating against corrosive materials, and the garb is porous to many other chemicals. For a contaminated patient, an emergency responder cart should be available.

Gough AR, Markus K: Hazardous materials protection in the ED practice: Laws and logistics. J Emerg Nurs 1989;15:476–480.

93.7. Answer: B Many chemicals, even in small amounts, may present a risk to medical practitioners if proper decontamination does not occur. However, because the amounts on a single contaminated victim are small, the decontamination and disposal of the waste can be safely handled in an ED if proper planning has already taken place.

Merritt NL, Anderson MJ: Malathion overdose: When one patient creates a departmental hazard. J Emerg Nurs 1989;15:463–465.

93.8. Answer: B The organization of a hazardous materials incident begins with the establishment of the hot zone with a decontamination zone and treatment zone subsequently safely established upwind to avoid injury to the responders.

Bronstein AC: Medical management of hazmat victims. In: Walter FG, Klein R, Thomas RG, ed: Advanced Hazmat Life Support Provider Manual, 2nf ed. Tucson, AZ, Arizona Board of Regents, 2000, pp. 49–65.

Leonard RB: Hazardous materials accidents: Initial scene assessment and patient care. Aviat Space Environ Med 1993;64: 546–551.

93.9. Answer: C Decontamination and protection of responders is the primary tenet of prehospital management. Inhalation is the most common route of exposure, and therefore, proper respiratory protective equipment as well as the training to use the equipment is important. Most incidents that involve the public are transporta-

tion related, occur in rural as well as urban areas, and are not related to manufacturing facilities.

Bronstein AC: Medical management of hazmat victims. In: Walter FG, Klein R, Thomas RG, ed: Advanced Hazmat Life Support Provider Manual, 2nf ed. Tucson, AZ, Arizona Board of Regents, 2000, pp. 49–65.

93.10. Answer: C With exposure to 75 to 125 rem, mild GI symptoms such as anorexia, nausea, and vomiting occur; acute radiation syndrome occurs with acute exposures of >500 rem. Chapter 99. Radiation.

CHAPTER 94

METHEMOGLOBINEMIA

94.1. Answer: C The *N*-hydroxylation of dapsone to its hydroxylamine metabolite is in part responsible for dapsone's methemoglobin production. This is a cytochrome P450 metabolite. Cimetidine, an inhibitor of this metabolic pathway, has been used to decrease the production of this methemoglobin-producing compound.

Rhodes LE, Tingle MD, Park BK, et al: Cimetidine improves the therapeutic/toxic ratio of dapsone in patients on chronic dapsone therapy. Br J Dermatol 1995;132:257–262.

94.2. Answer: B This slightly elevated level of methemoglobin may be related to well water consumption; however, the most common cause of cyanosis is hypoxia. This patient had a fever, responded to oxygen therapy, and had symptoms usually not found with this level of methemoglobin. Oxygen therapy is appropriate for both the hypoxia and methemoglobinemia causing the infant's cyanosis.

Comly HH: Cyanosis in infants caused by nitrates in well water. JAMA 1945;129:112–116.

Craun GF, Greathouse DG, Gunderson DH: Methemoglobin levels in young children consuming high nitrate well water in the United States. Int J Epidemiol 1981;10:309–317.

94.3. Answer: C A relatively small portion of the hemoglobin molecule is affected when methemoglobin is formed. The loss of an electron from the outer shell of iron in the center of the porphyrin ring profoundly alters oxygen affinity. Oxidant stress on the proteins in the red cell membrane may cause hemolysis, but this is unrelated to methemoglobinemia.

94.4. Answer: C Although it may be a cause of symptoms after fire injury, carbon monoxide toxicity alone is not associated with cyanosis. Increased levels of deoxygenated hemoglobin and in some cases methemoglobin may be the cause of cyanosis.

Hoffman RS, Sauter D: Methemoglobinemia resulting from smoke inhalation. Vet Hum Toxicol 1989;31:40–42.

94.5. Answer: E All of the substances mentioned have been associated with methemoglobin formation in infants. Infants under 4 months of age are particularly susceptible because of their low levels of NADH methemoglobin reductase activity.

Craun GF, Greathouse DG, Gunderson DH: Methemoglobin levels in young children consuming high nitrate well water in the United States. Int J Epidemiol 1981;10:309–317.

Dean BS, Lopez G, Krenzelok EP: Environmentally induced methemoglobin in an infant. J Toxicol Clin Toxicol 1992;30:127–133.

94.6. Answer: B   Patients generally tolerate methemoglobin levels of 15% quite well and exhibit a mild cyanosis. However, preexisting disease such as anemia, pneumonia, or cardiovascular disease may make this level of methemoglobin clinically stressful.

94.7. Answer: B   Metoclopramide has been associated with both methemoglobinemia and sulfhemoglobinemia.

Van Veldhuizen PJ, Wyatt A: Metoclopramide-induced sulfhemoglobinemia. Am J Gastroenterol 1995;90:1010–1011.

94.8. Answer: B   NADH methemoglobin reductase activity is low during the first 4 months of life. This contributes to the increased susceptibility of infants to methemoglobinemia.

Pollack ES, Pollack CV: Incidence of subclinical methemoglobinemia in infants with diarrhea. Ann Emerg Med 1994;24:652–656.

Yano SS, Danish EH, Hsia YE: Transient methemoglobinemia with acidosis in infants. J Pediatr 1982;100:415–418.

94.9. Answer: C   Small amounts (1.5 g/dL) of oxidized hemoglobin (methemoglobin) produce a detectable cyanosis. It takes 5 g/dL of reduced hemoglobin (deoxygenated hemoglobin) to produce the same cyanosis. Sulfhemoglobin produces detectable cyanosis with just 0.5 g/dL of this pigment present.

94.10. Answer: E   All of the compounds listed are electron donors capable of reducing oxidized hemoglobin. NADH generated in the Embden-Meyerhof glycolytic pathway is quantitatively the most important reducing agent. Individuals deficient in NADH methemoglobin reductase have elevated methemoglobin levels ranging from 10 to 50% even without oxidant stress provocation.

Beutler E: Methemoglobin and sulfhemoglobinemia. In: Williams JW, Beutler E, Ersleu AJ, Lichtman MA, eds: Hematology, 4th ed. New York, McGraw-Hill, 1990, pp. 379–388.

Hegesh E, Hegesh J, Kaftory A: Congenital methemoglobinemia with a deficiency of cytochrome b5. N Engl J Med 1985;314:757–761.

CHAPTER 95

SIMPLE ASPHYXIANTS AND PULMONARY IRRITANTS

95.1. Answer: C   Although it is possible to develop both ALI and MI simultaneously, heart failure during an MI commonly causes cardiogenic pulmonary edema or congestive heart failure. Acute lung injury is a spectrum ranging from very mild lung injury to ARDS. ALI is rarely fatal, although ARDS is associated with poor outcomes. ARDS requires the demonstration of severe pulmonary failure secondary to noncardiogenic pulmonary edema. ARDS may be caused by many clinical conditions, most commonly trauma or sepsis; toxin exposure is a relatively uncommon etiology. The more water-soluble gases tend to produce upper airway irritation, and the less soluble gases affect the lower airway and lung.

Bernard GR, Artigas A, Brigham KL, et al: The American-European Consensus Conference on ARDS: Definitions, mechanisms, relevant outcomes, and clinical trial coordination. Am J Respir Crit Care Med 1994;149:818–824.

Kimbell JS, Gross EA, Joyner DR, et al: Application of computational fluid dynamics to regional dosimetry of inhaled chemicals in the upper respiratory tract of the rat. Toxicol Appl Pharmacol 1993;121:253–263.

95.2. Answer: B   Simple asphyxiants produce their clinical toxicity by limiting the supply of available oxygen. Therefore, toxicity is directly related to the concentration of gas present and is independent of which gas it is. By definition they produce hypoxia (and a low Po_2 and O_2 saturation). A few asphyxiant gases produce clinical toxicity even in the absence of hypoxia. For example, carbon dioxide may produce a respiratory acidosis, and nitrogen may produce "nitrogen narcosis." Asphyxiant gases may not produce dyspnea or pulmonary edema because the patient's gas exchange (Pco_2) is initially normal, and they do not have pulmonary irritation. The finding of blood-tinged sputum should suggest pulmonary edema. Although uncommon, simple asphyxiation may occur outdoors, as in Lake Nyos, 1986.

Suruda A, Agnew J: Deaths from asphyxiation and poisoning at work in the United States, 1984–1986. Br J Ind Med 1989;46:541–546.

95.3. Answer: D   Water-soluble irritants typically produce rapid onset of upper airway irritation and prompt escape from the gas, limiting exposure. Although symptoms may progress for hours, they do not begin in a delayed fashion. Symptoms may develop in the eyes, nose, and mouth if they are exposed. The blood gas is typically normal because the lungs are not involved. Symptoms following inhalation of acid-forming gases, such as chloramine, may improve with nebulized dilute sodium bicarbonate. However, it is currently unclear whether the natural history of the disease is altered.

Vinsel PJ: Treatment of acute chlorine gas inhalation with nebulized sodium bicarbonate. J Emerg Med 1990;8:327–329.

95.4. Answer: C   Chloramine is a toxic product that results from the admixture of bleach and ammonia. Combustion of plastic may liberate phosgene, nitrogen dioxide, or cyanide as well as other toxic gases, depending on which type of plastic is burned. Silo filler disease is caused by the development of the oxides of nitrogen including nitrogen dioxide, which is generated by decomposing fertilizer and dirt. HF is irritating, but its lethality results from its chemical properties (eg, hypocalcemia, hyperkalemia).

Braun J, Stoss H, Zober A: Intoxication following the inhalation of hydrogen fluoride. Arch Toxicol 1984;56:50–54.

Douglas WW, Hepper NGG, Colby TV: Silo-filler's disease. Mayo Clin Proc 1989;64:291–304.

95.5. Answer: A   Reactive airways dysfunction syndrome (RADS), or "irritant-induced asthma," is a persistent asthmalike syndrome associated with acute exposure to a toxic gas. It appears that virtually any irritating gas may produce RADS. Helium is a nonirritating simple asphyxiant that has never been associated with RADS.

Brooks SM, Weiss MA, Bernstein IL: Reactive airways dysfunction syndrome. Case reports of persistent asthma syndrome after high level irritant exposure. Chest 1985;88:376–384.

Meggs WJ: RADS and RUDS: The toxic induction of asthma and rhinitis. J Toxicol Clin Toxicol 1994;32:487–501.

95.6. Answer: D   Although anecdotal cases support their utility, corticosteroids have never been proven beneficial. Because highly concentrated bicarbonate by nebulizer is irritating and may induce bronchospasm, dilute (2%) solutions should be used. Hypoxic patients need supplemental oxygen to fully oxygenate their hemoglobin (oxygen-carrying capacity is almost totally predicted by the hemoglobin saturation). Beyond that, little further improvement in oxygen delivery occurs, but there may be a risk of oxygen-induced worsening of the pulmonary damage. Hyperbaric oxygen therapy may be even more problematic because of the extremely high partial pressure of oxygen to which the patient is exposed. Surfactant therapy is still experimental.

Deneke SM, Fanburg BL: Normobaric oxygen toxicity of the lung. N Engl J Med 1980;303:76–86.

Meduri GU, Belenchia JM, Estes RJ, et al: Fibroproliferative phase of ARDS: clinical findings and effects of corticosteroids. Chest 1991;100:943–952.

95.7. Answer: D   Phosgene poisoning unfortunately still occurs as a result of fires and its use in industry. It has a pleasant odor ("freshly cut hay"), which accounts in part for its success as a war gas. Its dissolution in lung water is slow, but once dissolved, it generates acid products that incite an inflammatory response. Many agents, including *N*-acetylcysteine, have been used to limit the inflammatory influx, most without dramatic success.

Ghio AJ, Kennedy TP, Hatch GE, Tepper JS: Reduction of neutrophil influx diminishes lung injury and mortality following phosgene inhalation. J Appl Physiol 1991;71:657–665.

95.8. Answer: D   CN (chloroacetophenone) has been used as a riot-control agent, although it has largely been replaced by CS (2-chlorobenzylidenemalononitrile) and capsaicin. Ozone is not effective because it is not irritating acutely. MIC (methylisocyanate) and acrolein are highly toxic irritants and, like cyanide, too dangerous to use for riot control.

Hu H, Fine J, Epstein P, et al: Tear gas: Harassing agent or toxic chemical weapon? JAMA 1989;262:660–663.

95.9. Answer: B   A recurrent flulike illness (dyspnea, myalgia, headache) associated with fever in patients exposed to metal fumes essentially defines metal fume fever. The etiology is likely to be immunologic, and direct pulmonary toxicity does not occur. Patients generally have normal chest radiographs, and serum metal levels are not elevated. Interestingly, acute tolerance develops so that repeat daily exposure produces milder symptoms, but after a short work hiatus, such as a weekend, the tolerance is lost. Galvanized steel, which contains zinc, is most frequently implicated. The management of patients with metal fume fever is supportive and includes analgesics and antipyretics. There is no specific antidote, and chelation is unnecessary.

Blanc P, Wong H, Bernstein MS, Boushey HA: An experimental human model of metal fume fever. Ann Intern Med 1991;114:930–936.

Blount BW: Two types of metal fume fever: Mild vs. serious. Mil Med 1990;155:372–377.

95.10. Answer: C   Ammonia added to hypochlorous acid (bleach) forms chloramine gas (**A**). Chlorine dissolved in water liberates both acid and nascent oxygen, which is a potent oxidizer (**B**). Oxygen generates superoxide and other free radicals in the presence of transition metal catalysts such as iron (**D**). Sulfur dioxide forms sulfurous acid when exposed to water (**E**). Nitrogen (**C**) is inert and does not dissolve well in water; nitrous acid is not formed.

Hattis RP, Greer JR, Dietrich S, et al: Chlorine gas toxicity from mixture of bleach with other cleaning products—California. MMWR 1991;40;619–629.

Manahan SE: Toxicologic Chemistry, 2nd ed. Boca Raton, FL, Lewis Publishers, 1992.

CHAPTER **96**

SMOKE INHALATION

96.1. Answer: C   Disastrous fires are frequent reminders of the role of smoke inhalation injuries in fire deaths. In 1999, the National Fire Protection Agency reported 3570 fire deaths and 21,875 fire injuries in the United States. An estimated 50 to 80% of these fire deaths are from smoke inhalation injuries rather than dermal burns or trauma.

Bowes PC: Casualties attributed to toxic gas and smoke at fires: A survey of statistics. Med Sci Law 1976;16:104–110.

Harwood B, Hall JR: What kills in fires: Smoke inhalation or burns? Fire J 1989;84:29–34.

96.2. Answer: B   Cyanide is produced from combustion of many nitrogen-containing products such as plastics, polyurethanes, wool, silk, nylon, nitrocellulose, polyacrylonitriles, synthetic rubber, and paper. High concentrations of cyanide have been measured in air samples from fires, and elevated blood cyanide concentrations have been reported in both fire survivors and fire fatalities. In addition to cyanide, combustion of plastics produces HCl, aldehydes, ammonia, oxides of nitrogen, phosgene, and chlorine.

Orzel RA: Toxicologic aspects of firesmoke: Polymer pyrolysis and combustion. Occup Med 1993;8:414–429.

Shusterman D, Alexeeff G, Hargis C, et al. Predictors of carbon monoxide and hydrogen cyanide exposure in smoke inhalation patients. J Toxicol Clin Toxicol 1996;34:61–71.

96.3. Answer: E   Polyvinyl chloride (PVC) is widely used in a number of products including furnishings, floor coverings, and electrical insulation. Subsequently, the combustion products of PVC, carbon monoxide, hydrogen chloride, chlorine, and phosgene, are present in many fires.

Dyer RF, Esch VH: Polyvinyl chloride toxicity in fires: Hydrogen chloride toxicity in fire fighters. JAMA 1976;235:393–397.

Markowitz JS, Gutterman EM, Schwartz S, et al: Acute health effects among firefighters exposed to a polyvinyl chloride (PVC) fire. Am J Epidemiol 1989;129:1023–1031.

96.4. Answer: D   Water solubility is the most important chemical characteristic of an irritant toxin in determining the level of the respiratory tract injury. Highly water-soluble gases react with the upper airway mucosa to produce an intense inflammatory reaction. Unless irritant gas concentrations are extremely high or duration of exposure is prolonged, injury is limited to the mucosa of the upper airways. Conversely, chemicals with low water solubility do not react with the upper airway mucosa and reach the lung parenchyma.

Prien T: Toxic smoke compounds and inhalation injury—a review. Burns 1988;14:451–460.

96.5. Answer: D   Acrolein, ammonia, sulfur dioxide, phosgene, chlorine, and hydrogen chloride are all examples of irritant chemicals formed during combustion and found within smoke. Acrolein is one of the most common irritant gases generated in fires.

Davies JW: Toxic chemicals versus lung tissue—an aspect of inhalation injury revisited. J Burn Care Rehabil 1986;7:213–222.

96.6. Answer: C   There are four chemical asphyxiants: carbon monoxide, cyanide, hydrogen sulfide, and oxides of nitrogen, which may generate methemoglobinemia. Acrolein is one of the most common irritant gases found within smoke.

Becker CE: The role of cyanide in fires. Vet Hum Toxicol 1985; 27:487–490.

Birky MM, Clarke FB: Inhalation of toxic products from fires. Bull NY Acad Med 1981;57:997–1013.

96.7. Answer: E   Indications for early intubation in the burn victim include CNS depression, stridor, full-thickness circumferential neck burns, and oropharyngeal edema. Rapid clinical deterioration may occur in these patients, and upper airway patency must be established. Fiberoptic endoscopy is the preferred method, but when it is not available, prophylactic intubation is justified. Wheezing is indicative of bronchospasm and commonly encountered in fire victims. Inhaled albuterol is the treatment of choice for bronchospasm.

Haponik EF, Summer WR: Respiratory complications in burned patients: Diagnosis and management of inhalation injury. J Crit Care 1987;2:121–143.

96.8. Answer: E   The water solubility, concentration and particle size of the toxin, the duration of exposure to the toxin, and the respiratory rate, absence of protective reflexes, and presence of preexisting disease in the person exposed to the smoke all influence the level of the respiratory tract injury.

Prien T: Toxic smoke compounds and inhalation injury—a review. Burns 1988;14:451–460.

96.9. Answer: E   Tracheobronchial injuries are a result of inhaled particulates and toxic gases causing increased airway resistance from intraluminal debris, airway mucosal edema, inspissated secretions, and bronchospasm. Thermal injury is rare at this level unless steam is inhaled.

Prien T: Toxic smoke compounds and inhalation injury—a review. Burns 1988;14:451–460.

Wang CZ, Li A, Yang ZC: The pathophysiology of carbon monoxide poisoning and acute respiratory failure in a sheep model with smoke inhalation injury. Chest 1990;97:736–742.

96.10. Answer: E   Lactic acidosis, common in patients with smoke inhalation, is the result of pulmonary dysfunction resulting in hypoxia, carbon monoxide poisoning, cyanide poisoning, and/or tissue hypoperfusion. Hypoxia from any cause impairs aerobic metabolism and generates lactic acid.

Baud FJ, Barriot P, Toffis V, et al: Elevated blood cyanide concentrations in victims of smoke inhalation. N Engl J Med 1991; 325:1761–1766.

Sokal JA, Kralkowska E: The relationship between exposure duration, carboxyhemoglobin, blood glucose, pyruvate and lactate, and the severity of intoxication in 39 cases of acute carbon monoxide poisoning in man. Arch Toxicol 1985;57:196–199.

CHAPTER **97**

CARBON MONOXIDE

97.1. Answer: D   Methylene chloride is metabolized in the liver to CO.

Stewart RD, Hake CL: Paint remover hazard. JAMA 1976;235: 398–401.

97.2. Answer: E   In the presence of CO and the formation of carboxyhemoglobin, the remaining oxyhemoglobin offloads oxygen less readily. This is a leftward shift in the oxyhemoglobin dissociation curve.

Roughton FJW, Darling RC: The effect of carbon monoxide on the hemoglobin dissociation curve. Am J Physiol 1944;141:17–31.

97.3. Answer: E   Pulse oximetry results in a falsely elevated oxygen saturation measure, thereby causing failure to detect appreciable amounts of carboxyhemoglobin. Likewise, the oxygen saturation from an arterial blood gas will be falsely high because it is calculated based on dissolved oxygen rather than measured. Breath sampling will erroneously detect carbon monoxide in the presence of ethanol, a hydrocarbon that can activate the CO-detecting electrodes. The most reliable way to exclude carbon monoxide intoxication is to determine a carboxyhemoglobin level. Heparinized tubes of venous blood appear to be as reliable as arterial samples.

Buckley RG, Aks SE, Eshom JL, et al: The pulse oximetry gap in carbon monoxide intoxication. Ann Emerg Med 1994;24: 252–255.

Touger M, Gallagher EJ, Tyrell J: Relationship between venous and arterial carboxyhemoglobin levels in patients with suspected carbon monoxide poisoning. Ann Emerg Med 1995;25:481–483.

97.4. Answer: E All the listed sequelae have been reported in two large series of serious CO exposures that had long-term followup and did not receive hyperbaric oxygen therapy.

Choi HS: Delayed neurologic sequelae in carbon monoxide intoxication. Arch Neurol 1983;40:433–435.

Kim SK: A brain syndrome associated with delayed neuropsychiatric sequelae following acute carbon monoxide intoxication. Acta Psychiatr Scand 1986;73:80–86.

97.5. Answer: E Many exposures to CO during pregnancy result in apparently normal infants. But a few of these pregnancies result in stillbirths, or if the fetus survives, it may manifest a variety of neurologic disorders including mental retardation or cerebral palsy. Placental abruption has not been reported.

Koren G, Sharav T, Paastuszak A, et al: A multicenter, prospective study of fetal outcome following accidental carbon monoxide poisoning in pregnancy. Reprod Toxicol 1991;5:397–403.

97.6. Answer: A Carbon monoxide has a gas density of 0.968 relative to air. With diffusion, it should distribute readily in an enclosed environment.

97.7. Answer: A Leukocyte adherence to brain microvasculature appears to be an essential step that precedes lipid peroxidation of the brain in the rat model of serious CO intoxication.

Thom SR: Leukocytes in carbon monoxide–mediated brain oxidative injury. Toxicol Appl Pharmacol 1993;123:234–247.

97.8. Answer: D The globus pallidus and deep white matter are the most common areas showing low density on CT scanning after serious CO poisoning.

Choi IS, Kim SK, Choi YC, et al: Evaluation of outcome after acute carbon monoxide poisoning by CT. J Korean Med Sci 1993;8:78–83.

Tom T, Abedon S, Clark RI, et al: Neuroimaging characteristics in carbon monoxide toxicity. J Neuroimaging 1996;6:161–166.

97.9. Answer: D The elimination half-life clearance of carboxyhemoglobin is reduced from about 5 hours to slightly less than 1 hour on 100% face-mask oxygen.

Myers RAM, Jones DW, Britten JS: Carbon monoxide half life. In: Proceedings of the VIII International Congress on Hyperbaric Medicine, Long Beach, CA, 1987, p. 263.

Peterson JE, Stewart RD: Absorption and elimination of carbon monoxide by inactive young men. Arch Environ Health 1970;21: 165–171.

97.10. Answer: A An interval of unconsciousness after acute CO exposure is associated with a higher risk of morbidity and neurologic sequelae. Particular carboxyhemoglobin levels are not reliable enough to predict outcome.

Hardy KR, Thom SR: Pathophysiology and treatment of carbon monoxide poisoning. J Toxicol Clin Toxicol 1994;32:613–629.

CHAPTER 98

CYANIDE AND HYDROGEN SULFIDE

98.1. Answer: C Evidence supports both antidotal mechanisms. Nitrites oxidize hemoglobin to methemoglobin, a hemoglobin form that has a higher affinity for CN ion than cytochrome oxidase. In addition, nitrites are potent vasodilators that increase hepatic blood flow and enhance CN metabolism.

Smith L, Kruszyna H, Smith RP: The effect of methemoglobin on the inhibition of cytochrome c oxidase by cyanide, sulfide, or azide. Biochem Pharmacol 1977;26:2247–2250.

Sun P, Borowitz JL, Kanthasamy AG, Kane MD, Isom GE: Antagonism of cyanide toxicity by isosorbide dinitrate: Possible role of nitric oxide. Toxicology 1995;104:105–111.

98.2. Answer: D Hypotension is common as a result of nitric oxide–mediated vasodilation. Excessive methemoglobin formation is another adverse event that would result in cyanosis but not in lowered P_{O_2}.

Kiese M, Weger NP: Formation of ferrihemoglobin with aminophenols in the human for the treatment of cyanide poisoning. Eur J Pharmacol 1969;7:97–105.

98.3. Answer: C The CNS appears to be the organ system most sensitive to cyanide. CNS manifestations include headache, confusion, agitation, convulsions, and coma. Cardiac toxicity includes progressive failure with bradycardia and not ventricular dysrhythmias. Gastrointestinal symptoms are frequent following ingestion of cyanide or cyanogens. Cyanide interferes with oxygen utilization but not with the capacity of the blood to carry oxygen. Thus, cyanosis may occur, but it is uncommon and is seen in late toxicity when the patient has profound shock.

98.4. Answer: D There is substantial evidence that cyanide toxicity is multifactorial in nature. Cyanide promotes lipid peroxidation and inhibits antioxidant enzymes. Cyanide inhibits ctyochrome oxidase in the electron transport chain, thereby decreasing tissue oxygen utilization. Cyanide stimulation of CNS NMDA receptors leads to excessive free cytosolic calcium and subsequent neuronal death. The blood oxygen content and P_{O_2} are normal.

Johnson JD, Conroy WG, Burris KD, Isom GE: Peroxidation of brain lipids following cyanide intoxication in mice. Toxicology 1987;46:21–28.

Patel MN, Yim GKW, Isom GE: N-Methyl-D-aspartate receptors mediate cyanide-induced toxicity in hippocampal cultures. Neurotoxicology 1993;14:35–40.

Way JL: Cyanide intoxication and its mechanism of antagonism. Annu Rev Pharmacol Toxicol 1984;24:451–481.

98.5. Answer: B The basal ganglia (including the globus pallidus and putamen) are the brain structures most commonly damaged following cyanide poisoning.

Rosenow F, Herholz K, Lanfermann H, et al: Neurological sequelae of cyanide intoxication—The patterns of clinical, magnetic resonance imaging, and positron emission tomography findings. Ann Neurol 1995;38:825–828.

98.6. Answer: B Cyanide poisoning results in anion-gap metabolic acidosis caused by lactate accumulation. Central venous oxygen content increases as a result of diminished oxygen uptake by the peripheral tissues.

Johnson RP, Mellors JW: Arteriolization of venous blood gases: A clue to the diagnosis of cyanide poisoning. J Emerg Med 1988; 6:401–404.

98.7. Answer: E Cyanide is a significant cause of death in fire victims. Ingestion of nitriles and seeds of pitted fruits can lead to toxicity when gut enzymes release cyanide from the parent cyanogenic compound. Cyanide poisoning can occur iatrogenically when nitroprusside is used for a prolonged period in the presence of renal failure.

Baud FJ, Barriot P, Toffis V, et al: Elevated blood cyanide concentrations in victims of smoke inhalation. N Engl J Med 1991; 325:1761–1766.

Caravati EM, Litovitz TL: Pediatric cyanide intoxication from an acetonitrile-containing cosmetic. JAMA 1988;260:3470–3473.

98.8. Answer: C Olfactory paralysis occurs at >100 ppm, and coma typically at >700 ppm. Rescuers may misperceive failure to smell the rotten eggs as a sign that it is safe to enter a contaminated environment and expose themselves to more hazardous concentrations of hydrogen sulfide.

Reiffenstein RJ, Hulbert WC, Rother SH: Toxicology of hydrogen sulfide. Annu Rev Pharmacol Toxicol 1992;32:109–134.

98.9. Answer: B Hydrogen sulfide is a strong mucous membrane and pulmonary irritant. At higher concentrations, it causes central respiratory paralysis.

Burnett WW, King EG, Grace M: Hydrogen sulfide poisoning: Review of 5 years' experience. Can Med Assoc J 1977;117: 1277–1280.

98.10. Answer: D Hydrogen sulfide is a by-product of industrial processes such as paper production, leather production, vulcaniza-

tion of rubber, and natural gas refining. Hydrogen sulfide is a natural product of bacterial decomposition of protein-containing substances (sewage) and of volcanoes, sulfur springs, and underground gas deposits.

Smith RP, Gosselin RE: Hydrogen sulfide poisoning. J Occup Med 1979;21:93–97.

CHAPTER **99**

RADIATION

99.1. Answer: D Criticality refers to a chain reaction of fissions of fissionable material, such as ^{235}U or ^{239}Pu. As an efficient means of generating energy, the fission of 1 g of a nuclide material per day yields energy at a rate of 1 megawatt, which would otherwise require the combustion of 2.6 tons of coal. As in Los Alamos, New Mexico, and more recently in Tokaimura, Japan, criticality events may occur when too much fissionable material is placed in one area, such as a laboratory or storage tank. The "critical mass" then achieved refers to the increased probability that a stray neutron that can precipitate the reaction will be captured by the fissionable material instead of lost.

Halliday D, Resnick R, Edwards WF, Merrill J: Fundamentals of Physics, 2nd ed. New York, John Wiley & Sons, 1970, pp. 912–916.

99.2. Answer: A In September 1987, two men scavenged an abandoned radiotherapy clinic, eventually removing a 3×3 cm Cs pellet weighing 91.9 g. This pellet contained 50.9×10^{12} Bq of Cs. By comparison, the estimated amount or radioactivity released after the Chernobyl event was 1.2×10^{19} Bq, and the amount used in a thallium stress test is about 111×10^{6} Bq.

Oliveira AR, Hunt JG, Valverde NJL, et al: Medical and related aspects of the Goiânia accident: An overview. Health Phys 1991;60:17–24.

99.3. Answer: B All of these devices utilize electromagnetic radiation, which is mediated by photons of various energies as determined by their frequency. However, all of these signals are considered to consist of photons of insufficient energy to cause cellular injury. Studies are ongoing to determine the long-term effects of the various devices in our environment; however, the data regarding potential harm remain inconclusive to date.

99.4. Answer: C Of the natural products of decay, only neutrons may cause an exposed item to become radioactive. ^{24}Na, ^{36}Cl, and ^{32}P represent several radioactive isotopes that may be created following an exposure. This is the principle of radioactive fallout when a nuclear device is detonated. The dust and debris from the explosion are changed into radioactive materials and are dispersed over the blast site and carried in the atmosphere.

Saenger EL: Radiation accidents. Ann Emerg Med 1986;15: 1061–1066.

Shipman TL: Acute radiation death resulting from an accidental nuclear critical excursion. J Occup Med [Spec Suppl] 1961;3: 146–192.

99.5. Answer: B In general, radiosensitivity is directly related to the rate of proliferation and inversely with the degree of differentiation. However, the most radiosensitive cell type is the lymphocyte, which is a nondividing, mature cell. The various tissues' radiosensitivities are important in determining the severity and timing of a large radiation exposure where acute radiation syndrome results.

Reeves GI: Radiation injuries. Crit Care Clin 1999;2:457–473.

99.6. Answer: B Because water is the most abundant constituent of most cells, it is the molecule most commonly affected by radiation. Fortunately, conversion of water to hydrogen and hydroxyl ions is of little consequence in that most of these ions will recombine to form water. The statistical likelihood of any particular radiation resulting in an alteration in DNA and thus affecting subsequent cellular function or longevity is actually quite small, in comparison.

99.7. Answer: C Radon is the only gaseous radioactive uranium daughter. People with exposure to radioactive uranium-238 (through mining or residential exposure) inhale radioactive radon-222, which results from decay of the uranium. The radon then irradiates their lungs, resulting in an increased risk of carcinoma.

Pershagen G, Akerblom G, Axelson O, et al: Residential radon exposure and lung cancer in Sweden. N Engl J Med 1994; 330:159–164.

99.8. Answer: A A dose–response relationship has been established between radiation exposure in Nagasaki and thyroid disease. Survivors tended to have a high incidence of cancer, adenomatous goiter, adenoma, solid nodules, and nodules without histologic diagnosis. A concave dose–response relationship suggests an unclear relationship with relatively low-dose radiation.

Nagataki S, Shibata Y, Inoue S, et al: Thyroid diseases among atomic bomb survivors in Nagasaki. JAMA 1994;272:364–370.

99.9. Answer: E Children exposed in utero to radiation from the atomic bombs have higher incidences of mental retardation and microcephaly. However, first-generation offspring from bomb survivors who were not exposed in utero seem to have no increased incidence of cancer or these other disorders.

Yoshimoto Y: Cancer risk among children of atomic bomb survivors: A review of RERF epidemiologic studies. JAMA 1990; 264:596–600.

99.10. Answer: E Total body radiation doses in excess of 1000 rad (10 gy) are usually fatal, but with a delay of 1 to 2 weeks. Patients die of gastrointestinal fluid loss, bleeding, and subsequent infection. Doses in excess of 10,000 rad (100 gy) are immediately fatal, with death resulting from cerebral edema.

Fry RJM, Fry SA: Health effects of ionizing radiation. Med Clin North Am 1990;74:475–488.

CHAPTER **100**

CHEMICAL AND BIOLOGIC WEAPONS

100.1. Answer: E Of the nerve agents listed, VX has the least volatility and greatest persistence; it is an oily liquid at standard temperature and pressure. The concept of volatility does not apply to gaseous chemical agents such as phosgene (in essence, they are infinitely volatile under standard conditions).

Sidell FR, Borak J: Chemical warfare agents: II. Nerve agents. Ann Emerg Med 1992;21:865–871.

100.2. Answer: C Sulfur mustard is a vesicant, or blister agent. GD (soman) and VX are organic phosphorus nerve agents. Botulinum toxin is a bioweapon with no dermal activity. T-2 toxin, a tricothecene mycotoxin, is one of the few dermally active biologic agents but causes irritation and inflammation without vesiculation.

Mellor SG, Rice P, Cooper GJ: Vesicant burns. Br J Plast Surg 1991;44:434–437.

100.3. Answer: A Although nerve agents are extremely potent, acute treatment requires less atropine than for victims poisoned to a similar degree with organic phosphorus insecticides. The total dose of atropine required in nerve agent victims typically does not exceed 12 to 20 mg within the first 24 hours.

Okumura T, Takasu N, Ishimatsu S, et al: Report on 640 victims of the Tokyo subway sarin attack. Ann Emerg Med 1996;28:129.

100.4. Answer: B Although toxicity from inhaled botulinum toxin can result in diaphragmatic paralysis and respiratory failure, the pulmonary parenchyma is not affected, and so a true "pulmonary syndrome" does not occur. Phosgene induces delayed pulmonary edema from increased capillary–alveolar membrane permeability. Inhalational anthrax *(Bacillus anthracis)* and pneumonic plague *(Yersinia pestis)* produce fever, cough, and dyspnea that can rapidly progress to fatal results. Q fever *(Coxiella burnetti)* is characterized by fever, malaise, and cough that may be temporarily incapacitating.

Franz DR, Jahrling PB, Friedlander AM, et al: Clinical recognition and management of patients exposed to biological warfare agents. JAMA 1997;278:399–411.

100.5. Answer: D Agents with the greatest persistence are most likely to remain on victims, their clothing, and possessions, potentially contaminating other persons or objects. Sarin and soman are less persistent than sulfur mustard and VX. Victims contaminated with VX will almost certainly be symptomatic, if not already dead, providing clear clues to rescue and healthcare personnel that proper protective gear and decontamination will be necessary. Victims contaminated with sulfur mustard may initially have minimal or no symptoms, which can allow for lapses in contamination precautions. Aerosolized anthrax spores pose little risk of cross-contamination.

Brennan RJ, Waeckerle JF, Sharp TW, Lillibridge SR: Chemical warfare agents: Emergency medical and emergency public health issues. Ann Emerg Med 1999;34:191–204.

100.6. Answer: C Severe nerve agent and cyanide toxicity can present with sudden collapse and respiratory failure. Botulism may also cause victims to collapse from weakness and produce respiratory failure, although the symptoms will take many hours to days to develop. Mass-casualty victims from Lewisite exposure should present with dermal, ocular, and respiratory tract symptoms. The most severely poisoned Lewisite victims can develop shock and respiratory tract failure in a delayed fashion.

100.7. Answer: C The described toxidrome is typical for riot-control agents. Although nausea and vomiting are classic from Adamsite exposure, such systemic effects may also be produced by lacrimator agents such as chloroacetophenone. Nerve agents can produce a similar toxidrome, with increased secretions, GI upset, and eye pain from ciliary spasm. Sulfur mustard can irritate the eyes and mucous membranes, cause corneal damage and eye pain, and induce vomiting. Hydrogen cyanide, a weakly acidic compound, produces no mucous membrane irritation and rapid loss of consciousness.

100.8. Answer: A Release of botulinum toxin would be expected to result in fatal toxic effects in some victims and prolonged disability in others. Capsaicin is intended for short-term (minutes) incapacitation, whereas the effects of 3-quinuclidinyl benzilate last hours to a day. Q fever and inhaled staphylococcal enterotoxin B should result in a temporarily debilitating but nonlethal pulmonary syndrome.

100.9. Answer: D 3-Quinuclidinyl benzilate is an antimuscarinic incapacitating chemical agent that can reverse nerve agent toxicity in a similar manner to atropine. Pyridostigmine bromide can be used prophylactically to mitigate soman toxicity, but if given after nerve agent exposure, it would only exacerbate toxic effects. The other choices should have no beneficial effect on nerve agent toxicity. Sodium nitrite and 4-dimethylaminophenol may be used to treat cyanide toxicity by inducing methemoglobinemia, and 2,3-dimercaprol (BAL) would help with Lewisite toxicity.

100.10. Answer: B Although many organic phosphorus insecticides are reputed to smell like garlic, the organic phosphorus nerve agents do not. Tabun has a faint fruity odor, soman has a fruity or camphoraceous odor, and sarin and VX are effectively odorless. Sulfur mustard is a CW agent with a strong garliclike odor. The other associations are all correct.

Marrs TC, Maynard RL, Sidell FR: Chemical Warfare Agents. Toxicology and Treatment. Chichester; John Wiley & Sons; 1996.

CHAPTER **101**

SNAKES AND OTHER REPTILES

101.1. Answer: C Antivenom has little effect in reducing local tissue injury, but it consistently reverses coagulopathies. It has no effect on infection rates or pain. Although it may reduce CNS pathology, seizures are very rare, and its effect on seizures has not been studied.

Dart RC, McNally J: Efficacy, safety, and use of snake antivenoms in the United States. Ann Emerg Med 2001;37:181–188.

101.2. Answer: A Although the crotalines (pit vipers) are usually considered to have primary hematoxic venom and the elapids primary neurotoxic venom, there are important exceptions. The Mojave rattlesnake, *Crotalus scutulatus scutulatus,* may have primary neurotoxic signs and symptoms similar to the coral snakes and produce little or none of the edema and tissue destruction seen with most rattlesnake bites.

Burgess JL, Dart RC: Snake venom coagulopathy: Use and abuse of blood products in the treatment of pit viper envenomation. Ann Emerg Med 1991;20:795–780.

Simon TL, Grace TG: Envenomation coagulopathy in wounds from pit vipers. N Engl J Med 1981;305:443–447.

101.3. Answer: A Unfortunately there is no good way to estimate the dose of pit viper antivenin. The amount of venom that the snake injects is unknown, and therefore, the amount of antivenin needed to neutralize the venom is unknown. The victim's response to the antivenin is the only way to determine how much more antivenin is needed. A large snake has the potential to inject a large amount of venom but may inject little. A smaller patient may require more antivenin than a larger patient.

Otten EJ: Antivenin therapy in the emergency department. Am J Emerg Med 1983;1:83–94.

Wingert WA, Chan L: Rattlesnake bites in southern California and rationale for recommended treatment. West J Med 1988;148:37–44.

101.4. Answer: B Antivenom will correct most forms of coagulopathy, but its ability to correct, and maintain, platelet levels is problematic. The exact clinical significance of minor and persistent (up to weeks) thrombocytopenia is unclear and may not signify the need for additional interventoin. Antivenom is most effective in reversing systemic, multiorgan dysfunction. RBC hemolysis is very rare, and the effect of antivenom on this pathology is not known.

Dart RC, McNally J: Efficacy, safety, and use of snake antivenoms in the United States. Ann Emerg Med 2001;37:181–188.

101.5. Answer: C Although the systemic symptoms of pit viper envenomation are protean, many victims complain of weakness, nausea, and muscle fasciculations. Confusion and diplopia may be observed with Mojave rattlesnake and coral snake envenomation.

Butner AN: Rattlesnkae bites in northern California. West J Med 1983;139:179–183.

Dart RC, Hurlbut KM, Garcia R, et al: Validation of severity score for the assessment of crotalid snakebite. Ann Emerg Med 1996; 27:321–326.

101.6. Answer: A Most victims, even with minimal bites, complain of some degree of pain. Fangs rarely penetrate more than 1 to 2 cm. Compartment syndrome is quite rare; most of the swelling is subcutaneous. Copperhead bites commonly cause local edema but rarely cause a significant tissue necrosis.

Davidson TM, Schafer SF, Jones J: North American pit vipers. J Wilderness Med 1992;3:397–421.

Kunkel DB, Curry SC, Vance MV, et al: Reptile envenomations. J Toxicol Clin Toxicol 1983;21:503–526.

101.7. Answer: B Anaphylactic reactions are serious but uncommon problems associated with antivenin therapy. Serum sickness is very common in patients receiving more than 10 vials of antivenin, and a negative skin test is not predictive of which patients will have either an immediate or delayed allergic reaction. Patients with a history of allergic reactions to antivenin may still require antivenin therapy because of the magnitude of the envenomation.

Otten EJ, McKim D: Venomous snakebite in a patient allergic to horse serum. Ann Emerg Med 1983;12:624–627.

101.8. Answer: D Coral snakes have a primary neurotoxin component to their venom. Because of this, the manifestations of coral snake envenomation may be delayed until significant neurologic symptoms, including respiratory failure, occur.

Kitchens CS, VanMierop LHS: Envenomation by the eastern coral snake (*Micrurus fulvius fulvius*). JAMA 1987;258:1615–1618.

McCullough ND, Gennaro JF: Coral snake bites in the United States. J Fla Med Assoc 1963;49:968–970.

101.9. Answer: C Bites by the gila monster are quite rare, and fatalities have not been reported. Because the bites are so rare, no antivenin has been developed. The most common symptoms are pain and edema. The pain is out of proportion to physical findings, but the edema is usually mild compared with snakebite.

Mebs D: Clinical toxicology of helodermatidae lizard bites. In: Meier J, White J, eds: Handbook of Clinical Toxicology of Animal Venoms and Poisons. New York, CRC Press, 1995.

Russell FE, Bogart CM: Gila monster: Its biology, venom, and bite: a review. Toxicon 1981;19:341–359.

101.10. Answer: A In the presence of acute hypersensitivity, antivenom may still be given in life-threatening situations. Treatment of anaphylaxis will likely reverse signs of anaphylaxis, and after treatment with epinephrine, antihistamines, and steroids, antivenom can be carefully, and slowly reinstituted. Slowing the rate of infusion is often the most effective way to limit acute hypersensitivity reactions.

Otten EJ: Antivenin in the emergency department. Am J Emerg Med 1983;1:83–94.

CHAPTER **102**

ARTHROPODS

102.1. Answer: C Severe muscle cramps, nausea, weakness, and tremor can develop within several hours of a black widow spider envenomation. Only the female envenomates successfully; the male spider's fangs are too short to penetrate human skin. Significant local reactions are rare. The spider can be identified by a red to orange hourglass on the thorax. The antivenom is reserved for patients with severe cramps refractory to other therapy because it is an equine antivenom, and the risk of anaphylaxis and other complications is significant.

102.2. Answer: E The brown recluse is uncommon in the northern part of the country even in summer, and it is never found during the winter. The most common description is a purple papule that develops hours after a painless bite, and the victim may develop fever, arthralgias, hemolysis, and DIC. This latter syndrome is called loxoscelism.

102.3. Answer: D Victims may develop muscle fasciculations and cramps, seizures, renal failure, and, rarely, cardiovascular collapse after a scorpion sting. The *Centruroides* scorpion is found predominantly in the Southwestern states and Mexico. Mortality is rare. Mannitol can be used to treat ciguatera poisoning but not scorpion stings.

102.4. Answer: A Improvement in paralysis often occurs after the entire tick is removed from the skin. The tick must remain on the person for 5 to 6 days before symptoms occur. Young girls are reported to develop tick paralysis more commonly than young boys. Absent or decreased deep tendon reflexes may be the earliest sign and develop 24 to 48 hours after the bite.

Dworkin MS, Shoemaker PC, Anderson DE: Tick paralysis: 33 human cases in Washington State, 1946–1996. Clin Infect Dis 1999;29:1435–1439.

102.5. Answer: A Because the venom produced by wasps, hornets, and yellow jackets is almost identical, immunotherapy has been developed from a common venom. Delayed reactions occur 1 to 2 weeks after the sting. If subcutaneous epinephrine is to be used, the 1:1000 (1 mg/mL) concentration should be used. The body's reaction to bee venom is mediated by IgE (anaphylaxis). Autoinjectors should contain epinephrine, not diphenhydramine.

Annila I: Bee venom allergy. Clin Exp Allergy 2000;30:1682–1687.

102.6. Answer: C The funnel web spider is found in Queensland, New South Wales, Tasmania, and Victoria. The male spider is the more dangerous, containing high concentrations of a neurotoxin atraxotoxin (α-bungarotoxin is found in elapids). Fatalities have been reported in children. Treatment is supportive with use of a specific antivenom of rabbit origin. Atropine can be used to control secretions.

Gray RR: Getting to known funnel-webs. Aust Nat Hist 1981;20:256–258.

102.7. Answer: E All of the other substances listed are found in the venom of fire ants.

deShazo RD, Williams DF, Moak ES: Fire ant attacks on residents in health care facilities: A report of two cases. Ann Intern Med 1999;131:424.

Goddard J, Jarratt J, de Castro FR: Evolution of the fire ant lesion. JAMA 2000;284:2162.

102.8. Answer: E   The hobo spider *(Tegenaria agrestis)*, also known as the aggressive house spider, is native to Europe and was introduced into the northwestern United States in the 1920s. Unlike the black widow *(Latrodectus mactans)* and brown recluse spiders, the males of this species are more venomous than the females. None of the other arthropods in question produce necrotic lesions.

Vest DK, Keene WE, Heumann M: Necrotic arachnidism—Pacific Northwest, 1988–1996. MMWR 1996;45:433–436.

102.9. Answer: C   Tarantula bites, which are rare, usually cause minor localized histamine-related effects including localized pruritus, erythema, and swelling. Ocular irritation or damage from urticating hairs is the most common complaint. Oral exposure to tarantula hairs produces oropharyngeal irritation. These spiders are venomous but cannot envenomate humans.

Watts P, Mcpherson R, Hawksworth NR: Tarantula keratouveitis. Cornea 2000;19:393–394.

Editorial. The tarantula—poison spider or a case of mistaken identity? Adverse Drug React Toxicol Rev 1996;15:199–202.

102.10. Answer: B   Of the items listed only morphine relieves pain sufficiently and is the drug of choice. Other therapeutic interventions include *Latrodectus* antivenom, diazepam, methocarbamol, and calcium salts.

Clark RF, Wethem-Kestner S, Vance MV, Gerkin R: Clinical presentation and treatment of black widow spider envenomation: A review of 163 cases. Ann Emerg Med 1992;21:782–787.

CHAPTER **103**

MARINE ENVENOMATIONS

103.1. Answer: A   The lionfish is normally an extremely passive fish when found in the wild. It will not attack humans unless it is cornered. This is the accepted explanation for the envenomations that occur during the cleansing of home aquariums.

Kizer KW, McKinney HE, Auerbach PS: Scorpaenidae envenomation: A five-year poison center experience. JAMA 1985;253: 807–810.

103.2. Answer: B   The stonefish is the most dangerous of the Scorpaenidae family. It is an aggressive fish and will not swim away from man. It is a bottom dweller and typically produces injury to divers who step on the fish in deep water. The stonefish causes immediate muscle spasm and excruciating pain, which may prevent the diver from surfacing and gaining assistance.

Wiener S: Observations on the venom of the stonefish *(Synanceja trachynis)*. Med J Aust 1959;2:260–265.

103.3. Answer: A   A sheep-derived *Chironex* antivenom is available for victims of sea wasp envenomations (Commonwealth Serum Laboratory, Australia). The antivenom is best administered intravenously (one ampule, 20,000 units, diluted 1:5 to 1:10 in isotonic crystalloid) over a 5-minute period.

Bloom DA, Burnett JW, Hebel JR, et al: Effects of verapamil and CSL antivenom on *Chironex fleckeri* (box-jellyfish) induced mortality. Toxicon 1999;37:1621–1626.

103.4. Answer: E   *Linuche unguiculata*, the larvae of the jellyfish, cause a dermatitis by attaching to the fibers of bathing suits (seabather's eruption). The inflammatory reaction can be limited with the use of a topical corticosteroid.

Tomchik RS, Russell MT, Szmant AM, Black NA: Clinical perspectives on seabather's eruption, also known as sea lice. JAMA 1993;269:1669–1672.

103.5. Answer: B   The weeverfish has dorsal spines that are sharp enough and powerful enough to be thrust through a leather boot. Following envenomation the victim will experience a burning or crushing pain that increases in intensity as it spreads through the affected limb.

Halstead BW, Modglin FR: Weeverfish stings and venom apparatus of weever *(Trachinus)*. Z Tropenmed Parasitol 1958;9:129.

103.6. Answer: C   The third-generation cephalosporins provide broad coverage for all of the organisms commonly associated with marine envenomations.

Reed KC, Crowell MC, Castro MD, et al: Skin and soft-tissue infections after injury in the ocean: culture methods and antibiotic therapy for marine bacteria. Mil Med 1999;164:198–201.

103.7. Answer: D   The Portuguese man-of-war contains a neurotoxic venom capable of causing excruciating pain. The tentacles are usually about 10 feet long, number about 40, and remain active for many hours after they are detached. Most Portuguese man-of-war are found in the southern Atlantic Ocean and in the Caribbean Sea.

Stein MR, Marraccini JV, Rothschild NE: Fatal Portuguese man-of-war *(Physalia physalis)* envenomation. Ann Emerg Med 1989; 18:312–315.

103.8. Answer: C   Very few starfish are venomous. The crown-of-thorns is one of the few that contains venom sacs that surround the spines of the starfish. A brush with a crown-of-thorns can cause a painful puncture wound associated with nausea, vomiting, and muscular paralysis.

Taira E, Tananara N, Fanatsu M: Studies on the toxin in the spines of the starfish *Acanthaster planci*: 1. Isolation and properties of the toxin found in spines. Sci Bull Coll Agr Univ Ryukus 1975;22:203–212.

103.9. Answer: D   The spines of a sea urchin often break off and remain embedded in the skin following an exposure. The high calcium content of the spines makes them radiopaque.

Baden HP, Burnett JW: Injuries from sea urchins. South Med J 1977;23:459–460.

103.10. Answer: E   The venom isolated from the toxic sea snakes has been shown to alter both sodium and chloride permeability at peripheral nerve endings without affecting the Na^+-K^+-ATPase pump.

Tu AT: Biotoxicology of sea snake venoms. Ann Emerg Med 1987;16:1023–1028.

CHAPTER 104

USE OF THE INTENSIVE CARE UNIT FOR POISONED PATIENTS

104.1. Answer: A Criteria from a retrospective study defining high-risk patients were: need for intubation; unresponsiveness to verbal stimuli; seizures; $P_{CO_2} > 45$ mm Hg; systolic blood pressure < 80 mm Hg; QRS duration > 0.12 seconds; or any cardiac rhythm except normal sinus, sinus tachycardia, or sinus bradycardia. Patients were classified at low risk when none of the above criteria was present in the emergency department (ED). Retrospectively, none of the 151 patients considered low risk developed complications or required ICU interventions after admission.

Brett A, Rothchild N, Gray R, et al: Predicting the clinical course in intentional drug overdose. Arch Intern Med 1987;147:133–137.

104.2. Answer: C Often a patient may be admitted to the ICU not for intervention but for observation and monitoring. Placing patients in the ICU solely for observation is not an effective use of this expensive resource. The presence of certain signs or symptoms requires ICU observation or intervention, whatever the toxic exposure. This approach is most consistent with the philosophy of "treating the patient and not the poison."

Ron A, Aronne L, Kalb P, et al: The therapeutic efficacy of critical care units. Arch Intern Med 1989;149:338–341.

Zimmerman J, Knaus W, Judson J, et al: Patient selection for intensive care: A comparison of New Zealand and United States hospitals. Crit Care Med 1988;16:318–326.

104.3. Answer: E Studies concerning cyclic antidepressant overdoses suggest that patients may be safely discharged if they remain asymptomatic for a 6-hour observation period after presentation. Unique absorption, distribution, metabolism, or elimination characteristics of toxins may alter the time of onset of symptoms, duration of effects, and risk of complications. Patients with preexisting medical conditions may have an increased risk of developing toxicity.

Callaham M: Admission criteria for tricyclic antidepressant ingestion. West J Med 1982;137:425–429

104.4. Answer: E Severity-of-illness models are effective for stratifying risks in clinical research trials and comparing quality of care among ICUs. None of these models has included large numbers of patients with overdoses. Clinical outcome predictors used in scoring systems cannot be reliably applied to poisoned patients. Specifically, severe poisoning can mimic brain death yet have complete neurologic recovery. Despite negative predictors of outcome, aggressive resuscitative efforts are justified for most poisoned patients.

104.5. Answer: D Undoubtedly, an asymptomatic patient ingesting a highly toxic substance (LD_{50} = 10 mg/kg), a suicidal patient, or a rising serum drug level needs close observation. However, alternatives to placing the patient in the ICU may be equally appropriate. Signs of serious end-organ toxicity are the most important reason to admit poisoned patients to the ICU.

104.6. Answer: A Poisoning produces both anticipated and unanticipated complications that can prolong ICU care and decrease survival. Loss of airway protective reflexes in critically ill patients will be evident in the ED. Loss of airway protective reflexes leads to aspiration pneumonitis that can prolong ICU care. Other serious complications of poisoning include pulmonary compromise, rhabdomyolysis, compartment syndrome, and anoxic brain injury. Complications such as acute renal or fulminant hepatic failure may also prolong the ICU course. These complications may not be evident until the patient has spent several hours or days in the ICU.

104.7. Answer: D Diagnostic tests such as routine laboratory analysis, electrocardiography, and radiography should be used as indicators of the potential for serious toxicity. These diagnostic tests may suggest the need for more aggressive management or careful monitoring. Elevated serum levels of some drugs indicate an increased likelihood of serious toxicity. Serial serum levels show the benefits of GI decontamination and warn of increasing potential for serious toxic effects. Most often, decisions are made based on the patient's clinical status and not on a single test result. Therefore, relatively few patients should be admitted to the ICU based on the results of a single diagnostic test.

Curtis DL, Piibe R, Ellenhorn MJ, et al: Phenytoin toxicity: Predictors of clinical course. Vet Hum Toxicol 1989;31:162–163.

104.8. Answer: C In overdose, enteric-coated and sustained-release preparations may delay absorption and in turn delay onset of toxicity. Clinical effects may be delayed when toxicity depends on alteration of enzyme functions, cellular reproduction, or metabolic functions. Because of the delay in onset of severe toxicity, even if a patient is asymptomatic, a history of ingestion of MAOIs, sulfonylureas, or cholchicine requires prolonged, close monitoring. Shortly after fluoxetine's introduction many clinicians appropriately admitted fluoxetine overdosed patients to the ICU to observe for toxic effects. However, now that clinicians have experience with this drug and studies are available demonstrating few severe manifestations, ICU resources are seldom needed to treat a patient with a fluoxetine overdose.

104.9. Answer: B Complications of poisoning make it difficult to assess the suicidal risk of such patients adequately. Patients have an increased rate of suicide following discharge from an ICU for drug overdose. Until suicidal risks are adequately assessed, it must be assumed that a patient needs close observation. Monitoring policies for suicidal patients not on a psychiatric ward may differ among institutions. The ultimate goal of treatment for any suicidal patient is to provide a maximally safe environment, which may include admitting all patients with suicidal risks to the ICU, physically or chemically restraining a patient, or providing a patient with one-to-one observation. In many hospitals, the ICU is the safest place, but also the most expensive place, to observe a patient with suicidal risks until it is medically safe to transfer the patient to the psychiatric service.

Strom J, Thisted B, Krantz T, et al: Self-poisoning treated in an ICU: drug pattern, acute mortality and short term survival. Acta Anaesthesiol Scand 1986;30:148–153.

104.10. Answer: A Unlike many diseases managed in the ICU, toxicologic emergencies do not have a well-defined clinical course or predictable complications. More than almost any other disease managed in the ICU, uncertainties typify toxicologic emergencies. A patient's history is often unreliable with regard to the kind of poison ingested, time of ingestion, and amount ingested. The poison may have unknown or unpredictable toxic effects. The therapies, antidotes, and complications of acute poisoning may be unfamiliar to the ICU staff. These uncertainties challenge health care providers and influence decisions about admitting patients to the ICU.

CHAPTER 105

REPRODUCTIVE AND PERINATAL PRINCIPLES

105.1. Answer: A Analgesic agents are the most commonly ingested substances during pregnancy, and acetaminophen is the most commonly ingested analgesic agent. Acetaminophen is an FDA category B drug and is safe to use in pregnancy at standard doses. In overdose, acetaminophen may have effects that are toxic to the fetus.

Rayburn W, Aronow R, DeLancey B, Hogan MJ: Drug overdose during pregnancy: An overview from a metropolitan poison control center. Obstet Gynecol 1984;64:611–614.

Riggs BS, Bronstein AC, Kulig KW, et al: Acute acetaminophen overdose during pregnancy. Obstet Gynecol 1989;74:247–253.

105.2. Answer: B Ampicillin is an FDA category B drug and is considered safe for use during pregnancy. Tetracyclines cause staining of teeth from the fourth gestational month throughout the remainder of the pregnancy. Valproic acid can cause neural tube defects such as spina bifida. Warfarin is associated with a specific syndrome of malformations. Angiotensin-converting enzyme inhibitors may cause significant malformations during the later parts of gestation.

Beckman DA, Brent RL: Teratogenesis: Alcohol, angiotensin-converting-enzyme inhibitors, and cocaine. Curr Opin Obstet Gynecol 1990;2:236–245.

105.3. Answer: E Diaphoresis is part of the syndrome of neonatal opioid withdrawal. Other symptoms include wakefulness, poor feeding, hyperactivity, hyperreflexia, hypertonicity, and alkalosis.

American Academy of Pediatrics Committee on Drugs: Neonatal drug withdrawal. Pediatrics 1983;72:895–902.

Besunder JB, Blumer JL: Neonatal drug withdrawal syndromes. In: Koren G, ed: Maternal–Fetal Toxicology. New York, Marcel Dekker, 1994, pp. 321–352.

105.4. Answer: D Penicillamine use during pregnancy is associated with the development of cutis laxa and hyperflexibility of joints, although the risk is probably low. The other agents have been used clinically for acute episodes of poisoning during pregnancy. Hyperbaric oxygen and deferoxamine are associated with teratogenic effects in some animal models.

Tenenbein M: Poisoning in pregnancy. In: Koren G, ed: Maternal–Fetal Toxiclogy. New York, Marcel Dekker, 1994, pp. 223–252.

105.5. Answer: B Fetal alcohol syndrome (FAS) is characterized by (1) intrauterine or postnatal growth retardation; (2) facial dysmorphogenesis, particularly microcephaly, short palpebral fissures, epicanthal folds, maxillary hypoplasia, cleft palate, hypoplastic philtrum, and micrognathia; and (3) mental retardation or behavioral abnormalities. These effects are seen after consumption of the equivalent of 2 to 3 ounces of absolute ethanol (four to six drinks of hard liquor) per day throughout pregnancy. The craniofacial effects probably represent early teratogenic effects on the embryo, whereas the central nervous system abnormalities may result from adverse effects later in gestation. Benzodiazepines are the recommended therapy for neonatal alcohol withdrawal. The leading cause of birth defects is unknown, but FAS may be the leading preventable cause of mental retardation.

105.6. Answer: A Moderate coffee (caffeine) use is not associated with significant adverse effects during pregnancy. Heavy ethanol consumption during pregnancy is associated with fetal alcohol syndrome, although a safe lower limit is not yet defined. Smoking (nicotine) is associated with growth retardation and possibly SIDS. Cocaine is associated with premature delivery, abruptio placentae, and growth retardation and may be associated with certain malformations of the genitourinary tract. Isotretinoin is a well-known teratogen whose use is contraindicated in pregnancy.

105.7. Answer: E Carbon monoxide poisoning may lead to adverse fetal effects even when maternal toxicity is inconsequential. Peak fetal carboxyhemoglobin generally exceeds maternal levels and peaks at a later time. For this reason, it is recommended that oxygen therapy be continued for a period of time five times as long as it takes to lower the maternal level to normal. Lower fetal Po_2 and the greater affinity of fetal hemoglobin for carbon monoxide exacerbates the effects of carbon monoxide exposure. Hyperbaric therapy should be strongly considered for all cases of carbon monoxide poisoning in pregnancy. Therapy should follow standard treatment protocols for time and pressure.

Elkharrat D, Raphael JC, Korach JM, et al: Acute carbon monoxide intoxication and hyperbaric oxygen in pregnancy. Intensive Care Med 1991;17:282–292.

van Hoesen KB, Camporesi EM, Moon RE, et al: Should hyperbaric oxygen be used to treat the pregnant patient for acute carbon monoxide poisoning? A case report and literature review. JAMA 1989;261:1039–1043.

105.8. Answer: B The case literature suggests that maternal iron toxicity exceeds fetal toxicity, and fetal effects are related to maternal hemodynamic and physiologic status, not to fetal iron poisoning. Because iron crosses biologic membranes by a process of receptor-mediated endocytosis, little iron reaches the fetus. Concern about deferoxamine is related to references to teratogenic effects in animal models; however, deferoxamine may be used successfully and safely in human iron poisoning. Acetaminophen is the most commonly ingested pharmaceutical substance during pregnancy.

Curry S, Bond GR, Rashke R, et al: An ovine model of maternal iron poisoning in pregnancy. Ann Emerg Med 1990;19:632–638.

105.9. Answer: E   The benzodiazepines are not associated with specific adverse fetal effects, although there are reports suggesting possible associations with congenital anomalies. There may be sedative effects on the newborn when benzodiazepines are used close to the time of delivery, and there are reports of neonatal benzodiazepine withdrawal. Trimethadione is an anticonvulsant that is no longer used in the United States; it is a well-characterized teratogen. Carbamazepine is associated with some craniofacial defects. Valproic acid is associated with neural tube defects. Phenytoin is associated with the fetal hydantoin syndrome.

Pasturszak A, Koren G, Milich V, et al: Prospective assessment of pregnancy outcome following first trimester exposure to benzodiazepines. In: Koren G, ed: Maternal–Fetal Toxicology. New York, Marcel Dekker, 1994, pp. 77–88.

105.10. Answer: D   Treatment with an opioid agonist such as paregoric is more effective at preventing withdrawal seizures than sedative-hypnotic agents, which may help to control other withdrawal symptoms. Methadone withdrawal symptoms can occur later (days to weeks) than those from heroin (within 24 hours), although withdrawal from either substance usually occurs within 48 hours. Neonatal methadone withdrawal is associated with a plasma level of less than 0.06 mg/mL. Withdrawal is felt to be modulated by increased α-adrenergic activity in the locus ceruleus.

Besunder JB, Blumer JL: Neonatal drug withdrawal syndromes. In: Koren G, ed: Maternal–Fetal Toxicology. New York, Marcel Dekker, 1994, pp. 321–352.

Kandall SR, Doberczak TM, Mauer KR, et al: Opiate v CNS depressant therapy in neonatal drug abstinence syndrome. Am J Dis Child 1983;137:378–382.

CHAPTER 106

PEDIATRIC PRINCIPLES

106.1. Answer: E   Ingestion is the most common route of childhood poisoning exposures. Several characteristics of toddler ingestions differentiate them from adolescent or adult ingestions: (1) they are without suicidal intent, (2) there is usually only one substance involved, (3) the substances are frequently nontoxic, (4) the amount is usually small, and (5) children usually present for evaluation soon after the ingestion.

Bond GR: The poisoned child: Evolving concepts in care. Emerg Med Clin North Am 1995;13:343–355.

106.2. Answer: E   The use of cathartic agents to induce diarrhea is one of the techniques of gastrointestinal decontamination. Cathartic agents such as magnesium sulfate, magnesium citrate, and those containing phosphorus are frequently associated with fluid and electrolyte abnormalities, which complicate poisoning management. Sorbitol has fewer problems when a single dose is used but causes similar complications after multiple-dose use. Polyethylene glycol is a bowel-irrigating solution that was originally developed as a preparation for bowel surgery. It was subsequently incorporated into poison management schemes for sustained-release preparations and for agents that are not well adsorbed to activated charcoal.

Tuggle DW, Hoelzer DJ, Tunell WP, Smith EI: The safety and cost effectiveness of polyethylene glycol electrolyte solution bowel preparation in infants and children. J Pediatr Surg 1987; 22:513–515.

106.3. Answer: B   Children most frequently ingest nonpharmaceutic common household substances. This is most likely related to their easy availability as well as to the child's familiarity with the product. Analgesic agents are the most commonly ingested pharmaceutic substances.

McGuigan MA. Common culprits in childhood poisoning: epidemiology, treatment and parental advice for prevention. Paediatr Drugs 1999;1:313.

106.4. Answer: C   Carbon monoxide is the leading cause of poisoning deaths in children. Iron is the pharmaceutic agent with the highest mortality. Hydrocarbons, antidepressants, and cardiovascular agents are other significant causes of pediatric poisoning, morbidity, and mortality.

Litovitz T, Manoguerra A: Comparison of pediatric poisoning hazards: An analysis of 3.8 million exposure incidents. Pediatrics 1992;89:999–1006.

106.5. Answer: D   Factitious illness (Munchausen syndrome) by proxy (MSBP) is a condition in which a parent, usually the mother, fabricates a history of a nonexistent disease in a child or creates the signs and symptoms of disease in a child, for example by administering a medication such as syrup of ipecac to make the child vomit. This is usually a manifestation of the parent's complex psychiatric illness, which may include Munchausen syndrome itself. Several characteristics have been identified that may suggest the syndrome: (1) persistent or recurrent illness that cannot be explained; (2) a history of the disease that is not consistent with the child's health and appearance; (3) parent refusal to leave the child's bedside, even for a few minutes; (4) the parent developing close relations with medical staff; (5) signs and symptoms not recurring after separation of the child from the parent; (6) treatments being poorly tolerated and prescribed medications frequently leading to vomiting; (6) the working explanation of the signs and symptoms being a rare disease; (8) seizures frequently reported, never witnessed by medical staff, and reportedly not responsive to anticonvulsants; and (9) the parent frequently having some previous association with the healthcare field.

Hall DE, Eubanks L, Meyyazhagan LS, et al: Evaluation of covert video surveillance in the diagnosis of Munchausen syndrome by proxy: lessons from 41 cases. Pediatrics 2000;105:1305.

Souid AK, Keith DV, Cunningham AS: Munchausen syndrome by proxy. Clin Pediatr 1998;37:497.

106.6. Answer: C Child-resistant containers (CRCs) are believed to be responsible for the almost 90% decline in mortality from childhood poisonings over the past 30 years. CRCs are not 100% effective. Not all medications are required to be dispensed in CRCs. They are not designed to prevent all unwanted access, but they prevent the majority of young children from opening them. CRCs will not function properly if there is pill or liquid residue around the closure. Children often find pills outside of the CRC in which they were originally dispensed.

Lembersky RB, Nichols MH, King WD: Effectiveness of child-resistant packaging on toxin procurement in young poisoning victims. Vet Hum Toxicol 1996;38:380–383.

Walton WW: An evaluation of the Poison Prevention Packaging Act. Pediatrics 1982;69:363–370.

106.7. Answer: D Several agents such as oral hypoglyemic agents and diphenoxylate-atropine (Lomotil) may show the onset of significant toxicity long after the time of ingestion (12–18 hours). Similar delays may be expected after ingestion of sustained-release preparations of calcium channel blockers or β-adrenergic antagonists.

106.8. Answer: D Tetrahydrozoline is an imidazoline derivative associated with CNS depression in children. Chloramphenicol is associated with the "gray-baby" syndrome. Benzyl alcohol causes the "gasping" syndrome. Ethanol is associated with hypoglycemia. Acetaminophen is not associated with a specific syndrome in children.

Gershanik J, Boecler B, Ensley H, et al: The gasping syndrome and benzyl alcohol poisoning. N Engl J Med 1982;307:1384.

Mahieu LM, Rooman RP, Goosens E: Imidazoline intoxication in children. Eur J Pediatr 1993;152:944–946.

106.9. Answer: D The gray-baby syndrome is characterized by vomiting, metabolic acidosis, cyanosis, irregular respirations, hypotension, abdominal distension, hypothermia, and death.

Holt D, Harvey D, Hurley R: Chloramphenicol toxicity. Adverse Drug React Toxicol Rev 1993;12:83–85.

106.10. Answer: E A 6-month-old child does not have the developmental skills to get to the mother's purse, open it, and remove pills. When the history of the ingestion conflicts with the child's developmental abilities, child abuse must be suspected. **A** and **D** are typical toddler ingestion scenarios. **B** illustrates a common problem when a child wakes up early on the morning after a party and discovers some leftover alcohol that had not yet been cleaned up. **C** illustrates the problem of poison lookalikes, substances that resemble other tasty nontoxic substances with which the child is familiar.

Bays J: Child abuse by poisoning. In: Reece R, ed: Child Abuse: Medical Diagnosis and Management. Philadelphia, Lea & Febiger, 1994, pp. 69–106.

CHAPTER **107**

GERIATRIC PRINCIPLES

107.1. Answer: B Although the elderly account for only 5% of poisoning exposures, nearly 19% of deaths from poisoning occur among the elderly. This is likely because of the presence of underlying disease or physiologic change in various organ systems. Physiologic vulnerability leading to life-threatening complications from poisonings, as well as serious nontoxicologic illness, is what most likely accounts for the high rate of critical care admissions of elderly patients from emergency departments. The rate of completed suicides increases with age, particularly among white men, although most suicides among men are associated with firearms rather than drug overdose.

107.2. Answer D The suicide rate increases markedly with age, especially among white men, but remains relatively low among women of all ages. In contrast, suicide attempts are more common among women, but attempts increase with age among men. Completed suicides among men are most often by gunshot wounds, but among women they are more often by poisoning or inhalation.

Hall RCW, Platt DE, Hall RC: Suicide risk assessment: A review of risk factors for suicide in 100 patients who made severe suicide attempts. Psychosomatics 1999;40:18–27.

Meehan PJ, Saltzman LE, Sattini RW: Suicides among older United States residents: Epidemiologic characteristics and trends. Am J Public Health 1991;81:1198–1200.

107.3. Answer: C Very few people over the age of 75 are subjects in clinical trials of new drugs in the United States, but this probably is related to problems recruiting appropriate, disease-free elderly subjects, as there are no government regulations that would hinder their participation. Enhanced effects of many, but not all, substances increase the risk of serious adverse drug events among the elderly. Likewise, the elderly take more prescription and nonprescription drugs than do other age groups, increasing exposure to potentially harmful drugs as well as increasing the risk of clinically important drug–drug interactions. Pharmacokinetic changes may increase the risk; delayed elimination of active substances can delay peak action, so toxicity can be delayed, sometimes for days, when long-acting agents are ingested. Coexisting occult disease may first become manifest in conjunction with drug administration. Most commonly, occult brain disease increases the risk of drug-induced delirium and other potentially reversible cognitive disturbances.

Schwartz JB: Clinical pharmacology. In: Hazzard WR, Blass JP, Ettinger WH, et al, eds: Principles of Geriatric Medicine and Gerontology, 4th ed. New York, McGraw-Hill, 1999, pp. 303–311.

107.4. Answer: E Weakness or disorientation from drug toxicity can lead to a fall, which is also a common presentation of nontoxicologic illness among the elderly. Focal neurologic deficits may also occur, probably as a result of subclinical brain disease, such as a silent stroke, which is not manifest until illness or toxicity supervenes; in addition, drug toxicity itself could produce physiologic compromise leading to cerebral anoxia and focal deficits related to underlying cerebrovascular disease. Memory loss and more serious confusional states are a common presentation of drug toxicity, often related to therapeutic doses of prescribed drugs. Agitation can occur as a direct result of drug toxicity but is also a common secondary symptom of confusional states.

107.5. Answer: E Theophylline is dependent on hepatic oxidation for elimination. Age-related decline in hepatic oxidation may account in part for theophylline elimination. Although long-acting benzodiazepines, such as diazepam, are also metabolized in this way, active metabolites are renally eliminated, and the prolonged effect of these agents may be partly a result of this renal mechanism. Clearance of digoxin, gentamicin, and lithium is significantly affected by age-related decline in renal function. Serum creatinine clearance declines on the average by approximately 50% by age 75, although decline in renal function is by no means universal. It is uncertain if this decline is clinically important; however, when drugs that are cleared by the kidney are given, toxic levels can be attained unless dose adjustments are made. Renal function cannot be predicted by serum creatinine; serum creatinine does not rise with age because creatinine is produced by muscle, and muscle mass declines with age.

Brouwer K, Dukes G, Powel J: Influence of liver function on drug disposition. In: Evans W, Schentag J, Jusko W, eds: Applied Pharmacokinetics. Vancouver, Applied Therapeutics, 1992, pp. 1–59.

107.6. Answer: D Gastric alcohol dehydrogenase declines with age, possibly because of atrophy of the gastric mucosa. The resulting decrease of "gastric first-pass" metabolism leads to an enhanced effect of alcohol. Because alcohol distributes in water and there is an increase in the body's fat-to-lean ratio with age, alcohol has a decreased volume of distribution in late life, leading to a more rapid peak effect. The half-life of alcohol may actually decrease with age because of the smaller volume of distribution.

Pozzato G, Moretti M, Franzin F, et al: Ethanol metabolism and aging: the role of "first pass metabolism" and gastric alcohol dehydrogenase activity. J Gerontol 1995;50A:B135–B141.

107.7. Answer: D The fat-to-lean ratio increases with advancing age. Highly lipid-soluble drugs tend to have an increased volume of distribution. As a result, there may be a delay before steady state is reached, and peak effect and toxicity may be delayed. This mechanism may be part of the reason drugs such as diazepam and flurazepam have a prolonged half-life among otherwise healthy elderly patients.

Novak LP: Aging, total body potassium, fat-free mass, and cell mass in males and females between ages 18 and 85 years. J Gerontol 1972;27:428–443.

107.8. Answer: E All of the listed antidotes have been used to treat the elderly patient with an overdose appropriate for these drug therapies. Sodium bicarbonate may predispose the patient with underlying cardiovascular disease to congestive heart failure, pulmonary edema, and hypertension.

Puczynski MS, Cunningham DG, Mortimer JC: Sodium intoxication caused by baking soda as a home remedy. Can Med Assoc J 1983;128:821–822.

107.9. Answer: E All of the listed medications have a high hepatic extraction rate. Each will have a decreased clearance, as there is an age-related decline in hepatic blood flow. Additional drugs with high hepatic extraction rates include meperidine, metoprolol, verapamil, and triazolam.

Brouwer K, Dukes G, Powel J: Influence of liver function on drug disposition. In: Evans W, Schentag J, Jusko W, eds: Applied Pharmacokinetics. Vancouver, Applied Therapeutics, 1992, pp. 1–59.

107.10. Answer: C The aging process includes an increase in the percentage of body fat and the plasma protein α_1-acid glycoprotein. Simultaneously there is a decline in intracellular water and muscle mass.

Fox F, Auestad A: Geriatric emergency clinical pharmacology. Emerg Med Clin North Am 1990;8:221–223.

CHAPTER **108**

THE HIV-POSITIVE PATIENT—AIDS PHARMACOLOGY AND TOXICOLOGY

108.1. Answer: B Lamivudine, a nucleoside reverse transcriptase inhibitor, was approved to be used against HIV/AIDS only in combination with other antiviral agents such as zidovudine. The most common adverse effects found with lamivudine are gastrointestinal irritation, headache, fatigue, and rash.

Leeuwen VR, Lange JMA, Hussey E, et al: The safety and pharmacokinetics of a reverse transcriptase inhibitor, 3TC, in patients with HIV infection: A phase I study. AIDS 1992;6:1471–1475.

Threlkeld SC, Hirsch MS: Antiviral therapy: The epidemiology of HIV and AIDS: Current trends. Med Clin North Am 1996;80: 1263–1283.

108.2. Answer: B Zidovudine is a thymidine analogue. Cellular kinases convert zidovudine into its triphoshate form, which intracellularly inhibits viral reverse transcriptase.

Lacy C, Amstrong LL, Ingrim N, et al: Drug Information Handbook. Hudson, OH, Lexi-Comp, 1996–1997.

108.3. Answer: B AZT, ganciclovir, and amphotericin B can cause bone marrow toxicity. Therefore, concomitant use of these agents should be avoided because of the potential additive adverse effects.

Richman DD, Fischl MA, Grieco MH, et al: The toxicity of azidothymidine (AZT) in the treatment of patients with AIDS and AIDS-related complex. N Engl J Med 1987;317:192–197.

108.4. Answer: C Zidovudine (AZT) achieves high CSF concentration (50% of plasma). CSF concentrations are approximately 20% of serum level for ddC, ddI, d4T, and 3TC.

Kowacs JA: Efficacy of atovaquone in treatment of toxoplasmosis in patients with AIDS. Lancet 1992;2:637–638.

Yarchoan R, Thomas RV, Allain JP, et al: Phase I studies of 2′, 3′-dideoxycytidine in severe human immunodeficiency virus infection as a single agent and alternating with zidovudine (AZT). Lancet 1988;1:76–81.

108.5. Answer: D Invirase (saquinavir), Crixivan (indinavir), and Norvir (ritonavir) are protease inhibitors. Epivir (lamivudine) is a nucleoside reverse transcriptase inhibitor, and Viramune (nevirapine) is a nonnucleoside reverse transcriptase inhibitor.

Threlkeld SC, Hirsch MS: Antiviral therapy: The epidemiology of HIV and AIDS: current trends. Med Clin North Am 1996;80: 1263–1283.

108.6. Answer: C Hematologic toxicity is the major toxicity of ganciclovir. Ganciclovir is primarily used to treat CMV. It is available for oral and parenteral administration and is eliminated unmetabolized by the kidneys.

Buhles WC Jr, Mastre BJ, Tinker AJ, et al: Ganciclovir treatment of life- or sight-threatening cytomegalovirus infection: Experience in 314 immunocompromised patients. Rev Infect Dis 1988;10: S495–S506.

Drew WL: Antiviral therapy of CMV infection. AIDS Reader 1993;3:99–104.

108.7. Answer: B Indinavir is the only protease inhibitor listed. Nevirapine and delavirdine are both nonnucleoside reverse transcriptase inhibitors, and lamivudine is a nucleoside reverse transcriptase inhibitor. Ganciclovir inhibits viral replication.

Threlkeld SC, Hirsch MS: Antiviral therapy: The epidemiology of HIV and AIDS: current trends. Med Clin North Am 1996;80: 1263–1283.

108.8. Answer: B Pentamidine is used only for PCP, whereas sulfadiazine is used mainly as an adjunctive agent for toxoplasmosis and not PCP. Clarithromycin is not used in either PCP or toxoplasmosis; it is used mostly for *Mycobacterium avium complex* coverage in *HIV/AIDS patients. Ketoconazole is used to treat mucocutaneous candidiasis, coccidioidomycosis*, and histoplasmosis.

Carr A, Tindall B, Brew BS, et al: How does trimethoprim-sulfamethoxazole provide prophylaxis for toxoplasmic encephalitis in patients with AIDS? Ann Intern Med 1992;117:106–111.

108.9. Answer: C Pentamidine causes hypoglycemia followed by hyperglycemia. These effects are the direct result of toxic injury to the insulin-producing β cells of the pancreas.

Bouchard P, Sai P, Reach G, et al: Diabetes mellitus following pentamidine-induced hypoglycemia in humans. Diabetes 1982;31: 40–45.

108.10. Answer: B Dysrhythmias such as torsades de pointes can occur with concurrent administration of ketoconazole with terfenadine. Ketoconazole needs an acidic medium to be absorbed. Clarithromycin is not an antifungal agent. Amphotericin B is very nephrotoxic. Patients are often pretreated with a corticosteroid, NSAID, or antihistamine before receiving amphotericin B. An antiemetic would not be necessary.

Lacy C, Armstrong LL, Ingrim N, et al: Drug Information Handbook, Hudson, OH, Lexi-Comp, 1996–1997.

CHAPTER 109

SUBSTANCE USERS

109.1. Answer: C The absence of a murmur on presentation does not exclude endocarditis. All intravenous drug–using patients with a fever require hospital admission to exclude endocarditis and other infectious diseases. The transesophageal echocardiogram is the best imaging modality to identify valvular vegetations. Left-sided endocarditis requires higher doses of antibiotics for a longer period of time.

Cherubin CE, Sapira JD: The medical complications of drug addiction and the medical assessment of the intravenous drug abuser: 25 years later. Ann Intern Med 1993;119:1017–1028.

Weisse AB, Heller DR, Schimenti RJ, et al: The febrile parenteral drug abuser: A prospective study in 121 patients. Am J Med 1993; 94:274–280.

109.2. Answer: B It is not uncommon to find adulterants or contaminants in specimens of illicit drugs. They may be added to enhance the bulk of the drug (eg, mannitol) or to misrepresent the drug's purity (eg, lidocaine to produce the gum numbness of cocaine). Heavy metals are detected in specimens obtained from clandestine laboratories and have produced clinical toxicity. Law enforcement officers now receive hazardous materials training, as they must always assume the presence of toxic chemicals when investigating clandestine laboratories.

Allcott JV 3rd, Barnhart RA, Mooney LA: Acute lead poisoning in two users of illicit methamphetamine. JAMA 1987;258:510.

Klatt EC, Montgomery S, Namiki T, et al: Misrepresentation of stimulant street drugs: A decade of experience in an analysis program. J Toxicol Clin Toxicol 1986;24:441–450.

109.3. Answer: B The rate of illicit drug use by young individuals continues to increase, as has the use of heroin and marijuana by all age groups. Only emergency department and medical examiner data are collected by the Drug Abuse Warning Network.

Substance Abuse and Mental Health Services Administration/Office of Applied Studies: 1999 Annual Emergency Department Data. August 2000. Department of Health and Human Services, Rockville MD.

Substance Abuse and Mental Health Services Administration/Office of Applied Studies: 1999 National Household Survey on Drug Abuse. August 2000. Department of Health and Human Services, Rockville MD.

109.4. Answer: D Skin necrosis is a late finding in patients with necrotizing fasciitis. The femoral vasculature must be evaluated to rule out a pseudoaneurysm before drainage of a groin abscess is done. Parenteral drug users continue to strain their drug using cotton or cigarette filters before injection. Intranasal use carries the same substantial risk of dependence as intravenous heroin, although the populations that use these routes are demographically different, making comparison difficult.

Cherubin CE, Sapira JD: The medical complications of drug addiction and the medical assessment of the intravenous drug abuser: 25 years later. Ann Intern Med 1993;119:1017–1028.

109.5. Answer: A The Drug Abuse Warning Network usually underreports drug-related trauma. Substance use is a common cause of motor vehicle collisions in the elderly. Substance use is associated with both thermal injury and spinal cord injury. Cocaine was found in 27% of New York City residents who had fatal injuries.

Higgins JP, Wright SW, Wrenn KD: Alcohol, the elderly, and motor vehicle crashes. Am J Emerg Med 1996;14:265–267.

Mannenbach MS, Hargarten SW, Phelan MB: Alcohol use among injured patients aged 12 to 18 years. Acad Emerg Med 1997;4: 40–44.

109.6. Answer: A A reliable psychiatric diagnosis requires a 2-week period of abstinence. Inpatient care is preferable in patients with a dual diagnosis. The psychiatric history provided by a substance user is often inaccurate and must be supplemented by data from other individuals, the physical examination, and laboratory analysis.

109.7. Answer: C It is estimated that 21% of tax dollars in New York City cover substance abuse. The modified concept of dependence stresses the impaired control of substance use and applies to a variety of substances that do not produce physiologic dependence.

American Psychiatric Association: Diagnostic and Statistical Manual of Mental Disorders, 4th ed. Washington, DC, APA, 1994.

109.8. Answer: D The healthcare provider cannot distinguish in an intravenous drug user with a fever a trivial disease from endocarditis. Hospital admission is mandatory to rule out endocarditis and other important infectious diseases. Uncommon diseases occur in these patients with greater frequency than in the general poulation, and exotic diseases must always be considered.

Cherubin CE, Sapira JD: The medical complications of drug addiction and the medical assessment of the intravenous drug abuser: 25 years later. Ann Intern Med 1993;119:1017–1028.

109.9. Answer: A Drug use is a risk factor for tuberculosis even in patients not infected with the human immunodeficiency virus. Opioid withdrawal has been precipitated by rifampin administration in patients receiving methadone, and methadone users frequently do not take anti-HIV medications because of important drug interactions. There have been no proven drug therapies for cocaine addiction.

109.10. Answer: D The most common cause of viral transmission occurs when the substance user verifies placement in a vein by drawing blood into the syringe and then shares the needle. Nonsterile tap water is commonly used to dissolve drugs.

CHAPTER 110

HEALTHCARE WORKERS

110.1. Answer: A Most studies find that 1.0% glutaraldehyde is the minimum effective concentration when the intended use is as a high-level disinfectant.

Cole EC, Rutala WA, Nessen L, et al: Effect of methodology, dilution, and exposure time on the tuberculocidal activity of glutaraldehyde-based disinfectants. Appl Environ Microbiol 1990;56: 1813–1817.

110.2. Answer: C Although almost any patient or health care worker can become sensitized to latex following even brief exposures, those individuals who are repeatedly exposed in significant ways are at the highest risk. Children with spina bifida undergo frequent urinary bladder catheterizations and thus receive mucosal exposure to the latex present in catheters as well as to the rubber gloves worn by the operator performing the catheterization. The development of latex reactions in children with spina bifida is well recognized and well described.

Landwehr LP, Boguniewicz M: Current perspectives on latex allergy. J Pediatr 1996;128;305–312.

110.3. Answer: D Psyllium is implicated in the sensitization of exposed workers and associated with the development of occupationally-related asthma. The problem is probably more common in chronic care facilities, where the use of laxatives is widespread. As many as 18% of healthcare workers reported allergic reactions while handling psyllium-containing materials.

Freeman GL: Psyllium hypersensitivity. Ann Allergy 1994; 73:490–492.

Gillespie BF, Rathburn FJ: Adverse effects of psyllium. Can Med Assoc J 1994;146:16–17.

110.4. Answer: D Psychiatrists are the most likely group to self-report according to a study that surveyed a large group of New England doctors.

McAuliffe WE, Rohman M, Santangelo S, et al: Psychoactive drug use among practicing physicians and medical students. N Engl J Med 1986;315:805–810.

110.5. Answer: B Despite the fact that ribavirin has not been conclusively shown to exert adverse reproductive effects in humans, it has indeed been shown to be teratogenic in laboratory animals.

Chutaputti A: Adverse effects and other safety aspects of the hepatitis C antivirals. J Gastroenterol Hepatol 2000;15(Suppl): E156–E163.

110.6. Answer: E Formalin is "cidal" against all of the listed entities.

Pandey CK, Agarwal A, Baronia A, et al: Toxicity of ingested formalin and its management. Hum Exp Toxicol 2000;19:360–366.

110.7. Answer: A Laboratory animal allergy (LAA) is a clinical syndrome characterized by rhinitis, upper airway inflammation, and occasionally bronchospasm. It is important to note that the majority of workers suffering from LAA report symptoms associated with rhinitis and upper airway symptoms as opposed to asthmatic symptoms.

Eggleston PA, Wood RA: Management of allergies to animals. Allergy Proc 1992;13:289–292.

110.8. Answer: A Among resident physicians, the use of psychoactive substances was generally lower than it was among similar age groups in the general population, although, as among their older colleagues, the use of benzodiazepines was greater, with self-treatment generally being cited as the reason for such use.

Hughes PH, Conard SE, Baldwin DC, et al: Resident physician substance use in the United States. JAMA 1991;265:2069–2073.

110.9. Answer: A The broadest level of OSHA communication is the so-called Hazard Communication Standard, which requires all employers to inform their employees of the specific chemical hazards involved in their jobs. In the healthcare setting, this standard includes the preparation of drugs and medicines by pharmacists and nurses. In addition, this standard requires that employees be provided with written information (in the form of the Material Safety Data Sheet) describing the chemical hazards to which they may be exposed on the job.

Greenberg MI, Cone DC, Roberts JR: The material safety data sheet: A useful resource for the emergency physician. Ann Emerg Med 1996;27:347–352.

110.10. Answer: B Exposure to ethylene oxide has been associated with the development of cataracts after prolonged exposure. Lid edema and conjunctival irritation are possible at very high concentrations, but these levels are rarely, if ever, attained and maintained long enough during routine use to result in these effects. Hyphema is almost exclusively related to direct ocular trauma. Hordeolums do not form in response to ocular chemical irritation.

Bihari V, Srivastava AK, Gupta BN: Occupational health hazards among operating room personnel exposed to anesthetic gases: A review. J Environ Pathol Toxicol Oncol 1994;13:213–219.

CHAPTER **111**

FARM TOXICOLOGY

111.1. Answer: A A mixed motor and sensory peripheral neuropathy was described following triorthocresyl phosphate exposure as an adulterant of Jamaican ginger extract and occurs after exposures to numerous organic phosphorus compounds. Neuropsychiatric disability, including depression and memory deficits, has been widely reported following organic phosphorus compound poisoning and recently verified in controlled studies. Paralysis, including delayed bilateral recurrent laryngeal nerve paralysis, can occur 25 to 35 days after poisoning with chlorpyrifos, parathion, and methamidophos. Although parkinsonism has been reported,

Alzheimer disease is not expected or reported following organic phosphorus compound poisoning.

Steenland K, Jenkins B, Ames RG, et al: Chronic neurological sequela to organophosphate pesticide poisoning. Am J Public Health 1994;84:731–736.

111.2. Answer: C In a study of poisoning with agricultural chemicals in the United States, organic phosphorus pesticides were the leading recognized cause of hospitalizations and deaths. Paraquat, diquat, chlorophenoxy compounds, chlorinated hydrocarbons, carbamates, strychnine, arsenic, and anticoagulants were also associated with deaths.

Klein-Schwartz W, Smith GS: Agricultural and horticultural chemical poisonings: Mortality and morbidity in the United States. Ann Emerg Med 1997;29:232–238.

111.3. Answer: D Organic phosphorus and carbamate insecticides affect respiration via several mechanisms. Bronchospasm and bronchorrhea-associated pulmonary edema result from parasympathetic (muscarinic) stimulation. Weakness of the muscles of respiration through nicotinic stimulation and central depression of the respiratory drive center also occur. Acute lung injury implies structural damage to the endothelium; this does not occur with organic phosphorus pesticide poisoning.

Do Pico GA: Hazardous exposure and lung disease among farm workers. Clin Chest Med 1992;13:311–328.

Schenker M, Ferguson T, Gamsky T: Respiratory risks associated with agriculture. In: Cordes DH, Rea DF, eds: Occupational Medicine: State of the Art Reviews, vol 6. Philadelphia, Hanley & Belfus, 1991, pp. 415–428.

111.4. Answer: B Paraquat-induced pulmonary fibrosis has never been reported after inhalation exposure because doses are not sufficient to induce fibrosis. Pulmonary fibrosis most commonly occurs after ingestion of paraquat, although there have been reports of fibrosis after dermal absorption. Animal models routinely use parenteral routes, including the intraperitoneal route, to administer paraquat.

111.5. Answer: A Silo filler disease occurs from exposure to nitrogen dioxide gas, which is formed from the decay of silage in the silo. An acute illness with cough, dyspnea, bronchitis, and pulmonary edema can be followed by bronchiolitis obliterans after 2 to 6 weeks. Hydrogen cyanide is a metabolic toxin that produces rapid coma and death. Phosgene and hydrogen chloride are respiratory irritants created (among other ways) by the burning of chlorinated hydrocarbons such as polyvinylchloride. Endotoxin is released from certain microorganisms on grain and may subsequently be inhaled when the grain is disturbed.

Von Essen S, Donham K: Respiratory diseases related to work in agriculture. In: Langley RL, McLymore RL, Meggs WJ, Roberson GT: Safety and Health in Agriculture, Forestry and Fisheries. Rockville, MD, Government Institutes, 1997, pp. 352–384.

111.6. Answer: D Hydrogen sulfide is a metabolic poison similar to cyanide. Hydrogen sulfide levels in agitated manure may reach 400 to 500 ppm or more. At these levels, unconsciousness, convulsions, and sudden death may occur. The worker entering a closed space containing manure must wear a self-contained breathing apparatus. The individual should wear a lifeline and should have an observer outside the tank at all times. Unlike hydrogen sulfide, methane is a light gas that rapidly diffuses into the environment.

Morese D, Woodbury M: Death caused by fermenting manure. JAMA 1981;245:63–64.

111.7. Answer: D In a study of contact dermatitis among farmers, poison ivy/oak accounted for 63% of the cases, with poison oak accounting for 48% of these cases. Other plants (including weeds and flowers), leather, hides, fur, feathers, lumber, and wood products less commonly cause dermatitis. Agricultural chemicals caused 20% of cases.

Mathias CGT: Epidemiology of occupational skin disease in agriculture. In: Dosman JA, Crockfort DW, eds: Principles of Health and Safety in Agriculture. Boca Raton, CRC Press, 1989, pp. 285–287.

111.8. Answer: E Clinical effects of grain dust exposure include nasal stuffiness, rhinorrhea, acute bronchitis, asthma, chronic bronchitis, acute febrile syndrome, hypersensitivity pneumonitis, and eye and skin irritation. Infectious diseases, such as pneumonia, are not directly caused by grain dust.

Melbostad E, Eduard W: Organic dust-related respiratory and eye irritation in Norwegian farmers. Am J Ind Med 2001;39:209.

111.9. Answer: B Integrated pest management is an agricultural program that replaces routine spraying with pesticides with a surveillance program that applies pesticides to crops based on the amount and type of infestation. This program reduces both the cost and potential health hazards of pesticide use.

111.10. Answer: A Anhydrous ammonia is used as a fertilizer to increase nitrogen concentrations in soil. It is extremely caustic to the eye, and severe eye injuries including blindness can occur rapidly.

Helmers S, Top FH, Knapp LW: Ammonia injuries in agriculture. J Iowa Med Soc 1971;36:271–280

CHAPTER 112

SPORTS TOXICOLOGY

112.1. Answer: C Testosterone esters are water soluble and are injected intramuscularly. They are important for bridging therapy. They do not account for most of the side effects of anabolic androgenic steroids simply because the alkylated testosterone derivatives are more frequently utilized. Testosterone esters are detected with current laboratory methods, primarily gas chromatography. There is no known difference in efficacy dependent on the menstrual cycle.

Bagatell CJ, Bremner WJ: Androgens in men—uses and abuses. N Engl J Med 1996;334:707–714.

112.2. Answer: B Plateauing, stacking, and cycling refer to the use of androgenic anabolic steroids. "Plateauing" refers to the development of tolerance to any one drug's effect. "Cycling" is the use of steroids in regularly recurring time intervals. "Stacking" implies combining use of several steroids at one time, often involving both oral and intramuscular administration.

Wilson JD: Androgen abuse by athletes. Endocr Rev 1988;9(2): 181–199.

112.3. Answer: D Clenbuterol is a long-acting orally administered β-adrenergic agonist. It is a prohibited substance and is not allowed with a doctor's permission. It does not cause acne.

Zeman RJ, Ludemann R, Easton TG, Etlinger JD: Slow to fast alterations in skeletal muscle fibers caused by clenbuterol, a beta 2-receptor agonist. Am J Physiol 1988;254(6 Pt 1):E726–E732.

112.4. Answer: B Furosemide may be used as a masking agent. By causing dilute urine, it makes detection of small quatities of certain drugs more difficult. Furosemide is also used to cause weight loss in those sports with weight restrictions, such as wrestling and boxing.

www.olympic.org. International Olympic Committee, 2000.

112.5. Answer: D Bromontan is an amphetaminelike substance used as a masking agent. Most of the literature on bromontan is in Russian, as the substance was first described in Russia.

112.6. Answer: E Alkylated androgens may be administered orally because they are more resistant to hepatic metabolism. Alkylated androgens account for more of the complications associated with anabolic androgenic steroid use because they are most commonly used by athletes. Alkylated anabolic androgenic steroids are adminstered orally and are prohibited by the IOC. Testosterone propionate is the prototypic testosterone ester.

Wilson JD: Androgen abuse by athletes. Endocr Rev 1988;9(2): 181–199.

112.7. Answer: A Consuming carbohydrates with creatine supplements increases absorption of creatine and increases total creatine stores in skeletal muscle. This is why creatine is marketed in combination with carbohydrate. One of the primary results of creatine use is weight gain. Use of creatine may increase urinary creatinine excretion. Creatine is relatively inexpensive, costing about $9 per day. Gymnasium acne is caused by anabolic steroids, not creatine.

112.8. Answer: B Insulinlike growth factor may cause hypoglycemia. The other side effects of IGF-1 are similar to human growth hormone side effects and include acromegaly, headache, and jaw pain. IGF-1 does not cause virilization, and this may make it attractive to female athletes. IGF-1 is not known to cause testicular atrophy, a side effect reported for anabolic androgenic steroids. Weight loss is not reported with IGF-1.

Russell-Jones DL, Umpleby M: Protein anabolic action of insulin, growth hormone and insulin-like growth factor I. Eur J Endocrinol 1996;135:631–642.

Thissen JP, Ketelslegers JM, Underwood LE: Nutritional regulation of the insulin-like growth factors. Endocr Rev 1994;15:80–101.

112.9. Answer: D Perfluorocarbons cause a dose-related thrombocytopenia. Crossmatching is not required. Advantages of perfluorocarbons include the absence of infectious contaminants and no increase in the viscosity of blood. Because perfluorocarbons are perceived by the immune system as foreign substances, they are rapidly cleared by the reticuloendothelial system.

Clark LC Jr, Gollan F: Survival of mammals breathing organic liquids equilibrated with oxygen at atmospheric pressure. Science 1966;152:1755–1756.

Smith DJ, Lane TA: Effect of a high concentration perfluorocarbon emulsion on platelet function. Biomater Artif Cells Immobilization Biotechnol 1992;20:1045–1049.

112.10. Answer: E Chromium picolinate acts as a cofactor for insulin. It is reported to cause anemia in high doses. Renal insufficiency is a reported complication of use. Carbohydrate is thought to enhance chromium absorption. The use of chromium picolinate is not known to be associated with an increased incidence of colon cancer.

Davis JM, Welsh RS, Alerson NA: Effects of carbohydrate and chromium ingestion during intermittent high-intensity exercise to fatigue. Int J Sport Nutr Exerc Metab 2000;10:476–485.

Wasser WG, Feldman NS, D'Agati VD: Chronic renal failure after ingestion of over-the-counter chromium picolinate. Ann Intern Med 1997;126:410.

CHAPTER 113

PSYCHOSOCIAL PRINCIPLES IN ASSESSMENT AND INTERVENTION

113.1. Answer: D Hospitals are increasingly becoming part of primary care networks linked to community-based health and social services and providing a continuum of care.

Berkman B: The emerging health care world. Implications for social work practice and education. Social Work 1996;41:541–551.

113.2. Answer: B Psychosocial evaluation addresses the complex interaction of psychological and social factors in understanding individual functioning.

113.3. Answer: C Medical social work was formally established in 1905 with the introduction of social service workers at Massachusetts General Hospital in Boston and, shortly thereafter, at Bellevue Hospital in New York City.

113.4. Answer: B During the first decade of the 20th century there was growing awareness of the connection between disease and social environmental factors of poverty, substandard and overcrowded housing, and the impact of immigration on densely populated urban areas. Social service workers became an extension of the hospital into the community, making home visits, working with community agencies, and providing education and supportive casework services.

113.5. Answer: D Healthcare professionals should use all appropriate opportunities to provide clear, unambiguous, and nonjudgmental information to patients about the physical and social consequences of substance abuse and referrals for treatment.

Barber J: Working with resistant drug abusers. Social Work 1995; 40:17–23.

113.6. Answer: D Childhood sexual abuse and being a victim of domestic violence are factors associated with increased incidence of substance abuse in women.

Goldberg ME: Substance abusing women: False stereotypes and real needs. Social Work 1995;40:789–798.

113.7. Answer: E The correlation between substance abuse and maternal/child health, medical, and psychosocial risk supports the need for perinatal addiction programs that are coordinated with women's health and pediatric services.

113.8. Answer: C Substance abuse of parents is one of the most common reasons for children entering foster care placement.

Azzi-Lessing L, Olsen LJ: Substance abuse–affected families in the child welfare system: New challenges, new alliances. Social Work 1996;41:15–23.

113.9. Answer: C The special needs and concerns of women who abuse drugs or alcohol must be acknowledged by health care professionals in order for services to be responsive and effective. Among these concerns, fear of the child welfare system is prominent.

Abbott AA: A feminist approach to substance abuse treatment and service delivery. Social Work Health Care 1994;19:67–83.

113.10. Answer: E Social work staff, as members of interdisciplinary teams in emergency departments, contribute to comprehensive and effective assessment, management, and discharge planning for high-risk patients.

CHAPTER 114

PSYCHIATRIC PRINCIPLES

114.1. Answer: C As of 1993, the last year for which statistics are available, deliberate gunshot wounds are still the most common method for suicide in both sexes. Overdoses have decreased among women since the late 1970s.

US Department of Commerce: Statistical Abstracts of the United States, 116th ed. Washington DC. US Government Printing Office 1996.

114.2. Answer: D Two psychological autopsy studies examined clinical and demographic variables of persons who had completed suicide. Among these were the communication of suicidal intent. Intent was viewed as a direct statement about ending one's life or an indirect remark about "no longer being here" or being "better off dead." A review of 100 cases of suicide found that 55% of completed suicides gave some warning of their intention. A study of 134 cases of suicide found that 69% of completed suicides gave a warning.

Barraclough B, Bunch J, Nelson B, et al: A hundred cases of suicide: Clinical aspects. Br J Psychiatry 1974;125:355–373.

Robins E, Murphy GE, Wilkinson RH, et al: Some clinical considerations in the prevention of suicide based on a study of 134 successful suicides. Am J Public Health 1959;49:888–889.

114.3. Answer: E Major mental illness, including manic-depression, schizophrenia, alcoholism, drug addiction, and anxiety disorders, was found in more than 90% of persons who had completed suicide. The percentage is seen in other psychological autopsy studies as well.

Barraclough B, Bunch J, Nelson B, et al: A hundred cases of suicide: Clinical aspects. Br J Psychiatry 1974;125:355–373.

114.4. Answer: C Patients will not be "provoked" into suicidal crisis by a discussion of their suicidal ideation and thoughts about death. Many patients will be relieved that the physician is willing to speak openly with them about their distress.

Fawcett J, Clark DC, Busch KA: Assessing and treating the patient at risk for suicide. Psychiatr Ann 1993;23:244–255.

114.5. Answer: D In 1993 the age-adjusted suicide rate for men was 19.9/100,000 compared to 4.6/100,000 for women. White men have a higher suicide rate than black men. Adolescent suicide is increasing in this country. Among completed suicide in women, the suicide rate for white women is 5.0/100,000 compared to 2.1/100,000 for black women. Since 1980, the suicide rate in the United States has remained fairly constant at 12/100,000.

US Department of Commerce: Statistical Abstracts of the United States, 116th ed. Washington DC. US Government Printing Office 1996.

114.6. Answer: D Both benzodiazepines and antipsychotic are useful in the treatment of aggression. The use of barbiturates in aggression has largely fallen from favor because these medications can produce rapid tolerance, untoward drug–drug interactions, and lethal overdosage.

114.7. Answer: C Haloperidol and other antipsychotic drugs lower the seizure threshold and can promote seizure activity in vulnerable patients (cocaine intoxication, alcohol withdrawal, epilepsy).

Kane J, Marder SR: Psychopharmacologic treatment of schizophrenia. Schizophren Bull 1993;19:287–302.

114.8. Answer: B Seclusion is not an effective intervention for the delirious patient because the reduction in sensory stimuli may act to confuse the patient further and worsen his or her condition.

American Psychiatric Association: Clinician Safety (Task Force Report No. 33). Washington, DC, American Psychiatric Association, 1992.

114.9. Answer: C Confidentiality is a vital part of the physician–patient relationship. A patient's request for confidentiality should be honored unless the patient is a danger to self or others. Reasons for breaching confidentiality should be recorded in the patient's chart. In clinical situations when a patient is threatening to harm a person, the physician has a duty to warn the potential victim. This duty arose from the Tarsoff ruling of 1973.

Simon RI: Clinical Psychiatry and the Law, 2nd ed. Washington, DC, American Psychiatric Press, 1992, pp. 268–269, 319–320.

114.10. Answer: E Suicide is more common in men than in women. Past suicide attempts increase the risk of future attempts. Alcoholism is associated with an increased risk of suicide, as is the presence of depression.

Beck AT, Steer RA: Clinical predictors of eventual suicide: A 5–10 year prospective study of suicide attempters. J Affect Dis 1989;17:203–209.

CHAPTER **115**

NURSING PRINCIPLES

115.1. Answer: B The role of triage is to determine the relative priorities for medical treatment among a group of patients.

115.2. Answer: C As with any medical evaluation, the immediate assessment of a patient presenting for medical care includes attending to the patient's life-threatening problems. This is commonly prioritized as airway, breathing, and circulation. In this patient, the airway and breathing are maintained using a bag valve mask.

115.3. Answer: E Any patient with an altered mental status should be controlled before complete assessment to avoid injury to both the patient and the medical staff. Although the administration of thiamine, dextrose or a fingerstick glucose assessment, and oxygen should be considered early, an agitated patient should not be given naloxone or diphenhydramine. The sedative of choice is a benzodiazepine, such as diazepam, or perhaps haloperidol under certain circumstances.

115.4. Answer: A Orogastric lavage is reserved for patients with consequential overdoses or those patients already manifesting life-threatening symptoms.

115.5. Answer: D The poison center provides poisoning-specific medical advice to parents, patients, and medical care providers. In addition, as part of the public health network, the poison control centers collect epidemiologic and demographic data concerning poisoning and drug abuse. In general, the poison center does not provide direct care or intervene on interhospital transfers.

115.6. Answer: A   The left lateral decubitus position places the patient's stomach in a dependent position. This prevents ingested drug from moving through the pylorus, which would allow better absorption and prevent retreival during lavage.

115.7. Answer: B   Physical restraint is always temporary and should be reduced or removed when the patient is pharmacologically sedated.

115.8. Answer: A   Although tissue hypoxia may be substantial, pulse oximetry is usually normal with elevated carboxyhemoglobin levels. In the presence of other overdoses, pulse oximetry will usually be a reliable representation of patient oxygenation.

115.9. Answer: B   Patients should be humanely restrained with appropriate material such as padded cloth. The patient's legs should be tied together, and the individual's upper arms should be individually restrained.

115.10. Answer: C   Understanding antidotal therapy is critical. *N*-Acetylcysteine is the correct treatment for acetaminophen poisoning.

CHAPTER **116**

POISON INFORMATION CENTERS AND POISON EPIDEMIOLOGY

116.1. Answer: E   Multiple comparisons of TESS data with other existing databases clearly demonstrate that these systems fail to agree and that, under most circumstances, TESS underreports cases of significant exposure.

Blanc PD, Olson KR: Occupationally related illness reported to a regional poison control center. Am J Public Health 1986;76: 1303–1307.

Chafee-Bahamon C, Caplan DL, Lovejoy FH: Patterns in hospitals' use of a regional poison information center. Am J Public Health 1983;73:396–400.

Linakis JG, Frederick KA: Poisoning deaths not reported to the regional poison control center. Ann Emerg Med 1993;22:42–48.

116.2. Answer: C   Although it would be nice to think that utilization of poison services reduces morbidity and mortality following exposure, and this may actually be the case, the data only support that because many exposures are unlikely to result in toxicity, because timely use of poison centers prevents unnecessary use of ambulances and emergency departments by assuring parents that their children are unlikely to become ill, and by providing appropriate followup.

Chafee-Bahamon C, Lovejoy FH: Effectiveness of a regional poison center in reducing excess emergency room visits for children's poisonings. Pediatrics 1983;72:164–169.

116.3. Answer: A   According to the most recent data, poisoning ranks third as a cause of injury-related fatalities. This was behind only motor vehicle crashes and firearms-related fatality.

Fingerhut LA, Cox CS: Poisoning mortality, 1985–1995. Public Health Rep 1998;113:218–233.

116.4. Answer: E   In addition to the factors listed in the answer, the route of exposure should be defined, the quantity known, and the exposed individuals must be available for followup. Unless all of these factors can be met, the exposure should not be immediately labeled nontoxic.

Mofenson HC, Greensher J, Caraccio T: Ingestions considered nontoxic. Emerg Med Clin North Am 1984;2:159–174.

116.5. Answer: B   It costs approximately $35 for a poison center to answer a single call. When compared to the price of an ambulance response, emergency department visit, or visit to a physician's office, this value is clearly justified.

Youniss J, Litovitz T, Vilanueva P: Characterization of US poison centers: A 1998 survey conducted by the American Association of Poison Control Centers. Vet Hum Toxicol 2000;42:43–53.

CHAPTER **117**

ADVERSE DRUG EVENTS

117.1. Answer: E   There are preclinical (animal testing) and clinical (phase 1–4) trials performed in the development of a new drug. Marketing is not considered part of drug testing.

117.2. Answer: C   All are goals or functions of MedWatch except to provide funding.

117.3. Answer: C   A relationship based on biologic plausability is desirable but not necessary, given the multitude of potential toxicologic mechanisms and the lack of a complete understanding of many physiologic processes.

117.4. Answer: E   Carcinogenesis is rarely if ever the cause of a recall or withdrawal. The others are common.

117.5. Answer: D   Medical errors are common, and most are preventable. There are many reasons that they occur, suggesting that there is no simple solution.

117.6. Answer: C   An adverse event is any undesirable experience associated with the use of a medical product in a patient. Rectifying serious events may not be expensive and correcting relatively unimportant ones may be costly. Each of the other events is considered serious.

Edwards IR, Aronson JK: Adverse drug reactions: Definitions diagnosis and management. Lancet 2000;356:1255–1259.

117.7. Answer: B   The accelerated approval track has not changed the percent of drugs withdrawn, although since more drugs are approved, the absolute number of withdrawals has increased. The Orphan Drug Act of 1983 provides incentives to develop drugs that may be financially unrewarding because of the limited use of the drug, such as for the treatment of rare diseases. By charging for review of new drug applications, the FDA is able to speed the review process. The FDA has more limited authority over dietary supplements, but may remove those that are a serious risk to the public. MedWatch is a voluntary, spontaneous reporting system and there is not requirement to report. However, reporting is encouraged in order to allow the collection of initial and subsequent data regarding potential safety issues involving drugs.

MedWatch website: *http://www.fda.gov/medwatch/partner.htm*

117.8. Answer: D   Clinical and medical toxicologists are specifically trained to observe for potential and existent adverse drug effects. Through aggressive history-taking, a link between a disease entity and a prior or current medication exposure may be identified. The toxicology community educates primary care and specialty physicians of the mechanisms and clinical importance of drug interactions, adverse drug events, and poisoning. Although they are actively involved in preventing medical errors, elimination of such events requires more than clinical toxicologists; medication errors are a system wide and exceedingly complex problem that will only be solved thorugh a combination of provider education and administrative and mechanical controls.

Bates DW, Cullen DJ, Laird N, et al: Incidence of adverse drug events and potential adverse drug events. Implications for prevention. ADE Prevention Study Group. JAMA 1995;274:29–34.

117.9. Answer: B   The Food, Drug and Cosmetic Act of 1938 was in response to more than 100 deaths from the diethylene glycol diluent in the elixir of sulfanilamide, a sulfa antibiotic. The tragedy of thalidomide in Europe never occurred in the United States due to a strong regulatory stance by the FDA; it led to the Kefauver-Harris Act of 1968. Despite years of recognized toxicity, the manufacturer of terfenadine only removed the product from the market when a suitable substitute was approved. The report of the Institute of Medicine suggested that medication errors are a significant and growing problem. MedWatch is utilized for post-marketing surveillance.

Kohn LT, Corrigan JM, Donaldson MS: To Err is Human: Building a Safer Health System. Washington, DC, Committee on Quality of Health Care in America, Institute of Medicine, 2000.

Bren L: Frances Oldham Kelsey. FDA medical reviewer leaves her mark on history. FDA Consum 2001;35:24–29.

117.10. Answer: A   Fewer than 10% of cases are believed to be reported; this is because it is a voluntary, spontaneous system and not mandatory. It collects the "numerator" or the actual cases, and not the "denominator," which are the exposed cases. Thus it is a hypothesis generating system, but it cannot do accurate risk assessment. MedWatch is widely supported by nearly every medical organization.

MedWatch website. *http://www.fda.gov/medwatch/partner.htm*

CHAPTER **118**

RISK MANAGEMENT AND LEGAL PRINCIPLES

118.1. Answer: C   Patients suffering from toxicologic emergencies are often unable to give consent for treatment because of their impaired consciousness. Emergency physicians must recognize the legal responsibilities of the healthcare profession regarding patients with organic impairment and should not allow these patients to leave their emergency departments.

118.2. Answer: C   It is not necessary that patients understand exceptionally rare risks not commonly known in the medical community. An informed consent must include the potential risks of not receiving treatment, the potential risks of receiving treatment, and the possible alternative treatments.

118.3. Answer: D   Patients who refuse treatment should be questioned regarding their specific concerns. For example, a Jehovah's Witness may refuse blood transfusions even if the individual's life is in jeopardy. Patients without legitimate rationale for refusal of critical treatment should be evaluated for psychiatric and/or organic impairment.

118.4. Answer: B   The forcible restraint of a patient should be reserved for those patients with life-threatening conditions who have impaired judgment and an inability to comprehend the consequences of their actions. Even though the heroin user is now neurologically normal, these abilities are caused by a medical intervention known to have a limited duration of effect. The suspicion or admission of suicidality places an additional burden on the healthcare provider to prevent the patient from leaving the emergency department. The physician should document his or her assessment and all clinical findings that support the decision.

118.5. Answer: C   A well-documented medical record does not prove that a physician did not commit malpractice. The law is very clear on what constitutes malpractice, and documentation can only help to defend or support a claim.

118.6. Answer: D   Any time the practitioner uses subjective terms to describe a patient's condition or behavior, the medical record can be used to suggest that the physician has a less than caring attitude. Objective observations and vital signs are the most appropriate documentation for the medical record.

118.7. Answer: C   A patient who does not have a well-prepared Living Will or DNR order should be resuscitated. DNR orders need to be well documented. A simple reference or comment from the patient, family, or friend should never be accepted.

118.8. Answer: B   Any person who operates a motor vehicle is considered to have consented to a test to determine alcohol or drug ingestion. In addition, a blood test may be needed to evaluate the relationship between the patient's altered level of consciousness and a potential ingestion of drugs or alcohol.

118.9. Answer: D   It is acceptable to discharge patients with elevated blood alcohol levels provided there are no potential risks to the patient. Additionally, the chronic alcoholic usually has an elevated baseline blood alcohol level and can usually be discharged without any serious consequence.

118.10. Answer: E The physician should document only objective clinical findings. Any time the practitioner uses subjective terms to describe a patient's condition or behavior, the medical record can be used to suggest that the physician has a less than caring attitude. Additionally, practitioners should use caution when documenting presumptive diagnosis, especially in cases where alcohol or drugs may be involved.

CHAPTER 119

POSTMORTEM TOXICOLOGY

119.1. Answer: B Postmortem xenobiotic concentrations can fall if the agent undergoes postmortem metabolism, as is classically seen with cocaine, or postmortem glycolysis of glucose from peripheral blood. Bacteria can cause molecular breakdown of certain xenobiotics during putrefaction, causing a decreased recovery of the agent on sampling. Xenobiotics with a large V_d often redistribute from the tissues into the blood as the energy-dependent processes maintaining cellular integrity begin to fail. Such is the case with digoxin.

119.2. Answer: C Postmortem ethanol production is detected only in bodies in advanced stages of decomposition, where putrefactive changes are evident. It is unlikely that ethanol production will occur to substantial concentrations when there is no evidence of putrefaction; furthermore, the vitreous is only relatively protected for the early postmortem interval. Thus, in relatively intact bodies, vitreous concentrations of ethanol lower than that in blood suggest that the ethanol was consumed before death and was in the early stage of absorption. Vitreous concentrations equal to that in blood suggest a postabsorptive stage. A urine concentration, if available, would be helpful in determining if the patient was primarily in the elimination phase.

119.3. Answer: E Cause of death is the physiologic event necessary for death to occur. Accident and Homicide are classifications of manner of death, which distinguishes natural from nonnatural deaths.

119.4. Answer: C The vitreous humor is relatively protected in the early postmortem interval. Vitreous creatinine concentrations can be reasonably assumed to reflect antemortem concentrations, as little postmortem production, metabolism, or redistribution occurs for creatinine in this period. Potassium rises early as a result of intracellular release. Although it is possible that hyperkalemia was a cause of death, the evidence is not definitive because postmortem potassium redistribution may cause artifact.

119.5. Answer: B Phenobarbital has been identified in larvae obtained from exhumed bodies. Unlike ethanol, it is not produced as the postmortem interval progresses. Similarly, it is not present in embalming fluid or soil samples. Thus, phenobarbital must have been present in the body before death. Because of the inability to

determine antemortem serum concentrations and the inability to estimate physiologic tolerance, cause of death can not be established on this information alone.

119.6. Answer: C Arsenic can be naturally present in the water and soil and contaminate hair, nails, and other sample sites. In addition, embalming agents from many decades ago, sometimes contained heavy metals. Ideally, samples of soil both above and below the body are obtained to determine if the arsenic leached into the tissues from the soil. If the concentration of arsenic in the soil below the body is greater than the concentration of arsenic in the soil above the body, the metal is more likely to have been present in the body before death. Also, knowing when and if the body was embalmed provides information regarding potential contaminants. Newer techniques in washing and handling hair and nail samples may also help to make the distinction.

119.7. Answer: C Carboxyhemoglobin of 2% is close to a normal concentration. In a serious house fire it is uncommon to die without first inhaling some amount of carbon monoxide before death, even with a serious burn. Although carbon monoxide is a by-product of hemoglobin metabolism, it exists in small quantities and ceases to progress after death. All of this information raises suspicion that the individual was dead before the fire. This will cause an investigation into whether the fire was, in fact, arson in attempt to destroy other bodily evidence of murder. As per the other bodies, little can be presumed with this evidence alone.

119.8. Answer: D A recent ingestion of a therapeutic dose may have been at peak absorption before redistribution at the time of death from an unrelated cause. Tricyclic antidepressants have anticholinergic effects, which are expected to delay gastric emptying, so a large overdose resulting in death would likely result in some detectable drug amounts in the gastric contents at autopsy. Also, tricyclic antidepressants have a large V_d and are expected to redistribute back into the blood as the postmortem interval progresses.

119.9. Answer: C All of those listed are routinely or infrequently used except for fecal material, which except for meconium and bile, has little role in forensic testing.

119.10. Answer: D Even if a compilation of postmortem tissue concentrations was available, there are so many variables that affect the interpretation that it would be of limited value. For example, some drugs are stable postmortem while others are continually metabolized or redistributed. Thus the specialized knowledge of the medical examiner, forensic toxicologist, and clinical toxicologists are often necessary to interpret the laboratory value in a clinical context.

CHAPTER 120

PRINCIPLES OF EPIDEMIOLOGY AND RESEARCH DESIGN

120.1. Answer: C A screening test should be simple, safe, and inexpensive. High sensitivity is required to identify exposed individuals for more specific testing.

120.2. Answer: B Cases were separated from controls on the basis of outcome (seizures) and were subsequently examined for the presence of risk factors (electrocardiographic findings). In a cohort study the subjects and controls would have been recruited on the basis of the risk factor.

120.3. Answer: D In this instance, sensitivity refers to the proportion of TCA-exposed individuals with an abnormal T40msec-QRS. Therefore, 62% of TCA-exposed individuals had a normal T40msec QRS. Specificity refers to the number of unexposed individuals with a normal T40msec QRS.

120.4. Answer: B The 95% confidence interval around a study finding 0 outcomes in 20 exposures ranges from an incidence of 0 to 0.139 (~14%). A *p*-value is best reserved for hypothesis testing.

Jovanovic BD, Zalenski RJ: Safety evaluation and confidence intervals when number of observed events is small or zero. Ann Emerg Med 1997;30:301–306.

120.5. Answer: E Statistical power, artificially set by investigators before a clinical study, is the inverse of type II *(β)* error. Type II error is the likelihood that investigators will, by chance, fail to find a statistical difference between treatment groups even though a difference truly exists. Neither type I nor type II error can account for bias in a study.

120.6. Answer: B "Blinding" of data abstractors is a tool for reducing bias. Misclassification bias would refer to error in assigning subjects to either the physostigmine or diazepam groups. Selection bias refers to systematic error in the recruitment of study subjects.

120.7. Answer: A In this instance the observed association between coffee drinking and lung cancer resulted from another confounding variable (smoking). Luckily, investigators controlled for this potential confounder—that is not always the case.

120.8. Answer: C An odds ratio is a surrogate measure for relative risk. An odds ratio greater than 1.0 suggests that an exposure increases risk for disease; an odds ratio less than 1.0 suggests that an exposure is protective.

120.9. Answer: A A clinically significant difference between groups should be determined by investigators before the study, and power set accordingly. Trivial differences can be statistically significant if the sample size is very large.

120.10 Answer: E It is unlikely that deaths would be misclassified. However, there may be reasons that poison centers are not "selected" to receive calls about patient deaths.

INDEX

Page numbers followed by f and t indicate figures and tables, respectively. Page numbers followed by CS indicate pages in the Case Studies section of the text.

Primidone. *See also* Sedative-hypnotic(s)
  crystalluria from, 449
  with inducible porphyria, 387t
  on nursing infants, 1622t
  pharmacology of, 932t
Primin, 1155t, 1173
Primrose
  Evening *(Oenothera biennis),* 1136t, 1140,
    1146t
  family (Primulaceae), contact dermatitis
    from, 1173
  Primula obconica, 1155t
Proanthocyanidins, 1167
Probenecid
  hypoglycemic agent interactions of, 598t
  nephrotoxicity of, 356
Procainamide, 790. *See also* Antidysrhythmic
    agents, class I
  agranulocytosis from, 234
  antidotes in depth for (sodium bicarbonate),
    520t, 521 (*See also* Sodium bicarbonate)
  autoimmunity induction by, 236t
  cardiomegaly from, 106t, 107
  chemical structure of, 790f
  diagnostic imaging of, 95t
  hepatotoxicity of, 220t, 224t
  hypersensitivity hemolytic anemia from, 237t
  management of, 791
    antidotes in, 520t, 521, 1739t
    extracorporeal removal in, 64, 64t, 65
  neutropenia from, 390t
  pharmacokinetics and toxicokinetics of, 789t
  pleural effusions from, 106t
  systemic lupus erythematosus from, 236
  transmission neuropathy from, 298t
Procaine. *See also* Anesthetics, local
  chemical structure of, 825, 826f
  history of, 825
Procaine hydrochloride (KH-3), 1137t
Procarbazine, 887. *See also* Monoamine oxidase
    inhibitors (MAOIs)
  hepatotoxicity of, 224t
  infertility from, 441
  pharmacology of, 706t
Prochlorperazine. *See also* Antipsychotic agents
  akathisia from, 289t
  dystonia from, 289t
  pharmacology of, 876–878, 876t, 877t
  resting tremor from, 288t
Product identification, 40
Progestational drugs, hypertension from, 565t
Progesterone, 407
  erythema multiforme from, 436
  hyperventilation from, 304t
  on nursing infants, 1622t
Progestins, 406
  with inducible porphyria, 387t
  teratogenic effects of, 1611t
Progoitrin, 1154t
Proguanil, 672t, 677–678
Promethazine, 536f
Promotion, of carcinogenesis, 246
Proof spirits, 952–953. *See also* Alcohol(s),
    ethyl
Pro-opiomelanocortin (POMC), 404
Propafenone, 792–793
  management of, 794
  pharmacokinetics and toxicokinetics of, 789t
Pro-2-PAM, 1362
Propane
  as asphyxiant, 304t, 1454 (*See also* Asphyxi-
    ants)
  physical properties of, 199t
  as pulmonary irritant, 1456t (*See also* Pul-

monary irritants; Pulmonary toxic exposures)
Propanediols, 932t. *See also* Sedative-hyp-
    notic(s)
1-Propanol, 199t
Propentofylline, on adenosine, 162
Propionic acids, 531–532. *See also* Nonsteroidal
    antiinflammatory drugs (NSAIDs)
Propofol, 939–940. *See also* Sedative-hyp-
    notic(s)
  on GABA, 153
  as glycine agonist, 156t
  on glycinergic action, 155
  pharmacology of, 932t, 939
Proportionality constant (k), 176
Propoxyphene, 916
  acute lung injury from, 305
  antidotes for, 521, 1739t
    sodium bicarbonate, 521 (*See also* Sodium
      bicarbonate)
  cardiac conduction abnormalities/heart block
    from, 327t
  chemical structure of, 908f
  diabetes insipidus from, 372t
  dysrhythmias from, 330t
  hypoglycemic agent interactions of, 598t
  pharmacokinetics of, 172t
  pharmacology of, 911t
  testing for, 87t
Propranolol. *See also* Beta-adrenergic antago-
    nists
  chemical structure of, 741f
  ECG from, 127
  erectile dysfunction from, 443
  hypoglycemia from, 597–598
  hypothermia on, 266
  metabolism of, hypothermia on, 266
  on neuromuscular blocking agents, response
    to, 811t
  pharmacokinetics of, 172t
  pharmacology of, 744–745, 745t
Proprietary name, 194, 195t
Proprionitrile, cyanide from, 1499
Propylene glycol, 841–842, 841t, 981, 988t. *See
    also* Alcohol(s), toxic
  acid-base disturbances from, 842
  cardiovascular toxicity of, 841
  clinical manifestations of, 985
  drug interactions with, 842
  fluid and electrolyte disturbances from, 842
  metabolism of, 983, 984f, 985
  nephrotoxicity of, 354
  neurotoxicity of, 841
  ototoxicity of, 841–842
  pharmacokinetics of, 841
  thrombophlebitis from, 842
Propylhexedrine. *See also* Amphetamine(s)
  in nasal inhalers, 1024
  pharmacology of, 1024
Propylthiouracil (PTU), 404
  aplastic anemia from, 383t
  hepatotoxicity of, 219t, 220t
  myopathy from, 298t
  neutropenia from, 390t
  olfactory toxicity of, 423t
Prostaglandin E₁ (Alprostadil), for erectile dys-
    function, 444
Prostaglandins, oral, as abortifacient, 446
Protamine (sulfate)
  acute lung injury from, 305t
  as antidote, 39t
  as antidote in depth, 651–652
    adverse effects and risk factors with, 651
    alternatives to, 651–652

  availability of, 652
  chemistry of, 651
  dosing of, 652
    in cardiopulmonary bypass, 652
    heparin rebound and, 652
    in overdose setting, 652
  mechanism of action of, 651
  safety issues with, 651
Proteaceae, allergic contact dermatitis from,
    1173
Protease (proteinase) inhibitors, 1650t,
    1658–1659. *See also* specific agents
  amprenavir, 1659
  on fatty acid metabolism, 207, 207t
  HIV drug interactions with, 1655t–1656t
  in HIV-positive patients, 1650t
  indinavir, 1659
  mechanism of action of, 1648f, 1658
  nelfinavir, 1659
  ritonavir, 1659
  saquinavir, 1658
Protective equipment, personal, 1414–1415
Protein kinase A, 318, 743, 744f
Proteinase inhibitors. *See* Protease (proteinase)
    inhibitors
Proteins. *See also* specific proteins
  in plants, 1155t–1156t
Prothrombin time (PT), 637, 637t
Protoanemonin, 1154t, 1172, 1172f
Proto-oncogenes, 246–247
Protriptyline. *See* Antidepressants, cyclic; Anti-
    depressants, tricyclic
Proximal tubule, 346
Prunus, 1134t, 1150t, 1154t, 1162
  amygdalin in, 1499, 1499f
  cyanogenic glycosides in, 1132, 1154t,
    1163
  laboratory analysis and antidote for, 1133t
  P. amygdala (almond seeds), 1150t, 1154t
  P. armeniaca (apricot seeds), 1133t, 1134t,
    1150t, 1154t, 1163
  P. avium (cherry pits), 1132, 1150t, 1154t,
    1155t
  P. cerasus (cherry pits), 1132, 1150t, 1154t,
    1155t
  P. domestica (plum seeds), 1150t, 1154t,
    1163
  P. persica (peach seeds), 1132, 1150t, 1154t,
    1163
Pruritis, 435
Prussian blue (potassium fericyanoferrate), for
    thallium, 53, 1277
Psathyrella foenisecii, 1117t, 1121
Pseudoephedrine. *See also* Decongestants
  clinical manifestations of, 540
  hypertension from, 258t, 320t
  hyperthermia from, 263t
  pharmacology of, 537
  tachycardia from, 259t
Pseudotumor cerebri. *See* Idiopathic intracranial
    hypertension
Psilocybe (psilocybin mushrooms), 1048–1049,
    1117t, 1121. *See also* Psilocybin
  early use of, 10
  P. caerulescens, 1121
  P. caerulipes, 1117t
  P. cubensis, 1117t, 1121
  physical characteristics of, 1126t
Psilocybin, 10, 1048–1049
  chemical structure of, 1048f, 1121f
  history and epidemiology of, 1046–1047
  on serotonin, 150
  vs. serotonin, 1121f
  violence and, 1727

COMMON STANDARD LABORATORY VALUES

	Conventional Unit	SI Unit
Bicarbonate	18–24 mEq/L	18–24 mmol/L
BUN	7–18 mg/dL	2.5–6.4 mmol/L
Calcium	8.4–10.2 mg/dL	2.10–2.55 mmol/L
Chloride	98–106 mEq/L	98–106 mmol/L
Creatinine	0.6–1.2 mg/dL	0.053–0.106 mmol/L
Glucose	60–110 mg/dL	3.3–6.1 mmol/L
Lactate	<2 mEq/L	<2 mmol/L
Magnesium	1.3–2.1 mEq/L	0.65–1.05 mmol/L
P_{CO_2} (arterial)	35–45 mm Hg	4.7–6.0 kPa
P_{CO_2} (venous)	45–55 mm Hg	6.0–7.33 kPa
pH (arterial)	7.35–7.45	7.35–7.45
pH (venous)	7.33–7.40	7.33–7.40
P_{O_2} (arterial)	90–100 mm Hg	12–13.3 kPa
P_{O_2} (venous)	30–50 mm Hg	4.0–6.67 kPa
Potassium	3.5–5.0 mEq/L	3.5–5.0 mmol/L
Sodium	135–145 mEq/L	135–145 mmol/L

PERIODIC TABLE OF THE ELEMENTS

1 H 1.008																	2 He 4.003
3 Li 6.941	4 Be 9.012											5 B 10.81	6 C 12.011	7 N 14.007	8 O 15.999	9 F 18.998	10 Ne 20.179
11 Na 22.99	12 Mg 24.305											13 Al 26.981	14 Si 28.086	15 P 30.974	16 S 32.06	17 Cl 35.453	18 Ar 39.948
19 K 39.098	20 Ca 40.08	21 Sc 44.956	22 Ti 47.88	23 V 50.942	24 Cr 51.996	25 Mn 54.938	26 Fe 55.847	27 Co 58.933	28 Ni 59.69	29 Cu 63.546	30 Zn 65.38	31 Ga 69.72	32 Ge 72.59	33 As 74.922	34 Se 78.96	35 Br 79.904	36 Kr 83.80
37 Rb 85.468	38 Sr 87.62	39 Y 173.04	40 Zr 91.22	41 Nb 92.91	42 Mo 95.94	43 Tc 98	44 Ru 101.07	45 Rh 102.91	46 Pd 106.42	47 Ag 107.87	48 Cd 112.41	49 In 114.82	50 Sn 118.69	51 Sb 121.75	52 Te 127.60	53 I 126.90	54 Xe 131.29
55 Ca 132.91	56 Ba 137.33	* 57–71	72 Hf 178.49	73 Ta 180.95	74 W 183.85	75 Re 186.21	76 Os 190.2	77 Ir 192.22	78 Pt 195.08	79 Au 196.97	80 Hg 200.59	81 Tl 204.38	82 Pb 207.2	83 Bi 208.98	84 Po 209	85 At 210	86 Rn 222
87 Fr 223	88 Ra 226.03	† 89-103	104 Unq 261	105 Unp 262	106 Unh 263												

*	57 La 138.91	58 Ce 140.12	59 Pr 140.91	60 Nd 144.24	61 Pm 145	62 Sm 150.36	63 Eu 151.96	64 Gd 157.25	65 Tb 158.93	66 Dy 162.50	67 Ho 164.93	68 Er 167.26	69 Tm 168.93	70 Yb 173.04	71 Lu 174.97
†	89 Ac 227.03	90 Th 232.04	91 Pa 231.04	92 U 238.03	93 Np 237.05	94 Pu 244	95 Am 243	96 Cm 247	97 Bk 247	98 Cf 251	99 Es 252	100 Fm 257	101 Md 258	102 No 259	103 Lr 260